Measure	SI	Conventional (C)	C × CF = SI
Glucose tolerance test, 2-h postprandial plasma glucose			
Normal	<7.8 mmol/L	<140 mg/dL	0.05551
Impaired glucose tolerance	7.8–11.1 mmol/L	140–200 mg/dL	0.05551
Diabetes mellitus	>11.1 mmol/L	>200 mg/dL	0.05551
Gonadal steroids, plasma			
Androstenedione			
Women	3.5–7.0 nmol/L	1–2 ng/mL	3.492
Men	3.0–5.0 nmol/L	0.8–1.3 ng/mL	3.492
Estradiol			
Women: Basal	70–220 pmol/L	20–60 pg/mL	3.671
Ovulatory surge	>740 pmol/L	>200 pg/mL	3.671
Men	<180 pmol/L	<50 pg/mL	3.671
Dihydrotestosterone			
Women	0.17–1.0 nmol/L	0.05–3 ng/mL	3.467
Men	0.87–2.6 nmol/L	0.25–0.75 ng/mL	3.467
Progesterone			
Women: Luteal phase	6–64 nmol/L	2–20 ng/mL	3.180
Follicular phase	<6 nmol/L	<2 ng/mL	3.180
Men	<6 nmol/L	<2 ng/mL	3.180
Testosterone			
Women	<3.5 nmol/L	<1 ng/mL	3.467
Men	10–35 nmol/L	3–10 ng/mL	3.467
Prepubertal boys and girls	0.2–0.7 nmol/L	0.05–0.2 ng/mL	3.467
Gonadotropins, plasma			
Women, basal			
FSH	5–20 IU/L	5–20 mIU/mL	1.0
LH	5–25 IU/L	5–25 mIU/mL	1.0
Women, ovulatory peak			
FSH	12–30 IU/L	12–30 mIU/mL	1.0
LH	25–100 IU/L	25–100 mIU/mL	1.0
Men			
FSH	5–20 IU/L	5–20 mIU/mL	1.0
LH	5–20 IU/L	5–20 mIU/mL	1.0
Prepubertal boys and girls			
FSH	<5 IU/L	<5 mIU/mL	1.0
LH	<5 IU/L	<5 mIU/mL	1.0
Growth hormone, plasma			
After 100 g glucose orally	<5 µg/L	<5 ng/mL	1.0
After insulin-induced hypoglycemia	>9 µg/L	>9 ng/mL	1.0
Human chorionic gonadotropin, beta subunit, plasma			
Men and nonpregnant women	<3 IU/L	<3 mIU/mL	1.0
β-Hydroxybutyrate, plasma	<300 nmol/L	<3.0 mg/dL	96.05
Insulin, plasma			
Fasting	35–145 pmol/L	5–20 µU/mL	7.175
During hypoglycemia (plasma glucose <2.8 nmol/L [<50 mg/dL])	<35 pmol/L	<5 µU/mL	7.175
Insulin-like growth factor I (IGF I, somatomedin-C)			
Women	0.45–2.2 kU/L	0.45–2.2 U/mL	1.0
Men	0.34–1.9 kU/L	0.34–1.9 U/mL	1.0
Lactate, plasma	0.56–2.2 mmol/L	5–20 mg/dL	0.111
Magnesium, serum	0.8–1.20 mmol/L	1.8–3.0 mg/dL	0.4114
Osmolality, plasma	285–295 mmol/kg	285–295 mOsm/kg	1.0
Oxytocin, plasma			
Random	1–4 pmol/L	1.25–5 ng/L	0.80
Ovulatory peak in women	408 pmol/L	5–10 ng/L	0.80
Parathyroid hormone, serum (intact PTH using immuno-radiometric assay [IRMA])	10–65 ng/L	10–65 pg/mL	1.0
Phosphorus, inorganic, serum	1–1.5 mmol/L	3.0–4.5 mg/dL	0.3229
Potassium, serum	3.5–5.0 mmol/L	3.5–5.0 mEq/L	1.0
Prolactin, serum	2–15 µg/L	2–15 ng/mL	1.0
Pyruvate, blood	39–102 µmol/L	0.3–0.9 mg/dL	0.01129
Renin activity, plasma, normal-sodium diet			
Supine	3.2 ± 1 µg/L/h	3.2 ± 1.1 ng/mL/h	1.0
Standing	9.3 ± 4.3 µg/L/h	9.3 ± 4.3 ng/mL/h	1.0
Sodium, serum	136–145 mmol/L	136–145 mEq/L	1.0
Thyroid function tests			
Radioactive iodine uptake, 24 h	0.05–0.30	5–30%	—
Reverse triiodothyronine (rT$_3$), serum	0.15–0.61 nmol/L	10–40 ng/dL	0.01536
Thyrotropin (TSH), highly sensitive assay, serum	0.6–4.6 mU/L	0.6–4.6 µU/mL	1.0
Thyroxine (T$_4$), serum	51–42 nmol/L	4–11 µg/dL	12.87
Thyroxine-binding globulin, serum (as thyroxine)	150–360 nmol/L	12–28 µg/mL	12.87
Triiodothyronine (T$_3$), serum	1.2–3.4 nmol/L	75–220 ng/dL	0.01536
Triiodothyronine resin uptake, serum	0.25–0.35	25–35%	—
Triglycerides, plasma (as Triolein)	<1.80 mmol/L	<160 mg/dL	0.01129
Uric acid, serum	120–420 µmol/L	2–7 mg/dL	59.48
Vitamin D (as vitamin D$_3$, cholecalciferol), plasma			
1,25-Dihydroxycholecalciferol (1,25(OH)$_2$D)	36–144 pmol/L	15–60 pg/mL	2.400
25-Hydroxycholecalciferol (25-OHD)	20–100 nmol/L	8–40 ng/mL	2.496

WILLIAMS
TEXTBOOK
OF
ENDOCRINOLOGY

8th Edition

WILLIAMS
TEXTBOOK
OF
ENDOCRINOLOGY

Edited by

Jean D. Wilson, M.D.

Professor and Chief of the Division of Endocrinology and Metabolism
Department of Internal Medicine
The University of Texas Southwestern Medical Center at Dallas

Daniel W. Foster, M.D.

Professor and Chairman
Department of Internal Medicine
The University of Texas Southwestern Medical Center at Dallas

W. B. SAUNDERS COMPANY
Harcourt Brace Jovanovich, Inc.
Philadelphia   London   Toronto   Montreal   Sydney   Tokyo

W. B. SAUNDERS COMPANY
Harcourt Brace Jovanovich, Inc.

The Curtis Center
Independence Square West
Philadelphia, Pennsylvania 19106

Library of Congress Cataloging-in-Publication Data

Williams textbook of endocrinology / [edited by] Jean D. Wilson
and Daniel W. Foster.—8th ed.

    p. cm.

Includes bibliographical references.
Includes index.

ISBN 0–7216–9514–0

1. Endocrine glands—Diseases.   2. Endocrinology.
I. Williams, Robert Hardin.   II. Wilson, Jean D.
III. Foster, Daniel W.   IV. Title: Textbook of
endocrinology. [DNLM: 1. Endocrine Diseases.
2. Endocrine Glands. WK 100 W721]

RC648.T46 1992

616.4–dc20

DNLM/DLC   90-8913

Listed here is the latest translated edition of this book together with the language of the translation and the
publisher.

Polish *(3rd Edition)*—Lekarskich, Warsaw, Poland
Spanish *(5th Edition)*—Salvat Editores, Barcelona, Spain
French *(4th Edition)*—Flammarion, Paris, France
Italian *(5th Edition)*—Piccin Editore, Padova, Italy
Japanese *(5th Edition)*—Hirokawa Publishing Company, Tokyo, Japan
Serbo-Croatian *(4th Edition)*—Medicinska Knjiga, Belgrade, Yugoslavia

Editor: W. B. Saunders Staff

Designer: Maureen Sweeney

Cover Designer: Michelle Maloney

Production Manager: Ken Neimeister

Manuscript Editors: Judith Gandy and Mary Prescott

Illustration Specialist: Lisa Lambert

Indexer: Alexandra Nickerson

WILLIAMS TEXTBOOK OF ENDOCRINOLOGY   ISBN 0–7216–9514–0

Last digit is the print number: 9   8   7   6   5   4   3   2   1

CONTRIBUTORS

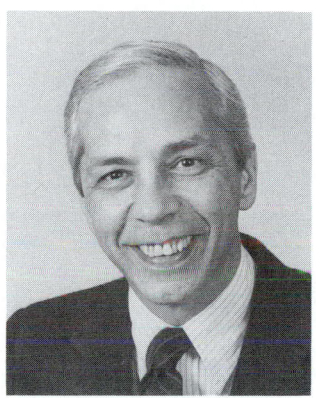

Thomas E. Andreoli

Professor and Chairman, Department of Internal Medicine, University of Arkansas College of Medicine, Little Rock

The Posterior Pituitary and Water Metabolism

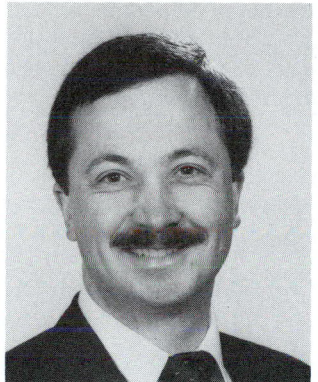

W. Scott Appleton

Post Doctoral Research Fellow, Department of Internal Medicine, University of Utah School of Medicine, Salt Lake City

Humoral Manifestations of Cancer

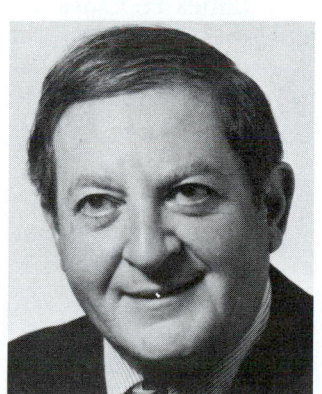

Gerald D. Aurbach

Chief, Metabolic Diseases Branch, National Institute of Diabetes and Digestive and Kidney Diseases, National Institutes of Health, Bethesda

Parathyroid Hormone, Calcitonin, and the Calciferols
Metabolic Bone Disease

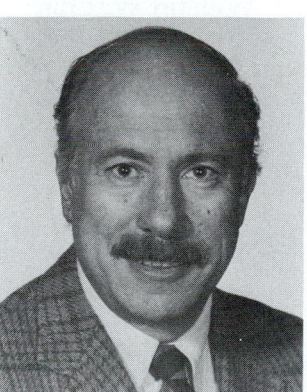

Edwin L. Bierman

Professor of Medicine and Head, Division of Metabolism and Endocrinology, University of Washington, Seattle

Disorders of Lipid Metabolism

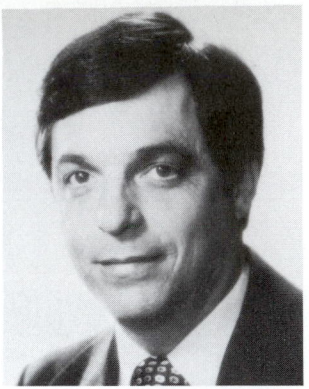

Bruce R. Carr

Paul C. MacDonald Professor of Obstetrics and Gynecology and Director, Division of Reproductive Endocrinology, The University of Texas Southwestern Medical Center at Dallas

Disorders of the Ovary and Female Reproductive Tract
Fertility Control and Its Complications

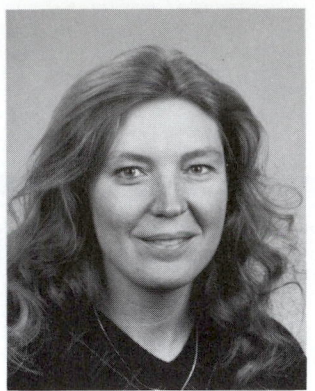

M. Linette Casey

Associate Professor, Cecil H. and Ida Green Center for Reproductive Biology Sciences, Departments of Biochemistry and Obstetrics-Gynecology, The University of Texas Southwestern Medical Center at Dallas

Endocrinological Changes of Pregnancy

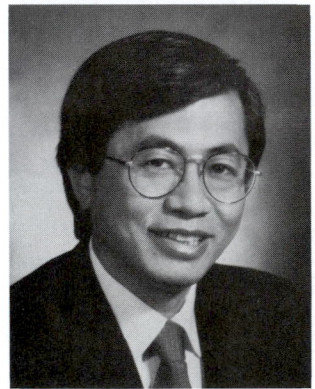

William W. Chin

Associate Professor of Medicine and Investigator, Howard Hughes Medical Institute, Harvard Medical School, Boston

Mechanism of Action of Hormones That Act at the Cell
Surface

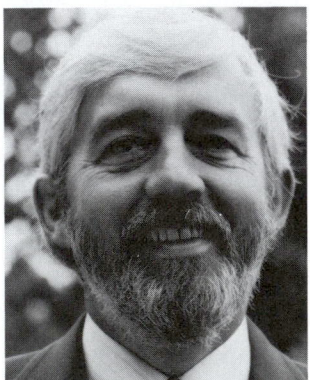

James H. Clark

Professor of Cell Biology, Baylor College of Medicine, Houston

Mechanisms of Action of Steroid Hormones

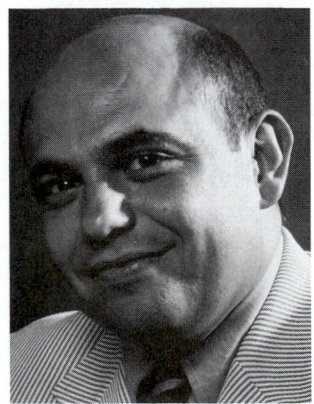

Felix A. Conte

Professor of Pediatrics, University of California, San Francisco

Disorders of Sex Differentiation

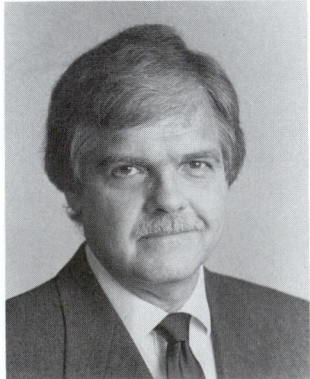

Philip E. Cryer

Professor of Medicine and Director, Division of Endocrinology, Diabetes and Metabolism, Washington University School of Medicine, St. Louis

Glucose Homeostasis and Hypoglycemia

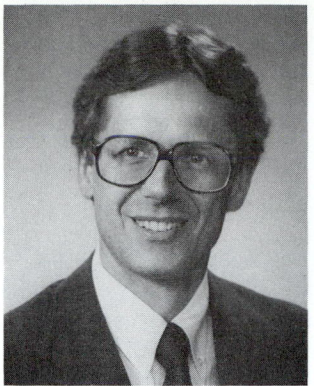

C. Rowan DeBold

Adult Endocrinologist, Park Nicolett Medical Center, Minneapolis

The Adrenal Cortex

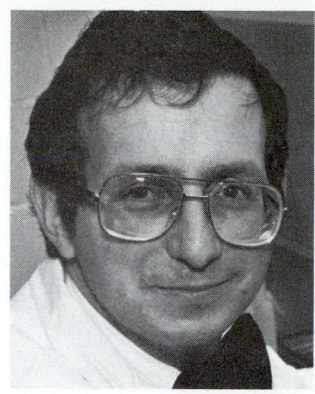

George S. Eisenbarth

Associate Professor of Medicine, Harvard Medical School; Chief, Section of Immunology and Immunogenetics, Joslin Diabetes Center, Boston

The Immunoendocrinopathy Syndromes

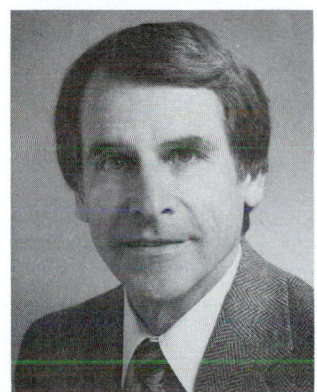

Delbert A. Fisher

Professor of Pediatrics and Medicine, University of California, Los Angeles, School of Medicine; Director, Walter Martin Research Center, Harbor-UCLA Medical Center, Torrance

Endocrinology of Fetal Development

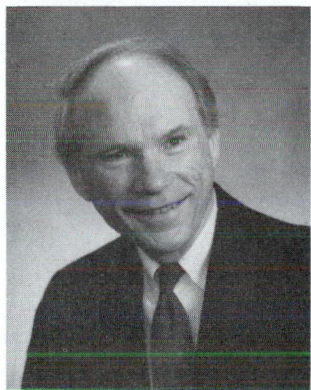

Daniel W. Foster

Donald W. Seldin Distinguished Chair in Internal Medicine and Chairman, Department of Internal Medicine, The University of Texas Southwestern Medical Center at Dallas

Diabetes Mellitus
Eating Disorders: Obesity, Anorexia Nervosa, and Bulimia Nervosa

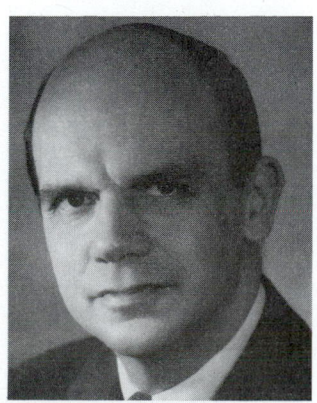

Andrew G. Frantz

Professor of Medicine, Columbia University College of Physicians and Surgeons, New York

Endocrine Disorders of the Breast

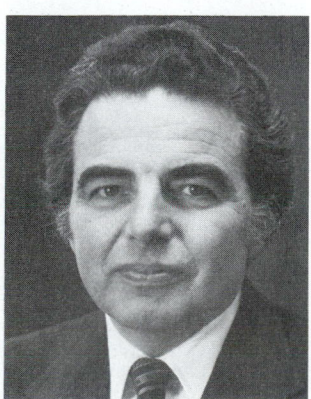

Norbert Freinkel

Late Kettering Professor of Medicine; Professor of Molecular Biology; Director, Center for Endocrinology, Metabolism and Nutrition; Chief, Section of Endocrinology, Metabolism and Nutrition, Northwestern University–McGaw Medical Center, Chicago

Metabolic Changes in Pregnancy

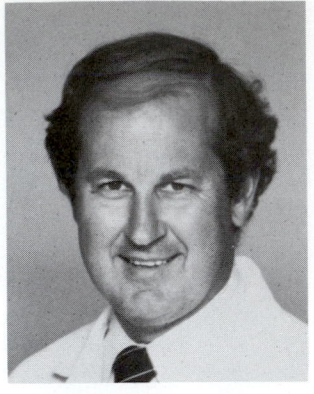

Robert F. Gagel

Associate Professor of Medicine and Cell Biology, Baylor College of Medicine; Clinical Investigator, Department of Veterans Affairs Medical Center, Houston

Multiple Endocrine Neoplasia

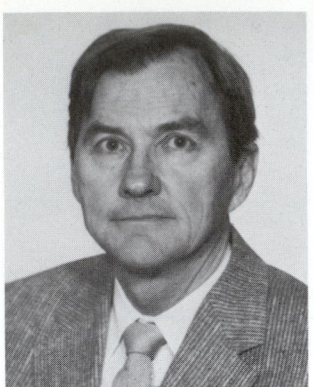

John A. Glomset

Professor of Medicine and Biochemistry, University of Washington, Seattle

Disorders of Lipid Metabolism

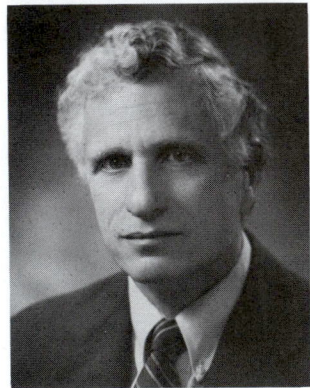

Phillip Gorden

Director, National Institute of Diabetes and Digestive and Kidney Diseases, National Institutes of Health, Bethesda

Radioreceptor and Other Functional Hormone Assays

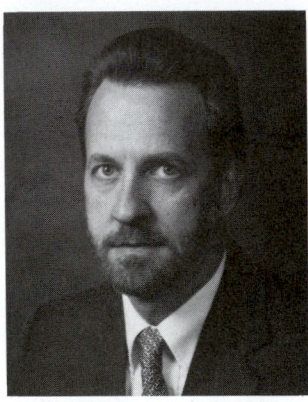

James E. Griffin

Professor of Internal Medicine, The University of Texas Southwestern Medical Center at Dallas

Disorders of the Testes and the Male Reproductive Tract
Fertility Control and Its Complications
Dynamic Tests of Endocrine Function

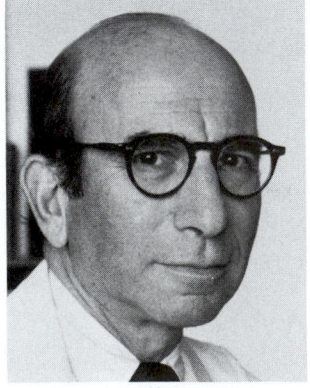

Melvin M. Grumbach

Edward B. Shaw Professor of Pediatrics, University of California, San Francisco

Disorders of Sex Differentiation
Puberty: Ontogeny, Neuroendocrinology, Physiology, and Disorders

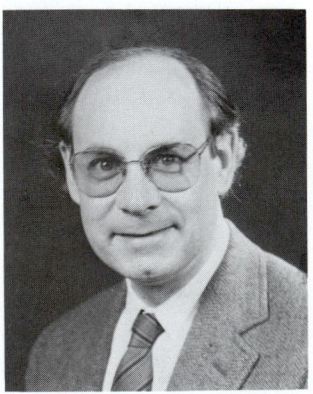

Joel F. Habener

Professor of Medicine, Harvard Medical School; Chief, Laboratory of Molecular Endocrinology, Massachusetts General Hospital, Boston

Genetic Control of Hormone Formation

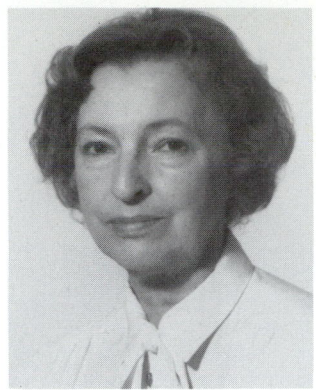

Eva Horvath

Associate Professor of Pathology, Department of Pathology, University of Toronto

The Anterior Pituitary

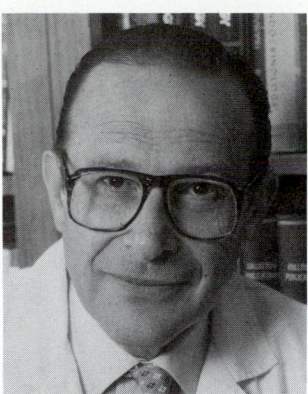

Sidney H. Ingbar

Late William Bosworth Castle Professor of Medicine, Harvard Medical School, Boston

The Thyroid Gland

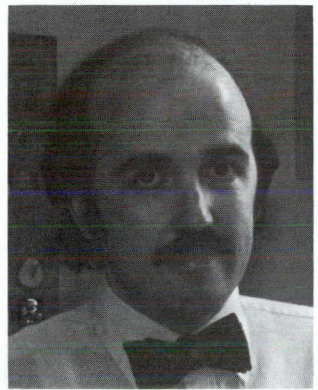

Richard A. Jackson

Assistant Professor of Medicine, Harvard Medical School, Boston

The Immunoendocrinopathy Syndromes

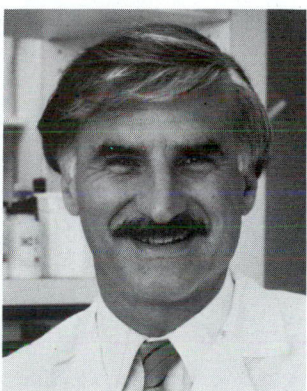

C. Ronald Kahn

Mary K. Iacocca Professor of Medicine, Harvard Medical School; Research Director, Joslin Diabetes Center, Boston

Mechanism of Action of Hormones That Act at the Cell Surface

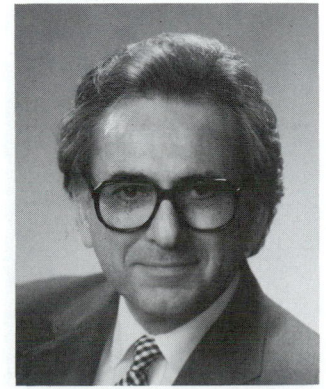

Norman M. Kaplan

Professor of Internal Medicine, The University of Texas Southwestern Medical Center at Dallas

Endocrine Hypertension

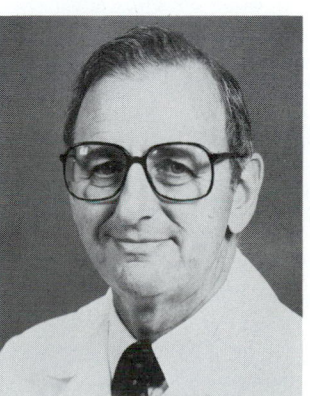

Stanley G. Korenman

Professor of Medicine-Endocrinology, School of Medicine, University of California, Los Angeles

Sexual Dysfunction

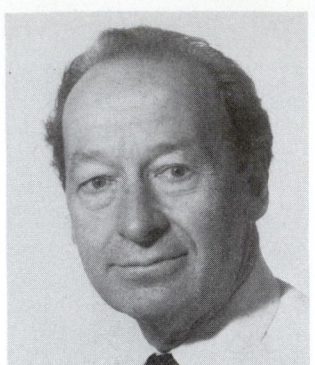

Kalman Kovacs

Professor of Pathology, Department of Pathology, University of Toronto

The Anterior Pituitary

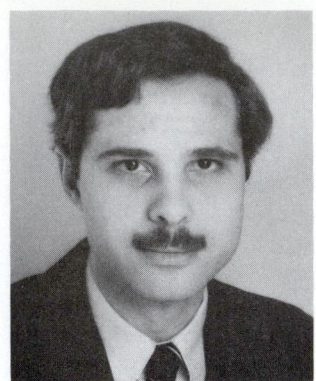

William J. Kovacs

Associate Professor of Medicine, Vanderbilt University School of Medicine, Nashville

The Adrenal Cortex

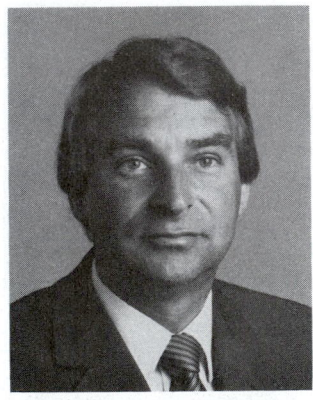

Guenter J. Krejs

Professor and Chairman, Department of Medicine, Karl Franzens University, Graz, Austria

Non–Insulin-Secreting Tumors of the Gastroenteropancreatic System

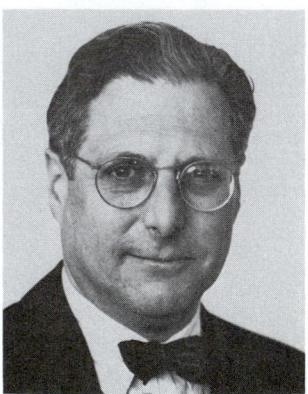

Lewis Landsberg

Cutter Professor and Chairman, Department of Medicine, and Director, Center for Endocrinology, Metabolism and Nutrition, Northwestern University Medical School, Chicago

Catecholamines and the Adrenal Medulla

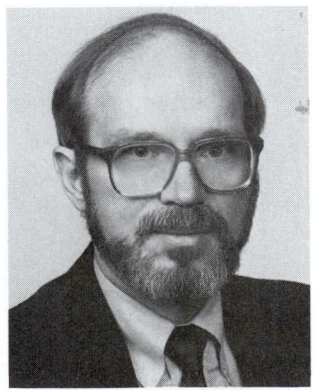

P. Reed Larsen

Professor of Medicine, Harvard Medical School, Boston

The Thyroid Gland

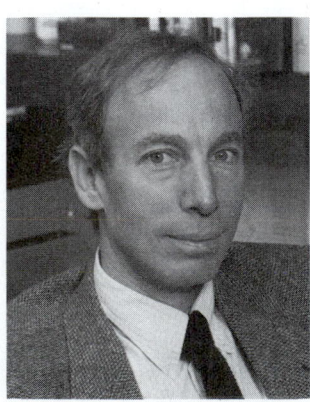

Marc E. Lippman

Professor of Medicine and Pharmacology and Director, Vincent T. Lombardi Cancer Research Center, Georgetown University Medical School, Washington, DC

Endocrine-Responsive Cancers of Humans

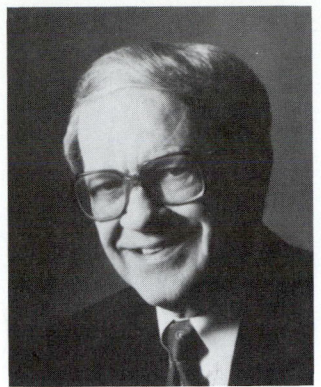

Paul C. MacDonald

Professor, Cecil H. and Ida Green Center for Reproductive Biology Sciences, Departments of Obstetrics-Gynecology and Biochemistry, The University of Texas Southwestern Medical Center at Dallas

Endocrinological Changes of Pregnancy

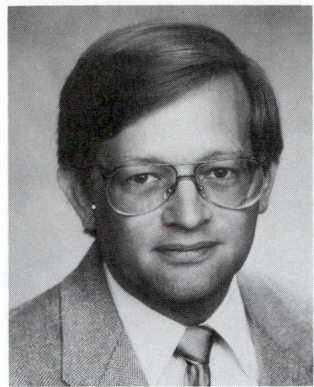

Stephen J. Marx

Chief, Mineral Metabolism Section, National Institute of Diabetes and Digestive and Kidney Diseases, National Institutes of Health, Bethesda

Parathyroid Hormone, Calcitonin, and the Calciferols
Metabolic Bone Disease

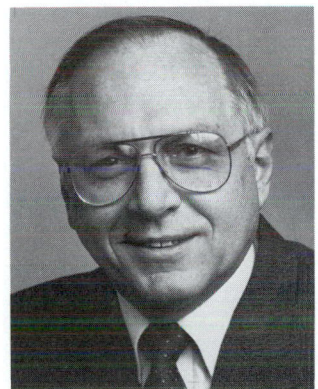

Boyd E. Metzger

Professor of Medicine and Acting Chief, Section of Endocrinology, Metabolism and Nutrition, Northwestern University Medical School, Chicago

Metabolic Changes in Pregnancy

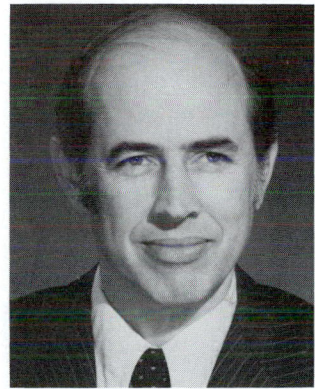

John A. Oates

Professor of Medicine and Pharmacology and Chairman, Department of Medicine, Vanderbilt University School of Medicine, Nashville

Disorders of Vasodilator Hormones: The Carcinoid Syndrome
and Mastocytosis

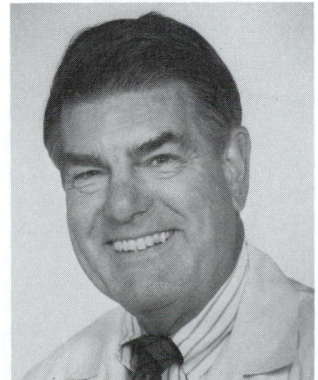

William D. Odell

Professor of Medicine and Physiology and Chairman, Department of Internal Medicine, University of Utah School of Medicine, Salt Lake City

Humoral Manifestations of Cancer

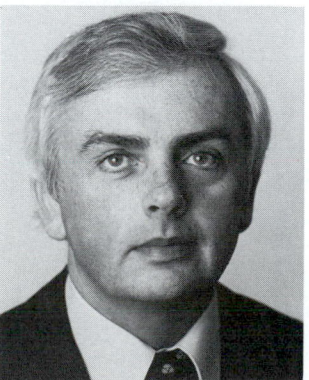

Bert W. O'Malley

Professor and Chairman, Department of Cell Biology, Baylor College of Medicine, Houston

Mechanisms of Action of Steroid Hormones

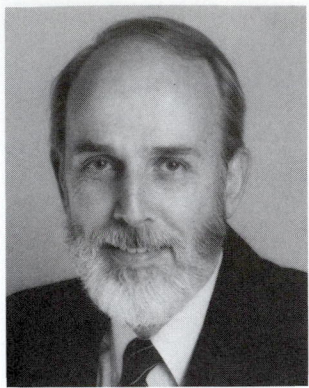

David N. Orth

Professor of Medicine, Professor of Molecular Physiology and Biophysics, and Director, Division of Endocrinology, Vanderbilt University School of Medicine, Nashville

The Adrenal Cortex

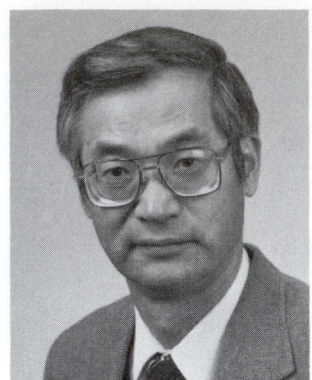

Charles Y. C. Pak

Professor of Medicine, The University of Texas Southwestern Medical Center at Dallas

Kidney Stones

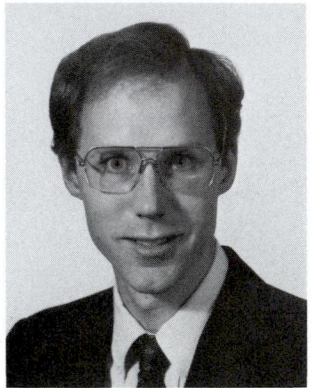

W. Brian Reeves

Assistant Professor of Internal Medicine, Division of Nephrology, University of Arkansas College of Medicine, Little Rock

The Posterior Pituitary and Water Metabolism

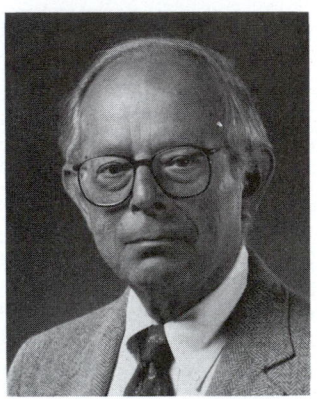

Seymour Reichlin

Professor of Medicine, Tufts University School of Medicine; Chief, Endocrine Division, New England Medical Center, Boston

Neuroendocrinology

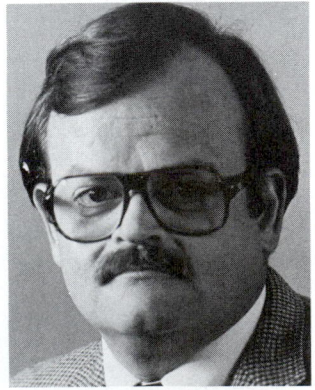

L. Jackson Roberts II

Professor of Pharmacology and Medicine, Vanderbilt University School of Medicine, Nashville

Disorders of Vasodilator Hormones: The Carcinoid Syndrome and Mastocytosis

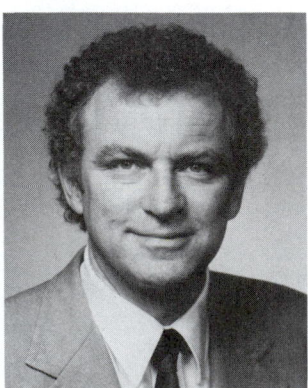

William T. Schrader

Professor of Cell Biology, Baylor College of Medicine, Houston

Mechanisms of Action of Steroid Hormones

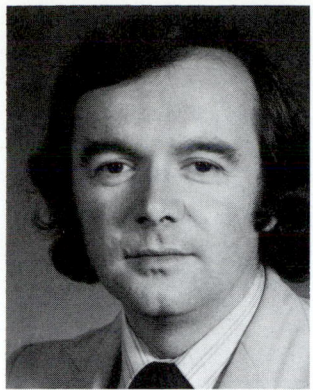

Evan R. Simpson

Professor, Cecil H. and Ida Green Center for Reproductive Biology Sciences, Departments of Obstetrics-Gynecology and Biochemistry, The University of Texas Southwestern Medical Center at Dallas

Endocrinological Changes of Pregnancy

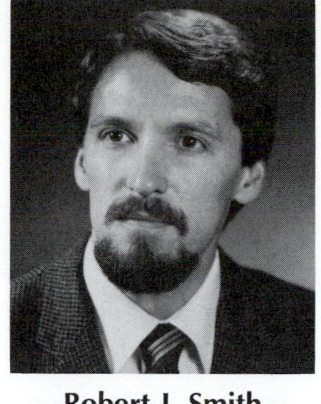

Robert J. Smith

Associate Professor of Medicine, Harvard Medical School; Assistant Director of Research, Head of Section on Metabolism, Joslin Diabetes Center, Boston

Mechanism of Action of Hormones That Act at the Cell Surface

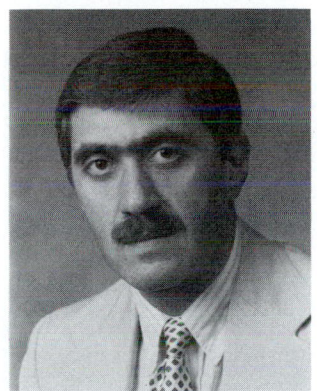

Allen M. Spiegel

Chief, Molecular Pathophysiology Branch, National Institute of Diabetes and Digestive and Kidney Diseases, National Institutes of Health, Bethesda

Parathyroid Hormone, Calcitonin, and the Calciferols
Metabolic Bone Disease

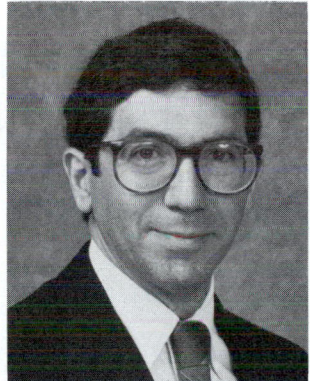

Dennis M. Styne

Professor and Chairman of Pediatrics, University of California, Davis

Puberty: Ontogeny, Neuroendocrinology, Physiology, and Disorders

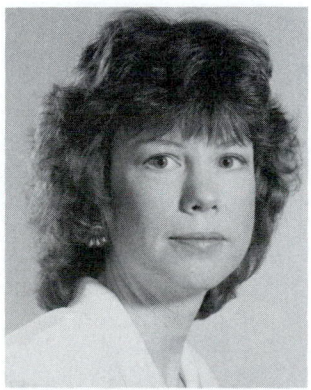

Sandra M. Swain

Assistant Professor of Medicine and Director, Comprehensive Breast Center, Vincent T. Lombardi Cancer Research Center, Georgetown University Medical School, Washington, DC

Endocrine-Responsive Cancers of Humans

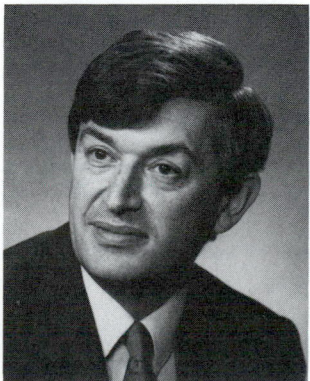

Michael O. Thorner

Kenneth R. Crispell Professor of Medicine and Head, Division of Endocrinology and Metabolism, Department of Internal Medicine, University of Virginia Medical School, Charlottesville

The Anterior Pituitary

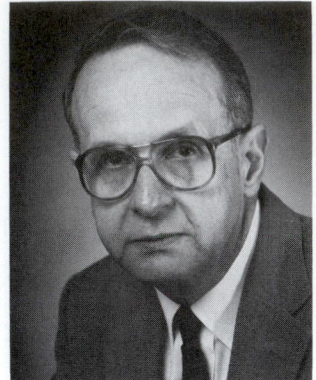

Louis E. Underwood

Professor of Pediatrics, University of North Carolina at Chapel Hill

Normal and Aberrant Growth

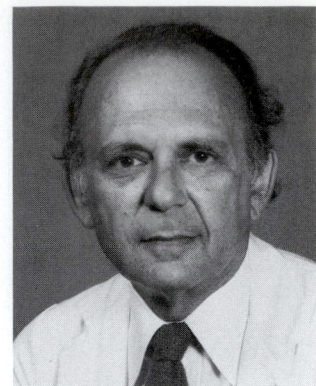

Roger H. Unger

Touchstone/West Distinguished Chair in Diabetes Research and Director, Gifford Laboratories for Diabetes Research, The University of Texas Southwestern Medical Center at Dallas; Senior Medical Investigator, Department of Veterans Affairs Medical Center, Dallas

Diabetes Mellitus

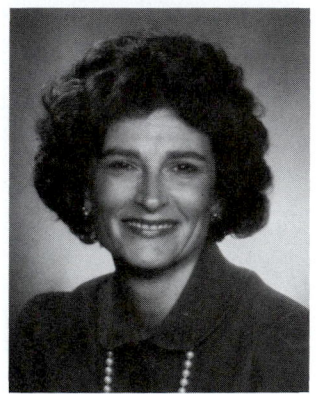

Mary Lee Vance

Associate Professor of Medicine, University of Virginia Medical School, Charlottesville

The Anterior Pituitary

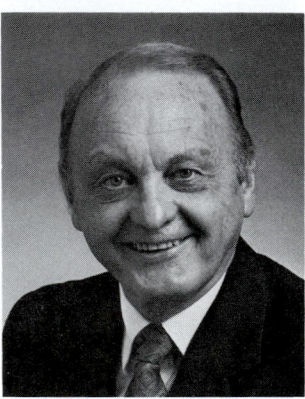

Judson J. Van Wyk

Kenan Professor of Pediatrics, University of North Carolina at Chapel Hill

Normal and Aberrant Growth

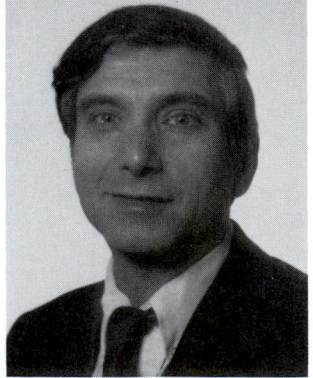

Bruce D. Weintraub

Chief, Molecular, Cellular and Nutritional Endocrinology Branch, National Institute of Diabetes and Digestive and Kidney Diseases, National Institutes of Health, Bethesda

Radioreceptor and Other Functional Hormone Assays

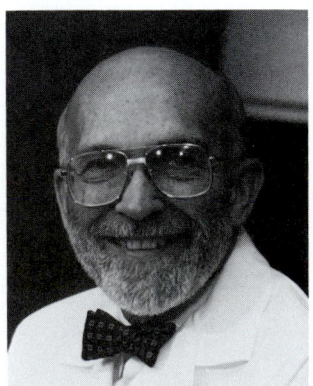

Jean D. Wilson

Charles C. Sprague Professor of Internal Medicine, The University of Texas Southwestern Medical Center at Dallas

Disorders of the Testes and the Male Reproductive Tract
Endocrine Disorders of the Breast

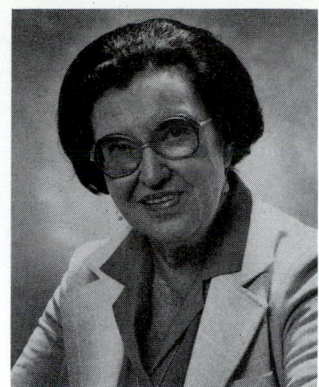

Rosalyn S. Yalow

Solomon A. Berson Distinguished Professor-at-Large, Mt. Sinai School of Medicine of City University of New York; Senior Medical Investigator, Department of Veterans Affairs Medical Center, Bronx

Radioimmunoassay of Hormones

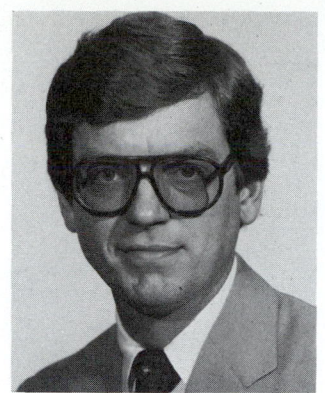

James B. Young

Professor of Medicine, Northwestern University Medical School, Chicago

Catecholamines and the Adrenal Medulla

PREFACE

The aim of *Williams Textbook of Endocrinology* continues to be to serve as a bridge between basic science and clinical endocrinology. This aim was clearly formulated in the preface to the first edition:

> *The rapidity and extent of advances in endocrinology have made it increasingly difficult for the student and physician to take full advantage of information available for the understanding, diagnosis and treatment of clinical disorders. It is the realization of these difficulties that prompted the writing of this book. The main objective is to provide a condensed and authoritative discussion of the management of clinical endocrinopathies, based upon the application of fundamental information obtained from chemical and physiologic investigations.*

Since the publication of the seventh edition, endocrinology has continued to change. The impact of molecular and cell biology has been to radically transform our understanding of endocrine physiology and endocrine pathology. Today in the approach to disease—no less than in basic endocrine science—the focus is more on how hormones act than on factors that influence hormone levels. Moreover, the recognition that many chemical mediators behave like hormones, even though they act by autocrine or paracrine mechanisms rather than via the circulation, has vastly broadened the scope of endocrinology. The technological change in clinical medicine, especially the imaging revolution, has given new power to diagnosis that was unknown at the time of the last edition and has expanded the therapeutic repertoire.

The eighth edition of *Williams Textbook of Endocrinology* has been carefully planned to reflect the rapidly advancing elements of modern endocrinology. Molecular biology and cell biology are in evidence in essentially every chapter. The introductory chapters on hormone action, which are rich with diagrams, make the basic principles readily understandable both to beginning students and to clinicians who trained before the new science appeared. We have also added new chapters on fetal endocrinology and on puberty and its disorders.

In organizing this edition, we faced the special problem of the dual system of laboratory unit nomenclature within the United States. Since 1988, virtually all medical journals have used the International System of Units (SI units) for clinical laboratory values, whereas most hospital laboratories in the United States have used conventional units. Thus one system is used in the medical literature and another in the hospital. We decided to use both systems in the text: SI units are given first and the conventional units follow in parentheses for all measurements except blood pressure, which is given only in millimeters of mercury; energy value of food, which is given in kilocalories; and quantities for which the numbers are the same in both systems (e.g., nanomoles per liter or milliequivalents per liter for sodium concentration and international units per liter or milli–international units per milliliter for luteinizing hormone). In most instances the conversion between SI and conventional units is straightforward. In other cases the optimal way to convert from one system to the other is not clear-cut because there are different ways to express values in both systems. It is imperative that each reader consult his or her own laboratory for normal values. Readers must be alert to units, not only in our text, but also in clinical practice.

A striking feature of this textbook has always been the fact that the contributors are at the forefronts of their disciplines, thereby ensuring the freshness of each edition. This feature remains true for the current edition. Those who wrote in previous editions have devoted an immense effort to updating material, and the new contributors have expended an equal or greater effort in formulating new chapters. Neither task is easy, and to our authors we say thank you.

The book could not have been edited without the dedicated help of the co-workers in our offices—Christy K. Gonzales, Brenda H. Hennis, and Rita A. Koger. We acknowledge the special contributions made by Judith Gandy, our manuscript editor at the W. B. Saunders Company. Her remarkable attention to detail and her pursuit of excellence have had a major impact on the editors and on the book.

JEAN D. WILSON
DANIEL W. FOSTER

CONTENTS

SECTION 11

ASSESSMENT OF ENDOCRINE FUNCTION

INTRODUCTION

Jean D. Wilson and Daniel W. Foster

The capacity of specialized tissues to function in integrated fashion as components of intact organisms is made possible in large part by three systems of extracellular communication: (1) the nervous system, which transmits electrochemical signals as two-way traffic between the brain and peripheral tissues or between tissues in reflex circuits; (2) the endocrine system, which releases chemical mediators termed hormones into the circulation for action away from their sites of origin; and (3) the immune system, which protects the organism against external (bacteria, viruses, fungi) and internal (malignancy) threats. The distinctive features of the endocrine system were clearly delineated by Starling in the Croonian Lectures for 1905, in which he described separate endocrine and neurogenic control mechanisms for the regulation of gastric function.[1] Endocrinology was defined as that branch of biological science that concerns itself with the actions of hormones and the organs in which the hormones are formed. Its boundaries included study of the anatomy and physiological function of the major endocrine organs, the secretory products of these organs, the mechanisms of hormone action, and the clinical manifestations of hormone dysfunction. It was subsequently recognized, however, that there is no sharp distinction between the endocrine and nervous systems. Thus the nervous system liberates chemical agents that can act as local mediators or true circulating hormones, and hormones of several types also act as neurogenic mediators within the central nervous system. Furthermore, at the level of the hypothalamus and the pituitary there is an intimate link between the nervous and endocrine systems that serves to integrate the two into one functional control unit (see Chapter 5). The traditional definition of endocrinology has become even more blurred by the recognition that circulating hormones can also have local effects in the cells in which they are synthesized (e.g., locally formed estrogen in the central nervous system) or in adjacent cells after diffusion (e.g., the role of testosterone in regulating spermatogenesis, the effects of cortisol on the adrenal medulla, and the regulation of glucagon secretion by insulin). The immune system, which was long considered to function autonomously, is now recognized as a regulated system, subject to endocrine and neural control. It, in turn, exerts a reciprocal controlling effect on neuroendocrine systems.[2] For these reasons, there is a certain artificiality in attempting to define a specific arena of knowledge as endocrinology.

Despite these theoretical problems, certain factors serve to unify the discipline. First, regardless of their sites of action or the complexity of interactions among the various control systems, the central focus of endocrinology is on hormones. Second, the synthesis of these hormones is controlled by similar types of regulatory mechanisms, namely, feedback control in which the concentration of the hormone signals the need for more or less production. Third, there is a tight coupling between the basic science of endocrinology and clinical medicine. Clinical phenomena are frequently of fundamental import to basic science, and virtually all advances in the basic science of endocrinology have clinical ramifications. The subjects covered in this book seem appropriate for this concept of endocrinology, even though they range from those central to the discipline to those at the periphery.

THE FUNCTION OF HORMONES

Hormonal function involves four broad domains—reproduction; growth and development; maintenance of the internal environment; and production, utilization, and storage of energy (Fig. 1–1).

REPRODUCTION. Hormones not only regulate gametogenesis but also control the dimorphic anatomical, functional, and behavioral development of males and females that is essential for sexual reproduction. It is of particular interest in this regard that no exclusive male or female hormones have been identified. All hormones characterized to date are present in both sexes, and both sexes have receptor mechanisms that allow response to all hormones. Sexual dimorphism is the result of differences in the amounts of individual hormones and differences in their patterns of secretion, rather than of their presence or absence. It follows that sexual reproduction requires a precise genetic programming that allows for the synthesis of an appropriate enzyme complement in the ovary or testis that in turn catalyzes the formation of appropriate amounts of hormones at the critical stages of life. Endocrinological control affects every phase of reproduction, including many behavioral aspects.

GROWTH AND DEVELOPMENT. Endocrine control is fundamental for growth and development and involves the interaction of hormones of all classes, including peptide, steroid, catecholamine, and thyroid hormones. Although hormones are necessary for normal growth and development, it is of equal importance that they are also required for the limitation of growth. For example, if closure of the epiphyses did not occur, skeletal growth would presumably continue for an indefinite period. Hormonal interactions involved in the regulation and control of growth are multiple. Many hormones probably influence growth by regulating a final common mediator, the somatomedin system.

MAINTENANCE OF THE INTERNAL ENVIRONMENT. Hormones are critical to maintenance of the internal environment necessary to sustain structure and function. Thus they are involved in regulating and stabilizing body fluids and their electrolyte content; blood pressure and heart rate; acid-base balance; body temperature; and mass of bone, muscle, and fat. These homeostatic mechanisms not only operate on a minute-to-minute basis but also make possible the adaptation to extreme environmental change. Of the major homeostatic systems, only respiration does not have a significant element of endocrine control.

ENERGY PRODUCTION, UTILIZATION, AND STORAGE. Hormones are the pre-eminent mediators of substrate flux and the conversion of food into energy production or storage. In the anabolic state that follows a meal, excess fuel is stored as glycogen and fat under the influence of insulin. In the catabolic state that occurs postprandially or after more prolonged fasting, glucagon and other counterregulatory hormones induce glycogen breakdown and mobilize amino acids and free fatty acids as substrates for gluconeogenesis and ketogenesis, respectively. Oxidation of fatty acids and ketones preserves the plasma glucose level in a safe range for functioning of the central nervous system.

INTERACTION OF HORMONES

The effects of hormones are complex (see Chapters 3 and 4). A single hormone can have different effects in various tissues and in the same tissue at different times of life. Similarly, some biological processes are under the control of single hormones, whereas others require complex interactions among several hormones (Fig. 1–2).

ONE HORMONE, MULTIPLE ACTIONS. An example of a hormone with multiple effects is testosterone. Its actions include fusion of the labioscrotal fold in the male embryo during embryogenesis, induction of male differentiation of the wolffian ducts, regression of the embryonic breast (in some species), growth of the male urogenital tract, induction of spermatogenesis, growth of beard and body hair, promotion of muscle growth, retention of nitrogen, increased synthesis of erythropoietin, temporal regression of scalp hair, hyperplasia of the sebaceous glands with increased sebum production, development of prostatic hyperplasia in aging males of several species, secretion of ejaculate, and virilization of the hypothalamus. It was originally believed that testosterone exerted these diverse effects by distinct mechanisms. However, one of the most important findings of modern molecular biology is that diverse effects can be modulated by a single mechanism. In the case of testosterone, most actions can be explained by binding of the hormone (or its active metabolite dihydrotestosterone) to a high-affinity cytoplasmic receptor protein, followed by attachment of the hormone-receptor complex to specific DNA-binding sites in the cell nucleus of target tissues where it promotes the synthesis of messenger RNAs. The diverse effects of the hormone are due in large part not to different mechanisms of action but rather to the fact that different cells at different stages of development are programmed to respond to the hormone-receptor complex in different ways. Occasionally, hormone effects can be due to "cross-talk" among receptors; for example, some actions of testosterone are due to its binding to the estradiol receptor and hence to action as an antiestrogen. It is also possible that testosterone at high concentrations exerts anabolic effects by binding to the glucocorticoid receptor, thus blocking glucocorticoid action. Still other hormonal effects may be indirect. Testosterone, for example, enhances erythropoietin formation, which stimulates erythropoiesis and causes the differences in hemoglobin concentration between men and women. The same pattern of many effects from limited modes of action is seen with most hormones, including peptides that act at the cell surface.

ONE FUNCTION, MULTIPLE HORMONES. It is commonplace to think of hormones and their actions in isolation, but virtually all complex processes under endocrine regulation are influenced by more than one hormone. A classic example is maintenance of the plasma glucose concentration within a narrow range: high enough to prevent dysfunction

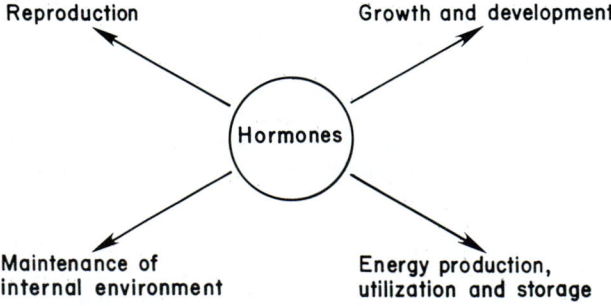

Figure 1–1. The four primary arenas of hormone action.

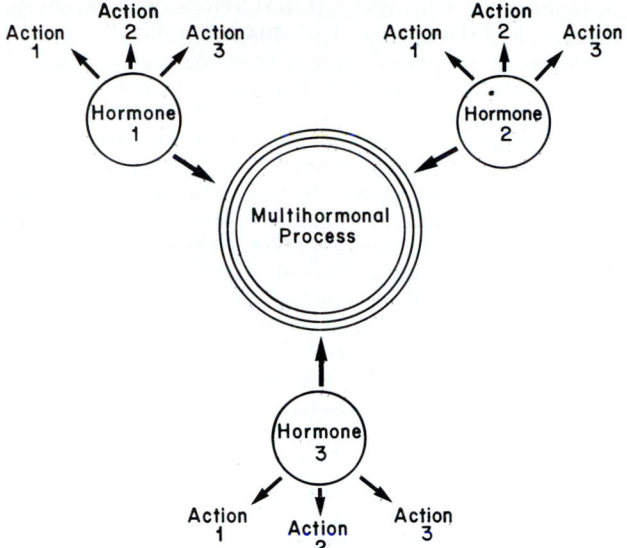

Figure 1–2. Actions of hormones. A single hormone may act independently or in concert with other hormones. For example, in this scheme the multihormone process might be maintenance of the plasma glucose level, hormone 1 being insulin; hormone 2, glucagon; and hormone 3, epinephrine. Each hormone may also act to control or influence more than one process.

of the central nervous system on the one hand, and low enough to prevent the detrimental effects of hyperglycemia on the other. Such regulation could not be accomplished smoothly by a single hormone, no matter how powerful. Primary control at the upper boundary of normality is exerted by insulin, which modulates hepatic glucose production and enhances glucose transport into cells for both utilization and storage, thereby protecting against hyperglycemia. The pre-eminent glucose-elevating hormone is glucagon, which stimulates glucose production in the liver via glycogen breakdown and enhances gluconeogenesis whenever plasma glucose approaches hypoglycemic levels, thus protecting the central nervous system against dysfunction related to substrate or energy depletion. Because hypoglycemia is a greater risk to life than hyperglycemia, a back-up set of glucose-raising hormones is released as the plasma glucose concentration falls to dangerous levels: epinephrine, norepinephrine, cortisol, and growth hormone. Thus at least six hormones play important roles in directly maintaining the plasma glucose level. This list is not exhaustive because other hormones influence the process indirectly: e.g., thyroxine, which influences appetite; somatostatin (SRIF, somatotropin release–inhibiting factor), which blocks insulin or glucagon release and slows nutrient absorption from the gut; and gastric inhibitory polypeptide, which enhances insulin release in response to glucose absorption. Another example of a process under multiple hormonal control is lactation, which involves (at a minimum) prolactin, placental lactogen, glucocorticoids, thyroxine, estrogen, progesterone, and oxytocin.

The existence of such complex control mechanisms has two major implications. First, there can be a remarkable degree of fine tuning: blood glucose levels can be maintained within normal limits under nutritional conditions that vary in the extreme. Second, complex control mechanisms for vital functions may provide safety insofar as alternative mechanisms can take over when one hormone in the series is deficient (a fail-safe function). Even in processes that are under predominant control by one hormonal system, other hormones commonly play permissive roles. For example, the differentiation and growth of the male external genitalia

is mediated predominantly by dihydrotestosterone, but growth hormone and thyroxine are essential for normal development of the genitalia during postnatal life.

THE CHEMICAL NATURE OF HORMONES

Hormones fall into two broad categories. The majority are peptides or amino acid derivatives, a category that includes complex polypeptides (luteinizing hormone [LH], chorionic gonadotropin), intermediate-sized peptides (insulin and glucagon), small peptides (thyrotropin-releasing hormone), dipeptides (thyroxine and triiodothyronine), and derivatives of single amino acids (catecholamines, serotonin, and histamine). The remainder are steroids, derivatives of cholesterol that are of two types: those with an intact steroid nucleus (adrenal steroids and gonadal steroids), and those in which the B ring of the steroid has been broken (vitamin D and its various metabolites).

The existence of diverse structures for chemical mediation implies that evolution of the mechanisms for chemical control must have taken place over a long time. However, there is no fixed relationship between hormones in primitive species and those in more advanced species. In some cases, such as estrogen, essentially the same molecule has wide distribution. Conversely, other hormones, such as the steroid hormone ecdysone of insects, have no known counterpart in humans. Occasionally, homologies between structures of different hormones (e.g., that between prolactin, placental lactogen, and growth hormone) or between the structures of hormone receptors (e.g., that between the receptors for prolactin and growth hormone) allow deductions to be drawn regarding patterns of evolution.

Regardless of their chemical structures or how they evolved, all hormones share several characteristics. First, they are present in the circulation at low concentration. The plasma concentration of steroid and thyroid hormones ranges between picomolar and micromolar, whereas that for peptide hormones is generally between 1 and 100 fM. Second, because they are present in such small amounts, they must be directed to sites of action by specific mechanisms. This direction commonly is accomplished by specific receptors in target tissues that recognize and bind the hormone with high affinity. There is considerable variability in the degree of restriction of the receptors; some, such as the insulin receptor, are present in virtually all tissues, whereas others, such as the mineralocorticoid receptor, appear to have a more limited distribution. Although receptors are essential for hormone response, they may not in themselves be sufficient. Thus some tissues possess receptors but lack some other molecule(s) necessary for hormone response. For example, insulin receptors are present on erythrocytes but the red blood cell does not exhibit typical insulin responses. It is generally true, nevertheless, that the principal target organs for a given hormone contain the largest complement of receptor molecules and that as a consequence the concentration of that hormone in the target tissue is higher than that in the circulation.

Another mechanism by which hormones can be directed to specific target tissues is by delivery within a restricted circulation. The liver is a major target tissue for insulin not because of unique receptor content but because the amount delivered to hepatic tissue through the portal circulation is higher than that reaching peripheral tissues through the systemic circulation. The same is true for the delivery of the various releasing factors from the hypothalamus to the pituitary through the hypophyseal-portal system and for the delivery of hormones from the adrenal cortex to the adrenal medulla. Because of dilution and the rapid clearance of these hormones from the systemic circulation, their concentrations in the circulation-restricted sites are higher than those achieved systemically.

A third means of targeting is by direct diffusion to adjacent sites. For example, testosterone synthesized in the Leydig cells of the testes diffuses into the adjacent spermatogenic tubule to achieve the high level of the hormone necessary to promote spermatogenesis; it is also released into plasma.

A fourth mechanism is local formation of hormone within a tissue from circulating precursors. One example is the formation of dihydrotestosterone from testosterone within androgen target tissues such as prostate. Similarly, estradiol can be formed from circulating androgenic precursors in target tissues such as the brain. Thus there are various means by which the action of hormones can be focused or magnified in specific tissues.

The concept of a target tissue, important as it is, should not be exaggerated. Consider, for example, insulin. By most criteria its major sites of action are liver, muscle, and adipose tissue. However, insulin has distinct or permissive effects in many tissues or systems, including pancreas, kidney, brain, lung, immune system, platelets, nervous system, and bone. The same type of gradation is true for the action of many, probably most, hormones. Thus the "targeting" of hormone action may actually influence the magnitude or amplitude of hormonal response rather than determine whether a response will occur. In rigorous terms, the all-or-none concept of a target tissue should be replaced by quantitative assessments, i.e., whether a tissue is a major or a minor site of hormone action.

HORMONE SYNTHESIS, STORAGE, AND RELEASE

The synthetic mechanisms that result in hormone formation are not unique. Thus peptide hormones are synthesized by the same biochemical pathways as other proteins and are subsequently processed by cleavage and/or chemical modification to form the active molecules. Often the initial product is a large molecule that is progressively shortened in distinct steps, e.g., pre-proparathyroid hormone → proparathyroid hormone → parathyroid hormone. Steroid hormones and catecholamines are synthesized from smaller precursors. In the case of steroid hormones the parent molecule, cholesterol, is modified by sequential hydroxylations and cleavages of carbon-carbon bonds to form the varied products. For many years it was assumed that endocrine organs possessed unique enzymatic capacities that allowed these reactions to take place. It is now known that hormone synthesis can occur in diverse tissues. Glucagon is formed in the wall of the gastrointestinal tract as well as in the pancreas, and many peptide hormones are formed in the central nervous system, the pituitary, and the gastrointestinal tract. Human chorionic gonadotropin appears to be synthesized in almost every tissue of the body. Even when hormones cannot be synthesized de novo in a tissue, they may be derived by transformation reactions. Estrogen, for example, can be formed from testosterone and androstenedione in ovary, brain, adipocytes, and hair follicles. The synthesis of the active forms of vitamin D is even more complicated. The prohormone, 7-dehydrocholesterol, or provitamin D_3, is synthesized in the skin and is converted there to cholecaliferol, which enters the circulation and is then sequentially hydroxylated in the liver (25-hydroxycholecaliferol) and the kidney (1,25-dihydroxycholecaliferol).

Although endocrine organs are not the sole sites of hormone formation, they synthesize and regulate these hormones more efficiently than do other tissues. Three fundamental characteristics distinguish endocrine organs from nonendocrine tissues that happen to make hormones. First, rates of synthesis are generally greater in the major endocrine organs. Thus the placenta produces far greater amounts of human chorionic gonadotropin per unit weight than does liver or testis. Second, appropriate processing machinery is available to complete conversion of prohormones to hormones. Pro-opiomelanocortin, for example, is efficiently converted to corticotropin (ACTH, adrenocorticotropin) in the pituitary but not in the brain. Third, endocrine glands contain mechanisms for the release of the hormone into the circulation, often but not always, by a regulated process.

The rate of release of hormone is determined ultimately by the rate of its synthesis. Most tropic hormones and regulatory factors act by controlling the rate of synthesis, although there are exceptions (e.g., thyrotropin enhances thyroxine release before enhancing thyroxine synthesis). In most instances only limited quantities of hormones are stored within the body. For example, the testicular testosterone content is invariably small so that the total amount must turn over several times each day to explain the daily production rate in normal men. Variable amounts of peptide hormones are stored in the pancreas and the pituitary; these stores serve a critical function in emergencies and periods of stress but are generally depleted within hours to days. The general rule is for continuous synthesis and turnover of hormones. Two major exceptions to the generalization of limited storage are thyroxine and 1,25-dihydroxycholecaliferol. In both instances, precursor forms of the actual hormone—thyroglobulin and either 7-dehydrocholesterol or cholecaliferol—are stored in large amounts to serve as a reservoir for potential hormone formation. The consequence is to provide a safeguard against long periods of iodine deficiency or absence of sunlight, respectively. In the case of most hormones, however, no such long-term safeguards exist.

TRANSPORT

Water-soluble hormones are transported in plasma in solution and require no specific transport mechanism. The more insoluble hormones require carrier mechanisms, namely, transport proteins. Because in most instances only the free or unbound hormone enters cells, the transport proteins act as reservoirs so that bound hormone is in dynamic equilibrium with a small amount of free hormone in the plasma. As unbound hormone enters cells, it is replaced by hormone newly released from the carrier protein. This process ensures that all cells have access to even the most insoluble of the hormones.[3] Transport proteins are of two types. Albumin and transthyretin (formerly termed prealbumin) bind many small ligands and can be considered general transport molecules. The specific transport proteins—thyroxine-binding globulin, testosterone-estrogen–binding globulin, and corticosteroid-binding globulin—have restricted binding sites of high affinity. They resemble intracellular receptor proteins in their specificities and binding characteristics.

These specific transport systems are nonexclusive because alternative systems can function in their absence. Thus, in hereditary deficiency of thyroxine-binding globulin, thyroid hormones are transported adequately by albumin and transthyretin. Likewise, in analbuminemia, hormones can be carried by other proteins. No situation is known in which transport of hormones ceases or abnormal transport by itself causes disease.

Several general features of transport proteins have been identified. First, they have a profound effect on clearance rates for hormones. In general, the greater the capacity for high-affinity binding of a hormone, the slower is its clearance rate.[3] This characteristic follows from the fact that the rate of metabolic clearance (usually by liver and/or kidney) is determined by the level of free (or readily available) hormone. Women, for example, have higher levels of testosterone-estrogen–binding globulin and clear hormones that are tightly bound to this binding globulin (testosterone and dihydrotestosterone) about half as rapidly as men.[4] Second, the transport proteins usually have binding capacities that are much higher than the physiological concentration of most hormones. This difference means that when hormones are overproduced or given in pharmacological amounts for therapy, enormous quantities of even the most insoluble hormones can be delivered to tissues. Third, because the rate of hormone production is ultimately determined by the level of free hormone, synthesis can be adjusted appropriately to compensate for changes in the concentration of the transport proteins. As a consequence, increases or decreases in the amounts of specific transport protein have little effect on endocrine control mechanisms in the steady state, although they may cause diagnostic confusion by altering total concentrations of hormone in plasma. To illustrate, an increase in corticosteroid-binding globulin would be followed by a transient decrease in the level of free cortisol, which in turn would be followed by an increase in cortisol production until corticosteroid-binding globulin is saturated sufficiently for the free hormone level to approximate normal. It follows that changes in transport proteins cause pathological endocrine conditions only if the regulatory feedback systems are impaired, which basically means that the endocrine gland is abnormal. The most common clinical problem involving transport proteins has to do with the increases in thyroxine-binding globulin that accompany estrogen therapy or pregnancy, for which measurement of total thyroxine may suggest hyperthyroidism in a euthyroid subject.

How hormones are transported across cell membranes has not been resolved completely. In the case of peptide hormones that bind to cell-surface receptors, the hormone-receptor complexes can be internalized by endocytosis.[5] This mechanism is active in the sense that energy is required, but because it has not been demonstrated to occur against a concentration gradient it is not usually defined as active transport. The internalization process may serve primarily to deliver the hormones to intracellular sites of degradation and hence function as a termination signal to limit hormone action. In the case of hormones with cytosolic receptors, it has been suggested that hormone that is bound to transport proteins might be selectively transported across the membranes of some cells, but the bulk of evidence suggests that free hormone diffuses passively across cell membranes down activity gradients.[4] The presence of intracellular proteins that bind the hormones may tend to keep the intracellular concentration of the free hormone low and thus favor the diffusion process.

FEEDBACK RELATIONSHIPS

The distinguishing characteristic of endocrine systems is the feedback control of hormone production. The paradigm for feedback control is the interaction of the pituitary gland with the thyroid, adrenals, and gonads. Hormones produced in peripheral endocrine organs feed back on the hypothalamic-pituitary system, thus regulating the production of the tropic hormones that control the peripheral endocrine glands (Fig. 1–3). Virtually all hormones are under some type of feedback control, some by cations (calcium on parathyroid hormone), some by metabolites (glucose on insulin and glucagon), some by other hormones (somatostatin on insulin and glucagon), and some by osmolality or extracellular fluid volume (vasopressin, renin, and aldosterone).

The feedback relationship is the reason that simultaneous assessment of hormone/effector pairs is almost always required for assessment of endocrine status. The plasma insulin level must be interpreted in terms of the plasma glucose level in a simultaneously drawn sample. Thyrotropin levels may be interpretable only in terms of the serum thyroxine level. The feedback relation is also the basis for most dynamic tests of endocrine function. Disturbances in these relationships are almost invariably involved in pathological states that perturb endocrine function. This concept is so pervasive in endocrinology that it can be argued that feedback control, rather than the hormones themselves, is the distinguishing feature of the endocrine system. Feedback control is not always operative, however. Thus estrogen production in men and testosterone production in women are not regulated in this manner. In both situations, gonadotropin production is controlled by the predominant steroids (testosterone in men and estradiol and progesterone in women). Estrogens in men are synthesized predominantly

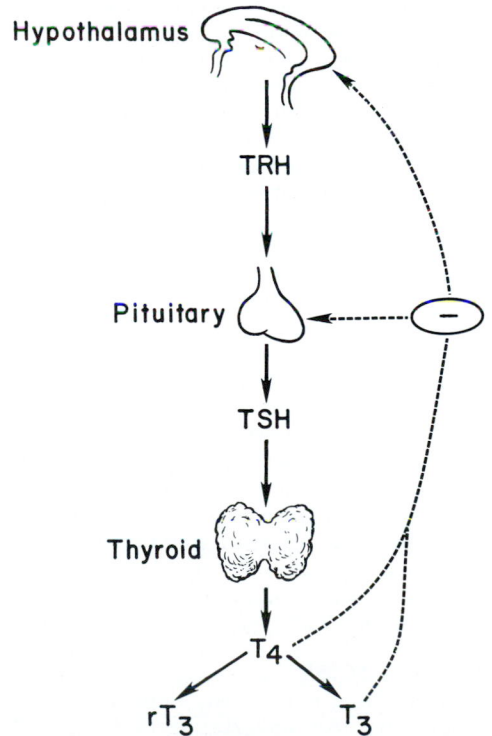

Figure 1–3. A classic feedback system: control of thyroid hormone release. When thyroid hormone levels are inadequate, the repressive effect of triiodothyronine (T_3) and thyroxine (T_4) on the hypothalamus and pituitary is removed. Thyrotropin-releasing hormone (TRH) release stimulates thyrotropin (TSH), which in turn activates thyroxine synthesis in the thyroid gland. When triiodothyronine and thyroxine levels are adequate, inhibition of release of thyrotropin-releasing hormone and thyrotropin occurs. Conversion of thyroxine, a prohormone, to triiodothyronine is probably also regulated.

in extraglandular tissue from circulating androgens, and under physiological conditions the amounts of estrogen formed do not influence the secretion of LH. In women, androgens are formed in the ovary under the control of LH but do not appear to participate in the regulation of LH secretion. In these two situations, considerable variability can occur in the formation (and expression) of the hormones without altering gonadotropin production. Feedback control mechanisms also do not appear to operate in the secretion of placental hormones; the production of these hormones is programmed to supply temporary needs but is not subject to ordinary moment-to-moment regulatory control. Finally, so-called ectopic hormone production is rarely under feedback control regardless of whether it is derived from a tumor or from nontumorous tissue. Renin production by the uterus, for example, does not respond to volume expansion and contraction.

BIORHYTHMS

Rhythms in the release of hormones are a common feature of almost all endocrine systems, and disturbance in the normal operation of cyclic release is a common cause of pathological endocrine changes.[6] These rhythms can vary over minutes to hours (the pulsatile secretion of LH and testosterone), days (the circadian variability in cortisol secretion), weeks (the menstrual cycle), or even longer periods (seasonal variability in thyroxine production). Patterns of release may differ at different stages of life. Thus the sleep-associated surges of gonadotropin secretion that herald the onset of puberty differ from the rhythms of gonadotropin release in adult life. Cyclic or pulsatile variations in hormone concentrations related to alterations in release are more apparent when the half-life of the hormone is short. For example, insulin, with a half-life of 5 to 6 min, shows extreme variations in concentration, whereas insulin-like growth factors (somatomedins) have a slow turnover and consequently have almost constant values in plasma throughout the day.

Hormonal rhythmicity is caused by a variety of factors. Some, such as sleep-associated alterations and stimulation of prolactin secretion by the suckling reflex, are due to neurogenic factors. Others, such as the circadian variability in glucocorticoid production, are controlled by environmental factors acting through uncertain mechanisms. The menstrual cycle is the result of a complex interplay between positive and negative feedback systems.

One of the most remarkable endocrine rhythms is that involved in the pulsatile secretion of hormones from the pituitary and the ensuing pulsatile release of hormones from the endocrine glands, e.g., the system linking luteinizing hormone–releasing hormone (LHRH), LH, and testosterone. In simplistic terms, such oscillations can be envisioned as initiating in the synchronous discharge by an ultradian pacemaker in the arcuate nucleus and the ensuing discharge of LHRH from LHRH-containing neurons. In the steady state, however, cyclic fluctuation of hormone levels in blood also requires inertia or time delay in the negative feedback system that controls its operation.[7] Inertia is the time required for a signal to pass along the whole of the feedback loop. For example, if the synthesis of testosterone requires x seconds, an increase in LH levels cannot be followed by an increase in testosterone production for x seconds. The resulting oscillation becomes magnified by the time required for plasma testosterone to influence LH production. At a minimum, then, the magnitude of the oscillations is a function of the pacemaker itself, the half-life of the effectors in plasma, and the inertia built into the system. Such oscillations

may be fundamental to the operation of feedback systems; indeed, the administration of LHRH by a constant infusion rather than in a pulsatile fashion results in inhibition rather than enhancement of LH secretion under some conditions.[8, 9] Furthermore, the frequency of pulsatile stimulation may alter the ratios of the gonadotropins released from the pituitary.[10] The mechanisms by which these rhythms operate, the reasons why attenuation does not occur in the steady state, and the physiological (and pathological) ramifications of the rhythms in endocrinology are still poorly understood.

ENDOCRINE PATHOLOGY

Endocrine disorders can be divided into six broad categories—subnormal hormone production, hormone overproduction, production of abnormal hormone, resistance to hormone action, abnormalities of hormone transport or metabolism, and multiple hormone abnormalities. There is considerable overlap among these groups. For example, impaired hormone production because of enzyme deficiency can lead to increased synthesis of another hormone, as in the overproduction of adrenal androgen in patients with cortisol deficiency related to a defect in steroid 21-hydroxylase. Hormone overproduction can accompany clinical evidence of deficient hormone action in the hormone resistance states. Finally, hormone overproduction, hormone underproduction, and resistance to hormone action may occur at different times in the course of a disease in a single individual, as is frequently seen with insulin in patients with non–insulin-dependent diabetes and obesity. Nevertheless, a categorization based on the fundamental defect provides a useful means of analyzing endocrine pathology.

SUBNORMAL HORMONE PRODUCTION. Diminished or absent hormone secretion can have several causes. Absence or malformation of endocrine organs can be due to defects in embryogenesis, as in the sublingual thyroid and in gonadal dysgenesis. Alternatively, the endocrine organ may develop but lack some enzyme essential for hormone synthesis, as in some forms of congenital goiter and in the various types of congenital adrenal hyperplasia. More commonly, a normal endocrine gland is destroyed by a secondary process. Such processes can include granulomatous or infectious agents as in tuberculosis of the adrenals; infarction as in the postpartum necrosis of the pituitary that leads to Sheehan syndrome; autoimmune disorders as in Hashimoto thyroiditis; chemical exposure as in testicular damage related to cancer chemotherapy; or a variety of forms of physical damage including radiation, surgical extirpation, and thermal injuries. Despite the multiple etiologies now recognized for hormone underproduction, the cause in many instances remains unknown. A common example is primary hypothyroidism without goiter, in which no evidence may exist for an autoimmune mechanism. In general, the results of hormone deficiency are well understood because it is possible to reproduce and study the manifestations of deficiency by removal or ablation of the appropriate endocrine organ in experimental animals.

HORMONE EXCESS. Hormone overproduction is less well understood than is hormone deficiency because fewer animal models exist for such disorders. Causes are diverse. Tumors, either benign or malignant, can affect an endocrine gland, as in Cushing syndrome arising from a carcinoma or an adenoma of the adrenal cortex. Tumors of nonendocrine tissues can secrete hormones such as corticotropin or human chorionic gonadotropin that drive target glands to hypersecrete and cause disease. The homeostatic mechanisms that control normal hormone secretion can be set at an abnormal level, as in Cushing disease with bilateral adrenal hyperplasia related to corticotropin-secreting pituitary microadenoma. Hyperplasia and autonomous tumor formation in some instances form a continuum; for example, prolonged hyperplasia of the parathyroid glands in renal insufficiency can lead eventually to true autonomous hyperparathyroidism or even adenoma formation. Stimulatory substances can be produced as part of an autoimmune reaction, for example, the production of thyroid-stimulating immunoglobulins in Graves disease. Overproduction can be permanent as in most of the above-mentioned illustrations or transient as may occur in viral thyroiditis. It is of particular interest that manifestations of hyperfunction do not occur for all hormones; no syndrome of testosterone excess in males has been characterized.

PRODUCTION OF ABNORMAL HORMONES. Most pathological states involve the production of too much or too little of hormones normally produced by endocrine glands, but in some circumstances abnormal hormones can be produced. A single-gene mutation may alter both structure and function. Thus a mild form of diabetes mellitus may be produced by an abnormal insulin molecule formed as the result of a single-gene mutation; the abnormal insulin does not bind well to the insulin receptor and thus is ineffective.[11] Occasionally immunoglobulins function as hormones, as in the thyroid-stimulating immunoglobulins that occur in hyperthyroidism (see Chapter 8) and the antibodies to the insulin receptor that can sometimes mimic the action of insulin (see Chapter 4). In other cases, hormone precursors or incompletely processed peptide hormones may be released into the circulation; this situation is common in the case of the so-called ectopic hormone production by many carcinomas (see Chapter 34). Finally, more than one gene specifies the structures for some hormones, some of which are not expressed normally but might be expressed in pathological states (see Chapter 2).

RESISTANCE TO HORMONE ACTION. Hormone resistance, which is defined as a defect in the capacity of normal target tissues to respond to a hormone, was first recognized by Albright and colleagues in their characterization of pseudohypoparathyroidism in 1942.[12] That disorder is now known to result from several hereditary defects, the most common of which resides in the guanosine triphosphate–binding protein in cell membranes (G_s) that activates the catalytic subunit of adenylate cyclase after binding of parathyroid hormone to its receptor (see Chapter 27). Syndromes of resistance have been described for many hormones and involve abnormalities in cell-surface and intracellular receptors, defects in hormone metabolism within cells, and abnormalities in other steps involved in normal hormone action.[13] Resistance can be hereditary (e.g., androgen resistance in the testicular feminization syndrome) or acquired (e.g., insulin resistance of obesity). Studies of hormone resistance states have been of particular importance in establishing the role of hormone receptors in normal hormone action and in the pathogenesis of disease. A common feature of such resistance is the presence of a normal or elevated level of the hormone in the circulation. This level is the consequence of the fact that most hormone production is under some type of regulatory feedback control so that failure of hormone action leads to increased hormone production. Because partial defects can be compensated for by an increased hormone concentration and have little clinical consequence, hormone resistance may go unrecognized. It should be suspected whenever hormone levels are inappropriately high in the face of either clinical normality or symptoms and signs of hormone deficiency.

Hereditary resistance to hormones that are essential for life (e.g., cortisol and corticotropin) is inevitably partial because severe or complete defects in the action of these hormones are incompatible with life. Fetuses with complete defects are probably eliminated as stillbirths or abortions. When severe defects exist (e.g., the absence of functional androgen receptor in complete testicular feminization), it can be assumed that the hormone is not essential for the life of the individual. It is interesting that neither resistance to estrogen action nor a hereditary defect in estrogen synthesis has been described, which implies that estrogen action in implantation of the blastocyst[14] may be essential for life, so that affected individuals do not survive for expression of the defect.

It is useful to consider hormone resistance as prereceptor, receptor, or postreceptor. More than one kind of resistance can be present, as with the insulin resistance of obesity, which has both receptor and postreceptor components. Prereceptor resistance is usually due to abnormal hormones or to antibodies to hormones. Abnormalities of receptors themselves can be either hereditary or acquired. Postreceptor hormone resistance is the category least well understood. In the case of hormones of the steroid/thyroid class, the general outline by which postreceptor action is mediated is clear, namely, through binding of the hormone-receptor complex to specific nucleotide sequences in the regulatory regions of genes called regulatory elements.[15] Similarly, in the case of the hormones that act via the guanosine triphosphate–regulatory proteins, the intracellular cascade of reactions that follow hormone binding are understood in outline.[16] In the case of other hormones such as insulin, the postreceptor events involved in hormone action are less clear, although mutations of the human insulin receptor are providing insight into the sequence of events after insulin binds to its receptor.[17] Elucidation of the mechanisms of postreceptor hormone resistance will constitute a major advance in physiology and medicine.

ABNORMALITIES OF HORMONE TRANSPORT OR METABOLISM. Under ordinary circumstances, abnormalities of hormone transport or metabolism do not result in endocrine pathology. For example, in two extreme situations—hereditary absence of thyroid-binding globulin and cirrhosis of the liver with a markedly diminished rate of cortisol catabolism—no endocrine pathology results because feedback control mechanisms compensate for the defects. Hormone production is controlled by the level of free hormone and consequently can be adjusted up or down as required. Abnormalities of this type most commonly cause deviation of laboratory parameters from normal but do not cause either hyper- or hypofunction. The important point is to recognize that unusual hormonal values do not necessarily imply functional pathological changes. Under some circumstances, however, such abnormalities may cause pathology. For example, administration of physiological replacement doses of glucocorticoid to an individual with cirrhosis of the liver may cause florid Cushing syndrome, because free hormone levels will be high in the face of diminished plasma binding and decreased rate of steroid catabolism. This is equivalent to unregulated entry of hormones into the circulation, as would occur with Cushing syndrome. Defects of hormone metabolism are more likely to cause endocrine pathology than are defects in transport because alternative mechanisms of transport exist for virtually all hormones.

MULTIPLE HORMONE ABNORMALITIES. The original paradigm for disorders involving multiple hormones is hypopituitarism. More important, familial disorders are now characterized that involve hyperfunction (the multiple endocrine neoplasia syndromes; see Chapter 30) or mixed patterns of hyperfunction and hypofunction of various endocrine glands (the polyglandular endocrinopathy syndromes; see Chapter 31). These syndromes are of importance out of all proportion to their frequency for at least two reasons. First, it is mandatory after the diagnosis is made to evaluate patients periodically for involvement of additional endocrine glands and to evaluate relatives at risk before the development of serious manifestations of the disorders. Second, analysis of the mechanisms by which these relatively rare single-gene defects predispose individuals to the development of these disorders may allow understanding of the pathogenesis of more common endocrine diseases.

SUMMARY

In this brief introduction we have attempted to outline some of the principles of endocrinology that will be covered much more extensively in the remainder of the book. Our purpose has been to show that endocrinology is in many ways an orderly clinical discipline, by which we mean that the general principles are usually informative whether applied to normal physiology or to endocrine disease.

REFERENCES

1. Starling EH. The Croonian Lectures on the chemical correlation of the functions of the body. Lancet 1905; 2:339–341, 423–425, 501–503, 579–583.
2. Bateman A, Singh A, Kral T, et al. The immune-hypothalamic-pituitary-adrenal axis. Endocr Rev 1989; 10:92–111.
3. Mendel CM. The free hormone hypothesis: a physiologically based mathematical model. Endocr Rev 1989; 10:232–274.
4. Rosner W. The functions of corticosteroid-binding globulin and sex hormone-binding globulin: recent advances. Endocr Rev 1990; 11:80–91.
5. Goldstein JL, Anderson RGW, Brown MS. Coated pits, coated vesicles, and receptor-mediated endocytosis. Nature 1979; 279:679–685.
6. Van Cauter E, Aschoff J. Endocrine and other biological rhythms. In: DeGroot LJ, et al., eds. Endocrinology, Vol 3. 2nd ed. Philadelphia: W. B. Saunders, 1989: 2658–2705.
7. Burgi H. I. General aspects of endocrinology. In: Labhart A, ed. Clinical Endocrinology Theory and Practice. New York: Springer-Verlag, 1974: 1–23.
8. Wickings EJ, Zaidi P, Brabant G, et al. Stimulation of pituitary and testicular functions with LH-RH agonist or pulsatile LH-RH treatment in the rhesus monkey during the non-breeding season. J Reprod Fertil 1981; 63:129–136.
9. Akhtar FB, Marshall GR, Wickings EJ, et al. Reversible induction of azoospermia in rhesus monkey by constant infusion of a gonadotropin-releasing hormone agonist using osmotic minipumps. J Clin Endocrinol Metab 1983; 56:534–540.
10. Gross KM, Matsumoto AM, Southworth MB, et al. The pattern of luteinizing hormone releasing hormone (LHRH) administration controls the relative secretion of follicle stimulating hormone (FSH) and luteinizing hormone (LH) in man. Clin Res 1984; 32:74A.
11. Haneda M, Chan SJ, Kwok SCM, et al. Studies on mutant human insulin genes: identification and sequence analysis of a gene encoding (Ser^{b24}) insulin. Proc Natl Acad Sci USA 1983; 80:6366–6370.
12. Albright F, Burnett CH, Smith PH, et al. Pseudohypoparathyroidism—an example of Seabright's bantam syndrome. Endocrinology 1942; 30:922–932.
13. Verhoeven GFM, Wilson JD. The syndromes of primary hormone resistance. Metabolism 1979; 28:253–289.
14. George FW, Wilson JD. Estrogen formation in the early rabbit embryo. Science 1978: 199:200–201.
15. Carson-Jurica MA, Schrader WT, O'Malley BW. Steroid receptor family: structure and functions. Endocr Rev 1990; 11:201–220.
16. Gilman AG. G proteins: transducers of receptor-generated signals. Annu Rev Biochem 1987; 56:615–649.
17. Kahn CR, Goldstein BJ. Molecular defects in insulin action. Science 1989; 245:13.

2

GENETIC CONTROL OF HORMONE FORMATION

Joel F. Habener

INTRODUCTION

Advances in the fields of molecular and cellular biology have provided new insights into the working of the cell. Recombinant DNA technology makes it possible to analyze the precise structure and functions of the genetic substance of life itself. The uncovering of the unique properties of DNA has provided the conceptual framework with which to begin a systematic investigation of the origin, development, and organization of life forms.[1]

The polypeptide hormones[1] constitute an important and diverse set of regulatory molecules whose function is to convey specific information among cells and organs. This type of communication arose early in the development of life and evolved into a complex system for the control of growth, development, and reproduction and for the maintenance of metabolic homeostasis. These hormones consist of approximately 100 small proteins ranging from as few as three amino acids (thyrotropin-releasing hormone, TRH) to 192 amino acids (growth hormone). In a broader sense these polypeptides function both as hormones in which their actions are mediated on distant organs by way of their transport through the bloodstream and as local cell-cell communicators (Fig. 2–1). This latter function of the polypeptide hormones is exemplified by their elaboration and secretion within neurons of the central, autonomic, and peripheral nervous systems, where they probably act as neurotransmitters. These multiple modes of expression of the peptide hormone genes have aroused great interest in the specific functions of these peptides and the mechanisms of their synthesis and release.

The purpose of this chapter is to review the structure and expression of genes encoding peptide hormones. The synthesis of nonpeptide hormones such as catecholamines, thyroid hormones, and steroid hormones involves the action of multiple enzymes, and hence the expression of multiple genes, and is discussed in the individual chapters devoted to such hormones.

DEVELOPMENT OF MOLECULAR ENDOCRINOLOGY AS A DISCIPLINE

The modern era in this field was inaugurated in the early 1950s with the determination by Popenoe and du

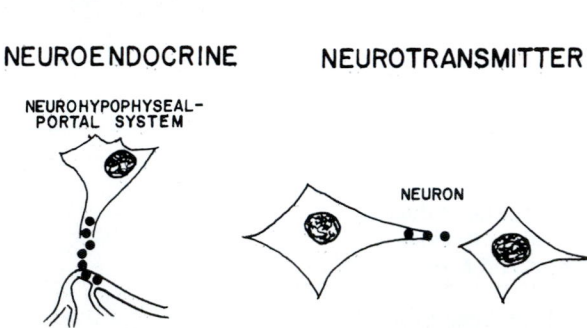

Figure 2–1. Different modes of utilization of polypeptide hormones in expression of their biological actions. Many of the peptide hormones are expressed in at least four ways in fulfilling their functions as cellular messenger molecules: (1) *endocrine* mode, for purposes of communication among organs; (2) *paracrine* mode, for communication among adjacent cells, often located within endocrine organs; (3) *neuroendocrine* mode, for synthesis and release of peptides from specialized peptidergic neurons for action on distant organs via the bloodstream— e.g., neuroendocrine peptides of hypothalamus; and (4) *neurotransmitter* mode, for action of peptides in concert with classic amino acid–derived aminergic transmitters in the neuronal communication network. Identical polypeptides are often utilized in the nervous system both as neuroendocrine hormones and as neurotransmitters. In many instances, the identical gene product is used in all four modes of expression.

Vigneaud[2] (and their co-workers) of the amino acid sequences of vasopressin and oxytocin. In ensuing years, the amino acid sequences of approximately 50 different polypeptide hormones and regulatory peptides were established. The structural analysis of the polypeptide hormones was made possible by advances in methods for the isolation of proteins and the development of automated techniques for their sequencing. A major breakthrough for studies of physiological and cellular endocrine regulation came with the application of the principle of the radioimmunoassay.[3] Exploitation of this technique provided insight into the workings of endocrine control mechanisms under physiological and pathological circumstances. The availability of both natural and synthetic peptides in homogeneous form allowed the production of specific antisera for use in radioimmunoassay and immunocytochemical studies. The purified peptides were also used to study receptors of hormones and for the construction of specific receptor assays. These studies led to the synthesis of numerous analogues that proved useful as potent agonists and antagonists.

Development of the powerful techniques for producing recombinant DNA resulted in an acceleration of studies of cellular control mechanisms. The successful cloning of the cDNAs for insulin[4] and growth hormone[5] established that the genetic engineering of recombinant DNA molecules can be utilized to determine the structures of proteins by way of decoding the nucleotide sequences. It is also possible with this technique to remove a segment of genetic material from its normal context and replicate it in high yield in microorganisms; this segment can then be reintroduced into a variety of cells, where it can be studied and manipulated under controlled circumstances.

To a large extent this technique of gene cloning has altered the approaches used to garner new information on the structure and function of polypeptide hormones. Instead of isolating minuscule amounts of peptide from large amounts of tissue and analyzing amino acid sequences, it is now possible to obtain DNA templates from the messenger RNAs (mRNAs) encoding the polypeptides. Recombinant DNA molecules prepared from these RNA templates can be cloned and amplified, thereby producing large amounts of DNA for nucleotide sequencing and deduction of the amino acid sequences. Genes have now been cloned for approximately 200 hormonal regulatory peptides, many of which are present in only trace amounts in the tissues from which they originate.

The expansion of technology for DNA sequencing raises the prospect that the primary structure of the entire mammalian genome may be known by the year 2000.[6, 7] At present, approximately 10^7 of the 10^9 base pairs of the mammalian genome have been determined. Continued efforts in the field of DNA sequencing and the likely development of even more rapid and efficient methods make it reasonable to expect that the rate of acquisition of sequence information will accelerate.

Determination of the structure of genes, however, provides only the foundation of information about how the expression of genes is controlled. As a consequence, scientists are just now gaining insight into the cellular mechanisms involved in the regulation of gene expression. Recombinant DNA molecules provide powerful probes with which to analyze the effects of regulatory molecules on gene transcription in intact animals and in cultured cells. Of greater potential importance is the ability to introduce specific DNA sequences that encode polypeptides into foreign cells and into the germ lines of animals. In addition the selective alteration of the sequences of genes by site-directed mutagenesis permits a molecular dissection of the structural aspects of the gene required for accurate control. After the mechanisms of gene control are understood, it may be possible to correct genetic defects in humans by specific engineering of DNA. Such gene transfer experiments have already been performed in laboratory animals. Introduction of foreign genes into the germ line of mice by microinjection of DNA into fertilized oocytes gives rise to expression of these foreign genes in the offspring. Current methods, however, do not allow for introduction of these genes into specific loci that are under physiological control.

EVOLUTION OF PEPTIDE HORMONES AND THEIR FUNCTIONS

Peptide hormones arose early in the evolution of life. Indeed, polypeptides that are structurally similar to mammalian peptides are present in lower vertebrates, insects, yeasts, and bacteria.[8] An example of the early evolution of regulatory peptides is the alpha-factor (mating pheromone) of yeast, which is similar in structure to mammalian luteinizing hormone–releasing hormone (LHRH, also called gonadotropin-releasing hormone, GnRH).[9] Other such examples are glucagon-like immunoreactivity in the corpus cardiacum of the tobacco hornworm; pancreatic polypeptide and vasoactive intestinal peptide–like substances in the earthworm; and cholecystokinin, neurotensin, and substance P in coelenterates (hydra and sea anemone). Insulin, corticotropin (ACTH, adrenocorticotropin), and somatostatin (SRIF, somatotropin release–inhibiting factor) are reported to exist in ciliated protozoa (*Tetrahymena*) and in various strains of *Escherichia coli*. Thus the genes encoding polypeptide hormones, and particularly regulatory peptides, evolved early in the development of life and initially fulfilled the function of cell-cell communication to cope with problems concerning nourishment, growth, development, and reproduction. As specialized organs connected by a circulatory system developed during evolution, similar, if not identical, gene products became hormones for purposes of organ-organ communication. Perhaps as a consequence of the development of the blood-brain barrier, the local cell-cell regulatory functions of the polypeptides in the brain may have been maintained apart from the endocrine functions of peptides in the rest of the body, thus explaining the presence of many peptide hormones in specific neuronal populations within the central nervous system. The peptidergic neurons that populate the hypothalamus may represent a transition between the cell-cell communication and organ-organ regulatory functions of the peptides.

The known regulatory peptides number in the hundreds, and additional peptide hormones will be found in the isolation of substances responsible for specific biological activities or by the decoding of gene sequences. The potential number of unique amino acid sequences that are possible is immense. For example, if all possible combinations of the 20 amino acids were utilized, 2×10^{11} different peptides, each of 10 amino acids, could exist. A typical mammalian cell expresses genes encoding between 5000 and 10,000 different proteins, and among differentiated cells the total repertoire is probably somewhere around 50,000 proteins. By searching for similarities among approximately 2000 known protein sequences, Doolittle[10] estimated that, when it is possible to identify subtle similarities among different proteins indicative of their common origin from ancestral proteins, there may be as few as 1000 fundamental proteins, each probably distinct with regard to its functional properties. For example, one may envision distinct amino acid sequences that are specific for binding sites of cellular receptors, chelation of heavy-metal ions, expression of proteolytic activity, structural components of membranes, and hydrolysis of ATP. The findings that the coding sequences of genes are separated into blocks (exons) by intervening DNA sequences (introns) and that the exons appear to constitute distinct functional domains lend credence to the hypothesis that specific protein-encoding gene segments have maintained a function essentially unchanged throughout evolution, presumably because of the special selective advantages of the function to the organisms.

STEPS IN EXPRESSION OF A PROTEIN-ENCODING GENE

The steps involved in transfer of information encoded in the polynucleotide language of DNA to the poly–amino acid language of biologically active protein involve transcription, post-transcriptional processing, translation, and post-translational processing. The expression of genes and protein synthesis can be considered in terms of several major processes, any one or more of which may serve as specific control points in the regulation of gene expression (Fig. 2–2):

1. *Rearrangements and transpositions of DNA segments.* These processes occur in evolution, with the exception that

STEPS IN PROTEIN SYNTHESIS

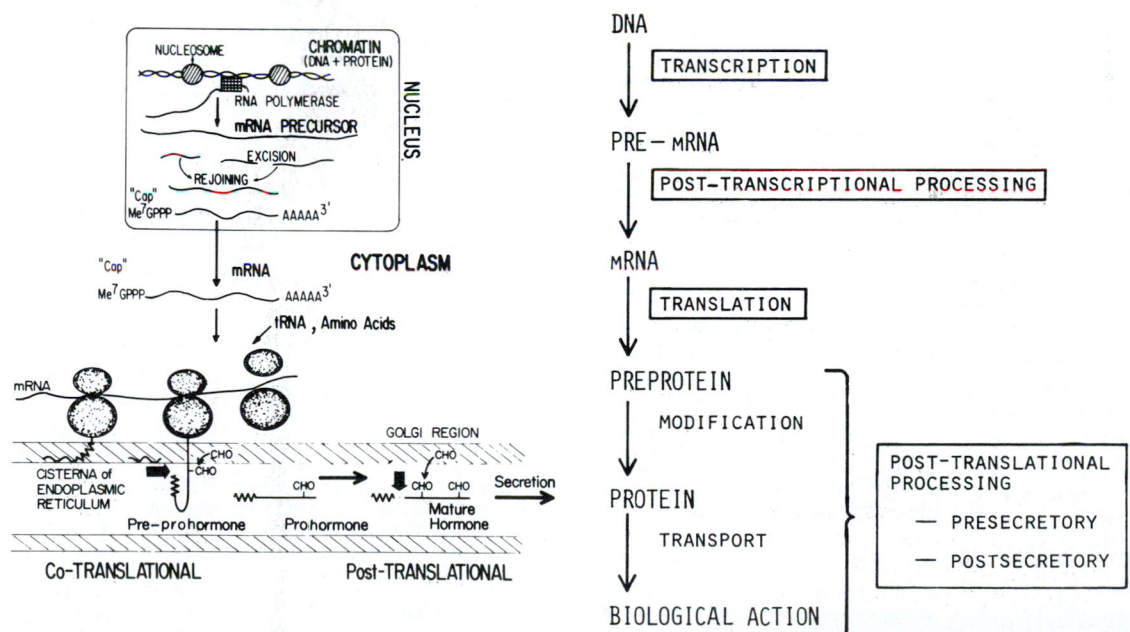

Figure 2–2. Steps in the cellular synthesis of polypeptide hormones. Steps that take place within the nucleus include transcription of genetic information into an mRNA precursor (pre-mRNA) followed by post-transcriptional processing, which includes RNA cleavage, excision of introns, and rejoining of exons, resulting in formation of mRNA. Ends of mRNA are modified by addition of methylguanine caps at the 5' end and addition of poly(A) tracts at the 3' ends. The cytoplasmic mRNA is assembled with ribosomes. Amino acids, carried by aminoacylated transfer RNAs (tRNAs), are then polymerized into a polypeptide chain. The final step in protein synthesis is that of post-translational processing. These processes take place both during growth of the nascent polypeptide chain (cotranslational) and after release of the completed chain (post-translational), and they include proteolytic cleavages of polypeptide chain (conversion of pre-prohormones or prohormones to hormones), derivatizations of amino acids (glycosylation, phosphorylation), and cross-linking and assembly of the polypeptide chain into its conformed structure. The diagram depicts post-translational synthesis and processing of a typical secreted polypeptide, which requires vectorial, or unidirectional, transport of the polypeptide chain across the membrane bilayer of the endoplasmic reticulum, thus resulting in sequestration of polypeptide in cisterna of the endoplasmic reticulum, a first step in export process of proteins destined for secretion from the cell (see Fig. 2–6). Most translational processing occurs within the cell as depicted (presecretory), and in some instances outside the cell, during which time further proteolytic cleavages or modifications of the protein may take place (postsecretory). CHO, carbohydrate.

such rearrangements take place in the immunoglobulin gene during the lifetime of an individual.

2. *Transcription.* Synthesis of RNA results in the formation of RNA copies of the two gene alleles and is catalyzed by RNA polymerase II.

3. *Post-transcriptional processing.* Specific modifications of the RNA include the formation of mRNA from the precursor RNA by way of excision and rejoining of RNA segments (introns and exons) and modifications of the 3′ end of the RNA by polyadenylation and of the 5′ end by addition of 7-methylguanine "caps."

4. *Translation.* Amino acids are assembled by base pairing of the nucleotide triplets (anticodons) of the specific "carrier" aminoacylated transfer RNAs to the corresponding codons of the mRNA bound to polyribosomes and are polymerized into the polypeptide chains.

5. *Post-translational processing and modification.* Final steps in protein synthesis involve one or more cleavages of peptide bonds, which result in the conversion of biosynthetic precursors, or prohormones, to intermediate or final forms of the protein, derivatization of amino acids (glycosylation, phosphorylation, acetylation), and the folding of the processed polypeptide chain into its native conformation.

Each of the specific steps of gene expression requires the integration of precise enzymatic and other biochemical reactions. These processes have developed to provide high fidelity in the reproduction of the encoded information and to provide control points for the expression of the specific phenotype of cells.

The post-translational processing of proteins creates diversity in gene expression through the modifications of the protein. Although the functional information contained in protein is ultimately encoded in the primary amino acid sequence, the specific biological activities are a consequence of the higher-ordered secondary, tertiary, and quaternary structures of the polypeptide. Given the wide range of possible specific modifications of the amino acids, such as glycosylation, phosphorylation, acetylation, and sulfation,[11] any one of which may affect the conformation of the protein, a single gene may ultimately encode a wide variety of specific proteins as a result of post-translational processes.

Polypeptide hormones are synthesized in the form of larger precursors that appear to fulfill several functions in biological systems (Fig. 2–3), including (1) intracellular signaling, by which the cell distinguishes among specific classes of proteins and directs them to their sites of action; and (2) the generation of multiple biological activities from a common genetically encoded protein by regulated or cell-specific variations in the post-translational modifications (Fig. 2–4).[12]

All the peptide hormones and regulatory peptides studied thus far contain signal or leader sequences at the NH₂ termini; these sequences are hydrophobic and recognize specific sites on the membranes of the rough endoplasmic reticulum, which results in the transport of nascent polypeptides into the secretory pathway of the cell (see Figs. 2–2 and 2–3).[12] The consequence of the specialized signal sequences of the precursor proteins is that proteins destined for secretion are selected from a great many other cellular proteins for sequestration and subsequent packaging into secretory granules and export from the cell.

In addition, most, if not all, of the smaller hormones and regulatory peptides are produced as a consequence of post-translational cleavages of the precursors within the Golgi complex of secretory cells.

SUBCELLULAR STRUCTURE OF CELLS THAT SECRETE PROTEIN HORMONES

Cells whose principal functions are the synthesis and export of proteins contain highly developed, specialized subcellular organelles for the translocation of secreted proteins and their packaging into secretory granules. The subcellular pathways utilized in protein secretion have been elucidated largely through the efforts of Palade[13] and colleagues. Secretory cells contain an abundance of endoplasmic reticulum, Golgi complexes, and secretory granules (Fig. 2–5). The proteins that are to be secreted from the cells are transferred during their synthesis into these subcellular organelles, which transport the proteins to the plasma membrane.

Protein secretion begins with translation of the mRNA encoding the precursor of the protein on the rough endoplasmic reticulum, which consists of polyribosomes attached to elaborate membranous saccules that contain cavities (cisternae). The newly synthesized, nascent proteins are discharged into the cisternae by transport across the lipid bilayer of the membrane. Within the cisternae of the endoplasmic reticulum, proteins are carried to the Golgi complex by mechanisms that are incompletely understood. The proteins gain access to the Golgi complex either by direct transfer from the cisternae, which are in continuity with the membranous channels of the Golgi complex, or by way of shuttling vesicles known as transition elements (see Fig. 2–5). Different secretory cells appear to use predominantly one or the other of these two mechanisms for transport of protein from the rough endoplasmic reticulum to the Golgi complex. Within the Golgi complex, the proteins are packaged into secretory vesicles or secretory granules by their budding from the Golgi stacks in the form of immature granules that undergo maturation through condensation of

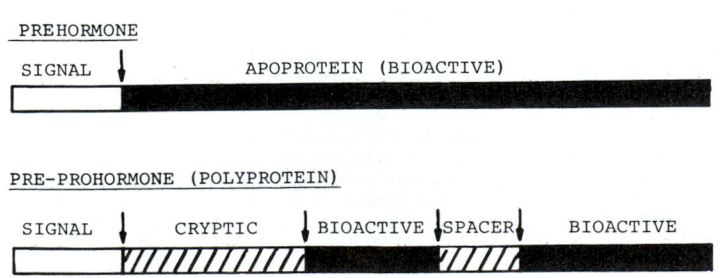

BIOSYNTHETIC PRECURSOR OF HORMONES

PREHORMONE

SIGNAL | APOPROTEIN (BIOACTIVE)

PRE-PROHORMONE (POLYPROTEIN)

SIGNAL | CRYPTIC | BIOACTIVE | SPACER | BIOACTIVE

Other peptides may serve as spacer sequences between two bioactive peptides, e.g., the C peptide of proinsulin. In instances in which bioactive peptide is located at the COOH terminus of the prohormone, the NH₂-terminal prohormone sequence may simply facilitate cotranslational translocation of polypeptide in endoplasmic reticulum (see Fig. 2–6).

Figure 2–3. Diagrammatic depiction of two configurations of precursors of polypeptide hormones. Diagrams represent polypeptide backbones of protein sequences encoded in mRNA. One form of precursor consists of the NH₂-terminal signal, or presequence, followed by the apoprotein portion of the polypeptide that needs no further proteolytic processing for activity. A second form of precursor is a pre-prohormone that consists of the NH₂-terminal signal sequence followed by a polyprotein, or prohormone, sequence consisting of several peptide domains linked together that are subsequently liberated by cleavages during post-translational processing of the prohormone. The reason for synthesis of polypeptide hormones in the form of precursors is only partly understood. Clearly, NH₂-terminal signal sequences function in the early stages of transport of polypeptide into the secretory pathway. Prohormones, or polyproteins, often serve to provide a source of multiple bioactive peptides (see Fig. 2–4). However, many prohormones contain peptide sequences that are cleaved out and have no known biological activity, and they are referred to as cryptic peptides.

Figure 2–4. Diagrammatic illustration of primary structures of several prohormones. Darkly shaded regions of prohormones denote regions of sequence that constitute known biologically active peptides after their post-translational cleavage from prohormones. Sequences indicated by hatching denote regions of precursor that alter biological specificity of that region of precursor. For example, the precursor contains the sequence of α-melanocyte-stimulating hormone (α-MSH), but when the latter is covalently attached to the clip peptide, it constitutes corticotropin (ACTH). Somatostatin-28 (SS-28) is an NH₂-terminally extended form of somatostatin-14 (SS-14) that has a higher potency than has somatostatin-14 on certain receptors. The neurophysin sequence linked to the COOH terminus of vasopressin (ADH) functions as a carrier protein for hormone during its transport down the axon of neurons in which it is synthesized. Precursor proenkephalin represents a polyprotein that contains multiple similar peptides within its sequence, either met-enkephalin (M) or leu-enkephalin (L), or a COOH-terminally extended form of met-enkephalin (M+). Procalcitonin and procalcitonin gene–related product (CGRP) share identical NH₂-terminal sequences but differ in their COOH-terminal regions as a result of alternative splicing during the post-transcriptional processing of the RNA precursor. GRP, glucagon-related peptide; γ-LPH, γ-lipotropin.

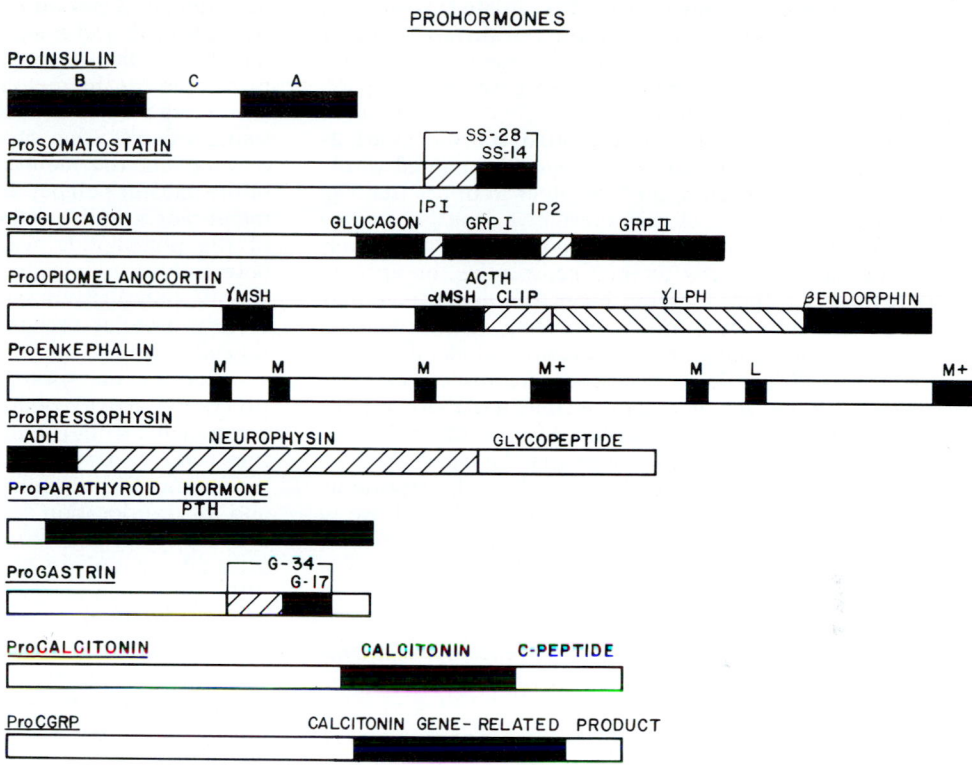

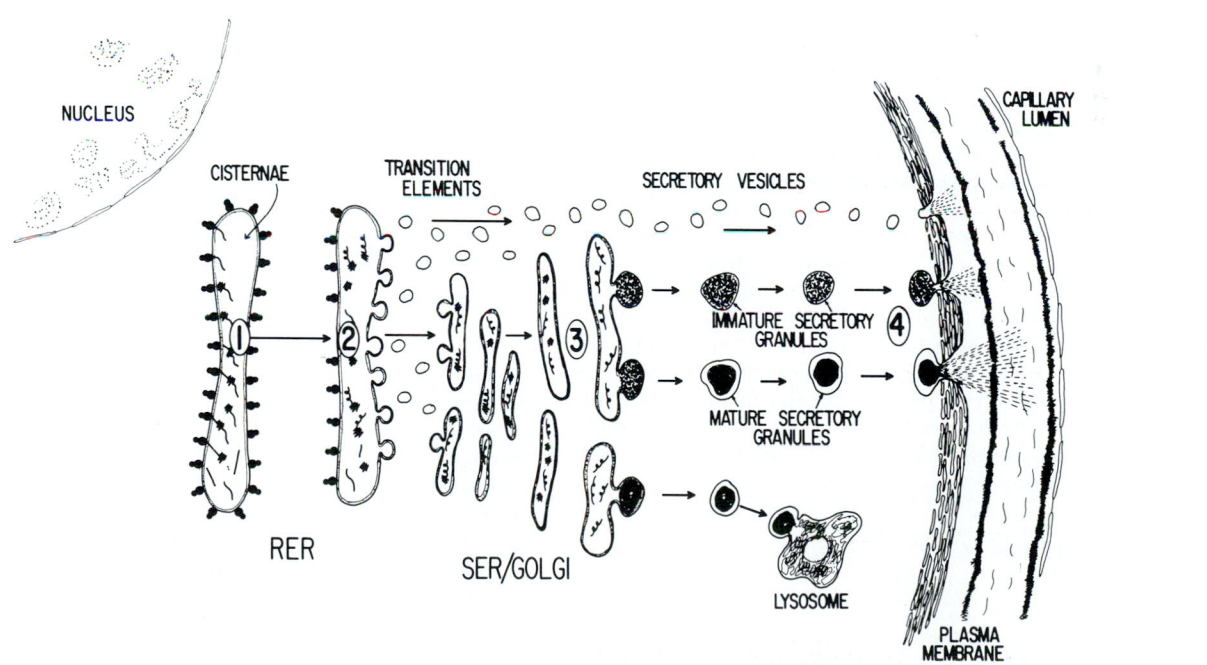

Figure 2–5. Schematic representation of subcellular organelles involved in transport and secretion of polypeptide hormones or other secreted proteins within a protein-secreting cell. (1) Synthesis of proteins on polyribosomes attached to endoplasmic reticulum (RER), and vectorial discharge of proteins through the membrane into the cisterna. (2) Formation of shuttling vesicles (transition elements) from endoplasmic reticulum followed by their transport to and incorporation by the Golgi complex. (3) Formation of secretory granules in the Golgi complex. (4) Transport of secretory granules to the plasma membrane, fusion with the plasma membrane, and exocytosis resulting in the release of granule contents into the extracellular space. Note that secretion may occur via transport of secretory vesicles and immature granules, as well as mature granules. Some granules are taken up and hydrolyzed by lysosomes (crinophagy). RER, rough endoplasmic reticulum; SER, smooth endoplasmic reticulum; Golgi, Golgi complex. (From Habener JF. Hormone biosynthesis and secretion. In: Felig P, Baxter JD, Broadus AE, et al., eds. Endocrinology and Metabolism. New York: McGraw-Hill, 1981: 29–59. Copyright © 1981 by McGraw-Hill, Inc. Used by permission of McGraw-Hill Book Company.)

the proteinaceous material and application of a second membrane around the initial Golgi membrane. On receiving the appropriate extracellular stimuli (regulated pathway of secretion), the granules migrate to the cell surface and fuse to become continuous with the plasma membrane, which results in the release of proteins into the extracellular space, a process known as exocytosis.

The second pathway of intracellular transport and secretion involves the migration of proteins contained within secretory vesicles and immature secretory granules (see Fig. 2–5). Although the use of this alternative vesicle-mediated transport pathway remains to be demonstrated conclusively (it is generally considered to be a constitutive, or unregulated, pathway), different extracellular stimuli may modulate hormone secretion differently, depending on the pathway of secretion. For example, in the parathyroid gland[14] and in the pituitary cell line derived from corticotropic cells (AtT-20), newly synthesized hormone is released more rapidly than is hormone synthesized earlier. These findings suggest that the newly synthesized hormone may be transported by way of a vesicle-mediated pathway without incorporation into mature storage granules. Furthermore, the release of newly synthesized hormone from these tissues is preferentially stimulated by analogues of cyclic AMP (cAMP).

INTRACELLULAR SEGREGATION AND TRANSPORT OF POLYPEPTIDE HORMONES

Specific amino acid sequences encoded in the proteins serve as directional signals in the sorting of proteins within subcellular organelles.[12, 15] A typical eukaryotic cell synthesizes an estimated 50,000 different proteins during its cycle.[16] These different proteins are synthesized by a common pool of polyribosomes. However, each of the different proteins is directed to a specific location within the cell, where its biological function is expressed. For example, specific groups of proteins are transported into mitochondria, into membranes, into the nucleus, or into other subcellular organelles where they serve as regulatory proteins, enzymes, or structural proteins. A subset of proteins is specifically designed for export from the cell, e.g., immunoglobulins, serum albumin, blood coagulation factors, and protein and polypeptide hormones. This process of directional transport of proteins involves sophisticated informational signals. Because the information for these translocation processes must reside either wholly or in part within the primary structure or in the conformational properties of the protein, sequential post-translational modifications may be crucial for specificity of protein function.

Signal Hypothesis

The early processes of protein secretion that result in the specific transport of exported proteins into the secretory pathway are now partly understood (reviewed in ref. 12). Initial clues to this process came from determinations of the amino acid sequences of the proteins programmed by the cell-free translation of mRNAs encoding secreted polypeptides.[17] With the possible exception of the egg white protein ovalbumin,[18] all secretory proteins are synthesized as precursors that are extended at their NH$_2$ termini by sequences of 15 to 30 amino acids, which are called signal or leader sequences. When translations of the mRNA encoding secretory polypeptides are carried out in cell-free systems containing cellular membranes, the signal sequences are not present on the translated proteins, which indicates that they have been cleaved during their synthesis in the presence of microsomal membranes.[17] These observations led to the conclusion that the signal sequence extension or its functional equivalent is required for vectorial transport of the protein across the membrane of the endoplasmic reticulum. On emergence of the signal sequence from the large ribosomal subunit, the ribosomal complex specifically makes contact with the membrane, which results in translocation of the nascent polypeptide across the endoplasmic reticulum membrane into the cisterna as the first step in the transport of the polypeptide within the secretory pathway. These observations initially left unanswered the question of how specific polyribosomes that translate mRNAs encoding secretory proteins recognize and attach to the endoplasmic reticulum (Fig. 2–6).

Because microsomal membranes could reproduce the processing activity of intact cells, it was possible to extract components from the microsomal membranes and reconstitute cell-free translation experiments, thereby identifying macromolecules responsible for processing of the precursor and for translocation activities.[19] The endoplasmic reticulum and the cytoplasm contain an aggregate of molecules, called a signal recognition particle complex, that consists of six different proteins and a 7S RNA.[19, 20] This complex, or particle, binds to the polyribosomes involved in the translation of mRNAs encoding secretory polypeptides when the NH$_2$-terminal signal sequence first emerges from the large subunit of the ribosome. The specific interaction of the signal recognition particle with the nascent signal sequence and the polyribosome arrests further translation of mRNA. The nascent protein remains in a state of arrested translation until it finds a high-affinity binding protein on the endoplasmic reticulum, the signal recognition particle receptor, or docking protein.[20] On interaction with the specific docking protein, the translational block is released, and protein synthesis resumes. The protein is then transferred across the membrane of the endoplasmic reticulum, presumably through a proteinaceous tunnel. At some point, near the termination of synthesis of the polypeptide chain, the NH$_2$-terminal signal sequence is cleaved from the polypeptide, presumably by a specific peptidase located on the cisternal surface of the endoplasmic reticulum membrane. The removal of the hydrophobic signal sequence frees the protein (prohormone) so that it may assume its characteristic secondary structure during transport through the endoplasmic reticulum and the Golgi apparatus.

This sequence in the directional transport of specific polypeptides ensures optimal cotranslational processing of secretory proteins, even when synthesis commences on free ribosomes. The presence of a cytoplasmic form of the signal recognition particle complex that blocks translation guarantees that the synthesis of the presecretory proteins is not completed in the cytoplasm; the efficient transfer of proteins occurs only after the contact has been made with the specific receptor or docking protein on the membrane. Although the identification of the signal recognition particle and the docking protein explains the specificity of the binding of ribosomes containing mRNAs encoding the secretory proteins, it does not explain the mode of translocation of the nascent polypeptide chain across the membrane bilayer. Further dissection and analysis of the membrane are necessary to identify other macromolecules that are responsible for the transport process.

Cellular Processing of Prohormones

Although the signal sequences of prehormones and preprohormones are involved in the transport of these mole-

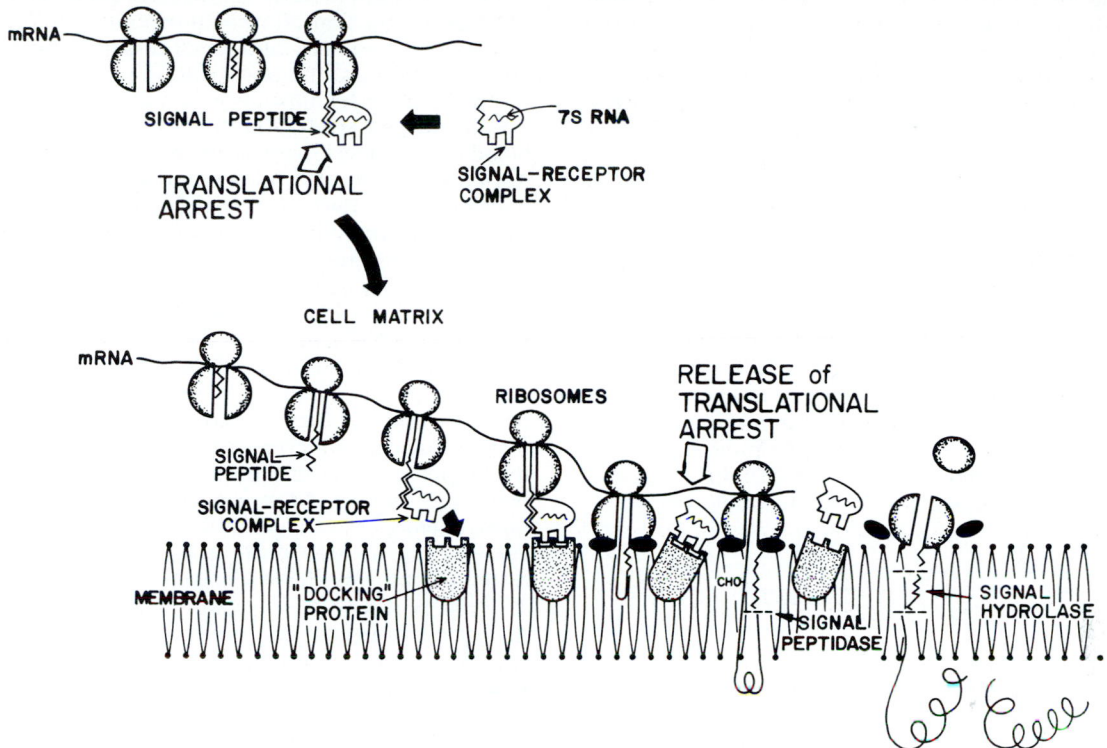

Figure 2–6. Diagram depicting cellular events in initial stages of synthesis of a polypeptide hormone according to the signal hypothesis. In this schema, a signal recognition particle, consisting of a complex of six proteins and an RNA (7S RNA), interacts with the NH$_2$-terminal signal peptide of the nascent polypeptide chain after approximately 70 amino acids are polymerized, which results in the arrest of further growth of the polypeptide chain. The complex of the signal recognition particle and the polyribosome nascent chain remains in a state of translational arrest until it recognizes and binds to a docking protein, which is a receptor protein located on the cytoplasmic face of the endoplasmic reticular membrane. This interaction of the signal recognition particle complex with docking protein releases translational block, and protein synthesis resumes. The nascent polypeptide chain is discharged across the membrane bilayer into the cisterna of the endoplasmic reticulum and is released from the signal peptide by cleavage with a signal peptidase located in the cisternal face of the membrane. In this model the signal peptide is cleaved from the polypeptide chain by signal peptidase before the chain is completed (cotranslational cleavage). The configuration of the polypeptide during transport across the membrane and the forces and mechanisms responsible for its translocation are unknown. The loop, or hairpin, configuration of the chain that is shown is an arbitrary model; other models are equally possible.

cules, the function of the intermediate hormone precursors (prohormones) is not fully understood. The conversion of prohormones to their final products takes place in the Golgi apparatus. For example, the time that elapses between the synthesis of pre-proparathyroid hormone and the first appearance of parathyroid hormone correlates closely with the time required for radioautographic grains to reach the Golgi apparatus.[21] Similarly, the conversion of proinsulin to insulin takes place about an hour after the synthesis of proinsulin is completed, and processing of proinsulin to insulin and C peptide takes place during the transport within the secretory granule.[22] The conversion of prohormones to hormones can also be blocked by inhibitors of cellular energy production such as antimycin A and dinitrophenol,[23] and by drugs that interfere with the functions of microtubules (vinblastine, colchicine).[24] Thus the translocation of the prohormone from the rough endoplasmic reticulum to the Golgi complex depends on metabolic energy and probably involves microtubules.

There is no evidence that sequences that are specific to the prohormone per se contribute to or are chemically involved in transport of the newly synthesized protein from the rough endoplasmic reticulum to the Golgi apparatus or that they are involved in the packaging of the hormone in the vesicles or granules. Analyses of the structures of the primary products of translation of mRNAs encoding secretory proteins indicate that many of these are not synthesized in the form of prohormone intermediates (see Fig. 2–3). It remains puzzling that some secretory proteins (e.g., parathy-

roid hormone, insulin, and serum albumin) are formed by way of intermediate precursors, whereas others (e.g., growth hormone, prolactin, and albumin) are not. Size constraints may be placed on the length of a secretory polypeptide. When the bioactivity of peptides resides at the COOH termini of the precursors (e.g., somatostatin, calcitonin, and gastrin), NH$_2$-terminal extensions may be required to provide sufficient "spacer" sequence to allow the signal sequence on the growing nascent polypeptide chain to emerge from the large ribosome subunit for interaction with the signal recognition particle and to provide adequate polypeptide length to span the large ribosomal subunit and the membrane of the endoplasmic reticulum during vectorial transport of the nascent polypeptide across the membrane (see Fig. 2–6). When the final hormonal product is 100 amino acids long or longer (e.g., growth hormone, prolactin, or the alpha and beta subunits of the glycoprotein hormones), there may be no requirement for a prohormone intermediate.

Although the exact functions of prohormones remain unknown, certain details of their cleavages have been established. Unlike the situation with prehormones, in which the amino acids at the cleavage site between the signal sequence and the remainder of the molecule (hormone or prohormone) vary from one prehormone to the next, the cleavage sites of the prohormone intermediates uniformly consist of the basic amino acids lysine or arginine, or both, usually two to three together. This sequence is preferentially cleaved by endopeptidases with trypsin-like activities. A breakthrough in understanding prohormone processing is the cloning from an insulinoma of a cDNA encoding a calcium-dependent serine protease that may be involved in the processing of proinsulin to insulin.[25] After endopeptidase cleavage, the remaining basic residues are selectively removed by exopeptidases with activity resembling that of carboxypeptidase B. In those instances in which the COOH-terminal residue of the peptide hormone is amidated, a process that appears to enhance the stability of a peptide by conferring resistance to carboxypeptidase, specific amidation enzymes in the Golgi complex work in concert with the cleavage enzymes for modification of the COOH terminal of the bioactive peptides.[26]

All proproteins and prohormones are probably cleaved by a common enzymatic process within the Golgi complex of cells of diverse origin. The significance of a general cleavage process of prohormones remains unknown, as does the reason for the existence of prohormone intermediates in some but not all secretory proteins. As indicated earlier, precursor peptides removed from the prohormones may have intrinsic biological activities as yet unrecognized.

PROCESSES OF HORMONE SECRETION

Specific extracellular stimuli control the secretion of polypeptide hormones. The stimuli consist of changes in homeostatic balance; the hormonal products released in response to the stimuli act on the respective target organs to re-establish homeostasis (Fig. 2–7). For example, an increase in the concentration of plasma electrolytes as a consequence of dehydration stimulates the release of vasopressin (AVP, also called antidiuretic hormone, ADH) in the neural lobe of the pituitary, and vasopressin in turn acts on the kidney to increase the reabsorption of water from the renal tubule, thereby readjusting serum electrolyte concentrations toward normal levels. Another example is the slight fall in blood calcium level that stimulates the release of parathyroid hormone, which acts on bone and kidney to promote fluxes of calcium back into the extracellular fluid. These regulatory processes commonly include inhibitory feedback loops in which the products elaborated by the target organs in response to the actions of a hormone inhibit further endocrine secretion. An example of such a negative feedback regulation is the control of the secretion of ACTH by the anterior pituitary. Increased ACTH stimulates the adrenal cortex to produce and secrete cortisol, which in turn feeds back to suppress further pituitary secretion of ACTH. In many instances endocrine regulation is complex and involves the responses of several endocrine glands and their respective target organs. After a meal, the release of a dozen or more hormones is triggered as a result of gastric distention, variations in the pH of the stomach, and increased concentrations of glucose, fatty acids, and amino acid in the blood. The rise in plasma glucose and amino acid levels stimulates the release of insulin and suppresses the release of glucagon from the pancreas. Both effects promote the net uptake of glucose by the liver; insulin increases cellular transport and uptake of glucose, and the lower blood levels of glucagon diminish the outflow of glucose because of diminished rates of glycogenolysis and gluconeogenesis.

The molecular mechanisms involved in the coupling of extracellular stimuli to the secretion of hormone, and ultimately to the biosynthesis of the new hormone required to replace that which is secreted, are incompletely understood.

RECOMBINANT DNA TECHNIQUES

The techniques for construction of recombinant DNAs make use of two classes of reagents. The first is the group of restriction endonucleases, polymerases, and ligases. These enzymes cleave DNA at specific sites, synthesize DNA from RNA and DNA templates, and join segments of DNA together. The second consists of bacterial plasmids and viruses, extrachromosomal organisms that replicate at high efficiency in their bacterial hosts. Through the application of these reagents, it is possible to synthesize DNAs from cellular mRNAs and to engineer these enzymatically synthesized DNAs in ways that permit their insertion into the genomes of bacterial plasmids and bacteriophages. The recombinant DNA can then be amplified by replication within the bacterial hosts, thus providing large quantities of the recombinant DNA for structural analyses, for use as hybridization probes, and for introduction into the genomes of mammalian cell lines for purposes of analyzing the structural properties of the DNA involved in the regulation of gene expression.

The two major breakthroughs that made the development of DNA technology possible were the discoveries of reverse transcriptase[27, 28] and restriction endonucleases.[29] Reverse transcriptase was found in the RNA of tumor viruses and is the means by which the virus makes DNA copies of the RNA templates. This enzyme allows the molecular biologist to copy mRNA into DNA, which is an essential step in the preparation of recombinant DNA for purposes of cloning. Restriction endonucleases cleave DNA at specific sequences, generally of four to six base pairs. Each of the many restriction endonucleases now isolated is specific for a

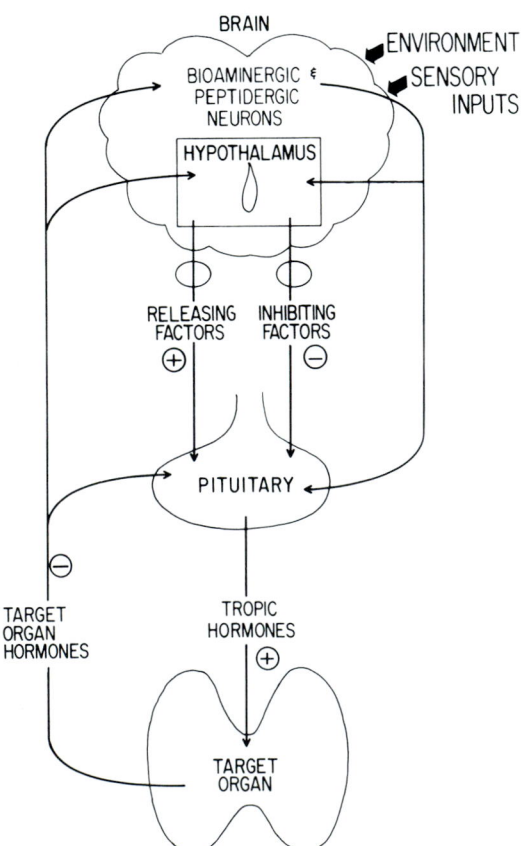

Figure 2–7. Regulatory feedback loops of the hypothalamic-pituitary-target organ axis. Being a combination of both stimulatory and inhibitory factors, hormones often act in concert to maintain homeostatic balance in the face of physiological or pathophysiological perturbations.

given sequence of nucleotides; these restriction endonucleases are the "trypsins" of polynucleotides. With these enzymes it is possible to cleave DNA reproducibly and predictably at specific sites, a property that is critical for the engineering of DNA segments.

In practice the analysis of a particular gene is begun by first preparing and cloning cDNAs from mRNAs of a particular cell (Fig. 2–8).[30–31] The cDNAs are prepared by "priming" the reverse transcription (reverse transcriptase) with short oligonucleotide fragments of oligodeoxyribothymidine, which preferentially binds to the 3'-polyadenylate, or poly(A), tract that is characteristic of cellular mRNAs. Double-stranded DNA is then prepared from the single-stranded cDNA by using DNA polymerase, and the cDNAs are inserted into bacterial plasmids that have been cleaved at a single site with a restriction endonuclease. To ensure a reasonably high efficiency of insertion of the foreign DNA into the plasmids, cohesive, or "sticky," ends are first prepared by adding short DNA sequences to the ends of the foreign DNA and to the plasmids. Vectors that are commonly used are derivatives of the plasmid pBR322, which was engineered specifically for the purposes of cloning DNA fragments (see Fig. 2–8). Foreign DNA is inserted into the unique site prepared by the endonuclease *Pst* I in which poly(dC) and poly(dG) homopolymers serve as the complementary, or cohesive, ends. This site is located within the gene that confers resistance to the antibiotic ampicillin. The plasmid also carries a gene for resistance to tetracycline. Thus bacteria containing the plasmids can be selected by their resistance to tetracycline; those specifically containing DNA inserts can be selected by their sensitivity to ampicillin because the ampicillinase gene is inactivated by the inserted foreign DNA. The recombinant plasmids containing DNA sequences that are complementary to the specific mRNAs of interest are identified by hybridizing recombinant plasmids to the initial mRNA preparations used in the cloning. The hybrid-selected mRNA is subsequently eluted and translated in a cell-free system appropriate for the protein under study.[32] Alternatively, specific inhibition of the translation of an mRNA can be used to identify the DNA of interest: DNA that is complementary to the mRNA being translated will bind the RNA, thus precluding translation and causing a reduced amount of the protein being synthesized.[33]

The techniques of hybridization selection and hybridization arrest in which cell-free translation is used as the assay system are often supplanted by hybridization of the bacterial colonies with synthetic oligonucleotide "probes" that are labeled with ³²P. Mixtures of oligonucleotides in the size range of 14 to 17 bases are prepared complementary to the nucleotide sequences predicted from the known amino acid sequences of segments of the protein encoded by mRNA. Because of the degeneracy in the genetic code (there are 61 amino acid codons and 20 amino acids), mixtures of from 24 to 48 oligonucleotides ordinarily represent all possible sequences complementary to a particular 14- to 17-base region of mRNA. Later-generation cDNA libraries have been prepared in bacterial phages (λ gt-11) or hybrids between plasmids and phages (phagemids), which have been engineered to allow the bacteria infected with the recombinant phages to translate mRNAs expressed from the cDNAs and thereby to produce the protein products encoded by the cDNAs. The desired sequence of interest can be selected at the protein level by screening the library of bacterial clones with an antiserum directed to the protein. When the desired product is a DNA-binding protein, the library can be screened with a labeled DNA duplex containing copies of the target sequence to which the protein binds.

The ability to prepare DNA by reverse transcription of mRNA was an important development in recombinant DNA technology, because there are more copies of mRNA in cells than there are genes that encode particular polypeptides. Usually, cells contain only two copies of the gene, whereas in cells in which the gene is expressed there may be 10,000 to 100,000 copies of the mRNA. Hence, it is easier to isolate recombinant DNAs by reverse transcription of RNA templates extracted from these cells than to isolate specific gene sequences. The complete natural gene sequences are subsequently isolated by hybridization with ³²P-labeled cloned recombinant cDNAs.

The techniques used in the cloning of genomic DNA are similar to those used for cloning cDNA, except that the genomic sequences are longer than the cDNA sequences

Figure 2–8. An approach used in construction and molecular cloning of recombinant DNA. *A,* Preparation of double-stranded DNA from an mRNA template. The enzyme reverse transcriptase is used to reverse transcribe a single-stranded DNA copy complementary to the mRNA primed with an oligonucleotide of polydeoxythymidylic acid hybridized to the poly(A) tract at the 3' end of mRNA. A complementary copy of the DNA strand is then prepared with DNA polymerase. Ends of double-stranded DNA are made flush by cleavage with the enzyme S₁ nuclease, and homopolymer extensions of deoxycytidine are synthesized at 3' ends of DNA with the enzyme terminal transferase. Oligo(dC) homopolymer extensions form sticky ends for purposes of insertion of DNA into a linearized bacterial plasmid on which complementary oligo(dG) homopolymer extensions have been synthesized. *B,* Insertion of foreign DNA into a bacterial plasmid for molecular cloning. A bacterial plasmid, typically pBR322 that has been specifically engineered for purposes of cloning DNA, is linearized by cleavage with restriction endonuclease *Pst* I. Poly(dG) homopolymer extensions are synthesized onto 3' ends of plasmid DNA. Foreign DNA with complementary poly(dC) homopolymer extensions is hybridized to and inserted into the plasmid. Recombinant plasmid DNA is transfected into susceptible host strains of bacteria in which plasmid replicates apart from bacterial chromosomal DNA. Bacteria are then grown on a plate containing tetracycline. Colonies that are resistant to tetracycline are tested for sensitivity to ampicillin. Because native plasmids contain genes encoding resistance to both tetracycline and ampicillin, and the gene encoding resistance to ampicillin is inactivated by insertion of a foreign DNA at the *Pst* I site, bacterial colonies harboring plasmids with DNA inserts are resistant to tetracycline and sensitive to ampicillin. Subsequent screening of tetracycline-resistant, ampicillin-sensitive clones containing specific DNA-inserted sequences is carried out by either DNA hybridization with labeled DNA probes or by other techniques such as hybridization arrest and cell-free translation.

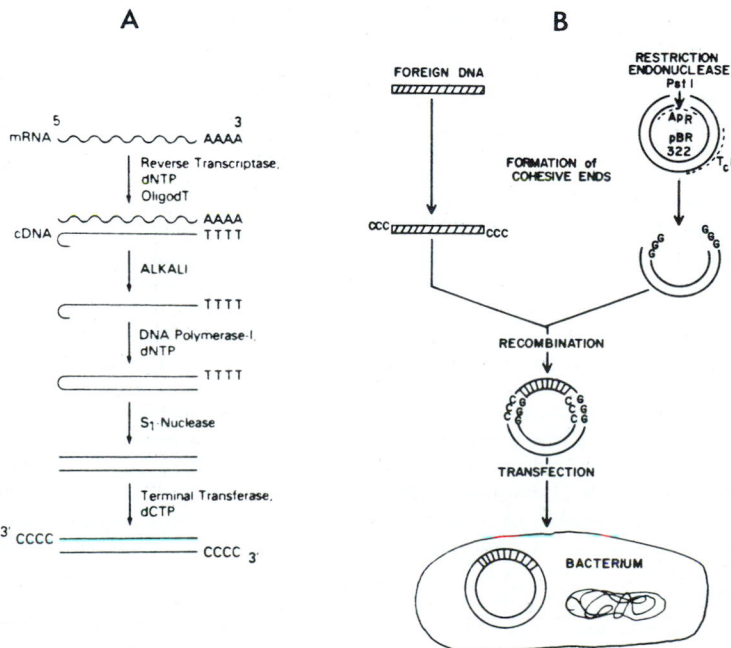

and that different cloning vectors are required. The common vectors are derivatives of the bacteriophage λ that can accommodate DNA fragments of from 10 to 20 kb. Certain hybrids of bacteriophages and plasmids, called *cosmids,* can accommodate inserts of DNA of up to 40 to 50 kb. In the cloning of genomic DNA, restriction fragments are prepared by partial digestion of unsheared DNA with a restriction endonuclease that cleaves the DNA into many fragments. DNA fragments of proper size are prepared by fractionation on agarose gels and are ligated to the bacteriophage DNA. The recombinant DNA is mixed with bacteriophage proteins, which results in the production of viable phage particles. The recombinant bacteriophages are grown on agar plates covered with growing bacteria. When the bacteria are infected by a phage particle, they lyse and form visible plaques. Specific phage colonies are transferred to nitrocellulose filters and are hybridized by cDNA probes labeled with ^{32}P. Libraries of genomic DNA fragments and tissue-specific cDNAs from various animal species cloned in plasmids and bacteriophages are available from a number of commercial laboratories.

Recombinant cDNAs are valuable for determination of the protein-encoding nucleotide sequences and as hybridization probes to measure cellular levels of mRNAs, mRNA precursors, and the numbers of gene copies contained in the genomes of animals. The last two measurements involve the separation either of the cellular RNA or of restriction endonuclease digests of genomic DNA on agarose gels, followed by transfer of the polynucleotide fragments to nitrocellulose filters and hybridization with ^{32}P-labeled cDNA probes. These procedures are known as Northern (RNA) transfer and Southern (DNA) transfer, respectively. It is sometimes possible to use labeled probes for hybridization directly to tissue slices or to spreads of metaphase chromosomes. For example, labeled cDNA encoding pro-opiomelanocortin, the precursor to ACTH, identified specific neurons containing pro-opiomelanocortin mRNA when hybridized to histological sections prepared from the medial basal hypothalamus of rats.[34] Similarly, the human insulin gene maps to the distal end of the short arm of chromosome 11 by hybridization of mitotic chromosome preparations from human lymphocytes in culture with a tritium-labeled recombinant plasmid encoding pre-proinsulin.[35] These powerful histohybridization techniques add a new dimension to molecular technology, inasmuch as it is possible to analyze individual cells for expression of specific genes.

The development of the technique for the rapid amplification of specific DNA sequences—the polymerase chain reaction[36, 37]—constitutes a breakthrough. This procedure relies on the unique properties of a thermal-stable DNA polymerase (Taq polymerase) to allow for sequential annealing of small oligonucleotide primers that bracket a DNA sequence of interest, which results in successive synthesis of the DNA strands. It is possible to amplify specific DNA sequences as short as 50 base pairs to several thousand base pairs over a million-fold in just a few hours by using an automated thermal cycler. The technique is so sensitive that DNA from a single cell can be so amplified. Indeed, a sample containing only a single target DNA molecule can be amplified.[37] The applications of this technique are diverse. Not only is it possible to amplify and clone rare sequences for detailed studies, but the technique has application in the fields of medical diagnosis and forensics. Detection of scarce viruses is possible in a drop of serum or urine or a single white blood cell. Genotyping can be done from a blood or semen stain, saliva, or a single hair. Paradoxically, a major drawback of the polymerase chain reaction is its exquisite sensitivity, which leaves open possibilities of producing false-positive results because of minute contaminations of the samples being tested. Thus extreme precautions must be taken to to avoid the introduction of contaminants.

APPLICATIONS OF SOMATIC CELL GENETICS AND GENE TRANSFER TECHNIQUES TO ANALYSIS OF GENE CONTROL

It is difficult to apply classic mammalian genetics to the analysis of genetic control and development. Many mutations that affect the developmental process and the regulation of genes are lethal and, as such, are difficult to propagate. These difficulties pose particular problems in humans in whom naturally occurring mutants are infrequent and may be inaccessible for study. Techniques are now available for the introduction of specifically engineered genes into the genomes of cultured cell lines and the germ cells of animals for study of the regulation of genes that determine development and cellular differentiation. For example, fragments containing strong promoters can be inserted adjacent to genes to enhance their expression. In addition, mutations in preselected regions, such as point and deletion mutations in 5'-flanking regions of expressed genes containing regulatory sequences, can be generated by treating a DNA fragment with a mutagen or by excising a segment of DNA with restriction endonucleases and assessing its functions after introduction into the genomes of living cells.

Several methods are available for the introduction of genetic material into mammalian cells in culture:[38] (1) fusion of two somatic cells to provide hybridomas; (2) gene transfer by DNA-mediated endocytosis; (3) transfection of cells with recombinant retroviruses containing covalently linked foreign DNA; and (4) microinjection of genes into cell nuclei.

Somatic Cell Fusion

Somatic cell fusion consists of fusion of two distinct somatic cell lines by incubation with a fusion-promoting agent such as inactivated Sendai virus or polyethylene glycol. The cells may be derived from different species of animals, e.g., human and mouse. Initially, a fused cell has two nuclei, each containing the chromosomes of one of the parent cells. In the course of cell division, the nuclear membranes disintegrate, and a single nucleus forms (heterokaryon) that contains chromosomes from both parent cells and that expresses certain genes from both parents. Appropriate genetic markers are used to select hybrid cells from parental cells. The large multiple genomes of the hybrids are unstable, and chromosomes are typically lost during successive cell divisions. Eventually, stable clones are isolated, each containing only one or a few different chromosomes from one of the specific parental cell lines. One advantage of the hybridomas is that libraries of hybrid cells can be collected, each of which contains a single chromosome from one animal species. For example, by cytological procedures the 24 human chromosomes (22 autosomal pairs plus X and Y chromosomes) can be identified and distinguished from the chromosomes of other species. Cell lines containing these chromosomes can be used to map the presence of particular genes. The assignment of genes to specific chromosomes is accomplished by analysis of the phenotypic expression of the function of the gene, e.g., an assay for a particular enzyme. The chromosomal localization of genes has been extended by combining somatic cell fusion with gene hybridization, which makes possible the detection of genes genotypically rather than phenotypically. In this approach, radiolabeled probes prepared from cloned cDNA or genomic fragments are used to detect complementary nucleotide sequences in the DNA of the cell hybrids by the Southern blotting technique. DNA is fragmented by restriction endonucleases, and the fragments are separated by electrophoresis, transferred onto nitrocellulose filters, and hybridized with the labeled polynucleotide probes. DNA fragments containing the complementary sequences are detected as labeled bands by autoradiography. A distinction is made between human and mouse genes by use of a sequence that hybridizes selectively to only one of the genes, or by identification of a restriction endonuclease fragment that is characteristic of the gene of one or the other of the two species. By these techniques, the chromosomal localizations of genes encoding several polypeptide hormones have been identified. For example, the human genes for growth hormone, placental lactogen (chorionic somatomammotropin), and a third growth hormone–like protein are located on chromosome 17,[39] and the gene for human prolactin is present on chromosome 6.[40]

Direct Transfer of Genes into Cells

DNA fragments carrying single genes can be inserted into living mammalian cells by DNA-mediated endocytosis. In this procedure, a purified DNA fragment carrying the desired gene is mixed with carrier DNA and calcium phosphate. The target cells are incubated with the DNA/calcium phosphate particles, which bind to the plasma membrane and enter the cells by endocytosis. Studies of the functions of gene promoters and regulatory DNA elements can be performed in transiently transfected cells during periods of from 24 to 96 h. The transfected DNA forms circular episomes within the nucleus and is subjected to regulatory influences that can closely mimic the regulation of the endogenous gene located within its natural chromosome. To facilitate studies of gene regulation, the regulatory sequences of interest are linked in cis to convenient "reporter" functions, such as the enzymes bacterial chloramphenicol acetyltransferase, alkaline phosphatase, or firefly luciferase. These enzymes are proteins with catalytic functions that (1) are stable when expressed in the host cells; (2) are entirely foreign (exogenous) to the host cells, i.e., have no endogenous background; and (3) have catalytic activities that are readily measured by simple assays. By using transient transfection assays it is possible to test tens to hundreds of different mutated sequences required for transcriptional expression. In addition, many different DNAs can be cotransfected simultaneously. For example, a trans expression vector encoding a transcription factor such as one encoding the cAMP response element–binding protein[41] or the glucocorticoid receptor[42] can be cotransfected with a cis element reporter vector containing the cAMP response element or the glucocorticoid response element. Thereby it is possible by mutational analyses to map regions of the expressed proteins that are important for transcriptional activation, binding of glucocorticoids, or phosphorylation that alters the functions of the proteins.

Although many (1 to 10%) of the cultured cells transiently take up DNA, only a small fraction, approximately 1 to 100 per million, subsequently stably express the transferred genetic information. The cells expressing the foreign gene are selected by particular markers that are cointroduced with the foreign gene, e.g., a gene encoding thymidine kinase or one encoding a protein that inactivates neomycin. The commonly used thymidine kinase method involves growth of cells in media containing hypoxanthine, aminopterin, and thymidine. Only cells to which thymidine kinase and the gene to be studied have been successfully transferred

will grow. Cells containing the gene for neomycin resistance are selected by growth in the presence of neomycin, which kills cells not expressing neomycin resistance. During the first few days after introduction of foreign DNA into cells, the DNA replicates as extrachromosomal DNA particles. In this stage, it is unstable and is often lost from the cells. However, on further cell divisions the foreign DNA becomes integrated into the chromosomal DNA of the host cell, thus forming a stable cell line. The transferred genes are integrated into one or a few sites in the host chromosomes; several copies of the gene may be integrated into one site.

Another method for introducing specific genes into the genome is to prepare recombinant DNAs between the gene of interest and the genomes of a virus such as simian virus 40.[43] After several cell divisions in the presence of the virus, the recombinant particles are also integrated into the host chromosome and carry the foreign DNA along with them.

An alternative technique of gene transfer is that of microinjection. With fine microcapillary pipettes, DNA solutions can be injected directly into the nucleus of a recipient cell. Several hundred copies of a DNA fragment may be introduced into each nucleus, and an expert operator can inject solution into 500 to 1000 cells/h. The advantage of the microinjection technique is that DNA fragments, which usually ligate to form chain-like concatemers, are rapidly integrated into the host chromosomes. The efficiency of cellular transformation obtained with this technique is higher than that obtained with the calcium phosphate procedure. In some instances up to 20% of microinjected cells form stable transformants.

The technique of microinjection has also been used to insert genetic material into one-cell mammalian embryos that are then allowed to develop (Fig. 2–9).[44] This approach allows analysis of the regulation of defined genes in the context of normal development of a complex organism. DNA is injected into the male pronucleus of fertilized mouse ova, followed by insertion of the ova into the reproductive tract of pseudopregnant foster mothers. The transgenic animals that develop from this procedure contain the foreign DNA integrated into one or more of the host chromosomes at an early stage of embryo development. As a consequence, the foreign DNA is generally transmitted to the germ line, and, in a number of instances, the foreign genes are expressed. Because the foreign DNA is injected at the one-cell stage, there is a good chance that the DNA will be distributed among all the progeny cells as development proceeds. This situation provides an opportunity to analyze and compare the qualitative and quantitative efficiencies of expression of the genes among various organs. The technique is quite efficient; more than half of postinjection embryos produce viable offspring, and of these approximately 10% carry the foreign genes.

For example, with this procedure the genes encoding growth hormone,[45] somatostatin,[46] and vasopressin[47] have been introduced into the germ lines of mice. These genes were expressed at high levels in most of the tissues analyzed. In several of the transgenic animals, levels of growth hormone in plasma were 100 to 1000 times higher than normal. The phenotypic changes in the mice bearing the foreign growth hormone genes were remarkable; they grew at a rate two to three times faster than normal littermates. The animals bearing and expressing the foreign somatostatin and vasopressin genes showed no phenotypic changes, although levels of bioactive hormones in the plasma were 100 to 200 times above normal. The absence of demonstrable phenotypic changes in these transgenic animals may be a consequence of down-regulation or uncoupling of receptors for the hormone in target organs. In the transgenic animals the foreign genes were passed on and expressed at high levels

PREPARATION OF TRANSGENIC MICE

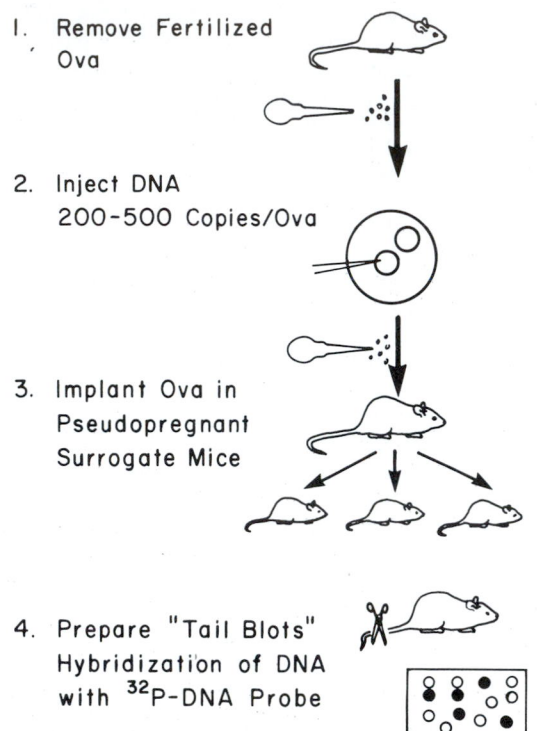

1. Remove Fertilized Ova

2. Inject DNA 200-500 Copies/Ova

3. Implant Ova in Pseudopregnant Surrogate Mice

4. Prepare "Tail Blots" Hybridization of DNA with ^{32}P-DNA Probe

Figure 2–9. Method for the integration of a foreign gene into the germ line of mice. DNA containing a specific foreign gene is microinjected into the male pronucleus of fertilized ova obtained from the oviduct of a mouse. Ova are then implanted into the uterus of pseudopregnant surrogate mothers. Progeny are analyzed for the presence of foreign genes by hybridization with a ^{32}P-labeled DNA probe and DNA prepared from a piece of tail of a mouse that has been immobilized on a nitrocellulose filter (tail blots).

in several generations of progeny. The practical implications of this technology of gene transfer are discussed later.

STRUCTURE OF A GENE ENCODING A POLYPEPTIDE HORMONE

Structural analyses of gene sequences have resulted in at least three major discoveries that are important to an understanding of the expression of peptide-encoding genes. First, sequences of all the known biological peptides are contained within larger precursors that often encode for other peptides, many of which are of unknown biological activity. Second, the coding regions of genes (exons) are interrupted by sequences (introns) that are transcribed but subsequently cleaved from the initial RNA transcripts during their nuclear processing and assembly into specific mRNAs. Third, specific regulatory sequences reside in the regions of DNA-flanking structural genes, and these DNA sequences constitute specific targets for the interactions of DNA-binding proteins.

The DNA of higher organisms is wound into a tightly and regularly packed chromosomal structure in association with a number of different proteins organized into elements called nucleosomes.[48] Nucleosomes are composed of four or five different histone subunits that form a core structure about which approximately 140 base pairs of genomic DNA are wound. Structures of histones are highly conserved

throughout evolution, which indicates their fundamental importance in the architecture of the nucleosome. The nucleosomes are arranged as beads on a string, and coils of nucleosomes form the fundamental organizational units of the eucaryotic chromosome. The nucleosomal structure serves several purposes. For example, nucleosomes enable the large amount of DNA (approximately 2×10^9 pairs) of the genome to be compacted into a small volume. Nucleosomes may also be involved in replication of DNA and gene transcription. In addition to histones, other proteins are associated with DNA, and the complex nucleoprotein structure may provide specific recognition sites for regulatory proteins and enzymes involved in DNA replication, rearrangements of DNA segments, and gene expression.

The topography of a typical protein-encoding gene consists of two functional units: (1) a transcriptional region and (2) a promoter or regulatory region (Fig. 2–10).

Transcriptional Regions

The transcriptional unit is the segment of gene that is transcribed into a mRNA precursor. Note that the nucleotide thymidine (T) in DNA is transcribed as uridine (U) in RNA. The coding sequence of the gene consists of the exon sequences that are spliced from the primary transcript during the post-transcriptional processing of the precursor RNA; these exons contain the code for the mRNA sequence that is translated into protein and for untranslated sequences at the 5'- and 3'-flanking regions. The 5' sequence begins typically with a methylated guanine residue known as the cap site. The 3'-untranslated region contains within it a short sequence, AATAAA, that signals the site of cleavage of the 3' end of the RNA and the addition of a poly(A) tract of 100 to 200 nucleotides located approximately 20 bases from the AATAAA sequence. Although the functions of these modifications of the ends of mRNAs are poorly understood, they enhance stability, perhaps through providing resistance to degradation by exonucleases. Likewise, the nature of the enzymatic mechanisms that result in the excision of intron-coded sequences and the rejoining of exon-coded sequences is incompletely understood. Short "consensus" sequences of nucleotides reside at the splice junctions, e.g., the bases GT and AG at the 5' and 3' ends of the introns, respectively.[49] A population of small nuclear RNAs, known as the U1 RNAs, contain short nucleotide sequences that are complementary to the splice junctions. These small RNAs may serve as templates that base-pair with the splice junctions, which provides secondary structure for specific endonucleolytic cleavages.[50] As indicated earlier, the protein-coding sequence of the mRNA begins with the codon AUG for methionine and ends with the codon immediately preceding one of the three nonsense, or stop, codons (UGA, UAA, and UAG). The protein-coding sequences of polypeptide hormones invariably encode precursor prehormones (or pre-prohormones) that then undergo specific post-translational cleavages during their passage through the secretory pathway.

Regulatory Regions

The regulation of expression of genes that encode polypeptides is now beginning to be understood. As a result of experiments involving the deletion of 5' sequences upstream from structural genes, followed by analyses of their expression after introduction into cell lines, several insights have been obtained. These regulatory sequences, termed promoters and enhancers, consist of short polynucleotide sequences (see Fig. 2–10). They can be divided into four groups with respect to their functions and distances from the transcriptional initiation site. First, the sequence TATAA

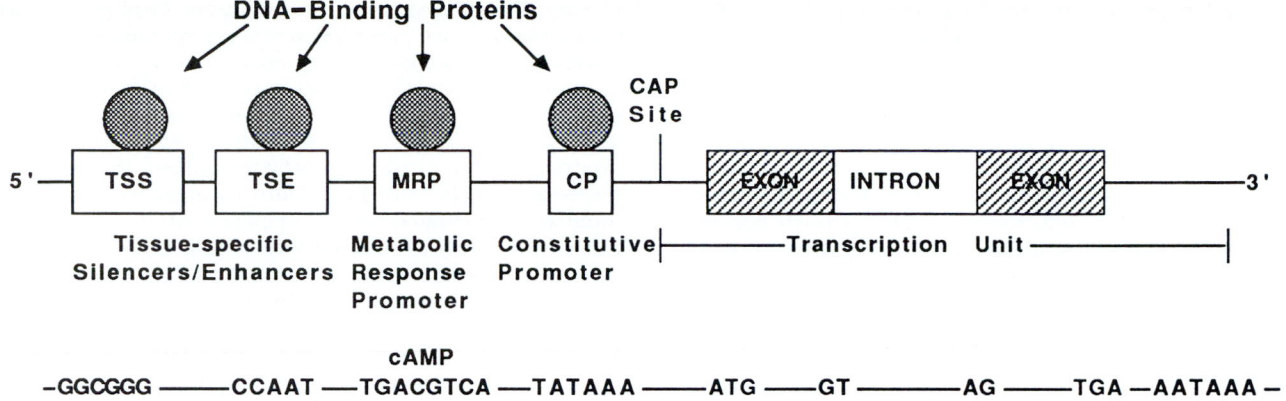

Figure 2–10. Diagrammatic structure of a "consensus" gene encoding a polypeptide hormone. Such a gene typically consists of a promoter region and a transcription unit. The transcription unit is that region of DNA composed of exons and introns that is transcribed into an mRNA precursor. Transcription begins at the cap site sequence in DNA and extends several hundred bases beyond the poly(A) addition site in the 3' region. During post-transcriptional processing of the RNA precursor, the 5' end of mRNA is capped by addition of methylguanosine residues. The transcript is then cleaved at the poly(A) addition site approximately 20 bases 3' to the AATAAA signal sequence, and the poly(A) tract is added to the 3' end of the RNA. Introns are cleaved from the RNA precursor, and exons are joined together. Dinucleotides GT and AG are invariably found at the 5' and 3' ends of introns. Translation of mRNA invariably starts with the codon ATG for methionine. Translation is terminated when the polyribosome reaches the stop codons TGA, TAA, or TAG. The promoter region of the gene located 5' to the cap site contains numerous short regulatory DNA sequences that are targets for interactions with specific DNA-binding proteins. These sequences consist of the basal constitutive promoter (TATA box), metabolic response promoters that modulate transcription, e.g., in response to cAMP, steroid hormone receptors, and thyroid hormone receptors, as well as tissue-specific enhancers and silencers that permit or prevent transcription of the gene, respectively. The enhancer and silencer elements direct expression of specific subsets of genes to cells of a given phenotype. Whether a gene will or will not be expressed in a particular cellular phenotype depends on complex interactions of the various DNA-binding proteins among themselves and, most important, with the TATA box proteins of the constitutive promoter.

(TATA, or Goldberg-Hogness, box) is present in the more proximal promoter within 25 to 30 nucleotides upstream from the point of transcriptional initiation. The integrity of the TATA sequence is required to ensure the accuracy of initiation of transcription at a particular site. The TATA box binds a complex of several proteins, including RNA polymerase II (Fig. 2–11). The proteins, which are referred to as TATA box factors, number about five or six transcription factors IIA to IIE and, along with RNA polymerase II, form the general or basal transcriptional machinery required for the initiation of RNA synthesis.[51] Upstream from the TATA sequence in the more distal promoter region resides a series of sequences that serve as amplifiers of the transcriptional response such as CCAAT or CCGCCC that bind the transcription factors CTF or SP-1, respectively. Located further upstream from the TATA box are sequences that function either as tissue- or cell-specific enhancers or suppressors and/or as metabolic response elements. These elements may be located close to or at a distance from the promoter elements. The tissue-specific elements confer latent transcriptional inducibility to a gene for expression in a given cellular phenotype but require stimulation by a metabolic response element (or elements). The metabolic response elements are the key sequences involved in the up- or down-regulation of transcription and are targets for the binding of important "third messengers," namely, DNA-binding proteins whose binding and transcriptional transactivation activities are regulated by the second messengers such as cAMP-dependent protein kinase A, diacylglycerol-dependent protein kinase C, calcium/calmodulin-dependent protein kinase, or steroid hormone– or thyroid hormone–bound receptors. Specific sequence elements have been identified that bind cAMP-regulated proteins such as the protein cAMP response element–binding protein that binds to a cAMP response element and the proteins jun and fos that bind to the tetradecanoylphorbol acetate response element.[52–54] Similarly, elements have been identified that bind receptors for the steroid and thyroid hormones and for retinoic acid. The cell-specific enhancer and metabolic response functions often are colocalized within the same DNA element. Combinations of elements with their cognate DNA-

binding proteins usually work in synergy to generate a transcriptionally productive holocomplex involving interactions with the TATA box factors of the basal promoter (see Fig. 2–11). The rapid progress that has been made in the identification of regulatory DNA elements and in the cloning of the genes that encode DNA-binding proteins will lead to a more complete understanding of gene control mechanisms.

Introns and Exons

The discovery that genes encoding proteins and ribosomal RNAs in eucaryotes are interrupted by intervening DNA sequences (introns) that separate them into coding blocks (exons) was unexpected.[55] In bacterial genes the nucleotide sequences of the chromosomal genes match precisely the corresponding sequences in the mRNAs. Interrup-

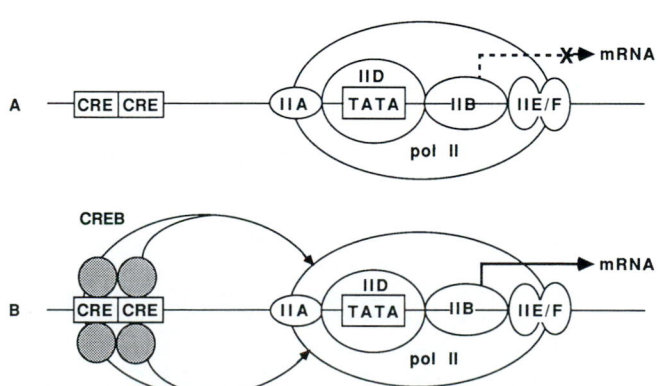

Figure 2–11. Diagrammatic depiction of the basal transcriptional proteins of the constitutive promoter (TATA box). A, In the absence of protein binding to enhancer or metabolic response promoter, e.g., the cAMP response element (CRE), the basal rate of transcription mediated by the TATA box factors TFII A–F and RNA polymerase II (pol II) is low. B, When specific proteins such as cAMP response element–binding proteins (CREBs) bind to the cAMP response element, the basal transcription complex is activated, which initiates the synthesis of mRNA. (Adapted from O'Malley BW. The steroid receptor superfamily: more excitement predicted for the future. Mol Endocrinol 1990; 4:363–369. © The Endocrine Society.)

tion of the continuity of genetic information appears to be unique to nucleated cells. The reasons for such interruption are not completely understood, but introns appear to separate exons into functional domains with respect to the proteins that they encode. An example is the gene for proglucagon, a precursor of glucagon in which five introns separate six exons, three of which encode glucagon and the two glucagon-related peptides contained within the precursor (Fig. 2–12).[56] A second example is the growth hormone gene, which is divided into five exons by four introns that separate the promoter region of the gene from the protein-coding region and the latter into three partly homologous repeated segments, two coding for the growth-promoting activity of the hormone and the third for its carbohydrate metabolic functions.[57] As a general rule the genes for the precursors of hormones and regulatory peptides contain introns at or about the region where the signal peptides join the apoproteins or prohormones, thus separating the signal sequences from the components of the precursor that are exported from the cell as hormones or peptides.

The existence of a genetic model in which the transcripts of active protein-encoding genes consist of a mosaic of introns and exons explains two aspects of the genetic structure of higher cells. Intron-coded sequences in transcripts account for a large part of the heterogeneous nuclear RNA, which has been recognized for some years in eucaryotic cells. Introns also explain the extra DNA that is present in the genomes of higher cells, the "selfish DNA" that is replicated but has no recognized function. Only 5 to 10% of eucaryotic DNA can be accounted for as coding sequences for proteins and RNAs. Another 10 to 15%, about which little is known, appears to contain highly reiterated sequences, called repetitive DNA, scattered throughout the genome. Thus approximately 70 to 80% of DNA sequences are without known function. On average, the intron sequences contain approximately 10 times the amount of DNA that is present in the exons.

Several functions have been proposed for introns.[55, 58] Topographic separations of exons encoding regions of proteins of specific functions may reflect the evolutionary processes of genetic recombination. The result of such recombination is the bringing together, within a single gene, of multiple functional components that are widely distributed within the genome, and the eventual creation of chimeric proteins with new functions. The existence of specific functional coding blocks of DNA separated by noncoding DNA sequences allows recombination to take place anywhere within the intron DNA without interruption of the reading frames of the exons, because during the enzymatic processing of the primary gene transcript the introns within which recombination occurred are excised.

Introns may also have other roles. Not only can specific recombinations between introns bring exons together into new transcriptional units to make special differentiated products, but the utilization of new splicing patterns could create new gene products. For example, differentiation could be determined by the appearance of a new splicing enzyme that utilizes existing intron sequences to make new exons, thereby providing additional coding information for new proteins. Introns may also serve as a repository for DNA sequences that serve as control, or regulatory, sequences. In fact, the glucocorticoid promoter region that regulates expression of the rat growth hormone gene resides within the second intron of that gene. Clearly, the genome is in a dynamic state of rearrangement. Transposable DNA elements (transposons), identified in plants by McClintock,[59] are also found in higher organisms.

Genetic rearrangement occurs not only by recombination but also by transposition of sequences via extrachromosomal mechanisms.[60] For example, pseudogenes, which are derived from the transcripts of expressed genes, are located throughout the genome.[61] These pseudogenes, although not functionally expressed in their own right, are believed to be derived from reverse transcription of RNA transcripts into DNA with reinsertion of the DNA back into the genome. Such a mechanism could provide a means for amplifying specific functional DNA sequences such as protein-encoding and -regulatory segments.

The functions of introns in the evolutionary processes of genetic recombination may explain the absence of introns in procaryotes. It is tempting to speculate that procaryotes represent an end product in the evolutionary process. It is possible that at one time the genomes of microorganisms contained introns, but as the organisms became highly differentiated the genomes reached an end point in evolution, becoming "frozen" after they had arranged themselves to provide the highest benefit to the organism. Subsequently, the introns were simply lost because they afforded no further benefit. Similar reasoning may explain the low frequency of introns in yeasts, which are highly differentiated eucaryotes. To obtain additional genetic information, bacteria and yeasts would have to rely on the acquisition of extra chromosomal DNA sequences in the form of viruses or plasmids. This hypothetical argument may explain the exceptions to the theory of "one exon, one function" in mammalian cells. The genes of many precursors of peptide hormones are not

RAT PRE-PROGLUCAGON GENE AND mRNA

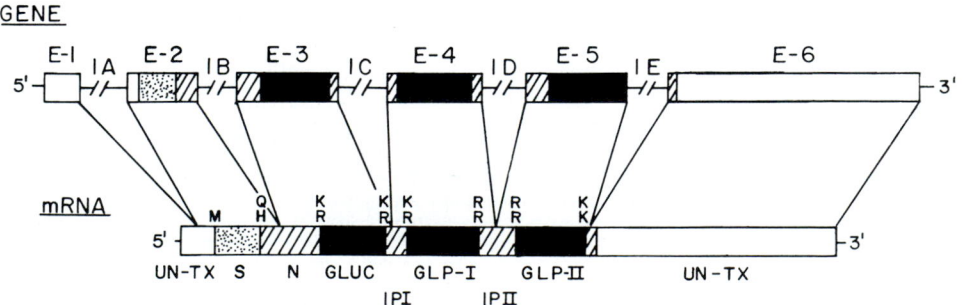

Figure 2–12. Diagram of the pancreatic glucagon gene and its encoded mRNA (cDNA). The glucagon gene is an example of a gene in which exons precisely encode separate functional domains. The gene consists of six exons (E1–E6) and five introns (1A–1E). mRNA encoding pre-proglucagon, the protein precursor of glucagon, consists of 10 specific regions: from left to right, a 5'-untranslated sequence (UN-TX, unshaded); a signal sequence (S, stippled); an NH$_2$-terminal extension sequence (N, hatched); glucagon (GLUC, shaded); a first intervening peptide (IP-I, hatched); a first glucagon-like peptide (GLP-I, shaded); a second intervening peptide (IP-II, hatched); a second glucagon-like peptide (GLP-II, shaded); a dilysyl dipeptide (hatched) after the glucagon-like peptide II sequence; and an untranslated region (UN-TX, unshaded). Exons from left to right encode the 5'-untranslated region; signal sequence; glucagon; glucagon-like peptide I; glucagon-like peptide II; and 3'-untranslated sequence. Letters shown above the mRNA denote amino acids located at positions in pre-proglucagon that are cleaved during cellular processing of precursor. Q, glutamine; H, histidine; K, lysine; R, arginine. M denotes the amino acid methionine, which marks the initiation of translation of mRNA into pre-proglucagon.

interrupted by introns in a manner that corresponds to the separation of the functional components of the precursor. Notable in this regard is the precursor pro-opiomelanocortin, from which the peptides ACTH, α-melanocyte-stimulating hormone, and β-endorphin are cleaved during the post-translational processing of the precursor. The protein-coding region of the pro-opiomelanocortin gene is devoid of introns. Likewise, no introns interrupt the protein-coding region of the gene for the proenkephalin precursor, which contains seven copies of the enkephalin sequences. It is possible that, in the past, introns separated each of these coding domains and were lost during the course of evolution. A precedent for the selective loss of introns appears to be exemplified by the rat insulin genes. The rat contains two nonallelic insulin genes: one contains two introns, and the other a single intron. The most likely explanation is that an ancestral gene containing two introns was duplicated, and in the process of duplication or sometime thereafter one of the introns was eliminated.

In summary, the precise roles that introns play in the evolution of the gene and in the control of gene expression remain to be determined. Elucidation of the molecular mechanisms by which introns are excised and exons are spliced together should provide insight into the evolution and function of this splicing mechanism.

REGULATION OF GENE EXPRESSION

The regulation of expression of genes encoding polypeptide hormones can take place at one or more levels in the pathway of hormone biosynthesis (Fig. 2–13):[62, 63] (1) DNA synthesis (cell growth and division), (2) transcription, (3) post-transcriptional processing of mRNA, (4) translation, and (5) post-translational processing. In different endocrine cells, one or more levels may serve as specific control points for regulation of production of a hormone.

Levels of Gene Control

Newly synthesized prolactin transcripts are formed within minutes after exposure of a prolactin-secreting cell line to TRH.[64] Cortisol stimulates growth hormone synthesis in both somatotropic cell lines and pituitary slices through increases in rates of gene transcription and by enhancement of the stability of mRNA.[65, 66] The time required for cortisol to enhance transcription of the growth hormone gene is 1 to 2 h, which is considerably longer than the time required for the action of TRH on prolactin gene transcription. Regulation of proinsulin biosynthesis appears to take place primarily at the level of translation.[67] Within minutes after raising the plasma glucose level, the rate of proinsulin biosynthesis increases 5- to 10-fold. Glucose acts either directly or indirectly to enhance the efficiency of initiation of translation of proinsulin mRNA. Regulation at the level of post-transcriptional processing of mRNA precursors is not yet clearly established. However, the fact that the primary RNA transcripts derived from the calcitonin gene are alternatively spliced to provide two or more mRNAs that encode chimeric protein precursors with both common and different amino acid sequences suggests that regulation might take place at the level of processing of the calcitonin gene transcripts. The regulation of the biosynthesis of parathyroid hormone by calcium takes place principally at the levels of DNA synthesis and cell division. Stimulation of the parathyroid gland by lowering calcium levels appears to have little effect on the rates of RNA synthesis but readily leads to hyperplasia of the gland.[68] In addition, a decrease

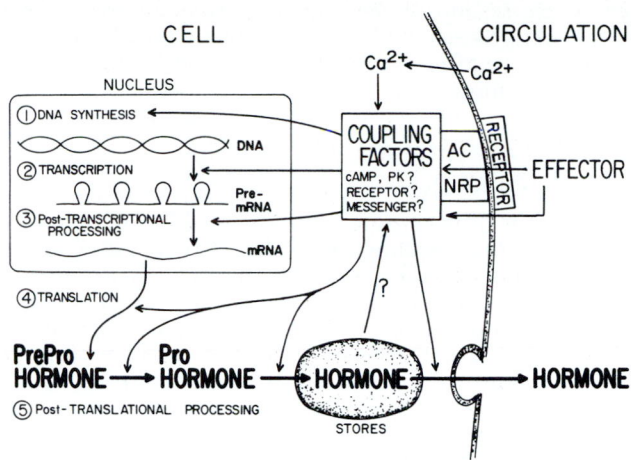

Figure 2–13. Diagram of an endocrine cell showing potential control points for regulation of gene expression in hormone production. Specific effector substances bind either to plasma membrane receptors (peptide effectors) or to cytosolic receptors (steroids), which leads to initiation of a series of events that couple the effector signal with gene expression. Peptide effector-receptor complex interactions appear to act initially via activation of adenylate cyclase (AC) coupled with a nucleotide regulatory protein (NRP). Coupling factors through which other effectors act, such as glucose, thyroid hormones, and cations, are unknown but probably involve, at least in part, activation of protein kinases (PK) and a series of phosphorylations of macromolecules. As discussed in the text, specific effectors for various endocrine cells appear to act at one or more of the indicated five levels of gene expression, with the possible exception of post-translational processing of prohormones, for which no definite examples of regulation have yet been found.

in intracellular turnover time of parathyroid hormone is caused by hypocalcemia.

In many instances the level of gene expression under regulatory control is optimal for meeting secretory and biosynthetic demands of the endocrine organ. For example, after a meal there is an immediate requirement for the release of large amounts of insulin. Because this release depletes insulin stores of the pancreatic beta cells within a few minutes, increasing the translational efficiency of pre-formed proinsulin mRNA provides additional hormone rapidly. In contrast, the release of parathyroid hormone remains almost constant at all times, and small fluctuations in secretion rate are adequate to maintain the levels of serum ionized calcium within a narrow range. Because of the importance of ionized calcium in the homeostatic maintenance of cells, a hormonal feedback system between ionized calcium and parathyroid hormone secretion is tightly regulated.[68, 69] The consequence is that prolonged stimulation of the parathyroid gland, as in chronic renal failure, results in marked hyperplasia; low levels of ionized calcium can thus be considered a "growth factor" for the parathyroid glands.

Although tissue-specific differences occur in the processing of prohormones, alterations in the rates of conversion of a prohormone to a hormone under physiological circumstances in a given tissue have not been identified as a point of cellular control. However, glucocorticoids appear to regulate the post-translational processing and compartmentalization of murine mammary tumor virus protein in hepatic carcinoma cells.[70] The mammary tumor virus encodes two major proteins, each of which is modified, cleaved, and compartmentalized in reactions similar to those that affect maturation of various classes of cellular proteins. At least two post-translational maturation pathways in production of viral proteins are regulated by glucocorticoids, one controlling glycoprotein processing by modification of carbohydrate residues and the other involved in phosphorylation of the proteins.[70] Thus in addition to regulating transcription of the mammary tumor virus gene, glucocorticoids affect the genetic expression of the mammary tumor virus proteins. These observations imply that the same or similar signaling molecules can affect expression of a gene long after it has been transcribed.

Coupling of Hormone Secretion to Gene Regulation

The biosynthetic processes expressed by genes must be coupled in some manner with the secretory processes of endocrine cells. Synthesis of new hormone is required to replace that which is released, and, conversely, when secretory demands decrease, synthesis of new hormone must also decrease to prevent overloading of the cell with hormone. Little is known about the cellular mechanisms that link secretory events to biosynthetic events, i.e., whether the extracellular stimulatory factors that regulate rates of secretion also directly affect rates of hormone biosynthesis, or whether the process of secretion somehow provides regulatory signals that are transmitted to the steps in biosynthesis. As indicated earlier, the closeness of coupling of secretory and biosynthetic activities in a particular endocrine gland may depend to a large degree on the relative magnitude of the amount of hormone that is present in stored form. A gland that has large stores of hormone can meet secretory demands for a longer time than a gland with a smaller store. Most endocrine cells store hormone to some extent, as evidenced by the presence of secretory granules. Such a storage system has probably evolved to provide a reservoir of hormone that can be called on to meet secretory demands over a very short time without the necessity for abrupt changes in rates of hormone biosynthesis.

Cis and Trans Mechanisms of Gene Regulation

Studies of gene regulation suggest several possible mechanisms of control. The first requirement is that the factors and structural components of a gene that allow expression be present in a given tissue. If present, regulatory mechanisms can then be brought into play.

Certain genes or sets of genes are expressed only in specific tissues. Two conceptually distinct mechanisms have been proposed for differential gene expression: cis and trans mechanisms (Fig. 2–14). It is likely that, when the processes involved in gene regulation are understood more completely, it will be found that both mechanisms are used. In the simpler cis mechanism, a specific signaling factor interacts with a sensor-receptor region of the gene to activate transcription of the structural gene. The cis mechanism probably works by inducing structural or conformational change in the chromatin.

The trans mechanism requires a second step of gene activation in which a diffusible intermediary product of a regulatory gene activates transcription of the producer gene. In this model the intracellular signal that arises as a consequence of activation of the cell interacts with the sensor region of a regulatory gene, which results in the transcription of an RNA from an associated integrator gene (acting in cis). The RNA either serves as an mRNA for the encoding of a protein that, in turn, interacts with the activator receptor responsible for initiating transcription of the producer gene or serves directly as an activator RNA. As discussed earlier, many so-called integrator genes encode a multitude of DNA-binding proteins, which, in turn, operate by direct interactions with DNA control elements of genes. The cis and trans models depicted in Figure 2–14 reflect the ideas of Britten and Davidson,[71, 72] who suggested that repetitive cis recognition sequences might provide the structural basis for the

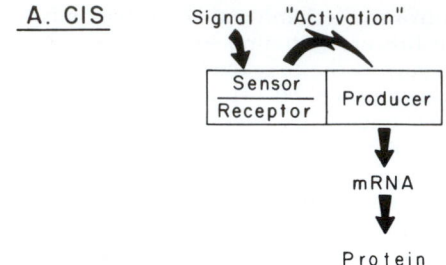

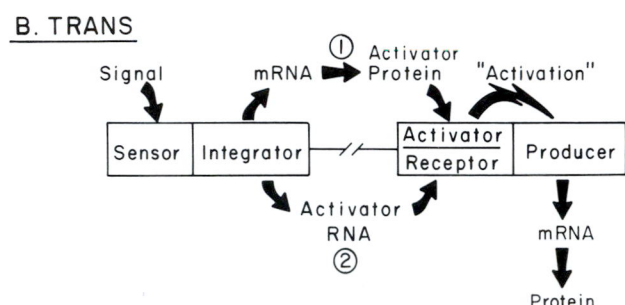

Figure 2–14. Hypothetical cis (A) and trans (B) models for activation of gene expression. In both models the specific intracellular signal interacts with a sensor-receptor on the gene. In the cis model, the sensor-receptor (activator) is adjacent to the producer gene, which is the transcriptional unit, leading to production of mRNA and protein. In the trans model, the sensor is separated from the activator-receptor, which is adjacent to the producer gene, and the activator substance, originating from the sensor, acts in trans by transport to the activator receptor. This activator substance may be either an RNA molecule or a protein activator translated from RNA. Activator binds or otherwise interacts with an activator-receptor sequence on the gene, which results in initiation of transcription. Thus far, experimental evidence indicates that activation of most genes involves a cis-acting mechanism; no trans-acting regulatory activators have been definitely identified.

coordinate induction of unlinked structural genes. This hypothesis arose from the observation that specific DNA sequences exist in multiple copies in the genomes of eucaryotic cells. For example, the so-called Alu sequences, which consist of highly homologous segments of approximately 300 bases, are present in 300,000 to 500,000 copies in the human genome.[73] The repeated DNA sequences are scattered throughout the genome, and many or all of them have, or have had, the capacity to transpose during evolution.[74] One mechanism for the evolution of new gene products is the diffusion within and around the genome of transposable cis regulatory sequences.[55, 75, 76] One can envision that transposable DNA sequence elements could occasionally carry with them and deposit specific control sequences in the right genomic environment, which would result in the display of specific receptor gene functions.

Although the functions for the Alu sequences are not known, it appears that the DNA-binding proteins that regulate the expression of genes are themselves encoded by superfamilies of sequence-related genes. So in essence, the hypothesis set forth by Britten and Davidson has proved to be correct: the genes encoding the DNA-binding proteins are the integrator genes, and the genes encoding other RNAs and cellular proteins are the producer genes. It appears, however, that the sensor and the activator receptors are similar; they respond alike to the interactions of DNA-binding proteins. This circumstance raises interesting questions regarding how so many genes can all be regulated by DNA-binding proteins whose genes are regulated by binding proteins, and so on. If there were an open-ended cascade of unique DNA-binding protein genes, the DNA sequences required to encode the proteins would predictably exceed the amount of DNA in the genome. The situation poses an apparent dilemma akin to that faced by immunologists a number of years ago in attempting to understand how the repertoire of some 10^6 different antibody proteins (preimmune repertoire) could be expressed when the total number of unique expressed genes in animal cells was estimated to be less than 10^5. The generation of antibody diversity turned out to be the utilization of a combinatorial process consisting of somatic recombination and mutation, i.e., gene rearrangement and point mutations followed by clonal selection of antibody-producing lymphocytes in response to a challenge by a specific antigen. The generation of diversity in the regulation of gene expression by DNA-binding proteins likewise almost certainly involves a combinatorial process. As envisioned, this process is not gene rearrangement but rather a number of different occurrences, including the formation of uniquely structured proteins by diversification at the various levels of gene expression (multiple-related genes, alternative patterns of RNA splicing, post-translational modifications) (see later under Generation of Biological Diversification), limited but distinct permissiveness in the formation of active protein dimers, and assembly of unique combinations of multiple protein-DNA interactions.

Tissue-Specific Gene Expression

Differentiated cells possess a remarkable capacity for selective expression of specific genes. In one cell type, a single gene may account for a large fraction of the total gene expression, and in another cell type the same gene may be expressed at undetectable levels.

The chromatin is more loosely arranged in genes that are capable of expression than it is in those same genes in a tissue in which they are never expressed. Thus the DNA within the chromatin of genes from tissues in which they are expressed is more susceptible to cleavage by DNase than is that in tissues in which the genes are quiescent.[77] This looseness may facilitate access of RNA polymerase to the gene for purposes of transcription. In addition, inactive genes appear to have a higher content of methylated cytosine residues than do the same genes in tissues in which they are expressed.[78]

Determinants for the tissue-specific transcriptional expression of genes exist in control sequences usually residing within 1000 base pairs of the 5'-flanking region of the transcriptional sequence. Enhancer sequences in animal cell genes were first described for immunoglobulin genes, a finding that extended the earlier observations of enhancer control elements in viral genomes.[79] However, the first clear demonstrations of the properties of these elements to direct transcription to cells of distinct phenotypes came from studies of the comparative expressions of two model genes, insulin and chymotrypsin, expressed in the endocrine and exocrine pancreas, respectively.[80]

Recombinant DNA techniques were used to link 5'-flanking regions of the insulin and chymotrypsin genes to the coding sequence of a chloramphenicol acetyltransferase gene. The latter serves as an enzymatic assay for detection of activity in the 5'-flanking sequences presumed to be gene control regions. When the recombinant insulin gene was introduced into pancreatic beta cells, acetylation of chloramphenicol took place. When placed in pancreatic exocrine cells, the insulin recombinant gene was quiescent, i.e., chloramphenicol acetyltransferase was not expressed. The reverse was true for the chymotrypsin recombinant: expression in the exocrine cell but not in the beta cell. These observations have been confirmed by studies of many additional genes in other tissues, and they have profound implications for an understanding of the nature of control elements in the tissue-specific expression of genes. It now appears that the specific and restricted expression of genes in a cell-specific manner is determined by the assembly of specific combinations of DNA-binding proteins on a predetermined array of control elements of the promoter regions of genes so as to create a transcriptionally active complex of proteins that includes the components of the general or basal transcriptional apparatus (TATA box factors).

Coupling of Effector Action to Cellular Response

Another mode of gene control consists of the induction and suppression of genes that are normally expressed within a specific tissue. These processes are at work in the minute-to-minute and day-to-day regulation of rates of production of the specific proteins produced by the cells, e.g., the production of polypeptide hormones in response to extracellular stimuli.

At least two classes of macromolecules, phosphoproteins and steroid hormone receptors, appear to be involved in the physiological regulation of hormone gene expression. These two types of macromolecules mediate the actions of peptide and steroid hormones, respectively. Peptide ligands bind to receptor complexes on the plasma membrane, which results in hydrolysis of phosphatidylinositol, mobilization of calcium, formation of phosphorylated nucleotide intermediates, activation of protein kinases, and phosphorylation of specific regulatory proteins.[81] Steroidal compounds, because of their hydrophobic composition, readily diffuse through the plasma membrane, bind to specific receptor proteins, and interact with other macromolecules in the nucleus, including specific domains on the chromatin located in and around the gene that is activated (see Chapter 3).[82–84] Phosphorylated nucleotides, as well as calcium, appear to have important functions in secretory processes. In particular, fluxes of calcium from the extracellular fluid into the cell and from intracellular organelles (e.g., mitochondria) into the cytosol are closely coupled to secretion.[85]

The cellular mechanism of protein phosphorylation often utilizes cAMP as a second messenger (Fig. 2–15).[52] In this model the stimulatory factor (ligand) interacts with a receptor located within the plasma membrane, and when bound to the plasma membrane receptor, activates adenylate cyclase, which results in the generation of cAMP, which in turn converts an inactive form of a protein kinase to an active form by way of dissociation of a regulatory (R) subunit from the active catalytic (C) subunit. The protein kinase (active subunit) catalyzes the phosphorylation of certain intracellular proteins, and the phosphoproteins thus formed function in the processes of gene activation and inactivation. As indicated earlier, one demonstration of the role of phosphorylated intermediates in the activation of gene expression of a peptide ligand is the stimulation of the transcription of the prolactin gene by TRH.[64] New gene transcription is detectable within minutes after interaction of TRH with its plasma receptor, and concomitant with the activation of transcription a specific subset of nuclear proteins is phosphorylated. The exact mechanisms by which phosphoproteins activate gene transcription are unknown.

Insight has been obtained into the identities of some of the phosphoproteins. As discussed earlier, a specific group of transcription factors, DNA-binding proteins, interacts with cAMP-responsive and phorbol ester–responsive DNA elements to stimulate gene transcription mediated by the cAMP–protein kinase A and diacylglycerol–protein kinase C signal transduction pathways (Fig. 2–16). These proteins are encoded by a complex family of genes and bind to the

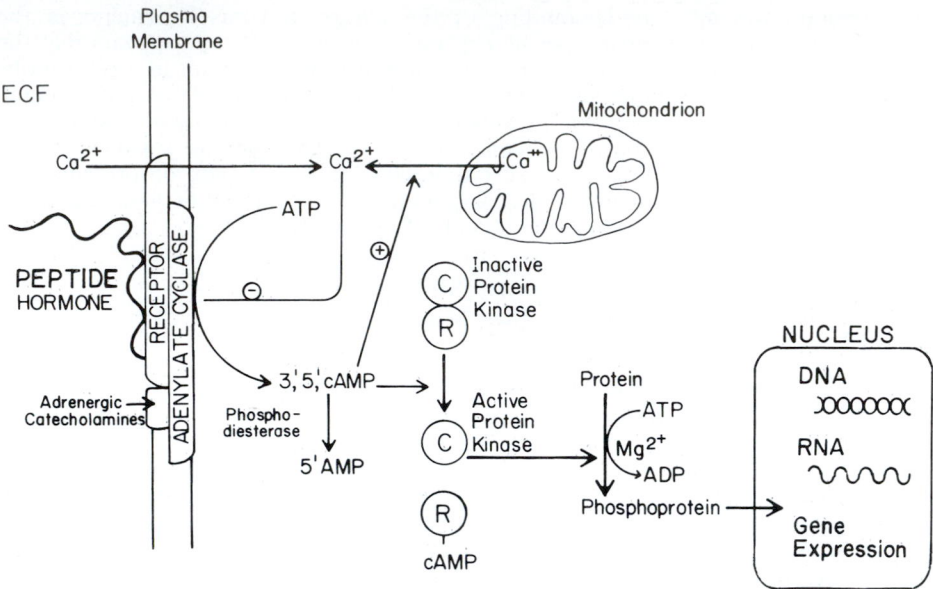

Figure 2–15. Proposed cellular mechanism through which a peptide hormone effector might activate gene expression of an endocrine cell. In the model shown, binding of peptide to plasma membrane receptor activates adenylate cyclase, which leads to formation of 3',5'-cAMP and a cascade of reactions resulting in conversion of inactive to active protein kinases; kinases then phosphorylate specific proteins. The presumed final active protein in this cascade of reactions is a phosphoprotein that interacts with regulatory sites on the gene, thereby activating gene transcription and expression. C and R refer to catalytic and regulatory (cAMP-receptor) subunits of protein kinase, respectively.

DNA elements in the form of heterodimers or homodimers via a coiled coil helical structure known as a leucine zipper motif.[53] There is evidence that phosphorylations of these proteins mediated by the signaling pathways first described modulate dimerization, DNA recognition and binding, and transcriptional transactivation activities. Phosphorylation of the protein substrates might change their conformations and thereby activate the proteins, which, in turn, could interact both with chromatin DNA element "receptors" and with TATA box factors, thereby allowing for RNA polymerase to initiate gene transcription.

In the regulation of gene expression by steroids (e.g., ACTH-secreting cells in the pituitary, which are regulated by cortisol), the steroids penetrate the plasma membrane by simple or facilitated diffusion. The steroids then bind to specific receptors located in the cytoplasm, and the hormone-receptor complexes bind to specific target sites on the chromatin (Fig. 2–17).[82–84] In the case of the glucocorticoid

estrogen and progesterone receptors, the translocation of the ligand-bound receptor from the cytoplasm to the nucleus first requires the dissociation of the receptor from a complex of proteins that includes the 90-kd heat shock protein (hsp-90). The mechanism of action of the thyroid hormones is similar, except that the receptors appear to be located predominantly in the nucleus so that thyroid hormone diffuses into the cell and is then transported to the nucleus for interactions with the chromatin-bound receptors.[84] By as-yet undefined processes, transcription of the gene takes place, followed by increased protein synthesis. Considerable progress has been made in the elucidation of gene activation by steroid and thyroid hormones, retinoic acids, and vitamin D. The cis-acting DNA-regulatory elements that bind the receptors for these ligands have been identified, and the structures of many of the receptors have been determined by cDNA cloning. The cis elements consist of typically short sequences of 15 to 20 base pairs that have a dyadic symmetry, so-called palindromic sequences, i.e., the ends of the sequences contain several bases that are complementary to each other and form a potential stem-loop structure. These palindromic sequences are characteristic of sequences in the control regions of many eucaryotic genes. Subtle substitution changes of two to three base pairs within these elements can change binding specificities for a given receptor, e.g., from binding a glucocorticoid receptor to an estrogen receptor. Serial repetitive arrays of these elements on a gene promoter give multiplicative, synergistic responses, a circumstance that probably reflects the cooperative protein-protein interactions among the receptors occupying the DNA binding sites.

The important structural characteristic of the receptors is that they consist of distinct DNA binding and hormone-ligand binding domains.[82–84] The DNA binding domains comprise metal binding sites, so-called zinc fingers that chelate zinc atoms and result in the formation of a higher-ordered helical structure that is important for binding to the DNA elements. In a poorly understood manner, the ligand binding domains mediate the transcriptional transactivation functions of the receptors in conjunction with the zinc finger region. Occupancy of the receptor by ligand is believed to lead to an allosteric conformational change in the receptor, thereby resulting in the formation of a transcriptionally competent protein capable of making productive interactions with the general or basal transcriptional apparatus (TATA box proteins).

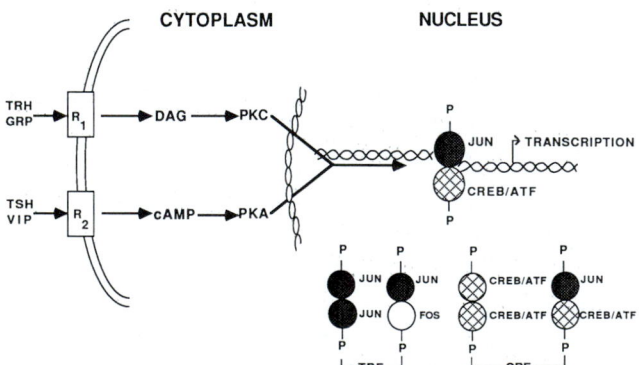

Figure 2–16. Diagram showing two cell-surface receptor–coupled signal transduction pathways involved in the activation of a superfamily of nuclear transcription factors. Peptide hormone ligands, e.g., TRH, gastrin-releasing peptide (GRP), thyroid-stimulating hormone (TSH), and vasoactive intestinal peptide (VIP), interact with receptors (R_1 and R_2) coupled to either the diacylglycerol (DAG)–protein kinase C (PKC) or the cAMP–protein kinase A (PKA) pathway. The protein kinases phosphorylate members of the CREB/ATF, jun/AP-1 and fos/fra families of DNA-binding proteins to modulate DNA-binding affinities and/or transcriptional activation. The various proteins bind as dimers determined by a poorly understood code that is not promiscuous inasmuch as only certain homodimer or heterodimer combinations are permissible. CRE, cAMP response element; TRE, tetradecanoylphorbol acetate response element.

Figure 2–17. Proposed mechanism of action of steroids (glucocorticoids, estrogens, progesterone) in activation of specific gene transcription. In this model the steroid (S) readily diffuses across the plasma membrane and binds to a cytosolic receptor (SR). In the absence of steroid, the receptor resides in the cytoplasm as an inactive complex with heat shock protein (HSP). When the steroid binds to the receptor, the HSP dissociates from it. The steroid-receptor complex is translocated to the nucleus, where it binds to a chromatin receptor consisting of the steroid receptor response DNA element (SRE), thereby activating the transcription of specific genes involved in steroid hormone action. RNA transcripts are translated into proteins that mediate changes in cell function. Some evidence suggests an alternative model in which steroid receptor resides in the nucleus and not in the cytoplasm. In this model, presumably, steroid diffuses through the cytoplasm into the nucleoplasm, where it binds to the receptor before gene activation occurs. (Adapted from Chan L, O'Malley BW. Mechanism of action of the sex steroid hormones. Reprinted, by permission of The New England Journal of Medicine, 294; 1322–1328, 1372–1382, 1429–1437, 1976.)

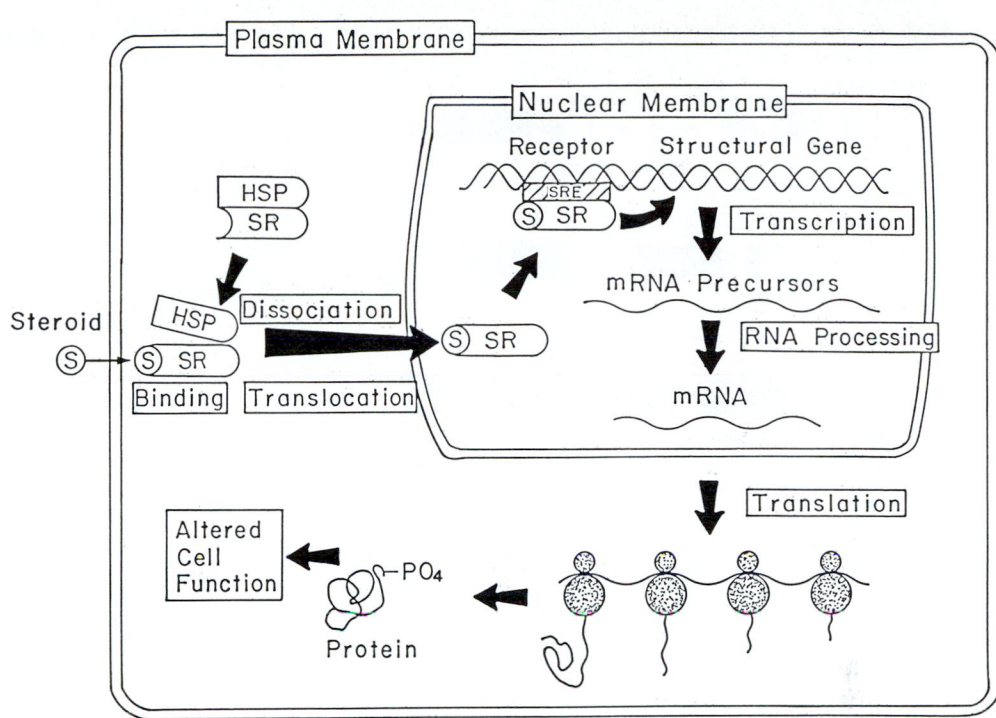

GENERATION OF BIOLOGICAL DIVERSIFICATION

In addition to providing control points for the regulation of gene expression, the various steps involved in transfer of information encoded in the DNA of the gene to the final bioactive protein are a means for diversification of information stored in the gene (Figs. 2–18 and 2–19).

At the level of DNA, diversification of genetic information comes about by way of gene duplication and amplification. Many of the polypeptide hormones are derived from families of multiple, structurally related genes. Examples include the growth hormone family, consisting of growth hormone, prolactin, and placental lactogen; the glucagon family, consisting of glucagon, vasoactive intestinal peptide, secretin, gastric-inhibitory peptide, and growth hormone–releasing hormone; and the glycoprotein hormones,

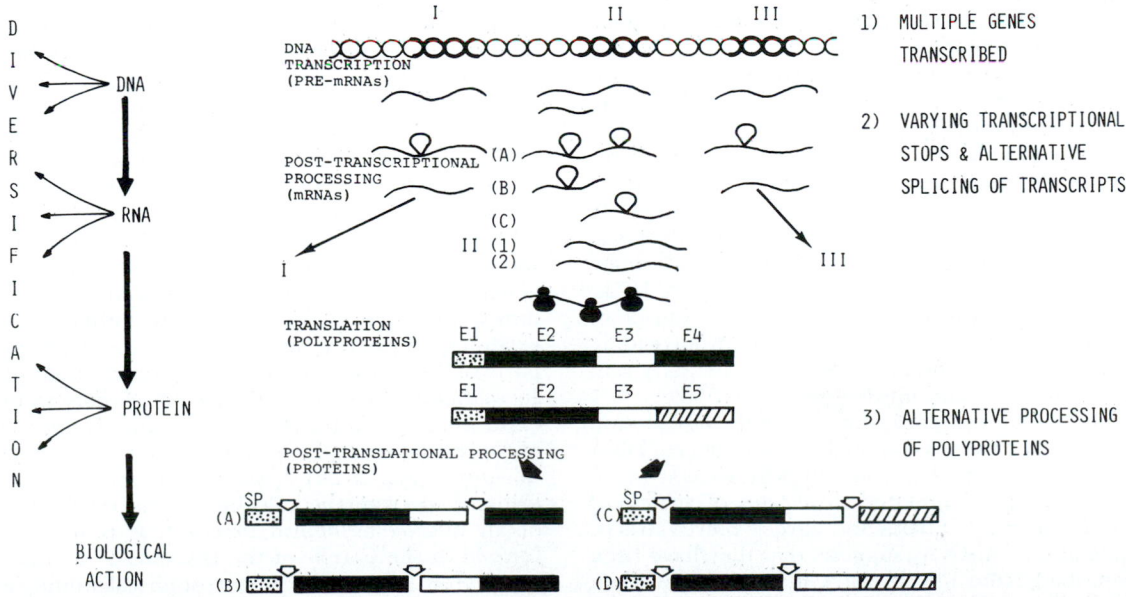

Figure 2–18. Schema indicating levels in expression of genetic information at which diversification of information encoded in a gene may take place. The three major levels of genetic diversification are (1) gene duplication, a process that occurs in terms of evolutionary time; (2) variation in the processing of RNA precursors, which results in formation of two or more mRNAs by way of alternative pathways of splicing of transcript (see Figs. 2–19 and 2–20); (3) use of alternative patterns in processing of protein biosynthetic precursors (polyproteins, or prohormones). These three levels in gene expression provide a means for diversification of gene expression at levels of DNA, RNA, or protein. One or more of a combination of these processes leads to formation of final biologically active peptide or hormone. In the diagram, loops depicted in transcripts denote introns; in diagrammatic structures of proteins, the stippled, shaded, and unshaded areas denote exons. SP, signal peptide. See text for details.

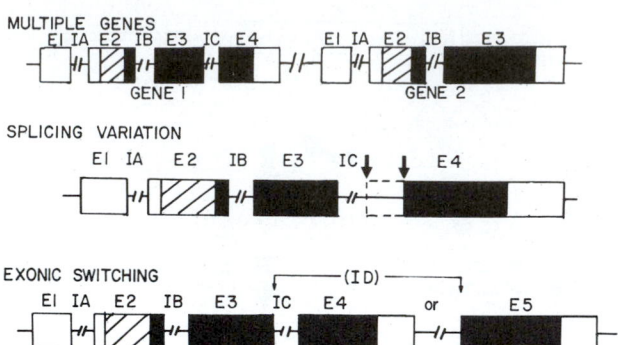

GENETIC and TRANSCRIPTIONAL ORIGIN of DIVERSITY

Figure 2–19. Genetic and transcriptional origin of biological diversity. This figure illustrates in greater detail the mechanisms of alternative splicing of RNA transcripts. The initial level of diversification arises from multiplication of genes, a process that occurs in the context of evolutionary time. Each of the genes consists of a series of exons (E1–E4) and introns (IA–ID). Variations at the site at which introns are cleaved from the primary transcript can lead to formation of two or more mRNAs with sequence deletions or insertions. When variations of splicing occur in the protein-coding sequence of RNA, they result in corresponding insertions or deletions of codons for amino acids. Such a splicing variation occurs in the human growth hormone gene, in which a minor transcribed mRNA lacks 15 codons in its central region, resulting in translation of a growth hormone that is 2 kd smaller than normal growth hormone. A second splicing variation, exonic switching, occurs in transcription of the calcitonin gene (see Fig. 2–20). By this mechanism of RNA splicing, an entire exon is substituted for another. In the illustration, exon 5 (E5) can be substituted for exon 4 (E4), and intron C (IC) and E4 become the functional equivalent of intron D (ID) of the second messenger. The shading scheme of the exons is as follows: untranslated regions of transcript, *unshaded;* signal sequence region and prohormone sequence, *shaded.*

thyrotropin, luteinizing hormone, follicle-stimulating hormone, and chorionic gonadotropin. Over the course of evolution an ancestral gene encoding a prototypic polypeptide representative of each of these families was duplicated one or more times and, through mutation and selection, the progeny proteins of the ancestral gene assumed different biological functions. As discussed earlier, the structural organization of the genome of higher animals lends itself to recombination, resulting in rearrangement of transcriptional units and regulatory sequences.[76]

One hypothesis to explain the mechanism by which new genetic information may arise suggests that mutations are introduced into DNA via RNA intermediates.[86] This hypothesis is based on two lines of evidence. First, the error frequency in DNA replication in mammalian eucaryotes is approximately one incorrect base incorporated for every 10^9 to 10^{11} bases polymerized during any one round of replication. In contrast, the error rate in synthesis of RNA molecules is on the order of one incorrect base for every 10^3 to 10^4 bases polymerized during synthesis. This circumstance comes about because during DNA synthesis proofreading enzymes correct misincorporated bases, whereas RNA synthesis has no such correction mechanism.

The second line of evidence comes from the observation that the mammalian genomes contain large numbers of DNA segments, called pseudogenes, that appear to consist of cDNAs that are partially mutated duplicates of structural genes, many of which lack introns and have 3'-poly(A) tracts. Their resemblance to mRNAs suggests that they have been reverse-transcribed from mRNA back into DNA and then reinserted into the genome. Such pseudogenes, or "processed" genes, have been observed for the alpha chain of hemoglobin, immunoglobulins, and α-tubulin and β-tubulin. Perhaps as much as 20% of the mammalian genome originated as RNA that was reverse-transcribed back to DNA.[76] If this is the mechanism for pseudogene formation, a rein-

tegration event must have occurred in the germ line for about 10% of genes within the last 10 to 20 million years, which corresponds to about 0.5 to 1% of genes per million years, or once for each gene every 100 to 200 million years. In evolutionary terms, this is a relatively high rate of introduction of new genetic information.

DNA that has been reverse-transcribed from mRNA may reinsert itself back into the genome by one of two known mechanisms. First, the RNA-derived DNA may donate its RNA-based mutations to the parent gene by gene conversion, a process that appears to take place quite frequently in the genomes of higher cells. If a cDNA reverse-transcribed from mRNA were matched against its original gene, conversion in one direction could imprint the restructured intron-deficient or intron-lacking sequence into its genomic homologue while leaving the promoter signal intact. This process would allow processed information to feed back into the genome in functional form.

The second possible mechanism is that RNA molecules transcribed from transposon-like elements may be reverse-transcribed into a heterogeneous pool of DNA particles, such as has been observed in the case of the Alu family of sequences. These DNA particles would be potentially transmissible through the germ line in a nonmendelian fashion without necessarily integrating into chromosomal DNA. Thus cells from a common ancestor may become polymorphic in those molecules that have passed through an RNA phase, while retaining rigorous sequence identity in the original DNA genes. In this way, new adaptive possibilities could occur without erasing the existing phenotype. These mechanisms for providing genetic diversification allow nuclear information occasionally to pass through a noisy RNA copier, which results in changes in the genetic information that can then be introduced back into the parent gene. It is also possible that rearrangement and amplification of genetic sequences encoding polypeptide hormones could take place during the life span of an individual animal. The enormous diversification of antibody molecules is a consequence largely of the rearrangement of genetic segments encoding regions of the immunoglobulins. Perhaps, as work progresses on the analysis of genes encoding receptor molecules, such a mechanism of gene rearrangement coupled with somatic mutation may be found to be involved in the generation of highly complex receptor proteins.

Identification of the mosaic structure of transcriptional units encoding polypeptide hormones and other proteins that consist of exons and introns that are spliced during post-transcriptional processing raised the possibility that the use of alternative pathways in RNA splicing could provide informationally distinct molecules. One can imagine that a wide variety of different translation sequences could be generated through the use of alternative splicing mechanisms. Different codes could arise either by inclusion or exclusion of specific exonic segments or by utilization of parts of introns in one mRNA as exons in another mRNA. In addition, differences in the splice sites would result in expression of new translational reading frames. An example of an alternative splicing mechanism is the gene encoding calcitonin (Fig. 2–20).[87] Alternative processing of the RNA transcribed from the calcitonin gene results in production of an mRNA in neural tissues that is distinct from that formed in the C cells of the thyroid. The mRNA found in the thyroid encodes a precursor to calcitonin, whereas the mRNA in the neural tissues generates a neuropeptide known as the calcitonin gene–related peptide (see Fig. 2–20). Immunocytochemical analyses of the distribution of the peptide in brain and other tissues suggest functions for the peptide in perception of pain, ingestive behavior, and modulation of the autonomic and endocrine systems.

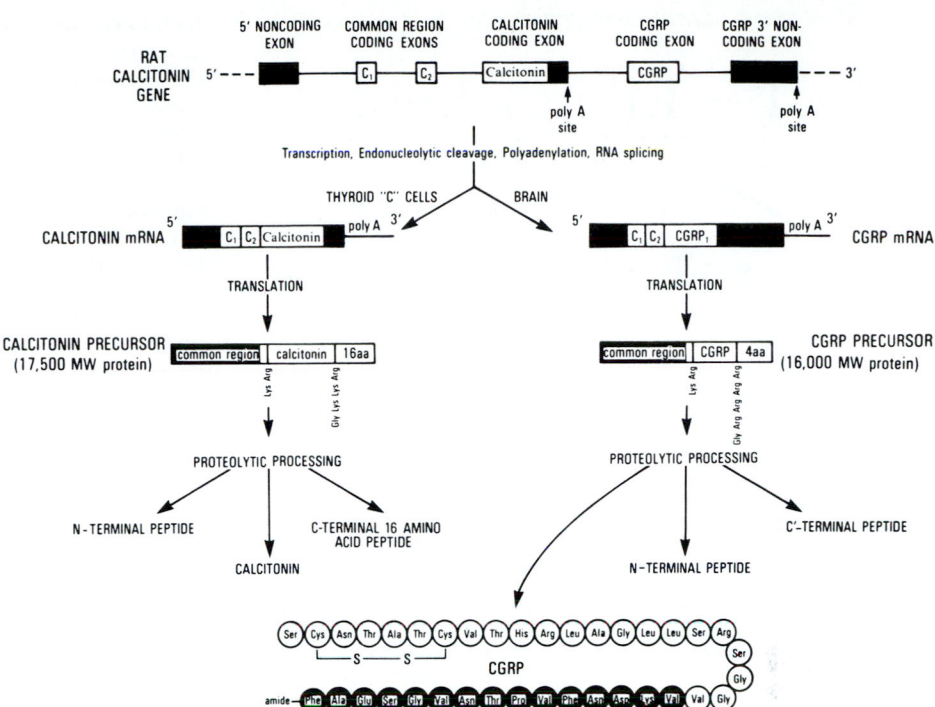

Figure 2–20. Alternative pathways in processing of RNA transcripts derived from the calcitonin gene. The rat calcitonin gene contains six exons and five introns. Two mRNAs result from transcriptional and post-transcriptional processing of transcripts. Each of two mRNAs is made up of five exons. They share in common the first three exons and differ in the last two exons. In one mRNA, the fourth exon encodes the peptide hormone calcitonin, and in the other mRNA the corresponding exon encodes a peptide termed CGRP, or calcitonin gene–related peptide. Both calcitonin and CGRP are liberated from the calcitonin precursor during post-translational processing of precursor. In addition to the novel aspect of exonic assembly of mRNAs, there is marked tissue specificity in expression of one or the other mRNAs. The mRNA containing the calcitonin sequence is expressed almost exclusively in thyroid C cells, whereas the mRNA containing the sequence for CGRP is expressed in the hypothalamus and in other extrahypothalamic regions of the brain. (From Rosenfeld MG, Mermod JJ, Amara SG, et al. Production of a novel neuropeptide encoded by the calcitonin gene via tissue-specific RNA processing. Reprinted by permission from Nature, vol. 304, pp. 129–136, Copyright © 1983 Macmillan Journals Limited.)

Other examples of genetic diversification arise from the programmed flexibility in the splicing of coding regions, which allows an array of coding sequences (exons) to be put together in a number of possible useful combinations. For example, the coding sequences of immunoglobulin heavy chains can be brought together in two different ways, one to include, another to exclude, an exonic coding sequence specifying part of the polypeptide chain that anchors an immunoglobulin molecule to the surface of a lymphocyte.[88] If mRNA splicing excludes the anchor's peptide sequence, a secreted rather than a surface immunoglobulin is produced.

The splicing of the RNA precursor that encodes substance P can take place in at least two ways.[89] One splicing pattern results in the mRNA that encodes substance P and another peptide called substance K in a common protein precursor. Other mRNAs are apparently spliced so as to exclude the coding sequence for substance K. An alternative RNA-splicing pattern also occurs in the processing of transcripts arising from the gene encoding bradykinin.[90] The high- and low-molecular-weight kininogens are translated from mRNAs that differ by the alternative use of 3'-end exons encoding the COOH termini of the prohormones, a situation similar to that found in the transcription of the calcitonin gene. The primary RNA transcript from the human growth hormone gene is processed in an alternative manner to provide some mRNAs that lack a portion of the third exon of growth hormone and that result in synthesis of a growth hormone lacking 15 amino acids from its central region.[57] Other examples of alternative splicing will probably be found in the processes that generate biological diversification.

A third level in gene expression at which diversification of biological information can take place is that of post-translational processing. Many precursors of polypeptide hormones, particularly those encoding small peptides, contain multiple peptides that are cleaved during post-translational processing of the prohormones. Certain polyprotein precursors, however, contain several copies of the peptide. Examples of prohormones that contain multiple identical peptides are the precursors encoding TRH[91] and the alpha-mating factor of yeast,[92] each of which contains four copies of the respective peptide. Polyproteins that contain several distinct peptides include proenkephalins,[93] pro-opiomelanocortin,[94] and proglucagon.[95]

In many instances biological diversification at the level of post-translational processing occurs in a tissue-specific manner. The processing of pro-opiomelanocortin differs markedly in the anterior compared with the intermediate lobe of the pituitary.[96] In the anterior pituitary the primary peptide products are ACTH and β-endorphin, whereas in the intermediate lobe of the pituitary one of the primary products is α-melanocyte-stimulating hormone. The smaller peptides produced are extensively modified by acetylation and phosphorylation of amino acid residues. The processing of proglucagon in the pancreatic A cells and that in the intestinal L cells are also different (Fig. 2–21).[56] In the pancreatic A cells the predominant bioactive product of the processing of proglucagon is glucagon itself; the two glucagon-like peptides are not processed efficiently from proglucagon in the A cells and are biologically inactive by virtue of having NH_2-terminal and COOH-terminal extensions. On the other hand, in the intestinal L cell the glucagon immunoreactive product is a molecule, called glicentin, which consists of the NH_2-terminal extension of the proglucagon plus glucagon and the small COOH-terminal peptide known as intervening peptide I. Glicentin has no glucagon-like biological activity, and therefore the bioactive peptide (or peptides) in the intestinal L cells must be one or both of the glucagon-like peptides. In fact glucagon-like peptide I in its shortened form of 31 amino acids, GLP-I(7–37), is a potent insulinotropic hormone in its actions of stimulating insulin release from pancreatic beta cells.[97] This peptide is released from the intestines into the bloodstream in response to oral nutrients and as such appears to be a potent intestinal "incretin" factor implicated in the augmented release of insulin in response to oral compared with systemic (intravenous) nutrients.

This potential for diversification of biological information provided by the alternative pathways of gene expression

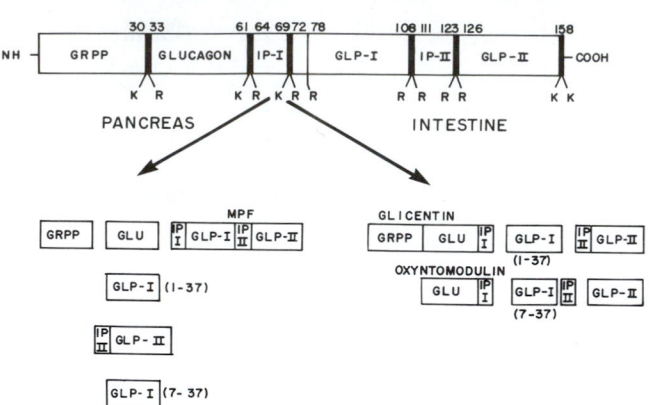

Figure 2–21. Alternative pathways of processing of proglucagon in gut and pancreatic islets. Pathways shown on the left and the right represent predicted patterns of processing of proglucagon in pancreatic islets and intestine, respectively. Processing of proglucagon occurs at pairs of basic amino acids, lysine (K) and arginine (R). In intestine the major glucagon-containing peptide is glicentin, which consists of glucagon in covalent linkages with NH_2-terminal and short COOH-terminal extensions, glucagon-related polypeptide (GRPP), and intervening peptide I (IP-I). Although not proved, it is likely that the two glucagon-related peptides, glucagon-like peptide I (GLP-I) in various forms and glucagon-like peptide II (GLP-II), are the major biologically active peptides liberated in the gut by processing of proglucagon. In pancreatic islets, the major glucagon peptide is glucagon itself. The COOH-terminal peptides resulting from cleavages that liberate glucagon are not further processed efficiently to glucagon-related peptides but rather remain as a major proglucagon fragment (MPF).

is impressive when one considers that these pathways can occur in multiple combinations.

POTENTIAL APPLICATIONS OF RECOMBINANT DNA TECHNOLOGY AND MOLECULAR GENETICS TO DIAGNOSIS AND TREATMENT OF ENDOCRINE DISEASES

The availability of recombinant molecular probes has led to the detection of mutations, gene deletions, and insertions by the use of either allele-specific probes (point mutations) or restriction fragment length polymorphisms as genetic markers of disease. The fact that foreign genes can be expressed in microorganisms (bacteria and yeasts) and mammalian cells provides the means to produce large amounts of specific gene products such as polypeptide hormones for use in therapy for endocrine deficiency diseases. As indicated earlier, the development of techniques for stable integration of foreign genes into cultured cells and into germ lines of experimental animals also introduces the feasibility of correcting defective genes by the introduction of correct genes.

Detection of Specific Genetic Defects by Molecular Probe Hybridization

Restriction fragment length polymorphisms arise as a fortuitous consequence of variations that normally occur in DNA sequences.[98] These variations, most often point mutations (base substitutions), are detectable because they either generate or eradicate specific sites that are cleaved by restriction endonucleases. Therefore, the restriction endonuclease fragments generated by enzymatic cleavage from the two alleles differ in length. Because fragments of different length can be separated by agarose gel electrophoresis and can be detected with specific DNA probes, it is possible to determine

which form of a polymorphic sequence is carried by any individual and through any family. The frequency of nucleotide site polymorphisms in the population is estimated to be 0.03 to 1%.[98, 99] Thus a nucleotide in a given position in the genome differs among individuals on the average of every 100 to 3000 base pairs. Therefore, the probability is 0.1 to 4.0% that a restriction endonuclease fragment defined by an enzyme recognizing a four-base sequence will differ in size. These restriction fragment length polymorphisms can be easily assayed in individuals, inasmuch as small volumes of peripheral blood or amniotic fluid provide sufficient cellular DNA for analysis by enzymatic cleavage, electrophoretic separation, and molecular probe hybridization. Because restriction fragment length polymorphisms are inherited as simple mendelian codominant markers, relationships can be established by pedigree analysis. Evaluation of many DNA marker loci allows recognition of well-spaced, highly polymorphic genetic markers and a correlation of the cosegregation of a specific fragment with a particular disease state. Analyses of large pedigrees are necessary, however, to find at least one and preferably several polymorphic loci that are close enough to the chromosomal locus responsible for the disease to minimize the chance that the marker locus and the disease locus will be separated by genetic recombination during formation of the gametes. Important advantages of this technique are that no specific gene isolation is required and the restriction fragment length polymorphisms can be random sequences, functionally unrelated and physically distant from the DNA encoding the locus responsible for the particular disease. To ensure cosegregation of the marker locus with the disease locus, the loci should be located no more than 20 centimorgans apart (20 million base pairs) on the genome. (One centimorgan represents a distance on the chromosome between two genes that will allow recombination with a frequency of 1%.) This technique has been used to isolate the genes (defective) responsible for chronic granulomatous disease, muscular dystrophy, and cystic fibrosis and to identify polymorphic loci linked to Huntington disease.[100] Thus the linked restriction fragment length polymorphisms can provide a means of detecting the presence of a mutation, even when the nature of the lesion is completely unknown.

The application of techniques for identification of restriction fragment length polymorphisms offers great potential in the future for diagnosis of many hereditary endocrine diseases such as polyglandular endocrinopathy, the multiple endocrine neoplasia syndromes, non–insulin-dependent (type II) diabetes mellitus, and so forth. Although this technique has not yet been applied to any endocrine diseases, a polymorphic locus located close to the insulin gene may be correlated with the development of non–insulin-dependent diabetes mellitus. A highly polymorphic region consisting of a family of randomly repeated nucleotides approximately 15 bases long is located approximately 400 base pairs upstream from the transcriptional start site of the insulin gene.[101, 102] Because this polymorphic locus is in or close to the region of the insulin gene involved in the regulation of gene transcription, and because non–insulin-dependent diabetes may be in part a result of relative insulin deficiency, it was suggested that this polymorphic variation in the region of the insulin gene might impair expression of the gene. The correlation of this polymorphism with non–insulin-dependent diabetes is incomplete, so alternative explanations are possible. Indeed, other studies have indicated that polymorphism near the insulin gene is not specific for non–insulin-dependent diabetes but may be found equally often in insulin-dependent diabetes.[103]

A second use of recombinant DNA techniques in detection of defective genes is the application of small, synthetic oligonucleotide probes to detect known point mutations in specific genes. Defective gene expression is often a consequence of a single point mutation in the transcriptional unit. Many of these would change a codon, which results in a substitution of an amino acid in the protein coded for by the gene. The fact that substitution of a single base can lead to profound changes was demonstrated as early as 1959 when Ingram[104] showed that a single amino acid change altered the phenotype of persons with sickle cell anemia. More than 130 separate point mutations have now been identified in the globin genes, all of which result in a defect in the rate of gene transcription or a defect in the hemoglobin itself.[105] Each of these globinopathies, or thalassemias, can be identified by hybridization-blotting techniques that utilize small oligonucleotide probes. One technique consists of the synthesis of two complementary oligonucleotides, one of which is complementary to a sequence in the normal allele and the other of which is complementary to the sequence in the mutated allele. Restriction endonuclease fragments prepared from white blood cells of the patients are separated by electrophoresis on an agarose gel, and, after transfer of the DNA fragments to nitrocellulose filters, the filters are hybridized sequentially with both oligonucleotide probes. Because of the short length of the probes, only the probe that is identical in sequence to the complement of either the normal or the mutant allele will hybridize. By this approach, the normal and the mutant alleles can be identified. Such techniques can be applied to any situation in which a specific base mutation is recognized.

The technique of oligonucleotide probe hybridization is probably applicable to certain genetically determined endocrine disorders. At least three point mutations have been identified in the coding region of the insulin gene. Two of these mutations, one resulting in a glycine instead of a phenylalanine[106] and another in a serine instead of a phenylalanine,[107] are in the region of the beta chain containing the phenylalanine at position 24, an amino acid that is critically important in receptor binding. These substitutions thus provide an explanation for the diabetes mellitus in these two kindreds. The third point mutation was identified in the codon for arginine at position 65 of the proinsulin gene.[108] This substitution blocks conversion of proinsulin to insulin, which results in impairment of production of biologically active insulin at the level of post-translational processing of proinsulin.

The application of the polymerase chain reaction for the rapid amplification of DNA sequences to the diagnosis of genetic diseases has accelerated understanding of the structural basis of several endocrine diseases. The detection of base mutations or deletions and resultant translocation of aberrant, biologically defective proteins has enabled the identification of the genetic lesions in vitamin D receptors[109] and thyroid hormone receptors[110] in patients with syndromes of vitamin D and thyroid hormone resistance, respectively. After the target gene sequence is identified, the genetic locus of concern can be analyzed by amplification and sequencing of DNA from as little as a milliliter of blood. The power of this technique for the amplification and analysis of DNA opens the way for generalized genetic screening of the population.

Gene Transfer

Recombinant DNA research provides the prospect for the transfer of genes into individuals who suffer from defects in the expression of specific genes.[111, 112] As described earlier, foreign genes can be introduced and expressed in cultured cells and laboratory animals. It is now feasible to introduce genes encoding hormones into commercially valuable animals. For example, the fact that the integration of the growth hormone gene into the germ line of mice results in marked acceleration of growth suggests a practical means for accelerating the growth of livestock.[45] The benefit would accrue from shorter production time and possibly from increased efficiency in food utilization. Additional growth hormone derived from the introduced gene might increase the size and therefore the yield of usable meat in cattle, swine, and fowl. Furthermore, valuable hormones might be commercially produced by extraction from the blood of the animal expressing the specific hormone genes. The growth hormone levels in the blood of the transgenic mice expressing transferred genes are as high as 1 mg/mL of plasma and are within the range of feasibility for the harvest of growth hormone, much as one harvests antisera from animals that are immunized.

Biologically important proteins are now being produced by genes introduced into cultured cells. Both human growth hormone and human insulin produced by bacterial cultures are available for use in patients. Intensive work is taking place in the preparation of interferons and proteins involved in the coagulation pathway.

Many approaches can be envisioned for correction of gene defects in humans by introduction of specific genes. For example, one might obtain a biopsy of skin or liver and use this to prepare cultured cells into which the appropriate foreign gene can be transferred. The cells may then be transplanted back into the patient, under the skin or in some other readily accessible region. Such an isologous graft could provide the source of the missing protein (hormones). An additional, albeit highly speculative, possibility is the introduction of genes into fertilized ova resulting from the union of germ cells in a case in which both parents carry defective alleles. This procedure will achieve the purpose of allowing the propagation of the parental germ lines in a stably corrected phenotype. Oocytes fertilized in vitro have been successfully transplanted into the uteri of surrogate mothers, which resulted in successful pregnancies. An alternative approach that would eliminate gene defects in progeny would be the development of a technique for specific selection of ova and sperm containing the normal parental allele. This would be possible only if one of the parents were normal or if they both were heterozygotes for the genetic defect.

Before gene transfer experiments can be undertaken in humans, it will be necessary to obtain additional information about the regulation of the expression of genes. Because the expression of genes encoding polypeptide hormones is characteristically regulated by products of target organs of the hormone, it will be desirable if not essential to include the regulatory elements along with the transcriptional units in the genes that are transferred, and to target integration of the genes into a region of genome in which no deleterious consequences would occur. For example, it would be important not to interrupt or inactivate a gene that has essential biological functions or to activate otherwise quiescent genes such as proto-oncogenes.

REFERENCES

1. Watson JD, Crick FHC. Molecular structure of nucleic acids. Nature 1953; 171:737–738.
2. Popenoe EA, du Vigneaud V. A partial sequence of amino acids in performic acid–oxidized vasopressin. J Biol Chem 1954; 206:353–360.
3. Yalow RS. Radioimmunoassay: a probe for the fine structure of biologic systems. Science 1978; 200:1236–1245.
4. Ullrich A, Shine J, Chirgwin J, et al. Rat insulin genes: construction of plasmids containing the coding sequences. Science 1977; 196:1313–1319.
5. Seeburg PH, Shine J, Martial JA, et al. Nucleotide sequence and amplification in bacteria of structural gene for rat growth hormone. Nature 1977; 270:486–490.

6. Gilbert W. DNA sequencing and gene structure. Science 1981; 214:1305–1312.

7. Sanger F. Determination of nucleotide sequences in DNA. Science 1981; 214:1205–1210.

8. Roth J, LeRoith D, Shiloach J, et al. The evolutionary origins of hormones, neurotransmitters, and other extracellular chemical messengers. N Engl J Med 1982; 306:523–527.

9. Loumaye E, Thorner J, Catt KJ. Yeast mating pheromone activates mammalian gonadotrophs: evolutionary conservation of a reproductive hormone? Science 1982; 218:1323–1325.

10. Doolittle RF. Similar amino acid sequences: chance or common ancestry? Science 1981; 214:149–159.

11. Uy R, Wold F. Post-translational covalent modification of proteins. Science 1977; 198:890–896.

12. Lingappa VR. Intracellular traffic of newly synthesized proteins. J Clin Invest 1989; 83:739–751.

13. Palade G. Intracellular aspects of the process of protein synthesis. Science 1975; 189:347–358.

14. Morrissey JJ, Cohn DV. Regulation of secretion of parathormone and secretory protein-I from separate intracellular pools by calcium, dibutyryl cyclic AMP, and l-isoproterenol. J Cell Biol 1979; 82:93–102.

15. Blobel G. Intracellular protein topogenesis. Proc Natl Acad Sci USA 1980; 77:1496–1500.

16. Lehninger AL. Biochemistry. 2nd ed. New York: Worth, 1975.

17. Blobel G, Dobberstein B. Transfer of proteins across membranes. II. Reconstitution of functional rough microsomes from heterologous components. J Cell Biol 1975; 67:852–862.

18. Palmiter RD, Gagnon J, Walsh KA. Ovalbumin: a secreted protein without a transient hydrophobic leader sequence. Proc Natl Acad Sci USA 1978; 75:94–98.

19. Walter P, Blobel F. Signal recognition particle contains a 7S RNA essential for protein translocation across the endoplasmic reticulum. Nature 1982; 299:691–698.

20. Meyer DI, Krause E, Dobberstein B. Secretory protein translocation across membranes—the role of the "docking protein." Nature 1982; 297:647–650.

21. Habener JF, Amherdt M, Ravazzola M, et al. Parathyroid hormone biosynthesis. J Cell Biol 1979; 80:715–731.

22. Orci L, Like AA, Amherdt M, et al. Monolayer cell culture of neonatal rat pancreas: an ultrastructural and biochemical study of functioning endocrine cells. J Ultrastruct Res 1973; 43:270–297.

23. Chu LLH, MacGregor RR, Cohn DV. Energy-dependent intracellular translocation of proparathormone. J Cell Biol 1977; 72:1–10.

24. Kemper B, Habener JF, Rich A, et al. Microtubules and the intracellular conversion of proparathyroid hormone to parathyroid hormone. Endocrinology 1975; 96:903–912.

25. Smeekens SP, Steiner DF. Identification of a human insulinoma cDNA encoding a novel mammalian protein structurally related to the yeast dibasic processing protease Kex2. J Biol Chem 1990; 265:2997–3000.

26. Bradbury AF, Finnie MDA, Smyth DG. Mechanism of C-terminal amide formation by pituitary enzymes. Nature 1982; 298:686–688.

27. Baltimore D. Viruses, polymerases, and cancers. Science 1976; 192:632–636.

28. Temin HM. The DNA provirus hypothesis. Science 1976; 192:1075–1080.

29. Nathans D, Smith HO. Restriction endonucleases in the analysis and restructuring of DNA molecules. Annu Rev Biochem 1975; 44:273–293.

30. Wu R, ed. Recombinant DNA (part A). Methods Enzymol 1979; 68.

30a. Wu R, Grossman L, eds. Recombinant DNA (part B). Methods Enzymol 1983; 100.

30b. Wu R, Grossman L, Moldave K, eds. Recombinant DNA (part C). Methods Enzymol 1983; 101.

31. Maniatis T, Fritsch EF, Sambrook J. Molecular Cloning—A Laboratory Manual. Cold Spring Harbor, NY: Cold Spring Harbor Laboratory, 1989.

32. Riccardi RP, Miller JS, Roberts BE. Purification and mapping of specific mRNAs by hybridization-selection and cell-free translation. Proc Natl Acad Sci USA 1979; 76:4927–4931.

33. Chin WC, Kronenberg HM, Dee PC, et al. Nucleotide sequence of mRNA encoding the pre-alpha-subunit of mouse thyrotropin. Proc Natl Acad Sci USA 1981; 78:5329–5333.

34. Gee CE, Chen CL, Roberts JL, et al. Identification of proopiomelanocortin neurones in rat hypothalamus by in situ cDNA-mRNA hybridization. Nature 1983; 306:374–376.

35. Harper ME, Ullrich A, Saunders GF. Localization of the human insulin gene to the distal end of the short arm of chromosome II. Proc Natl Acad Sci USA 1981; 78:4458–4460.

36. Frohman MA, Dush MK, Martin GR. Rapid production of full-length cDNAs from rare transcripts: amplification using a single gene-specific oligonucleotide primer. Proc Natl Acad Sci USA 1988; 85:8998–9002.

37. Eisenstein BI. The polymerase chain reaction: a new method of using molecular genetics for medical diagnosis. N Engl J Med 1990; 322:178–183.

38. Ruddle FH. Applications of somatic cell genetics and gene transfer techniques for the analysis of genetic control and development. In: Schmitt FO, Bird ST, Bloom FE, eds. Molecular Genetic Neuroscience. New York: Raven, 1982: 63–72.

39. Owerbach D, Rutter WJ, Martial JA, et al. Genes for growth hormone, chorionic somatomammotropin, and growth hormone–like gene on chromosome 17 in humans. Science 1980; 209:289–292.

40. Owerbach D, Rutter WJ, Cooke NE, et al. The prolactin gene is located on chromosome 6 in humans. Science 1981; 212:815–816.

41. Gonzalez GA, Montminy MR. Cyclic AMP stimulates somatostatin gene transcription by phosphorylation of CREB at serine 133. Cell 1989; 59:675–680.

42. Brasier AR, Tate EJ, Ron D, et al. Synergistic enhansons located within an acute phase responsive enhancer modulate glucocorticoid induction of angiotensinogen gene transcription. Mol Endocrinol 1990; 4:1921–1933.

43. Berg P. Dissections and reconstructions of genes and chromosomes. Science 1981; 213:296–303.

44. Brinster RL, Chen HY, Trumbauer M, et al. Somatic expression of herpes thymidine kinase in mice following injection of a fusion gene into eggs. Cell 1981; 27:223–231.

45. Palmiter RD, Brinster RL, Hammer RE, et al. Dramatic growth of mice that developed from eggs microinjected with metallothionein–growth hormone fusion genes. Nature 1982; 300:611–615.

46. Low MJ, Goodman RH, Brinster RL, et al. Tissue-specific post-translational processing of rat pre-prosomatostatin encoded by a metallothionein-somatostatin fusion gene expressed in transgenic mice. Cell 1985; 41:211–219.

47. Habener JF, Cwikel BJ, Hermann H, et al. Transgenic mice express a vasopressin-metallothionein fusion gene in the magnocellular neurons of the brain and manifest a syndrome of mild nephrogenic diabetes insipidus. J Biol Chem 1989; 264:18844–18852.

48. Kornberg RD, Klug A. The nucleosome. Sci Am 1981; 244(2):52–64.

49. Sharp PA. Speculations on RNA processing. Cell 1981; 23:643–646.

50. Rogers J, Wall R. A mechanism for RNA splicing. Proc Natl Acad Sci USA 1980; 77:1877–1879.

51. Buratowski S, Hahn S, Guarente L, et al. Five intermediate complexes in transcription initiation by RNA polymerase II. Cell 1989; 56:549–561.

52. Roesler WJ, Vanderbork GR, Hanson RW. Cyclic AMP and the induction of eukaryotic gene expression. J Biol Chem 1988; 263:9063–9066.

53. Habener JF. Cyclic AMP response element binding proteins—a cornucopia of transcription factors. Mol Endocrinol 1990; 4:1087–1094.

54. Curran T, Franza RB Jr. Fos and Jun: the AP–1 connection. Cell 1988; 55:395–397.

55. Crick F. Split genes and RNA splicing. Science 1979; 204:264–271.

56. Mojsov S, Heinrich G, Wilson IB, et al. Preproglucagon gene expression in pancreas and intestine diversifies at the level of post-translational processing. J Biol Chem 1986; 261:11880–11889.

57. Miller W, Eberhardt NL. Structure and evolution of the growth hormone gene family. Endocr Rev 1983; 4:97–130.

58. Gilbert W. Why genes in pieces? Nature 1978; 271:501.

59. McClintock B. Genes and mutations. Cold Spring Harbor Symp Quant Biol 1951; 16:13–47.

60. Calos MP, Miller JH. Transposable elements. Cell 1980; 20:579–595.

61. Hollis GF, Hieter PA, McBride OW, et al. Processed genes: a dispersed human immunoglobulin gene bearing evidence of RNA-type processing. Nature 1982; 296:321–325.

62. Darnell JE. Variety in the level of gene control in eukaryotic cells. Nature 1982; 297:365–371.

63. Brown DD. Gene expression in eukaryotes. Science 1981; 211:667–674.

64. Murdoch GH, Franco R, Evans RM, et al. Polypeptide hormone regulation of gene expression. J Biol Chem 1983; 258:15329–15335.

65. Wegnez M, Schachter BS, Baxter JD, et al. Hormonal regulation of growth hormone mRNA. DNA 1982; 1:145–153.

66. Baxter JD, Ivarie RD. Regulation of gene expression by glucocorticoid hormones: studies of receptors and responses in cultured cells. Receptors Horm Action 1978; 2:251–284.

67. Itoh N, Okamoto H. Translational control of proinsulin synthesis by glucose. Nature 1980; 283:100–102.

68. Habener JF, Jacobs JW. Biosynthesis and control of secretion of the calcium-regulating peptides. In: Parsons JA, ed. Endocrinology of Calcium Metabolism. New York: Raven, 1982: 143–181.

69. Habener JF. Regulation of parathyroid hormone secretion and biosynthesis. Annu Rev Physiol 1981; 43:211–223.

70. Firestone GI, Farhang P, Yamamoto KR. Glucocorticoid regulation of protein processing and compartmentalization. Nature 1982; 300:221–225.

71. Britten RF, Davidson EH. Gene regulation for higher cells: a theory. Science 1969; 165:349–357.

72. Davidson EH, Britten RF. Regulation of gene expression: possible role of repetitive sequences. Science 1979; 204:1052–1059.

73. Schmidt CW, Jelinek WR. The Alu family of dispersed repetitive sequences. Science 1982; 216:1065–1070.

74. Sharp PA. Conversion of RNA to DNA in mammals. Alu-like elements and pseudogenes. Nature 1983; 301:471–472.

75. Davidson EH, Jacobs HT, Britten RJ. Very short repeats and coordinate induction of genes. Nature 1983; 301:468–470.

76. Dover G. Molecular drive: a cohesive mode of species evolution. Nature 1982; 299:111–117.
77. Wu C, Gilbert W. Tissue-specific exposure of chromatin structure at the 5' terminus of the preproinsulin II gene. Proc Natl Acad Sci USA 1981; 78:1577–1580.
78. Razin A, Riggs AD. DNA methylation and gene function. Science 1980; 210:604–610.
79. Marx JL. Immunoglobulin genes have enhancers. Science 1983; 221:735–757.
80. Walker MD, Edlund T, Boulet AM, et al. Cell-specific expression controlled by the 5'-flanking region of insulin and chymotrypsin genes. Nature 1983; 306:557–561.
81. Cohen P. The role of protein phosphorylation in neural and hormonal control of cellular activity. Nature 1982; 296:613–620.
82. Beato M. Gene regulation by steroid hormones. Cell 1989; 56:335–344.
83. O'Malley B. The steroid receptor superfamily: more excitement predicted for the future. Mol Endocrinol 1990; 4:363–369.
84. Evans RM. The steroid and thyroid hormone receptor superfamily. Science 1988; 240:889–896.
85. Rubin RP. The role of calcium in the release of neurotransmitter substances and hormones. Pharmacol Rev 1970; 22:389–428.
86. Reanney D. Genetic noise in evolution. Nature 1984; 307:318–319.
87. Rosenfeld MG, Mermod JJ, Amara SG, et al. Production of a novel neuropeptide encoded by the calcitonin gene via tissue-specific RNA processing. Nature 1983; 304:129–135.
88. Leder P, Max EE, Seidman JF. The organization of immunoglobulin genes and the origin of their diversity. In: Fougerau M, Dausset J, eds. 4th International Congress of Immunology: Immunology Eighty. London: Academic, 1981: 34–47.
89. Nawa H, Hirose T, Takashima H, et al. Nucleotide sequences of cloned cDNAs for two types of bovine brain substance P precursor. Nature 1983; 306:32–36.
90. Kitamura N, Takagaki Y, Furuto S, et al. A single gene for bovine high molecular weight and low molecular weight kininogens. Nature 1983; 305:545–549.
91. Lechan RM, Wu P, Jackson IMD, et al. Thyrotropin-releasing hormone precursor: characterization in rat brain. Science 1986; 231:159–161.
92. Kurjan J, Herskowitz I. Structure of a yeast pheromone gene (MFα): a putative α-factor precursor contains four tandem copies of mature α-factor. Cell 1982; 30:933–943.
93. Noda M, Teranishi Y, Yakahashi T, et al. Isolation and structural organization of the human preproenkephalin gene. Nature 1982; 297:431–434.
94. Nakanishi S, Inoue A, Kita T, et al. Nucleotide sequence of cloned cDNA for bovine corticotropin-β-lipotropin precursor. Nature 1979; 278:423–427.
95. Heinrich G, Fros P, Lund PK, et al. Pre-proglucagon messenger RNA: nucleotide and encoded amino acid sequences of the rat pancreatic cDNA. Endocrinology 1984; 115:2176–2181.
96. Zakarian S, Smyth DG. β-Endorphin is processed differently in specific regions of rat pituitary and brain. Nature 1982; 296:250–252.
97. Mojsov S, Weir GC, Habener JF. Insulinotropin: glucagon-like peptide I(7–37) coencoded in the glucagon gene is a potent stimulator of insulin release in perfused rat pancreas. J Clin Invest 1987; 79:616–619.
98. Bostein D, White RL, Skolnick M, et al. Construction of a genetic linkage map in man using restriction fragment length polymorphisms. Am J Hum Genet 1980; 32:314–331.
99. McConkey EH. Molecular evolution, intracellular organization, and the quinary structure of proteins. Proc Natl Acad Sci USA 1982; 79:3236–3240.
100. Gusella JF, Wexler NS, Conneally PM. A polymorphic DNA marker genetically linked to Huntington's disease. Nature 1983; 306:234–237.
101. Bell GI, Selby MJ, Rutter WJ. The highly polymorphic region near the human insulin gene is composed of simple tandemly repeating sequences. Nature 1982; 295:31–35.
102. Rotwein PS, Chirgwin J, Provincer M, et al. Polymorphism in the 5'-flanking region of the human insulin gene: a genetic marker for noninsulin-dependent diabetes. N Engl J Med 1983; 308:65–71.
103. Bell GI, Horita S, Karam JH. A polymorphic locus near the human insulin gene is associated with insulin-dependent diabetes mellitus. Diabetes 1984; 33:176–183.
104. Ingram VM. Abnormal haemoglobins III. The chemical difference between normal and sickle cell haemoglobins. Biochim Biophys Acta 1959; 36:402–411.
105. Treisman R, Orkin SH, Maniatis T. Specific transcription and RNA splicing defects in five cloned β-thalassaemia genes. Nature 1983; 302:591–596.
106. Kwok SCM, Steiner DF, Rubenstein AH, et al. Identification of a point mutation in the human insulin gene giving rise to a structurally abnormal insulin (insulin Chicago). Diabetes 1983; 32:872–875.
107. Haneda M, Chan SJ, Kwok SCM, et al. Studies on mutant human insulin genes: identification and sequence analysis of a gene encoding [Ser^{824}]insulin. Proc Natl Acad Sci USA 1983; 80:6366–6370.
108. Robbins DC, Blix PM, Ruberstein AH, et al. A human proinsulin variant at arginine 65. Nature 1981; 291:679–681.
109. Hughes MR, Malloy PJ, Kieback DG, et al. Point mutations in the human vitamin D receptor gene associated with hypocalcemic rickets. Science 1988; 242:1702–1705.
110. Usala SJ, Tennyson GE, Bale AE, et al. A base mutation of the c-erb A beta thyroid hormone receptor in a kindred with generalized thyroid hormone resistance: molecular heterogeneity in two other kindreds. J Clin Invest 1990; 85:93–100.
111. Motulsky AG. Impact of genetic manipulation on society and medicine. Science 1983; 219:135–140.
112. Cocking EC, Davey MR, Pental D, et al. Aspects of plant genetic manipulation. Nature 1981; 293: 265–270.

GENERAL READING

Alberts B, Bray D, Lewis J, et al. Molecular Biology of the Cell. 2nd ed. New York: Garland, 1989.

Antonarakis SE. Diagnosis of genetic disorders at the DNA level. N Engl Med 1989; 320: 153–163. (Erratum: 1989; 321:56.)

Darnell J, Lodish H, Baltimore D. Molecular Cell Biology. New York: W. H. Freeman, 1986.

Habener JF, ed. Molecular Cloning of Hormone Genes. Clifton, NJ: Humana, 1987.

Lewin B. Genes IV. 4th ed. New York: John Wiley & Sons, 1990.

Maniatis T, Goodbourn S, Fischer JA. Regulation of inducible and tissue-specific gene expression. Science 1987; 236:1237–1244.

Mitchell PJ, Tjian R. Transcriptional regulation in mammalian cells by sequence-specific DNA binding proteins. Science 1989; 245:371–378.

Ptashne M. How eukaryotic transcriptional activators work. Nature 1988; 335:683–689.

Walson JD, Tooze J, Kurtz DT. Recombinant DNA—A Short Course. New York: W. H. Freeman, 1983.

3

MECHANISMS OF ACTION OF STEROID HORMONES

James H. Clark, William T. Schrader, and Bert W. O'Malley

INTRODUCTION

Steroid hormones have effects at all levels of biological organization. Not only steroid hormones but also calcitriol, thyroid hormone, and retinoic acid act via remarkably similar mechanisms to produce the same general effects, i.e., the induction of RNA and protein synthesis. Therefore, we will present a generalized model of their action at the molecular and cellular levels.

Steroid hormones enter most cells by diffusion, although in some cases active uptake may be involved (Fig. 3–1). In target cells (i.e., cells sensitive to hormone) the steroid binds to macromolecules called receptors. These molecules are relatively large proteins that have specific binding sites for the hormone and are found in both the cytoplasmic and nuclear fractions of the cell. Binding of the steroid to its receptor molecule results in ill-defined conformational (al-

losteric) changes in structure that convert the receptor from an inactive to an active conformation. These changes result in the formation of an "activated" or "transformed" receptor-steroid complex that has a high affinity for various nuclear binding sites. In Figure 3–1 the receptor-steroid complexes are shown binding to regulatory DNA sequences in the 5' end of a responsive gene. Receptor-hormone complexes also bind to other nuclear sites such as the nuclear matrix, nonhistone proteins, and nuclear membranes. In the past it was thought that the activation or transformation step occurred in the cytoplasm (this possibility is shown in Fig. 3–1); however, this process may occur also in the nuclear compartment (also shown in Fig. 3–1). The binding of the receptor-hormone complex to regulatory elements usually results in gene activation, i.e., transcription of the gene by RNA polymerase to produce messenger RNA (mRNA). The mRNA is translated on cytoplasmic ribosomes to produce

Molecular Pathway of Steroid Hormone Action

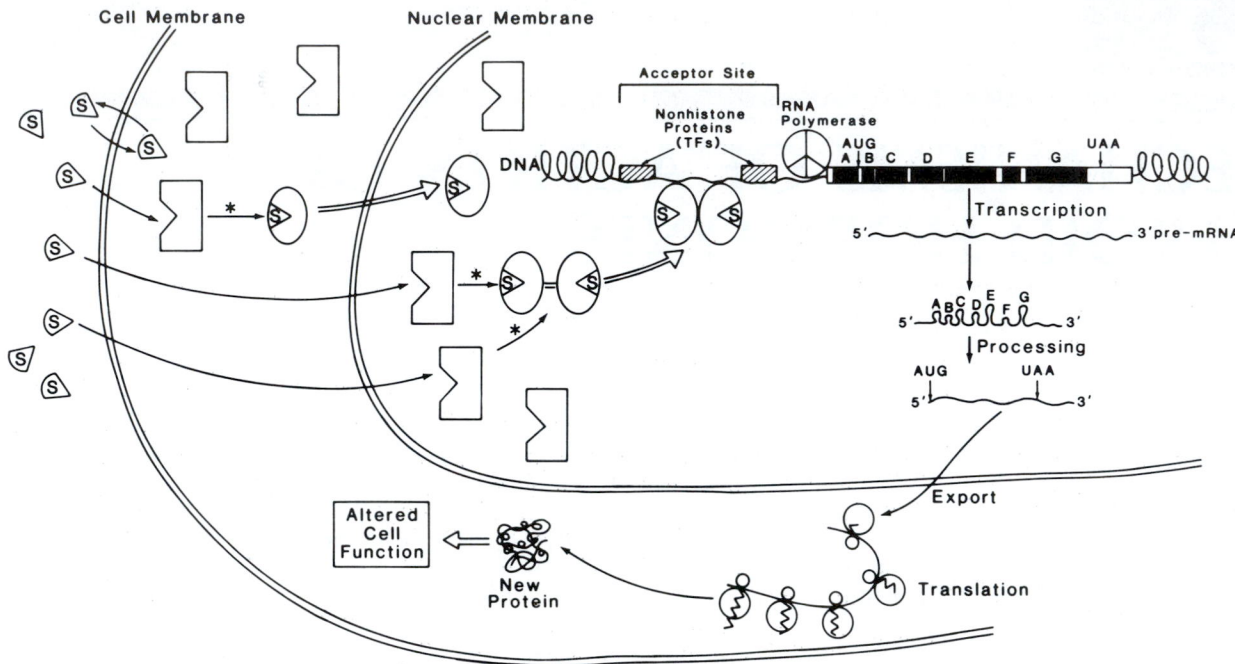

Figure 3–1. A complete understanding of the relationship between steroid receptor binding and the mechanism of hormone action depends on valid characterization and accurate measurement of steroid receptors.[1] In this section the criteria and methods by which this can be accomplished are described to provide the necessary background for the discussions presented later in the chapter.

the appropriate protein, which alters cell function, growth, or differentiation. In some cases receptor-gene interaction causes gene activity to be decreased rather than increased.

Once the receptor-hormone complex has interacted with a gene, the protein undergoes reactions that are not well understood but that result in the reestablishment of unoccupied receptor (recycling) and elimination of the steroid from the cell. These steps may involve dissociation of the steroid from the receptor and conversion of the receptor to a form that can subsequently bind hormone again and recycle. The steroid may be metabolized to forms that do not bind tightly to the receptor and hence diffuse out of the cell.

STEROID RECEPTORS: DEFINITION AND MEASUREMENT

A complete understanding of the relationship between steroid receptor binding and the mechanism of hormone action depends on characterization and measurement of steroid receptors.[1]

Receptor Criteria

FINITE BINDING CAPACITY. The biological response to steroid hormones is a saturable phenomenon. Assuming that the formation of receptor-hormone complexes is obligatory for the production of biological responses, then the number of receptors per unit mass of tissue should be limited; hence there should be a finite number of receptor sites. This criterion is met by the demonstration that the steroid-binding system under study can be saturated. This is usually accomplished by exposing the receptor to various concentrations of radioactive steroid and subsequently measuring the

amount of bound and/or free steroid after equilibrium is achieved. This would be a simple process if there existed only a single class of binding sites for a given steroid. Unfortunately, such is seldom the case. Most systems display multiple binding components, each with its own affinity and capacity for the steroid under study. These complexities will be discussed further in the following sections.

HIGH AFFINITY. Steroid receptors should possess a high affinity for their respective hormones. This is expected because the circulating levels of steroid are usually 10^{-10} to 10^{-8} M. The existence of receptor-mediated responses of physiological importance demands that the receptor have an affinity for the hormone that is in the range of these blood levels; otherwise the response would not occur. These considerations are true for a variety of target tissue receptors but do not preclude receptor interactions of weaker affinity if blood or tissue levels of steroids or receptors are elevated.

STEROID SPECIFICITY. Generally speaking, receptors display high affinities for a specific hormone or class of hormones. This specificity enables a given target cell to respond to a hormonal signal without interference from other signals. Thus hormones of the same class, as well as their agonists and antagonists, should compete effectively for a given class of receptor while not affecting other receptor systems. Nevertheless, receptor sites do not display absolute stereospecificity; that is, the binding site on the receptor has a limited capacity for recognition and differentiation of various ligand structures. This point will be discussed in more detail later.

TISSUE OR CELLULAR SPECIFICITY. As explained in the introduction, only specific cell types or tissues respond to given steroid hormones. Because the response is thought to be mediated via receptors, receptors should exist in these cell types and not in others. This criterion has been applied successfully to receptor systems for hormones. For instance, only certain tissues are stimulated by gonadal steroids, and these tissues are referred to as target organs; examples are uterus, vagina, and mammary gland in the case of estrogen receptor. If one compares such targets with nontargets, such as diaphragm or spleen, the density of estrogen receptor is higher per unit mass of target tissue.

CORRELATION WITH BIOLOGICAL RESPONSE. Implicit in all studies of macromolecules that bind steroid hormones and meet the foregoing criteria is the assumption that this binding results in a biological response. Thus binding of hormone to receptors must precede or accompany tissue responses, and the extent of response should be related to receptor occupancy. This criterion, the demonstration of receptor-dependent hormonal response, is not often met and is difficult to establish. The relationships that have been observed in some systems will be discussed later.

Analysis of Single-Component Systems

In most cases, steroid receptors exist in the presence of other binding components that complicate the analysis of receptor binding parameters. However, for the purpose of illustration we will consider a system that contains only one receptor site. In such a system, the total amount of receptor (R_t) is determined under equilibrium conditions by adding steroid (S) until saturation or near-saturation is obtained (Fig. 3–2). The amount of bound ligand (RS) in this system can be related mathematically to free ligand(s), total receptor (R_t), and the dissociation constant (K_d) of the receptor-ligand complex in the following way:

$$[RS] = \frac{[R_t][S]}{K_d + [S]}$$

This is the formulation of rapid equilibrium kinetics employed in the derivation of the Michaelis-Menten equation and applies equally well to ligand binding as long as conditions of equilibrium exist. As steroid is added to the system, the receptor sites become saturated. The actual point of saturation is equal to the number of receptor sites (n) or R_t. The dissociation constant (K_d) is the concentration of steroid at which 50% of the receptor sites are bound. This value in Figure 3–2 is 1 nM. Although one can make reasonable estimates of R_t and K_d from saturation plots, these parameters should be obtained by Scatchard analysis,[2] as shown in Figure 3–2B.

Analysis of Multiple-Component Systems

The simple system described in the preceding section does not exist unless the receptor has been purified and has only one class of binding sites. Additional binding sites are

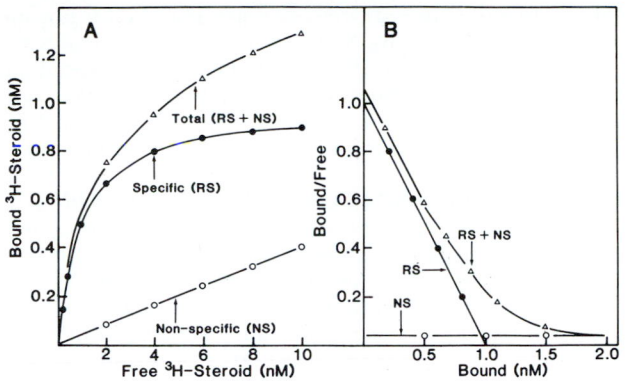

Figure 3–3. Saturation (A) and Scatchard (B) analyses of specific and nonspecific binding.

usually present and complicate the measurement of receptors. In this section we will describe some of the complications and attempt to explain how they can be manipulated so that receptor parameters can still be ascertained.

SPECIFIC AND NONSPECIFIC BINDING. As discussed earlier, the binding of a ligand to its receptor is stereospecific and thus is defined as specific. Nonspecific binding is the result of the ligand binding to nonreceptor sites, which are usually of low affinity and high capacity relative to the receptor. The total amount of steroid bound in such a system (RS + NS) is the sum of that bound to receptor sites (RS) and that bound to nonspecific sites (NS, Fig. 3–3A).

The data from Figure 3–3A are plotted according to the method of Scatchard in Figure 3–3B. The RS/S ratio is a curvilinear function of the amount of ligand bound (RS). This curve represents the summation of specific and nonspecific components, both of which are plotted individually as well and appear as linear functions in this graph. These components can be resolved by use of competitive inhibitors or by geometric fitting procedures described later.

A direct assessment of the amounts of specific and nonspecific binding can be made by the use of competitive inhibition of labeled-steroid binding by nonlabeled steroid. In practice, the receptor is exposed to multiple concentrations of radioactive steroid in the presence or absence of excess nonradioactive steroid. Under these conditions data similar to those shown in Figure 3–3A are obtained. The line designated as RS + NS represents the amount of ^{3}H-labeled ligand that is bound to both receptor (or "specific") sites and nonspecific sites and thus contains both saturable and nonsaturable components. Nonspecific binding sites (NS) are measured as the radioactive steroid bound in the presence of excess unlabeled competitive ligand. The competing nonlabeled ligand occupies essentially all high-affinity receptor sites but does not interfere appreciably with the binding of ^{3}H-labeled ligand to nonspecific sites. Receptor sites are estimated by subtracting NS from RS + NS. The number of receptor sites and the K_d can be determined from a direct plot of these data (see Fig. 3–3B).

The use of inhibition to determine receptor-binding parameters is based on the assumption that the nonlabeled steroid is a competitive inhibitor. If the nonlabeled ligand is identical to the radioactive ligand, this will be true. In some cases, however, it is necessary to use a nonidentical inhibitor, and the assumption of competitive inhibition must be verified by the methods discussed later. In addition, the use of competitive inhibition to determine receptor parameters is based on the assumption that nonspecific binding sites are of low affinity and high capacity relative to the receptor system. This is true for many receptor systems but must be

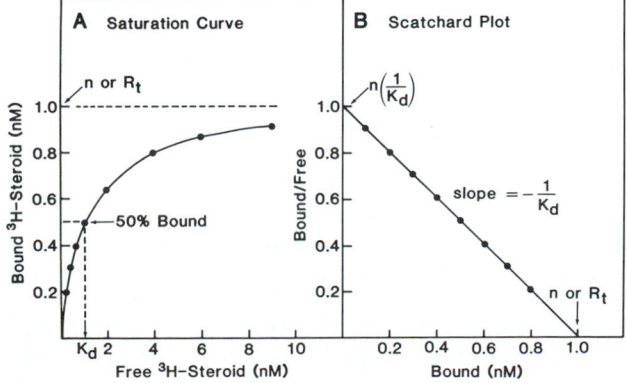

Figure 3–2. Saturation and Scatchard analyses of receptor steroid binding. n or R_t, number of receptor sites; K_d, dissociation constant.

validated by the demonstration of a straight line for nonspecific binding, as in Figure 3–3A, or by Scatchard analysis.

For receptor assays, the use of the term nonspecific to describe nonreceptor binding is adequate. However, nonspecific actually means nondisplaceable by a competitive steroid in the concentration range of ^{3}H-labeled steroid used in the assay.

COMPETITIVE INHIBITION OF RECEPTOR BINDING. To use the displacement method just discussed for the measurement of receptor parameters, the appropriate concentration of unlabeled steroid must be chosen and the displacement must be due to competitive inhibition. Inhibition of steroid binding to receptor sites may occur by either competitive or noncompetitive means, that is, by mechanisms that involve mutually exclusive binding of ligands (competitive) or by mechanisms in which ligand inactivates (either reversibly or irreversibly) the ligand-binding capacity of the receptor (noncompetitive). Competitive inhibitors decrease steroid binding to receptor sites by combining with the receptor in such a manner that the labeled steroid can no longer be bound—as when ligand and inhibitor compete for the same or adjacent and overlapping sites. The mutually exclusive nature of steroid and inhibitor binding in such systems results in data such as those shown in Figure 3–4, which are analyzed by saturation and Scatchard analyses. Note that increasing concentrations of inhibitor alter the apparent K_d for the receptor-steroid complex but do not change the number of sites.

In contrast to the effects of a competitive inhibitor on receptor steroid-binding parameters, noncompetitive inhibitors do not alter the apparent K_d of the interaction but decrease the apparent number of receptor sites (Fig. 3–5). Thus the demonstration of suppression of ^{3}H-labeled steroid binding to receptors is not sufficient to establish competitive inhibition. Noncompetitive inhibition may occur for many reasons. For example, the inhibitor may precipitate or denature the receptor or its active site; alternatively, the inhibitor may bind to a second site on the receptor and in so doing alter the active site of the receptor.

Another technique used to study the specificity and relative binding affinity of steroid receptors is shown in Figure 3–6. In this method the concentration of ^{3}H-labeled steroid is held constant and the concentration of inhibiting steroid is varied. The relative binding affinity (RBA) is determined by comparing the point at which 50% inhibition is observed for S (the nonlabeled steroid that is identical to the ^{3}H-labeled steroid) and for X (the test compound). It can be seen from Figure 3–6 that 50% inhibition occurs for S at 10 nM and for X at 100 nM; therefore, the relative

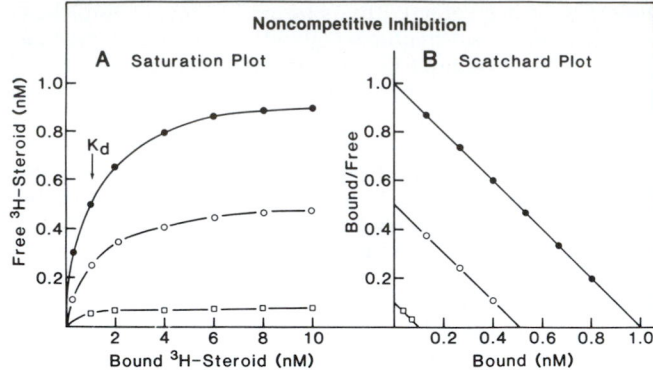

Figure 3–5. Noncompetitive inhibition of receptor binding. ●, no inhibitors added; ○, inhibitor added at 1 nM; □, inhibitor added at 10 nM.

affinity of the receptor for X is 0.1 of that for S. Although this method is useful, the determination of RBA is valid only when the slopes of the two curves are parallel, as is the case for S and X in Figure 3–6. If the slopes are not parallel, as shown for compounds Y and Z in Figure 3–6, no determination of RBA can be made. In fact, the inhibition is not occurring by a competitive mechanism. Therefore, the observed inhibition must involve a noncompetitive mechanism, and this will require further study using the methods shown in Figures 3–4 and 3–5.

ASSOCIATION AND DISSOCIATION OF RECEPTOR-STEROID COMPLEXES. The equilibrium constant (K_d) for the receptor-steroid complex is a function of the rate of association (on reaction) and the rate of dissociation (off reaction) of the steroid. Receptor sites that bind hormone at a high rate and release it at a low rate have high affinities. The rate of association can be assessed by exposing the receptor to labeled hormone and measuring the amount of hormone bound as a function of time. The rate of dissociation is measured by adding a large excess of nonlabeled hormone to solution containing labeled hormone–receptor complexes. The excess nonlabeled hormone blocks reassociation of labeled hormone with the receptor during the dissociation process. Aliquots of the mixture are removed and assayed

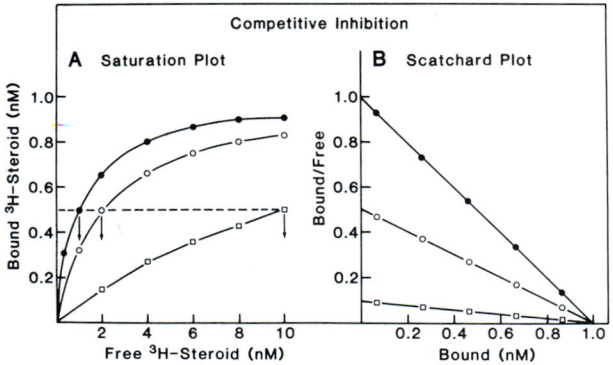

Figure 3–4. Competitive inhibition of receptor binding. ●, no competing steroid added; ○, competing steroid added at a concentration of 1 nM; □, competing steroid added at a concentration of 10 nM; dashed line in A marks point at which 50% of total specific binding is achieved; arrow indicates apparent shift in K_d.

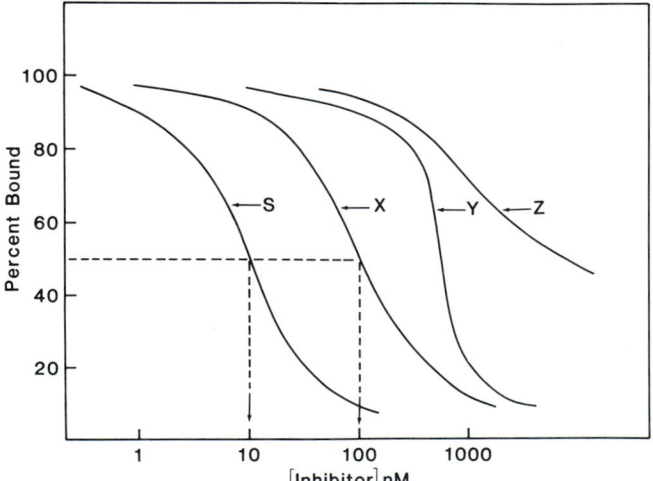

Figure 3–6. Competitive inhibition analysis and relative binding affinity. Concentrations of receptor and ^{3}H-labeled steroid are 1 nM and 10 nM, respectively. S, steroid identical to the ^{3}H-labeled steroid; X, steroid with a relative affinity of 0.1; Y and Z, noncompetitive inhibitors. Horizontal dashed line indicates point of 50% inhibition; vertical dashed lines indicate concentration of competing steroid that inhibits 50% of binding of ^{3}H-labeled steroid to receptor.

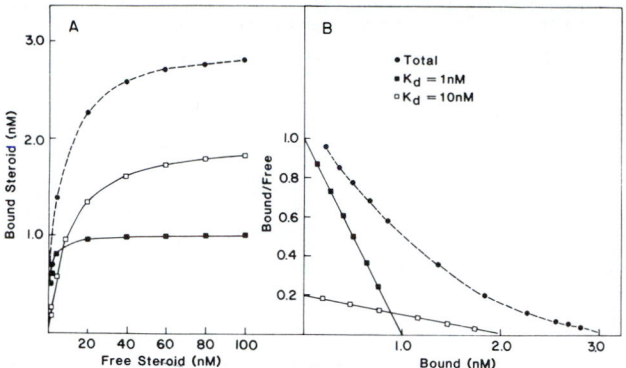

Figure 3–7. Saturation *(A)* and Scatchard *(B)* analyses of two specific binding sites of identical concentrations but different affinities. ●, total specific binding; ■, specific binding related to binding site with K_d of 1 nM; □, specific binding related to binding site with K_d of 10 nM.

for the amount of unbound labeled hormone as a function of time. A single semilogarithmic plot of this value versus time yields a straight line whose slope is the rate constant for dissociation. The half-life of the complex can be determined as the time needed for the concentration of free hormone to double in value. Such a measurement reveals that particularly active steroids may be characterized by long half-lives of the receptor-steroid complex.

MULTIPLE SPECIFIC COMPONENTS. In addition to non-specific binding sites for steroid hormones, many receptor systems contain two or more specific sites that bind the same steroid with high affinities. This condition could produce the theoretical situations shown in Figures 3–7 and 3–8. In these examples, the nonspecific binding component has been eliminated for convenience and will be discussed later. These mixtures of binding sites produce saturation curves that do not appear by casual inspection to be composed of two binding components; however, the Scatchard analyses (see Figs. 3–7B and 3–8B) clearly demonstrate their presence. The usual saturation analysis might include only the lower range of ligand concentration; thus extrapolation of an apparent straight line would yield an improper estimate of the number of binding sites. In addition, it would be concluded falsely that only one specific binding component was present. Errors of this type are more exaggerated when the binding component with lower affinity is in excess over the higher-affinity component (see Fig. 3–8). In such cases binding analyses at low concentrations of ligand lead to gross overestimates of the number of sites and an underestimate of their affinity for the steroid.

Another situation is shown in Figure 3–9. In this example two different types of specific binding are represented: one that displays the usual saturation curve, which is a rectangular hyperbola, and a second that is represented by a sigmoid function.[3] These two sites yield a Scatchard plot with linear (type I) and curvilinear (type II) components. When such complex curves are present, failure to perform complete saturation analysis or direct extrapolation of the linear portion of the Scatchard plot will result in overestimates of the first site. In addition, the false conclusion would be drawn that only a single specific binding component exists. The curvilinear portion of the curve is often mistakenly considered to be a straight line and is equated to nonspecific binding or binding of no significance. It should be noted that the nonspecific binding component in these analyses has been subtracted and is not shown in Figure 3–9. The resolution of these mixed binding systems into their components is discussed in the following section.

RESOLVING MIXED BINDING SYSTEMS. The ideal approach to mixed binding systems such as those just discussed is physical separation of the various components by purification procedures so that each can be studied as an isolated system. However, this is usually not feasible because of the limited quantities of tissue available. In the simplest case, the system is composed of one specific or saturable component and one nonspecific component (as in Fig. 3–3) and competitive inhibition can be used to determine these components. It is also possible to use graphic analysis of curvilinear Scatchard plots as shown in Figure 3–10. Such curved plots can be resolved into two straight lines, which, when summed point by point in a vectorial manner, reproduce the original curve. The data shown in Figure 3–10 are identical to those shown in Figure 3–8. Note that sections determined by two independent components must sum to the curve. Usually the data from steroid-binding studies are limited and the Scatchard curves are imprecisely determined so that the resolution of more than two components is not possible by this method.

Analytical methods employing geometric or parametric procedures such as those discussed earlier are useful if complete and detailed steroid-binding data can be obtained. Often this is not the case because of limitations in biological material, and other methods must be found to cope with the problem. Differential inhibition of ligand binding has been employed to measure a given component in a number of mixed systems. The use of [³H]estradiol and diethylstilbestrol (DES) for the assay of estrogen receptors in the presence of α-fetoprotein (α-FP) is a good example. α-FP is present in large quantities in the neonatal rat and has a high

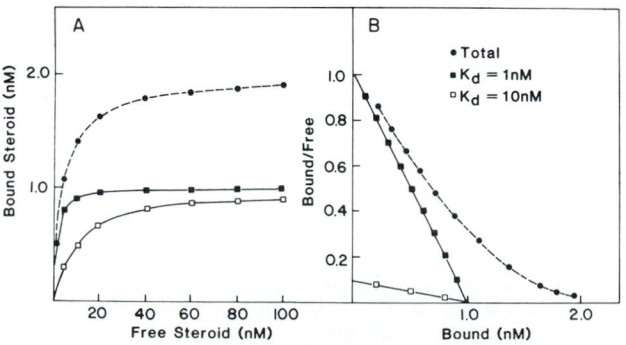

Figure 3–8. Saturation *(A)* and Scatchard *(B)* analyses of two specific binding sites of dissimilar concentrations and affinities. ●, total specific binding; ■, specific binding related to binding site with K_d of 1 nM and concentration of 1 nM; □, specific binding related to binding site with K_d of 10 nM and concentration of 2 nM.

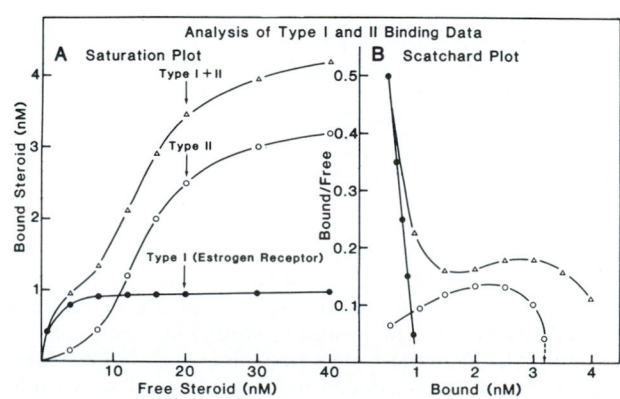

Figure 3–9. Saturation and Scatchard analyses of type I and II binding sites. △, total specific binding; ●, binding related to type I site (estrogen receptor); ○, specific binding related to type II sites; arrow in *B* indicates number of type II sites.

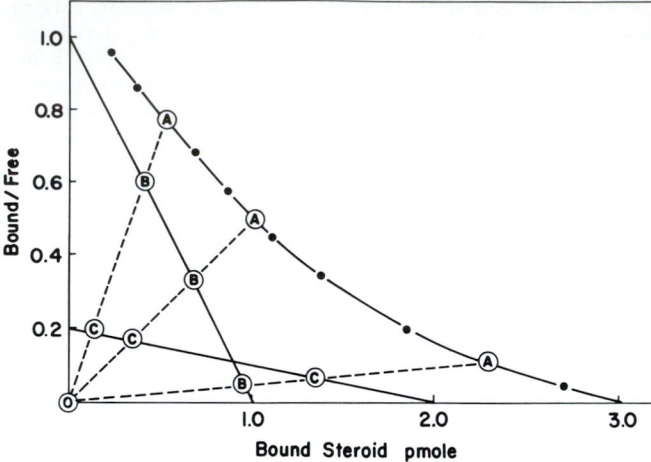

Figure 3–10. Resolution of two binding sites by vectorial analysis of a curved Scatchard plot. Each point A of the Scatchard plot is the vectorial sum of points B and C for each of the binding components (solid straight lines). These two linear components can be resolved by adjusting their slopes until OC + OB = A for all dashed lines drawn from the origin (O) to points A on the Scatchard plot.

affinity for estradiol ($K_d = 10^{-9}$ to 10^{-10} M), approximating that of the receptor. The amount of receptor is measured by taking advantage of the fact that DES binds with low affinity to α-FP but competes effectively with [³H]estradiol for estrogen receptor binding sites. Thus the binding of labeled estradiol to R can be determined by subtracting the amount of [³H]estradiol bound in the presence of DES from the amount bound in the absence of DES.

In addition to the approaches already discussed, in some receptor systems it is possible to eliminate one of the binding components and measure the receptor without interference. For instance, the addition of a reducing agent, such as dithiothreitol, to nuclear exchange assays causes the disappearance of type II binding sites and permits independent assessment of the estrogen receptor (type I site; see Fig. 3–9 for representative plot of these two types of sites and ref. 3 for details).

Exchange Assays

Most biological systems contain receptors in occupied and unoccupied states. The measurement of both forms is obligatory if an accurate picture of the relationship between receptor binding and physiology is to emerge. To measure the occupancy state of receptors, exchange assays must be used. These assays employ methods that result in dissociation of the endogenous steroid from occupied receptor sites and association of a labeled steroid. The conditions by which this is accomplished vary; however, in general, the theoretical considerations are the same.

As an example, we will discuss the estradiol exchange assay.[4, 5] In this procedure the cytosolic or nuclear fraction to be assayed is warmed to 30°C for 30 min in the presence of varying concentrations of [³H]estradiol. At this temperature endogenous (nonlabeled) steroid dissociates from occupied sites (RS, Fig. 3–11) and the added labeled steroid (S) is exchanged. Unoccupied sites (R) will also be bound by the labeled steroid. The resulting complexes (RS) can then be analyzed by Scatchard plots (see Fig. 3–11). Nonexchange receptor methods that detect only unoccupied sites underestimate the total amount of receptor present; in this example, the number of sites is reduced to one half of that observed with the exchange method.

BIOCHEMISTRY AND MOLECULAR BIOLOGY OF STEROID RECEPTORS

Introduction

Steroid receptors represent a class of ligand-activated transcription factors that includes, among others, the thyroid hormone and vitamin D receptors.[6] Many of the known steroid receptors have been cloned, and as a result we now know a great deal about the structure of steroid receptors (progesterone receptor,[7–9] estrogen receptor,[10, 11] androgen receptor,[12, 13] glucocorticoid receptor,[14–16] mineralocorticoid receptor,[17, 18] thyroid receptor,[19–21] retinoic acid receptor,[22–25] and vitamin D₃ receptor;[6, 26, 27] see refs. 21, 28, and 29 for reviews). Steroid receptors mediate all known activities of steroid hormones. Modulation of the effective concentration of these proteins is probably the first step in control of cellular responses.

CONTROL OF FUNCTIONAL RECEPTOR ACTIVITY. Receptor proteins, like other regulatory proteins and enzymes, may exist in both active and inactive states. There are two hypothetical classes of activation: (1) steroid site activation and (2) functional activation. In this section we consider only the first case. Because the responsiveness of a cell to a hormone will be related in some way to the cell's effective receptor concentration, factors that affect the steroid binding site will be able to influence the cell's sensitivity. Receptor regulation involves phosphorylation of the receptor protein itself.[30, 31] In the case of glucocorticoids, receptor dephosphorylation appears to cause destruction of a functional hormone binding site. Readdition of ATP in the presence of protein kinase causes restoration of the site. This reversible activation-deactivation reaction can be seen in living cells. Mouse thymus cells in primary culture, for example, lose detectable amounts of glucocorticoid receptor when

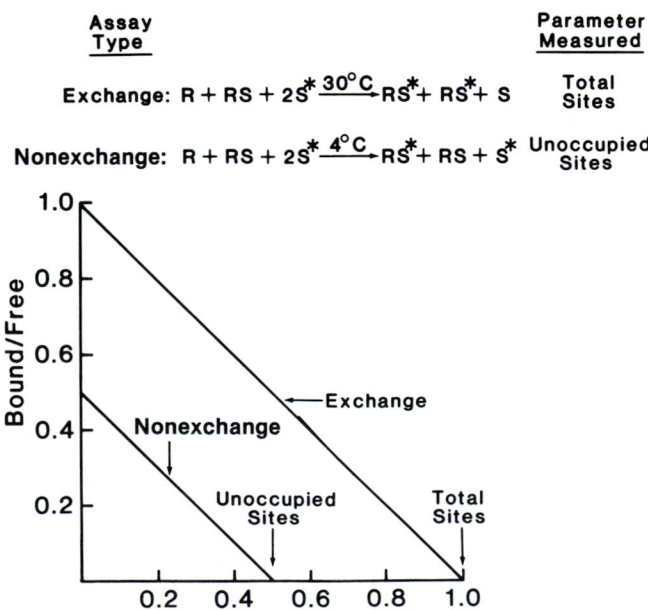

Figure 3–11. Determination of receptor binding by exchange and nonexchange assays. Results of these two procedures are plotted by the Scatchard method in lower portion of figure. R, unoccupied receptor sites; RS, occupied receptor sites; S*, ³H-labeled steroid; RS*, receptor–³H-labeled steroid complex.

their intracellular ATP pools are depleted (as by uncouplers of oxidative phosphorylation or by oxygen deprivation). Receptor activity is restored in minutes by replenishment of ATP. The extent to which this type of regulation occurs in normal tissues is not known. Evidence from antibody assays for receptor proteins suggests that intracellular pools of inactive receptor exist.

Other possible mechanisms for affecting receptor-steroid interactions also exist. One that has attracted a great deal of interest involves endogenous "antihormones," i.e., competitors or modulators of the hormone-binding activity. Whole-cell extracts have been fractionated in various ways to obtain low-molecular-weight factors able to block or reduce binding of radioactive steroids to receptors in vitro. At this writing, no such compound has been purified or characterized. The action of such factors would be difficult to distinguish from nonspecific receptor destruction, as by proteases.

Finally, the authentic hormone itself can regulate the effective receptor titer in the cell. Three pathways for this effect have been described. The first, called down-regulation, is seen as a reduction in receptor hormone-binding activity after acute treatment of an animal with the hormone. Uterine progesterone receptor levels, for example, are decreased within 1 h after administration of progesterone to rabbits. Similarly, glucocorticoids down-regulate their receptor levels. Receptor genes lack DNA sequences known to respond to hormone receptors, so the pathway remains to be established. A second means of regulation is to augment the receptor titer. In castrated rats, estrogen administration causes a net increase in measurable estrogen receptor levels in the uterus, generally between 12 and 24 h after injection. Similarly, estradiol administration increases progesterone receptor levels over the same time frame. In both of these examples, it is assumed that de novo receptor synthesis is increased, although other possibilities such as activation cannot be excluded at present. Finally, the hormone can alter the receptor protein's ligand site by some type of induced-fit mechanism. Estradiol-17β, when bound to its receptor from rat uterus, promotes receptor dimerization or aggregation and causes a dramatic increase in the half-life of the hormone-receptor complexes. This pathway has not been observed in other receptor systems.

STRUCTURAL ORGANIZATION OF RECEPTOR PROTEINS. Because of the interest in steroid receptors both as gene regulatory proteins and for their clinical significance in endocrine-related disease, these proteins have been studied intensively. They are present in only small amounts in cells, ranging in abundance from about 0.001% (aldosterone receptor) to 0.1% (progesterone receptors) of total soluble protein. Thus their purification for structural studies has been difficult and yields are small, typically 1 μg of pure receptor per kg of starting tissue. Receptor proteins for most steroid hormones have now been purified to apparent homogeneity. Target tissue can be used directly, but research is also being done with receptors overexpressed in bacteria[32, 33] and in yeast.[34, 35]

Various purification methods have been employed. The most elegant is steroid affinity chromatography, in which a derivative of the natural hormone is immobilized on beads of Sepharose and used as a column. Receptors containing a functional hormone binding site should adsorb, whereas other macromolecules lacking affinity for the hormone are not retarded. The method has been used successfully, but proteins unable to bind the hormone frequently are adsorbed as well. Other methods involve ion-exchange, adsorption, and gel-filtration chromatography. In all cases the desired receptor is labeled with radioactive steroid, and the

hormone-receptor complex is followed through the various steps in this manner.

Purified proteins such as receptors may, of course, be altered from their in situ condition by such factors as removal of cofactors, partial proteolysis, subunit disassembly, or denaturation. Thus considerable work on receptor structure has been done with unpurified cytoplasmic extracts that have been subjected to minimal experimental manipulation.

Sequence comparisons of the cloned receptors reveal three regions of consensus homology, referred to as C1, C2, and C3, shown in Figure 3–12. The C1 region is the most highly conserved and is a cysteine-rich DNA binding domain. C2 and C3 are less highly conserved, yet still have significant homology. The COOH-terminal region is associated with ligand binding, transcriptional activation, and potential protein-protein interactions with other steroid receptors as well as potential inhibitory factors. These structural observations suggest that the steroid receptor supergene family represents an old family of regulatable transcription factors. One can speculate that the early forms of these receptors were regulated by intracellular metabolic ligands in an intracrine fashion.[29] Some of the receptors may have lost the ligand binding domain and hence become constitutive transcription factors, such as v-erb A.[36] Other receptors may have acquired ligand specificity for steroids, thyroid hormones, retinoic acid, and perhaps even other unidentified ligands. Low-stringency Southern blot hybridization analysis with the DNA binding domain of the glucocorticoid receptor suggests the existence of an abundance of related receptor proteins.[37] Some of these receptor proteins have been cloned, but the ligands are yet to be identified.[37–39] These "orphan receptors" may represent primitive forms of the steroid receptor gene family.

One of the fascinating observations to evolve from the cloning of these cDNAs is the unexpected large size of the

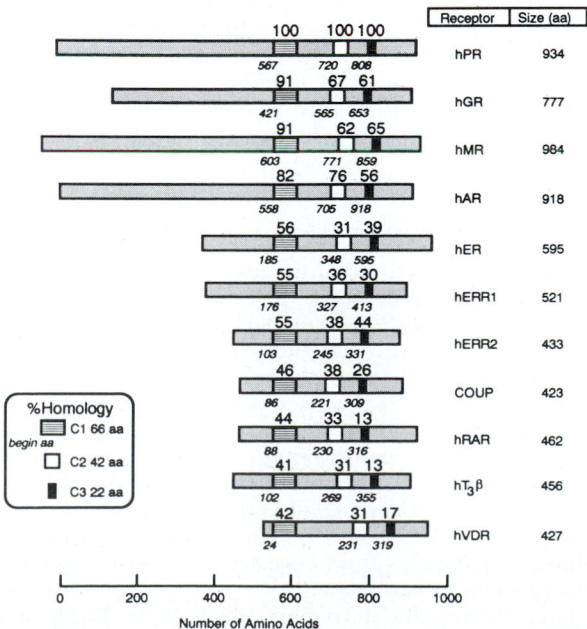

Figure 3–12. Homology of the steroid receptor supergene family. There are three regions of homology, referred to as C1, C2, and C3. C1 has been identified as the DNA-binding domain. The functional significance of the homologies in C2 and C3 remains to be determined.

steroid receptor superfamily of related genes. After elucidation of the receptors for the more traditional members of this family (glucomineralocorticoids, gonadal steroids, thyroid hormone, vitamin D_3, and retinoic acid), a large number of cloned receptor isotypes or variants were discovered.[21] These molecules can be considered to be orphan receptors in search of a function and a ligand. Because they were cloned by cDNA cross-hybridization screening using cDNA probes, we have little clue to their cellular physiology. A function is implicit, however, because they are expressed in cells as fully processed cytoplasmic mRNAs.

A number of orphan receptor sequences have been published.[37, 40–43] They are recognized by extensive amino acid sequence homology in the DNA binding region (C1) and strict conservation of the two zinc finger motifs. These orphan receptors may represent the earliest forms of the steroid receptor gene family. One member of this family that has a known function has been identified. The protein is a transcription factor that binds upstream of several hormone-regulated genes and participates in their regulation. The chicken ovalbumin gene, for example, contains within its upstream promoter the DNA sequence GTGTCAAAGGTCAAA, termed the chicken ovalbumin upstream promoter (COUP) element. A DNA-binding protein in oviduct nuclear extracts binds specifically to the COUP sequence.[44, 45] The protein, named COUP–transcription factor (COUP-TF), is found in HeLa, chicken oviduct, HIT, and many other cell types.[44–47] Its cDNA was cloned, and the protein is structurally related to the steroid receptor proteins. The DNA binding domain of COUP-TF is a 66-amino-acid zinc finger motif in which all 20 invariant amino acids of the receptor superfamily are conserved and 11 out of 12 conserved residues are identical.[38] In addition to the zinc finger motif, two regions in the probable ligand binding domain share significant similarity among members of this superfamily. Comparison with different members of the steroid receptor superfamily shows that COUP-TF is most homologous to hERR-1 and hERR-2, two orphan receptors whose functions and ligands have yet to be defined.

A *Drosophila* homologue of COUP-TF, the Seven-up gene, was identified.[48] This gene's product is required for photoreceptor cell formation during eye development in the fruit fly. *Drosophila* Seven-up gene and human COUP-TF are virtually identical (93% identical) in the DNA binding and COOH-terminal putative ligand binding regions. This striking conservation suggests that both might be regulated by the same ligand.

The Steroid Receptor Gene Family

A number of structural features are similar in all members of the steroid receptor gene family, suggesting that they are considered rightly as members of a class of regulatory proteins. These features include (1) a structurally separate hormone binding site that is a fraction of the total receptor polypeptide chain, (2) the presence of a high-affinity DNA binding site distinct from the hormone site, (3) a tendency to aggregate at low ionic strength to form either dimers or tetramers of the subunits, and (4) enhanced affinity for the cell nucleus in the presence of bound hormone. These four characteristics can be observed in both crude extracts and purified preparations and hence are probably characteristics of the proteins in situ.

Even before the steroid receptors were cloned, it was clear that they were organized into functional domains. Proteolytic cleavage analysis first revealed receptor fragments in which DNA-binding activity was separated from steroid binding.[49, 50] Once the receptors were cloned, these domains were better defined.[51–56] Functionally, the steroid receptors interact with inhibitory proteins such as heat shock protein hsp90 (see later), bind to ligand, dimerize, bind to specific sequences of DNA with high affinity, and activate transcription. These various functions ascribed to receptor proteins will be discussed by structure and putative locations.

GENERAL FEATURES. Steroid receptor proteins have molecular masses of about 80 to 100 kd. Each monomeric unit binds a single steroid molecule, but the receptors dimerize when bound to the genes they regulate. They are acidic, asymmetric, and present in low abundance in cells. With the exception of phosphate, no covalent post-translational modifications are known. There is no evidence for lipid, carbohydrate, or nucleic acid in their structures and no confirmed evidence that any receptor has intrinsic enzymatic activity. Rather, the proteins function primarily by virtue of their DNA-binding activity (see later).

MOLECULAR PARAMETERS OF STEROID RECEPTOR SUBUNITS. The subunits are asymmetric, rather than globular, proteins with axial ratios (long axis/short axis) of about 10:1. This asymmetry is not as evident in the receptor 8S aggregate, suggesting an arrangement of subunits lying with their long axes parallel to each other. The hormone-binding properties are sometimes perturbed by dissociation to individual subunits, as in the case of estrogen receptor, for which the binding constant changes about twofold at high ionic strength. However, the chicken progesterone receptor's hormone site is unaffected by subunit dissociation. Glucocorticoid receptor in the unliganded state loses its hormone-binding activity when the 8S cytoplasmic complex is dissociated in vitro by high ionic strength or warming. Loss of the nonreceptor hsp90 occurs under these circumstances and is thought to be responsible for destruction or destabilization of the ligand binding region. Thus one proposed role for hsp90 is to stabilize (or create) the hormone binding site of glucocorticoid receptor.

DNA Sequences Mediating Steroid Hormone Regulation of Genes

Most steroid-regulated genes share one important structural feature, the presence of steroid receptor binding sites referred to as steroid response elements (SREs). SREs have all of the characteristics of a classic enhancer element.[57] They are independent of position and orientation, and their presence has a profound effect on transcriptional activity when stimulated by hormone.[58, 59]

Receptor interactions with specific DNA sequences have been observed in numerous ways. DNA sequences of potential interest are defined by deletion studies and gene transfection into cells in culture or by comparison with known response elements. Then the DNA to be evaluated is synthesized in vitro and labeled with ^{32}P. Examples of such synthesized sequences are shown in Figure 3–13A. After chicken progesterone receptor is mixed with all three DNAs, an antibody to receptor is added to precipitate [^{32}P]DNA. Figure 3–13B shows specific binding of the progesterone response element (PRE) sequence but not a randomized DNA of the same base composition or an estrogen response element (ERE). Binding to the SRE DNA sequence involves receptor dimerization on the DNA, as detected by gel retardation assays like that shown in Figure 3–14. Either intact receptors or cloned fragments can be used in such an experiment.

Coordinate regulation of gene networks is achieved through the appropriate combination of SREs, silencers, tissue-specific promoter elements, and basal promoter elements for each individual gene.[60–62] Thus different genes can be regulated to varying extents in the same cell by a single concentration of activated steroid receptors. Tran-

A

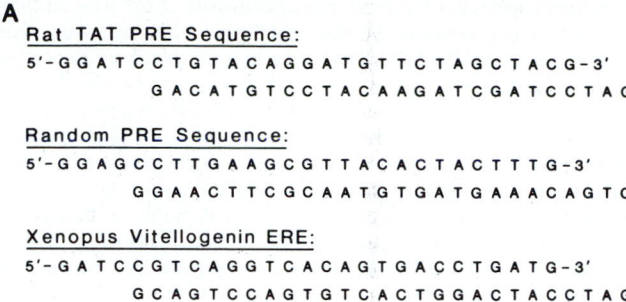

Rat TAT PRE Sequence:

5'-G G A T C C T G T A C A G G A T G T T C T A G C T A C G-3'
      G A C A T G T C C T A C A A G A T C G A T C C T A G

Random PRE Sequence:

5'-G G A G C C T T G A A G C G T T A C A C T A C T T T G-3'
      G G A A C T T C G C A A T G T G A T G A A A C A G T C

Xenopus Vitellogenin ERE:

5'-G A T C C G T C A G G T C A C A G T G A C C T G A T G-3'
      G C A G T C C A G T G T C A C T G G A C T A C C T A G

B

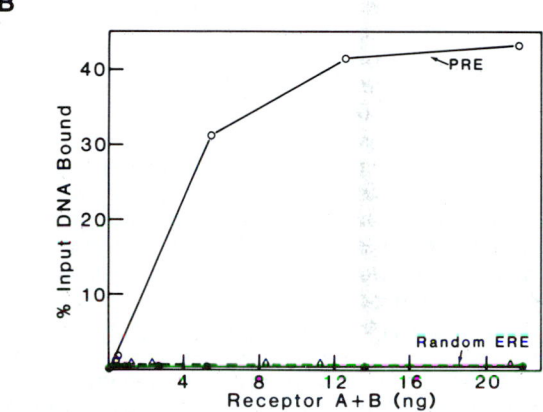

Figure 3–13. A, Oligonucleotides used for DNA-binding studies of chicken progesterone receptors. TAT PRE, progesterone response element detected in the rat tyrosine aminotransferase gene; ERE, estrogen response element sequence from vitellogenin gene. B, Immunoprecipitation of receptor-[32P]DNA complexes. Cytosol from oviducts of estrogenized chicks was incubated with a specific monoclonal antibody, then immunoprecipitated with protein A–Sepharose. Each immunoprecipitate was then incubated with [32P]DNA having the sequences shown in A. The complexes were washed and collected by centrifugation.

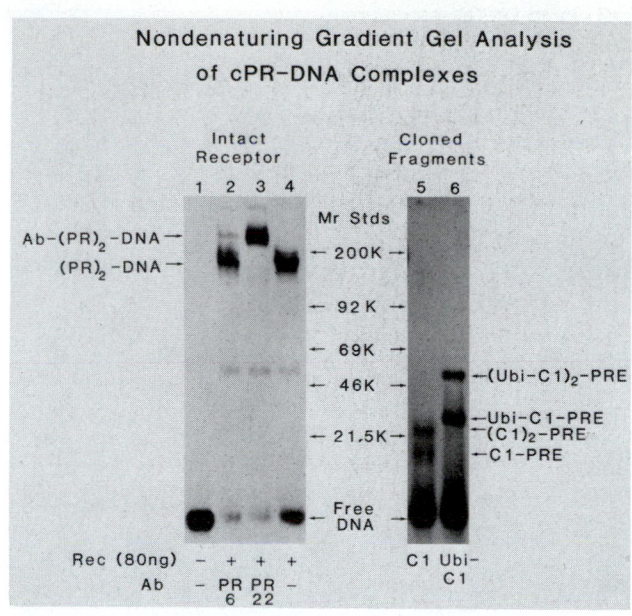

Figure 3–14. Gel retardation method for detecting receptor-DNA specificity. Autoradiogram of nondenaturing gradient gel electrophoretic analysis of PRE-receptor complexes. Left, intact purified receptor; right, receptor DNA-binding fragment expressed as fusion protein in Escherichia coli. Lane 1, free [32P]PRE DNA; lanes 2–4, wild-type PR + DNA; lanes 5 and 6, cloned receptor fragment + DNA. Lane 2 shows lack of reaction when using unreactive antibody. Lane 3 shows further upshift of receptor-DNA band by reactive antibody. Molecular weights were determined from migration of protein standards in adjacent lanes.

scriptional response to steroids in different tissues and cells is also controlled by limiting the tissue-specific expression and concentration of the various steroid receptors.[63]

SREs have been described for each of the known ligand-activated nuclear receptors. Figure 3–15 outlines the major SREs according to common structural characteristics. In general, SREs are characterized by an imperfect hexanucleotide palindrome separated by a spacer, suggesting that receptors bind these sequences as functional dimers.[64] The classic reproductive and adrenal steroid receptors have a trinucleotide spacer, but the thyroid hormone receptor and vitamin D$_3$ receptor family have a less stringent spacing requirement. These receptors can vary from having no spacers at all to having as many as six nucleotides separating the palindromic half-sites. Negatively regulated steroid response elements (nSREs) have also been described. In most cases, however, nSREs appear to be SREs that have been positioned so that binding of a steroid receptor sterically prevents the formation of an active transcription complex.[65–67]

The first SREs identified were the glucocorticoid response elements (GREs) of the mouse mammary tumor virus (MMTV) long terminal repeat[68–70] and of the chick lysozyme gene.[71] Figure 3–16 shows an electron micrograph of glucocorticoid receptors bound to the MMTV GRE. As more GREs were discovered,[72–74] a common consensus sequence emerged, and it became apparent that the same sequences that confer steroid responsiveness to glucocorticoids could also function as response elements for progesterone,[75, 76] mineralocorticoids,[17] and androgens[77, 78] but not estrogen.[79] The ERE[80, 81] is similar to but structurally distinct from the canonical GRE.[82] The consensus ERE is more closely related

to the thyroid hormone response element (TRE).[83] The sequences are identical except that the ERE contains a trinucleotide spacer in the center of the recognition sequence. Similarly, the retinoic acid receptor is capable of stimulating transcription from what was originally described as a thyroid hormone response element.[84, 85] The physiological implications of this overlapping enhancer specificity are not clear. Unliganded thyroid hormone receptor acts as an inhibitor of thyroid hormone– and retinoic acid–responsive genes, and the unliganded retinoic acid receptor appears to lack this ability. Thus by coordinating the levels of thyroid hormone and retinoic acid, a large range of hormone responsiveness may be achieved.

Steroid Receptor Organization of Functional Elements

ORGANIZATION OF THE HORMONE BINDING DOMAIN. The structure of the hormone binding site on a receptor protein has not been determined by x-ray crystallography or other precise means. Rather, measurements of the relative binding activity of both agonists and antagonists have been used. When a large number of substituted steroids

CLASS	RECEPTOR	P BOX	D BOX	STEROID RESPONSE ELEMENT	SOURCE
I	GR, PR, MR AR	GSCKV GSCKV	AGRND ASRND	GGTACA-N$_3$-TGTTCT	Consensus
II A	ER	EGCKA	PATNQ	AGGTCA-N$_3$-TGACCT	Consensus
II B	TR-alpha TR-beta	EGCKG EGCKG	KYDSC KYEGK	AGGTCA——TGACCT	Consensus
				GATCA-N$_6$-TGACC	rGH
II C	RAR (alpha, beta, & gamma)	EGCKG	HRDKN	GATCA-N$_5$-TGACG	rGH
				GTTCAC-N$_5$-GTTCAC	RAR-beta
II D	VDR	EGCKG	PFNGD	GACTCA——TGAACG	hOsteocalcin

Figure 3–15. The SREs of the various steroid hormone receptors.

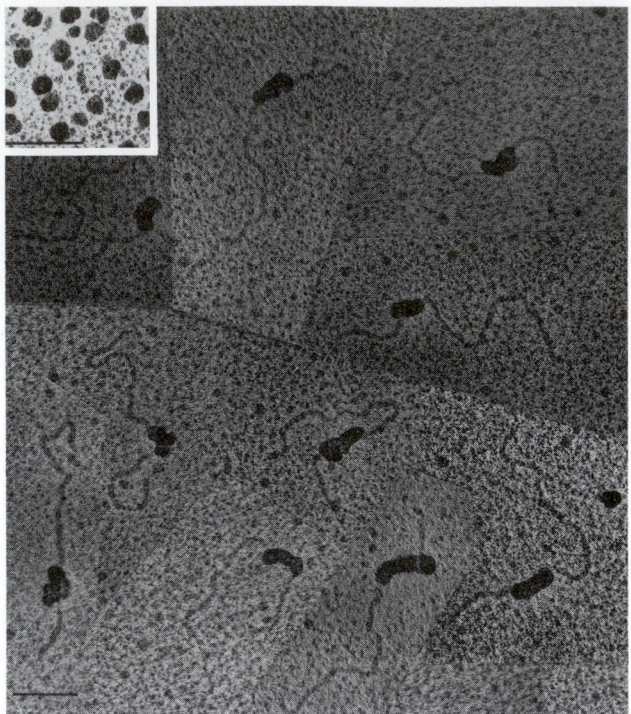

Figure 3–16. Electron micrographs of glucocorticoid receptors bound to DNA. Purified rat liver glucocorticoid receptors were bound in vitro to a 1453-base-pair DNA containing the region flanking the start of the MMTV proviral sequence. Multiple glucocorticoid receptors are bound, giving a globular appearance. Bar at lower left is 100 nm. *Inset:* Receptors alone without DNA. (From Payvar F, DeFranco D, Firestone GL, et al. Sequence-specific binding of glucocorticoid receptor to MTV DNA at sites within and upstream of the transcribed region. Cell 1983; 35:381–392. Copyright © by Cell Press.)

of a particular class is tested, a pattern of preferred structures and side groups can be discerned.

A hormone binding site consists of a hydrophobic pocket that is generally in contact with the steroid A ring with great precision and, with greater structural flexibility, the D-ring end of the molecule. Substituents at the latter end are also recognized. Progesterone and testosterone, for example, differ only at the D ring, but each hormone's receptor is selective for the proper hormone. No cofactors are known to participate in the hormone site. Use of metal chelators, exhaustive dialysis, or other treatments such as partial denaturation that are likely to dislodge such cofactors does not reduce hormone-binding activity.

Unlike the DNA binding domain, the steroid binding domain is less well localized and has only limited homology among the various receptors. Early proteolytic studies with affinity-labeled receptors suggested that steroid-binding activity resides in so-called meroreceptor polypeptides of 27 to 34 kd.[86–89] Progesterone, glucocorticoid, estrogen, and vitamin D receptor mutants that lack COOH-terminal residues are unable to bind steroid, suggesting that this steroid binding domain is at the COOH terminus.[8, 14, 51, 90–93] More direct evidence was obtained by insertional mutagenesis studies,[94, 95] which revealed that mutations in roughly the last 200 to 250 amino acids of the glucocorticoid and progesterone receptors abolish steroid-binding activity. Moreover, chimeric proteins involving these COOH-terminal residues fused to E1A[96] and to c-*myc*[97] conferred hormone-dependent regulation of transcription and transformation, respectively.

STUDIES USING COVALENT ATTACHMENT OF LABELED HORMONES. Steroids containing a Δ^4–3-keto group (progestogens, androgens, glucocorticoids) form highly re-

active free radicals on ultraviolet radiation. The free radical can attach to a protein at the hormone binding site. This strategy was used to label both chick progesterone receptor proteins. Results of such an experiment are shown in Figure 3–17. Labeling of either protein A or protein B was observed by [3H] fluorography of the dried gel after sodium dodecyl sulfate–polyacrylamide gel electrophoresis (SDS-PAGE). Simultaneous addition of excess nonradioactive progesterone blocked the photocoupling. Crude extracts can be analyzed because the high specificity and affinity of the receptor permit most of the covalent label to be coupled to the desired receptor and not to contaminants. From such an experiment, molecular weights of receptor polypeptides were determined. Similar photolabeling of mammalian progesterone and glucocorticoid receptors has been accomplished. An alternative approach was to use an estrogen antagonist, tamoxifen aziridine, as an affinity probe. This compound couples to estrogen receptor with an efficiency approaching 100%. Finally, steroid derivatives bearing alkylating substituents have been utilized for glucocorticoid receptor. The reagent dexamethasone 21-mesylate couples without ultraviolet radiation.

Proteolytic digestion in vitro of covalently labeled receptors has allowed detailed mapping of the proteins in many cases. In chicken progesterone receptor, for example, a unique progestogen-labeled peptide fragment (9.5 kd) has been isolated from both progesterone receptor subunits. Proteolysis under mild nondenaturing conditions reveals a series of progessively smaller receptor fragments bearing the hormone. Because discrete partial digests are produced, it is deduced that steroid receptors consist of a relatively protease-resistant hormone site linked to regions of the polypeptide that are relatively sensitive to proteases.

Affinity labeling of glucocorticoid receptor with [3H]dexamethasone mesylate forms covalent bonds via sulfhydryl groups at C-21 of the steroid. Using this approach, it was determined that Cys-656 of the rat glucocorticoid receptor[98, 99] and the corresponding Cys-644 of the murine glucocorticoid receptor[100] interact with the mesylate

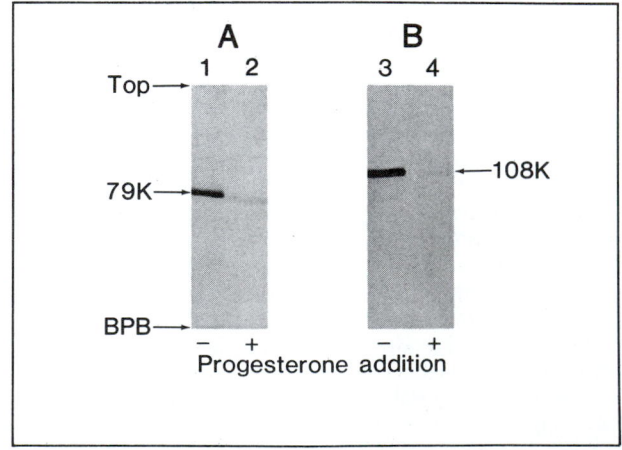

Progesterone Receptor Subunit Photoaffinity Labeling by [3H] R5020

Figure 3–17. Photoaffinity labeling of chick oviduct progesterone receptor and analysis by SDS-PAGE. After electrophoresis, gel was soaked in fluor and fluorography performed on x-ray film. Receptors were complexed in the crude state with [3H]promegestone (R 5020), a synthetic progesterone. Ultraviolet-induced photocoupling was done for each sample; reaction was blocked completely in lanes in which the sample also received an excess of cold progesterone. (From Birnbaumer M, Schrader WT, O'Malley BW. Photoaffinity labeling of the chick progesterone receptor proteins. J Biol Chem 1983; 258:1637–1644.)

group of dexamethasone 21-mesylate. Similarly, Cys-530 of the human estrogen receptor forms a covalent adduct with the affinity-labeling estrogens ketonestrol aziridine and tamoxifen aziridine.[101] Photoaffinity labeling by ultraviolet radiation of glucocorticoid receptor–[³H]triamcinolone acetonide complexes creates covalent adducts that interact with the A ring of the glucocorticoid receptor. Both Met-622 and Cys-754 interact with the A ring of triamcinolone acetonide.

Digestion of unliganded (no hormone present) rat glucocorticoid receptor with low concentrations of trypsin generates a 16-kd polypeptide fragment that binds dexamethasone mesylate with 23-fold lower affinity than does wild-type receptor.[102, 103] This cleavage peptide maps to Thr-537–Arg-673 and probably forms the core of the steroid-binding domain extending from Thr-537 to Lys-795. The core of the steroid-binding domain appears to have a highly conserved hydropathy profile and contains the sites of two known point mutations that abolish steroid binding, as well as two directly interacting residues. The "specific" portion of the steroid binding domain is conserved between the glucocorticoid receptor and the progesterone receptor, both of which bind to ligands with identical A rings.[104, 105] However, this region is markedly divergent in the estrogen receptor, which differs at the A ring. Consistent with this model of steroid-binding specificity, affinity labeling of the estrogen receptor showed a contact site within the specific portion of the steroid binding domain.

The molecular genetic approach of generating steroid-binding mutants has been less informative than the analogous DNA-binding experiments. The primary difficulty is that there is no way to distinguish active mutations that directly disrupt steroid interactions from mutations that disturb receptor structure globally. This problem is compounded by the fact that steroid-binding mutants occur over a broad range of the COOH terminus. For example, an S49 cell murine glucocorticoid receptor mutant with a single amino acid substitution at position 546 completely abolishes steroid-binding activity,[103] suggesting that the steroid binding domain is at least 240 amino acids long. However, a synthetic rat glucocorticoid receptor polypeptide extending from 547 to 795 (with a mass of 31 kd), which corresponds to positions 535 to 783 of the murine glucocorticoid receptor, has little affinity for the synthetic glucocorticoid dexamethasone. Mutations in the 31-kd portion of the receptor abolish ligand binding. Thus this region is necessary but not sufficient for ligand-binding activity. Similarly, a point mutation at position 400 in the human estrogen receptor causes a temperature-sensitive loss of steroid-binding activity.[106]

THE RECEPTOR DNA BINDING DOMAIN. Sequence comparisons of the earliest cloned steroid receptors suggested that the conserved 66- to 68-amino-acid C1 region coded for the DNA binding domain.[90, 105, 106] However, direct evidence was not obtained until receptor chimeras were constructed in which the 66-amino-acid DNA binding domain of the human glucocorticoid receptor was cloned in place of the homologous sequence of the human estrogen receptor.[23, 107, 108] This estrogen receptor–glucocorticoid receptor chimera was stimulated by estrogen to activate a glucocorticoid-responsive reporter gene but was unable to stimulate an estrogen-inducible gene. These experiments verified that the C1 domain contained all the information necessary for the sequence-specific recognition of target DNA. Alignment of the various C1 domains of the steroid receptors, as shown in Figure 3–18, reveals the high degree of homology. There are nine invariant cysteine residues with the potential to coordinate Zn^{2+} in a structure analogous to that of the protein transcription factor TFIIIA.[109] The technique of EXAFS (extended x-ray absorption fine structure) spectroscopy has demonstrated the coordination of Zn^{2+} or

Cd^{2+} by a tetrahedral arrangement of four cysteines in the glucocorticoid receptor.[110] Others have demonstrated by titration experiments that Zn^{2+} is required for maintenance of the DNA-binding activity[111] of certain steroid receptors. This type of arrangement predicts the occurrence of two fingers, as shown at the bottom of Figure 3–18, separated by a linker region of 15 to 17 amino acids. Unlike TFIIIA, which coordinates Zn^{2+} by a pair of cysteines and a pair of histidines, steroid receptors coordinate Zn^{2+} only with cysteines. Substitution of cysteine pairs with histidine pairs results in the inactivation of DNA binding,[112] and nonpaired substitution of cysteines with histidines partially inactivates DNA binding.[113] The ninth highly conserved cysteine appears to be nonessential for DNA binding, eliminating the possibility of an alternative finger structure involving this cysteine. These results underscore the structural differences between the fingers of TFIIIA and those of steroid receptors. Interestingly, genomic cloning of some of the steroid receptors reveals that the two Zn^{2+} fingers are coded in separate introns;[113–117] these fingers are sufficiently different in structure that if they arose by duplication, they have since diverged considerably.

Once it was established that DNA binding occurs through the specific arrangement of two Zn^{2+} fingers, experiments were directed at elucidating the structural features of these fingers that determine DNA-binding specificity (see ref. 118 for a review). The approach taken was analogous to that of studies of the *lac* repressor interaction with the *lac* operator sequence[119]—the generation of "change-of-specificity" mutations. Early experiments, performed by swapping individual fingers of the estrogen and glucocorticoid receptors,[120] suggested that the first finger is largely responsible for DNA sequence specificity. This result was unexpected because naturally occurring mutations in the tip of either finger in the vitamin D receptor cause hypocalcemic rickets.[6] In addition, other zinc finger proteins have a basal DNA-binding activity separable from other functions such as DNA sequence specificity and transcriptional activation.[121, 122] Several large-scale point mutation projects were initiated independently to identify which of the amino acids of the two zinc fingers determined target gene specificity.[123–125] A discussion of all the results of these experiments is beyond the scope of this chapter, but one set of revealing mutations is shown in Figure 3–19. The general strategy of these experiments was to start with a given steroid receptor and convert its target gene specificity by a series of stepwise mutations. In the experiment shown, human glucocorticoid receptor was converted to a "promiscuous receptor" that activated both glucocorticoid- and estrogen-responsive elements by a single Gly-to-Glu conversion in the second "knuckle" of the first finger (experiment 2). An additional conversion of the adjacent Ser to a Gly resulted in a hybrid receptor that activated a GRE reporter construct only weakly while activating the ERE reporter strongly (experiment 3). Almost complete conversion of glucocorticoid receptor to estrogen receptor was accomplished by the additional conversion of a Phe to a Gly. The amino acids required for this change in specificity are located in the proximal portion of the first finger, and hence this region is referred to as a P box (see Fig. 3–15). To complete the change in specificity from a glucocorticoid receptor to an estrogen receptor, an additional series of conversions (not shown) was necessary in the first knuckle of the distal finger, referred to as the D box (see Fig. 3–15).

These experiments reveal a class heterogeneity in the structure of steroid receptor DNA-binding fingers, also outlined in Figure 3–15. Two major classes of receptors differ primarily in the three variant amino acids of the P box. The first class includes the glucocorticoid, progesterone,

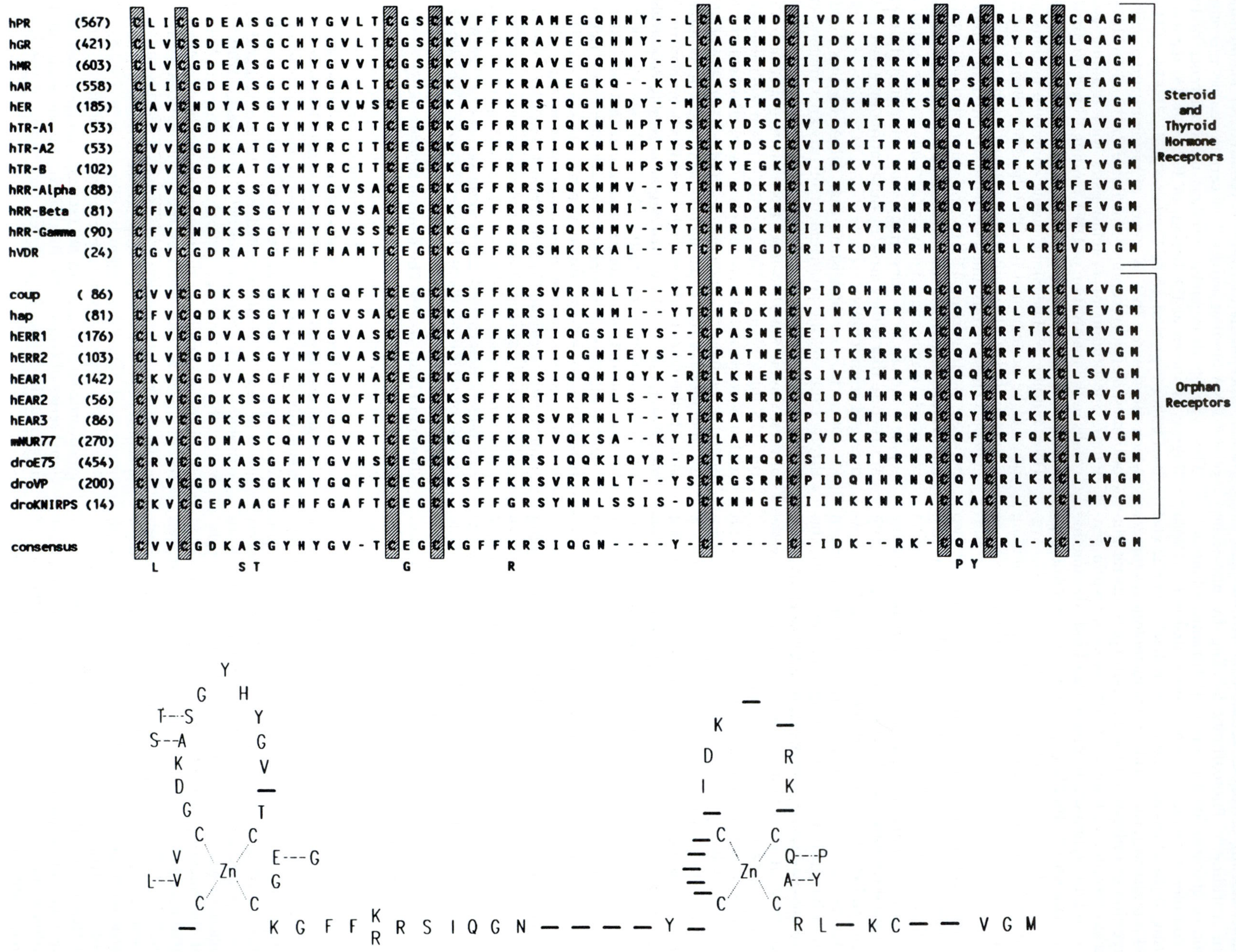

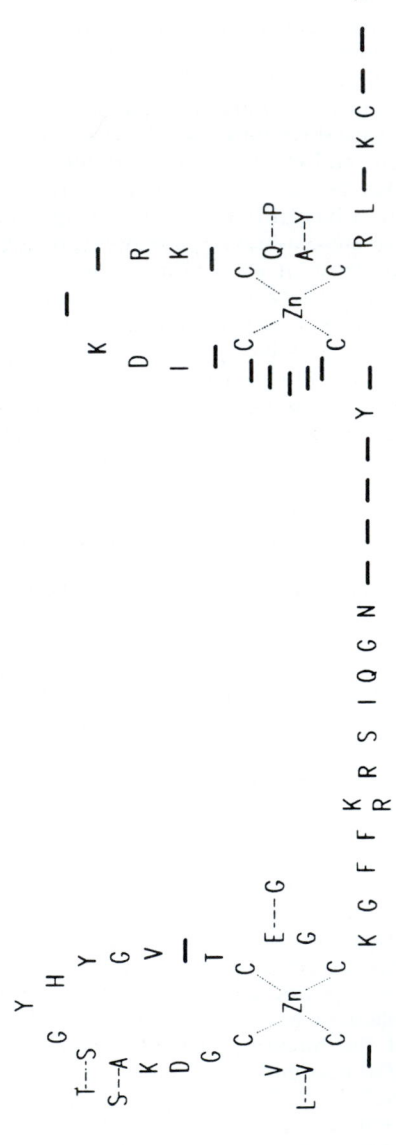

Figure 3–18. Sequence alignment of the DNA-binding domain (C1) of the various steroid receptors. There are nine invariant cyteines, which form the basis of two zinc coordinating finger structures.

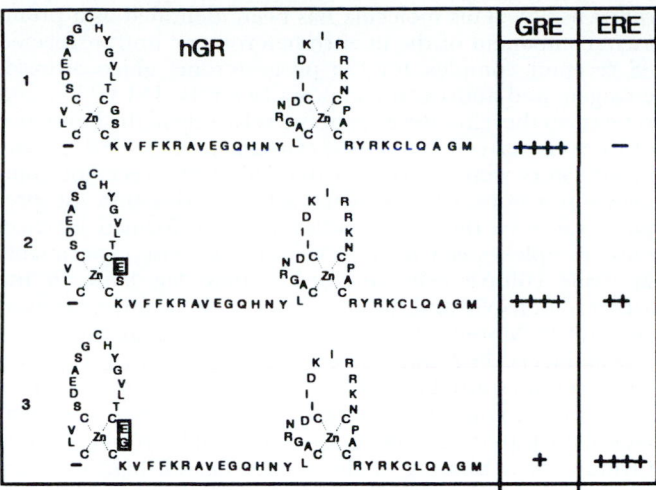

	GRE	ERE
hGR 1	++++	−
2	++++	++
3	+	++++

Figure 3–19. Summary of change-of-specificity studies. Boxed residues represent mutations to the wild-type receptor. Such experiments have defined two regions of the receptors that are largely responsible for sequence specificity.

mineralocorticoid, and androgen receptors, which are all capable of stimulating the same steroid response element as discussed earlier. The second class of receptors has similar P boxes but divergent D boxes. Thus each of these receptors can be broken down into subclasses. In this arrangement, the estrogen receptor exists in a class related to the thyroid hormone receptors. This interpretation is supported by the observation mentioned earlier that the ERE and the TRE differ only by a trinucleotide spacer. The thyroid hormone receptors also stimulate the rat growth hormone (rGH)-TRE, which contains a six-nucleotide spacer. As described earlier, the same TRE is also stimulated by the retinoic acid receptors and bears some resemblance to the retinoic acid response element found upstream of the retinoic acid beta gene.[126] Finally, the vitamin D receptor stimulates a response element that is also structurally similar to the consensus TRE. The vitamin D response element also lacks any spacer nucleotides. Although certain receptors may recognize the same or similar response elements within a class grouping, there are subtle differences in the mode of interaction with the target DNA.[127–129] These differences emphasize the role of additional amino acids in determining the final mode and outcome of receptor-DNA interactions.

TRANSCRIPTION ACTIVATION REGIONS. The ultimate function of receptors is to modulate specific effects at the transcriptional level. This function has been analyzed extensively in vivo using receptor-deficient cell lines into which expression vectors are introduced. These vectors contain cDNAs encoding receptors together with a receptor vector containing specific response elements linked to a gene whose product is readily assayable, such as chloramphenicol acetyltransferase or luciferase. Using these analyses, the regions of the receptor responsible for gene activation can be defined. For example, mutations that affect conserved cysteines in the C1 region result in loss of glucocorticoid receptor trans-activation function.[130] In the rat glucocorticoid receptor an 86-amino-acid region including the DNA binding region (C1) is sufficient to mediate gene activation in stably and transiently transfected cells.[131] Similar results were reported for the human glucocorticoid[132] and progesterone[133] receptors. However, in some cases the activation capacity of mutant receptors was low compared with that of wild-type receptors. A mutant of the human estrogen receptor that lacked the hormone binding domain exhibited only 5% of activity.[108] For several receptors, deletion of amino acids in the NH$_2$ terminus results in reduced activation capacity.[8, 108, 132–134] Thus multiple regions of receptors, both NH$_2$ terminal and COOH terminal, are involved in the transcriptional activation process.

With the exception of one point mutant of the human glucocorticoid receptor,[135] it has not been possible to separate the gene activation and DNA-binding functions of receptor molecules. However, functional hybrid proteins composed of the DNA binding domains from unrelated transcription factors linked to receptor hormone binding domains allow analysis of portions of the receptor molecules for activation potential independent of receptor DNA-binding activity. Trans-activation domains of several receptors have been identified using these chimeric receptor constructs. A trans-activation domain is defined as a portion of the protein that, when combined with DNA-binding activity, produces an increase in transcriptional initiation.[136, 137] Chimeric proteins containing the hormone binding domain of the human estrogen or glucocorticoid receptor and the DNA binding domain of the yeast transcription factor GAL4, which itself has no intrinsic activation function, exhibited hormone-dependent activation of a GAL4-responsive reporter gene.[138] These results indicate the presence of an activation domain in the hormone binding region of the estrogen and glucocorticoid receptors. This trans-activation domain in the human glucocorticoid receptor is in a 30-amino-acid region (tau2; amino acids 526 to 556) in the COOH terminus of the molecule.[139] A second trans-activation domain (tau1; 185 amino acids in length—amino acids 77 to 262) was identified in the NH$_2$-terminal region of the protein. Both sequences appear to function independently of their position in the molecule and are acidic in character. In the rat glucocorticoid receptor, an enhancer region, enh2, is located in the NH$_2$ terminus from amino acid 106 to 318.[140] This region is further localized to an 82-amino-acid region (amino acids 237 to 318) and is not analogous in sequence to the enhancer region defined for the human glucocorticoid receptor.[141] Thus receptors contain two or more activation domains. These regions are indicated in Figure 3–20.

The chicken and human progesterone receptors provide a unique system in which to analyze the function of the NH$_2$ terminus of the protein because the A protein lacks more than 100 amino acids, including a highly acidic region found in the NH$_2$ terminus of the B protein. Differential activation of transcription was reported for the chicken progesterone

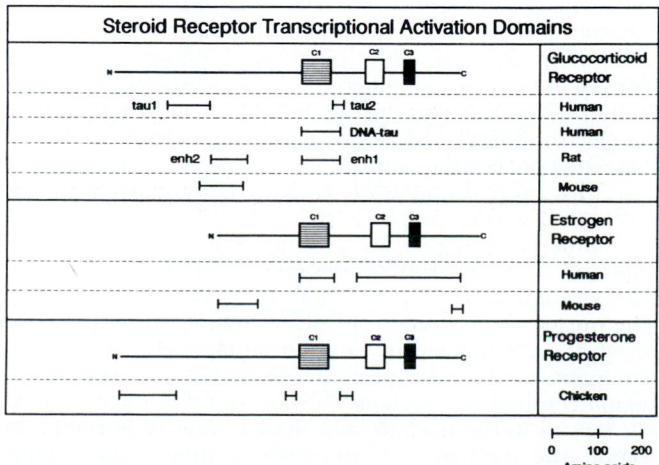

Figure 3–20. Steroid receptor trans-activation domains. Horizontal bars below each receptor schematic show boundaries of the receptor required for retention of the function.

receptor. The receptor A protein but not the B protein was able to activate transcription from the ovalbumin promoter, whereas both proteins activated transcription from a reporter plasmid containing a GRE or PRE fused to the thymidine kinase promoter and the chloramphenicol acetyltransferase gene.[142, 143] The lack of activation of ovalbumin by protein B was further investigated using a chimera of the human estrogen receptor and the NH$_2$-terminal 128 amino acids of the progesterone receptor B protein. This fusion protein did not induce ovalbumin gene transcription, whereas the estrogen receptor alone did.[143] These results suggest an inhibitory role for the NH$_2$-terminal domain that is independent of DNA-binding specificity. In addition, this region may help to determine gene specificity.

Regulatory elements do not exist as isolated pieces of DNA in vivo but rather are arranged in complex chromatin structures. It is probable that to achieve appropriate gene activation, receptors must interact with other transcription factors or with structural components of chromatin. However, little is known about these interactions.

Interactions of Receptors with Other Proteins

RECEPTOR DIMERIZATION. Although dimerization of the estrogen receptor has been known for more than a decade,[88, 89] the relevance of this phenomenon for the other steroid receptors has only recently been determined. That is, dimerization facilitates the binding of steroid-receptor complexes to target DNA enhancer sequences.[144] However, receptor monomers are equally capable of binding to nonspecific DNA sequences such as calf thymus DNA.[145] The first demonstrations of functional receptor dimer–DNA complexes were accomplished by mixing experiments with receptor mutants of various sizes.[146, 147] The formation of receptor heterodimer–DNA complexes generated an intermediate band in the gel retardation assays, confirming that two molecules of receptor bind to a single DNA response element. However, because the end point of the assays was based on DNA-binding activity, these experiments were unable to determine whether the receptors dimerized before binding DNA or bound cooperatively on a DNA template. A 2:1 stoichiometry of receptor protein molecules to DNA has been established using a combination of glycerol gradient sedimentation and double labeling.[148] In addition, gluteraldehyde cross-linking, which stabilizes receptor monomers as dimers, had no effect on the apparent Stokes radius determined by gel filtration. This result suggests that the glucocorticoid receptor is a homodimer in the absence of binding DNA. More direct evidence for receptor dimerization in the absence of DNA was obtained for the progesterone receptors by both chemical cross-linking and nondenaturing gradient gel electrophoresis.[149] In these experiments receptor homodimers were shown to exist in the absence of steroid ligand, and they were capable of binding quantitatively to the progesterone DNA response element.

Some clues suggesting a dimerization motif have also emerged from experiments designed to analyze the nuclear translocation signals of the rabbit progesterone receptor.[150] The nuclear translocation signals of the rabbit progesterone receptor were defined by deletion mutagenesis. A constitutive signal was found at position 638 to 642. Deletion of this region resulted in a mutant that was found in the cytoplasm but moved to the nucleus with the addition of hormone. A second site (663 to 930) suggested a dimerization signal because a nuclear monomer mutant was able to facilitate the nuclear translocation of a cytoplasmic monomer mutant.

INTERACTIONS WITH NONRECEPTOR PROTEINS. Certain steroid receptors bind to a 90-kd heat shock protein called hsp90. This molecule has been identified as a prominent component of the in vitro heteromeric untransformed 8S receptor complex for the progesterone, glucocorticoid, estrogen, and androgen receptors (see refs. 151 to 154 and references therein). Because of the relatively high abundance of hsp90 in the cell (1 to 2% of cytosolic proteins[155, 156]), many investigators were concerned that the hsp90-receptor complex was a nonspecific in vitro artifact. Although the preponderance of the early studies were performed in vitro, these complexes can form in vivo. Pulse-chase experiments in tissue culture cells revealed a time lag between the synthesis of hsp90 and the association with the glucocorticoid receptor.[157] Moreover, chemical cross-linking of the receptors in intact cells resulted in covalent association of hsp90.[158] Thus, certain steroid receptors can interact with hsp90 under physiological conditions. When a steroid receptor is complexed to hsp90, the 8S complex is unable to bind to calf thymus DNA. Binding of the steroid ligand, high salt concentrations, high temperature, and various other treatments facilitate the dissociation of this 8S complex to the 4S to 5S receptor forms. One physiological implication is that hsp90 may be involved in the hormone-induced activation of certain steroid receptors, but this remains to be proved.

Deletion mutagenesis mapping studies have been performed on the glucocorticoid and progesterone receptors to try to determine the hsp90 interaction site.[159, 160] Both studies have localized a fairly large COOH-terminal region that includes a large portion of the steroid binding domain. Interestingly, small deletions created throughout this entire region do not disrupt the formation of an 8S complex.[160] Thus the receptor may have multiple hsp90 contact sites. Monospecific polyclonal antibodies generated against peptide fragments within the DNA binding domain[161, 162] and the linker region[163] are sterically prohibited from binding when the receptor is in the 8S form.

In addition to hsp90, a number of other proteins have been described in association with the untransformed 8S receptor complex. A 59-kd protein, p59, is associated with the progesterone, estrogen, androgen, and glucocorticoid receptors.[164] Although less is known about p59, it does appear to be predominantly an intranuclear phosphoprotein.[165]

Another nonreceptor component of the untransformed 8S complex is hsp70.[166] hsp70 is a highly conserved protein in all cells from bacteria to higher eucaryotes. Normally hsp70 is found in the cytoplasm. However, under stress it is concentrated in the nucleus of the cell, where it activates certain target genes in the heat shock response.[167] Unlike hsp90, hsp70 binds ATP and may be a member of the energy-dependent chaperonin class of proteins that are thought to be involved in protein folding.[168] Although salt and heat treatment alone are not sufficient to cause hsp70 to dissociate from the progesterone receptor, high concentrations of ATP do cause dissociation.[166] The role, if any, of hsp70 in mediating steroid receptor function is still unknown.

RECEPTOR ACTIVITY MODIFICATIONS BY PHOSPHORYLATION. All steroid receptors studied to date are phosphoproteins. This type of post-translational covalent modification is another potential pathway for control of hormone action, particularly if a phosphorylation is hormone dependent. However, the functional significance of steroid receptor phosphorylation has yet to be determined.

Phosphorylation has been implicated in the hormone-binding capacity of the androgen,[169] estrogen,[170] and glucocorticoid[171] receptors. Phosphatase studies of the androgen receptor suggest that hormone binding is enhanced by the presence of phosphotyrosine.[172] In the case of the estrogen receptor, hormone-binding activity requires the presence of phosphotyrosine.[173] Moreover, treatment of estrogen receptor synthesized in vitro with a purified tyrosine kinase increases the hormone-binding capacity from 1–4% to near-maximal levels.[174] Other work has shown no evidence for this pathway. In contrast, the progesterone receptor appears to be phosphorylated exclusively on serine residues,[175] and the glucocorticoid receptor contains 89% phosphoserine and 11% phosphotyrosine.[176] Thus it is not clear that the phosphorylation-dependent hormone-binding requirements of the estrogen and androgen receptors can be extended to all steroid receptors.

Hormone-dependent phosphorylation of the steroid receptors results in a characteristic decrease of mobility by SDS-PAGE.[177] This characteristic upshift has been used successfully as a means of correlating receptor modification with function. The human progesterone B receptor in breast tumor cells in culture has a nascent molecular mass of 114 kd. About 6 to 10 h after hormone treatment of the cells, the receptor undergoes a phosphorylation maturation step that results in increased apparent molecular masses of 117 and 120 kd by SDS-PAGE.[178] Studies using [35S]methionine pulse-chase labeling and immunoaffinity purification demonstrated that the phosphorylation maturation is not necessary for hormone-binding activity.[179] Similarly, progesterone receptor purified from hormone-treated cells can be used for DNA-binding filter assays. In that analysis, the hormone-induced phosphorylation of the progesterone receptor had no effect on the absolute affinity for DNA.[180] In contrast, other studies of hormone-dependent receptor processing have indicated that crude preparations of the progesterone receptor from cells treated with hormone have an enhanced affinity for DNA.[181, 182] Because similar hormone treatments increase the phosphorylation of the progesterone[183–185] and glucocorticoid[186] receptors, it is widely held that phosphorylation may regulate the DNA-binding and/or transcriptional activation functions of steroid receptors.[187]

Receptor Localization in the Cell

ANTIBODIES TO RECEPTOR PROTEINS. Monoclonal and polyclonal antibodies that recognize specific receptors for each steroid have been obtained. In no case have receptor antibodies cross-reacted with the receptor for a different hormone. However, some monoclonal antibodies are reactive against the same receptor from other species. Thus the proteins are distinctly different for each hormone but are conserved to some degree among species extending at least from birds to mammals. Receptor antibodies have now been used to develop sensitive assays not dependent on hormone binding.

IMMUNOCYTOCHEMISTRY. Immunocytochemical localization of receptor proteins within cells has been used to measure receptors in tissues, in cells in culture, and in solid-tumor biopsy specimens. These studies have had two interesting results. First, estrogen receptor and progesterone receptor have been identified in nuclei of cells whether hormone is present or not. This finding suggests that the original view of receptors as exclusively cytoplasmic proteins until hormone is present may be based on an artifact of cell fractionation techniques.

Second, comparison of estrogen receptor–rich human breast tumor sections with receptor-poor specimens (as shown by biochemical analysis) shows that receptor-poor tumors contain foci of cells containing the normal high receptor titer interspersed with cells appearing to lack receptor in this assay. Thus within a tissue—be it tumor or normal—cell heterogeneity will be reflected in varying receptor titers. This finding may contribute to our understanding of how cell sensitivity to hormones may be regulated through alterations in receptor levels.

The intracellular localization of steroid receptors has been studied extensively in broken cell preparations. Glucocorticoid, progesterone, and estrogen receptors are readily isolated in cellular cytosols in the absence of hormone, whereas after hormone treatment receptors are extractable only at high salt levels. Thus it was proposed that cytoplasmic receptors bind hormone and rapidly translocate into the nucleus.[188–190] With the production of specific antireceptor antibodies and the development of immunocytochemical techniques, progesterone, estrogen, and androgen receptors were found to be primarily nuclear in the absence of hormone treatment.[191, 192] Nevertheless, several studies revealed immunoreactive glucocorticoid receptors in the cytoplasm of cells[193–196] in which progesterone receptor was exclusively nuclear. Part of this difference may be due to the use of antibodies that are characterized only partially with respect to reactivity with structural determinants of the native receptors. It remains unclear whether the histochemistry reflects epitope exposure or cellular localization. Fixation conditions, as with any immunocytochemical question, also alter the results to some degree. This aspect is particularly vexing with detection of very low levels of a protein, as for the steroid receptors.

Immunofluorescence analysis using a β-galactosidase–specific antibody revealed that glucocorticoid receptor–galactosidase fusion proteins are almost exclusively cytoplasmic in the absence of dexamethasone.[197] Fluorescent signals become nuclear with the addition of hormone. In contrast, detection of cytoplasmic native glucocorticoid receptor results from diffusion of the receptor from the nucleus in the absence of hormone.[198] The rate of glucocorticoid receptor diffusion from the liver cell nuclei of adrenalectomized rats is higher in the presence than in the absence of dexamethasone and is higher than the diffusion rate of progesterone receptor. These data suggest that glucocorticoid receptors may be primarily nuclear regardless of the hormonal state. Thus the cellular localization of glucocorticoid receptors in the absence of hormone remains uncertain. It is clear, however, that all receptors reside in the nucleus after hormone administration.

Nuclear localization of proteins occurs by two mechanisms: diffusion of proteins through the nuclear membrane and interaction of proteins with the nuclear pore, a process mediated by a translocation signal in the protein.[199] In the former case, the exclusion limit for spherical proteins is a molecular mass of 67 kd,[200] although the elliptical shape of steroid receptors[201] might facilitate their diffusion despite their larger size.

Amino acid sequences that bear strong homology to the nuclear translocation signal of simian virus 40 T antigen[202, 203] are present in several steroid receptors. These sequences, shown in Figure 3–21, are located on the COOH-terminal side of the DNA-binding (C1) region. Nearly identical sequences are found in the glucocorticoid, progesterone, androgen, and mineralocorticoid receptors from various species. In contrast, sequences in this region of the estrogen, vitamin D, thyroid, and retinoic acid receptors do not exhibit strong homology to the T antigen nuclear localization signal. Vitamin D and thyroid receptors are tightly associated with the nucleus even in the absence of hormone and therefore may differ from the larger receptors in their subcellular localization mechanisms.[204–206]

Receptor sequences have been shown to function as nuclear translocation signals in the rabbit progesterone[207] and rat glucocorticoid receptors by analyses of deletion mutants.[197, 208] For the rabbit progesterone receptor this

"Nuclear Localization" Sequences of the Steroid Receptors and SV40 T antigen								
Protein	1st. AA	Sequence						
SV40 T Ag.		P	K	K	K	R	K	V
GR	491	R	K	T	K	K	K	I	K
MR	673	R	K	S	K	K	L	G	K
AR	628	R	K	L	K	K	L	G	N
PR	637	R	K	F	K	K	F	N	K
ER	256	R	K	D	R	R	G	G	R
T3Rβ	179	K	R	L	A	K	R	K	L
RAR	162	R	K	A	H	Q	E	T	F
VDR	102	R	K	R	E	M	I	L	L

Figure 3–21. Nuclear localization sequences determined by comparison with a known sequence of this type present in simian virus 40 (SV40).

sequence is the primary signal, but a second minor signal requires activation of the DNA binding domain to function. Unlike the case of the progesterone receptor, the primary signal for nuclear localization of rat glucocorticoid receptor deletion mutants is located in the steroid binding domain of the molecule and is unrelated to sequences found in T antigen.[21, 54]

HORMONAL CONTROL OF GENE EXPRESSION

Hormone Effects on Protein and RNA Synthesis

Hormones regulate growth, differentiation, and metabolic activity in most tissues. The regulation of protein synthesis is undoubtedly the principal action of steroid hormones, although certain metabolic processes are exceptions to this rule. Early experiments suggested that general protein synthesis could be stimulated by steroid hormones, and studies with antibodies to specific proteins confirmed this concept. Because RNAs play a central role in the control of protein synthesis in microorganisms, a large body of experimental evidence accumulated suggesting that animal hormones also regulate the amount of cell enzymes and secretory proteins via RNA mediators. Studies in the 1960s revealed that all major RNA fractions are stimulated by steroid hormones.[208–210] These observations cast some doubt on the specificity of the role of new RNA molecules. The early evidence favoring mRNA accumulation as the mechanism for regulating protein synthesis was based on general observations such as hormonal stimulation of nuclear RNA polymerase activity and inhibition of steroid effects on protein synthesis by the RNA synthesis inhibitor dactinomycin (actinomycin D).[208, 211–213] The concept was stimulated further by nearest-neighbor analysis (dinucleotide composition analysis) of RNA synthesized from the chromatin template isolated from tissues before and after gonadal steroid hormone administration, which showed a qualitative hormone-mediated change in nuclear gene transcription.[213, 214] The advent of nucleic acid hybridization methods permitted studies showing that either estrogen or progesterone stimulated the production of new RNA species. These findings suggested strongly that steroid hormones could exert a qualitative influence on DNA transcription.[214]

REGULATION OF MESSENGER RNA LEVELS. The initial indication that steroid hormones lead to elevated cellular mRNA levels was the result of studies of the chicken oviduct using RNA translated in vitro with ribosomes from rabbit reticulocytes. The synthesis of radiolabeled ovalbumin is dependent on prior administration of estrogen.[210, 215–218] After purification of the ovalbumin mRNA to near-homogeneity, a radioactive cDNA probe was synthesized using reverse transcriptase and employed in hybridization studies to quantify the number of ovalbumin mRNA molecules per cell. The data are summarized in Table 3–1.[9] In the absence of hormone, oviduct cells contained less than five copies of ovalbumin mRNA. Within 4 h after stimulation with DES, the mRNA reached levels greater than 2000 molecules per cell, and by 24 h the level approached 20,000 molecules per cell. The accumulation curves are consistent with an effect of steroid hormones on ovalbumin gene transcription.

HORMONES INCREASE THE RATE OF MESSENGER RNA SYNTHESIS. Although these and other results were consistent with the primary effect of steroid hormones being at the level of gene transcription, it could be argued that the rate of transcription remains relatively constant during induction and that the accumulation of mRNA is due simply to the prevention of RNA degradation by steroid hormone. In fact, evidence exists that in certain cases steroid hormones can indeed decrease the turnover of mRNA. Definitive answers to these questions required synthetic analyses of pulse-labeled RNA obtained in nuclear runoff assays.

In the chick oviduct, nuclei were obtained before and after hormonal stimulation of target cells. The nuclei were incubated with radioactive precursors to RNA, and the labeled RNA was hybridized to cloned ovalbumin cDNA or natural gene fragments. In the absence of hormone, no synthesis of radiolabeled mRNA was detected, but within 1 h after the exposure of cells to steroid hormones an induction of synthesis was observed. Under these conditions, an accurate assessment of the rate of mRNA synthesis could be obtained.[216, 219] In similar studies, induction of MMTV transcription was observed when liver tumor cells were exposed to glucocorticoids.[220–222] The intracellular concentration of viral RNA was increased 100-fold. Subsequent studies in the same system revealed that the rate of MMTV gene transcription is near maximal within 15 min of exposure of tissue culture cells to dexamethasone. This extremely rapid response was consistent with a more direct effect of the hormone-receptor complex on DNA transcription rather than with a complex set of intermediate reactions or with a requirement for a newly synthesized intermediate protein.

TABLE 3–1. Induction of Ovalbumin mRNA During Acute Estrogen Administration*

Hormonal Status	Number of Ovalbumin mRNA Molecules/Cell
Withdrawn	4
0.5 h × DES	9
1 h × DES	50
4 h × DES	2300
8 h × DES	5100
29h × DES	17,000
7 d × DES	43,000
Egg-laying hen	147,000

*Chicks were treated with DES for 10 d and then withdrawn from hormone for 11 or 12 d. The animals were then injected with a single dose of DES for the times indicated. Molecules of ovalbumin mRNA per cell were calculated from cDNA hybridization data.

Reprinted with permission from Harris SE, Rosen JM, Means AR, et al. Use of a specific probe for ovalbumin mRNA to quantitate estrogen-induced gene transcripts. Biochemistry 1975; 14:2072. Copyright 1975 American Chemical Society.

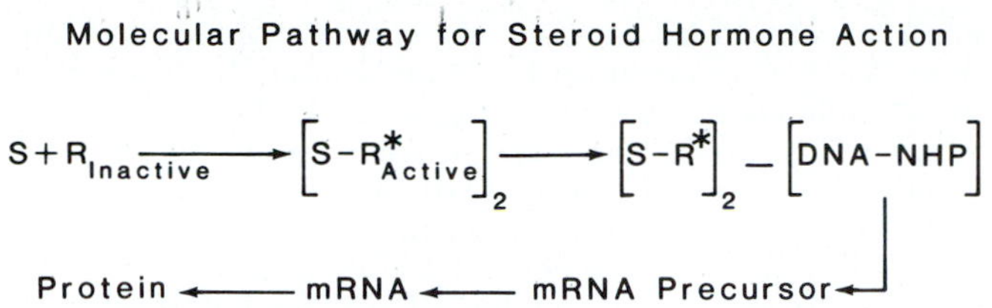

Molecular Pathway for Steroid Hormone Action

$$S + R_{Inactive} \longrightarrow \left[S - R^*_{Active}\right]_2 \longrightarrow \left[S - R^*\right]_2 - \left[DNA-NHP\right]$$

$$Protein \longleftarrow mRNA \longleftarrow mRNA\ Precursor \longleftarrow$$

Figure 3–22. Steroid hormone (S) enters the cell and binds to an inactive receptor (Rinactive) in nucleus (or cytoplasm). The receptor is activated and binds to nuclear DNA as a dimer. This activated dimer complex binds upstream of genes to regulatory sites (DNA-NHP) composed of DNA and nonhistone chromosomal protein (NHP). This interaction leads to synthesis of mRNA precursor, which is processed to mature mRNA before exiting the nucleus. The mRNA is then transported to the cytoplasm, where it is translated on polysomes to produce the induced protein.

These results were subsequently confirmed for the actions of additional steroid hormones on the synthesis of a variety of mRNAs in other systems.[223, 224] The molecular pathway for steroid hormone action is summarized in Figure 3–22.[225–229] It should be noted, however, that not all steroid responses at the level of DNA may be inductive. For example, evidence exists that glucocorticoid actions on pro-opiomelanocortin mRNA and prolactin mRNA and on thymus cell function may be inhibitory; that is, transcription of specific mRNAs is decreased in the presence of hormone. Nevertheless, the totality of studies has provided definitive evidence that the major effect of steroid hormones is to induce the accumulation of specific mRNAs in target cells, and for the most part the effect is at the level of gene transcription.

HORMONES REGULATE MESSENGER RNA STABILITY. The majority of inducible proteins are synthesized from inducible mRNAs. In the case of steroid hormones, for instance, it is rare for increased protein levels not to result from increased mRNA levels via stimulation of gene transcription. If such mRNAs and proteins were totally stable, they would soon reach an infinite concentration. Therefore, differential stability is a fundamental property of mRNAs and proteins that makes biological regulation possible.[230] Average half-lives of eucaryotic mRNAs range from 8 to 20 h; the average half-life for protein is about 48 to 72 h. Labile mRNAs contain structural features that make them unstable in cells via nuclease degradation. Although various sequence motifs exist, one common feature of labile mRNAs consists of uridine residues interspersed with occasional adenine residues, denoted by $(U)_nA$. These structures occur most commonly in 3'-nontranslated regions of unstable mRNAs and are thought to be sites of attack for endonucleases. Deletion of these residues leads to stabilization of the mRNA.[231] In addition to their well-known effects on gene transcription, hormones can coordinately lead to stabilization of mRNA and protein products emanating from their target genes. This is a powerful combination in that a 5-fold increase in transcription coupled with a 5-fold increase in both mRNA and protein half-lives can result in a 125-fold increase in the protein product of that gene. One of the most dramatic illustrations of mRNA stability occurs in *Xenopus* liver cells under the influence of estrogen. In the absence of steroid hormone, vitellogenin mRNA has a half-life of 16 h; in the presence of estrogen its half-life is 500 h.[232] The half-life of total poly(A) mRNA in these cells is unaffected by hormone. These data on mRNA stabilization were established by constructing a minivitellogenin gene containing 5'- and 3'-untranslated regions of the mRNA that lacked over 5000 nucleotides of internal coding sequence and transfecting it into cells.[231] The mini-mRNA was stabilized by estrogen, and the stabilization was dependent

on the presence of estrogen-receptor complex. Evidence such as this argues that the mRNA stabilization occurs via a receptor-dependent process and involves information contained in 5'- and 3'-untranslated regions of the molecule.

Gene Structure and Evolution

The advent of recombinant DNA technology led to a revolution in our ideas about the structure and evolution of eucaryotic genes. We realized for the first time that genes are split into pieces and that the protein-coding information is assembled at the RNA level. This information changed our theories about the evolution of eucaryotes and humans in particular.[233–236]

GENE STRUCTURE. In eucaryotic cells, the structure of genes is characterized by the peptide-coding information lying in noncontiguous segments along the DNA.[237, 238] The DNA regions that correspond to sequences expressed in the mature message are referred to as *structural sequences* or *exons*. Exons include both the coding regions that are translated into protein and the nontranslated regions that appear in the mature mRNA. The regions of DNA within the native gene, as defined genetically, but between segments that encode parts of the mature RNA product, we call *intervening sequences* or *introns*. The gene is thus an alternating series of exons and introns, the introns being eliminated from the mature cytoplasmic RNA by splicing reactions within the nucleus of eucaryotic cells. Figure 3–23 is a schematic representation of a simple eucaryotic gene containing two exons and a single intron. This amazing genetic structure was first observed for the genes in adenovirus, followed closely by similar documentation for a large number of eucaryotic genes such as those for the globins, the immunoglobulin light chains, ovalbumin, immunoglobulin heavy chains, ovomucoid, and insulin. Only a limited number of genes, such as those coding for the histones and for adrenergic receptors, are devoid of intervening sequences. The majority of eucaryotic structural genes contain intervening sequences ranging from as few as one (an insulin gene) to as many as 50 (a collagen gene).[234, 235, 239, 240]

INTRONS. The lengths of introns are variable, ranging from as short as 50 bases to as long as 10,000 or more bases. Introns occur in both the coding region and the untranslated parts of the ultimate mRNA. Introns for the most part are different in sequence with the exception of a few general homologies such as a CAGG tetranucleotide at each of the two ends of introns. There is an absolute requirement for a GT at the 5' end and an AG at the 3' end of all the intron sequences. The intron sequences are generally pyrimidine rich, especially at the 3' end. The combined length of the intron sequences of a gene is greater than the combined length of the exons, causing the gene to spread across the genomic DNA to a greater length than the final coding capacity would require. In other words, genes are not

Structure of a Simple Eucaryotic Gene

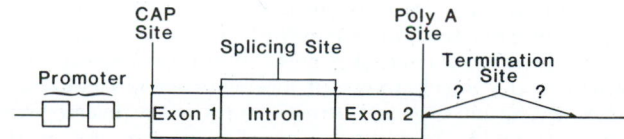

Figure 3–23. Most genes are composed of exons (structural sequences retained in mature mRNA) and introns (intervening sequences removed during splicing of pre-mRNA). Transcription begins at CAP site and ends at poly(A) site. Exact point of termination is variable among genes. Initiation of transcription by RNA polymerase is controlled at promoter region.

An Evolutionary Hypothesis for the Origin of Intervening Sequences

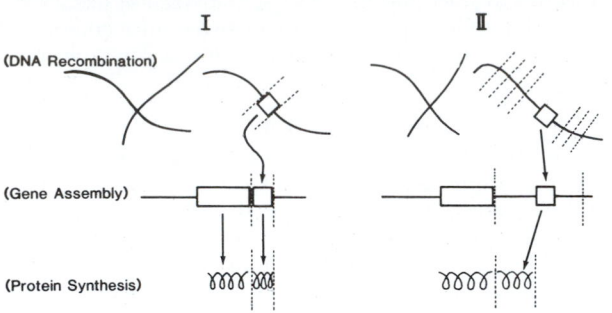

Figure 3–24. Column I depicts gene assembly from diverse exon elements in a manner that would not account for introns. Column II represents a more likely method of gene assembly that accounts for the generation of introns. See text for details.

compressed exact structural counterparts of their mRNAs but instead exist as entities many times longer than required to code for these protein products. The existence in genes of intervening sequences or introns is a feature of eucaryotic organisms and is not found in procaryotic organisms such as bacteria.[235, 237]

GENE EVOLUTION. Since the recognition of the structure of eucaryotic genes, a number of roles have been postulated for introns. They have been suggested to be (1) protective elements that prevent recombination by unequal crossing over between families of closely related genes, (2) adventitious structural features of genes reminiscent of random insertions in DNA by transposition, (3) regulatory elements that control either the production of biologically active mRNA or its export to the cytoplasm, or (4) remnants of the evolutionary construction of genes. The evolutionary hypothesis for the origin of intervening sequences is now more generally accepted. A hypothesis for the probable origin of intervening sequences is shown in Figure 3–24. The open boxes represent coding regions of DNA (exons), and the thin solid lines represent either introns or flanking DNA sequences. Column I shows gene assembly from diverse exon elements without the benefit of introns, and column II represents the alternative method of gene assembly in which introns are generated. It is statistically unlikely that large eucaryotic genes coding for peptides would arise by simple point mutations that eventually become arranged in a continuous appropriate sequence to code for amino acid assembly into protein. It is more likely that genes evolved by the assembly of blocks of coding sequence during DNA recombination. Column I shows the problem inherent in the assembly of complex genes from diverse exon segments. The recombination must occur at precise sites at either end of the exon. Otherwise, the reading frame of the resulting mRNA would be altered and the functional integrity of the resulting polypeptide possibly destroyed. Because the recombination process itself is random, a requirement for absolute precision in breakage (or excision) of the segments of DNA to be reassembled makes the event an occurrence of low probability. Thus the evolutionary process would be lengthened greatly. Column II depicts the same event as it is now thought to have occurred, leading to the development of modern complex eucaryotic genes. Recombination, to bring together the diverse exon segments, could occur at any one of numerous sites in the flanking DNA sequence on either side of the exon sequences. This model greatly facilitates genetic evolution because the probability of occurrence is orders of magnitude greater than for the model depicted in column I. In this manner,

eucaryotes could have a faster genetic development per unit time. As shown in column II, recombination by this mechanism would create an intervening sequence between the two exons. This would pose no problem provided an early mechanism existed (or developed) for splicing these introns out of the primary RNA transcripts. Such a process would allow the rapid development of a diverse functional gene. Evidence from a large number of sources has shown that such RNA-splicing enzymes do exist and that introns do not provide a barrier to functional gene expression. Once assembled, the introns would provide two additional evolutionary advantages to the organism. Recombination of exons from separate genes could occur. Such exon shuffling could permit the rapid assembly of new combinations of coding sequences, which, if they provided a selective advantage to the organism, could be held constant. In addition, homologous recombination would be facilitated by the extra length of the intron existing between exon units. This would allow proteins to duplicate their own exons and grow in length. If this argument is correct, the introns should be located within eucaryotic genes in specific sites separating functional domains for the protein. This has proved to be the case for a number of proteins, such as immunoglobulins, myoglobin, ovomucoid, globin, glyceraldehyde-phosphate dehydrogenase, proinsulin, and α-FP.

A theoretical example of the evolution of a complex gene coding for a secretory protein is shown in Figure 3–25. In an early stage of evolution a primitive gene existed that coded for a functionally inefficient protein a. A second exon coding for a peptide b that complemented peptide a was brought into the genetic unit via recombination. Because peptide b provided peptide a with increased functional efficiency, the recombination was stabilized by positive selection. With time, an intragenic duplication of the gene occurred via unequal crossing over to provide exons a′ and b′. This led to a larger, even more efficient protein and the duplication was stabilized. This event provided more evolutionary flexibility because exons a′ and b′ were now free to undergo small "trial mutations" without disrupting the basic function of exons a and b, thereby eventually providing a broader range of activity for the gene product as a whole. Finally, to provide advantageous secretory capacity for the protein, a "signal" exon was acquired by a fortuitous but stabilized recombination event. The final resulting gene

Evolution of a Multidomain Secretory Protein

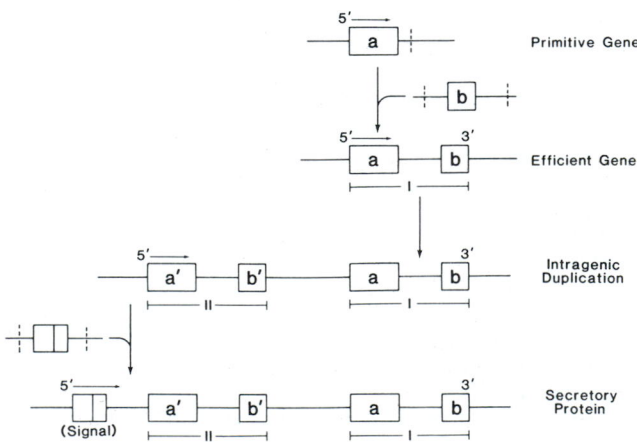

Figure 3–25. A primitive gene (exon a) evolves by a recombination event, which brings a new exon (b) into the gene unit. At this point the gene is composed of two exons and one intron. An intragenic duplication event occurs, probably by unequal crossing over, followed by addition of a final exon, which acts as a signal sequence for secretion. Final gene unit contains five exons and four introns.

structure is displayed in Figure 3–25. This general structure is not uncommon among structural genes. The question arises of how the splicing reaction evolved. It appears that the earliest RNA molecules were capable of self-splicing; that is, no enzyme protein was required for removal of introns or nonsense sequences. This fascinating observation was first proved in *Tetrahymena,* in which splicing of a ribosomal RNA precursor was observed in the absence of protein.[241] In this instance, GTP acts as an attacking group to break the RNA chain at the correct phosphodiester site and eliminate the intron as an RNA circle, followed by religation of the exons. This reaction of RNA catalysis is inefficient, and with time enzyme-RNA complexes termed *splicesomes* evolved, which improve the accuracy and efficiency of this process. These functional complexes are composed of proteins and small nuclear RNAs and are located in the nuclear compartment.

Processing of Messenger RNA Precursors

During the transcription reaction, the entire gene (exons plus introns) is transcribed 5′ to 3′ (left to right, Fig. 3–26) as one high-molecular-weight precursor that exactly represents the genetic sequence. In this form the precursor mRNA is inactive biologically (nontranslatable) for the production of protein. For translation to be possible, the introns must be removed to produce the smaller biologically active cytoplasmic mRNA that consists only of a series of contiguous exons joined together in the order in which they are represented in DNA. This means that colinearity of gene and protein exists between the individual exons and the corresponding parts of the protein chain.[242–248]

PRECURSOR MESSENGER RNA. The primary transcript (pre-mRNA) is acted on by the splicing or processing enzyme that recognizes and removes the intervening-sequence RNA. it. The enzymatic splicing reaction requires two independent steps: (1) excision of the intron and (2) ligation of the adjacent exons to form an uninterrupted coding sequence. When cytoplasmic and nuclear RNA is extracted from a chick oviduct, run on denaturing gels, and analyzed by hybridization to a cloned [32P]cDNA probe of ovomucoid, the results shown in Figure 3–27 are obtained. In the cytoplasm, a single ovomucoid mRNA species of 1100 nucleotides (NT) represents the biologically active mature mRNA. When the nuclear RNA is examined, a series of

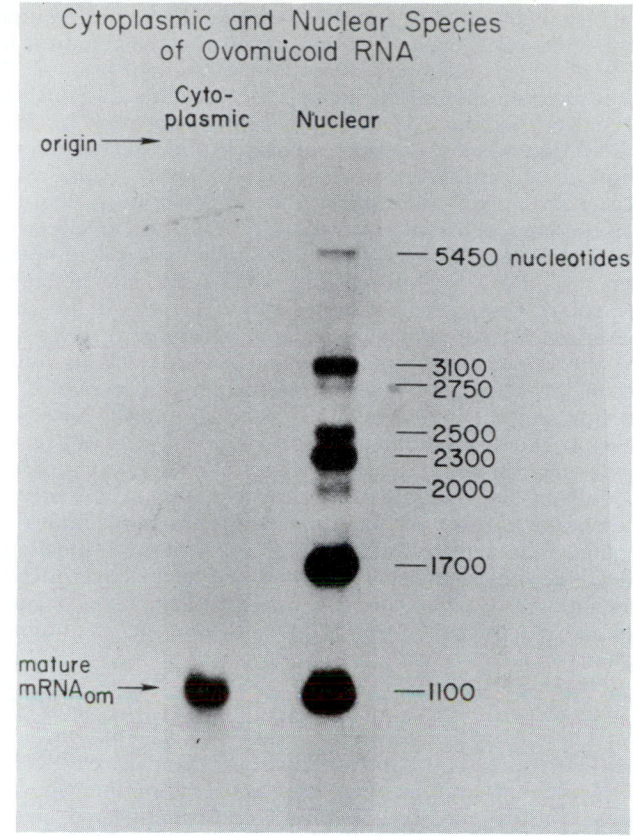

Figure 3–27. Northern blot hybridization to detect mRNA precursors. RNA has been extracted from cytoplasm and from purified nuclei of oviduct cells. RNA is separated according to size on a denaturing gel, and ovomucoid RNA is detected by hybridizing to a [32P]ovomucoid DNA probe. Cells were washed and subjected to autoradiography. Film shows dark bands in all regions where ovomucoid RNA exists. As shown, cytoplasm contains only mature mRNA devoid of introns. In contrast, nucleus contains high-molecular-weight species of ovomucoid RNA, representing primary transcript (5450 nucleotides) and various processing intermediates.

discrete bands is noted. This suggests that splicing occurs via preferred pathways rather than in a random manner. The largest band of nuclear RNA (5450 NT) corresponds to the size of the gene and represents the primary transcript that contains the RNA complement of eight exons and seven introns. The smaller band is again the mature mRNA devoid of introns. In between, each band represents a particular precursor intermediate from which some but not other of the introns have been removed. For instance, the intermediate of size 1700 NT contains only one remaining intron of 600 NT (see Fig. 3–27). The general conclusion implicit to these analyses is that the conformation of the RNA may influence the accessibility of the splicing junctions to the enzyme.[246–251] The excision of introns in pre-mRNA may occur on small nuclear RNA templates in combination with protein (small nuclear RNA particles, SNRPs).[242] Probably with the aid of the SNRP template, the splicing enzyme recognizes the 5′ beginning (donor site) and the 3′ end (acceptor site) of the intron and positions itself so that it can excise accurately the intron sequence from the pre-mRNA.[252, 253] The 5′ and 3′ junctions of introns from different genes share a common but imperfect homology (e.g., CAGGT) called a *consensus sequence.* In the RNA introns *always* begin (5′ end) with a G-U base pair and end (3′ end) with an A-G base pair. Excision usually occurs between a G-G base pair. After excision of an intron, the adjacent exon ends are ligated in a reaction that is likely to require ATP. No evidence exists that exons of different RNA molecules

Transcription of the Natural Ovomucoid Gene

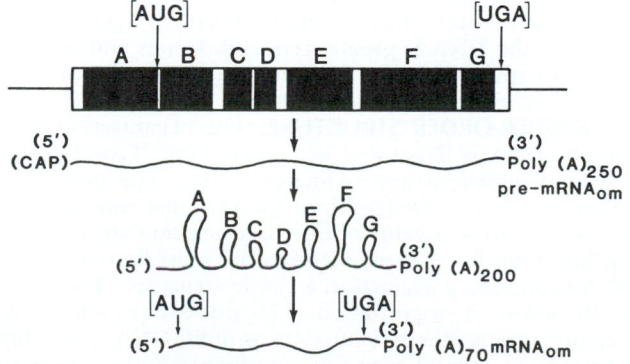

Figure 3–26. Ovomucoid gene of chicken contains eight exons and seven introns. Primary transcript contains a continuous RNA copy of the entire gene. It receives a CAP at the 5′ end, and poly(A) is added to the 3′ end. It attaches to nuclear matrix, where a complex splicing enzyme system removes all intron sequences (labeled A to G). When transcript is free of introns, it detaches from matrix and is transported to cytoplasm, where it can be translated.

can be joined together. Introns are removed in a preferential order and occasionally a single intron may be removed in several steps. It is thought that the processing of pre-mRNA takes place on the nuclear matrix because almost all nuclear pre-mRNA is bound to the matrix whereas mature nuclear mRNA does not demonstrate such a preferential attachment. Unprocessed mRNA precursor is not found in the cytoplasm, most likely because its release from the matrix requires removal of all introns. The splicing involved in removal of introns from pre-mRNA may be a rate-limiting step for mRNA generation and could serve as a potential control reaction for regulating mRNA levels in the cell. Nevertheless, the available evidence does not support the hypothesis that hormones regulate mRNA levels by influencing processing of mRNA precursors. The existence of introns and the requirement for their removal, however, have provided the etiological basis for a new series of genetic diseases. Gene mutations occurring in the middle of individual introns are generally without effect because the introns are not part of the mRNA. In contrast, mutations in intron sequences immediately adjacent to the intron-exon junctions interfere with their splicing and create an inactive mRNA containing a residual intron. A number of examples of such mutations have been reported in diseases such as human thalassemias.

MATURE CYTOPLASMIC MESSENGER RNA. A typical structure of a eucaryotic mRNA is shown in Figure 3–28. The CAP site is defined by the first nucleotide (+1) of the mRNA precursor (and consequently the mature mRNA), which is generally a purine followed by a pyrimidine. Shortly after synthesis of pre-mRNA, a hypermethylated pyrophosphate containing nucleotide (guanine) is added to the structural nucleotides (e.g., N_1, N_2) so that a final average 5' end of an mRNA molecule can be represented as $M^7G(5')ppp(5')N_1mp-N_2p...$, with m representing the methyl groups. The CAP site is often followed by an untranslated leader region followed by a ribosome binding site approximately 40 bases long that includes the initiation codon (AUG or GUG) for translation. If the mRNA codes for a secreted protein, the subsequent region contains a signal sequence that codes for a short processed peptide (15 to 30 amino acids) and provides the means for ribosomes translating the mRNA to attach to the intracisternal membranes as a complex. In this manner, secreted proteins can be channeled into the appropriate cytoplasmic compartments and membranes. The coding sequence is followed by a termination codon (UAA, UAG, and UGA), which ends protein synthesis and causes release of the mRNA from ribosomes. The termination codon is followed by an untranslated region that is variable in size and sequence among mRNAs.[235, 236] The 3' terminus of eucaryotic mRNA contains a string of 30 to 150 adenylic acid residues. The poly(A) sequence is not coded in the DNA but is added in the nucleus after transcription. This poly(A) tail may aid in stabilization and/or in export of the mRNA to the cytoplasm. The hexanucleotide AAUAAA at the 3' end of all mRNAs about 25 nucleotides before the poly(A) tail appears to act as a polyadenylation signal for the poly(A) polymerase. It is

important to note that transcription need not end at the last nucleotide of the last exon. In fact, in certain cases gene transcription may terminate thousands of nucleotides downstream from the exon terminus. In each case, however, the extra nucleotides are removed in concert with the addition of poly(A) to the last nucleotide of the terminal exon. Although transcription termination and poly(A) addition are potential regulation sites for expression of viral genes, no such evidence has evolved for native eucaryotic genes to date.

Organization of Eucaryotic Chromosomes

The human cell contains 3×10^9 base pairs of DNA and contains information for about 100,000 functional genes. This extraordinary length of DNA must fit into the nucleus of a cell whose diameter may be only 6 μm. In addition, most (90%) of the DNA in most cells is not called into action for cellular functions. For these reasons, it seems logical for the cell to package most of its DNA into inaccessible higher-order chromosomal structures such that the length of the DNA is greatly reduced. Genes and segments of DNA expressed in the lifetime of a given cell must be in a more accessible structure.[254–259]

HIGHER-ORDER STRUCTURE. The organization of eucaryotic DNA is illustrated in Figure 3–29. Free DNA has a fiber diameter of approximately 2 nm. The ratio of the length of DNA to the length of the unit that contains it can be normalized to a value of one. Because an extremely high packing ratio for the genetic material must be reached, the DNA cannot be packaged in a single structure. There must be *hierarchies* of organization. The nuclear proteins play a role in forming this structure, so protein-DNA interactions form a fundamental basis for the organization of eucaryotic DNA. The primary structural interaction for the formation of eucaryotic chromosomes is that between histone and DNA.[256, 260, 261] There are five basic histones (H1, H2A, H2B, H3, and H4). All the histones except H1 interact directly with DNA to form a first-level organization of particles in

Higher Order Level of Chromatin Organization

Structure	Fiber Diameter (nm)	Compaction Ratio
Free DNA	2.5	1
Strand of Nucleosomes	10	6
"Solenoid"	30	40
Interphase Chromosome		1,000
Mitotic Chromosome		10,000

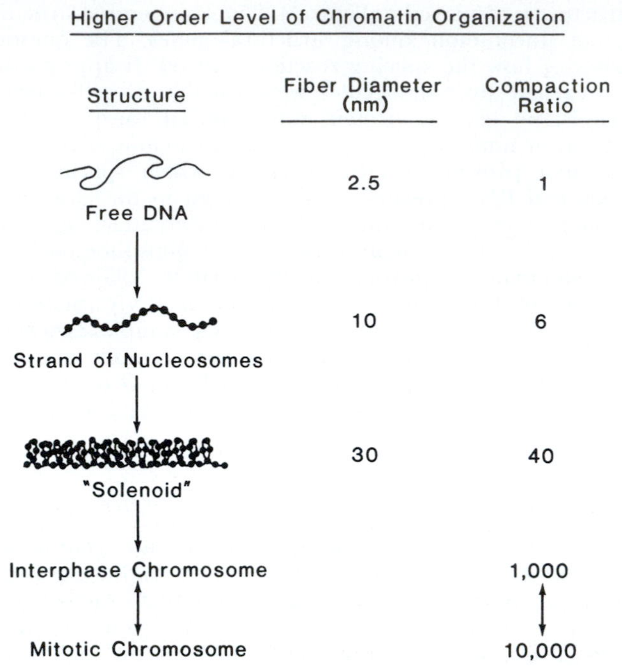

Figure 3–29. Free DNA is successively packaged into higher levels of organization by complex supercoiling. At each level, the length of the DNA is reduced by a factor approximating the compaction ratio. This packaging is due primarily to interactions with histones.

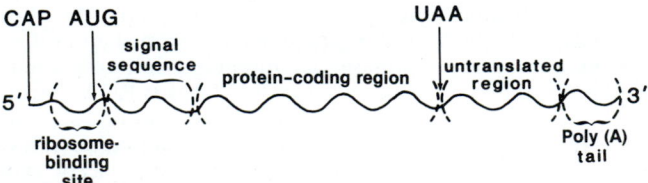

Figure 3–28. Functional regions of mature (cytoplasmic) mRNA. See text for details.

chromatin. This basic level of organization of chromatin is the histone octamer, which in combination with about 200 base pairs of DNA forms bead-like structures (nucleosomes) along the DNA, increasing the fiber width to 10 nm and creating a length compaction ratio of 6 (see Fig. 3–29). The DNA is wound around the outside of the core histone particles and may be available to interact with regulatory proteins or RNA polymerase. This nucleosomal level of organization is now supercoiled on itself, like a giant "Slinky," into a structure referred to as a solenoid.[262, 263] Histone H1 plays a critical role in linking the nucleosomal strands to produce the solenoid. The fiber now becomes thicker (30 nm) and the length compaction ratio reaches approximately 40. The final structural organization of chromatin is not well understood but probably involves a further supercoiling of the solenoid to achieve a final length compaction ratio of approximately 1000 in interphase chromosomes. The mitotic chromosomes are packaged even more tightly to a length compaction ratio of approximately 10,000. The second group of proteins involved in chromosomal organization are the nonhistone proteins.[263, 264] There are probably hundreds of different species of nonhistone proteins. They include all of the proteins necessary for replicating and transcribing DNA, in addition to the enzymes involved in structural and covalent modifications or degradations. Most important, however, are the regulatory proteins, which play an important role in determining the appropriate structures for gene expression and in aiding or retarding the initiation of transcription. This group of proteins is the object of intense experimentation.[259, 264, 265]

ACTIVE DOMAINS IN CHROMOSOMES. Expressible genes are packaged into chromatin differently than are regions of the DNA that are genetically repressed.[264, 266, 267] In particular, genes that are transcriptionally active or have the potential for rapid expression in response to appropriate inducers are more susceptible to cleavage by nucleases. Such genes include globin, ovalbumin, vitellogenin, insulin, immunoglobulin, histone, and a variety of integrated genes for viral proteins. It is thought that nuclease sensitivity is simply the result of accessibility to the enzyme because the DNA exists in a more unraveled or "open" superstructure. Considering the variety of genes and systems studied and the fact that no expressible gene has been reported to exist in a nuclease-resistant state in the cell in which it will be expressed, acquisition of a nuclease-sensitive structure appears to be a general prerequisite to the potentiation of eucaryotic gene expression. It is possible to define the borders of nuclease sensitivity around expressible genes with cloned DNA fragments as specific hybridization probes.[264] Using the technique in which isolated nuclei are digested with DNase I to render 15% of the DNA acid soluble, it is possible to show that the DNase I–sensitive conformation extends well beyond the boundaries of the transcription units of genes into the sequences that flank the 5' and 3' ends of the genes. The DNase I sensitivity appears to reflect a region of more accessible chromatin structure that is related to the developmental capacity of a cell to express the gene in question. It can be viewed as a necessary but not wholly sufficient step in the prior commitment of the cell to allow a given gene to be transcribed (Fig. 3–30). Such a mechanism would make it possible for individual cell types to respond to a single inducer in an individual and distinctive manner.[267, 268] In the chicken, the size of these chromosomal DNase I–sensitive domains ranges from 20 kb for the glyceraldehyde-phosphate dehydrogenase gene to over 100 kb for the three ovalbumin gene family members. The domain containing the constitutive glyceraldehyde-phosphate dehydrogenase gene is sensitive to DNase I in all cells because it is expressed in all cells. In the case of a domain containing hormone-

Relationship Between Cell Differentiation and DNase I Sensitivity of Tissue-Specific Genes – A Working Model

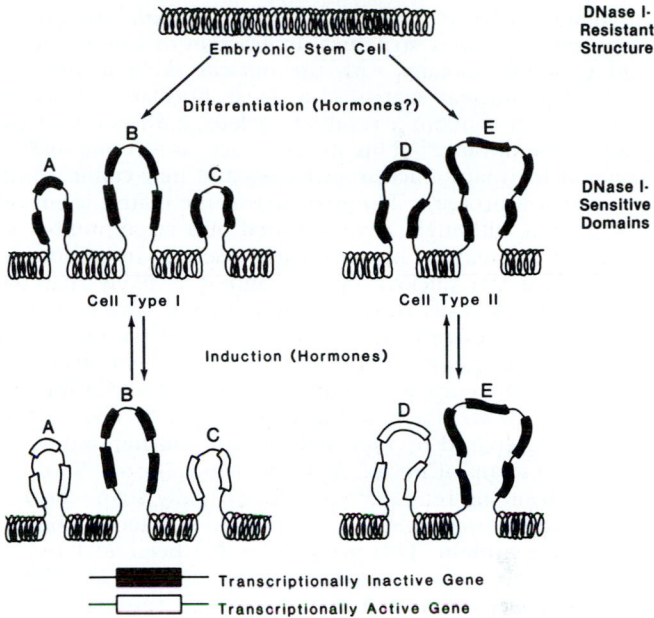

Figure 3–30. At early stages of differentiation, much of DNA is packaged into higher-order structure with histones and is unavailable to interact with either biochemical probes such as DNase I or regulatory molecules such as steroid receptors and RNA polymerase. During differentiation, regions of genomic DNA that contain potentially expressible genes are converted to "open" or uncoiled structures, which are now accessible to regulatory molecules and RNA polymerase. This structure is necessary but not sufficient for expression. Hormone-receptor complexes now bind to these regions and activate the genes.

regulatable genes such as the ovalbumin gene family, the genes are sensitive to DNase I only in the oviduct target cells in which these genes are expressed. Furthermore, when the transcription of ovalbumin X and Y genes is eliminated by the withdrawal of hormone from estrogen-stimulated chickens, the entire domain remains in a DNase I–sensitive configuration. For this reason DNase I–sensitive domains may provide the chromosomal structural capacity required for gene expression, and they appear to be a result of the differentiation process because they are cell specific and contain all of the potentially expressible genes of that cell type (see Fig. 3–30). Sequences called dominant control regions are present at the borders of these large chromosomal domains.[269] They are thought to maintain the domain structure, perhaps by binding certain proteins and preventing the packaging of the DNA into the solenoid structure and repression of the included genes. Such sequences are likely to be repetitive in nature and may be composed of cis elements (e.g., enhancers) that bind cellular transcription factors and prevent the folding and packaging of protein-free DNA by histones at the time of DNA replication. In other words, all genes that are capable of transcription in a given cell must be contained within these accessible regions of chromatin at the time of terminal differentiation. The chromosomal domains appear to be related to molecular differentiation because they both tissue specific and irreversible. In the absence of functioning dominant control region complexes, the DNA that is not contained in these domains appears to be passively packaged into a more complex and inaccessible chromatin structure by histones. The DNA in such higher-order structures—most of the DNA in each cell type—is unavailable for subsequent interactions with regulatory molecules. In contrast, DNA in an "expressible" domain contains genes accessible to regulatory factors such as hormone-receptor complexes (see Fig. 3–30).[267, 268]

NUCLEAR MATRIX. It is appropriate to conclude a discussion of higher-order structure by consideration of an even more complex structural interaction of cellular genes and genomic domains with the nuclear skeleton (matrix) itself. The nuclear matrix is a dense fibrillar network of proteins that contains a residual nucleus and lies within the nuclear membrane.[270] This structure acts as a framework or skeleton for many nuclear processes and may connect with cytoskeleton proteins. The structure of the matrix is not yet understood, although it is composed of a large number of different proteins. The chromatin itself is intermittently attached to the nuclear matrix, and it is likely that the primary RNA transcripts of genes become attached soon after or even during their transcription. RNA processing also may take place on the matrix. The salient structural features of the eucaryotic matrix, as defined by Coffey and collaborators, are illustrated in Figure 3–31.[270] The nuclear matrix is prepared by repeated low-salt and high-salt (2 M NaCl) extraction of nuclei. Approximately 10 to 15% of the nuclear proteins remain.[270, 271] This virtually strips the nucleus of all histone and a great deal of the loosely bound nonhistone protein. This preparation has been analyzed by electron microscopy and sedimentation analysis. The dehistonized and uncoiled DNA is attached to the residual protein matrix in short regions interspersed with unattached "loops" of DNA that average 30 to 100 kb in length (not shown in Fig. 3–31). If the dehistonized and unattached DNA in the loops is digested with a site-specific restriction endonuclease, 85% of the DNA can be released from the preparation. The residual matrix-bound DNA, representing 15% of the total, can be purified and analyzed for the presence of specific sequences. In the chicken, all actively transcribed genes are firmly bound to the proteinaceous nuclear matrix.[271, 272] All genes not expressed are in the released DNA fraction after restriction enzyme treatment because they are not attached to the matrix. Specific hormone-regulatable genes such as the ovalbumin gene are attached to matrix during hormonal stimulation. In contrast, when hormone is withdrawn and ovalbumin gene transcription ceases, the gene is no longer attached to the matrix. Constitutively expressed genes are always attached to the matrix, and the attachment is inde-

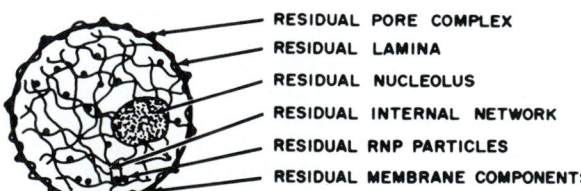

NUCLEAR MATRIX
(RESIDUAL NUCLEAR SKELETON)

RESIDUAL PORE COMPLEX
RESIDUAL LAMINA
RESIDUAL NUCLEOLUS
RESIDUAL INTERNAL NETWORK
RESIDUAL RNP PARTICLES
RESIDUAL MEMBRANE COMPONENTS

- LIPID FREE
- REPRESENTS ONLY 10% OF TOTAL NUCLEAR PROTEINS. CONTAINS RELATED PROTEINS
- SITE OF ATTACHMENTS OF DNA LOOPS
- CONTAINS FIXED SITES FOR DNA SYNTHESIS
- ASSOCIATED WITH HnRNA
- SPECIFIC BINDING OF HORMONES
- PROTEINS PHOSPHORYLATED
- MAY HAVE DYNAMIC PROPERTIES

Figure 3–31. Major structural features of nuclear matrix. (Courtesy of Dr. Donald S. Coffey, Johns Hopkins School of Medicine.)

Determinants for Hormonal Induction of Gene Expression

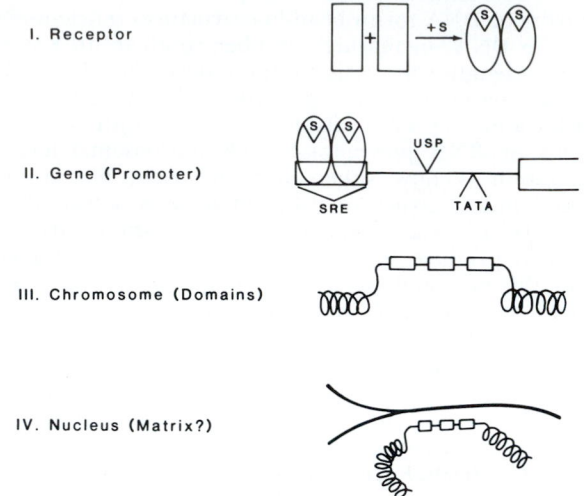

I. Receptor

II. Gene (Promoter)

III. Chromosome (Domains)

IV. Nucleus (Matrix?)

Figure 3–32. Major structural levels of control are (I) steroid-receptor interaction; (II) regulatory sequences around (or in) structural genes; (III) chromosomal structure, including "expressible domains"; and (IV) interactions of chromosomal genes with nuclear matrix.

pendent of the absolute rate of transcription. This close relationship between the transcription of genes and their association with the nuclear matrix indicates that the nuclear matrix is a likely site for cellular DNA transcription. This conclusion is consistent with the idea that the nucleus is a highly organized organelle and that transcription does not occur free in solution in the eucaryotic nucleus but rather occurs on a fixed protein skeleton. Such attachment to the matrix could either facilitate transcription of DNA by RNA polymerase or be a concomitant of transcription. Cessation of transcription in the presence of dactinomycin does not itself lead to release of genes from the matrix.

Steroid hormone receptors have also been found associated with the nuclear matrix. On hormonal withdrawal, the cellular receptors are no longer associated with the nuclear matrix. Although receptors may play some role in the attachment of inducible genes to the nuclear matrix, it appears unlikely that the hormone receptor is the sole protein responsible for binding an active gene to the matrix.

STRUCTURAL REQUIREMENTS FOR GENE EXPRESSION. The cellular forces involved in steroid hormone induction of transcription are complex indeed. These parameters are summarized in Figure 3–32. At a minimum, there are several major structural determinants for induction of gene expression:

1. The steroid receptor is activated by hormone, dimerizes, and binds DNA. The receptor is the obligatory and active intermediate required for steroid hormone action and acts as a transducer to transfer the informational signal inherent in a steroid hormone molecule to the regulatable gene. Steroid hormone receptors are members of a larger, as yet undefined, class of nuclear transcription factors.

2. The primary sequence of the gene to be expressed contains not only the inherited structural code for the protein but also distinct promoter and enhancer elements, both of which bind transcription factors and receptors and determine the maximal rate of hormone-induced gene expression. An enhancer element is the cognate DNA binding site for the receptor dimer.

3. Inducible genes are contained within large structurally distinct (DNAse I–sensitive) domains that are an index

of molecular differentiation and probably maintain the capacity of genes to respond to inductive influences.

4. The chromatin itself undergoes a specific attachment to the nuclear matrix so that the actively expressed regions of these domains appear to be more firmly bound and perhaps more easily transcribed by the nuclear transcription apparatus.

This picture is complicated by other potentially important levels of substructure such as modification of primary DNA sequence (e.g., methylation and Z-DNA, a left-handed coil of DNA)[224] and chromatin fine structure (nuclease hypersensitivity).[265, 273] Only by obtaining more precise structural and functional information about each of these levels of regulation can we understand completely the molecular mechanism for steroid hormone action. To accomplish this task continued application of the combined technologies of molecular biology and cellular biology is required.

Regulatory Elements Located Adjacent to Genes

During the transcription of eucaryotic genes, RNA polymerase must initiate and terminate at specific sites on DNA. The initiation reaction requires the formation of a tightly bound complex between RNA polymerase and DNA at a site that surrounds the first base to be transcribed into RNA. There is a limited amount of RNA polymerase in eucaryotic cells, ranging from 5×10^4 to 10^5 molecules per cell. When one considers that as many as 10^4 genes may be expressed in a given cell type, it is obvious that this enzyme is not in great excess. For this reason, the cellular genes are in competition for RNA polymerase and must seduce the enzyme to their respective regulatory regions to be transcribed. The region of DNA that is necessary for the formation of the initiation complex with RNA polymerase is called the promoter-enhancer region. It may include the DNA sequence that is stably bound in the initiation complex as well as other sequences in the vicinity whose recognition is necessary but which are not an integral part of the stable binding site (Fig. 3–33). The promoter appears to act as a thermostat to regulate the rate and accuracy of transcription. Additional regulatory elements adjacent to the promoter region may act as enhancers to activate further (or alternatively to "silence") functional promoters. Hormone control elements are one example of the enhancer class of regulators.[274–279]

PROMOTERS. The basic promoter for eucaryotic genes transcribed by RNA polymerase II appears to consist of two main parts (see Fig. 3–33). Beginning at −30 nucleotides (30 bases upstream) before the start site of transcription is the proximal promoter, a 7 base pair AT-rich sequence called the TATA box. A consensus sequence for all TATA boxes can be described as TATAT/AAT/A. The TATA box may contain either an A or a T in positions 5 and 7, and in a minority of cases a G-C pair is present within the box. This sequence is required absolutely for accurate and efficient initiation of transcription at nucleotide +1 of the structural gene. Changing only one interior nucleotide pair in the sequence to a GC residue is usually sufficient to eliminate 80% of the appropriate transcription from that gene.[280] Further upstream (to the left) of the structural gene is an additional sequence within the promoter that has been conserved in many instances. This distal element lies at approximately −80 nucleotides from the gene itself and consists of a series of subfamilies related in sequence. This sequence is commonly referred to as an upstream promoter (USP) element and is thought to be important in modifying the basal *rate* of transcription as determined for a given promoter (see Fig. 3–33). The proximal (TATA box) and distal (USP) elements of the promoter function as a unit to encourage RNA polymerase to bind and initiate transcription.[281]

ENHANCERS AND SILENCERS. Enhancer elements are short (about 15 base pairs) sequences that lead to an increased rate of transcription of adjacent genes. They are located usually in the 5'-flanking region of eucaryotic genes but are position and orientation independent to a large degree (see Fig. 3–33). Genes that are expressed at high levels may have multiple enhancers. In contrast, silencers are cis elements that work in an opposite fashion to regulate genes negatively. They act to decrease or silence transcription of genes in the absence of strong positive regulation (see Fig. 3–33). For example, if a silencer is present the adjacent gene has a low or zero basal rate of transcription in the absence of enhancer activation. Both enhancer and silencer elements are activated by cognate trans-acting factors that bind with specificity and high affinity to the core recognition sequences.[282] Enhancers may be of two general classes: regulatable and nonregulatable (see Fig. 3–33). In relation to the field of endocrinology, we may consider them as steroid hormone–regulatable or steroid hormone–independent enhancers. The steroid-regulatable enhancer or SRE is activated when it is bound by hormone-receptor complexes.[69, 82, 283] Steroid-independent sites require specific interactions with other trans-acting factors. Each steroid receptor type has a strong affinity for its cognate SRE sequence. This affinity is over 1000 times greater than the receptor's affinity for nonspecific DNA sequences. The receptor's affinity for an SRE is a dominant force in the protein's ability to find these small (15 base pair) SRE regulatory sequences among the 3 billion base pairs of DNA in the human genome. This reaction is of prime importance for selective regulation of genes by steroid hormones. We have learned only recently how the steroid-activated receptor molecule binds to its SRE. The SRE is composed of two half-sites, each of which binds one molecule of steroid receptor.[146, 147, 284] This dimer of receptor is bound tightly and stably and has a significant ability to stimulate gene transcription. Stability is important in this instance because the length of receptor residence time on the SRE should be related to the potency for stimulation of transcription. In fact, optimal stability seems to be provided when a second dimer binds to another nearby enhancer and the two dimers touch each other. Two SREs have a much greater effect (>10-fold) on gene expression than does one; in this case 1 + 1 = 10, not 2. It is thought that if the two SREs are located at a distance from one another, the DNA can bend in such a way that the receptor dimers come into proximity with each other and couple (Fig. 3–34). This type of "protein-protein touching" seems to be a general mechanism whereby trans factors are stabilized at their respective cis elements and gene expression is thereby stimulated. Ptashne,[285] in an elegant series of studies of microorganisms and yeast, has highlighted the mechanism and importance of protein-protein contacts for trans-factor function. Many of these principles

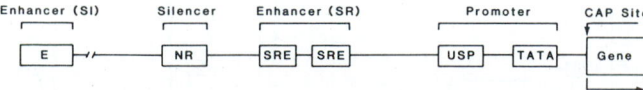

Figure 3–33. Typical combination of regulatory elements for a tightly controlled gene. CAP site is located at +1 base pair in the gene. Promoter is usually located within −100 base pairs upstream from the gene. Enhancers, of which SREs are one type, may be located anywhere surrounding the gene (or within an intron). Silencers or negative regulators (NR) are also position independent, as are steroid-independent (SI) enhancers.

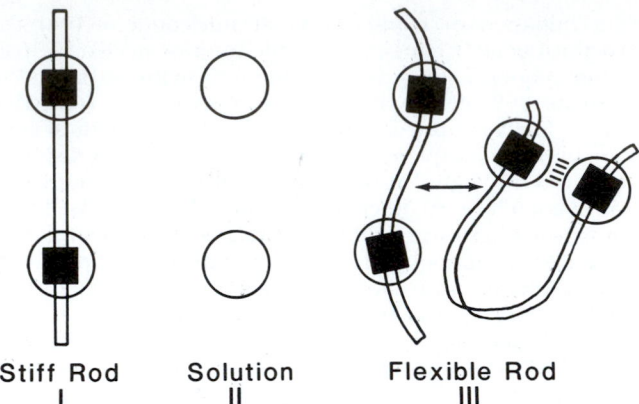

Figure 3–34. Schematic model for protein-protein interactions between transcription factors. Proteins bound to separate sites on a stiff rod are unable to interact (I). Proteins can interact in solution, depending on their concentration and diffusion rates (II). Proteins bound to sites on a flexible rod can fold back (looping out intervening DNA) and form a stable protein-protein complex (III). At low concentrations of DNA-binding protein, reaction III is most advantageous. Genomic DNA is a flexible rod.

appear to hold for animal cells as well. Because steroid hormones may occasionally inhibit gene transcription, we can speculate how this might occur. For instance, if SRE binding sites overlap with a promoter recognition sequence, occupation of the SRE by a receptor dimer could interfere with binding of a promoter trans factor required for gene expression (Fig. 3–35).[66, 286] Such protein-protein interference could occur also any time a negative regulatory factor binds within the transcriptional control region and interferes with the combinatorial coupling reactions among positive regulatory factors. Such mechanisms would allow cells to use the same regulatory protein to stimulate transcription of some genes and to down-regulate the expression of other genes. The pattern of expression would be determined by the architecture of the cis elements located in the 5'-flanking sequence of the genes (see Fig. 3–35).

COMBINATIONS OF CIS ELEMENTS PROVIDE TRANSCRIPTIONAL SPECIFICITY. To understand how steroid receptors might regulate gene function in a variety of fashions we must first review the result of various combinations of cis elements assembled within the regulatory region of genes. A typical array of regulatory components for a steroid hormone–regulated gene is shown at the top of Figure 3–36. The structural gene contains the information transcribed into mRNA and later into the protein product of the gene. The mRNA is not synthesized, however, unless the regulatory elements of the gene are intact and "activated." These elements are linked to the gene and located near the beginning (5' end) of the gene; they are termed cis elements because they are linked to the same strand of DNA (gene unit). The cis elements that regulate expression of steroid-controlled genes are classified into four main groups: (1) promoters, (2) steroid-responsive enhancers, (3) silencers, and (4) steroid-independent enhancers. The manner in which these four types of cis elements cooperate to achieve precise regulation of expression of a gene is summarized schematically in Figure 3–36. In the presence of a promoter, a gene is transcribed at a constant (constitutive) rate (Fig. 3–36, panel 1). If the promoter is a "strong" one, the rate of transcription is high; if the promoter is "weak," it is expressed at a lower rate. In this case, the transcription of the gene is not subject to stimulation (or suppression) by steroid hormones. In contrast, the existence of a nearby SRE (enhancer) allows the gene to be placed under control of steroid hormones, as shown in Figure 3–36, panel 2. For example, hormone stimulation might increase the rate of transcription another fivefold over the basal level. If a silencer element is then added to the regulatory cassette, the basal level is decreased to near zero but the maximal attainable level after hormone stimulation remains unaltered. This combination would then permit a 10-fold level of stimulation by hormone (Fig. 3–36, panel 3). Finally, the addition of one or more steroid-independent enhancers leads to synergistic increases in the maximal level of expression in response to hormone

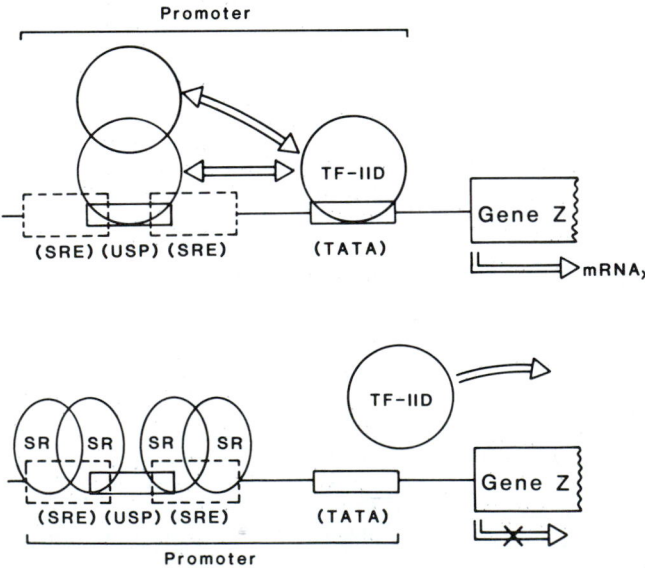

Figure 3–35. A hypothesis for down-regulation of gene transcription mediated by steroid receptors. A protein complex binds to a promoter (USP) and activates transcription via interactions with TATA proteins (e.g., TFIID). In this region of the transcription unit, SREs overlap with the USP site. Consequently, when steroid receptors bind to the SREs they displace the USP complex and thereby remove the USP-mediated stabilization of TATA proteins, shutting down transcription.

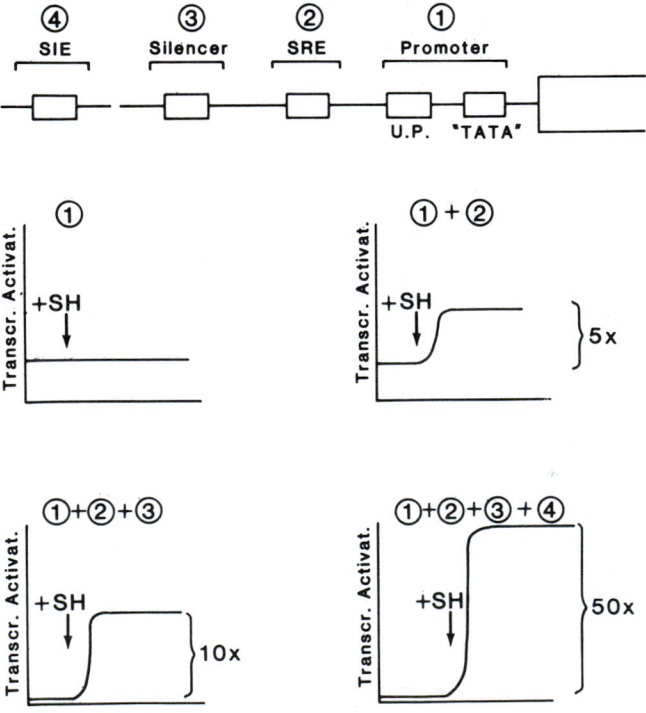

Figure 3–36. Evolution of a tightly controlled gene with a marked inductive response to steroid hormones (SH). See text for explanation.

(Fig. 3–36, panel 4) but does not influence the basal level of transcription in the absence of hormone. Such combinations of regulatory cis elements have been assembled around genes over thousands of millions of years of evolution. The process of evolution allows each gene to gather and retain the particular combination of cis elements that suits its own cellular needs. Assembly of these elements occurs by random DNA recombination, and retention occurs by positive evolutionary selection. That is, when a cis element "jumps" into the vicinity of a gene, it is retained in the gene's regulatory cassette if it provides a selective advantage for the cell's function and survival. There is no particular reason why a given gene may not have multiple similar or identical copies of each type of cis element. This would simply magnify the quantitative effect of each type of response. The ovalbumin gene of the chicken is an example of the type of gene portrayed in Figure 3–36, panel 4. It has a strong promoter, is totally silent in the absence of hormone, and is induced to an extremely high rate of expression by steroid hormones because of the presence of a particularly efficient combination of SREs and steroid-independent enhancers. Delineation of regulatory sequences around eucaryotic promoters has been accomplished by using two separate methodologies. The first involves in vitro transcription of cloned gene fragments in the presence of RNA polymerase and crude cellular transcription factors. This type of analysis can be carried out effectively to determine the specific nucleotide requirements within the TATA box. The modifier element (USP) located further upstream also lends itself to effective analysis in vitro. Promoter functions of cloned genes have also been studied by transferring them back into cells in culture using transfection techniques. The cloned genes are thus expressed in an environment that more closely resembles their in vivo state. In such typical experiments, deletion of upstream 5'-flanking sequences to position -95 (i.e., only 95 base pairs are retained) generally has no effect on promoter function; deletion to -75 reduces transcription to approximately 50% of the wild-type level; and deletion to -50 reduces the level to about 5%, because only the TATA element remains. Using such techniques, the promoter element of a gene can be mapped and the relative importance of specific internal sequences can be assessed.

Models for Regulating the Expression of Gene Sets

Hormonal regulation of gene expression at the level of DNA transcription is well documented in the case of gonadal steroid regulation of genes for egg white proteins and glucocorticoid regulation of viral (MMTV) gene expression. It is too early to draw firm conclusions about whether gene expression is an automatic process once it has begun or whether control by hormones can be exerted at additional levels. It is possible to distinguish at least five potential control points. These sequential steps can be separately defined as (1) structural activation of genes, (2) initiation of transcription, (3) precursor mRNA processing and export to cytoplasm, (4) translation of mRNA, and (5) degradation of mRNA and protein. At present there is good evidence for the existence of control at steps 1, 2, and 5 but no evidence for selective control by hormones at steps 3 and 4. Of perhaps equal interest for future investigation is the question of how gene expression is coordinated between different loci of the genome. The members of a set of coordinately expressed genes required to generate specific cell functions are often distributed at distant loci throughout the genome. Major remaining questions are how each cell activates the appropriate set of genes to produce its pheno-

type and how, within a given cell, the appropriate gene sets are coordinately regulated to produce a given function. It is possible that each gene is present in multiple copies and that only one copy is activated in each cell in which it is expressed or, alternatively, that the regulatory element associated with each gene is subjected to multiple controls. Although both mechanisms are probably employed at times, many eucaryotic genes are present in a single copy and are therefore likely to be subject to multiple controls. In procaryotes there are operons in which coordinate control of a group of genes is accomplished by placing them together in a single unit of transcription under a single control element. This is not possible in eucaryotes, in which individual genes usually exist in independent transcription units and often on separate chromosomes. Consequently, it appears that each gene has its own control element. If a set of genes that are unrelated and evolved separately from each other are under a common control, it seems unlikely statistically that they have developed the same control element independently. How then can such evolution take place at the molecular level? Given the current evidence that the eucaryotic genome is fluid and changing constantly by recombinations and translocations, we now have a logical solution to the problem. All that is needed is a translocation event in which the hormone control elements of genes are duplicated and distributed to the transcription units of other genes. Because we have already reviewed evidence for the existence of control elements that are separate and distinguishable from the basal promoters of eucaryotic genes, it is easier to visualize the mechanics of the process.

Consider the example shown in Figure 3–37. Two genes, X and Y, exist on separate chromosomes. Each gene has its own promoter element (p) and one or more control elements. Gene X is under control of inducers a and b, and gene Y is under control of inducer c. For instance, a, b, and c could represent the binding sites for receptors for three different steroid hormones. As evolution proceeds to stage 2, the DNA sequence containing the a element undergoes a translocation so that a replicate copy is now located in the 5'-flanking region of gene Y. Thus gene Y now comes under control of receptors for both hormones a and c. By accepted theory, genomic translocations and recombinations are occurring continually. When such an event leads to some selective advantage for the organism, the genomic rearrangement is "locked in" and becomes permanent. In this way, a single hormone can control many genes if each gene locus contains a copy of the appropriate control element. Also, a single gene may have acquired the appropriate control elements for a number of different hormone recep-

Evolution of Co-ordinate Gene Control

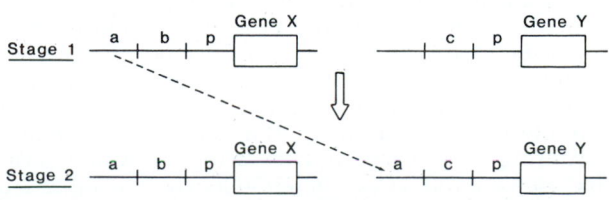

Figure 3–37. In an early stage of evolution (stage 1), gene X is under control of hormones because it contains regulatory sites (a and b) that interact with receptors for hormones and allow the promoter (p) to function. Gene Y is under constitutive synthesis (c). At stage 2, hormone control element a has been duplicated in the genome and has been translocated to the 5'-flanking region of gene Y. This now brings gene Y under hormonal control by virtue of its proximity to the promoter of gene Y. In this manner, a group of genes located anywhere on the genome can be brought under control of a single regulatory molecule. See text for details.

tors. All of the genes containing a common control element for hormone a would be coordinately activated in response to the same hormonal stimulus (see Fig. 3–37). The overall result is equivalent to that of a bacterial operon in that a set of genes are expressed coordinately under the direction of a common regulatory element. The only difference in the case of eucaryotes is that the control elements are repetitive DNA sequences present in multiple copies and associated with spatially separate genes whose coordinate expression provides some biological advantage to the organism. Such a grouping of genes might specify proteins with related functions, such as the set of enzymes in a metabolic pathway. A classic example of both coordinate control and multihormonal control of gene sets can be found again in the chicken oviduct system. The genes for ovalbumin, ovomucoid, conalbumin, and lysozyme are all under coordinate control for steroid hormones such as estrogen. This is of obvious selective advantage to the laying hen as each of the proteins must be available to produce the white of eggs. This could be accomplished easily if each gene had at least one copy of a common control element and thus each gene could be responsive to estrogenic regulation. This concept could easily be extended to coordinate regulation of enzyme metabolic pathways or other gene sets by cellular inducers.[267, 278] The mechanisms employed for the evolutionary, developmental, and transient actions of hormones represent a classic example of the logic and efficiency of the structural and functional organization of the eucaryotic genome.

Trans-Acting Factors and Gene Expression

The assembly of appropriate cis elements around eucaryotic genes is necessary but not sufficient for expression. A cell must also contain the appropriate complement of trans-acting factors to bind to these sequence-specific DNA elements and activate transcription. If the cell is deficient in one or more requisite trans-acting factors, expression will be poor to nonexistent. Each DNA-regulatory cis element may bind as few as one or as many as five (TATA box) different transcription factors. There is a limited number of such factors—perhaps 50 as a guess—and they are in low concentration even in cells in which they function. Also, multiple individual factors must be bound simultaneously within the 5'-flanking region of genes for transcriptional regulation to occur. For example, a given gene may have five cis elements that bind as many as 12 different factors. Multimeric protein complexes form at each DNA element; communication occurs between different elements via protein-protein interactions among bound transcription factors. In a manner that is not clearly understood at present, an appropriate mixture of trans-acting factors provides an "activation surface" or alters chromatin structure in a way that leads to recruitment of RNA polymerase to that gene for initiation of transcription.[285] Many genes are in competition for a limited amount of polymerase, and the genes with the most effective array of factors and the most stable array of factors are transcribed repetitively and at a high rate. Transcription can be subdivided into four general steps: (1) a "template commitment" step during which transcription factors bind and form a stable complex with DNA, (2) a step in which a "rapid-start" complex is formed that poises factors and RNA polymerase for RNA synthesis when ribonucleotide substrates are provided, (3) initiation of transcription, and (4) elongation of RNA chains and termination of transcription.

TRANS ACTIVATION OF THE PROXIMAL PROMOTER (TATA BOX). Multiple general transcription factors, TFIID, IIA, IIB, IIE, and IIF and RNA polymerase II bind to the

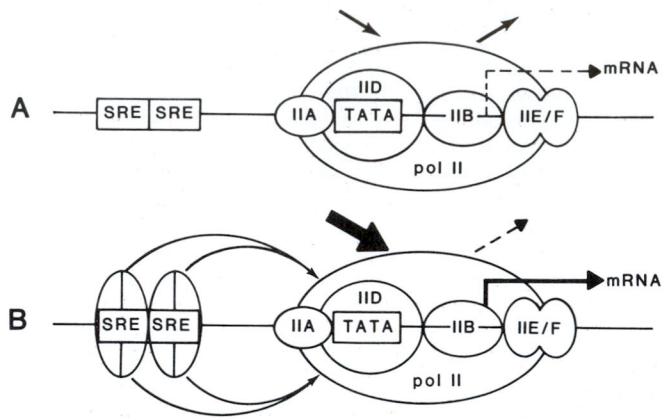

Steroid Receptor Stabilizes the Preinitiation Complex for Transcription

Figure 3–38. Steroid receptors act by stabilizing the preinitiation complex formed at the proximal promoter (TATA box). A reversible association of IID, IIA, IIB, Pol II (polymerase), and IIE/F is shown schematically (A). Only when all factors are present can Pol II initiate RNA synthesis. When upstream SREs are occupied by receptor dimers, the resulting tight-binding tetramer of receptor exerts a stabilizing effect on proximal promoter factors to generate a committed complex that allows Pol II to effect rapid-start RNA synthesis (B). This stabilization by receptor promotes repeated initiations of transcription.

TATA box and are required for initiation of transcription.[287–290] The primary DNA-binding protein required to form this complex is TFIID.[291] TFIIA then binds and stabilizes IID, followed by IIB, which encourages RNA polymerase into the complex. TFIIE and TFIIF then bind and promote initiation of transcription and perhaps unwinding of DNA (Fig. 3–38). Transcription will not occur if this complex of proteins is not in residence at the TATA box. Because these factors are in short supply in eucaryotic nuclei and bind only weakly to the TATA element, help in recruitment and stabilization of these factors at the TATA element must be provided by factors bound to other upstream elements.

UPSTREAM PROMOTER FACTORS. The upstream (distal) promoter is located near (about 50 base pairs away from) the TATA box and is more heterogeneous in sequence. Each sequence (e.g., CAAT box, SP1 site, and COUP box) binds a selected subset of factors. Once bound to the USP site, these factors aid in recruiting and stabilizing TATA factors in a manner that promotes transcriptional initiation by polymerase. It has been demonstrated that adenovirus major late transcription factor and ATF protein both bind to upstream sequences, stabilize TFIID, and enhance TATA-dependent transcription.[292–294] As with other cis elements, more than one protein may bind at the USP. In the case of COUP (chicken ovalbumin upstream promoter), a trans-acting factor (COUP-TF) binds with high affinity and specificity.[44, 45, 239] COUP-TF is active in directing initiation of transcription in a cell-free transcription assay that includes a target gene and general transcription factors.[295]

ENHANCER FACTORS. Again, a wide variety of enhancer elements each bind subsets of transcription factors to enhance transcription. Because these elements may be located at great distances (e.g., about 2000 base pairs) from the promoter, they must somehow fold back and interact with promoter factors, again via protein-protein bonding. This appears to be accomplished by "looping out" of the intervening DNA so that the proteins touch each other.[276] One of the best-studied groups of enhancer regulatory proteins is the steroid receptor superfamily. These powerful trans activators of gene expression provide a good model for mechanistic studies of enhancer function.

Molecular Mechanism of Steroid Receptor Action

The pathway of steroid receptor activation has been known since about 1980 (Fig. 3–39). It is generally accepted that the primary regulatory interactions occur at the level of nuclear DNA. A large number of mutational analyses using cloned receptor cDNAs have been carried out to determine the structure-function relationships of steroid hormone receptors. A more precise description of the mechanism(s) of receptor action, however, required in vitro studies of receptor function in a cell-free (reconstituted) transcription system. Until recently, such a system was not available.

THE ROLE OF STEROID RECEPTOR IN TRANS ACTIVATION OF TARGET GENES. Hormone-dependent transcription of the vitellogenin gene was first observed in crude extracts of *Xenopus* nuclei.[296] Subsequently, bacterially expressed truncated glucocorticoid receptor fragment[297] and native progesterone receptor[298, 299] were shown to be capable of enhancing RNA synthesis in an in vitro transcription assay. After many years of experimentation, the steroid receptor–mediated regulation of target gene transcription can be demonstrated directly in cell-free systems. As expected, enhancement of transcription by progesterone-receptor complexes depends on the presence of PREs in the template[298] and is inhibited by addition of competitor DNA containing authentic PREs. Test constructs containing two PREs yield 30-fold induction of levels of transcription in the presence of chicken progesterone receptor while the transcription of test genes lacking PREs is unaffected by addition of receptor. To elucidate the molecular mechanism by which steroid hormone receptors interact with core promoter factors to enhance the initiation of gene transcription, we examined whether the progesterone receptor is essential for formation of a template-committed preinitiation complex of factors at target gene promoters. The results indicate that in the presence of general transcription factors provided by

HeLa cell extracts, progesterone receptor directs the formation of a stable preinitiation complex (see Fig. 3–38).[298] Further analyses of the requirements for general transcription factors indicate that TFIID and TFIIE/F together with progesterone receptor are sufficient to confer template commitment to PRE-containing promoters. This result suggests that progesterone receptor bound to a PRE can interact primarily with TFIID and TFIIE/F to facilitate the enhancement of gene transcription. In separate studies, receptors were shown to interact with proteins at the USP site, which in turn interact with and stabilize factors at the TATA box. These findings suggest that enhancer-binding proteins may interact with one or a subset of general transcription factors to recruit and stabilize the formation of preinitiation complexes at proximal promoters and thus enhance the initiation of transcription. Preliminary investigations using other steroid receptors (e.g., glucocorticoid and estrogen) indicate that this may be a general mechanism by which all receptors act to regulate the expression of their respective target genes.

MULTIPLE HORMONE RESPONSE ELEMENTS MEDIATE TRANSCRIPTION SYNERGISTICALLY. SREs are often found in multiple copies in the 5'-flanking regions of hormone-responsive genes.[81, 129, 299–301] Transient transfection studies demonstrate that deletion or mutation of one of two SREs leads to a dramatic decrease in the inducibility of a target gene, suggesting that the SREs cooperate with one another to confer synergistic induction (see Fig. 3–39). Cooperative binding of receptors to PREs appears to contribute to the hormone-induced synergism in gene expression observed in vivo. Using the in vitro transcription assay to analyze levels of transcription of test genes containing various copy numbers of PREs, we showed that one copy of PRE enhances receptor-dependent transcription 4-fold and two copies enhance transcription 30-fold. These results indicate that two copies of PRE function cooperatively under our in vitro transcription conditions. Similar regulation through cooperative interactions has been observed between other DNA-binding proteins such as glucocorticoid receptor,[302] heat shock transcription factor,[303] and Oct-2 factor.[304] In addition

Molecular Mechanism of Steroid Activation of Receptor

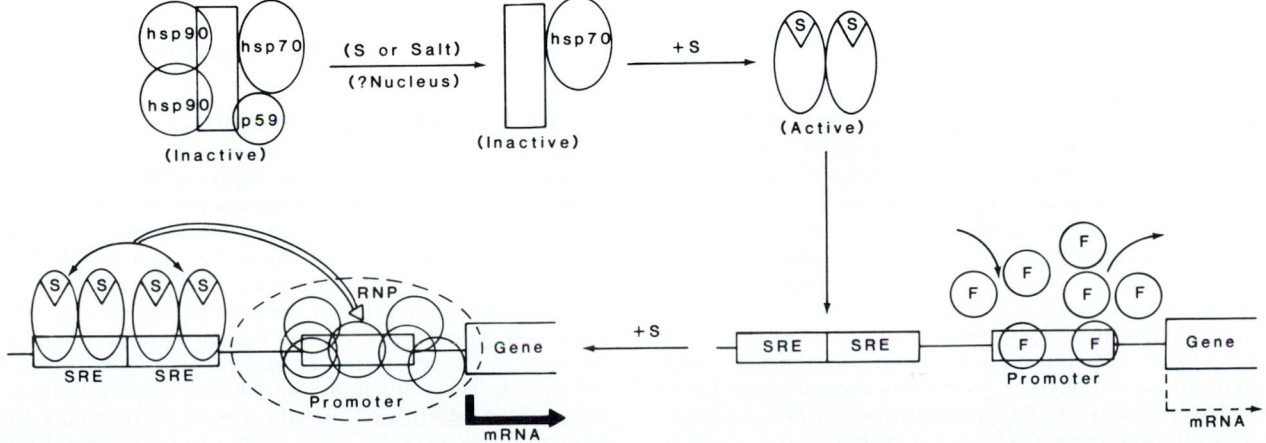

Figure 3–39. Before binding hormone, the inactive receptor is complexed with heat shock proteins, e.g., hsp90, hsp70, and p59. High salt levels, and perhaps the nuclear environment, can lead to dissociation of hsp90 and p59. Hormone induces dissociation of all proteins, including hsp70, from receptor and encourages a conformational (allosteric) change in the molecule. Cooperative enhancement of transcription proceeds from stable occupation of an SRE by steroid receptors. After receptor activation, binding of a monomer to an SRE is very weak but a dimer binds to an SRE sufficiently strongly to exert a stabilizing effect on promoter complexes. If two SREs are upstream and interact cooperatively, the binding is very strong and exerts a much greater recruitment and/or stabilizing effect on promoter transcription factors. When promoter transcription factors are bound stably because of interactions with receptors, RNA polymerase will repeatedly initiate transcription at the target gene, leading to a high output of mRNA.

to cooperativity induced by two similar response elements, synergism has been demonstrated with heterologous response elements such as a GRE with nuclear factor 1 (NF$_1$) in the promoter region of MMTV,[305] a GRE with a CACA promoter element, and others. We have carried out studies of in vitro transcription with complex regulatory regions containing SREs and different USPs and TATA elements. Using transcription competition assays, it was observed that glucocorticoid receptor, bound to GREs, cooperates with NF$_1$ to confer high levels of expression to the MMTV promoter; glucocorticoid receptor or NF$_1$ alone provides only low levels of expression. Interestingly, progesterone receptors purified from either chicken oviduct or T47D cells failed to enhance high levels of expression from an MMTV promoter, resembling the results obtained in vivo.[306] Based on these observations, we suggest that glucocorticoid and progesterone receptors possess qualitatively different types of activation domains. The activation surfaces of glucocorticoid receptors can interact well with NF$_1$, but those of progesterone receptor are less effective. On the other hand, both activation domains can function equally well in conjunction with COUP-TF bound to its USP. Using mixed elements, synergism appears to be dependent on both cooperative binding and overall conformation. High levels of induction can also be achieved by placing a combination of heterologous elements, such as estrogen and PREs, upstream of a promoter. This synergistic induction is due not to cooperative binding but to combinatorial interactions between different activation domains in the heterologous receptor complex. Taken together, these results demonstrate that complex regulation of eucaryotic gene expression can be achieved by assembling unique subsets of cis elements. Through either cooperative binding or cooperative interactions of specific activation domains with other transcription factors at target genes, expression of a given gene can be regulated over a wide range.

THE ROLE OF LIGAND IN STEROID RECEPTOR FUNCTION. Steroid receptor–mediated induction of target gene expression in vivo is dependent on the presence and concentration of steroid hormone.[307–309] Consistent with this model, specific hypersensitive sites, which correlate with the state of expression of hormone-responsive genes, are detected in and around the SREs in the presence of the cognate hormone.[310] A nuclear genomic footprint demonstrating receptor binding to the PRE/GRE element of the tyrosine aminotransferase gene is observed only in the presence of hormone.[311] Furthermore, estrogen[147] or progesterone[312] receptors in crude nuclear extracts bind to their respective SRE DNAs only when the extracts are prepared from hormone-treated cells. In vitro transcription experiments have revealed that highly purified progesterone receptors bind and function to enhance the expression of PRE-containing target genes in a hormone-independent manner. In contrast, less pure nuclear extracts from T47D cells contain ligand-free progesterone receptors that do not bind to PRE sites; these receptors also fail to enhance transcription of PRE-containing test genes. Upon treatment with progesterone ligand, either in vitro or in vivo, the receptors in such extracts bind specifically to their respective PREs and enhance transcription of PRE-containing test genes (see Fig. 3–39).[46] This transcriptional stimulation is specific for progestogens and is inhibited by 70% when the antiprogestogen 17β-hydroxy-11β-[4-(dimethylamino)phenyl]-17α-(1-propynyl)estra-4,9-dien-3-one (RU 486) is added to the reaction. High-salt extraction of receptor converts the unliganded progesterone receptor to a 4S form, as determined by sucrose gradient centrifugation. The 4S form of receptor does not contain hsp90 or 59-kd protein but is still inactive

in the cell-free transcription assay. Clearly, conversion of the 8S complex to 4S form, accompanied by the release of hsp90 and 59-kd protein by salt treatment, is not sufficient to activate the receptor. Two additional events must occur: hsp70 must be removed before receptor dimerization, and the receptor must assume the appropriate "active conformation" to interact with and stabilize requisite promoter factors (see Fig. 3–39). This novel inactive 4S form of receptor (free of hsp90) could have been detected and defined only in cell-free studies. These results are consistent with the observations that neither thyroid hormone nor vitamin D receptors are associated with heat shock protein in their native unliganded state but are still inactive. Such evidence leads us to suggest that hormone is needed to effect an additional structural alteration(s) in the receptor molecule, an event not induced completely by antihormones or steroid antagonists. In situ, this event could involve dissociation of additional inhibitory proteins (e.g., hsp70), induction of a specific conformational change in the receptor via covalent modifications such as phosphorylation, or a combination of these effects. After such an alteration, the receptor gains the capacity to bind and activate hormone-responsive genes. Steroid antagonists are inefficient in effecting this process. In highly purified forms of receptor, this active conformation may be achieved via the purification process itself.

In summary, steroid-activated receptor dimers bind to SREs and further stabilize crucial transcription factors bound at the distal and proximal promoter elements. Receptor tetramers, bound to two SREs, are most efficient in this process. When these transcription factors are bound stably, they are able to recruit RNA polymerase repeatedly to that gene and a high rate of transcription is achieved. Results of experiments of this type[313] are shown schematically in Figure 3–39.

PHYSIOLOGICAL CONSIDERATIONS IN STEROID HORMONE ACTION

The actions of steroid hormones with their respective target cells depend on interactions that occur at various levels of biological organization. In this section we will examine them at the physiological level and relate these actions to the known biochemical and molecular mechanisms.

Role of Metabolism and Blood Binding in Steroid Hormone Action

STEROID BINDING IN THE BLOOD. The interactions of steroid hormones with receptors are dependent on the delivery of the steroids to the target tissue. This is accomplished by the blood, which transports steroids in a bound state and an unbound (free) state. The unbound steroid is generally considered to be the active or available form of the hormone; however, the uptake of bound steroid may play an important role in the interactions of steroids with some cell types.[314] Also, there is considerable discussion of the role of hormone uptake and target organ transit time, the specificity of hormone uptake and intracapillary hormone dissociation, and specific tissue permeability to hormone-binding proteins.[315, 316] The affinity of blood binding proteins for steroids varies from very weak ($K_d = 10^{-3}$ M) to very strong (10^{-10} to 10^{-8} M). Frequently these proteins are present in high concentrations and can restrict the amount of free hormone available for receptor binding, so they may be important in the control of steroid hormone action. One such binding molecule is the gonadal hormone–binding globulin that binds testosterone and estradiol with equal affinity ($K_d = 10^{-10}$ M).[317] Another important blood component that binds estrogens but not androgens is α-FP, which is present in both the pregnant and neonatal rat. During neonatal and prepubertal life of the rat, α-FP levels gradually decrease from high values in the newborn to low values just before and after puberty.[318] Therefore, the quantity of free gonadal steroid gradually increases as the concentration of α-FP decreases. In this manner increasing concentrations of steroid are available for cellular interactions. These observations have led several investigators to suggest that α-FP plays a protective role in the fetus and neonate and may be involved in the onset of puberty.

Corticosteroid-binding globulin (CBG) is also of special interest and importance.[319] CBG binds glucocorticoids and progesterone with a K_d of 10^{-7} to 10^{-6} M at 37°C and therefore may be important in the control of free hormone. This is even more important when one considers that levels of CBG can be elevated by estrogens. Therefore, estrogens may control the availability of free progesterone and glucocorticoids. This concept is speculative because no experimental evidence has been presented, but it is suggestive of the profound and complex influences that hormone binding in blood may have in the control of steroid hormone effects. It has also been suggested that CBG increases the specificity of adrenocortical steroids by targeting these hormones to specific organs where CBG is recognized and accumulated.[314]

Binders of gonadal steroids that do not demonstrate pharmaco- or stereospecificity also may play significant roles in reproductive physiology. Serum albumin has a relatively weak affinity for estrogen ($K_d = 10^{-4}$ to 10^{-5} M) but is a significant estrogen binder. The concentration of serum albumin in blood is about 4% (7×10^{-4} M); at this concentration serum albumin may become a significant competitor for estrogen binding.[319]

METABOLISM AND STEROID BINDING. The quantity of steroid available in vivo for receptor binding depends not only on blood-binding relationships but also on the rate of metabolism and excretion of the hormone. Therefore, the metabolic clearance rate, or the volume of blood processed per unit time to remove the administered hormone from the body, is important in considerations of biological activity. A hormone with a high affinity for its receptor and thus with a predicted high potency also may have a high metabolic clearance rate. Hence, the exposure time of the hormone to a target cell is short, and the prediction of high potency may be incorrect. This is exemplified by the weak estrogenic potency of estriol after a single injection.[320] The anticipated potency would be 0.1 that of estradiol if estrogenic potency were dependent solely on the affinity of the estrogen receptor for the hormone. However, uterine growth after administration is far greater for estradiol than for estriol, partly because estriol is cleared from the blood in approximately 10 min compared with 30 min for estradiol. Conversely, a hormone with a low metabolic clearance rate and a relatively low affinity may display unexpectedly high biological activity. This is the case for the long-acting estrogen agonists-antagonists, such as tamoxifen or clomiphene. The affinity of the estrogen receptor for these drugs is only 1/20 to 1/30 that for estradiol; however, their effects are much more long-lasting because of the long-term retention of the antagonist-receptor complex by the nucleus of uterine cells and very long half-life of these drugs. Therefore, their biological effectiveness is much greater than that of estradiol when response time parameters are considered.

The actions of estrogen receptor and progesterone receptor do not usually depend on the metabolic conversion

of these steroids to active forms.[321, 322] Therefore, once receptor-steroid binding has occurred as a result of steroid entry into the cell, the receptor-steroid complex is functionally active. Metabolism is important in some cases; for instance, the conversion of testosterone to 5α-dihydrotestosterone (5α-DHT) is a requirement for androgen action in some male accessory sex structures. In addition, the aromatization of testosterone to estradiol is required for masculinization of the central nervous system. These metabolic conversions of androgens will be discussed in detail later in this section. Estradiol and estrone undergo extensive interconversion in human endometrium, where estradiol is metabolized to estrone before it is released from the tissue. This conversion of estradiol to estrone may be a mechanism for lowering the level of estradiol in the tissue and thereby controlling the level of functional estrogen-receptor complexes in cells. This metabolism may also be involved in the dissociation of receptor-hormone complex from nuclear binding sites. Progesterone is rapidly converted to 5α-pregnane-3,20-dione in the chick oviduct.[323] This steroid competes effectively with progesterone for binding to the progesterone receptor and is as potent as progesterone in the stimulation of avidin synthesis. 5α-Pregnane-3,20-dione is also capable of stimulating luteinizing hormone (LH) release in the rat and hamster. However, this compound is not active as a uterotropic agent, which correlates with its lack of binding to the progesterone receptor in the rat uterus. Thus the metabolism of progesterone to 5α-pregnane-3,20-dione and other inactive metabolites in the uterus may play an important regulatory role by reducing the effectiveness of progesterone, thereby providing the tissue with yet another control mechanism for hormone-induced responses.

Target Organ Responses to Steroid Hormones

Steroid hormones control many metabolic and biosynthetic events in virtually every tissue and organ in the body. These various responses appear to be regulated by the binding of steroids to their respective receptors.

ESTROGEN AND PROGESTERONE ACTIONS. Estrogen and progesterone interact to control the growth, development, and physiology of the female reproductive tract and other organ systems.

Uterus: Early and Late Uterotropic Responses. Many hormones induce responses within minutes after hormone exposure.[324] The relationship between these early responses and later events that culminate in cellular hypertrophy and hyperplasia (true growth) has received considerable study. Uterotropic responses to estrogen will be used as an example of such relationships. Other growth-promoting hormones also stimulate similar pleiotropic response patterns (reviewed by Tata[325]). Uterotropic responses to estrogen can be classified according to their time of appearance and functional relationship (Tables 3–2 and 3–3). Early responses include both biosynthetic and metabolic activities. The relationship between these events can be visualized in the following way. Hyperemia, calcium influx, histamine release, eosinophil infiltration, increased DNA and protein precursor uptake, and enhanced glucose oxidation are due to the ability of estrogen to mobilize many physiological functions to enhance biosynthetic activity. Early responses also include increased synthesis of RNA and protein, which are components of the biosynthetic machinery that eventually causes the uterus to grow. However, as discussed later, the stimulation of these biosynthetic events is not necessarily obligatory in the stimulation of uterine growth. Late responses, some of which are simply extensions of those begun during the early period, include increased and sustained RNA and protein synthesis.

TABLE 3–2. Early Uterotropic Responses to Estrogen

Supportive or Metabolic
Hyperemia
Histamine mobilization
Eosinophil infiltration
Water imbibition
Albumin accumulation
Increased electrolyte levels
Lysosome labilization
Increased cyclic nucleotide and prostaglandin levels and associated enzyme activation
Increased glucose metabolism and associated enzyme activity
Increased uptake of RNA
Calcium influx
Ornithine decarboxylase
Biosynthetic
Increased lipid synthesis
Increased activity of RNA
Synthesis of the induced protein and its mRNA
Increased synthesis of glucose-6-phosphate dehydrogenase
Increased chromatin template activity and RNA polymerase initiation sites
Increased synthesis of histone and nonhistone proteins

This biosynthetic activity results in cellular hypertrophy and eventual DNA synthesis and hyperplasia. These late responses are considered to be true growth responses of the uterus. Obviously, true growth occurs most readily in an environment in which substrate availability is optimal. This environment is provided by the increased blood flow and other supportive events listed in Tables 3–2 and 3–3.

Rapid elevations in cyclic AMP levels are demonstrable after estrogen treatment in the uterus, and it has been suggested that cyclic AMP is a mediator of estradiol effects.[326] Estrogen treatment in vivo and in vitro also stimulates cyclic GMP accumulation in the rat uterus.[327] This response appears to depend on RNA and protein synthesis because it can be blocked by cycloheximide and dactinomycin administration. Tchernitchin and Tchernitchin[328] have suggested that estrogen causes eosinophils to be attracted to uterine capillaries, where they migrate into the extracellular spaces of the uterus. The eosinophils then release hydrolytic enzymes that depolymerize the uterine ground substance. Eosinophils may also cause mast cells to release histamine, and this release, coupled with the hydrolysis of mucopolysaccharides, increases vascular permeability and creates an osmotic environment that favors water imbibition and precursor uptake.

It has been suggested that uterine growth is mediated by estrogen-induced histamine release that causes increased capillary permeability and hyperemia.[329] Although these events undoubtedly enhance the ability of the uterus to grow, most investigators do not consider them as primary events. Eosinophil infiltration and its attendant responses can be blocked with glucocorticoids without any significant effect on DNA, RNA, and protein synthesis in the uterus.[330] Early uterotropic responses can be induced by estradiol in rats pretreated with nafoxidine, an antiestrogen that blocks late responses; however, no stimulation of late responses is observed.[331] Estrogen-induced uterine growth is independent of cyclic AMP, prostaglandins, and beta-adrenergic action.[332] Even when the estrogen-induced elevation in the activity of ornithine decarboxylase, an enzyme assumed to be involved in cell proliferation, is blocked, estrogen-induced uterine growth still takes place.[333]

Additional evidence that these early events are not primary in stimulating true uterine growth comes from the observation that estriol and other short-acting estrogens do not cause true uterine growth after a single injection.[324, 334, 335] Estriol causes transient nuclear binding of the estrogen receptor and stimulates all the early uterotropic responses but does not stimulate uterine hyperplasia and growth. Estriol apparently fails in this regard because it does not maintain the estrogen receptor in an occupied state for a sufficient length of time, so it does not maintain the necessary biosynthetic events (late responses) that culminate in cell proliferation and growth. From these results it is concluded that early uterotropic responses are supportive but are not obligatory for the stimulation of uterine hypertrophy and hyperplasia. It is likely that separate regulatory mechanisms are involved in the control of some early and late events in the rat uterus.

The sustained stimulation of RNA and protein synthesis that culminates in cell proliferation appears to depend on nuclear occupancy by 10 to 20% of estrogen receptors for longer than 4 to 6 h.[324, 336] This long-term nuclear occupancy by receptor is correlated with elevations in total cellular RNA levels, sustained RNA polymerase I and II activity, sustained chromatin template activity, DNA synthesis, and cellular growth (Fig. 3–40). Sustained levels of estrogen are required for mRNA stability and continued synthesis of several proteins.[337, 338] Long-term nuclear occupancy by estrogen receptors is also associated with an elevation of nuclear type II estrogen binding sites, which is correlated with the late uterotropic growth responses.[339]

The results indicate that a sustained occupancy of estrogen receptors is required for the complete sequence of events that ultimately produce uterine hypertrophy and hyperplasia. Therefore, the examination of initial binding interactions of hormone-receptor complexes with acceptor sites may give only a limited amount of information about the full sequence of events necessary to elicit growth responses. Also, the minimal number of receptor-acceptor sites appears to be small and involves only 10 to 20% of the total number of receptors available. These facts will also eventually have to be integrated into the overall scheme of binding and response studies at the molecular level.

Progesterone acts to modify and redirect the cellular growth and biosynthetic activity of the uterus. Progesterone inhibits further endometrial proliferation induced by estrogen and converts the endometrium to the secretory type. The endometrial glands become irregular and convoluted, the glycogen content of the epithelium increases, and the stroma becomes edematous. In this progestational or secretory state, the endometrium is now ready for implantation of the blastocyst and subsequent maintenance of pregnancy. The functions of progesterone are dependent on prior elevation of its receptor levels by estrogen. Progesterone affects certain biosynthetic processes discussed later and decreases levels of both estrogen receptor and its own receptor (termed down-regulation).

In addition to the direct hormone-receptor pathway that leads to changes in cellular function and proliferation, indirect pathways may account for some of the actions of ovarian steroids. For example, it has been proposed that a factor from the pituitary is necessary to obtain a full growth response of the oviduct and uterus on the basis of experiments in which a single injection of estradiol failed to stimulate the complete growth response in the absence of

TABLE 3–3. Late Uterotropic Responses to Estrogen

Supportive or Metabolic
Many of the functions that are listed in Table 3–2 continue for many hours after estrogen administration
Biosynthetic
Increased general and specific protein and RNA synthesis
Continued stimulation of RNA polymerase activity
DNA synthesis and mitosis
Cellular hypertrophy and hyperplasia
Increased synthesis of or changes in histone and nonhistone proteins

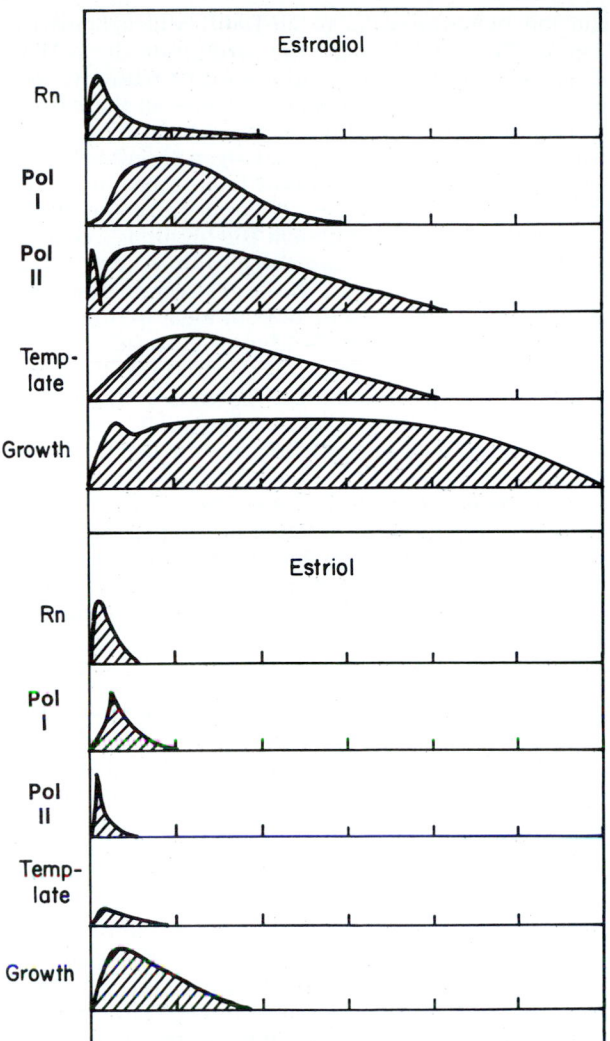

Figure 3–40. Effects of estradiol and estriol on estrogen receptor binding and uterotropic responses. Hormones were injected at time zero in equal quantities (1 μg) and the following responses were monitored as a function of time (each interval on the x axis equals 12 h): quantity of estrogen-receptor complexes in nucleus (Rn), RNA polymerase I activity (Pol I), RNA polymerase II activity (Pol II), chromatin template activity (Template), and uterine net weight (Growth).

the pituitary.[340, 341] However, a full uterotropic response can be obtained in hypophysectomized rats if estradiol is given for several days.[342] Therefore, it seems that the pituitary plays a permissive role, probably because pituitary hormones are required to maintain the integrity of the metabolic machinery and obtain a maximal response to a single estrogen injection. Other experimental results indicating that pituitary factors are unlikely to be involved include the stimulation of epithelial proliferation after direct local application of estrogen to the vagina.

It has also been proposed that the liver responds to estrogen and acts as an intermediary in the stimulation of the quail oviduct.[343] In these experiments estradiol was infused into the hepatoportal circulation and was completely metabolized by the liver. Under these circumstances no estrogen receptor accumulation by oviduct nuclei was observed, yet the DNA content of the oviduct was elevated to the same extent as in animals receiving systemic treatment with estradiol. Although these are interesting findings, the same investigators did not observe a similar liver-mediated effect on the rat uterus.[344] Therefore, the general applicability of a liver-mediated effect is questionable. It has also

been proposed that estrogens stimulate the synthesis of polypeptide growth factors that act as mitogens on estrogen-responsive cells.[345] These growth factors are thought to act in one of three ways: (1) as endocrine factors that are secreted into the circulation, (2) as paracrine factors that are produced by cells in proximity to the target cell, or (3) as autocrine factors produced by the cell in which they act. There is evidence for a paracrine function of uterine stromal tissue on the epithelium of this organ,[346] but whether these stromal-epithelial interactions involve peptide growth factors remains to be determined. Epidermal growth factor (EGF) and its receptor are present in the uterus of several species and in the mammary gland of the mouse.[347, 348] Although the role of EGF in the uterus is not known, EGF is known to be mitogenic in many cell types.

The stimulation of autocrine or paracrine factors by estradiol in the uterus seems much more likely to be of physiological significance than the stimulation of endocrine factors. As mentioned earlier, local application of estrogen to the vagina causes cellular proliferation and cornification. These experiments were first done by Robson and Adler,[349] who surgically formed two separate vaginal sacs in mice. They placed small amounts of estradiol in one vaginal sac and observed typical epithelial proliferation and cornification. No estrogenic effect was observed in the untreated vaginal sac. Thus they concluded that estradiol had a direct effect on the vaginal cells and did not act systemically in some indirect way. Several investigators have applied estradiol locally to the vagina and uterus and have drawn similar conclusions. Although these experiments rule out an endocrine or systemic effect of estradiol, they do not rule out cell-cell interactions (paracrine) or autocellular stimulation (autocrine). It seems likely that ovarian steroids act via cellular receptors to stimulate cellular growth directly as well as by elevating the local production of growth factors that may act on surrounding cells or on the cell producing them.

Chick Oviduct. Estrogen causes the growth and differentiation of the immature chick oviduct as shown diagrammatically in Figure 3–41.[345, 350] These processes include the stimulation of epithelial cells to invaginate and form tubular glands. Tubular glands when fully developed constitute 90% of the cell population of the oviduct and are responsible for the synthesis of ovalbumin, conalbumin, lysozyme, ovomucoid, and various other egg white proteins. As discussed earlier, estrogen stimulates the synthesis of these proteins by increasing the transcription of the specific mRNAs. The increased transcriptional activity is preceded by the binding of receptor-estrogen complexes to gland cell nuclei.

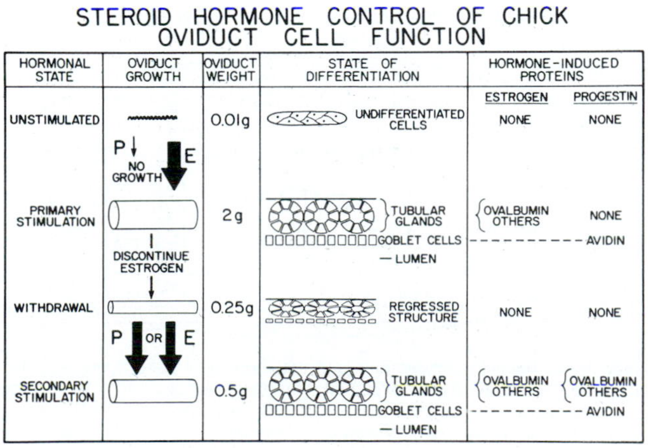

STEROID HORMONE CONTROL OF CHICK OVIDUCT CELL FUNCTION

HORMONAL STATE	OVIDUCT GROWTH	OVIDUCT WEIGHT	STATE OF DIFFERENTIATION	HORMONE-INDUCED PROTEINS	
				ESTROGEN	PROGESTIN
UNSTIMULATED		0.01g	UNDIFFERENTIATED CELLS	NONE	NONE
	P↓ ↑E NO GROWTH				
PRIMARY STIMULATION		2g	TUBULAR GLANDS GOBLET CELLS — LUMEN	OVALBUMIN OTHERS	NONE AVIDIN
	↓ DISCONTINUE ESTROGEN				
WITHDRAWAL		0.25g	REGRESSED STRUCTURE	NONE	NONE
	P↓ OR ↓E				
SECONDARY STIMULATION		0.5g	TUBULAR GLANDS GOBLET CELLS — LUMEN	OVALBUMIN OTHERS	OVALBUMIN OTHERS AVIDIN

Figure 3–41. Differentiation and development of chick oviduct.

The initial stimulation of protein synthesis and growth of the oviduct is caused exclusively by estrogen; however, if the estrogen is withdrawn from the animal, other steroid hormones can mimic the effect of estrogen on protein synthesis. After withdrawal of estrogens, the synthesis of egg white proteins decreases; however, the oviduct retains tubular gland cells. Secondary stimulation of the animal by estrogen, progesterone, or glucocorticoid results in a resumption of egg white protein synthesis. In this endocrine state, all of these hormones induce mRNA synthesis for these genes by the molecular events described earlier. However, why nonestrogenic hormones can function during secondary but not during primary stimulation is not known.

Liver. Estrogen controls the synthesis of many different proteins by the liver; the type of protein depends on the species. In birds and amphibians, estrogen stimulates the synthesis of large quantities of proteins that are carried by the blood and deposited in the developing oocytes as yolk. The synthesis of these proteins (vitellogenin and very-low-density lipoprotein) is correlated with the nuclear binding of estrogen-receptor complexes and appears to involve the enhanced transcription of specific genes that code for these proteins.[351]

The binding of the estrogen-receptor complexes with nuclear sites in avian liver is somewhat different from that observed in the uterus. After an injection of estrogen in the chicken, estrogen-receptor complexes appear in the nuclear fraction, as would be expected; however, there is no evidence that they are depleted from the cytosol or that there are unoccupied sites in the nuclear fraction. The cytosol of chicken liver contains few, if any, detectable receptor sites; therefore the appearance of nuclear-bound hormone-receptor complexes after estrogen exposure results from activation of receptor sites or de novo synthesis. Because protein inhibitors block the appearance of nuclear receptors, it is assumed that receptor synthesis is involved.

ANDROGENS. The tissues and organs that are regulated by androgens are very diverse.[340] In addition, and in contrast to most other steroids, androgens may undergo metabolic activation before binding to the receptor. Therefore, this section begins with a discussion of metabolism in relation to hormone action and follows with examination of androgen actions in the male reproductive tract and other tissues.

Metabolism in Target Tissues. The metabolism of androgens by target tissues is of major physiological importance. Testosterone may act directly via its binding to the androgen receptor, or it may be metabolized to steroids that are more androgenic, estrogenic, or not active at all. As shown in Figure 3–42, one of these metabolic pathways involves the

reduction of testosterone to 5α-DHT, which binds to the receptor. In the adult male, the production of 5α-DHT in the reproductive tract and skin is a major pathway, and 5α-DHT is the primary androgenic hormone in these tissues.

Testosterone may also be converted in the brain to estrogens that function via the estrogen receptor.[352, 353] This metabolic conversion is of utmost importance in many species because it results in the development of the male-type brain. During early development the brain, as well as other organs of the body, is bipotential with regard to sexual development. In the male, the testes secrete testosterone, which acts as a signal to cause development to proceed down the male pathway. Figure 3–42 also illustrates how in the brain the male testosterone signal paradoxically functions via the formation of a female hormone, estradiol. The mechanism by which estradiol switches on the male pathway in the brain is not known, but the estrogen receptor is involved.

Reproductive Tract Structures. Androgens regulate the growth and physiological function of the prostate and seminal vesicles.[352] In castrated rats, androgen treatment stimulates DNA synthesis and cell proliferation of the prostate. When the number of cells reaches the normal intact level, DNA synthesis slows or stops and cell proliferation is curtailed. After this time androgen stimulates the synthesis and secretion of prostatic proteins. Withdrawal of androgens is followed by atrophy of the prostate, which involves autophagic processes.

The major effect of androgenic stimulation of the adult prostate and seminal vesicle is the synthesis of large quantities of secretory proteins. Forty percent of all proteins synthesized are secreted into the ejaculatory ducts. The functions of most of these proteins are known; however, along with the spermatozoa, they are the major components of the seminal fluid. In the rat, one of these proteins is responsible for forming the vaginal plug after coitus; such proteins are often called coagulation proteins. The prostate secretes proteins that bind steroids and are thus functionally analogous to the androgen-binding protein synthesized by the Sertoli cells of the testes.

Testosterone, in concert with follicle-stimulating hormone (FSH), regulates spermatogenesis. Both of these hormones promote the synthesis of androgen-binding protein by Sertoli cells of the testes. Androgen-binding protein is secreted into the fluid by the seminiferous tubules and is found in large quantities in the epididymis. Its function appears to be to transport testosterone and maintain high concentrations of the hormone in the epididymis. These high concentrations promote the viability and maturation of the spermatozoa.

Target Organs Other Than Reproductive Tract. Androgens control and regulate the biosynthetic and enzymatic activity of several organs and tissues that are not a part of the reproductive apparatus.

Kidney. The males of many species have larger kidneys than the females.[352] This size difference is attributed to androgens in the male, which cause hypertrophy of the cells of the Bowman capsule and the proximal convoluted tubules. This effect depends on the continued presence of androgens, because castration leads to a decrease in size of the kidney and androgen treatment causes the kidney to grow. Thus this male-female difference is not analogous to the organizational effects of early hormone exposure, which cause the fixation of male or female developmental pathways. Androgens interact with renal cells in much the same fashion as they do with reproductive tract cells. Androgen-receptor complexes are found in the nucleus within minutes after exposure to the hormone. This is followed by a stim-

Metabolism and Receptor Interactions of Androgens

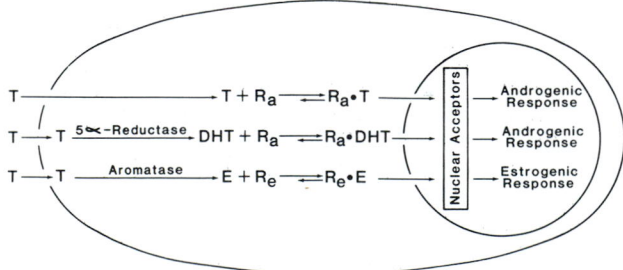

Figure 3–42. Receptor interactions and metabolism of testosterone in a target cell. T, testosterone; R_a, unoccupied androgen receptor; $R_a \cdot T$, androgen receptor–testosterone complex; DHT, dihydrotestosterone; $R_a \cdot DHT$, androgen receptor–dihydrotestosterone complex; E, estradiol; R_e, unoccupied estrogen receptor; $R_e \cdot E$, estrogen receptor–estradiol complex.

ulation of RNA and protein synthesis that culminates in cellular hypertrophy. At least one specific enzyme (β-glucuronidase) is induced in the kidney by androgens.

Liver. Hormone-regulated or -controlled sexual differences exist in the liver of many species. These differences involve enzymes of drug and steroid metabolism, neonatal or fetal organizational effects, and secretory proteins such as alpha-2u–globulin. The steroid hydroxylases, which are involved in the metabolism of steroid hormones, are dependent on androgen because their activities decrease after castration. These effects of androgen on enzymatic activity are thought to occur via androgen-receptor interactions because they are absent in animals that lack androgen receptors and are blocked by antiandrogens. However, it should be noted that androgens stimulate an increase in liver weight and microsomal protein content in animals that do not have functional androgen receptors (Tfm mouse). Thus it appears that this response is indirect and probably involves other unknown mechanisms. Neonatal exposure to androgen has an organizational effect on steroid metabolism that results in establishment of the male pattern of liver metabolism. The mechanisms involved in this effect are not known, but they appear to involve the hypothalamic-hypophyseal system.

Androgens regulate the synthesis of certain urinary proteins in rodents. These proteins are synthesized by the liver, secreted into the blood, and excreted in the urine by the kidney. One of these proteins, alpha-2u–globulin, is found exclusively in male rats and is clearly regulated by androgens. Urinary proteins which are found in mice are also regulated by androgens; however, they are found in females as well as males.

Muscle. Stimulation of skeletal muscle growth is a major action of androgens. The magnitude of their acute effect on muscle is small compared with that in the reproductive tract; however, the long-term low-level effects of androgens account for the difference in muscle mass between males and females. Testosterone appears to be the active androgen in stimulation of muscle growth because muscle has a limited capacity to form 5α-DHT. Androgen receptors are present in muscle, and it is presumed that the hormone functions via these receptors. However, androgens bind to glucocorticoid receptors in muscle, and some anabolic action may occur because they block the catabolic effect of glucocorticoids.[354]

Hemoglobin Synthesis. Androgens stimulate erythropoietin synthesis by the kidney and are thus involved in the control of hemoglobin synthesis.[54] The 5β-androgens apparently also stimulate hemoglobin synthesis in the bone marrow by a direct effect not involving the stimulation of erythropoietin. This 5β-steroid effect is mediated by a specific receptor that preferentially binds 5β-steroids, as opposed to 5α-steroids or testosterone. These observations, which have been made in many species, indicate that the stem cell population of the bone marrow has evolved a unique androgen receptor mechanism that allows it to respond to 5β-steroids.

GLUCOCORTICOIDS. Glucocorticoids influence virtually every organ and tissue in the body. The responses span the physiological spectrum from effects on behavior to effects on carbohydrate metabolism by the liver. These hormones also have the capacity to both stimulate and inhibit the functions of many biological systems. For the most part, the relationship between these physiological effects and the mechanism of action of glucocorticoids is not established. Therefore, in this section we will present only the physiological actions that have been examined in relation to the mechanisms involved.

Stimulatory Responses. The concentration and activity of several liver enzymes are increased by glucocorticoid treatment.[355] These increases appear to result from the binding of glucocorticoids to the receptor, which stimulates the transcription of specific mRNAs that code for the synthesis of these enzymes. The binding of glucocorticoid-receptor complexes to nuclear sites is closely correlated with the level of enzymatic stimulation. Thus, occupancy of the receptor by hormone is closely coupled with the response, indicating that there are no "spare receptors" present in the system. This is in contrast to the ability of some hormones to elicit a maximal response yet occupy only a portion of the receptors.

The induction of enzyme activity in cells in culture by glucocorticoids is a cell cycle–dependent process. Glucocorticoids stimulate the activity of tyrosine aminotransferase during the late G_1 and S phases but not during G_2, M, or early G_1. The concentration of cytosol receptors ranges from 10,000 to 40,000 sites per cell during the cell cycle, but no correlation seems to exist between the number of cytosol receptors per cell and enzyme induction. However, the level of nuclear receptor binding and response is correlated. High levels of nuclear receptor are maintained in late G_1 and S phases, and lower levels are found in G_2, M, and early G_1.

Inhibitory Responses. Although there are clear-cut examples of the stimulatory (anabolic) effects of glucocorticoids, these hormones also have inhibitory or catabolic effects in many systems. These include the suppression of DNA synthesis; the promotion of protein breakdown in muscle; the suppression of immunological and inflammatory responses; and the inhibition of cell proliferation in lymphoid, fibroblastic epithelial, and bone cells. Although the mechanism of action of glucocorticoids in these inhibitory responses is not known, it appears to involve hormone-receptor interactions. Glucocorticoid killing of lymphoid cells involves only cells containing functional receptors. The anti-inflammatory activity of glucocorticoids similarly parallels their affinity for receptors and can be blocked by the glucocorticoid antagonist RU 486.[356]

Although receptor steroid binding is generally associated with stimulatory or tropic effects, inverse effects can also occur via gene regulatory mechanisms. Thus the binding of glucocorticoid-receptor complexes to specific gene sites could stimulate the synthesis of mRNAs that encode proteins that turn off or inhibit cell function. Receptors might also bind to DNA and block transcription.

MINERALOCORTICOIDS. Mineralocorticoids, such as aldosterone, regulate electrolyte balance in the kidney, salivary glands, sweat glands, and gastrointestinal tract. Aldosterone augments the transport of sodium across the epithelium by stimulating the synthesis of proteins that are involved in increased apical membrane permeability to sodium and in the energy metabolism of the cell. Aldosterone receptors are present in target organs for mineralocorticoids, such as the kidney and toad urinary bladder. These receptors form activated nuclear-bound complexes similar to those of other steroids. As shown in Figure 3–43, the mechanism by which aldosterone controls sodium transport probably involves the synthesis of proteins involved in the function of the sodium channel and energy production (ATP). Aldosterone stimulates an increase in the number of sodium-specific apical membrane channels and increases the activities of at least four mitochondrial enzymes. Therefore, the major effect of aldosterone is to increase the activities of enzymes that are involved in the generation of ATP. The increased ATP acts as an energy source for sodium pumps and also may increase their number. Aldosterone also stimulates phospholipase activity, fatty acid synthesis, and acyltransferase activity. These actions are involved in altering the membrane functions in the renal cell and probably result in the stimulation

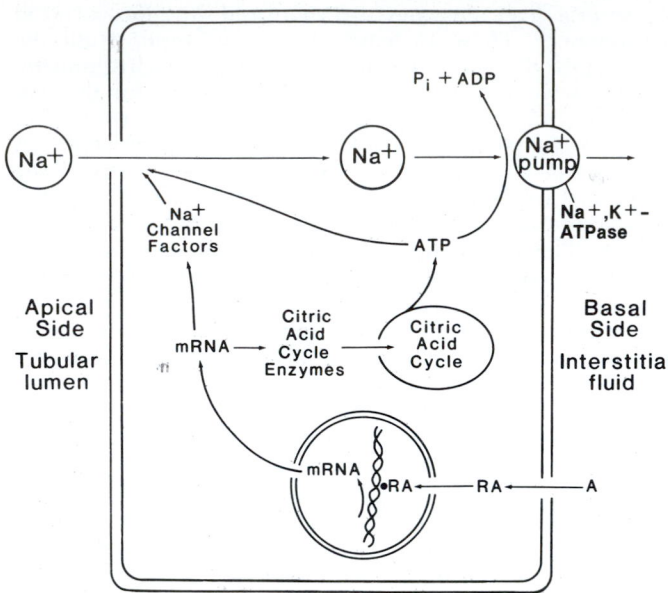

Figure 3–43. Aldosterone action and sodium transport. A, aldosterone; RA, receptor-aldosterone complex.

of specific mRNAs for the proteins involved in the control of sodium transport.

It has been difficult to explain how aldosterone could bind to its receptor when the concentration of glucocorticoids is several orders of magnitude higher than that of aldosterone and the receptor binds both classes of hormones with equal affinity.[357] Aldosterone specificity appears to be the result of the action of 11β-hydroxysteroid dehydrogenase, an enzyme present in the kidneys that converts glucocorticoids to metabolites for which the receptor has low affinity. Because 11β-hydroxysteroid dehydrogenase has no effect on the concentration of aldosterone in the kidney, aldosterone is readily available for binding to the receptor.

Control of Steroid Receptor Concentration

The intracellular concentration of steroid receptors is an important factor in determining the responsive state of the target cells. As before, the term cytosolic receptor is used for the soluble unoccupied form of the receptor regardless of its actual cellular localization. The control of the cellular concentration of steroid receptors is influenced by several interacting factors. After transformation and nuclear binding, receptor regulation may occur in at least three ways (Fig. 3–44). The receptor-steroid (RS) complex may stimu-

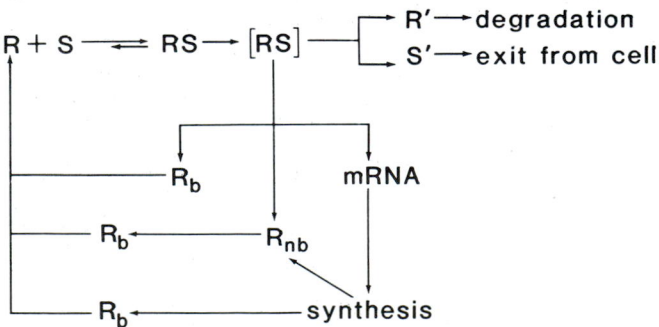

Figure 3–44. Pathways for receptor regulation.

late mRNA transcription that will result in the synthesis of new receptor molecules. These may be either hormone-binding forms (R_b) or non–hormone-binding forms (R_{nb}) that must be converted to R_b. The RS complex may be reutilized either by being converted to a nonbinding form that is subsequently activated to a binding form or by being recycled directly as an activated binding form. In addition to these replenishment mechanisms, the receptor may undergo degradation to an inactive form (R'). Associated with each of these receptor pathways is the loss or elimination of the steroid from the cell (S').

ESTROGEN RECEPTOR CONCENTRATION. Estrogen-responsive cells in the uterus of a castrated rat maintain levels of receptor that enable it to respond to administered estrogen. This basal level of receptor is probably controlled by genetic mechanisms that are programmed for the constitutive synthesis of the receptor. Thus estrogen target tissues can usually detect and respond to estrogens. This is also true of estrogen target tissues in the male animal, which respond readily to exogenous estrogen and have estrogen receptor levels equal to those of the female.[358–360]

Although estrogen target cells appear capable of maintaining a constitutive level of cytosolic receptor, this does not imply that gonadal hormones have no influence on the level of cytosolic receptor. To the contrary, steroid receptor levels are influenced by endogenous and exogenous steroids. As pointed out earlier, an injection of estradiol causes a rapid depletion of cytosolic receptors, which bind tightly in the nucleus as estrogen-receptor complexes. This is followed by a period during which the cytosolic receptor is replenished by at least two processes: the reactivation or reutilization of nuclear-bound receptor and the de novo synthesis of receptor molecules. In tissues that do not grow in response to hormone, replenishment may involve only reactivation or recycling, as first suggested by Munck and colleagues[361] for glucocorticoid receptors in thymus cells. Replenishment of cytosolic receptors for glucocorticoids does not depend on protein and RNA synthesis.[362]

A nonbinding form of the estrogen receptor in the chick oviduct can be reactivated.[363] The Y form (K_d = 1.0 nM) exists in a binding and a nonbinding form in oviduct cytosol. Addition of ATP or ADP to the nonbinding form converts it to the binding form, and this process can be reversed by dialysis. How these interconversions are related to replenishment of the estrogen receptors is not known, but they suggest that such interactions may occur in vivo.

In tissues that grow in response to hormone stimulation, such as uterus, vagina, and mammary gland, both reaction and synthesis may be involved in the replenishment process. It follows that synthesis of more cytosolic receptor molecules is required in cells that will undergo division after hormone stimulation. In this manner a constant amount of receptor per cell is maintained. Cells that grow in size and do not divide may also require receptor synthesis to counteract the dilution brought about by cellular hypertrophy. The involvement of protein synthesis in the replenishment process has been suggested by experiments in which protein synthesis inhibitors, such as cycloheximide, partially block replenishment of the estrogen receptor. These results are subject to question, because long periods of cycloheximide exposure are required to produce observed inhibitory effects, and nonspecific toxic side effects of this drug cannot be ruled out. Kassis and Gorski[364] demonstrated that the short-acting estrogen estradiol-16α causes complete replenishment of cytosolic receptor within 4 h after injection, a replenishment that is not blocked by cycloheximide. Thus, reutilization or recycling of the estrogen receptor can occur when short-acting estrogens cause nuclear accumulation. Such short-acting estrogens do not cause true uterine growth and therefore may not stimulate the biosynthetic events associated with cell hypertrophy and hyperplasia. This point will be discussed in more detail under Steroid Hormone Antagonism.

The replenishment of cytosolic receptors after hormone-induced depletion is important in determining the ability of the uterus to respond to hormone stimulation. Within the first 6 h after an injection of estradiol, a time during which very little replenishment has taken place, a second injection of estradiol does not stimulate uterotropic responses above those obtained with the first injection.[365] A second injection at 12 h, however, when cytosolic receptors are replenished, causes nuclear accumulation of the newly replenished receptor and enhanced uterotropic responses.

CONTROL OF THE PROGESTERONE RECEPTOR BY ESTROGEN. The uterus is relatively insensitive to progesterone unless first exposed to estrogen. Thus progesterone treatment in the nonestrogenized uterus does not produce a secretory uterine epithelium;[364] however, after estrogen priming, progesterone treatment has dramatic effects on the production of secretory responses.[366] These observations may be explained by assuming that estrogen priming stimulates the synthesis of the progesterone receptor, thereby enhancing the ability of the uterus to respond to progesterone. Several studies have shown that estrogen treatment does increase the quantity of progesterone receptors.[11] These effects occur in both the endometrium and myometrium of the guinea pig uterus.[367] Estradiol also increases the level of the cytosolic progesterone receptor in the neurons of hypothalamus.[368]

Estrogen treatment not only increases the quantity of cytosolic progesterone receptor but also causes a shift in the sedimentation coefficient. Castrated animals contain primarily the 4S form of the receptor, and estrogen treatment causes a shift to the 7S to 8S form. This phenomenon occurs in endometrium and myometrium of the monkey,[369, 370] the human uterus,[371] the guinea pig uterus,[372] and the chick oviduct.[373] From these observations it can be concluded that estrogen stimulates the uterus to produce qualitative, as well as quantitative, changes in the cytosolic progesterone receptor. This increase in the quantity of progesterone receptor results from an increased rate of protein synthesis and a concomitant increase in receptor mRNA concentrations.[374, 375] Thus estrogen sets the stage for the binding of progesterone, a prerequisite for progesterone action.

EFFECTS OF PROGESTERONE ON THE PROGESTERONE RECEPTOR. Progesterone has the paradoxical effect of causing a rapid decrease in the quantity of cytosolic progesterone receptor in the guinea pig uterus.[376–378] This loss of receptor is due to a decrease in the rate of progesterone receptor gene transcription. This decreased transcription, coupled with the fact that the mRNA for progesterone receptor is short-lived, causes a rapid decline in receptor levels.[379]

It should be remembered that the presence of estrogen is required to maintain progesterone receptor levels. If rats are maintained on estrogen, no decrease of progesterone receptor levels occurs after progesterone administration, whereas in estrogen-withdrawn animals a rapid decrease takes place. Estrogen withdrawal implies a lack of estrogen action, which could result from either decreasing serum levels of estrogen or decreasing levels of estrogen receptor. Because progesterone suppresses the synthesis of the estrogen receptor (see later) and the synthesis of the progesterone receptor is dependent on the action of estrogens via the estrogen receptor, progesterone may suppress the synthesis of its own receptor by desensitizing the uterus to estrogen. The level of cytosolic progesterone receptor correlates with the ability of the uterus to respond to progesterone. When cytosolic progesterone receptor levels are low, an injection

of progesterone has no antagonistic effect on estrogen-induced early uterotropic events. Thus the ability of the uterus to respond to progesterone depends on the presence of its receptor.

CONTROL OF THE ESTROGEN RECEPTOR BY PROGESTERONE. Progesterone acts on the estrogen-primed uterus to alter cell function and reproductive competence. Often this ability of progesterone is considered to be antagonistic to estrogen; however, it probably should be considered a modifier of estrogen action. Nevertheless, progesterone reduces the ability of estrogens to cause uterine growth and vaginal cornification.[342, 380] This ability of progesterone to modify or antagonize estrogen action is generally considered to involve receptor mechanisms.

Progesterone does not interfere with the initial binding of estradiol to the cytosolic estrogen receptor or with the subsequent nuclear binding of the complex. Instead, progesterone decreases the cytosolic estrogen receptor concentration.[381] This decrease in receptor level correlates with a decreased ability of estradiol to stimulate uterine growth.[382] In addition, in the hamster uterus progesterone reduces the level of nuclear-bound estrogen-receptor complexes.[383, 384] This reduction in nuclear-bound estrogen-receptor complexes may be due to the induction of an estrogen receptor–regulatory factor by progesterone.[385] Such a factor may be involved in the dephosphorylation-inactivation mechanisms.[386] Under conditions of continuous exposure of the animal to estrogen, progesterone causes a temporary reduction of the level of nuclear estrogen-receptor complexes, followed by a return to elevated levels.[387] The control of estrogen receptor levels by progesterone and other proposed antagonistic functions of progesterone are discussed in more detail later under Steroid Hormone Antagonism.

Acute administration of progesterone to estrogen-stimulated chicks causes a preferential destruction of the Y form ($K_d \sim 1.0$ nM) of the estrogen receptor in the oviduct but has no effect on the X form ($K_d \sim 0.1$ nM).[388] This alteration is accompanied by an interruption of ovalbumin gene expression. Because both X and Y forms of the receptor are thought to be necessary for estrogen action, it is possible that progesterone antagonizes estrogenic effects by this mechanism.

NONRECEPTOR BINDING PROTEINS. Several nonreceptor proteins that bind estrogen and progesterone are found in both cytosolic and nuclear fractions.

Cytosolic Nonreceptor Binding Sites. The cytosol from immature rat uteri contains a proteinaceous macromolecule that is observed with saturation analysis by [³H]estradiol exchange. These type II estrogen binding sites have a sedimentation coefficient of 4S on postlabeled sucrose density gradients, but, unlike the estrogen receptor, they do not undergo translocation to the nucleus.[389, 390] That is, an injection of estradiol that causes cytoplasmic depletion and concomitant nuclear accumulation of the estrogen receptor does not deplete type II sites from the cytosol. Type II sites have a lower affinity ($K_d \sim 20$ nM) than does the receptor ($K_d \sim 1$ nM), but the number of type II sites may exceed that of type I sites. Type II sites display stereospecificity for estrogens and are present in other estrogen targets such as the vagina, mouse and human mammary tumors, MCF-7 cells, rabbit endometrial cells, and müllerian ducts of the chick embryo. Similar secondary binding sites have been observed in the prostate,[391, 392] seminal vesicle,[393] and rabbit corpus luteum.[394] Thus the presence of secondary binding sites for estrogenic hormones appears to be a general phenomenon.

Although the function of type II sites is not known, their presence complicates the interpretation of receptor assays. The quantity of these sites may range from 2 to 10 times the quantity of estrogen receptor. The influence of these variations on the determination of the type I receptor can be significant. As the quantity of type II sites increases, the error introduced in the estimation of the K_d and of the number of type I sites progressively increases. This becomes apparent only when saturation analysis is determined over a wide range of hormone concentrations. Consequently, assays limited to a single concentration of hormone (1 to 10 nM) measure both sites and may lead to overestimates of the affinity and number of type I sites. These points have been discussed in detail by Clark and Peck.[1, 324]

A steroid-binding protein that is similar to cytosol type II sites is present in chick oviduct.[395] This protein, which is called the Z protein, does not display stereospecificity for estrogen but instead binds estrogens, progestogens, and androgens with similar affinities. Therefore, the Z protein is different from cytosol type II sites; however, it is similar in that it does not undergo translocation to the nucleus and has approximately the same affinity for estradiol ($K_d = 20$ nM). Also the Z protein is in excess (~15-fold) of the estrogen receptor in the oviduct cytosol.[396]

The relationship of the Z protein to steroid receptor is unknown; however, the two classes of protein have certain characteristics in common. These include a sedimentation coefficient of about 8S, tissue specificity, stabilization by molybdate, and similar chromatographic behavior on diethylaminoethyl (DEAE) cellulose. Thus it is possible that this protein is a precursor of other gonadal steroid receptors in the oviduct. Alternatively, the Z protein could act as a general mechanism for concentrating steroids in oviduct tissues. This function has also been suggested for type II sites. However, it is currently thought that type II sites are more likely involved in binding an endogenous ligand that is concerned with the control of cell proliferation (see the section on physiological estrogen antagonists for a discussion of this point).

Nuclear Type II Estradiol Binding Sites. In addition to nuclear-bound estrogen receptor (type I sites), a second estrogen binding site is found in nuclei of various tissues. These type II nuclear estradiol binding sites are located on the nuclear matrix.[397, 398] The relationship between cytosolic and nuclear type II sites is not known; however, as explained earlier, cytosolic type II sites do not appear to undergo nuclear translocation, so the cytosolic and nuclear sites may be separate forms of related macromolecules. Nuclear type II sites are specific for estrogenic molecules, and their levels are increased by estrogen treatment.

Nuclear type II sites appear to bind estrogen in a cooperative manner and display a sigmoid saturation curve. Figure 3–9 shows an example of this type of curve and its relationship to the type of curve obtained with the estrogen receptor (type I). Type I sites display the usual saturation curve, which has the shape of a rectangular hyperbola and can be analyzed by use of a Scatchard plot to yield a linear component. Nuclear type II sites, however, have a more complex binding curve, which is sigmoidal and curvilinear by saturation and Scatchard analysis, respectively (see Fig. 3–9A and B). Complex curves such as these are difficult to resolve into their individual components: however, we have observed that dithiothreitol exposure causes the disappearance of type II sites and permits the independent measurement of the estrogen receptor.[399] The physiological role of nuclear type II sites and their relationship to cytosolic type II sites are discussed later in the section on physiological estrogen antagonists.

Hypothalamic-Hypophyseal Interactions

Receptors for steroid hormones are found in various specific loci in the brain that are known to be associated with the actions of steroid hormones.[1, 400] Pituitary cells contain various steroid receptors, localized in cell types that are thought to be responsive to the respective hormone; i.e., gonadotropes contain estrogen receptors, corticotropes contain glucocorticoid receptors, and so on. Thus the brain, particularly the hypothalamus and pituitary, contains response systems for steroid hormones. The steroid receptors in brain and pituitary tissue are similar to those in other tissues and are thought to act via similar mechanisms. Although steroid hormones do not cause cellular proliferation in the brain, as some do in other tissues, they do stimulate protein synthesis. These proteins are thought to be involved in the processes by which the neurons in the brain control gonadotropin secretion by the pituitary.

Estrogen stimulates the synthesis of progesterone receptors in the hypothalamus in much the same way as it does in other target tissues. This increase in progesterone receptor levels appears to be required for the induction of sexual behavior by progesterone, which occurs during the estrous cycle. Thus steroid hormones interact with the hypothalamic-hypophyseal system to control ovulation and reproductive behavior in a carefully timed fashion.

Glucocorticoid receptors in the brain and pituitary are also thought to be involved in the control of corticotropin (ACTH, adrenocorticotropin) release and behavior. The distribution of glucocorticoid receptors in the rat brain differs greatly from that for estrogen and androgen receptors. Glucocorticoid receptors are concentrated in the neurons of hippocampus, septum, and amygdala. Glucocorticoid receptors in the pituitary appear to function in the delayed or long-term negative feedback effects of glucocorticoids on corticotropin secretion; however, the functional relationships between neuronal activity and receptor hormone binding have not been established.

Some of the responses to steroid hormones in the brain occur rapidly and are not likely to be the result of gene-level stimulation. Instead, they are thought to result from steroid-membrane interactions.[401] Diencephalic neuronal discharge rates increase within seconds after iontophoretic administration of estradiol 17β-hemisuccinate. Likewise, cortisol administration alters the response of hypothalamic neurons. The release of corticotropin-releasing hormone is rapidly inhibited by application of glucocorticoids to hypothalamic fragments or synaptosomes in vitro. These effects may be related to the observation that glucocorticoid treatment in vivo has a rapid negative feedback effect on corticotropin, followed by a delayed, long-term negative feedback.

Steroid Receptors and the Reproductive Cycle

The assumption that steroid hormone binding is causally related to steroid response is difficult to prove; however, certain predictions and corollaries can be stated if this assumption is correct. Fluctuation of the free hormone concentration in the blood should be accompanied by concomitant receptor binding and target tissue stimulations. Because the blood levels of steroid hormones at various reproductive stages are well known, it should be possible to correlate receptor occupation with these levels under various physiological conditions.

RECEPTOR BINDING IN THE OVARY. The ovary is responsive to exogenous estrogens. Estrogen-induced maturation of follicular development involves complex mechanisms and does not simply involve estradiol sensitization of follicular cells to gonadotropin stimulation. Estradiol treatment of the hypophysectomized rat does not increase the number of FSH receptors per granulosa cell but does increase the number of its own receptors.[402] Estrogen also increases the number of granulosa cells and hence increases the quantity of FSH binding by the ovary. FSH treatment likewise increases the quantity of FSH receptors. Both hormones in concert increase the LH receptor levels of granulosa cells and hence enhance the sensitivity of these cells to the ovulatory effect of LH. Follicular atresia is associated with loss of receptors for estrogen, FSH, and LH.

STEROID RECEPTORS IN THE UTERUS. The concentration of nuclear estrogen receptor in the uterus correlates with the level of estrogen in the blood of the rat.[403] The number of nuclear complexes is at a minimum during estrus and metestrus (1000 sites per cell), increases between metestrus and diestrus (3500 sites per cell), and reaches a maximum at proestrus (5000 sites per cell). Uterine weight, protein content, and the ratio of protein to DNA are higher in proestrus than in metestrus or diestrus, suggesting that fluctuations in protein synthetic activity of the uterus occur throughout the estrous cycle. Thus maximal estrogenic responses are accompanied by peak concentrations of nuclear complexes in the proestrus uterus. Similar observations have been made in the oviduct and uterus in the cat. The quantity of nuclear-bound receptor in both organs correlates with ciliation and cell height in the oviduct during the estrous cycle.

The level of cytosolic progesterone receptor varies during the estrous cycle in all species, and estrogen appears to control its synthesis. During the follicular phase of the cycle, the level of cytosolic progesterone receptor is relatively low, and as estrogen blood levels increase, the quantity of receptor is elevated. This increase in progesterone receptor levels is probably a requisite for the actions of progesterone during pregnancy and during the luteal phase of the cycle.

Elevated levels of serum progesterone cause the usual depletion of cytosolic progesterone receptors and accumulation of nuclear receptor-progesterone complexes, but the situation differs from that of estrogen in that an eventual decrease in total progesterone receptor concentration occurs after progesterone injection. Cytosolic progesterone receptor levels are increased before the preovulatory peak in plasma progesterone receptor synthesis and subsequently decrease as the corpus luteum produces high levels of progesterone. The receptor level also remains low during pregnancy in the guinea pig. Similar changes occur during the estrous cycle in the hamster, rat, and mouse and in human endometrial tissue. The quantity of cytosolic progesterone receptor increases gradually during the menstrual cycle, reaching high levels at midcycle followed by a decline during the luteal phase.

The decrease in cytosolic progesterone receptor level under the influence of elevated progesterone levels in the blood is not the result of nuclear accumulation but is an actual decrease in the total number of receptors. This suppression of cytosolic progesterone receptor probably results from the serial inhibition phenomenon discussed earlier; i.e., progesterone, via its inhibition of estrogen receptor synthesis, suppresses the synthesis of its own receptor. Alternatively, this decrease may result from a combination of low estrogen levels and a change in relative abundance of receptors among specific cell types that constitute a small number of the total cell population. Although progesterone receptors are present in both endometrial and myometrial tissues of guinea pig, sheep, and human, this does not rule out the possibility of differential cell effects of progesterone.

In general, estrogen acts to promote uterine growth and to increase the tissue content of progesterone receptor, whereas progesterone antagonizes the action of estrogen by decreasing tissue levels of estrogen receptor. Thus the interaction of these ovarian hormones at the receptor level provides a basis for the cyclic changes observed in uterine tissues during the estrous cycle of the rat.

HYPOTHALAMIC-PITUITARY INTERACTIONS. As discussed earlier under Hypothalamic-Hypophyseal Interactions, the hypothalamic neurons and cells of the pituitary contain estrogen and progesterone receptors.[1] These receptors accumulate in the nuclear fraction of both tissues after hormone exposure. This relation can also be observed in the cycling rat during the various phases of the estrous cycle. The quantity of nuclear estrogen receptor in the pituitary and hypothalamus increases before and during proestrus in the rat. This change corresponds to the increased nuclear binding of the receptor in the uterus mentioned earlier and probably reflects the interaction of estrogen with the hypothalamic-pituitary cells that control gonadotropin secretion. The precise relationships between the quantity of nuclear-bound receptor and the positive and negative effects of estrogen on gonadotropin secretion have not been established. However, negative effects may be mediated by nuclear receptor accumulation in the pituitary at low levels of circulating estrogen, and positive effects may be controlled by the hypothalamic binding that occurs only at high levels of estrogen in the blood.

PREGNANCY AND LACTATION. *Uterus.* The fluctuations in number and compartmentalization of uterine steroid hormone receptors during pregnancy have received little study.[1] The complexities of examining each of the various organs and tissues involved as pregnancy progresses obviously make such work difficult. One time period in which such studies are not complicated by the presence of the placenta is the first few days after conception in the rat. This period is of special interest because of implantation of the blastocyst is estrogen dependent. Blood levels of estradiol are transiently elevated in the pregnant rat between days 1 and 4 of pregnancy. At this time the quantity of nuclear estrogen complexes in the uterus increases significantly (days 2 and 3 of the implantation period) and then decreases (on day 4). These data suggest that elevated blood levels of estradiol cause nuclear accumulation of the hormone-receptor complex, which in turn may stimulate the events that lead to blastocyst implantation. The reduction of estrogen receptor levels may also be linked to rising progesterone levels at this time. Alternatively, both decreasing levels of estrogen and increasing titers of progesterone may bring about this effect.

The quantity of cytosolic progesterone receptor gradually increases during pregnancy in the rat to high levels, whereas nuclear levels of receptor accumulate and then decrease just before parturition. The number of cytoplasmic sites available for nuclear binding is large compared with the quantity of nuclear sites measured. The reason for this distribution is not clear because blood levels of progesterone are high during pregnancy. Either the receptor sites are not all measured in these studies or the metabolic conversion of progesterone to 5α-reduced steroids results in apparent discrepancies. The ability of the rat uterus to form 5α-pregnane-3,20-dione and 3α-hydroxy-5α-pregnan-20-one increases substantially between days 11 and 21 of pregnancy. Thus, although blood levels of progesterone are high at these times, tissue levels may be much lower. This metabolic sequence could produce a cellular environment wherein the concentration of progesterone is gradually lowered during pregnancy and hence fewer estrogen-receptor complexes are formed. Elevated levels of cytoplasmic progesterone receptor during the last few days of pregnancy in the rat could be due to elevated levels of estrogen at this time. The decrease in nuclear levels of progesterone receptor before birth is probably an important mechanism for decreasing the control of the uterus by progesterone and increasing its sensitivity to estrogen. This shift would provide a nonquiescent uterus capable of contracting and would result in parturition.

Progesterone receptors during pregnancy have also been studied in guinea pig, hamster, and mouse. In contrast to the results for the rat, levels of cytosolic progesterone receptor either change little, as in the mouse, or are depressed, as in the guinea pig. Additional work is required to understand these species differences.

Ovary. The corpus luteum of the rabbit requires estrogen for its maintenance and contains cytosolic estrogen receptors similar to those in other tissues.[404] Control of cytosolic estrogen receptor levels by luteolytic factors from the uterus may be important in the maintenance of corpus luteum function. The level of nuclear-bound estrogen-receptor complexes in the corpus luteum of the rat increases between days 2 and 12 of pregnancy. After day 12 the total amount of receptor per cell gradually decreases, despite the continuing elevated levels of estrogen. However, because the ovary is the source of estradiol, blood measurements need not reflect the concentration of estrogen in the corpus luteum. In addition, administration of estradiol to hypophysectomized pregnant rats causes maintenance of cytosolic estrogen receptors in luteal tissue. The relationship between these observations and luteotropic control by estradiol is not clear.

Mammary Gland. The mammary gland is a target organ for several hormones, and steroids stimulate the development and growth of this tissue. Estrogen, progesterone, and glucocorticoid receptors in the tissue appear to be similar to those in other target tissues. During pregnancy, the receptor levels increase and the sedimentation pattern gradually shifts from the 4S form to an 8S form.[405] These qualitative and quantitative changes appear to be controlled by prolactin. However, because the cellular composition of the gland changes during pregnancy, this elevation may be due to an increased number of epithelial cells per unit mass of tissue.

In the lactating rat, the concentration of cytoplasmic estrogen receptor increases dramatically by day 10 and is even higher by day 21.[406] In contrast, nuclear estrogen-receptor complexes remain low throughout lactation because estrogen levels in the blood are low. The low quantities of nuclear estrogen-receptor complexes do not result from a failure of the translocation process, because an injection of estradiol promotes the accumulation of nuclear estrogen-receptor complexes. The elevation of cytoplasmic receptor number in lactating tissue does not depend on the presence of the ovary. The physiological function of the elevated cytoplasmic receptor level remains to be determined.

Placenta. Estrogen receptors are present in the maternal placenta during pregnancy in the rat.[407] The basal zone of the rat placenta contains large numbers of cytosolic estrogen receptors during a limited period of midpregnancy. The number of cytosolic receptors on day 9 of pregnancy is 30,000 per cell, while levels of nuclear receptor are relatively low (3400 per cell). This distribution of receptors is probably due to the low concentration of estrogens in the blood at this time. However, the reason for such high levels of cytoplasmic receptor during early pregnancy in this tissue is unknown. By day 15 of pregnancy the levels of receptor decrease to 600 and 200 sites per cell for cytoplasmic and nuclear receptors, respectively. The reason for the decrease in estrogen receptor level during this time period is not evident. However, the secretion of progesterone by trophoblastic giant cells may bring about this decline.

Receptors and Development

Steroid receptors are present in their respective target organs before the maturation of the endocrine glands that secrete the effector hormones. In the guinea pig, estrogen receptors are present in the fetal uterus and are fully capable of responding to exogenous estrogen administration to the mother.[408] In the rat, which has a short gestational period, estrogen receptors in the uterus are synthesized during the first 10 d of life.[409] The concentration of estrogen receptors in the neonatal rat or fetal guinea pig is either equal to or greater than that in the adult animal. Early appearance of estrogen receptors during neonatal life in the rat also occurs in the hypothalamus and pituitary. The development of receptors in these organs and tissues does not appear to depend on steroid hormone stimulation but is an autonomous developmental property of the reproductive target organs that prepares them for subsequent responses to tropic hormones.

In contrast to the situation in the mammal, oviduct development in the chicken appears to be dependent on the presence of estrogen. In most birds, the right müllerian duct regresses in the female and the left duct develops into the oviduct and shell gland of the mature bird. The development of the left oviduct and regression of the right duct are estrogen dependent. The quantity of cytosolic receptors increases from day 8 to day 12 of embryonic development, and the quantity of nuclear estrogen-receptor complexes increases dramatically between days 10 and 18. This nuclear accumulation of receptor probably results from endogenous estrogens present in the yolk.

Receptors and Aging

In the preceding section it was pointed out that steroid receptors appear in target tissues before the maturation of the gonads, thus setting the stage for the appropriate response of the tissue to hormones. It has been proposed that aging might be caused by the reverse of this developmental pathway; i.e., receptors may decrease in numbers or affinity for their tropic hormones and thereby render systems less sensitive to hormonal stimulation, leading to decreased function and aging. Some support for this concept has been obtained from studies in the rat, which gradually loses its regular 4- to 5-d estrous cycle and enters a stage of persistent estrus at approximately 1 to 1.5 y of age.[410] This is usually followed by periods of persistent diestrus. During these periods the estrogen receptor concentration decreases but there is no decrease in binding affinity for estrogens. Thus it is possible that receptor loss is associated with aging; however, whether it is a cause-effect relationship is unknown.

In the male, levels of certain urinary proteins under the control of androgens decrease with age. In the young adult male rat, androgen regulates the synthesis of alpha-2u–globulin by the liver.[411] This protein is secreted into the blood and is excreted in the urine. Although the function of alpha-2u–globulin is not known, it is an excellent marker for aging in the rat. In the senescent (750-d-old) rat, this protein is absent from the urine and androgen treatment does not restore its synthesis and excretion. Associated with this androgen insensitivity is a shift in the normal sedimentation value of the liver androgen receptor from 8S to 3.5S. This shift may be associated with structural changes in the androgen receptor with age and may render the animal insensitive to androgens.[412]

STEROID HORMONE ANTAGONISM

Compounds that block the action of a given steroid hormone are called antagonists or antihormones. Most of these act by binding to receptors and interfering with their normal function. However, this generalization requires qualification, depending on the specific hormone.

Antiestrogens

Antiestrogens can be divided into three groups: (1) short-acting antagonists, such as estriol; (2) long-acting antagonists, such as tamoxifen and clomiphene; and (3) physiological antagonists, such as progesterone, androgens, and glucocorticoids.

SHORT-ACTING ANTAGONISTS. Short-acting estrogens such as estriol and estradiol-17α are actually time-dependent mixed agonists-antagonists (Fig. 3–45). They stimulate early uterotropic responses but have little effect on true uterine hypertrophy and hyperplasia when injected in saline.[1, 413] This explains why they have no antagonistic action when examined by short-term uterotropic assays but display partial antagonism when long-term uterine growth assays are used. This dichotomy may be understood by examining the idealized data shown in Figure 3–46. The response patterns for estradiol and estriol at three dose levels are plotted as a function of time after a single injection. If uterotropic responses are measured at 6 h after an injection of either estradiol or estriol, they are identical (see Fig. 3–46B), and therefore no antagonism will be noted. However, measurements made at 24 h do show antagonism (see Fig. 3–46C). This inhibition is shown in the form of dose-response curves and results from the reduced capacity of estriol to stimulate true uterine growth. When estradiol and estriol are administered simultaneously the overall uterotropic effect is reduced at 24 h.

The short-acting agonists do cause nuclear binding of the hormone-receptor complex for short periods of time and thus they are able to stimulate early uterotropic events. However, they are unable to maintain the receptor in the nucleus for a sufficient period of time to cause true uterine growth. The antagonistic actions of these compounds result from competition between estradiol-receptor and estriol-receptor complexes for functional nuclear sites. The competition reduces the number of effective estrogen-receptor complexes retained in the nuclear compartment and thus

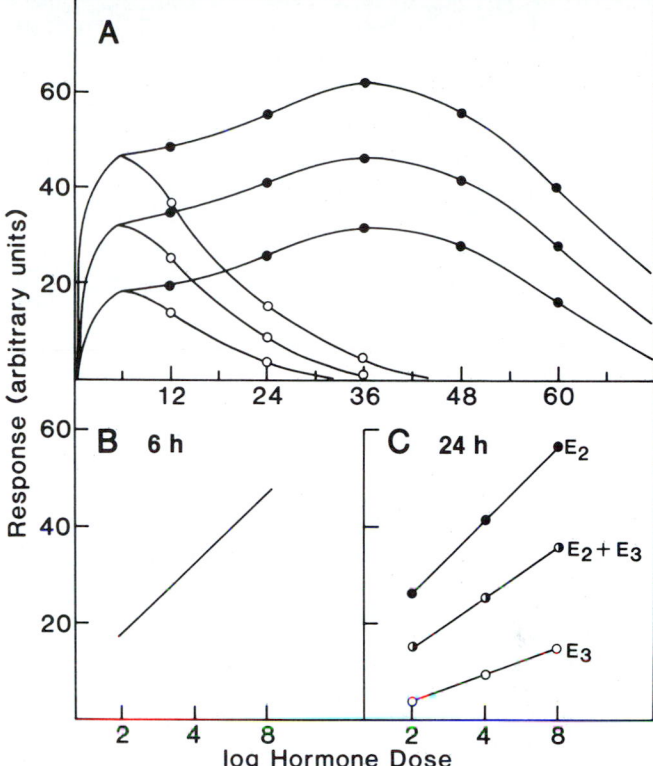

Figure 3–46. Effects on long-acting and short-acting estrogens on uterotropic response in rat. Uterotropic response (growth) in *A* is measured as a function of time after an injection of three dose levels of estradiol (●) or estriol (○). Identical dose response at 6 h for both hormones is shown in *B*. Dose-response curves at 24 h for estradiol (E_2), estriol (E_3), and a combination of these hormones are shown in *C*.

reduces the long-term uterotropic stimulation. When short-acting estrogens are administered via a pellet implant to cause continuous release of hormones and continuous occupancy of the receptor, no antagonism is observed. Thus the biological response with short-acting estrogens is dependent on the conditions of administration and is the consequence of receptor occupancy.

Why short-acting estrogens occupy nuclear-bound receptors for short periods after an injection is not completely clear. The rate of dissociation of estriol from the receptor is higher than that of estradiol,[414] leading to the suggestion that this difference in dissociation rate accounts for short-term nuclear retention.[415] Estriol is also cleared from the body more rapidly than is estradiol.[416] Therefore, the equilibrium between tissue and blood levels results in more rapid dissociation of nuclear-bound estriol-receptor complexes. It is also possible that estriol-receptor complexes dissociate from their nuclear binding sites more rapidly than do estradiol-receptor complexes. This could result in faster turnover or processing of receptor and loss of hormone from the tissues.

LONG-ACTING ANTAGONISTS. Triphenylethylene derivatives, such as tamoxifen or clomiphene (Fig. 3–47), are mixed agonists-antagonists of estrogen action.[417] Mixed agonism-antagonism is common among the anti–steroid hormones. An agonist is a compound that stimulates a response (Fig. 3–48A), whereas an antagonist completely inhibits the action of an agonist. A mixed agonist-antagonist partially inhibits the action of an agonist, but because it has inherent agonistic properties it partially mimics the response of the agonist. The degree of agonist or antagonist activity observed depends on the species, organ, tissue, or cell type that is

Estrogen Structures

Long Acting

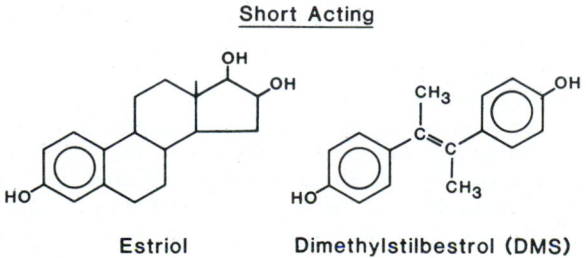

Estradiol   Diethylstilbestrol (DES)

Short Acting

Estriol   Dimethylstilbestrol (DMS)

Figure 3–45. Chemical structures of long-acting and short-acting estrogens.

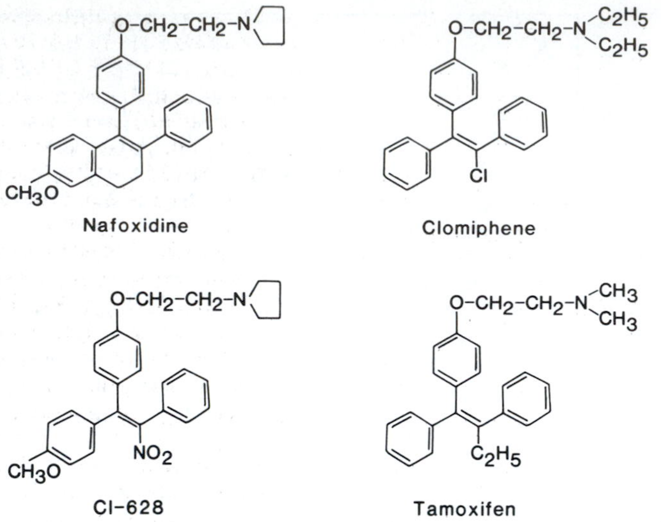

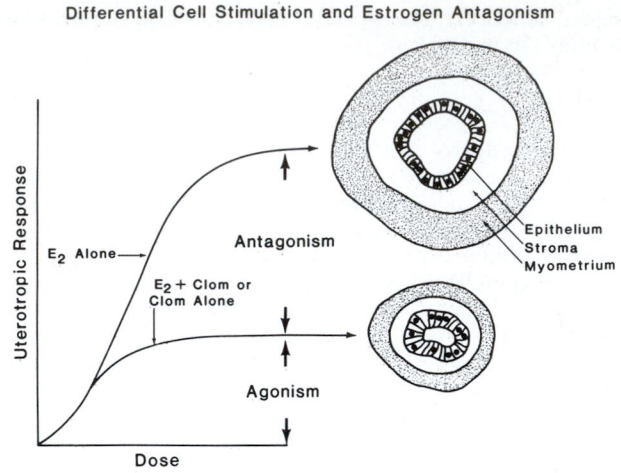

Differential Cell Stimulation and Estrogen Antagonism

Figure 3–49. The agonistic and antagonistic effects of estradiol and clomiphene on uterine growth and histology. E_2, estradiol; Clom, clomiphene.

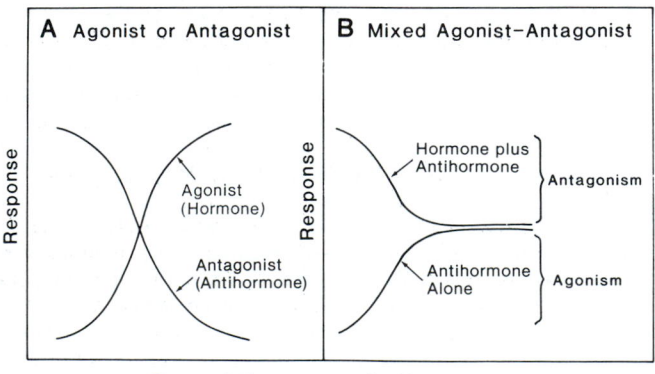

Figure 3–47. Antiestrogens of triphenylethylene type.

being examined and on the end-point assay chosen. Clomiphene and tamoxifen cause growth of the rat uterus when administered alone but inhibit the growth-promoting effects of estradiol when given simultaneously (Fig. 3–49). These stimulatory and inhibitory functions are the result of the ability of these drugs to stimulate hypertrophy of the epithelial cells of the endometrium while having little effect on the stromal or myometrial compartments. Estradiol, on the other hand, stimulates cellular hypertrophy and hyperplasia in all three tissue layers and hence produces a larger uterus than clomiphene alone. The elevation in uterine weight caused by clomiphene or tamoxifen alone is due primarily to the hypertrophy of epithelial cells and slight stimulation of the stroma and myometrium. The inhibition of estradiol action on uterine growth results from the antagonism of cellular growth in the stromal and myometrial compartments. Therefore, triphenylethylene drugs act like partial estrogen agonists in the epithelial cells and as estrogen antagonists in other uterine cells.

The mechanisms by which long-acting estrogen antagonists block estrogen action in some cell types, yet stimulate estrogen responses in others, are not fully understood. However, these drugs bind to the estrogen receptor and cause nuclear accumulation of antagonist-receptor complexes. This accumulation is accompanied by long-term depletion of cytosolic receptors and altered nuclear processing of the antagonist-receptor complex. All of these altered receptor functions may be involved in the mechanism by which the antagonists block estrogen action.

Subtle differences have been reported in the physicochemical characteristics of antiestrogen-receptor and estradiol-receptor complexes.[418, 419] However, it is not clear how such differences are related to hormone antagonism. No difference between antiestrogen-receptor and estradiol-receptor complexes has been found with respect to their recognition by monoclonal antibodies to the receptor or their binding to DNA or polynucleotides.[420, 421] Evans and colleagues[422] showed that estradiol-receptor complexes bind more tightly to calf thymus DNA than do antiestrogen-receptor complexes. Perhaps this observation relates to the finding that nuclear-bound antiestrogen-receptor complexes can be readily extracted by high salt concentrations, whereas a portion of the estrogen-receptor complexes cannot.[423] These salt-extracted forms of the receptor do not differ significantly from those of the estradiol-receptor complex.[424] Differential extraction of estrogen-receptor and tamoxifen-receptor complexes has also been observed with the nonionic detergent Nonidet P-40.[425] All of the nuclear tamoxifen-receptor complex from MCF-7 cells is extracted with this detergent and sediments as 7S and 5S peaks on sucrose density gradients. In contrast, nuclear estradiol-receptor complexes resist extraction. These results suggest that the interactions of these two receptor complex forms with chromatin differ in some way.

Understanding the mechanism of action of long-acting agonists-antagonists is complicated further by interspecies variation. In contrast to the mixed agonistic-antagonistic function of nonsteroidal antiestrogens in the rat, in the adult mouse these compounds are estrogenic with little if any antiestrogenic activity.[426] In the chick oviduct and liver, however, these compounds are estrogen antagonists and have virtually no detectable agonist activity under most circumstances.[351, 427] However, tamoxifen, when administered with progesterone, induces cytodifferentiation of oviduct tubular gland cells and stimulates the synthesis of conalbumin and ovalbumin, whereas tamoxifen alone has no effect. The interactions that bring about these effects are not known. In primates, clomiphene and tamoxifen are primarily antiestrogenic; however, estrogenicity has been noted depending on the species and end point used.[428, 429] The effects of clomiphene at the hypothalamic-hypophyseal level in primates are discussed in the next section. Other species manifest a broad spectrum of agonistic-antagonistic responses to nonsteroidal antiestrogens, discussion of which

Figure 3–48. Effects of agonists, antagonists, and mixed agonists-antagonists on response.

goes beyond the scope of this chapter (for reviews see refs. 428 and 430).

These species differences in response to nonsteroidal antiestrogens essentially disappear in cell culture. Tamoxifen and 4-hydroxytamoxifen block the estrogen-stimulated increases in several specific proteins in MCF-7 cells and have no agonistic activity.[431] Tamoxifen and nafoxidine inhibit [³H]thymidine incorporation and DNA polymerase activity and reduce cell number in MCF-7 cell cultures.[432] Estrogen-stimulated prolactin synthesis is inhibited by tamoxifen, and no agonistic effect is seen with the drug alone.[433, 434]

These drugs may act in part via indirect mechanisms that do not involve the estrogen receptor at all. Triphenylethylene antiestrogen binding sites (TABSs) that bind tamoxifen and clomiphene with high affinity ($K_d \sim 1$ nM) are present in estrogen target and nontarget tissues.[435, 436] In addition, somewhat similar sites with lower affinity ($K_d \sim 10$ nM) are associated with low-density lipoprotein (LDL) in rat serum.[437] The binding specificity of TABS spans a rather broad range; however, triphenylethylene derivatives that contain the alkylaminoethoxy side chain are bound with the highest affinity and steroids are not bound by these sites. Other compounds, such as chlorpromazine, ketocholesterol, and cholesterol, have a reduced affinity; however, as discussed later, these may be significant.[483]

The subcellular localization of TABS appears to vary with species and/or cell type. TABSs have been characterized in cytosols of the chick oviduct, guinea pig and rat uterus, human mammary carcinoma, and nontarget human tissues.[439–441] Cytosolic and nuclear localization has been reported in the guinea pig uterus by Gulino and Pasqualini,[440] and the level of these sites may be modulated by estradiol and progesterone.[437, 442] Nuclear localization has also been reported in human breast cancer tissue and in chicken and rat liver.

The physiological functions of TABSs have not been defined, and although it is tempting to suggest that they are antiestrogen receptors, in general the data do not support this hypothesis. The estrogenic and antiestrogenic properties of nonsteroidal antiestrogens correlate with their relative binding affinities for the estrogen receptor and not for TABS.[443] The cis and trans isomers of clomiphene bind to TABS with similar affinities but have dissimilar agonist-antagonist profiles. Tamoxifen resistance has been described in a line of MCF-7 breast cancer cells that contained extremely low levels of TABS and normal levels of estrogen receptor. However, it has not been possible to relate the levels of TABS to tamoxifen sensitivity.[443]

The possible involvement of TABS in the mechanism of action of antiestrogen is suggested by the observation that estrogen administration and the physiological state of the ovary influence the level of TABS in both liver and uterus.[444] At the time of puberty, the liver TABS concentration increases in the female. TABS levels in rat uterine cytosol also increase in mature females, and both uterine and liver TABS levels fluctuate throughout the estrous cycle and reach a peak approximately on the day of estrus. Treatment of ovariectomized rats with physiological amounts of estradiol causes a twofold increase in TABS levels in the uterus, mimicking the midcycle peak of TABS. Gulino and Pasqualini[442] have shown that the level of TABS in the guinea pig uterus is modulated by estradiol and progesterone.

The presence of TABS associated with the serum LDL fraction from the rat is of interest because LDL cholesterol is involved in the control of cellular cholesterol synthesis. Triphenylethylene antiestrogens are inhibitors of cholesterol synthesis, and tamoxifen inhibits cholesterol synthesis in MCF-7 cells.[445] 7-Ketocholesterol may act as an endogenous ligand for TABS.[446] This compound is a potent inhibitor of cholesterol synthesis and cell growth in human fibroblasts, and its half-maximal concentration (1 nM) for inhibition is in the range of its binding affinity for TABS.[445] These results suggest that TABSs may be involved in some aspect of cholesterol synthesis or metabolism. Because cellular growth is dependent on cholesterol synthesis, it is possible that these sites are somehow involved. However, triparanol is a potent inhibitor of cholesterol synthesis, yet it has little to no antiestrogenic action.

The binding of 7-ketocholesterol to TABS may be fortuitous, because many other compounds inhibit the binding of [³H]tamoxifen with the same relative affinities. Cholesterol, chlorpromazine, various ligands, and W13, a calmodulin inhibitor, act as competitive inhibitors of the binding of [³H]tamoxifen to TABS. The inhibition by W13 is of special interest because tamoxifen is an inhibitor of calmodulin-mediated phosphodiesterase activity.[447] Calmodulin is thought to be involved in the control of cell proliferation, and inhibitors of calmodulin block the cell cycle at the G_1 phase.[448] Because nonsteroidal antiestrogens block cellular proliferation, calmodulin inhibition may be involved in this effect. However, such an inhibition of cell proliferation appears to occur primarily in estrogen-responsive cells and therefore must somehow be linked to estrogen sensitivity.

PURE ANTIESTROGENS. All of the compounds discussed previously have been mixed estrogen agonists-antagonists. Another class of drugs appear to be pure antagonists.[449] ICI 164384 is a 7α-alkylamide analogue of estradiol that lacks agonist activity for uterine growth in both rats and mice and is unable to induce the progesterone receptor in the immature rat. ICI 164384 binds to the estrogen receptor with an affinity similar to that of estradiol; however, its ability to inhibit estrogen-induced mRNA synthesis is 50- to 150-fold less than predicted.[449] Similar discrepancies have been noted for tamoxifen and hydroxytamoxifen[450] and may result from a differential ability of these compounds to enter cells or from binding interactions with nonreceptor proteins.

PHYSIOLOGICAL ESTROGEN ANTAGONISTS. Fluctuation of blood levels of estrogen during the reproductive cycle is accompanied by changing levels of estrogen-receptor binding. Thus the effects of estrogen wax and wane as a result of these changes in ovarian secretion of estrogens. In addition, other hormones act to alter the actions of estrogen at the cellular level and modify estrogen-directed functions.

Progesterone. Progesterone acts on the estrogen-primed uterus to alter cell function and reproductive competence. Often this action of progesterone is considered to be antagonistic to estrogen; however, progesterone probably should be referred to as a modifier of estrogen action rather than an antagonist. Nevertheless, progesterone reduces the ability of estrogens to cause uterine growth and vaginal cornification. This ability of progesterone to modify estrogen action is generally considered to involve receptor mechanisms that have been discussed previously under Control of Steroid Receptor Concentration. These effects of progesterone involve decreases in the number of cytosolic and nuclear-bound estrogen-receptor complexes. Such reductions in receptor number correlate with a reduced sensitivity of the uterus to estradiol.[451]

Most of the studies concerned with progesterone effects on estrogen receptor levels have been done under nonphysiological circumstances. However, in the elegant studies of Brenner and colleagues,[452] physiological conditions were maintained by creating artificial menstrual cycles in ovariectomized rhesus monkeys. Under these conditions estradiol blood levels were maintained constant throughout the cycle and the progesterone level was elevated during the second half of the cycle. Cytosolic estrogen receptor levels were elevated during the first half of the cycle and dramatically decreased during the second half. These data suggest that progesterone does lower cytosolic estrogen receptor levels even when estradiol is present. Although nuclear estrogen receptors were not examined in this study, progesterone decreases the level in the hamster uterus under physiological circumstances. In the pig endometrium progesterone induces estrogen sulfotransferase, an enzyme that inactivates estradiol, these interfering with the estrogen-dependent replenishment of the estrogen receptor.[453] Therefore, several mechanisms exist whereby progesterone can decrease the level of estrogen receptor and reduce the ability of a tissue to respond to estrogen.

Modulated estrogen receptor levels correlate with striking changes in the morphology of the uterine luminal epithelium.[1] When nuclear receptor levels are elevated, the epithelium is hypertrophied and mitotic, whereas the epithelium is atrophied and shows degenerative changes when receptor levels are suppressed. Such changes in morphology and functional state of uterine cells probably reflect the normal cyclic interaction of estrogen and progesterone in the reproductive tract.

Progesterone also inhibits the stimulation of nuclear type II estrogen binding sites. This inhibition is correlated with a reduced uterotropic response to estrogen and does not appear to be related to any effects of progesterone on estrogen receptor levels. The inhibitory effects of progesterone do appear to be mediated by the progesterone receptor, because estrogen priming is necessary to observe the inhibitory effects of progesterone.

Androgens. Androgenic steroids inhibit the actions of estrogen on the growth of estrogen target tissues.[454] Indeed, androgen therapy has been used in the treatment of estrogen-dependent breast cancer. This treatment is based on the rationale that androgens should block or antagonize the estrogen-stimulated growth of breast cancer cells. The mechanisms by which androgens antagonize estrogenic functions are not known; however, it is known that androgen receptors are present in estrogen target tissues.[455] Physiological concentrations of androgens do not cause growth or stimulate other known functions of MCF-7 breast cancer cells, even though nuclear binding of the androgen-receptor complex is readily observed.[456] Likewise, in the rat uterus there appears to be no biological response to nuclear binding of the androgen-receptor complex. However, chronic exposure to physiological levels of androgens in the rat depresses uterine weight, an indication that androgens are antiestrogenic by some mechanism.

In contrast, high doses of androgens stimulate growth of the rat uterus, mammary tumors, and MCF-7 cells.[457] Thus androgens appear to have the capacity to inhibit and stimulate estrogen target tissues, depending on the dose used. The low-dose inhibition may be mediated directly by the androgen receptor or may occur indirectly via interactions at the hypothalamic-pituitary level or some other pathway. The high-dose stimulation effect is mediated by the estrogen receptor, because high concentrations of androgens bind to the estrogen receptor, cause nuclear accumulation, and produce an estrogen-like response.[458]

Type II Estrogen Binding Sites and Estrogen Antagonism. One of the pleiotropic events stimulated by exposure to estrogen is an elevation of type II estrogen binding sites. These sites are present in the cytosol and nuclei and are different from the estrogen receptor (type I). Nuclear type II receptors are occupied by an endogenous ligand that appears to be an inhibitor of cell proliferation and, as such, may constitute a new class of antiestrogen.[459] Estrogen-induced uterine cell proliferation is observed only when levels of nuclear type II sites are elevated, which may mean

that the inhibitory ligand has dissociated from these sites. Such dissociation would open up sites that are measured by the binding of labeled estradiol. Nuclear type II sites are tightly associated with the nuclear matrix and may be coupled to the regulatory components involved in DNA synthesis. Therefore, the dissociation of an inhibitory ligand from these sites may act as a positive regulatory signal to initiate DNA synthesis and cell proliferation.

Glucocorticoids. Glucocorticoids inhibit several of the early uterotropic responses induced by estrogen. These include water imbibition, histamine mobilization, eosinophil infiltration, and vasodilation, which are all components of the support pathway facilitating uterine growth. When these estrogen-induced responses are blocked by glucocorticoid administration, the biosynthetic ability of estrogen is not blocked; however, estrogen-mediated uterine growth is reduced, possibly because of the reduced availability of substrates to the growing uterus. The mechanisms involved in the antagonism of early uterotropic responses are not known, but they involve such uterine components as the vasculature, mast cells (histamine release), and eosinophil infiltration. Uterine cells contain glucocorticoid receptors, but their functional relationships to estrogen antagonism is not known.

Antiprogestogens

Although there are several exogenous and endogenous antiestrogens, few antiprogestational compounds have been developed. Many progesterone derivatives have been synthesized, but only one compound appears to have antagonistic properties. RU 486 interrupts the luteal phase of the menstrual cycle and terminates pregnancy in women.[460] RU 486 induces early onset of vaginal bleeding when administered during the luteal phase to cycling monkeys.[461, 467] Such actions are due to a direct antagonistic effect of RU 486 at the receptor level in the uterine endometrium. This compound binds to progesterone receptors in the rabbit uterus and to glucocorticoid receptors in the thymus, where it acts as an antiglucocorticoid. In T47D cells RU 486 binds to the progesterone receptor and inhibits cellular proliferation, as does R5020, a synthetic progestogen.[463] Thus RU 486 is an agonist by this criterion, but it does antagonize the stimulation of insulin receptors by R5020. Agonistic properties have also been observed in T47D cells, which grow in response to RU 486.[464] Therefore, in T47D cells RU 486 manifests mixed agonistic-antagonistic properties.

RU 486 binds well to all mammalian progesterone receptors except those of the hamster,[465] a species in which the drug has no antiprogestational effects. Progesterone receptors from the chick oviduct display a low affinity for RU 486. Such reduced affinity in the chicken and loss of affinity in the hamster indicate structural differences in the receptors in these animals.

The mechanism by which RU 486 exerts its antagonistic activity does not involve any differences in activation and transformation of the drug-receptor complex.[466, 467] Both progesterone and RU 486 form complexes that bind to hormone response elements in a qualitatively and quantitatively similar manner. The only difference appears to be in the sedimentation and gel retardation characteristics of the two receptor–hormone response element complexes. Thus the binding of the receptor–RU 486 complex to hormone response elements probably results in a conformation that is different from that of the receptor-progesterone complex. This different conformation does not permit the protein-protein interactions necessary for induction of gene transcription.

As pointed out earlier for antiestrogens, the actions of

anti–steroid hormone drugs in vitro are not necessarily identical to their actions in vivo. More work in vivo is needed on this important class of antiprogestogens before definitive statements can be made regarding their mechanism of action and their true pharmacological and physiological effects.

An inhibitor of progesterone-receptor binding has been described in the cytosol from rat placenta.[468] This inhibitor is a macromolecule that decreases the affinity of the receptor for progesterone but has no effect on the number of receptor sites. The function of this inhibitor is not known; however, inhibitory activity in trophoblast cytosol is greatest on days 9 and 12 of pregnancy and decreases thereafter. By day 18 inhibitory activity is no longer detectable, and this coincides with a sharp decrease in progesterone receptor concentration. Such inhibitors have not been described in other systems, but their potential significance in the regulation of progesterone action is considerable.

Antiandrogens

Androgen antagonists are a diverse group of compounds that inhibit the growth-stimulating actions of androgens. The structures of two of the best-known antiandrogens, cyproterone acetate and flutamide, are shown in Figure 3–50. Even though these two drugs lack structural similarity, they both bind to the androgen receptor and act as competitive inhibitors of androgen binding. In addition, administration of these drugs in vivo decreases the nuclear accumulation of androgen-receptor complexes. Thus antiandrogens appear to antagonize the action of androgens by blocking or interfering with nuclear accumulation of active hormone-receptor complexes.[469] Another possibility is that antagonist-receptor complexes accumulate in the nucleus but are so loosely bound that they are dissociated during the homogenization or nuclear preparation for the assay.

Progestogens also act as antiandrogens; however, their interactions are complex, and in some cases they mimic and even potentiate the action of androgens. The mechanism of action of progestogens as antiandrogens is not known. Progestogens bind to the androgen receptor with less affinity than does testosterone, and in competitive binding assays they cannot be distinguished from androgenic compounds. Presumably, progestogens bind to the androgen receptor

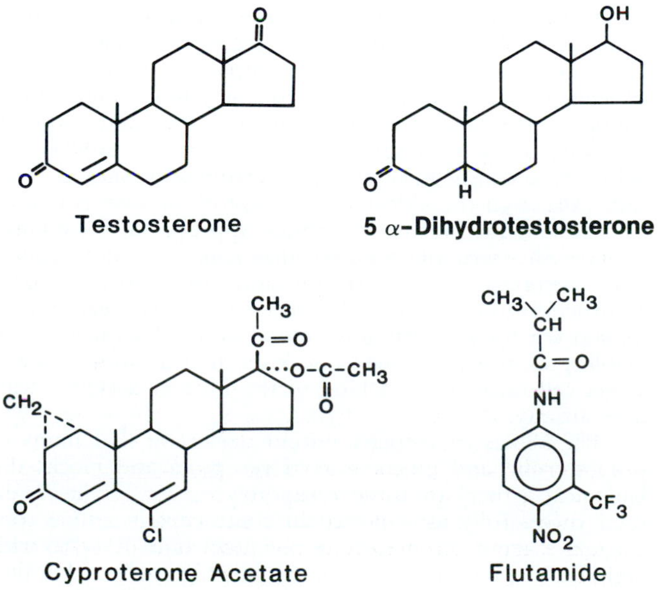

Figure 3–50. Chemical structures of androgens and antiandrogens.

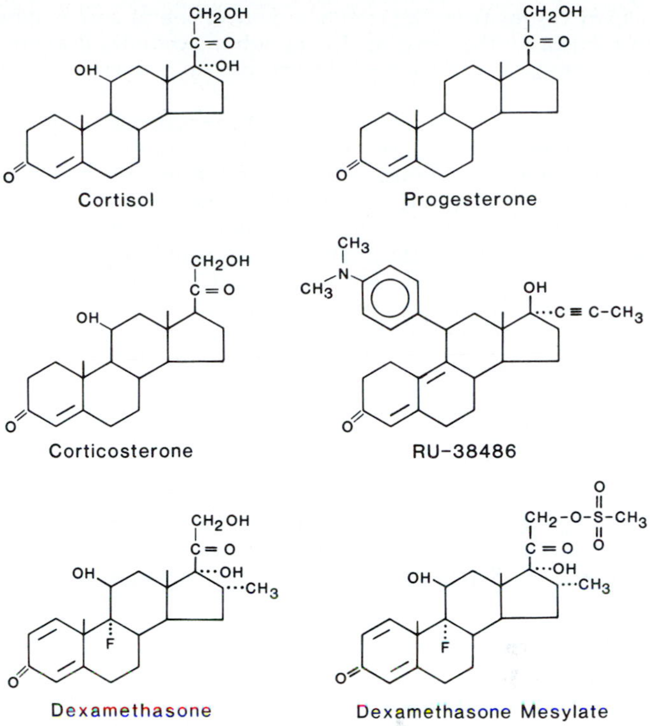

Figure 3–51. Chemical structures of glucocorticoids and antiglucocorticoids.

and hold it in a conformational state different from that of the testosterone-receptor complex.

Antiglucocorticoids

Glucocorticoid antagonists can be divided into two groups: (1) 4-pregnene or 4-androstene derivatives with modifications on the 11β-hydroxy group and (2) derivatives of cortisol or dexamethasone with alterations of the side chain located in the 17 position (Fig. 3–51). The antagonistic activity of these compounds is readily demonstrated in cells in culture.[470] However, when the same compounds are examined in vivo, they have mixed agonistic-antagonistic effects. Therefore, the subject of antiglucocorticoid drugs will be divided into two sections.[471]

IN VITRO OBSERVATIONS. Progesterone is an antagonist of the induction of tyrosine aminotransferase by dexamethasone in rat hepatoma cells. This antagonism is thought to result from the formation of a progesterone–glucocorticoid receptor complex that does not undergo nuclear binding. It is also possible that nuclear binding of the complex occurs but the complex is readily dissociated from these sites. 11-Desoxy-17-hydroxycorticosterone (cortexolone) competes for glucocorticoid receptor binding sites and blocks the effect of glucocorticoids on the uptake of 2-deoxyglucose in rat thymocytes. This antagonistic effect appears to result from the inability of the receptor-cortexolone complexes to bind to nuclear sites. Mixed agonists-antagonists, such as deoxycorticosterone, cause only partial nuclear accumulation and submaximal stimulation of tyrosine aminotransferase activity. Full antagonistic activity is readily demonstrated in vitro for RU 486, dexamethasone 21-mesylate, and dexamethasone oxetanone; yet this is not the case when these compounds are tested in vivo.

IN VIVO OBSERVATIONS. It is difficult to extrapolate from the in vitro ligand binding results just discussed to the in vivo situation. For example, cortexolone is an excellent antagonist of glucocorticoid action in vitro but it acts as a full agonist in most tests in the intact animal. This agonistic activity results from the metabolic conversion of cortexolone to cortisol by the adrenal. In the adrenalectomized animal cortexolone is a full antagonist because no conversion takes place.

The antagonistic actions of antiglucocorticoids are tested by two types of bioassays: (1) acute assays are done within a few hours after administration of the hormone (e.g., elevation in liver glycogen level or liver tyrosine aminotransferase or tryptophan oxygenase activity), and (2) chronic assays are done several days after hormone exposure (e.g., growth suppression, reduced adrenal weight, reduced thymus weight, and suppression of the inflammatory reaction).

Many antagonists in acute assays prove to be mixed agonists-antagonists in chronic assays. Thus the interpretation of relative agonistic-antagonistic properties depends on the test being used. A further complication results from the unexplained biphasic nature of chronic assays; i.e., at low doses a compound can be a partial antagonist and at higher doses become a full agonist. These complications are probably related to indirect actions that are not presently understood. However, it is clear that much more work is required before we understand antiglucocorticoid action in vivo.

Antimineralocorticoids

The action of aldosterone is inhibited by spironolactone and progesterone (Fig. 3–52). Both of these compounds are competitive inhibitors of the binding of [³H]aldosterone to the receptor and appear to form complexes that are inactive and do not bind to nuclear acceptor sites. Thus they reduce the effective level of aldosterone-receptor complexes and thereby reduce the response to the hormone.

CLINICAL AND BIOMEDICAL CONSIDERATIONS

Major improvements in our knowledge of the mode of action of the gonadal steroids can now be related to medical theory and practice of medicine. The resulting concepts are important to an understanding of medical pharmacology, physiology, pathology, diagnosis, and therapy.

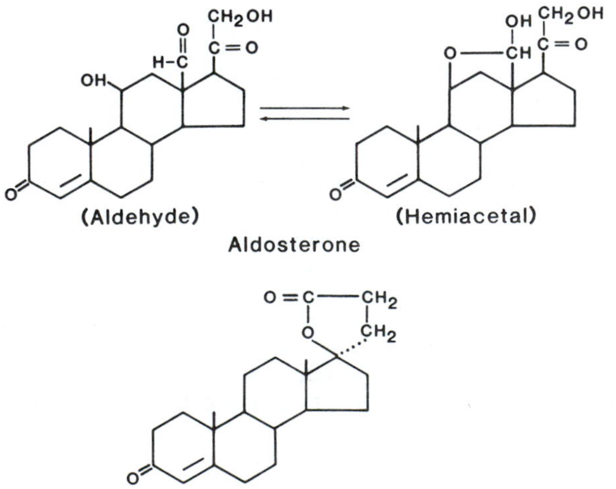

Figure 3–52. Chemical structures of aldosterone and the antimineralocorticoid spironolactone.

Pharmacological Concepts

Hormone antagonists have played an important part in the elucidation of the mechanism of action of the gonadal steroids. Conversely, understanding of the basic biochemical actions of hormones makes it possible to postulate and document the existence of several types of hormonal antagonists. Any agent that interferes with steroid hormone action may do so through one of the following mechanisms: (1) depletion or down-regulation of the specific steroid hormone receptor, (2) inhibition of the nuclear binding or alteration of the conformation of the steroid hormone–receptor DNA complex, (3) perturbation of the receptor cycle, and (4) inhibition of steroid hormone–induced gene transcription.

DEPLETION OF GONADAL STEROID HORMONE RECEPTORS. If the intracellular concentration of active receptor molecules is depleted, the cell will not show a normal response to the hormone. One way of permanently occupying, and thereby depleting, available steroid receptor binding sites is by affinity labeling with steroid derivatives. Affinity labeling (i.e., site-directed irreversible binding) depends on the formation of a covalent bond between the steroid derivative and amino acid residues present at the hormone receptor binding site. If a true covalent bond is formed, the binding is irreversible and the steroid is not capable of leaving the site. Such a compound would theoretically occupy the site for the "life" of the receptor, precluding binding for the natural hormone. Affinity-labeling steroids are useful for the characterization of steroid binding sites on receptor molecules. At present these compounds are experimental and have not been used clinically. They are also potentially useful as antihormones and for disorders like hirsutism and acne. They probably will have to be applied locally because of their highly reactive groups.

INHIBITION OF THE NUCLEAR BINDING OR ALTERATION OF THE CONFORMATION OF THE STEROID HORMONE–RECEPTOR DNA COMPLEX. Cortexolone, an antiglucocorticoid, and spironolactone, an antimineralocorticoid, are examples of this type of hormone antagonist.[470, 471] Because other anti–steroid hormones acting through analogous mechanisms will probably be uncovered, we shall briefly describe these two model systems. In rat thymocytes, cortexolone competes for binding to glucocorticoid receptors and blocks the effect of triamcinolone acetonide on 2-deoxyglucose uptake. Whereas the triamcinolone-receptor complex readily undergoes a temperature-dependent translocation to the nucleus, the cortexolone-receptor complex fails to do so. Thus cortexolone is an antagonist because of its maintenance of receptors in the extranuclear compartment. However, as explained under Steroid Hormone Antagonism, in the intact animal cortexolone is metabolized to cortisol and is not an antagonist. The spironolactone dicirenone (SC-26304) and aldosterone compete for the same cytoplasmic sites in renal cells. Although the aldosterone-receptor complex is readily translocated to the nucleus under appropriate conditions, the cytosolic spironolactone-receptor complex is not. Apparently, cortexolone and spironolactone function as antiglucocorticoid and antimineralocorticoid, respectively, rather than as the corresponding hormone agonists because of the inability of the hormone complexes to translocate to the target cell nucleus or to bind to the nuclear acceptor with high affinity.

RU 486 is a synthetic steroid derivative that binds to progesterone and glucocorticoid receptors and blocks the biological activity of these hormones.[461, 472, 473] It has been used successfully as a postcoital contraceptive and a contragestive agent. Progesterone receptors bind RU 486 with high affinity, and the complex exhibits high-affinity binding to nuclei. The receptor-antagonist complex also binds tightly to the steroid response sequences. Thus the mechanism by which RU 486 antagonizes the action of progesterone must involve the interactions of the receptor-antagonist complex and other transcription factors. Although the binding of the receptor-antagonist complex to DNA is normal, it is possible that the conformation of the complex is sufficiently different from that of the receptor-agonist complex when bound to DNA to result in a failure of the complex to interact appropriately with other transcription factors. This failure would result in reduced or blocked gene expression.

PERTURBATION OF THE RECEPTOR CYCLE. After an injection of estrogen in the rat, the uterine soluble receptor is depleted and bound in the nucleus as a hormone-receptor complex. Maximal depletion of soluble receptor occurs at 1 to 4 h. During the period when the concentration of soluble receptor is reduced, the uterus is insensitive to additional exogenous estrogen. This state is followed by replenishment and eventual overshoot in the number of binding sites. Any agent that interferes with this replenishment process is a potential antiestrogen.

As discussed under Steroid Hormone Antagonism, progesterone may be considered an estrogen antagonist. Simultaneous administration of the two hormones results in inhibition or modification of estrogen-induced growth and differentiation of target organs. Progesterone does not compete for the estrogen receptor binding site, and it does not interfere with the binding of the estrogen-receptor complex to the nucleus. However, progesterone does interfere with the replenishment of soluble estrogen receptors and decreases the level of estrogen-receptor complexes in the nuclei of the uterus. Thus progesterone acts to decrease estrogen responsiveness by depressing estrogen receptor function.

INHIBITION OF STEROID HORMONE–INDUCED GENE TRANSCRIPTION. Various metabolic inhibitors such as actinomycin D inhibit steroid hormone–induced gene transcription. These effects are nonspecific, however, and because of general toxicity, such metabolic inhibitors are not suitable for use as antihormones.

Pathological and Diagnostic Considerations

Molecular studies of steroid hormone action have provided an understanding of many endocrine syndromes that were previously perplexing from a pathogenetic and diagnostic point of view. In addition, such studies have suggested treatment regimens for some of these diseases.

STEROID 5α-REDUCTASE DEFICIENCY. This type of male pseudohermaphroditism, also called pseudovaginal perineoscrotal hypospadias, is inherited as an autosomal recessive trait. Affected males are usually classified as female at birth because of severe hypospadias and the presence of an underdeveloped vagina. However, the testes and male wolffian duct structures (epididymis, vas deferens, and seminal vesicles) are present. Tissues derived from the urogenital sinus and from the anlage of the external genitalia, on the other hand, are female in character. Nevertheless, partial virilization occurs at the time of puberty, and there is no breast development. The primary defect in this syndrome is a deficiency in dihydrotestosterone formation. Testosterone appears to be the hormone responsible for the differentiation of the wolffian duct into the epididymis, the vas deferens, and the seminal vesicle, whereas dihydrotestosterone is responsible for the virilization of the urogenital sinus and tubercle into the male external genitalia, urethra, and prostate. A deficiency of dihydrotestosterone may be responsible for the lack of virilization of the urogenital sinus and tubercle into the male external genitalia, urethra, and prostate. Such a deficiency of dihydrotestosterone would be expected to lead to failure of masculinization of the structures derived from the urogenital sinus and urogenital tubercle—the observed distinctive defect in this syndrome. Furthermore, a marked deficiency in the formation of dihydrotestosterone from testosterone has been demonstrated in fibroblasts from either the foreskin or the inner aspect of the arm of patients affected.

ANDROGEN RESISTANCE (TESTICULAR FEMINIZATION SYNDROME). The term testicular feminization applies to patients who are genetic males and present with a spectrum of developmental abnormalities ranging from a complete external female phenotype to partially masculinized ambiguous genitalia.[474] This disorder is X linked, and affected patients include some infertile males with apparently normal genitalia but defective spermatogenesis.[475]

In the investigation of the primary defect leading to unresponsiveness to dihydrotestosterone, two animal models have been useful: the Tfm mouse and the Tfm rat. The Tfm mouse is insensitive to androgen, whereas the Tfm rat seems to respond to pharmacological doses of testosterone. Defects in androgen production or metabolism cannot account for the lack of end-organ responsiveness.[476] Because these animals do not have a prostate or seminal vesicles, other androgen-sensitive tissues such as the preputial gland, kidney, and submandibular gland were examined. In normal rats, androgens stimulate DNA, RNA, and protein synthesis in the preputial gland. Likewise, the kidney of the normal rat and mouse responds to testosterone by both growth and induction of enzymes, such as β-glucuronidase. The normal mouse submandibular gland also responds by producing certain proteins, including cathepsin D, nerve growth factor, and EGF. All of these normal responses are absent in the Tfm animals. A deficiency in the nuclear binding of androgens has been demonstrated in the kidney, preputial gland, and submandibular gland in these animals. This deficiency of nuclear binding is due to deficiency of functional unoccupied androgen receptors, which renders the animal resistant to androgens.

Mutations in the androgen receptor have long been thought to be responsible for complete androgen insensitivity in the human. Human skin fibroblasts obtained from normal subjects contain receptors that bind dihydrotestosterone with the usual high affinity. Conversely, fibroblasts from some patients with testicular feminization had no detectable specific dihydrotestosterone binding. This finding was the first piece of evidence that a deficiency of the dihydrotestosterone receptor may be the basis for this androgen resistance in the human. Studies of cultured human fibroblasts allowed the determination of the exact mode of inheritance of this disorder in humans. Fibroblasts were obtained from an obligate heterozygote, the mother of three patients with the disease. Specific dihydrotestosterone binding was found to be within the normal range in these cells. However, a substantial population of clones from heterozygotes had deficient receptor activity, a finding compatible with inactivation of one X-linked allele at this locus. This observation provides definitive proof that the androgen resistance in testicular feminization results from a mutation of an X-linked gene specifying a dihydrotestosterone receptor. The resolution of the factors involved in the testicular feminization syndrome offers an excellent example of the role that our basic knowledge of cellular and molecular mechanisms plays in solving the underlying causes of disease.

Androgen resistance has also been analyzed at the molecular level in the human. One family has been described in which the receptor lacks the hormone binding region of the molecule.[477] Because in vivo receptor activity depends on hormone binding, these individuals are completely androgen resistant. Other mutations are less severe and involve single amino acid alterations in the hormone binding region of the receptor.[478] The precise relationships between reduced affinity of these mutated receptors for androgens and the level of androgen resistance has not been determined.

VITAMIN D RESISTANCE. Vitamin D resistance in humans leads to a form of rickets. Patients with this disease hydroxylate vitamin D to the active form, and the receptors bind the hormone normally in vitro. However, receptors from these patients do not bind to DNA with high affinity as do receptors from normal people. This was the clue that led to the idea that mutations might exist in the DNA-binding portion of the receptor. Abnormal DNA was taken from skin cells of the parents of affected children and analyzed for mutations by sequence analysis. Point mutations were found in the DNA-binding zinc fingers of each parent's genes.[479] Thus the alteration of one amino acid in the zinc finger region of the gene is sufficient to reduce the affinity of the receptor for its respective response element on the target gene. Such weak interactions between hormone-receptor complexes and their response elements on target genes apparently do not stimulate normal gene expression and thus produce deficiency disease states.

GLUCOCORTICOID RESISTANCE. In the human with cortisol resistance circulating levels of plasma cortisol are high but there is no evidence of Cushing syndrome. Glucocorticoid receptors from these individuals display reduced affinity for cortisol.[480, 481] Sequence analysis of the glucocorticoid receptor cDNA from one of these patients has identified a single base substitution at position 2054 that alters an amino acid in the hormone binding domain. This area of the hormone binding domain is associated with the glucocorticoid-binding cavity. Thus a single mutation in this region of the receptor may account for the resistance to cortisol.

New World monkeys also have very high blood levels of cortisol and receptors with reduced affinities.[481] These monkeys seem to suffer no ill effects from this condition. However, in the severe form of this disease in the human, levels of the sodium-retaining steroids (corticosterone and deoxycorticosterone) are elevated manyfold and produce hypertension and hypokalemic alkalosis. The overproduction of these sodium-retaining steroids appears to be due to corticotropin hyperstimulation of the adrenal cortex. In the New World monkeys, evolution and selection pressures seem to have favored the development of a zona fasciculata that can hypersecrete cortisol without secreting steroid precursors with sodium-retaining activity.

New World monkeys also have very high blood levels of estrogen, progesterone, aldosterone, and testosterone. However, in contrast to the cortisol resistance state just described, the receptors for estrogen, progesterone, and aldosterone are reduced in number and not in affinity. Thus the normal physiology of New World monkeys is characterized by decreased steroid receptor quantities or decreased receptor affinities and very high levels of steroid hormones. Old World monkeys have much lower blood levels of steroid hormones, normal receptor numbers, and normal affinities. High blood levels of steroid hormones in New World monkeys may have evolved as a compensatory response to a receptor mutation(s) that lowered the affinity and/or number of steroid receptors for their respective hormones. This mutation probably occurred after the geographic separation of the New World and Old World primates, which occurred approximately 60 million years ago.

GENERAL COMMENTS ON MOLECULAR GENETICS AND HORMONE RESISTANCE DISEASE. Elucidation of the pathophysiology of steroid hormone resistance syndromes has been important in providing insight into the normal pathway of nuclear receptor action. Each new type of resistance that is recognized and each new mutation that is uncovered behind that process provide an opportunity for defining the nature of a specific reaction essential for the action of the hormone. How does the receptor affinity for DNA affect transcriptional regulation? How does ligand binding alter receptor conformation and activity at the genome? What additional functional domains and requisite trans-acting factors are yet to be defined for the receptor molecule? Site-directed point mutagenesis of the various receptors has provided many clues to amino acids that contribute significantly to receptor function. The interpretation of such studies has, in many instances, been difficult because of limitations in the cis-trans cotransfection assay. In this assay, the receptors are expressed in heterologous cells together with a steroid response element linked to a reporter gene such as the chloramphenicol acetyltransferase or luciferase gene. Much of the data and most of the structure-function conclusions drawn from these studies have relied on this method of measuring receptor activity. However, a number of biological differences exist between cotransfected endogenous genes. For instance, cotransfected genes exist as episomes and are unlikely to exist in a native chromatin structure. Furthermore, transfection efficiencies are low, so only a fraction of the cells acquire the DNA. Because receptors are often overexpressed in this subpopulation of cells, transfected cells may contain wild-type or mutant receptors in vast excess over the levels that occur naturally. Although this type of assay should reflect the gross functional state of the nascent mutagenized protein, more subtle assessments regarding functionality may be difficult to make.

Further characterization of the defects in patients with steroid-resistant disorders should provide important insight into how these proteins function in target cells. In contrast to random in vitro mutagenesis, appropriate selection of genetic diseases of hormone resistance in humans and animals should permit the investigation of subtle mutations that result in decreased function under physiological conditions in vivo. Study of nature's mutational experiments has been invaluable in understanding human disease conditions as well as normal physiological processes. Study of the mutations producing tissue resistance to nuclear receptors will improve our knowledge of the mechanisms by which these proteins regulate cellular transcription.

HORMONE-RESPONSIVE HYPERPLASIA AND NEOPLASIA. Several disease states such as benign prostatic hyperplasia, leukemia, and cancer of the prostate, breast, and uterus respond to antihormone therapy. Anti–steroid hormone drugs work by blocking the binding of the hormone agonist to the receptor and thereby reduce the response of the tissue to hormonal stimulation. The principles and mechanisms of antihormone function are covered in other sections of this chapter, and the hyperplastic and neoplastic disease states are covered elsewhere in the volume.

Steroid Hormones and Reproductive Toxicology

The normal maturation and reproductive capacity of the female animal depend on the secretion of steroid hormones by the ovary. Yet inappropriate exposure to steroid hormones can disrupt the normal flow of maturational events and cause reproductive dysfunction. Thus steroid hormones are physiological agents that can be toxic under certain circumstances.

NEONATAL EXPOSURE TO STEROID HORMONES AND THE CYCLIC NATURE OF THE REPRODUCTIVE SYSTEM. The maturation of the mechanisms that control reproductive cycles and ovulation results in the cyclic release of luteinizing

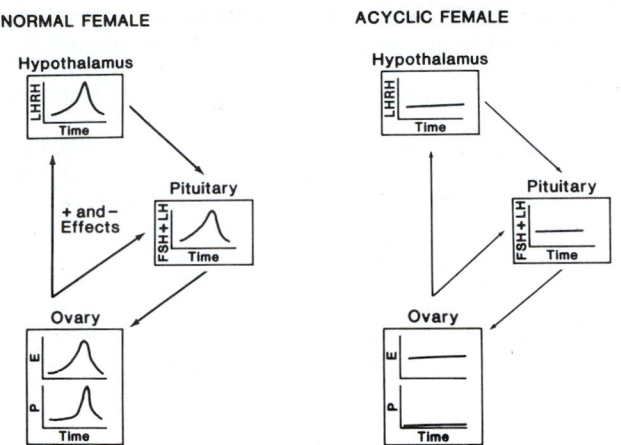

NORMAL FEMALE

ACYCLIC FEMALE

Figure 3–53. Hormone cycles in the normal female compared with the (acyclic) animal with persistent estrus. LHRH, luteinizing hormone–releasing hormone; FSH, follicle-stimulating hormone; LH, luteinizing hormone; P, progesterone; E, estrogen.

hormone–releasing hormone (LHRH, also called gonadotropin-releasing hormone, GnRH), from the hypothalamus (Fig. 3–53). This cyclic secretion of LHRH causes cyclic release of FSH and LH from the pituitary. These hormones stimulate the synthesis and secretion of estrogen and progesterone in a cyclic fashion. In addition, the action of FSH and LH on the ovary causes the cyclic release of eggs. Estrogen and progesterone interact with the hypothalamus and pituitary via negative and positive feedback mechanisms and influence the cyclic secretion of LHRH, FSH, and LH.

Exposure of female rats to androgens or estrogens during fetal or neonatal life results in disruption of the mechanisms that control cyclic secretion of the various hormones shown in Figure 3–53.[482] This leads to the development of the persistent estrus syndrome, which is characterized by lack of reproductive cyclicity and infertility. Such animals may display masculine behavior and masculinized external genitalia.

This effect of estrogen or androgen takes place only if the animal is exposed during the critical period of development that extends from day 18 of pregnancy to days 8 to 10 of life in the rat. During this period, the hypothalamic structures thought to be involved in control of normal cyclic hormone secretion are undergoing neuronal maturation. Disruption or modification of hypothalamic maturation has a permanent effect that results in an acyclic pattern of hormone release and infertility. Data for the rodent should be extrapolated to other species with caution.

In the rat and other rodent species, the persistent estrus syndrome appears to result from the action of estrogens on hypothalamic development. Even the effects of androgens are thought to occur by their metabolic conversion to estrogens. Physiological estrogens, such as estradiol, estriol, and estrone, and nonphysiological estrogens, such as DES, chlordecone (Kepone), mitotane (*o,p'*-DDD), and clomiphene, are known to cause this acyclic syndrome in the rat. Both physiological and nonphysiological estrogens bind to estrogen receptors and stimulate biosynthetic events that appear to be identical.

NEONATAL EXPOSURE TO STEROID HORMONES AND REPRODUCTIVE TRACT ABNORMALITIES. In addition to the effects on the reproductive cycle just discussed, exposure of rats and other rodents to gonadal steroids during neonatal life causes abnormalities in the reproductive system. Neonatal exposure of mice, rats, and hamsters to estrogens of various types results in preneoplastic and neoplastic changes

in the vagina, uterus, pituitary, and mammary gland.[483] Neonatal androgen treatment causes squamous metaplasia and reorientation of stromal collagen in rat uteri and persistent vaginal estrus in mice. These effects of androgen may result from conversion of androgens to estrogens in extraglandular sites or from continuous exposure to ovarian estrogens as the result of persistent estrus during adult life.

Nonphysiological estrogens, such as DES and clomiphene, also cause the development of reproductive tract abnormalities in rodents. Other estrogenic agents, such as chlordecone and mitotane, have adverse effects on reproductive function, but little is known about the teratogenic effect of these agents. Many of the reproductive tract abnormalities, both nonneoplastic and neoplastic, can be reproduced in the adult by chronic exposure to estrogens. Therefore, the occurrence of these abnormalities does not depend on a critical period of exposure, as does the persistent estrus syndrome.

The mechanisms that control the development of the cyclic nature of the female reproductive cycle in humans and other primates appear to be different and/or less sensitive to toxic hormonal influences. In the rat, androgens secreted by the testes during development are converted to estrogens in the hypothalamus. These estrogens act to defeminize the hypothalamus and produce a typical acyclic male pattern of hormone secretion. However, these mechanisms do not appear to operate in primates; instead, testosterone is converted to dihydrotestosterone, which is the active androgen. Therefore, exposure to estrogenic toxins is not likely to lead to defeminized patterns of secretion of gonadotropins or infertility. This also appears to be the case for exposure to androgenic substances. It is possible to produce pseudohermaphroditic female monkeys by injecting the mothers with testosterone propionate during gestation; however, no changes were observed in the adult menstrual cycle of the offspring. This insensitivity of the hypothalamic control centers to androgens is also exemplified by the congenital adrenal hyperplasia syndrome. This disease is characterized by production of large amounts of adrenal androgens that masculinize the external genitalia of females; however, the reproductive cycle is not affected to any great extent.

Even though it seems unlikely that either estrogenic or androgenic insult during development in the human is detrimental to the cyclic nature of the female reproductive system, masculinization of behavior patterns is produced in rhesus monkeys by exposure to androgens during pregnancy. In addition, DES exposure during pregnancy may be associated with menstrual irregularity and subfertility. However, not all investigators agree on this point.

SHORT-ACTING ESTROGENS AND TOXICITY. Some estrogens, such as estriol, dimethylstilbestrol, and estradiol-16α, are classified as short-acting because they are rapidly cleared from the body and from estrogen receptor sites after a single injection (see under Steroid Hormone Antagonism for more discussion of this point). Consequently, when they are administered by a single injection, these hormones fail to elicit full estrogenic responses in organs such as the uterus. However, if such hormones are supplied to receptor sites in a continuous fashion, by either a series of injections or implants, they stimulate full estrogenic responses.[1] Hence, these short-acting estrogens, previously called weak or impeded estrogens, are fully competent to elicit estrogenic responses. This concept is important because some investigators have considered estriol to have protective effects against the ability of estradiol to induce mammary carcinoma. This proposal was based on the concept that estriol was a weak or impeded estrogen, a concept that was in turn based on the evidence derived from experiments that employed a single injection of hormone. However, because estriol is present in a continuous fashion under physiological circumstances, it is unlikely that this hormone can reduce the effectiveness of other estrogens. Instead, it adds more estrogenicity to the system. In addition, estriol exposure during the neonatal period causes reproductive dysfunction and is equal to estradiol in its ability to facilitate the onset of mammary cancer in mice. Likewise, both estradiol and estriol implants in adult rats cause multiple abnormalities of the reproductive tract and related systems.

Thus the ability of estriol to express its toxicity is related to the way in which it is administered and reflects the pharmacokinetic and receptor dynamics of the compound. These properties should be considered in evaluating the reproductive toxicological potential of any compound.

LONG-ACTING ESTROGEN AGONISTS-ANTAGONISTS.

As discussed under Steroid Hormone Antagonism, clomiphene and tamoxifen are mixed estrogen agonists-antagonists with long-lasting estrogenic and antiestrogenic effects. When these drugs are administered to rats during the perinatal period, they cause early vaginal opening and growth of the uterus.[483] These estrogenic effects are similar to those seen with estradiol or DES and are correlated with nuclear occupancy of the estrogen receptor. Such animals exhibit a syndrome as adults that is similar to the persistent estrus condition described earlier. They also have reproductive tract abnormalities, including uterine metaplasia and hyperplasia, cystic hyperplasia, atrophic ovaries, pyometra, and inflamed oviducts. The persistent estrus syndrome that results from the neonatal exposure to clomiphene appears to be responsible for the development of reproductive tract abnormalities, because ovariectomy eliminates such abnormal development.

Because clomiphene is used to induce ovulation in women, the fact that clomiphene is estrogenic in the fetal and neonatal rat has been of some concern with respect to human development. However, no reproductive tract abnormalities have been reported in controlled studies of clomiphene-treated women or their children. This fortunate circumstance may be due to the low level of estrogen agonistic activity of clomiphene in humans. That is, clomiphene is primarily an antiestrogen in women and therefore has little or no ill effects on the human fetus. In addition, humans do not manifest a syndrome comparable with the persistent estrus condition, even when exposed to DES during pregnancy. Therefore, even if the human fetus were exposed to the estrogenic effects of clomiphene in utero, it is unlikely that reproductive tract abnormalities would result.

DIETHYLSTILBESTROL AND REPRODUCTIVE TOXICOLOGY.

DES is an estrogen often considered to act by different mechanisms from those of physiological estrogens. This idea originated from the observation that the incidence of vaginal adenosis is increased in young women whose mothers were treated with DES during pregnancy.[484] Physiological estrogens are elevated to high levels during pregnancy with no adverse effects on the fetus, so it was reasoned that DES must be different from physiological estrogens. It is currently thought that this is not the case but that inappropriate exposure of the fetus to any estrogen during early pregnancy would cause similar adverse effects. The critical period for the development of vaginal adenosis is during the early months of pregnancy (first trimester), a period during which the urogenital tract is differentiating and endogenous estrogen levels are relatively low. DES exposure during this time increases the estrogenic load of the mother and fetus and probably causes an inappropriate stimulation of the urogenital tract that predisposes the fetus to subsequent development of vaginal abnormalities. The mechanism is thought to involve stimulation of the müllerian duct, resulting in retention of müllerian duct derivatives within the upper third of the vagina. The residual müllerian duct tissue has the capacity to develop uterine glands, and these appear at puberty as adenosis in the upper vagina.

MECHANISM OF ACTION OF ESTROGENS: RELATIONSHIPS AMONG ESTROGENICITY, TOXICITY, AND CARCINOGENICITY.

As discussed earlier, estrogens can cause abnormal development of the reproductive tract and neoplasia. These adverse effects occur because of either inappropriate exposure to estrogens during some critical period of development or continuous exposure to estrogens. In rodents, exposure during a critical period results in the persistent estrus syndrome, which is characterized by continuous ovarian secretion of estrogens during adult life. This continuous exposure to estrogens results in the development of reproductive tract abnormalities and neoplasia. Similar adverse effects can be obtained in adult rats by implanting estrogen-containing pellets that hyperestrogenize the animal. Continuous exposure to estrogens also causes similar adverse effects in humans. Endometrial hyperplasia and cancer occur in women who have been exposed to either endogenous or exogenous estrogens for prolonged periods of time. Such instances include women with ovarian tumors that produce estrogens, women who fail to ovulate and as a result are exposed to estrogen without the normal intervention of the luteal phase of the cycle, and women who have taken estrogens for many years because they lack functional ovaries.

These adverse effects caused by continuous exposure to estrogens are probably due to the lack of normal cyclic elevations in progesterone. Progesterone antagonizes and modifies the ability of estrogen to act on estrogen target tissues. As discussed under Physiological Considerations in Steroid Hormone Action, this probably occurs because progesterone decreases the concentration of estrogen receptors and thereby decreases the ability of estrogen to stimulate the target tissues.

The biochemical or molecular mechanisms by which estrogens elicit carcinogenic effects are not known. However, physiological as well as nonphysiological estrogens, such as DES, clomiphene, chlordecone, and mitotane, bind to estrogen receptors and exert their actions at the level of gene transcription. Such interactions at the gene level are normally modulated by the presence of other hormones, such as progesterone. When these modulating influences are absent, the continuous stimulation of estrogen-controlled biosynthetic events may lead to disruption of normal cell function. Such disruption could increase the probability of the expression of events and to neoplastic development.

REFERENCES

1. Clark JH, Peck EJ Jr. Female sex steroids: receptors and function. Monogr Endocrinol 1979; 14:4–36.
2. Scatchard G. The attractions of proteins for small molecules and ions. Ann NY Acad Sci 1949; 51:660–672.
3. Markaverich BM, Williams M, Upchurch S, et al. Heterogeneity of nuclear estrogen binding sites in the rat uterus: a simple method for the quantitation of type I and II sites by [³H]estradiol exchange. Endocrinology 1981; 109:62–68.
4. Anderson JN, Clark JH, Peck EJ Jr. Estrogen and nuclear binding sites: determination of specific sites by [³H]estradiol exchange. Biochem J 1972; 126:561–567.
5. Katzenellenbogen J, Johnson HJ, Carlson KE. Studies on the uterine cytoplasmic estrogen binding protein, thermal stability and ligand dissociation rate. An assay of empty and filled sites by exchange. Biochemistry 1973; 12:4092–4099.
6. Hughes MR, Malloy PJ, Kieback DG, et al. Point mutations in the human vitamin D receptor gene associated with hypocalcemic rickets. Science 1988; 242:1702–1705.
7. Conneely OM, Sullivan WP, Toft DO, et al. Molecular cloning of the chicken progesterone receptor. Science 1986; 233:767–770.

8. Gronemeyer H, Turcotte B, Quirin-Stricker C, et al. The chicken progesterone receptor: sequence, expression and functional analysis. EMBO J 1987; 6:3985–3994.

9. Misrahi M, Atger M, d'Auriol L, et al. Complete amino acid sequence of the progesterone receptor deduced from cloned cDNA. Biochem Biophys Res Commun 1987; 143:740–748.

10. Koike S, Masaharu S, Maramatsu M. Molecular cloning and characterization of rat estrogen receptor cDNA. Nucleic Acids Res 1987; 15:2499–2513.

11. Walter PW, Green S, Greene G, et al. Cloning of the human estrogen receptor cDNA. Proc Natl Acad Sci USA 1985; 82:7889–7893.

12. Chang C, Kokontis J, Liao S. Molecular cloning of human and rat complementary DNA encoding androgen receptors. Science 1988; 240:324–327.

13. Lubahn DB, Joseph DR, Sullivan PM, et al. Cloning of human androgen receptor complementary DNA and localization to the X chromosome. Science 1988; 240:327–330.

14. Hollenberg SM, Weinberger C, Ong ES, et al. Primary structure and expression of a functional human glucocorticoid receptor cDNA. Nature 1985; 318:635–641.

15. Miesfeld R, Rusconi S, Godowski PJ, et al. Genetic complementation of a glucocorticoid receptor deficiency by expression of cloned receptor cDNA. Cell 1986; 46:389–399.

16. Murray JC, Smith RF, Ardinger HA, et al. RFLP for the glucocorticoid receptor (GRL) located at 5q11–5q13. Nucleic Acids Res 1987; 15:6765.

17. Arriza JL, Weinberger C, Cerelli G, et al. Cloning of human mineralocorticoid receptor complementary DNA: structural and functional kinship with the glucocorticoid receptor. Science 1987; 237:268–274.

18. Patel PD, Sherman TG, Goldman DJ, et al. Molecular cloning of a mineralocorticoid (type I) receptor complementary DNA from rat hippocampus. Mol Endocrinol 1989; 3:1877–1885.

19. Thompson CC, Weinberger C, Lebo R, et al. Identification of a novel thyroid hormone receptor expressed in the mammalian central nervous system. Science 1987; 237:1610–1614.

20. Benbrook D, Pfahl M. A novel thyroid hormone receptor encoded by a cDNA clone from a human testis library. Science 1987; 238:788–791.

21. Evans RE. The steroid and thyroid hormone receptor superfamily. Science 1988; 240:889–895.

22. Giguere V, Ong ES, Segui P, et al. Identification of a receptor for the morphogen retinoic acid. Nature 1987; 330:624–629.

23. Petkovich M, Brand NJ, Krust A, et al. A human retinoic acid receptor which belongs to the family of nuclear receptors. Nature 1987; 330:444–450.

24. Zelent A, Krust A, Petkovich M, et al. Cloning of murine alpha and beta retinoic acid receptors and a novel receptor gamma predominantly expressed in skin. Nature 1989; 339:714–717.

25. Krust A, Kastner P, Petkovich M, et al. A third human retinoic acid receptor, hRAR-gamma. Proc Natl Acad Sci USA 1989; 86:5310–5314.

26 McDonnell DP, Mangelsdorf DJ, Pike JW, et al. Molecular cloning of cDNA encoding the avian receptor for vitamin D. Science 1987; 235:1214–1217.

27. Baker AR, McDonnell DP, Hughes M, et al. Cloning and expression of full length cDNA encoding human vitamin D receptor. Proc Natl Acad Sci USA 1988; 85:3294–3298.

28. Green S, Chambon P. A superfamily of potentially oncogenic hormone receptors. Nature 1986; 324:615–617.

29. O'Malley BW. Did eucaryotic steroid receptors evolve from intracrine gene regulators? Endocrinology 1989; 125:1119–1120.

30. Mendel DB, Orti E, Smith LI, et al. Evidence for a glucocorticoid receptor cycle and nuclear dephosphorylation of the steroid binding protein. Prog Clin Biol Res 1990; 322:97–117.

31. Orti E, Mendel DB, Smith LI, et al. A dynamic model of glucocorticoid receptor phosphorylation and cycling in intact cells. J Steroid Biochem 1989; 34:85–96.

32. Bonifer C, Dahlman K, Stromstedt PE, et al. DNA binding of glucocorticoid receptor protein A fusion protein expressed in E. coli. J Steroid Biochem 1989; 32:5–11.

33. Power RF, Conneely OM, McDonnell DP, et al. High level expression of a truncated chicken progesterone receptor in Escherichia coli. J Biol Chem 1990; 265:1419–1424.

34. Mak P, McDonnell DP, Weigel NL, et al. Expression of functional chicken oviduct progesterone receptors in yeast (Saccharomyces cerevisiae). J Biol Chem 1989; 264:21613–21618.

35. Metzger D, White JH, Chambon P. The human oestrogen receptor functions in yeast. Nature 1988; 334:31–36.

36. Debuire B, Henry C, Banaissa M, et al. Sequencing the erb A gene of avian erythroblastosis virus reveals a new type of oncogene. Science 1984; 224:1456–1459.

37. Giguere V, Yang N, Segui P, et al. Identification of a new class of steroid hormone receptors. Nature 1988; 331:91–94.

38. Wang LH, Tsai SY, Cook RG, et al. COUP transcription factor is a member of the steroid receptor superfamily. Nature 1989; 340:163–166.

39. Watson MA, Milbrandt J. The NGFI-B gene, a transcriptionally inducible member of the steroid receptor gene superfamily: genomic structure and expression in rat brain after seizure induction. Mol Cell Biol 1989; 9:4213–4219.

40. de Thé H, Marchio A, Tiollais P, et al. A novel steroid thyroid hormone receptor–related gene inappropriately expressed in human hepatocellular carcinoma. Nature 1987; 330:667–670.

41. Nauber U, Pankratz MJ, Kienlin A, et al. Abdominal segmentation of the Drosophila embryo requires a hormone receptor–like protein encoded by the gap gene knirps. Nature 1988; 336:489–492.

42. Oro AE, Ong ES, Margolis JS, et al. The Drosophila gene knirps-related is a member of the steroid receptor gene superfamily. Nature 1988; 336:493–496.

43. Lazar MA, Hodin RA, Darling DS, et al. A novel member of the thyroid/steroid hormone receptor family is encoded by the opposite strand of the rat c-erb A alpha transcriptional unit. Mol Cell Biol 1989; 9:1128–1136.

44. Sagami I, Tsai SY, Wang H, et al. Identification of two factors required for transcription of the ovalbumin gene. Mol Cell Biol 1986; 6:4259–4267.

45. Wang LH, Tsai SY, Sagami I, et al. Purification and characterization of COUP transcription factor from HeLa cells. J Biol Chem 1987; 262:16080–16086.

46. Bagchi MK, Tsai MJ, O'Malley BW. Purification and characterization of chicken ovalbumin gene upstream promoter transcription factor from homologous oviduct cells. Mol Cell Biol 1987; 7:4151–4158.

47. Hwung YP, Crowe DT, Wang L-H, et al. The COUP transcription factor binds to an upstream promoter element of the rat insulin II gene. Mol Cell Biol 1988; 8:2070–2077.

48. Mlodzik M, Hiromi Y, Weber U, et al. The Drosophila Seven-up gene, a member of the steroid receptor gene superfamily, controls photoreceptor cell fates. Cell 1990; 60:211–224.

49. Vedeckis WV, Schrader, WT, O'Malley BW. Progesterone-binding components of chick oviduct: analysis of receptor structure by limited proteolysis. Biochemistry 1980; 2:343–349.

50. de Boer W, Bolt J, Kuiper GG, et al. Analysis of steroid- and DNA-binding domains of the calf uterine androgen receptor by limited proteolysis. J Steroid Biochem 1987; 28:9–19.

51. Rusconi S, Yamamoto KR. Functional dissection of the hormone and DNA binding activities of the glucocorticoid receptor. EMBO J 1987; 6:1309–1315.

52. Green S, Kumar V, Krust P, et al. Structural and functional domains of the estrogen receptor. Cold Spring Harbor Symp Quant Biol 1986; 51:751–758.

53. Carlstedt-Duke J, Stromstedt P-E, Wrange O, et al. Domain structure of the glucocorticoid receptor protein. Proc Natl Acad Sci USA 1987; 84:4437–4440.

54. Maxwell BL, McDonnell DP, Conneely OM, et al. Structural organization and regulation of the chicken estrogen receptor. Mol Endocrinol 1987; 1:25–35.

55. White R, Lees JA, Needham M, et al. Structural organization and expression of the mouse estrogen receptor. Mol Endocrinol 1987; 1:735–744.

56. Haussler MR, Mangelsdorf DJ, Yamaoka K, et al. Molecular characterization and actions of the Vitamin D hormone receptor. Recent Prog Horm Res 1988; 44:263–305.

57. Maniatis T, Goodbourn S, Fischer JA. Regulation of inducible and tissue-specific gene expression. Science 1987; 236:1237–1244.

58. Chandler VL, Maler BA, Yamamoto KR. DNA sequences bound specifically by glucocorticoid receptor in vitro render a heterologous promoter hormone responsive in vivo. Cell 1983; 33:489–499.

59. Ponta H, Kennedy N, Skroch P, et al. Hormonal response region of the mouse mammary tumor virus long terminal repeat can be dissociated from the proviral promoter and has enhancer properties. Proc Natl Acad Sci USA 1985; 84:1020–1024.

60. Bradshaw MS, Tsai M-J, O'Malley BW. A steroid response element can function in the absence of a distal promoter. Mol Endocrinol 1988; 2:1286–1293.

61. Dynan WS. Modularity in promoters and enhancers. Cell 1989; 58:1–4.

62. Tremea F, de Medeiros SRB, Heggeler-Bordier BT, et al. Identification of two steroid-responsive promoters of different strength controlled by the same estrogen-responsive element in the 5′ end region of the Xenopus laevis vitellogenin gene A1. Mol Endocrinol 1989; 3:1596–1609.

63. Vanderbilt JN, Miesfeld R, Maler BA, et al. Intracellular receptor concentration limits glucocorticoid-dependent enhancer activity. Mol Endocrinol 1987; 1:68–74.

64. Chalepakis G, Postma JPM, Beato M. A model for hormone receptor binding to the mouse mammary tumour virus regulatory element based on hydroxyl radical footprinting. Nucleic Acids Res 1988; 16:10237–10247.

65. Drouin J, Chamberland M, Charron J, et al. Pro-opiomelanocortin gene: a model for negative regulation of transcription by glucocorticoids. J Cell Biochem 1987; 35:293–304.

66. Akerblom IE, Slater EP, Beato M, et al. Negative regulation by glucocorticoids through interference with a cAMP responsive enhancer. Science 1988; 241:350–353.

67. Sakai DD, Helms S, Carlstedt-Duke J, et al. Hormone-mediated repression: a negative glucocorticoid response element from the bovine prolactin gene. Genes Dev 1988; 2:1144–1154.

68. Payvar F, Wrange O, Carstedt-Duke J, et al. Purified glucocorticoid receptors bind selectively in vitro to a cloned DNA fragment whose transcription is regulated by glucocorticoids in vivo. Proc Natl Acad Sci USA 1981; 78:6628–6632.

69. Scheidereit C, Geisse S, Westphal HM, et al. The glucocorticoid receptor binds to defined nucleotide sequences near the promoter of mouse mammary tumor virus. Nature 1983; 304:749–752.

70. Bronnegard M, Poellinger L, Okret S, et al. Characterization and sequence-specific binding to mouse mammary tumor virus DNA of purified activated human glucocorticoid receptor. Biochemistry 1987; 26:1697–1704.

71. Renkawitz R, Schutz G, von der Ahe D, et al. Sequences in the promoter region of the chicken lysozyme gene required for steroid regulation and receptor binding. Cell 1984; 37:503–510.

72. Struhe U, Klock G, Schutz G. A DNA sequence of 15 base pairs is sufficient to mediate both glucocorticoid and progesterone induction of gene expression. Proc Natl Acad Sci USA 1987; 84:7871–7875.

73. Danesch U, Gloss B, Schmid W, et al. Glucocorticoid induction of the rat tryptophan oxygenase gene is mediated by two widely separated glucocorticoid-response elements. EMBO J 1987; 6:625–630.

74. Scheidereit C, Westphal HM, Carlson C, et al. Molecular model of the interaction between the glucocorticoid receptor and the regulatory elements of inducible genes. DNA 1986; 5:383–391.

75. Cato ACB, Miksicek R, Schutz G, et al. The hormone regulatory element of mouse mammary tumour virus mediates progesterone induction. EMBO J 1986; 5:2237–2240.

76. von der Ahe D, Janich S, Scheidereit C, et al. Glucocorticoid and progesterone receptors bind to the same sites in two hormonally regulated promoters. Nature 1985; 313:706–09.

77. Parker MG, Webb P, Needham M, et al. Identification of androgen response elements in mouse mammary tumour virus and the rat prostate C3 gene. J Cell Biochem 1987; 35:285–292.

78. Ham J, Thomson A, Needham M, et al. Characterization of response elements for androgens, glucocorticoids, and progestins in mouse mammary tumour virus. Nucleic Acids Res 1988; 16:5263–5276.

79. Otten AD, Sanders MM, McKnight GS. The MMTV LTR promoter is induced by progesterone and dihydrotestosterone but not by estrogen. Mol Endocrinol 1988; 2:143–147.

80. Peale FV, Ludwig LB, Zain S, et al. Properties of a high-affinity DNA binding site for estrogen receptor. Proc Natl Acad Sci USA 1988; 85:1038–1042.

81. Klein-Hitpass L, Tsai SY, Greene GL, et al. Specific binding of estrogen receptor to the estrogen response element. Mol Cell Biol 1989; 9:43–49.

82. Klock G, Struhle U, Schutz G. Oestrogen and glucocorticoid responsive elements are closely related but distinct. Nature 1987; 329:734–736.

83. Brent GA, Harney JW, Chen Y, et al. Mutations of the rat growth hormone promoter which increase and decrease response to thyroid hormone define a consensus thyroid hormone response element. Mol Endocrinol 1989; 3:1996–2004.

84. Umesono K, Giguere V, Glass CK, et al. Retinoic acid and thyroid hormone induce gene expression through a common responsive element. Nature 1988; 336:262–265.

85. Graupner G, Wills KN, Tzukerman M, et al. Dual regulatory role for thyroid-hormone receptors allows control of retinoic-acid receptor activity. Nature 1989; 340:653–656.

86. Reichman ME, Foster CM, Eisen LP, et al. Limited proteolysis of covalently labeled glucocorticoid receptors as a probe of receptor structure. Biochemistry 1984; 23:5376–5384.

87. Wrange O, Okret S, Radojcic M, et al. Characterization of the purified activated glucocorticoid receptor from rat liver cytosol. J Biol Chem 1984; 259:4534–4541.

88. Weichman BM, Notides AC. Estradiol-binding kinetics of the activated and nonactivated estrogen receptor. J Biol Chem 1977; 252:8856–8862.

89. Gorden MS, Notides AC. Computer modeling of estradiol interactions with the estrogen receptor. J Steroid Biochem 1986; 25:177–181.

90. Kumar V, Green S, Staub A, et al. Localisation of the oestradiol-binding and putative DNA-binding domains of the human oestrogen receptor. EMBO J 1986; 5:2231–2236.

91. Dobson ADW, Conneely OM, Beatie W, et al. Mutational analysis of the chicken progesterone receptor. J Biol Chem 1989; 264:4207–4211.

92. Carson MA, Tsai M-J, Conneely OM, et al. Structure-function properties of the chicken progesterone receptor A synthesized from complementary deoxyribonucleic acid. Mol Endocrinol 1987; 1:791.

93. McDonnell DP, Scott RA, Kerner SA, et al. Functional domains of the human vitamin D$_3$ receptor regulate osteocalcin gene expression. Mol Endocrinol 1989; 3:635–644.

94. Giguere V, Hollenberg SM, Rosenfeld MG, et al. Functional domains of the human glucocorticoid receptor. Cell 1986; 46:645–652.

95. Conneely OM, Dobson AD, Carson MA, et al. Structure-function relationships of the chicken progesterone receptor. Biochem Soc Trans 1988; 16:683–687.

96. Picard D, Salser SJ, Yamamoto KR. A movable and regulable inactivation function within the steroid binding domain of the glucocorticoid receptor. Cell 1988; 54:1073–1080.

97. Eilers M, Picard D, Yamamoto KR, et al. Chimearas of Myc oncoprotein and steroid receptors cause hormone-dependent transformation of cells. Nature 1989; 340:66–68.

98. Simons SS Jr, Pumphrey JG, Rudikoff S, et al. Identification of cysteine 656 as the amino acid of hepatoma tissue culture cell glucocorticoid receptors that is covalently labeled by dexamethasone 21-mesylate. J Biol Chem 1987; 262:9676–9680.

99. Carlstedt-Duke J, Stromstedt P-E, Persson B, et al. Identification of hormone-interacting amino acid residues within the steroid-binding domain of the glucocorticoid receptor in relation to other steroid hormone receptors. J Biol Chem 1988; 263:6842–6846.

100. Smith LI, Bodwell JE, Mendell DB, et al. Identification of cysteine–644 as the covalent site of attachment of dexamethasone 21-mesylate to murine glucocorticoid receptors in WEHI-7 cells. Biochemistry 1988; 27:3747–3753.

101. Harlow KW, Smith DN, Katzenellenbogen JA, et al. Identification of cysteine 530 as the covalent attachment site of an affinity-labeling estrogen (ketonanestrol aziridine) and antiestrogen (tamoxifen aziridine) in the human estrogen receptor. J Biol Chem 1989; 264:17476.

102. Simons SS Jr, Sistare FD, Chakraborti PK. Steroid binding activity is retained in a 16-kDa fragment of the steroid binding domain of rat glucocorticoid receptors. J Biol Chem 1989; 264:14493–14497.

103. Danielson M, Northrop JP, Ringold GM. The mouse glucocorticoid receptor: mapping of functional domains by cloning, sequencing and expression of wildtype and mutant receptor proteins. EMBO J 1986; 5:2513–2522.

104. Tora L, Mullick A, Metzger D, et al. The cloned human estrogen receptor contains a mutation which alters its hormone binding properties. EMBO J 1989; 8:1981–1986.

105. Conneely OM, Dobson ADW, Carson MA, et al. Structure-function relationships of the chicken progesterone receptor. Biochem Soc Trans 1988; 16:683–687.

106. Weinberger C, Hollenberg SM, Rosenfeld MG, et al. Domain structure of human glucocorticoid receptor and its relationship to the v-*erb*-A oncogene product. Nature 1985; 318:668–672.

107. Green S, Chambon P. Oestradiol induction of a glucocorticoid-responsive gene by a chimaeric receptor. Nature 1987; 325:75–78.

108. Kumar V, Green S, Stack G, et al. Functional domains of the human estrogen receptor. Cell 1987; 51:941–951.

109. Miller J, McLachlan AD, Klug A. Repetitive zinc-binding domains in the protein transcription factor IIIA from *Xenopus* oocytes. EMBO J 1985; 4:16091614.

110. Freedman LP, Luisi BF, Korszun ZR, et al. The function and structure of the metal coordination sites within the glucocorticoid receptor DNA binding domain. Nature 1988; 334:543–546.

111. Medici N, Minucci S, Nigro V, et al. Metal binding sites of the estradiol receptor from calf uterus and their possible role in the regulation of receptor function. Biochemistry 1989; 28:212–219.

112. Green S, Chambon P. Chimeric receptors used to probe the DNA-binding domain of the estrogen and glucocorticoid receptors. Cancer Res 1989; 49(Suppl):2282s–2285s.

113. Severne Y, Wieland, S, Schaffner W, et al. Metal binding 'finger' structures in the glucocorticoid receptor defined by site-directed mutagenesis. EMBO J 1988; 7:2503–2508.

114. Huckaby C, Conneely O, Beattie WG, et al. Structure of the chromosomal chicken progesterone receptor gene. Proc Natl Acad Sci USA 1987; 84:8380–8384.

115. Misrahi M, Loosfelt H, Atger M, et al. Organisation of the entire rabbit progesterone receptor mRNA and of the promoter and 5' flanking region of the gene. Nucleic Acids Res 1988; 16:5459–5472.

116. Ponglikitmongkol M, Green S, Chambon P. Genomic organization of the human oestrogen receptor gene. EMBO J 1988; 7:3385–3388.

117. Green S, Chambon P. Nuclear receptors enhance our understanding of transcription regulation. Trends Genet 1988; 4:309–314.

118. Berg JM. DNA binding specificity of steroid receptors. Cell 1989; 57:1065–1068.

119. Lehming N, Sartorius J, Oehler S, et al. Recognition helices of lac and lambda repressor are oriented in opposite directions and recognize similar sequences. Proc Natl Acad Sci USA 1988; 85:7947–7951.

120. Green S, Kumar V, Theulaz I, et al. The N-terminal DNA-binding 'zinc finger' of the osestrogen and glucocorticoid receptors determines target gene specificity. EMBO J 1988; 7:3037–3044.

121. Corton JC, Johnston SA. Altering DNA-binding specificity of GAL4 requires sequences adjacent to the zinc finger. Nature 1989; 340:724–727.

122. Kim KS, Guarente L. Mutations that alter transcriptional activation but not DNA binding in the zinc finger of yeast activator HAPI. Nature 1989; 342:200–203.

123. Mader S, Kumar V, de Verneuil H, et al. Three amino acids of the oestrogen receptor are essential to its ability to distinguish an oestrogen from a glucocorticoid responsive element. Nature 1989; 338:271–274.

124. Danielsen M, Hinck L, Ringold GM. Two amino acids within the knuckle of the first zinc finger specify DNA response element activation by the glucocorticoid receptor. Cell 1989; 7:1131–1138.

125. Umesono K, Evans RM. Determinants of target gene specificity for steroid thyroid hormone receptors. Cell 1989; 57:1139–1146.

126. de Thé H, del Mar Vivanco-Ruiz M, Tiollais P, et al. Identification of a retinoic acid responsive element in the retinoic acid receptor β3 gene. Nature 1990; 343:177–180.

127. von der Ahe D, Renoir J-M, Buchou T, et al. Receptors for glucocorticoid and progesterone recognize distinct features of a DNA regulatory element. Proc Natl Acad Sci USA 1986; 83:2817–2821.

128. Gowland PL, Buetti E. Mutations in the hormone regulatory element of mouse mammary tumor virus differentially affect the response to progestins, androgens, and glucocorticoids. Mol Cell Biol 1989; 9:3999–4008.

129. Chalepakis G, Arnemann J, Slater E, et al. Differential gene activation by glucocorticoids and progestins through the hormone regulatory element of mouse mammary tumor virus. Cell 1988; 53:371–382.

130. Severne Y, Wieland S, Schaffner W, et al. Metal binding 'finger' structures in the glucocorticoid receptor defined by site-directed mutagenesis. EMBO J 1988; 7:2503–2508.

131. Wrange O, Erikson P, Perlmann T. The purified activated glucocorticoid receptor is a homodimer. J Biol Chem 1989; 64:5253–5259.

132. Hollenberg SM, Giguere V, Segui P, et al. Co-localization of DNA-binding and transcriptional activation functions in the human glucocorticoid receptor. Cell 1987; 49:39–46.

133. Rossini GP, Wikstrom AC, Gustafsson JA. Glucocorticoid receptor complexes are associated with small RNA in vitro. J Steroid Biochem 1989; 32:633–641.

134. Danielsen M, Northrop JP, Ringold GM. The mouse glucocorticoid receptor: mapping of functional domains by cloning, sequencing and expression of wild-type and mutant receptor proteins. EMBO J 1986; 5:2513–22.

135. Miesfeld R, Godowski PJ, Maler BA, et al. Glucocorticoid receptor mutants that define a small region sufficient for enhancer activation. Science 1987; 236:423–427.

136. Guarente L. UASs and enhancers: common mechanism of transcriptional activation in yeast and mammals. Cell 1988; 52:303–305.

137. Sigler PB. Transcriptional activation, acid blobs and negative noodles. Nature 1988; 333:210–212.

138. Webster NJ, Green S, Jin JR, et al. The hormone-binding domains of the estrogen and glucocorticoid receptors contain an inducible transcription activation function. Cell 1988; 54:199–207.

139. Hollenberg SM, Evans RM. Multiple and cooperative trans-activation domains of the human glucocorticoid receptor. Cell 1988; 55:899–906.

140. Godowski PJ, Picard D, Yamamoto KR. Signal transduction and transcriptional regulation by glucocorticoid receptor-lexA fusion proteins. Science 1988; 241:812–816.

141. Sabbah M, Redeuilh G, Secco C, et al. The binding activity of estrogen receptor to DNA and heat shock protein (M_r 90,000) is dependent on receptor-bound metal. J Biol Chem 1987; 262:8631–8635.

142. Tora L, Gronemeyer H, Turcotte B, et al. The N-terminal region of the chicken progesterone receptor specifies target gene activation. Nature 1988; 333:185–188.

143. Conneely OM, Kettelberger D, Tsai M-J, et al. Promoter specific activating domains of the chicken progesterone receptor. In: Roy AK, Clark JH, ed. Gene Regulation by Steroid Hormones IV. New York: Springer-Verlag, 1989: 221.

144. Eriksson P, Wrange O. Protein-protein contacts in the glucocorticoid receptor homodimer influence its DNA binding properties. J Biol Chem 265:3535–3542.

145. de Boer W, Bolt J. Transformation (4S–5S) of the nuclear estrogen receptor is reversible, but not accompanied by a change in the affinity for DNA. J Steroid Biochem 1988; 31:931–937.

146. Tsai SY, Carlstedt-Duke J, Weigel NL, et al. Molecular interactions of steroid hormone receptor with its enhancer element: evidence for receptor dimer formation. Cell 1988; 55:361–369.

147. Kumar V, Chambon P. The estrogen receptor binds tightly to its responsive element as a ligand induced homodimer. Cell 1988; 55:145–156.

148. Wrange O, Erikson P, Perlmann T. The purified activated glucocorticoid receptor is a homodimer. J Biol Chem 1989; 64:5253–5259.

149. Rodriguez R, Weigel NL, O'Malley BW, et al. Dimerization of the chicken progesterone receptor: evidence for a hormone independent dimerization domain. Mol Endocrinol 1990; 4:1782–1790.

150. Guiochon-Mantel A, Loosefelt H, Lescop P, et al. Mechanisms of nuclear localization of the progesterone receptor: evidence for interaction between monomers. Cell 1989; 57:1147–1154.

151. Joab I, Radanyi C, Renoir M, et al. Common non-hormone binding component in nontransformed chick oviduct receptors of four steroid hormones. Nature 1984; 308:850–853.

152. Schuh S, Yonemoto W, Brugge J, et al. A 90,000-dalton binding protein common to both steroid receptors and the Rous sarcoma virus transforming proteins, pp60v-src. J Biol Chem 1985; 260:14292–14296.

153. Aranyi P, Radanyi C, Renoir M, et al. Covalent stabilization of the nontransformed chick oviduct cytosol progesterone receptor by chemical cross-linking. Biochemistry 1988; 27:1330–1336.

154. Baulieu E-E. Steroid hormone antagonists at the receptor level: a role

155. for the heat-shock protein MW 90,000 (hsp90). J Cell Biochem 1987; 35:161–174.

155. Craig EA. The heat shock response. CRC Crit Rev Biochem 1985; 18:239–280.

156. Riehl RM, Sullivan WP, Vroman BT, et al. Immunological evidence that the nonhormone binding component of avian steroid receptors exists in a wide range of tissues and species. Biochemistry 1985; 24:6586–6591.

157. Howard KJ, Distelhorst CW. Evidence for intracellular association of the glucocorticoid receptor with the 90-kDa heat shock protein. J Biol Chem 1988; 263:3474–3481.

158. Rexin M, Busch W, Gehring U. Chemical cross-linking of heteromeric glucocorticoid receptors. Biochemistry 1988; 27:5593–5601.

159. Pratt WB, Jolly DJ, Pratt DV, et al. A region in the steroid binding domain determines formation of the non-DNA-binding, 9S glucocorticoid receptor complex. J Biol Chem 1988; 263:267–273.

160. Carson-Jurica MA, Lee AT, Dobson AW, et al. Interaction of the chicken progesterone receptor with heat shock protein (HSP)–90. J Steroid Biochem 1989; 34:1–8.

161. Smith DF, McCormick DJ, Toft DO. Studies with antibodies against the conserved cysteine region of progesterone receptor. J Steroid Biochem 1988; 30:1–7.

162. Smith DF, Lubahmn DB, McCormick DJ, et al. The production of antibodies against the conserved cysteine region of steroid receptors and their use in characterizing the avian progesterone receptor. Endocrinology 1988; 122:2816–2825.

163. Weigel NL, Schrader WT, O'Malley BW. Antibodies to chicken progesterone receptor peptide 523–536 recognize a site exposed in receptor–deoxyribonucleic acid complexes but not in receptor–heat shock protein–90 complexes. Endocrinology 1989; 125:2494–2501.

164. Tai PK, Maeda Y, Nakao K, et al. A 59-kilodalton protein associated with progestin, estrogen, androgen, and glucocorticoid receptor. Biochemistry 1986; 25:5269–5275.

165. Gasc JM, Renoir JM, Faber LE, et al. Nuclear localization of 2 steroid receptor–associated proteins, hsp90 and p59. Exp Cell Res 1990; 186:362–367.

166. Kost SL, Smith DF, Sullivan WP, et al. Binding of heat shock proteins to the avian progesterone receptor. Mol Cell Biol 1989; 9:3829–3838.

167. Velazquez JM, Lindquist S. hsp70: nuclear concentration during environmental stress and cytoplasmic storage during recovery. Cell 1984; 36:655–662.

168. Cheng MY, Hart F-U, Martin J, et al. Mitochondrial heat shock protein hsp60 is essential for assembly of proteins imported into yeast mitochondria. Nature 1989; 337:620–625.

169. Liao S, Rossini GP, Hiipakka RA, et al. Factors that can control the interaction of the androgen-receptor complex with the genomic structure in the rat prostate. In: Bresciani F, ed. Perspectives in Steroid Receptor Research. New York: Raven, 1980: 99–112.

170. Auricchio R, Migliaccio A, Castoria G, et al. Direct evidence of in vivo phosphorylation-dephosphorylation of the estradiol-17β receptor. Role of Ca^{2+}-calmodulin in the activation of hormone binding sites. J Steroid Biochem 1984; 20:31–35.

171. Grandics P, Miller A, Schmidt TJ, et al. Phosphorylation in vivo of rat hepatic glucocorticoid receptors. Biochem Biophys Res Commun 1984; 120:59–65.

172. Goldsteyn EJ, Graham JS, Goren HJ, et al. Phosphorylation status of nuclear and cytosolic androgen receptors in the rat ventral prostate. Prostate 1989; 14:91–101.

173. Auricchio F, Migliaccio A, Castoria G, et al. Phosphorylation of estradiol receptor on tyrosine and interaction of estradiol and glucocorticoid receptors with antiphosphotyrosine antibodies. Adv Exp Med Biol 1988; 231:519–539.

174. Migliaccio A, Di Domenicio M, Green S, et al. Phosphorylation on tyrosine of in vitro synthesized human estrogen receptor activates its hormone binding. Mol Endocrinol 1989; 3:1061–1069.

175. Sheridan PL, Evans RM, Horwitz KB. Phosphotryptic peptide analysis of human progesterone receptors. New phosphorylated sites formed in nuclei after hormone treatment. J Biol Chem 1989; 264:6520–6528.

176. Rao KV, Fox CF. Epidermal growth factor stimulates tyrosine phosphorylation of human glucocorticoid receptor in cultured cells. Biochem Biophys Res Commun 1987; 144:512–519.

177. Logeat F, Le Cunff M, Pamphile R, et al. The nuclear-bound form of the progesterone receptor is generated through a hormone-dependent phosphorylation. Biochem Biophys Res Commun 1985; 131:421–427.

178. Horwitz KB, Alexander PS. In situ photolinked nuclear progesterone receptors of human breast cancer cells: subunit molecular weights after transformation and translocation. Endocrinology 1983; 113:2195–2201.

179. Sheridan PL, Francis MD, Horwitz KB. Synthesis of human progesterone receptors in T47D cells. Nascent A- and B-receptors are active without a phosphorylation-dependent post-translational maturation step. J Biol Chem 1989; 264:7054–7058.

180. Bailly A, Le Page C, Rauch M, et al. Sequence-specific DNA binding of the progesterone receptor to the uteroglobin gene: effects of hormone, antihormone, and receptor phosphorylation. EMBO J 1986; 5:3235–3241.

181. Edwards DP, Kuhnel B, Estes PA, et al. Human progesterone receptor binding to mouse mammary tumor virus deoxyribonucleic acid: dependence on hormone and nonreceptor nuclear factor(s). Mol Endocrinol 1989; 3:381–391.

182. Denner LA, Weigel NL, Schrader WT, et al. Hormone-dependent regulation of chicken progesterone receptor deoxyribonucleic acid binding and phosphorylation. Endocrinology 1989; 125:3051–3058.

183. Sullivan WP, Madden BJ, McCormick DJ, et al. Hormone-dependent phosphorylation of the avian progesterone receptor. J Biol Chem 1989; 263:14717–14723.

184. Sullivan WP, Smith DF, Beato TG, et al. Hormone-dependent processing of the avian progesterone receptor. J Cell Biochem 1988; 36:103–119.

185. Denner LA, Bingman WE, Greene GL, et al. Phosphorylation of the chicken progesterone receptor. J Steroid Biochem 1987; 27:235–243.

186. Hoeck W, Rusconi S, Groner B. Down-regulation and phosphorylation of glucocorticoid receptor in cultured cells. Investigations with a monospecific antiserum against a bacterially expressed receptor fragment. J Biol Chem 1989; 264:14296–14402.

187. Sheridan PL, Krett NL, Gorden JA, et al. Human progesterone receptor transformation and nuclear down-regulation are independent of phosphorylation. Mol Endocrinol 1988; 2:1329–1342.

188. Gorski J, Toft D, Shyamala G, et al. Hormone receptors: studies on the interaction of estrogen with the uterus. Recent Prog Horm Res 1986; 24:45–80.

189. Jensen EV, Suzuki T, Kawashima T, et al. A two-step mechanism for the interaction of estradiol with rat uterus. Proc Natl Acad Sci USA 1986; 59:632–638.

190. Siiteri PK, Schwarz BE, Moriyama I, et al. Estrogen binding in the rat and human. In: O'Malley BW, Means AR, eds. Receptors for Reproductive Hormones. New York: Plenum, 1973: 97–112.

191. Perrot-Applanat M, Groyer-Picard M-T, Lorenzo F, et al. Immunocytochemical study with monoclonal antibodies to progesterone receptor in human breast tumors. Cancer Res 1987; 47:2652–2661.

192. King WJ, Greene GL. Monoclonal antibodies localize estrogen receptor in the nuclei of target cells. Nature 1984; 307:745–747.

193. Wikstrom AC, Bakke O, Okret S, et al. Intracellular localization of the glucocorticoid receptor; evidence for cytoplasmic and nuclear localization. Endocrinology 1987; 120:1232–1242.

194. Fuxe K, Harfstrand A, Agnati LF, et al. Immunocytochemical studies on the localization of glucocorticoid receptor immunoreactive nerve cells in the lower brain stem and spinal cord of the male rat using a monoclonal antibody against rat liver glucocorticoid receptor. Neurosci Lett 1985; 60:1–6.

195. Antakly T, Thompson EB, O Donnell D. Demonstration of the intracellular localization and up-regulation of glucocorticoid receptor by in situ hybridization and immunocytochemistry. Cancer Res 1989; 49(Suppl):2230s–2234s.

196. Qi M, Hamilton BJ, DeFranco D. v-mos oncoproteins affect the nuclear retention and re-utilization of glucocorticoid receptors. Mol Endocrinol 1989; 3:1279–1288.

197. Picard D, Yamamoto KR. Two signals mediate hormone-dependent nuclear localization of the glucocorticoid receptor. EMBO J 1987; 6:3333–3340.

198. Gasc JM, Delahaye F, Baulieu E-E. Compared intracellular localization of the glucocorticosteroid and progesterone receptors: an immunocytochemical study. Exp Cell Res 1989; 181:492–504.

199. Dingwall C, Laskey RA. Protein Import into the nucleus. Annu Rev Cell Biol 1986; 2:367–390.

200. Paine PL, Moore LC, Horowitz SB. Nuclear envelope permeability. Nature 1975; 254:109–114.

201. Sherman MR, Corvol Pl, O'Malley BW. Progesterone-binding components of chick oviduct. J Biol Chem 1970; 245:6085–6096.

202. Kalderon D, Roberts BL, Richardson WD, et al. A short amino acid sequence able to specify nuclear location. Cell 1984; 39:499–509.

203. Lanford RE, Kanda P, Kennedy RC. Induction of nuclear transport with a synthetic peptide homologous to the SV40 antigen transport signal. Cell 1986; 46:575–582.

204. Clemens TL, Garrett KP, Zhou XY, et al. Immunocytochemical localization of the 1,25-dihydroxyvitamin D_3 receptor in target cells. Endocrinology 1988; 122:1224–1230.

205. Oppenheimer JH. Thyroid hormone action at the cellular level. Science 1979; 203:971–979.

206. Walters MR, Hunziker W, Norman AW. 1,25-Dihydroxyvitamin D_3 receptors: intermediates between triiodothyronine and steroid hormone receptors. Trends Biochem Sci 1981; 6:268–271.

207. Picard D, Salser SJ, Yamamoto KR. A movable and regulatable inactivation function within the steroid binding domain of the glucocorticoid receptor. Cell 1988; 54:1073–1080.

208. Gorski J, Noteboom WD, Nicollette JA. Estrogen control of the synthesis of RNA and protein in the uterus. J Cell Comp Physiol 1965; 66(Suppl 1):91.

209. Hastie ND, Bishop JO. The expression of three abundance classes of mRNA in mouse tissues. Cell 1976; 9:761–774.

210. Means AR, Comstock JP, Rosenfeld GC, et al. Ovalbumin messenger RNA of chick oviduct: partial characterization, estrogen dependence and translation in vitro. Proc Natl Acad Sci USA 1972; 69:1146.

211. Chambon P. Eucaryotic nuclear RNA polymerase. Annu Rev Biochem 1975; 44:613–638.

212. Tata JR. Hormones and the synthesis and utilization of ribonucleic acid. Prog Nucleic Acid Res Mol Biol 1966; 5:191–207.

213. Williams-Ashman HG, Liao S, Hancock RL, et al. Testicular hormones and the synthesis of ribonucleic acids and proteins in the prostate gland. Recent Prog Horm Res 1964; 20:247–301.

214. O'Malley BW, McGuire WL, Middleton PA. Altered gene expression during differentiation: population changes in hybridizable RNA after stimulation of the chick oviduct with oestrogen. Nature 1968; 218:1249.

215. Chan L, O'Malley BW. Mechanism of action of the sex steroid hormones. N Engl J Med 1976; 294:1322–1328, 1372–1381, 1430–1437.

216. LeMeur M, Glanville N, Mandell JL, et al. The ovalbumin gene family: hormonal control of X and Y gene transcription and mRNA accumulation. Cell 1981; 23:561–571.

217. McKnight GS, Palmiter RD. Transcriptional regulation of the ovalbumin and conalbumin genes by steroid hormones in chick ovodict. J Biol Chem 1979; 254:9050–9058.

218. Rhoads RE, McKnight GS, Schimke RT. Synthesis of ovalbumin in a rabbit reticulocyte cell-free system programmed with hen oviduct ribonucleic acid. J Biol Chem 1971; 246:7407–7410.

219. Swaneck GE Nordstrom JL, Kreutzaler F, et al. Effect of estrogen on gene expression in chicken oviduct: evidence for transcriptional control of ovalbumin gene. Proc Natl Acad Sci USA 1979; 76:1049–1053.

220. Ringold GM, Yamamoto KR, Bishop JM, et al. Glucocorticoid-stimulated accumulation of mouse mammary tumor virus RNA: increased rate of synthesis of viral RNA. Proc Natl Acad Sci USA 1977; 74:2879–2883.

221. Parks WP, Scolnick EM, Kozikowski EH. Dexamethasone stimulation of murine mammary tumor virus expression: a tissue culture source of virus. Science 1974; 184:158–160.

222. Ringold G, Lasfargues EY, Bishop, JM et al., Production of mouse mammary tumor virus by cultured cells in the absence and presence of hormones: assay by molecular hybridization. Virology 1975; 65:135–147.

223. Tomkins GM, Gelehrter TD, Granner D, et al. Control of specific gene expression in higher organisms. Science 1969; 166:1474–1478.

224. Zubay G. Biochemistry. Reading, MA: Addison-Wesley, 1983.

225. Anderson JE. The effect of steroid hormones on gene transcription. In: Goldberger RF, Yamamoto KR, eds. Biological Regulation and Development. New York: Plenum, 1984: 169–212.

226. O'Malley BW, Means AR. Female steroid hormones and target cell nuclei. Science 1974; 183:610–620.

227. O'Malley BW, McGuire WL, Kohler PO, et al. Studies of the mechanism of steroid hormone regulation of synthesis of specific proteins. Recent Prog Horm Res 1969; 25:105–160.

228. Roy AK, Clark JH. Gene Regulation by Steroid Hormones II. New York: Springer-Verlag, 1983.

229. Spindler SR, Mellon SH, Baxter JD. Growth hormone gene transcription is regulated by thyroid and glucocorticoid hormones in cultured rat pituitary tumor cells. J Biol Chem 1982; 257:11627–11632.

230. Hargrove JL, Schmidt FH. The role of mRNA and protein stability in gene expression. FASEB J 1989; 3:2360–2370.

231. Shapiro DJ, Blume JE, Nielsen DA. Regulation of messenger RNA stability in eukaryotic cells. Bioessays 1987; 6:221–226.

232. Brock ML, Shapiro DJ. Estrogen stabilizes vitellogenin mRNA against degradation. Cell 1983; 34:207–214.

233. Alberts B, Bray D, Lewis J, et al. Molecular Biology of the Cell. New York: Garland, 1983.

234. Brown DD. Developmental biology using purified genes. In: Proceedings of ICN-UCLA Symposia on Molecular Cellular Biology. Vol XXII. New York: Academic, 1981.

235. Lewin B. Genes. New York: Wiley, 1983.

236. May LL. Genetics: A Molecular Approach. New York: Macmillan, 1981.

237. Breathnack R, Chambon P. Organization and expression of eucaryotic split genes coding for proteins. Annu Rev Biochem 1981; 50:349–383.

238. O'Malley BW, Stein JP, Means AR. The evaluation of a complex eucaryotic gene. Metabolism 1982; 31:646–653.

239. Axel R, Maniatis T, Fox CF. Eucaryotic gene regulation. In: Proceedings of ICN-UCLA Symposia on Molecular and Cellular Biology. Vol XIV. New York: Academic, 1979.

240. Gilbert W. Introns and exons: playgrounds of evolution. In: Axel R, Maniatis T, Fox M, eds. Eucaryotic Gene Regulation. Vol XIV. New York: Academic, 1979: 1–12.

241. Cech TR. RNA as an enzyme. Sci Am 1986; 255(5):64–75.

242. Padgett RA, Grabowski PJ, Konarska MM, et al. Splicing of messenger RNA precursors. Annu Rev Biochem 1986; 55:1119–1150.

243. Crick F. Split genes and RNA splicing. Science 1979; 204:264–271.

244. Darnell JE Jr. Variety in the level of gene control in eucaryotic cells. Nature 1982; 297:365–371.

245. Darnell JE Jr. Transcription units for mRNA production in eukaryotic cells and their DNA viruses. Prog Nucleic Acid Res Mol Biol 1979; 22:327–353.

246. Lewin B. Eucaryotic genomes. In: Gene Expression 2. New York: John Wiley & Sons, 1980.

247. Perry RP. Processing of RNA. Annu Rev Biochem 1976; 45:605–629.

248. Ziff EB. Transcription and RNA processing by the DNA tumor viruses. Nature 1980; 287:491–499.

249. Tsai M-J, Ting AC, Nordstrom JL, et al. Processing of high molecular weight ovalbumin and ovomucoid precursor RNA to messenger RNA. Cell 1980; 22:219–230.
250. Perry RP. RNA processing comes of age. J Cell Biol 1981; 91:28s–38s.
251. Tilghmen SM, Curtis PJ, Tiemeier DC, et al. The intervening sequence of a mouse β-globin gene is transcribed with in the 15s β-globin mRNA precursor. Proc Natl Acad Sci USA 1978; 1309–1313.
252. Nevins JR, Darnell JE Jr. Steps in the processing of Ad 2 mRNA: poly(A)+ nuclear sequences are conserved and poly(A) addition precedes splicing. Cell 1978; 15:1477–1493.
253. Lerner MR, Steitz JA. Snurps and scyrps. Cell 1981; 25:298–300.
254. Fawcett DW. The Cell. 2nd ed. Philadelphia: WB Saunders, 1981: 266–302.
255. Kornberg RD. Structure of chromatin. Annu Rev Biochem 1977; 46:931–954.
256. Kornberg RD, Klug A. The nucleosome. Sci Am 1981; 244(2):52–64.
257. Miller OL. The nucleolus, chromosomes, and visualization of genetic activity. J Cell Biol 1981; 91:15s–27s.
258. Watson JD. Molecular Biology of the Gene. 3rd ed. Menlo Park, CA: Benjamin/Cummings, 1976.
259. Weisbrod S. Active chromatin (a review). Nature 1982; 297:289–295.
260. Klug A, Rhodes D, Smith J, et al. A low resolution structure for the histone core of the nucleosome. Nature 1980; 287:509–516.
261. Laskey RA, Earnshaw WC. Nucleosome assembly. Nature 1980; 286:763–767.
262. McGhee JD, Rau DC, Charney E, et al. Orientation of the nucleosome within the higher order structure of chromatin. Cell 1980; 22:87–96.
263. McGhee JD, Felsenfeld G. Nucleosome structure. Annu Rev Biochem 1980; 49:1115–1156.
264. Weintraub H, Groudine M. Chromosomal subunits in active genes have an altered conformation. Science 1976; 193:848–856.
265. Elgin SCR. DNase I–hypersensitive sites of chromatin. Cell 1981; 27:413–415.
266. Lamb MM, Daneholt B. Characterization of active transcription units in Balbiani rings of Chronomus tentans. Cell 1979; 17:835–848.
267. Lawson GM, Knoll BJ, March CJ, et al. Definition of 5′ and 3′ structure boundaries of the chromatin domain containing the ovalbumin multigene family. J Biol Chem 1981; 257:1501–1507.
268. O'Malley BW. Gene Regulation. In: Proceedings of UCLA Symposia on Molecular and Cellular Biology. Vol XXVI. New York: Academic, 1982:507–521.
269. Grosveld F, van Assendelft GB, Greaves DR, et al. Position-independent, high-level expression of the human β-globin gene in transgenic mice. Cell 1987; 51:975–985.
270. Barrack ER, Coffey DS. Biological properties of the nuclear matrix: steroid hormone binding. Recent Prog Horm Res 1982; 28:133–195.
271. Ciejek EM, Tsai M-J, O'Malley BW. Actively transcribed genes are associated with the nuclear matrix. Nature 1983; 306:607–609.
272. Robinson SI, Nelkin BD, Vogelstein B. The ovalbumin gene is associated with the nuclear matrix of chicken oviduct cells. Cell 1982; 28:99–106.
273. Razin A, Riggs AD. DNA methylation and gene function. Science 1980; 210:604–610.
274. Ptashne M, Jeffrey A, Johnson AD, et al. How the λ repressor and Cro work. Cell 1980; 19:1–11.
275. Brown DD. Gene expression in eucaryotes. Science 1981; 211:667–674.
276. McKnight SL, Gavis ER, Kingsbury R. Analysis of transcriptional regulatory signals of the HSV-thymidine kinase gene: identification of an upstream control region. Cell 1981; 25:385–398.
277. McKnight SL, Kingsbury R. Transcriptional control signals of a eucaryotic protein-coding gene. Science 1982; 217:316–324.
278. Ptashne M, Gilbert W. Genetic repressors. Sci Am 1970; 222(4):36–44.
279. Rodriguez RL, Chamberlin MJ. Promoters: Structure and Function. New York: Praeger, 1982.
280. Corden, J, Wasylyk B, Buchwalder A, et al. Promoter sequences of eukaryotic protein-coding genes. Science 1980; 209:1406–1414.
281. Serfling E, Jasin M, Schaffner W. Enhancers and eukaryotic gene transcription. Trends Genet 1985; 1:224–230.
282. Darnell J, Lodish H, Baltimore D. Molecular Cell Biology. 2nd ed. New York: Scientific American Books, 1990.
283. Payvar F, DeFranco D, Firestone GL, et al. Sequence-specific binding of glucocorticoid receptor to MTV DNA at sites within and upstream of the transcribed region. Cell 1983; 35:381.
284. Tsai SY, Tsai M-J, O'Malley BW. Cooperative binding of steroid hormone receptor contributes to transcriptional synergism at target enhancer elements. Cell 1989; 57:443.
285. Ptashne M. How gene activators work. Sci Am, 1989; 260(1):40–47.
286. Charron J, Drouin J. Glucocorticoid inhibition of transcription from episomal proopiomelanocortin gene promoter. Proc Natl Acad Sci USA 1986; 83:8903–8904.
287. McKnight SL, Lane MD, Gluecksohnwaelsch S. Is CCAAT enhancer-binding protein a central regulator of energy metabolism? Genes Dev 1989; 3:2021–2024.
288. Hawley DK, Roeder R.G. Separation and partial characterization of three functional steps in transcriptional initiation by human RNA polymerase II. J Biol Chem 1985; 260:8163–8172.
289. Reinberg D, Horikoshi M, Roeder RG. Factors involved in specific transcription in mammalian RNA polymerase II. Functional analysis of initiation factors IIA and IID and identification of a new factor operating at sequences downstream of the initiation site. J Biol Chem 1987; 262:3322–3330.
290. Buratowski S, Hahn S, Guarente L, et al. Five intermediate complexes in transcription initiation by RNA polymerase II. Cell 1989; 56:549–561.
291. Van Dyke MW, Sawadogo M, Roeder RG. Stability of transcription complexes on class II genes. Mol Cell Biol 1989; 9:342–344.
292. Sawadogo M, Roeder RG. Interaction of a gene-specific transcription factor with the adenovirus major late promoter upstream of the TATA box region. Cell 1985; 43:165–175.
293. Hai T, Horikoshi M, Roeder RG, et al. Analysis of the role of the transcription factor ATF in the assembly of a functional preinitiation complex. Cell 1988; 54:1043–1051.
294. Horikoshi M, Hai T, Lin YS, et al. Transcription factor ATF interacts with the TATA factor to facilitate establishment of a preinitiation complex. Cell 1988; 54:1033–1042.
295. Tsai SY, Sagami I, Wang H, et al. Interactions between a DNA-binding transcription factor (COUP) and a non-DNA binding factor (S300-II). Cell 1987; 50:701–709.
296. Corthesy B, Hispking R, Theulaz I, et al. Estrogen-dependent in vitro transcription from the vitellogenin promoter in liver nuclear extracts. Science 1988; 239:1137–1139.
297. Freedman L, Yoshinaga S, Vanderbilt J, et al. In vitro transcription enhancement by purified derivatives of the glucocorticoid receptor. Science 1989; 245:298–300.
298. Klein-Hitpass L, Tsai SY, Weigel NL, et al. The progesterone receptor stimulates cell-free transcription by enhancing the formation of a stable preinitation complex. Cell 1990; 60:247–257.
299. Bagchi MK, Tsai SY, Weigel NL, et al. Regulation of in vitro transcription by progesterone receptor—characterization and kinetic studies. J Biol Chem 1990; 265:5129–5134.
300. Glass CK, Holloway JM, Devary OV, et al. The thyroid hormone receptor binds with opposite transcriptional effects to a common sequence motif in thyroid hormone and estrogen response elements. Cell 1988; 54:313–323.
301. Jantzen K, Fritton HP, Igo-Kemenes T, et al. Partial overlapping of binding sequences for steroid hormone receptors and DNase I hypersensitive sites in the rabbit uteroglobin gene region. Nucleic Acids Res 1987; 15:4535–4552.
302. Schmid W, Strahle U, Schutz G, et al. Glucocorticoid receptor binds cooperatively to adjacent recognition sites. EMBO J 1989; 2257–2263.
303. Topol J, Ruder DM, Parker CS. Sequences required for in vitro transcriptional activation of a Drosophila hsp70 gene. Cell 1985; 42:527–537.
304. Poellinger L, Yoza BK, Roeder RG. Functional cooperativity between protein molecules bound at two distinct sequence elements of the immunoglobulin heavy chain promoter. Nature 1989; 337:573–576.
305. Schule R, Muller M, Kaltschmidt C, et al. Many transcription factors interact synergistically with the steroid receptors. Science 1988; 242:1418–1420.
306. Nordeen SK, Kunhnel B, Lawler-Heavener J, et al. A quantitative comparison of dual control of a hormone response element by progestins and glucocorticoids in the same cell line. Mol Endocrinol 1989; 3:1270–1278.
307. O'Malley BW, Roop DR, Lai EC, et al. The ovalbumin gene: organization, structure, transcription and regulation. Recent Prog Horm Res 1979; 35:1–46.
308. Yamamoto KR. Steroid receptor–regulated transcription of specific genes and gene networks. Annu Rev Genet 1985; 19:209–252.
309. Beato M. Gene regulation by steroid hormones. Cell 1989; 56:335–344.
310. Fritton HP, Igo-Kemenes TI, Nowock J, et al. Alternative sets of DNaseI-hypersensitive sites characterize the various functional states of the chicken lysozyme gene. Nature 1984; 311:163–165.
311. Becker PB, Gloss B, Schmid W, et al. In vivo protein DNA interactions in a glucocorticoid response element require the presence of the hormone. Nature 1986; 324:686–688.
312. Bagchi MK, Elliston JF, Tsai SY, et al. Steroid hormone–dependent interaction of human progesterone with its target enhancer element. Mol Endocrinol 1988; 2:1221–1229.
313. O'Malley BW. The steroid receptor superfamily: more excitement predicted for the future. Mol Endocrinol 1990; 4:363–369.
314. Siiteri PK, Mura JT, Hammond GL, et al. The serum transport of steroid hormones. Recent Prog Horm Res 1982; 38:457–510.
315. Pardridge WM. Transport of protein bound hormones into tissues in vivo. Endocrinol Rev 1981; 2:102–123.
316. Ekins R, Edwards P, Sinha A. Organ-specific regulation of hormone efflux from tissue capillaries: a physiological role for hormone binding proteins? Steroids 1988; 52:369–370.
317. Soloff MS, Creange JE, Potts GO. Unique estrogen-binding properties of rat pregnancy plasma. Endocrinology 1971; 88:427–432.
318. Raynaud JP. Influence of rat estradiol binding plasma protein (EBP) on uterotrophic activity. Steroids 1973; 21:249–258.
319. Westphal U. Steroid-Protein Interactions. New York: Springer-Verlag, 1971.

320. Anderson JN, Peck EJ Jr, Clark JH. Nuclear receptor estrogen complex: in vivo and in vitro binding of estradiol and estriol as influenced by serum albumin. J Steroid Biochem 1974; 5:103–107.

321. Jensen EV, Jacobson HI. Basic guides to the mechanism of estrogen action. Recent Prog Horm Res 1962; 18:387–414.

322. Schrader WT, Toft DO, O'Malley BW. Progesterone binding protein of chick oviduct. VI. Interaction of purified progesterone receptor components with nuclear constituents. J Biol Chem 1972; 247:2401–2407.

323. O'Malley BW, Strott CA. The mechanism of action of progesterone. In: Greep RO, Astwood EB, eds. Handbook of Physiology. Sect 7: Endocrinology. Vol II. Female Reproductive System. Part 1. Washington, DC: American Physiological Society, 1973: 591–602.

324. Clark JH, Peck EJ Jr. Steroid hormone receptors: basic principles and measurement. In: O'Malley BW, Birnbaumer L, eds. Receptors and Hormone Action. Vol 1. New York Academic, 1977: 383–410.

325. Tata JR. The action of growth and developmental hormones: evolutionary aspects. In: Goldberger RF, Yamamoto KR, eds. Biological Regulation and Development. New York: Plenum, 1984: 1–58.

326. Szego CM, Davis JS. Adenosine 3′5′-monophosphate in rat uterus: acute elevation by estrogen. Proc Natl Acad Sci USA 1967; 58:1711–1718.

327. Flandroy L, Fastrez-Boute A, Galand P. Oestrogen induced changes in uterine cGMP: relationship with other parameters of hormonal stimulation. Arch Int Physiol Biochim 1976; 84:1072–1078.

328. Tchernitchin A, Tchernitchin X. Characterization of the estrogen receptors in the uterine and blood eosinophil leukocytes. Experientia 1977; 32:1240–1242.

329. Szego CM, Lawson DA. Influence of histamine on uterine metabolism: stimulation of incorporation of radioactivity from amino acids into protein, lipid and purines. Endocrinology 1977; 74:372–381.

330. Tchernitchin A, Roorijck J, Tchernitchin X, et al. Effects of cortisol on uterine eosinophilia and other oestrogenic responses. Mol Cell Endocrinol 1976; 2:331–337.

331. Galand P, Mairesse N, Roorijck J, et al. Differential blockade of estrogen induced uterine responses by the antiestrogen nafoxidine. J Steroid Biochem 1983; 19:1259–1263.

332. Zor U, Koch Y, Lamprecht SA, et al. Mechanism of oestradiol action on the rat uterus: independence of cyclic AMP, prostaglandin E₂ and β-adrenergic mediation. J Endocrinol 1973; 58:525–533.

333. Rorke EA, Katzenellenbogen BS. Dissociated regulation of growth and ornithine decarboxylase activity by estrogen in the rat uterus. Biochem Biophys Res Commun 1984; 122:1186–1193.

334. Anderson JN, Peck EJ Jr, Clark JH. Estrogen-induced uterine responses and growth: relationship to receptor estrogen binding by uterine nuclei. Endocrinology 1975; 96:160–167.

335. Harris J, Gorski J. Evidence for a discontinuous requirement for estrogen in stimulation of deoxyribonucleic acid synthesis in the immature rat uterus. Endocrinology 1978; 103:240–245.

336. Anderson JN, Clark JH, Peck EJ Jr. The relationship between nuclear receptor estrogen binding and uterotrophic responses. Biochem Biophys Res Commun 1972; 48:1460–1468.

337. Guyette WA, Matusik RJ, Rosen JM. Prolactin-mediated transcriptional and post-transcriptional control of casein gene expression. Cell 1979; 17:1013–1023.

338. Palmiter RD. Quantitation of parameters that determine the rate of ovalbumin synthesis. Cell 1975; 4:189–197.

339. Markaverich BM, Clark JH. Two binding sites for estradiol in rat uterine nuclei: relationship to uterotropic response. Endocrinology 1979; 105:1458–1462.

340. Kirkland JL, Gardner RM, Ireland JS, et al. The effect of hypophysectomy on the uterine response to estradiol. Endocrinology 1977; 101:403–410.

341. Sonnenschein C, Soto AM. Pituitary uterotropic effect in the estrogen-dependent growth of the rat uterus. J Steroid Biochem 1978; 9:533–537.

342. Huggins C, Jensen EV. The depression of estrone-induced uterine growth by phenolic estrogens with oxygenated functions at positions 6 or 16: the impeded estrogens. J Exp Med 1955; 102:334–346.

343. Langier C, Pageaux JF, Soto AM, et al. Mechanisms of estrogen action: indirect effect of estradiol on proliferation of quail oviduct cells. Proc Natl Acad Sci USA 1983; 80:1621–1625.

344. Schatz R, Soto AM, Sonnenschein C. Estrogen induced cell multiplication: direct or indirect effect on rat uterine cells? Endocrinology 1984; 115:501–506.

345. Sirbasku DA, Benson RH. Estrogen-inducible growth factors that may act as mediators (estromedins) of estrogen promoted tumor cell growth. Cold Spring Harbor Conf Cell Proliferation 1988; 6:477–497.

346. Cunha GR, Chung LWK, Shannon JM, et al. Hormone induced morphogenesis and growth: role of mesenchymal-epithelial interactions. Recent Prog Horm Res 1983; 39:559–598.

347. Edery M, Pang K, Larson L et al. Epidermal growth factor receptor levels in mouse mammary glands in various physiological states. Endocrinology 1985; 117:405–411.

348. Mukku VR, Stancel GM. Receptors for epidermal growth factor in rat uterus. Endocrinology 1985; 117:149–154.

349. Robson JM, Adler J. Site of action of oestrogens. Nature 1940; 212:146–160.

350. O'Malley BW, McGuire WL, Kohler PO, et al. Studies on the mechanism of steroid hormone regulation of synthesis of specific proteins. Recent Prog Horm Res 1969; 25:105–160.

351. Snow LD, Eriksson H, Hardin JW, et al. Nuclear estrogen receptor in the avian liver: correlation with biologic response. J Steroid Biochem 1978; 9:1017–1026.

352. Janne CO, Bardin W, Jacob ST. DNA-dependent RNA polymerase I and II from kidney. Effect of polyamines on the in vitro transcription of DNA and chromatin. Biochemistry 1975; 14:3589–3597.

353. Naftolin F, Ryan KJ, Petro Z. Aromatization of androstenedione by the anterior hypothalamus of adult male and female rats. Endocrinology 1972; 90:295–298.

354. Danhaive PA, Rousseau GG. Evidence for sex-dependent anabolic response to androgenic steroids mediated by muscle glucocorticoid receptors in the rat. J Steroid Biochem 1988; 29:575–581.

355. Cidlowski JA, Cidlowski NB. Glucocorticoid receptors and the cell cycle. Endocrinology 1982; 110:1653–1662.

356. Laue L, Kawai S, Brandon OD et al. Receptor mediated effects of glucocorticoids on inflammation: enhancement of the inflammatory response with a glucocorticoid antagonist. J Steroid Biochem 1988; 28:591–598.

357. Funder JW. How can aldosterone act as a mineralocorticoid? Endocr Res 1989; 15:227–238.

358. Anderson JN, Peck EJ, Clark JH. Nuclear receptor estrogen complex: accumulation, retention and localization in the hypothalamus and pituitary. Endocrinology 1973; 93:711–717.

359. Cidlowski JA, Muldoon TG. Sex-related differences in the regulation of cytoplasmic estrogen receptor levels in responsive tissues of the rat. Endocrinology 1976; 94:833–841.

360. Clark JH, Campbell PS, Peck EJ Jr. Receptor estrogen complex in the nuclear fraction of the pituitary and hypothalamus of male and female immature rats. Neuroendocrinology 1972; 77:218–228.

361. Munck A, Wira C, Young DA, et al. Glucocorticoid-receptor complexes and the earliest steps in interaction of glucocorticoids on thymus cells. J Steroid Biochem 1972; 4:567–578.

362. Rousseau GG, Baxter JD, Higgins SJ, et al. Steroid-induced nuclear binding of glucocorticoid receptors in intact hepatoma cells. J Mol Biol 1973; 79:539–544.

363. Raymoure WJ, McNaught RW, Smith RG. Reversible activation of non-steroid binding oestrogen receptor. Nature 1985; 313:745–747.

364. Kassis JA, Gorski J. Estrogen receptor replenishment: evidence for receptor recycling. J Biol Chem 1984; 256:738–7382.

365. Anderson JN, Peck EJ Jr, Clark JH. Nuclear receptor estradiol complex: a requirement for uterotropic responses. Endocrinology 1974; 95:174–178.

366. Reynolds SRM. Determinants of uterine growth and activity. Physiol Rev 1951; 31:244–273.

367. Luu Thi MT, Baulieu EE, Milgrom E. Comparison of the characteristics and of the hormonal control of endometrial and myometrial progesterone receptors. J Endocrinol 1975; 66:349–356.

368. McEwen BS. Gonadal steroid receptors in neuroendocrine tissues. In: O'Malley BW, Birnbaumer L, eds. Receptors for Hormones. Vol II. New York: Academic, 1983: 353–400.

369. Elsner CW, Illingworth DV, De Groot K, et al. Cytosol and nuclear estrogen receptor in the genital tract of the rhesus monkey. J Steroid Biochem 1977; 8:151–155.

370. Illingworth DV, Elsner C, De Groot K, et al. A specific progesterone receptor of myometrial cytosol from the rhesus monkey. J Steroid Biochem 1977; 8:157–160.

371. Junne O, Kontula K, Vihko R. Progestin receptors in human tissues: concentrations and binding kinetics. J Steroid Biochem 1976; 7:1061–1068.

372. Freifeld ML, Feil PD, Bardin CW. The in vivo regulation of the progesterone "receptor" in guinea pig uterus: dependence on estrogen and progesterone. Steroid 1974; 23:93–103.

373. Toft D, O'Malley BW. Target tissue receptors for progesterone: the influence of estrogen treatment. Endocrinology 1972; 9:1041–1045.

374. Narduli AM, Greene GL, O'Malley BW, et al. Regulation of progesterone receptor messenger ribonucleic acid and protein levels in MCG–7 cells by estradiol: analysis of estrogen's effect on progesterone receptor synthesis and degradation. Endocrinology 1988; 122:935–944.

375. Loosfelt H, Atger M, Misrahi M, et al. Cloning and sequence analysis of rabbit progesterone-receptor complementary DNA. Proc Natl Acad Sci USA 1986; 83:9045–9049.

376. Milgrom E, Atger M, Baulieu EE. Progesterone in uterus and plasma. IV. Progesterone receptors in guinea pig uterus cytosol. Steroids 1970; 16:741–764.

377. Freifeld ML, Feil PD, Bardin CW. The in vivo regulation of the progesterone "receptor" in guinea pig uterus: dependence on estrogen and progesterone. Steroids 1974; 23:93–103.

378. Milgrom E, Thi L, Atger M, et al. Mechanisms regulating the concentration and the conformation of progesterone receptors in the uterus. J Biol Chem 1973, 248:6366–6377.

379. Alexander IE, Clarke CL, Shine J, et al. Progestin inhibition of progesterone receptor gene expression in human breast cancer cells. Mol Endocrinol 1989; 3:1377–1386.

380. Lerner LJ. Hormone antagonists: inhibitors of specific activities of estrogen and androgen. Recent Prog Horm Res 1964; 20:435–490.

381. Hsueh AJ, Peck EJ Jr, Clark JH. Control of uterine estrogen receptor levels by progesterone. Endocrinology 1976; 98:438–444.

382. Hsueh AJ, Peck EJ Jr, Clark JH. Progesterone antagonism of the oestrogen receptor and oestrogen-induced uterine growth. Nature 1975; 254:337–339.

383. Okulicz WC, Evans RW, Leavitt WW. Progesterone regulation of estrogen receptor in the rat uterus: a primary inhibitory influence on the nuclear fraction. Steroids 1981; 37:463–470.

384. Okulicz WC, Evans RW, Leavitt WW. Progesterone regulation of the occupied form of nuclear estrogen receptor. Science 1981; 213:1503–1505.

385. MacDonald RG, Okulicz WD, Leavitt WW. Progesterone-induced inactivation of nuclear estrogen receptor in the hamster uterus is mediated by acid phosphatase. Biochem Biophys Res Commun 1982; 104:570–576.

386. Aurrichio F, Migliaccio A, Castoria G, et al. Direct evidence of in vitro phosphorylation-dephosphorylation of the estradiol–17β receptor, role of Ca^{2+}calmodulin in the activation of hormone binding sites. J Steroid Biochem 1984; 20:31–35.

387. Okulicz WC. Temporal limitation of progesterone inhibition of occupied nuclear estrogen receptor retention in the rat uterus. Endocr Soc Abstr 1985; 81.

388. McNaught RW, Raymoure WJ, Smith RG. Separation and progesterone regulation of two chick estrogen receptors. Endocrinology 1983; 112(Suppl):342.

389. Eriksson H, Upchurch S, Hardin JW, et al. Heterogeneity of estrogen receptors in the cytosol and nuclear fractions of the rat uterus. Biochem Biophys Res Commun 1978; 81:1–7.

390. Clark JH, Hardin JW, Upchurch S, et al. Heterogeneity of estrogen binding sites in the cytosol of the rat uterus. J Biol Chem 1978; 253:433–437.

391. Ekman P, Barrack ER, Greene GL, et al. Estrogen receptors in human prostate: evidence for multiple binding sites. J Clin Endocrinol Metab 1983; 57:166–176.

392. Swaneck GE, Alvarez JM, Sufrin G. Multiple species of estrogen binding sites in the nuclear fraction of the rat prostate. Biochem Biophys Res Commun 1982; 106:1441–1447.

393. Weinberger MJ. Heterogeneity and distribution of estrogen binding sites in guinea pig seminal vesicle. J Steroid Biochem 1984; 20:1327–1332.

394. Yuh KC, Keyes PL. Properties of nuclear and cytoplasmic estrogen receptor in the rabbit corpus luteum: evidence for translocation. Endocrinology 1979; 105:690–696.

395. Taylor RN, Smith RG. Identification of a novel sex steroid binding protein. Proc Natl Acad Sci USA 1982; 79:1742–1746.

396. Ruh MF, Toft DO. Characterization of an unusual sex steroid binding component from the chicken oviduct. J Steroid Biochem 1984; 21:1–8.

397. Clark JH, Markaverich BM. Heterogeneity of estrogen binding sites and the nuclear matrix. In: Manul B, ed. The Nuclear Envelope and the Nuclear Matrix. New York: Alan R. Liss, 1982: 259–269.

398. Markaverich BM, Clark JH. Two binding sites for estradiol in rat uterine nuclei: relationship to uterotropic response. Endocrinology 1979; 105:1458–1462.

399. Markaverich BM, Upchurch S, Clark JH. Progesterone and dexamethasone antagonism of nucleus growth: a role for a second nuclear binding site for estradiol in estrogen action. J Steroid Biochem 1981; 14:125–132.

400. Pfaff DW, McEwen BS. Actions of estrogen and progestins on nerve cells. Science 1981; 219:808–814.

401. Rousseau GG, Baxter JD. Glucocorticoid receptors. In: Baxter JD Rousseau GG, eds. Glucocorticoid Hormone Action. New York: Springer-Verlag, 1979: 49–77.

402. Richards JS. Content of nuclear estradiol receptor complex in rat corpora lutea during pregnancy: relationship to estrogen concentration and cytosol receptor availability. Endocrinology 1975; 96:227–230.

403. Clark JH, Anderson J, Peck EJ Jr. Receptor estrogen complex in the nuclear fraction of the rat uterus during the estrous cycle. Science 1972; 176:528.

404. Scott RS, Rennie PI, An estrogen receptor in the corpora lutea of the pseudopregnant rabbit. Endocrinology 1971; 89:297–301.

405. Muldoon TG. Mouse mammary tissue estrogen receptors: ontogeny and molecular heterogeneity. In: Hamilton TH, Clark JH, Sadler W, eds. Ontogeny of Receptors and Molecular Mechanism of Reproductive Hormone Action. New York: Raven, 1978:212–236.

406. Hseuh AJW, Peck EJ Jr, Clark JH. Oestrogen receptors in the mammary gland of the lactating rat. J Endocrinol 1973; 58:503–511.

407. McCormack SA, Glasser SR. Ontogeny and regulation of a rat placental estrogen receptor. Endocrinology 1978; 102:273–280.

408. Pasqualini JR, Sumida C, Gelly C, et al. Specific [³H]estradiol binding in the fetal uterus and testis of guinea pig. Quantitative evolution of [³H]estradiol receptors in the different fetal tissues (kidney, lung, uterus and testis) during fetal development. J Steroid Biochem 1976; 7:1031–1038.

409. Clark JH, Gorski J. Ontogeny of the estrogen receptor during early uterine development. Science 1970; 169:76–76.

410. Roth GS, Hess GD. Changes in the mechanism of hormone and neurotransmitter action during ageing: current status of the role of receptor and post-receptor alterations. A review. Mech Ageing Dev 1982; 20:175–194.

411. Mulvihill ER, LePennec JP, Chambon P. Chicken oviduct progesterone receptor: location of specific regions of high-affinity binding in cloned DNA fragments of hormone-responsive genes. Cell 1982; 24:621–632.

412. Milin B, Roy AK. Androgen receptor in rat liver: cytosol receptor deficiency in pseudohermaphrodite male rats. Nature New Biol 1973; 242:248–250.

413. Clark JH, Markaverich BM. The agonistic and antagonistic effects of short acting estrogens: a review. Pharmacol Ther 1982; 21:429–453.

414. Brecher PI, Wotiz HH. Stereospecificity of the uterine nuclear hormone receptors. Proc Soc Exp Biol Med 1968; 128:470–473.

415. Bouton M, Raynaud JP. The relevance of interaction kinetics in determining biological responses to estrogens. Endocrinology 1979; 105:509–515.

416. Jensen EV, Jacobson HI, Flesher JW, et al. Estrogen receptors in target issues. In: Nakao T, Tait JF, eds. Steroid Dynamics. New York: Academic, 1966: 133–157.

417. Clark JH, Markaverich BM. The agonistic-antagonistic properties of clomiphene: a review. Pharmacol Ther 1966; 15:467–519.

418. Tate AC, Greene GL, DeSombre ER, et al. Differences between estrogen- and antiestrogen-estrogen receptor complexes from human breast tumors identified with an antibody raised against the estrogen receptor. Cancer Res 1984; 44:1012–1018.

419. Tate AC, Jordan VC. Nuclear [³H]4-hydroxytamoxifen (4-OHTAM)- and [³H]estradiol (E_2)-estrogen receptor complexes in the MCF-7 breast cancer and GH3 pituitary tumor cell lines. Mol Cell Endocrinol 1984; 36:211–219.

420. Murphy LC, Sutherland RL. Antitumor activity of clomiphene analogs in vitro: relationship to affinity for the estrogen receptor and another high affinity antiestrogen-binding site. J Clin Endocrinol Metab 1983; 57:373–379.

421. Tate AC, DeSombre ER, Greene GL, et al. Interaction of [³H]monohydroxytamoxifen-estrogen receptor complexes with a monoclonal antibody. Breast Cancer Res Treat 1983; 3:267–277.

422. Evans E, Baskevitch PP, Rochefort H. Estrogen receptor DNA interactions: difference between activation by estrogen and antiestrogen. Eur J Biochem 1982; 128:185–191.

423. Ruh TS, Baudendistel LJ. Different nuclear binding sites for antiestrogen and estrogen receptor complexes. Endocrinology 1977; 100:420–426.

424. Ruh TS, Ruh MF. The agonistic and antagonistic properties of the high affinity antiestrogen H1285. Pharmacol Ther 1983; 21:247–264.

425. Ikeda M, Omukai Y, Hosokawa K, et al. Differences in extractability of estradiol and tamoxifen receptor complex in the nuclei from MCF-7 cells with Nonidet P-40. Steroids 1984; 43:481–489.

426. Terenius L. Structure-activity relationships of anti-oestrogens with regard to interaction with 17β-oestradiol in the mouse uterus and vagina. Acta Endocrinol 1971; 66:431–447.

427. Binart N, Catelli MH, Geynet G, et al. Monohydroxytamoxifen: an antiestrogen with high affinity for the chick oviduct oestrogen receptor. Biochem Biophys Res Commun 1979; 91:812–818.

428. Clark JH, Markaverich BM. Agonist and antagonist properties of clomiphene: a review. Pharmacol Ther 1982; 15:467–519.

429. Natrajan PK, Greenblat RB. Clomiphene Citrate: Induction of Ovulation. Philadelphia: Lea & Febiger, 1979: 35–76.

430. Furr BJA, Jordan VC. The pharmacology and clinical uses of tamoxifen. Pharmacol Ther 1984; 25:127–205.

431. Westley BR, Rochefort H. Estradiol-induced proteins in the MCF-7 human breast cancer cell line. Biochem Biophys Res Commun 1979; 90:410–416.

432. Coezy E, Borgna JL, Rochefort H. Tamoxifen and metabolites in MCF-7 cells: correlations between binding to estrogen and cell growth inhibition. Cancer Res 1982; 42:317–323.

433. Lieberman ME, Gorski J, Jordan VC. An estrogen receptor model to describe the regulation of prolactin synthesis by antiestrogens in vitro. J Biol Chem 1983; 258:4741–4745.

434. Lieberman ME, Jordan VC, Fritsch M, et al. Direct and reversible inhibition of estradiol-stimulated prolactin synthesis by antiestrogen in vitro. J Biol Chem 1983; 258:4734–4740.

435. Sutherland RL. Estrogen antagonists in chick oviduct: antagonist activity of eight synthetic triphenylethylene derivatives and their interactions with cytoplasmic and nuclear estrogen receptors. Endocrinology 1981; 109:2061–2068.

436. Sutherland RL, Murphy LC, Foo MS, et al. High affinity anti-oestrogen binding site distinct from the oestrogen receptor. Nature 1980; 288:273–275.

437. Winneker RC, Clark JH. Estrogen stimulation of the antiestrogen specific binding site in rat uterus and liver. Endocrinology 1983; 112:1910–1915.

438. Murphy PR, Breckenridge WC, Lazier CB. Binding of oxygenated

cholesterol metabolites to antiestrogen binding sites from chicken liver. Biochem Biophys Res Commun 1985; 127:786–792.

439. Faye JC, Lasserre B, Bayard F. Antiestrogen specific, high affinity saturable binding sites in rat uterine cytosol. Biochem Biophys Res Commun 1980; 93:1225–1231.

440. Gulino A, Pasqualini JR. Heterogeneity of binding sites for tamoxifen and tamoxifen derivatives in estrogen target and nontarget fetal organs of guinea pig. Cancer Res 1982; 42:1913–921.

441. Kon OL. An antiestrogen-binding protein in human tissues. J Biol Chem 1983; 258:3173–3177.

442. Gulino A, Pasqualini JR. Modulation of tamoxifen specific binding sites and estrogen receptors by estradiol and progesterone in the neonatal uterus of guinea pig. Endocrinology 1983; 112:187–1873.

443. Miller MA, Katzenellenbogen BS. Characterization and quantitation of antiestrogen binding sites in estrogen receptor–positive and –negative human breast cancer cell lines. Cancer Res 1983; 43:3094–3100.

444. Winneker RC, Clark JH. Estrogen stimulation of the antiestrogen specific binding site in rat uterus and liver. Endocrinology 1983; 112:1910–1915.

445. Tabacik C, Cypriani B, Alian S et al. Cholesterol biosynthesis in MCF-7 cell line in relation to cell division: stimulation by estradiol and inhibition by tamoxifen. In: Bresciani F, King RJB, Lippman ME, et al., eds. Progress in Cancer Research and Therapy. Vol 31. New York: Raven, 1984:213–222.

446. Murphy PR, Breckenridge WC, Lazier CB. Binding of oxygenated cholesterol metabolites to antiestrogen binding sites from chicken liver. Biochem Biophys Res Commun 1985; 127:786–792.

447. Lam PHY. Tamoxifen is a calmodulin antagonist in the activation of cAMP phosphodiesterase. Biochem Biophys Res Commun 1984; 118:27–32.

448. Chafouleas JG, Lagace L, Boulton WE, et al. Changes in calmodulin and its mRNA accompany re-entry of quiescent (G0) cells in the cell cycle. Cell 1984; 36:73–81.

449. Wiseman LR, Wakelin AE, May FEB, et al. Effects of the antioestrogen, ICI 164,384 on oestrogen induced RNAs in MCF–7 cells. J Steroid Biochem 1989; 33:1–6.

450. May FEB, Westley BR. Effects of tamoxifen and 4-hydroxytamoxifen on the pNR–1 and pNR–2 estrogen-regulated RNAs in human breast cancer cells. J Biol Chem 1987; 262:15894–15899.

451. Clark JH, Paszko Z, Peck EJ Jr. Nuclear binding and retention of the receptor estrogen complex: relation to the agonistic and antagonistic properties of estriol. Endocrinology 1977; 100:91–96.

452. Brenner RM, Resko JA, West NB. Cyclic changes in oviductal morphology and residual cytoplasmic estradiol binding capacity induced by sequential estradiol-progesterone treatment of spayed rhesus monkeys. Endocrinology 1974; 95:1094–1104.

453. Saunders DE, Lozon MM, Corombos JD, et al. Role of porcine endometrial estrogen sulfotransferase in progesterone mediated down regulation of estrogen receptors. J Steroid Biochem 1989; 32:749–757.

454. Rochefort H, Garcia G. The estrogenic and antiestrogenic activities of androgens in female target tissues. Pharmacol Ther 1984; 23:193–216.

455. Garcia M, Rochefort H. Evidence and characterization of the binding of two ^{3}H androgens to the estrogen receptor. Endocrinology 1979; 104:1797–1804.

456. Rochefort H, Garcia G. The estrogenic and antiestrogenic activities of androgens in female target tissues. Pharmacol Ther 1984; 23:193–216.

457. Garcia M, Rochefort H. Androgen effects mediated by estrogen receptor in 7,12-dimethylbenz(a)anthracene-induced rat mammary tumors. Cancer Res 1978; 48:3922–3929.

458. Rochefort H, Lignon F, Capony F. Formation of estrogen nuclear receptor in uterus: effects of androgen, estrone and nafoxidine. Biochem Biophys Res Commun 1972; 47:662–670.

459. Markaverich BM, Robert RR, Finney RW, et al. Preliminary characterization of an endogenous inhibitor of [^{3}H]estradiol binding in rat uterine nuclei. J Biol Chem 1983; 258:11663–11671.

460. Herrmann W, Wyss R, Riondel A, et al. The effects of an antiprogesterone steroid in women: interruption of the menstrual cycle and of early pregnancy. C R Acad Sci [III] 1982; 294:933–938.

461. Asch RH, Rojas FJ. The effects of RU 486 on the luteal phase of the rhesus monkey. J Steroid Biochem 1985; 22:227–230.

462. Healy DL, Baulieu EE, Hodgen GD. Induction of menstruation by an antiprogesterone steroid (RU 486) in primates: site of action, dose-response relationships, and hormonal effects. Fertil Steril 1983; 40:253–257.

463. Horwitz KB. The antiprogestin RW 38486: receptor-mediated progestin versus antiprogestin actions screened in estrogen-insensitive T47D human breast cancer cells. Endocrinology 1985; 116:2236–2245.

464. Bowden RT, Hissom JR, Moore MR. Growth stimulation of T47D human breast cancer cells by the anti-progestin RU 486. Endocrinology 1989; 124:2642–2644.

465. Gray OG, Leavitt WW. RU 486 is not an antiprogestin in the hamster. J Steroid Biochem 1987; 28:493–497.

466. El-Ashry D, Onate SA, Nordeen SK, et al. Human progesterone receptor complexed with the antagonist RU 486 binds to hormone response elements in a structurally altered form. Mol Endocrinol 1989; 3:1545–1558.

467. Bagchi MK, Tsai SY, Tsai M-J, et al. Progesterone-dependent cell free transcription: identification of a functional intermediate in receptor activtion. Nature 1990; 345:547–550.

468. Olge FF. Kinetic and physiochemical characteristics of an endogenous inhibitor to progesterone-receptor binding in rat placenta cytosol. Biochem J 1981; 199:371–381.

469. Tindall DJ, Chang CH, Lobl TJ, et al. Androgen antagonists in androgen target tissue. Pharmacol Ther 1984; 24:367–400.

470. Rousseau GG, Baxter JD, Higgins SI, et al. Steroid induced nuclear binding of glucocorticoid receptors in intact hepatoma cells. J Mol Biol 1973; 29:539–554.

471. Chrousos GP, Cutler CG Jr, Sauer M, et al. Development of glucocorticoid antagonists. Pharmacol Ther 1983; 20:263–281.

472. Healy DL, Baulieu EE, Hodgen GD. Induction of menstration by an antiprogesterone steroid (RU 486) in primates: site of action, dose-response relationship and hormonal effects. Fertil Steril 1983; 40:253.

473. Baulieu, EE. RU 486: an antiprogestin steroid with contragestive activity in women. In: Baulieu EE, Segal SI, eds. The Antiprogestin Steroid RU486 and Human Fertility Control. New York: Plenum, 1985: 1.

474. French FS, Van Wyk JJ, Baggett B, et al. Further evidence of a target organ defect in the syndrome of testicular feminization. J Clin Endocrinol Metab 1986; 26:493–503.

475. Ainman J, Griffin JE, Gazak JM, et al. Androgen insensitivity as a cause of infertility in otherwise normal men. N Engl J Med 1979; 300:223–227.

476. Bardin CW, Catterall JF. Testosterone: a major determinant of extragenital sexual dimorphism. Science 1981; 211:1285–1294.

477. Brown TR, Lubahn DB, Wilson EM, et al. Deletion of the steroid-binding domain of the human androgen receptor gene in one family with complete androgen insensitivity syndrome: evidence for further genetic heterogeneity in this syndrome. Proc Natl Acad Sci USA 1988; 85:8151–8155.

478. Lubahn DB, Brown TR, Simental JA, et al. Sequence of the intron/exon junctions of the coding region of the human androgen receptor gene and identification of a point mutation in a family with complete androgen insensitivity. Proc Natl Acad Sci USA 1989; 86:9534–9538.

479. Hughes MR, Malloy PJ, Kieback DG, et al. Point mutation in the human vitamin D receptor gene associated with hypocalcemic rickets. Science 1988; 382:1702.

480. Chrousos GP, Renquist D, Brandon D, et al. Glucocorticoid hormone resistance during primate evolution: receptor mediated mechanisms. Proc Natl Acad Sci USA 1982; 79:2031–2040.

481. Brandon DD, Markwick AJ, Chrousos GP, et al. Glucocorticoid resistance in humans and nonhuman primates. Cancer Res 1989; 49:2203s–2213s.

482. MacLusky NJ, Naftolin F. Sexual differentiation of the central nervous system. Science 1981; 211:1294–1303.

483. Clark JH. Sex steroids and maturation in the female. Banbury Report 11. Cold Spring Harbor, NY: Cold Spring Harbor Laboratory, 1982: 315–328.

484. Herbst AL, Poskanzer DC, Robboy SF, et al. Prenatal exposure to stilbestrol: a prospective comparison of exposed female offspring with unexposed controls. N Engl J Med 1971; 292:334–339.

MECHANISM OF ACTION OF HORMONES THAT ACT AT THE CELL SURFACE

C. Ronald Kahn, Robert J. Smith, and William W. Chin

INTRODUCTION

Hormone Systems and Intercellular Communication

Regulation of metabolic processes, control of cell growth and differentiation, and appropriate integration of normal physiological function in multicellular organisms depend on communication among cells. Cell-cell communication is mediated, in large part, by the action of informational molecules of the endocrine, paracrine, autocrine, and neurotransmitter systems. In the endocrine system, the primary signals of cellular communication are hormones and growth factors. These substances can be divided chemically into peptides, steroids, iodothyronines, prostaglandins and prostacyclins, and catecholamines.

Humans and other higher mammals possess more than 100 different hormones with the capability of interacting with the even larger number of different cell types distrib-uted in tissues throughout the body. This poses a tremendous challenge to any system of information exchange in terms of both specificity and sensitivity. The specificity of informational transfer between cells is governed by the concentration and type of hormonal mediator and by the capacity of each target cell to respond to some of these signals but not to others. In addition, specificity is controlled by the volume of distribution of the active substance. Some hormones act on cells located at a distance (an endocrine effect), whereas other hormones and growth factors act on adjacent cells (paracrine effect) or on the secretory cell itself (autocrine effect). Hormones acting by paracrine or autocrine mechanisms, as well as many neurotransmitters, may be able to stimulate multiple tissues, but their action is limited by the fact that the concentrations required for a biological response are achieved only within the limited space of a synapse or on cells that are adjacent to the same extracellular space.

The major factor determining the response of a tissue to a hormone is the presence of a cellular receptor for the hormone and the postreceptor machinery to which that hormone receptor is coupled. For peptide hormones, growth factors, neurotransmitters, and prostaglandins, the receptors are present on the plasma membrane of the cell. For steroid hormones and iodothyronines, the receptors and initial sites of action are in the cytoplasm or the nucleus of the cell. All hormone receptors serve two critical functions: (1) recognition of the hormone as an entity distinct from all other substances present in blood or extracellular fluid. This recognition is accomplished by specific, high-affinity binding. (2) Transformation of this binding into a signal that ultimately modifies cellular metabolism and/or growth. Although many of the concepts of hormone action are similar for membrane-active and nuclear-active hormones, in this chapter we focus on the mechanism of action of hormones that act at the cell surface and the nature of some of the proteins involved in this action. The mechanism of action of steroid and thyroid hormones is discussed in Chapter 3.

Development of the Receptor Concept

The concept that cells possess specific receptors for hormones and other molecules derives from studies in the early 1900s by J. N. Langley[1] on the actions of nicotine and curare and by Paul Ehrlich[2] on the actions of certain toxins and antitrypanocidal drugs. Although the idea of an endocrine system had not yet been developed and the concept of hormones had not yet been introduced, these investigators concluded that certain drugs and toxins have a specificity of action that is governed by the presence of specific "receptive substances" on or in the target cell. This idea was quickly captured by pharmacologists as a model for the effects of drugs, but early attempts to demonstrate receptors for hormones were largely inconclusive. It remained uncertain whether cells possessed specific receptors for hormones and, if they did, whether these receptors were in or on the cell.

The first convincing evidence that some hormones may act via surface membrane receptors came from indirect studies that revealed that antibodies to peptide hormones, such as thyrotropin (TSH) and insulin, can reverse the actions of these hormones after they have begun.[3] This result was consistent with the idea that the hormone was on the cell surface and accessible to the antibody at the time of biological action. In contrast, antibodies to steroid hormones do not block their actions after initiated, because by that time the steroid hormone has entered the cell to interact with its receptor and is inaccessible. Similar conclusions were reached in studies showing that treatment of cells with proteolytic enzymes, at concentrations that did not disrupt cell integrity, specifically blocked the action of some peptide hormones.[4] Also, experiments suggested that peptide hormones remained active after being covalently coupled to large polymeric beads that prevented their entrance into the cell,[5] although the latter studies were subsequently challenged because of possible technical artifacts.[6] Most important, however, was the discovery by Sutherland and coworkers of the first intracellular messenger of hormone action, cyclic AMP (cAMP).[7–9] On the basis of the preceding studies, these workers proposed the second messenger concept of hormone action. In this scheme, the hormone is the first messenger of intercellular communication and is secreted into the bloodstream where it is free to interact with surface membrane receptors on target cells. This interaction results in generation of a second, intracellular messenger that mediates the hormone's effects on intracellular enzymes, gene expression, and even on the cell membrane itself (Fig. 4–1). The second messenger may be a small organic molecule, such as cAMP, cyclic GMP (cGMP), or an inositol phosphate; it may be an ion, such as calcium or

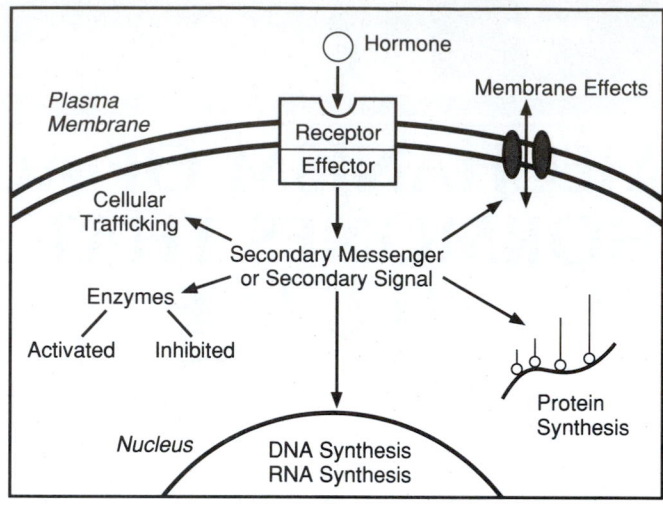

Figure 4–1. A general model for the action of peptide hormones, catecholamines, and other membrane-active hormones. The hormone in the extracellular fluid interacts with the receptor and activates an associated effector system (which may or may not be in the same molecule). This activation results in generation of an intracellular signal or second messenger that, through a variety of common and branched pathways, produces the final effects of the hormone on metabolic enzyme activity, protein synthesis, membrane transport, cellular trafficking, DNA and RNA synthesis, and cellular growth and differentiation.

hydrogen; or it may be the process of activation of a protein kinase, which results in covalent modification of intracellular proteins by phosphorylation, with a resulting change in their activity. This model represents the paradigm on which all concepts of peptide hormone action are built.

Although the specific details of the hormone-receptor interaction and the mechanism of peptide hormone action are best characterized at the cellular and molecular levels, this process can be visualized at the whole body level through studies of hormone distribution and fate in intact animals by use of native or radiolabeled hormone. The latter approach has been utilized for a number of peptide hormones and neurotransmitters, usually by determining the tissue uptake of a radiolabeled hormone followed by dissection of the target organs or autoradiography[10, 11] or by using noninvasive techniques such as external scintillation scanning with high-energy gamma emitters (e.g., ^{123}I)[12] or photoemission tomography.[13]

An example of a study evaluating the biokinetics of insulin by scintillation scanning is illustrated in Figure 4–2. After intravenous injection, the hormone is rapidly cleared from the bloodstream as it is distributed into the extracellular fluid space and is bound to receptors on liver, muscle, and adipose tissue. Within the first 15 min, most of the insulin is bound, internalized, and degraded. In addition, some uptake of hormone and of degradation fragments occurs in nontarget tissues, such as the kidney and the spleen, through receptor-independent mechanisms. By 30 min after the injection, all that remains are some degradation fragments of the hormone in the kidney and the bladder. Although the exact details of the distribution may vary between injected and physiologically secreted insulin, because the latter first enters the portal rather than the systemic circulation, the basic principles are the same. It is important to remember that compared with these distribution kinetics there is a lag in both the onset and the offset of hormone action. This lag is determined by the time required for distribution of the hormone; by the time required for the hormone to exit the vascular space and enter the extracellular fluid space, where it may interact with its target tissues;[14] by the time required to bind to receptors; and by the half-life of the proteins or

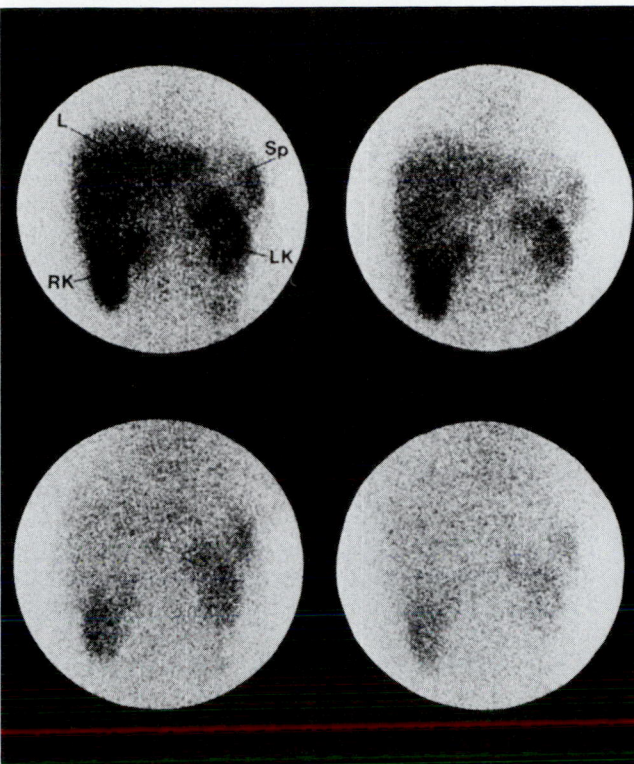

Figure 4–2. Scintiscans obtained 3 min *(upper left)*, 10 min *(upper right)*, 20 min *(lower left)*, and 30 min *(lower right)* after antecubital vein injection of 0.84 mCi of labeled insulin into a normal female volunteer (age 25, weight 63 kg, height 168 cm). L, liver; RK, right kidney; LK, left kidney; Sp, spleen. (From Sodoyez JC, Sodoyez-Goffaux F. Studies of insulin receptors in vivo using ^{131}I-insulin and scintillation scanning. In Venter C, Harrison LC, eds. Receptor Biochemistry and Methodology. Vol 12B. New York: Alan R. Liss, 1988: 149. Copyright © 1988 Alan R. Liss. Reprinted by permission of Wiley-Liss, a division of John Wiley and Sons, Inc.)

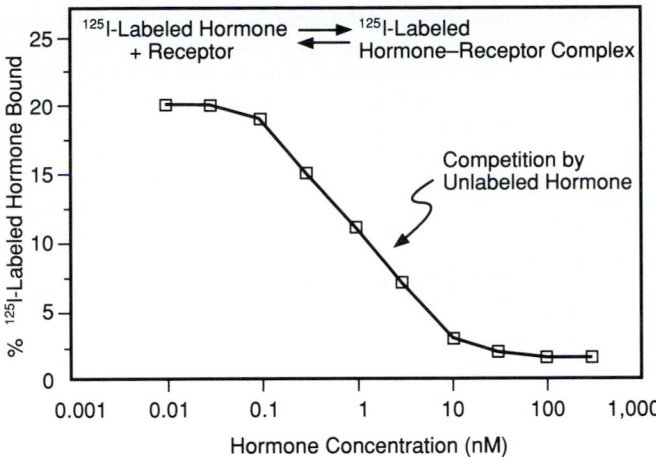

Figure 4–3. A typical hormone-binding study. ^{125}I-labeled hormone is incubated with receptor and increasing concentrations of unlabeled hormone. After separation of bound and free hormone, the percentage of bound ^{125}I is calculated and plotted against the total hormone concentration (labeled plus unlabeled hormone). The result is a competition (or inhibition) curve. Note that even at extremely high concentrations, there is some binding of hormone. This binding is considered to be nonspecific and is subtracted from the total to give the specific binding.

other secondary mediators of hormone action generated by the initial signal.

PROPERTIES OF THE HORMONE-RECEPTOR INTERACTION

Direct Studies of Membrane Receptors

Direct studies of the interaction of peptide hormones with their receptors were first achieved in 1969 with angiotensin[15] and corticotropin (ACTH, adrenocorticotropin)[16] and soon thereafter with insulin[17] and glucagon.[18] Hormone-binding studies have now been performed for virtually all of the peptide hormones, neurotransmitters, and many prostaglandins. The basic approach involves incubation of a suitable radioactively labeled hormone (usually with ^{125}I or ^{3}H) and isolated intact cells or cell membranes as a source of receptors in the presence or absence of unlabeled hormone until equilibrium is obtained.[19–21] The receptor-bound hormone is then separated from the free hormone by centrifugation, precipitation, or other methods, and the percentage of hormone bound to the receptor is determined by counting the radioactive tracer in a gamma or scintillation counter. Unlabeled hormone competes with the labeled hormone for binding, and a competition, or inhibition, curve is produced (Fig. 4–3). Binding of labeled hormone to receptors is a saturable process, and the residual binding in the presence of a large excess of unlabeled hormone is

considered to be nonspecific. Although ideally the tracer hormone is identical with the native hormone except for the addition or substitution of the radioactive atom, in some cases it is necessary to use hormone analogues, particularly if the native hormone is difficult or impossible to label radioactively, if it has a low affinity for the receptor, or if it is rapidly degraded. For some receptors, especially neurotransmitter receptors, the labeled ligand may be a receptor antagonist, because the antagonist binds to the receptor with higher affinity and specificity than the normal agonist.[22, 23] Antireceptor antibodies have also been used as ligands for receptor detection.[24, 25] Such antibodies may recognize domains of the receptor distinct from the hormone binding domain and thus allow detection of receptors with altered regions of ligand binding. Such assays are particularly valuable in assessing receptor alterations in disease.[25]

The basic technique of radioreceptor assay is similar to that of radioimmunoassay (see Chapter 36) but differs in several important respects. Because the interaction of hormone and receptor requires biological specificity (rather than immunological specificity), it is critical that the hormone is labeled in a manner that does not alter its integrity or bioactivity. In addition, because the receptors are part of a cell membrane, the receptor is usually in a particulate or cell-associated form rather than in aqueous solution, i.e., limited to a two-dimensional rather than three-dimensional space. Solubilization of the receptors requires detergent treatment. By using these systems appropriately, however, many of the properties of hormone-receptor interaction have been characterized.

Hormone-Receptor Interaction

For most membrane-active hormones, the interaction between the hormone and the receptor is rapid and reversible, thus serving the physiological need for rapid initiation and rapid termination of hormone action.[19–21] On any cell there are a finite number of receptors for each hormone to which the cell responds, the number varying from fewer than 100 to more than 1 million per cell. Although the classic target cells for hormone action usually possess a higher number of receptors than do nontarget cells—a relation consistent with the specificity requirements of the endocrine system—this arrangement is not always the case. For example, insulin receptors are present in relatively high concentration not only on liver, muscle, and fat cells but also on lymphocytes, gonadal cells, and even brain cells.[26] Similarly, TSH receptors are found on both thyroid cells and adipocytes,[27] and prolactin receptors are present on mammary cells and hepatocytes.[28] The presence of receptors for a hormone on a cell that is thought not to be a target has often led to discovery of previously unrecognized hormone actions on these cells.

RECEPTOR AFFINITY. Hormones bind to their receptors with high affinity and specificity. Because most peptide hormones are present in the circulation at low concentrations (picomolar to nanomolar, i.e., 10^{-12} to 10^{-9} M), receptors must have appropriately high affinities (10^{-12} to 10^{-8} M^{-1}) to achieve significant binding at physiological concentrations. Receptor affinity may be calculated from the kinetics of association and dissociation, or from equilibrium-binding data (Fig. 4–4). The most common method of analysis is the Scatchard plot, in which the bound/free ratio of hormone at equilibrium is plotted against the total hormone bound.[29] If the hormone is a monomer (most are) and if there is a single class of noninteracting receptor sites (many are not), the Scatchard plot results in a straight line (Fig. 4–5). The slope of the line represents the negative value of the equilibrium binding constant $-K_{eq}$, and the intercept on the abscissa corresponds to the total receptor concentration R_0. Many receptors exhibit two or more classes of binding sites of different affinity and capacity, e.g., a high-affinity, low-capacity site and a low-affinity, high-capacity site; others exhibit negative or positive interactions between receptors (see Fig. 4–5). Both phenomena can result in curvilinear Scatchard plots and complex kinetics of interaction.[30-33]

RECEPTOR SPECIFICITY. The characteristic and essential feature of the hormone-receptor interaction is the specificity of binding. At a first level of consideration, this specificity means that each hormone binds to its specific receptor, e.g., glucagon binds only to glucagon receptors, insulin to insulin receptors. At a more subtle level, specificity implies that a hormone or a hormone antagonist binds to its receptor with an affinity that is directly related to its bioactivity (Fig. 4–6). Human insulin is about 50 times as potent in stimulating the metabolism of isolated fat cells as human proinsulin and binds to the insulin receptor with 50 times the affinity of proinsulin.[17] Insulin-like growth factor I (IGF I, also called somatomedin-C) has an even lower affinity for the insulin receptor and even lower insulin-like activity. Most of the differences observed in potency of various hormone analogues or derivatives are due to differences in binding affinity of the receptor. Hormones may also differ in their ability to initiate signal transduction after binding, i.e., their intrinsic activity, although this is less common. Competitive antagonists are ligands that bind to the receptor with high affinity but have no intrinsic activity. Some weak agonists may act as antagonists under certain conditions.

The structural features of hormones that define receptor affinity and intrinsic activity are only partially understood. For some simple peptide hormones such as corticotropin, glucagon, angiotensin, and many gastrointestinal hormones, the binding affinity and intrinsic activity of the receptor appear to be governed by small linear domains of the molecule.[34, 35] For these molecules it is usually possible to produce peptide fragments that retain bioactivity and competitive antagonists that bind to the receptor but lack intrinsic activity. For hormones with a complex three-dimensional structure, such as insulin, the domains for ligand binding

$$H + R \underset{k_R}{\overset{k_F}{\rightleftharpoons}} HR \qquad \textit{Hormone-Receptor Equilibrium Reaction}$$

$$K_{eq} = \frac{[HR]}{[H]\,[R]} = \frac{k_F}{k_R} \qquad \textit{Equilibrium Equation}$$

$$\frac{[HR]}{[H]} = K\,[R] \qquad \textit{Rearranged Equilibrium Equation}$$

$$\frac{[HR]}{[H]} = K\,(R_0 - HR) = K\,[R_0] - K\,[HR]$$

$$\frac{B}{F} = K\,[R_0] - K\,(B) \qquad \textit{Scatchard Equation}$$

Figure 4–4. Analysis of hormone-receptor interactions: deriving the Scatchard equation. This analysis assumes a simple bimolecular interaction with a monomer hormone, a monomeric receptor, and no cooperative interactions. Often the system is more complex, with two or more classes of receptors that differ in affinity or that exhibit cooperative interactions.

H = free hormone concentration

R = free receptor concentration

HR = concentration of hormone-receptor complexes

k_F = forward reaction rate

k_R = reverse reaction rate

K_{eq} = equilibrium constant

R_0 = total receptor concentration

B = amount of hormone bound

F = amount of hormone free

Figure 4–5. Scatchard analysis of hormone-receptor interaction. When the bound/free ratio is plotted against the bound hormone for a single class of noninteractive sites (an ideal bimolecular reversible reaction), a straight line is obtained *(left)*. The slope of the line is the negative value of the equilibrium constant ($-K_{eq}$), and the intercept on the abscissa is the total receptor concentration (R_0). Curvilinear Scatchard plots may arise as the result of two classes of sites *(middle)* or the presence of negative cooperativity *(right)*. In the two-class model, the curve is the sum of two straight lines representing a high-affinity, low-capacity site (K_1, R_1) and a low-affinity, high-capacity site (K_2, R_2). In the negative cooperativity model, there is a single class of interactive sites. The total receptor concentration is R_0. The high-affinity state is K_e (the affinity of the empty receptor). As the sites are filled, the affinity falls, eventually reaching a low-affinity state K_{fl} (the affinity of the filled receptor).

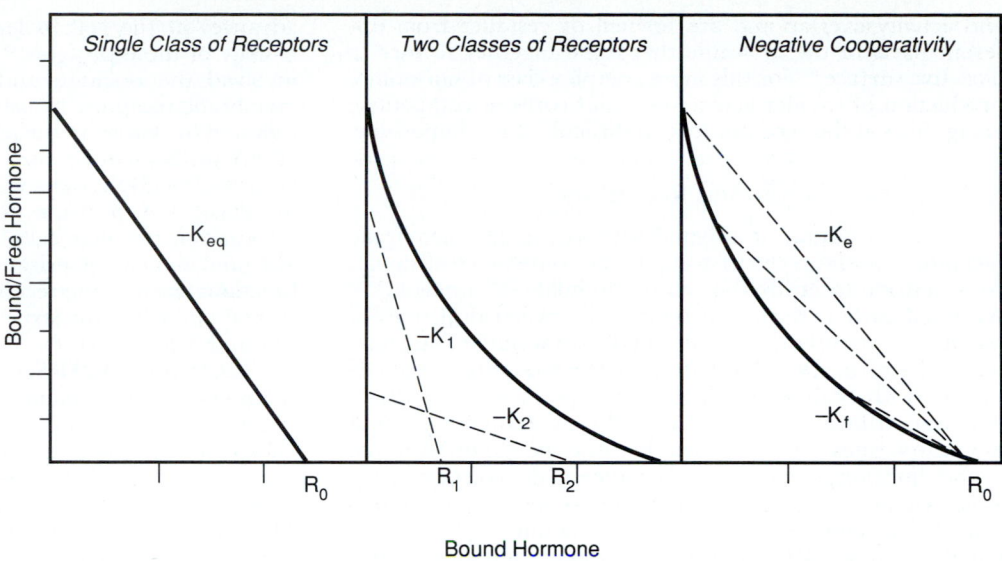

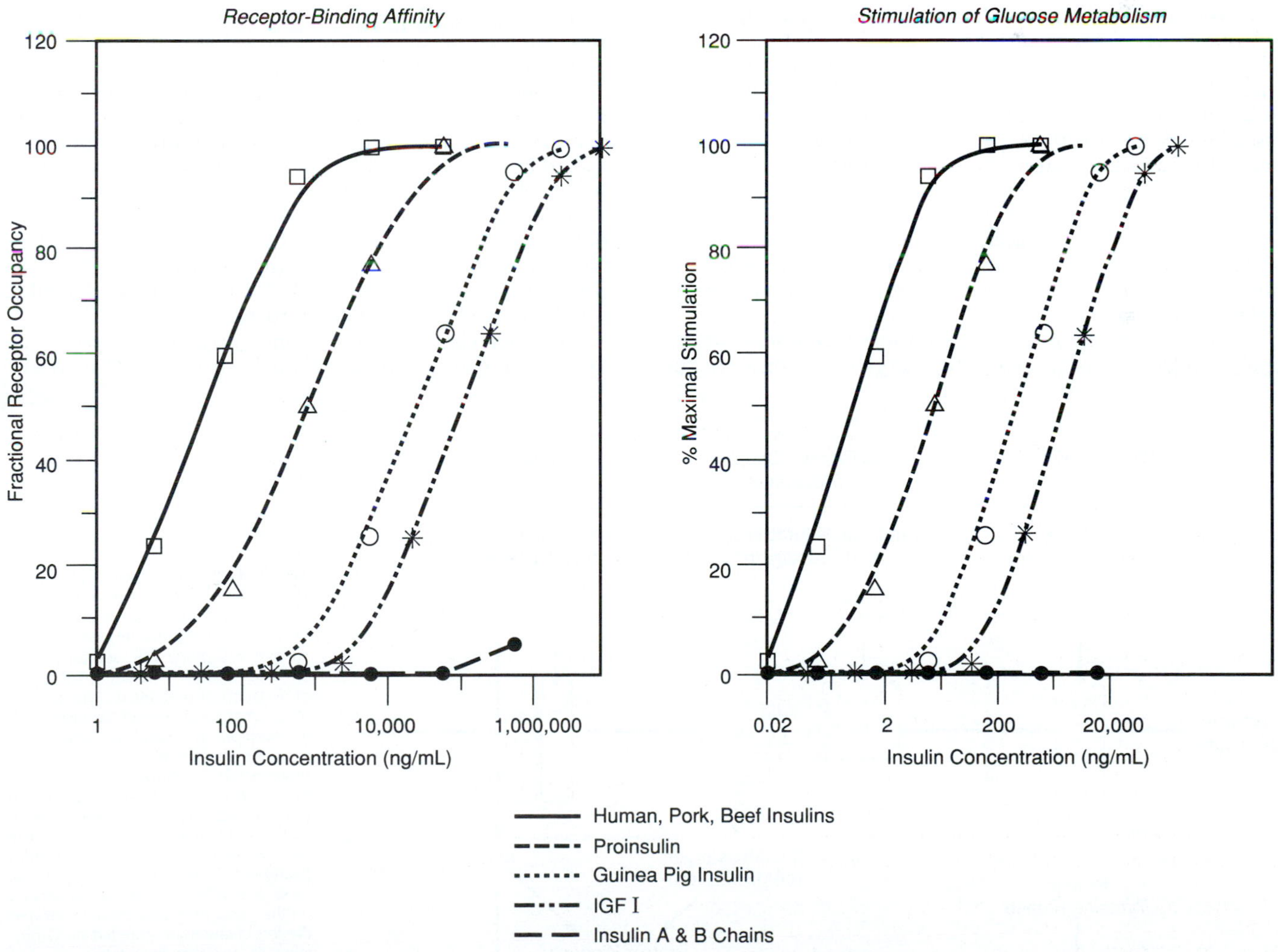

Figure 4–6. Correlation between binding and bioactivity. The left panel shows the binding of a series of insulin analogues to the receptor in rat liver plasma membranes. The right panel shows the ability of the same analogues to stimulate glucose metabolism in isolated adipocytes. Note the almost perfect correlation between receptor affinity *(left)* and relative bioactivity *(right)*. Also, note that the bioactivity scale reflects increased insulin sensitivity because of the presence of spare receptors. IGF I, insulin-like growth factor I. To convert insulin values from nanograms per milliliter to picomoles per liter, multiply by 1.722×10^5. (Adapted from Freychet P, Roth J, Neville DM Jr. Insulin receptors in the liver: specific binding of [^{125}I]-insulin to the plasma membrane and its relation to insulin bioactivity. Proc Natl Acad Sci USA 1971; 68:1833–1837.)

and activity overlap and are formed by residues from different parts of the molecule that come together to form a bioactive surface.[36] For this more complex class of hormones, production of smaller active molecular cores or competitive antagonists at the receptor level is difficult, if not impossible.

Structure of Membrane Receptors

The interaction of a ligand with its cognate membrane receptor represents the first step in the conveyance of signals from outside to inside the cell to modulate its function.[37–42] As noted earlier, this event defines the two critical roles of membrane receptors: (1) to bind extracellular signaling molecules or ligands, present in minute amounts, at the cell surface with both high affinity and specificity; and (2) to relay the information inherent in this ligand-binding event to multiple sites within the cell. Because the members of the ligand hormone superfamily include small molecules such as catecholamines and neuropeptides as well as large molecules such as complex-carbohydrate–containing glycoprotein hormones (e.g., TSH and gonadotropins [luteinizing hormone and follicle-stimulating hormone]), the binding domains of the receptors vary significantly to accommodate this range of ligands. The initial signal produced by hormone binding is transduced intracellularly via effector pathways that may be multiple and interactive. The effector systems involve cAMP, cGMP, arachidonic acid, inositol 1,4,5-trisphosphate (IP$_3$), Ca^{2+}, and other ions as second messengers and are produced by enzymes (such as adenylate and guanylate cyclases and phospholipases A$_2$ and C) and ion channels. In many cases the hormone-receptor complexes do not interface directly with these effectors but act via an intermediate modulating signal transducer, often a guanine nucleotide–binding regulatory protein (G protein). This situation results in production of intracellular signals that are receptor specific and amplified, generate a variety of secondary and tertiary effects on cellular function, and have the potential to allow direct and indirect interactions in related pathways.

The structures of many membrane receptors in mammalian cells have been elucidated, largely as a result of the advances in the cell biology, biochemistry, and molecular biology of these proteins.[43] In many cases the approach has involved the isolation and partial characterization of the membrane receptors by using classic biochemical techniques, followed by partial amino acid sequence analysis. From these, cDNA probes can be prepared and used to screen specific libraries for cDNAs encoding the membrane receptor apoproteins.[44, 45] Expression cloning by using *Xenopus laevis* oocytes and mammalian cells has also allowed the identification, isolation, and characterization of cDNAs and genes encoding functional membrane receptors.[46] Such studies have revealed several motifs for the structure of membrane receptors (Fig. 4–7 and Table 4–1).

RECEPTOR MOTIFS. The largest family of membrane receptors uses G proteins to couple to specific intracellular effector systems,[39, 43–45, 47] such as the adenylate cyclase or phosphatidylinositol turnover pathways. Its members include alpha- and beta-adrenergic, dopaminergic, serotoninergic, muscarinic cholinergic, and peptidergic receptors. These receptors are characteristically glycosylated and contain seven transmembrane domains. Each transmembrane domain consists of approximately 20 to 30 hydrophobic amino acid residues, possesses predominantly alpha-helical secondary structure, and is long enough (approximately 30 nm) to span the lipid membrane bilayer. The transmembrane domains are connected by three extracellular and three intracellular hydrophilic loops. A cytoplasmic tail contains potential phosphorylation sites that may be targets for regulation of receptor activity.

A second class of membrane receptors contains the effector activity as an intrinsic part of the structure.[48, 49] For instance, protein tyrosine kinase–containing receptors, as typified by the insulin, IGF I, epidermal growth factor (EGF), and platelet-derived growth factor (PDGF) receptors, possess inherent enzyme activity. Each of these membrane receptors contains an extracellular ligand binding domain, a single transmembrane spanning domain, and an intracellular kinase domain. The insulin and IGF I receptors are linked to form biologically active dimeric forms.

Another class of self-contained signaling receptors includes the ligand-gated ion channels, of which there are two

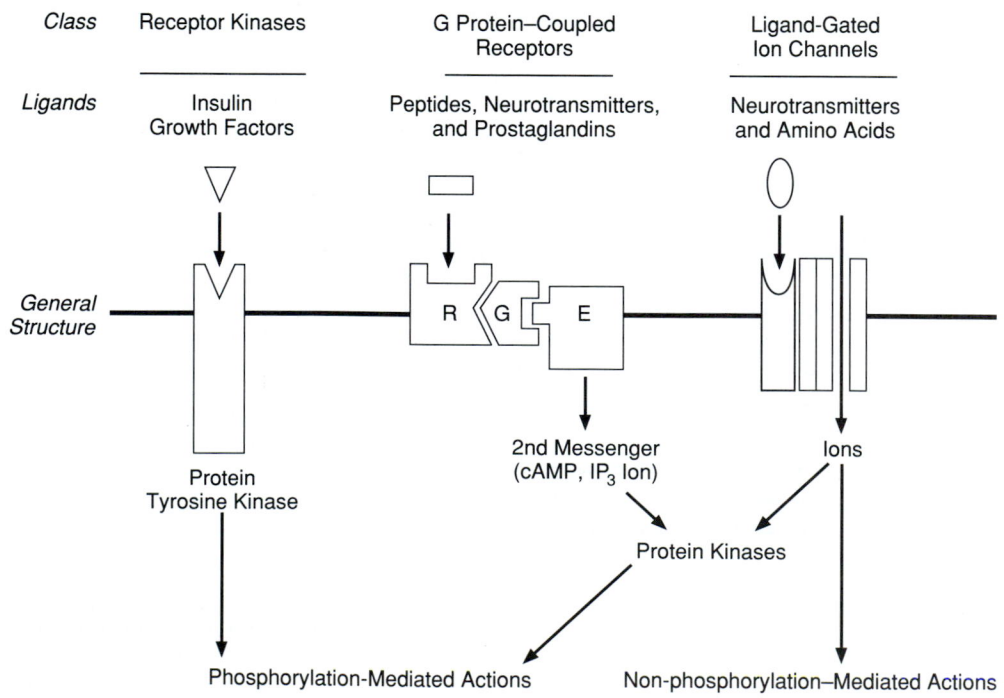

Figure 4–7. Three major classes of membrane receptors exist for hormones and neurotransmitters. Many growth factors, including insulin, bind to cell-surface receptors that act as protein tyrosine kinases stimulating the phosphorylation of proteins on tyrosine residues. A second class of agonists binds to receptors (R), which are coupled to separate effector (E) molecules by G proteins (G). Effectors may be enzymes that produce second messengers that in turn can activate distinct protein (generally serine/threonine) kinases. The third major class of receptors includes ligand-gated ion channels. Some of these are self-contained, as illustrated on the right. In others the receptor and the ion channel are coupled by G proteins, as shown in the center.

TABLE 4–1. Classification of Hormone Receptors and Effectors

Adenylate Cyclase
  Corticotropin
  Beta-adrenergic catecholamines
  Luteinizing hormone and human chorionic gonadotropin
  Follicle-stimulating hormone
  Glucagon
  Prostaglandins
  Parathyroid hormone
  TSH
  Alpha-adrenergic (inhibition)
  Somatostatin (inhibition)
Guanylate Cyclase
  Atrial peptide (AP, also called atrial natriuretic factor)
Receptor Protein Tyrosine Kinases
  Insulin
  Insulin-like growth factor (somatomedin-C)
  Epidermal growth factor
  Colony-stimulating factor 1
  Fibroblast growth factor
Phosphoinositol Turnover and Calcium Flux
  Acetylcholine receptor (muscarinic)
  Alpha-adrenergic catecholamines
  Angiotensin
  Luteinizing hormone–releasing hormone
  Thyrotropin-releasing hormone
  Vasopressin
Ion Channels
  Acetylcholine receptor (nicotinic)
  γ-Aminobutyric acid
Unknown Effector System
  Growth hormone
  Prolactin
  Erythropoietin
  Interleukins
  Nerve growth factor
  T cell receptor

known subtypes.[50–60] One subtype includes the nicotinic acetylcholine, γ-aminobutyric acid (GABA), glycine, and kainate receptors, all of which possess four transmembrane spanning domains.[50–52] The other includes the ligand-gated ion channels that encode specific conduits for sodium, calcium, and potassium cations and possess multiple subunits, each containing six transmembrane spanning domains. These form homo- or heteromultimers.[53–60]

Finally, there are membrane receptors for growth hormone (GH), prolactin, granulocyte-macrophage colony-stimulating factor (GM-CSF), and cytokines (interleukin [IL] 2, IL 4, IL 6, and IL 7).[61, 62] These receptors are similar in structure to the receptor kinases and contain a single transmembrane spanning domain. However, they have no known intrinsic activity, and the specific associated effector systems are not yet defined. Of note, several members of this receptor family may also be expressed in a circulating, non–membrane-associated form, as a result of alternative splicing of an exon encoding the membrane spanning domain. These circulating receptor forms act as serum-binding proteins for these ligands.

DOMAIN STRUCTURE. All membrane-associated hormone receptors can be viewed as possessing multiple functional domains. Experiments utilizing in vitro mutagenesis to form chimeric receptors that possess specific domains derived from different receptors have provided a better understanding of overall receptor structure and function. In general, membrane receptors contain specific domains that (1) bind ligand; (2) interact with effector systems, either indirectly (i.e., via G proteins) or directly (ligand-coupled ion channels); (3) possess inherent enzyme activity (i.e., tyrosine kinases); and (4) determine membrane localization and internalization. The NH₂ terminus of the peptide chain is generally extracytoplasmic and contains a domain that can interact directly with ligands.[44, 45] These regions are often extensively glycosylated and may contain sulfate and phos-

phate groups. They may also have sites of fatty acid acylation, as well as complex disulfide linkages. The "center" of the receptor consists of one or more transmembrane spanning domains. In addition to serving as anchors to the membrane, these transmembrane domains may play important roles in both signal transduction and, in some cases, interactions with ligands. For example, the fourth transmembrane spanning domain of the beta-2–adrenergic receptor is critical for interactions with agonists.[63]

The COOH-terminal intracellular domain may be the direct effector domain of the molecule, as in the case of the tyrosine kinases, or may play a role in modulation of receptor activity and/or internalization. In receptors with multiple transmembrane segments, such as the adrenergic receptor, the intracytoplasmic loops also serve as the site of interaction with the G proteins.[64] The ability of receptors to bind to different ligands and to transduce these signals by yet other sets of effectors resides in structural subtleties of the specific domains. More detailed discussion of receptor structure-function relationships is presented under Receptor-Effector Systems.

Families of Membrane Receptors

Although most hormones have distinct receptor sites on the membrane and separate pathways of action, certain hormones have overlapping structural features and/or biological activities. Examples include the prolactin, GH, and placental lactogen family of hormones; the insulin and insulin-like growth factor (IGF) family; the families of secretin-like and gastrin-like gastrointestinal hormones, luteinizing hormone, and human chorionic gonadotropin; and corticotropin, melanocyte-stimulating hormone, and other derivatives of pro-opiomelanocortin. Many of these families of hormones are related evolutionarily and are derived from similar or identical precursors.

Many of these related hormones interact with families of related receptors. For example, the prolactin and GH receptors have an approximate 30% overall similarity, with four highly homologous regions in the extracellular domain and one in the cytoplasmic domain.[65, 66] The receptors for insulin and IGF I are virtually identical in overall structure and have about 80% sequence identity throughout their length[67] (see under Receptor-Effector Systems).

Structural similarities of hormone receptors may extend beyond the families of hormones with which they interact and include the use of similar effector pathways. The receptors for insulin, IGF I, EGF, and PDGF have highly homologous intracellular tyrosine kinase domains, which possess the enzymatic activity required for signal transduction, but quite different extracellular domains, which are responsible for ligand binding. Likewise, receptors that act through G proteins have similar overall structures with seven transmembrane segments, although the ligands they bind are quite different, ranging from large glycoproteins such as luteinizing hormone and human chorionic gonadotropin to catecholamines. In the case of receptors coupled to G proteins, the signal transduction mechanisms are similar, but the final effects of the hormones are quite different.

There are some striking exceptions to the general rule that homologous hormones have structurally related receptors. For example, IGF II is a peptide growth factor with a structure closely related to that of insulin and IGF I, but the primary receptor for IGF II is a large single chain polypeptide that bears no resemblance to the tetrameric receptors for IGF I and insulin.[68] Furthermore, unlike the receptors for IGF I and insulin, the IGF II receptor has no intrinsic tyrosine kinase activity, nor is it phosphorylated on tyrosine residues. In fact, the IGF II receptor appears to be of a class different from that of the insulin and IGF I receptors, possessing two functional binding sites—one for IGF II and one for a large variety of glycoproteins containing mannose-6-phosphate. The primary function of the IGF II/mannose-6-phosphate receptor appears to be to transport these ligands to lysosomes for degradation.

A single hormone or neurotransmitter may also interact with receptors that differ in structure. Acetylcholine binds to a nicotinic receptor composed of four different subunits that form an ion channel and a muscarinic receptor coupled to phospholipid turnover through a G protein. In addition, many neurotransmitter receptors and some peptide hormone receptors are present as multiple, closely related receptor isotypes that may be products of distinct genes and have ligand binding sites that differ slightly in affinity for the various related ligand agonists and antagonists.[69]

The existence of families of related hormones and receptors has physiological and pathological significance, which is evidenced, for example, by the almost interchangeable biological effects of luteinizing hormone and human chorionic gonadotropin and by the similar effects of GH and prolactin on breast tissue. Other examples of overlapping hormone action include circumstances in which one hormone is elevated to pathologically high levels and mimics the action of another hormone by binding to its receptor with low affinity, a phenomenon termed *specificity spillover* (see under Membrane Receptors and Disease).

LIFE CYCLE OF THE HORMONE-RECEPTOR COMPLEX

Biosynthesis and Turnover of Membrane Receptors

Like all components of the cell, membrane receptors are in a constant state of turnover. Receptor synthesis begins on the rough endoplasmic reticulum.[70–72] In the endoplasmic reticulum, proteins destined for the plasma membrane are sorted from other proteins by the presence of a signal sequence and other conformational determinants. The endoplasmic reticulum also provides a form of quality control, by sorting out incompletely folded or misfolded proteins, unassembled protein subunits, and proteins whose transport is post-translationally regulated. The immature receptors then pass through the Golgi complex where they are modified by glycosylation, fatty acid acylation, disulfide bond formation, and, in some cases, cleavage into subunits. The mature receptors are inserted into the plasma membrane by a poorly understood process.

After the receptors are inserted into the plasma membrane, they are available for ligand binding and signal transduction. In the basal state, most hormone receptors are distributed diffusely over the surface of the cell exposed to the plasma or the extracellular milieu. After binding to hormone, receptors tend to aggregate.[73–75] The initial aggregates are small (most likely dimers) and may be important in signal generation (see later). Larger aggregates are eventually formed and undergo internalization. For most receptors, internalization occurs through specialized regions of the membrane lined on the intracellular surface with the protein clathrin. These regions are termed *coated pits*.[76] The coated pits invaginate and pinch off to form endosomal vesicles, which are surrounded by a cage-like structure formed by clathrin (Fig. 4–8). Eventually these receptor-containing endosomes, or receptosomes, are acidified and fuse with lysosomes. In this acidic environment the ligand usually dissociates from the receptor and undergoes degradation, and the receptor is recycled to the cell surface where it is again available for hormone binding.[77–79] The receptor may make 50 cycles or more into the cell and back to the surface membrane before it undergoes degradation. Thus, whereas the hormone is degraded in minutes, the half-time for degradation of receptors varies from a few hours to about a day.

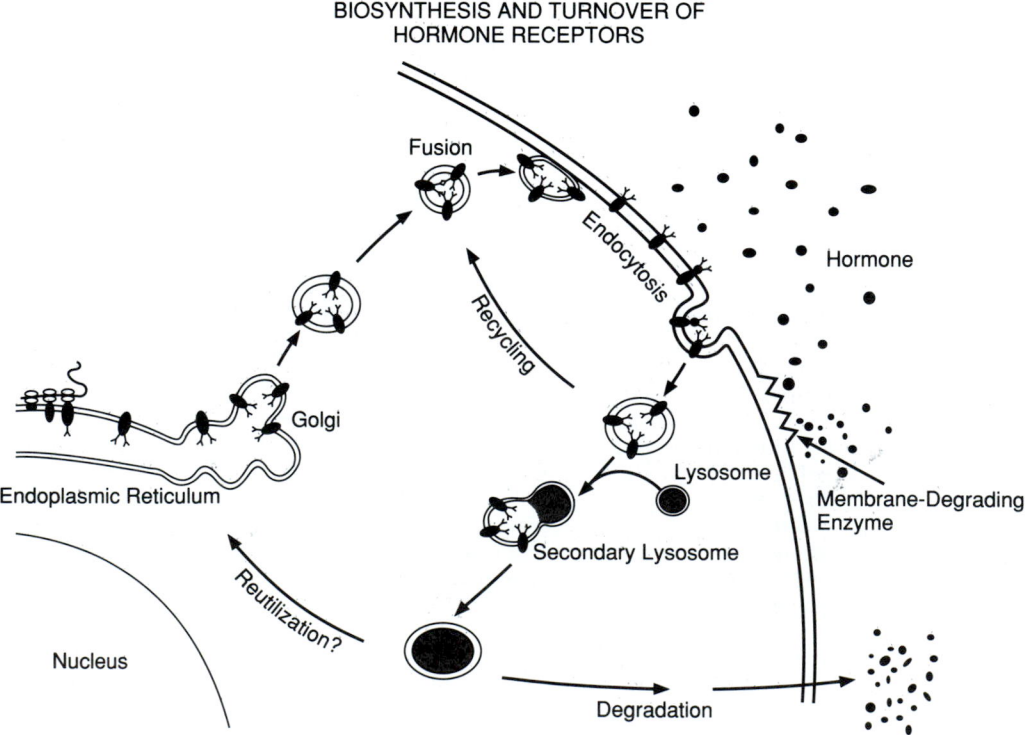

BIOSYNTHESIS AND TURNOVER OF HORMONE RECEPTORS

Fusion
Endocytosis
Recycling
Golgi
Hormone
Endoplasmic Reticulum
Lysosome
Reutilization?
Membrane-Degrading Enzyme
Secondary Lysosome
Nucleus
Degradation

Figure 4–8. A general model for the life cycle of the hormone receptor. Membrane receptors are synthesized in the rough endoplasmic reticulum, glycosylated in the Golgi apparatus, and inserted into the membrane, probably by a process involving membrane fusion. After binding the hormone, the receptors aggregate and are internalized by either coated or noncoated pits. The endosome containing the hormone-receptor complex may fuse with lysosomes, resulting in degradation of both the hormone and the receptor, or, more likely, the hormone is degraded and the receptor recycles to the membrane.

TABLE 4–2. Classification of Receptors by Mechanisms of Internalization

	Class I	Class II
Ligand	Peptide hormones, neurotransmitters	Nutrients (e.g., low-density lipoprotein, transferrin)
Internalization		
Rate	Low	High
Mechanism	Ligand stimulated	Constitutive
Primary function	Signaling	Internalization
Membrane localization	Diffuse or microvilli	Coated pits

RECEPTOR AGGREGATION AND INTERNALIZATION.

Aggregation and internalization are common features of ligand-receptor interactions and occur for a variety of membrane receptors, including hormone receptors, immunoglobulin receptors, and nutrient receptors. Internalization, rather than cellular signaling, is the primary function of receptors for ligands serving a nutrient function, such as low-density lipoprotein, cyanocobalamin, and transferrin[80, 81] (Table 4–2). The relative degree of internalization appears to be governed by factors intrinsic and extrinsic to the receptor itself. Low-density lipoprotein and other nutrient receptors are preferentially localized in coated pits (which favors internalization), whereas most hormone receptors are distributed over the surface of the cell and localize in coated pits only after ligand binding. In addition, some receptors possess a specific amino acid sequence (Gln-Pro-X-Tyr, where X is any amino acid) that is located in the region of the protein just inside the cell membrane and that seems to be critical for internalization.[82] For some receptors, covalent modification by enzymes, such as phosphorylation of threonine, serine, and tyrosine residues, may also play a role in stimulating internalization.[83]

Under normal circumstances the half-time for receptor synthesis matches the half-time for degradation so that the receptor pool remains in steady state. Alterations in synthesis or degradation rate can result in changes in receptor number and an altered biological response. Such changes may play a critical role in certain pathophysiological states.

HORMONE DEGRADATION AND HORMONE TRANSPORT.

Hormone degradation may occur via receptor-mediated and receptor-independent mechanisms. Receptor-mediated degradation is a by-product of the internalization process and occurs when the hormone is released in the strong degradative environment of the lysosome. Receptor-independent mechanisms include degradation by circulating proteases and degradation by membrane-associated enzymes distinct from the receptor. The extent to which receptor-mediated and receptor-independent pathways play a role in degradation varies considerably from hormone to hormone. For insulin, for example, the majority of degradation is receptor mediated; for glucagon, circulating and receptor-independent membrane proteases play an important role.[84, 85] In certain specialized cells, such as endothelial cells, the receptor internalization process may be modified and used to carry the hormone across the vascular barrier to the extracellular space.[86, 87] This transendothelial transport may be important in bringing the hormone to the receptor on the target cell, because in many tissues the capillary network possesses tight junctions that block access of the hormone to its target cell.[14] In the endothelial cell during the process of transcytosis, there is little or no fusion of the endosome bearing the hormone-receptor complex with lysosomes and thus little or no degradation. The exact mechanisms that govern the fate of internalized hormones, receptor recycling, and transendothelial transport are the subject of much current research.

MEMBRANE LIPIDS, RECEPTOR AGGREGATION, AND CELL SIGNALING.

Peptide hormone receptors on the cell surface are integrated into the phospholipid bilayer of the plasma membrane, and the properties of this lipid environment may have important influences on hormone action. Although the membrane limits the movement of receptors to a two-dimensional, rather than a three-dimensional, space, in general the protein receptors appear to be freely mobile in this lipid environment.[88] In addition the membrane lipid serves as a barrier between the ligand binding domain outside the cell and the signal transduction domain in the membranous or intracellular portions of the receptor.

After ligand binding the receptors aggregate or cluster.[63, 64, 89] This microaggregation or dimerization may play a critical role in receptor signaling, as evidenced by the fact that divalent antireceptor antibodies that bind to and cross-link receptors often mimic hormone action, whereas monovalent antibodies that bind to receptors but cause no aggregation do not[90, 91] (Fig. 4–9). Most hormonal ligands also induce receptor aggregation, although they appear to bind only monovalently. It seems likely that in addition to aggregation, many receptors undergo some type of conformational change that is propagated across the membrane and is important in cell signaling.

Because many membrane receptors require aggregation for normal signaling, diseases that result in simultaneous production of abnormal and normal receptors, such as a heterozygous genetic defect in which one allele codes for a mutant receptor and the other allele codes for a normal receptor, may produce profound alterations in signal-

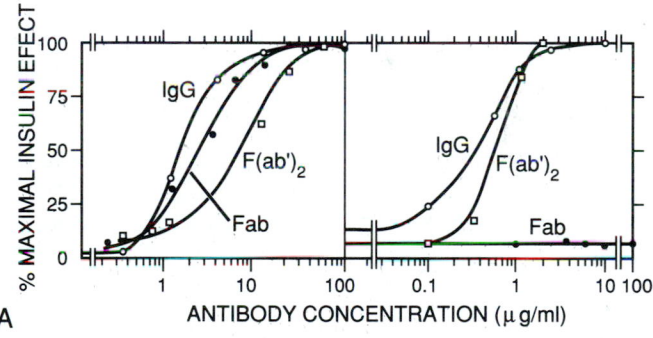

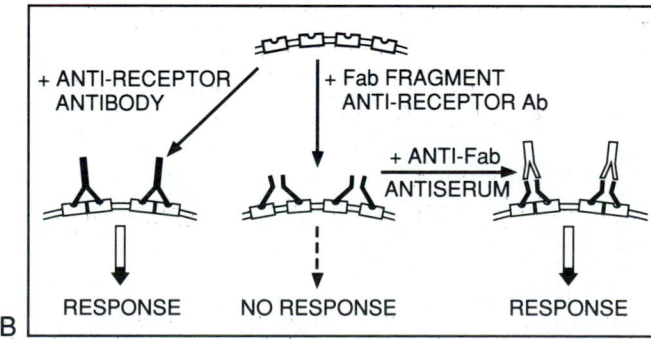

Figure 4–9. *A,* The role of valence in the action of antibodies to the insulin receptor. *Left,* Inhibition of ^{125}I-labeled insulin binding to isolated adipocytes by antireceptor immunoglobulin F(ab')$_2$, and Fab. *Right,* Ability of the same preparations to stimulate glucose oxidation in these cells. Note that both monovalent (Fab) and bivalent (F(ab')$_2$ and immunoglobulin G) antibodies inhibit insulin binding, but only bivalent antibodies mimic insulin action. This is depicted schematically in *B.* These data, and other data indicating that hormones also stimulate receptor aggregation, have suggested an important role for receptor aggregation in cellular signaling. (From Kahn CR, Baird KL, Jarrett DB, et al. Direct demonstration that receptor cross-linking or aggregation is important in insulin action. Proc Natl Acad Sci USA 1978; 75:4209–4213.)

ing.[92, 93] Alterations in the physical properties of plasma membrane, such as a change in phospholipid content or lipid saturation, can also augment or inhibit receptor mobility and aggregation. It is not surprising, therefore, that alterations in membrane lipid composition affect receptor binding and transmembrane signaling in cells in tissue culture.[94] The pathophysiological significance of similar alterations in human disease, however, has not been fully explored.

INTEGRATION AND CONTROL OF RECEPTOR SIGNALS

Signal Amplification and the Relationship Between Receptor Occupancy and Bioeffect

Because the concentration of peptide hormones in the circulation is usually between 10^{-12} and 10^{-9} M, target cells must not only recognize a hormone with high affinity and specificity but also amplify the hormone signal to regulate cellular metabolic processes that operate on substrates in the millimolar (10^{-3} M) concentration range. This process of amplification occurs at both the receptor and the postreceptor levels.

SPARE RECEPTORS AND COUPLING. At the level of the receptor, many peptide hormones produce a maximal biological response with only a fraction of the total cell-surface receptors occupied (Fig. 4–10A). For example, insulin stimulation of glucose transport in adipocytes is maximal when only about 2% of all insulin receptors are occupied.[95, 96] Similar observations have been made for the actions of corticotropin on glucocorticoid production in the adrenal and of gonadotropins on steroidogenesis in the ovary and the testis.[97] This phenomenon has given rise to the term *spare receptors*. The concept of spare receptors implies that the maximal hormone response occurs with less than maximal receptor occupancy. This formulation does not mean, however, that some receptors are active and others inactive. In all cases that have been studied, it appears that all receptors are active and that the occupancy of any small fraction is sufficient to produce the bioeffect.

A second, more subtle dissociation between occupancy and action is termed *nonlinear coupling*. In this case there is amplification of the signal such that the half-maximal effect occurs with less than 50% of the occupancy required for a maximal effect. Nonlinear coupling and spare receptors may exist together.

These phenomena play important physiological roles in both the kinetics of hormone action and the potential for regulation in disease states. Because the affinity of most receptors for hormone is lower than the circulating concentration of the hormone, the binding of hormone to receptor would proceed slowly if it were not for the relative excess of receptors on the cell surface. These excess receptors drive the reaction forward, especially at low hormone concentrations. Likewise, as the concentration of hormone in the blood begins to fall, the occupation of spare receptors by hormone allows the signal to persist beyond the circulating half-life of the hormone.

Similar types of signal amplification occur at postreceptor steps in the hormone action pathway.[96] For example, hormones that act through stimulation of adenylate cyclase and accumulation of cAMP usually produce more cAMP than is required for maximal activation of cAMP-dependent protein kinase. Likewise, cAMP-dependent protein kinase is usually activated beyond the level required for maximal substrate phosphorylation. Thus a series of increasingly sensitive dose-response curves amplify the hormone signal at each step in the action pathway (see Fig. 4–10B).

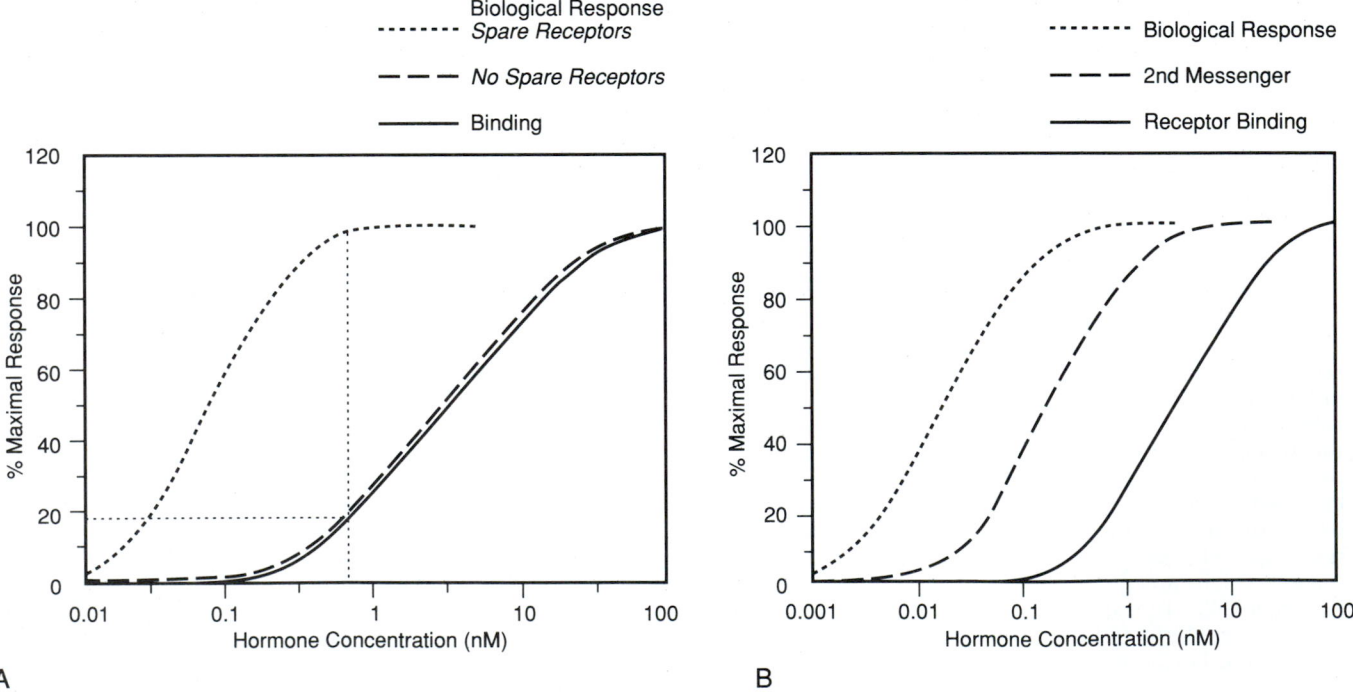

Figure 4–10. Correlation between hormone binding and biological response. *A,* Effect of spare receptors to amplify signal. The solid line represents a hormone binding to its receptor. The dashed line indicates a biological response in which there are no spare receptors. The dotted line indicates a response for which there are spare receptors. In the last case, the maximal biological response occurs with less than 20% receptor occupancy. *B,* Amplification of hormonal signaling. When it is possible to measure intermediate steps in hormonal signaling, there is often progressive signal amplification as one goes from receptor binding to second messenger to final biological response.

HORMONE-RESISTANT STATES. Spare receptors and signal amplification influence hormone response patterns in physiological and pathological states in which one or more steps in the hormone action pathway is altered. In a system with no spare receptors or postreceptor amplification, a 50% decrease in receptor number or any postreceptor step would result in a parallel 50% decrease in the final biological response. In contrast, a 50% fall in receptor number in a system with many spare receptors produces only a small (twofold) rightward shift in the dose-response curve for hormone action and no change in the maximal response. A decrease in the maximal response occurs only when receptor concentration falls to extremely low levels (Fig. 4–11).

Analysis of the relationship between hormone concentration and hormone action in a pathological state provides important insights into the mechanism of the altered hormone response (Fig. 4–12). In states of hormone resistance there may be decreased sensitivity to the hormone, i.e., a rightward shift in the dose-response curve with no change in maximal response.[98] This response implies a defect in hormone action at some step that is not rate-limiting. This defect is often at the level of the receptor in cells with spare receptors but may also be at a postreceptor step involved in amplification. In states of decreased sensitivity, increasing the hormone concentration overcomes the resistance and eventually produces a normal biological response. In some states of hormone resistance, there is a decrease in the maximal response, i.e., decreased responsiveness, with or without a concomitant decrease in sensitivity. Decreased responsiveness implies a defect at some rate-limiting step in the hormone action pathway. Usually, but not always, this step is a postreceptor site. In such states, increasing hormone concentrations produces increasing bioresponse only up to a point, but the maximal response is never normal.

Integration and Control of Hormone Signals

The classic concept of endocrinology that a single hormone acts on a single type of receptor to produce a single type of postreceptor signal and biological response is no longer valid. At every step in the pathway, there is an opportunity for interacting signals to amplify or attenuate the action of a hormone (Fig. 4–13). At the level of receptor binding, many peptide hormones are members of families of related hormones interacting with families of related receptors. In turn, each of these receptors may produce several independent or interrelated signals. Some receptor systems, for example, interact with several different types of second messenger systems. In the case of G protein–coupled receptors, the G protein may interact with multiple receptors and effector systems. Even the apparently self-contained tyrosine kinase receptors (the insulin, IGF I, EGF, PDGF, and CSF-1 receptors) may produce multiple postreceptor signals. For example, with in vitro mutagenesis it has been possible to produce mutant insulin and PDGF receptors that retain the ability to stimulate some metabolic processes but lose growth-stimulating activity.[99–101] Other mutations may produce the converse. Although the exact mechanism of such divergent effects remains unknown, these findings clearly indicate the complexity of the signaling pathway. In addition each individual pathway may contain multiple levels of both positive and negative feedback.

Interaction between separate hormones or pathways may take a variety of forms. At the most simple level, these forms may represent synergistic or antagonistic effects of two hormones on a single effector system or enzyme, such as the interplay between insulin and glucagon on glycogenolysis and glycogen synthesis. Such interactions may occur

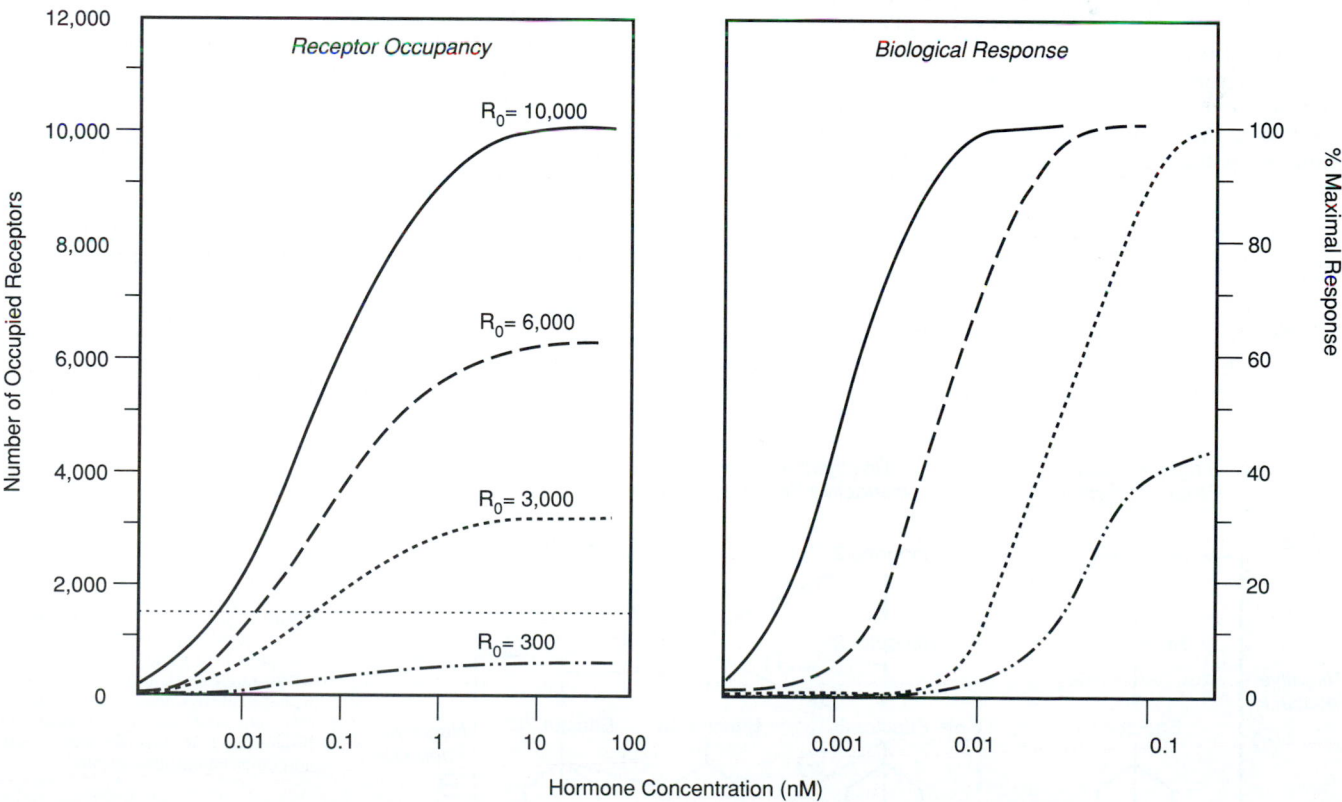

Figure 4–11. Effect of spare receptors on signaling after a loss of receptors. The original curve (solid line) represents the binding curve and biological response curve for $K_d = 0.1$, total receptor sites = 10,000 per cell, and a capacity of cell to respond to 10,000 occupied receptors. When only the number of receptor sites per cell is reduced, there is at each hormone concentration a proportional reduction in the concentration of the hormone-receptor complex and in biological response and a shift in the dose-response curve to the right. Because only about 18% receptor occupancy is needed to achieve a maximal response, this maximal response is reduced only when the total receptor concentration R_0 falls below 1800.

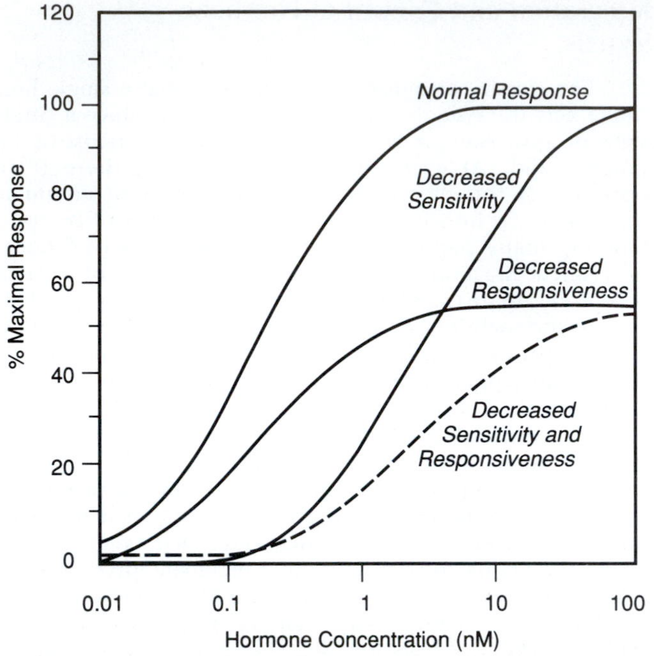

Figure 4–12. Types of resistance to hormone action. In hormone-resistant states there may be a rightward shift of the dose-response curve (decreased sensitivity), a decrease in maximal response (decreased responsiveness), or a combination of the two. Decreased sensitivity indicates a defect at a non–rate-limiting step (often the receptor), whereas decreased responsiveness indicates a defect at a rate-limiting step (usually postreceptor). (Adapted from Kahn CR. Insulin resistance, insulin insensitivity and insulin unresponsiveness: a necessary distinction. Metabolism 1978; 27[Suppl 2]:1893–1902.)

TABLE 4–3. Mechanisms of Regulation of Hormone Receptors and Their Signals

Hormone binding
   Receptor concentration
     Down-regulation
     Up-regulation
Receptor signaling
   Receptor phosphorylation
   Altered membrane lipids
   Other mechanisms of desensitization
     Conformational changes
Postreceptor alterations

regulated, or potentially regulated, by a variety of factors (Table 4–3). A large number of physiological and pathological factors can affect binding affinity, receptor number, signal transmission ability of membrane receptors, or postreceptor steps in hormone action and thus play a role in normal physiology or in disease. These regulators of receptor binding and signal transduction may result in desensitization or in hypersensitization of a hormone response. The regulatory response may be classified by the site of regulatory action—i.e., factors that alter receptor binding versus factors that affect receptor or postreceptor signaling—and by the nature of the regulatory factor—homologous regulation referring to effects of the hormone itself and heterologous regulation related to effects of other hormones or drugs.

The best-characterized regulator of receptor function is the hormone itself. In many endocrine cells, hormone binding increases the rate of internalization of the receptor,[80, 83, 89] which produces an increase in the fraction of receptors both inside the cell and undergoing degradation.[102–106] Ultimately, the accelerated degradation of receptors leads to down-regulation of receptor number on the cell surface.[107, 108] This example of negative homologous regulation can be viewed teleologically as a simple negative feedback loop that functions to reduce receptor concentration when hormone concentrations are chronically elevated, thus protecting the cell against the excessive hormone action. In reality the regulation process is often imperfect, with a small increase in hormone concentration producing a relatively large amount of down-regulation, thus leading to a hormone-resistant state. For example, in obesity and in type II diabetes, hyperinsulinemia produces down-regulation of the insulin receptor and contributes to insulin resistance.

Although most hormones produce down-regulation of their receptors, a few hormones, such as prolactin, may act as positive homologous regulators.[109] In this case the exposure of liver cells to prolactin increases receptor synthesis. This increase, in turn, results in increased receptor number

via heterologous receptor regulation or via interaction of postreceptor signals. At a more subtle level, one branch of a signal pathway for hormone A may act synergistically with a pathway of action of hormone B, while other divergent branches of these pathways may antagonize one another. In its entirety the endocrine signaling system should be considered as a series of convergent and divergent pathways interacting through feedback control to maintain a delicate homeostatic balance.

RECEPTOR REGULATION AND MECHANISMS OF DESENSITIZATION

Homologous Receptor Regulation

To achieve the delicate balance required for normal endocrine homeostasis, every step of hormone action is

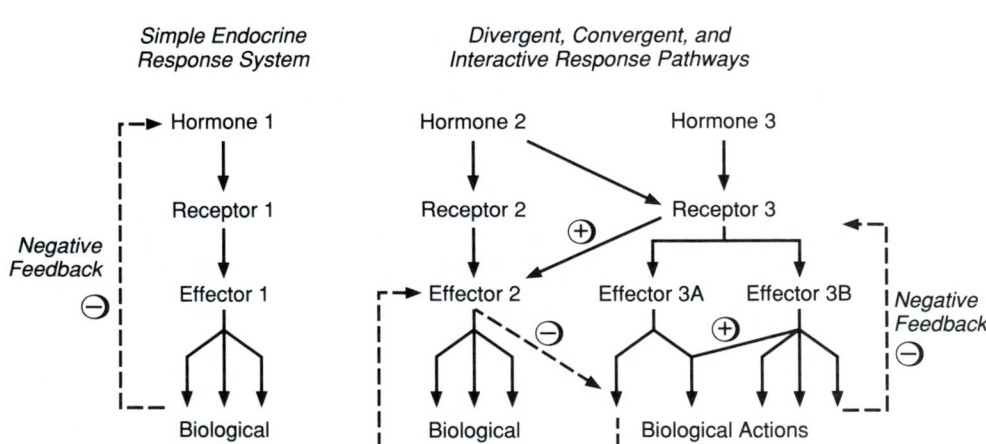

Figure 4–13. Interaction between hormone-signaling pathways. *Left,* A simple (idealized) signal response system, which rarely exists in nature. Most signaling pathways contain a multitude of divergent and convergent pathways, positive and negative feedback loops, and other interactions *(right).*

and enhanced cellular responsiveness to the hormone and provides a positive feedback loop in hormone response.

In addition to direct receptor regulation, hormone binding can be associated with other forms of homologous regulation at the receptor level, the postreceptor level, or both. For example, catecholamine binding to the beta-adrenergic receptor results in phosphorylation of the beta-receptor by a specific serine protein kinase, the beta-adrenergic receptor kinase, inside the cell.[110] This kinase recognizes only the agonist-occupied beta-receptor and phosphorylates it on serine residues. This phosphorylation event alters the subsequent association of the receptor with G proteins and leads to disruption in signal transduction or desensitization to beta-agonists. Not all phosphorylation of receptors produces a negative effect. Hormone binding to insulin receptor also results in phosphorylation of the receptor. In this case, however, phosphorylation is a direct action of protein kinase intrinsic to the insulin receptor, occurs in tyrosine residues, and enhances insulin receptor kinase activity toward cellular substrates, hence potentiating insulin action.[111, 112]

Heterologous Receptor Regulation

There are many examples in which positive heterologous regulation plays an essential role in the complex interactions characteristic of endocrine regulation. Follicle-stimulating hormone stimulates the production of luteinizing hormone receptors in the ovary, which leads to normal maturation of the ovum.[113] Prolactin also potentiates luteinizing hormone action in the Leydig cell, in part, by increasing the number of luteinizing hormone receptors.[114] Thyroid hormone augments the expression of beta-adrenergic receptors, which accounts for some of the findings of a hyperadrenergic state in hyperthyroid patients.[115] Estrogens cause an increase in the number of oxytocin receptors in the uterus[116] and also augment the effect of prolactin to increase expression of prolactin receptor number in mammary tissues.[117] Negative heterologous regulation also occurs. One of the most frequent examples involves hormones that stimulate protein kinase C (such as adrenergic agents). Stimulation of protein kinase C alters insulin receptor signaling and down-regulates the EGF receptor.[118] Down-regulation of the EGF receptor also occurs after stimulation of cells by PDGF through protein kinase C–independent mechanisms.[119] Some hormones exert both positive and negative effects by acting at different points in the hormone action cascade and thus produce a complex combination of effects. Glucocorticoids, for example, lower the binding affinity of insulin receptors in adipose tissue but increase receptor expression at a transcriptional level in lymphoid tissue.[120, 121] Glucocorticoids also increase the synthesis of many insulin counterregulatory enzymes at the transcriptional level.[122] A variety of other factors, including membrane lipid composition, the state of cell growth and differentiation, drugs, and viral infection, may also alter receptor binding and signal transduction properties (Table 4–4). Although knowledge of receptor regulation is incomplete, signal transduction in the endocrine system is regulated as much at the level of the target cell as by alterations in hormone synthesis or secretion.

CELLULAR MECHANISMS OF PEPTIDE HORMONE ACTION

Protein Phosphorylation in Hormone Action

The cellular actions of peptide hormones, whether mediated by cell-surface receptors possessing an intrinsic enzyme or ion channel activity or whether linked via a G protein with generation of cAMP or some other form of second messenger, ultimately are coupled to the metabolic machinery of the cell. This process occurs by covalent modification of some enzyme or protein critical to an intracellular pathway, stimulation of a transport process, or regulation of transcription of a gene for some protein involved in the hormone action cascade. The most common mechanism is covalent modification by phosphorylation of the regulated protein through transfer of phosphate groups from ATP to specific hydroxy amino acids (usually serine, but occasionally threonine or tyrosine) (Fig. 4–14A). Thus phosphorylation and dephosphorylation of serine represent important and often final steps in the transmission of peptide hormone signals. Many key regulatory enzymes exist in alternative phosphorylated and dephosphorylated states that differ markedly in their catalytic activity (Table 4–5). In some cases phosphorylation activates the enzyme; in others it inactivates the enzyme. The level of enzyme phosphorylation is determined by the activities of two types of enzyme: protein kinases that catalyze phosphorylation and phosphoprotein phosphatases that catalyze dephosphorylation (Fig. 4–14B). Kinases and phosphatases may be limited in their actions to a single target enzyme or may act on multiple regulatory proteins.

SERINE PHOSPHORYLATION PATHWAYS. Serine phosphorylation control mechanisms are involved in the actions of cAMP-dependent protein kinase, calmodulin-sensitive pathways, protein kinase C–mediated actions, and many other regulatory processes.[123] The regulation of a single biological response, such as the rate of flux into and out of tissue glycogen stores, can involve the interrelated effects of multiple hormones, distinct postbinding mechanisms, and modification of rates of both phosphorylation and dephosphorylation reactions.

The complexity and precision of regulation that result from these phosphorylation and dephosphorylation mechanisms are perhaps best illustrated by the pathways involved in the regulation of gluconeogenesis by insulin and glucagon (see Fig. 4–14C). During the normal daily transitions between fed and fasted states, the maintenance of normal

---

Table 4–4. Factors Affecting Receptor Concentration or Affinity and Postreceptor Signaling

Homologous hormone
Heterologous hormones
Ions and other small molecules
Drugs
Membrane lipid composition
Cell growth and differentiation
Viral infection
Antibodies to the receptor
Covalent modifications (e.g., phosphorylation, glycosylation)

TABLE 4–5. Selected Enzymes and Proteins Regulated by Phosphorylation and Dephosphorylation

Activated Enzyme or Protein	Inhibited Enzyme or Protein
Pyruvate kinase	Glycogen synthase
Phosphorylase kinase	Pyruvate kinase
Phosphorylase	Beta-adrenergic receptor
Triglyceride lipase	Insulin receptor (serine
ATP citrate lyase	or threonine
Ribosomal S6 kinase	phosphorylation)
Insulin receptor (tyrosine phosphorylation)	

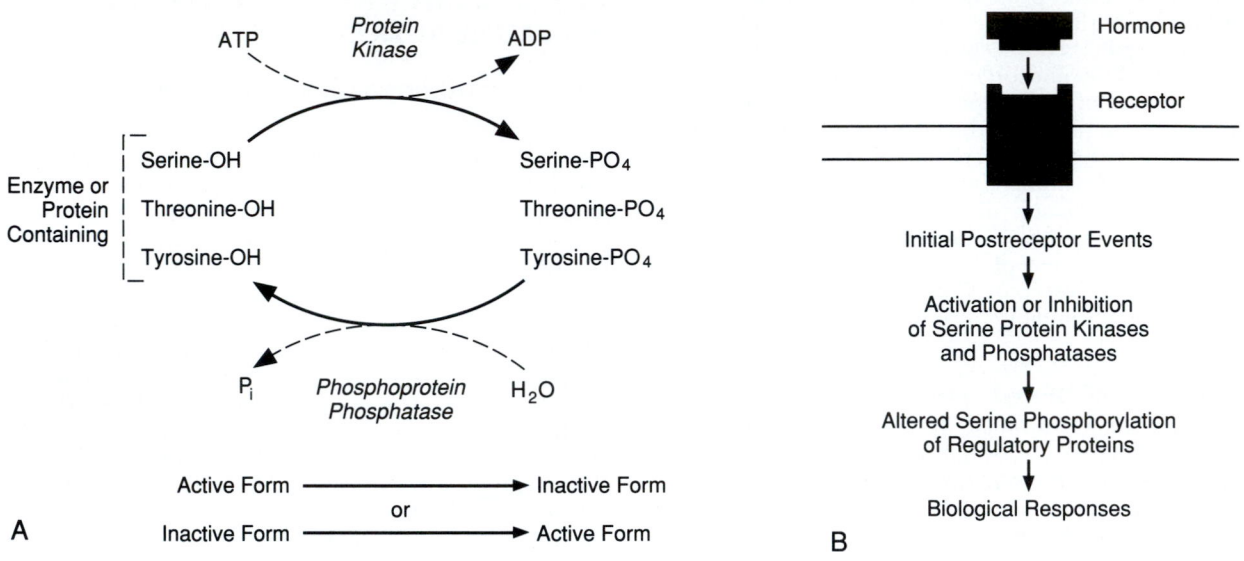

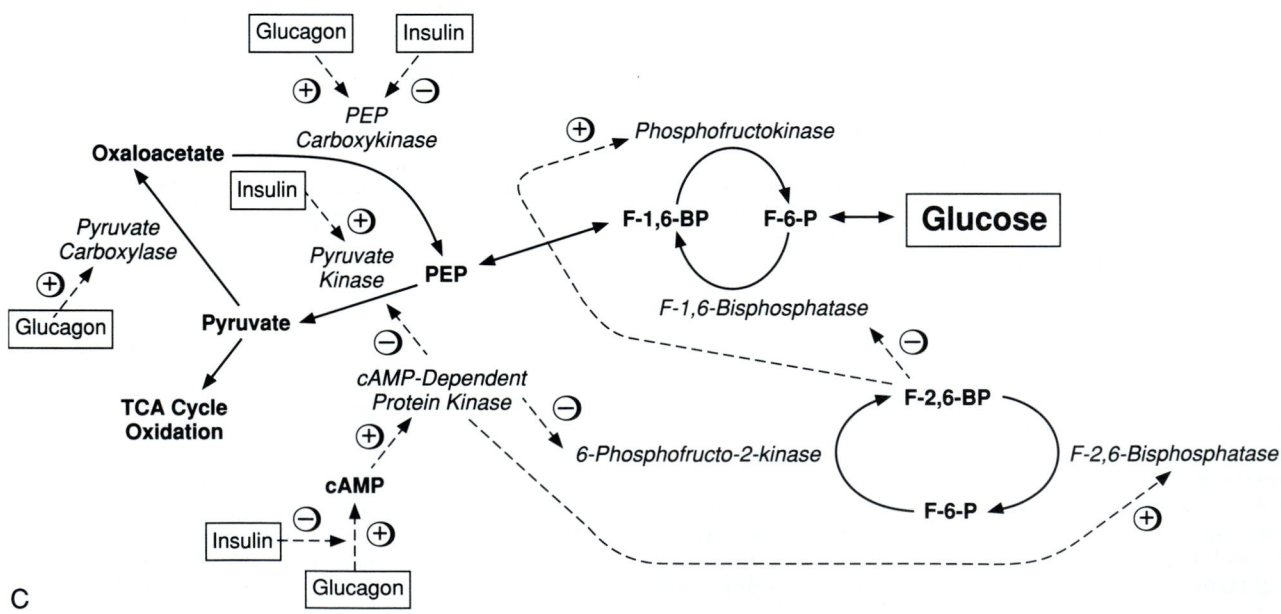

Figure 4–14. *A,* Regulation of enzymes and other proteins by phosphorylation and dephosphorylation. In phosphorylation of a protein, a protein kinase stimulates the transfer of a phosphate group from ATP to a hydroxyl group on the side chain of a serine, threonine, or tyrosine residue. The phosphate group can be removed by the action of phosphoprotein phosphatases. This process usually results in conversion of an active protein or enzyme to an inactive form or vice versa (see Table 4–5). *B,* Role of phosphorylation and dephosphorylation of serine in mediating the effects of peptide hormones on metabolic pathways. *C,* Regulation of gluconeogenesis by insulin and glucagon: + indicates a positive regulatory effect and − an inhibitory effect. F-6-P, fructose-6-phosphate; F-1,6-BP, fructose-1,6-bisphosphate; PEP, phosphoenolpyruvate; TCA, tricarboxylic acid.

blood glucose levels depends in part on regulated increases and decreases in flux through hepatic gluconeogenic pathways. The rate of gluconeogenesis is determined by the hormonally regulated delivery of precursors such as amino acids and glycerol from peripheral tissues[124] and by the counterbalancing effects of insulin and glucagon on hepatic metabolic pathways. Glucagon stimulates gluconeogenesis by increasing flux through the rate-limiting step in the glucose synthetic pathway, the conversion of pyruvate to phosphoenolpyruvate. This occurs through several different phosphorylation-linked mechanisms and via effects of glucagon on gene expression. After glucagon binds to its specific receptors on hepatocytes, adenylate cyclase is activated as a result of the effects of the glucagon hormone-receptor complex on a GTP-regulatory protein, and intracellular cAMP levels increase.[125–128] Acting as a second messenger, cAMP binds to the regulatory subunit of inactive cAMP-dependent protein kinase and releases the active protein kinase catalytic subunits[129, 130] (Fig. 4–15). This active cAMP kinase phosphorylates specific serine residues in pyruvate kinase and converts it from an inactive to an active form and increases the net conversion of pyruvate to phosphoenolpyruvate.[131] This process is further enhanced by glucagon-stimulated increases in phosphoenolpyruvate carboxykinase and pyruvate carboxylase activities that occur through cAMP-mediated actions on gene expression.[132, 133] The glucagon-stimulated rise in cAMP also results in serine phosphorylation of a bifunctional enzyme that contains both 6-phosphofructo-2-kinase and fructose-2,6-bisphosphatase activities.[134, 135] Serine phosphorylation modifies this protein so that fructose-2-6-bisphosphate concentrations decrease, thus favoring substrate flow toward increased gluconeogenesis.[134, 136–138] Insulin opposes each of these actions of glucagon, in part by inhibiting cAMP generation and cAMP-dependent protein kinase activity[139, 140] and in part by inhibiting transcription of phosphoenolpyruvate carboxykinase and stimulating transcription of pyruvate kinase.[133, 141] The net effect is that the rate of hepatic glucose production is appropriate for body requirements. The central role of regulation of key enzymes by serine phosphorylation coupled with phosphorylation-independent mechanisms, including regulation of enzyme content at the level of gene expression and regulation of substrate content by control of membrane transport, is typical for the effect of many peptide hormones on metabolic pathways.

TYROSINE PHOSPHORYLATION AND OTHER PHOSPHORYLATION EVENTS. With the recognition that some peptide hormone receptors possess an intrinsic protein tyrosine kinase activity, whereas others are linked to an increase in serine/threonine kinase activity via increases in cellular calcium or phosphoinositol turnover, the number of recognized protein kinases involved in peptide hormone action continues to increase. In some cases it is not yet evident how these early events are linked to the final pathways of hormone regulation. For example, although the insulin receptor is itself a tyrosine kinase, insulin action involves increased serine phosphorylation of some enzymes and decreased phosphorylation of others, presumably through the action of one or more insulin-stimulated serine kinases and phosphatases, which act to switch the signal from tyrosine phosphorylation to serine phosphorylation.[142] Some of the kinases have been defined and are known to phosphorylate the receptor itself or other proteins and thereby initiate a cascade of serine phosphorylation that changes cellular metabolism.[142, 143] Additional serine kinases and phosphoprotein phosphatases have been only partially defined and may be equally important components of the postbinding response. Serine kinases may also modify gene expression at the level of protein synthesis. For example, a

specific insulin-stimulated serine kinase appears to cause phosphorylation and activation of ribosomal protein S6.[144] This activation, in turn, may lead to the increased synthesis of many cellular proteins that is seen in response to insulin. A challenge for future investigation is to determine the nature of the molecular interactions between early postbinding events and the biological responses produced by all peptide hormones.

Regulation of Membrane Transport by Membrane Receptors

An important action of many peptide hormones is to regulate the interaction of the cell with its environment by governing the entry and exit of nutrients and ions into and out of the cell. The control of ion transport may be directly affected by receptors that act as ligand-gated ion channels, whereas the control of influx of nutrients, such as glucose and amino acids, involves actions of the hormones on specific transport systems for these molecules (Fig. 4–16).

AMINO ACID TRANSPORT. At least five different carrier systems for amino acids are present in the plasma membrane of mammalian cells.[145] Each is believed to depend on the function of a specific transport protein that recognizes a group of closely related amino acids. Most of these amino acid transporters function as cotransport systems, or symports, bringing in Na^+ together with the amino acid. Not all amino acid transport systems are hormonally regulated. The neutral amino acid transport system, which shows preference for alanine, glycine, and proline, termed *system A*, is the most active of the hormonally regulated systems and responds to insulin, glucagon, and glucocorticoids, as well as to other peptide hormones.[145, 146]

Regulation of amino acid metabolism by hormones has three components: (1) hormone-stimulated transport into the target cell; (2) hormone-regulated metabolism of the intracellular amino acid; and (3) hormone control of protein degradation and amino acid metabolism (reviewed in ref. 145). The effect of a given hormone is observed specifically in target cells bearing the requisite receptor. Thus amino acid transport is increased by corticotropin in adrenal, by glucagon in liver, by luteinizing hormone in ovary, and by insulin in muscle, liver, fat, and a number of other tissues. Although the exact steps involved in hormone stimulation of transport remain uncertain, in all cases this event appears to be a mediated, rather than a direct receptor, one. Thus there is usually a lag of 5 to 15 min before the increase in transport is observed, and then the cell is committed to the increase in transport (for some period), even if the hormone is removed.[147] In the case of hormones known to act via cAMP, the effect of the hormone in stimulating transport can be mimicked in isolated cells by cAMP analogues. As with many other effects, there is nonlinear coupling between receptor occupancy and transport activation so that half the effect may be observed with 5 to 20% receptor occupancy. In most cases the increase in transport activity is associated with an increase in the V_{max} of the transporter. Possible mechanisms for this increase in V_{max} include de novo synthesis of the transporter molecules, post-translational conversion of inactive transporters to an active form, translocation of transporters from an intracellular pool to a membrane pool, or some effect secondary to an increase in membrane potential that might secondarily increase transport as a result of the dependence of these systems on the cotransport of sodium ions (see Fig. 4–16).

GLUCOSE TRANSPORT. Hormone regulation of sugar transport, especially glucose transport, has long been recognized as an important effect of insulin.[148] In contrast to the effect of insulin and other hormones on amino acid

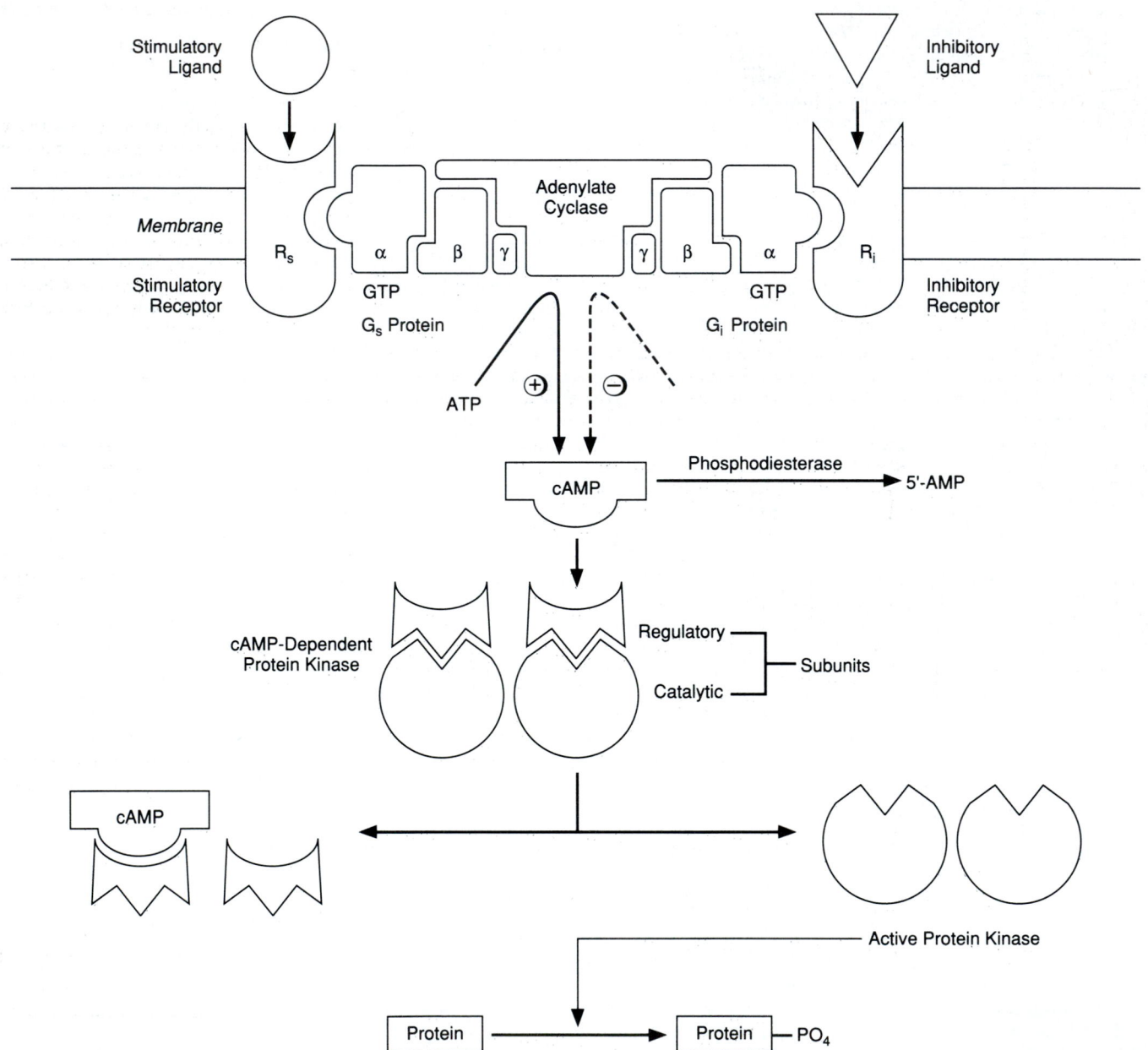

Figure 4–15. Schematic depiction of the adenylate cyclase system. Stimulatory ligands (H$_s$) and inhibitory ligands (H$_i$) interact with their respective receptors (R$_s$ and R$_i$). The H$_s$-R$_s$ complex then activates adenylate cyclase via interaction with the regulatory coupling protein G$_s$. In the process G$_s$ binds GTP and hydrolyzes it to GDP. The H$_i$-R$_i$ complex inhibits adenylate cyclase via a homologous regulatory protein G$_i$. When the catalytic component of adenylate cyclase is activated, ATP is converted to cAMP, which in turn activates cAMP-dependent protein kinase and results in substrate phosphorylation. cAMP-dependent protein kinases consist of four subunits, two catalytic subunits (C) and a dimer regulatory subunit (R-R), which can bind two molecules of cAMP. When cAMP binds to the regulatory dimer of the holoenzyme, the two catalytic subunits are released and become fully active. With removal of cAMP, the regulatory dimer reassociates with catalytic subunits, inactivating the latter. Recent data indicate that a total of four cAMP molecules bind to the regulatory dimer.

Note that R is widely used as an abbreviation for receptor as well as for regulatory components, especially for the regulatory component of cAMP-dependent protein kinases. Also note that C is widely used as an abbreviation for a catalytic component of an enzyme, especially for adenylate cyclase and cAMP-dependent protein kinase.

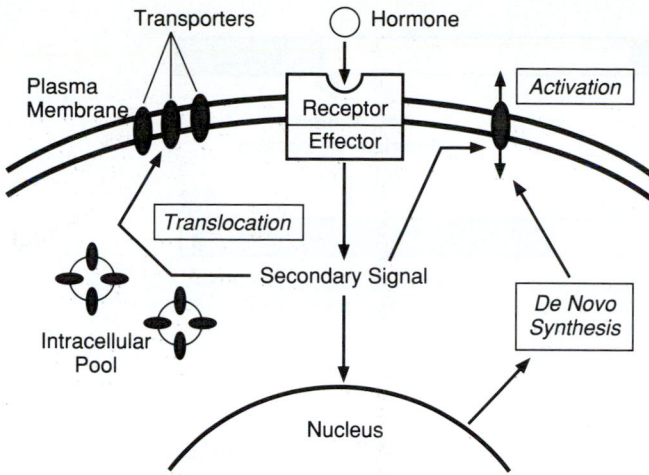

Figure 4–16. Possible mechanisms of hormone stimulation of membrane transport. Hormones act on amino acid and glucose transport by a number of mechanisms, which include de novo synthesis, activation, and translocation of transporters from an intracellular pool to the plasma membrane.

transport, this effect appears to be independent of changes in cAMP levels and occurs quite rapidly, within seconds, of hormone administration. Seven distinct mammalian glucose transporters have been identified by cDNA cloning and sequencing.[148–153] All of the transporters are proteins of 45 to 50 kd and possess 12 membrane spanning domains. One is the Na^+,glucose cotransporter involved in active transport of glucose by intestinal epithelium and renal tubular cells; six transporters are involved in Na^+-independent facilitative diffusion of glucose into cells. Only one of these transporters appears to be hormonally sensitive: the so-called insulin-sensitive transporter present in skeletal muscle, cardiac muscle, and adipose tissue.[150–153] The glucose transporters in red blood cells, brain, kidney, liver, and so on have a different sequence and do not respond to hormone stimulation.

Hormone stimulation of glucose transport appears to involve a unique translocation mechanism.[154] Under basal conditions, most glucose transporters are in an intracellular pool associated with microsomal membranes. Insulin causes a rapid translocation of these transporters to the plasma

membrane, where they take up glucose from the extracellular milieu. Although the major effects of insulin on glucose transport can be explained by this translocation, there may also be an activation of the transporters so that each transporter can take up more glucose, especially in response to other stimulators of transport. Insulin also stimulates translocation of IGF II receptors and low-density lipoprotein receptors to the plasma membrane, where they may be active in the uptake of the ligands and nutrients.

Regulation of Gene Expression by Membrane Receptors

In addition to the effects of hormone binding to membrane receptors—to stimulate phosphorylation and transport phenomena—some peptide hormones act at the genomic level to regulate gene expression.[155, 156] Peptide hormone action at the nucleus and the tertiary messengers of membrane receptors that regulate gene expression are poorly understood. The best-characterized examples are the cAMP response element–binding protein (CREB)[157] and a protein that appears to mediate protein kinase C action on gene expression.[158]

A general model for peptide hormone regulation of gene expression is shown in Figure 4–17. In this model the interaction of hormone, receptor, and effector results in stimulation of a cytoplasmic protein kinase such as cAMP kinase or protein kinase C. This kinase then phosphorylates a regulatory protein capable of entering the nucleus and binding to a specific sequence in the control regions (generally the 5′-flanking sequences) of the gene to be regulated. This sequence is usually only 6 to 10 nucleotides long but may be repeated more than once so that the regulatory protein can bind as a dimer. Such hormone response elements are members of a family of DNA sequences known as enhancers, which may be both orientation and position independent. They bind nuclear transcription factors to result in the modulation of the overall rate of gene transcription. Binding of this regulatory protein to the hormone response element results in an increase or a decrease in transcription of the regulated gene and a consequent increase or decrease in its respective messenger RNA (mRNA) and protein products. Peptide hormones may also regulate

Figure 4–17. General scheme of peptide hormone regulation of gene expression. Interaction of hormone (H) with its target cell surface receptor (R) results ultimately in the production of second messengers. These molecules may activate cytoplasmic kinases that, in turn, can phosphorylate transcription factors (TFs). Such modified TFs (PO_4-TFs) can then act in the nucleus to modulate gene expression by binding to hormone response elements (HREs) in gene-regulatory regions, often as dimers (as shown). Altered rates of gene transcription may lead to changes in steady-state levels of corresponding mRNA and protein.

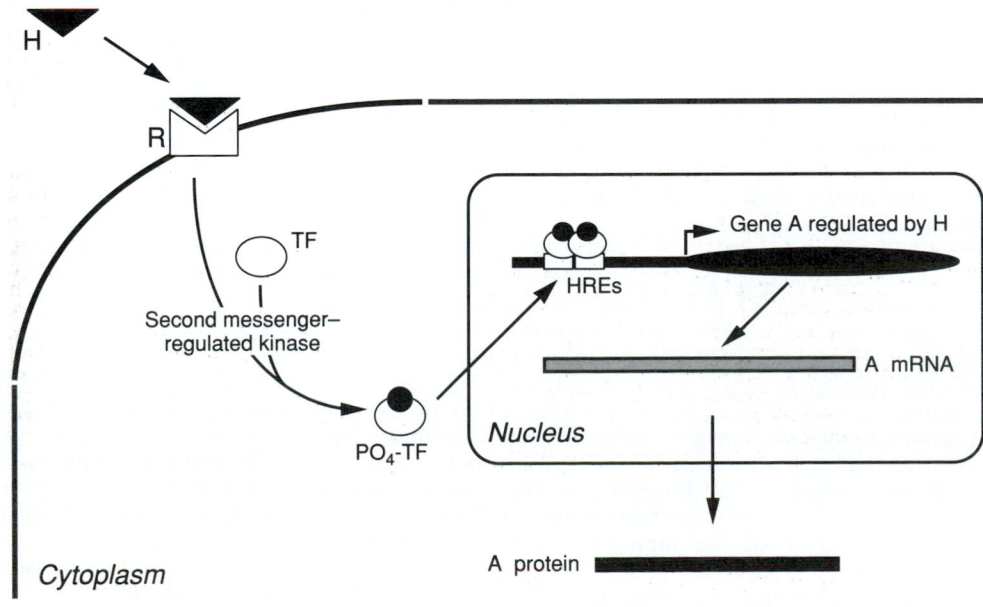

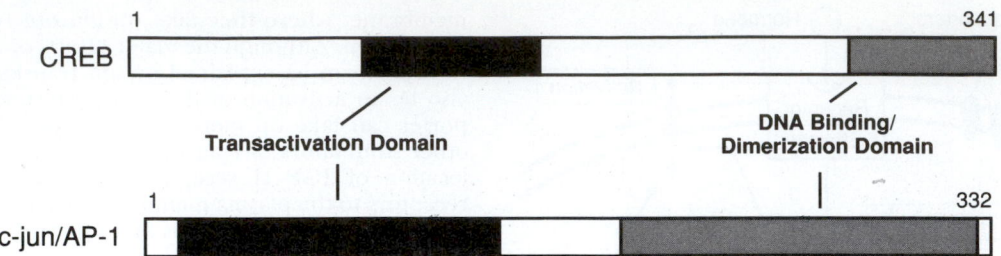

Figure 4–18. Schematic diagram of two transcription factors that mediate peptide hormone signal transduction. These proteins act via the cAMP and Ca^{2+}/protein kinase C pathways, i.e., CREB and c-*jun*/AP-1, respectively. NH_2-terminal transactivation domains, often with multiple phosphorylation sites, and COOH-terminal DNA binding domains, with leucine zipper dimerization motifs, are depicted. The sizes of these proteins in amino acid residues are shown.

gene expression by influencing mRNA translation, mRNA half-life or stability, and protein processing and/or degradation.

cAMP REGULATION OF GENE EXPRESSION. A palindromic octamer DNA sequence TGACGTCA (cAMP response element) is present in the 5' region of several cAMP-responsive genes, including those encoding somatostatin (SRIF, somatotropin release–inhibiting factor), phosphoenolpyruvate carboxykinase, vasoactive intestinal peptide, and the alpha subunit of glycoprotein hormones.[159] This sequence mediates cAMP stimulation of gene expression in the presence of either a homologous or a heterologous promoter. A 43-kd protein in nuclear extracts of cells responsive to cAMP binds to this palindromic sequence with high affinity. This protein has been termed the *cAMP response element–binding protein*. Phosphorylation of nuclear extracts containing CREB by the catalytic subunit of cAMP-dependent protein kinase results in a greater than 10-fold increase in cAMP response element–dependent transcription without an apparent effect on DNA affinity. Although both monomer and dimer forms bind the cAMP response element, only the dimer appears to possess transcriptional activity.

cDNAs encoding CREB and a CREB-like protein in rats and humans provide some insights into the nature of these proteins.[157, 160] CREB is a protein of 341 amino acids that contains three functional regions: (1) a transactivation domain with a number of potential phosphorylation sites; (2) a DNA binding domain with a high content of basic amino acid residues; and (3) a "leucine zipper" dimerization domain (Fig. 4–18). The DNA binding domain of CREB involves a stretch of basic amino acids located near its COOH terminus that shares some sequence similarity with the cellular proto-oncogene c-*jun*. This proto-oncogene also contains a leucine zipper dimerization domain, which suggests the possibility that CREB can form heterodimers with the proto-oncogenes containing a similar domain, such as c-*fos* and c-*jun*, leading to coordinate regulation of gene expression and a yet higher level of complexity in the cAMP regulation pathway.

PROTEIN KINASE C AND AP-1. Another transcriptional factor involved in the regulation of gene expression by peptide hormones is AP-1. AP-1 can interact with a heptamer sequence TGACTCA found in phorbol ester/protein kinase C–regulated genes.[161] This sequence is similar to the cAMP response element except for the absence of a central G residue. The product of the proto-oncogene c-*jun* and a related protein in yeast called GCN4 represent the major components of AP-1. c-*jun* is a transcription factor that contains a DNA binding domain possessing basic amino acid residues and a leucine zipper dimerization domain similar to that described for CREB (see Fig. 4–18). Another nuclear transcription factor that interacts at the AP-1 site is c-*fos*. c-*fos* is a member of the family of early response genes activated in the conversion of quiescent serum-starved 3T3 fibroblasts to growing cells. However, c-*fos* can bind to DNA only in the presence of c-*jun*. Hence only the heterodimer, and not the c-*fos* homodimer, can stimulate transcription. Furthermore, the c-*fos*/c-*jun* heterodimer has higher affinity for the AP-1–regulatory sites than the c-*jun* homodimer. Thus hormones acting to stimulate protein kinase C act indirectly at the genomic level by phosphorylating, and hence activating, c-*jun* and other proteins, in analogy to the regulation of CREB by protein kinase A.

The identification of additional nuclear protein factors that are targets for cellular kinases in the membrane receptor–signaling pathway is anticipated. For example, insulin regulates the expression of a number of genes at the transcriptional level, but the insulin response element in DNA and its regulatory protein have not been defined (reviewed in ref. 122). A multitude of such DNA-binding factors are believed to play intricate and interactive roles in the regulation of gene expression. Some of these peptide hormone–regulatory factors, such as c-*jun* and c-*fos*, may also be involved in interactions with the nuclear ligand-regulated receptors such as the vitamin A (retinoic acid) and vitamin D receptors.[162]

RECEPTOR-EFFECTOR SYSTEMS

General Features

Receptors and signal transduction systems for membrane-active hormones encompass a broad spectrum of biochemical structures. Membrane receptors can be categorized on the basis of structural and functional characteristics that include intrinsic tyrosine kinase activity, linkage via G proteins to adenylate cyclase or phosphatidylinositol turnover, or association with ion channels (see Table 4–1). For several receptors the effector systems remain unknown. Most peptide hormones can be viewed as ultimately exerting their effects by alterations in either protein phosphorylation or gene expression, or by activation of one or more transport pathways. In this section we consider some of the structural features of each of the receptor classes and their mechanisms of linkage to these final response pathways.

Receptors Linked to Adenylate Cyclase

cAMP-LINKED RECEPTORS. cAMP is the prototypical second messenger. Intracellular levels of cAMP are determined, in large part, by ligand-receptor interactions. This physiological event involves the interaction of three cellular components located near the plasma membrane: the ligand receptor, a signal transducer (G protein), and the effector enzyme (adenylate cyclase)[163–171] (Figs. 4–15 and 4–19). In vitro reconstitution studies with purified receptors, G proteins, and adenylate cyclase introduced into phospholipid

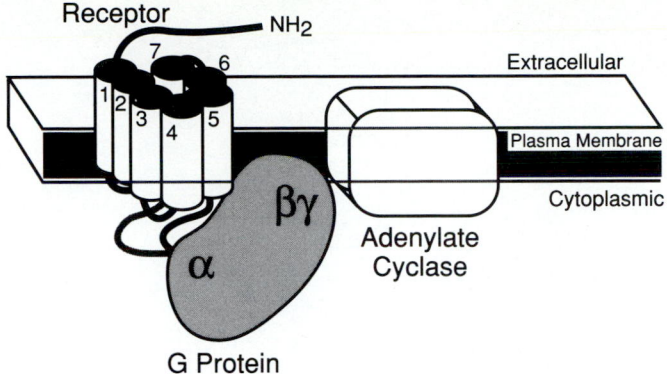

Figure 4–19. Schematic diagram of the locations of receptor, G protein (αβγ heterotrimer), and adenylate cyclase within the plasma membrane.

vesicles have shown that only these three components are required for ligand stimulation of cAMP production. In this fashion, this second messenger is produced by the interaction of three *functional cassettes.* Signal diversity, as well as specificity, is governed primarily by heterogeneity in the first two components, i.e., the existence of multiple receptors and G proteins, whereas the final effector adenylate cyclase appears to be unique.

Studies of adrenergic receptors have provided great insight into the mechanisms by which receptors are linked to G proteins and adenylate cyclase.[64] Among the adrenergic receptors, there are examples of receptors that either stimulate or inhibit adenylate cyclase. Interaction of the beta-1 and beta-2 subtypes with their cognate ligands results in increased cAMP levels, whereas alpha-2–adrenergic receptor–ligand interaction results in decreased cAMP levels. The molecular cloning of the adrenergic receptor cDNAs and genes has provided valuable information about their amino acid structure and possible mechanisms for specificity of action (Fig. 4–20).

The adrenergic receptors share considerable protein sequence homology.[64, 69] Each is a single polypeptide chain with an approximate molecular size of 64 to 80 kd. These receptors are similar to the visual pigment receptor rhodopsin. The human beta-1– and beta-2–adrenergic receptors are 477 and 413 amino acid residues in size, respectively. The domains of the isolated polypeptide chain have been identified by utilizing in vitro mutagenesis and reconstitution experiments. On the basis of the deduced protein sequence, the beta-adrenergic receptor appears to possess seven hydrophobic, alpha-helical regions that correspond to the seven transmembrane domains, similar to those previously seen in rhodopsin. In the human beta-1– and beta-2–receptors these domains are more conserved than is the overall molecule (71 versus 54%, respectively). Comparison of transmembrane domains between beta-adrenergic and muscarinic cholinergic receptors suggests that the most conserved regions involve the half of each alpha helix closest to the cytoplasm. The great variability in these helices near the external (extracytoplasmic) region between different receptors suggests a functional role, probably in ligand binding.

The identification of functional domains among the adrenergic receptors has been facilitated by the ability to produce chimeric receptor forms by combining various regions of the different adrenergic receptor subtypes. For example, although ligands interact with transmembrane regions 2 to 7, adrenergic agonist specificity is determined primarily in transmembrane region 4. In contrast, antagonist interactions may involve transmembrane regions 6 and 7.[63] The NH$_2$ terminus, COOH terminus, and the large third intracytoplasmic domain are not involved in ligand interac-

tions, as shown by deletion-mutagenesis and protease digestion studies. Thus the catecholamine appears to interact with its receptor primarily via a pocket formed by the transmembrane domains as they appear at the extracytoplasmic face.

An equally important domain for functioning of this class of receptors is the domain required for G protein coupling. This domain appears to be located in the second and third cytoplasmic loops and in the COOH-terminal tail of the receptor. Yet another domain mediates receptor desensitization, a process in which a rapid diminution of effector response is observed after exposure of receptor to agonist. In the adrenergic receptor system, homologous desensitization (see earlier) requires the cytoplasmic enzymes cAMP-dependent protein kinase and beta-adrenergic receptor kinase to phosphorylate serine/threonine kinase targets in regions of the COOH-terminal tail or the third cytoplasmic loop of the receptor to uncouple the receptor from its associated G protein.[110, 172] A molecule known as β-arrestin may further modulate the interaction between the beta-adrenergic receptor and beta-adrenergic receptor kinase.[172] All of the genes encoding the adrenergic receptors lack introns within the protein coding regions. This lack is somewhat surprising in view of the receptors' apparent domain organization, because in many eucaryotic genes exons encode specific functional domains.

G PROTEINS. The G proteins are the critical signal transducers between the receptor and the effector in the plasma membrane, both topologically and functionally (see Figs. 4–15 and 4–19). The G protein family is extensive, with over 30 members described to date. These proteins share structural homology and the ability to bind GDP and GTP with relatively high affinity. The G proteins can be divided into two groups based on molecular size. Smaller G proteins (20 to 25 kd) are present in both higher and lower eucaryotes.[43] The best-characterized protein in this class is the p21 or *ras* proto-oncogene. Larger G proteins (80 to 90 kd) are more relevant to hormone action pathways. The latter share structural homology with a number of regulators of protein synthesis, including elongation factor Tu.

High-molecular-weight G proteins exist as heterotrimers consisting of three different subunits: α, β, and γ[168–171, 173–176] (Fig. 4–21). The α subunits are activated by binding GTP in the presence of Mg^{2+} and then can interact with the appropriate effector system such as adenylate cyclase. The β and γ subunits are not easily dissociable from each other and serve as a functional dimer that can interact with the α subunit. Multiple G proteins may serve different signal

TABLE 4–6. Selected Features of G Protein Subunit Structure and Function

Subunit	Feature
α subunits	Are unique for each G protein
	Are approximately 39–52 kd
	Bind guanine nucleotides; act as GTPase
	Are substrates for bacterial toxin ADP-ribosylation
	Bind to receptors, effectors, and β/γ complex
β/γ complex	Binds to an α subunit; may function as inhibitor of G protein activation
	Is probably required for G protein–receptor interaction but not for effector interaction
β subunits	May be identical for all G proteins
	Are 36 kd (an additional 35-kd form, structurally distinct from the 36-kd form, also copurifies with some G proteins)
	Bind tightly, but not covalently, to the γ subunit (β/γ complex dissociates only under denaturing conditions)
γ subunits	That of transducin differs from those of other G proteins
	Structure of other G protein γ subunits not yet known
	Are small (about 8–11 kd)
	May be involved in G protein membrane attachment

Adapted from Spiegel AM. Guanine nucleotide binding proteins and signal transduction. Vitam Horm 1988; 44:47–101.

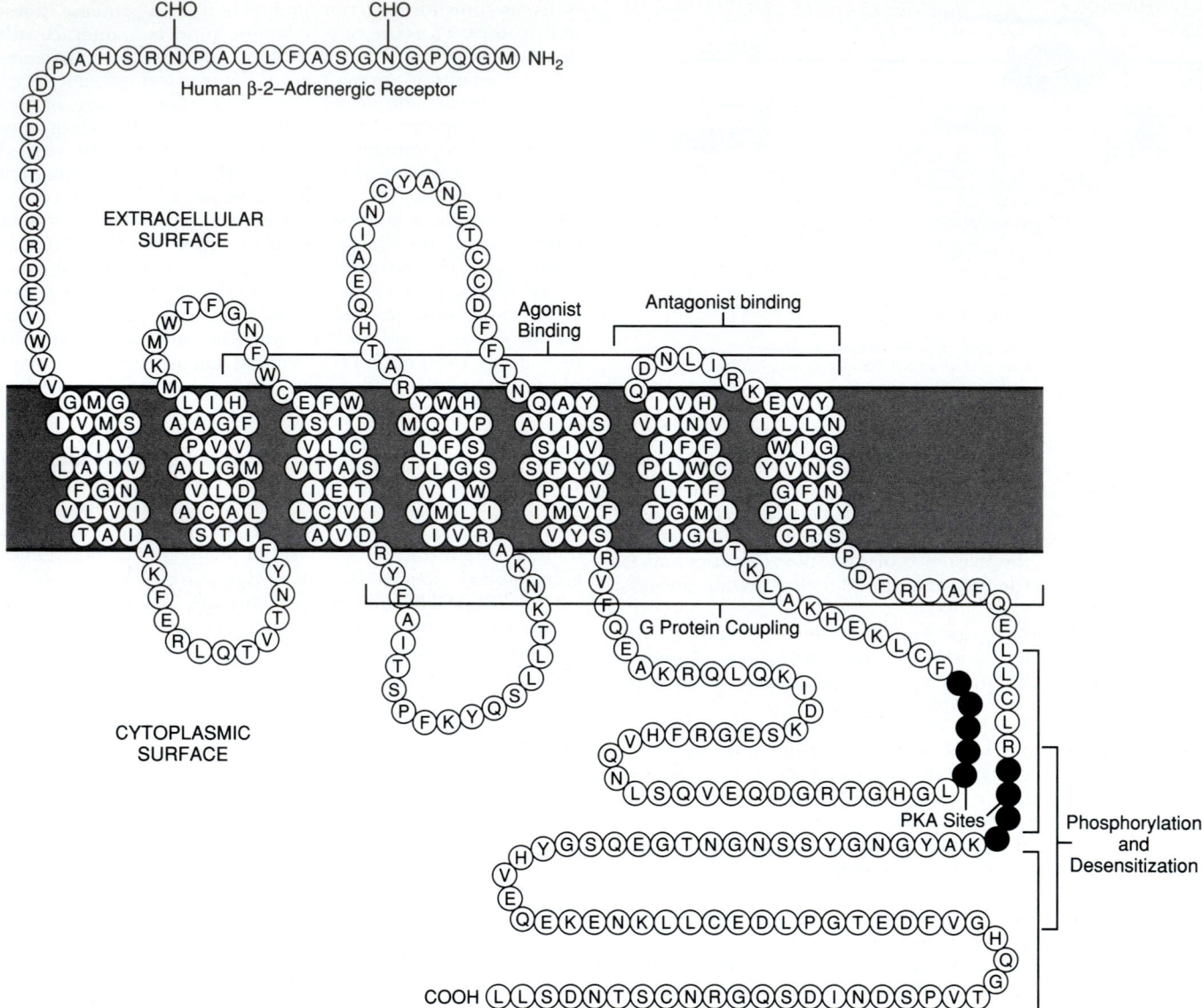

Figure 4–20. Structure of the beta-2–adrenergic receptor. A model of the human beta-2–adrenergic receptor, based on its deduced amino acid sequence, is shown. The CHO indicates probable glycosylation sites in the extracellular domain of the receptor. The residues indicated in the shaded circles represent probable phosphorylation (by protein kinase A [PKA]) sites in the intracellular domain of the receptor. The clusters of residues between the two horizontal lines delimiting the plasma membrane represent hydrophobic, alpha-helical membrane spanning domains. Domains of putative agonist and antagonist binding, G protein coupling, and phosphorylation (involved in desensitization) are shown. (Modified with permission from Dohlman HG, Caron MG, Lefkowitz RJ. A family of receptors coupled to guanine nucleotide regulatory proteins. Biochemistry 1987; 26:2657–2664. Copyright 1987 American Chemical Society.)

	G_s Protein	G_s Protein	Transducin
Receptors	Beta-adrenergic Glucagon ACTH and Others	Alpha-adrenergic Muscarinic Somatostatin and Others	Rod and Cone Opsins
Effectors	Adenylate Cyclase Ca^{2+} Channels	Adenylate Cyclase K^+ and Ca^{2+} Channels	cGMP Phosphodiesterase
ADP-Ribosylation	Cholera Toxin	Pertussis Toxin	Cholera Toxin Pertussis Toxin

Figure 4–21. Structure and properties of G proteins and transducin. Subunits are α, β, and γ.

transduction functions. For example, the ability of the adrenergic receptor subtypes either to stimulate or to decrease cAMP production resides in the interaction of beta-1– and beta-2–adrenergic receptors with stimulatory G proteins (G_s) and of alpha-2–adrenergic receptor with an inhibitory G protein (G_i). G proteins are located near the plasma membrane, although the precise interaction of the trimer with the lipid bilayer is not well known. The α subunits are more variable in structure than the $\beta\gamma$ subunits (Table 4–6). At least nine genes encoding the α subunit have been elucidated. These α subunits show considerable structural homology and have molecular sizes that range from 39 to 52 kd. There are four α_s (α_{s1-4}) subunits derived from the alternative splicing of exon 3 in the α_s gene. This splicing results in long and short forms that differ by 15 amino acid residues. The long form has a lower affinity and faster dissociation rate for GDP than the short form, which suggests functional heterogeneity among G proteins formed with these different α_s variants. The α_i subunit exists in at least three forms, each derived from a different gene. When present in the $\alpha\beta\gamma$ heterotrimer, α_i results in a G protein that mediates the inhibition of adenylate cyclase. α_i may also couple some receptors to K^+ and Ca^{2+} channels. Other α subunits include α_o, derived largely from brain, α_t or α-transducin found in association with the visual pigment rhodopsin, and other less well characterized forms. α_s is present in nearly all cells, but not all α_i subunits are present in every cell.

Again, the molecular cloning of the cDNAs for the α subunits provided insight into the domain organization of G protein subunits. Each α subunit has at least five domains including (1) a Mg^{2+}-dependent GTP binding site, (2) a GTPase domain, (3 and 4) receptor binding and effector interaction domains located in the COOH-terminal end,[177] and (5) a domain involved in $\beta\gamma$ interaction near the NH_2-terminal region. In some cultured cell lines, mutations in the COOH-terminal end of the α subunit of G_s result in uncoupling of the receptors from the G proteins.[178] These mutants have been termed *unc*. Additional evidence regarding the domain involved in receptor interaction comes from the ability of pertussis toxin to ADP-ribosylate and α_s subunit on a cysteine residue located in the COOH-terminal end of the molecule and to uncouple α_i, and α_o and α_t from the receptors. Similar conclusions have been reached from analyses of α_s/α_i chimeras.

The β subunit is found in two highly related 36- and 35-kd forms and is likely encoded by two different genes.[168, 169, 173] The γ subunits are more heterogeneous, with apparent molecular sizes of 6 to 10 kd, and are visualized as three bands by denaturing gel electrophoresis.[168, 169, 173] The β and γ subunits are usually observed in tight association, with formation of a $\beta\gamma$ dimer. Both β and γ subunits can also apparently function as homodimers rather than heterodimers, as evidenced from studies with yeast mutants lacking one or the other subunit. The $\beta\gamma$ subunits are required for regulation of the α subunit by hormone-receptor complexes and may serve to anchor the G proteins to plasma membranes. Furthermore, the affinity of $\beta\gamma$ for α suggests that this dimer may inhibit the action of α subunits and thus suggests a potential independent regulatory role of the $\beta\gamma$ dimer.

ACTIVATION OF ADENYLATE CYCLASE. The general mechanism of G protein linked–hormone activation of adenylate cyclase is well understood[173, 179] (Fig. 4–22). In the absence of ligand, the hormone receptor interacts directly with the heterotrimer G protein. In this state the rate of GDP dissociation from the α subunit is low and limits GTPase activity of the G protein complex. The presence of the hormone ligand results in formation of the hormone-recep-

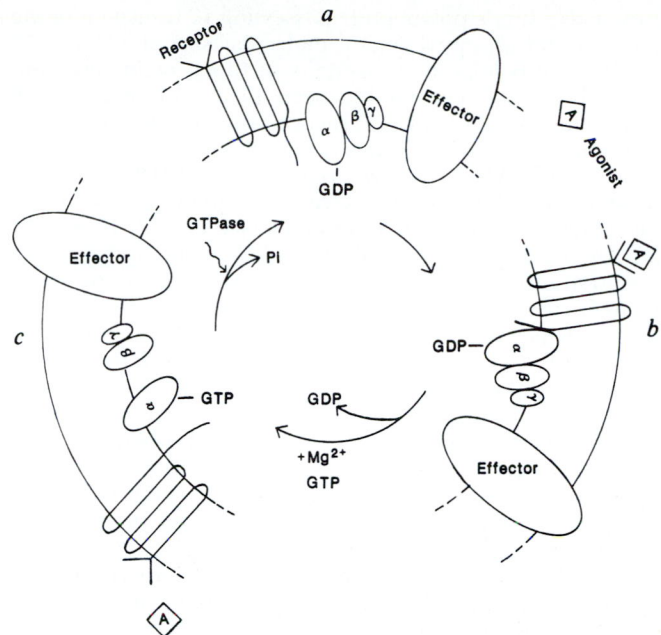

Figure 4–22. G protein signal transduction. In the absence of ligand binding to the receptor (a), the heterotrimer G protein binds GDP via its α subunit but apparently does not interact with either receptor or effector. Formation of the ligand-receptor complex (b) results in interaction of receptor and G protein, and subsequent replacement of GDP with GTP in the presence of Mg^{2+}. At this point, the GTP-bound, activated α subunit dissociates from the $\beta\gamma$ subunits (c). Then either one or both contact effectors and modulate their activities. Simultaneously, the inherent GTPase activity of the α subunit hydrolyzes the GTP to GDP to terminate peptide hormone signaling. (From Neer EJ, Clapham DE. Roles of G protein subunits in transmembrane signaling. Reprinted by permission from Nature vol. 333 pp. 129–134 Copyright © 1988 Macmillan Magazines Ltd.)

tor complex, which in turn promotes GDP dissociation from the α subunit of the heterotrimer and allows intracellular GTP to bind to the α subunit. This binding results in (1) dissociation of the α subunit from $\beta\gamma$; (2) lowering of the affinity of the receptor for the ligand; (3) production of an activated α subunit that can interact with an effector molecule such as adenylate cyclase; and (4) induction of the inherent GTPase activity in the α subunit. Like many signaling events, the presence of ligand results in a rapid but short-lived intracellular response. The increased ability of the "activated" α subunit to break down GTP and thus to increase GDP/GTP ratios gradually favors GDP rather than GTP binding to the G protein complex and results in a brake on the activation process. Thus a G protein signal transduction cycle can be produced and regulated.

In contrast to the role of the α subunit, the role of the $\beta\gamma$ dimer in the signal transduction process is less clear. The $\beta\gamma$ dimer, in the absence of α, may either directly or indirectly (via stimulation of phospholipase A_2) activate the M-type potassium channel in the heart.[168] In addition, a yeast mutant lacking the α subunit responds to yeast mating factor (a cAMP-linked response), which suggests that $\beta\gamma$ serves a stimulatory role with respect to this effector system.[168] Also, the $\beta\gamma$ may serve a regulatory role by inhibiting α_s activity. In this model, G_i inhibits adenylate cyclase by providing excess $\beta\gamma$ subunits, which then rapidly bind the relatively small amounts of α_s within a cell to limit stimulatory activity. In this indirect manner, effector activity is inhibited by the hormone-receptor complex.

The "activated" α subunit modulates the activity of adenylate cyclase, the ultimate effector enzyme in this system. Adenylate cyclase is an integral membrane glycoprotein present as a single polypeptide possessing 12 transmembrane domains and an approximate molecular size of 115 to 150 kd.[180] There is microheterogeneity of this protein, although generally a single enzyme has been assumed to exist for all cyclase-linked receptors. Interaction with activated α_s results in augmented enzyme activity, rapidly converting ATP to cAMP. The cAMP, in turn, reacts with cAMP-dependent protein kinase (kinase A), a tetramer containing two each of the regulatory and catalytic subunits (see Figs. 4–15 and 4–23). In the absence of cAMP, regulatory subunits prevent activation of the catalytic subunit. However, in the presence of cAMP, the regulatory subunits dissociate from the catalytic subunit, which unmasks its enzyme activity. This kinase then may phosphorylate other proteins within the cell to produce secondary and tertiary messengers.

A special feature of this signal transduction system is the heterogeneity of structure and function allowed by the cassette design (see Figs. 4–7, 4–15, and 4–19). For example, multiple G proteins may interact with a single receptor-hormone complex to result in activation and inhibition of different effector systems in response to a single agonist, as illustrated in Figure 4–13. Similarly, multiple receptors may interact with a single G protein. Thus flexibility of interaction at the receptor–G protein and G protein–effector interfaces results in a complex regulatory network. Examples of such heterogeneity lie in the observations that the beta-adrenergic receptor, in reconstitution studies, can activate G_s and G_i, and that G_s can interact with both adenylate cyclase and calcium channels in atrial tissues. Because various G proteins

are expressed in a tissue-specific fashion and because their levels may be hormonally regulated, there is a significant opportunity for regulation of these pathways at every step, both physiologically and pathologically.

Another important feature of this signal transduction system is its ability to amplify signals. Because activation of G proteins results in dissociation of the G proteins from bound complexes, a single hormone-receptor complex can activate multiple G proteins. For instance, in the beta-adrenergic receptor system, one agonist-receptor interaction can activate up to 20 G proteins (Fig. 4–23). Similarly, light activation of rhodopsin can result in a 1000-fold increase in the stimulation of G_t.

EFFECTS OF BACTERIAL TOXINS ON G PROTEINS. Two bacterial toxins interact with G proteins and alter cellular cAMP levels[173] (Table 4–7). Pertussis toxin (derived from B pertussis) causes ADP-ribosylation of α_i, α_o, and α_t at a cysteine residue near the COOH-terminal end. This reaction results in receptor uncoupling from G_i, constitutive activation of adenylate cyclase, and increase in cellular cAMP levels. Inhibition of G_i may account for the pertussis-associated increase in sensitivity to histamines and for pertussis-associated hypoglycemia by blocking the inhibitory effect of alpha-adrenergic influences on histamine-mediated pathways and on insulin secretion.

Cholera toxin, by comparison, ADP-ribosylates α_s at an internal arginine residue, which results in a decreased α association with $\beta\gamma$ and effective stabilization of α_s in the GDP-bound conformation. The final result is an inhibition

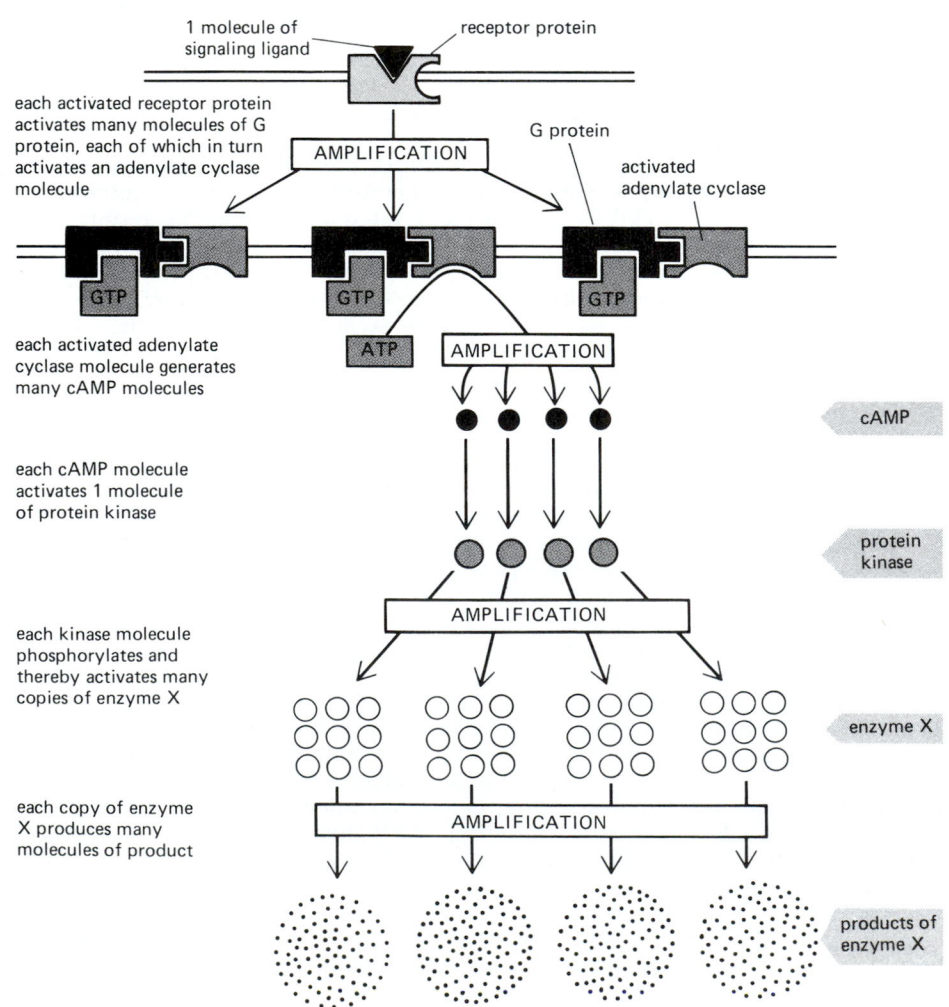

Figure 4–23. Amplification of cellular signaling after stimulation of a cAMP-linked receptor. (From Alberts B, Bray D, Lewis J, et al. Molecular Biology of the Cell. New York: Garland, 1983: 750.)

TABLE 4–7. Interaction of Bacterial Toxins with G Proteins and Cyclase Systems

Parameter	Cholera Toxin	Pertussis Toxin
Cellular receptor	Gangliosides	?
G protein target for ADP-ribosylation	α_s, α_i	α_i, α_t, α_o
Effects		
G proteins	Activates G_s	Inactivates G_p, G_o
cAMP	Increases	Variable increases
Final biological effects	Increased ion flux in GI tract	Increased insulin secretion and lipolysis; bronchoconstriction, decreased neutrophil response

of GTPase activity, prolonged ability of α_s to stimulate effector systems, and increased cAMP levels. The severe diarrhea that is characteristic of infection with *Vibrio cholerae* and the analogous symptoms produced by some toxin-producing strains of *Escherichia coli* are thought to be due to continuous activation of the adenylate cyclase. The interdiction of GDP hydrolysis in a number of hormone systems by the use of a nonhydrolyzable GTP analogue or aluminum fluoride results in persistent G protein activation and ligand-receptor dissociation.

Receptor Tyrosine Kinases

GENERAL STRUCTURAL FEATURES. Although the earliest studies of the mechanism of peptide hormone action focused on indirect second messenger systems, such as those involving cAMP, the role of receptors as direct catalysts of phosphorylation reactions has been a subject of intense investigation after the recognition that several receptors contain an intrinsic hormone-activated tyrosine kinase activity. The first such evidence came from studies of the EGF receptor.[181–183] A receptor-associated protein kinase is activated by EGF and differs from most known cellular protein kinases in that it phosphorylates proteins on *tyrosine* rather than serine residues. This tyrosine protein kinase activity was similar to several oncogene-associated tyrosine kinase activities and was ultimately shown to be intrinsic to the EGF receptor. A number of other peptide hormone receptors have subsequently been shown to contain hormone-activated tyrosine kinase activities. These receptors include those for insulin,[184–186] IGF I,[186, 187] PDGF,[188, 189] CSF-1,[190, 191] and fibroblast growth factor[192] (see Table 4–1). In spite of the existence of multiple receptors and of oncogene products with tyrosine kinase activity, phosphorylation of cellular proteins on tyrosine residues is less common than serine phosphorylation, representing less than 1% of all protein phosphorylation in the cell under normal conditions.

Each of the known tyrosine kinase–containing peptide hormone receptors has been cloned at the cDNA level, and the complete amino acid sequences have been deduced from the cDNA sequences. By comparison of the individual structures, the receptors can be divided into three classes (Fig. 4–24).[193] The highly homologous insulin and IGF I receptors are the most complex, with a heterotetrameric structure consisting of two α and two β subunits joined by disulfide cross-bridges. The α subunits are entirely extracellular and contain a cysteine-rich region that is believed to be involved in hormone binding. The β subunits possess an extracellular domain, a transmembrane domain, and an intracellular domain that contains an ATP binding site and a catalytic kinase domain. The α and β subunits are synthesized as part of a single precursor molecule that undergoes proteolytic processing to form the two subunits in a manner analogous to synthesis of insulin from proinsulin.[194]

The second class is represented by the EGF receptor, which differs from the first class in that the domains for hormone binding and tyrosine kinase are contained in a single transmembrane protein chain.[183] The configurations of the ATP binding site and the tyrosine kinase domain are generally similar to those of the insulin and IGF I receptors, and there are also cysteine-rich domains that appear to be important for hormone binding, although these domains

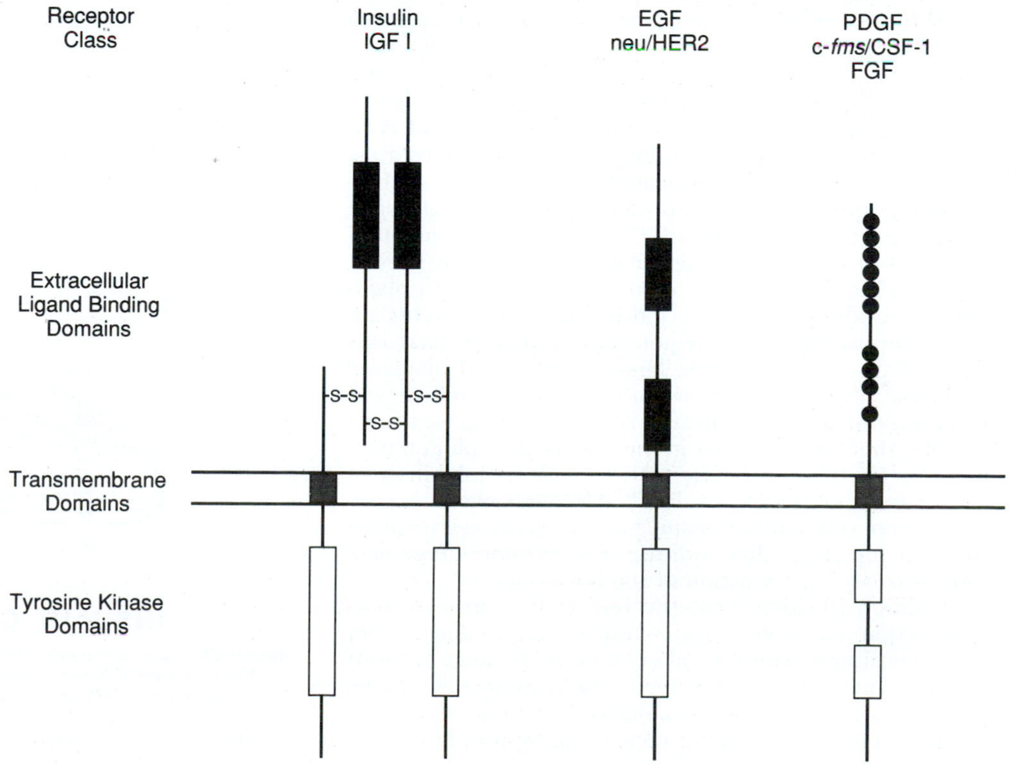

Figure 4–24. Structural features of different subclasses of tyrosine kinase receptors. The black rectangles represent cysteine-rich repeat regions and the circles represent conserved cysteine residues. Disulfide bonds in these regions are thought to have an important role in establishing the structure of the hormone binding site. The white rectangles represent the tyrosine kinase domain, which is an interrupted sequence in PDGF and related receptors.

Receptor Class: Insulin IGF I | EGF neu/HER2 | PDGF c-*fms*/CSF-1 FGF

Extracellular Ligand Binding Domains

Transmembrane Domains

Tyrosine Kinase Domains

exist in two interrupted regions in the EGF receptor. The EGF receptor appears to be inactive in the monomeric form, and transmission of the hormone signal requires the dimerization of receptors.[195] In this dimerized form, the EGF receptor resembles the insulin and IGF I receptors, except that the two receptor halves are noncovalently, rather than covalently, associated.

The PDGF, fibroblast growth factor, and CSF-1 receptors form a third structural class of tyrosine kinase receptors. They contain binding and tyrosine kinase activities in a single peptide chain but possess a different type of extracellular cysteine-rich structure that is believed to form immunoglobulin G–like repeats. In addition the tyrosine kinase domain is interrupted by about 100 amino acids that are unrelated to other tyrosine kinases.[188–193] The significance of the structural similarities and differences of the tyrosine kinase receptors is not known, although these features probably have importance in regard to both receptor evolution and function.

INVOLVEMENT OF RECEPTOR TYROSINE KINASE ACTIVITY IN HORMONE ACTION. For each receptor in this class, the tyrosine kinase activity is the only known intrinsic catalytic activity. The enzyme is activated immediately after hormone binding, as evidenced by rapid receptor autophosphorylation, which is initiated within seconds and is maximal within several minutes. Although the specific molecular events that lead from tyrosine phosphorylation to hormone action have not been established, there is considerable experimental evidence in support of a role for the tyrosine kinase activity in mediating some or all of the actions of the hormones. This evidence is reviewed here for the insulin receptor, because this tyrosine kinase receptor is most closely linked to the classic endocrine system.

With the isolation of cDNA for the insulin receptor, it is possible to modify individual regions of the receptor, including regions of the β subunit that are important for tyrosine kinase activity, by site-directed mutagenesis. The resulting mutant receptors can then be expressed at high levels in cells that normally have few insulin receptors by the process of transfection, and the consequences of the receptor mutation on hormone action can be studied. When normal insulin receptors are transfected and overexpressed in Chinese hamster ovary cells, which have low numbers of endogenous insulin receptors, insulin can be shown to stimulate a number of biological responses (Fig. 4–25). If the transfected insulin receptors are mutated at the site of ATP binding, they retain insulin-binding activity but lack tyrosine kinase activity and fail to stimulate biological actions including glucose uptake, ribosomal protein S6 activation, glycogen synthesis, and DNA synthesis.[196, 197] Likewise, replacement of one or more of the tyrosine autophosphorylation sites at positions 1146, 1150, and 1151 in the β subunit with phenylalanine residues by site-directed mutagenesis prevents autophosphorylation in this region and results in decreased effects of insulin on tyrosine kinase activity and biological responses.[99, 190, 198] Similarly, when monoclonal antibodies to the kinase domain of the insulin receptor are microinjected into cells, there is a decrease in the effects of insulin on both the receptor tyrosine kinase activity and an inhibition of biological responses to insulin.[199] Although these experiments do not reveal how tyrosine phosphorylation is involved in insulin signaling, they indicate that tyrosine kinase activation is necessary for action of the hormone.

Additional evidence for the role of the kinase in hormone action has come from studies of signaling under physiological and pathological conditions. In some patients with the type A syndrome of insulin resistance,[200] insulin binding is normal, but there is a marked decrease in receptor tyrosine kinase activity and in receptor autophosphorylation

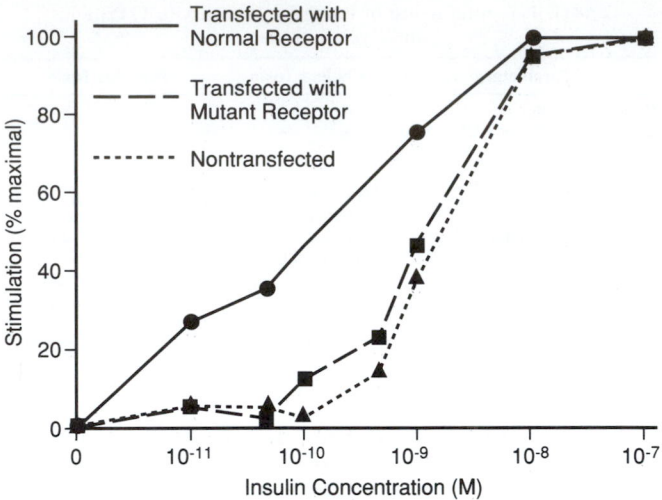

Figure 4–25. Effect of insulin on thymidine incorporation into DNA (DNA synthesis) in Chinese hamster ovary (CHO-K1) fibroblasts transfected with normal human insulin receptors or mutant insulin receptors with alanine substituted for lysine in the region of ATP binding (amino acid 1018). The nontransfected CHO cells have a much lower number of insulin receptors than either of the transfectants. (Adapted from Chou CK, Dull TJ, Russel DS, et al. Human insulin receptors mutated at the ATP-binding site lack protein tyrosine kinase activity and fail to mediate postreceptor effects of insulin. J Biol Chem 1987; 262:1842–1847.)

(Fig. 4–26).[201, 202] Similarly, in type II diabetes, insulin resistance is associated with decreased receptor tyrosine kinase activity.[203–205] The association between receptor tyrosine kinase activity and alterations in insulin action in other human insulin resistance states is discussed later in detail. Taken together, these observations suggest that insulin-stimulated tyrosine kinase activity and receptor autophosphorylation are necessary for insulin action. Studies with site-directed mutants of other tyrosine kinase receptors, such as the EGF,[83, 206, 207] PDGF,[208] and CSF-1 receptors,[209] have shown similar associations between active receptor tyrosine kinases and hormone action.

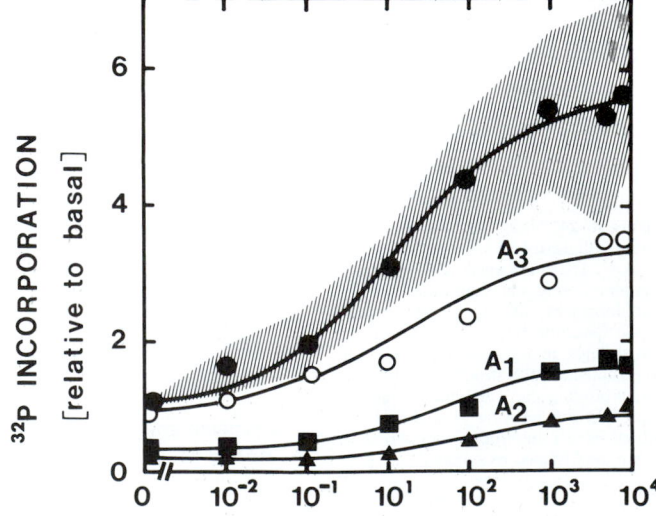

Figure 4–26. Insulin stimulation of phosphorylation of isolated erythrocyte insulin receptors from normal control subjects (shaded area) and three patients with type A syndrome of insulin resistance. (Adapted from Grigorescu F, Flier JS, Kahn CR. Defect in insulin receptor phosphorylation in erythrocytes and fibroblasts associated with severe insulin resistance. J Biol Chem 1984; 259:15003–15006.)

Peptide hormones bind to the extracellular portions of transmembrane receptors, and the extracellular binding domains are responsible for both the affinity and the specificity of the receptors. This selective binding mechanism appears to be adequate under most circumstances to ensure specificity of hormone action, e.g., preventing insulin from activating EGF-sensitive pathways. In spite of the generally similar structural and catalytic properties of the intracellular receptor tyrosine kinases, specificity of hormone action may also be determined by differences in structure of the intracellular domains. It is possible to create receptors with the extracellular binding domain of one receptor and the intracellular tyrosine kinase of a different receptor by combining portions of the cDNAs for the two different receptors and then expressing the chimeric receptors in transfected cells.[210] By this method, receptors have been constructed that contain the extracellular domain of the insulin receptor and the intracellular tyrosine kinase domain of the EGF receptor or the tyrosine kinase of the oncogene v-*ros* (Fig. 4–27).[211] The hybrid receptors bind insulin with high affinity, and insulin is able to activate the v-*ros* or EGF kinase domains. In contrast to cells transfected with intact insulin receptors, however, insulin does not stimulate glucose uptake or DNA synthesis and produces EGF-like effects via the insulin-EGF receptor chimera. Thus the cellular response appears to be governed by specific features of the intracellular domain. Activation of the tyrosine kinase activity is not sufficient. These features may include a failure of the v-*ros* or EGF receptor tyrosine kinase to phosphorylate specific proteins that are substrates for only the insulin receptor (enzymatic substrate specificity) or a failure to initiate tyrosine kinase–independent responses that are required for normal insulin action.

REGULATION OF RECEPTOR TYROSINE KINASE ACTIVITY. For each of the known peptide hormone receptors containing tyrosine kinase, the earliest intracellular events after hormone binding are increased tyrosine kinase catalytic activity and autophosphorylation of the receptor. The tyrosine kinase receptors behave like classic allosteric enzymes in which the primary role of the domain or subunit for ligand binding is to suppress the kinase activity intrinsic to the intracellular domain. For example, in the case of the insulin receptor, the α subunit may be viewed as the ligand-binding regulatory subunit and the β subunit as the catalytic kinase subunit, very much in analogy with cAMP-dependent protein kinase. Ligand binding to the receptor or removal of the ligand binding domain by proteolysis or in vitro mutagenesis results in constitutive activation of the kinase. It is not clear exactly how the binding of hormone to an extracellular portion of the receptor results in derepression of the tyrosine kinase because the receptor remains intact; however, the derepression probably results from a binding-induced conformational change in the receptor and/or from receptor-receptor aggregation. In the case of the insulin receptor, hormone binding leads to changes in accessibility of the receptor to chemicals and enzymes and to changes in chromatographic properties that can be best explained by a shift in conformation.[212, 213]

REGULATION BY MULTISITE PHOSPHORYLATION. For all of the receptors that have been studied, autophosphorylation occurs on multiple tyrosine residues.[193] The functional significance of each of these phosphorylation sites has not been determined, but autophosphorylation at certain sites may have a positive or a negative regulatory effect on the tyrosine kinase catalytic activity. For example, autophosphorylation of tyrosine residues within the tyrosine kinase domain of the insulin receptor appears to both increase and stabilize the catalytic activity of the kinase so that activity remains even after dissociation of the bound hormone.[111, 112] The analogous tyrosine residue in the EGF receptor is not

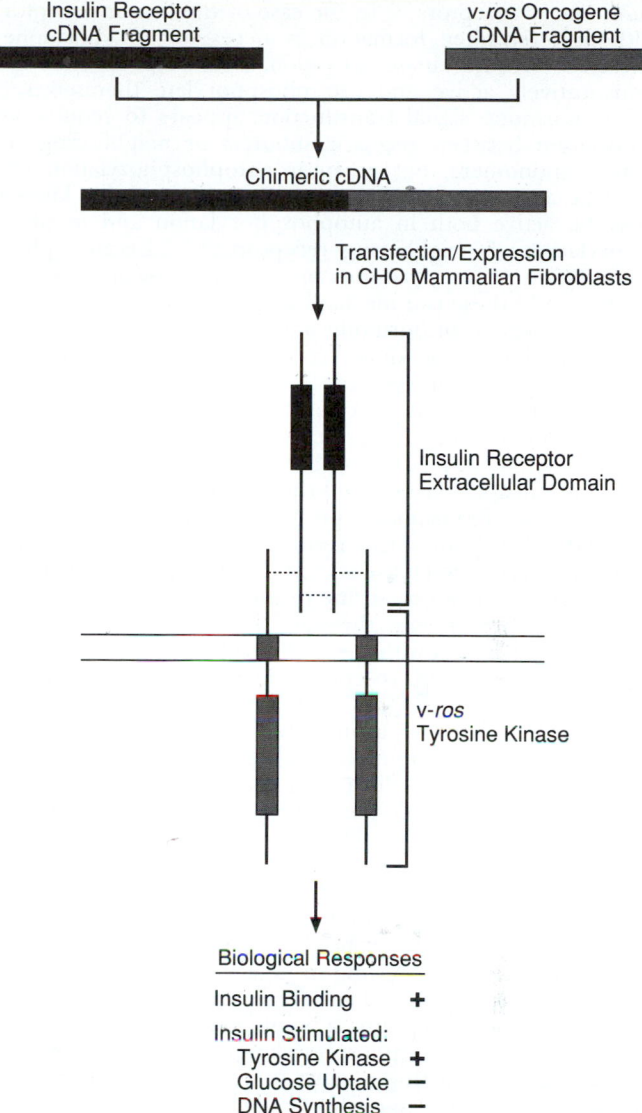

Figure 4–27. Use of chimeric receptor constructs to investigate the role of specific receptor domains in mediating hormone action. A hybrid receptor cDNA can be created by combining a fragment of the insulin receptor cDNA corresponding to the α subunit and extracellular portion of the β subunit with cDNA corresponding to the transmembrane and intracellular domains of the v-*ros* oncogene. When expressed in mammalian cells (e.g., Chinese hamster ovary [CHO] fibroblasts), the resulting hybrid receptor binds insulin with high affinity and undergoes insulin-stimulated autophosphorylation. Although the receptor tyrosine kinase has thus been activated, insulin-stimulated glucose uptake and DNA synthesis are not observed. See text for further details.

phosphorylated, but autophosphorylation at a site within the COOH-terminal tail of the receptor may increase kinase activity.[214] Specific structural features of the kinase and specific aspects of the autophosphorylation may be important for the divergent signals generated during the signal cascade. Mutation of the insulin receptor at Tyr-1146 alters the growth-stimulating potential of the receptor but not its metabolic activity,[100] whereas mutation of Tyr-1150 and Tyr-1151 produces the opposite effect.[198] Deletion of the intervening sequence in the kinase domain of the PDGF receptor alters its ability to stimulate mitogenesis but not its acute effects on phosphatidylinositol turnover or ion influx.[208]

Studies with several different tyrosine kinase receptors have shown that hormone binding and tyrosine kinase activation require the association of αβ dimers into tetramers[215, 216] or the formation of oligomers in the case of monomeric receptors.[217] In the case of the insulin receptor, although tetramer formation is necessary for hormone-directed tyrosine kinase activation, isolated β subunits are constitutively active and can phosphorylate themselves.[218] Thus hormone signal transduction appears to require an association between receptor subunits or neighboring receptor monomers, but receptor autophosphorylation can then be an intramolecular event. Receptor tyrosine kinases may be active both in autophosphorylation and in phosphorylation of neighboring receptors.[218–220] Because phosphorylation of key tyrosines may increase receptor kinase activity,[111, 112] these two mechanisms could each have roles in the amplification of hormone signaling.

Several tyrosine kinase receptors are phosphorylated not only on tyrosine residues but also on serine and threonine residues by cellular kinases extrinsic to the receptor. The extent of receptor serine phosphorylation appears to be modulated, and this phosphorylation may decrease tyrosine autophosphorylation and the tyrosine kinase activity of the receptors. For example, protein kinase C phosphorylates the EGF receptor on serine residues and decreases the EGF-stimulated tyrosine kinase activity.[221] The insulin receptor is also phosphorylated on serine residues in response to phorbol esters, presumably through their effects on protein kinase C activity. As with the EGF receptor, serine phosphorylation of the insulin receptor is associated with decreased tyrosine kinase activity and decreased insulin action.[222] Prolonged stimulation with insulin itself, in addition to its effects on tyrosine autophosphorylation, leads to increased phosphorylation of the insulin receptor on serine residues,[223, 224] and this serine phosphorylation may have a role in modulating or turning off insulin action. As with the beta-adrenergic receptor kinase, a specific insulin receptor–associated serine kinase may be present,[225] although this enzyme has not been well characterized. As for the possible role of insulin-stimulated serine phosphorylation in reversing hormone action, it is interesting to note that insulin-stimulated serine phosphorylation of insulin receptors does not occur in cells transfected with mutant receptors that cannot undergo tyrosine autophosphorylation.[226] Thus the normal insulin-signaling pathway must be intact to allow insulin stimulation of serine phosphorylation.

In addition to the role of serine phosphorylation in receptor regulation, the COOH-terminal tail of the insulin receptor β subunit may regulate receptor signaling by folding into the catalytic site and thus blocking receptor tyrosine kinase activity.[193] It is speculated that phosphorylation of tyrosine residues in the COOH terminus may cause the molecule to unfold, thus increasing the susceptibility of the catalytic region to activating tyrosine phosphorylation and also increasing the access of substrates. A regulatory response of this type would provide a mechanism to decrease basal kinase activity and thus make possible a greater increase in signaling with hormone activation. Figure 4–28 summarizes some of these modulators of insulin receptor kinase activity. Similar mechanisms have been suggested for the EGF receptor. Other possible modulators include proteins and peptides within the cell that may modify hormone responsiveness by either activating or inhibiting receptor tyrosine kinase activity.

SUBSTRATES FOR RECEPTOR TYROSINE KINASES. Because a number of peptide hormone receptors contain intrinsic, hormone-activated tyrosine kinase activity, there have been extensive efforts to identify substrates for the kinases that may explain the molecular mechanism of hormone action. The receptors themselves often represent one of the best substrates for their own kinase activity leading to receptor autophosphorylation. This autophosphorylation, in turn, appears to have a role in the regulation of receptor

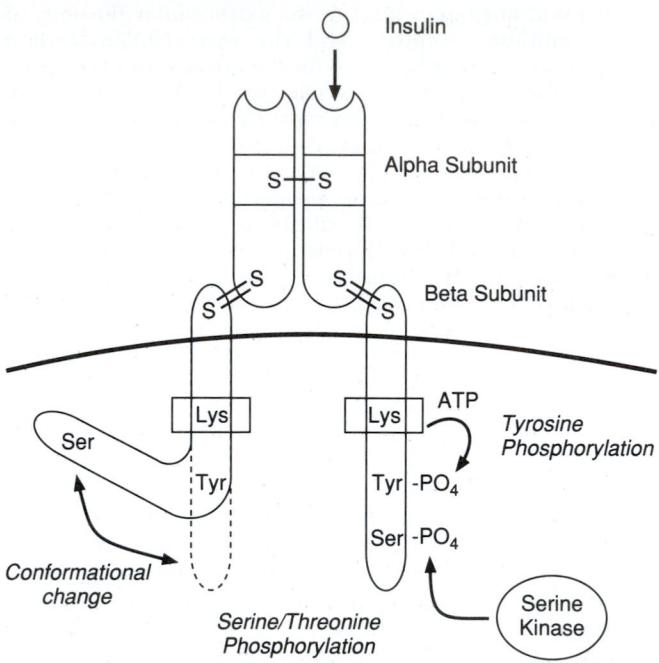

Figure 4–28. Potential mechanisms for modulation of insulin receptor kinase activity. These mechanisms include tyrosine autophosphorylation, which is stimulatory; serine/threonine phosphorylation by protein kinase C and cAMP kinase, which is inhibitory; and conformational changes, which could produce positive or negative effects.

kinase activity toward other substrates. Receptors not only phosphorylate themselves but also may cross-phosphorylate receptors for other hormones. For example, in cultured skeletal muscle cells, the insulin receptor phosphorylates unoccupied IGF I receptors, possibly leading to IGF I–like effects[219] (Fig. 4–29). The EGF receptor also appears both to phosphorylate other EGF receptors in oligomeric complexes[217] and to phosphorylate the proto-oncogene *neu*.[220] Such cross-phosphorylation of receptors may contribute to the diversity of biological actions of hormones such as insulin and also provides another mechanism for the amplification of hormone signals.

Because protein substrates for tyrosine kinases are rare, identification of the proteins has been challenging. One approach to identification of cellular substrates of the tyrosine kinases involves the use of antibodies that recognize phosphorylated tyrosine residues in proteins with high affinity and specificity.[227, 228] With such antibodies it is possible to immunoprecipitate phosphotyrosine-containing proteins from extracts of cells and tissues. By comparing immunoprecipitates from cells equilibrated with [32P]orthophosphate and then incubated in the presence or absence of peptide hormones, a number of different proteins have been demonstrated that undergo hormone-stimulated tyrosine phosphorylation (Fig. 4–30). These proteins range in molecular size from 15 kd to more than 200 kd and generally are phosphorylated rapidly after the addition of hormone.[229–236] It is suspected that some of these proteins have functional activities that are altered by tyrosine phosphorylation and mediate the transfer of hormone signals from the receptors to the cellular machinery, in analogy with serine phosphorylation mechanisms. Some of the phosphoproteins appear to be common substrates for the kinases of different receptors, possibly explaining overlapping actions of different hormones. For example, a phosphoprotein of 185 kd, designated pp185, is phosphorylated in response to both insulin and IGF I;[232, 234, 235, 237, 238] pp240 is phosphorylated in response to insulin, IGF I, and EGF;[235] and pp36 is responsive to EGF

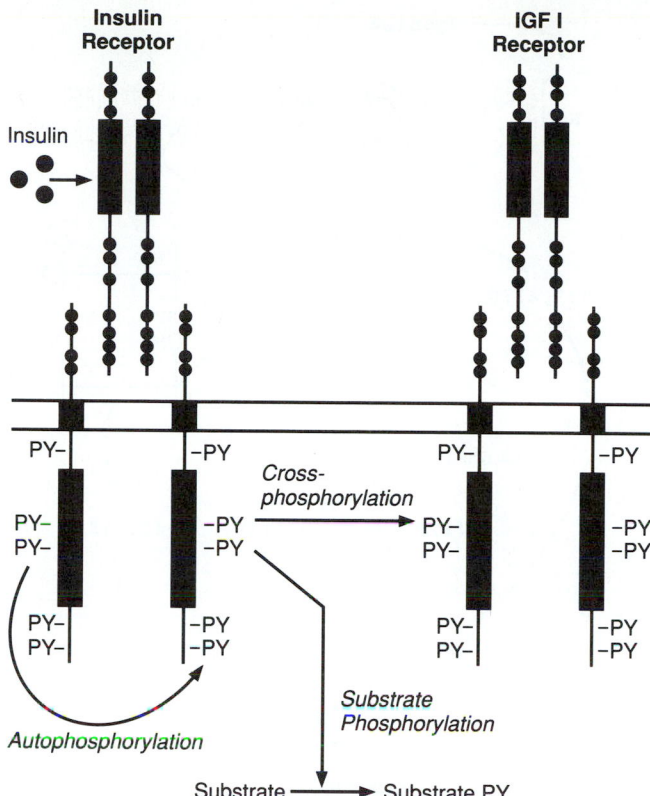

Figure 4—29. Tyrosine phosphorylation pathways activated after binding of insulin to insulin receptor. The receptor may tyrosine phosphorylate itself, other receptors, including the IGF I receptor, and nonreceptor substrates. PY represents phosphotyrosine residues.

and PDGF.[229,230] Other substrate phosphorylation events may be specifically associated with individual receptors and mediate unique actions of individual hormones. In spite of the potential importance of these in vivo substrates for the receptor kinases, the structure and function of most of the proteins have not been established, and their roles in hormone action remain uncertain.

A second approach to the search for substrates for peptide hormone receptor tyrosine kinases has been based on reconstitution experiments in which known proteins are allowed to interact with isolated receptors in vitro. This method led to the identification of several potential mediators of peptide hormone action, such as a serine kinase designated MAP2,[239] calmodulin,[240] and several cytoskeletal proteins.[239] Although these proteins are known and their biological activities are at least partially understood, none has been proved to be an important substrate for the receptors in vivo. In future experimental work, it is hoped that the results of these two different methods of studying tyrosine phosphoproteins can be brought together and that individual proteins with activities in the pathways of hormone action can identified that are substrates for one or more of the receptors both in vivo and in vitro.

In considering the role of tyrosine phosphorylation in peptide hormone action, it is important to recognize that the pleiotropic actions of hormones such as insulin may depend on multiple postreceptor pathways. Tyrosine phosphorylation may be an initial step in all pathways or may represent only one of several specific biochemical mechanisms that lead to different hormone-induced biological responses.

POSSIBLE MEDIATORS OF RECEPTOR KINASE SYSTEMS. In addition to regulation of cellular metabolism by tyrosine phosphorylation, insulin and other growth factors may con-

trol synthesis of second messengers that could mediate some hormone actions on intracellular enzymes. Some of these mediators are members of the inositol phosphate family discussed later. In addition, insulin may cause activation of a phosphatidylinositol-glycan–specific phospholipase C (reviewed in ref. 241). This phospholipase is thought to hydrolyze a membrane-associated substrate to produce the phosphatidylinositol-glycan and 1,2-diacylglycerol (DAG), which then modulates the activities of several intracellular enzymes. Because these products are apparently released outside the cell, they may be taken up back into cells to exert their effects. Although this hypothesis is interesting, confirmation of the structure and activities of these mediators has not been obtained. Thus their role in insulin action remains to be defined.

Receptors Associated with Guanylate Cyclase

Guanylate cyclase catalyzes the formation cGMP from GTP, in analogy with adenylate cyclase.[242] Guanylate cyclase,

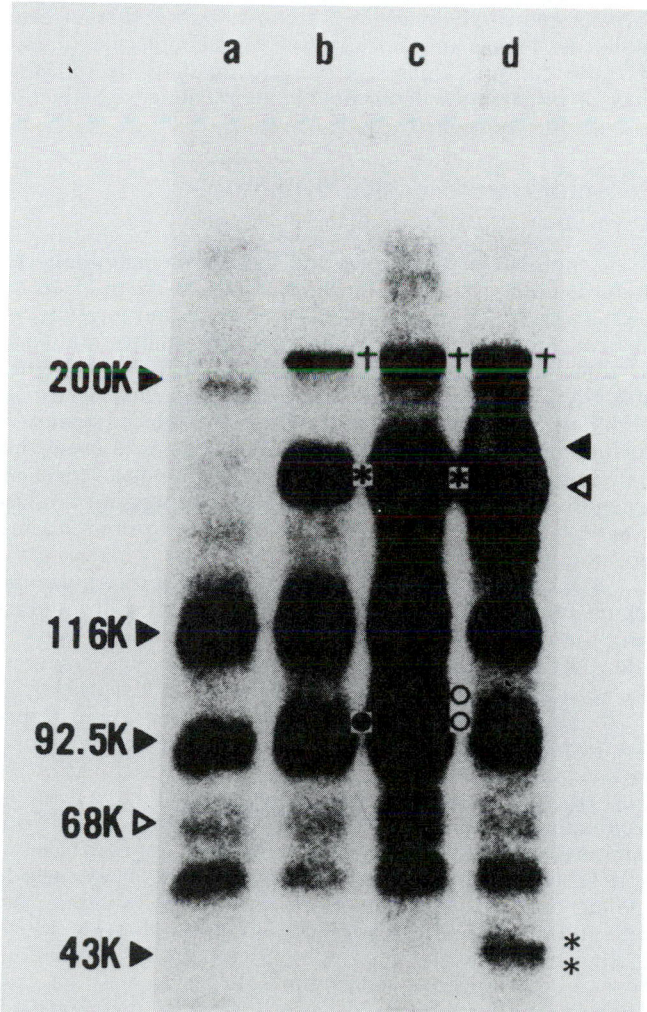

Figure 4—30. Phosphotyrosine-containing proteins from [^{32}P]orthophosphate-labeled KB cells. ^{32}P-labeled cells were incubated in the absence of hormone (a) or with 10^{-7} M insulin (b), 10^{-7} M IGF I (c), or 10^{-8} M EGF (d). Tyrosine phosphoproteins were immunoprecipitated with antiphosphotyrosine antibody, separated by polyacrylamide gel electrophoresis, and visualized by autoradiography. Hormone-stimulated proteins include ●, pp92 (insulin receptor); ○, pp98/pp92 (IGF I receptors); ◁, pp175 (EGF receptor); *, pp185; ◀, pp190; †, pp240; and *, pp48. (From Kadowaki T, Koyasu S, Nishida E, et al. Tyrosine phosphorylation of common and specific sets of cellular proteins rapidly induced by insulin, insulin-like growth factor I, and epidermal growth factor in an intact cell. J Biol Chem 1987; 262:7342–7350.)

however, exists in cells in both soluble and membrane-associated forms. The membrane-associated form is regulated by hormones and other ligands. Like the tyrosine kinases and unlike adenylate cyclase, guanylate cyclase may directly serve receptor and effector functions.

Sea urchin egg proteins (resact and speract) and atrial naturietic peptides appear to activate guanylate cyclase by binding directly to its membrane-associated forms. The deduced amino acid sequence of guanylate cyclase derived from cloned cDNAs predicts a single transmembrane domain, similar to that of the tyrosine kinases. The COOH-terminal domain is intracellular and is highly conserved in sea urchins and mammals. In contrast, the extracellular domain is variable, contains the NH_2 terminus, and may serve as a ligand binding domain. The deduced protein sequence suggests that the membrane-associated guanylate cyclase is a member of a family of proteins that include the low-molecular-weight receptor for atrial natriuretic peptides and the cytoplasmic form of the guanylate cyclase. Rat brain guanylate cyclase has been expressed in mammalian cells by DNA transfection and has been shown to bind and be activated by atrial natriuretic peptides. Thus the membrane form of guanylate cyclase is both a receptor and an effector molecule. This is another example of one molecule, like the receptor tyrosine kinases, serving to mediate the complete flow of information from ligand interaction to production of a second messenger.

Receptors and Phosphatidylinositol Turnover

A number of hormones and ligands mediate their cellular actions via calcium ions and DAG as second messengers[37, 243-247] (see Table 4–1). The second messengers, in turn, modulate the activity of protein kinases regulated by calcium binding–regulatory protein (e.g., calmodulin), and DAG activates protein kinase C. These enzymes phosphorylate specific intracellular proteins, which results in further hormone action. Examples of hormones using this signaling system in specific tissues include alpha-1–adrenergic and muscarinic cholinergic agents, vasopressin (V_1), histamine (H_1), cholecystokinin, LHRH, thyrotropin-releasing hormone, angiotensin II, and oxytocin.

ROLE OF G PROTEINS. In general, the various hormone ligands that stimulate phosphoinositide turnover interact with the receptors that activate G proteins, as described for adenylate cyclase.[248, 249] These activated G proteins, however, are coupled to stimulation of phospholipase C activity.[37, 243, 245-247] This enzyme fosters the conversion of membrane-bound phosphatidylinositol 4,5-bisphosphate to the second messenger form, inositol 1,4,5-trisphosphate (IP_3) (Fig. 4–31). IP_3 then interacts with an intracellular compartment containing calcium stores (Fig. 4–32). Evidence that G proteins are coupled to receptors involved in changes in calcium and DAG levels comes from various results. They include the fact that pertussis toxin blocks calcium activation in mast cells and neutrophils. In addition, aluminum fluoride, which is known to activate G proteins, increases IP_3 formation. Several hormones coupled to this pathway, such as thyrotropin-releasing hormone and vasopressin, also increase GTP hydrolysis, and a nonhydrolyzable analogue of GTP (GTPγS) decreases agonist binding to receptors for alpha-1–adrenergic agents, muscarinic nicotinic agonists, and angiotensin II.

EFFECTS ON INTRACELLULAR CALCIUM. The hormones involved in regulation of phosphatidylinositol turnover also regulate intracellular calcium levels.[37, 243, 245-247] Calcium inside cells is maintained at a concentration of approximately 10^{-7} M, whereas extracellular calcium levels are about 10^{-3} M.

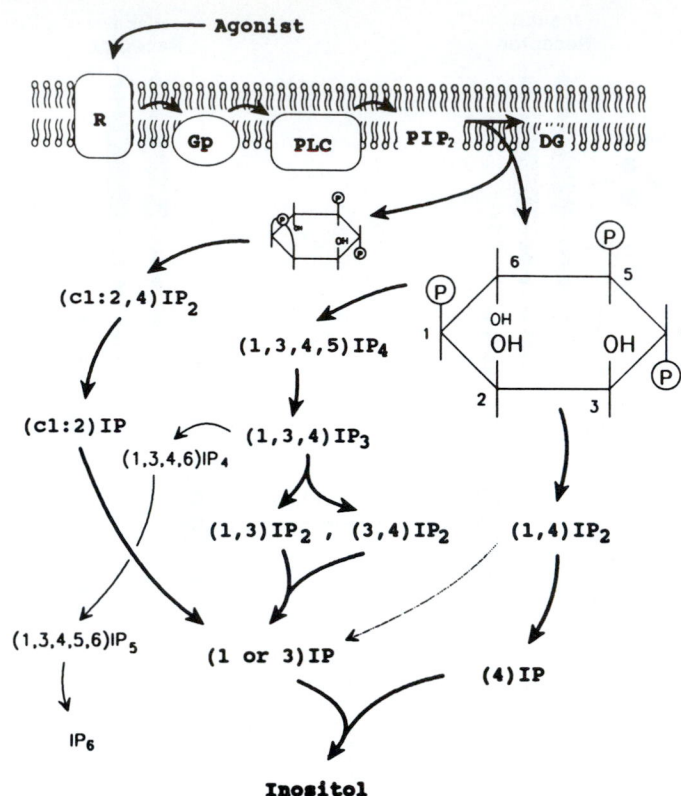

Figure 4–31. Pathways in the synthesis and metabolism of phosphatidylinositol. Ligand-receptor (R) interaction results in the activation of phospholipase C (PLC) via a G protein (Gp). Phospholipase C hydrolyzes membrane-bound phosphatidylinositol 4,5-bisphosphate (PIP$_2$) and active second messengers, inositol 1,4,5-trisphosphate (IP$_3$) and diacylglycerol (DG). Known metabolic pathways of IP$_3$ are shown. (From Putney JW Jr, Takemura H, Hughes AR, et al. How do inositol phosphates regulate calcium signaling? FASEB J 1989; 3:1899–1905.)

Thus there is a 10,000-fold concentration gradient across the two sides of the cell's plasma membrane. This gradient is maintained by a number of plasma membrane–based calcium pumps, channels, and transporters that are largely either voltage gated or not regulatable (see Fig. 4–32). There is also an internal releasable calcium pool in a nonmitochondrial, non–endoplasmic reticulum intracellular compartment. This compartment involves small membrane vesicles termed *calciosomes* that are similar to those in the sarcoplasmic reticulum of muscle. This internal releasable pool of calcium is the major means by which IP_3 regulates cytoplasmic calcium levels. About 50% of the calcium in this compartment is releasable on IP_3 stimulation, and the remainder is discharged only in the presence of ionophores. The intracellular IP_3 generated by interactions of ligand, membrane, receptor, and G protein induces this calcium release by binding to an IP_3 receptor (approximately 260 kd in size) in the calciosome.[250] The IP_3 receptor and calcium channel activities may reside in the same protein.

In addition to transient increases in intracellular calcium levels induced by IP_3, calcium waves initiated by the IP_3 interaction may be further propagated by a calcium-sensitive, IP_3-insensitive calcium pool[251] (see Fig. 4–32). The action of IP_3 is attenuated by metabolism of IP_3 to an inactive inositol bisphosphate (see Fig. 4–31). IP_3 may also be converted to inositol 1,3,4,5-tetrakisphosphate via the action of IP_3 kinase, which phosphorylates IP_3 in the presence of ATP. Inositol 1,3,4,5-tetrakisphosphate, however, may not be inactive and may serve to augment the effect of IP_3 by increasing the transfer of calcium among intracellular pools.[252] Thus ave-

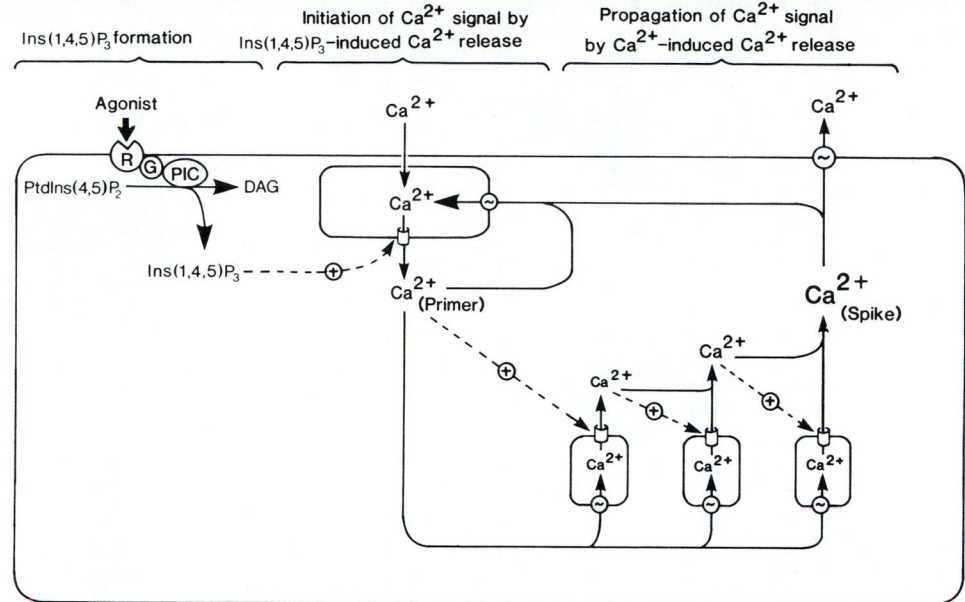

Figure 4–32. Calcium (Ca^{2+}) signaling initiated by the generation of IP_3. Activation of phospholipase C results in an increase in cellular levels of IP_3 ($Ins(1,4,5)P_3$ in figure). IP_3 then releases calcium from a cytosolic, P_3-sensitive pool and promotes influx of external calcium. Transient elevations in cytosolic calcium may trigger or prime the further release of calcium from P_3-insensitive pools to result in intracellular calcium waves and oscillations. (From Berridge MJ, Irvine RF. Inositol phosphates and cell signalling. Reprinted by permission from Nature vol. 341 pp. 197–204 Copyright © 1989 Macmillan Magazines Ltd.)

nues for both augmentation and reduction in signal activity are inherent in the phosphatidylinositol turnover pathway.

CALCIUM-DEPENDENT KINASE. Ultimately both the inositol phosphate derivatives and calcium interact with specific protein kinases and produce phosphorylation-mediated actions.[253] Calcium/calmodulin-dependent protein kinases exist in at least five forms in mammalian systems.[254] These forms serve to mediate calcium-dependent changes in kinase activity. The action of phospholipase C on phosphatidylinositol 4,5-bisphosphate also results in the production of DAG, which serves to activate protein kinase C.[247, 255] DAG, like the tumor-promoting phorbol esters, greatly augments the ability of protein kinase C to bind calcium and phosphatidylserine and thus allows activation of the enzyme at low intracellular calcium levels.[256] Calcium further augments the ability of DAG to activate protein kinase C, perhaps by altering the specificity of phospholipase C to cleave phosphatidylinositol monophosphate, as well as phosphatidylinositol 4,5-bisphosphate, thereby increasing the production of DAG. In addition, calcium may sensitize protein kinase C to DAG activation. The protein kinase C then continues to phosphorylate other intracellular proteins in a fashion similar to calcium/calmodulin-dependent protein kinases. Together these act on a wide variety of metabolic pathways in both the cytosol and the nucleus.

PROTEIN KINASE C. Part of the diversity of this pathway comes from the fact that protein kinase C is not a single enzyme but a family of related isozymes. The enzymes are approximately 80 kd in size and are encoded by at least three (and probably six or seven) different genes.[257, 258] Furthermore, alternative splicing may result in even greater complexity of these forms. These protein kinase C isozymes are expressed in a tissue-specific fashion and thus may play a role in the differential effects of DAG stimulation of protein kinase C in different tissues. Protein kinase C may also be stimulated by substances other than DAG, including unsaturated fatty acids, such as arachidonic acid, which is derived from the breakdown of phosphatidylcholine, and related compounds via the phospholipase A_2–phosphatidylcholine system, again providing a mechanism for interaction between different signaling pathways.

The DAG activation of protein kinase C may also help intracellular calcium levels return to normal by stimulating calcium pump activity and/or by decreasing IP_3 production.

Another interesting aspect of IP_3 and DAG interactions involves the ability of membrane potential changes within cells to alter IP_3 metabolism.[247, 255] Furthermore, stimulation of IP_3 can augment cAMP generation via adenylate cyclase–linked receptors and vice versa. Also, the activity of DAG can be attenuated by the conversion of DAG to phosphatidate via DAG kinase. This interaction results in the resynthesis of phosphatidylinositols and a reduction in intracellular protein kinase C activity. The structure of DAG kinase has been elucidated.[259] Like protein kinase C, it is 80 kd in size and possesses an ATP binding site and two cysteine-rich zinc finger–like motifs. It also contains two motifs that are typical of calcium-binding proteins, called E-F hand motifs. DAG kinase activity is increased in the presence of calcium. A number of protein tyrosine kinases may also stimulate phosphatidylinositol kinase activity, which leads to activation of the calcium-DAG pathway. This pathway remains to be elucidated in greater detail.

Receptors and Ion Channels

Ion channels including those that control potassium, sodium, and calcium fluxes at the plasma membrane level may be regulated by charge gradients across the cell membrane, i.e., voltage gated, or by binding of hormones and neurotransmitters to the channel or associated receptors, i.e., ligand gated.[260–262] The ligand-gated ion changes represent a distinct class of membrane receptors and may or may not require G proteins for signal transduction. The ligand-gated ion channels include the nicotinic cholinergic, $GABA_a$, glycine, glutamate, and kainic acid receptors.

The best studied of the ligand-gated ion channels is the nicotinic cholinergic receptor, which was first described for *Torpedo californica*.[52] This receptor consists of five glycosylated subunits, two of which are identical (Fig. 4–33). The interaction of nicotinic cholinergic agonists with the receptor activates a cation channel inherent in the receptor structure. The subunits of the nicotinic cholinergic receptor are encoded by separate genes. The molecular sizes of the α, β, γ, and δ subunits are 40, 48, 58, and 64 kd, respectively. Each receptor subunit possesses a high degree of similarity, including four transmembrane spanning domains. The second transmembrane spanning domain may form the lining for the ion pore. As a pentameric complex, the $α_2βγδ$ ligand-

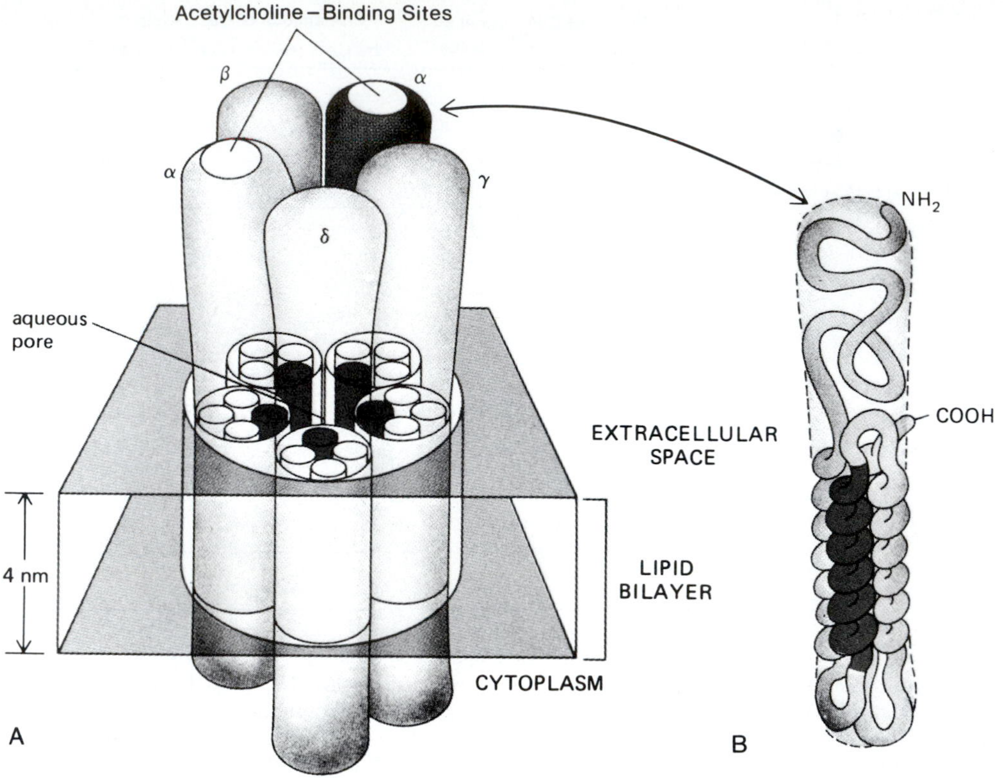

Figure 4–33. Schematic diagram of the nicotinic acetylcholine receptor. *A*, The receptor is composed of five subunits arranged in a pentagonal array to form the aqueous pore. The two α subunits interact with ligand. *B*, Each subunit contains alpha-helical regions that span the plasma membrane with four hydrophobic domains. In addition, there is along NH$_2$-terminal extracellular region, and one of the transmembrane regions in each subunit serves to line the pore.

gated ion channel has a molecular size of approximately 250 kd. Each receptor requires two agonist molecules, each binding to an α subunit, to induce a rapid conductance change.

The basic subunit structures of the other known ligand-gated ion channels are homologous to the nicotinic receptor. The GABA$_a$ and glycine receptors, which mediate inhibitory activity in the central nervous system, contain structurally similar subunits. The α subunits of the GABA$_a$ receptor have 75% homology to the acetylcholine receptor, whereas the α, β, γ, and δ subunits are 30 to 40% homologous. In addition, the GABA$_a$ α subunit shares 35% homology with the similar subunit of the glycine receptor. Thus the ligand-gated ion channels appear to be derived from a common ancestral gene.

Each subunit of the ligand-gated channel receptors contains an extensive extracellular NH$_2$-terminal domain with multiple sites of glycosylation. This structure is reminiscent of that in a number of G protein–linked receptors. There is a large intracytoplasmic loop located between trans-membrane regions 3 and 4 that contains multiple sites for phosphorylation, which suggests a role for regulation by cellular protein kinases. The COOH terminus of most subunits is short and is located in the cytoplasmic space.

Some ligand-gated ion channels require the involvement of G proteins as signal transducers.[248, 263–266] For instance, the muscarinic cholinergic–regulated potassium channel and the beta-adrenergic–gated calcium channel in the heart involve the participation of poorly characterized G proteins.

Receptors of Unknown Effector Function

A number of peptide hormones and growth factors bind to membrane receptors whose signaling mechanism remains poorly understood.

GROWTH HORMONE AND PROLACTIN RECEPTOR SYSTEMS. GH is a pleiotypic hormone that is thought to act primarily by stimulating the synthesis and release into the circulation of insulin-like growth factors (IGF I and IGF II) by liver and other tissues.[267] Although the GH receptor may be tyrosine phosphorylated and may possess tyrosine kinase activity,[268] the elucidation of its primary structure by purification and cDNA cloning has not supported this hypothesis.[65] In rabbit liver the GH receptor is a 130-kd protein different in structure from all of the classes of receptors described earlier. It consists of 620 amino acids divided into a 246-residue extracellular domain, a single transmembrane domain of 24 amino acids, and an intracellular domain of about 350 residues (Fig. 4–34). The extracellular domain possesses several potential sites of *N*-linked and *O*-linked glycosylation, as in most membrane receptors, but there are no cysteine-rich regions or obvious repeating structures. Likewise, the intracellular domain bears no resemblance to receptors of known functional type. The difference between the apparent molecular size (130 kd) and the predicted size by amino acid composition (70 kd) is thought to be due to a high level of glycosylation and covalent association of the receptor with ubiquitin. When expressed in mammalian cells, the human GH receptor binds only human GH, whereas the rabbit receptor binds human GH, bovine GH, and ovine prolactin.[65] This result correlates with the known species specificity of GH.[269]

The prolactin receptor in liver is also a single transmembrane polypeptide with 210 amino acids on the extracellular face but only 58 amino acids in the cytoplasm.[66] It has four homologous regions in the extracellular domain, but only one homologous region in the intracellular domain (see Fig. 4–34). Like the GH receptor, the prolactin receptor has no known functional signaling elements. In mammary tissue there is a larger form of the prolactin receptor, highly homologous to the GH receptor, which is probably the product of alternative splicing. Also, as a result of alternative splicing, secretory forms of both the GH and the prolactin receptors exist that contain no transmembrane or intracellular domains.[65, 66]

NERVE GROWTH FACTOR RECEPTOR. The nerve

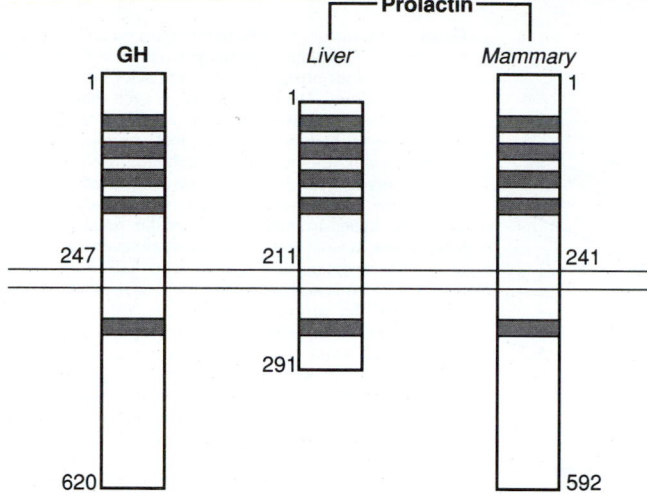

Figure 4–34. Comparison of structures for the prolactin and GH receptors. The hatched areas represent homologous regions. (Data from Leung DW, Spencer SA, Cachianes G, et al. Growth hormone receptor and serum binding protein: purification, cloning and expression. Nature 1987; 330:537–543; Boutin JM, Jolicoeur C, Okamura H, et al. Cloning and expression of the rat prolactin receptor, a member of the growth hormone/prolactin receptor gene family. Cell 1988; 53:69–77; and personal communication, P. Kelley.)

growth factor receptor is a unique protein but has some features in common with other growth factor receptors.[270] The extracellular domain has a cysteine-rich region similar to that of EGF and insulin receptors. The cytoplasmic domain is much shorter than that of the other growth factor receptors (about 152 amino acids), lacks an ATP binding domain, and is not homologous to any of the tyrosine kinase– or G protein–coupled receptors. Although phosphorylation of the nerve growth factor receptor on serine and threonine residues has been reported, this phosphorylation appears to be insensitive to nerve growth factor. The mechanism of signal transduction by this receptor remains unknown.

MEMBRANE RECEPTORS AND DISEASE

Receptor Regulation and Desensitization

Both the number and affinity of peptide hormone receptors, as well as postbinding steps in hormone action, are regulated by a number of physiological factors that have important roles in coordinating receptor activity with the overall metabolic state of the cell and in limiting hormone action. In a variety of pathological states, regulatory responses of receptors can lead to abnormalities in hormone responsiveness that cause or contribute to clinical disorders. Most of these disease states are characterized by decreased hormone action or hormone resistance, rather than increased hormone responsiveness. Because physiological and pathological insulin receptor regulation has been most extensively studied, we review this regulation in detail here (summarized in Table 4–8). It should be considered, however, simply as a model system that is representative of peptide hormone receptors in general. In addition we consider disorders of G protein–mediated responses and GH receptors and disorders mediated by specificity spillover or antireceptor antibodies.

Insulin Receptor Regulation

The pathways involved in regulation of insulin receptors have been discussed in detail in the foregoing sections of this chapter. The cell-surface receptor number is down-regulated in response to extracellular insulin, apparently as a result of the internalization of insulin-receptor complexes, with subsequent degradation to some degree of both insulin and the receptor.[103, 107] The binding affinity of the insulin receptor is affected by many factors including extracellular insulin,[107] other hormones such as glucocorticoids,[271] fasting,[272] exercise,[273] and diet composition[274] (see Table 4–4). In contrast to changes in receptor number, which appear to derive from modifications in the normal pathways of receptor synthesis and degradation, the molecular mechanisms that lead to altered binding affinity are less well defined. Binding affinity of the insulin receptor is inversely related to plasma membrane fluidity,[275] and some of the physiological regulation of binding affinity may result from altered physical properties of the membrane.[276] Even less is known about insulin receptor regulation at the postbinding level, although serine phosphorylation and possibly other modifications in the receptor may alter tyrosine kinase activity and the intrinsic activity of the receptor itself.

OBESITY. Insulin resistance is common in obesity[277] and appears to result from alterations in both receptor number and postbinding receptor activity.[278–283] Lower numbers of insulin binding sites are present in monocytes and adipocytes from obese patients[279, 280] and in a variety of animal models of obesity.[281] Characteristically, circulating insulin levels are elevated and correlate inversely with insulin receptor number[272] (Fig. 4–35). If insulin levels are lowered, for

TABLE 4–8. Involvement of Insulin Receptors in Disorders of Glucose Tolerance and Insulin Sensitivity

I. Target cell dominates (i.e., plasma hormone concentration discordant with clinical state)
  A. Insulin resistance
    1. Moderate resistance
      a. Clinical
        (1) Obesity
        (2) Diabetes mellitus, obese and thin
        (3) Acromegaly
        (4) Glucocorticoid excess
      b. Experimental animals
        (1) Glucocorticoid excess
        (2) GH excess
        (3) Uremia
    2. Extreme resistance
      a. Immunological (antireceptor antibodies)
        (1) Type B
        (2) Ataxia telangiectasia
        (3) Immunoglobulin A or E deficiency
        (4) New Zealand obese mouse
      b. Not immunological (? genetic)
        (1) Type A
        (2) Leprechaunism
        (3) Lipoatrophic diabetes
        (4) Rabson-Mendenhall syndrome
  B. Insulin supersensitivity
      (1) Anorexia nervosa
      (2) Glucocorticoid deficiency (in experimental animals)
      (3) GH deficiency
II. Hormone dominates (i.e., plasma hormone concentration concordant with clinical state)
  A. Insulin deficiency
      a. Clinical
        (1) Type I (insulin-dependent) diabetes mellitus
        (2) Pancreatic diabetes (e.g., chronic pancreatitis)
      b. Experimental animals
        (1) Streptozocin-induced hypoinsulinemia
        (2) Hypoinsulinemic diabetic Chinese hamster
  B. Insulin excess
      (1) Insulinoma
      (2) Infants of diabetic mothers
      (3) Other hypoglycemias in newborns
      (4) Chronic insulin excess in experimental animals
  C. Disorders of receptor design (specifically spillover)
      (1) Infants of diabetic mothers
      (2) Non–islet cell tumors with hypoglycemia

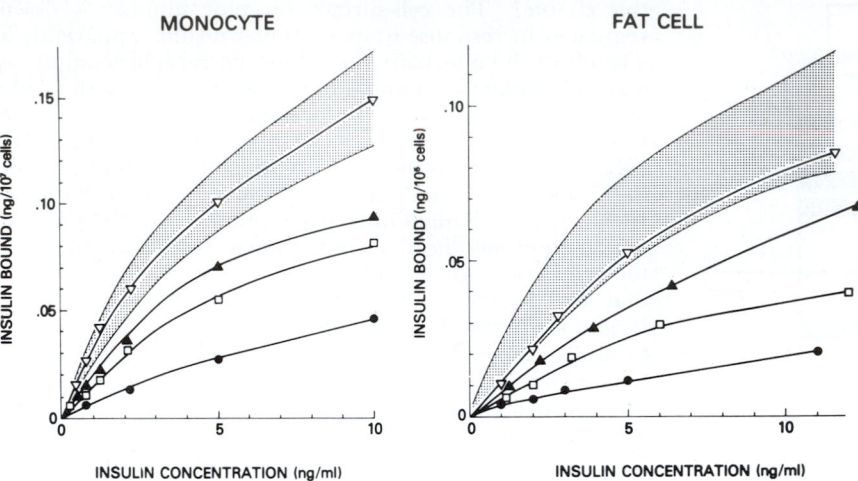

Figure 4–35. Insulin binding to receptors on cells of obese patients. *A*, Circulating monocytes. *B*, Adipocytes. For each graph, four obese patients were selected to show a range of findings. The upper curve in each represents an obese patient who was indistinguishable from normal; these patients had normal receptors, normal levels of plasma insulin, and normal sensitivity to insulin. The two middle curves in each graph show a moderate decrease in receptor concentration, which was associated with moderate hyperinsulinemia and insulin resistance. The lower curve in each graph shows a more severe deficiency of insulin receptors in a patient who had more severe hyperinsulinemia and insulin resistance. Dietary treatment (600 kcal/d) for several weeks (not shown) is associated with restoration of receptor concentration to normal (or near-normal) levels. To convert insulin values from nanograms per milliliter to picomoles per liter, multiply by 1.722×10^5. (From Bar RS, Harrison LC, Muggeo M, et al. Regulation of insulin receptors in normal and abnormal physiology in humans. Adv Intern Med 1978; 24:23–52.)

example by diet or drugs that interfere with insulin secretion, the receptor number returns to normal even though the degree of obesity may not be significantly changed.[282] This change suggests that the decreased number of insulin receptors in insulin-resistant obese patients may result from the effects of excess insulin on normal pathways of receptor down-regulation. In addition, coexistent postbinding defects in insulin action can be demonstrated in euglycemic clamp studies.[284, 285] These defects may have their basis in postbinding pathways of receptor signaling, or in true postreceptor sites, such as in the glucose transport system. The exact mechanism of the latter has not been identified. The observation that insulin receptor number can be restored to normal if insulin levels are decreased in obese patients suggests that the changes in receptor number are secondary to the insulin resistance and not a primary causal factor. Possibly, the postbinding alterations in insulin action in obesity initiate resistance to the hormone, insulin levels rise as a compensatory response, and this increase results in a decrease in insulin receptor number and more profound insulin resistance.

TYPE II DIABETES MELLITUS. Type II diabetes mellitus is characterized by resistance to insulin in both obese and nonobese individuals.[283] Many type II diabetics have low levels of insulin by the time disease is fully manifested, but some patients have elevated insulin levels in association with glucose intolerance, presumably reflecting insulin resistance. The cellular abnormalities associated with insulin resistance of type II diabetes in patients with elevated insulin levels are similar to those in obesity, with both decreased receptor number and impaired postbinding insulin action.[284, 285] In patients who do not have elevated insulin levels, receptor number is not markedly decreased, and insulin resistance appears to result primarily from postbinding abnormalities. Because the majority of type II diabetics are obese, the common occurrence of insulin resistance is not unexpected, and a similar underlying abnormality may exist in both obesity and type II diabetes mellitus. This parallel with obesity cannot explain all insulin resistance in type II diabetes, however, because nonobese diabetics may also be insulin resistant.[283] Independent of obesity, defects in insulin action in type II diabetes may result from both decreased receptor tyrosine kinase activity (Fig. 4–36) and defects in postreceptor steps in insulin action.[286–289] Thus the insulin resistance of type II diabetes mellitus represents a complex of a number of altered hormone action pathways. Which, if any, of these alterations is primary remains to be determined.

OTHER DISORDERS. With the exception of insulin-resistant states associated with antireceptor antibodies (see later), most other acquired disorders of insulin responsiveness appear to be explained by alterations in postreceptor pathways with or without some alteration in receptor function (see Table 4–8). These other disorders include states of glucocorticoid excess[290–292] and GH excess,[293] uremia,[294] and diabetic ketoacidosis.[295] For a more complete discussion of these disorders, the reader is referred to Chapter 24.

Genetic Defects in Receptors

SYNDROMES OF INSULIN RESISTANCE. At least three syndromes of severe insulin resistance appear to result from genetic defects in the insulin receptor or insulin action pathways. These disorders include the type A syndrome of insulin resistance, leprechaunism, and lipoatrophic diabetes.

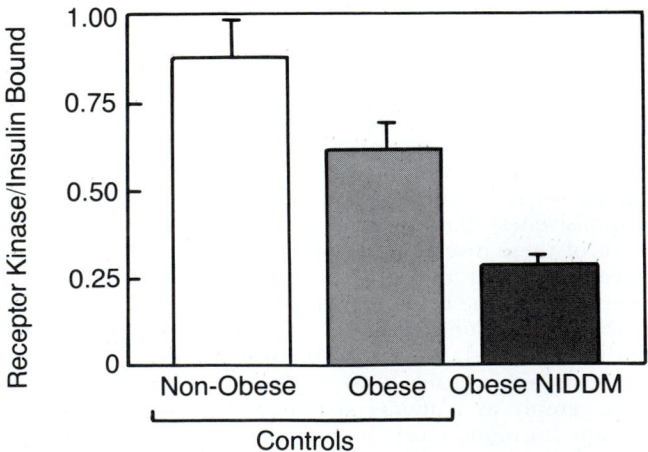

Figure 4–36. Insulin receptor tyrosine kinase activity in liver biopsy specimens from normal and obese humans and those with type II diabetes mellitus (Obese NIDDM). The data are expressed as kinase activity per insulin bound to correct for the decrease in receptor number. Note that kinase activity is still decreased in type II diabetes even allowing for this change. (From Caro JF, Ittoop O, Pories WJ, et al. Studies on the mechanism of insulin resistance in the liver from humans with noninsulin-dependent diabetes. Reproduced from the Journal of Clinical Investigation, 1986, vol. 78, pp. 249–258 by copyright permission of the American Society of Clinical Investigation.)

TABLE 4–9. Clinical Syndromes of Extreme Insulin Resistance That Result from Genetic Defects in the Insulin Receptor or Insulin Action Pathways

Syndrome	Clinical Features
Type A syndrome	Glucose intolerance, acanthosis nigricans, hyperandrogenism
Lipoatrophic diabetes	Glucose intolerance, atrophy of subcutaneous fat, hypertriglyceridemia, acanthosis nigricans, hyperandrogenism
Leprechaunism	Intrauterine growth retardation, "leprechaun" facies, paradoxical fasting hypoglycemia, mild hirsutism, and hyperandrogenism

In addition to insulin resistance and glucose intolerance or overt diabetes, these syndromes share a number of common features including variable degrees of acanthosis nigricans and hyperandrogenism (Table 4–9). Until recently, understanding of genetic disorders of insulin resistance has been primarily descriptive, but, with the development of new techniques for molecular cloning, multiple specific defects in insulin receptors have been defined for these patients.

Type A Syndrome. The type A syndrome of insulin resistance has been described as including extreme insulin resistance, acanthosis nigricans, and hyperandrogenism occurring in the absence of obesity or lipoatrophy.[200] It is distinguished from type B insulin resistance by the lack of antibodies to the insulin receptor or other evidence of autoimmune disease. Even before the identification of specific molecular defects in patients with type A insulin resistance, biochemical evidence suggested that this group of disorders is heterogeneous. Patients usually have a decreased number of insulin receptors, presumably as a result of a defect in receptor biosynthesis.[200, 296] In some patients, however, receptor levels are normal, and receptor tyrosine kinase activity is decreased[201, 202, 297] (see Fig. 4–26). In others, an abnormal, unprocessed insulin receptor has been demonstrated.[298] Even in patients with decreased receptor number, insulin receptor mRNA levels vary from decreased to normal.[296] This heterogeneity is the result of specific mutations in the insulin receptor gene.

Several such mutations have been described (Fig. 4–37). In one patient, a genetic recombination event appears to have occurred, with a resulting loss of the complete tyrosine kinase domain of the insulin receptor coded for by one of the two alleles.[299] In another patient, a point mutation resulted in the substitution of valine for glycine in a critical part of the ATP binding site of the receptor β subunit;[300] this mutation produces a marked decrease in tyrosine kinase activity of the receptor.[300] Both of these patients also have decreased receptor number, which suggests that there may be an abnormality in the second insulin receptor allele or a suppressive effect of the mutant receptor on normal receptor expression. In a third patient with the type A syndrome of insulin resistance, a point mutation converted the sequence of the prorecptor cleavage site from Arg-Lys-Arg-Arg to Arg-Lys-Arg-Ser.[298, 301] This change results in the accumulation of unprocessed receptor. This prorecptor binds insulin ineffectively and also has reduced insulin-stimulated kinase activity. Additional mutational defects are being defined in the insulin receptors of patients with the type A syndrome of insulin resistance. It is also likely, however, that some patients have defects in proteins other than the receptor in the insulin action pathway that modify either receptor function or postreceptor pathways.

Leprechaunism. The syndrome of leprechaunism is also likely due to heterogeneous genetic defects. In addition to insulin resistance and other features shared with patients with the type A syndrome (see Table 4–9), patients with leprechaunism have intrauterine and neonatal growth retardation and a clinical course complicated by fasting hypoglycemia that is frequently fatal within the first year of life.[302] In one of these patients, insulin resistance was shown to result from a compound heterozygous state with two mutant insulin receptor alleles.[303] In one allele a missense mutation converts Lys-460 to Glu-460 in the receptor α subunit, and in the second allele a nonsense mutation in the α subunit leads to chain termination.

The specific mechanisms through which mutations in the insulin receptor lead to the leprechaun phenotype have not been defined. The prominent growth retardation in these patients suggests that growth and metabolic regulation pathways are affected by the genetic defects. In some pa-

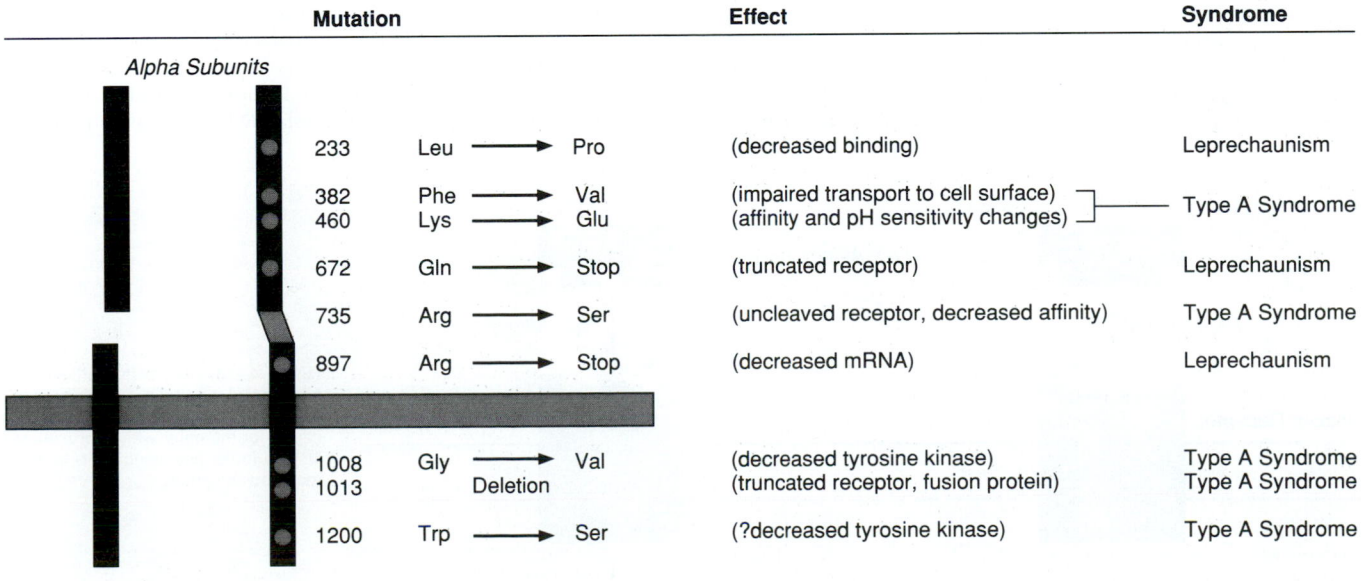

Figure 4–37. Mutations in the insulin receptor associated with clinical syndromes of insulin resistance. Note that the two mutations Val-382 and Glu-460 occur in a single patient (compound heterozygote). See text for further description.

tients the responses to IGF I, EGF, and other growth factors are decreased, which suggests a defect in common postreceptor pathways.[304] Alternatively, abnormal insulin receptors may somehow interact with other receptors and modulate their function.[219, 305] It is certain that additional genetic defects will be defined in patients with type A insulin resistance, leprechaunism, and also lipoatrophic diabetes. An understanding of such specific genetic abnormalities will provide insights into normal receptor and postreceptor events in insulin action, in addition to explaining the basis for these rare disorders.

PSEUDOHYPOPARATHYROIDISM. Pseudohypoparathyroidism is an inherited disorder of parathyroid hormone (PTH) resistance that was initially described in 1942.[306] At that time, Fuller Albright hypothesized that the disorder is the result of target organ unresponsiveness to hormone, although this hypothesis was made before the identification of cell-surface receptors and effector systems for any hormone.[306] It is now recognized that the prototypical features of PTH resistance and hereditary osteodystrophy occur in only a subset of affected individuals and that other individuals manifest PTH resistance with different phenotypic and biochemical expression (see Chapter 27).

Patients with pseudohypoparathyroidism type Ia have diminished levels of G_s that is necessary for coupling the PTH receptor to the catalytic subunit of adenylate cyclase.[307–309] Levels of the α subunit of G_s mRNA are also reduced in affected subjects.[310] This protein is shared by a number of adenylate cyclase–coupled receptors, and, as expected, patients with G_s deficiency characteristically exhibit resistance to multiple hormones including TSH, glucagon, and gonadotropins. Another subgroup of patients with pseudohypoparathyroidism may have a defect in the catalytic subunit of adenylate cyclase.[311] As in insulin resistance, it is likely that the clinical syndrome of pseudohypoparathyroidism will ultimately be attributable to the effects of heterogeneous genetic abnormalities affecting the PTH receptor, coupling mechanisms, and postreceptor pathways.

LARON-TYPE DWARFISM. The syndrome of Laron-type dwarfism is characterized by decreased somatic growth evident from the first months of life and clinical features similar to those in patients with isolated GH deficiency.[312, 313] In contrast to GH-deficient patients, however, circulating levels of GH are elevated in patients with Laron-type dwarfism, and instead the GH-dependent somatomedins appear to be deficient.[314] The GH molecule itself is normal, which suggests that GH receptors may be defective.[315, 316] Subsequently, GH receptors were shown to be markedly deficient in hepatic tissue of most affected subjects.[317] Subjects with Laron-type

dwarfism also have decreased levels of a circulating GH-binding protein that is thought to be derived from the cell-surface receptor.[318] This finding is most consistent with a mutation that leads to either decreased synthesis or accelerated degradation of the receptor protein. On the basis of expanding knowledge of inherited peptide hormone receptor defects, it can be predicted that Laron-type dwarfism will prove to be due to a mutated GH receptor and that heterogeneous mutations in different patients will lead to similar but slightly different clinical phenotypes. It can also be predicted that similar defects will be described for other peptide hormone receptors. Some of these may produce significant clinical symptoms, whereas others may have minor clinical consequences.

Specificity Spillover Syndromes

Peptide hormone receptors provide mechanisms for transduction of hormone signals and also for specificity of biological responses through the high-affinity binding of the respective hormones. Because the receptors interact with intracellular pathways, under most circumstances the receptor plays a more important role than does the hormone in determining the pattern of biological responses. As evident from the foregoing sections of this chapter, receptors for different hormones and the peptide hormones themselves can be classified into families with structural similarities that reflect evolution from common ancestral molecules. These structural homologies can result in the binding of a given hormone to the receptors for another hormone, albeit with lower affinity. This crossover of hormone binding is illustrated for insulin, IGF I, and their respective receptors in Figure 4–38. In diseases in which there are elevated hormone levels, syndromes of specificity spillover can result from the activation of receptors for one hormone via low-affinity binding of another hormone.[319]

Several examples of specificity spillover syndromes are described in Table 4–10. In acromegaly, high levels of GH lead to abnormal tissue growth through the activation of GH receptors. In a significant number of patients, there is also evidence of excess prolactin activity, with resulting galactorrhea, amenorrhea, and infertility. In some cases these changes result from concurrent elevations of both GH and prolactin levels, but in others prolactin levels are normal and the apparent hyperprolactinemia syndrome is best explained by binding of GH to prolactin receptors.[320] Similar hormone-receptor cross-reactivity appears to explain the occurrence of hyperthyroidism in some patients with trophoblastic tumors.[321, 322] Trophoblastic tumor tissue produces

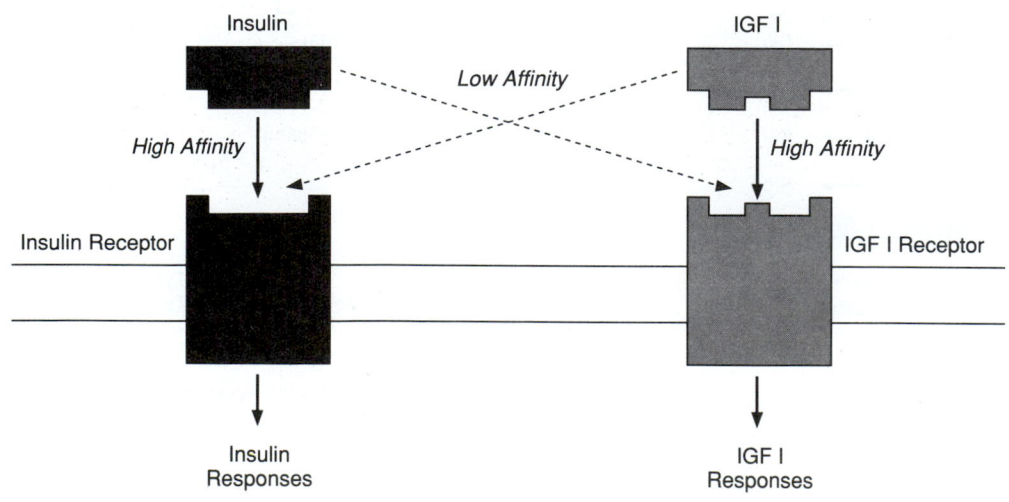

Figure 4–38. Specificity spillover between insulin and IGF I. Each hormone binds to and activates the specific receptor for the other with approximately 10-fold lower potency than its own homologous receptor.

TABLE 4–10. Specificity Spillover Syndromes Involving Peptide Hormones

Hormone	Cross-Reacting Receptor	Clinical Syndrome
GH	Prolactin	Galactorrhea (with acromegaly)
Human chorionic gonadotropin	TSH	Hyperthyroidism (with trophoblastic tumors)
Insulin	IGF I (in ovary)	Hyperandrogenism (with insulin resistance)
Insulin	IGF I (?)	Macrosomia (in newborn infants of diabetic mothers)
IGF II	Insulin and/or IGF I	Hypoglycemia (with certain tumors)

large quantities of human chorionic gonadotropin, which can bind with low affinity to the TSH receptor, but, in addition, in other cases variants of human chorionic gonadotropin are produced that exhibit even greater affinity for TSH receptors than does the human chorionic gonadotropin of normal pregnancy.[323] Nonpancreatic neoplasms that produce large quantities of IGF II can lead to significant specificity spillover and hypoglycemia, although it is not clear whether this results from the binding of IGF II to insulin receptors, IGF I receptors, or both.[324–326] Other disorders that may be due to specificity spillover include the hyperandrogenism of certain forms of severe insulin resistance (cross-reactivity of insulin with ovarian IGF I receptors)[327] and possibly macrosomia in infants of diabetic mothers (insulin cross-reactivity with IGF I receptors in somatic tissues).[328] Additional specificity spillover syndromes will probably be recognized as knowledge of peptide hormone receptors increases.

Antireceptor Antibodies

Immunological abnormalities are associated with a broad spectrum of endocrine disorders. Antibodies against endocrine tissue components have been demonstrated in a number of endocrine deficiency states, including type I diabetes mellitus,[329] adrenal insufficiency,[330] Hashimoto thyroiditis,[331–332] and some forms of gonadal insufficiency.[332–333] These antibodies provide valuable clues to the existence of specific endocrine disorders, often before hormone deficiency can be detected, but in most cases the role of specific antibodies in endocrine tissue destruction has not been clearly established. Thus it is not certain whether specific anti–endocrine tissue antibodies are markers of disease or whether they have a pathogenetic role.

In a subgroup of autoimmune endocrine disorders antireceptor antibodies play an important role in the development of clinical states of deficient or excess hormone action.[333] Disorders resulting from antireceptor antibodies have been described for peptide hormone receptors (insulin, TSH), for beta-adrenergic receptors, and for neurotransmitter receptors (acetylcholine) and are summarized in Table 4–11. In experimental systems, antibodies have been generated against additional receptors (prolactin, EGF) that may provide models for yet undescribed human diseases. These antibodies may mimic the action of the normal hormone ligand or may inhibit ligand action by blocking receptor binding, accelerating receptor turnover, or inducing receptor or postreceptor desensitization (Fig. 4–39). Although the basis for the antireceptor endocrine disorders has not been defined, it is likely related to some alteration in specific immune response genes because some patients exhibit more than one type of autoimmune disease.

INSULIN RECEPTOR ANTIBODIES. Antibodies to the insulin receptor were first identified in patients with severe insulin resistance and a cluster of other clinical findings termed the type B syndrome of insulin resistance.[334, 335] This syndrome is characterized by glucose intolerance and diabetes mellitus, insulin levels 10 to 100 times higher than normal in both basal and stimulated states, and resistance to injected insulin. In addition these patients commonly have a skin disorder termed acanthosis nigricans, in which there is dermal thickening and hyperpigmentation in the axillae and skin folds in other body regions. Acanthosis may result from the effects of insulin on cutaneous tissues. Patients with type B insulin resistance typically are middle-aged women with other evidence of autoimmune disease that may include alopecia, vitiligo, Raynaud phenomenon, arthralgias and arthritis, splenomegaly, antinuclear and anti-DNA antibodies, and elevated erythrocyte sedimentation rate.

Most patients have high levels of polyclonal immunoglobulin antibodies that bind to the insulin receptor and block hormone binding. Studies in vitro have shown that antibody binding to the receptor is followed initially by metabolic effects that mimic the response to insulin binding.[90, 336, 337] Subsequently, the antibodies appear to induce receptor internalization, down-regulation, and postbinding desensitization, thus resulting in hormone unresponsiveness. A chronic down-regulated and desensitized state appears to predominate in vivo and thus explain the clinically evident insulin resistance.

The investigation of antibody-receptor interactions in type B insulin resistance provided insight into the mechanisms of receptor activation. These antibodies mimic hormone effects only when present in a bivalent form.[90] Monovalent (Fab) antibody fragments bind to receptors and block hormone binding but do not stimulate postreceptor responses (see Fig. 4–9). This finding indicates the potentially important role for the association of receptors and receptor-receptor interactions in the initiation of tissue responses. In some patients, anti–insulin receptor antibodies result in excess receptor stimulation and hypoglycemia rather than insulin resistance.[337, 338] Hypoglycemia can be the presenting finding or can evolve in the course of a disease that initially presents with insulin resistance. The spectrum of clinical

TABLE 4–11. Clinical Syndromes Associated with Naturally Occurring Antibodies to Cell-Surface Receptors

Syndrome	Receptor	Clinical Features
Type B insulin resistance	Insulin	Insulin-resistant diabetes, acanthosis nigricans, other evidence of autoimmune disease (e.g., vitiligo, alopecia)
Ataxia telangiectasia	Insulin	Insulin-resistant diabetes, progressive ataxia, telangiectasia
Graves disease	TSH	Thyrotoxicosis (stimulatory antibody, possible passage through phases of hypothyroidism secondary to inhibitory antibodies)
Asthma (some cases)	Beta-adrenergic	Bronchospasm
Myasthenia gravis	Acetylcholine	Muscle weakness

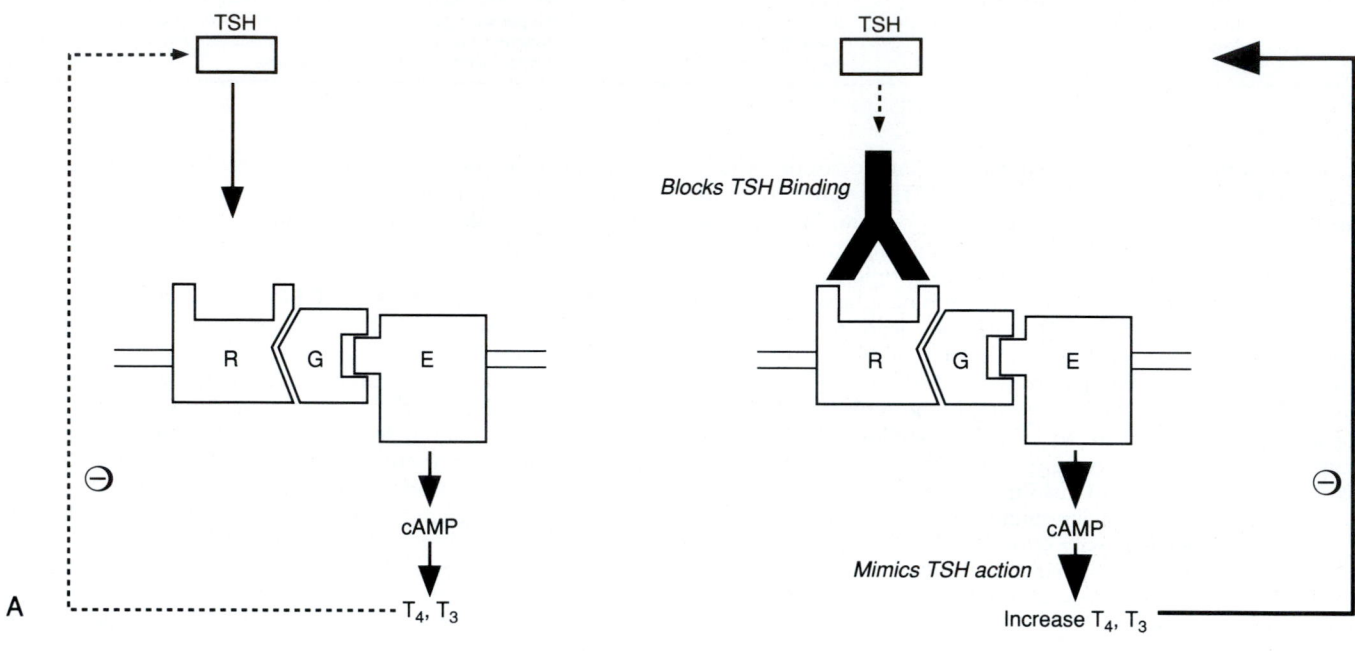

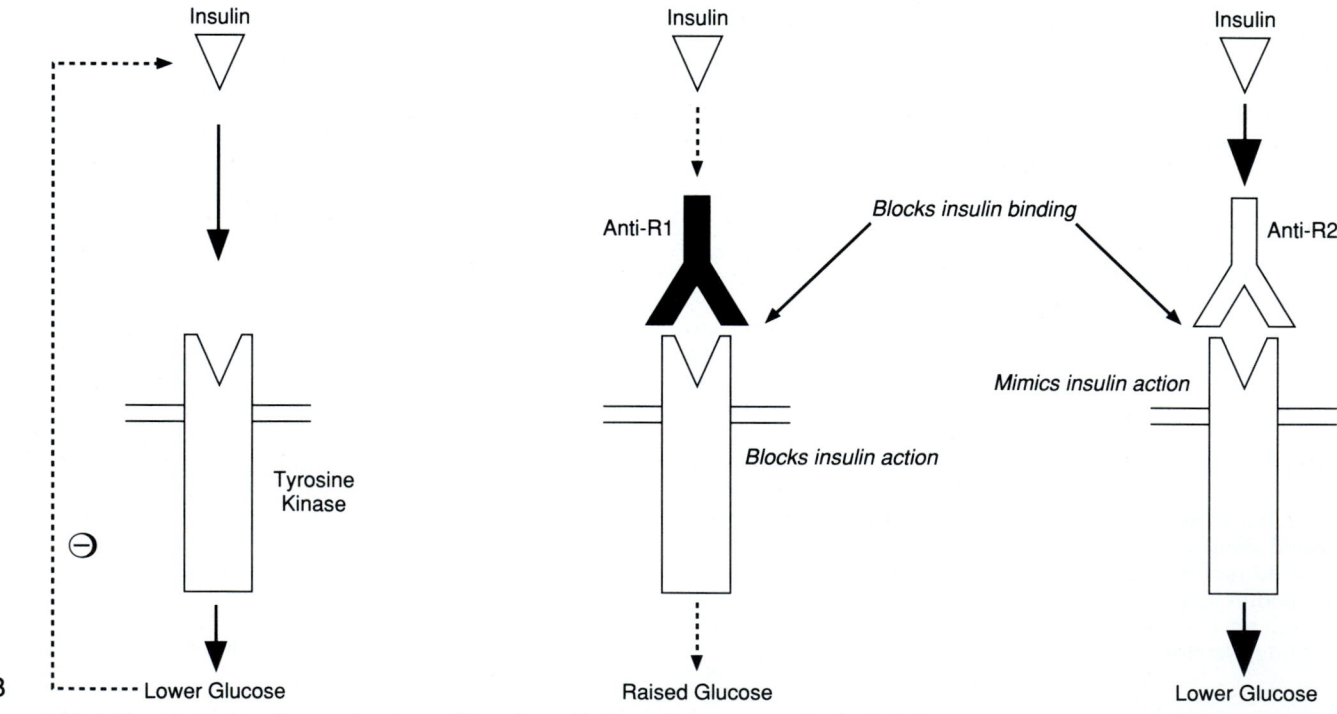

Figure 4–39. *A,* Thyroid stimulators in normal persons and in patients with Graves disease. In normal individuals the pituitary releases TSH, which binds to its specific receptors (R) on the surface of thyroid cells and stimulates intracellular events that lead to release of triiodothyronine (T_3) and thyroxine (T_4). Thyroid hormones, among their many effects, act on the hypothalamus and the pituitary to reduce TSH secretion (negative feedback). In patients with Graves disease, autoantibodies bind to the TSH receptor and stimulate the same intracellular pathways as TSH, which results in release of thyroid hormones (triiodothyronine, thyroxine) even in the absence of TSH. Typically, elevated levels of thyroid hormones suppress TSH secretion but have no effect on circulating levels of thyroid-stimulating immunoglobulins. *B,* Insulin receptor autoantibodies block insulin binding and may block or mimic insulin action. These antibodies may produce hyperglycemia or hypoglycemia and may be associated with low, normal, or high plasma insulin levels.

findings from insulin resistance to hypoglycemia reflects the properties of specific antibodies that are predominant at a given point in time.

A second form of insulin resistance secondary to anti–insulin receptor antibodies has been described in patients with ataxia telangiectasia.[339, 340] This disorder is autosomal recessive, with multisystem disease including progressive ataxia, telangiectasia, immune system abnormalities, increased incidence of neoplasia, and insulin-resistant diabetes mellitus. Most patients have decreased or undetectable levels of immunoglobulins and A and E, and the antireceptor antibodies belong to an unusual low-molecular-weight form of immunoglobulin M.

Anti–insulin receptor antibodies have also been described in some patients with new-onset type I diabetes mellitus.[341] In this case, the antibodies may occur as an anti-idiotype response to anti-insulin antibodies in the circulation. These antireceptor antibodies are of low titer and probably play no clinically significant role.

TSH RECEPTOR ANTIBODIES. The most common endocrine disorder in which antireceptor antibodies play an important role is Graves disease (see Chapter 8). As part of an autoimmune process, patients with Graves disease have circulating antibodies that recognize diverse thyroid cell surface antigens and in many cases stimulate cell growth and thyroid hormone synthesis and release.[342] An enigmatic serum factor termed *long-acting thyroid stimulator*, or LATS, which was originally described more than 30 years ago in patients with Graves disease,[343] is now known to consist of various types of anti-TSH receptor and antithyroid antibodies. Stimulatory activity of these LATS immunoglobulins results, in most, but not all, patients, from the interaction of the immunoglobulin with the TSH receptor or with cell-surface gangliosides closely associated with the receptor.[344, 345] In contrast to anti–insulin receptor antibodies, which usually lead to insulin resistance, anti–TSH receptor antibodies usually activate the receptor and thus contribute to the thyrotoxicosis of Graves disease. In occasional patients, anti–TSH receptor antibodies are inhibitory rather than stimulatory and lead to hypothyroidism.

In the course of the disease in a single patient, the nature of receptor antibodies in the circulating pool can shift from stimulatory to inhibitory and back to stimulatory.[346] This change in activity results from the expression of antibodies that recognize different domains of the receptors and may ultimately give insight into the mechanism of receptor signaling. Because the antireceptor antibodies block hormone binding, receptor activation must result directly from antibody binding.

Anti–TSH receptor antibodies are important not only in explaining the pathogenesis of hyperthyroidism in Graves disease but also in monitoring the response to therapy.[347, 348]

Treatment with antithyroid drugs (propylthiouracil or methimazole) frequently induces a remission, so that further therapy is not required for prolonged periods. High anti–TSH receptor antibody levels are a good predictor of relapse in these patients and thus can be followed periodically to assess the status of the remission and the requirement for further therapy.

RECEPTORS AND ONCOGENES

Specific genes play a role in the initiation and maintenance of the malignant state. Studies of genes in oncogenic viruses and of genes in the genome of some tumor cells that can transform normal 3T3 fibroblasts have led to the identification and characterization of *oncogenes*.[349] More than 50 separate oncogenes have been described. Oncogenes usually have cellular counterparts that play key roles in normal growth control and differentiation. These genes are called cellular or *proto-oncogenes*.[349] It is likely that certain viruses have developed cell transformation capabilities by virtue of acquiring a proto-oncogene.

A major challenge is the determination of the molecular mechanisms involved in altered function of a given proto-oncogene that leads to tumorigenesis. For example, a proto-oncogene under the control of viral elements may be abnormally regulated, leading to abnormal levels of the corresponding protein product and ultimate cellular dysfunction. Alternatively, mutations of the proto-oncogene could result in altered function of the encoded protein.

In view of the critical role of membrane receptors in the regulation of cellular activities including growth and development, it is not surprising that proto-oncogenes may encode important components of the receptor-signal transduction pathway.[350] Table 4–12 and Figure 4–40 illustrate the diverse proto-oncogenes that may be involved in cellular signaling. Some encode receptors with intrinsic kinase activity, and others are GTP-binding proteins that may be membrane associated. Several encoded proteins are located in the cytoplasm and possess tyrosine or serine/threonine kinase functions or may be secreted as autocrine or paracrine factors. Last, proto-oncogenes can encode nuclear proteins, some of which may exhibit transcriptional activity.

An example of a proto-oncogene that serves a receptor function is the EGF receptor.[351, 352] The EGF receptor is a single polypeptide with one transmembrane domain, an extracellular ligand binding region, and tyrosine kinase activity. EGF mediates a potent mitogenic response in appropriate cells, and uncontrolled EGF activity could result in abnormal cell growth. The avian erythroblastosis virus, which can transform erythroid and fibroblast cells, contains

TABLE 4–12. Hormone-Receptor Signal Transduction and Oncogenes*

Proto-oncogene	Hormone/Receptor Analogue	Location	Function
erb B	EGF-R	Transmembrane	Tyrosine kinase
neu/Her-2	EGF-R	Transmembrane	Tyrosine kinase
fms	GM-CSF-R	Transmembrane	Tyrosine kinase
src	pp60	Membrane-associated	Tyrosine kinase
ras	p21	Membrane-associated	Small GTP-binding protein
sis	PDGFβ	Cytoplasmic, ? secreted	Growth factor
int-2	FGF	Cytoplasmic, ? secreted	Growth factor
erb A	T_3-R	Nuclear	Transcription factor
jun	AP-1	Nuclear	Transcription factor
fos	Heterodimer with *jun*	Nuclear	Transcription factor

*Proto-oncogenes related to the signal transduction pathway are listed. The abbreviations used are R, receptor; EFG, epidermal growth factor; GM-CSF, granulocyte-macrophage colony-stimulating factor; PDGF, platelet-derived growth factor; FGF, fibroblast growth factor; T_3, triiodothyronine.

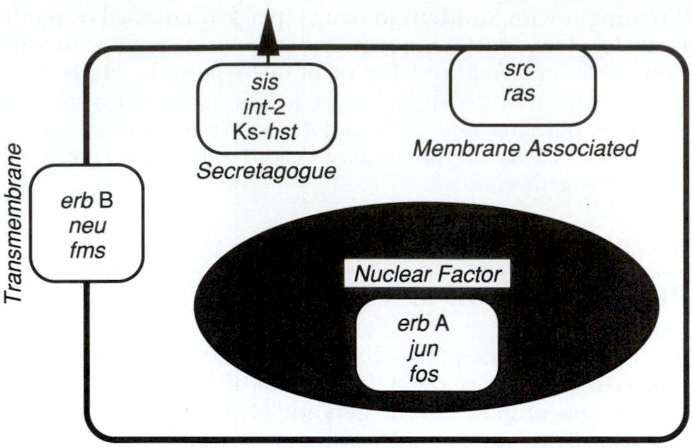

Figure 4–40. Cellular localization of proto-oncogenes. There are four major categories of cellular oncogenes: transmembrane (receptors with inherent tyrosine kinase activity), secretagogue (growth factors produced as potential autocrine regulators), membrane-associated (small GTP-binding protein *[ras]* or tyrosine kinase *[src]*), and nuclear transcription factors.

a viral oncogene, v-*erb* B. v-*erb* B encodes a form of EGF receptor that is truncated both in the NH₂-terminal, extracellular domain and in the COOH-terminal, cytoplasmic tail and consequently is active in the *absence* of the ligand. It is the constitutive action of EGF receptor that apparently contributes to cellular transformation.

Two key types of proto-oncogenes encode products that are membrane associated: one is *src*, which encodes a tyrosine kinase function, and the other is *ras*, which is a member of the low-molecular-weight GTP-binding protein family.[353, 354] Mutants of *ras* often possess altered intrinsic GTPase activity and participate in tumorigenesis, either alone or in concert with other oncogenes. These *ras* forms may malfunction by being maintained in the GTP-bound, active state. Several GH-producing pituitary tumors harbor a defect in the α_s subunit of the G protein,[355] and a number of adrenal and ovarian malignancies contain an abnormal α_i subunit.[356]

Yet other proto-oncogenes may encode growth factors or other secretagogues that can influence cell growth and differentiation. As an example, v-*sis* encodes the β subunit of PDGF. This subunit may form an active dimer that can stimulate cell growth.[49, 357] Similarly, *int*-2 and KS-*hst* encode growth factors in the fibroblast growth factor family. Alternatively, proto-oncogenes may encode cytosolic proteins with kinase properties. For example, *raf*-1 encodes a serine/threonine kinase activity located in the cytoplasm. However, its physiological function is unclear.[358]

A number of nuclear proteins, some capable of binding specific DNA sequences, are the products of members of the oncogene family. These transcription regulatory proteins are critical for the distal part of the hormone signaling pathway. Some early growth response genes such as *jun* and *fos* appear to bind specific, hormone-dependent, enhancer DNA sequences in gene-regulatory regions (AP-1 sites).[359] Another major example is v-*erb* A, the second gene in the avian erythroblastosis virus and one that collaborates with v-*erb* B. c-*erb* A encodes the thyroid hormone receptor and is a member of a large family of ligand-dependent transcription factors that include the steroid hormone, retinoic acid, and vitamin D receptors[156] (see Chapter 3). v-*erb* A is a mutant *erb* A whose gene product cannot bind thyroid hormone. As such, it may function to repress thyroid hormone action via unclear mechanisms. Such novel activity may represent an example of dominant negative regulation by oncogene products.[360]

Finally, fusion of normal and malignant cells occasionally results in extinguishing the malignant phenotype, which

suggests the existence of an "oncogene" that results in tumorigenic activity only in the absence of its expression. The best-studied example of recessive oncogenes is the retinoblastoma (Rb) gene.[361] The absence of both Rb genes in a particular somatic cell increases its susceptibility to transformation. The Rb product is a 105-kd nuclear DNA-binding protein that likely participates in the regulation of the cell cycle. Furthermore, the action of the oncogenes in several well-known DNA tumor viruses may be manifest by the ability of their products to counteract Rb function by direct binding. It is likely that other examples of cellular oncogenes encoding factors that participate in cellular signaling will be forthcoming.

REFERENCES

1. Langley JN. On nerve endings and on special excitable substances. Proc R Soc Lond 1906; 78:170–194.
2. Ehrlich P. Nobel lecture (1908) on partial functions of the cell. In: Himmelwert M, Marquardt M, Dale H, eds. The Collected Papers of P. Ehrlich. Vol 3. Oxford: Pergamon, 1956: 183–194.
3. Pastan I, Roth J, Macchia V. Binding of hormone to tissue: the first step in polypeptide hormone action. Proc Natl Acad Sci USA 1966; 56:1802–1809.
4. Kono T. Destruction of insulin effector system of adipose tissue cells by proteolytic enzymes. J Biol Chem 1969; 244:1772–1778.
5. Cuatrecasas P. Interaction of insulin with the cell membrane: the primary action of insulin. Proc Natl Acad Sci USA 1969; 63:450–454.
6. Butcher RW, Crofford OB, Gammeltoft S, et al. Insulin activity: the solid matrix. Science 1973; 182:396–397.
7. Sutherland EW. Studies on the mechanism of hormone action. Science 1972; 177:401–408 (Nobel lecture).
8. Ross EM, Gilman AG. Biochemical properties of hormone-sensitive adenylate cyclase. Annu Rev Biochem 1980; 49:533–565.
9. Auerbach GD. Polypeptide and amine hormone regulation of adenylate cyclase. Annu Rev Physiol 1982; 44:653–666.
10. Zeleznik AJ, Roth J. Demonstration of the insulin receptor in vivo in rabbits and its possible role as a reservoir for the plasma hormone. J Clin Invest 1978; 61:1363–1367.
11. Rouleau MF, Mitchell J, Goltzman D. In vivo distribution of parathyroid hormone receptors in bone: evidence that a predominant osseous target cell is not the mature osteoblast. Endocrinology 1988; 123:187–191.
12. Sodoyez JC, Sodoyez-Goffaux F, Giullaume M, et al. ¹²³I-insulin metabolism in normal rats and humans: external detection by a scintillation camera. Science 1983; 219:865–867.
13. Eckelman WC, Reba RC, Rzeszotarski WJ, et al. External imaging of cerebral muscarinic acetylcholine receptors. Science 1984; 223:291–293.
14. Bergman RN. Toward physiological understanding of glucose tolerance. Minimal-model approach. Diabetes 1989; 38:1512–1517.
15. Lin SY, Goodfriend TL. Angiotensin receptors. Am J Physiol 1970; 218:1319–1328.
16. Lefkowitz RJ, Roth J, Pricer W, et al. ACTH receptors in the adrenal: specific binding of ACTH-¹²⁵I and the relation to adenyl cyclase. Proc Natl Acad Sci USA 1970; 65:745–752.
17. Freychet P, Roth J, Neville DM, Jr. Insulin receptors in the liver: specific binding of [¹²⁵I]-insulin to the plasma membrane and its relation to insulin bioactivity. Proc Natl Acad Sci USA 1971; 68:1833–1837.
18. Rodbell M, Krans HMJ, Pohl SL, et al. The glucagon-sensitive adenyl cyclase system in plasma membranes of rat liver. III. Binding of glucagon: method of assay and specificity. J Biol Chem 1971; 246:1861–1871.
19. Kahn CR. Membrane receptors for hormones and neurotransmitters. J Cell Biol 1976; 70:261–286.
20. Hollenberg MD, Nexo E. Receptor binding assays. In: Jacobs S, Cuatrecasas P, eds. Receptors and Recognition. Series B. Vol II. London: Chapman & Hall, 1981: 1–31.
21. Venter C, Harrison LC, eds. Receptor Biochemistry and Methodology. Vols 1–12. New York: Alan R. Liss, 1980–1989.
22. Matozaki T, Goke B, Tsunoda Y, et al. Two functionally distinct cholecystokinin receptors show different modes of action on Ca²⁺ mobilization and phospholipid hydrolysis in isolated rat pancreatic acini. Studies using a new cholecystokinin analog JMV-180. J Biol Chem 1990; 265:6247–6254.
23. Pitschner HF, Schlepper M, Schulte B, et al. Selective antagonists reveal different functions of M cholinoreceptor subtypes in humans. Trends Pharmacol Sci Suppl 1989; 92–96.
24. Maron R, Taylor SI, Jackson R, et al. Analysis of insulin receptors on human lymphoblastic cell lines by flow cytometry. Diabetologia 1984; 22:118–129.
25. Katoh M, Raguet S, Zachwieja J, et al. Hepatic prolactin receptors in the rat: characterization using monoclonal antireceptor antibodies. Endocrinology 1987; 120:739–749.

26. LeRoith D, Lowe WL Jr, Shemer J, et al. Development of brain insulin receptors. Int J Biochem 1988; 20:225–230.

27. Konishi J, Iida Y, Kasagi K, et al. Adipocyte TSH receptor related antibodies in Graves' disease detected by immunoprecipitation. Endocrinol Jpn 1982; 29:219–226.

28. Boutin JM, Edery M, Shirota M, et al. Identification of a cDNA encoding a long form of prolactin receptor in human hepatoma and breast cancer cells. Mol Endocrinol 1989; 3:1455–1461.

29. Scatchard G. The attraction of proteins for small molecules and ions. Ann NY Acad Sci 1949; 51:660–672.

30. Kahn CR, Freychet P, Neville DM Jr, et al. Quantitative aspects of the insulin-receptor interaction in liver plasma membranes. J Biol Chem 1974; 249:2249–2257.

31. Boeyaems JM, Dumont JE. The two-step model of ligand-receptor interaction. Mol Cell Endocrinol 1977; 7:33–47.

32. DeLean A, Rodbard D. Kinetics of cooperative binding. In: O'Brien J, ed. The Receptor. Vol II. New York: Plenum, 1970; 143–192.

33. DeMeyts P, Bianco AR, Roth J. Site-site interactions among insulin receptors: characterization of the negative cooperativity. J Biol Chem 1976; 241:1877–1888.

34. Hoffman K, Wingender W, Finn FM. Correlation of adrenocorticotropic activity of ACTH analogues with degree of binding to an adrenal cortical particulate preparation. Proc Natl Acad Sci USA 1970; 67:829–836.

35. Rorstad OP, Wanke I, Coy DH, et al. Selectivity of binding of peptide analogs to vascular receptors for vasoactive intestinal peptide. Mol Pharmacol 1990; 37:971–977.

36. Blundell T, Wood S. The conformation, flexibility, and dynamics of polypeptide hormones. Annu Rev Biochem 1982; 51:123–154.

37. Hokin LE. Receptors and phosphoinositide-generated second messengers. Annu Rev Biochem 1985; 54:202–235.

38. Cuatrecasas P. Hormone receptors, membrane phospholipids, and protein kinases. Harvey Lect 1984; 80:89–128.

39. Raymond JR, Hantowich M, Lefkowitz RJ, et al. Adrenergic receptors: models for regulation of signal transduction processes. Hypertension 1990; 15:119–131.

40. Muldoon TG, Evans AC Jr. Hormones and their receptors. Arch Intern Med 1988; 148:961–967.

41. Yip CC. Cell-membrane hormone receptors: some perspectives on their structure and function relationship. Biochem Cell Biol 1988; 66:549–556.

42. Michell RH. How do receptors at the cell surface send signals to the cell interior? Br Med J 1987; 295:1320–1323.

43. Strader CD, Sigal IS, Dixon RA. Genetic approaches to the determination of structure-function relationships of G protein–coupled receptors. Trends Pharmacol Sci 1989; 10:346–348.

44. McFarland KC, Sprengel R, Phillips HS, et al. Lutropin-choriogonadotropin receptor: an unusual member of the G protein–coupled receptor family. Science 1989; 245:494–499.

45. Loosfelt H, Misrahi M, Atger M, et al. Cloning and sequencing of porcine LH-hCG receptor cDNA: variants lacking transmembrane domain. Science 1989; 245:525–528.

46. Masu Y, Nakayama K, Tamaki H, et al. cDNA cloning of bovine substance K receptor through oocyte expression system. Nature 1987; 329:836–838.

47. Hinkle PM. Pituitary TRH receptors. Ann NY Acad Sci 1989; 560:176–187.

48. Waterfield MD. Growth factor receptors. Br Med Bull 1989; 45:541–553.

49. Williams LT. Signal transduction by the platelet-derived growth factor receptor. Science 1989; 243:1564–1570.

50. Dingledine R, Myers SJ, Nicholas RA. Molecular biology of mammalian amino acid receptors. FASEB J 1990; 4:2636–2645.

51. Schimerlik MI. Structure and regulation of muscarinic receptors. Annu Rev Physiol 1989; 51:217–227.

52. Changeux JP. The acetylcholine receptor: its molecular biology and biotechnological prospects. Bioessays 1989; 10:48–54.

53. Jan LY, Jan YN. Voltage-sensitive ion channels. Cell 1989; 56:13–25.

54. Krueger BK. Toward an understanding of structure and function of ion channels. FASEB J 1989; 3:1906–1914.

55. Bolton TB, Beech DJ, Komori S, et al. Voltage- and receptor gated channels. Prog Clin Biol Res 1990; 327:229–243.

56. Salemme FR. Structural polymorphism in transmembrane channels. Science 1988; 241:229–230.

57. Nicoll RA. The coupling of neurotransmitter receptors to ion channels in the brain. Science 1988; 241:545–551.

58. Montal M. Molecular anatomy and molecular design of channel proteins. FASEB J 1990; 4:2623–2635.

59. Lester HA. Heterologous expression of excitability proteins: route to more specific drugs? Science 1988; 241:1057–1063.

60. Catterall WA. Structure and function of voltage-sensitive ion channels. Science 1988; 242:50–61.

61. Goodwin RG, Friend D, Ziegler SF, et al. Cloning of the human and murine interleukin-7 receptors: demonstration of a soluble form and homology to a new receptor superfamily. Cell 1990; 60:941–951.

62. Leung DW, Spencer SA, Cachianes G, et al. Growth hormone receptor and serum binding protein: purification, cloning and expression. Nature 1987; 330:537–543.

63. Frielle T, Daniel KW, Caron MG, et al. Structural basis of β-adrenergic receptor subtype specificity studied with chimeric β_1/β_2-adrenergic receptors. Proc Natl Acad Sci USA 1988; 85:9494–9498.

64. O'Dowd BR, Lefkowitz RJ, Caron MG. Structure of the adrenergic and related receptors. Annu Rev Neurosci 1989; 12:67–83.

65. Witters LA. Protein phosphorylation and dephosphorylation. Curr Opin Cell Biol 1990; 2:212–220.

66. Boutin JM, Jolicoeur C, Okamura H, et al. Cloning and expression of the rat prolactin receptor, a member of the growth hormone/prolactin receptor gene family. Cell 1988; 53:69–77.

67. Rechler MM, Nisley SP. The nature and regulation of receptors for insulin-like growth factors. Annu Rev Physiol 1985; 47:425–552.

68. Morgan DO, Edman JC, Standring DN, et al. Insulin-like growth factor II receptor as a multifunctional binding protein. Nature 1987; 329:301–307.

69. Caron MG. The guanine nucleotide regulatory protein–coupled receptors for nucleosides, nucleotides, amino acids and amine neurotransmitters. Curr Opin Cell Biol 1989; 1:159–166.

70. Goldstein JL, Brown MS. Regulation of low-density lipoprotein receptors: implications for pathogenesis and therapy of hypercholesterolemia and atherosclerosis. Circulation 1987; 76:504–507.

71. Hedo JA, Kahn CR, Hayashi M, et al. Biosynthesis and glycosylation of the insulin-receptor evidence for a single-polypeptide precursor of the two major subunits. J Biol Chem 1983; 258:10020–10026.

72. Ronnett GV, Knutson VP, Kohanski RA, et al. Role of glycosylation in the processing of the newly translated insulin proreceptor in 3T3-L1 adipocytes. J Biol Chem 1984; 259:4566–4572.

73. Schlessinger J, Schechter Y, Willingham MC, et al. Direct visualization of binding, aggregation and internalization of insulin and epidermal growth factor on living fibroblastic cells. Proc Natl Acad Sci USA 1978; 75:2659–2663.

74. Carpentier JL, Fehlmann M, Van Obberghen E, et al. Redistribution of ^{125}I-insulin on the surface of rat hepatocytes: as a function of dissociation time. Diabetes 1985; 34:1002–1007.

75. Bergeron JJ, Lai WH, Kay DG, et al. The endosomal apparatus and transmembrane signalling. Adv Exp Med Biol 1988; 234:213–224.

76. Pearse BMF, Bretscher MS. Membrane recycling by coated vesicles. Annu Rev Biochem 1981; 50:85–101.

77. Ascoli M. Lysosomal accumulation of the hormone-receptor complex during receptor-mediated endocytosis of human choriogonadotropin. J Cell Biol 1984; 99:1242–1250.

78. Pastan IH, Willingham MC. Receptor-mediated endocytosis of hormones in cultured cells. Annu Rev Physiol 1981; 43:239–250.

79. Marshall S. Kinetics of insulin receptor internalization and recycling in adipocytes. J Biol Chem 1985; 260:4136–4144.

80. Goldstein JL, Anderson RG, Brown MS. Receptor mediated endocytosis and the cellular uptake of low density lipoprotein. Ciba Found Symp 1982; 92:77–95.

81. Enns CA, Larrick JW, Suomalainen H, et al. Co-migration and internalization of transferrin and its receptor on K562 cells. J Cell Biol 1983; 97:579–585.

82. Chen WJ, Goldstein JL, Brown MS. NPXY, a sequence often found in cytoplasmic tails, is required for coated pit–mediated internalization of the low density lipoprotein receptor. J Biol Chem 1990; 265:3116–3123.

83. Glenney JR Jr, Chen WS, Lazar CS, et al. Ligand-induced endocytosis of the EGF receptor is blocked by mutational inactivation and by microinjection of anti-phosphotyrosine antibodies. Cell 1988; 52:675–684.

84. Duckworth WC. Insulin degradation: mechanisms, products and significance. Endocr Rev 1988; 9:319–345.

85. Tsubouchi H, Miyazaki H, Gohda E, et al. Degradation of [^{125}I]iodoglucagon by normal rat plasma in radioimmunoassay mixture containing aprotinin and its prevention by p-chloromercuriphenyl sulfonate and leupeptin. Endocrinology 1986; 119:1137–1145.

86. King GL, Johnson SM. Receptor-mediated transport of insulin across endothelial cells. Science 1985; 227:1583–1586.

87. Dernovsek K, Bar R, Ginsberg B, et al. Rapid transport of biologically intact insulin through cultured endothelial cells. J Clin Endocrinol Metab 1984; 58:761–765.

88. Jacobson K, Ishihara A, Inman R. Lateral diffusion of proteins in membranes. Annu Rev Physiol 1987; 49:167–175.

89. Posner BI, Khan MN, Kay DG, et al. Internalization of hormone receptor complexes: route and significance. Adv Exp Med Biol 1986; 205:185–201.

90. Kahn CR, Baird KL, Jarrett DB, et al. Direct demonstration that receptor cross-linking or aggregation is important in insulin action. Proc Natl Acad Sci USA 1978; 75:4209–4213.

91. Ishizaka T, Ishizaka K. Triggering of histamine release from rat mast cells by divalent antibodies against IgE-receptors. J Immunol 1978; 120:800–805.

92. Becker AB, Roth RA. Insulin receptor structure and function in normal and pathological conditions. Annu Rev Med 1990; 41:99–115.

93. McClain DA. Insulin action in cells expressing truncated or kinase-defective insulin receptors. Dissection of multiple hormone-signalling pathways. Diabetes Care 1990; 13:302–316.

94. Simon I, Brown TJ, Ginsberg BH. Modification of membrane physical properties, biological response and insulin binding in Friend cells by low serum concentration. Biochim Biophys Acta 1987; 896:165–172.

95. Kono T, Barham FW. The relationship between the insulin binding capacity of fat cells and the cellular response to insulin. J Biol Chem 1971; 246:6210–6216.

96. Gliemann J, Gammeltoft S, Vinten J. Time course of insulin receptor binding and insulin-induced lipogenesis in isolated rat fat cells. J Biol Chem 1975; 250:3368–3374.

97. Dufau ML. Endocrine regulation and communicating functions of the Leydig cell. Annu Rev Physiol 1988; 50:483–508.

98. Kahn CR. Insulin resistance, insulin insensitivity and insulin unresponsiveness: a necessary distinction. Metabolism 1978; 27(Suppl 2):1893–1902.

99. Debant A, Ponzo G, Clauser E, et al. Replacement of insulin receptor tyrosine residues 1162 and 1163 does not alter the mitogenic effect of the hormone. Proc Natl Acad Sci USA 1988; 85:8032–8036.

100. Wilden PA, Backer JM, Kahn CR, et al. The insulin receptor with phenylalanine replacing tyrosine 1146 provides evidence for separate signals regulating cellular metabolism and growth. Proc Natl Acad Sci USA 1990; 87:3358–3362.

101. Escobedo JA, Williams LT. A PDGF receptor domain essential for mutagenesis but not for many other responses to PDGF. Nature 1988; 335:85–87.

102. Kasuga M, Kahn CR, Hedo JA, et al. Insulin-induced receptor loss in cultured lymphocytes is due to accelerated receptor degradation. Proc Natl Acad Sci USA 1981; 78:6917–6921.

103. Ronnott GV, Knutson VP, Lane MD. Insulin-induced down-regulation of insulin receptors in 3T3-L1 adipocytes. Altered rate of receptor inactivation. J Biol Chem 1982; 257:4285–4291.

104. Hartzell HC, Frambrough DM. Acetylcholine receptor production and incorporation into membranes of developing muscle fibers. Dev Biol 1973; 30:153–165.

105. Bockaert J, Roy C, Rajerison R, et al. Specific binding of [³H]lysine-vasopressin to pig kidney plasma membranes: relationship of receptor occupancy to adenylate cyclase activation. J Biol Chem 1973; 248:5922–5931.

106. Hinkle DM, Tashijian AH Jr. Thyrotropin-releasing hormone regulates the number of its own receptors in GH₃ strain of pituitary cells in culture. Biochemistry 1975; 14:3845–3851.

107. Gavin JR III, Roth J, Neville DM Jr, et al. Insulin dependent regulation of insulin receptor concentrations: a direct demonstration in cell culture. Proc Natl Acad Sci USA 1974; 71:84–88.

108. Hauger RL, Aguilera G, Catt KJ. Angiotensin II regulates its receptor sites in the adrenal glomerulosa zone. Nature 1978; 271:176–177.

109. Posner BI, Kelley PA, Friesen HG. Prolactin receptor in rat liver: possible induction by prolactin. Science 1978; 188:57–59.

110. Benovic JL, Bouvier M, Caron MG, et al. Regulation of adenylyl cyclase–coupled beta and adrenergic receptors. Annu Rev Cell Biol 1988; 4:405–420.

111. White MF, Shoelson SE, Keutmann H, et al. A cascade of tyrosine phosphorylation in the β-subunit activates the phosphotransferase activity of the insulin receptor. J Biol Chem 1988; 264:2969–2980.

112. Rosen OM, Herrera R, Olowe Y, et al. Phosphorylation activates the insulin receptor tyrosine protein kinase. Proc Natl Acad Sci USA 1983; 80:3237–3240.

113. Nimrod A, Tsafriri A, Linder HR. In vitro induction of binding sites for HCG in rat granulosa cells by FSH. Nature 1977; 267:632–633.

114. Williams LT, Lefkowitz RJ, Watanabe AM, et al. Thyroid hormone regulation of beta-adrenergic receptor number. J Biol Chem 1977; 252:2787–2789.

115. Hammond HK, White FC, Buxton IL, et al. Increased myocardial beta-receptors and adrenergic responses in hyperthyroid pigs. Am J Physiol 1987; 252:H283–H290.

116. Soloff M. Uterine receptor for oxytocin: effects of estrogen. Biochem Biophys Res Commun 1975; 65:205–212.

117. Posner BI, Kelley PA, Friesen HG. Induction of lactogenic receptor in rat liver: influence of estrogen and the pituitary. Proc Natl Acad Sci USA 1974; 71:2407–2410.

118. Zachary I, Sinnett-Smith SW, Rozengart E. Early events elicited by bombesin and structurally related peptides in quiescent Swiss 3T3 cells. I. Activation of protein kinase C and inhibition of epidermal growth factor binding. J Cell Biol 1986; 102:2211–2222.

119. Wrann M, Fox CF, Ross R. Modulation of epidermal growth factor receptors on 3T3 cells by platelet-derived growth factor. Science 1980; 210:1363–1365.

120. Goldfine ID, Kahn CR, Neville DM Jr, et al. Decreased binding of insulin to its receptors in rats with hormone induced insulin resistance. Biochem Biophys Res Commun 1973; 53:852–857.

121. McDonald AR, Goldfine ID. Glucocorticoid regulation of insulin receptor gene transcription in IM9 cultured lymphocytes. J Clin Invest 1988; 81:499–504.

122. O'Brien RM, Granner DK. PEPCK gene is a model of inhibitory effects of insulin on gene transcription. Diabetes Care 1990; 13:327–339.

123. Cohen P. The role of protein phosphorylation in the hormonal control of enzyme activity. Eur J Biochem 1985; 151:439–448.

124. Smith RJ. Biological actions and interactions of insulin and glucagon. In: DeGroot LJ, Besser GM, Cahill GF Jr, et al., eds. Endocrinology. Vol 2. 2nd ed. Philadelphia: W.B. Saunders, 1989:1333–1345.

125. Sonne O, Berg T, Christoffersen T. Binding of ¹²⁵I-labelled glucagon and glucagon-stimulated accumulation of adenosine 3′:5′-monophosphate in isolated intact rat hepatocytes: evidence for receptor heterogeneity. J Biol Chem 1978; 253:3203–3210.

126. Goldberg ND, Dietz SB, O'Toole AG. Cyclic guanosine 3′,5′-monophosphate in mammalian tissues and urine. J Biol Chem 1969; 244:4458–4466.

127. Exton JH, Robison GA, Sutherland EW, Park CR. Studies on the role of adenosine 3′,5′-monophosphate in the hepatic actions of glucagon and catecholamines. J Biol Chem 1971; 246:6166–6177.

128. Liljenquist JE, Bomboy JD, Lewis SB, et al. Effect of glucagon on net splanchnic cyclic AMP production in normal and diabetic men. J Clin Invest 1974; 53:198–204.

129. Brostrom MA, Reimann EM, Walsh DA, et al. A cyclic 3′,5′-AMP-stimulated protein kinase from cardiac muscle. Adv Enzyme Regul 1970; 8:191–203.

130. Corbin JD, Sugden PH, West L, et al. Studies on the properties and mode of action of the purified regulatory subunit of bovine heart adenosine 3′:5′-monophosphate-dependent protein kinase. J Biol Chem 1978; 253:3997–4003.

131. Feliu JE, Hue L, Hers HG. Hormonal control of pyruvate kinase activity and of gluconeogenesis in isolated hepatocytes. Proc Natl Acad Sci USA 1976; 73:2762–2766.

132. Claus TH, Park CR, Pilkis SJ. Glucagon and gluconeogenesis. In: Lefebre PJ, ed. Glucagon. Vol I. Berlin: Springer-Verlag, 1983: 315–360.

133. Beale E, Andreone T, Koch S, et al. Insulin and glucagon regulate cytosolic phosphoenolpyruvate carboxykinase (GTP) mRNA in rat liver. Diabetes 1984; 33:328–332.

134. Claus TH, El-Maghrabi MR, Regen DM, et al. The role of fructose 2,6-bisphosphate in the regulation of carbohydrate metabolism. Curr Top Cell Regul 1984; 23:57–86.

135. Pilkis SJ, Chrisman T, Burgress B, et al. Rat hepatic 6-phosphofructo-2-kinase/fructose 2,6-bisphosphatase: a unique bifunctional enzyme. Adv Enzyme Regul 1983; 21:147–173.

136. Van Schaftingen E, Davies DR, Hers HG. Fructose-2,6-bisphosphatase from rat liver. Eur J Biochem 1982; 124:143–149.

137. Van Schaftingen E, Hue L, Hers HG. Fructose 2,6-bisphosphate, the probable structure of the glucose- and glucagon-sensitive stimulator of phosphofructokinase. Biochem J 1980; 192:897–901.

138. Van Schaftingen E, Hers HG. Inhibition of fructose-1,6-bisphosphatase by fructose 2,6-bisphosphate. Proc Natl Acad Sci USA 1981; 78:2861–2863.

139. Castano JG, Nieto A, Feliu JE. Inactivation of phosphofructokinase by glucagon in rat hepatocytes. J Biol Chem 1979; 254:5576–5579.

140. Claus TH, Pilkis SJ. Hormonal control of hepatic gluconeogenesis. In: Litwack G, ed. Biochemical Actions of Hormones. Vol 8. New York: Academic, 1981: 209–271.

141. Noguchi T, Inoue H, Tanaka T. Regulation of rat liver L-type pyruvate kinase mRNA by insulin and by fructose. Eur J Biochem 1982; 128:583–588.

142. Sale GJ. Recent progress in our understanding of the mechanism of action of insulin. Int J Biochem 1988; 20:897–908.

143. Yu KT, Khalaf N, Czech MP. Insulin stimulates a membrane-bound serine kinase that may be phosphorylated on tyrosine. Proc Natl Acad Sci USA 1987; 84:3972–3976.

144. Avruch J, Nemenoff RA, Pierce M, et al. Protein phosphorylations as a mode of insulin action. In: Czech MP, ed. Molecular Basis of Insulin Action. New York: Plenum, 1985: 263–296.

145. Shotwell MA, Kilberg MS, Oxender DL. The regulation of neutral amino acid transport in mammalian cells. Biochim Biophys Acta 1983; 737:267–284.

146. Cariappa R, Kilberg MS. Hormone-induced system A amino acid transport activity in rat liver plasma membrane and Golgi vesicles. J Biol Chem 1990; 265:1470–1475.

147. Fehlmann M, LeCam A, Freychet P. Insulin and glucagon stimulation of amino acid transport in isolated rat hepatocytes. J Biol Chem 1979; 254:10431–10437.

148. Levine R, Goldstein MS. On the mechanism of action of insulin. Recent Prog Horm Res 1955; 11:343–380.

149. Mueckler M, Caruso C, Baldwin SA, et al. Sequence and structure of a human glucose transporter. Science 1985; 229:941–945.

150. Birnbaum MB. Identification of a novel gene encoding an insulin-responsive glucose transport protein. Cell 1989; 57:305–315.

151. Charron MJ, Brosius FC III, Alper SL, et al. A glucose transport protein expressed predominately in insulin responsive tissues. Proc Natl Acad Sci USA 1989; 86:2535–2539.

152. James DR, Brown R, Navarro J, et al. Insulin regulatable tissues express

a unique insulin sensitive glucose transport protein. Nature 1988; 333:183–185.

153. Fukumoto H, Seino S, Imura H, et al. Sequence, tissue distribution, and chromosomal localization of mRNA encoding a human glucose transporter–like protein. Proc Natl Acad Sci USA 1988; 85:5434–5438.

154. Simpson IA, Cushman SW. Hormonal regulation of mammalian glucose transport. Annu Rev Biochem 1986; 55:1059–1089.

155. Johnson PF, McKnight SL. Eukaryotic transcriptional regulatory proteins. Annu Rev Biochem 1989; 58:799–839.

156. Evans RM. The steroid and thyroid hormone receptor superfamily. Science 1988; 240:889–895.

157. Montminy MR, Gonzalez GA, Yamamoto KK. Regulation of cAMP inducible genes by CREB. Trends Neurosci 1990; 18:184–188.

158. Angel P, Allegretto EA, Okino ST, et al. Oncogene *jun* encodes a sequence-specific trans-activator similar to AP-1. Nature 1988; 332:166–169.

159. Montminy MR, Sevarino KA, Wagner JA, et al. Identification of a cyclic-AMP responsive element within the rat somatostatin gene. Proc Natl Acad Sci USA 1986; 83:6682–6686.

160. Hoeffler JP, Meyer TE, Yun Y, et al. Cyclic AMP-responsive DNA-binding protein: structure based on a cloned placental cDNA. Science 1988; 242:1430–1432.

161. Angel P, Imagawa M, Chiu R, et al. Phorbol ester–inducible genes contain a common cis element recognized by a TPA-modulated trans-acting factor. Cell 1987; 49:729–739.

162. Schule R, Umesono K, Mangelsdorf DJ, et al. Jun-fos and receptors for vitamins A and D recognize a common response element in the human osteocalcin gene. Cell 1990; 61:497–504.

163. Robishaw JD, Foster KA. Role of G-proteins in the regulation of the cardiovascular system. Annu Rev Physiol 1989; 51:229–244.

164. Firtel RA, van Haastert PJ, Kimmel AR, et al. G protein linked signal transduction pathways in development: dictyostelium as an experimental system. Cell 1989; 58:235–239.

165. Johnson GL, Dhanasekaran N. The G-protein family and their interaction with receptors. Endocr Rev 1989; 10:317–331.

166. Lochrie MA, Simon MI. G protein multiplicity in eukaryotic signal transduction systems. Biochemistry 1988; 27:4957–4965.

167. Gilman AG. G-proteins and regulation of adenylyl cyclase. JAMA 1989; 262:1819–1825.

168. Neer EJ, Clapham DE. Roles of G protein subunits in transmembrane signalling. Nature 1988; 333:129–134.

169. Ross EM. Signal sorting and amplification through G protein coupled receptors. Neuron 1990; 5:141–152.

170. Birnbaumer L, Codina J, Mattera R, et al. Signal transduction by G proteins. Kidney Int Suppl 1987; 23:S14–S42.

171. Spiegel AM. Signal transduction by guanine nucleotide binding proteins. Mol Cell Endocrinol 1987; 49:1–16.

172. Hausdorff WP, Caron MG, Lefkowitz RJ. Turning off the signal: desensitization of β-adrenergic receptor function. FASEB J 1990; 4:2881–2889.

173. Casey PJ, Gilman AG. G protein involvement in receptor-effector coupling. J Biol Chem 1988; 263:2577–2580.

174. Gilman AG. G proteins: transducers of receptor-generated signals. Annu Rev Biochem 1987; 56:615–649.

175. Casey PJ, Graziano MP, Freissmuth M, et al. Role of G proteins in transmembrane signalling. Cold Spring Harb Symp Quant Biol 1988; 53:203–208.

176. Freissmuth M, Casey PJ, Gilman AG. G proteins control diverse pathways of transmembrane signalling. FASEB J 1989; 3:2125–2131.

177. Masters SB, Sullivan KA, Millre RT, et al. Carboxyl terminal domain of $G_s\alpha$ specifies coupling of receptors to stimulation of adenylyl cyclase. Science 1988; 241:448–451.

178. Gupta SK, Diez E, Heasley LE, et al. A G protein mutant that inhibits thrombin and purinergic receptor activation of phospholipase A_2. Science 1990; 249:662–666.

179. Limbird LE. Receptors linked to inhibition of adenylate cyclase: additional signaling mechanisms. FASEB J 1988; 2:2686–2695.

180. Salter RS, Krinks MH, Klee CB, et al. Calmodulin activates the isolated catalytic subunit of brain adenylate cyclase. J Biol Chem 1981; 256:9830–9833.

181. Ushiro H, Cohen S. Identification of phosphotyrosine as a product of epidermal growth factor–activated protein kinase in A-431 cell membranes. J Biol Chem 1980; 255:8363–8365.

182. Hunter T, Cooper JA. Tyrosine protein kinases and their substrates: an overview. Adv Cyclic Nucleotide Protein Phosphorylation Res 1984; 17:443–455.

183. Ullrich A, Coussens L, Hayflick JS, et al. Human epidermal growth factor receptor cDNA sequence and aberrant expression of the amplified gene in A431 epidermoid carcinoma cells. Nature 1984; 309:418–425.

184. Kasuga M, Karlsson FA, Kahn CR. Insulin stimulates the phosphorylation of the 95,000-dalton subunit of its own receptor. Science 1982; 215:185–187.

185. Ullrich A, Bell JR, Chen EY, et al. Human insulin receptor and its relationship to the tyrosine kinase family of oncogenes. Nature 1985; 313:756–761.

186. Jacobs S, Kull FC Jr, Earp HS, et al. Somatomedin-C stimulates the phosphorylation of the β-subunit of its own receptor. J Biol Chem 1983; 258:9581–9584.

187. Ullrich A, Gray A, Tam AW, et al. Insulin-like growth factor I receptor primary structure: comparison with insulin receptor suggests structural determinants that define functional specificity. EMBO J 1986; 5:2503–2512.

188. Escobedo JA, Navankasatussas S, Cousens LS, et al. A common PDGF receptor is activated by homodimeric A and B forms of PDGF. Science 1988; 240:1532–1544.

189. Yarden Y, Escobedo JA, Kuang WJ, et al. Structure of the receptor for platelet-derived growth factor helps define a family of closely related growth factor receptors. Nature 1986; 323:226–232.

190. Sherr CJ, Rettenmier CW, Sacca R, et al. The c-*fms* proto-oncogene product is related to the receptor for the mononuclear phagocyte growth factor CSF-1. Cell 1985; 41:665–676.

191. Coussens L, Van Beveren C, Smith D, et al. Structural alteration of viral homologue of receptor proto-oncogene *fms* at carboxyl terminus. Nature 1986; 320:277–280.

192. Lee PL, Johnson DE, Cousens LS, et al. Purification and complementary DNA cloning of a receptor for basic fibroblast growth factor. Science 1989; 245:57–60.

193. Yarden Y, Ullrich A. Growth factor receptor tyrosine kinases. Annu Rev Biochem 1988; 57:443–478.

194. Olson TS, Bamberger MJ, Lane MD. Post-translational changes in tertiary and quaternary structure of the insulin proreceptor. Correlation with acquisition of function. J Biol Chem 1990; 263:7342–7351.

195. Schlessinger J. The epidermal growth factor receptor as a multifunctional allosteric protein. Biochemistry 1988; 27:3119–3123.

196. Chou CK, Dull TJ, Russel DS, et al. Human insulin receptors mutated at the ATP-binding site lack protein tyrosine kinase activity and fail to mediate postreceptor effects of insulin. J Biol Chem 1987; 262:1842–1847.

197. Ebina Y, Araki E, Taira M, et al. Replacement of lysine residue 1030 in the putative ATP-binding region of the insulin receptor abolishes insulin- and antibody-stimulated glucose uptake and receptor kinase activity. Proc Natl Acad Sci USA 1987; 84:704–708.

198. Ellis L, Clauser E, Morgan DO, et al. Replacement of insulin receptor tyrosine residues 1162 and 1163 compromises insulin-stimulated kinase activity and uptake of 2-deoxyglucose. Cell 1986; 45:721–732.

199. Morgan DO, Roth RA. Acute insulin action requires insulin receptor kinase activity: introduction of an inhibitory monoclonal antibody into mammalian cells blocks the rapid effects of insulin. Proc Natl Acad Sci USA 1987; 84:41–45.

200. Kahn CR, Flier JS, Bar RS, et al. The syndromes of insulin resistance and acanthosis nigricans: insulin-receptor disorders in man. N Engl J Med 1976; 294:739–745.

201. Grunberger G, Zick Y, Gorden P. Defect in phosphorylation of insulin receptors in cells from an insulin-resistant patient with normal insulin binding. Science 1984; 223:932–934.

202. Grigorescu F, Flier JS, Kahn CR. Defect in insulin receptor phosphorylation in erythrocytes and fibroblasts associated with severe insulin resistance. J Biol Chem 1984; 259:15003–15006.

203. Kadowaki T, Kasuga M, Akanuma Y, et al. Decreased autophosphorylation of the insulin receptor-kinase in streptozotocin-diabetic rats. J Biol Chem 1984; 259:14208–14216.

204. Freidenberg GR, Henry RR, Klein HH, et al. Decreased kinase activity of insulin receptors from adipocytes of non–insulin-dependent diabetic subjects. J Clin Invest 1987; 79:240–250.

205. Comi RJ, Grunberger G, Gorden P. Relationship of insulin binding and insulin-stimulated tyrosine kinase activity is altered in type II diabetes. J Clin Invest 1987; 79:453–462.

206. Honegger AM, Dull TJ, Felder S, et al. Point mutation at the ATP binding site of EGF receptor abolishes protein-tyrosine kinase activity and alters cellular routing. Cell 1987; 51:199–209.

207. Honegger AM, Szapary D, Schmidt A, et al. A mutant epidermal growth factor receptor with defective protein tyrosine kinase is unable to stimulate proto-oncogene expression and DNA synthesis. Mol Cell Biol 1987; 7:4568–4571.

208. Escobedo JA, Barr PJ, Williams LT. Role of tyrosine kinase and membrane spanning domains in signal transduction by the platelet derived growth factor receptor. Mol Cell Biol 1988; 8:5126–5131.

209. Roussel MF, Downing JR, Rettenmeir CW, et al. A point mutation in the extracellular domain of the human CSF-1 receptor (c-*fms*) proto-oncogene product 1 activates its transforming potential. Cell 1988; 55:979–988.

210. Riedel H, Dull TJ, Honegger AM, et al. Cytoplasmic domains determine signal specificity, cellular routing characteristics and influence ligand binding of epidermal growth factor and insulin receptors. EMBO J 1989; 8:2943–2954.

211. Ellis L, Morgan DO, Clauser E, et al. Mechanisms of receptor-mediated transmembrane communication. Cold Spring Harb Symp Quant Biol 1986; 51:773–784.

212. Pilch PF, Czech MP. Hormone binding alters the conformation of the insulin receptor. Science 1980; 210:1152–1153.

213. Maturo JM III, Hollenberg MD, Aglio LS. Insulin receptor: insulin-modulated interconversion between distinct molecular forms involving disulfide-sulfhydryl exchange. Biochemistry 1983; 22:2579–2586.

214. Bertics PJ, Gill GN. Self-phosphorylation enhances the protein-tyrosine kinase activity of the epidermal growth factor receptor. J Biol Chem 1985; 260:14642–14647.

215. Böni-Schnetzler M, Kaligian A, DelVecchio R, et al. Ligand-dependent intersubunit association within the insulin receptor complex activates its intrinsic kinase activity. J Biol Chem 1988; 263:6822–6828.

216. Sweet LJ, Morrison BD, Wilden PA, et al. Insulin-dependent intermolecular subunit communications between isolated alpha beta heterodimeric insulin receptor complexes. J Biol Chem 1987; 262:16730–16738.

217. Honegger AM, Kris RM, Ullrich A, et al. Evidence that autophosphorylation of solubilized receptors for epidermal growth factor is mediated by intermolecular cross-phosphorylation. Proc Natl Acad Sci USA 1989; 86:925–929.

218. Shoelson SE, Böni-Schnetzler M, Pilch PF. Autophosphorylation occurs within individual β-subunits of the insulin receptor. Diabetes 1988; 37(Suppl 1):8A.

219. Beguinot F, Smith RJ, Kahn CR, et al. Phosphorylation of insulin-like growth factor I receptor by insulin receptor tyrosine kinase in intact cultured skeletal muscle cells. Biochemistry 1988; 27:3222–3228.

220. Stern DF, Kamps MP. EGF-stimulated tyrosine phosphorylation of p185[neu]: a potential model for receptor interactions. EMBO J 1988; 7:995–1001.

221. Cochet C, Gill GN, Meisenhelder J, et al. C-kinase phosphorylates the epidermal growth factor receptor and reduces its epidermal growth factor–stimulated tyrosine protein kinase activity. J Biol Chem 1984; 259:2553–2558.

222. Takayama S, White MF, Lauris V, et al. Phorbol esters modulate insulin receptor phosphorylation and insulin action in cultured hepatoma cells. Proc Natl Acad Sci USA 1984; 81:7797–7801.

223. Gazzano H, Kowalski A, Fehlmann M, et al. Two different protein kinase activities are associated with the insulin receptor. Biochem J 1983; 216:575–582.

224. White MF, Takayama S, Kahn CR. Differences in the sites of phosphorylation of the insulin receptor in vivo and in vitro. J Biol Chem 1985; 260:9470–9478.

225. Smith DM, King MJ, Sale GJ. Two systems in vitro that show insulin-stimulated serine kinase activity towards the insulin receptor. Biochem J 1988; 250:509–519.

226. Russell DS, Gherzi R, Johnson EL, et al. The protein-tyrosine kinase activity of the insulin receptor is necessary for insulin-mediated receptor down-regulation. J Biol Chem 1987; 262:11833–11840.

227. Pang DT, Sharma BR, Shafer JA. Purification of the catalytically active phosphorylated form of insulin receptor kinase by affinity chromatography with o-phosphotyrosyl-binding antibodies. Arch Biochem Biophys 1985; 242:176–186.

228. Kamps MP, Sefton BM. Identification of multiple novel polypeptide substrates of the v-src, v-yes, v-fps, v-ros, and v-erb-B oncogenic tyrosine kinases utilizing antisera against phosphotyrosine. Oncogene 1988; 2:305–315.

229. Cooper JA, Hunter T. Similarities and differences between the effects of epidermal growth factor and Rous sarcoma virus. J Cell Biol 1981; 91:878–883.

230. Cooper JA, Bowen-Pope DF, Raines E, et al. Similar effects of platelet-derived growth factor and epidermal growth factor on the phosphorylation of tyrosine in cellular proteins. Cell 1982; 31:263–273.

231. Rees-Jones RW, Taylor SI. An endogenous substrate for the insulin receptor–associated tyrosine kinase. J Biol Chem 1985; 260:4461–4467.

232. White MF, Maron R, Kahn CR. Insulin rapidly stimulates tyrosine phosphorylation of a M_r 185,000 protein in intact cells. Nature 1985; 318:183–186.

233. Häring HU, White MF, Machicao F, et al. Insulin rapidly stimulates phosphorylation of a 46-kDa membrane protein on tyrosine residues as well as phosphorylation of several soluble proteins in intact fat cells. Proc Natl Acad Sci USA 1987; 84:113–117.

234. Izumi T, White MF, Kadowaki T, et al. Insulin-like growth factor I rapidly stimulates tyrosine phosphorylation of a M_r 185,000 protein in intact cells. J Biol Chem 1987; 262:1282–1287.

235. Kadowaki T, Koyasu S, Nishida E, et al. Tyrosine phosphorylation of common and specific sets of cellular proteins rapidly induced by insulin, insulin-like growth factor I, and epidermal growth factor in an intact cell. J Biol Chem 1987; 262:7342–7350.

236. Yu KT, Khalaf N, Czech MP. Insulin stimulates the tyrosine phosphorylation of a M_r = 160,000 glycoprotein in rat adipocyte plasma membranes. J Biol Chem 1987; 262:7865–7873.

237. Condorelli G, Formisano P, Villone G, et al. Insulin and insulin-like growth factor I (IGF I) stimulate phosphorylation of a M_r 175,000 cytoskeleton-associated protein in intact FRTL5 cells. J Biol Chem 1989; 264:12633–12638.

238. Beguinot F, Kahn CR, Moses AC, et al. Differentiation-dependent phosphorylation of a 175,000 molecular weight protein in response to insulin and insulin-like growth factor-I in L6 skeletal muscle cells. Endocrinology 1989; 125:1599–1605.

239. Kadowaki T, Fujita-Yamaguchi Y, Nishida E, et al. Phosphorylation of

240. Häring HU, White MF, Kahn CR, et al. Interaction of the insulin receptor kinase with serine/threonine kinases in vitro. J Cell Biochem 1985; 28:171–182.

241. Low MG, Saltiel AR. Structural and functional roles of glycosyl-phosphatidylinositol in membranes. Science 1988; 239:268–275.

242. Schulz S, Chinkers M, Garbers DL. The guanylate cyclase/receptor family of proteins. FASEB J 1989; 3:2026–2035.

243. Catt KJ, Balla T. Phosphoinositide metabolism and hormone action. Annu Rev Med 1989; 40:487–509.

244. Williamson JR, Monck JR. Hormone effects on cellular Ca^{2+} fluxes. Annu Rev Physiol 1989; 51:107–124.

245. Exton JH. Signalling through phosphatidylcholine breakdown. J Biol Chem 1990; 265:1–4.

246. Putney JR Jr. Formation and actions of calcium-mobilizing messenger, inositol 1,4,5-trisphosphate. Am J Physiol 1987; 252:G149–G157.

247. Berridge MJ. Inositol trisphosphate and diacylglycerol: two interacting second messengers. Annu Rev Biochem 1987; 56:159–193.

248. Brown AM, Yatani A, Imoto Y, et al. Direct G-protein regulation of Ca^{2+} channels. Ann NY Acad Sci 1989; 560:373–386.

249. Birnbaumer L, Brown AM. G proteins and the mechanism of action of hormones, neurotransmitters, and autocrine and paracrine regulatory factors. Am Rev Respir Dis 1990; 141:S106–S114.

250. Supattapone S, Worley PF, Baraban JM, et al. Solubilization, purification, and characterization of an inositol trisphosphate receptor. J Biol Chem 1988; 263:1530–1534.

251. Putney JW Jr. The molecular heterogeneity of protein kinase C and its implications for cellular regulation. Nature 1988; 334:661–665.

252. Morris AP, Gallacher DV, Irvine RF, et al. Synergism of inositol trisphosphate and tetrakisphosphate in activating Ca^{2+}-dependent K^+ channels. Nature 1987; 330:653–655.

253. Manalan AS, Klee CB. Calmodulin. Adv Cyclic Nucleotide Protein Phosphorylation Res 1984; 18:227–278.

254. Hanks SK, Quin AM, Hunter T. The protein kinase family: conserved features and deduced phylogeny of the catalytic domains. Science 1988; 241:42–52.

255. Bell RM. Protein kinase C activation by diacylglycerol second messengers. Cell 1986; 45:631–632.

256. Nishizuka Y. The molecular heterogeneity of protein kinase C and its implications for cellular regulation. Nature 1988; 334:661–665.

257. Panayotou G, Waterfield MD. Cell surface receptors for polypeptide hormones, growth factors and neuropeptides. Curr Opin Cell Biol 1990; 1:167–176.

258. Blackshear PJ, Nairn AC, Kuo JF. Protein kinases 1988: a current perspective. FASEB J 1988; 2:2957–2969.

259. Sakane F, Yamada K, Kanoh H, et al. Porcine diacylglycerol kinase sequence has zinc finger and E-F hand motifs. Nature 1990; 344:345–358.

260. Rosenthal W, Hescheler J, Trautwein W, et al. Receptor- and G-protein–mediated modulations of voltage-dependent calcium channels. Cold Spring Harb Symp Quant Biol 1988; 53:247–254.

261. Levitan ED, Schofield PR, Burt DR, et al. Structural and functional basis for GABA$_A$ receptor heterogeneity. Nature 1988; 328:221–227.

262. Birnbaumer L, Codina J, Yatani A, et al. Molecular basis of regulation of ionic channels by G-proteins. Recent Prog Horm Res 1989; 45:121–206.

263. Rosenthal W, Hescheler J, Trautwein W, et al. Control of voltage-dependent Ca^{2+} channels by G-protein coupled receptors. FASEB J 1988; 2:2784–2790.

264. Kurachi Y. Regulation of G protein gated K^+ channels. News Physiol Sci 1989; 4:158–161.

265. Meldolesi J, Pozzan T. Pathways of Ca^{2+} influx at the plasma membrane: voltage-, receptor-, and second messenger–operated channels. Exp Cell Res 1987; 171:271–283.

266. Hallam TJ, Rink TJ. Receptor-mediated Ca^{2+} entry: diversity of function and mechanism. Trends Pharmacol Sci 1989; 10:8–10.

267. Daughaday WH, Rotwein P. Insulin-like growth factors I and II. Peptide, messenger ribonucleic acid and gene structures, serum and tissue concentrations. Endocr Rev 1989; 10:68–91.

268. Carter-Su C, Stubbart JR, Wang XY, et al. Phosphorylation of highly purified growth hormone receptors by a growth hormone receptor–associated tyrosine kinase. J Biol Chem 1989; 264:18654–18661.

269. Lesniak MA, Gorden P, Roth J. Reactivity of non-primate growth hormones and prolactins with human growth hormone receptors on cultured human lymphocytes. J Clin Endocrinol Metab 1977; 44:838–849.

270. Radke MJ, Misko TP, Hsu C, et al. Gene transfer and molecular cloning of the rat nerve growth factor receptor. Nature 1987; 325:593–597.

271. Grunfeld C, Baird K, Van Obberghen E, et al. Glucocorticoid-induced insulin resistance in vitro: evidence for both receptor and postreceptor defects. Endocrinology 1981; 109:1723–1730.

272. Bar RS, Gorden P, Roth J, et al. Fluctuations in the affinity and concentration of insulin receptors on circulating monocytes of obese patients. J Clin Invest 1976; 38:1123–1135.

273. Pedersen O, Beck-Nielsen H, Heding L. Increased insulin receptors

after exercise in patients with insulin-dependent diabetes mellitus. N Engl J Med 1980; 302:886–892.

274. Kolterman OG, Greenfield M, Reaven GM, et al. Effect of a high carbohydrate diet on insulin binding to adipocytes and on insulin action in vivo in man. Diabetes 1979; 28:731–736.

275. Ginsberg BH, Brown TJ, Simon I, et al. Effect of the membrane lipid environment on the properties of insulin receptors. Diabetes 1981; 30:773–780.

276. Neufeld ND, Ezrin C, Corbo L, et al. Effects of caloric restriction and exercise on insulin receptors in obesity: association with changes in membrane lipids. Metabolism 1986; 34:580–587.

277. Rabinowitz D. Some endocrine and metabolic aspects of obesity. Annu Rev Med 1970; 21:241–258.

278. Truglia JA, Livingston JN, Lockwood DH. Insulin resistance: receptor and post-binding defects in human obesity and non–insulin dependent mellitus. Am J Med 1985; 79:13–22.

279. Archer JA, Gorden P, Roth J. Defect in insulin binding to receptors in obese man: amelioration with caloric restriction. J Clin Invest 1975; 55:166–174.

280. Adams M, LeRoith D, Simon J, et al. Effect of altered nutritional states on insulin receptors. Annu Rev Nutr 1988; 8:144–166.

281. Soll AS, Kahn CR, Neville DM Jr, et al. Insulin receptor deficiency in genetic and acquired obesity. J Clin Invest 1975; 56:769–780.

282. Wigand JP, Blackard WG. Down-regulation of insulin receptors in obese man. Diabetes 1979; 28:287–291.

283. Reaven GM. Insulin-independent diabetes mellitus: metabolic characteristics. Metabolism 1980; 29:445–454.

284. Olefsky JM, Reaven GM. Insulin binding in diabetes: relationships with plasma insulin levels and insulin sensitivity. Diabetes 1977; 26:680–688.

285. Kolterman OG, Gray RS, Griffin J, et al. Receptor and postreceptor defects contribute to the insulin resistance in non–insulin-dependent diabetes mellitus. J Clin Invest 1981; 68:957–969.

286. Freidenberg GR, Reichart D, Olefsky JM, et al. Reversibility of defective adipocyte insulin receptor kinase activity in non–insulin-dependent diabetes mellitus. J Clin Invest 1988; 82:1398–1406.

287. Caro JF, Ittoop O, Pories WJ, et al. Studies on the mechanism of insulin resistance in the liver from humans with noninsulin-dependent diabetes. J Clin Invest 1986; 78:249–258.

288. Arner P, Pollare T, Lithell H, et al. Defective insulin receptor tyrosine kinase in human skeletal muscle in obesity and type 2 (non–insulin-dependent) diabetes mellitus. Diabetologia 1987; 30:437–440.

289. Häring H, Obermaier-Kusser B. Insulin receptor kinase defects in insulin-resistant tissues and their role in the pathogenesis of NIDDM. Diabetes Metab Rev 1989; 5:431–441.

290. Truglia JA, Hayes GR, Lockwood DH. Intact adipocyte insulin-receptor phosphorylation and in vitro tyrosine kinase activity in animal models of insulin resistance. Diabetes 1988; 37:147–153.

291. Karasik A, Kahn CR. Dexamethasone-induced changes in phosphorylation of the insulin and epidermal growth factor receptors and their substrates in intact rat hepatocytes. Endocrinology 1988; 123:2214–2222.

292. Block NE, Buse MG. Effects of hypercortisolemia and diabetes on skeletal muscle insulin receptor function in vitro and in vivo. Am J Physiol 1989; 256:E39–E48.

293. Hansen I, Tsalikian E, Beaufrere B, et al. Insulin resistance in acromegaly: defects in both hepatic and extrahepatic insulin action. Am J Physiol 1986; 250:E269–E273.

294. Cecchin F, Ittoop O, Sinha MK, et al. Insulin resistance in uremia: insulin receptor kinase activity in liver and muscle from chronic uremic rats. Am J Physiol 1988; 254:E394–E401.

295. Van Putten JPM, Wieringa T, Krans HMJ. Low pH and ketoacids induce insulin receptor binding and postbinding alterations in cultured 3T3 adipocytes. Diabetes 1985; 34:744–750.

296. Taylor SI. Insulin action and inaction. Clin Res 1986; 35:459–472.

297. Fukushima N, Matsuura N, Nohara Y, et al. A case of insulin resistance associated with acanthosis nigricans. Tohoku J Exp Med 1984; 144:129–138.

298. Yoshimasa Y, Seino S, Whittaker J, et al. Insulin-resistant diabetes due to a point mutation that prevents insulin proreceptor processing. Science 1988; 240:784–787.

299. Taira M, Taira M, Hashimoto N, et al. Human diabetes associated with a deletion of the tyrosine kinase domain of the insulin receptor. Science 1989; 245:63–66.

300. Odawara M, Kadowaki T, Yamamoto R, et al. Human diabetes associated with a mutation in the tyrosine kinase domain of the insulin receptor. Science 1989; 245:66–68.

301. Kobayashi M, Sasaoka T, Takata Y, et al. Insulin resistance by unprocessed insulin proreceptors. Point mutation at the cleavage site. Biochem Biophys Res Commun 1988; 153:657–663.

302. Schilling EE, Rechler MM, Grunfeld C, et al. Primary defect of insulin receptors in skin fibroblasts cultured from an infant with leprechaunism and insulin resistance. Proc Natl Acad Sci USA 1979; 76:5877–5881.

303. Kadowaki T, Bevins CL, Cama A, et al. Two mutant alleles of the insulin receptor gene in a patient with extreme insulin resistance. Science 1988; 240:787–790.

304. Kaplowitz PB, d'Ercole AJ. Fibroblasts from a patient with leprechaunism are resistant to insulin, epidermal growth factor, and somatomedin C. J Clin Endocrinol Metab 1982; 55:741–748.

305. Moxham CP, Duronio V, Jacobs S. Insulin-like growth factor I receptor β-subunit heterogeneity: evidence for hybrid tetramers composed of insulin-like growth factor I and insulin receptor heterodimers. J Biol Chem 1989; 264:13238–13244.

306. Albright F, Burnett C, Smith PH, et al. Pseudohypoparathyroidism—an example of "Seabright-Bantam" syndrome. Endocrinology 1942; 30:922–932.

307. Farfel Z, Brickman AS, Kaslow HR, et al. Defect of receptor-cyclase coupling protein in pseudohypoparathyroidism. N Engl J Med 1980; 303:237–242.

308. Levine MA, Downs RW, Singer M, et al. Deficient activity of guanine nucleotide regulatory protein in erythrocytes from patients with pseudohypoparathyroidism. Biochem Biophys Res Commun 1980; 94:1319–1324.

309. Spiegel AM, Gierschik P, Levine MA, et al. Clinical implications of guanine nucleotide–binding proteins as receptor-effector couplers. N Engl J Med 1985; 312:26–33.

310. Carter A, Bardin C, Collings R, et al. Reduced expression of multiple forms of G_s-alpha in pseudohypoparathyroidism type Ia. Proc Natl Acad Sci USA 1987; 84:7266–7269.

311. Barrett D, Breslau NA, Wax MB, et al. New form of pseudohypoparathyroidism with abnormal catalytic adenylate cyclase. Am J Physiol 1989; 257:E277–E283.

312. Laron Z, Pertzelan A, Mannheimer S. Genetic pituitary dwarfism with high serum concentration of growth hormone. A new inborn error of metabolism? Isr J Med Sci 1966; 2:152–155.

313. Laron Z, Pertzelan A, Karp M. Pituitary dwarfism with high serum levels of growth hormone. Isr J Med Sci 1968; 4:883–894.

314. Daughaday WH, Laron Z, Pertzelan A, et al. Defective sulfation factor generation: a possible etiological link in dwarfism. Trans Assoc Am Physicians 1969; 82:129–138.

315. Laron Z, Kowadlo-Silbergeld A, Eshet R, et al. Growth hormone resistance. Ann Clin Res 1980; 12:269–277.

316. Elders MJ, Garland JT, Daughaday WH, et al. Laron's dwarfism: studies on the nature of the defect. J Pediatr 1973; 83:253–263.

317. Eshet R, Laron Z, Pertzelan A, et al. Defect of human growth hormone receptors in the liver of two patients with Laron-type dwarfism. Isr J Med Sci 1984; 20:8–11.

318. Daughaday WH, Trivedi B. Absence of serum growth hormone binding protein in patients with growth hormone receptor deficiency (Laron dwarfism). Proc Natl Acad Sci USA 1987; 84:4636–4640.

319. Fradkin JE, Eastman RC, Lesniak MA, et al. Specificity spillover at the hormone receptor—exploring its role in human disease. N Engl J Med 1989; 320:640–645.

320. DePablo F, Eastman RC, Roth J, et al. Plasma prolactin in acromegaly before and after treatment. J Clin Endocrinol Metab 1981; 53:344–352.

321. Carayon P, Lefort G, Nisula B. Interaction of human chorionic gonadotropin and human luteinizing hormone with human thyroid membranes. Endocrinology 1980; 106:1907—1916.

322. Nisula BC, Taliadouros GS, Carayon P. Primary and secondary biologic activities intrinsic to the human chorionic gonadotropin molecule. In: Segal SJ, ed. Chorionic Gonadotropin. New York: Plenum, 1980:17–35.

323. Mann K, Schneider N, Hoermann R. Thyrotropic activity of acidic isoelectric variants of human chorionic gonadotropin from trophoblastic tumors. Endocrinology 1986; 118:1558–1566.

324. Gorden P, Hendricks CM, Kahn CR, et al. Hypoglycemia associated with non–islet-cell tumor and insulin-like growth factors: a study of the tumor types. N Engl J Med 1981; 305:1452–1455.

325. Hyodo T, Megyesi K, Kahn CR, et al. Adrenocortical carcinoma and hypoglycemia: evidence for production of nonsuppressible insulin-like activity by the tumor. J Clin Endocrinol Metab 1977; 44:1175–1184.

326. Daughaday WH, Emanuele MA, Brooks MH, et al. Synthesis and secretion of insulin-like growth factor II by a leiomyosarcoma with associated hypoglycemia. N Engl J Med 1988; 319:1434–1440.

327. Taylor SI, Dons RF, Hernandez E, et al. Insulin resistance associated with androgen excess in women with autoantibodies to the insulin receptor. Ann Intern Med 1982; 97:851–855.

328. Milner RDG, Hill DJ. Fetal growth control: the role of insulin and related peptides. Clin Endocrinol 1984; 21:415–433.

329. Wilson K, Eisenbarth GS. Immunopathogenesis and immunotherapy of type I diabetes. Annu Rev Med 1990; 41:497–508.

330. Neufeld M, Maclaren NK, Blizzard RM. Two types of autoimmune Addison's disease associated with different autoimmune (PGA) syndromes. Medicine 1981; 60:355–362.

331. Dussault JH, Rousseau F. Immunologically mediated hypothyroidism. Endocrinol Metab Clin North Am 1987; 16:417–429.

332. Neufeld M, Maclaren N, Blizzard R. Autoimmune polyglandular syndromes. Pediatr Ann 1980; 9:154–162.

333. Blecher M. Receptors, antibodies, and disease. Clin Chem 1984; 30:1137–1156.

334. Flier JS, Kahn CR, Roth J, et al. Antibodies that impair insulin receptor

binding in an unusual diabetic syndrome with severe insulin resistance. Science 1975; 190:63–65.

335. Kahn CR, Flier JS, Bar RS, et al. The syndromes of insulin resistance and acanthosis nigricans. Insulin-receptor disorders in man. N Engl J Med 1976; 294:739–745.

336. Grunfeld C, Van Obberghen E, Karlsson FA, et al. Antibody-induced desensitization of the insulin receptor: studies of the mechanism of desensitization in 3T3-L1 fatty fibroblasts. J Clin Invest 1980; 66:1124–1134.

337. Flier JS, Bar RS, Muggeo M, et al. The evolving clinical course of patients with insulin receptor autoantibodies: spontaneous remission or receptor purification with hypoglycemia. J Clin Endocrinol Metab 1978; 47:985–995.

338. Taylor SI, Grunberger G, Marcus-Samuels B, et al. Hypoglycemia associated with antibodies to the insulin receptor. N Engl J Med 1982; 307:1422–1426.

339. Bar RS, Levis WR, Rechler MM, et al. Extreme insulin resistance in ataxia telangiectasia: defect in affinity of insulin receptors. N Engl J Med 1978; 298:1164–1171.

340. Blecher M. Receptors, antibodies and disease. Clin Chem 1984; 30:1137–1156.

341. Maron R, Elias D, deJongh BM, et al. Autoantibodies to the insulin receptor in juvenile onset insulin-dependent diabetes. Nature 1983; 303:817–818.

342. Smith BR, McLachlan SM, Furmaniak J. Autoantibodies to the thyrotropin receptor. Endocr Rev 1988; 9:106–121.

343. Adams DD. The presence of an abnormal thyroid stimulating hormone in the serum of some thyrotoxic patients. J Clin Endocrinol Metab 1958; 18:699–712.

344. Beckner SK, Brady RO, Fishman PH. Reevaluation of the role of gangliosides in the binding and action of thyrotropin. Proc Natl Acad Sci USA 1981; 78:4848–4852.

345. Yavin E, Yavin Z, Schneider MD, et al. Monoclonal antibodies to the thyrotropin receptor: implications for receptor structure and the action of autoantibodies in Graves' disease. Proc Natl Acad Sci USA 1981; 78:3180–3184.

346. Furmaniak J, Nakajima Y, Hashim FA, et al. The TSH receptor: structure and interaction with autoantibodies in thyroid disease. Acta Endocrinol Suppl 1987; 281:157–165.

347. Madec AM, Laurent MC, Lorcy Y, et al. Thyroid stimulating antibodies: an aid to the strategy of treatment of Graves' disease? Clin Endocrinol 1984; 21:247–255.

348. Rapoport B, Greenspan FS, Filetti S, et al. Clinical experience with a human thyroid cell bioassay for thyroid stimulating immunoglobulin. J Clin Endocrinol Metab 1984; 58:332–338.

349. Bishop JM. The molecular genetics of cancer. Science 1987; 235:305–311.

350. Hunter T. The functions of oncogene products. Prog Clin Biol Res 1989; 288:25–34.

351. Margolis B, Rhee S, Felder S, et al. EGF induces tyrosine phosphorylation of phospholipase C-II: a potential mechanism for EGF receptor signaling. Cell 1989; 57:1101–1107.

352. Kraux MH, Pierce JH, Fleming TP, et al. Mechanisms by which genes encoding growth factors and growth factor receptors contribute to malignant transformation. Ann NY Acad Sci 1988; 551:320–335.

353. McCormick F. ras GTPase activating protein: signal transmitter and signal terminator. Cell 1989; 56:5–8.

354. Burgoyne RD. Small GTP-binding proteins. Trends Biochem Sci 1989; 14:394–396.

355. Landis CA, Masters SB, Spada A, et al. GTPase inhibiting mutations activate the α chain of G_s and stimulate adenyl cyclase in human pituitary tumors. Nature 1989; 340:692–696.

356. Lyons J, Landis CA, Harsh G, et al. Two G protein oncogenes in human endocrine tumors. Science 1990; 249:655–659.

357. Doolittle RF, Hunkapiller MW, Hood LE, et al. Simian sarcoma virus onc gene, v-sis, is derived from the gene (or genes) encoding a platelet-derived growth factor. Science 1983; 221:275–277.

358. Morrison DK, Kaplan DF, Escobedo JA, et al. Direct activation of the serine/threonine kinase Raf-1 through tyrosine phosphorylation by the PDGF beta-receptor. Cell 1989; 58:649–657.

359. Kouzarides T, Ziff E. Leucine zippers of fos, jun, and GCN4 dictate dimerization specificity and thereby control DNA binding. Nature 1989; 340:568–571.

360. Damm K, Thompson CC, Evans RM. Protein encoded by v-erbA functions as a thyroid-hormone receptor antagonist. Nature 1989; 339:593–597.

361. Weinberg RA. Oncogenes, antioncogenes and the molecular basis of multistep carcinogenesis. Cancer Res 1989; 49:3713–3721.

5

NEUROENDOCRINOLOGY

Seymour Reichlin

INTRODUCTION

The endocrine and nervous systems regulate almost all metabolic and homeostatic activities of the organism, determine the pace of growth and development, influence many forms of behavior, and control reproduction. The two regulatory systems interact: the rate of most endocrine secretions is influenced directly or indirectly by the brain, and virtually all hormones can influence brain activity. The basic functional unit of the nervous system is the neuron, which provides an organized network of point-to-point connections. The basic functional unit of the endocrine system is the secretory cell, which provides its regulatory influence through the circulating blood. Nerve cells and endocrine cells have many attributes in common. Nerve cells have a secretory function as well as a capacity to propagate action potentials, and endocrine cells have electric potentials as well as a secretory capacity. Neurons, in common with endocrine glands, activate their target cells through chemical mediators that react with specific cell receptors.[1] Several kinds of peptides and neurotransmitters that are synthesized by nerve cells are identical with those secreted by endocrine glands and appear to have their evolutionary origin as cell-regulatory factors of primitive, single-cell organisms.[2, 3] Many of the regulatory peptide hormones of the gastrointestinal tract are also found in neurons of both the central and the peripheral nervous systems (gut-brain peptides).

For these reasons, traditional distinctions between neural and hormonal control have become blurred, and the field of neuroendocrinology, which was traditionally defined as the study of the relationship between the nervous system and the endocrine system, has been expanded to include the study of the secretions of the brain regardless of whether they enter the bloodstream.[4–6] As a generalization, specificity of circulating hormone action is endowed by the presence of receptors on target tissues, whereas neuronal specificity comes from receptor distribution and anatomical connections (which are sometimes referred to as "hard wiring").

The immune system is now recognized to be a third integrative system that interacts with both the endocrine system and the nervous system. Neural and endocrine factors can influence various elements of the immune response, and, in turn, various aspects of the immune response (which are mediated by cytokines, the soluble secretions of activated lymphocytes) modulate both neural and endocrine functions. Viewed from a neuroendocrine perspective the lymphocyte population is a foreign protein recognition system, which responds to antigen invasion by secreting specialized hormonal factors.[7]

This chapter deals with the pathophysiological basis of the diseases that arise from disturbed neural regulation of endocrine secretion. This chapter also deals with the function of brain peptides, with the secretions of the brain, and with the interaction of the brain and the immune system. These topics are considered in other chapters as well: the anterior pituitary in Chapter 6; the adrenal medulla and the sympathetic nervous system in Chapter 10; the reproductive system in Chapters 12, 13, 14, and 18; and the role of the neurohypophysis in water balance in Chapter 7. The development of the field of neuroendocrinology has been recorded in a number of historical reviews,[8–17] and current knowledge in the field is summarized in textbooks, monographs, and review volumes.[18–33]

NEURAL CONTROL OF GLANDULAR SECRETION

Secretory cells were traditionally classified into two general types: *exocrine cells*, which release their products to the exterior of the body or into a hollow lumen that communicates with the exterior; and *endocrine cells*, which secrete their products into the circulation. The discovery of neurosecretion added a third category of secretory cells: *neurohormonal cells*, which are nerve cells that release their products into the general circulation. With few exceptions, exocrine and endocrine glands are regulated directly or indirectly by neural impulses: exocrine cells by *secretomotor fibers*; pituitary-dependent target glands by the hypothalamic *neurosecretory fibers*; and neurosecretory cells, in turn, by *neurotransmitters*. Although circulating lymphocytes do not receive a direct nerve supply, the thymus, the lymph nodes, and the spleen are innervated by autonomic nerve fibers. Virtually all glands are influenced by circulating hormones and metabolic factors, in addition to neural regulation (Fig. 5–1). Circulating hormones and local neural innervation, in turn, can interact with each other and with local *(paracrine)* mediators.

Secretomotor Control

Secretomotor control is mediated through nerves that end directly on secretory cells in defined synapses that bear a resemblance to the nerve terminals on muscles.[34–41] Examples of secretomotor control are regulation of the flow of saliva, tears, sweat, sebum, and gastric juice; secretion of epinephrine and melatonin; and control of the function of juxtaglomerular cells and pancreatic islets. Analogous nerve

---

SUPRAOPTICOHYPOPHYSEAL

RELEASES VASOPRESSIN (AVP) AND OXYTOCIN INTO THE PERIPHERAL CIRCULATION.

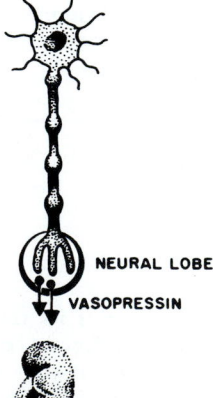

NEURAL LOBE

VASOPRESSIN

HYPOPHYSEOTROPIC

RELEASES HYPOPHYSEOTROPIC HORMONES INTO INTERSTITIAL SPACE OF MEDIAN EMINENCE OF HYPOTHALAMUS, THENCE THE RELEASING FACTORS REACH THE PITUITARY VIA THE HYPOPHYSEAL-PORTAL VESSELS.

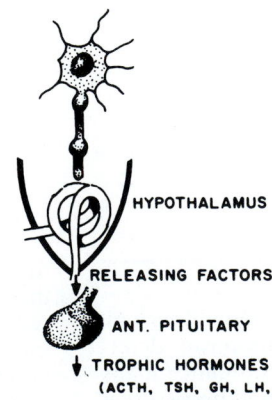

HYPOTHALAMUS

RELEASING FACTORS

ANT. PITUITARY

TROPHIC HORMONES (ACTH, TSH, GH, LH, FSH, PROLACTIN)

NEUROMODULATORS

Figure 5–1. Three types of neurosecretory cells. *Left,* A supraopticohypophyseal cell that secretes vasopressin (AVP). The cell body, which is located in the hypothalamus, projects its neuronal process into the neural lobe, and neurohormone is released from nerve endings. Similar peptidergic neurons are located in the medial basal hypothalamus *(center).* Neurohormones in this case are released into the specialized blood supply to the pituitary to regulate its secretion. Although the distance involved is small, the secretion can be termed a neurohormone because it enters the circulating blood. Similar in plan are neurosecretory neurons that terminate in relation to another neuron *(right).* Such neurosecretions may serve as neurotransmitters or neuromodulators. ACTH, corticotropin; TSH, thyrotropin; GH, growth hormone; LH, luteinizing hormone; FSH, follicle-stimulating hormone.

terminals are involved in regulation of cardiac contraction and gastrointestinal motor activity. Secretomotor nerve fibers are part of the sympathetic and the parasympathetic nervous systems and thus can be controlled directly by central nervous system pathways. Secretomotor effects often interact with hormonal influences. Secretomotor control has been traditionally attributed to the release at nerve endings of norepinephrine (sympathetic nerves) and acetylcholine (cholinergic nerves); however, neuropeptide transmitters usually coexist in the same fibers as the catecholamines and acetylcholine, and the effects of nerve stimulation are often due to the synergistic action of more than one transmitter. An excellent example of synergistic relationships of neurotransmitters is the parasympathetic neuronal control of the parotid gland, which is mediated by both acetylcholine and vasoactive intestinal peptide (VIP).[39] Stimulation of the nerve supply to the parotid (the chorda tympani) releases both factors. When administered alone, acetylcholine stimulates secretion of enzyme-rich saliva; VIP by itself has little effect on salivary production but stimulates parotid blood flow. When administered together, VIP and acetylcholine bring about an increase in salivary secretion much greater than that caused by acetylcholine alone.

Preganglionic sympathetic fibers that terminate in sympathetic ganglia, which were traditionally classified as cholinergic, may also contain biologically active peptides. For example, preganglionic sympathetic nerve stimulation in higher vertebrates releases both VIP and acetylcholine. Two or more kinds of neurotransmitters can also be present in the same central neurons (see later).

Neurosecretion

The term *neurosecretion* refers to the release of a hormone into the circulation from a nerve terminal.[42] The idea that a neuron could possess secretory functions was proposed by Scharrer in the 1930s on the basis of the morphological study of hypothalamic cells of fish.[43] Later, he and his colleagues observed analogous structures in the mammalian hypothalamus, recognized that the appearance of certain groups of neurons was modified by changes in state of hydration, and showed that extracts of the hypothalamus contained bioassayable antidiuretic hormone. They proposed that the secretions of the neural lobe actually arose in the hypothalamus. The clues that led to the acceptance of this view were the discovery of the phenomenon of axoplasmic flow (the transport of constituents of cytoplasm and organelles from the body of the nerve cell to the axon terminal)[44-46] and the demonstration that secretory products of the neurohypophysis accumulate proximal to section or ligation of the pituitary stalk.

An example of a typical neurosecretory gland in the mammal is the neurohypophysis. Neurosecretions (vasopressin [AVP, also called antidiuretic hormone, ADH] and oxytocin) that are formed in cell bodies located in the hypothalamus and are transported to the neural lobe by axoplasmic flow are released into the blood as true hormones; they regulate the function of organs at remote sites. Neurosecretions of this type are called *neurohormones*. Because neurons that are analogous to those of the neurohypophysis can terminate in synapses on other neurons *within* the neuroaxis, the concept of neurosecretion has now been expanded to include the release of any neuronal secretory product from a nerve ending; the secretion can serve as either a neurotransmitter or a neuromodulator (see Fig. 5–1).[47] Neurotransmitters are released into the synaptic cleft and stimulate (or inhibit) postsynaptic neurons with a brief latency. The distinction between a neurotransmitter and a neuromodulator is not absolute, but neuromodulators tend

to have a longer latency of effect and persist for a longer period. They function mainly to modify the responsiveness of the target neuron to the action of a neurotransmitter.[48] Because communication within the nervous system is almost exclusively through chemical messengers, neurosecretion is a fundamental property of all neurons. The ultimate route that is taken by the secretory product of an axon and its site of action depend on its anatomical relationships to other structures.

Discovery of the endogenous opioids and of the widespread distribution of extrahypothalamic peptidergic neuron systems has led to recognition that many important brain functions are modulated by the secretions of specific neurons. Guillemin referred to this insight as "the new endocrinology of the neuron."[47] The role of neuropeptides in brain function is reviewed later.

Peptide secretions, which are the products of *peptidergic* neurons, are synthesized on the endoplasmic reticulum, as is the case for more obviously glandular cells such as those of the parathyroid gland or pancreatic islet cells (see Chapters 2 and 3). Synthesis is directed by the genetic program of the cell so that the secretory product is packaged into granules in the Golgi apparatus and is transported by axoplasmic flow to nerve endings (Fig. 5–2). Release occurs by reverse pinocytosis in response to a propagated action po-

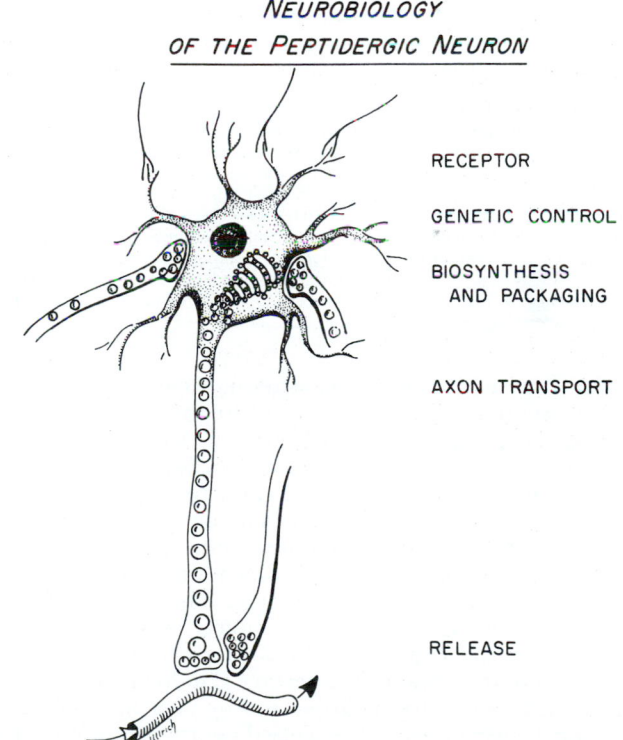

NEUROBIOLOGY OF THE PEPTIDERGIC NEURON

RECEPTOR

GENETIC CONTROL

BIOSYNTHESIS AND PACKAGING

AXON TRANSPORT

RELEASE

Figure 5–2. Neurobiology of the peptidergic neuron. Neurosecretory neurons can be regarded as having secretory functions in many ways analogous to those of glandular cells. A secretory product, which is formed on the endoplasmic reticulum under the direction of messenger RNA, is packaged in granules and is transported along the axon by axoplasmic flow to reach nerve terminals, where they are released. Virtually all neurons carry out similar functions: some secrete neurotransmitters, such as acetylcholine or norepinephrine; others, such as motor nerves, secrete myotrophic factors. In all neurons there is a constant orthograde (forward) flow of cytoplasm and formed elements such as mitochondria. Retrograde flow also takes place to bring substances that enter nerve endings back to the body of the cell. In typical neurotransmitter neurons the neurotransmitters are synthesized by enzymes and are packaged into secretory granules. These granules are transported similarly to neuropeptide-containing granules. In many neurons cosecretion of one or two peptides may occur in association with secretion of a classic neurotransmitter. (From Reichlin S. Summarizing comments. In: Gotto AM Jr, Peck EJ Jr, Boyd AE III, et al., eds. Brain Peptides: A New Endocrinology. New York: Elsevier/North-Holland, 1979: 379–403.)

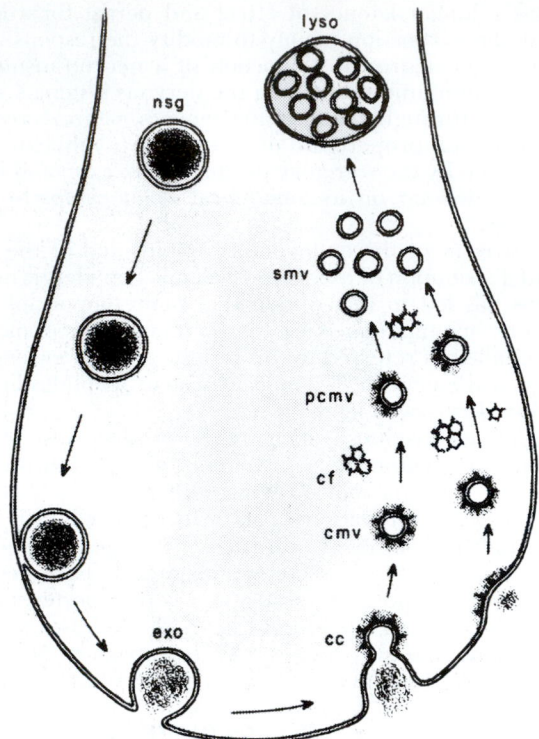

Figure 5–3. Release of stored neurosecretory granules from nerve terminals in the neural lobe. According to Douglas and collaborators, exocytosis (exo) takes place by fusion of neurosecretory granule (nsg) membrane and cell membrane, with extrusion of the granule contents into the extracellular space. The granule membrane is retrieved from the terminal's surface by micropinocytosis-like activity (vesiculation), which produces coated caveolae (cc) that pinch off as coated microvesicles (cmv) and then shed coat fragments (cf) to become partially coated microvesicles (pcmv) and, finally, smooth (synaptic) microvesicles (smv). These microvesicles, in turn, are incorporated in lysosome bodies (lyso), where presumably they are degraded, and contents are recycled. (From Douglas WW. Mechanism of release of neurohypophysial hormones: stimulus-secretion coupling. In: Greep RO, Astwood EB, Knobil E, et al., eds. Handbook of Physiology. Sect 7: Endocrinology. Vol IV. The Pituitary Gland and Its Neuroendocrine Control. Part 1. Washington, DC: American Physiological Society, 1974: 191–224.)

tential (Fig. 5–3).[45, 46] Neurosecretory cells, regardless of their location, retain functional and structural properties of neurons. They display typical neuronal electrophysiological characteristics, have neuron-type organelles, are acted on by other neurons through synapses, and react to neurotransmitter substances such as acetylcholine. The specialized neural structures that secrete hormones into the blood serve as one of the major links by which the brain regulates metabolic and reproductive activities. The term *neuroendocrine transducer* has been applied to nerve cells of this type,[49] because they are capable of translating neural activity into hormonal output. Neurons affecting glandular function are governed by still other neurons and by their metabolic and hormonal environments. Specialized neuronal receptors that react to changes in both the internal and the external environments can thus modulate endocrine function. These receptors also serve to generate adaptive and sexual behaviors. At the highest level the central nervous system integrates the varied neural and hormonal mechanisms to maintain the integrity of the individual organism and to perpetuate the species.

THE HYPOTHALAMIC-PITUITARY UNIT
Overview

Pituitary function depends on hypothalamic neurosecretion; the anatomical organization of the hypothalamic-

pituitary unit reflects this close relationship. In most vertebrates the pituitary is divided into three clearly defined lobes: the anterior lobe (also called the adenohypophysis, the pars distalis, or the pars glandularis), the neural lobe (also called the posterior pituitary or the infundibular process), and the intermediate lobe (also called the pars intermedia) (Figs. 5–4, 5–5, and 5–6). Only rudimentary vestiges of the intermediate lobe are apparent in adult humans, the bulk of intermediate lobe cells being distributed diffusely in the anterior and the posterior lobes. However, during fetal life and in pregnant women, an intermediate lobe is evident. The functional significance of the intermediate lobe in these two situations is unknown.

The *neurohypophysis* includes the neural stalk, the neural lobe, and the specialized neural tissue at the base of the hypothalamus forming the crucial region for the transfer of pituitary-regulating neurosecretions to the *anterior* pituitary. Viewed grossly, the neurohypophyseal portion of the hypothalamus (which forms the base of the third ventricle) looks like a funnel (Fig. 5–7). This resemblance is so striking that Vesalius, who first described these structures, proposed that the infundibulum (funnel) drained cerebrospinal fluid (CSF) as pituita (mucus) through the pituitary gland into the nose.

The central region of the base of the hypothalamus forms a mound (called the *median eminence of the tuber cinereum*) from which the pituitary stalk arises. It is enveloped from below by a delicate anterior extension of anterior pituitary tissue termed the *pars tuberalis*. This entire structure is penetrated by numerous capillary loops from the primary portal plexus of the hypophyseal-portal circulation. This neurovascular complex forms a small but conspicuous structure.[50, 51]

Neurohypophysis

ANATOMY. The neural lobe develops embryologically as a down-growth from the ventral diencephalon and retains its neural character in adult life. It is composed of dilated terminals of two major hypothalamic nerve tracts; capillaries; and supportive, glia-like nonsecreting cells (termed *pituicytes*). Unlike most brain capillaries, which form a barrier to diffusion (the blood-brain barrier), neural lobe capillaries resemble those of other endocrine glands in being fenestrated, thus permitting diffusion of secretions into the circulation.[52–56]

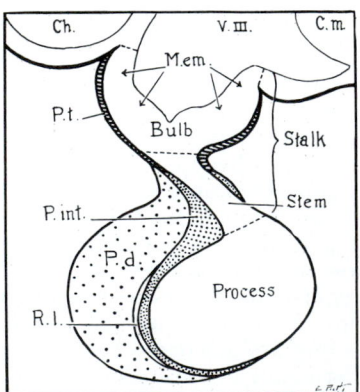

Figure 5–4. Structure and standard nomenclature of the hypothalamic-pituitary unit are outlined in this diagram of the hypophysis of a macaque monkey (*Macaca mulatta*). Bulb, "bulb" of "infundibulum," Ch., optic chiasma; C.m., mamillary body; M.em., median eminence; P.d., pars distalis; P.t., pars tuberalis; P.int., pars intermedia; Process, infundibular process (neural lobe); R.l., residual lumen; Stem, infundibular stem; V.III., third ventricle. (Reproduced from Rioch DM, Wislocki GB, O'Leary JL, et al. Précis of preoptic, hypothalamic and hypophyseal terminology with atlas. Assoc Res Nerv Ment Dis Proc [1939] 1940; 20:3–30, © 1940, The Williams & Wilkins Co., Baltimore.)

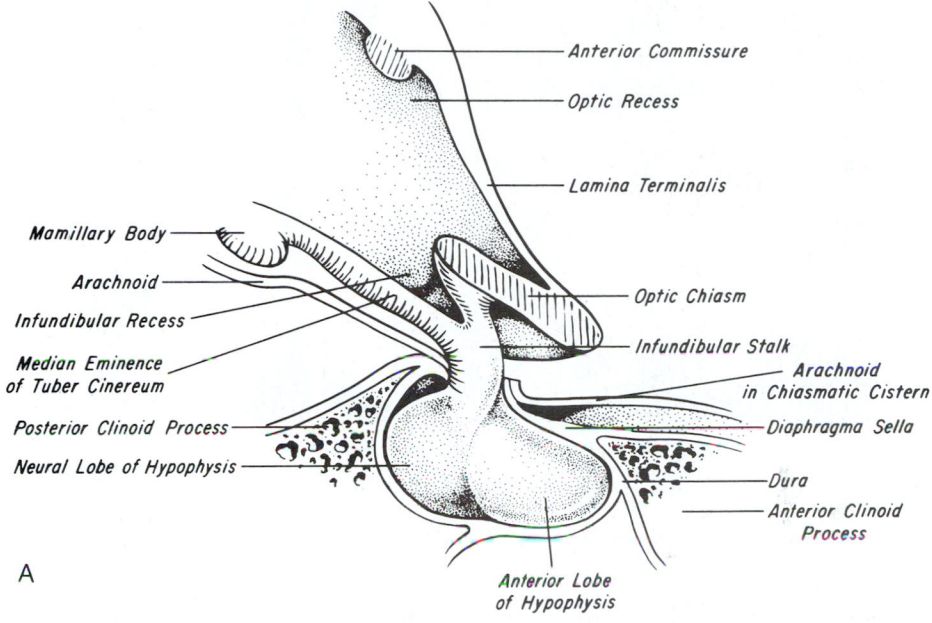

Anterior Commissure

Optic Recess

Lamina Terminalis

Mamillary Body

Arachnoid

Infundibular Recess

Median Eminence
of Tuber Cinereum

Posterior Clinoid Process

Neural Lobe of Hypophysis

Optic Chiasm

Infundibular Stalk

Arachnoid
in Chiasmatic Cistern

Diaphragma Sella

Dura

Anterior Clinoid
Process

A

Anterior Lobe
of Hypophysis

Figure 5–5. *A,* Human hypothalamic-pituitary unit showing the relationship to the sella turcica, brain membranes, and optic chiasm. *B,* Midsagittal nuclear magnetic resonance scan of the brain of a normal woman, which corresponds to the diagram in *A.* Note the location of the pituitary stalk, the intense signal from the posterior pituitary, and the anatomical relationship to the optic commissure and the optic nerve. See also Figure 5–7A. (Scan kindly provided by Dr. Samuel Wolpert.)

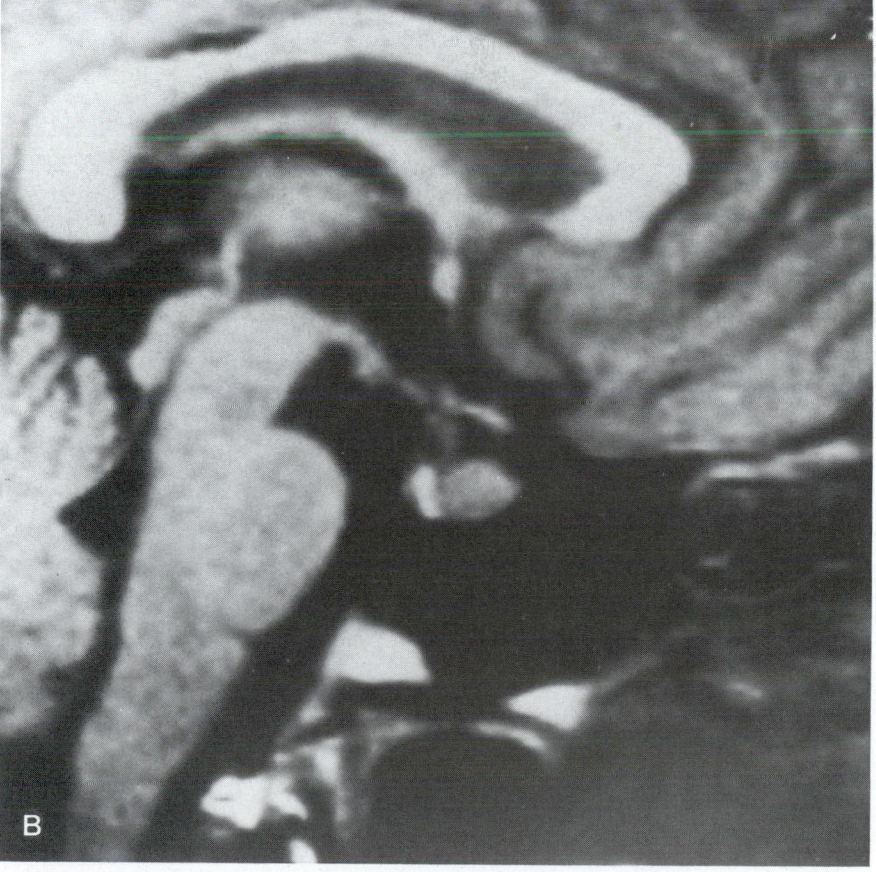

B

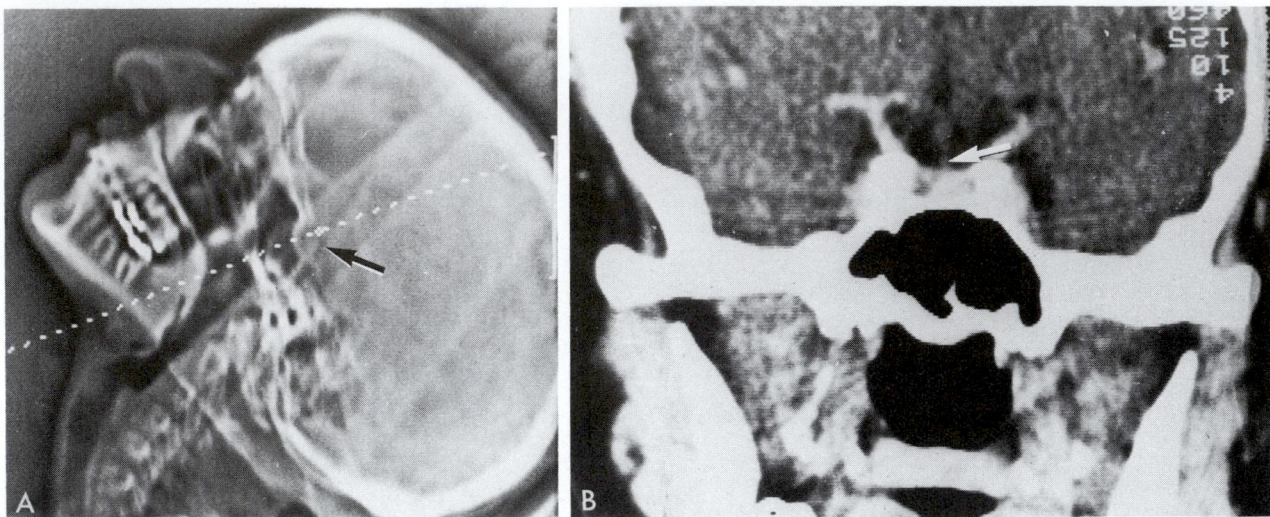

Figure 5–6. Computed tomographic (CT) scan of a coronal section of the human brain showing the relationship of the pituitary stalk and the pituitary to the sella turcica. *A,* Lateral scan with dotted line to indicate the plane of the CT scan through the pituitary; the arrow points to the posterior clinoid. *B,* Frontal scan taken 15 to 20 s after rapid intravenous injection of contrast material. By this method the first structures to contain contrast material are the blood vessels of the circle of Willis and the vascularized pituitary stalk *(point of arrow).* Lateral radiolucent areas on each side of the pituitary correspond to the cavernous sinus, which has not yet been filled with contrast material. (By kind permission of Dr. Samuel Wolpert.)

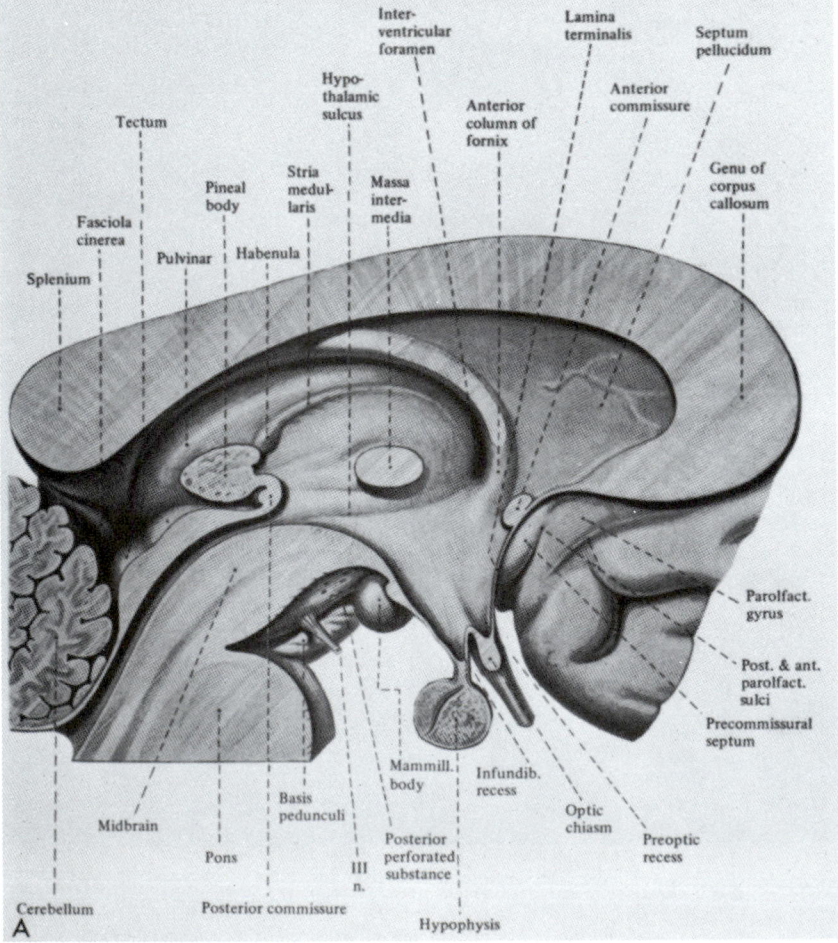

Figure 5–7. *A,* Midsagittal view of the human brain showing the hypothalamus and neighboring structures.

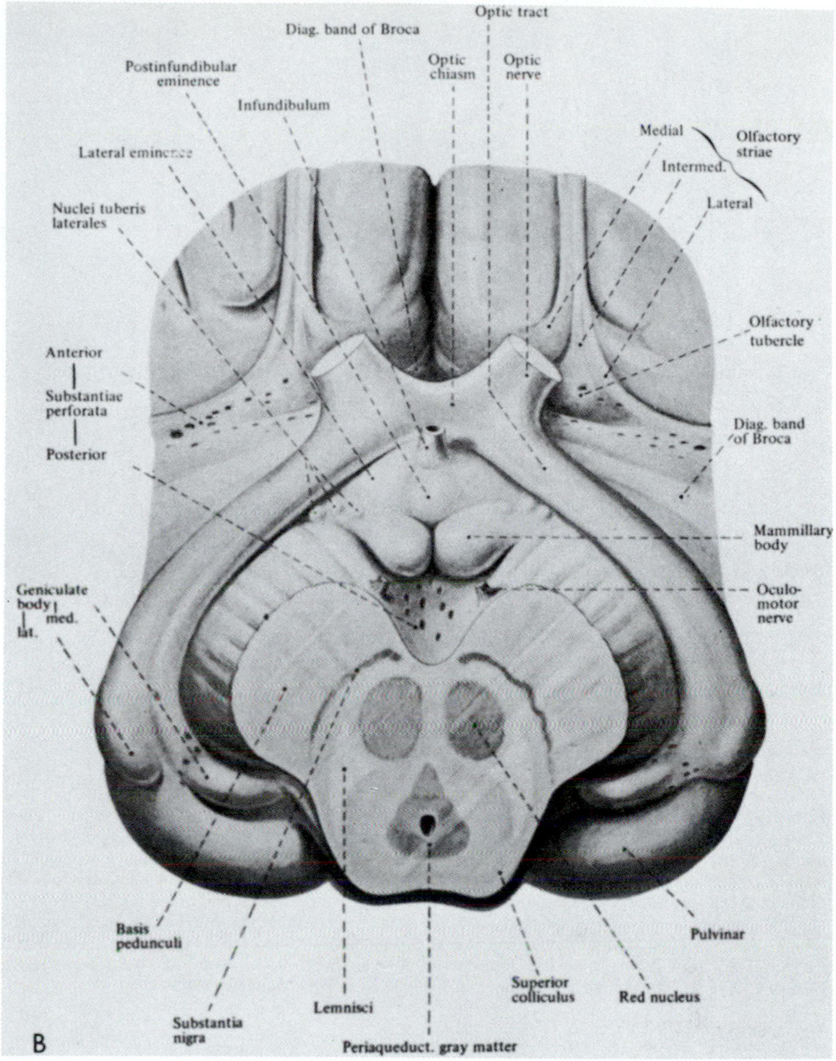

Optic tract
Diag. band of Broca
Postinfundibular eminence
Optic chiasm
Optic nerve
Infundibulum
Lateral eminence
Medial
Intermed.
Olfactory striae
Lateral
Nuclei tuberis laterales
Anterior
Substantiae perforata
Posterior
Olfactory tubercle
Diag. band of Broca
Geniculate body med. lat.
Mammillary body
Oculomotor nerve
Basis pedunculi
Pulvinar
B
Substantia nigra
Lemnisci
Superior colliculus
Red nucleus
Periaqueduct. gray matter

Figure 5–7 *Continued B,* Base of the human brain, showing the hypothalamus and neighboring structures. Several landmarks outline the hypothalamus on gross inspection. It is bounded anteriorly by the optic chiasm, laterally by the sulci formed with the temporal lobes, and posteriorly by the mamillary bodies (in which are located the mamillary nuclei). Dorsally, the hypothalamus is delineated from the thalamus by the hypothalamic sulcus. The smooth, rounded base of the hypothalamus is the tuber cinereum; the pituitary stalk descends from its central region, termed the *median eminence.* The median eminence stands out from the rest of the tuber cinereum because of its dense vascularity, which is formed by the primary plexus of the hypophyseal-portal system. The long portal veins run along the ventral surface of the pituitary stalk. (From Nauta WJ, Haymaker W. Hypothalamic nuclei and fiber connections. In: Haymaker W, Anderson E, Nauta WJ, eds. The Hypothalamus. Springfield, IL: Charles C Thomas, 1969: 136–209.)

The major nerve tracts of the neurohypophysis arise from relatively large-celled (hence termed *magnicellular*) paired nuclei: the supraoptic nucleus, which is located above the optic tract, and the paraventricular nucleus, which is located on each side of the ventricle (Figs. 5–8 and 5–9). Both tracts (the supraopticohypophyseal and the paraventriculohypophyseal) are unmyelinated and descend through the infundibulum and neural stalk to terminate in the neural lobe. Some fibers also terminate in the median eminence, where they are involved in regulation of the anterior lobe. Their principal secretions are AVP and oxytocin, but smaller populations of neurons terminating in the neural lobe contain other neuropeptides, including thyrotropin-releasing hormone (TRH), corticotropin-releasing hormone (CRH), VIP, and neurotensin. In some fibers two different peptides are colocalized, as is the case for CRH-AVP fibers arising in the paraventricular nucleus.[33]

AVP- and oxytocin-containing fibers are also distributed widely within the neuroaxis. Paraventricular AVP cells project to the brain stem, the spinal cord, and brain regions that are associated with emotional expression and higher functions including memory. Within the spinal cord they terminate on cells of the autonomic nervous system and can influence blood pressure; within the brain stem they end in the sensory nuclei of the vagus and glossopharyngeal nerves to which they convey information about blood pressure and blood volume.[53, 56] Vasopressinergic fibers also terminate on the choroid plexus, where they influence water and salt

exchange between the brain and the CSF.[57] Central fibers of these vasopressinergic and oxytocinergic pathways function independently of those that innervate the neurohypophysis. This situation has been shown by comparing the pattern of

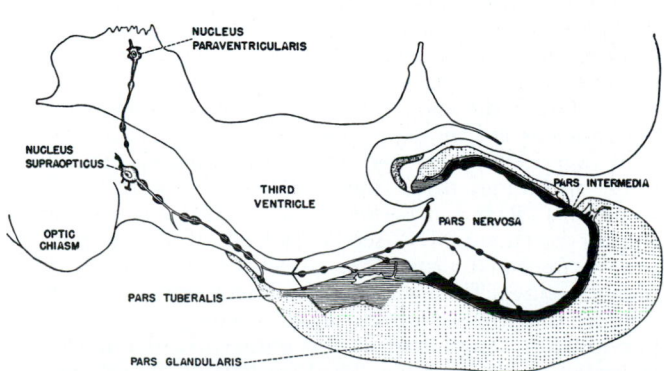

NUCLEUS PARAVENTRICULARIS
NUCLEUS SUPRAOPTICUS
THIRD VENTRICLE
PARS INTERMEDIA
PARS NERVOSA
OPTIC CHIASM
PARS TUBERALIS
PARS GLANDULARIS

Figure 5–8. Course of the neurosecretory substance from the hypothalamic cell body, along the neural stalk to the neurohypophysis. This diagram illustrates the concept of cell body formation of oxytocin and AVP and passage of the material down the stalk to a storage site in the neural lobe. The dilated areas on the axons were previously thought to represent extraneuronal accumulation of neurosecretory material. Electron microscopy now shows that all of the neurosecretory material is within the axon itself. (From Bargmann W, Scharrer E. The site of origin of the hormones of the posterior pituitary. Z Zellforsch Mikrosk Anat 1951; 39:255–259.)

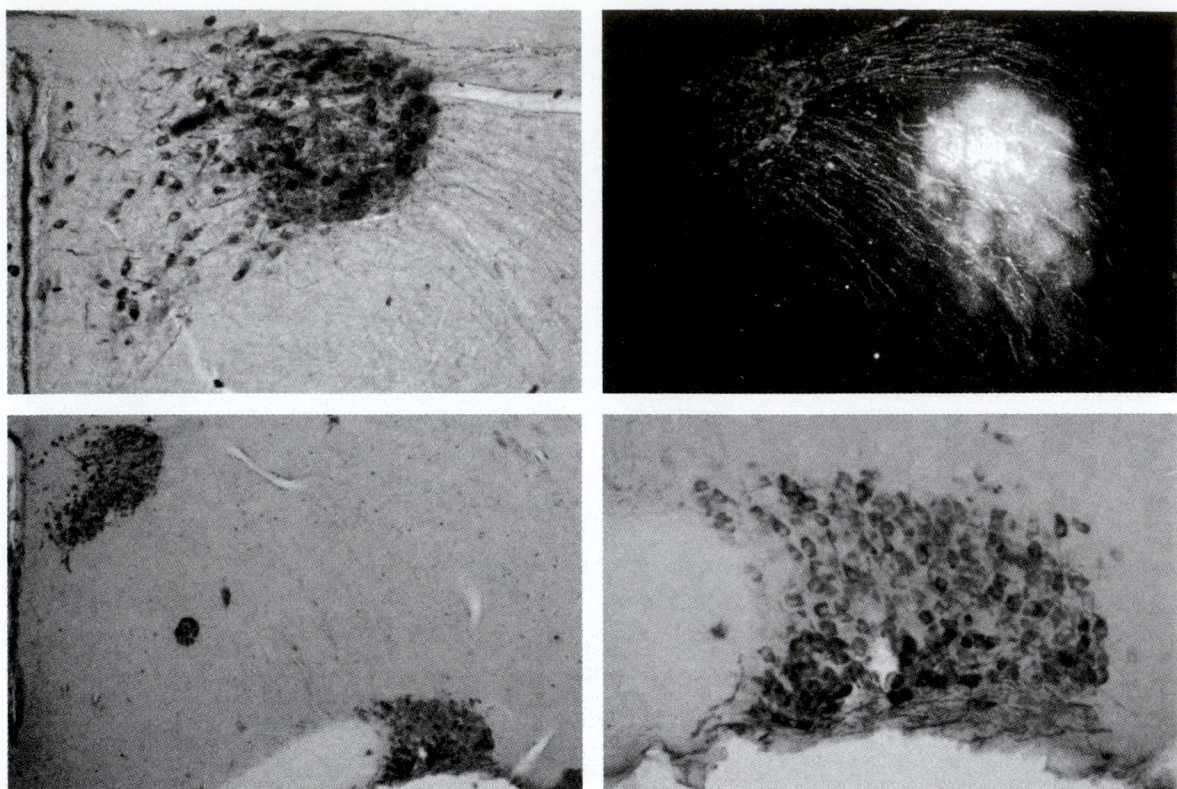

Figure 5–9. Photomicrographs of coronal sections of rat hypothalamus immunostained with antibodies to AVP and to oxytocin to show the paraventricular and supraoptic nuclei. *Lower left,* Both nuclei are immunostained, the paraventricular nucleus forming a wing-like structure lateral to the third ventricle, the supraoptic nucleus in this level appearing at the extreme lateral margin of the optic tract. *Upper left,* Higher magnification of the paraventricular nucleus. AVP-staining neurons form a central core in the lateral magnicellular group rimmed by oxytocin-containing neurons. *Lower right,* Higher magnification of the supraoptic nucleus. AVP-containing neurons (staining darker) are more concentrated in the ventral part of the nucleus at this level. *Upper right,* Dark-field photomicrograph of the paraventricular nucleus reacted only with monoclonal antibody specific to AVP. Numerous beaded axonal fibers project laterally from cell bodies through and around the fornix, which shows here as a white mass in the lateral hypothalamus. (Photographs by Alfred T. Lamme, FBPA. Illustrations published with permission of Plenum Publishing Corporation. From Zimmerman EA, Hou-Yu A, Nilaver G, et al. Anatomy of pituitary and extrapituitary vasopressin secretory systems. In: Reichlin S, ed. The Neurohypophysis: Physiological and Clinical Aspects. New York: Plenum, 1984: 5–33.)

CSF level of AVP with the peripheral AVP level. Central AVP levels show a circadian rhythm independent of the state of hydration.[58] In contrast, peripheral AVP levels, which reflect the secretion of the neurohypophysis, do not follow a circadian pattern and are related to blood volume and plasma osmolarity. Oxytocin levels in CSF also follow a time-dependent pattern that is dissociated from blood levels.[59] Most of the cell bodies in the supraoptic nucleus contain AVP, but some contain oxytocin. A somewhat smaller percentage (but still the majority) of cells in the paraventricular nucleus contain AVP.[60]

Although the magnicellular neurons of the paraventricular nucleus are most prominent, the small-celled component (parvicellular neurons) secretes additional neuropeptides, including those that control thyrotropin (TSH) secretion (TRH) and corticotropin (ACTH, adrenocorticotropin) secretion (CRH) (see later). Cells of this nucleus also receive neuronal projections directly and indirectly from higher centers, from visceral regulating centers, and from regions that determine circadian rhythms.[33] Indeed, the parvicellular component of the paraventricular nucleus is regarded by many as the "head nucleus of the neuroendocrine system," which generates neural signals that modulate anterior lobe secretion and integrate it with other neurally driven homeostatic functions.

SECRETIONS OF THE NEUROHYPOPHYSIS. The significance of the neurohypophysis as an organ of water conservation first came to light as the result of clinical investigation of patients with diabetes insipidus (DI).[52] The association of

pathological conditions of the neural stalk and pituitary with this syndrome prompted Farini and Von den Velden, working independently, to postulate that DI is a deficiency disease. They reported in 1913 that neural lobe extracts given to patients restored water balance. In 1924 Starling and Verney identified the site of action of posterior pituitary extracts on water excretion by perfusing the isolated kidney and demonstrating an antidiuretic effect. In the early 1930s Verney demonstrated the influence of hyperosmolar stimuli on antidiuresis by perfusing the carotid artery with hypertonic saline, and the neuroanatomical basis of neurohypophyseal secretion was established by Fisher and collaborators. Extensive efforts to identify the active principles of the neural lobe led to the elucidation of the structure of oxytocin in 1950 and of vasopressin in 1954. These nonapeptides were the first peptides and/or protein hormones to be sequenced and synthesized.

The principal biologically active substances from neural lobes are classified as having antidiuretic (water-conserving) activity and oxytocic (uterus-contracting) activity. Vasopressin raises blood pressure through vasoconstriction when given in relatively large doses. Oxytocin is the principal oxytocic substance. Both vasopressin and oxytocin are nonapeptides, i.e., contain nine amino acids; both have a Cys-Cys bridge in the 1-6 position (Table 5–1). Most submammalian vertebrates have only one neurohypophyseal peptide, arginine vasotocin,[61] which is a peptide that is probably the phylogenetic precursor of both oxytocin and vasopressin. A single-point mutation in vasotocin in position 8 (arginine to

TABLE 5–1. Sequences of the Principal Peptides of the Neurohypophysis

	1 2 3 4 5 6 7 8 9	1 2 3 4 5 6 7 8 9
Mammals (except pig)	Cys-Tyr-Ile-Gln-Asn-Cys-Pro-Leu-Gly-NH₂ Oxytocin	Cys-Tyr-Phe-Gln-Asn-Cys-Pro-Arg-Gly-NH₂ Arginine vasopressin
Pig	Cys-Tyr-Ile-Gln-Asn-Cys-Pro-Leu-Gly-NH₂ Oxytocin	Cys-Tyr-Phe-Gln-Asn-Cys-Pro-Lys-Gly-NH₂ Lysine vasopressin
Birds, reptiles, amphibians, lungfishes	Cys-Tyr-Ile-Gln-Asn-Cys-Pro-Ile-Gly-NH₂ Mesotocin	Cys-Tyr-Ile-Gln-Asn-Cys-Pro-Arg-Gly-NH₂ Vasotocin
Bony fishes (palcopteryglans and neopteryglans)	Cys-Tyr-Ile-Ser-Asn-Cys-Pro-Ile-Gly-NH₂ Isotocin	Cys-Tyr-Ile-Gln-Asn-Cys-Pro-Arg-Gly-NH₂ Vasotocin

leucine) gives rise to oxytocin. A single-point mutation in position 3 (leucine to phenylalanine) gives rise to vasopressin. The prohormones for oxytocin and vasopressin also share extensive homology, which suggests that the two peptides originated from a common gene.[62] Vasotocin is also found in the pineal gland but probably not in the neurohypophysis of mammals.[63] Mammalian vasopressins, with the exception of the pig, have identical amino acid sequences (AVP); in swine, arginine in position 9 is replaced by lysine. In keeping with a common evolutionary origin, vasopressin possesses minimal oxytocic activity; oxytocin exhibits minimal antidiuretic activity. Two somewhat overlapping classes of vasopressin receptors have been identified: V_1 receptors, which are located on vascular smooth muscle cells where they raise blood pressure, and V_2 receptors, which are located in the renal tubule where they promote water reabsorption.[64] A

TABLE 5–2. Neuroactive Materials in the Paraventricular Nucleus and the Arcuate Nucleus

Paraventricular Nucleus
Magnicellular Division
Angiotensin II
Cholecystokinin
Glucagon
Oxytocin
Peptide 7B2
Proenkephalin B (dynorphin, rimorphin, α-neoendorphin)
Vasopressin
Parvicellular Division
γ-Aminobutyric acid
Angiotensin II
Atrial natriuretic factor
Cholecystokinin
Corticotropin-releasing hormone
Dopamine
Follicle-stimulating hormone–releasing factor
Galanin
Glucagon
Neuropeptide Y
Neurotensin
Peptide 7B2
Proenkephalin A (met-enkephalin, leu-enkephalin, BAM 22P, metorphamide, met-enkephalin-Arg⁶-Phe⁷, met-enkephalin-Arg⁶-Gly⁷-Leu⁸)
Somatostatin
Thyrotropin-releasing hormone
Vasopressin
Vasoactive intestinal peptide/peptide-histidine-isoleucine (PHI)
Arcuate Nucleus
Acetylcholine (?)
γ-Aminobutyric acid
Dopamine
Galanin
Growth hormone–releasing hormone
Neuropeptide Y
Neurotensin
Pancreatic polypeptide
Proenkephalin A
Prolactin
Pro-opiomelanocortin (ACTH, β-lipotropin, γ-melanocyte-stimulating hormone, β-endorphin)
Somatostatin
Substance P

Modified from Lechan RM. Neuroendocrinology of pituitary hormone regulation. Endocrinol Metab Clin North Am 1987; 16:475–502.

synthetic peptide that is a relatively selective type V_2 agonist, desmopressin, is useful in the treatment of DI (see Chapter 7).

Other biologically active substances in the neurohypophysis include somatostatin (SRIF, somatotropin release–inhibiting factor), TRH, substance P, luteinizing hormone–releasing hormone (LHRH, also termed gonadotropin-releasing hormone, GnRH), dopamine, serotonin, histamine, and β-melanocyte-stimulating hormone (β-MSH).[65] Dynorphin A 1–8, an opioid peptide, is present in AVP-containing neurons and appears to be located in the same neurosecretory vesicles as AVP.[66] CRH colocalizes in most paraventricular vasopressinergic neurons; the two hormones act synergistically to release ACTH (see later). Other neuroactive materials in the paraventricular nucleus are given in Table 5–2. AVP and oxytocin are each associated with distinct peptides termed *neurophysins*. Neurophysins are part of the respective prohormones propressophysin and prooxyphysin (Fig. 5–10).[67-69] The neurophysins are released simultaneously with their respective neurohypophyseal peptides. Factors regulating the secretion of AVP and oxytocin also regulate the secretion of the respective neurophysins.[70, 71]

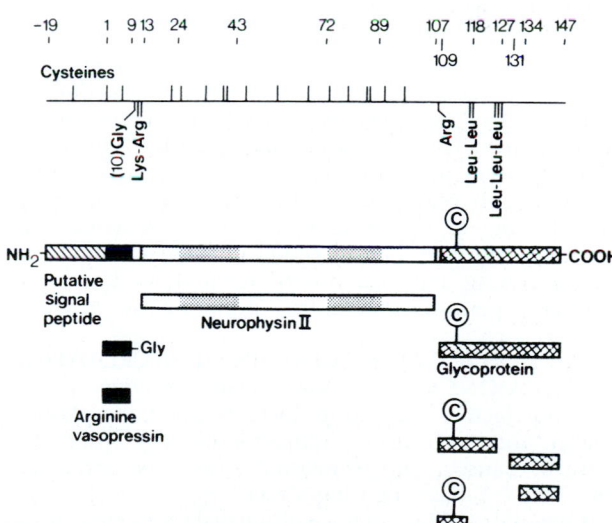

Figure 5–10. Schematic representation of the structure of bovine AVP–neurophysin II precursor, based on recombinant DNA analysis. Sequence coding for AVP is located immediately after the signal peptide, followed by sequence coding for neurophysin II. Following the neurophysin region is a glycoprotein segment. The top line illustrates the amino acid number. The second line from top shows the crucial amino acid sequence at which post-translational processing of the peptide takes place in secretory granules. The indication of glycine in position 10 is a characteristic extension in peptide hormones that contain a terminal amide. Glycine is exchanged for NH₂ during processing. Lys-Arg sequences at positions 11 and 12 are typical enzymatic cleavage sites, as is Arg in position 107. In the neurohypophyseal system, the entire prohormone is packaged in secretory granules, processed during axoplasmic transport, and AVP (a nonapeptide) is secreted in equimolar amounts as neurophysin II. (From Land H, Schütz G, Schmale H, et al. Nucleotide sequence of cloned cDNA encoding bovine arginine vasopressin–neurophysin II precursor. Reprinted by permission from Nature, Vol. 295, pp. 299–303. Copyright © 1982 Macmillan Journals Ltd.)

HORMONE SYNTHESIS, TRANSPORT, AND SECRETION.
Vasopressin and its related neurophysin (designated neurophysin II) and oxytocin and its related neurophysin (neurophysin I) are synthesized as prohormones in the cell bodies of the supraoptic and paraventricular neurons (see Fig. 5–9). The prohormones are transported in membrane-bound vesicles through the axons to the neural lobe, where they are stored and later released. Processing of the prohormone to the secreted products AVP, oxytocin, and the two neurophysins takes place in the vesicles during the course of transport.

Nerve action potentials arising in the cell body are propagated along the axon and trigger the hormone discharge. The neurohypophyseal hormones are secreted together with the neurophysins in fixed ratio.

The function of neurohypophyseal neurons is directly controlled by cholinergic and noradrenergic neurotransmitters[54, 72] and by several neuropeptides including angiotensin II, atrial peptide (AP, also called atrial natriuretic factor, ANF), and the endorphins (see later). Acetylcholine stimulation releases AVP (thus explaining the antidiuretic effects of tobacco smoking, which results in a response to nicotinic acid receptor stimulation). Acetylcholine also stimulates oxytocin secretion. Application of acetylcholine onto single supraoptic neurons markedly accelerates their firing rate. Adrenergic influences, in contrast, are inhibitory to oxytocin secretion through beta-adrenergic receptors. The stress-induced inhibition of the milk let-down reflex, which is well known from both animal husbandry and human nursing experience, is likely due to beta-adrenergic inhibition of oxytocin release. AVP secretion is also inhibited by beta-adrenergic fibers.

These neurons are also regulated by certain peptides. Angiotensin II releases AVP[73] and stimulates drinking behavior.[74] AP, which is also localized in the hypothalamus, inhibits AVP release and blocks the effects of angiotensin II, as well as effects of hypertonic saline on AVP release and on drinking behavior (see later).[75] Neurohypophyseal neurons are also stimulated by endogenous opioids (endorphins).[76] The antidiuretic action of morphine is due to the release of AVP, an effect that can be duplicated by intracerebroventricular administration of β-endorphin. The possibility that the endorphins may be involved in regulation of AVP secretion regulation is supported by the observation that naloxone, an opiate antagonist, can reverse neurogenically inappropriate AVP secretion in some situations.[77] Oxytocin-secreting neurons are innervated by a specialized brain stem pathway that utilizes inhibin as its neurotransmitter.[78]

PHYSIOLOGICAL REGULATION OF NEUROHYPOPHYSEAL HORMONE RELEASE. *Vasopressin Secretion*. The most important factors regulating AVP secretion are plasma osmolality and "effective" circulating blood volume. Blood pressure, nausea, and emotional stress also influence its release[54, 76, 79, 80] (also see Chapter 7).

Osmolality. Maintenance of normal water concentration in blood is the major homeostatic function of the neurohypophysis. Blood osmolality is zealously kept to within a relatively narrow range (± 1.8%). The mean set point of plasma osmolality for normal individuals is about 282 mmol/kg, and AVP release that is initiated after infusion of hypertonic saline causes an increase to about 287 mmol/kg, a level termed the *osmotic threshold*.[77–81] Above this value, AVP secretion increases rapidly and progressively with increasing plasma osmolality (Fig. 5–11). Water loading inhibits AVP release.

This osmotic regulatory system operates through a hypothalamic osmoreceptor neuron system. Intracarotid perfusion with hypertonic saline leads to antidiuresis,[82] a finding

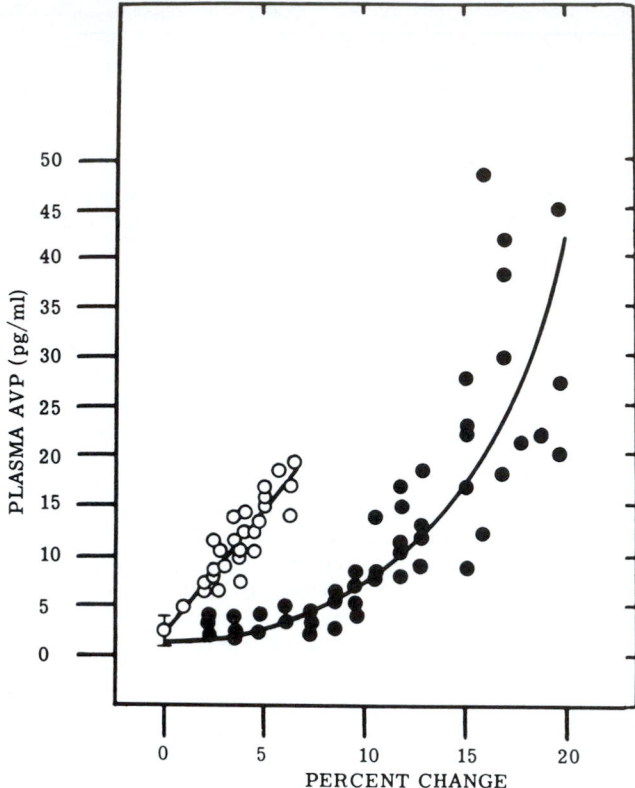

Figure 5–11. Relationship of plasma AVP level to the percent *increase* in blood osmolality (O) or *decrease* in blood volume (●) in conscious rats. The plasma AVP level is a linear function of the percent change in blood volume; virtually no change in AVP is detectable until there has been a 10 to 15% change in blood volume. To convert AVP values to picomoles per liter, multiply by 0.99. (From Dunn FL, Brennan TJ, Nelson AE, et al. The role of blood osmolality and volume in regulating vasopressin secretion in the rat. Reproduced from the Journal of Clinical Investigation, 1973, vol. 52, pp. 3212–3219 by copyright permission of the American Society of Clinical Investigation.)

indicating that some form of osmoreceptor exists within the perfusion area of the carotid. However, the precise mechanisms of osmoreceptor control have not been established. Neurons in both supraoptic and paraventricular nuclei, including some that project directly to the neural lobe (and hence are hormone-secreting), show an increased frequency of electric discharge immediately after intracarotid injections of hypertonic saline.[54] Thus the supraopticohypophyseal and paraventriculohypophyseal neurons may be intrinsically osmoreceptive. Alternatively, another population of anatomically closely related osmoreceptor cells may activate the AVP-secreting cells transynaptically. Clinical observations may provide some insight into this question. Some patients with hypothalamic disease lose osmoreceptor control of AVP secretion while retaining other regulatory responses such as those to cholinergic stimuli. In others, osmoreceptor control of AVP can be retained while the thirst sensation is lost. These findings suggest that there may be separate populations of osmoreceptor, AVP-secreting, and thirst-generating neurons, although there may be some overlap in these functions. The neuronal nature of the osmoreceptive process is uncertain. The effect is not specific for certain ions; any osmotically active particle (such as sucrose) that does not enter nerve cell bodies can stimulate AVP release. Vasopressinergic neurons receive abundant and diverse neuronal input from local and remote regions of the brain.

Volume Regulation. Hemorrhage or decrease in blood volume, if sufficient in degree, is followed by release of AVP. The change in volume (as contrasted with the change in osmolarity) must be relatively large. For example, phlebotomy that reduces blood volume by 6 to 9% or the assumption of the upright posture that reduces central blood volume by 10 to 15% has no effect on AVP release.[80] On the other hand, a change of blood volume of more than 10%, which can be produced by the combination of phlebotomy and assumption of the erect position, brings about this release. Under usual conditions, plasma osmolality is the prime determinant of AVP secretion, but severe volume depletion can override the osmoreceptor control. With less severe degrees of volume change, osmotic control is precisely exerted, but there is a shift of the osmotic set point, so that a lower osmotic threshold is required to trigger AVP secretion in the volume-depleted animal.

Glucocorticoids modulate the set point of neurohypophyseal control. Adrenocortical insufficiency lowers the set point and thereby induces a relative increase in AVP secretion,[83] which contributes to the low serum sodium level in both primary and secondary adrenocortical deficiency.[84] Glucocorticoid effects on AVP secretion are mediated by changes in AVP gene transcription. Glucocorticoids acting on specific receptors[85] lower the concentration of AVP messenger RNA (mRNA), and glucocorticoid deficiency brings about an increase in AVP mRNA (as do changes in osmolality).[86] These changes in AVP secretion reflect the importance of secretion of this neurohormone in the regulation of ACTH release (see later).

Receptors for volume control are located in the left atrium and in the baroreceptors of the carotid sinus, and perhaps elsewhere. Modest degrees of volume depletion that are insufficient to lower blood pressure activate the atrial receptors, whereas depletion that is sufficient to cause hypotension mobilizes baroreceptor reflexes. Because even high doses of vasopressin do not cause hypertension in humans, the neurohypophysis probably has only a modest role in blood pressure regulation in normal persons, but vasopressin plays a complex role in cardiovascular regulation under conditions such as shock and volume depletion.[87]

Neural impulses that are involved in volume and blood pressure sensors reach the brain stem by way of cranial nerve afferents terminating in the midbrain, ascend through multisynaptic pathways, and impinge on the nuclei of the neurohypophyseal system. Presumably the principal activating pathways are mediated by cholinergic neurotransmitters, but other pathways could be involved in view of the wealth of potential neurotransmitters and neuropeptides in the paraventricular and supraoptic nuclei.

Atrial Peptides. The left atrium plays an endocrine role in control of blood volume (which is separate from the role of the left atrial neural volume receptors in regulation of AVP release and drinking behavior). A family of peptides with potent natriuretic activity, termed *atrial peptides,* have been isolated from atrial muscle and shown to be part of a homeostatic feedback mechanism for regulation of intravascular volume (Fig. 5–12).[75, 88–90] Expansion of the left atrium through effects on muscle stretch receptors induces the release of APs from atrial myocyte neurosecretory granules; APs then act through the circulation on the kidney tubule to increase sodium excretion.

In addition to their role as circulating peptides, APs are found in an extensive central nervous system network, particularly in areas that are crucial to the regulation of blood volume through changes in drinking behavior and alterations in AVP release.[75, 89, 90] Most striking is the presence of AP and AP receptors in the anterior tip of the third ventricle in the region of the subfornical organ (SFO). Injections of AP in this region inhibit AVP release and inhibit drinking both in normal animals and in animals in which these functions have been stimulated by angiotensin II injections. The SFO, like other periventricular organs (see

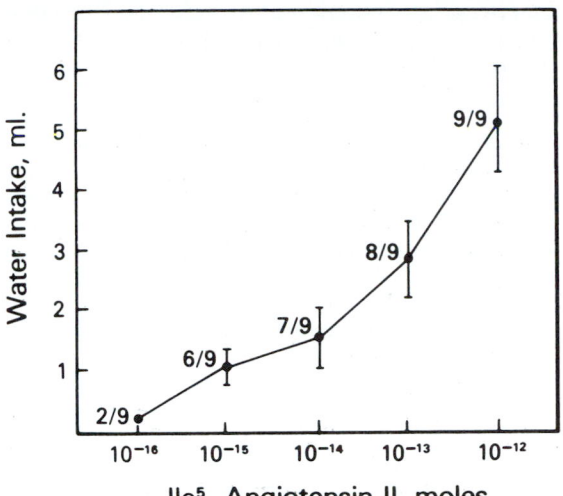

Figure 5–12. Dose-response curve of drinking produced by injection of angiotensin II directly into the subfornical organ, a structure located in the dorsal anterior wall of the third ventricle. (From Simpson J, Epstein JN, Camardo JS Jr. The localization of receptors for the dipsogenic action of angiotensin II in the subfornical organ of rat. J Comp Physiol Psychol 1978; 92:581–608. Copyright 1978 by the American Psychological Association. Reprinted by permission.)

later), lacks a blood-brain barrier. AP is also present in the neural pathways that convey peripheral volume information to central homeostatic regulating areas of the hypothalamus. Thus the peripheral and central AP systems are integrated for the defense of blood volume. A distinct atrionatriuretic-like peptide has been isolated from pig brain (which is now designated *brain natriuretic peptide,* BNP[89]), and two different genes coding for AP receptors have been identified in brain and kidney.[90] These differences reflect evolutionary responses to different functions of related regulatory molecules.

Several lines of evidence suggest an important role for AP in neuroendocrine regulation of the anterior pituitary. AP is present in many neuronal endings in the median eminence, and AP stimulates the formation of cyclic guanosine monophosphate (cGMP) in isolated pituitary cells and is probably synthesized in a subpopulation of anterior pituitary cells. However, its function is not established. The functions of APs and angiotensin II are considered further in sections on drinking behavior and periventricular organs.

Stress and Nausea. The secretion of AVP is affected by inputs from various parts of the "visceral brain" and the reticular activating system, regions that are involved in maintenance of consciousness and in emotional expression. Nausea is accompanied by intense AVP release, presumably by reflex stimulation from the medullary vomiting center (area postrema).

When Verney began his studies of water regulation in dogs, he was struck by the marked effect of emotional stress on antidiuretic activity. It has been generally believed that humans and rats also release AVP in response to emotional stress, but Robertson[80] showed that pain or other stresses that are incidental to human physiological experiments rarely influence plasma AVP concentrations. The same is true for deliberately applied severe stress in rats. Nevertheless, the influence of "higher" neural centers on AVP secretion can be demonstrated by experimental induction of diuresis or antidiuresis by hypnotic suggestion in humans or by psychological conditioning of dogs. Other examples of neurogenic disturbance in regulation of AVP secretion are the disturbed control of water excretion in patients with anorexia nervosa[91] and in some schizophrenics who have succeeded in overhydrating themselves to the point of water intoxication.[92]

Inappropriate Secretion of Antidiuretic Hormone. The syndrome of excessive and inappropriate secretion of antidiuretic hormone (SIADH) is most commonly due to ectopic hormone secretion by malignancies of several kinds (see Chapter 34) but can be induced by certain drugs (see Chapter 7) and can arise in brain disorders in humans.[93] Such cases are probably due to loss of normal tonic inhibitory influences on the neurohypophyseal neurons. Experimentally induced lesions involving the anterior margin of the supraoptic nucleus increase neuronal activity in the supraopticohypophyseal pathway and give rise to inappropriate antidiuretic hormone release.[94] Acute neurological lesions such as intraventricular hemorrhage are commonly associated with SIADH (see Chapter 7).

Relation Between Vasopressin Secretion and Drinking Behavior. Drinking behavior, like AVP secretion, is regulated by plasma osmolality and circulating blood volume, is integrated by hypothalamic mechanisms, and is designed to maintain the constancy of the internal water milieu.[73, 74, 95–97] The sensation of thirst (as contrasted with the sensation of dry mouth) results from an internally perceived signal arising from the hypothalamus. As with AVP secretion, thirst can be generated by severe hemorrhage or by inducing local hyperosmolality in the hypothalamus with hypertonic saline microinjections. The thirst mechanism is integrated with the AVP-controlling mechanism; both are activated by hypothalamic osmoreceptors. Drinking behavior and AVP release can be activated by intrahypothalamic administration of acetylcholine analogues, which suggests that there may be a common neuromediator pathway for the two functions. The hypothalamic angiotensin II system may also be important in AVP regulation, as it is in drinking behavior. All of the biochemical components and enzyme systems for the formation of angiotensin II are present in the hypothalamus, and angiotensin II–containing neurons and angiotensin II receptors have been demonstrated in the region.[73, 74, 98] Angiotensin II–containing neurons project from the SFO to the paraventricular nucleus. mRNA coding for angiotensinogen is also present in the brain.[99]

Injection of angiotensin II into the third ventricle stimulates drinking in the rat in dose-related fashion. Drinking by dehydrated rats is blocked by local administration of saralasin, which is an angiotensin II receptor antagonist. Central angiotensin receptors respond to angiotensin II synthesized outside the brain, thus accounting at least in part for the severe thirst that is sometimes seen in renovascular hypertension and hypovolemic shock. Drinking is also influenced by a specialized periventricular structure of the brain—the SFO—through which circulating angiotensin II may gain entry and bypass the blood-brain barrier (see later). This anatomical region is also rich in AP-containing neurons. In humans hyperosmolarity mobilizes both drinking and AVP release, but a few rare cases have been described in which AVP osmoregulation is normal but drinking is deficient, thus causing chronic hypernatremia.

Oxytocin Secretion. **Milk Let-Down Reflex.** An infant who begins to nurse does not obtain milk immediately. Rather, milk appears at the nipple after a delay of half a minute or so. This response is termed milk *let-down*.[100, 101] The stimulus of suckling initiates a neurogenic reflex that is transmitted from afferent nerve endings in the nipple and is conducted through the spinal cord, the midbrain, and finally the hypothalamus, where it triggers release of oxytocin from the neurohypophysis (Fig. 5–13). A central peptidergic neuronal pathway containing inhibin conducts impulses from the midbrain to the oxytocin-secreting cell bodies.[78] In the breast oxytocin causes contraction of the myoepithelial cells that encircle mammary acini, thereby expelling the milk into the milk ducts and thence into the

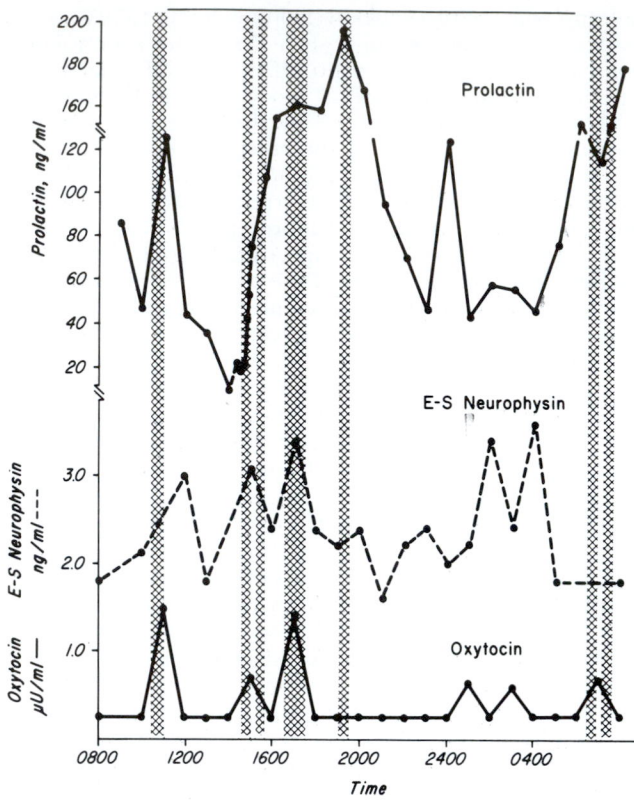

Figure 5–13. Patterns of release of prolactin, oxytocin, and oxytocin-related neurophysin (E-S neurophysin) in a postpartum woman. Each vertical bar corresponds to a suckling episode. Neurophysin release parallels oxytocin release. Some episodes of hormone release, at night, are spontaneous and unrelated to nursing. (From J. Stern, J. D'Amico, A.G. Robinson, et al., unpublished).

nipple. In the absence of this reflex contraction, milk cannot be obtained, even from a full breast. Nursing rats, for example, cannot obtain milk from mothers previously subjected to removal of the neural lobe but can do so after injections of oxytocin are given. The milk let-down reflex is accompanied by changes in hypothalamic neuronal function and can be blocked by specific neural lesions and by certain types of neural stimuli. In cows the let-down reflex can be abolished by a strange or threatening environment. Pain or fright inhibits milk let-down in the rabbit through adrenergic stimulation. In women, milk let-down occurs in response to suckling and in some can be conditioned by the crying of a hungry infant. Milk let-down can be inhibited by emotional stress and can be triggered by sexual excitement and orgasm. Oxytocin has been administered therapeutically in some women with failure of normal milk let-down, but most women with DI appear to nurse normally.[102]

Oxytocin in Labor. Although the uterus-contracting property of oxytocin has been used to induce labor and manage obstetrical hemorrhage, a role for the hormone in initiation and maintenance of normal labor in humans has not been established with certainty[100–102] (see Chapter 16). Local changes in uterine responsivity to oxytocin rather than changes in oxytocin secretion may be a determinant of the timing of the onset of labor. Concentrations of oxytocin receptors increase in the uterus at term.[103] Labor is relatively normal in women with DI, even in those in whom oxytocin deficiency can be demonstrated.[101, 102] After labor has begun in normal women, maternal oxytocin secretion, which takes place in spurts, increases and reaches a maximum at the time of delivery.[101] Reflexes arising from the contracting uterus trigger additional oxytocin release, thus providing an amplifying mechanism for labor.

Secretion of AVP and secretion of oxytocin are independent. For example, in lactating women, AVP secretion can be stimulated by hypertonic saline infusion without producing let-down, and the suckling stimulus induces let-down without accompanying antidiuresis.

Intermediate Lobe

The intermediate lobe of the pituitary, derived embryologically from the posterior wall of the Rathke pouch (the adenohypophysis is derived from the anterior wall), is well developed in most vertebrates, including the human fetus, but in the human adult it is vestigial, its cells being dispersed throughout the anterior and neural lobes.[51] Much of the research on the function of the intermediate lobe has been carried out in organisms such as amphibians, in which the lobe regulates skin pigmentation by secretion of MSH.[104, 105] MSH increases skin pigmentation by stimulating the dispersal of melanin granules in melanocytes; this function is the basis of environmentally adaptive pigmentation in frogs and salamanders. In rodents the intermediate lobe is innervated by a direct dopamine-secreting neural pathway from the hypothalamus that exerts tonic suppression of MSH secretion.[106] Hypertrophy of the intermediate lobe follows pituitary stalk section. The nature of hypothalamic control of the intermediate lobe in humans is not known, but it could be dopaminergic.[106] It was previously believed that intermediate lobe function was regulated by hypothalamic releasing factors,[104, 105] but this view is no longer held in light of current understanding of the chemical nature and origin of the intermediate lobe peptides and of the direct nerve supply to this region.

The MSHs of the intermediate lobe are synthesized as part of a large prohormone, designated pro-opiomelanocortin (POMC), which is also the precursor of ACTH, β-lipotropin (β-LPH), and β-endorphin in the anterior pituitary and of a number of ACTH-related peptides in hypothalamic neurons[107–109] (Fig. 5–14) (see Chapter 6). Although the prohormone sequence is identical in anterior lobe, intermediate lobe, and hypothalamic neurons, the formation of the active hormones in these sites differs owing to variations in enzymatic post-translational processing. In the intermediate lobe the initial proteolytic cleavages appear to be the same as those in anterior pituitary corticotropes, but in addition almost all the β-LPH that is present is processed to γ-lipotropin and β-endorphin.[109] β-Endorphin is converted to a variety of endorphin-related products that are not detectable in the anterior lobe. In the intermediate lobe,

ACTH is broken down to form α-MSH and a fragment corresponding to ACTH 18–39 (designated corticotropin-like intermediate lobe peptide, CLIP). Many of the forms are acetylated. It is important to recognize (as is the case for a number of other neuropeptides) that the same gene can be expressed and regulated differently in different tissues. For example, the formation of POMC by the intermediate lobe is regulated primarily by dopamine and serotonin, whereas the principal regulation of POMC gene expression in the anterior lobe is by glucocorticoids[108] and CRH (see later).[110] In the brain the expression of POMC is not regulated by glucocorticoids.

The intermediate lobe does not appear to be of much importance in humans under normal circumstances, although administered MSH does increase skin pigmentation. Intermediate lobe POMC cells may give rise to basophilic adenomas in Cushing disease in humans, as also appears to be the case in dogs and horses.[111] The biological behavior of such tumors is different from that of tumors of anterior lobe corticotropes.[112, 113]

Median Eminence, and Tuberoinfundibular and Tuberohypophyseal Neurons

ANATOMY. The median eminence of the hypothalamus is the site at which hypothalamic neurons that regulate the anterior pituitary release their secretions in anatomical relation to the primary plexus of the hypophyseal-portal system. This region is also the site through which neurons that end in the neural lobe and intermediate lobe of the pituitary pass. These complex functions have been extensively studied[9, 17, 33, 50, 114–124] (Figs. 5–15 to 5–25). Three components of this structure can be identified: *neural*, consisting of nerve terminals and neurons in passage; *vascular*, consisting of the primary capillary plexus and the portal veins; and *epithelial*, consisting of the pars tuberalis of the anterior pituitary gland. Special features of this region are the densely packed nerve endings, capillaries with conspicuous perivascular spaces, supporting cells, and ependymal cells, including one variety, the tanycyte, that traverses the median eminence from the lumen of the third ventricle to the outer mantle plexus. The nerve endings are the terminals of the tuberohypophyseal neurons, which arise chiefly in the ventral hypothalamus. The capillaries form the primary plexus of the portal circulation.

Two kinds of tuberohypophyseal neurons project to the median eminence. Most are peptidergic (e.g., TRH, LHRH,

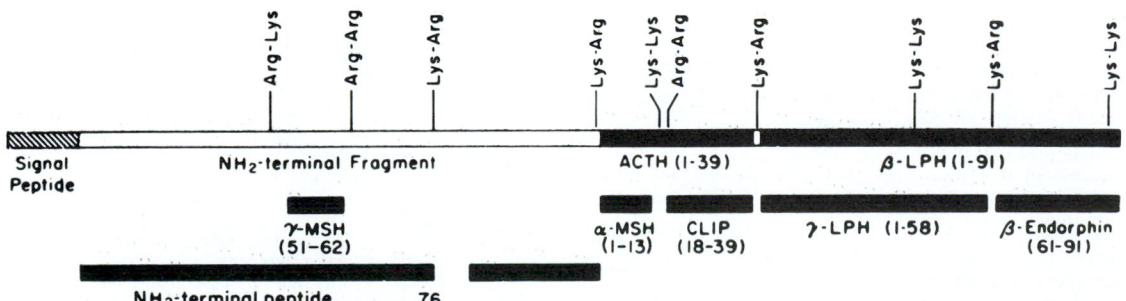

Figure 5–14. Organization of POMC, the precursor hormone of ACTH, β-LPH, and related peptides. The precursor protein contains a leader sequence (signal peptide), followed by a long fragment that includes sequence 51–62 corresponding to γ-MSH. This fragment is cleaved at Lys-Arg bonds to form ACTH 1–39, which in turn includes the sequences for α-MSH (ACTH 1–13) and corticotropin-like intermediate lobe peptide (CLIP) (ACTH 18–39), and a sequence corresponding to β-LPH (1–91) that includes γ-LPH (γ-LPH 1–58), and β-endorphin (61–91). The β-endorphin sequence also includes a sequence corresponding to met-enkephalin (see later). As outlined by Krieger,[109] the precursor molecule in the anterior lobe of the pituitary is processed predominantly to ACTH and β-LPH. In the intermediate pituitary lobe (in the rat), ACTH and β-LPH are further processed into α-MSH and a β-endorphin–like material. In all extrapituitary tissues, post-translational processing of the prohormone resembles that in the intermediate lobe. Hypothalamic processing is similar but not identical with that in the intermediate lobe. In the intermediate lobe, β-endorphin and α-MSH are present predominantly in their acetylated forms. (See also Fig. 5–60 for a more detailed description of met-enkephalin, which makes up the first five amino acids of β-endorphin 61–91.)

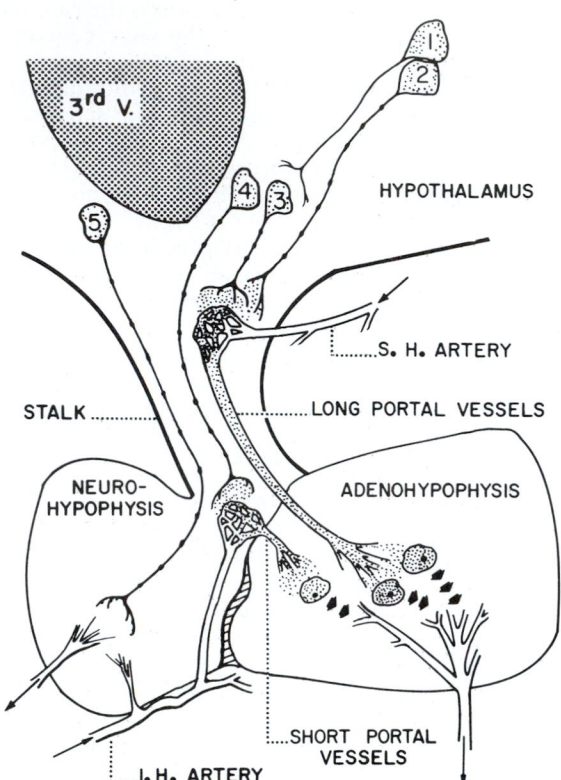

Figure 5–15. Neural control of the pituitary gland. This figure summarizes the types of neural input into pituitary regulation. Neuron 5 represents the peptidergic neurons of the supraopticohypophyseal and paraventriculohypophyseal tracts with hormone-producing cell bodies in the hypothalamus and nerve terminals in the neural lobe. Neurons 4 and 3 are the neurons of the tuberoinfundibular tract that secrete the hypophyseotropic hormones into the substance of the median eminence in anatomical relationship to the primary plexus. Neuron 1 represents a monoaminergic neuron ending in relation to the cell body of the peptidergic neuron. Neuron 2 represents a monoaminergic neuron ending on terminals of the peptidergic neuron to give axoaxonic transmission. Neurons 1 and 2 are the functional links between the remainder of the brain and the peptidergic neuron. Not shown are the fibers of the tuberohypophyseal tract. These fibers in certain animal species, but not in humans, arise in the arcuate nucleus of the hypothalamus and terminate on the cells of the intermediate lobe. In adult humans the intermediate lobe is vestigial. (From Gay VL. The hypothalamus: physiology and clinical use of releasing factors. Fertil Steril 23:51, 1972. Reproduced with permission of the publisher, The American Fertility Society.)

Figure 5–16. Diagrammatic representation of a number of peptides and neurotransmitters that terminate in the median eminence, together with their origin. ACh, acetylcholine; ACTH, corticotropin; ANF, atrionatriuretic factor; ANG II, angiotensin II; CCK, cholecystokinin; CGRP, calcitonin gene-related peptide; CLIP, corticotropin-like intermediate lobe peptide; CRH, corticotropin-releasing hormone; DA, dopamine; DYN, dynorphin; β-END, β-endorphin; ENK, enkephalin; EP, epinephrine; 5HT, 5-hydroxytryptamine; GABA, γ-aminobutyric acid; GAL, galanin; GRF, growth hormone–releasing factor (hormone); HIS, histamine; LHRH, luteinizing hormone–releasing hormone; Mot, motilin; α MSH, α-melanocyte-stimulating hormone; n., nucleus; NE, norepinephrine; NPY, neuropeptide Y; NT, neurotensin; OT, oxytocin; ovlt-pom, organum vasculosum of the lamina terminalis–preoptic medial nucleus; PHI, peptide-histidine-isoleucine; POMC, pro-opiomelanocortin; PRL, prolactin; SP, substance P; SRIF, somatostatin; TRH, thyrotropin-releasing hormone; VIP, vasoactive intestinal peptide; VP, vasopressin; ZE, zona exterior; ZI, zona interior; ZL, zona lateralis. (From Jacobowitz DM. Multifactorial control of pituitary hormone secretion: the "wheels" of the brain. Synapse 1988; 2:186–192.)

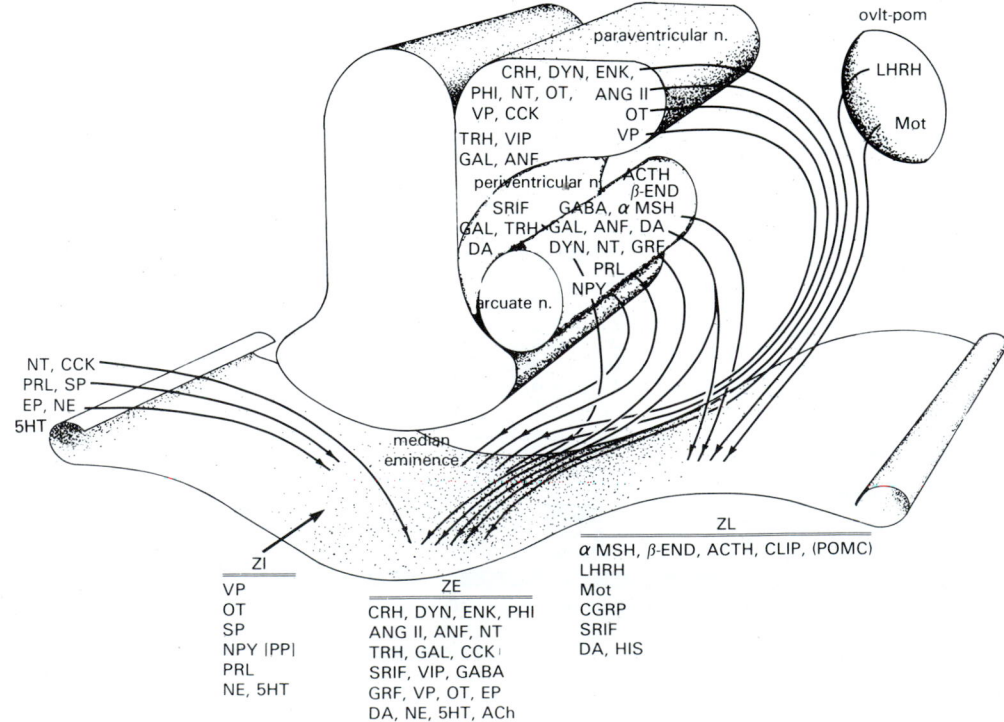

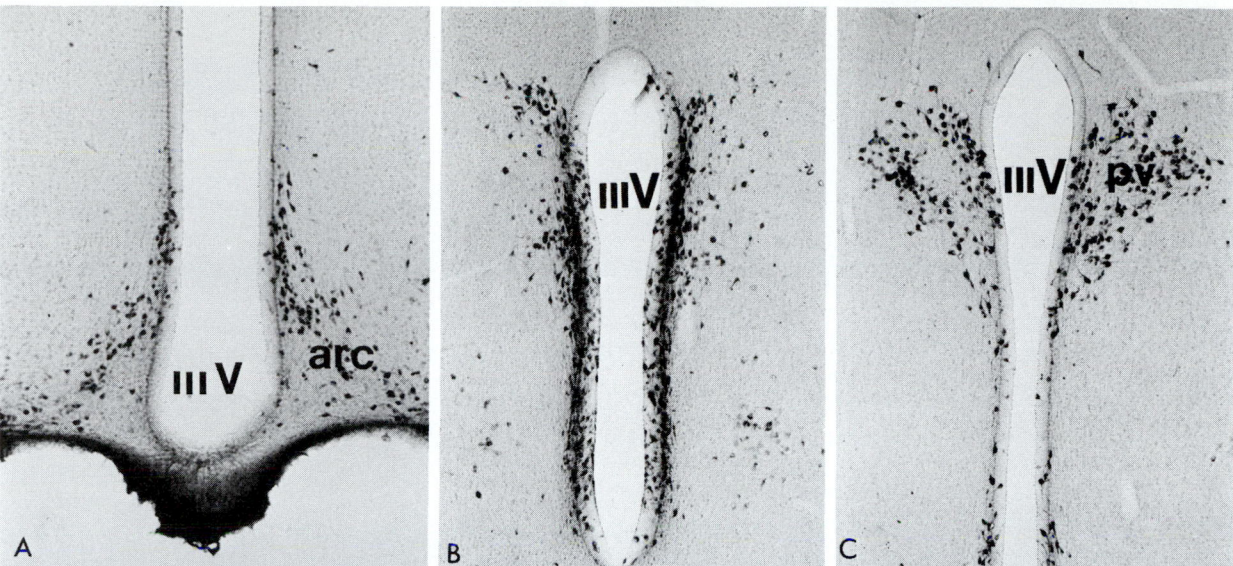

Figure 5–17. The tuberoinfundibular neuron system revealed by retrograde transport of wheat germ agglutinin. The location of cell bodies of neurons projecting to the median eminence of the hypothalamus can be traced (as in this study by Lechan and colleagues[120]) by injecting a small tracer dose of wheat germ agglutinin into the median eminence of the rat *(A)*. Tracer, which is a lectin, binds to carbohydrate groups on nerve endings, is taken up into the cell by endocytosis, and is transported in retrograde fashion to be localized in cell bodies. Principal groups are the arcuate nucleus (arc); periventricular nucleus (which forms a feltwork of fibers and cells around the third ventricle) (IIIV) *(B)*; and *(C)* the small cell division of the paraventricular nucleus (pv). Note that the distribution of cell bodies in the paraventricular nucleus differs somewhat from that shown for the neurohypophyseal peptides (see Fig. 5–9). Those projecting to the neural lobe are larger, are located laterally in the nucleus, and do not contain the retrograde tracer that was injected into the median eminence. (From Lechan RM, Nestler JL, Jacobson S. The tuberoinfundibular system of the rat as demonstrated by immunohistochemical localization of retrogradely transported wheat germ agglutinin [WGA] from the median eminence. Brain Res 1982; 245:1–15.)

and somatostatin); others are bioaminergic, the most important being dopaminergic.

The anatomical relationships of nerve endings, basement membrane, interstitial space, and capillary wall are identical with those in the neural lobe, and the release of neuropeptides can be stimulated by depolarizing conditions such as exposure to a high K^+ concentration in the presence of Ca^{2+}. Thus the process of secretion at median eminence terminals is analogous to the stimulus-secretion mechanism of the neurohypophysis. The large contact area of the perivascular space and the special vessels in this region, which have fenestrations that are typical of those seen in ordinary endocrine glands, account for the observation that the neurohypophysis, including the median eminence, unlike most of the brain, is permeable to molecules such as thyroxine (T_4), trypan blue, and growth hormone (GH). No morphologically demonstrable synapses or axons have been identified in the median eminence; hence these structures can be regarded as "presynaptic."[121] Joseph and Knigge[116] noted that

The extracellular and perivascular space of the median eminence would appear to be a medium of remarkable composition . . . large pools of nerve terminals and nonneuronal elements are bathed in an interstitial fluid containing a multitude of hormones and excitatory and inhibitory neurotransmitters.

A representation of the complexity of neurochemical factors reaching the pituitary from the brain is shown in Figure 5–16.

Although most axons of the supraopticohypophyseal and paraventriculohypophyseal tracts pass *through* the median eminence on their way from cells of origin in the hypothalamus to terminate in the neural lobe, a population of paraventricular neurons projects to the median eminence. In this location they have anterior pituitary–regulatory roles, especially for ACTH and prolactin (PRL) secretion.

The form of the blood vessels in the primary plexus varies somewhat among species. In humans the capillaries form loops that are part of complex spiral structures termed *gomitoli*. These capillaries penetrate the infundibulum and stalk. Arterioles of the stalk and median eminence of humans have highly muscular walls, which suggests that hemodynamic changes in these vessels might affect pituitary function, but evidence to support this point of view is lacking. Reflex constriction of these vessels after postpartum hemorrhage might be a factor in the genesis of pituitary infarction.

Blood reaches the plexus of the median eminence and upper stalk by way of the superior hypophyseal artery, which is a branch of the internal carotid artery (see Fig. 5–23). This plexus is drained by the long portal veins that run along the stalk and drain into the pituitary sinusoids. The capillary plexus in the lower portion of the stalk is supplied by the inferior hypophyseal artery and is drained by short portal veins that enter the pituitary almost directly. Although the direction of blood flow in the long portal vessels is predominantly from the hypothalamus to the pituitary, reverse flow from the pituitary to the median eminence can also occur by way of the short portal vessels that drain both anterior and posterior pituitary.[122] One consequence of this circular flow is that the hypothalamus could be exposed to high concentrations of the secretions of both anterior and posterior pituitary lobes. However, dynamic studies indicate that reverse flow of blood from the pituitary to the brain is not significant.[123]

The third component of the median eminence, the pars tuberalis, is a thin glandular sheath around the infundibulum and pituitary stalk. In some animals the epithelial component may make up as much as 10% of the total glandular tissue of the pituitary and contains pituitary tropic hormones including luteinizing hormone (LH) and TSH. These findings notwithstanding, the pars tuberalis probably does not have an important physiological function but serves mainly as the structure through which arteries and veins of the hypophyseal-portal circulation are conducted.

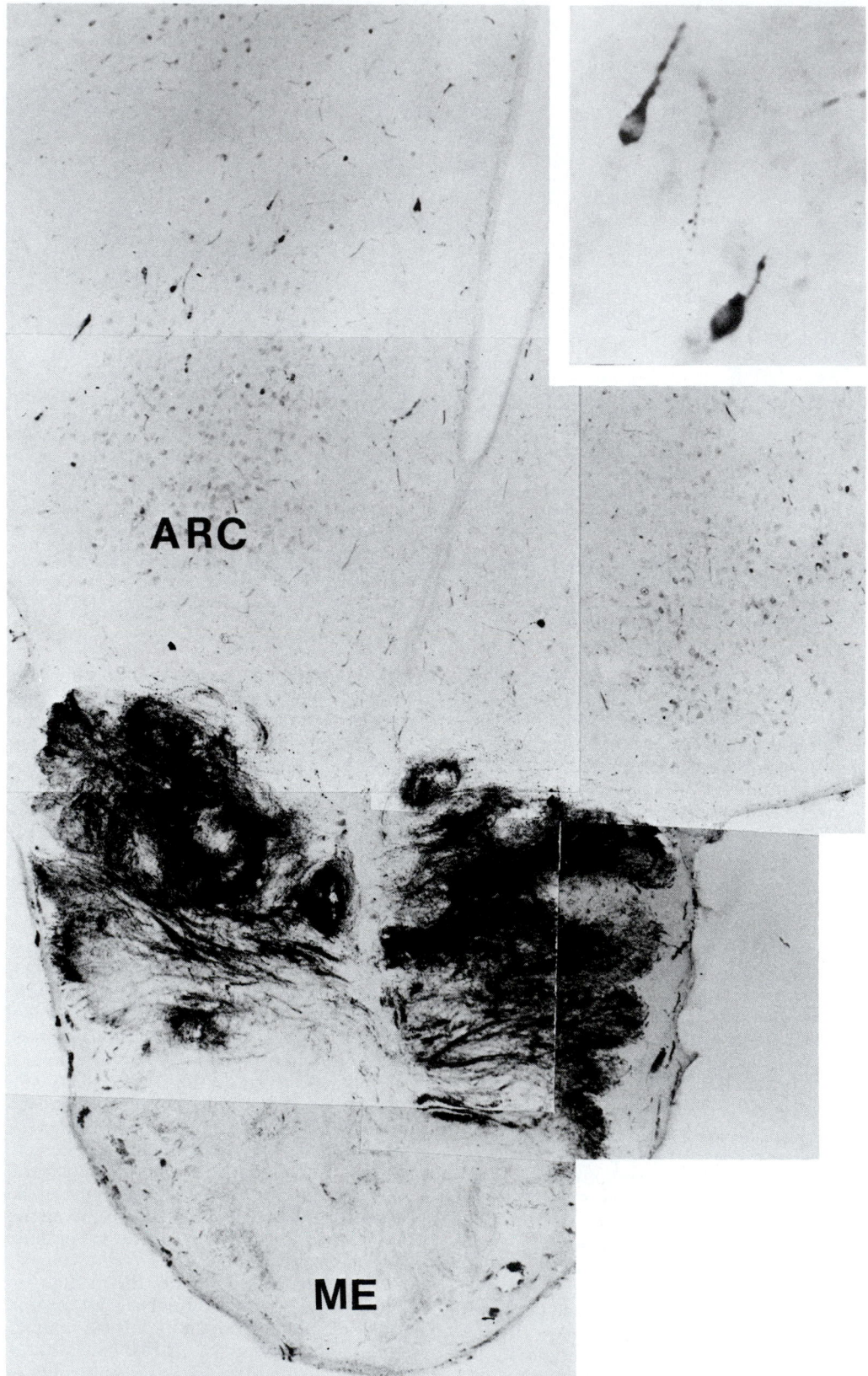

Figure 5–18. Anatomy of growth hormone–releasing hormone (GHRH) in rhesus monkey delineated by immunohistochemical staining with an antibody directed against GHRH 1–44-NH$_2$. Note the heavy distribution of fibers in the lateral margins of the median eminence (ME) and the scattering of cells in the arcuate nucleus (ARC). Inset shows cell bodies of GHRH cells in the arcuate nucleus. (From Lechan R, Lin HD, Ling N, et al. Distribution of immunoreactive growth hormone releasing factor [1–44]NH$_2$ in the tuberoinfundibular system of the rhesus monkey. Brain Res 1984; 309:55–61.)

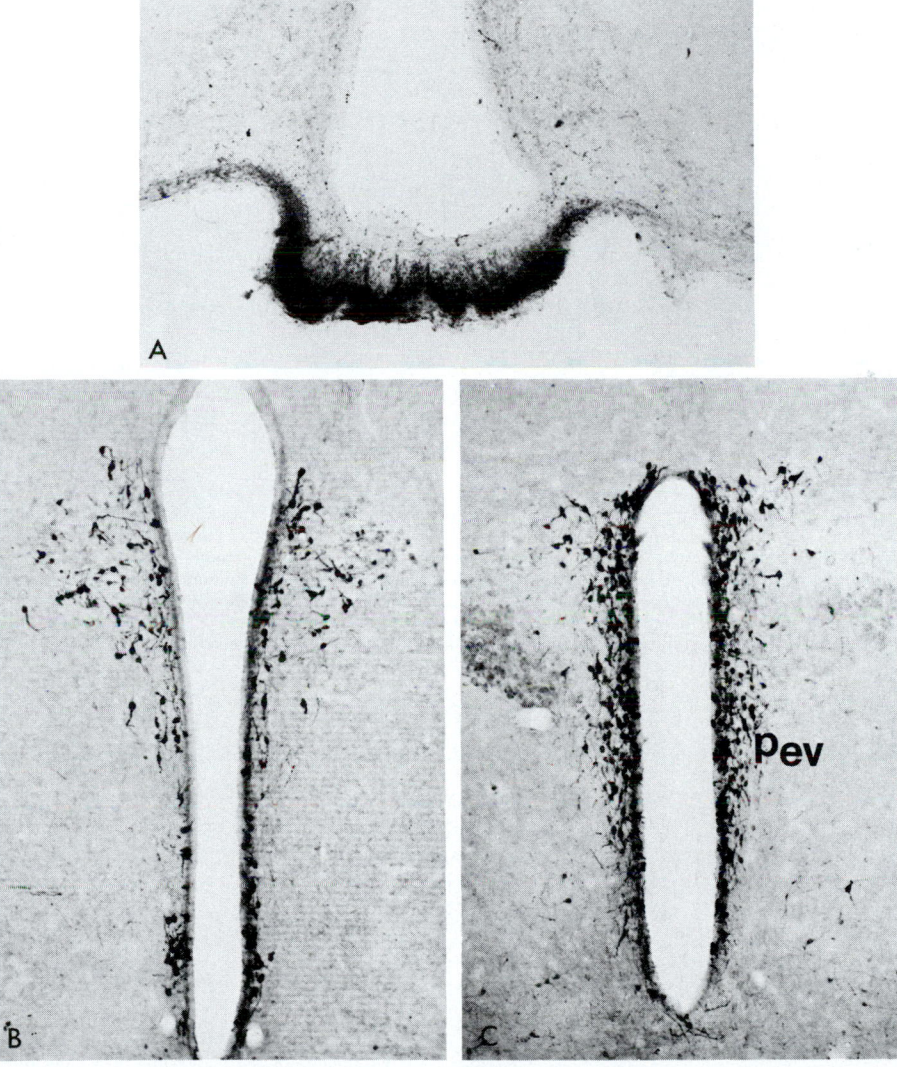

Figure 5–19. *A*, External median eminence of the rat, showing immunoreactive somatostatin in nerve terminals. (Courtesy of Dr. Ronald M. Lechan. From Lechan RM, Goodman RH, Rosenblatt M, et al. Prosomatostatin-specific antigen in rat brain: localization by immunocytochemical staining with an antiserum to a synthetic sequence of preprosomatostatin. Proc Natl Acad Sci USA 1983; 80:2780–2784.)

B, Periventricular plexus (Pev) of somatostatin-containing cells in the anterior hypothalamus of the rat. The distribution corresponds well with the location of the periventricular plexus that contains retrogradely transported wheat germ agglutinin (see Fig. 5–17).

C, The medial division of the paraventricular nucleus contains many somatostatin-positive cells. Note again the close similarity of these cells to those that project to the median eminence (see Fig. 5–17).

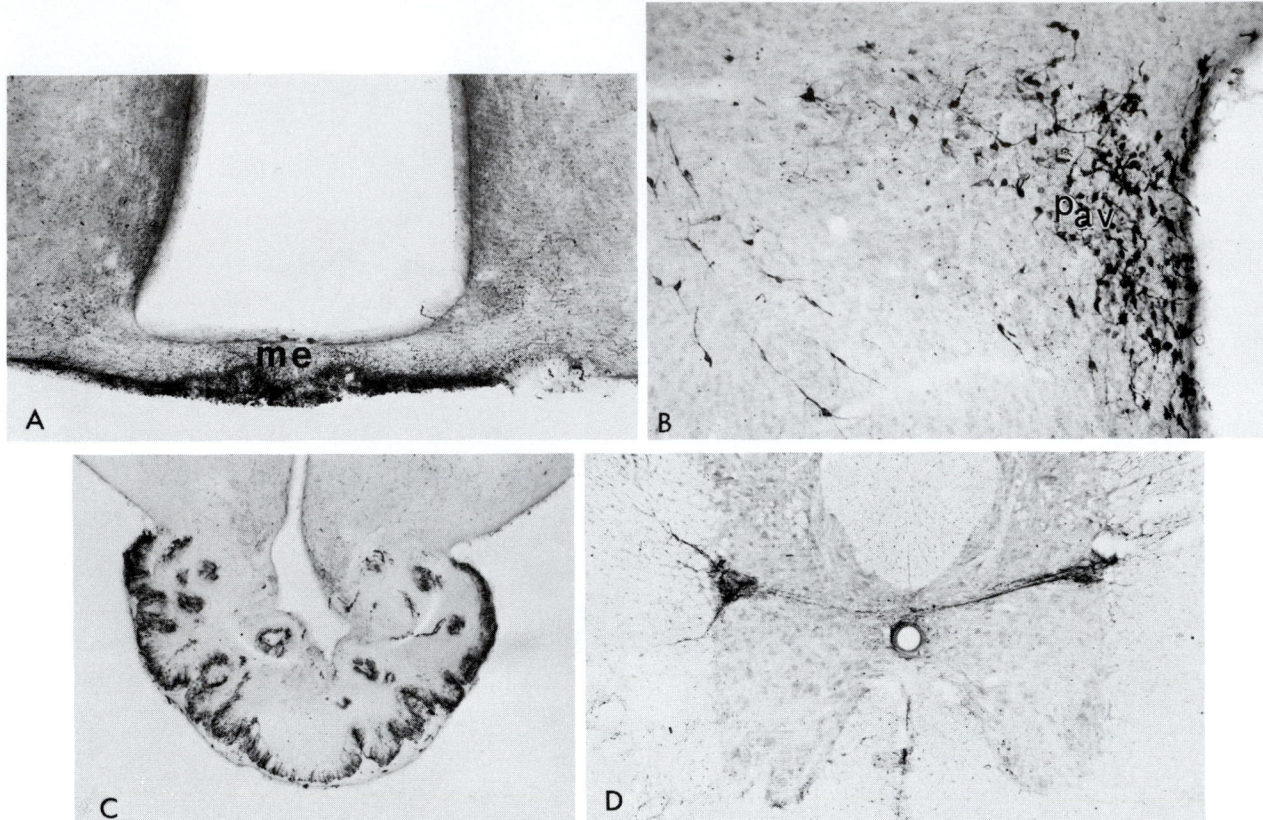

Figure 5–20. *A,* Distribution of TRH immunoreactivity in the stalk–median eminence (me) of the rat. *B,* TRH-immunoreactive cell bodies in the medial division of the paraventricular nucleus (Pav) of the rat. *C,* TRH-immunoreactive nerve endings in the median eminence of the rhesus monkey. *D,* Transverse section of the upper thoracic spinal cord of the rat showing the distribution of TRH-immunoreactive fibers terminating in the intermediolateral column (site of the preganglionic sympathetic nervous system). (All figures courtesy of Dr. Ronald M. Lechan. *A* and *B* from Lechan RM, Jackson IM. Immunohistochemical localization of thyrotropin-releasing hormone in the rat hypothalamus and pituitary. Endocrinology 1982; 111:55–65. Copyright 1982, The Endocrine Society. *C* from Lechan R, Lin HD, Ling N, et al. Distribution of immunoreactive growth hormone releasing factor [1–44]NH$_2$ in the tuberoinfundibular system of the rhesus monkey. Brain Res 1984; 309:55–61. *D* from Jackson IM. Thyrotropin-releasing hormone. Reprinted, by permission of the New England Journal of Medicine 306; 145–155, 1982.)

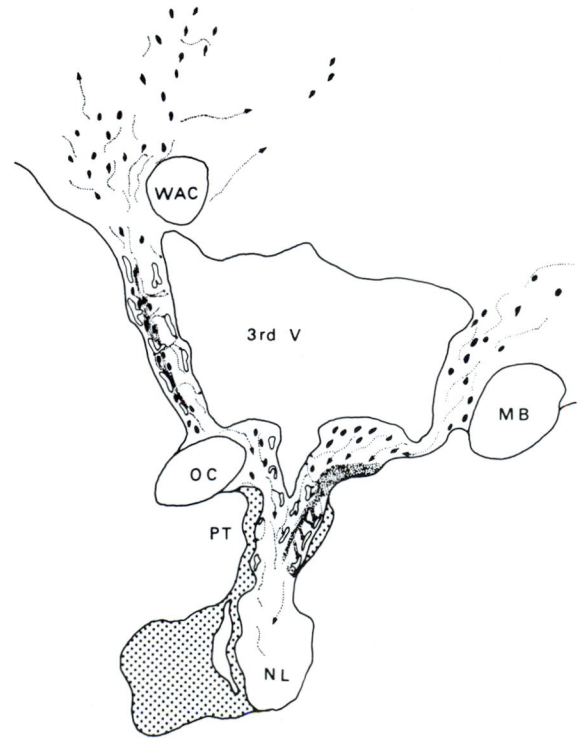

Figure 5–21. Distribution of cell bodies and fiber trajectories containing immunoreactive LHRH in the human fetus. Note the heavy concentration in the septum and preoptic area and anterior commissure. PT, pars tuberalis; NL, neural lobe; OC, optic chiasm; MB, mamillary body; WAC, anterior commissure. (From Bugnon C, Bloch H, Lenys D, et al. Cytoimmunochemical study of the LHRH neurons in humans during fetal life. In: Scott DE, Kozlowski GP, Weindl A, eds. Neural Hormones and Reproduction. Basel: S. Karger, 1978: 183–196.)

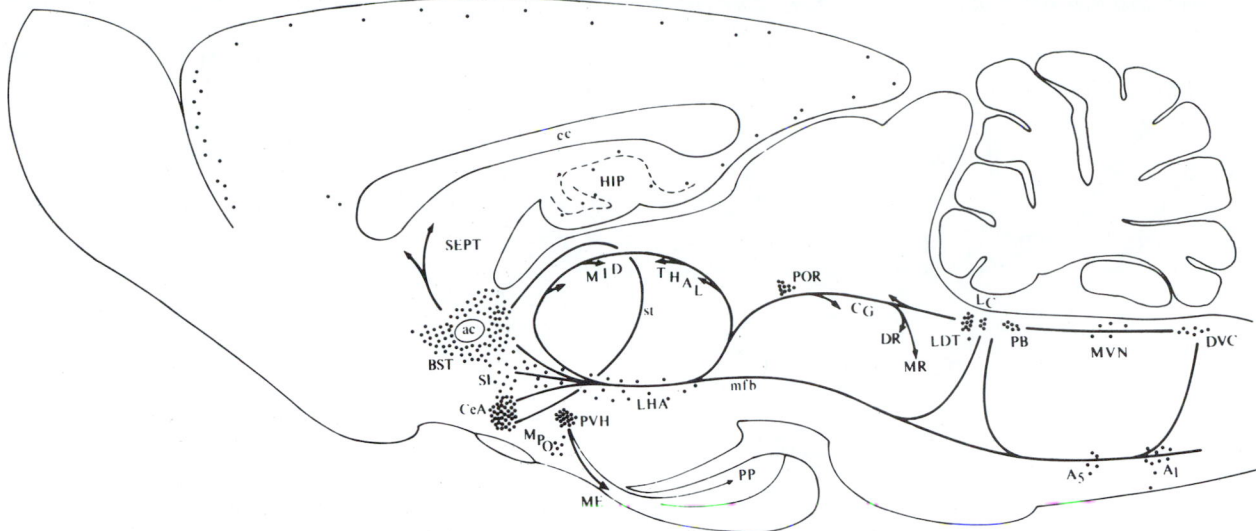

Figure 5–22. Major CRH-immunoreactive cells in the rat brain. The principal fibers regulating the anterior pituitary are shown as arising from the paraventricular nucleus (PVH), but there is an extensive distribution elsewhere, especially around the hypothalamus. A_1, noradrenergic cell group 1; A_5, noradrenergic cell group 5; ac, anterior commissure; BST, bed nucleus of the stria terminalis; cc, corpus callosum; CeA, central nucleus amygdala; CG, central gray; DR, dorsal raphe; DVC, dorsal vagal complex; HIP, hippocampus; LC, locus coeruleus; LDT, laterodorsal tegmental nucleus; LHA, lateral hypothalamic area; ME, median eminence; MID THAL, midline thalamic nuclei; mfb, medial forebrain bundle; MPO, medial preoptic area; MR, medial raphe; MVN, medial vestibular nucleus; PB, parabrachial nucleus; POR, perioculomotor nucleus; PP, posterior pituitary; PVH, periventricular nucleus; SEPT, septal region; SI, substantia innominata; st, stria. (From Swanson LW, Sawchenko PE, Rivier J, et al. Organization of ovine corticotropin-releasing factor immunoreactive cells and fibers in the rat brain: an immunohistochemical study. Neuroendocrinology 1983; 36:165–186.)

SPECIFIC TUBEROINFUNDIBULAR PATHWAYS. Elucidation of the chemical structures of the hypophyseotropic hormones and their availability as antigens has made possible the development of specific antisera for localization of the principal releasing hormones of the hypothalamus. The cells of origin of each regulatory peptide have distinct distributions, but all converge on the median eminence, where they come into contact with the capillaries of the hypophyseal-portal plexus. The cells projecting to the median eminence have been demonstrated by retrograde transport methods (see Fig. 5–17).[120] Localization of these neurons is illustrated in Figures 5–18 to 5–22.[33, 114–118, 124–137]

Figure 5–23. In this drawing of a pituitary vascular cast, the posterior portion of the infundibulum has been removed. The arrows demonstrate the potential efferent routes from the neurohypophysis: (1) portal vessels may convey blood to the adenohypophysis; (2) confluent pituitary veins may carry blood to the cavernous sinus; (3) blood may flow from the infundibulum to the hypothalamus via connecting capillaries; (4) tanycytes may transport some substances into the ventricle; (5) substances may leak through the endothelial fenestrations of portal vessels into the subarachnoid space; (6) certain hypophyseal arteries may under certain conditions serve as efferent vascular channels; and (7) retrograde axonal flow may carry substances from the neurohypophysis to the hypothalamus. Five of these routes are directed toward the brain. Follow-up studies indicate that in sheep there is little or no significant retrograde flow of blood above the median eminence. (From Bergland RM, Page RB. Can the pituitary secrete directly to the brain? [affirmative anatomical evidence]. Endocrinology 102, 1325–1338, 1978, © by The Endocrine Society.)

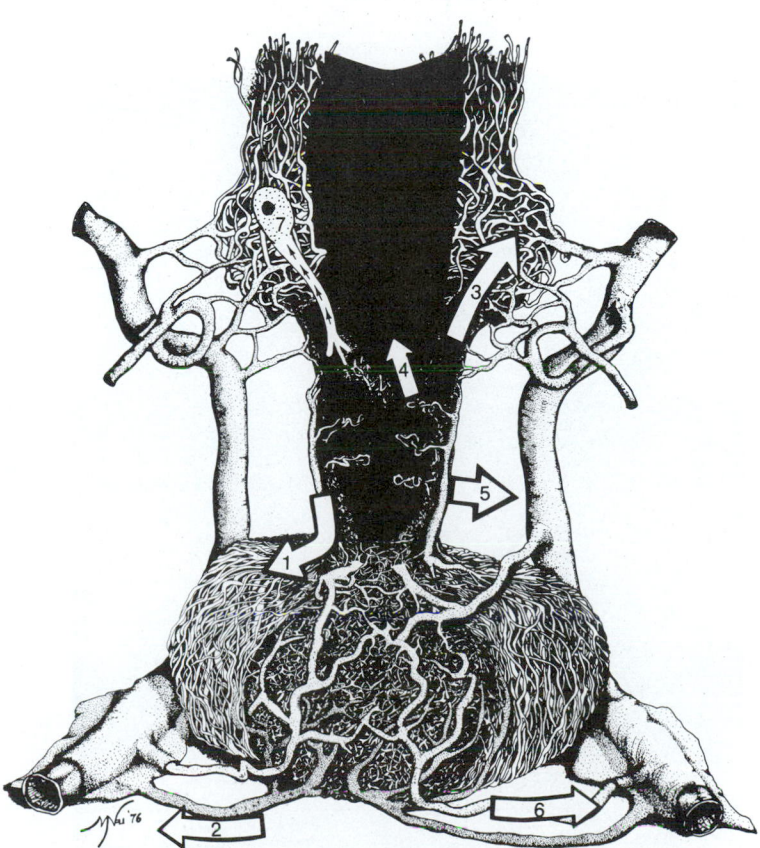

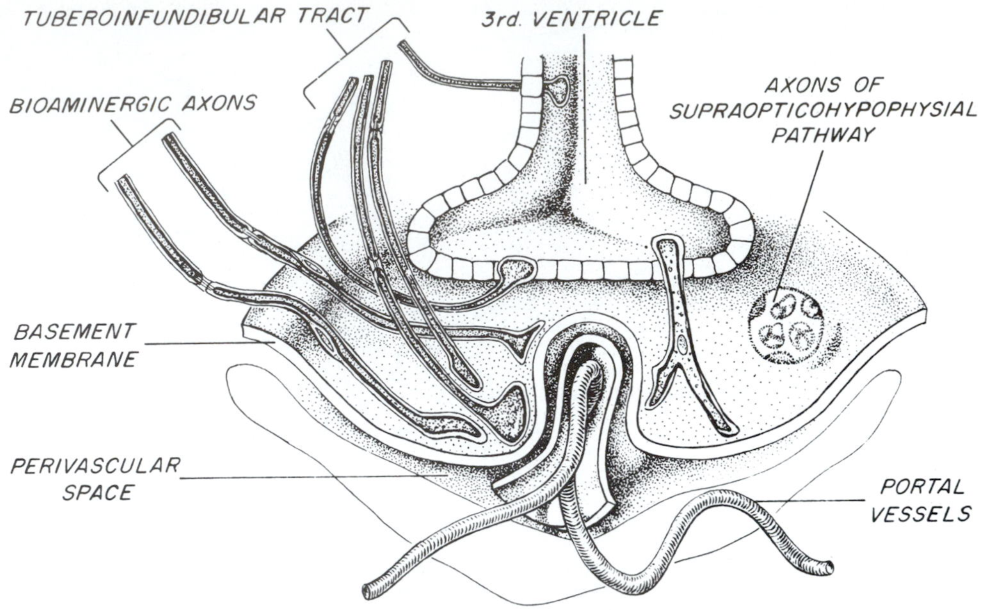

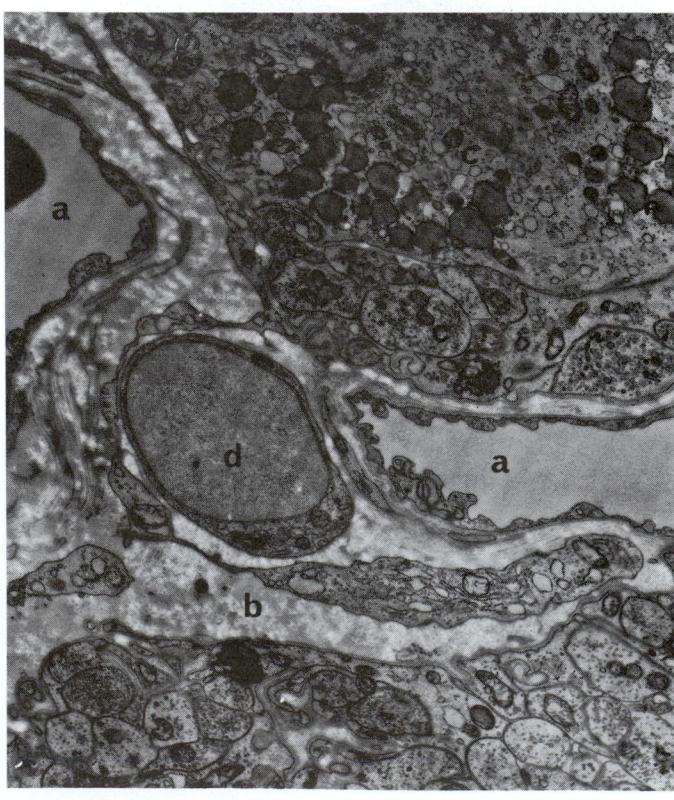

TUBEROINFUNDIBULAR TRACT   3rd. VENTRICLE

BIOAMINERGIC AXONS

AXONS OF
SUPRAOPTICOHYPOPHYSIAL
PATHWAY

BASEMENT
MEMBRANE

PERIVASCULAR
SPACE

PORTAL
VESSELS

Figure 5–24. Diagram of anatomical relationships of important secretory structures in the median eminence, visualized as if one were looking rostrally at a cut section. The interstitial space in which all the nerve endings terminate is a free pool without a blood-brain barrier. It is separated from the lumen of the third ventricle by ependyma, whose tight junctions prevent direct diffusion from medial eminence to third ventricle lumen. Tuberoinfundibular neurons, some peptidergic, some bioaminergic, end in the interstitial space; many, but not all, end directly on capillary loops. Few if any true axoaxonic synapses are found here. Stretching between lumen and outer third of median eminence are tanycytes, which are specialized cells that may have transport functions. The supraopticohypophyseal pathway is shown as a cut section of fibers in passage, but it should be recognized that some of the neurohypophyseal neurons end in the median eminence.

PORTAL VESSEL–CHEMOTRANSMITTER CONTROL. The hypophyseal–portal vessel–chemotransmitter hypothesis of pituitary control provides an explanation of how the anterior pituitary gland, which is devoid of secretomotor nerve fibers, is influenced by the nervous system.

By the mid-1940s several workers had postulated a neurohumoral control system for the anterior pituitary,[138, 139] but Green and Harris[140] provided the modern formulation of this theory.[14, 16, 17, 141–143] Their studies of the function of the vascular component of the pituitary stalk supported the concept of a hypophyseal–portal vessel–chemotransmitter system and stimulated a wealth of physiological and anatomical experiments. The first hypophyseo-

tropic hormone to be chemically defined was TRH. Its discovery in 1969 by Guillemin and Schally and their collaborators was crucial to the validation of the hypophyseal–portal vessel–chemotransmitter hypothesis and to the development of the field of neuroendocrinology (see refs. 142, 143).

Hypophyseotropic Hormones of the Hypothalamus

The search for hypothalamic neurohormones with anterior pituitary–regulating properties focused on extracts of stalk median eminence and hypothalamus. Such hypophy-

Figure 5–25. Electron micrograph of hamster median eminence, which is made up of densely packed nerve endings distributed in relation to the perivascular space of the primary portal capillaries in a schema resembling in principle the distribution of nerve endings in the neurohypophysis. The nerve endings shown here in cross-sectional profiles contain a variety of vesicles, both large and small, of different electron density; some contain neurosecretions and others are thought to be recycled membrane vessels (see Fig. 5–3). Mitochondria are also found. Note that nerves end in close relation to a basement membrane. The path of secretion is from nerve endings through axon basement membrane and finally endothelium. This arrangement is characteristic of glandular cells throughout the endocrine system. a, capillary lumen; b, perivascular space; c, nerve endings; d, nucleus of supporting (connective tissue) cell. (Courtesy of Karl M. Knigge, unpublished, 1966.)

seotropic materials were called *releasing factors*, after the initial designation of corticotropin-releasing factor (now known as CRH). This factor was extracted from hypothalamic tissues that stimulated the release of ACTH from pituitary fragments maintained in organ culture.[142] As currently used the term *releasing factor* is applied to hypothalamic substances of unknown chemical nature, whereas substances with established chemical identity are referred to as *releasing hormones*.

Chemical structures of all of the classic releasing factors have now been established. All are peptides with one important exception, dopamine, which is the principal PRL release–inhibitory factor. Further, the mode of biosynthesis of all of these peptides has been established, and all are now available for human investigational and clinical use. Their structures are shown in Tables 5–3 and 5–4. In addition to regulating hormone release, the hypophyseotropic factors regulate pituitary cell differentiation, proliferation, and hormone synthesis.

The original idea that there would be a single stimulatory factor corresponding to each anterior pituitary hormone now appears to be naive. Certain hypothalamic factors exert significant inhibitory actions on anterior pituitary function. Inhibitory factors interact with the respective releasing factor to exert dual control of the secretion of PRL, GH, and TSH. Further, the actions of hypophyseotropic hormones are not limited strictly to a single pituitary hormone. For example, TRH is a potent releaser of PRL as well as TSH and, under some circumstances, releases ACTH and GH. LHRH releases both LH and follicle-stimulating hormone (FSH). Somatostatin inhibits the secretion of GH, TSH, and a wide variety of other nonpituitary hormones. The principal inhibitor of PRL secretion, dopamine, also inhibits TSH, gonadotropin, and (under certain conditions) GH secretion.

TABLE 5–3. Structural Formulas of Principal Human Hypothalamic Peptides Related Directly to Pituitary Secretion

Vasopressin

Cys-Tyr-Phe-Gln-Asn-Cys-Pro-Arg-Gly-NH₂ (MW* 1084.38)

Oxytocin

Cys-Tyr-Ile-Gln-Asn-Cys-Pro-Leu-Gly-NH₂ (MW 1007.35)

Thyrotropin-Releasing Hormone

pGlu-His-Pro-NH₂ (MW 362.42)

Luteinizing Hormone–Releasing Hormone (Gonadotropin-Releasing Hormone)

pGlu-His-Trp-Ser-Tyr-Gly-Leu-Arg-Pro-Gly-NH₂ (MW 1182.39)

Corticotropin-Releasing Hormone (Human, Rat)

Ser-Glu-Glu-Pro-Pro-Ile-Ser-Leu-Asp-Leu-Thr-Phe-His-Leu-Leu-Arg-Glu-Val-Leu-Glu-Met-Ala-Arg-Ala-Glu-Gln-Leu-Ala-Gln-Gln-Ala-His-Ser-Asn-Arg-Lys-Leu-Met-Glu-Ile-Ile-NH₂ (MW 4758.14)

Growth Hormone–Releasing Hormone (GHRH 1–40, 1–44-NH₂, Human)

Tyr-Ala-Asp-Ala-Ile-Phe-Thr-Asn-Ser-Tyr-Arg-Lys-Val-Leu-Gly-Gln-Leu-Ser-Ala-Arg-Lys-Leu-Leu-Gln-Asp-Ile-Met-Ser-Arg-Gln-Gln-Gly-Glu-Ser-Asn-Gln-Glu-Arg-Gly-Ala (MW 4544.73), [-Arg-Ala-Arg-Leu-NH₂] (MW 5040.4)

Somatostatin

Ala-Gly-Cys-Lys-Asn-Phe-Phe-Trp-Lys-Thr-Phe-Thr-Ser-Cys (MW 1638.12)

Somatostatin-28

Ser-Ala-Asn-Ser-Asn-Pro-Ala-Met-Ala-Pro-Arg-Glu-Arg-Lys-Ala-Gly– Cys-Lys-Asn-Phe-Phe-Trp-Lys-Thr-Phe-Thr-Ser-Cys (MW 3149.00)

Somatostatin-28 (1–12)

Ser-Ala-Asn-Ser-Asn-Pro-Ala-Met-Ala-Pro-Arg-Glu (MW 1244.49)

Vasoactive Intestinal Peptide (Human, Pig, Rat)

His-Ser-Asp-Ala-Val-Phe-Thr-Asp-Asn-Tyr-Thr-Arg-Leu-Arg-Lys-Gln-Met-Ala-Val-Lys-Lys-Tyr-Leu-Asn-Ser-Ile-Leu-Asn-NH₂ (MW 3326.26)

*MW, molecular weight.

TABLE 5–4. Structural Formulas of Several Gut-Brain Peptides of Neuroendocrine Importance

Angiotensin I (Human)

Asp-Arg-Val-Tyr-Ile-His-Pro-Phe-His-Leu (MW* 1296.7)

Angiotensin II (Human)

Asp-Arg-Val-Tyr-Ile-His-Pro-Phe (MW 1046.3)

α-Atrial Natriuretic Polypeptide 1–28 (Human, Dog)

Ser-Leu-Arg-Arg-Ser-Ser-Cys-Phe-Gly-Gly-Arg-Met-Asp-Arg-Ile-Gly-Ala-Gln-Ser-Gly-Leu-Gly-Cys-Asn-Ser-Phe-Arg-Tyr (MW 3080.31)

Brain Natriuretic Peptide-32 (Human)

Ser-Pro-Lys-Met-Val-Gln-Gly-Ser-Gly-Cys-Phe-Gly-Arg-Lys-Met-Asp-Arg-Ile-Ser-Ser-Ser-Ser-Gly-Leu-Gly-Cys-Lys-Val-Leu-Arg-Arg-His (MW 3461.74)

Human Calcitonin

Cys-Gly-Asn-Leu-Ser-Thr-Cys-Met-Leu-Gly-Thr-Tyr-Thr-Gln-Asp-Phe-Asn-Lys-Phe-His-Thr-Phe-Pro-Gln-Thr-Ala-Ile-Gly-Val-Gly-Ala-Pro-NH₂ (MW 3418.41)

Calcitonin Gene–Related Peptide (Human)

Ala-Cys-Asp-Thr-Ala-Thr-Cys-Val-Thr-His-Arg-Leu-Ala-Gly-Leu-Leu-Ser-Arg-Ser-Gly-Gly-Val-Val-Lys-Asn-Asn-Phe-Val-Pro-Thr-Asn-Val-Gly-Ser-Lys-Ala-Phe-NH₂ (MW 3789.16)

Cholecystokinin Octapeptide (26–33)

Asp-Tyr(SO₃)-Met-Gly-Trp-Met-Asp-Phe-NH₂ (MW 1142.31)

Galanin (Rat)

Gly-Trp-Thr-Leu-Asn-Ser-Ala-Gly-Tyr-Leu-Leu-Gly-Pro-His-Ala-Ile-Asp-Asn-His-Arg-Ser-Phe-Ser-Asp-Lys-His-Gly-Leu-Thr-NH₂ (MW 3162.56)

Gastrin I (Human)

pGlu-Gly-Pro-Trp-Leu-Glu-Glu-Glu-Glu-Glu-Ala-Tyr-Gly-Trp-Met-Asp-Phe-NH₂ (MW 2098.49)

Glucagon (Human)

His-Ser-Gln-Gly-Thr-Phe-Thr-Ser-Asp-Tyr-Ser-Lys-Tyr-Leu-Asp-Ser-Arg-Arg-Ala-Gln-Asp-Phe-Val-Gln-Trp-Leu-Met-Asp-Thr (MW 3550)

Katacalcin

Asp-Met-Ser-Ser-Asp-Leu-Glu-Arg-Asp-His-Arg-Pro-His-Val-Ser-Met-Pro-Gln-Asn-Ala-Asn (MW 2436.92)

Motilin (Pig)

Phe-Val-Pro-Ile-Phe-Thr-Tyr-Gly-Glu-Leu-Gln-Arg-Met-Gln-Glu-Lys-Glu-Arg-Asn-Lys-Gly-Gln (MW 2699.45)

NPY (Neuropeptide Y)

Tyr-Pro-Ser-Lys-Pro-Asp-Asn-Pro-Gly-Glu-Asp-Ala-Pro-Ala-Glu-Asp-Leu-Ala-Arg-Tyr-Tyr-Ser-Ala-Leu-Arg-His-Tyr-Ile-Asn-Leu-Ile-Thr-Arg-Gln-Arg-Tyr-NH₂ (MW 4254.21)

Neurotensin

pGlu-Leu-Tyr-Glu-Asn-Lys-Pro-Arg-Arg-Pro-Tyr-Ile-Leu (MW 1673.15)

Pancreatic Polypeptide (Human)

Ala-Pro-Leu-Glu-Pro-Val-Tyr-Pro-Gly-Asp-Asn-Ala-Thr-Pro-Glu-Gln-Met-Ala-Gln-Tyr-Ala-Ala-Asp-Leu-Arg-Arg-Tyr-Ile-Asn-Met-Leu-Thr-Arg-Pro-Arg-Tyr-NH₂ (MW 4184.28)

Peptide-Histidine-Methionine-27 (Human)

His-Ala-Asp-Gly-Val-Phe-Thr-Ser-Asp-Phe-Ser-Lys-Leu-Leu-Gly-Gln-Leu-Ser-Ala-Lys-Lys-Tyr-Leu-Glu-Ser-Leu-Met-NH₂ (MW 2985.87)

Peptide YY

Tyr-Pro-Ala-Lys-Pro-Glu-Ala-Pro-Gly-Glu-Asp-Ala-Ser-Pro-Glu-Glu-Leu-Ser-Arg-Tyr-Tyr-Ala-Ser-Leu-Arg-His-Tyr-Leu-Asn-Leu-Val-Thr-Arg-Gln-Arg-Tyr-NH₂ (MW 4241.22)

Secretin (Porcine)

His-Ser-Asp-Gly-Thr-Phe-Thr-Ser-Glu-Leu-Ser-Arg-Leu-Arg-Asp-Ser-Ala-Arg-Leu-Gln-Arg-Leu-Leu-Gln-Gly-Leu-Val-NH₂ (MW 3055.87)

Substance P

Arg-Pro-Lys-Pro-Gln-Gln-Phe-Phe-Gly-Leu-Met-NH₂ (MW 1347.80)

Gastrin-Releasing Peptide (Porcine Bombesin-Like)

Ala-Pro-Val-Ser-Val-Gly-Gly-Gly-Thr-Val-Leu-Ala-Lys-Met-Tyr-Pro-Arg-Gly-Asn-His-Trp-Ala-Val-Gly-His-Leu-Met-NH₂ (MW 2805.81)

*MW, molecular weight.

c DNA

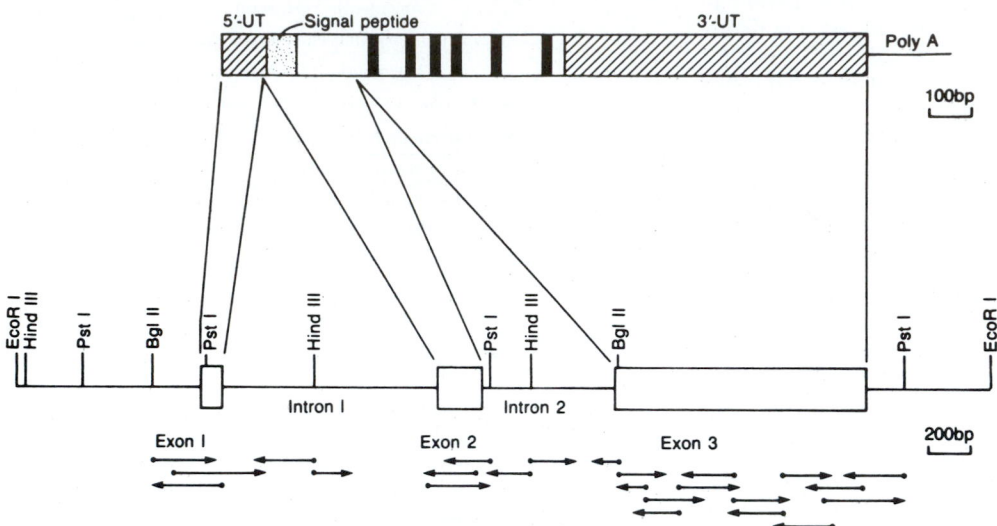

Figure 5–26. Structure of human TRH gene, showing six repeating codons for the TRH sequence. (From Yamada M, Radovick S, Wondisford FE, et al. Cloning and structure of human genomic DNA and hypothalamic cDNA encoding human preprothyrotropin-releasing hormone. Mol Endocrinol 1990; 4:551–556.)

Genomic DNA

In a synergistic way, the secretion of ACTH is regulated by CRH, AVP, and epinephrine (the last derived from the general circulation). The actions of GH-releasing hormone (GHRH) and CRH are relatively specific, although GHRH has weak PRL-releasing potency. There are a number of candidate PRL-releasing factors (PRFs). Secretion of the releasing hormones is regulated by local neurotransmitters and neuropeptides, which interact with the effects of circulating hormones such as glucocorticoids, gonadal steroids, and thyroid hormone. There is also evidence for feedback effects of anterior pituitary hormones (short-loop feedback control) and of hypophyseotropic factors themselves (ultra-short-loop feedback control).

THYROTROPIN-RELEASING HORMONE. *Chemistry and Effects on the Pituitary*. TRH is a tripeptide pyroGlu-His-Pro-NH$_2$ (Fig. 5–26).[143–145] An intact amide and the cyclized glutamic acid terminus are essential for activity.[146, 147] TRH is synthesized as part of a large prohormone, which contains five repeating sequences in the rat and six in the human. The prohormone undergoes extensive post-translational processing, including enzymatic cleavage, cyclization of NH$_2$-terminal glutamic acid, and exchange of an amide for the COOH-terminal glycine in the nascent molecule (see Fig. 5–26).[148, 149, 149a]

After intravenous injection of TRH in humans, serum TSH levels rise within a few minutes (Fig. 5–27).[150–155] The surge of TSH leads to a readily detected rise in serum triiodothyronine (T$_3$) level; there is an increase in T$_4$ release, but a change in steady-state blood levels of T$_4$ is usually not demonstrable. The clinical applications of TRH testing are covered in Chapter 8,[150–155] and its role in neuroendocrine regulation of TSH secretion is discussed later.

TSH action on the pituitary is blocked by previous treatment with thyroid hormone. In fact, the interaction of the negative feedback action of thyroid hormone on the pituitary with the stimulating effects of TRH is the main basis of the integrated neuroendocrine control system of TSH secretion.

As noted earlier, TRH is a potent PRF (Fig. 5–28).[150–152, 154, 155] The time course of response of blood PRL levels to TRH, dose-response characteristics, and suppressibility by thyroid hormone pretreatment (all of which parallel changes in TSH secretion) suggest that TRH is probably involved in the regulation of PRL secretion. However, the role of TRH as a physiological regulator of PRL secretion is not established.[156, 157] In women the PRL response to nursing is unaccompanied by changes in plasma TSH levels.[158] Nevertheless, the PRL release–stimulating actions of TRH may be responsible for the occasional occurrence of hyperprolactinemia (with or without galactorrhea) in patients with hypothyroidism.

In normal individuals TRH has no influence on secretion of pituitary hormones other than TSH and PRL. Under special circumstances, however, it exerts other effects, including the release of ACTH in some patients who have

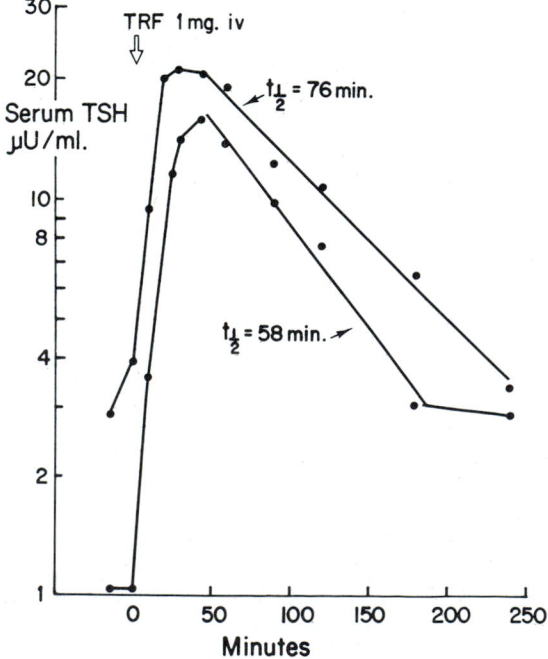

Figure 5–27. Effect of intravenous injection of TRH on serum TSH levels in humans. (From Hershman JM, Pittman JA Jr. Control of thyrotropin secretion in man. N Engl J Med 1971; 285:997–1006. Reprinted by permission of The New England Journal of Medicine.)

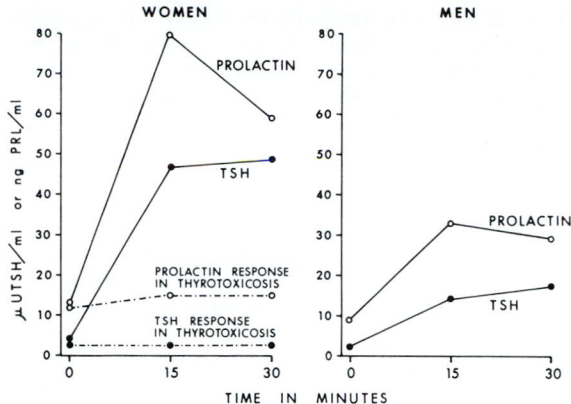

Figure 5–28. PRL- and TSH-secretory responses to intravenous injection of 800 μg of TRH in humans. This figure shows that TRH induces discharge of both PRL and TSH, that the effect in females is greater than that in males (presumably owing to estrogen sensitization of the pituitary), and that thyrotoxicosis inhibits the response of both PRL and TSH to TRH. An inhibitory effect on the TRH response is noted at the upper limit of the normal range of thyroid hormone levels and is a sensitive test of minor degrees of thyroid hormone excess. Although TRH is a potent PRF, there is evidence that there is another PRF physiologically connected to PRL regulation. (Replotted from data of Bowers S, Friesen HG, Hwang P, et al. Prolactin and thyrotropin release in man by synthetic pyroglutamylhistidyl-prolinamide. Biochem Biophys Res Commun 1971; 45:1033–1041.)

Cushing disease and the release of GH in some patients with acromegaly. The responses in acromegaly were first thought to be due to the presence on pituitary cell membranes of TRH receptors that were ordinarily obscured by the normal regulatory processes of the pituitary or that appeared as a consequence of "derepression" of the adenoma to a more primitive cell resembling an ancestral pituitary stem cell. However, prolonged stimulation of the normal pituitary with GHRH can sensitize it to the GH-releasing effects of TRH.[159, 160] TRH also causes release of GH in some patients with uremia, hepatic disease, anorexia nervosa, and psychotic depression.[153, 155] The same is true in children with hypothyroidism. TRH inhibits sleep-induced GH release through the central nervous system.

Mechanism of Action of TRH. Stimulatory effects of TRH are initiated by binding of the peptide to specific receptors on the plasma membrane of the pituitary cell.[161] TRH action is exerted on the membrane and does not depend on internalization, although the latter does take place. The receptor is specific, and neither thyroid hormone nor somatostatin, which antagonize the biological effects of TRH, do so by interfering with its binding. TRH was originally thought to act by activating membrane adenylate cyclase with the formation of cyclic 3',5'-AMP (cAMP).[155] TRH does indeed stimulate cAMP formation, and cAMP stimulates TSH secretion. However, cAMP may not increase under all conditions of TRH-induced TSH release, and certain situations in which the intracellular cAMP concentration is increased may not be associated with increased TSH secretion. It is now widely accepted that TRH action is mediated mainly through hydrolysis of phosphatidylinositol, with phosphorylation of key protein kinases[162, 163] as the crucial step in postreceptor activation. TRH effects can be mimicked by exposure to a Ca^{2+} ionophore and are partially abolished by a Ca^{2+}-free medium. The mechanism of action of TRH on tissues other than the pituitary, in particular the nervous system, has not been elucidated. TRH stimulates the formation of mRNA coding for PRL (in a TRH-responsive pituitary tumor cell line),[164] thus confirming that this peptide is a true trophic factor as well as a releasing factor. Thyroid hormone reduces the number of TRH receptors on the thyrotrope cell.

Extrahypothalamic Distribution and Neuromodulator Function of TRH. TRH is present in brain tissue outside of the classic "thyrotrophic area" of the hypothalamus.[155] It has been identified by immunoassay or immunohistochemistry in virtually all parts of the brain: cerebral cortex, circumventricular structures, neurohypophysis, pineal gland, and spinal cord (see Fig. 5–20).[155, 165–168] TRH is also present in pancreatic islet cells and in various parts of the gastrointestinal tract. It has a characteristic pattern of ontogenesis in the developing mammal.[169] Although present in low concentrations outside the hypothalamus, the total amount in extrahypothalamic tissues far exceeds the total amount in the hypothalamus. As the phylogenetic scale is descended, the concentration of TRH in neural tissues outside the hypothalamus increases, so that in the frog, for example, the concentration in the extrahypothalamic brain is fully half that in the hypothalamus. In some species of frogs, TRH is found in the skin in concentrations higher than those found in the hypothalamus, an association presumed to be related to the embryological origin of both skin and brain from neuroectoderm. TRH is present in primitive vertebrates (the larval form of the lamprey), in *Amphioxus* (a provertebrate), and in nerve ganglia of the snail. Because the lamprey probably does not synthesize TSH and because *Amphioxus* and snails lack a pituitary gland, it seems that the TRH molecule appeared in evolutionary development as a primitive neurosecretion before the evolution of TSH and that the pituitary "co-opted" TRH as its regulatory hormone. The increasing specialization of regulatory factors as the phylogenetic scale is ascended is a general feature of the evolution of neuropeptides and neurotransmitters.

The extensive extrahypothalamic distribution of TRH, its localization in nerve endings, and the presence of TRH receptors in brain tissue suggest that TRH serves as a neurotransmitter or neuromodulator outside the hypothalamus. Neural effects of TRH are summarized in Table 5–5. TRH has a general stimulant activity.[155, 170–172] It induces hyperthermia on intracerebroventricular injection, which suggests a role in central thermoregulation (see later). A beneficial psychological effect of TRH has been reported in depressed patients in some but not all studies.[173] Although the role of TRH in depression is unclear, the pituitary TSH response to TRH is blunted in many depressed patients, and changes in responsiveness correlate with clinical

TABLE 5–5. Central Nervous System–Mediated Actions of Thyrotropin-Releasing Hormone

Increases spontaneous motor activity
Alters sleep patterns
Produces anorexia
Inhibits conditioned avoidance behavior
Causes head-to-tail rotation
Opposes actions of barbiturates on sleeping time, hypothermia, lethality
Opposes actions of ethanol, chloral hydrate, chlorpromazine, and diazepam on sleeping time and hypothermia
Enhances convulsion time and lethality of strychnine
Increases motor activity in morphine-treated animals
Potentiates DOPA-pargyline effects
Ameliorates human behavioral disorders?
Causes central inhibition of morphine-mediated secretion of GH and PRL
Alters brain cell membrane electric activity
Increases norepinephrine turnover
Releases norepinephrine and dopamine from synaptosomal preparations
Enhances disappearance of norepinephrine from nerve terminals
Potentiates excitatory actions of acetylcholine on cerebral cortical neurons
Increases blood pressure
Protects against spinal shock
Improves motor function in lower motor neuron disease (amyotrophic lateral sclerosis)

Modified from Vale W, Rivier C, Brown M. Regulatory peptides of the hypothalamus. Annu Rev Physiol 1977; 39:473–527. Reproduced, with permission, from the Annual Review of Physiology, Vol. 39, © 1977 by Annual Reviews Inc.

course.[173] The importance of TRH as a neuropharmacological therapeutic agent is being evaluated for two types of disorder: shock and spinal muscle atrophy, including amyotrophic lateral sclerosis. TRH administration to experimental animals reduces the severity of spinal shock[155, 174] and septic shock related to gram-negative infections. These effects may be due to stimulation of TRH receptors on the cells of the intermediolateral column of the spinal cord, which is the site of origin of preganglionic sympathetic nerve cells. TRH is distributed to nerve terminals in this region, and when administered to normal animals and humans it increases blood pressure.

Because TRH administered to experimental animals increases muscle tone and the intensity of spinal reflexes, it was tried for the treatment of spinal muscle disease. Transient improvement in strength was reported in patients with spinal motor atrophy[175] and amyotrophic lateral sclerosis.[176–178] Because only small amounts of TRH enter the CSF after systemic injection, it has also been given by intrathecal infusion.[177] The earlier suggestion that amyotrophic lateral sclerosis might be associated with a deficiency of spinal cord TRH[176] has not been supported by studies of spinal cords at autopsy.[179] Consequently, TRH might be acting as a trophic factor rather than as a replacement of a spinal cord deficiency.

Although TRH that is added to in vitro spinal cord cultures exerts a trophic effect on motor neurons,[179a] the combined experience of researchers at many centers who use a variety of treatment protocols failed to provide unequivocal evidence of efficacy.[178]

Metabolic Degradation Products of TRH. TRH is enzymatically degraded to acid TRH and to a dipeptide, histidylprolineamide, that cyclizes nonenzymatically to histidylproline diketopiperazine (cyclic His-Pro).[155, 180] Acid TRH has some behavioral effects in rats similar to those of TRH but no other proven biological actions. Cyclic His-Pro is reported to act as a PRF and to have other neural effects, including reversal of ethanol-induced sleep (TRH is also effective in this system), elevation of brain cGMP levels, increase in stereotypical behavior, modification of body temperature, and inhibition of eating behavior. Some of the effects of TRH may be mediated through cyclic His-Pro.

LUTEINIZING HORMONE–RELEASING HORMONE.
Chemistry and Effects on the Pituitary. McCann and colleagues showed by bioassay in 1960 that the systemic injection of acid extracts of the hypothalamus released LH from the pituitary of the rat.[181] Campbell and colleagues in the laboratory of Harris observed that intrapituitary injection of hypothalamic extracts induced ovulation in the rabbit, a response attributable to the release of LH.[182] This biological activity was shown by Matsuo and colleagues in 1971 to reside in a decapeptide (see Table 5–3).[183] LHRH, like other neuropeptides, is synthesized as part of a large prohormone that is enzymatically cleaved and further modified within secretory granules. The amino acid sequence of pre-pro-LHRH from human placenta was elucidated by Seeburg and Adelman[184] by recombinant DNA techniques (Fig. 5–29).

During the early research on LHRH, it appeared that two different hypothalamic factors regulated the secretion of gonadotropins, one stimulating LH secretion and the other stimulating the release of FSH. This view is still held by McCann and colleagues, who have summarized evidence that supports this contention.[185] Other workers[186–188] believe that all situations in which LH and FSH secretion are dissociated can be explained by differences in the way in which the two types of gonadotropin-secreting cells respond to secretory patterns of LHRH, to the gonadal steroid milieu, and to the secretion of inhibin, which is a peptide secretion of the gonads that has a selective inhibitory effect on FSH secretion.[189] The rate at which LHRH pulses are administered can alter the pattern of LH and FSH secretion, fast frequencies lowering secretion of both LH and FSH, slower frequencies increasing FSH relative to LH, and constant infusions suppressing secretion of both LH and FSH.[190] Administration of antisera against LHRH inhibits secretion of both gonadotropins. Further, complete restoration of male and female gonadal function in patients with hypothalamic LHRH deficiency has been accomplished by using only LHRH in appropriate doses in a pulsatile manner. For these reasons, the unitarian view that there is only one hormone that releases gonadotropin is widely held.

Because the hypothalamic hypophyseotropic factors act in all species of animals and because TRH has an identical structure throughout the animal kingdom, it was initially assumed that the chemical structure of LHRH would also be identical across species. However, this proved not to be true. There are structural differences among species,[191] and even within the same species more than one form of LHRH can be found at different sites. For example, the LHRH in frog sympathetic ganglia appears to be different from that in frog brain, which resembles mammalian LHRH.[192] Fish brain LHRH differs from that of the mammal by two amino acid substitutions.[193] Indeed, the structures of all releasing hormones larger than TRH (a tripeptide) display species differences, and in some instances they are coded for by more than one gene in the same species.

After a single intravenous injection, LHRH brings about a prompt dose-related increase of LH and FSH levels in all vertebrate species (Fig. 5–30). The onset of FSH release after a single bolus injection is delayed in comparison with that of LH secretion, and the values peak at 10 to 30 min after injection. The response to LHRH is influenced by the previous LHRH-secretory state, by the steroid milieu, by the patient's sex, by the stage of sexual development, and by the time course of administration of the hormone. As noted earlier, sustained high levels of LHRH suppress LH and FSH secretion; a normal pattern can be restored by intermittent injections. Under appropriately defined conditions, LHRH can induce spermatogenesis and testosterone production in men with hypothalamic hypogonadotropic hypogonadism,[194] ovulation in women with hypothalamic amenorrhea,[187, 188] and puberty in both boys and girls with delayed or arrested puberty.[195] LHRH analogues in high doses can suppress gonadal function in patients with pre-

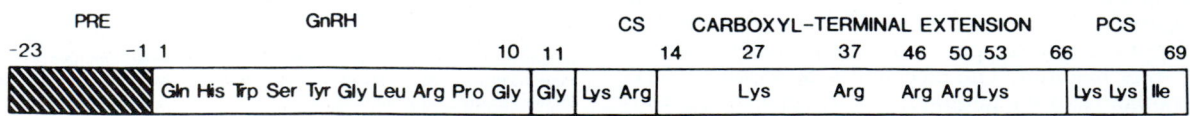

Figure 5–29. Schematic diagram of the structure of the precursor of human placental LHRH (GnRH in figure), as determined by nucleic acid sequencing of the corresponding cDNA (Seeburg and Adelman).[184] The precursor consists of a signal sequence (PRE) of 23 amino acids followed immediately by the LHRH decapeptide sequence. Cleavage of the signal peptide reveals an NH₂-terminal Gln, which cyclizes (enzymatically or spontaneously) to pyroGlu. The LHRH sequence is followed by a Gly, which is the donor for the COOH-terminal amide of LHRH, and Lys-Arg, which is a conventional dibasic amino acid cleavage site (CS). A peptide of 53 amino acids follows. The 53-amino-acid sequence includes a fragment that has been designated GAP (gonadotropin-releasing hormone–associated peptide), which has been reported to have effects on PRL secretion, although these results are controversial. PCS, potential cleavage site. (From Miller RP, King JA. Structural and functional evolution of gonadotropin-releasing hormone. Int Rev Cytol 1987; 106:149–182.)

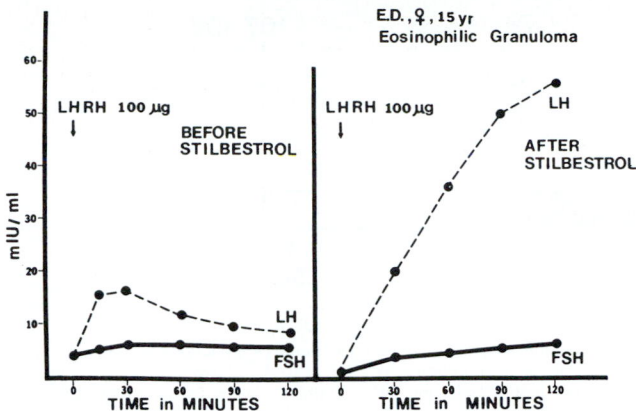

Figure 5–30. Gonadotropin-secretory response to an LHRH bolus injection (100 μg) in a patient with hypothalamic hypopituitarism. Note that the LH response is greater than the FSH response and that the peak response is somewhat delayed. After estrogen treatment, there was marked sensitization of the LH response, which is characteristic of the "positive" feedback effect of estrogens on hypothalamic-pituitary gonadotropin secretion. (From Reichlin S. Regulation of the endocrine hypothalamus. Med Clin North Am 1978; 62:235–250.)

cocious puberty[196] as well as in normal men[197, 198] and women.[187, 199, 200] The role of LHRH in gonadotropin regulation is discussed later.

The potential clinical usefulness of LHRH as a contraceptive, as a regulator of fertility, and as an agent for the treatment of abnormal sexual development has led to the synthesis of analogues with both agonist and antagonist properties.[201] For example, the insertion of D-amino acids at sites that are normally cleaved by proteases markedly prolongs activity. Two general types of analogues are now available: "super agonists" that have prolonged action and true antagonists that bind to LHRH receptors and block hormone action. Because the pattern of delivery of LHRH determines its effects on the pituitary, super agonists can inhibit gonadotropin secretion, as do true antagonists.

Extrahypothalamic Distribution and Function of LHRH. Almost all the LHRH in mammalian brain is present in the hypothalamus and related neural structures. It is found outside the hypothalamus in a number of regions of the limbic system, including the hippocampus, cingulate cortex, and olfactory bulb.[202] This distribution is potentially important because these structures are responsible for emotional expression and because LHRH has been implicated in sexual drive.[203] An LHRH-like peptide in frog sympathetic ganglia is thought to be an important neurotransmitter.[204] LHRH is secreted into milk[205] (as is TRH), which suggests that the breast, a dermal-derived structure, may have embryological origins analogous to the primitive neuroectoderm, which is the source of neuroendocrine cells. LHRH is also present in the placenta,[202] and mRNA coding for LHRH was first isolated from this tissue. LHRH can enhance or depress electric activity of certain nerve cells. Despite the fact that the peptide is located in only a restricted area, responding cells are present in many other areas of the brain. The most important neural effects appear to be those involved in regulation of mating behavior.[202, 203, 206] Direct injection of LHRH into the hypothalamus enhances female sexual responsivity in rats, even in animals without a pituitary and hence incapable of responding with gonadal activation. Trials of LHRH as a stimulator of sex drive in humans were inconclusive.[206]

Mechanism of Action of LHRH. LHRH action on the pituitary is initiated by binding to specific cell-surface receptors, which leads, in turn, to an increased free intracellular calcium concentration, hydrolysis of inositol phosphates, and phosphorylation of protein kinase C.[207] Increased release and increased synthesis of gonadotropins follow exposure to LHRH. Changes in membrane LHRH receptors are an important means by which gonadotropin secretion is regulated. Estrogens (which sensitize the pituitary to LHRH) increase and androgens decrease the number of LHRH receptors. The reduced number of LHRH receptors resulting from constant infusion of LHRH or from the use of super agonists probably explains the reduced secretion of gonadotropins that follows such treatment. These changes in receptor number are the basis of agonist treatment of precocious puberty and the blockade of ovulation.[208]

LHRH receptors are also present in the ovary and testis of the rat[202] and in human ovary.[209] Although LHRH stimulates the release of steroid hormones (androstenedione and progesterone) from isolated rat ovaries,[210] it is doubtful whether circulating LHRH has a physiological role in gonadal function because the concentration of this peptide in blood is so low.

GROWTH HORMONE–REGULATING FACTORS. *Growth Hormone–Releasing Hormone.* Because alterations in growth rate are expressed over relatively long periods compared with other endocrine-related phenomena, the idea that GH secretion is regulated by the brain appeared late in the history of neuroendocrinology.[211] The first convincing evidence of neural control of GH secretion came from studies of its regulation in animals with lesions of the hypothalamus and from the demonstration that hypothalamic extracts stimulate the release of GH from the pituitary. When it was shown that GH is released episodically, follows a circadian rhythm, responds rapidly to stress and electric stimulation of specific regions of the brain, and is blocked by pituitary stalk section, the concept of neural control of GH secretion became a certainty.[211] However, two decades of efforts to characterize the GH-stimulating factor from hypothalamic extracts were unsuccessful. It was only with the discovery of the paraneoplastic syndrome of ectopic GHRH secretion by pancreatic adenomas in humans that sufficient material became available for sequencing.[212] The structure was elucidated by Guillemin and co-workers[213] and Rivier and collaborators.[214] The materials isolated from human pancreatic tumors are identical to those isolated from hypothalamus (see Table 5–3). The term *somatocrinin* was proposed to replace the term GHRH, but it has not been widely accepted. Three molecular forms of GHRH are designated GHRH 1–44-NH₂, GHRH 1–40-OH, and GHRH 1–37-OH. Recombinant DNA techniques have been applied to elucidate the sequence of the precursors to GHRH in human pancreatic tumors. A single prohormone was isolated from one tumor, and two prohormones different by only one amino acid were isolated from another (Fig. 5–31).[213–215] As is the case for all other neuropeptides, the various forms of GHRH are derived by selective post-translational enzymatic cleavage of the respective prohormones. The NH₂-terminal tyrosine of GHRH is essential for action; all three forms of GHRH in the hypothalamus are biologically active. In humans the two larger forms are equipotent, and the smaller is less active. Fragments as short as 1–29-NH₂ are still active, but GHRH 1–27-NH₂ is without effect. As is the case for LHRH, there are species differences among GHRHs.

Ectopic secretion of GHRH is a rare cause of acromegaly (see Chapter 6). Less than 1% of patients with acromegaly have elevated serum levels of this peptide.[216] Approximately 20% of pancreatic adenomas and 5% of carcinoid tumors contain immunoreactive GHRH[217, 218] but are clinically silent.

When GHRH is given to individuals with normal pituitaries, it brings about a prompt increase in serum GH, followed by a rapid return to basal levels (Fig. 5–32).[219–221] Sustained infusions over several hours cause a *decrease* in

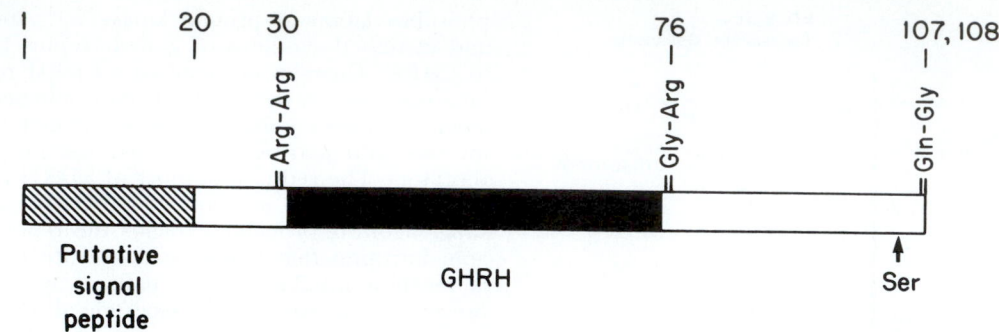

Figure 5–31. Diagram of the amino acid sequence of human GHRH derived by recombinant techniques from a pancreatic adenoma of a patient who had acromegaly related to ectopic secretion of GHRH. Following a signal sequence and an intervening sequence is the region coding for GHRH 1–44, followed by a glycine that will be exchanged for NH₂ during post-translational processing. In the particular tumor studied, two different prohormones were identified, one with 107 and the other with 108 amino acids. (Drawn from data of Gubler U, Monahan JJ, Lomedico PT, et al. Cloning and sequence analysis of cDNA for the precursor of human growth hormone–releasing factor, somatocrinin. Proc Natl Acad Sci USA 1983; 80:4311–4314.)

GH levels, which suggests that GHRH, like LHRH, depends on pulsatile secretion for its physiological effect. Administration of GHRH as repeated boluses stimulates the formation of insulin-like growth factor I (IGF I, also called somatomedin-C), which accounts for its potential usefulness as a therapeutic agent in individuals with hypothalamic forms of GH deficiency.[220, 221] Clinical trials are under way to determine the relative usefulness of synthetic GHRH compared with recombinant GH. A number of GHRH analogues with more favorable characteristics (e.g., duration of action, molecular size) have been synthesized.

The effects of a single injection of GHRH are almost completely specific for GH secretion, although there is a minimal change in PRL. It has no effect on known gut peptide hormones.[219] The response to GHRH is strongly influenced by age. Most men older than age 40 have either low or absent responses to GHRH.[222] This finding is compatible with previous work indicating that older individuals have lower 24-h secretion of GH, a kind of physiological GH deficiency in the elderly. As noted, patients with hypothalamic deficiency of GHRH (Fig. 5–33) respond to GHRH, as do most, but not all, patients with acromegaly. The latter occasionally are hyper-responsive.[220, 223]

GHRH exerts a number of actions on somatotropes.[224–227] After binding to pituitary cell membranes, it stimulates GH secretion by a Ca²⁺-dependent mechanism and activates adenylate cyclase with the accumulation of cAMP. It also activates the phosphatidylinositol cycle and may have a direct action within the cell via phosphorylation of a secretory granule–linked enzyme. GHRH also increases formation of new GH by stimulating transcription of specific GH mRNA.[228] The effects of GHRH are blocked by somatostatin and are enhanced by glucocorticoids[229] and by estrogen.[230] Transgenic mice bearing GHRH cDNA coupled to a suitable promoter develop marked somatotrope hyperplasia,[231] thus demonstrating the growth-stimulating effect of this factor on the pituitary.

***Somatostatin.* History and Chemistry.** During efforts to isolate GHRH from hypothalamic extracts, Krulich and colleagues[232] discovered a factor that *inhibited* GH release

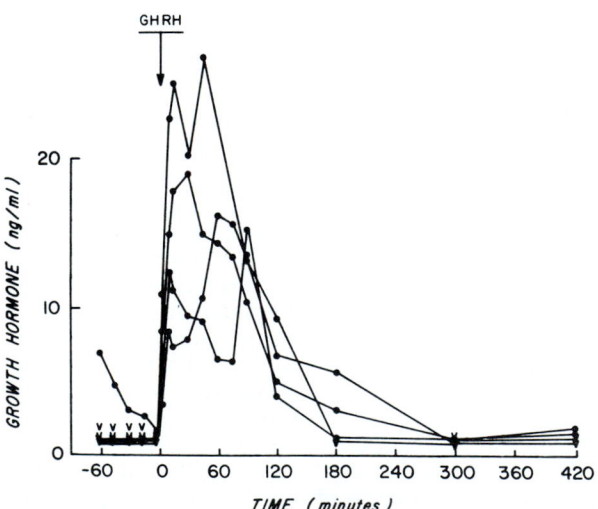

EFFECT OF GHRH ON GH SECRETION IN NORMAL ADULTS

Figure 5–32. Response of normal men to GHRH administered by intravenous injection. Note the prompt release of GH, followed by a rather prolonged fall in hormone level, in some cases associated with a double peak. (From Thorner MO, Rivier J, Speiss J, et al. Human pancreatic growth-hormone–releasing factor selectively stimulates growth-hormone secretion in man. Lancet 1983; 1:24–28.)

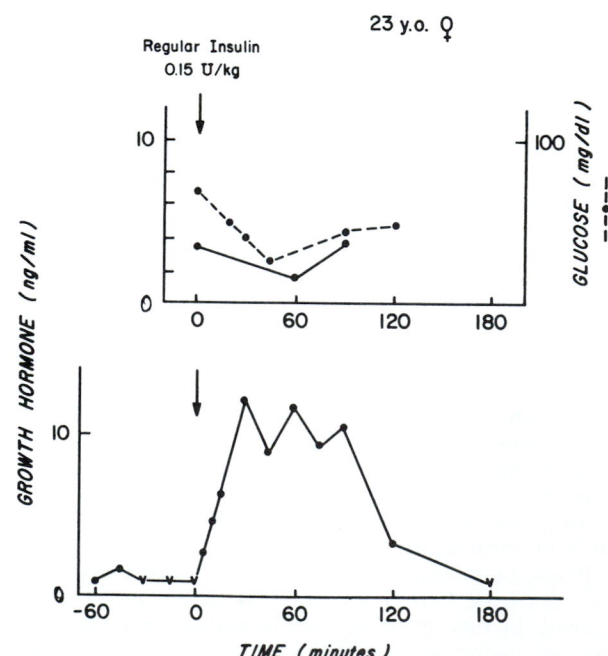

Figure 5–33. GH responses to GHRH in a patient with hypothalamic GH failure related to eosinophilic granuloma of the hypothalamus, and comparison with the response to insulin-induced hypoglycemia. This figure illustrates the failure of the GH response to a physiological stimulus involving the hypothalamus *(top)* and the normal response to direct pituitary stimulation *(bottom)*. GHRH was given as a bolus *(arrow, bottom)*. To convert glucose values to millimoles per liter, multiply by 0.055510. (From J. Goldman, M.E. Molitch, S. Reichlin, unpublished, 1984.)

RAT SOMATOSTATIN GENE

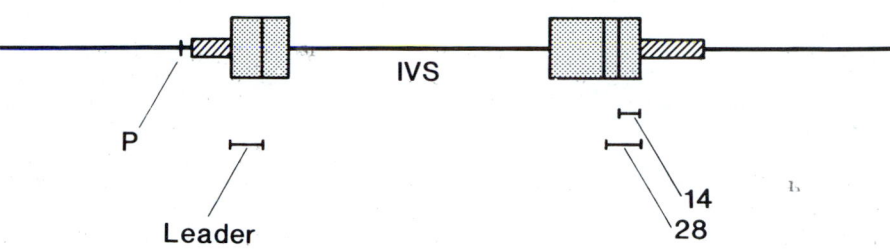

Figure 5–34. Diagram of gene sequence coding for somatostatin in the rat, which was characterized from recombinant bacteriophage libraries prepared from rat liver DNA. IVS, intervening sequence; P, promoter. (From Montminy MR, Goodman RH, Horovitch SJ, et al. Primary structure of the gene encoding rat preprosomatostatin. Proc Natl Acad Sci USA 1984; 81:3337–3340.)

from pituitary incubates in vitro. They named the factor growth hormone–release inhibiting factor and postulated that GH secretion was regulated by a dual control system, one stimulatory and the other inhibitory. At about the same time, Hellman and Lernmark[233] described a factor in pancreatic islet extracts that inhibited insulin secretion and proposed that this activity was part of a local secretory control system. In retrospect, these biological activities are known to be mainly due to somatostatin. Growth hormone–release inhibitory factor was rediscovered, isolated, and sequenced in Guillemin's laboratory.[234] The work in this area and its clinical application have been summarized in many reviews.[235–244]

The term *somatostatin* was originally applied to the cyclic peptide containing 14 amino acids (see Table 5–3). Somatostatin-like peptides are now known to constitute a family of related molecules. In mammals they include the originally identified peptide, designated somatostatin-14 (S-14), NH$_2$-terminal–extended somatostatin (S-28), a fragment corresponding to the first 12 amino acids of somatostatin-28 (S28 [1–12]), and still larger forms that vary in molecular size in different locations and different species from 11.5 to 15.7 kd. The larger forms are secreted; because they possess biological activity, they can be classified as both hormone and prohormone. There is some degree of functional specificity of the two forms in that somatostatin-14 is the predominant form in the brain, whereas somatostatin-28 predominates in the gastrointestinal tract, especially the colon. The term somatostatin is descriptively inaccurate because the molecule also inhibits TSH secretion, is distributed widely in cells throughout the nervous system, and is present in many extraneural tissues including the gut and pancreas, where it exerts effects on a wide range of structures including epithelia, endocrine tissue, and exocrine glands. In its function as a pituitary regulator it is a true neurohormone, i.e., a neuronal secretory product that enters the blood (hypophyseal-portal circulation) to affect cell function at remote sites. In the gut and the pancreas, somatostatin influences the function of adjacent cells and is thus a paracrine secretion. It also can influence its own secretion (an *autocrine* function), and because it can affect gut secretion by intraluminal action, it has been classified as a *lumone*. In short, somatostatin is secreted by different kinds of cells and serves different functions. Because of its wide distribution, broad spectrum of regulatory effects, and evolutionary history, this peptide can be regarded as an archetype of a gut-brain peptide.

The complete sequence of the pre-prohormone in humans[245] and rats[246] has been elucidated (Fig. 5–34). Comparative investigations of somatostatin have demonstrated its ancient lineage because it has been identified in the single-celled protozoan *Tetrahymena pyriformis*. During evolution the amino acid sequence of somatostatin-14 has undergone little change, mammalian somatostatin and one of the two an-

glerfish somatostatins being identical. Mammals and anglerfish are thought to be separated in evolution by at least 400 million years. The other regions of somatostatin-28 also show considerable homology. At least seven genes for somatostatin may exist in the animal kingdom; in anglerfish, for example, there are two separate prohormones, one for each of the somatostatins. The biosynthesis of the peptides conforms to the general rules governing peptide synthesis. Extensive studies of the structure and function of somatostatins have been published,[235, 242, 243, 247] and novel "mini-somatostatins" have been synthesized that are potentially useful in therapy.[242–244]

The function of somatostatin in GH and TSH regulation and in the extrahypothalamic brain is considered here. Its function in pancreatic islet cell regulation is described in Chapter 24, and the manifestations of somatostatin excess are described in Chapter 32. Its therapeutic uses are also summarized here.

Actions of Somatostatin. In the pituitary, somatostatin inhibits GH and TSH secretion and, under certain conditions, PRL and ACTH also. It exerts inhibitory effects on virtually all endocrine and exocrine secretions of the pancreas, gut, and gallbladder (Table 5–6). Somatostatin inhibits secretion by the salivary glands and under some conditions the secretion of parathyroid hormone and of calcitonin. Somatostatin blocks hormone release in many endocrine-secreting tumors including insulinomas, glucagonomas, VIPomas, and carcinoid tumors.

As is the case for the other hypophyseotropic hormones, somatostatin acts by first binding to receptors on plasma membranes of pituitary cells (and of other target cells such as pancreatic islets and neurons). At least two classes of receptors have been identified, which are organ specific. Receptor binding leads to activation of one or more membrane-bound guanine nucleotide–binding proteins, which in

TABLE 5–6. Biological Actions of Somatostatin Outside the Central Nervous System

Inhibits Hormone Secretion by	Inhibits Other Gastrointestinal Actions
Pituitary gland	Gastric acid secretion
TSH, GH	Gastric secretion
Gastrointestinal tract	Gastric emptying
Gastrin	Pancreatic bicarbonate secretion
Secretin	Pancreatic enzyme secretion
Gastrointestinal polypeptide	Intestinal absorption
Motilin	Gastrointestinal blood flow
Glicentin (enteroglucagon)	AVP-stimulated water transport
VIP	Bile flow
Pancreas	
Insulin	
Glucagon	
Somatostatin	
Genitourinary tract	
Renin	

TABLE 5–7. Therapeutic Uses of the Long-Acting Somatostatin Analogue Octreotide

Neuroendocrine tumor hyperfunction
  VIPoma*
  Carcinoid tumors*
  Glucagonoma
  Insulinoma
  Nisidioblastosis
  GHRHomas (ectopic GHRH)
  Gastrinoma†
Pituitary tumor
  Somatotropinoma (acromegaly)
  Thyrotropinoma
Gut disease
  Diarrhea
    Diabetic neuropathy
    Ileostomy
    Idiopathic diarrhea of childhood
    AIDS associated
  Pancreatic fistula
  Bleeding esophageal varices, bleeding peptic ulcer†
Postural hypotension
Miscellaneous
  Migraine headache
  Psoriasis
  ?Meningioma

*Approved for use in the United States by the Food and Drug Administration in 1989.
†H_2 blockers are superior or equivalent.

turn lower the cAMP and intracellular free Ca^{2+} concentrations. The effects of lowered cAMP can account only in part for the observed effects of somatostatin because this peptide also blocks the effects of cAMP-induced secretion and thus must be acting "downstream" from cAMP. It is more likely that changes in Ca^{2+} concentration are the crucial determinant of somatostatin action in blocking the secretion and synthesis of cellular proteins. The lowering of Ca^{2+} level is not a direct effect but is probably secondary to an increase in K^+ conductance and membrane hyperpolarization.[248]

Clinical Applications of Somatostatin Analogues. The potential therapeutic usefulness of somatostatin has generated much effort to synthesize analogues that resist degradation and that have a longer duration of action than the few minutes characteristic of native peptide. A number of such analogues have been introduced into clinical trials. One designated octreotide has been approved in the United States for treatment of carcinoid tumors and VIPomas (pancreatic cholera, Werner-Morrison syndrome)[242–244] (see Chapter 32). The actions of this agent illustrate the general potential of somatostatin in therapy (Tables 5–6 and 5–7). It controls excess secretion of GH in acromegaly in the majority of patients and actually shrinks tumors in about one third of cases and is useful in the management of many forms of

diarrhea (acting on salt and water excretion mechanisms in the gut). Octreotide has been used to reduce external secretions in pancreatic fistulas (thus permitting healing) and to treat functioning neuroendocrine tumors, particularly VIPoma, carcinoid, glucagonoma, and insulinoma. It is not useful for treatment of gastrinoma; H_2 blockers are more practical and equally effective. A decrease in blood flow to the gastrointestinal tract is the physiological basis of its use in bleeding from esophageal varices and peptic ulcers and in the treatment of postprandial orthostatic hypotension.[249]

CORTICOTROPIN-RELEASING HORMONE. The idea that the brain controlled ACTH secretion was established by the 1940s,[14, 110, 142, 250] and in conformity with the portal vessel–chemotransmitter hypothesis of Harris, control through hypothalamic factors was postulated. In 1955 Saffran and colleagues[251] showed that the addition of an extract of neurohypophysis to pituitary incubates led to the release of ACTH, and they coined the term CRF (corticotropin-releasing factor). Guillemin and Rosenberg[252] in the same year showed that the addition of a hypothalamic fragment to explant cultures of anterior pituitaries restored ACTH secretion. However, it was not until 1981 that the chemical structure of this factor, now designated CRH, was identified in ovine hypothalamic tissue and a biologically active peptide was synthesized.[110] The delay was due to many factors: the peptide is present in minute amounts; it is a relatively large molecule (41 amino acids); and hypothalamic extracts also contain authentic ACTH, which confounded earlier bioassays. Furthermore, median eminence extracts contain other factors that have CRH activity (or that synergize with CRH), including AVP and epinephrine.[110] This confusion has been cleared with the isolation of ovine CRH 1–41-NH_2 and of human CRH 1–41-NH_2[253] (see Table 5–3), which differs from the ovine sequence by seven amino acids (Fig. 5–35).

As with other neuropeptides, CRH is synthesized as part of a prohormone and undergoes enzymatic modification to the amidated form. Mammalian CRH has homologies with two peptides found in lower animal forms, the peptide sauvagine (derived from the skin of a certain species of frog) and urotensin 2 (the secretion of the caudal gland of a fish). Both of these homologues have potent CRH activity.[110, 254]

Structure-function activities of CRH have received much attention because of the importance of developing agonist and antagonist analogues. The NH_2 terminus is not essential for action, but removal of the terminal amide reduces activity.

CRH injection in humans and experimental animals causes a prompt increase in the release of ACTH into the blood, followed by the secretion of cortisol (Fig. 5–36).[255–258] The effect is specific to ACTH release and is inhibited by glucocorticoids. High cortisol levels reduce or abolish CRH

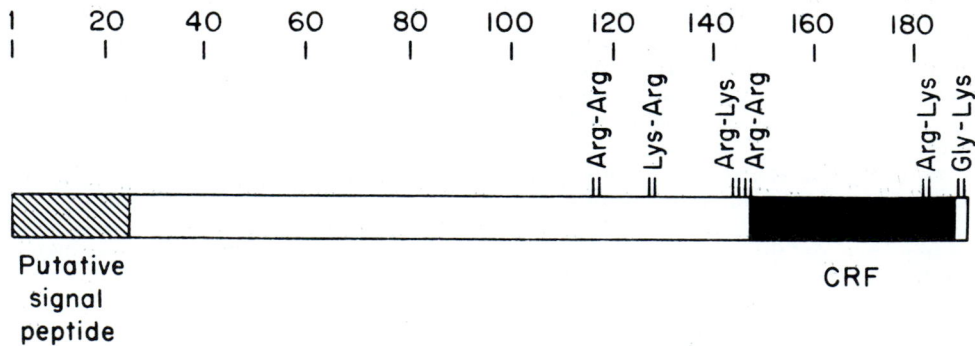

Figure 5–35. Sequence of human CRH (CRF in figure) pre-prohormone derived by recombinant DNA techniques. The sequence coding for CRH occurs at the terminus of the prohormone. Cleavage sites and the terminal Gly position is shown. (Redrawn from data of Shibahara S, Morimoto Y, Furutani Y, et al. Isolation and sequence analysis of the human corticotropin-releasing factor precursor gene. EMBO J 1983; 2:775–779.)

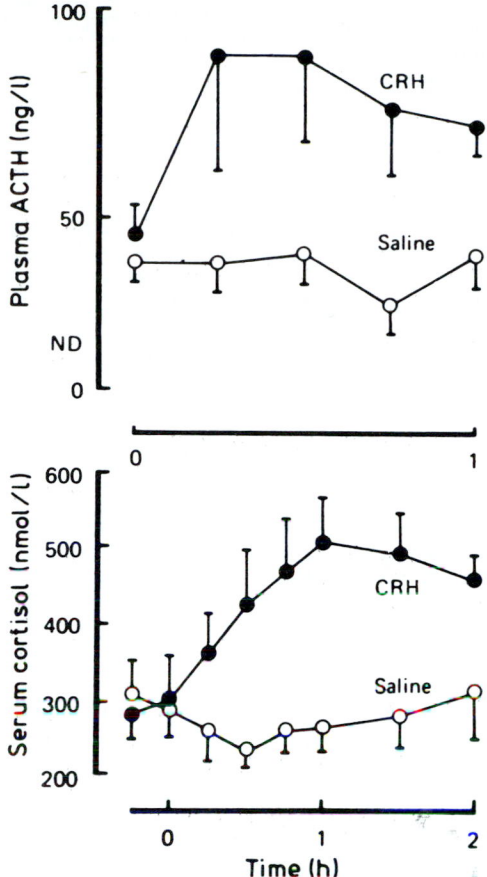

Figure 5–36. Changes in plasma levels of ACTH and serum levels of cortisol after intravenous injection of CRH (●) in a group of six normal men. The initial prompt response in ACTH is followed by a somewhat delayed secondary change in cortisol. Also shown are stable control periods (○). To convert ACTH values to picomoles per liter, multiply by 0.2202. To convert cortisol values to millimoles per liter, multiply by 27.59. (From Grossman A, Kruseman ACN, Perry L, et al. New hypothalamic hormone, corticotropin-releasing factor, specifically stimulates the release of adrenocorticotropic hormone and cortisol in man. Lancet 1982; 1:921–922.)

action on the pituitary (Fig. 5–37). CRH has been used as a diagnostic tool to differentiate causes of hypercortisolism[255-258] but has no established therapeutic role.

CRH acts by binding to specific receptors on corticotropes[110, 257, 259, 260] and stimulates hormone release only in the presence of Ca^{2+}. The concentration of cAMP in the tissue is increased in parallel with the biological effect; the stimulating effect of CRH on cAMP production is reduced by glucocorticoids. The suppressive effects of glucocorticoids are not complete, however, because they can be overcome by adding sufficiently large amounts of CRH. The rate of transcription of mRNA coding for ACTH and its prohormone POMC is also enhanced by CRH,[261] which supports the concept that CRH is a true trophic factor as well as a releasing hormone.

Detailed studies of the interaction of CRH with other hypothalamic factors that have CRH activity have helped to clarify the neural control of ACTH secretion in stress (discussed later).

Extrapituitary Functions of CRH. In the brain CRH has an extensive distribution outside of tuberoinfundibular cells: it is found in the hypothalamus, in the cerebral cortex, and in the limbic system, as well as in the spinal cord. This localization is believed to be the basis of the wide range of neural effects of CRH, which include increased sympathetic nervous system activity, hypertension, tachycardia, suppression of the hypothalamic component of gonadotropin regulation, suppression of GH, inhibition of eating, and general arousal.[262, 263] The complex of physiological and behavioral responses that are induced by central injections of CRH in rats and monkeys led Vale and colleagues[262] to suggest that responses to stress, including psychological changes and dysphoria, are mediated by central CRH pathways.

CRH is also found outside of the brain in the lung, the liver, and the gastrointestinal tract. The functional significance of extraneural CRH is unknown, but this localization makes it easier to understand how ectopic CRH-secreting tumors may arise. Human placenta has the highest concentration of CRH outside of the hypothalamus, and during the second and third trimesters of pregnancy the plasma levels of CRH rise.[264] These changes may contribute to the activation of the pituitary-adrenal axis during labor and of fetal pituitary-adrenal function.

PROLACTIN-REGULATORY FACTORS. ***Prolactin-Inhibiting Factor.*** In contrast to the secretion of other pituitary hormones, the secretion of PRL is *increased* in the absence of hypothalamic influences. This finding led to the idea of early researchers that the hypothalamus releases a PRL release–inhibitory factor. Indeed, extracts of whole hypothalamus inhibit PRL release in vitro.[265] This bioactivity was termed *prolactin-inhibiting factor* (PIF).[266-268] Dopamine, the most important PIF, is the secretory product of the tuberoinfundibular dopaminergic pathways and is present in hypophyseal–portal vessel blood in sufficient concentration to inhibit PRL release. γ-Aminobutyric acid (GABA), which is a constituent of hypothalamic extracts, is also an active PIF. However, all of the known PRL-inhibitory functions of the hypothalamus can be explained by dopamine alone, despite the presence of nondopamine PIF activity of hypothalamic extracts.

After administration of dopamine, levodopa (which is converted to dopamine in both peripheral tissues and the brain), or dopamine agonists such as bromocriptine, PRL levels drop sharply in normal individuals and in persons with hyperprolactinemia. TSH secretion is also inhibited by dopamine.

Dopamine suppresses virtually all aspects of PRL secretion.[267, 269, 270] It acts on the lactotrope via specific receptors to inhibit release and biosynthesis of PRL, to inhibit cell division and DNA synthesis, and to bring about the loss of stored PRL in granules by stimulating *crinophagy* (autodigestion of secretory product). Dopamine inhibits formation of cAMP (a stimulator of PRL secretion), synthesis of phosphoinositol, phospholipid turnover, and release of arachidonic acid. These actions are responsible for the therapeutic effect of dopamine agonists such as bromocriptine in hyperprolactinemic states, including prolactinomas.

Prolactin-Releasing Factors. The predominant effect of the hypothalamus on PRL secretion is to inhibit basal function. However, several stimuli bring about PRL release, not merely by disinhibition of PIF effects but by causing release of one or more PRFs.[271-273] Hypothalamic extracts contain several substances with PRF activity. The most important of the putative PRFs are TRH, AVP, VIP, oxytocin, PHI-27 (peptide-histidine-isoleucine-27), and the as-yet uncharacterized neurointermediate lobe factor.[272] As described earlier, administration of TRH stimulates PRL release with the same dose-response characteristics as stimulation of TSH release. TRH secretion into the hypophyseal-portal blood supply is increased by nipple stimulation in rats, and in some experiments the administration of anti-TRH antisera partially blocks suckling-induced PRL release. However, suckling does not release TSH in humans as would be expected if TRH was the mediator of PRL release.

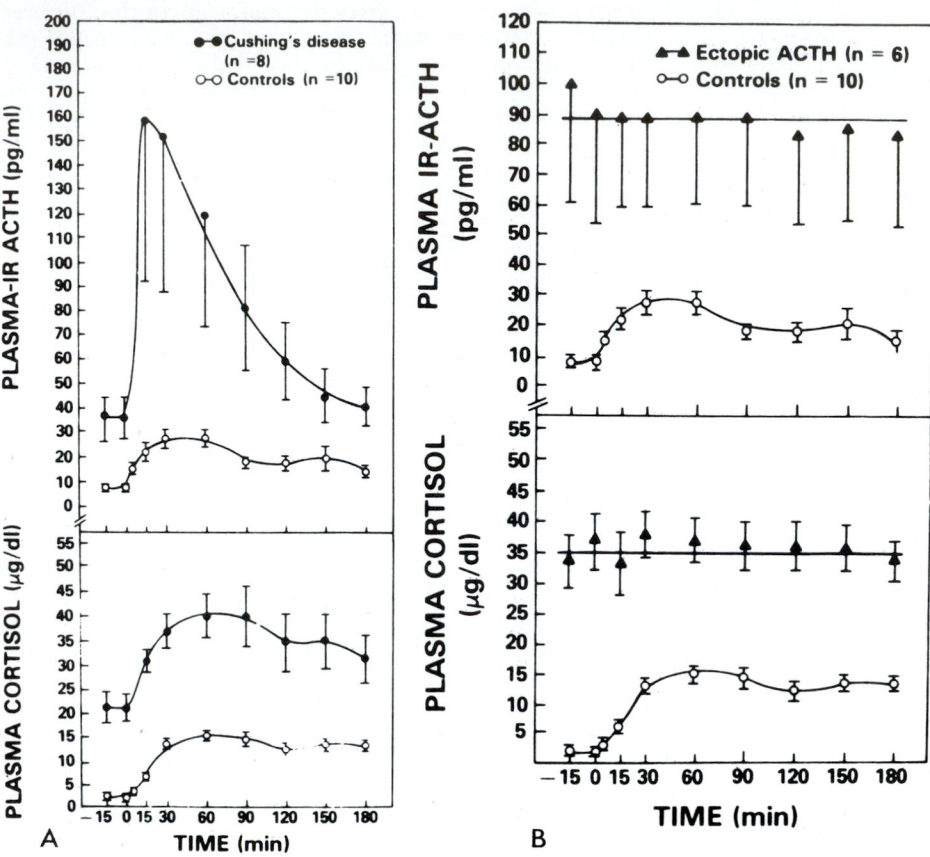

Figure 5–37. Plasma ACTH and cortisol responses to CRH in patients with Cushing disease *(left)* and hypercortisolism related to ectopic ACTH secretion *(right)*. Patients with Cushing disease show hyper-responsiveness to CRH; those with ectopic secretion show unchanged plasma ACTH levels. These data demonstrate the suppressive effect of ACTH-cortisol excess on pituitary responsiveness. Similar results are obtained in patients with adrenal adenoma. To convert ACTH values to picomoles per liter, multiply by 0.2202. To convert cortisol values to millimoles per liter, multiply by 27.59. (From Chrousos GP, Schulte HM, Oldfield EH, et al. The corticotropin-releasing factor stimulation test: an aid in the evaluation of patients with Cushing's syndrome. Reprinted, by permission of the New England Journal of Medicine, 310; 622–626, 1984.)

AVP also stimulates PRL release and cannot be excluded as a physiological PRF. It is present in hypophyseal-portal blood and is released during stress and shock, as is PRL.

VIP, when added directly to the pituitary, stimulates PRL secretion. Concentrations of VIP in hypophyseal-portal blood are sufficient to produce effects in vivo, and its release is stimulated by serotonin, an agent that increases PRL secretion. Moreover, anti-VIP antiserum given to rats blocks stress-induced PRL release and reduces the elevated PRL levels of nursing mothers. However, anatomical studies of the hypothalamus are not in accord with reports that VIP is present in hypophyseal-portal blood; VIP-containing nerve endings make only a minimal contribution to the neurons of the tuberoinfundibular system. Another candidate PRF is PHI.[274] This peptide releases PRL,[275] is colocalized with CRH in a population of paraventricular neurons, and is presumably released by the same stimuli that release ACTH, such as stress.[276] PHI has structural homology with VIP and is synthesized as part of the VIP prohormone. Suckling-induced PRL release (in the rat) is mediated by the neuro-intermediate lobe. Removal of this structure blocks suckling-induced PRL release, and exposure of the anterior pituitary to intermediate lobe extracts (devoid of VIP, AVP, and other known PRFs) stimulates PRL secretion.[272] The particular neuropeptides or neurotransmitters that mediate PRL release appear to be stimulus specific and anatomically distinct.[271-273]

MSH-REGULATORY FACTORS. MSH secretion is controlled by the nervous system. At one time it was postulated that this control is mediated by hypothalamic factors analogous to those that regulate other pituitary hormones. One peptide that was isolated from the hypothalamus, Pro-Leu-Gly-NH$_2$ (so-called MSH-inhibitory factor [MIF], an enzymatic degradation product of oxytocin), is a potent inhibitor of MSH secretion.[104, 105] However, MSH activity of the intermediate lobe in species such as the rat is attributable to α-

MSH and β-MSH, peptides that are encoded in POMC. Secretion of POMC-derived peptides by the intermediate lobe is tonically suppressed by a direct dopaminergic secretomotor nerve supply that arises in the arcuate nucleus of the hypothalamus, and there is no evidence of hypophyseal-portal control.

Although MIF is no longer considered to be a physiologically important MSH regulator, it does have many effects in the central nervous system.[277] Furthermore, because oxytocin has an extensive extrahypothalamic distribution, this factor may be a central neurotransmitter or neuromodulator. MSH itself is probably more important as a central neuropeptide than as a pituitary hormone. α-MSH is synthesized in the hypothalamus, and MSH receptors are widely distributed in the brain.[278] In addition to behavioral changes, α-MSH blocks central pyrogen-induced fever.[279]

REGULATION OF SECRETION OF TUBEROHYPOPHYSEAL NEURONS

As outlined in previous sections, the tuberohypophyseal neurons are the "final common pathway" of neural control of the anterior pituitary. This group of neurons is acted on by neurotransmitters; by the feedback effects of hormones secreted by target glands, such as the gonadal steroids, thyroid hormone, and cortisol; by pituitary peptide hormones (short-loop feedback control); and by neuropeptide modulators.

Secretion by the tuberoinfundibular neurons is influenced by many factors, including most neurotransmitters and neuropeptides. These substances interact within the hypothalamus and perhaps within the median eminence with circulating hormones and metabolic factors.

Few areas in biology have undergone such dramatic increases in knowledge as those dealing with identification of neurotransmitters, their anatomical distribution, molecular structure, distribution of receptors, mode of regulation, and mechanisms of action. Interest in this subject is enhanced by the relevance of neuropharmacology to understanding emotion, memory, and development of psychotropic drugs. Many studies of the effects of agonists and antagonists of the classic neurotransmitters on anterior pituitary function have been carried out, but many of the drugs used are not entirely specific, may act at more than one level in the neuroaxis, and may affect secretion of both excitatory and inhibitory hypophyseotropic hormones. Hence, studies that assess only changes in pituitary function are indirect indicators of the neurotransmitters that regulate secretion of the tuberoinfundibular system, the final common pathway from hypothalamus to pituitary.

Neurotransmitters fall into several classes, each with its own mode of biosynthesis, anatomical distribution, and regulatory system. The best understood are acetylcholine and the biogenic amines: dopamine, norepinephrine, serotonin, epinephrine, and histamine.[280-299] In addition, hypophyseotropic neurons are influenced by the excitatory amino neurotransmitters: glutamate (with all its subtypes), glycine,

TABLE 5–8. Summary of Function of Central Catecholaminergic Neurons and Sites of Action of Neuropharmacological Agents

Step 1:	Uptake of amino acids into aminergic neurons: tyrosine, precursor of dopamine, norepinephrine, epinephrine.
Drug:	No drug is known to interfere with tyrosine uptake.
Step 2:	Enzymatic synthesis.
	Tyrosine is hydroxylated by tyrosine hydroxylase to form L-dopa. L-Dopa is decarboxylated to form dopamine, which in turn is hydroxylated to form norepinephrine. Norepinephrine is methylated to form epinephrine.
Drug:	α-Methyltyrosine blocks L-dopa synthesis. Disulfiram (Antabuse) blocks dopamine conversion to norepinephrine.
Step 3:	Storage phase.
	Norepinephrine, dopamine, and epinephrine are stored in specific granules within nerve terminals.
Drug:	Reserpine blocks storage of norepinephrine, dopamine, and epinephrine.
Step 4:	Release of preformed granules.
	In response to neuronal depolarization, granules are extruded from nerve ending.
Drug:	Amphetamines may act, at least in part, on release of norepinephrine.
Step 5:	Interaction of catecholamine with receptor located on postsynaptic neuron.
	Extruded bioamine binds to specific receptors.
Drug:	Noradrenergic effects are duplicated by alpha-receptor agonist clonidine, beta-receptor agonist isoproterenol; alpha-receptors are blocked by phentolamine, beta-receptors by propranolol.
	Dopamine effects are duplicated by agonists apomorphine and bromocriptine and are blocked by antagonists phenothiazines and pimozide.
Step 6:	Reuptake process.
	After release of preformed hormone, free neurotransmitter in synaptic cleft that has not reacted with receptor is taken up into presynaptic nerve ending.
Drug:	Cocaine and tricyclic antidepressants make norepinephrine more available by blocking reuptake.
Step 7:	Degradation of neurotransmitter and dopamine.
	Norepinephrine bound to postsynaptic membranes or free in the presynaptic nerve ending is destroyed by the enzyme monoamine oxidase.
	The enzyme catechol O-methyltransferase is also responsible for inactivating these amines.
Drug:	Monoamine oxidase inhibitors (pargyline, isocarboxazid, tranylcypromine) make more neurotransmitter available to the postsynaptic cell.

Adapted from Cooper JR, Bloom FE, Roth RH. The Biochemical Basis of Neuropharmacology. 3rd ed. New York: Oxford University Press, 1978; and Martin JB, Reichlin S, eds. Clinical Neuroendocrinology. 2nd ed. Philadelphia: F. A. Davis, 1987.

TABLE 5–9. Neurotransmitters and Anterior Pituitary Secretion*†

	NE	DA	5-HT	ACh	H	GABA
ACTH‡	↑↓	↓→	↑	↑	↑	↓
TSH	↑	↓	↓	→	↑	—
LH-FSH	↑	↑↓	↓→	↑	↑	↑
GH	↑	↑	↑	→	→	↑
PRL	↑↓	↓	↑	↓↓	↑	↓↓

*The effects of various neurotransmitters are inferred from neuropharmacological studies using agonists, antagonists, and precursors. It must be *emphasized* that *there are many inconsistencies and contradictions in the literature,* which are due in part to species differences, previous functional status, lack of specificity of some drugs, and direct pituitary effects differing from hypothalamic effects.

†Symbols: ↑, increase; ↓, decrease; →, no change; —, not known. NE, norepinephrine; DA, dopamine; 5-HT, 5-hydroxytryptamine; ACh, acetylcholine; H, histamine; GABA, γ-aminobutyric acid.

‡ Central alpha-1—receptors activate CRH release.

Adapted from Müller EE, Nistico G, Scapagnini U, eds. Neurotransmitters and Anterior Pituitary Function. New York: Academic, 1977; and Weiner RI, Ganong WF. Role of brain monoamines and histamine in regulation of anterior pituitary secretion. Physiol Rev 1978; 58:905–976.

aspartic acid, taurine, and the inhibitory amino acid GABA. Many neuropeptides (in mammalian brain, 50 or more), several cytokines (interleukin 1 [IL 1], interleukin 2, and interleukin 6), and neurotrophic factors influence tuberoinfundibular neurons. Indeed, this enormously rich repertoire of regulatory factors enables the pituitary to respond to homeostatic and regulatory needs. The function of central catecholaminergic neurons and sites of action of some standard neuropharmacological agents are summarized in Table 5–8, and the overall effects of these agents on pituitary function are summarized in Table 5–9.

Dopaminergic Pathways

Central dopamine-secreting neural pathways make up a complex system that carries on diverse functions. The dopamine-containing fibers concerned with pituitary regulation arise chiefly in the arcuate nucleus of the hypothalamus (Fig. 5–38). From this nucleus, fibers project to the median eminence (tuberoinfundibular pathway) and, in species with a defined intermediate lobe, into this structure as well (tuberohypophyseal pathway). The arcuate nuclear cells make up only a small fraction of the central dopaminergic pathways. Most of the neurons that synthesize dopamine arise in the midbrain and project to the forebrain. The neurons projecting to the basal ganglia (nigrostriatal) are involved in extrapyramidal control; deficits in this system give rise to Parkinson disease. Dopaminergic fibers are also directed to various parts of the cerebral cortex and limbic system (mesolimbic-cortical pathways); dysfunction of these fibers has been postulated to be a cause of schizophrenia.

Although all of these groups of neurons synthesize dopamine by identical mechanisms, they are not identical functionally.[282, 288, 289] Alterations in pituitary function related to changes in dopamine secretion by tuberoinfundibular neurons do not necessarily reflect alterations in the other central dopaminergic systems. For example, tuberoinfundibular neurons (in contrast to the other dopaminergic neurons) do not possess dopamine receptors but do have PRL receptors. Tuberoinfundibular neurons are components of the short-loop feedback control of PRL secretion by PRL.[288, 289] Dopamine agonist and antagonist drugs thus act directly on the mesolimbic and nigrostriatal systems and on the pituitary, but not on the tuberoinfundibular system. These differences deserve emphasis because of the interest in the use of neuroendocrine techniques for the study of psychiatric disease.[289]

Noradrenergic Pathways

Almost all noradrenergic cells originate from nuclei in the midbrain locus coeruleus and adjacent regions and project to the forebrain (including the cerebral cortex), the hypothalamus, the limbic system, the brain stem, and the spinal cord (see Fig. 5–38).[290–292] The principal components that regulate the anterior pituitary project either to the median eminence (where they come into contact with nerve endings of the tuberoinfundibular system) or to the tuberoinfundibular cells. The other components of central noradrenergic systems play essential roles in visceral homeostasis and adaptive behaviors, including regulation of sleep, appetite, eating, blood pressure, and spontaneous physical activity. The central noradrenergic system is the site of action of amphetamines and antidepressant drugs. Deficiency in this system has been implicated in the pathogenesis of depression. Several of the pathways are believed to be activated selectively by physiological stimuli, but the diffuseness of the central noradrenergic pathways makes it difficult to localize the sites of such functions.

Central Adrenergic Pathways

Of the central pathways concerned with biogenic amines, those in which epinephrine is a neurotransmitter are among the least plentiful.[293] Like the noradrenergic system, cell bodies of origin in the midbrain have an extensive distribution, including the hypothalamus and the median eminence. Certain aspects of GH secretion depend on this neurotransmitter.[287]

Central Serotoninergic Pathways

Almost all the neurons that synthesize serotonin (5-hydroxytryptamine, 5-HT) originate from two nuclei in the midbrain, the raphe nuclei (see Fig. 5–38).[291, 292, 294, 295] From these nuclei, fibers ascend through several pathways to innervate virtually all parts of the forebrain and diencephalon. Serotoninergic fibers involved in pituitary control terminate in several sites of the hypothalamus, including the paraventricular nucleus, the median eminence, and the lumen of the third ventricle itself. Raphe nuclei also project downward into the brain stem and spinal cord.[295] A proportion of these cells cocontain peptide neurotransmitters as well as serotonin. For example, many downstream projecting fibers contain both TRH and substance P and form extensive

projections to the intermediolateral column of the spinal cord (the site of origin of the sympathetic nerves) and to the motor horn cells of the ventral spinal cord. Some serotoninergic fibers projecting to the forebrain contain both substance P and enkephalin.[295]

Central Cholinergic Pathways

Acetylcholine-responsive cells, containing both muscarinic and nicotinic receptors, are found throughout the brain, including the hypothalamus.[296] Certain pituitary secretions, especially AVP, ACTH, and GH, are under cholinergic control. However, the location of the bodies of the cholinergic cells that control pituitary secretion is not known with certainty. One central cholinergic pathway arises in the nucleus basalis of the forebrain and is distributed to the hippocampus. Loss of these neurons is a hallmark of Alzheimer disease. Certain groups of cells in the hippocampus are particularly vulnerable to aging, to neurotoxins, and to the damaging effects of glucocorticoids.[297]

Amino Acid Neurotransmitters

Excitatory amino acids (glutamate, aspartate, glycine) and the inhibitory GABA are found in hypothalamic neurons and can modify tuberohypophyseal function.[280, 298–300] Glutamate receptor subtypes in the hypothalamus have been well characterized,[280, 299] and the damaging effects of glutamate administration to immature rodents and primates have been demonstrated.[300] Early postnatal exposure to glutamate produces a characteristic pattern of neuronal destruction in the hypothalamus. Most of the cells of the medial basal hypothalamus are destroyed, which leads to hypothalamic hyperphagia, loss of spontaneous ovulation, and impaired secretion of GH. Glutamate poisons neurons by causing hyperpolarization, which leads in turn to excessive intracellular concentrations of calcium.

GABA appears to play two different roles. In tuberohypophyseal neurons it tonically inhibits neuronal function. In addition, GABA secreted into the hypophyseal-portal blood may serve as a PRF.

Central Peptidergic Pathways Involved in Pituitary Regulation

The functional relevance of many of the neuropeptides as controllers of the secretion of the tuberoinfundibular

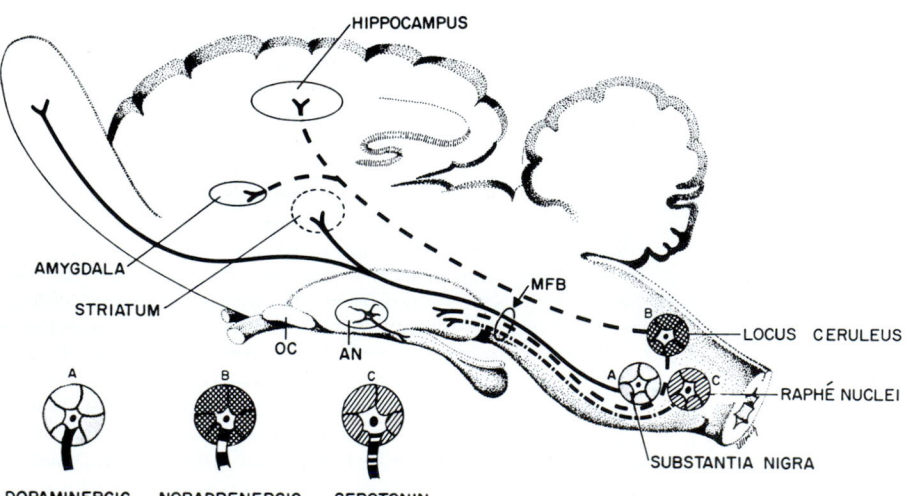

Figure 5–38. Simplified diagram showing the major distribution of the ascending monoaminergic pathways in mammalian brain. The principal source of all three major biogenic amines in the brain is nuclei in the brain stem: the locus coeruleus, the source of most noradrenergic fibers; the raphe nucleus, the source of most serotoninergic fibers; and the substantia nigra, the source of most dopaminergic fibers. An important dopaminergic pathway arises in the arcuate nucleus of the hypothalamus and is the principal source of dopamine to the hypophyseal circulation. Epinephrinergic fibers arise from the region of the locus coeruleus in a pattern similar to that of norepinephrine. OC, optic chiasm; AN, arcuate nucleus; MFB, medial forebrain bundle. (From Martin JB, Reichlin S, Brown GM. Hypothalamic control of anterior pituitary secretion. In: Clinical Neuroendocrinology. Philadelphia: F. A. Davis, 1977: 13–44.)

TABLE 5–10. Effects of Neuropeptides on Pituitary Hormone Release

Peptide	ACTH	PRL	GH	TSH	FSH	LH
Effects Mediated Through Central Nervous System						
Cholecystokinin	+	+	+	−	0	−
Gastrin		−	+	−	0	−
VIP		+	+	0	0	+
Substance P		?+	+	0	0	+
Neurotensin		−	+	0	0	−
Opioids	+	+	+	−	−	−
Bradykinin		−	0	0	−	0
Angiotensin II	+	−	−	0	−	0
Bombesin		+	+			
Somatostatin		0	+	−	−	−
Vasotocin		−		−		0
Inhibin					−	0
Galanin			+			
Neuropeptide Y						−
CRH			+		−	−
Effects Mediated Directly at Pituitary Level						
Cholecystokinin		0	0	0	0	0
Gastrin		0	0	−	0	0
VIP		+	0	0	0	0
Substance P		+	0	0	0	0
Neurotensin		+	0	+	0	0
Opioids		0	0	0	0	0
Bradykinin		0	?−	0	?−	0
Angiotensin II		+	+	+	0	+
Bombesin		0	0			
Vasotocin		+			+	+
Inhibin					−	0
Galanin			+			
Neuropeptide Y					+	+

Adapted from McCann SM. The role of several hypothalamic peptides in the control of anterior pituitary hormone secretion. In: Müller EE, MacLeod RM, eds. Neuroendocrine Perspectives. Vol 1. New York: Elsevier Biomedical, 1982: 1–22.

neurons is under active study.[301, 302] The most intensively investigated are the endogenous opioid peptides (discussed later). The overall effects of the various classes of neurotransmitters and other hypothalamic regulators on anterior pituitary regulation are summarized in Tables 5–8 and 5–9. Many of the findings are not uniform in all studies, for all species, and under all conditions. Direct effects of some neuropeptides may be exerted at the level of the pituitary, as well as in the hypothalamus (Table 5–10).

NEUROENDOCRINE CONTROL OF INDIVIDUAL PITUITARY HORMONES

General Considerations: Feedback Concepts in Neuroendocrinology

For each pituitary control system, one can identify hormonal feedback effects exerted on the pituitary and the hypothalamus and interactions with behavioral and homeostatic functions. Servoengineering concepts and formulations have been applied to the description of endocrine control systems. A simplified account of feedback control is presented in this section as it relates to endocrine regulation.

Most hormonal systems form part of a feedback loop in which the controlled variable (generally the blood hormone level or some effect of the hormone) determines the rate of secretion of the hormone.[303–305] These systems are generally negative feedback control systems, but positive feedback control does occur. All of the negative and positive feedback systems in which the pituitary is involved have nervous system inputs that either alter the set point of the feedback control system or introduce an open-loop element of control.

Some terms used in feedback control models are defined here (as adapted from DiStefano and colleagues[303]):

A *system* is a set of components related in such a way as to act as a unit.

A *control system* is arranged so as to regulate itself or another system.

An *input* is the stimulus applied to a control system from a source outside the system so as to produce a specified response from the control system.

An *output* is the actual response of a control system.

A *closed-loop control system* is one in which the control action depends on (is a function of) output.

A *negative feedback system* is a closed-loop control system in which the output accelerates the control action.

All endocrine negative feedback systems have a controlled variable, i.e., the hormone or substance that the system is designed to maintain. For example, thyroid hormone levels are the controlled variable of the pituitary-thyroid axis, the blood calcium level is the controlled variable of the parathyroid-calcitonin-skeletal axis, and the blood glucose level is one of the controlled variables of the pancreas-liver axis.

In engineering formulations of feedback, three elements of "executive" control of the controlled variable can be identified: a sensing element, which detects the concentration of the controlled variable; a reference input, which defines the proper control levels; and an error signal. The error signal is a function of the difference between what the sensor senses and what the reference is. The error signal determines the output of the system. The reference input can be considered the set point of the system. An example of these terms can be found in a description of the common household thermostat. The sensor is a thermometer that detects the actual room temperature. The reference input is the preferred temperature setting of the thermostat. When the temperature sensed by the detector is different from the reference input, the furnace is turned either off or on until the error signal is minimized. In simple feedback applications, the error signal is either off or on; in more complex systems the error signal might determine output in a more sophisticated way. For example, a large error signal might call for a large initial burst of heat, and a small error signal might call for a small burst of heat; thus the rate of heating may be programmed as a complex function.

Hormonal feedback control systems resemble engineering analogues in that the concentration of the hormone in the blood (or some function of the hormone) regulates the output of the controlling gland. Hormonal feedback control systems differ from engineering systems in that the sensor element and the reference input element are not readily distinguishable. Rather than having a reference input signal with which the controlled variable is compared (thus providing an error signal to determine gland output), the controlled variable has a more or less direct regulatory influence on the secretory process, such as regulation of the rate of an enzyme activity. The set point of the controlled variable is thus determined by a complex cascade beginning with the kinetics of binding to a receptor, and the kinetics of successive intermediate messengers. Sophisticated models incorporating control elements, compartmental analysis, and hormone production and clearance rates have been developed for many systems. Examples of classic feedback formulations that have been developed are for the hypothalamic-pituitary-thyroid and hypothalamic-pituitary-adrenal axes.[303]

Endocrine Rhythms

Virtually all organized functions of living animals (regardless of their position on the evolutionary scale) are subject to periodic or cyclic changes, many of which are influenced mainly by the nervous system.[306-319] Some periodic changes are free-running, i.e., they are brought about by an intrinsic mechanism within the organism independent of the environment. Some free-running rhythms can be coordinated (entrained) by external signals (cues), such as light-dark changes, cycles of the lunar periods, or the ratio of the length of day to the length of night. External signals of this type are termed *zeitgebers* (time givers); they do not bring about the rhythm but rather provide the synchronizing time cue. Many endogenous rhythms have a period of approximately 24 h and therefore are called *circadian* (about a day). Rhythms that occur more frequently than once a day are referred to as *ultradian* rhythms. Some periodic phenomena have a longer period, as in the approximately 28-d human menstrual cycle; the breeding pattern of many animals is seasonal (about a year), and some plants and animals have growth cycles of more than a year.

Circadian rhythms are characteristic of most endocrine functions. With respect to the human pituitary gland, the secretion of GH and PRL is maximal shortly after an individual has gone to sleep, and that of cortisol is maximal between 2 and 4 AM. TSH secretion is lowest in the morning between 9 AM and 12 noon and is maximal between 8 PM and midnight. Gonadotropin secretion in developing adolescents is maximal at night.[317]

Superimposed on the circadian cycle are ultradian bursts of hormone secretion. Gonadotropin secretion during adolescence is characterized by rapid high-amplitude pulsations, especially at night, whereas in sexually mature individuals, episodes of secretion are lower in amplitude and occur throughout the 24 h.[317] PRL, GH, and ACTH[318] are also secreted in brief, fairly regular pulses. The short-term fluctuations in hormonal secretion have important functional significance. In the case of gonadotropins, the normal endogenous rhythm of pituitary secretion reflects the pulsatile release of LHRH. The period of approximately 90 min between the peak of pulses corresponds to the optimal timing to induce maximal pituitary stimulation. Episodic secretion of GH also enhances its biopotency. On the basis of the finding that nocturnal hypersecretion of PRL persists in lactating women, it has been proposed that circadian PRL rhythms evolved to provide nocturnal secretion of PRL in the absence of nocturnal suckling.[320] That hormonal cycles have persisted throughout the evolutionary scale argues that they serve an important function, but for most rhythms the teleological implications are not clear.

Most homeostatic activities are also rhythmical, including body temperature, water balance, and blood volume.

From a practical point of view it is important to know about these rhythms; adequate assessment of endocrine function must take into account the variability of hormone levels in the blood, and appropriately obtained samples at different times of day or night may provide useful dynamic indicators of hypothalamic-pituitary function. For example, loss of diurnal rhythm of GH secretion may be an early sign of hypothalamic dysfunction. Furthermore, the optimal timing for administration of glucocorticoids to suppress ACTH secretion (as in therapy for congenital adrenal hyperplasia) must take into account the varying suppressibility of the pituitary at different times of the day.

All endocrine rhythms are regulated by the brain. Best understood of the neural structures responsible for circadian rhythms in higher vertebrates is the suprachiasmatic (SC) nucleus, a paired structure located in the anterior hypothalamus just above the optic chiasm (Fig. 5–39).[306, 308, 309, 311] This nucleus is organized to permit reciprocal neuron-neuron interactions through direct synaptic contacts. It possesses

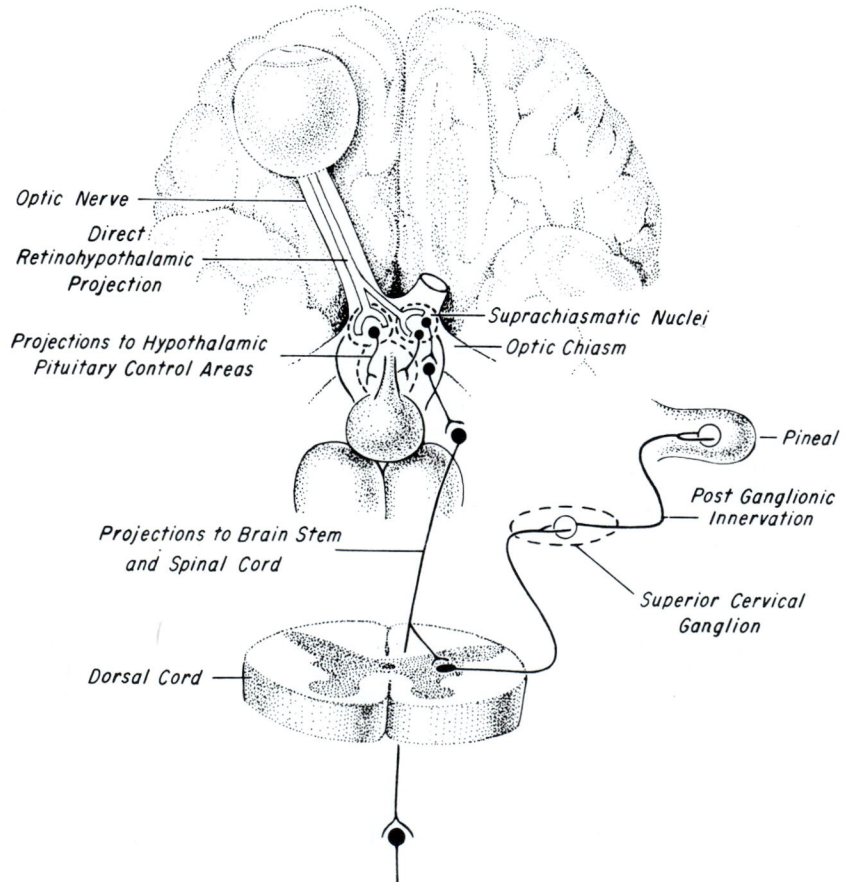

Figure 5–39. Schematic diagram of neural structures regulating circadian hormone rhythms. The SC nucleus, a paired nucleus located in the hypothalamus, generates a spontaneous rhythm roughly 24 h long that modifies anterior pituitary function through its projections to the hypothalamus and alters pineal function through its projection to the sympathetic nervous system. Sympathetic nerves to the pineal regulate secretion of pineal hormones. Endogenous rhythms are entrained to the light-dark cycle by stimuli that reach the SC from the eye by way of a direct retinohypothalamic projection. Light cycles thus act as a zeitgeber (time giver). (Adapted from Moore RY. Central neural control of circadian rhythms. In: Ganong WF, Martini L, eds. Frontiers in Neuroendocrinology. Vol 5. New York: Raven, 1978: 185–206.)

Optic Nerve

Direct Retinohypothalamic Projection

Projections to Hypothalamic Pituitary Control Areas

Suprachiasmatic Nuclei

Optic Chiasm

Pineal

Post Ganglionic Innervation

Projections to Brain Stem and Spinal Cord

Superior Cervical Ganglion

Dorsal Cord

intrinsic rhythmicity, even in vitro, and receives neuronal input from many parts of the brain and from a direct, nonvisual projection from the retina. This retinohypothalamic pathway is the route by which the nucleus is cued by light-dark changes.[306, 308] The SC nucleus is especially rich in cells and nerve terminals that contain neuropeptides, including somatostatin, VIP, neuropeptide Y, and neurotensin. Circadian rhythms are peptide regulated. For example, microinjections of neuropeptide Y into the SC nucleus reset the timing cycle of some circadian rhythms in hamsters.[312] The SC nucleus also responds to the secretion of the pineal gland because it has a uniquely rich concentration of melatonin receptors.[321] It has been proposed that maternal secretion of melatonin, which is the principal hormone of the pineal, could influence the development of circadian rhythms in the fetus. For example, fetal rats display light-driven changes in metabolism of the SC nucleus, and fetal sheep show a light-driven circadian rhythm in PRL secretion.[310]

Dramatic changes in metabolic and secretory activities accompany circadian rhythms in the SC nucleus, such as increased uptake of 2-deoxyglucose and increased concentration of VIP.[309] This nucleus projects to the pineal gland by way of the autonomic nervous system (see later under The Pineal Gland) and regulates its activity. However, most, but not all, biological rhythms that are controlled by the brain are mediated by mechanisms independent of the pineal secretions.

In addition to determining patterns of pituitary secretion, the circadian "pacemaker" influences many homeostatic and activity levels. In humans the alteration of sleep that is brought about by jet lag and by shift work has profound effects on the sense of well-being and on efficiency and may be a factor in the pathogenesis of seasonal affective disorder.

Although it had been thought (on the basis of light-induced changes in melatonin secretion) that the human circadian oscillator was responsive only to intense illumination,[322] normal illumination also determines the time setting of the pacemaker.[323] In humans, triazolam, a short-acting benzodiazepine, can shift the pacemaker.[324]

Thyrotropin Regulation

The secretion of TSH is regulated by two interacting elements: negative feedback by thyroid hormone and open-loop neural control by hypothalamic hypophyseotropic factors (see Fig. 5–38). TSH secretion is also modified by other hormones, particularly estrogens and glucocorticoids, and may be influenced by GH. Aspects of the pituitary-thyroid axis are also considered in Chapter 8. Neuroendocrine mechanisms are emphasized in this chapter.[325–333]

PITUITARY-THYROID AXIS. As early as 1851, Nièpce noted that the pituitaries from cretins that were seen at autopsy were grossly enlarged; the contemporary clinician can demonstrate enlargement of the sella turcica in patients with hypothyroidism of long-standing.[325]

The "pituitary-thyroid axis," as it was first christened by Salter, is a typical example of a negative feedback system. Hoskins described the system in 1949 as follows (see ref. 325):

When the titer of circulating thyroxine rises, the anterior pituitary is selectively inhibited and the discharge of thyrotropin is thereby decreased. Contrariwise, episodic or persistent thyroxine deficiency, if sufficient in degree, results in augmented thyrotropin production with resulting tendency for the production of more thyroid hormone.

This concept, supplemented by more recent views about neural control and the tissue-effective form of the circulating thyroid hormone, is a fundamental principle of endocrinology.

In the context of a feedback system the thyroid hormone level in blood or the concentration of its unbound fraction can be looked on as the controlled variable. The set point of pituitary-thyroid function is the normal resting level of plasma thyroid hormone. Maintenance of this level requires a specific concentration of TSH. Secretion of TSH is inversely regulated by the level of thyroid hormone, so that deviations from the set point of control lead to appropriately graded changes in the rate of TSH secretion (Fig. 5–40). Additional factors determine the rate of TSH secretion required to maintain a given level of thyroid hormone. These factors include the rate of peripheral degradation of both TSH and thyroid hormone and the conversion of T_4 to T_3. Disappearance times for both TSH and thyroid hormones are affected by changes in peripheral tissue metabolic activity. Peripheral metabolic factors determine the rate of TRH degradation.

Feedback control by thyroid hormone at the pituitary level is remarkably precise. Small doses of T_3 and T_4, administered daily for 3 to 4 wk to normal individuals in amounts insufficient to raise plasma thyroid hormone levels significantly, nevertheless inhibit the TSH response to TRH.[334] As a complementary finding, barely detectable decreases in plasma thyroid hormone levels produced by administration of sodium iodide are sufficient to sensitize the pituitary to TRH.[335] These results indicate that the fine adjustment of TSH secretion can be mediated at the pituitary level by the feedback effect of the thyroid hormones. Effects of TRH are almost immediate; increases in plasma TSH

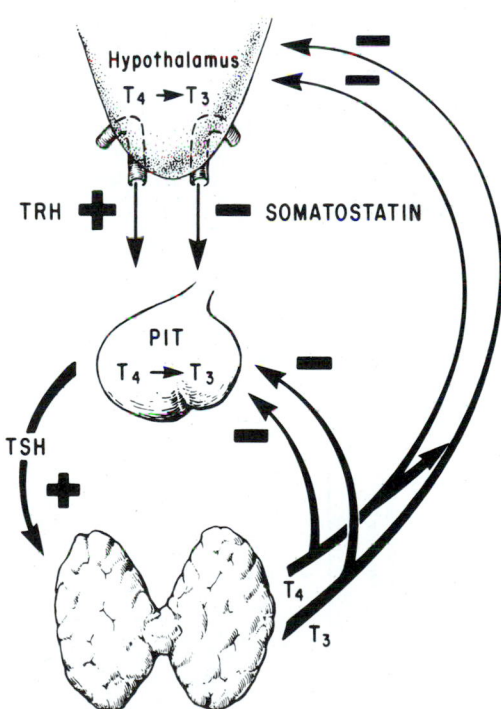

HYPOTHALAMIC – PITUITARY – THYROID AXIS

Figure 5–40. TSH from the pituitary stimulates the secretion of both T_4 and T_3. These act at the pituitary level to control secretion of TSH by a negative feedback mechanism. In addition, T_4 is degraded to the much more potent T_3 within the pituitary by a monoiodinase. Secretion of TSH is stimulated by TRH from the hypothalamus and inhibited by somatostatin and to a lesser extent by dopamine. Hypothalamic factors thus interact at the pituitary level to determine the secretion rate. Thyroid hormone acts at the hypothalamus to stimulate secretion of somatostatin (this stimulating effect acts as a negative signal to the pituitary). The effect of thyroid hormones on secretion of TRH has not been determined precisely. Finally, within the hypothalamus, T_4 is also degraded to T_3, and this degradation may play a role in feedback control.

levels are detectable within 1 or 2 min after intravenous administration of TRH in animals and in humans. On the other hand, inhibition of TSH secretion after T_4 and T_3 administration shows a lag period of several hours. The cellular and molecular bases of thyroid hormone regulation of the pituitary (and brain) are considered later.

NEURAL CONTROL OF PITUITARY-THYROID FUNCTION. The nervous system plays a major role in the regulation of the pituitary-thyroid axis. In situations in which the pituitary is deprived of input from the median eminence, TSH secretion is markedly reduced. This situation occurs after section of the pituitary stalk, after transplantation of the pituitary to a remote site, after the production of lesions of the "thyrotropic area" of the hypothalamus, and in pituitary cells in culture.

Although basal secretion of TSH is reduced when the pituitary is deprived of hypothalamic input, appropriate secretory responses are elicited by alterations in thyroid hormone concentration. For example, in response to thyroidectomy animals with lesions of the thyrotropic area show increased TSH levels but at a reduced level. Thyroid hormone administration to such animals is followed by inhibition of TSH secretion (Fig. 5–41).

The hypothalamus functions in pituitary-thyroid regulation to determine the set point of feedback control around which the usual feedback regulatory responses are elicited. This view was originally based on the observation that lesions of the thyrotropic area lower the set point and make the pituitary more sensitive to inhibition by thyroid hormone. With the demonstration that constant high doses of TRH can raise TSH and thyroid hormones (T_4 and T_3) levels for prolonged periods (in humans), it is now apparent that TRH can determine the set point over the full range of hormone levels from low to high.[336]

Although secretion of the hypothalamic factors determines the set point of feedback control of pituitary TSH secretion in a classic negative loop, hypothalamic factors can also influence TSH secretion by an open-loop mechanism. For example, in experimental animals and in human newborns, exposure to cold causes a sharp increase in TSH release[337, 338] because of TRH hypersecretion. This means that TRH has "broken through" the negative feedback control system or has changed the set point of control. However, TRH cannot overcome thyroid hormone–induced inhibition if thyroid hormone levels are sufficiently elevated, as is the case, for example, in Graves disease.

Hypothalamic regulation of TSH secretion is also mediated by somatostatin, which inhibits TSH secretion (see Fig. 5–40). The importance of somatostatin has been shown in rats by immunoneutralization studies. Antisomatostatin increases basal TSH levels and potentiates the response to stimuli that normally induce TSH release, such as cold exposure and TRH administration.[339, 340] Thyroid hormone also inhibits the release of somatostatin, a finding that suggests a coordinated, reciprocal regulation by thyroxine of the two major hypothalamic regulatory peptides.[341] GH also regulates somatostatin synthesis[342] and thereby influences TSH secretion indirectly. However, the importance of somatostatin in regulation of TSH secretion in humans is not known.

Dopamine also inhibits TSH release. Its importance has been shown in humans by administration of drugs that block pituitary dopamine receptors. One such drug, domperidone, stimulates TSH secretion, but the magnitude of the response is small.[328]

The secretion of TSH is influenced by central neurotransmitters acting on the TRH and somatostatinergic neurons.[280, 283, 287, 326–329, 343] Most data suggest that beta-adrenergic stimuli enhance TSH release (presumably by stimulating TRH secretion) and that serotoninergic stimuli inhibit TSH secretion, but contrary data can be cited to indicate that serotonin stimulates TSH release.[343] The central opioid pathways appear to inhibit TSH secretion by inhibiting TRH release.[344]

CELLULAR AND MOLECULAR BASIS OF THYROID HORMONE ACTION. The mechanism of thyroid hormone control of the hypothalamus and the anterior pituitary has been clarified by the elucidation of the role of conversion of T_4

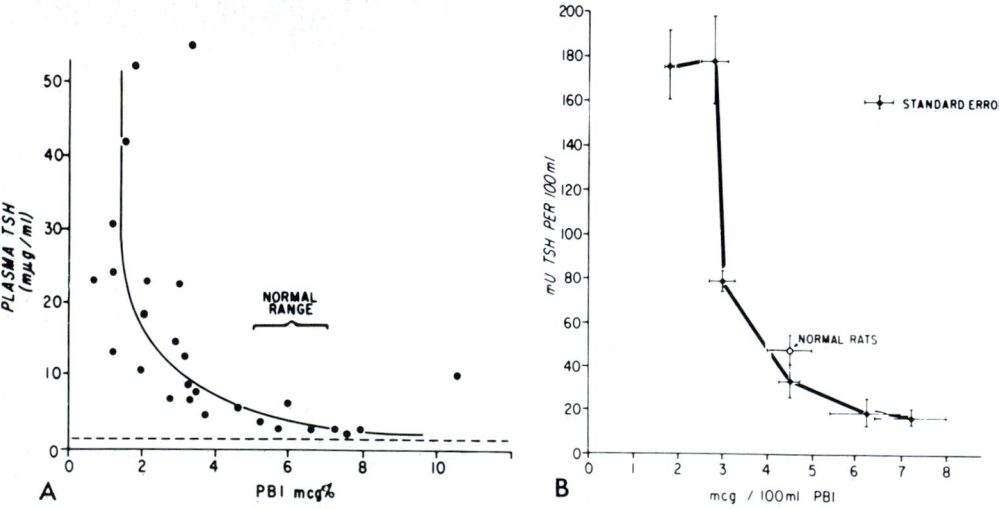

Figure 5–41. The relationship between plasma TSH levels and thyroid hormone as determined by plasma protein-bound iodine (PBI) measurements in humans and rats. These curves illustrate in the human (A) and the rat (B) that plasma TSH levels are a curvilinear function of plasma thyroid hormone level. Human studies were carried out by giving myxedematous patients successive increments of thyroxine at approximately 10-d intervals. Each point represents simultaneous measurements of plasma PBI and plasma TSH at various times in the six patients studied. The rat studies were done by treating thyroidectomized animals with various doses of T_4 for 2 wk before assay of plasma TSH and plasma PBI. These curves illustrate that the secretion of TSH is regulated over the entire range of thyroid hormone levels. At the normal set point for T_4, the small changes above and below the control level are followed by appropriate increases or decreases in plasma TSH. (A from S Reichlin, RD Utiger. Regulation of the pituitary thyroid axis in man: relationship of TSH concentration to concentration of free and total thyroxine in plasma, J Clin Endocrinol Metab 27, 251–255, 1967, © by The Endocrine Society. B from Reichlin S, Martin JB, Boshans RL, et al. Measurement of TSH in plasma and pituitary of the rat by a radioimmunoassay utilizing bovine TSH: effect of thyroidectomy or thyroxine administration on plasma TSH levels. Endocrinology 87, 1022–1031, 1970, © by The Endocrine Society.)

to T_3,[345] of the structure of the gene that encodes mammalian TRH,[148, 149, 332, 333] and of the structures of the thyroid receptors and their relationship to the oncogene c-*erb* A.[346–349] (See also Chapters 3 and 8.) Thyroid hormone regulates both the hypothalamus and the pituitary.

Two classes of thyroid hormone receptors encoded by different genes are termed the alpha and beta subtypes.[348] The type designated beta (for rat) is distributed in the anterior pituitary (the only type found in this structure[348]) and in the parvicellular component of the paraventricular nucleus of the hypothalamus where TRH-synthesizing neurons (and many other hypophyseotropic neurons) are found.[347] T_3 binds to its receptor and causes an altered configuration of the receptor, which then enables it to bind to one or more well-defined regulatory sequences (hormone response elements) in cellular genes. These hormone response elements, in turn, modify the rate of gene transcription. In the pituitary, binding of T_3-receptor complexes to genetic control elements alters the synthesis and processing of the constituent alpha and beta units of TSH.[350] The direct effect of T_3 on the pituitary is well established on the basis of physiological[325] and binding studies,[346] but the question of whether thyroid hormone directly affects the hypothalamus has been resolved only by showing inhibitory changes in levels of TRH mRNA and TRH prohormone after administration of T_3 to hypothyroid animals[332] and by direct introduction of T_3 into the hypothalamus[333] (Fig. 5–42).

BRAIN REGIONS INVOLVED IN TSH REGULATION AND THEIR HOMEOSTATIC FUNCTIONS. Individual tuberoinfundibular neuron populations that secrete TRH, somatostatin, and dopamine have been localized in the hypothalamus by immunohistochemical techniques (see Fig. 5–20), which clarified earlier studies that utilized ablation and electric stimulation. The principal TRH-secreting cells are in the paraventricular nucleus, and the principal somatostatin-secreting cells are in the anterior periventricular area and the paraventricular nucleus. The principal dopamine-secreting cells arise in the arcuate nucleus.

Other regions of the brain influence TSH secretion. The supraoptic area is the site of temperature-sensitive neurons that mediate body temperature and body heat homeostasis. Local cooling of the preoptic area in experimental animals mobilizes heat defense mechanisms: shivering, catecholamine discharge from the adrenal medulla and sympathetic nervous system, peripheral vasoconstriction, increased eating (presumably to provide additional calories for heat production), and TSH release.[351] Local heating of this region inhibits heat conservation mechanisms and suppresses TSH release. The increased secretion of TSH in animals after exposure to a cold environment is brought about by release of TRH[337] secondary to signals from temperature receptors in the skin. The preoptic region integrates cold signals received from the skin with brain temperature. TRH, acting as a central neurotransmitter in the preoptic region, increases body temperature.[351] Central TRH pathways that arise in the midbrain raphe nuclei and project downstream to the spinal cord have as one of their major targets the cells of origin of the sympathetic nervous system in the intermediolateral column, which regulates catecholamine secretion. Catecholamines are important determinants of heat production, especially in animals with brown fat such as the rat. From a teleological viewpoint, TRH thus appears to influence body heat homeostasis at three levels: as a neurohormone that releases TSH and thereby activates the thyroid gland, as a central temperature-regulating neurotransmitter in the hypothalamus, and as a central transmitter in the brain stem and the spinal cord that regulates sympathetic nerve activity.

It has been difficult to document in humans that body temperature and environmental temperature regulate TSH secretion. For example, exposure to cold ambient temperature or central hypothalamic cooling by means of ice ingestion does not modify pituitary-thyroid function in adults.[352] On the other hand, exposure of infants to cold at the time of delivery brings about a sharp increase in blood TSH level, which may be due in part to alterations in the turnover and degradation of the thyroid hormones induced by delivery.[353] Blood thyroid hormone levels are reportedly higher in the winter than in the summer in individuals in cold climates,[354] but not in other populations.[338] Most studies with humans indicate that the sympathetic nervous system and shivering are more important in temperature regulation than is the thyroid response.[338]

Two other aspects of TSH secretion undoubtedly reflect altered neuronal control of the tuberoinfundibular cells that secrete TSH and somatostatin: circadian rhythms of TSH secretion and the response to stress. Because circadian rhythms are determined by the function of the SC nucleus, it is likely that this region, which is known to project axons to the hypothalamus, modulates secretion of TRH. The 24-h plasma TSH profile in humans is characterized by a circadian periodicity, with a maximum between 9 PM and 5:30 AM and a minimum between 4 PM and 7 PM.[355] Superimposed on the circadian pattern are smaller TSH peaks occurring every 2 to 4 h. These ultradian rhythms have been attributed to TRH release, but the role of somatostatin (which is released in an ultradian fashion in the rat) is unknown.

Stress is also an important regulator of TSH secretion.[325, 329, 355–357] Stressful stimuli in animals inhibit the release of both TSH and GH. In the rat this effect is due at least in part to release of somatostatin,[358] possibly the consequence of central CRH mobilization.[359, 360] In humans, severe physical stress also probably inhibits TSH release, as indicated by the finding that in the euthyroid sick syndrome low T_3 and T_4 levels are not accompanied by compensatory elevated TSH levels, as would be predicted from studies of nonstressed individuals.[356, 357]

The molecular basis of infection- or inflammation-induced TSH suppression is now reasonably well established (see also later under Neuroimmunomodulation). Sterile abscesses or the injection of IL 1β (endogenous pyrogen, a secretory peptide of activated lymphocytes) leads to inhibition of TSH secretion,[361] and IL 1β stimulates the secretion of somatostatin.[362] Tumor necrosis factor, which is a cytokine released during inflammation, inhibits TSH secretion directly.[363] The possibility of autocrine and paracrine regulation of TSH also exists because the pituitary contains interleukin 1β, some of which is localized in thyrotropes.[364] It is likely, therefore, that the TSH inhibition in animal models of the sick euthyroid syndrome are due to cytokine-induced changes in hypothalamic and pituitary function. Whether this is true for human disease is not known. IL 1β also stimulates CRH release, which may be the basis of infection-induced ACTH discharge.[365]

Transient elevation of T_4 levels occurs in some patients who are admitted to psychiatric hospitals,[329] which suggests that psychological factors act in general through the limbic system, and a well-defined system of neurons connects the hypothalamus to the rest of the limbic system.[366]

Several other brain regions have been implicated in the regulation of thyroid function, including the pineal, which is reported to inhibit thyroid function by some[367] but not all[368] workers. The pineal contains TRH, and in the frog it shows changes in content with the season and with changes in light and dark cycles independent of hypothalamic TSH.[369] The extrapyramidal system is also a regulatory area.[325, 329]

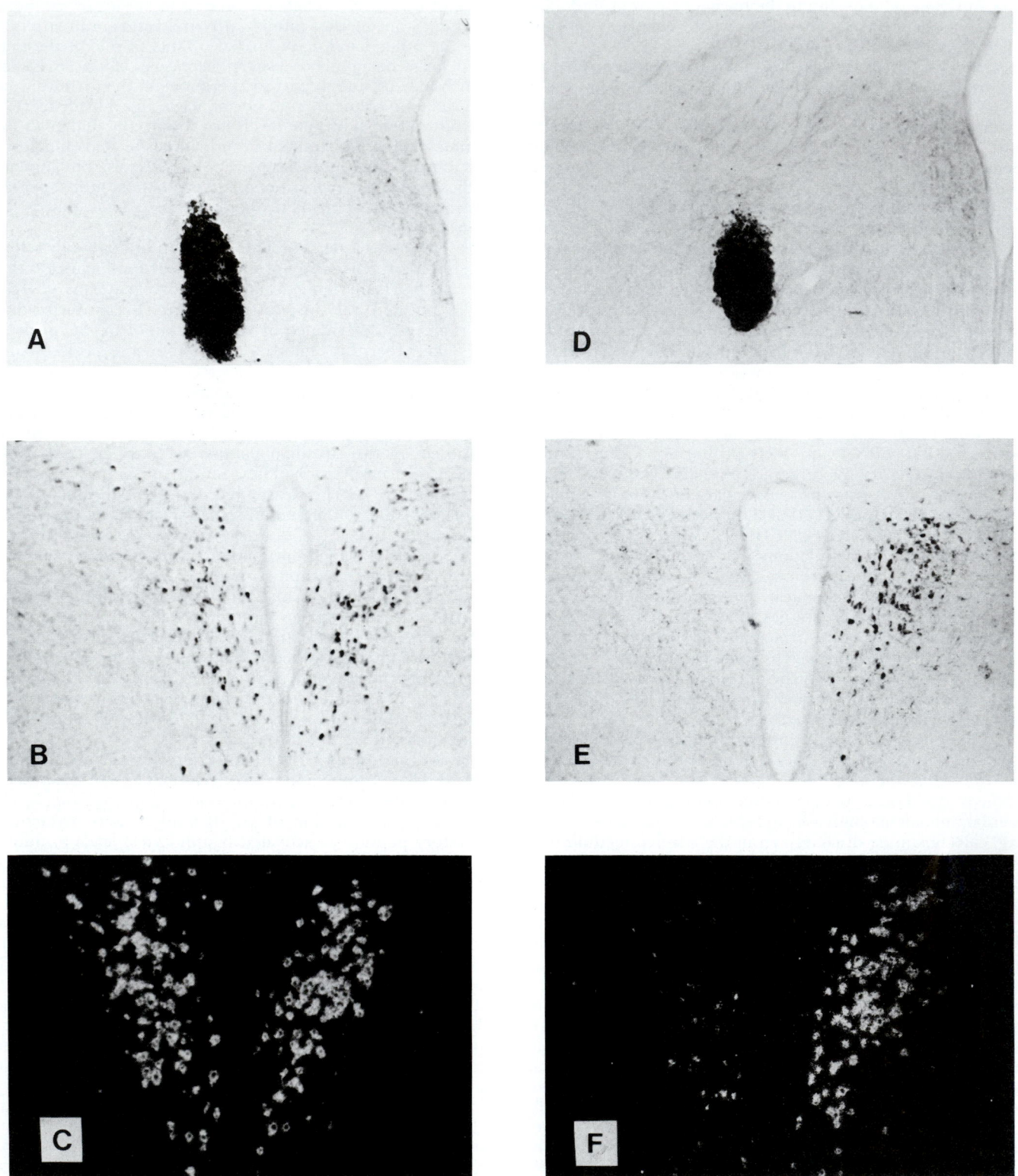

Figure 5–42. Direct effects of T_3 on TRH synthesis in the rat hypothalamic paraventricular nucleus (parvicellular division) were shown in this experiment by immunohistochemical detection of pre-proTRH (25–50) and of proTRH mRNA (by in situ hybridization) after implantation of a pellet of either T_3 (D) or of inactive diiodotyrosine (T_2) as a control (A). The T_2 pellet had no effect on the concentration of pre-proTRH (B) or on the concentration of proTRH mRNA (C). In contrast, both the TRH prohormone (E) and the proTRH mRNA (F) concentrations were markedly reduced. These studies indicate that thyroid hormone regulates the hypothalamic component of the pituitary-thyroid axis, as well as the pituitary thyrotroph itself. Original magnification ×40 in A and D; ×79 in B, C, E, and F. (Photographs courtesy of Dr. R. M. Lechan. From Dyess EM, Segarson TP, Liposits Z, et al. Triiodothyronine exerts direct cell-specific regulation of thyrotropin-releasing hormone gene expression in the hypothalamic paraventricular nucleus. Endocrinology 123, 2291–2297, 1988, © by The Endocrine Society.)

Corticotropin Secretion

Any theory designed to explain how ACTH secretion is regulated must account for several important aspects of pituitary-adrenal function. These features include open-loop control elements: (1) the occurrence of a circadian rhythm entrained to both sleep-wake and light-dark cycles, (2) spontaneous bursts of release (ultradian rhythm), and (3) the release induced by stress. The system also includes closed-loop feedback elements: (1) inhibition by glucocorticoid administration and (2) enhanced secretion after adrenalectomy (see Chapter 10) (Fig. 5–43).[110, 256, 257, 370, 371]

Feedback effects of glucocorticoids are directed at both pituitary corticotropes and the hypothalamic ACTH-regulating hypophyseotropic neurons that secrete CRH and AVP. The pituitary and neuronal glucocorticoid receptors have been well characterized,[338, 349, 372] and the distribution of neuronal glucocorticoid receptor has been studied by immunohistochemical and binding techniques.[373, 374] In both sites the glucocorticoid effects appear to be mediated by binding of the steroid-hormone complex to specific gene sequences. In the pituitary the glucocorticoids inhibit the

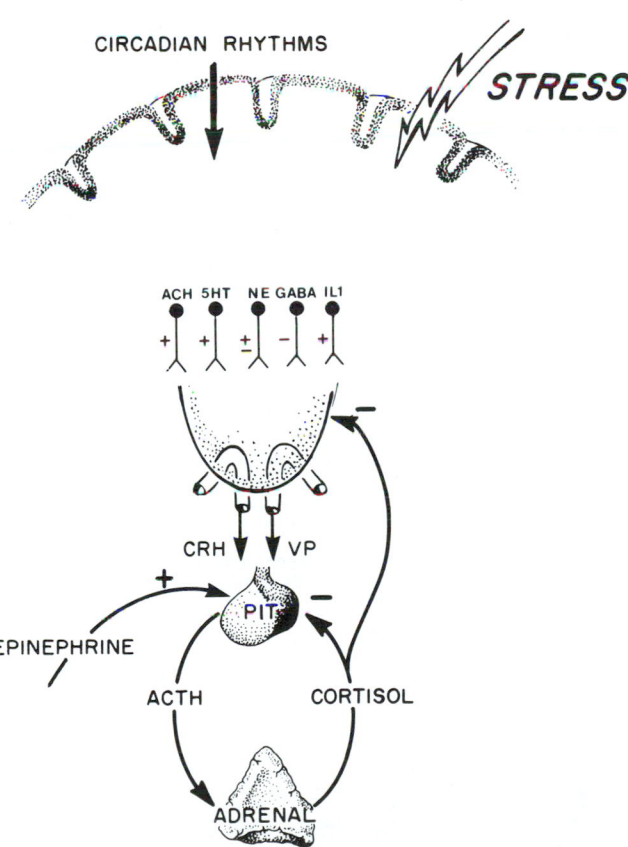

Figure 5–43. Schematic outline of function of the hypothalamic-pituitary-adrenal axis. ACTH stimulates the adrenal cortex to release cortisol, which in turn exerts a negative feedback effect on the anterior pituitary (PIT). Secretion of ACTH is stimulated by CRH, which acts in concert with AVP (VP in figure). Stress-induced epinephrine in circulating blood potentiates the effects of AVP and CRH. Feedback effects of glucocorticoids are exerted directly on the pituitary and also on the synthesis and secretion of CRH and AVP. Within the hypothalamus, CRH and AVP secretion is also regulated by an array of neurotransmitters and neuropeptides, only the most important of which are portrayed here. Of the classic neurotransmitters, excitatory effects are exerted by acetylcholine (ACH) and serotonin (5HT), inhibitory effects by GABA. Catecholamines can exert both inhibitory and excitatory effects.[389] In an earlier formulation of this control system, serotonin was thought to act through acetylcholine. More recent work suggests that serotonin can act directly on the CRH neuron.[388] NE, norepinephrine; IL1, interleukin 1. (From Martin JB, Reichlin S. Clinical Neuroendocrinology. 2nd ed. Philadelphia: F. A. Davis, 1987: 160.)

synthesis of POMC mRNA; in the hypothalamus the mRNAs for both CRH and AVP are reduced by glucocorticoids.

The criterion of the time it takes for infused glucocorticoids to block stress-induced ACTH release has been used to propose two and perhaps three different mechanisms of feedback suppression. One has a short latency (less than 30 min), one has a latency of 30 to 120 min, and the third mediates long-term suppression.[375] In addition, glucocorticoids may induce changes in neuronal membrane excitability within a few seconds.[376] These time differences may indicate different forms of control, some genomic and others nongenomic. With the exception of the immediate neuronal effects, all feedback is initiated by binding of the steroid to regulator gene elements.[377] Either type of glucocorticoid receptor, type I (mineralocorticoid) or type II (glucocorticoid), can mediate feedback suppression.

Two forms of glucocorticoid receptor in brain have been identified by using ligand-binding methods and cloning techniques.[349, 372] Although glucocorticoid receptors are involved in feedback regulation of ACTH secretion, most glucocorticoid target neurons lie outside the hypothalamus in the hippocampus, septum, and amygdala.[297, 373, 378] These structures are part of the "visceral brain" and are involved in manifestations of emotional state that occur in hyper- and hypocortisolism. Hippocampal glucocorticoid receptors also determine the set point for cortisol feedback.[297]

Glucocorticoid effects on cerebrovascular permeability and choroidal transport of water and electrolytes are important in regulating CSF synthesis and brain volume. Advantage is taken of this mechanism in the treatment of brain edema with high-dose glucocorticoids. Interestingly, adrenal insufficiency (particularly in children) can be accompanied by brain edema.

Although most steroids in brain are derived from the circulation, some steroids (and their synthesizing enzymes) arise in the brain endogenously. These steroids, called *neurosteroids*, include estradiol, pregnenolone, and dehydroepiandrosterone.[379] Most neurosteroids are located in oligodendroglia, and a few are present in neurons; their role in brain function has not been defined.

BRAIN REGIONS INVOLVED IN CORTICOTROPIN REGULATION. The CRH-secreting neurons have been identified by immunohistochemical techniques (see Fig. 5–22). Those neurons involved in anterior pituitary regulation arise in cells in the paraventricular nucleus and project to the median eminence. AVP and norepinephrine are synergistic with CRH in regulation of the stress response,[110, 371, 380–382] and CRH neurons cocontain AVP. The CRH neurons receive regulatory signals from many parts of the brain. Important excitatory inputs are from the SC nucleus (the regulator of circadian rhythms), the amygdala, and the raphe nuclei of the brain stem. The anatomy of afferent control has been studied extensively.[383–386] Inhibitory inputs on CRH secretion arise in the hippocampus and in the locus coeruleus of the midbrain. These anatomical inputs are neurotransmitter coded; excitatory influences are cholinergic, serotoninergic, or noradrenergic. Inhibitory influences are noradrenergic as well (see Fig. 5–43).[387–389]

A plausible model of the integration of neural and feedback factors influencing ACTH secretion is analogous to the way in which the pituitary-thyroid axis operates. The set point of plasma cortisol feedback is determined by the central nervous system through modulation of the rate of CRH and AVP release. In the presence of high CRH levels, high concentrations of cortisol are required to inhibit ACTH secretion. Contrariwise, when CRH secretion is low (as in the late afternoon or in individuals with hypothalamic lesions), the brain-pituitary controlling mechanism is highly susceptible to steroid suppression. The brain thus deter-

TABLE 5–11. Factors That Influence Serum Prolactin Levels in Humans

Physiological	Pathological	Pharmacological
Increase in Serum Prolactin Levels		
Pregnancy	PRL-secreting pituitary tumors	TRH
Postpartum states	Hypothalamic-pituitary disorders	Psychotropic drugs
Non-nursing mothers (days 1–7)	("Functional"?)	Phenothiazines
Nursing mothers after suckling	Tumors (craniopharyngioma),	Reserpine
Nipple stimulation (males and females)	metastases	Oral contraceptives
Coitus (some subjects)	Histiocytosis X	Estrogen therapy
Stress	Inflammation-sarcoidosis	Methyldopa
Exercise	Pituitary stalk section	
Neonatal period (2–3 mo)	Hypothyroidism	
Sleep	Renal failure	
	Ectopic production by malignant tumors	
Decrease in Serum Prolactin Levels		
Water loading	Isolated pituitary PRL deficiency	Levodopa
		Apomorphine
		Bromocriptine

From Martin JB, Reichlin S. Clinical Neuroendocrinology. 2nd ed. Philadelphia: F. A. Davis, 1987: 45–63.

mines the set point of the "adrenostats" that are located both in the pituitary and in part of the brain.

Unlike the case of the secretion of TSH, which becomes completely unresponsive to TRH if thyroid hormone levels are sufficiently high, severe neurogenic stress and large amounts of CRH can break through the feedback inhibition by glucocorticoids.

In addition to the feedback effects exerted by glucocorticoids on ACTH secretion, a short-loop feedback effect is exerted on ACTH secretion by ACTH itself. Administration of ACTH to adrenalectomized animals maintained on a fixed dose of glucocorticoid suppresses ACTH secretion;[390] i.e., ACTH inhibits its own secretion.

Endorphinergic pathways also play a role in ACTH regulation. Acute administration of morphine stimulates the release of ACTH, and chronic administration blocks ACTH release induced by a wide variety of stresses.[391] These observations suggest that endorphinergic fibers are part of the stress pathway. Because opiate antagonists do not block stress-induced ACTH release, the endorphin system is only *one* of the inputs into ACTH regulation rather than the sole mediator. CRH, via its actions as an ACTH regulator and a centrally active neurotransmitter, may be an integrative stress response mediator. Intrahypothalamic injections of CRH inhibit gonadotropin secretion[392] and induce a characteristic pattern of behavior that suggests severe emotional distress.[359]

Prolactin Regulation

The secretion of PRL, like that of GH and ACTH, responds to a variety of external stimuli, including suckling, mating, emotional and physical stresses, and internal rhythms related to the sleep cycle (Table 5–11).[266–272, 393–396] In contrast to other anterior pituitary secretions, the predominant effect of the hypothalamus on PRL secretion is that of tonic suppression (see earlier). Secretion of PRL also responds to alterations in the hormonal milieu of the pituitary, especially to the stimulatory action of estrogenic hormones (Fig. 5–44).

NEURAL CONTROL. Hypothalamic control of PRL secretion is mediated by several regulatory hormones synthesized by tuberohypophyseal neurons. The set point of regulation is mainly determined by the secretion of dopamine (a PIF), as suggested by the finding that section of the pituitary stalk or administration of dopamine receptor antagonists induces sharp increases in basal PRL secretion.

Superimposed on the tonic dopamine inhibition are several factors that increase PRL release: stress, suckling, circadian rhythms, and, in some animals, mating and preovulatory neural signals. Effects of stress on PRL release are probably mediated through the release of VIP and PHI, as indicated by studies in which immunoneutralization of these peptides leads to blockade of stress-induced PRL release in the rat. The effects of suckling may be mediated through a different neuronal pathway because treatment with anti-VIP and anti-PHI have only modest effects, whereas posterior lobectomy (in the rat) blocks suckling-induced PRL release completely. The posterior lobe secretes several peptides with PRL-releasing activity. These peptides include oxytocin, AVP, and TRH. However, PRF activity in neural lobe extracts cannot be attributed to any of these peptides and is probably due to an as-yet uncharacterized neural lobe factor arising from the intermediate lobe.[272] Mating in rats induces

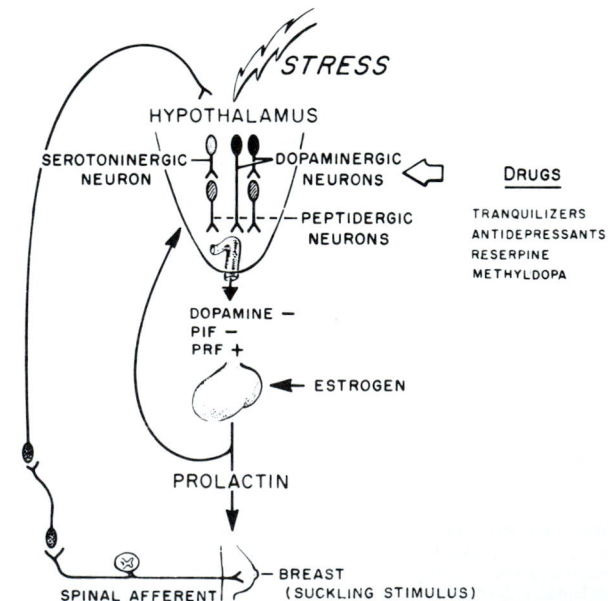

Figure 5–44. Hypothalamic regulation of PRL secretion. The predominant effect of the hypothalamus is inhibitory, an effect mediated principally by dopamine secreted by the tuberohypophyseal dopaminergic neuron system. One or more PRFs probably mediate acute release of PRL as in suckling and stress. There are several candidate PRFs, including TRH and VIP. The central dopaminergic system appears to be under methyldopa control, and PRF is controlled by serotonin. Estrogen sensitizes the pituitary to release PRL. PRL feeds back on the pituitary to regulate its own secretion (short-loop feedback) and also influences gonadotropin secretion by suppressing release of LHRH. Short-loop feedback is probably mediated indirectly by modifications of hypothalamic catecholamine secretion and turnover.

PRL secretion,[396] an effect mediated by both oxytocin and VIP.[273] PRL release is mediated by a host of stimulus-specific neurotransmitter pathways.

Although detailed knowledge of tuberohypophyseal coding of PRFs is still lacking, PRL secretion is determined by neurotransmitter influences impinging on the hypothalamus. Central dopaminergic pathways inhibit PRL release, whereas central serotoninergic pathways are excitatory. PRL secretion is also determined by central neuropeptide pathways, including the endorphinergic system that stimulates PRL release (see Table 5–9).

PRL secretion is regulated by both open- and closed-loop stimuli. Suckling and stress involve open-loop control. PRL itself exerts negative feedback loop control by decreasing the hypophyseal-portal dopamine concentration and increasing dopamine turnover in the tuberoinfundibular neurons.[288] PRL acting in the hypothalamus, in addition to regulating its own secretion, inhibits secretion of LHRH, thus accounting in part for the gonadotropin inhibition that is characteristic of hyperprolactinemic states. Inhibition of LHRH secretion is also responsible in part for the gonadotropin inhibition in women who are nursing and in patients with PRL-secreting adenomas of the pituitary.

External and internal stimuli that modify PRL release converge on the tuberohypophyseal neurons that secrete PIFs and PRFs. Pathways involved in the suckling reflex arise in nerves innervating the nipple, enter the spinal cord by way of spinal afferent neurons, ascend the spinal cord through spinothalamic tracts to the midbrain, and enter the hypothalamus by way of the median forebrain bundle. For the greatest part of the pathway, neurons regulating the milk let-down response accompany those involved in PRL regulation; at the level of the paraventricular nuclei, fibers influencing oxytocin release separate. The suckling reflex brings about a release of PRFs, as well as inhibition of PIF activity.

The development of PRL release and the milk let-down reflex provide a mechanism by which the infant can regulate the mother's milk production and milk delivery. The complementary sucking reflex of the infant, a response to tactile stimulation of the lips, presumably developed in parallel fashion. It has been argued that the nocturnal rise in PRL secretion in nursing women as well as in non-nursing women (and in men) evolved as a mechanism of PRL (and hence milk) maintenance during prolonged nonsuckling periods at night.[397] These behavioral and neuroendocrine mechanisms involving mother and infant are essential for successful survival of the species. The PRL-secretory response to breast stimulation also has major implications for human ecology. In many societies, lactation-induced suppression of ovulation is the principal means by which pregnancies are spaced.[398] Inhibition of gonadotropins by suckling not only is mediated by the feedback effects of high PRL levels but also occurs in nursing monkeys whose PRL levels are reduced by bromocriptine.[399] PRL secretion in humans is stimulated by food ingestion,[400] a teleologically inexplicable phenomenon.

The PRL-regulatory system and its bioaminergic control have been scrutinized in detail because of the frequent occurrence of syndromes of PRL hypersecretion (see Chapters 6 and 15).[395, 396, 401–405] Both pituitary and hypothalamus have PRL-inhibitory dopamine receptors; unfortunately the response to dopamine receptor stimulation and blockade does not distinguish between central and peripheral actions of the drug, and no pharmacological tests definitively identify the etiology of PRL hypersecretion.

Many commonly used neuroleptic drugs also influence PRL secretion. Reserpine (a catecholamine depletor) and phenothiazines such as chlorpromazine and haloperidol bring about the release of PRL by disinhibition of tonic

dopamine action on the pituitary. Lactation and amenorrhea occur in some patients. Indeed, the PRL response is an excellent predictor of the antipsychotic effects of phenothiazines.[406]

In the management of drug-induced hyperprolactinemia it must be remembered that the major antipsychotic neuroleptic agents act on brain dopamine receptors in the mesolimbic system. Attempts to treat such patients with dopamine agonist drugs such as bromocriptine can reverse the psychiatric benefits of such drugs. Bromocriptine can also induce schizophrenic psychosis in a small proportion of individuals with no history of mental disorder.[407]

Growth Hormone Regulation

Secretion of GH is modified by external stimuli, by endogenous neural rhythms, and by the feedback effects of GH itself (Fig. 5–45, Table 5–12).[211, 220, 221, 408–412] The important triggers of GH release are exercise, physical and emotional stresses, high intake of protein (mediated by amino acids) and intake of carbohydrate-rich meals (during the falling phase of blood glucose level). Endogenous modifications of GH release include surges of secretion within an hour or two of falling asleep and random changes throughout the day and night unrelated to any identifiable extrinsic or internal event. An ultradian rhythm in humans is similar to but of lower magnitude than that in the rat.[413] These

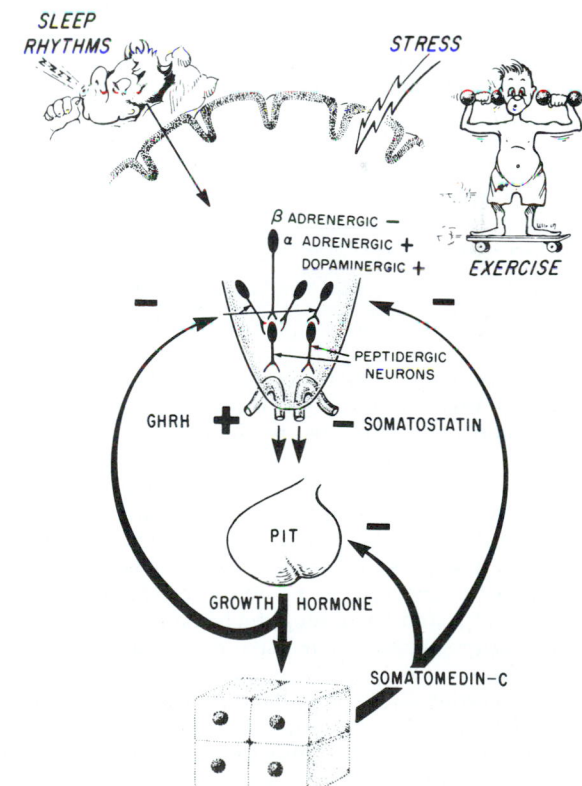

HYPOTHALAMIC – GROWTH HORMONE – SOMATOMEDIN AXIS

Figure 5–45. Regulation of GH secretion. GH secretion by the pituitary (PIT) is stimulated by GHRH and is inhibited by somatostatin. Negative feedback control of the pituitary is exerted at the pituitary level by IGF I. IGF I also acts on the hypothalamus to stimulate secretion of somatostatin. On the basis of indirect pharmacological data, it appears that release of GHRH is stimulated by acetylcholine, alpha-adrenergic, and dopaminergic stimuli and is inhibited by beta-adrenergic stimuli. Secretion of somatostatin, studied by direct assay in vitro, is stimulated by acetylcholine and VIP and is inhibited by GABA. Secretion of GH is modified by endogenous sleep rhythms, by stress, and by exercise.

TABLE 5–12. Factors That Stimulate or Inhibit Growth Hormone Secretion in Primates

Physiological	Hormones and Neurotransmitters	Pathological
	Stimulatory Factors	
Episodic, spontaneous release	Insulin hypoglycemia	Acromegaly
Exercise	2-Deoxyglucose	TRH
Stress	Amino acid infusions, e.g.,	LHRH
Physical	Arginine	Glucose
Psychological	Leucine	Arginine
Sleep	Lysine	Interleukins 1, 2, 6
Postprandial glucose decline	Small peptides	Protein depletion
	GHRH	Fasting and starvation
	AVP	Anorexia nervosa
	α-MSH	
	ACTH 1–24	
	Glucagon	
	Galanin	
	Monoaminergic stimuli	
	Epinephrine, alpha-receptor stimulation	
	Levodopa	
	Apomorphine	
	Bromocriptine	
	Clonidine	
	5-Hydroxytryptophan	
	Fusaric acid (dopamine β-hydroxylase inhibitor)	
	Propranolol	
	Melatonin	
	Nonpeptide hormones	
	Estrogens	
	Diethylstilbestrol	
	Potassium infusion	
	Dibutyryl cAMP	
	Inhibitory Factors*†	
Postprandial hyperglycemia	Somatostatin	Acromegaly
Elevated free fatty acid levels	Melatonin	Levodopa
Elevated GH levels	Serotonin antagonists	Apomorphine
	Methysergide	Phentolamine
	Cyproheptadine	Bromocriptine
	Phentolamine	Hyperthyroidism
	Chlorpromazine	Hypothyroidism
	Morphine	
	Cosyntropin	
	Progesterone	
	Theophylline	

*In many instances, the inhibition can be demonstrated only as a suppression of GH release induced by a pharmacological stimulus.

†Modified from Martin JB, Brazeau P, Tannenbaum GS, et al. Neuroendocrine organization of growth hormone regulation. In: Reichlin S, Baldessarini RJ, Martin JB, eds. The Hypothalamus. Vol 56. New York: Raven, 1978: 329–357.

functional changes in GH secretion are determined by the central nervous system acting through the hypothalamus. GH secretion is also modified by the hormonal milieu of the pituitary: enhanced in the presence of estrogens,[230] progesterone, testosterone, and thyroid hormone and suppressed by high levels of glucocorticoids. One can infer that the inhibitory effects of glucocorticoids are mediated at the level of the hypothalamus because glucocorticoids act directly on the pituitary to sensitize its response to GHRH.[229] Gonadal steroids and thyroid hormone, which stimulate GH synthesis, act through specific gene sequences in the somatotrope.[348, 349]

GH secretion is also regulated by three inhibitory peptides: GH itself, somatostatin,[414] and IGF I.[415–417] Direct GH influences on the hypothalamus can be considered as short-loop feedback control systems, whereas those involving IGF I are long-loop systems and thus analogous to pituitary-target systems such as the pituitary-thyroid and pituitary-adrenal axes. Control of GH secretion thus includes two closed-loop systems (GH and IGF I) and one open-loop regulatory system (neural).

When injected into the hypothalamus, both GH and IGF I inhibit GH release[415] by stimulating somatostatin release.[416] IGF I reduces the direct stimulatory effects of GHRH on the pituitary,[414, 417] whereas GH has no direct action at the pituitary level. These feedback influences probably account for the finding that in conditions in which circulating levels of IGF I are low, such as anorexia nervosa,[418] kwashiorkor,[419] and Laron dwarfism,[420] blood GH levels are elevated. Somatostatin deficiency may be the neuroendocrine basis of syndromes of inappropriate GH hypersecretion (see later).

The predominant influence of the hypothalamus on GH release is stimulatory, as evidenced by the fact that damage to the hypothalamic pituitary connection, such as that occurring with section of the pituitary stalk or lesions of the basal hypothalamus, is followed by inhibition of both basal and induced GH release. When the inhibitory somatostatinergic component is inactivated (e.g., by antisomatostatin antibody injection), basal GH levels are higher than normal, and responses to the usual provocative stimuli are exaggerated. The paradoxical release of GH that follows glucose injection in some patients with optic nerve glioma (a lesion compressing the anterior hypothalamus) or with various forms of metabolic encephalopathy, including uremia and hepatic coma, may be due to inactivation of the somatostatinergic inhibitory control system.

BRAIN AREAS INVOLVED IN GH REGULATION. Somatostatin-containing nerve fibers that inhibit GH secretion are located mainly in the anterior hypothalamic periventricular system. GHRH-containing nerve fibers arise principally from the arcuate nucleus and to a lesser extent from the ventro-

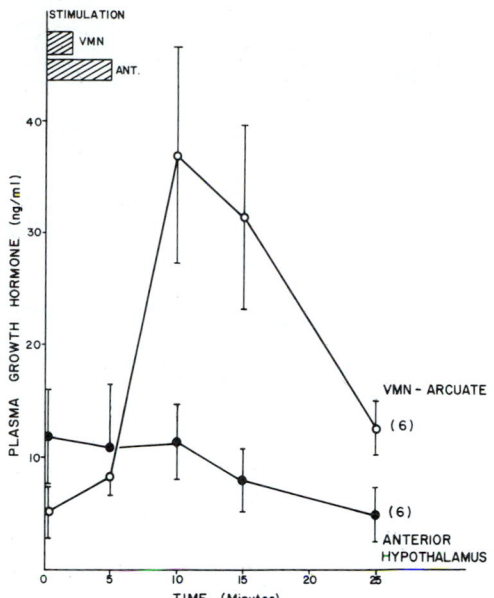

Figure 5–46. Effect on plasma GH level of electric stimulation of the ventromedial hypothalamic nucleus (VMN) of the rat. This figure shows the marked increase in plasma GH levels that follows electric stimulation of this nucleus. The ventromedial nucleus and ventral-basal hypothalamus are the only regions of the hypothalamus that are capable of this response, although certain extrahypothalamic sites may also cause this change. Note the short latent period of the response. The ventromedial nucleus is also important in that it has an effect on insulin secretion and satiety sensation and is the site of glucoreceptors. (From Martin JB. Plasma growth hormone [GH] response to hypothalamic or extrahypothalamic electric stimulation. Endocrinology 91, 107–115, 1972, © by The Endocrine Society.)

medial nucleus. The neuronal systems regulating GHRH and somatostatin release receive a variety of neural inputs (Figs. 5–46 and 5–47). The systems arising in the hippocampus (presumed to be linked to the sleep cycle) are excitatory,

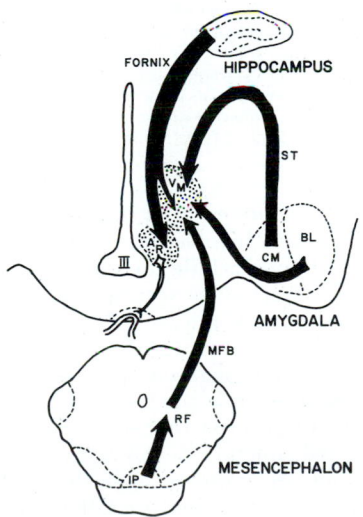

Figure 5–47. Neural pathways involved in GH regulation. This diagram illustrates the varied pathways by which impulses from the limbic system (visceral brain) ultimately impinge on the ventromedial nucleus, which in turn is capable of stimulating GH release through the mediation of GHRH. Pharmacological blocking studies show that the pathways between the extrahypothalamic regions and the ventromedial nucleus are catecholaminergic, whereas those between the ventromedial nucleus and stalk–median eminence region are not catecholaminergic. AR, arcuate nucleus; BL, basolateral nucleus; CM, corticomedial; IP, interpeduncular; MFB, medial forebrain bundle; RF, reticular formation; ST, stria terminalis; VM, ventromedial nucleus; III, third ventricle. (From Martin JB. Plasma growth hormone [GH] response to hypothalamic or extrahypothalamic electric stimulation. Endocrinology 91, 107–115, 1972, © by The Endocrine Society.)

whereas those arising in the amygdaloid nuclei can be both excitatory (basolateral amygdala) and inhibitory (corticomedial amygdala).[409, 411] The amygdala is a part of the visceral brain involved in emotion and responses to stress; it is probably a component of the pathways responsible for stress-induced GH release. Inhibitory inputs activate somatostatin release through the anterior hypothalamus. The stimulatory pathway involves both ventromedial and arcuate nuclei.

The association of the ventromedial nucleus with GH release is relevant to the neural regulation of fat and carbohydrate metabolism.[421] This nucleus is the site of glucoreceptors capable of influencing insulin secretion and GH release; it also generates a behavioral satiety signal. Insulin and somatostatin receptors and insulin-sensitive nerve pathways are located in this region. Thus the hypothalamus, especially the ventromedial nucleus, probably integrates the secretion of important glucoregulatory hormones with eating.

Both GHRH and somatostatin are regulated by a host of central neurotransmitters and neuropeptides. The demonstration that GH secretion in humans is stimulated by administration of the dopamine precursor L-dopa was the first evidence that releasing factors in humans are controlled by classic neurotransmitters.[422] Certain kinds of induced GH release are blunted by alpha-adrenergic blockers[280, 423] and are stimulated by beta-2–adrenergic agonists such as clonidine.[280, 424] Clonidine has been advocated for the treatment of neuroendocrine GH dysfunction,[425] but therapeutic benefits are controversial.[426] It is potentially useful in a diagnostic test of GH reserve, however.[427] The regulatory neuronal system for GH receives impulses from the four principal ascending monoaminergic systems—dopaminergic, noradrenergic, adrenergic, and serotoninergic—and from cholinergic fibers. Control attributed to the hippocampus and the amygdala is mediated via the aminergic systems. Dopamine is believed to stimulate GHRH both by direct action on central dopamine receptors and by stimulation of alpha-adrenergic receptors after conversion to norepinephrine. Norepinephrine, acting centrally, is a potent GH release stimulator, as is serotonin. Epinephrine may also be a link in the neural control of GH secretion,[287] as is acetylcholine.[428–430] Neurotransmitters may be specific to particular physiological stimuli of GH secretion. For example, sleep-induced GH release is mediated mainly by serotoninergic fibers and possibly by cholinergic fibers. Spontaneous endogenous ultradian rhythmical discharge of GH is blocked by drugs that inhibit epinephrine synthesis, which suggests that this component of control involves epinephrine interaction with alpha-adrenergic receptors. The latter are also involved in hypoglycemia- and exercise-induced GH release. A cholinergic link has been demonstrated for GH responses to glucagon, arginine,[428] and opiates.[429] In humans, anticholinergic drugs reduce or block all GH-stimulatory responses, with the exception of the response to hypoglycemia.[280] Anticholinergics also block the direct effects of GHRH on GH release.[430] One or more mechanisms may underlie this effect. In some situations acetylcholine inhibits somatostatin release;[431] anticholinergics may thus reverse tonic somatostatin inhibition. In addition, acetylcholine can act directly on the pituitary to inhibit GH release,[432] and some pituitary cells themselves secrete acetylcholine, which suggests the operation of a paracrine cholinergic control system within the pituitary.[432] The relative importance of the aminergic control system differs among species, as does the character of response to specific stimuli such as hypoglycemia and stress. Results of studies with rats and monkeys therefore cannot necessarily be extrapolated to humans.

Several central peptidergic neuron nets are also involved in GH regulation.[391, 433, 434] Endorphin receptor stimulation, either by administration of morphine or its analogues or by injection of β-endorphin into the third ventricle, stimulates GH release. Because these agents have no direct effect on the pituitary, the action appears to be secondary to activation of the GHRH neuronal system. Other peptides simulating GH release are VIP, neurotensin, and galanin.[435] Because VIP-secreting[436] and galanin-secreting[437] cells are intrinsic to the pituitary, both paracrine and neuroendocrine effects are probably mediated by these peptides. Substance P inhibits GH release when injected into the third ventricle by inducing somatostatin secretion. TRH has paradoxical effects on GH secretion. When introduced directly into the brain, TRH inhibits GH release, and likewise after systemic injection into humans it inhibits the secretory surge of GH that normally follows early sleep.[438] Thus central TRH pathways are generally inhibitory. However, under several circumstances, such as malnutrition and acromegaly, TRH acts directly on the pituitary to stimulate GH secretion.

Neuroendocrine Aspects of Reproduction and Sexual Function

Every component of reproductive activity of vertebrates depends on an interplay between neural and endocrine events.[439–448] Perpetuation of a species requires that overt mating behavior be correlated with the internal events of gametogenesis in the ovary and the testis. This correlation of behavior and readiness for insemination is achieved by neuroendocrine mechanisms involving the brain, pituitary, and gonadal hormones.[187, 189, 190, 449–453] Beyond the regulation of pituitary-gonadal function and the integration of reproductive behavior and the production of reproductive cycles, the nervous system plays additional roles in reproduction. The brain determines the timing of the onset of puberty,[454–459] regulates the initiation and maintenance of lactation, and controls parenting behavior.

Human sexual function is influenced by the brain in diverse ways. Pseudocyesis (false pregnancy) and menstrual abnormalities in psychologically disturbed women are examples of that influence. Spontaneously occurring disease of the hypothalamus is a cause of gonadal insufficiency, and neuroleptic agents interfere with ovulation. In rodents sex-specific mating behaviors are hormone determined, but a role for gonadal steroids in human sexual orientation is not established (see later).

Pituitary-gonadal function is regulated by the feedback effects of gonadal hormones and by the hypothalamus (Figs. 5–48 and 5–49). All three classes of steroid secretions of the gonad—estrogens, progestogens, and androgens—bind to specific receptors in the pituitary and influence gonadotropin secretion directly. Steroid receptors are also demonstrable in a wide distribution of brain cells, where they are involved in regulation of sexual behavior, regulation of LHRH secretion, and differentiation of the brain. Steroid receptors also are found on glial supporting cells and in ependyma (cells lining the ventricles).

The anatomical localization of steroid hormones, their mechanism of binding to specific receptors, and their metabolic transformation in brain have received extensive study.[460–469] Mechanisms that govern localization, binding, and degradation of steroid hormones are generally the same as those in peripheral target tissues, but modulation by previous endocrine status, influence of stage of maturation, and great anatomical specificity of affected cell populations are special features of steroid hormone metabolism in brain. Catechol estrogens (so called because ring A bears two hydroxyl groups) occur exclusively in the brain,[468] and the so-called neurosteroids are synthesized de novo in brain by glia.[379]

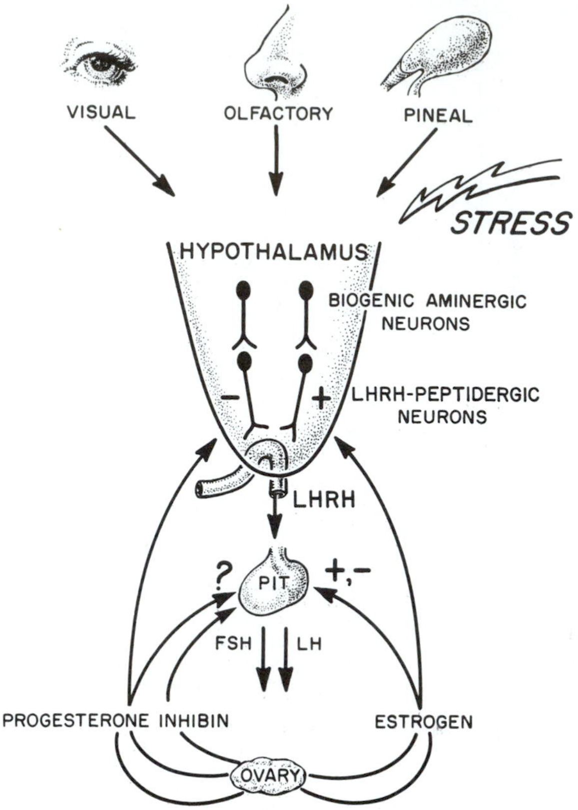

Figure 5–48. Regulation of gonadotropin secretion in the human female. Schematic diagram of gonadotropin control systems in the female, showing the interactions of neural and hormonal feedback controls. The development of the ovarian follicle is largely under the control of FSH. Ovulation is brought about by LH. Estrogenic hormones have complex effects on the feedback control mechanism of LH and FSH secretion. Depending on dose, time course, and previous hormonal status, estrogens can either inhibit or stimulate the secretion of LH through effects at both negative and positive feedback controls. Progesterone also can either stimulate or inhibit LHRH secretion, depending on the setting in which it is given, but its effects at the pituitary level are relatively insignificant. Secretions of the LHRH peptidergic neurons are in turn regulated by the biogenic aminergic system, through which a variety of nonhormonal signals can influence reproductive function. Visual stimuli in many lower animals can influence the onset of sexual function (as in seasonal breeders). Olfactory signals through pheromones influence estrous cycles in many rodents and may do so in women as well. Pineal factors in lower animals delay the onset of puberty. (From Martin JB, Reichlin S, Brown GM. Neuroendocrinology of reproduction. In: Clinical Neuroendocrinology. Philadelphia: F. A. Davis, 1977: 93–128.)

A number of hormones other than gonadal steroids and gonadotropins are also involved in the regulation of reproductive function. These include the inhibins and the activins, which are peptide hormones secreted by the gonads;[189, 470] PRL, which inhibits the release of LHRH;[471] dopamine, which under some circumstances directly inhibits LH secretion;[472] and VIP, which is secreted by the ovarian sympathetic neurons.[473] A few neurons in the hypothalamus secrete LH[474] or PRL,[475] but it is not known whether these neurons exert a specifically sexual function in this area.

Gonadotropins may also act directly on the hypothalamus to modulate gonadotropin secretion (short-loop feedback), and LHRH may influence its own secretion (ultra-short-loop feedback).[476]

Imposed on the steroid-regulatory inputs from the gonads are neural influences on the secretion of LHRH that are derived from several parts of the brain; these influences mediate reflex gonadotropin secretion and neurogenic amenorrhea.

Neuroendocrine control of gonadotropin secretion can be considered in three categories: (1) negative feedback, (2) positive feedback, and (3) neural open-loop components.

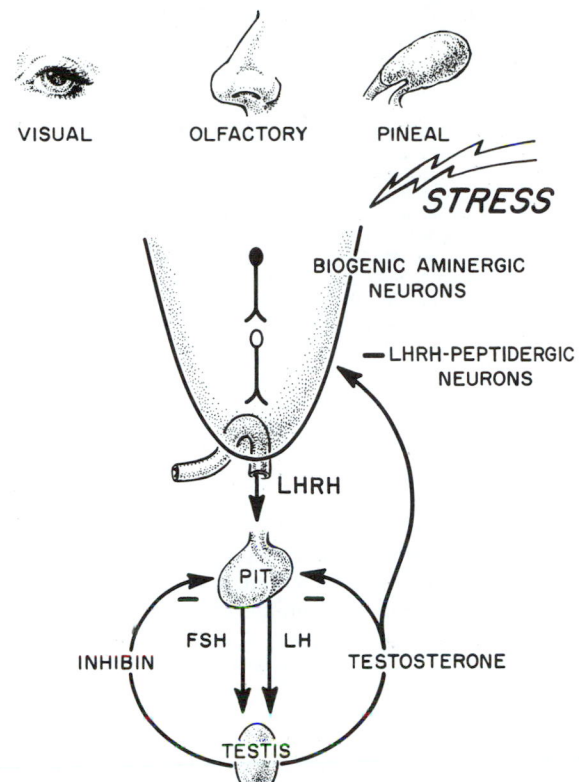

Figure 5—49. Regulation of gonadotropin secretion in the human male. Schematic diagram of gonadotropin control system in the male, showing the interaction of neural and hormonal feedback controls. Pituitary and testis are connected by a negative feedback link. Secretion of testosterone by the testis is stimulated by LH, whereas maturation and growth of the tubule cells are stimulated by FSH. The secretion of testosterone in turn inhibits the secretion of LH and FSH. It is likely that the major target of negative feedback is the hypothalamus; testosterone administration in humans does not interfere with the effectiveness of LHRH (pituitary sensitivity is relatively unaltered). A peptide secretion of the testis, inhibin, is believed to be secreted by tubular epithelium and to exert a direct inhibitory effect on FSH secretion. It is not known whether inhibin affects the hypothalamus directly. The LHRH peptidergic neurons are in turn regulated by a biogenic aminergic system that links gonadotropin regulation to the remainder of the brain. Through this system a wide variety of impulses can be exerted on reproductive function. Stimuli affecting male gonadotropic secretion have been well demonstrated in experimental animals, although they are not as well worked out in the human. Visual influences include light-induced changes in seasonal breeders such as domestic cattle, deer, and birds. Olfactory signals in male rats influence gonadal function. The pineal gland in many species of animals inhibits gonadotropin secretion by direct effects of pineal secretions on either the hypothalamus or the pituitary. The role of the pineal in human reproduction control has not been established. (From Martin JB, Reichlin S, Brown GM. Neuroendocrinology of reproduction. In: Clinical Neuroendocrinology. Philadelphia: F. A. Davis, 1977: 93–128.)

NEGATIVE FEEDBACK BY STEROIDS AND INHIBIN. In the presence of a normally functioning hypothalamus, the secretion of LH and FSH by both sexes is suppressed by administration of constant doses of estrogens and androgens, and it is increased after castration (or administration of antiestrogenic or antiandrogenic drugs) (Fig. 5–50). Negative feedback effects involve both the pituitary and the hypothalamus. If the hypothalamic component of control is inactivated (e.g., by destruction of the medial basal hypothalamus, by pituitary stalk section, or by transplantation of the pituitary away from the brain), basal gonadotropin secretion falls dramatically and the pituitary hypersecretory response to castration is blunted or abolished. Thus a functioning hypothalamus is necessary for the expression of normal pituitary response to gonadectomy. In castrated animals LHRH secretion is increased, as shown by alterations

in the concentration of LHRH mRNA,[477] which proves that the hypothalamus is a target of gonadal steroids.

Suppression of pituitary secretion by gonadal steroids involves both neural and pituitary targets, is sex specific, and is influenced by both dosage and time-dependent variables. In women with normal menstrual cycles, administration of physiological doses of estrogens suppresses basal levels of both LH and FSH. For the first 1 to 3 d after initiation of treatment, pituitary responsiveness to LHRH is reduced, which indicates that the suppressive effects of the estrogen are exerted, at least in part, by direct inhibition of the pituitary. The secretion of FSH is more sensitive to the inhibitory effects of estrogen than is the secretion of LH.[478] After approximately 3 d (and despite the fact that basal levels of LH and FSH remain depressed), the pituitary becomes *sensitized* to test doses of LHRH. In men treated with estrogens the plasma levels of LH and FSH are also reduced, but, in contrast to women, responsivity to LHRH remains suppressed.[479] These findings indicate that negative feedback effects of estrogen in men are exerted mainly at the level of the pituitary, whereas in women the primary site is the hypothalamus. Testosterone treatment in men causes a fall in basal gonadotropin secretion unassociated, at least initially, with a change in pituitary responsivity to LHRH.[479] These findings imply that testosterone negative feedback under these circumstances largely involves the hypothalamus. In both sexes the long-term administration of estrogens or testosterone lowers gonadotropin secretion and suppresses pituitary responsiveness to LHRH, indicating a major effect on the pituitary.

Negative feedback, directed mainly at the pituitary FSH-secreting cell, is also exerted by the inhibins, which are peptide hormones derived from germinal cells of the ovary and the testis.[189, 480] When germinal activity is reduced (as in normal prepubertal children or after cyclophosphamide destruction of the germinal epithelium of the testis and the ovary), plasma FSH levels are disproportionately elevated compared with LH levels, and the FSH-secretory response to LHRH is exaggerated.

POSITIVE FEEDBACK BY ESTROGENS: MIDCYCLE OVULATORY SURGE, THE LHRH PACEMAKER, AND THE FEMALE BRAIN. As just noted, gonadotropin secretion is increased in the presence of low blood estrogen or androgen levels and is suppressed when levels of estrogens or androgens are raised. These responses are manifestations of the negative feedback control of gonadotropin secretion. This type of control does not explain all the responses in the course of normal ovulatory cycling. The characteristic surge of gonadotropin secretion in adult women at midcycle, which is responsible for inducing ovulation, is brought about by a preovulatory surge of estrogens secreted by the developing ovum. In this setting, estrogens act as a positive feedback signal, largely by increasing the sensitivity of the pituitary gonadotrophs to endogenous LHRH. Prerequisites for this response are a normal intrinsic pulsatile LHRH rhythm and a pulse of estrogen superimposed on a background of sustained low levels of estrogen (Fig. 5–51). This formulation is based on a number of observations: during the early follicular stage of the cycle, surges of LH and FSH release are induced by administration of amounts of estrogen that approximate the normal preovulatory rise;[481–483] this hypersecretory state is accompanied by marked sensitization of the pituitary to injections of LHRH.[479] In women with hypothalamic amenorrhea (and in female rhesus monkeys with experimentally induced hypothalamic lesions), normal ovulatory LH surges can be induced by estrogens only if exogenous LHRH is supplied in an appropriate pulsatile fashion that approximates the normal intrinsic LH rhythm (Fig. 5–52).[483–485]

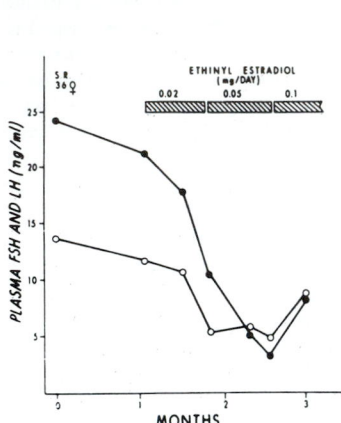

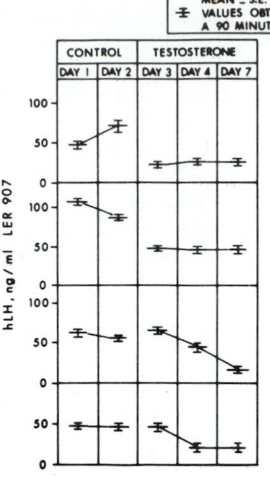

MEAN ± S.E. OF 10 hLH
VALUES OBTAINED DURING
A 90 MINUTE PERIOD

Figure 5–50. Inhibitory effects of gonadal steroids on LH secretion. Administration of estrogen to hypogonadal (menopausal) women *(left)* or of testosterone to men *(right)* results in a fall in plasma LH level, which demonstrates negative feedback control. To convert LH values to international units per liter, multiply by 0.664. To convert FSH values to international units per liter, multiply by 0.002. *Left,* (●) FSH; (○) LH. (Left from Schalch DS. Gonadotropin secretion in the human. In: Mack HC, Sherman AE, eds. Neuroendocrinology of Human Reproduction. Springfield, IL: Charles C Thomas, 1971: 127–145.)

The normal endogenous LHRH rhythm is supplied by an intrinsic mechanism termed by Knobil the hypothalamic "GnRH pulse generator," which provides an LHRH pulse into the hypophyseal-portal vessels at approximately 90-min intervals;[483] the menstrual cycle is timed by the monthly development of the ovum under the influence of normal gonadotropin secretion. The aphorism of Knobil that "the ovulatory clock is in the pelvis"[439] means that the ripening ovary signals the hypothalamic-pituitary axis that it is ready

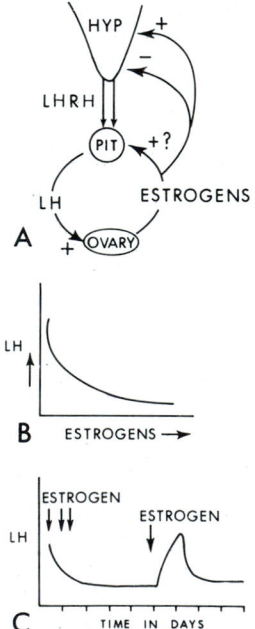

Figure 5–51. Pituitary-gonadal axis: closed-loop negative feedback system with positive feedback elements and open-loop neural transients. *A,* Negative feedback. The level of estrogen in plasma controls LH secretion. When plasma estrogen levels are elevated, LH secretion is inhibited. When plasma estrogen levels are low, secretion of LH is enhanced *(B).* The precise target for estrogen in bringing out this negative inhibition is still not firmly established, but most work indicates that the effect is mediated at the hypothalamic level (here designated as a [−]), presumably through inhibition of the secretion of LHRH. *C,* Positive feedback. Estrogen transients (such as occur after administration of estrogens in animals or humans and in the spontaneous phases of the estrous cycle) are capable of stimulating the release of LH. The site of action of the positive hormone transient has not been fully established. There is evidence that the positive feedback element is exerted at the level of the pituitary (by sensitizing the LH-releasing mechanism to estrogen) and may be exerted at the hypothalamic level. In addition, the secretion of LHRH by the hypothalamus is subject to open-loop neural transients, such as sexual stimulation, which in some species, including the human, can alter LH secretion.

to be stimulated by an ovulatory surge of gonadotropins. In addition, there may be a hypothalamic effect of estrogen as well: LHRH secretion is stimulated by preovulatory release of estrogens in the rat, monkey, and perhaps the human.[486]

Abnormalities of ovulatory patterns can thus be induced by any interference with the normal patterns of intrinsic hypothalamic cyclicity or dysfunction of the pituitary or the ovaries.

The rhythmicity of the LHRH pulse generator is regulated to some extent by the hormonal milieu.[483] Testosterone, in physiological amounts, slows the intrinsic rate of discharge; this hypothalamic effect is the main mechanism by which testosterone inhibits gonadotropin release.[487] Progesterone also slows the pacemaker. In contrast, estrogen appears to have no effect on the pacemaker.

The capacity to develop an increase in LH secretion, i.e., the positive feedback response, is characteristic of females of all species. In rodents, the organism in which most neuroendocrine research has been done, the female pattern of responsivity of pituitary and hypothalamus to estrogens is prevented if the newborn female is exposed to androgens during a critical developmental period (in rats this period extends from birth to the fifth postnatal day[445, 450, 453, 488]). Not only is the capacity for positive hormone feedback prevented by androgens in rats, but the ability to display adult female patterns of sexual behavior are lost, even if hormonal balance is restored in adult life. These observations have led to the concept that the "male" brain and the "female" brain are determined by the hormonal milieu at a critical developmental stage. This concept is supported by the clear-cut neuroanatomical differences between male and female rats, particularly in so-called sexually dimorphic regions of the hypothalamus and the spinal cord,[453] and by the demonstration that brain transplantation of androgenized preoptic regions of the hypothalamus into the preoptic region of neonatal females leads to male mating behavior.[488]

The striking effects of early hormonal milieu on gonadotropin secretion and sexual behavior in rats have led to speculation about similar functions in humans.[489–490] Indeed, human male-female differences have been described in mathematical ability and the incidence of left-handedness, brain asymmetry, and dyslexia.[489] Moreover, behavioral differences between normal women and women who had been exposed to androgens in utero have been reported.[489] Pituitary regulation in men also differs from that in women in that short-term estrogen exposure does not sensitize the pituitary to exogenous LHRH.[479]

These minor sex differences in the human notwithstanding, differences in gonadotropin regulation between

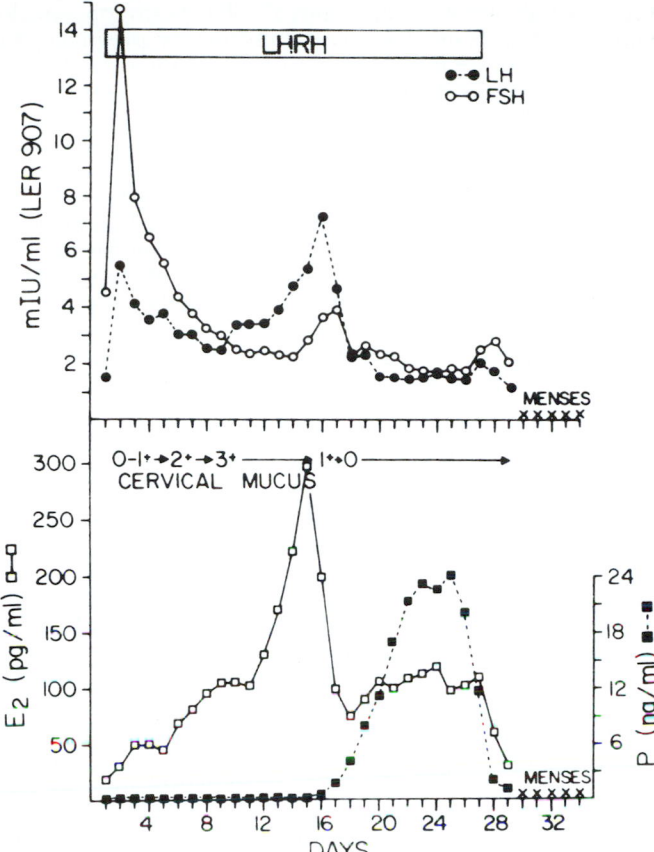

Figure 5–52. In this patient with hypothalamic LHRH deficiency related to Kallmann syndrome, pulsatile administration of synthetic LHRH (by means of a programmed pump) stimulated ovulation. Shown are the blood levels of LH and FSH (demonstrating a normal ovulatory surge), a normal preovulatory estradiol (E_2) surge, and a normal postovulation rise in serum progesterone (P) level. Ultrasound examination was reported to demonstrate a single follicle in the right ovary on day 13 of treatment. This study demonstrates that the normal sequence of hormone secretion, including typical patterns for gonadotropins and ovarian hormones, can be induced by the administration of constant amounts of LHRH in a pulsatile fashion. To convert estradiol values to picomoles per liter, multiply by 3.671. To convert progesterone values to nanomoles per liter, multiply by 3.180. See Figure 5–50 for conversions of FSH and LH values. (From WF Crowley Jr, JW McArthur. Stimulation of the normal menstrual cycle of Kallman's syndrome by pulsatile administration of luteinizing hormone–releasing hormone [LHRH], J Clin Endocrinol Metab, 51, 173–175, 1980, © by The Endocrine Society.)

men and women are not due to fundamental differences in hypothalamic function: men and women display spontaneous LH and FSH ultradian rhythms of approximately the same duration;[484, 487, 490] this pacemaker rhythm is slowed in both men and women by exposure to testosterone or progesterone;[487] in the absence of the testis, male monkeys release LH and FSH when given an estrogen pulse;[481–483] and the exposure of female humans and female monkeys in utero to masculinizing doses of androgen does not influence later menstrual cycling.[487] Thus there does not appear to be a male or a female brain pattern of gonadotropin regulation in the higher primates. Hormonal "imprinting" is thought to be of minimal importance in human gender orientation.[490a]

It is not clear, however, why normal women release LH in response to estrogen, whereas men do not. One possibility is that estrogen effects are blocked by testosterone (in the male). This possibility is probably not the explanation, however, because estrogen induces LH secretion in castrated male monkeys whether or not the animal has been treated with testosterone.[482] The fact that the presence of a normal testis abolishes the stimulating effects of estrogen suggests

that a nontestosterone testicular hormone (or hormones) blocks estrogen effects. Because both LH secretion and FSH secretion are blocked, this blocking hormone cannot be inhibin (which acts only on FSH release). Another substance may be involved.

NEUROTRANSMITTER CONTROL OF GONADOTROPINS. Neurons controlling LHRH secretion receive innervation from other neural sites capable of either stimulation or inhibition. Through these inputs, gonadal function responds to changes in light-dark cycle, emotional stress, and (in some species) sexual stimuli that are visual or olfactory or result from uterine cervical stimulation. Various parts of the visceral brain, including the hippocampus and the amygdala, project to the LHRH pathways. In addition, LHRH-containing neurons receive an important noradrenergic pathway from the midbrain locus coeruleus nucleus.[491]

From a historical standpoint, efforts to identify neurotransmitters controlling gonadotropin secretion led to the first convincing evidence of neuropharmacological control of the anterior pituitary. The administration of acetylcholine directly onto the pituitary induces constant estrus in the rat,[492] and atropine, which is a cholinergic (muscarinic) blocker, blocks reflex ovulation in the rabbit.[493] The normal endogenous estrous rhythm of the rat is delayed by exactly 1 d after administration of pentobarbital but only when this agent is given during a critical period in the afternoon of the day of proestrus.[494]

Other neurotransmitters in addition to cholinergic factors modify central control of gonadotropins.[280, 284, 445, 495] Most important is the noradrenergic input (alpha-adrenergic). Injection of norepinephrine into the medial basal hypothalamus triggers LH release in the rat: alpha-adrenergic blockers prevent the usual ovulatory response of both rat and rabbit, and drugs that block alpha-adrenergic control can prevent ovulation in women. A population of *inhibitory* beta-adrenergic neurons has been identified. Feedback effects on estrogen are mediated in part by effects on central catecholaminergic fibers projecting to the hypothalamus,[496] and estrogens modify catecholamine synthesis in the brain.

Endorphins and other endogenous opioids can influence LHRH secretion. Morphine and its analogues inhibit ovulation, whereas the opiate antagonist naloxone can induce ovulation in some patients with hyperprolactinemia.[497]

NEUROGENIC CONTROL OF THE TIMING OF PUBERTY. Long before the onset of puberty, the pituitary, the gonads, and the secondary sex accessories are all capable of being stimulated. Puberty does not begin, however, until the appearance of pulsatile LHRH secretion by the hypothalamus. This change is analogous to other maturational brain changes that include enhancement of intellectual capacity and alterations in behavior and personality.[454–459, 498] Clinical analysis of patients with hypothalamic disease[499] and studies of the effects of destruction of various parts of the brain in animals have shown that certain regions of the hypothalamus tonically inhibit gonadotropin secretion before puberty. The fundamental change during puberty may thus be a reduction in tonic hypothalamic inhibition of LHRH release. In the presence of low LHRH secretion in prepubertal children, the pituitary is much more sensitive to suppression by the negative feedback effects of gonadal steroids. Only the negative feedback effect of gonadal steroids can be demonstrated before puberty; positive feedback in the female occurs after puberty is well advanced.

Hypothalamic-pituitary stimulation of gonadal secretion occurs in late fetal life and during the first few months of infancy. Some sexual development, albeit at a low level, occurs even in the prepubertal period.

The time of onset of pubertal brain function is influenced by genetic and environmental factors. In humans the trend toward decreasing age at onset of puberty over the past century and comparisons of different population groups suggest that an important trigger for puberty is related to body size.[500-502] This effect probably explains why improved nutrition and freedom from disease have been followed by decreasing age at onset of menarche. Moderately obese girls have earlier puberty than do girls of normal weight, and individuals (or rats) with malnutrition fail to develop normal pituitary-ovarian function. Body fat mass (or some function of fat mass) is believed to be the crucial trigger for female puberty. A body fat mechanism may also be responsible for gonadal suppression in patients with anorexia nervosa and for its return with refeeding.[502-504]

EFFECT OF GONADAL STEROIDS ON THE BRAIN. Feedback action of gonadal steroids on the central nervous system plays an important role both in regulating gonadotropin secretion and in controlling sexual behavior (see Chapters 12 and 13).[449-453, 462-469, 505, 506] After castration, female cats will not mate and the genital tract becomes atrophic, both responses resulting from lack of estrogen and both readily reversed by estrogen replacement treatment. The estrogen effect on behavior is mediated centrally. Minute implants of estrogen in the hypothalamus restore normal sexual behavior without reversing the atrophic genital changes.[506] Cat brain is thus shown to be sensitive to the erotogenic actions of estrogens, and local brain stimulation is capable of inducing the full range of sexual behavior. Estrogen chemoreceptor function of the hypothalamus has been demonstrated by radioautographic localization of labeled hormones after systemic administration, estrogen concentrating in areas in which local estrogen implantations cause physiological effects. Specific receptors for estrogen have been identified in these regions, localized both in the cell nucleus and in other parts of the cell body.[460-464] The generation of sex drive by a neural signal from an estrogen receptor within the hypothalamus is analogous to the generation of hunger drive in hypoglycemia, thirst after hyperosmolarity, and temperature-safeguarding behavior after central cooling and heating.

Neurophysiological studies indicate that progesterone acts on certain hypothalamic neurons to decrease the rate of spontaneous firing and to elevate the threshold of excitability to reflex stimulation from the uterine cervix. Progesterone in humans also acts on the hypothalamus to raise body temperature. This mechanism is responsible for the postovulatory rise in basal body temperature that is commonly used as an index of ovulation. The hypothalamus is not the only structure in which excitability is decreased by progesterone. Spontaneous and electrically or pharmacologically stimulated contractions of the uterus are also inhibited by progesterone.

PHEROMONES AND SEXUAL FUNCTION. The female dog in heat emits a scent that is attractive to male dogs. This phenomenon is an example of a response mediated by a *pheromone,* the term defined as a chemical substance secreted by one animal that arouses either behavioral or hormonal changes in a member of the same species.[507, 508] In nonvertebrates such as moths, pheromones are potent sex attractants. In sheep and goats the onset of estrus and ovulation is accelerated if males are placed with the flock. In the female mouse the gonadotropic function is altered by the presence of a male. Female mice housed in cages without males tend to have irregular and prolonged estrous cycles. In the presence of the male, sexual cycles become synchronized, and on the third night after contact with the male, estrous behavior and mating occur. This response can be induced merely by exposing the females to the urine-contaminated bedding of the male. Female mouse urine contains a factor that stimulates LH release when it is applied to the vomeronasal organ of male mice.[509] Furthermore, female mice mated with familiar males fail to carry pregnancy to term if they come into contact with the urine of a strange male. Female rats deprived of their olfactory bulbs do not build nests for their young or retrieve them. In monkeys the fatty acids that are formed in the vagina at estrus, presumably as a consequence of hormonally altered bacterial flora, arouse grooming behavior in the male. The vaginal discharge of the hamster contains a protein (151 amino acid residues; 17 kd) that elicits copulatory behavior in the male.[510] This substance, to which the euphonious term *aphrodisin* has been applied, may act as a carrier protein for other, as-yet unrecognized, olfactants.

Two primary classes of pheromones have been defined.[508] The first class includes the *releasing or signaling* pheromones, those that seem to cause either the initiation of particular behaviors or changes in behavior pattern. These pheromones include those used in territorial marking, those eliciting or inhibiting agonist responses, those serving for sexual recognition and attraction, and those maintaining contact between mothers and young.

The second class includes the *priming* pheromones, those that induce changes in endocrine or neuroendocrine activity in the receiving organism. Most consequences of such pheromones are related to reproductive functioning and include effects on estrous cyclicity, the onset of puberty, and the maintenance of pregnancy. Olfactory function depends on specific binding of olfactants to the cilia of olfactory neurons located, in humans, mainly above the first turbinate in the region of the ethmoid plate. Olfactory neurons are unique among mammalian neurons in that they are constantly renewed from stem cells. Olfactory thresholds are regulated by hormonal status—by gonadal steroids and by adrenocortical hormones.

Little is known about the role of pheromones in human sexual activity. Several of the ingredients that are commonly used in human perfumes (musk and civet) are obtained from the glands of animals that utilize these secretions as sexual attractants. The ability to detect certain kinds and amounts of smells is hormone dependent in women and is heightened at midcycle. There is a correlation between the timing of the menstrual cycle in women living together as roommates compared with that of those who are separated.[511] The basis of this synchronization of cycles is unknown, but pheromones may play a role. Pheromones may act without the individual's being consciously aware of the stimulus, and the role of pheromones in human function may prove to be more important than is now recognized.

THE PINEAL GLAND AND CIRCUMVENTRICULAR ORGANS

Lining the ventricles of the brain and the central canal of the spinal cord are ependymal cells that form cuboidal, usually ciliated, epithelium. In several areas of the third and fourth ventricles, the simple single-layered lining is modified into secretory structures that are of known or presumptive neuroendocrine function (Fig. 5-53).[512, 513] Most important of these is the pineal gland, which is derived from ependymal cells of the roof of the third ventricle. Other structures in the third ventricle are the subcommissural organ (SCO), the subfornical organ (SFO), the organum vasculosum of the lamina terminalis (OVLT), and the specialized ependyma of the median eminence. At the posterior margin of the lip of the roof of the fourth ventricle is another periventricular organ, the area postrema. All of these structures have interstitial tissue spaces into which relatively large molecules

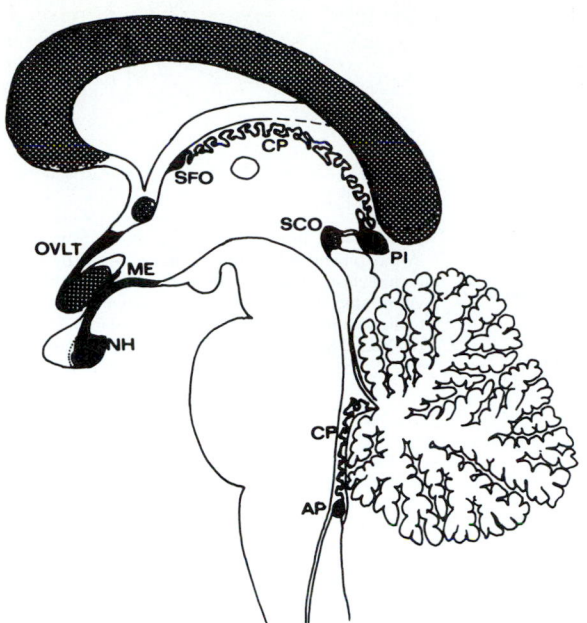

Figure 5–53. Median sagittal section through the human brain to show the circumventricular organs *(in black)*: AP, area postrema; ME, median eminence; NH, neurohypophysis; OVLT, organum vasculosum of the lamina terminalis; PI, pineal body; SFO, subfornical organ; SCO, subcommissural organ; CP, choroid plexus. (From Weindl A. Neuroendocrine aspects of circumventricular organs. In: Ganong WF, Martini L, eds. Frontiers in Neuroendocrinology. Vol 3. New York: Oxford University Press, 1973: 3–32.)

circulating in the blood can penetrate, thus revealing that this region lacks the usual blood-brain barrier. In these regions the nerve endings, with their associated blood vessels, form neurohemal organs. Despite their contiguity with the ventricles, the periventricular organs (with the exception of the SCO; see later) probably do not secrete their products into the CSF. This inference is based on electron microscopic demonstration of tight junctions at the ventricular boundary. Rather, these structures permit brain secretions to enter peripheral blood and have been called, somewhat fancifully, "windows to the brain."

The Pineal Gland

STRUCTURE OF THE PINEAL GLAND. The pineal gland (which in humans weighs only 0.10 to 0.18 g) is separated by the relatively thin tectal plate from the aqueduct of Sylvius, as it lies in the groove between the superior colliculi (see Fig. 5–7). The pineal (so called because it resembles a pinecone) has been believed from the time of antiquity to be associated with mental functions.[514, 515] The pineal is a true secretory structure; it contains an extraordinary number of biologically active substances, and it is occasionally the site of significant human disease.

The pineal gland is made up of cells with ultrastructural features suggesting neurosecretory functions. In lower vertebrates such as fish and amphibia, pineal cells form a true eye-like, light-sensitive structure; in higher vertebrates, including mammals, all vestiges of light-receptive function have disappeared (except for the residual expression of some retinal chemical markers), and the secretory activities emerge as the dominant feature. Early in phylogenetic development (when the pineal is still a light-sensitive organ), the pineal is connected to the roof of the brain (epithalamus) by sensory nerves, but in mammals all direct nerve connection of the pineal to the brain is lost and is replaced by a

circuitous innervation, a postganglionic sympathetic nerve supply from the superior cervical ganglia (see Fig. 5–39).[516, 517] Preganglionic fibers in the superior sympathetic chain arise in the lateral cell column of the spinal cord. These sympathetic nerve cells are regulated by descending nerve impulses, some of which arise (either directly or via intermediate synapses) from a paired nucleus located in the hypothalamus just above the optic chiasm termed the *suprachiasmatic nucleus* (see earlier under Endocrine Rhythms). The SC nucleus receives a direct nerve input from the retina, the retinohypothalamic tract, that conveys information about light and dark independent of conscious perception. It is by way of this neural pathway that external light regulates pineal activity. In the absence of light input, pineal rhythms persist (driven by the SC pacemaker), but they are no longer entrained to the external light-dark cycle. Light-dark shifts are the most important cues for pineal rhythm.

Crucial to the regulation of pineal function is its sympathetic nerve innervation, which consists of noradrenergic fibers that end in the interstitial space of the gland or on the plasma membrane of pinealocytes.[514, 516, 518] Pinealocytes are true secretory cells, organized into cords and resting on a basement membrane in relationship to an interstitial space.

The endothelium of the pineal gland is fenestrated, thus permitting the entry and exit of relatively large molecules to and from the interstitial space of the gland. In this regard the pineal differs from the bulk of brain in not having a blood-brain barrier, but it resembles other periventricular organs such as the median eminence, SFO, and SCO.

All neuroendocrine functions of the pineal parenchymal cells are regulated by beta-adrenergic receptors. Section of the sympathetic innervation or use of beta-adrenergic antagonists inhibits pineal metabolic activity.[518–522]

PHYSIOLOGICAL FUNCTION OF THE PINEAL GLAND. Most research on the function of the pineal has dealt with a possible role in regulation of sexual function and sexual development.[523–582] In rodents the secretion of gonadotropin is suppressed by the pineal gland under certain well-defined circumstances.[523, 533–536] Extirpation of the pineal gland leads to precocious puberty in several species, but the effect is modest. More convincingly, pinealectomy reverses the gonadal involution that follows exposure to constant darkness or shortened photoperiods in both rats and hamsters. If blinded or exposed to constant darkness, male rats show a reduction in testicular weight and testosterone deficiency. In female rats, gonadotropin secretion and ovarian growth are also impaired by blindness. These effects are reversed by pinealectomy, which indicates that darkness generates some kind of pineal signal. Section of neural pathways to the pineal produces the same effects as pinealectomy. These findings indicate that pineal secretions can affect the timing of puberty, and most data point to melatonin as the most important pineal mediator of this effect (see later under Secretions of the Pineal Gland). Melatonin may "set" the SC nucleus cycling mechanism, this area being uniquely rich in melatonin receptors.[321] In humans exposure to bright light at certain time intervals, a procedure known to suppress melatonin secretion, can reset the internal clock mechanism[323] (see earlier under Endocrine Rhythms).

On the other hand, a role for the pineal in regulating the onset of puberty in the human is not established. On the basis of animal work, it would be anticipated that if melatonin suppresses onset of puberty, levels in blood would fall with the onset of puberty. Some[527] but not all[528] studies have shown that melatonin secretion falls as anticipated. An alternative hypothesis is that melatonin reduction at puberty is instead *secondary* to gonadal steroid secretion. For example, in one study of delayed puberty the excretion of melatonin

Tryptophan

5-Hydroxytryptophan

Serotonin

N-Acetylserotonin

Melatonin

Figure 5–54. Biosynthesis of melatonin from tryptophan in the pineal gland. Step 1 is catalyzed by tryptophan hydroxylase; step 2 by aromatic-L-amino acid decarboxylase; step 3 by N-acetylating enzyme; and step 4 by hydroxyindole-O-methyltransferase. (From Wurtman RJ, Axelrod J, Kelly DE. Biochemistry of the pineal gland. In: The Pineal. New York: Academic, 1968: 47–75.)

in urine fell when puberty was initiated by treatment with LHRH.[537]

Other actions of the pineal, as inferred from removal studies in animals, are less clear-cut. Changes in PRL, GH, adrenal, and thyroid function have been observed inconsistently.[535]

SECRETIONS OF THE PINEAL GLAND. Biologically active substances in the pineal include biogenic amines (norepinephrine, serotonin, histamine, melatonin and other related indolamines, dopamine, and octopamine) and peptides (LHRH, TRH, somatostatin, and vasotocin, which is an analogue of oxytocin).[520, 525, 536] The pineal also contains the inhibitory neurotransmitter GABA, a protein that resembles neurophysin, and a protein termed epiphysin. In addition, other as-yet uncharacterized peptide factors may mediate the gonadotropin-inhibitory actions of the pineal.

Melatonin was the first biologically active compound that was identified in the pineal gland. This discovery was the result of an effort to isolate from mammalian pineal glands the factor that caused lightening of amphibian skin.[538] Melatonin is synthesized from tryptophan within pineal parenchymal cells (Fig. 5–54).[518–522] The formation of N-acetylserotonin from serotonin (by serotonin-N-acetyltransferase) is the principal rate-limiting step in formation of melatonin, but the final synthetic reaction involving O-methylation by hydroxyindole-O-methyltransferase may also be rate-limiting.[519–522] Hydroxyindole-O-methyltransferase is also present in the retina, the harderian glands (orbital structures of unknown function in rodents), and red blood cells.[520, 536] The extent to which nonpineal sources contribute to melatonin blood levels is unknown, but the presence of this enzyme outside the pineal may explain the fact that melatonin excretion persists at about 25% of basal levels after pinealectomy.[520]

During the night (with lights off), when melatonin secretion is highest, the content of melatonin in the pineal gland is high and that of serotonin (its precursor) is low. When melatonin secretion is high, the concentration of N-acetyltransferase is high; the reverse is also true. Changes in N-acetyltransferase content are dramatic—increases of 25- to 100-fold are evident within a few minutes of light deprivation. Administration of beta-adrenergic blocking agents or exposure to light causes a sharp decline in enzyme activity (half-life of 3.5 min). Beta-adrenergic activation is mediated by cAMP and a cascade of protein transcription and translation.[519–522]

FACTORS THAT INFLUENCE PINEAL SECRETION. Activation of the sympathetic nervous system by immobilization or hypoglycemic stress can increase the concentration of melatonin-synthesizing enzymes in the pineal and thereby enhance the secretion of melatonin. Administration of L-dopa, a precursor of L-dopamine, also increases melatonin synthesis in rats.

Melatonin is released into the general circulation (Fig. 5–55).[520, 530, 531, 537, 539, 540] In humans and animals, secretion is activated almost immediately after exposure to darkness and is stopped on exposure to light. There also are occasional bursts of secretion that are unrelated to changes in lighting or stress.[540] The rhythm in melatonin excretion in urine can be entrained by the light-dark cycle and by other factors such as sleep, diet, posture, and activity.[521] Characteristic rhythms are unaffected by sleep deprivation or by short-term exposure to sustained light, but a group of women trained to sleep at odd hours were capable of shifting melatonin-secretory patterns.

The route by which melatonin reaches the pituitary and hypothalamus (its targets) is unclear. Anatomical study of the mammalian pineal gland led Kappers and colleagues[517]

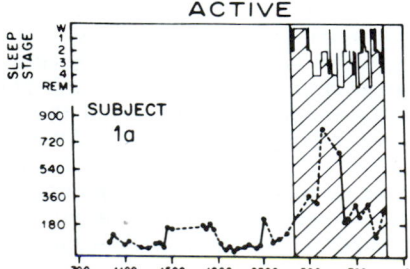

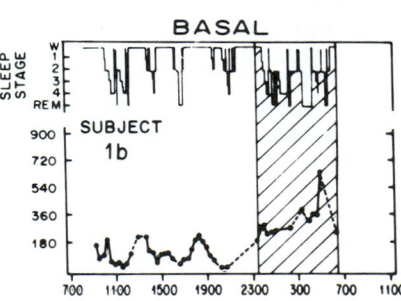

Figure 5–55. Pattern of melatonin secretion in a normal subject when active and at rest. The condition of lights off, striped area, brought about a release of melatonin. Note also that spontaneous release of melatonin also takes place. To convert melatonin values to picomoles per liter, multiply by 4.5. (From U Weinberg, RD D'Eletto, ED Weitzman, et al., Circulating melatonin in man: episodic secretion throughout the light-dark cycle, J Clin Endocrinol Metab, 48, 114–118, 1979, © by The Endocrine Society.)

to conclude that all secretions must leave by way of venous drainage into the peripheral circulation. They pointed out that there is no direct conduit from the pineal to the third ventricle and that the pineal, although partly located in the subarachnoid space, has a fairly thick capsule that would not favor direct subarachnoid release. On the other hand, anatomical differences exist among species, and in primates the pineal forms part of the roof of the third ventricle. In calves and children the concentration of melatonin in CSF is higher than that in blood, but in adult humans and monkeys the reverse is true.[520, 522] These findings suggest that in adult primates melatonin enters the CSF from blood. The relative concentrations are attributable to the distribution of a melatonin-binding protein, which has a higher level in blood than in CSF.

When injected into the hypothalamus, melatonin inhibits gonadotropin secretion, but a direct effect on the pituitary has also been shown.[541] Thus melatonin may act on both hypothalamus and pituitary to inhibit gonadotropin secretion. Melatonin receptors are very dense in the SC nucleus. They are also present in the ovary.

Failure to demonstrate that melatonin injection duplicates the effects of functional activation of the pineal has led to efforts to identify other inhibitory substances. Pineal extracts that are free of melatonin produce gonadal inhibition in a number of assay systems.[523, 533] Vasotocin, reported to be a constituent of mammalian pineal glands, is a candidate inhibitory hormone for gonadotropins, but it has not been proved that the doses used to produce an effect are equivalent to the levels found under physiological circumstances. Vasotocin is a normal constituent of the posterior lobe of the pituitary in birds, but its presence in mammals has been strongly challenged.[535] Pineal extracts from which both melatonin and vasotocin have been removed still retain potent gonad-inhibitory effects. Thus the nature of pineal gonadotropin-inhibitory factors (if not melatonin) remains uncertain.

Serotonin is synthesized in pineal parenchymal cells and is taken up by sympathetic nerve endings in the gland. Dopamine and norepinephrine are also present in sympathetic nerve endings. The physiological function of these and other biologically active substances in the pineal is unknown. It is likewise unknown whether TRH, somatostatin, and LHRH, which are present in the pineal of some species of animals, are secreted by this structure into the blood.

EFFECTS OF MELATONIN IN HUMANS. Melatonin administration to normal subjects causes a lowering of plasma LH levels and suppresses GH secretion. It induces sleepiness; changes in the electroencephalogram (mainly an increase in the number of alpha waves); increases in rapid eye movement sleep; and, in a few cases, "a sensation of well-being and moderate elation."[542, 543] Relatively large amounts may produce headaches and abdominal cramps. Because melatonin is secreted in response to darkness, an attractive (although unproven) hypothesis is that it contributes to drowsiness when the lights are turned down. When administered to depressed patients, melatonin increases self-ratings of depression and, paradoxically, increases the degree of insomnia.[542] The administration of melatonin by mouth has been reported to ameliorate jet lag in air travelers,[544] presumably by resetting the internal SC time clock. The relevance of any of these findings to normal or abnormal brain function is unknown. Melatonin has no beneficial effect on patients with depression, schizophrenia, parkinsonism, or Huntington chorea. However, melatonin levels are said to be low in depressed patients, possibly a reflection of decreased adrenergic "tone."[542] A link has also been reported between pineal function and the course of experimental

breast cancer in mice,[545] but the physiological basis of such a response is unknown.

CALCIFICATION OF THE PINEAL GLAND. The pineal is important as a marker of the midline of the brain because it becomes calcified. Calcification begins early in childhood and becomes increasingly evident radiographically, beginning in the second decade of life.[513] The prevalence of calcification is different among several racial groups. Calcification has no known effect on pineal function, as inferred from the fact that the concentrations of characteristic enzymes of the pineal (hydroxy-O-methyltransferase, monoamine oxidase, and histamine N-methyltransferase) are relatively constant throughout life. An apatite form of calcium phosphate crystals is laid down in a matrix of ground substance secreted by pinealocytes to form nodules termed acervuli. Calcium deposition may be related to cell function because section of the nerves to the pineal of the hamster reduces the growth rate of acervuli.[523]

Circumventricular Organs

SUBCOMMISSURAL ORGAN. The SCO has persisted throughout evolutionary development from fish to human.[512] It is a collection of columnar cells lining the roof of the caudal end of the third ventricle, where it enters the aqueduct connecting the third and fourth ventricles. This region is beneath the habenular commissure and is adjacent to the pineal recess (to the apex of which is attached the pineal gland). Cells of the SCO differ from the usual ependymal cell in being taller and containing secretory granules that stain selectively with various histochemical reagents. A peculiarity of the SCO is that the cells secrete a relatively insoluble substance into the lumen of the aqueduct. This secretion forms a cord-like structure in some species (Reissner fiber) that is extruded through the aqueduct, the fourth ventricle, and the spinal cord lumen to terminate in the caudal spinal canal.[546]

Reissner fiber contains mucopolysaccharides and apparently breaks down at its termination in the sacral spinal cord, but in some species, such as the rat, the tip of the fiber forms a coil much as a rope would under similar mechanical circumstances. In humans the intracellular secretory granules are identifiable in the SCO, but Reissner fiber is absent. The SCO secretion in humans is therefore presumed to be more soluble than that in other animals and is absorbed directly from the CSF. In addition to drainage into the CSF, which is characteristic of ependyma in general, there may be drainage into regional capillaries. The SCO has no direct nerve supply.

SUBFORNICAL ORGAN. The SFO is another neurohemal ependymal structure[512, 513, 547] that contains both neurosecretory neurons and modified ependymal cells (see Fig. 5–53). It is located at the junction between the lamina terminalis and the tela choroidea of the third ventricle. Its name is derived from its location under the fornices. The neurons of the SFO receive cholinergic innervation from the midbrain and contain several neuropeptides, including angiotensin II[548] and atriopeptin.[549] Its structure suggests that it is a neurosecretory gland. The intensity of staining of the neurosecretory material is modified by anesthesia, stress, hyperosmotic challenge, alcohol injection, and estrogen administration. The SFO plays an important role in salt and water regulation. Injection of angiotensin II or hypertonic saline into the SFO leads to release of AVP and stimulation of drinking. The effects of angiotensin II are potentiated by saline. The endothelium of this region (as in other parts of the brain) contains the enzyme that converts angiotensin I to angiotensin II, and local neurons contain mRNA coding for angiotensinogen, the precursor to angiotensin I.[550] Angiotensinergic neurons project to the paraventricular nucleus, thus providing a neural pathway by which stimuli arising in the SFO can regulate AVP secretion. The SFO is an important sensor that regulates and integrates drinking and AVP release in the defense of serum osmolality.

ORGANUM VASCULOSUM OF THE LAMINA TERMINALIS. The OVLT (supraoptic crest) lies in the midline of the lamina terminalis of the third ventricle, between the anterior commissure and the optic chiasm[512, 513] (see Fig. 5–53). Its external surface is in contact with the CSF of the prechiasmatic cistern, and its internal surface is in contact with the CSF of the brain. Large molecules are prevented from entering the CSF by the presence of tight junctions between the ependymal cells, a finding analogous to that of the median eminence. The structure has its own arterial and venous circulations independent from those of other circumventricular organs. Large molecules readily penetrate the OVLT, which indicates that the blood-brain barrier is absent here. The OVLT is richly innervated by nerve endings containing LHRH, somatostatin, and neurophysin. The region of the OVLT in the rat is the site of estrogen receptor neurons, and direct application of estrogen or electric stimulation at this site is capable of stimulating ovulation through LHRH-containing neurons that project to the median eminence. Injection of LHRH in the same area is reported to increase sexual drive in hypophysectomized and normal rats. This region therefore may be involved in regulating behavior in the rat. Its function in primates is unknown. The OVLT may also be the site of entry of interleukin 1 (IL 1) into thermoregulatory regions of the brain.[551]

NEUROENDOCRINE DISEASE

Depending on the site of the lesion and its rate of development, disease of the hypothalamus can result in abnormal mental function, disturbed visceral regulation, abnormal behavior, and altered pituitary function.[18, 21, 33, 552-557] Hypothalamic lesions can cause pituitary insufficiency by damaging the tuberohypophyseal neurons. Clinical manifestations of pituitary insufficiency related to hypothalamic dysfunction are generally similar to those related to primary pituitary lesions, with some exceptions. Decreased secretion is the usual finding, but a hypothalamic deficit may be manifested as a hypersecretory state because of the loss of a usual inhibitory control. Examples of the latter occurrence are hypersecretion of PRL after damage to the PIF control system and precocious puberty caused by the loss of normal restraint over gonadotropin maturation. Deficits in inhibitory control of the neurohypophysis at a supranuclear level can lead to SIADH (see earlier and Chapter 7). More subtle abnormalities in secretion may take place owing to selective impairment of the control system. For example, loss of the normal circadian rhythm of ACTH secretion may occur before loss of pituitary-adrenal secretory reserve,[558] and paradoxical responses to the usual physiological stimuli sometimes occur. Because there is no direct way to measure hypophyseotropic hormone secretion in humans and because most pituitary hormones are regulated by complex, multilayered controls, the measurement of pituitary hormones in blood does not necessarily give a meaningful picture of events at hypothalamic and higher levels.

The clinician should approach hypothalamic or pituitary disease by considering three important aspects: the anatomical extent of the lesion, the physiological impact of the lesion, and the specific etiology. All elements must be taken into account in assessment and management of the patient.

The etiology of hypothalamic disorders is summarized in Tables 5–13 and 5–14, and symptoms and signs of hypothalamic disease are summarized in Table 5–15. Disorders of the hypothalamic-pituitary unit result from lesions at several levels of function. At the lowest level, defects can arise from

TABLE 5–13. Etiology of Hypothalamic Disease by Age

Premature Infants and Neonates
Intraventricular hemorrhage
Meningitis: bacterial
Tumors: glioma, hemangioma
Trauma
Hydrocephalus, kernicterus
1 mo–2 y
Tumors
  Glioma, especially optic glioma
  Histiocytosis X
  Hemangioma
Hydrocephalus
Meningitis
Familial disorders
  Laurence-Moon-Biedl
  Prader-Labhart-Willi
2–10 y
Neoplasms
  Craniopharyngioma
  Glioma, dysgerminoma, hamartoma, histiocytosis X, leukemia
  Ganglioneuroma, ependymoma, medulloblastoma
Meningitis
  Bacterial
  Tuberculous
Encephalitis
  Viral
  Exanthematous demyelinating
Familial
  Diabetes insipidus
X-ray therapy
Diabetic ketoacidosis
10–25 y
Tumors
  Craniopharyngioma
  Glioma, hamartoma, dysgerminoma
  Histiocytosis X, leukemia
  Dermoid, lipoma, neuroblastoma
Trauma
Vascular
  Subarachnoid hemorrhage
  Aneurysm
  Arteriovenous malformation
Inflammatory disease
  Meningitis
  Encephalitis
  Sarcoidosis
  Tuberculosis
Structural brain defect
  Chronic hydrocephalus
  Increased intracranial pressure
25–50 y
Nutritional: Wernicke disease
Tumors
  Glioma, lymphoma, meningioma
  Craniopharyngioma, pituitary tumors
  Angioma, plasmacytoma, colloid cysts
  Ependymoma, sarcoma, histiocytosis X
Inflammatory disease
  Sarcoidosis
  Tuberculosis, viral encephalitis
Subarachnoid hemorrhage, vascular aneurysm, arteriovenous malformation
Damage from pituitary radiation therapy
50 y and Older
Nutritional: Wernicke disease
Tumors
  Sarcoma, glioblastoma, lymphoma
  Meningioma, colloid cysts, ependymoma, pituitary tumors
Vascular disease
  Infarct, subarachnoid hemorrhage
  Pituitary apoplexy
Inflammation: encephalitis, sarcoidosis, meningitis
X-ray therapy for nasopharygeal carcinoma

Adapted from Plum F, Van Uitert R. Nonendocrine diseases and disorders of the hypothalamus. In: Reichlin S, Baldessarini RJ, Martin JB, eds. The Hypothalamus. Vol 56. New York: Raven, 1978: 415–473.

TABLE 5–14. Etiology of Endocrine Syndromes of Hypothalamic Origin

Hypophyseotropic Hormone Deficiency
  Surgical pituitary stalk section
  Basilar meningitis and granuloma, sarcoidosis, tuberculosis, sphenoid osteomyelitis, eosinophilic granuloma
  Craniopharyngioma
  Hypothalamic tumor
    Infundibuloma
    Teratoma (ectopic pinealoma)
    Neuroglial tumor, particularly astrocytoma
  Maternal deprivation syndrome, psychosocial dwarfism
  Isolated GHRH deficiency
  Hypothalamic hypothyroidism
  Panhypophyseotropic failure
Disorders of Regulation of LHRH Secretion
  Female
    Precocious puberty
    Delayed puberty
    Neurogenic amenorrhea
    Pseudocyesis
    Anorexia nervosa
    "Functional" amenorrhea
    "Functional" oligomenorrhea
    Drug-induced amenorrhea
  Male
    Precocious puberty
    Fröhlich syndrome
    Olfactory-genital dysplasia (Kallmann syndrome)
Disorders of Regulation of PRL-Regulating Factors
  Tumor
  Sarcoidosis
  Drug-induced
  Reflex
  Herpes zoster of chest wall
  Post-thoracotomy
  Nipple manipulation
  Spinal cord tumor
  "Psychogenic"
  Hypothyroidism
  Carbon dioxide narcosis
Disorders of Regulation of CRH
  Paroxysmal ACTH discharge (Wolff syndrome)
  Loss of circadian variation
  Depression

destruction of the pituitary (as by tumor, infarct, or inflammation) or from a genetically determined deficiency of a particular pituitary cell, as in rare cases of isolated FSH or GH deficiency. The selective loss of thyroid hormone receptors in the pituitary can give rise to increased TSH secretion and thyrotoxicosis. At a higher anatomical level, disorders may arise through disruption of the stalk–median eminence vascular contact zone, the stalk itself, or the nerve terminals of the tuberohypophyseal system. Such destruction of the final common pathway of anterior pituitary regulation occurs after surgical stalk section, in tumors of the stalk region, and in some inflammatory diseases. At a still higher level, that of input into the tuberoinfundibular system, tonic

TABLE 5–15. Symptoms and Signs of Hypothalamic Disease*

Symptoms and Signs	No. of Cases
Sexual abnormalities (hypogonadism or precocious puberty)	43
Diabetes insipidus	21
Psychic disturbance	21
Obesity or hyperphagia	20
Somnolence	18
Emaciation, anorexia	15
Thermodysregulation	13
Sphincter disturbance	5

*From a review of 60 autopsy-proven cases.
Adapted from HG Bauer, Endocrine and other clinical manifestations of hypothalamic disease: a survey of 60 cases with autopsies, J Clin Endocrinol Metab, 14, 13–31, 1954, © by The Endocrine Society.

inhibitory and excitatory inputs can be lost, as manifested by a loss of circadian rhythms or development of precocious puberty. At the highest level of control, symbolic stress and emotional disorders can activate the stress response and suppress normal gonadotropin secretion (e.g., psychogenic amenorrhea)[559] or inhibit GH secretion (e.g., psychosocial dwarfism)[560] (see Chapter 21). These various levels of deficit are considered in the following section. Intrinsic disease of the anterior pituitary is reviewed in Chapter 6, and disturbances in neurohypophyseal function are discussed in Chapter 7.

Pituitary Isolation Syndrome

Destructive lesions of the pituitary stalk, such as rupture after head injury, surgical transection, or spontaneous disease (tumor, granuloma), produce a characteristic pattern of pituitary dysfunction. Diabetes insipidus (DI) develops in approximately 80% of cases, the crucial factor in its occurrence being the level at which the stalk has been sectioned.[561, 562] If the stalk is cut close to the hypothalamus, DI is almost always produced, whereas if the section is low on the stalk the incidence is less. The extent to which neurohypophyseal nerve terminals in the upper stalk are preserved determines the clinical course. The classic triphasic syndrome of initial polyuria, followed by normal water control and then by AVP deficiency,[563] occurring over a period of approximately 1 wk to 10 d, is seen in about half the patients.[561, 562, 564] The sequence is attributed to an initial loss of neurogenic control of the neural lobe, followed by autolysis of the neural lobe with release of AVP into the circulation, and finally by complete loss of AVP. DI may develop after stalk injury without an overt transitional phase. Injury to the neurohypophysis or stalk, such as may occur during the course of surgical exploration of the pituitary, can sometimes give rise to transient SIADH. When DI occurs after head injury or operative trauma, recovery can take place even after months or years.[562] Full expression of polyuria requires adequate cortisol levels; if ACTH is deficient, AVP deficiency may be present with minimal polyuria.

Although head injury, granulomas, and tumors are the most common causes of acquired DI, a proportion of cases develop in the absence of any clear-cut etiological factor.[556, 565] Some cases may be due to autoimmune disease of the hypothalamus, as suggested by the finding of autoantibodies to neurohypophyseal cells in 11 of 30 cases of "idiopathic DI" in one series.[566] In a few cases, atrophy of the supraopticohypophyseal cells was reported at autopsy.[557, 565]

DI in humans can be part of a hereditary disorder. An animal model of this disorder is the Brattleboro rat, in which an autosomal recessive genetic defect leads to defective production of AVP but not of oxytocin.[567, 568] The defect has been identified by genetic recombinant techniques as a frameshift in coding of the gene sequence.[568]

Menses cease after either stalk section[569] or hypophysectomy. Unlike the situation after hypophysectomy, gonadotropins may still be detectable in urine after stalk section. Plasma hydroxysteroid levels and urinary excretion of 17-hydroxysteroids and 17-ketosteroids fall after both hypophysectomy and stalk section, but the change is slower after stalk section.[570, 571] A transient increase may occur in adrenocortical secretion, which is postulated to be due to release of preformed stores of ACTH. The ACTH response to the lowering of blood corticoid levels is markedly reduced in pituitary isolation syndrome, but release of ACTH after stress may be retained in some patients,[572] possibly the result of release into the blood of CRH from other parts of the brain. CRH has a wide distribution in the extrahypothalamic brain and in the gastrointestinal tract (see earlier). Thyroid function is also reduced by stalk section and approaches the deficits observed after hypophysectomy.[573, 574] GH secretion falls in similar fashion.[573]

The most striking difference between patients with section of the pituitary stalk and those with hypophysectomy relates to the secretion of PRL. Stalk-sectioned monkeys[575] and humans[576] consistently have hyperprolactinemia, and some develop galactorrhea.[576, 577] Pituitary PRL responses to hypoglycemia and to TRH are blunted.[576] Blunted PRL responses to hypoglycemia are due in part to loss of neural connections with the hypothalamus. However, because the poor response to direct stimulation of the pituitary with TRH is also blunted, the impaired response cannot be attributed solely to loss of hypothalamic control. PRL-secretory dynamics and responses to dopamine agonists and antagonists in pituitary isolation syndrome are indistinguishable from those in the majority of patients with prolactinomas.[576] Spontaneously arising disease in the region of the median eminence also causes the stalk interruption syndrome, and a partial interruption may result from distortions of this region in the empty sella syndrome.[576, 578]

Anterior pituitary failure after stalk section is due in part to loss of specific neural and vascular links to the hypothalamus and in part to variable degrees of pituitary infarction.[579, 580] The pattern of cell damage is related to the distribution of minor blood vessels that enter the pituitary below the level of section.

Hypophyseotropic Hormone Deficiency

Selective pituitary failure can arise from deficiency of specific pituitary cell types or of one or more hypothalamic hormones. Deficiency of TRH secretion gives rise to the syndrome of hypothalamic hypothyroidism, also called tertiary hypothyroidism. This condition may be seen in any form of hypothalamic disease and rarely also as an isolated defect of hypothalamic function.[33, 555, 581, 582] Hypothalamic causes can be distinguished from pituitary causes of TSH deficiency by a consideration of the anatomical site of the lesion, by the pattern of other pituitary deficits, and, to a limited extent, by the TRH test.[581, 582] The typical pituitary response to TRH administration in patients with TRH deficiency is an enhanced and somewhat delayed peak (Fig. 5–56), whereas the response to TRH in patients with intrinsic pituitary TSH failure is subnormal.[582] The hypothalamic response has been attributed to an associated GH deficiency

that sensitizes the pituitary to TRH,[583] but GH also affects peripheral T_4 metabolism, which may alter pituitary responses as well.[584] Deficient TRH secretion leads to altered TSH synthesis by the pituitary, including changes in glycosylation. Poorly glycosylated TSH has low biological activity; dissociation of bioassayable from immunoassayable TSH can lead to the apparently paradoxical finding of normal or even elevated levels of TSH in hypothalamic hypothyroidism.[585] In actual practice the responses in hypothalamic and pituitary disease overlap substantially. Patterns in an individual case, therefore, cannot be used in the absence of other data to classify the type of TSH failure. Persistent failure to demonstrate responses to TRH is good evidence for the presence of intrinsic pituitary disease, but a response does not mean that the pituitary is normal. In summary, the diagnosis of true hypothalamic hypothyroidism is difficult to establish, and some cases in the literature may be misclassified.

Isolated LHRH deficiency is the most common hypophyseotropic hormone deficiency. In Kallmann syndrome (gonadotropin deficiency with associated hyposmia),[586–591] hereditary agenesis of the olfactory lobe is the major neuroanatomical defect. Magnetic resonance imaging scans can be used to document this abnormality in living patients.[592] Defective development of the LHRH neuronal system appears to arise from defective migration of the LHRH-containing neurons from the olfactory nasal epithelium in early embryological life.[593] Unlike the mouse model of isolated deficiency, the amino acid sequence of LHRH in Kallmann syndrome is normal.[594]

Malformations of the midline structures, such as absent septum pellucidum, are also associated with defects in gonadotropin regulation, the most common of which is hypogonadotropic hypogonadism,[595] but precocious puberty has also been observed.[596] The LHRH test often gives seemingly inappropriate results in patients with hypothalamic hypogonadism.[597–600] One would predict that such patients would show normal gonadotropin secretory responses, because the pituitary itself is preserved. In fact almost all patients show little or no response to an initial test dose, and only after repeated injection does pituitary response return to normal (see Fig. 5–48). This slow response has been attributed to the loss of LHRH receptors after long-term LHRH deficiency and to the fact that LHRH sensitizes the pituitary to LHRH. In gonadotropin deficiency related to intrinsic pituitary disease, the response to LHRH may be absent or

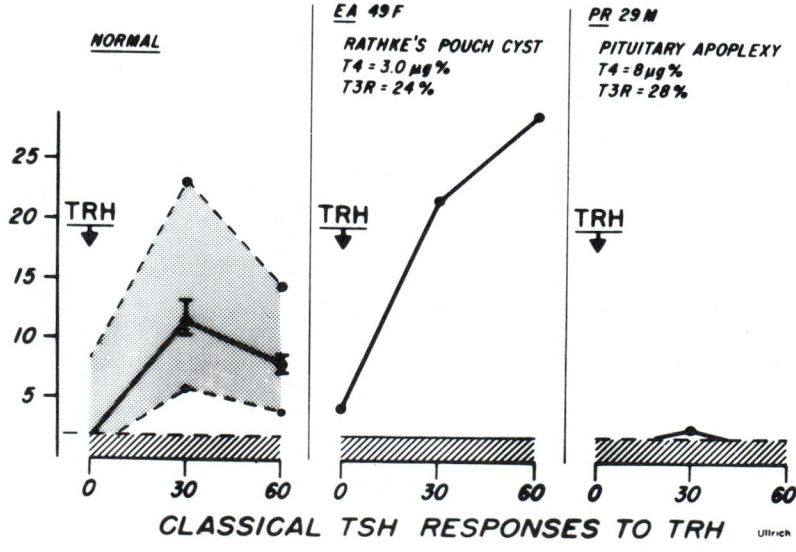

NORMAL

EA 49 F
RATHKE'S POUCH CYST
T4 = 3.0 µg %
T3R = 24 %

PR 29 M
PITUITARY APOPLEXY
T4 = 8 µg %
T3R = 28 %

CLASSICAL TSH RESPONSES TO TRH

Ullrich

Figure 5–56. Typical pituitary response to TRH administration in patients with hypothalamic-pituitary disease that has caused hypothyroidism. If there is intrinsic pituitary damage, the response is abnormally low. If there is hypothalamic damage, the response is normal or exaggerated. It must be emphasized that some patients with hypothalamic disease may not respond to TRH and that some patients with pituitary disease may respond to TRH. (From Jackson IMD. Diagnostic tests for the evaluation of pituitary tumors. In: Jackson IMD, Reichlin S, eds. The Pituitary Adenoma. New York: Plenum, 1980: 219–238.)

may be within the normal range. Because of these variations in response, a single injection of LHRH does not constitute an adequate means of distinguishing between hypothalamic and pituitary disorders. Prolonged infusions or repeated injections of LHRH agonists or gonadal steroid priming, on the other hand, may lead to more precise diagnosis.[600]

GHRH deficiency appears to underlie the GH deficit in most patients with idiopathic dwarfism, which agrees with the observation that most children with idiopathic hypopituitarism show normal pituitary responses to TRH,[601] LHRH, and GHRH,[602] as do patients with hypothalamic disease of established cause (Fig. 5–57).[603] The frequent association of hypophyseotropic deficiency with abnormal electroencephalographic results and a history of birth trauma suggests an analogy with other forms of birth injury.[604] Furthermore, magnetic resonance imaging scans show that most children with idiopathic GH deficiency have a torn pituitary stalk,[605] which is presumed evidence for birth trauma as an etiological factor. GH secretion is the most vulnerable of all anterior pituitary functions to damage of the pituitary stalk (and to radiation[606]).

Deficiency of PIF secretion leads to hyperprolactinemia.[573, 576, 607] Although PRL levels are elevated by lesions that isolate the pituitary from the hypothalamus, values of serum PRL are usually less than 56 μg/L and rarely as high as 120 μg/L. Adrenal insufficiency is a common manifestation of hypothalamic disease, attributed in some cases to CRH deficiency[608] or to isolated autoimmune destruction of adrenotropes.[608a] The usefulness of the CRH test in distinguishing hypothalamic from pituitary failure is not established.

Hypophyseotropic Hormone Hypersecretion

With the availability of immunohistochemical techniques for identification of hypophyseotropic peptides in histological preparations, it is now known that pituitary hypersecretion can be induced (albeit rarely) by neurogenic tumors of the hypothalamus. Most common are the LHRH-secreting hamartomas discussed later as a cause of precocious puberty,[609] CRH-secreting gangliocytomas that can cause Cushing syndrome,[610] and GHRH-secreting gangliocytomas of the hypothalamus that cause acromegaly.[611] Although they do not arise from the hypothalamus, paraneoplastic syndromes can also cause pituitary hypersecretion, as with CRH-secreting tumors[612] and GHRH-secreting tumors of the bronchi and pancreas.[159, 220]

Neuroendocrine Disorders of Gonadotropin Regulation

PRECOCIOUS PUBERTY. Of all hypothalamic-pituitary disorders, those involving gonadotropin secretion are the most varied and complex. The term *precocious puberty* is used when normal pituitary-gonadal function appears at an abnormally early age.[613, 614] In boys this means the onset of androgen secretion and spermatogenesis before the age of 9 or 10, and in girls the onset of estrogen secretion and cyclic ovarian activity before the age of 8. Neurogenic causes of precocious puberty are considered in this section. True precocious puberty always arises from disturbed neural function, which may or may not have an identifiable structural basis. Pseudoprecocious puberty refers to premature sexual development that is due to excessive secretion of androgens or estrogenic hormones by tumors (both gonadal and extragonadal) and is discussed in Chapters 12, 13, and 22.

Idiopathic Sexual Precocity. This category is the largest of true precocious puberty. Familial occurrence is uncommon, but there is a hereditary form that is largely confined to males. In one study[604] girls with true precocity were found to have a high incidence of abnormal electroencephalograms and behavioral disturbances, which suggests the presence of underlying or associated brain damage. In another report idiopathic precocious puberty was unaccompanied by brain changes.[613] The pathogenesis of this disorder is obscure, but the crucial factor may be related to hypothalamic development. Many cases previously thought to be idiopathic are due to hypothalamic hamartomas. For example, in the series of Pescovitz and co-workers,[609] 14 of 95 cases in girls and 10 of 34 cases in boys were due to this disorder (see later for further discussion of hamartomas). This conclusion was based on the use of high-resolution computed tomographic scanning.

Neurogenic Precocious Puberty. The site of hypothalamic lesions that influence the timing of puberty in the human is not well established. Approximately two thirds of the cases in which pathological correlations can be made have destruction of the posterior hypothalamus,[499] but by the time most patients come to autopsy, damage is extensive. Precocious puberty in the rat is produced by localized lesions in the preoptic hypothalamus. Electric stimulation of the amygdala delays puberty, which suggests that in the rodent the timing of puberty is determined by a dual control system—hypothalamic and extrahypothalamic. Specific lesions recognized to cause precocity include craniopharyngioma (although delayed puberty is more common), astrocytoma, pineal tumors, encephalitis, miliary tuberculosis, tuberous sclerosis, the Sturge-Weber syndrome, porencephaly, craniostenosis, microcephaly, hydrocephalus, and Tay-Sachs disease.

Hamartoma of the hypothalamus is an exception to the generalization that tumors of the brain cause precocious puberty by destructive effects on regions that normally suppress gonadotropin secretion (although occasionally hamartomas can cause hypothalamic damage). A hamartoma is a tumor-like collection of normal nerve tissue lodged in

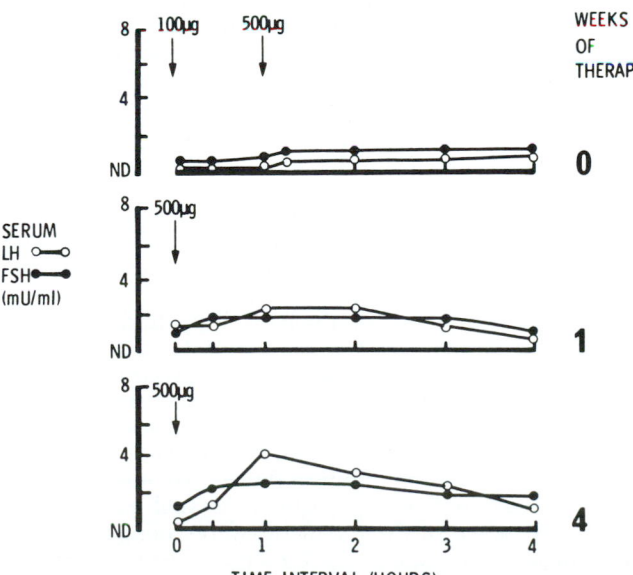

Figure 5–57. Demonstration of increasing responsivity of gonadotropin secretion to LHRH after repeated administration of the hormone in a prepubertal boy with a craniopharyngioma. The hormone was given subcutaneously, 500 μg twice daily for 4 wk, and responsiveness was tested with intravenous doses. There was little or no response initially, but after a period of treatment, responsivity gradually rose. (From Mortimer CH. Gonadotropin-releasing hormone. In: Martini L, Besser GM, eds. Clinical Neuroendocrinology. New York: Academic, 1977: 213–236.)

an abnormal location. One type of hypothalamic hamartoma consists of a sharply encapsulated nodule of nerve tissue attached to the posterior hypothalamus at a point between the anterior portion of the mamillary body and the posterior region of the tuber cinereum.[615] The hypothalamic hamartoma grows into the cisternal space between the cerebral peduncles, adapts to the pyramidal shape of the cisterna, and may produce precocious puberty before other neural effects occur. Until the use of high-resolution scanning techniques,[609] tumors of this type were considered to be rare, fewer than 50 having been reported up to 1972. But miniature hamartomatous nodular formations of the tuber cinereum are discovered at autopsy. As noted earlier, hamartomas are recognized with some frequency in patients previously considered to have idiopathic disease. Precocious puberty is believed to occur when the cells of the hamartoma make connections with the median eminence and thus serve as an "accessory hypothalamus."[616, 617] Bierich[613] found LHRH in the CSF of three such patients and hypothesized that the tumors may secrete LHRH. This hypothesis has been supported by direct demonstration of LHRH peptidergic nerve endings in excised hamartomas.[616, 617] Secretion by ectopically placed LHRH peptidergic neurons is probably not subject to the normal restraining influences of the anterior hypothalamus, and early pubertal development is likely the consequence of unrestrained LHRH secretion.

The manifestations in patients with hamartomas are similar to those of other known cerebral causes of precocity. Hamartomas occur in both sexes and may occur in infants as young as 3 mo. In the past most cases were thought to be fatal before the age of 20, although one patient surviving into the seventh decade has been reported. Now it is recognized that these lesions may cause no brain damage and need not be excised in many cases.[618] The interpeduncular fossa of the brain is difficult to approach, and surgical experience is somewhat limited. Early in the course of illness, precocity and seizures may occur; the epilepsy may present as "brief, repetitive, steretyped attacks of laughter,"[619] which may provide a clue to the disease. Late in the disease, hypothalamic damage can cause severe neurological damage.

Hypothyroidism. Hypothyroidism is considered to be a possible cause of neurogenic precocious puberty without proof that the disordered gonadotropin secretion is due to hypothalamic disturbance.[620, 621] This condition, sometimes associated with hyperprolactinemia and galactorrhea, is a "functional" disorder of gonadotropin regulation that is reversible with thyroid hormone replacement. One explanation proposed is that there is cross-reactivity in negative feedback control of TSH, LH, and FSH, which are all glycoprotein hormones secreted by basophilic cells.[620] According to this view, low levels of thyroid hormone would simultaneously activate TSH, LH, and FSH release. Alternatively, hypothyroidism could cause hypothalamic encephalopathy, with resultant deficits in the usual tonic-suppressing actions of the hypothalamus on gonadotropin release. The high PRL levels that sometimes accompany this disorder may be due to a deficiency in PIF secretion, or to increased secretion of TRH and/or to increased sensitivity of the pituitary to tonic TRH secretion.

Tumors of the Pineal Gland. Pineal tumors are uncommon, composing 0.2 to 1% of brain neoplasms in the United States and 4% of brain tumors in Japan.[622, 623] The various types of lesions that are found in the pineal region (including the posterior third ventricle) are summarized in Table 5–16. The term *pinealoma* refers to a tumor of the pineal parenchymal cell and can be a pineoblastoma or pineocytoma, according to its degree of differentiation.[624] In one series of pineal tumors, only 9 of 53 were pinealomas; there were 13 glial tumors, including astrocytomas and glioblas-

TABLE 5–16. Classification of Tumors of Pineal Region

A. Germ Cell Tumors
1. Germinoma
   a. Posterior third ventricle and pineal lesions
   b. Anterior third ventricle, suprasellar or intrasellar lesions
   c. Combined lesions in anterior and posterior third ventricle, apparently noncontiguous, with or without foci of cystic or solid teratoma
2. Teratoma
   a. Evidencing growth along two or three germ lines in varying degrees of differentiation
   b. Dermoid and epidermoid cysts with or without solid foci of teratoma
   c. Histologically malignant forms with or without differentiated foci of benign, solid, or cystic teratoma—teratocarcinoma, chorioepithelioma, embryonal carcinoma (endodermal-sinus tumor or yolk-sac carcinoma), combinations of these with or without foci of germinoma, chemodectoma

B. Pineal Parenchymal Tumors
1. Pinealocytes
   a. Pineocytoma
   b. Pineoblastoma
   c. Ganglioglioma and chemodectoma
   d. Mixed forms exhibiting transitions between these
2. Glia
   a. Astrocytoma
   b. Ependymoma
   c. Mixed forms and other less frequent gliomas (e.g., glioblastoma, oligodendroglioma)

C. Tumors of Supporting or Adjacent Structures
1. Meningioma
2. Hemangiopericytoma

D. Non-neoplastic Conditions of Neurosurgical Importance
1. "Degenerative" cysts of pineal lined by fibrillary astrocytes
2. Arachnoid cysts
3. Cavernous hemangioma

From DeGirolami U. Pathology of tumors of the pineal region. In: Schmidek HH, ed. Pineal Tumors. New York: Masson, 1977: 1–19.

tomas.[625] The most common tumors of the pineal region are germinomas (a form of teratoma), so designated because of their presumed origin in germ cells. Some germinomas, which are histologically indistinguishable from those of the pineal region, may arise in the anterior hypothalamus or the floor of the third ventricle. They have traditionally been classified as atypical teratomas or as ectopic pinealomas (germinoma-like lesions arising outside the pineal).[624] They have also been called seminomatous pinealomas by pathologists because they resemble testicular tubules. Identical tumors can be found in the testis and anterior mediastinum. Intracranial germinomas have a tendency to spread locally, infiltrate the hypothalamus, metastasize to the spinal cord (or other brain regions), and appear in CSF.[626–629] Even extracranial metastases (to the skin, lung, or liver) have been observed rarely.[627] Teratomas containing structures derived from two or more germ cell layers are also found in the pineal region. Chorionic tissue in such teratomas may secrete human chorionic gonadotropin (hCG) in sufficient amounts to cause gonadal maturation.[630–634] A possible viral cause for pinealoma was proposed on the basis of the finding of virus-like particles in one case.[635]

The relationship of pineal tumors to precocious puberty has been much studied in an effort to determine whether the pineal is truly involved in regulation of sexual function in humans (see earlier under The Pineal Gland). Precocious puberty is not common in pineal disease. In one series of 65 pineal tumors, not a single case of sexual precocity was noted; only seven of these patients were younger than age 11.[636] In another study of 177 patients, 56 were younger than age 15, and of these only one third had sexual precocity.[637] Neuroanatomical evidence pointed in that series to extensive damage beyond the pineal region in all cases of precocious puberty. Thus precocious puberty is probably due to the effects of tumor on function of the adjacent hypothalamus; additional evidence of hypothalamic involvement, such as DI, polyphagia, somnolence, obesity, or behavioral disturbance, is present in most. It is likely, therefore, that pineal neoplasms cause precocious puberty by mechanisms similar to those of other types of brain lesions. Pineal tumors cause other types of endocrine abnormalities as well.[630, 638]

Choriocarcinoma of the pineal is associated with high plasma levels of hCG and decreased or normal FSH serum levels.[626, 629–634] hCG can stimulate testosterone secretion from the testis but does not stimulate estrogen secretion from the ovary. It would be expected, therefore, that precocious puberty caused by pineal tumors would be seen almost exclusively in males.[630, 634] This situation is in fact the case, although the syndrome has been reported in a 5-y-old female in whom specific immunoassays documented the presence of high plasma hCG levels, normal FSH levels in serum, and hCG in tumor extracts.[631] The prevalence of gonadotropin secretion in patients with pineal tumors causing precocious puberty is unknown, but the occurrence of this phenomenon further challenges the argument proposed by Kitay[639] that nonparenchymal tumors cause precocious puberty by damage to normally functioning pineal tissue. Furthermore, the fact that the pineal contains LHRH suggests another potential (although not proven) mechanism by which a pineal tumor could stimulate gonadotropin secretion.

Rarely, delayed puberty is attributable to a pineal tumor. Parenchymal tumors were responsible for 20 of 30 cases of pineal tumor–related hypogonadism found in the literature.[640] It is in this group that the postulation of a gonadotropin-inhibitory hormone of pineal origin is most reasonable. As yet, no studies of gonadotropin-inhibitory factors or circulating melatonin have been reported in such cases, but in two instances (not necessarily associated with delayed puberty), assays of tumor tissue have demonstrated melatonin-forming enzymes.[641]

Because other signs of pituitary insufficiency, including DI, are common in patients with pineal tumors, it is likely that some, if not most, such patients have tumor-induced hypothalamic lesions rather than an intrinsic pineal-secretory disorder.

Germinomas of the floor of the third ventricle (sometimes inaccurately referred to as ectopic pineal germinomas) give rise to a characteristic clinical triad: DI, visual impairment, and hypopituitarism.[642] Tumors of identical morphological structure may arise in the region of the pineal, and tumors of the pineal can spread to the base of the brain. More than half of these germinomas can be diagnosed by measurements of hCG in CSF or blood.

Pinealomas cause a variety of neurological disorders (Tables 5–17 and 5–18). The most characteristic is Parinaud syndrome, which consists of paralysis of upward gaze, pupillary areflexia (to light) and paralysis of convergence, and wide-based gait (see Tables 5–17 and 5–18). Gait disturbances also occur because of brain stem or cerebellar compression. Classic Parinaud syndrome occurs in about half of the cases of pinealoma.

Management of tumors in the pineal region is not straightforward. The earlier literature emphasized the danger involved in biopsy and attempted removal, and operative mortality rates of 14 to 37% have been reported.[643] On the other hand, an aggressive approach to the pineal region has been advocated by Stein,[644] who emphasizes the need for making a histological diagnosis, the variety of pathological disorders found in this region, the possibility of removal of an encapsulated lesion, and the possible use of cytotoxic chemotherapeutic agents for certain lesions such as germinoma and choriocarcinoma. In another series in which microsurgical techniques were used, four of six pineal tumors were completely excised; one death occurred in 20 patients who underwent craniotomy.[645] More than 70% of tumors in the posterior third ventricle are radiosensitive and should respond to adequate radiation therapy within 3 to 6 mo.[646] Radiation therapy may be combined with shunting procedures when hydrocephalus is present.

Ectopic pinealomas in the chiasmal region generally should be explored surgically (if assays of CSF are inconclusive; see later), the tumor debulked if possible, and a biopsy diagnosis made. This recommendation is based on the relative safety of these procedures and the occurrence of lesions that are not radiosensitive but are amenable to surgical removal. Germinomas are radiosensitive, in contrast to most other tumors in the region of the third ventricle. In the series of 18 cases studied by Takeuchi and collaborators, 15 underwent radiation; of these, 4 survived 10 y or more and 8 others (with shorter follow-up periods) were still alive.[647] These lesions are potentially curable.[648] The diagnosis can often be made by cytological study of CSF, by radioimmunoassay of CSF for hCG, or by specific serum radioimmunoassays that will show high β-hCG levels. A tumor revealed by computed tomographic scanning and demonstration of hCG in CSF makes surgical biopsy unnecessary and is an indication for x-ray therapy. The use of prophylactic whole skull and spine x-ray therapy must be considered in patients with intracranial germinomas because of the high

TABLE 5–18. Ocular Symptoms and Signs in 22 Cases of Pinealoma

Symptoms and Signs	No. of Patients
Symptoms	
Diplopia	7
"Blurred vision"	4
Reading difficulty	1
Signs	
Upward gaze palsy	12
Pupils: Areflexic to light, near response retained	13
Accommodative control disorder	3
Convergent-retraction nystagmus	10
Convergence paresis	3
Downward gaze palsy	0
Collier sign	0
Skew deviation	5
Third nerve palsy	0
Fourth nerve palsy (bilateral)	1
Sixth nerve palsy	3
Fundi: Normal	8
Papilledema	10
Optic atrophy	4
Vision: Reduced acuity	8
Visual fields: Normal	15
Constricted	3
Bitemporal	4

From Wray SH. The neuro-ophthalmic and neurologic manifestations of pinealomas. In: Schmidek HH, ed. Pineal Tumors. New York: Masson, 1977: 61–77.

TABLE 5–17. Pinealomas: Frequency (%) of Presenting Symptoms and Signs

1. Increased intracranial pressure	85
2. Spasticity	35
3. Ataxia	30
4. Parinaud syndrome	25
5. Cerebellar-type nystagmus	25
6. Syncope	20
7. Vertigo	20
8. Cranial nerve palsy (other than cranial nerves VI, VIII)	20
9. Intention tremor	15
10. Scotoma	10
11. Tinnitus	10
12. Other	10

From Brady WL. The role of radiation therapy. In: Schmidek HH, ed. Pineal Tumors. New York: Masson, 1977: 99–113.

incidence of seeding of the neuroaxis. Chemotherapeutic approaches are now being evaluated, but recorded literature is based on a few case reports. Among the agents advocated are bleomycin, vinblastine, and cisplatin.[649] Clinicians dealing with such cases should consult with oncologists who are expert in management of germ cell tumors.

Approach to the Patient with Precocious Puberty. In the child with precocious secondary sexual characteristics, the most important diagnostic question is whether mature germ cells are being formed. If they are, the case can be classified as true, meaning neurogenic precocity, and the work-up is directed at the function of the hypothalamic-pituitary system. If gonadal maturation has not occurred, the disorder is due to abnormalities of the gonads or adrenals (also see Chapter 22).

In boys the presence of adult-sized testes (appropriate to the stage of development) is an important clue to the diagnosis of true precocity. However, adult-sized testicles can occur in a few rare situations other than true precocity: growth of intratesticular adrenal rests,[650] ectopic secretion of hCG (as from a teratoma), or a manifestation of gonadotropin-independent familial sexual precocity (also termed familial testotoxicosis).[651] Laboratory tests readily identify these rare causes of testicular enlargement, and the demonstration of sperm in an overnight urine specimen or in urine after seminal vesicular massage is evidence of true maturation. Excessive secretion of androgenic hormones by adrenal or other tumors usually leads to small, prepubertal-sized testes.

After the diagnosis of male neurogenic precocity is made, the patient must undergo complete neurological evaluation. Computed tomographic or magnetic resonance imaging scans of the brain are essential. CSF should be examined for the presence of hCG and for cells immunoreactive with anti-hCG, which will permit diagnosis of germinoma. Pituitary function should be evaluated to identify the DI and other hormonal deficiencies. If no abnormalities are noted on the computed tomographic scan, the diagnosis of idiopathic precocious puberty is warranted, but continued, regular follow-up is indicated.

In girls the appearance of regular menses suggests a normal pituitary-gonadal axis: evaluation of the central nervous system is also indicated but is less likely to reveal a structural abnormality.

Management of Sexual Precocity. Identifiable causes of non-neurogenic precocity can be treated by specific measures directed at the cause, e.g., removal of androgen-secreting adenomas or ovarian tumors, or suppression of adrenal steroid hypersecretion in adrenal hyperplasia (see Chapters 12, 13, and 22). Structural disease of the hypothalamus, when indicated, is dealt with by neurosurgical and/or radiotherapeutic approaches. Symptomatic idiopathic or neurogenic precocity is best treated with LHRH superagonists[652] and if these fail by inhibitors of gonadal steroid biosynthesis such as ketoconazole.[653] Precocious puberty is stressful to both the child and the parents, and it is essential to provide psychological support.[654–657]

PSYCHOGENIC AMENORRHEA. Cessation of normal menstrual cycles in young, nonpregnant women who have no demonstrable structural abnormalities of the brain, the pituitary, or the ovary occurs in several situations:[658, 659] pseudocyesis (false pregnancy), anorexia nervosa, a loose collection of conditions called psychogenic or functional amenorrhea, and hyperprolactinemia related to an occult microadenoma of the pituitary or some other cause (Table 5–19). Functional amenorrhea, which is the largest single cause of secondary amenorrhea excepting pregnancy, can be associated with gross psychopathology or with minor degrees of psychic stress. It is often temporary. Depending on the degree and type of gonadotropin deficiency present,

TABLE 5–19. Incidence (%) of Various Causes of Secondary Amenorrhea in 106 Cases Studied After Referral

Functional	34.0
Postpill	27.4
Prolactinoma	16.0
Anorexia nervosa	8.5
Polycystic ovary	4.7
Premature menopause	3.8
Asherman syndrome*	2.8
Phenothiazine	1.9
Ovarian tumor	0.9

*Post–dilatation and curettage destruction of endometrial lining, endocrinologically normal.

From Barnea ER, Naftolin F, Tolis G, et al. Hypothalamic amenorrhea syndromes. In: Givens JR, ed. The Hypothalamus. Chicago: Year Book Medical, 1984: 147–170.

the ovarian abnormality ranges from a short luteal phase through failure of ovulation to severe estrogen loss. These disorders probably arise from functional abnormalities in the hypothalamic gonadotropin-regulating areas. Psychogenic amenorrhea may be due to excessive endogenous opioid activity because naloxone (an opiate receptor blocker) can induce ovulation in some patients with this disorder.[660]

Exercise amenorrhea may be a variant of psychogenic amenorrhea but may also be due to loss of body fat.[501–504, 661, 662] The syndrome is associated with intense and prolonged physical exertion such as competitive running, swimming, and ballet dancing. Patients are always below ideal body weight and have low stores of fat. If this activity is begun before puberty, normal sexual maturation can be delayed for many years. The mass of fat may be a regulator of gonadotropin secretion,[502] and dietary composition also may play a role.[503] Exercise-induced or hypothalamic amenorrhea can have significant adverse effects because of the associated estrogen deficiency. Significant osteopenia is found in the majority[663] (also see Chapter 28).

NEUROGENIC HYPOGONADISM IN MALES. From the historical point of view any discussion of neurogenic hypogonadism in males should begin with an account of Fröhlich syndrome (adipose genital dystrophy). As first reported in 1901 (see refs. 664 and 665), the affected boy had hypogonadism and obesity related to a pituitary tumor. It took an additional decade and a half for the pathological studies of Erdheim to show that this disorder could be due to a pituitary tumor that damages the hypothalamus (causing obesity), or as a primary hypothalamic disorder that damages crucial areas that regulate gonadotropins. Efforts to understand the pathogenesis of Fröhlich syndrome gave the first emphasis to studies of the role of the brain in regulation of anterior pituitary function. It is now established that either hypothalamic or pituitary dysfunction can cause this disorder; the presence of obesity implies that there is damage to the food-regulating regions of the hypothalamus. A wide variety of organic lesions of the hypothalamus can cause this disorder, including tumors, encephalitis, microcephaly, Friedreich ataxia, and demyelinating disorders.

As noted earlier under Hypophyseotropic Hormone Deficiency, an important cause of hypogonadotropic hypogonadism is Kallmann syndrome, a disorder that is apparently caused by failure of LHRH-containing neurons to migrate normally. The animal model of Kallmann syndrome, the LHRH-deficient mouse, is the result of a gene deletion[666] and can be treated either via intrahypothalamic brain transplants[667] or by transgenic introduction of a normal LHRH gene.[666] The transplanted LHRH-containing neurons make proper connections within the hypothalamus and support normal ovulatory cycles. In Kallmann syndrome in the human, the gene for LHRH appears to be normal; the defect thus must arise from developmental abnormalities.

Most men with delayed sexual development do not have serious neurological conditions. For example, the majority of obese boys with delayed sexual development have no structural damage to the hypothalamus. In most of these boys the problem can be classified as constitutional delayed puberty, which is commonly associated with obesity. Whether there is a functional disorder of the hypothalamus in these cases is not known.

It is believed that brain maturation depends on the presence of androgens. For this reason it is important to treat male hypogonadism (regardless of cause) by the middle teen years (15 y old at the latest), because serious emotional and personality consequences may otherwise ensue.[656]

Several forms of functional impairment of gonadotropin secretion have been recognized in adult men. Hypogonadism (including reduced spermatogenesis) can be induced by emotional stress[668] and by severe exercise,[669] but this abnormality seldom reaches clinical awareness because the symptoms are more subtle than changes in the menstrual cycle. Excessive exercise in men can be associated with anorexia,[669] which suggests a similarity to anorexia nervosa in women. Another neurogenic cause of hypogonadism in men is disease of the spinal cord, such as post-traumatic paraplegia.[670-672]

Neurogenic Disorders of Prolactin Regulation

One of the most significant developments in clinical endocrinology over the past decades has been recognition of the frequency of hyperprolactinemia and PRL-secreting microadenomas (see Chapters 6 and 12) (Table 5–20). Important neurogenic causes of hyperprolactinemia include irritative lesions of the chest wall (herpes zoster, after thoracotomy), which are presumed to act by chronic stimulation of afferent nerves of the nipple; excessive tactile stimulation of the nipple; and lesions within the spinal cord such as ependymoma. Prolonged mechanical stimulation of the nipples by suckling or the use of a breast pump can initiate lactation in some women who are not pregnant. Any lesions that can interrupt the hypothalamic-pituitary connection can also cause hyperprolactinemia. The use of neuroleptic agents such as phenothiazines, reserpine, and methyldopa must be excluded in all cases.

The possible role of psychogenic factors in the pathogenesis of hyperprolactinemia is not established, and, in view of the frequency of microadenoma, the existence of hyperprolactinemia as a psychogenic disorder is now in question. Nevertheless, a number of patients, perhaps one third or more, have unexplained hyperprolactinemia for many years and never manifest roentgenographic evidence of an adenoma.[3951]

Because the nervous system exerts profound effects on PRL secretion, it has been postulated that patients with hyperprolactinemia (including those with adenomas) may have a deficit of PIF or an excess of PRF activity. A number of studies of PRL-secretory dynamics have now been performed with patients who were apparently cured of hyperprolactinemia by removal of a pituitary microadenoma.[404, 673] In some studies, regulatory abnormalities reportedly persisted in most patients,[674] but in other series[675, 676] patients who were cured showed a return toward normal in all dynamic tests of PRL secretion. This result would suggest that most cases do not show underlying hypothalamic dysregulation. The cause of the persistent hyperprolactinemia and secretory disturbance in those patients who were unsuccessfully treated by surgery is unresolved. Does this group represent incomplete removal (as is likely for larger tumors),

abnormal function of the remaining part of the gland, or underlying hypothalamic dysregulation?[673, 676, 677]

Neurogenic Disorders of Growth Hormone Secretion

HYPOTHALAMIC HYPOSOMATOTROPINEMIA. Loss of GH-secretory responses to provocative stimuli and of the normal nocturnal increase in GH secretion occurs early in the course of hypothalamic disease of any cause and is usually the most sensitive endocrine indicator of hypothalamic dysfunction. As noted earlier under Hypophyseotropic Hormone Deficiency, anatomical malformations of midline cerebral structures have been documented in which GH secretion is abnormal, presumably owing to failure to develop normal GH-regulatory structures. Such disorders include optic nerve dysplasia and midline prosencephalic malformations (absence of the septum pellucidum, abnormal third ventricle, and abnormal lamina terminalis). Idiopathic

TABLE 5–20. Differential Diagnosis of Galactorrhea and/or Hyperprolactinemia*

A. Structural Hypothalamic Lesions with Damage to Ventral Hypothalamus or Pituitary Stalk

Craniopharyngioma	Metastatic neoplasms
Sarcoidosis	Rathke pouch cyst
Encephalitis	Surgical stalk section
Irradiation	Ectopic pinealoma
Head trauma	Histiocytosis X
Ectopic pinealoma	

B. Structural Pituitary Lesions

PRL-producing pituitary tumors	Pituitary angiosarcoma
Empty sella syndrome	Acromegaly
Combined PRL/GH-producing pituitary tumors	
Cushing disease	

C. Drug-Induced Disorders

Prochlorperazine†	Trifluoperazine†	Sulpiride	Amphetamines
Chlorpromazine†	Thioridazine†	Fluphenazine	Amitriptyline
Cyproheptadine	Reserpine	Methyldopa	Pimozide
Metoclopramide	Prostaglandins	Estrogens	Androgens
Meprobamate			

D. Endocrine-Metabolic Disorders

Hypothyroidism (50% with myxedema have increased PRL but only 5% have galactorrhea, usually with amenorrhea)

Addison disease	Nelson syndrome	Sheehan syndrome
Adrenocarcinoma	Adrenal hyperplasia	Diabetes mellitus
Liver disease	Chronic renal failure	

E. Irritative Lesions of Chest Wall

Herpes zoster	Thoracotomy	Thoracic burns
Tight garments	Mastectomy	Cystic breast disease
Chest trauma	Atopic dermatitis	Mammoplasty

F. Hypothalamic Biochemical Lesions with Presumed Decrease of PIF or Increase of PRF‡

G. Other Described Causes

Pseudotumor cerebri	Syringomyella	Pseudocyesis
Tabes dorsalis	Male hypogonadism	Pneumoencephalo-gram
Chorioepithelioma of testis	Stein-Leventhal syndrome	Intrauterine device use
Hysterectomy	Ovarian resection	
Dilatation and curettage	Neck surgery	

H. Lesions of Upper Spinal Cord

Extrinsic tumors	Cervical ependymoma

I. Ectopic PRL Production

Bronchogenic cancer	Hypernephroma

*Compiled by Dr. Bruce Biller.

†Twenty-five percent of psychiatric patients taking phenothiazine derivatives have galactorrhea, but many have normal PRL levels; amenorrhea may also occur and both may persist for several years after medication is stopped.

‡Diagnosis of exclusion: patients may still have a biochemical and radiologically undetectable PRL-producing pituitary tumor that will become apparent only as time goes on.

hypopituitarism with GH deficiency was considered earlier in this chapter.

Maternal Deprivation Syndrome and Psychosocial Dwarfism. GH-secretory impairment can occur in infants (maternal deprivation syndrome) and children (psychosocial dwarfism) with growth failure occurring in a setting of severe emotional disturbance (also see Chapter 21).[678-681] Deficient GH release occurs in response to stimuli such as insulin-induced hypoglycemia or arginine infusion. In some patients there is also deficiency in release of ACTH and gonadotropins. This disorder is rapidly reversed by placing a child in a supportive hospital milieu, after which growth and neuroendocrine GH responses return rapidly to normal.

In the human the characteristic GH-secretory response to physical or emotional stress is generally a marked *increase* in secretion, thus suggesting that patterns of GH response in children with the maternal deprivation syndrome may be determined by more subtle psychological stimuli. On the other hand, inhibition of GH release is the usual pattern of response to stress in several species;[211] in rats the effects of stress are blocked by treatment with antisera to somatostatin.[682] It is believed, therefore, that stress in rats brings about release of somatostatin. The extent to which the increase in somatostatin secretion and the suppression of GHRH secretion are involved in the human response to deprivation is unknown.

It has been suggested that malnutrition related to stress rather than psychological factors causes growth failure[680] in children with the maternal deprivation syndrome, and each case should be carefully evaluated from this point of view. It is also possible that growth retardation in deprived children is a function of stress-induced sleep disturbance.[683] Sleep deprivation presumably leads to GH deficiency because most GH is secreted during the night. Higher cerebral functions are also impaired in children with the maternal deprivation syndrome, who improve after resocialization.[684]

Neuroregulatory Growth Hormone Deficiency. The availability of biosynthetic GH for treatment of children with short stature has brought into focus a group of patients who grow at low rates (below the third percentile), who may have low serum levels of IGF I, but who have a normal GH-secretory reserve (to hypoglycemia, exercise, levodopa, or clonidine). Under earlier guidelines for therapy with cadaver-derived GH, such children would have been diagnosed as having constitutional short stature and would not have been eligible for GH therapy. Detailed studies of 24-h GH-secretory dynamics indicate that some children can respond normally to provocative tests of GH-secretory reserve but do not show normal spontaneous GH-secretory patterns (abnormal ultradian and circadian rhythms and decreased number and/or amplitude of secretory bursts). It has been postulated by Bercu and collaborators[685, 686] that these children have a functional or neuroendocrine regulatory disorder of the hypothalamus; when given GH some of these children grow at a normal rate. There is, however, considerable uncertainty about the criteria for diagnosis of neuroregulatory GH deficiency. In studies of GH-secretory patterns, many normally growing children have profiles of GH secretion that are indistinguishable from those in children with postulated syndrome.[687] Patterns of GH secretion do not predict which child will benefit from therapy, and there is poor correlation between GH secretion and growth. The prevalence of a GH-neuroregulatory deficiency syndrome is thus unclear, and other considerations govern the decision to treat short children with GH[688] (see Chapter 21).

NEUROGENIC HYPERSECRETION OF GROWTH HORMONE. ***Diencephalic Cachexia.*** Children and infants with tumors in and around the third ventricle frequently develop diencephalic cachexia, which may include elevated GH levels,

TABLE 5–21. Clinical Features of Diencephalic Syndrome (Pooled Data of 67 Anatomically Defined Tumors)

Clinical Feature	%
Emaciation	100
Alert appearance	87
Increased vigor and/or hyperkinesis	72
Vomiting	68
Euphoria	59
Pallor	55
Nystagmus	55
Irritability	32
Hydrocephalus*	33
Optic atrophy	24
Tremor	23
Sweating	15
Large hands/feet	5
Large genitals	5
Polyuria	5
Papilledema	5
Positive pneumoencephalogram results	98
Endocrine anomalies†	90
CSF protein	64
CSF abnormal cells	23

*Hydrocephalus includes clinical plus pneumoencephalographic findings.
†Positive in 9 of 10 with adequately recorded investigation. (Occasionally, patients had electrolyte and blood pressure anomalies and eosinophilia.)
From Burr IM, Slonim AE, Danish RK, et al. Diencephalic syndrome revisited. J Pediatr 1976; 88:439–444.

often with paradoxical responses to administration of glucose and of insulin.[689, 690] GH hypersecretion may be due to a hypothalamic regulatory abnormality or may be secondary to malnutrition. Deficits of pituitary-adrenal regulation are seen. A striking feature in most children is the alert appearance and seeming euphoria despite the wasted state. A variety of associated neurological abnormalities have been identified (Table 5–21), and the various types of tumor producing this syndrome have been summarized by Burr and colleagues[689] (Table 5–22).

Syndrome of Inappropriate Growth Hormone Hypersecretion. In a number of clinical situations apparently inappropriate GH hypersecretion occurs.[410, 411, 691] By analogy with SIADH, these disorders can be termed *syndrome of inappropriate somatotropin secretion.*[691] These conditions include poorly controlled diabetes mellitus, hepatic failure, uremia, anorexia nervosa, and protein-calorie malnutrition. Nutritional factors are probably important in this response because obesity inhibits and fasting in normal persons stimulates episodic GH hypersecretion.[692] Best studied of these hypersecretory states is diabetes mellitus, in which cholinergic blockers reverse the abnormality,[693] possibly by inhibiting hypothalamic somatostatin secretion. One interpretation of this finding is that metabolic abnormalities may act in the hypothalamus on the neuroendocrine control of the releasing

TABLE 5–22. Histology of Tumors Producing Diencephalic Syndrome

Tumor	No. of Patients	
Gliomas	56	
Astrocytoma		37
Not subclassified		10
Spongioblastoma		5
Astroblastoma		1
Oligodendroglioma		1
Mixed astrocytoma/spongioblastoma		1
Mixed astrocytoma/oligodendroglioma		1
Ependymoma	2	
Ganglioglioma	1	
Dysgerminoma	1	
No histology	10	

From Burr IM, Slonim AE, Danish RK, et al. Diencephalic syndrome revisited. J Pediatr 1976; 88:439–444.

factors that regulate GH secretion. Loss of IGF I inhibition of GH secretion at the pituitary or the hypothalamic level may also play a role because most disorders in which this syndrome occurs are associated with low IGF I levels.

Role of the Hypothalamus in the Etiology of Acromegaly. The possible role of the hypothalamus in the pathogenesis of acromegaly has been the subject of studies and reviews.[694–698] The main points at issue are whether patients who have no x-ray evidence of adenoma have occult pituitary lesions and whether increased GHRH secretion can lead to adenoma formation. Although acromegaly can be caused by ectopic secretion of GHRH by pancreatic or other neuroendocrine tumors (see earlier under Growth Hormone–Releasing Hormone), or by hypothalamic gangliocytoma,[611] these disorders are rare and usually cause pituitary hyperplasia rather than adenoma formation. The demonstration of abnormalities in the structure of membrane regulatory proteins in about half of patients (see discussion earlier under Growth Hormone–Releasing Hormone) suggests that the disease begins as a clonal mutation and hence is a primary pituitary disorder.

Neurogenic Disorders of Corticotropin Regulation

Hypothalamic CRH hypersecretion is the likely cause of pituitary-adrenal hyperfunction in at least three situations. Most striking of these is the rare form of Cushing syndrome caused by CRH-secreting gangliocytoma of the hypothalamus.[699] This disorder is analogous to the form of precocious puberty related to LHRH-secreting hamartoma of the hypothalamus and to acromegaly related to GHRH-secreting gangliocytoma.

Patients with severe depression often show pituitary-adrenal abnormalities, including inappropriately elevated ACTH levels, abnormal cortisol circadian rhythms, and relative resistance to dexamethasone suppression.[700] In contrast to patients with Cushing disease, patients with depression show diminished responses to the administration of CRH, which was interpreted by Gold and colleagues[700] to indicate that depressed individuals are CRH hypersecretors.

Another syndrome of ACTH hypersecretion likely caused by disordered central nervous system function has been described under the name of periodic hypothalamic discharge. The patient had a recurring cyclic disorder characterized by high fever, paroxysms of glucocorticoid hypersecretion, and electroencephalographic abnormalities.[701] When first seen at age 14, the boy had cushingoid features, dilatation of the left lateral ventricle, and cortical atrophy. To inhibit central neurotransmitters regulating CRH secretion, he was given chlorpromazine, which induced a complete remission. During a follow-up period of more than 25 y, the patient remained in remission as long as he continued to take chlorpromazine. There is no evidence of progressive neurological abnormality (personal communication, Sheldon Wolff).

The question is still unresolved as to whether the usual case of Cushing disease is due to hypersecretion of CRH.[696–698, 702, 703] The weight of evidence favors a primary pituitary clonal defect in most cases. The possibility that the glucocorticoid receptor that mediates feedback inhibition is defective has not been supported by study of the pituitary adenoma glucocorticoid receptor.[704]

Nonendocrine Manifestations of Hypothalamic Disease

When considering the clinical manifestations of hypothalamic disease, it is well to keep in mind that the hypo-

TABLE 5–23. Neurological Manifestations of Nonendocrine Hypothalamic Disease

Disorders of Temperature Regulation	**Periodic Disease of Hypothalamic Origin**
Hyperthermia	Diencephalic epilepsy
Hypothermia	Kleine-Levin syndrome
Poikilothermia	Periodic discharge syndrome of Wolff
Disorders of Food Intake	
Hyperphagia (bulimia)	**Disorders of Autonomic Nervous System**
Anorexia, aphagia	
Disorders of Water Intake	Pulmonary edema
Compulsive water drinking	Cardiac arrhythmias
Adipsia	Sphincter disturbance
Essential hypernatremia	**Hereditary Hypothalamic Disease**
Disorders of Sleep and Consciousness	Laurence-Moon-Biedl syndrome
Somnolence	**Miscellaneous**
Sleep rhythm reversal	Prader-Willi syndrome
Akinetic mutism	Diencephalic syndrome of infancy
Coma	Cerebral gigantism
Disorders of Psychic Function	
Rage behavior	
Hallucinations	

thalamus is involved in the regulation of visceral functions and behavior (Table 5–23).[10, 15, 21, 705–707] Psychic abnormalities are common in hypothalamic disease, including attacks of rage, laughing, and crying; disturbed sleep patterns; excessive sexuality; antisocial behaviors; and hallucinations. Both somnolence (with posterior lesions) and pathological wakefulness (with anterior lesions) have been observed, as have bulimia and profound anorexia. The abnormal eating patterns in humans are analogous to the syndromes of hyperphagia and loss of food drive produced in rats by destruction of the ventromedial nucleus and lateral hypothalamus, respectively. Patients with hypothalamic damage may show hyperthermia, hypothermia, and unexplained fluctuations in body temperature. Rarely, they may present as having fever of unknown origin. Disturbances of sweating, acrocyanosis, and loss of sphincter control can also occur, and diencephalic epilepsy is a rare manifestation. One of the most distressing aspects of hypothalamic damage is the loss of recent memory, believed to require intact mamillothalamic pathways. The impact of hypothalamic damage on higher brain functions is important to physicians who deal with pituitary problems, because severe memory loss, obesity, and personality changes (apathy, loss of ability to concentrate, aggressive antisocial behavior) may follow suprasellar extension of tumors, hypothalamic radiation, or damage incurred by surgical attempts to remove parasellar tumors. Behavioral changes frequently occur after removal of suprasellar tumors. These potential consequences should be weighed carefully with the neurosurgeon, patient, and patient's family in planning the therapeutic approach. For example, the occurrence of these adverse effects has led to more conservative surgical guidelines for treatment of craniopharyngioma.[708]

Hypothalamic lesions grow slowly and may reach a large size without producing much disturbance of behavior or visceral homeostasis, but acute surgical manipulation of much less extent can produce striking immediate functional abnormalities. Presumably this is because the slowly developing lesions permit compensatory responses to take place.

NEUROPEPTIDES IN THE BRAIN

The role of peptides as pituitary-regulating factors has been considered in previous sections. Outside of the pituitary-regulatory areas, a variety of peptides are distributed in specific pathways in the central nervous system (Fig. 5–58). Although much is known about their anatomical pat-

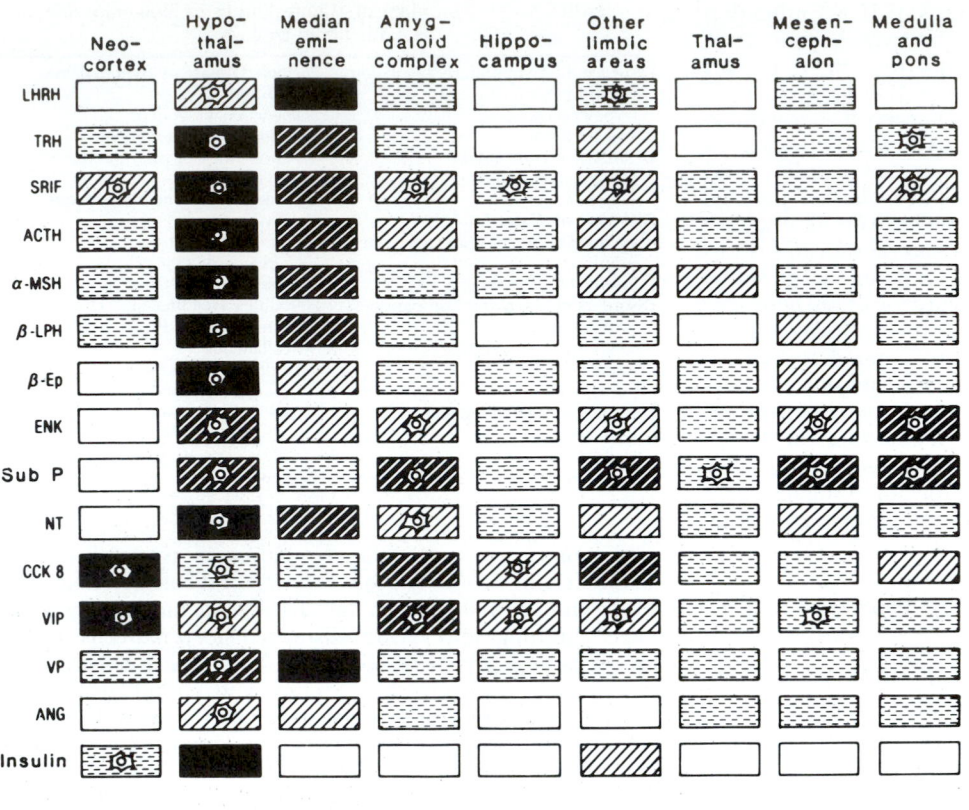

Figure 5–58. Regional distribution of neuropeptides in the mammalian central nervous system. This compilation is intended to show the selectivity of some peptides, which presumably is related to specific functions. The hypothalamus contains the highest concentrations of most peptides, with the exception of cholecystokinin (CCK) and vasoactive intestinal peptide (VIP). Not shown is the distribution of peptide Y, which is present in the cortex in the highest concentration of any peptide. LHRH, luteinizing hormone–releasing hormone; TRH, thyrotropin-releasing hormone; SRIF, somatostatin; ACTH, corticotropin; MSH, melanocyte-stimulating hormone; LPH, lipotropin; Ep, endogenous pyrogen; ENK, enkephalin; Sub P, substance P; NT, neurotensin; VP, vasopressin; ANG, angiotensin. (From Krieger DT. Brain peptides: what, where, and why? Science 1983; 222:975–985. Copyright 1983 by the American Association for the Advancement of Science.)

tern, mode of biosynthesis, regulation, receptors, and mechanism of action, their actual functions, with but few exceptions, are poorly understood. They may have important influences on behavior, homeostasis, pain perception, memory, learning, eating and drinking behaviors, body temperature regulation, and sleep.[21, 29, 282, 709–714] More than 50 different peptides have been localized to specific neurons, and new peptides and new activities are being described each year (see Tables 5–2 to 5–4). Because neuropeptides are formed as part of larger prohormones, many other peptides are formed in the course of post-translational processing whose functions, if any, are unknown. The likelihood that some may be important is suggested by the fact that certain established prohormones such as POMC and procalcitonin give rise to more than one active hormone.[715] Most plentiful in brain are neuropeptide Y, cholecystokinin, VIP, and somatostatin.

At the time of their discovery, most peptides are given trivial names, usually related to the first of the known activities of the compound. A more systematic method of naming peptides designates them by the first and last amino acid (in the single-letter code) and the number of amino acids. For example, PHI-27 (peptide-histidine-isoleucine-27) is the peptide cosecreted with VIP.[716]

Some peptides are found in long tracts and in local circuit neurons. They may act as neurotransmitters or as neuromodulators, i.e., factors that modulate neuronal responses to neurotransmitters. In most neurons one or more neuropeptides coexist with a neurotransmitter[717–719] (see earlier discussion of secretomotor control). Neurons also interact with regulatory peptides, such as cytokines, derived from supportive glia (see later under Neuroimmunomodulation) and growth factors such as brain growth factor.

Pain and Endogenous Opioids

CHEMISTRY. The term *endorphin* (endogenous morphine-like) at first was used to designate a general class of substances postulated to occur in the brain and was subsequently applied to a particular class of compounds related to the enkephalins; the term *endogenous opioid* is now used to describe any peptide with morphine-like activity of known or unknown sequence.[720–722] The search for these compounds was instituted in several laboratories when it was established that morphine and its analogues bind to specific receptors in the brain and in peripheral target tissues. It was reasoned that the presence of morphine binding sites could not be a fortuitous occurrence and must be associated with the presence of an endogenous ligand to be bound by the receptor. This idea was supported by the observation that the antinociceptive (antipain) effects of electric stimulation of certain regions of the midbrain were reversed by administration of the morphine antagonist naloxone.[720] The concept that the presence of a specific receptor in the brain is a marker of an endogenous ligand has been generalized and led to the discovery of endogenous digitalis-like compounds,[723] endogenous benzodiazepines,[724] and adenosines as neurotransmitters.[725]

The first endogenous opioids to be isolated from brain extracts were pentapeptides, designated met-enkephalin and leu-enkephalin.[720, 726] The amino acid sequence of met-enkephalin corresponds to an identical sequence in a pituitary hormone, β-lipotropin (β-LPH), that had been isolated previously by Li and colleagues[727] in 1964 (Figs. 5–14 and 5–59) and whose function at the time was unknown.

β-LPH is the prohormone of several endogenous opioids (see Figs. 5–14 and 5–59), the most potent of which

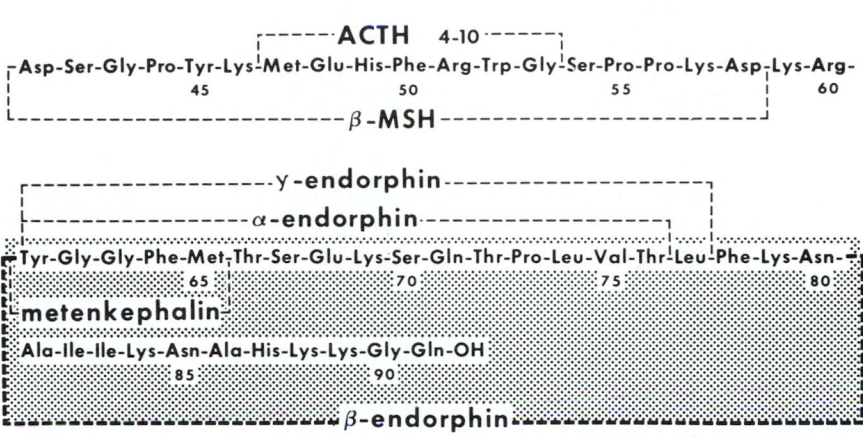

H-Glu-Leu-Thr-Gly-Glu-Arg-Leu-Glu-Gln-Ala-Arg-Gly-Pro-Glu-Ala-Gln-Ala-Glu-Ser-Ala-

Ala-Ala-Arg-Ala-Glu-Leu-Glu-Tyr-Gly-Leu-Val-Ala-Glu-Ala-Glu-Ala-Ala-Glu-Lys-Lys-

Figure 5–59. Homologies in structures of sheep β-LPH with ACTH fragment (4–10), β-MSH (41–58), met-enkephalin (61–65), α-endorphin (61–76), γ-endorphin (61–77), and β-endorphin (61–91). (From Martin JB, Reichlin S, Brown GM. Effects of hormones on the brain. In: Clinical Neuroendocrinology. Philadelphia: F. A. Davis, 1977: 275–303.)

is designated β-endorphin. Two other endorphins have been described, α-endorphin and γ-endorphin. β-LPH also includes a sequence corresponding to β-MSH. The entire molecule is synthesized together with ACTH in a large prohormone, POMC.[109, 722–729] The pattern of peptide processing is organ specific, with ACTH being the final product in the anterior pituitary and larger forms being products in brain and intermediate lobe.

Although the leu-enkephalin sequence is contained within the POMC molecule, the distribution of immunoreactive leu-enkephalin in the brain does not correspond to the distribution of immunoreactive POMC-related peptides.

This discrepancy and other observations led to a search for additional leu-enkephalin precursors. It now appears that the leu-enkephalin isolated from brain (and also from the adrenal medulla) arises from two additional prohormone precursors, one designated pre-proenkephalin A[730, 731] and the other, pre-proenkephalin B (Fig. 5–60).[732–734] Pre-proenkephalin A contains four base sequences coding for met-enkephalin and one coding for leu-enkephalin. Within this same prohormone are sequences coding for additional opioids containing the enkephalin sequence. Pre-proenkephalin B codes for the sequence of leu-enkephalin and in addition codes for several other potent opioids including

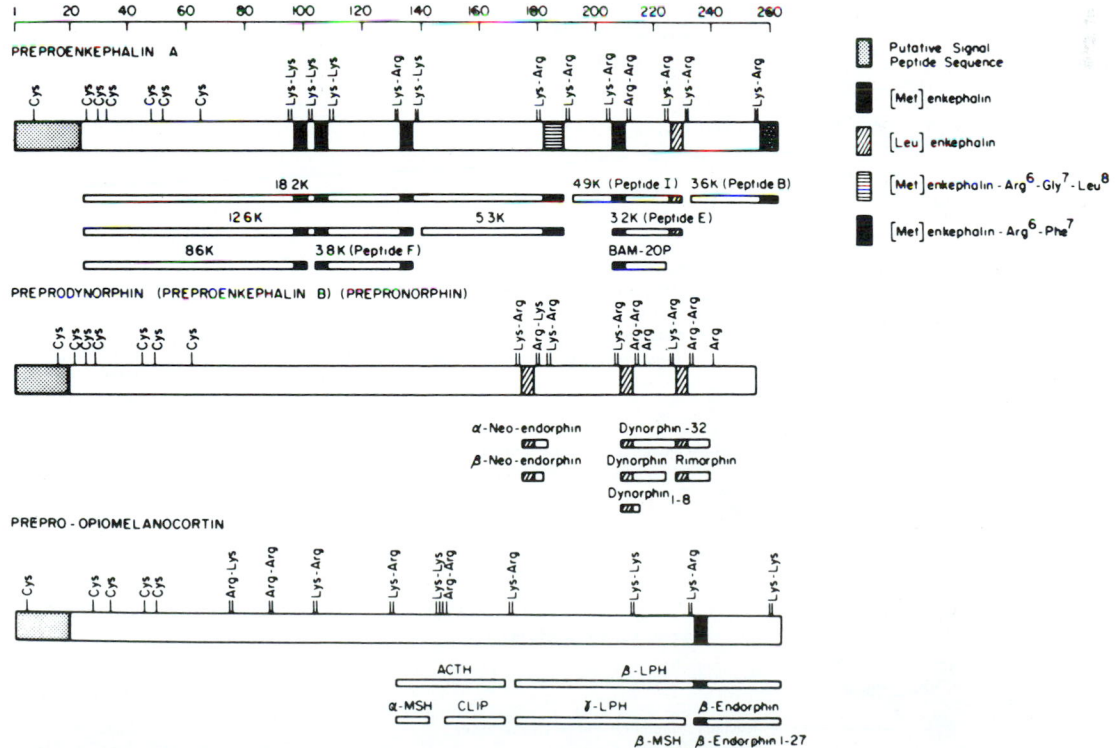

Figure 5–60. Biological relationship between the three prohormones coding for enkephalins. Met-enkephalin is derived from POMC (where it is represented by a single sequence) and from pre-proenkephalin A (where it is represented by four sequences). Leu-enkephalin is not part of the POMC prohormone but is represented as a single sequence in pre-proenkephalin A and as three sequences in pre-proenkephalin B. Various enkephalin-containing fragments, larger than the enkephalin pentapeptides, are also formed from the prohormone; some, such as dynorphin, have even higher opioid potency than the enkephalins. (Courtesy of DT Krieger. From Krieger DT. The multiple faces of pro-opiomelanocortin, a prototype precursor molecule. Clin Res 1983; 31:342–353.)

TABLE 5–24. Various Classes of Opioid Receptors, Principal Tissues, Principal Endogenous Ligands, and Relationship to Naloxone Antagonism

	Mu	Delta	Kappa	Epsilon	Sigma
Bioassay	Guinea pig ileum	Mouse vas deferens	Rabbit vas deferens	Rat vas deferens	—
Naloxone antagonism	Sensitive	Resistant	Resistant	Sensitive	Highly resistant
Probable endogenous ligand	? Endorphin	Met/leu-enkephalin	Dynorphin	Endorphin	?
Principal location	Periaqueductal gray Hypothalamus	Limbic system Basal ganglia	Substantia nigra Posterior pituitary	?	?

From Grossman A. Brain opiates and neuroendocrine function. Clin Endocrinol Metab 1983; 12:725–746.

dynorphin and β-neoendorphin (see Fig. 5–60). Several of these are much more potent as opioids than the earliest recognized enkephalins.

Leu-enkephalin and met-enkephalin thus arise from three different prohormones (POMC and the two proenkephalins) and are present in functionally distinct neurons in the brain and in cells of the pituitary and the adrenal medulla (Fig. 5–61). On the basis of the finding of similar sequences in all three genes, it appears likely that all three may have arisen from a single ancestral gene.[733]

Other endogenous opioids have been isolated but not characterized chemically. One from blood has been named anodynin,[735] one from CSF has been designated humoral endorphin,[736] and a third in brain has been identified by its reactivity with an antibody directed against morphine.[737, 738]

Additional complexity is added to the physiology of endogenous opioids by the finding that there are several types of opioid receptor, which are to some extent region, peptide, and drug specific (Table 5–24).[739]

LOCALIZATION OF ENDOGENOUS OPIOIDS AND THEIR FUNCTION. Enkephalin-containing neurons, which account for the bulk of endogenous opioids, are distributed in regions correspondingly rich in opiate receptors.[134, 740] Regional concentrations of the endorphins correspond to regionally specialized functions (see Fig. 5–61). In the spinal cord, opioid receptors and enkephalins are present in highest concentration in the dorsal gray matter, which corresponds to the centrally directed nerve endings of primary sensory neurons. Enkephalins are believed to modulate pain perception at the cord level and to suppress the release of substance P from central sensory nerve endings that arise in sensory ganglia.[741] Vagal nuclear localization corresponds to the emetic effects of morphine and its antitussive properties. Localization of enkephalins in the locus coeruleus (the principal site of origin of ascending noradrenergic fibers) may account for the euphoria-producing actions of morphine and, through projections to the hypothalamus, for the regulation of some pituitary functions. The amygdala is also

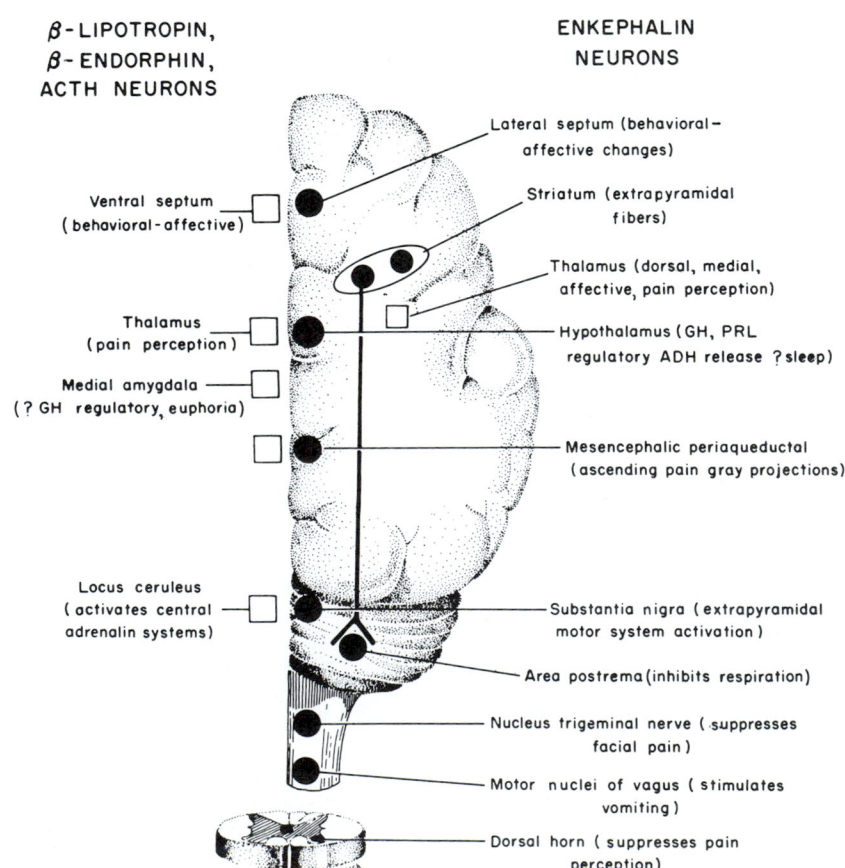

SCHEMATIC DISTRIBUTION OF ENDORPHINS AND RELATED PEPTIDES IN RAT BRAIN

β-LIPOTROPIN, β-ENDORPHIN, ACTH NEURONS

ENKEPHALIN NEURONS

Ventral septum (behavioral-affective)
Thalamus (pain perception)
Medial amygdala (? GH regulatory, euphoria)
Locus ceruleus (activates central adrenalin systems)

Lateral septum (behavioral-affective changes)
Striatum (extrapyramidal fibers)
Thalamus (dorsal, medial, affective, pain perception)
Hypothalamus (GH, PRL regulatory ADH release ? sleep)
Mesencephalic periaqueductal (ascending pain gray projections)
Substantia nigra (extrapyramidal motor system activation)
Area postrema (inhibits respiration)
Nucleus trigeminal nerve (suppresses facial pain)
Motor nuclei of vagus (stimulates vomiting)
Dorsal horn (suppresses pain perception)

Figure 5–61. Regional concentrations of endorphins in the central nervous system. (Modified from Barchas JD, Akil H, Elliott GR. Behavioral neurochemistry: neuroregulators and behavioral states. Science 1978; 200:964–973. Copyright 1978 by the American Association for the Advancement of Science.)

considered a prime site for morphine-generated euphoria. Rich concentrations of enkephalin and opiate receptors in the hypothalamus and in the locus coeruleus may account for the effects of endorphins on stimulation of release of PRL and GH and on suppression of TSH and gonadotropin release.[739]

In contrast, the principal localization of β-endorphin is in the pituitary, especially in the intermediate lobe. Less is found in the hypothalamus, and still smaller amounts are present elsewhere in the brain. Brain homogenates can break down β-LPH of pituitary origin to form β-endorphin, but the content of brain β-LPH and of POMC mRNA is unaltered by hypophysectomy or by adrenal status, which indicates that β-endorphin originates in the brain and that it is independent of pituitary β-LPH.

Enkephalins are widely distributed in the gut in neurons and in secretory cells. The presence of a rich population of opiate receptors in the intestine, together with the well-known effects of morphine in inhibiting gut motility, suggests an important role for these compounds in intestinal function. Enkephalins are also present in the peripheral nervous system; are cocontained in catecholaminergic neurons not only in the sympathetic nervous system but also in the carotid body;[742] and, as noted earlier, are found in the adrenal medulla, where they are located in the same secretory granules that contain epinephrine.[743–746] They are also synthesized and secreted by pheochromocytomas.[747] Endorphins are present in a population of intestinal cells (as part of the POMC complex) and also in the pineal gland, kidney, eye, and placenta.

The endogenous opioids raise the threshold of pain, produce sedation, and influence extrapyramidal motor activity. Electric stimulation of the periaqueductal gray of the spinal cord causes analgesia in humans and is associated with an increase in the concentration of enkephalins in CSF.[748] Contrariwise, pain-prone individuals have lower than normal concentrations of bioassayable opioids in the CSF.[749]

MECHANISM OF ACTION OF OPIOID PEPTIDES. As in the case of other peptides, activity of opioid peptides is initiated by binding to specific cell membrane receptors. Several classes of opioid receptors have been described (see Table 5–24). Commonly used morphine antagonists do not block all classes of receptors to the same extent. Therefore, the use of naloxone (for example) to determine whether a given disturbance (endocrine or psychological) is mediated by endogenous opioid activity may give misleading results.

Morphine effects, including addiction and tolerance, appear to be region specific.[750] In isolated systems, morphine inhibits cAMP generation initially, but levels soon return to normal, a state postulated to be the basis of tolerance. Withdrawal of the drug leads to cAMP rebound.[751] Region-specific changes in synthesis of G proteins[752] and in c-*fos* oncogene[753] are induced by morphine.

The mechanism of addiction to morphine is not fully understood. Exogenous opiates may exert a feedback effect, either on production and release of endogenous opioids or on receptor number or postreceptor second messengers. When the addicted individual is deprived of the drug, a deficiency of the opioid effect is induced. Withdrawal syndromes can be thus looked on as related to the loss of the normal endogenous opioid basal state in regions of the brain that generate affects and regulate autonomic functions.

ENDOCRINE ASPECTS OF ENDOGENOUS OPIOIDS. Paraneoplastic secretion of ACTH is associated with the formation of other compounds of the POMC molecule, including β-endorphin (see Chapter 34). In conformity with their presence in normal adrenal medulla, met-enkephalin and β-LPH and their respective mRNAs are present in pheochromocytomas and other tumors of the sympathetic nervous system,[743–746] and they may even be released into the blood.[747]

Administration of morphine or its analogues brings about a number of endocrine responses, including release of GH and PRL and inhibition of the release of gonadotropins and TSH.[739, 754–756] Naloxone, an opiate antagonist, has been reported to reinitiate menses in some women with hypothalamic amenorrhea, which suggests that excess opioid activity could play a role in the regulation of LHRH secretion.[757, 758] GH release that is induced by exercise and arginine is blunted by naloxone, whereas hypoglycemia-induced GH release is not.[759] Morphine induces AVP release,[755] and in one study naloxone reversed SIADH, which suggests that this disorder could be brought about by excessive secretion of endogenous opioids in the neurohypophyseal system.[77]

Peptides in Memory and Learning

Personality disorder, impaired mentation, depression, and even delirium occur in some individuals with hypopituitarism, which are changes traditionally attributed to the combined secondary deficiencies of adrenocortical and thyroid hormones. A direct primary effect of pituitary hormones on the brain was first demonstrated in hypophysectomized rats that showed defects in the acquisition of behaviors and a more rapid rate of extinction of learned behaviors.[760–762] An extensive literature implicates deficiency in both AVP- and ACTH-related peptides in such disturbances. Intracerebral or systemic injection of vasopressin or certain of its analogues restores learning and memory in rats with DI; similarly, injection of ACTH, of ACTH analogues that have no adrenal cortex–stimulating activity, and of certain enkephalin-related peptides also restores learning ability. Contrariwise, administration of antivasopressin antiserum impairs learning in the rat. In humans, results of studies of the effects of ACTH-related peptides on memory are conflicting,[762] but vasopressin itself and certain vasopressin analogues that have no antidiuretic action may improve long-term memory in aging individuals.[761] Central vasopressinergic and oxytocinergic neuronal systems completely independent of the neurohypophysis are widely distributed in many parts of the brain, including the cerebral cortex and the limbic system, as are corticotropinergic (ACTH-containing) neurons.[763] Vasopressin and oxytocin have direct electrophysiological effects, as do their breakdown products.[24, 764, 765]

On the other hand, a number of unexplained aspects have led to skepticism about the biological significance of a central vasopressinergic system for memory consolidation. Most of the work in animals has utilized pain-aversive conditioning and therefore may not represent all types of learning. Hypophysectomy, the model associated with abnormal memory function, does not affect the concentration of AVP or of POMC-related peptides in the brain, both of which are present in extensive intrinsic neuronal networks. Furthermore, the blood-brain barrier excludes entry of all but minute amounts of peptide, and systemic administration of such peptides does not have a demonstrable effect on the concentration of intrinsic brain peptides.[766, 767] It has been difficult, therefore, to explain how peptides injected systemically could influence behavior or why hypophysectomy should. The role of the blood-brain barrier in central effects of peptides is considered in detail by Partridge and Frank,[766] Meisenberg and Simons,[767] and Partridge.[768] Nevertheless, behavioral changes do occur after systemic injection of peptides; these changes are sufficiently marked to warrant the tentative conclusion that they are physiologically important.[769]

Eating Behavior and Neuropeptides

Eating behavior is regulated by an interplay of metabolites in blood (including glucose, lipids, glycerol, and amino acids), neural signals from the mouth and gastrointestinal tract, circulating hormones, and higher cerebral activities.[770, 771] Appetite and nausea are powerfully influenced by chemoreceptors in the area postrema (a circumventricular neurohemal structure located in the floor of the fourth ventricle).[772] Like other circumventricular organs, the blood-brain barrier is lacking in this region, thus permitting access to the brain of chemicals that can sense nauseants. One or more gut peptides may provide satiety signals (Table 5–25). Among the candidate satiety peptides are glucagon, cholecystokinin (CCK), bombesin (the mammalian analogue is gastrin-releasing peptide), pancreatic polypeptide, somatostatin, and TRH.[770–775] Several cytokines that circulate during inflammation (IL 1, IL 2, and tumor necrosis factor) are powerful appetite suppressors (see later under Neuroimmunomodulation). The claim that a specific peptide (pyroGlu-His-Gly-OH) that has been isolated from the urine of patients with anorexia nervosa[776] is an anorexogenic peptide[776, 777] has not been confirmed.[778]

In contrast to the response to anorexogenic peptides, eating is *increased* by injections of some peptides.[771] The injection of neuropeptide Y directly into the hypothalamus is the most potent known stimulator of eating.[775]

All established peptides that influence eating in animals are present in specific hypothalamic neural pathways; peripheral gut peptides are postulated to interact with central peptide receptors involved in appetite regulation.

The most extensive work on appetite regulation by neuropeptides is that dealing with CCK, which is released from the small bowel when food, particularly lipid, from the stomach enters the duodenum. Indeed, the CCK hypothesis of satiety, first proposed by Smith and co-workers,[773] is a widely tested model of peptide appetite regulation. Administration of CCK to rats and monkeys reduces eating and induces the behaviors that accompany satiety, but the agent has equivocal effects in humans.[773] Because vagal nerve section abolishes the satiety effects of CCK, the peptide probably acts on receptors in the gut. A reasonable explanation of the local effects of CCK on the intestine has been proposed by McHugh and colleagues,[779, 780] who showed that CCK receptors are present in circumferential muscular fibers in the pylorus that contract to prevent gastric emptying. They postulate that CCK modulates the rate at which food enters the small bowel and that the CCK-induced satiety

signal is an afferent neural signal from the distended stomach. However, in the rat peripheral CCK receptors do not appear to be important in regulating food intake. Administration of a peripheral CCK antagonist does not modify eating behavior, whereas central CCK blockers delay satiety.[781]

In the regulation of eating, central peptides interact with bioaminergic neurotransmitters such as dopamine and norepinephrine, whose effects are both site and receptor specific within the hypothalamus.[782, 783] Anorexogenic drugs, such as amphetamines, act through these receptors.[782, 783] Patterns of central neurotransmitter turnover can be modified by altering patterns of food intake or by modifying the amino acid content of the diet. Control of macronutrient intake (carbohydrate vs. lipid preference) is neurotransmitter specific as well.[782, 783] Amino acids also play a role in regulating GH, insulin, and glucagon secretion, and PRL secretion in humans is influenced by the pattern of food intake.[784]

Multiple factors that influence eating and satiety have been described, but it is not possible to provide a comprehensive model of the way in which these factors interact to govern behavior and to integrate them with metabolic and neuroendocrine regulation.

Drinking Behavior and Neuropeptides

Many similarities exist between neural control of drinking and that of eating. The goal of both behaviors is to maintain homeostasis—of blood volume and osmolality in the case of fluid intake and of metabolic function in the case of food ingestion. As with eating, drinking behavior is an integrated function of neural signals arising largely from volume receptors in the carotid sinus and left atrium, and with central receptors sensitive to changes in brain electrolytes. Central neuropeptides that play an important role in regulating water conservation responses are analogous to or identical with those that have the same function in the periphery. The best characterized of the water- and salt-regulating neuropeptides are AVP, angiotensin II, and the atriopeptins. These peptides were discussed earlier in the section on control of the posterior pituitary.[785–788] The angiotensinergic system of peptides and receptors in the brain has been well characterized.[789–791]

Peptides and Thermoregulation

Body temperature is regulated by the interaction of heat-dissipating and heat-producing mechanisms—neural, autonomic, and endocrine—that are integrated in the hypothalamus by a temperature-sensitive system. The neuronal substrate of this system includes several neurotransmitter pathways, the principal ones being adrenergic and serotoninergic.[792] In addition, a number of neuropeptide transmitters are involved in thermoregulation. The injection of TRH directly into the brain raises body temperature, and several peptides lower body temperature or counteract the effects of pyrogens. Temperature-lowering peptides of this type include gastrin-releasing hormone, neurotensin, and AVP; α-MSH is the most potent antipyretic central neuropeptide.[793]

The induction of fever by inflammation is brought about through the action of endogenous pyrogens that are released from activated immunocompetent cells. Several cytokines can induce fever through direct neuronal action, the most important being IL 1α and IL 1β, IL 2, and tumor necrosis factor (cachectin). It is believed that they act by stimulating prostaglandin formation[794, 795] in the hypothalamus,[796] thus accounting for the antipyretic action of aspirin and nonste-

TABLE 5–25. Peptides and Neurotransmitters That Influence Eating Behavior

Stimulate Eating	Inhibit Eating
Opioids	Insulin
Neuropeptide Y	TRH
Galanin	Somatostatin
GHRH	Cholecystokinin
Alpha-2–noradrenergic	Calcitonin
Serotonin (in median raphe)	Bombesin
GABA	VIP
Diazepam	CRH
	Neurotensin
	CGRP
	Glucagon
	IL 1
	Cachectin
	Beta-adrenergic
	Serotonin (in paraventricular nucleus)
	Prostaglandins

Adapted from Morley JE. Neuropeptide regulation of appetite and weight. Endocr Rev 1987; 8:256–287.

roidal anti-inflammatory drugs. Circulating ILs are excluded from the brain by the blood-brain barrier; they may induce fever by coming in contact with the temperature-regulating area through the OVLT, a circumventricular organ located in the anterior wall of the third ventricle[797] (also see earlier under Circumventricular Organs). As noted later under Neuroimmunomodulation, ILs also act on the hypothalamus to regulate anterior pituitary secretion.

Sleep Peptides

The CSF of sleeping animals contains one or more substances that bring about sleep when infused into the CSF of assay animals.[798–800] One such peptide has been isolated from CSF, and a second has been identified in human urine, but proof that these substances are released during normal sleep or are contained in specific neuronal pathways has not been provided. The first of the peptides to be isolated is a nonapeptide, Trp-Ala-Gly-Gly-Asp-Ala-Ser-Gly-Glu (DSIP, delta sleep-inducing peptide).[798] The second sleep-inducing peptide[799] causes sleep in the rabbit and is a muramyl dipeptide N-acetylglucosaminyl-N-acetylanhydromuramylal-anylglutamyldiaminopimelylalanine.[800] Antisera prepared against this material is immunoreactive with rabbit brain extracts.[801] Most muramyl peptides are not represented in animals but are characteristic of certain bacteria. It has been hypothesized that the material found in urine and brain is the product of bacterial action that is utilized by the host organism as a synthetic reagent, much as a vitamin is incorporated into cofactors.[801] A variety of muramyl peptides induce sleep when introduced into the third ventricle.[799]

As reviewed by Borbely and Tobler,[802] a large number of endogenous substances in brain can induce sleep. It is not clear, however, whether any of them, including the naturally occurring benzodiazepine ligands, mediate normal sleep.

Peptides in Sexual Function and Behavior

Although the gonadal steroids appear to be the most important hormonal factors that regulate sexual behavior in animals, central and peripheral peptidergic neuronal systems may also be involved. As mentioned previously, LHRH appears to have a stimulating effect on mating behavior in rats, and antagonistic analogues and antisera to LHRH appear to inhibit mating behavior (studies with humans have been inconclusive).[203, 206] ACTH has also been reported to stimulate sexual behavior. In contrast, a number of peptides, when introduced directly into the brain, inhibit or reduce sexual receptivity in the rat. These include β-endorphin, AVP, and CRH.[803] CRH also inhibits gonadotropin release and may be responsible for stress-induced hypogonadism.[804]

VIP plays an important role in erection. The genitalia of both men and women are richly innervated by VIP-containing neurons, which are especially concentrated in erectile tissue.[805, 806] Corresponding to this extensive genital VIP distribution is a dense concentration of VIP-containing neurons in the sacral cord of rats and humans.[807, 808] VIP is involved in the erection response because it relaxes penile smooth muscle and levels of VIP are increased in plasma from the deep dorsal vein and cavernous body during sexual arousal.[808] Anticholinergic drugs do not prevent the erection produced by stimulation of the pelvic nerves, which indicates that cholinergic stimuli are not the sole mediators of the sacral outflow regulation of penile function. The number of penile VIPergic neurons in experimental diabetes mellitus and in a human diabetic with impotence have been reported to be reduced.[809] The complex neurotransmitter control of erection has been reviewed in detail.[810]

In the female, VIP inhibits uterine smooth muscle activity and increases myometrial blood flow. Clitoral stimulation increases peripheral plasma levels of VIP.[811] It is reasonable to propose, therefore, that the increased vaginal secretion and pelvic congestion that accompany sexual excitement may be due to release of VIP from nerve endings in the vagina and pelvic mucosa. The nose is also innervated by VIPergic fibers, which are presumably involved in regulation of tumescence of the nasal turbinates.[812]

NEUROIMMUNOMODULATION

The immune system is one of the major adaptive systems of animals and is capable of recognizing foreign proteins, viruses, and bacteria as *nonself* and of mounting cellular reactions that defend the integrity of the host. In response to foreign molecules, specific lymphocyte receptors are synthesized, and immunocompetent cells are stimulated to secrete an extraordinary range of regulatory peptides whose function is to neutralize, to inactivate, and to sequester these invading substances.[813] Lymphocyte secretions include the immunoglobulins and the lymphokines. Because some lymphokines are secreted by other types of cells as well, they have also been called cytokines. Lymphokines regulate differentiation, proliferation, and function of other lymphocytes and in addition exert powerful effects on other tissues, such as induction of fever, alterations in protein and lipid metabolism in muscle, and modulation of neuroendocrine function.[794, 795, 814] In addition, endocrine and neural cells may also synthesize cytokines that may serve paracrine functions as well. The pathogenesis of autoimmune disease of the endocrine glands is reviewed in Chapter 31; this section deals with the neuroendocrine function of cytokines.

The function of the immune system is subject to neural and hormonal modulation; many of the same neuropeptides, protein hormones, and hormone receptors are expressed in nerve cells, endocrine cells, and lymphocytes; and the products of lymphocytes can influence neuroendocrine function.[7, 794, 795, 815, 816] An emerging literature, albeit controversial, suggests that stress, both emotional and physical, can modulate the immune response, at least in part by neuroendocrine mechanisms.[817] Thus the functions of the three major regulatory systems may be integrated. An important generalizing concept, proposed by Blalock,[7] is that the peripheral lymphocyte provides a sensing mechanism by which foreign substances are recognized and thereby mobilize neuroendocrine adaptive responses.

These insights have spawned several new research disciplines. *Neuroimmunology* is the study of immune reactions involving the brain, nerves, and muscles, e.g., autoimmune allergic encephalitis, multiple sclerosis, and myasthenia gravis. In the past this term was also applied to the study of neural modulation of the immune response, but a more specific term for the interaction of nervous and immune systems is *neuroimmunomodulation*. To emphasize the role of neuroendocrine mechanisms, the term *neuroendocrineimmunology* has been coined.[817] This section will consider the effects of hormones and peptides on immune responses, the effects of lymphokines on neuroendocrine function, and the hormones and neuropeptides produced by the immune system.

Neuroendocrine Regulation of the Immune Process

The nervous system can influence immune function through the classic route of hypothalamic-pituitary secretion.[818] The most important hormonal factors influencing immune reactions are the glucocorticoids that inhibit most aspects of the immune response, including the proliferation of lymphocytes; the production of immunoglobulins, cytokines, and the inflammatory mediators that follow antigen-antibody binding; and the cellular toxicity including the production of inflammatory leukotrienes.[819] These inhibitory reactions (which form the basis of the anti-inflammatory actions of glucocorticoids (see Chapter 9) occur within the range of values induced by stress or by inflammation. It is the contention of Munck and colleagues[819] that the pituitary-adrenal response to stress serves to modulate the intensity of the immune response and its inflammatory components, including changes in vascular tone and vascular permeability. Loss of this function makes adrenocorticoid-deficient animals vulnerable to inflammation. The fact that the products of inflammation such as IL 1 can activate the hypothalamic-pituitary-adrenal axis (see later) suggests the operation of a negative feedback control loop that regulates the intensity of inflammation.

Because pituitary-adrenal function is almost completely controlled by the brain, this system is an excellent example of neuroimmunomodulation. Studies of experimental autoimmune arthritis have shown high vulnerability in a strain of rats with genetically determined CRH deficiency,[820] a finding best explained by loss of the postulated feedback control of inflammation by the adrenal cortex.

The physiological effects of other neurally controlled anterior pituitary hormones on the immune response are more subtle. GH-deficient mice show thymic atrophy, involution of lymphatic tissue, and T cell impairment, abnormalities that are reversible by GH treatment.[821] In addition, the characteristic decrease in GH secretion in aging may be responsible for the decline in immune function because thymic atrophy in the aging rat is reversed by GH treatment.[822] The presence of GH receptors on lymphocytes further supports the view that these cells are GH regulated. PRL can also stimulate immune function.[823–826] Human T and B lymphocytes bear PRL receptors, as do certain lymphoma cells; the immunoincompetent state in hypophysectomized mice is corrected by PRL administration; antibodies to PRL inhibit lymphocyte proliferation in several cell lines; and cyclosporine, an immunosuppressant drug, blocks the lymphocyte-stimulating effects of PRL.[826] Lymphocyte PRL dependency may be a manifestation not only of a response to pituitary-derived PRL but also of a response to an autocrine or paracrine system because lymphocytes can also synthesize and secrete PRL[7] (see later). The effects of hyperprolactinemia and of drug-induced PRL suppression on human immune function have not been elucidated.

TABLE 5–26. Immunoregulatory Effects of Several Hormones and Neuropeptides*

Hormone/Neuropeptide	Effect
ACTH	Suppression of Ig and IFN-γ synthesis Augmentation of B cell proliferation Suppression of IFN-γ—mediated macrophage activation
Glucocorticoids	Inhibition of all aspects of lymphokine synthesis and effects
Estrogens	Stimulation of a number of lymphocyte functions
GH	Enhancement of generation of T cells
PRL	Stimulation of thymulin secretion Stimulation of lymphocyte proliferation
TSH	Enhancement of Ig synthesis
hCG	Suppression of T_c and NK cell activity Suppression of T cell proliferation Suppression of mixed lymphocyte reactions Generation of T_s cells
α-Endorphin	Suppression of Ig synthesis and secretion Suppression of antigen-specific helper T cell
β-Endorphin	Enhancement of Ig and IFN-γ synthesis Modulation of T cell proliferation Enhancement of generation of T_c cells Enhancement of NK cell activity Chemotactic for monocytes and neutrophils
Leu- or met-enkephalin	Suppression of Ig synthesis Enhancement of IFN-γ synthesis Enhancement of NK cell activity Chemotactic for monocytes
Substance P	Augmentation of T cell proliferation Degranulation of mast cells and basophils Enhancement of macrophage phagocytosis Elicitation of O_2, H_2O_2, and thromboxane B_2 production
AVP and oxytocin	Replacement of IL 2 requirement for IFN-γ synthesis
Somatostatin	Suppression of histamine and leukotriene D_4 release from basophils Suppression of T cell proliferation
VIP	Inhibition of mitogen-stimulated T cells through cAMP link Inhibition of release of T lymphocytes from popliteal nodes Inhibition of migration of T lymphocytes into mesenteric nodes
α-MSH	Suppression of IL 1 stimulated fever Suppression of monocyte secretion of IL 2 Suppression of fibroblast production of prostaglandins Suppression of neutrophil migration

*Ig, immunoglobulin; IFN-γ, interferon-γ; NK cells, natural killer T cells; T_s cells, T suppressor cells; T_c cells, cytotoxic T cells.
Adapted from Blalock JE. A molecular basis for bidirectional communication between the immune and neuroendocrine systems. Physiol Rev 1989; 69:1–32.

A role for pituitary-gonadal function as a modulator of the immune process has been suspected because of the sex differences in the prevalence of all the autoimmune diseases—Graves disease, rheumatoid arthritis, and systemic lupus erythematosus.[827] The sex ratio for patients with Hashimoto thyroiditis, for example, is as high as 25:1 in favor of women. The course of systemic lupus erythematosus is also influenced by estrogens; women given contraceptive steroids may show an exacerbation, as is also true for mouse models of the disease.[827] Estradiol potentiates mitogen-induced B cell stimulation in men.[828] Lymphocyte function varies during the menstrual cycle, reduction in activity of T lymphocytes being greatest in the first half of the cycle.[829]

Other pituitary hormones can bind to specific receptors on lymphocytes. This list of potential regulators include AVP, oxytocin, the endorphins, α-MSH, and LH.[7] Table 5–26 summarizes some of the immunoregulatory effects of these substances. Several of these substances appear to act both centrally and peripherally in mediating responses to inflammation. As noted in the previous section, both AVP and α-MSH are potent inhibitors of pyrogen-induced fever;[792, 793, 830] nerve endings containing these peptides are localized in the brain to temperature-regulating areas,[793] and in the periphery α-MSH counteracts several effects of IL 1 on monocyte and fibroblast function.[831–833]

Other neuropeptides that influence the immune response include substance P, somatostatin, and VIP. The concentrations required for biological effect are seemingly too high to be physiologically relevant. However, these peptides may be released locally in high concentration from sensory nerve endings;[834, 835] it has been postulated that arthritis may be potentiated by substance P released from sensory neurons in the joint.[834, 835] Moreover, some of the peptides may be secreted by the lymphocytes themselves. Substance P and its cosecretion substance K (both derived from the same prohormone) have vasodilating properties and are mediators of the wheal-and-flare response to tissue injury.[836] Somatostatin can inhibit immunoglobulin E–dependent stimulation of basophils and the in vitro proliferation of T and B lymphocytes.[837] VIP is generally inhibitory to all aspects of lymphocyte function and may act by modifying patterns of lymphocyte secretion from lymph nodes, a novel form of immunomodulation.[838]

Neuroendocrine Effects of the Lymphokines (Table 5–27)

Evidence is clear-cut that lymphokines act on the brain.[794, 795, 830, 839] Bacterial pyrogen administration or bacterial infection activates a lymphokine cascade including release of IL 1, IL 6, and tumor necrosis factor.[794, 795, 814, 840] IL 1 leads to fever (through anterior hypothalamic effects, as noted earlier) and also causes anorexia, drowsiness, increased slow-wave sleep, and various levels of central nervous system disturbance ranging from malaise to frank delirium and coma. Neuroendocrine responses to pyrogens (or to injections of purified IL 1β or IL 2) include activation of the pituitary-adrenal axis[841–844] and the release of PRL and GH in humans.[844] Inflammatory cytokines inhibit the release of TSH[845] and GH (in the rat).[846]

Regulatory pathways by which these effects are mediated have also been studied. IL 1β stimulates the release of CRH by a direct action on the hypothalamus;[843] it may act on the pituitary as well.[842] TSH and GH suppression by IL 1 (in the rat) is attributable (in part) to enhanced hypothalamic somatostatin synthesis.[847] IL 6 (also released during inflammation) stimulates several anterior pituitary hormones in vitro.[848] Many of the details of these regulatory responses remain to be worked out, but the essential point of this line

TABLE 5–27. Neuroendocrine Effects of Lymphokines and Monokines*

Lymphokine/ Monokine	Effect
IL 1	Causes fever
	Results in slow-wave sleep
	Causes CRH release
	Causes ACTH and endorphin release
	Elevates glucocorticoid levels
	Stimulates GH and PRL (in humans)
	Inhibits TSH release (in rats)
	Stimulates somatostatin secretion
	Inhibits TRH synthesis
	Stimulates AVP release
	Stimulates IL 6 production
IL 2	Stimulates release of ACTH, glucocorticoids, PRL, and GH
	Stimulates synthesis of TNF and IL 1
IL 6	Stimulates release of ACTH, glucocorticoids, GH, and PRL (present in folliculostellate pituitary cells)
TNF	Inhibits GH release (directly)
	Stimulates ACTH adrenocortical secretion
	Inhibits TSH, T_4, and T_3 secretion
	Inhibits thyroid response to TSH
	Increases PRL release
IFN-α and/or β	Induction of adrenal steroidogenesis
	Increases iodine uptake by thyroid cells
	Excites neurons
	Suppresses morphine withdrawal symptoms
	Causes catalepsy, analgesia
Thymosin	Elevates ACTH and glucocorticoid levels

*TNF, tumor necrosis factor; IFN-α or IFN-β, interferon-α or interferon-β.
Adapted from Blalock JE. A molecular basis for bidirectional communication between the immune and neuroendocrine systems. Physiol Rev 1989; 69:1–32.

of work is that the inflammatory response can regulate neuroendocrine function through circulating cytokines acting on the brain and/or the pituitary.

Additional sites of cytokine control have been documented: pituitary folliculostellate cells contain[849] and release[849, 850] IL 6, and one or more secretory cell types of the pituitary contain IL 1β.[851] Furthermore, neuronal pathways in the medial basal hypothalamus of humans[852] and rat[853] contain IL 1β and IL 6.[854] The potential thus exists for regulation of anterior pituitary function via endocrine effects (circulating lymphokines from activated lymphocytes), neuroendocrine effects (exerted by the hypothalamus through the classic tuberoinfundibular portal vessel system), and paracrine control within the pituitary itself.

In addition to the pituitary hormone changes induced by lymphokines, IL 1 and tumor necrosis factor are responsible in part for the acute-phase response, which has widespread effects including switching liver production of albumin to acute-phase glycoprotein, tissue sequestration of iron and copper, marked negative nitrogen balance, and loss of the ability to store fat.[794, 795] Negative catabolic effects of tumor necrosis factor on lipid metabolism led to the initial designation of this activity as *cachexin*.[814]

Hormones and Peptides Produced by the Immune System

Sensitive immunochemical and molecular methods have shown that immunocompetent cells secrete many peptides and hormones classically associated with endocrine or neural activity (Table 5–28).[7] Lymphocyte-secreted pituitary hormone is reportedly regulated by the same factors that regulate the pituitary. For example, ACTH secretion by lymphocytes is suppressed by glucocorticoids and is stimulated by CRF; TSH immunoreactivity of lymphocytes is stimulated by TRH and is suppressed by thyroid hormone, and lymphocyte GH is stimulated by GHRH and is suppressed by somatostatin.[7]

TABLE 5–28. Neuroendocrine Peptides Produced by the Immune System

Peptide	Cell or Tissue Source	Comments
ACTH	Lymphocytes and macrophages	Stimulated by CRH; inhibited by glucocorticoids
GH	Lymphocytes	Stimulated by GHRH; inhibited by somatostatin
TSH	T cells	Stimulated by TRH; inhibited by thyroid hormone
PRL	Lymphocytes	
hCG	T cells	
Enkephalins	T_h cells	
VIP	Mononuclear leukocytes, mast cells	
Somatostatin	Mononuclear leukocytes, mast cells, and polymorphonuclear leukocytes	
AVP	Thymus	
Oxytocin	Thymus	
Neurophysin	Thymus	

Adapted from Blalock JE. A molecular basis for bidirectional communication between the immune and neuroendocrine systems. Physiol Rev 1989; 69:1–32.

Although hormone secretion by lymphocytes is established, there is still uncertainty as to its biological significance. For example, the claim that the lymphocytes of hypophysectomized mice infected with Newcastle virus can synthesize enough ACTH to stimulate the adrenal cortex (one of the seminal claims in this field)[855] has been criticized on methodological grounds.[856] However, a case of Cushing syndrome apparently related to ACTH secretion by a large inflammatory mass was reported,[857] and a patient with adrenal failure caused by ACTH receptor deficiency was shown to lack lymphocyte ACTH receptors.[858]

Psychoneuroimmunology

Research efforts to identify neural pathways of immune regulation just summarized were initiated largely because of an extensive literature that asserts that psychological stress and depression can change human immune function,[817] that immune responses in animals can be conditioned in a classic pavlovian paradigm,[817, 859] and that specific neural lesions can inhibit various aspects of the immune response.[860] These changes could affect immune surveillance and have implications for the course of cancer, for the course of acquired immunodeficiency syndrome (AIDS), and for the initiation or aggravation of autoimmune diseases including those associated with the endocrine system (Graves disease and infiltrative exophthalmopathy, and insulin-dependent diabetes mellitus). The extent to which such influences, if present, are mediated through known neuroendocrine pathways is unknown. Alternative regulatory pathways from the central nervous system to the immune system include the catecholamines (and cosecreted neuropeptides) of the autonomic nervous system that innervate lymph nodes, spleen, and thymus;[861] adrenomedullary catecholamines; and the hormones that influence secretion of thymosin and other lymphocyte-regulating thymic hormones.[862]

REFERENCES

Introduction and Reviews

1. Snyder SH. Drug and neurotransmitter receptors in the brain. Science 1984; 224:22–31.
2. Roth J, LeRoith D, Shiloach J, et al. The evolutionary origins of hormones, neurotransmitters, and other extracellular chemical messengers. N Engl J Med 1982; 306:523–527.
3. Roth J, LeRoith D, Shiloach J, et al. Intercellular communication: an attempt at a unifying hypothesis. Clin Res 1983; 31:354–363.
4. Krieger DT, Martin JB. Brain peptides. N Engl J Med 1981; 304:876–885, 944–951.
5. Buchanan KD. Gut hormones and the brain. In: Besser GM, Martini L, eds. Clinical Neuroendocrinology. Vol II. New York: Academic, 1982: 332–359.
6. Krieger DT. Brain peptides: what, where, and why? Science 1983; 222:975–985.
7. Blalock JE. A molecular basis for bidirectional communication between the immune and neuroendocrine systems. Physiol Rev 1989; 69:1–32.
8. The Hypothalamus. Proceedings of Association for Research in Nervous and Mental Disease. New York: Hafner Publishing, 1940 (reprinted in 1966).
9. Harris GW. Neural control of the pituitary. Physiol Rev 1948; 28:139–179.
10. Friedgood HB. Neuroendocrinology. In: Williams RH, ed. Textbook of Endocrinology. 2nd ed. Philadelphia: W. B. Saunders, 1955.
11. Reichlin S. Medical progress. Neuroendocrinology. N Engl J Med 1963; 269:1246–1250, 1296–1303.
12. Szentágothai J, Flerkó B, Mess B. Hypothalamic Control of the Anterior Pituitary. New York: Grune & Stratton, 1968.
13. Heller H. History of neurohypophysial research. In: Greep RO, Astwood EB, Knobil E, et al., eds. Handbook of Physiology. Sect 7: Endocrinology. Vol IV. The Pituitary Gland and Its Neuroendocrine Control. Part 1. Washington, DC: American Physiological Society, 1974: 103–117.
14. Anderson E, Haymaker W. Breakthroughs in hypothalamic and pituitary research. Prog Brain Res 1974; 41:1–60.
15. Haymaker W, Anderson E, Nauta WJH. The Hypothalamus. Springfield, IL: Charles C Thomas, 1969.
16. Meites J, Donovan BT, McCann SM, eds. Pioneers in Neuroendocrinology. Vols I and II. New York: Plenum, Vol 1, 1975; Vol 2, 1978.
17. Flerko B. The hypophysial portal circulation today. Neuroendocrinology 1980; 30:56–63.
18. Martini L, Ganong WF, eds. Neuroendocrinology. New York: Academic, Vol 1, 1966; Vol 2, 1967.
19. Martini L, Ganong WF, eds. Frontiers in Neuroendocrinology. New York: Oxford University Press, Vol 1 (Ganong, Martini), 1969; Vol 2 (Martini, Ganong), 1971; Vol 3 (Martini, Ganong), 1973; New York: Raven, Vol 4 (Martini, Ganong), 1976; Vol 5 (Ganong, Martini), 1978; Vol 6 (Martini, Ganong), 1980; Vol 7 (Ganong, Martini), 1982; Vol 8 (Martini, Ganong), 1984; Vol 9 (Martini, Ganong), 1986; Vol 10 (Martini, Ganong), 1988.
20. Greep RO, Astwood EB, Knobil E, et al., eds. Handbook of Physiology. Sect 7: Endocrinology. Vol IV. The Pituitary Gland and Its Neuroendocrine Control. Part 1. Washington, DC: American Physiological Society, 1974.
21. Martin JB, Reichlin S, Brown GM. Clinical Neuroendocrinology. 2nd ed. Philadelphia: F. A. Davis, 1987.
22. Besser GM, Martini L, eds. Clinical Neuroendocrinology. New York: Academic, Vol I, 1977; Vol II, 1982.
23. Jeffcoate SL, Hutchinson JSM, eds. The Endocrine Hypothalamus. London: Academic, 1978.
24. Jackson IMD, Vale WW, eds. Extrapituitary functions of hypothalamic hormones. Fed Proc 1981; 49:2543–2544.
25. Krieger DT, Hughes JC, eds. Neuroendocrinology. Sunderland, MA: Sinauer Associates, 1980.
26. Müller EE, MacLeod RM, eds. Neuroendocrine Perspectives. Amsterdam: Elsevier Biomedical, Vol 1, 1982; Vol 2, 1983; Vol 3, 1984; Vol 4, 1985; Vol 5, 1986. New York: Springer-Verlag, Vol 6, 1987.
27. Scanlon MR, ed. Clinics in Endocrinology and Metabolism. London: W. B. Saunders, 1988.
28. Givens JR, ed. The Hypothalamus. Chicago: Year Book Medical, 1984.
29. Müller EE, Nistico G. Brain Messengers and the Pituitary. New York: Academic, 1989.
30. Nemeroff CB, Loosen PT. Handbook of Clinical Psychoneuroendocrinology. New York: Guilford, 1987.
31. Halbreich MD, ed. Hormones and Depression. New York: Raven, 1987.
32. Brown WA, ed. Endocrinology of neuropsychiatric disorders. Endocrinol Metab Clin North Am 1988; 17:1–239.
33. Lechan RM. Neuroendocrinology of pituitary hormone regulation. Endocrinol Metab Clin North Am 1987; 16:475–501.

Neural Control of Glandular Secretion

34. Schultzberg M, Hökfelt T, Lundberg JM. Peptide neurons in the autonomic nervous system. Adv Biochem Psychopharmacol 1980; 25:341–348.
35. Hökfelt T, Lundberg JM, Schultzberg M, et al. Coexistence of peptides and putative transmitters in neurons. Adv Biochem Psychopharmacol 1980; 22:1–23.
36. Hökfelt T, Johansson O, Ljungdahl A, et al. Peptidergic neurons. Nature 1980; 284:515–521.
37. Schultzberg M, Hökfelt T, Lundberg JM. Coexistence of classical transmitters and peptides in the central and peripheral nervous systems. Br Med Bull 1982; 38:309–313.
38. Lundberg JM, Hökfelt T, Änggard A, et al. Organizational principles

in the peripheral sympathetic nervous system: subdivision by coexisting peptides (somatostatin-, avian pancreatic polypeptide– and vasoactive intestinal polypeptide–like immunoreactive materials). Proc Natl Acad Sci USA 1982; 79:1303–1307.

39. Lundberg JM, Änggard A, Fahrenkrug J, et al. Vasoactive intestinal polypeptide in cholinergic neurons of exocrine glands: functional significance of coexisting transmitters for vasodilation and secretion. Proc Natl Acad Sci USA 1980; 77:1651–1655.

40. Lundberg JM, Änggard A, Fahrenkrug J. Complementary role of vasoactive intestinal polypeptide (VIP) and acetylcholine for cat submandibular gland blood flow and secretion. Acta Physiol Scand 1982; 3:329–337.

41. Ip NY, Perlman RL, Zigmond RE. Acute transsynaptic regulation of tyrosine 3-monoxygenase activity in the rat superior cervical ganglion: evidence for both cholinergic and noncholinergic mechanisms. Proc Natl Acad Sci USA 1983; 80:2081–2085.

42. Bern HA, Knowles FGW. Neurosecretion. In: Martini L, Ganong WF, eds. Neuroendocrinology. Vol 1. New York: Academic, 1966: 139–186.

43. Scharrer E, Scharrer B. Secretory cells within the hypothalamus. In: The Hypothalamus. Association for Research on Nervous and Mental Disease. New York: Hafner, 1940: 170–194.

44. Ochs S. Axoplasmic transport in peripheral nerve and hypothalamo-neurohypophyseal systems. In: Porter JC, ed. Hypothalamic Peptide Hormones and Pituitary Regulation. New York: Plenum, 1977: 13–40.

45. Pickering BT. The neurosecretory neurone: a model system for the study of secretion. Essays Biochem 1978; 14:45–81.

46. Livett BG. Axonal transport and neuronal dynamics: contributions to the study of neuronal connectivity. In: Porter R, ed. Neurophysiology II. Vol 10. Baltimore: University Park Press, 1976: 37–124.

47. Guillemin R. Peptides in the brain: the new endocrinology of the neuron (Nobel lecture). Science 1978; 202:390–402.

48. Bloom FE. Contrasting principles of synaptic physiology: peptidergic and non-peptidergic neurons. In: Fuxe K, Hökfelt T, Luft R, eds. Central Regulation of the Endocrine System. New York: Plenum, 1979: 173–187.

49. Wurtman RJ, Anton-Tay F. The mammalian pineal as a neuroendocrine transducer. Recent Prog Horm Res 1969; 25:493–522.

The Hypothalamic-Pituitary Unit

50. Everett JW. The mammalian hypothalamo-hypophysial system. In: Jeffcoate SL, Hutchinson JSM, eds. The Endocrine Hypothalamus. London: Academic, 1978: 1–34.

51. Wingstrand KG. Microscopic anatomy, nerve supply and blood supply of the pars intermedia. In: Harris GW, Donovan BT, eds. The Pituitary Gland. London: Butterworths, 1966: 1–27.

Neurohypophysis

52. Lederis K. Neurosecretion and the functional structure of the neurohypophysis. In: Greep RO, Astwood EB, Knobil E, et al., eds. Handbook of Physiology, Sect 7: Endocrinology. Vol IV. The Pituitary Gland and Its Neuroendocrine Control. Part 1. Washington, DC: American Physiological Society, 1974: 81–102.

53. Zimmerman EA, Hou-Yu A, Lilaver G, et al. Anatomy of pituitary and extrapituitary vasopressin secretory systems. In: Reichlin S, ed. The Neurohypophysis. New York: Plenum, 1984: 5–27.

54. Hayward JN. Functional and morphological aspects of hypothalamic neurons. Physiol Rev 1977; 57:574–658.

55. Reichlin S, ed. The Neurohypophysis. New York: Plenum, 1984.

56. Sofroniew MV, Weindl A. Extrahypothalamic neurophysin-containing perikarya, fiber pathways and the clusters in the rat brain. Endocrinology 1978; 102:334–337.

57. Raichle ME. Hypothesis: a central neuroendocrine system regulates brain ion homeostasis and volume. In: Martin JB, Reichlin S, Bick KL, eds. Neurosecretion and Brain Peptides. New York: Raven, 1981: 329–336.

58. Perlow MJ, Reppert SM, Artman HA, et al. Oxytocin, vasopressin, and estrogen-stimulated neurophysin: daily patterns of concentration in cerebrospinal fluid. Science 1982; 216:1416–1418.

59. Amico JA, Tenicela R, Johnston J, et al. A time dependent peak of oxytocin exists in the cerebrospinal fluid but not in the plasma of humans. J Clin Endocrinol Metab 1982; 57:947–951.

60. Dierickx K, Vandesande F. Immunocytochemical demonstration of separate vasopressin-neurophysin and oxytocin-neurophysin in neurons in the human hypothalamus. Cell Tissue Res 1979; 196:203–212.

61. Acher R. Chemistry of neurohypophysial hormones: an example of molecular evolution. In: Greep RO, Astwood EB, Knobil E, et al., eds. Handbook of Physiology, Sect 7: Endocrinology. Vol IV. The Pituitary Gland and Its Neuroendocrine Control. Part 1. Washington, DC: American Physiological Society, 1974: 119–130.

62. Ruppert S, Scherer G, Schütz G. Recent gene conversion involving bovine vasopressin and oxytocin precursor genes suggested by nucleotide sequence. Nature 1984; 308:554–557.

63. Blask DE, Vaughan MK, Reiter RJ. Pineal peptides and reproduction.

In: Relkin R, ed. The Pineal Gland. New York: Elsevier Biomedical, 1983: 201–223.

64. Manning M, Sawyer WH. Development of selective agonists and antagonists of vasopressin and oxytocin. In: Schrier RW, ed. Vasopressin. New York: Raven, 1985: 131–144.

65. Pelletier G. Immunohistochemical localization of somatostatin. Prog Histochem Cytochem 1980; 12:1–41.

66. Whitnall MH, Gainer H, Cox BM, et al. Dynorphin-A-(1-8) is contained within vasopressin neurosecretory vesicles in rat pituitary. Science 1983; 222:1137–1139.

67. Brownstein MJ, Russell JT, Gainer H. Synthesis, transport, and release of posterior pituitary hormones. Science 1980; 207:373–378.

68. Land H, Schutz G, Schmale H, et al. Nucleotide sequence of cloned cDNA encoding bovine arginine vasopressin–neurophysin II precursor. Nature 1982; 295:299–301.

69. Gainer H. Biosynthesis of vasopressin and neurophysin. In: Reichlin S, ed. The Neurohypophysis. New York: Plenum, 1984: 35–49.

70. Robinson AG. Neurophysins. In: Martini L, Besser GM, eds. Clinical Neuroendocrinology. New York: Academic, 1977: 585–602.

71. Robinson AG. The contribution of measured secretion of neurophysins to our understanding of neurohypophysial function. In: Reichlin S, ed. The Neurohypophysis. New York: Plenum, 1984: 65–93.

72. Sladek JR, Sladek GD. Neurological control of vasopressin release. Fed Proc 1985; 44:66–71.

73. Ramsey DJ. Effect of circulating angiotensin II on the brain. In: Ganong WF, Martini L, eds. Frontiers in Neuroendocrinology. Vol 7. New York: Raven, 1982: 263–286.

74. Ganten D, Fuxe K, Phillips MI, et al. The brain isorenin-angiotensin system: biochemistry, localization, and possible role in drinking and blood pressure regulation. In: Ganong WF, Martini L, eds. Frontiers in Neuroendocrinology. Vol 5. New York: Raven, 1978: 61–100.

75. Standaert DG, Needleman P, Saper CB. Atriopeptin: neuromediator in the central regulation of cardiovascular function. In: Martini L, Ganong WF, eds. Frontiers in Neuroendocrinology. Vol 10. New York: Raven, 1988: 63–78.

76. Edwards CRW. Vasopressin. In: Martini L, Besser GM, eds. Clinical Neuroendocrinology. New York: Academic, 1977: 527–567.

77. Miller M, Moses AM. Clinical states due to alteration of ADH release and action. In: Neurohypophysis. International Conference, Key Biscayne, Florida, 1976. White Plains, NY: A. J. Phiebig (Basel: S. Karger), pp. 153–166, 1977.

78. Sawchenko PE, Plotsky PM, Pfeiffer SW, et al. Is inhibin β in central neural pathways involved in the control of oxytocin secretion? Nature 1988; 334:615–617.

79. Moses AM. Diabetes insipidus and ADH regulation. In: Krieger DT, Hughes JC, eds. Neuroendocrinology. Sunderland, MA: Sinauer Associates, 1980: 141–148.

80. Robertson GL. The regulation of vasopressin function in health and disease. Recent Prog Horm Res 1977; 33:333–385.

81. Moses AM. Clinical and laboratory features of central and nephrogenic diabetes insipidus and primary polydipsia. In: Reichlin S, ed. The Neurohypophysis. New York: Plenum, 1984: 115–138.

82. Verney EB. The antidiuretic hormone and the factors which determine its release. Proc R Soc Lond 1947; 135:23–106.

83. Aubry Rh, Nankin HR, Moses AM, et al. Measurement of the osmotic threshold for vasopressin release in human subjects, and its modification by cortisol. J Clin Endocrinol Metab 1965; 25:1481–1492.

84. Oelkers W. Hyponatremia and inappropriate secretion of vasopressin (antidiuretic hormone) in patients with hypopituitarism. N Engl J Med 1989; 321:492–496.

85. Evans RM, Arriza JL. A molecular framework for the actions of glucocorticoid hormones in the nervous system. Neuron 1989; 2:1105–1112.

86. Swanson LW, Simmons DM. Differential steroid hormone and neural influences on peptide mRNA levels in CRH cells of the paraventricular nucleus: a hybridization histochemical study in the rat. J Comp Neurol 1989; 285:413–435.

87. Share L. Vasopressin and cardiovascular regulation. Symposium. Fed Proc 1984; 43:78–106.

88. Largh JH. Atrial natriuretic hormone, the renin-aldosterone axis, and blood pressure–electrolyte homeostasis. N Engl J Med 1985; 313:1330–1340.

89. Sudoh T, Kangwa K, Minamino N, et al. A new natriuretic peptide in porcine brain. Nature 1988; 332:78–80.

90. Chang MS, Lowe DG, Lewis M, et al. Differential activation by atrial and brain natriuretic peptides of two different receptor guanylate cyclases. Nature 1989; 341:68–72.

91. Gold PW, Kaye W, Robertson GL, et al. Abnormalities in plasma and cerebrospinal-fluid arginine vasopressin in patients with anorexia nervosa. N Engl J Med 1983; 308:1117–1123.

92. Goldman MB, Luchins DJ, Robertson GL. Mechanisms of altered water metabolism in psychotic patients with polydipsia and hyponatremia. N Engl J Med 1988; 318:397–403.

93. Hou S. Syndrome of inappropriate antidiuretic hormone secretion. In: Reichlin S, ed. The Neurohypophysis. New York: Plenum, 1984: 165–189.

94. Andersson B, Leksell LG, Lishajko F. Perturbations in fluid balance induced by medially placed forebrain lesions. Brain Res 1975; 99:261–275.

95. Fitzsimmons JT. Thirst. Physiol Rev 1972; 52:468–561.

96. Fitzsimmons JT. Some historical perspectives in the physiology of thirst. In: Epstein AN, Kissileff HR, Stellar E, eds. The Neurophysiology of Thirst. Washington, DC: V. H. Winston & Sons, 1973: 3–33.

97. Brody MJ, Johnson AK. Role of the anteroventral third ventricle region in fluid and electrolyte balance, arterial pressure regulation and hypertension. In: Martini L, Ganong WF, eds. Frontiers in Neuroendocrinology. Vol 6. New York: Raven, 1980: 249–292.

98. Phillips MI, Felix D. Specific angiotensin II receptive neurons in the cat subfornical organ. Brain Res 1976; 109:531–540.

99. Ohkubo H, Kageyama R, Ujihara M, et al. Cloning and sequence analysis of cDNA for rat angiotensinogen. Proc Natl Acad Sci USA 1983; 80:2196–2200.

100. Bissett GW. Milk ejection. In: Greep RO, Astwood EB, Knobil E, et al., eds. Handbook of Physiology. Sect 7: Endocrinology. Vol IV. The Pituitary Gland and Its Neuroendocrine Control. Part 1. Washington, DC: American Physiological Society, 1974: 493–520.

101. Chard T. Oxytocin. In: Martini L, Besser GM, eds. Clinical Neuroendocrinology. New York: Academic, 1977: 569–583.

102. Amico JA. Diabetes insipidus and pregnancy. Front Horm Res 1985; 13:266–277.

103. Fuchs AR, Fuchs F, Husslein P, et al. Oxytocin receptors and human parturition: a dual role for oxytocin in the initiation of labor. Science 1982; 215:1396–1398.

Intermediate Lobe

104. Kastin AJ, Viosca S, Schally AV. Regulation of melanocyte-stimulating hormone release. In: Greep RO, Astwood EB, Knobil E, et al., eds. Handbook of Physiology. Sect 7: Endocrinology. Vol IV. The Pituitary Gland and Its Neuroendocrine Control. Part 2. Washington, DC: American Physiological Society, 1974: 551–562.

105. Taleisnik S. Control of melanocyte-stimulating hormone (MSH) secretion. In: Jeffcoate SL, Hutchinson J, eds. The Endocrine Hypothalamus. New York: Academic, 1978: 421–438.

106. Moore KE, Johnston CA. The median eminence: aminergic control mechanisms. In: Müller EE, MacLeod RM, eds. Neuroendocrine Perspectives. Vol 1. Amsterdam: Elsevier Biomedical, 1982: 23–68.

107. Herbert E, Roberts J, Phillips M, et al. Biosynthesis, processing, and release of corticotropin, β-endorphin, and melanocyte-stimulating hormone in pituitary cell culture systems. In: Martini L, Ganong F, eds. Frontiers in Neuroendocrinology. Vol 6. New York: Raven, 1980: 67–102.

108. Roberts JL, Chen CLC, Eberwine JH, et al. Glucocorticoid regulation of proopiomelanocortin gene expression in rodent pituitary. Recent Prog Horm Res 1982; 38:227–256.

109. Krieger DT. The multiple faces of pro-opiomelanocortin, a prototype precursor molecule. Clin Res 1983; 31:342–353.

110. Vale W, Rivier C, Brown MR, et al. Chemical and biological characterization of corticotropin releasing factor. Recent Prog Horm Res 1983; 39:245–270.

111. Krieger DT. Physiopathology of Cushing's disease. Endocr Rev 1983; 4:22–43.

112. Lamberts SWJ, DeLange SA, Stefanke SZ. Adrenocorticotropin-secreting pituitary adenomas originate from the anterior or the intermediate lobe in Cushing's disease: differences in the regulation of hormone secretion. J Clin Endocrinol Metab 1982; 54:286–291.

113. Daughaday WH. Cushing's disease and basophilic microadenoma. N Engl J Med 1984; 310:919–929.

Median Eminence, and Tuberoinfundibular and Tuberohypophyseal Neurons

114. Gay VL. The hypothalamus: physiology and clinical use of releasing factors. Fertil Steril 1972; 23:50–63.

115. Knigge KM, Silverman AJ. Anatomy of the endocrine hypothalamus. In: Greep RO, Astwood EB, Knobil E, et al., eds. Handbook of Physiology. Sect 7: Endocrinology. Vol IV. The Pituitary Gland and Its Neuroendocrine Control. Part 1. Washington, DC: American Physiological Society, 1974: 1–32.

116. Joseph SA, Knigge KN. The endocrine hypothalamus: recent anatomical studies. In: Reichlin S, Baldessarini RJ, Martin JB, eds. The Hypothalamus. Vol 56. New York: Raven, 1978:15–47.

117. Hökfelt T, Elde R, Fuxe K, et al. Aminergic and peptidergic pathways in the nervous system with special reference to the hypothalamus. In: Reichlin S, Baldessarini RJ, Martin JB, eds. The Hypothalamus. Vol 56. New York: Raven, 1978: 69–135.

118. Jacobowitz DM. Multifactorial control of pituitary hormone secretion: the "wheels" of the brain. Synapse 1988; 2:186–192.

119. Swanson LW, Sawchenko PE. Hypothalamic integration: organization of the paraventricular and supraoptic nuclei. Annu Rev Neurosci 1983; 6:269–324.

120. Lechan RM, Nestler JL, Jacobson S. The tuberoinfundibular system of the rat as demonstrated by immunohistochemical localization of retrogradely transported wheat germ agglutinin (WGA) from the median eminence. Brain Res 1982; 245:1–15.

121. Negro-Vilar A. The median eminence as a model to study presynaptic regulation of neural peptide release. Peptides 1982; 3:305–310.

122. Oliver C, Mical RS, Porter JC. Hypothalamic-pituitary vasculature: evidence for retrograde blood flow in the pituitary stalk. Endocrinology 1977; 101:598–604.

123. Page RB. Directional pituitary blood flow: a microcinephotographic study. Endocrinology 1983; 112:157–165.

124. Lechan RM, Jackson IMD. Immunohistochemical localization of thyrotropin-releasing hormone in the rat hypothalamus and pituitary. Endocrinology 1982; 111:55–65.

125. Anthony EL, King JC, Stopa EG. Immunocytochemical localization of LHRH in the median eminence, infundibular stalk, and neurohypophysis. Evidence for multiple sites of releasing hormone secretion in humans and other mammals. Cell Tissue Res 1984; 236:5–14.

126. Lechan RM, Lin HD, Ling N, et al. Distribution of immunoreactive growth hormone releasing factor (1–44)NH$_2$ in the tuberoinfundibular system of the rhesus monkey. Brain Res 1984; 309:55–61.

127. Alpert LC, Brawer JR, Patel YC, et al. Somatostatinergic neurons in anterior hypothalamus: immunohistochemical localization. Endocrinology 1976; 98:255–258.

128. Krisch B. Hypothalamic and extrahypothalamic distribution of somatostatin-immunoreactive elements in the rat brain. Cell Tissue Res 1978; 195:499–513.

129. Bennett-Clarke C, Romagnano MA, Joseph SA. Distribution of somatostatin in the rat brain: telencephalon and diencephalon. Brain Res 1980; 188:473–486.

130. Swanson LW, Sawchenko PE, Rivier J, et al. Organization of ovine corticotropin-releasing factor immunoreactive cells and fibers in the rat brain: an immunohistochemical study. Neuroendocrinology 1983; 36:165–186.

131. Kahn D, Abrams GM, Zimmerman EA, et al. Neurotensin neurons in the rat hypothalamus: an immunohistochemical study. Endocrinology 1980; 107:47–54.

132. Vanderhaeghen JJ, Lotstra F, Demey J, et al. Immunohistochemical localization of cholecystokinin- and gastrin-like peptides in the brain and hypophysis of the rat. Proc Natl Acad Sci USA 1980; 77:1190–1194.

133. Hökfelt T, Fahrenkrug J, Tatemoto K, et al. The PHI (PHI-27)/corticotropin-releasing factor/enkephalin immunoreactive hypothalamic neuron: possible morphological basis for integrated control of prolactin, corticotropin, and growth hormone secretion. Proc Natl Acad Sci USA 1983; 80:895–898.

134. Barchas JD, Akil H, Elliott GR, et al. Behavioral neurochemistry: neuroregulators and behavioral states. Science 1978; 200:964–973.

135. Watson SJ, Khachaturian H, Taylor L, et al. Pro-dynorphin peptides are found in the same neurons throughout rat brain: immunohistochemical study. Proc Natl Acad Sci USA 1983; 80:891–894.

136. Quinlan JT, Phillips MI. Immunoreactivity for an angiotensin II–like peptide in the human brain. Brain Res 1981; 205:212–218.

137. Conlon JM, Samson WK, Dobbs RE, et al. Glucagon-like polypeptides in canine brain. Diabetes 1979; 28:700–702.

138. Hinsey JC, Markee JE. Pregnancy following bilateral section of the cervical sympathetic trunks in the rabbit. Proc Soc Exp Biol NY 1933; 31:270–271.

139. Friedgood HB. Studies on the sympathetic nervous control of the anterior hypophysis with special reference to a neuro-humoral mechanism. Symposium on endocrine glands. Harvard Tercentennial Celebration, 1936, reprinted in J Reprod Fertil 1970; 10:3–14.

140. Green JD, Harris GW. Neurovascular link between neurophysis and adenohypophysis. J Endocrinol 1947; 5:136–146.

141. Fink G. The development of the releasing factor concept. Clin Endocrinol 1976; 5:245s–260s.

142. Saffran M. Chemistry of hypothalamic hypophysiotropic factors. In: Greep RO, Astwood EB, Knobil E, et al., eds. Handbook of Physiology. Sect 7: Endocrinology. Vol IV. The Pituitary Gland and Its Neuroendocrine Control. Part 2. Washington DC: American Physiological Society, 1974: 563–586.

143. Reichlin S. TRH: historical aspects. Ann NY Acad Sci 1989; 553:1–6.

Hypophyseotropic Hormones

144. Bowers CY, Schally AV, Enzmann F, et al. Porcine thyrotropin releasing hormone is (pyro)glu-his-pro(NH$_2$). Endocrinology 1970; 86:1143–1153.

145. Burgus R, Dunn TF, Desiderio D, et al. Structure moléculaire du facteur hypothalamique hypophysiotrope TRF d'origine ovine: mise en évidence par spectrométrie de masse de la séquence PCA-His-Pro-NH$_2$. C R Acad Sci D 1969; 269:1870–1873.

146. Vale W, Rivier C, Brown M. Pharmacology of thyrotropin releasing factor (LRF) and somatostatin. In: Porter JC, ed. Hypothalamic Peptide Hormones and Pituitary Regulation. New York: Plenum, 1977: 123–156.

147. Sandow J, König W. Chemistry of the hypothalamic hormones. In:

Jeffcoate SL, Hutchinson JS, eds. The Endocrine Hypothalamus. London: Academic, 1978: 150–212.

148. Lechan RM, Segerson TP. Pro-TRH gene expression and precursor peptides in rat brain. Observations by hybridization analysis and immunocytochemistry. Ann NY Acad Sci 1989; 553:29–59.

149. Lee SL, Stewart K, Goodman RH. Structure of the gene encoding rat thyrotropin releasing hormone. J Biol Chem 1988; 263:16604–16609.

149a. Yamada M, Radovick S, Wondisford FE, et al. Cloning and structure of human genomic DNA and hypothalamic cDNA encoding human preprothyrotropin-releasing hormone. Mol Endocrinol 1990; 4:551–556.

150. Bowers CY, Friesen HG, Hwang P, et al. Prolactin and thyrotropin release in man by synthetic pyroglutamyl-histidyl-prolinamide. Biochem Biophys Res Commun 1971; 45:1033–1041.

151. Hershman JM. Use of thyrotropin-releasing hormone in clinical medicine. Med Clin North Am 1978; 62:313–325.

152. Snyder JJ, Jacobs LS, Rabello MM, et al. Diagnostic value of thyrotropin-releasing hormone in pituitary and hypothalamic disease: assessment of thyrotropin and prolactin in 100 patients. Ann Intern Med 1974; 81:751–757.

153. Burger HG, Patel YC. TSH and TRH: their physiological regulation and the clinical applications of TRH. In: Martini L, Besser GM, eds. Clinical Neuroendocrinology. New York: Academic, 1977: 67–132.

154. Frohman LA. Newer understanding of human hypothalamic-pituitary disease obtained through the use of synthetic hypothalamic hormones. In: Reichlin S, Baldessarini RJ, Martin JB, eds. The Hypothalamus. Vol 56. New York: Raven, 1978: 387–413.

155. Jackson IMD. Thyrotropin-releasing hormone. N Engl J Med 1982; 306:145–155.

156. Fink G, Koch Y, Ben Aroya N, et al. Release of thyrotropin releasing hormone into hypophysial portal blood is high relative to other neuropeptides and may be related to prolactin secretion. Brain Res 1982; 243:186–189.

157. Reichlin S. Neuroendocrine regulation of prolactin secretion. Adv Biosci 1988; 69:277–292.

158. Gautvik KM, Tashjian AH Jr, Kourides IA, et al. Thyrotropin-releasing hormone is not the sole physiologic mediator of prolactin release during suckling. N Engl J Med 1974; 290:1162–1165.

159. Thorner MO, Perryman RL, Cronin MJ, et al. Somatotroph hyperplasia: successful treatment of acromegaly by removal of a pancreatic islet tumor secreting a growth hormone–releasing factor. J Clin Invest 1982; 70:965–977.

160. Borges JL, Uskavitch DR, Kaiser DL, et al. Human pancreatic growth hormone–releasing factor-40 (hpGRF-40) allows stimulation of GH release by TRH. Endocrinology 1983; 113:1519–1521.

161. Halpern J, Hinkle PM. Direct visualization of receptors for thyrotropin-releasing hormone with a fluorescein-labeled analog. Proc Natl Acad Sci USA 1981; 78:587–591.

162. Tashjian AH Jr, Heslop JP, Berridge MJ. Subsecond and second changes in inositol polyphosphates in GH4C1 cells induced by thyrotropin-releasing hormone. Biochem J 1987; 243:305–308.

163. Winiger BP, Schlegel W. Rapid transient elevations of cytosolic calcium triggered by thyrotropin releasing hormone in individual cells of the pit line GH3B6. Biochem J 1988; 255:161–167.

164. Rosenfeld MG, Amara SG, Birnberg NC, et al. Prolactin and growth hormone gene expression as model systems for the characterization of neuroendocrine regulation. Recent Prog Horm Res 1983; 39:305–352.

165. Johannsson O, Hökfelt T, Pernow B, et al. Immunohistochemical support for three putative transmitters in one neuron: coexistence of 5-hydroxytryptamine, substance P, and thyrotropin-releasing hormone–like immunoreactivity in medullary neurons projecting to the spinal cord. Neuroscience 1981; 6:1857–1881.

166. Lechan RM, Snapper SC, Jackson IMD. Evidence that spinal cord TRH is independent of the paraventricular nucleus. Neurosci Lett 1983; 43:61–65.

167. Lechan RM, Snapper SC, Jacobson S, et al. The distribution of thyrotropin-releasing hormone (TRH) in the rhesus monkey spinal cord. Peptides 1984; 5(Suppl 1):185–194.

168. Lechan RM, Adelman LS, Forte S, et al. Organization of thyrotropin-releasing (TRH) immunoreactivity in the human spinal cord. Soc Neurosci Abstr 1984; 431.

169. Engler D, Scanlon MF, Jackson IMD. Thyrotropin releasing hormone in the systemic circulation of the neonatal rat is derived from the pancreas and other extraneural tissues. J Clin Invest 1981; 67:800–808.

170. Reichlin S. Neural functions of TRH. Acta Endocrinol 1986; 112:21–33.

171. Griffiths EC, Bennett GW, eds. Thyrotropin-Releasing Hormone. New York: Raven, 1983.

172. Jackson IMD, Metcalf G, eds. TRH. Ann NY Acad Sci 1989; 553:1–631.

173. Loosen PT, Prange AJ Jr. The serum thyrotropin (TSH) response to thyrotropin-releasing hormone in psychiatric patients: a review. Am J Psychiatry 1982; 139:405–416.

174. Faden AI, Jacobs TP, Holaday JW. Thyrotropin-releasing hormone improves neurologic recovery after spinal trauma in cats. N Engl J Med 1981; 305:1063–1067.

175. Sobue I, Takayanagi T, Nakanishi T, et al. Controlled trial of thyrotropin-releasing hormone tartrate in ataxia of spinocerebellar degenerations. J Neurol Sci 1983; 61:235–248.

176. Engel WK, Siddique T, Nicoloff JT. Effect on weakness and spasticity in amyotrophic lateral sclerosis of thyrotropin-releasing hormone. Lancet 1983; 2:73–75.

177. Munsat TL, Lechan R, Taft JM, et al. TRH and diseases of the motor system. Ann NY Acad Sci 1989; 553:388–398.

178. Brooks BR. A summary of the current position of TRH in ALS therapy. Ann NY Acad Sci 1989; 553:431–461.

179. Jackson IM, Adelman LS, Munsat TL, et al. Amyotrophic lateral sclerosis: thyrotropin-releasing hormone and cerebrospinal fluid. Neurology 1986; 36:1218–1223.

179a. Askanas V, Engel WK, Eagelson K, et al. Influence of TRH and TRH analogues RGH-2202 and DN-1417 on cultured ventral spinal cord neurons. Ann NY Acad Sci 1989; 553:325–336.

180. Peterkofsky A, Battaini F, Koch Y, et al. Histidyl-proline diketopiperazine: its biological role as a regulatory peptide. Mol Cell Biochem 1982; 42:45–63.

181. McCann SM, Taleisnik S, Friedman HM. LH-releasing activity in hypothalamic extracts. Proc Soc Exp Biol Med 1960; 104:432–434.

182. Campbell HJ, Feuer G, Harris GW. The effect of intrapituitary infusion of median eminence and other brain extracts on anterior pituitary gonadotrophic secretion. J Physiol (Lond) 1974; 170:474–486.

183. Matsuo H, Baba Y, Nair RMB, et al. Structure of the porcine LH- and FSH-releasing hormone. 1. The proposed amino acid sequence. Biochem Biophys Res Commun 1971; 43:1334–1339.

184. Seeburg PH, Adelman JP. Characterization of cDNA for precursor of human luteinizing hormone releasing hormone. Nature 1984; 311:666–668.

185. McCann SM, Mizunuma H, Samson WK. Differential hypothalamic control of FSH secretion: a review. Psychoneuroendocrinology 1983; 8:299–308.

186. Wise PM, Rance N, Barr GD. Further evidence that luteinizing hormone–releasing hormone also is follicle-stimulating hormone–releasing hormone. Endocrinology 1979; 104:940–947.

187. Marshall LA, Monroe SE, Jaffe RB. Physiologic and therapeutic aspects of GnRH and its analogs. In: Martini L, Ganong WF, eds. Frontiers in Neuroendocrinology. Vol 10. New York: Raven, 1988: 239–278.

188. Sandow J. The regulation of LHRH action at the pituitary and gonadal receptor level: a review. Psychoneuroendocrinology 1983; 8:277–297.

189. Ying SY. Inhibins and activins. In: Martini L, Ganong WF, eds. Frontiers in Neuroendocrinology. Vol 10. New York: Raven, 1988: 167–184.

190. Marshall JC, Kelch RP. Gonadotropin-releasing hormone: role of pulsatile secretion in the regulation of reproduction. N Engl J Med 1986; 315:1459–1468.

191. Millar RP, King JA. Evolution of gonadotropin-releasing hormone: multiple usage of a peptide. News Physiol Sci 1988; 3:49–53.

192. Eiden LE, Loumaye E, Sherwood N, et al. Two chemically and immunologically distinct forms of luteinizing hormone–releasing hormone are differentially expressed in frog neural tissues. Peptides 1982; 3:323–327.

193. Sherwood N, Eiden L, Brownstein M, et al. Characterization of a teleost gonadotropin-releasing hormone. Proc Natl Acad Sci USA 1983; 80:2794–2798.

194. Hoffman AR, Crowley WF Jr. Induction of puberty in men by long-term pulsatile administration of low-dose gonadotropin-releasing hormone. N Engl J Med 1982; 307:1237–1241.

195. Stanhope R, Brook CGD, Pringle PJ, et al. Induction of puberty by pulsatile gonadotropin releasing hormone. Lancet 1987; 2:552–555.

196. Mansfield MJ, Beardsworth DE, Loughlin JS, et al. Long-term treatment of central precocious puberty with a long-acting analogue of luteinizing hormone–releasing hormone. N Engl J Med 1983; 309:1286–1290.

197. Borgmann V, Hardt W, Schmidt-Gollwitzer M, et al. Sustained suppression of testosterone production by the luteinising-hormone releasing-hormone agonist buserelin in patients with advanced prostate carcinoma. A new therapeutic approach? Lancet 1982; 1:1097–1099.

198. Labrie F, Dupont A, Belanger A, et al. New hormonal treatment in cancer of the prostate: combined administration of an LHRH agonist and an antiandrogen. J Steroid Biochem 1983; 19:999–1007.

199. Rabin D, McNeil LW. Pituitary and gonadal desensitization after continuous luteinizing hormone–releasing hormone infusion in normal females. J Clin Endocrinol Metab 1980; 51:873–876.

200. Schally AV, Arimura A, Coy DH. Recent approaches to fertility control based on derivatives of LH-RH. Vitam Horm 1980; 38:257–323.

201. Sandow J. Gonadotropic and antigonadotropic actions of LH-RH analogues. In: Müller EE, MacLeod RM, eds. Neuroendocrine Perspectives. Vol 1. Amsterdam: Elsevier Biomedical, 1982: 339–396.

202. Hsueh AJW, Jones BC. Extrapituitary actions of gonadotropin-releasing hormone. Endocr Rev 1981; 2:437–461.

203. Moss RL. Actions of hypothalamic-hypophysiotropic hormones on the brain. Annu Rev Physiol 1979; 41:617–631.

204. Kuffler SW, Sejnowski TJ. Peptidergic and muscarinic excitation at amphibian sympathetic synapses. J Physiol (Lond) 1983; 341:257–278.

205. Amarant T, Fridkin M, Koch Y. Luteinizing hormone–releasing hormone and thyrotropin-releasing hormone in human and bovine milk. Eur J Biochem 1982; 127:647–650.

206. Ehrensing RH, Kastin AJ, Schally AV. Behavioral and hormonal effects of prolonged high doses of LHRH in male impotency. Peptides 1981; 2(Suppl 1):115–121.

207. Conn PM. The molecular basis of gonadotropin-releasing hormone action. Endocr Rev 1986; 7:3–10.

208. Clayton RN, Catt KJ. Gonadotropin-releasing hormone receptors: characterization, physiological regulation, and relationship to reproductive function. Endocr Rev 1981; 2:186–209.

209. Popkin R, Bramley TA, Currie A, et al. Specific binding of luteinizing hormone releasing hormone to human luteal tissue. Biochem Biophys Res Commun 1983; 114:750–756.

210. Popkin R, Fraser HM, Jonassen J. Stimulation of androstenedione and progesterone release by LHRH and LHRH agonist from isolated rat preovulatory follicles. Mol Cell Endocrinol 1983; 29:169–179.

211. Reichlin S. Regulation of somatotrophic hormone secretion. In: Greep RO, Astwood EB, Knobil E, et al., eds. Handbook of Physiology. Sect 7: Endocrinology. Vol IV. The Pituitary Gland and Its Neuroendocrine Control. Washington, DC: American Physiological Society, 1974: 405–448.

212. Frohman LA, Szabo M, Berelowitz M, et al. Partial purification and characterization of a peptide with growth hormone–releasing activity from extrapituitary tumors in patients with acromegaly. J Clin Invest 1980; 65:43–54.

213. Guillemin R, Barazeau P, Bohlen P, et al. Growth hormone–releasing factor from a human pancreatic tumor that caused acromegaly. Science 1981; 218:585–587.

214. Rivier J, Speiss J, Thorner M, et al. Characterisation of a growth hormone–releasing factor from a human pancreatic islet tumour. Nature 1982; 300:276–278.

215. Mayo KE, Vale W, Rivier J, et al. Expression-cloning and sequence of a cDNA encoding human growth hormone–releasing factor. Nature 1983; 306:86–88.

216. Thorner MO, Frohman LA, Leong DA, et al. Extrahypothalamic growth hormone–releasing factor (GRF) is a rare cause of acromegaly: plasma GRF levels in 177 acromegalic patients. J Clin Endocrinol Metab 1984; 59:846–849.

217. Asa SL, Kovacs K, Thorner MO, et al. Immunohistological localization of growth hormone–releasing hormone in human tumors. J Clin Endocrinol Metab 1985; 60:423–427.

218. Dayal Y, Lin HD, Tallberg K, et al. Immunocytochemical demonstration of growth hormone–releasing factor in gastrointestinal and pancreatic endocrine tumors. Am J Clin Pathol 1986; 85:13–20.

219. Thorner MO, Rivier J, Spiess J. Human pancreatic growth hormone–releasing factor selectively stimulates growth hormone secretion in man. Lancet 1983; 1:24–28.

220. Frohman LA, Jansson JO. Growth hormone–releasing hormone. Endocr Rev 1986; 7:223–253.

221. Vance ML, Thorner MO. Some clinical considerations of growth hormone and growth hormone–releasing hormone. In: Martini L, Ganong WF, eds. Frontiers in Neuroendocrinology. Vol 10. New York: Raven, 1988: 279–294.

222. Shibasaki T, Shizume K, Nakahara M, et al. Age-related changes in plasma growth hormone response to growth hormone–releasing factor in man. J Clin Endocrinol Metab 1984; 58:212–214.

223. Shibasaki T, Shizume K, Masuda A, et al. Plasma growth hormone response to growth hormone–releasing factor in acromegalic patients. J Clin Endocrinol Metab 1984; 58:215–217.

224. Brazeau P, Ling N, Esch F, et al. Somatocrinin (growth hormone–releasing factor) in vitro bioactivity: Ca^{++} involvement, cAMP mediated action and additivity of effect with PGE_2. Biochem Biophys Res Commun 1982; 109:588–594.

225. Michel D, Lefevre G, Labrie F. Interactions between growth hormone–releasing factor, prostaglandin E_2 and somatostatin on cyclic AMP accumulation in rat adenohypophysial cells in culture. Mol Cell Endocrinol 1983; 33:255–264.

226. Canonico PL, MacLeod RM. The role of phospholipids in hormonal secretory mechanisms. In: Müller EE, MacLeod RM, eds. Neuroendocrine Perspectives. Vol 2. Amsterdam: Elsevier Biomedical, 1983: 123–172.

227. Lewin MJ, Reyl-Desmars F, Ling N. Somatocrinin receptor coupled with cAMP-dependent protein kinase on anterior pituitary granules. Proc Natl Acad Sci USA 1983; 80:6538–6541.

228. Barinaga M, Yamonoto G, Rivier C, et al. Transcriptional regulation of growth hormone gene expression by growth hormone–releasing factor. Nature 1983; 306:84–85.

229. Wehrenberg WB, Baird A, Ling N. Potent interaction between glucocorticoids and growth hormone–releasing factor in vivo. Science 1983; 221:556–558.

230. Dawson-Hughes B, Stern D, Goldman J, et al. Regulation of growth-hormone and somatomedin-C secretion in postmenopausal women: effect of physiological estrogen replacement. J Clin Endocrinol Metab 1986; 63:424–432.

231. Mayo KE, Hammer RE, Swanson LW, et al. Dramatic pituitary hyperplasia in transgenic mice expressing a human growth hormone–releasing factor gene. Mol Endocrinol 1988; 2:606–612.

232. Krulich L, Dhariwal AP, McCann SM. Stimulatory and inhibitory effects of purified hypothalamic extracts on growth hormone release from rat pituitary in vitro. Endocrinology 1968; 83:783–790.

233. Hellman B, Lernmark A. Inhibition of the in vitro secretion of insulin by an extract of pancreatic A_1 cells. Endocrinology 1969; 84:1484–1487.

234. Brazeau P, Vale W, Burgus R, et al. Hypothalamic polypeptide that inhibits the secretion of immunoreactive pituitary growth hormone. Science 1973; 179:77–79.

235. Gerich JE. Somatostatin. In: Brownlee M, ed. Handbook of Diabetes Mellitus. Vol 1. New York: Garland STPM, 1978: 297–354.

236. Reichlin S. Somatostatin. In: Krieger DT, Brownstein M, Martin JB, eds. Brain Peptides. New York: John Wiley & Sons, 1983:711–752.

237. Reichlin S. Somatostatin. N Engl J Med 1983; 309:1495–1501, 1556–1563.

238. Patel YC, Tannenbaum GS, eds. Somatostatin. New York: Plenum, 1984.

239. Patel YC, Srikant CB. Somatostatin mediation of adenohypophysial secretion. Annu Rev Physiol 1986; 48:551–567.

240. Reichlin S, ed. Somatostatin. New York: Plenum, 1986.

241. Patel YC, Tannenbaum GS, eds. Somatostatin: basic and clinical aspects. Metabolism 1990; 39(Suppl 2):1–192.

242. Lamberts SWJ. Non-pituitary actions of somatostatin: a review on the therapeutic role of SM 201-995 (Sandostatin). Acta Endocrinol 1986; 276(Suppl):41–55.

243. Gorden P, Comi RJ, Maton PM, et al. NIH conference: somatostatin and somatostatin analog (SMS 201-995) in treatment of hormone-secreting tumors of the pituitary and gastrointestinal tract and non-neoplastic diseases of the gut. Ann Intern Med 1989; 110:35–50.

244. Octreotide. Lancet 1989; 2:541 (editorial).

245. Shen LP, Rutter WJ. Sequence of human somatostatin I gene. Science 1984; 224:168–171.

246. Montminy MR, Goodman RH, Horovitch SJ, et al. Primary structure of the gene encoding rat pre-prosomatostatin. Proc Natl Acad Sci USA 1984; 81:3337–3340.

247. Nutt RF, Veber DR, Curley PE, et al. Somatostatin analogs which define the role of the lysine-9 amino group. Int J Pept Protein Res 1983; 21:66–73.

248. Schonbrunn A. Somatostatin action in pituitary cells involves two independent transduction mechanisms. Metabolism 1990; 39(Suppl 2):96–100.

249. Hoeldtke RD, Israel BC. Treatment of orthostatic hypotension with octeotide. J Clin Endocrinol Metab 1989; 68:1051–1059.

250. Makara GB, Antoni FA, Stark E, et al. Hypothalamic organization of corticotropin releasing factor (CRF) producing structures. In: Müller EE, MacLeod RM, eds. Neuroendocrine Perspectives. Vol 3. Amsterdam: Elsevier Biomedical, 1984: 71–119.

251. Saffran M, Schally AV, Benfey BG. Stimulation of the release of corticotropin from the adenohypophysis by a neurohypophysial factor. Endocrinology 1955; 57:439–444.

252. Guillemin R, Rosenberg B. Humoral hypothalamic control of anterior pituitary: study with combined tissue cultures. Endocrinology 1955; 57:599–607.

253. Shibahara S, Morimoto Y, Furutani Y, et al. Isolation and sequence analysis of the human corticotropin-releasing factor precursor gene. EMBO J 1983; 2:775–779.

254. Erspamer V, Melchiorri P. Actions of amphibian skin peptides on the central nervous system and the anterior pituitary. In: Müller EE, MacLeod RM, eds. Neuroendocrine Perspectives. Vol 2. Amsterdam: Elsevier Biomedical, 1983: 37–106.

255. Müller OA, Stalla GK, von Werder K. Corticotropin releasing factor: a new tool for the differential diagnosis of Cushing's syndrome. J Clin Endocrinol Metab 1983; 57:227–229.

256. Chrousos GP, moderator. Clinical applications of corticotropin-releasing factor. Ann Intern Med 1985; 102:344–358.

257. Taylor AL, Fishman LM. Corticotropin-releasing hormone. N Engl J Med 1988; 319:213–222.

258. Chrousos GP, Schulte HM, Oldfield EH, et al. The corticotropin-releasing factor stimulation test. N Engl J Med 1984; 310:622–626.

259. Wynn PC, Aguilera G, Morell J, et al. Properties and regulation of high-affinity pituitary receptors for corticotropin-releasing factor. Biochem Biophys Res Commun 1983; 110:602–608.

260. Leroux P, Pelletier G. Radioautographic study of binding and internalization of corticotropin-releasing factor by rat anterior pituitary corticotrophs. Endocrinology 1984; 114:14–21.

261. Abou-Samra AB, Harwood JP, Catt KJ, et al. Mechanisms of action of CRF and other regulators of ACTH release in pituitary corticotrophs. Ann NY Acad Sci 1987; 512:67–84.

262. Rivier C, Rivier J, Vale W. Stress-induced inhibition of reproductive functions: role of endogenous corticotropin-releasing factor. Science 1989; 245:607–609.

263. Lenz HG. Extrapituitary effects of corticotropin-releasing factor. Horm Metab Res Suppl 1987; 16:17–23.

264. Petraglia F, Sawchenko PE, Rivier J, et al. Evidence for local stimulation of ACTH secretion by corticotropin-releasing factor in human placenta. Nature 1987; 328:717–719.

265. Pasteels JL. Prolactin regulatory factors. Premiers résultats de culture combinée in vitro d'hypophyse et d'hypothalamus dans le but d'en

apprecier la sécrétion de prolactine. C R Acad Sci (Paris) 1961; 253:3074–3075.

266. Neill JD. Prolactin: its secretion and control. In: Greep RO, Astwood EB, Knobil E, et al., eds. Handbook of Physiology. Sect 7: Endocrinology. Vol IV. The Pituitary Gland and Its Neuroendocrine Control. Part 2. Washington DC: American Physiological Society, 1974: 469–488.

267. MacLeod RM. Regulation of prolactin secretion. In: Martini L, Ganong WF, eds. Frontiers in Neuroendocrinology. Vol 4. New York: Raven, 1976: 169–194.

268. Neill JD. Neuroendocrine regulation of prolactin secretion. In: Martini L, Ganong WF, eds. Frontiers in Neuroendocrinology. Vol 6. New York: Raven, 1980: 129–155.

269. Cronin MJ. The role and direct measurement of the dopamine receptor(s). In: Müller EE, MacLeod RM, eds. Neuroendocrine Perspectives. Vol 1. Amsterdam: Elsevier Biomedical, 1982: 169–210.

270. Judd AM, Koike K, Schettini G, et al. Dopamine decreases prolactin secretion induced by increases in calcium mobilization in the 7315a pituitary tumor, but not the MtTW 15 pituitary tumor. In: MacLeod RM, Thorner MO, Scapagnini V, eds. Prolactin, Basis and Clinical Correlates. Padua: Livania, 1985: 205–212.

271. Reichlin S. Neuroendocrine regulation of prolactin secretion. Adv Biosci 1988; 69:277–292.

272. Ben-Jonathan N. Prolactin releasing and inhibiting factors in the posterior pituitary. In: Müller EE, MacLeod RM, eds. Neuroendocrine Perspectives. Vol 8. New York: Springer-Verlag, 1990: 1–38.

273. Arey BJ, Freeman ME. Oxytocin, vasoactive intestinal peptide and serotonin regulate the mating-induced surges of prolactin secretion in the rat. Endocrinology 1990; 126:279–284.

274. Itoh N, Obata K, Yanaihara N, et al. Human preprovasoactive intestinal polypeptide contains a novel PHI-27–like peptide, PHM-27. Nature 1983; 304:547–549.

275. Werner S, Hulting AL, Hökfelt T, et al. Effect of the peptide PHI-27 on prolactin release in vitro. Neuroendocrinology 1983; 37:476–478.

276. Hökfelt T, Fahrenkrug J, Tatemoto K, et al. The PHI (PHI-27)/corticotropin-releasing factor/enkephalin immunoreactive hypothalamic neuron: possible morphological basis for integrated control of prolactin, corticotropin, and growth hormone secretion. Proc Natl Acad Sci USA 1983; 80:895–898.

277. Sandman CA, Kastin AJ, Miller LH. Central nervous system actions of MSH and related pituitary peptides. In: Martini L, Besser GM, eds. Clinical Neuroendocrinology. New York: Academic, 1978: 443–469.

278. Tatro JB, Reichlin S. Specific receptors for alpha-melanocyte–stimulating hormone are widely distributed in tissues of rodents. Endocrinology 1987; 121:1900–1907.

279. Lipton JM, Clark WG. Neurotransmitters in temperature control. Annu Rev Physiol 1986; 48:613–623.

Regulation of Secretion of Tuberohypophyseal Neurons

280. Müller EE, Nistico G. Brain Messengers and the Pituitary. San Diego, CA: Academic, 1988.

281. Renaud LP, Blume HW, Pittman QJ. Neurophysiology and neuropharmacology of the hypothalamic tuberoinfundibular system. In: Ganong F, Martini L, eds. Frontiers in Neuroendocrinology. Vol 5. New York: Raven, 1978: 135–162.

282. Palkovits M. Topography of chemically identified neurons in the central nervous system: progress in 1981–1983. In: Müller EE, MacLeod RM, eds. Neuroendocrine Perspectives. Vol 3. Amsterdam: Elsevier Biomedical, 1984: 1–69.

283. Weiner RL, Ganong WF. Role of brain monoamines and histamine in regulation of anterior pituitary secretion. Physiol Rev 1978; 58:905–976.

284. Delitala G. Neurotransmitter control of anterior pituitary hormone secretion and its clinical implications in man. In: Besser GM, Martini L, eds. Clinical Neuroendocrinology. Vol II. New York: Academic, 1982: 68–139.

285. Cooper JR, Bloom FE, Roth RH. The Biochemical Basis of Neuropharmacology. 5th ed. New York: Oxford University Press, 1986.

286. Barraclough CA, Wise PM. The role of catecholamines in the regulation of pituitary luteinizing and follicle-stimulating hormone secretion. Endocr Rev 1983; 4:91–119.

287. Terry LC. Neuropharmacologic regulation of anterior pituitary hormone secretion in man. In: Givens JR, ed. Hormone-Secreting Pituitary Tumors. Chicago: Year Book Medical, 1982: 27–44.

288. Moore KE, Demarest KT. Tuberoinfundibular and tuberohypophysial dopaminergic neurons. In: Ganong F, Martini L, eds. Frontiers in Neuroendocrinology. Vol 7. New York: Raven, 1982: 211–230.

289. Thorner M. Is prolactin a marker for brain dopamine function? In: Brown GM, Koslow SH, Reichlin S, eds. Neuroendocrinology and Psychiatric Disorders. New York: Plenum, 1984: 55–66.

290. Moore RY, Bloom FE. Central catecholamine neuron systems. Anatomy and physiology of the norepinephrine and epinephrine systems. Annu Rev Neurosci 1979; 2:113–168.

291. Iversen LL, Iversen SD, Snyder SH, eds. Chemical pathways in the brain. In: Handbook of Psychopharmacology. Vol 9. New York: Plenum, 1978.

292. Bowker RM, Westlund KN, Sullivan MC, et al. Transmitters of the raphe-spinal complex: immunocytochemical studies. Peptides 1982; 3:291–298.

293. Swanson LW, Hartman BK. The central adrenergic system. An immunofluorescence study of the location of cell bodies and their efferent connections in the rat utilizing dopamine-β-hydroxylase as a marker. J Comp Neurol 1975; 163:467–505.

294. Steinbusch HW, Nieuwenhuys R. Distribution of serotonin-immunoreactivity in the central nervous system and pituitary of the rat with special references to the innervation of the hypothalamus. Adv Exp Med Biol 1981; 133:7–35.

295. Bowker RM, Westlund KN, Sullivan MC, et al. Descending serotonergic, peptidergic and cholinergic pathways from the raphe nuclei: a multiple transmitter complex. Brain Res 1983; 288:33–48.

296. Armstrong DM, Saper CB, Levey AI, et al. Distribution of cholinergic neurons in rat brain demonstrated by the immunocytochemical localization of choline acetyltransferase. J Comp Neurol 1983; 216:53–68.

297. Sapolsky RM, Krey LC, McEwen BS. The neuroendocrinology of stress and aging: the glucocorticoid cascade hypothesis. Endocr Rev 1986; 7:284–301.

298. Vincent SR, Hökfelt T, Wu JY. GABA neuron systems in hypothalamus and the pituitary gland. Neuroendocrinology 1982; 34:117–125.

299. Masotto C, Wisnewski G, Negro-Villar A. Different gamma-aminobutyric acid receptor subtypes are involved in the regulation of opiate-dependent and -independent luteinizing hormone–releasing hormone secretion. Endocrinology 1989; 125:548–553.

300. Badger TM, Millard WJ, Martin JB, et al. Hypothalamic-pituitary function in adult rats treated neonatally with monosodium glutamate. Endocrinology 1982; 111:2031–2038.

301. Clement-Jones V, Rees LH. Neuroendocrine correlates of the endorphins and enkephalin. In: Besser GM, Martini L, eds. Clinical Neuroendocrinology. Vol II. New York: Academic, 1982: 140–204.

302. McCann SM. The role of brain peptides in the control of anterior pituitary hormone secretion. In: Müller EE, MacLeod RM, eds. Neuroendocrine Perspectives. Vol 1. Amsterdam: Elsevier Biomedical, 1982: 1–22.

Neuroendocrine Control of Individual Pituitary Hormones

303. DiStefano JJ III, Stubberud AR, Williams IJ. Theory and Problems of Feedback and Control Systems. New York: Schaum Publishing, 1967.

304. Yates FE. Modeling periodicities in reproductive, adrenocortical and metabolic systems. In: Ferin M, Halberg F, Richart RM, et al., eds. Biorhythms and Human Reproduction. New York: John Wiley & Sons, 1974: 133–142.

305. Houk JC. Control strategies in physiological systems. FASEB J 1988; 2:97–107.

306. Moore RY. Central neural control of circadian rhythms. In: Ganong WF, Martini L, eds. Frontiers in Neuroendocrinology. Vol 5. New York: Raven, 1978: 185–206.

307. Zucker I. Light, behavior, and biologic rhythms. In: Krieger DR, Hughes JC, eds. Neuroendocrinology. Sunderland, MA: Sinauer Associates, 1980: 93–101.

308. Moore RY. Organization and function of a central nervous system circadian oscillator: the suprachiasmatic hypothalamic nucleus. Fed Proc 1983; 42:2783–2789.

309. Albers HE, Minamitani N, Stopa E, et al. Light selectively alters vasoactive intestinal peptide and peptide histidine isoleucine immunoreactivity within the rat suprachiasmatic nucleus. Brain Res 1987; 437:189–192.

310. Ebling FJP, Wood RI, Suttie JM, et al. Prenatal photoperiod influences neonatal prolactin secretion in the sheep. Endocrinology 1989; 125:384–391.

311. Kafka MD, ed. Central nervous system control of mammalian circadian rhythms. Fed Proc 1983; 42:2782–2814.

312. Albers HE, Ferris CF, Leeman SE, et al. Avian pancreatic polypeptide phase shifts hamster circadian rhythms when microinjected into the suprachiasmatic region. Science 1984; 223: 833–835.

313. Moore-Ede MC. The circadian timing system in mammals: two pacemakers preside over many secondary oscillators. Fed Proc 1983; 42:2802–2808.

314. Krieger DT, ed. Endocrine Rhythms. New York: Raven, 1979.

315. Aschoff J. Circadian rhythms: general features and endocrinologic aspects. In: Krieger DT, ed. Endocrine Rhythms. New York: Raven, 1979: 1–61.

316. Aschoff J. The circadian system in man. In: Krieger DT, Hughes JC, eds. Neuroendocrinology. Sunderland, MA: Sinauer Associates, 1980: 77–84.

317. Boyar RM. Sleep-related endocrine rhythms. In: Reichlin S, Baldessarini RJ, Martin JB, eds. The Hypothalamus. Vol 56. New York: Raven, 1978: 373–386.

318. Iranmanesh A, Lizarralde G, Johnson ML, et al. Circadian, ultradian, and episodic release of β-endorphin in men, and its temporal coupling with cortisol. J Clin Endocrinol Metab 1989; 68:1019–1026.

319. Czeisler CA, Johnson MP, Duffy JF, et al. Exposure to bright light and darkness to treat physiologic maladaptation to night work. N Engl J Med 1990; 322:1253–1259.

320. Stern JM, Reichlin S. Prolactin circadian rhythm persists throughout lactation in women. Neuroendocrinology 1990; 51:31–37.
321. Weaver DR, Rivkees SA, Reppert SM. Localization and characterization of melatonin receptors in rodent brain by in vitro radioautography. J Neurosci 1989; 9:2581–2590.
322. Lewy AJ. Biochemistry and regulation of mammalian melatonin production. In: Relkin R, ed. The Pineal Gland. New York: Elsevier Biomedical, 1983: 77–128.
323. Czeisler CA, Kronauer RE, Allan JS, et al. Bright light induction of strong (type O) resetting of the human circadian pacemaker. Science 1989; 244:1328–1333.
324. Turek FW, Van Reeth O. Altering the mammalian circadian clock with the short-acting benzodiazepine, triazolam. Trends Neurosci 1988; 11:535–541.

Thyrotropin Regulation

325. Reichlin S. Control of thyrotropic hormone secretion. In: Martini L, Ganong WF, eds. Neuroendocrinology. Vol 1. New York: Academic, 1966: 445–536.
326. Reichlin S, Martin JB, Jackson IMD. Regulation of thyroid-stimulating hormone (TSH) secretion. In: Jeffcoate SL, Hutchinson JSM, eds. The Endocrine Hypothalamus. New York: Academic, 1978: 239–270.
327. Burger HG, Patel YC. TSH and TRH: their physiological regulation and the clinical applications of TRH. In: Martini L, Besser GM, eds. Clinical Neuroendocrinology. New York: Academic, 1977: 67–131.
328. Scanlon MF, Lewis M, Weightman DR, et al. The neuroregulation of human thyrotropin secretion. In: Martini L, Ganong F, eds. Frontiers in Neuroendocrinology. Vol 6. New York: Raven, 1980: 333–380.
329. Morley JE. Neuroendocrine control of thyrotropin secretion. Endocr Rev 1981; 2:396–436.
330. Larsen PR. Thyroid-pituitary interaction. N Engl J Med 1982; 306:23–32.
331. Reichlin S. Regulation of thyrotropin and gonadotropin secretion. In: Black P, Ridgeway C, Martin JB, et al., eds. Pituitary Adenoma. New York: Plenum, 1984: 309–326.
332. Segerson TP, Kauer J, Wolfe HC, et al. Thyroid hormone regulates TRH biosynthesis in the paraventricular nucleus of the rat hypothalamus. Science 1987; 238:78–80.
333. Dyess EM, Segerson TP, Liposits Z, et al. Triiodothyronine exerts direct cell-specific regulation of thyrotropin-releasing hormone gene expression in the hypothalamic paraventricular nucleus. Endocrinology 1988; 123:2291–2297.
334. Snyder PJ, Utiger RD. Inhibition of thyrotropin response to thyrotropin releasing hormone by small quantities of thyroid hormones. J Clin Invest 1972; 51:2077–2084.
335. Vagenakis AG, Rapoport B, Azizi F, et al. Hyper-response to thyrotropin releasing hormone accompanying small decreases in serum thyroid hormone concentration. J Clin Invest 1974; 54:913–918.
336. Kaplan MM, Taft JA, Reichlin S, et al. Sustained rises in serum thyrotropin, thyroxine, and triiodothyronine during long term, continuous thyrotropin-releasing hormone treatment in patients with amyotrophic lateral sclerosis. J Clin Endocrinol Metab 1986; 63:808–814.
337. Arancibia S, Tapai-Arancibia L, Assenmacher I, et al. Direct evidence of short-term cold-induced TRH release in the median eminence. Neuroendocrinology 1983; 37:225–228.
338. Galton VA. Environmental effects. In: Ingbar SH, Braverman LE, eds. Werner's the Thyroid. Philadelphia: J. B. Lippincott, 1986: 407–413.
339. Arimura A, Schally AV. Increases in basal and thyrotropin releasing hormone (TRH)-stimulated secretion of thyrotropin (TSH) by passive immunization with antiserum to somatostatin in rats. Endocrinology 1976; 98:1069–1072.
340. Ferland L, Labrie F, Jobin M, et al. Physiologic role of somatostatin in the control of growth hormone and thyrotropin secretion. Biochem Biophys Res Commun 1976; 68:149–151.
341. Berelowitz M, Maeda K, Harris S, et al. The effect of alterations in the pituitary-thyroid axis on hypothalamic content and in vitro release of somatostatin-like immunoreactivity. Endocrinology 1980; 107:24–29.
342. Rogers KV, Vician L, Steiner RA, et al. The effect of hypophysectomy and growth hormone administration on pre-prosomatostatin messenger ribonucleic acid in the periventricular nucleus of the rat hypothalamus. Endocrinology 1988; 122:586–591.
343. Smythe GA, Bradshaw JE, Cai WY, et al. Hypothalamic serotoninergic stimulation of thyrotropin secretion and related brain-hormone and drug interactions in the rat. Endocrinology 1982; 111:1181–1191.
344. Tapia-Arancibia L, Astier H. Opiate inhibition of K+-induced TRH release from superfused mediobasal hypothalami in rats. Neuroendocrinology 1985; 37:166–168.
345. Kaplan MM. The role of thyroid hormone deiodination in the regulation of hypothalamo-pituitary function. Neuroendocrinology 1984; 38:254–260.
346. Hinkle PM, Perrone MH, Schonbrunn A. Mechanisms of thyroid hormone inhibition of thyrotropin-releasing hormone action. Endocrinology 1981; 108:199–205.
347. Bradley DJ, Young WS 3rd, Weinberger C. Differential expression of alpha and beta thyroid hormone receptor genes in rat brain and pituitary. Proc Natl Acad Sci USA 1989; 86:7250–7254.
348. Hodin RA, Lazar MA, Wintman BI, et al. Identification of a thyroid hormone receptor that is pituitary-specific. Science 1989; 244:76–79.
349. Evans RM. The steroid and thyroid hormone receptor superfamily. Science 1988; 240:889–895.
350. Burnside J, Darling DS, Carr FE, et al. Thyroid hormone regulation of the rat glycoprotein hormone alpha-subunit gene promoter activity. J Biol Chem 1989; 264:6886–6891.
351. Brown MR. Thermoregulation. In: Brownstein MJ, Martin JB, eds. Brain Peptides. New York: John Wiley & Sons, 1983: 301–314.
352. Berg GR, Utiger RD, Schalch DS, et al. Effect of central cooling in man on pituitary-thyroid function and growth hormone secretion. J Appl Physiol 1966; 21:1791–1794.
353. Sack J, Fisher DA, Wang CC. Serum thyrotropin, prolactin and growth hormone levels during the early neonatal period in the human infant. J Pediatr 1976; 89:298–300.
354. DuRuisseau J. Seasonal variation of PBI in healthy Montrealers. J Clin Endocrinol Metab 1965; 25:1513–1515.
355. Burger HG, Patel YC, TSH and TRH: their physiological regulation and the clinical applications of TRH. In: Martini L, Besser GM, eds. Clinical Neuroendocrinology. New York: Academic, 1977: 67–131.
356. Wartofsky L, Burman KD. Alterations in thyroid function in patients with systemic illness: the "euthyroid sick syndrome." Endocr Rev 1982; 3:164–217.
357. Peters JR, Foord SM, Diequez C, et al. TSH neuroregulation and alterations in disease states. Clin Endocrinol Metab 1983; 12:669–695.
358. Arimura A, Smith W, Schally AV. Blockade of the stress-induced decrease in blood GH by anti-somatostatin serum in rats. Endocrinology 1976; 98:540–543.
359. Sutton RE, Koob GF, LeMoal M, et al. Corticotropin releasing factor produces behavioral activation in rats. Nature 1982; 297:331–333.
360. Peterfreund RA, Vale WW. Ovine corticotropin-releasing factor stimulates somatostatin secretion from cultured brain cells. Endocrinology 1983; 112:1275–1278.
361. Dubuis JM, Dayer JM, Siegrist-Kaiser CA, et al. Human recombinant interleukin-1β decreases plasma thyroid hormone and thyroid stimulating hormone levels in rats. Endocrinology 1988; 123:2175–2181.
362. Scarborough DE, Lee SL, Dinarello CA, et al. Interleukin-1 beta stimulates somatostatin biosynthesis in primary cultures of fetal rat brain. Endocrinology 1989; 124:549–551.
363. Pang XP, Hershman JM, Mirell CJ, et al. Impairment of hypothalamic-pituitary-thyroid function in rats treated with human recombinant tumor necrosis factor-alpha (cachectin). Endocrinology 1989; 125:76–84.
364. Koenig J, Snow K, Clark B, et al. Intrinsic pituitary interleukin-1b is induced by bacterial lipopolysaccharide. Endocrinology 1990; 126:3053–3058.
365. Sapolsky R, Rivier C, Yamamoto G, et al. Interleukin-1 stimulates the secretion of hypothalamic corticotropin-releasing factor. Science 1987; 238:522–524.
366. Palkovits M, Zaborsky L. Neural connections of the hypothalamus. In: Morgane PJ, Panksepp J, eds. Handbook of the Hypothalamus. New York: Marcel Dekker, 1979: 379–510.
367. Relkin R. Pineal-hormonal interactions. In: Relkin R, ed. The Pineal Gland. New York: Elsevier Biomedical, 1983: 225–246.
368. Brammer GL, Morley JE, Geller E, et al. Hypothalamus-pituitary-thyroid axis interactions with pineal gland in the rat. Am J Physiol 1979; 236:E416–E420.
369. Jackson IMD, Sapirstein R, Reichlin S. Thyrotropin releasing hormone (TRH) in pineal and hypothalamus of the frog: effect of season and illumination. Endocrinology 1977; 100:97–100.

Corticotropin Secretion

370. Imura H, Yoshikatsu N, Kazuwa N, et al. Control of biosynthesis and secretion of ACTH, endorphins and related peptides. In: Müller EE, MacLeod RM, eds. Neuroendocrine Perspectives. Vol 1. Amsterdam: Elsevier Biochemical, 1982: 137–167.
371. Antoni FA. Hypothalamic control of adrenocorticotropin secretion: advances since the discovery of 41-residue corticotropin-releasing factor. Endocr Rev 1986; 7:351–378.
372. Arriza JL, Simerly RB, Swanson LW, et al. The neuronal mineralocorticoid receptor as a mediator of glucocorticoid response. Neuron 1988; 1:887–900.
373. Fuxe K, Wikstrom AC, Okret S, et al. Mapping of glucocorticoid receptor immunoreactive neurons in the rat tel- and diencephalon using a monoclonal antibody against rat liver glucocorticoid receptor. Endocrinology 1985; 117:1803–1812.
374. Liposits ZS, Uht RM, Harrison RW, et al. Ultrastructural localization of glucocorticoid receptor (GR) in hypothalamic paraventricular neurons synthesizing corticotropin releasing factor (CRF). Histochemistry 1987; 87:407–412.
375. Keller-Wood MB, Dallman MF. Corticosteroid inhibition of ACTH secretion. Endocrin Rev 1984; 5:1–24.
376. Hua SY, Chen YZ. Membrane receptor-mediated electrophysiological effects of glucocorticoid on mammalian neurons. Endocrinology 1989; 124:687–691.

377. Dayanithi G, Antoni FA. Rapid as well as delayed inhibitory effects of glucocorticoid hormones on pituitary adrenocorticotropic hormone release are mediated by type II glucocorticoid receptors and require newly synthesized messenger ribonucleic acid as well as protein. Endocrinology 1989; 125:308–313.

378. McEwen BS, Davis PG, Parsons B, et al. The brain as a target for steroid hormone action. Annu Rev Neurosci 1979; 2:65–112.

379. Le Gascogne C, Robel P, Gouézou M, et al. Neurosteroids: cytochrome P-450 in rat brain. Science 1987; 237:1212–1215.

380. Feek CM, Marante DJ, Edwards CRW. The hypothalamic-pituitary-adrenal axis. Clin Endocrinol Metab 1983; 12:597–618.

381. Axelrod J, Reisine TD. Stress hormones: their interaction and regulation. Science 1984; 224:452–459.

382. Rivier C, Vale W. Modulation of stress-induced ACTH release by corticotropin-releasing factor, catecholamines and vasopressin. Nature 1983; 305:325–327.

383. Maran JW, Carlson DE, Grizzle WE, et al. Organization of the medial hypothalamus for control of adrenocorticotropin in the cat. Endocrinology 1978; 103:957–970.

384. Ward DG, Bolton MG, Gann DS. Inhibitory and facilitatory areas of the ventral midbrain mediating release of corticotropin in the cat. Endocrinology 1978; 102:1147–1154.

385. Carlson DE, Dornhorst A, Gann DS. Organization of the lateral hypothalamus for control of adrenocorticotropin release in the cat. Endocrinology 1980; 107:961–969.

386. Dornhorst A, Carlson DE, Seif SM, et al. Control of release of adrenocorticotropin and vasopressin by the supraoptic and paraventricular nuclei. Endocrinology 1981; 108:1420–1424.

387. Jones MT, Hillhouse EW, Burden J. Effect of various putative neurotransmitters on the secretion of corticotrophin-releasing hormone from the rat hypothalamus in vitro—a model of the neurotransmitters involved. J Endocrinol 1976; 69:1–10.

388. Calogero AE, Bernardini R, Gold PW, et al. Regulation of rat hypothalamic corticotropin-releasing hormone secretion in vitro: potential clinical implications. Adv Exp Med Biol 1988; 245:167–181.

389. Al-Damluji S. Adrenergic mechanisms in the control of corticotrophin secretion. J Endocrinol 1988; 119:5–14.

390. Kitay JI, Holub N, Jailer JW. Inhibition of pituitary ACTH release: an extra-adrenal action of exogenous ACTH. Endocrinology 1959; 64:475–482.

391. Grossman A. Brain opiates and neuroendocrine function. Clin Endocrinol Metab 1983; 12:725–746.

392. Rivier C, Rivier J, Vale W. Stress-induced inhibition of reproductive functions—role of endogenous corticotropin-releasing factor. Science 1986; 231:607–609.

Prolactin Regulation

393. Meites J. Control of mammary growth and lactation. In: Ganong WF, Martini L, eds. Neuroendocrinology. Vol 1. New York: Academic, 1966: 669–707.

394. Thorner MO. Prolactin: clinical physiology and the significance and management of hyperprolactinemia. In: Martini L, Besser GM, eds. Clinical Neuroendocrinology. New York: Academic, 1977: 320–361.

395. Molitch ME, Reichlin S. Hyperprolactinemic disorders. DM 1982; 28:1–58.

396. Gunnett JW, Freeman ME. The mating-induced release of prolactin: a unique neuroendocrine response. Endocr Rev 1983; 4:44–61.

397. Stern JM, Reichlin S. Prolactin circadian rhythm persists throughout lactation in women. Neuroendocrinology 1990; 51:31–37.

398. Short RV. Breast feeding. Sci Am 1984; 250:35–41.

399. Schallenberger E, Richardson DW, Knobil E. Role of prolactin in the lactational amenorrhea of the rhesus monkey (Macaca mulatta). Biol Reprod 1981; 25:370–374.

400. Ishizuka B, Quigley ME, Yen SSC. Pituitary hormone release in response to food ingestion: evidence for neuroendocrine signals from gut to brain. J Clin Endocrinol Metab 1957; 57:1111–1116.

401. Müller EE, Genazzani AR, Murru S. Nomifensine: diagnostic test in hyperprolactinemic states. J Clin Endocrinol Metab 1978; 47:1352–1357.

402. Cocchi D, Locatelli V, Cella S, et al. Antidepressant drugs as a tool to investigate CNS–anterior pituitary interactions. Adv Biochem Psychopharmacol 1982; 32:317–328.

403. Webb CB, Thominet JL, Barowsky H, et al. Evidence for lactotroph dopamine resistance in idiopathic hyperprolactinemia. J Clin Endocrinol Metab 1983; 56:1089–1093.

404. Reichlin S, Molitch ME. Neuroendocrine aspects of pituitary adenoma. In: Camanni F, Müller EE, eds. Pituitary Hyperfunction: Physiopathology and Clinical Aspects. New York: Raven, 1984: 47–70.

405. Faglia G, Spada A, Moriondo P, et al. What is the role of dopamine in the pathogenesis of prolactinomas? In: Camanni F, Müller EE, eds. Pituitary Hyperfunction: Physiopathology and Clinical Aspects. New York: Raven, 1984: 279–288.

406. Creese I, Burt DR, Snyder SH. Dopamine receptor binding predicts clinical and pharmacological potencies of antischizophrenic drugs. Science 1976; 192:481–483.

407. Turner TH, Cookson JC, Wass JAH, et al. Psychotic reactions during treatment of pituitary tumours with dopamine agonists. Br Med J 1984; 289:1101–1103.

Growth Hormone Regulation

408. Reichlin S. Regulation of somatotropic hormone secretion. In: Greep RO, Astwood EB, Knobil E, et al., eds. Handbook of Physiology. Sect 7: Endocrinology. Vol IV. The Pituitary Gland and Its Neuroendocrine Control. Part 2. Washington, DC: American Physiological Society, 1974: 405–447.

409. Martin JB, Brazeau P, Tannenbaum GS. Neuroendocrine organization of growth hormone regulation. In: Reichlin S, Baldessarini RJ, Martin JB, eds. The Hypothalamus. Vol 56. New York: Raven, 1978: 329–357.

410. Wass JAH. Growth hormone neuroregulation and the clinical relevance of somatostatin. Clin Endocrinol Metab 1983; 12:695–724.

411. Martin JB. Regulation of growth hormone secretion. In: Raiti S, Tolman RA, eds. Human Growth Hormone. New York: Plenum, 1986: 303–324.

412. Tannenbaum GS, Ling N. The interrelationship of growth hormone (GH)–releasing factor and somatostatin in generation of the ultradian rhythm of GH secretion. Endocrinology 1984; 115:1952–1957.

413. Drobny EC, Amburn K, Baumann G. Circadian variation of basal growth hormone in man. J Clin Endocrinol Metab 1983; 57:524–528.

414. Wehrenberg WB, Ling H, Bohlen P, et al. Physiological roles of somatocrinin and somatostatin in the regulation of growth hormone secretion. Biochem Biophys Res Commun 1982; 109:562–567.

415. Abe H, Molitch ME, Van Wyk JJ, et al. Human growth hormone and somatomedin C suppress the spontaneous release of growth hormone in unanesthetized rats. Endocrinology 1983; 113:1319–1324.

416. Berelowitz M, Szabo M, Frohman LA, et al. Somatomedin-C mediates growth hormone negative feedback by effects on both the hypothalamus and the pituitary. Science 1981; 212:1279–1281.

417. Brazeau P, Guillemin R, Ling N, et al. Somatomedin inhibition of the growth hormone secretion stimulated by the hypothalamic factor somatocrinin or the synthetic peptide hpGRF. C R Acad Sci III 1982; 295:651–654.

418. Vigersky RA, Loriaux DL, Anderson AE, et al. Anorexia nervosa: behavioral and hypothalamic aspects. Clin Endocrinol Metab 1976; 5:517–535.

419. Gunoz H, Neyz O, Sencer E, et al. Growth hormone secretion in protein energy malnutrition. Acta Paediatr Scand 1981; 70:521–526.

420. Underwood LE, Van Wyk JJ. Hormones in normal and aberrant growth. In: Williams RH, ed. Textbook of Endocrinology. 6th ed. Philadelphia: W. B. Saunders, 1981: 1149–1191.

421. Frohman LA. Glucoregulation. In: Krieger DT, Brownstein MJ, Martin JB. Brain Peptides. New York: John Wiley & Sons, 1983: 281–300.

422. Boyd AE, Lebovitz HE, Pfeiffer JB. Stimulation of growth hormone secretion by L-dopa. N Engl J Med 1970; 283:1425–1429.

423. Heidingstelder S, Blackard WH. Adrenergic control mechanisms for vasopressin induced plasma growth hormone response. Metabolism 1968; 17:1019–1024.

424. Delitala G. Neurotransmitter control of anterior pituitary hormone secretion and its clinical implications in man. In: Besser GM, Martini L, eds. Clinical Neuroendocrinology. Vol II. New York: Academic, 1982: 68–139.

425. Loche S, Lampis A, Cella SG, et al. Clonidine treatment in children with short stature. J Endocrinol Invest 1988; 11:763–767.

426. Pescovitz OH, Tan E. Lack of benefit of clonidine treatment for short stature in a double-blind, placebo-controlled trial. Lancet 1988; 2:874–877.

427. Laron Z, Gil-Ad T, Topper E, et al. Oral dose of clonidine: an effective screening test for growth hormone deficiency. Acta Paediatr 1982; 71:847–848.

428. Delitala G, Frulio T, Pacifico A, et al. Participation of cholinergic muscarinic receptors in glucagon- and arginine-mediated growth hormone secretion in man. J Clin Endocrinol Metab 1982; 55:1231–1233.

429. Delitala G, Grossman A, Besser GM. Opiate peptides control growth hormone through a cholinergic mechanism in man. Clin Neuroendocrinol 1983; 18:401–405.

430. Massara F, Ghigo E, Demislis K, et al. Cholinergic involvement in the growth hormone releasing hormone–induced growth hormone release: studies in normal and acromegalic subjects. Neuroendocrinology 1986; 43:670–675.

431. Richardson SB, Hollander CS, D'Eletto R, et al. Acetylcholine inhibits the release of somatostatin from rat hypothalamus in vitro. Endocrinology 1980; 107:122–129.

432. Carmeliet P, Denef C. Immunocytochemical and pharmacological evidence for an intrinsic cholinomimetic system modulating prolactin and growth hormone release in rat pituitary. Endocrinology 1988; 123:1128–1139.

433. McCann SM. The role of brain peptides in the control of anterior pituitary hormone secretion. In: Müller EE, MacLeod RM, eds. Neuroendocrine Perspectives. Vol 1. New York: Elsevier Biomedical, 1982: 1–22.

434. Clement-Jones V, Rees LH. Neuroendocrine correlates of the endor-

phins and enkephalins. In: Besser GM, Martini L, eds. Clinical Neuroendocrinology. Vol II. New York: Academic, 1982: 140–204.

435. Davis TM, Burrin JM, Bloom SR. Growth hormone (GH) release in response to GH-releasing hormone in man is 3-fold enhanced by galanin. J Clin Endocrinol Metab 1987; 65:1248–1252.

436. Lam KS, Lechan RM, Minamitani N, et al. Vasoactive intestinal peptide in the anterior pituitary is increased in hypothyroidism. Endocrinology 1989; 124:1077–1084.

437. Vrontakis ME, Yamamoto T, Schroedter IC, et al. Estrogen induction of galanin synthesis in the rat anterior pituitary gland demonstrated by in situ hybridization and immunohistochemistry. Neurosci Lett 1989; 100:59–64.

438. Chihara K, Kato Y, Maeda K, et al. Effects of thyrotropin-releasing hormone on sleep and sleep-related growth hormone release in normal subjects. J Clin Endocrinol Metab 1977; 44:1094–1100.

Neuroendocrine Aspects of Sexual Function

439. Knobil E, Plant TM. The hypothalamic regulation of LH and FSH secretion in the rhesus monkey. In: Reichlin S, Baldessarini RJ, Martin JB, eds. The Hypothalamus. Vol 56. New York: Raven, 1978: 359–372.

440. Knobil E, Neill JD, eds. The Physiology of Reproduction. New York: Raven, 1988.

441. Knobil E. The neuroendocrine control of the menstrual cycle. Recent Prog Horm Res 1980; 36:53–88.

442. Plant TM. Gonadal regulation of hypothalamic gonadotropin-releasing hormone release in primates. Endocr Rev 1986; 7:75–88.

443. Bardin CW. The neuroendocrinology of male reproduction. In: Krieger DT, Hughes JC, eds. Neuroendocrinology. Sunderland, MA: Sinauer Associates, 1980: 239–248.

444. Pohl CR, Knobil E. The role of the central nervous system in the control of ovarian function in higher primates. Annu Rev Physiol 1982; 44:571–593.

445. Kalra SP, Kalra PS. Neural regulation of luteinizing hormone secretion in the rat. Endocr Rev 1983; 4:311–351.

446. Belchetz PE. Gonadotropin regulation and clinical applications of GnRH. Clin Endocrinol Metab 1983; 12:619–640.

447. Fink G, Stanley HF, Watts AG. Central nervous control of sex and gonadotropin release: peptide and nonpeptide transmitter interactions. In: Krieger DT, Brownstein MJ, Martin JB, eds. Brain Peptides. New York: John Wiley & Sons, 1983: 423–435.

448. Shivers BD, Harlan RE, Pfaff DW. Reproduction: the central nervous system role of luteinizing hormone releasing hormone. In: Krieger DT, Brownstein MJ, Martin JB, eds. Brain Peptides. New York: John Wiley & Sons, 1983: 389–412.

449. Davidson JM. Hormones and sexual behaviour in the male. In: Krieger DT, Hughes JC, eds. Neuroendocrinology. Sunderland, MA: Sinauer Associates, 1980: 232–238.

450. Gorski RA. Sexual differentiation of the brain. In: Krieger DT, Hughes JC, eds. Neuroendocrinology. Sunderland, MA: Sinauer Associates, 1980: 215–222.

451. Michael RP. Hormones and sexual behavior in the female. In: Krieger DT, Hughes JC, eds. Neuroendocrinology. Sunderland, MA: Sinauer Associates, 1980: 223–232.

452. Wilson JD, Griffin JE, George FW, et al. The role of gonadal steroids in sexual differentiation. Recent Prog Horm Res 1981; 37:1–40.

453. Gorski RA. Steroid-induced sexual characteristics in the brain. In: Müller EE, MacLeod RM, eds. Neuroendocrine Perspectives. Vol 2. Amsterdam: Elsevier Biomedical, 1983: 1–35.

454. Donovan BT, van der Werff ten Bosch JJ. Physiology of Puberty. Baltimore: Williams & Wilkins, 1965.

455. Reiter EO, Grumbach MM. Neuroendocrine control mechanisms and the onset of puberty. Annu Rev Physiol 1982; 44:595–613.

456. Styne DM, Grumbach MM. Puberty in the male and female: its physiology and disorders. In: Yen SSC, Jaffe RB, eds. Reproductive Endocrinology: Physiology, Pathophysiology and Clinical Management. 2nd ed. Philadelphia: W. B. Saunders, 1986: 313–384.

457. Job JC. The neuroendocrine system and puberty. In: Martini L, Besser GM, eds. Clinical Neuroendocrinology. New York: Academic, 1978: 488–501.

458. Grumbach MM. The neuroendocrinology of puberty. In: Krieger DT, Hughes JC, eds. Neuroendocrinology. Sunderland, MA: Sinauer Associates, 1980: 249–258.

459. Ojeda SR, Andrews WW, Advis JP, et al. Recent advances in the endocrinology of puberty. Endocr Rev 1980; 1:228–257.

460. McEwen BS, Biegon A, Davis PG, et al. Steroid hormones: humoral signals which alter brain cell properties and functions. Recent Prog Horm Res 1982; 38:41–83.

461. Koch M, Ehret G. Immunocytochemical localization and quantitation of estrogen-binding cells in the male and female (virgin, pregnant, lactating) mouse brain. Brain Res 1989; 489:101–112.

462. Sheridan PJ. Androgen receptors in the brain: what are we measuring? Endocr Rev 1983; 4:171–178.

463. Pfaff DW, McEwen BS. Actions of estrogens and progestins on nerve cells. Science 1983; 219:808–814.

464. Martini L. The 5α-reduction of testosterone in the neuroendocrine structures: biochemical and physiological implications. Endocr Rev 1983; 4:1–25.

465. Challis JRG, Nartolin F, Davies IJ, et al. Endogenous steroids in neuroendocrine tissues. In: Naftolin F, Ryan KJ, Davies IJ, eds. Subcellular Mechanisms in Reproductive Neuroendocrinology. Amsterdam: Elsevier Scientific, 1976: 247–261.

466. Davies IJ, Naftolin F, Ryan KJ, et al. Specific binding of steroids by neuroendocrine tissues. In: Naftolin F, Ryan KJ, Davies IJ, eds. Subcellular Mechanisms in Reproductive Neuroendocrinology. Amsterdam: Elsevier Scientific, 1976: 263–275.

467. McEwen B. Steroid receptors in neuroendocrine tissues: topography, subcellular distribution, and functional implications. In: Naftolin F, Ryan KJ, Davies IJ, eds. Subcellular Mechanisms in Reproductive Neuroendocrinology. Amsterdam: Elsevier Scientific, 1976: 277–304.

468. Paul SM, Hoffman AR, Axelrod J. Catechol estrogens: synthesis and metabolism in brain and other endocrine tissues. In: Martini L, Ganong WF, eds. Frontiers in Neuroendocrinology. Vol 6. New York: Raven, 1980: 203–207.

469. Jouan P, Samperez S. Metabolism of steroid hormones in the brain. In: Motta M, ed. The Endocrine Functions of the Brain. New York: Raven, 1980: 95–115.

470. Mason AJ, Berkemeier LM, Schmelzer CH, et al. Activin B: precursor sequences, genomic structure and in vitro activities. Mol Endocrinol 1989; 3:1352–1358.

471. Evans WS, Cronin MJ, Thorner MO. Hypogonadism in hyperprolactinemia: proposed mechanisms. In: Ganong WF, Martini L, eds. Frontiers in Neuroendocrinology. Vol 7. New York: Raven, 1982: 77–122.

472. Quigley ME, Rakoff JS, Yen SS. Increased luteinizing hormone sensitivity to dopamine inhibition in polycystic ovary syndrome. J Clin Endocrinol Metab 1981; 52:231–234.

473. Dees WL, Ahmed CE, Ojeda SR. Substance P and vasoactive intestinal peptide–containing fibers reach the ovary by independent routes. Endocrinology 1986; 119:638–641.

474. Emanuele NV, Kostka D, Wallock L, et al. Hypothalamic luteinizing hormone increases dramatically following intracerebroventricular injection of colchicine. Neuroendocrinology 1985; 41:526–528.

475. Emanuele NV, Metcalfe L, Wallock L, et al. Hypothalamic prolactin: characterization by radioimmunoassay and bioassay and response to hypophysectomy and restraint stress. Neuroendocrinology 1986; 44:217–221.

476. Motta M, Piva F, Martini L. The hypothalamus as the center of endocrine feedback mechanisms. In: Martini L, Motta M, Fraschini F, eds. The Hypothalamus. New York: Academic, 1970: 463–490.

477. Zoeller RT, Seeburg PH, Young WS 3rd. In situ hybridization histochemistry for messenger ribonucleic acid (mRNA) encoding gonadotropin-releasing hormone (GnRH): effect of estrogen on cellular levels of GnRH mRNA in female rat brain. Endocrinology 1988; 122:2570–2577.

478. Marshall JC, Case GD, Valk TW, et al. Selective inhibition of follicle-stimulating hormone secretion by estradiol. Mechanism for modulation of gonadotropin responses to low dose pulses of gonadotropin-releasing hormone. J Clin Invest 1983; 71:248–257.

479. Seyler LE Jr, Graze K, Canalis E, et al. Effects of sex-steroid priming on pituitary responses to LH-RH. In: Beling CG, Wentz AC, eds. The LH-Releasing Hormone. New York: Masson, 1980: 87–112.

480. Ling N, Ueno N, Ying SY, et al. Inhibins and activins. Vitam Horm 1988; 44:1–46.

481. Karsch FJ, Dierschke DJ, Knobil E. Sexual differentiation of pituitary function: apparent difference between primates and rodents. Science 1973; 179:484–486.

482. Westfahl PK, Stadelman HL, Horton LE, et al. Experimental induction of estradiol positive feedback in intact male monkeys: absence of inhibition by physiologic concentrations of testosterone. Biol Reprod 1984; 31:856–862.

483. Knobil E, Hotchkiss J. The menstrual cycle and its neuroendocrine control 1971–1984. In: Knobil E, Neill JD, eds. The Physiology of Reproduction. New York: Raven, 1988: 1143–1160.

484. Hoffman AR, Crowley WF Jr. Chronic administration of low-dosage pulsatile GnRH in idiopathic hypogonadotropic hypogonadism. In: Givens JR, ed. The Hypothalamus. Chicago: Year Book Medical, 1984: 204–214.

485. Santoro N, Filicori M, Crowley WF Jr. Hypogonadotropic disorders in men and women: diagnosis and therapy with pulsatile gonadotropin-releasing hormone. Endocr Rev 1986; 17:11–23.

486. Elkind-Hirsch K, Ravnikar V, Tulchinsky D, et al. Episodic secretory patterns of immunoreactive luteinizing hormone–releasing hormone (IR-LH-RH) in the systemic circulation of normal women throughout the menstrual cycle. Fertil Steril 1984; 41:56–61.

487. Spinder T, Spijkstra JJ, Gooren J, et al. Effects of long-term testosterone administration on gonadotropin secretion in agonadal female to male transsexuals compared with hypogonadal and normal women. J Clin Endocrinol Metab 1989; 68:200–207.

488. Arendash GW, Gorski RA. Enhancement of sexual behavior in female rats by neonatal transplantation of brain tissue from males. Science 1982; 217:1276–1278.

489. Schumacher M, Legros JJ, Balthazart J. Steroid hormones, behavior, and sexual dimorphism in animals and men: the nature-nurture controversy. Exp Clin Endocrinol 1987; 90:129–156.

490. Gooren L. The neuroendocrine response of luteinizing hormone to estrogen administration in heterosexual, homosexual, and transsexual subjects. J Clin Endocrinol Metab 1986; 63:583–588.

490a. Gooren L. The endocrinology of transsexualism: a review and commentary. Psychoneuroendocrinology 1990; 15:3–14.

491. Barraclough CA, Wise PM. The role of catecholamines in the regulation of pituitary luteinizing hormone and follicle-stimulating hormone secretion. Endocr Rev 1982; 3:91–119.

492. Taubenhaus M, Soskin S. Release of luteinizing hormone from the anterior hypophysis by an acetylcholine-like substance from the hypothalamic region. Endocrinology 1941; 29:958–964.

493. Sawyer CH, Markee JE, Townsend BF. Cholinergic and adrenergic components in the neurohumoral control of the release of LH in the rabbit. Endocrinology 1949; 44:18–37.

494. Everett JW, Sawyer CH. A 24-hour periodicity in the "LH-release apparatus" of female rats, disclosed by barbiturate sedation. Endocrinology 1950; 47:198–218.

495. Weiner RI, Findell PR, Kordon C. Role of classic and peptide neuromediators in the neuroendocrine regulation of LH and prolactin. In: Knobil E, Neill JD, eds. The Physiology of Reproduction. New York: Raven, 1988: 1143–1160.

496. Shivers BD, Harlan RE, Morrell JI, et al. Absence of oestradiol concentration in cell nuclei of LHRH-immunoreactive neurons. Nature 1983; 304:345–347.

497. Quigley ME, Sheehan KL, Casper RF, et al. Evidence for an increased opioid inhibition of luteinizing hormone secretion in hyperprolactinemic patients with pituitary microadenoma. J Clin Endocrinol Metab 1980; 50:427–430.

Timing of Puberty

498. Ojeda SR, Smith (Wright) SS, Urbanski HF, et al. Onset of female puberty: underlying neuroendocrine mechanisms. In: Müller EE, MacLeod RM, eds. Neuroendocrine Perspectives. Vol 3. Amsterdam: Elsevier Biomedical 1984: 225–278.

499. Weinberger LM, Grant FC. Precocious puberty and tumors of the hypothalamus. Arch Intern Med 1941; 67:762–792.

500. Wyshak G, Frisch RE. Evidence for a secular trend in age at menarche. N Engl J Med 1982; 306:1033–1035.

501. Frisch RE. Fatness, menarche, and female fertility. Perspect Biol Med 1985; 28:611–633.

502. Frisch RE. Body fat, menarche, fitness and fertility. Prog Reprod Biol Med 1990; 14:1–26.

503. McArthur JW, Beitins IZ, Bullen BA. Motility, nutrition and reproduction: recent clues to an ancient relationship. In: Givens JR, ed. The Hypothalamus. Chicago: Year Book Medical, 1984: 171–188.

504. Bates GW, Whitworth NS. Effects of body weight on female reproductive function. In: Givens JR, ed. The Hypothalamus. Chicago: Year Book Medical, 1984: 97–115.

505. Crowley WR, Zemlan FP. The neurochemical control of mating behavior. In: Adler NT, ed. Neuroendocrinology of Reproduction. New York: Plenum, 1981: 451–484.

506. Michael RP. Estrogen-sensitive neurons and sexual behavior in female cats. Science 1962; 136:322–323.

507. Aron C. Mechanisms of control of the reproduction function of olfactory stimuli in female mammals. Physiol Rev 1979; 59:229–284.

508. Leshner AI. Pheromonal and ultrasonic communication. In: An Introduction to Behavioral Endocrinology. New York: Oxford University Press, 1978: 114–145.

509. Singer AG, Clancy AN, Macrides F, et al. Chemical properties of a female mouse pheromone that stimulates gonadotropin secretion in males. Biol Reprod 1988; 38:193–199.

510. Henzel WJ, Rodriguez H, Singer AG, et al. The primary structure of aphrodisin. J Biol Chem 1988; 263:16682–16687.

511. McClintock MK. Menstrual synchrony and suppression. Nature 1971; 229:244–245.

The Pineal Gland and Circumventricular Organs

512. Weindl A, Joynt RJ. The median eminence as a circumventricular organ. In: Knigge K, Scott DE, Weindl A., eds. Brain-Endocrine Interaction: I. Median Eminence: Structure and Function. Proceedings, International Symposium on Brain-Endocrine Interactions, Munich, 1971. White Plains, NY: AJ Phiebig (Basel: S. Karger), 1972: 280–297.

513. Weindl A, Sofroniew MV. Relation of neuropeptides to mammalian circumventricular organs. Adv Biochem Psychopharmacol 1981; 28:303–320.

514. Wurtman RJ, Axelrod J, Kelly DE. The Pineal. New York: Academic, 1968.

515. Rolleston HD. The Endocrine Organs in Health and Disease with an Historical Review. New York: Oxford University Press, 1936: 452.

516. Pévet P. Anatomy of the pineal gland of mammals. In: Relkin R, ed. The Pineal Gland. New York: Elsevier Biomedical, 1983: 1–76.

517. Kappers JA, Smith AR, De Vries RAC. The mammalian pineal gland and its control of hypothalamic activity. Prog Brain Res 1974; 41:149–174.

518. Wurtman RJ, Axelrod J. The pineal gland. Sci Am 1965; 213:50–60.

519. Klein DC. The pineal gland: a model of neuroendocrine regulation. In: Reichlin S, Baldessarini RJ, Martin JB, eds. The Hypothalamus. Vol 56. New York: Raven, 1978: 303–327.

520. Lewy AJ. Biochemistry and regulation of mammalian melatonin production. In: Relkin R, ed. The Pineal Gland. New York: Elsevier Biomedical, 1983: 77–128.

521. Wurtman RJ, Moskowitz MA. The pineal organ. N Engl J Med 1977; 296:1329–1333, 1383–1386.

522. Reppert SM, Klein DC. Mammalian pineal gland: basic and clinical aspects. In: Motta M, ed. The Endocrine Functions of the Brain. New York: Raven, 1980: 327–372.

523. Reiter RJ. The pineal and its hormones in the control of reproduction in mammals. Endocr Rev 1980; 1:109–131.

524. Moskowitz MA, Wurtman RJ. Pathological states involving the pineal. In: Martini L, Besser GM, eds. Clinical Neuroendocrinology. New York: Academic, 1977: 503–526.

525. Axelrod L. Endocrine dysfunction in patients with tumors of the pineal region. In: Schmidek HH, ed. Pineal Tumors. New York: Masson, 1977: 61–77.

526. Silman RE, Leone RM, Hooper RJ, et al. Melatonin, the pineal gland and human puberty. Nature 1979; 282:301–303.

527. Waldhauser F, Weiszenbacher G, Frisch H, et al. Fall in nocturnal serum melatonin during prepuberty and pubescence. Lancet 1984; 1:362–365.

528. Fevre M, Segel T, Marks JF, et al. LH and melatonin secretion patterns in pubertal boys. J Clin Endocrinol Metab 1978; 47:1383–1386.

529. Ehrenkranz JR, Tamarkin L, Comite F, et al. Daily rhythms of plasma melatonin in normal and precocious puberty. J Clin Endocrinol Metab 1982; 55:307–310.

530. Tetsuo M, Poth M, Markey SP. Melatonin metabolite excretion during childhood and puberty. J Clin Endocrinol Metab 1982; 55:311–313.

531. Penny R. Melatonin excretion in normal males and females: increase during puberty. Metabolism 1982; 8:816–823.

532. Klein DC. Melatonin and puberty. Science 1984; 224:6.

533. Cardinali DP. Melatonin: a mammalian pineal hormone. Endocr Rev 1981; 2:327–346.

534. Reiter RJ, Richardson BA, King TS. The pineal gland and its indole products: their importance in the control of reproduction. In: Relkin R, ed. The Pineal Gland. New York: Elsevier Biomedical, 1983: 151–201.

535. Relkin R. Pineal-hormonal interactions. In: Relkin R, ed. The Pineal Gland. New York: Elsevier Biomedical, 1983: 225–246.

536. Blask DE, Vaughn MK, Reiter RJ. Pineal peptides and reproduction. In: Relkin R, ed. The Pineal Gland. New York: Elsevier Biomedical, 1983: 201–224.

537. Arendt J, Labib MH, Bojkowski C, et al. Rapid decrease in melatonin production during successful treatment of delayed puberty. Lancet 1989; 1:1326 (letter).

538. Lerner AB, Case JD, Heinzelman RV. Structure of melatonin. J Am Chem Soc 1959; 81:6084–6085.

539. Wetterberg L. Melatonin in humans: physiological and clinical studies. J Neural Transm 1978; 13:289.

540. Weinberg U, Eletto RD, et al. Circulating melatonin in man: episodic secretion throughout the light-dark cycle. Clin Endocrinol Metab 1979; 48:114–118.

541. Martin JE, McKellar S, Klein DC. Melatonin inhibition of the in vivo pituitary response to luteinizing hormone–releasing hormone in the neonatal rat. Neuroendocrinology 1980; 31:13–17.

542. Watson SJ, Maden J. IV. Melatonin and other pineal substances: psychiatric and neurological implications. In: Usdin E, Hamburg DA, Barchas JD, eds. Neuroregulators and Psychiatric Disorders. New York: Oxford University Press, 1977: 193–200.

543. Lerner AB, Norlund JH. Melatonin: clinical pharmacology. J Neural Transm 1978; 13:339–347.

544. Arendt J, Aldhous M, Marks V. Alleviation of jet lag by melatonin: preliminary results of controlled double blind trial. Br Med J 1986; 292:1170.

545. Hill SM, Blask DE. Effects of the pineal hormone melatonin on the proliferation and morphological characteristics of human breast cancer cells (MCF-7) in culture. Cancer Res 1988; 48:6121–6126.

546. Losecke W, Naumann W, Sterba G. Preparation and discharge of secretion in the subcommissural organ of the rat. An electron-microscopic immunocytochemical study. Cell Tissue Res 1984; 235:201–206.

547. Akert K. The mammalian subfornical organ. J Neurovasc Relat 1969; 9(Suppl):78–93.

548. Pickel VM, Chan J, Ganten D. Dual peroxidase and colloidal gold-labeling study of angiotensin converting enzyme and angiotensin-like immunoreactivity in the rat subfornical organ. J Neurosci 1986; 6:2457–2469.

549. Standaert DG, Saper CB. Origin of the atriopeptin-like immunoreactive innervation of the paraventricular nucleus of the hypothalamus. J Neurosci 1988; 8:1940–1950.

550. Hellman W, Suzuki F, Ohkubo H, et al. Angiotensinogen gene expres-

sion in extrahepatic rat tissues: application of a solution hybridization assay. Naunyn-Schmiedebergs Arch Pharmacol 1988; 338:327–331.

551. Blatteis CM, Hales JR, McKinley MJ, et al. Role of the anteroventral third ventricle region in fever in sheep. Can J Physiol Pharmacol 1987; 65:1255–1260.

Neuroendocrine Disease

552. Riddoch G. Clinical aspects of hypothalamic disease. In: Le Gros Clark WE, Beattie J, Riddoch G, et al., eds. NM. The Hypothalamus. Edinburgh: Oliver and Boyd, 1938: 101–130.

553. Daniel PM, Treip CS. The pathology of the hypothalamus. Clin Endocrinol Metab 1977; 6:3–19.

554. Plum F, Van Uitert R. Nonendocrine diseases and disorders of the hypothalamus. In: Reichlin S, Baldessarini RJ, Martin JB, eds. The Hypothalamus. Vol 56. New York: Raven, 1978: 415–473.

555. Krieger DT. The hypothalamus and neuroendocrine pathology. In: Krieger DT, Hughes JC, eds. Neuroendocrinology. Sunderland, MA: Sinauer Associates, 1980: 13–22.

556. Kovacs K, Bilbao JM, Asa SL. The pathology of parasellar and hypothalamic lesions. In: Givens JR, ed. The Hypothalamus. Chicago: Year Book Medical, 1984: 17–38.

557. Kovacs K. Pathology of the neurohypophysis. In: Reichlin S, ed. The Neurohypophysis. New York: Plenum, 1984: 95–138.

558. Krieger DT, Glick S, Silverberg A, et al. A comparative study of endocrine tests in hypothalamic disease. Circadian periodicity of plasma 11-OHCS and growth hormone response to insulin hypoglycemia and metyrapone responsiveness. J Clin Endocrinol Metab 1968; 28:1589–1598.

559. Barnea ER, Naftolin F, Tolis G, et al. Hypothalamic amenorrhea syndromes. In: Givens JR, ed. The Hypothalamus. Chicago: Year Book Medical, 1984: 147–170.

560. Green WH, Campbell M, David R. Psychosocial dwarfism: a critical review of the evidence. J Am Acad Child Psychiatry 1984; 1:39–48.

Pituitary Isolation Syndrome

561. Randall RV, Clark EC, Dodge HW, et al. Polyuria after operation for tumors in the region of the hypophysis and hypothalamus. J Clin Endocrinol Metab 1960; 20:1614–1621.

562. Moses AM. Long-standing posttraumatic diabetes insipidus. Med Grand Rounds 1983; 2:117–128.

563. Fisher C, Ingram WR, Ranson SW. Diabetes Insipidus and the Neurohormonal Control of Water Balance. Ann Arbor, MI: Edwards Brothers, 1938.

564. Hollinshead WH. The interphase of diabetes insipidus. Mayo Clin Proc 1964; 39:92–100.

565. Green JR, Buchan GC, Alvord EC Jr. Hereditary and idiopathic types of diabetes insipidus. Brain 1967; 90:707–714.

566. Scherbaum WA, Bottazzo GF. Autoantibodies to vasopressin cells in idiopathic diabetes insipidus: evidence for an autoimmune variant. Lancet 1983; 1:897–901.

567. Valtin H, Stewart SHW. Genetic control of the production of posterior pituitary principles. In: Greep RO, Astwood EB, Knobil E, et al., eds. Handbook of Physiology. Sect 7: Endocrinology. Vol IV. The Pituitary Gland and Its Neuroendocrine Control. Part 1. Washington, DC: American Physiological Society, 1974: 131–171.

568. Schmale H, Richter D. Single base deletion in the vasopressin gene is the cause of diabetes insipidus in Brattleboro rats. Nature 1984; 308:705–709.

569. Dugger GS, Van Wyk JJ, Newsome JF. The effect of pituitary-stalk section on thyroid function and gonadotropic-hormone secretion in women with mammary carcinoma. J Neurosurg 1962; 19:589–593.

570. Van Wyk JJ, Dugger GS, Newsome JF, et al. The effect of pituitary stalk section on the adrenal function of women with cancer of the breast. J Clin Endocrinol Metab 1960; 20:157–172.

571. Lipsett MB, West CD, MacLean JP, et al. Adrenal function after hypophysectomy in man. J Clin Endocrinol Metab 1957; 17:356–363.

572. Hökfelt T, Luft R. The effect of suprasellar tumours on the regulation of adrenocortical function. Acta Endocrinol 1959; 32:177.

573. Anthony GJ, Van Wyk JJ, French FS. Influence of pituitary stalk section on growth hormone, insulin and TSH secretion in women with metastatic breast cancer. J Clin Endocrinol Metab 1969; 29:1238–1250.

574. Li MC, Rall JE, MacLean JP, et al. Thyroid function following hypophysectomy in man. J Clin Endocrinol Metab 1955; 15:1228–1238.

575. Vaughan L, Carmel PW, Dyrenfurth I. Section of the pituitary stalk in the rhesus monkey. 1. Endocrine studies. Neuroendocrinology 1980; 30:70–75.

576. Molitch ME, Reichlin S. Hypothalamic hyperprolactinemia: neuroendocrine regulation in man. In: MacLeod RM, Thorner MO, Scapagnini V, eds. Prolactin, Basis and Clinical Correlates. Padua: Liviana, 1985: 709–719.

577. Ehni G, Eckles NE. Interruption of the pituitary stalk in the patient with mammary cancer. J Neurosurg 1959; 16:628–652.

578. Haney AF, Kramer RS, Wiebe RH, et al. Hypothalamic-pituitary function and radiographic evaluation of women with hyperprolactinemia and an "empty" sella turcica. Am J Obstet Gynecol 1979; 134:917–924.

579. Adams JH, Daniel PM, Prichard MM. Some effects of transection of the pituitary stalk. Br Med J 1964; 2:1619–1625.

580. Adams JH, Daniel PM, Prichard MM. Transection of the pituitary stalk in man: anatomical changes in the pituitary glands of 21 patients. J Neurol Neurosurg Psychiatry 1966; 29:545–555.

Hypophyseotropic Hormone Deficiency

581. Snyder PJ, Jacobs LS, Rabello MM, et al. Diagnostic value of thyrotropin-releasing hormone in pituitary and hypothalamic diseases: assessment of thyrotropin and prolactin secretion in 100 patients. Ann Intern Med 1974; 81:751–757.

582. Lamberton RP, Jackson IMD. Investigation of hypothalamic-pituitary disease. Clin Endocrinol Metab 1983; 12:509–534.

583. Cobb WE, Reichlin S, Jackson IMD. Growth hormone secretory status is a determinant of the thyrotropin response to thyrotropin releasing hormone (TRH) in euthyroid patients with hypothalamic-pituitary disease. J Clin Endocrinol Metab 1981; 52:324–329.

584. Jorgensen JOL, Pederson SA, Laurberg P, et al. Effects of growth hormone therapy on thyroid function of growth hormone–deficient adults with and without concomitant thyroxine-substituted central hypothyroidism. J Clin Endocrinol Metab 1989; 69:1127–1132.

585. Beck-Peccoz P, Amr S, Menezes-Ferriera M, et al. Decreased receptor binding of biologically inactive thyrotropin in central hypothyroidism. N Engl J Med 1985; 312:1085–1090.

586. Tagatz G, Fialkow PJ, Smith D, et al. Hypogonadotropic hypogonadism associated with anosmia in the female. N Engl J Med 1970; 283:1326–1329.

587. Boyar RM. The effect of clomiphene citrate in anosmic hypogonadotrophism. Ann Intern Med 1969; 71:1127–1131.

588. Santen RJ, Paulsen CA. Hypogonadotropic enuchoidism. I. Clinical study of the mode of inheritance. J Clin Endocrinol Metab 1973; 36:47–54.

589. Weinstein RL, Reitz RE. Pituitary-testicular responsiveness in male hypogonadotropic hypogonadism. J Clin Invest 1974; 53:408–415.

590. Lieblich JM, Rogol AD, White BJ, et al. Syndrome of anosmia with hypogonadotropic hypogonadism (Kallmann syndrome): clinical and laboratory studies in 23 cases. Am J Med 1982; 73:506–519.

591. Iba K, Hamada N, Sowa E, et al. A female case of Kallmann's syndrome. Endocrinol Jpn 1977; 23:289–293.

592. Klinmuller D, Dewes W, Krahe T, et al. Magnetic resonance imaging of the brain in patients with anosmia and hypothalamic hypogonadism (Kallman's syndrome). J Clin Endocrinol Metab 1987; 65:581–584.

593. Schwanzel-Fukuda M, Bick D, Pfaff DW. Luteinizing hormone–releasing hormone (LHRH)-expressing cells do not migrate normally in an inherited hypogonadal (Kallmann) syndrome. Mol Brain Res 1989; 6:311–326.

594. Weiss J, Crowley WF Jr, Jameson JL. Normal structure of the gonadotropin-releasing hormone (GnRH) gene in patients with GnRH deficiency and idiopathic hypogonadotropic hypogonadism. J Clin Endocrinol Metab 1989; 69:299–303.

595. Krause Brucker W, Gardner DW. Optic nerve hypoplasia associated with absent septum pellucidum and hypopituitarism. Am J Ophthalmol 1980; 89:113–120.

596. Fitz CR. Holoprosencephaly and related entities. Neuroradiology 1983; 25:225–238.

597. Mortimer CH, Besser GH, McNeilly AS, et al. The luteinizing hormone and follicle stimulating hormone–releasing hormone test in patients with hypothalamic-pituitary-gonadal dysfunction. Br Med J 1974; 4:73–77.

598. Mortimer CH. Gonadotropin-releasing hormone. In: Martini L, Besser GM, eds. Clinical Neuroendocrinology. New York: Academic, 1977: 213–236.

599. Roth JC, Grumbach MM, Kaplan SL. Effect of synthetic luteinizing hormone–releasing factor on serum testosterone and gonadotropins in prepubertal, pubertal and adult males. J Clin Endocrinol Metab 1973; 37:680–686.

600. Beling CG, Wentz AC. The LH-Releasing Hormone. New York: Masson, 1980.

601. Costom BH, Grumbach MM, Kaplan SL. Effects of thyrotropin-releasing factor on serum thyroid stimulating hormone: an approach to distinguishing hypothalamic from pituitary forms of idiopathic hypopituitary dwarfism. J Clin Invest 1971; 50:2219–2225.

602. Schriock EA, Lustig RH, Rosenthal SM, et al. Effect of growth hormone (GH)–releasing hormone (GRH) on plasma GH in relation to magnitude and duration of GH deficiency in 26 children and adults with isolated GH deficiency or multiple pituitary hormone deficiencies: evidence for hypothalamic GRH deficiency. J Clin Endocrinol Metab 1984; 58:1043–1049.

603. Grossman A, Savage MO, Wass JA, et al. Growth-hormone–releasing factor in growth hormone deficiency: demonstration of a hypothalamic defect in growth hormone release. Lancet 1983; 2:137–138.

604. Liu N, Grumbach MM, de Napoli RA. Prevalence of electroencephalographic abnormalities in idiopathic precocious puberty and premature pubarche: bearing on pathogenesis and neuroendocrine regulation of puberty. J Clin Endocrinol Metab 1965; 25:1296–1308.

605. Kikuchi K, Fujisawa I, Momoi T, et al. Hypothalamic-pituitary function in growth hormone–deficient patients with pituitary stalk transection. J Clin Endocrinol Metab 1988; 67:817–823.

606. Brauner R, Rappaport R, Prevot C, et al. A prospective study of the development of growth hormone deficiency in children given cranial irradiation, and its relation to statural growth. J Clin Endocrinol Metab 1989; 68:346–351.

607. Stewart C, Castro-Magana M, Sherman J, et al. Septo-optic dysplasia and median cleft face syndrome in a patient with isolated growth hormone deficiency and hyperprolactinemia. Am J Dis Child 1983; 137:484–487.

608. Stacpoole PW, Interland JW, Nicholson WE, et al. Isolated ACTH deficiency: a heterogeneous disorder. Critical review and report of four new cases. Medicine (Baltimore) 1982; 61:13–24.

608a. Sauter NP, Toni R, McLaughlin CD, et al. Isolated adrenocorticotropin deficiency associated with an autoantibody to a corticotroph antigen that is not adrenocorticotropin or other proopiomelanocortin–derived peptides. J Clin Endocrinol Metab 1990; 70:1391–1397.

Hypophyseotropic Hormone Hypersecretion

609. Pescovitz OH, Comite F, Hench K, et al. The NIH experience with precocious puberty: diagnostic subgroups and response to short-term luteinizing hormone analogue therapy. J Pediatr 1986; 108:47–54.

610. Asa SL, Kovacs K, Tindall GT, et al. Cushing's disease associated with an intrasellar gangliocytoma producing corticotrophin-releasing factor. Ann Intern Med 1984; 101:789–793.

611. Asa SL, Scheithauer BW, Bilbao JM, et al. A case for hypothalamic acromegaly: a clinicopathological study of six patients with hypothalamic gangliocytomas producing growth hormone–releasing factor. J Clin Endocrinol Metab 1984; 58:796–803.

612. Hashimoto K, Suemaru S, Hattori T, et al. Multiple endocrine neoplasia with Cushing's syndrome due to paraganglioma producing corticotropin-releasing factor and adrenocorticotropin. Acta Endocrinol 1986; 113:189–195.

Neuroendocrine Disorders of Gonadotropin Regulation

613. Bierich JR. Sexual precocity. J Clin Endocrinol Metab 1975; 4:107–142.

614. Wilkins L. The Diagnosis and Treatment of Endocrine Disorders in Childhood and Adolescence. 3rd ed. Springfield, IL: Charles C Thomas, 1965.

615. Richter RB. True hamartoma of the hypothalamus associated with pubertas praecox. J Neuropathol 1951; 10:368.

616. Judge DM, Kulin HE, Page R, et al. Hypothalamic hamartoma. A source of luteinizing-hormone–releasing factor in precocious puberty. N Engl J Med 1977; 296:7–10.

617. Hochman HI, Judge DM, Reichlin S. Precocious puberty and hypothalamic hamartoma. Pediatrics 1981; 67:236–244.

618. Comite F, Pescovitz OH, Rieth KG, et al. Luteinizing hormone–releasing hormone analog treatment of boys with hypothalamic hamartoma and true precocious puberty. J Clin Endocrinol Metab 1984; 59:888–892.

619. Berkovic SF, Andermann F, Melanson D, et al. Hypothalamic hamartomas and ictal laughter: evolution of a characteristic epileptic syndrome and diagnostic value of magnetic resonance imaging. Ann Neurol 1988; 23:429–439.

620. Van Wyk JJ, Grumbach MM. Syndrome of precocious menstruation and galactorrhea in juvenile hypothyroidism: an example of hormonal overlap in pituitary feedback. J Pediatr 1960; 57:416–435.

621. Wood LC, Olichney M, Locke H, et al. Syndrome of juvenile hypothyroidism associated with advanced sexual development: report of two new cases and comment on the management of an associated ovarian mass. J Clin Endocrinol Metab 1965; 25:1289–1295.

622. Moskowitz MA, Wurtman RJ. Pathological states involving the pineal. In: Martini L, Besser GM, eds. Clinical Neuroendocrinology. New York: Academic, 1977: 503–526.

623. DeGirolami U. Pathology of tumors of the pineal region. In: Schmidek HH, ed. Pineal Tumors. New York: Masson, 1977: 1–19.

624. Russell DS, Rubinstein LJ. Pathology of Tumours of the Nervous System. 5th ed. Baltimore: Williams & Wilkins, 1989: 380–394.

625. DeGirolami U, Schmidek HH. Clinicopathological study of 53 tumors of the pineal region. J Neurosurg 1973; 39:455–462.

626. Bagshawe KD, Harland S. Immunodiagnosis and monitoring of gonadotropin-producing metastases in the central nervous system. Cancer 1976; 38:112–118.

627. Tompkins VN, Haymaker W, Campbell EH. Metastatic pineal tumors. J Neurosurg 1950; 7:159–160.

628. Castleman B, McNeely BU. Case 25-1971 (germinoma). Case records of the Massachusetts General Hospital. N Engl J Med 1971; 284:1427–1434.

629. Spiegel AM, DiChiro G, Gorden P, et al. Diagnosis of radiosensitive hypothalamic tumors without craniotomy. Endocrine and neuroradiologic studies of intracranial atypical teratomas. Ann Intern Med 1976; 85:290–293.

630. Axelrod L. Endocrine dysfunction in patients with tumors of the pineal region. In: Schmidek HH, ed. Pineal Tumors. New York: Masson, 1977: 61–77.

631. Kubo O, Yamasaki N, Kamjo Y, et al. Human chorionic gonadotropin produced by ectopic pinealoma in a girl with precocious puberty. J Neurosurg 1977; 47:101–105.

632. Giovannelli G. Pineal region tumors: endocrinological aspects. Childs Brain 1982; 9:267–273.

633. Ahmed SR, Shalet SM, Price DA, et al. Human chorionic gonadotropin secreting pineal germinoma and precocious puberty. Arch Dis Child 1983; 58:743–745.

634. Sklar CA, Conte FA, Kaplan SL, et al. Human chorionic gonadotropin–secreting pineal tumor: relation to pathogenesis and sex limitation of sexual precocity. J Clin Endocrinol Metab 1981; 53:656–660.

635. Kurmado K, Mori W. Virus-like particles in human pinealoma. Acta Neuropathol (Berl) 1976; 37:273–276.

636. Ringertz N, Nordestam H, Flyger G. Tumors of the pineal region. J Neuropathol 1954; 13:540–561.

637. Bing JF, Globus JH, Simon H. Pubertas praecox: a survey of the reported cases and verified anatomical findings. Mt Sinai J Med NY 1938; 4:935–965.

638. Sklar CA, Grumbach MM, Kaplan SL, et al. Hormonal and metabolic abnormalities associated with central nervous system germinoma in children and adolescents and the effect of therapy: report of 10 patients. J Clin Endocrinol Metab 1981; 52:9–16.

639. Kitay JI. Pineal lesions and precocious puberty: a review. J Clin Endocrinol Metab 1954; 14:622–625.

640. Kitay JI, Altschule MD. The Pineal Gland. Cambridge, MA: Harvard University Press, 1954.

641. Wurtman RJ, Kammer H. Melatonin synthesis by an ectopic pinealoma. N Engl J Med 1966; 274:1233–1237.

642. Wray SH. The neuro-ophthalmic and neurologic manifestations of pinealomas. In: Schmidek HH, ed. Pineal Tumors. New York: Masson, 1977: 61–77.

643. Schmidek HH. Surgical management of pineal region tumors. In: Schmidek HH, ed. Pineal Tumors. New York: Masson, 1977: 99–113.

644. Stein BM. Supracerebellar-infratentorial approach to pineal tumors. Surg Neurol 1979; 11:331–337.

645. Neuwelt EA, Glasberg M, Frenkel E, et al. Malignant pineal region tumors. A clinico-pathological study. J Neurosurg 1979; 51:597–607.

646. Brady LW. The role of radiation therapy. In: Schmidek HH, ed. Pineal Tumors. New York: Masson, 1977: 99–113.

647. Takeuchi J, Handa H, Nagata I. Suprasellar germinoma. J Neurosurg 1978; 49:41–48.

648. Rubin P, Kramer S. Ectopic pinealoma: a radiocurable neuroendocrinologic entity. Radiology 1965; 85:512–523.

649. Allen JC, Helson L, Jereb B. Preradiation chemotherapy for newly diagnosed childhood brain tumors. A modified phase II trial. Cancer 1983; 51:2001–2006.

650. Wilson BE, Netzloff ML. Primary testicular abnormalities causing precocious puberty. Leydig cell tumor, Leydig cell hyperplasia, and adrenal rest tumor. Ann Clin Lab Sci 1983; 13:315–320.

651. Rosenthal SM, Grumbach MM, Kaplan SL. Gonadotropin-independent familial sexual precocity with premature Leydig and germinal cell maturation (familial testotoxicosis): effect of a potent luteinizing hormone–releasing factor agonist and medroxyprogesterone acetate therapy in four cases. J Clin Endocrinol Metab 1983; 57:571–579.

652. Mansfield MJ, Beardsworth DE, Loughlin JS, et al. Long-term treatment of central precocious puberty with a long-acting analogue of luteinizing hormone releasing hormone. N Engl J Med 1983; 309:1286–1290.

653. Holland FJ, Fishman L, Bailey JD, et al. Ketoconazole in the management of precocious puberty not responsive to LHRH-analogue therapy. N Engl J Med 1985; 312:1023–1028.

654. Money J, Hampson JG. Idiopathic sexual precocity in the male. Management: report of a case. Psychosom Med 1955; 17:1–15.

655. Money J, Alexander D. Psychosexual development and absence of homosexuality in males with precocious puberty. J Nerv Ment Dis 1969; 148:111–123.

656. Ehrhardt AA, Meyer-Bahlburg HFL. Psychologic correlates of abnormal pubertal development. Clin Endocrinol Metab 1975; 4:207–222.

657. Hampson JG, Money J. Idiopathic sexual precocity in the female. Report of 3 cases. Psychosom Med 1955; 17:16–35.

658. Ihalainen O. Psychosomatic aspects of amenorrhoea. Acta Psychiatr Scand 1975; 262(Suppl):1–139.

659. Barnea ER, Naftolin F, Tolis G, et al. Hypothalamic amenorrhea syndromes. In: Givens JR, ed. The Hypothalamus. Chicago: Year Book Medical, 1984: 147–170.

660. Khoury SA, Reame NE, Kelch RP, et al. Diurnal patterns of pulsatile luteinizing hormone secretion in hypothalamic amenorrhea: reproducibility and responses to opiate blockade and an alpha 2–adrenergic agonist. J Clin Endocrinol Metab 1987; 64:755–762.

661. Rebar RW. Effects of exercise on reproductive function in females. In: Givens JR, ed. The Hypothalamus. Chicago: Year Book Medical, 1984: 245–262.

662. Frisch RE. Menarche and fatness: re-examination of the critical body composition hypothesis. Reply to the technical comment of J. Trussell. Science 1978; 200:1509–1513.

663. Klibanski A, Biller BM, Rosenthal DI, et al. Effects of prolactin and estrogen deficiency in amenorrheic bone loss. J Clin Endocrinol Metab 1988; 67:124–130.

664. Reichlin S. Introduction. In: Reichlin S, Baldessarini RJ, Martin JB, eds. The Hypothalamus. Vol 56. New York: Raven, 1978: 1–14.

665. Reichlin S. Overview of the anatomical and physiologic basis of anterior pituitary regulation. In: Tolis G, Labrie F, Martin JB, et al., eds. Clinical Neuroendocrinology. New York: Raven, 1979: 1–14.

666. Mason AJ, Pitts SL, Nikolics K, et al. The hypogonadal mouse: reproductive functions restored by gene therapy. Science 1986; 234:1372–1378.

667. Gibson MJ. Role of the preoptic area in the neuroendocrine regulation of reproduction: an analysis of functional preoptic homografts. Ann NY Acad Sci 1986; 474:53–63.

668. Kreuz LE, Rose RM, Jennings JR, et al. Suppression of plasma testosterone levels and psychological stress. Arch Gen Psychiatry 1972; 26:479–482.

669. Yates A, Leehey K, Shisslak CM. Running—an analogue of anorexia? N Engl J Med 1983; 308:251–255.

670. Morley JE, Melmed S. Gonadal dysfunction in systemic disorders. Metabolism 1979; 10:1051–1073.

671. Young RJ, Strachan RK, Seth J, et al. Is testicular endocrine function abnormal in young men with spinal cord injuries? Clin Endocrinol 1982; 3:303–306.

672. Cortes-Gallegos V, Castaneda G, Alonso R, et al. Diurnal variations of pituitary and testicular hormones in paraplegic men. Arch Androl 1982; 8:221–226.

Neurogenic Disorders of Prolactin Regulation

673. Reichlin J, Molitch M. Neuroendocrine aspect of pituitary adenoma. In: Cammanni F, Muller EE, eds. Pituitary Hyperfunction: Physiopathology and Clinical Aspects. New York: Raven, 1984: 47–70.

674. Tucker HS, Lankford HV, Gardner DF, et al. Persistent defect in regulation of prolactin secretion after successful pituitary tumor removal in women with galactorrhea-amenorrhea syndrome. J Clin Endocrinol Metab 1980; 51:968–971.

675. Barbarino A, Marinis LDE, Menini E, et al. Pre- and postoperative pituitary function tests in patients with prolactin-secreting pituitary adenoma. In: Camanni F, Müller EE, eds. Pituitary Hyperfunction: Physiopathology and Clinical Aspects. New York: Raven, 1984: 333–342.

676. Molitch ME, Reichlin S. Neuroendocrine studies of prolactin secretion in hyperprolactinemic states. In: Mena F, Valverde-Rodriguez S, eds. Frontiers and Perspectives in Prolactin Secretion: A Multidisciplinary Approach. New York: Academic, 1984: 393–421.

677. Faglia G, Spada A, Moriondo P, et al. What is the role of dopamine in the pathogenesis of prolactinomas. In: Camanni E, Müller EE, eds. Pituitary Hyperfunction: Physiopathology and Clinical Aspects. New York: Raven, 1984: 279–288.

Neurogenic Disorders of Growth Hormone Secretion

678. Powell GF, Brasel JA, Blizzard RM. Emotional deprivation and growth retardation simulating idiopathic hypopituitarism. II. Endocrinologic evaluation of the syndrome. N Engl J Med 1967; 267:1279–1283.

679. Krieger L, Mellinger RC. Pituitary function in the deprivation syndrome. J Pediatr 1971; 79:216–225.

680. Whitten CF, Petit MG. Evidence that growth failure from maternal deprivation is secondary to undereating. JAMA 1969; 209:1675–1682.

681. Underwood LE, Van Wyk JJ. Hormones in normal aberrant growth. In: Williams RH, ed. Textbook of Endocrinology. 6th ed. Philadelphia: W. B. Saunders, 1981: 1149–1191.

682. Tannenbaum GS, Epelbaum J, Colle E, et al. Antiserum to somatostatin reverses starvation-induced inhibition of growth hormone but not insulin secretion. Endocrinology 1978; 102:1909–1914.

683. Wolff G, Money J. Relationship between sleep and growth in patients with reversible somatotropin deficiency (psychosocial dwarfism). Psychol Med 1973; 3:18–27.

684. Money J, Annecillo C, Kelley JF. Growth of intelligence: failure and catchup associated respectively with abuse and rescue in the syndrome of abuse dwarfism. Psychoneuroendocrinology 1983; 8:309–319.

685. Bercu BB, Shulman D, Root AW, et al. Growth hormone (GH) provocative testing frequently does not reflect endogenous GH secretion. J Clin Endocrinol Metab 1986; 63:709–716 (erratum 1987; 64:382).

686. Bercu BB, Diamond FB, Jr. Growth hormone neurosecretory dysfunction. Clin Endocrinol Metab 1986; 15:537–590.

687. Lin TH, Kirkland RT, Sherman BM, et al. Growth hormone testing in short children and their response to growth hormone therapy. J Pediatr 1989; 115:57–63.

688. Grumbach MM. Growth hormone therapy and the short end of the stick. N Engl J Med 1988; 319:238–241 (editorial).

689. Burr IM, Slonim AE, Danish RK, et al. Diencephalic syndrome revisited. J Pediatr 1976; 88:439–444.

690. Drop SL, Guyda HJ, Colle E. Inappropriate growth hormone release in the diencephalic syndrome of childhood: case report and 4 year endocrinological follow-up. Clin Endocrinol 1980; 13:181–187.

691. Reichlin S. Neuroregulatory abnormalities of growth hormone secretion. In: Müller EE, Cocchi D, Locatelli V, eds. Advances in Growth Hormone and Growth Factor Research. Rome: Pythagora, 1989: 445–464.

692. Ho KY, Veldhuis JD, Johnson ML, et al. Fasting enhances growth hormone secretion and amplifies the complex rhythms of growth hormone secretion in man. J Clin Invest 1988; 81:968–975.

693. Atiea JA, Cregagh F, Page M, et al. Early-morning hyperglycemia in IDDM. Acute effects of cholinergic blockade. Diabetes Care 1989; 12:443–448.

694. Daughaday WH, Cryer PE, Jacobs LS. The role of the hypothalamus in the pathogenesis of pituitary tumors. In: Kohler PO, Ross GT, eds. Diagnosis and Treatment of Pituitary Tumors. Amsterdam: Excerpta Medica, 1973: 26–34.

695. Reichlin S. Etiology of pituitary adenomas. In: Post K, Jackson IMD, Reichlin S, eds. Pituitary Adenomas. New York: Plenum, 1980: 29–46.

696. Reichlin S. Functional aspects of endocrine neoplasms. In: Kovacs K, Asa S, eds. Functional Endocrine Pathology. Boston: Blackwell Scientific, 1991: 898–913.

697. Molitch M. Pathogenesis of pituitary tumors. Endocrinol Metab Clin North Am 1987; 16:503–528.

698. Faglia G, Spada A, Ambrosi B, et al. What's the role of the hypothalamus in pituitary adenoma formation? In: Melmed S, Robbins RJ, eds. Molecular and Clinical Advances in Pituitary Disorders. Boston: Blackwell Scientific, 1991:213–228.

Neurogenic Disorders of Corticotropin Regulation

699. Asa SL, Kovacs K, Tindall GT, et al. CRF-producing hypothalamic gangliocytoma associated with pituitary corticotropin cell hyperplasia: evidence for a hypothalamic etiology of Cushing's disease. Endocrinology 1983; 112(Suppl):191.

700. Gold PW, Goodwin FK, Chrousos GP. Clinical and biochemical manifestations of depression. Relation to the neurobiology of stress. N Engl J Med 1988; 319:348–353, 413–420.

701. Wolff SM, Adler RC, Buskirk ER, et al. A syndrome of periodic hypothalamic discharge. Am J Med 1964; 36:956–967.

702. Krieger DT. Physiopathology of Cushing's disease. Endocr Rev 1983; 4:22–43.

703. Daughaday WH. Cushing's disease and basophilic microadenomas. N Engl J Med 1984; 310:919–920.

704. Lamberts SW, Bons EG, Uitterlinden P. Studies on the glucocorticoid-receptor blocking action of RU 38386 in cultured ACTH-secreting human pituitary tumour cells and normal rat pituitary cells. Acta Endocrinol 1985; 109:64–69.

Nonendocrine Manifestations of Hypothalamic Disease

705. Plum FC, Uitert RV. Nonendocrine diseases and disorders of the hypothalamus. In: Reichlin S, Baldessarini RJ, Martin JB, eds. The Hypothalamus. Vol 56. New York: Raven, 1978: 415–474.

706. Krieger DT. The hypothalamus and neuroendocrine pathology. In: Krieger DT, Hughes JC, eds. Neuroendocrinology. Sunderland, MA: Sinauer Associates, 1980: 13–22.

707. Morgane PJ, Panksepp J. The Handbook of the Hypothalamus. Behavioral Studies of the Hypothalamus. Vol 3, Parts A and B. New York: Marcel Dekker, 1980, 1981.

Neuropeptides in the Brain

708. Fischer EG, Welch K, Belli JA, et al. Treatment of craniopharyngiomas in children. J Neurosurg 1985; 62:496–501.

709. Krieger DT, Martin JB. Brain peptides. N Engl J Med 1981; 304:876–885, 944–951.

710. Krieger DT, Brownstein M, Martin JB. Brain Peptides. New York: John Wiley & Sons, 1983.

711. Martin JB, Brownstein MJ, Krieger DT, eds. Brain Peptides Update. Vol 1. New York: John Wiley & Sons, 1987.

712. Krieger DT. Brain peptides: what, where and why? Science 1983; 222:975–985.

713. Erspamer V, Melchiorri P, Eroccardo M, et al. The brain-gut-skin triangle: new peptides. Peptides 1981; 2:7–16.

714. Newmark P. An embarrassment of peptides. Nature 1983; 303:655.

715. Rosenfeld MG, Mermod JJ, Amara SG, et al. Production of a novel neuropeptide encoded by the calcitonin gene via tissue-specific RNA processing. Nature 1983; 304:129–135.

716. Tatemoto K, Mutt V. Isolation and characterization of the intestinal peptide porcine PHI (PHI-27), a new member of the glucagon-secreting family. Proc Natl Acad Sci USA 1981; 78:6603–6607.

717. Cooper JR, Bloom FE, Roth RH. The Biochemical Basis of Neuropharmacology. 5th ed. New York: Oxford University Press, 1986.

718. Vincent SR, Johansson O, Hökfelt T, et al. Neuropeptide coexistence in human cortical neurons. Nature 1982; 298:65–67.

719. Hökfelt T, Rehfeld JF, Skirboll L, et al. Evidence for coexistence of dopamine and CCK in meso-limbic neurons. Nature 1980; 285:476–478.

Pain and Endogenous Opioids

720. Kosterlitz HW. Endogenous opioid peptides: historical aspects. In: Hughes J, ed. Centrally Acting Peptides. Baltimore: University Park Press, 1978: 157.

721. Garfield E. Current comments. Controversies over opiate receptor research typify problems facing awards committees. Current Contents 1979; 20:5–18.

722. Uhl GR, Childers SR, Snyder SH. Opioid peptides and the opiate receptor. Front Neuroendocrinol 1978; 5:289–328.

723. Kelly RA, Smith TW. The search for the endogenous digitalis: an alternative hypothesis. Am J Physiol 1989; 256:C937–C950.

724. Müller EE, Nistico G. Benzodiazepines. In: Muller EE, Nistico G, eds. Brain Messengers and the Pituitary. San Diego, CA: Academic, 1989: 159–161.

725. Snyder SH. Adenosine as a neuromodulator. Annu Rev Neurosci 1985; 8:103–124.

726. Goodman RR, Fricker LD, Snyder SH. Enkephalins. In: Krieger DT, Brownstein MJ, Martin JB, eds. Brain Peptides. New York: John Wiley & Sons, 1983: 827–850.

727. Li CH, Barnafi L, Chrétien M, et al. Isolation and amino acid sequence of β-LPH from sheep pituitary glands. Nature 1975; 208:1093–1094.

728. Goldstein A. Opioid peptides (endorphins) in pituitary and brain. Science 1976; 193:1081–1086.

729. Krieger D. Endorphins and enkephalins. DM 1982; 28:1–53.

730. Noda M, Furutani Y, Takahashi H, et al. Cloning and sequence analysis of cDNA for bovine adrenal preproenkephalin. Nature 1982; 295:202–206.

731. Noda M, Teranishi Y, Takahashi H, et al. Isolation and structural organization of the human preproenkephalin gene. Nature 1982; 197:431–434.

732. Kakidani H, Furutani Y, Takahashi H, et al. Cloning and sequence analysis of cDNA for porcine β-neo-endorphin/dynorphin precursor. Nature 1982; 298:245–249.

733. Horikawa S, Takai T, Toyosato M, et al. Isolation and structural organization of the human preproenkephalin B gene. Nature 1983; 306:611–614.

734. Comb M, Seeburg PH, Adelman J, et al. Primary structure of the human met- and leu-enkephalin precursor and its mRNA. Nature 1982; 295:663–666.

735. Pert CB, Pert A, Tallman JF. Isolation of a novel endogenous opiate analgesic from human blood. Proc Natl Acad Sci USA 1976; 73:2226–2230.

736. Sarne Y, Weissman BA, Keren O, et al. Humoral endorphin: a new endogenous factor with opiate-like activity. Life Sci 1981; 28:673–680.

737. Gintzler AR, Levy A, Spector S. Antibodies as a means of isolating and characterizing biologically active substances: presence of a nonpeptide, morphine-like compound in the central nervous system. Proc Natl Acad Sci USA 1976; 73:2132–2136.

738. Gintzler AR, Gershon MD, Spector S. A nonpeptide morphine-like compound: immunocytochemical localization in the mouse brain. Science 1978; 199:447–448.

739. Grossman A, Clement-Jones V, Besser GM. Clinical implications of endogenous opioid peptides. In: Müller EE, MacLeod RM, Frohman LA, eds. Neuroendocrine Perspectives. Vol 4. Amsterdam: Elsevier Biomedical, 1985: 243–294.

740. Gee CE, Chen CL, Roberts JL, et al. Identification of proopiomelanocortin neurons in rat hypothalamus by in situ cDNA-mRNA hybridization. Nature 1983; 306:374–376.

741. Mudge AW, Leeman SE, Fischbach G. Enkephalin inhibits release of substance P from sensory neurons in culture and decreases action potential duration. Proc Natl Acad Sci USA 1979; 76:526–530.

742. Varndell I, Tapia F, DeMey J, et al. Electron immunocytochemical localization of enkephalin-like material in catecholamine-containing cells of the carotid body, the adrenal medulla, and in pheochromocytomas of man and other mammals. J Histochem Cytochem 1982; 30:682–690.

743. Comb M, Herbert E, Crea R. Partial characterization of mRNA that codes for enkephalins in bovine adrenal medulla and human pheochromocytoma. Proc Natl Acad Sci USA 1982; 79:360–364.

744. Rossier J, Dean D, Livett B, et al. Enkephalin congeners and precursors are synthesized and released by primary cultures of adrenal chromaffin cells. Life Sci 1981; 28:781–789.

745. Eiden L, Giraud P, Hotchkis A, et al. Enkephalins and VIP in human pheochromocytomas and bovine adrenal chromaffin cells. In: Costa E, Trabucchi M, eds. Regulatory Peptides: From Molecular Biology to Function. New York: Raven, 1982: 387–395.

746. Yoshimasa T, Nakao K, Ohtsuke H, et al. Methionine-enkephalin and leucine-enkephalin in human sympathoadrenal system and pheochromocytoma. J Clin Invest 1982; 69:643–650.

747. Yoshimasa T, Nakao K, Li S, et al. Plasma methionine-enkephalin and leucine-enkephalin in normal subjects and patients with pheochromocytoma. J Clin Endocrinol Metab 1983; 57:706–712.

748. Akil H, Richardson DE, Barchas JD, et al. Appearance of beta-endorphin–like immunoreactivity in human ventricular cerebrospinal fluid upon analgesic electrical stimulation. Proc Natl Acad Sci USA 1978; 75:5170–5172.

749. Terenius L, Wahlstrom A. Physiological and clinical relevance of endorphins. In: Hughes J, ed. Centrally Acting Peptides. Baltimore: University Park Press, 1978: 161–178.

750. Bozarth MA, Wise RA. Anatomically distinct opiate receptor fields mediate reward and physical dependence. Science 1984; 224:516–517.

751. Sharma SK, Klee WA, Nirenberg M. Dual regulation of adenylate cyclase accounts for narcotic dependence and tolerance. Proc Natl Acad Sci USA 1975; 72:3092–3096.

752. Nestler EJ, Erdos JJ, Terwilliger R, et al. Regulation of G proteins by chronic morphine in the rat locus coeruleus. Brain Res 1989; 476:230–239.

753. Chang SL, Squinto SP, Harlan RE. Morphine activation of c-fos expression in rat brain. Biochem Biophys Res Commun 1988; 157:698–704.

754. Morley JE. Neuroendocrine effects of endogenous opioid peptides in human subjects: a review. Psychoneuroendocrinology 1983; 8:361–379.

755. Grossman A. Brain opiates and neuroendocrine function. Clin Endocrinol Metab 1983; 12:725–746.

756. Rossier J. Functions of β-endorphin and enkephalins in the pituitary. In: Ganong F, Martini L, eds. Frontiers in Neuroendocrinology. Vol 7. New York: Raven, 1982: 191–209.

757. Quigley ME, Sheehan KL, Casper RF, et al. Evidence for increased dopaminergic and opioid activity in patients with hypothalamic hypogonadotropic amenorrhea. J Clin Endocrinol Metab 1980; 50:949–954.

758. Blankstein J, Reyes FI, Winter JS, et al. Endorphins and the regulations of the human menstrual cycle. Clin Endocrinol 1981; 14:287–294.

759. Spiler IJ, Molitch ME. Lack of modulation of pituitary hormone stress response by neural pathways involving opiate receptors. J Clin Endocrinol Metab 1980; 50:516–520.

Peptides in Memory and Learning

760. DeWeid D. Hormonal influences on motivation, learning, memory, and psychosis. In: Krieger DT, Hughes JC, eds. Neuroendocrinology. Sunderland, MA: Sinauer Associates, 1980: 194–205.

761. van Wiermsma Greidanus TB, van Raee JM, de Wied D. Vasopressin and memory. Pharmacol Ther 1983; 20:437–458.

762. Audibert A, Moeglen JM, Lancranjan I. Central effects of vasopressin in man. Int J Neurol 1980; 14:162–174.

763. Krieger DT, Liotta AS, Brownstein MJ, et al. ACTH, beta-lipotropin, and related peptides in brain, pituitary, and blood. Recent Prog Horm Res 1980; 36:277–344.

764. Burbach JPH, Kovacs GL, de Weid D, et al. A major metabolite of arginine vasopressin in the brain is a highly potent neuropeptide. Science 1983; 221:1310–1312.

765. Dyball RE, Paterson AT. Neurohypophysial hormones and brain function: the neurophysiological effects of oxytocin and vasopressin. Pharmacol Ther 1983; 20:419–436.

766. Partridge WM, Frank HJL. Mechanisms of peptide transport from blood to brain. In: Müller EE, MacLeod RM, eds. Neuroendocrine Perspectives. Vol 2. Amsterdam: Elsevier Biomedical, 1983: 107–122.

767. Meisenberg G, Simmons WH. Minireview. Peptides and the blood-brain barrier. Life Sci 1983; 32:2611–2623.

768. Partridge WM. Receptor-mediated peptide transported through the blood-brain barrier. Endocr Rev 1986; 7:314–330.

769. Koob G, Bloom FE. Memory, learning, and adaptive behaviors. In: Krieger DT, Brownstein MJ, Martin JKB, eds. Brain Peptides. New York: John Wiley & Sons, 1983: 369–388.

Eating Behavior and Neuropeptides

770. Schneider BS, Friedman JM, Hirsch J. Feeding behavior. In: Krieger DT, Brownstein MJ, Martin JB, eds. Brain Peptides. New York: John Wiley & Sons, 1983: 251–279.

771. Morley JE. Neuropeptide regulation of appetite and weight. Endocr Rev 1987; 8:256–287.

772. Borison HL. History and status of the area postrema. Fed Proc 1984; 43:2937–2940.

773. Smith GP, Gibbs J, Jerome C, et al. The satiety effect of cholecystokinin: a progress report. Peptides 1981; 2:57–59.

774. Baile CA, Della-Fera MA, McLaughlin CL. Hormones and feed intake. Proc Nutr Soc 1983; 42:113–127.

775. Stanley BG, Kyrkouli SE, Lampert S, et al. Neuropeptide Y chronically injected into the hypothalamus: a powerful neurochemical inducer of hyperphagia and obesity. Peptides 1986; 7:1189–1192.

776. Reichelt KL, Foss I, Trygstad O, et al. Humoral control of appetite—II. Purification and characterization of an anorexogenic peptide from human urine. Neuroscience 1978; 3:1207–1211.

777. Nance DM, Coy DH, Kastin AJ. Experiments with a reported anorexigenic tripeptide: Pyro-Glu-His-Gly-OH. Pharmacol Biochem Behav 1979; 11:733–735.

778. Blavet N, DeFeudis FV, Clostre F. Lack of effect of the peptide pyro-Glu-His-Gly-OH on food consumption in mice and rats. Gen Pharmacol 1982; 13:173–176.

779. McHugh PR. The control of gastric emptying. J Autonom Nerv Syst 1983; 9:221–231.

780. Smith GT, Moran TH, Coyle JT, et al. Anatomic localization of chole-

cystokinin receptors to the pyloric sphincter. Am J Physiol 1984; 246:R127–R130.

781. Dourish CT, Rycroft W, Iversen SD. Postponement of satiety by blockade of brain cholecystokinin (CCK-B) receptors. Science 1989; 245:1509–1511.

782. Leibowitz SF. Brain neurotransmitters and appetite regulation. Psychopharmacol Bull 1985; 21:412–418.

783. Leibowitz SF. Hypothalamic neurotransmitters in relation to normal and disturbed eating patterns. Ann NY Acad Sci 1987; 499:137–143.

784. Ishizuka B, Quigley ME, Yen SS. Pituitary hormone release in response to food ingestion: evidence for neuroendocrine signals from gut to brain. J Clin Endocrinol Metab 1983; 57:1111–1116.

Drinking Behavior and Neuropeptides

785. Fitzsimmons JT, Epstein AN, Johnson AK. The peptide specificity of receptors for angiotensin-induced thirst. In: Buckley JP, Ferrario CM, eds. Central Actions of Angiotensin and Related Hormones. New York: Plenum, 1977: 405–415.

786. Ramsay DJ, Ganong WF. CNS regulation of salt and water balance. In: Krieger DT, Hughes JC, eds. Neuroendocrinology. Sunderland, MA: Sinauer Associates, 1980: 123–130.

787. Ramsay DJ. Effects of circulating angiotensin II on the brain. In: Ganong F, Martini L, eds. Frontiers in Neuroendocrinology. Vol 7. New York: Raven, 1982: 263–285.

788. Ganong WF. The brain renin-angiotensin system. In: Krieger DT, Brownstein MJ, Martin JB, eds. Brain Peptides. New York: John Wiley & Sons, 1983: 805–826.

789. Ganten D, Mullins J, Lindpaintner K. The tissue renin-angiotensin system: a target for angiotensin-converting enzyme inhibitors. J Hum Hypertens 1989; 3(Suppl 1):63–70.

790. Jin M, Wilhelm MJ, Lang RE, et al. Endogenous tissue renin-angiotensin systems. From molecular biology to therapy. Am J Med 1988; 84:28–36.

791. Unger T, Badoer E, Ganten D, et al. Brain angiotensin: pathways and pharmacology. Circulation 1988; 77:140–154.

Peptides and Thermoregulation

792. Brown MM. Thermoregulation. In: Krieger DT, Brownstein MJ, Martin JB, eds. Brain Peptides. New York: John Wiley & Sons, 1983: 301–314.

793. Lipton JM, Glyn JR, Zimmer JA. ACTH and α-melanotropin in central temperature control. Fed Proc 1981; 40:2760–2764.

794. Dinarello CA, Mier JW. Lymphokines. N Engl J Med 1987; 317:940–945.

795. Dinarello CA. Biology of interleukin 1. FASEB J 1988; 2:108–115.

796. Coceani F, Bishai I, Lees J, et al. Prostaglandin E₂ and fever: a continuing debate. Yale J Biol Med 1986; 59:169–174.

797. Blatteis CM. Neural mechanisms in the pyrogenic and acute-phase responses to interleukin-1. Int J Neurosci 1988; 38:223–232.

Sleep Peptides

798. Schoenenberger GA, Maier PF, Tobler HJ, et al. The delta EEG (sleep)-inducing peptide (DSIP). XI. Amino-acid analysis, sequence, synthesis and activity of the nonapeptide. Pfluegers Arch 1978; 376:119–129.

799. Krueger JM, Pappenheimer JR, Karnovsky ML. Sleep-promoting effects of muramyl peptides. Proc Natl Acad Sci USA 1982; 79:6102–6106.

800. Martin SA, Karnovsky ML, Krueger JM, et al. Peptidoglycans as promoters of slow-wave sleep. I. Structure of the sleep-promoting factor isolated from human urine. J Biol Chem 1984; 259:12652–12658.

801. Chedid L. Muramyl peptides as possible endogenous immunopharmacological mediators. Microbiol Immunol 1983; 27:723–732.

802. Borbely AA, Tobler I. Endogenous sleep-promoting substances and sleep regulation. Physiol Rev 1989; 69:605–670.

Peptides in Sexual Function and Behavior

803. Rivier C, Rivier J, Vale W. Stress-induced inhibition of reproductive functions: role of endogenous corticotropin-releasing factor. Science 1986; 231:607–609.

804. Sirinathsinghji DJ, Rees LH, Rivier J, et al. Corticotropin-releasing factor is a potent inhibitor of sexual receptivity in the female rat. Nature 1983; 305:232–235.

805. Polak JM, Gu J, Mina S, et al. Vipergic nerves in the penis. Lancet 1981; 2:217–219.

806. Dall WG, Moll MA, Weber K. Localization of vasoactive intestinal polypeptide in penile erectile tissue and in the major pelvic ganglion of the rat. Neuroscience 1983; 101:1379–1386.

807. Anand P, Gibson SJ, McGregor GP, et al. A VIP-containing system concentrated in the lumbosacral region of human spinal cord. Nature 1983; 305:143–145.

808. Dixson AF, Kendrick KM, Blank MA, et al. Effects of tactile and electrical stimuli upon release of vasoactive intestinal polypeptide in the mammalian penis. J Endocrinol 1984; 100:249–252.

809. Crowe R, Lincoln J, Blacklay PF, et al. Vasoactive intestinal polypeptide–like immunoreactive nerves in diabetic penis. A comparison between streptozotocin-treated rats and man. Diabetes 1983; 32:1075–1077.

810. Krane RJ, Goldstein I, Saenz-de-Tejada I. Impotence. N Engl J Med 1989; 321:1648–1659.

811. Ottesen B, Ulrichsen H, Fahrenkrug J, et al. Vasoactive intestinal polypeptide and the female genital tract: relationship to reproductive phase and delivery. Am J Obstet Gynecol 1982; 143:414–420.

812. Anggard A, Lundberg JM, Lundblad L. Nasal autonomic innervation with special reference to peptidergic nerves. Eur J Respir Dis 1983; 128:143–149.

Neuroimmunomodulation

813. Paul WE, ed. Fundamental Immunology. New York: Raven, 1989.

814. Tracey KJ, Lowry SF, Cerami A. Cachectin: a hormone that triggers acute shock and chronic cachexia. J Infect Dis 1988; 157:413–420.

815. Goetzl EJ, Sreedharan SP, Harkonen WS. Pathogenetic roles of neuroimmunologic mediators. Immunol Allergy Clin North Am 1988; 8:183–200.

816. Payan DG, McGillis JP, Goetzl EJ. Neuroimmunology. Adv Immunol 1986; 39:299–323.

817. Ader R, ed. Psychoneuroimmunology. New York: Academic, 1981.

818. MacLean D, Reichlin S. Neuroendocrinology and the immune process. In: Ader R, ed. Psychoneuroimmunology. New York: Academic, 1981: 475–520.

819. Munck A, Guyre PM, Holbrook NJ. Physiological functions of glucocorticoids in stress and their relation to pharmacological actions. Endocr Rev 1984; 5:25–44.

820. Sternberg EM, Young WS III, Bernardini R, et al. A central nervous system defect in biosynthesis of corticotropin-releasing hormone is associated with susceptibility to streptococcal cell wall–induced arthritis in Lewis rats. Proc Natl Acad Sci USA 1989; 86:4771–4775.

821. Ahlqvist J. Hormonal influences on immunologic and related phenomena. In: Ader R, ed. Psychoneuroimmunology. New York: Academic, 1981: 355–403.

822. Goff BL, Roth JA, Arp LH, et al. Growth hormone treatment stimulates thymulin production in aged dogs. Clin Exp Immunol 1987; 68:580–587.

823. Hartman DP, Holaday JW, Bernton EW. Inhibition of lymphocyte proliferation by antibodies to prolactin. FASEB J 1989; 3:2194–2202.

824. Cross RJ, Roszman TL. Neuroendocrine modulation of immune function: the role of prolactin. PNEI 1989; 2:17–20.

825. Bernton EW. Prolactin and immune host defenses. PNEI 1989; 2:21–29.

826. Hiestand PC, Mekler P, Nordmann R, et al. Prolactin as a modulator of lymphocyte responsiveness provides a possible mechanism of action for cyclosporine. Proc Natl Acad Sci USA 1986; 83:2599–2603.

827. Schwartz RS, Datta SK. Autoimmunity and autoimmune disease. In: Paul WE, ed. Fundamental Immunology. New York: Raven, 1989: 819–866.

828. Kalman B, Olsson O, Link H, et al. Estradiol potentiates poke-weed mitogen–induced B cell stimulation in multiple sclerosis and healthy subjects. Acta Neurol Scand 1989; 79:340–346.

829. Ressel M, Kohler G, Straub W. Verhalten der T-lymphozyten im normalen mensuaellen Zyklus. Zentralbl Gynakol 1988; 110:619–622.

830. Opp MR, Obal F Jr, Krueger JM. Effects of α-MSH on sleep, behavior, and brain temperature: interactions with IL-1. Am J Physiol 1988; 255:R914–R922.

831. Cannon JG, Tatro JB, Reichlin S, et al. α-Melanocyte stimulating hormone inhibits immunostimulatory and inflammatory actions of interleukin 1. J Immunol 1986; 137:2232–2236.

832. Mason MJ, Van Epps D. Modulation of IL-1, tumor necrosis factor, and C5a-mediated murine neutrophil migration by α-melanocyte-stimulating hormone. J Immunol 1989; 1142:1646–1651.

833. Daynes RA, Robertson BA, Cho BH, et al. α-Melanocyte-stimulating hormone exhibits target cell selectivity in its capacity to affect interleukin 1–inducible responses in vivo and in vitro. J Immunol 1987; 139:103–109.

834. Lotz M, Vaugn JH, Carson DA. Effect of neuropeptides on production of inflammatory cytokines by human monocytes. Science 1988; 241:1218–1221.

835. Kidd BL, Mapp PI, Gibson SJ, et al. A neurogenic mechanism for symmetrical arthritis. Lancet 1989; 2:1128–1130.

836. Aronin N, DiFiglia M, Leeman SE. Substance P. In: Krieger DT, Brownstein MJ, Martin JB, eds. Brain Peptides. New York: John Wiley & Sons, 1983: 783–804.

837. Sreedharan SP, Kodama KT, Peterson KE, et al. Distinct subsets of somatostatin receptors on cultured human lymphocytes. J Biol Chem 1989; 264:949–952.

838. Ottaway CA. Vasoactive intestinal peptide as a modulator of lymphocyte and immune function. Ann NY Acad Sci 1988; 527:486–500.

839. Scarborough DE, Reichlin S. Cytokines, the brain and aging. PNEI 1988; 1:10–15.

840. Waage A, Brandtzaeg P, Halstensen A, et al. The complex pattern of cytokines in serum from patients with meningococcal septic shock. Association between interleukin 6, interleukin 1, and fatal outcome. J Exp Med 1989; 169:333–338.

841. Besedovsky J, del Rey A, Sorkin E, et al. Immunoregulatory feedback

between interleukin-1 and glucocorticoid hormones. Science 1986; 233:652–654.

842. Bernton EW, Beach JE, Holaday JW, et al. Release of multiple hormones by a direct action of interleukin-1 on pituitary cells. Science 1987; 238:519–521.

843. Sapolsky R, Rivier C, Yamamoto G, et al. Interleukin-1 stimulates the secretion of hypothalamic corticotropin-releasing factor. Science 1987; 238:522–524.

844. Atkins MB, Gould JA, Allegretta M, et al. Phase I evaluation of recombinant interleukin-2 in patients with advanced malignant disease. J Clin Oncol 1986; 4:1380–1391.

845. Dubois JR, Dayer JM, Siegrist-Kaiser CA, et al. Human recombinant interleukin-1 decreases plasma thyroid hormone and thyroid stimulating hormone levels in rats. Endocrinology 1988; 123:2175–2181.

846. Kasting NW, Martin JB. Altered release of growth hormone and thyrotropin induced by endotoxin in the rat. Am J Physiol 1982; 243:E332–E337.

847. Scarborough DE, Lee SL, Dinarello CA, et al. Interleukin-1 beta stimulates somatostatin biosynthesis in primary cultures of fetal rat brain. Endocrinology 1989; 124:544–551.

848. Spangelo B, Judd AM, Isakson PC, et al. IL-6 stimulates anterior pituitary hormone release in vitro. Endocrinology 1989; 125:575–577.

849. Vankelecom H, Carmeliet P, Van Damme J, et al. Production of interleukin-6 by folliculo-stellate cells of the anterior pituitary gland in a histiotypic cell aggregate culture system. Neuroendocrinology 1989; 49:102–106.

850. Romero L, Lechan R, Dinarello CA, et al. Pituitary IL-6 is stimulated in vitro by bacterial lipopolysaccharide. 72nd Annual Meeting of The Endocrine Society, Atlanta GA. 1990: Abstract 775.

851. Koenig JI, Snowe K, Clark BD, et al. Intrinsic pituitary interleukin 1-β is induced by bacterial lipopolysaccharide. Endocrinology 1990; 126:3053–3058.

852. Breder CD, Dinarello CD, Saper CB. Interleukin-1 immunoreactive innervation of the human hypothalamus. Science 1988; 240:321–324.

853. Lechan RM, Toni R, Clark BD, et al. Immunoreactive interleukin-1beta localization in the rat forebrain. Brain Res 1990; 514:135–140.

854. Spangelo BL, Login IS, Judd AM, et al. Release of interleukin-6 from rat hypothalamus. Soc Neurosci Abstr 1989; 8.

855. Smith EM, Meyer WJ, Blalock JE. Virus-induced corticosterone in hypophysectomized mice: a possible lymphoid adrenal axis. Science 1982; 218:1311–1312.

856. Dunn AJ, Powell ML, Moreshead WV, et al. Effects of Newcastle disease virus administration to mice on the metabolism of cerebral biogenic amines, plasma corticosterone and lymphocyte proliferation. Brain Behav Immun 1987; 1:216–230.

857. Dupont AGG, Somers AC, Van Steviteghem AC, et al. Ectopic adrenocorticotropin production: disappearance after removal of inflammatory tissue. J Clin Endocrinol Metab 1984; 58:654–658.

858. Smith EM, Brosnan P, Meyer WJ, et al. An ACTH receptor on human mononuclear leukocytes. Relation to adrenal ACTH-receptor activity. N Engl J Med 1987; 317:1266–1269.

859. Lysle DT, Cunnick JE, Fowler H, et al. Pavlovian conditioning of shock-induced suppression of lymphocyte reactivity: acquisition, extinction, and preexposure effects. Life Sci 1988; 42:2185–2194.

860. Stein M, Schleifer SJ, Keller SE. Hypothalamic influences on immune responses. In: Ader R, ed. Psychoneuroimmunology. New York: Academic, 1981: 429–447.

861. Felten DL, Felten SY, Carlson SL, et al. Noradrenergic and peptidergic innervation of lymphoid tissue. J Immunol 1985; 135:755s–765s.

862. Dardenne M, Savino W, Gagnerault MC, et al. Neuroendocrine control of thymic hormonal production. I. Prolactin stimulates in vivo and in vitro the production of thymulin by human and murine thymic epithelial cells. Endocrinology 1989; 125:3–12.

THE ANTERIOR PITUITARY

Michael O. Thorner, Mary Lee Vance, Eva Horvath,
and Kalman Kovacs

INTRODUCTION

The anterior pituitary gland regulates various endocrine organs by integrating the signals from the brain and the feedback effects of peripheral hormones to stimulate intermittently hormone release by a particular gland. The pituitary is the source of at least six hormones that regulate growth, development, and function of the thyroid gland, adrenal cortex, gonads, and breasts. Peripheral nonendocrine tissues are also the target for some pituitary hormones. Thus disorders of pituitary function may produce selective overstimulation of one target gland, such as the adrenal gland in Cushing's disease, or cause pituitary hormone deficiency, which may or may not be selective. By virtue of the anatomical location of the pituitary in the sella turcica, expanding lesions of the gland may give rise to visual disturbances, cavernous sinus syndrome(s), and headaches.

The function and importance of the pituitary were recognized in the second half of the 19th century, although its existence was known for more than 2000 y. The name pituitary originates from the Greek *ptuo* (to spit) and the Latin *pituita* (mucus). It was thought that mucus, produced by the brain, was excreted through the nose by the pituitary. The term hypophysis is derived from Greek (*hypo*: under; *physis*: growth) and was first used by von Soemmening in 1798.

The beginning of pituitary endocrinology is often dated to 1886, when Pierre Marie, the French neurologist, described pituitary enlargement in acromegaly and postulated that the pituitary plays an important role in the pathogenesis of this disease. Marie's contribution was fundamental because it focused attention on the pituitary and initiated research to gain insight into the structure and function of the pituitary in health and disease.

During this century the hormones of the hypothalamus and pituitary have been isolated, characterized, and sequenced, and their physiological roles have been defined. The importance of hypothalamic regulation of the anterior pituitary via secretion of hypothalamic regulatory hormones into the hypothalamic-hypophyseal portal circulation has been established. The clinical features associated with excessive or deficient secretion of the various anterior pituitary hormones have been characterized. The study of these conditions and the clinical evaluation of patients with pituitary disease were revolutionized by the development of sensitive, specific, and reliable radioimmunoassays for the pituitary hormones and the hormones secreted by the target glands. This advance has been complemented by a similar revolution in noninvasive imaging techniques such as magnetic resonance imaging (MRI) and computed tomographic (CT) scanning that allow precise anatomical evaluation of the hypothalamus, pituitary, and surrounding structures. Finally, the application of modern histochemical techniques—including immunocytochemistry, electron microscopy, and in situ hybridization—has permitted the identification of different pituitary cell types and development of a logical framework for classification of pituitary tumors.

Similar advances have been made in treatment of hypothalamic and pituitary disease with the development of synthetic replacement therapy for the hormones secreted by the target glands or by the pituitary and/or hypothalamus. The advent of transsphenoidal pituitary microsurgery has made operative intervention safer, simpler, and more effective. Similarly, the use of medical therapy to control certain types of pituitary tumors has improved therapeutic results and precluded the need for surgery in many patients.

PITUITARY MORPHOLOGY

Embryology

The pituitary is derived from two sources.[1-4] The epithelial portion, which includes the pars distalis, intermediate lobe, and pars tuberalis, originates from evagination of the stomodeal ectoderm, Rathke's pouch, named after its discoverer. The neural portion, which includes the infundibulum, the neural stalk, and the posterior lobe, arises in the saccus infundibuli, a part of the diencephalon. Rathke's pouch is apparent in the 3-mm embryo during the third week of pregnancy. Initially it is composed of a small, thin-walled vesicle in the roof of the primitive buccal cavity, termed the stomodeum, and subsequently expands in the direction of the saccus infundibuli and adheres to it. After the attachment of the two parts, the distal end narrows and forms the craniopharyngeal canal, a hollow stalk that usually is obliterated in the 17-mm embryo. In some embryos, however, it remains patent until the end of intrauterine life and may persist until after birth. Nests of adenohypophyseal tissue may be deposited along the route of its fetal development. A resulting pharyngeal hypophysis[5,6] is capable of hormone synthesis and may also give rise to ectopic adenomas. The cells at the distal end of Rathke's pouch gradually disappear, whereas those at the proximal end begin to proliferate at about the third month of gestation. Cell proliferation occurs at the attachment site of the two primordia, the ectoderm and the neural tube; cell accumulation is more rapid and extensive at the anterior wall than at the posterior wall. The anterior wall gives rise to the pars distalis of the adenohypophysis, and the posterior wall develops into the intermediate lobe. In the human adult the latter remains rudimentary, constituting only a small part of the anterior lobe. At approximately the fifth week of gestation the anterolateral portion of Rathke's pouch extends upward bilaterally, fuses in front of the infundibulum, and forms the pars tuberalis.

By the end of the third month of gestation the gross compartments of the pituitary are recognizable. The infundibulum elongates, and the pituitary becomes embedded deeper in the sella turcica that is formed by the sphenoid bone. Thus the close proximity of the pituitary and the infundibulum is lost. The neurohypophysis differentiates into the proximally located median eminence and the distal posterior lobe, connected to the median eminence by the pituitary stalk.

The timing of the onset of pituitary hormone synthesis and release by the embryo has been extensively investigated by using various methods such as histology, immunocytochemistry, electron microscopy, hormone measurements by in vitro techniques such as the reverse hemolytic plaque assay, and hybridization histochemistry.[1,2,4,7,8] Acidophilic cells are present in the anterior lobe of the human embryo around the third month of gestation; basophilic cells become detectable somewhat later. Cells that produce growth hormone (GH) and corticotropin (ACTH, adrenocorticotropin) are identifiable at about 9 wk of gestation, as shown by immunocytochemistry. The synthesis of these hormones is followed by the production of the alpha subunit and subsequently the beta subunits of the glycoprotein hormones. At about the eighth week of gestation connective tissue and blood vessels grow into the anterior lobe, establishing a direct neurohormonal link between the anterior lobe and the hypothalamus. The neurosecretory material in the posterior lobe is demonstrable at about the fifth month of gestation. The last anterior pituitary cell type to become manifest in the anterior lobe is the lactotrope. These cells are recognizable at about the fifth month of gestation. The functional activity of the pituitary in embryonic life is not understood in every regard (also see Chapter 20). It is clear that the hormone-producing cells can develop without hypothalamic stimulation, a reflection of the intrinsic property of cellular maturation. Commencement of hormone synthesis in the embryonic pituitary in the absence of hypothalamic stimulation has been conclusively documented in several in vitro studies. In addition, in anencephaly all adenohypophyseal cell types, with the exception of corticotropes, develop and are capable of some degree of hormone synthesis and release.

Anatomy

The pituitary is located in the sella turcica or hypophyseal fossa of the skull, under the brain.[3,4] It is protected by the sphenoid bone, which surrounds it bilaterally and inferiorly and is covered by the dura, a dense layer of connective tissue that lines the sella turcica. Superiorly it is covered by the diaphragma sellae, or sellar diaphragm, a dural sheath that forms the roof of the sella. The diaphragma sellae has a 5-mm-wide central opening that is penetrated by the hypophyseal stalk. In some subjects this opening is wider and is thought to allow transmission of pulsations of cerebrospinal fluid (CSF) pressure leading to the development of the empty sella syndrome or cisternal herniation.

The pituitary is an oval, bean-shaped, bilaterally symmetrical, brownish-red organ. It averages 13 mm transversely, 9 mm anteroposteriorly, and 6 mm vertically. At birth, pituitary weight is approximately 100 mg. The weight of the pituitary varies in adults, averaging 0.6 g (range 0.4 to 0.9 g). The pituitary weighs somewhat more in women than in men. During pregnancy, it enlarges and may weigh 0.9 to 1.0 g.[9] The pituitary is usually heavier in multiparous than in nulliparous women and decreases in weight with advancing age. In senescence, connective tissue accumulates in the anterior lobe; although fibrosis and loss of parenchymal cells can be substantial, pituitary hormone production is preserved.

The anterior lobe is larger than the posterior lobe and constitutes 80% of the gland. The two lobes are clearly demarcated and are distinguishable with the naked eye; the cut surface of the anterior lobe is brownish-red and that of the posterior lobe is grayish-brown.

The pituitary is close to several structures that may be affected by enlargement of the gland. Space-occupying lesions can compress neighboring structures and give rise to clinically significant manifestations. The lateral walls of the sella are close to the cavernous sinuses containing the internal carotid arteries and the oculomotor (III), trochlear (IV), and abducens (VI) nerves and the V_1 and V_2 divisions of the trigeminal (V) nerve. The sphenoid sinus is anterior and inferior to the pituitary and is separated from it by the inferior portion of the sella, a thin layer of bone. When a pituitary tumor enlarges, the thin bone may be resorbed and eroded, allowing tumor extension into the sphenoid sinus. The optic chiasm lies directly above the diaphragma sellae in front of the hypophyseal stalk; suprasellar growth of a pituitary tumor may compress the chiasm and cause visual compromise. The tuber cinereum of the hypothalamus and the third ventricle of the brain lie above the roof of the sella. Space-occupying lesions in or above the pituitary may compress and compromise the tuber cinereum, causing hypthalamic-hypophyseal dysfunction, usually manifested as hypopituitarism associated with mild hyperprolactinemia.

Minor anatomical variations frequently occur in the shape and size of the pituitary and in the width of the opening of the diaphragma sellae.[10, 11] These differences do not affect pituitary function but may cause confusion in the interpretation of imaging studies.

The pituitary is divided into the anterior and posterior lobes. The anterior lobe is composed of three divisions: pars distalis, pars intermedia, and pars tuberalis.[3, 4] The pars distalis is the largest and is the site of the hormone-producing cells. The pars intermedia is poorly developed in the human and consists of a few dilated cavities lined by a single layer of cuboidal or columnar epithelium and filled with an amorphous proteinaceous material often containing cell debris. The pars tuberalis is the upward extension of the anterior lobe and is attached to the pituitary stalk. It contains a few small groups of cells that produce mainly glycoproteins and may contain squamous cell nests.

The neurohypophysis or posterior pituitary consists of three parts:[10, 12] the median eminence of the tuber cinereum, the infundibular stem or hypophyseal stalk, and the infundibular process or posterior lobe or neural lobe.

The hypophyseal circulation is complex[13–16] and plays an important role in the hypothalamic regulation of the anterior pituitary. The pituitary receives blood from two paired arteries: the superior and the inferior hypophyseal arteries that originate from the internal carotid arteries. Some branches of the superior hypophyseal arteries terminate in the infundibulum. The superior hypophyseal arteries end in the gomitoli or the adjacent capillaries. The gomitoli, central arteries with a well-developed muscular layer and surrounded by many capillaries, are approximately 1 to 2 mm long and 50 to 100 µm wide and are present in large numbers in the infundibulum and proximal part of the hypophyseal stalk. Their function has not been fully established, but they may influence blood flow to adjacent capillaries and the adenohypophysis and thereby regulate the transport of hypothalamic hormones, neuropeptides, and neurotransmitters to the anterior pituitary. The hypothalamic hormones are produced in neurons that originate in various parts of the hypothalamus and terminate at the infundibulum, where they permeate through fenestrations in the perigomitolar capillaries to enter the portal circulation. The large parallel veins, the portal veins or portal vessels, consist of a confluence of the capillaries. High concentrations of hypothalamic hormones are present in the portal blood, which transports the hormones to the capillaries in the anterior pituitary. The long portal vessels arise in the infundibulum and proximal part of the pituitary stalk, and the short portal vessels originate in the posterior lobe and distal portion of the pituitary stalk. The short portal vessels provide a direct vascular connection between the posterior and anterior lobes of the pituitary.

The portal circulation provides approximately 80 to 90% of the blood supply to the anterior lobe. The adenohypophysis also receives blood from extraportal sources. The capsular arteries carry blood to a few superficial cell layers of the adenohypophysis. In addition, bilateral arteries bypass the infundibulum to carry arterial blood directly from the superior hypophyseal arteries, providing 10 to 20% of the blood supply to the pituitary. The superior hypophyseal arteries arise from the peripheral circulation, and the blood is relatively devoid of hypothalamic hormones. The capsular arteries arise from the inferior hypophyseal arteries and provide blood to the hypophyseal fibrous capsule; they also penetrate the superficial layers of the anterior lobe and supply the superficial cell rows with arterial blood.

The neurohypophysis receives its blood supply from the inferior hypophyseal arteries. These arteries do not supply blood to the anterior lobe, except through the capsular arteries. Venous blood leaves the pituitary through adjacent venous sinuses to enter the internal jugular veins bilaterally.

Unidirectional blood flow from the hypothalamus to the anterior pituitary has been assumed, but under certain circumstances the direction of the blood flow may be reversed. The reversal of blood flow could have important functional implications that have yet to be determined. If under certain conditions the direction of circulation is reversed and the blood flows through the short portal vessels from the anterior lobe to the neural lobe and through the long portal vessels from the anterior lobe to the median eminence, the adenohypophyseal hormones may affect the functional activity of several neural centers, producing ultrashort-loop feedback.

Neovascularization of the anterior pituitary has been described and is of unknown significance. Weiner and associates[17, 18] suggested that in the pituitaries of some subjects arteries are formed to carry arterial blood from the peripheral circulation directly to the anterior lobe. This blood contains extremely low levels of hypothalamic regulatory hormones compared with portal blood. Thus lactotrope cells are not exposed to the suppressive effect of hypothalamic dopamine and, as a consequence, they may proliferate; hyperplasia could ultimately be transformed into an adenoma. Thus arteriogenesis and neovascularization may play a fundamental role in the genesis of prolactin-producing adenomas; this remains to be proved. Although arteries carrying extraportal blood may be present in large adenomas, neovascularization does not precede adenoma formation; in addition, arteriogenesis occurs in adenomas other than prolactinomas.[18, 19]

The structure of the adenohypophyseal capillaries has been analyzed by electron microscopy. These capillaries are lined by a single layer of fenestrated endothelial cells with a well-defined subendothelial space and basement membrane. The hormones secreted by the adenohypophyseal cells have to pass through the cell membrane, the basement membrane of the cell and the capillary, the subendothelial layer, and the endothelium before they are secreted into the blood. The hormone-containing secretory granules become undetectable, with presently available morphological techniques, after they are discharged from the cells. Thus the process of hormonal transport from the adenohypohyseal cell to the capillary and the factors that affect the transfer cannot be fully investigated by morphological methods.

Despite its proximity to the brain, the anterior lobe has no direct innervation except for a few sympathetic nerve fibers that reach the tissue along the blood vessels. The nerve fibers contain several peptides and may influence blood circulation but presumably have no major importance in the control of hormone synthesis or release. Hypothalamic regulation is exerted via the neurohormonal link, the hypothalamic regulatory peptides reaching the pituitary via the portal vessels.

The posterior lobe possesses a rich nerve supply. The innervation of the neurohypophysis is discussed in Chapter 7. Unmyelinated nerve fibers enter the posterior lobe via the pituitary stalk. These fibers originate in the supraoptic and paraventricular nuclei and other areas of the hypothalamus. They not only affect the posterior lobe by neural influences but also contain vasopressin (AVP, also called antidiuretic hormone, ADH) and oxytocin and their respective neurophysins or carrier proteins. These two neurohypophyseal hormones are synthesized in the hypothalamus, transported and stored in the posterior lobe, and released into the peripheral circulation. Neurohypophyseal structure and function depend on this innervation. When the pituitary stalk is sectioned and innervation is interrupted, the posterior lobe becomes atrophic with loss of neurohypophyseal hormones. Clinically, this defect is manifested by the development of diabetes insipidus.

Cytology of the Normal Anterior Pituitary Gland

The "normal" human pituitary is one of the least studied organs. Compounding the inaccessibility of the tissue, the pituitary consists of several hormone-producing cell types, whose number, endocrine activity, and morphology are affected by changes in the endocrine milieu. The morphological responses to stimulatory and inhibitory influences differ among cell types, further complicating studies of pituitary cytology. The following summary is based chiefly on the study of more than 1000 pituitaries obtained at autopsy and on histological, immunohistological, and electron microscopic observations of pituitary tissues removed surgically either for therapeutic hypophysectomy or in conjunction with adenomectomy.[20]

The five pituitary cell types of the human anterior pituitary gland have a remarkable regional distribution. In horizontal cross-section the adenohypophysis is composed of two lateral wings and a central mucoid wedge (median wedge). The cytology of each cell type will be considered in the discussion of the principal hormone it secretes.

PITUITARY HORMONES

Hypothalamic-Pituitary Regulation

Each pituitary hormone is regulated by hypothalamic regulatory hormones synthesized in the hypothalamus and transported from the median eminence to the anterior pituitary via the hypothalamic-pituitary portal circulation. Hypothalamic hormones bind to specific high-affinity cell membrane receptors of the individual pituitary cell type to regulate hormone secretion from that cell. With the possible exception of prolactin, all of the anterior pituitary hormones are also under feedback regulation by the hormones secreted by the target glands on which the pituitary hormones act. Thus there is an interaction and integration of signals from the brain and the periphery to regulate pituitary hormone secretion to maintain a normal endocrine state. If a target gland fails, there is a reduction in negative feedback that leads to augmented secretion of the tropic hypothalamic hormone (and also reduced secretion of any tonic hypothalamic inhibiting hormone). This results in enhancement of pituitary responsiveness to the hypothalamic tropic stimulus. Thus negative feedback occurs at both the pituitary and hypothalamic levels (Table 6–1). In addition, pituitary hormones are probably transported back to the hypothalamus, which is called short-loop feedback, to inhibit secretion of the pituitary hormone by reducing the hypothalamic stimulation (Fig. 6–1).

All anterior pituitary hormones are secreted in a pulsatile fashion. Thus measurement of a single random sample

TABLE 6–1. Relationship Between Hypothalamic, Pituitary, and Target Gland Secretion*

Hypothalamic Hormone	Pituitary Hormone	Target Gland	Feedback Hormone
TRH	TSH	Thyroid	T_4 and T_3
LHRH	LH	Gonad	E_2 (women), T (men)
	FSH	Gonad	Inhibin and (?) E_2 and T
SS	GH	Multiple	IGF I
GHRH	GH	Multiple	IGF I
DA	Prolactin	Breast	?
CRH	ACTH	Adrenal	Cortisol
AVP	ACTH	Adrenal	Cortisol

*ACTH, corticotropin; AVP, arginine vasopressin; CRH, corticotropin-releasing hormone; DA, dopamine; E_2, estradiol; FSH, follicle-stimulating hormone; GH, growth hormone; GHRH, growth hormone–releasing hormone; IGF I, insulin-like growth factor I; LH, luteinizing hormone; LHRH, luteinizing hormone–releasing hormone; SS, somatostatin; T, testosterone; T_3, triiodothyronine; T_4, thyroxine; TRH, thyrotropin-releasing hormone; TSH, thyrotropin.

may not provide adequate assessment of hormone secretion, and more frequent measurements may be necessary for research and often for clinical purposes. The development of computer algorithms to identify hormone pulses and calculate the quantitative characteristics has facilitated such studies. Two examples of such programs are Cluster[21] and Ultra.[22] With adequate frequency of peripheral blood sampling it is possible to characterize the profile of hormone secretion in normal subjects and in patients with various

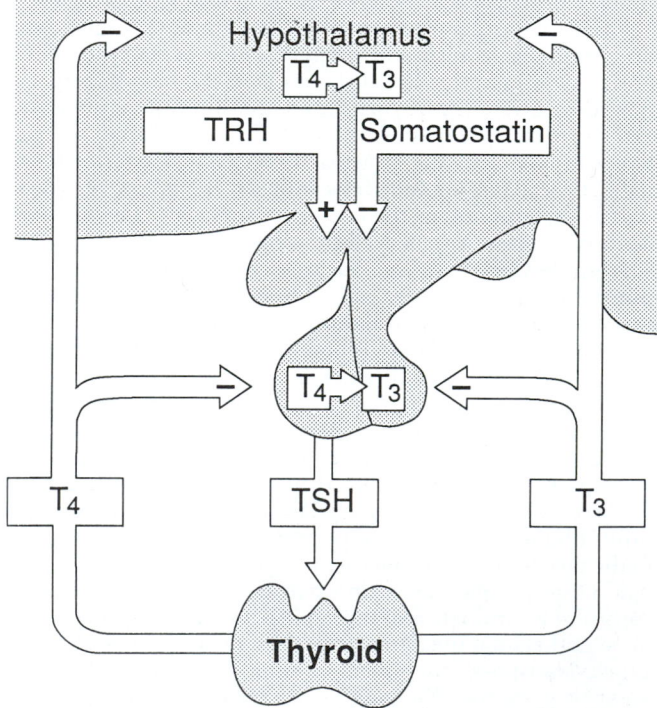

Figure 6–1. Schematic representation of the hypothalamic-pituitary-target gland axis. Hypothalamic hormones regulate secretion of pituitary hormones, which in turn stimulate target gland hormone production. Peripheral hormones feed back on the hypothalamus and pituitary to modulate secretion in a classic negative fashion. For example, hypothalamic thyrotropin-releasing hormone (TRH) stimulates pituitary release of thyrotropin (TSH), which stimulates thyroid hormone release. Thyroid hormones inhibit TRH and TSH in the hypothalamus and pituitary, respectively. In addition, there is a "short loop" by which the pituitary hormone feeds back at the hypothalamic level to inhibit hypothalamic stimulation of pituitary hormone secretion. T_3, triiodothyronine; T_4, thyroxine. (Modified from Reichlin S. Neuroendocrine control of pituitary function. In: Besser GM, Cudworth AG, eds. Clinical Endocrinology: An Illustrated Text. London: Gower Medical, 1987: 1.1–1.14.)

TABLE 6–2. Anterior Pituitary Hormones: Pituitary Content and Metabolic Characteristics in Normal Adult Men

Hormone	Pituitary Content (mg)	Production (μg/24 h)	Metabolic Clearance Rate (mL/min/m²)	Half-Life (min)*		
				Mono	*Alpha*	*Beta*
ACTH	0.25	25–50		8		
GH	5–10	1000–2000	100–150	20	3.5	21
Prolactin	0.1	200	45	20		
TSH	0.1–0.15	50–200	50			
LH	700 IU	1000 IU	34	47	18	90
FSH	200 IU	200 IU	4–12	220	100	500

*Mono, monoexponential decay; alpha, first component of biexponential decay; beta, second component of biexponential decay.

pituitary disorders. The pulsatile pattern of pituitary hormone release is important for efficient and effective signaling of target tissues so that the effects of intermittently generated endocrine signals are prolonged despite ongoing metabolic clearance of the hormone. The degree to which a signal is prolonged presumably reflects differential requirements of specific target tissues for biologically active serum concentrations of different hormones. Specific pituitary hormone production and clearance rates are illustrated in Table 6–2. The study of pituitary hormone secretion has been facilitated by development of a variety of deconvolution methods that mathematically remove the effect of metabolic clearance and calculate the underlying hormone-secretory rates.[23–25] By using this methodology, it is estimated that 95% of luteinizing hormone (LH) secretion occurs during approximately 27% of the day even though serum LH concentrations are consistently detectable because of the slow metabolic clearance.[23] In contrast, although 95% of GH secretion occurs during 37% of the day, serum GH concentrations are undetectable in conventional assays during approximately half of the day because of rapid clearance of GH from the plasma.[26] Alterations in the pulsatile pattern of pituitary hormone release have adverse effects on the target tissues, as exemplified by Cushing's disease, in which the circadian pattern of pulsatile ACTH release is altered,[27] and acromegaly, in which serum GH concentrations remain detectable throughout the day.[28]

Corticotropin*

ACTH stimulates the adrenal cortex to secrete cortisol, adrenal androgens, and mineralocorticoids. Pituitary ACTH secretion is regulated by hypothalamic corticotropin-releasing hormone (CRH) and AVP, which stimulate ACTH secretion. The feedback loop is closed by the negative feedback of cortisol on AVP, CRH, and ACTH secretion. In addition, ACTH acts via a short-loop feedback to suppress CRH secretion (for review see ref. 29).

STRUCTURE OF ACTH, RELATED PEPTIDES, AND PRO-OPIOMELANOCORTIN GENE. ACTH, a 39-amino-acid peptide, is synthesized as part of a large, 241-amino-acid precursor molecule, pro-opiomelanocortin (POMC). The human POMC gene is located on chromosome 2 and has three exons; exon 2 codes for the signal sequence and 18 amino acids of the NH₂ terminus of the molecule, and exon 3 codes for the remaining translated portion of the molecule.[30] POMC undergoes considerable post-translational processing, including glycosylation, enzymatic cleavage and phosphorylation, NH₂-terminal acetylation, and COOH-terminal amidation of certain cleaved peptides. This processing is species and tissue specific. In the human anterior pituitary gland POMC is enzymatically cleaved at dibasic amino acids, predominantly into β-lipotropin (β-LPH), ACTH, joining

peptide, and an NH₂-terminal peptide. In the human the intermediate lobe is vestigial except during fetal life and at the end of pregnancy. In the intermediate lobe of humans, ACTH is cleaved into α-melanocyte-stimulating hormone (ACTH(1–13)) and ACTH-like peptide (ACTH(18–39)), and β-LPH is split into LPH and β-endorphin.

The first 18 amino acids of ACTH have full biological activity, and the first 24 amino acids are identical across species. Synthetic ACTH(1–24) has a longer half-life than native ACTH(1–18) and is useful in clinical evaluations.

Because the peptides produced by the corticotrope are derived from the same precursor molecule, they are secreted in equimolar amounts. However, the circulating concentrations of the peptides do not vary in tandem because the half-lives are different. Because the half-life of β-LPH is longer than that of ACTH, the β-LPH/ACTH ratio increases after administration of hydrocortisone, which inhibits secretion of both ACTH and β-LPH. The β-LPH/ACTH ratio increases because of the more rapid clearance of ACTH. Similarly, β-LPH concentrations increase in renal failure because of slower metabolic clearance. The hyperpigmentation in ACTH-hypersecretory states and in uremia is not a result of secretion of intermediate-lobe peptides; melanocyte-stimulating hormone–like activity of β-LPH and ACTH themselves produces hyperpigmentation.

CORTOCOTROPE CELLS AND ACTH CONTENT. Corticotrope cells reside primarily in the median wedge. Their relative abundance is estimated to be 10%, but no reliable cell counts are available. The human pituitary contains approximately 250 μg of ACTH. The corticotrope cell may represent only one subtype of the POMC-producing cell line. Other POMC-producing cell populations, the putative sources of silent "corticotrope" adenoma subtypes 1 and 2, may have morphological features similar to those of corticotrope cells. The typical corticotrope cell is medium sized, ovoid or angular, and displays basophilia, bright periodic acid–Schiff (PAS) positivity, and immunoreactivity for ACTH and other POMC-derived peptides, such as endorphins, β-LPH, and NH₂-terminal fragment. Electron microscopy reveals ovoid or angular cells with relatively electron-dense cytoplasm containing numerous secretory granules in the size range 150 to 450 nm. The granules are morphologically distinctive, being spherical, dented, heart shaped and drop shaped, often with variable electron density. The specific markers of the human corticotrope cell are type 1 filaments,[31] which represent cytokeratin.[31, 32] Crooke's hyalinization is the morphological appearance of keratin-positive type 1 filaments associated with loss of rough endoplasmic reticulum (RER) and Golgi membranes, a finding unique to the human corticotrope cell. It occurs when there is functional suppression of corticotrope cells, as in the nontumorous (and sometimes tumorous) areas of pituitaries harboring corticotrope adenomas, in subjects with ectopic ACTH production or adrenal adenoma, or with chronic administration of large doses of glucocorticoid. These changes are reversible with treatment of the primary disease.

*For a detailed discussion of the hypothalamic-pituitary-adrenal axis see Chapter 9.

REGULATION OF ACTH SECRETION. CRH stimulates ACTH secretion by binding to high-affinity CRH receptors on the corticotrope and by stimulating the accumulation of cyclic AMP (cAMP), which activates protein kinase A. ACTH and related peptides are rapidly released by CRH, which also increases POMC gene transcription and synthesis. Administration of exogenous CRH stimulates ACTH and cortisol secretion; the magnitude of the response is dependent on the time of day and the level of circulating glucocorticoids. The cortisol response is greater in the afternoon than in the morning.[33] Exogenous glucocorticoids inhibit both the ACTH and cortisol responses to CRH. Conversely, lowering endogenous cortisol levels with metyrapone enhances the ACTH and cortisol responses to CRH.[34] AVP alone is a weak secretagogue of ACTH but acts synergistically with CRH to regulate ACTH release.[35] Many other peptides and neurotransmitters have been implicated in the control of CRH, AVP, and ACTH secretion, but only CRH has been demonstrated to be essential.

ACTH SECRETION. ACTH is secreted in bursts that cause similar sharp peaks in plasma cortisol concentrations. The ACTH-secretory bursts increase in frequency after 3 to 5 h of sleep and are maximal in the last hours before awakening and the hour thereafter. ACTH secretion is also under a circadian control that is regulated by a number of factors, one of the most important being light. Blind people have a free-running ACTH rhythm of about 25 h.[36, 37] In normal subjects ACTH concentrations decline over the morning and reach a nadir in the evening. The rhythm is established after the first year of life; the timing of the peak level (acrophase) shifts to 3 h earlier in the elderly. The circadian rhythm is resilient and is unaffected by short-term sleep deprivation, continuous feeding, prolonged bed rest, or even night shift work if a normal sleep pattern is preserved on weekends. The rhythm can be disrupted by a major time shift, as occurs with transmeridian jet travel. In that circumstance, it usually takes several days for the rhythm to be restored to normal.[38]

Stresses, both psychological and physical, activate the hypothalamic-pituitary-adrenal axis with an increase in both ACTH and cortisol secretion. Stressors include trauma, major surgery, fever, hypoglycemia, and burn injury. Hypoglycemia and fever both activate the hypothalamic-pituitary axis, the former by direct action at the basomedial hypothalamus[39] and the latter indirectly through the release of the cytokines interleukin 1, interleukin 2, and interleukin 6. These cytokines act predominantly in the hypothalamus to release CRH.[40] Hypercortisolism also occurs during psychological stress, which may vary from anticipation of physical activity to intense mental activity. Hypercortisolism also occurs in patients with anorexia nervosa and depression but is not a feature of either schizophrenia or chronic anxiety.

Glucocorticoids act at multiple sites within the corticotrope to inhibit ACTH secretion by inhibiting the ACTH response to CRH and by inhibiting ACTH synthesis via blockade of POMC gene transcription and synthesis. At the hypothalamus, glucocorticoids inhibit CRH and AVP synthesis and release.

ACTH ACTIONS. The actions of ACTH on the adrenal are mediated through specific high-affinity cell membrane receptors with a dissociation constant (K_d) of approximately 1.6 nmol/L. Extracellular calcium is required for the binding of ACTH to its receptor. The actions of ACTH are mediated by activation of adenylate cyclase, which leads to accumulation of intracellular cAMP and thus increased protein kinase A activity and phosphorylation of a number of important proteins. ACTH stimulates cortisol synthesis and secretion; only small amounts of cortisol are stored in the adrenal. The actions of ACTH are both acute and prolonged.[41] The acute effects, which occur within minutes, involve stimulation of the initial, rate-limiting step of cholesterol conversion to pregnenolone. In addition, there is an increase in the supply of free cholesterol ester. The prolonged effects of ACTH promote maintenance (and growth) of adrenal size by increasing protein synthesis, including synthesis of the enzymes involved in steroid hormone biosynthesis. Although ACTH has actions in other tissues, the physiological significance of most of these actions is uncertain. In Nelson's syndrome and in Addison's disease, circulating ACTH concentrations are extremely high and both ACTH and β-LPH are thought to act on melanocytes to increase skin pigmentation.

Prolactin–Growth Hormone Family

Because of shared amino acid homologies, human GH, prolactin, and placental lactogen (hPL, also called human chorionic somatomammotropin, hCS) are related and are thought to have had a common ancestral gene.[42] The genes for these three hormones also have a common structural organization; their nucleotide homologies are greater than the sequence homology of the proteins they encode.[43, 44] Each gene has four introns separating five coding exons.[45, 46] The introns occur at homologous sites in the coding regions despite enormous differences in the gene sizes. The prolactin gene is greater than 10 kb in length and is located on chromosome 6;[47] the GH gene is less than 2.5 kb in length and is located on chromosome 17.[48]

The prolactin-GH family may be divided into prolactin and GH subfamilies based on homologies and chromosomal segregation. In the human a single prolactin gene is present on chromosome 6. However, in rodent species several prolactin genes are expressed at different times during gestation, and cDNAs have been cloned that code for placental lactogens, prolactin-like proteins, proliferin, and prolactin-related proteins (for review see ref. 49). These various peptides are also likely to exist in the human but await identification. Most GH genes in different mammalian species evolved from a presumed common precursor. Primate GH and its receptor have relatively little homology with other mammalian GHs, so the GHs of other species are biologically inactive in humans. The human GH subfamily consists of five members, all of which are located on a 78-kb section of chromosome 17. They include the normal GH gene, a GH variant gene, two expressed hPL genes, and an incompletely characterized hPL-like gene, which is thought not to be expressed, i.e., is a pseudogene.[50] The gene for the GH variant protein codes for a protein that differs from GH by 13 amino acids and has two additional amino acids that are different in the leader sequence. The genes in this GH subfamily all have greater amino acid and nucleotide homology than they do with prolactin.

PROLACTIN STRUCTURE. Prolactin was identified in animal species as a distinct anterior pituitary hormone in 1928[51] and was purified and named in 1932;[52–54] human prolactin was purified and shown to be different from GH in 1971.[55, 56] The genes for human prolactin and GH were isolated, sequenced, and defined as members of the same family in the early 1980s.

Human prolactin consists of 199 amino acids and has three intramolecular disulfide bonds, one more than human GH. Only 16% of the amino acids of prolactin are homologous with those of GH. Prolactin circulates in blood predominantly in a monomeric form ("little prolactin," 23 kd), but also exists in dimeric ("big" prolactin, 48 to 56 kd) and polymeric (>100 kd) forms.[57–62] Glycosylated forms of prolactin also exist.[63] The biological significance of these different forms is unclear, although the larger forms may have reduced receptor-binding affinity and biological activity.[59, 61, 63, 64] Monomeric prolactin may be cleaved to liberate 8- and 16-kd forms.[65] The biological significance of the cleaved forms is unknown, but they may be mitogenic for mammary cells.[66]

LACTOTROPE CELLS AND PITUITARY PROLACTIN CONTENT. Lactotrope cells have a wide distribution throughout the pars distalis. This arrangement is not completely random; they account for most of the cells in the posterolateral rim of the pars distalis. The number of lactotrope cells is widely variable (10 to 30%); it is lowest in men and highest in multiparous women.[67] Lactotrope cells in the normal pituitary gland are small, polyhedral, and sparsely granulated with fine multiple cytoplasmic processes and a well-developed RER and Golgi complex. With immunohistochemistry, the Golgi complex is represented by positive streaks and strands located in the juxtanuclear area. The scant, small secretory granules contribute little to the immunopositivity. Densely granulated lactotrope cells, which exhibit strong, diffuse cytoplasmic immunopositivity, are rare, particularly in the pituitaries of older subjects. Knowledge of these densely granulated lactotrope cells is sketchy because of their rarity and the inadequate amount of material for study. In contrast to the apparently stable somatotrope, the lactotrope demonstrates marked changes in its fine structure depending on secretory activity.[20] Pleomorphic secretory granules within Golgi sacculi and secretory granule extrusions occur predominantly at the vascular surface of the cells and are useful markers of lactotrope cells. The development of lactotrope hyperplasia during pregnancy, during estrogen treatment, or in some cases of Cushing's disease and primary hypothyroidism results in progressive cellular enlargement, accumulation of highly organized RER with formation of concentric whorls (nebenkern), and prominence of immature granules within the Golgi complex. Because of enhanced exocytic discharge of secretory material, stimulated lactotrope cells contain few cytoplasmic storage granules. In contrast, suppressed lactotrope cells adjacent to a tumorous prolactinoma are reduced in size with a decrease in the quantity of RER and Golgi membranes. Suppressed lactotrope cells can be distinguished from null cells (cells that contain scant secretory granules but no other morphological markers indicating their derivation and differentiation) only by occasional granule extrusions.

The normal pituitary contains 100 µg of prolactin, 50 times less than the pituitary content of GH. Thus the pituitary prolactin pool turns over more rapidly than the GH pool.

REGULATION OF PROLACTIN SECRETION. Prolactin secretion varies under different physiological conditions. Prolactin, like all anterior pituitary hormones, is secreted in an episodic manner. Its secretion is regulated by the hypothalamic prolactin-inhibiting hormone dopamine and by various prolactin-releasing factors. Prolactin is unique among the anterior pituitary hormones in that it is under tonic hypothalamic inhibition by dopamine produced by tuberoinfundibular dopamine neurons. Dopamine acts by stimulating the lactotrope D_2 receptor to inhibit adenylate cyclase and consequently inhibits both prolactin release and prolactin synthesis. The putative prolactin-releasing factors include thyrotropin-releasing hormone (TRH), vasoactive intestinal peptide (VIP), and PHM-27, a peptide with structural homology to VIP (see Chapter 5). The physiological significance of prolactin-releasing factors in humans is unknown, and it is not known which prolactin-releasing factor is predominant. VIP is produced in the anterior pituitary gland cells and has been proposed to act as the autocrine or paracrine hormone that regulates prolactin secretion.[68–70] If large quantities of VIP are secreted in the anterior pituitary and normal lactotropes are responsive, disorders of pituitary VIP secretion might cause hyperprolactinemia, lactotrope hyperplasia, or adenoma formation.

Normal baseline serum prolactin levels are less than 20 µg/L in adults and usually less than 10 µg/L in men. Prolactin is secreted in an episodic manner with a distinct 24-h pattern.[71, 72] Circulating prolactin levels are lowest at midday, and a modest increase occurs during the afternoon. A marked increase in prolactin levels occurs shortly after onset of sleep, although peak levels are seen during the middle to end of the night.[73–76] Studies involving either sleep deprivation or jet lag have demonstrated that there is also an important circadian component.[77] In normal men there are approximately 14 pulses of prolactin secretion per day with an average interpulse interval of 95 min.[76] Prolactin release in young men appears to have a close temporal coupling with LH release.[78] Enhanced prolactin secretion during the night is due to increased pulse amplitude rather than increased pulse frequency.[78]

Prolactin synthesis is also regulated by effects of estrogen on prolactin gene expression, so that serum prolactin levels are higher in normal premenopausal women than in men. Similarly, prolactin levels rise in girls during menarche[79] and rise during pregnancy in both the mother and the fetus[80] (Fig. 6–2). After delivery, serum prolactin levels in the mother decline into the normal range over the course of the first 3 mo if breast-feeding does not occur. With suckling maternal prolactin levels rise; this response is greatest early after delivery. If breast-feeding is intermittently supplemented with bottle-feeding, the suckling-induced increase in the mother's serum prolactin level wanes. However, normal mean prolactin levels are sufficient to sustain established lactation. Prolactin levels increase in women during stimulation of the nipple and also during orgasm. In both men and women prolactin levels rise in response to stress.

Disruption of the hypothalamus or of the hypothalamic-hypophyseal stalk or administration of drugs that interfere with dopamine synthesis or action can cause hyperprolactinemia. In some patients with primary hypothyroidism, mild hyperprolactinemia may result from increased hypothalamic TRH secretion. In such patients thyroid hormone replacement lowers thyrotropin (TSH) concentrations, although it may require months for prolactin levels to reach normal.

PROLACTIN SECRETION. Prolactin is synthesized by the fetal anterior pituitary from the fifth week of gestation,[81] although specific lactotrope cells are not distinguishable until the fifth month. From the 10th week until term there are progressive increases in the weight of the pituitary and the prolactin content such that at term the pituitary contains approximately 2 µg of prolactin.[82] Serum prolactin levels in the fetus remain low until approximately week 26 and rise progressively to levels in excess of 150 µg/L at term. The adult human pituitary contains about 100 µg of prolactin, compared with 5 to 10 mg of GH.

Circulating fetal prolactin presumably originates from the fetal pituitary. In contrast, amniotic fluid prolactin is 50% glycosylated and originates from decidual cells. Maximal amniotic fluid prolactin levels are 100-fold higher than those of fetal or maternal blood and occur at midtrimester, whereas maximal serum levels occur at term in both the fetus and the mother.[83] Decidual prolactin, which is also produced by decidualized endometrial cells from days 22 to 28 of the menstrual cycle, is not under tonic dopaminergic inhibition but is instead stimulated by progesterone.[84, 85] Messenger RNA (mRNA) for prolactin is present in chorion and decidua, and a prolactin cDNA cloned from human term decidua is identical with pituitary prolactin except for four silent nucleotide changes.[86, 87]

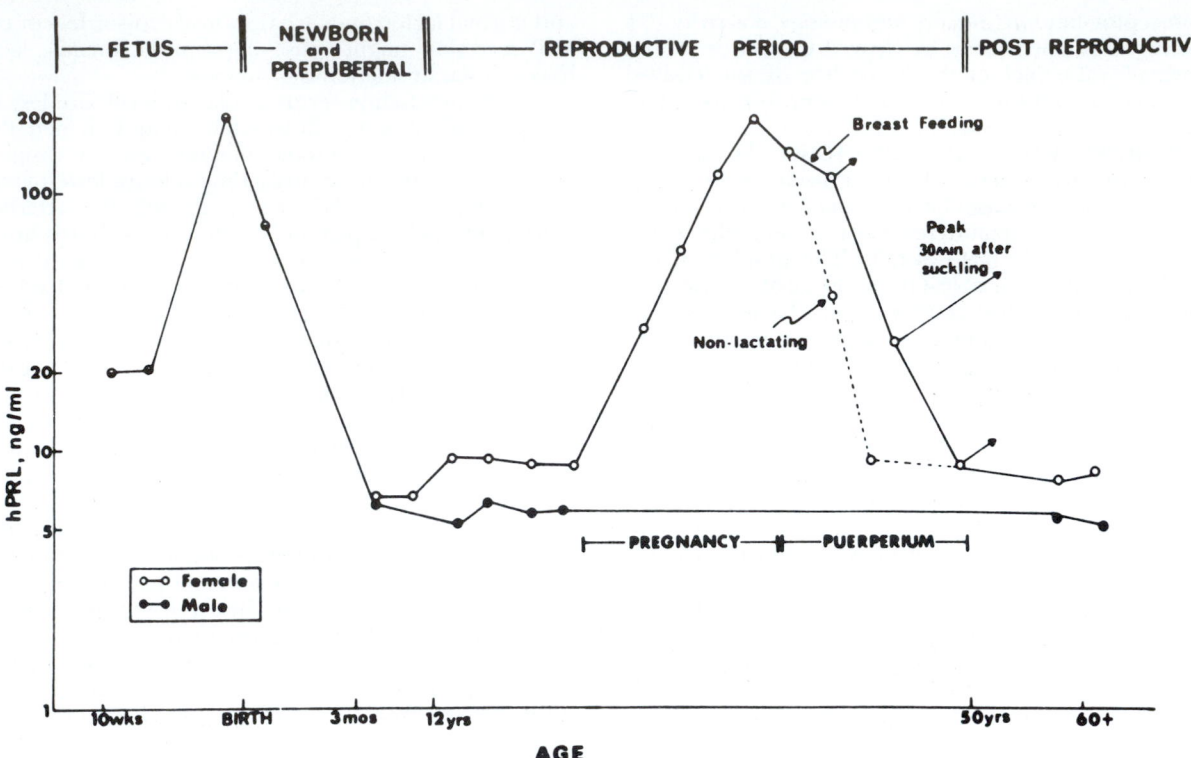

Figure 6–2. Average serum prolactin levels during various periods of life in men and women. The length of the arrows for nursing women indicates the magnitude of increase in serum prolactin level after each episode of suckling. To convert prolactin (hPRL) values to micrograms per liter, multiply by 1.0. (From Friesen HG. Human prolactin. Ann R Coll Physicians Surg Can 1978; 11:275–281.)

PROLACTIN ACTIONS. Prolactin acts through specific prolactin receptors in multiple tissues including breast, liver, ovary, testis, and prostate (also see Chapter 4). In the human these receptors are also stimulated by GH with equal potency. The prolactin receptor has been isolated, and its cDNA has been cloned; there is homology between the prolactin and GH receptors and homology with a number of cytokine receptors.[88] The receptors are not linked to G proteins, nor do they have tyrosine kinase activity. Different forms of the prolactin receptor differ in the length of the cytoplasmic domains.

The main site of prolactin action is the mammary gland. Prolactin initiates and maintains lactation. During pregnancy the breast undergoes considerable development of the secretory apparatus through an interaction of several hormones (see Chapter 15). Insulin, cortisol, and thyroid hormone are all required, but the major stimuli for development are from estrogen, progesterone, prolactin, and placental mammotropic hormones, probably including GH (or its placental variant). Lactation is inhibited during pregnancy by the high levels of estrogen and progesterone. After delivery there is a rapid fall in estrogen and progesterone concentrations, enabling prolactin to initiate lactation. If prolactin secretion is inhibited after delivery with a dopamine agonist, lactation is prevented.

Prolactin acts at sites other than the breast, but the physiological function of these actions is poorly characterized. Prolactin also acts in the hypothalamus to regulate dopamine turnover and influence gonadotropin secretion. Physiological hyperprolactinemia during pregnancy and lactation and pathological hyperprolactinemia are associated with suppression of the hypothalamic-pituitary-gonadal axis. This probably results from prolactin-mediated inhibition of pulsatile secretion of luteinizing hormone–releasing hormone (LHRH, also called gonadotropin-releasing hormone,

GnRH), which results in impaired gonadotropin secretion and inhibition of gonadal function.

GROWTH HORMONE STRUCTURE. Human GH is a nonglycosylated, single chain, 191-amino-acid, 22-kd protein with two intramolecular disulfide bonds. Approximately 75% of pituitary GH is in this form, and 5 to 10% is a 20-kd form. The 20-kd form is produced by alternate splicing of the second coding exon that deletes the codons for amino acids 32 to 46 from the RNA.[89, 90] GH is present in several different forms in the anterior pituitary. Additional forms have been described, some of which result from analytical artifacts[91] (Table 6–3).

The 20-kd form is to be distinguished from the human GH variant (hGH-V) secreted by the placenta during pregnancy; the latter is a 22-kd protein that is not produced by the anterior pituitary.[92–95] hPL, like human GH and the GH variant, contains 191 amino acids, 161 of which are identical with those of human GH, and has two S-S bonds located in

TABLE 6–3. Human Growth Hormone Variants and Their Abundance in the Pituitary

Variant	Abundance (%)*
Monomeric	
22-kd form	75
20-kd form	5–10
Desamido–human GH (Gln-137 and Asn-152)	5
N-acylated human GH	5
Dimeric	
Dimers (noncovalent and disulfide dimers)	5–10
Oligomers	5

*Values represent an average.

From Baumann G. Molecular variants of human growth hormone in serum and circulating growth hormone binding proteins. In: Frisch H, Thorner MO, eds. Hormonal Regulation of Growth. Serono Symposia Publications. Vol 58. New York: Raven, 1989: 175–184.

the same position as in human GH. hPL has only about 0.001 of the growth-promoting activity of GH.

SOMATOTROPE CELL AND PITUITARY GROWTH HORMONE CONTENT. The somatotrope cells that secrete GH make up about 50% of the hormone-producing cells of the anterior pituitary and occupy the lateral wings; a minority of somatotropes are scattered throughout the median section. There are several types of somatotropes. The ovoid, middle-sized cells exhibit strong immunoreactivity for GH,[20, 96] although some GH-producing cells may contain prolactin or alpha subunit as well, suggesting the existence of subsets of somatotropes. Electron microscopy demonstrates numerous, large (500 nm or greater) secretory granules and uncommon small granules (150 to 200 nm). Sparsely granulated variants of the GH-secreting cell are also present.[20] The derivation and physiological and functional activity of the latter subpopulation are unknown.

Somatotrope cells are remarkably stable, and the number, morphology, and immunoreactivity are unchanged by age or disease. No significant changes are observed in nontumorous somatotropes in pituitaries harboring somatotrope adenomas that cause acromegaly. In somatotrope hyperplasia, which occurs in response to chronic stimulation by ectopically produced growth hormone–releasing hormone (GHRH), the most characteristic alteration is hypertrophy of the Golgi complex.[97] The consistent appearance of somatotropes, determined chiefly by the abundance of large secretory granules, may mask fluctuations in secretory activity. Quantification of subcellular organelles may be required to detect morphological evidence of changes in secretory function.

The human adenohypophysis contains 5 to 10 mg of GH, synthesized and stored in somatotropes; GH in the secretory granules accounts for as much as 30% of the protein in the cells.

GROWTH HORMONE VARIANTS, GROWTH HORMONE RECEPTOR, AND BINDING PROTEIN. Human GH circulates in several forms, including a 22-kd form, a 20-kd form, and at least one acidic form (Table 6–4). A mixture of GH oligomers (up to a pentamer) is also detectable in peripheral blood. Two thirds of the oligomers are noncovalently bound, and one third are linked by intermolecular disulfide bonds; it is likely that they are secreted in these forms.[98, 99] The nature of the secretory stimulus (i.e., its magnitude, duration, and mechanism) does not affect the relative proportions of the mixture of circulating GH forms, nor sex, age, or pathological disorders.[100–102] Fragments of 16 and 12 kd are detectable during periods of low secretory activity;[103] it is not known whether these are secreted or are produced in the periphery by degradation. Their biological function, if any, is unknown.

The proportions of the GH variants in the circulation are similar to those in the pituitary except that the 20-kd form and oligomeric forms are more predominant in the

TABLE 6–4. Human Growth Hormone Variants in the Circulation*

Variant	Percent
22 kd	76
20 kd	16
Acidic GH (desamido-, *N*-acyl-)	8
Monomeric	55
Dimeric	27
Tri-, tetra-, and pentameric	18
Complexed 22 kd	45
Complexed 20 kd	25

*During the second and third trimesters of pregnancy the variant form becomes the predominant form of GH in the maternal circulation and the pituitary forms decrease.[93]

From Baumann G. Molecular variants of human growth hormone in serum and circulating growth hormone binding proteins. In: Frisch H, Thorner MO, eds. Hormonal Regulation of Growth. Serono Symposia Publications. Vol 58. New York: Raven, 1989: 175–184.

circulation because of their slower metabolic clearance (see Table 6–4).

Growth Hormone Receptor. The elucidation of the structure of the rabbit GH receptor was achieved by purification of the receptor from liver and the binding protein from serum followed by partial amino acid sequence analysis.[104] The NH$_2$-terminal amino acid sequence of the binding protein is identical with that of the receptor, and it is now clear that the structures of the binding protein and the extracellular domain of the GH receptor are identical. This work was followed by cloning of the cDNA for the receptor and subsequent expression of the receptor from these clones.[105] The rabbit cDNA clones were then used to screen a human cDNA library to obtain similar clones encompassing the human GH receptor. The rabbit and human receptor clones contain a single long open reading frame encoding 638 amino acids (Fig. 6–3). The NH$_2$-terminal sequence is preceded by 18 amino acids that constitute the signal peptide. A stretch of 24 hydrophobic amino acids in the middle of the protein probably represents the transmembrane domain and divides the molecule into extracellular and intracytoplasmic domains of approximately equal size. The rabbit and human receptors have 620 amino acids and considerable homology (84% amino acid identity). The translated molecular size of the receptor is 70 kd, which is smaller than the originally isolated receptor (130 kd), a difference largely accounted for by glycosylation. The prolactin receptor has also been cloned and sequenced and shown to have homology with the GH receptor.[106] This family of receptors is unrelated to known tyrosine kinase growth factor receptors and G protein–linked receptors but is related to various cytokine receptors.[88]

In one patient with Laron dwarfism, analysis of GH receptor gene RNA transcripts revealed a thymidine-to-cytosine substitution that generated a serine instead of a phenylalanine at position 96 in the extracellular coding domain of the mature receptor. This substitution replaces a

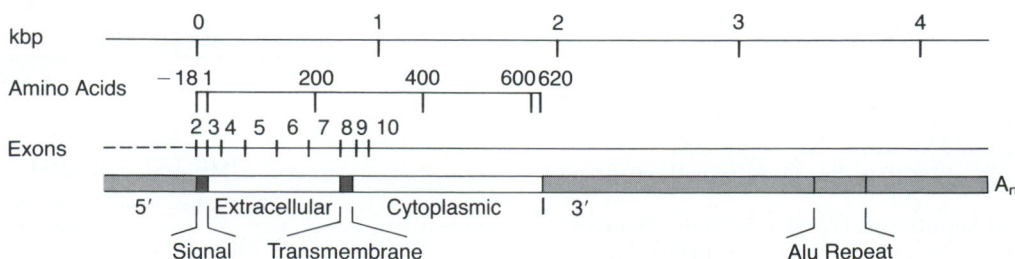

Figure 6–3. Schematic representation of the GH receptor mRNA and protein. Scales of nucleotides and amino acids, the locations of the exon boundaries, and the major features of the protein and mRNA are illustrated. (Modified from Gowdowski PJ, Leung DW, Meacham LR, et al. Characterization of the human growth hormone receptor gene and demonstration of a partial gene deletion in two patients with Laron-type dwarfism. Proc Natl Acad Sci USA 1989; 86:8083–8087.)

nonpolar amino acid with a polar one and may affect the binding site for GH. The importance of this mutation is supported by the finding that this region of the molecule is highly conserved across species. However, a nonglycosylated, recombinant-derived portion of this mutant receptor does bind GH.[107] This mutation was not found in another family with Laron dwarfism or in six unrelated patients with Laron dwarfism. In a separate study, a partial gene deletion was documented in two of nine patients with Laron dwarfism. These two patients had a deletion of a large part of the extracellular hormone binding domain, accounting for absence of the binding protein and resistance to GH action. In the other seven patients no changes were observed in the genomic blots, which can detect major gene deletions but do not exclude point mutations. Mutations may arise in other genes that encode proteins required for expression of the receptor or for transduction of the GH signal; the phenotypic expression of these defects is that of Laron dwarfism. It is, therefore, certain that the molecular defects that alter the function of the GH receptor are heterogeneous.

Growth Hormone–Binding Protein. When radiolabeled monomeric GH is incubated with human plasma, two high-molecular-weight forms can be identified. This phenomenon is due to the presence of a binding protein that is identical in amino acid sequence with the extracellular domain of the human GH receptor.[90, 104, 105] Absence of the binding protein in the plasma of Laron dwarfs, in whom there is a functional deficiency of the GH receptor, supports the relationship between the GH-binding protein and receptor.[108, 109] The principal binding protein binds 22-kd GH with high affinity (association constant K_a of 50 nmol/L) and limited binding capacity, i.e., a limited number of binding sites per molecule of human GH–binding protein. Its affinity for 20-kd GH is somewhat lower. The binding protein is a 61-kd glycoprotein with an apparent molecular mass of 80 to 85 kd when complexed with GH. The complex coelutes on Sephadex columns with "big" and "big, big" GH. Thus, "big" GH forms consist of both GH oligomers and GH complexed with its binding protein. Another GH-binding protein of 100 kd in human plasma has saturable, specific binding for GH, although the binding affinity is less than that of the 61-kd binding protein. The 100-kd binding protein is present in patients deficient in the GH receptor, suggesting that it may not be related to the GH receptor. Further characterization of this binding protein is necessary.

Forty-five percent of 22-kd GH and 25% of 20-kd GH are complexed with the binding proteins, and the high-affinity binding protein accounts for 85% of this binding.[103] When circulating GH concentrations are consistently above 10 to 20 μg/L, a progressively smaller proportion is bound to the binding protein.

The association rate of GH and its binding protein is such that the complex forms in the circulation.[99] Administration of monomeric, recombinant-derived, 22-kd GH to normal young men with suppressed endogenous GH secretion results in binding similar to that observed in vitro with the mixing of radiolabeled GH and normal human plasma.[99] Thirty-eight percent of the GH is bound to binding protein at plasma GH levels of 32 to 59 μg/L, and 46% is bound at a serum GH concentration of 7 μg/L. The proportions bound to the high-affinity and low-affinity binding proteins are similar in vivo and in vitro. No oligomeric GH forms were observed, suggesting that the pituitary is the source of these forms.

The biological significance of the binding proteins is unclear. Protein-bound GH is metabolized differently from monomeric GH and persists 10 times longer in plasma. The volume of distribution of protein-bound GH is twice the intravascular compartment, whereas the volume of distri-

bution of monomeric GH is the extracellular space.[110, 111] These two effects of protein binding may enhance the biological activity of GH. Alternatively, the enhancement may be neutralized because the high-affinity binding protein competes with receptor for the binding of GH.[112]

The plasma concentrations of the binding proteins appear to remain fairly constant in an individual but vary widely among individuals. Levels of binding proteins are low prenatally and at birth and increase during the first year of life; the levels of the high-affinity protein increase throughout childhood.[103, 113] Levels of the low-affinity binding protein increase during pregnancy when there is no change in the concentration of high-affinity binding protein. Binding is decreased in Laron dwarfism and in Pygmies, during prolonged fasting, and with uremia.[103, 108, 109]

REGULATION OF GROWTH HORMONE SECRETION. The pulsatile secretion of GH is regulated by two hypothalamic regulatory hormones, GHRH and somatostatin (SRIF, somatotropin release–inhibiting factor). GHRH controls GH synthesis by regulating transcription of GH mRNA via control of cAMP levels.[114] Somatostatin appears to determine the timing and amplitude of GH pulses but has no effect on GH synthesis. The neuroendocrine regulation of GHRH and somatostatin secretion is discussed in Chapter 5.

The mechanisms of action of GHRH and somatostatin have been studied by using primary cultured rat anterior pituitary cells, clonal cell lines, and, occasionally, human pituitary cells. The rat somatotrope has spontaneous intracellular calcium oscillations (Fig. 6–4). Binding of somatostatin to its receptor inhibits GH release by decreasing intracellular calcium concentrations and inhibiting adenylate cyclase.[115] These effects are mediated by a G protein that is sensitive to pertussis toxin, although the exact molecular mechanisms have not been established.[116–118] GHRH interacts with a cell membrane receptor to stimulate adenylate cyclase, leading to an increase in intracellular cAMP levels.[119–122] Intracellular calcium concentrations are also increased by GHRH.[116] When cells are exposed to both somatostatin and GHRH, somatostatin exerts the dominant effect; intracellular calcium concentration decreases, and GH release is inhibited (Fig. 6–5). There is significant interaction among the various intracellular second messenger pathways, and it is likely that the phospholipase C–diacylglycerol–protein kinase C pathway is also involved in regulation of GH secretion both by modulating intracellular calcium concentrations and by activating protein kinase C.[122]

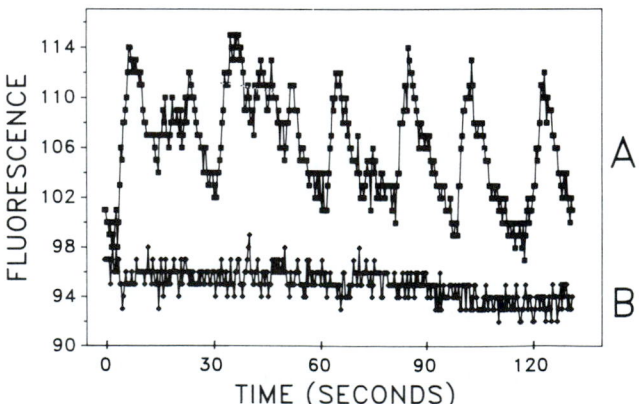

Figure 6–4. Pattern of calcium oscillations in a rat somatotrope (A) and nonsomatotrope pituitary cell (B) in the same field. Fluorescence intensity (arbitrary units) was measured every 300 ms from a continuous recording (excitation at 340 nm) that allows high temporal resolution and qualitative changes in cytosolic calcium concentrations. (From Holl RW, Thorner MO, Mandell GL, et al. Spontaneous oscillations of intracellular calcium and growth hormone secretion. J Biol Chem 1988; 263:9682–9685.)

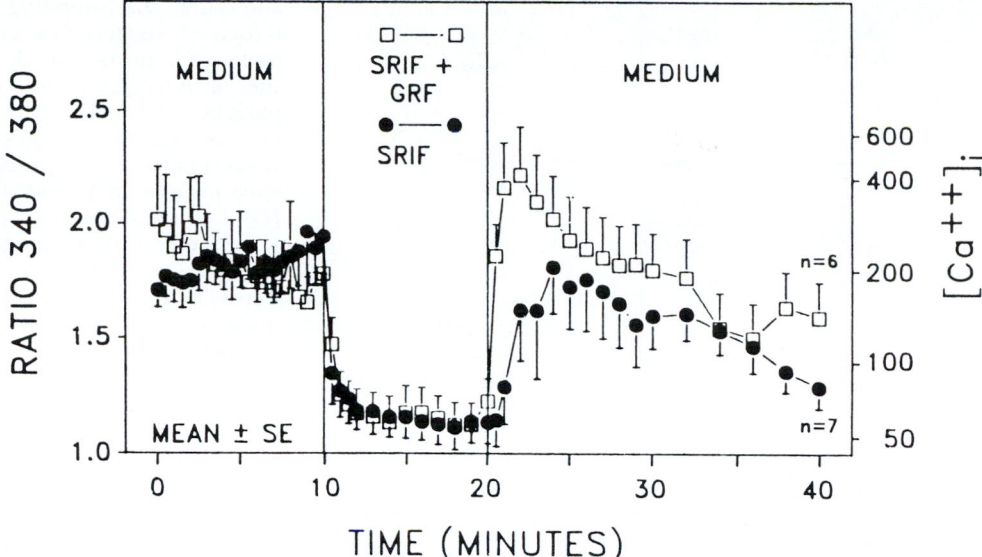

Figure 6–5. Identical reduction of intracellular calcium concentration ($[Ca^{2+}]_i$) in normal rat somatotropes treated with somatostatin (SRIF) plus GHRH (GRF) and cells exposed to somatostatin alone. Recordings of $[Ca^{2+}]_i$ were made every 30 s. Basal recordings were made for 10 min, followed by the addition of either 10 nmol/L GHRH or 1 nmol/L somatostatin. After an additional 10 min, the regulatory peptides were replaced by medium alone. Data points represent the mean ± SE of a group of six or seven somatotropes, respectively, as identified by reverse hemolytic plaque assay. The ratio of fluorescence with excitation at 340 and 380 nm is given on the left axis; the corresponding free cytosolic calcium concentration is shown on the right axis. (From RW Holl, MO Thorner, DA Leong, Intracellular calcium concentration and growth hormone secretion in individual somatotropes: effects of growth hormone–releasing factor and somatostatin, Endocrinology, 122, 2927–2932, 1988, © by The Endocrine Society.)

An overview of the regulation of GH secretion is shown in schematic form in Figure 6–6. In addition to the hypothalamic influences, the somatotrope is regulated by negative feedback by circulating somatomedins such as insulin-like growth factor I (IGF I, also called somatomedin-C) at the pituitary and hypothalamic levels and by short-loop feedback by GH itself on the hypothalamus (also see Chapter 5).

GH is detectable in fetal serum at the end of the first trimester, and its concentration increases rapidly thereafter to reach a peak of 100 to 150 µg/L at about 20 wk of gestation.[81] GH is not thought to be essential for normal intrauterine development and growth. Premature infants have higher serum GH levels than full-term infants. Mean levels subsequently decrease to about 30 µg/L in cord serum, and GH concentrations continue to fall during the early postnatal months. The amount of GH secreted is greatest during adolescence and decreases with age (Fig. 6–7). Premenopausal women have higher GH production rates than do young men.[123]

The pattern of GH secretion depends on a number of factors, including stage of development, nutritional state, sleep stage, stress, and exercise. Metabolic clearance may also vary. Characteristic profiles of GH concentrations in normal men and women are shown in Figure 6–8.

The mean half-life of exogenously administered GH in normal subjects ranges from 9 to 27 min.[124–127] The monoexponential half-life of endogenous GH has been determined by deconvolution analysis (17 ± 1.7 min) and by sequential administration of intravenous boluses of GHRH and somatostatin, followed by a somatostatin infusion (18 ± 0.8 min).[26, 128] The latter technique made possible the delineation of two components of GH disappearance: a distribution (alpha) phase of 3.5 ± 0.7 min and a metabolic clearance

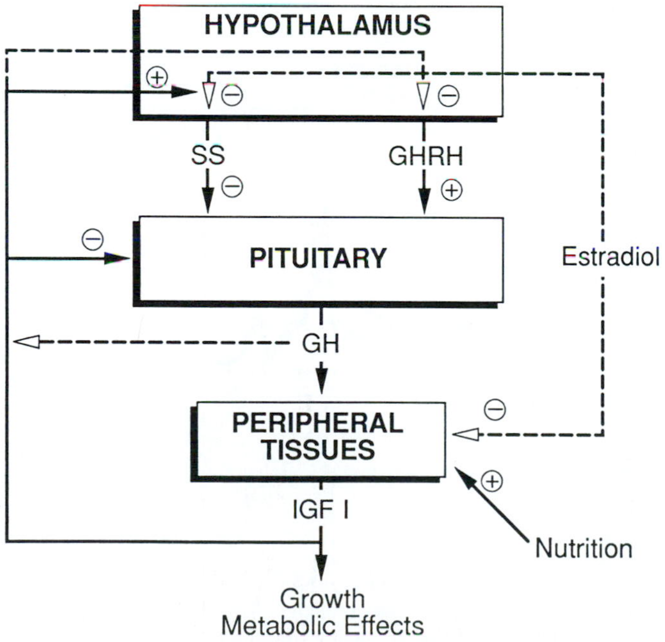

Figure 6–6. Schematic illustration of regulation of serum GH secretion. GH is secreted in a pulsatile fashion under coordinate regulation by hypothalamic somatostatin (SS) and GHRH. GH acts on multiple tissues to regulate metabolic functions and growth. Peripheral tissues produce IGF I, which is secreted into the circulation and acts as a paracrine factor. Circulating and hypothalamic- or pituitary-derived IGF I may also inhibit GH secretion at the pituitary and/or hypothalamic levels. GH also regulates its own secretion by short-loop feedback. Estrogen stimulates GH secretion in humans; the mechanism of action is unclear, but the effect may be either to inhibit the action of GH peripherally or stimulate GH secretion at the hypothalamic level.

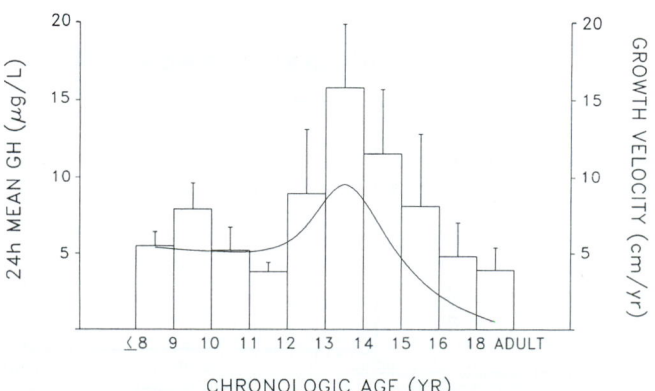

Figure 6–7. Histogram of the 24-h mean (± SE) concentration of GH (bars) from sixty 24-h GH profiles by chronological age. An idealized growth velocity curve (50th percentile values) (solid line) for North American boys[829] is superimposed (right axis). (From PM Martha Jr, AD Rogol, JD Veldhuis, et al, Alterations in the pulsatile properties of circulating growth hormone concentrations during puberty in boys, J Clin Endocrinol Metab 69, 563–570, 1989, © by The Endocrine Society.)

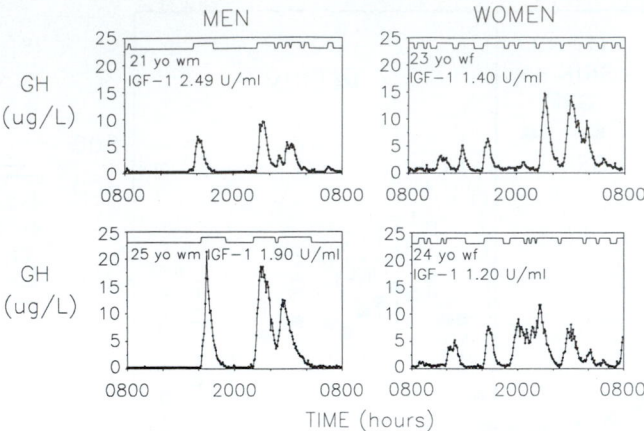

Figure 6–8. Representative 24-h serum GH concentration profiles of two normal men and two normal women. Blood sampling was performed every 5 min for 24 h. The continuous schematized line in the upper portion of each panel identifies individually significant GH pulses detected by cluster analysis. (From ML Hartman, JD Veldhuis, ML Vance, et al., Somatotropin pulse frequency and basal concentrations are increased in acromegaly and are reduced by successful therapy, J Clin Endocrinol Metab, 70, 1375–1384, 1990, © by The Endocrine Society.)

(beta) phase of 20.7 ± 0.7 min.[128] Reported endogenous 24-h GH production rates for adult men range from 0.25 to 0.52 mg/m² surface area[26, 129, 130] as determined by deconvolution analysis and by infusions of radiolabeled GH.

The effects of age and sex on GH release have been studied by measuring GH concentrations in samples drawn every 20 min for 24 h from young men, young women, older men, and older women. In stepwise regression analysis, serum estradiol but not testosterone levels correlated with the 24-h integrated GH concentration.[123] When the effects of estradiol were removed from the analysis, neither age nor sex influenced the integrated GH concentration. This study

and others characterizing the increased GH secretion during puberty[131] suggest that gonadal steroids, particularly estradiol, are important in the regulation of GH secretion. The site of estrogen action is unknown but may be in the periphery or at the pituitary or hypothalamic level. Studies in rats suggest that gonadal steroids affect GHRH and somatostatin gene expression.[132, 133] Estrogens may also influence peripheral factors such as synthesis of IGF I and/or IGF I– and GH-binding proteins.

Studies using frequent sampling and sensitive assays for GH have modified our understanding of GH physiology. Between bursts of GH release, serum GH concentrations are undetectable in conventional assays (<0.2 μg/L). In adults, as during early childhood and puberty, GH is secreted in volleys of multiple secretory bursts. These complex volleys probably arise from multiple GHRH-secretory bursts into the hypophyseal-portal blood during periods of reduced somatostatin secretion.[26] Regardless of nutritional state, the amplitude of GH-secretory bursts is maximal during the night. The most consistent period of GH secretion in both children and young adults (and possibly other age groups) is with the onset of the first slow wave sleep (stages III and IV), which usually occurs within the first hour of sleep. Delay in the onset of deep sleep usually delays the onset of the major GH peak. GH levels are highest during slow wave sleep and lowest during rapid eye movement (REM) sleep. Plasma levels of glucose, fatty acids, and insulin do not change with the burst of GH secretion, although resistance to exogenous insulin and decreased glucose tolerance develop after the peak of GH secretion. REM sleep may be responsible for the termination of sleep-related GH secretion. Similar observations have been made with GHRH administration during different stages of sleep, at different times during the night, and with sleep deprivation.[134] These studies support the hypothesis that decreased hypothalamic somatostatin secretion initiates GH-secretory bursts. Sleep studies suggest that there is a circadian rhythm for GH

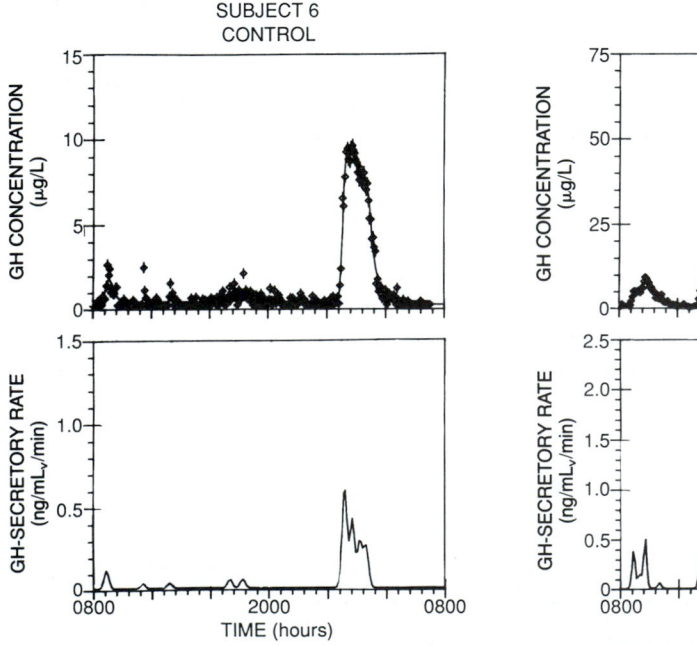
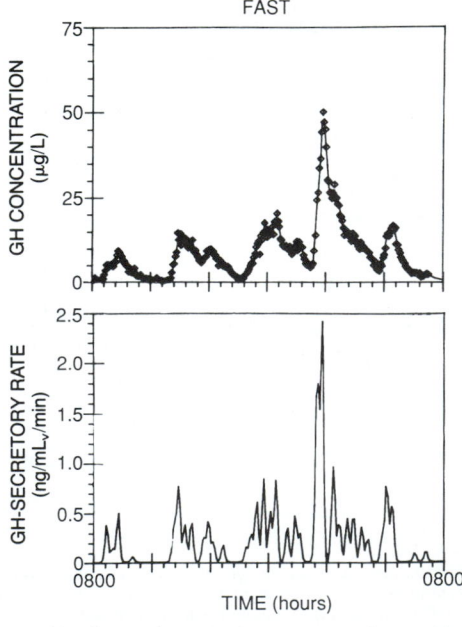

Figure 6–9. Profiles (24 h) of serum GH concentrations and GH-secretory rates as determined by deconvolution analysis in a normal 25-y-old man from a control (fed) day *(left)* and the second day of a fast *(right)*. The upper panels show serum GH concentrations measured every 5 min over 24 h with continuous fitted curves predicted by the deconvolution model. Intrasample standard deviations are denoted by vertical marks through individual values. In the lower panels, the calculated GH-secretory rate is plotted vs. time (ng/mL$_v$/min, where mL$_v$ = mL of distribution volume). Fasting increases the frequency and amplitude of GH-secretory bursts, so that serum GH concentrations are increased throughout the day compared with the fed state. The half-life of GH disappearance, calculated by deconvolution analysis, was unchanged by fasting. Different scales are used for the vertical axes because of the wide range of serum GH concentrations and secretory rates. To convert the GH-secretory rate to micrograms per liter of distribution volume per minute, multiply by 1.0. (Unpublished observations, courtesy of M. L. Hartman, J. D. Veldhuis, and M. O. Thorner.)

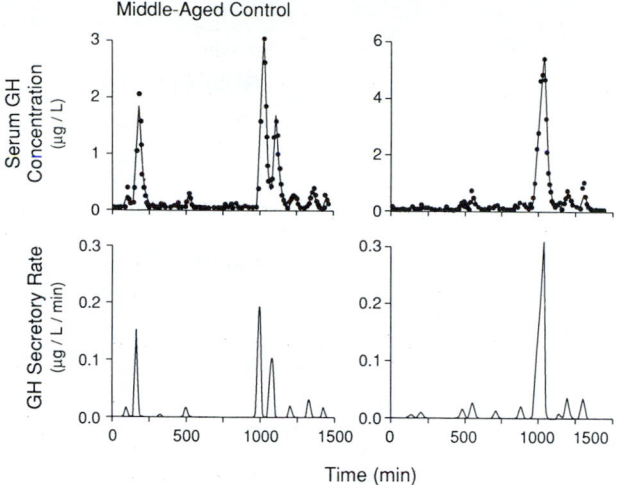
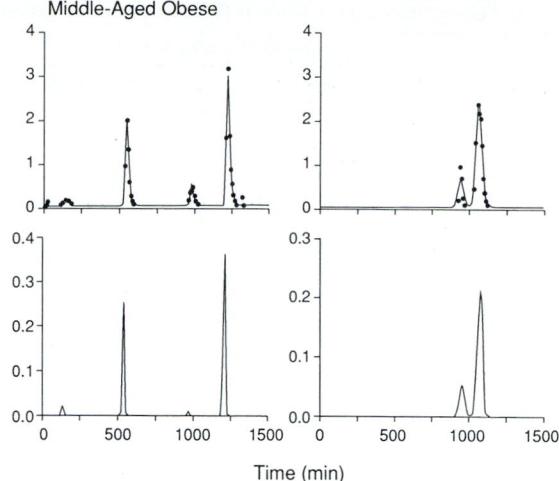

Figure 6–10. Profiles (24 h) of serum GH concentrations and GH-secretory rates as determined by deconvolution analysis in a normal-weight middle-aged man *(left)* and a healthy obese middle-aged man *(right).* The upper panels illustrate serial serum GH concentrations measured every 5 min over 24 h with continuous fitted curves predicted by the deconvolution model; the lower panels demonstrate the calculated GH-secretory rates plotted vs. time. The obese subject had fewer GH-secretory bursts over 24 h, but the amplitudes of these secretory bursts are similar to those of the age-matched nonobese subject. (From JD Veldhuis, A Iranmanesh, KK Ho, et al., Dual defects in pulsatile growth hormone secretion and clearance subserve the hyposomatotropism of obesity in man, J Clin Endocrinol Metab, 72, 51–59, 1991, © by The Endocrine Society.)

secretion in humans and that variations of somatostatin secretion may account for differences in sensitivity to GHRH during different phases of sleep. Thus slow wave sleep may be associated with low levels of hypothalamic somatostatin secretion, and REM sleep may be associated with high levels.

Fasting increases the number and amplitude of secretory bursts[135] (Fig. 6–9). It has been proposed that fasting causes decreased hypothalamic somatostatin secretion. In contrast, GH secretion is decreased in obese subjects; the number of GH-secretory bursts is reduced, but the amplitude of these secretory bursts is similar to those of age-matched subjects of normal weight (Fig. 6–10). The metabolic clearance rate of GH is accelerated in obesity, which contributes to the hyposomatotropism.[136] The diminished GH release in obesity may be due to high levels of somatostatin secretion. Attributes of GH secretion in humans as determined by deconvolution analysis are shown in Table 6–5. Studies of patients with GHRH-secreting tumors and of normal adults given intravenous GHRH infusions support the concept of somatostatin as the zeitgeber (time giver) for pulses of GH secretion.

The significance of pulsatile GH secretion is not established. However, as discussed earlier, the pattern of secretion may determine tissue responses. Pulsatile GH secretion may be particularly important for growth and the multiple effects of the hormone on metabolism (for review see ref. 137).

GH secretion is also influenced by a number of neurogenic, metabolic, and hormonal influences (Table 6–6). These factors may act only in the acute situation. For example, hyperglycemia in normal subjects acutely suppresses GH secretion,[138] whereas in poorly controlled diabetics GH levels are increased.[139] Similarly, although acute increases in free fatty acid concentrations inhibit GH release, fatty acid levels are increased during starvation when GH secretion is augmented. GH secretion appears to be inversely related to insulin concentrations. Thus GH secretion is augmented in fasting, anorexia nervosa, insulin-dependent diabetes mellitus, and hepatic cirrhosis when circulating insulin levels are low. In contrast, in obesity hyperinsulinemia is present and GH secretion is suppressed. Certain amino acids, particularly arginine and leucine, stimulate GH secretion (Fig. 6–11).

Whereas exercise, stress, and some neurogenic factors stimulate GH secretion, emotional deprivation can inhibit its release in children and lead to diminished linear growth.[140, 141] Central alpha-adrenergic agonists (norepinephrine) stimulate GH secretion (for review see ref. 142); clonidine, a central alpha-adrenergic agonist, stimulates GH secretion in this manner. Beta-adrenergic antagonists augment the efficacy of various stimuli for GH secretion. Dopamine agonists stimulate GH secretion in normal subjects by stimulating dopamine receptors. Acetylcholine agonists stimulate[143, 144] and agents that lower acetylcholine tone suppress GH release. Stimulation of GH release by dopamine agonists, alpha-adrenergic agonists, glucagon, and amino acids is inhibited by pirenzepine, a cholinergic muscarinic blocking drug.[145–148] In addition, sleep-induced GH secretion is blocked by the cholinergic blocking agent methscopolamine. These agents are thought to act at the level of the hypothalamus or the median eminence. GH-secretory responses

TABLE 6–5. Growth Hormone Secretion in Men as Determined by Deconvolution Analysis

	GH Secreted (µg/24 h)*	Secretory Bursts	Mass of GH Secreted per Burst (µg)*	Half-Life (min)
Normal young men[830]†	540 ± 44	12 ± 1.2	45 ± 3.7	17 ± 1.7
Fasted men[831]†	2171 ± 333	32 ± 2.4	64 ± 9.4	18 ± 2.2
Obese men[136]‡	77 ± 20	3.2 ± 0.5	24 ± 4.6	12 ± 1.6
Normal middle-aged men[136]‡	196 ± 65	9.7 ± 0.7	20 ± 6.3	16 ± 0.8

*Assuming mean GH volume of distribution of 7.9% of body weight.
†Samples obtained at 5-min intervals; age of subjects, 22 to 28 y; body mass index (BMI), 21 to 29 kg/m².
‡Samples obtained at 10-min intervals; mean age of obese subjects, 40 ± 3.1 y; mean age of normal subjects, 48 ± 4.7 y; mean BMI of obese subjects, 46 ± 1.6 kg/m²; mean BMI of normal subjects, 28 ± 1.3 kg/m².

TABLE 6–6. Factors Influencing Normal Growth Hormone Secretion

Factor	Growth Hormone Secretion	
	Augmented	*Inhibited*
Neurogenic	Stages III and IV sleep	REM sleep
	Stress (traumatic, surgical, inflammatory, psychogenic)	Emotional deprivation
	Alpha-adrenergic agonist	Alpha-adrenergic antagonist
	Beta-adrenergic antagonist	Beta-adrenergic agonist
	Dopamine agonist	
	Acetylcholine agonist	Acetylcholine antagonist
Metabolic	Hypoglycemia	Hyperglycemia
	Fasting	
	Falling fatty acid level	Rising fatty acid level
	Amino acids	
	Uncontrolled diabetes mellitus	Obesity
	Uremia	
	Hepatic cirrhosis	
Hormonal	GHRH	Somatostatin
	Low IGF I level	High IGF I level
	Estrogens	Hypothyroidism
	Glucagon	High glucocorticoid levels
	AVP	

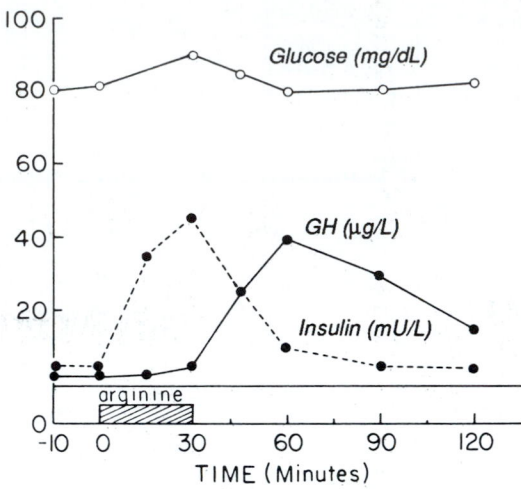

Figure 6–11. Effects of intravenous arginine (0.5 g/kg body weight) on plasma glucose, GH, and insulin concentrations. To convert plasma glucose values to millimoles per liter, multiply by 0.0555. To convert insulin values to picomoles per liter, multiply by 7.175.

to a number of stimuli are augmented after treatment with estrogens (e.g., diethylstilbestrol 3 mg/d for 3 d). The role of serotonin in human GH secretion is unclear (see ref. 142), and histamine does not appear to play a role. Endogenous opiates probably do not directly influence GH secretion, because spontaneous GH secretion is not modified by naloxone. Morphine and β-endorphin do not affect GH secretion, but nalorphine and an enkephalin analogue (DAMME, FK33824) stimulate GH secretion through naloxone-sensitive mechanisms.[149] The pharmacological agent GH-releasing peptide[150] is a potent stimulator of GH release; this hexapeptide was developed from an enkephalin series of peptides. The mechanism of action is unknown, but it does not act through characterized GHRH, somatostatin, or enkephalin receptors.

GROWTH HORMONE ACTIONS. There are two theories regarding the actions of GH: the GH hypothesis and the somatomedin hypothesis[151, 152] (see Chapter 21). Figure 6–12 illustrates the various proposed sites of direct actions of GH. The need to invoke the existence of somatomedins came from observations that growth and mitotic activity of cartilage in vivo are dependent on GH but that direct addition of growth hormone in vitro is ineffective in promoting either action. Cartilage proliferation from hypophysectomized rats is stimulated by serum from normal rats but not by serum from GH-deficient rats. GH treatment of GH-deficient individuals restores the stimulatory effect of the serum within 24 to 48 h. The active components of the serum are two closely related peptides, IGF I and IGF II. They are both single chain peptides that exhibit a high degree of homology with human proinsulin. Serum IGF I concentrations are markedly elevated in acromegaly and reduced in GH deficiency; IGF II levels are unchanged in acromegaly and

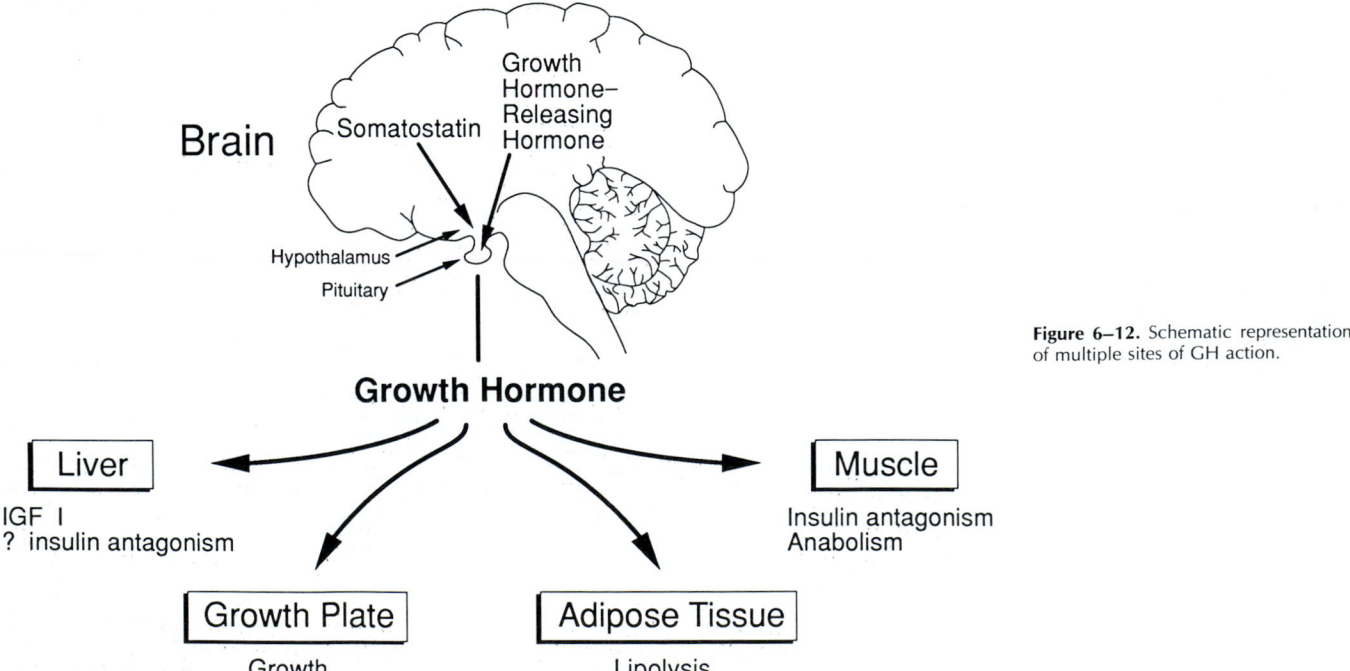

Figure 6–12. Schematic representation of multiple sites of GH action.

modestly reduced in GH deficiency. These observations suggest that IGF I is the important mediator of GH action, and the fact that IGF I feeds back to inhibit GH secretion lends support to this hypothesis.[153–156] The site of IGF I production in relation to its biological action and the significance of circulating levels have been difficult to establish. Insight into this issue came from an experiment in which tissue concentrations of IGF I were measured in normal and in hypophysectomized rats. After accounting for the serum IGF I concentration, it was found that a striking reduction in IGF I occurred after hypophysectomy in all tissues except the brain. After GH administration, tissue IGF I concentrations increased many hours before the increase in circulating levels, providing a satisfactory explanation for the several hours delay in the restoration of serum IGF I levels after GH administration and for the lack of a clear relationship between IGF I levels and growth response during GH treatment (Table 6–7).

Based on studies of GH action in a preadipocyte cell line, a dual-effector model of GH action has been proposed (Fig. 6–13). GH first stimulates precursor cells to undergo differentiation, and somatomedins then act as mitogens to stimulate clonal growth of the differentiated cells.[157] Evidence supporting this hypothesis comes from experiments in which GH was injected into the epiphyseal plate of hypophysectomized rats;[94, 158, 159] this therapy stimulated growth only in the injected limb, and the effect was prevented by passive immunization with IGF I antibodies.[160] Immunoreactive IGF I is present in the proliferative chondrocytes of rat epiphyseal growth plates,[161] as well as other extrahepatic organs, including skeletal muscle.[162] In addition, IGF I concentration increases in response to GH in many of these tissues.[161, 162] Thus locally produced IGF I, under GH regulation, contributes to the stimulatory effects of GH, particularly the stimulation of longitudinal growth.[163, 164] Administration of IGF I to hypophysectomized rats does not promote growth equivalent to that achieved with GH.[165, 166]

Metabolic Actions of Growth Hormone. Many GH actions have been described in isolated tissues and organs (Table 6–8). These GH effects must be interpreted with the knowledge that studies in isolated tissues and organs are subject to all the limitations inherent in in vitro studies.

Growth Hormone Action in Vivo. The effects of GH on metabolism are the subject of intensive study in humans and

TABLE 6–7. Extractable Tissue IGF I Concentrations in Normal and Hypophysectomized Male Rats

	IGF I (µg/g)		
		Hypophysectomized	
Tissue	Normal Rats*	Rats*	% of Normal
Serum	28.7 ± 0.98	0.74 ± 0.12	2.6
Liver	1.91 ± 0.23	0.23 ± 0.08	12.0
Lung	2.04 ± 0.86	0.57 ± 0.13	27.9
Kidney	2.59 ± 0.80	0.77 ± 0.29	29.7
Heart	0.92 ± 0.33	0.48 ± 0.14	52.2
Muscle (iliopsoas)	0.42 ± 0.05	<0.08	<19.1
Brain	0.26 ± 0.09	0.28 ± 0.04	107.7
Testes	1.88 ± 0.42	0.52 ± 0.32	27.7
Prostate	1.06	0.40	37.7
Thymus	0.33	0.10	30.3
Lymph nodes	0.48	0.08	16.7
Cartilage (sternum)	0.67	0.53	79.1
Fat pad (perirenal)	0.67 ± 0.19	0.25 ± 0.10	37.3
Submaxillary gland	1.73	0.78	45.1

*Values are mean ± SD.
From D'Ercole AJ, Stiles AD, Underwood LE. Tissue concentrations of somatomedin C: further evidence for multiple sites of synthesis and paracrine or autocrine mechanisms of action. Proc Natl Acad Sci USA 1984; 81:935–939.

animals because of the potential for promoting protein synthesis and either lipolysis or reduced fat deposition. The availability of biosynthetic human GH produced by recombinant DNA technology and the development of precise methods for assessing subtle metabolic changes make it possible to define the role of this hormone in human metabolism. GH is described as anabolic, lipolytic, and diabetogenic. These characterizations are derived primarily from in vitro studies of isolated tissues deprived of the normal hormonal milieu and from in vivo studies involving administration of pharmacological amounts of GH either acutely or in a nonphysiological manner.

Effects of Growth Hormone in Animals. Administration of GH to growing animals causes improved nutrient "partitioning" and utilization. Administration of pharmacological GH doses to growing pigs and cattle causes increased nitrogen retention, improved feed efficiency, and alteration of carcass composition (reduced fat and increased protein content).[167–169] For example, barrows (castrated male pigs) treated with porcine GH for 35 d had increased feed efficiency, a 25% decrease in carcass lipid, and a 16%

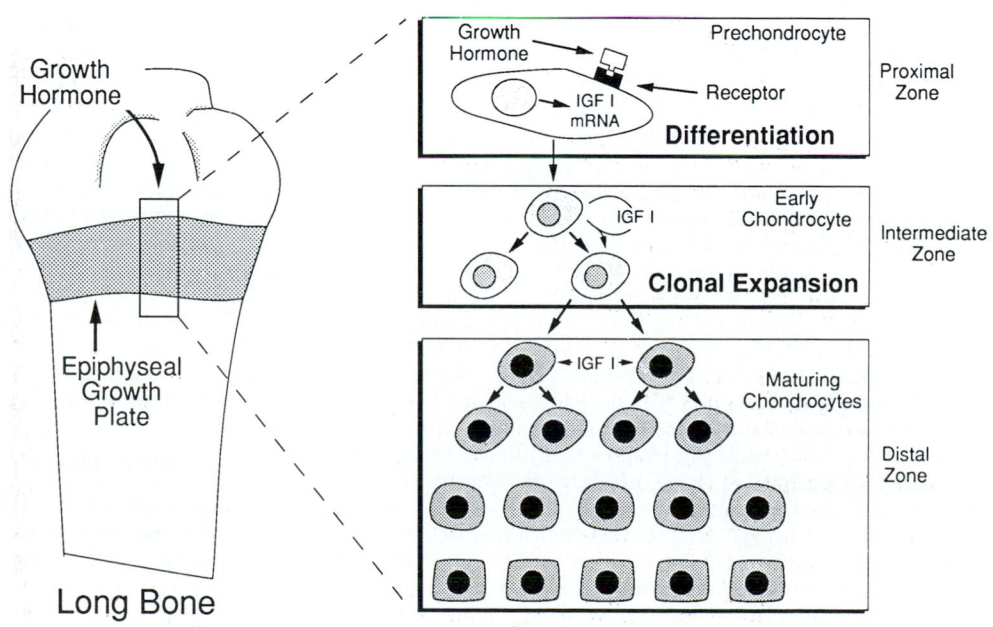

Figure 6–13. Schematic representation of the dual-effector hypothesis proposed by Green.[157] GH acts directly at the epiphyseal plate to stimulate linear growth. GH stimulates differentiation of prechondrocytes into early chondrocytes, which then secrete IGF I. In turn, IGF I stimulates clonal expansion and maturation of chondrocytes. (Modified from Isaksson OGP, Isgaard J, Nilsson A, et al. Direct action of growth hormone. In: Bercu BB, ed. Basic and Clinical Aspects of Growth Hormone. New York: Plenum, 1988: 199–211.)

TABLE 6–8. Direct Actions of Growth Hormone on Isolated Tissues and Organs

Tissue or Organ	Action
Liver	
Perfusion	RNA synthesis[832]
	Plasma protein synthesis[833]
	Somatomedin release[834]
Cell culture	Replication[835]
Muscle	
Isolated rat diaphragm incubation	Amino acid transport and incorporation[836]
Rat heart perfusion	Amino acid transport and incorporation[837]
Human vascular smooth muscle cell culture	Outgrowth[838]
Rat adipocyte incubations	Amino acid incorporation[839]
	Lipolysis[840]
Human fibroblast culture	Somatomedin production[841]
Rabbit and rat chondrocytes	DNA synthesis[842]
	Sulfate incorporation[842]
Hematopoietic cell culture	
Rat thymic lymphocyte culture	Mitosis[843]
Human leukemic lymphoblast culture	[³H]Thymidine, [³H]uridine, and [³H]leucine incorporation[844]
Human erythrogenic precursors	[³H]Thymidine uptake[845]
Isolated rat hypothalamus	Somatostatin secretion[154]

increase in carcass muscle compared with controls.[170] This partitioning effect of GH has yet to be demonstrated in humans. GH effects cannot be extrapolated from one species to another, but studies in animals provide a rationale for studies in humans. In addition, the studies in animals have been performed during the growth phase, and the effects may differ in the adult.

Effects of Growth Hormone in Humans. The metabolic effects of GH administration on various aspects of metabolism have been documented in normal, diabetic, and GH-deficient subjects. Most studies either involved intermittent (once daily) pharmacological administration or were of limited duration and designed to study only the acute effects of GH on a specific aspect of metabolism.

The effects of GH on serum glucose, insulin, and fatty acid levels vary among individuals and among different study protocols. Continuous intravenous infusion of GH that produces serum concentrations of 6 to 10 μg/L causes lipolysis and ketosis in diabetics but not in normal subjects.[171] Continuous intravenous GH infusion in normal subjects, producing serum GH concentrations of 10 to 50 μg/L, causes hyperinsulinemia without hyperglycemia, ketonemia, or consistent changes in lipid concentrations. More prolonged GH infusion produces fasting hyperglycemia, hyperinsulinemia, and increased nonesterified fatty acid concentrations without ketonemia or change in serum glycerol concentrations.[172] Eight hours of continuous GH infusion in normal men (serum GH concentrations 30 to 35 μg/L) increases serum nonesterified fatty acid, ketone, and insulin concentrations and causes glucose intolerance but no change in fasting glucose level.[173] GH induction of insulin resistance at a postreceptor site may be the mechanism for these effects, as suggested by studies involving pharmacological amounts of GH[174] and studies employing euglycemic insulin and hyperglycemic clamp techniques.[175] Hyperglycemic clamp studies with a continuous 14-h GH infusion suggest that the site of insulin resistance is the liver.[176] In summary, despite minor differences in study designs, either continuous GH exposure or pharmacological GH doses produce alterations in carbohydrate and lipid utilization.

Administration of GH to GH-deficient children produces positive nitrogen balance, decreased urea production, redistributed body fat, and reduced carbohydrate utilization but not development of diabetes mellitus. A single dose of GH decreases free fatty acid, blood glucose, and amino acid concentrations for only a few hours. Similar effects may also occur in normal subjects, albeit to a lesser extent.[177]

Increased nitrogen retention occurs during short-term (1 to 3 wk) GH administration, daily or on alternate days, to normal and obese subjects during caloric restriction and to older adults during surfeit nutrition;[178–180] this effect does not persist during more prolonged treatment (5 wk) in obese subjects.[181]

Growth Hormone and Aging. GH secretion in men and women declines with age.[123, 182–185] Both integrated and pulsatile GH secretion decreases, accompanied by a decline in serum IGF I concentration. Other changes in metabolism with aging include alteration in body composition with loss of muscle mass and increased fat composition despite maintenance of normal weight.[186, 187] Six months of daily or three times weekly GH administration to older adults with diminished GH secretion or to GH-deficient adults causes an increase in serum IGF I concentrations to those of young healthy subjects. Changes in body composition during GH treatment include a 10% increase in lean body mass, a 15% decrease in adipose tissue, and a 2% increase in vertebral bone density. These changes were associated with an increase in fasting serum glucose and insulin concentrations.[188, 189] It is not known whether improvements in exercise capacity or marked changes in carbohydrate, lipid, and protein metabolism occur with chronic GH treatment of the elderly.

Growth Hormone in Catabolic Illness. Burn injury and surgery are associated with a catabolic state despite surfeit nutritional support and treatment of associated complications such as infection and anemia. Serum GH concentrations are inappropriately low. A study of seven postoperative patients receiving a hypocaloric diet of 400 kcal/d as 5% dextrose demonstrated that the median serum GH level was 3 μg/L (range 3 to 22 μg/L) and did not change when oral nutrition was introduced.[190] Although "stress" is an effective stimulus for GH release, the low concentrations in catabolic patients may be a result of hypercaloric and high-carbohydrate diets.

Studies involving administration of large doses of GH to burn patients have focused primarily on the nitrogen-sparing effect. In several studies, GH, given over a 4- to 12-d period, decreased urinary nitrogen excretion, suggesting that GH exerts an "anabolic" effect.[191–194] A limitation of these studies was the presumption that the decrease in nitrogen excretion reflected increased protein synthesis, because this methodology cannot distinguish between an anabolic effect and a decrease in catabolism. Burn patients treated with GH also have increased basal plasma insulin concentrations without development of glucose intolerance.[194] Effects of GH on glucose and lipid turnover are less well defined, but indirect calorimetry studies suggest that lipid utilization is increased by GH because oxygen consumption increased and the respiratory quotient fell.[193]

Administration of pharmacological doses of glucocorticoids produces a catabolic state by promoting protein wasting. Seven days of GH treatment prevents glucocorticoid-induced protein catabolism in normal volunteers, suggesting that GH has a distinctly anabolic effect.[195] These findings have wide-ranging implications for potential applications of GH treatment of a variety of patients with catabolic illnesses.

Glycoprotein Hormone Family*

The three anterior pituitary glycoprotein hormones are thyroid-stimulating hormone (thyrotropin, TSH), luteinizing hormone (lutropin, LH), and follicle-stimulating hormone

---

*For reviews see refs. 196 and 197.

(follitropin, FSH). Each consists of two noncovalently bound subunits, alpha and beta. The alpha subunit is common to all three hormones, but the beta subunit is unique for each hormone and confers biological specificity.[198] The subunits are synthesized as separate peptides from distinct mRNAs.[199–201] Microheterogeneity of the carbohydrate constituents of the individual hormones causes heterogeneity in receptor affinity, biological potency, and metabolic clearance.

The alpha subunit peptide is more abundant than the unique beta subunit of peptides. Free serum alpha subunits are secreted and are present in concentrations equivalent to the combined concentration of TSH, LH, and FSH. Free serum beta subunit concentrations are lower, usually below the level of detectability in conventional assays.[202–204] The overabundance of alpha subunit has led to the speculation that regulation of beta subunit synthesis is the rate-limiting step in modulating the levels of TSH, LH, and FSH. Although most studies have concentrated on regulation of peptide synthesis, the glycosylation step is probably also regulated.[205]

Alpha Subunit

The alpha subunits are approximately 20 to 22 kd, have 92 amino acid residues in the human and 96 amino acid residues in other species, and contain two N-linked carbohydrate groups. The human, cow, mouse, and rat alpha subunit genes are similar. The human gene is located on chromosome 6q21.1-q23,[206] is 13.5 kb in size, and consists of four exons and three introns. The 5'-untranslated region is encoded by exon 1 and by 14 base pairs of exon 2. A large first intron, approximately 6.4 kb (in humans), interrupts this 5'-untranslated region. The coding portion of the gene is present in exons 2, 3, and 4, and the 3'-untranslated region is contained entirely within exon 4. The alpha subunit has a single transcriptional start site. All species have a single mRNA species that is between 730 and 800 bases long. This mRNA encodes the precursor of the alpha subunit and a leader sequence of an average of 24 amino acids. In all species except the human, intron 2 interrupts the coding sequence after the first nucleotide of codon +10; in the human it interrupts the codon +6 after its first nucleotide. In the human a four-codon deletion at the beginning of exon 3[207–213] accounts for an apoprotein with 92 amino acids in the human versus 96 in other species.

Thyrotropin Beta Subunit

The TSH beta subunit is approximately 18 kd, consists of 110 amino acids, and contains one N-linked complex carbohydrate.[198] The human TSH beta subunit gene is located on chromosome 1p22[214] and consists of three exons separated by two introns of 3.9 and 0.45 kb.[215] The genes for the beta subunit of TSH of mouse,[216, 217] rat,[210, 218] and cow[219] and portions of the human TSH beta gene[215, 220, 221] have been cloned. Each mRNA is approximately 700 bases in length, with minor variations. The TSH beta mRNA encodes the precursor TSH beta subunit with a 20-amino-acid leader sequence and a 117- or 118-amino-acid coding region. There is at least 80 to 89% homology at the amino acid level among the sequences of rat, mouse, and bovine species, and at the nucleotide level there is 91% homology between rat and mouse.

Unlike the rat and mouse genes, the human gene may have only one transcriptional start site. Two transcriptional start sites, a major one and a minor one, have been observed in a human TSH-secreting tumor, similar to the observation in TSH beta genes of other species.[222] A point mutation in the TSH beta subunit gene that causes a glycine-to-arginine substitution caused a congenital isolated TSH deficiency in two siblings.[223, 224] It is believed that this mutation impairs the formation of the αβ dimers.

Although both the alpha and beta subunits of TSH are negatively regulated by thyroid hormone, there is no consensus sequence in the 5'-flanking regions of each gene that would suggest a common thyroid hormone response element. Nevertheless, thyroid hormone receptors do bind to the 5'-flanking regions of the alpha and beta subunit genes. Which thyroid hormone receptor is responsible and whether it acts directly or by interacting with transacting factors remain to be elucidated.

THYROTROPE CELLS AND THYROTROPIN CONTENT. Thyrotrope cells account for only about 5% of anterior pituitary cells and are located in the anteromedial portion of the gland. These fairly large cells display angular outlines and cytoplasmic processes in immunohistochemical studies. By electron microscopy, normal active thyrotrope cells have a spherical nucleus, well-developed and somewhat dilated RER, and a global Golgi complex with numerous vesicles. The secretory granules range from 50 to 300 nm but are usually 200 to 300 nm in diameter. Large lysosomes are common. Less typical, sparsely granulated cells may be identifiable only by immunoelectron microscopy. Sustained stimulation of the thyrotrope cell, as occurs in primary hypothyroidism, results in development of "thyroid deficiency" cells and thyrotrope hyperplasia.[225] The thyroid deficiency cells are massively enlarged with extensive well-developed, dilated RER. In thyrotoxicosis the thyrotropes are small and densely granulated by light microscopy, but the fine structure has not been defined. The human pituitary contains approximately 100 to 150 μg of TSH.

REGULATION OF THYROTROPIN SECRETION. (For a review see ref. 196.) Studies with intact pituitaries and transplantable thyrotrope tumors in mice have demonstrated that mRNAs that encode alpha and TSH beta subunits are regulated by thyroid hormone; the degree of suppression is greater for TSH beta than for the alpha subunit.[217] The response to triiodothyronine (T_3) is rapid (1 h). In the hypothyroid rat the amount of TSH beta mRNA increases up to 10-fold. However, the ratios of mRNAs for alpha and beta are relatively constant. In vivo or in vitro studies of the euthyroid, hypothyroid, and T_3-treated states, the ratios were 1.1 to 1.7, 0.4 to 1.3, and 2 to 3, respectively. These studies demonstrate that T_3 feedback occurs at the level of the thyrotrope.[217, 226, 227] The reduction in steady-state mRNA levels in response to thyroid hormone is mediated by a reduction in transcription that is demonstrable within 30 min.[228] The mRNAs coding for the subunits appear to have a short half-life in hyperthyroid animals, but it is not known whether the half-life is altered during hypothyroidism. The occupancy, time course of binding of the T_3 receptor, and suppression of TSH gene transcription are correlated.[227, 229, 230] Protein synthesis is apparently not required for suppression of TSH gene expression in response to thyroid hormone, suggesting a direct action of the thyroid hormone receptor with specific DNA motifs in the promoter region of the alpha and TSH beta subunit genes.

TRH increases TSH alpha and beta mRNA levels within 30 min and levels decline thereafter.[231, 232] The extent of stimulation is similar for both alpha and beta, in contrast to the more profound reduction of TSH beta mRNA levels after thyroid hormone administration. Dopamine can inhibit TSH secretion, reducing both basal and TRH-stimulated TSH secretion by more than 50%. In vitro, dopamine decreases mRNA levels for both subunits and suppresses transcription by 60 to 75%. Effects are demonstrable within 15 min and are maximal after 30 min.[231] The mode of action of dopamine is unknown.

After injection, radiolabeled TSH is distributed in a space slightly larger than the plasma volume. The plasma half-life is approximately 50 min; the relatively slow clearance is due to glycosylation of the hormone. The secretion rate of TSH in euthyroid individuals is 50 to 200 μg/d and increases up to fivefold during hypothyroidism.

THYROTROPIN SECRETION. Secretion of TSH is regulated by both hypothalamic hormones and circulating thyroid hormones. The hypothalamic tripeptide TRH stimulates TSH release.[233] If the hypothalamic pituitary stalk is interrupted, secondary hypothyroidism develops and TSH secretion is reduced but not absent. Somatostatin and dopamine can inhibit TSH secretion, but it is not clear whether these actions are important in the physiological regulation of thyrotropin. They may influence the circadian rhythm of TSH secretion, which is preserved during constant TRH infusions in humans.

The principal regulator of TSH secretion is feedback by thyroid hormones. Thyroid hormone acts at the hypothalamic level to inhibit TRH synthesis[234, 235] and at the pituitary to inhibit TSH secretion. Intracellular T_3 in the thyrotrope regulates TSH secretion, although plasma thyroxine (T_4) levels correlate better with TSH levels than do T_3 levels in normal subjects and in hypothyroid patients. When T_4 levels decline to the lower normal range, TSH levels rise exponentially, as shown in Figure 6–14. This is because the thyrotrope has a potent intracellular 5'-deiodinase that converts T_4 to T_3.[236] Approximately three quarters of intracellular T_3 in the pituitary is derived from conversion of T_4, and the remainder is derived from the circulation. In contrast, in hypothyroid patients receiving hormone replacement with T_4, the serum T_3 level correlates better with suppression of TSH levels than does the serum T_4 level.[237]

TSH is measured by either radioimmunoassay or immunoradiometric assay (IRMA). The IRMAs for TSH are more sensitive, have fewer cross-reacting substances, and are better able to distinguish between normal and low TSH levels, which was often not possible with radioimmunoassays.

TSH is secreted in a pulsatile fashion with low-amplitude peaks[238] and in a circadian fashion. TSH levels are low during the day and increase at approximately 8 PM; higher levels are present during the night and decrease in the early hours of the morning. During sleep deprivation the nighttime increase in TSH secretion is enhanced.[238] Although pharmacological doses of glucocorticoids inhibit TSH secretion,[239] the normal circadian change in plasma cortisol level is probably not an important regulator of TSH secretion.[240]

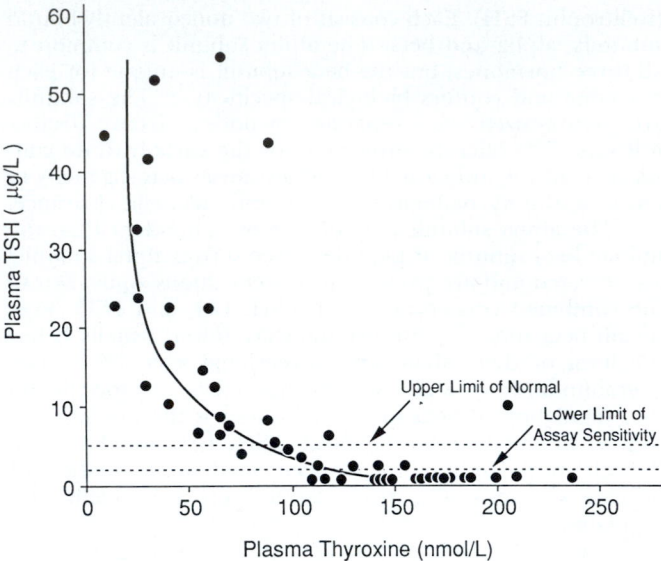

Figure 6–14. Relationship between plasma T_4 and plasma TSH levels. When the plasma T_4 value decreases below 100 nmol/L, plasma TSH concentration increases above normal. (Modified from S Reichlin, RD Utiger, Regulation of the pituitary-thyroid axis in man: relationship of TSH concentration to concentration of free and total thyroxine in plasma, J Clin Endocrinol Metab, 27, 251–255, 1967, © by The Endocrine Society.)

During the night circulating T_4 and T_3 levels decline as a consequence of the posture-related decline in plasma proteins.[240]

The IRMAs have resulted in improved sensitivity so that it is now possible to distinguish between a normal serum TSH value and a suppressed value in hyperthyroidism[241] (Fig. 6–15). To interpret TSH levels simultaneous thyroid hormone levels must be measured. In thyroid failure serum TSH levels may rise before the serum thyroid hormone levels decline to below the normal range; this is often considered to be a harbinger of incipient hypothyroidism, as occurs in Hashimoto's thyroiditis. Both serum TSH and T_4 levels should be measured to exclude hypothyroidism, because in hypothalamic-pituitary disease the TSH level may be in the "normal" range (for euthyroid thyroid hormone levels) but be inappropriately low for the measured thyroid hormone level.

As a diagnostic test for TSH reserve, TRH can be

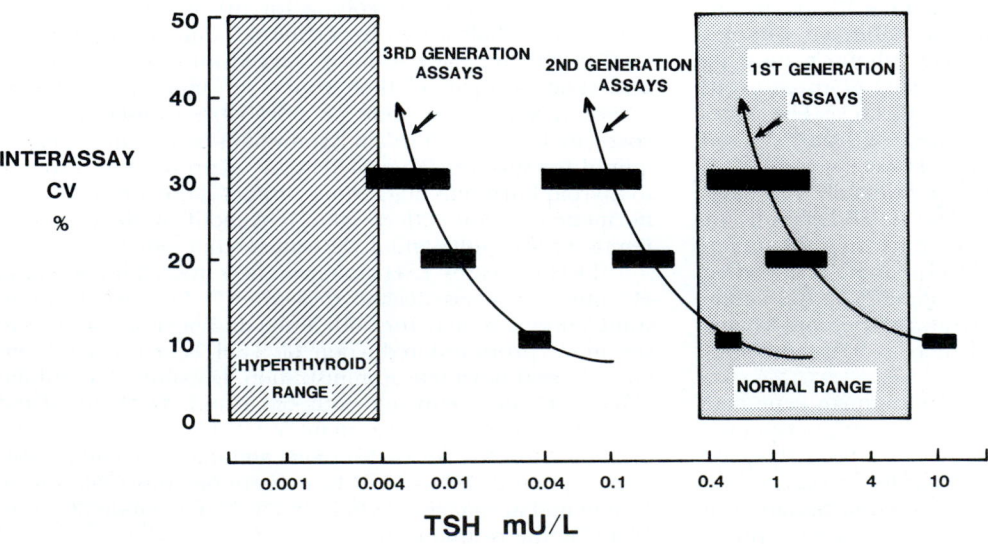

Figure 6–15. With the development of modern TSH assays with greater sensitivity, it is possible to distinguish between normal TSH concentrations and the suppressed values of hyperthyroidism.[846] Each generation of assays represents a 10-fold improvement in functional sensitivity (20% interassay coefficient of variation value). The black bars denote the 95% confidence limits of measurement at different TSH concentrations. (From JT Nicoloff, CA Spencer, Clinical review 12: the use and misuse of the sensitive tyrotropin assays, J Clin Endocrinol Metab, 71, 553–558, 1990, © by The Endocrine Society.)

administered to amplify the TSH signal in order to distinguish between low, normal, and high TSH levels and to assess feedback inhibition by peripheral thyroid hormone levels. Figure 6–16 shows the TSH responses to TRH in normal subjects and in patients with primary hypothyroidism and pituitary and hypothalamic hypothyroidism. Patients with thyrotoxicosis have no response to TRH, reflecting negative feedback by thyroid hormone. The need for this test to exclude hyperthyroidism has been largely eliminated with the development of the sensitive IRMA for TSH. However, the TRH test is still helpful in two areas. In the patient with elevated thyroid hormone levels and "normal" TSH levels, the absence of a TSH response is compatible with either hyperthyroidism or a thyrotrope adenoma (see later), and the presence of a response may suggest pituitary resistance to thyroid hormone. TRH is also administered to distinguish between pituitary and hypothalamic hypothyroidism in which the peripheral thyroid hormone level is low and the TSH level is normal or low. If the TSH response to TRH is adequate, the abnormality is most likely hypothalamic in origin; in this case the 60-min TSH level is often higher than the 20-min level. An absent TSH response to TRH is more likely to reflect pituitary failure, often associated with other pituitary hormone deficiencies.

THYROTROPIN ACTIONS. TSH binds to specific thyroid cell plasma membrane receptors. Specific TSH binding also occurs in other cells, including adipocytes, but the physiological significance of the extrathyroidal binding sites is unknown. The TSH receptor also binds human thyroid-stimulating immunoglobulins (see Chapter 8). The binding of TSH to its receptor activates adenylate cyclase, which increases intracellular cAMP levels and activation of protein kinase A, leading to phosphorylation of proteins that regulate the thyroid cells.

TSH regulates both synthesis and secretion of thyroid hormones by increasing the size and the vascularity of the gland. TSH increases the height of the follicular epithelium and decreases the amount of colloid. The consequences are increased iodide transport, thyroglobulin synthesis, iodotyrosine and iodothyronine formation, thyroglobulin proteolysis, and T_4 and T_3 release.

Gonadotropins

BETA SUBUNITS OF LH, FSH, AND hCG. The beta subunits of both LH and FSH are composed of 115 amino acids and have two carbohydrate side chains. The structure of the beta subunit of LH is similar to that of human chorionic gonadotropin (hCG) except that the hCG beta subunit has an additional 32 amino acids and additional carbohydrate residues on the COOH end. A terminal sialic acid is frequently present on the carbohydrate side chains of the beta subunit of hCG and FSH. Sialic acid is not necessary for receptor binding but decreases the metabolic clearance of these hormones compared with that of TSH and LH (which do not have sialic acid side chains).

The human LH beta subunit gene is located on chromosome 19q13.32 and is close to the hCG beta genes.[206] Each of the glycoprotein beta subunits is coded for by a single gene except for hCG beta. There are at least seven hCG beta genes and pseudogenes, and only primates and horses are known to have these genes. The LH and hCG beta genes are approximately 1.5 kb in size and consist of three exons and two introns. The LH beta gene encodes a protein with a 24-amino-acid leader sequence and a mature protein of 121 amino acids. Intron 1 interrupts the region of the gene that encodes the signal peptide (between amino acids -15 and -16), and intron 2 interrupts the mature protein between amino acids $+41$ and $+42$. The hCG beta protein differs from the other beta subunits in having a 24-amino-acid COOH-terminal extension. In addition, the 5'-untranslated portion of the molecule has 366 bases, in contrast to the 9-base 5'-untranslated portion of LH beta. The 5'-flanking region of the LH beta gene contains a putative estrogen response element with a high degree of homology to estrogen response elements in prolactin and vitellogenin genes.

The human FSH beta gene is located on chromosome 11p13.[242] It has three exons and two introns. The nucleotide and amino acid sequences of the coding regions of the rat and human FSH beta subunits show 79 and 80% homology, respectively. In contrast to a single mRNA in rat and cow, the human FSH beta subunit gene is transcribed into four mRNA species. This diversity is brought about by an alternate splicing site in exon 1 and two polyadenylation sites.[243]

GONADOTROPE CELLS AND PITUITARY LH AND FSH CONTENT. Gonadotrope cells are ovoid, medium sized or smaller, and widely distributed throughout the pars distalis of the pituitary;[20, 244] their prevalence in the human gland is unknown. The morphology and immunoreactivity of gonadotrope cells vary with different hormonal states. The gonadotrope cell is bihormonal and elaborates both FSH and LH; during the menstrual cycle the secretion of these hormones varies, and their concentrations in the gonadotrope cell change. The cells have a large interface with capillary basement membranes.[20] They are often close to lactotrope cells, raising the possibility of a paracrine interaction between the two.[245] Gonadotrope cells have a spherical, conspicuously euchromatic nucleus and low-density cytoplasm that contains well-developed, mildly dilated RER and a prominent Golgi apparatus. In women, the secretory granules tend to be larger (200 to 600 nm) with marked differences in electron density. However, no specific histological changes occur with physiological hormonal variations. In men, the small (< 200 nm) secretory granules are usually more numerous. In nontumorous human gonadotrope cells "light bodies,"[246] thought to be markers for gonadotrope cells in the rat

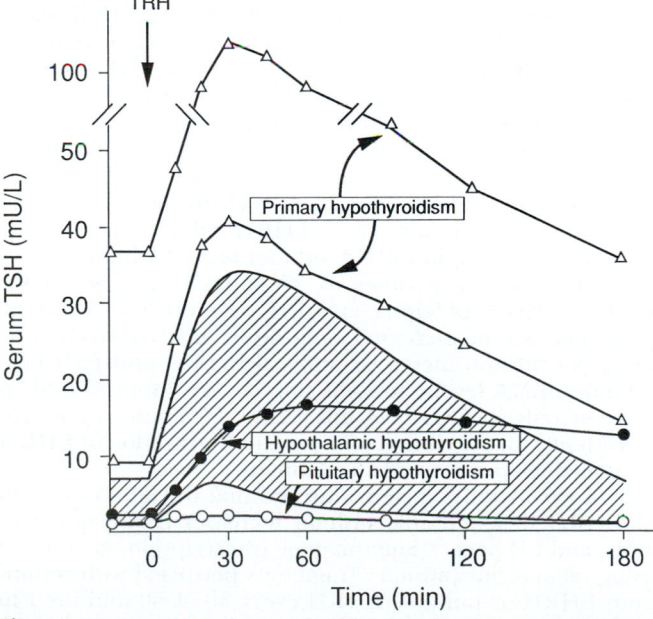

Figure 6–16. Serum TSH changes after TRH administration in normal subjects (shaded area) and in patients with primary hypothyroidism, hypothalamic disease, and pituitary hypothyroidism. Patients with hypothalamic disease may have a delayed TSH response to TRH. (Modified from Utiger RD. Tests of the hypothalamic-pituitary-thyroid axis. In: Ingbar SH, Braverman LE, eds. The Thyroid. 5th ed. Philadelphia: J. B. Lippincott, 1986: 515.)

pituitary, are rare. Chronic sustained stimulation of gonadotrope cells, such as after castration, results in the development of "castration cells" that are massively enlarged with abundant, markedly dilated RER, a prominent Golgi complex, and few granules.[247] The morphology of inactive gonadotrope cells is poorly studied. Such inactive gonadotropes occur in hypogonadotropic hypogonadism or nontumorous parts of pituitaries that harbor gonadotrope cell adenomas.[248] The inactive gonadotrope cells are small and ovoid and have heterochromatic nuclei, scant membranous organelles and secretory granules, and several large, compartmentalized lysosomes.

The content of gonadotropins is low in the pituitaries of prepubertal children. In men and in menstruating women, the pituitary contains approximately 700 IU of LH and 200 IU of FSH. After menopause, the content of pituitary LH rises to approximately 1700 IU but there is no change in FSH content. hCG was previously thought to originate only from the placenta and from trophoblastic tumors but is now known to be present in small amounts in the pituitary, testis, and other nonplacental tissues.[249–251]

REGULATION OF LH AND FSH SECRETION. Secretion from the gonadotrope is regulated by integration of the LHRH signal and feedback effects of gonadal steroids and peptides (e.g., inhibin). LHRH interacts with a membrane receptor to regulate both LH and FSH release and synthesis and is necessary for gonadotrope function; gonadal steroids and peptides are ineffective alone in stimulating release. However, once LHRH is present, the effects of gonadal steroids and inhibin are demonstrable. There is uncertainty regarding the mechanism of LHRH action (for review see ref. 252). Interaction of LHRH with the gonadotrope membrane receptor leads to receptor microaggregation, which in turn regulates the number of receptors and the cellular response. Gonadotropin secretion is initiated by mobilization of intracellular calcium followed by mobilization of extracellular calcium. Synergism between the calcium-calmodulin system and the inositol trisphosphate–diacylglycerol–protein kinase C cascade allows optimal gonadotropin secretion. cAMP is also likely to have a role in the regulation of gonadotropins, although it is not the primary second messenger for the action of the hormone. Gonadal steroids act by binding to gonadotrope nuclear receptors that affect transcription of various genes by binding to appropriate response elements on DNA.[253, 254] In addition, gonadal peptides affect gonadotropin synthesis by binding to cell-surface receptors and indirectly regulating hormone synthesis (see later).

Regulation of gonadotropin synthesis can be assessed by measuring incorporation of labeled amino acids in the glycoproteins or by measuring gonadotropin subunit mRNA synthesis. The results of such experiments correlate with in vivo studies of gonadotropin secretion in humans.

Estradiol. Transcription of alpha and LH beta and FSH beta subunit mRNAs from ovariectomized rats is increased 2.5-, 10-, and 3.5-fold over that in intact rats, and estradiol treatment causes a decline in the synthesis of the three subunit mRNAs (alpha, 70%; LH beta, 88%; and FSH beta, 74%).[255] The estrogen effects appear to be mediated indirectly through the hypothalamus. For example, hypothalamic estradiol implants have selective effects in gonadectomized rats to prevent the development of castration cells. In addition, in ovariectomized monkeys the LHRH pulse generator is slowed by injection of estradiol.[256] These studies do not exclude additional effects of estradiol at the pituitary level, and such a pituitary site of action has been demonstrated in lower species and in primates.[257] The negative effects of estradiol on pituitary gonadotropin secretion ap-

pear to be mediated by modulation of LHRH action at the pituitary rather than by a direct effect on transcription of subunit mRNAs.[196] The inhibition by estradiol of LH secretion may be a membrane effect. Although a membrane receptor for estrogen has not been described, a membrane receptor for progesterone is present in *Xenopus laevis* oocytes.[258, 259] Estradiol also acts in a positive manner to enhance LH secretion, probably as a result of effects at the pituitary level,[257] for example, to increase transcription of LH beta subunit mRNA,[254] and at the level of the hypothalamus to enhance LHRH secretion.[260, 261]

Progesterone regulates gonadotropin secretion at the hypothalamus to slow the LHRH pulse generator. Thus during the luteal phase of the menstrual cycle LH pulse frequency is decreased.[262–264]

Androgens suppress LHRH secretion by the hypothalamus.[265] In vivo, androgens decrease levels of alpha and LH beta mRNAs by suppressing LHRH secretion but have no effect on FSH beta mRNA.[266] In vitro, androgens increase levels of FSH beta mRNA by a direct effect on the pituitary.[197, 266] Androgen feedback is best exemplified by the study of patients with testicular feminization syndrome who have androgen resistance because of a defect in the androgen receptor. In these patients the mean LH levels are elevated, and there is an increase in the number of LH-secretory episodes per day.[267] Gonadotropin levels in these patients are not suppressed by elevated endogenous testosterone levels or by administration of nonaromatizable androgens.

LHRH is essential for gonadotropin secretion, and the timing of LHRH delivery is crucial in the regulation of LH and FSH secretion. In ovariectomized sheep, each LH pulse is preceded by a pulse of LHRH release as measured in the hypothalamic-pituitary portal blood. Gonadotropin secretion can be restored in monkeys with hypothalamic lesions and in humans with isolated gonadotropin deficiency (actually LHRH deficiency) by pulsatile LHRH administration.[268–270] The frequency and amplitude of LHRH pulses are important in regulating LH and FSH secretion differentially. The pulsatile secretion of both LH and FSH is maintained with one LHRH pulse per hour; more frequent LHRH pulses initially increase the frequency of LH pulses and mean LH concentrations.[271, 272] In contrast, when the LHRH pulse frequency is decreased to once per 3 h, FSH secretion is preferentially stimulated.[271, 273] The effect of LHRH alterations on gonadotrope mRNA levels has been studied. In gonadectomized sheep and rats either surgical separation of the hypothalamus from the pituitary or suppression of the hypothalamus by administration of testosterone[265] resulted in a progressive decline in mRNA levels for alpha, LH beta, and FSH beta subunits.[274–277] LHRH administration prevented this decline in mRNA subunit levels. Administration of LHRH to rats at doses of 75 and 25 ng/pulse causes increased levels of alpha and LH beta mRNA.[277–279] One pulse per 8 min increased only alpha mRNA levels; one pulse per 30 min increased alpha, LH beta, and FSH beta subunit mRNA levels; and one pulse every 2 h produced an increase only in FSH beta mRNA levels. These results are consistent with the clinical effects of administration of LHRH on gonadotropin secretion in humans.

In vitro studies have confirmed that the administration of LHRH in a pulsatile fashion increases transcription of alpha and LH beta.[280] Subunit gene transcription was studied using rat anterior pituitary fragments perifused with continuous LHRH or pulsatile LHRH every 30 or 60 min for 1 to 6 h. During continuous LHRH exposure only alpha subunit mRNA synthesis was stimulated (threefold). During pulsatile LHRH administration LH beta transcription was increased 2- to 2.5-fold at 1 h and 3- to 4-fold after 3 or 6 h, FSH beta mRNA synthesis was increased only 2-fold at 1 h, and alpha subunit gene transcription was increased 2-fold at 1 h and 4- to 5-fold at 3 or 6 h.

Gonadal Peptides. Peptides produced in the gonad have important feedback effects on secretion of gonadotropin and possibly other pituitary hormones. Inhibin plays an important role in the regulation of FSH secretion, but most physiological data in this regard are indirect because of inadequate methods for measurement of circulating inhibin. Gonadal secretion of inhibin is regulated by gonadotropins, growth factors, and gonadal steroids. Gonadectomy is followed by increased FSH secretion, indicating that the gonad produces factors that inhibit FSH secretion. Gonadal steroids (in physiological concentrations) lower LH levels to normal, but FSH levels remain elevated.[281, 282]

Inhibin is a member of a larger inhibin family of glycoprotein hormones and growth factors that includes antimüllerian hormone (AMH, also known as müllerian-inhibiting factor, MIF) transforming growth factor β, an erythroid differentiation factor, and an insect protein that plays an important role in cellular differentiation. The isolation and cloning of the cDNA that encodes inhibin were expected to answer the question of selective control of FSH secretion by gonadal feedback. However, FSH regulation is complex. The two forms of inhibin[283–285] are heterodimers that have a common alpha subunit and one of two distinct beta subunits, type A or type B. Both forms of inhibin, types $\alpha\beta_A$ and $\alpha\beta_B$, inhibit FSH secretion. However, the two beta subunits, as heterodimers or homodimers ($\beta_A\beta_A$, $\beta_B\beta_B$, or $\beta_A\beta_B$), stimulate FSH secretion in vitro (activin or FSH-releasing protein).[286, 287] It remains to be determined whether this phenomenon is of physiological significance. Inhibin is synthesized by Sertoli cells of the testis, granulosa cells of the ovary, the placenta,[288] pituitary gonadotropes,[289] and the brain.[290, 291] Thus inhibin may regulate LHRH and gonadotropin secretion not only as a hormone but also by local production and as an autocrine or paracrine factor. In the juvenile monkey (*Macaca mulatta*), puberty is accelerated by administering pulsatile LHRH at 3-h intervals (selective for FSH). The administration of a similar regimen to 2-d post-orchiectomized monkeys causes a two- to threefold increase in FSH levels. Passive immunization of intact monkeys with an antibody directed at the alpha subunit of inhibin produces an additional two- to threefold increase in FSH levels after LHRH administration.[292] Passive immunization to endogenous inhibin in the diestrous female rat also increases FSH release. In addition, frequency and amplitude of LH pulsatile secretion are enhanced and responsiveness to exogenous LHRH is increased. In vivo and in vitro studies indicate that inhibin selectively reduces mRNA levels for FSH beta subunit, and in vitro studies suggest that activin selectively increases FSH beta subunit mRNA levels.[293–295]

Follistatin is a single chain glycosylated polypeptide produced by the ovary and is not a member of the inhibin family.[296, 297] However, it selectively decreases levels of FSH beta mRNA and inhibits FSH secretion in vitro, as does inhibin.[294]

Menstrual and Estrous Cycles. During menstrual and estrous cycles there is dissociated regulation of LH and FSH secretion. Steady-state mRNA levels or transcription of RNA encoding the alpha, LH beta, and FSH beta subunits has not been measured in primates during the menstrual cycle, but changes in both the steady-state levels[298, 299] and transcription rates occur during the rat estrous cycle.[254] The proestrous LH surge at 7 PM is preceded by an increase in LH beta mRNA levels at 6 PM (Fig. 6–17). A rapid increase in FSH beta mRNA level occurs at 8 PM immediately after the LH surge, and there are no changes in alpha subunit mRNA

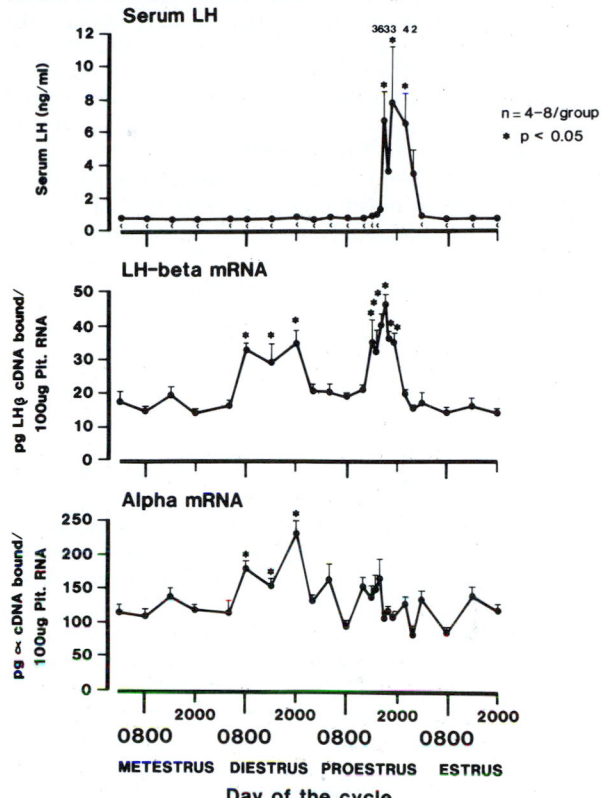

ALPHA AND LH-BETA mRNA DURING THE RAT ESTROUS CYCLE

Figure 6–17. Changes in serum LH concentrations and subunit mRNA levels during the rat estrous cycle. Serum LH and pituitary alpha and LH beta mRNA levels from individual pituitaries were measured at various times during the rat estrous cycle. Mean (± SEM) serum LH, LH beta, and alpha mRNA levels are shown in the upper, middle, and lower panels, respectively. < denotes undetectable LH levels. Asterisks denote significant increases over values observed at metestrus. (Modified from SM Zmeili, SS Papavasiliou, MO Thorner, et al., Alpha and luteinizing hormone beta subunit messenger ribonucleic acids during the rat estrous cycle, Endocrinology, 119, 1867–1869, © by The Endocrine Society.)

level at the time of the preovulatory LH surge. A modest increase occurs in both alpha and LH beta levels at 8 PM in diestrus. In addition, FSH beta mRNA levels increase from 11 PM in estrus until 5 PM in diestrus. Similarly, transcription rates for LH beta mRNA are twofold higher on the afternoon of proestrus compared with metestrus, and FSH beta mRNA transcription is increased at proestrus and continues to increase until the morning of metestrus.

LH AND FSH SECRETION. Circulating concentrations of gonadotropins as measured by immunological and bioassay techniques are not always closely correlated.[300] After a single injection of LH in men, the half-time of the first phase of biexponential kinetics was 18 ± 5 min and that of the second phase was 90 ± 15 min for immunoreactive LH. Corresponding values for bioactive LH were 32 ± 8 and 85 ± 7 min.[301] In a monoexponential model, immunoreactive and bioactive LH half-times were 47 ± 7 and 65 ± 5 min, respectively. The prolonged bioactive half-lives of LH and FSH are a result of their oligosaccharide content. Asialoglycoproteins (i.e., proteins stripped of sialic acid) are cleared rapidly by the liver.[302] The LH volume of distribution is approximately 3 L in a 70-kg man. The metabolic clearance rate for bioactive LH is 26 ± 3 mL/min/m² and for immunoreactive LH is 34 ± 3 mL/min/m².[301] The half-time of immunoreactive FSH is greater than that of LH. With a monoexponential model the half-time was 3.7 h, and with a two-compartment model it was 1.7 h for the first component and 8.3 h for the second component. Similarly, metabolic clearance of FSH is less than that of LH, being 6 to 14 mL/min in women and 4 to 12 mL/min in men.[303] Gonadal function does not affect the metabolic clearance rate.[300, 304, 305] Circulating LH and FSH are degraded by the liver and kidneys; small amounts of intact LH and FSH are excreted in the urine (e.g., 3 to 5% for FSH).

Estimates of production of immunoreactive LH and FSH are shown for normal men in Table 6–9. The production rates of LH and FSH increase 3- to 15-fold in women after menopause.

The two principal functions of the gonads in men and women are to produce gonadal steroids and gametes. These activities are regulated precisely by coordinated secretion of LH and FSH, which in turn are regulated by hypothalamic LHRH secretion and feedback effects of gonadal steroids and peptides. These hormones are also responsible for the timing and control of pubertal development. With aging, some reduction in gonadal function may occur in men; this reduction may be centrally mediated (a reduction of bioactive LH levels) and is different from the primary ovarian failure of female menopause. Menopause in women also differs from development of anestrus in older female rats, which is hypothalamic, not ovarian, in origin.

The regulation of LH and FSH secretion is unique in that the pulsatile patterns of gonadotropin and LHRH secretion are necessary for normal gonadal stimulation. Destruction of the arcuate nucleus in the monkey results in reduction in gonadotropin secretion.[306] Studies in primates have provided insight into gonadotropin secretion. The cells responsible for generating pulsatile LHRH secretion (the LHRH pulse generator) reside in the mediobasal hypothalamus. In the female rhesus monkey, deafferentation of the mediobasal hypothalamus (i.e., disconnection of the mediobasal hypothalamus from the rest of the brain) does not interfere with the menstrual cycle. Studies of gonadectomized monkeys with electrolytic destruction of the mediobasal hypothalamus showed that the mode of LHRH administration (continuous or intermittent) is critical. Continuous LHRH infusion initially stimulates LH and FSH secretion; after 7 to 10 d the response diminishes and LH and FSH concentrations return to baseline, essentially undetectable levels. In contrast, intermittent pulsatile administration of LHRH every hour stimulates gonadotropin secretion indefinitely in ovariectomized animals; in animals with ovaries and mesiobasal hypothalamic lesions, pulsatile administration of LHRH sustains the menstrual cycle. Variation in the frequency of LHRH administration to gonadectomized animals alters the ratio of LH to FSH; increasing the interval between LHRH pulses from 1 to 3 h preferentially increases FSH secretion. These findings have been the basis for many human studies, particularly in subjects with isolated gonadotropin deficiency (Kallmann's syndrome). Kallmann's syndrome involves either disordered LHRH secretion or defi-

ciency of LHRH neuronal development or migration. In one fetus with this condition, lack of migration of LHRH neurons from the fetal olfactory pit was demonstrated.[307] Pulsatile administration of LHRH reverses human hypothalamic hypogonadism of either congenital or acquired etiology.[308] Long-acting LHRH agonist analogues are administered to simulate continuous administration. As in the monkey, this mode of administration initially increases gonadotropin secretion, but within 14 d gonadotropin secretion is inhibited and gonadal function ceases. This therapy is useful for controlling gonadotropin-dependent precocious puberty; for inhibiting ovarian function, for example, in endometriosis; and for treating metastatic prostatic cancer ("medical gonadectomy"). Effective LHRH antagonists may replace the LHRH agonists in the future. They have the advantage of immediately suppressing, rather than initially stimulating, gonadotropin secretion. Antagonists, in contrast to agonists, do not require receptor down-regulation to suppress gonadotropin secretion.

The exact secretory profile of LHRH in the portal circulation of humans is unknown, but in other species LHRH pulses have brief duration and high amplitude.[309–312] A number of neurotransmitters influence LHRH secretion and mediate the effects of gonadal steroids on LHRH secretion (Table 6–10). For example the suppressive effects of estradiol and dihydrotestosterone on LH secretion are blocked by opiate antagonists. Androgens exert negative feedback by suppressing the frequency of LHRH pulsatile secretion and may also reduce the release of bioactive LH. Estrogen administration to men reduces the amplitude, but not the frequency, of LH pulsations and may also reduce the ratio of bioactivity to immunological activity. Positive feedback by estradiol is responsible for the midcycle LH surge in women, and positive feedback by estradiol is not normally operative in men. The ontogeny of gonadotropin secretion in humans has been reviewed by Grumbach and Kaplan.[313] A schematic representation of the components and interactions of the hypothalamic-pituitary-gonadal axis and their respective characteristics are shown in Figure 6–18.

TABLE 6–9. Production Rates of Immunoradiometric Luteinizing Hormone and Follicle-Stimulating Hormone Determined by Deconvolution Analysis

Subjects	LH (IU/24 h)*	FSH (IU/24 h)*
Men	230[847]†	53 ± 12.8[848]
Ovulating women	200[264]‡	NA§
Postmenopausal women	3500[849]†	NA

*Assuming mean volume of distribution of 2.5 L.
†The bioactive LH production rate is considerably higher at 2400 IU/24 h[850] in men and 10,000 IU/24 h in postmenopausal women.[849]
‡Immunoreactive LH production rates do not vary significantly with various stages of the menstrual cycle.[264]
§NA, not available.

TABLE 6–10. Effects of Various Factors on Secretion of Luteinizing Hormone and Follicle-Stimulating Hormone in Men

Factor	LH		FSH	
	Frequency	Amplitude	Frequency	Amplitude
Androgen (nonaromatized)	↓	None	None	↓
Estrogen	↓ *	↓ *	None (decreases half-life)	
Opiate antagonist†	↑ *	↑ *	NT‡	
Alpha-adrenergic antagonist	None in men		NT	

*Demonstrated in women also, in whom stage of the menstrual cycle influences the exact nature of the response.
†Effect dependent on adequate negative feedback by gonadal steroids.
‡NT, not tested.

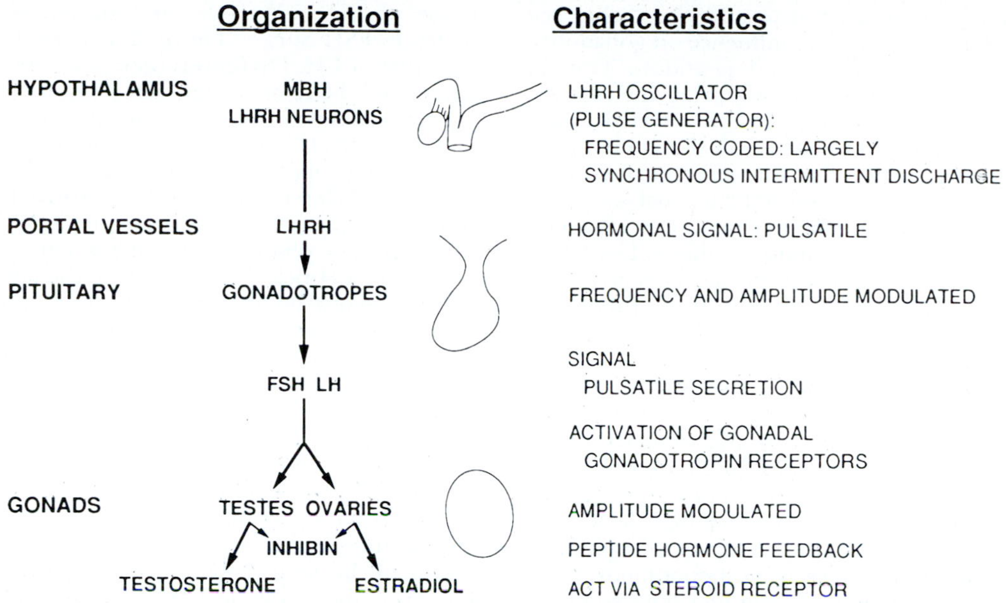

Organization   ## Characteristics

Figure 6–18. Organization and characteristics of the hypothalamic-pituitary-gonadal axis. The medial basal hypothalamus (MBH) contains the LHRH neurons, which translate neural signals into a periodic, oscillatory chemical signal, LHRH. This MBH complex functions as an oscillator (LHRH pulse generator), which is frequency coded and releases LHRH from its axon terminals at the median eminence into the hypothalamic-hypophyseal portal circulation with synchronous intermittent discharge. The LHRH pulse generator is influenced by neurotransmitters, peptidergic neuromodulators, neuroexcitatory amino acids, and neural pathways. During the follicular phase in adult women and men, an LHRH pulse occurs approximately every 90 to 120 min throughout the day. Changes in the frequency and amplitude of the LHRH-secretory episodes modulate the pattern of LH and FSH secretion. Circulating inhibin and gonadal steroids influence the secretion of gonadotropins by acting on both the hypothalamus and the pituitary. (Modified from Grumbach MM, Kaplan SL. The neuroendocrinology of human puberty: an ontogenetic perspective. In: Grumbach MM, Sizonenko PC, Aubert ML, eds. Control of the Onset of Puberty. Baltimore: Williams & Wilkins, 1990: 1–68. © 1990, the Williams & Wilkins Co., Baltimore.)

Gonadal maturation is regulated by gonadotropin. True precocious puberty can occur as early as the first months of life because the onset of puberty is not limited by the hypothalamic LHRH neurons, pituitary gland, gonads, or gonadal steroid target organs from infancy to the normal pubertal age. Before puberty, the release of FSH is greater than that of LH; this relation is reversed at puberty.[314] The prepubertal pattern can be overridden in primates by pulsatile chemical stimulation of the hypothalamus to activate LHRH neurons[283] or by pulsatile LHRH administration to stimulate the pituitary;[315] an adult pattern of gonadotropin secretion is induced and puberty follows. However, if exogenous LHRH is discontinued, gonadotropin secretion regresses to the prepubertal pattern and puberty will commence at the appropriate time. Thus the pubertal response to LHRH likely reflects the hormonal input rather than the stage of development. The differential release of LH or FSH is not well understood but may reflect inhibin secretion. The major restraint on prepubertal LHRH secretion originates in the central nervous system (CNS). Grumbach and Kaplan[313] have postulated the ontogeny of development of the human hypothalamic–pituitary gonadotropin–gonadal axis and divided the process into five stages: fetus, early infancy, late infancy and childhood, late prepubertal period, and puberty. (Also see Chapter 22.)

Fetus. By day 80 of gestation the mediobasal hypothalamic LHRH neurons (pulse generator) are operative and stimulate pulsatile LH and FSH secretion. From days 100 to 150 of gestation LHRH secretion is unrestrained. Development of negative feedback by gonadal steroids occurs by day 150 of gestation. After day 150 suppression of LHRH appears to be greater in the male fetus, a phenomenon attributed to the effect of testosterone.

Early Infancy. At term, the secretion of LHRH is low, and after delivery levels of plasma hCG, alpha subunit, and placental steroids decline in both sexes and testosterone levels decline in the male. Hypothalamic LHRH pulsatile secretion is active by 12 d of age, and prominent FSH and LH episodic discharges occur until approximately 6 mo of age in boys and 12 mo of age in girls. Transient increases in plasma testosterone and estradiol occur in boys and girls, respectively.

Late Infancy and Childhood. A proposed intrinsic CNS inhibition of hypothalamic LHRH secretion becomes functional, and by 4 y of age inhibition of LHRH is maximal. The negative feedback of LH and FSH secretion is sensitive to gonadal steroids (low set point). LHRH pulsatile secretion is inhibited, and the amplitude and frequency of LHRH discharges are low with resulting minimal secretion of FSH, LH, and gonadal steroids.

Late Prepubertal Period. The intrinsic CNS inhibitory influences and the sensitivity of the hypothalamus and pituitary to gonadal steroids decrease concomitantly, resulting in an increased set point and an increased amplitude and frequency of LHRH pulses. Initially these pulses are most prominent during sleep. There are an increase in gonadotrope sensitivity to LHRH, increased secretion of FSH and LH, and increased gonadal responsiveness to FSH and LH, with consequent increase in gonadal hormone secretion.

Puberty. A further decrease occurs in both the CNS restraint of the hypothalamic "LHRH pulse generator" and the sensitivity to negative feedback by gonadal steroids. The prominent sleep-associated increase in episodic secretion of LHRH gradually changes to the adult pattern of one pulse approximately every 90 min throughout the day; the pulsatile pattern of LH follows this LHRH pattern. Progressive development of secondary sexual characteristics occurs, and spermatogenesis is initiated in boys. In girls, at middle to late puberty, the capacity for estrogen positive feedback develops, culminating in a midcycle LH surge and ovulation.

This schema provides a logical explanation for the changes in gonadotropin levels that are observed, not only during puberty but also in agonadal children. Agonadal children have relatively low levels of LH and FSH at birth.

During the first 2 y of life, according to the model just outlined, the predominant negative influence on gonadotropin secretion is gonadal steroids (and peptides). Thus in these children LH and FSH levels rise during the first 2 y of life to levels similar to those observed in castrated adults. At 2 to 4 y of age there is a progressive decline in both LH and FSH levels, reflecting the maturation of intrinsic CNS inhibition. This decrease persists until the normal age of the late prepubertal period, when the intrinsic CNS inhibition declines and LH and FSH levels similar to those of castrated adults are once more observed. Furthermore, central precocious puberty is considered to result from premature cessation of or inadequate development of the intrinsic CNS inhibition of pulsatile secretion.

Menstrual Cycle. The minimal requirements for the complicated changes in gonadotropin secretion during the menstrual cycle can be generated by the pituitary under invariant pulsatile LHRH stimulation (e.g., LHRH pump therapy at one fixed dose administered hourly for the full cycle of 28 d). This suggests that the feedback effects of gonadal steroids and peptides can occur at the pituitary level. It is likely that under physiological conditions, there are additional levels of regulation, including the hypothalamus. During the menstrual cycle, changes occur in the frequency and amplitude of LHRH bursts secreted into the portal circulation.

During the normal menstrual cycle characteristic changes occur in the serum concentrations of LH and FSH. Figure 6–19 shows gonadotropin, 17-hydroxyprogesterone, progesterone, and basal body temperature changes during a normal menstrual cycle synchronized around the day of the midcycle preovulatory peak. LH levels rise slightly during the follicular phase, peak at the time of the midcycle surge, and then decrease during the luteal phase of the cycle. The serum FSH concentration begins to rise during the late luteal phase, increases during the early follicular

phase of the next cycle, and decreases just before the midcycle FSH surge. The midcycle FSH surge is smaller than that of LH. FSH levels then decrease during the luteal phase and increase again before the next menses. This profile is based on results from groups of normal women sampled daily. Gonadotropin secretion has also been studied by sampling subjects at frequent intervals, e.g., every 10 or 20 min, at different stages of the menstrual cycle.[316–318] These studies demonstrate that the frequency of LH peaks varies with different phases of the menstrual cycle. The greatest number of LH peaks occurs during the late follicular phase, and the fewest occur during the luteal phase of the cycle, with an intermediate number during the early follicular phase. LH secretion has been calculated using deconvolution analysis, which demonstrated that the number (mean ± SEM) of LH-secretory bursts per 24 h is maximal in the late follicular phase (27 ± 1.6), minimal in the midluteal phase (10 ± 1), and intermediate in the early follicular phase (18 ± 1.4).[264] There is no evidence of tonic (i.e., intersecretory burst) LH secretion during any phase of the menstrual cycle, and no differences have been documented in the LH half-life or in the total daily secretion of LH during the cycle. However, the midcycle LH surge was not studied. These studies suggest that the mode of pulsatile LH secretion is the distinct signal for the ovary because the total amount of LH secreted over 24 h is the same in early follicular, late follicular, and luteal phases of the menstrual cycle. These studies also suggest that if the LH pulses reflect hypothalamic LHRH pulsatility, variations in the frequency of LHRH secretion also occur during the menstrual cycle. In sheep, concordance has been demonstrated between peripheral LH concentration peaks and peaks of LHRH in the hypothalamic-pituitary portal blood.[309]

LH AND FSH ACTIONS.* LH is primarily responsible for the regulation of gonadal steroid production by Leydig cells of the testis and by the ovarian follicles. The preovulatory LH surge in women produces rupture and luteinization of the follicle. FSH stimulates gametogenesis. In the male FSH stimulates Sertoli cells, which have an important role in spermatogenesis, and in the female FSH is important for follicular development. FSH also stimulates the production of LH receptors on the Leydig cell.

hCG is produced primarily by the placenta, but small amounts are synthesized by the pituitary and other tissues. hCG has a longer half-life than LH, but the two have similar actions. hCG is the most important hormone involved in maintaining the corpus luteum during pregnancy. Because it can easily be extracted in large quantities from the urine of pregnant women, hCG is used as replacement therapy for LH to treat delayed puberty or infertility.

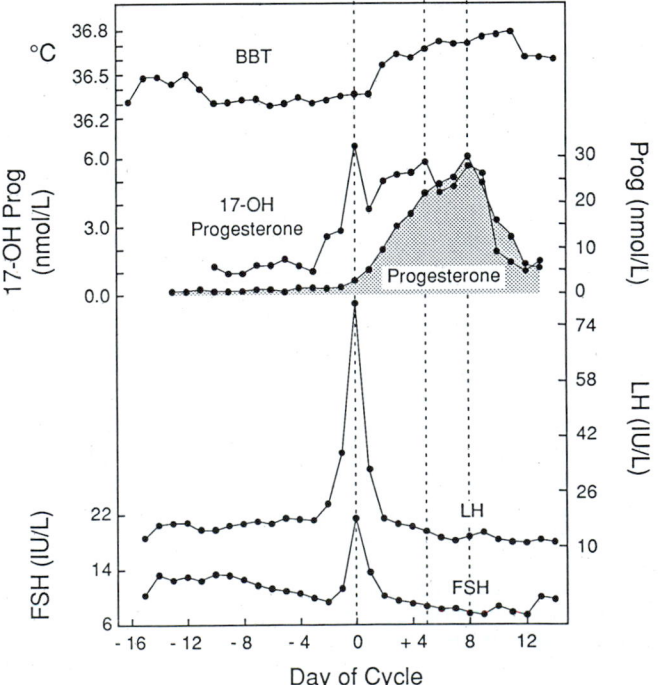

Figure 6–19. Mean daily plasma FSH, LH, progesterone, and 17-hydroxyprogesterone concentrations and basal body temperature (BBT) during 16 presumptive ovulatory cycles in 15 young women. (Modified from Ross GT, Cargille CM, Lipsett MB, et al. Pituitary and gonadal hormones in women during spontaneous and induced ovulatory cycles. Recent Prog Horm Res 1970; 26:1–62.)

UNSOLVED PROBLEMS IN PITUITARY FUNCTION

The classification of pituitary cell types and the hormones that are secreted by a given cell provide a limited explanation for the genealogy of pituitary tumors. The identification of tumor cells that secrete several classes of hormones, e.g., GH, prolactin, and TSH, is difficult to reconcile with our understanding of the lineage of different pituitary cell types. The characterization of transcription factors in the pituitary may provide new insights into the ontogeny.

Cloning of cDNAs encoding various hypothalamic hor-

---

*For more detail see Chapters 12 and 13.

mones, pituitary hormones, and receptors will provide insight into the evolution of different members of a hormone family and into the pathogenesis of various inherited endocrinopathies. For example, the demonstration that defects in the gene encoding the GH receptor are associated clinically with GH resistance (i.e., Laron dwarfism) provided insight into the pathogenesis of the disorder and into the function of the normal receptor.[107, 319, 320] The structures of many complex molecules have been determined with the application of molecular biology. Examples relevant to the anterior pituitary are the elucidation of the structure of inhibin and receptors for dopamine (D_2), GH, LH, insulin, and IGF I, and for at least one hypothalamic hormone, TRH.[320a]

Anterior Pituitary Ontogeny

Immunohistochemical studies indicate that five phenotypically distinct cell types appear during anterior pituitary ontogeny in a characteristic order that appears to be species independent. The expression of the α-glycoprotein subunit before the formation of Rathke's pouch heralds the onset of pituitary organogenesis.[321] The order of appearance of distinct cell types is: corticotropes producing POMC, thyrotropes producing TSH, gonadotropes producing LH and FSH, somatotropes producing GH, and lactotropes producing prolactin. The coexpression of GH and prolactin in precursor cells before the appearance of the mature lactotrope cell and in a subpopulation of mature anterior pituitary cells suggests that prolactin and GH genes are regulated by related factors. Studies in transgenic mice, using as the reporter gene as few as 181 base pairs of the rat GH promoter linked to the human GH gene, revealed that the human GH gene is expressed primarily in somatotrope cells but also in a subset of cells that produce TSH and prolactin, suggesting a functional relationship between activation of expression of the GH, prolactin, and TSH genes.[322]

The ontogeny of cells that produce GH and prolactin has been analyzed by using the approach of gene-directed ablation in transgenic mice. Transgenic mice were created that carried either the herpesvirus 1–thymidine kinase (HSV1-TK) gene or the diphtheria toxin A chain (DT-A) gene under control of the rat GH or prolactin gene promoter. Cells expressing the HSV1-TK gene acquire pharmacological sensitivity to synthetic nucleosides whose metabolites kill dividing cells.[323] Expression of DT-A results in ADP-ribosylation of elongation factor 2, which inhibits protein synthesis.[324] Data from gene-directed ablation studies in transgenic mice demonstrate that most lactotrope cells are derived from the presomatotrope (or mammosomatotrope) line. Expression of HSV1-TK linked to the GH promoter causes dwarfism with nearly complete obliteration of GH- and prolactin-producing cells; expression of ACTH, TSH, LH, and FSH was unaffected. In contrast, animals carrying HSV1-TK coupled to the prolactin promoter have anatomically and physiologically normal pituitaries, suggesting that prolactin expression and lactotrope cell differentiation are postmitotic events (because HSV1-TK expression is toxic only to dividing cells). Delaying the onset of treatment with synthetic nucleosides results in a graded increase in the number of somatotrope cells, but the lactotrope cell population remains repressed, suggesting that postmitotic somatotrope cells cannot progress toward lactotrope cells. When animals are treated with nucleosides and allowed to recover, a rebound in somatotrope cell number and an increase in body weight are observed; partial recovery in lactotrope cell number occurs. Therefore, it appears that a replicating and potentially self-renewing GH-expressing cell (the stem somatotrope cell) is a common precursor of the terminally differentiated somatotrope and lactotrope cells, supporting a model of direct descent.[323]

Transcription Factors and the Anterior Pituitary

The factors that regulate differentiation of the five phenotypic cell types and the expression of specific hormones in specific cell types are incompletely understood. In 1988 a 33-kd protein that binds cell-specific DNA elements in the rat prolactin and GH genes, referred to as Pit-1 (or GHF-1), was characterized.[325–327] The Pit-1 gene transcript is initially detected during embryonic day 15 of the rat in most cells of the anterior pituitary. Although all five phenotypically pituitary cell types express the Pit-1 gene transcript, the Pit-1 protein is detected in the nuclei only of thyrotrope, lactotrope, and somatotrope cells. The absence of the protein in gonadotrope and corticotrope cells probably reflects a specific inhibitory mechanism preventing translation of Pit-1 mRNA or alternate splicing of the gene transcript. The COOH terminus of Pit-1 shows homology with some Drosophila developmental genes, and it is likely that both types of protein are members of a family of transcription factors. Pit-1 binds to two specific regions of the 5'-flanking promoter regions of the GH and prolactin genes. This binding permits full basal and hormonally regulated tissue expression. When transfected into nonpituitary cells, Pit-1 permits expression of GH or prolactin fusion genes. Pit-1 and other (to be identified) transcription factors are believed to be responsible for tissue-specific expression. If transcription factors regulate hormone secretion by pituitary cells, it is also conceivable that they regulate pituitary cell differentiation. For example, some human pituitary tumors are immunopositive for GH, prolactin, and TSH; Pit-1 is found in thyrotrope cells, as well as in somatotrope and lactotrope cells, and its expression in thyrotrope cells may explain why these three hormones can be produced by the same cell. This hypothesis also provides a conceptual framework for explaining the high frequency of expression of multiple genes encoding unrelated pituitary hormones in a single pituitary tumor cell. The hypothesis is supported by observations in dwarf mice. In mutant strains of dwarf mice, including the Jackson, Snell, and Ames strains, there is no development of thyrotrope, lactotrope, or somatotrope cells. The Jackson mouse has a major deletion in the Pit-1 gene, the Snell has a point mutation in the Pit-1 gene, and the Pit-1 gene appears to be normal in the Ames mouse (ref. 328 and personal communication, M. G. Rosenfeld).

The expression in pituitary of Pit-1 on embryonic day 15 (of rat) precedes activation of the prolactin and GH genes. Pit-1 appears to be required for initial activation of both genes, but additional transcription factors are required to achieve full expression. Interactions between the prolactin promoter and the distal enhancer region, which contains an estrogen response element, are critical for prolactin gene expression;[329] the estrogen receptor probably acts in concert with Pit-1 to regulate prolactin transcription.[321] Because lactotrope cells appear to arise from stem somatotrope cells, secondary mechanisms must restrict GH expression. The expression of Pit-1 in thyrotrope cells suggests that other mechanisms prevent the expression of GH and prolactin in that cell type.[321, 329] Similarly, in somatotrope cells restrictive mechanisms must inhibit expression of prolactin and TSH. Post-transcriptional factors also influence the physiological patterns of gene expression that define the distinct pituitary cell types.[328]

Molecular Defects and Tumorigenesis

Insight into pituitary tumor development has come from study of somatotrope adenomas. cAMP is an intracellular second messenger for several tropic hormones. Landis and associates[330] have described mutations in four of eight GH-secreting human pituitary tumors. The point mutations cause constitutive activation of α_s, the GTP-binding subunit of the stimulatory regulator of adenylate cyclase, G_s, by inhibition of GTPase.[330] This mutation was present only in the pituitary tumor cells and not in leukocytes from the same patients.

Pituitary tumors also occur in multiple endocrine neoplasia type 1 (MEN 1). MEN 1 is an inherited disorder associated with parathyroid hyperplasia and tumors of the endocrine pancreas and anterior pituitary. The gene for MEN 1 has been assigned to chromosome 11q13.[331, 332] Insulinomas appear to be caused by unmasking of a recessive mutation in the MEN 1 locus. In examining whether a similar mechanism may apply for development of pituitary adenomas, Werner and colleagues demonstrated retention of the constitutional genotype on chromosome 11 in 27 sporadic pituitary adenomas (ref. 333 and personal communication, S. Werner). The DNA patterns of 27 pituitary adenomas were examined for any allele losses; 5 of 27 tumors had loss of alleles, but only 2 had losses of segments of chromosome 11 associated with MEN 1 development. One notably aggressive adenoma had allele losses related to five different chromosomes. Aneuploidy was present in 3 of 27 tumors, all of which were secretory and also affected by allele losses.

Clonality of Human Pituitary Tumors

It is possible under certain circumstances to determine whether tumors result from polyclonal proliferation or monoclonal expansion of a single aberrant cell. This is determined by assessing X-linked restriction fragment length polymorphisms (RFLPs) at genes for two enzymes, phosphoglycerate kinase and hypoxanthine phosphoribosyltransferase. Maternal and paternal X chromosomes can be distinguished by using such RFLPs and a methylation-sensitive restriction enzyme to identify allelic X inactivation patterns.

In polyclonal tissues in females the two X chromosomes should be randomly inactivated, whereas in monoclonal tumors only one of the two is inactivated, and this pattern persists through each cell cycle. By analyzing the pattern of X chromosome inactivation, several pituitary tumors have been demonstrated to be monoclonal in origin, including "nonfunctioning" tumors, somatotrope adenomas, prolactinomas, and corticotrope adenomas.[334, 335] Whether all pituitary tumors are monoclonal is not known.

Chromosomal Location of Human Genes Related to Anterior Pituitary Function

Whereas several cDNAs coding for hypothalamic and pituitary hormones and their receptors have been cloned, relatively few hypothalamic-pituitary diseases have been demonstrated to be caused by single gene defects. Inherited TSH deficiency results from a point mutation in TSH beta subunit, and some cases of Laron dwarfism are a result of either a point mutation or partial deletion of the gene coding for the human GH receptor. Table 6–11 shows the known chromosomal locations of some of the relevant genes.

APPROACH TO PITUITARY DISEASE

Pituitary tumors account for 10 to 15% of intracranial tumors in surgical specimens and 6 to 23% of intracranial tumors in unselected adult autopsy series.[336] Pituitary tumors are usually classified as microadenomas (diameter < 10 mm) and macroadenomas (diameter > 10 mm). The patient with a pituitary tumor presents with symptoms of a mass lesion, endocrine dysfunction, or both. Endocrine dysfunction may be either hyperfunction or hypofunction or a combination of the two.

Clinical Manifestations

PITUITARY MASS. The manifestations of a sellar mass (Fig. 6–20) include headache and symptoms secondary to compression of intracranial nerves, i.e., visual field distur-

TABLE 6–11. Chromosomal Location of Human Genes Related to Anterior Pituitary and Associated Clinical Disorders

Hormone	Chromosome	MIM Number*	Clinical Disorder†
Hypothalamic			
Somatostatin	3q28	18245	
LHRH	8p21-q11.2	15276	Kallmann's syndrome
CRH	8q13	12256	Isolated ACTH deficiency
AVP	20	19234	Diabetes insipidus
GHRH	20	13919	GH deficiency
Oxytocin	20	16705	Absent milk let-down reflex
Pituitary			
POMC	2p25	17683	ACTH deficiency
Prolactin	6p22.2-q21.3	17676	Prolactin deficiency
Alpha subunit	6q21.1-q23	11885	Glycoprotein hormone deficiency
VIP	6q26-q27	19232	
FSH beta	11p13	13653	Isolated FSH deficiency
GH/prolactin	17q22-q24	13925	GH and PL deficiency
CG beta‡	19q13.32	11886	Infertility
LH beta	19q13.32	15278	Isolated LH deficiency
TSH beta	1p22	18854	TSH deficiency[851, 852]
Other Relevant Genes			
GH receptor	5p13.1-p12		Laron dwarfism[853]
LH receptor			Resistant gonad syndrome
			Delayed puberty
D_2 receptor			Hyperprolactinemia
TRH receptor			Secondary hypothyroidism

*MIM number is the entry number in Mendelian Inheritance in Man and its on-line version (OMIM).
†Only referenced clinical disorders have been proved to give rise to these clinical disorders.
‡CG, chorionic gonadotropin.

Headaches

(a) stretching of dura
    by tumor

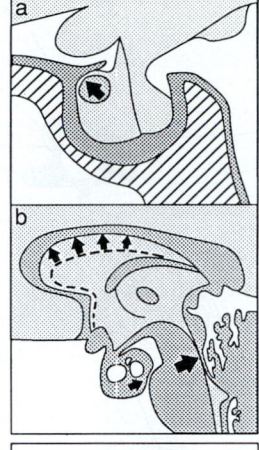

(b) hydrocephalus (rare)

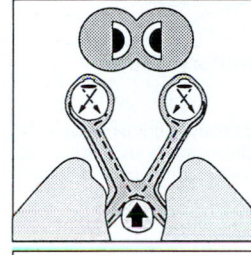

Visual Field Defects

nasal retinal fibers
compressed by tumor

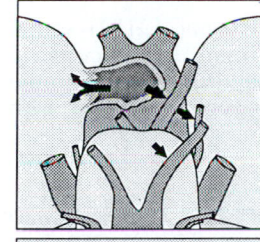

**Cranial Nerve Palsies
and Temporal Lobe
Epilepsy**

lateral extension of
tumor

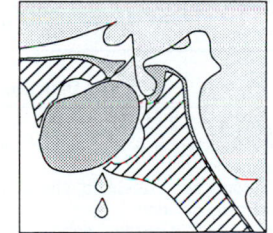

**Cerebrospinal Fluid
Rhinorrhea**

downward extension of
tumor

Figure 6–20. Various symptoms of a pituitary tumor. Headaches are rarely caused by hydrocephalus. Visual field defects caused by extension of the tumor are plotted by using the Goldmann perimeter. (From Wass JAH. Hypopituitarism. In: Besser GM, Cudworth AG, eds. Clinical Endocrinology: An Illustrated Text. London: Gower Medical, 1987: 2.1–2.14.)

bances, ophthalmoplegia, and, occasionally, compression of the first or second branch of the trigeminal nerve, giving rise to facial pain. The extent of abnormality depends on the size of the tumor and its anatomical position. Thus microadenomas may be asymptomatic except for producing endocrine dysfunction. A macroadenoma that extends inferiorly may also be asymptomatic other than causing headache, and a tumor extending superiorly and abutting the optic chiasm may produce visual field defects. The extent of the visual field defect varies. The classic finding with suprasellar extension of a pituitary adenoma is bitemporal hemianopsia, but any visual disturbance can occur, depending on the extent of suprasellar extension and the location of the optic chiasm, i.e., whether it is prefixed or postfixed (see Fig. 6–27). A pituitary tumor can cause diminished visual acuity, scotoma, quadrantic defects, and total blindness of one or both eyes.[337] The fibers of the optic nerve course along a precise path, depending on the site of origin in the retina. Thus fibers from the temporal halves of the retina (for nasal vision) do not cross but course posteriorly along the ipsilateral optic tract. The fibers from the nasal half of the retina (for temporal vision) cross in the chiasm and course posteriorly along the contralateral optic tract. Bitemporal hemianopsia, when present, is often asymmetrical.

Headache from pituitary tumor can be variable and nonspecific. It may be occipital, but retro-orbital pain or bitemporal headaches are more typical, are sometimes worse on awakening, and generally improve over the course of the day. The headache is often ameliorated by aspirin or other analgesics. The pathogenesis of the headache is unknown, but it may result from stretching of the dura mater (i.e., diaphragma sellae) above the pituitary fossa. Very large pituitary tumors or suprasellar hypothalamic tumors, e.g., craniopharyngioma, may extend sufficiently superiorly or posteriorly to compress either the foramen of Monro or the aqueduct of Sylvius. The former leads to obstruction of the lateral ventricles and the latter to obstruction of the CSF flow from the third ventricle to the fourth ventricle. This leads to hydrocephalus involving the lateral ventricles or the lateral and third ventricles, respectively.

The relationship of the pituitary gland to the cavernous sinus is shown in Figure 6–21. Extensive lateral extension of a pituitary tumor may produce dysfunction of cranial nerves III, IV, V_1, V_2, and VI.

The frequency of headache and visual disturbance in patients with pituitary tumors is not clear. Patients with macroadenomas usually have marked symptoms from the mass lesion, although large tumors may be discovered incidentally during evaluation for another medical complaint. In a series of 1000 pituitary tumors, described by Hollenhorst and Younge,[338] symptoms of visual disturbance occurred during the course in 61% of the patients. Loss of vision was the presenting complaint in 42%, and diplopia was the presenting complaint in less than 1%. If the tumor extends inferiorly the patient may have no symptoms or may develop sphenoid sinusitis. Rare complications include CSF rhinorrhea (the fluid discharged contains glucose) and recurrent meningitis from erosion of the sella turcica and loss of the barrier between the CSF and the exterior. Giant tumors may extend into the temporal lobes and cause temporal lobe epilepsy and occasionally can extend to the cerebral peduncles and give rise to motor and/or sensory disturbances.

MANIFESTATIONS OF ANTERIOR PITUITARY HORMONE DEFICIENCY. Total or selective hypopituitarism may occur in patients with pituitary adenomas, those with parasellar diseases (see later), those who have undergone pituitary surgery or radiation (including cranial radiation for intracranial malignancies), or those who have had head injury. The anterior pituitary secretes six major hormones (LH, FSH, GH, TSH, ACTH, and prolactin), and deficiency of any or all can occur. The most common symptom in both men and women is cessation of gonadal function. The secondary hypogonadism may result from LH and FSH deficiency but may also occur with hyperprolactinemia. The classic finding is progressive loss of pituitary hormone secretion in the following order: gonadotropin (LH, FSH), GH, TSH, ACTH. However, variations occur, and some patients have ACTH and/or TSH deficiency as the presenting feature. Prolactin deficiency is uncommon and is usually caused by pituitary infarction. In children, cessation of growth and delayed puberty are common presentations.

GROWTH HORMONE DEFICIENCY. GH deficiency in adults is not recognized as a pathological syndrome. However, GH has a number of important physiological actions, including partitioning of nutrients and energy and maintenance of muscle mass, and it is possible that GH deficiency

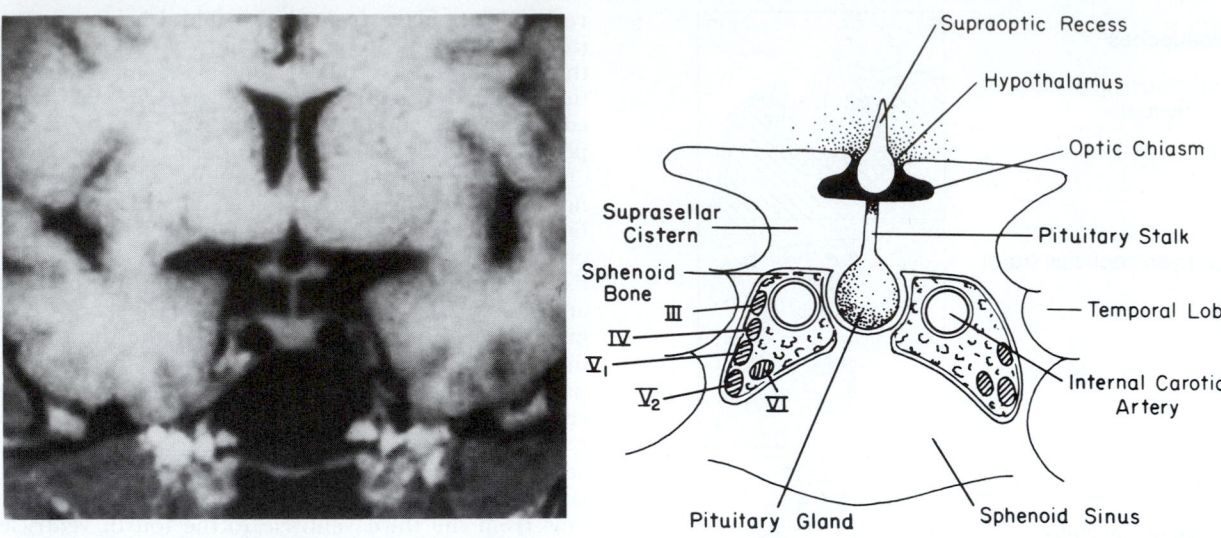

Figure 6–21. MRI scan *(left)* and schematic diagram *(right)* of the normal pituitary fossa. The pituitary is bordered laterally by the cavernous sinus, which contains the internal carotid artery and cranial nerves III, IV, V₁, V₂, and VI. The optic chiasm lies immediately above the pituitary gland and is separated from it by a CSF-filled cistern. Note the location of the sphenoid sinus and temporal lobes. (From Lechan RM. Neuroendocrinology of pituitary hormone regulation. Endocrinol Metab Clin North Am 1987; 16:475–502.)

may cause symptoms in the adult. Studies of short-term GH administration to GH-deficient adults indicate that such replacement may be beneficial for restoration of muscle mass, skinfold thickness, and nutrient utilization.[188, 189, 339]

The manifestations of GH deficiency in children depend on the age of onset. GH deficiency in children is associated with short stature, relatively good nutrition (weight for height), and reduced growth velocity. Neonatal GH deficiency is characterized by hypoglycemia that is particularly severe in infants with other anterior pituitary failure but also occurs with isolated GH deficiency. GH is not required for normal intrauterine growth, so that GH-deficient children are usually of normal weight and length at birth; during the first 2 y growth velocity decreases, with a decline in the height and growth velocity percentiles. Weight is normal for length or height, and bone age is frequently delayed. It is important to measure the growth velocity as well as the height and weight percentiles because height reflects only the cumulative growth. For example, a child starting off in the 70th percentile would have had a prolonged reduction in growth velocity before being observed to be in the third percentile for height.

GH deficiency in children can be either congenital or acquired (for a detailed discussion see Chapter 21). Idiopathic GH deficiency is most often a result of deficiency of hypothalamic GHRH, and mutations of the GH gene itself are rare. Other causes of GH deficiency are associated with developmental abnormalities such as aplasia or hypoplasia of the pituitary and midline brain abnormalities. Acquired causes include tumors of the hypothalamus or pituitary, other intracranial tumors such as optic nerve glioma, hypopituitarism secondary to cranial radiation, head injury (including injury at birth), and infection or inflammation. GH deficiency may also occur in the setting of severe psychosocial deprivation. The incidence of different causes of GH deficiency depends on the population studied. Table 6–12 shows the incidence of the various causes of GH deficiency in a large central pediatric growth clinic in Paris, France. In contrast to experience in the United States, the majority of the French children had radiation-induced GH deficiency.

GONADOTROPIN DEFICIENCY. Gonadotropin deficiency results from either a pituitary defect or deficiency of

hypothalamic LHRH stimulation of the gonadotrope. Gonadotropin deficiency may occur because of hypothalamic disease, disease of the pituitary stalk, or a functional abnormality such as occurs with hyperprolactinemia, anorexia

TABLE 6–12. Causes of Growth Hormone Deficiency and Their Relative Incidence in 369 Cases (1970–1981), Hôpital des Enfants Malades, Paris, France

GH Deficiency	Relative Incidence
Idiopathic, n = 82 (22%)	
Sporadic (isolated or part of multiple anterior pituitary deficiencies)	64
Familial (only two associated with absence of GH because of GH gene deletion)	10
Associated with idiopathic diabetes insipidus	8
Organic, n = 287 (78%)	
Secondary to cranial radiation[854–856] (n = 191)	
Acute lymphocytic leukemia	77
Retinoblastoma	18
Medulloblastoma	35
Other head and neck tumors	21
Optic glioma	40
Secondary tumors (before or after surgery) (n = 49)	
Craniopharyngioma	35
Other tumors in hypothalamic-pituitary area	14
Associated with cranial malformations (n = 25)	
Suprasellar arachnoid cyst	6
Hydrocephalus	2
Cleft lip and palate or single incisor and other midline defects	17
Associated with cranial trauma	1
Associated with various diseases (n = 21)	
Diabetes insipidus with histiocytosis X	6
Thalassemia major	1
Diabetes mellitus, insulin dependent	3
Athyroidism	1
Gonadal dysgenesis	1
Nephroblastoma	1
Renal hypoplasia	1
Constitutional bone dysplasia	1
Gastrointestinal tract, facial malformations with omphalocele	2
William-Beuren syndrome	1
Blackfan-Diamond syndrome	1
Mitochondrial defect	1
Dandy-Walker syndrome	1

Personal communication, R. Rappaport.

nervosa, secondary adrenal insufficiency, or secondary hypothyroidism.

Gonadotropin deficiency often occurs early in the course of development of hypopituitarism. In adolescents, it causes delayed or arrested puberty. In women it is manifested by infertility, menstrual disorders, or amenorrhea. The resulting low serum estradiol levels are in the range of those of the follicular phase of the menstrual cycle. Hypoestrogenemia is often associated with lack of libido and dyspareunia; long-standing estrogen deficiency produces breast atrophy. However, in women who are hypogonadal from hyperprolactinemia, breast atrophy is not observed. Long-standing estrogen deficiency of any etiology causes development of osteopenia. In men, the hypogonadism may be undiagnosed because the syndrome develops slowly and the diminished libido and impotence may be discounted as a function of "age." More often hypogonadism is diagnosed retrospectively when the patient presents with the symptoms of a mass lesion. Even if the patient is unaware of deficiencies, his sexual partner may provide a more accurate and objective assessment of the onset of sexual dysfunction. As in women, gonadotropin deficiency in men may result from hyperprolactinemia (see later). Low gonadotropin concentrations result in serum testosterone levels in the prepubertal range, and testicular size may decrease; testicular consistency may be soft. Acquired gonadotropin deficiency is a rare cause of male infertility. Spermatogenesis is often well preserved, and the principal abnormality of the semen analysis is a reduced ejaculate volume, which is a function of the serum testosterone concentration. Beard growth and muscle bulk may also be reduced, and osteopenia also develops with long-standing hypogonadism. Hypogonadal men and women often develop fine wrinkling of the skin of the face, particularly around the mouth and eyes.

THYROTROPIN DEFICIENCY. Secondary hypothyroidism usually occurs relatively late in the course of hypopituitarism and is characterized by failure to thrive, weight gain, lack of energy, cold intolerance, and constipation. The degree of hypothyroidism depends on the duration of TSH deficiency but is rarely as severe as that of primary hypothyroidism.

ACTH DEFICIENCY. Secondary adrenal failure may occur as an isolated deficiency or in the course of the development of panhypopituitarism. The symptoms are essentially the same as those of primary adrenal insufficiency (see Chapter 9) but differ in two important respects. Secondary adrenal insufficiency results from lack of ACTH stimulation of the adrenal and therefore affects only adrenal steroids under predominant ACTH regulation, namely cortisol and adrenal androgen. Mineralocorticoid secretion, primarily regulated by renin and angiotensin, is preserved, although it may not be optimal. Because of preserved mineralocorticoid secretion, these patients may not experience an adrenal crisis. More commonly the symptoms are malaise, loss of energy, anorexia, weight loss, postural hypotension, and orthostatic dizziness. Such patients may be misdiagnosed as malingerers. Women tend to lose secondary sexual hair and libido, but men have preserved secondary sexual hair unless there is coexistent gonadotropin deficiency. In contrast to patients with primary adrenal insufficiency, these patients have a pale and sometimes slightly sallow complexion; ACTH levels are low, and there is no hyperpigmentation. Severe cortisol deficiency may result in hypoglycemia and hyponatremia; hyperkalemia usually occurs only with aldosterone deficiency. These patients, particularly those with panhypopituitarism, may deteriorate gradually, and a relatively trivial illness may precipitate vascular collapse, coma, or hypoglycemia-induced seizure. Adrenal insufficiency, regardless of the cause, is a medical emergency.

Morphological Classification of Pituitary Adenomas

The old tinctorial classification of pituitary adenomas, originating at the beginning of this century, has survived into the era of electron microscopy and immunohistochemistry despite the fact that not all acidophilic adenomas produce GH and the fact that more than half of chromophobic adenomas are endocrinologically active. Before 1970 there were few ultrastructural studies of adenomas associated with well-defined endocrine syndromes such as acromegaly or Cushing's disease.[340-342] Introduction of modern imaging techniques, development of improved hormone assays, and renewed interest in transsphenoidal pituitary surgery created an increasing volume of material for morphologists. Additional methods include the use of electron microscopy and immunohistochemistry.[343]

The functional classification of pituitary adenomas required histological, immunohistochemical, and electron microscopic investigation of surgical pituitary specimens and the attempt to characterize every normal and adenomatous cell type. Morphological findings are correlated with the clinical and laboratory information. This approach allows the morphological classification of tumors with known hormonal secretion and the delineation of several previously unknown entities. For example, three types of ultrastructurally distinct and, as judged by their features, hormonally active adenomas are now recognized that are not related to the known cell types.[344-346] These findings suggest that the cytological mapping of the pituitary is not yet complete and that additional cell types are likely to be discovered. Table 6–13 shows the functional morphological classification of pituitary adenomas and their prevalence in unselected surgical specimens.

This classification,[347] which has gained wide acceptance, is useful for predicting the biological behavior, natural history, growth pattern, and age-related occurrence of various adenoma types. Electron microscopy is eminently suitable for investigating the effect of drugs, such as dopamine agonists and somatostatin analogues, on the structure of adenomas and correlating morphology with clinical results.

Progress in the field has resolved old questions, opened new avenues, and created new problems. Application of immunohistochemical testing led to discovery of plurihormonality[347-349] in pituitary adenomas. It became obvious that more than one hormone can be produced by the same tumor and by the same cells within a tumor; this was first demonstrated in acidophil stem cell adenoma[350] and later in monomorphous-bihormonal mammosomatotrope adenomas.[351] In addition, many (densely granulated) GH cell adenomas express alpha subunit, TSH, and sometimes even FSH and LH.[352] Glycoprotein hormone–producing adenomas often display minor immunoreactivity for GH and,

TABLE 6–13. Prevalence of Pituitary Adenoma Types in Unselected Surgical Material

Adenoma Type	Prevalence (%)
GH-producing adenoma	13.3
Prolactin-producing adenoma	27.3
GH- and prolactin-producing adenoma	7.5
Corticotrope adenoma	10.1
Silent corticotrope adenoma, subtypes 1, 2, 3	5.1
Thyrotrope adenoma	1.0
Gonadotrope adenoma	9.0
Null cell adenoma, including oncocytoma	25.6
Plurihormonal adenoma	1.1

Unpublished data, courtesy of E. Horvath and K. Kovacs.

rarely, for prolactin.[348] Thus immunohistochemistry, instead of sharply defining entities, created a certain degree of ambiguity in the classification of some tumors. Until the nature and significance are clarified, a prudent approach should be adopted toward the plurihormonal phenomena. Instead of creating new subgroups and expanding the classification, plurihormonality should be accommodated within the existing, well-characterized categories. The diagnosis of a plurihormonal adenoma is warranted only if clinical findings and/or multiple morphological phenotypes are compatible with overproduction of more than one hormone.

In the study of plurihormonality the most important question is whether the presence of multiple hormones in adenomas represents abnormal gene expression or is an abnormal amplification of genes that are normally expressed at a low level in the non-neoplastic phenotypes. It is not possible to provide an unequivocal solution to this problem. It is notable that colocalizations of GH and prolactin and of GH and alpha subunit have been demonstrated in normal human pituitary cells.[20] Furthermore, in lactotrope hyperplasia during pregnancy or lactation many cells express both prolactin and GH genes, strongly suggesting the participation of GH cells in the process.[353] In rats, estrogen-induced lactotrope hyperplasia is also often bihormonal.[354] In addition, a subset of somatotropes in the rat pituitary are capable of transforming into bihormonal thyroidectomy cells in experimentally induced hypothyroidism.[355] Thus a new perception of the pituitary gland is emerging; the seemingly homogeneous populations of five (or more) cell types is not really uniform but consists of subsets of cells with one primary function and the potential of producing other hormone(s). Proof of such a possibility may mean that plurihormonality in adenomas represents not abnormal gene expression but a deregulation and amplification of genes expressed in the mother cell that gave rise to the tumor.

Evaluation of Suspected Pituitary Disease

Therapy for pituitary tumors is dictated by the tumor type and the extent of growth. The evaluation of the patient with a pituitary tumor should determine (1) presence and type of hormone hypersecretion, (2) any hormonal deficiencies and need for replacement therapy, (3) presence of any visual abnormalities, and (4) pituitary anatomy including presence of extrasellar extension. Each of these areas needs to be evaluated before therapeutic intervention.

Assessment of Hypothalamic Pituitary Function

For each hyperfunctioning pituitary adenoma, specific tests are performed to confirm the clinical suspicion. In assessment of pituitary function a number of factors must be considered. These include (1) interpretation of the level of the pituitary hormone in relation to the level of the target hormone; (2) pulsatile secretion of anterior pituitary hormones; and (3) specific factors that affect the concentration of each of the pituitary hormones, e.g., time of day, stress, nutritional status (fed or fasting), whether the patient is asleep or awake, and stage of development. In general, screening for hyperfunction and hypofunction can usually be achieved by taking a history, performing a physical examination, and drawing a single basal blood sample for assessment of pituitary and target organ hormone levels. More subtle abnormalities require more sophisticated studies.

Table 6–14 shows the pituitary hormones and the target gland hormones. Normal ranges are not listed because they

TABLE 6–14. Pituitary and Target Hormones

Pituitary Hormone	Target Gland	Feedback Hormone
ACTH	Adrenal	Cortisol
TSH	Thyroid	T_4, T_3
LH	Gonad	Testosterone (men)
		Estradiol (women)
FSH	Gonad	Testosterone (men)
		Estradiol (women)
		Inhibin
GH	Liver, bone, adipocytes, and other tissues	IGF I
Prolactin	Breast	Unknown

vary from assay to assay. Each laboratory should provide a normal range of values for each test.

Interpretation of hormone concentrations requires consideration of several issues. Currently, hormone concentrations are measured by radioimmunoassay or by IRMA. The IRMAs are usually more specific and more sensitive and have a wider working concentration range than do radioimmunoassays. Precise results are more readily and rapidly available with the IRMA than with previous techniques, because the samples rarely need to be diluted. A limitation of IRMAs is that they are subject to matrix effects and may also give artifactual results, as do radioimmunoassays, when heterophile antibodies are present.[356–358] Binding proteins, precursors, and metabolites may also interfere with both radioimmunoassays and IRMAs and theoretically produce spuriously low values, particularly in IRMAs.

Plasma ACTH

This hormone is uncommonly measured. Many commercial kits are unsatisfactory in regard to precision of measurement at lower concentrations. Measurement of ACTH is probably required only in the evaluation of adrenal failure or Cushing's syndrome (see Chapter 9). Additional problems include the short plasma half-life of ACTH, which requires sample collection into a cold syringe, placement in an EDTA tube, immediate centrifugation at 4°C, and immediate storage of plasma in a freezer. If these precautions are not followed the peptide will be degraded and the results uninterpretable. ACTH secretion is pulsatile with a circadian rhythm and increases during stress. Therefore, ACTH results also must be interpreted with knowledge of time of sample collection, whether the sample was drawn from an indwelling cannula (in place for at least 2 h), whether the patient was stressed, and whether exogenous synthetic glucocorticoids were administered. A simultaneously obtained plasma cortisol sample is necessary to interpret the appropriateness of the plasma ACTH concentration. Practically, much information is obtained from a plasma cortisol measurement alone. Because ACTH is the prime regulator of cortisol secretion, the plasma cortisol level is an index of hypothalamic-pituitary-adrenal function. An 8 AM cortisol value between 10 and 20 μg/dL effectively excludes adrenal insufficiency, although it does not assess ACTH reserve.

Serum Thyrotropin

Ultrasensitive IRMAs have greatly improved the utility of TSH assays, which now distinguish among low, normal, and high levels. Older radioimmunoassays could distinguish only between normal and high levels. The ultrasensitive TSH assay has decreased the need for dynamic function tests, particularly the TRH test. If the TSH concentration is in the normal range in association with normal serum thyroid hormone levels, the patient is euthyroid and requires no further testing. If the serum thyroid hormone levels are low and the TSH level is normal (but inappropriately low for the prevailing thyroid hormone levels) or low, the patient has secondary thyroid failure. Distinction between pituitary and hypothalamic failure can be attempted by administering TRH, but in long-standing TSH deficiency of hypothalamic etiology a single dose of TRH may not stimulate intrinsically normal, but quiescent, thyrotropes.

Serum Growth Hormone

GH is secreted in a pulsatile fashion, and values in a normal subject may vary from undetectable (during an interpulse interval) to more than 40 μg/L. GH secretion is affected by ingestion of food; it is suppressed by hyperglycemia and stimulated by amino acids and hypoglycemia. Sleep stages III and IV, slow wave sleep, are associated with increased GH secretion, particularly in young adults and children. For these reasons, a random serum GH measurement is usually unhelpful. If GH deficiency is suspected, a stimulation test is required (Table 6–15). If GH hypersecretion is suspected, a suppression test (i.e., the oral glucose tolerance test) is employed. Because the bursts of spontaneous GH secretion may occur at any time of day, the timing of the sample is not helpful. GH, like ACTH and prolactin, is a stress hormone, and secretion increases in response to psychogenic or physical stress or to pain. Therefore, evaluation of spontaneous GH secretion requires measurement of multiple samples over time via an indwelling venous cannula.[359] GH secretion can also be estimated by measuring urinary excretion. However, less than 1% of circulating GH is excreted, and urinary measurement requires a sensitive assay.[360, 361] In addition, urinary GH assays are subject to interfering substances, and concentrations are affected by glomerular disease. Consequently, measurement of urinary GH is a research procedure and not used in clinical practice. The serum IGF I level provides an overall index of GH secretion and is particularly useful as a screening test for acromegaly. GH secretion is influenced by nutritional status and is increased by fasting for 24 h.[362] GH secretion is also increased in type I diabetes mellitus,[139] in anorexia nervosa,[363] and in hepatic failure and is reduced in obesity.[136] GH secretion increases during puberty and is greater in girls than in boys; this increase is accompanied by an increase in the serum IGF I concentration. Thus at puberty the diagnosis of acromegaly may be difficult. During pregnancy, GH secretion is progressively suppressed by the human GH variant secreted by the placenta, which presumably feeds back on the maternal hypothalamus and pituitary to suppress GH secretion. However, serum IGF I concentrations are increased, indicating a biological effect of the variant GH.

Serum Luteinizing Hormone and Follicle-Stimulating Hormone

Serum LH and FSH are secreted in a pulsatile fashion. In men the levels of these hormones, despite pulsatile secretion, are within a fairly narrow range; therefore, marked abnormalities of secretion are easily diagnosed from a pool of three blood samples drawn at 20-min intervals, particularly when interpreted with the clinical findings, simultaneous testosterone level, and possibly semen analysis.

In women the situation is more complex because of marked changes in gonadotropin secretion during different phases of the menstrual cycle. Clinically, measurement of serum LH and FSH in a woman who is not taking an oral contraceptive and who has regular menstrual cycles begs the

TABLE 6–15. Provocative Tests of Growth Hormone Secretion

1. Insulin 0.15 U/kg body weight causes a peak GH response in 45–60 min. A physician should be in attendance. Severe hypoglycemic symptoms should be reversed with IV glucose.

2. Arginine hydrochloride, 0.5 g/kg body weight in normal saline, is administered IV over 30 min. GH peak occurs at 45–60 min.

3. Levodopa (>30 kg body weight, 500 mg; 15–30 kg, 250 mg; <15 kg, 125 mg) is given by mouth. Transient nausea is common and vomiting may occur. Side effects are minimized if patient is kept in a supine position in a quiet room. Peak GH response usually occurs between 45 and 90 min.

4. Glucagon, 1 mg, is given intramuscularly. Peak GH response usually occurs 2–3 h later. Nausea and vomiting may result.

question; a normal menstrual cycle with documentation of a normal luteal phase serum progesterone concentration effectively excludes significant gonadotropin dysfunction.

In amenorrheic women measurement of serum LH and FSH, estradiol, prolactin, and hCG concentrations can provide insight into the following diagnoses: (1) primary ovarian failure with resulting increases in LH and FSH levels (FSH > LH) and usually normal or low serum prolactin levels; (2) hyperprolactinemia with normal or follicular phase LH, FSH, and estradiol levels; and (3) pregnancy with positive hCG test, normal or high serum prolactin level, high serum LH level (if hCG cross-reacts in the assay), and high serum estradiol level.

Serum Prolactin

Prolactin is also secreted in a pulsatile fashion. Prolactin secretion is increased in the early hours of the morning, particularly just before awakening. Prolactin is a stress hormone, and levels rise in response to psychological and physical stress, including pain. Levels also rise in response to nipple stimulation and may increase during sexual intercourse. Prolactin secretion is increased in response to estrogens, and during pregnancy serum levels may reach 200 to 500 μg/L.

Clinically, a random serum prolactin determination is useful if the level is normal or markedly elevated. If the serum prolactin concentration is greater than 250 μg/L it is almost certain that the patient harbors a prolactinoma and further prolactin measurements are unnecessary. However, mild elevation of serum prolactin level, e.g., 25 μg/L, likely reflects the stress of venipuncture or of the physical examination, including the examination of the breasts. In this situation, it is necessary to repeat the measurement once or twice. Alternatively, samples can be obtained from an indwelling venous cannula after a rest period of 2 h; samples should be obtained at 20-min intervals over the ensuing 2 h.[364] If the prior elevation was a result of stress, samples obtained with this procedure are usually normal. Although prolactin concentrations vary during the day, being lower in the afternoon, the time of sampling is usually not critical. Similarly, although changes in prolactin secretion can occur with eating, the magnitude of the changes is so small that for clinical purposes fasting is not necessary.

Interpretation of Hormone Levels During Pregnancy

Pregnancy is associated with several alterations in hormonal balance, primarily because the placenta is a pleiotropic endocrine gland. During pregnancy estrogen levels rise many hundredfold. In response, prolactin secretion is increased, and pituitary gonadotropes are suppressed. The high estrogen concentration stimulates the production by the liver of binding proteins for thyroid hormone, cortisol, and androgens (and estrogens) such that total serum T_4, T_3, and cortisol concentrations are elevated, although the free (unbound) levels are normal.

During the first 2 wk of pregnancy hCG levels increase progressively, reach a peak at about 10 wk, and then decline to a nadir at about 120 d. Many modern LH assays do not cross-react with hCG, but if cross-reactivity occurs serum LH levels are spuriously elevated, whereas FSH levels are low (in contrast to changes at midcycle, when both are high).

The placenta produces a number of prolactin- and GH-like hormones in addition to prolactin, two different hPLs, and a human GH variant. (Also see Chapter 20.) The human GH variant appears to suppress maternal pituitary GH secretion. The GH variant is thought to be responsible for the high levels of IGF I during normal pregnancy. In contrast to the hPLs, the human GH variant has GH-like biological activity.

Posterior Pituitary Failure

Diabetes insipidus is discussed in detail in Chapter 7. AVP is synthesized in the magnicellular neurons that arise from the supraoptic nucleus and paraventricular nuclei. AVP neurons terminate in the posterior pituitary for AVP storage and direct secretion into the peripheral circulation. AVP acts on the renal distal tubule to enhance reabsorption of free water. In patients who have hypothalamic tumors or a history of trauma to the pituitary stalk or who have undergone pituitary surgery, diabetes insipidus is common. However, in cases in which the nuclei are not involved the condition is usually temporary. Diabetes insipidus is unusual in primary anterior pituitary disease.

Diabetes insipidus is characterized by polyuria and polydipsia that persist throughout 24 h. Patients may have a craving for iced water and typically drink large amounts of water at night. Patients with combined ACTH (or cortisol) deficiency and AVP deficiency may not manifest diabetes insipidus until after cortisol is replaced, because in the absence of cortisol renal free water excretion is decreased. Thus before patients are tested for diabetes insipidus it is essential to document normal adrenal function or adequate glucocorticoid replacement. A diagnosis of diabetes insipidus is confirmed by simultaneous measurement of plasma and urine osmolality and, if necessary, a water deprivation test (see Chapter 7). Typically, patients with diabetes insipidus have a plasma osmolality greater than 287 mmol/kg with a simultaneous urine osmolality less than 200 mmol/kg. The hallmark of diabetes insipidus is inappropriately dilute urine for plasma osmolality.

Dynamic Tests of Pituitary Function

COMBINED ANTERIOR PITUITARY TEST. Simultaneous administration of four hypothalamic releasing hormones and measurement of the response of target pituitary hormone concentrations permits assessment of pituitary reserve in an ambulatory care setting.

Rationale. Pituitary hormone responses depend on the presence of specific pituitary cell types; the previous exposure of these cells to endogenous hypothalamic hormones, which "prime" the cells, enabling them to respond to the exogenous hypothalamic hormone; and the feedback effects of target cell hormones on the hypothalamus and pituitary.

Indication. The combined anterior pituitary (CAP) test is a screening test in suspected pituitary dysfunction. If there is a clinical indication of a deficiency, definitive testing is performed, e.g., insulin hypoglycemia or metyrapone administration for suspected ACTH deficiency. The CAP test

may be useful in assessing pituitary function after pituitary surgery or radiation.

Test Procedure. The four hypothalamic hormones, GHRH, CRH, LHRH, and TRH, are administered intravenously (sequentially) over 20 s. The doses are LHRH, 100 µg; TRH, 200 µg; CRH, 1 µg/kg body weight; and GHRH, 1 µg/kg body weight. The normal pituitary hormone response ranges have been established.[365] More than 300 patients with various hypothalamic-pituitary diseases have been studied before and/or after therapy. Samples are drawn at −30, 0, 15, 30, 60, 90, and 120 min for measurement of ACTH, TSH, LH, FSH, GH, and prolactin. Results must be interpreted in the light of the baseline levels of the target gland hormones. Baseline samples are obtained at 8 AM for cortisol, T_4, T_3 resin uptake, estradiol (amenorrheic women), testosterone (men), and IGF I.

Interpretation. Results of administration of the hypothalamic hormones may be of limited utility, but pituitary reserve is likely to be normal if the pituitary hormone response is normal in the setting of an appropriate peripheral target hormone level. The CAP test is useful for amplifying the abnormalities; thus if the TSH level is low, together with low peripheral T_4 levels, there is a high probability of secondary hypothyroidism; an absent TSH response to TRH confirms the suspicion. An absent response to a hypothalamic hormone may be a result of absent or dysfunctional pituitary cells or of increased negative feedback by the peripheral hormone. An example of the latter situation is an absent TSH response to TRH in thyrotoxicosis. An absent or diminished pituitary response may also result from lack of priming because of insufficient exposure to the hypothalamic hormone, as in isolated gonadotropin deficiency, which in most instances results from LHRH deficiency. Administration of CRH may also be useful in distinguishing between ectopic ACTH production and Cushing's disease. However, exceptions occur, and differentiating between these two conditions still remains difficult (see Chapter 9). GHRH has been administered to presumably GH-deficient children. More than 70% of GH-deficient children have an increase of serum GH level of more than 7 µg/L; in those with an initial subnormal response the GH response may become normal after repeated GHRH injections. Thus a single injection of GHRH is not useful in identifying the etiology of GH deficiency, which is usually a result of a hypothalamic GHRH deficiency. However, a deficient GH response to GHRH makes a diagnosis of GH deficiency likely.

The CAP test is useful in documenting the presence of a specific type of functional cell in the anterior pituitary. It is not diagnostic of hypopituitarism or hyperpituitarism but may aid in defining pituitary function, for example, after pituitary surgery, pituitary or cranial radiation, or pituitary infarction before administering chronic replacement therapy. Patients receiving chronic hormone replacement therapy may also be reassessed after hormone withdrawal for documentation of the extent of hypopituitarism.

INSULIN TOLERANCE TEST. The insulin tolerance test is the test most widely used to determine ACTH and GH reserve.[366, 367]

Rationale. Insulin-induced hypoglycemia activates hypothalamic neurons to stimulate pituitary secretion of ACTH, GH, and prolactin.

Indication. To test ACTH and GH reserve in a patient suspected of having hypothalamic-pituitary dysfunction.

Test Procedure. If the test is performed by knowledgeable, well-trained, and experienced personnel in a properly equipped facility, it is effective and safe. Contraindications to the insulin tolerance test include an 8 AM plasma cortisol level less than 140 nmol/L (<5 µg/dL) or a history of a seizure disorder, altered mental status, or ischemic heart disease. If the 8 AM plasma cortisol is less than 140 nmol/L (<5 µg/dL) the patient has adrenal failure and requires a test to distinguish primary from secondary adrenal failure, i.e., a plasma ACTH value measured simultaneously with plasma cortisol and a short ACTH (cosyntropin) test followed by a 48-h ACTH (cosyntropin) infusion (see Chapter 9). Hypoglycemia may precipitate seizures in a patient with a seizure disorder or myocardial infarction in a patient with ischemic heart disease. If a patient has a seizure disorder or ischemic heart disease, an alternative test such as metyrapone administration should be performed (see Chapter 9).

The test must be performed only when a physician is present. Before insulin administration a history, physical examination, and electrocardiography must be performed and interpreted, and the 8 AM plasma cortisol level must be documented to be above 140 nmol/L (>5 µg/dL). The test and symptoms of hypoglycemia are explained in detail to the patient. The patient must fast from midnight but may take water ad libitum. A heparin-lock venous cannula is placed about 1 h before beginning the test, which should take place in the morning. Blood is drawn for plasma glucose, plasma cortisol (and, if indicated, ACTH), prolactin, and GH determination at −30, 0, 30, 45, 60, and 90 min. At 0 min, 0.15 U/kg body weight of regular insulin is injected intravenously (IV). Pulse rate and blood pressure are measured and clinical observations are made at the times of blood sampling. During the initial 30 min after the injection symptoms are not usually present, but between 30 and 45 min sweating, tachycardia, drowsiness, and hunger usually occur. If there are no signs of hypoglycemia and the plasma glucose level does not decrease to less than 2.2 mmol/L (40 mg/dL), a second dose of regular insulin, 0.3 U/kg body weight, is administered. In the event of adverse effects, such as seizure, the hypoglycemia is reversed with intravenous glucose, and 1 mg dexamethasone is administered IV. Sampling should continue until the end of the test because it is likely that the hypothalamic-pituitary-adrenal axis will have been activated. In patients known to have insulin resistance (e.g., in those with acromegaly) a dose of 0.3 U/kg body weight may be used initially. However, if doubt exists, it is safer to start with the standard dose and then double it.

There is no point repeating the same dose, because it is unlikely to induce hypoglycemia if initially unsuccessful.

Interpretation (Fig. 6–22). Clinical signs of hypoglycemia and a plasma glucose level less than 2.2 mmol/L (40 mg/dL) are required for the interpretation of ACTH and GH levels. If these two criteria are fulfilled, the plasma cortisol level should rise to more than 580 nmol/L (21 µg/dL) and the GH level should increase to more than 11 µg/L.[366, 367] If these levels are not achieved, ACTH and/or GH deficiency is present.

GLUCOSE TOLERANCE TEST. Rationale. GH secretion is inhibited by acute hyperglycemia. The test is performed to diagnose or exclude acromegaly.

Indication. Suspected acromegaly.

Test Procedure. The patient fasts from midnight and is allowed to take water ad libitum. A heparin-lock cannula is placed in a forearm vein 1 h before beginning the test. Blood samples for plasma glucose (serum insulin) and serum GH are obtained at −30, 0, 30, 60, 90, and 120 min. Glucose (75 g) is dissolved in iced orange- or lemon-flavored water and ingested by the patient immediately after the 0-min blood sample is obtained.

Interpretation. Serum GH level, as determined by a sensitive IRMA, should decrease to less than 1 µg/L (<2 mU/L) after oral glucose ingestion.[138] The development of ultrasensitive GH assays that measure GH concentrations as low as 0.01 µg/L will probably make it necessary to re-evaluate the normal GH response to oral glucose. In routine GH radioimmunoassays, the GH concentration responds to oral glucose ingestion by decreasing to less than 2 µg/L. In acromegaly serum GH concentrations remain unchanged, are partially lowered, or increase paradoxically.

Pituitary Imaging

Skull x-ray films, hypocycloidal sellar tomography, cerebral arteriography, and pneumoencephalography were previously used to assess pituitary gland anatomy indirectly. These techniques provide limited visualization of the gland and its relationship to surrounding structures. In addition, arteriography and pneumoencephalography are associated

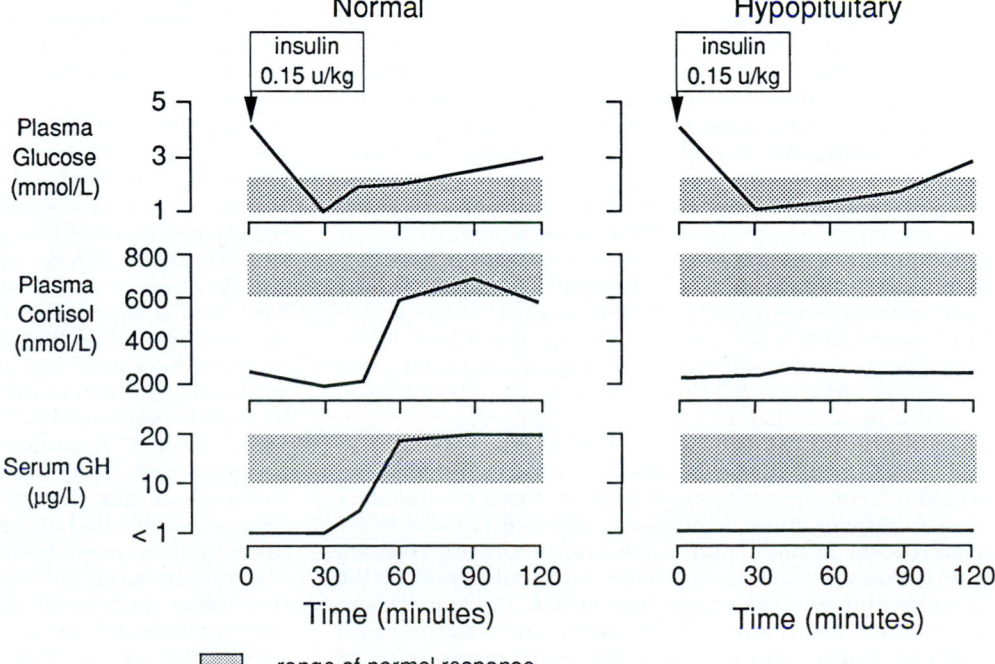

Figure 6–22. The insulin hypoglycemia test in the diagnosis of hypopituitarism. Plasma glucose, cortisol, and serum GH concentrations in a normal subject (left) and a subject with hypopituitarism (right) are shown. GH levels should rise to a minimum of 10 µg/L, and cortisol levels should increase to 580 nmol/L (21 µg/dL) with achievement of adequate hypoglycemia, namely a blood glucose concentration less than or equal to 2.2 mmol/L (40 mg/dL). (Modified from Wass JAH. Hypopituitarism. In: Besser GM, Cudworth AG, eds. Clinical Endocrinology: An Illustrated Text. London: Gower Medical, 1987: 2.1–2.14.)

Normal

Hypopituitary

insulin 0.15 u/kg

insulin 0.15 u/kg

Plasma Glucose (mmol/L)

Plasma Cortisol (nmol/L)

Serum GH (µg/L)

Time (minutes)

Time (minutes)

range of normal response

with risk and discomfort. CT and MRI techniques provide a noninvasive means of imaging the pituitary gland directly and, with MRI, the structures surrounding the pituitary gland. Consequently, the evaluation of a patient with suspected pituitary or hypothalamic disease is best done with an MRI or CT scan. X-ray films of the skull, sellar tomography, cerebral arteriography, and pneumoencephalography are rarely indicated. For example, because pituitary enlargement may occur without enlargement of the sella, a normal skull x-ray film or sellar tomogram does not exclude a pituitary mass. Unless specific visualization of the bone anatomy surrounding the pituitary gland is required, a skull x-ray film or sellar tomogram is of little value in the evaluation of pituitary anatomy. Cerebral angiography may occasionally be required in some patients before surgical intervention but also has no place in the initial evaluation of such patients. In most situations the best method for visualization of hypothalamic-pituitary anatomy is the MRI scan; the second best method is a high-resolution coronal CT scan. The reason for the superiority of MRI is that the optic chiasm is easily visualized and can be distinguished from the diaphragma sellae, vascular structures are defined, and lateral tumor extension can be delineated.

NORMAL PITUITARY ANATOMY. The high-resolution CT scan provided major insight into pituitary anatomy, particularly with respect to variability of gland size and the presence of focal hypodense or hyperdense lesions in normal glands. Routine axial images of 5-mm thickness do not provide adequate visualization of the pituitary unless a large lesion is present and thus can lead to a misdiagnosis of "normal." Direct coronal images, every 1.5 mm through the pituitary fossa, after contrast administration IV provide optimal visualization (Fig. 6–23). If the patient cannot hyperextend the neck for a coronal study, sagittal and coronal reconstructions of 1.5-mm images are usually adequate.

The height of a normal pituitary gland ranges from 3 to 9 mm, with the average being 6 to 7 mm.[368, 369] Larger glands may occur in young women of reproductive age but do not correlate with the serum prolactin concentration. Similarly, the superior margins of the gland are convex more often in younger (18 to 36 y) than in older (37 to 70 y) women,[368] and gland density is heterogeneous, described as "mottled," in the majority of women of all ages. Focal hypodense areas occur in 13 to 36% of normal women,[368, 369] and hyperdense focal areas are present in 9% of normal women. An empty or partially empty sella, defined as a gland height of less than 4 mm, may be present in up to 18% of normal women.[368] The pituitary gland normally enlarges during the second and third trimesters of pregnancy.

Visualization of hypothalamic and pituitary anatomy is best accomplished by using MRI after administration of gadolinium diethylenetriaminepentaacetic acid (Gd-DTPA) to enhance lesions such as an adenoma. Gland size on MRI scans correlates with both CT and autopsy findings. Approximately 75% of the pituitary is the anterior lobe, which is usually isointense with brain white matter on most pulse sequences, although heterogeneity may be present. The posterior pituitary has a high signal intensity that is thought to reflect fatty substances within the AVP-containing neurons; this high signal may be absent in patients with diabetes insipidus. The optic chiasm is directly above the pituitary fossa in 80% of subjects and is usually well visualized; the hypothalamic infundibulum is posterior to the optic chiasm. The cavernous sinus is isointense with and lateral to the pituitary and contains cranial nerves III, IV, and VI and the V_1 and V_2 divisions of V; the nerves are lower in signal intensity than the pituitary. The low signal intensity (signal void) in the cavernous sinus reflects blood flow in the internal

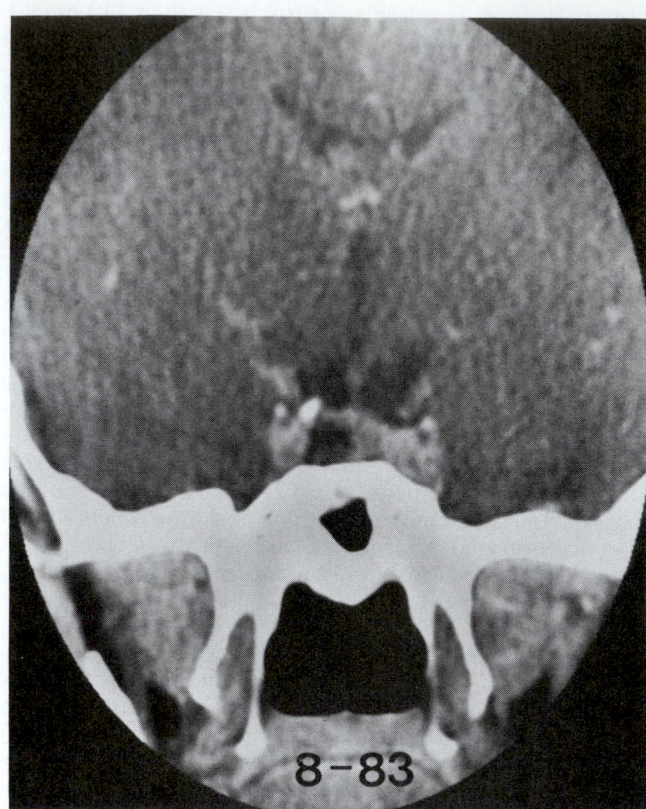

Figure 6–23. Coronal CT scan with intravenous contrast enhancement demonstrating a 1-cm adenoma of low density. Note the elevation of the diaphragma sellae and deviation of the pituitary stalk.

carotid artery. Incidental hemorrhage is occasionally present. A partially empty sella may be observed in normal subjects.[370]

Hemorrhage into the brain, and presumably into a pituitary tumor, has a characteristic appearance, depending on the age of the hemorrhage and disruption of the blood-brain barrier. An acute hemorrhage less than 1 wk old, consisting of deoxyhemoglobin, is isointense with the gland on T1-weighted images and has low signal intensity on T2-weighted images. A subacute hemorrhage, 1 to 4 wk old, contains methemoglobin that forms from the periphery to the central region and is of high signal intensity on both T1-weighted and T2-weighted images. A hemorrhage of greater than 4 wk produces a homogeneously high signal on both T1-weighted and T2-weighted images; hemosiderin appears as a ring around the hemorrhage and is of low signal intensity on T1-weighted and T2-weighted images.[371]

PITUITARY MASS. Although CT and MRI scans are equally effective in identifying large pituitary tumors, the MRI scan is superior in defining the full extent and relationship to surrounding structures (Fig. 6–24) and is more accurate in identifying small lesions. In patients with a surgically proven microadenoma the MRI scan detected and located the lesion in 100%; identification with CT scans was made in half.[372] A pituitary microadenoma on an MRI scan is round and hypointense to the normal gland on T1-weighted images; lesions, best demonstrated on coronal images, exhibit higher signals on T2-weighted scans. The infundibulum may deviate from the side of the tumor. Macroadenomas (>10 mm) tend to have signal characteristics similar to those of the normal gland but may contain cystic or hemorrhagic areas[370] (Fig. 6–25). Intravenous administration of Gd-DTPA produces enhancement of the normal pituitary that is maximal after approximately 30

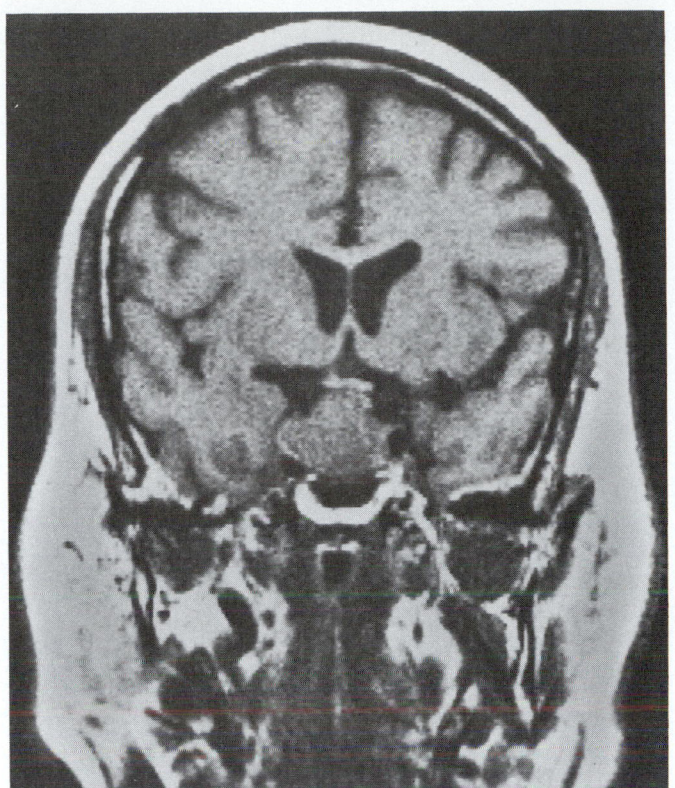
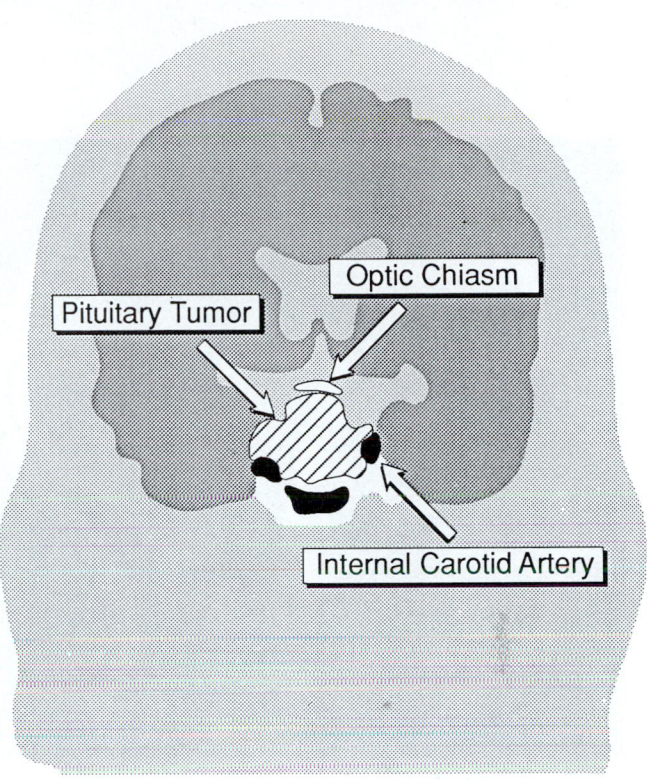

Figure 6–24. Coronal MRI scan and schematic drawing demonstrating a large pituitary tumor extending laterally into both cavernous sinuses and superiorly abutting the optic chiasm.

min; compared with normal glands, adenomas are enhanced more slowly, and the enhancement persists for a longer period. Gd-DTPA and coronal images increase the probability of identifying small lesions and should be used when a pituitary tumor is suspected.[373] MRI may also identify nonpituitary intrasellar masses such as a meningioma or an internal carotid artery aneurysm (Fig. 6–26). Although MRI is the most sensitive method for identification of microadenomas, very small tumors may not be detectable. This is particularly true for patients with Cushing's disease, in whom only 83% of the tumors are detectable by MRI.[373]

Neuro-ophthalmological Evaluation

Every patient with a suspected or documented pituitary macroadenoma should undergo a complete ophthalmological examination before therapeutic intervention and, if abnormalities are present, careful follow-up during and after treatment. Use of the MRI scan has greatly aided in assessment of the anatomical relationship between the pituitary and the optic chiasm. A distinct separation between the mass and the optic chiasm and absence of tumor invasion into the cavernous sinus suggest that the ophthalmological examination will be normal. The CT scan cannot provide this information.

Visual acuity and visual fields should be assessed at the initial examination either with the use of a Snellen chart or with estimation of visual fields by confrontation. Confrontational screening is performed by finger counting or comparison of two targets. The patient is asked to identify the number of fingers or the appearance of paired objects in each quadrant of one field. Confrontational testing with a red object (e.g., tip of a pen) may detect color desaturation when the patient is able to identify the object, thus revealing subtle visual field loss.

Although suprasellar extension of a pituitary macroadenoma may produce visual field abnormalities obvious to the patient and examiner, a normal confrontational examination does not exclude subtle abnormalities detectable only with perimetry. Manual perimetry requires a skilled technician; automated perimetry does not require as much technical expertise, and a standardized strategy is utilized for each field. All types of visual field measurements require cooperation by the patient. An adequate instrument should test both central and peripheral fields, automatically retest missed points, monitor the patient's fixation, and calibrate the background and target luminance.[374]

Development of visual field abnormality depends on the extent of compression of the optic chiasm or optic tract and the position of the chiasm in relation to the pituitary gland. In approximately 80% of persons the chiasm lies directly over the pituitary gland, in 15% the chiasm is anterior to the pituitary and lies above the tuberculum sella (prefixed chiasm), and in the remaining 5% the chiasm is posterior to the pituitary or the dorsum sella (postfixed chiasm)[337] (Fig. 6–27). The optic chiasm is separated from the tuberculum sella, diaphragma sella, and dorsum sella by the basal cistern of the subarachnoid space, the height of the cistern ranging between 0 and 10 mm. The infundibulum and hypothalamus are posterior and superior to the optic chiasm.

The pattern of visual field loss caused by a pituitary tumor depends on the location of the chiasm, the course of the optic nerves, and the degree of nerve compression. Permanent loss of vision and visual field defect(s) usually result from long-standing nerve compression; however, the exact relation between duration of compression and permanent damage is not known. If one eye is normal, the patient may fail to notice an abnormality or may describe the vision as dim or foggy. Vision is usually lost gradually, except when there is significant hemorrhage into the tumor

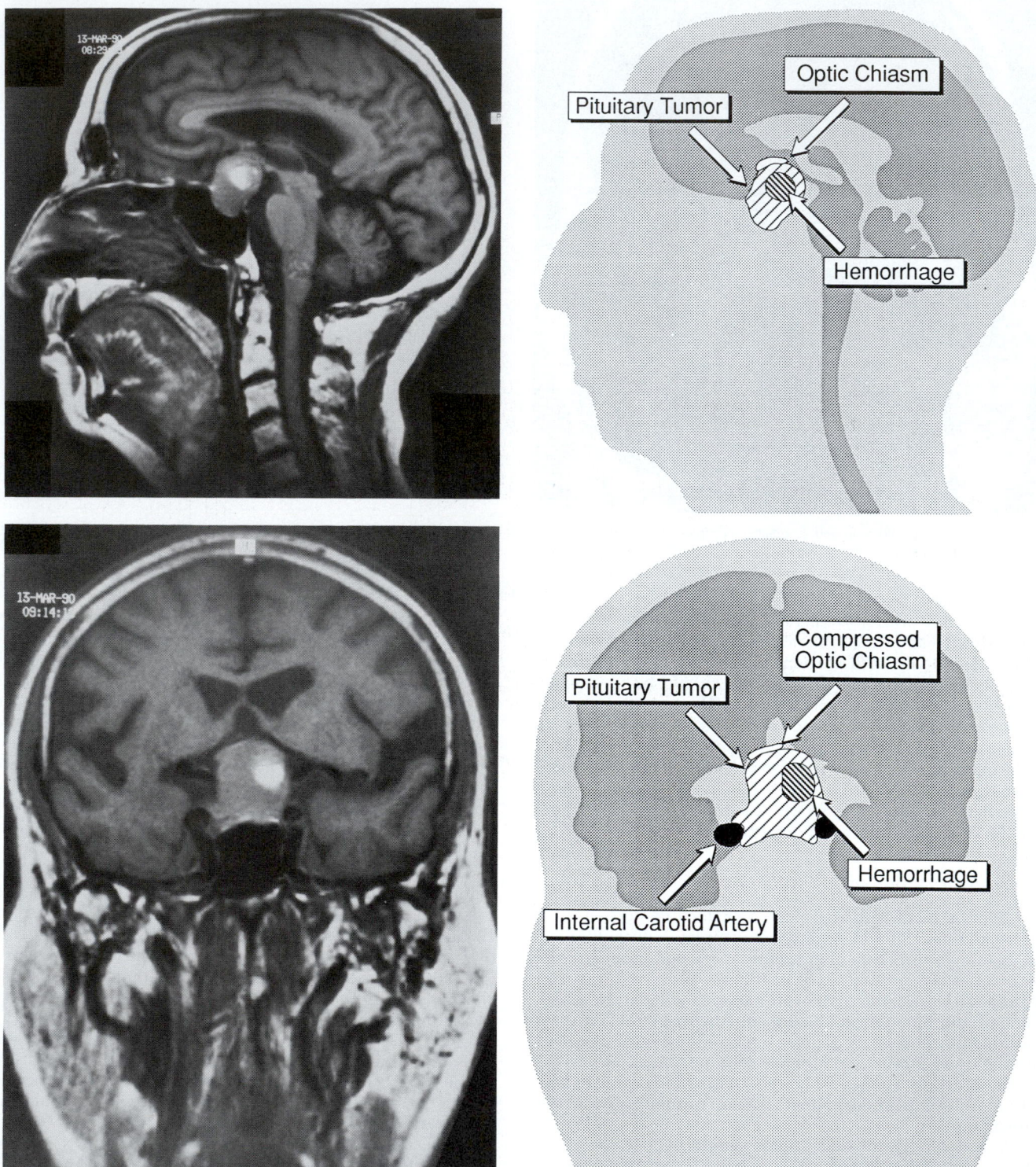

Figure 6–25. Saggital *(top left)* and coronal *(bottom left)* MRI scans and corresponding schematic drawings of a patient with a macroadenoma with superior extension compressing the optic chiasm and inferior extension into the sphenoid sinus. Note area of high signal intensity suggestive of hemorrhage. (Unpublished observations, courtesy of M. O. Thorner.)

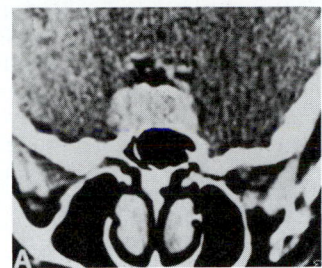 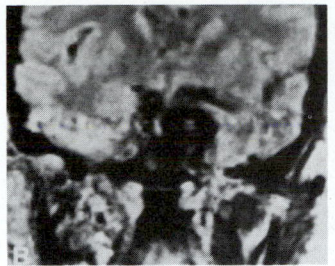 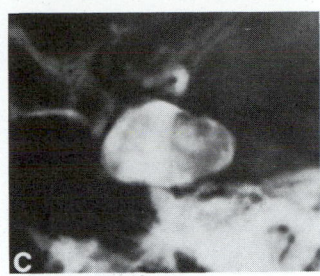

Figure 6–26. *A*, Coronal CT scan with contrast enhancement of a large pituitary mass. *B*, Coronal MRI scan of the pituitary mass with a signal void from free-flowing blood. *C*, Lateral cerebral arteriogram demonstrating an internal carotid artery aneurysm mimicking a pituitary tumor on CT scan. (Unpublished observations, courtesy of M. L. Vance.)

(pituitary apoplexy). In pituitary apoplexy, visual impairment may be sudden with loss of central vision and development of bitemporal field defects, ophthalmoplegia, and changes in mental function. Visual acuity may range from normal to near or complete blindness. Loss of perception of color, particularly red, and a decreased pupillary light reaction may accompany decreased visual acuity. If the optic nerve is compromised for at least 6 wk, as occurs in 33 to 70% of patients with large tumors, the optic discs may be pallid.[338, 375–377]

Although less common, ophthalmoplegia may occur if the tumor extends laterally. Lateral extension of the tumor into the cavernous sinus is present in up to 15% of patients but is usually not clinically apparent. Symptoms include diplopia and/or ptosis or altered facial sensation. Depending on the degree of cavernous sinus invasion, cranial nerves III, IV, and VI and the V_1 and V_2 divisions of V may be impaired. The most common abnormality is impaired third nerve function.

Five characteristic patterns of visual field loss and changes in visual acuity result from pituitary tumors (Fig. 6–28).[378, 379] Compression of an optic nerve by anterior and superior tumor extension produces decreased central acuity and a normal contralateral visual field. This pattern is characteristic of optic neuropathy and may be confused with optic neuritis. A junctional syndrome—contralateral superotemporal field loss and ipsilateral decreased acuity—results from compression of inferonasal fibers from the contralateral eye that form a loop into the proximal optic nerve (Wilbrand's knee) at its junction with the chiasm. Superior bitemporal field loss, with normal acuity, occurs when the chiasm is compressed from below, involving the crossing inferior nasal retinal fibers. This may progress to complete bitemporal loss with further chiasmal compression. Compression of the posterior portion of the chiasm produces a bitemporal scotomatous pattern of loss with central bitemporal defects and normal acuity. A homonymous hemianopia with normal acuity results from compression of an optic tract in the setting of a prefixed chiasm or tumor extension superiorly and posteriorly. The last two patterns of visual field loss also occur with hypothalamic tumors such as craniopharyngioma, hypothalamic glioma, and germinoma.

Successful decompression of the optic nerves and chiasm by either surgical resection or tumor shrinkage with medical therapy (e.g., in prolactinoma or acromegaly) is often accompanied by improvement in visual function. Surgical removal is associated with improvement in visual abnormalities and visual acuity in 62 to 80% of patients.[338, 376, 380] The improvement is usually evident within hours or days of surgery and may continue for months. In a minority of patients, 4 to 10%, visual abnormalities worsen after surgical decompression.[338, 380] Risk of visual deterioration appears to be less with the transsphenoidal approach. Prognostic factors for visual improvement include absence of optic atrophy and short duration of abnormalities. Improvement in visual acuity occurs in almost all eyes with a preoperative visual acuity of 20/100 or better and in approximately 60% with acuity worse than 20/100.[337, 376]

Careful ophthalmological examination, in conjunction with imaging studies, must be performed after surgery and after institution of medical therapy to assess the efficacy of treatment and to allow early detection of tumor recurrence. An ophthalmological examination should be performed shortly after the operation or institution of medical therapy and at least at 6-mo intervals for the first year. Objective assessment of visual fields requires that the patient be alert and cooperative. The frequency of follow-up examinations is determined by the individual abnormalities, type of treatment, and presence of residual tumor on imaging studies. Changes in visual acuity and fields may indicate tumor recurrence even when imaging studies are unchanged, emphasizing the need for regular ophthalmological examination.

Hormone Replacement Therapy

Replacement therapy usually consists of administering the hormones produced by the target glands. The exceptions are GH administration for GH deficiency (discussed in detail in Chapter 21), gonadotropin therapy for induction of

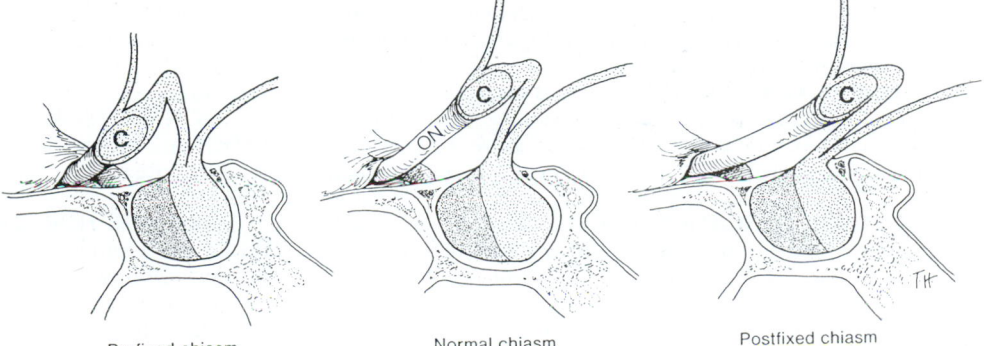

Figure 6–27. Three different positions of the chiasm in relation to the pituitary gland. C, chiasm; ON, optic nerve. (From Miller NR. Anatomy and physiology of the optic chiasm. In: Miller NR, ed. Walsh and Hoyt's Clinical Neuroophthalmology. Baltimore: Williams & Wilkins, 1982: 60–69. © 1982, the Williams & Wilkins Co., Baltimore.)

Prefixed chiasm   Normal chiasm   Postfixed chiasm

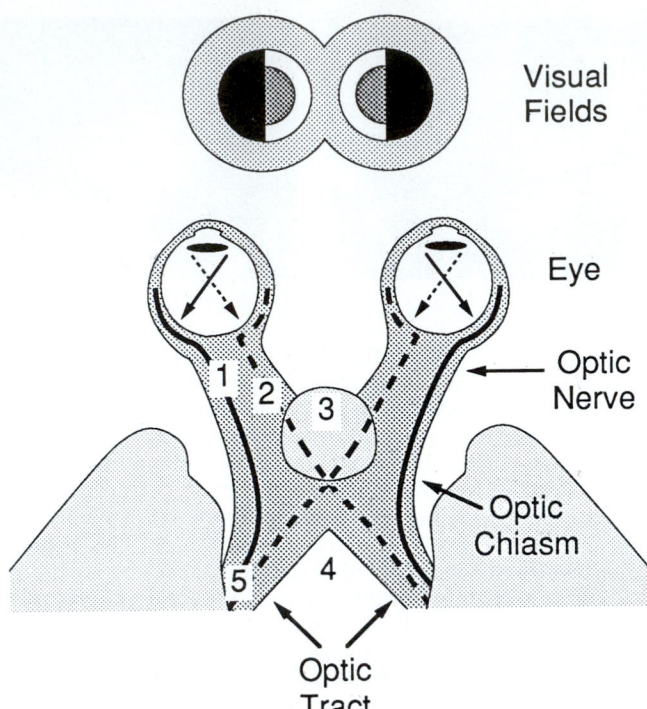

Figure 6–28. The most common visual field defect, bitemporal hemianopia (black areas of visual fields) is caused by compression of the posterior aspect of the chiasm (4) from below. Visual disturbances resulting from compression of the optic nerves, chiasm, and tracts are listed below. The site of lesion is indicated by number.

Pattern	Visual Field/Acuity	Anatomical Correlate
1. Optic neuropathy	Normal contralateral field; decreased central acuity	Postfixed chiasm/anterior extension
2. Junctional syndrome	Contralateral superotemporal field cut; decreased acuity	Junction of Wilbrand knee
3. Bitemporal	Superior bitemporal desaturation; normal acuity	Inferior fibers cross first
4. Bitemporal scotoma	Relative central bitemporal defect; normal acuity	Relative macular involvement related to posterior compression
5. Tract	Homonymous hemianopia: normal acuity	Prefixed chiasm/posterior extension

(Figure modified from Wass JAH. Hypopituitarism. In: Besser GM, Cudworth AG, eds. Clinical Endocrinology: An Illustrated Text. London: Gower Medical, 1987: 2.1–2.14. Table from Newman SA. Advances in diagnosis and treatment of pituitary tumors. Int Ophthalmol Clin 1986; 26:285–300.)

ovulation in women and treatment of infertility in men, and desmopressin for treatment of diabetes insipidus.

Replacement therapy must be tailored to the individual hormone deficiency and if possible should not be instituted until the hypothalamic-pituitary-adrenal axis has been assessed. For example, thyroid hormone replacement before institution of glucocorticoid therapy in a cortisol-deficient subject may precipitate an adrenal crisis.

MEDICAL ALERT (MEDIC ALERT) BRACELET. Every patient receiving adrenal or posterior pituitary (and/or thyroid hormone) replacement therapy should have and wear an identifying necklace or bracelet in the event of an emergency.

CORTISOL DEFICIENCY. Cortisol deficiency is usually treated by oral administration of 20 mg hydrocortisone on awakening and 10 mg at 6 PM. This is the simplest way to simulate the circadian rhythm of cortisol secretion. Some patients require an additional 10 mg at lunch time, and others, particularly very small patients, may require a lower dose. Alternatively, synthetic glucocorticoids may be used—either a prednisone dose of 5 mg on awakening and 2.5 mg at 6 PM or 0.5 mg dexamethasone on awakening. The choice of the appropriate replacement dose usually is determined clinically; in patients receiving hydrocortisone, measurement of plasma cortisol through the day may be helpful, but urinary free cortisol levels are not helpful. During stress, whether psychological or physical; fever; and illness, the dose is usually increased to an equivalent of 20 mg hydrocortisone every 6 to 8 h. If parenteral administration is required, 100 mg hydrocortisone is given IV every 4 h or intramuscularly (IM) every 6 h. Alternatively, dexamethasone is given IV or IM at a dose of 1 mg every 12 h; this regimen is frequently used in patients undergoing surgery.

THYROID HORMONE DEFICIENCY. Thyroid hormone deficiency is treated with levothyroxine; the oral dose usually ranges from 0.075 to 0.15 mg once daily. The dose is adjusted according to the clinical response, and the serum T_3 level should be in the middle to upper part of the normal range. Measurement of serum TSH is of no value in assessing response to levothyroxine in patients with hypothalamic/pituitary disease.

GONADAL STEROIDS. Testosterone enanthate for hypogonadal men is usually administered IM, 200 mg every 2 wk or 300 mg every 3 wk.[381] Testosterone replacement via the transdermal route is under trial; an adherent testosterone-impregnated patch is applied to the scrotum daily and normal adult serum testosterone concentrations are maintained throughout the day.[381, 382] Some patients have an increase in serum dihydrotestosterone concentration to above normal, presumably because of scrotal skin 5α-reductase activity. Advantages of transdermal testosterone administration include avoidance of wide fluctuations in serum testosterone concentrations and avoidance of intramuscular injection. When initiating testosterone therapy IM it is advisable to begin with a low dose and gradually increase the dose; an initial dose of 50 mg testosterone enanthate is given IM and the dose is doubled every 2 wk until the final dose is reached. Adequacy of therapy is assessed by measuring serum testosterone concentration just before the scheduled injection. (See also Chapter 13.)

There are numerous regimens for estrogen replacement in hypogonadal women. Estrogen replacement therapy is given to improve the woman's sense of well-being, to maintain and/or promote feminization, and to prevent bone loss. If the uterus has not been removed, estrogens are administered cyclically with appropriate progestogens. This is easily achieved by administering one of the several low-dose oral contraceptive preparations containing 30 μg ethinyl estradiol. These preparations are conveniently packaged and do not require the patient to remember when to take the progestogen and when to stop the tablets. Alternatively, estrogen can be given for 3 wk out of 4 and a small dose of progestogen administered for the third week. One such regimen consists of conjugated estrogens at 0.625 mg/d for 3 wk together with medroxyprogesterone acetate at 5 or 10 mg/d for the last 7 or 10 d. A withdrawal menses should occur within a few days of stopping the medications during the fourth week of the cycle.

GONADOTROPINS AND LHRH. Gonadotropins and LHRH are administered to initiate puberty and to restore fertility. (Regimens are discussed in detail in Chapters 12 and 13.)

GROWTH HORMONE. Two recombinant DNA–produced preparations are available in the United States; one has an additional methionyl group at the COOH terminus of the molecule, and the other contains only the natural sequence. Both preparations are equally effective. GH is administered subcutaneously at a dose of 0.043 mg/kg/d (0.3

mg/kg/wk). In the past, GH was administered three times weekly. Three times weekly and daily GH administrations result in similar increases in linear growth during the first 6 to 12 mo, but during the second and third years of treatment the daily regimen minimizes the decline in growth velocity (see Chapter 21).

GROWTH HORMONE–RELEASING HORMONE. GHRH has been administered to GH-deficient children by twice-daily injections and by pulsatile subcutaneous administration.[383] Additional experience is needed to determine whether chronic GHRH treatment is equivalent to or has advantages over GH treatment.

VASOPRESSIN. Treatment of central diabetes insipidus is discussed in detail in Chapter 7. The major drug for this purpose is desmopressin, an analogue of vasopressin that is 1000 times more potent in increasing distal tubular water reabsorption and has 1000 times less vasopressor activity. It is administered by nasal spray, 10 µg once or twice daily. If nasal insufflation is inappropriate, e.g., after transsphenoidal surgery, the agent is given by subcutaneous administration, 1 or 2 µg every 12 or 24 h. This analogue has improved the therapy of central diabetes insipidus.

Pituitary Surgery

Modern pituitary surgery offers the possibility of selective resection of pituitary adenomas, leaving the normal pituitary intact. Harvey Cushing pioneered the transsphenoidal technique but abandoned it in favor of the transcranial approach in 1927. Modern transsphenoidal pituitary surgery was developed by Gerard Guiot and Jules Hardy.[384] Use of intraoperative fluoroscopy to confirm entry into the sella turcica and avoid the risk of being in the wrong plane (which could lead to catastrophic consequences) and use of the operating microscope to visualize the sella contents made it possible to identify and selectively remove the tumor and leave the normal gland intact and functional.[385] By decompressing the pituitary fossa from below, a defect results in the sellar floor that usually allows any recurrent tumor growth to extend inferiorly instead of laterally or superiorly. Other advantages include minimal disturbance of the brain, absence of external scars, and no requirement to shave the head. The operation is often well tolerated by the elderly or frail patient, who may not be able to survive a craniotomy. Blood loss is minimal, and transfusion is usually not required. It must be recognized, however, that transsphenoidal surgery requires great skill and experience. Published studies indicate that the better outcomes, in terms of cure and limitation of complications, usually occur when the surgeon performs the operation frequently and has done several hundred such operations.

It is beyond the scope of this chapter to provide a detailed analysis of transcranial versus transsphenoidal surgery. The guiding principle is that, unless contraindicated, the approach to the pituitary is transsphenoidal. Major contraindications to transsphenoidal surgery include (1) anatomical features that prevent the approach, such as lack of pneumatization of the sphenoid sinus or hyperostosis; (2) suprasellar extension that precludes removal from below; and (3) ambiguity regarding the type of lesion, such as aneurysm or meningioma that cannot be resected transsphenoidally.

INDICATIONS FOR PITUITARY SURGERY. *Pituitary Apoplexy.* Minor pituitary hemorrhage into a pituitary tumor probably occurs frequently and may be clinically insignificant; many such cases are probably not diagnosed. However, a severe hemorrhage leading to prostration, visual disturbance, profound headache, and coma is a neurosurgical emergency. If sudden visual compromise occurs, neurosurgical intervention is mandatory. The usual approach is by the transsphenoidal route.

Pituitary Tumor. If pituitary tumors hypersecrete or if they are large enough to produce mass effects, therapy is indicated. With the exception of prolactin-secreting pituitary adenomas, transsphenoidal surgery is usually the treatment of choice. Extirpation of the tumor theoretically, and often practically, cures the hypersecretion of the pituitary hormone(s) and leads to decompression of any involved structures such as the optic chiasm and cavernous sinus. An exception is lateral extension of the tumor into the cavernous sinus, for which a transcranial approach may be required.

Failure of Other Therapies. Patients in whom previous therapy has failed are candidates for surgery. For example, children with Cushing's disease and adults with acromegaly that has not been cured by pituitary radiation are candidates for surgery. Patients with prolactinomas whose prolactin levels have been restored to normal but whose "tumor" continues to grow are also candidates for surgery. In this situation two lesions may occur simultaneously; for example, in a patient with a prolactinoma and a meningioma, although the growth of the prolactinoma was controlled by bromocriptine, the apparent growth of the tumor was due to the growth of the meningioma.[386] Intolerance to bromocriptine or other dopamine agonist drugs may also be an indication for surgical removal of the tumor. Prolactinomas are not always fully responsive to dopamine agonist therapy, such that the prolactin does not return to normal, gonadal function is not restored, and the tumor does not adequately decrease in size. In such a case surgery may reduce the bulk of the tumor and allow better control with medical therapy.

RESULTS OF PITUITARY SURGERY. Because most pituitary tumors are benign, the results of surgery are usually gratifying, particularly in patients with suprasellar extension and visual abnormalities. Improvement in visual field abnormalities occurs in 80% of such patients, progression of visual disturbance is arrested in 16%, and visual deterioration occurs in 4%.[380, 387]

The results of pituitary surgery for hyperfunctioning tumors are discussed in the relevant sections of this chapter. However, the same issues determine the results: (1) the experience and expertise of the surgeon, (2) the size of the tumor, (3) tumor invasion of bone or dura, and (4) previous therapy.

The complications of pituitary surgery in large series are few. However, every operation carries a risk. Mortality rates of 0.86, 0.27, and 2.5% have been reported in patients with macroadenomas, microadenomas, and macroadenomas previously treated by other modalities, respectively.[388] The complication rate is lower in patients with microadenomas and higher in patients who have had previous therapy (i.e., cases of recurrent or persistent tumor). For patients with previous treatments or microadenomas, respectively, visual loss occurred in 2.5 and 0.1%, CSF leak in 5.7 and 1.3%, stroke or vascular injury in 1.3 and 0.2%, meningitis or abscess in 1.3 and 0.1%, and oculomotor palsy in 0.6 and 0.1%.[388] The incidence of postoperative hypopituitarism is about 3% in patients with microadenomas and increases with invasiveness of the tumor.

Pituitary Radiation

Before improvement in microsurgical techniques and development of medical therapies, pituitary radiation was the only treatment for many patients with pituitary tumors. Pituitary radiation usually prevents further tumor growth and eventually results in a reduction in hormone hypersecretion. However, prompt reduction in either tumor size or hormone hypersecretion is rare. In addition, hypopituitarism, either total or partial, is a risk. Currently, pituitary radiation is reserved for patients with residual disease after surgery and patients who cannot undergo surgical resection.

Types of radiotherapy include conventional supervoltage therapy, yttrium implantation, stereotactic radiosurgery using alpha particles or proton beam therapy, and single high-dose focused radiation from the gamma unit. The type of radiation treatment administered must be individualized according to the tumor size and location (proximity to the optic chiasm and cavernous sinus) and the availability of the radiation source. The most commonly used radiation is conventional supervoltage therapy administered in daily fractions 5 d/wk over 4 or 5 wk to provide a total dose of 45 to 50 Gy. This type of treatment is used in patients with large or small pituitary tumors. Yttrium implantation involves surgical placement of radioactive ^{90}Y seeds in the pituitary and is available in few centers. Alpha particle or proton beam radiotherapy can be used only to treat small tumors and requires a cyclotron for the energy source, thus limiting availability. Focused radiation from the gamma unit is also limited to treatment of small tumors and is of limited availability.

Each method of radiation has advantages and limitations. The results of these treatments are, in general, similar with the exception of gamma unit therapy, about which information is inadequate for comparison with other techniques. In most studies few patients have progression of disease after radiotherapy, but the recurrence rate was 10% in one series.[389] Reduction in hormone hypersecretion may occur within 3 to 6 mo of therapy, but attainment of normal values usually requires at least 5 y and often 10 y.[390–392]

Development of hypopituitarism is a common consequence of radiotherapy; it may be partial or complete and may occur at any time after treatment. In one study, half of the patients treated with conventional supervoltage radiation developed hypopituitarism within 26 mo of therapy.[393] In other series at least a third of patients develop pituitary deficiencies within 2 to 3 y. The incidence of hypopituitarism increases with length of follow-up, and consequently all patients treated with pituitary radiation should be monitored long term with appropriate hormone measurements and dynamic studies as indicated for early detection of pituitary gland failure.

Other complications of radiotherapy include damage to the optic chiasm and/or optic nerve(s) and cranial nerves with consequent visual loss or ophthalmoplegia; vascular damage causing cerebral ischemia; seizures; and development of a pituitary or brain malignancy.[389, 394, 395] The incidence of these complications varies among centers and with the type of radiation administered. Complications of radiotherapy occur more frequently in patients who have received prior surgery.[396] As with surgical excision of tumors, radiotherapy should be performed in centers with expertise in these techniques.

PITUITARY DISORDERS

Prolactinoma

Hyperprolactinemia—excessive prolactin production by the lactotropes—is the most common anterior pituitary disorder. The causes of increased prolactin production are numerous, including a prolactin-secreting pituitary adenoma or prolactinoma, the most common type of secretory pituitary tumor.

NATURAL HISTORY. The natural history of development and progression of a prolactinoma is not known precisely, but the majority of these tumors grow slowly, over years. Autopsy studies demonstrate that 23 to 27% of individuals have pituitary microadenoma;[11, 397] the vast majority of such individuals have no antemortem evidence of endocrine dysfunction, and 40% of the tumors are positive for prolactin by immunocytochemical staining.[11] Serial observations of untreated patients with a microadenoma indicate that a minority have a significant increase in serum prolactin concentration and/or in tumor size and that most have a decrease in serum prolactin levels over time. Table 6–16 summarizes the course in untreated patients. The factors responsible for tumor enlargement and further increases in prolactin in a subset of individuals are not known.

ETIOLOGIES. Several theories of the genesis of prolactinomas have been proposed. Administration of estrogen in the form of an oral contraceptive has been suggested as a cause of prolactinoma formation,[398, 399] but studies of large numbers of women who used oral contraceptives document no association between use of oral contraceptives, particularly those with lower estrogen doses, and development of a prolactinoma.[400–405] The development of prolactinomas in a strain of rats sensitive to estrogen is thought to result from estrogen-induced stimulation of the development of new nonhypothalamic (systemic) arteries that provide dopamine-deficient blood to the anterior pituitary and result in loss of dopaminergic tone and adenoma formation.[17] Abnormalities of hypothalamic regulation have also been postulated as the cause of prolactinoma formation; this hypothesis is based primarily on abnormal prolactin responses to stimulatory agents (e.g., TRH, dopamine antagonists) and inhibitory agents (e.g., dopamine agonists). Responses to these agents are inconsistent, both before and after "curative" resection, so that a unitary hypothesis as to the pathogenesis cannot be proved. In all likelihood, prolactinomas arise de novo and are not a result of hypothalamic dysfunction.[406] Clonal analysis of tumor DNA indicates that prolactinomas are monoclonal in origin.[335]

CLINICAL FEATURES. The clinical presentation of hyperprolactinemia varies with age and sex, duration of hyperprolactinemia, and the size of the tumor, if one is present. Men and postmenopausal women usually come to medical attention because of symptoms of a pituitary mass such as headache and visual abnormalities, including decreased visual acuity, visual field deficits, and/or ophthalmoplegia. The most common visual abnormality is bitemporal hemianopsia secondary to compression of the optic chiasm.

Hypogonadism is an almost invariable consequence of hyperprolactinemia. Women of reproductive age commonly seek medical attention because of delayed menarche or disturbance of menstrual function, including amenorrhea, oligomenorrhea, or regular menses with infertility. Galactorrhea is present in 30 to 80% of these women and may be related to the duration of gonadal dysfunction; women with long-standing amenorrhea are less likely to have galactorrhea, which probably reflects prolonged estrogen deficiency. Other features of estrogen deficiency may include decreased libido, vaginal dryness, and dyspareunia. The majority of premenopausal, hyperprolactinemic women have a microadenoma.

In men hypogonadism may be complete or partial, producing decreased libido, complete or partial impotence, and/or infertility. Many hyperprolactinemic men report "normal" sexual function and realize that there was a problem only after successful treatment of the hyperprolactinemia. With long-standing hypogonadism, beard and body hair may be decreased and the testes are usually soft but of normal size (>12 mL in volume). Galactorrhea occurs in 14 to 33% of men with marked hyperprolactinemia;[407, 408] demonstration may require vigorous breast manipulation. Gy-

TABLE 6–16. Natural History of Untreated Prolactin-Secreting Microadenomas

Author, Year	Number of Patients	Mean Duration of Observation (y)	Serum Prolactin Level		
			Unchanged	Decreased	Increased
March et al., 1981[857]	43	4	38	3	2
von Werder et al., 1983[858]	30	3–6	26	2	2
Koppelman et al., 1984[859]	20	5.3	2	14	4
Martin et al., 1985[860]	41	5.5	11	23	7
Sisam et al., 1987[861]	38	4.2	5	21	12

necomastia is uncommon; the breasts may appear enlarged, usually because of fatty tissue. In the circumstance of arrested puberty, a female body habitus may be evident and the testes are small (<12 mL in volume) and soft. Symptoms in men with prolactinomas include decreased libido (83%), adiposity (69%), apathy (63%), and headache (63%).[409] The decreased libido and headaches are explained by the tumor itself; however, the reasons for apathy and increased appetite are less clear. Although for most men seeking treatment for sexual dysfunction there is a psychogenic etiology, as many as 8% of such men are hyperprolactinemic, emphasizing the importance of measuring the serum prolactin concentration.[410]

In addition, a pituitary tumor may be incidentally imaged when a CT or MRI scan is obtained because of head trauma or for evaluation of headaches. A less common presentation is that of severe headache and/or prostration secondary to hemorrhage into a previously undiagnosed pituitary tumor. This may cause hypopituitarism, including secondary adrenal insufficiency and hypothyroidism, which requires evaluation and treatment.

COMPLICATIONS. Complications of a prolactin-secreting pituitary tumor may be categorized as those related to tumor size and those produced by hyperprolactinemia. Because a microadenoma is, by definition, an intrasellar tumor, visual abnormalities do not occur. However, headache occurs more often (50%) than in normal subjects (27%).[411] A larger tumor that extends beyond the confines of the sella turcica most commonly produces headache and visual abnormalities. The classic presentation is bitemporal hemianopsia from compression of the optic chiasm by a tumor that has extended superiorly. If the chiasm is prefixed or if the tumor extends posteriorly, compression of a single optic tract occurs, producing a homonymous visual field defect. Lateral extension into the cavernous sinus can cause impaired oculomotor function involving cranial nerves III, IV, and VI and the V_1 and V_2 divisions of V, either singly or in combination. Occasionally, large tumors may extend into the temporal lobe of the brain and cause seizures.

Patients with a large tumor are at risk for compromise of other anterior pituitary function by compression of normal pituitary tissue, producing GH, ACTH, LH, FSH, or TSH deficiency, singly or in combination. GH deficiency is probably the most common, but this has not been studied systematically. Hyperprolactinemia is associated with impaired pulsatile gonadotropin (LH, FSH) release, most likely via alteration in hypothalamic LHRH secretion. The diminished pulsatile LH and FSH release is restored toward normal during infusions of an opiate antagonist, naloxone, suggesting that increased endogenous opiate tone plays a role in the abnormalities of gonadotropin secretion.[412–414] Gonadal insufficiency results from altered pituitary LH and FSH release and is reversible with reduction of prolactin levels.

Decreased bone density is characteristic of both men and women with chronic hyperprolactinemia.[415–418] In men, suppression of hyperprolactinemia and restoration of gonadal function are accompanied by an increase in radial shaft bone density and little change in vertebral bone density; suppression of hyperprolactinemia without restoration of gonadal function does not produce an increase in bone density.[417] In hyperprolactinemic, amenorrheic women, bone mineral content is decreased compared with that in both amenorrheic women with normal serum prolactin and eugonadal women, suggesting that prolactin itself may have a direct effect on bone metabolism.[416]

BIOCHEMICAL EVALUATION. Any patient with a suspected or documented pituitary tumor requires studies to determine whether hypersecretion of one or more hormones is present and whether other pituitary function is normal. Before embarking on extensive, and frequently expensive, testing, a thorough history of drug ingestion should be obtained, because numerous medications may produce hyperprolactinemia. Some causes of pathological hyperprolactinemia are listed in Table 6–17.

In evaluating a patient with a suspected or documented pituitary tumor, the investigations should be focused on the clinical findings, such as evidence of Cushing's syndrome, acromegaly, or TSH-induced hyperthyroidism. If these conditions are not evident, screening studies should include measurement of serum prolactin, alpha subunit, LH, FSH, IGF I (to exclude coexistent excessive GH secretion), β-hCG (in women, to exclude pregnancy), T_4, and TSH (to exclude primary hypothyroidism). A single prolactin measurement may be sufficient to diagnose a prolactinoma if the value is greater than 200 μg/L. Because prolactin is secreted in a pulsatile fashion and in response to breast manipulation, a

TABLE 6–17. Causes of Hyperprolactinemia

Hypothalamic disease
  Tumor, e.g., metastases, craniopharyngioma, germinoma, cyst, glioma, hamartoma
  Infiltrative disease, e.g., sarcoidosis, tuberculosis, histiocytosis X, granuloma
  Pseudotumor cerebri
  Cranial radiation
Pituitary disease
  Prolactinoma
  Acromegaly
  Cushing's disease
  Pituitary stalk section
  Empty sella syndrome
  Other tumors, e.g., metastases, nonsecretory, gonadotrope adenoma, meningioma
  Intrasellar germinoma
  Infiltrative disease, e.g., sarcoidosis, giant cell granuloma, tuberculosis
Drugs
  Dopamine receptor antagonists, e.g., chlorpromazine, fluphenazine, haloperidol, perphenazine, promazine, domperidone, metoclopramide, sulpiride
  Other drugs
    Antihypertensives, e.g., methyldopa, reserpine, verapamil
    Estrogens
    Opiates
    Cimetidine
Primary hypothyroidism
Chronic renal failure
Cirrhosis
Neurogenic, e.g., breast manipulation, chest wall lesions, spinal cord lesions
Stress, e.g., physical, psychological
Idiopathic

mildly increased concentration of 20 to 60 μg/L may be difficult to interpret; in this situation it is prudent to obtain several measurements before making the diagnosis of pathological hyperprolactinemia. A morning cortisol concentration is used as a screen for adrenal function. However, a normal morning cortisol concentration does not assess hypothalamic-pituitary reserve, and a stimulatory test such as insulin-induced hypoglycemia or metyrapone administration is necessary to determine whether the hypothalamic-pituitary-adrenal axis is functionally intact. Induction of hypoglycemia can also be used to determine GH reserve. Additional helpful studies include measurement of plasma testosterone (men) and estradiol (women).

An increased serum prolactin concentration must be interpreted in conjunction with the anatomical findings (MRI and CT scans) to determine whether the hyperprolactinemia is a result of a prolactinoma or is a secondary phenomenon. A serum prolactin concentration of 200 μg/L or greater, in the presence of a macroadenoma (>10 mm), is most likely to be due to a prolactinoma. Conversely, a serum prolactin concentration of less than 200 μg/L in the setting of a large pituitary tumor most likely indicates secondary hyperprolactinemia resulting from the mechanical effects of a non–prolactin-secreting tumor that causes pituitary stalk compression or interference with dopamine transport from the hypothalamus to the anterior pituitary. This distinction is particularly important in selecting appropriate therapy; dopamine agonist drugs reduce serum prolactin levels in both instances, but shrinkage of the tumor is unlikely with secondary hyperprolactinemia.[419] Patients with a prolactin-secreting microadenoma usually have serum prolactin concentrations of less than 200 μg/L. Hyperprolactinemia can also be caused by nonpituitary intracranial lesions; serum prolactin concentrations may be increased, usually to less than 100 μg/L, in the setting of a craniopharyngioma, meningioma, ectopic pinealoma, metastatic tumor, or third ventricle tumor.[420]

Several stimulatory tests have been proposed to determine whether the elevated prolactin concentration is a result of a prolactinoma; these include administration of TRH, dopamine antagonists (e.g., sulpiride, chlorpromazine), and other drugs that act through diverse mechanisms (e.g., cimetidine and dextroamphetamine). For example, patients with prolactinomas have a diminished prolactin response to TRH, but this response is not consistent and cannot be used to diagnose or exclude a tumor or to distinguish between hypothalamic or pituitary disease.[421] Thus these tests are nonspecific and not particularly useful in evaluating a patient with a suspected prolactinoma.

PATHOLOGY. The lactotrope adenoma is the most common pituitary adenoma in surgical series.[347] Its frequency was as high as 31% before the introduction of dopamine agonist therapy and is now approximately 26%. With the exception of rare acidophilic tumors, lactotrope adenomas are chromophobic or slightly acidophilic with a diffuse histological pattern. Small tumors may rarely be papillary. Immunohistochemistry substantiates prolactin production in the form of strong positivity in the Golgi region of adenoma cells. Diffuse cytoplasmic immunostaining is noted in the rare, densely granulated variant. Accumulation of spherical calcified bodies (calcospherites) in these tumors[422–424] is an important marker because, with the exception of craniopharyngioma and meningioma, calcification is uncommon in sellar tumors. A form of endocrine amyloid may be present intra- and extracellularly.[347, 425]

The ultrastructural appearance of the sparsely granulated lactotrope adenoma is highly characteristic.[347, 426, 427] The middle-sized, polyhedral adenoma cells have nuclei with large dense nucleoli. The ample cytoplasm contains abundant, highly organized RER and a prominent Golgi apparatus with pleomorphic, immature secretory granules (Fig. 6–29). The cytoplasmic storage granules are sparse, are between 120 and 300 nm in size, and are invariably involved in exocytosis. The number of granule extrusions varies widely among tumors. The electron microscopic features of the rare, densely granulated variant are similar to those of densely granulated somatotrope adenomas, including the similar size of the secretory granules (400 to 700 nm). A distinguishing feature is the presence of granule extrusions in the lactotrope. It is important to note that the wide range of biological behavior displayed by lactotrope adenomas is not reflected in the light microscopic or electron microscopic features of these tumors.

The variable clinical response[428–430] of lactotrope adenomas to dopaminergic agonists is reflected in the light microscopic and electron microscopic appearance of these tumors.[426, 431] Optimally, a dopaminergic agonist produces a significant decrease or return to normal of serum prolactin concentration and a reduction in tumor volume. The lactotrope tumor that has been suppressed by dopamine agonists is cellular and contains scant, sometimes barely detectable, prolactin immunoreactivity. By electron microscopy the tumor tissue consists of small cells with markedly heterochromatic, multiply indented nuclei and a small rim of cytoplasm containing involuted RER and Golgi membranes (Fig. 6–30). Secretory granules vary in number, and granule extrusions are present[432–434] (Fig. 6–31). In addition, some tumors contain a mixed population of suppressed cells and cells

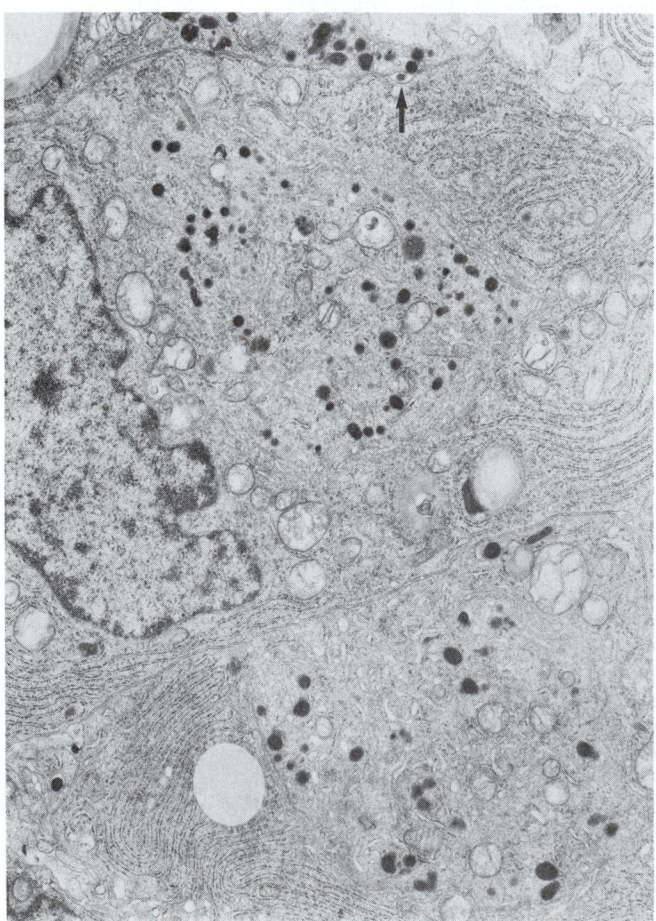

Figure 6–29. Typical sparsely granulated prolactin cell adenoma with abundant RER, prominent Golgi apparatus with numerous immature secretory granules, and granule extrusion *(arrow)*. Magnification × 11,800.

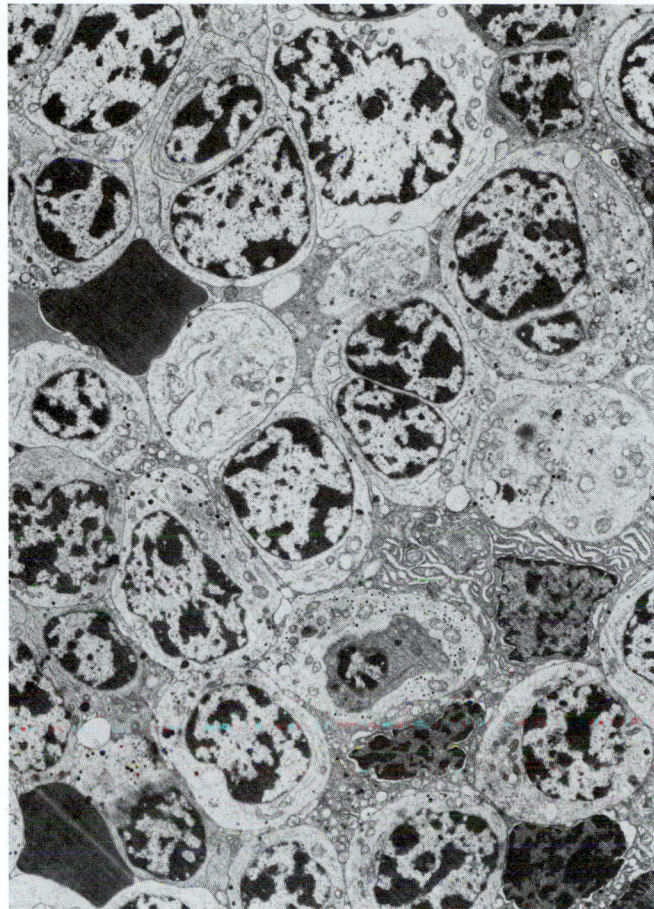

Figure 6–30. Marked bromocriptine effect in a sparsely granulated prolactin cell adenoma. Note the irregular, heterochromatic nuclei and the tiny rim of cytoplasm containing few membranous organelles and secretory granules. Magnification × 4450.

displaying varying degrees of synthetic activity.[426, 431] Conversely, in a minority of tumors under dopaminergic agonist influence, neither a significant decrease in the serum prolactin concentration nor morphological signs of suppression are noted.[431]

The variability of responsiveness to dopaminergic agonists is also evident after withdrawal of drug treatment.[431] Under such conditions the original structure of cells may be restored within 2 wk, but in some lactotrope adenomas groups of suppressed cells are still present 1 mo or more after cessation of medical treatment. This phenomenon may partly explain why serum prolactin concentrations do not always return to pretreatment values.[435]

The morphological findings indicate that individual prolactin-producing adenomas respond in different ways to dopaminergic drugs.[436] A significant reduction of the serum prolactin level and tumor volume represents a decrease in gene expression and thus in hormone synthesis.[436] Mild or moderate decreases in serum prolactin concentration without morphological signs of suppression probably occur because of tissue insensitivity to dopamine.

Protracted medical treatment of prolactinomas may lead to marked calcification, deposition of endocrine amyloid, and perivascular and interstitial fibrosis.[437–440] The latter, if extensive, may decrease the chance for successful surgery.[438, 441] Prolactin cell carcinoma is rare, and only a few cases have been published.[442–444]

Lactotrope hyperplasia, as the sole demonstrable pathological lesion responsible for hyperprolactinemia, is rare in surgical material, but on occasion there may be an increase in the number of lactotropes in the nontumorous pituitary adjacent to the prolactinoma.[347, 445] Overactivity and hyperplasia of prolactin cells may also develop in association with thyrotrope hyperplasia secondary to untreated long-standing hypothyroidism,[446] and increased activity and hyperplastic proliferation of lactotropes may be present in glands harboring corticotrope adenomas.[447] Because of limited availability of tissue, prolactin cell hyperplasia is probably underreported in surgical specimens; even when observed, the extent has not been established and the etiology is unknown.

GOALS OF TREATMENT. The therapeutic objectives for a prolactinoma and for other types of tumors are well defined. Treatment should promote reduction in hormonal hypersecretion to normal, reduction in tumor size, and correction of visual and/or cranial nerve abnormalities; should restore any abnormal pituitary function, and, if possible, should preclude the need for chronic hormone replacement therapy. These objectives are the ideal, but in the case of very large tumors, only partial achievement of these goals may be possible.

Successful treatment of a prolactinoma is most often and easily accomplished with administration of a dopamine agonist drug. Over the past 20 y dopamine agonist drugs have undergone extensive evaluation, and the results indicate that the therapeutic goals are most successfully accomplished with medical therapy. In addition to medical and surgical treatments, pituitary radiation is also employed, most often as adjunctive therapy. A minority of patients

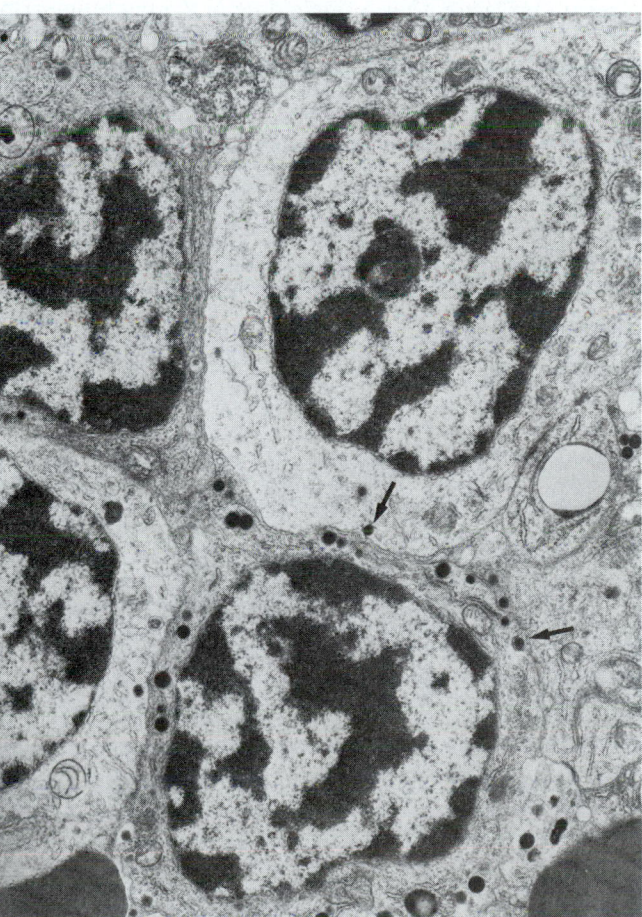

Figure 6–31. Same prolactin cell adenoma as depicted in Figure 6–30. Despite bromocriptine-induced involution of cytoplasmic organelles, granules are still being extruded (arrows). Magnification × 13,200.

require more than one type of treatment to effect reduction in prolactin concentration to normal and a decrease in tumor size.

MEDICAL THERAPY. An orally active dopamine agonist, the semisynthetic ergot alkaloid bromocriptine, was introduced in 1971 for treatment of hyperprolactinemia. The development of this and other dopamine agonists provided a medical approach to the treatment of hyperprolactinemia and prolactinomas. During the ensuing years numerous studies have documented the effectiveness of these drugs in lowering serum prolactin concentrations, in reducing tumor size, in improving visual field and cranial nerve abnormalities, and in restoring gonadal function.

A dopamine agonists lower serum prolactin concentrations in the majority of patients, but the degree of prolactin suppression varies (Fig. 6–32). In 13 reported series of 286 hyperprolactinemic women, bromocriptine lowered serum prolactin levels to normal in 64 to 100%, galactorrhea was improved in 57 to 100%, and menses and ovulation returned in 57 to 100%.[448] Suppression of prolactin secretion is dependent on the number and affinity of adenoma dopamine receptors as demonstrated by studies correlating the clinical response to bromocriptine with in vitro measurement of the number and affinity of dopamine receptors on the surgically resected adenomas. The adenomas from patients with the greatest suppression of serum prolactin by bromocriptine contained the largest number of dopamine receptors, and receptor binding activity was greater in these adenomas than in those from patients less responsive to bromocriptine.[449] As an example of the variable response, earlier studies demonstrated either partial or almost complete suppression of serum prolactin after a single dose of 2.5 mg bromocriptine. Serum prolactin was suppressed for 9 h by 47 to 97%; chronic treatment produced a further decrease in serum prolactin concentration.[430, 450] In addition, although patients with markedly increased serum prolactin concentrations, such as 1000 µg/L, have reductions in prolactin with dopamine agonist administration, suppression to normal may not occur as rapidly as in patients with lesser degrees of elevation; this variability may be related to the number of adenoma cells.

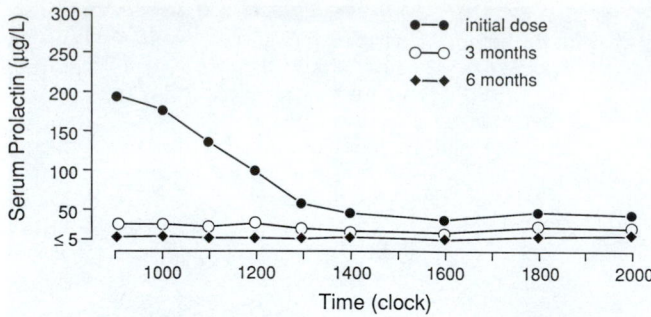

Figure 6–32. Effects of bromocriptine in vivo. After a single 2.5-mg dose of bromocriptine administered at 9 AM, prolactin secretion was inhibited within 2 h and reached a nadir at 7 h. With chronic treatment (2.5 mg three times daily) of 3 and 6 mo, prolactin levels were maintained within the normal range throughout a 24-h period. (Modified from Thorner MO. Hyperprolactinaemia. In: Besser GM, Cudworth AG, eds. Clinical Endocrinology: An Illustrated Text. London: Gower Medical, 1987: 4.1–4.12.)

The results of dopamine agonist treatment of patients with macroadenomas are similar to those of patients with microadenomas except that patients with large tumors may require a longer time to achieve the desired outcome of lowering serum prolactin level to normal (Fig. 6–33). Nevertheless, reduction in tumor size with improvement in visual abnormalities and 60 to 80% suppression of serum prolactin usually occur before achievement of a normal serum prolactin level. In a prospective study of 27 patients with a macroadenoma treated with bromocriptine, 67% had suppression of prolactin concentration to normal during 15 mo of treatment, all had a reduction in tumor size, and 9 of 10 had improvement in visual field defects.[430] In 38 patients treated with either lisuride or bromocriptine for 30 to 88 mo, 79% had reduction of prolactin level to normal and 76% had a decrease in tumor size.[451] In patients in whom serum prolactin concentration does not return to normal there is usually a substantial reduction in the serum level. Patients with visual field defects may have improvement in these abnormalities before a demonstrable decrease in tumor

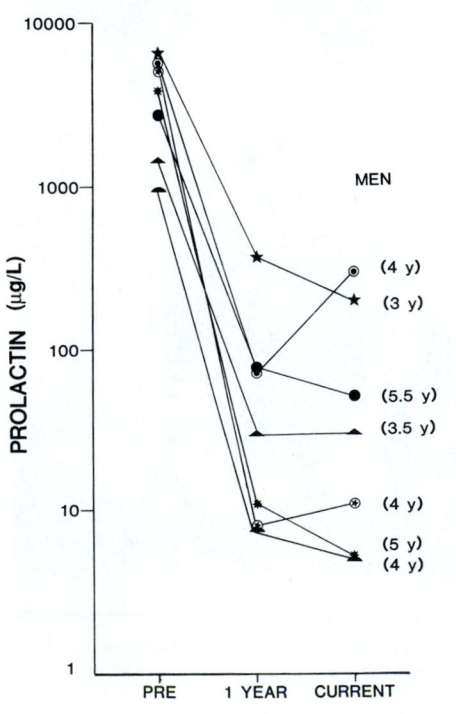

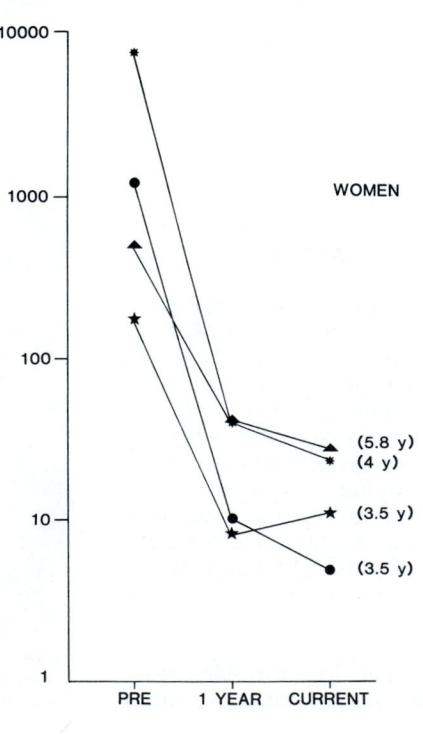

Figure 6–33. Serum prolactin concentrations in patients with prolactin-secreting macroadenomas before and after long-term treatment with bromocriptine, 2.5 mg three times a day. Note continued suppression of prolactin over time. Values are plotted on a semilogarithmic scale. (Unpublished observations, courtesy of M. L. Vance.)

size by CT or MRI studies; this emphasizes the fact that careful monitoring of vision and visual fields is a more sensitive indicator of tumor response than imaging studies.

The usual dose of bromocriptine is 2.5 mg three times daily. In patients who achieve a normal serum prolactin level, the dose may be reduced to 2.5 mg twice daily; continued suppression may continue with the reduced dose. Some patients have been given larger bromocriptine doses (e.g., 20 to 30 mg/d) in an attempt to suppress prolactin concentration to normal, but there is no conclusive evidence that a larger dose is any more effective than the standard regimen. The standard dose of lisuride is 0.2 mg three times daily. In 30 patients treated with either bromocriptine or lisuride, 21 had continued suppression of prolactin level to normal and no increase in tumor size after reduction of the dose.[451]

Available dopamine agonists include bromocriptine (the only drug approved in the United States for treatment of hyperprolactinemia), lisuride, pergolide, metergoline, and an experimental nonergot preparation, CV 205–502. Figure 6–34 shows the results of treatment of a macroprolactinoma with CV 205–502. These drugs act by direct stimulation of neuronal and pituitary cell membrane dopamine receptors (D_2); both in vitro and in vivo, prolactin secretion is inhibited.[452–454] A single dose of 2.5 mg bromocriptine suppresses serum prolactin level for up to 14 h,[428, 455] and although the drug is not measurable in the serum[428, 456] the biological effect may persist up to 24 h in some patients. The most common side effects of dopamine agonists are nausea and orthostatic hypotension, which occur commonly on initiation of treatment and can be minimized by beginning with a small dose administered with food and by increasing the dose gradually over 1 to 2 wk. Less common side effects include headache, fatigue, nasal stuffiness, abdominal cramping, and constipation.[448] Despite taking the medication

with food, some patients have gastrointestinal intolerance. Administration of bromocriptine intravaginally to women suppresses prolactin levels with fewer side effects.[457] Hallucinations and psychosis have also been observed. The incidence of psychosis was 1.3% in one study of 600 patients; the symptoms included auditory hallucinations, delusions, and mood changes that abated when the dopamine agonist was discontinued.[458] Concomitant alcohol ingestion may exacerbate the symptoms of nausea and abdominal discomfort.[459] Patients usually develop tolerance to the side effects, but there is no loss of effectiveness in suppressing prolactin secretion.

A dopamine agonist is usually given chronically and thus functions as a hormone "replacement" because, for whatever reason, these patients have a functional pituitary dopamine deficiency. Withdrawal of treatment usually results in an increase in serum prolactin concentrations (Fig. 6–35) and re-expansion of the tumor.[429, 448, 454, 460] Occasionally, a patient with a microadenoma or no demonstrable tumor has no increase in prolactin concentration after stopping dopamine agonist therapy. Whether spontaneous infarction of the tumor occurred is not known. If medication is discontinued, the patient should be followed closely with measurement of the serum prolactin concentration; if it increases, medical therapy should be restarted.

Suppression of serum prolactin level to normal and resumption of ovulatory menses occur in 80 to 90% of hyperprolactinemic women during bromocriptine therapy.[448, 461] The fertility rate of these patients should be identical with that of other women of the same age. A standard recommendation for women attempting to become pregnant is that barrier contraception be used until the patient has had two or three regular cycles, so that cycle length can be determined. After discontinuation of mechanical contraception, a serum β-hCG measurement is made to

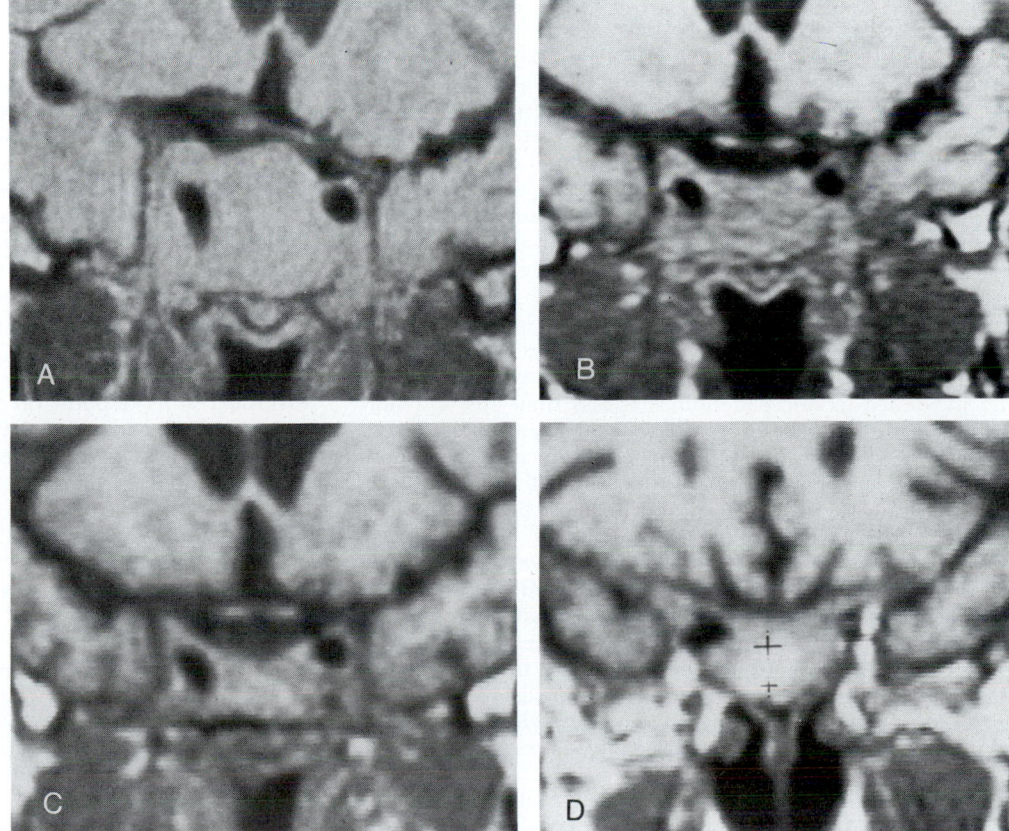

Figure 6–34. T1-weighted coronal MRI scan of a 67-y-old man treated with the dopamine agonist CV 205-502. *A,* Homogeneous tumor extending to the optic chiasm and into the cavernous sinus bilaterally, serum prolactin level 15,000 μg/L. *B,* After 8 wk of treatment, the height of the tumor decreased by 20 mm. *C,* After 24 wk of treatment, gland height decreased by 30 mm from baseline, serum prolactin level 11 μg/L. *D,* After 24 wk of treatment, more anterior image demonstrating an area of high signal consistent with hemorrhage that was not present on previous scans. (From Vance ML, Lipper M, Klibanski A, et al. Treatment of prolactin-secreting pituitary macroadenomas with the long-acting non-ergot dopamine agonist CV 205-502. Ann Intern Med 1990; 112:668–673.)

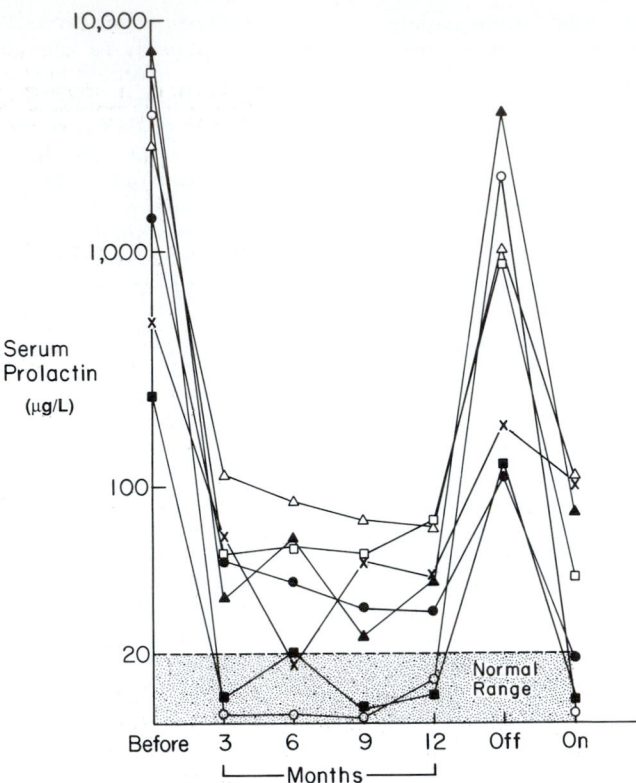

Figure 6–35. Serum prolactin concentrations in seven patients with prolactin-secreting macroadenomas before and during treatment with bromocriptine, 2.5 mg three times a day, and after discontinuation and reinstitution of treatment. Bromocriptine reduces serum prolactin concentrations; withdrawal of treatment results in an increase toward pretreatment values. Serum concentrations decrease with reinstitution of therapy. Values are plotted on a semilogarithmic scale. (From Vance ML, Evans WS, Thorner MO. Drugs five years later. Bromocriptine. Ann Intern Med 1984; 100:78–91.)

confirm pregnancy as soon as there is a delay in expected menses. This regimen makes possible early diagnosis of pregnancy and early discontinuation of dopamine agonist therapy. Surveillance of more than 2000 pregnancies indicates that bromocriptine use is not associated with an increased risk of multiple pregnancies, spontaneous abortions, ectopic pregnancy, trophoblastic disease, or congenital malformations.[462–466] Complications related to tumor expansion during pregnancy may occur, particularly in women with macroadenomas. The incidence of clinically significant tumor enlargement during pregnancy is 1.4% in women with microadenomas and approximately 16% in women with macroadenomas.[461] Both of these percentages are likely overestimates resulting from observer bias. In our experience the incidence in microadenomas is less than 1% and may even be less than 0.1%. Therapies in the event of significant tumor enlargement include surgical resection, high-dose glucocorticoid therapy, and reinstitution of bromocriptine. Bromocriptine is effective and is the most benign therapy. Patients with macroadenomas treated with bromocriptine continuously during pregnancy do not have tumor-related complications. Similarly, those given bromocriptine after tumor expansion had occurred experienced improvement or resolution of headaches and of visual field defects.[467–471] Because of the risk of tumor expansion in women with macroadenomas, a thorough ophthalmological examination, including visual field testing, is recommended before conception is attempted so that baseline values can be documented.

After cyclic menses have been restored, the need for contraception for those not desiring pregnancy should be addressed. Because estrogens stimulate prolactin synthesis and lactotrope mitotic activity, there is a theoretical risk of promoting enlargement of a prolactinoma with oral contraceptive use. However, in hyperprolactinemic women who have had suppression of prolactin concentration to normal with bromocriptine, addition of an oral contraceptive is not associated with an increase in serum prolactin level.[472] Thus the use of an oral contraceptive containing a low dose of estrogen after suppression of prolactin to normal is a reasonable regimen as long as dopamine agonist treatment is continued.

Men treated with a dopamine agonist have improvement in libido and potency as the serum testosterone concentration increases. Some men note marked improvement in function early in treatment before the testosterone concentration becomes normal. The semen analysis (sperm count and semen volume) improves with lowering of prolactin level to normal and restoration of normal pulsatile gonadotropin (LH and FSH) secretion. A large number of such men have not been surveyed, but individual reports have documented such improvements.[467]

Although the majority of patients have a favorable response to dopamine agonist treatment, some have a partial response or are unresponsive. The clinical response to bromocriptine and the number and affinity of tumor dopamine receptors are correlated. Surgically resected adenomas from bromocriptine-responsive patients have twice as many dopamine receptors and approximately 50% higher binding affinity for dopamine than adenomas from bromocriptine-resistant patients.[449] These observations probably explain tumor growth during bromocriptine therapy, loss of responsiveness, and occasional metastasis of tumors.[442, 473–475] Fortunately, resistance to bromocriptine is uncommon, but all patients should be closely monitored during medical therapy. If a patient fails to respond to medical treatment, surgical resection should be considered.

The nonergot long-acting dopamine agonist CV 205–502 has been used to treat microadenomas and macroadenomas. This compound, an octahydrobenzyl(q)quinolone, is given once daily and may be useful in patients intolerant of bromocriptine and other ergot derivatives. The suppression of serum prolactin, restoration of gonadal function, and decrease in tumor size with this drug are comparable to those with other dopamine agonists.[476–478]

SURGICAL THERAPY. Before the development of medical therapy, surgery was the most effective treatment for a prolactinoma. Transsphenoidal resection of the adenoma is frequently employed and is associated with better results and less morbidity than other surgical approaches. Although surgical resection offers the potential for cure, in fact a cure is effected in a minority of patients with large tumors and is associated with a risk of recurrence in all patients. The surgical results depend on the skill and experience of the surgeon. Patients with microadenomas (<10 mm) treated with surgery at centers where the procedure is performed frequently have a normal postoperative serum prolactin concentration 60 to 80% of the time; a normal serum prolactin level is achieved in 0 to 40% of patients with macroadenomas (>10 mm).[479–484] The most important factors predictive of successful surgery are the preoperative serum prolactin concentration and the tumor size. Of 266 women with a prolactinoma, a normal postoperative serum prolactin level was achieved in 86% when the preoperative prolactin concentration was 20 to 250 μg/L, in 48% when the preoperative concentration was 250 to 500 μg/L, and in 6% when the preoperative concentration was greater than 1000 μg/L; similar results have been obtained in 55 hyperprolactinemic men.[484] A summary of reports of surgical series is shown in Table 6–18.

TABLE 6–18. Surgical Results in Patients with Prolactinomas

Author, Year	Number of Patients*	Normal Postoperative Prolactin (%)	Percent Recurrence (Time, y)
Aubourg et al., 1980[862]	90		NR†
	23 micro	57	
	67 macro	39	
Chang et al., 1977[480]	33		NR
	17 micro	59	
	6 macro	0	
Charpentier et al., 1985[863]	347		17 (1.5 ± 0.4)
	PRL < 100	89	
	PRL < 200	72	
	PRL > 200	21	
Ciric et al., 1983[864]	41		NR
	41 macro	27	
Faria and Tindall, 1982[865]	100		
	72 PRL < 200	76	13 (0.6–7)
	28 PRL > 200	46	36 (0.6–7)
Grisoli et al., 1980[866]	20		NR
	PRL < 100	100	
	PRL > 100	25	
Hardy et al., 1978[481]	80		NR
	PRL < 200	87	
	PRL > 200	19	
Keye et al., 1979[867]	43	85	NR
Landolt, 1981[868]	70		NR
	PRL < 200	88	
	PRL > 200	18	
Nelson et al., 1983[485]	40	63	36 (1.3 ± 0.2)
Parl et al., 1986[490]	24		
	13 micro	100	31 (5.2, mean)
	11 macro	100	91 (5.2, mean)
Post et al., 1979[483]	30		NR
	17 micro	82	
	13 macro	46	
Randall et al., 1983[869]	100		NR
	54 micro	69	
	36 macro	34	
Rawe et al., 1980[870]	30		NR
	21 micro	81	
	9 macro	33	
Rodman et al., 1984[488]	65		
	42 micro	88	17 (4.2 ± 0.3)
	23 macro	39	20 (4.2 ± 0.3)
Schlechte and Sherman, 1981[871]	67	43	NR
Thomson et al., 1985[489]	69		
	61 micro	75	10 (5)
	8 macro	50	50 (5)
Tindall et al., 1978[482]	37		NR
	26 prolactin < 200	73	
	11 prolactin > 200	27	
Tucker et al., 1981[486]	45		12 (3.2)
	27 micro	74	
	15 macro	53	
Woosley et al., 1982[487]	36		
	22 micro	72	5 (0.3–3)
	14 macro	29	0 (0.3–3)

*Characterization of patients: micro, tumor less than 10 mm in diameter; macro, tumor greater than 10 mm in diameter. PRL < or > indicates preoperative prolactin level, in µg/L.
†NR, not reported.

Although surgery is effective in debulking large tumors and may be curative for small tumors, the potential for recurrent hyperprolactinemia and presumptive tumor regrowth must be taken into account when considering this treatment. Recurrence rates in up to 5 y of follow-up range from 10 to 50% in patients with a microadenoma and from 0 to 91% in those with a macroadenoma.[485–490] There is a very low risk of mortality with transsphenoidal surgery (<1%);[491] complications include CSF rhinorrhea, diabetes insipidus, infection, damage to the visual system (less common with transsphenoidal surgery than with craniotomy), and anterior pituitary insufficiency. The cumulative risk for these complications is on the order of 2% for patients with microadenomas and 14% for patients with macroadenomas.[491] The risk of morbidity is increased in patients subjected to a second surgical procedure; in a heterogeneous group of 158 patients who had received prior surgical and/or medical therapy, 35% with pituitary hypersecretion had a successful surgical outcome, 59% with visual disturbances improved, and 74% had successful repair of CSF rhinorrhea. However, 32% had new complications after surgery, including stroke or vascular injury, hemorrhage, visual loss, meningitis, CSF rhinorrhea, cranial nerve palsy, permanent diabetes insipidus, hypopituitarism, nasal septal perforation, and four deaths.[492] Thus surgical resection of a microadenoma offers the greatest potential for cure; the usual outcome for patients with a large tumor is partial resection with residual tumor and persistent hyperprolactinemia requiring additional therapy.

RADIATION THERAPY. Pituitary radiation as primary treatment of a prolactinoma is effective in preventing further growth of the tumor but is less effective in promoting a prompt reduction of the serum prolactin concentration. Patients given pituitary radiation as primary therapy have a progressive reduction in serum prolactin concentration over time, but rapid lowering of the hormone concentration is rare. Of 28 patients treated with radiation, only 2 had a normal serum prolactin level 2 to 10 y (mean 4.2 y) after treatment;[493] in another group of 6 followed for 13 to 72 mo (mean 32.2 mo) the prolactin level was reduced by 94% but none became normal.[479] In another group of 14 patients, 3 had a decrease in prolactin concentration to normal within 21 to 33 mo, and a single patient had a normal prolactin level 6 y after treatment.[494] Of 26 patients who were treated with radiation, 3 had reduction of prolactin level to normal, the duration of observation ranging from 1 mo to 6 y.[390] Combined therapy with a dopamine agonist and radiotherapy was given to 36 women with small prolactinomas; 28 were later evaluated when the dopamine agonist was withdrawn. Prolactin concentration decreased in 25, and 8 became normal 2 to 8 y after radiotherapy. The fertility rate in these women was 73% in those who desired pregnancy, and the apparent ovulation rate was 94%. The restoration of fertility was most likely a result of the dopamine agonist treatment because 92% of those who conceived did so within 4 mo of combined dopamine agonist and radiation therapy. None had a significant increase in tumor size during pregnancy.[495]

The recommended radiation dose is a total of 45 Gy administered as 1.8 Gy/d over 25 d. A high-energy linear accelerator, rather than a ^{60}Co teletherapy apparatus, combined with a rotational arc technique provides maximal limitation of the high-dose region and usually produces little or no hair loss.[496] A total radiation dose of less than 40 Gy results in poor tumor control, and total doses greater than 50 Gy or daily doses greater than 2 Gy are associated with higher complication rates and no demonstrable improvement in the overall results.[389] Complications of pituitary radiation include hypopituitarism, optic chiasm and/or optic nerve injury, vascular damage with stroke, brain necrosis, and carcinogenesis (fibrosarcoma, osteosarcoma). Radiation-induced hypopituitarism has been best documented in acromegalic patients treated with radiotherapy, and the incidence increases with time after radiotherapy. Of the pituitary hormone deficiencies, gonadotropin deficiency is most common, occurring in 47 to 70% of patients treated with either radiation alone or surgery and radiation. Second most common is ACTH deficiency (15 to 67%), followed by TSH deficiency (15 to 55%).[396, 497, 498] There have been no adequate studies of GH secretion after radiotherapy, but random measurements in these patients frequently reveal undetectable plasma GH.

Acromegaly

In 1886 Pierre Marie used the term acromegaly in describing two patients and reviewed eight previously published papers describing patients with presumed acromegaly.[499] Minkowsky, in 1887, deduced a relationship between a pituitary tumor and the development of acromegaly.[500] Four years later the New Sydenham Society published a translation of Marie's original paper and a review by de Souza-Leite of 48 patients.[501]

The exact prevalence of acromegaly in the United States is unknown. Information on acromegaly in hospital populations does not reflect a general population. In Newcastle-upon-Tyne in England the estimated prevalence of acromegaly was 38 per million with an annual incidence of 3 per million.[502] In Göteborg, Sweden the prevalence and annual incidence were estimated to be 69 per million and 3.3 per million, respectively.[503] The percentages of acromegalics in two large pituitary surgical series, each of more than 1000 pituitary tumors, were 13.7 and 17.1%, respectively.[504, 505]

Acromegaly occurs with equal frequency in men and women and may occur at any age but is most frequent in the fourth and fifth decades. When it occurs before puberty, gigantism results—a rare syndrome that accounts for less than 5% of acromegalics (derived from data in ref. 504). Acromegaly may occur as a part of MEN 1 syndrome; the prevalence of MEN 1 in the Mayo Clinic surgical series was 15 of 254 (5.9%) acromegalic patients.[504] The MEN 1 syndrome most commonly includes parathyroid adenoma (hyperparathyroidism), pancreatic islet cell tumor (insulinoma), and pituitary adenomas, of which prolactinoma is the most common type.

ETIOLOGIES. Table 6–19 lists the various causes of acromegaly. Over 99% of cases result from a primary pituitary adenoma.[506] Excessive production of GHRH causing somatotrope hyperplasia and possibly tumor formation accounts for less than 1% of cases. GHRH secretion occurs in gangliocytomas (eutopic, either hypothalamic or pituitary) or peripheral tumors (ectopic).[507] Ectopic GH secretion by a pancreatic islet cell tumor has been described.[508]

Whether development of somatotrope adenomas is primarily a pituitary disease or the result of hypothalamic dysregulation is unresolved. However, most evidence suggests that it is a primary pituitary disease. Somatotrope adenomas are circumscribed tumors; the remaining pituitary is normal without evidence of somatotrope hyperplasia. With successful tumor removal and reduction of GH concentration to normal, recurrence is rare. If acromegaly were a hypothalamic disease, recurrence would be expected to be common. Reichlin wrote in 1986, "In my view, the etiology of most cases [of acromegaly] will more likely be found in the genetic analysis of clonal tumors that encode chromosomal growth factors, an insight we have gained from the study of oncogene pathogenesis of cancer."[509] This prediction has been fulfilled in part by the description of a point mutation in an α_s, the GTP-binding subunit of the stimulatory regulator of adenylate cyclase (G_s), in several somatotrope tumors that causes adenylate cyclase to be activated constitutively.[330] Somatotrope tumors appear to be monoclonal in origin.[335]

Ectopic GHRH production is probably more common than is indicated by most series. Approximately 20% of neuroendocrine tumors, including carcinoids, pancreatic endocrine tumors, medullary carcinoma of the thyroid, small cell carcinoma of the lung, and pheochromocytoma, are positive for GHRH when examined with immunocytochemistry,[510, 511] and approximately 60% are positive when tissue is subjected to radioimmunoassay.[512, 513] The elaboration of GHRH by these tumors may be common, but clinical expression is rare for three reasons: (1) somatostatin is often also present in these tumors and is presumably cosecreted, minimizing stimulation of the somatotrope;[514–516] (2) the tumor mass and the synthetic efficiency for GHRH may be inadequate to produce circulating levels that stimulate pituitary GH secretion; and (3) symptoms of acromegaly may be mild, and the patient's life span may be too short for the condition to be detected clinically. With highly malignant tumors, death can occur before the condition is evident.

TABLE 6–19. Etiology of Acromegaly

Gangliocytoma—hypothalamic or pituitary[507]
Pituitary adenoma—pure somatotrope, mammosomatotrope, mixed
Ectopic GHRH-secreting tumors[872]
    59% carcinoid: bronchus (55%), gastrointestinal/pancreas (25%), undetermined (20%)
    21% pancreatic islet tumor
    7% small cell carcinoma
    3% adrenal adenoma
Ectopic GH secretion (one case)[508]

CLINICAL FEATURES. (Table 6–20.) Patients with acromegaly have a gradual progression of symptoms and signs. Thus the diagnosis is often delayed for as many as 15 to 20 y. The symptoms usually begin insidiously, and the changes in the body occur gradually and go unnoticed until complications develop (Figs. 6–36 and 6–37). Symptoms and signs may be a result of the pituitary tumor itself, hypopituitarism, excessive GH secretion, or a combination of features.

The tumor mass may produce headaches and or visual disturbances including a visual field defect or diplopia from ophthalmoplegia. Hypopituitarism may occur if the tumor is large; gonadal dysfunction is more common than hypothyroidism or secondary adrenal insufficiency.

The most common presentation is due to the manifestations of excessive secretion of GH. If the condition occurs before puberty, excessive linear growth causes gigantism. Gigantism is not a trivial problem; the following description from the obituary of Ella Ewing, a 19th-century giant, is quoted to emphasize the major physical, social, and personal problems that giants experience. It should also be noted that Ms. Ewing died prematurely at the age of 40 y, exemplifying the increased morbidity and mortality of untreated gigantism and acromegaly.

Miss Ella Ewing, who died yesterday at her home near Gorin, Scotland County, Missouri, was said to have been the tallest woman in the world. Miss Ewing was 8 feet 4 inches tall. She was 40 years old.

The extraordinary part of Miss Ewing's unusual growth was from the time she was 7 years old until she was 10. At the former age she was a normal little girl. Soon after her seventh birthday anniversary, she began to grow rapidly, and when 10 years old she measured 6 feet 9 inches. She still had the tastes of a child of her age and her life became miserable. She was denied the pleasures of games other children played, because her presence robbed the games of their best while the other children stared at her. She became the butt of their thoughtless jests, and being timid their gibes brought her to tears and drove her away from associates of her own age.

At school desks and seats of great size were constructed for her, and an exceptionally long bed for her was necessary. She was forced to stoop on entering ordinary doors, and the home in which her father and mother were comfortable was like a cage to her. The care of the young giantess became a burden to her father, who was a man of meager means.

But a visit to the county fair solved the financial problem. While she went about the fair grounds in ecstacies at the wonders she saw—prize stock, giant vegetables and the mysteries described by the

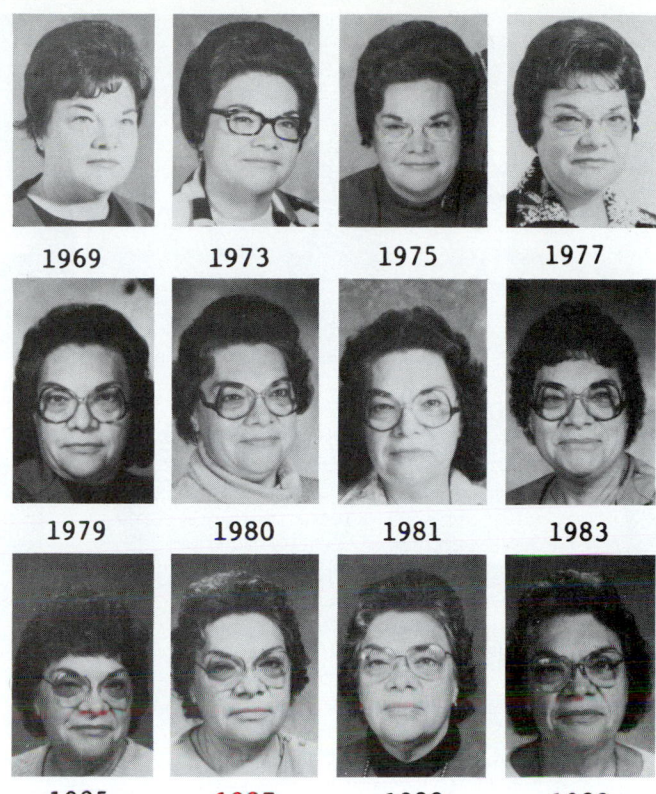

1969   1973   1975   1977

1979   1980   1981   1983

1985   1987   1988   1989

Figure 6–36. Photographs taken over 20 y of a woman with acromegaly from 1969 (age 41) through 1989 (age 61). Note progressive coarsening of facial features. Other characteristics of acromegaly included bilateral carpal tunnel syndrome (1973), hypertension (1975), arthralgias (1979), colonic polyps (1987), and diabetes mellitus (1988). (Unpublished observations, courtesy of M. L. Vance.)

sideshow spielers, she herself was the chief attraction to the others who followed her about, staring at her in wonderment. A museum manager approached her father with an offer of a good salary for her as a museum attraction. It was arranged that her mother should accompany her, and she accepted the offer. Being heralded as a freak stung her sensitive feelings at first but she eventually learned to look upon her extreme size philosophically. That attitude was made more easy by the big receipts.

Subsequently she entered a contract with P. T. Barnum and for several years was an attraction of the big circus, traveling over Europe and America. The dream of her girlhood to own a home where she would be comfortable, at last was realized. In her travels she never had been comfortable. Beds and berths were too short, tables and doors and ceilings too low. She couldn't find comfortable chairs. Life for her was a succession of makeshifts. She saved her salary received from Barnum and after accumulating what she believed to be sufficient to last her, she left the show business and built a home near Gorin. The doors to this house are ten feet tall. The ceilings are fifteen feet. The beds are as long as she chose. Her bathtub was 6 feet long, and a specially made hammock on her veranda was 15 feet long. Clothes closets are the size of ordinary bedrooms and her dining table is 4½ feet high. A peculiarity of Miss Ewing's growth was that above the waistline she remained almost normal, except that her arms grew in proportion to the growth of her legs. Her feet required specially made shoes, No. 24, and she wore No. 24 gloves. Thirty yards of goods were required to make a dress for her. After building a home to her measure, the giantess again became a show attraction, but traveled only in states near her home. She never married. At one time she was engaged to Edward Beaupre, a French-Canadian of Butte, Montana, himself 2 inches taller than his fiancee, but the engagement was "broken off."

Another romance of Miss Ewing's life involved Louis Wilkins of Enid, Oklahoma who measured 8 feet 2 inches in height. He was a suitor for her hand years ago. Both had then just signed contracts with the Barnum show.

TABLE 6–20. Clinical and Laboratory Findings in 57 Patients with Acromegaly

Finding	Present/Total
Recent acral growth	57/57
Arthralgias	41/57
Excessive sweating	52/57
Weakness	50/57
Malocclusion	39/57
New skin tags	33/57
Hypertension (blood pressure > 150/95)	21/57
Carpal tunnel syndrome	25/57
Fasting blood glucose > 6 mmol/L	17/57
Abnormal glucose tolerance test (blood glucose > 6.1 mmol/L [>110 mg/dL])	39/57
Heel pad thickness > 22 mm	48/53
Serum prolactin > 25 µg/L	8/51
Serum phosphorus > 1.5 mmol/L (>4.5 mg/dL)	26/54
Sella volume > 1300 mm³	55/57
Serum T_4 < 53 nmol/L (<4.1 µg/dL)	0/57*
Serum testosterone (men) < 10 nmol/L (<3 ng/mL)	7/30
8 AM serum cortisol < 200 nmol/L (<8 µg/dL)	2/57

*Eleven patients were receiving T_4 replacement at the time of the study.
From Clemmons DR, Van Wyk JJ, Ridgway EC, et al. Evaluation of acromegaly by radioimmunoassay of somatomedin-C. Reprinted, by permission of The New England Journal of Medicine, 301; 1138–1142, 1979.

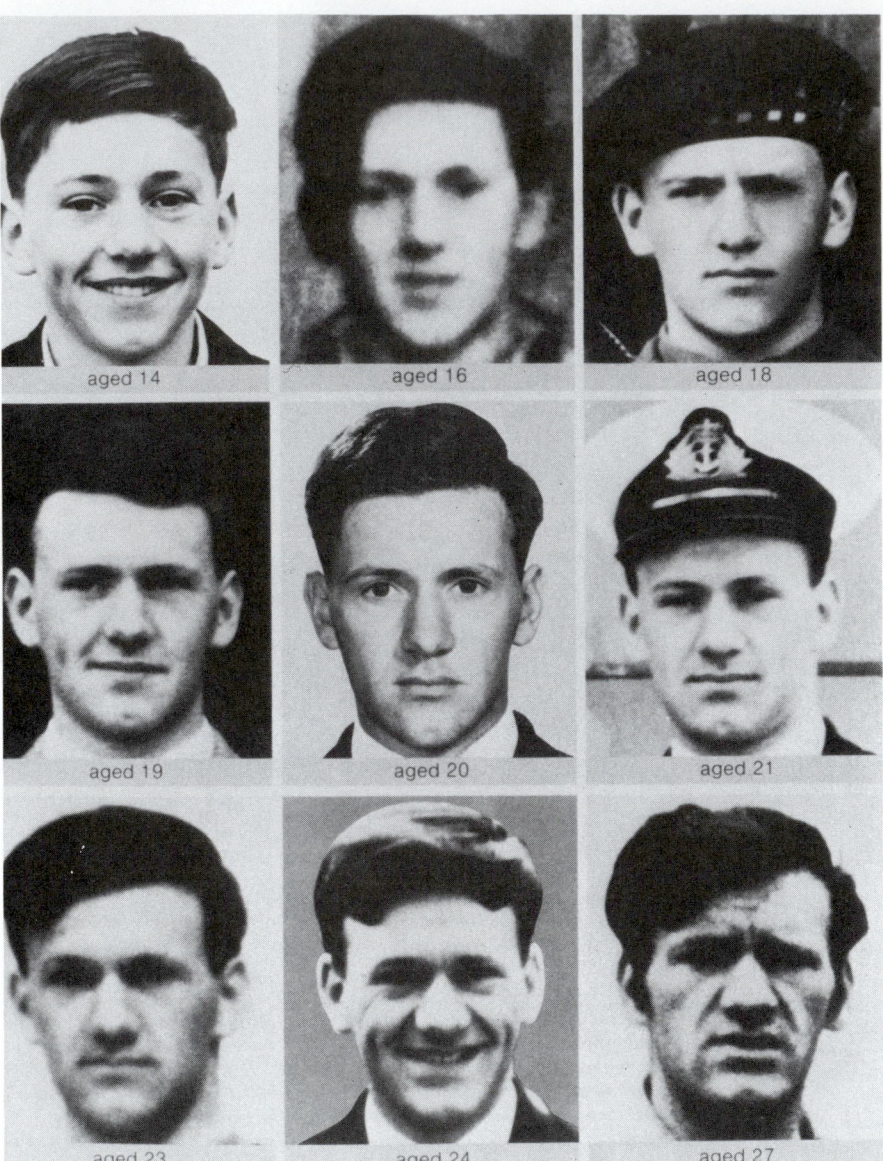

aged 14   aged 16   aged 18

aged 19   aged 20   aged 21

aged 23   aged 24   aged 27

Figure 6–37. Change in facial appearance of a patient with acromegaly over a 13-y period. The development of an acromegalic appearance is seen with enlargement of the supraorbital ridges and nose, thickening of the lips, and generalized coarsening of the features. (From Wass JAH. Acromegaly. In: Besser GM, Cudworth AG, eds. Clinical Endocrinology: An Illustrated Text. London: Gower Medical, 1987: 3.1–3.12.)

Wilkins's suit was unsuccessful. He quit the show business in America and spent years following Miss Ewing's refusal in Germany and Austria. He returned several times to visit his parents, and always on those trips brought some gift for Miss Ewing. Wilkins died about six years ago in Chicago. (Kansas City Times Obituary of Miss Ella Ewing, January 11, 1913.)

More commonly, the condition occurs after puberty, resulting in acromegaly. Thickening and oiliness of the skin, particularly of the face, occur. Facial changes include thick lips, exaggerated nasolabial folds, thickening of the scalp giving rise to the development of deep folds, cutis verticis gyrata, that are visible on skull x-ray film or CT scan. Acanthosis nigricans may occur. The vocal cords thicken, which, in conjunction with sinus enlargement, results in a characteristically deep and resonant voice. The overall appearance and deep voice give acromegalic women a rather masculinized appearance. Women often develop mild hirsutism. The hands and feet enlarge; rings become tighter, cannot be removed, and may have to be cut off. The increased hand and finger size may cause difficulty with performing fine tasks such as picking up a pin; glove size also increases. The foot increases in both length and width. Head size increases because of increases in both soft tissue and skull mass. The calvarium of the skull thickens; hyperostosis frontalis and expansion of the frontal sinuses result in protrusion of the brows (frontal bossing). The zygomatic

arch enlarges to produce prominence of the cheek bones and relative hollowness of the temporal fossae. This feature is particularly evident after successful treatment when the soft tissues regress. The mandible grows in length and breadth, leading to protrusion of the lower jaw, malocclusion, and development of temporomandibular arthritis. The changes in the lower jaw and the temporomandibular arthritis are sometimes the initial feature leading to the diagnosis.

Joint pain resulting from accelerated osteoarthrosis may also be the presenting symptom and may be misdiagnosed as arthritis. In addition to changes in the soft tissues, the shafts of the metacarpals, metatarsals, and phalanges and of the articular cartilages thicken. Tufting of the terminal phalanges develops, and exostoses occur in the bones of the hands and feet. Arthralgias occur in 62 to 75% of acromegalic patients, and arthropathy is present in 16 to 62%. Between 10 and 40% of patients have joint symptoms severe enough to limit daily activities. The knees, hips (main weight-bearing joints), and shoulders are frequently affected; elbows and ankles are relatively spared. The spine may also be affected, most commonly in the lumbosacral region. The initial symptom is joint stiffness, particularly in the hands, which may reflect the increase of subcutaneous tissue that is reversible with reduction of circulating GH concentrations.

Early in the course of the disease joint spaces are

increased secondary to cartilage proliferation. The synovial and periarticular swelling produces joint swelling without effusion. Weight bearing on proliferating cartilage in joints leads to ulceration and development of osteoarthritis. Cartilage degeneration is irreversible.[517, 518] This is often so disabling as to require artificial joint replacement. The arthropathy is often severe at the time of diagnosis and is usually irreversible. However, if acromegaly is treated before the articular cartilage is destroyed, then joint symptoms are reversible.[519, 520]

Backache is associated with dorsal kyphosis. Disc spaces are increased, and anterior osteophytes are common. The spinal mobility is normal or increased because the discs are resilient and paraspinal ligaments become hypertrophied and lax.[517, 518]

Patients with acromegaly often develop a characteristic barrel chest. This is caused by a combination of the changes in the vertebrae and the ribs. The vertebral bodies become elongated and widened by periosteal apposition of bone along the anterior and lateral surfaces. The intervertebral discs in the cervical and lumbar region thicken, and discs in the thoracic area become thin, resulting in development of kyphosis.[521] Because the epiphyses of the osteochondral junctions fail to close, the ribs elongate,[522] which causes an increase in the anteroposterior diameter of the chest. Thus rib elongation and the thoracic kyphosis contribute to the development of a barrel chest.

High levels of GH are associated with excessive sweating, particularly of the face, head, hands, and feet; hyperhidrosis may be a presenting symptom. The increase in soft tissue mass may produce median nerve compression and carpal tunnel syndrome. Carpal tunnel syndrome is a common presentation of acromegaly, and this possibility should be considered in patients with newly diagnosed carpal tunnel syndrome.

Galactorrhea often occurs in acromegalic women but is rare in men. Hyperprolactinemia may be present in up to 40% of acromegalics, but galactorrhea can occur in the absence of hyperprolactinemia, possibly as a result of the lactogenic effects of GH.[523] Between 32 and 87% of acromegalic women under the age of 45 have menstrual abnormalities, and decreased libido and impotence occur in 27 to 46% of men.[524] Gonadal dysfunction can be due to hyperprolactinemia or to the lactogenic effects of GH.

Physical examination demonstrates the typical facial appearance with soft tissue thickening, greasiness of the skin, coarse features, increased breadth of the nose, thickening of the lips, macroglossia, and prognathism. The growth of the lower jaw may produce increased spaces between the teeth. In women, mild hirsutism may be present. The hands are usually spade-like with sausage-shaped fingers (Fig. 6–38). There may be thenar wasting, weakness of thumb abduction, and loss of pinprick sensation in the distribution of the median nerve. The chest may be kyphotic. Generalized organomegaly may be present, including thyroid gland enlargement and palpable thyroid nodules. The skinfold thickness is increased, and the skin, particularly the palms of the hands and soles of the feet, is moist. Multiple skin tags correlate with the occurrence of colonic polyps. Galactorrhea is common in women. The testes may be enlarged. There are often signs of arthritis, particularly in the knees and hips. The feet have soft tissue thickening and an increase in the heel pad thickness. The relative frequencies of these clinical findings are shown in Table 6–20.

COMPLICATIONS. Many of the clinical features of acromegaly are a result of the effects of long-standing overproduction of GH. Some of the complications can be serious.

Metabolic and Endocrine. Hypersecretion of GH induces insulin resistance and glucose intolerance in 29 to 45% and overt diabetes mellitus in 10 to 20%.[524] In nondiabetic acromegalics excessive GH secretion is associated with an exaggerated insulin response to intravenous glucose. In those with impaired glucose tolerance or diabetes mellitus, the insulin response is inadequate to overcome the insulin resistance. The human leukocyte antigen (HLA) phenotype, family history of diabetes mellitus, and duration of acromegaly do not appear to be major risks for development of overt diabetes mellitus.[525]

Hypertriglyceridemia occurs in 19 to 44% of acromegalic patients.[526, 527] There is a positive correlation between the serum insulin response to glucose and increased serum triglyceride concentrations. Hepatic triglyceride lipase and lipoprotein lipase activities are decreased in acromegaly. After successful lowering of GH levels, the activities of these enzymes rise. No consistent abnormalities of cholesterol have been observed.

Respiratory. Pulmonary complications of acromegaly account for some of the risk of premature mortality. A threefold increase in respiratory deaths occurred in the study reported by Wright and colleagues.[528] Abnormal pulmonary

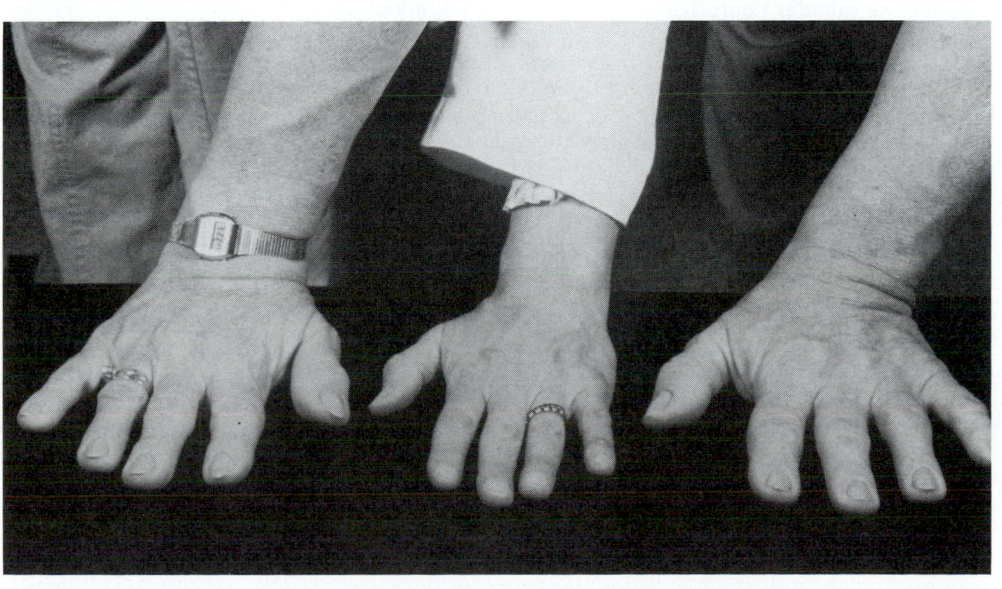

Figure 6–38. Hands of a 49-y-old acromegalic woman (*right and left*) compared with the hand of a normal woman (*middle*). (Unpublished observations, courtesy of M. L. Vance.)

function tests are observed in both acromegalic men and women; increased total lung capacity is present in 81% of men and 56% of women, 36% have small airway narrowing, and 26% have upper airway narrowing.[529, 530] It is likely that airway narrowing accounts for the increased morbidity and mortality of the disease. Airway obstruction caused by exacerbation of upper airway narrowing during upper respiratory tract infections may result in acute dyspnea and stridor. Intubation may be difficult during induction of anesthesia, and the airway may be obstructed by an enlarged tongue after extubation. The risks of anesthesia can be minimized by proper preparation, use of fiberoptic laryngoscopy, and careful monitoring.

Many acromegalic patients have the obstructive sleep apnea syndrome. Symptoms include excessive daytime sleepiness, habitual snoring, and apneic episodes during sleep; the syndrome is diagnosed by polysomnography studies during sleep because pulmonary function tests when the subject is awake are not helpful. Sleep apnea is said to be present if more than 5 apneic episodes occur per hour of sleep or more than 30 apneic episodes occur during the night. The overall prevalence of obstructive sleep apnea was 38%, with men being more commonly affected than women.[531–533] Both the prolapse of an enlarged tongue and the inspiratory collapse of the hypopharynx have been implicated in the pathogenesis of this disorder.[534, 535] Cure of acromegaly does not necessarily correct the sleep apnea.[533, 535] In short-term studies of somatostatin analogue (6 d) or bromocriptine therapy (3 mo), 41 and 75%, respectively, fewer apneic episodes occurred.[536, 537]

Cardiovascular. The major cardiovascular complications of acromegaly are increased prevalence of death from cardiovascular causes, hypertension, and cardiomyopathy. The precise nature of acromegaly-associated heart disease is not clear, but cardiovascular disease is the most common cause of death in acromegalics.[503, 528] The coexistence of hypertension and/or diabetes mellitus makes it difficult to determine whether the cardiac disease is secondary to these disorders or is directly related to GH excess; indeed, there is controversy as to whether a specific acromegalic cardiomyopathy exists. The problem is exemplified by the results of a prospective study of 57 patients;[538] 9 had symptoms of heart disease, but other disorders contributing to the heart disease were identified in 7 of the 9, including hypertension, coronary heart disease, and hyperthyroidism.[538] Of 256 patients studied retrospectively, 10 had heart disease without evidence of hypertension, diabetes mellitus, thyroid disease, or coronary or valvular heart disease.[539] No specific pathological findings have been demonstrated at autopsy.[540] Myocardial hypertrophy occurred in 93%, interstitial fibrosis in 85%, and lymphomononuclear myocarditis in 59% of 27 cases. However, in approximately 80% of acromegalic patients, cardiac enlargement, usually an increase of left ventricular mass, can be detected by echocardiography and is independent of hypertension or ischemic heart disease.[541–545] Impaired left ventricular function is present in some patients. Although the severity of these abnormalities does not consistently correlate with GH levels, the duration of the disease may be an important determinant.[543–545] Increased left ventricular mass, end-systolic wall stress (afterload), fractional shortening, and abnormal cardiac index were documented in 12 acromegalic patients (39 ± 5 y of age) with a relatively short duration of disease (6 ± 3 y). These patients did not have hypertension or cardiac disease.

A model of expanded blood volume and increased peripheral blood flow leading to left ventricular hypertrophy and a hyperkinetic left ventricle has been proposed. With prolonged disease, hypertension develops, and left ventricular function declines. The cardiac abnormalities may persist in some patients after restoration of normal GH levels; in others restoration of normal GH levels is associated with significant improvement. A specific acromegalic cardiomyopathy is unproved.

Hypertension occurs in 18 to 41% of acromegalics;[524, 538, 540, 546–549] the pathophysiology is poorly understood, but it is of the low-renin type. Sodium retention, extracellular fluid volume expansion, and suppression of renin-angiotensin-aldosterone secretion occur in both hypertensive and normotensive acromegalic patients. Overactivity of the sympathetic nervous system has been suggested as a possible etiological factor.[550] Hypertension has been associated with higher mean GH concentrations and longer duration of acromegaly; it is usually mild and uncomplicated and responds to conventional antihypertensive medications. Rarely, the hypertension may result from other endocrine causes, such as pheochromocytoma,[551] primary hyperparathyroidism, or an aldosterone-secreting adenoma.[552]

Calcium and Bone Metabolism. Serum 1,25-dihydroxycholecalciferol concentrations are increased in acromegaly, whereas 25-hydroxycholecalciferol levels are low and serum parathyroid hormone and calcitonin levels are normal. The increase in 1,25-dihydroxycholecalciferol concentrations is a result of GH stimulation of renal 1α-hydroxylase activity. The consequence is an increase in intestinal calcium absorption and hypercalciuria; serum calcium levels are normal unless coincidental hyperparathyroidism is present. GH increases tubular phosphate reabsorption with resulting hyperphosphatemia in approximately half of acromegalics. The metabolic consequences are reversed with lowering of serum GH levels to normal. Urolithiasis occurs in 6 to 12.5%. Acromegaly is associated with increased bone turnover and increased bone density; osteoporosis does not occur unless hypogonadism is also present.[553–555]

Neuromuscular. Although acromegalics have a muscular appearance, they are usually weak. The weakness may be due to a myopathy,[556, 557] but this relation has not been confirmed.[558]

The bony changes of the vertebral column may cause nerve root compression at the vertebral foramina and lumbar radiculopathy. Spinal stenosis and an amyotrophic-like syndrome may occur.[559, 560] Carpal tunnel syndrome was present in 35% of one series of 100 patients[561] and in 43% of another group of 57 acromegalic patients.[562]

Colonic Polyps and Malignancies. A prospective study identified an increased incidence of colonic polyps in acromegalic patients (9 of 17 had polyps), raising the concern that these patients may be at increased risk for development of colon cancer. A retrospective review of 44 acromegalic patients by the same authors identified four cases of colon cancer.[563] Two other studies have suggested an increased incidence of gastrointestinal malignancies in acromegalics. In one series 3 of 12 had colon cancer,[564] and 2 of 48 acromegalic patients had carcinoma of the stomach and 3 had colon cancer.[565] However, a large survey of mortality in acromegaly (194 patients) did not reveal an increased mortality from malignant neoplasms;[528] similar findings have been obtained in other studies of the prevalence of malignant disease in acromegalic patients.[566, 567]

PROGNOSIS. No studies establish that treatment of acromegaly leads to a reduction in morbidity and mortality. A priori, one would predict that reversal of the adverse metabolic effects of excessive GH secretion does prevent progression of the disease and probably leads to regression, as manifested by reduced soft tissue swelling, diminished sweating, and restoration of normal glucose tolerance. Increased awareness of the early symptoms and signs of acromegaly, ease of diagnosis, ability to determine the correct etiology, results of modern transsphenoidal pituitary microsurgery (which demonstrate that the smaller the tumor at the time of operation, the better the outcome), and results of radiotherapy and medical therapies all suggest that patients with acromegaly are more likely to be cured today than in the past.

BIOCHEMICAL EVALUATION. The clinical diagnosis of acromegaly is confirmed by biochemical tests that should be performed before imaging studies are undertaken.

Growth Hormone Secretion in Acromegaly. Serum GH concentrations are elevated but fluctuate widely in acromegaly.[568, 569] The quantitative features of pulsatile and periodic GH secretion in acromegaly have been determined. Frequent venous sampling over 24 h (every 5 or 20 min) and use of objective pulse detection algorithms are adequate methods for characterizing GH release[28, 570] (Fig. 6–39). Acromegalics have a 10- to 15-fold increase in 24-h integrated GH concentrations. The increase in integrated GH concentrations is accounted for by an increase in the nonpulsatile fraction. The number of discrete GH pulses over 24 h is 2- to 3-fold higher than that in normal subjects, and basal GH concentrations are increased 16- to 20-fold above normal. There is an associated attenuation of the underlying 24-h rhythm, which may be secondary to the intrinsic pathology of adenomatous somatotropes and/or effects of altered hypothalamic regulation. During biochemical remission after therapy, acromegalics have GH profiles that resemble those of normal subjects.

A single random serum GH measurement may not be helpful for diagnosing or excluding acromegaly because a "normal" value may be a nadir level in an acromegalic; conversely, a "high" value may be a peak value in a normal subject. It is necessary to measure GH values frequently, probably every 5 or 10 min over 24 h, to characterize GH secretion, an assessment that can be carried out only in a research setting. However, the diagnosis of acromegaly can be made readily in an outpatient setting with two biochemical tests.

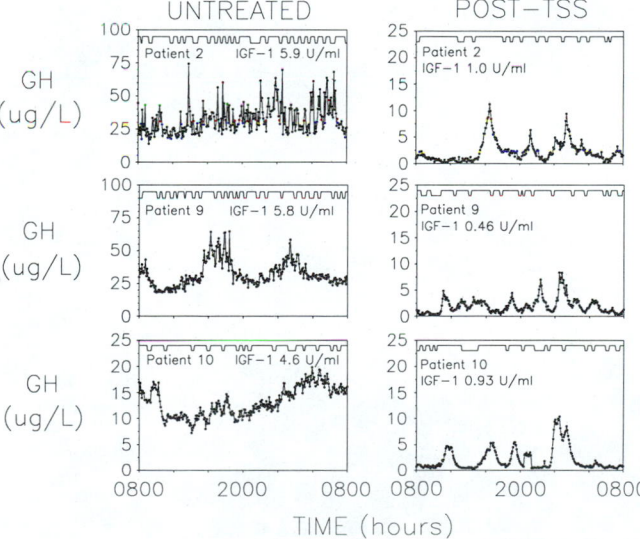

Figure 6–39. Serum GH concentration profiles (24 h) of three acromegalic patients before and after transsphenoidal surgery that induced biochemical and clinical remission. Samples were measured every 5 min over 24 h. The continuous schematized line in the upper portion of each panel defines the individually significant GH pulses detected by cluster analysis. Different scales are used for the vertical axes because of the wide range of serum GH concentrations. After surgery the serum GH concentrations were reduced, and the pattern of GH release closely resembled that of the normal young subjects shown in Figure 6–8. (From ML Hartman, JD Veldhuis, ML Vance, et al., Somatotropin pulse frequency and basal concentrations are increased in acromegaly and are reduced by successful therapy, J Clin Endocrinol Metab, 70, 1375–1384, 1990, © by The Endocrine Society.)

Serum IGF I Concentration. The serum IGF I concentration is the best screening test for acromegaly; an elevated value suggests excessive GH secretion except during pregnancy or puberty, when IGF I levels are appropriately increased. Serum IGF I levels are considered to reflect overall GH secretion during the previous 24 h. Serum IGF I concentrations vary minimally over 24 h and thus provide a reliable indicator of GH secretion. In studies correlating the serum IGF I concentration with clinical activity of acromegaly and a fasting GH concentration, some investigators report excellent correlation,[562, 571, 572] whereas others dispute this relation.[573, 574] The circulating IGF I concentration does, however, correlate with the 24-h integrated serum GH level when GH is measured at frequent intervals (every 5 or 20 min).[28, 570] IGF I assays are variable in reliability and problems related to IGF I binding to various IGF I–binding proteins. Proper interpretation of the values requires knowledge of details of the assay, such as whether the serum is pretreated to remove the binding proteins. The predominant IGF I binding protein is positively regulated by GH (see Chapter 21). Serum IGF I concentration should be measured as an initial screen, as an index of activity of disease, and to assess efficacy of therapy.

Oral Glucose Tolerance Test. The definitive test for the diagnosis of acromegaly is failure of serum GH level to decrease to less than 2 µg/L after ingestion of glucose.[138] In acromegaly, the serum GH level may decrease partially, remain unchanged, or increase paradoxically. The dose of oral glucose ranges from 50 to 100 g; in normal subjects the serum GH level decreases to less than 2 µg/L with as little as 50 g.[568, 569, 575–577] It is anticipated that the dose of oral glucose will be standardized in the near future, probably at 75 g. The oral glucose test should be performed after an overnight fast. In the morning, a heparin-lock cannula is placed in a forearm vein for blood sampling; 1 h later a −30-min sample is obtained, followed 30 min later by a 0-min sample, at which time the patient drinks a flavored iced drink containing 75 g of glucose. The flavoring and addition of ice reduce the sweet taste of the glucose. Blood samples are obtained through the cannula 30, 60, 90, and 120 min after glucose ingestion, and serum GH, plasma glucose, and, if indicated, serum insulin levels are measured.[569] As noted, in patients with acromegaly the serum GH level does not decrease to less than 2 µg/L.

Other tests have been proposed for diagnosis of acromegaly, including administration of TRH, LHRH, levodopa, and other dopamine agonists.[578–582] These compounds produce different (paradoxical) effects in acromegalic patients compared with normal subjects. In normal subjects, GH concentrations are unaffected by TRH or LHRH, whereas in many acromegalic patients GH secretion is stimulated by these agents. These responses are not as uniform as is the abnormal response to oral glucose and therefore are not routinely used. Levodopa and dopamine agonists stimulate GH secretion in normal subjects; GH secretion is acutely inhibited by these agents in 50 to 70% of acromegalics.[582, 583]

Administration of the two physiological hypothalamic regulators of GH secretion, somatostatin and GHRH, does not discriminate between normal and excessive GH secretion. Both normal subjects and patients with acromegaly have an increase in GH concentrations after GHRH administration and a decrease in GH release during somatostatin infusion.[577, 584]

Insulin-induced hypoglycemia is used in acromegalic patients to evaluate the hypothalamic-pituitary-adrenal axis.[366, 367] Patients with acromegaly have insulin resistance and frequently require higher doses of regular insulin to decrease the blood glucose level to below 2.2 mmol/L (40 mg/dL). Until the degree of insulin resistance is known, however, the usual intravenous dose of regular insulin, 0.15 U/kg body weight, is administered. If there is insufficient reduction in serum glucose or absence of hypoglycemic symptoms within 45 min, a second dose of insulin, 0.3 U/kg body weight, is administered. If after another 45 min the response is inadequate, the dose is again increased, to 0.6 U/kg body weight. Results are interpretable when the blood glucose level has decreased to below 2.2 mmol/L (40 mg/dL), which is associated with hypoglycemic symptoms such as tachycardia, palpitations, diaphoresis, somnolence, or hunger. The plasma cortisol level should increase to greater than 580 nmol/L (20 μg/dL); serum GH levels also increase, even in acromegalic patients, to greater than 20 μg/L.

The differential diagnosis of acromegaly includes a primary pituitary adenoma, either a microadenoma or a macroadenoma, and GH hypersecretion from a hyperplastic pituitary gland that is hyperstimulated by eutopic (hypothalamic tumor) or ectopic (peripheral tumor) GHRH.[97, 507] There is only one documented case of acromegaly associated with ectopic GH secretion from a pancreatic tumor.[508] More than 99% of acromegalics have a primary pituitary tumor. However, it is important to make the correct diagnosis because initial therapy is directed to the primary lesion. Unfortunately, radiological studies cannot distinguish between an enlarged pituitary with an adenoma and an enlarged hyperplastic gland.[97, 585] To date, no patient with hypothalamic acromegaly associated with a GHRH-secreting hypothalamic tumor has been diagnosed ante mortem, but patients with a presumed pituitary adenoma have been retrospectively recognized as having extension into the pituitary of hypothalamic gangliocytoma neurons that produce surrounding somatotrope hyperplasia.[507] Theoretically, a mass lesion in the hypothalamus in association with acromegaly presumptively suggests eutopic GHRH secretion by a hypothalamic tumor as indicated by pathological studies.[507] Ectopic GHRH secretion is more common than eutopic secretion, but very few cases of ectopic GHRH production have been diagnosed prospectively.[586] A patient with acromegaly and elevated circulating GHRH levels should be suspected as having ectopic GHRH secretion.[506, 586, 587] Plasma GHRH levels in normal subjects are less than 100 ng/L; in contrast, patients with acromegaly resulting from ectopic GHRH secretion have plasma GHRH levels of micrograms per liter. If a patient has an elevated GHRH level, a peripheral or hypothalamic tumor should be sought. However, because GHRH may be secreted even by tumors in a pulsatile fashion, a normal or only modestly elevated GHRH level may not exclude ectopic GHRH secretion. The most likely peripheral sites are the pancreas, lung, thymus, adrenal (in association with pheochromocytoma), or gastrointestinal tract. A whole body CT or MRI scan should be obtained. Occasionally, no ectopic source can be found.[587]

PATHOLOGY. Histological, immunocytochemical, and ultrastructural investigation of a large number of pituitary tumors removed at surgery or autopsy revealed a variety of histological findings in patients with acromegaly or gigantism:[347, 588-590] (1) densely granulated somatotrope adenoma; (2) sparsely granulated somatotrope adenoma; (3) mixed somatotrope-lactotrope adenoma; (4) acidophilic stem cell adenoma; (5) mammosomatotrope adenoma; (6) plurihormonal adenoma producing GH and one or more glycoprotein hormones, principally alpha subunit; (7) somatotrope carcinoma; (8) somatotrope hyperplasia; and (9) no distinct morphological change. Densely granulated somatotrope adenomas and sparsely granulated somatotrope adenomas are the most commonly occurring tumors in patients with acromegaly; bihormonal somatotrope-lactotrope adenomas and

mammosomatotrope adenomas occur most often in young individuals with gigantism.

Densely granulated somatotrope adenomas are acidophilic, PAS-negative tumors with immunoreactivity for GH. Sparsely granulated somatotrope adenomas are chromophobic on hematoxylin and eosin–stained sections, exhibit no PAS positivity, and have distinct GH immunopositivity. Ultrastructural analysis reveals that densely granulated somatotrope adenomas are composed of well-differentiated cells that resemble somatotropes of the nontumorous adenohypophysis and contain numerous spherical, or ovoid, homogeneously electron-dense secretory granules 150 to 600 nm in diameter[347, 588-593] (Fig. 6–40).

Cells of sparsely granulated somatotrope adenomas differ from nontumorous somatotropes and contain a few randomly distributed secretory granules up to 250 nm in diameter.[347, 589, 591, 592, 594, 595] Sparsely granulated somatotrope adenomas often contain fibrous bodies or cytoplasmic filamentous aggregates (Fig. 6–41). These formations consist of keratin-positive intermediate filaments, trapping mitochondria, centrioles, and secretory granules. The genesis and functional significance of these cytoplasmic fibrous bodies, most often located adjacent to the concave nucleus, are obscure.

Densely granulated somatotrope adenomas and sparsely granulated somatotrope adenomas do not produce different clinical or biochemical alterations. Endocrine amyloid may occur in both variants.[425, 596, 597] However, they differ in

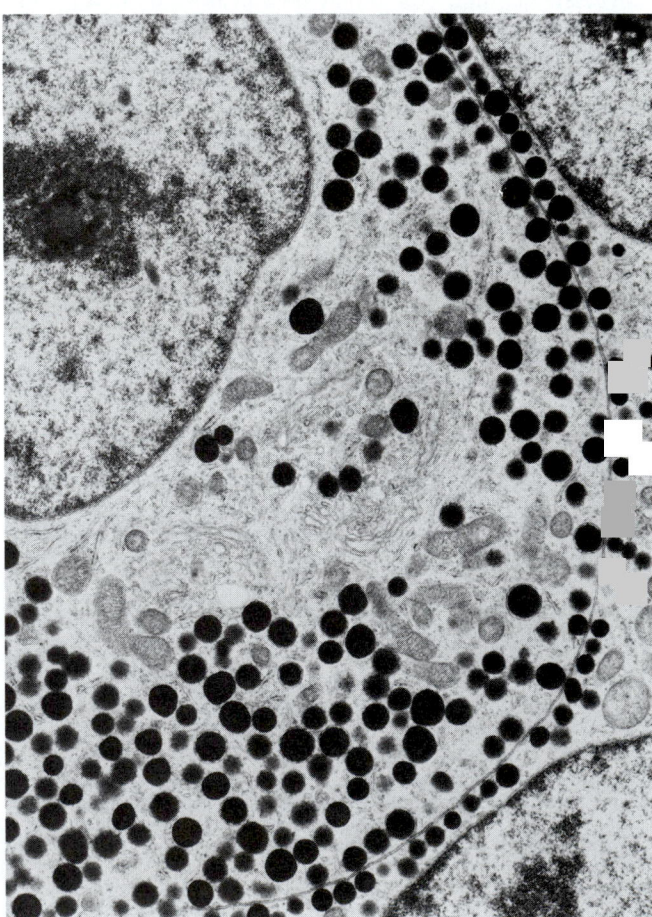

Figure 6–40. Densely granulated GH cell adenoma with well-developed membranous organelles and numerous large secretory granules. Magnification × 12,700.

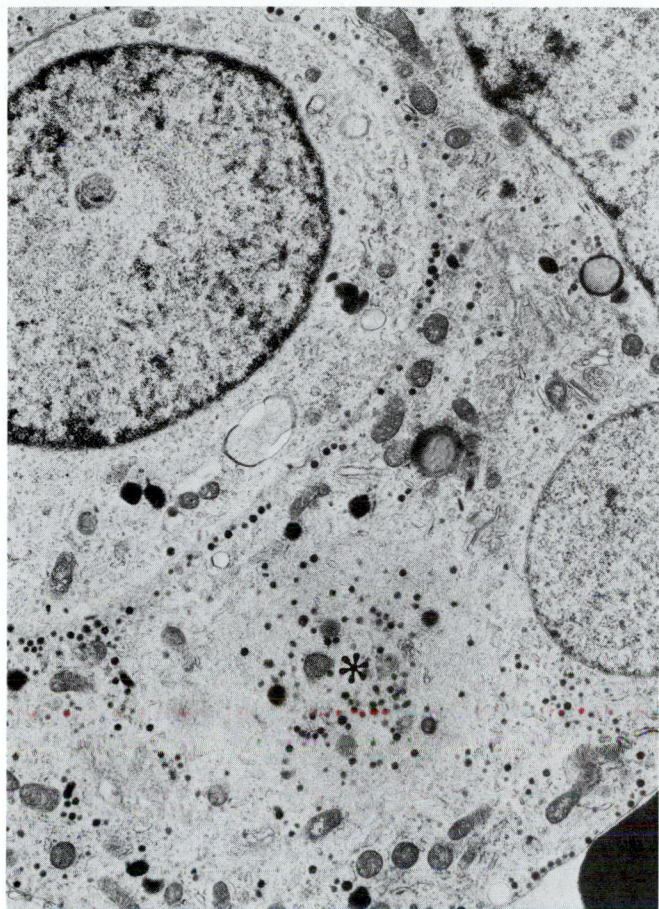

Figure 6–41. Typical features of a sparsely granulated GH cell adenoma. Note the small (less than 200 nm), scant secretory granules and the fibrous body (asterisk) trapping secretory granules, mitochondria, and a few lysosomes. Magnification × 12,150.

biological behavior, emphasizing the importance of precise pathological identification. In contrast to densely granulated somatotrope adenomas, the sparsely granulated tumors occur in somewhat younger individuals, grow faster, are usually larger and more difficult to remove, and recur more often.

Mixed somatotrope-lactotrope adenomas,[598] acidophilic stem cell adenomas,[350] and mammosomatotrope adenomas[351] are bihormonal tumors that produce both GH and prolactin.[598, 599] They are bimorphous tumors consisting of two separate cell types, resembling somatotropes and lactotropes, respectively. Hematoxylin and eosin–stained sections are either acidophilic or chromophobic or consist of an admixture of acidophilic and chromophobic cells. Electron microscopy reveals densely granulated or sparsely granulated somatotropes and lactotropes[598, 599] (Fig. 6–42). Although these tumors consist principally of two distinct cell types, as evidenced by light microscopic immunocytochemistry and ultrastructural analysis, studies using the immunogold technique with double labeling demonstrate that bihormonal cells containing both GH and prolactin may also be present.[600–603]

Acidophilic stem cell adenomas are chromophobic or slightly acidophilic tumors exhibiting no PAS positivity.[350] Clinically, patients rarely exhibit features of acromegaly. The most characteristic finding is hyperprolactinemia of various degrees; serum GH levels may be elevated or within the normal range. This tumor is monomorphous and bihor-

monal, consisting of one cell type that produces both GH and prolactin. Acidophilic stem cell adenomas are assumed to originate in the alleged common precursor cell of somatotropes and lactotropes. These tumors usually occur in younger individuals and grow faster than other tumors arising from the acidophilic cell line. By electron microscopy the sparsely granulated, often oncocytic, tumors have features of both somatotropes and lactotropes, including fibrous bodies and misplaced exocytosis of secretory granules (Fig. 6–43).

Mammosomatotrope adenomas[351] are associated with acromegaly and varying degrees of hyperprolactinemia. They are acidophilic, PAS negative, monomorphous, bihormonal tumors in which the same cells are immunoreactive for both GH and prolactin.[604] By electron microscopy the densely granulated tumor cells are well differentiated and contain numerous large secretory granules, some of which are engaged in misplaced exocytosis (Fig. 6–44). The tumors grow slowly and occur more frequently than was previously thought.

Plurihormonal adenomas produce GH and one or more glycoprotein hormones, primarily alpha subunit.[348, 352, 605–608] Patients have acromegaly and elevated serum GH levels; the serum alpha subunit levels may also be elevated. Hyperthyroidism rarely occurs. In these patients serum thyroid hormone levels are increased in the presence of inappropriately elevated serum TSH levels. Histologically the tumors are predominantly monomorphous and acidophilic. Less commonly, they may consist of more than one morphological

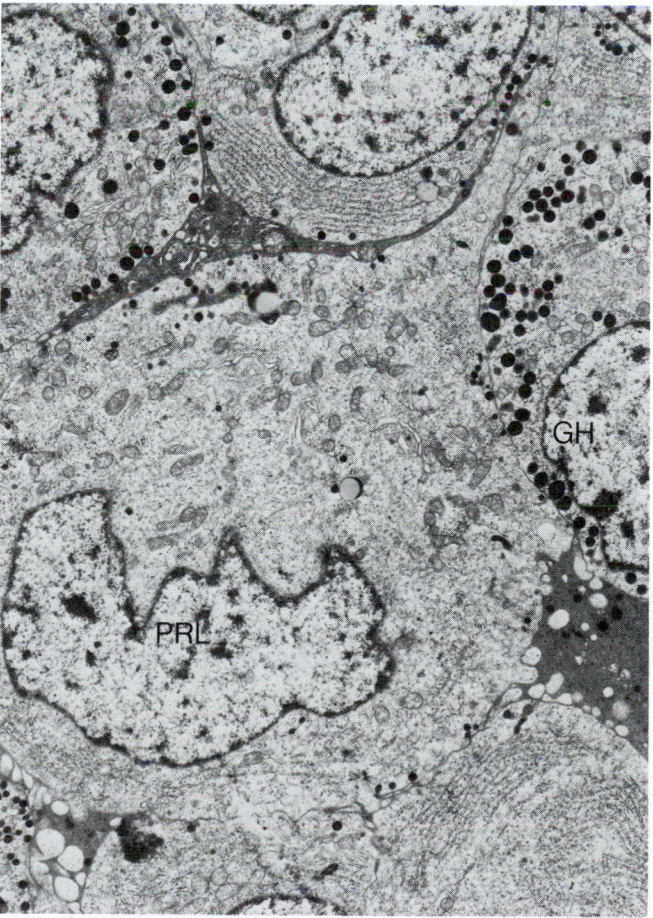

Figure 6–42. Mixed adenoma consisting of sparsely granulated prolactin cells (PRL) and densely granulated GH cells (GH). Magnification × 6500.

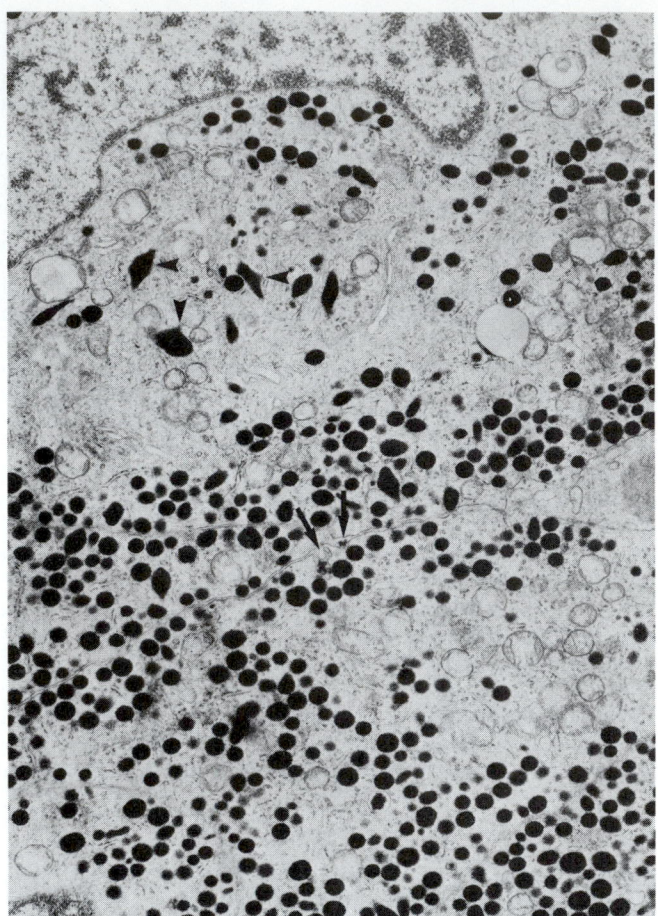

Figure 6–43. The appearance of this mammosomatotrope adenoma is similar to that of densely granulated GH cell adenomas with the added feature of granule extrusions *(arrows)*. Note the geometrically shaped secretory granules seen chiefly in the Golgi area *(arrowhead)*, which sometimes occur in GH-producing adenomas. Magnification × 11,550.

somatotrope hyperplasia is stimulated by excessive GHRH secretion by extrapituitary tumors, including pancreatic, pheochromocytoma, bronchial, thymic, and intestinal carcinoids; medullary carcinoma of the thyroid; and small cell carcinoma of the lung. A hypothalamic gangliocytoma may also secrete GHRH and produce somatotrope hyperplasia. In some cases GHRH immunopositivity of the peripheral tumor cells is not associated with increased serum levels of GHRH, GH, and IGF I. However, when large quantities of GHRH are released from the tumors, pituitary somatotropes are stimulated with resulting GH hypersecretion and acromegaly or giantism. Somatotrope hyperplasia can result in pituitary enlargement as assessed by various imaging techniques. It is not known whether hyperplasia can transform into adenoma. However, in some cases the pituitary lesion is indistinguishable from adenoma. It is not clear whether this is a continuous process or whether protracted chronic stimulation results in neoplastic growth. According to the multistep theory of tumorigenesis, protracted GHRH stimulation does not initiate tumor growth but does promote it. Alternatively, GHRH may increase the susceptibility of somatotropes to oncogenic stimulation, with hyperplastic somatotropes becoming more prone to undergo neoplastic transformation.

In a few patients with acromegaly, no significant morphological changes have been observed in the pituitary;[612] however, immunohistochemistry and electron microscopy were not performed. The diagnosis of no pathological abnormality is acceptable only if the entire pituitary is studied

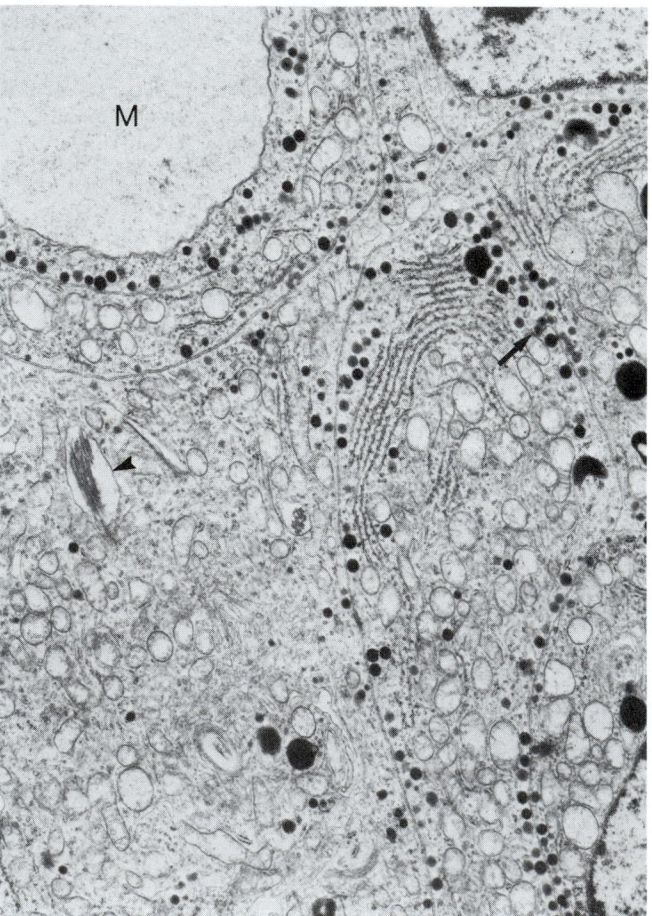

Figure 6–44. Acidophilic stem cell adenoma displaying the characteristic oncocytic change with development of giant mitochondria (M) and occurrence of intramitochondrial electron-dense tubular structures *(arrowhead)*. Note granule extrusion site *(arrow)*. Magnification × 11,550.

cell type. Immunocytochemistry demonstrates the presence of cells producing GH and alpha subunit, TSH, FSH, or rarely LH. By electron microscopy the tumors are chiefly monomorphous and less often bimorphous or trimorphous. In bimorphous tumors one cell type represents densely granulated somatotropes and the other cell type is the sparsely granulated glycoprotein hormone–producing cell. However, in plurihormonal adenomas the results obtained by light microscopic immunocytochemistry, electron microscopy, and immunoelectron microscopy are not always in agreement. The cytogenesis of these tumors is not clear. They may arise from a precursor cell that undergoes multidirectional differentiation so that it is capable of producing several hormones or from plurihormonal clones that have been identified in the normal pituitary.

Only a few documented cases of somatotrope carcinomas have been reported.[609, 610] However, some somatotrope adenomas are pleomorphic, contain multiple mitotic figures, are invasive, and have a high growth rate. These tumors are considered to be pleomorphic or invasive adenomas and not carcinomas. The diagnosis of carcinoma is accepted only when distant metastases are identified. Somatotrope carcinomas may be acidophilic or chromophobic, and the cells are pleomorphic and contain GH as evaluated by immunocytochemistry. Sites of distant metastases include lymph nodes, liver, brain, heart, and bones.

Somatotrope hyperplasia is rare.[97, 506, 611] The number of somatotropes is normally constant in the pituitary, and

by examination of serial sections. GH hypersecretion and acromegaly in patients with normal pituitary morphology raise intriguing questions; more cases must be studied by modern morphological methods before definite conclusions can be drawn.

Tumor recurrence after "successful" surgery depends on whether tumor tissue was left behind during surgery. Somatotrope adenomas are practically never associated with somatotrope hyperplasia (except in cases of GHRH-producing extrapituitary tumors), and the theory that new tumors develop from proliferating hyperplastic cells after surgery is not tenable.

Morphological changes after radiotherapy include vascular changes, interstitial fibrosis, cell loss, and degenerative features such as oncocytic change and nuclear pleomorphism. Bizarre nuclei may be present in multinucleated cells.

Demonstration that somatotrope adenoma cells have dopamine and/or somatostatin receptors raises the possibility that these tumors could be treated effectively with dopamine agonists or long-acting somatostatin analogue(s). Somatotrope adenomas are not affected morphologically by dopamine agonist treatment even when large doses of the drug are administered for long periods of time (months to years). The adenoma cells are not damaged; no shrinkage, involution, necrosis, fibrosis, or vascular changes are present. The only abnormality is accumulation of mitochondria in a few adenoma cells, but because oncocytic change may occur without medical treatment the significance of mitochondrial accumulation in somatotrope adenomas during dopamine agonist treatment is uncertain.

Treatment with a somatostatin analogue also produces no consistent morphological changes.[613–615] In some tumors, the cells and the cytoplasm appear smaller than in untreated tumors.[615, 616] Mitochondrial accumulation, amyloid formation, lysosomal accumulation, crinophagy, and increases in the size and number of secretory granules have also been reported. In some cases in which there are clinical and biochemical responses, no morphological changes are observed even with electron microscopic examination.

GOALS OF TREATMENT. The goals of treatment are to effect a cure such that GH secretion is normal, clinical symptoms and signs abate, mass effects of the tumor such as headache and/or visual abnormalities are reversed, and other anterior pituitary function is preserved. The definition of cure is a reduction of the serum IGF I concentration to normal for age and sex and a normal GH response to oral glucose, i.e., reduction of GH level to less than 2 μg/L after ingestion of 75 or 100 g of glucose. In many reports of surgical results a single postoperative GH concentration of less than 10 or less than 5 μg/L was considered indicative of "cure." A serum GH level less than 10 μg/L is not normal and is not a valid indication of successful surgery. Studies of frequent GH measurements over 24 h suggest that even when postoperative IGF I concentration and GH response to oral glucose are normal, the pattern of pulsatile GH release may not be completely normal, so that some acromegalics have persistent elevation of basal GH concentrations.[28] This observation is of unknown significance and requires long-term follow-up.

The treatments of GH-secreting pituitary adenomas include surgical resection, pituitary radiation, and medical therapies with dopamine agonists or somatostatin analogues. Many patients, particularly those with large tumors, require more than one type of treatment to produce clinical improvement and reduction in serum GH concentrations.

SURGICAL THERAPY. The preferred surgical approach is the transsphenoidal route because it permits visualization of the tumor, usually avoids contact with the optic chiasm and nerves, potentially allows complete resection, and is

TABLE 6–21. Results of Transsphenoidal Surgery for Acromegaly: Patients with Postoperative Serum Growth Hormone < 5 μg/L and Normal Oral Glucose Tolerance Test (OGTT)*

Author, Year	Number of Patients	Basal GH < 5 μg/L	OGTT GH < 2 μg/L†
Arafah et al., 1980[621]	28	20 (78%)	13 (46%)
Tucker et al., 1980[622]	32	24 (75%)	22 (71%)
Quabbe, 1982[623]	152		
114 micro‡		68 (60%)	39 (39%)
38 macro		13 (40%)	9 (26%)
Grisoli et al., 1985[873]	100	60 (60%)	43 (43%)
Serri et al., 1985[874]	25		
8 micro		8 (100%)	8 (100%)
17 macro		14 (82%)	13 (76%)

*GH < 2 μg/L after glucose ingestion.
†Percentage based on number of patients tested.
‡When possible, results are presented according to preoperative tumor size; micro, intrasellar tumor; macro, extrasellar extension or invasion of dura or bone.

associated with less morbidity than the transcranial approach. As with any type of pituitary tumor, the surgical outcome depends on two factors: the size of the tumor and the expertise of the surgeon. An intrasellar microadenoma (<10 mm in diameter) offers the greatest possibility for a surgical cure. The presence of a macroadenoma (>10 mm in diameter), particularly with suprasellar extension or extension into the cavernous sinus, decreases the probability of a surgical cure. Nevertheless, surgery may result in a substantial reduction in tumor mass and immediate improvement in visual abnormalities, headaches, and symptoms of excessive GH and is the preferred initial therapy.

As shown in Tables 6–21 and 6–22, the results of transsphenoidal surgery, although variable, are fairly consistent in that a basal postoperative GH concentration of less than 5 μg/L is achieved in approximately 60% of patients, with the best outcome occurring in those with a small tumor. These results are representative of medical centers in which transsphenoidal surgery is performed frequently. Although a basal serum GH concentration of less than 5 μg/L may be indicative of successful surgery, dynamic studies, particularly the oral glucose tolerance test, are more accurate for evaluating postoperative GH secretion. As shown in Table 6–21, when suppression of GH to less than 2 μg/L after oral glucose ingestion is used as the criterion, some patients with a postoperative serum GH level of less than 5 μg/L do not have suppression to less than 2 μg/L. Furthermore, in patients with a preoperative paradoxical GH response to TRH and/or LHRH, a postoperative lowering of basal GH concentration to less than 5 μg/L may occur despite a persistently abnormal GH response to TRH and/or LHRH.

The serum IGF I concentration should be measured before and after surgery. However, the serum IGF I level does not decrease as rapidly as GH concentrations after tumor removal. Clearance of IGF I, complexed with a

TABLE 6–22. Results of Transsphenoidal Surgery for Acromegaly: Patients with Postoperative Serum Growth Hormone < 5 μg/L

Author, Year	Number of Patients	Basal GH < 5 μg/L (%)
Williams et al., 1975[618]	59	39 (66%)
Richards and Thomas, 1980[624]	34	27 (80%)
Balagura et al., 1981[875]	132	76 (58%)
Laws et al., 1985[876]	75	40 (53%)
Roelfsema et al., 1985[625]	60	37 (62%)
Fahlbusch and Buchfelder, 1988[877]	38	21 (55%)
Ross and Wilson, 1988[878]	214	117 (54%)
van't Verlaat et al., 1988[619]	25	14 (56%)

binding protein, may require several days and thus does not reflect an immediate change in circulating GH concentrations. A potentially useful method of assessing somatotrope function after surgery is measurement of serum GH concentration after administration of GHRH. An absent GH response to GHRH may be indicative of a cure; an increase is difficult to interpret because nonadenomatous somatotropes release GH in response to GHRH. Even if all tests of GH secretion are normal postoperatively, some patients develop late recurrence of acromegaly, emphasizing the need for careful follow-up and monitoring. The incidence of recurrence is not known, but after an average follow-up of 2 to 3.5 y recurrence rates ranged from 0 to 13%.[498, 617–619]

Surgical mortality is low. Particular care must be taken with intubation and extubation because airway obstruction by an enlarged tongue is a risk. Common surgical complications include transient diabetes insipidus and CSF rhinorrhea in less than 5% of patients. Other complications include meningitis, sinusitis, hematoma, and cranial nerve palsy in less than 1%.[498, 620] The incidence of postsurgical anterior pituitary dysfunction is variable and is dependent on the amount of tissue removed. The reported incidence of postoperative anterior pituitary insufficiency ranges from 2 to 67% for ACTH, 5 to 61% for TSH, and 3 to 58% for the gonadotropins.[498, 618, 619, 621–625] Permanent diabetes insipidus occurs in 1 to 9% of patients.[498, 620, 624–626]

RADIATION THERAPY. Before the development of transsphenoidal surgery, radiation was the primary treatment for acromegaly and other types of pituitary tumors. Now pituitary radiation is usually reserved for persistent disease after surgery in an attempt to prevent tumor growth and reduce hormone hypersecretion. Limitations of radiotherapy include inability to effect a prompt reduction in tumor size and in hormone hypersecretion. This is particularly important for patients with visual abnormalities and severe manifestations of acromegaly. Several types of radiotherapy are available, including conventional high-dose therapy, yttrium implantation, stereotactic radiosurgery with alpha particles or proton beam therapy, and single high-dose administration of focused radiation using the gamma unit.

Conventional supervoltage pituitary radiation consists of administration of a total dose of 45 to 50 Gy in daily fractions 5 d/wk over 4 or 5 wk. Lower or higher radiation doses are associated with suboptimal control of the disease and an increased risk of complications, respectively. Of 43 acromegalic patients treated with only pituitary radiation, 16 (37%) had a reduction in serum GH concentrations to less than 5 µg/L; this reduction required 2 yr in 4, 5 y in 8, and 10 y in 4 patients. None had evidence of tumor enlargement; 5 of 39 (13%) developed secondary hypothyroidism and 11 of 40 (28%) required glucocorticoid replacement.[391] Of 27 acromegalic patients given conventional radiation as primary treatment, 5 (19%) required glucocorticoid replacement and 7 (26%) required thyroid hormone replacement; the recurrence rate was 10%, and radiation-induced visual abnormalities occurred in 13%.[389] In another study, radiation-induced hypopituitarism occurred in 50% of patients at a mean follow-up of 26 mo, emphasizing the need for close monitoring of any patient given radiotherapy.[393] Other complications include visual loss secondary to optic nerve damage, cerebral ischemia, and development of a pituitary or brain malignancy. Of 139 patients given 40 to 60 Gy, 3 developed radiation necrosis of the brain, 10 developed cerebral ischemia, and 1 developed a glioblastoma of the temporal lobe.[395] The development of partial or complete hypopituitarism after radiotherapy occurs more frequently in patients previously treated with pituitary surgery.[396]

Alpha particle pituitary radiotherapy, using a cyclotron as the energy source, delivers a maximal tumor dose of 90 Gy. This treatment is usually given on one occasion. Reduction of serum GH concentrations to less than 5 µg/L occurs approximately 5 y after therapy in patients with macroadenomas and approximately 3 y after treatment in those with microadenomas. Anterior pituitary deficiency developed in approximately one third, with 34% requiring glucocorticoid replacement, 33% requiring thyroid hormone replacement, and 25% requiring gonadal steroid replacement. Complications of alpha particle therapy include development of visual field abnormalities (29%), cranial nerve palsy (43%), and temporal lobe epilepsy (29%); these complication occurred only in patients who had received prior photon beam therapy. The incidence of CNS complications in patients treated solely with alpha particle radiation was less than 1%.[394]

Proton beam radiation, generated by a cyclotron, delivers up to 120 Gy to the tumor mass and is administered as a single treatment. Of 435 acromegalic patients given proton beam therapy, 30% had a serum GH concentration below 5 µg/L 2 y after treatment, 50% achieved this result after 5 y, 78% after 10 y, and 88% after 20 y. The median time for development of hypopituitarism was 2.8 y after treatment, with 10% requiring thyroid replacement, 9% requiring glucocorticoid replacement, and 7% requiring gonadal steroids. Other complications of proton beam therapy included temporal lobe seizures in three, an arachnoid cyst in one, pituitary carcinoma in two, and a CNS sarcoma in one patient.[392]

Surgical implantation of radioactive ^{90}Y seeds into the pituitary is another method for treating acromegaly. Of 22 patients given these implants, 11 had a reduction in serum GH level to less than 5 µg/L, 3 to 11 mo after treatment. Complications of the surgical implantation included transient cranial nerve palsy in 2 and fever in 2. Seven of 22 required hormone replacement therapy, including glucocorticoid therapy in 6, gonadal steroid replacement in 4, levothyroxine in 2, and vasopressin in 1. Dynamic testing after yttrium therapy revealed an impaired TSH response to TRH in 16 of 23, an impaired LH response to LHRH in 6 of 16, and an impaired cortisol response to hypoglycemia in 4 of 14 patients. Limitations of this treatment include exclusion of patients with tumor extension into the sphenoid sinus, significant suprasellar extension, a partially empty sella, carotid arteries in proximity to the midline, and poor general health.[627] Although this method of administering radiation therapy appears to be effective in reducing GH secretion, it has not achieved widespread use.

Stereotactic radiotherapy using the gamma unit employs a heavily shielded central body containing approximately 200 sources of ^{60}Co. The radiation sources are radially distributed over a segment of a sphere, and the beams are individually collimated toward the center of the lesion.[628] This method of delivery of radiation has been applied to a variety of intracranial lesions, including brain tumors, acoustic neuromas, ateriovenous malformations, aneurysms, craniopharyngiomas, and pituitary tumors. Results of this method of radiotherapy for the treatment of acromegaly are not available. However, in one series of 29 patients with Cushing's disease, 22 (76%) achieved complete remission 1 to 3 y after the treatment.[628] This procedure is usually limited to patients with microadenomas because of the potential for damage to the optic chiasm, optic nerves, and structures in the cavernous sinus.

MEDICAL THERAPY. Bromocriptine, an orally active dopamine agonist used to treat hyperprolactinemia, also reduces serum GH concentrations in acromegalic patients and has been used to treat acromegaly since 1974.[582] Most patients have improvement in clinical symptoms (70 to 90%) and a reduction in serum GH concentrations during chronic bromocriptine therapy (approximately 70%). However, as shown in Table 6–23, reduction of serum GH concentration to less than 5 μg/L occurs rarely. Other effects of bromocriptine include reduction in urinary hydroxyproline excretion, improvement of control of overt diabetes mellitus or glucose intolerance, resolution of hyperprolactinemia (if present), and improvement in visual field abnormalities. A larger bromocriptine dose is required to treat acromegaly than to treat hyperprolactinemia; acromegalic patients usually require 10 to 20 mg/d (or more) in divided doses four times per day. As noted in the discussion of dopamine agonist treatment of hyperprolactinemia, bromocriptine treatment should be initiated with a small dose followed by a gradual increase to minimize side effects.

Although suppression of GH secretion may be incomplete during bromocriptine therapy, this drug is useful for symptomatic treatment of patients with residual postoperative disease or until radiation therapy is effective.

Somatostatin Analogue. Somatostatin is a 14-amino-acid cyclic peptide in the brain, hypothalamus, pancreas, and gastrointestinal tract.[629] In the hypothalamus, somatostatin functions as the GH release–inhibiting hormone and, in conjunction with GHRH, produces the episodic GH release. Intravenous administration of somatostatin produces a prompt reduction in serum GH concentrations in normal subjects and in patients with acromegaly. After cessation of the infusion, there is a rapid rise in serum GH level, and a rebound hypersecretion occurs in some acromegalics.[577] Somatostatin must be administered by continuous intravenous infusion because its half-life is less than 3 min, which makes it impractical for clinical use. Octreotide is an 8-amino-acid cyclic peptide analogue of somatostatin that has a serum half-life of approximately 90 min and that suppresses GH release for up to 8 h in normal and acromegalic subjects.[630, 631] This peptide, administered subcutaneously, is 20 times more suppressive of GH release than the native peptide and is 22 times more suppressive of GH release than of insulin release. Despite its greater selectivity for GH, insulin release is decreased for approximately 3 h after administration, and postprandial hyperglycemia may occur.[630, 631]

Octreotide has been used in clinical trials to treat acromegaly and other hypersecretory endocrine tumors since 1984. Studies of limited numbers of acromegalic patients, usually treated briefly, indicate that most patients have improvement in symptoms and signs of disease and a reduction in serum GH and IGF I concentrations.[616, 632–656] A small number of patients have had a reduction in pituitary tumor size.[616, 656] Reduction in serum GH concentrations occurs within an hour of administration and continues for 6 to 8 h in most patients; insulin release is partially inhibited for less than 3 h after administration.[632] Whereas some patients have suppression of GH and IGF I concentrations to normal, others have only a partial suppression of GH release. This heterogeneity of response is most likely dependent on the density of somatostatin receptors in the adenoma and variable binding affinities for octreotide. In patients who were given octreotide and subsequently underwent surgical resection of the adenoma, the patients with the greatest degree of GH suppression with octreotide had a higher density of homogeneously distributed somatostatin receptors on the tumors than did patients with a poor response.[657]

The recommended octreotide dose is 100 μg every 8 h; however, some patients have adequate GH suppression with 100 μg/d, and others require as much as 1500 μg/d in divided doses.[652] Some patients have a better response to continuous subcutaneous octreotide infusion than to intermittent injections.[638, 639, 643, 658] A small number of patients have greater GH suppression with the combination of octreotide and bromocriptine.[635, 637, 656] The precise dose and frequency of administration should be adjusted according to the response.

Octreotide inhibits gallbladder contractility and may facilitate formation of gallstones,[659] although the true incidence of gallstone formation and symptomatic cholelithiasis during octreotide therapy is unknown. Because postprandial gallbladder motility is decreased by octreotide, a potential method of decreasing the risk of gallstone formation is administration of the drug 2 to 3 h after meals.

In addition to treating patients not cured by or unresponsive to other therapy, octreotide may be useful for reducing pituitary tumor size before surgical resection. In 10 patients studied by Barkan and colleagues, pituitary tumor size decreased by 20 to 54% when octreotide was administered for 3 to 30 wk before surgery.[616] It is not yet known whether preoperative octreotide therapy produces improved surgical resection and an increase in the rate of cure.

Ectopic GHRH Secretion. Somatotrope stimulation by a tumor secreting GHRH is the cause of less than 1% of cases of acromegaly.[506] If an ectopic GHRH-secreting tumor is identified, therapy consists of resection of the tumor. In the absence of metastases, surgical resection is curative. Patients with metastatic disease are responsive to octreotide therapy, which lowers circulating GHRH and GH concentrations.[660, 661] Differential sensitivity to octreotide is observed, with greater suppression of GH than of GHRH.[658]

Treatment of acromegaly frequently involves more than

TABLE 6–23. Results of Bromocriptine Therapy for Acromegaly

Author, Year	Total	Suppression of GH	Normal GH*	↓ Sweating	↓ Ring Size	Dose (mg/d)
Thorner et al., 1975[583]	11	9/11 (82)	0/11	11/11	6/11 (55)	20
Thorner and Besser, 1976[879]	25	10/15 (67)	Not reported	24/25 (96)	17/18 (94)	15–60
Wass et al., 1977[880]	73	58/73 (79)	15/73 (21)	60/63 (95)	30/34 (88)	10–60
Belforte et al., 1977[881]	30	17/30 (57)	6/30 (21)	"Most"	5/14 (36)†	10–20
Halse et al., 1977[882]	8	7/8 (88)	0/8	7/7	7/7	10–20
Eskildsen et al., 1978[883]	14	10/14 (71)‡	10/14 (71)§	7/9 (78)	7/11 (64)	30–55
Lundin et al., 1978[884]	11	9/11 (82)	1/11 (9)	7/11 (64)	10/11 (91)	15–40
Besser et al., 1980[885]	101	78/101 (77)	NR‖	59/63 (94)	17/19 (89)	20–60
Lindholm et al., 1981[886]	18	6/18 (33)	0/18	NR	NR	20
Moses et al., 1981[574]	7	6/7 (86)	2/7 (29)	NR	6/7 (86)¶	10–40

*Normal GH level < 5 μg/L.
†Reduction in hand volume.
‡24-h urinary levels.
§Urinary excretion < 100 μg/24 h.
‖NR, not reported.
¶Decrease in shoe size.
From Vance ML, Evans WS, Thorner MD. Drugs five years later. Bromocriptine. Ann Intern Med 1984; 100:78–91.

one approach, including surgery, radiation, and medical treatment. Because uncontrolled acromegaly is associated with premature mortality and significant morbidity, all of these therapies should be considered in an attempt to reduce GH secretion to normal.

Cushing's Disease

Cushing's syndrome that is caused by an adenoma of the corticotrope cells of the anterior pituitary or, more rarely, by corticotrope hyperplasia is referred to as Cushing's disease. The first detailed description of patients with this disease was in a monograph by Harvey Cushing.[662] The disease has a female-to-male preponderance of 3–8 to 1; it commonly occurs in women of childbearing age but may occur at any age. It accounts for approximately 70% of all cases of spontaneous (endogenous) Cushing's syndrome, excluding those with ectopic ACTH syndrome. The latter syndrome is frequently characterized by weight loss, hypokalemic alkalosis, and hyperglycemia secondary to ACTH secretion by a malignant peripheral tumor. Spontaneous, endogenous Cushing's syndrome is usually ACTH dependent. Causes include pituitary adenoma (Cushing's disease) and ectopic ACTH production, of which the common causes are oat cell carcinoma, bronchial and foregut (including thymus) carcinoid tumors, pancreatic islet cell tumors (many of which are carcinoid tumors), pheochromocytoma, and rarely, ovarian tumors (<1%). Rarely, ectopic CRH production may cause Cushing's syndrome. The non–ACTH-dependent causes include adrenal adenomas and carcinomas.

In this section Cushing's disease is discussed in outline form because a detailed discussion is included in Chapter 9.

ETIOLOGIES. The diagnosis of Cushing's *syndrome* is usually straightforward. However, once the diagnosis of Cushing's syndrome has been made, the etiology must be ascertained to determine appropriate therapy. Cushing's syndrome is either ACTH dependent or ACTH independent. In this section we consider only the ACTH-dependent causes, including Cushing's disease, ectopic ACTH secretion, and the rare disorder of ectopic or eutopic production of CRH. Separation of Cushing's disease from other ACTH-dependent causes of the syndrome is rarely straightforward. Perhaps the most difficult distinction is between chronic ectopic ACTH secretion by a relatively benign tumor (e.g., bronchial carcinoid) and Cushing's disease.

Whether Cushing's disease is primarily a pituitary or a hypothalamic disease is controversial; this is discussed in detail in Chapter 9. There is little evidence that Cushing's disease is hypothalamic in origin; current information supports a pituitary etiology. Thus selective removal of the adenoma leads to return to normal hypothalamic-pituitary-adrenal function and a low rate of recurrence. The often prolonged delay in recovery of the hypothalamic-pituitary-adrenal axis (months) is incompatible with a hypothalamic etiology; if hypothalamic stimulation were the cause, removal of the adenoma should allow the remaining normal corticotropes to respond rapidly to the continued hypothalamic CRH stimulation. Furthermore, if the etiology were hypothalamic, corticotrope hyperplasia would be expected, whereas this is rare.

CLINICAL FEATURES. The clinical features of Cushing's syndrome are a result of chronic exposure to elevated cortisol concentrations. Signs include weight gain, centripetal obesity, moon facies, violaceous striae, easy bruisability, proximal myopathy, and psychiatric disturbances.

Although the florid case of Cushing's syndrome is easy to diagnose, the more subtle case presents a diagnostic challenge. In children and prepubertal adolescents the presentation is usually one of obesity and growth retardation.

Adult women may have mild weight gain, menstrual irregularities, and mild depression. Occasionally patients have only skin manifestations, particularly thinning, bruising, and poor wound healing. Similarly, the diagnosis may be made incidentally by x-ray findings of healed fractures (e.g., rib) with no history of fracture. Because of the severe pain normally associated with a rib fracture, a painless rib fracture should always raise the question of Cushing's syndrome.

Symptoms and signs usually involve almost every system in the body, which may be obvious only after the diagnosis is made. In patients who diet or exercise regularly, it is possible to have Cushing's syndrome without obesity. Hypertension is present in most.

Skin changes include thinning of the epidermis and purple striae that are often more than 1 cm wide. This contrasts with the striae of rapid weight gain or pregnancy, which are narrower and either very pale or pink. In severe Cushing's syndrome the skin is so thinned that the skin of the back of the hand is paper thin and is easily peeled off or torn (e.g., by removing adhesive tape). Women with Cushing's disease typically have fine downy facial lanugo hair and may have acne, hirsutism, and temporal scalp hair regression secondary to increased adrenal androgen secretion. Superficial fungal infections, particularly tinea versicolor, are common. The shins often show signs of lacerations that have healed poorly and may be hyperpigmented. Patients with Cushing's disease often have had the disease for 3 to 6 y before diagnosis, and it may be possible to date the onset of the condition by determining which scars are pigmented. Pigmented scars develop after the onset of the condition (an effect of excessive secretion of ACTH and other melanotropins).

Virtually all patients with Cushing's disease have neuropsychiatric manifestations. The most common is depression, but psychotic and manic behavior may occur. Depression may be so severe that the patient is suicidal.

Women with Cushing's disease have disturbed menstruation because of several abnormalities. Adrenal androgen secretion is increased as a result of the increased ACTH secretion and may adversely affect the development of the ovarian follicles. Both the increased androgens and cortisol exert a negative feedback on gonadotropin secretion. Men often have decreased libido, which may be a result of decreased gonadotropin secretion and/or depression.

Because the diagnosis of Cushing's disease is often delayed, significant osteopenia and/or vertebral collapse or other fractures may be present. The osteopenia is unlike other forms of osteoporosis in that it is reversible with cure of the Cushing's disease. Although complaints of muscle weakness are present in only about half of patients, proximal myopathy is demonstrable in the majority; such patients are unable to rise from a deep knee bend or to rise unassisted from a seated position.

Excessive glucocorticoid levels cause insulin resistance and glucose intolerance in 75% of patients but overt diabetes mellitus in only 8 to 10%. Hypercalciuria results in an increased incidence of renal calculi.

Patients with small cell lung carcinoma with ectopic ACTH production usually have a fulminating form of Cushing's syndrome. ACTH levels are high, and cortisol production rates may be increased more than 10-fold. Because the condition is acute in onset and progresses rapidly, weight is lost instead of gained, and a severe proximal myopathy is present. Common features include pigmentation (from the very high plasma ACTH and other melanotropin hormones), severe electrolyte disturbances (especially hypokalemia), and hyperglycemia with insulin resistance that may lead to overt diabetes mellitus. Hypokalemic alkalosis results from the mineralocorticoid effects of very high plasma cortisol levels. The hypokalemic alkalosis may be a medical emergency; untreated patients can die from hypokalemia. This syndrome is different from that of the patient with typical Cushing's syndrome resulting from chronic ectopic ACTH production by a relatively benign tumor such as a carcinoid.

BIOCHEMICAL EVALUATION. The evaluation of patients with Cushing's syndrome is designed to confirm the diagnosis and determine the etiology of the excessive cortisol production. This is discussed in detail in Chapter 9. It cannot be stressed too strongly that the differential diagnosis is primarily addressed by functional studies; radiological imaging of the adrenal glands and the pituitary does not have a role at this stage of the evaluation because imaging provides information on anatomy, not function, and "nonfunctioning" adenomas in the pituitary and adrenal gland are common. Thus without the biochemical tests the results of imaging studies may be misleading.

Establishing the Diagnosis of Cushing's Syndrome. The evaluation of Cushing's syndrome can be done on an outpatient basis. The disorder is most commonly a result of iatrogenic administration of excessive quantities of synthetic glucocorticoids for treatment of other disorders. Therefore, the first step is to determine whether the patient is receiving such medication(s), including prior intramuscular injections of dexamethasone or other synthetic glucocorticoids that can have effects lasting over many months.[663] This condition is suspected if the patient has clinical evidence of Cushing's syndrome but has undetectable urinary or plasma cortisol. Having excluded iatrogenic Cushing's syndrome, the next step is to determine if the 24-h secretion of glucocorticoids is elevated. This can be achieved most easily by performing a 24-h urine collection for measurement of urinary cortisol.[664] Usually two baseline collections are obtained, with measurement of total volume and creatinine to assess the adequacy of the collections and to correct for body mass. If the 24-h urinary cortisol excretion is elevated, a standard dose of the synthetic glucocorticoid dexamethasone is administered to test the sensitivity of the hypothalamic-pituitary-adrenal axis to suppression. Dexamethasone does not cross-react to a significant degree in the radioimmunoassays for plasma and urinary cortisol. Many investigators use the overnight dexamethasone suppression test (1 mg given at 11 PM with measurement of plasma cortisol at 8 AM), but this is associated with significant false-positive and false-negative results.[665] False-positive results (lack of suppression) occur most frequently in hospitalized patients, so the test is best reserved as an outpatient *screening* test. The standard dexamethasone dose (0.5 mg every 6 h for 48 h) is equivalent to approximately four times the normal cortisol production. In normal individuals, this amount of dexamethasone exerts a negative feedback on the hypothalamus and pituitary to suppress ACTH secretion. Thus adrenal cortisol secretion ceases. The standard low-dose dexamethasone suppression test is performed by administering 0.5 mg orally at 8 AM, 2 PM, 8 PM, and 2 AM for 2 d. Doses for children are corrected on the basis of weight.[666] Urine collections are made from 8 AM through 8 AM for each of the 2 baseline days and 2 dexamethasone test days. The criterion for normal suppression for the low-dose test is a plasma cortisol level 6 h after the last dose of dexamethasone of less than 138 nmol/L (<5 μg/dL) or a urinary cortisol level of less than 55 nmol/d (<20 μg/24 h).[667] In patients with Cushing's syndrome, regardless of etiology, neither plasma cortisol nor urinary cortisol excretion is suppressed in response to 2 d of dexamethasone. Patients who metabolize dexamethasone rapidly may also not have suppressed excretion; this can be determined by measuring a plasma dexamethasone level. Six hours after the last 0.5-mg dose in the low-dose test, the

plasma dexamethasone level should be 5.1 to 15 nmol/L (200 to 600 ng/dL), with a mean of 9.4 nmol/L (370 ng/dL). Six hours after the last 2-mg dose in the high-dose test, the plasma dexamethasone level should be 18 to 51 nmol/L (700 to 2000 ng/dL), with a mean of 35 nmol/L (1350 ng/dL).[668, 669] This assessment is particularly important in patients receiving drugs such as carbamazepine, phenobarbital, or other drugs that stimulate the cytochrome P-450 system of the liver. This measurement also helps document patient compliance with the regimen.

Distinction of ACTH-Dependent from ACTH-Independent Causes. The cornerstone for determining whether the syndrome is ACTH dependent or ACTH independent is measurement of the plasma ACTH concentration. ACTH levels are suppressed in patients with adrenal adenoma or adrenal carcinoma, whereas levels are easily detectable, but may overlap with the normal range, in patients with ectopic ACTH syndrome, Cushing's disease, or ectopic CRH syndrome (Fig. 6–45).

Distinction of Pituitary from Nonpituitary Sources of ACTH. Once the syndrome is determined to be ACTH dependent, it is necessary to determine the origin of the ACTH: the pituitary gland or an ectopic source. An empirical observation is that hypokalemic alkalosis is rare in Cushing's disease. If hypokalemic alkalosis occurs in the absence of diuretic ingestion, ectopic ACTH secretion should be suspected. The rationale for tests to distinguish between pituitary and ectopic ACTH production is that in pituitary-dependent disease, the pituitary gland is responsive to high levels of glucocorticoid and to marked reductions in circulating glucocorticoid concentrations. The sensitivity to the negative feedback effect of high glucocorticoid concentra-

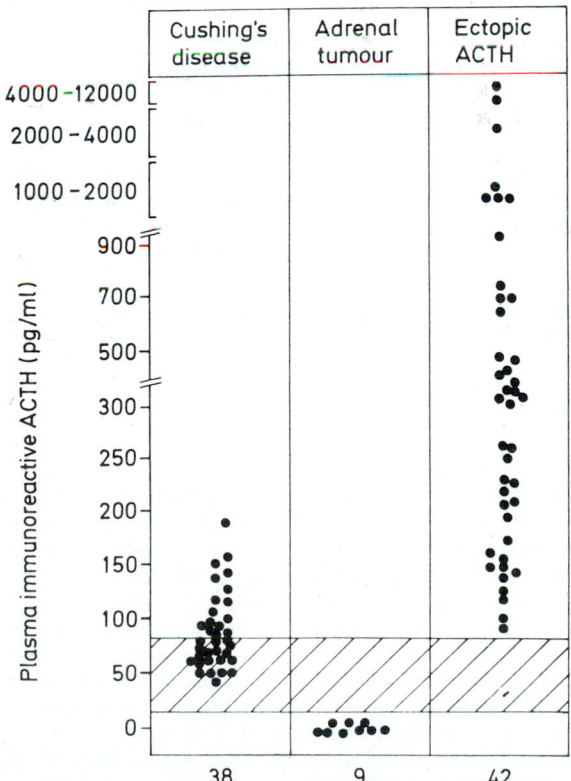

Figure 6–45. Plasma ACTH concentrations in patients with excessive cortisol production of different etiologies. To convert ACTH values to picomoles per liter, multiply by 0.2202. (Modified from Rees LH, Holdaway IM, Phenekos C, et al. ACTH secretion and clinical investigations. In: Some Aspects of Hypothalamic Regulation of Endocrine Functions. Symposium Vienna June 3–6, 1973. Stuttgart: Schattauer Verlag, 1974.)

tions is present but is reset at a higher than normal level. Thus administration of a high dose of dexamethasone produces suppression of ACTH production by a pituitary adenoma with a resulting decrease in adrenal cortisol secretion. Peripheral tumors that produce ACTH are generally unresponsive to high doses of dexamethasone. The standard high-dose dexamethasone suppression test of 2 mg every 6 h for 48 h (8 mg/d) is used to distinguish between a pituitary and an ectopic source of ACTH. Consistent reduction in urinary excretion of 17-hydroxycorticosteroid concentrations to 50% or more of the baseline value usually occurs in patients with pituitary-dependent disease.[670] This 50% suppression has been adopted as a required value by some investigators, but this criterion is probably incorrect (see Chapter 9). An additional measurement of urinary free cortisol excretion is helpful because any reproducible suppression of cortisol is indicative of pituitary-dependent disease. If a pituitary cause is suspected and adequate suppression of urinary steroids does not occur with usual high-dose dexamethasone administration, it is prudent to retest the patient using a total dexamethasone dose of 16, 32, or 64 mg/d, because a few patients with a pituitary adenoma responded to these higher doses. The same criteria as for the 8 mg/d test for suppression of urinary steroid excretion are used. If there is no suppression of adrenal cortisol production, even with the highest dexamethasone doses, it can be assumed that a peripheral tumor is the source of ACTH.

The metyrapone test is also used to distinguish between a pituitary and an ectopic ACTH source and is complementary to the high-dose dexamethasone test. An ACTH-producing pituitary adenoma (and the normal pituitary gland) responds to a marked decrease in circulating cortisol concentrations produced by inhibition of cortisol synthesis by metyrapone. In normal subjects and in patients with pituitary-dependent disease, inhibition of cortisol synthesis by metyrapone results in increased pituitary ACTH secretion; this does not occur with an ectopic ACTH-producing tumor. Metyrapone inhibits cortisol synthesis at several steps, the most prominent being inhibition of the conversion of 11-deoxycortisol to cortisol. The commencement of the test should be delayed at least 48 h, and preferably longer, after the high-dose dexamethasone suppression test, for two reasons: (1) dexamethasone must be metabolized and its biological effects eliminated so that reduction of endogenous cortisol synthesis during metyrapone administration is detected by the pituitary; and (2) 48 h of high-dose dexamethasone may suppress ACTH such that the adrenals are transiently unresponsive to ACTH stimulation during metyrapone administration (because of reduction of steroidogenic enzymes; personal communication, David Orth). In patients with ectopic ACTH secretion, hypothalamic-pituitary function is chronically suppressed and cannot be reactivated by a short-term (24-h) reduction in plasma cortisol concentrations such as occurs with metyrapone. Conversely, patients with pituitary-dependent disease remain responsive to a sudden reduction in circulating cortisol levels, and ACTH secretion increases. This additional ACTH stimulation of the adrenal glands produces an increase in levels of circulating cortisol precursors, with plasma 11-deoxycortisol being the most frequently measured. The metyrapone test consists of oral administration of 750 mg every 4 h (with food to minimize development of nausea) for 24 h (six doses) and measurement of the plasma 11-deoxycortisol concentration before and 4 h after the last metyrapone dose. Plasma cortisol is also measured 4 h after the last metyrapone dose to assess the adequacy of 11β-hydroxylase blockade.[671] Patients with pituitary-dependent disease have an increase in plasma 11-deoxycortisol level to more than 144 nmol/L (>5

μg/dL) in the setting of an undetectable plasma cortisol concentration. Urinary 17-hydroxysteroid excretion may also be measured to distinguish between a pituitary and an ectopic ACTH etiology. Twenty-four-hour urine collections must be obtained on the day before, during, and on the day after metyrapone administration. Because the cortisol precursors are metabolized and excreted as urinary 17-hydroxysteroids, a two- to threefold increase in 17-hydroxysteroid excretion occurs in pituitary-dependent disease. With an ectopic ACTH tumor or an adrenal tumor, CRH and ACTH function is suppressed, and no increase in adrenal steroid synthesis occurs during metyrapone administration. However, this ACTH suppression does not always mean that these tumors cannot respond to exogenous ACTH. Furthermore if the ectopic ACTH syndrome is of recent onset, the hypothalamic-pituitary-adrenal axis may not be completely suppressed, resulting in either an attenuated or a normal response to metyrapone.

CRH administration has been used in the diagnostic evaluation of Cushing's syndrome and was initially believed to be useful in distinguishing between pituitary-dependent disease and ectopic ACTH syndrome. It appeared that CRH administration to patients with a pituitary adenoma stimulated ACTH release, whereas in the ectopic ACTH syndrome there was no increase in ACTH release.[672] Additional studies demonstrated that exceptions occur; some patients with ectopic ACTH syndrome have an increase in ACTH release in response to CRH.[673] CRH has also been administered during petrosal sinus catheterization with measurement of petrosal sinus and peripheral ACTH concentrations.[674] This technique allows definitive identification of a pituitary source of ACTH and may indicate which side of the pituitary contains the adenoma. Several investigators recommend that this procedure be performed in every ACTH-dependent patient to confirm the diagnosis of Cushing's disease and to aid in localization of the tumor.[675] A limitation of this study is that in patients with recent onset of ectopic ACTH syndrome, the pituitary may still respond to CRH. In this case, there is usually no gradient in ACTH concentration between the left and right petrosal samples after CRH. In patients in whom the diagnosis is clear from the noninvasive studies, this procedure is usually not necessary, but it should be performed if there is doubt about the source of ACTH. Petrosal sinus sampling should be performed by an experienced interventional radiologist who is skilled in this technique.

Summary of Evaluation. A logical strategy for evaluating a patient with Cushing's syndrome has been outlined (Table 6–24). Because a small number of patients with Cushing's syndrome, of all etiologies, have cyclic disease, it is possible to be misled by the results of either the dexamethasone or the metyrapone test when the results are due to spontaneous cyclic variation. However, both tests should be performed, and if the results are consonant with each other greater certainty in the diagnosis is achieved.

Based on our knowledge of feedback mechanisms, ectopic CRH causing Cushing's syndrome would be expected to respond in a manner identical with that of Cushing's disease. In the few cases described, the response is similar to that in ectopic ACTH syndrome. These ectopic tumors often secrete both ACTH and CRH. The best-studied case of ectopic CRH production causing Cushing's syndrome was in a patient with prostatic carcinoma metastatic to the median eminence.[676]

Hypothalamic CRH-producing gangliocytoma causing Cushing's syndrome has been recognized only retrospectively at pathological examination; the responses to dynamic function tests are unknown. Again, this is an extremely rare cause of Cushing's syndrome. It is anticipated that these

TABLE 6–24. Test Results in Patients with Cushing's Syndrome of Various Etiologies

Etiology	Low-Dose Dexamethasone*	Plasma ACTH	High-Dose Dexamethasone†	Metyrapone‡
Pituitary	No or partial	Normal or elevated	Suppression	Increase in serum 11-deoxycortisol More than doubling urinary 17-hydroxycorticosteroid
Ectopic ACTH	No suppression	Normal or elevated	No suppression§	No change
Adrenal	No suppression	Low	No suppression	Fall

*Normal response: plasma cortisol < 138 nmol/L (<5 µg/dL) at 48 h; urinary free cortisol < 55 nmol/d (<20 µg/24 h).
†24-h urinary 17-hydroxycorticosteroid decreases reliably.
‡24-h urinary 17-hydroxycorticosteroid and plasma deoxycortisol.
§5% suppressed; approximately 50% of bronchial carcinoid tumors suppressed.

patients would respond with a similar pattern to those with Cushing's disease.

RADIOLOGICAL EVALUATION. Once the diagnosis of Cushing's disease is established, the therapeutic strategy must be defined. In most instances, unless there is a contraindication, transsphenoidal surgery will be performed, and the surgeon will be aided if the location and size of the pituitary tumor are defined by either a high-resolution CT scan or an MRI scan. MRI scanning does not show the bony structures but is excellent for demonstrating vascular structures and the optic chiasm, nerves, and cavernous sinuses. Only about half of adenomas causing Cushing's disease are detectable by CT or MRI because these tumors may be very small.[677, 678] The findings vary from upward bulging of the diaphragma sellae to a low-density or enhancing area that represents the microadenoma. Macroadenomas are a rare cause of Cushing's disease and are usually invasive and difficult to cure. It should be remembered that patients with ectopic ACTH syndrome may have incidental non–ACTH-secreting adenomas, such as nonfunctioning adenomas or prolactinomas; this emphasizes the importance of making the correct diagnosis based on the biochemical tests.[679]

Because a few patients with ectopic ACTH secretion from bronchial or thymic carcinoids respond with suppression during dexamethasone administration, it is mandatory that patients thought to have Cushing's disease have a CT or MRI scan of the chest to exclude a bronchial or thymic tumor. If this test is negative, it is probably worthwhile to obtain an abdominal CT scan to search for pancreatic islet tumor or pheochromocytoma. These studies identify approximately 90% of tumors that cause chronic ectopic ACTH secretion, but some lesions are too small to be detected and may take as long as 18 y to manifest themselves.[680]

In contrast, the patient with biochemical evidence suggesting ectopic ACTH syndrome may in fact have an aggressive pituitary adenoma. Occasionally, malignant, aggressive ACTH-secreting pituitary tumors are not under negative feedback by glucocorticoids. Thus in all patients with Cushing's disease a CT or MRI scan of the pituitary should be obtained to exclude this unlikely possibility.

PATHOLOGY. In Cushing's disease the most frequent anatomical finding is an ACTH-producing microadenoma, measuring less than 1.0 cm in diameter, in the anterior lobe. It is not surprising that some of these adenomas are difficult or impossible to localize preoperatively even using sensitive and sophisticated methods such as MRI and petrosal sinus catheterization with CRH stimulation and measurement of ACTH concentrations. In some cases the adenoma is not visible on gross examination of the resected tissue. In these cases serial histological sections of the removed tissue must be examined to identify an adenoma.

The tumor cells are basophilic and stain positively with the PAS method.[347, 681] Immunocytochemistry demonstrates the presence of ACTH and other POMC-related peptides such as endorphins and lipotropin in the cytoplasm of adenoma cells.[347, 681–683] Corticotrope adenomas are most often monomorphous and monohormonal. Rarely, they may exhibit immunoreactivity for alpha subunit, LH,[684] or prolactin.[685]

The findings on electron microscopy of corticotrope adenomas are characteristic and diagnostic.[347, 681–683] The adenoma cells are elongate or angular with ovoid nuclei that manifest some indentation. The cytoplasm is abundant and has prominent RER membranes, free ribosomes and polysomes, a prominent Golgi complex, a few bundles of type 1 filaments, and many secretory granules in the size range of 150 to 450 nm. The granules are spherical, indented, and heart shaped and vary in electron density (Fig. 6–46). In some cases corticotrope adenomas are large and invade adjacent structures. These adenoma cells may exhibit varying degrees of pleomorphism, and mitotic figures may be present. The immunocytochemical features of these tumor cells do not differ and in many cases are indistinguishable from those of corticotrope microadenomas.

Another variant is the chromophobic pituitary adenoma with mild or no PAS positivity and usually scant immunoreactivity for ACTH and other POMC-related peptides.[347] By electron microscopy, chromophobic tumors contain fewer and smaller secretory granules and may contain more free ribosomes and mitochondria and few type 1 filaments.[347] The small basophilic tumors usually grow slowly but are hormonally very active. The chromophobic tumors are larger, often invasive, hormonally less active despite larger size, and grow rapidly. It is not clear whether these two types of tumors that differ in morphology and biological behavior arise from the same cell type and differentiate or dedifferentiate after neoplastic transformation, originate from two different clones, or undergo mutation. In brief, it is not clear if the morphological and functional differences represent examples of tumor cell heterogeneity or tumor cell variability.

Another rare morphological variant is the so-called Crooke's cell adenoma.[686, 687] It was once thought that Crooke's hyalinization, the morphological indicator of functional suppression of corticotropes, occurs only in nontumorous corticotropes and not in the adenoma cells. However, in some adenomas various degrees of Crooke's hyaline change may occur, suggesting that such tumors are not fully autonomous. The hyaline change is an accumulation of keratin-positive intermediate filaments.[32, 688] On electron microscopy the hyaline change is easily identified because it consists of bundles of 7-nm-wide type 1 filaments that have no periodicity, are not membrane bound, and are located in the perinuclear areas.[347, 681–683] In advanced forms the filaments almost completely occupy the cytoplasm, and only a few secretory granules are present, predominantly under the plasmalemma and the Golgi area (Fig. 6–47). Clinically, Crooke's cell adenomas cause heterogeneous effects. Some produce severe Cushing's disease; others produce more subtle disease.[687] The reason for these differences is not understood.

Nelson's syndrome develops in patients with pre-existing

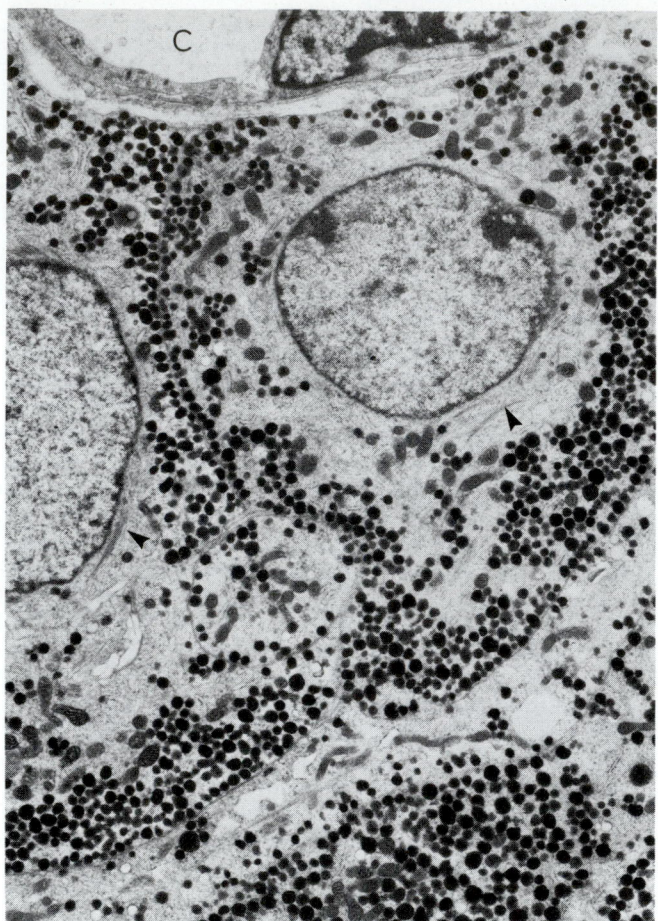

Figure 6–46. Corticotrope cell adenoma with numerous irregular, dented, and heart-shaped secretory granules. Note bundles of type 1 filaments (*arrowheads*). C, capillary. Magnification × 8150.

cretory pituitary tumor. However, morphologically these tumors are indistinguishable from those of Cushing's disease, and the tumor cells are immunoreactive for ACTH and other POMC-related peptides. On electron microscopy there is no difference between a silent corticotrope adenoma and the clinically functional ACTH-secreting tumor. The silent corticotrope adenoma contains large amounts of POMC mRNA; thus the POMC gene is expressed in these tumors, but the gene product is probably processed differently,[690] explaining the absence of clinical symptoms and signs of hypercortisolism.

Corticotrope hyperplasia is a controversial issue, although there is no doubt that non-neoplastic accumulation of corticotropes may be responsible for pituitary Cushing's disease.[347, 681–683, 691–699] However, the pathological diagnosis of corticotrope hyperplasia in the usually fragmented surgical biopsy specimens is difficult and in some cases impossible. Because corticotrope hyperplasia and adenoma may rarely coexist, serial sectioning of all available tissue is required in suspected cases of hyperplasia. Corticotrope hyperplasia may be diffuse, but most commonly it is present in a combination of the diffuse and nodular forms.[697] The light microscopic and electron microscopic features of corticotropes with diffuse hyperplasia resemble those of Crooke's cells, whereas the smaller, angular cells of corticotrope nodules are somewhat similar to those of adenomatous corticotropes. Corticotrope hyperplasia has been observed in CRH-producing gangliocytoma,[699] CRH-producing extrapituitary tumors,[676, 700–702] and pituitaries of patients with Addison's disease.[703]

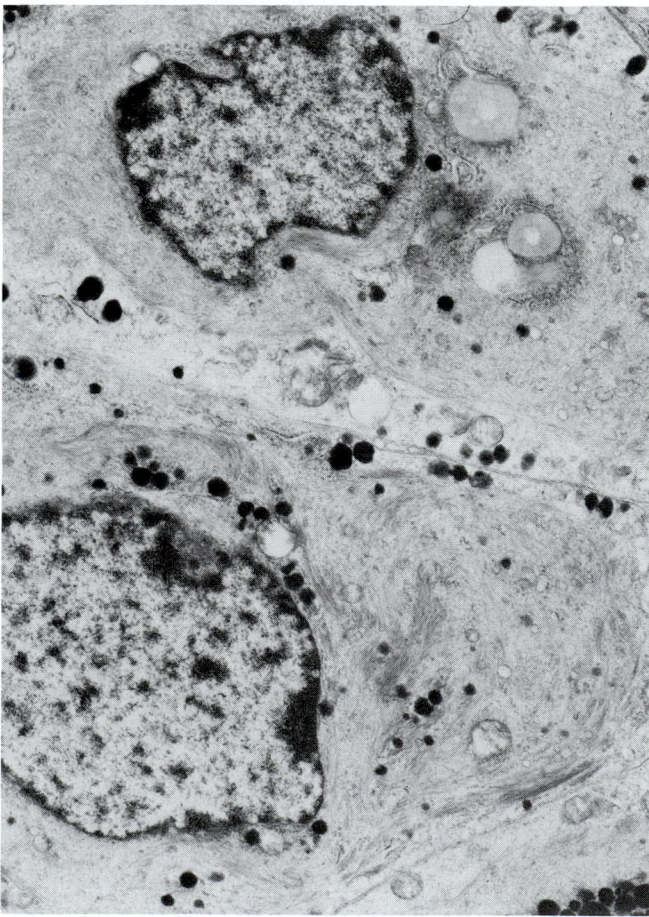

Figure 6–47. Corticotrope cell adenoma displaying advanced Crooke's hyalinization. Most of the cytoplasm is occupied by a thick ring of type 1 filaments displacing secretory granules to the cell periphery. Magnification × 12,550.

Cushing's disease who underwent bilateral adrenalectomy. Nelson's syndrome is now uncommon because patients with Cushing's disease usually undergo pituitary surgery instead of bilateral adrenalectomy. Patients with Nelson's syndrome have rapidly growing and often invasive basophilic and PAS-positive adenomas.[347, 681] The tumor cells are immunoreactive for ACTH and other POMC-related peptides. The electron microscopic features of the tumor cells are indistinguishable from those of patients with Cushing's disease and intact adrenal glands. The only ultrastructural difference is the scarcity or absence of type 1 filaments in the adenoma of Nelson's syndrome. This finding is further evidence that glucocorticoid hormones are probably essential for the formation of cytoplasmic type 1 filaments. Another difference between Nelson's syndrome and Cushing's disease is that in Nelson's syndrome the tumors are usually larger, grow more rapidly, are frequently invasive, and have nuclear and cellular pleomorphism; mitotic figures are more frequent. These differences are consistent with the hypothesis that corticotrope adenomas are not completely autonomous but are responsive tumors whose secretory activity and growth rate can be suppressed or modulated by glucocorticoid hormones.

Another tumor type that should be mentioned is the silent "corticotrope" adenoma, subtype 1.[344, 345, 347, 681–683, 689] These tumors are not associated with clinical or biochemical evidence of ACTH hypersecretion, and patients with the tumor are diagnosed as having a nonfunctioning or nonse-

Corticotrope carcinomas are rare; only a few cases have been described.[347, 704, 705] The diagnosis is accurate only when invasion and distant metastases are present. These tumors, which may cause Cushing's disease, exhibit considerable nuclear and cytoplasmic pleomorphism and many mitotic figures. The tumor cells are often chromophobic and either PAS negative or slightly PAS positive. However, basophilic, PAS-positive tumors may also behave as carcinomas; the tumor cells are immunoreactive for ACTH and other POMC-related peptides. Electron microscopy shows rather poorly differentiated pleomorphic corticotropes that are usually sparsely granulated.

In some cases the pituitary appears normal in patients with biochemical evidence of Cushing's disease, except that Crooke's hyaline change is present. These cases are difficult to interpret. An adenoma may have been present, but either it was not removed or, if removed, it was too small for detection. Alternatively, corticotropes may have been hyperactive without an increase in the cell mass.

Cushing's syndrome includes all patients with hypercortisolism who have no primary pituitary abnormalities. In patients with a nonpituitary cause of Cushing's syndrome, the pituitary shows various degrees of Crooke's hyaline change; no adenoma or corticotrope hyperplasia is present. However, the Crooke's hyaline change is a valuable morphological indicator of glucocorticoid excess. There is substantial individual variation among subjects, and the degree of Crooke's hyaline change does not indicate the degree or duration of glucocorticoid excess. The Crooke's hyaline change is reversible; after cessation of glucocorticoid excess the corticotropes regain normal morphology.

In some cases, the morphology of corticotropes does not permit distinction between Cushing's disease and Cushing's syndrome. In CRH excess caused by a CRH-producing extrahypothalamic tumor, Crooke's hyaline change and corticotrope hyperplasia are both present. In the ectopic ACTH syndrome, Crooke's hyaline change may be marked, but the number of corticotropes is normal and no corticotrope adenoma is found. In Nelson's syndrome and Addison's disease, Crooke's hyaline change is not present.

There is evidence suggesting that some corticotrope adenomas may arise in the pars intermedia corticotropes.[706] This concept is controversial and has not been confirmed.[707]

ACTH immunoreactivity is rarely present in plurihormonal adenomas. These ACTH-immunoreactive plurihormonal pituitary tumors will not be discussed here because they are not clearly defined.

TREATMENT. In this section the therapeutic strategy for Cushing's disease is discussed; the strategy for other types of Cushing's syndrome is discussed in Chapter 9.

The diagnosis of Cushing's disease should be made after a thorough evaluation, and there should be little doubt that the patient has an ACTH-secreting pituitary adenoma. The therapeutic objective is to cure the patient without causing permanent adrenal or other pituitary insufficiency. The ideal approach is to direct therapy toward the problem and selectively remove the pituitary adenoma. In the past, the treatment was total bilateral adrenalectomy. The advantages of pituitary surgery are that it restores normal physiology, obviates the risk of developing Nelson's syndrome, and avoids bilateral adrenalectomy, which is associated with greater morbidity and mortality and requires chronic glucocorticoid and mineralocorticoid replacement.

Surgical Therapy. Selective pituitary adenoma removal can be achieved by transsphenoidal surgery. Other than standard contraindications to surgery, such as cardiac or severe pulmonary disease, the specific contraindications to transsphenoidal surgery include a pituitary gland that is inaccessible because of abnormal bone structures or because a dural venous complex surrounds the pituitary. In patients with microadenomas operated on by a surgeon experienced with transsphenoidal microadenectomy, a cure rate of approximately 80% can be expected.[708–711] If a tumor is not visible after careful exploration of the gland, either a total hypophysectomy (in a patient without the capacity or desire for reproduction) or a hemihypophysectomy is usually performed. If a tumor is not visualized on imaging studies, petrosal sampling with attempts to lateralize the side of ACTH production makes hemihypophysectomy more rational. The operative results are less successful if dural invasion is present; a success rate of about 25% can be expected. These poor results reflect inability to remove the tumor totally because of invasion of bone and/or dura.

The patient with Cushing's disease is treated as any patient with a pituitary tumor. The evaluation includes determination of all anterior pituitary function and assessment of visual fields before surgery. If there are marked clinical effects of excessive cortisol production and if there is concern about operative morbidity, medical therapy to inhibit cortisol synthesis (metyrapone) should be initiated before surgery. Replacement glucocorticoids should be administered before surgery, and "stress" doses should be given before induction of anesthesia and continued through surgery and during the postoperative period. If surgery is successful, replacement glucocorticoid therapy may need to be continued for several months until the hypothalamus and residual corticotrope cells resume function. Dexamethasone, 1 mg every 12 h, is often given preoperatively because it is long-acting and can be given by the oral or parenteral route. This regimen is continued for 48 h and is then changed to hydrocortisone, 20 mg on waking and 10 mg at 6 PM. Hydrocortisone has the advantage of being short-acting and thus permits recovery of the hypothalamic-pituitary axis. Patients may have symptoms of steroid withdrawal after successful surgery, even with adequate replacement. The longer the delay in recovery of the hypothalamic-pituitary-adrenal axis, the better the prognosis for cure; total recovery may take as long as 18 mo.

Radiation Therapy. Another treatment of Cushing's disease is external pituitary radiation. Usually 45 to 50 Gy is administered over a 5-wk period. This is successful in about 80% of cases of childhood Cushing's disease[712] but is successful in only 15 to 20% of adults.[713] Pituitary radiation (for acromegaly) carries a risk of development of anterior pituitary dysfunction that may occur 10 y or more after treatment.[391] It is unlikely that patients with Cushing's disease are immune to this effect. Less common complications of radiotherapy include damage to the optic nerves or chiasm, damage to the vascular system, and development of brain tumors. Other forms of radiation therapy including alpha particle and proton beam therapy are contraindicated in tumors with extrasellar extension (suprasellar or lateral extension). They also carry a significant risk of hypopituitarism and cranial nerve injury. Gamma knife therapy (single high-dose, focused radiation) has not been adequately evaluated.

Radiation therapy is recommended routinely for patients who undergo bilateral adrenalectomy for Cushing's disease to avoid the risk of development of Nelson's syndrome, the aggressive growth of the pituitary adenoma after bilateral adrenalectomy.[713]

Because radiation therapy and transsphenoidal surgery produce similar results in children, it is difficult to be dogmatic about the best approach. However, in a center with excellent transsphenoidal surgery, this procedure is recommended with the hope of curing the patient and avoiding hypopituitarism. The surgeon will be more conservative in a child than in an adult, and if no tumor is found a hemihypophysectomy will often be performed. If the patient is not cured, postoperative radiation therapy remains an option.

Medical Therapy. Medical therapy for Cushing's disease is only adjunctive. Medical therapy to reduce cortisol production is helpful in preparing an extremely ill patient for surgery and can be used to maintain normal plasma cortisol levels after radiation while awaiting its full effects. The goal is to inhibit the enzymes responsible for cortisol synthesis with drugs such as metyrapone, aminoglutethimide, and ketoconazole. Metyrapone and aminoglutethimide have been the standard therapy, and when the two agents are used in combination side effects may be decreased. Steroid synthesis may be completely inhibited so that replacement glucocorticoid therapy is required. Because aminoglutethimide stimulates hepatic enzymes that degrade dexamethasone, hydrocortisone should be used for replacement therapy. Ketoconazole, a broad-spectrum antimycotic drug, inhibits adrenal steroid biosynthesis at several sites, including side-chain cleavage and 11β-hydroxylation.[714, 715] It is administered at 800 to 1200 mg/d until normal plasma cortisol levels are achieved, after which the dose may be adjusted to maintain that state. All of these drugs are expensive and have significant side effects.

Other medical therapies, such as use of cyproheptadine and bromocriptine to reduce pituitary ACTH secretion, are effective in few patients. Those who respond to bromocriptine may have intermediate-lobe tumors,[706] but this clinical entity is unconfirmed.[707]

Nelson's Syndrome

Nelson's syndrome is due to the development of an aggressive ACTH-secreting pituitary adenoma in patients who have undergone bilateral adrenalectomy for Cushing's disease.[716] These patients develop symptoms of a mass, including headaches, visual field defects, and external ophthalmoplegia. The high ACTH levels cause hyperpigmentation similar to that in Addison's disease. Because the patient initially had a pituitary tumor secreting ACTH, this syndrome presumably represents enhancement of the tumor growth by the removal of the negative feedback of excessive cortisol from the adrenal glands. The estimated incidence of Nelson's syndrome varies from 10 to 50%. Some studies suggest that this syndrome is preventable by external pituitary irradiation[712, 713] before or at the time of adrenalectomy, although others dispute this.[717, 718]

The condition is suspected from the characteristic history and physical findings. Plasma ACTH levels are extremely high, often ranging from 220 pmol/L (1000 pg/mL) to 2200 pmol/L (10,000 pg/mL) or higher. However, the level of ACTH does not accurately reflect the size or aggressiveness of the tumor. The presence of the tumor is confirmed by CT or MRI scan. In contrast to the tumors of Cushing's disease, these tumors are usually macroadenomas.

Nelson's syndrome is preventable. Currently, bilateral adrenalectomy is rarely used to treat Cushing's disease. Because pituitary microsurgery is the preferred initial treatment, this condition is likely to become of historical interest. Once the diagnosis of Nelson's syndrome is made, the treatment should be aggressive, as these tumors are locally invasive and grow rapidly. Pituitary surgery is the preferred treatment. Most neurosurgeons approach the tumor by the transsphenoidal route and resect as much as possible. If residual tumor is known to be present, the patient should undergo pituitary radiation, particularly if the tumor was not previously radiated.[646] The ACTH secretion by the tumor is responsive to endogenous CRH and AVP. Thus by optimizing negative feedback to the hypothalamus by using

a long-acting glucocorticoid and judiciously timing its administration to reverse the normal glucocorticoid rhythm, hypothalamic stimulation of the tumor can be minimized; a suggested regimen is 0.5 mg dexamethasone on retiring. This approach has not been demonstrated to be superior but is logical and is used by several groups.

Glycoprotein-Producing Adenomas

Glycoprotein adenomas produce LH, FSH, TSH, or the alpha subunit, either alone or in combination, and may or may not result in increased serum concentrations of the protein. When the serum hormone concentrations are normal, glycoprotein hormone production may be detectable by in vitro studies such as radioimmunoassay of medium from pituitary tumor cell cultures, detection of specific mRNAs in tumor extracts, or immunocytochemical staining of surgical specimens. Identification of hormone production by serum measurements and by in vitro techniques indicates that glycoprotein-producing adenomas may occur in as many as 24% of surgical specimens.[719] These tumors appear to arise spontaneously without an identifiable cause.[720] One hypothesis about the origin of FSH-secreting tumors is that gonadotrope hyperplasia can develop into an adenoma in the setting of primary gonadal failure. Another theory is that increased FSH production results from a nonsecretory adenoma that impairs LH but not FSH secretion. These theories do not explain the clinical and biochemical features associated with gonadotrope-producing tumors.[721] Also, the gonadal failure of female menopause is not associated with an increase in the incidence of this tumor type in this age group.

Patients with glycoprotein-producing adenomas most commonly come to medical attention because of symptoms and/or signs of a mass lesion or, in the case of a TSH-secreting tumor, because of hyperthyroidism. Most of these tumors are diagnosed in middle-aged men (mean age 55) with symptoms of headache, visual disturbance, and acquired hypogonadism. These tumors are uncommon in women of reproductive age, and the prevalence in postmenopausal women is unknown because serum LH and FSH concentrations are appropriately increased. However, in some, the gonadotropin concentrations are depressed. Mild hyperprolactinemia (<100 µg/L) may result from stalk compression. Men often have a subnormal serum testosterone concentration associated with low, normal, or increased LH and FSH concentrations. The reasons for hypogonadism are unclear, and it has been attributed to depressed bioactive LH secretion, secretion of abnormally glycosylated gonadotropins, or abnormal pulsatile gonadotropin secretion.[720]

THYROTROPE ADENOMA. The TSH adenoma is the least common type of pituitary tumor, representing less than 1% of the total, and is the only glycoprotein tumor producing a characteristic clinical syndrome.[722] Common clinical features include symptoms referable to the pituitary mass lesion and/or hyperthyroidism with goiter. The tumor also frequently secretes free alpha subunit, which is increased in concentration in more than 80% of patients.[723, 724] The molar ratio of alpha subunit to TSH may be helpful in distinguishing a TSH-secreting adenoma from other forms of hyperthyroidism; an alpha subunit/TSH ratio greater than 1 is common in TSH tumors. Other secretory products of thyrotrope adenomas include GH and prolactin. The diagnosis of acromegaly or hyperprolactinemia may be evident only when the patient seeks medical care for symptoms of hyperthyroidism. The hyperthyroxinemia is associated with an inappropriately normal or elevated serum TSH concentration. Because use of a sensitive TSH assay distinguishes between normal and suppressed values, the diagnosis of a

TSH-secreting adenoma should be easy, thus facilitating appropriate treatment of the pituitary tumor. Although this tumor is uncommon, it should be excluded by measurement of the serum TSH concentration in patients with hyperthyroidism or hyperthyroxinemia. Serum TSH concentrations may be markedly increased, but approximately one third of patients with a TSH-secreting adenoma have values less than 10 mU/L.[720, 725] As noted, measurement of the serum alpha subunit concentration is helpful for the diagnosis of a TSH-secreting adenoma. It also aids in excluding the syndrome of pituitary resistance to thyroid hormone, in which serum TSH concentrations are inappropriately increased in the setting of hyperthyroxinemia. (See Chapter 8.) Serum alpha subunit concentrations are not increased in the syndrome of pituitary resistance to thyroid hormone. Administration of TRH may also distinguish between a TSH-secreting adenoma and the syndrome of pituitary resistance to thyroid hormone. Administration of TRH to patients with TSH-secreting tumors does not produce an increase in serum TSH concentration, but patients with pituitary resistance to thyroid hormone may have an exaggerated increase in serum TSH level.[723]

The initial treatment of a TSH-secreting adenoma is surgical. As with all large pituitary tumors, however, complete resection may not be possible. Preliminary reports indicate that medical treatment with octreotide may lower serum TSH concentrations, resulting in a euthyroid state.[726] Postoperative pituitary radiation may be employed for residual tumor. If hyperthyroidism persists, treatment with antithyroid drugs may be necessary.

Pathology of Thyrotrope Tumors. Tumors composed of thyrotropes may be associated with hyperthyroidism,[727-730] hypothyroidism,[731-733] or euthyroidism. Morphologically, TSH-secreting tumors are indistinguishable despite different clinical effects. Thus the morphological features of these tumors do not reflect the endocrine milieu. No conclusions can be drawn regarding hormone secretion and the functional activity of the pituitary-thyroid axis from morphological studies.

Thyrotrope adenomas are chromophobic tumors that may contain a few PAS-positive granules or larger globules, especially in patients with prolonged primary hypothyroidism.[347] Densely granulated tumors with cytoplasmic basophilia are rare. By immunocytochemistry the adenoma cells have positive immunostaining for the beta subunit of TSH and the alpha subunit of TSH. The tumor cells are polyhedral, elongated, and sometimes tall columnar, forming pseudorosettes around vessels. The adenomas have a distinct border and the tumor cells show no major pleomorphism. By electron microscopy,[347, 732, 734, 735] the tumor cells are elongated and polar and have long cytoplasmic processes, a spherical or ovoid nucleus, and prominent nucleoli. The RER and Golgi complexes are moderately or well developed, and cytoplasmic microtubules often form a rich network. The secretory granules are small and spherical, vary slightly in electron density, most commonly measure between 50 and 200 nm, and are frequently arranged under the plasmalemma in a single row. Exocytosis is not observed (Fig. 6-48).

Autopsy studies indicate that in the nontumorous area of the hypophysis harboring a TSH-producing adenoma, the various other cell types are normal.[736] In hyperthyroidism, thyrotropes are normal or small, suggesting functional inhibition. In patients with prolonged primary hypothyroidism the thyrotropes are numerous and large with abundant cytoplasm ("thyroidectomy cells"), and the mass of the pituitary may be increased clinically, simulating a pituitary adenoma. In the thyrotrope tumor the large hypothyroid-associated (thyroidectomy) cells are very rare.

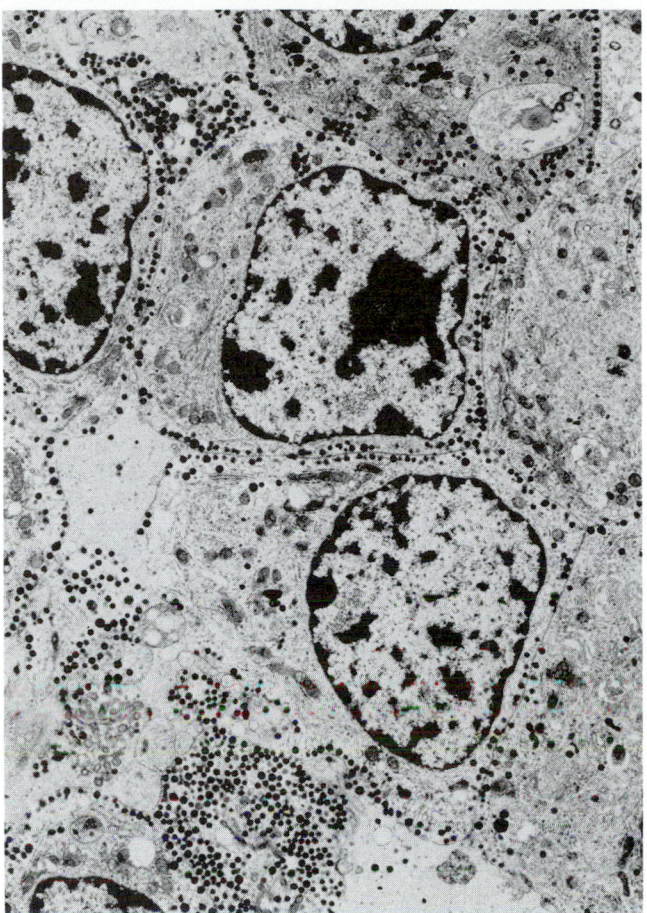

Figure 6–48. Thyrotrope cell adenoma. The angular shape of cells is accentuated by the peripheral localization of small secretory granules. Magnification × 6650.

Some plurihormonal tumors produce several hormones, including TSH.[347, 348] Synthesis of TSH is not uncommon in plurihormonal adenomas, and densely granulated somatotrope adenomas often contain TSH-positive cells.[352] Few of these plurihormonal tumors are accompanied by hyperthyroidism, and instead the TSH-producing component is usually clinically silent. Thus structural features and functional activity are not always correlated.

Thyrotrope hyperplasia is a well-defined pathological entity. It occurs and is easily recognizable in patients with long-standing primary hypothyroidism.[737, 738] Other conditions causing thyrotrope hyperplasia have not been identified. Morphologically, thyrotrope hyperplasia consists of markedly enlarged, stimulated thyrotropes or thyroid deficiency cells.[225, 446] In some cases, overactivity of lactotropes and even frank lactotrope hyperplasia are also present.[446] Whether hyperplastic thyrotropes can undergo neoplastic transformation, are the predecessors of a thyrotrope adenoma, and are more susceptible to neoplastic transformation than normal thyrotropes have not been clarified.

Thyrotrope carcinoma has not been described.

GONADOTROPE ADENOMA. Gonadotrope adenomas are identified either by increased serum LH, FSH, and/or alpha subunit concentrations or by in vitro studies including immunocytochemistry, electron microscopy, or tumor cell culture studies.

The prevalence of gonadotrope adenomas is unknown. In one series of 139 men with untreated macroadenomas, 24% had gonadotrope tumors; 17% had hypersecretion of FSH, either alone or in combination with alpha, LH beta, and FSH beta subunits, and 7% had hypersecretion of only the alpha subunit.[719] The majority of these men, 87%, presented with visual impairment indicative of a large tumor. In two studies of surgical specimens, gonadotrope adenomas were present in 3.5 and 4.1% of cases, respectively.[739, 740]

The most commonly observed glycoprotein hormone secreted is FSH, which appears by gel filtration chromatography to be intact FSH.[741] This may be accompanied by an increase in circulating alpha subunit concentrations, as also occurs in association with tumors producing the LH beta subunit. Hypersecretion of intact LH occurs less commonly than does secretion of intact FSH or free FSH beta or alpha subunits. However, a raised serum LH level may also be a result of assay cross-reactivity with free alpha subunit or LH beta subunit; gel filtration chromatography is necessary for precise identification of the secretory product. In most men, the serum testosterone concentration is either normal or below normal because intact LH is not produced. Thus, by hormone measurements, inappropriately normal serum LH concentrations are observed in the setting of reduced testosterone production. When intact LH is produced, the serum testosterone concentration is above normal. Administration of TRH may be helpful in the diagnosis because approximately half of patients with a gonadotrope adenoma have an increase in LH or FSH level after TRH stimulation.[719] The FSH and LH responses to exogenous LHRH are variable; approximately 50% of patients with an FSH-secreting tumor have an increase in serum FSH concentration, whereas an increase in serum LH concentration occurs less frequently.[742–751]

Gonadotrope adenomas are most commonly diagnosed in middle-aged men (mean age 45) who report normal sexual function but who seek medical attention because of visual abnormality or headaches.[719] It is not known whether these tumors occur more frequently in men or are more difficult to diagnose in women, as exemplified by a postmenopausal woman with a pituitary adenoma and increased serum LH and FSH concentrations. The distinction between a nonsecretory adenoma and a gonadotrope adenoma may not be possible clinically or biochemically and may require electron microscopic or immunocytochemical studies of the excised tumor.

A history of normal pubertal development, sexual function, and fertility, particularly in men with hypersecretion of FSH, suggests that a gonadotrope tumor developed spontaneously and did not result from primary hypogonadism. Most tumors do not hypersecrete intact LH, and the serum testosterone concentration in men may be normal or subnormal. Diagnostic difficulty arises when the serum testosterone level is below normal and the serum immunoreactive LH level is increased because of increased free alpha subunit or LH beta subunit secretion with assay cross-reactivity; an increased immunoreactive serum LH concentration may erroneously suggest the diagnosis of primary gonadal failure. In this circumstance, it is prudent to consider the possibility of a gonadotrope tumor, particularly if there is a history of headache or change in vision. In a man with a subnormal serum testosterone level and an inappropriately normal serum LH concentration, the diagnosis of secondary hypogonadism is evident. A pituitary tumor, gonadotrope or other type, cannot be excluded without an appropriate imaging study.

The initial treatment of a gonadotrope tumor is surgical resection, particularly if visual function is abnormal. Transsphenoidal surgery improves vision in most patients and may correct hormonal hypersecretion, hypogonadism, and the abnormal gonadotropin response to TRH.[752] Persistent hormonal hypersecretion and the presence of residual tumor may require postoperative pituitary radiation treatment.

Medical treatment of gonadotrope adenomas has involved use of the dopamine agonist bromocriptine, the somatostatin analogue octreotide, and long-acting LHRH agonist and antagonist analogues. Dopamine and its agonists may decrease basal and LHRH-stimulated gonadotropin secretion and free alpha subunit concentrations.[720] Some patients treated with bromocriptine have a reduction in hormone hypersecretion, improvement in visual abnormalities, and a decrease in tumor size.[748, 753] However, this is not a consistent finding; some patients have no response to bromocriptine, indicating variable responsiveness to dopamine.[439, 754, 755]

Somatostatin inhibits gonadotropin secretion in vitro and in vivo. A somatostatin infusion decreases serum alpha subunit, LH, and FSH concentrations by 40 to 60% in patients with gonadotrope tumors.[720] Administration of octreotide has been reported to decrease serum LH concentrations in a patient with an LH- and alpha subunit–secreting adenoma.[756] Octreotide treatment in another patient had variable effects on residual tumor mass and serum alpha subunit concentrations.[757] More extensive studies of a larger number of patients treated with octreotide are necessary before the efficacy can be determined.

Another experimental medical treatment for gonadotrope adenomas is administration of long-acting LHRH agonist and antagonist analogues to inhibit gonadotropin secretion. LHRH agonists are not consistently successful in reducing hormone hypersecretion or tumor size and frequently cause an increase in serum alpha subunit concentrations.[758–761] The LHRH antagonist Nal-Glu GnRH has been administered to five patients with FSH-secreting adenomas; preliminary results indicate that this antagonist decreases serum FSH concentrations in the majority.[762]

In summary, the medical treatment of gonadotrope adenomas is not established but is used in an attempt to reduce hormone hypersecretion and tumor size after unsuccessful surgery and while awaiting the full effects of pituitary radiation. Because efficacy has not been determined in a suitably large number of patients, close and careful medical evaluations are necessary.

Pathology of Gonadotrope Adenoma. Gonadotrope adenoma was the last type of pituitary tumor characterized.[744, 763] Its frequency in surgical specimens ranged from less than 1 to 10% between 1979 and 1989. Gonadotrope adenomas are not as well defined as other types of pituitary tumors. They were the first tumor type showing sex-related ultrastructural dichotomy;[740] several quantitative differences also exist between tumors from men and women, and these features will be discussed separately.

Preoperative diagnosis of gonadotrope adenoma in men is based on the finding of inappropriately high gonadotropin levels.[719, 764–768] These tumors, however, may also be associated with local symptoms of a mass causing visual disturbances, nausea, headaches, and cranial nerve palsies. Gonadotrope adenomas in men[740, 744] are chromophobic or slightly to moderately acidophilic. The histological pattern is most commonly sinusoidal with pseudorosette formation around vessels, or it may be diffuse. Strong immunoreactivity for FSH, LH, or both is a fairly consistent feature and the best diagnostic marker in men. Some adenomas, however, exhibit modest immunoreactivity for FSH and/or LH, not exceeding that of many null cell adenomas. The alpha subunit, which is a fairly consistent clinical marker in gonadotrope adenomas,[745, 769] is not a reliable morphological indicator. The electron microscopic appearance, which in general is helpful in diagnosing other adenoma types, is variable in gonadotrope adenomas of men.[739, 740, 770] These differences include a well-differentiated tumor consisting of elongate, polar cells with uniform nuclei; well-developed, slightly dilated RER;

and a prominent Golgi complex (Fig. 6–49) with sparse secretory granules, 200 nm in diameter, unevenly distributed and more numerous in the basal part of the cytoplasm. Another type of adenoma has the uncharacteristic appearance of null cell adenomas.[740, 744] Intermediate forms with cells displaying features of varying degrees of functional differentiation are common. There is no correlation between serum FSH or LH levels and immunoreactivity or ultrastructure. Because of these uncertainties, one method may not be sufficient for diagnosis.

In women, gonadotrope adenomas are rarely associated with markedly elevated serum FSH or LH levels; in most patients the gonadotropin levels are within normal limits for age.[740] The morphology of gonadotrope adenoma in women is enigmatic. The well-differentiated, nontumorous, chromophobe adenomas display scant, if any, immunoreactivity for gonadotropins; strong generalized immunostaining is rare. However, by electron microscopy these sparsely granulated tumors are characterized by a unique morphological marker, the "honeycomb Golgi complex" (Fig. 6–50). The sacculi of Golgi apparatus transform into clusters of spheres containing low-density proteinaceous substance. Few if any immature secretory granules are present in these membrane systems, probably indicating impaired packaging of secretory material, which, in turn, may be the cause of sparse immunoreactivity in these tumors.

No gonadotropin-producing carcinoma has been reported.

Hyperplasia of gonadotrope cells is rare and poorly

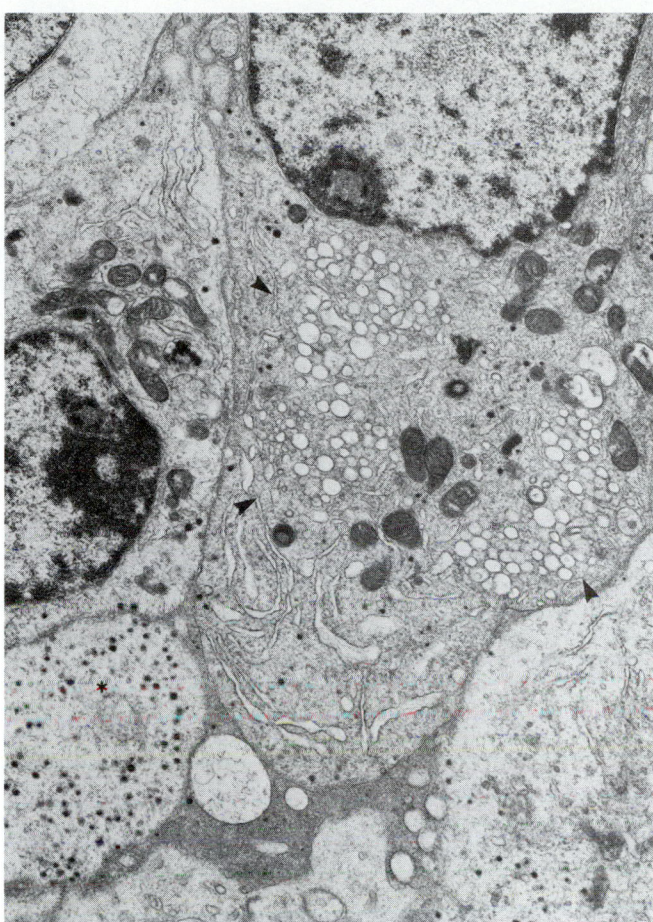

Figure 6–50. Gonadotrope adenoma, female type, containing "honeycomb Golgi complex," the diagnostic marker of the tumor type *(arrowheads)*. Most of the small (150-nm) secretory granules collect in cytoplasmic processes *(asterisk)*. Magnification × 12,750.

studied. At autopsy, one case of diffuse, massive gonadotrope hyperplasia was associated with Klinefelter's syndrome.

Nonsecretory Adenoma

A nonsecretory or nonfunctioning pituitary tumor, sometimes called a chromophobe adenoma, is characterized by the absence of a particular clinical syndrome and the absence of increased serum hormone concentrations. The tumor is classified as nonsecretory in 25 to 30% of patients. However, on morphological examination, these tumors often contain secretory granules suggesting hormone synthesis and storage.[771] Immunocytochemical and electron microscopic studies have identified many of these tumors as gonadotrope, alpha subunit, or corticotrope tumors. In addition, a tumor may be immunopositive for more than one hormone, with combinations including hCG alpha, LH beta, FSH beta, TSH beta, and ACTH.[772] In vitro studies of cultured cells and techniques using specific oligonucleotide cDNAs for hybridization confirmed that these tumors may produce alpha subunit, LH beta subunit, and hCG beta subunit.[773] The absence of increased serum hormone concentrations has been attributed to abnormal post-translational processing or unavailability of specific glycoprotein subunit assays. With increased availability of specific glycoprotein subunit assays, more presumptive nonfunctioning tumors will probably be recognized as glycoprotein-producing tumors.

The majority of patients are seen because of symptoms of a macroadenoma (headache, visual disturbance) or symp-

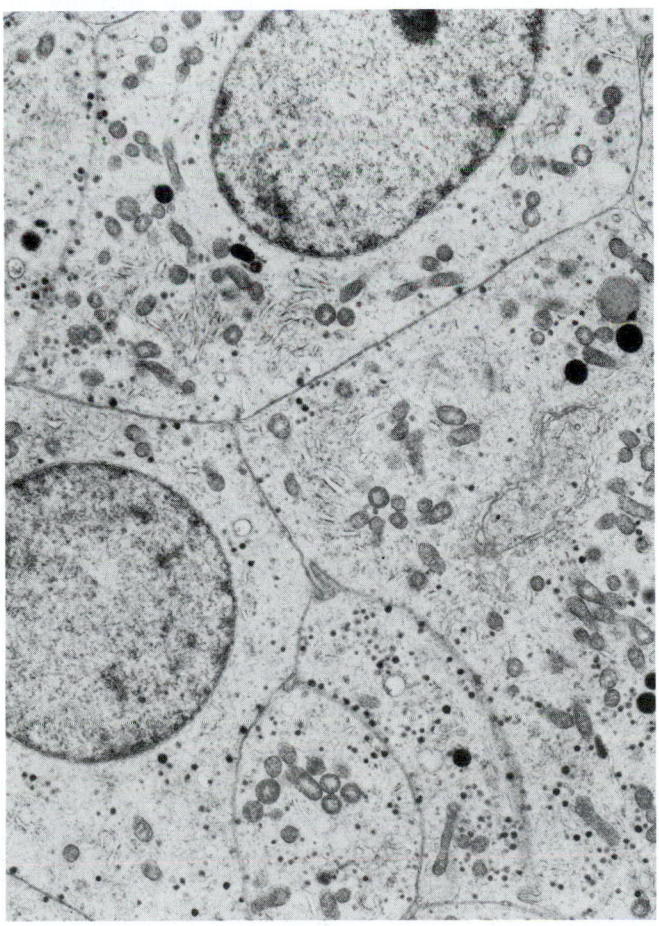

Figure 6–49. Gonadotrope adenoma, male type, featuring uniform euchromatic nuclei, slightly dilated RER, a prominent Golgi complex with regular appearance, and small, unevenly distributed secretory granules. Magnification × 10,000.

toms of hypopituitarism such as adrenal insufficiency, hypothyroidism, or, more commonly, hypogonadism. These tumors occur most commonly in men and in postmenopausal women. A mild or moderate elevation of serum prolactin concentration (<100 μg/L) is common and is thought to reflect stalk compression. Despite an increase in serum prolactin level, a large tumor with a mild hyperprolactinemia is not a prolactinoma.

Pretreatment evaluation includes evaluation of pituitary function, including measurement of serum prolactin, IGF I (as a measure of GH secretion), LH, FSH, TSH, and alpha subunit concentrations. If assays are available, LH beta, FSH beta, and TSH beta subunit concentrations should also be measured. The need for hormone replacement, particularly cortisol and T_4, should be assessed by measuring basal levels of T_4, cortisol and testosterone (men). If these values are abnormal, replacement is necessary. A normal morning cortisol concentration is not sufficient to exclude impairment of the hypothalamic-pituitary-adrenal axis; a stimulatory test such as insulin-induced hypoglycemia or the metyrapone test is required for accurate assessment. The ophthalmological examination includes funduscopy, ocular motility determination, visual acuity, and quantitative assessment of visual fields. Anatomical evaluation should consist of a gadolinium-enhanced MRI scan or a coronal CT scan with contrast.

The recommended treatment for a nonsecretory tumor is surgical excision, usually via the transsphenoidal approach. A large tumor with extrasellar extension may not be completely resectable, but removal of a substantial portion of the tumor may produce improvement in visual abnormalities or minimize the potential for future loss. The transfrontal approach is rarely indicated because it is associated with higher rates of morbidity and mortality; unless most of the tumor is suprasellar, producing signs of brain compression, the transsphenoidal approach is preferable. Transsphenoidal resection usually results in improvement in visual abnormalities and amelioration of headaches. In one study significant residual tumor or recurrence of tumor after 1 y was present in 20% of patients. Tumor recurred in 18% who received postoperative radiotherapy and 12% who did not. However, because radiotherapy was administered to those with known or suspected residual disease, it is difficult to compare the two groups directly.[774]

Residual tumor is usually treated with postoperative conventional supervoltage radiation. If the patient is unable to undergo surgery or if the tumor is asymptomatic and intrasellar (uncommon) and vision is normal, pituitary radiation with careful monitoring of pituitary function, tumor size, and vision is an alternative primary therapy. The response to pituitary radiation is similar to that of other pituitary tumors; prompt reduction in tumor size is rare, but additional tumor growth may be inhibited.

Medical treatment of nonsecretory tumors with the dopamine agonist drugs has been used in a small number of patients. Nonsecretory tumors have fewer high-affinity membrane-bound dopamine receptors than are found in prolactin-secreting tumors.[775] Despite isolated reports of reduction in tumor size with bromocriptine, dopamine agonist treatment is unsuccessful in a majority of patients.[441, 755, 775–777] However, because a few patients are responsive to dopamine agonist treatment, a trial of bromocriptine may be warranted in the patient who is unwilling or unable to undergo surgery.

The postoperative management is identical with that of any patient undergoing pituitary surgery and should include assessment of the visual system and assessment of the need for hormone replacement. Anatomical assessment should include an MRI or CT scan within a month of surgery and 6 and 12 mo postoperatively. If there is evidence of residual tumor, pituitary radiation is usually given to prevent an increase in the tumor size. If no tumor is visible on the postoperative or on the 6- and 12-mo scans, the anatomical study can be performed at yearly intervals.

PATHOLOGY OF NONFUNCTIONING PITUITARY ADENOMAS. These adenomas represent approximately 25% of pituitary tumors in surgical material.[347] They do not secrete hormones in excess and are not associated with any hypersecretory syndrome. Mild hyperprolactinemia may develop in those with large tumors because of the so-called stalk section effect; i.e., the growing suprasellar mass impairs the hypothalamic synthesis, release, or transport of dopamine and other prolactin-inhibiting factors.

The pathology of nonfunctioning pituitary adenomas was confusing for many years and several names were used for these tumors.[347] They were called chromophobic, nonfunctioning, undifferentiated, precursor cell, fetal, and embryonic adenomas. However, none of these names satisfactorily expresses their real nature. The name null cell adenoma[778, 779] reflects the main characteristic of these tumors, the lack of morphological, immunocytochemical, or ultrastructural markers that reveal their cellular origin. Null cell is a useful name for the majority of apparently nonfunctioning pituitary adenomas. Nonfunctioning pituitary adenomas can be divided into two groups: null cell adenomas including oncocytomas and silent adenomas.

Null cell adenomas are histologically chromophobic or slightly acidophilic, PAS-negative tumors.[347, 349, 778–780] Either immunocytochemistry yields negative results for anterior pituitary hormones or, more frequently, groups of adenoma cells are immunoreactive for one or more pituitary hormones, most frequently FSH and/or the alpha subunit, less frequently TSH and LH, and occasionally GH, prolactin, or ACTH. Hormone secretion by null cell adenomas does occur, as shown by in vitro studies in which hormones were measured in the culture media by radioimmunoassay and by the reverse hemolytic plaque assay.[781, 782] mRNA for glycoprotein hormones can be demonstrated in many of these tumors,[773] and in another study ACTH and prolactin mRNAs were also documented.[783] By electron microscopy null cell adenomas contain secretory granules signifying endocrine differentiation.[347, 778, 779] The hormone-producing machinery of the cells, however, is poorly developed, resulting in very low hormonal activity (Fig. 6–51). The secretory granules are sparse and small, 50 to 200 nm in diameter, and no exocytosis can be observed. Some of the null cell adenomas have immunoreactivity for neuron-specific enolase, chromogranin, and/or synaptophysin.[779]

Null cell adenomas can be divided into nononcocytic and oncocytic tumors;[347, 778, 779] oncocytomas contain large numbers of mitochondria.[784–787] Because of mitochondrial accumulation, the cytoplasm is granular and may take up acidic dyes. Oncocytomas also show focal immunostaining for one or more anterior pituitary hormones, mainly FSH and the alpha subunit.[779] They produce hormones in vitro; release mainly FSH and alpha subunit,[781] as shown also by the reverse hemolytic plaque assay; and express mRNA primarily for glycoprotein hormones.[773] The cause of mitochondrial accumulation is not known. Oncocytomas are characteristic on electron microscopy because the abundant cytoplasm contains numerous mitochondria, often showing morphological abnormalities[787] (Fig. 6–52). In the oncocytic variant, mitochondrial cytoplasmic volume density may reach 40 to 45%. Despite the marked mitochondrial abundance, RER membranes, Golgi complexes, and secretory granules are always recognized.

Null cell adenomas contain various receptors, including

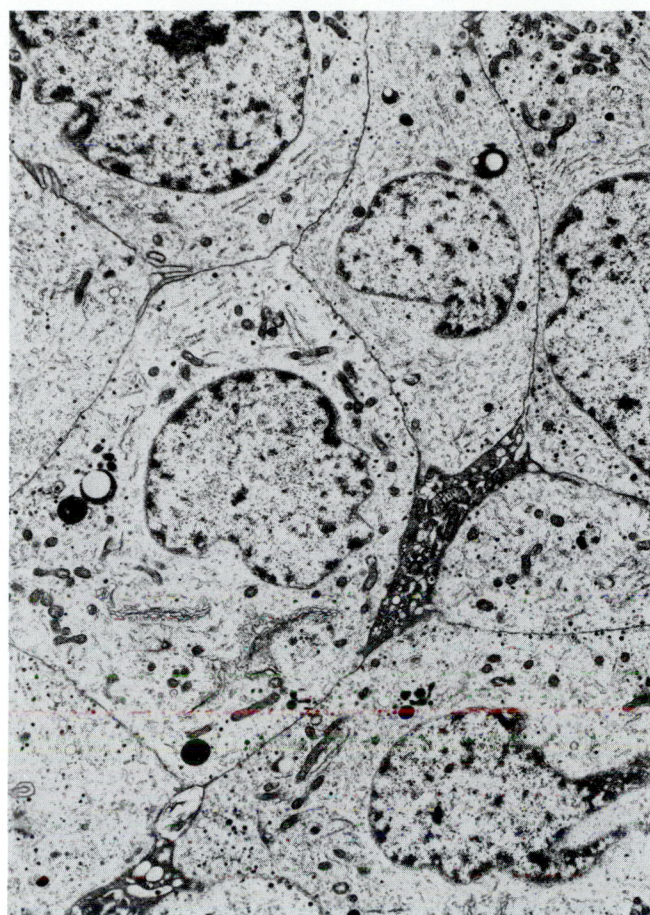

Figure 6–51. Null cell adenoma with poorly developed RER and Golgi complex and scant secretory granules. Magnification × 6850.

those for dopamine[775] and somatostatin.[788] The presence of these receptors raises the hope that null cell adenomas will be responsive to medical treatment.

Similarities have been drawn between null cell adenomas and gonadotrope adenomas.[740, 779, 781, 789] The histological and ultrastructural features are indistinguishable in some cases in men,[740] and the immunocytochemical profile may also be similar. Both null cell adenomas and gonadotrope adenomas may be immunoreactive for FSH and the alpha subunit.[781, 787, 789] The FSH, LH, and alpha subunit genes are also expressed in both tumor types.[773] Thus the question arises whether one should distinguish between null cell adenomas and gonadotrope adenomas or consider null cell adenomas as a variant of gonadotrope adenomas.

However, some null cell adenomas are not immunoreactive for glycoprotein hormones and do not express their genes, whereas others are immunoreactive and express genes for additional hormones such as prolactin or ACTH,[783] clearly indicating the heterogeneity of the null cell adenoma-oncocytoma. With refinement of diagnostic techniques, some null cell adenomas will find their place among functioning tumors. Derivation of others may remain undetermined because of the absence of endocrine activity; these are usually slowly growing large tumors that cause local symptoms such as visual defects.

Silent adenomas are three morphological subtypes of well-differentiated tumors that have characteristic ultrastructural appearances, which are distinct in two of the subtypes from those of other adenomas.[344–346, 689] Clinically, these adenomas are apparently functionless and, apart from possible

mild hyperprolactinemia,[689] are not associated with elevated serum levels of known pituitary hormones. Although the cause of the apparent lack of function is not established, it is assumed that silent adenomas are derived from pituitary cell types not yet characterized and elaborate hormones that do not cause conspicuous clinical syndromes.

Silent "corticotrope" adenoma subtype 1 is morphologically indistinguishable from corticotrope adenomas associated with Cushing's disease.[344, 345, 689, 690] The tumors are macroadenomas at the time of diagnosis, and approximately 40% are associated with symptoms of recent hemorrhage.[347] The type is somewhat more common in women. By electron microscopy, lysosomal accumulation and follicle formation may be seen as additional features.[344] These structural markers are common in the pars intermedia and posterior lobe basophils that may be the precursor cell of the tumor type. In all tested cases, in situ hybridization detects strong expression of the POMC gene.[690] The post-translational processing of the gene product is not known.

Silent "corticotrope" adenoma subtype 2 is clinically similar to a nonfunctional macroadenoma.[345, 347] This tumor type displays a marked (4:1) male preponderance. Histologically these tumors are chromophobes or show mild basophilia and PAS positivity. Varying degrees of immunoreactivity for ACTH and other POMC-derived peptides are present. Ultrastructurally the adenomas are well differentiated and consist of polyhedral cells without polarity (Fig. 6–53). The secretory granules are similar morphologically to corticotrope granules, including numerous drop-shaped forms, but are smaller (less than 400 nm, chiefly 200 to 300

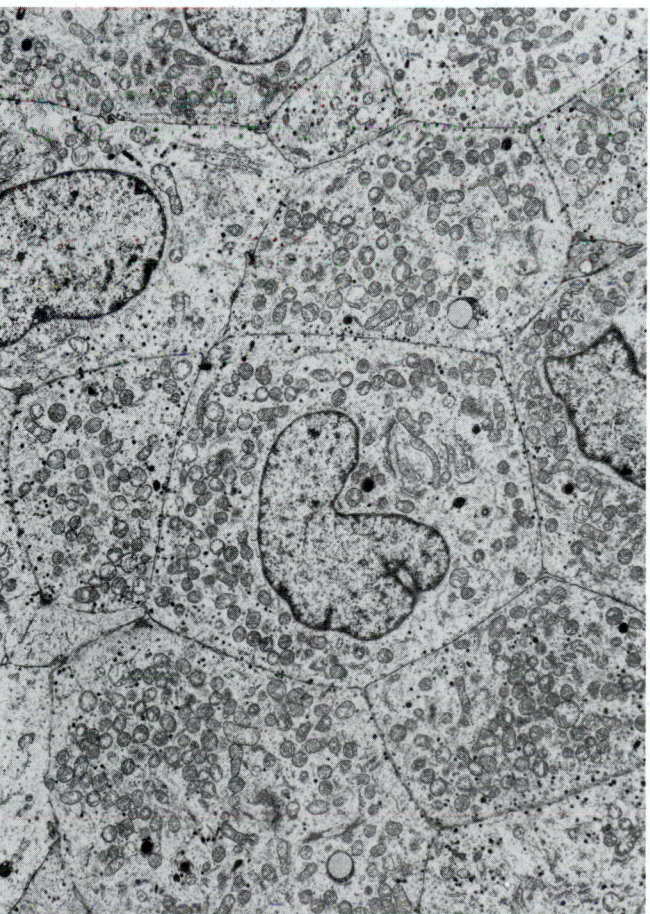

Figure 6–52. Pituitary oncocytoma showing abundance of mitochondria. Magnification × 5050.

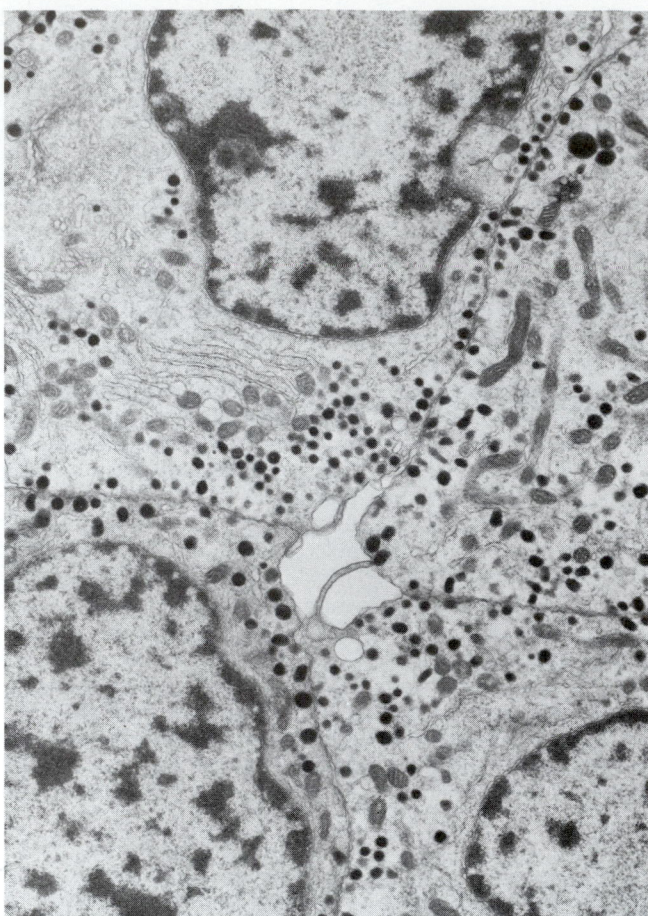

Figure 6–53. Silent "corticotrope" adenoma, subtype 2. The rather small, polyhedral cells contain irregular nuclei, moderately developed RER and Golgi complex, and numerous, often drop-shaped, rod-shaped, or dented secretory granules. Magnification × 11,900.

nm). Unlike subtype 1 adenomas, subtype 2 tumors contain no type 1 filaments. Morphological studies suggest that the tumor also produces POMC and an active hormone as yet unknown. The cell of derivation is unknown. Cells morphologically similar to cells of silent corticotrope adenoma subtype 2 are present in normal, nontumorous pituitary gland.

Subtype 3 silent adenomas[345, 347] were originally thought to consist of POMC-producing cells because several tumors showed variable immunoreactivity for ACTH and other POMC-related peptides. However, several such tumors were immunonegative for ACTH. Scattered adenoma cells are immunoreactive for GH, prolactin, or one or more glycoprotein hormones.[346] By electron microscopy these tumors are composed of cells that resemble well-differentiated active glycoprotein hormone–producing cells (Fig. 6–54). They are composed of large irregular polar cells with abundant cytoplasm containing well-developed RER and often smooth endoplasmic reticulum membranes and prominent Golgi complexes. The secretory granules are sparse, more numerous in cell processes, and measure about 200 nm. Ultrastructural studies suggest that these cells are in a hyperactive state, but the hormonal product is unknown. There is no sex predilection for this tumor type. In young women, the tumors may be mistaken for prolactin-producing adenomas because of the associated mild to moderate hyperprolactinemia. Treatment with a dopamine agonist reduces serum prolactin levels without effect on tumor size, and the excess prolactin appears to be secreted by nontumorous prolactin cells. Because hyperprolactinemia is present when the tumor

is still small, stalk compression is not likely to play a role. One possibility is that the tumor produces a prolactin-stimulating substance that increases prolactin release from nontumorous lactotropes.

Silent tumors also occur among adenomas with known cell derivation. Several gonadotrope adenomas and a few thyrotrope tumors are not associated with clinical manifestations of hormone overproduction. A few examples of sparsely granulated GH cell adenomas may also be clinically silent.[790] Such tumors have a typical ultrastructure but GH immunoreactivity is sparse or almost absent. However, in situ hybridization shows expression of the GH gene in a variable number of tumor cells. This finding indicates that the GH gene is transcribed, but either the message is not translated or the gene product is not processed into an immunoreactive and biologically active form of hormone in sufficient amounts to be clinically detectable.

Plurihormonal adenomas also have silent component(s).[347, 348] With the exception of mixed GH cell–prolactin cell adenomas, in most of these one morphological cell type is predominant. The corresponding hormone is oversecreted, leading to a hypersecretory syndrome, while other hormones are detectable only in trace quantities.

The silent adenomas raise intriguing conceptual questions. The discrepancy between morphology and endocrine activity is difficult to explain. In reality, many silent adenomas are pseudosilent. As judged by their ultrastructure, all three subtypes of silent adenomas produce and release

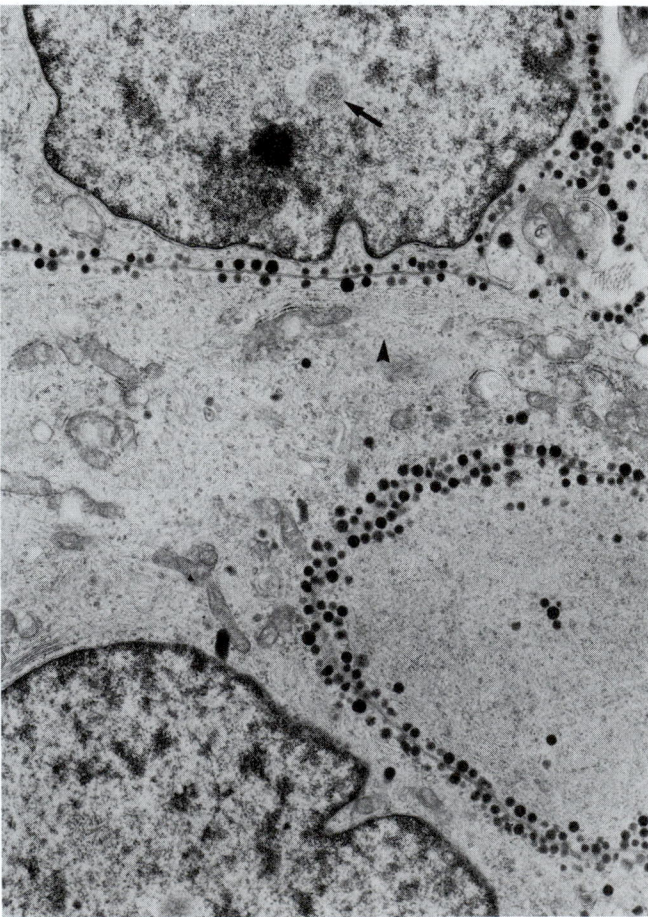

Figure 6–54. Silent adenoma subtype 3. The large cytoplasm is filled with arrays of delicate, partly rough and partly smooth endoplasmic reticulum *(arrowhead)* and Golgi membranes. The small secretory granules are often located at the cell periphery. Note prominent nuclear inclusion (spheridium) *(arrow)*. Magnification × 12,550.

hitherto unknown hormones that cause no visible symptoms. The silence of some GH adenomas may be explained by the lack of bioactivity of the product or subtlety of the clinical features. The silent component (or components) of plurihormonal adenomas is probably produced and released, but in small quantities that do not produce an elevated hormone level. The same circumstance may also explain the lack of function in cases of null cell adenomas and oncocytomas.

Nonpituitary Sellar Mass

A number of lesions in the region of the hypothalamus and pituitary are not pituitary tumors. These include craniopharyngioma, hypophysitis, apoplexy, germinoma, Rathke's pouch cyst, arachnoid cyst, chordoma, optic nerve glioma, reticulosis, meningioma, and secondary deposits. Only the first four will be discussed, as the management of the others follows standard medical lines. It is important to make the correct diagnosis because therapies are often quite different. Specifically, the transsphenoidal approach can be disastrous for some lesions such as an internal carotid artery aneurysm. The advent of modern imaging techniques has facilitated diagnosis before therapeutic intervention.

CRANIOPHARYNGIOMA. A craniopharyngioma or Rathke's pouch tumor arises from embryonic squamous cell rests that persist after the upward migration of stomodeal epithelium to the anterior pituitary. Because a tumor may arise from any position along the craniopharyngeal canal, it may be intrasellar or extrasellar. The tumor is usually well encapsulated and composed of cystic and solid components.[791–793] The cysts may be multiloculated and contain dark brown, oily fluid. These tumors may occur at any age but are most common in children, accounting for 5 to 10% of primary brain tumors in children. Approximately one quarter are diagnosed after the age of 40.[791, 794]

Clinical Presentation. Children are usually diagnosed because of growth failure or because of symptoms of increased intracranial pressure (headache, vomiting, somnolence). Sixty percent of children have visual disturbances, and growth retardation is usual.[793] Eighty percent of adults present with complaints of visual disturbance, but on examination more than 90% have visual abnormalities.[795] Disturbance of intellectual function, which may include dementia, occurs in approximately 30% of adults.[794, 796]

A prospective study of endocrine function in 20 patients with craniopharyngioma (6 adults and 14 children and adolescents) revealed a variable degree of hypopituaritism.[797] GH and gonadotropin deficiencies were most common, occurring in 19 of 20. Sixty-five percent had secondary hypothyroidism, and half had corticotropin deficiency; none had diabetes insipidus. Clinically, diabetes insipidus is common after surgical resection of the tumor.

Assessments of hypothalamic-pituitary function and vision and anatomical evaluation are identical with those of any patient with a pituitary or suprasellar mass. Craniopharyngiomas are characteristically suprasellar. They may extend inferiorly into the sella turcica, causing destruction of bony margins of the sella and dorsum sellae. They may also extend superiorly into the third ventricle, producing hydrocephalus by block at the foramen of Monro.[791] The CT scan appearance may be helpful in suggesting the diagnosis preoperatively. Calcification of the tumor occurs in 70 to 90% of children and in 40 to 60% of adults; calcification is detectable on a CT scan but not on an MRI scan. The solid portion of the tumor may appear enhanced on a CT scan after administration of intravenous contrast agent. The high cholesterol content of cyst fluid produces a characteristic MRI signal that may also aid in the diagnosis.[798, 799]

Therapy. The primary treatment of a craniopharyngioma is surgical resection.[791, 800] Surgery is associated with considerable morbidity and mortality, usually from the standard surgical approach (craniotomy) and from diabetes insipidus and other hypothalamic-pituitary dysfunction.[801] Tumor recurrence is a definite risk. Because these tumors are relatively radioresistant and grow slowly, it is difficult to assess the efficacy of radiotherapy.[802]

With the use of CT and MRI scans to evaluate patients with complaints referable to the cranium, more asymptomatic patients with a craniophyaryngioma are being diagnosed. These patients are a therapeutic dilemma. The preferred approach is surgical resection, but a craniotomy is associated with greater risk; thus if the patient is asymptomatic, an argument can be made for an anticipatory approach with careful follow-up, including a repeat imaging study at 6 mo or 1 y. The interval between scans may be doubled if there has been no increase in tumor size or tumor symptoms.

LYMPHOCYTIC HYPOPHYSITIS. Lymphocytic infiltration of the pituitary gland is associated with complete or partial hypopituitarism, a pituitary mass, and occurrence exclusively in women, often during pregnancy or in the postpartum period. The maternal death rate associated with this entity has been approximately 50%, most likely because of unrecognized secondary adrenal failure, emphasizing the need for consideration of the diagnosis in a pregnant or postpartum woman with symptoms of headache, visual disturbance, weakness, and fatigue.

Lymphocytic hypophysitis was first described in an autopsy specimen in 1962; fewer than 30 cases have been reported subsequently.[803–814] Seventy percent of women were in the second or third trimester of pregnancy or up to 7 mo post partum; in 30% there was no temporal relationship with pregnancy. The clinical presentation is one of symptoms and signs of pituitary dysfunction, frequently hypocortisolism, and a pituitary mass. Pituitary deficiencies include ACTH, TSH, LH, FSH, and AVP, either alone or in combination; an increased serum prolactin concentration occurs in half. The most common symptoms and signs of a mass are headache in the majority and visual field loss in 32%. In patients who had imaging studies, suprasellar extension of the mass was present in 64%.[807] Although the majority of women had permanent destruction of all or part of the pituitary and required chronic hormone replacement therapy, one patient had transient hypopituitarism of 12 mo duration, suggesting that total pituitary destruction may not always occur.[809] Thus these patients should probably be evaluated at regular intervals to determine the necessity for continued hormone replacement. The etiology is unknown. However, several studies have suggested an autoimmune cause. Antipituitary antibodies were present in the sera of some women, and others had other autoimmune endocrine disorders, including thyroiditis and adrenalitis. Another proposed etiology is virus-induced autoimmune destruction of the gland as suggested by studies in animals. The common association with pregnancy has been attributed to increased exposure to pituitary antigens or changes in maternal immunological status.

Although the diagnosis may be suspected in a pregnant or postpartum woman with the typical clinical features, confirmation requires surgical biopsy and histological examination of the tissue. Diffuse infiltration with lymphocytes and plasma cells, some areas of follicles with germinal centers, and destruction of normal pituitary cells are the characteristic morphological changes on light and electron microscopy. Immunoperoxidase staining is positive for all pituitary cell types that remain intact.[806] The differential diagnosis based on light microscopic findings includes sarcoidosis, histiocytosis, syphilis, tuberculosis, granulomatous hypophysitis, and postpartum hemorrhagic infarction. Examination of the specimen with electron microscopy is helpful in demonstrating the characteristic interdigitation of lymphocytes and pituitary cells, fusion of lysosomes and secretory granules, and swollen mitochondria indicative of oncocytic transformation. Evidence of vascular injury or immune complex deposition was not present in the cases examined with electron microscopy.[806, 807]

SUPRASELLAR GERMINOMA (ECTOPIC PINEALOMA). This highly malignant tumor has no sex preponderance[815, 816] and appears to have an increased prevalence in Japan. It has been diagnosed in patients 6 to 41 y of age but is rare after age 30. The tumor is of hypothalamic origin and is usually curable by radiotherapy. It is vital to make the correct diagnosis and thus avoid an unnecessary and likely destructive operation.

The tumor may originate in the ventral region of the hypothalamus, in association with a pineal tumor (either metastatic or of multifocal origin), in the anterior third ventricle, or, more rarely, in the pituitary fossa and mimic a pituitary tumor.[817] Because of rapid growth and large size it often compresses the optic nerves and chiasm and extends inferiorly into the pituitary and sella. Extension into the third ventricle produces hydrocephalus.

Clinical Presentation.[816] The most common initial symptom is diabetes insipidus, which occurs in 50% of patients. Other symptoms include visual disturbance, symptoms of increased intracranial pressure (headaches, nausea, vomiting), and obesity. At the time of diagnosis, diabetes insipidus is present in 83%, visual disturbance in 78%, headache in 50%, and endocrine abnormalities including growth retardation in 39% and hypogonadism in 17%. Other systemic symptoms include anorexia in 28% and nausea and vomiting in 11%, which likely reflect hydrocephalus, electrolyte disturbances, and/or secondary adrenal or thyroid failure. This tumor is malignant, often multifocal, and may metastasize within or outside the CNS. For these reasons, staging is very important.

The radiological appearances are not distinctive.[799] Usually a large mass in the third ventricle extends superiorly and inferiorly. It may be enhanced with intravenous contrast agent on a CT scan. A suprasellar germinoma should be considered if there is a hypothalamic mass, particularly if diabetes insipidus is present. This is an unusual presentation for either a pituitary tumor or a craniopharyngioma.

In addition to the tests that would be performed for a patient with a pituitary tumor, a number of other studies are necessary. The serum β-hCG level should be measured quantitatively and is suggestive of a germinoma if elevated. If β-hCG is undetectable, germinoma is not excluded and a CSF sample should be obtained for cytological examination and measurement of glucose, protein, β-hCG, and α-fetoprotein levels. Expected results are malignant cells, elevated serum protein levels, and increased concentrations of hCG and α-fetoprotein. Elevation of either tumor marker in CSF is sufficient to make the diagnosis.[818] The diagnosis is confirmed by rapid reduction in the size of the lesion with as little as 5 Gy of radiation.

Therapy. The first step is to correct any hormone deficiencies. If there is likely to be a delay in obtaining the results, glucocorticoid and thyroid hormone replacement should be given. These can always be discontinued if the results are normal. If present, diabetes insipidus should be promptly treated with desmopressin. If the thirst center is intact and if the patient is alert, he or she will usually be able to drink an adequate amount of fluid. Water should never be restricted in a patient suspected of having diabetes insipidus.

Because of the location of this tumor and its propensity to metastasize in the CNS, surgery is not likely to effect a cure. Surgery may be required to relieve hydrocephalus, but the risk of seeding tumor cells must be considered; surgery should be performed if high-dose steroids and radiation therapy have failed. Any surgery of the hypothalamus can potentially damage remaining hypothalamic centers. If the diagnosis is uncertain, a therapeutic trial of 5 Gy of radiation may be administered. If within 14 d the tumor decreases in size, the diagnosis is confirmed because other types of masses are not that sensitive to radiation therapy. A full course of radiation therapy to the whole brain and spinal cord is then recommended. If there is evidence of peripheral metastases, chemotherapy may also be indicated.[816]

An alternative approach is administration of chemotherapy before radiation. Effective regimens include single therapy with cyclophosphamide or combination therapy with cyclophosphamide, vinblastine, bleomycin, and cisplatin. If remission occurs with chemotherapy, the radiotherapy dose can be reduced without compromising long-term survival.[819]

PITUITARY APOPLEXY. Pituitary apoplexy is classically defined as an acute, life-threatening infarction of the pituitary gland. Hemorrhagic infarction most commonly occurs in the presence of a pituitary tumor but may also occur spontaneously in a normal gland, after obstetric hemorrhage (Sheehan's syndrome), or in the setting of increased intracranial pressure or systemic anticoagulation therapy. Other predisposing factors include diabetes mellitus, bleeding disorders, pituitary radiation, pneumoencephalography, carotid angiography, mechanical ventilation, trauma, and upper respiratory tract infection.[820–824]

Pituitary infarction usually produces anterior pituitary dysfunction that may be permanent or transient, with the degree of impairment being dependent on the amount of tissue destruction. Deficient hormones include GH (88%), gonadotropins (58 to 76%), and ACTH (66%). Secondary hypothyroidism occurs in 42 to 53%, and abnormal prolactin secretion is present in 67 to 100%. Diabetes insipidus is uncommon, occurring in 2 to 3% of patients.[825] The precise incidence of pituitary infarction and hemorrhage is unknown. In unselected autopsy studies, infarction of more than 25% of the gland was present in 1 to 3% of specimens. The frequency of apoplexy in patients with a known pituitary tumor was 17% in one series of 560 patients undergoing pituitary surgery; 8% had no clinical symptoms of hemorrhage.[824] Imaging studies of patients with a known pituitary tumor with CT and MRI scans indicate that intratumoral hemorrhage can occur without clinical evidence of apoplexy.[478] Of 12 patients with radiographically proven hemorrhage, only 3 had clinical evidence of apoplexy.[826]

Apoplexy may occur in a nontumorous pituitary gland in postpartum women who had excessive blood loss during delivery. After a period of complete ischemia, revascularization and vascular congestion with thrombosis of the anterior lobe are observed.[820] Spontaneous hemorrhage also occurs in pituitary tumors. Hemorrhage occurs in all types of pituitary tumors and may range from a catastrophic to an asymptomatic event.

The pattern of tumor growth, the size of the tumor, and the amount of hemorrhage and edema in the gland determine the symptoms. Infarction with hemorrhage and edema may cause rapid expansion of the lesion, compression of surrounding structures, and abnormal neurological function. In a conscious patient, the initial symptom is usually a severe retro-orbital headache, frequently accompanied by nausea and vomiting. Extravasation of blood or necrotic tissue into the subarachnoid space may cause meningeal irritation, fever, clouding of consciousness, or coma. Superior expansion produces compression of the optic chiasm and/or optic nerve(s) with visual field loss and/or decreased visual acuity. Lateral expansion into the cavernous sinus produces cranial nerve dysfunction that may involve cranial nerves III, IV, and VI and the first division of cranial nerve V. The most common abnormality is unilateral involvement of the third cranial nerve with ophthalmoplegia (impaired medial and downward gaze), diplopia, ptosis, and mydriasis. If expansion causes mechanical compression of the carotid siphon against the anterior clinoid process, hemispheric dysfunction, including seizures and hemiplegia, may result. Hemispheric dysfunction may also be due to vasospasm secondary to irritation by subarachnoid hemorrhage.

Clinical evaluation of the patient with a sudden change in sensorium, headache, ophthalmoplegia, visual loss, or prostration should include an immediate imaging study of the pituitary area and orbits, either a non–contrast-enhanced CT scan or an MRI scan. If a CT scan is performed, thin (1.5-mm) sections should be obtained through the pituitary in the coronal plane to identify the lesion; an unenhanced scan is necessary to identify hemorrhage, and contrast agent may be administered IV after initial images are obtained. Increased intensity, signifying hemorrhage, is also seen on a T1-weighted MRI scan. A CT scan may be superior for visualizing intratumoral hemorrhage within the first few days of the event, but the MRI scan is more sensitive in detecting and following the hemorrhage in the subacute stage.[826]

If pituitary apoplexy is suspected, the patient should be presumed to have anterior pituitary insufficiency and treated accordingly. Blood should be obtained for measurement of serum cortisol and T_4 levels, and glucocorticoid should be administered immediately. The glucocorticoid dose must be adequate for the stress of the illness and for presumptive cerebral edema (e.g., dexamethasone 2 mg every 6 h). Ophthalmological examination is performed to determine the nature and extent of deficits. If significant visual deficits or altered sensorium is present, emergent neurosurgical intervention is required. Immediate surgical decompression of the hemorrhage and tumor can result in recovery of visual deficits and alleviation of increased intracranial pressure. After recovery from surgery the patient should undergo a complete endocrinological evaluation to determine the nature and degree of hormone deficits. Because hormone deficits may be transient, function should also be re-evaluated several months after the event.[827, 828] Evidence for hormone hypersecretion should also be sought. Surgical decompression may not be necessary in the setting of normal sensorium and visual function. The patient should be hospitalized, treated with glucocorticoid replacement, and given serial ophthalmological and imaging examinations. Complete endocrine evaluation may be performed after recovery to assess the need for hormone replacement. With modern imaging techniques, objective assessment of the visual system, prompt hormone replacement, and surgical decompression as indicated, mortality caused by pituitary gland apoplexy is unusual.

REFERENCES

Pituitary Morphology

1. Asa SL, Kovacs K. Functional morphology of the human fetal pituitary. Pathol Annu 1984; 19(Pt 1):275–315.
2. Asa SL, Kovacs K, Laszlo FA, et al. Human fetal adenohypophysis. Histologic and immunocytochemical analysis. Neuroendocrinology 1986; 43:308–316.
3. Ikeda H, Suzuki J, Sasano N, et al. The development and morphogenesis of the human pituitary gland. Anat Embryol (Berl) 1988; 178:327–336.
4. Goodyer CG. Ontogeny of pituitary hormone secretion. In: Collu R, Ducharme JR, Guyda HJ, eds. Pediatric Endocrinology. New York: Raven, 1989: 125–169.
5. Boyd JD. Observations on human pharyngeal hypophysis. J Endocrinol 1956; 14:66–77.
6. McGrath P. Volume and histology of the human pharyngeal hypophysis. Aust NZ J Surg 1967; 37:16–27.
7. Frawley LS, Miller HA. Ontogeny of prolactin secretion in the neonatal rat is regulated posttranscriptionally. Endocrinology 1989; 124:3–6.
8. Lugo DI, Roberts JL, Pintar JE. Analysis of proopiomelanocortin gene expression during prenatal development of the rat pituitary gland. Mol Endocrinol 1989; 3:1313–1324.
9. Scheithauer BW, Sano T, Kovacs K, et al. The pituitary gland in pregnancy: a clinicopathologic and immunohistochemical study of 69 cases. Mayo Clin Proc 1990; 65:461–474.
10. Sheehan HL, Kovacs K. Neurohypophysis and hypothalamus. In: Bloodworth JMB Jr, ed. Endocrine Pathology. Baltimore: Williams & Wilkins, 1982: 45–99.
11. Burrow GN, Wortzman G, Rewcastle NB, et al. Microadenomas of the pituitary and abnormal sellar tomograms in an unselected autopsy series. N Engl J Med 1981; 304:156–158.
12. Scheithauer BW. The hypothalamus and neurohypophysis. In: Kovacs K, Asa SL, eds. Functional Endocrine Pathology. Vol 1. Boston: Blackwell Scientific, 1991: 170–244.
13. Stanfield JP. The blood supply of the human pituitary gland. J Anat 1960; 94:257–273.
14. Sheehan HL, Stanfield JP. The pathogenesis of post-partum necrosis of the anterior lobe of the pituitary gland. Acta Endocrinol 1961; 37:479–510.
15. Bergland RM, Page RB. Pituitary-brain vascular relations: a new paradigm. Science 1979; 204:18–24.
16. Gorczyca W, Hardy J. Arterial supply of the human anterior pituitary gland. Neurosurgery 1987; 20:369–378.
17. Elias KA, Weiner RI. Direct arterial vascularization of estrogen-induced prolactin-secreting anterior pituitary tumors. Proc Natl Acad Sci USA 1984; 81:4549–4553.
18. Schechter J, Goldsmith P, Wilson C, et al. Morphological evidence for the presence of arteries in human prolactinomas. J Clin Endocrinol Metab 1988; 67:713–719.
19. Racadot J, Gremain J, Kujas M, et al. Involvement of arterial vessels in the blood supply to adenomas of the human pituitary, functional implications. Bull Assoc Anat (Nancy) 1986; 70:5–12 (in French).
20. Horvath E, Kovacs K. Fine structural cytology of the adenohypophysis in rat and man. J Electron Microsc Tech 1988; 8:401–432.

Pituitary Hormones

Hypothalamic-Pituitary Regulation

21. Veldhuis JD, Johnson ML. Cluster analysis: a simple, versatile, and robust algorithm for endocrine pulse detection. Am J Physiol 1986; 250:E486–E493.
22. Van Cauter E. Estimating false-positive and false-negative errors in analyses of hormonal pulsatility. Am J Physiol 1988; 254:E786–E794.
23. Veldhuis JD, Carlson ML, Johnson ML. The pituitary gland secretes in bursts: appraising the nature of glandular secretory impulses by simultaneous multiple-parameter deconvolution of plasma hormone concentrations. Proc Natl Acad Sci USA 1987; 84:7686–7690.
24. Polonsky KS, Licinio Paixao J, Given BD, et al. Use of biosynthetic human C-peptide in the measurement of insulin secretion rates in normal volunteers and type I diabetic patients. J Clin Invest 1986; 77:98–105.
25. Polonsky KS, Given BD, Van Cauter E. Twenty-four-hour profiles and pulsatile patterns of insulin secretion in normal and obese subjects. J Clin Invest 1988; 81:442–448.
26. Hartman ML, Faria ACS, Vance ML, et al. Temporal structure of in vivo growth hormone secretory events in man. Am J Physiol 1991; 260:E101–E110.
27. Van Cauter E, Refetoff S. Evidence for two subtypes of Cushing's disease based on the analysis of episodic cortisol secretion. N Engl J Med 1985; 312:1343–1349.
28. Hartman ML, Veldhuis JD, Vance ML, et al. Somatotropin pulse frequency and basal concentrations are increased in acromegaly and are reduced by successful therapy. J Clin Endocrinol Metab 1990; 70:1375–1384.

Corticotropin

29. Jones MT, Gillham B. Factors involved in the regulation of adrenocorticotropic hormone/beta-lipotropic hormone. Physiol Rev 1988; 68:743–818.
30. Lundblad JR, Roberts JL. Regulation of proopiomelanocortin gene expression in pituitary. Endocr Rev 1988; 9:135–158.
31. Kovacs K, Horvath E, Stratmann IE, et al. Cytoplasmic microfilaments in the anterior lobe of the human pituitary gland. Acta Anat (Basel) 1974; 87:414–426.
32. Neumann PE, Horoupian DS, Goldman JE, et al. Cytoplasmic filaments of Crooke's hyaline change belong to the cytokeratin class. An immunocytochemical and ultrastructural study. Am J Pathol 1984; 116:214–222.

33. DeCherney GS, DeBold CR, Jackson RV, et al. Diurnal variation in the response of plasma adrenocorticotropin and cortisol to intravenous ovine corticotropin-releasing hormone. J Clin Endocrinol Metab 1985; 61:273–279.

34. DeBold CR, Jackson RV, Kamilaris TC, et al. Effects of ovine corticotropin-releasing hormone on adrenocorticotropin secretion in the absence of glucocorticoid feedback inhibition in man. J Clin Endocrinol Metab 1989; 68:431–437.

35. DeBold CR, Sheldon WR, DeCherney GS, et al. Arginine vasopressin potentiates adrenocorticotropin release induced by ovine corticotropin-releasing factor. J Clin Invest 1984; 73:533–538.

36. Moore-Ede MC, Czeisler CA, Richardson GS. Circadian timekeeping in health and disease. Part 1. Basic properties of circadian pacemakers. N Engl J Med 1983; 309:469–476.

37. Orth DN, Besser GM, King PH, et al. Free-running circadian plasma cortisol rhythm in a blind human subject. Clin Endocrinol 1979; 10:603–617.

38. Desir D, Van Cauter E, Fang VS, et al. Effects of "jet lag" on hormonal patterns. I. Procedures, variations in total plasma proteins, and disruption of adrenocorticotropin-cortisol periodicity. J Clin Endocrinol Metab 1981; 52:628–641.

39. Widmaier EP, Plotsky PM, Sutton SW, et al. Regulation of corticotropin-releasing factor secretion in vitro by glucose. Am J Physiol 1988; 255:E287–E292.

40. Bateman A, Singh A, Kral T, et al. The immune-hypothalamic-pituitary-adrenal axis. Endocr Rev 1989; 10:92–112.

41. Simpson ER, Waterman MR. Regulation of the synthesis of steroidogenic enzymes in adrenal cortical cells by ACTH. Annu Rev Physiol 1988; 50:427–440.

Prolactin–Growth Hormone Family

42. Niall HD, Hogan ML, Sauer R, et al. Sequences of pituitary and placental lactogenic and growth hormones: evolution from a primordial peptide by gene reduplication. Proc Natl Acad Sci USA 1971; 68:866–870.

43. Cooke NE, Coit D, Weiner RI, et al. Structure of cloned DNA complementary to rat prolactin messenger RNA. J Biol Chem 1980; 255:6502–6510.

44. Cooke NE, Baxter JD. Structural analysis of the prolactin gene suggests a separate origin for its 5' end. Nature 1982; 297:603–606.

45. Cooke NE, Coit D, Shine J, et al. Human prolactin. cDNA structural analysis and evolutionary comparisons. J Biol Chem 1981; 256:4007–4016.

46. Truong AT, Duez C, Belayew A, et al. Isolation and characterization of the human prolactin gene. EMBO J 1984; 3:429–437.

47. Owerbach D, Rutter WJ, Cooke NE, et al. The prolactin gene is located on chromosome 6 in humans. Science 1981; 212:815–816.

48. Owerbach D, Rutter WJ, Martial JA, et al. Genes for growth hormone, chorionic somatomammotropin, and growth hormone-like gene on chromosome 17 in humans. Science 1980; 209:289–292.

49. Cooke NE. Prolactin: normal synthesis, regulation, and actions. In: DeGroot LJ, Besser GM, Cahill GF Jr, et al. eds. Endocrinology. 2nd ed. Philadelphia: W. B. Saunders, 1989: 384–407.

50. Barsh GS, Seeburg PH, Gelinas RE. The human growth hormone gene family: structure and evolution of the chromosomal locus. Nucleic Acids Res 1983; 11:3939–3958.

51. Stricker S, Grueter F. Action du lobe antérieur de l'hypophyse sur la montée laiteuse. C R Soc Biol (Paris) 1928; 99:1978–1980.

52. Riddle O, Braucher PF. Studies on the physiology of reproduction in birds. XXX. Control of the special secretion of the crop-gland in pigeons by anterior pituitary hormones. Am J Physiol 1931; 97:617–625.

53. Riddle O, Bates RW, Dykshorn SW. The preparation, identification and assay of prolactin—a hormone of the anterior pituitary. Am J Physiol 1933; 105:191–216.

54. Riddle O, Bates RW, Dykshorn SW. A new hormone of the anterior pituitary. Proc Soc Exp Biol Med 1932; 29:1211–1215.

55. Lewis UJ, Singh RN, Seavey BK. Human prolactin: isolation and some properties. Biochem Biophys Res Commun 1971; 44:1169–1176.

56. Hwang P, Guyda H, Friesen H. Purification of human prolactin. J Biol Chem 1972; 247:1955–1958.

57. Sinha YN, Gilligan TA, Lee DW. Detection of a high molecular weight variant of prolactin in human plasma by a combination of electrophoretic and immunologic techniques. J Clin Endocrinol Metab 1984; 58:752–754.

58. Suh HK, Frantz AG. Size heterogeneity of human prolactin in plasma and pituitary extracts. J Clin Endocrinol Metab 1974; 39:928–935.

59. Farkouh NH, Packer MG, Frantz AG. Large molecular size prolactin with reduced receptor activity in human serum: high proportion in basal state and reduction after thyrotropin-releasing hormone. J Clin Endocrinol Metab 1979; 48:1026–1032.

60. Benveniste R, Helman JD, Orth DN, et al. Circulating big human prolactin: conversion to small human prolactin by reduction of disulfide bonds. J Clin Endocrinol Metab 1979; 48:883–886.

61. Whittaker PG, Wilcox T, Lind T. Maintained fertility in a patient with hyperprolactinemia due to big, big prolactin. J Clin Endocrinol Metab 1981; 53:863–866.

62. Soong YK, Ferguson KM, McGarrick G, et al. Size heterogeneity of immunoreactive prolactin in hyperprolactinaemic serum. Clin Endocrinol 1982; 16:259–265.

63. Lewis UJ, Singh RN, Sinha YN, et al. Glycosylated human prolactin. Endocrinology 1985; 116:359–363.

64. Andersen AN, Pedersen H, Djursing H, et al. Bioactivity of prolactin in a woman with an excess of large molecular size prolactin, persistent hyperprolactinemia and spontaneous conception. Fertil Steril 1982; 38:625–628.

65. Sinha YN, Gilligan TA, Lee DW, et al. Cleaved prolactin: evidence for its occurrence in human pituitary gland and plasma. J Clin Endocrinol Metab 1985; 60:239–243.

66. Mittra I. A novel "cleaved prolactin" in the rat pituitary: Part II. In vivo mammary mitogenic activity of its N-terminal 16K moiety. Bichem Biophys Res Commun 1980; 95:1760–1767.

67. Asa SL, Penz G, Kovacs K, et al. Prolactin cells in the human pituitary. A quantitative immunocytochemical analysis. Arch Pathol Lab Med 1982; 106:360–363.

68. Lam KS, Lechan RM, Minamitani N, et al. Vasoactive intestinal peptide in the anterior pituitary is increased in hypothyroidism. Endocrinology 1989; 124:1077–1084.

69. Nagy G, Mulchahey JJ, Neill JD. Autocrine control of prolactin secretion by vasoactive intestinal peptide. Endocrinology 1988; 122:364–366.

70. Hagen TC, Arnaout MA, Scherzer WJ, et al. Antisera to vasoactive intestinal polypeptide inhibit basal prolactin release from dispersed anterior pituitary cells. Neuroendocrinology 1986; 43:641–645.

71. Nokin J, Vekemans M, L'Hermite M, et al. Circadian periodicity of serum prolactin concentration in man. Br Med J 1972; 3:561–562.

72. Parker DC, Rossman LG, Vander L. Sleep-related, nychthermeral and briefly episodic variation in human plasma prolactin concentrations. J Clin Endocrinol Metab 1973; 36:1119–1124.

73. Sassin JF, Frantz AG, Weitzman ED, et al. Human prolactin: 24-hour pattern with increased release during sleep. Science 1972; 177:1205–1207.

74. Sassin JF, Frantz AG, Kapen S, et al. The nocturnal rise of human prolactin is dependent on sleep. J Clin Endocrinol Metab 1973; 37:436–440.

75. Parker DC, Rossman LG, Vanderlaan EF. Relation of sleep-entrained human prolactin release to REM-nonREM cycles. J Clin Endocrinol Metab 1974; 38:646–651.

76. Van Cauter E, L'Hermite M, Copinschi G, et al. Quantitative analysis of spontaneous variations of plasma prolactin in normal man. Am J Physiol 1981; 241:E355–E363.

77. Desire D, Van Cauter E, L'Hermite M, et al. Effects of "jet lag" on hormonal patterns. III. Demonstration of an intrinsic circadian rhythmicity in plasma prolactin. J Clin Endocrinol Metab 1982; 55:849–857.

78. Veldhuis JD, Johnson ML. Operating characteristics of the hypothalamo-pituitary-gonadal axis in men: circadian, ultradian, and pulsatile release of prolactin and its temporal coupling with luteinizing hormone. J Clin Endocrinol Metab 1988; 67:116–123.

79. Thorner MO, Round J, Jones A, et al. Serum prolactin and oestradiol levels at different stages of puberty. Clin Endocrinol 1977; 7:463–468.

80. Friesen HG. Human prolactin. Ann R Coll Physicians Surg Can 1978; 11:275–281.

81. Gluckman PD, Grumbach MM, Kaplan SL. The neuroendocrine regulation and function of growth hormone and prolactin in the mammalian fetus. Endocr Rev 1981; 2:363–395.

82. Suganuma N, Seo H, Yamamoto N, et al. Ontogenesis of pituitary prolactin in the human fetus. J Clin Endocrinol Metab 1986; 63:156–161.

83. Tyson JE, Hwang P, Guyda H, et al. Studies of prolactin secretion in human pregnancy. Am J Obstet Gynecol 1972; 113:14–20.

84. Maslar IA, Riddick DH. Prolactin production by human endometrium during the normal menstrual cycle. Am J Obstet Gynecol 1979; 135:751–754.

85. Riddick DH, Daly DC. Decidual prolactin production in human gestation. Semin Perinatol 1982; 6:229–237.

86. Clements J, Whitfeld P, Cooke N, et al. Expression of the prolactin gene in human decidua-chorion. Endocrinology 1983; 112:1133–1134.

87. Takahashi H, Nabeshima Y, Ogata K, et al. Molecular cloning and nucleotide sequence of DNA complementary to human decidual prolactin mRNA. J Biochem (Tokyo) 1984; 95:1491–1499.

88. Goodwin RG, Friend D, Ziegler SF, et al. Cloning of the human and murine interleukin-7 receptors: demonstration of a soluble form and homology to a new receptor superfamily. Cell 1990; 60:941–951.

89. Cooke NE, Ray J, Watson MA, et al. Human growth hormone gene and the highly homologous growth hormone variant gene display different splicing patterns. J Clin Invest 1988; 82:270–275.

90. DeNoto FM, Moore DD, Goodman HM. Human growth hormone DNA sequence and mRNA structure: possible alternative splicing. Nucleic Acids Res 1981; 9:3719–3730.

91. Baumann G. Molecular variants of human growth hormone in serum and circulating growth hormone binding proteins. In: Frisch H, Thomer MO, eds. Hormonal Regulation of Growth. Serono Symposia Publications. Vol 58. New York: Raven, 1989: 175–184.

92. Frankenne F, Rentier Delrue F, Scippo ML, et al. Expression of the

growth hormone variant gene in human placenta. J Clin Endocrinol Metab 1987; 64:635–637.

93. Frankenne F, Closset J, Gomez F, et al. The physiology of growth hormones (GHs) in pregnant women and partial characterization of the placental GH variant. J Clin Endocrinol Metab 1988; 66:1171–1180.

94. Isgaard J, Nilsson A, Lindahl A, et al. Effects of local administration of GH and IGF-1 on longitudinal bone growth in rats. Am J Physiol 1986; 250:E367–E372.

95. Igout A, Scippo ML, Frankenne F, et al. hGH V gene: specific placental expression, isolation and structure of the related cDNA. Endocr Soc Abstr 1988; 303.

96. Pelletier G, Robert F, Hardy J. Identification of human anterior pituitary cells by immunoelectron microscopy. J Clin Endocrinol Metab 1978; 46:534–542.

97. Thorner MO, Perryman RL, Cronin MJ, et al. Somatotroph hyperplasia. Successful treatment of acromegaly by removal of a pancreatic islet tumor secreting a growth hormone–releasing factor. J Clin Invest 1982; 70:965–977.

98. Stolar MW, Baumann G. Big growth hormone forms in human plasma: immunochemical evidence for their pituitary origin. Metabolism 1986; 35:75–77.

99. Baumann G, Vance ML, Shaw MA, et al. Plasma transport of human growth hormone in vivo. J Clin Endocrinol Metab 1990; 71:470–473.

100. Stolar MW, Baumann G, Vance ML, et al. Circulating growth hormone forms after stimulation of pituitary secretion with growth hormone–releasing factor in man. J Clin Endocrinol Metab 1984; 59:235–239.

101. Baumann G, Stolar MW. Molecular forms of human growth hormone secreted in vivo: nonspecificity of secretory stimuli. J Clin Endocrinol Metab 1986; 62:789–790.

102. Baumann G, Winter RJ, Shaw M. Circulating molecular variants of growth hormone in childhood. Pediatr Res 1987; 22:21–22.

103. Baumann G, Shaw MA, Merimee TJ. Decreased growth hormone–binding protein in pygmy plasma. Clin Res 1988; 36:551A (abstract).

104. Leung DW, Spencer SA, Cachianes G, et al. Growth hormone receptor and serum binding protein: purification, cloning and expression. Nature 1987; 330:537–543.

105. Spencer SA, Hammonds RG, Henzel WJ, et al. Rabbit liver growth hormone receptor and serum binding protein. Purification, characterization, and sequence. J Biol Chem 1988; 263:7862–7867.

106. Boutin JM, Jolicoeur C, Okamura H, et al. Cloning and expression of the rat prolactin receptor, a member of the growth hormone/prolactin receptor gene family. Cell 1988; 53:69–77.

107. Bass S, Wells J. Growth hormone-receptor gene in Laron dwarfism. N Engl J Med 1990; 332:854–855.

108. Baumann G, Shaw MA, Winter RJ. Absence of the plasma growth hormone–binding protein in Laron-type dwarfism. J Clin Endocrinol Metab 1987; 65:814–816.

109. Daughaday WH, Trivedi B. Absence of serum growth hormone binding protein in patients with growth hormone receptor deficiency (Laron dwarfism). Proc Natl Acad Sci USA 1987; 84:4636–4640.

110. Baumann G, Amburn KD, Buchanan TA. The effect of circulating growth hormone–binding protein on metabolic clearance, distribution, and degradation of human growth hormone. J Clin Endocrinol Metab 1987; 64:657–660.

111. Baumann G, Shaw MA, Buchanan TA. In vivo kinetics of a covalent growth hormone–binding protein complex. Metabolism 1989; 38:330–333.

112. Herington AC, Ymer S, Stevenson J. Identification and characterization of specific binding proteins for growth hormone in normal human sera. J Clin Invest 1986; 77:1817–1823.

113. Daughaday WH, Trivedi B, Andrews BA. The ontogeny of serum GH binding protein in man: a possible indicator of hepatic GH receptor development. J Clin Endocrinol Metab 1987; 65:1072–1074.

114. Barinaga M, Yamonoto G, Rivier C, et al. Transcriptional regulation of growth hormone gene expression by growth hormone–releasing factor. Nature 1983; 306:84–85.

115. Holl RW, Thorner MO, Mandell GL, et al. Spontaneous oscillations of intracellular calcium and growth hormone secretion. J Biol Chem 1988; 263:9682–9685.

116. Holl RW, Thorner MO, Leong DA. Intracellular calcium concentration and growth hormone secretion in individual somatotropes: effects of growth hormone–releasing factor and somatostatin. Endocrinology 1988; 122:2927–2932.

117. Dorflinger LJ, Schonbrunn A. Somatostatin inhibits vasoactive intestinal peptide–stimulated cyclic adenosine monophosphate accumulation in GH pituitary cells. Endocrinology 1983; 113:1541–1550.

118. Koch BD, Blalock JB, Schonbrunn A. Characterization of the cyclic AMP–independent actions of somatostatin in GH cells. I. An increase in potassium conductance is responsible for both the hyperpolarization and the decrease in intracellular free calcium produced by somatostatin. J Biol Chem 1988; 263:216–225.

119. Cronin MJ, Rogol AD, Dabney LG, et al. Selective growth hormone and cyclic AMP stimulating activity is present in human pancreatic islet cell tumor. J Clin Endocrinol Metab 1982; 55:381–383.

120. Cronin MJ, Hewlett EL, Evans WS, et al. Human pancreatic tumor growth hormone (GH)–releasing factor and cyclic adenosine 3',5'-

monophosphate evoke GH release from anterior pituitary cells: the effects of pertussis toxin, cholera toxin, forskolin, and cycloheximide. Endocrinology 1984; 114:904–913.

121. Schettini G, Cronin MJ, Hewlett EL, et al. Human pancreatic tumor growth hormone–releasing factor stimulates anterior pituitary adenylate cyclase activity, adenosine 3',5'-monophosphate accumulation, and growth hormone release in a calmodulin-dependent manner. Endocrinology 1984; 115:1308–1314.

122. Holl RW, Thorner MO, Leong DA. Cytosolic free calcium in normal somatotropes: effects of forskolin and phorbol ester. Am J Physiol 1989; 256:E375–E379.

123. Ho KY, Evans WS, Blizzard RM, et al. Effects of sex and age on the 24-hour profile of growth hormone secretion in man: importance of endogenous estradiol concentrations. J Clin Endocrinol Metab 1987; 64:51–58.

124. Hendricks CM, Eastman RC, Takeda S, et al. Plasma clearance of intravenously administered pituitary human growth hormone: gel filtration studies of heterogeneous components. J Clin Endocrinol Metab 1985; 60:864–867.

125. Hindmarsh PC, Matthews DR, Brain CE, et al. The half-life of exogenous growth hormone after suppression of endogenous growth hormone secretion with somatostatin. Clin Endocrinol 1989; 30:443–450.

126. Owens D, Srivastava MC, Tompkins CV, et al. Studies on the metabolic clearance rate, apparent distribution space and plasma half-disappearance time of unlabelled human growth hormone in normal subjects and in patients with liver disease, renal disease, thyroid disease and diabetes mellitus. Eur J Clin Invest 1973; 3:284–294.

127. Parker ML, Utiger RD, Daughaday WH. Studies on human growth hormone. II. The physiological disposition and metabolic rate of human growth hormone in man. J Clin Invest 1962; 41:262–268.

128. Faria AC, Veldhuis JD, Thorner MO, et al. Half-time of endogenous growth hormone (GH) disappearance in normal man after stimulation of GH secretion by GH-releasing hormone and suppression with somatostatin. J Clin Endocrinol Metab 1989; 68:535–541.

129. MacGillivray MH, Frohman LA, Doe J. Metabolic clearance and production rates of human growth hormone in subjects with normal and abnormal growth. J Clin Endocrinol Metab 1970; 30:632–638.

130. Thompson RG, Rodriguez A, Kowarski A, et al. Growth hormone: metabolic clearance rates, integrated concentrations, and production rates in normal adults and the effect of prednisone. J Clin Invest 1972; 51:3193–3199.

131. Martha PM Jr, Rogol AD, Veldhuis JD, et al. Alterations in the pulsatile properties of circulating growth hormone concentrations during puberty in boys. J Clin Endocrinol Metab 1989; 69:563–570.

132. Zeitler P, Argente J, Chowen-Breede JA, et al. Growth hormone releasing hormone messenger ribonucleic acid in the hypothalamus of the adult male rat is increased by testosterone. Endocrinology 1990; 127:362–368.

133. Werner H, Koch Y, Baldino F, et al. Steroid regulation of somatostatin mRNA in the rat hypothalamus. J Biol Chem 1988; 263:7666–7671.

134. Van Cauter E, Kerkhofs M, Van Onderbergen A, et al. Modulation of spontaneous and GHRH-stimulated GH secretion by sleep. Endocr Soc Abstr 1989; 220.

135. Fiddes JC, Goodman HM. The gene encoding the common alpha subunit of the four human glycoprotein hormones. J Mol Appl Gene 1981; 1:3–18.

136. Veldhuis JD, Iranmanesh A, Ho KK, et al. Dual defects in pulsatile growth hormone secretion and clearance subserve the hyposomatotropism of obesity in man. J Clin Endocrinol Metab 1991; 72:51–59.

137. Jansson JO, Isaksson OG, Eden S, et al. Effects of plasma GH pattern on growth factors and body growth. In: Frisch H, Thorner MO, eds. Hormonal Regulation of Growth. Serono Symposia Publications. Vol 58. New York: Raven, 1989: 185–199.

138. Stewart PM, Smith S, Seth J, et al. Normal growth hormone response to the 75 g oral glucose tolerance test measured by immunoradiometric assay. Ann Clin Biochem 1989; 26:205–206.

139. Asplin CM, Faria AC, Carlsen EC, et al. Alterations in the pulsatile mode of growth hormone release in men and women with insulin-dependent diabetes mellitus. J Clin Endocrinol Metab 1989; 69:239–245.

140. Silver HK, Finkelstein M. Deprivation dwarfism. J Pediatr 1967; 70:317–324.

141. Powell GF, Brasel JA, Blizzard RM. Emotional deprivation and growth retardation stimulating idiopathic hypopituitarism. I. Clinical evaluation of the syndrome. N Engl J Med 1967; 276:1271–1278.

142. Delitala G. Clinical neuropharmacology in the management of disorders of the pituitary and hypothalamus. In: DeGroot LJ, Besser GM, Cahill GF Jr, eds. Endocrinology. 2nd ed. Philadelphia: W. B. Saunders, 1989: 454–473.

143. Soulairac A, Schaub C, Franchimont P, et al. A study of the pharmacological activation of the central pole of the hypothalamo-hypophyseal axis. Ann Endocrinol (Paris) 1968; 29:45–54.

144. Salvadorini F, Galeone F, Nicotere M. Clinical evaluation of CDP-choline: efficacy as antidepressant treatment. Curr Ther Res Clin Exp 1968; 18:513–520.

145. Mendelson WB, Sitaram N, Wyatt RJ, et al. Methoscopolamine inhibition

of sleep-related growth hormone secretion. Evidence for a cholinergic secretory mechanism. J Clin Invest 1978; 61:1683–1690.

146. Delitala G, Frulio T, Pacifico A, et al. Participation of cholinergic muscarinic receptors in glucagon- and arginine-mediated growth hormone secretion in man. J Clin Endocrinol Metab 1982; 55:1231–1233.

147. Delitala G, Grossman A, Besser GM. Opiate peptides control growth hormone through a cholinergic mechanism in man. Clin Endocrinol 1983; 18:401–405.

148. Delitala G, Maioli M, Pacifico A, et al. Cholinergic receptor control mechanisms for L-dopa, apomorphine, and clonidine-induced growth hormone secretion in man. J Clin Endocrinol Metab 1983; 57:1145–1149.

149. Stubbs WA, Delitala G, Jones A, et al. Hormonal and metabolic responses to an enkephalin analogue in normal man. Lancet 1978; 2:1225–1227.

150. Bowers CY, Reynolds GA, Durham D, et al. Growth hormone (GH)–releasing peptide stimulates GH release in normal men and acts synergistically with GH-releasing hormone. J Clin Endocrinol Metab 1990; 70:975–982.

151. Salmon WD Jr, Daughaday WH. A hormonally controlled serum factor which stimulates sulfate incorporation by cartilage in vitro. J Lab Clin Med 1957; 49:825.

152. Daughaday WH, Reeder C. Synchronous activation of DNA synthesis in hypophysectomized rat cartilage by growth hormone. J Lab Clin Med 1966; 68:357–368.

153. Abe H, Molitch ME, Van W, et al. Human growth hormone and somatomedin C suppress the spontaneous release of growth hormone in unanesthetized rats. Endocrinology 1983; 113:1319–1324.

154. Berelowitz M, Szabo M, Frohman LA, et al. Somatomedin-C mediates growth hormone negative feedback by effects on both the hypothalamus and the pituitary. Science 1981; 212:1279–1281.

155. Brazeau P, Guillemin R, Ling N, et al. Inhibition par les somatomédines de la sécrétion de l'hormone de croissance stimulée par le facteur hypothalamique somatocrinine (GRF) ou le peptide de synthèse hpGRF. C R Seances Acad Sci [III] 1982; 295:651–654.

156. Melmed S, Yamashita S. Insulin-like growth factor-I action on hypothyroid rat pituitary cells: suppression of triiodothyronine-induced growth hormone secretion and messenger ribonucleic acid levels. Endocrinology 1986; 118:1483–1490.

157. Green H, Morikawa M, Nixon T. A dual effector theory of growth-hormone action. Differentiation 1985; 29:195–198.

158. Isaksson OG, Jansson JO, Gause IA. Growth hormone stimulates longitudinal bone growth directly. Science 1982; 216:1237–1239.

159. Russell SM, Spencer EM. Local injections of human or rat growth hormone or of purified human somatomedin-C stimulate unilateral tibial epiphyseal growth in hypophysectomized rats. Endocrinology 1985; 116:2563–2567.

160. Schlechter NL, Russell SM, Spencer EM, et al. Evidence suggesting that the direct growth-promoting effect of growth hormone on cartilage in vivo is mediated by local production of somatomedin. Proc Natl Acad Sci USA 1986; 83:7932–7934.

161. Nilsson A, Isgaard J, Lindahl A, et al. Regulation by growth hormone of number of chondrocytes containing IGF-I in rat growth plate. Science 1986; 233:571–574.

162. D'Ercole AJ, Stiles AD, Underwood LE. Tissue concentrations of somatomedin C: further evidence for multiple sites of synthesis and paracrine or autocrine mechanisms of action. Proc Natl Acad Sci USA 1984; 81:935–939.

163. Isaksson OG, Eden S, Jansson JO. Mode of action of pituitary growth hormone on target cells. Annu Rev Physiol 1985; 47:483–499.

164. Isaksson OG, Lindahl A, Nilsson A, et al. Mechanism of the stimulatory effect of growth hormone on longitudinal bone growth. Endocr Rev 1987; 8:426–438.

165. Skottner A, Clark RG, Robinson IC, et al. Recombinant human insulin–like growth factor: testing the somatomedin hypothesis in hypophysectomized rats. J Endocrinol 1987; 112:123–132.

166. Guler HP, Zapf J, Scheiwiller E, et al. Recombinant human insulin–like growth factor I stimulates growth and has distinct effects on organ size in hypophysectomized rats. Proc Natl Acad Sci USA 1988; 85:4889–4893.

167. Bauman DE, Eisemann JH, Currie WB. Hormonal effects on partitioning of nutrients for tissue growth: role of growth hormone and prolactin. Fed Proc 1982; 41:2538–2544.

168. Muir LA, Wien S, Duquette PF, et al. Effects of exogenous growth hormone and diethylstilbestrol on growth and carcass composition of growing lambs. J Anim Sci 1983; 56:1315–1323.

169. Evock CM, Etherton TD, Chung CS, et al. Pituitary porcine growth hormone (pGH) and a recombinant pGH analog stimulate pig growth performance in a similar manner. J Anim Sci 1988; 66:1928–1941.

170. Etherton TD, Wiggins JP, Evock CM, et al. Stimulation of pig growth performance by porcine growth hormone: determination of the dose-response relationship. J Anim Sci 1987; 64:433–443.

171. Gerich JE, Lorenzi M, Bier DM, et al. Effects of physiologic levels of glucagon and growth hormone on human carbohydrate and lipid metabolism. Studies involving administration of exogenous hormone during suppression of endogenous hormone secretion with somatostatin. J Clin Invest 1976; 57:875–884.

172. Metcalfe P, Johnston DG, Nosadini R, et al. Metabolic effects of acute and prolonged growth hormone excess in normal and insulin-deficient man. Diabetologia 1981; 20:123–128.

173. Sherwin RS, Schulman GA, Hendler R, et al. Effect of growth hormone on oral glucose tolerance and circulating metabolic fuels in man. Diabetologia 1983; 24:155–161.

174. Rosenfeld RG, Wilson DM, Dollar LA, et al. Both human pituitary growth hormone and recombinant DNA–derived human growth hormone cause insulin resistance at a postreceptor site. J Clin Endocrinol Metab 1982; 54:1033–1038.

175. Bratusch-Marrain PR, Smith D, DeFronzo RA. The effect of growth hormone on glucose metabolism and insulin secretion in man. J Clin Endocrinol Metab 1982; 55:973–982.

176. Orskov L, Schmitz O, Jorgensen JO, et al. Influence of growth hormone on glucose-induced glucose uptake in normal men as assessed by the hyperglycemic clamp technique. J Clin Endocrinol Metab 1989; 68:276–282.

177. Frohman LA. Diseases of the anterior pituitary. In: Felig P, Baxter JD, Broadus AE, et al., eds. Endocrinology and Metabolism. New York: McGraw-Hill, 1981: 151–231.

178. Manson JM, Wilmore DW. Positive nitrogen balance with human growth hormone and hypocaloric intravenous feeding. Surgery 1986; 100:188–197.

179. Clemmons DR, Snyder DK, Williams R, et al. Growth hormone administration conserves lean body mass during dietary restriction in obese subjects. J Clin Endocrinol Metab 1987; 64:878–883.

180. Binnerts A, Wilson JH, Lamberts SW. The effects of human growth hormone administration in elderly adults with recent weight loss. J Clin Endocrinol Metab 1988; 67:1312–1316.

181. Snyder DK, Clemmons DR, Underwood LE. Treatment of obese, diet-restricted subjects with growth hormone for 11 weeks: effects on anabolism, lipolysis, and body composition. J Clin Endocrinol Metab 1988; 67:54–61.

182. Carlson HE, Gillin JC, Gorden P, et al. Absence of sleep-related growth hormone peaks in aged normal subjects and in acromegaly. J Clin Endocrinol Metab 1972; 34:1102–1105.

183. Finkelstein JW, Boyar RM, Roffwarg HP, et al. Age-related change in the twenty-four-hour spontaneous secretion of growth hormone. J Clin Endocrinol Metab 1972; 35:665–670.

184. Dudl RJ, Ensinck JW, Palmer HE, et al. Effect of age on growth hormone secretion in man. J Clin Endocrinol Metab 1973; 37:11–16.

185. Rudman D, Kutner MH, Rogers CM, et al. Impaired growth hormone secretion in the adult population: relation to age and adiposity. J Clin Invest 1981; 67:1361–1369.

186. Young VR, Uauy R, Winterer JC. Protein metabolism and needs in elderly people. In: Rockstein M, Sussman ML, eds. Nutrition, Longevity and Aging. New York: Academic, 1976: 67–102.

187. Forbes GB, Reina JC. Adult lean body mass declines with age: some longitudinal observations. Metabolism 1970; 19:653–663.

188. Rudman D, Feller AG, Nagraj HS, et al. Effects of human growth hormone in men over 60 years old. N Engl J Med 1990; 323:1–6.

189. Salomon F, Cuneo RC, Hesp R, et al. The effects of treatment with recombinant human growth hormone on body composition and metabolism in adults with growth hormone deficiency. N Engl J Med 1989; 321:1797–1803.

190. Ward HC, Halliday D, Sim AJ. Protein and energy metabolism with biosynthetic human growth hormone after gastrointestinal surgery. Ann Surg 1987; 206:56–61.

191. Soroff HS, Pearson E, Green NL, et al. The effect of growth hormone on nitrogen balance at various levels of intake in burned patients. Surg Gynecol Obstet 1960; 111:259–273.

192. Liljedahl SO, Gemzell CA, Plantin LO, et al. Effect of human growth hormone in patients with severe burns. Acta Chir Scand 1961; 122:1–14.

193. Soroff HS, Rozin RR, Mooty J, et al. Role of human growth hormone in the response to trauma. I. Metabolic effects following burns. Ann Surg 1967; 166:739–752.

194. Wilmore DW, Moylan JA Jr, Bristow BF, et al. Anabolic effects of human growth hormone and high caloric feedings following thermal injury. Surg Gynecol Obstet 1974; 138:875–884.

195. Horber FF, Haymond MV. Human growth hormone prevents the protein catabolic side effects of prednisone in humans. J Clin Invest 1990; 86:265–272.

Glycoprotein Hormone Family

196. Shupnik MA, Ridgway EC, Chin WW. Molecular biology of thyrotropin. Endocr Rev 1989; 10:459–475.

197. Gharib SD, Wierman ME, Shupnik MA, et al. Molecular biology of the pituitary gonadotropins. Endocr Rev 1990; 11:177–199.

198. Pierce JG, Parsons TF. Glycoprotein hormones: structure and function. Annu Rev Biochem 1981; 50:465–495.

199. Vamvakopoulos NC, Kourides IA. Identification of separate mRNAs coding for the alpha and beta subunits of thyrotropin. Proc Natl Acad Sci USA 1979; 76:3809–3813.

200. Giudice LC, Weintraub BD. Evidence for conformational differences

between precursor and processed forms of thyroid-stimulating hormone beta subunit. J Biol Chem 1979; 254:12679–12683.

201. Godine JE, Chin WW, Habener JF. Luteinizing and follicle-stimulating hormones. Cell-free translations of messenger RNAs coding for subunit precursors. J Biol Chem 1980; 255:8780–8783.

202. Blackman MR, Gershengorn MC, Weintraub BD. Excess production of free alpha subunits by mouse pituitary thyrotropic tumor cells in vitro. Endocrinology 1978; 102:499–508.

203. Kourides IA, Landon MB, Hoffman BJ, et al. Excess free alpha relative to beta subunits of the glycoprotein hormones in normal and abnormal human pituitary glands. Clin Endocrinol 1980; 12:407–416.

204. Ross DS, Downing MF, Chin WW, et al. Changes in tissue concentrations of thyrotropin, free thyrotropin beta, and alpha-subunits after thyroxine administration: comparison of mouse hypophyroid pituitary and thyrotropic tumors. Endocrinology 1983; 112:2050–2053.

205. Weintraub BD, Stannard BS, Magner JA, et al. Glycosylation and posttranslational processing of thyroid-stimulating hormone: clinical implications. Recent Prog Horm Res 1985; 41:577–606.

206. Fiddes JC, Talmadge K. Structure, expression, and evolution of the genes for the human glycoprotein hormones. Recent Prog Horm Res 1984; 40:43–78.

207. Chin WW, Kronenberg HM, Dee PC, et al. Nucleotide sequence of the mRNA encoding the pre-alpha-subunit of mouse thyrotropin. Proc Natl Acad Sci USA 1981; 78:5329–5333.

208. Schorr Toshav NL, Gurr JA, Catterall JF, et al. Thyrotropin and alpha-subunit in the brain: evidence for biosynthesis within the pituitary. Endocrinology 1983; 112:1434–1440.

209. Godine JE, Chin WW, Habener JF. α subunit of rat pituitary glycoprotein hormones. Primary structure of the precursor determined from the nucleotide sequence of cloned cDNAs. J Biol Chem 1982; 257:8368–8371.

210. Croyle ML, Maurer RA. Thyroid hormone decreases thyrotropin subunit mRNA levels in rat anterior pituitary. DNA 1984; 3:231–236.

211. Nilson JH, Thomason AR, Cserbak MT, et al. Nucleotide sequence of a cDNA for the common alpha subunit of the bovine pituitary glycoprotein hormones. Conservation of nucleotides in the 3′-untranslated region of bovine and human pre-alpha subunit mRNAs. J Biol Chem 1983; 258:4679–4682.

212. Erwin CR, Croyle ML, Donelson JE, et al. Nucleotide sequence of cloned complementary deoxyribonucleic acid for the alpha subunit of bovine pituitary glycoprotein hormones. Biochemistry 1983; 22:4856–4860.

213. Fiddes JC, Goodman HM. Isolation, cloning and sequence analysis of the cDNA for the alpha-subunit of human chorionic gonadotropin. Nature 1979; 281:351–356.

214. Dracopoli NC, Rettig WJ, Whitfield GK, et al. Assignment of the gene for the beta subunit of thyroid-stimulating hormone to the short arm of human chromosome 1. Proc Natl Acad Sci USA 1986; 83:1822–1826.

215. Wondisford FE, Radovick S, Moates JM, et al. Isolation and characterization of the human thyrotropin beta-subunit gene. Differences in gene structure and promoter function from murine species. J Biol Chem 1988; 263:12538–12542.

216. Gurr JA, Catterall JF, Kourides IA. Cloning of cDNA encoding the pre-beta subunit of mouse thyrotropin. Proc Natl Acad Sci USA 1983; 80:2122–2126.

217. Chin WW, Shupnik MA, Ross DS, et al. Regulation of the alpha and thyrotropin beta-subunit messenger ribonucleic acids by thyroid hormones. Endocrinology 1985; 116:873–878.

218. Chin WW, Muccini JA Jr, Shin L. Evidence for a single rat thyrotropin-beta-subunit gene: thyroidectomy increases its mRNA. Biochem Biophys Res Commun 1985; 128:1152–1158.

219. Maurer RA, Croyle ML, Donelson JE. The sequence of a cloned cDNA for the beta subunit of bovine thyrotropin predicts a protein containing both NH₂- and COOH-terminal extensions. J Biol Chem 1984; 259:5024–5027.

220. Hayashizaki Y, Miyai K, Kato K, et al. Molecular cloning of the human thyrotropin-beta subunit gene. FEBS Lett 1985; 188:394–400.

221. Whitfiled GK, Powers RE, Gurr JA, et al. Isolation of a gene encoding human thyrotropin beta subunit. In: Medeiros-Neto G, Gaitan E, eds. Frontiers in Thyroidology. New York: Plenum, 1986: 173–176.

222. Samuels MH, Wood WM, Gordon DF, et al. Clinical and molecular studies of a thyrotropin-secreting pituitary adenoma. J Clin Endocrinol Metab 1989; 68:1211–1215.

223. Miyai K, Hayashizaki Y, Matsubara K. Familial hypothyroidism due to thyrotropin gene abnormality. Int Congr Endocrinol (Jpn) 1988; 1:545–550.

224. Hayashizaki Y, Hiroaka Y, Endo Y, et al. Thyroid-stimulating hormone (TSH) deficiency caused by a single base substitution in the CAGYC region of the beta subunit. EMBO J 1989; 8:2291.

225. Khalil A, Kovacs K, Sima AA, et al. Pituitary thyrotroph hyperplasia mimicking prolactin-secreting adenoma. J Endocrinol Invest 1984; 7:399–404.

226. Gurr JA, Kourides IA. Ratios of alpha to beta TSH mRNA in normal and hypothyroid pituitaries and TSH-secreting tumors. Endocrinology 1984; 115:830–832.

227. Shupnik MA, Ridgway EC. Thyroid hormone control of thyrotropin gene expression in rat anterior pituitary cells. Endocrinology 1987; 121:619–624.

228. Shupnik MA, Chin WW, Habener JF, et al. Transcriptional regulation of the thyrotropin subunit genes by thyroid hormone. J Biol Chem 1985; 260:2900–2903.

229. Shupnik MA, Ardisson LJ, Meskell MJ, et al. Triiodothyronine (T₃) regulation of thyrotropin subunit gene transcription is proportional to T₃ nuclear receptor occupancy. Endocrinology 1986; 118:367–371.

230. Gershengorn MC. Thyroid hormone regulation of thyrotropin production and interaction with thyrotropin-releasing hormone in thyrotropic cells in culture. In: Oppenheimer JH, Samuels HH, eds. Molecular Basis of Thyroid Hormone Action. San Diego: Academic, 1983: 387–411.

231. Shupnik MA, Greenspan SL, Ridgway EC. Transcriptional regulation of thyrotropin subunit genes by thyrotropin-releasing hormone and dopamine in pituitary cell culture. J Biol Chem 1986; 261:12675–12679.

232. Lippman SS, Amr S, Weintraub BD. Discordant effects of thyrotropin (TSH)-releasing hormone on pre- and posttranslational regulation of TSH biosynthesis in rat pituitary. Endocrinology 1986; 119:343–348.

233. Reichlin S. TRH: historical aspects. Ann NY Acad Sci 1989; 553:1–6.

234. Dyess EM, Segerson TP, Lipositis Z, et al. Triiodothyronine exerts direct cell-specific regulation of thyrotropin-releasing hormone gene expression in the hypothalamic paraventricular nucleus. Endocrinology 1988; 123:2291–2297.

235. Lechan RM. Neuroendocrinology of pituitary hormone regulation. Endocrinol Metab Clin North Am 1987; 16:475–502.

236. Larsen PR. Thyroid-pituitary interaction: feedback regulation of thyrotropin secretion by thyroid hormones. N Engl J Med 1982; 306:23–32.

237. Fish LH, Schwartz HL, Cavanaugh J, Replacement dose, metabolism, and bioavailability of levothyroxine in the treatment of hypothyroidism. Role of triiodothyronine in pituitary feedback in humans. N Engl J Med 1987; 316:764–770.

238. Parker DC, Rossman LG, Pekary AE, et al. Effect of 64-hour sleep deprivation on the circadian waveform of thyrotropin (TSH): further evidence of sleep-related inhibition of TSH release. J Clin Endocrinol Metab 1987; 64:157–161.

239. Brabant G, Brabant A, Ranft U, et al. Circadian and pulsatile thyrotropin secretion in euthyroid man under the influence of thyroid hormone and glucocorticoid administration. J Clin Endocrinol Metab 1987; 65:83–88.

240. Chan V, Jones A, Liendo-Ch P, et al. The relationship between circadian variations in circulating thyrotrophin, thyroid hormones and prolactin. Clin Endocrinol 1978; 9:337–349.

241. Nicoloff JT, Spencer CA. Clinical review 12: the use and misuse of the sensitive thyrotropin assays. J Clin Endocrinol Metab 1990; 71:553–558.

242. Watkins PC, Eddy R, Beck AK, et al. DNA sequence and regional assignment of the human follicle-stimulating hormone beta-subunit gene to the short arm of human chromosome 11. DNA 1987; 6:205–212.

243. Jameson JL, Becker CB, Lindell CM, et al. Human follicle-stimulating hormone beta-subunit gene encodes multiple messenger ribonucleic acids. Mol Endocrinol 1988; 2:806–815.

244. Pelletier G, Leclerc R, Labrie F. Identification of gonadotropic cells in the human pituitary by immunoperoxidase technique. Mol Cell Endocrinol 1976; 6:123–128.

245. Denef C. Paracrine interactions in the anterior pituitary. Clin Endocrinol Metab 1986; 15:1–32.

246. Holck S, Albrechtsen R, Wewer UM. Laminin in the anterior pituitary gland of the rat. Laminin in the gonadotrophic cells correlates with their functional state. Lab Invest 1987; 56:481–488.

247. Kovacs K, Horvath E. Gonadotrophs following removal of the ovaries: a fine structural study of human pituitary glands. Endokrinologie 1975; 66:1–8.

248. Kovacs K, Sheehan HL. Pituitary changes in Kallmann's syndrome: a histologic, immunocytologic, ultrastructural, and immunoelectron microscopic study. Fertil Steril 1982; 37:83–89.

249. Braunstein GD, Rasor J, Wade ME. Presence in normal human testes of a chorionic-gonadotropin–like substance distinct from human luteinizing hormone. N Engl J Med 1975; 293:1339–1343.

250. Chen HC, Hodgen GD, Matsuura S, et al. Evidence for a gonadotropin from nonpregnant subjects that has physical, immunological, and biological similarities to human chorionic gonadotropin. Proc Natl Acad Sci USA 1976; 73:2885–2889.

251. Odell WD, Griffin J. Pulsatile secretion of human chorionic gonadotropin in normal adults. N Engl J Med 1987; 317:1688–1691.

252. Conn PM. GnRH regulation of gonadotropin release and target cell responsiveness. In: DeGroot LJ, Besser GM, Cahill GF Jr, et al., eds. Endocrinology. 2nd ed. Philadelphia: W. B. Saunders, 1989: 284–295.

253. Shupnik MA, Weinmann CM, Notides AC, et al. An upstream region of the rat luteinizing hormone beta gene binds estrogen receptor and confers estrogen responsiveness. J Biol Chem 1989; 264:80–86.

254. Shupnik MA, Gharib SD, Chin WW. Divergent effects of estradiol on gonadotropin gene transcription in pituitary fragments. Mol Endocrinol 1989; 3:474–480.

255. Shupnik MA, Gharib SD, Chin WW. Estrogen suppresses rat gonadotropin gene transcription in vivo. Endocrinology 1988; 122:1842–1846.

256. Yamaji T, Dierschke DJ, Bhattacharya AN, et al. The negative feedback control by estradiol and progesterone of LH secretion in the ovariectomized rhesus monkey. Endocrinology 1972; 90:771–777.

257. Knobil E. The neuroendocrine control of the menstrual cycle. Recent Prog Horm Res 1980; 36:53–88.

258. Blondeau JP, Baulieu EE. Progesterone receptor characterized by photoaffinity labelling in the plasma membrane of *Xenopus laevis* oocytes. Biochem J 1984; 219:785–792.

259. Baulieu EE, Godeau F, Schorderet M, et al. Steroid-induced meiotic division in *Xenopus laevis* oocytes: surface and calcium. Nature 1978; 275:593–598.

260. Clarke IJ, Cummins JT. Increased gonadotropin-releasing hormone pulse frequency associated with estrogen-induced luteinizing hormone surges in ovariectomized ewes. Endocrinology 1985; 116:2376–2383.

261. Neill JD, Patton JM, Dailey RA, et al. Luteinizing hormone releasing hormone (LHRH) in pituitary stalk blood of rhesus monkeys: relationship to level of LH release. Endocrinology 1977; 101:430–434.

262. Marshall JC, Kelch RP. Gonadotropin-releasing hormone: role of pulsatile secretion in the regulation of reproduction. N Engl J Med 1986; 315:1459–1468.

263. Soules MR, Steiner RA, Clifton DK, et al. Progesterone modulation of pulsatile luteinizing hormone secretion in normal women. J Clin Endocrinol Metab 1984; 58:378–383.

264. Sollenberger MJ, Carlsen EC, Johnson ML, et al. Specific physiological regulation of LH secretory events throughout the human menstrual cycle: new insights into the pulsatile mode of gonadotropin release. J Neuroendocrinol 1990; 2:845–852.

265. Steiner RA, Bremner WJ, Clifton DK. Regulation of luteinizing hormone pulse frequency and amplitude by testosterone in the adult male rat. Endocrinology 1982; 111:2055–2061.

266. Wierman ME, Gharib SD, LaRovere JM, et al. Selective failure of androgens to regulate follicle stimulating hormone beta messenger ribonucleic acid levels in the male rat. Mol Endocrinol 1988; 2:492–498.

267. Boyar RM, Moore RJ, Rosner W, et al. Studies of gonadotropin-gonadal dynamics in patients with androgen insensitivity. J Clin Endocrinol Metab 1978; 47:1116–1122.

268. Belchetz PE, Plant TM, Nakai Y, et al. Hypophysial responses to continuous and intermittent delivery of hypothalamic gonadotropin-releasing hormone. Science 1978; 202:631–633.

269. Valk TW, Corley KP, Kelch RP, et al. Hypogonadotropic hypogonadism: hormonal responses to low dose pulsatile administration of gonadotropin-releasing hormone. J Clin Endocrinol Metab 1980; 51:730–738.

270. Hoffman AR, Crowley WF Jr. Induction of puberty in men by long-term pulsatile administration of low-dose gonadotropin-releasing hormone. N Engl J Med 1982; 307:1237–1241.

271. Pohl CR, Richardson DW, Hutchison JS, et al. Hypophysiotropic signal frequency and the functioning of the pituitary-ovarian system in the rhesus monkey. Endocrinology 1983; 112:2076–2080.

272. Clarke IJ, Cummins JT, Findlay JK, et al. Effects on plasma luteinizing hormone and follicle-stimulating hormone of varying the frequency and amplitude of gonadotropin-releasing hormone pulses in ovariectomized ewes with hypothalamo-pituitary disconnection. Neuroendocrinology 1984; 39:214–221.

273. Wildt L, Hausler A, Marshall G, et al. Frequency and amplitude of gonadotropin-releasing hormone stimulation and gonadotropin secretion in the rhesus monkey. Endocrinology 1981; 109:376–385.

274. Mercer JE, Clements JA, Funder JW, et al. Luteinizing hormone–beta mRNA levels are regulated primarily by gonadotropin-releasing hormone and not by negative estrogen feedback on the pituitary. Neuroendocrinology 1988; 47:563–566.

275. Hamernik DL, Crowder ME, Nilson JH, et al. Measurement of messenger ribonucleic acid for luteinizing hormone beta-subunit, alpha-subunit, growth hormone, and prolactin after hypothalamic pituitary disconnection in ovariectomized ewes. Endocrinology 1986; 119:2704–2710.

276. Hamernik DL, Nett TM. Gonadotropin-releasing hormone increases the amount of messenger ribonucleic acid for gonadotropins in ovariectomized ewes after hypothalamic-pituitary disconnection. Endocrinology 1988; 122:959–966.

277. Papavasiliou SS, Zmeili S, Khoury S, et al. Gonadotropin-releasing hormone differentially regulates expression of the genes for luteinizing hormone alpha and beta subunits in male rats. Proc Natl Acad Sci USA 1986; 83:4026–4029.

278. Haisenleder DJ, Katt JA, Ortolano GA, et al. Influence of gonadotropin-releasing hormone pulse amplitude, frequency, and treatment duration on the regulation of luteinizing hormone (LH) subunit messenger ribonucleic acids and LH secretion. Mol Endocrinol 1988; 2:338–343.

279. Dalkin AC, Haisenleder DJ, Ortolano GA, et al. The frequency of gonadotropin-releasing-hormone stimulation differentially regulates gonadotropin subunit messenger ribonucleic acid expression. Endocrinology 1989; 125:917–924.

280. Shupnik MA. Effects of gonadotropin-releasing hormone on rat gonadotropin gene transcription in vitro: requirement for pulsatile administration of luteinizing hormone beta gene stimulation. Mol Endocrinol 1990; 4:1444–1450.

281. Abeyawardene SA, Plant TM. Bilateral orchidectomy and concomitant testosterone replacement in the juvenile male rhesus monkey (*Macaca mulatta*) receiving an invariant intravenous gonadotropin-releasing hormone (GnRH) infusion results, as in the hypothalamus lesioned GnRH-driven adult male, in a selective hypersecretion of follicle-stimulating hormone. Endocrinology 1989; 125:257–259.

282. Dubey AK, Zeleznik AJ, Plant TM. In the rhesus monkey (*Macaca mulatta*), the negative feedback regulation of follicle-stimulating hormone secretion by an action of testicular hormone directly at the level of the anterior pituitary gland cannot be accounted for by either testosterone or estradiol. Endocrinology 1987; 121:2229–2237.

283. Plant TM, Gay VL, Marshall GR, et al. Puberty in monkeys is triggered by chemical stimulation of the hypothalamus. Proc Natl Acad Sci USA 1989; 86:2506–2510.

284. Ying SY. Inhibins and activins: chemical properties and biological activity. Proc Soc Exp Biol Med 1987; 186:253–264.

285. de Jong FH. Inhibin. Physiol Rev 1988; 68:555–607.

286. Vale W, Rivier J, Vaughan J, et al. Purification and characterization of an FSH releasing protein from porcine ovarian follicular fluid. Nature 1986; 321:776–779.

287. Ling N, Ying SY, Ueno N, et al. Pituitary FSH is released by a heterodimer of the beta-subunits from the two forms of inhibin. Nature 1986; 321:779–782.

288. Petraglia F, Sawchenko P, Lim AT, et al. Localization, secretion, and action of inhibin in human placenta. Science 1987; 237:187–189.

289. Roberts V, Meunier H, Vaughan J, et al. Production and regulation of inhibin subunits in pituitary gonadotropes. Endocrinology 1989; 124:552–554.

290. Ramasharma K, Li CH. Human seminal alpha-inhibins: detection in human pituitary, hypothalamus, and serum by immunoreactivity. Proc Natl Acad Sci USA 1986; 83:3484–3486.

291. Sawchenko PE, Plotsky PM, Pfeiffer SW, et al. Inhibin beta in central neural pathways involved in the control of oxytocin secretion. Nature 1988; 334:615–617.

292. Medhamurthy R, Abeyawardene SA, Culler MD, et al. Immunoneutralization of circulating inhibin in the hypophysiotropically clamped male rhesus monkey (*Macaca mulatta*) results in a selective hypersecretion of follicle-stimulating hormone. Endocrinology 1990; 126:2116–2124.

293. Mercer JE, Clements JA, Funder JW, et al. Rapid and specific lowering of pituitary FSH beta mRNA levels by inhibin. Mol Cell Endocrinol 1987; 53:251–254.

294. Carroll RS, Corrigan AZ, Gharib SD, et al. Inhibin, activin, and follistatin: regulation of follicle-stimulating hormone messenger ribonucleic acid levels. Mol Endocrinol 1989; 3:1969–1976.

295. Attardi B, Keeping HS, Winters SJ, et al. Rapid and profound suppression of messenger ribonucleic acid encoding follicle-stimulating hormone beta by inhibin from primate Sertoli cells. Mol Endocrinol 1989; 3:280–287.

296. Ueno N, Ling N, Ying SY, et al. Isolation and partial characterization of follistatin: a single-chain M_r 35,000 monomeric protein that inhibits the release of follicle-stimulating hormone. Proc Natl Acad Sci USA 1987; 84:8282–8286.

297. Ying SY, Becker A, Swanson G, et al. Follistatin specifically inhibits pituitary follicle stimulating hormone release in vitro. Biochem Biophys Res Commun 1987; 149:133–139.

298. Zmeili SM, Papavasiliou SS, Thorner MO, et al. Alpha and luteinizing hormone beta subunit messenger ribonucleic acids during the rat estrous cycle. Endocrinology 1986; 119:1867–1869.

299. Ortolano GA, Haisenleder DJ, Dalkin AC, et al. Follicle-stimulating hormone beta subunit messenger ribonucleic acid concentrations during the rat estrous cycle. Endocrinology 1988; 123:2149–2151. (Erratum 1988; 123:2942.)

300. Veldhuis JD. Hypothalamic pituitary-testicular axis. In: Yen SSC, Jaffe RB, eds. Reproduction Endocrinology. 3rd ed. Philadelphia: W. B. Saunders (in press).

301. Veldhuis JD, Fraioli F, Rogol AD, et al. Metabolic clearance of biologically active luteinizing hormone in man. J Clin Invest 1986; 77:1122–1128.

302. Van Hall EV, Vaitukaitis JL, Ross GT, et al. Effects of progressive desialylation on the rate of disappearance of immunoreactive HCG from plasma in rats. Endocrinology 1971; 89:11–15.

303. Urban RJ, Veldhuis JD. Kinetics of distribution and metabolic clearance of human FSH in men. Tenth Annual NIH Testis Workshop 1988; 34 (abstract).

304. Coble YD, Kohler PO, Cargille CM, et al. Production rates and metabolic clearance rates of human follicle-stimulating hormone in premenopausal and postmenopausal women. J Clin Invest 1969; 48:359–363.

305. Amin HK, Hunter WM. Human pituitary follicle-stimulating hormone: distribution, plasma clearance and urinary excretion as determined by radioimmunoassay. J Endocrinol 1970; 48:307–317.

306. Plant TM, Krey LC, Moossy J, et al. The arcuate nucleus and the control of gonadotropin and prolactin secretion in the female rhesus monkey (*Macaca mulatta*). Endocrinology 1978; 102:52–62.

307. Schwanzel-Fukuda M, Bick D, Pfaff DW. Luteinizing hormone–releasing hormone (LHRH)–expressing cells do not migrate normally in an inherited hypogonadal (Kallmann) syndrome. Brain Res Mol Brain Res 1989; 6:311–326.

308. Crowley WF Jr, Filicori M, Spratt DI, et al. The physiology of gonadotropin-releasing hormone (GnRH) secretion in men and women. Recent Prog Horm Res 1985; 41:473–531.

309. Clarke IJ, Cummins JT. The temporal relationship between gonadotropin releasing hormone (GnRH) and luteinizing hormone (LH) secretion in ovariectomized ewes. Endocrinology 1982; 111:1737–1739.

310. Clarke IJ, Thomas GB, Yao B, et al. GnRH secretion throughout the ovine estrous cycle. Neuroendocrinology 1987; 46:82–88.

311. Levine JE, Pau KY, Ramirez VD, et al. Simultaneous measurement of luteinizing hormone–releasing hormone and luteinizing hormone release in unanesthetized, ovariectomized sheep. Endocrinology 1982; 111:1449–1455.

312. Levine JE, Ramirez VD. Luteinizing hormone–releasing hormone release during the rat estrous cycle and after ovariectomy, as estimated with push-pull cannulae. Endocrinology 1982; 111:1439–1448.

313. Grumbach MM, Kaplan SL. The neuroendocrinology of human puberty: an ontogenetic perspective. In: Grumbach MM, Sizonenko PC, Aubert ML, eds. Control of the Onset of Puberty. Baltimore: Williams & Wilkins, 1990: 1–68.

314. Germak JA, Knobil E. Control of puberty in the rhesus monkey. In: Grumbach MM, Sizonenko PC, Aubert ML, eds. Control of the Onset of Puberty. Baltimore: Williams & Wilkins, 1990: 69–81.

315. Wildt L, Marshall G, Knobil E. Experimental induction of puberty in the infantile female rhesus monkey. Science 1980; 207:1373–1375.

316. Santen RJ, Bardin CW. Episodic luteinizing hormone secretion in man. Pulse analysis, clinical interpretation, physiologic mechanisms. J Clin Invest 1973; 52:2617–2628.

317. Reame N, Sauder SE, Kelch RP, et al. Pulsatile gonadotropin secretion during the human menstrual cycle: evidence for altered frequency of gonadotropin-releasing hormone secretion. J Clin Endocrinol Metab 1984; 59:328–337.

318. Filicori M, Santoro N, Merriam GR, et al. Characterization of the physiological pattern of episodic gonadotropin secretion throughout the human menstrual cycle. J Clin Endocrinol Metab 1986; 62:1136–1144.

Unsolved Problems in Pituitary Function

319. Amselem S, Duquesnoy P, Attree O, et al. Laron dwarfism and mutations of the growth hormone–receptor gene. N Engl J Med 1989; 321:989–995.

320. Godowski PJ, Leung DW, Meacham LR, et al. Characterization of the human growth hormone receptor gene and demonstration of a partial gene deletion in two patients with Laron-type dwarfism. Proc Natl Acad Sci USA 1989; 86:8083–8087.

320a. Straub RE, Frech GC, Joho RH, et al. Expression cloning of a cDNA encoding the mouse pituitary thyrotropin-releasing hormone receptor. Proc Natl Acad Sci USA 1990; 87:9514–9518.

321. Simmons DM, Voss JW, Ingraham HA, et al. Pituitary cell type phenotypes involve cell-specific Pit-1 mRNA translation and synergistic interactions with other classes of transcription factors. Genes Dev 1990; 4:696–711.

322. Lira SA, Crenshaw EB, Glass CK, et al. Identification of rat growth hormone genomic sequences targeting pituitary expression in transgenic mice. Proc Natl Acad Sci USA 1988; 85:4755–4759.

323. Borrelli E, Heyman RA, Arias C, et al. Transgenic mice with inducible dwarfism. Nature 1989; 339:538–541.

324. Behringer RR, Mathews LS, Palmiter RD, et al. Dwarf mice produced by genetic ablation of growth hormone–expressing cells. Genes Dev 1988; 2:453–461.

325. Ingraham HA, Chen RP, Mangalam HJ, et al. A tissue-specific transcription factor containing a homeodomain specifies a pituitary phenotype. Cell 1988; 55:519–529.

326. Castrillo JL, Bodner M, Karin M. Purification of growth hormone–specific transcription factor GHF-1 containing homeobox. Science 1989; 243:814–817.

327. Mangalam HJ, Albert VR, Ingraham HA, et al. A pituitary POU domain protein, Pit-1, activates both growth hormone and prolactin promoters transcriptionally. Genes Dev 1989; 3:946–958.

328. Crenshaw EB III, Li S, Simmons DM, et al. The role of Pit-1 in phenotypic development in the anterior pituitary. Endoc Soc Abstr 1990; 17.

329. Crenshaw EB, Kalla K, Simmons DM, et al. Cell-specific expression of the prolactin gene in transgenic mice is controlled by synergistic interactions between promoter and enhancer elements. Genes Dev 1989; 3:959–972.

330. Landis CA, Masters SB, Spada A, et al. GTPase inhibiting mutations activate the alpha chain of Gs and stimulate adenylyl cyclase in human pituitary tumours. Nature 1989; 340:692–696.

331. Larsson C, Skogseid B, Oberg K, et al. Multiple endocrine neoplasia type 1 gene maps to chromosome 11 and is lost in insulinoma. Nature 1988; 332:85–87.

332. Bystrom C, Larsson C, Blomberg C, et al. Localization of the MEN1 gene to a small region within chromosome 11q13 by deletion mapping in tumors. Proc Natl Acad Sci USA 1990; 87:1968–1972.

333. Werner S, Bystrom C, Askensten U, et al. Retained constitutional genotype on chromosome 11 in 26 sporadic pituitary adenomas. J Endocrinol Invest 1989; 12:52 (abstract).

334. Alexander JM, Biller BMK, Bikkal H, et al. Clinically nonfunctioning pituitary tumors are monoclonal in origin. J Clin Invest 1990; 86:336–340.

335. Herman I, Gonsky R, Fagin J, et al. Clonal origin of secretory and nonsecretory pituitary tumors. Clin Res 1990; 38:296A (abstract).

336. Kovacs K, Horvath E. Pathology of pituitary tumors. Endocrinol Metab Clin North Am 1987; 16:529–551.

337. Melen O. Neuro-ophthalmologic features of pituitary tumors. Endocrinol Metab Clin North Am 1987; 16:585–608.

338. Hollenhorst RW, Younge BR. Ocular manifestations produced by adenomas of the pituitary gland: analysis of 1000 cases. In: Kohler PO, Ross GT, eds. Diagnosis and Treatment of Pituitary Tumors. New York: American Elsevier, 1973: 53–64.

339. Jorgensen JOL, Pedersen SA, Thuesen L, et al. Beneficial effects of growth hormone treatment in GH-deficient adults. Lancet 1989; 1:1221–1225.

Approach to Pituitary Disease

Morphological Classification of Pituitary Adenomas

340. Foncin JF, LeBeau J. Light and electron microscope study of a pituitary tumor with adrenocorticotropic function. C R Soc Biol (Paris) 1963; 157:249–252.

341. Cardell RR Jr, Knighton RS. The cytology of a human pituitary tumor: an electron microscopic study. Trans Am Microsc Soc 1966; 85:58–78.

342. Peake GT, McKeel DW, Jarett L, et al. Ultrastructural, histologic and hormonal characterization of a prolactin-rich human pituitary tumor. J Clin Endocrinol Metab 1969; 29:1383–1393.

343. Nakane PK. Classifications of anterior pituitary cell types with immunoenzyme histochemistry. J Histochem Cytochem 1970; 18:9–20.

344. Kovacs K, Horvath E, Bayley TA, et al. Silent corticotroph cell adenoma with lysosomal accumulation and crinophagy. A distinct clinicopathologic entity. Am J Med 1978; 64:492–499.

345. Horvath E, Kovacs K, Killinger DW, et al. Silent corticotropic adenomas of the human pituitary gland: a histologic, immunocytologic, and ultrastructural study. Am J Pathol 1980; 98:617–638.

346. Horvath E, Kovacs K, Smyth HS, et al. A novel type of pituitary adenoma: morphological features and clinical correlations. J Clin Endocrinol Metab 1988; 66:1111–1118.

347. Kovacs K, Horvath E. Tumors of the pituitary gland. In: Hartmann, WH, ed. Atlas of Tumor Pathology. Fascicle 21. 2nd series. Washington, DC: Armed Forces Institute of Pathology, 1986: 1–264.

348. Scheithauer BW, Horvath E, Kovacs K, et al. Plurihormonal pituitary adenomas. Semin Diagn Pathol 1986; 3:69–82.

349. Heitz PU, Landolt AM, Zenklusen HR, et al. Immunocytochemistry of pituitary tumors. J Histochem Cytochem 1987; 35:1005–1011.

350. Horvath E, Kovacs K, Singer W, et al. Acidophil stem cell adenoma of the human pituitary: clinicopathologic analysis of 15 cases. Cancer 1981; 47:761–771.

351. Horvath E, Kovacs K, Killinger DW, et al. Mammosomatotroph cell adenoma of the human pituitary: a morphologic entity. Virchows Arch [A] 1983; 398:277–289.

352. Horvath E, Kovacs K, Scheithauer BW, et al. Pituitary adenomas producing growth hormone, prolactin, and one or more glycoprotein hormones: a histologic, immunohistochemical, and ultrastructural study of four surgically removed tumors. Ultrastruct Pathol 1983; 5:171–183.

353. Stefaneanu L, Kovacs K, Lloyd RV, et al. The pituitary in pregnancy. A morphologic study including immunocytochemistry and in situ hybridization. FASEB J 1991; 5:A1391 (abstract).

354. Stratmann IE, Ezrin C, Sellers EA. Estrogen-induced transformation of somatotrophs into mammotrophs in the rat. Cell Tissue Res 1974; 152:229–238.

355. Horvath E, Lloyd RV, Kovacs K. Propylthiouracyl-induced hypothyroidism results in reversible trans-differentiation of somatotrophs into thyroidectomy cells. A morphologic study of the rat pituitary including immunoelectron microscopy. Lab Invest 1990; 63:511–520.

Evaluation of Suspected Pituitary Disease

356. Felder RA, Holl RW, Martha P Jr, et al. Influence of matrix on concentrations of somatotropin measured in serum with commercial immunoradiometric assays. Clin Chem 1989; 35:1423–1426.

357. Boscato LM, Stuart MC. Heterophilic antibodies: a problem for all immunoassays. Clin Chem 1988; 34:27–33.

358. Boscato LM, Stuart MC. Incidence and specificity of interference in two-site immunoassays. Clin Chem 1986; 32:1491–1495.

359. Evans WS, Faria AC, Christiansen E, et al. Impact of intensive venous sampling on characterization of pulsatile GH release. Am J Physiol 1987; 252:E549–E556.

360. Winer LM, Shaw MA, Baumann G. Urinary growth hormone excretion rates in normal and acromegalic man: a critical appraisal of its potential clinical utility. J Endocrinol Invest 1989; 12:461–467.

361. Hattori N, Kato Y, Murakami Y, et al. Urinary growth hormone levels measured by ultrasensitive enzyme immunoassay in patients with renal insufficiency. J Clin Endocrinol Metab 1988; 66:727–732.

362. Ho KY, Veldhuis JD, Johnson ML, et al. Fasting enhances growth hormone secretion and amplifies the complex rhythms of growth hormone secretion in man. J Clin Invest 1988; 81:968–975.
363. Hurd HP, Palumbo PJ, Gharib H. Hypothalamic-endocrine dysfunction in anorexia nervosa. Mayo Clin Proc 1977; 52:711–716.
364. Jeffcoate SL. Diagnosis of hyperprolactinaemia. Lancet 1978; 2:1245–1247.
365. Sheldon WR Jr, DeBold CR, Evans WS, et al. Rapid sequential intravenous administration of four hypothalamic releasing hormones as a combined anterior pituitary function test in normal subjects. J Clin Endocrinol Metab 1985; 60:623–630.
366. Landon J, Greenwood FC, Stamp TC, et al. The plasma sugar, free fatty acid, cortisol, and growth hormone response to insulin, and the comparison of this procedure with other tests of pituitary and adrenal function. II. In patients with hypothalamic or pituitary dysfunction or anorexia nervosa. J Clin Invest 1966; 45:437–449.
367. Greenwood FC, Landon J, Stamp TC. The plasma sugar, free fatty acid, cortisol, and growth hormone response to insulin. I. In control subjects. J Clin Invest 1966; 45:429–436.
368. Wolpert SM, Molitch ME, Goldman JA, et al. Size, shape, and appearance of the normal female pituitary gland. AJR 1984; 143:377–381.
369. Swartz JD, Russell KB, Basile BA, et al. High-resolution computed tomographic appearance of the intrasellar contents in women of childbearing age. Radiology 1983; 147:115–117.
370. Chakeres DW, Curtin A, Ford G. Magnetic resonance imaging of pituitary and parasellar abnormalities. Radiol Clin North Am 1989; 27:265–281.
371. Gomori JM, Grossman RI, Zimmerman RA, et al. Intracranial hematomas: imaging by high-field MRI. Radiology 1985; 157:87–93.
372. Kulkarni MV, Lee KF, McArdle CB, et al. 1.5-T MR imaging of pituitary microadenomas: technical considerations and CT correlation. AJNR 1988; 9:5–11.
373. Dwyer AJ, Frank JA, Doppman JL, et al. Pituitary adenomas in patients with Cushing disease: initial experience with Gd-DTPA–enhanced MR imaging. Radiology 1987; 163:421–426.
374. Beck RW. Automated perimetry: principles and practice. Int Ophthalmol Clin 1986; 26:163–174.
375. Chamlin F, Davidoff LM, Feiring EH. Ophthalmologic changes produced by pituitary tumors. Am J Ophthalmol 1955; 40:353–368.
376. Cohen AR, Cooper PR, Kupersmith MJ, et al. Visual recovery after transsphenoidal removal of pituitary adenomas. Neurosurgery 1985; 17:446–452.
377. Wilson P, Falconer MA. Patterns of visual failure with pituitary tumors: clinical and radiological correlations. Br J Ophthalmol 1968; 52:94–110.
378. Wass JAH. Hypopituitarism. In: Besser GM, Cudworth AG, eds. Clinical Endocrinology: An Illustrated Text. Philadelphia: J. B. Lippincott, 1987: 2.1–2.14.
379. Newman SA. Advances in diagnosis and treatment of pituitary tumors. Int Ophthalmol Clin 1986; 26(4):285–300.
380. Trautmann JC, Laws ER Jr. Visual status after transsphenoidal surgery at the Mayo Clinic, 1971–1982. Am J Ophthalmol 1983; 96:200–208.

Hormone Replacement Therapy

381. Snyder PJ, Lawrence DA. Treatment of male hypogonadism with testosterone enanthate. J Clin Endocrinol Metab 1980; 51:1335–1339.
382. Carey PO, Howards SS, Vance ML. Transdermal testosterone treatment of hypogonadal men. J Urol 1988; 140:76–79.
383. Thorner MO, Rogol AD, Blizzard RM, et al. Acceleration of growth rate in growth hormone–deficient children treated with human growth hormone–releasing hormone. Pediatr Res 1988; 24:145–151.

Pituitary Surgery

384. Guiot G. Transsphenoidal approach in surgical treatment of pituitary adenomas: general principles and indications in nonfunctioning adenomas. In: Kohler PO, Ross GT, eds. Diagnosis and Treatment of Pituitary Tumors. New York: American Elsevier, 1973: 159–178.
385. Hardy J. Transphenoidal microsurgery of the normal and pathological pituitary. Clin Neurosurg 1969; 16:185–217.
386. Zentner J, Gilsbach J. Pituitary adenoma and meningioma in the same patient. Report of three cases. Eur Arch Psychiatry Neurol Sci 1989; 238:144–148.
387. Laws ER Jr, Trautmann JC, Hollenhorst RW Jr. Transsphenoidal decompression of the optic nerve and chiasm. Visual results in 62 patients. J Neurosurg 1977; 46:717–722.
388. Laws ER Jr. Pituitary surgery. Endocrinol Metab Clin North Am 1987; 16:647–665.

Pituitary Radiation

389. Bloom B, Kramer S. Conventional radiation therapy in the management of acromegaly. In: Black PM, Zervas NT, Ridgway EC, et al., eds. Secretory Tumors of the Pituitary Gland. Progress in Endocrine Research and Therapy. Vol 1. New York: Raven, 1984: 179–190.
390. Frantz AG, Cogon PH, Chang CH, et al. Long-term evaluation of the results of transsphenoidal surgery and radiotherapy in patients with prolactinoma. In: Crosignan PG, Rubin BL, eds. Endocrinology of Human Infertility: New Aspects. New York: Grune & Stratton, 1981: 161–170.
391. Eastman RC, Gorden P, Roth J. Conventional supervoltage irradiation is an effective treatment for acromegaly. J Clin Endocrinol Metab 1979; 48:931–940.
392. Kliman B, Kjellberg RN, Swisher B, et al. Proton beam therapy of acromegaly: a 20-year experience. In: Black PM, Zervas NT, Ridgway EC, et al., eds. Secretory Tumors of the Pituitary Gland. Progress in Endocrine Research and Therapy. Vol 1. New York: Raven, 1984: 191–211.
393. Nelson PB, Goodman ML, Flickenger JC, et al. Endocrine function in patients with large pituitary tumors treated with operative decompression and radiation therapy. Neurosurgery 1989; 24:398–400.
394. Linfoot JA. Alpha particle pituitary irradiation in the primary and post-surgical management of pituitary microadenomas. In: Faglia G, Giovanelli MA, McLeod RM, eds. Pituitary Microadenomas. London: Academic, 1978: 515–529.
395. Hashimoto N, Handa H, Yamashita J, et al. Long-term follow-up of large or invasive pituitary adenomas. Surg Neurol 1986; 25:49–54.
396. Snyder PJ, Fowble BF, Schatz NJ, et al. Hypopituitarism following radiation therapy of pituitary adenomas. Am J Med 1986; 81:457–462.

Pituitary Disorders

Prolactinoma

397. Costello RT. Subclinical adenoma of the pituitary gland. Am J Pathol 1936; 12:205–215.
398. Abu Fadil S, DeVane G, Siler TM, et al. Effects of oral contraceptive steroids on pituitary prolactin secretion. Contraception 1976; 13:79–85.
399. Dericks Tan JS, Taubert HD. Elevation of serum prolactin during application of oral contraceptives. Contraception 1976; 14:1–8.
400. Jacobs HS, Knuth UA, Hull MG, et al. Post-"pill" amenorrhoea—cause or coincidence? Br Med J 1977; 2:940–942.
401. Coulam CB, Annegers JF, Abboud CF, et al. Pituitary adenoma and oral contraceptives: a case-control study. Fertil Steril 1979; 31:25–28.
402. Wingrave SJ, Kay CR, Vessey MP. Oral contraceptives and pituitary adenomas. Br Med J 1980; 280:685–686.
403. Franks S. Regulation of prolactin secretion by oestrogens: physiological and pathological significance. Clin Sci 1983; 65:457–462.
404. Franks S, Jacobs HS, Hull MGR. The oral contraceptive and hyperprolactinemic amenorrhea. In: Molinatti GM, Crosignani PG, Muller EE, eds. Pituitary Hyperfunction: Physiopathology and Clinical Aspects. New York: Raven, 1984: 175–178.
405. Davis JR, Selby C, Jeffcoate WJ. Oral contraceptive agents do not affect serum prolactin in normal women. Clin Endocrinol 1984; 20:427–434.
406. Molitch ME. Pathogenesis of pituitary tumors. Endocrinol Metab Clin North Am 1987; 16:503–527.
407. Thorner MO, Edwards CRW, Hanker JP, et al. Prolactin and gonadotropin interaction in the male. In: Troen P, Nankin H, eds. The Testis in Normal and Infertile Men. New York: Raven, 1977: 351–366.
408. Carter JN, Tyson JE, Tolis G, et al. Prolactin-screening tumors and hypogonadism in 22 men. N Engl J Med 1978; 299:847–852.
409. Cohen LM, Greenberg DB, Murray GB. Neuropsychiatric presentation of man with pituitary tumors (the 'four A's'). Psychosomatics 1984; 25:925–928.
410. Schwartz MF, Bauman JE, Masters WH. Hyperprolactinemia and sexual disorders in men. Biol Psychiatry 1982; 17:861–876.
411. Kemmann E, Jones JR. Hyperprolactinemia and headaches. Am J Obstet Gynecol 1983; 145:668–671.
412. Quigley ME, Sheehan KL, Casper RF, et al. Evidence for an increased opioid inhibition of luteinizing hormone secretion in hyperprolactinemic patients with pituitary microadenoma. J Clin Endocrinol Metab 1980; 50:427–430.
413. Lightman SL, Jacobs HS, Maguire AK, et al. Constancy of opioid control of luteinizing hormone in different pathophysiological states. J Clin Endocrinol Metab 1981; 52:1260–1263.
414. Grossman A, Moult PJ, McIntyre H, et al. Opiate mediation of amenorrhoea in hyperprolactinaemia and in weight-loss related amenorrhoea. Clin Endocrinol 1982; 17:379–388.
415. Klibanski A, Neer RM, Beitins IZ, et al. Decreased bone density in hyperprolactinemic women. N Engl J Med 1980; 303:1511–1514.
416. Schlechte JA, Sherman B, Martin R. Bone density in amenorrheic women with and without hyperprolactinemia. J Clin Endocrinol Metab 1983; 56:1120–1123.
417. Greenspan SL, Neer RM, Ridgway EC, et al. Osteoporosis in men with hyperprolactinemic hypogonadism. Ann Intern Med 1986; 104:777–782.
418. Jackson JA, Kleerekoper M, Parfitt AM. Symptomatic osteoporosis in a man with hyperprolactinemic hypogonadism. Ann Intern Med 1986; 105:543–545.
419. Boulanger CM, Mashchak CA, Chang RJ. Lack of tumor reduction in hyperprolactinemic women with extrasellar macroadenomas treated with bromocriptine. Fertil Steril 1985; 44:532–535.

420. Balagura S, Frantz AG, Housepian EM, et al. The specificity of serum prolactin as a diagnostic indicator of pituitary adenoma. J Neurosurg 1979; 51:42–46.

421. Klijn JG, Lamberts SWJ, de Jong FH, et al. The value of the thyrotropin-releasing hormone test in patients with prolactin-secreting pituitary tumors and suprasellar non-pituitary tumors. Fertil Steril 1981; 35:155–161.

422. Landolt AM, Rothenbuhler V. Pituitary adenoma calcification. Arch Pathol Lab Med 1977; 101:22–27.

423. Rilliet B, Mohr G, Robert F, et al. Calcifications in pituitary adenomas. Surg Neurol 1981; 15:249–255.

424. Mukada K, Ohta M, Uozumi T, et al. Ossified prolactinoma: case report. Neurosurgery 1987; 20:473–475.

425. Landolt AM, Kleihues P, Heitz PU. Amyloid deposits in pituitary adenomas. Differentiation of two types. Arch Pathol Lab Med 1987; 111:453–458.

426. Horvath E, Kovacs K. Pathology of prolactin cell adenomas of the human pituitary. Semin Diagn Pathol 1986; 3:4–17.

427. Saeger W, Mohr K, Caselitz J, et al. Light and electron microscopical morphometry of pituitary adenomas in hyperprolactinemia. Pathol Res Pract 1986; 181:544–550.

428. Thorner MO, Schran HF, Evans WS, et al. A broad spectrum of prolactin suppression by bromocriptine in hyperprolactinemic women: a study of serum prolactin and bromocriptine levels after acute and chronic administration of bromocriptine. J Clin Endocrinol Metab 1980; 50:1026–1033.

429. Thorner MO, Perryman RL, Rogol AD, et al. Rapid changes of prolactinoma volume after withdrawal and reinstitution of bromocriptine. J Clin Endocrinol Metab 1981; 53:480–483.

430. Molitch ME, Elton RL, Blackwell RE, et al. Bromocriptine as primary therapy for prolactin-secreting macroadenomas: results of a prospective multicenter study. J Clin Endocrinol Metab 1985; 60:698–705.

431. Horvath E, Kovacs K, Killinger DW, et al. Diverse ultrastructural response to dopamine agonist's medication in human pituitary prolactin cell adenomas. In: Hoshino K, ed. Prolactin Gene Family and Its Receptors. Amsterdam: Elsevier, 1988: 307–311.

432. Tindall GT, Kovacs K, Horvath E, et al. Human prolactin-producing adenomas and bromocriptine: a histological, immunocytochemical, ultrastructural, and morphometric study. J Clin Endocrinol Metab 1982; 55:1178–1183.

433. Bassetti M, Spada A, Pezzo G, et al. Bromocriptine treatment reduces the cell size in human macroprolactinomas: a morphometric study. J Clin Endocrinol Metab 1984; 58:268–273.

434. Saitoh Y, Mori S, Arita N, et al. Cytosuppressive effect of bromocriptine on human prolactinomas: stereological analysis of ultrastructural alterations with special reference to secretory granules. Cancer Res 1986; 46:1507–1512.

435. Arita K, Uozumi T, Ohta M. A case of large prolactinoma supposed to be cured by bromocriptine therapy. Endocrinol Jpn 1988; 35:503–509.

436. Maurer RA. Transcriptional regulation of the prolactin gene by ergocryptine and cyclic AMP. Nature 1981; 294:94–97.

437. Gen M, Uozumi T, Ohta M, et al. Necrotic changes in prolactinomas after long term administration of bromocriptine. J Clin Endocrinol Metab 1984; 59:463–470.

438. Landolt AM, Osterwalder V. Perivascular fibrosis in prolactinomas: is it increased by bromocriptine? J Clin Endocrinol Metab 1984; 58:1179–1183.

439. Esiri MM, Bevan JS, Burke CW, et al. Effect of bromocriptine treatment on the fibrous tissue content of prolactin-secreting and nonfunctioning macroadenomas of the pituitary gland. J Clin Endocrinol Metab 1986; 63:383–388.

440. Hallenga B, Saeger W, Ludecke DK. Necroses of prolactin-secreting pituitary adenomas under treatment with dopamine agonists: light microscopical and morphometric studies. Exp Clin Endocrinol 1988; 92:59–68.

441. Bevan JS, Adams CB, Burke CW, et al. Factors in the outcome of transsphenoidal surgery for prolactinoma and non-functioning pituitary tumour, including pre-operative bromocriptine therapy. Clin Endocrinol 1987; 26:541–556.

442. Martin NA, Hales M, Wilson CB. Cerebellar metastasis from a prolactinoma during treatment with bromocriptine. J Neurosurg 1981; 55:615–619.

443. U HS, Johnson C. Metastatic prolactin-secreting pituitary adenoma. Hum Pathol 1984; 15:94–96.

444. Scheithauer BW, Randall RV, Kramer S, et al. Prolactin cell carcinoma of the pituitary: clinicopathologic, immunohistochemical and ultrastructural study of a case with cranial and extracranial metastases. Cancer 1985; 55:598–604.

445. Landolt AM, Minder H. Immunohistochemical examination of the paraadenomatous "normal" pituitary. An evaluation of prolactin cell hyperplasia. Virchows Arch [A] 1984; 403:181–193.

446. Pioro EP, Scheithauer BW, Kramer S, et al. Combined thyrotroph and lactotroph cell hyperplasia simulating prolactin-secreting pituitary adenoma in long-standing primary hypothyroidism. Surg Neurol 1988; 29:218–226.

447. Wowra B, Peiffer J. An immunoperoxidase study of a human pituitary adenoma associated with Cushing's syndrome. Pathol Res Pract 1984; 178:349–354.

448. Vance ML, Evans WS, Thorner MO. Drugs five years later. Bromocriptine. Ann Intern Med 1984; 100:78–91.

449. Pellegrini I, Rasolonjanahary R, Gunz G, et al. Resistance to bromocriptine in prolactinomas. J Clin Endocrinol Metab 1989; 69:500–509.

450. Thorner MO, McNeilly AS, Hagan C, et al. Long-term treatment of galactorrhoea and hypogonadism with bromocriptine. Br Med J 1974; 2:419–422.

451. Liuzzi A, Dallabonzana D, Oppizzi G, et al. Low doses of dopamine agonists in the long-term treatment of macroprolactinomas. N Engl J Med 1985; 313:656–659.

452. Hokfelt T, Fuxe K. On the morphology and the neuroendocrine role of the hypothalamic catecholamine neuron. In: Knigge KM, Jacobs HS, Weindl A, eds. Brain-Endocrine Interaction. Median Eminence: Structure and Function. Basel: S. Karger, 1972: 181–223.

453. Corrodi H, Fuxe K, Hökfelt T, et al. Effect of ergot drugs on central catecholamine neurons: evidence for a stimulation of central dopamine neurons. J Pharm Pharmacol 1973; 25:409–412.

454. Calabro MA, MacLeod RM. Binding of dopamine to bovine anterior pituitary gland membranes. Neuroendocrinology 1978; 25:32–46.

455. Muller EE, Panerai AE, Cocchi D, et al. Endocrine profile of ergot alkaloids. Life Sci 1977; 21:1545–1558.

456. Schran HF, Bhuta SI, Schwarz HJ, et al. The pharmacokinetics of bromocriptine in man. Adv Biochem Psychopharmacol 1980; 23:125–139.

457. Kletzky OA, Vermesh M. Effectiveness of vaginal bromocriptine in treating women with hyperprolactinemia. Fertil Steril 1989; 51:269–272.

458. Turner TH, Cookson JC, Wass JA, et al. Psychotic reactions during treatment of pituitary tumours with dopamine agonists. Br Med J 1984; 289:1101–1103.

459. Ayres J, Maisey MN. Alcohol increases bromocriptine's side effects. N Engl J Med 1980; 302:806 (letter).

460. Werder K, Fahlbusch R, Landgraf R, et al. Treatment of patients with prolactinomas. J Endocrinol Invest 1978; 1:47–58.

461. Molitch ME. Pregnancy and the hyperprolactinemic woman. N Engl J Med 1985; 312:1364–1370.

462. Mornex R, Orgiazzi J, Hugues B, et al. Normal pregnancies after treatment of hyperprolactinemia with bromoergocryptine, despite suspected pituitary tumors. J Clin Endocrinol Metab 1978; 47:290–295.

463. Lamberts SWJ, Klijn JG, de Lange SA, et al. The incidence of complications during pregnancy after treatment of hyperprolactinemia with bromocriptine in patients with radiologically evident pituitary tumors. Fertil Steril 1979; 31:614–619.

464. Turkalj I, Braun P, Krupp P. Surveillance of bromocriptine in pregnancy. JAMA 1982; 247:1589–1591.

465. Krupp P, Turkalj I. Surveillance of Parlodel (bromocriptine) in pregnancy and offspring. In: Jacobs HS, Harrison RF, Bonnar J, et al., eds. Prolactinomas and Pregnancy. Lancaster: MTP, 1983: 45–50.

466. Raymond JP, Goldstein E, Konopka P, et al. Follow-up of children born of bromocriptine-treated mothers. Horm Res 1985; 22:239–246.

467. Thorner MO, Martin WH, Rogol AD, et al. Rapid regression of pituitary prolactinomas during bromocriptine treatment. J Clin Endocrinol Metab 1980; 51:438–445.

468. Canales ES, Garcia IC, Ruiz JE, et al. Bromocriptine as prophylactic therapy in prolactinoma during pregnancy. Fertil Steril 1981; 36:524–526.

469. van Roon E, van der Vijver JCM, Gerretsen G, et al. Rapid regression of a suprasellar extending prolactinoma after bromocriptine treatment during pregnancy. Fertil Steril 1981; 36:173–177.

470. Konopka P, Raymond JP, Merceron RE, et al. Continuous administration of bromocriptine in the prevention of neurological complications in pregnant women with prolactinomas. Am J Obstet Gynecol 1983; 146:935–938.

471. Maeda T, Ushiroyama T, Okuda K, et al. Effective bromocriptine treatment of a pituitary macroadenoma during pregnancy. Obstet Gynecol 1983; 61:117–121.

472. Moult PJ, Dacie JE, Rees LH, et al. Oral contraception in patients with hyperprolactinaemia. Br Med J 1982; 284:868.

473. Breidahl HD, Topliss DJ, Pike JW. Failure of bromocriptine to maintain reduction in size of a macroprolactinoma. Br Med J 1983; 287:451–452.

474. Gasser RW, Finkenstedt G, Skrabal F, et al. Multiple intracranial metastases from a prolactin secreting pituitary tumour. Clin Endocrinol 1985; 22:17–27.

475. Plangger CA, Twerdy K, Grunert V, et al. Subarachnoid metastases from a prolactinoma. Neurochirurgia (Stuttg) 1985; 28:235–237.

476. Newman CB, Hurley AM, Kleinberg DL. Effect of CV 205–502 in hyperprolactinaemic patients intolerant of bromocriptine. Clin Endocrinol 1989; 31:391–400.

477. Vance ML, Cragun JR, Reimnitz C, et al. CV 205–502 treatment of hyperprolactinemia. J Clin Endocrinol Metab 1989; 68:336–339.

478. Vance ML, Lipper M, Klibanski A, et al. Treatment of prolactin-secreting pituitary macroadenomas with the long-acting non-ergot dopamine agonist CV 205–502. Ann Intern Med 1990; 112:668–673.

479. Antunes JL, Housepian EM, Frantz AG, et al. Prolactin-secreting pituitary tumors. Ann Neurol 1977; 2:148–153.

480. Chang RJ, Keye WR Jr, Young JR, et al. Detection, evaluation, and treatment of pituitary microadenomas in patients with galactorrhea and amenorrhea. Am J Obstet Gynecol 1977; 128:356–363.

481. Hardy J, Beauregard H, Robert F. Prolactin-secreting pituitary adenomas: transsphenoidal microsurgical treatment. In: Robyn C, Harter M, eds. Progress in Prolactin Physiology and Pathology. Developments in Endocrinology. Vol 2. Amsterdam: Elsevier/North-Holland, 1978: 361–370.

482. Tindall GT, McLanahan CS, Christy JH. Transsphenoidal microsurgery for pituitary tumors associated with hyperprolactinemia. J Neurosurg 1978; 48:849–860.

483. Post KD, Biller BJ, Adelman LS, et al. Selective transsphenoidal adenomectomy in women with galactorrhea-amenorrhea. JAMA 1979; 242:158–162.

484. Hardy J. Transsphenoidal microsurgery of prolactinomas. In: Black PM, Zervas NT, Ridgway EC, et al., eds. Secretory Tumors of the Pituitary Gland. Progress in Endocrine Research and Therapy. Vol 1. New York: Raven, 1984: 73–81.

485. Nelson PB, Goodman M, Maroon JC, et al. Factors in predicting outcome from operation in patients with prolactin-secreting pituitary adenomas. Neurosurgery 1983; 13:634–641.

486. Tucker HS, Grubb SR, Wigand JP, et al. Galactorrhea-amenorrhea syndrome: follow-up of forty-five patients after pituitary tumor removal. Ann Intern Med 1981; 94:302–307.

487. Woosley RE, King JS, Talbert L. Prolactin-secreting pituitary adenomas: neurosurgical management of 37 patients. Fertil Steril 1982; 37:54–60.

488. Rodman EF, Molitch ME, Post KD, et al. Long-term follow-up of transsphenoidal selective adenomectomy for prolactinoma. JAMA 1984; 252:921–924.

489. Thomson JA, Teasdale GM, Gordon D, et al. Treatment of presumed prolactinoma by transsphenoidal operation: early and late results. Br Med J 1985; 291:1550–1553.

490. Parl FF, Cruz VE, Cobb CA, et al. Late recurrence of surgically removed prolactinomas. Cancer 1986; 57:2422–2426.

491. Zervas NT. Surgical results for pituitary adenomas: results of an international survey. In: Black PM, Zervas NT, Ridgway EC, et al., eds. Secretory Tumors of the Pituitary Gland. Progress in Endocrine Research and Therapy. Vol 1. New York: Raven, 1984: 377–385.

492. Kramer S, Fode NC, Redmond MJ. Transsphenoidal surgery following unsuccessful prior therapy. An assessment of benefits and risks in 158 patients. J Neurosurg 1985; 63:823–829.

493. Sheline GE, Grossman A, Jones AE, et al. Radiation therapy for prolactinomas. In: Black PM, Zervas NT, Ridgway EC, et al., eds. Secretory Tumors of the Pituitary Gland. Progress in Endocrine Research and Therapy. Vol 1. New York: Raven, 1984: 93–108.

494. Nabarro JD. Pituitary prolactinomas. Clin Endocrinol 1982; 17:129–155.

495. Grossman A, Cohen BL, Charlesworth M, et al. Treatment of prolactinomas with megavoltage radiotherapy. Br Med J 1984; 288:1105–1109.

496. Halberg FE, Sheline GE. Radiotherapy of pituitary tumors. Endocrinol Metab Clin North Am 1987; 16:667–684.

497. Feek CM, McLelland J, Seth J, et al. How effective is external pituitary irradiation for growth hormone–secreting pituitary tumors? Clin Endocrinol 1984; 20:401–408.

498. Ross DA, Wilson CB. Results of transsphenoidal microsurgery for growth hormone–secreting pituitary adenoma in a series of 214 patients. J Neurosurg 1988; 68:854–867.

Acromegaly

499. Marie P. Sur deux cas d'acromégalie. Hypertrophie singulière non congénitale des extrémités supérieures, inférieures et céphaliques. Rev Med 1886; 6:297–333.

500. Minkowski O. Uber einen Fall von Akromegalie. Berl Klin Wochenschr 1887; 24:371–374.

501. Marie P, de Souze-Leite JD. Essays on Acromegaly. London: New Sydenham Society, 1891.

502. Alexander L, Appleton D, Hall R, et al. Epidemiology of acromegaly in the Newcastle region. Clin Endocrinol 1980; 12:71–79.

503. Bengtsson BA, Eden S, Ernest I, et al. Epidemiology and long-term survival in acromegaly. A study of 166 cases diagnosed between 1955 and 1984. Acta Med Scand 1988; 223:327–335.

504. Randall RV. Acromegaly and gigantism. In: DeGroot LJ, Besser GM, Cahill GF Jr, et al., eds. Endocrinology. 2nd ed. Philadelphia: W. B. Saunders, 1989: 330–350.

505. Wilson CB. A decade of pituitary microsurgery. The Herbert Olivecrona lecture. J Neurosurg 1984; 61:814–833.

506. Thorner MO, Frohman LA, Leong DA, et al. Extrahypothalamic growth-hormone-releasing factor (GRF) secretion is a rare cause of acromegaly: plasma GRF levels in 177 acromegalic patients. J Clin Endocrinol Metab 1984; 59:846–849.

507. Asa SL, Scheithauer BW, Bilbao JM, et al. A case for hypothalamic acromegaly: a clinicopathological study of six patients with hypothalamic gangliocytomas producing growth hormone–releasing factor. J Clin Endocrinol Metab 1984; 58:796–803.

508. Melmed S, Ezrin C, Kovacs K, et al. Acromegaly due to secretion of growth hormone by an ectopic pancreatic islet-cell tumor. N Engl J Med 1985; 312:9–17.

509. Reichlin S. Etiology of acromegaly from the neuroendocrine point of view: a historical perspective. In: Robbins RJ, Melmed S, eds. Acromegaly. A Century of Scientific and Clinical Progress. New York: Plenum, 1987: 7–15.

510. Asa SL, Kovacs K, Thorner MO, et al. Immunohistological localization of growth hormone–releasing hormone in human tumors. J Clin Endocrinol Metab 1985; 60:423–427.

511. Dayal Y, Lin HD, Tallberg K, et al. Immunocytochemical demonstration of growth hormone–releasing factor in gastrointestinal and pancreatic endocrine tumors. Am J Clin Pathol 1986; 85:13–20.

512. Frohman LA. Growth hormone–releasing factor: a neuroendocrine perspective. J Lab Clin Med 1984; 103:819–832.

513. Christofides ND, Stephanou A, Suzuki H, et al. Distribution of immunoreactive growth hormone–releasing hormone in the human brain and intestine and its production by tumors. J Clin Endocrinol Metab 1984; 59:747–751.

514. Frohman LA, Thominet JL, Szabo M. Ectopic growth hormone releasing factor syndromes. In: Raiti S, Tolman R, eds. Human Growth Hormone. New York: Plenum, 1986: 347–360.

515. Frohman LA, Szabo M, Berelowitz M, et al. Partial purification and characterization of a peptide with growth hormone–releasing activity from extrapituitary tumors in patients with acromegaly. J Clin Invest 1980; 65:43–54.

516. Guillemin R, Brazeau P, Bohlen P, et al. Growth hormone–releasing factor from a human pancreatic tumor that caused acromegaly. Science 1982; 218:585–587.

517. Bluestone R, Bywaters EG, Hartog M, et al. Acromegalic arthropathy. Ann Rheum Dis 1971; 30:243–258.

518. Detenbeck LC, Tressler HA, O'Duffy JD, et al. Peripheral joint manifestations of acromegaly. Clin Orthop 1973; 91:119–127.

519. Dons RF, Rosselet P, Pastakia B, et al. Arthropathy in acromegalic patients before and after treatment: a long-term follow-up study. Clin Endocrinol 1988; 28:515–524.

520. Layton MW, Fudman EJ, Barkan A, et al. Acromegalic arthropathy. Characteristics and response to therapy. Arthritis Rheum 1988; 31:1022–1027.

521. Steinbach HL, Feldman R, Goldberg MB. Acromegaly. Radiology 1959; 72:535–549.

522. Jones DR, Bahn RC, Randall RV, et al. The human costochondral junction. II. Patients with acromegaly. Mayo Clin Proc 1969; 44:330–334.

523. Fradkin JE, Eastman RC, Lesniak MA, et al. Specificity spillover at the hormone receptor—exploring its role in human disease. N Engl J Med 1989; 320:640–645.

524. Jadresic A, Banks LM, Child DF, et al. The acromegaly syndrome. Relation between clinical features, growth hormone values and radiological characteristics of the pituitary tumours. Q J Med 1982; 51:189–204.

525. Wass JA, Cudworth AG, Bottazzo GF, et al. An assessment of glucose intolerance in acromegaly and its response to medical treatment. Clin Endocrinol 1980; 12:53–59.

526. Nikkila EA, Pelkonen R. Serum lipids in acromegaly. Metabolism 1975; 24:829–838.

527. Takeda R, Tatami R, Ueda K, et al. The incidence and pathogenesis of hyperlipidaemia in 16 consecutive acromegalic patients. Acta Endocrinol 1982; 100:358–362.

528. Wright AD, Hill DM, Lowy C, et al. Mortality in acromegaly. Q J Med 1970; 39:1–16.

529. Evans CC, Hipkin LJ, Murray GM. Pulmonary function in acromegaly. Thorax 1977; 32:322–327.

530. Harrison BD, Millhouse KA, Harrington M, et al. Lung function in acromegaly. Q J Med 1978; 47:517–532.

531. Perks WH, Horrocks PM, Cooper RA, et al. Sleep apnoea in acromegaly. Br Med J 1980; 280:894–897.

532. Hart TB, Radow SK, Blackard WG, et al. Sleep apnea in active acromegaly. Arch Intern Med 1985; 145:865–866.

533. Pekkarinen T, Partinen M, Pelkonen R, et al. Sleep apnoea and daytime sleepiness in acromegaly: relationship to endocrinological factors. Clin Endocrinol 1987; 27:649–654.

534. Mezon BJ, West P, MaClean JP, et al. Sleep apnea in acromegaly. Am J Med 1980; 69:615–618.

535. Cadieux RJ, Kales A, Santen RJ, et al. Endoscopic findings in sleep apnea associated with acromegaly. J Clin Endocrinol Metab 1982; 55:18–22.

536. Chanson P, Timsit J, Benoit O, et al. Rapid improvement in sleep apnoea of acromegaly after short-term treatment with somatostatin analogue SMS 201–995. Lancet 1986; 1:1270–1271 (letter).

537. Ziemer DC, Dunlap DB. Relief of sleep apnea in acromegaly by bromocriptine. Am J Med Sci 1988; 295:49–51.

538. McGuffin WL Jr, Sherman BM, Roth F, et al. Acromegaly and cardio-

vascular disorders. A prospective study. Ann Intern Med 1974; 81:11–18.

539. Hayward RP, Emanuel RW, Nabarro JD. Acromegalic heart disease: influence of treatment of the acromegaly on the heart. Q J Med 1987; 62:41–58.

540. Lie JT. Pathology of the heart in acromegaly: anatomic findings in 27 autopsied patients. Am Heart J 1980; 100:41–52.

541. Jonas EA, Aloia JF, Lane FJ. Evidence of subclinical heart muscle dysfunction in acromegaly. Chest 1975; 67:190–194.

542. Savage DD, Henry WL, Eastman RC, et al. Echocardiographic assessment of cardiac anatomy and function in acromegalic patients. Am J Med 1979; 67:823–829.

543. Luboshitzki R, Hammerman H, Barzilai D, et al. The heart in acromegaly: correlation of echocardiographic and clinical findings. Isr J Med Sci 1980; 16:378–383.

544. O'Keefe JC, Grant SJ, Wiseman JC, et al. Acromegaly and the heart—echocardiographic and nuclear imaging studies. Aust NZ J Med 1982; 12:603–607.

545. Csanady M, Gaspar L, Hogye M, et al. The heart in acromegaly: an echocardiographic study. Int J Cardiol 1983; 2:349–361.

546. Gordon DA, Hill FM, Ezrin C. Acromegaly: a review of 100 cases. Can Med Assoc J 1962; 87:1106–1109.

547. Hejtmancik MR, Bradfield JY Jr, Herrmann GR. Acromegaly and the heart: a clinical and pathologic study. Ann Intern Med 1951; 34:1445–1456.

548. Balzer R, McCullagh EP. Hypertension in acromegaly. Am J Med Sci 1959; 237:449–452.

549. Hamwi GJ, Skillman TG, Tufts KC. Acromegaly. Am J Med 1960; 29:690–699.

550. Sowers JR, Tuck ML. Hypertension associated with diabetes mellitus, hypercalcaemic disorders, acromegaly and thyroid disease. Clin Endocrinol Metab 1981; 10:631–656.

551. Anderson RJ, Lufkin EG, Sizemore GW, et al. Acromegaly and pituitary adenoma with phaeochromocytoma: a variant of multiple endocrine neoplasia. Clin Endocrinol 1981; 14:605–612.

552. Rioperez E, Botella JM, Valdivieso L, et al. Conn's syndrome in a patient with acromegaly. Horm Metab Res 1981; 13:186–187.

553. Riggs BL, Randall RV, Wahner HW, et al. The nature of the metabolic bone disorder in acromegaly. J Clin Endocrinol Metab 1972; 34:911–918.

554. Seeman E, Wahner HW, Offord KP, et al. Differential effects of endocrine dysfunction on the axial and the appendicular skeleton. J Clin Invest 1982; 69:1302–1309.

555. Diamond T, Nery L, Posen S. Spinal and peripheral bone mineral densities in acromegaly: the effects of excess growth hormone and hypogonadism. Ann Intern Med 1989; 111:567–573.

556. Mastaglia FL, Barwich DD, Hall R, Myopathy in acromegaly. Lancet 1970; 2:907–909.

557. Mastaglia FL. Pathological changes in skeletal muscle in acromegaly. Acta Neuropathol 1973; 24:273–286.

558. Pickett JB, Layzer RB, Levin SR, et al. Neuromuscular complications of acromegaly. Neurology 1975; 25:638–645.

559. Epstein N, Whelan M, Benjamin V. Acromegaly and spinal stenosis. Case report. J Neurosurg 1982; 56:145–147.

560. McCullagh EP, Hewlett JS. Acromegaly with amyotrophic lateral sclerosis of the amyotrophic type. J Clin Endocrinol 1947; 7:636–643.

561. O'Duffy JD, Randall RV, MacCarty CS. Median neuropathy (carpal-tunnel syndrome) in acromegaly. Ann Intern Med 1973; 78:379–383.

562. Clemmons DR, Van Wyk JJ, Ridgway EC, et al. Evaluation of acromegaly by radioimmunoassay of somatomedin-C. N Engl J Med 1979; 301:1138–1142.

563. Klein I, Parveen G, Gavaler JS, et al. Colonic polyps in patients with acromegaly. Ann Intern Med 1982; 97:27–30.

564. Ituarte EM, Petrini J, Hershman JM. Acromegaly and colon cancer. Ann Intern Med 1984; 101:627–628.

565. Pines A, Rozen P, Ron E, et al. Gastrointestinal tumors in acromegalic patients. Am J Gastroenterol 1985; 80:266–269.

566. Evans HM, Briggs JH, Dixon JS. The physiology and chemistry of growth hormone. In: Harris GW, Donovan BT, eds. The Pituitary Gland. Vol 1. Berkeley: University of California Press, 1966: 439–491.

567. Mustacchi P, Shimkin MB. Occurrence of cancer in acromegaly and hypopituitarism. Cancer 1957; 10:100–104.

568. Cryer PE, Daughaday WH. Regulation of growth hormone secretion in acromegaly. J Clin Endocrinol Metab 1969; 29:386–393.

569. Jaquet P, Guibout M, Jaquet C, et al. Circadian regulation of growth hormone secretion after treatment in acromegaly. J Clin Endocrinol Metab 1980; 50:322–328.

570. Barkan AL, Stred SE, Reno K, et al. Increased growth hormone pulse frequency in acromegaly. J Clin Endocrinol Metab 1989; 69:1225–1233.

571. Wass JA, Clemmons DR, Underwood LE, et al. Changes in circulating somatomedin-C levels in bromocriptine-treated acromegaly. Clin Endocrinol 1982; 17:369–377.

572. Rieu M, Girard F, Bricaire H, et al. The importance of insulin-like growth factor (somatomedin) measurements in the diagnosis and surveillance of acromegaly. J Clin Endocrinol Metab 1982; 55:147–153.

573. Stonesifer LD, Jordan RM, Kohler PO. Somatomedin C in treated

574. Moses AC, Molitch ME, Sawin CT, et al. Bromocriptine therapy in acromegaly: use in patients resistant to conventional therapy and effect on serum levels of somatomedin. J Clin Endocrinol Metab 1981; 53:752–758.

575. Beck P, Parker ML, Daughaday WH. Paradoxical hypersecretion of growth hormone in response to glucose. J Clin Endocrinol Metab 1966; 26:463–469.

576. Earll JM, Sparks LL, Forsham PH. Glucose suppression of serum growth hormone in the diagnosis of acromegaly. JAMA 1967; 201:628–630.

577. Besser GM, Mortimer CH, McNeilly AS, et al. Long-term infusion of growth hormone release inhibiting hormone in acromegaly: effects on pituitary and pancreatic hormones. Br Med J 1974; 4:622–627.

578. Lawrence AM, Goldfine ID, Kirsteins L. Growth hormone dynamics in acromegaly. J Clin Endocrinol Metab 1970; 31:239–247.

579. Irie M, Tsushima T. Increase of serum growth hormone concentration following thyrotropin-releasing hormone injection in patients with acromegaly or gigantism. J Clin Endocrinol Metab 1972; 35:97–100.

580. Hanew K, Kokubun M, Sasaki A, et al. The spectrum of pituitary growth hormone responses to pharmacological stimuli in acromegaly. J Clin Endocrinol Metab 1980; 51:292–297.

581. Liuzzi A, Chiodini PG, Botalla L, et al. Inhibitory effect of L-dopa on GH release in acromegalic patients. J Clin Endocrinol Metab 1972; 35:941–943.

582. Liuzzi A, Chiodini PG, Botalla L, et al. Decreased plasma growth hormone (GH) levels in acromegalics following CB 154 (2-Br-alpha ergocryptine) administration. J Clin Endocrinol Metab 1974; 38:910–912.

583. Thorner MO, Chait A, Aitken M, et al. Bromocriptine treatment of acromegaly. Br Med J 1975; 1:299–303.

584. Gelato MC, Merriam GR, Vance ML, et al. Effects of growth hormone–releasing factor on growth hormone secretion in acromegaly. J Clin Endocrinol Metab 1985; 60:251–257.

585. Ramsay JA, Kovacs K, Asa SL, et al. Reversible sellar enlargement due to growth hormone–releasing hormone production by pancreatic endocrine tumors in a acromegalic patient with multiple endocrine neoplasia type I syndrome. Cancer 1988; 62:445–450.

586. Barth RJ, Constant RB, Parker MW, et al. Preoperative diagnosis of acromegaly by growth hormone releasing factor radioimmunoassay. Milit Med 1991; 156:375–378.

587. Penny ES, Penman E, Price J, et al. Circulating growth hormone releasing factor concentrations in normal subjects and patients with acromegaly. Br Med J 1984; 289:453–455.

588. Melmed S, Braunstein GD, Horvath E, et al. Pathophysiology of acromegaly. Endocr Rev 1983; 4:271–290.

589. Kovacs K, Horvath E. Pathology of growth hormone–producing tumors of the human pituitary. Semin Diagn Pathol 1986; 3:18–33.

590. Scheithauer BW, Kovacs K, Randall RV, et al. Pathology of excessive production of growth hormone. Clin Endocrinol Metab 1986; 15:655–681.

591. Trouillas J, Girod C, Lheritier M, et al. Morphological and biochemical relationships in 31 human pituitary adenomas with acromegaly. Virchows Arch [A] 1980; 389:127–142.

592. Kanie N, Kageyama N, Kuwayama A, et al. Pituitary adenomas in acromegalic patients: an immunohistochemical and endocrinological study with special reference to prolactin-secreting adenoma. J Clin Endocrinol Metab 1983; 57:1093–1101.

593. Saeger W, Rubenach Gerz K, Caselitz J, et al. Electron microscopical morphometry of GH producing pituitary adenomas in comparison with normal GH cells. Virchows Arch [A] 1987; 411:467–472.

594. Horvath E, Kovacs K. Morphogenesis and significance of fibrous bodies in human pituitary adenomas. Virchows Arch [B] 1978; 27:69–78.

595. Neumann PE, Goldman JE, Horoupian DS, et al. Fibrous bodies in growth hormone–secreting adenomas contain cytokeratin filaments. Arch Pathol Lab Med 1985; 109:505–508.

596. Mori H, Mori S, Saitoh Y, et al. Growth hormone–producing pituitary adenoma with crystal-like amyloid immunohistochemically positive for growth hormone. Cancer 1985; 55:96–102.

597. Saitoh Y, Mori H, Matsumoto Y, et al. Accumulation of amyloid in pituitary adenomas. Acta Neuropathol 1985; 68:87–92.

598. Corenblum B, Sirek AM, Horvath E, et al. Human mixed somatotrophic and lactotrophic pituitary adenomas. J Clin Endocrinol Metab 1976; 42:857–863.

599. Bassetti M, Spada A, Arosio M, et al. Morphological studies on mixed growth hormone (GH)– and prolactin (PRL)-secreting human pituitary adenomas. Coexistence of GH and PRL in the same secretory granule. J Clin Endocrinol Metab 1986; 62:1093–1100.

600. Halmi NS. Occurrence of both growth hormone- and prolactin-immunoreactive material in the cells of human somatotropic pituitary adenomas containing mammotropic elements. Virchows Arch [A] 1983; 398:19–31.

601. Zurschmiede C, Landolt AM. Distribution of growth hormone and prolactin in secretory granules of the normal and neoplastic human adenohypophysis. Virchows Arch [B] 1987; 53:308–315.

602. Bassetti M, Arosio M, Spada A, et al. Growth hormone and prolactin

secretion in acromegaly: correlations between hormonal dynamics and immunocytochemical findings. J Clin Endocrinol Metab 1988; 67:1195–1204.

603. Beckers A, Courtoy R, Stevenaert A, et al. Mammosomatotropes in human pituitary adenomas as revealed by electron microscopic double gold immunostaining method. Acta Endocrinol 1988; 118:503–512.

604. Felix IA, Horvath E, Kovacs K, et al. Mammosomatotroph adenoma of the pituitary associated with gigantism and hyperprolactinemia. A morphological study including immunoelectron microscopy. Acta Neuropathol 1986; 71:76–82.

605. Kovacs K, Horvath E, Ezrin C, et al. Adenoma of the human pituitary producing growth hormone and thyrotropin. A histologic, immunocytologic and fine-structural study. Virchows Arch [A] 1982; 395:59–68.

606. Carlson HE, Linfoot JA, Braunstein GD, et al. Hyperthyroidism and acromegaly due to a thyrotropin- and growth hormone–secreting pituitary tumor. Lack of hormonal response to bromocriptine. Am J Med 1983; 74:915–923.

607. Beck-Peccoz P, Bassetti M, Spada A, et al. Glycoprotein hormone alpha-subunit response to growth hormone (GH)–releasing hormone in patients with active acromegaly. Evidence for alpha-subunit and GH coexistence in the same tumoral cell. J Clin Endocrinol Metab 1985; 61:541–546.

608. Beck-Peccoz P, Piscitelli G, Amr S, et al. Endocrine, biochemical, and morphological studies of a pituitary adenoma secreting growth hormone, thyrotropin (TSH), and alpha-subunit: evidence for secretion of TSH with increased bioactivity. J Clin Endocrinol Metab 1986; 62:704–711.

609. Asai A, Matsutani M, Funada N, et al. Malignant growth hormone–secreting pituitary adenoma with hematogenous dural metastasis: case report. Neurosurgery 1988; 22:1091–1094.

610. Mountcastle RB, Roof BS, Mayfield RK, et al. Pituitary adenocarcinoma in an acromegalic patient: response to bromocriptine and pituitary testing: a review of the literature on 36 cases of pituitary carcinoma. Am J Med Sci 1989; 298:109–118.

611. Horvath E, Scheithauer BW, Kovacs K. Morphologic aspects of growth hormone–producing pituitary adenomas with emphasis on novel concepts. In: Ludecke DK, Tolis G, eds. Growth Hormone, Growth Factors, and Acromegaly. New York: Raven, 1987: 107–114.

612. Kovacs K. The relation of the endocrine system to tumors of non-endocrine organs. Dtsch Gesundheitswes 1966; 21:1105–1108 (in German).

613. Landolt AM, Osterwalder V, Stackmann G. Preoperative treatment of acromegaly with SMS 201-995: surgical and pathological observations. In: Ludecke DK, Tolis G, eds. Growth Hormone, Growth Factors, and Acromegaly. New York: Raven, 1987: 229–244.

614. George SR, Kovacs K, Asa SL, et al. Effect of SMS 201-995, a long-acting somatostatin analogue, on the secretion and morphology of a pituitary growth hormone cell adenoma. Clin Endocrinol 1987; 26:395–405.

615. Beckers A, Stevenaert A, Kovacs K, et al. The treatment of acromegaly with SMS 201-995. Adv Biosci 1988; 69:227–228.

616. Barkan AL, Lloyd RV, Chandler WF, et al. Preoperative treatment of acromegaly with long-acting somatostatin analog SMS 201-995: shrinkage of invasive macroadenomas and improved surgical remission rate. J Clin Endocrinol Metab 1988; 67:1040–1048.

617. Kramer S, Piepgras DG, Randall RV, et al. Neurosurgical management of acromegaly. Results in 82 patients treated between 1972 and 1977. J Neurosurg 1979; 50:454–461.

618. Williams RA, Jacobs HS, Kurtz AB, et al. The treatment of acromegaly with special reference to transsphenoidal hypophysectomy. Q J Med 1975; 44:79–98.

619. van't Verlaat JW, Nortier JW, Hendriks MJ, et al. Transsphenoidal microsurgery as primary treatment in 25 acromegalic patients: results and follow-up. Acta Endocrinol 1988; 117:154–158.

620. Black PM, Zervas NT, Candia GL. Incidence and management of complications of transsphenoidal operation for pituitary adenomas. Neurosurgery 1987; 20:920–924.

621. Arafah BU, Brodkey JS, Kaufman B, et al. Transsphenoidal microsurgery in the treatment of acromegaly and gigantism. J Clin Endocrinol Metab 1980; 50:578–585.

622. Tucker HS, Grubb SR, Wigand JP, et al. The treatment of acromegaly by transsphenoidal surgery. Arch Intern Med 1980; 140:795–802.

623. Quabbe HJ. Treatment of acromegaly by trans-sphenoidal operation, 90-yttrium implantation and bromocriptine: results in 230 patients. Clin Endocrinol 1982; 16:107–119.

624. Richards SH, Thomas JP. Treatment of acromegaly by transethmoidal hypophysectomy. Q J Med 1980; 49:21–31.

625. Roelfsema F, van Dulken H, Frolich M. Long-term results of transsphenoidal pituitary microsurgery in 60 acromegalic patients. Clin Endocrinol 1985; 23:555–563.

626. Quabbe HJ. Acromegaly: an overview. In: Lamberts SWJ, Tilders FJH, Van der Veen EA, et al., eds. Trends in Diagnosis and Treatment of Pituitary Adenomas. Amsterdam: Free University Press, 1984: 247–256.

627. Cassar J, Doyle FH, Banks LM, et al. Interstitial pituitary irradiation with ^{90}Y for the treatment of acromegaly. A reappraisal. Acta Endocrinol 1981; 96:295–300.

628. Leksell DG. Special stereotactic techniques: stereotactic radiosurgery. In: Heilbrun MP, ed. Stereotactic Neurosurgery. Vol 2. Concepts in Neurosurgery. Baltimore: Williams & Wilkins, 1988: 195–209.

629. Reichlin S. Somatostatin. N Engl J Med 1983; 309:1495–1501.

630. Davies RR, Miller M, Turner SJ, et al. Effects of somatostatin analogue SMS 201-995 in normal man. Clin Endocrinol 1986; 24:665–674.

631. Plewe G, Beyer J, Krause U, et al. Long-acting and selective suppression of growth hormone secretion by somatostatin analogue SMS 201-995 in acromegaly. Lancet 1984; 2:782–784.

632. Lamberts SW, Oosterom R, Neufeld M, et al. The somatostatin analog SMS 201-995 induces long-acting inhibition of growth hormone secretion without rebound hypersecretion in acromegalic patients. J Clin Endocrinol Metab 1985; 60:1161–1165.

633. Verschoor L, Lamberts SWJ, Uitterlinden P, et al. Glucose tolerance during long term treatment with a somatostatin analogue. Br Med J 1986; 293:1327–1328.

634. Lamberts SWJ, Zweens M, Verschoor L, et al. A comparison among the growth hormone–lowering effects in acromegaly of the somatostatin analog SMS 201-995, bromocriptine, and the combination of both drugs. J Clin Endocrinol Metab 1986; 63:16–19.

635. Wass JA, Lytras N, Besser GM. Somatostatin octapeptide (SMS 201-995) in the medical treatment of acromegaly. Scand J Gastroenterol Suppl 1986; 119:136–140.

636. Chiodini PG, Cozzi R, Dallabonzana D, et al. Medical treatment of acromegaly with SMS 201-995, a somatostatin analog: a comparison with bromocriptine. J Clin Endocrinol Metab 1987; 64:447–453.

637. Christensen SE, Weeke J, Orskov H, et al. Continuous subcutaneous pump infusion of somatostatin analogue SMS 201-995 versus subcutaneous injection schedule in acromegalic patients. Clin Endocrinol 1987; 27:297–306.

638. Ducasse MC, Tauber JP, Tourre A, et al. Shrinking of a growth hormone–producing pituitary tumor by continuous subcutaneous infusion of the somatostatin analog SMS 201-995. J Clin Endocrinol Metab 1987; 65:1042–1046.

639. George SR, Hegele RA, Burrow GN. The somatostatin analogue SMS 201-995 in acromegaly: prolonged, preferential suppression of growth hormone but not pancreatic hormones. Clin Invest Med 1987; 10:309–315.

640. Lamberts SWJ, Uitterlinden P, del Pozo E. SMS 201-995 induces a continuous decline in circulating growth hormone and somatomedin-C levels during therapy of acromegalic patients for over two years. J Clin Endocrinol Metab 1987; 65:703–710.

641. Pieters GF, van Liessum PA, Smals AG, et al. Long-term treatment of acromegaly with Sandostatin (SMS 201-995). Normalization of most anomalous growth hormone responses. Acta Endocrinol Suppl 1987; 286:9–18.

642. Timsit J, Chanson P, Larger E, et al. The effect of subcutaneous infusion versus subcutaneous injections of a somatostatin analogue (SMS 201-995) on the diurnal GH profile in acromegaly. Acta Endocrinol 1987; 116:108–112.

643. Beckers A, Stevenaert A, Hennen G. A new therapy for acromegaly. Rev Med Liege 1988; 43:429–432 (in French).

644. Cozzi R, Liuzzi A, Dallabonzana D, et al. Clinical use of the somatostatin analog SMS 201-995 in endocrinology. J Endocrinol Invest 1988; 11:737–740.

645. Garcia-Luna PP, Leal del Cerro A, Montero C, et al. A rare cause of acromegaly: ectopic production of growth hormone–releasing factor by a bronchial carcinoid tumor. Surg Neurol 1987; 27:563–568.

646. Halberg FE, Sheline GE. Radiotherapy of pituitary tumors. Endocrinol Metab Clin North Am 1987; 16:667–684.

647. Gavilan I, Santos C, Garcia-Luna PP, et al. Response of growth hormone to the acute test using GH-releasing factor 1–29 in acromegaly. Comparison in the baseline situation and under treatment with prolonged-action somatostatin. Rev Clin Esp 1988; 182:187–191 (in Spanish).

648. Tolis G. Long-term management of acromegaly with sandostatin. Horm Res 1988; 29:112–114.

649. van Liessum PA, Pieters GF, Hermus AR, et al. Successful treatment of ophthalmoplegia in acromegaly with the somatostatin analogue SMS 201-995. Neth J Med 1988; 32:289–292.

650. Chanson P, Timsit J, Masquet C, et al. Heart failure responding to octreotide in patient with acromegaly. Lancet 1989; 1:1263–1264 (letter).

651. Quabbe HJ, Plockinger U. Dose-response study and long term effect of the somatostatin analog octreotide in patients with therapy-resistant acromegaly. J Clin Endocrinol Metab 1989; 68:873–881.

652. Sassolas G, Fossati P, Chanson P, et al. Experience of a six-month treatment with Sandostatin at increasing doses in acromegaly. Horm Res 1989; 31:51–54.

653. Tauber JP, Babin T, Tauber MT, et al. Long term effects of continuous subcutaneous infusion of the somatostatin analog octreotide in the treatment of acromegaly. J Clin Endocrinol Metab 1989; 68:917–924.

654. Harris AG, Prestele H, Herold K, et al. Long-term efficacy of Sandostatin (SMS 201-995, octreotide) in 178 acromegalic patients. In: Lamberts SWJ, ed. Sandostatin in the Treatment of Acromegaly. Berlin: Springer-Verlag, 1988:117–125.

655. Barnard LB, Grantham WG, Lamberton P, et al. Treatment of resistant

acromegaly with a long-acting somatostatin analogue (SMS 201-995). Ann Intern Med 1986; 105:856–861.

656. Reubi JC, Landolt AM. The growth hormone responses to octreotide in acromegaly correlate with adenoma somatostatin receptor status. J Clin Endocrinol Metab 1989; 68:844–850.

657. Kvols LK, Moertel CG, O'Connell MJ, et al. Treatment of the malignant carcinoid syndrome. Evaluation of a long-acting somatostatin analogue. N Engl J Med 1986; 315:663–666.

658. Moller DE, Moses AC, Jones K, et al. Octreotide suppresses both growth hormone (GH) and GH-releasing hormone (GHRH) in acromegaly due to ectopic GHRH secretion. J Clin Endocrinol Metab 1989; 68:499–504.

659. van Liessum PA, Hopman WP, Pieters GF, et al. Postprandial gallbladder motility during long term treatment with the long-acting somatostatin analog SMS 201-995 in acromegaly. J Clin Endocrinol Metab 1989; 69:557–562.

660. Barkan AL, Shenker Y, Grekin RJ, et al. Acromegaly from ectopic growth hormone–releasing hormone secretion by a malignant carcinoid tumor. Successful treatment with long-acting somatostatin analogue SMS 201-995. Cancer 1988; 61:221–226.

661. von Werder K, Losa M, Muller OA, et al. Treatment of metastasising GRF-producing tumour with a long-acting somatostatin analogue. Lancet 1984; 2:282–283 (letter).

Cushing's Disease

662. Cushing H. The basophil adenomas of the pituitary body and their clinical manifestations. Bull Johns Hopkins Hosp 1932; 50:137–195.

663. Hughes JM, Hichens M, Booze GW, et al. Cushing's syndrome from the therapeutic use of intramuscular dexamethasone acetate. Arch Intern Med 1986; 146:1848–1849.

664. Crapo L. Cushing's syndrome: a review of diagnostic tests. Metabolism 1979; 28:955–977.

665. Connoly CK, Gore MBR, Stanley N, et al. Single-dose dexamethasone suppression in normal subjects and hospital patients. Br Med J 1968; 2:665–667.

666. Streeten DH, Stevenson CT, Dalakos TG, et al. The diagnosis of hypercortisolism. Biochemical criteria differentiating patients from lean and obese normal subjects and from females on oral contraceptives. J Clin Endocrinol Metab 1969; 29:1191–1211.

667. Burke CW, Beardwell CG. Cushing's syndrome: an evaluation of the clinical usefulness of urinary free cortisol and other urinary steroid measurements in diagnosis. Q J Med 1973; 165:175–204.

668. Meikle AW, Lagerquist LG, Tyler FH. Apparently normal pituitary-adrenal suppressibility in Cushing's syndrome: dexamethasone metabolism and plasma levels. J Lab Clin Med 1975; 86:472–478.

669. Meikle AW. Dexamethasone suppression tests: usefulness of simultaneous measurement of plasma cortisol and dexamethasone. Clin Endocrinol 1982; 16:401–408.

670. Liddle GW. Tests of pituitary-adrenal suppressibility in the diagnosis of Cushing's syndrome. J Clin Endocrinol Metab 1960; 20:1539–1560.

671. Sindler BH, Griffing GT, Melby JC. The superiority of the metyrapone test versus the high-dose dexamethasone test in the differential diagnosis of Cushing's syndrome. Am J Med 1983; 74:657–662.

672. Chrousos GP, Schulte HM, Oldfield EH, et al. The corticotropin-releasing factor stimulation test. An aid in the evaluation of patients with Cushing's syndrome. N Engl J Med 1984; 310:622–626.

673. Lytras N, Grossman A, Perry L, et al. Corticotrophin releasing factor: responses in normal subjects and patients with disorders of the hypothalamus and pituitary. Clin Endocrinol 1984; 20:71–84.

674. Oldfield EH, Chrousos GP, Schulte HM, et al. Preoperative lateralization of ACTH-secreting pituitary microadenomas by bilateral and simultaneous inferior petrosal venous sinus sampling. N Engl J Med 1985; 321:100–103.

675. Aron DC, Findling JW, Tyrrell JB. Cushing's disease. Endocrinol Metab Clin North Am 1987; 16:705–730.

676. Carey RM, Varma SK, Drake CR Jr, et al. Ectopic secretion of corticotropin-releasing factor as a cause of Cushing's syndrome. A clinical, morphologic, and biochemical study. N Engl J Med 1984; 311:13–20.

677. Pojunas KW, Daniels DL, Williams AL, et al. Pituitary and adrenal CT of Cushing syndrome. AJR 1986; 146:1235–1238.

678. Chandler WF, Schteingart DE, Lloyd RV, et al. Surgical treatment of Cushing's disease. J Neurosurg 1987; 66:204–212.

679. Findling JW, Tyrrell JB. Occult ectopic secretion of corticotropin. Arch Intern Med 1986; 146:929–933.

680. Yamashina M. An 18-year history of a corticotropin-secreting spindle cell carcinoid in the lung. Arch Pathol Lab Med 1985; 109:673–675.

681. Robert F, Hardy J. Human corticotroph cell adenomas. Semin Diagn Pathol 1986; 3:34–41.

682. Charpin C, Hassoun J, Oliver C, et al. Immunohistochemical and immunoelectron-microscopic study of pituitary adenomas associated with Cushing's disease. A report of 13 cases. Am J Pathol 1982; 109:1–7.

683. Lloyd RV, Chandler WF, McKeever PE, et al. The spectrum of ACTH-producing pituitary lesions. Am J Surg Pathol 1986; 10:618–626.

684. Berg KK, Scheithauer BW, Felix I, et al. Pituitary adenomas producing ACTH and alpha subunit: a clinicopathologic, immunohistochemical, ultrastructural and immunoelectron microscopical study in nine cases. Neurosurgery 1990; 26:397–403.

685. Sherry SH, Guay AT, Lee AK, et al. Concurrent production of adrenocorticotropin and prolactin from two distinct cell lines in a single pituitary adenoma: a detailed immunohistochemical analysis. J Clin Endocrinol Metab 1982; 55:947–955.

686. Felix IA, Horvath E, Kovacs K. Massive Crooke's hyalinization in corticotroph cell adenomas of the human pituitary. A histological, immunocytological, and electron microscopic study of three cases. Acta Neurochir (Wien) 1981; 58:235–243.

687. Horvath E, Kovacs K, Josse R. Pituitary corticotroph cell adenoma with marked abundance of microfilaments. Ultrastruct Pathol 1983; 5:249–255.

688. Halliday WC, Asa SL, Kovacs K, et al. Intermediate filaments in the human pituitary gland: an immunohistochemical study. Can J Neurol Sci 1990; 17:131–136.

689. Serri O, Robert F, Pelletier G, et al. Hyperprolactinemia associated with clinically silent adenomas: endocrinologic and pathologic studies; a report of two cases. Fertil Steril 1987; 47:792–796.

690. Lloyd RV, Fields K, Jin L, et al. Analysis of endocrine active and clinically silent corticotropic adenomas by in situ hybridization. Am J Pathol 1990; 137:479–488.

691. Ludecke D, Kautzky R, Saeger W, et al. Selective removal of hypersecreting pituitary adenomas? An analysis of endocrine function, operative and microscopical findings in 101 cases. Acta Neurochir (Wien) 1976; 35:27–42.

692. Lamberts SWJ, Stefanko SZ, de Lange SA, et al. Failure of clinical remission after transsphenoidal removal of a microadenoma in a patient with Cushing's disease: multiple hyperplastic and adenomatous cell nets in surrounding pituitary tissue. J Clin Endocrinol Metab 1980; 50:793–795.

693. Schnall AM, Kovacs K, Brodkey JS, et al. Pituitary Cushing's disease without adenoma. Acta Endocrinol 1980; 94:297–303.

694. McNicol AM. Patterns of corticotropic cells in the adult human pituitary in Cushing's disease. Diagn Histopathol 1981; 4:335–341.

695. McKeever PE, Koppelman MC, Metcalf D, et al. Refractory Cushing's disease caused by multinodular ACTH-cell hyperplasia. J Neuropathol Exp Neurol 1982; 41:490–499.

696. Saeger W, Ludecke DK. Pituitary hyperplasia. Definition, light and electron microscopical structures and significance in surgical specimens. Virchows Arch [A] 1983; 399:277–287.

697. Horvath E. Pituitary hyperplasia. Pathol Res Pract 1988; 183:623–625.

698. Young WF Jr, Scheithauer BW, Gharib H, et al. Cushing's syndrome due to primary multinodular corticotrope hyperplasia. Mayo Clin Proc 1988; 63:256–262.

699. Asa SL, Kovacs K, Tindall GT, et al. Cushing's disease associated with an intrasellar gangliocytoma producing corticotrophin-releasing factor. Ann Intern Med 1984; 101:789–793.

700. Belsky JL, Cuello B, Swanson LW, et al. Cushing's syndrome due to ectopic production of corticotropin-releasing factor. J Clin Endocrinol Metab 1985; 60:496–500.

701. Schteingart DE, Lloyd RV, Akil H, et al. Cushing's syndrome secondary to ectopic corticotropin-releasing hormone–adrenocorticotropin secretion. J Clin Endocrinol Metab 1986; 63:770–775.

702. Zarate A, Kovacs K, Flores M, et al. ACTH and CRF-producing bronchial carcinoid associated with Cushing's syndrome. Clin Endocrinol 1986; 24:523–529.

703. Scheithauer BW, Kovacs K, Randall RV. The pituitary gland in untreated Addison's disease. A histologic and immunocytologic study of 18 adenohypophyses. Arch Pathol Lab Med 1983; 107:484–487.

704. Fachnie JD, Zafar MS, Mellinger RC, et al. Pituitary carcinoma mimics the ectopic adrenocorticotropin syndrome. J Clin Endocrinol Metab 1980; 50:1062–1065.

705. Gabrilove JL, Anderson PJ, Halmi NS. Pituitary pro-opiomelanocortin–cell carcinoma occurring in conjunction with a glioblastoma in a patient with Cushing's disease and subsequent Nelson's syndrome. Clin Endocrinol 1986; 25:117–126.

706. Lamberts SWJ, de Lange SA, Stefanko SZ. Adrenocorticotropin-secreting pituitary adenomas originate from the anterior or the intermediate lobe in Cushing's disease: differences in the regulation of hormone secretion. J Clin Endocrinol Metab 1982; 54:286–291.

707. McNicol AM, Teasdale GM, Beastall GH. A study of corticotroph adenomas in Cushing's disease: no evidence of intermediate lobe origin. Clin Endocrinol 1986; 24:715–722.

708. Bigos ST, Somma M, Rasio E, et al. Cushing's disease: management by transsphenoidal pituitary microsurgery. J Clin Endocrinol Metab 1980; 50:348–354.

709. Boggan JE, Tyrrell JB, Wilson CB. Transsphenoidal microsurgical management of Cushing's disease. Report of 100 cases. J Neurosurg 1983; 59:195–200.

710. Salassa RM, Kramer S, Carpenter PC, et al. Transsphenoidal removal of pituitary microadenoma in Cushing's disease. Mayo Clin Proc 1978; 53:24–28.

711. Tyrrell JB, Brooks RM, Fitzgerald PA, et al. Cushing's disease: selective transsphenoidal resection of pituitary adenomas. N Engl J Med 1976; 295:1137–1138.

712. Jennings AS, Liddle GW, Orth DN. Results of treating childhood Cushing's disease with pituitary irradiation. N Engl J Med 1977; 297:957–962.

713. Orth DN, Liddle GW. Results of treatment in 108 patients with Cushing's syndrome. N Engl J Med 1971; 285:243–247.

714. Pont A, Graybill JR, Craven PC, et al. High-dose ketoconazole therapy and adrenal and testicular function in humans. Arch Intern Med 1984; 144:2150–2153.

715. Sonino N, Boscaro M, Merola G, et al. Prolonged treatment of Cushing's disease by ketoconazole. J Clin Endocrinol Metab 1985; 61:718–722.

716. Nelson DH, Meakin JW, Dealy JB, et al. ACTH-producing tumor of the pituitary gland. N Engl J Med 1958; 259:161–164.

717. Moore TJ, Dluhy RG, Williams GH, et al. Nelson's syndrome: frequency, prognosis, and effect of prior pituitary irradiation. Ann Intern Med 1976; 85:731–734.

718. Findling JW, Aron DC, Tyrell JB. Cushing disease. In: Imura H, ed. The Pituitary Gland. New York: Raven, 1985: 441.

Glycoprotein-Producing Adenomas

719. Snyder PJ. Gonadotroph cell adenomas of the pituitary. Endocr Rev 1985; 6:552–563.

720. Oppenheim DS, Klibanski A. Medical therapy of glycoprotein hormone–secreting pituitary tumors. Endocrinol Metab Clin North Am 1989; 18:339–358.

721. Snyder PJ. Gonadotroph cell pituitary adenomas. Endocrinol Metab Clin North Am 1987; 16:755–764.

722. Weintraub BD, Gershengorn MC, Kourides IA, et al. Inappropriate secretion of thyroid-stimulating hormone. Ann Intern Med 1981; 95:339–351.

723. Kourides IA, Weintraub BD, Rosen SW, et al. Secretion of alpha subunit of glycoprotein hormones by pituitary adenomas. J Clin Endocrinol Metab 1976; 43:97–106.

724. Ridgway EC. Glycoprotein hormone production by pituitary tumors. Prog Endocr Res Ther 1984; 1:343.

725. Smallridge RC. Thyrotropin-secreting pituitary tumors. Endocrinol Metab Clin North Am 1987; 16:765–792.

726. Comi RJ, Gesundheit N, Murray L, et al. Response of thyrotropin-secreting pituitary adenomas to a long-acting somatostatin analogue. N Engl J Med 1987; 317:12–17.

727. Afrasiabi A, Valenta L, Gwinup G. A TSH secreting pituitary tumour causing hyperthyroidism: presentation of a case and review of the literature. Acta Endocrinol 1979; 92:448–454.

728. Hill SA, Falko JM, Wilson CB, et al. Thyrotrophin-producing pituitary adenomas. J Neurosurg 1982; 57:515–519.

729. Cravioto H, Fukaya T, Zimmerman EA, et al. Immunohistochemical and electron-microscopic studies of functional and non-functional pituitary adenomas including one TSH secreting tumor in a thyrotoxic patient. Acta Neuropathol 1981; 53:281–292.

730. Grisoli F, Leclercq T, Winteler JP, et al. Thyroid-stimulating hormone pituitary adenomas and hyperthyroidism. Surg Neurol 1986; 25:361–368.

731. Samaan NA, Osborne BM, Mackay B, et al. Endocrine and morphologic studies of pituitary adenomas secondary to primary hypothyroidism. J Clin Endocrinol Metab 1977; 45:903–911.

732. Katz MS, Gregerman RI, Horvath E. Thyrotroph cell adenoma of the human pituitary gland associated with primary hypothyroidism: clinical and morphological features. Acta Endocrinol 1980; 95:41–48.

733. Wajchenberg BL, Tsanaclis AM, Marino J. TSH-containing pituitary adenoma associated with primary hypothyroidism manifested by amenorrhoea and galactorrhoea. Acta Endocrinol 1984; 106:61–66.

734. Saeger W, Ludecke DK. Pituitary adenomas with hyperfunction of TSH. Frequency, histological classification, immunocytochemistry and ultrastructure. Virchows Arch [A] 1982; 394:255–267.

735. Girod C, Trouillas J, Claustrat B. The human thyrotropic adenoma: pathologic diagnosis in five cases and critical review of the literature. Semin Diagn Pathol 1986; 3:58–68.

736. Scheithauer BW, Kovacs K, Randall RV, et al. Pituitary gland in hypothyroidism. Histologic and immunocytologic study. Arch Pathol Lab Med 1985; 109:499–504.

737. Vagenakis AG, Dole K, Braverman LE. Pituitary enlargement, pituitary failure, and primary hypothyroidism. Ann Intern Med 1976; 85:195–198.

738. Farley JD, Toth EL, Ryan EA. Primary hypothyroidism presenting as growth delay and pituitary enlargement. Can J Neurol Sci 1988; 15:35–37.

739. Trouillas J, Girod C, Sassolas G, et al. Human pituitary gonadotropic adenoma; histological, immunocytochemical, and ultrastructural and hormonal studies in eight cases. J Pathol 1981; 135:315–336.

740. Horvath E, Kovacs K. Gonadotroph adenomas of the human pituitary: sex-related fine-structural dichotomy. A histologic, immunocytochemical, and electron-microscopic study of 30 tumors. Am J Pathol 1984; 117:429–440.

741. Snyder PJ, Johnson J, Muzyka R. Abnormal secretion of glycoprotein alpha-subunit and follicle-stimulating hormone (FSH) beta-subunit in men with pituitary adenomas and FSH hypersecretion. J Clin Endocrinol Metab 1980; 51:579–584.

742. Snyder PJ, Sterling FH. Hypersecretion of LH and FSH by a pituitary adenoma. J Clin Endocrinol Metab 1976; 42:544–550.

743. Koide Y, Kugai N, Kimura S, et al. A case of pituitary adenoma with possible simultaneous secretion of thyrotropin and follicle-stimulating hormone. J Clin Endocrinol Metab 1982; 54:397–403.

744. Kovacs K, Horvath E, Van Loon GR, et al. Pituitary adenomas associated with elevated blood follicle-stimulating hormone levels: a histologic, immunocytologic, and electron microscopic study of two cases. Fertil Steril 1978; 29:622–628.

745. Borges JL, Ridgway EC, Kovacs K, et al. Follicle-stimulating hormone–secreting pituitary tumor with concomitant elevation of serum alpha-subunit levels. J Clin Endocrinol Metab 1984; 58:937–941.

746. Wide L, Lundberg PO. Hypersecretion of an abnormal form of follicle-stimulating hormone associated with suppressed luteinizing hormone secretion in a woman with a pituitary adenoma. J Clin Endocrinol Metab 1981; 53:923–930.

747. Berezin M, Olchovsky D, Pines A, et al. Reduction of follicle-stimulating hormone (FSH) secretion in FSH-producing pituitary adenoma by bromocriptine. J Clin Endocrinol Metab 1984; 59:1220–1223.

748. Vance ML, Ridgway EC, Thorner MO. Follicle-stimulating hormone– and alpha-subunit–secreting pituitary tumor treated with bromocriptine. J Clin Endocrinol Metab 1985; 61:580–584.

749. Friend JN, Judge DM, Sherman BM, et al. FSH-secreting pituitary adenomas: stimulation and suppression studies in two patients. J Clin Endocrinol Metab 1976; 43:650–657.

750. Cunningham GR, Huckins C. An FSH and prolactin-secreting pituitary tumor: pituitary dynamics and testicular histology. J Clin Endocrinol Metab 1977; 44:248–253.

751. Demura R, Kubo O, Demura H, et al. FSH and LH secreting pituitary adenoma. J Clin Endocrinol Metab 1977; 45:653–657.

752. Harris RI, Schatz NJ, Gennarelli T, et al. Follicle-stimulating hormone–secreting pituitary adenomas: correlation of reduction of adenoma size with reduction of hormonal hypersecretion after transsphenoidal surgery. J Clin Endocrinol Metab 1983; 56:1288–1293.

753. Klibanski A, Deutsch PJ, Jameson JL, et al. Luteinizing hormone–secreting pituitary tumor: biosynthetic characterization and clinical studies. J Clin Endocrinol Metab 1987; 64:536–542.

754. Barrow DL, Tindall GT, Kovacs K, et al. Clinical and pathological effects of bromocriptine on prolactin-secreting and other pituitary tumors. J Neurosurg 1984; 60:1–7.

755. Grossman A, Ross R, Charlesworth M, et al. The effect of dopamine agonist therapy on large functionless pituitary tumours. Clin Endocrinol 1985; 22:679–686.

756. Vos P, Croughs RJ, Thijssen JH, et al. Response of luteinizing hormone secreting pituitary adenoma to a long-acting somatostatin analogue. Acta Endocrinol 1988; 118:587–590.

757. Sassolas G, Serusclat P, Claustrat B, et al. Plasma alpha-subunit levels during the treatment of pituitary adenomas with the somatostatin analog (SMS 201–995). Horm Res 1988; 29:124–128.

758. Chapman AJ, MacFarlane IA, Shalet SM, et al. Discordant serum alpha-subunit and FSH concentrations in a woman with a pituitary tumour. Clin Endocrinol 1984; 21:123–129.

759. Roman SH, Goldstein M, Kourides IA, et al. The luteinizing hormone-releasing hormone (LHRH) agonist [D-Trp[6]-Pro[9]-NEt]LHRH increased rather than lowered LH and alpha-subunit levels in a patient with an LH-secreting pituitary tumor. J Clin Endocrinol Metab 1984; 58:313–319.

760. Sassolas G, Lejeune H, Trouillas J, et al. Gonadotropin-releasing hormone agonists are unsuccessful in reducing tumoral gonadotropin secretion in two patients with gonadotropin-secreting pituitary adenomas. J Clin Endocrinol Metab 1988; 67:180–185.

761. Zarate A, Fonseca ME, Mason M, et al. Gonadotropin-secreting pituitary adenoma with concomitant hypersecretion of testosterone and elevated sperm count. Treatment with LRH agonist. Acta Endocrinol 1986; 113:29–34.

762. Daneshdoost L, Molitch ME, Snyder PJ. Inhibition of follicle stimulating hormone secretion from gonadotroph adenomas by repetitive administration of a GnRH antagonist. Endoc Soc Abstr 1990; 366.

763. Kovacs K, Horvath E, Rewcastle NB, et al. Gonadotroph cell adenoma of the pituitary in a women with long-standing hypogonadism. Arch Gynecol 1980; 229:57–65.

764. Nicolis GL, Modhi G, Gabrilove JL. Gonadotropin producing pituitary adenomas. A case report and review of the literature. Mt Sinai J Med 1982; 49:297–304.

765. Beckers A, Stevenaert A, Mashiter K, et al. Follicle-stimulating hormone–secreting pituitary adenomas. J Clin Endocrinol Metab 1985; 61:525–528.

766. Miura M, Matsukado Y, Kodama T, et al. Clinical and histopathological characteristics of gonadotropin-producing pituitary adenomas. J Neurosurg 1985; 62:376–382.

767. Snyder PJ. Gonadotroph cell pituitary adenomas. Endocrinol Metab Clin North Am 1987; 16:755–764.

768. Nicolis G, Shimshi M, Allen C, et al. Gonadotropin-producing pituitary

adenoma in a man with long-standing primary hypogonadism. J Clin Endocrinol Metab 1988; 66:237–241.

769. Demura R, Jibiki K, Kubo O, et al. The significance of alpha-subunit as a tumor marker for gonadotropin-producing pituitary adenomas. J Clin Endocrinol Metab 1986; 63:564–569.

770. Trouillas J, Girod C, Sassolas G, et al. The human gonadotropic adenoma: pathologic diagnosis and hormonal correlations in 26 tumors. Semin Diagn Pathol 1986; 3:42–57.

Nonsecretory Adenoma

771. Klibanski A. Non-secretory pituitary tumors. Endocrinol Metab Clin North Am 1987; 16:793–804.

772. Heshmati HM, Turpin G, Kujas M, et al. The immunocytochemical heterogeneity of silent pituitary adenomas. Acta Endocrinol 1988; 118:533–537.

773. Jameson JL, Klibanski A, Black PM, et al. Glycoprotein hormone genes are expressed in clinically nonfunctioning pituitary adenomas. J Clin Invest 1987; 80:1472–1478.

774. Ebersold MJ, Quast LM, Laws ER Jr, et al. Long-term results in transsphenoidal removal of nonfunctioning pituitary adenomas. J Neurosurg 1986; 64:713–719.

775. Bevan JS, Burke CW. Non-functioning pituitary adenomas do not regress during bromocriptine therapy but possess membrane-bound dopamine receptors which bind bromocriptine. Clin Endocrinol 1986; 25:561–572.

776. D'Emden MC, Harrison LC. Rapid improvement in visual field defects following bromocriptine treatment of patients with non-functioning pituitary adenomas. Clin Endocrinol 1986; 25:697–702.

777. Johnston DG, Hall K, McGregor A, et al. Bromocriptine therapy for "nonfunctioning" pituitary tumors. Am J Med 1981; 71:1059–1061.

778. Kovacs K, Horvath E, Ryan N, et al. Null cell adenoma of the human pituitary. Virchows Arch [A] 1980; 387:165–174.

779. Kovacs K, Asa SL, Horvath E, et al. Null cell adenomas of the pituitary: attempts to resolve their cytogenesis. In: Lechago J, Kameya T, eds. Endocrine Pathology Update. Vol 1. Philadelphia: Field & Wood, 1990: 17–31.

780. Martinez AJ. The pathology of nonfunctional pituitary adenomas. Semin Diagn Pathol 1986; 3:83–94.

781. Asa SL, Gerrie BM, Singer W, et al. Gonadotropin secretion in vitro by human pituitary null cell adenomas and oncocytomas. J Clin Endocrinol Metab 1986; 62:1011–1019.

782. Yamada S, Asa SL, Kovacs K, et al. Analysis of hormone secretion by clinically nonfunctioning human pituitary adenomas using the reverse hemolytic plaque assay. J Clin Endocrinol Metab 1989; 68:73–80.

783. Sakurai T, Seo H, Yamamoto N, et al. Detection of mRNA of prolactin and ACTH in clinically nonfunctioning pituitary adenomas. J Neurosurg 1988; 69:653–659.

784. Kovacs K, Horvath E. Pituitary "chromophobe" adenoma composed of oncocytes. A light and electron microscopic study. Arch Pathol 1973; 95:235–239.

785. Landolt AM, Oswald UW. Histology and ultrastructure of an oncocytic adenoma of the human pituitary. Cancer 1973; 31:1099–1105.

786. Gunzl HJ, Saeger W, Diehl S, et al. Immunohistochemical analyses of oncocytic and chromophobe pituitary adenomas. Exp Clin Endocrinol 1988; 92:51–58.

787. Yamada S, Asa SL, Kovacs K. Oncocytomas and null cell adenomas of the human pituitary: morphometric and in vitro functional comparison. Virchows Arch [A] 1988; 413:333–339.

788. Peillon F, Le D, Garnier P, et al. Receptors and neurohormones in human pituitary adenomas. Horm Res 1989; 31:13–18.

789. Asa SL, Gerrie BM, Kovacs K, et al. Structure-function correlations of human pituitary gonadotroph adenomas in vitro. Lab Invest 1988; 58:403–410.

790. Kovacs K, Lloyd R, Horvath E, et al. Silent somatotroph adenomas of the human pituitary. A morphologic study of three cases including immunocytochemistry, electron microscopy, in vitro examination, and in situ hybridization. Am J Pathol 1989; 134:345–353.

Nonpituitary Sellar Mass

791. Carmel PW. Craniopharyngiomas. In: Wilkins RH, Rengachary SS, eds. Neurosurgery. Vol 1. New York: McGraw-Hill, 1985: 905–916.

792. Hunt WE, Sayers MP, Yashon D. Tumor of the sellar and parasellar area. In: Youmans JR, ed. Neurological Surgery. 2nd ed. Philadelphia: W. B. Saunders, 1973: 1412–1431.

793. Matson DD. Neurosurgery of Infancy and Childhood. Springfield, IL: Charles C Thomas, 1969.

794. Ross-Russell RW, Pennybaker JB. Craniopharyngioma in the elderly. J Neurol Neurosurg Psychiatry 1961; 24:1–13.

795. Baskin DS, Wilson CB. Surgical management of craniopharyngiomas. J Neurosurg 1986; 65:22–27.

796. Bartlett JR. Craniopharyngiomas—a summary of 85 cases. J Neurol Neurosurg Psychiatry 1971; 34:37–41.

797. Jenkins JS, Gilbert CJ, Ang V. Hypothalamic-pituitary function in

patients with craniopharyngiomas. J Clin Endocrinol Metab 1976; 43:394–399.

798. Daniels DL, Williams AL, Thornton RS, et al. Differential diagnosis of intrasellar tumors by computed tomography. Radiology 1981; 141:697–701.

799. Naidich TP, Pinto RS, Kushner MJ, et al. Evaluation of sellar and parasellar masses by computed tomography. Radiology 1976; 120:91–99.

800. Streja D, Teichner F, Marliss EB. Fifty-year survival after surgery for craniopharyngioma. JAMA 1975; 234:510–512.

801. Lyen KR, Grant DB. Endocrine function, morbidity, and mortality after surgery for craniopharyngioma. Arch Dis Child 1982; 57:837–841.

802. Lichter AS, Wara WM, Sheline GE, et al. The treatment of craniopharyngiomas. Int J Radiat Oncol Biol Phys 1977; 2:675–683.

803. Miyamoto M, Sugawa H, Mori T, et al. A case of hypopituitarism due to granulomatous and lymphocytic adenohypophysitis with minimal pituitary enlargement: a possible variant of lymphocytic adenohypophysitis. Endocrinol Jpn 1988; 35:607–616.

804. Mayfield RK, Levine JH, Gordon L, et al. Lymphoid adenohypophysitis presenting as a pituitary tumor. Am J Med 1980; 69:619–623.

805. Hassoun P, Anayssi E, Salti I. A case of granulomatous hypophysitis with hypopituitarism and minimal pituitary enlargement. J Neurol Neurosurg Psychiatry 1985; 48:949–951.

806. Asa SL, Bilbao JM, Kovacs K, et al. Lymphocytic hypophysitis of pregnancy resulting in hypopituitarism: a distinct clinicopathologic entity. Ann Intern Med 1981; 95:166–171.

807. McDermott MW, Griesdale DE, Berry K, et al. Lymphocytic adenohypophysitis. Can J Neurol Sci 1988; 15:38–43.

808. Jensen MD, Handwerger BS, Scheithauer BW, et al. Lymphocytic hypophysitis with isolated corticotropin deficiency. Ann Intern Med 1986; 105:200–203.

809. McGrail KM, Beyerl BD, Black PM, et al. Lymphocytic adenohypophysitis of pregnancy with complete recovery. Neurosurgery 1987; 20:791–793.

810. Meichner RH, Riggio S, Manz HJ, et al. Lymphocytic adenohypophysitis causing pituitary mass. Neurology 1987; 37:158–161.

811. Vanneste JA, Kamphorst W. Lymphocytic hypophysitis. Surg Neurol 1987; 28:145–149.

812. Gal R, Schwartz A, Gukovsky Oren S, et al. Lymphoid hypophysitis associated with sudden maternal death: report of a case review of the literature. Obstet Gynecol Surv 1986; 41:619–621.

813. Wild RA, Kepley M. Lymphocytic hypophysitis in a patient with amenorrhea and hyperprolactinemia. A case report. J Reprod Med 1986; 31:211–216.

814. Okamoto T, Moriyama E, Mizukawa N. Lymphoid adenohypophysitis. Acta Pathol Jpn 1986; 36:751–756.

815. Camins MB, Mount LA. Primary suprasellar atypical teratoma. Brain 1974; 97:447–456.

816. Takeuchi J, Handa H, Nagata I. Suprasellar germinoma. J Neurosurg 1978; 49:41–48.

817. Ghatak NR, Hirano A, Zimmerman HM. Intrasellar germinomas: a form of ectopic pinealoma. J Neurosurg 1969; 31:670–675.

818. Neuwelt EA, Frenkel EP, Smith RG. Suprasellar germinomas (ectopic pinealomas): aspects of immunological characterization and successful chemotherapeutic responses in recurrent disease. Neurosurgery 1980; 7:352–358.

819. Allen JC, Kim JH, Packer RJ. Neoadjuvant chemotherapy for newly diagnosed germ-cell tumors of the central nervous system. J Neurosurg 1987; 67:65–70.

820. Reid RL, Quigley ME, Yen SSC. Pituitary apoplexy. Arch Neurol 1985; 42:712–719.

821. Cardoso ER, Peterson EW. Pituitary apoplexy: a review. Neurosurgery 1984; 14:363–373.

822. Jacobi JD, Fishman LM, Daroff RB. Pituitary apoplexy in acromegaly followed by partial pituitary insufficiency. Arch Intern Med 1974; 134:559–561.

823. Markowitz S, Sherman L, Kolodny HD, et al. Acute pituitary vascular accident (pituitary apoplexy). Med Clin North Am 1981; 65:105–116.

824. Wakai S, Fukushima R, Teramoto A, et al. Pituitary apoplexy: its incidence and clinical significance. J Neurosurg 1981; 55:187–193.

825. Veldhuis JD, Hammond JM. Endocrine function after spontaneous infarction of the human pituitary: report, review, and reappraisal. Endocr Rev 1980; 1:100–107.

826. Ostrov SG, Quencer RM, Hoffman JC, et al. Hemorrhage within pituitary adenomas: how often associated with pituitary apoplexy syndrome? AJR 1989; 153:153–160.

827. Pelkonen R, Kuusisto A, Salmi J, et al. Pituitary function after pituitary apoplexy. Am J Med 1978; 65:773–778.

828. Wright RL, Ojemann RG, Drew JH. Hemorrhage into pituitary adenomata. Arch Neurol 1965; 12:326–331.

Miscellaneous References

829. Tanner JM, Davies PS. Clinical longitudinal standards for height and height velocity for North American children. J Pediatr 1985; 107:317–329.

830. Hartman ML, Faria ACS, Vance ML, et al. Temporal structure of in vivo growth hormone secretory events in man. Am J Physiol 1991; 260:E101–E110.

831. Hartman ML, Veldhuis JD, Thorner MO. Augmented growth hormone (GH) secretory burst frequency and amplitude mediate enhanced GH secretion during a two day fast in normal men. Second International Pituitary Congress, Palm Desert, CA, 1989 (abstract P-13).

832. Jefferson LS, Korner A. A direct effect of growth hormone on the incorporation of precursors into proteins and nucleic acids of perfused rat liver. Biochem J 1967; 104:826–832.

833. Griffin EE, Miller LL. Effects of hypophysectomy of liver donor on net synthesis of specific plasma proteins by the isolated perfused rat liver. Modulation of synthesis of albumin, fibrinogen, alpha 1–acid glycoprotein, alpha 2-(acute phase)–globulin, and haptoglobin by insulin, cortisol, triiodothyronine, and growth hormone. J Biol Chem 1974; 249:5062–5069.

834. McConaghey P, Sledge CB. Production of "sulphation factor" by the perfused liver. Nature 1970; 225:1249–1250.

835. Moon HD, Jentoft VL, Li CH. Effect of human growth hormone on growth of cells in tissue culture. Endocrinology 1962; 70:31–38.

836. Kostyo JL, Hotchkiss J, Knobil E. Stimulation of amino acid transport in isolated diaphragm by growth hormone added in vitro. Science 1959; 130:1653–1654.

837. Hjalmarson A, Isaksson O, Ahmen K. Effects of growth hormone and insulin on amino acid transport in perfused rat heart. Am J Physiol 1969; 217:1795–1802.

838. Ledet T. Growth hormone stimulating the growth of arterial medial cells in vitro. Absence of effect of insulin. Diabetes 1976; 25:1011–1017.

839. Goodman HM. Multiple effects of growth hormone on lipolysis. Endocrinology 1968; 83:300–308.

840. Fain JN, Kovacev VP, Scow RO. Effect of growth hormone and dexamethasone on lipolysis and metabolism in isolated fat cells of the rat. J Biol Chem 1965; 240:3522–3529.

841. Atkison PR, Weidman ER, Bhaumick B, et al. Release of somatomedin-like activity by cultured WI-38 human fibroblasts. Endocrinology 1980; 106:2006–2012.

842. Madsen K, Makower AM, Friberg U, et al. Effect of human growth hormone on proteoglycan synthesis in cultured rat chondrocytes. Acta Endocrinol 1985; 108:338–342.

843. Whitfield JF, MacManus JP, Rixon RH. Stimulation by growth hormone of deoxyribonucleic acid synthesis and proliferation of rat thymic lymphocytes. Horm Metab Res 1971; 3:28–33.

844. Desai LS, Lazarus H, Li CH, et al. Human leukemic cells. Effect of human growth hormone. Exp Cell Res 1973; 81:330–332.

845. Golde DW, Bersch N, Li CH. Growth hormone: species-specific stimulation of erythropoiesis in vitro. Science 1977; 196:1112–1113.

846. Spencer CA. Thyroid profiling for the 1990's: free T_4 estimate or sensitive TSH measurement. J Clin Immunol 1989; 12:82–89.

847. Veldhuis JD, Johnson ML. In vivo dynamics of luteinizing hormone secretion and clearance in man: assessment by deconvolution mechanics. J Clin Endocrinol Metab 1988; 66:1291–1300.

848. Urban RJ, Dahl KD, Padmanabhan V, et al. Specific regulatory actions of dihydrotestosterone and estradiol on the dynamics of FSH secretion and clearance in man. J Androl 1991; 12:27–35.

849. Urban RJ, Veldhuis JD, Dufau ML. Estrogen regulates the gonadotropin-releasing-hormone stimulated secretion of biologically active luteinizing hormone. J Clin Endocrinol Metab 1991; 72:661–668.

850. Veldhuis JD, Johnson ML, Dufau ML. Physiological attributes of endogenous bioactive luteinizing hormone secretory bursts in man. Am J Physiol 1989; 256:E199–E207.

851. Miyai K, Hayashizaki Y, Matsubara K. Familial hypothyroidism due to thyrotropin gene abnormality. Int Congr Endocrinol (Jpn) 1988; 1:545–550.

852. Hayashizaki Y, Hiroaka Y, Endo Y, et al. Thyroid-stimulating hormone (TSH) deficiency caused by a single base substitution in the CAGYC region of the beta subunit. EMBO J 1989; 8:2291.

853. Godowski PJ, Leung DW, Meacham LR, et al. Characterization of the human growth hormone receptor gene and demonstration of a partial gene deletion in two patients with Laron-type dwarfism. Proc Natl Acad Sci USA 1989; 86:8083–8087.

854. Brauner R, Malandry F, Rappaport R, et al. Growth and endocrine disorders in optic glioma. Eur J Pediatr 1990; 149:825–828.

855. Rappaport R, Brauner R. Growth and endocrine disorders secondary to cranial irradiation. Pediatr Res 1989; 25:561–567.

856. Sulmont V, Brauner R, Fontoura M, et al. Response to growth hormone treatment and final height after cranial or craniospinal irradiation. Acta Paediatr Scand 1990; 79:542–549.

857. March CM, Kletzky OA, Davajan V, et al. Longitudinal evaluation of

858. patients with untreated prolactin-secreting pituitary adenomas. Am J Obstet Gynecol 1981; 139:835–844.

858. von Werder K, Fahlbusch R, Rjosk H-K. Macroprolactinomas: clinical and therapeutic aspects. In: Tolis G, Stefanis C, Mountokalakis T, et al., eds. Prolactin and Prolactinomas. New York: Raven, 1983: 415–429.

859. Koppelman MC, Jaffe MJ, Rieth KG, et al. Hyperprolactinemia, amenorrhea, and galactorrhea. A retrospective assessment of twenty-five cases. Ann Intern Med 1984; 100:115–121.

860. Martin TL, Kim M, Malarkey WB. The natural history of idiopathic hyperprolactinemia. J Clin Endocrinol Metab 1985; 60:855–858.

861. Sisam DA, Sheehan JP, Sheeler LR. The natural history of untreated microprolactinomas. Fertil Steril 1987; 48:67–71.

862. Aubourg PR, Derome PJ, Peillon F, et al. Endocrine outcome after transsphenoidal adenomectomy for prolactinoma: prolactin levels and tumor size as predicting factors. Surg Neurol 1980; 14:141–143.

863. Charpentier G, de Plunkett T, Jedynak P, et al. Surgical treatment of prolactinomas. Short- and long-term results, prognostic factors. Horm Res 1985; 22:222–227.

864. Ciric I, Mikhael M, Stafford T, et al. Transsphenoidal microsurgery of pituitary macroadenomas with long-term follow-up results. J Neurosurg 1983; 59:395–401.

865. Faria MA Jr, Tindall GT. Transsphenoidal microsurgery for prolactin-secreting pituitary adenomas. J Neurosurg 1982; 56:33–43.

866. Grisoli F, Vincentelli F, Jaquet P, et al. Prolactin secreting adenoma in 22 men. Surg Neurol 1980; 13:241–247.

867. Keye WR Jr, Chang RJ, Monroe SE, et al. Prolactin-secreting pituitary adenomas in women. II. Menstrual function, pituitary reserves, and prolactin production following microsurgical removal. Am J Obstet Gynecol 1979; 134:360–365.

868. Landolt AM. Surgical treatment of pituitary prolactinomas: postoperative prolactin and fertility in seventy patients. Fertil Steril 1981; 35:620–625.

869. Randall RV, Kramer S, Abboud CF, et al. Transsphenoidal microsurgical treatment of prolactin-producing pituitary adenomas. Results in 100 patients. Mayo Clin Proc 1983; 58:108–121.

870. Rawe SE, Williamson HO, Levine JH, et al. Prolactinomas: surgical therapy, indications and results. Surg Neurol 1980; 14:161–167.

871. Schlechte JA, Sherman BM. Abnormal regulation of prolactin secretion after successful surgery for prolactin-secreting pituitary tumours. Clin Endocrinol 1981; 15:165–174.

872. Frohman LA, Downs TR. Ectopic GRH syndromes. In: Robbins RJ, Melmed S, eds. Acromegaly. A Century of Scientific and Clinical Progress. New York: Plenum, 1987: 115–125.

873. Grisoli F, Leclercq T, Jaquet P, et al. Transsphenoidal surgery for acromegaly—long-term results in 100 patients. Surg Neurol 1985; 23:513–519.

874. Serri O, Somma M, Comtois R, et al. Acromegaly: biochemical assessment of cure after long term follow-up of transsphenoidal selective adenomectomy. J Clin Endocrinol Metab 1985; 61:1185–1189.

875. Balagura S, Derome P, Guiot G. Acromegaly: analysis of 132 cases treated surgically. Neurosurgery 1981; 8:413–416.

876. Laws ER, Scheithauer BW, Carpenter S, et al. The pathogenesis of acromegaly: clinical and immunocytochemical analysis in 75 patients. J Neurosurg 1985; 63:35–38.

877. Fahlbusch R, Buchfelder M. Transsphenoidal surgery of parasellar pituitary adenomas. Acta Neurochir 1988; 92:93–99.

878. Ross DA, Wilson CB. Results of transsphenoidal microsurgery for growth hormone–secreting pituitary adenoma in a series of 214 patients. J Neurosurg 1988; 68:854–867.

879. Thorner MO, Besser GM. Successful treatment of acromegaly with bromocriptine. Postgrad Med J 1976; 52(1):71–74.

880. Wass JA, Thorner MO, Morris DV, et al. Long-term treatment of acromegaly with bromocriptine. Br Med J 1977; 1:875–878.

881. Belforte L, Camanni F, Chiodini PG, et al. Long-term treatment with 2-Br-alpha-ergocryptine in acromegaly. Acta Endocrinol 1977; 85:235–248.

882. Halse J, Haugen HN, Bohmer T. Bromocriptine treatment in acromegaly: clinical and biochemical effects. Acta Endocrinol 1977; 86:464–472.

883. Eskildsen PG, Svendsen PA, Vang L, et al. Long-term treatment of acromegaly with bromocriptine. Acta Endocrinol 1978; 87:687–700.

884. Lundin L, Ljunghall S, Wide L, et al. Bromocriptine therapy in eleven patients with acromegaly. Acta Endocrinol Suppl 1978; 216:207–216.

885. Besser GM, Wass JAH, Thorner MO. Bromocriptine in the medical management of acromegaly. In: Goldstein M, Calne DB, Lieberman A, et al., eds. Ergot Compounds and Brain Function: Neuroendocrine and Neuropsychiatric Aspects. New York: Raven, 1980: 191–198.

886. Lindholm J, Riishede J, Vestergaard S, et al. No effect of bromocriptine in acromegaly: a controlled trial. N Engl J Med 1981; 304:1450–1454.

THE POSTERIOR PITUITARY AND WATER METABOLISM

W. Brian Reeves and Thomas E. Andreoli

INTRODUCTION

The anatomy, the function, and the pathophysiology of the posterior pituitary neurohypophyseal system are considered in this chapter. Dysfunction of the neurohypophysis is most apparent clinically as a failure to regulate the osmolality of body fluid. Sudden alterations in body fluid osmolality may have lethal consequences as the result of abrupt changes in the volume of the central nervous system (CNS) that occur when the osmotic disturbance is acute: brain shrinkage in the hypertonic syndromes and brain swelling in the hypotonic syndromes. Therefore the coordinated responses involving vasopressin (AVP, also called antidiuretic hormone, ADH), thirst, and the kidney, which maintain osmotic homeostasis, are described here.

A convenient way of introducing osmoregulatory disorders is to consider briefly two of the cardinal physiologic processes in osmotic homeostasis: the water repletion reaction and the cell volume–regulatory response. The former provides a frame of reference for understanding the pathogenesis of these disorders, and the latter provides a means of considering the changes in brain volume that can attend osmoregulatory disorders.

The Water Repletion Reaction

In normal individuals the serum osmolality is virtually constant from day to day, and the serum sodium concentration is an accurate index of body water osmolality. The ranges of normal values for serum sodium concentrations and osmolality values in healthy individuals depend on small differences among individuals rather than on variations in the solute/water ratio of body fluids in a given individual.

Figure 7–1 presents a brief analysis of the key elements in water homeostasis. The solid lines indicate mechanisms that are activated by changes in effective extracellular fluid (ECF) osmolality and consequently by changes in cell volume; the dashed lines indicate mechanisms activated by changes in effective circulating volume; and the dotted lines indicate negative feedback limbs. Figure 7–1 illustrates the sensor elements that adjust water balance. Osmoreceptors, both for AVP release and for thirst, respond to small changes in

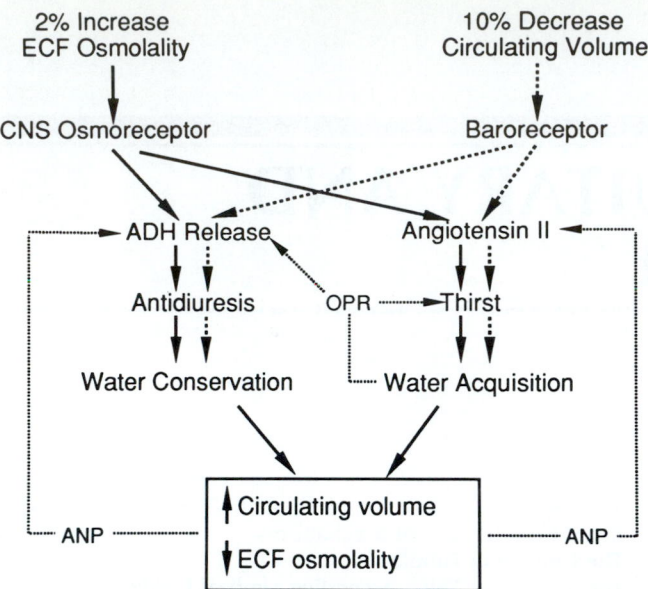

Figure 7–1. A schematic illustration of the water repletion reaction. Solid lines indicate osmotically stimulated pathways and dashed lines indicate volume-stimulated pathways. The dotted lines indicate negative feedback pathways. ANP, atrial natriuretic peptide; AVP, vasopressin; CNS, central nervous system; ECF, extracellular fluid; OPR, oropharyngeal reflex.

effective ECF osmolality, whereas baroreceptors respond to changes in effective circulating volume. As little as a 2% increase in effective ECF osmolality causes shrinkage of osmoreceptor cells and stimulation of both AVP release from the posterior pituitary and thirst. A second way of stimulating both AVP release and thirst involves volume-mediated stimuli that can operate independently of changes in plasma osmolality. When the effective circulating volume is reduced by approximately 10%, these volume-dependent mechanisms stimulate AVP release.

It was previously thought that increases in plasma osmolality and in plasma volume directly suppress water repletion. It now seems likely, however (see Fig. 7–1), that suppression of thirst and of AVP release depends on two factors: the oropharyngeal reflex and the release of atrial natriuretic peptide (ANP), the latter occurring, in all likelihood, both systemically and in the CNS. These issues are discussed later.

When considered in these terms, certain features of the water repletion reaction are particularly noteworthy. First, redundant mechanisms, namely, thirst and the antidiuretic effect, protect osmotic homeostasis. Second, the water repletion reaction operates at varying levels of sensitivity. That is, osmotic release of AVP and osmotic stimuli of thirst require rather small changes in effective ECF osmolality, whereas nonosmotic stimuli of thirst and of AVP release occur only in association with rather large reductions, approximately 10%, in effective circulating volume.

Cell Volume Regulation

The goals of fluid transport between extracellular and intracellular compartments are to maintain constancy of cell volume and to maintain a negligible hydrostatic pressure gradient between the cells and the ECF. Because cell membranes are freely permeable to water, the two goals are achieved when the ECF osmolality is normal and when intracellular and extracellular osmolality values are identical. The water repletion reaction (see Fig. 7–1) functions to maintain a normal ECF osmolality. The general mechanism

for maintaining identical osmolality in intracellular fluid and ECF involves the balance between the tendency for dissipative processes (i.e., ionic "leak" processes) to reach equilibrium and the action of the ubiquitous Na⁺,K⁺-ATPase to extrude Na⁺ from cells while pumping K⁺ into cells.

More specifically, sodium leakage from the ECF into cells and potassium leakage out of cells into the ECF are counterbalanced exactly by active outward sodium transport coupled to active inward potassium transport, which are both mediated by Na⁺,K⁺-ATPase. These active transport events maintain the intracellular cation (and therefore osmolar) content equal to that of ECF.

These considerations indicate that cation transport that is mediated by Na⁺,K⁺-ATPase is the major factor regulating cell volume when the effective ECF osmolality is normal. Thus it may be argued that in normal individuals the Na⁺,K⁺-ATPase maintains the equality of intracellular cation concentrations, whereas the water repletion reaction (see Fig. 7–1) determines the solute/water ratio in body fluids.

Finally, when the effective ECF osmolality is increased or decreased, additional processes maintain the constancy of cell volume. When cells are exposed to an elevated extracellular osmolality, the initial response is the loss of cell water with an increase in the *concentration* of solutes within the cell.[1] Conversely, extracellular hypotonicity causes water movement into cells and a dilution of the cell contents. Thus, acutely, cells establish osmotic equilibrium with their surroundings at the expense of cell volume.

Many cells also possess osmoregulatory mechanisms that enable the cells either to gain solute, as is the case in hypertonicity, or to lose solute, as is the case in hypotonicity, and thereby to return cell volume toward normal (Fig. 7–2). The nature of the transport processes that are responsible for this gain or loss of solute varies from tissue to tissue. In the kidney medulla, for instance, in which large changes in extracellular osmolality are common, cells adjust to hypertonicity in two phases. In the early phase, cell volume is increased as a result of NaCl transport into cells.[2] In the second phase, NaCl is replaced by organic solutes, or osmolytes, such as betaine, sorbitol, and glycerol phosphorylcholine, which are less perturbing to cell function.[1, 3]

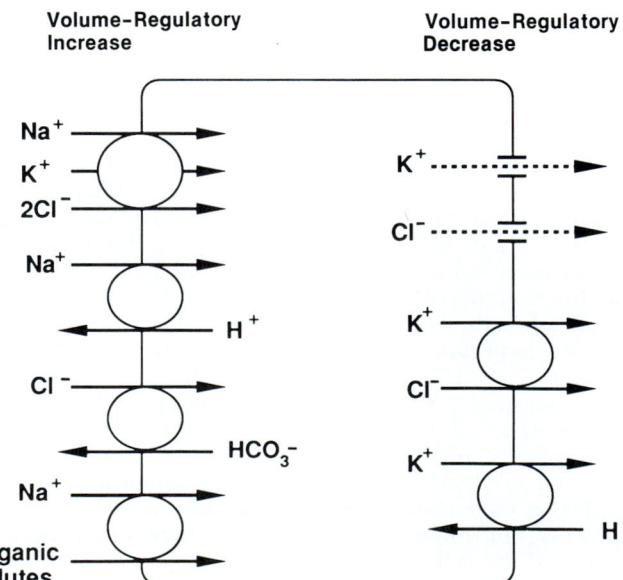

Figure 7–2. A schematic representation of some of the cell membrane transport systems that help to regulate cell volume. Cell shrinkage stimulates solute uptake pathways (*left*) and results in an increase in cell volume. Cell swelling activates solute loss, primarily via conductive pathways for K⁺ and Cl⁻.

The Clinical Syndromes: Definitions

Derangements in osmotic homeostasis, either hypertonic or hypotonic, depend on derangements in the operation of the water repletion reaction. The clinical manifestations of these disorders are due to alterations in cell volume, particularly in the CNS; changes in effective circulating volume; and, in the case of central diabetes insipidus, local disturbances produced, for example, by an intracranial neoplasm.

The *hypertonic* syndromes develop when the ratio of solutes to water in body fluids is increased. These disorders occur when water intake is less than the sum of renal plus extrarenal water losses; in the steady state, the net water balance may be zero.

The *hypotonic* syndromes occur when the ratio of solutes to water in body fluids is reduced, and the serum osmolality and serum sodium concentration are both reduced in parallel. The hypotonic syndromes develop when water intake exceeds the sum of renal plus extrarenal water losses; in chronic hyponatremia, however, water intake and water output may be equal.

The pathophysiology, clinical manifestation, and management of these disorders are discussed in detail in subsequent sections of this chapter.

THE NEUROHYPOPHYSIS

Historical Perspectives

The continuity of cell bodies of hypothalamic neurons that are located in the supraoptic nucleus (SON) and the paraventricular nucleus (PVN) with unmyelinated fibers that terminate in the posterior pituitary gland was established by Ramon y Cajal.[4] The notion that the CNS might be involved in the control of renal water excretion was introduced with Claude Bernard's observation[5] in 1859 that a piqûre in the vicinity of the corpus restiforme resulted in a persistent, nonglycosuric water diuresis that was distinct from the glycosuric diuresis associated with more posterior lesions. Subsequent reports noted the association of polyuria with basilar skull fractures,[6] bitemporal hemianopia,[7,8] and gunshot wounds to the pituitary.[9]

A different line of evidence implicating the posterior pituitary gland as a modulator of renal water excretion originated in the demonstration by Magnus and Schäfer[10] that the administration of posterior pituitary extracts to experimental animals regularly produced a diuresis. This effect, which was subsequently shown to be due to an alteration in renal hemodynamics, established the erroneous concept that the posterior pituitary contained a diuretic substance. Cushing[11] observed transient polyuria after experimental canine hypophysectomies and also noted polyuria and polydipsia in patients with pituitary tumors. He attributed the polyuria to "the excessive elaboration of the hormone . . . which activates renal secretion," although he admitted that "there is some difficulty in satisfactorily explaining the diuresis which may accompany hypopituitarism."[11]

The discovery of the antidiuretic effect of posterior pituitary extraction is credited to Farini[12] and von den Velden.[13] Working independently, these two clinicians were struck by the evidence of pathological pituitary destruction in patients with diabetes insipidus and concluded, contrary to the prevailing view at the time, that diabetes insipidus resulted from a deficiency of a posterior pituitary hormone. They provided confirmation of this view by documenting that extracts of the posterior pituitary gland diminished the polyuria in patients with diabetes insipidus.[12,13]

In 1920 Camus and Roussy[14] produced a variety of lesions at the base of the brain in dogs and demonstrated that polyuria regularly followed disruption of the optopeduncular tract at the hypophyseal infundibulum. An interesting observation made by these experimentalists was that a "clean" removal of the pituitary gland without injury to the hypothalamus did not produce polyuria. These workers thus declared emphatically: "the lesion which determines polyuria in no way concerns the pituitary body."

Using an elaborate preparation of heart, lung, and kidney, Verney[15] subsequently demonstrated that the exaggerated urine flow from an isolated perfused kidney returned toward normal if the blood that was perfusing the kidney passed through the cephalic circulation of a living dog; perfusion with blood that was circulated through the hindquarters of the dog did not affect urine flow, and perfusion with blood from the cephalic circulation of a hypophysectomized dog was equally ineffective in diminishing urine flow. He concluded that an intact pituitary added a factor to the circulation that tonically regulated urine volume. In 1929 Verney[15] reviewed the arguments that related the neurohypophysis and renal water excretion. After noting the observation by Priestley[16] that the rapid consumption of water led to a measurable decrease in the electrical conductivity of the serum, Verney concluded that "diabetes insipidus is due to the divorce of the pituitary body from the kidney whilst water ingestion in all probability leads to a temporary inhibition in the function of the pituitary, and so to the release of the kidney from its anti-diuretic influence."

The work that would finally establish the functional relations among the hypothalamic nuclei, the posterior pituitary, and the modulation of renal water excretion began with Broers in 1933.[17] Using a stereotactic apparatus to produce lesions in the brains of cats, Broers showed that selective destruction of the SON, the infundibulum, or the pituitary stalk could lead to a polyuric state and that the induced lesion was, in each case, associated with atrophy of both the SON, and the PVN. Fisher and co-workers[18] subsequently expanded this work by showing that bilateral, but not unilateral, lesions of the supraopticohypophyseal tract produced a polyuric state and that both the SON and the PVN atrophied on the same side as that of the tract lesion. Furthermore, the posterior pituitary showed atrophy in relation to the lesions of the hypothalamic nuclei: bilateral nuclear destruction caused complete posterior pituitary atrophy and unilateral nuclear lesions caused partial, unilateral posterior pituitary atrophy.

In 1936 Fisher and Ingram[19] added a final anatomical note that set the stage for studies of the origin of the antidiuretic hormone. They demonstrated that atrophied tissue remaining in the posterior pituitary fossa after destruction of the supraopticohypophyseal tract contained no pressor or antidiuretic activity; this finding was interpreted to indicate that the posterior pituitary axons were carriers of the antidiuretic substance.

Structure of the Neurohypophysis

The neurohypophysis consists of a set of hypothalmic nuclei that house the perikarya of the magnicellular neurons that are responsible for synthesis of oxytocin and AVP; the axonal processes of these neurons, which form the supraopticohypophyseal tract; and the termini of these neurons within the posterior lobe of the pituitary. The posterior pituitary gland also contains small cells known as pituicytes, which are glial elements apparently unrelated to the neuroendocrine function of the gland.

The locations of the neurohypophyseal nuclei, first

identified by Gomori-positive staining characteristics, are shown schematically in Figure 7–3. The SON is situated along the proximal half of the optic tract, whereas PVN lies vertically within the anterolateral wall of the third ventricle; scattered neurons bridge the two principal nuclei in some species, thus forming the internuclear group. The SON consists almost entirely of magnicellular neurons, all of which project to the posterior pituitary;[20] the PVN contains magnicellular neurons that project to the posterior pituitary, as well as parvicellular neurons that project to the median eminence or to autonomic centers in the brain stem.[21] By using specific antibodies to AVP and oxytocin or to their respective neurophysins (see later), immunocytochemical staining has demonstrated cells containing AVP and oxytocin in both nuclei.[22, 23] However, the hormones are located in different cells.[23, 24] In several species, including humans, AVP-containing magnicellular neurons occupy the more ventral aspects of the SON and are located more centrally within the PVN, whereas oxytocin-containing magnicellular neurons tend to be in the dorsal portion of the SON and in the periphery of the PVN.[25] AVP is also found in certain parvicellular neurons in the PVN and in some magnicellular neurons near the organum vasculosum of the lamina terminalis (OVLT).[26] AVP secretion by parvicellular neurons, which terminate in the hypophyseal-portal capillary bed, accounts for the high concentration of AVP in portal blood.[27, 28] These cells also secrete corticotropin-releasing hormone (CRH), and after adrenalectomy the number of neurons that stain for both CRH and AVP increases dramatically.[29, 30] AVP secretion into the portal blood may potentiate the effect of CRH on corticotropin (ACTH, adrenocorticotropin) secretion.[27] The physiological role of AVP release at the OVLT is unknown.

The axons of the magnicellular neurons are unmyelinated fibers that average less than 1 μm in diameter, but they include numerous varicosities (Herring bodies), approximately 20 μm in diameter, that contain clusters of Gomori-positive granules.[31] Microtubules can be traced down the length of the axons but do not appear to radiate into the granule-filled dilations. These axons terminate in the posterior lobe (pars nervosa) of the pituitary gland; they make up about 40% of the bulk of the gland.

The axonal nerve endings are distinctive in two respects.[31] First, terminal sacculations contain electron-lucent vesicles, and preterminal dilations do not contain vesicles but do contain Gomori-positive granules. Second, the terminal sacculations abut directly onto basement membranes that are separated by a perivascular space from basement membranes of capillaries originating in the inferior hypophyseal artery, and the preterminal dilations are removed from capillary contact.

The ability to secrete AVP or oxytocin in response to appropriate stimuli requires that the neurosecretory cells in the PVN and SON receive information from various sensor elements. For example, information from low-pressure baroreceptors is carried to the brain stem by cranial nerves IX and X. These afferents relay in the nucleus tractus solitarius and a noradrenergic nucleus (A_1) before ultimately projecting to the magnicellular regions of the PVN and SON.[32] Additional noradrenergic afferents arise from the locus coeruleus (A_6) and solitary tract and project to the AVP and CRH parvicellular neurons of the medial PVN.[33] Cholinergic innervation of the SON is provided by cholinergic neurons that are situated immediately adjacent to the SON.[34, 35] Nicotinic and muscarinic receptors are present in the SON and PVN, respectively, and stimulation of these receptors increases AVP secretion.[36]

Two circumventricular organs, the subfornical organ (SFO) and the OVLT, also provide input to the AVP neurons of the SON and PVN. These organs lie outside of the blood-brain barrier and therefore may be important for osmoreception and interaction with blood-borne hormones, such as angiotensin II (AII).[37] Both the anatomy and the physiology of the afferent pathways to the PVN and the SON are poorly defined.

Hormone Biosynthesis, Transport, and Metabolism

Kamm and co-workers[38] isolated from whole posterior pituitary extracts one agent with oxytocic but no pressor activity, and a second agent with antidiuretic and pressor activity but little uterus-stimulating activity. Because of the basic nature of both hypophyseal compounds, Kamm termed them *hypophamines.* Taking as a lead the cysteine content of the compounds that were isolated by Kamm, du Vigneaud[39] began a project that led to the isolation and amino acid sequencing of oxytocin from ox pituitary and of lysine vasopressin from hog pituitary. This effort culminated in 1954 with the first synthetic production of a polypeptide hormone, oxytocin; the synthesis of lysine vasopressin occurred in 1957 and that of AVP, in 1958.[40]

The hormones that are elaborated by most mammalian neurohypohyses are oxytocin and AVP. As shown in Figure 7–4, both oxytocin and AVP are octapeptides with a molecular mass of approximately 1.1 kd. In both molecules, a sulfhydryl bond between the cysteine residues at positions 1 and 6 forms a single cystine moiety, yielding a ring comprising 20 atoms. At least nine neurohypophyseal octapeptides have been isolated from vertebrates.[39] AVP is the antidiuretic hormone in all mammals except hogs and other members of the suborder Suina, in which lysine vasopressin (containing lysine rather than arginine in position 8) occurs. The antidiuretic hormone among lower vertebrates is arginine vasotocin, which contains the same three COOH-terminal acyclic amino acids as AVP but the "tocin" ring structure of oxytocin (see Fig. 7–4).

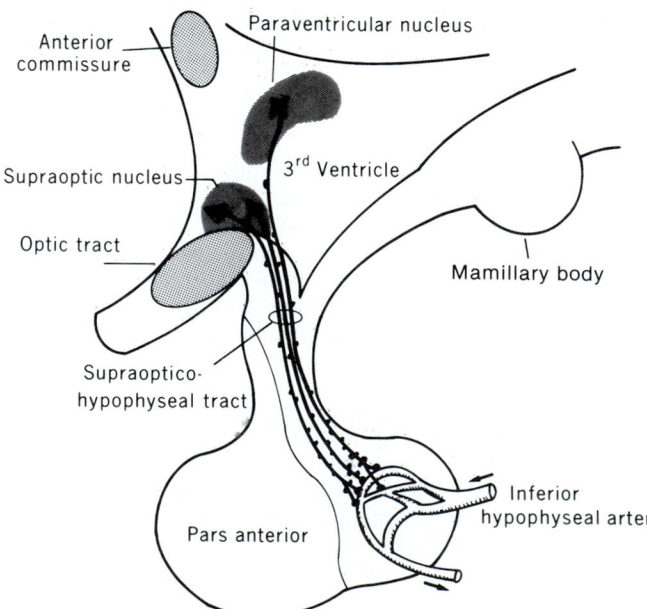

Figure 7–3. A schematic illustration of the neurohypophysis showing hypothalamic magnicellular nuclei, the supraopticohypophyseal tract with Herring bodies, and nerve endings forming on capillaries of the posterior pituitary.

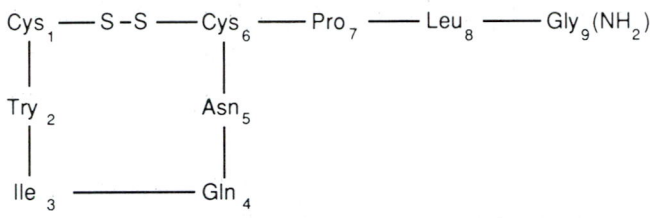

**Arginine Vasopressin
(AVP)**

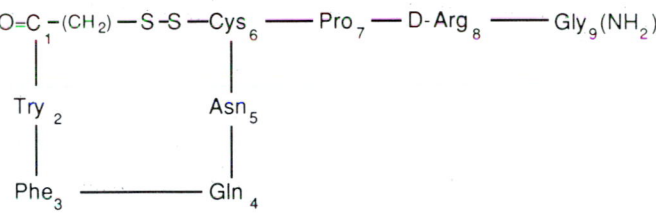

Oxytocin

O=C -(CH₂)—S—S —Cys₆ —— Pro₇ — D-Arg₈ —— Gly₉(NH₂)

**1-Desamino-8-D-Arginine Vasopressin
(Desmopressin)**

Figure 7–4. Chemical structures of the major posterior pituitary hormones.

The Neurophysins

The association of AVP with a binding protein derives from the work of van Dyke and co-workers[41] and Pickering and Jones,[42] who described the protein in extracts of bovine posterior pituitary. This "van Dyke protein," a cystine-rich protein complex of approximately 30 kd, had all the biological activity of the crude extract. Acher and colleagues[43] isolated a pure protein, which they termed *neurophysine*, from the protein complex and showed that mixing the soluble protein with AVP formed a noncovalently linked complex that was precipitable by NaCl.

The neurophysins are sulfur-rich proteins with molecular masses of 9 to 10 kd; they are soluble in 10% NaCl solutions at acid pH (3.9) and form insoluble, ionic complexes with added neurohypophyseal hormones.[42] Neurophysins contain 92 to 95 amino acid residues with conservation of the central portion of molecules from all species;[42] a high content of cysteine residues results in extensive disulfide binding within the molecule. The high cysteine content of neurophysin also accounts for the Gomori staining characteristics of neurosecretory granules (NSGs). The wide variety of molecular weights determined for different neurophysins has led to the suggestion that neurophysins are transported as polymeric aggregates within NSGs, thereby reducing the osmotic activity of the intravesicular protein.[42, 44]

Separate hormone-specific neurophysins exist for vasopressin and oxytocin in each species.[45] The nomenclature for the neurophysins, which is based on electrophoretic mobility, is not uniform. In the cow and the pig the vasopressin-associated neurophysin is designated as NpII, and the oxytocin-associated neurophysin, NpI. In humans the AVP-associated neurophysin is designated as the nicotine-stimulated neurophysin, and the oxytocin-associated neurophysin, the estrogen-stimulated neurophysin. A third neurophysin, which has been detected in certain species, is a truncated form of one of the two major neurophysins.[45]

Hormone Biosynthesis

Figure 7–5 summarizes the cardinal steps in hormone biosynthesis. Sachs and colleagues[46, 47] initiated studies that elucidated the biosynthetic origins of the neurohypophyseal hormones and that confirmed the existence of a common precursor for the two species. After an 8- to 36-h infusion of [35S]-labeled cysteine into the third ventricle of dog brain, AVP from the hypothalamus showed a two- to threefold greater incorporation of label than AVP from posterior pituitary; labeled AVP failed to appear in the posterior pituitary when the pituitary stalk was sectioned. Furthermore, hypothalamus–median eminence slices incorporated [35S]cysteine into AVP in vitro, whereas pituitary stalk and posterior pituitary tissue was incapable of such synthesis.[46, 48]

After ventricular injection of [35S]cysteine, AVP was rapidly labeled at the level of the SON, appeared in the median eminence after about 1 h, and was present in the posterior pituitary after about 1½ h; the appearance of labeled AVP in the posterior pituitary was abolished by

Figure 7–5. Flow diagram for the pathway of posterior pituitary hormone biosynthesis.

Form	Molecular Weight	Synthetic Step
Pre-prohormone	≃ 21,000	Protein synthesis; magnicellular neuron ribosomes
Prohormone	≃ 23,000	Glycosylation and membrane packaging; magnicellular neuron Golgi apparatus
Neurosecretory granule (NSG)	$(23,000)_n$	Transport down supraopticohypophyseal tract as osmotically inactive granules
Neurophysin	≃ 10,000	Storage in posterior pituitary; cleavage within NSG
+		
Hormone	≃ 1,100	

colchicine.[49] These observations suggest that axonal transport of hormone from the SON to the posterior pituitary is an active process.

The labeled precursors that were isolated from the SON were larger than and had different isoelectric points from either neurophysin or AVP. In vitro trypsin digestion of the larger labeled proteins yielded 10-kd peptides identical with neurophysin, as well as smaller 1-kd peptides that comigrated with AVP on gel filtration and were bound by antibodies to AVP.[49, 50]

These results indicated that AVP and neurophysin are derived from a common precursor. Further proof has come from analysis of the AVP gene.[51, 52] The organization of the AVP precursor peptide and the AVP gene of the rat are illustrated in Figure 7–6. The hormone precursor contains three peptide regions: a signal peptide and AVP at the NH_2 terminus, a neurophysin II region, and a COOH-terminal glycoprotein region of unknown significance.[53] Each of these regions of the precursor protein is, in turn, coded for by one of three exons of the AVP precursor gene. The human AVP gene is on chromosome 20.[54]

Thus the main steps in the biosynthesis of AVP are as follows: transcription of the AVP precursor messenger RNA (mRNA); translation of the mRNA to a pre-prohormone of 166 amino acids; removal of the signal peptide sequence while the peptide is still attached to the ribosome, to yield the prohormone; and conversion of the prohormone peptide into AVP and neurophysin II. This final step occurs within the NSG during its transport to the neurohypophysis.[55] The extrahypothalamic mRNA is shorter than the hypothalamic mRNA because of differences in the length of the poly(A) tail.

These types of studies have yielded an interesting insight into the possible pathogenesis of hereditary central diabetes insipidus. The Brattleboro rat lacks the ability to produce hypothalamic AVP and therefore is a useful model for the study of central diabetes insipidus. In the Brattleboro rat, the defect is due to a single base deletion in the exon encoding neurophysin II.[56] Although the AVP-containing region of the precursor is translated normally, the frameshift that results from the nucleotide deletion causes misreading of the COOH-terminal codons, including the stop codon, so that translation proceeds to the extreme 3′ end of the poly(A) tail of the mRNA. The resulting protein is not processed normally into AVP and neurophysin II so that no hormone is detectable in the pituitary, even though AVP mRNA is present in relatively normal amounts in the hypothalamus nuclei.[56]

Neurosecretory Cells

The concept of a neurosecretory cell derives largely from the work of Scharrer and Scharrer,[57] who identified "gland-nerve" cells by the content of Gomori-stainable granules and drops of colloid alongside classic Nissl bodies, the long axonal processes of the cells, and the close association of the cells with an intricate capillary bed. NSGs approximately 160 nm in diameter that appear to be identical with those present in cell bodies of the SON and PVN are present along the length of the supraopticohypophyseal tract leading to the posterior pituitary[25] and in nerve endings located in the posterior pituitary. The neurosecretory material is depleted in proportion to the reduction in AVP content of posterior pituitary gland after dehydration, whereas repletion of NSGs in the posterior pituitary occurs with hydration.[57] These observations led Scharrer and Scharrer to conclude that the posterior pituitary is a storage depot for AVP that is produced in hypothalamic cells and transported via the axons in NSGs.[57] Subsequent studies have shown

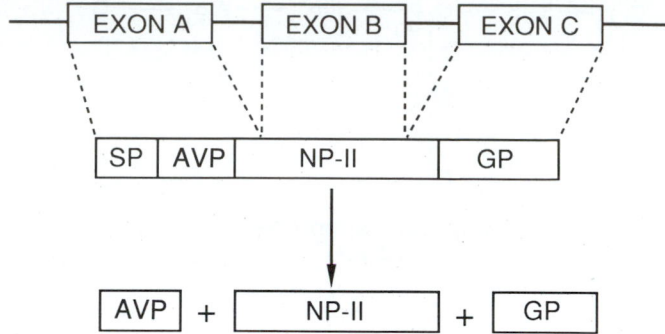

Figure 7–6. A schematic representation of the organization of the AVP gene and its relation to the pre-prohormone and final peptide products. GP, glycoprotein; NP-II, neurophysin II; SP, signal peptide.

axonal NSG transport rates of about 200 mm/d, in contrast to approximately 4 mm/d for axonal protoplasmic flow, a finding that indicates facilitated axonal transport of NSGs.[31] Furthermore, NSG transport is inhibited by the microtubule disrupter colchicine,[31] which suggests that microtubules participate in NSG movement. The presence of AVP in NSGs was demonstrated by Weinstein and co-workers,[58] who isolated granules from dog posterior pituitary and showed that the isolated particles are morphologically identical with in situ NSGs (100 to 200 nm in diameter, surrounded by a single membrane) and that isolated granules contained active AVP that could be released by treatments that disrupt the granule membrane. Finally, studies of NSGs from bovine posterior pituitary[59] indicated that NSGs are packets of hormone and an associated binding protein.

Neuropeptide Release

Evidence for the relation between electrical activity of the hypothalamohypophyseal axis and release of posterior pituitary hormones was first provided by Harris,[60] who implanted electrodes in the vicinity of the supraoptic nucleus of rabbits and demonstrated that electrical stimulation of the neurohypophysis in these animals causes inhibition of urine flow. Magnicellular neurons secreting AVP respond to osmotic stimulation by firing in a characteristic phasic pattern, with bursts of 5 to 15 Hz separated by silent periods. Stimulation of AVP-secreting neurons by dehydration causes a progressive recruitment of neurons into phasic activity,[61] which suggests a titration of hormone release relative to the magnitude of osmolar derangement.

Although cells of the SON generate action potentials after application of hyperosmotic solutions in vitro,[62] the magnicellular neurons are believed to be at least one synapse removed from the osmoreceptors.[63] Cholinergic stimuli, such as nicotine, release AVP directly.[64, 65] The microiontophoretic application of acetylcholine in the presence of selective nicotinic or muscarinic receptor blockers has suggested that excitatory nicotinic receptors and inhibitory muscarinic receptors modulate activity in the SON.[64] Acetylcholine may be the synaptic transmitter between osmoreceptor and magnicellular neurons.

Neurohypophyseal secretion is believed to occur by exocytosis, which is a quantal process.[64] The exocytotic events involve fusion of membranes from NSGs with plasma membranes; granule opening at the site of fusion; and release of granule material, including AVP and neurophysin II, into the extracellular space. Because all of the AVP-neurophysin complexes within the posterior pituitary gland are not readily available for release, AVP and neurophysin II may be segregated into two pools: a readily released pool and a storage pool.[66] The readily released pool is composed of AVP-neurophysin complexes within NSGs that are located adjacent to plasma membranes, and the storage pool contains AVP-neurophysin complexes in granules that are remote from plasma membranes.

Exocytosis of the NSGs is triggered by neurotransmitter-induced depolarization of the AVP-producing hypothalamic magnicellular neurons. The control of AVP-producing neuron electrical activity by various neurotransmitters and afferent pathways is discussed later. The partial depolarization that is caused by these neurotransmitters, however, results in the generation and propagation of a sodium-dependent, tetrodotoxin-sensitive[67] action potential. Voltage-sensitive calcium channels, which are opened by the membrane depolarization, allow calcium to flow into the nerve endings.[64, 68, 69] The calcium entry, in turn, activates, by an as-yet unidentified mechanism, exocytosis of NSGs and release of AVP and neurophysin II into the circulation. The rate of AVP secretion depends on both the rate and the pattern of neuron firing. For example, stimulation of AVP-producing neurons in rapid, intermittent bursts results in greater AVP secretion than does the same degree of stimulation delivered at regular intervals.[70]

Distribution and Metabolism

Lysine vasopressin or AVP entering the circulation is distributed in a volume approximately equal to the extracellular space.[71] Nearly all of the hormone in the plasma of dogs and humans exists in an unbound form,[71] which, because of its relatively low molecular weight, permeates peripheral and glomerular capillaries readily. In humans the total clearance time of AVP, which represents both metabolic degradation and renal excretion, is in the range of 30 to 40 min.[72, 73] These observations[71, 73, 74] indicate that, in humans, suppression of endogenous AVP release results in a detectable change from the antidiuretic to the water diuretic state after approximately 30 min.

Metabolic degradation of AVP appears to be mediated through binding of biologically active AVP to specific hormone receptors.[72–75] At least four sites of proteolytic cleavage for the hormone have been identified. AVP (see Fig. 7–4) may undergo cleavage: within the liver, by rupture of the 1,6-disulfide bond;[76, 77] within the brain, by cleavage at position 6,7 and by subsequent hydrolysis of 9-glycinamide from the tripeptide;[78] within a variety of tissues, by hydrolysis of the peptide bond between the hemicystine residue in position 1 and the tyrosine in position 2;[78, 79] and within the kidney, by proteolysis of the peptide bond between residues 8 and 9, which results in glycinamide release.[80] A peptidase of 442 kd, which cleaves glycinamide and results in biological inactivation, has been isolated from renal plasma membranes.[81] Renal excretion is the second method for elimination of circulating hormone and accounts for about one fourth of total metabolic clearance.[71, 82]

Chemistry

The hormones that are elaborated by most mammalian neurohypophyses include oxytocin and AVP. Figure 7–4 shows the structure of AVP and that of a commonly used analogue, 1-desamino-8-D-arginine vasopressin (desmopressin, DDAVP; see later). There are many synthetic analogues of AVP. The vast majority of these agents possess various degrees of antidiuretic, vasopressor, and uterotonic activities. There also exist analogues that function as competitive antagonists of both the vasopressor and antidiuretic action of the hormone.

AVP acts via tissue receptors classified as V_1 receptors in smooth muscle and V_2 receptors in renal epithelia; only the latter receptors activate adenylate cyclase.[83] Antidiuretic activity in the intact animal depends on the ability of a peptide to bind to the renal receptor, to stimulate the adenylate cyclase system, and to resist metabolic degradation. Thus peptides that activate adenylate cyclase poorly may still produce a maximal antidiuretic response in the intact animal.[84, 85] In many cases synthetic analogues of AVP with reduced receptor affinity and reduced ability to activate adenylate cyclase in vitro exhibit potent and specific antidiuretic activity in the intact animal.[86–88] Given these apparent discrepancies between in vitro and in vivo observations, it is clear that metabolic stability plays an important role in determining in vivo antidiuretic activity.

Deamination at position 1 reduces receptor affinity and so renders the compound more resistant to metabolic degradation. As a result, 1-desamino-arginine vasopressin (dAVP) possesses antidiuretic activity fourfold higher than that of AVP. Substitution of D-arginine for L-arginine at position 8 decreases the pressor activity so that the product, DAVP, has an antidiuretic/pressor activity ratio of 28.[88] Deamination at position 1 combined with substitution of D-arginine for L-arginine at position 8 yields a compound (desmopressin) that has a long duration of action and an antidiuretic/pressor ratio of approximately 3000.[88] Desmopressin is the most widely used synthetic AVP analogue. Further substitution of the hydrophobic amino acid valine for glutamine at position 4 (dDVAVP) prolongs the duration of action and abolishes the pressor effects, thus making the compound the most specific antidiuretic agonist reported.[88]

Selective antagonists have also been developed to the antidiuretic effects of AVP. The first such compound contains a pentamethylene ring at position 1, an O-ethyltyrosine substitution at position 2, and a valine substitution for glutamine at position 4.[89] This compound, d(CH_2)$_5$ Tyr (ET)VAVP, is a potent AVP antagonist for both V_1 and V_2 receptors. Manning and Sawyer[90] showed that selective modification of d(CH_2)$_5$ Tyr (ET)VAVP can yield compounds with enhanced antidiuretic antagonist activity and increased selectivity for antidiuretic over antivasopressor activity. The substitution of the L-Tyr (ET) at position 2 of d(CH_2)$_5$ Tyr (ET)VAVP by aliphatic D-amino acids, such as D-isoleucine, D-leucine, or D-valine, results in increased antidiuretic/antivasopressor selectivity.[91] Further substitution at position 4 with aminobutyric acid, isoleucine, or alanine leads to even greater antidiuretic/antivasopressor selectivity.[92] Finally, the COOH-terminal glycine-NH_2 may be deleted or substituted by a variety of amino acid amides with full retention of antagonist activity.[93] Although they promote an initial, brief antidiuresis, these analogues competitively inhibit the antidiuretic response to exogenous and endogenous vasopressin and result in a water diuresis in normally hydrated rats that is equal in intensity to that seen in AVP-deficient Brattleboro rats.[89] These antagonists competitively inhibit lysine vasopressin binding and adenylate cyclase activation in renal medullary membrane preparations.[94–96]

In isolated segments of collecting ducts and medullary thick ascending limbs, these antagonists inhibit the AVP-induced increase in adenylate cyclase activity but do not affect the response to other agonists such as glucagon or parathyroid hormone.[97] In isolated perfused collecting duct segments[97] and in toad urinary bladder,[98] d(CH_2) Tyr (ET)VAVP completely prevents the AVP-induced increase in water permeability but has no effect on the response to forskolin, an agent that directly activates the catalytic subunit of adenylate cyclase. In other words, these agents antagonize the effect of AVP by preventing the binding of AVP to its receptor and thus preventing the subsequent activation of adenylate cyclase.[95] These antagonists are useful for analyzing the physiology of the system and may ultimately be useful clinically in the management of acute water intoxication that is associated with the syndrome of inappropriate antidiuretic hormone (SIADH) (see later).

THE CONTROL OF VASOPRESSIN RELEASE

To maintain plasma osmolality at a constant level, AVP secretion from the posterior pituitary must vary in response to small changes in plasma osmolality. However, AVP may also be released when the plasma osmolality is less than normal, if the effective circulating volume is released.

Osmotic Regulation of Vasopressin Release

Studies by Verney[99] of the relation between changes in plasma osmolality and AVP release showed that injections of hypertonic NaCl or sucrose, but not urea solutions, provided prompt antidiuresis. He postulated the presence of osmoreceptors, located in the distribution of the internal carotid arteries, that stimulated AVP release when plasma osmolality is raised by solutes to which osmoreceptors are impermeable. The failure of hypertonic urea injections to provoke antidiuresis was interpreted as indicating that these osmoreceptors are freely permeable to urea. McKinley and co-workers[100] showed in addition that carotid infusion of hypertonic urea solutions leads to a higher cerebrospinal fluid sodium concentration than infusion of either hypertonic saline or sucrose, yet it produces only minor antidiuresis compared with these two solutions. They postulated that the osmoreceptors must be located in an area of the brain lacking an effective blood-brain barrier.

The precise location of the osmoreceptors is still debated. Leng[101] showed that the neurons of the SON are themselves osmosensitive in that microinjections of hypertonic saline into the SON produce a depolarization of the membrane potential and increased frequency of action potentials. He and co-workers argued that the SON itself is the most important site of osmoreception.[102]

Other evidence, however, suggests that the osmoreceptor is separate from the SON. First, studies of McKinley and colleagues[100] and of Thrasher and co-workers[103] indicated that the osmoreceptor lies outside of the blood-brain barrier. Second, the observation that neurotransmitter antagonists block osmotically induced AVP release[104] suggests a need for neural afferents in the process. Third, lesions of the OVLT, which reside outside of the blood-brain barrier (see earlier), impair AVP secretion.[104] Finally, interruption of the pathways between the region of the anteroventral aspect of the third ventricle (AV3V), which includes the OVLT, and the SON produces hypernatremia in rats.[105, 106] Thus afferent fibers, probably from the OVLT, play an important role in the osmotic stimulation of AVP secretion.

Because normal individuals are not ordinarily in a state of water diuresis, it is generally believed that the maintenance of normal plasma osmolality requires the tonic secretion of AVP. It is instructive in this regard to consider the relationship between serum osmolality and plasma AVP concentrations determined by radioimmunoassay.[107] As shown in Figure 7–7, for plasma osmolalities below 280 mmol/kg, plasma AVP levels are in the range of 0.45 to 1.4 pmol/L (0.5 to 1.5 ng/L); for those above 280 mmol/kg, plasma AVP levels rise in proportion to plasma osmolality according to the following relation: plasma AVP = 0.38 (plasma osmolality − 280).[108–110] Thus a plasma osmolality

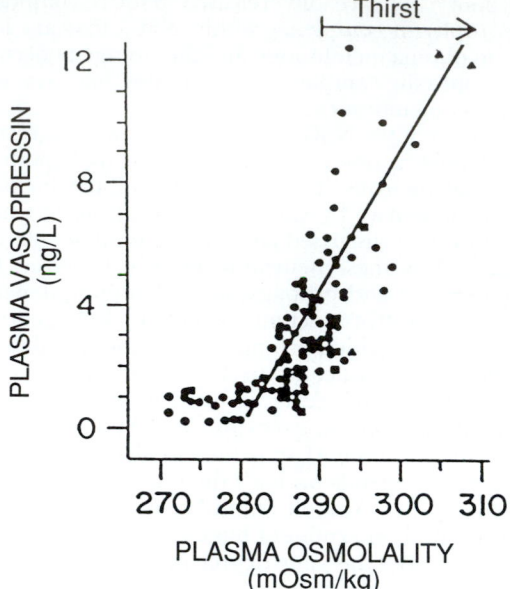

Figure 7–7. The relationship between plasma osmolality and plasma AVP level. To convert AVP values to picomoles per liter, divide by 1.1. (Adapted from Robertson GL, Berl T. Water metabolism. In: Brenner BM, Rector FC Jr, eds. The Kidney. 3rd ed. Philadelphia: W. B. Saunders, 1986: 385–432.)

of 280 mmol/kg is considered to be the osmotic threshold for AVP release, a view that coincides well with Verney's deduction that maintenance of normal plasma osmolality depends on the tonic secretion of AVP. In practical terms, a 0.9 pmol/L (1 ng/L) rise in the level of plasma AVP translates into an increase in urine osmolality of about 200 mmol/kg. This "gain" factor means that maximal urine concentrations are produced at a plasma osmolality of about 290 to 292 mmol/kg and a plasma AVP level of 4.6 to 5.5 pmol/L (5 to 6 ng/L).

Nonosmotic Regulation of Vasopressin Release

In 1935 Peters[111] recognized the role of ADH in volume regulation by commenting that "in subjects who have become dehydrated . . . volume of body fluids seems to become more important than . . . osmotic pressure as a determinant of renal activity." A large body of evidence now indicates that volume-mediated release of AVP may occur as a consequence of stimuli arising from "volume receptors," or baroreceptors. Gauer and Henry[112] termed loci in the venous bed of the systemic circulation, the right side of the heart, and the left atrium the *low-pressure* baroreceptors, and loci within the systemic arterial system of the carotid sinus and aortic arch the *high-pressure* baroreceptors. The electrical activity of the baroreceptor is related to the degree of stretch in the vessel wall. Increases in pressure and wall tension cause an increase in the rate of firing of the receptor. Conversely, decreases in blood pressure or blood volume result in a decrease in the electrical activity of the baroreceptor.[113]

The afferent pathways for the atrial and carotid bifurcation baroreceptors appear to be the vagus and the glossopharyngeal nerves, respectively. Following synapses in the nucleus tractus solitarius, noradrenergic projections relay baroreceptor input to the PVN and the SON.[63, 113] Baroreceptors exert an inhibitory influence on AVP secretion under resting conditions, and severing of all baroreceptor afferents results in a marked increase in plasma AVP levels. In addition, stimulation of baroreceptors by balloon distention of either the left atrium or the carotid bifurcation inhibits electrical activity in the SON.[63] This inhibitory influence is abolished by sections of the vagus nerve or local anesthesia of the carotid bifurcation.

Although each of the baroreceptors can influence AVP secretion, the most important one seems to be the left atrial baroreceptor.[113] Thus atrial baroreceptors respond to smaller changes in blood volume than do arterial receptors;[114, 115] balloon distention of the left atrium inhibits AVP secretion more effectively than does distention of the right atrium; and cardiac denervation markedly attenuates the secretion of AVP in response to hemorrhage.[116]

Specific radioimmunoassays for AVP have provided a measure of the sensitivity of the baroreceptor mechanism (Fig. 7–8). In humans acute reductions in arterial blood pressure exceeding 5 to 10% cause an exponential rise in AVP secretion.[110] Likewise, volume depletion in humans[117] and in a variety of animal species[118–120] produces little elevation in plasma AVP levels until blood volume decreases by more than 8 to 10%. Further volume depletion results in exponential increases in plasma AVP levels.

Further interplay between osmotic and nonosmotic stimuli for AVP release was demonstrated by Quillen and Cowley[119] in studies of conscious dogs whose left atrial pressure was manipulated and whose response of plasma AVP levels to osmotic stimulation was measured. They found that decreases in left atrial pressure reduced the osmotic threshold and increased the sensitivity for osmotic AVP release, whereas increases in left atrial pressure raised the threshold and dampened the sensitivity for osmotic AVP release (Fig. 7–9). This change in set point was confirmed by the demonstration that adequate water loading can suppress AVP secretion further even in the presence of hyponatremia.[118, 121] The resetting of the osmotic threshold in response to nonosmotic stimuli may involve opioid-secretory neurons and can be abolished by opioid antagonists.[121]

Chemical Mediators of Vasopressin Release

Another dimension of complexity to understanding nonosmotic mechanisms for AVP release has been added with recognition that AVP release can also be modulated by agents that have either systemic hemodynamic effects or CNS actions. Table 7–1 provides some drugs, neurotransmitters, and other chemical agents that modulate the regulation of AVP release either via peripheral nervous system or CNS effects.

Catecholamines

Schrier and colleagues[122] have summarized the results of studies that provide evidence for a hemodynamic role of alpha- and beta-adrenergic agents in mediating AVP release as the primary means of affecting renal water excretion. The beta-agonist isoproterenol causes antidiuresis in normal rats, whereas the alpha-agonist norepinephrine reduces urine osmolality. Neither agent has an effect on Brattleboro rats lacking AVP. These results indicate that the effects on water excretion are secondary to stimulation (beta-agonists) or suppression (alpha-agonists) of endogenous AVP release.[123]

Adrenergic agents may also stimulate central release of AVP through a neurotransmitter function. An abundance of nerve terminals containing norepinephrine has been demonstrated in both the SON and the PVN through histochemical and immunocytochemical fluorescence techniques.[65, 124] Central norepinephrine fibers stimulate AVP

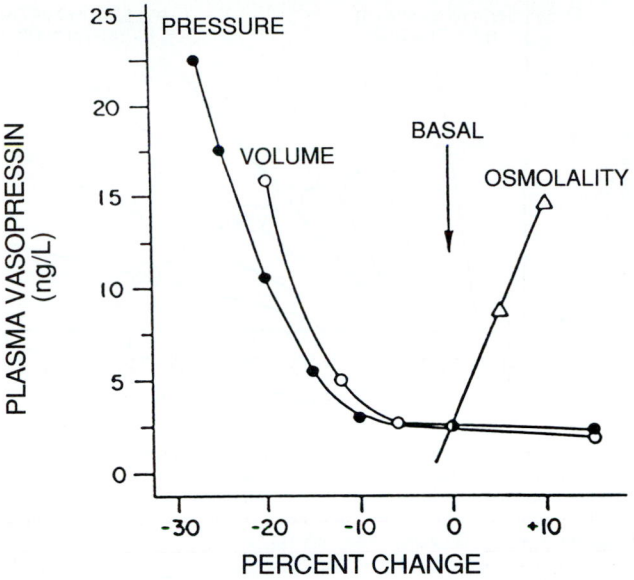

Figure 7–8. The relationship between plasma AVP and changes in plasma osmolality, blood volume, and mean arterial pressure in humans. To convert AVP values to picomoles per liter, divide by 1.1. (Adapted from Robertson GL, Berl T. Water metabolism. In: Brenner BM, Rector FC Jr, eds. The Kidney. 3rd ed. Philadelphia: W. B. Saunders, 1986: 385–432.)

secretion via alpha-1—receptors located on the AVP-producing neurons.[125–127]

Angiotensin II

The renin-angiotensin system also participates in the regulation of AVP release. Nerve cells and fibers that contain AII have been detected in the SFO and in the magnicellular division of the PVN and SON.[128] Likewise, AII stimulates the electrical activity of many neurons in the SFO, PVN, and SON.[129] The SFO lies outside of the blood-brain barrier and may be responsible for conveying blood-borne signals to the hypothalamic nuclei. Peripherally or centrally administered AII, for instance, increases AVP secretion in the rat.[130, 131] This response can be abolished by lesions of the SFO[130] or by transection of the SFO efferents.[132]

Electrophysiological evidence also indicates that AII modulates AVP release. Neurons in the SFO with efferent projections to the PVN, identified by antidromic stimulation, are stimulated by intravenously administered AII.[132] In addition, in rat brain slices AII directly stimulates AVP-producing cells in the SON.[129] Thus AII may stimulate AVP

TABLE 7–1. Agents That Alter Vasopressin Release

Agents That Enhance Release	Agents That Suppress Release
Prostaglandin E$_2$	Phenytoin
Morphine and narcotic analogues	Alcohol
Nicotine	Alpha-adrenergic agents
Beta-adrenergic agents	Atrial natriuretic peptide
Angiotensin II	
Anesthetic agents	
Hypoxia	
Hypercapnia	
Vincristine	
Cyclophosphamide	
Clofibrate	
Carbamazepine	
Barbiturates	
Acetylcholine	
Histamine	
Metoclopramide	

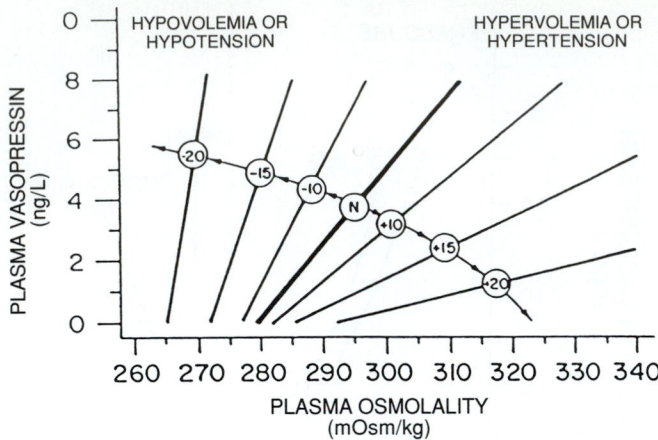

Figure 7–9. The effect of changes in blood volume or arterial pressure on the relation between plasma osmolality and plasma AVP activity. To convert AVP values to picomoles per liter, divide by 1.1. (Modified from Robertson GL, Berl T. Water metabolism. In: Brenner BM, Rector FC Jr, eds. The Kidney. 3rd ed. Philadelphia: W. B. Saunders, 1986: 385–432.)

release through a direct action on AVP-producing neurons and by stimulating afferent pathways from other regions of the brain. In humans the intravenous infusion of AII stimulates AVP release,[133] and reduction of AII by the converting enzyme inhibitor captopril inhibits AVP release.[134] In one study, however, in which plasma AII levels were increased fivefold by sodium depletion, no change in plasma AVP levels was detected.[135]

Opiates

It has long been known that morphine induces antidiuresis. The demonstration of the presence of endogenous opiates within the neurohypophysis and the association of leu-enkephalin (see Chapter 5) with AVP-containing nerve terminals[136] have led to a reinvestigation of the relation between opiates and AVP release. Studies with isolated rat neurohypophyses[126, 137] and with conscious dogs[138] and rats[139, 140] have demonstrated that opioids, acting through kappa-receptors,[117, 140] inhibit rather than stimulate AVP secretion. In addition to direct effects on AVP-producing cells, opioids also appear to suppress AVP secretion by inhibiting the release of norepinephrine from neurohypophyseal nerve terminals.[126] As mentioned earlier, norepinephrine stimulates AVP secretion.

Prostaglandins

Endogenous CNS prostaglandins may modulate the response of AVP release to osmotic stimulation. Intraventricular infusions of E prostaglandins[65] raise plasma AVP levels in the absence of changes in systemic hemodynamics. In close agreement with these results, Hoffman and co-workers[141] found that intraventricular prostaglandin synthesis inhibition by indomethacin attenuated AVP release to an osmotic stimulus, although release could be effected by exogenous prostaglandin E_2 (PGE_2) even with indomethacin present.

Anesthetics

Although anesthesia commonly causes antidiuresis, Forsling and Ullmann[142] found that only halothane anesthesia leads to a persistent antidiuretic state. These results coincide with those of studies with humans undergoing anesthesia for surgery, in whom plasma AVP levels rise only after the initiation of the surgical procedure.[142]

Chemoreceptors

A fall in arterial oxygen tension (PaO_2) to below 60 mm Hg has been associated with a rise in mean arterial pressure and with a marked rise in plasma AVP concentrations; the catecholamine-depleting agent guanethidine almost totally eliminated the rise in plasma AVP levels.[142] The latter result is consistent with arguments that propose an adrenergic step in the stimulation of AVP release. Electrophysiological studies[63] of the SON showed increased activity of SON neurons when the PcO_2 of arterial blood was elevated. Local anesthesia of the carotid bodies eliminated this response, which indicates that arterial chemoreceptors also influence the secretion of AVP from the neurohypophysis.

Atrial Natriuretic Peptide

As indicated in Figure 7–1, ANP may provide negative feedback for the release of AVP. AVP, principally through its vasopressor action, may stimulate the release of ANP.[143] ANP, in turn, may inhibit both the release of AVP and the effect of AVP on the permeability of the renal collecting duct to water.[144]

ANP-containing nerve cell bodies have been detected in the AV3V region of the brain.[145] This region, which surrounds the third ventricle and includes the OVLT and connections to the SFO, plays an important role in the control of body fluid homeostasis. Injection of ANP into the cerebral ventricles of rats in vivo[146, 147] or superfusion of hypothalamus-pituitary explants with ANP in vitro[146, 148, 149] inhibits the secretion of AVP.

Oropharyngeal Stimulation

As noted in Figure 7–1, a second level of feedback control of AVP release involves the oropharyngeal reflex. This term refers to the prompt suppression of AVP secretion after the ingestion of water. In both animals and humans[150–153] suppression occurs before the absorption of the ingested water and precedes any fall in the plasma osmolality. That is, the inhibition of AVP secretion is an anticipatory response to the subsequent absorption of water and fall in plasma osmolality. Indeed, suppression of AVP secretion occurs even if the ingested water is diverted from the stomach through a fistula.[150] Moreover, the ingested fluid need not be hypotonic. Ingestion of isotonic[150] and even hypertonic[154] solutions (but not solid foods[152]) also suppress AVP release, at least transiently. Cold liquids appear to elicit a stronger oropharyngeal reflex than warm liquids.[153] This finding may explain the curious preference of patients with diabetes insipidus for ice water. The rapidity with which AVP secretion and hypothalamic electrical activity are suppressed[155] and the lack of a requirement for the gastric absorption of fluid suggest that neural mechanisms mediate the response. The similarities between the oropharyngeal suppression of AVP release and the anticipatory control of drinking are striking and may indicate a common mediator, e.g., intracerebral ANP.

THIRST

The acquisition of water to preserve body fluid tonicity is governed by the sense of thirst, which, in turn, is regulated by many of the same factors that determine AVP release. The response of thirst to osmotic (hypertonic) stimuli is sufficiently powerful that significant hypertonicity does not develop even in the total absence of AVP in conscious individuals who have free access to water. The osmotic threshold for thirst stimulation in humans and other primates is reached with a 2 to 3% increase in plasma osmolality, a value about 10 mmol/kg higher than the value that stimulates AVP release.[151, 156, 157] Thirst-mediated water intake also attends pronounced falls in effective ECF volume and often continues, as in severe loss of gastrointestinal fluids, decompensated cirrhosis with ascites, and severe congestive heart failure, despite significant diminution in body fluid osmolality.

Osmotic Regulation of Thirst

In 1881 Nothnagel[158] first suggested the existence of a thirst center in the CNS based on his observation of a patient who developed severe thirst after a head injury. Following the work of Verney,[99] Andersson and Rundgren[159] demonstrated that injections of hypertonic NaCl into the medial hypothalamus elicited excessive drinking in water-replete goats, which suggests osmoreceptor involvement in the regulation of water intake. Ablation of tissue surrounding the OVLT in the midline of the anterior wall of the optic recess of sheep significantly reduced the water intake subsequent to intracarotid infusion of hypertonic NaCl.[160] This work suggests that an osmoreceptor mechanism for thirst stimulation is located in or close to the OVLT, just as osmoregulation of AVP seems to be controlled from this region of the brain.[104–106] The specificities of the osmoregulation of thirst and of AVP release are also similar: hypertonic NaCl stimulates both thirst and AVP release, whereas hypertonic urea or glucose stimulates neither. In spite of the functional similarities of the osmoregulation of thirst and AVP secretion, electrophysiological studies indicate that they are mediated by two distinct, but adjacent, osmoreceptors. Andersson and McCann[161] found that immediate drinking could be induced in animals by electrical stimulation of the anterior wall of the third ventricle. Stimulation at the SON or PVN did not elicit drinking but caused antidiuresis, whereas anterior stimulation in the internuclear region caused both drinking and antidiuresis.

AII is a potent dipsogenic agent when injected directly into the third ventricle[162] and may also mediate osmotically stimulated thirst. Intraventricular infusion of the AII inhibitor saralasin slowed the onset of drinking in one group of dehydrated animals but had no effect on water consumption in another group.[162, 163] However, the addition of the cholinergic inhibitor atropine to saralasin suppressed drinking in the latter group.[163] Thus there may be parallel pathways for thirst regulation, with AII being more important in the response to a nonosmotic stimulus. A further association between AII and osmotic thirst stimulation has been shown by the presence of AII receptors on the OVLT and by the ablation of the dipsogenic effect of intraventricularly administered AII when the OVLT is destroyed.[162]

Volume-Mediated Thirst

Alterations in baroreceptor function, such as those that occur with underfilling of the low-pressure thoracic circulation, elicit drinking,[159] and crushing of the left atrial appendage in sheep abolishes the drinking response to hypovolemia while leaving intact the response to hyperosmolality.[164] This response is mediated via nerve traffic along the vagus nerve. On the other hand, although it is apparent that hypovolemia stimulates the renin-angiotensin system, there is still controversy as to whether blood-borne AII has access to the thirst centers and as to whether peripherally generated AII participates in the hypovolemic thirst response. The dipsogenic effects of AII may be mediated via a nerve-stimulated renin-angiotensin system within the brain.[159]

Satiation of Thirst

There appear to be two major patterns of water repletion in response to hypertonic dehydration, an observation first made in 1938 by Dill[165] on the basis of his experiments with himself and his dog as test subjects in a desert environment. When given access to water, dogs, sheep, goats, and camels drink an amount that closely approximates the amount lost during dehydration.[166] Passage of water through the pharynx and out an esophageal fistula only temporarily suppresses drinking, as does distention of the stomach by a balloon, yet drinking halts before any water might be absorbed into the bloodstream.[167] The second pattern, exhibited by rats, rabbits, and humans, involves replenishment of about half of the water lost in 10 to 12 min, which is about the time required for ingested water to arrive at body tissues;[166] further water intake takes place over another 20 to 30 min.

Ramsay and co-workers[167] demonstrated that, in animals with hypertonic volume depletion, intracarotid infusions of water that are sufficient to restore the osmolality of the carotid circulation to normal, but not to affect osmolality outside the CNS, caused a 70% decrease in drinking. Restoration of the ECF volume deficit in these animals with intravenous isotonic NaCl, which does not ameliorate the plasma hypertonicity, reduced drinking by about 30%. In contrast, thirst in primates depends almost totally on hyperosmolality, with minimal dependence on ECF volume contraction.[157] These findings coincide with observations that left atrial stretch receptors do little to regulate AVP release in primates[168] and have led to the suggestion that decreased dependence of thirst on volume stimuli is an adaptive correlate to the upright posture of primates.[157, 168] In humans the ingestion of water is an even more complex process, which is influenced by pharyngeal, gastrointestinal, thermal, chemical, and social factors, but "permanent" satisfaction of thirst occurs only when the volume of water ingested is sufficient to return body fluid osmolality to normal levels.[159]

OXYTOCIN

General

Oxytocin is the second cyclic octapeptide hormone that is produced in magnicellar nuclei and is stored in the posterior pituitary. Oxytocin, like AVP, appears to be synthesized as a single 20-kd peptide molecule, termed prooxyphysin, which consists of the 1-kd peptide hormone and its specific, nonglycosylated 10-kd carrier protein, type I neurophysin.[42] Neurons capable of synthesizing oxytocin occur in both the SON and the PVN, with a tendency for oxytocin-containing cells to cluster in more rostral aspects of these nuclei. Oxytocin is packaged in secretory granules, is stored in the posterior pituitary, and, like AVP, seems to enter the portal system of the neurohypophysis by calcium-dependent exocytosis of the membrane-bound granules on nerve cell stimulation. However, oxytocin secretion is characterized by distinct bursts of electrical activity superimposed on a background of continuous firing activity.[63] This pattern is to be compared with the phasic electrical discharge and progressive recruitment of AVP-secreting neurons.[63]

Oxytocin Release

The primary stimuli for oxytocin release are mechanical distention of the reproductive tract (vagina) and stimulation of the nipples by suckling; both stimuli act through neural pathways to effect this release. Like AVP release, oxytocin release is stimulated by plasma hypertonicity. In conscious dogs and rats, the rise in the plasma concentration of oxytocin is comparable to that of AVP at any given rise in plasma osmolality.[169, 170] Likewise, isotonic volume contraction causes an increase in plasma oxytocin levels, although less than that of AVP.[169]

As noted in a previous section, the magnicellular neurons of the hypothalamus receive extensive input from structures within the AV3V region. Electrical stimulation of the AV3V region increases the firing rate of oxytocin-secreting neurons and causes oxytocin release. Lesions in the AV3V region abolish the release of oxytocin in response to hyperosmolality but not in response to suckling or parturition.[171] The pattern of electrical activity of oxytocin-secreting neurons, and thus of hormone secretion, depends on the physiological stimulus: suckling causes firing in brief, synchronized bursts; parturition causes bursts of activity superimposed on a background of increased activity; and hyperosmolality causes a gradual increase in the rate of firing.[171]

Like AVP secretion, the secretion of oxytocin is modulated by a number of centrally acting chemical mediators (Table 7–2). Endogenous opioids inhibit the secretion of oxytocin.[126, 172–174] This inhibition is mediated both at the level of the cell body to reduce electrical activity and at the neurosecretory terminals to reduce the amount of hormone secretion.[126] In addition to their direct, receptor-mediated effects on oxytocin-secreting neurons, opioids may modulate oxytocin secretion by inhibiting norepinephrine release from neurohypophyseal terminals.[127, 173] Different classes of opioid receptors may mediate the inhibition in response to different stimuli of oxytocin secretion.[174]

Intraventricular injection of AII stimulates oxytocin secretion in the rat.[140] Perfusion of rat brain slices with AII evokes excitatory responses in oxytocin-secreting neurons in the SON and in cells of the AV3V and SFO.[129] These regions may be important pathways for the conveyance of blood-borne signals to the hypothalamic nuclei.[175]

Nausea, satiety, and cholecystokinin, each acting through a vagal afferent pathway, stimulate oxytocin secretion.[176] A role for oxytocin in regulating food intake has not been established.

Relaxin, which is an ovarian peptide hormone that acts primarily to suppress uterine contraction and to relax pelvic connective tissue during parturition,[177] may also affect oxytocin secretion. Intravenous or intraventricular injection of relaxin suppresses reflex milk ejection in lactating rats,[178] and, in isolated neural lobes and neurosecretory terminals, relaxin exerts a dual effect on oxytocin release. Relaxin inhibits the basal release of oxytocin and AVP but potentiates their release in response to electrical stimulation.[179] It is not known if the effects on oxytocin release are due to locally produced or circulating relaxin.

TABLE 7–2. Factors That Influence Oxytocin Secretion

Physiological	Chemical
Parturition	*Stimulatory*
Suckling/breast stimulation	Angiotensin II
ECF hypertonicity	Cholecystokinin
Nausea	Vasoactive intestinal peptide
Volume contraction	Norepinephrine
Satiety	*Inhibitory*
	Opioids
	Relaxin
	ANP

Actions of Oxytocin

Oxytocin stimulates uterine contractions at parturition and stimulates smooth muscle contraction in the mammary gland during suckling. It also promotes maternal behavior.[180] Oxytocin may have other endocrine and paracrine functions in a wide variety of tissues; for example, oxytocin, oxytocin mRNA, or both are present in several nonhypothalamic sites such as ovary, uterus, placenta, testis, renal medulla, thymus, and anterior pituitary (reviewed in ref. 181). The physiological roles of locally produced oxytocin in these tissues are not yet well defined (Table 7–3).

Finally, oxytocin and AVP have similarities with regard to water homeostasis. That oxytocin can influence water metabolism is well documented in anuran epithelia,[182] in which oxytocin binds to high-affinity receptors, stimulates cellular accumulation of cyclic AMP (cAMP), and increases the natriferic and hydro-osmotic responses of the tissue. These actions are analogous to the action of AVP on either anuran epithelia or mammalian renal tubules. Although oxytocin production and release are not necessarily impaired in central diabetes insipidus in humans,[183] the effects of oxytocin secretion on water homeostasis in normal individuals are unknown. However, pharmacological doses of oxytocin, such as those used for pregnancy termination and, occasionally, for induction of labor, alter the metabolism of water by the kidney.[184] One unit of oxytocin, as defined by uterotonic activity, has about 0.01 IU of antidiuretic activity. Severe water intoxication can occur in women who receive infusions of oxytocin at high rates, usually greater than 20 mIU/min, and who are simultaneously given hypotonic fluids, usually in excess of 3.5 L.[183–185] A definite antidiuresis is notable at infusion rates of 15 mIU/min and is near maximal at 30 mIU/min, with the antidiuretic effect becoming apparent 10 to 15 min after the onset of infusion and continuing 10 to 15 min after its cessation.

THE RENAL CONTRIBUTION TO OSMOTIC HOMEOSTASIS

Renal Countercurrent Mechanisms

From the evolutionary standpoint, the ability to concentrate urine coincides with the appearance of the loop of Henle. This structure consists of three anatomically and functionally distinct regions interposed between proximal and distal tubules: the thin descending limb, the thin ascending limb, and the thick ascending limb. Although all mammalian nephrons possess this structure, the maximal level to which the urine can be concentrated depends, in a general way, on the fraction of nephrons whose loops of Henle dip deep into the papilla, the so-called long loops of Henle. The average adult kidney contains about 1 million nephrons, and approximately 15% of these are long looped.

Modern views of renal concentrating and diluting mechanisms have their origin in the work of Kuhn and Ryffel,[186] who considered the descending and ascending limbs of Henle as parallel tubes that are joined by a hairpin turn; oppositely directed flows in the two tubes permitted small differences in osmolality between fluid in the descending and ascending limbs at any level of the renal medulla (the so-called single effect) to be amplified many-fold along the length of the loop of Henle. Gottschalk and colleagues provided confirmation of the countercurrent hypothesis: urine in the loop of Henle at the papillary tip is as concentrated as that in the collecting duct during antidiuresis, fluid

TABLE 7–3. Localization of Oxytocin in Peripheral Tissues

Tissue	Immunoreactive Oxytocin	Oxytocin mRNA	Possible Function
Ovary	+	+	Modulation of uterine prostaglandin release
Uterus	+	–	?
Placenta	+	–	Uterine contraction
Testis	+	+	Modulation of seminiferous tubule contraction
Adrenal	+	+	Modulation of steroidogenesis and/or catecholamine secretion
Thymus	+	+	Lymphokine production
Anterior Pituitary	+	+	Regulation of corticotropin and prolactin secretion

Modified from Clements JA, Funder JW. Arginine vasopressin and oxytocin in organs outside the nervous system. In: Martini L, Ganong WF, eds. Frontiers in Neuroendocrinology. Vol 10. New York: Raven, 1988: 117–152.

entering the early distal convolution is hypotonic to plasma in both the absence and the presence of AVP,[187] and approximately 20% of the glomerular filtrate is absorbed in the loop of Henle.[188] Because proximal tubular fluid absorption is an isotonic process, Gottschalk[188] reasoned that the combination of fluid absorption in the loop of Henle and early distal tubular fluid hypotonicity meant that, during transit through the loop, more solute than water was removed from tubular fluid and therefore that the factor driving the countercurrent multiplier was solute abstraction from ascending limbs.

The active transport properties of the thick ascending limb of Henle (TALH) were investigated by Burg and Green[189] and Rocha and Kokko,[190] who confirmed that the thick ascending limb of the loop of Henle is impermeable to water and transported solute actively, thus providing both for dilution of the urine leaving the loop of Henle and for the active step (single effect) in countercurrent multiplication. Because the cortical and the outer medullary collecting ducts are relatively impermeable to water in the absence of AVP but are highly permeable to water in the presence of AVP, the fate of the dilute tubular fluid leaving the loop of Henle—and therefore final urine osmolality—depends on the presence or absence of AVP.

These data have been integrated[191] into a model that provides two spatially distinct sites for countercurrent multiplication: an active step in the outer medulla and a passive step in the inner medulla (Fig. 7–10). The first multiplication step depends on NaCl efflux from water-impermeable thick ascending limbs; thus fluid entering the distal tubule is both hypotonic and salt poor. During antidiuresis, AVP-enhanced water abstraction from urea-impermeable cortical and outer medullary collecting ducts results in accumulation of urea in fluid entering papillary collecting ducts. Because these ducts are permeable to urea, passive urea transport down a chemical gradient from tubular fluid to medullary interstitium contributes to medullary hypertonicity, thereby providing a second, but in this case passive, multiplication step. Simultaneously, osmotic equilibration of papillary collecting duct fluid with the medullary interstitium results in the formation of hypertonic urine.

Kokko and Rector[191] rationalized the progressive concentration and dilution of tubular fluid in, respectively, descending and ascending thin limbs entirely in terms of passive flow. Consider, for example, a medulla whose osmolality ranges from 300 mmol/kg at the corticomedullary junction to 1400 mmol/kg at the papillary tip (see Fig. 7–10). In keeping with tissue analyses,[192] approximately half of the medullary hypertonicity is due to NaCl and the remainder is due to urea. Isotonic fluid containing 280 mmol/kg of NaCl entering the highly water-permeable, but urea- and Na$^+$-impermeable, thin descending limb is concentrated almost entirely by water abstraction, so that fluid entering the thin ascending limb has a higher NaCl concentration and a lower urea concentration than the medullary interstitium. These passive driving forces between lumen and interstitium, coupled with the fact that the thin ascending limb is more permeable to NaCl than to urea, poise the system for fluid dilution. As fluid moves up the water-impermeable thin ascending limb, passive NaCl efflux from lumen to interstitium exceeds passive urea influx from interstitium to tubular fluid and, concomitantly, urea recycling from papillary collecting ducts through the interstitium to thin ascending limbs. Finally, the process begins again by active NaCl transport from the thick ascending limb.

The Vascular Countercurrent Exchange

Maintenance of a hypertonic medullary interstitium requires that the rate of solute removal by medullary blood flow be reduced sufficiently to prevent equilibration of medullary interstitial fluid with isotonic plasma. These requirements are satisfied by countercurrent exchange processes within medullary capillary loops.

The medullary vasa recta form a counterflow system. In descending vasa recta, water leaves the blood and solute enters, so that the osmolality at the bend of the vasa recta is the same as that of the tip of the loop of Henle, and presumably also the same as that of the medullary interstitium, at the same point.[193] As blood flows from the tip of the vasa recta back to venules in the inner cortex, it gains water and loses NaCl to the progressively less hypertonic medullary interstitium. The net effect of this countercurrent

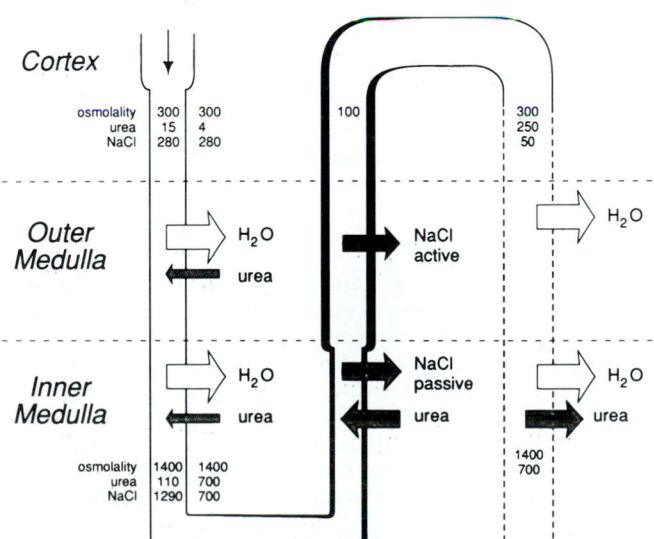

Figure 7–10. Schematic illustration of the model of Kokko and Rector[198] for the renal concentrating mechanism. (From Reeves WB, Andreoli TE. Nephrogenic diabetes insipidus. In: Scriver CR, Beaudet AL, Sly WS, et al., eds. The Metabolic Basis of Inherited Disease. 6th ed. New York: McGraw-Hill, 1989: 1985–2011. Copyright © 1989 by McGraw-Hill, Inc. Used by permission of McGraw-Hill Book Co.)

exchange in the vasa recta is to reduce the rate of solute loss from the medulla, with respect to a linear blood flow system.

Effects of Filtration Rate and Solute Excretion

Factors in addition to AVP and counterflow processes within the renal medulla also affect concentration and dilution of urine. For example, the permeability of the collecting duct to water, even in the absence of AVP, is clearly finite. Thus by varying the rate of fluid delivery to collecting ducts, and hence the time available for water efflux from these ducts, the rate of glomerular filtration (GFR) can influence the final osmolality of urine. This effect has been documented in animals lacking circulating AVP.[194, 195] Presumably, in the presence of low urine flow rates in the collecting duct, there is at least partial osmotic equilibration of urine with the medullary interstitium. Conversely, increased GFRs that are produced by sustained expansion of the ECF volume can cause a hypo-osmotic urine, even when high levels of AVP are maintained by infusion.

In clinical terms, the nature and rate of solute excretion have a greater influence on urine osmolality than GFR. The effect of osmotic diuresis on urine composition may be viewed by considering solute excretion in terms of the osmolar clearance (C_{osm}, in milliliters per minute), which can be regarded as the urine flow rate that is required to produce a urine isotonic to plasma. In antidiuresis, a volume of solute-free water, termed *negative free water clearance*, is removed from urine, and the urine flow rate is less than C_{osm}. In water diuresis, the urine flow rate exceeds C_{osm}; the difference between the urine flow rate and C_{osm}, termed *positive free water clearance*, is the amount of solute-free water that is excreted. During progressive osmotic diuresis, an increasingly greater volume of isotonic fluid containing nonabsorbed solute escapes proximal tubular absorption and is delivered to the loop of Henle. As a consequence the C_{osm} becomes sufficiently large that, even if the magnitude of either positive (during water diuresis) or negative (during antidiuresis) free water clearance stays unchanged, urine osmolality approaches isotonicity.

Figure 7–11 provides a schematic illustration of this argument. At relatively low rates of solute excretion, the urine may be either concentrated maximally or diluted maximally. However, as urine solute excretion increases, that is, as C_{osm} increases, the osmolality of either hypotonic or hypertonic urine approaches isotonicity.[196] Stated in another way, during a massive solute diuresis, the ability of the renal concentrating or diluting mechanisms to modify the osmolality of proximal tubular fluid becomes progressively blunted (Fig. 7–11A). Even though the urine osmolality may approach isotonicity during progressive solute diuresis, the absolute free water clearance continues to rise (Fig. 7–11B). Thus for C_{osm} values as high as 20 mL/min, the formation of free water, i.e., salt absorption in the thick ascending limb, is not saturable.[197] In addition, the urine osmolality in a solute diuresis does not approach isotonicity until the solute excretion rate exceeds approximately 8000 mmol/d. By comparison, a healthy individual eating a normal diet excretes 600 to 800 mmol/d.

The Collecting Tubule

The major contribution of AVP to the renal antidiuretic response is to increase the water permeability of terminal nephron segments, specifically, the cortical collecting duct, the outer medullary collecting duct, and the papillary collecting duct. The increase in the water permeability of these nephron segments augments osmotic water flow from tubular lumen into a hypertonic medullary interstitium, thus

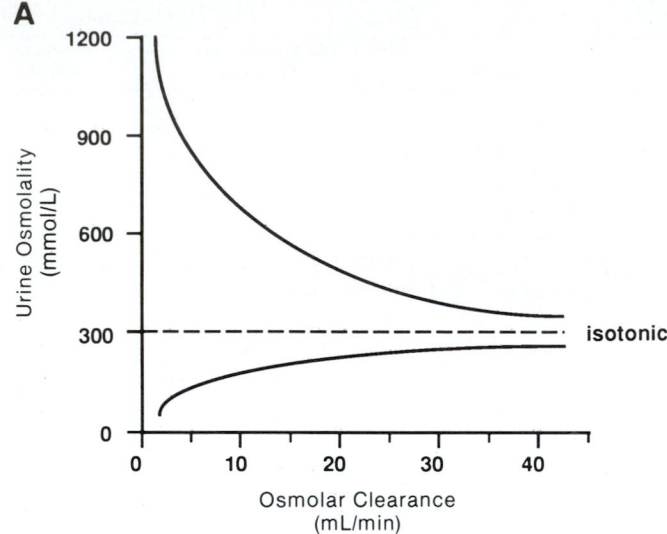

A

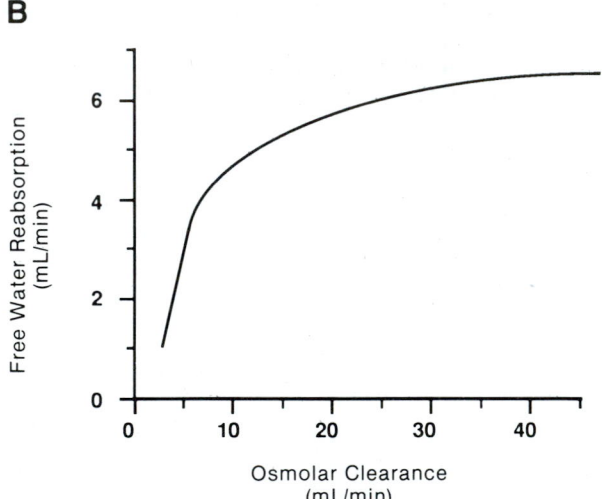

B

Figure 7–11. The effect of varying rates of urine osmolar clearance (C_{osm}) on urine osmolality (*A*) and free water reabsorption (*B*). As C_{osm} increases, hypertonic urine becomes progressively diluted and approaches isotonicity; hypotonic urine becomes less dilute and also approaches isotonicity. In spite of the approach to isotonicity, free water reabsorption continues to increase as C_{osm} increases (*B*). (From data in Rapoport S, Brodsky WA, West CD, et al. Urinary flow and excretion of solutes during osmotic diuresis in hydropenic man. Am J Physiol 1949; 156:433–442; and Goldberg M, McCurdy DK, Foltz EL, et al. Effects of ethacrynic acid (a new saluretic agent) on renal diluting and concentrating mechanisms: evidence for site of action in the loop of Henle. J Clin Invest 1964; 43:201–216.)

providing for maximal urine concentration during antidiuresis. Virtually all information about the effects of AVP on water transport in collecting duct segments or in other hormone-responsive epithelia derives from analyses of the effects of AVP on water and solute transport, from assessments of the effects of AVP on the energetic requirements for water and solute transport (i.e., from activation energy measurements), and from studies of the effects of AVP on the morphological characteristics of hormone-responsive epithelia.

Water and Solute Permeability Measurements

AVP increases the water permeability of apical plasma membranes in hormone-responsive epithelia.[198, 199] In general, two methods may be used to assess this increase in water permeability.

In one method, net water flux is measured when either a hydrostatic or an osmotic pressure gradient exists across the membrane. In accord with the Starling hypothesis, net water flow across the membrane is linearly related to the driving force by P_f (in micrometers per second), the permeability coefficient for net water flow; thus P_f may be computed from the relation between net water flux and hydrostatic or osmotic pressure. In the second method, the flux of tracer water, e.g., tritiated water, is measured at zero net volume flow: both solutions bathing a membrane are at the same hydrostatic pressure and are identical in composition. Tracer water molecules in one solution exchange at random (by diffusion) across the membrane with unlabeled water molecules in the other solution, but there is no net water flux. From Fick's first law of diffusion and the tracer appearance rate in the nonlabeled solution, one may compute P_{Dw} (in micrometers per second), the permeability coefficient for water diffusion across the membrane.

The most widely used method for the study of the response of nephron water permeability to AVP utilizes in vitro microperfusion of isolated tubule segments. Grantham and Burg[200] observed that freshly dissected rabbit cortical collecting duct segments have a high initial water permeability that declines temporarily and reaches a minimum in approximately 180 min; when AVP is introduced into the bathing solution, the water permeability rises to its initial high value. These observations have been confirmed.[201, 202] Table 7–4 lists P_f and P_{Dw} values measured in this nephron segment at 23°C. P_f is more than 4-fold higher than P_{Dw} in the absence of AVP and more than 13-fold higher in the presence of the hormone.[200–202]

The stability of the AVP-dependent hydro-osmotic effect depends on the species studied and the experimental condition. In perfused rabbit cortical collecting duct,[203] the water permeability reaches a peak about 10 min after the addition of AVP, followed by a gradual decline to baseline values at 37°C even in the continued presence of hormone. The diffusional water permeability P_{Dw} follows the same pattern. When the rabbit collecting duct is perfused at 25°C, however, the AVP-induced increase in water permeability is sustained.[203] In the rat[204] the hydro-osmotic effect of AVP on the cortical collecting duct is sustained even at 37°C.

In spite of the dramatic increase in both the diffusional and the osmotic water permeability coefficients observed with AVP in the cortical collecting duct, this epithelium remains virtually impermeable to even the smallest hydrophilic nonelectrolytes (see Table 7–4).[200, 205, 206] The same conclusion, namely, that cortical collecting ducts are virtually impermeable to small hydrophilic solutes in either the presence or the absence of AVP, also obtains from solute reflection coefficient measurements in this nephron segment.

Thus either in the presence or in the absence of AVP, urea, NaCl, and sucrose all have reflection coefficients of unity in cortical collecting ducts.[206] Stated in another way, for cortical collecting ducts, the antidiuretic response involves a profound increase in the water permeability of an epithelium that can discriminate more than 1000-fold between water and hydrophilic solutes, such as urea, that have effective radii less than twice as large as that of a water molecule. These biophysical data have been interpreted as evidence of water movement through narrow (radius of 2 Å) pores.[207]

Morphological Studies of the Vasopressin Response

The final site of AVP action on water permeability is at the apical epithelial surface. Moreover, the bulk of water flow across the collecting tubule proceeds through epithelial cells rather than through the junctional complexes, and the water permeability change that is induced by AVP occurs in the apical membranes of the collecting duct cells.[208]

Structural studies of AVP-responsive anuran epithelia (principally toad and frog urinary bladders) have demonstrated that a number of ultrastructural changes occur in the apical membranes of granular cells in association with the application of serosal AVP. Chevalier and co-workers[209] reported the aggregation of apical membrane intramembranous particles in frog urinary bladder that was treated with oxytocin, and Kachadorian and colleagues[210, 211] described similar apical membrane aggregates in toad urinary bladder that was exposed to AVP.

These aggregates are believed to represent AVP-induced water channels.[212] Thus freeze-fracture electron microscopy has demonstrated aggregates in the apical membrane of AVP-stimulated but not unstimulated toad bladders.[210, 213] The appearance of aggregates is induced by serosal, but not mucosal, application of AVP, and by cAMP or forskolin;[210, 213, 214] it is independent of an imposed osmotic gradient[213] and can be inhibited by drugs that inhibit the AVP-induced increase in water flow.[215] Furthermore, in most circumstances the number of membrane aggregates is proportional to the AVP-induced increase in water permeability.[210, 211, 216]

In the absence of AVP, aggregates are seen in the walls of small vacuoles situated beneath the apical membranes of granular cells in both toad and frog urinary bladders.[217] These vacuoles, commonly known as aggrephores, have a tubular shape and measure 1 to 2 μm long and 0.1 μm in diameter. The walls of the aggrephores are densely packed with particles arranged in a helical array. At one or both ends of the aggrephore in toad bladder is a spherical head that appears to be coated with clathrin.[218] The significance of this clathrin coat is unknown. In the presence of AVP, the number of these aggregate-containing vacuoles decreases while the number of aggregates in the apical membrane increases. Occasionally, aggrephores can be seen fusing with the apical membrane. The frequency of these so-called fusion events correlates with the accumulation of aggregates in the apical membrane.[215] These observations have led to the hypothesis that the water permeation sites are "shuttled" from the membranes of these aggrephores to the apical membrane under the influence of AVP (Fig. 7–12).[212, 217, 219]

However, correlation between the frequency of formation of intramembranous particle aggregates and water permeability is not proof that the particle aggregates actually mediate water transport. In some studies the frequency of particle aggregates has been dissociated from the AVP-induced increase in water permeability. For example, in time course studies of aggregate accumulation after AVP appli-

---

TABLE 7–4. The Effect of Vasopressin on Water and Solute Permeation in Cortical Collecting Ducts*

Variable	Zero AVP	250 U/L AVP
P_f (μm/s)	20	186
P_{Dw} (μm/s)	4.7	14.2
P_f/P_{Dw}	4	13
P_{Durea} (μm/s)	0.03	0.02
$P_{Dthiourea}$ (μm/s)	0.03	0.02

*P_f, osmotic water permeability; P_{Dw}, diffusional water permeability coefficient; P_{Durea}, $P_{Dthiourea}$, diffusional permeability coefficients for urea and thiourea, respectively.

Data from Hebert SC, Schafer JA, Andreoli TE. The effects of antidiuretic hormone (ADH) on solute and water transport in the mammalian nephron. J Membr Biol 1981; 58:1–19; and Hebert SC, Andreoli TE. Water permeability of biological membranes. Lessons from antidiuretic hormone–responsive epithelia. Biochim Biophys Acta 1982; 650:267–280.

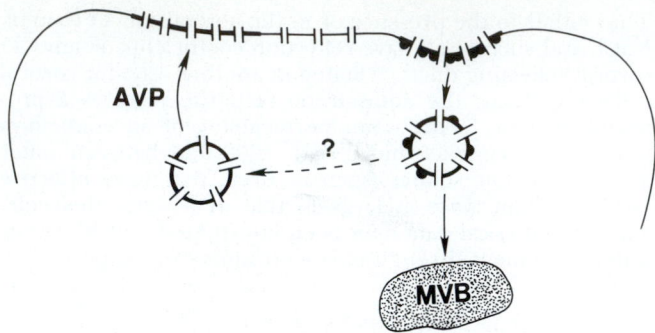

Figure 7–12. A schematic model of the shuttle mechanism for the action of AVP in the collecting tubule. In the absence of AVP, water channels are located in vesicles, or endosomes, beneath the apical membrane. On stimulation by AVP, these endosomes fuse with the apical membrane delivering water channels to the cell surface. Water channels are retrieved from the cell surface by endocytonin of clathrin-coated vesicles. MVB, multivesicular bodies.

cation in toad urinary bladder, aggregate accumulation was maximal before osmotic water flow peaked,[220] and when the AVP-stimulated water flow declined after 60 min of hormone exposure, the aggregate number did not decline.[221] Also, when a comparison was made of the effects of AVP, cAMP, and forskolin (a nonhormonal stimulator of the catalytic subunit of adenylate cyclase) on aggregate frequency and osmotic water permeability in toad bladder, cAMP caused the same degree of aggregate appearance but only half the water permeability as AVP. Likewise, forskolin caused the same frequency of aggregate appearance but twice as high a water permeability as AVP.[214] These results suggest that AVP has an effect on postapical membrane barriers to water flow. Strange and Spring,[222, 223] however, found no effect of AVP in the collecting duct on the water permeability of the basolateral membrane.

Some caution must be used in attempting to correlate quantitatively aggregate frequency and water permeability. Aggregate frequency is measured in freeze-fracture sections of the apical membrane, but such methods do not generally assess aggregate frequency in subapical membranes that may be associated with the luminal membrane. As discussed earlier, aggregates are carried into the apical membranes on tubulovesicular structures called aggrephores. These aggrephores have a higher density of aggregates than the flat apical membrane surface, even after fusion increases the water permeability. Therefore, the density of aggregates in the apical membrane itself must be assumed to reflect a constant proportion of those present in the fused aggrephores.

The termination of the AVP-induced increase in water permeability is effected by retrieval of the aggregates from the apical membrane.[224, 225] When the toad urinary bladder is exposed to AVP in the presence of a large osmotic gradient, there is an initial, but transient, large flow of water that is proportional to the magnitude of the imposed osmotic gradient. The initial rate of water flow, however, rapidly attenuates even in the continued presence of both AVP and the osmotic gradient. This phenomenon of decreasing water permeability in the presence of transepithelial osmotic gradients has been termed *flux inhibition*. Flux inhibition is not seen if the osmotic gradient is small or absent. Likewise, the number of particle aggregates and of aggrephore fusion is decreased in toad bladders that are stimulated with AVP in the presence of an osmotic gradient compared with bladders that are stimulated with AVP in the absence of a gradient. Flux inhibition, with its associated decrease in water permeability and loss of membrane particle aggregates, is due to retrieval of apical membrane.[225, 226]

The retrieval of apical membrane during flux inhibition or after the removal of AVP from the serosal solution has been studied by observing the incorporation of enzymatic, electron-dense, or fluorescent markers from the mucosal solution into cytoplasmic tubular vesicles. The uptake of markers into tubular vesicles occurs during retrieval of fused aggrephores from apical membrane. When toad bladders are stimulated with AVP under isosmotic conditions and are exposed to a hypotonic mucosal solution, the uptake of the marker is increased compared with bladders that are exposed to isosmotic solutions throughout.[225, 226] Conversely, the uptake of marker into cytoplasmic vacuoles is inhibited by exposing the bladder to an osmotic gradient for 15 min before adding the marker molecules.[225] Thus transepithelial volume flow regulates apical membrane water permeability by stimulating the retrieval of aggrephores from the apical membrane.

On removal of AVP from the basolateral solution, the water permeability of the toad bladder decreases, and aggregates and aggrephore fusion sites disappear from the apical membrane. Early after AVP is removed, fluid-phase markers, such as horseradish peroxidase or fluorescent dextran, become localized to cytoplasmic tubular vacuoles that resemble aggrephores.[224, 227] After about 20 min, the markers label multivesicular bodies. These results indicate that the AVP-induced increase in apical water permeability in the toad urinary bladder is terminated through the retrieval of aggregates and aggrephores from the apical membrane and their subsequent incorporation into multivesicular bodies. It is not known if aggrephores cycle into and out of the apical membrane without some intervening modification step.

Structural studies of mammalian collecting ducts indicate that the general scheme of AVP action in the anuran bladder, namely, insertion of water channels into the apical membrane and their subsequent retrieval, also occurs in mammalian collecting ducts.[219] Thus apical intramembranous particle aggregates are present in rat medullary collecting ducts (Fig. 7–13)[228–230] and in outer medullary and cortical collecting ducts of rabbits, in which the aggregates are confined to the apical membranes of principal cells.[231] There are slight differences in the way the anuran urinary bladder and the mammalian collecting duct respond to AVP. For example, the particle aggregates in these mammalian tubules are similar to, but not identical with, those of anuran epithelia. Furthermore, cytoplasmic aggrephores or fused tubular vesicular structures that are typical of the anuran bladder have not been found in mammalian collecting ducts. Rather, morphological and functional evidence indicates that the movement of aggregates, i.e., water channels, into and out of the apical membrane of collecting duct cells may be mediated by the exocytosis and endocytosis of clathrin-coated vesicles.[228, 232, 233]

Endocytotic vesicles in the mammalian collecting tubule contain water channels,[234] and AVP stimulates the movement of water channels between the apical membrane and the endosomal compartments.[234] In addition, Verkman and co-workers[235] showed that clathrin-coated vesicles from bovine renal medulla have a high water permeability that is inhibited by mercurial diuretics and that has a low activation energy. That is, the clathrin-coated vesicles probably contain functional water channels and may be involved in the cycling of water channels between the apical membrane and an intracellular compartment.

Intracellular Mediators of Vasopressin Action

The effects of AVP on transport processes in renal epithelia are mediated primarily by the intracellular second messenger cAMP.[236] AVP binds to specific receptors, the V_2

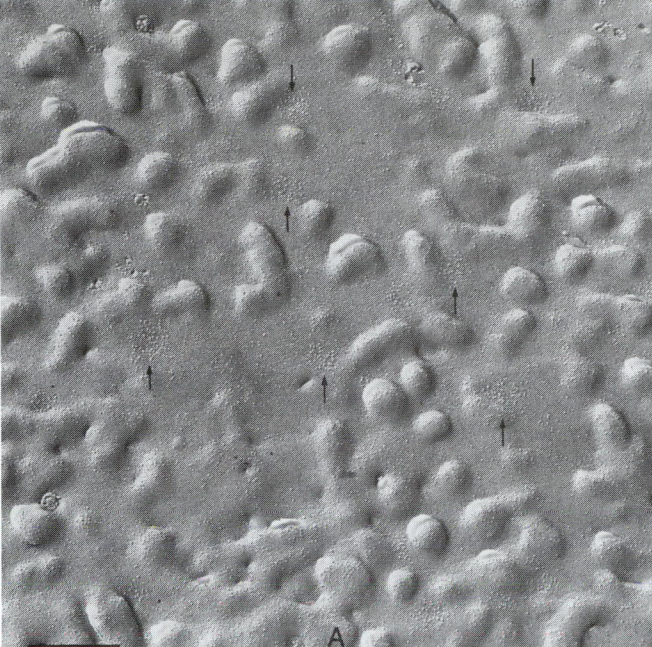

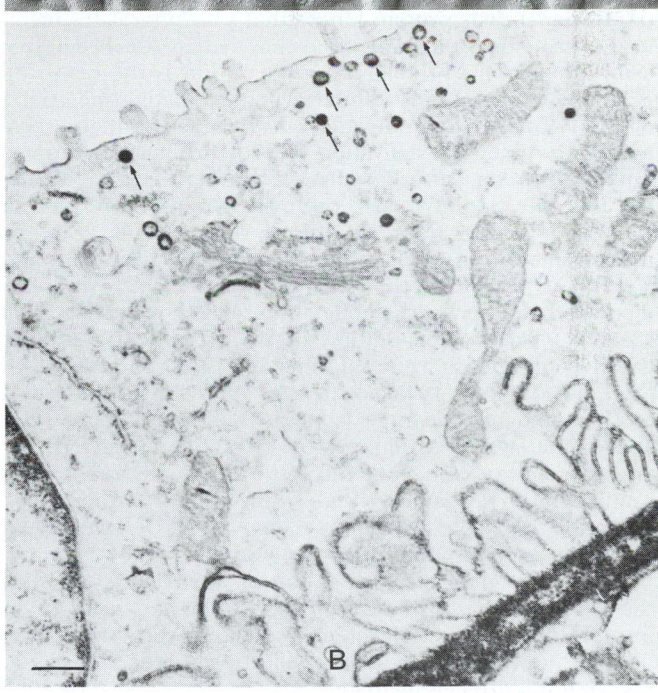

Figure 7–13. Electron micrographs of collecting duct principal cells. *A,* Freeze-fracture electron micrograph of the apical plasma membrane P face of a principal cell from a normal mouse. Numerous clusters of intramembranous particles (*arrows*) are visible on this membrane. The clusters of intramembranous particles are the hallmark of the AVP-induced water permeability response in these apical plasma membranes. The rounded projections that are also visible on this membrane are stubby microvilli that characterize these cells. Bar = 0.5 μm. (From Brown D, Shields GI, Valtin H, et al. Lack of intramembranous particle clusters in collecting ducts of mice with nephrogenic diabetes insipidus. Am J Physiol 1985; 249:F582–F589.) *B,* Thin section of a principal cell from a normal Long-Evans rat that was injected with 6 mg/mL horseradish peroxidase 15 min before fixation. Many vesicles loaded with horseradish peroxidase–diaminobenzidine reaction product are present in the cytoplasm, where they are concentrated below the apical plasma membrane (*arrows*). Most of the peroxidase-labeled endocytotic vesicles are smooth (noncoated), which is consistent with the known rapid decoating of clathrin-coated vesicles after they detach from the plasma membrane. (From Brown D, Weyer P, Orci L. Vasopressin stimulates endocytosis in kidney collecting duct principal cells. Eur J Cell Biol 1988; 46:336–341.)

receptors, on basolateral membrane surfaces of hormone-responsive epithelial cells and activates membrane-associated adenylate cyclase to catalyze cAMP generation from ATP (also see Chapter 4). Adenylate cyclase is a multicomponent enzyme system (Fig. 7–14) in which the catalytic subunit is under regulation by two guanosine triphosphate (GTP)–binding proteins, G_s and G_i.[237] G_s and G_i require GTP binding for activity and, when activated, stimulate or inhibit the activity of the catalytic subunit, respectively.[238] Consequently, these proteins, which are generally referred to as guanine nucleotide–binding proteins or G proteins, are responsible for the transduction of hormone-receptor interactions into changes in cAMP formation.[239] In tissues in which hormone action is mediated by cAMP, the hormone-receptor complex activates the G_s subunit of the adenylate cyclase enzyme; this G_s subunit may also be activated by cholera toxin.[238] The

activated, GTP-bound G_s then stimulates the catalytic subunit (C) of adenylate cyclase to produce more cAMP. Hormones that antagonize the tissue effects of cAMP bind to receptors that are coupled to the G_i subunit. Activation of G_i by these hormone-receptor complexes inhibits the activity of the catalytic subunit of adenylate cyclase; the G_i subunit may be inactivated by pertussis toxin.[238] Because the effects of AVP on epithelia are mediated by cAMP, it is believed that the V_2 receptor is associated with the G_s-regulatory subunit.

Studies with individual nephron segments have identified vasopressin-stimulated adenylate cyclase in the medullary TALH (mTALH) and along the entire collecting duct.[239] The intimate relation between hormone binding and adenylate cyclase activation was firmly established by Jard and co-workers,[240] who described a close correlation between binding of analogues of lysine vasopressin and adenylate cyclase activation, as well as comparable half-times of lysine vasopressin binding and adenylate cyclase activation. Their work[240] and that of others[241] have led to the suggestion that binding of neurohypophyseal hormones to only a small fraction of receptors is necessary to activate sufficient adenylate cyclase for a maximal physiological response.

The role of G_s and G_i units in AVP-responsive renal epithelia has been demonstrated through stimulation of AVP-dependent transport processes in the mouse mTALH with cholera toxin, a G_s-specific agent, or with forskolin, a cyclase-specific agent,[242] in the absence of AVP.[243] Likewise, in the rabbit cortical collecting tubule, cholera toxin and forskolin increase hydraulic water permeability in the absence of AVP.[244] The presence of G_s and G_i proteins has also been demonstrated directly in microdissected segments of the mouse and rabbit TALH,[245] in the cortical collecting tubule,[246] and in medullary collecting tubules.[245] Intracellular cAMP, probably acting via a cell-specific protein kinase, effects an alteration in transport processes at the luminal membrane of renal epithelia to augment water transport in the collecting duct cell, and NaCl transport in the mTALH cell. Finally, the level of cAMP within the cell may be reduced through enzymatic cleavage to 5'-AMP by cytosolic phosphodiesterase, a process that terminates hormone action.

The finding that the bovine renal medulla contains a cAMP-dependent protein kinase that phosphorylates membrane proteins from that tissue has led to the belief that cAMP-dependent protein phosphorylation is the next step in the sequence of intracellular events mediating the effects of AVP on renal epithelial transport.[247] In intact renal medullary tissue the activation of protein kinase is proportional to the concentration of AVP bathing the tissue and to the concentration of cAMP within the tissue.[248]

Using a fluorescent technique that permits real-time measurement of osmotic water permeability, Kuwahara and Verkman[249] examined the initial phases of the AVP-induced increase in water permeability in isolated collecting duct segments. After the addition of AVP to the peritubular bathing solution, there was a time lag of approximately 23 s (Fig. 7–15) before P_f began to rise. With the addition of a cAMP analogue, the time lag was reduced to 11 s. Thus approximately 12 s is required for AVP to bind to its receptor and to generate sufficient intracellular cAMP, and 11 s is required for the more distal steps in the cascade (e.g., activation of protein kinase A, activation of cytoskeletal elements, and insertion of water channels).

In addition to the stimulation of adenylate cyclase via the V_2 receptor, AVP produces a spike-like increase in intracellular calcium level in rabbit cortical collecting tubule[250] and in rat medullary collecting tubule.[251] It is not known if this effect is mediated by V_2 receptors, V_1 receptors, or oxytocin receptors. However, the concentration of AVP

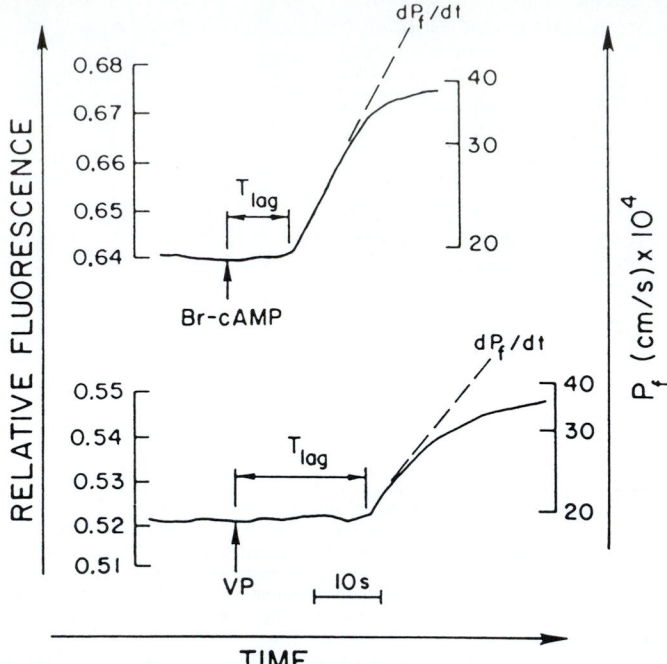

Figure 7–15. The early time course of the AVP response in cortical collecting tubules measured by using a fluorescent technique capable of providing rapid time resolution. P_f began to increase 23 ± 3 s after the addition of AVP (VP on figure) and only 11 ± 2 s after the addition of Br-cAMP. (From Kuwahara M, Verkman AS. Pre–steady state analysis of the turn-on and turn-off of water permeability in the kidney collecting tubule. J Membr Biol 1989; 110:57–65.)

that is required to elicit an increase in intracellular calcium concentration exceeds the physiological range, and it is unlikely that changes in intracellular calcium level mediate the hydro-osmotic effects of AVP.[250, 251]

The molecular details explaining how AVP regulates apical membrane transport processes are uncertain. As noted earlier, stimulation of amphibian urinary bladder or mammalian collecting ducts with AVP leads to the insertion of patches of membrane that contain water channels into the apical membrane.[219, 252] The insertion of these membrane units depends on the integrity of the cytoskeleton.[253] Treatment of amphibian bladders with agents that disrupt microtubules and microfilaments decreases the number of fusion events between aggrephores and the apical membrane, the number of aggregates appearing on the cell surface, and the hydro-osmotic response to AVP.[221, 253]

These findings suggest that AVP, working via cAMP and protein kinase, alters water transport in hormone-responsive epithelia by causing the microtubule-dependent insertion of specialized membrane units within the apical plasma membranes of these cells. In other tissues, such as the mTALH, AVP may act by different mechanisms to increase the functional number of $Na^+,K^+,2Cl^-$ cotransport units and K^+ channels in apical membranes.

Modulation of Vasopressin Action

ALPHA-ADRENERGIC AGENTS. In addition to their effects on AVP secretion, alpha-adrenergic agents modulate water excretion at the level of the collecting duct. In isolated collecting ducts that are stimulated with AVP, the alpha-adrenergic agonist phenylephrine decreases water permeability.[254] This effect is blocked by alpha-adrenergic antagonists and is not observed in tubules that are stimulated with cAMP, which indicates that the point of modulation of alpha-

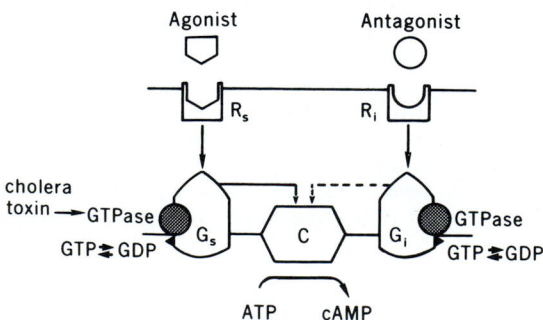

Figure 7–14. A schematic model for the regulation of adenylate cyclase activity by G_s and G_i guanine nucleotide–regulatory subunits.

agonists is at the generation of cAMP. Moreover, the inhibitory effects of the alpha-adrenergic agonists clonidine and epinephrine are attenuated by preincubation of collecting ducts with pertussis toxin,[245, 246] an agent that inactivates the inhibitory guanine-regulatory protein G_i. Thus alpha-adrenergic agonists inhibit AVP action in the collecting duct by activating the G_i subunit and by decreasing cAMP formation.

ATRIAL NATRIURETIC PEPTIDE. This agent inhibits the hydro-osmotic effect of AVP in isolated rabbit cortical collecting tubules. This inhibition apparently occurs at a site proximal to the catalytic subunit of adenylate cyclase because ANP has no effect on cAMP- and forskolin-stimulated water flow.[144]

PROSTAGLANDINS. Locally generated renal prostaglandins play a role in modulating the actions of AVP on renal epithelial transport processes. In the mammalian cortical collecting tubule, in the medullary interstitial cell, and in the toad urinary bladder, AVP stimulates the production of PGE_2,[255, 256] and inhibition of prostaglandin production with prostaglandin synthase inhibitors such as indomethacin or meclofenamate increases the rate of Na^+ transport and the rate of osmotic water permeation.[256] In both the rabbit cortical collecting tubule and the toad urinary bladder, prostaglandins inhibit AVP-stimulated accumulation of cAMP within the cell and exert little or no inhibitory action on transport events beyond the accumulation of cAMP within the cell.[201, 244, 257] Thus the AVP effects on transport in these tissues are modulated by an inhibitor that is synthesized in situ, whose production is stimulated by AVP, and whose action reduces the ability of AVP to elevate cellular levels of cAMP.

The locus for this PGE_2-mediated inhibition of cAMP formation has been defined. PGE_2 does not inhibit the hydro-osmotic effect of the nonhormonal catalytic subunit activator forskolin, but it does inhibit the stimulation of water flow by cholera toxin, which activates adenylate cyclase by irreversible binding to G_s, the stimulatory guanine nucleotide–binding subunit of adenylate cyclase. Thus it is likely that PGE_2 inhibits AVP-stimulated generation of cAMP in the cortical collecting tubule by interacting with G_i, the inhibitory guanine nucleotide–binding subunit of adenylate cyclase.[244] An identical pattern of interactions has been reported for prostaglandin-mediated inhibition of NaCl transport in isolated mTALH.[243, 245] It is noteworthy in this connection that AVP appears to stimulate PGE_2 synthesis in medullary interstitial cells[255, 258] and in medullary collecting duct cells,[259] although some studies have failed to show this effect.[260–262]

CALCIUM. Hypercalcemia causes an AVP-resistant decrease in maximal urine osmolality. The mechanism by which hypercalcemia interferes with renal concentrating ability is not well understood. Studies with the toad urinary bladder[263, 264] demonstrated that the hydro-osmotic effect of AVP is inhibited by high concentrations of calcium in the serosal solutions. There was no effect of calcium on the cAMP-induced hydro-osmotic effect, which suggests that the high serosal calcium concentration interferes with the generation of cAMP. In contrast, Goldfarb[265] found, in the rabbit collecting duct, that an increase in the peritubular calcium concentration enhances the hydro-osmotic effect of AVP but not cAMP. Furthermore, increasing the peritubular calcium concentration from 1 to 5 mM does not inhibit AVP-dependent cAMP production in the mouse collecting duct.[245] In the mTALH, however, high peritubular calcium concentrations do inhibit AVP-induced cAMP generation.[245, 266] Preincubation of tubule segments with pertussis toxin abolishes this inhibition, which indicates that the inhibition of cAMP generation by high calcium levels is mediated through activation of G_i.[245] Although high extracellular calcium concentrations appear to have little effect on cAMP generation,

increases in intracellular calcium concentration produced by the calcium ionophore A23187[267] or by permeabilization of the cell membrane markedly inhibit AVP-induced cAMP accumulation in the collecting duct.

PROTEIN KINASE C. The action of AVP in the collecting duct is mediated by intracellular cAMP. In other tissues, such as hepatocytes and vascular smooth muscle cells, AVP activates a V_1 receptor leading to phosphoinositide turnover, and the phosphoinositide–protein kinase C pathway may down-regulate the activation by AVP through protein kinase A of the water transport pathway. In toad urinary bladder,[268] frog skin,[269] and rabbit cortical collecting tubule,[267, 270] compounds such as phorbol esters that activate protein kinase C inhibit the hydro-osmotic effect of AVP. The studies with the toad[268] and the frog[269] indicate an effect on the generation of cAMP because the phorbol esters did not inhibit the response to exogenous cAMP, whereas in the rabbit collecting duct a "post-cAMP" effect has been proposed.[267]

The Medullary Thick Ascending Limb of Henle

The concept that AVP might regulate renal concentrating power by modulating the rate of NaCl absorption in the mTALH was set forth by Wirz and co-workers.[271] Subsequently, Morel provided strong support for this view with the demonstration that AVP increases adenylate cyclase activity in isolated mTALH segments (see ref. 272 for a general review).

Figure 7–16 presents a general model for net NaCl absorption in the mTALH based on current experimental data on this nephron segment in mammalian species, notably the mouse and the rabbit. Net transepithelial Cl^- absorption in the TALH involves a secondary active transport process in which luminal Cl^- entry into cells is mediated by an electroneutral $Na^+,K^+,2Cl^-$ cotransport mechanism.[273, 274] Studies assessing either the uptake of radioactive Na^+ and Cl^- [275, 276] or the binding of the radiolabeled loop diuretic [³H]bumetanide by apical membrane vesicles from mTALH

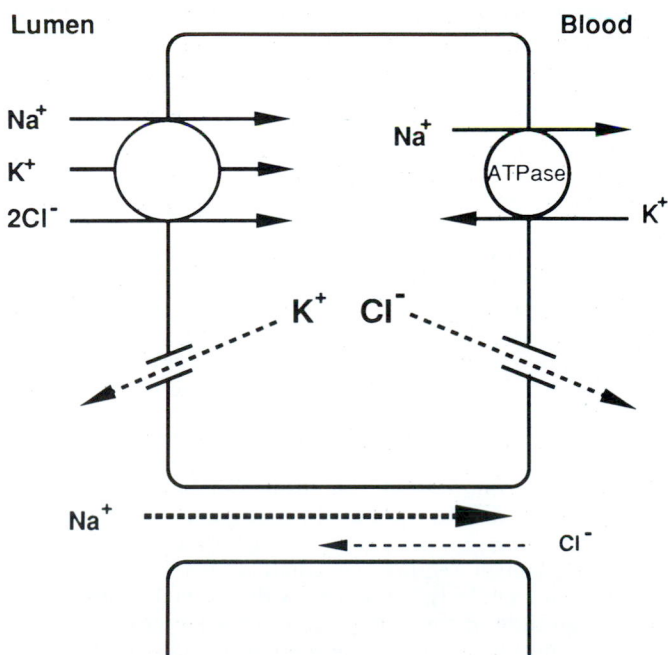

Figure 7–16. A model for salt absorption in mouse mTALH. The solid lines denote conservative (primary or secondary) processes, and the dashed lines denote dissipative processes.

segments[277] have confirmed the dependence of Cl⁻ uptake on both Na⁺ and K⁺ in this nephron segment.

No measurements have yet been made of the electrochemical gradient for ion cotransport across apical membranes of the mammalian TALH. However, in the *Amphiuma* diluting segment, there is a favorable integrated chemical gradient for entry of neutral Na⁺,K⁺,2Cl⁻ units from luminal fluids into cells;[278] this favorable driving force for Cl⁻ entry across the apical membrane is provided by the Na⁺ electrochemical gradient, which is maintained by basolateral membrane Na⁺,K⁺-ATPase. Thus maneuvers that inhibit Na⁺,K⁺-ATPase, such as addition of ouabain to or removal of K⁺ from peritubular solutions, abolish NaCl absorption and the transepithelial voltage.[189, 190]

Cl⁻ exit from the cell across the basolateral membrane of the TALH appears to be primarily conductive.[279] This notion derives in part from the observations that net Cl⁻ absorption accounts for about 90% of the equivalent short-circuit current in both the mouse mTALH[280] and the rabbit cortical TALH.[281] The large intracellular negative voltage of -40 to -70 mV (cell with respect to bath) provides a portion of the driving force for conductive transport of Cl⁻ across the basolateral membrane in these nephron segments.[280, 281] A large fraction of Cl⁻ uptake into basolaterally enriched renal medullary vesicles proceeds through conductive pathways.[282] These pathways have been identified as Cl⁻ channels by incorporating vesicles into planar lipid bilayers. The channels have a conductance of 90 pS, exhibit voltage-dependent conductance properties (analogous to Goldman-type rectification), and are more active at depolarizing voltages, i.e., when intracellular Cl⁻ concentrations increase.[283] As discussed later, these characteristics may account for the rise in basolateral membrane Cl⁻ conductance in AVP-stimulated TALH segments.

Apical membranes of diluting segments, either mammalian[273, 284] or amphibian,[178] also contain Ba^{2+}-sensitive K⁺ conductances that account almost entirely for the electrical conductance of apical membranes. These K⁺ channels exhibit many of the characteristics of K⁺ channels in excitable tissues and other epithelia, such as voltage dependence, concentration dependence, and Ba^{2+}/K^+ competition effects on electrical conductance. These channels also constitute the route for the active K⁺-secretory pathway in renal tubular diluting segments.[280, 285] However, the majority of K⁺ that is secreted from cells to lumen is recycled into cells via the Na⁺,K⁺,2Cl⁻ cotransport process. Thus the rate of net K⁺ secretion constitutes less than 10% of the rate of net Cl⁻ absorption, whereas the calculated K⁺ current across apical membranes is approximately 60% of the rate of net Cl⁻ absorption.[280]

Two classes of K⁺ channels have been identified in patch-clamp studies of the apical membrane of TALH cells. Guggino and co-workers[286,287] characterized in detail a large, Ca^{2+}-activated "maxi" K⁺ channel in cultured TALH cells. This channel is probably not a significant pathway for apical membrane K⁺ recycling during salt absorption but may play a role in cell volume regulation.[288] A 10- to 20-pS K⁺ channel identified by Wang and colleagues[289] is not Ca^{2+} activated, is Ba^{2+} sensitive, and is inhibited by ATP.

Because dilution of the urine by the TALH occurs through the net absorption of equal quantities of Na⁺ and Cl⁻, a stoichiometry of 1Na⁺:2Cl⁻ for the transcellular transport mechanism requires that half of net Na⁺ absorption occurs paracellularly. In accord with this view, estimates of the magnitude of the Na⁺-permselective shunt conductance in the mouse mTALH[279] indicate that the magnitudes of the lumen-positive transepithelial voltage and the calculated Na⁺ conductance of the shunt pathway are sufficient to drive a

quantity of Na⁺ through the paracellular route equal to about half of the rate of net Cl⁻ absorption.

Finally, the model for NaCl absorption in the TALH shown in Figure 7–16 appears to have at least two general implications. First, about half of the total net Na⁺ absorption occurs through the paracellular route. In other words, the combination of a lumen-positive transepithelial voltage and a high shunt conductance reduces—with respect to exclusively transcellular, active Na⁺ absorption—the metabolic energy expenditure for net Na⁺ absorption. Second, the regulatory mechanisms in epithelial cells promote the rapid adjustment of the rate of Na⁺ entry into cells to equal the rate of Na⁺ exit from cells, thus avoiding large and potentially lethal changes in cell volume ("flush through" effect) when net Na⁺ absorption is varied.[290] The flush through effect is also minimized in diluting segments in which half of net Na⁺ absorption proceeds through the paracellular route.

The Effect of Vasopressin on Net Salt Absorption

AVP increases both the net rate of salt absorption and the spontaneous transepithelial voltage in isolated mouse mTALH segments.[274, 291] This stimulating effect on net salt absorption occurs at peritubular hormone concentrations found in the plasma of mammalian species during ordinary antidiuresis, and cAMP analogues produce the same effect on mouse mTALH segments.[291] Moreover, AVP also increases the rate of salt absorption from the mTALH of homozygous Brattleboro rats with central diabetes insipidus.[292]

THE MECHANISM OF THE VASOPRESSIN EFFECT. Simultaneous to increasing the net rate of salt absorption and transepithelial voltage in the mouse mTALH, AVP increases the transepithelial electrical conductance and the rate of net K⁺ secretion in that nephron segment.[279, 280] Moreover, these effects on net salt transport and on transepithelial electrical conductance are probably linked; a synopsis of the argument in favor of this suggestion is as follows.

A primary effect of AVP in increasing salt absorption in the mTALH appears to depend on a hormone-mediated increase in the functional number of conductive K⁺ channels in apical plasma membranes. Thus in membrane vesicles from outer renal medulla, exposure to cAMP-dependent protein kinase in vitro resulted in a 50% increase in barium-sensitive K⁺ uptake.[276] This increase in apical membrane K⁺ channels may also account for AVP- or cAMP-mediated increases in the rate of net K⁺ secretion.[284]

AVP also produces an increase in transepithelial conductance and in the Cl⁻ conductance of basolateral membranes.[293, 294] However, the AVP-dependent increase in basolateral Cl⁻ conductance is abolished when furosemide is used to inhibit net salt absorption.[294] The latter observation has been rationalized by assuming that cell Cl⁻ activity increases pari passu with AVP-mediated increases in the rate of net Cl⁻ absorption, and that the increase in cell Cl⁻ activity is responsible for the AVP-dependent increase in basolateral conductance.[284, 294] In this regard, the activity of Cl⁻ channels in basolateral medullary membrane vesicles is increased both by depolarizing the basolateral membrane and by increasing intracellular Cl⁻ activity.[283] AVP may activate basolateral Cl⁻ channels directly.[293, 294]

AVP also appears to increase the functional number of Na⁺,K⁺,2Cl⁻ cotransport units in apical membranes.[284, 295] Obviously, because AVP increases net Cl⁻ absorption in the mouse mTALH, the rate of Cl⁻ flux across apical membranes is greater with hormone than without hormone. But as noted earlier, it is likely that cell Cl⁻ concentrations rise in the presence of AVP. Consequently, the chemical driving force for electroneutral Na⁺,K⁺,Cl⁻ cotransport (see Fig. 7–16) from lumen to cell may be less in the presence of AVP than in its absence. According to this view, AVP increases the functional number of Na⁺,K⁺,2Cl⁻ cotransport units as well as K⁺ conductance units in apical plasma membranes.[284, 294, 295]

Modulation of the Thick Ascending Limb of Henle Function

The actions of AVP on NaCl absorption in the TALH can be modulated by a number of factors, including increases in peritubular osmolality and prostaglandins. In isolated mouse mTALH segments, increases in peritubular osmolality, produced either with permeant solutes such as urea or with impermeant solutes such as mannitol, rapidly and reversibly inhibit the AVP-stimulated rate of net Cl⁻ absorption.[296, 297] This inhibition of transcellular NaCl absorption occurs at a locus beyond the generation of cAMP, because supramaximal concentrations of either AVP or cAMP are unable to reverse the hypertonicity-mediated effect. Thus increasing the absolute magnitude of interstitial osmolality provides a negative feedback signal, which can reduce AVP-dependent NaCl absorption by the mTALH.

PGE₂ also participates in a local negative feedback system in the renal medulla that modulates the rate of net NaCl absorption by the mTALH.[298–300] In the in vitro mouse mTALH,[243, 301] PGE₂ has no effect on NaCl absorption when AVP is absent. In the presence of AVP, PGE₂ reduces the AVP-dependent values for transepithelial voltage and net NaCl absorption to AVP-independent values. Likewise, reported biochemical studies with the mTALH[302] indicate that PGE₂ has no effect on cellular cAMP concentrations in the absence of AVP and that PGE₂ markedly inhibits the AVP-dependent stimulation of cytosolic cAMP concentrations.

PGE₂ does not inhibit the component of NaCl transport in the mouse mTALH that is stimulated by the nonhormonal catalytic subunit activator forskolin, but PGE₂ does inhibit transport stimulation by cholera toxin, which activates adenylate cyclase specifically and irreversibly at G_s.[243] Thus PGE₂ probably inhibits AVP-stimulated generation of cAMP in the mTALH by activating G_i.

The significance of these interactions of prostaglandins, AVP, and concentrating ability has been affirmed by a number of in vivo studies. Inhibition of endogenous renal prostaglandin synthesis, either with indomethacin or with meclofenamate, causes antinatriuresis and an enhanced urine concentrating ability in response to administration of AVP.[303, 304] In addition, an increase in medullary NaCl content follows prostaglandin synthesis inhibition even in the absence of any discernible change in papillary blood flow.[305]

PGE₂ is synthesized in the medullary collecting duct and in interstitial cells. Craven and DeRubertis[258] have shown that PGE₂ synthesis by medullary interstitial cells can be modulated both by AVP and by increases in osmolality produced with urea or NaCl. These agents appear to function in acute experiments by affecting the calcium-dependent acyl hydrolase activity that regulates the availability of arachidonic acid in these cells. Finally, increases in local osmolality in the renal medulla, produced by AVP-mediated increases in NaCl absorption from the mTALH and the consequent enhancement in countercurrent multiplication, might be expected to play a major role in PGE₂ synthesis in vivo. For example, hypertonic NaCl stimulates PGE₂ release from medullary cells, and hypertonic urea suppresses this effect, as well as the PGE₂ release that is mediated directly by pharmacological concentrations of AVP.

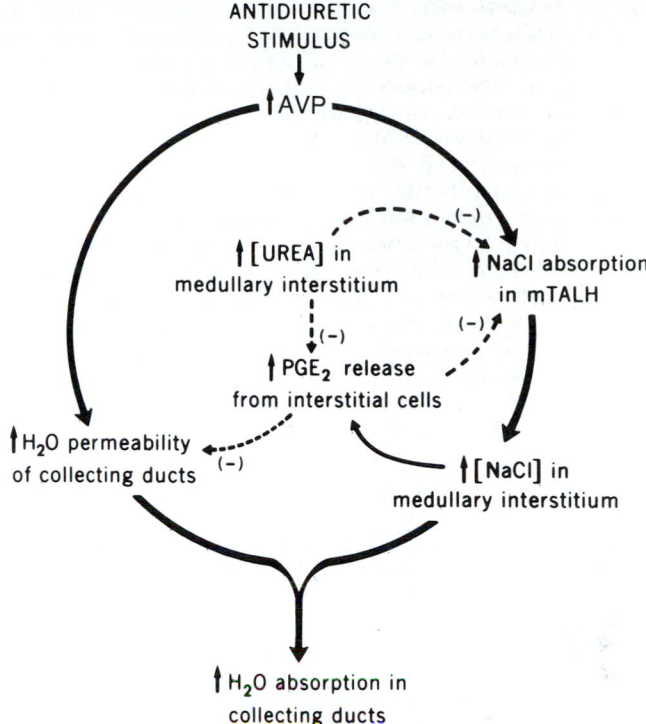

Figure 7–17. Model for the feedback regulation of renal concentrating mechanisms. (From Hebert SC, Andreoli TE. Control of NaCl transport in the thick ascending limb. Am J Physiol 1984; 246:F745–F756.)

Integration of Vasopressin Action on Concentration of Urine

The in vivo and in vitro data summarized in this section can be integrated into a model for the modulation of renal concentrating mechanisms (Fig. 7–17). AVP-stimulated NaCl absorption by the mTALH is regulated by two negative feedback loops (the dashed lines in Fig. 7–17), each of which depends on increases in interstitial osmolality produced by the enhancement of countercurrent multiplication. During the early stages of antidiuresis, an AVP-mediated increase in NaCl absorption by the mTALH leads to a rapid rise in the interstitial NaCl concentration. This increase in interstitial osmolality stimulates the release of PGE₂ from interstitial cells, which, in turn, decreases the rate of AVP-stimulated NaCl absorption. Later during antidiuresis, a rise in medullary interstitial urea concentration tends to inhibit PGE₂ release from interstitial cells and the AVP-mediated increase in NaCl absorption from the mTALH.[279]

Thus the direct inhibition by interstitial hyperosmolality on AVP-dependent NaCl absorption by the mTALH is coupled to PGE₂ production, which modulates AVP action through the second messenger cAMP; the net effect is a negative feedback loop on AVP-dependent NaCl addition to the medullary interstitium. A similar negative feedback loop operates at the level of the collecting duct, where endogenous PGE₂ production, stimulated by AVP, decreases the AVP-induced increase in water permeability at the level of cellular cAMP accumulation.

CLINICAL DERANGEMENTS OF WATER BALANCE

The control of plasma osmolality and its primary determinant, the plasma sodium concentration, is achieved through AVP-mediated water conservation and thirst-induced water acquisition (see Fig. 7–1). Likewise, abnormal plasma osmolality, i.e., hypo- or hypernatremia, is generally the result of a derangement in water balance rather than salt balance. The integrated actions of the two effector limbs of the water repletion reaction are required: water conservation and water intake.

As illustrated in Figure 7–7, the principal physiological stimulus for AVP secretion is plasma osmolality.[306] At low plasma osmolalities, AVP secretion is suppressed, but when plasma osmolality exceeds the threshold value, usually about 280 mmol/kg, AVP secretion increases in a linear fashion. AVP, in turn, produces urine concentration. Figure 7–18 depicts the relation, at a given solute excretion rate, between the plasma AVP level and urine osmolality. A comparison of Figures 7–7 and 7–18 indicates that, at a plasma osmolality of 290 mmol/kg, 10 mmol/kg above the AVP threshold, the plasma AVP concentration, approximately 4 to 5 pmol/L (4 to 5 ng/L), is sufficient to cause maximal urine concentration. Conversely, at a plasma osmolality of 280 mmol/kg, the plasma AVP level is completely suppressed, and the urine is maximally dilute. In other words, a 3% increase in plasma osmolality converts a normal individual from a state of maximal diuresis to one of maximal antidiuresis.

The urine flow rate varies inversely with the urine osmolality. Thus when plasma AVP is suppressed to levels that allow maximal urine dilution, the rate of water excretion increases dramatically. At solute excretion rates of 800 to 900 mmol/d, for example, the free water clearance can approach 20 L/d. That is, a normal individual can ingest up to 20 L of water daily and not risk water intoxication.

The osmotic threshold for thirst is roughly 290 mmol/kg, 10 mmol/kg above the AVP threshold. Small increases in plasma osmolality above the thirst threshold result in intense thirst and a large increase in water intake. Thus the thresholds for AVP and thirst form the lower and upper boundaries, respectively, for plasma osmolality. A fall in plasma osmolality toward the AVP threshold causes a large water diuresis with a subsequent increase in plasma osmolality. An increase in plasma osmolality past the thirst threshold, on the other hand, causes a large increase in water intake with a subsequent fall in plasma osmolality. It should also be apparent that, within the range defined by these thresholds, the plasma osmolality is determined primarily by AVP-mediated changes in urine concentration.

THE HYPERTONIC SYNDROMES

As discussed in the introductory section, increases in effective ECF osmolality are caused by substances to which cell membranes are relatively impermeable (such as NaCl, mannitol, and, in the case of insulin deficiency, glucose). The hypertonic syndromes are defined by an increased ratio of an effectively impermeable solute to water in the ECF and are directly associated with cellular dehydration and shrinkage. Because body fluids are in osmotic equilibrium, the plasma osmolality is determined by the ratio of total body solutes to total body water. The major extracellular and intracellular solutes are salts of sodium and potassium, respectively. Accordingly, hypertonicity can result from an increase in total body sodium or potassium, or both, or from a decrease in total body water.

Hypertonicity that is associated with increased total body sodium most often results from the administration of hypertonic sodium bicarbonate during cardiopulmonary resuscitation. Hyperkalemia is lethal before the development of significant hypertonicity resulting from increases in total body potassium. Hypertonicity can also result from increases in the concentration of solutes other than sodium and potassium, for example, mannitol or glycerol. In these cases the serum sodium concentration may be normal or even depressed. However, as the solute is excreted with its obligate water load, the serum sodium concentration may become elevated. This phenomenon is discussed later in more detail under Osmotic Diuresis.

In practice, hypertonic syndromes result from decreases in total body water that are due to either renal or extrarenal water losses in the face of inadequate water replacement.

Classification

With reference to Figure 7–1, failure of water homeostasis may result from inadequacy of either AVP-dependent water conservation or thirst-mediated water acquisition. On the basis of the underlying pathophysiology, the clinical circumstances that lead to hypernatremia may be grouped into the general categories that are given in Table 7–5.

Total deficiency of renal concentrating mechanisms will not lead to hypertonicity if free access to water is ensured. Most commonly, clinically significant hypertonic volume depletion is seen in the very young or the very old, in whom either physical immaturity or debility prevents the translation of thirst into water-acquiring behavior, and in individuals who are unable to communicate thirst, for example, trauma victims and comatose patients. In a small group of

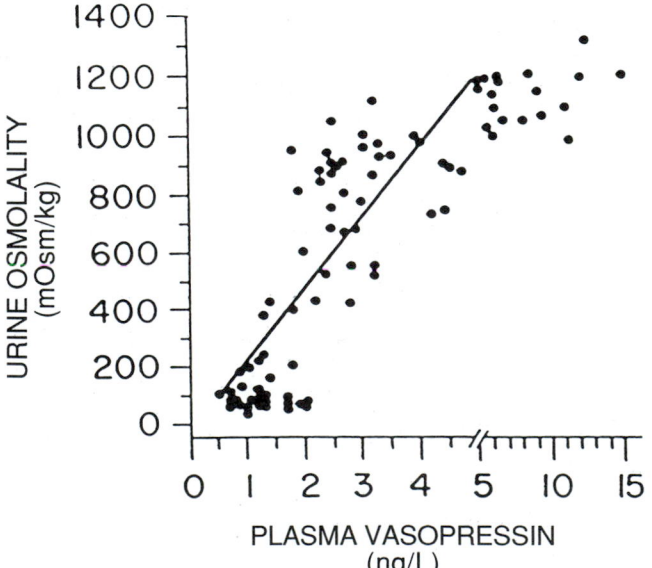

Figure 7–18. The relation between plasma AVP concentrations and urine osmolality. (Adapted from Robertson GL, Berl T. Water metabolism. In: Brenner BM, Rector FC Jr, eds. The Kidney. 3rd ed. Philadelphia: W. B. Saunders, 1986: 385–432.)

TABLE 7–5. Major Causes of Hypernatremia

Impaired Thirst	Solute Diuresis
Coma	Glucose
Essential hypernatremia	Diabetic ketoacidosis
Excessive Water Losses	Nonketotic hyperosmolar coma
Renal	Other
Central diabetes insipidus	Mannitol administration
Nephrogenic diabetes insipidus	Glycerol adminstration
Impaired medullary	**Sodium Excess**
hypertonicity	Administration of hypertonic NaCl
Extrarenal	Administration of hypertonic NaHCO₃
Sweating	
Osmotic diarrhea	
Burns	

patients, those with essential hypernatremia, the osmoregulatory centers are diseased, and osmotic stimulation of both AVP release and thirst is impaired.

Central diabetes insipidus is characterized by the failure of appropriate osmotic, volume, or chemical stimuli to evoke antidiuresis and by a prompt response to exogenous vasopressin to diminish urine volume and to raise urine osmolality. Congenital nephrogenic diabetes insipidus is identified by polyuria present since birth, generally in males, and by persistent unresponsiveness to exogenous vasopressin. Acquired nephrogenic diabetes insipidus is recognized by unresponsiveness to vasopressin combined with a history of exposure to agents, such as lithium, demeclocycline, or methoxyflurane anesthesia, that antagonize the action of AVP on collecting ducts. The history and laboratory data are adequate to identify disorders such as sickle cell disease or interstitial nephritis, both of which impair the ability to generate a hypertonic medullary interstitium. Finally, routine laboratory screening readily identifies the presence of hypercalcemia or hypokalemia.

Disorders such as diabetes mellitus, which produces a solute diuresis, are characterized by an isotonic urine and by glycosuria. Therapeutic administration of mannitol or glycerol for reduction of intracranial pressure is likewise associated with production of large volumes of a relatively isotonic urine. In other words, hypertonic disorders that are associated with solute diuresis are characterized by high rates of solute excretion (i.e., by a high C_{osm}; see Fig. 7–11), whereas the central or nephrogenic diabetes insipidus syndromes are characterized by defects in water conservation with normal rates of solute excretion. Rarely, hypernatremia is due to therapeutic administration of hypertonic NaCl.

The Clinical Syndromes

Essential Hypernatremia

A number of patients have been described[307, 308] with chronic hypernatremia in a setting of euvolemia, normal renal function, decreased thirst perception, and a normal renal response to exogenous vasopressin; this disorder is generally referred to as *essential hypernatremia*. Despite marked elevations of serum sodium concentrations and ECF osmolalities, these patients exhibit hypodipsia and an inappropriately dilute urine.[307, 308] This disorder might be due to a resetting of the threshold sensitivity of osmoreceptors in the CNS.[307, 308] However, Halter and co-workers[309, 310] showed that the osmotic threshold for AVP release is normal but that the release of AVP at any level of plasma osmolality is markedly attenuated. The syndrome of essential hypernatremia has been reported in association with CNS histiocytosis, with pineal tumors, with surgery for craniopharyngioma, and with head trauma.[300, 307, 308]

A common finding in these patients has been a normal response of AVP release, measured either as a rise in urine osmolality[307, 308] or as an increase in plasma AVP levels measured by radioimmunoassay,[309, 310] to effective baroreceptor stimulation. This finding has been interpreted to indicate adequate AVP production and storage associated with a dissociation between the osmoreceptor and the remainder of the neurohypophysis.

Given the association of a diminished sensation of thirst and a diminished release of AVP in response to osmotic stimulation, it is likely that essential hypernatremia represents a more or less specific ablation of hypothalamic osmoreceptor function. Forced hydration does not consistently correct the hypernatremia in these patients, but chlorpropamide, a drug that augments the antidiuretic effect of low levels of circulating AVP,[311] has been useful in restoring osmotic homeostasis.[307, 308]

Central Diabetes Insipidus

Central diabetes insipidus AVP is a polyuric syndrome that results from a lack of sufficient AVP to concentrate the urine for water conservation. The disease is identified by three primary findings: the persistence of an inappropriately dilute urine in the presence of strong osmotic or nonosmotic stimuli for AVP secretion; the absence of intrinsic renal disease; and a rise in urine osmolality on the administration of AVP.

ETIOLOGY. The spectrum of etiological factors causing central diabetes insipidus (Table 7–6) has changed over time. In 1928 Fink[7] reviewed necropsy data from 107 recorded cases of central diabetes insipidus and found 63% of cases to be associated with tumors of the basilar surface of the brain, 11% to be secondary to head trauma, and 25% to be associated with inflammation of the basal meninges; of the last group, half were syphilitic and one fifth were tuberculous. In contrast, of 92 patients with central diabetes insipidus who were studied by Moses and Notman[312] in 1972 to 1980, 30% of cases were idiopathic, 25% were related to malignant or benign tumors of either the brain or the pituitary fossa, 16% were secondary to head trauma, and 20% followed cranial surgery for tumor or hypophysectomy.

Primary intracranial tumors that are associated with diabetes insipidus are often craniopharyngiomas, and metastatic tumors are most often from lung or breast. The appearance of local hypothalamic disease may be delayed up to 10 y after the onset of diabetes insipidus.[313, 314] Periodic follow-up of patients who are diagnosed as having idiopathic central diabetes insipidus is recommended to detect delayed intracranial lesions. Finally, histiocytosis (either eosinophilic granuloma or Hand-Schüller-Christian disease), encephalitis or meningitis, sarcoidosis, and intraventricular hemorrhage can cause central diabetes insipidus.[312, 315]

A rare, hereditary form of the disorder is transmitted as an autosomal dominant trait, has equal occurrence in males and females, displays father-to-son transmission, and shows variable expression among affected individuals.[316, 317] These patients may maintain a persistently hypotonic urine even when hyperosmolality is induced by dehydration or infusion of hypertonic saline, or when hypotension is induced pharmacologically; yet, all patients respond to exogenous vasopressin with a reduction in urine volume and elevation of urine osmolality. This disorder therefore is different from familial nephrogenic diabetes insipidus, in which vasopressin administration is ineffective in inducing antidiuresis.[318] Some patients with familial central diabetes insipidus exhibit increased plasma AVP levels in response to strong osmotic or nonosmotic stimuli of AVP release.[317, 319] This finding, plus the observations of neuronal degeneration and gliosis in the SON and the PVN and the fact that symptoms of polyuria and polydipsia are not usually present at birth, has suggested that the disorder is due to a degenerative process of magnicellular neurons.[316, 319] Finally, central diabetes insipidus has been reported in about one third

TABLE 7–6. Causes of Central Diabetes Insipidus

Familial (autosomal dominant) etiology
Acquired etiology
  Idiopathic disorder
  Traumatic or postsurgical cause
  Neoplastic disease: craniopharyngioma, lymphoma, meningioma, metastatic carcinoma
  Ischemic or hypoxic disorder: Sheehan syndrome, aneurysms, cardiopulmonary arrest, aortocoronary bypass, shock, brain death
  Granulomatous disease: sarcoidosis, histiocytosis
  Infections: viral encephalitis, bacterial meningitis
  Autoimmune disorder

of patients with the inherited DIDMOAD (Wolfram) syndrome: diabetes insipidus, diabetes mellitus, optic atrophy, and deafness.[320, 321]

PATHOPHYSIOLOGY. Two features associated with the development of diabetes insipidus after injury to the neurohypophyseal system are noteworthy: the first relates to the site and degree of injury necessary to reduce AVP levels to lower than those that are required for normal water homeostasis; and the second is the characteristic triphasic response of neurohypophyseal function to injury.

Removal of the posterior pituitary gland does not necessarily lead to diabetes insipidus.[14] Rather, persistent polyuria develops only after an injury that is sufficiently high in the supraopticohypophyseal tract to cause bilateral neuron degeneration in the SON and the PVN.[19] Heinbecker and White[322] compared the degree of injury in the SON and the PVN of dogs by counting the number of intact residual cells after high section of the supraopticohypophyseal tract and by correlating these results with the magnitude of the ensuing permanent polyuria. Preservation of as few as 15% of magnicellular neurons prevented polyuria entirely, whereas fully evident diabetes insipidus occurred when only 6 to 8% of the neurons remained.

A similar estimate of the number of functional cells that are required for normal water metabolism in humans was made by Rasmussen and Gardner,[323] who found only 15% of the normal number of cells in the SONs of a patient with surgical trauma to the hypothalamus but no symptoms of diabetes insipidus. These studies are consistent with the observation that anterior pituitary tumors compress the posterior pituitary but rarely cause diabetes insipidus.[315, 324] In addition, diabetes insipidus occurs uncommonly in patients with spontaneous, hemorrhagic infarction of the anterior pituitary gland, that is, Sheehan syndrome.[325, 326] In short, although transient diabetes insipidus may accompany any injury to the neurohypophysis, permanent diabetes insipidus usually follows neurohypophyseal damage only high in the pituitary stalk.

Diabetes insipidus after surgery to the pituitary or hypothalamus may exhibit one of three patterns: transient, permanent, or triphasic. Transient diabetes insipidus usually has an abrupt onset within the first postoperative day and resolves within several days. Permanent or prolonged diabetes insipidus also has an abrupt and early onset but persists for weeks or may be permanent. This form of diabetes insipidus follows damage to the neurohypophyseal stalk or hypothalamus. In the triphasic pattern, shown in Figure 7–19, there is an immediate postinjury increase in urine volume and a concomitant fall in urine osmolality, which lasts 4 to 5 d; an intervening period of 5 to 7 d (the interphase) during which urine flow falls abruptly and urine osmolality rises; and a final phase consisting of permanent, hyposthenuric polyuria. This triphasic pattern also occurs after destruction of the supraopticohypophyseal tract in cats.[19] A similar response may take place in patients who are subjected to ablative pituitary surgery.

The initial diuresis of the triphasic response has been assumed to be due to an injury-related neuronal shock during which time no hormone release occurs.[315, 324] Alternatively, release of biologically inactive precursors from the damaged neurohypophysis may inhibit the renal actions of AVP.[327] The interphase appears to be due to the leak of hormone from degenerating neurons, because the urinary excretion of water cannot be altered either by water loading or by hypotonic saline infusions[328] and because complete removal of the posterior pituitary together with hypothalamic nuclei of the neurohypophyseal system prevents the appearance of an interphase.[315]

Patients who develop central diabetes insipidus postop-

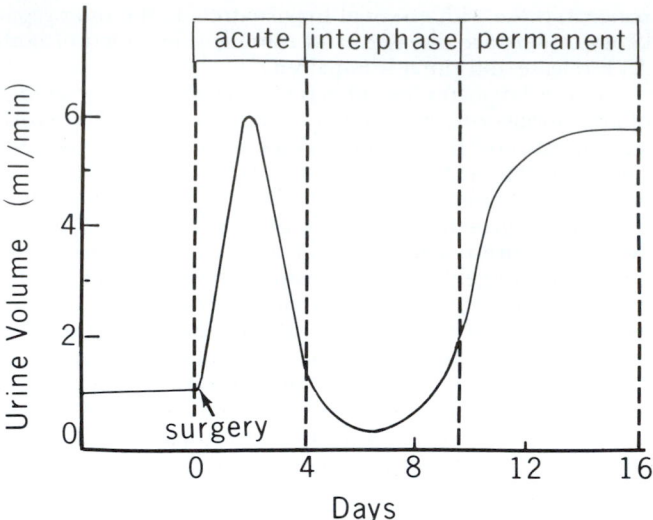

Figure 7–19. Triphasic response of urine volume after injury to the supraopticohypophyseal tract. (From C Fisher, WR Ingram, The effect of interruption of the supraoptico-hypophyseal tracts on the antidiuretic, pressor and oxytocic activity of the posterior lobe of the hypophysis, Endocrinology 20, 762–768, 1936, © by The Endocrine Society.)

eratively can osmoregulate effectively despite these extreme fluctuations in AVP levels, as long as they control water intake through thirst. However, severe water intoxication can develop during the phase of autonomous AVP release if infusion of hypotonic fluids, which is often initiated during the initial polyuric phase, is continued. Urine and serum osmolalities should be monitored carefully in patients after surgery in the area of the neurohypophysis.

CLINICAL MANIFESTATIONS. The primary symptoms of diabetes insipidus are persistent polyuria and its constant companions, thirst and polydipsia. Willis in 1670 made a clear distinction between the saccharine nature of the urine in the polyuria of diabetes mellitus and the odorless, tasteless urine in the polyuric state that is now known as diabetes insipidus. A thorough description of the clinical manifestations can be found in the 1883 edition of Quain's A Dictionary of Medicine[329] under the title "Polyuria":

Regarding the clinical history of polyuria . . . thirst and watery urine are the two prime symptoms, for there may be little wasting, and the general health may be good. As long as drink is supplied in plenty, the condition of the patients is very tolerable, were it not for the broken sleep caused by the increased thirst and the desire to pass water; but any attempt to restrict the quantity of fluid gives rise to intense discomfort. . . . The urine is inordinate in its quantity, and of a specific gravity little above that of spring water . . . persistently at 1.001. If the drink be restricted, more will be passed than is consumed, by the abstraction of water from the body.

When circumstances may prevent it [the bladder] from being emptied with sufficient frequency, thickening of the walls of the bladder, dilation of the ureters, and sacculations of the kidney have been described.

Osler[330] added to this description by noting that patients with pituitary diabetes insipidus "may pass 20–40 pints of urine daily, having a specific gravity from 1.001–1.005, and lacking sugar, albumen or sediment." He also noted that "perspiration in these patients was slight; the skin, harsh; the saliva, small; and the mouth was dry." He concluded, "Death usually takes place from some intercurrent affliction."

Little need be added to these descriptions. The volume of urine excreted may vary from only a few liters per day, in the case of a partial hormone deficiency, to a maximum of about 18 L/d, the average volume of glomerular filtrate that is delivered to collecting ducts, in the case of a total absence of AVP. Thus patients with partial central diabetes insipidus may be so little inconvenienced as to ignore their symptoms, with the disorder being noticed only when they are deprived of water. Nocturia is almost invariably present in patients with diabetes insipidus, as opposed to patients with primary polydipsia, in whom nocturia is uncommon.

Most cases of central diabetes insipidus have a rather abrupt onset of polyuria and polydipsia, in contrast to the onset of polyuria syndromes that are due to alterations in the renal handling of water. The central diabetes insipidus that follows intracranial surgery usually shows a triphasic pattern (see earlier), with permanent polyuria commencing 10 to 14 d after surgery.

Patients with central diabetes insipidus usually show a particular predilection for cold or iced drinks to quench thirst. The most striking clinical manifestations occur if access to water is interrupted and hypertonic volume depletion develops. This condition, described later, is characterized by CNS manifestations beginning with irritability, followed by mental dullness, and progressing to coma with secondary signs of ataxia, hyperthermia, and hypotension. Finally, in patients with diabetes insipidus that is due to intracranial lesions, neurological symptoms of the primary lesion may be prominent.

LABORATORY MANIFESTATIONS. Persistent hyposthenuria, with a urine specific gravity of 1.005 or less and a urine osmolality less than 200 mmol/kg, is the hallmark of diabetes insipidus.[312, 315] Partial deficiency of AVP may be recognized only as an inappropriately dilute urine in the face of an elevated serum osmolality.[331] In euvolemic patients, the GFR is normal.[312, 315] Because patients with diabetes insipidus ingest water in response to plasma hypertonicity, random plasma osmolality determinations in these patients are, on the average, above the usual normal value of 287 mmol/kg.[332] The serum sodium concentrations are also elevated and account for the increases in plasma osmolality. In contrast, individuals with primary polydipsia have a primary aberration of the thirst mechanism and ingest water independent of physiological stimuli. These patients often have mild dilutional hyponatremia.[332] In patients in whom diabetes insipidus, either central or nephrogenic in origin, begins in childhood, considerable dilation of the urinary bladder, ureters, and renal pelvis may lead to renal damage.[333, 334]

DIAGNOSIS. With reference to Table 7–5, central diabetes inspidus must be separated from other polyuria states, such as solute diuresis, impaired renal concentrating ability, or nephrogenic diabetes insipidus. Measurement of serum and urine solute concentrations should disclose osmotic diuretics (glucose, mannitol, urea), and measurements of serum creatinine and serum electrolyte levels identify GFR reductions, hypokalemia, and hypercalcemia. A history of recent head trauma, intracranial surgery, or neurological deficits (bitemporal hemianopsia) that suggest midline tumors obviously points to central diabetes insipidus as a cause of the polyuric state.

A more difficult diagnostic problem is the separation of patients with partial or complete deficiency of AVP from those with primary polydipsia.[331, 332, 335] Certain factors suggest the most likely diagnosis. For example, a 24-h urine volume greater than 18 L, a random plasma osmolality determination lower than 285 mmol/kg, and a history of episodic polyuria all suggest compulsive water drinking as the underlying disorder. A history of head trauma or neoplasm, a history of sudden onset of unrelenting polyuria, and a random plasma osmolality determination higher than 290 mmol/kg suggest central diabetes insipidus. These distinguishing features depend on the fact that patients with central diabetes insipidus ingest water only in response to

appropriate physiological stimuli and therefore do not ingest water to the point of becoming hyponatremic.

The basis of all tests for central diabetes insipidus rests on the ability of the kidney to excrete a hypertonic urine after an osmotic stimulus. The simplest maneuver is to produce hypertonicity of body fluids by water deprivation. The absolute level of urine concentration with water deprivation is nondiagnostic, because maximal concentrating ability depends on the degree of medullary hypertonicity as well as on the presence of adequate amounts of AVP. For example, Miller and co-workers[331] found the maximal urine osmolality that was produced by water deprivation in a group of randomly selected hospitalized patients to be 764 mmol/kg compared with 1067 mmol/kg in healthy volunteers. Presumably, the lower value for maximal concentrating ability in hospitalized patients reflects a reduction in medullary interstitial hypertonicity compared with that in normal volunteers.

However, even in patients with reduced medullary interstitial tonicity, the maximal urine osmolality that is achieved with water deprivation depends on maximal degrees of endogenous AVP release in response to dehydration. Therefore, in individuals with intact AVP production and release, the administration of exogenous vasopressin does not produce an increase in the maximal urine osmolality that is achieved via water deprivation. This rationale forms the framework for a test scheme,[312, 331] which is illustrated in Figure 7–20, for distinguishing complete or partial central diabetes insipidus from other polyuria syndromes.

In patients with mild polyuria, water deprivation may begin the night preceding the test; patients with severe polyuria should have water restricted during the day to allow for close observation. The test begins with paired measurements of osmolality of urine and plasma. All water intake is then withheld, and hourly measurements of urine osmolality and body weight are made. When two sequential urine osmolality values vary by less than 30 mmol/kg, or when 3 to 5% of body weight is lost, 5 U of aqueous vasopressin is injected subcutaneously. A final urine osmolality measurement is taken 60 min later. It is particularly important that this test be carried out under careful supervision to avoid water intoxication in patients with primary polydipsia related to continued ingestion of water in association with parenteral vasopressin administration.

The combined water restriction–vasopressin administration test may be interpreted as follows. The time that is required to achieve maximal urine concentration varies from 4 to 18 h.[312] In normal individuals the water deprivation results in a urine osmolality two to four times greater than that of plasma. More important, the subsequent administration of exogenous vasopressin results in less than 9% further increase in urine osmolality. Patients with primary polydipsia, who have a reduced medullary interstitial tonicity as a result of prolonged water diuresis, may concentrate urine only slightly after water deprivation. However, they too have maximally enhanced endogenous AVP release and exhibit a less than 9% rise in urine osmolality with supplemental vasopressin.

Patients with complete central diabetes insipidus do not increase urine osmolality above plasma osmolality in response to water deprivation but do show a greater than 50% increase in urine osmolality in response to injection of vasopressin.[312, 331] Patients with partial central diabetes insipidus may concentrate the urine to some degree in response to water deprivation, but they also increase urine osmolality by at least 10% after vasopressin injection.[312, 331] Patients with partial central diabetes insipidus often show a peak urine osmolality that decreases with further water restriction, which suggests a limited reserve of neurohypophyseal hor-

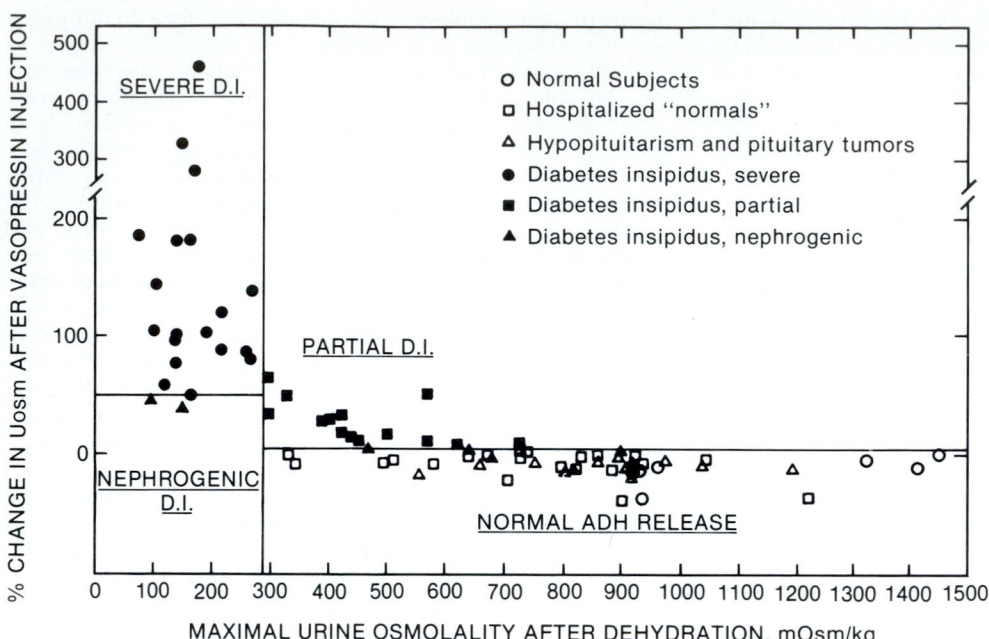

Figure 7–20. Response of urine osmolality to water deprivation and vasopressin injection in normal subjects, in patients with central or nephrogenic diabetes insipidus, and in patients with hypopituitarism. (Reproduced with permission, from Miller M, Dalakos T, Moses AM, et al. Recognition of partial defects in antidiuretic hormone secretion. Ann Intern Med 1970; 73:721–729.)

mone that becomes depleted after an initial secretory burst. Finally, deprivation of water in patients with nephrogenic diabetes insipidus fails to increase urine osmolality above plasma osmolality even when exogenous vasopressin is given.

When a diagnosis of central diabetes insipidus is made, a careful evaluation for neoplasms involving the hypothalamus or the neurohypophyseal tract is mandatory. Computed tomography or magnetic resonance imaging of the head has helped to reveal not only small mass lesions of the hypothalamic region but also an empty posterior sella, which results from posterior pituitary atrophy.[336]

Levels of circulating AVP have heretofore been measured by radioimmunoassay only for research purposes. A commercial assay is marketed for clinical use, but its general applicability is undefined. Zerbe and Robertson[335] compared the diagnostic accuracy of the indirect test for AVP release described earlier with actual measurements of plasma AVP levels by radioimmunoassay. The diagnosis of severe central diabetes insipidus or nephrogenic diabetes insipidus that was made by the indirect test was confirmed in every case by direct measurements of plasma AVP levels. In contrast, two patients who were diagnosed as having partial diabetes insipidus by the indirect test had normal plasma AVP levels when subjected to dehydration; one patient had primary polydipsia, the other, nephrogenic diabetes insipidus. Finally, 3 of 10 patients who were classified as having primary polydipsia by the indirect test had plasma AVP levels that were consistent with partial central diabetes insipidus. These authors concluded that direct measurement of plasma AVP levels can improve the diagnostic accuracy of indirect tests for diagnosis of the polyuria syndromes, but care must be taken in interpreting results from currently available radioimmunoassays.[335]

Hypertonic saline infusion has also been utilized to test for release of AVP.[312] In this procedure hypertonic saline is briefly infused to raise the serum sodium concentration to between 145 and 150 mmol/L and one or more blood samples are obtained for measurement of serum osmolality and AVP concentration. Patients with primary polydipsia or nephrogenic diabetes insipidus exhibit normal stimulation of AVP release in response to the hypertonicity. Patients with central diabetes insipidus, however, have little or no rise in plasma AVP levels. This procedure may be hazardous

in patients with limited cardiac reserve, in whom volume expansion may precipitate cardiac decompensation.

Nicotine, which is a nonosmotic stimulus of AVP secretion (see under The Control of Vasopressin Release), has been used to elicit antidiuresis in patients with essential hypernatremia, who release AVP in response to volume contraction but not in response to hypertonicity. A preferable diagnostic approach in these patients is to assess the antidiuretic response to mild volume contraction.[308, 310]

THERAPY

Estimation of Free Water Deficit. Patients with diabetes insipidus, either central pituitary or nephrogenic, may require emergency treatment for hypertonic encephalopathy consequent to polyuria and inadequate water intake. The goal in treating hypertonic encephalopathy is to replenish body water, thereby restoring osmotic homeostasis and repleting cell volume at a rate that avoids significant complications. Because the brain adjusts to hypertonicity, at least in part, by increasing the intracellular solute content via the accumulation of "idiogenic osmoles"[337, 338] (see later), the rapid repletion of body water with ECF dilution causes translocation of water into cells to achieve osmotic equilibrium. The result of this water movement is cell swelling and cerebral edema. Accordingly, seizures may occur in up to 40% of patients who were treated for severe hypernatremia by rapid infusions of hypotonic solutions.[339] If slower water repletion is undertaken, brain cells lose the accumulated intracellular solutes, and osmotic equilibration can occur without cell swelling. Consequently, a good rule of thumb is to administer fluids at a rate that reduces the serum sodium concentration by about 1 mmol/L every 2 h.

The magnitude of acute water loss in disorders such as central or nephrogenic diabetes insipidus, in which hypernatremia is due to water loss exclusively, can be estimated by using the assumption that the total ECF sodium content has remained nearly constant. A quantitative statement of this argument is

$$\text{Body water}_N \times [\text{Na}^+]_N = \text{body water}_H \times [\text{Na}^+]_H$$

where the subscript N denotes total body water and serum sodium concentration in the normal state and the subscript

H denotes the same values in the hypertonic state. Because body water is approximately 60% of body weight in kilograms, this equation can be rearranged to obtain

$$\text{Water deficit} = 0.6 \times \text{body weight} (1 - 140/[\text{Na}^+])$$

where body weight is estimated as the initial weight in kilograms, before hypertonicity develops, 140 is the normal serum sodium concentration, and $[\text{Na}^+]$ is the serum sodium concentration in millimoles per liter. As stressed earlier, this formulation is most applicable when there is no deficit in total ECF sodium content. In hypernatremic states that are associated with net sodium deficits, the formulation underestimates the total water deficit.

The choice of fluid to be administered in diabetes insipidus depends on three factors: the extent to which circulatory collapse may be present; the rate at which hypernatremia has developed; and the magnitude of the hypernatremia. Hypotonic NaCl solutions or oral fluids are best used as initial therapy in patients with modest volume contraction and only modest elevations of serum sodium concentrations, that is, less than 160 mmol/L. However, in patients with more advanced hypernatremia, particularly if the hypernatremia has developed gradually, that is, over a period more than 24 h, and is accompanied by circulatory collapse, a more prudent initial therapy is to administer normal saline solutions. The reasons for this choice are twofold: in advanced hypernatremia, a normal saline solution is dilute relative to body fluid osmolality and thus will dilute the latter while minimizing the risk of iatrogenic cerebral swelling; at the same time, normal saline provides an effective means of volume expansion.

Finally, 5% glucose solutions may be used to replenish body water in acute hypernatremia in the absence of significant circulatory collapse. However, the glucose infusion rate must be less than the rate of glucose metabolism to avoid glycosuria. Otherwise, the resulting osmotic diuresis will thwart attempts to replenish body free water.

Chronic Therapy. Because the most troublesome effects of central diabetes insipidus are persistent polyuria, inevitable nocturia, and constant thirst, the goal of treatment is to reduce the daily volume of urine excretion. Patients with partial hormonal deficiency and urine volumes of 2 to 6 L daily may require no treatment as long as they are assured access to water. The specific therapy for central diabetes insipidus is some form of vasopressin replacement. Hormone preparations differ in the mode of administration and the duration of biological effect (Table 7–7).

Early preparations of dried posterior pituitary extract, termed *pituitary snuff*, were given by nasal insufflation, had an effective biological life of only a few hours, and inevitably produced chronic rhinitis, which often led to inadequate absorption of hormone.[312] Pulmonary hypersensitivity reactions have also occurred with this preparation;[340] it is no longer used. Aqueous vasopressin is active for only a few hours and is thus not practical, although nasal sprays of aqueous lysine vasopressin may provide intermittent relief of polyuria.[312, 315] Neither of these preparations is effective in preventing nocturia.

A widely used preparation in the past was vasopressin tannate in oil, given intramuscularly. As little as 1.5 U (0.3 mL) daily may provide adequate hormone for 24 to 48 h.[312, 315] Great care must be exercised in preparing the injection by careful warming and mixing of the ampule so as to suspend the hormone uniformly in the oil. Failure to do so may result in injection of the oil vehicle alone and thus in apparent vasopressin resistance. Pain at injection sites and sterile abscesses are frequent and recurrent abdominal pain from the effect of vasopressin on intestinal motility may occur.

A synthetic analogue of vasopressin, desmopressin (see earlier), provides antidiuretic activity for 8 to 20 h with negligible pressor effect, can be taken as a nasal formulation, and is the drug of choice for both adults and children.[312, 315, 341] The drug is best started at night to find the lowest dose that prevents nocturia. This dose, usually 5 to 10 μg, can be given twice daily or can be doubled as a single morning dose. A nasal catheter is calibrated for convenient dosing in the 5- to 20-μg range. Headache may be a troublesome side effect with large doses but usually disappears with a reduction of dosage.[342] A parenteral formulation is available for patients who are unable to take the drug by nasal insufflation. The parenteral route is also used when desmopressin is used for its hemostatic effects in patients with uremia or von Willebrand disease. Desmopressin can also be effective when administered orally.[343] The doses that are required for oral administration are higher than those for the nasal route. The oral preparation is not available in the United States.

For patients having some residual AVP production, the oral hypoglycemic agent chlorpropamide may provide adequate amelioration of symptoms. Studies with normal, water-loaded subjects, in whom chlorpropamide administration

TABLE 7–7. Therapy of Central Diabetes Insipidus

Type of Therapy	Dose	Route	Duration of Action (h)	Usage/Comments
AVP replacement				
Aqueous vasopressin	5–10 U	SC, IM	4–6	Useful for diagnostic testing; acute management after trauma or surgery.
Vasopressin tannate in oil	1.5–5 U	IM	24–72	Long-term management failures can be due to improper mixing of emulsion. Side effects include smooth muscle contraction, angina, abdominal cramps.
Lysine vasopressin	5–10 U	Nasal spray	4–6	Short-acting, relatively nonirritating.
Desmopressin	5–20 μg	Nasal drops	12–24	Preferred drug. Side effects are few.
Adjunctive therapy				
Thiazide diuretics, e.g., hydrochlorothiazide	50–100 mg/d	PO	12–24	Also useful in nephrogenic diabetes insipidus. Na$^+$ loading diminishes effectiveness.
Chlorpropamide	250–750 mg/d	PO	24–36	Useful only in partial central diabetes insipidus. Hypoglycemia is not uncommon.
Clofibrate	250–500 mg every 6–8 h	PO	6–8	Useful only in partial central diabetes insipidus. Side effects are frequent.

caused increased urine AVP excretion, led to the suggestion that the drug stimulates AVP release.[344] Studies using specific radioimmunoassays in humans and rats have failed to demonstrate a rise in either AVP or its related neurophysin with chlorpropamide treatment.[341] There is now general agreement[312, 315, 344, 345] that chlorpropamide enhances the action of small amounts of AVP on renal tubules to augment urine-concentrating ability.

The exact mechanism of the potentiating effect of chlorpropamide on the action of AVP in the kidney is unclear. Chlorpropamide may enhance AVP stimulation of renal medullary cAMP by augmenting adenylate cyclase sensitivity to AVP or by inhibiting phosphodiesterase.[315] Inhibition of PGE_2 synthesis, thereby removing an antagonist of AVP, has also been proposed as a mechanism for chlorpropamide potentiation.[315] Finally, in microdissected tubules from normal and AVP-deficient Brattleboro rats, vasopressin-stimulated cAMP accumulation is enhanced in mTALH of chlorpropamide-treated animals.[346] The corticopapillary gradient of interstitial hypertonicity is also increased, predominantly through NaCl accumulation, in chlorpropamide-treated animals. Thus chlorpropamide treatment might augment AVP-dependent NaCl absorption in mTALH, thereby increasing the driving force for water absorption in collecting ducts.

Doses of 250 to 750 mg chlorpropamide daily are sufficient to reduce polyuria in most patients with partial central diabetes insipidus; between 50 and 80% of patients with central diabetes insipidus respond to this dosage with varying degrees of antidiuresis.[315] The side effect of hypoglycemia, which is especially common in children and in patients taking more than 500 mg daily of the drug, limits its usefulness.

The hypolipidemic agent clofibrate[347] and the anticonvulsant carbamazepine[348] may also curtail polyuria in patients with partial central diabetes insipidus. Both drugs seem to work by directly stimulating the release of AVP from the hypothalamus. In addition, carbamazepine may increase the sensitivity of the kidney to AVP.[349] The combination of clofibrate and chlorpropamide is useful for some patients.[315]

Finally, thiazide diuretics may reduce the volume of urine in patients with any form of diabetes insipidus, that is, either central or nephrogenic, by causing mild salt depletion. This depletion results in a secondary increase in isotonic proximal tubular fluid absorption and a decrease in the volume of fluid delivered to the collecting duct. The effect is produced by 50 to 100 mg of hydrochlorothiazide daily, is sustained by salt restriction, and can be abolished by salt loading even with continued diuretic administration.[350]

Nephrogenic Diabetes Insipidus

Nephrogenic diabetes insipidus is a polyuric disorder that is identified by the presence of normal rates of renal filtration and solute excretion, a persistently hypotonic urine, normal or high levels of plasma AVP, and a failure of exogenous vasopressin to raise urine osmolality or to reduce urine volume. Some of the conditions that are associated with a failure of the renal tubule to respond to vasopressin are noted in Table 7–8.

FAMILIAL DISEASE: HISTORY. In 1892 McIlraith[351] described three generations of individuals with diabetes insipidus: males were affected with "extreme thirst," females were "slightly affected," and male offspring of "slightly affected" females suffered from "extreme thirst." He concluded that this form of diabetes insipidus involved "a heredity occurring chiefly in males on the female side of the house." In a report of a family with hereditary diabetes insipidus involving four generations, deLange[352] observed a

TABLE 7–8. Causes of Nephrogenic Diabetes Insipidus

Familial (X-linked) etiology
Acquired etiology
  Hypokalemia
  Hypercalcemia
  Postobstruction
  Drugs: lithium, demeclocycline, methoxyflurane
  Sickle cell trait or disease
  Amyloidosis
  Pregnancy

lack of male-to-male transmission and noted that administration of posterior pituitary extracts did not reduce urine volume or increase urine specific gravity in affected patients.

In 1945 Forssman[353] published a review of hereditary diabetes insipidus and new data on five different kindreds involving 32 possible male patients. He established that male-to-male transmission does not occur, that descendants of phenotypically normal males are healthy, that polyuria invariably has its onset in infancy, that daily urine volumes in adults exceed 4 L, that urine specific gravity values after water deprivation are in the range 1.003 to 1.008, and that female carriers frequently have unusual thirst, nocturnal water consumption, and impaired urine-concentrating ability after water deprivation. In three affected men from one kindred, water deprivation combined with injections of posterior pituitary extracts failed to reduce urine volume or increase urine specific gravity. In 1947 Williams and Henry[354] applied the term *nephrogenic diabetes insipidus* to the disease; they stressed the fact that renal tubular insensitivity to AVP was the primary pathophysiological disturbance. The abnormal gene in this disorder is localized to the Xq28 region on the long arm of the X chromosome.[355] The close linkage of the gene with a number of X chromosome markers may provide a means for prenatal diagnosis of the disorder.[356]

CLINICAL MANIFESTATIONS. The narrative by Waring and co-workers[357] summarizes eloquently and succinctly the main clinical and pathophysiological features of the disease:

The syndrome is characterized by onset shortly after birth . . . polydipsia and polyuria which do not respond to pitressin . . . high values for serum sodium and chloride . . . rapid dehydration if fluids are reduced or withheld . . . inability to excrete urine of high specific gravity . . . familial incidence and occurrence in boys only (?).

The presenting complaints were unexplained fever, failure to gain weight and constipation.

Pitressin was given until toxic reactions were seen without any alteration in fluid intake or output.

Renal clearances done under good conditions of hydration showed normal values for mannitol, urea, phosphates and para-aminohippuric acid at high and low levels. . . . Only 70 to 80% of filtered water, as against 99.5 percent of the filtered sodium and 98.8 percent of the chloride, was reabsorbed in the renal tubules.

In short, the picture in dehydrated patients with nephrogenic diabetes insipidus is one of volume contraction, hypernatremia, and hyperthermia, attended by potentially lethal effects, particularly on the CNS. Because of the nonspecific nature of symptoms in early stages, the disorder may be difficult to identify in the first few months of life. Mental and physical retardation may occur, or children with the disorder may have normal intelligence and physical maturation. Inadequate caloric ingestion associated with incessant water intake accounts for growth retardation, and repeated bouts of hypernatremia may lead to mental impairment.[318]

RENAL FUNCTION. The cardinal abnormality is the failure of collecting ducts to increase water permeability in response to AVP, which results in the excretion of urine that is hypotonic to plasma. Williams and Henry[354] showed clearly that the concentrating defect is due to end-organ refractoriness to AVP, because doses of vasopressin that were sufficient to cause abdominal cramps and cutaneous blanching had no effect on urine volume and concentration.

Striking dilatation of the urinary tract may occur, as in some patients with central diabetes insipidus.[333] The dilatation may progress to massive hydroureter, hydronephrosis, and a urinary bladder capacity of more than 1 L.

SERUM VASOPRESSIN CONCENTRATIONS. Using a specific radioimmunoassay for AVP, Robertson and associates[107, 108] showed that, both in normal subjects and in patients with nephrogenic diabetes insipidus, serum osmolality values higher than 280 mmol/kg result in near-linear increments in serum AVP concentrations, whereas in patients with central diabetes insipidus, plasma AVP concentrations change negligibly or not at all in response to an osmotic challenge (Fig. 7–21). Second, normal subjects and patients with central diabetes insipidus exhibit a near-linear relationship between urine osmolality and plasma AVP concentrations, whereas patients with nephrogenic diabetes excrete a consistently hypotonic urine despite 15-fold variations in plasma AVP levels. These observations strongly support the hypothesis that familial nephrogenic diabetes insipidus is due to end-organ unresponsiveness to AVP.

PATHOPHYSIOLOGY. Hereditary vasopressin-unresponsive diabetes insipidus occurs in an inbred strain of mice termed DI $^{+/+}$ severe.[358] Stimulation of renal medullary adenylate cyclase activity by vasopressin is reduced in these mice. Because the basal level of renal medullary adenylate cyclase activity is normal and the stimulation of renal cortical adenylate cyclase by parathyroid hormone is normal,[354] the defect appears to be specific. Further studies with these mice indicate that vasopressin-stimulated adenylate cyclase activity is modestly reduced in medullary collecting duct and is severely reduced in medullary ascending limb compared

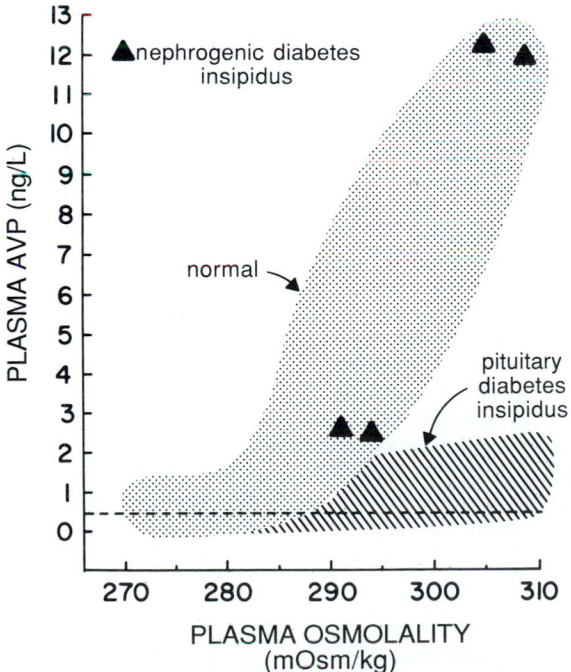

Figure 7–21. Relation between plasma AVP levels and serum osmolality in normal subjects, in patients with central diabetes insipidus, and in patients with nephrogenic diabetes insipidus. (Adapted from Robertson GL, Mahr EA, Athar S, et al. Development and clinical application of a new method for the radioimmunoassay of arginine vasopressin in human plasma. Adapted from the Journal of Clinical Investigation, 1973, vol. 52, pp. 2340–2352 by copyright permission of the American Society of Clinical Investigation; and Robertson GL. Vasopressin in osmotic regulation in man. Adapted, with permission, from the Annual Review of Medicine, Vol. 25, © 1974 by Annual Reviews Inc.)

with activity in normal mice.[360] In the medullary collecting duct, cAMP phosphodiesterase activity is markedly higher in DI $^{+/+}$ mice than in normal mice. The defect in cAMP accumulation in collecting duct segments is partially corrected by phosphodiesterase inhibitors alone, and in the presence of a phosphodiesterase inhibitor, the combination of AVP and forskolin results in normal cAMP accumulation.[361] These data indicate that elevated phosphodiesterase activity and a defect in the coupling of the AVP receptor to the catalytic subunit of adenylate cyclase may contribute to the concentrating defect in DI $^{+/+}$ mice.

The significance of these studies for the pathogenesis of human familial nephrogenic diabetes insipidus is uncertain. In normal individuals or patients with central diabetes insipidus, administration of exogenous vasopressin increases the rate of urinary cAMP excretion. In the majority of patients with familial nephrogenic diabetes insipidus, however, vasopressin and desmopressin have little or no effect on cAMP excretion.[362–364] The specificity of the defect is demonstrated by the ability of epinephrine to stimulate cAMP excretion normally in these individuals.[364] Thus the defect is specific to AVP responses and appears to reside at a pre-cAMP locus.

The lack of response to vasopressin in these patients appears to be restricted to the responses mediated by the V_2 receptor. V_1 receptor–mediated effects, such as vasoconstriction and enhancement of corticotropin release and renal prostaglandin production, are preserved in patients with familial nephrogenic diabetes insipidus.[365, 366] The V_2 receptor defect appears to be generalized and not restricted to the renal action of the hormone. Extrarenal effects that are mediated by V_2 receptors include an increase in levels of von Willebrand factor and factor VIII, a fall in diastolic blood pressure, and stimulation of renin release. In most patients with familial nephrogenic diabetes insipidus these extrarenal V_2 receptor–mediated responses are absent, which indicates a generalized defect in the V_2 receptor signal transduction pathway.[364, 367] Obligate carriers of the disorder, e.g., mothers of affected patients, demonstrate intermediate extrarenal responses to the administration of the selective V_2 agonist desmopressin. In occasional patients extrarenal V_2 receptor–mediated responses are preserved.[368, 369]

DRUG-INDUCED NEPHROGENIC DIABETES INSIPIDUS. Vasopressin-unresponsive hyposthenuria can occur in patients receiving demeclocycline; both the concentrating defect and the unresponsiveness to vasopressin are reversible and disappear after discontinuing the drug.[370] In toad urinary bladder, serosal demeclocycline inhibits the increase in water permeability produced by either vasopressin or cAMP.[370] In human renal medulla, demeclocycline noncompetitively inhibits basal adenylate cyclase activity, AVP-stimulated adenylate cyclase activity, and cAMP-dependent protein kinase activity but does not affect cyclic nucleotide phosphodiesterase activity.[371] These in vitro observations suggest that demeclocycline-induced nephrogenic diabetes insipidus may be due to inhibition of both cAMP accumulation and the action of cAMP on urinary membranes.[370]

Methoxyflurane anesthesia may also be followed by a vasopressin-resistant polyuria and hyposthenuria. Both fluoride and oxalic acid, which are metabolic products of methoxyflurane, contribute to the nephrotoxicity. However, the polyuric state is related to the increased serum concentration and urinary excretion of inorganic fluoride.[370] Sodium fluoride causes a vasopressin-resistant polyuria in dogs,[372] and in rats fluoride reduces collecting duct water permeability without affecting salt transport in the ascending limb.[373]

Finally, serum lithium concentrations of 0.5 to 1.5 mmol/L, which are in the therapeutic range for affective disorders, can produce vasopressin-resistant diabetes insipidus in 12 to 30% of patients receiving the drug; the disorder is usually reversible, and urine-concentrating ability returns toward normal when lithium is discontinued.[370]

In toad urinary bladder, lithium (11 mmol/L) inhibits the stimulation of water transport produced by vasopressin but not that produced by cAMP.[374] Furthermore, lithium specifically inhibits AVP-activated adenylate cyclase in mammalian renal medulla.[375] This inhibition is seen in both mTALH and medullary collecting ducts after acute administration of lithium but only in medullary collecting ducts in animals chronically treated with lithium.[376] Accordingly, lithium-induced polyuria that is observed clinically may be the consequence of inhibition of AVP-stimulated cAMP formation in collecting ducts.

DIAGNOSIS. The diagnostic characteristics of familial nephrogenic diabetes insipidus include onset during infancy; a positive family history; persistent thirst, polyuria, and hyposthenuria that are unresponsive to administration of vasopressin; and serum AVP levels that vary appropriately with changes in serum osmolality (see Fig. 7–21). In the absence of dehydration, renal function is normal. Likewise, acquired drug-induced nephrogenic diabetes insipidus is characterized by vasopressin-resistant polyuria. In the water deprivation test described earlier (see Fig. 7–20), urine osmolality in patients with nephrogenic diabetes insipidus achieved at maximal dehydration is further increased by less than 10% after administration of vasopressin.

TREATMENT. There is no specific therapy. Adequate hydration is easily achieved by oral intake in children and adults but sometimes requires parenteral supplementation in infants. Hydration is essential to prevent the damaging effects of hypernatremia and circulatory collapse, particularly in children. Although polyuria may be minimized by reducing solute intake, this measure is rarely necessary except in children. Neither vasopressin nor its analogues lysine vasopressin and desmopressin have any effect on the disease. Likewise, drugs that stimulate endogenous AVP release, such as clofibrate,[347] or that enhance AVP action, such as chlorpropamide,[346] are also ineffective. Inhibition of prostaglandin synthesis with ibuprofen, indomethacin, or aspirin reduces urine volume and slightly increases urine osmolality in patients with nephrogenic diabetes insipidus.[377–380] The effect appears to be secondary to a reduction in delivery of solute to the distal tubule and not to a reduction of prostaglandin antagonism to the tubular action of AVP.

The most effective therapy for nephrogenic diabetes insipidus is to attempt to reduce urine volume and hence to minimize nocturia and dilation of the urinary bladder and ureters. The most widely used approach is the combination of thiazide diuretics and mild salt depletion.[350] Amiloride is particularly effective in limiting the polyuria in lithium-induced diabetes insipidus.[381, 382] By blocking sodium channels in the collecting duct cell, amiloride may limit the entry of lithium into these cells. Amiloride is also less likely to produce hypokalemia and its associated concentrating defect than are thiazides.[383]

Mineralocorticoid Excess

Mild hypernatremia (serum sodium concentration > 145 mmol/L) often occurs in syndromes of primary mineralocorticoid excess. The hypernatremia is due to an increase in the osmotic threshold for AVP release in response to chronic hypervolemia (see Fig. 7–9). Reduction of the effective circulating volume with diuretics corrects the hypernatremia. Hypokalemia related to mineralocorticoid excess can impair renal concentrating ability, as discussed later, and can contribute to hypernatremia.

Electrolyte Disorders

Both potassium depletion and hypercalcemia can cause concentrating defects; in both circumstances the disorder is manifested primarily as a limitation in maximal renal concentrating ability rather than as persistent hyposthenuria. In hypokalemia, the defect in concentrating ability usually occurs when both GFR and urine-diluting ability are near normal; hence, it is difficult to argue that inadequate rates of solute absorption in the distal tubule are responsible for the concentrating defect.

Several factors may contribute to the genesis of hypokalemic polyuria. The Na^+ concentrations and osmolalities of the renal medulla and papilla are both decreased.[384] The polyuria is also associated with an increased excretion of PGE_2, and the administration of indomethacin, which inhibits prostaglandin synthesis, can partially correct the concentrating defect.[385] It thus appears that prostaglandin E inhibition of adenylate cyclase activation by AVP[256] contributes to the pathogenesis of hypokalemic polyuria. In addition, Berl and co-workers[386] suggested that potassium depletion results in polydipsia, thus accentuating polyuria independently of the concentrating defect.

In hypercalcemic states, the concentrating defect is ordinarily accompanied by a reduction in GFR. Additional factors that may contribute to the concentrating defect of hypercalcemia include the reduction in medullary solute content[387] and the inhibitory effect of calcium on adenylate cyclase activation by vasopressin in hormone-sensitive epithelia.[388] As mentioned previously, increases in extracellular calcium level inhibit AVP-sensitive adenylate cyclase activity in the mTALH.[245] Increases in intracellular (but not extracellular) calcium level also inhibit the AVP-induced cAMP accumulation in the collecting duct.[245,267]

Pregnancy

Diabetes insipidus is a rare complication of pregnancy.[389–392] This disorder, which has features of both central and nephrogenic diabetes insipidus, is thought to be caused by the degradation of circulating AVP by the enzyme vasopressinase.[389, 390, 392] The polyuria usually begins in the third trimester and resolves spontaneously after delivery. Plasma AVP levels are low, but the polyuria may not respond to exogenous vasopressin. In contrast, desmopressin promptly controls the polyuria.[389, 391] The serum contains high levels of vasopressinase.[389] This enzyme, which is a cysteine aminopeptidase, degrades AVP but not desmopressin, which accounts for the difference in therapeutic efficacy. Serum vasopressinase activity falls after delivery. In pregnant women the turnover rate of AVP normally increases during the later stages of pregnancy, presumably because of the high activity of vasopressinase in the placenta.[393]

True nephrogenic diabetes insipidus has also been reported during pregnancy. This condition, which is characterized by high plasma AVP levels and no response to either exogenous vasopressin or desmopressin, also remits after delivery. The pathogenesis is not known.[394]

Osmotic Diuresis

A type of vasopressin-resistant polyuria that can be confused with nephrogenic diabetes insipidus is osmotic diuresis. This syndrome is commonly iatrogenic and is typically seen in patients in an intensive care unit or in the postoperative state who receive infusions of large volumes of colloid or saline and in patients with uncontrolled diabetes mellitus. Analysis of the fluid therapy and measurement of the urine solute excretion rate generally are sufficient to diagnose this problem.

In diabetes insipidus, either nephrogenic or central, the polyuria represents a true water diuresis, and the solute excretion rate is normal. In contrast, the urine during an osmotic diuresis is nearly isotonic and the solute excretion rate is elevated. Thus the finding of an isotonic or a hypertonic urine in a polyuric patient usually indicates an osmotic diuresis. The reason for this is that the excretion of normal solute load ($\cong$ 800 mmol/d) in an isotonic urine (300 mmol/d) obligates only 2.7 L of urine daily. Urine volumes more than 3 L/d therefore require either an increased solute excretion rate or a hypotonic urine. Treatment is achieved by reducing the rate of solute administration.

Osmotic diuresis also affects the plasma sodium concentration. The accumulation of either exogenous solutes, e.g., glycerol or mannitol, which are given to reduce intracranial pressure, or endogenous solutes, e.g., glucose in uncontrolled diabetes mellitus, can result in plasma hypertonicity. The serum sodium concentration, however, may be normal or even reduced in the face of an elevated measured serum osmolality. Comparison of the measured osmolality and the calculated osmolality provides a clue to the diagnosis of these disorders.

Osmotic diuresis may also be associated with true hypernatremia (see Table 7–5). In the initial phases of an osmotic diuresis, patients are hypertonic, because of accumulation of nonsodium solutes, but are not hypernatremic. As the nonsodium solutes are excreted, the plasma osmolality falls slightly, because of a positive free water balance (see Fig. 7–11B), whereas sodium is left to represent an increasing fraction of the plasma osmolality. That is, as the nonsodium osmolality decreases, the sodium osmolality increases. When examined in these terms it can be said that the osmotic diuresis per se does not cause hypertonicity but results in the conversion of a normonatremic hypertonic state to a hypernatremic hypertonic state.

Hypertonic Encephalopathy

The consequences of the hypertonic syndromes—more specifically, disorders in which ECF osmolality is increased with solutes that are excluded from cells—include hypertonic encephalopathy and volume contraction. Virtually all cells, including those of the CNS, are permeable to water. Accordingly, an increase in the effective ECF osmolality inevitably results in osmotic equilibration between cells and ECF and, consequently, in an increase in intracellular osmolality. This equilibration may occur in one of three ways: in acute hypertonic states water is lost from cells, and the acute shrinkage in brain volume results in hypertonic encephalopathy; in chronic hypertonic states CNS cells accumulate solutes, and brain shrinkage is minimized so that CNS symptoms are also minimized; or a combination of these two processes may occur.[337] In other words, the rela-

tions among increases in effective ECF osmolality, changes in brain volume, and the occurrence of hypertonic encephalopathy depend on the magnitude of the ECF osmolality increase, the duration of the increase, and the solute responsible for the osmolality increase.

Hypernatremia may cause irreversible damage to the CNS, particularly in infants. An example of this phenomenon occurred in 1962 when infants were inadvertently given a nursery formula containing salt rather than sugar and developed hypernatremic encephalopathy with more than a 50% fatality rate.[395] In rabbits that are subjected to hypernatremia, neurological symptoms commence when the serum osmolality value reaches 350 to 375 mmol/kg; nystagmus and ataxia occur at a serum osmolality value of 375 to 400 mmol/kg; and coma, stupor, and death occur when the serum osmolality value is in the range of 400 to 435 mmol/kg.[396]

Because hypernatremic encephalopathy and death occur in animals in the absence of pathological changes in the CNS other than brain shrinkage and an increase in brain NaCl content,[397] it is reasonable to conclude that the combination of hyperosmolality and cellular shrinkage are the major factors responsible for hypertonic encephalopathy.[337] This hypothesis coincides with the clinical observation that, for a given elevation of serum osmolality, cerebral symptoms are more severe in patients with hypernatremia, diabetic ketoacidosis, or nonketotic hyperglycemic coma than in those with azotemia.

Cell Volume Adjustments to ECF Hypertonicity

The adjustments in brain cell volume and in the cellular content of osmotically active solutes that occur during acute (1 to 2 h) and chronic (2 h to 2 wk) increases in osmolality produced by endogenous and exogenous solutes are shown in Table 7–9. Although these data derive from experiments involving animals,[337, 398] similar changes are believed to occur in humans during the development of hypertonic states. The term *idiogenic osmoles* refers to osmotically active solutes measured as the difference between total cell osmolality and the sum of the osmolalities of Na^+, K^+, and Cl^-.[399]

During acute increases in osmolality caused by any of these endogenous or exogenous solutes, osmotic equilibrium between intracellular and extracellular water is achieved almost completely by cell water loss (see Table 7–9). In this case, increases in intracellular Na^+, K^+, and Cl^- concentrations account for the increase in cell osmolality, and idiogenic osmoles are therefore absent. This rapid change in brain cell volume appears to account for the severity of CNS symptoms and the high mortality from acute increases in effective ECF osmolality (see earlier).

In chronic hypertonic states, brain cell volume returns

TABLE 7–9. Brain Volume Adjustment During Hyperosmolality

Variable	Adjustment for Endogenous Solutes			Adjustment for Exogenous Solutes
	Na+	Glucose	Urea	Mannitol, Glycerol, Sucrose
Acute (1–2 h) hyperosmolality				
Brain water	↓↓	↓↓	↓↓	↓↓
Electrolyte content	Normal	Normal	Normal	Normal
Idiogenic osmoles	Absent	Absent	Absent	Absent
Chronic (2 h–2 wk) hyperosmolality				
Brain water	Normal	Normal	Normal	↓↓
Electrolyte content	↑	↑	Normal	Normal
Idiogenic osmoles	↑↑↑	↑↑	↑	Absent

Data from Arieff AI, Guisado R, Lazarowitz VC. The pathophysiology of hyperosmolar states. In: Andreoli TE, Grantham JJ, Rector FC, eds. Disturbances in Body Fluid Osmolality. Bethesda: American Physiological Society, 1977: 227–250; and Chan PH, Fishman RA. Elevation of rat brain amino acids and idiogenic osmoles induced by hyperosmolality. Brain Res 1979; 161:293–301.

toward normal (volume-regulatory increase) when the increase in osmolality is produced by endogenous solutes such as Na^+, glucose, and urea, but not with exogenous solutes such as glycerol, mannitol, and sucrose (see Table 7–9).[337] Why the exogenous solutes do not produce a brain cell volume–regulatory increase is not understood, but this result provides a rationale for the use of these solutes to reduce brain volume during episodes of cerebral edema.

The extent to which brain cell volume regulation occurs by solute or electrolyte uptake or by accumulation of organic idiogenic osmoles differs for each of the endogenous solutes. About 50 to 60% of the brain osmoles that are responsible for brain cell volume regulation during chronic hypernatremia are amino acids.[337,338] The remaining 40 to 50% of cell volume regulation during hypernatremia results from the cellular accumulation of Na^+, K^+, and Cl^-. The transport mechanism mediating intracellular accumulation of these ions has not been defined but may be similar to the coupled $Na^+,K^+,2Cl^-$ cotransport process (see Fig. 7–2) that is responsible for hypertonic volume regulation in several other cell types.[400] Finally, it should be emphasized that dissipation of the hypernatremia-induced organic osmoles after returning to the isotonic state is not rapid but takes hours to a day.

During hyperglycemia, brain volume regulation is due to insulin-independent cellular uptake of glucose (20%), to electrolyte uptake, and to accumulation of idiogenic osmoles. These osmoles, however, are not amino acids, and their nature is unknown. In contrast to the hypernatremia-induced amino acids, the idiogenic osmoles that accumulate during hyperglycemia dissipate rapidly with decreasing plasma glucose levels.[337] This difference may account for the clinical axiom that rapid reduction in serum sodium concentrations in diabetes insipidus patients with chronic hypernatremia commonly elicits seizures, whereas reductions in plasma glucose concentrations during a 6- to 8-h period in patients with nonketotic hyperglycemic coma are less hazardous.

THE HYPOTONIC SYNDROMES

The hypotonic syndromes include disorders in which the water repletion reaction (see Fig. 7–1) is deranged so that free water is not excreted at a rate sufficient to maintain the serum sodium concentration and the body fluid osmolality at normal rather than subnormal values. According to the general outline for water repletion mechanisms that was illustrated in Figure 7–1, such a circumstance might occur for any of the following reasons: (1) ingestion of a quantity of water that exceeds the capacity of the normal kidney to excrete it (primary polydipsia); (2) diminished capacity to excrete a water load because of inadequate solute delivery to the diluting segment; and (3) diminished capacity to excrete a water load because of sustained, nonosmotic release of AVP.

Classification

In principle, hyponatremia can develop if the rate of water intake exceeds the normal ability of the kidney to excrete free water. In fact, the hyponatremia that occurs in primary polydipsia is generally slight, with serum sodium concentrations generally being in the range of 135 mmol/L.[332] The usual reason for clinically insignificant hyponatremia in primary polydipsia may be inferred from Figure 7–10. In normal individuals, salt abstraction in the TALH results in the formation of a dilute distal tubular fluid with an osmolality of approximately 50 mmol/kg and a

TABLE 7–10. The Hypotonic Syndromes

Excessive water ingestion
Decreased water excretion
  Decreased solute delivery to diluting segments
    Starvation
    Beer potomania
  AVP excess
    Syndrome of inappropriate antidiuretic hormone
    Drug-induced AVP secretion
  AVP excess with decreased distal solute delivery
    Congestive heart failure
    Cirrhosis of the liver
    Nephrotic syndrome
    Cortisol deficiency
    Hypothyroidism
    Diuretic use
Renal failure

volume of about 18 L, or approximately 10% of the GFR.[187] Thus because patients with primary polydipsia generally ingest approximately 5 to 15 L of water daily, they are ordinarily safe from profound hyponatremia.

In contrast, the most common reason for clinically significant hyponatremia is a disturbance in the rate of water excretion resulting from an inability of the kidney to excrete a maximally dilute urine. This inability may occur (1) because of a reduction in the rate of salt delivery to the diluting segment; (2) because of sustained nonosmotic AVP release; or (3) because of a combination of these factors. Table 7–10 presents a summary of the commonly encountered hyponatremic states based on this classification. Although the primary derangement in these disorders is a defect in the rate of renal free water excretion, the development of hyponatremia in these conditions also requires that free water intake exceed the rate of free water excretion. In other words, the development of hyponatremia in the disorders listed in Table 7–10 also requires that factors other than cellular shrinkage stimulate thirst.

The Clinical Syndromes

Increased Water Ingestion

As noted, because of the large capacity of the kidney to excrete free water, primary polydipsia alone rarely causes significant hyponatremia. However, polydipsia may contribute to severe hyponatremia in individuals with some underlying psychiatric illness.[401–403] Episodic polydipsia and hyponatremia occur in 3 to 5% of institutionalized patients with mental illness and polyuria occurs in more than 60% of institutionalized patients.[402] The cause of the polydipsia and the hyponatremia is uncertain. Most patients have, in addition to polydipsia, some abnormality in water excretion, such as excessive AVP secretion.[403–405] Carbamazepine, which is sometimes used to control agitation in psychotic patients, may also cause hyponatremia.[406,407]

Reduced Salt Delivery to the Diluting Segment

A reduced rate of salt delivery to the TALH and, consequently, a reduction in the volume of dilute urine formed may be the primary pathogenic mechanism responsible for hyponatremia in patients with euvolemic disorders such as beer potomania;[408,409] the same mechanism plays a major role in the hyponatremia that is associated with volume-contracted states such as adrenal insufficiency and with edematous disorders such as congestive heart failure or cirrhosis. An elegant analysis of hyponatremia in association with sodium depletion was provided by McCance,[410] who showed that salt depletion induced by sweating regularly led to hyponatremia after a net loss of about 150 to 200 mmol of sodium. Harrington[411] evaluated the contribution of AVP to this derangement by comparing the hyponatremic response to sodium depletion in control rats and rats with hypothalamic diabetes insipidus. Figure 7–22, which is adapted from his data, shows that the hyponatremic response to sodium depletion is similar in the two groups of animals. One may infer that water retention during sodium depletion can occur without AVP and that water ingestion in association with hyponatremia is driven by nonosmotic, volume-mediated factors.

Berliner and Davidson[412] subsequently showed that a diminished rate of sodium delivery to the diluting segment could result in urine concentration in the absence of AVP, and Edwards and co-workers[195] showed that this effect occurred with relatively small changes in GFR. Because renal sodium avidity is provoked[413] by an ECF volume loss as small as 200 mL (which corresponds to a sodium loss of approximately 28 mmol), one may infer that even small sodium losses may partially compromise the renal excretion of free water.

Beer potomania is the prototypical example of hyponatremia resulting from a reduction in distal solute delivery. Individuals with beer potomania can develop profound hyponatremia with urine osmolality values in the range of 70 mmol/kg and no significant weight loss.[408, 409] Thus the defect in free water excretion need not be in the degree to which urine is diluted maximally but rather in the amount of maximally dilute urine that is formed. Patients with beer potomania derive a large part of their caloric intake from the ingestion of large volumes of beer, which contains little salt or protein. Because sodium and urea are the major solutes in normal urine, dietary sodium restriction increases the fractional rate of proximal sodium absorption, diminishes the rate of salt delivery to diluting segments, and in turn limits the daily rate of formation of dilute urine. The relationship between daily solute excretion and the formation of dilute urine is depicted in Figure 7–23. As the daily urine solute excretion falls, the maximal rate of dilute urine formation is also reduced. Moreover, partial equilibration of reduced volumes of collecting duct fluid with the renal medullary interstitium further impairs the daily excretion of dilute urine. Hyponatremia related to reduced solute intake is not restricted to individuals with beer potomania;

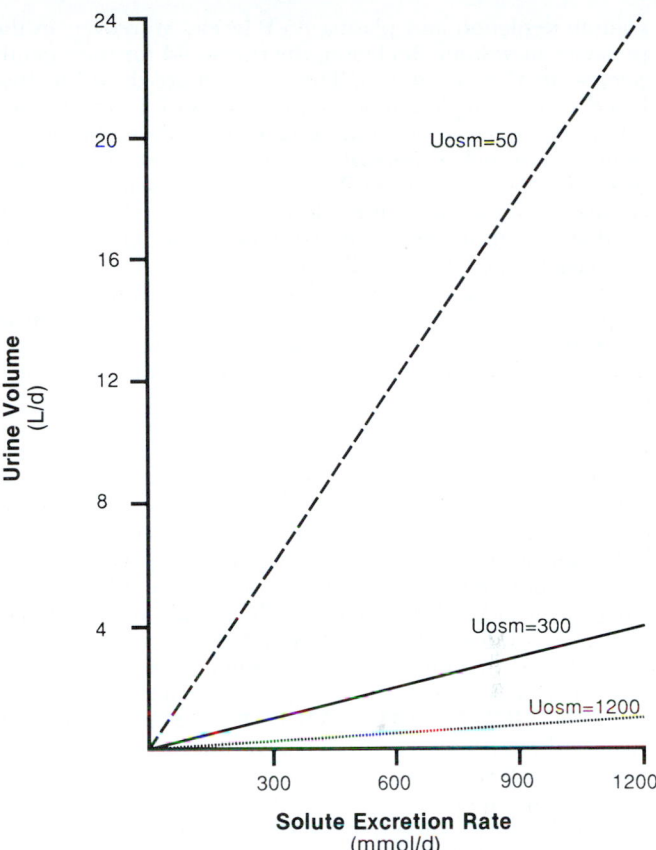

Figure 7–23. The relationship among daily solute excretion rate, urine osmolality (U$_{osm}$), and urine volume.

it may occur during starvation, particularly in the elderly, when solute intake may be dramatically reduced without parallel reductions in water intake.

It can be concluded that reduced solute intake may predispose subjects with primary polydipsia to the development of hyponatremia. With regard to Figure 7–23, consider, for example, a polydipsic patient who excretes 800 mmol/d of solute. This patient could excrete up to 16 L of dilute (50 mmol/kg) urine daily. If the solute excretion rate were reduced to 400 mmol/d, this same patient could excrete only 8 L of dilute urine. If more than this volume of water were ingested, the excess would be retained and hyponatremia would ensue.

Mixed Derangements: Nonosmotic Vasopressin Release and Reduced Distal Solute Delivery

Hyponatremia occurs commonly in states of true volume contraction and in edematous states such as congestive heart failure and cirrhosis. The former disorders include those in which both the ECF volume and total body water are reduced; the latter group includes states with deranged Starling forces, such as local or systemic increases in venous pressure that result in inadequate filling of the arterial tree. In both types of disorders, two factors may contribute, individually or in unison, to a renal defect in water excretion: (1) nonosmotic, volume-mediated AVP release and (2) reductions in the rate of sodium delivery to the diluting segment.

As indicated in Figure 7–8, there is a linear relation between increases in plasma osmolality and increases in plasma AVP levels, but a nonlinear relation between blood

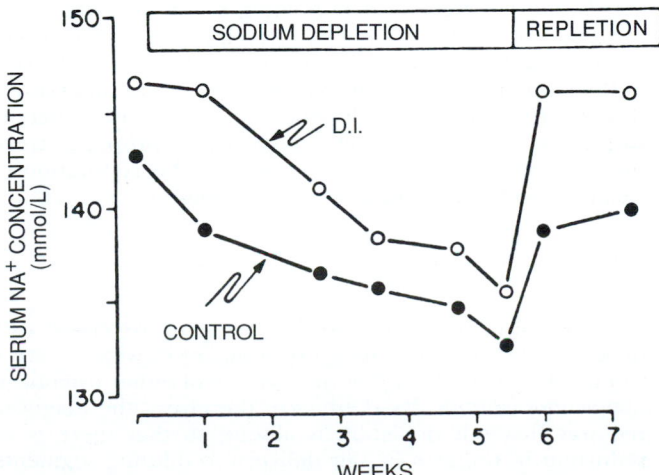

Figure 7–22. Hyponatremic response of normal and Brattleboro rats with diabetes insipidus (D.I.) to salt depletion. (Adapted from Harrington AR. Hyponatremia due to sodium depletion in the absence of vasopressin. Am J Physiol 1972; 222:768–774.)

volume depletion and plasma AVP levels. Moreover, in the presence of volume depletion, the threshold for the osmotic release of AVP is reduced. Thus when more than 7 to 10% blood volume depletion occurs, plasma AVP levels rise and can produce an antidiuretic effect even when the plasma osmolality is below normal.[107, 108] In other words, volume-mediated, nonosmotic AVP release occurs primarily when circulatory dynamics are moderately to severely advanced; in that circumstance, volume-mediated stimuli modulate osmotically mediated AVP release so that hyponatremia ensues. However, as shown in Figure 7–9, sufficient degrees of plasma hypotonicity can suppress AVP release even in the presence of volume depletion. Accordingly, low urine osmolality does not exclude the possibility of volume-mediated AVP release in a hyponatremic patient.

A second factor that accounts for hyponatremia in volume-contracted states is the inability to dilute urine because the rate of sodium delivery to diluting segments in the TALH is reduced.[195, 408–414] The significance of volume contraction in this type of hyponatremia can be gauged, as indicated earlier, by noting that hyponatremia occurs during volume contraction in Brattleboro rats with hypothalamic diabetes insipidus.[411, 414] Finally, the hyponatremia in volume-contracted states requires that water ingestion continue in the face of hypotonicity. Presumably, volume-mediated mechanisms account for thirst in such circumstances.

VOLUME-EXPANDED STATES. Hyponatremia occurs in advanced stages of disorders characterized by edema formation and a reduced effective circulating volume, particularly in intractable heart failure and hepatic cirrhosis with ascites. As noted earlier, reduced rates of salt delivery to diluting segments in these disorders contribute to the impairment in water excretion. Limited measurements of plasma AVP levels in patients with heart failure or severe ascites indicate that the plasma concentrations are inappropriately high with respect to the plasma osmolality.[415] Furthermore, because nonosmotic AVP release occurs only with significant reductions in blood volume (see Fig. 7–8), hyponatremia when there is congestive failure or cirrhosis indicates profound arterial underfilling. This observation correlates well with the ominous prognosis of hyponatremia in patients with these disorders.

VOLUME-CONTRACTED STATES. The hyponatremia in volume-contracted states may be rationalized most readily, as indicated earlier, in terms of a reduction in sodium delivery rates to the loop of Henle and, consequently, a reduction in the rate of renal free water formation. Thus hyponatremia commonly accompanies prolonged administration of diuretics.[408, 416] In this regard, two factors warrant particular consideration.

First, the most commonly used diuretics in clinical practice today include loop diuretics such as furosemide, bumetanide, and ethacrynic acid and terminal nephron diuretics such as the thiazides, triamterene, spironolactone, and amiloride. Because agents like furosemide inhibit salt absorption in the mTALH,[189, 190] they inhibit both renal concentrating and diluting power[417] (see Fig. 7–10). In contrast, thiazide diuretics inhibit salt absorption in cortical rather than medullary diluting segments and consequently inhibit renal diluting power but not concentrating power.[417] Accordingly, the risk of diuretic-induced hyponatremia is greater with thiazides than with furosemide.

Second, Fichman and colleagues[418] have described a group of patients in whom diuretic-associated hyponatremia referable to thiazide diuretics persisted even after correction of sodium depletion but was corrected with the repair of potassium depletion. These authors postulated that potassium depletion per se may have been responsible for sustained AVP release, because approximately half of the pa-

tients had rather hypertonic urine. Alternatively, a portion of the hyponatremia may have been due to the polydipsia that accompanies potassium depletion.[386]

It is often impossible to distinguish between volume contraction and normovolemia on the basis of physical examination and review of the history. In these cases the most reliable indicators of volume contraction are a low urine sodium concentration (<30 mmol/L) and a response to saline administration.[419] Thus in patients with hyponatremia it is useful to assess volume status. Patients who are either volume expanded or volume contracted tend to have mixed disorders, whereas normovolemic patients usually have excess AVP as the primary pathogenic factor. Volume-expanded states can usually be detected on the basis of the history and the physical examination.

ADRENAL INSUFFICIENCY. Hyponatremia may complicate untreated adrenal insufficiency. In mineralocorticoid deficiency, the combination of ECF volume contraction, GFR reduction, enhanced proximal tubular salt absorption, and volume-mediated, nonosmotic AVP release appears to be responsible for an inability to handle water loads.[408, 416] In Brattleboro rats with hypothalamic diabetes insipidus, bilateral adrenalectomy causes hyponatremia that can be partially reversed by the concomitant administration of glucocorticoids and salt;[416] thus in hypoadrenalism, volume depletion can cause hyponatremia even in the absence of AVP. Glucocorticoids are also required for the complete correction of the defect in water excretion in adrenal insufficiency.[408, 416] A glucocorticoid-mediated impairment of cardiac function also contributes to the reduction in effective circulating volume in adrenal insufficiency.[420]

Finally, nonosmotic AVP release may contribute to water retention.[421] Glucocorticoid-deficient rats have inappropriately high plasma AVP levels and an inability to excrete a water load.[421, 422] Specific AVP antagonists largely correct the deficit in water excretion.[423] As noted earlier, AVP and CRH are coproduced by certain parvicellular neurons in the PVN,[26] and both hormones are under negative feedback controlled by cortisol. After adrenalectomy the number of cells in this region that contain immunoreactive AVP increases dramatically.[29] In situ hybridization with probes for the AVP mRNA confirms that AVP synthesis is increased in the absence of glucocorticoids.[30]

HYPOTHYROIDISM. The cause for the hyponatremia that is occasionally seen in hypothyroid patients is not clear. Hyponatremia in myxedema might occur because of sustained AVP release[424] or because of a "reset osmostat,"[408] that is, normal modes for regulating plasma osmolality but at reduced plasma osmolality levels. Alternatively, De-Rubertis and co-workers[425] have inferred that salt delivery to the loop of Henle is reduced in hypothyroidism and that this effect accounted for the defect in free water excretion. Regardless of the mechanism involved, appropriate treatment of myxedema is accompanied by the restoration of renal concentrating and diluting capacities.[426]

Syndrome of Inappropriate Antidiuretic Hormone: Vasopressin Excess

The third group of disorders that are associated with hyponatremia includes those disturbances in which there is sustained release of AVP in the absence of either osmotic or nonosmotic stimuli. By definition, therefore, the diagnosis requires that salt depletion is absent, so that there is no reduction in the rate of salt delivery to diluting segments, and that effective circulating volume is not reduced, so that volume-mediated, nonosmotic stimuli for AVP release are absent. In general, a primary excess of AVP occurs in two settings: in the syndrome of inappropriate antidiuretic hormone (SIADH) and as a consequence of drugs that enhance AVP release or action. Measurements of AVP levels in patients with hyponatremia indicate that SIADH is the single most common cause of hyponatremia in hospitalized and, particularly, postoperative patients.[427-430] Overall, excessive, nonosmotic release of AVP is present in more than 95% of hospitalized patients with hyponatremia.[427, 428, 430]

SIADH. Studies by Leaf and co-workers[431] in 1953 provided convincing evidence that the increments in urine salt excretion that accompany exogenous vasopressin administration are the result of hormone-induced volume expansion related to water retention rather than to a direct effect of AVP on renal tubular salt absorption (Fig. 7–24).

As illustrated in Figure 7–24, the administration of vasopressin, coupled with unrestricted fluid intake, initially results in hyponatremia, urine concentration and antidiuresis, and a weight gain of approximately 3 kg. After 3 d, body weight and serum sodium concentration approach a steady state, and a natriuresis occurs; this natriuresis is termed *sodium escape.* Moreover, when fluid is restricted, hyponatremia is corrected, body weight declines, and urine sodium excretion falls, even in the face of continued vasopressin administration. Thus the natriuresis seen after 3 d of vasopressin administration is the consequence of volume expansion related to water retention. The natriuresis that is observed with volume expansion, either hypotonic or isotonic, is due, in part, to a reduction in the fractional rate of proximal tubular salt absorption, that is, to a resetting of glomerulotubular balance.[432] After prolonged vasopressin administration, there may also be a partial escape from vasopressin action.[433]

In 1957 Schwartz and co-workers[434] provided the first clear account of the occurrence of SIADH in a patient with bronchogenic carcinoma. Subsequently, SIADH has been observed in a variety of disorders, particularly pulmonary diseases, notably bronchogenic carcinoma, and cranial disorders.

In most patients with SIADH, there is persistent production of AVP or an AVP-like peptide despite body fluid hypotonicity and an expanded effective circulating volume.[416, 435, 436] Zerbe and colleagues[435] documented four kinds of responses of serum AVP levels to osmotic and nonosmotic stimuli in patients with SIADH:

1. The most common derangement (40%) is wide fluctuations of AVP levels independent of osmotic or nonosmotic control.

2. About a third of patients have an abnormally low osmotic threshold for AVP release, but at higher osmolalities there is a normal correlation between plasma AVP levels and plasma osmolality. These patients can produce a maximally dilute urine if they are sufficiently hyponatremic.

3. In a fifth of patients, AVP release is sustained ("AVP leak") below serum osmolality values of 278 mmol/kg, and AVP release is normal in response to osmotic stimuli.

4. Approximately a sixth of patients have no detectable abnormality of AVP levels but a failure to dilute urine maximally. This type of SIADH therefore has a poorly understood pathogenesis.

The fluid and electrolyte abnormalities that are observed in SIADH follow exactly from those illustrated in Figure 7–24. Specifically, as a result of the sustained release of AVP or AVP-like substances, patients retain ingested water and become hyponatremic, become modestly volume expanded, and generally increase body weight by 5 to 10%. The volume expansion results in reduced rates of proximal tubular sodium absorption and consequently in a natriuresis, albeit at a total expansion of total body weight. Increased levels of ANP also contribute to the natriuresis. Because aldosterone secretion is stimulated by hyponatremia, secretion of this mineralocorticoid may also contribute to reducing renal sodium losses in volume-expanded hyponatremic patients. There are also increased urinary losses of substances like uric acid, whose excretion rates vary directly with effective circulating volume and with rates of sodium excretion. Consequently, hypouricemia is common in SIADH. The GFR is normal, as is adrenal and thyroid function.

PHARMACOLOGICAL STIMULI. Hyponatremia may also result from drug therapy. As indicated earlier, diuretics can cause hyponatremia because of volume contraction, or less commonly, because of potassium depletion.[418] Certain agents (see Table 7–1) may either stimulate AVP release from the posterior pituitary or, as in the case of chlorpropamide, potentiate the effects of AVP on renal tubules. Thus each of these two classes of agents can result in an SIADH-like clinical syndrome, that is, sustained hyponatremia in the absence of a reduction in effective circulating volume.

Finally, as indicated earlier (see Fig. 7–17), renal medullary prostaglandins, particularly of the E series, inhibit salt absorption in the mTALH and antagonize the effects of AVP on collecting tubules. Furthermore, prostaglandins aid in the maintenance of glomerular blood flow during volume contraction.[437] Accordingly, aspirin or other nonsteroidal anti-inflammatory drugs might, by interfering with prostaglandin synthesis, lead to hyponatremia, particularly in volume-contracted patients.[438-440]

Pseudohyponatremia

In all of the disorders just discussed, plasma hyponatremia is accompanied by parallel decreases in plasma osmolality, that is, they are true hypotonic syndromes. In some patients, however, plasma hyponatremia may be associated with a normal or even an increased plasma osmolality. This situation, which can be detected by measurement of plasma osmolality, has been referred to as *pseudohyponatremia* (Table 7–11). The importance of detecting pseudohyponatremia lies in the fact that attempts to increase the plasma sodium concentrations are contraindicated. In severe hyperlipidemia or hyperproteinemia, the fractional volume of plasma that is composed of water may fall from a normal range of 93 to 95% to 70 to 75%. Because sodium is confined to the aqueous

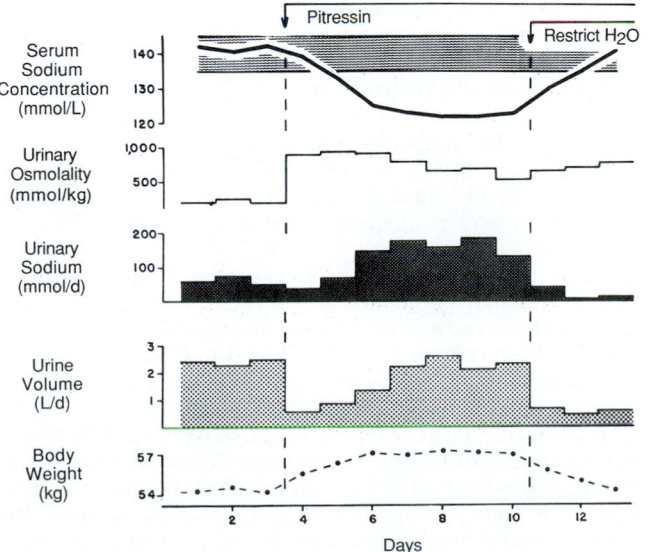

Figure 7–24. The role of volume expansion in vasopressin (Pitressin)–induced natriuresis. (Adapted from Goldberg M. Abnormalities in renal excretion of water. Med Clin North Am 1963; 47:915–933.)

TABLE 7–11. Causes of Pseudohyponatremia

Normal plasma osmolality
  Hyperproteinemia
  Hyperlipidemia
  Prostate surgery, with use of irrigant fluid containing glycine or sorbitol
Elevated plasma osmolality
  Hyperglycemia
  Mannitol
  Glycerol

phase, the sodium content of whole plasma, in millimoles per liter of plasma, falls in parallel with the fall in plasma water content. The plasma osmolality and the sodium concentration of the plasma water remain normal. Another reason for a falsely depressed sodium concentration in hyperproteinemia relates to hyperviscosity. With severe hyperviscosity, as in multiple myeloma, resistance to flow may limit the delivery of plasma to automated flame photometers.

Pseudohyponatremia related to hyperlipidemia or hyperproteinemia is becoming less common, not because of a decline in the incidence of the underlying conditions but rather because of advances in laboratory medicine.[441] The plasma sodium concentration has traditionally been determined by using flame photometry. This method measures the sodium content in a specified volume of whole plasma and is thus susceptible to changes in the water content of plasma or to errors in sample delivery. Plasma sodium concentration can now be measured by using sodium-selective electrodes. This method assesses directly the activity of sodium dissolved in the aqueous phase of plasma and is not susceptible to the errors introduced by hyperlipidemia and hyperproteinemia.

Pseudohyponatremia may also occur after urological procedures, typically transurethral prostatectomy.[442, 443] In these instances, the hyponatremia is due to the absorption of large amounts of isotonic irrigant fluid containing glycine or sorbitol. Absorption of the isotonic irrigant solution lowers the plasma sodium concentration but not the plasma osmolality. Hence a comparison of the measured plasma osmolality and the calculated osmolality reveals an elevated osmolar gap (see later).[443]

As discussed in the section on osmotic diuresis, nonsodium solutes, such as glucose or mannitol, may create hypertonicity with a normal or low plasma sodium concentration. When these poorly permeable solutes are added to the ECF, an osmotic gradient is created that draws water out of cells and into the extracellular space and results in a dilutional hyponatremia. Indeed, this effect accounts for the therapeutic efficacy of mannitol and glycerol in the treatment of increased intracranial pressure. Again, measurement of plasma osmolality discloses these conditions. Except in hyperglycemia, the measured plasma osmolality exceeds the calculated osmolality to produce an osmolar gap. The other common causes of an increased osmolar gap, e.g., ethanol, methanol, isopropanol, and ethylene glycol, are solutes that are freely permeable through cell membranes and do not cause shifts of water and hyponatremia.

Water Intoxication

An early description of water intoxication in humans was provided in 1920 by Wier and co-workers[444] as follows:

One of our patients at our solicitation continued, after the administration of pituitary extract, to take water . . . in a period of eight hours he ingested 5.25 liters, and excreted 800 cc of urine. . . . He became very ill, was nauseated and developed severe headache. . . .

The syndrome of water intoxication varies in severity depending on two major factors: the degree of hyponatremia and the duration of hyponatremia. In acute hyponatremia with serum sodium concentrations of less than 120 mmol/L, the syndrome is characterized by somnolence, seizures, coma, and mortality rates as high as 50%.[445, 446] The autopsy findings are those of cerebral edema.[446] In experimental animals that are subject to acute hyponatremia, there is also a significant reduction in brain electrolyte concentrations and in brain osmolality and a mortality rate of approximately 85%.[446]

Chronic hyponatremia in humans differs from the acute form in two important respects:[445] (1) approximately half of patients with chronic hyponatremia are asymptomatic, even with serum sodium concentrations less than 125 mmol/L; (2) the fatality rate is nearly 0 in asymptomatic patients and is approximately 10 to 15% in symptomatic patients. In experimental animals, chronic hyponatremia results in a greater decrease in brain sodium, potassium, and chloride levels, for a given reduction in serum sodium concentration, than in acute hyponatremia.[445] Consequently, in chronic hyponatremia, there is less of an increase in brain water content, for a given reduction in serum Na$^+$ concentration, than in acute hyponatremia, and a correspondingly lower mortality rate.[445, 446]

These observations can be interpreted as follows: First, the water permeability of the blood-brain barrier and of brain cells is sufficiently high that the brain approaches osmotic equilibrium with plasma quickly. Second, in acute hyponatremia the approach to osmotic equilibrium between brain cells and the ECF involves primarily water gain; this water gain accounts both for the cerebral edema and, in large part, for the high fatality rate of acute hyponatremia. Finally, for a given reduction in serum Na$^+$ level, brain electrolyte concentrations and brain water content are lower in chronic than in acute hyponatremia. In other words, when chronic hyponatremia occurs, homeostatic mechanisms are activated to extrude solutes from cells, so that osmotic equilibration between the brain and the ECF occurs with smaller increases in brain volume. Concomitantly, the fatality rate of chronic hyponatremia is less than that of acute hyponatremia.

A wide variety of cell types exhibit a volume-regulatory decrease (VRD) in response to a hypotonic ECF environment, that is, an initial period of cellular swelling, in which the cell acts as an osmometer, and a subsequent period of cellular shrinkage accompanied by solute loss, principally of electrolytes. The VRD response probably involves the loss of intracellular electrolytes through the activation of membrane transport processes other than Na$^+$,K$^+$-ATPase, whose role in the VRD response is largely permissive. The nature of these solute efflux processes differs among various cell types (see ref. 447 for a thorough review). In brain the VRD response involves principally a loss of intracellular KCl and NaCl.[446–448]

The occurrence of a VRD response in the setting of chronic hyponatremia has major therapeutic implications. The rapid correction of chronic hyponatremia to normal serum sodium concentrations will lead to CNS disturbances, particularly in children. The reason for such an occurrence follows from a consideration of the VRD response. Thus if the brain electrolyte content is adaptively reduced in chronic hyponatremia, the rapid correction of serum sodium concentrations to normal levels will, in effect, result in an acute hypertonic encephalopathy. It is important to note that central pontine myelinolysis can follow the rapid correction of hyponatremia both in experimental animals[449] and in humans.[450–452]

Diagnosis and Treatment

The diagnosis of hyponatremia is most commonly made from routine laboratory findings. Hyponatremia should also be considered whenever there is a sudden deterioration in CNS function, particularly in circumstances such as intractable heart failure, hepatic cirrhosis with ascites, or the administration of large volumes of intravenous fluids.

The history and physical examination are generally adequate for recognizing disorders such as beer potomania or compulsive water ingestion and for noting the ingestion of drugs that stimulate AVP release or enhance AVP action. The presence of edema is characteristic of individuals in whom hyponatremia occurs because of a reduced effective circulating volume coupled to ECF volume expansion. In hypothyroidism and adrenal insufficiency typical clinical and laboratory findings are generally present.

The most difficult differential diagnosis among hyponatremic disorders involves the distinction between patients who are modestly volume contracted and those who have SIADH. In both circumstances the serum sodium level and the serum osmolality are reduced, and the urine osmolality is inappropriately high with respect to the reduced serum osmolality. Nonosmotic water conservation in SIADH and in volume contraction is recognized by the presence of a urine osmolality value higher than 120 to 150 mmol/kg in association with a reduced serum osmolality.

Patients who are volume contracted may provide a history of volume losses or of diuretic ingestion and exhibit the signs of ECF volume contraction. When the volume losses are due to extrarenal causes, the urine sodium concentration is less than 10 to 15 mmol/L, and the fractional excretion of sodium is generally less than 1%. The presence of hyperuricemia and azotemia is also a useful index to ECF volume contraction. In contrast, patients with SIADH are generally normovolemic or slightly volume expanded and therefore exhibit none of the signs of volume contraction. The serum blood urea nitrogen and creatinine values are normal, and the serum uric acid level is generally reduced. The urine sodium concentration usually exceeds 30 mmol/L, and the fractional excretion of sodium is greater than 1%. Tests of adrenal function are normal.

The above-mentioned studies usually discriminate between SIADH and extrarenal volume contraction. However, when ECF volume contraction is due to renal salt wasting, urine sodium losses generally persist unless volume contraction is profound. A useful diagnostic and therapeutic maneuver in this situation is to observe the results of water restriction. When water intake is restricted to 600 to 800 mL daily, patients with SIADH exhibit a highly characteristic response: a 2- to 3-kg weight loss is accompanied by correction of hyponatremia and cessation of salt wasting, usually over a period of 2 to 3 d. If weight loss fails to correct both hyponatremia and urine sodium wasting simultaneously, the diagnosis of SIADH is doubtful. Rather, renal sodium wasting with ECF volume contraction, related to adrenal insufficiency or the other renal salt-losing disorders listed in Table 7–10, is the more probable diagnosis.

Therapy

The goal of treatment is to correct body water osmolality and to restore cell volume to normal by raising the ratio of sodium to water in the ECF. The increase in ECF osmolality draws water from cells and therefore reduces their volume. The therapeutic approach, as well as whether net sodium and water balance is adjusted to be positive or negative during therapy, depends on the serum sodium concentration, the rate at which hyponatremia has developed, the clinical status, and the underlying disorder.

SYMPTOMATIC HYPONATREMIA. Severe hyponatremia that is associated with a serum sodium concentration below 120 to 125 mmol/L and CNS manifestations requires immediate therapy. In volume-contracted states, the treatment of choice is to raise the serum sodium level to 125 mmol/L by administering hypertonic (3 to 5%) saline. Because the desired effect is to correct body water osmolality, the amount of sodium that is administered must be sufficient to raise total body water osmolality to approximately 250 mmol/kg, that is, to approximately twice the desired serum sodium concentration. A convenient formula for calculating this sodium requirement is

$$[125 - \text{measured serum Na}] \times 0.6 \text{ body weight} = \text{required mmol of Na}$$

The serum sodium concentration is in millimoles per liter and the body weight is in kilograms. Because 60% of body weight is water, the formula allows an estimate of the amount of sodium required to raise body water osmolality to 250 mmol/kg.

The administration of hypertonic saline is hazardous in volume-expanded, salt-retaining states such as congestive heart failure. Furthermore, in SIADH that is associated with volume expansion and sodium wasting, the administration of hypertonic saline alone may be ineffective in correcting hyponatremia because the administered salt is excreted promptly in a relatively concentrated urine. In such circumstances, normal saline or hypertonic saline solutions may be used in combination with furosemide (Fig. 7–25).[453] The diuretic induces urine salt loss and therefore reduces the risk of ECF volume expansion. Moreover, as illustrated in Figure 7–25, the diuresis that is induced by furosemide is characterized by the excretion of urine with an osmolality that is lower than the plasma osmolality. Consequently, the combination of intravenously administered normal or hypertonic saline, coupled with a furosemide-induced diuresis of urine that is dilute with respect to plasma, provides an effective way of raising the serum sodium level in SIADH or other volume-expanded states. By adjusting the rates of salt administration to be less than urine salt losses, reductions in ECF volume can be produced simultaneously.

As indicated in the preceding section, the rapid elevation of serum sodium concentrations to levels higher than 125 mmol/L is potentially hazardous. Because loss of brain solute represents one of the compensatory mechanisms for preserving brain cell volume in dilutional states,[445–448] a serum

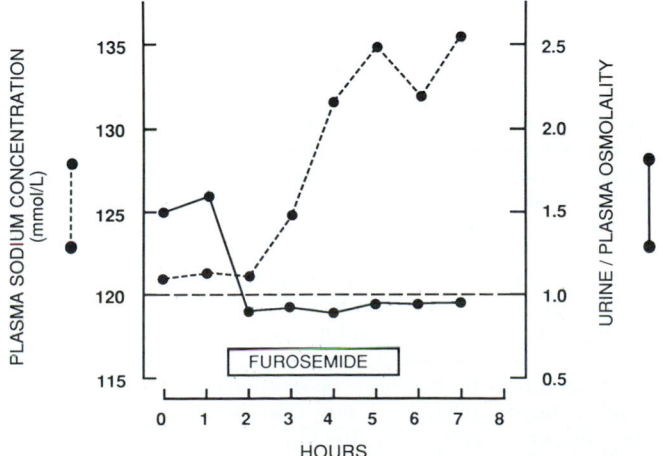

Figure 7–25. Effect of furosemide plus saline in treatment of hyponatremia in SIADH. (Modified from Hartman D, Rossier B, Fohlman R, et al. Rapid correction of hyponatremia in the syndrome of inappropriate secretion of antidiuretic hormone. Ann Intern Med 1973; 78:870–875.)

sodium level of 140 mmol/L is relatively hypertonic to brain cells that have become partially depleted of solute as a result of hyponatremia. Consequently, raising the serum sodium level rapidly to higher than 120 to 125 mmol/L can cause CNS damage such as central pontine myelinolysis.[447-452] Raising the serum sodium concentration to higher than 120 mmol/L is not only hazardous but unnecessary.

The major, and still unresolved, controversy surrounding the treatment of hyponatremia concerns the rate at which hyponatremia should be corrected.[454] Advocates of rapid correction point to the high mortality rate of hyponatremia, as high as 86% in one series. Advocates of slow correction caution that the rapid correction of hyponatremia itself may produce central pontine myelinolysis.

Mortality rates for severe hyponatremia of 33 to 86% have been cited in support of prompt correction of hyponatremia. These estimates, however, derive largely from single case reports and small, often retrospective and selective, series of patients. Thus these data may overestimate the mortality from hyponatremia. In a prospective study of 33 patients with symptomatic hyponatremia, there were no deaths.[455] Likewise, a retrospective analysis of all patients with severe hyponatremia (serum sodium level less than 110 mmol/L) at two hospitals found a mortality rate of only 8%, with most deaths attributed to underlying diseases.[456] In this series, slow or delayed correction of hyponatremia was not associated with higher mortality or with neurological complications. Indeed, the risk of developing neurological complications was greatest in patients whose serum sodium concentrations were corrected at a rate greater than 0.6 mmol/L/h (14 mmol/d).[456] In part, the discrepant mortality rates may relate to differences in the patient populations under study. Arieff and others[454, 455, 457, 458] have reported on more than 50 healthy young women who developed symptomatic hyponatremia after elective surgery and subsequently died or suffered permanent brain damage. Likewise, acutely hyponatremic female animals suffer a higher mortality rate than males.[459, 460] This apparent increased susceptibility of females to the neurological complications of hyponatremia may be related to impairment of brain cell volume-regulatory mechanisms and to impairment of high-energy phosphate production.[460] In contrast, the patients reported in the prospective studies tend to be older men and have underlying illnesses or are receiving diuretics. In these patients the hyponatremia does not carry as grave a prognosis as in young women.

As just noted, it is believed rapid correction of hyponatremia may lead to central pontine myelinolysis. Central pontine myelinolysis is a demyelinating lesion of the pons with destruction of myelin sheaths but sparing of the axis cylinders and nerve cells. The majority of patients in whom it has been described have had debilitating disease, malnutrition, or alcoholism and, occasionally, hyponatremia. The clinical characteristics include flaccid quadriplegia or paraplegia, facial weakness, dysphagia, dysarthria, and coma. The possible role of the rate of correction of hyponatremia in the development of central pontine myelinolysis remains uncertain.[454] For example, the incidence of this disorder in hyponatremia is low, and the rate of correction in patients who develop the complication is no faster than in those who do not.[455] Patients who develop central pontine myelinolysis generally have additional risk factors, such as alcoholism or malnutrition, which could be responsible for the lesion. Finally, the neurological lesion that develops in hyponatremic patients is often not myelinolysis but rather a diffuse lesion that may be caused by anoxia.[457] In rats rapid correction of severe hyponatremia to normonatremic levels results in diffuse necrotic brain lesions, whereas rapid correction to mildly hyponatremic levels (serum sodium concentration 139

mmol/L) does not.[461] Thus the extent of correction, as well as the rate of correction, may be important in the development of neurological complications.

On the basis of available data, we believe that it is prudent to correct the sodium concentration at a rate of 0.5 mmol/L/h until the serum sodium concentration reaches 120 to 125 mmol/L. However, young women with acute symptomatic hyponatremia are at risk for respiratory arrest, severe neurological sequelae, and death. It is reasonable to treat these patients with hypertonic saline to raise the serum sodium concentration to 125 mmol/L at a rate of 1 to 2 mmol/L/h. At this point, the patient should be asymptomatic and the serum sodium concentration can be returned to normal gradually over several days with water restriction. Overcorrection of the serum sodium concentration (to higher than 130 mmol/L) is unnecessary and potentially harmful. Even in acutely developing hyponatremia, symptoms and CNS signs are uncommon until the serum sodium concentration falls below 120 mmol/L. Patients with chronic hyponatremia may tolerate well even greater degrees of hyponatremia.

ASYMPTOMATIC HYPONATREMIA. Mild, asymptomatic chronic hyponatremia is generally managed by correction of the underlying disorder when the hyponatremia occurs in volume contraction or in salt-regaining states such as congestive heart failure or hepatic cirrhosis with ascites. Chronic hyponatremia in SIADH may be easily corrected by restricting water intake to 800 to 1000 mL daily, provided that patients can adhere to the program of water restriction.

An alternative approach involves the use of agents such as lithium or demeclocycline, which interfere with the renal tubular effects of AVP. However, the response to lithium is variable, and lithium itself causes multiple side effects, including renal tubular acidosis, cardiotoxicity, and thyroid dysfunction.[370, 374, 376, 380, 381, 462] In contrast, demeclocycline reproducibly inhibits renal concentrating ability in SIADH patients.[462, 463] However, demeclocycline should be used cautiously in patients with coexisting liver disease because of the risk of toxic nephropathy produced by accumulation of the drug.[465] As another alternative, some workers[465] have recommended reducing renal concentrating ability by administering oral urea loads that are sufficient to produce osmotic diuresis. A maneuver that is effective in patients who are not edematous, hypertensive, or in congestive heart failure is to administer oral furosemide (see Fig. 7–25) in association with a high-salt diet. Finally, the competitive antagonists of vasopressin binding to renal tubular receptors[94] may be useful in the treatment of acute water intoxication.

REFERENCES

1. Burg MB, Kador PF. Sorbitol, osmoregulation, and the complications of diabetes. J Clin Invest 1988; 81:635–640.
2. Blumenfeld JD, Grossman EB, Sun AM, et al. Sodium-coupled ion cotransport and the volume regulatory increase response. Kidney Int 1989; 36:434–440.
3. Bagnasco SM, Uchida S, Balaban RS, et al. Induction of aldose reductase and sorbitol in renal inner medullary cells by elevated extracellular NaCl. Proc Natl Acad Sci USA 1987; 84:1718–1720.
4. Ramon y Cajal S. Histologie du système nerveux de l'homme et des vertébrés. Paris: Maloine, 1911.
5. Bernard C. Leçon sur les propiertés physiologiques et les alterations pathologiques des liquides de l'organisme. Vol. 2. Paris: 1859.
6. Kahler O. Die dauernde Polyurie als cerebrales Herdsymptom. Z Heilk 1886; 7:105–220.
7. Fink EB. Diabetes insipidus. Arch Pathol Lab Med 1928; 6:102–120.
8. Spanbock A, Steinhaus J. Ueber das Zusammentreffen von bitemporaler Hemianopsie und Diabetes insipidus. Dtsch Med Wochenschr 1898; 24:828–830.
9. Frank E. Ueber Beziehungen der Hypophyse zum Diabetes insipidus. Berl Klin Wochenschr 1912; 49:393–397.

10. Magnus R, Schäfer EA. The action of pituitary extracts upon the kidney. J Physiol (Lond) 1901; 27:ix–x.

11. Cushing H. Concerning diabetes insipidus and the polyurias of hypophysial origin. Boston Med Surg J 1913; 168:901–910.

12. Farini F. Diabete insipido et opoterapia. Gass Osp Clin 1913; 34:1135–1139.

13. von den Velden R. Die Nierenwirkung von Hypophysenextrakten beim Menschen. Berl Klin Wochenschr 1913; 50:2083.

14. Camus J, Roussy G. Experimental researches on the pituitary body. Endocrinology 1920; 4:507–522.

15. Verney EB. Polyuria associated with pituitary dysfunction. Lancet 1929; 216:539–546.

16. Priestley BM. The regulation of excretion of water by the kidneys. J Physiol (Lond) 1916; 50:304–311.

17. Broers H. Experimentelle diabetes insipidus. Arch Sci Biol 1933; 18:83.

18. Fisher C, Ingram WR, Ranson SW. Relation of hypothalamico-hypophyseal system to diabetes insipidus. Arch Neurol Psychiatry 1935; 34:124–163.

19. Fisher C, Ingram WR. The effect of interruption of the supraoptico-hypophyseal tracts on the antidiuretic, pressor and oxytocic activity of the posterior lobe of the hypophysis. Endocrinology 1936; 20:762–768.

20. Morris JF. Organization of neural inputs to the supraoptic and paraventricular nuclei: anatomical aspects. Prog Brain Res 1983; 60:3–18.

21. Sawchenko PE, Swanson LW. The organization and biochemical specificity of afferent projections to the paraventricular and supraoptic nuclei. Prog Brain Res 1983; 60:19–29.

22. Vandesande F, Dierickx K. Identification of the vasopressin producing and of the oxytocin producing neurons in the hypothalamic magnocellular neurosecretory system of the rat. Cell Tissue Res 1975; 164:153–162.

23. Zimmerman EA, Robinson AG. Hypothalamic neurons secreting vasopressin and neurophysin. Kidney Int 1976; 10:12–24.

24. Morris JF, Sokol HW, Valtin H. One neuron—one hormone? In: Moses AM, Share L, eds. Neurohypophysis. Basel: S. Karger, 1977: 58–66.

25. Zimmerman EA, Defendi R. Hypothalamic pathways containing oxytocin, vasopressin and associated neurophysins. In: Moses AM, Share L, eds. Neurohypophysis. Basel: S. Karger, 1977: 22–29.

26. Sawchenko PE, Swanson LW, Vale WW. Co-expression of corticotropin-releasing factor and vasopressin immunoreactivity in parvocellular neurosecretory neurons of the adrenalectomized rat. Proc Natl Acad Sci USA 1984; 81:1883–1887.

27. Zimmerman EA, Silverman AJ. Vasopressin and adrenal cortical interactions. Prog Brain Res 1983; 60:493–504.

28. Whitnall MH, Mezey E, Gainer H. Co-localization of corticotropin-releasing factor and vasopressin in median eminence neurosecretory vesicles. Nature 1985; 317:248–252.

29. Kiss JZ, Mezey E, Skirboll L. Corticotropin-releasing factor—immunoreactive neurons of the paraventricular nucleus become vasopressin-positive after adrenalectomy. Proc Natl Acad Sci USA 1984; 81:1854–1858.

30. Davis LG, Arentzen R, Reid JM, et al. Glucocorticoid sensitivity of vasopressin mRNA levels in the paraventricular nucleus of the rat. Proc Natl Acad Sci USA 1986; 83:1145–1149.

31. Cross BA, Dyball REJ, Dyer RG, et al. Endocrine neurons. Recent Prog Horm Res 1975; 31:243–294.

32. Carter DA, Lightman SL. Neuroendocrine control of vasopressin secretion. In: Baylis PH, Padfield PL, eds. The Posterior Pituitary. Hormone Secretion in Health and Disease. New York: Marcel Dekker, 1985: 53–118.

33. Sawchenco PE, Swanson LW. Central noradrenergic pathways for the integration of hypothalamic neuroendocrine and autonomic responses. Science 1981; 214:685–687.

34. Saper CB, Standaert DG, Currie MG, et al. Atriopeptin-immunoreactive neurons in the brain: presence in cardiovascular regulatory areas. Science 1985; 227:1047–1049.

35. Johnson AK, Cunningham JT. Brain mechanisms and drinking: the role of lamina terminalis–associated systems in extracellular thirst. Kidney Int 1987; 32:S35–S42.

36. Iitake K, Share L, Ouchi Y, et al. Central cholinergic control of vasopressin release in conscious rats. Am J Physiol 1986; 251:E146–E150.

37. Russell JA, Blackburn RE, Leng G. The role of the AV3V region in the control of magnocellular oxytocin neurons. Brain Res Bull 1988; 20:803–810.

38. Kamm O, Aldrich TB, Grote IW, et al. The active principles of the posterior lobe of the pituitary gland. J Am Chem Soc 1928; 50:573–601.

39. du Vigneaud V. Hormones of the mammalian posterior pituitary gland and their naturally occurring analogues. Johns Hopkins Med J 1969; 124:53–65.

40. du Vigneaud V. Experiences in the polypeptide field: insulin to oxytocin. Ann NY Acad Sci 1960; 88:537–548.

41. van Dyke HB, Chow BF, Greep RO, et al. The isolation of a protein from the pars neuralis of the ox pituitary with constant oxytocic, pressor and diuresis-inhibiting activities. J Pharmacol Exp Ther 1942; 74:190–209.

42. Pickering BT, Jones CW. Neurophysins. In: Li CH, ed. Hormonal Proteins and Peptides. Vol. 5. New York: Academic, 1978: 103–158.

43. Archer R, Manoussos G, Olivry G. Sur les relations entre l'oxytocine et la vasopressine d'une part et la protéine de van Dyke d'autre part. Biochim Biophys Acta 1955; 16:155–156.

44. Robinson AG. Radioimmunoassay of neurophysin proteins: utilization of specific neurophysin assays to demonstrate independent secretion of different neurophysins in vivo. Ann NY Acad Sci 1975; 248:246–256.

45. Robinson AG. The neurophysins. In: Reichlin S, ed. The Neurohypophysis. Physiological and Clinical Aspects. New York: Plenum, 1984: 65–93.

46. Sachs H, Fawcett P, Takabatake Y, et al. Biosynthesis and release of vasopressin and neurophysin. Recent Prog Horm Res 1969; 25:447–484.

47. Sachs H, Takabatake Y. Evidence for a precursor in vasopressin biosynthesis. Endocrinology 1964; 75: 943–948.

48. Takabatake Y, Sachs H. Vasopressin biosynthesis. III. In vitro studies. Endocrinology 1964; 75:934–942.

49. Brownstein MJ, Russell JT, Gainer H. Synthesis, transport and release of posterior pituitary hormones. Science 1980; 207:373–378.

50. Russell JT, Brownstein MJ, Gainer H. Time course of appearance and release of [^{35}S]cysteine labelled neurophysins and peptides in the neurohypophysis. Brain Res 1981; 205:299–311.

51. Land H, Schuetz G, Schmale H, et al. Nucleotide sequence of cloned cDNA encoding bovine arginine vasopressin–neurophysin II precursor. Nature 1982; 295:299–303.

52. Schmale H, Heinsohn S, Richter D. Structural organization of the rat gene for the arginine vasopressin–neurophysin II precursor. EMBO J 1983; 2:763–767.

53. Schmale H, Fehr S, Richter D. Vasopressin biosynthesis: from gene to peptide hormone. Kidney Int 1987; 32:S8–S13.

54. Riddell DC, Mallonee R, Phillips JA, et al. Chromosomal assignment of human sequences encoding arginine vasopressin–neurophysin II and growth hormone releasing factor. Somatic Cell Mol Genet 1985; 11:189–195.

55. Gainer H, Sarne Y, Brownstein MJ. Neurophysin biosynthesis: conversion of a putative precursor during axonal transport. Science 1977; 195:1354–1356.

56. Schmale H, Richter D. Single base deletion in the vasopressin gene is the cause of diabetes insipidus in Brattleboro rats. Nature 1984; 308:705–709.

57. Scharrer E, Scharrer B. Hormones produced by neurosecretory cells. Recent Prog Horm Res 1954; 10:183–240.

58. Weinstein H, Malamed S, Sachs H. Isolation of vasopressin-containing granules from the neurohypophysis of the dog. Biochim Biophys Acta 1961; 50:386–389.

59. Russell JT, Brownstein MJ, Gainer H. Biosynthesis of vasopressin, oxytocin and neurophysins: isolation and characterization of two common precursors (propressophysin and prooxyphysin). Endocrinology 1980; 107:1880–1891.

60. Harris GW. The innervation and actions of the neurohypophysis: an investigation using the method of remote-control stimulation. Philos Trans Soc Lond [Biol] 1947; 232:425–439.

61. Wakerly JB, Poulain DA, Brown D. Comparison of firing patterns in oxytocin- and vasopressin-releasing neurones during progressive dehydration. Brain Res 1978; 148:425–440.

62. Hatton GI, Armstrong WE, Gregory WA. Spontaneous and osmotically-stimulated activity in slices of rat hypothalamus. Brain Res Bull 1978; 3:497–508.

63. Poulain DA, Wakerley JB. Electrophysiology of hypothalamic magnocellular neurones secreting oxytocin and vasopressin. Neuroscience 1982; 7:773–808.

64. Dreifuss JJ. A review on neurosecretory granules: their contents and mechanisms of release. Ann NY Acad Sci 1975; 248:184–201.

65. Sklar AH, Schrier RW. Central nervous system mediators of vasopressin release. Physiol Rev 1983; 63:1243–1280.

66. Sachs H, Haller EW. Further studies on the capacity of the neurohypophysis to release vasopressin. Endocrinology 1968; 83: 251–262.

67. Dreifuss JJ, Kalnins I, Kelly JS, et al. Action potentials and release of neurohypophyseal hormones in vitro. J Physiol (Lond) 1971; 215:805–817.

68. Nordmann JJ. Stimulus-secretion coupling. Prog Brain Res 1983; 60:281–304.

69. Nordmann JJ, Dyball REJ. Effects of veratridine on Ca fluxes and the release of oxytocin and vasopressin from the isolated rat neurohypophysis. J Gen Physiol 1978; 72:297–304.

70. Nordmann JJ, Diayanithi G, Cazalis M. Coupling between the bioelectrical activity of a neurosecretory cell and the release at its terminals of neuropeptides. In: Schrier RW, ed. Vasopressin. New York: Raven, 1985: 375–383.

71. Bauman G, Dingman JF. Distribution, blood transport, and degradation of antidiuretic hormone in man. J Clin Invest 1976; 57:1109–1116.

72. Weitzman RE, Fisher DA. Arginine vasopressin metabolism in dogs. I. Evidence for a receptor-mediated mechanism. Am J Physiol 1978; 235:E591–E597.

73. Czaczkes JW, Kleeman CR, Koenig M. Physiologic studies of antidiuretic

hormone by its direct measurement in human plasma. J Clin Invest 1964; 43:1625–1640.

74. Nitschke U, Balzar H. Die Inaktivierung von infundiertem Vasopressin bei Diabetes insipidus-Probanden. Acta Endocrinol 1969; 62:270–282.

75. Wilson KC, Weitzman RE, Fisher DA. Arginine vasopressin metabolism in dogs. II. Modeling and systems analysis. Am J Physiol 1978; 235:E598–E605.

76. Barth T, Krejci I, Kupkova B, et al. Pharmacology of cyclic analogues of deamino-oxytocin not containing a disulphide bond (carba analogues). Eur J Pharmacol 1973; 24:183–188.

77. Koida M, Glass JD, Schwartz IL, et al. Mechanism of inactivation of oxytocin by rat kidney enzymes. Endocrinology 1971; 88:633–643.

78. Marks N, Abrash L, Walter R. Degradation of neurohypophyseal hormones by brain extracts and purified brain enzymes. Proc Soc Exp Biol Med 1973; 142:455–460.

79. Cort JH, Schück O, Stribrna J, et al. Role of the disulfide bridge and the C-terminal tripeptide in the antidiuretic action of vasopressin in man and the rat. Kidney Int 1975; 8:292–302.

80. Walter R, Bowman RH. Mechanism of inactivation of vasopressin and oxytocin by the isolated perfused rat kidney. Endocrinology 1973; 92:189–193.

81. Nardacci NJ, Mukhopadhyay S, Campbell BJ. Partial purification and characterization of the antidiuretic hormone–inactivating enzyme from renal plasma membranes. Biochim Biophys Acta 1975; 377:146–157.

82. Shade RE, Share L. Renal vasopressin clearance with reductions in renal blood flow in the dog. Am J Physiol 1977; 232:F341–F347.

83. Sawyer WH. Evolution of neurohypophyseal hormones and their receptors. Fed Proc 1977; 36:1842–1847.

84. Butlen D, Guillon G, Rajerison RM, et al. Structural requirements for activation of vasopressin-sensitive adenylate cyclase, hormone binding, and antidiuretic actions: effects of highly potent analogues and competitive inhibitors. Mol Pharmacol 1978; 14:1006–1017.

85. Barth T, Rajerison MR, Roy C, et al. Activation of rat kidney adenylate cyclase by vasopressin analogues: lack of correlation with antidiuretic activity. Mol Cell Endocrinol 1975; 2:69–80.

86. Hechter O, Terada S, Nakahara T, et al. Neurohypophyseal hormone-responsive adenylate cyclase. II. Relationship between hormonal occupancy of neurohypophyseal hormone receptor sites and adenylate cyclase activation. J Biol Chem 1978; 253:3219–3229.

87. Roy C, Barth T, Jard S. Vasopressin-sensitive kidney adenylate cyclase. Structural requirements for attachment to the receptor and enzyme activation: studies with vasopressin analogues. J Biol Chem 1975; 250:3144–3156.

88. Sawyer WH, Acosta M, Balaspiri L, et al. Structural changes in the arginine vasopressin molecule that enhance antidiuretic activity and specificity. Endocrinology 1974; 94:1106–1115.

89. Sawyer WH, Pang PKT, Seto J, et al. Vasopressin analogs that antagonize antidiuretic responses by rats to the antidiuretic hormone. Science 1981; 212:49–51.

90. Manning M, Sawyer WH. Synthesis and receptor specificities of vasopressin antagonists. J Cardiovasc Pharmacol 1986; 8:S29–S32.

91. Manning M, Klis WA, Olma A, et al. Design of more potent and selective antagonists of the antidiuretic responses to arginine vasopressin. J Med Chem 1982; 25:414–419.

92. Manning M, Nawrocka E, Misicka A, et al. Potent and selective antagonists of the antidiuretic responses to arginine vasopressin based on modification of [1-(β-mercapto-β, β-cyclopentamethylenepropionic acid) 2-D-isoleucine, 4-valine] arginine vasopressin at position 4. J Med Chem 1984; 27: 423–429.

93. Manning M, Sawyer WA. Development of selective agonists and antagonists of vasopressin and oxytocin. In: Schrier RW, ed. Vasopressin. New York: Raven, 1985: 131–144.

94. Stassen FL, Heckman GD, Schmidt DB, et al. Actions of vasopressin antagonists: molecular mechanisms. In: Schrier RW, ed. Vasopressin. New York: Raven, 1985: 145–154.

95. Kinter LB, Huffman WF, Stassen FL. Antagonists of the antidiuretic activity of vasopressin. Am J Physiol 1988; 254:F165–F177.

96. Stassen FL, Erickson RW, Huffman WF, et al. Molecular mechanisms of novel antidiuretic antagonists: analysis of the effects on vasopressin binding and adenylate cyclase activation in animal and human kidney. J Pharmacol Exp Ther 1982; 223:50–54.

97. Kim JK, Schrier RW. Cellular effect of arginine vasopressin antagonist on the isolated renal tubule. In: Schrier RW, ed. Vasopressin. New York: Raven, 1985: 155–158.

98. Mann WA, Kinter LB, Stassen F, et al. Mechanism of action and structural requirements of vasopressin analog inhibition of transepithelial water flow in toad urinary bladder. J Pharmacol Exp Ther 1986; 238:401–406.

99. Verney EB. The antidiuretic hormone and the factors which determine its release. Proc Soc Lond [Biol] 1947; 135:25–105.

100. McKinley MJ, Denton DA, Weisinger RS. Sensors for antidiuresis and thirst—osmoreceptors or CSF sodium detectors? Brain Res 1978; 141:89–103.

101. Leng G. Rat supraoptic neurones: the effects of locally applied hypertonic saline. J Physiol (Lond) 1980; 304:405–414.

102. Leng G, Dyball REJ, Mason WT. Electrophysiology of osmoreceptors. In: Schrier RW, ed. Vasopressin. New York: Raven, 1985: 333–342.

103. Thrasher TN, Brown CJ, Keil LC, et al. Thirst and vasopressin release in the dog: an osmoreceptor or sodium receptor mechanism? Am J Physiol 1980; 238: R333–R339.

104. Thrasher TN, Keil LC, Ramsay DJ. Lesions of the organum vasculosum of the lamina terminalis (OVLT) attenuate osmotically-induced drinking and vasopressin secretion in the dog. Endocrinology 1982; 110:1837–1839.

105. Bealer SL, Crofton JT, Share L. Hypothalamic knife cuts alter fluid regulation, vasopressin secretion and natriuresis during water deprivation. Neuroendocrinology 1983; 36:364–370.

106. Honda K, Negoro H, Higuchi H, et al. Activation of neurosecretory cells by osmotic stimulation of anteroventral third ventricle. Am J Physiol 1987; 252:R1039–R1045.

107. Robertson GL, Mahr EA, Athar S, et al. Development and clinical application of a new method for the radioimmunoassay of arginine vasopressin in human plasma. J Clin Invest 1973; 52:2340–2352.

108. Dunn FL, Brennan JT, Nelson AE, et al. The role of blood osmolality and volume in regulating vasopressin secretion in the rat. J Clin Invest 1973; 52:3212–3219.

109. Robertson GL. Vasopressin in osmotic regulation in man. Annu Rev Med 1974; 25:315–322.

110. Robertson GL, Berl T. Water metabolism. In: Brenner BM, Rector FC Jr, eds. The Kidney. 3rd ed. Philadelphia: W.B. Saunders, 1986: 385–432.

111. Peters JP. Body Water. The Exchange of Fluids in Man. Springfield, IL: Charles C Thomas, 1935: 274–313.

112. Gauer OH, Henry JP. Circulatory basis of fluid volume control. Physiol Rev 1963; 43:423–481.

113. Sved AF. Central neural pathways in baroreceptor control of vasopressin secretion. In: Schrier RW, ed. Vasopressin. New York: Raven, 1985: 443–453.

114. Share L. Vasopressin, its bioassay and the physiological control of its release. Am J Med 1967; 42:701–712.

115. Gupta PD, Henry JP, Sinclair R, et al. Responses of atrial and aortic baroreceptors to nonhypotensive hemorrhage and to transfusion. Am J Physiol 1966; 211:1429–1437.

116. Wang BC, Sundet WD, Hakumäki MOK, et al. Vasopressin and renin responses to hemorrhage in conscious, cardiac-denervated dogs. Am J Physiol 1983; 245:H399–H405.

117. Caillens H, Pruszczynski W, Meyrier A, et al. Relationship between change in volemia at constant osmolality and plasma antidiuretic hormone. Miner Electrolyte Metab 1980; 4:161–171.

118. Stricker EM, Verbalis JG. Interaction of osmotic and volume stimuli in regulation of neurohypophyseal secretion in rats. Am J Physiol 1986; 250:R267–R275.

119. Quillen EW, Cowley AW. Influence of volume changes on osmolality-vasopressin relationships in conscious dogs. Am J Physiol 1983; 244:H73–H79.

120. Ross MG, Ervin MG, Leake RD, et al. Continuous ovine fetal hemorrhage: sensitivity of plasma and urine arginine vasopressin response,. Am J Physiol 1986; 251: E464–E469.

121. Robertson GL. Physiology of ADH secretion. Kidney Int 1987; 32:S20–S26.

122. Schrier RW, Berl T, Anderson RJ, et al. Non-osmotic regulation of renal water excretion. Trans Am Clin Climatol Assoc 1976; 87:161–169.

123. McDonald KM, Kuruvila KC, Aisenbrey GA, et al. Effect of alpha and beta adrenergic stimulation on renal water excretion and medullary cyclic AMP in intact and diabetes insipidus rats. Kidney Int 1977; 12:96–103.

124. Sladek JR, McNeill TH. Simultaneous monoamine histofluorescence and neuropeptide immunocytochemistry. IV. Verification of catecholamine-neurophysin interactions through single section analysis. Cell Tissue Res 1980; 210:181–190.

125. Willoughby JO, Jervois PM, Menadue MF, et al. Noradrenaline, by activation of alpha-1-adrenoceptors in the region of the supraoptic nucleus, causes secretion of vasopressin in the unanesthetized rat. Neuroendocrinology 1987; 45:219–226.

126. Zhao BG, Chapman C, Brown D, et al. Opioid-noradrenergic interactions in the neurohypophysis. II. Does noradrenaline mediate the actions of endogenous opioids on oxytocin and vasopressin release? Neuroendocrinology 1988; 48:25–31.

127. Zhao BG, Chapman C, Bicknell RJ. Opioid-noradrenergic interactions in the neurohypophysis. I. Differential opioid receptor regulation of oxytocin, vasopressin and noradrenaline release. Neuroendocrinology 1988; 48:16–24.

128. Lind RW, Swanson LW, Ganten D. Organization of angiotensin II immunoreactive cells and fibers in the rat central nervous system. Neuroendocrinology 1985; 40:2–24.

129. Okuya S, Inenaga K, Kaneko T, et al. Antiotensin II sensitive neurons in the supraoptic nucleus, subfornical organ and anteroventral third ventricle of rats in vitro. Brain Res 1987; 402:58–67.

130. Iovino M, Steardo L. Vasopressin release to central and peripheral

angiotensin II in rats with lesion of the subfornical organ. Brain Res 1984; 322:365–368.

131. Knepel W, Nutto D, Meyer DK. Effects of transection of subfornical organ efferent projections on vasopressin release induced by angiotensin or isoprendaline in the rat. Brain Res 1982; 248:180–184.

132. Tanaka J, Kaba H, Saito H, et al. Electrophysiological evidence that circulating angiotensin II sensitive neurons on the subfornical organ alter the activity of hypothalamic paraventricular neurohypophyseal neurons in the rat. Brain Res 1985; 342:361–365.

133. Usberti M, Federico S, Cianciaruso B, et al. Effects of angiotensin II on plasma ADH, PGE_2 synthesis and water excretion in normal man. Am J Physiol 1985; 248:F254–F259.

134. Usberti M, DiMinno G, Ungaro B, et al. Angiotensin II inhibition with captopril on plasma ADH, PG synthesis, and renal function in humans. Am J Physiol 1986; 250:F986–F990.

135. Morton JJ, Connell JM, Hughes MJ, et al. The role of plasma osmolality, angiotensin II and dopamine in vasopressin release in man. Clin Endocrinol 1985; 23:129–138.

136. Martin R, Voigt KH. Enkephalins co-exist with oxytocin and vasopressin in nerve terminals of rat neurohypophysis. Nature 1981; 289:502–504.

137. Iversen LL, Iversen SD, Bloom FE. Opiate receptors influence vasopressin release from nerve terminals in rat neurohypophysis. Nature 1980; 284:350–351.

138. Matsui K, Kimura T, Ota K, et al. Attenuation of the osmotic release of vasopressin by enkephalins in dogs. Am J Physiol 1989; 256:E270–E276.

139. Yamada T, Nakao K, Itoh H, et al. Inhibitory action of leumorphin on vasopressin secretion in conscious rats. Endocrinology 1988; 122:985–990.

140. Oiso Y, Iwasaki Y, Kondo K, et al. Effect of the opioid kappa-receptor agonist U50488H on the secretion of arginine vasopressin. Study on the mechanism of U50488H-induced diuresis. Neuroendocrinology 1988; 48:658–662.

141. Hoffman PK, Share L, Crofton JT, et al. The effect of intracerebroventricular indomethacin on osmotically stimulated vasopressin release. Neuroendocrinology 1982; 34:132–139.

142. Forsling ML, Ullmann EA. Non-osmotic stimulation of vasopressin release. In: Moses AM, Share L, eds. Neurohypophysis. Basel: S. Karger, 1977:128–135.

143. Manning PT, Schwartz D, Katsube NC, et al. Vasopressin-stimulated release of atriopeptin: endocrine antagonists in fluid homeostasis. Science 1985; 229:395–397.

144. Dillingham MA, Anderson RJ. Inhibition of vasopressin action by atrial natriuretic factor. Science 1986; 231:1572–1573.

145. Zimmerman EA, Ma L-Y, Nilaver G. Anatomical basis of thirst and vasopressin secretion. Kidney Int 1987; 32:S14–S19.

146. Poole CJM, Carter DA, Vallejo M, et al. Atrial natriuretic factor inhibits the stimulated in vivo and in vitro release of vasopressin and oxytocin in the rat. J Endocrinol 1987; 112:97–102.

147. Iitake K, Share L, Crofton JT, et al. Central atrial natriuretic factor reduces vasopressin secretion in the rat. Endocrinology 1986; 119:438–440.

148. Obana K, Natuse M, Inagami T, et al. Atrial natriuretic factor inhibits vasopressin secretion from rat posterior pituitary. Biochem Biophys Res Commun 1985; 132:1088–1094.

149. Crandall ME, Gregg CM. In vitro evidence for an inhibitory effect of atrial natriuretic peptide on vasopressin release. Neuroendocrinology 1986; 44:439–445.

150. Thrasher TN, Nistal-Herrera JF, Keil LC, et al. Satiety and inhibition of vasopressin secretion after drinking in dehydrated dogs. Am J Physiol 1981; 240:E394–E401.

151. Geelen G, Keil LC, Kravik SE, et al. Inhibition of plasma vasopressin after drinking in dehydrated humans. Am J Physiol 1984; 247:R968–R971.

152. Thrasher TN, Keil LC, Ramsay DJ. Drinking, oropharyngeal signals, and inhibition of vasopressin secretion in dogs. Am J Physiol 1987; 253:R509–R515.

153. Salata RA, Verbalis JG, Robinson AG. Cold water stimulation of oropharyngeal receptors in man inhibits release of vasopressin. J Clin Endocrinol Metab 1987; 65:561–567.

154. Seckl JR, Williams TDM, Lightman SL. Oral hypertonic saline causes transient fall of vasopressin in humans. Am J Physiol 1986; 251:R214–R217.

155. Arnauld E, duPont J. Vasopressin release and firing of supraoptic neurosecretory neurones during drinking in the dehydrated monkey. Pflügers Arch 1982; 394:195–201.

156. Robertson GL, Shelton RL, Athar S. The osmoregulation of vasopressin. Kidney Int 1976; 10:25–37.

157. Wood RJ, Rolls ET, Rolls BJ. Physiological mechanisms for thirst in the nonhuman primate. Am J Physiol 1982; R423–R428.

158. Nothnagel H. Durst und Polydipsie. Virchows Arch Pathol Anat Physiol 1881; 86:435–447.

159. Andersson B, Rundgren M. Thirst and its disorders. Annu Rev Med 1982; 33:231–239.

160. McKinley MJ, Denton DA, Leksell LG, et al. Osmoregulatory thirst in sheep is disrupted by ablation of the anterior wall of the optic recess. Brain Res 1982; 236:210–215.

161. Andersson B, McCann SM. Drinking, antidiuresis and milk ejection from electrical stimulation within the hypothalamus of the goat. Acta Physiol Scand 1956; 35:191–201.

162. Phillips MI, Hoffman WE, Bealer SL. Dehydration and fluid balance: central effects of angiotensin. Fed Proc 1982; 41:2520–2527.

163. Hoffman WE, Ganten U, Phillips MI, et al. Inhibition of drinking in water-deprived rats by combined central angiotensin II and cholinergic receptor blockade. Am J Physiol 1978; 234:F41–F47.

164. Zimmerman MB, Blaine EH, Stricker EM. Water intake in hypovolemic sheep: effects of crushing the left atrial appendage. Science 1981; 211:489–491.

165. Dill DB. Life, Heat and Altitude. Cambridge: Harvard University Press, 1938.

166. Adolph, EF. Termination of drinking: satiation. Fed Proc 1982; 41:2533–2535.

167. Ramsay DJ, Rolls BJ, Wood RJ. Thirst following water deprivation in dogs. Am J Physiol 1977; 232:R93–R100.

168. Gilmore JP, Zucker IH. Failure of left atrial distension to alter renal function in the nonhuman primate. Circ Res 1978; 42:267–270.

169. Weitzman RE, Glatz TH, Fisher DA. The effect of hemorrhage and hypertonic saline upon plasma oxytocin and arginine vasopressin in conscious dogs. Endocrinology 1978; 103:2154–2160.

170. Landgraf R, Neumann I, Schwarzberg H. Central and peripheral release of vasopressin and oxytocin in the conscious rat after osmotic stimulation. Brain Res 1988; 457:219–225.

171. Russell JA, Blackburn RE, Leng G. The role of the AV3V region in the control of magnocellular oxytocin neurons. Brain Res Bull 1988; 20:803–810.

172. Hartman RD, Rosella-Dampman LM, Emmert SE, et al. Inhibition of release of neurohypophyseal hormones by endogenous opioid peptides in pregnant and parturient rats. Brain Res 1986; 382:352–359.

173. Bicknell RJ, Zhao BG, Chapman C, et al. Opioid inhibition of secretion from oxytocin and vasopressin nerve terminals following selective depletion of neurohypophyseal catecholamines. Neurosci Lett 1988; 93:281–286.

174. Carter DA, Lightman SL. Opioid control of oxytocin secretion: evidence of distinct regulatory actions of two opiate receptor types. Life Sci 1987; 40:2289–2296.

175. Johnson AK. The periventricular anteroventral third ventricle (AV3V): its relationship with the subfornical organ and neural systems involved in maintaining body fluid homeostasis. Brain Res Bull 1985; 15:595–601.

176. Verbalis, JG, McCann MJ, McHale CM, et al. Oxytocin secretion in response to cholecystokinin and food: differentiation of nausea from satiety. Science 1986; 232:1417–1419.

177. Bradshaw JMC, Downing SJ, Moffatt A, et al. Demonstration of some of the physiological properties of rat relaxin. J Reprod Fertil 1981; 63:145–153.

178. Summerlee AJS, O'Byrne KT, Paisley AC, et al. Relaxin affects the central control of oxytocin release. Nature 1984; 309:372–374.

179. Dayanithi G, Cazalis M, Nordmann JJ. Relaxin affects the release of oxytocin and vasopressin from the neurohypophysis. Nature 1987; 325:813–816.

180. Rosenblatt JS, Mayer AD, Giodano AL. Hormonal basis during pregnancy for the onset of maternal behavior in the rat. Psychoneuroendocrinology 1988; 13:29–46.

181. Clements JA, Funder JW. Arginine vasopressin and oxytocin in organs outside the nervous system. In: Martini L, Ganong WF, eds. Frontiers in Neuroendocrinology. Vol 10. New York: Raven, 1988: 117–152.

182. Rajerison RM, Montegut M, Jard S, et al. The isolated frog skin epithelium: permeability characteristics and responsiveness to oxytocin, cyclic AMP and theophylline. Pflügers Arch 1972; 332:302–312.

183. Balment RJ, Brimble MJ, Forsling ML. Oxytocin release and renal actions in normal and Brattleboro rats. Ann NY Acad Sci 1982; 394:241–253.

184. Ahmad AJ, Clark EH, Jacobs HS. Water intoxication associated with oxytocin infusion. Postgrad Med J 1975; 51:249–252.

185. Feeney JG. Water intoxication and oxytocin. Br Med J 1982; 285:243.

186. Kuhn W, Ryffel K. Herstellung konzentrierter Lösungen aus verdünnten durch blosse Membranwirkung. Ein Modellversuch zur Funcktion der Niere. Z Physiol Chemie 1942; 276:145–178.

187. Gottschalk CW, Mylle M. Micropuncture study of the mammalian urinary concentrating mechanism: evidence for the countercurrent hypothesis. Am J Physiol 1959; 196:927–936.

188. Gottschalk CW. Osmotic concentration and dilution of the urine. Am J Med 1964; 36:670–685.

189. Burg MB, Green N. Function of the thick ascending limb of Henle's loop. Am J Physiol 1973; 224:659–668.

190. Rocha AS, Kokko JP. Sodium chloride and water transport in the medullary thick ascending limb of Henle. Evidence for active chloride transport. J Clin Invest 1973; 52:612–623.

191. Kokko JP, Rector FC Jr. Countercurrent multiplication system without active transport in inner medulla. Kidney Int 1972; 2:214–223.

192. Valtin H. Sequestration of urea and nonurea solutes in renal tissues of rats with hereditary hypothalamic diabetes insipidus: effect of vasopressin and dehydration on the countercurrent mechanism. J Clin Invest 1966; 45:337–345.

193. Stephenson JL. Concentration of urine in a central core model of the renal counterflow system. Kidney Int 1972; 2:85–94.

194. Gellai M, Edwards BR, Valtin H. Urinary concentrating ability during dehydration in the absence of vasopressin. Am J Physiol 1979; 237:F100–F104.

195. Edwards BR, Gellai M, Valtin H. Concentration of urine in the absence of ADH with minimal or no decrease in GFR. Am J Physiol 1980; 239:F84–F91.

196. Rapoport S, Brodsky WA, West CD, et al. Urinary flow and excretion of solutes during osmotic diuresis in hydropenic man. Am J Physiol 1949; 156:433–442.

197. Goldberg M, McCurdy DK, Foltz EL, et al. Effects of ethacrynic acid (a new saluretic agent) on renal diluting and concentrating mechanisms: evidence for site of action in the loop of Henle. J Clin Invest 1964; 43:201–216.

198. Hebert SC, Schafer JA, Andreoli TE. The effects of antidiuretic hormone (ADH) on solute and water transport in the mammalian nephron. J Membr Biol 1981; 58:1–19.

199. Hebert SC, Andreoli TE. Water permeability of biological membranes. Lessons from antidiuretic hormone–responsive epithelia. Biochim Biophys Acta 1982; 650:267–280.

200. Grantham JJ, Burg MB. Effect of vasopressin and cyclic AMP on permeability of isolated collecting tubules. Am J Physiol 1966; 211:255–259.

201. Grantham JJ, Orloff J. Effect of prostaglandin E₁ on the permeability response of the isolated collecting tubule to vasopressin, adenosine 3′,5′-monophosphate and theophylline. J Clin Invest 1968; 47:1154–1161.

202. Schafer JA, Andreoli TE. Cellular constraints to diffusion: the effect of antidiuretic hormone on water flows in isolated mammalian collecting tubules. J Clin Invest 1972; 51:1264–1278.

203. Hall DA, Grantham JJ. Temperature effect on ADH response of isolated perfused rabbit collecting tubules. Am J Physiol 1980; 239:F595–F601.

204. Reif MC, Troutman SL, Schafer JA. Sustained response to vasopressin in isolated rat cortical collecting tubules. Kidney Int 1984; 26:725–732.

205. Burg MB, Helman S, Grantham JJ, et al. Effect of vasopressin on the permeability of isolated rabbit cortical collecting tubules to urea, acetamide, and thiourea. In: Schmidt-Neilsen B, ed. Urea and the Kidney. Amsterdam: Excerpta Medica, 1970: 193–208.

206. Schafer JA, Andreoli TE. The effect of antidiuretic hormone on solute flows in mammalian collecting tubules. J Clin Invest 1972; 51:1279–1286.

207. Hebert SC, Andreoli TE. Interactions of temperature and ADH on transport processes in cortical collecting tubules: evidence for ADH-induced narrow aqueous channels in apical membranes. Am J Physiol 1980; 238:F470–F480.

208. Verkman AS. Mechanisms and regulation of water permeability in renal epithelia. Am J Physiol 1989; 257:C837–C850.

209. Chevalier J, Bourguet J, Hugon JJ. Membrane-associated particles: distribution in frog urinary bladder epithelium at rest and after oxytocin treatment. Cell Tissue Res 1974; 152:129–140.

210. Kachadorian WA, Wade JB, DiScala VA. Vasopressin: induced structural change in toad bladder luminal membranes. Science 1975; 190:67–69.

211. Kachadorian WA, Wade JB, Uiterwyk CC, et al. Membrane structural and functional responses to vasopressin in toad urinary bladder. J Membr Biol 1977; 30:381–401.

212. Wade JB. Membrane structural studies of the action of vasopressin. Fed Proc 1985; 44:2687–2692.

213. Kachadorian WA, Levine SD, Wade JB, et al. Relationship of aggregated intramembranous particles to water permeability in vasopressin-treated toad urinary bladder. J Clin Invest 1977; 59:576–581.

214. Kachadorian WA, Coleman RA, Wade JB. Water permeability and particle aggregates in ADH-, cAMP-, and forskolin-treated toad bladder. Am J Physiol 1987; 253:F14–F20.

215. Muller J, Kachadorian WA, DiScala VA. Evidence that ADH-stimulated intramembrane particle aggregates are transferred from cytoplasmic to luminal membranes in toad bladder epithelial cells. J Cell Biol 1980; 85:83–95.

216. Levine SD, Kachadorian WA. Barriers to water flow in vasopressin-treated toad urinary bladder. J Membr Biol 1981; 61:135–139.

217. Wade JB, Stetson DL, Lewis SA. ADH action: evidence for a membrane shuttle mechanism. Ann NY Acad Sci 1981; 372:106–117.

218. Franki N, Ding G, Quintana N, et al. Evidence that heads of ADH-sensitive aggrephores are clathrin-coated vesicles: implications for aggrephore structure and function. Tissue Cell 1986; 18:803–807.

219. Brown D. Membrane recycling and epithelial cell function. Am J Physiol 1989; 256:F1–F12.

220. Dratwa M, Tisher C, Sommer JR, et al. Intramembranous particle aggregation in toad urinary bladder after vasopressin stimulation. Lab Invest 1979; 40:46–54.

221. Kachadorian WA, Muller J, Rudich S, et al. Temperature dependence of ADH-induced water flow and intramembranous particle aggregates in toad bladder. Science 1979; 205:910–913.

222. Strange K, Spring KR. Absence of significant cellular dilution during ADH-stimulated water reabsorption. Science 1987; 235:1068–1070.

223. Strange K, Spring KR. Cell membrane water permeability of rabbit cortical collecting duct. J Membr Biol 1987; 96:27–43.

224. Harris HW, Wade JB, Handler JS. Fluorescent markers to study membrane retrieval in ADH treated toad urinary bladder. Am J Physiol 1986; 251:C274–C284.

225. Harris HW, Wade JB, Handler JS. Transepithelial water flow regulates apical membrane and retrieval on ADH-stimulated toad urinary bladder. J Clin Invest 1986; 78:703–712.

226. Masur SK, Cooper S, Rubin MS. Effect of an osmotic gradient on antidiuretic hormone–induced endocytosis and hydroösmosis in the toad urinary bladder. Am J Physiol 1984; 247:F370–F379.

227. Muller J, Kachadorian WA. Aggregate-carrying membranes during ADH stimulation and washout in toad bladder. Am J Physiol 1984; 247:C90–C98.

228. Brown D, Orci L. Vasopressin stimulates formation of coated pits in rat kidney collecting ducts. Nature 1983; 302:253–255.

229. Harmanci MC, Kachadorian WA, Valtin H, et al. Antidiuretic hormone-induced intramembranous alteration in mammalian collecting ducts. Am J Physiol 1978; 235:F440–F443.

230. Harmanci MC, Stern P, Kachadorian WA, et al. Vasopressin and collecting duct intramembranous particle clusters: a dose-response relationship. Am J Physiol 1980; 239:F560–F564.

231. Harmanci MC, Lorenzen M, Kachadorian WA. Vasopressin-induced intramembranous particle aggregates in isolated rabbit collecting duct. Kidney Int 1982; 21:275A.

232. Strange K, Willingham MC, Handler JS, et al. Apical membrane retrieval via clathrin-coated pits is stimulated by removal of ADH from isolated perfused rabbit cortical tubule. J Membr Biol 1988; 103:17–28.

233. Brown D, Weyer P, Orci L. Vasopressin stimulates endocytosis in kidney collecting duct principal cells. Eur J Cell Biol 1988; 46:336–341.

234. Verkman AS, Lencer WI, Brown D, et al. Endosomes from kidney collecting tubule cells contain the vasopressin-sensitive water channel. Nature 1988; 333:268–269.

235. Verkman AS, Weyer P, Brown D, et al. Functional water channels are present in clathrin-coated vesicles from bovine kidney but not from brain. J Biol Chem 1989; 264:20608–20613.

236. Dousa TP. Cyclic nucleotides in the cellular action of neurohypophyseal hormones. Fed Proc 1977; 36:1867–1871.

237. Hildebrandt J, Sekura R, Codina J, et al. Stimulation and inhibition of adenyl cyclases mediated by distinct regulatory proteins. Nature 1983; 302:706–709.

238. Gilman AG. Guanine nucleotide–binding regulatory proteins and dual control of adenylate cyclase. J Clin Invest 1984; 73:1–4.

239. Rodbell M. The role of hormone receptors and GTP-regulatory proteins in membrane transduction. Nature 1980; 284:17–22.

240. Jard S, Roy C, Barth T, et al. Antidiuretic hormone–sensitive kidney adenylate cyclase. Adv Cyclic Nucleotide Res 1975; 5:31–52.

241. Eggena P, Schwartz IL, Walter R. Threshold and receptor reserve in the action of neurohypophyseal peptides. A study of synergists and antagonists in the hydroosmotic response on the toad urinary bladder. J Gen Physiol 1970; 56:250–271.

242. Seamon KB, Daly JW. Forskolin, cyclic AMP and cellular physiology. Trends Pharmacol Sci 1983; 4:120–123.

243. Culpepper RM, Andreoli TE. PGE₂, forskolin, and cholera toxin interactions in modulating NaCl transport in mouse mTALH. Am J Physiol 1984; 247:F784–F792.

244. Nadler SP, Hebert SC, Brenner BM. PGE₂, forskolin, and cholera toxin interaction in rabbit cortical collecting tubule. Am J Physiol 1986; 250:F127–F135.

245. Takaichi K, Kurokawa K. Inhibitory guanosine triphosphate–binding protein-mediated regulation of vasopressin action in isolated single medullary tubules of mouse kidney. J Clin Invest 1988; 82:1437–1444.

246. Ribeiro CP, Ribeiro-Neto F, Field JB, et al. Prevention of α₂-adrenergic inhibition on ADH action by pertussis toxin in rabbit CCT. Am J Physiol 1987; 253:C105–C112.

247. Dousa TP, Valtin H. Cellular actions of vasopressin in the mammalian kidney. Kidney Int 1976; 10:46–63.

248. Dousa TP, Barnes LD, Kim JK. The role of cyclic AMP-dependent protein phosphorylations and microtubules in the cellular action of vasopressin in mammalian kidney. In: Moses AM, Share L, eds. Neurohypophysis. Basel: S. Karger, 1977: 220–235.

249. Kuwahara M, Verkman AS. Pre–steady state analysis of the turn-on and turn-off of water permeability in the kidney collecting tubule. J Membr Biol 1989; 110:57–65.

250. Yasuhiro A, Breyer MD, Jacobson HR. Dose-dependent heterogenous actions of vasopressin in rabbit cortical collecting ducts. Am J Physiol 1989; 256:F556–F562.

251. Star RA, Nonoguchi H, Balaban R, et al. Calcium and cyclic adenosine monophosphate as second messengers for vasopressin in the rat inner medullary collecting duct. J Clin Invest 1988; 81:1879–1888.

252. Wade JB. Dynamics of apical membrane responses to ADH in amphibian bladder. Am J Physiol 1989; 257:R998–R1003.

253. Valenti G, Hugon JS, Bourguet J. To what extent is microtubular network involved in antidiuretic response? Am J Physiol 1988; 255:F1098–F1106.

254. Krothapalli RK, Duffy WB, Senekjian HO, et al. Modulation of the hydroösmotic effect of vasopressin on the rabbit cortical collecting tubule by adrenergic agents. J Clin Invest 1983; 72:287–294.

255. Beck TR, Dunn MJ. The relationship of antidiuretic hormone and renal prostaglandins. Miner Electrolyte Metab 1981; 6:46–59.

256. Handler JS. Vasopressin-prostaglandin interactions in the regulation of epithelial cell permeability to water. Kidney Int 1981; 19:831–838.

257. Orloff J, Handler JS, Bergstrom S. Effect of prostaglandin (PGE-1) on the permeability response of toad bladder to vasopressin, theophylline and adenosine 3′,5′,-monophosphate. Nature 1965; 205:397–398.

258. Craven PA, DeRubertis FR. Effects of vasopressin and urea on Ca^{2+}-calmodulin-dependent renal prostaglandin E. Am J Physiol 1981; 241:F649–F658.

259. Wuthrich RP, Loup R, Favre L, et al. Dynamic response of PG synthesis to peptide hormones and osmolality in renal tubular cells. Am J Physiol 1986; 250:F790–F797.

260. Sato M, Dunn MJ. Interaction of vasopressin, prostaglandins and cAMP in rat papillary collecting tubule cells in culture. Am J Physiol 1984; 247:F423–F433.

261. Schlondorff D, Satriano JA, Schwartz GJ. Synthesis of prostaglandin E_2 in different segments of isolated collecting tubules from adult and neonatal rabbits. Am J Physiol 1985; 248:F134–F144.

262. Portilla D, Shayman JA, Morrison AR. Vasopressin does not hydrolyze polyphosphoinositides in rabbit collecting tubule cells. Biochim Biophys Acta 1987; 928:305–311.

263. Argy WP, Handler JS, Orloff J. Ca^{++} and Mg^{++} effects on toad bladder response to cyclic AMP, theophylline and ADH analogues. Am J Physiol 1967; 213:803–808.

264. Peterson MJ, Edelman IS. Calcium inhibition of the action of vasopressin on the urinary bladder of toad. J Clin Invest 1964; 43:583–594.

265. Goldfarb S. Effects of calcium on ADH action in the cortical collecting tubule perfused in vitro. Am J Physiol 1982; 243:F481–F486.

266. Takaichi K, Uchida S, Kurokawa K. High Ca^{2+} inhibits AVP-dependent cAMP production in thick ascending limbs of Henle. Am J Physiol 1986; 250:F770–F776.

267. Ando Y, Jacobson HR, Breyer MD. Phorbol ester and A23187 have additive but mechanistically separate effects on vasopressin action in rabbit collecting tubule. J Clin Invest 1988; 81:1578–1584.

268. Schlondorff D, Levine SD. Inhibition of vasopressin-stimulated water flow in toad bladder by phorbol myristate acetate, dioctanoylglycerol and RHC-80267. J Clin Invest 1985; 76:1071–1078.

269. Casavola V, Iacovelli L, Svelto M. Phorbol ester effect on the hydroösmotic response to vasopressin in frog skin. Pflügers Arch 1987; 408:318–320.

270. Ando Y, Jacobson HR, Bryer MD. Phorbol myristate acetate, dioctanoylglycerol and phosphatidic acid inhibit the hydroösmotic effect of vasopressin on rabbit cortical collecting tubule. J Clin Invest 1987; 80:590–593.

271. Wirz VH, Hargitay B, Kuhn W. Lokalisation des Konzentrierungsprozesses in der Niere durch direkte Kryoskopie. Helv Physiol Acta 1951; 9:196–207.

272. Morel F. Regulation of kidney functions by hormones: a new approach. Recent Prog Horm Res 1983; 39:271–304.

273. Greger R, Schlatter E. Properties of the lumen membrane of the cortical thick ascending limb of Henle's loop of rabbit kidney. Pflügers Arch 1983; 396:315–324.

274. Molony DA, Reeves WB, Andreoli TE. $Na^+:K^+:2Cl^-$ cotransport and the thick ascending limb. Kidney Int 1989; 36:418–426.

275. Eveloff J, Kinne R. Sodium-chloride transport in the medullary thick ascending limb of Henle's loop: evidence for a sodium-chloride cotransport system in plasma membrane vesicles. J Membr Biol 1983; 72:173–181.

276. Reeves WB, McDonald GA, Mehta P, et al. Activation of K^+ channels in renal medullary vesicles by cAMP-dependent protein kinase. J Membr Biol 1989; 109:65–72.

277. Forbush B, Palfrey HC. ^{3}H/Bumetanide binding to membranes isolated from dog kidney outer medulla. J Biol Chem 1983; 258:11787–11792.

278. Oberleithner H, Guggino W, Giebisch G. Mechanism of distal tubular chloride transport in Amphiuma kidney. Am J Physiol 1982; 242:F331–F339.

279. Hebert SC, Andreoli TE. Control of NaCl transport in the thick ascending limb. Am J Physiol 1984; 15:F745–F756.

280. Hebert SC, Friedman PA, Andreoli TE. The effects of antidiuretic hormone on cellular conductive pathways in mouse medullary thick ascending limbs of Henle. I. ADH increases transcellular conductance pathways. J Membr Biol 1984; 80:201–219.

281. Greger R, Schlatter E. Properties of the basolateral membrane of the cortical thick ascending limb of Henle's loop of rabbit kidney: a model for secondary active chloride transport. Pflügers Arch 1983; 396:325–334.

282. Bayliss JM, Reeves WB, Andreoli TE. Cl^- transport in basolateral renal medullary vesicles: I. Cl^- transport in intact vesicles. J Membr Biol 1990; 113:49–56.

283. Reeves WB, Andreoli TE. Cl^- transport in basolateral renal medullary vesicles: II. Cl^- channels in planar lipid bilayers. J Membr Biol 1990; 113:57–65.

284. Hebert SC, Andreoli TE. Effects of antidiuretic hormone on cellular conductive pathways in mouse medullary thick ascending limbs of Henle. II. Determinants of the ADH-mediated increases in transepithelial voltage and in net Cl^- absorption. J Membr Biol 1984; 80:221–233.

285. Stokes JB. Consequences of potassium recycling in the renal medulla. Effects on ion transport by the medullary thick ascending limb of Henle's loop. J Clin Invest 1982; 70:219–229.

286. Guggino SE, Suarez-Isla BA, Guggino WB, et al. Forskolin and antidiuretic hormone stimulate a Ca^{2+}-activated K^+ channel in cultured kidney cells. Am J Physiol 1985; 249:F448–F455.

287. Cornejo M, Guggino SE, Guggino WB. Ca^{2+}-activated K^+ channels from cultured renal medullary thick ascending limb cells: effects of pH. J Membr Biol 1989; 110:49–55.

288. Taniguchi J, Guggino WB. Membrane stretch: a physiological stimulator of Ca^{2+}-activated K^+ channels in thick ascending limb. Am J Physiol 1989; 257:F347–F352.

289. Wang W, White S, Giebel J, et al. A potassium channel in the thick ascending limb of Henle's loop of rabbit kidney. Am J Physiol 1990; 258:F244–F253.

290. Schultz, SG. Homocellular regulatory mechanisms in sodium-transporting epithelia: avoidance of extinction by "flush-through." Am J Physiol 1981; 241:F579–F590.

291. Hebert SC, Culpepper RM, Andreoli TE. NaCl transport in mouse medullary thick ascending limbs. I. Functional nephron heterogeneity and ADH-stimulated NaCl cotransport. Am J Physiol 1981; 241:F412–F431.

292. Work J, Galla JH, Booker BB, et al. Effect of ADH on chloride reabsorption in the loop of Henle of the Brattleboro rat. Am J Physiol 1985; 249:F698–F703.

293. Schlatter E, Greger R. cAMP increases the basolateral Cl^--conductance in the isolated perfused medullary thick ascending limb of Henle's loop of the mouse. Pflügers Arch 1985; 405:367–376.

294. Molony DA, Reeves WB, Hebert SC, et al. ADH increases apical $Na^+,K^+,2Cl^-$ entry in mouse medullary thick ascending limbs of Henle. Am J Physiol 1987; 252:F177–F187.

295. Molony DA, Mehta PS. cAMP dependent protein kinase stimulates directly conductive Cl^- efflux from basolateral membrane vesicles of the rabbit medullary thick ascending limb. Kidney Int 1990; 37:567.

296. Hebert SC, Culpepper RM, Andreoli TE. NaCl transport in mouse medullary thick ascending limbs. III. Modulation of the ADH effect by peritubular osmolality. Am J Physiol 1981; 241:F443–F451.

297. Molony DA, Andreoli TE. Diluting power of thick ascending limbs of Henle. I. Peritubular hypertonicity blocks basolateral Cl^- channels. Am J Physiol 1988; 255:F1128–F1137.

298. Higashihara E, Stokes JB, Kokko JP, et al. Cortical and papillary micropuncture examination of chloride transport in segments of the rat kidney during inhibition of prostaglandin production. J Clin Invest 1979; 64:1277–1287.

299. Kauker ML. Prostaglandin E_2 effect from the luminal side on renal tubular ^{22}Na efflux: tracer microinjection studies. Proc Soc Exp Biol Med 1977; 154:274–277.

300. Stokes JB. Effect of prostaglandin E_2 on chloride transport across the rabbit thick ascending limb of Henle. J Clin Invest 1979; 64:495–502.

301. Culpepper RM, Andreoli TE. Interactions among prostaglandin E_2, antidiuretic hormone, and cyclic adenosine monophosphate in modulating Cl^- absorption in single mouse medullary thick ascending limbs of Henle. J Clin Invest 1983; 71:1588–1601.

302. Torikai S, Kurokawa K. Effect of PGE_2 on vasopressin-dependent cell cAMP in isolated single segments. Am J Physiol 1983; 245:F58–F66.

303. Fejes-Tóth G, Magyar A, Walter J. Renal response to vasopressin after inhibition of prostaglandin synthesis. Am J Physiol 1977; 232:F416–F423.

304. Berl T, Raz A, Wald H, et al. Prostaglandin synthesis inhibition and the action of vasopressin: studies in man and rat. Am J Physiol 1977; 232:F529–F537.

305. Ganguli M, Tobian L, Azar S, et al. Evidence that prostaglandin synthesis inhibitors increase the concentration of sodium and chloride in rat renal medulla. Circ Res 1977; 40(Suppl 1):I135–I139.

306. Robertson GL, Athar S, Shelton RL. Osmotic control of vasopressin function. In: Andreoli TE, Grantham JJ, Rector FC, eds. Disturbances in Body Fluid Osmolality. Bethesda: American Physiological Society, 1977: 125–148.

307. Mahoney JH, Goodman AD. Hypernatremia due to hypodipsia and elevated threshold for vasopressin release. N Engl J Med 1968; 279:1191–1196.

308. DeRubertis FR, Michelis MF, Beck N, et al. "Essential" hypernatremia due to ineffective osmotic and intact volume regulation of vasopressin secretion. J Clin Invest 1971; 50:97–111.

309. Halter JB, Goldbert AP, Robertson GL, et al. Selective osmoreceptor dysfunction in the syndrome of chronic hypernatremia. J Clin Endocrinol Metab 1977; 44:609–616.

310. Fernandez CM, Vendrell SJM, Ricard W, et al. Arginine-vasopressin in essential hypernatremia. J Endocrinol Invest 1986; 9:331–335.

311. Miller M, Moses AM. Potentiation of vasopressin action by chlorpropamide in vivo. Endocrinology 1970; 86:1024–1027.
312. Moses AM, Notman DD. Diabetes insipidus and syndrome of inappropriate antidiuretic hormone secretion (SIADH). Adv Intern Med 1973; 27:73–100.
313. Randall RV, Clark EC, Bahn RC. Classification of the causes of diabetes insipidus. Mayo Clin Proc 1959; 34:299–302.
314. Sherwood MC, Stanhope R, Preece MA, et al. Diabetes insipidus and occult intracranial tumours. Arch Dis Child 1986; 61:1222–1224.
315. Weitzman RE, Kleeman CR. The clinical physiology of water metabolism. Part II: renal mechanisms for urinary concentration; diabetes insipidus. West J Med 1979; 131:486–515.
316. Martin MR. Familial diabetes insipidus. Q J Med 1959; 28:573–582.
317. Baylis PH, Robertson GL. Vasopressin function in familial cranial diabetes insipidus. Postgrad Med J 1981; 57:36–40.
318. Reeves WB, Andreoli TE. Nephrogenic diabetes insipidus. In: Schriver CR, Beaudet AL, Sly WS, et al., eds. Metabolic Basis of Inherited Disease. New York: McGraw-Hill, 1989: 1985–2011.
319. Kaplowitz PB, D'Ercole AJ, Robertson GL. Radioimmunoassay of vasopressin in familial central diabetes insipidus. J Pediatr 1982; 100:76–81.
320. Dreyer M, Rüdiger HW, Bujara K, et al. The syndrome of diabetes insipidus, diabetes mellitus, optic atrophy, deafness, and other abnormalities. Klin Wochenschr 1982; 60:471–475.
321. Blasi C, Pierelli F, Rispoli E, et al. Wolfram's syndrome: a clinical, diagnostic, and interpretative contribution. Diabetes Care 1986; 9:521–528.
322. Heinbecker P, White HL. Hypothalamico-hypophysial system and its relation to water balance in the dog. Am J Physiol 1944; 133:582–593.
323. Rasmussen AT, Gardner WJ. Effects of hypophysial stalk resection on the hypophysis and hypothalamus of man. Endocrinology 1940; 27:219–226.
324. Lipsett MB, MacLean JP, West CD, et al. An analysis of the polyuria induced by hypophysectomy in man. J Clin Endocrinol Metab 1956; 16:183–195.
325. Velhuis JD, Hammond JM. Endocrine function after spontaneous infarction of the human pituitary: report, review, and reappraisal. Endocr Rev 1980; 1:100–107.
326. Jialal E, Desai RK, Rajput MC. An assessment of posterior pituitary function in patients with Sheehan's syndrome. Clin Endocrinol 1987; 27:91–95.
327. Seckl JR, Dunger DB, Lightman SL. Neurohypophyseal peptide function during early postoperative diabetes insipidus. Brain 1987; 110:737–746.
328. Mudd RH, Dodge HW, Clark EC, et al. Experimental diabetes insipidus: a study of the hormal interphase. Proc Staff Meet Mayo Clin 1957; 32:94–108.
329. Quain R. Polyuria. In: Quain R, ed. A Dictionary of Medicine. New York: D. Appleton, 1883: 1239–1241.
330. Osler W. The Principles and Practice of Medicine. New York: D. Appleton, 1893.
331. Miller M, Dalakos T, Moses AM, et al. Recognition of partial defects in antidiuretic hormone secretion. Ann Intern Med 1970; 73:721–729.
332. Barlow E, deWardener HE. Compulsive water drinking. Q J Med 1959; 28:235–258.
333. Manson AD, Yalowitz PA, Randall RV, et al. Dilatation of the urinary tract associated with pituitary and nephrogenic diabetes insipidus. J Urol 1970; 103:327–331.
334. Streitz JM Jr, Streitz JM. Polyuric urinary tract dilatation with renal damage. J Urol 1988; 139:784–785.
335. Zerbe RL, Robertson GL. A comparison of plasma vasopressin measurements with a standard indirect test in the differential diagnosis of polyuria. N Engl J Med 1981; 305:1539–1546.
336. Marano GD, Horton JA, Vazquez AM. Computed tomography in diabetes insipidus: posterior empty sella. Br J Radiol 1981; 54:263–265.
337. Arieff AI, Guisado R, Lazarowitz VC. The pathophysiology of hyperosmolar states. In: Andreoli TE, Grantham JJ, Rector FC, eds. Disturbances in Body Fluid Osmolality. Bethesda: American Physiological Society, 1977: 227–250.
338. Chan PH, Fishman RA. Elevation of rat brain amino acids and idiogenic osmoles induced by hyperosmolality. Brain Res 1979; 161:293–301.
339. Morris-Jones PH, Houston IB, Evans RC. Prognosis of the neurological complications of acute hyponatremia. Lancet 1967; 2:1385–1389.
340. Mahon WE, Scott DJ, Ansell G, et al. Hypersensitivity to pituitary snuff with miliary shadowing of the lungs. Thorax 1967; 22:13–20.
341. Robertson GL, Harris A. Clinical use of vasopressin analogues. Hosp Pract 1989; 24:114–139.
342. Cobb WE, Spare S, Reichlin S. Neurogenic diabetes insipidus: management with dDAVP (1-desamino-8-D arginine vasopressin). Ann Intern Med 1978; 88:183–188.
343. Cunnah D, Ross G, Besser GM: Management of cranial diabetes insipidus with oral desmopressin (dDAVP). Clin Endocrinol 1986; 24:253–257.
344. Moses AM, Numann P, Miller M. Mechanism of chlorpropamide-induced antidiuresis in man: evidence for release of ADH and enhancement of peripheral action. Metab Clin Exp 1973; 22:59–66.
345. Pokracki FJ, Robinson AG, Seif SM. Chlorpropamide effect: measurement of neurophysin and vasopressin in humans and rats. Metabolism 1981; 30:72–78.
346. Kusano E, Braun-Werness JL, Vick DJ, et al. Chlorpropamide action on renal concentrating mechanism in rats with hypothalamic diabetes insipidus. J Clin Invest 1983; 72:1298–1313.
347. Moses AM, Howanitz J, van Gemert M, et al. Clofibrate-induced antidiuresis. J Clin Invest 1973; 52:535–542.
348. Kimura T, Matsui K, Sato T, et al. Mechanism of carbamazepine (Tegretol)–induced antidiuresis: evidence for release of antidiuretic hormone and impaired excretion of a water load. J Clin Endocrinol Metab 1974; 38:356–362.
349. Gold PW, Robertson GL, Ballenger JC, et al. Carbamazepine diminishes the sensitivity of the plasma arginine vasopressin response to osmotic stimulation. J Clin Endocrinol Metab 1983; 57:952–957.
350. Crawford JD, Kennedy GC. Clinical results of treatment of diabetes insipidus with drugs of the chlorothiazide series. N Engl J Med 1960; 262:737–742.
351. McIlraith CH. Notes on some cases of diabetes insipidus with marked family and hereditary tendencies. Lancet 1892; 2:767.
352. deLange C. Über erblichen Diabetes insipidus. Jahrb Kinderheilk 1935; 145:1.
353. Forssman H. On hereditary diabetes insipidus. Acta Med Scand 1945; 121(Suppl 159):3–196.
354. Williams RH, Henry C. Nephrogenic diabetes insipidus: transmitted by females and appearing during infancy in males. Ann Intern Med 1947; 27:84–95.
355. Kambouris M, Dlouhy SR, Trofatter JA, et al. Localization of the gene for X-linked nephrogenic diabetes insipidus to Xq28. Am J Med Genet 1988; 29:239–246.
356. Knoers N, van der Heyden H, van Oost BA, et al. Three-point linkage analysis using multiple DNA polymorphic markers in families with X-linked nephrogenic diabetes insipidus. Genomics 1989; 4:434–437.
357. Waring AJ, Kajdi L, Tappan V. A congenital defect of water metabolism. Am J Dis Child 1945; 69:323–324.
358. Naik DV, Valtin H. Hereditary vasopressin-resistant urinary concentrating defects in mice. Am J Physiol 1969; 217:1183–1190.
359. Dousa TP, Valtin H. Cellular action of antidiuretic hormone in mice with inherited vasopressin-resistant urinary concentrating defects. J Clin Invest 1974; 54:753–762.
360. Jackson BA, Edwards RM, Valtin H, et al. Cellular action of vasopressin in medullary tubules of mice with hereditary nephrogenic diabetes insipidus. J Clin Invest 1980; 66:110–122.
361. Kusano E, Yusufi ANK, Murayama N, et al. Dynamics of nucleotides in distal nephron of mice with nephrogenic diabetes insipidus. Am J Physiol 1986; 250:F151–F158.
362. Fichman MP, Brokker G. Deficient renal cyclic adenosine 3',5' monophosphate production in nephrogenic diabetes insipidus. J Clin Endocrinol Metab 1972; 35:35–47.
363. Bell NH, Clark CM Jr, Avery S, et al. Demonstration of a defect in the formation of adenosine 3',5'-monophosphate in vasopressin-resistant diabetes insipidus. Pediatr Res 1974; 8:223–230.
364. Bichet DG, Razi M, Arthus M–F, et al. Epinephrine and dDAVP administration in patients with congenital nephrogenic diabetes insipidus. Evidence for a pre-cyclic AMP V_2 receptor defective mechanism. Kidney Int 1989; 36:859–866.
365. Orr FR, Filipich RL. Studies with angiotensin in nephrogenic diabetes insipidus. Can Med Assoc J 1967; 97:841–845.
366. Moses AM, Scheinman SJ, Schroeder ET. Antidiuretic and PGE_2 responses to AVP and dDAVP in subjects with central and nephrogenic diabetes insipidus. Am J Physiol 1985; 248:F354–F359.
367. Bichet DG, Razi M, Lonergan M, et al. Hemodynamic and coagulation responses to 1-desamino/8-D-arginine vasopressin in patients with congenital nephrogenic diabetes insipidus. N Engl J Med 1988; 318:881–887.
368. Brenner B, Seligsohn U, Hochberg Z. Normal response of factor VIII and von Willebrand factor to 1-deamino-8D-arginine vasopressin in nephrogenic diabetes insipidus. J Clin Endocrinol Metab 1988; 67:191–193.
369. Moses AM, Miller JL, Levine MA. Two distinct pathophysiological mechanisms in congenital nephrogenic diabetes insipidus. J Clin Endocrinol Metab 1988; 66:1259–1264.
370. Singer I, Forrest JN. Drug-induced states of nephrogenic diabetes insipidus. Kidney Int 1976; 10:82–95.
371. Dousa TP, Wilson DM. Effects of demethylchlortetracycline on cellular action of antidiuretic hormone in vitro. Kidney Int 1974; 5:279–284.
372. Frascino JA, O'Flaherty J, Olmo C, et al. Effect of inorganic fluoride on the renal concentrating mechanism. Possible nephrotoxicity in man. J Lab Clin Med 1972; 79:192–203.
373. Wallin JD, Kaplan RA. Effect of sodium fluoride on concentrating and diluting ability in the rat. Am J Physiol 1977; 232:F335–F340.
374. Singer I, Rotenberg D, Puschett JB. Lithium-induced nephrogenic diabetes insipidus: in vivo and in vitro studies. J Clin Invest 1972; 51:1081–1091.
375. Dousa TP. Interaction of lithium with vasopressin-sensitive cyclic AMP system of human renal medulla. Endocrinology 1974; 95:1359–1366.

376. Jackson BA, Edwards RM, Dousa TP. Lithium-induced polyuria: effect of lithium on adenylate cyclase and adenosine 3′,5′-monophosphate phosphodiesterase in medullary ascending limb of Henle's loop and in medullary collecting tubules. Endocrinology 1980; 107:1693–1698.

377. Usberti M, Decaux M, Guillot M, et al. Renal prostaglandin E_2 in nephrogenic diabetes insipidus: effects of inhibition of prostaglandin synthesis in indomethacin. J Pediatr 1980; 97:476–478.

378. Blachar Y, Zadik Z, Shemesh M, et al. The effect of inhibition of prostaglandin synthesis on free water and osmolar clearances in patients with hereditary nephrogenic diabetes insipidus. Int J Pediatr Nephrol 1980; 1:48–52.

379. Delaney V, de Pertuz Y, Nixon D, et al. Indomethacin in streptozocin-induced nephrogenic diabetes insipidus. Am J Kidney Dis 1987; 9:79–83.

380. Allen HM, Jackson RL, Winchester MD, et al. Indomethacin in the treatment of lithium-induced nephrogenic diabetes insipidus. Arch Intern Med 1989; 149:1123–1126.

381. Kosten TR, Forrest JN. Treatment of severe lithium-induced polyuria with amiloride. Am J Psychiatry 1986; 143:1563–1568.

382. Batlle DC, von Riotte AB, Gaviria M, et al. Amelioration of polyuria by amiloride in patients receiving long-term lithium therapy. N Engl J Med 1985; 312:408–414.

383. Alon U, Chan JCM. Hydrochlorothiazide-amiloride in the treatment of congenital nephrogenic diabetes insipidus. Am J Nephrol 1985; 5:9–13.

384. Manitius A, Levitin H, Beck D, et al. On the mechanisms of impairment of renal concentrating ability in potassium deficiency. J Clin Invest 1960; 39:684–692.

385. Galvez OG, Roberts BW, Bay WH, et al. Studies on the mechanism of polyuria with hypokalemia. Kidney Int 1976; 10:583A.

386. Berl T, Linas SL, Aisenbery GA, et al. On the mechanism of polyuria in potassium depletion. J Clin Invest 1977; 60:620–625.

387. Manitius A, Levitin H, Beck D, et al. On the mechanism of impairment of renal concentrating ability in hypercalcemia. J Clin Invest 1960; 39:693–697.

388. Campbell BJ, Woodward G, Broberg V. Calcium-mediated interactions between the antidiuretic hormone and renal plasma membranes. J Biol Chem 1972; 247:6167–6175.

389. Durr JA, Hoggard JG, Hunt JM, et al. Diabetes insipidus in pregnancy associated with abnormally high circulating vasopressinase activity. N Engl J Med 1987; 316:1070–1074.

390. Barron WM, Cohen LH, Ulland LA, et al. Transient vasopressin-resistant diabetes insipidus of pregnancy. N Engl J Med 1984; 310:442–444.

391. Hughes JM, Barron WM, Vance ML. Recurrent diabetes insipidus associated with pregnancy: pathophysiology and therapy. Obstet Gynecol 1989; 73:462–464.

392. Shah SV, Thakur V. Vasopressinase and diabetes insipidus of pregnancy. Ann Intern Med 1988; 109:435–436.

393. Davison JM, Sheills EA, Barron WM, et al. Changes in the metabolic clearance of vasopressin and in plasma vasopressinase throughout human pregnancy. J Clin Invest 83:1313–1318.

394. Ford SM Jr. Transient vasopressin-resistant diabetes insipidus of pregnancy. Obstet Gynecol 1986; 68:288–289.

395. Finberg L, Kiley S, Lettrell CN. Mass accidental salt poisoning in infancy. JAMA 1963; 184:187–190.

396. Dodge PR, Sotos JF, Gamstorp I, et al. Neurophysiologic disturbances in hypertonic dehydration. Trans Am Neurol Assoc 1962; 87:33–36.

397. Sotos JF, Dodge PR, Meara P, et al. Studies in experimental hypertonicity: pathogenesis of the clinical syndrome, biochemical abnormalities and cause of death. Pediatrics 1960; 26:925–937.

398. Holliday MA, Kalayci MN, Harrah J. Factors that limit brain volume changes in response to acute and sustained hyper- and hyponatremia. J Clin Invest 1968; 47:1916–1928.

399. Arieff AI, Guisado R. Effects on the central nervous system of hypernatremic and hyponatremic states. Kidney Int 1976; 10:104–116.

400. Cala PM. Volume regulation by red blood cells: mechanisms of ion transport. Mol Physiol 1983; 4:33–52.

401. Cronin RE. Psychogenic polydipsia with hyponatremia: report of eleven cases. Am J Kidney Dis 1987; 4:410–416.

402. Victor W, Vieweg R, Godleski LS, et al. Failure of antipsychotic drug dose to explain abnormal diurnal weight gain among 129 chronically psychotic inpatients. Prog Neuropsychopharmacol Biol Psychiatry 1989; 13:709–723.

403. Kramer DS, Drake ME. Acute psychosis, polydipsia, and inappropriate secretion of antidiuretic hormone. Am J Med 1983; 75:712–714.

404. Levine S, McManus BM, Blackbourne BD, et al. Fatal water intoxication, schizophrenia, and diuretic therapy for systemic hypertension. Am J Med 1987; 82:153–155.

405. Goldman MB, Luchins DJ, Robertson GL. Mechanisms of altered water metabolism in psychotic patients with polydipsia and hyponatremia. N Engl J Med 1988; 318:397–403.

406. Vieweg V, Glick JL, Herring S, et al. Absence of carbamazepine-induced hyponatremia among patients also given lithium. Am J Psychiatry 1987; 144:943–947.

407. Yassa R, Iskandar H, Nastase C, et al. Carbamazepine and hyponatremia in patients with affective disorder. Am J Psychiatry 1988; 145:339–342.

408. Fanestil DA. Hyposmolar syndromes. In: Andreoli TE, Grantham JJ, Rector FC, eds. Disturbances in Body Fluid Osmolality. Bethesda: American Physiological Society, 1977:267–284.

409. Hilden T, Svendsen TL. Electrolyte disturbances in beer drinkers: a specific "hypo-osmolality syndrome." Lancet 1975; 2:245–246.

410. McCance RA. Experimental sodium chloride deficiency in man. Proc R Soc Lond [Biol] 1936; 119:245–268.

411. Harrington AR. Hyponatremia due to sodium depletion in the absence of vasopressin. Am J Physiol 1972; 222:768–774.

412. Berliner RW, Davidson DG. Production of hypertonic urine in the absence of pituitary antidiuretic hormone. J Clin Invest 1957; 36:1416–1427.

413. Kassirer JP, Berkman PM, Lawrenz DR, et al. The critical role of chloride in the correction of hypokalemic alkalosis in man. Am J Med 1965; 38:172–189.

414. Valtin H, Sokol HW, Sunde D. Genetic approaches to the study of the regulation and actions of vasopressin. Recent Prog Horm Res 1975; 31:447–486.

415. Szatalowicz VL, Arnold PE, Chaimovitz C, et al. Radioimmunoassay of plasma arginine vasopressin in hyponatremic patients with congestive heart failure. N Engl J Med 1981; 305:263–266.

416. Weitzman RE, Kleeman CR. The clinical physiology of water metabolism. III. The water depletion (hyperosmolar) and water excess (hyposmolar) syndromes. West J Med 1980; 132:16–38.

417. Seldin DW, Eknoyan G, Suki WN, et al. Localization of diuretic action from the pattern of water and electrolyte excretion. Ann NY Acad Sci 1966; 139:328–343.

418. Fichman MP, Vorherr H, Kleeman CR, et al. Diuretic-induced hyponatremia. Ann Intern Med 1971; 75:853–863.

419. Chung H-M, Kluge R, Schrier RW, et al. Clinical assessment of extracellular fluid volume in hyponatremia. Am J Med 1987; 83:905–908.

420. Schrier RW, Linas SL. Mechanisms of the defect in water excretion in adrenal insufficiency. Miner Electrolyte Metab 1980; 4:1–7.

421. Raff H. Glucocorticoid inhibition of neurohypophysial vasopressin secretion. Am J Physiol 1987; 252:R635–R644.

422. Linas SL, Berl T, Robertson GL, et al. Role of vasopressin in the impaired water excretion of glucocorticoid deficiency. Kidney Int 1980; 18:58–67.

423. Ishikawa S-E, Kim JK, Schrier RW. Effects of arginine vasopressin antidiuretic and vasopressor antagonists in glucocorticoid and mineralocorticoid deficient rats. In: Schrier RW, ed. Vasopressin. New York: Raven, 1985: 171–180.

424. Chinitz A, Turner FL. The association of primary hypothyroidism and inappropriate secretion of the antidiuretic hormone. Arch Intern Med 1965; 116:871–874.

425. DeRubertis FR, Mechelis MF, Bloom ME, et al. Impaired water excretion in myxedema. Am J Med 1971; 51:41–53.

426. DiScala VA, Kinney MJ. Effects of myxedema on the renal diluting and concentrating mechanism. Am J Med 1971; 50:325–335.

427. Anderson RJ, Chung H-M, Kluge R, et al. Hyponatremia: a prospective analysis of its epidemiology and the pathogenetic role of vasopressin. Ann Intern Med 1985; 102:164–168.

428. Chung H-M, Kluge R, Schrier RW, et al. Postoperative hyponatremia: a prospective study. Arch Intern Med 1986; 146:333–336.

429. Gross PA, Pehrisch H, Rascher W, et al. Pathogenesis of clinical hyponatremia: observations of vasopressin and fluid intake in 100 hyponatremic medical patients. Eur J Clin Invest 1987; 17:123–129.

430. Gross P, Pehrisch H, Rascher W, et al. Vasopressin in hyponatremia: what stimuli? J Cardiovasc Pharmacol 1986; 8:S92–S95.

431. Leaf A, Bartter FC, Santos RF, et al. Evidence in man that urinary electrolyte loss induced by polydipsia is a function of water retention. J Clin Invest 1953; 32:868–871.

432. Gertz KH, Boylan J. Glomerulotubular balance. In: Orloff J, Berliner RW, eds. Handbook of Physiology. Sect 8: Renal Physiology. Bethesda: American Physiological Society, 1973: 763–790.

433. Chan WY. A study on the mechanism of vasopressin escape: effects of chronic vasopressin and overhydration on renal tissue osmolality and electrolytes in dogs. J Pharmacol Exp Ther 1973; 184:244–252.

434. Schwartz WB, Bennett W, Curelop S, et al. A syndrome of renal sodium loss and hyponatremia probably resulting from inappropriate secretion of antidiuretic hormone. Am J Med 1957; 23:529–542.

435. Zerbe R, Stropes L, Robertson G. Vasopressin function in the syndrome of inappropriate diuresis. Annu Rev Med 1980; 31:315–327.

436. Goldberg M. Abnormalities in the renal excretion of water. Med Clin North Am 1963; 47:915–933.

437. Clive DM, Stoff JS. Renal syndromes associated with nonsteroidal antiinflammatory drugs. N Engl J Med 1984; 310:563–572.

438. Blum M, Aviram A. Ibuprofen induced hyponatremia. Rheumatol Rehabil 1980; 19:258–259.

439. Reeves WB, Foley RJ, Weinman EJ. Nephrotoxicity from non-steroidal anti-inflammatory drugs. South Med J 1985; 78:318–321.

440. Petersson I, Nilsson G, Hansson BG, et al. Water intoxication associated with non-steroidal anti-inflammatory drug therapy. Acta Med Scand 1987; 221:221–223.

441. Weisberg LS. Pseudohyponatremia: a reappraisal. Am J Med 1989; 86:315–318.

442. Rao PN. Fluid absorption during urological endoscopy. Br J Urol 1987; 60:93–99.
443. Campbell HT, Fincher ME, Sklar AH. Severe hyponatremia without severe hypoösmolality following transurethral resection of the prostate (TURP) in end-stage renal disease. Am J Kidney Dis 1988; 12:152–155.
444. Weir JF, Larson EE, Rowntree LG. Studies in diabetes insipidus, water balance and water intoxication. Arch Intern Med 1922; 29:321–330.
445. Arieff AI, Llach F, Massry SG. Neurological manifestations and morbidity of hyponatremia: correlation with brain water and electrolytes. Medicine 1976; 55:121–129.
446. Pollock AS, Arieff AI. Abnormalities of cell volume regulation and the functional consequences. Am J Physiol 1980; 239:F195–F205.
447. Grantham J, Linshaw M. The effect of hyponatremia on the regulation of intracellular volume and solute composition. Circ Res 1984; 54:483–491.
448. Sterns RH, Thomas DJ, Herndon RM. Brain dehydration and neurologic deterioration after rapid correction of hyponatremia. Kidney Int 1989; 35:69–75.
449. Kleinschmidt-DeMasters BK, Norenberg MD. Rapid correction of hyponatremia causes demyelination: relation to central pontine myelinolysis. Science 1981; 211:1068–1070.
450. Telfer AB, Miller EM. Central pontine myelinolysis following hyponatremia, demonstrated by computerized tomography. Ann Neurol 1979; 6:455–456.
451. Norenberg MD, Leslie KO. Correction of hyponatremia and central pontine myelinolysis. Am J Med 1982; 73:882.
452. Sterns RH. Neurological deterioration following treatment for hyponatremia. Am J Kidney Dis 1989; 13:434–437.
453. Hantman D, Rossier B, Zohlman R, et al. Rapid correction of hyponatremia in the syndrome of inappropriate secretion of antidiuretic hormone. Ann Intern Med 1973; 78:870–875.
454. Arieff AI. Hyponatremia associated with permanent brain damage. Adv Intern Med 1987; 32:325–344.
455. Ayus JC, Krothapalli RK, Arieff AI. Treatment of symptomatic hyponatremia and its relation to brain damage: a prospective study. N Engl J Med 1987; 317:1190–1195.
456. Sterns RH. Severe symptomatic hyponatremia: treatment and outcome. Ann Intern Med 1987; 107:656–664.
457. Fraser CL, Arieff AI. Fatal central diabetes mellitus and insipidus resulting from untreated hyponatremia: a new syndrome. Ann Intern Med 1990; 112:113–119.
458. Arieff AI. Hyponatremia, convulsions, respiratory arrest, and permanent brain damage after elective surgery in healthy women. N Engl J Med 1986; 314:1529–1535.
459. Ayus JC, Krothapalli RK, Arieff AI. Sexual difference in survival with severe symptomatic hyponatremia. Kidney Int 1988; 33:180.
460. Fraser CL, Kucharczyk J, Arieff AI, et al. Sex differences result in increased morbidity from hyponatremia in female rats. Am J Physiol 1989; 256:R880–R885.
461. Ayus JC, Krothapalli RK, Armstrong DL. Rapid correction of severe hyponatremia in the rat: histopathological changes in the brain. Am J Physiol 1985; 248:F711–F719.
462. Forrest JN Jr, Cox M, Hong C, et al. Superiority of demeclocycline over lithium in the treatment of chronic syndrome of inappropriate secretion of antidiuretic hormone. N Engl J Med 1978; 298:173–177.
463. Dias N, Hocken AG. Oliguric renal failure complicating lithium carbonate therapy. Nephron 1972; 10:246–249.
464. Schrier RW. New treatments for hyponatremia. N Engl J Med 1978; 298:214–215.
465. Decaux G, Brimioulle S, Genette F, et al. Treatment of the syndrome of inappropriate secretion of antidiuretic hormone by urea. Am J Med 1980; 69:99–106.

Section 3
THYROID

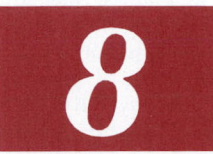

THE THYROID GLAND

P. Reed Larsen and Sidney H. Ingbar

INTRODUCTION

Several textbooks deal exclusively with thyroid disease.[1-4] The reader may find these useful in supplementing the discussions of biochemical processes and experimental thyroid physiology.

PHYLOGENY

In its phylogeny, its embryogenesis, and certain aspects of its function, the thyroid gland reveals its primitive relation to the gastrointestinal tract.

The capacity of the thyroid to metabolize iodine and incorporate it into a variety of organic compounds is found widely throughout the animal and plant kingdoms. Monoiodotyrosine (3-monoiodo-L-tyrosine, MIT) and diiodotyrosine (3,5-diiodo-L-tyrosine, DIT) are present in a variety of invertebrate fauna, including mollusks, crustaceans, coelenterates, annelids, and insects, as well as in certain marine algae. In these lower forms, however, no recognizable thyroid tissue is present. Thyroid tissue is confined to the vertebrates and is present in all species thereof. A close link to the thyroid of higher vertebrates is evident in the ammocoete, the larval form of the lamprey. Here the endostyle is capable of carrying out iodinations, but before metamorphosis a protease appears in the endostyle that can hydrolyze the iodoprotein formed. Presumably this permits the endostyle to lose its connection with the pharynx, as occurs during metamorphosis, and to assume its adult function as an endocrine organ that secretes iodothyronines, including 3,5,3',5'-tetraiodo-L-thyronine (thyroxine, T_4) and 3,5,3'-triiodo-L-thyronine (T_3). (Figure 8–1 shows the structural formulas of the thyroid hormones, their precursors, and certain of their metabolites.)

Except perhaps in some lower vertebrates, control of thyroid function is mediated by a pituitary thyrotropin (thyroid-stimulating hormone, TSH). In higher vertebrates, control of TSH secretion is, in turn, influenced by a thyrotropin-releasing hormone (TRH) of hypothalamic origin. In many lower vertebrates, a functional response of the pituitary-thyroid axis to TRH cannot be elicited, although TRH is clearly present within the brain.

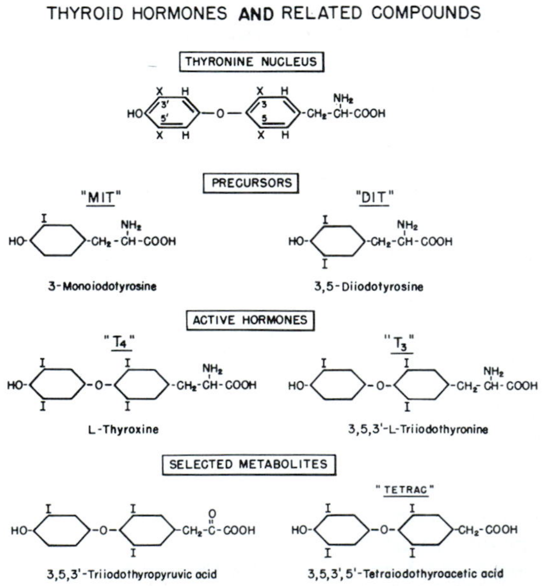

The phylogenetic association of the thyroid gland and the gastrointestinal tract is evident in several functional respects. Thus the salivary and gastric glands, like the thyroid, are capable of concentrating iodide in their secretions, although iodide transport in these sites is not responsive to stimulation by TSH. In the rare form of goitrous hypothyroidism that is due to lack of the thyroid iodide transport mechanism, salivary transport of iodide is also defective. The salivary gland contains enzymatic mechanisms that are capable of iodinating tyrosine when provided with hydrogen peroxide. Although the salivary gland forms insignificant quantities of iodoproteins under normal circumstances, when completely thyroidectomized rats are given large doses of iodide, stigmata of hypothyroidism are reversed and synthesis of DIT and T_4 occurs, probably within a protein matrix. Such iodoproteins may be formed in gastrointestinal structures, pass into the lumen, and be digested, and the iodinated amino acids may well be absorbed. The similarity of function to that found in prevertebrates and in the ammocoete is thus apparent.

ANATOMICAL AND FUNCTIONAL EMBRYOLOGY

The human thyroid anlage is first recognizable about 1 mo after conception, when the embryo is approximately 3.5 to 4.0 mm in length. The primordium begins as a thickening of epithelium in the pharyngeal floor, which later forms a diverticulum. With continuing development, the median diverticulum undergoes relative caudal displacement and the primitive stalk connecting the primordium with the pharyngeal floor undergoes elongation (thyroglossal duct). During its caudal displacement, the primordium assumes a more bilobate shape, coming into contact and fusing with the ventral aspect of the fourth pharyngeal pouch. Normally the thyroglossal duct undergoes dissolution and fragmentation by about the second month after conception, leaving at its point of origin a small dimple at the junction of the middle and posterior thirds of the tongue, the foramen cecum. Cells of the lower portion of the duct differentiate into thyroid tissue, forming the pyramidal lobe of the gland. Concomitantly, histological alterations occur. Complex interconnecting cord-like arrangements of cells interspersed with vascular connective tissue replace the solid epithelial mass. These transform to tubule-like structures at about the third month of fetal life, and shortly thereafter follicular arrangements devoid of colloid appear, followed by colloid-filled follicles.

The functional development of the thyroid has been studied in various species. Thyroprotein resembling thyroglobulin appears just before or at the time when follicular structure is first apparent. Evidently this antecedes by a short period the capacity to collect iodine, although results of some studies suggest that early iodine accumulation is virtually concurrent with the appearance of MIT, DIT, T_4, and T_3. Other results suggest that iodide transport, organic binding (binding of iodine to tyrosine), and iodotyrosine-coupling functions appear in sequence. The continued anatomical and functional development of the thyroid after these functions have begun, and perhaps even before, is dependent on TSH. The origin of the thyroid is necessarily fetal because the placenta is impermeable to maternal TSH.

THYROID HORMONES AND RELATED COMPOUNDS

Figure 8–1. Structural formulas of thyroid hormones and related compounds. The structure of the thyronine nucleus of the hormonally active iodinated amino acids, T_4 and T_3, is shown above. Iodinated thyronines are formed through the oxidative coupling of the precursor iodotyrosines, MIT and DIT, in varying combination. 3,5,3'-Triiodothyropyruvic acid is derived by oxidative deamination from T_3. Tetrac is derived from T_4 by oxidative deamination followed by decarboxylation.

Despite obvious difficulties in studying this problem, the ontogeny of thyroid function and its regulation in the human fetus are fairly well defined.[5] The capacity of future follicular cells to form thyroglobulin is established as early as the 29th day of gestation. Nonetheless, the capacities to concentrate iodide and to synthesize T_4 are delayed until about the 11th week. Significant accumulation of radioactive iodine given to the mother begins soon thereafter. Early growth and development of the thyroid do not seem to be TSH dependent, because the capacity of the pituitary to synthesize and secrete TSH is not apparent until the 10th to 12th week. After this, rapid changes in pituitary and thyroid function take place. Probably as a consequence of hypothalamic maturation and increasing secretion of TRH, the serum TSH concentration increases rapidly from about 18 to 26 wk, after which it remains largely unchanged at levels higher than those found in the mother. The higher levels may reflect a higher set point of the negative feedback control of TSH secretion during fetal life than during maturity. In the fetal rat and lamb the capacity of T_3 to inhibit the response to TRH is diminished, and in the human the fetal response to TRH is greater than that in the adult.[6] Thyroxine-binding globulin (TBG), the major thyroid hormone–binding protein in plasma, is detectable in the serum by the 10th gestational week and increases in concentration progressively to term. This increase in TBG concentration doubtless accounts in part for the progressive increase in the serum T_4 concentration in the second and third trimesters, but increased secretion of T_4 must also play a role because the concentration of unbound or free T_4 also rises.

The peripheral metabolism of T_4 in the human fetus differs markedly from that in the adult in both quantitative and qualitative senses. Overall, on the basis of unit body mass, rates of production and degradation of T_4 greatly exceed those found in the adult. In addition, in all species thus far studied, the specific enzymatic pathways by which T_4 is metabolized differ from those in the adult, favoring the formation of 3,3′,5′-triiodo-L-thyronine (reverse T_3, rT_3) at the expense of T_3.

Several aspects of fetal thyroidology are worthy of note from the clinical standpoint. Rarely, thyroid tissue may develop from remnants of the thyroglossal duct near the base of the tongue. Such lingual thyroid tissue may be the sole functioning thyroid present; its surgical removal will then lead to hypothyroidism. More commonly, elements of the thyroglossal duct may persist and later give rise to thyroglossal cysts, or thyroid tissue progenitors may migrate with adjacent cardiovascular structures to occupy a place within the mediastinum.

The fetal pituitary-thyroid axis functions as a unit that is essentially independent of that of the mother. Transplacental passage of TSH from mother to fetus is negligible or nearly so, but the same is not true of maternal T_4. In infants with congenital hypothyroidism caused by either thyroid peroxidase deficiency or athyreosis, serum concentrations of T_4 in cord blood are approximately one third to one half of normal.[7] Thus, at least when the maternal/fetal concentration gradient is high, there is significant transfer of T_4 to the fetal circulation. This transfer may have considerable significance given the capacity of the fetal brain to increase the efficiency of T_4-to-T_3 conversion. Maternal T_4 plus these compensatory adjustments might account for the apparent lack of clinical symptomatology and the normal intellectual function of infants with congenital hypothyroidism who are identified through screening programs and given adequate levothyroxine treatment before the appearance of symptoms. Thyroid hormones almost certainly condition late-phase skeletal maturation, influence late prenatal maturation of the lung, and are required for normal development of the brain and intellectual function, either before birth or soon thereafter, making the diagnosis of neonatal hypothyroidism extremely urgent. However, neonatal hypothyroidism is extremely difficult to detect by physical examination. For this reason the disease, which occurs at least once in every 4000 to 5000 newborns throughout the world, must be sought with measurements of the serum T_4 or TSH concentration.

ANATOMY AND HISTOLOGY

The thyroid is one of the largest of the endocrine organs, weighing approximately 20 g in North American adults. Moreover, the potential of the thyroid for growth is tremendous. Goiters weighing many hundreds of grams are not rare. The normal thyroid is made up of two lobes joined by a thin band of tissue, the isthmus. The latter is approximately 0.5 cm thick, 2 cm wide, and 2 cm high. The individual lobes normally have a rather pointed superior pole and a poorly defined, blunt inferior pole merging medially with the isthmus. Each lobe is approximately 2.0 or 2.5 cm in thickness and width at its largest diameter and is approximately 4.0 cm in length. Occasionally, especially when the remainder of the gland is goitrous, a pyramidal lobe is discernible as a finger-like projection directed upward from the isthmus, generally just lateral to the midline, usually on the left. The right lobe of the thyroid is normally more vascular than the left, is often the larger of the two, and tends to enlarge more in disorders associated with a diffuse increase in size.

The thyroid is closely affixed to the anterior and lateral aspects of the trachea by loose connective tissue. The upper margin of the isthmus generally lies just below the cricoid cartilage, which therefore provides a convenient landmark for locating the gland. Lying between the thyroid gland and the subcutaneous tissue are the thin infrahyoid muscles. Lateral to the gland are the carotid sheaths and sternocleidomastoid muscles, and the recurrent laryngeal nerves lie in the grooves between the lateral lobes and the trachea. Two pairs of parathyroid glands are normally situated on or beneath the posterior surface of the thyroid lobes.

Two main pairs of vessels constitute the major arterial blood supply. The superior thyroid artery, arising from the external carotid artery, and the inferior thyroid artery, arising from the subclavian artery, enter their respective poles. The gland is well vascularized. Estimates of thyroid blood flow range from 4 to 6 mL/min/g, well in excess of the blood flow to the kidney (3 mL/min/g). In diffuse toxic goiter blood flow rates greater than 1 L/min may occur. Increased flow is evidenced clinically by the presence of a thrill or audible bruit over the gland or in its immediate vicinity. There is rich lymphatic drainage. Its function relative to the endocrine activity of the gland is uncertain, but the lymph contains a higher concentration of newly released radioiodine than does thyroid venous blood, probably in the form of iodoprotein.

The thyroid is innervated by both adrenergic and cholinergic nervous systems via fibers arising from the cervical ganglia and the vagus nerve, respectively. Afferent fibers pass through the laryngeal nerves and regulate an active vasomotor system. One function of neurogenic stimuli is to regulate blood flow to the thyroid. Although acute changes in blood flow do not appear to alter the rate of hormonal release, the rate of perfusion influences the delivery of TSH, iodide, and metabolic substrates and may eventually influence glandular function and growth.

In addition to vasomotor innervation, there is a network of adrenergic fibers that terminates near the basement membrane of the follicular wall. Moreover, specific saturable adrenergic receptors are present in thyroid plasma membranes. These findings, together with the capacity of adrenergic (and other) amines to affect iodine and intermediary metabolism of the thyroid in vitro and in vivo, indicate that the adrenergic nervous system can influence thyroid function through a direct effect on the follicle cell, as well as by changing glandular blood flow.

The thyroid is invested with a thin fibrous capsule that penetrates the gland, forming irregular pseudolobules. The gland itself is firm yet resilient. The cut surface of a normal gland has a spotted beefy red appearance. Minute vesicles (the follicles) from which the amber-colored, sticky colloid exudes are distributed throughout.

With light microscopy, the gland is seen to be composed of closely packed sacs, called acini or follicles, which are invested with a rich capillary network. The interior of the follicle is filled with the clear proteinaceous colloid, which normally is the major constituent of the total thyroid mass. The diameter of the follicles varies considerably, even within a single gland, but averages about 200 μm. The iodine-accumulating function of the individual follicle varies with its surface area. The wall of the follicle is lined by a single layer of closely packed cuboidal cells, approximately 15 μm high. The cells of the acinar epithelium vary in height with the degree of glandular stimulation, becoming columnar when active and flat when inactive. The epithelium rests on a basement membrane that stains with reagents for mucopolysaccharides and separates the follicular cells from the surrounding capillaries. From 20 to 40 follicles are demarcated by connective tissue septa to form a lobule supplied by a single artery. The function of an individual lobule may vary from that of its neighbors.

With electron microscopy, the thyroid is seen to have many features in common with other secretory cells, but some are peculiar to the thyroid. From the apical aspect of the follicular cell, numerous microvilli extend into the colloid. It is at or near this surface of the cell that iodination, exocytosis, and the initial phase of hormone secretion, namely, colloid resorption, occur.[8] The nucleus of the follicular cell has no distinctive features. The cytoplasm contains an extensive endoplasmic reticulum laden with microsomes. The endoplasmic reticulum is distinctive in being composed of a network of wide irregular tubules that contain the precursor of thyroglobulin. The carbohydrate component of thyroglobulin is probably added to this precursor in the Golgi apparatus, which is located apically. Lysosomes and mitochondria are scattered throughout the cytoplasm. Stimulation by TSH results in enlargement of the Golgi apparatus, formation of pseudopodia at the apical surface, and appearance in the apical portion of the cell of many droplets that contain colloid taken up from the follicular lumen. A description of scanning electron microscopic studies of various thyroid diseases has been published.[9]

The thyroid also contains a population of other cells, termed parafollicular or C cells, that are the source of the calcium-lowering hormone calcitonin. These cells arise during embryonic development from the last pair of pharyngeal pouches but ultimately come to rest either among the cells of the follicular epithelium or in the thyroid interstitium. They differ from the cells of the follicular epithelium in never bordering on the follicular lumen and in being rich in both mitochondria and α-glycerophosphate dehydrogenase. C cells undergo hyperplasia early in the syndrome of familial medullary carcinoma of the thyroid and give rise to this tumor in both its familial and sporadic forms. (See Chapter 30.)

IODINE METABOLISM: SYNTHESIS, SECRETION, AND METABOLISM OF THYROID HORMONES

In the most general sense the function of the thyroid is to secrete such quantities of hormone as are necessary to meet the demands of the peripheral tissue.

Extrathyroidal Metabolism of Iodide

Formation of normal quantities of thyroid hormone ultimately depends on the availability of adequate quantities of exogenous iodine. Although there are efficient mechanisms for conserving iodine in the presence of iodine deficiency, they do not entirely succeed in preventing depletion of iodine stores; ultimately this may lead to insufficient hormone production. Normally iodine balance is maintained from dietary sources, i.e., food and water, but iodine may enter the body via medications, diagnostic agents, and dietary supplements and as a result of the use of iodine by the food-processing industry. Increases in available iodine modify both the metabolism of iodine and the clinical tests by which it is assessed.

It is difficult to assign normal limits to the daily dietary intake of iodine because it varies widely throughout the world, depending on the iodine content of soil and water and on culturally established dietary preferences. Even in a single area, considerable variation in iodine intake can be expected between different individuals and in the same individual from day to day. In most areas of the United States, for example, the dietary iodine intake is in the range of 500 μg daily, and in Japan, where large quantities of foods rich in iodine are characteristically consumed, intakes as high as several milligrams per day have been commonplace. In western Europe iodine intakes lower than those in the United States are tolerated without widespread overt thyroid dysfunction. The resulting marginal iodine deficiency does, however, predispose to development of hyperthyroidism upon exposure to sources of additional iodine.

As with pharmacologically induced alterations in iodine intake, variations in dietary iodine intake, when sustained, are reflected in differences in the kinetics of iodine metabolism and hence must be taken into account in assigning normal limits to tests designed to evaluate thyroid function. Figure 8–2 is a schema of the major pathways of overall iodine metabolism, summarizing the movement of iodine into, out of, and among the various compartments of body iodine. The numerical values presented are approximations of the normal means in the United States, but even here variations are encountered. Iodine used in the synthesis of thyroid hormone is drawn from the inorganic iodide of the extracellular fluid. The iodide thereby cleared is partly replenished both by iodide lost from the thyroid into the blood (iodide leak) and by iodide liberated through deiodination of thyroid hormones in peripheral tissues. Ultimately, however, the diet is the most important source of iodide. Iodine is ingested in both inorganic and organically bound forms. The rapidity of absorption of organically bound iodine and the form in which it is absorbed are uncertain, but eventually it is made available as inorganic iodide. Iodide itself is rapidly and efficiently absorbed from the gastrointestinal tract, and little is lost in the stool.

In the body, iodide is largely confined to the extracellular fluid. It is also found, however, within the red blood cell and is concentrated in the intraluminal fluids of the gastrointestinal tract, notably the saliva and gastric juice, from which it is ultimately reabsorbed and reenters the extracellular fluid. Until oxidized and bound to tyrosyl

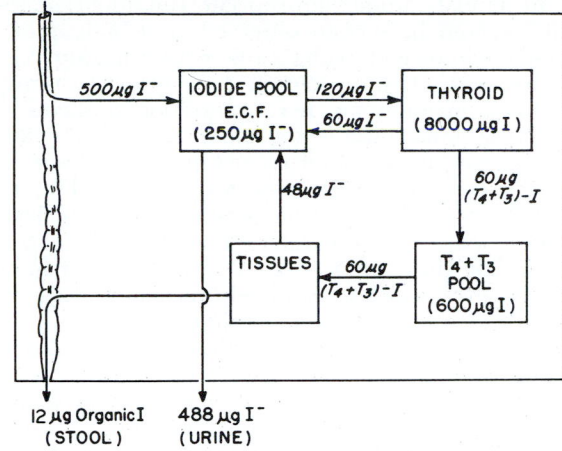

Figure 8–2. Diagram depicting normal pathways of iodine metabolism in a state of iodine balance. Note that most (approximately 90%) of body iodine store is present in the thyroid (chiefly in the organic form). Approximately 10% is present as iodide. Arrows indicate daily flux of iodine from one compartment to another. In this example, one fifth of the iodide entering the iodide space (120/608) is accumulated by the thyroid. Peak thyroid uptake of I* should be 20%, and the rate of turnover of thyronine-iodine peripherally 10%/d.

residues in thyroglobulin, iodide brought into the thyroid by active transport is in essence a portion of the extracellular iodide, because, like iodide in the other two extensions of the extracellular iodide space, it is in rapid equilibrium with the main compartment. The concentration of iodide in the extracellular fluid is normally approximately 10 to 15 μg/L and the content of the peripheral pool is approximately 250 μg. Thus only a very small percentage of total body iodine is present in the iodide compartment, and this is turned over several times daily.

There are two main avenues for the removal of iodide from the extracellular fluid. Small quantities are lost in expired air and through the skin, but the major clearance of iodine occurs via the thyroid and the kidneys. Renal removal of iodide determines the availability of iodide to the thyroid (and vice versa). Although iodide is almost completely filterable at the glomerulus, the renal clearance rate in adults is normally approximately 30 to 40 mL/min. Thus filtered iodide is largely reabsorbed, but reabsorption is passive rather than active. In humans, unlike other animals, the renal iodide clearance rate is unaffected by the excretion of chloride or other anions and is apparently independent of the plasma iodide concentration and hence the filtered load. Iodide clearance is minimally affected by the rate of urine flow per se and is uninfluenced by physiological agents, such as TSH, or drugs that alter thyroidal iodide transport. As with other urinary components that are passively reabsorbed, the renal clearance of iodide varies with changes in glomerular filtration rate, the iodide clearance increasing or decreasing disproportionately when the glomerular filtration rate is suddenly increased or decreased, respectively. Thus the kidneys are passive participants in iodide metabolism, not really sharing in the physiological adjustments designed to maintain thyroid homeostasis under abnormal circumstances.

Normally about 500 μg of iodine is cleared into the urine daily, almost entirely in the inorganic form. This quantity is only slightly smaller than the average daily dietary intake, reflecting the scant loss of iodine through other avenues. Among these, the gastrointestinal tract is the most important, about 12 μg of iodine being lost in the stool daily, mainly in the organic form. Under abnormal circumstances substantial losses of iodine may occur. In nephrosis or other proteinuric states, T_4 and T_3 are excreted in the urine in

association with their transport proteins. Metabolites of iodotyrosines are lost in the urine in the rare familial disorder in which the enzyme iodotyrosine dehalogenase is lacking from both the thyroid and peripheral tissues. Fecal loss of organic iodine may be excessive when gastrointestinal absorption is impaired, as in chronic diarrheal states or under the influence of certain dietary constituents, such as soybean products, or of cholestyramine. Finally, notable losses of iodine may occur through lactation.

The second major site of removal of iodide from the extracellular fluid is the thyroid. Iodide removed from the plasma by the thyroid is not irreversibly lost, however, because ultimately it is secreted into the circulation either as iodinated thyronines T_4 and T_3, whose iodine is largely returned to the extracellular fluid after peripheral deiodination, or as inorganic iodide. The thyroid contains the largest pool of body iodine, under normal circumstances approximately 8000 μg, most of which is in the form of iodinated amino acids. Normally this pool of iodine turns over slowly (about 1%/d).

Synthesis and Secretion of Thyroid Hormones

The structures of the thyroid hormones, their precursors, and several related compounds are shown in Figure 8–1, and the major steps in their synthesis and secretion are shown in Figure 8–3. The metabolism of iodine leading to the biosynthesis of thyroid hormones occurs in three sequential stages: active transport of iodide into the thyroid, oxidation of iodide and iodination of tyrosyl residues within thyroglobulin to yield the hormonally inactive iodotyrosines, and coupling of iodotyrosines to form the hormonally active iodothyronines, notably T_4 and T_3. The hormones thus formed are held in peptide linkage within the specific thyroprotein, thyroglobulin, which is the major component of the intrafollicular colloid. Release of hormones involves two additional groups of reactions: hydrolysis of thyroglob-

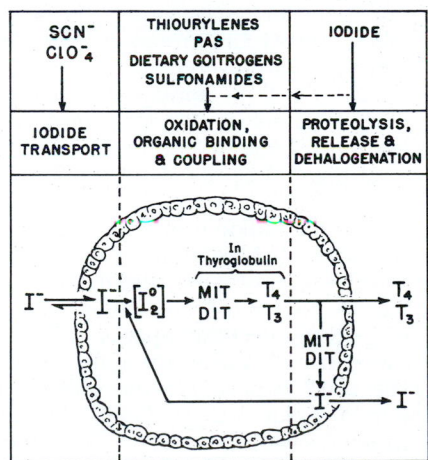

Figure 8–3. Diagram of the major steps in thyroid hormone biosynthesis. In this diagram, the follicular outline is intended merely to differentiate the intrathyroid from the interstitial compartment and should not be construed as indicating that the reactions shown necessarily occur in the follicular lumen. Note that the concentration of intrathyroid iodide maintained by the iodide transport mechanism is greater than that in the extracellular fluid. The processes of iodide oxidation, organic binding, and coupling of iodotyrosines are grouped together because they appear to be closely related oxidative reactions. The precise proportions of the iodide liberated from iodotyrosines by dehalogenation that are reused or released into the extracellular fluid are unknown. Shown above are the major inhibitors of the several steps in hormone biosynthesis. Large quantities of iodide inhibit organic binding and coupling (*dashed lines*), but this effect is usually transient. Although not shown, the lithium ion, like iodide, is an inhibitor of proteolysis and release.

ulin by a thyroid protease and by peptidases, liberating free iodinated amino acids, and passage of iodothyronines into the blood, while the iodotyrosines undergo intrathyroidal deiodination, with salvage of most of the resulting free iodide for reutilization.

Iodide Transport

Except when the plasma concentration of inorganic iodide is greatly increased, synthesis of adequate quantities of hormone requires that iodide enter the thyroid more rapidly than would be possible by simple diffusion from the extracellular fluid. The thyroid contains a transport mechanism (the iodide-concentrating, -transporting, or -trapping mechanism) that subserves this end and provides sufficient iodide substrate for subsequent steps in hormone formation. Iodide transported into the gland either is oxidized and organified or is free to diffuse back into the extracellular fluid. Under normal circumstances the rate of inward clearance of iodide exceeds the combined rates of organic binding* and back diffusion, with the result that intrathyroid concentration gradients in excess of unity are maintained within the gland. Such gradients are often referred to as thyroid/plasma or thyroid/serum ratios. Although most of the inorganic iodide within the thyroid is located within the follicular lumen, the iodide-concentrating mechanism is located within the acinar cell itself. The interior of the cell maintains a negative electrical potential with respect to both the interstitium and the follicular lumen. Presumably iodide is actively transported into the cell against this negative potential and then diffuses along the electrochemical gradient into the luminal area.

The biochemical mechanism of active iodide transport is unknown. However, like other active transport mechanisms, thyroid iodide transport is an energy-requiring process, dependent on continued generation of phosphate bond energy. In addition, active iodide transport is closely related to the function of the Na^+,K^+-ATPase system, and a mechanism for the cotransport of sodium and iodide has been proposed. Although TSH increases the activity of both the iodide transport and ATPase systems, the two do not respond in parallel in other circumstances. Hence the precise nature of their relationship remains uncertain. ATPase, acting on ATP at the cell membrane, may make phosphate bond energy available for iodide transport. Alternatively, reversible exchange of iodide for phosphate in a specific carrier may take place. The nature of the iodide carrier is unknown.

The activity of the iodide transport mechanism is influenced by a variety of physiological factors, the most important of which is the level of TSH stimulation. Iodide transport is enhanced by TSH and decreased by hypophysectomy. This relationship may reflect the capacity of TSH to increase cyclic AMP concentration within the follicular cell, because dibutyryl cyclic AMP reproduces the effects of TSH on iodide transport in isolated thyroid cells. The other major factor that influences iodide transport is an internal autoregulatory system through which the intrinsic activity of the iodide transport mechanism and its responsiveness to TSH stimulation vary inversely with the glandular content of organic iodine. This may reflect an autoregulatory effect on the cotransport of iodide and sodium.[10] As a result of these influences, thyroid/plasma ratios can be high when the thyroid is depleted of organic iodine or is stimulated by

TSH. In animals, under appropriate conditions, ratios of several hundred have been observed, and high ratios are also common in patients with thyroid hyperfunction, regardless of its cause. The capacity of the thyroid to transport iodide and to maintain iodide concentration gradients vis-à-vis the extracellular fluid is not unlimited, however. Rather there exists a maximal rate of inward iodide transport. Thus progressive increases in the concentration of iodide in the extracellular fluid are associated with progressively decreasing values of the thyroid/plasma ratio, while the concentration of iodide that has been actively transported into the gland rises progressively, ultimately reaching a maximum. Absolute values of both the thyroid/plasma ratio and the iodide transport maximum vary with the functional state of the gland.

The thyroid mechanism for concentrating iodide is shared by other monovalent anions, including perchlorate and pertechnetate. These act as competitive inhibitors of iodide transport, a property that may be related to the similarity of their partial specific molecular volumes. Thiocyanate, another monovalent anion that inhibits iodide transport, is not concentrated within the thyroid and may act by uncoupling thyroid oxidative phosphorylation. The capacity of perchlorate and thiocyanate to inhibit iodide transport is the basis of their use in the perchlorate- or thiocyanate-discharge test for defects in the thyroid organic-binding mechanism, and concentration of the radioactive anion pertechnetate makes this a valuable agent for thyroid imaging (see later section on thyroid function tests).

The capacity of the thyroid to concentrate iodide is shared by other tissues of endodermal origin, notably the salivary and gastric glands. The effect of metabolic inhibitors and inhibitory anions on iodide transport in these other tissues is similar to that on iodide transport in the thyroid. A rare disorder arises from the absence of an effective thyroid iodide transport mechanism. In patients with this disorder the salivary and gastric iodide concentration mechanisms are also lacking. Whether the result of disease or of the action of pharmacological agents, inadequate iodide transport results in goiter and hypothyroidism. Both can be overcome, however, by administering additional iodine.[11] Iodine administration increases the iodide concentration in plasma and permits sufficient iodine for hormone synthesis to enter the gland by simple diffusion.

In addition to iodide brought into the thyroid by active transport from the extracellular fluid, iodide is generated in the thyroid by the deiodination of iodotyrosines liberated during the hydrolysis of thyroglobulin. A portion of this iodide is reorganified, and the remainder is lost from the gland as the so-called iodide leak.

Oxidation of Iodide and Organic Iodinations

After its transport into or regeneration within the thyroid, iodide enters into a series of reactions that ultimately lead to the synthesis of the active thyroid hormones. The first of these reactions involves oxidation of iodide and incorporation of the resulting intermediate into the hormonally inactive iodotyrosines, MIT and DIT. Iodide thus metabolized is removed from the iodide pool and can no longer be discharged by thiocyanate, perchlorate, or other inhibitors of iodide transport. Oxidation of iodide is normally rapid. After administration of radioiodine (I*),† the

---

*For brevity, "organic binding," "organic iodine," "organified," and similar terms are often used. These expressions signify that iodide is bound to organic compounds, chiefly as iodotyrosine.

†The abbreviation I* is employed to denote any of the radioactive isotopes of iodine, which cannot be distinguished from one another physiologically or biochemically. When a specific isotope of iodine is referred to, it will be appropriately designated.

isotope is almost immediately found in organic combination, mainly in soluble thyroprotein, principally thyroglobulin, and to a limited extent in subcellular particulate proteins, lipids, and nucleic acids. These iodinated products are probably the result of random rather than specifically directed iodinations.

The iodinations that lead to formation of iodotyrosines occur within a preformed thyroprotein molecule rather than in free amino acids that are then incorporated into protein. Oxidation of thyroidal iodide is mediated by thyroid peroxidase. The cDNAs for both human and porcine thyroid peroxidase have been cloned, and the amino acid sequences of both have been deduced. Human thyroid peroxidase contains 933 amino acids and has a molecular size of 103 kd. It contains a putative membrane-spanning region near the COOH terminus and bears a striking homology to the porcine protein.[12, 13] Recognition that it is the major thyroid microsomal antigen allowed the cloning of this protein. Monoclonal antibody staining indicates that thyroid peroxidase is localized predominately at the apical border of the thyroid cell. Human follicular carcinomas show variable staining; papillary carcinomas exhibit weak or absent staining, consistent with the generally poor organification process in these tumors.[13] Peroxidase is a heme protein, which accounts for the requirement of organic iodinations for molecular oxygen and the inhibition of iodination by cyanide and azide. In vitro, thyroid peroxidase, when afforded a source of hydrogen peroxide, readily iodinates thyroglobulin as well as other proteins. The reaction catalyzed by peroxidase in vitro has many properties of the iodination reaction in vivo, including inhibition by antithyroid agents and by high concentrations of iodide (Wolff-Chaikoff effect). The evanescent product of the peroxidation of iodide, i.e., the active iodinating form, is uncertain but may be free hypoiodous acid.[14] The hydrogen peroxide that serves as the oxidant of iodide is generated through the auto-oxidation of flavin enzymes acting as NADH and particularly NADPH oxidases. In this way, generation of hydrogen peroxide is linked to electron transfers consequent to substrate oxidations within the thyroid.

Radioautographic and histochemical evidence, as well as the demonstration that thyroid cell ghosts that are virtually devoid of intracellular contents are capable of carrying out organic iodination, suggests that the reactions occur at the cell-colloid interface.[15] As judged from studies in vitro, soluble inhibitors of organic iodinations, principally ascorbic acid and reduced glutathione, exist in thyroid tissue. These may inhibit iodinations either by reducing the oxidized form of iodine or by reducing hydrogen peroxide itself. Thus mitochondrial systems provide a source of hydrogen peroxide and cell membranes possess the iodide peroxidase, while the cytoplasmic fraction may contain regulatory inhibitors of organic iodinations.

Organic iodinations are conditioned by the extent of thyroid stimulation by TSH. They are retarded in the hypophysectomized rat and are promptly increased by administration of TSH. Iodinations are susceptible to inhibition by a number of pharmacological agents, including the usual antithyroid drugs, most of which are inhibitors of peroxidase and also have intrinsic reducing activity. Iodinations are also inhibited by freezing, cooling, or storage of the thyroid tissue. Defects in the organic-binding mechanism in humans lead to the development of goitrous hypothyroidism or, if less severe, to goiter without hypothyroidism. In some instances the thyroid is lacking in peroxidase.[7] In others, peroxidase is present and the defect may reside in inadequate production of hydrogen peroxide or abnormalities in thyroglobulin that render it less readily iodinated.

Formation of Iodothyronines

Formation of MIT and DIT, via oxidation and organic binding of iodide, is followed by synthesis of the hormonally active iodothyronines, T_4 and T_3. Because noniodinated thyronine cannot be demonstrated in thyroglobulin, T_4 and T_3 must arise from iodinated precursors. Synthesis of T_4 from DIT requires the fusion of two DIT molecules to yield a structure with two diiodinated rings linked by an ether bridge. Concomitantly there occurs a net loss of the alanine side chain from the ring that ultimately contains the phenolic hydroxyl group (beta or outer ring). This reaction is termed the coupling reaction. In aqueous media, this or analogous reactions take place when DIT or derivatives of DIT are allowed to stand under oxidative conditions. Nevertheless, the manner in which T_4 is synthesized in vivo remains uncertain. Two general hypotheses have received major consideration.

The first hypothesis is that T_4 and T_3 are formed by the interaction of a peptide-bound DIT with an oxidation product of DIT or MIT, respectively. In the case of DIT, the suggested product is 3,5-diiodo-4-hydroxyphenylpyruvic acid (DIHPPA). In vitro, DIHPPA is a product of oxidative systems that yield T_4 from DIT. Moreover, when DIHPPA is added to solutions of DIT, T_4 is formed, with pyruvic acid and ammonia as by-products. Additional studies in vitro have revealed formation of labeled T_4 when thyroglobulin is incubated with labeled DIHPPA. Because small quantities of DIHPPA and its monoiodinated analogue, MIHPPA, the suggested precursor of T_3, are present in thyroid tissue, this mechanism of synthesis of iodothyronines in vivo is attractive. It does not require the extensive structural alterations in the thyroglobulin molecule during iodothyronine synthesis required by the alternative hypothesis.

The most commonly held view concerning the synthesis of T_4 and T_3 differs from that just described in that it requires the coupling of two iodotyrosines, both of which are initially held in a peptide bond within the thyroglobulin molecule. A free radical mechanism whereby two molecules of DIT yield T_4 via a quinol ether intermediate has been proposed, but, whatever the intermediates in the reaction may be, coupling of two peptide-bound iodotyrosines requires disruption of the peptide bonds holding the iodotyrosyl group that yields the beta ring of the thyronine nucleus. This requires substantial changes in the structure of thyroglobulin as iodothyronines are formed. Such rearrangements are possible, however, because T_4 can be formed in vitro during iodination of thyroglobulin or even of proteins that are not normally iodinated, such as casein, insulin, or albumin. Moreover, both in vivo and in vitro, the enhanced synthesis of iodothyronines that accompanies increasing iodination of thyroglobulin is associated with an increase in the sedimentation constant of the protein and its stability under conditions that induce dissociation. These changes are consistent with the occurrence of a major change in the structure of the protein consequent to the synthesis of T_4 and T_3.

THYROGLOBULIN. The amino acid sequence of thyroglobulin has also been deduced from its cDNA. In addition, the chromosomal gene has been cloned and is very large (greater than 260 kb).[16] The 3' portion of approximately 220 kb contains a number of intervening sequences, up to 60 kb in size, and is highly conserved. The human thyroglobulin gene is localized on chromosome 8 close to the oncogene c-myc. The thyroglobulin messenger RNA (mRNA) is 8 to 8.5 kb in length, and the analysis of its sequence has permitted a number of insights into the formation of T_4 and T_3. There are 140 tyrosine residues in the dimer of molecular size 660 kd. Only about one fourth of these tyrosines can be iodinated, and four specific portions of the molecule are involved in formation of thyroid hormones. The primary T_4 acceptor tyrosine is at residue 5, and in rabbit thyroglobulin this tyrosine may be the source of 40% of the T_4 in the molecule.[17] Two other acceptor tyrosine residues are near the COOH terminus. Interestingly, the third residue from the COOH terminus is the major T_3-forming site and accounts for over 50% of this hormone. There are approximately three to four T_4 molecules per mole of human thyroglobulin under conditions of normal iodination, but only about one in five molecules of human thyroglobulin contains a T_3 residue.[18] In thyroglobulin from patients with untreated Graves disease, however, the content of T_4 residues remains approximately the same but the number of T_3 residues doubles to an average of 0.4 per molecule. This effect is independent of the iodination state of the thyroglobulin.

Synthesis of iodothyronines requires oxidative conditions. It is thought that the coupling reaction is mediated by a peroxidase, perhaps the same peroxidase that mediates the initial oxidation of iodide, because there are interesting similarities between the two reactions. Virtually all agents that inhibit organic binding also inhibit coupling. In addition, cell-free particulate fractions can yield T_4 from free DIT when provided with a source of hydrogen peroxide. Moreover, synthesis of labeled iodothyronines from prelabeled iodotyrosines is demonstrable when prelabeled thyroglobulin is incubated with thyroid peroxidase and a source of hydrogen peroxide in the absence of free iodide. Despite this evidence that peroxidase may mediate both the organic-binding and the coupling mechanisms, there are certain physiological differences between the two. The coupling reaction is more sensitive to a variety of factors. Inhibition of coupling with continued generation of MIT and DIT occurs in response to small doses of antithyroid agents or during the acute response to large amounts of iodide.

Because the coupling reaction requires two molecules of iodotyrosine, the bimolecular combination would be expected to be reduced to 25% of its normal rate in situations in which iodination is reduced by one half, as appears to be the case. Iodine deficiency and a reduction in TSH also impair the synthesis of iodothyronines more than that of iodotyrosines, presumably for similar reasons. In certain forms of human goitrous hypothyroidism, iodotyrosines do not form T_4 even though such residues are present. Structural abnormalities of the gene could explain such impaired hormonogenesis without postulating the need for accessory proteins separate from peroxidase for carrying out this reaction. Here, inadequate secretion of iodothyronines occurs, and although the thyroid contains ample iodotyrosines, only minimal amounts of T_4 and T_3 are found. It is thus uncertain whether the organic-binding and coupling reactions are separate or whether they are mediated by a similar mechanism.

Storage and Release of Hormones

The thyroid is unique among the endocrine glands by virtue of the large store of hormone it contains and the low overall rate at which the hormone normally turns over. This aspect of thyroid hormone economy has homeostatic value in that the large hormone reservoir provides prolonged protection against depletion of circulating hormone should synthesis cease. In normal humans the administration of blocking doses of antithyroid agents for as long as 2 wk results in little lowering of the serum T_4 concentration, and plasma concentrations of TSH are not increased. Thus an important aspect of hormone economy is the storage func-

tion of the thyroid. As noted earlier, the normal thyroid contains about 8000 µg of iodine, of which as much as 10% may be inorganic. Analyses of human thyroids performed when iodine intake was generally lower indicated that the organic iodine is constituted as follows: MIT, 17 to 28%; DIT, 24 to 42%; T_4, 35%; T_3, 5 to 8%. More recent analyses show that the T_4/T_3 ratio is approximately 13:1.[18]

Although it had been thought that thyroglobulin is excluded completely from the peripheral blood, immunochemical analyses suggest that the protein is present in the plasma of normal individuals. The lymphatics are the avenue through which thyroglobulin normally enters the blood. It is very unlikely, however, that peripheral hydrolysis of thyroglobulin contributes significantly to the T_4 and T_3 in the circulation. Rather, T_4 and T_3 enter the blood directly after their liberation from thyroglobulin by proteolytic cleavage within the follicular cell.

The mechanisms of this cleavage have been investigated by submicroscopic, histochemical, and biochemical techniques. The sequence is best observed after stimulation of the resting thyroid by TSH. Within a few minutes after such stimulation, formation of pseudopodia is evident at the apical surface of the follicular cell, followed by endocytosis of colloid to yield multiple vesicles (colloid droplets). That these vesicles contain colloid is evident in that they are periodic acid–Schiff (PAS)–positive and contain ^{14}C-labeled amino acids or radioiodine previously allowed to accumulate in the luminal contents. The process of endocytosis apparently involves destabilization of the apical membrane, because membrane stabilizers, such as chlorpromazine, inhibit this process. Endocytosis is not confined to thyroglobulin; isolated thyroid cells are capable of accumulating latex particles, and the accumulation is stimulated by factors that enhance the endocytosis of colloid. Concomitantly with endocytosis, dense bodies, rich in esterases and acid phosphatase and apparently identical with lysosomes, migrate from the basal toward the apical end of the cell. Fusion of lysosomes with colloid droplets occurs. The resulting "phagolysosomes" have histochemical characteristics of both particles and are likely the site of the physiologically active protease. The latter is an acid hydrolase similar in properties to cathepsin D. Hydrolysis of thyroglobulin is thought to occur in the phagolysosomes, which gradually regain the ultrastructural properties and basal location of lysosomes as hydrolysis is completed. Microtubular and microfilamentous structures are apparently involved because inhibitors of both the former (vincristine, vinblastine, colchicine) and the latter (cytochalasin B) block the secretory process.

Studies in vitro with subcellular fractions of thyroid tissue containing phagolysosomes have shed light on the biochemical processes by which thyroglobulin is hydrolyzed. Hydrolysis of thyroglobulin is facilitated by reduction of disulfide bonds effected by a transhydrogenase that utilizes reduced glutathione. The availability of reduced glutathione in turn, depends on the activity of a second enzyme, glutathione reductase, that uses NADPH to reduce oxidized glutathione. If true, the proposed mechanism would link the secretory process to intermediary metabolism and biological oxidations within the gland.

The thyroid is capable of deiodinating both T_4 and T_3 and generating the latter from the former. However, the contribution of thyroidal T_4 deiodination to T_3 secretion under normal conditions is not known. The ratio of T_4 to T_3 in human thyroglobulin is about 13:1, and the T_4/T_3 ratio of the secreted hormones is about 10:1. One can attribute this modest difference to T_4 deiodination. In the rat TSH increases the type 1 deiodinase activity of the thyroid, and in Graves disease thyroidal type 1 deiodinase activity is higher than normal. Therefore, this process may play a role in the enhanced thyroidal T_3 contribution in patients with Graves disease.[19-21]

Iodotyrosines liberated from thyroglobulin are subject to the action of a microsomal iodotyrosine dehalogenase, an NADPH-dependent enzyme found in the peripheral tissues as well as in the thyroid. This enzyme liberates iodide from MIT and DIT and normally prevents their entry into the blood in appreciable quantities. It is inactive against peptide-bound iodotyronines or free iodothyronines, and hence the mechanism differs from that for T_4 deiodination already described. Activity of the thyroid iodotyrosine deiodinase system is enhanced by TSH administration, possibly because of increased NADPH generation, rather than an increase in enzyme concentration. Iodide liberated from MIT and DIT is partly used for hormone synthesis and partly lost from the gland as iodide leak.

The thyroid does not function as a single homogeneous unit. Radioautographic studies reveal variations among different areas of the gland and in different follicles. In addition, the thyroid contains at least two pools of organic iodine, which turn over at different rates. One pool, representing more newly iodinated materials, is smaller but turns over more rapidly than the other, larger pool of older hormone (last come–first served). This difference may result from the contiguity of the sites for iodination and colloid resorption. In truth, there may be many iodine pools in the thyroid turning over at different rates, just as there are many subtle differences in the thyroglobulin molecules within a single thyroid.

The storage function of the thyroid is not perfectly maintained, even under normal conditions. As already noted some thyroglobulin can be detected by radioimmunoassay in the blood of most normal individuals, and the frequency of detection is increased by pregnancy. Increased concentrations are present in the serum of patients with nontoxic goiter, in whom there is a correlation between the serum thyroglobulin level and goiter size, and in patients with hyperthyroidism, in whom there is a correlation with the degree of hyperfunction. Serum thyroglobulin concentrations are often increased in patients with differentiated thyroid tumors but do not distinguish benign from malignant forms. Serum thyroglobulin concentrations decrease when the tumor is removed, and, in patients with thyroid cancer, later elevation is a useful indicator of metastatic recurrence. Large quantities of thyroglobulin are released into the blood during surgical manipulation of the thyroid, in radiation thyroiditis, and in patients with subacute thyroiditis as well.[22] In both forms of thyroiditis, serum T_4 and T_3 concentrations may be increased sufficiently to produce thyrotoxicosis.

Uncertainty exists concerning the extent to which iodotyrosines are normally released into the blood. Some contribution may be made by the peripheral tissues, which are capable of cleaving the ether link of T_4 and T_3.[23,24] Large quantities of iodotyrosines are lost from the thyroid in the inherited form of goitrous hypothyroidism that results from a lack of iodotyrosine dehalogenase in both the thyroid and peripheral tissues. Here, iodotyrosines both leak from the gland and escape deiodination in the periphery. As a consequence, they are excreted into the urine, either intact or as their keto-acid metabolites. The resulting losses of iodine produce a state of iodine deficiency that is in large part responsible for the development of the goiter and can be overcome by dietary iodine supplementation.[3] A similar syndrome can be produced in animals by administration of an inhibitor of iodotyrosine dehalogenase, mononitrotyrosine or dinitrotyrosine. The extent to which mild forms of the disorder are responsible for sporadic nontoxic goiter in humans is unknown.

The processes of proteolysis and release are inhibited by several agents. Most important among these is iodine. Inhibition of hormone release is responsible for the rapid improvement in thyrotoxicosis that iodine induces in hyperthyroid patients. The complete mechanism by which this effect is mediated is uncertain, but iodine inhibits the stimulation of thyroid adenylate cyclase produced by TSH and by the stimulatory immunoglobulins of Graves disease. Increasing iodination of thyroglobulin also increases its resistance to hydrolysis by the thyroid acid protease. Lithium also inhibits thyroid hormone release although its mechanism of action is poorly understood and may differ from that of iodine. It inhibits both the increase in adenylate cyclase activity produced by TSH and the stimulation of I* release from prelabeled thyroid produced by dibutyryl cyclic AMP.

Transport, Turnover, and Metabolism of Thyroid Hormones

The transport and metabolism of the thyroid hormones occupy an important place in clinical and experimental thyroidology. At any level of thyroid function the concentrations of thyroid hormones in the blood are determined in large measure by their association with thyroid hormone–binding proteins. Consequently, in measuring such concentrations as an aid to diagnosis, one must be cognizant of the hormone-protein binding interaction. The metabolic transformations of thyroid hormones that take place in peripheral tissues influence their biological potency and perhaps the nature of their biological effect. Consequently, an understanding of thyroid physiopathology demands knowledge of thyroid hormone metabolism.

Hormones and Their Binding Proteins in Blood

A wide variety of iodothyronines and their metabolic derivatives exist in plasma. Of these, T_4 is highest in concentration and is the only one that arises solely by direct secretion from the thyroid gland. In normal humans T_3 is secreted to a slight extent from the thyroid, but most of the T_3 in the plasma is derived from the peripheral tissues, where it is generated by the enzymatic removal of a single iodine atom (monodeiodination) from T_4. The remaining iodothyronines and their derivatives are almost entirely generated in the peripheral tissues from T_4 and T_3. Principal among them are rT_3 and 3,3'-diiodo-L-thyronine ($3,3'$-T_2). Trace concentrations of other diiodothyronines, monoidothyronines, and conjugates thereof with glucuronic or sulfuric acid are also present. Deaminated derivatives of T_4 and T_3 which bear an acetic acid rather than an alanine side chain, are also present in very low concentrations. (See Figs. 8–1 and 8–4 for structural formulas.)

Although these derivatives, including T_3, can enter the plasma from the peripheral tissues, it is uncertain to what extent they are degraded in situ and whether they exert a metabolic action locally prior to their exit into the blood or their local degradation. T_4, T_3, and rT_3 are the components of greatest import.

EXTRACELLULAR BINDING PROTEINS. Upon entering the blood, the major secretory products of the normal thyroid gland, T_4 and T_3, as well as the products of peripheral T_4 and T_3 metabolism, are bound in a firm but reversible bond to several proteins, all of which are synthesized in the liver.[25] Much of what is known about the specific binding of the thyroid hormones, including its initial demonstration, has been derived from study of serum enriched with labeled hormone by the technique of zonal electrophoresis on filter

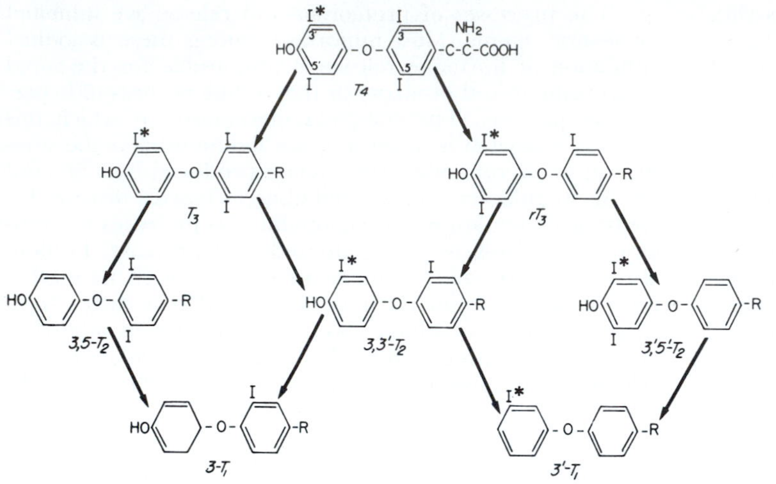

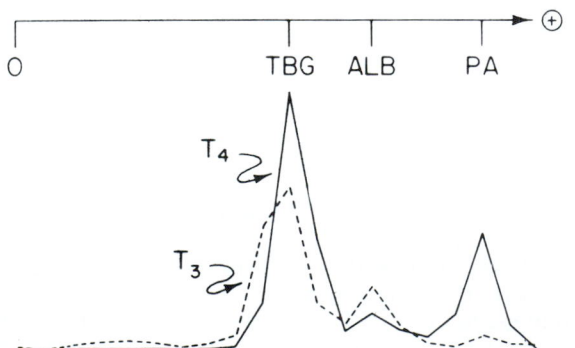

Figure 8–4. Pathways of the sequential monodeiodination of T_4 and its derivatives. Asterisk indicates which compounds would contain radioactive iodine if the original T_4 were labeled in its outer ring. Arrows pointing to left indicate 5'-monodeiodination, and arrows pointing to right, 5-monodeiodination. Not shown is deiodination of 3'-T_1 and 3-T_1 to thyronine. (From Sakurada T, Rudolph M, Fang SL, et al. Evidence that triiodothyronine and reverse triiodothyronine are sequentially deiodinated in man. J Clin Endocrinol Metab 1978; 46:916–922. © 1978, The Endocrine Society.)

paper, starch, agar, or polyacrylamide gels. The electrophoretic technique results in some distortions of the hormone-protein interactions, but these are quantitative rather than qualitative. Electrophoretic studies have disclosed two plasma proteins with which T_4 is mainly associated, a T_4-binding inter-α globulin (TBG) and T_4-binding prealbumin (TBPA, also termed transthyretin). To a limited extent, T_4 is also bound to albumin; T_3 is bound mainly by TBG and, to a small extent, by albumin (Fig. 8–5). For practical purposes, T_3 is not bound by TBPA. In view of the fact that TBG binds both T_4 and T_3, a more appropriate designation than the commonly employed T_4-binding globulin would be *thyronine-binding globulin*, a term that would not necessitate altering the universally accepted abbreviation TBG.

TBG is a glycoprotein with a molecular mass of about 54 kd, about 20% of which is carbohydrate. The cDNA for the gene has been cloned.[26] The cDNA encodes a 450-amino-acid protein with a 20-amino-acid signal peptide. The molecular mass is 44 kd and four glycosylation sites are present. As recognized from inheritance patterns, the gene coding for the protein is on the X chromosome. The nucleotide sequence of TBG resembles that coding for the serine antiproteases alpha-1 antichymotrypsin and alpha-1 antitrypsin. Because there is one iodothyronine binding site per TBG molecule, the binding capacity of TBG in normal human serum is equivalent to its concentration. Its concentration in human plasma is approximately 260 nmol/L (15 μg/mL). Its half-time in plasma is about 5 d; and its metabolic clearance rate is approximately 800 mL/d.

The glycosylation of TBG has a major influence on its clearance from the plasma and on its behavior during isoelectric focusing.[27, 28] Four to six bands are present after isoelectric focusing but after exposure to neuraminidase these differences are lost, indicating that they are due to differences in the number of sialic acid residues. In estrogen-treated patients there is an increase in the prevalence of the more anodally migrating (acidic) bands of TBG.[27] The more highly sialylated TBG is cleared more slowly from plasma than is the more positively charged TBG, which suggests that the reason for the long-recognized increase in serum TBG concentration with estrogen exposure is an alteration in the degree of TBG sialylation. Increased sialylation is a well-recognized mechanism for prevention of hepatic uptake of glycoproteins. Further studies have shown that sera from pregnant patients, women receiving oral contraceptives, and patients with acute hepatitis have increased fractions of acidic TBG. Patients with inherited TBG excess do not have this change, nor do nonpregnant women or men. Thus it appears that estrogen, by causing an increase in the degree of sialylation of the TBG molecule, impairs its hepatic clearance.[27, 28] Consistent with this hypothesis, estrogen has no effect on TBG synthesis in HEP G2 human hepatoma cells.

Other abnormalities of TBG may alter its susceptibility to heat denaturation and its capacity to bind thyroid hormone. One such variant has been well described in the Australian aborigines. Another, a TBG with increased heat lability, is found in American blacks.[29] All of these abnormalities are inherited in an X-linked fashion. L-Asparaginase blocks the synthesis of TBG in HEP G2 cells, which explains the etiology of the low TBG concentrations in patients receiving this agent.[30, 31] Studies of six families with inherited TBG deficiency have not revealed gross structural defects in the 4.2-kb TBG gene.[32] The overall frequency of TBG deficiency based on newborn screening tests is about 1 in 5000. Additional studies will be needed to demonstrate the putative point mutations in the gene that are probably responsible for the formation of proteins with abnormal binding or abnormal stability.

TBPA exists in part as a complex with retinol (vitamin A)–binding protein. It consists of four identical polypeptide chains whose total molecular mass is approximately 55 kd. Its complete amino acid sequence and three-dimensional structure, as well as the relation of the latter to hormone binding, have been determined.[33] Its concentration in plasma is approximately 4 mmol/L (250 μg/mL). Each mole of TBPA can bind 1 mol of T_4 with high affinity, although a second T_4 molecule is bound as well at much higher concentrations of T_4. Binding of T_4 by prealbumin is independent of the association with retinol-binding protein. TBPA is devoid of

Figure 8–5. Diagram depicting the electrophoretic migration of radioiodine-labeled T_4 and T_3 in normal human serum. T_4 is bound predominantly by TBG, to a lesser extent by TBPA, and to a slight extent by albumin. T_3 is bound by TBG and by albumin, but little, if at all, by TBPA. TBG, thyronine-binding globulin; ALB, albumin; PA, prealbumin, also known as T_4-binding prealbumin (TBPA).

carbohydrate but rich in tryptophan. Its half-time in plasma is about 2 d. Its concentration falls rapidly during illness. A curious aspect of TBPA has been the high level of its expression in the choroid plexus. The rat choroid plexus contains about 25 times more TBPA mRNA than does an equivalent quantity of liver.[34] It has been speculated that choroid plexus could be an important site for T_4 concentration in the brain.[35] T_3 enters the brain poorly, and given the higher affinity of TBPA for T_4 than for T_3, this is an intriguing possibility. Another curious aspect of TBPA is the association of variant forms of TBPA protein with familial amyloidotic polyneuropathy.[36] In these families the TBPA monomer has any of several different point mutations and TBPA accumulates in the amyloid tissue deposits. Neither thyroid dysfunction nor altered vitamin A metabolism has been reported, although there is a reduced affinity for thyroxine in some of the mutant proteins. Two types of patients have been reported with abnormalities in total thyroxine levels associated with abnormalities in TBPA. One type, found to date in only a few families, has a TBPA of high affinity. The other, also found in a few families, has increased TBPA concentrations.[37]

Although both TBG and TBPA are capable of binding T_4, avidly, their binding sites exhibit different properties. The TBG molecule appears to have one thyronine binding site. Its affinity for T_3 is less than that for T_4, the equilibrium constant for the latter reaction being about 10^{10} L/mol. TBG is the main binding protein for rT_3, but its affinity for rT_3 is lower than that for T_3. TBG binds the dextro isomer of T_4 as well as the naturally occurring levo isomer form. Deamination of the iodothyronine molecule greatly reduces the binding to TBG; the acetic and propionic acid analogues of T_4 and T_3 are bound by TBG little if at all. Binding by TBG is inhibited by a variety of medicinal and other organic compounds, including phenytoin, salicylate, barbital, furosemide, anilinonaphthalenesulfonic acid, and mitotane. The affinity of these compounds for TBG binding is weaker than that of T_4 or T_3, but their concentration is plasma is sufficient to have these effects.

Like TBG, the TBPA molecule has one major binding site, the equilibrium constant for the interaction with T_4 being about 10^8 L/mol. A second binding site of much lower affinity is apparently present. D-Thyroxine is not bound appreciably by TBPA, and deamination of the alanine side chain yields products that interact much more strongly than do the parent compounds. Thus tetraiodothyroacetic acid (tetrac) and tetraiodothyropropionic acid are bound to TBPA more strongly than is T_4. Moreover, the triiodinated analogues, unlike T_3 itself, are bound by TBPA quite strongly. A variety of organic compounds are potent inhibitors of the T_4-TBPA interaction; these include barbital, salicylate and some of its congeners, 2,4-dinitrophenol, and penicillin.

Small quantities of T_4 and T_3 are bound to human plasma lipoproteins. Such binding accounts for between 3 and 6% of the circulating T_4 and T_3. The T_4-binding protein is 27 kd in size on gel electrophoresis and in serum is present as a dimer.[38] The affinity of T_4 for this protein is lower than that for TBG ($K_a \sim 7.5 \times 10^7$). The protein is as yet of unknown physiological significance but could have a specific role in targeting T_4 delivery to specific tissues.

TBG is normally responsible for the transport of most of the T_4 (about 77%) and, with the serum T_4 concentration, is the major determinant of the free T_4. TBPA plays a lesser role, except when TBG is lacking, and even then rather marked variations in TBPA influence the concentration and turnover of T_4 only slightly. Much effort has been directed toward the elucidation of the function of the T_4-binding

proteins. Certain conclusions seem indisputable. As a result of their interaction with the transport proteins, the iodinated amino acids acquire macromolecular properties that alter their metabolism. The negligible urinary excretion of T_3 and T_4 is almost certainly due to the limited filterability of the hormone-binding protein complexes at the glomerulus. The volume of distribution and rate of turnover of the hormones are also affected by their protein associations, so that they resemble more closely those of the plasma proteins rather than those of unbound amino acids. In vitro, the interaction between the thyroid hormones and their binding proteins conforms to a reversible binding equilibrium that can be expressed by conventional equilibrium equations. For the formulations that follow, T_4 is used as the prototype, with the understanding that similar interactions apply in the case of T_3. TBG is used as the prototypic binding protein, in view of the predominant role that it normally plays in hormone transport. The interaction between T_4 and TBG can be expressed as follows:

$$T_4 + TBG \overset{k}{\rightleftharpoons} T_4 \cdot TBG$$

Here TBG represents the unoccupied binding sites of the protein; k, the equilibrium constant for the interaction; and $T_4 \cdot TBG$, the binding sites on TBG occupied by T_4. This interaction can also be expressed by the mass action relationship, wherein

$$\frac{T_4 \cdot TBG}{(T_4)(TBG)} = k$$

Rearranging

$$\frac{T_4}{T_4 \cdot TBG} = \frac{1}{(TBG)k}$$

and

$$T_4 = \frac{T_4 \cdot TBG}{(TBG)k}$$

These expressions predict that T_4 exists in the plasma in both the bound and free forms, and this has been shown to be the case by direct analysis. It is now possible to measure the free T_4 concentration in serum by indirect radioimmunoassay[39] but it is most commonly measured by the dialysis technique. With the aid of I*-labeled T_4, the proportion that is unbound by protein is determined and the concentration of free T_4 can then be calculated as the product of the total hormone concentration and the fraction that is free. In normal serum, the free T_4 is approximately 0.02% of the total (about 20 pmol/L).

It is also evident from the preceding formulas that the proportion of free hormone is inversely related to the concentration of unoccupied binding sites and their binding affinity for the hormone in question. The product of the two latter functions can be considered as an indication of the net binding affinity (of TBG) for T_4, and it is to the net binding affinity for T_4 that the proportion of free T_4 is inversely related. In whole serum the overall net binding affinity is the sum of the individual binding affinities of the various proteins that bind T_4, but in normal serum this is conditioned mainly by TBG. For example, the approximately 10-fold lower affinity of TBG for T_3 results in a proportion of free T_3 (0.30%) that is about 15 times that of T_4. Further, the absolute concentration of free T_4 is a direct function of the ratio of the concentrations of occupied and unoccupied binding sites on TBG.

Studies in vitro in which T_4 has been allowed to interact with both plasma and tissues have led to an expansion of the formulation as follows:

$$T_4 \begin{array}{c} + \text{TBG} \overset{k_1}{\rightleftharpoons} T_4 \cdot \text{TBG} \\[2ex] + \text{CBP} \underset{k_2}{\rightleftharpoons} T_4 \cdot \text{CBP} \overset{k_3}{\rightarrow} \end{array}$$

Here CBP represents the unoccupied binding sites on cellular binding proteins; k_2, their affinity for T_4; $T_4 \cdot$ CBP, occupied binding sites on CBP; and k_3, the rate at which T_4 in the cell is irreversibly metabolized to other products, such as T_3, rT_3, tetrac, or conjugates.

This formulation indicates that it is the free hormone that is available to the tissues and that can induce metabolic effects and undergo degradation. The bound form of the hormone acts merely as a metabolically inert reservoir. It follows that the concentration of the free hormone acts as an important determinant of the metabolic state and is defended by homeostatic mechanisms. In the presence of an increase in the overall net binding affinity for T_4, a normal free T_4 concentration can be maintained only if the bound T_4 concentration increases. This is true whether the causative factor is an increase in the concentration of TBG or the appearance of abnormal T_4-binding proteins.

It is useful to examine the effects of hormone binding not only on the static concentrations of free and bound hormone in the blood but also on the dynamic aspects of hormone metabolism. Two factors influence the plasma concentration of T_4: its rate of entry into the plasma, usually by secretion from the thyroid, and the efficiency of the processes that lead to its removal from plasma. A convenient means of expressing the latter is as a metabolic clearance rate, which relates the quantity of T_4 removed from the plasma per unit time to the quantity available for removal, i.e., its plasma concentration. Thus

$$\text{MCR} = D/[P]$$

where MCR is the metabolic clearance rate (volume/time), D is the absolute disposal or removal rate (amount/time), and [P] is the plasma concentration (amount/volume). Transposing,

$$[P] = D/\text{MCR}$$

However, under steady-state conditions, the production rate of T_4, PR, and the disposal rate, D, are equal. Hence,

$$[P] = \text{PR/MCR}$$

This relationship simply indicates that for any level of T_4 production, be it increased, normal, or decreased, the total plasma T_4 concentration varies inversely with its MCR. However, if only the free T_4 is readily able to leave the plasma and enter the cells, while the bound T_4 is largely confined to the intravascular space, then changing the fraction of total T_4 that is free, by changing the fraction that is available to the tissues, changes the MCR in a parallel manner. This would explain why a primary increase in hormone binding without any change in thyroid function will increase the plasma total T_4 concentration and why a decrease in hormone binding will have the converse effect. (See Fig. 8–6.)

This formulation, which has come to be known as the *free thyroxine hypothesis*, is better termed the *free thyroid hormone hypothesis*, in view of the fact that it is equally applicable to other thyromimetic compounds, including T_3.[40] If it is free hormone that diffuses into the tissue, a potential rate-limiting step could be the rate at which hormone dissociates

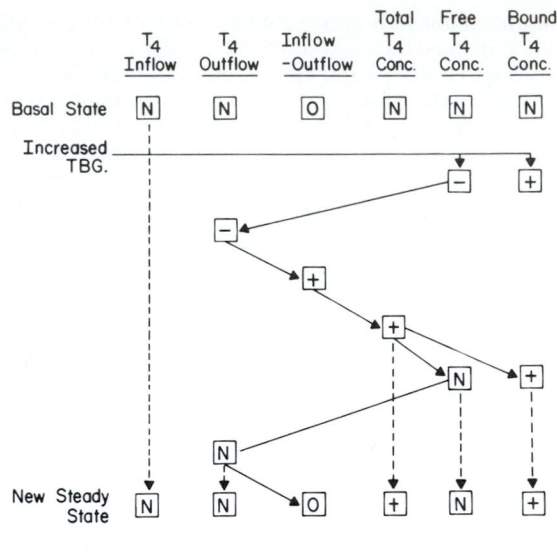

Figure 8–6. The sequence of events after an increase in TBG: its effects on the turnover of T_4 and on the serum concentration of total and free T_4. Converse consequences would follow a decrease in TBG.

from its binding proteins. If dissociation of hormone from binding proteins is slow relative to the rate of tissue uptake, this event would determine the rate of hormone entry into the cells,[41] and studies to test the hypothesis have been performed.[42-44] These studies showed that if a protein-free solution containing tracer T_4 is perfused through rat liver via the portal vein, there is a steep concentration gradient with a decreasing quantity of T_4 in cells as the distance from the center of the portal lobule increases. Virtually all of the T_4 is taken up by periportal cells. In contrast, if 4% serum albumin is added to the perfusate, the distribution of tracer is uniform throughout the lobule with only 46% of the tracer removed from the bolus. The uptake of free hormone is extremely rapid, as would be expected from its hydrophobic nature, suggesting that plasma hormone-binding proteins may function to ensure uniform distribution of hydrophobic ligands such as T_4 throughout the circulatory system and within various organs. In contrast, in similar studies T_3 dissociates rapidly from protein;[44] the pool of free T_3 is rapidly replenished in plasma, and free hormone can account for all the T_3 taken up by the liver. It may be concluded then that intracellular T_3 is in equilibrium with free T_3 pool in plasma, consistent with the free hormone hypothesis. This is true whether or not an active transport mechanism exists at the cell border because this system is not saturable at ambient free hormone concentrations. In summary the rate of T_3 and T_4 metabolism, not the dissociation rate from protein, determines the net removal of T_3 from plasma.

TRANSPORT OF THYROID HORMONES INTO CELLS. The cellular uptake of T_4 and T_3 is difficult to study because of the high but nonspecific affinity of thyroid hormones for plasma membrane. Nonetheless, there is carrier mediated transport of thyroid hormone into hepatocytes, human fibroblasts, rat skeletal muscle cells, and neuroblastoma cells.[45-53] The carrier transport system of T_3 and T_4 is saturable, is stereospecific, and requires cellular ATP, but the mechanisms for T_3 and T_4 uptake may be different in that the two iodothyronines do not compete for uptake. Extracellular sodium is required, and sodium ionophore increases the uptake of thyroid hormone by rat skeletal muscle.[50] Agents that interfere with the uptake process include iopanoic acid, monodansylcadaverine, phenytoin, phloretin, antimycin, and oligomycin.

In patients on a low-calorie diet for 1 wk, T_3 and T_4 uptake into both rapidly and slowly equilibrating pools is decreased. Thus inhibition of T_4 transport into liver could contribute to low production of T_3 in the serum of calorically deprived individuals.[54]

CELLULAR BINDING PROTEINS. The free thyroid hormone hypothesis implies the existence within the cell or on its surface of sites with which T_4 and T_3 engage in a reversible binding interaction. The characterization of such sites is still incomplete. Proteins that bind T_4 and T_3 have been identified in the cytosol of many tissues of different species, including human liver. Some studies suggest that the cytosol binding proteins for T_4 and T_3 are distinct from one another, whereas other studies do not. In the earlier view, entry of hormone into the cell would be conditioned by a simple competitive binding equilibrium between intracellular and extracellular, extravascular binding proteins.

In intact rats intracellular free T_3 concentration can be estimated by evaluating the binding affinity of intracellular binding proteins and by measuring the T_3 concentration in cytosol,[55] and such analyses suggested that there is a free hormone gradient of two- to threefold across the cell membrane in several tissues. These concentration gradients, however, are not as high as those calculated for the nuclear/cytosolic ratios in liver, kidney, heart, and brain, which are 50:1 to 250:1. Thus there may also be a specific transport system for concentration of T_3 into the nucleus. This appears to account for the discrepancy between the affinities of nuclear receptors for T_3 estimated from in vivo saturation studies ($K_d \sim 10^{-10}$ M) and those found with isolated nuclei ($K_d \sim 10^{-9}$ M).

Pathways of Hormone Metabolism

QUALITATIVE AND QUANTITATIVE ASPECTS. The most important pathway for metabolism of T_4 is its conversion to the active hormone T_3.[56] The other deiodination reactions of T_4 and T_3 all lead to inactive products; the reactions are complex and appear to be highly regulated (see Fig. 8–4).[57] There are three general classes of deiodinases in both rat and human tissues. The characteristics of the common deiodinase activities in rat tissue are summarized in Table 8–1. Similar reactions have been observed in human tissues[57, 58] as well as in other species. Two deiodinases, types 1 and 2, have the capacity to remove an iodine from the outer ring of T_4 and therefore produce the more active hormone T_3. However, this is the only similarity between these two activities. In the rat, and probably in humans, the type 1 enzyme appears to provide T_3 to the plasma and to deiodinate 3,3',5'-triiodothyronine (rT_3) to produce 3,3'-diiodothyronine ($3,3'-T_2$). Because rT_3 has no recognized biological effect, its deiodination has uncertain physiological significance. The apparent K_m for T_4 is relatively high for the type 1 enzyme, indicating that at the concentrations of T_4 present in the body this enzyme is not saturated. It is sensitive to inhibition by propylthiouracil, probably through the formation of a mixed disulfide between propylthiouracil and the putative sulfhydryl-containing active site on the enzyme. This enzyme activity is increased in hyperthyroidism and decreased in hypothyroidism. The increased activity in hyperthyroidism may explain why propylthiouracil is so effective in decreasing serum T_3 in hyperthyroid patients.[59] Because methimazole does not share this property, propylthiouracil is the drug of choice for the acute treatment of severe hyperthyroidism. The type 1 enzyme can also remove an inner-ring iodine from either T_4 or T_3. Sulfation of the phenolic hydroxyl of any of the substrates for the type 1 enzyme, a reaction that occurs in liver, will reduce the K_m and in the case of T_3 markedly increase the V_{max}.[60–62]

The requirement for a sulfhydryl-containing cytosolic cofactor is a critical aspect of all the deiodination reactions. For the type 1 enzyme, this cytosolic cofactor appears to depend on NADPH for regeneration. Because the hexose monophosphate shunt pathway is a major source of this pyridine nucleotide, fasting reduces both T_4 and rT_3 deiodination. The fraction of plasma T_3 derived from the type 1 enzyme in liver and kidney may not be as high in the human as in the rat. For example, propylthiouracil administration causes a marked inhibition of rT_3 deiodination in humans but causes only a modest decrease in total body T_3 production.[63] As mentioned, this is not the case in hyperthyroidism, in which propylthiouracil causes a rapid 50% fall in serum T_3 with a marked decrease in the ratio of T_3 to T_4.[59] The activity of type 1 deiodinase in the thyroid is increased by TSH in the rat and is higher in patients with Graves disease than in normal humans.[19, 20]

Type 2 deiodinase is present in the pituitary gland, central nervous system, brown fat, and placenta (see Table 8–1). The apparent K_m is three orders of magnitude lower than for the type 1 enzyme, and the type 2 enzyme can deiodinate only the outer ring of iodothyronines and is relatively resistant to inhibition by propylthiouracil.[64] The type 2 enzyme acts to maintain intracellular T_3 concentrations at constant levels in the tissues in which it is present.[65] Thus a reduction in serum T_4 concentration leads to an increase in the activity of this enzyme and vice versa.[66, 67] This regulation of type 2 deiodinase is not related to the metabolic potency of the iodothyronine involved. T_4 and even rT_3 are more effective as regulators of type 2 deiodinase than is T_3. The mechanism of the regulation of type 2 deiodinase by iodothyronine substrates is not understood.

As mentioned, the type 2 deiodinase may also provide

TABLE 8–1. Iodothyronine Deiodinases

Parameter	Type 1 (5')	Type 2 (5')	Type 3 (5)
Physiological role	Provide T_3 to plasma in rat (? human)	Provide intracellular T_3 (? plasma T_3 in human)	Inactivate T_3 and T_4
Tissue location	Liver, kidney, thyroid, central nervous system, pituitary	Central nervous system, pituitary, brown fat, placenta	Central nervous system, placenta, skin
Substrate preference	$rT_3 \gg T_4 > T_3$	$T_4 \geq rT_3$	$T_3 > T_4$
K_m for T_4 (apparent)	1×10^{-6} M	1×10^{-9} M	6×10^{-9} M (T_3), 37×10^{-9} M (T_4)
Deiodination site	Outer and inner ring	Outer ring	Inner ring
Kinetic mechanism	Ping-pong	Sequential	Sequential
Dithiothreitol	Stimulates	Stimulates	Stimulates
Apparent K_i for propylthiouracil	5×10^{-7} M (sensitive)	4×10^{-3} M (resistant)	? ($>10^{-3}$ M) (resistant)
Iopanoic acid	Inhibit	Inhibit	Inhibit
Hypothyroidism	Decrease	Increase	Decrease
Hyperthyroidism	Increase	Decrease	Increase

some of the plasma T_3 in humans, although the tissue or tissues responsible for propylthiouracil-insensitive T_3 production have not been identified. However, the type 2 deiodinase does provide the mechanism whereby the thyrotropic cells of the pituitary can monitor the concentration of T_4.[68] As shown in Figure 8–7, type 2 deiodinase is necessary for T_4 to suppress TSH release from the pituitary gland. If type 2 deiodinase is inhibited by an agent such as iopanoic acid, T_4 is a less effective inhibitor of TSH release.[69] This suggests a mechanism whereby the hypothalamic-pituitary axis could recognize a decrease in serum T_4 concentrations. The consequent increase in serum TSH serves to maintain serum T_3 concentrations at a stable level by altering the ratio of T_3 to T_4 in thyroid hormone secretion. This sequence is consistent with observations made in areas in which goiter is endemic and in animal models of iodine deficiency.[70]

The role of the type 3 enzyme is not as clear. Its increased activity in hyperthyroidism (see Table 8–1) suggests that it is part of a homeostatic mechanism for protecting the brain, and perhaps the fetus, from excess quantities of the active hormone, T_3. It also inactivates T_4 by converting it to rT_3, and this enzyme may be more important than type 1 enzyme as a source of plasma rT_3.

Ultimately, monoiodothyronines lose their iodine, leaving for excretion in the urine the iodine-free thyronine ring and its metabolites. The deaminated and decarboxylated derivatives of T_4 and T_3, tetrac and triac, are also formed and, having entered the blood, are rapidly metabolized by deiodination and conjugation, followed by biliary excretion (see Fig. 8–4).

About 80% of T_4 is degraded by deiodination; the remainder is eliminated in organic form by fecal excretion, which probably comprises a mixture of T_4, T_3, and their various conjugated and unconjugated derivatives. Deamination and decarboxylation reactions lead to the production of tetrac and triac in relatively small quantities, accounting for 5% or less of daily T_4 disposal.

About 40% of the T_4 secreted in normal humans is deiodinated to yield T_3, and about 40% is deiodinated to yield rT_3. Hence, with a normal T_4 production rate of 100 nmol (78 µg) daily, approximately 40 nmol (26 µg) of T_3 and rT_3 is produced by peripheral deiodinations. When these values are compared with the estimated total daily production rate for T_3 (Table 8–2), nearly all (at least 80%) of normal T_3 production (and all of rT_3 production) can be accounted for by peripheral generation from T_4 rather than direct thyroid secretion. The conclusion that the normal thyroid secretes little if any T_3 and essentially no rT_3 is

TABLE 8–2. Comparison of T_3 and T_4 in Humans

	T_3	T_4
Production rate (nmol/d)	50	100
Fraction from thyroid	0.2	1.0
Relative metabolic potency	1.0	0.3
Serum concentration		
Total (nmol/L)	1.8	100
Free (pmol/L)	5	20
Fraction of total hormone in free form ($\times 10^{-2}$)	0.3	0.02
Distribution volume (L)	40	10
Fraction intracellular	0.64	0.15
Half-life (d)	0.75	7.0

To convert T_4 from nmol/L to µg/dL (total) or pmol/L to ng/dL (free), divide by 12.87. To convert T_3 from nmol/L to ng/dL (total) or pmol/L to pg/dL (free), multiply by 65.1.

consonant with the concentration of these iodothyronines relative to that of T_4 within the thyroid gland. Although some of the T_3 and rT_3 produced from T_4 in the peripheral tissues leaves those tissues and enters the blood, it is uncertain to what extent T_3 and rT_3 are degraded locally before they enter the blood or whether they may be retained intact at their sites of origin, sequestered in pools that exchange only slowly with the plasma compartment. As pointed out, in pituitary and brain the T_3 bound to cell nuclei is derived to a large extent from local T_3 generation rather than from the blood.[65] Thus the foregoing estimates of the rate of conversion of T_4 to T_3 and rT_3, having been made solely on the basis of measurements in blood, must be considered minimal values. T_3 is metabolized mainly by 5-monodeiodination and rT_3 is metabolized principally by 5'-monodeiodination; both processes yield 3,3'-T_2.

PHYSIOLOGICAL IMPLICATIONS. Considering the tissue distribution of the various deiodinases and their different K_m values and the special characteristics of iodothyronine tissue uptake systems, it might be anticipated that various tissues would obtain the active thyroid hormone, T_3, from different sources. This does turn out to be the case and is important for the understanding of thyroid hormone action in different tissues.[65] Because the T_3 specifically bound to the nuclear receptors is likely to have the greatest effect on thyroid hormone-regulated processes (see discussion later), it is especially relevant to compare the quantity and source of this nuclear T_3 in various tissues of the rat (Fig. 8–8). There are two general patterns. In the kidney, liver, skeletal muscle, and heart, virtually all of the nuclear T_3 is derived directly from plasma T_3. Stated in other terms, these tissues depend on the circulating T_3 for the supply of active thyroid

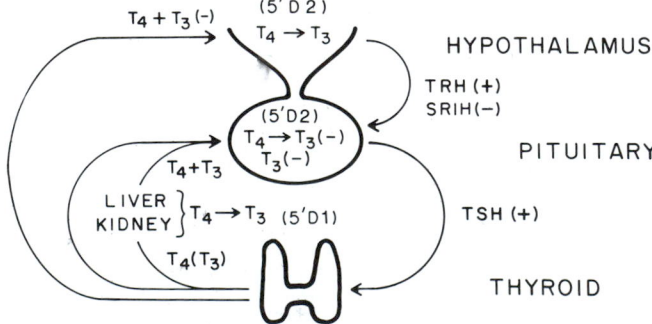

Figure 8–7. Schematic diagram of the role of T_4 and T_3 in the feedback regulation of TRH and TSH secretion. T_4, the secretory product of the thyroid gland, must be converted to T_3 to produce its effects. This conversion may take place in tissues such as the liver and kidney via a propylthiouracil-sensitive iodothyronine 5'-deiodinase (5'D1) or via intracellular T_3 production by the propylthiouracil-insensitive deiodinase (5'D2) in the pituitary and central nervous system.

QUANTITY AND SOURCE OF NUCLEAR T_3 IN VARIOUS TISSUES

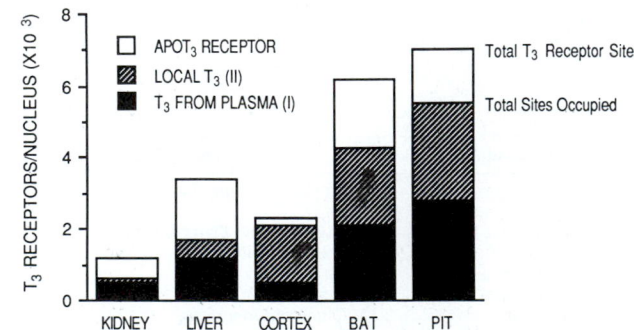

Figure 8–8. Schematic diagram of the origin of the specifically bound nuclear T_3 in various tissues of the rat. Data are derived from studies in which the sources of specifically bound nuclear T_3 were estimated using double-isotope labeling techniques. In tissues in which the receptor saturation is significantly greater than 50%, the additional T_3 is provided by the type 2 iodothyronine 5'-deiodinase. T_3 in rat plasma is derived largely via the action of the propylthiouracil-sensitive type 1 iodothyronine deiodinase (1).

hormone. The cerebral cortex, pituitary, and brown fat, all of which contain type 2 deiodinase, have a different pattern in that half or more of intracellular T_3 is generated locally from T_4 within the tissue. The tissues that depend on type 2 deiodinase activity for nuclear T_3 are those in which a constant supply of thyroid hormone is critical for either normal development (cerebral cortex), growth (pituitary), or survival during the cold stress of the newborn period (brown adipose tissue). These tissues are also characterized by a high degree of saturation of the nuclear T_3 receptors so that the ratio of occupied to unoccupied receptors is quite high. In the liver, kidney, and heart, on the other hand, nuclear receptor sites are only about 50% occupied at normal serum T_3 concentrations. This arrangement allows multiple levels of regulation of thyroid hormone supply. The supply of T_3 to tissues such as kidney, liver, or heart can be decreased by reducing the conversion of T_4 to the T_3 that appears in plasma. For example, starvation, surgical stress, glucocorticoid therapy, and diabetes mellitus all decrease type 1 deiodinase activity (Table 8–3). Some of these effects may be due to reduced levels of the cytosolic cofactor for type 1 deiodination. In humans, serum T_3 decreases to about a third of its normal value after overnight fasting, possibly acting to conserve protein and reduce metabolic rate as rapidly as possible.[71] This decrease would not affect the major source of T_3 supply to the brain or pituitary. Alternatively, the inverse relationship between the type 2 enzyme and the serum T_4 allows nuclear T_3 in the brain to remain at near-normal levels despite a fall in serum T_4 concentrations. This, plus the transplacental passage of maternal T_4, may account for the normal brain development in athyrotic infants if they are identified soon after birth and treated adequately. It is also critical to point out that only in specific tissues is it possible to predict the nuclear T_3 concentration from the concentration of this hormone in the plasma.

In regard to thyromimetic actions, T_3 is several times more active than T_4. Because approximately one third of all T_4 is converted to T_3 during the course of its metabolism, the question arises whether all the metabolic activity of T_4 can be ascribed to the T_3 that it gives rise to, i.e., whether T_4 is merely a prohormone for T_3, as thyroglobulin is for T_4. The question of whether T_4 has intrinsic biological activity cannot be answered unequivocally, but there is no evidence that it has independent physiological effects as long as T_4-to-T_3 conversion can occur.

The fact that rT_3 has no known metabolic effect, together with evidence that outer- or inner-ring T_4 deiodination can vary independently, has given rise to the concept that these two pathways cause either hormone activation or hormone inactivation. In situations such as fasting, when the plasma appearance of T_3 is reduced, rT_3 production is not increased but remains constant. As discussed previously, the abrupt rise in rT_3 concentrations during illness or fasting is due to impaired clearance of this triiodothyronine because of the reduced activity of the type 1 deiodinase. The hypo-

thalamic-pituitary axis is not nearly as affected by the fall in plasma T_3 concentration because of its dependence on T_4 and type 2 deiodination (see Fig. 8–7). This phenomenon may explain the absence of an increase in TSH in patients whose serum T_3 concentrations fall precipitously.

Finally, consideration must be given to the possibility that the metabolites of T_4 that are now considered to be metabolically inactive (rT_3, the various monoiodothyronines and diiodothyronines, tetrac, and triac) are not truly lacking in thyromimetic activity. Traditionally, tests for the bioactivity of such compounds almost always involved their systemic administration and were predicated on the assumption that they could be present in tissues only as a result of delivery from the blood. Because the derivatives of T_4, without exception, are cleared from the blood and degraded more rapidly than T_4 (some extremely so), their access to tissues may have been extremely limited in both amount and time, making them appear to be inactive. Further, the relative metabolic potency of various thyroid hormone analogues differs according to the particular action being considered. What is needed are studies to determine whether the various physiological derivatives of T_4 have particular metabolic actions in the tissues within which they are being generated.

HORMONE TURNOVER. The availability of radioiodine-labeled thyroid hormones and their derivatives has made possible studies of their overall metabolism in humans and experimental animals in vivo that have provided useful information concerning this aspect of thyroid hormone economy in normal and disease states. With few exceptions, these studies have involved administration of compounds labeled with radioiodine in their 3' position, either by a single intravenous injection or by continuous infusion, followed by serial measurements of the concentration of administered compound in the blood. When subjected to appropriate kinetic analysis, the data permit calculation of the metabolic clearance rate of the administered compound and often of its component functions, the volume of distribution and the fractional rate of turnover. Such studies can also provide quantitative evidence of the fate of the labeled iodine atoms and occasionally have been used to provide qualitative information concerning pathways of hormone metabolism, but they yield no evidence of the fate of the unlabeled compounds that remain when the radioiodine is removed. Nevertheless, in a state of physiological equilibrium, the quantity of hormone degraded or excreted per unit time must equal the rate of hormone secretion, which can be measured indirectly in this manner. Furthermore, in a homeostatically regulated system, the rate of hormone disposal may well determine the requisite rate of hormone manufacture. T_4 in the normal adult has a volume of distribution of approximately 10 L; that is the extrathyroid amount of T_4 is equivalent to the quantity that would be contained in 10 L of plasma (see Table 8–2). Because the normal concentration of T_4 in plasma is approximately 100 nmol/L (8 µg/dL), the extrathyroid pool of T_4 is approximately 1 µmol. In the young or middle-aged adult, the fractional rate of turnover of T_4 in the periphery is normally about 10%/d (half-time, 6.7 d). Thus about 1.1 L of the peripheral T_4 distribution space is cleared of hormone daily, a volume that contains approximately 110 nmol (85 µg) of T_4. The fractional rate of turnover and rate of clearance of T_4 are much smaller than those of most hormones. The slower turnover of T_4 is doubtless a reflection of the predominant extent to which T_4 is bound, leaving only a small fraction free for metabolic turnover. If only the free T_4, which is about $\frac{1}{5000}$ of the total, were available for metabolic turnover, the rate of clearance of free T_4 would be at least 5500 L/d.

The kinetics of T_3 metabolism differ greatly from those

TABLE 8–3. Factors That Impair Peripheral Conversion of T_4 to T_3

Physiological
Fetal and early neonatal life
Old age?

Pathological
Fasting, malnutrition
Hepatic or renal dysfunction
Systemic illness
Trauma, postoperative state

Pharmacological
Drugs (propylthiouracil, glucocorticoids, propranolol, amiodarone)
Oral cholecystographic agents

of T_4, partly because of differences in the intensity of their binding to TBG. A single dose of T_3 is rapidly cleared from the plasma as a result of both widespread distribution and rapid cellular metabolism. The volume of distribution of T_3 in the normal adult is about 40 L and its fractional turnover rate is about 60%/d. Hence, the MCR of T_3 is about 24 L/d. At a mean normal serum T_3 concentration of 1.8 nmol/L (120 ng/dL), this indicates a normal daily production rate for T_3 of approximately 50 nmol (36 µg).

The distribution and metabolism of rT_3 are exceedingly rapid. A large metabolic clearance rate of rT_3 and a very low concentration in plasma (0.3 nmol/L [25 ng/dL]) combine to yield daily production rates for rT_3 of about 45 nmol. The turnover and metabolism of $3,3'-T_2$ are even faster than those of rT_3. Its production rate in normal individuals is uncertain because of lack of agreement concerning its concentration in plasma.

Alterations in Transport, Turnover, and Metabolism of Thyroid Hormones

The free thyroid hormone hypothesis assigns to the concentration of free hormones a role as a major determinant of the quantity of hormone available to the cells and, hence, the absolute rate of hormone turnover and the metabolic state of the patient. It assigns to the proportion of free hormone a role as a major determinant of the proportionate distribution and metabolism of hormone. In addition, the hypothesis encompasses the operation of cellular factors that may influence the distribution, effectiveness, and metabolism of the hormone, independently of alterations in extracellular binding. These factors have been brought into prominence by studies of specific pathways of thyroid hormone metabolism and the manner in which they are altered in various abnormal states.

EXTRACELLULAR ABNORMALITIES. Abnormalities in the interaction between the thyroid hormones and their binding proteins are of two types: those that result primarily from a change in the number or affinity of available binding sites and those that result primarily from a change in the concentration of the hormone. The static, kinetic, and physiological consequences of these two types of change differ and can best be appreciated by considering the sequential perturbations that follow abnormalities of each type. Consider first the consequences that would follow from an increase in the concentration of TBG in plasma. (See Fig. 8–6.) Initially, the number of unoccupied binding sites would increase, resulting in a shift of hormone from the free to the bound state, a decrease in its MCR, and a decrease in the quantity of hormone removed from the plasma. With a normal or perhaps increased influx of T_4 into the plasma, the total concentration of hormone would increase progressively until the concentration of free hormone was restored to normal. At this time the total and bound concentrations of hormone, which are numerically almost equal, would be increased; hence, the proportion of free hormone and the MCR would remain decreased. The plasma concentration of T_4 would have risen sufficiently to counterbalance the decrease in the proportion of free T_4 and decrease in MCR, so that both the absolute concentration of free T_4 and its dependent variable, the rate of hormone disposal to the tissues, would be normal. The patient would remain euthyroid. This sequence is almost precisely that which has been observed for both T_4 and T_3 in states associated with an increased TBG level in plasma. The converse consequences have been observed in states associated with decreased levels of TBG (Table 8–4).

Thus, although primary alterations in TBG alter the total concentrations of hormone in plasma and the kinetics

TABLE 8–4. Circumstances Associated with Alterations in Binding of T_4 by TBG

Increased Binding	Decreased Binding
Pregnancy	Androgenic or anabolic steroids
Neonatal state	Large doses of glucocorticoids
Estrogens and hyperestrogenemic states	Active acromegaly
Tamoxifen	Nephrotic syndrome
Oral contraceptives	Major systemic illness
Acute intermittent porphyria	Genetic determination
Infectious and chronic active hepatitis	Asparaginase
Biliary cirrhosis	
Genetic determination	
Perphenazine	
HIV infection	

of T_4 metabolism, they do not ultimately influence the absolute quantity of hormone that enters the cell, acts, and is degraded per unit time. Therefore, they do not influence the total turnover of hormone or the metabolic state of the patient. These remain a function of the rate of hormone production or supply, and when homeostatic mechanisms are normal, hormone production and the metabolic state of the patient will be normal too.

Far different consequences follow a primary alteration in the rate of hormone supply. (See Fig. 8–9.) For example, in hyperthyroid states, hypersecretion of hormone leads to an increase in total hormone concentration. As a result, the concentration of unoccupied binding sites on TBG decreases and the concentrations of both free and bound hormone rise. As a consequence of the fixed quantity of TBG available, the mass action expression dictates that the concentration of free hormone would increase to a disproportionately great extent and that the proportion of free hormone would therefore rise. In vivo these changes would be reflected in an increase in the MCR of T_4, an increase in the rate of hormone disposal to the tissues, and a hypermetabolic state. Converse consequences occur when the supply of hormone is decreased, as in hypothyroidism. Here, as in the case of primary alterations in hormone binding, the flux of hormone to the tissues and the metabolic state of the patient are again determined by the rate of hormone production. In the final analysis, barring metabolically wasteful loss of hormone, the metabolic state of the patient over any prolonged period is

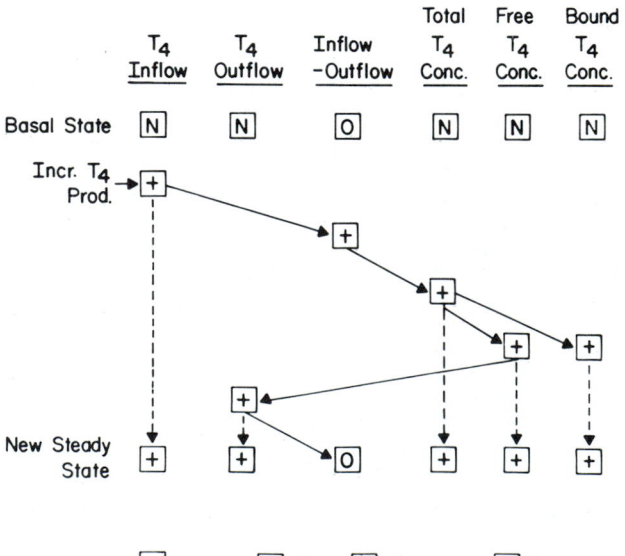

			Total	Free	Bound
T_4 Inflow	T_4 Outflow	Inflow –Outflow	T_4 Conc.	T_4 Conc.	T_4 Conc.
Basal State N	N	O	N	N	N
Incr. T_4 Prod. +					
New Steady State +	+	O	+	+	+

N Normal O Zero + Increased – Decreased

Figure 8–9. The sequence of events after a sustained increase in T_4 secretion: its effects on the turnover of T_4 and on the serum concentration of total and free T_4. Converse consequences follow a decrease in T_4 secretion.

determined by the rate of hormone production. The effect of alterations in binding is merely to change the plasma concentration, partition, and clearance rate of the hormone for a given rate of hormone production.

Alterations in the extracellular binding of T_4 and T_3 can also occur because of the presence in blood of abnormal binding proteins. A syndrome associated with abnormal binding of T_4 in serum has come to be known as familial dysalbuminemic hyperthyroxinemia (FDH). The syndrome has an autosomal dominant mode of transmission and is not especially rare. Patients with this disorder are euthyroid. They display, however, an elevation of serum total T_4 concentration, although the free T_4 concentration is normal, owing to the presence in serum of increased concentrations of an albumin that is present in normal serum, but only in minute amounts, and that has an unusually high affinity for T_4. Because the protein has a relatively low affinity for T_3, serum T_3 concentration and the assessments of binding sites in plasma using radioactive T_3 in vitro are normal. The abnormal protein has not been isolated or characterized. (For additional discussion of FDH, see later under States Associated with Abnormal Hormone Concentrations in Blood.)

CELLULAR ABNORMALITIES. As is consonant with the free thyroid hormone hypothesis, factors intrinsic to the cell can, in certain circumstances, play a primary role in mediating alterations in the overall rate of hormone metabolism, with or without changes in the specific pathways by which hormone metabolism proceeds. This was first demonstrated in the case of phenobarbital, an agent known to induce hypertrophy of the smooth endoplasmic reticulum. In rats, phenobarbital produces an increase in the liver/plasma concentration ratio for T_4 but not for T_3. The peripheral clearance of the two hormones is increased, that for T_4 resulting from an increase in both fecal and deiodinative removal and that for T_3 from an increase in the fecal component alone. Despite these losses of T_4, its concentration in plasma is maintained as a result of compensatory hyperfunction of the thyroid. These changes occur without a net change in extracellular hormone binding, indicating that they are cellular in origin. The response to phenobarbital typifies the effect of an increase in the cellular disposal of T_4 in which disposal is not associated with altered metabolic action and in which the pituitary and hypothalamus do not appear to be primarily affected.

Phenytoin, like phenobarbital, accelerates the peripheral metabolism of T_4 in the rat and in the human.[72] Here, too, the effect cannot be ascribed to an alteration in the extracellular binding of hormone. Indeed, the concentrations of total and free T_4 are subnormal while the total T_4 secretion rate is unchanged. There is no uniformity of data concerning the effect of phenytoin on serum T_3 and TSH concentrations. Some data suggest, however, that phenytoin accelerates the peripheral conversion of T_4 to T_3, thereby maintaining the serum T_3 concentration and obviating the need for increased TSH secretion, despite the subnormal serum concentrations of total and free T_4. If this is the case, it would represent an example of diversion of the T_4 metabolism into pathways that enhance its metabolic effectiveness. Phenytoin may also have thyromimetic activity at least at the level of the pituitary.[73] This would raise the possibility that the reduction in free T_4 concentration during phenytoin treatment is pathological rather than a compensatory physiological change. Any such effects, however, are minor, and there is no indication for administering supplemental levothyroxine to otherwise normal patients receiving this drug.

Alterations in thyroid status themselves induce changes in cellular mechanisms for T_4 disposal. In patients with thyrotoxicosis, the metabolic clearance rates of T_4 and T_3 are increased, and the converse is true in patients with hypothyroidism. These changes are partly due to alterations in extracellular binding of the hormones, but cellular factors operate as well. In experimental thyrotoxicosis and hypothyroidism in the rat, overall degradation of T_4 in liver preparations in vitro is accelerated or retarded, respectively, both 5'- and 5-monodeiodinases varying in concentration with the metabolic state. In the pituitary, in contrast, the rate of 5'-monodeiodination of T_4 varies inversely with the metabolic state (see Table 8–1).

As discussed earlier the conversion of T_4 to T_3 is impaired in conditions that have come to be known collectively as the low-T_3 syndrome, the euthyroid sick syndrome,[74] or nonthyroidal illness. Clinical circumstances that can lead to the syndrome are listed in Table 8–3. In addition to a reduction in serum T_3 concentration and in T_3 production rates, the serum rT_3 level rises because of impairment of outer-ring deiodination of this compound. In experimental circumstances in which T_4-to-T_3 conversion is blocked pharmacologically, e.g., by administration of iopanoic acid or propylthiouracil in animals, hypothyroidism is produced to a variable degree. In the subject with a normal hypothalamic-pituitary-thyroid axis, a compensatory increase in the production of the prohormone T_4 occurs. A clear-cut clinical example of this phenomenon is seen in individuals receiving the antiarrhythmic agent amiodarone, which partially blocks T_4-to-T_3 conversion.[75, 76] The physiological response to the administration of this agent is to increase TSH secretion and, consequently, serum T_4 until a new equilibrium is established, at which point the TSH level returns to normal. At this time all tests of thyroid hormone economy indicate a euthyroid state despite the reduced T_3/T_4 ratio and elevated serum T_4 concentration. It is not known whether amiodarone inhibits both type 1 and type 2 deiodinases or how much of its effect is due to inhibition of pituitary T_4-to-T_3 conversion in the thyrotrope as opposed to impairment of type 1 deiodination in liver and kidney. Whatever the cause, if amiodarone is given to an individual who is hypothyroid and receiving exogenous T_4, the requirement for levothyroxine may increase. Similar effects have been demonstrated in humans using the oral cholecystographic agent iopanoic acid.[77]

Another important cause of impaired T_4-to-T_3 conversion is illness or trauma (see Table 8–3).[74] Whether ill patients with serum T_3 concentrations less than one third of normal are hypothyroid is unclear, because of a paucity of sensitive tests to assess peripheral thyroid hormone action in the intact subject. The problem is further compounded by the dual TSH regulation by serum T_3 and intrapituitary T_4-to-T_3 conversion (see Fig. 8–7). Thus the most sensitive index of primary hypothyroidism, TSH production, is not valid. Because of these complexities, it cannot be stated unequivocally that the hypothyroidism that would be expected when the serum T_3 level is reduced is, in fact, present. Administration of T_4 or T_3 does not change the outcome in seriously ill patients.[78, 79] We are, therefore, unable to address the issue of whether it is appropriate to circumvent this abnormality, even in severely ill patients in whom serum T_3 concentrations may be virtually unmeasurable.

Peripheral iodothyronine metabolism in the fetus is grossly different from that in the mother or in other adults. In general, 5'-monodeiodination of T_4 is retarded, so the rate of T_3 neogenesis is low. Concomitantly 5-monodeiodinations are accelerated, so both rT_3 formation and the degradation of any T_3 formed are increased. At about the time of delivery, iodothyronine metabolism switches to a more mature pattern. This general pattern of fetal iodothyronine metabolism has been observed in all the vertebrate species thus far studied.[80]

REGULATION OF THYROID FUNCTION

As with other endocrine organs, the function of the thyroid gland is closely regulated. Figure 8–7 is a schema of regulatory mechanisms affecting the thyroid. Like the gonads and adrenal cortices, the thyroid participates with the hypothalamus and pituitary in a classic type of feedback control. In addition, intrinsic regulatory mechanisms create an inverse relationship between the glandular organic iodine level and the rate of hormone formation. Such autoregulatory mechanisms subserve an important purpose because the rate of hormone synthesis is potentially susceptible to acute fluctuations in the availability of a requisite substrate such as iodine. Compared with the effects of other hormones on metabolic processes (e.g., insulin, glucocorticoids, parathyroid hormone), the effects of thyroid hormones, although less dramatic, are longer-lasting. Hence, it is homeostatically important that fluctuation in hormone secretion be prevented, if possible, rather then merely compensated for after it has occurred. Prevention is achieved in part by the large intraglandular store of hormone that buffers the effect of acute increases or decreases in hormone synthesis. Autoregulatory mechanisms within the gland, in turn, tend to maintain the constancy of the thyroid hormone pool. Finally, the classic feedback mechanism senses variations in the availability of thyroid hormones and their metabolic impact at the periphery; it is generally concerned, therefore, with correcting abnormalities in the effective concentration of thyroid hormones in the blood, however small, once they have occurred.

Hypothalamic-Pituitary-Thyroid Complex

Abundant evidence in animals and humans indicates a close functional relationship between the anterior pituitary gland and the thyroid gland. The concept of an independent pituitary-thyroid axis has been extended to accommodate evidence of a similar nature with respect to the hypothalamus, leading to the concept of a hypothalamic-pituitary-thyroid complex, whose function is modified by still higher centers in the brain. Thus there is evidence for secretion by the pituitary of a thyroid stimulator and secretion by the hypothalamus of a stimulator of the pituitary, the function of the entire complex being modified in a typical negative feedback manner by the availability of the thyroid hormones. These observations culminated in the isolation and characterization of the respective simulators, TSH and TRH (Fig. 8–10). Subsequently radioimmunoassays for TSH and TRH and chemical synthesis of the latter led to an extensive understanding of the mechanism by which secretion of TSH is regulated in humans and animals and provided tools for use in the diagnosis of thyroid disease.

Regulation of TSH secretion results from a complex interaction, mainly or entirely at the level of the pituitary thyrotropic cell, in which TRH acts to stimulate first the release and later the synthesis of TSH, while thyroid hormones inhibit these functions. These inhibitory effects are not merely a direct antagonism of the effects of TRH; they can be observed when the hypothalamic source of TRH is destroyed or the pituitary gland is separated from it in vivo or in vitro. Moreover, the degree of thyroid hypofunction that results from destruction of the appropriate areas of the hypothalamus is less severe than that which follows hypophysectomy, and residual thyroid function in the former circumstance can be varied by raising or lowering the concentration of thyroid hormones in the blood. Thus thyroid hormones mediate the feedback regulation of TSH secretion and TRH determines its set point. Measurements of the mRNA coding the proTRH molecule in the paraventricular nuclei of hypothalamus indicate that thyroid hormone administration suppresses TRH as well as TSH production.[81-83]

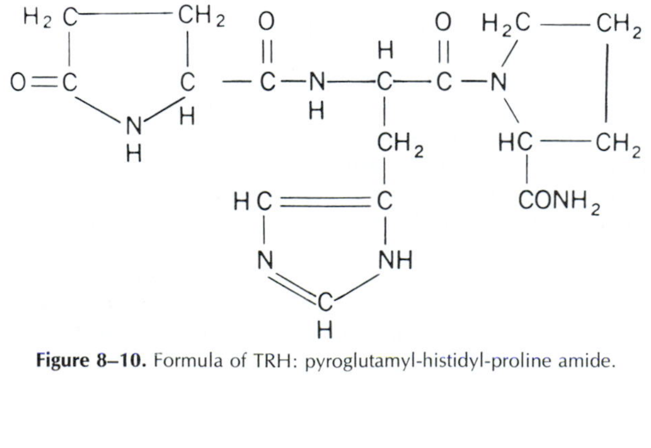

TRH, a modified tripeptide (pyroglutamyl-histidylproline amide), is synthesized by peptidergic neurons in the supraoptic and paraventricular nuclei of the hypothalamus, whence it is transported to and stored in the median eminence. From here, TRH enters the hypophyseal portal venous system, in which it traverses the pituitary stalk and is carried to the cells of the anterior pituitary gland. TRH probably causes TSH release by more than one mechanism.[84, 85] The acute effect is to increase the entry of extracellular calcium into the thyrotrope due to the opening of cellular calcium channels. A more chronic effect may be a consequence of the activation of phospholipase C by TRH leading to a cascade of phosphatidylinositol hydrolysis, inositol 1,4,5-trisphosphate (IP_3) formation, and an increase in the intracellular calcium concentration by interaction of the IP_3 with the endoplasmic reticulum calcium stores. In addition, the diacylglycerol formed during phosphatidylinositol hydrolysis activates protein kinase C, which in turn leads to phosphorylation of unknown proteins that facilitate TSH release.[84] TRH also activates adenylate cyclase in the pituitary, but this is not an important mechanism for induction of TSH or prolactin release by TRH.

The mechanism by which thyroid hormones inhibit the synthesis and secretion of TSH and effectively antagonize the action of TRH remains problematic. It is clear from circumstances in which hormone binding by TBG is abnormal that feedback regulation of TSH secretion is more closely related to the concentrations of free T_4 and free T_3 than to the concentrations of their bound counterparts, presumably because it is the former and not the latter that have access to the tissue.

The intricate relationship between serum T_4 and T_3 levels in the regulation of pituitary TSH release is demonstrated in Figure 8–7. All of the acute inhibition of TSH release by T_4 can be accounted for by the T_3 produced there from within the pituitary gland.[68] If T_4-to-T_3 conversion is blocked, T_4 no longer has this effect.[69] Nonetheless, the mechanism by which the nuclear binding of T_3 leads within minutes to an acute inhibition of TSH release remains to be determined. This effect occurs before the inhibition of synthesis of TSH and before the decrease in TSH mRNA level. A decrease in the serum T_3 or T_4 level leads to an increased TSH release. Likewise, if the serum T_3 concentration is increased twofold above normal, there is no longer a requirement for intracellular T_4-to-T_3 conversion for inhibition of TSH secretion. An important clinical implication of these concepts is that exogenous T_4 is a very effective suppressor of TSH secretion because it is converted to plasma T_3 and also serves as the prohormone for T_3 in the pituitary gland. Because only the T_3 that appears in the plasma affects the tissues that depend on circulating T_3 (see

Figure 8–10. Formula of TRH: pyroglutamyl-histidyl-proline amide.

Fig. 8–8), it may be possible to suppress TSH without causing a similar degree of hormonal effects in the heart. This may be of therapeutic advantage when TSH suppression is desired for treatment of thyroid carcinoma or a thyroid nodule. It follows that the suppression of TSH by any concentration of serum T_3 is greater if the T_3 is supplied via T_4 than if T_3 is administered directly.

Some degree of regulation of TSH secretion may also occur at the level of the TRH receptor on the surface of the thyrotropic cell. Thyroid hormone may decrease receptor density, an effect that would lessen the response to TRH.[87] Estrogens, in contrast, increase receptor density and increase the response to TRH.

One aspect of the regulatory control of TSH secretion that has important clinical implications is the delicate poise of the pituitary feedback mechanism and its sensitivity to extremely small alterations in the availability of thyroid hormone. Small doses of thyroid hormones, sufficient only to produce small alterations in their plasma concentrations, greatly diminish the response to exogenous TRH. By contrast, in euthyroid subjects large doses of iodide inhibit hormone release and produce very slight decreases in serum T_4 and T_3 concentrations. Although all values remain within the normal range, this is uniformly accompanied by increases in the basal serum TSH concentration and the response to TRH (Fig. 8–11).

Although TRH and thyroid hormones are the major regulators of TSH secretion, other factors play a role as well. Somatostatin (SRIF, somatotropin release–inhibiting factor) decreases the response to TRH in vitro and in vivo, and the infusion of antisomatostatin antiserum into rats enhances both basal serum TSH concentrations and the response to TRH. Prolonged administration of levodopa decreases the basal serum TSH concentration in hypothyroid patients and decreases the response to TRH. Similar effects follow dopamine infusion and the administration of bromocriptine, a stimulator of the dopamine receptor. Conversely, blockade of the dopamine receptor by metoclopramide increases the basal serum TSH concentration in both euthyroid and hypothyroid patients and increases the response to TRH. These findings leave little doubt that dopamine is a physiological inhibitor of TSH secretion, but its mechanism of action is unknown. Pharmacological doses of glucocorticoids inhibit the release of TSH in response to TRH and may decrease secretion of TRH as well.

Several aspects of the physiology of TRH, apart from its role in TSH secretion, are of importance. Exogenous TRH elicits the secretion of prolactin at threshold doses that are the same as those for stimulation of TSH secretion. As with TSH, the prolactin response to TRH is modified by the prevailing levels of thyroid hormones, although not to as marked an extent. The role of TRH as a physiological modulator of prolactin secretion is uncertain, however. In women, nursing increases the serum prolactin concentration but the serum TSH concentration is unchanged. TRH may also act as a neurotransmitter. It is found in areas of brain apart from the hypothalamus, in spinal cord, in cerebrospinal fluid, and in portions of the gastrointestinal tract. Application of TRH has a depressing effect in single-neuron preparations, and administration of TRH produces a variety of behavioral effects in animals.

Exogenous TRH elicits the secretion of growth hormone in patients with renal failure and in some patients with acromegaly. The basis for these anomalous responses is unknown.[88]

Thyroid Autoregulation

The changes in thyroid iodine content and intermediary metabolism, size, and histological features that accompany variations in the secretion of TSH suggest that TSH is the major regulator of thyroid structure and function. The thyroid is also the seat of a group of intrinsic responses that modify several aspects of its own function, most importantly its responsiveness to TSH. In contrast to the feedback control effected via TSH, which seeks to maintain the plasma or tissue concentrations of the thyroid hormones, these so-called autoregulatory mechanisms seek to maintain constancy of thyroid hormone stores. They are, therefore, most clearly evident in situations in which thyroid iodine content is varied by changes in iodine ingestion or by abnormalities in thyroid iodine utilization. The extent to which these autoregulatory responses are operative in diverse states of thyroid function is uncertain. Nevertheless, their participation as a first line of defense of thyroid homeostasis is likely. In humans, increases in iodine ingestion are not accompanied by increased serum hormone or decreased TSH concentrations. Hence, the decreased efficiency of thyroid iodide extraction manifested in the lowered thyroid uptake of radioactive iodine (RAIU) that follows excessive iodine ingestion is mediated by autoregulatory inhibition of iodide transport. Conversely, acute iodide depletion is associated with an enhanced autoregulatory response. Similarly, in both sporadic nontoxic goiter and the goiter associated with moderate iodine deficiency, the serum TSH concentration is usually normal. Such findings support the hypothesis that, by enhancing the morphological and functional response to TSH, autoregulatory mechanisms play a major role in the capacity of the thyroid to overcome factors that impair hormone synthesis.

Operationally, autoregulatory responses are those that are demonstrable when the level of TSH is constant, i.e., when TSH either is totally lacking or is provided in standard quantities. Although a variety of intrathyroid processes are influenced by iodine (see section on the pharmacology of iodine), the typical autoregulatory response is that which affects the activity of the thyroid iodide transport mechanism, as judged from both thyroid/serum iodide concentration ratios and iodide transport maxima. In the hypophysectomized rat, regardless of whether standard doses of TSH are administered, variations in the dietary iodine intake are associated with inverse changes in iodide transport activity. However, the inhibition of iodide transport induced by supplemental iodine, whether given chronically or acutely,

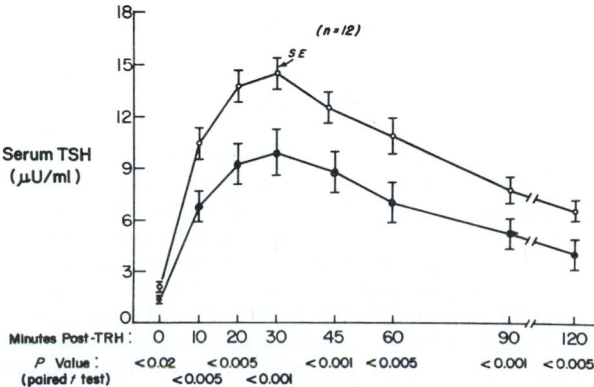

Figure 8–11. Increased response of the serum TSH concentration to administration of TRH in euthyroid volunteers given iodide (190 mg/twice daily for 10 d). During iodide administration, mean serum T_4 concentration decreased from 8.0 to 6.6 μg/dL and mean serum T_3 concentration from 128 to 110 ng/dL. (From Vagenakis AG, Rappoport B, Azizi F, et al. Hyperresponse to thyrotropin-releasing hormone accompanying small decreases in serum thyroid hormone concentrations. Reproduced from the Journal of Clinical Investigation, 1974, vol. 54, pp. 913–918 by copyright permission of the American Society of Clinical Investigation.)

is abolished if administered iodide is prevented from binding to tyrosine by the concomitant administration of propyl-thiouracil. This and other evidence indicate that it is organic rather than inorganic iodine that exerts an autoregulatory influence on iodide transport. Although an iodinated inhibitor of iodide transport has been postulated as the responsible agent, no such inhibitor has been specifically demonstrated; it is possible that autoregulatory inhibition of iodide transport and of other intrathyroid processes influenced by iodine results from the iodination and consequent inactivation of some reactant critical to the processes affected.

The organic iodine content of the thyroid also influences glandular morphology. Thyroids of hypophysectomized rats subjected to prolonged iodine deficiency are larger than those of iodine-sufficient hypophysectomized controls. Moreover, in hypophysectomized rats, depletion of thyroid iodine greatly increases the growth response of the thyroid to standard doses of TSH.

FACTORS THAT INFLUENCE THYROID HORMONE ECONOMY

The widespread metabolic role of the thyroid hormones; the diverse processes involved in the synthesis, secretion, and metabolism of the hormones; and the complex mode of regulation of thyroid function indicate that a great many factors could influence one or more aspects of thyroid hormone economy. In general, the factors can be considered in the following categories: endogenous variables, pharmacological agents, environmental alterations, and dysfunction or diseases of other organ systems.

Thyrotropin (Thyroid-Stimulating Hormone)

TSH is the major regulator of the morphological and functional state of the thyroid. Removal of TSH stimulation is followed by hypovascularity and atrophy of the gland, accompanied by decreased synthesis and secretion of hormone, whereas converse effects are produced by stimulatory doses of TSH. As indicated earlier, it is not certain that all adjustments in thyroid function in response to a variety of stimuli are mediated by changes in the rate of TSH secretion. Intrinsic autoregulatory mechanisms may be the first sensors of changes in the rate of hormone synthesis and may respond appropriately to alter thyroid sensitivity to constant degrees of TSH stimulation. If this response is inadequate to maintain continued secretion of requisite quantities of hormone, modification of the rate of TSH secretion follows.

TSH is a glycoprotein hormone secreted by a specific cell type, the thyrotropic cell, located principally in the anteromedial portion of the adenohypophysis. TSH is composed of two subunits: an alpha subunit of about 14 kd that is common to luteinizing hormone (LH), follicle-stimulating hormone (FSH), and human chorionic gonadotropin (hCG), and a beta subunit that confers specificity to these tropic molecules, which in the case of human TSH is a 112-amino-acid protein.[89] Transcription of both the alpha glycoprotein and the beta subunit is suppressed by thyroid hormone, although the effect on the beta subunit is greater.[90, 91] The genes are located on different chromosomes. Even in thyrotrope tumors, synthesis of alpha subunit is in excess, so beta subunit is rate limiting for TSH secretion. T_3 suppresses transcription of the mRNAs for these subunits without the requirement for an intermediate protein. Thus cycloheximide does not inhibit the effect of T_3 on transcriptional

regulation of the alpha and beta subunits, although it does inhibit the T_3 blockage of TSH release. TRH increases the transcription of both alpha and beta subunits, and dopamine inhibits this process.[92]

The glycosylation aspect of glycoprotein hormone synthesis occurs sequentially, involving addition of preformed asparagine-linked oligosaccharides in rough endoplasmic reticulum, successive modifications in proximal and distal Golgi apparatus, and finally the appearance of the intact folded hormone in the secretory granules. Thyroid status, possibly through changes in TRH secretion, may alter the glycosylation pattern of TSH. The glycosylation of the subunits protects them from intracellular degradation and permits normal folding of the protein chains so that internal disulfide linkages are correctly formed. In addition, glycosylation is required for full biological activity and sialylation of the oligosaccharide units may protect the circulating TSH from interaction with hepatic galactose receptors, thus increasing its half-life.[93–95]

Cytochemical bioassays of serum TSH from patients with pituitary tumors or hypothalamic disorders with hypothyroidism but TSH detectable by radioimmunoassay have shown that the biological activity of this TSH is inappropriately low compared with immunological activity, suggesting the formation of an abnormal product. Long-term administration of TRH enhances the biological activity of TSH in some patients with hypothalamic hypothyroidism and leads to increased thyroid hormone levels.[94] Thus TRH may not only provide the tonic regulation for alpha and beta TSH subunit synthesis but also regulate proper post-translational processing.

Normally only intact hormone and serum alpha subunit are detectable in the circulation. Levels of alpha subunit range from 0.5 to 2μg/L but are increased in postmenopausal women. In normal human serum, TSH is present at concentrations between 0.5 and 5 μU/L. It is increased in hypothyroidism and reduced in hyperthyroidism (see later). The plasma half-life of TSH is about 30 min, and production rates in humans are 40 to 150 mU/d.[96] (See ref. 96 for a discussion of TSH and subunit kinetics.)

TSH in serum displays both episodic and circadian variations. The former is characterized by fluctuations at 1- to 2-h intervals, suggesting that TSH is secreted in a pulsatile manner. The circadian variation is characterized by a nocturnal surge that antecedes the onset of sleep and appears not to be determined by the cortisol rhythm or by fluctuations in the serum T_4 and T_3 concentrations. When the onset of sleep is delayed, the nocturnal TSH surge is accentuated and prolonged, whereas the early onset of sleep results in a surge of lesser magnitude and shorter duration. These observations suggest that secretion of TSH is subject to a fundamental circadian rhythm that is modulated by sleep-associated inhibitory influences. A qualitatively similar variation in serum TSH concentration occurs in patients with mild primary hypothyroidism. In patients with severe hypothyroidism, the circadian variation may disappear. The circadian variation in TSH secretion does not appear to be related to changes in TRH secretion because it persists during prolonged TRH infusion; instead it may reflect fluctuations in dopaminergic inhibitory influences.

Although TSH is capable of inducing lipolysis in vitro, its major effects in vivo are on the structure and function of the thyroid gland. The effect of TSH on intrathyroid iodine metabolism is to enhance essentially all processes leading to the synthesis and secretion of hormone. Abolition of TSH secretion by hypophysectomy or suppression is followed by decreased activity of the thyroid iodide transport mechanism. In addition, organic binding is inhibited, as indicated both by kinetic analysis and by an increase in the proportion of newly accumulated intrathyroid iodine present in the organic form. A decreased fraction of organified iodine is present as iodothyronines, indicating a decrease in the rate of coupling of iodotyrosines. In the intact animal the fractional release of glandular I* is retarded, indicating a decrease in proteolysis of thyroglobulin. After administration of TSH, iodide transport activity is increased, apparently owing to the induction of specific protein, possibly the iodide carrier. Organic-binding reactions are also enhanced, and a prompt stimulation of the coupling reaction occurs. Proteolysis of thyroglobulin and release of glandular iodine are accelerated. Finally, the rate of iodotyrosine dehalogenation is increased, possibly because of increased availability of NADPH rather than an increase in concentration of the enzyme. Clinically the effects of TSH on iodine metabolism are evident in an increased RAIU and thyroid iodide clearance rate, an increase in the rate of release of glandular I*, and an increase in serum T_4 and T_3 concentrations.

In view of suggestive evidence that the several stages in thyroid hormone synthesis may be closely linked to or dependent on thyroid energy metabolism, considerable interest has centered on the effects of TSH on glandular intermediary metabolism. In brief, TSH stimulates thyroid oxygen consumption, glucose assimilation, and glucose oxidation via the hexose monophosphate shunt and glycolytic and tricarboxylic acid cycles. As a consequence, production of carbon dioxide and lactate from exogenous glucose is increased. Oxygen consumption and carbon dioxide production are increased by TSH in the absence of exogenous glucose, indicating increased oxidation of endogenous substrate. TSH rapidly increases the total thyroid content of NADP and increases the $NADP^+/NADPH$ ratio. TSH also has a rapid effect on phospholipid metabolism. Accelerated turnover of thyroid phospholipids is evident, particularly among the phosphomonoinositides, changes in phosphatidic acid and phosphatidylserine being less prominent. Incorporation of glucose and glycerol carbon into thyroid phospholipids is accelerated. The glandular concentration of inorganic phosphate is increased by TSH, reflecting hydrolysis of organic phosphates. This may serve as a stimulus to oxidative metabolism. TSH stimulates the synthesis of purine and pyrimidine precursors and their incorporation into nucleic acids. Uptake of α-aminoisobutyrate by thyroid cells is enhanced by TSH, and leucine incorporation is accelerated in the thyroid of rats given TSH. Thus TSH stimulates both catabolic and anabolic processes in the thyroid, the former presumably supplying energy requisite for the latter.

Cyclic AMP is the intracellular mediator of many of the effects of TSH on the thyroid. Activation of adenylate cyclase by TSH requires binding of the hormone to a specific receptor on the plasma membrane of the thyroid cell and may involve membrane phospholipids as the coupling mechanism. The TSH receptor has been partly characterized and contains gangliosides that may be important in the binding interaction. Prostaglandins can mimic many of the effects of TSH on the thyroid. However, indomethacin, an inhibitor of prostaglandin synthesis, does not block the effects of TSH, indicating that prostaglandins are not obligatory intermediates in TSH action.

Iodine

In addition to its role as a substrate for thyroid hormone biosynthesis, iodine participates in a number of clinically important interactions with the thyroid.[97]

Effects on Thyroid Hormone Synthesis

The effect of iodine on the rate of thyroid hormone synthesis depends on the amount of iodine and duration of administration. When administered acutely, small to moderate amounts of stable iodine do not influence the percentage of thyroid uptake of concomitantly administered I*. Direct analysis reveals little change in the fraction of accumulated iodine that has undergone organification or in the proportions of the several iodinated amino acids formed. Hence, these small acute doses result in an increased rate of thyroid hormone synthesis, at least for a time.

With progressively larger acute doses of iodide, more complex consequences result. The quantity of iodine that undergoes organification displays a biphasic response to increasing doses of iodide, at first increasing and then decreasing as a result of at least a relative blockade of organic binding. This decreasing yield of organic iodine from increasing doses of iodide is termed the acute Wolff-Chaikoff effect.[98] The mechanism of the effect is uncertain, but it depends on the establishment within the thyroid of a sufficiently high concentration of inorganic iodide. Under these conditions the reactive form of iodine generated by oxidative mechanisms may complex with iodide to yield a form that is relatively inefficient in iodinating tyrosine. In common with other situations in which the proportionate rate of organic binding is decreased, as when propylthiouracil is administered, qualitative changes in hormone synthesis also occur. Of the iodine that is bound to organic compounds, little if any is incorporated into T_4 and T_3, a subnormal proportion appears as DIT, and MIT becomes the major product formed. It is unlikely that organic iodinations are completely inhibited during the acute Wolff-Chaikoff effect, but from chromatographic evidence it appears that synthesis of the hormonally active iodothyronines is abolished. Thus the thyroid rejects both quantitatively and qualitatively the large quantity of iodide acutely administered, and the massive increase in thyroid hormone formation that would otherwise occur is prevented. (See Fig. 8–12 for a schematic representation of the Wolff-Chaikoff effect.)

Susceptibility to the Wolff-Chaikoff effect is increased either by stimulation of the iodide-trapping mechanism, as occurs in patients with Graves disease or after TSH administration, or by impairment of organic iodine formation, as may occur after radioiodine therapy, during propylthiouracil treatment, or in patients with Hashimoto disease. Such patients may develop goiter or hypothyroidism if given iodides for long periods.

When moderate or large doses of iodide are administered repeatedly, the relative inhibition of organic binding and inhibition of iodothyronine formation are at least partly relieved. This "escape" or "adaptation" phenomenon occurs

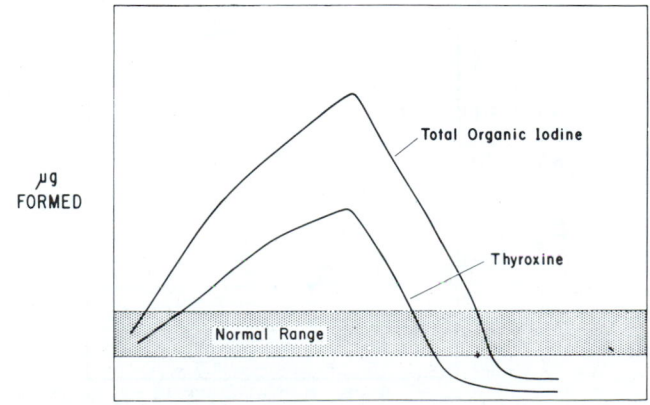

Figure 8–12. Schema of the Wolff-Chaikoff effect. Progressively increasing doses of iodide, given acutely, are associated with an increase and then a decrease in total organic iodinations and in T_4 synthesis. It is uncertain whether values really fall below the normal level in normal subjects.

because, with continued iodine administration, iodide transport activity decreases and the thyroid iodide concentration becomes insufficient to maintain a full Wolff-Chaikoff effect. This response is demonstrable in the hypophysectomized animal and hence is a manifestation of the thyroid autoregulatory inhibition of iodide transport discussed earlier. It allows synthesis of iodothyronines to resume, despite continued iodide administration, and thereby forestalls the development of goitrous hypothyroidism. The reduction in iodide transport that permits adaptation reduces the thyroid iodide clearance rate and hence the RAIU. Nonetheless, the quantity of iodine accumulated and organified is well in excess of normal, although the rate of secretion of T_4 is not enhanced. Thus during prolonged iodine administration the thyroid forms and releases noncalorigenic forms of iodine. Probably much of the iodine lost from the gland in this manner is iodide. In normal individuals the magnitude of this iodide leak varies directly with the dietary iodine intake. In unusual circumstances, adaptation does not occur and synthesis of hormone is chronically inhibited, leading to the development of goiter and hypothyroidism (iodide myxedema). This disorder, to which patients with Hashimoto disease, certain patients with Graves disease, patients who have undergone hemithyroidectomy, and patients with cystic fibrosis are prone, is discussed more fully in the section dealing with disorders that lead to hypothyroidism.

Effects on Thyroid Hormone Release

In the clinical setting the most important effect of pharmacological doses of iodine on the thyroid is a prompt inhibition of hormone release. When the thyroid iodine is labeled with I* and large doses of antithyroid agents are administered to prevent recycling of I* released from the gland, administration of iodine is followed soon thereafter by a decrease in the rate of disappearance of I* from the gland (Fig. 8–13). This effect is most clearly evident in hyperfunctioning thyroids but can also be demonstrated in the normal thyroid. Iodine not only decreases the fractional turnover of thyroid radioiodine but also decreases the actual T_4 secretion rate.

This effect is the mechanism whereby iodine rapidly lowers the serum T_4 concentration and quickly alleviates thyrotoxicity in the patient with diffuse toxic goiter. The response to iodine in this disorder cannot be ascribed to the

persistence of an acute Wolff-Chaikoff effect with inhibition of T_4 synthesis, because the ameliorative effect is more rapid than that produced by large doses of an antithyroid agent. Neither can the response to iodine be ascribed to an effect on the peripheral metabolism or the metabolic effectiveness of T_4, because none can be demonstrated. In most patients with otherwise untreated diffuse toxic goiter, the decrease in the serum T_4 concentration during iodine administration does not continue into the hypothyroid range but rather stabilizes at a normal or high-normal value. The reason for this stabilization is uncertain, but in normal individuals the decrease in serum T_4 and T_3 concentrations induced by iodine appears to elicit an increase in TSH secretion that counteracts the effect of iodine. Operation of a comparable mechanism in patients with diffuse toxic goiter is unlikely, because the TSH-secretory mechanism is suppressed by the hyperthyroid state and may remain so for weeks or months after a euthyroid state is restored.

The mechanism by which iodide inhibits secretion of T_4 is unknown. Clearly the effect is mediated at the thyroid level rather than through an action on TSH, in view of its occurrence in Graves disease. Moreover, the effect is demonstrable in the autonomously hyperfunctioning thyroid nodule, in which secretion of TSH is also lacking. The effect of iodine on the secretory mechanism is not confined to an effect on the release of T_4 but likely includes blockage of proteolysis, because iodine promptly inhibits iodide leak. The capacity of glandular iodine enrichment to inhibit hormone release mechanisms may result from an inhibition of the adenylate cyclase response to stimulation; this effect is more marked in the thyroid of patients with Graves disease than in the normal gland.[99] The increased resistance to proteolysis of thyroglobulin that is enriched in iodine content may also play a role.

Involution of Thyroid Hyperplasia

One of the most important and most enigmatic effects of iodine on the thyroid is that of diminishing the hypervascularity and hyperplasia that characterize the diffuse toxic goiter of Graves disease.[100] This effect, which greatly facilitates surgical therapy of this disorder, is not an obligatory action of iodide on the thyroid, because intense hyperplasia characterizes the thyroid gland of patients with iodide myxedema. In the latter disorder, pharmacological quantities of iodide inhibit hormone synthesis, whereas in Graves disease some binding of iodine to organic compounds doubtless occurs, even during treatment with antithyroid agents. The involuting effect of iodine may reflect an autoregulation of thyroid intermediary metabolism, because enrichment of the thyroid with iodine retards the incorporation of glucose carbon into CO_2, lipid, and especially lactate; decreases incorporation of precursors into nucleic acids; and reduces the incorporation of amino acids into protein. Decreased energy metabolism in the thyroid may retard anabolic processes necessary for maintenance of hyperplasia, whereas decreased production of acid metabolites may be responsible for the reduction in vascularity that iodine produces.

Adrenergic Nervous System and Bioactive Amines

The extent of adrenergic innervation of the thyroid varies from species to species and with the age of the animal. In the human and the mouse, abundant adrenergic fibers terminate in the thyroid in relation to both arterioles and follicle cells. Stimulation of the cervical sympathetic trunks in mice whose thyroid glands have been prelabeled with I* and then suppressed by exogenous T_4 induces formation of

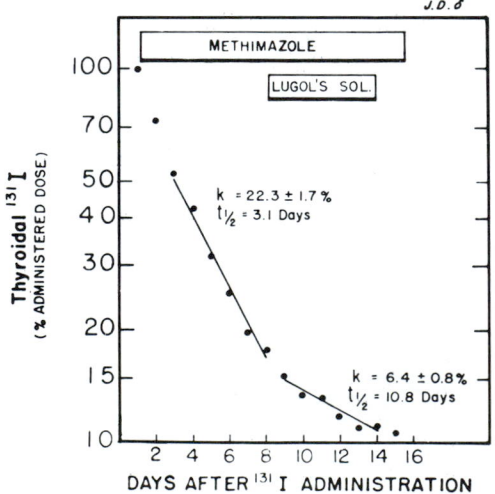

Figure 8–13. Effect of iodine on the thyroid turnover of ^{131}I in a patient with Graves disease. Initial turnover rate of 22.3%/d is much faster than that observed in normal patients and is abruptly slowed by administration of Lugol iodine.

colloid droplets and an increase in the blood I* concentration. Unilateral stimulation induces colloid droplet formation only within the distribution of the stimulated nerve. Moreover, a direct stimulatory effect of catecholamines on thyroid hormone secretion is indicated by the demonstration that exogenous norepinephrine, epinephrine, and dopamine induce release of I* from the prelabeled and T_4-suppressed thyroid of the mouse. Direct stimulatory effects of these catecholamines on iodine and intermediary metabolism have also been demonstrated. In common with TSH, the catecholamines exert their effects through activation of the adenylate cyclase–cyclic AMP system. In contrast to the effects of TSH, however, their stimulatory effects on adenylate cyclase activity and on thyroid hormone synthesis and secretion are inhibited by adrenergic antagonists.

The effects of catecholamines on thyroid hormone economy in humans have been less well defined. Depending on the magnitude and timing of the dose, the initial administration of epinephrine may either increase or decrease the RAIU, and thyroid function is normal in most patients with pheochromocytoma. No significant alterations in thyroid function or serum T_4 concentration are seen in patients given the usual pharmacological doses of adrenergic blocking agents, although propranolol (but not other beta-adrenergic agonists) may impair, to a modest extent, the peripheral conversion of T_4 to T_3.

Peptidergic influences may also be operative. Nerves containing vasoactive intestinal peptide (VIP) are found in the thyroid of humans and animals, and administration of VIP to the animal increases thyroid hormone release, an effect that is additive to that of TSH.[101]

Antithyroid Drugs

A wide variety of chemical agents have the capacity to inhibit one or more reactions required in the synthesis of thyroid hormones. When the effect of such agents is sufficient to reduce the secretion of thyroid hormones to subnormal levels, secretion of TSH is increased and goiter ensues. Hence such agents are commonly termed goitrogens. In clinical practice, goitrogenic agents are encountered as drugs used in the treatment of hyperthyroidism, as pharmacological agents used for other purposes, and as agents occurring naturally in foodstuffs. The present section will provide a classification of several varieties of antithyroid agents and their mode of action. Because the use of antithyroid drugs in the treatment of hyperthyroidism is discussed in a later section, special attention will be given here to agents that are not used in the control of hyperthyroidism but may nonetheless be encountered clinically.

From the standpoint of the aspects of iodine metabolism that they inhibit, antithyroid agents can be grouped into two classes: agents that inhibit thyroid iodide transport and those that inhibit the complex of reactions involved in organic binding and coupling processes. Inhibitors of iodide transport are monovalent anions; of these, thiocyanate and perchlorate have been used clinically. Because of their toxicity, neither thiocyanate nor perchlorate is now used in the treatment of hyperthyroidism, although they are usually effective agents in this respect. Inhibitors of iodide transport decrease hormone synthesis by limiting thyroid/plasma concentration ratios of iodide, thereby reducing the intrathyroid iodide concentration. This inhibition is effective when the plasma iodide concentration is normal or low; however, should the patient be exposed to excessive amounts of iodine, hormone overproduction will resume. Thus control may be unpredictable and, furthermore, these agents cannot be used with iodine in preparing patients for subtotal thyroidectomy.

The second class of antithyroid agents consists of compounds that inhibit the thyroid organic binding and coupling reactions. Compounds that exert this effect can be classified into three main groups, according to their basic chemical structure: thionamides, aminoheterocyclic compounds, and substituted phenols (Fig. 8–14). In the case of the thionamides, it was initially thought that these agents exert their antithyroid action solely by inhibiting the initial oxidation and binding of iodide in the thyroid. Later it was learned that the inhibitory action is directed, in order of decreasing sensitivity, at the coupling of iodotyrosines, the iodination of MIT to form DIT, and, lastly, the formation of MIT. Subsequent studies have shown a similar order of sensitivity in the action of all agents that ultimately (at their highest doses) inhibit organic binding per se.

As a class, the thionamide compounds are the most potent inhibitors of thyroid hormone formation and are characterized by the following substituent grouping:

$$S = C \left\langle \begin{array}{c} N- \\ R- \end{array} \right.$$

in which R may be a sulfur, oxygen, or nitrogen atom. In contrast to the action of agents that inhibit thyroid iodide transport, the action of the thionamides is not prevented by large doses of iodide, although it is decreased somewhat.

The aminoheterocyclic compounds are less potent than the thionamides and are not used in the treatment of hyperthyroidism. Their effects on the thyroid are sometimes manifest, however, during their use in the treatment of other disease. Para-aminosalicylic acid, formerly used as an antituberculosis agent, is goitrogenic in rats, lowers RAIU in humans, and occasionally produces goiter with or without hypothyroidism. The hypoglycemic sulfonylureas, tolbutamide and especially carbutamide, decrease RAIU in humans, although they are not sufficiently potent to be goitrogenic. The goitrogenic effect of para-aminosalicylic acid and the sulfonylureas, like that of the thionamides, is decreased by large amounts of iodine. An additional group of agents in this class is the sulfonamides. Although they have not been shown to be goitrogenic in humans, their goitrogenic potency is usually increased by supplemental iodine. This and other

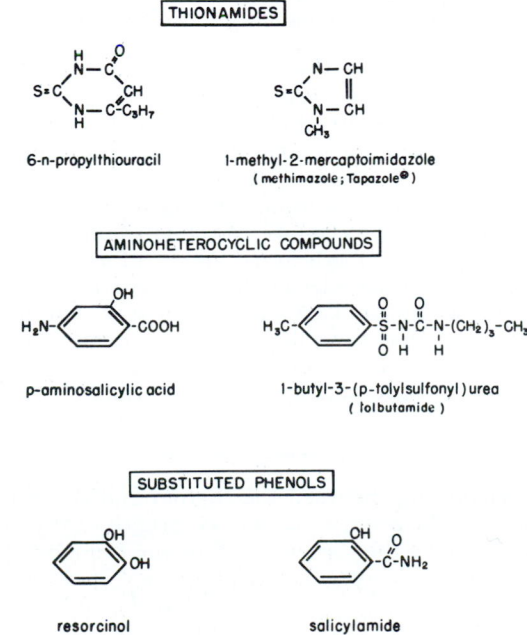

Figure 8–14. Structural formulas of some representative antithyroid compounds.

evidence indicate that the mechanism of action of the sulfonamides differs from that of the thionamides and of other aminoheterocyclic compounds. Another major category of antithyroid agents that inhibit organic binding is the substituted phenols. Agents of interest in this group include resorcinol, a cutaneous antiseptic that has produced goitrous hypothyroidism. Closely related to resorcinol are the congeners of salicylic acid. Salicylic acid itself is devoid of antithyroid action, although it does inhibit the protein binding of T_4 and T_3 by TBG and TBPA.[102]

A number of other agents of diverse chemical nature also have antithyroid activity. Phenylbutazone decreases the thyroid uptake of I* and has been reported to produce goitrous hypothyroidism in humans. Antithyroid activity has also been ascribed to ethionamide and 6-mercaptopurine, both of which contain the thionamide grouping.[103, 104]

Goiter, with or without hypothyroidism, is sometimes encountered in patients being treated with lithium, usually for bipolar manic-depressive psychosis. Like iodide, lithium inhibits thyroid hormone release, and, in high concentrations, can inhibit organic binding reactions. At least acutely, iodide and lithium act synergistically in the latter respect. The mechanism underlying the several effects of lithium is uncertain. Also uncertain is what differentiates patients who develop goiter during lithium therapy from those who do not. Underlying autoimmune thyroiditis may be at least one factor.[105]

Antithyroid agents also occur naturally in foods. These are widely distributed in the family Cruciferae or Brassicaceae, particularly in the genus *Brassica*. Included are cabbages, turnips, kale, kohlrabi, rutabaga, mustard, and a number of plants that are not eaten by humans but serve as animal fodder. It is likely that some thiocyanate is present in such plants (particularly cabbage), especially in the leaves. In addition, the seeds, roots, and perhaps leaves contain another variety of potential goitrogens or *progoitrins* in the form of various thioglycosides. The progoitrins are themselves not goitrogenic but become so when acted upon either by a heat-labile thioglycosidase, myrosinase, also present in the plant, or by the glycosidases liberated by intestinal bacteria. In the case of turnips, the active goitrogen is L-5-vinyl-2-thiooxazolidone. Actively goitrogenic isothiocyanates have been isolated from other plants of the same family. Cassava meal, a dietary staple in many regions of the world, contains linamarin, a cyanogenic glycoside whose metabolism leads to the formation of thiocyanate. Ingestion of cassava is a major factor in accentuating goiter formation in areas of endemic iodine deficiency. Except for thiocyanate, dietary goitrogens influence thyroid iodine metabolism in the same manner as do the thionamides, which they resemble chemically. The role of dietary goitrogens in the induction of disease in humans is uncertain; their effect may depend on the concomitant iodine intake. Although humans rarely if ever eat goitrogenic foods in quantities sufficient to lead to goiter, sufficient quantities of the goitrogen to cause goiter may be present in milk. An important contribution is the demonstration that water-borne, sulfur-containing goitrogens of mineral origin contribute to the development of endemic goiter in certain areas of the world.[106, 107]

Gender and Gonadal Steroids

A relationship between the thyroid and the gonads is suggested by the more frequent occurrence of thyroid disorders in women than in men and by the common appearance of goiter during puberty, pregnancy, and the menopause. This apparent relationship has engendered many studies to assess the effect of sex and of the administration of sex hormones on thyroid function.

Thyroid function and the peripheral metabolism of the thyroid hormones appear to be essentially independent of gender. There is no appreciable variation in RAIU during different phases of the menstrual cycle. The normal ranges for the serum T_4 and T_3 concentrations are the same in nonpregnant women and men. A clear difference between men and women exists, however, in the response of the serum TSH concentration to the administration of TRH. Responses are greater in women than in men, especially in individuals over the age of 40. Estrogens appear to enhance the response to TRH, probably by increasing the number of TRH receptors in the thyrotropic cell, but responses to TRH do not vary materially during the menstrual cycle. Nonetheless, an enhancing effect of estrogen and a possible depression of responsiveness to TRH by androgenic steroids may explain a somewhat greater responsiveness to TRH in women than in men.[88] The basal metabolic rate (BMR) tends to be somewhat higher in men than in women, probably because of the relatively greater muscle mass in men.

Pregnancy and the Newborn State

Pregnancy affects virtually all aspects of thyroid hormone economy. The thyroid gland is enlarged, and a bruit, reflecting the increased blood flow, may be present. The RAIU and thyroid iodide clearance rate are increased. These alterations are due in part to the iodine deficiency state that occurs during pregnancy as a consequence of the increase in renal iodide clearance.

The serum T_4 concentration may rise to reach levels that are twice those of nonpregnant individuals. Total serum T_3 level also increases to approximately the same extent.[108] A significant portion of this increment is due to the increase in TBG concentration in the first few weeks of pregnancy. This in turn is due to the enhancement by estrogen of sialylation of TBG, which increases its half-life in the serum.[27, 28] Nonetheless, free T_4 and free T_3 concentrations increase during the first trimester. Free hormone concentrations return to normal by about 20 wk of gestation and remain normal until the time of delivery. This pattern coincides with that of hCG activity, which is the probable cause of the change in free hormone levels.[109–111] A decrease in the concentration of TSH occurs during the first trimester, indicating that the increases in free T_4 and T_3 are not due to TSH. TBG continues to increase somewhat throughout pregnancy, although most of the increase has already occurred at 3 to 4 mo of gestation. As will be discussed later, these changes must be kept in mind when interpreting the results of thyroid function tests during pregnancy.

The capacity for hCG to stimulate thyroid function is especially important for patients with hydatidiform moles and choriocarcinomas. In these patients, modest increases in serum free T_4 and T_3 levels may cause clinical thyrotoxicosis; serum TSH is suppressed, indicating the nonpituitary source of the thyroid stimulator. The hyperthyroidism of molar pregnancy is usually not severe and is relieved by evacuation of the mole. One other clinical situation in which the effects of hCG in early pregnancy may play an important role is *hyperemesis gravidarum*. Such patients may have elevated free T_4 levels and, at times, free T_3 levels during the acute phase of their illness.[112] Because they may also have impairment of T_4 metabolism, continued stimulation of the thyroid by hCG may contribute to the inappropriately high free T_4 level, which might otherwise fall during this illness. Because hyperemesis occurs during the first trimester, when the hCG concentration is highest, this explanation is consistent; the serum TSH level is reduced, and the response to TRH is impaired in such patients, similar to the situation in Graves disease.

During the second and third trimesters, the serum TSH concentration is not appreciably different from that in the nonpregnant state, but the TSH response to TRH is accentuated relative to the nonpregnant state, very likely as a result of the hyperestrogenemia that is present.

The BMR increases during the second trimester, and values of +20 to +30 are common at term. The increase in BMR is due to the increase in the total mass of body tissue consequent to the pregnancy. The characteristic changes of pregnancy, together with the decreased peripheral vascular resistance, vasodilatation, and modest tachycardia, may suggest hyperthyroidism. It is important to appreciate that these are physiological changes, especially when treating hyperthyroidism in the pregnant patient.

In the authors' experience, an increased dose of levothyroxine is required for pregnant women with primary hypothyroidism to maintain a normal TSH concentration. After delivery, continuation of this elevated dose causes suppression of TSH below previous levels. One possible explanation for this phenomenon is an increased rate of T_4 deiodination or conjugation. However, it has not been possible to demonstrate a change in the metabolic clearance of T_4 during pregnancy.[113] Alternatively, absorption of levothyroxine may be reduced during pregnancy or the sensitivity of the hypothalamic-pituitary axis may be altered. Although it is not possible to distinguish among these various possibilities, from a practical standpoint, TSH should be monitored during pregnancy to document whether levothyroxine doses must be altered.

Mean total T_4 concentrations in cord serum average 150 nmol/L (12 μg/dL). Serum TBG concentrations are increased, but the increase is not as great as it is in the maternal serum. Free T_4 concentrations at term are slightly less than those in maternal serum. As a manifestation of the low activity of the type 1 deiodinase in fetal life, the serum T_3 concentrations are low, and those of rT_3 are elevated in cord serum. Because any thyroid hormone that traverses the placenta would do so in the unbound or free form, these concentration differentials bespeak a limited transplacental passage of T_4 and T_3 in either direction. Nonetheless, some maternal T_4 can cross the placenta when the fetus has no functioning thyroid. The amounts are sufficient to provide about one third to one half of the normal serum T_4 at the time of birth.[7]

After delivery, the serum TSH concentration in the neonate increases rapidly to a peak at 30 min of extrauterine life, returning to its initial value within 48 h. This neonatal surge of TSH is thought to be due in part to the cooling that follows emergence into the extrauterine environment. Serum T_4 and T_3 concentrations increase rapidly during the first few hours after delivery and are in the hyperthyroid range by 24 h of life. The increase in serum T_4 concentration can be accounted for by the surge in TSH secretion. Although the TSH surge doubtless contributes to the increase in serum T_3 concentration, enhancement of the extrathyroid conversion of T_4 to T_3 is the major factor responsible. Glucocorticoids may play a role in stimulating the conversion of T_4 to T_3 during the perinatal period. In addition, the marked stimulation of T_4-to-T_3 conversion in brown adipose tissue may contribute to the rapidly rising serum T_3 concentration during the first few hours of extrauterine life.[114]

In contrast to T_4 and T_3 the elevated serum rT_3 concentration displays little change during the first 24 h of postnatal life but decreases to normal values by the fifth postnatal day. By the 10th day or so, the serum T_4 and T_3 concentrations are lower but still exceed normal adult values. (See review in ref. 5.)

The serum T_3 concentrations are similarly increased in the first year of life but gradually fall to the normal adult range. Nevertheless, thyroid hormone production rates are higher per unit of body weight in children than in adults. Treatment of congenital hypothyroidism in newborns often requires a dose of 50 μg to maintain serum T_4 concentrations greater than 130 nmol/L (10 μg/dL).[115] When expressed on the basis of body weight, the levothyroxine requirement is about 10 μg/kg in the newborn and decreases progressively to about 1.6 μg/kg in the adult population. Requirements remain stable, except for the increase during pregnancy, until the seventh to eighth decade, when the T_4 production rate decreases 10 to 20%.[116]

Age

The increased serum T_4 concentrations in the neonate gradually decrease, reaching the normal adult range toward the end of the first year. Serum T_3 concentrations remain higher through early adolescence than they are later in life. Early suggestions that serum T_3 concentrations are systematically lower in the seventh and eighth decades (Fig. 8–15) have not been confirmed. In retrospect, this suggestion appears to have been due to the selection of individuals with various types of chronic illness as opposed to entirely asymptomatic individuals in this age group who have normal thyroid function. There appears to be a systematic decrease in the increment of serum TSH in response to TRH in men over the age of 40, which has no clinical significance. Free T_4 concentrations in the aged are somewhat low, on the average, and free T_3 concentrations are at the lower end of the normal range for younger individuals. The RAIU, thyroid clearance rate, and turnover rate decrease slightly with age, resulting in part from the decrease in the total daily disposal of T_4 that occurs with age and in part from an age-dependent decrease in renal iodide clearance. (For a comprehensive review of the effects of aging on thyroid hormone economy, see ref. 116.)

Glucocorticoids

Both corticotropin (ACTH, adrenocorticotropin), through its action on the adrenal cortex, and glucocorticoids influence thyroid function. Pharmacological doses of these agents decrease the thyroid RAIU, clearance rate, and turnover rate. These alterations could be reversed by the administration of exogenous TSH, suggesting that these agents can suppress pituitary TSH secretion. This was confirmed by studies showing that the administration of pharmacological doses of glucocorticoid reduces serum TSH concentrations in both normal and hypothyroid patients. When glucocorticoids are withdrawn, the serum TSH concentration rebounds to values in excess of pretreatment values. With continued administration of glucocorticoids, there occurs an escape from the suppression of serum TSH concentration in some patients. Decreased responses to TRH are also seen in patients with Cushing syndrome[117] and glucocorticoid increases may play a role in the genesis of the inappropriately low serum TSH concentrations during acute illness. The decrease in thyroid secretory rate resulting from the suppression of pituitary TSH secretion is in all likelihood responsible for the slight decrease in the serum T_4 concentration that glucocorticoids induce in normal subjects, because no change in the serum T_4 concentration is seen in hypothyroid patients maintained on a constant daily dose of exogenous hormone. On the other hand, pharmacological doses of glucocorticoid induce a prompt and significant decrease in the serum T_4 concentration in hyperthyroid patients; the mechanism underlying this effect has not been ascertained.[118]

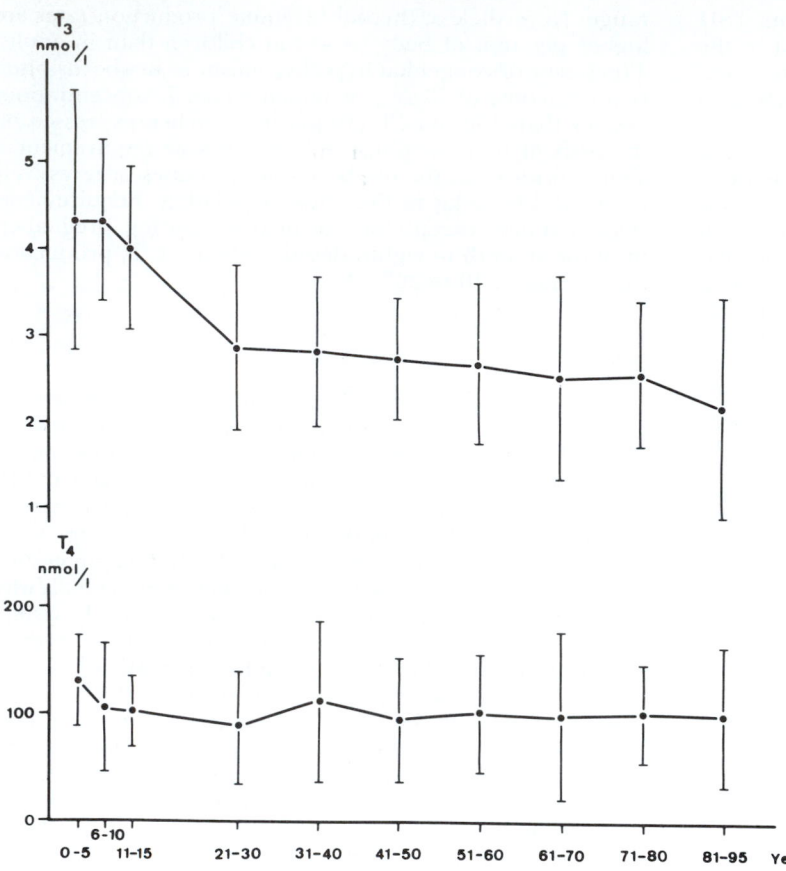

Figure 8–15. Changes with age in serum concentrations of T_3 and T_4. (From Westgren U, Burger A, Ingermansson S, et al. Blood levels of 3,5,3'-triiodothyronine and thyroxine: differences between children, adults, and elderly subjects. Acta Med Scand 1976; 200:493–495.)

Significant decreases in the serum T_3 concentration are induced by pharmacological doses of glucocorticoid in both normal and hyperthyroid patients. This phenomenon also occurs in hypothyroid patients maintained on replacement doses of exogenous T_4. The latter finding, as well as the fact that the decrease in serum T_3 concentration is accompanied by an increase in serum rT_3 concentration, provides compelling evidence that glucocorticoids inhibit monodeiodination of the outer ring of T_4 (and probably rT_3) in extrathyroid tissues. This is the converse of what is seen during the perinatal period, when glucocorticoids appear to result in an enhancement of the extrathyroid conversion of T_4 to T_3.

Pharmacological doses of glucocorticoids decrease the concentration in serum of TBG and increase that of TBPA but do not affect the proportion or absolute concentration of free T_4. Consistent with the latter finding is the observation that glucocorticoids do not induce significant alterations in the metabolic disappearance of T_4. However, they do retard the distributive disappearance of T_4, probably by decreasing the hepatic binding of hormone.

A deficiency of glucocorticoid may also affect thyroid function. Idiopathic Addison disease can be associated with reduced serum T_4 and elevated serum TSH concentrations, suggesting the coexistence of primary hypothyroidism. Surprisingly, treatment of the adrenal insufficiency can lead to complete resolution of the abnormalities in thyroid function, suggesting that they are a consequence of glucocorticoid deficiency rather than primary thyroid disease.[119]

Environmental Temperature

Exposure of human subjects to cold for several days results in an increase in the serum T_4 concentration, which is evident by 24 h and which reaches a maximum by 3 d. The RAIU and clearance rate also increase. These alterations

may represent a compensatory response to a depletion of the peripheral hormone pool, resulting from an increased rate of T_4 metabolism by the peripheral tissues. Short-term exposure to cold is not accompanied by an increased serum TSH concentration in adult subjects. In the newborn, on the other hand, brief cooling provokes an increase in serum TSH concentration, suggesting that the hypothalamus is initially responsive to the cold stimulus but becomes refractory with age.

Small seasonal variations in serum T_4 and T_3 concentrations have been noted in normal subjects. The values for both hormones appear to vary inversely with environmental temperature and are lowest in the summer.[120]

Nutritional Influences

Alterations in nutritional state, whether short-term or chronic, and whether the result of underfeeding, overfeeding, or merely a change in substrate mix, affect various aspects of thyroid hormone economy, especially peripheral hormone metabolism. When euthyroid lean or obese subjects are starved, the serum total and free T_3 concentrations decrease abruptly, often into the clearly hypothyroid range. By contrast, the serum total T_4 concentration remains essentially unchanged although the free T_4 concentration may increase slightly because of a modest decrease in the intensity of iodothyronine binding. Kinetic studies have demonstrated clearly that the decrease in the serum T_3 concentration reflects a decrease in the peripheral generation of T_3 from T_4 rather than a change in its metabolic clearance rate. As serum T_3 concentrations decrease concentrations of rT_3 increase reciprocally, usually to values about twice normal. This is the result not of a major increase in the production of rT_3 but rather of a decrease in its clearance rate. These changes have been ascribed to a selective inhibition of the outer-ring monodeiodination of both T_4 and rT_3, leading to decreased generation of T_3 from T_4 and increased accumulation of rT_3, as noted earlier. (See Fig. 8–4.)

These aspects of peripheral iodothyronine metabolism are exquisitely sensitive to changes in the carbohydrate content of the diet. The abnormal T_3 and rT_3 concentrations in serum are quickly restored to normal, not only by refeeding with a balanced diet but also by administration of small quantities (800 kcal) of pure carbohydrate. Similar quantities of protein have no effect on the serum T_3 level but may lower the serum rT_3 level. Calories given as fat are ineffective. Other evidence of these relationships is that patients receiving hypocaloric diets composed principally of carbohydrate display little or no change in the serum T_3 and rT_3 concentrations.

Despite the decrease in free T_3 concentration that occurs during starvation, the basal serum TSH concentration is unchanged, and the response to TRH is also unaffected or slightly depressed. Several factors could explain this apparent discordance. The pituitary may be responding to the normal or slightly increased concentration of free T_4. Alternatively, starvation may somehow alter the set point of the feedback mechanism or may enhance the sensitivity of the feed back mechanism to T_3. Finally, there is a possibility, supported by studies in the rat, that feedback regulation of TSH secretion is largely conditioned by intrapituitary generation of T_3 from T_4 by the type 2 deiodinase and that this continues unchanged during starvation (Fig. 8–7).

Although measurements of the serum TSH concentration provide no evidence that the peripheral tissues of the starved subject experience a lack of thyroid hormone, other evidence suggests that they do. Basal oxygen consumption and heart rate decline, negativity of the nitrogen balance ultimately decreases, and peripheral steroid metabolism shifts toward the pattern seen in hypothyroidism. These changes are at least partly reversed by administration of exogenous T_3 while fasting continues. It is intriguing to speculate that the decrease in T_3 neogenesis that occurs during fasting is a beneficial, energy- and nitrogen-sparing adaptation and that the mechanism that permits TSH secretion to remain normal, despite the decrease in serum T_3 concentration, allows this adaptation to persist.[71] A decrease in the concentration of T_3 receptors in the liver of the fasted rat may also contribute to this adaptation[121] (see review in ref. 74).

Chronic malnutrition, as in protein-calorie malnutrition, and undernutrition, as in anorexia nervosa, are also associated with a decreased serum T_3 concentration. Serum T_4 concentrations tend to be slightly decreased, but serum TSH concentrations and their response to exogenous TRH are generally normal.

Overfeeding, particularly with carbohydrate, increases the T_3 production rate, increases the serum T_3 concentration, lowers the serum rT_3 concentration, and induces an increase in basal thermogenesis,[122] an apparent converse of the adaptation to starvation.

Nonthyroidal Illness

Diverse abnormalities in thyroid hormone economy, some of them profound, can occur in patients with nonthyroidal illness. Certain of these are common to any type of illness or other physiological insult; others depend on the specific organ system involved. Most consistent are abnormalities in the transport and peripheral metabolism of the thyroid hormones and in their total and free concentrations in the blood. Although the physiological significance of these changes is uncertain, they have major implications for the diagnosis of thyroid disease in patients with moderate or severe intercurrent illness.[74, 123, 124]

A spectrum of abnormalities in peripheral thyroid hormone concentrations and metabolism occurs in euthyroid patients with nonthyroidal illness (see Fig. 8–16). Common to all is a decrease in the serum T_3 concentration, sometimes to extremely low levels and usually accompanied by an increase in the serum concentration of rT_3, the low-T_3 syndrome discussed earlier under the subject of T_4 deiodination pathways. These changes are similar to those that occur during starvation and, like them, have been ascribed to a coordinate reduction in the 5'-monodeiodination of T_4 and rT_3. In patients with cirrhosis and chronic renal disease, kinetic studies have shown this to be the case. Despite a reduction in the intensity of iodothyronine binding, the free T_3 concentration is also subnormal, owing to the marked reduction in total T_3 concentration (see Table 8–3).

Changes of this type in serum T_3 and rT_3 concentrations evidently can be elicited by any physiological stress of sufficient intensity, because they have been reported in many otherwise differing states. Among acute illnesses included are febrile illnesses of all types, acute myocardial infarction, acute respiratory failure, uncontrolled diabetes, and diabetic ketoacidosis; such changes also occur following surgery and the administration of anesthesia. The same changes occur in chronic illness of moderate or severe degree. The more severe the illness, the lower the serum T_3 concentration.

Because the decrease in serum T_3 concentration and increase in serum rT_3 concentration are common to all sick patients, the degree of illness is reflected by the serum total T_4 concentration. Most often this is not appreciably changed. Characteristically, the fraction of free T_4 is increased, especially if measured using an equilibrium dialysis or equivalent technique.[125–127] Because values for the in vitro estimates of the free fraction are often less increased than is the true free fraction, free T_4 indices calculated in the conventional manner may be subnormal.[123, 125] (See the section on diagnostic testing.)

The group of patients most confusing to the endocrinologist are those who are severely ill, often those who are hospitalized in the intensive care unit. In these patients, the severe illness may be complicated by a number of medications including glucocorticoids, anticonvulsants such as phenytoin, and dopamine. In such patients, serum T_4 concentrations are often reduced to less than 30 nmol/L (2 μg/dL) (Fig. 8–16). Serum T_3 is usually undetectable; the serum rT_3 level may be elevated, but, because it is derived from T_4, which is markedly reduced in concentration, it may not be extremely elevated. Even though the free fraction of T_4 is increased, at times the total serum T_4 concentration is so low that the free T_4 level is slightly subnormal. Such patients are generally extremely ill, and some studies have demonstrated that serum T_4 concentrations below 50 nmol/L (4 μg/dL) are associated with a poor prognosis for recovery from the acute illness. In these patients, as in those with illness of less severity, the serum TSH concentration is usually normal or modestly elevated.[127, 128] If dopamine or glucocorticoids are being given, their independent effects to suppress TSH release may partially explain the absence of a TSH elevation.[129] However, in most patients the lack of an appropriate TSH rise in response to a reduced free T_3 level is due to unidentified factors. It may be difficult to distinguish such patients from those with hypothalamic-pituitary hypothyroidism. In some situations, documentation of normal serum cortisol will indicate that global pituitary failure is not present. However, patients in this group are often too sick for thorough pituitary evaluation. In such circumstances, empirical temporary treatment with both glucocorticoid and

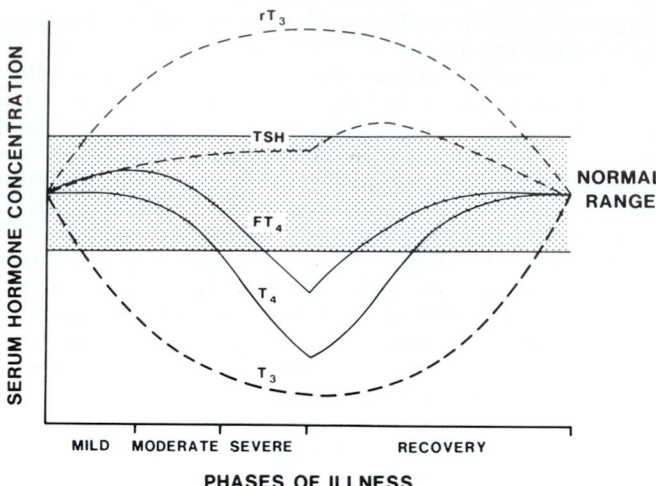

Figure 8–16. The spectrum of thyroid hormone concentrations in ill individuals. The most common abnormalities are a reduction in serum T_3 concentration and an elevation in serum rT_3 concentration, presumably as a consequence of inhibition of the propylthiouracil-sensitive iodothyronine 5'-deiodinase (type 1). Although the total T_4 level may fall, the free T_4 level is generally normal except in extremely ill patients, especially if they are receiving pharmacological doses of glucocorticoid or dopamine. Serum TSH concentration generally remains in the normal range, but it may be suppressed in the very sick patient or by dopamine or glucocorticoid. In some patients, particularly during the recovery phase, the TSH level may transiently rise above normal in patients who have no evidence of permanent thyroid dysfunction. (From Brent GA, Hershman JM. Effects of nonthyroidal illness on thyroid function tests. In: Van Middlesworth L, ed. The Thyroid Gland: A Practical Clinical Treatise. Chicago: Year Book Medical, 1986: 83–110.)

thyroid hormone replacement may be undertaken. In several studies in which thyroid hormone (either T_3 or T_4) has been given to such patients, no significant improvements were seen.[78, 79] Thus, subnormal free T_4 and T_3 levels do not appear to be deleterious in and of themselves.

As indicated, serum TSH concentrations in hospitalized patients without primary thyroid disease are usually normal or reduced. However, a systematic increase in TSH above the normal range occurs as patients recover from severe illness.[130] It seems as if an as yet unidentified endogenous suppressor of hypothalamic-pituitary thyroid function has disappeared, allowing the system to recognize the severe biochemical hypothyroid state and respond appropriately. The elevation in TSH concentration may persist until circulating free T_4 and T_3 levels return to normal. This can be confusing in that occasional patients are recognized in whom the elevated TSH concentration is associated with the still-reduced concentrations of free T_4 and T_3. Such patients meet all diagnostic criteria for primary hypothyroidism with the exception that the symptoms are not usually convincing. Except when the history is strongly suggestive, it is appropriate to follow such patients for 1 wk or more without instituting therapy to ascertain the course of thyroid axis recovery.

A fourth category of patients with illness is less common. These patients are generally thought to be intrinsically euthyroid with systemic illness; their serum T_3 concentrations are subnormal and serum T_4 concentrations are increased during their illness but return to normal thereafter.[131-133] Such patients generally have an elevation in the free T_4 level and free T_4 index (FT_4I) and a reduction in the free T_3 index (FT_3I). This pattern may occur during pregnancy and in patients with hyperemesis gravidarum.[112] It may also occur in patients with acute psychosis. In the latter group, the serum T_3 level may also be increased. The serum TSH concentration or its response to TRH infusion is also generally reduced. Nonetheless, when these patients

recover from acute illness, thyroid function usually returns to normal. In the authors' opinion, a number of such patients may have underlying subtle evidence of autonomous thyroid function that could cause persistent T_4 secretion despite an impairment of T_4 metabolic clearance related to illness. hCG may be involved in the patient with hyperemesis. In other situations, such patients may be very difficult to differentiate from those with T_4 thyrotoxicosis or Graves disease complicated by serious illness. The degree of suppression of the serum free T_3 concentration may be helpful in deciding. In those without intrinsic hyperthyroidism, serum T_3 concentrations tend to be reduced to less than 1 nmol/L (60 ng/dL), whereas patients with hyperthyroidism have higher levels.[131]

Virtually nothing is known of the peripheral metabolic state of the patient with the sick euthyroid syndrome or whether the changes in thyroid hormone metabolism are beneficial, detrimental, or neither.

As mentioned earlier, a decreased concentration of TBG in plasma is often found in patients with severe chronic illness, particularly those with nephrosis and alcoholic cirrhosis. By contrast, an increased concentration of TBG in plasma, with a resulting increase in the serum T_4 concentration, may be seen in patients with acute hepatitis, chronic active hepatitis, or biliary cirrhosis (see Table 8–4).

LABORATORY TESTS OF THYROID HORMONE ECONOMY

In considering the patient with known or suspected thyroid disease, the physician should seek to arrive at two types of diagnosis, an etiological or anatomical diagnosis and a functional diagnosis. The one encompasses an appreciation of the underlying cause or nature of the disorder, as well as the associated pathological change in the gland. The other involves a decision whether the physiological and metabolic state of the patient is being conditioned by an excess, normal, or insufficient supply of thyroid hormone. In many instances the one diagnosis facilitates or influences the other. For example, a patient with a single nonfunctioning nodule in otherwise normal gland is likely to be euthyroid, whereas a patient with a nodule that feels similar but who has clinical and laboratory evidence of thyroid hormone excess is likely to have a benign autonomous adenoma. On the other hand, many ambiguities are possible. An anatomical diagnosis of chronic thyroiditis is consistent with a metabolic state of hypothyroidism, euthyroidism, or thyrotoxicosis, either in different patients or in the same patient at different times. Conversely, clinical and laboratory evidence of thyrotoxicosis may follow from any of a great many causes. Consequently, a complete diagnosis in patients with thyroid disease, which is requisite for proper therapy, recognizes and exploits the interplay between the history, symptoms, and signs; the findings on palpation or biopsy of the thyroid gland; and the results of laboratory tests.

In this section, the laboratory tests employed as aids in the diagnosis of thyroid disease will be discussed. The reasons for this emphasis are many. For one, the fact that so many tests are available is in itself a source of confusion (see classification of tests in Table 8–5). More important, procedures of increasing specificity and sensitivity make possible the detection of thyroid dysfunction in patients in whom clinical findings are marginal or are obscured by coincidental nonthyroidal disorders. Further, even when the clinical picture seems clear and the diagnosis straightforward, the physician often seeks both the reassurance of confirmatory laboratory findings and the advantage of ob-

TABLE 8–5. Commonly Employed Laboratory Tests of Thyroid Hormone Economy

Direct Tests of Thyroid Function
Thyroid radioiodine uptake

Tests Related to Concentration and Binding of Thyroid Hormones in Blood
Measurements of hormone concentration
  Serum total T_4
  Serum total T_3
  Serum free T_4
Measurements of hormone binding
  Free fraction of T_4 or T_3
  In vitro uptake tests
  Thyroid hormone–binding ratio and free hormone index
  Thyroid-binding globulin

Tests That Assess Metabolic Impact of Thyroid Hormones
Basal metabolic rate
Serum cholesterol concentration
Specific serum enzyme concentration
Systolic time intervals

Tests That Assess Mechanisms for Regulating Thyroid Function
Serum TSH concentration
TRH stimulation test
Thyroid suppression test

Miscellaneous Tests
TSH stimulation test
Antithyroid antibodies
Serum thyroglobulin concentration
Immunoglobulins of Graves disease
External scintiscanning
Ultrasonography
Thyroid biopsy

taining pretreatment values. Finally, the profusion of testing procedures indicates that each procedure has inherent limitations. None is uniformly reliable in all disorders of thyroid function, and virtually all are subject to alteration by endogenous or exogenous factors that complicate their interpretation. Such factors may cause the several indices to diverge from their expected values in a confusing or conflicting way. Nevertheless, it is usually possible, through careful selection and interpretation, to achieve a thorough understanding of the physiopathological aberration present. To emphasize this dependence of clinical interpretation on an understanding of the physiological features, laboratory procedures are not discussed after the description of the disease states but after a review of the physiology and biochemistry of the thyroid and its hormones.

Laboratory procedures can be divided into five major categories: (1) direct tests of thyroid function that provide quantitative or qualitative information or both about hormone synthesis and secretion; (2) tests related to the concentration and binding of the thyroid hormones and other iodinated materials in the blood; (3) tests that assess the impact of the thyroid hormones on the tissues (metabolic indices); (4) tests that assess the mechanisms for regulating thyroid function; and (5) miscellaneous tests that do not fit into the other categories.

Direct Tests of Thyroid Function: Radioiodine Uptake

Although many tests exist from which the state of thyroid function can be inferred, it is only by means of in vivo procedures that employ a radioactive isotope of iodine as a tag for the body's stable form of iodine, ^{127}I, that the function of the thyroid gland can be directly measured. Among the many tests of this general type that have been devised, the most common by far is the measurement of the fractional uptake by the thyroid of a tracer (chemically inconsequential) dose of radioiodine, the thyroid RAIU. In the past, the RAIU was frequently employed as a major aid in the diagnosis of hyperthyroidism or hypothyroidism, but several factors have combined to make this less frequently the case. The first is the improvement in indirect methods for assessing thyroid status, either through specific measurement of the thyroid hormones in the blood or through assessment of the mechanisms for regulating thyroid function. The second is the progressive decrease in normal values for thyroid radioiodine uptake consequent to the widespread increase in daily dietary iodine intake. The latter has greatly reduced the usefulness of measurements of thyroid radioiodine uptake in the diagnosis of hypothyroid states.

Two radioactive isotopes of iodine, ^{131}I and ^{123}I, are most commonly employed in a clinical setting. ^{125}I is extensively used as a tracer for in vitro procedures, such as radioimmunoassays, because of its long half-life (60 d) and the consequent long shelf life of reagents labeled with it. ^{131}I (half-life 8.1 d) and ^{123}I (half-life 0.55 d) are both emitters of gamma radiation, which permits their external detection and quantitation at sites of accumulation, such as the thyroid. Physiologically these isotopes are indistinguishable, not only from one another but also from the naturally occurring stable isotope of iodine, ^{127}I, which permits their use as valid tracers. Although ^{131}I has been the radioisotope predominantly used for decades, the shorter half-life of ^{123}I makes it preferable because the radiation delivered to the thyroid per microcurie of administered ^{123}I is only about one hundredth of that delivered by ^{131}I.

Measurements of Thyroid Iodine Accumulation

PHYSIOLOGICAL BASIS. When tracer quantities of inorganic radioiodine are administered either orally or intravenously, the isotope quickly becomes uniformly mixed with the endogenous stable iodide within the extracellular fluid. Immediately on its entrance into the extracellular fluid, I* begins to be removed by its two major sites of clearance, the thyroid and the kidneys. As this process continues, the plasma concentration of I* decreases exponentially. Normally, low values are reached by 24 h and inorganic I* is virtually undetectable in the plasma by 72 h after its administration. Because the quantity of I* that enters the thyroid (or urine) during any time period is proportional to the concentration of I* in the plasma, the thyroid content of I* increases rapidly during the early hours, then at a decreasing rate until a virtual plateau is reached. The proportion of administered I* ultimately accumulated by the thyroid is a function of the relative rates of clearance of iodide by the thyroid and kidneys. The relation is simply expressed as follows:

$$\text{RAIU at plateau} = \frac{C_T}{C_T + C_K}$$

where C_T represents the thyroid iodide clearance rate and C_K the renal iodide clearance rate. The normal thyroid iodide clearance rate is approximately 0.4 L/h and the renal iodide clearance rate is 2.0 L/h, so the ultimate uptake of I* normally approximates 0.17 of the administered dose (range, approximately 0.05 to 0.25).

Measurements of the percent RAIU are generally made at 24 h not only as a matter of convenience but also because the value at 24 h is usually near its plateau except in unusual circumstances to be noted. Usually measurements of the RAIU are taken to indicate the rate of thyroid hormone synthesis and, by inference, the ongoing rate at which thyroid hormones are being released into the blood. In most instances this is justified.

RAIU. The 24-h uptake procedure is the most commonly used isotopic procedure for the assessment of thyroid function per se. It is not necessary that uptake be determined at precisely 24 h. Little difference will be noted if the uptake is measured at any time during the day following the day on which the isotope was administered. In some abnormal states associated with marked hyperactivity, measurements should be made earlier.

Because of the varying sensitivity of different counting devices to scattered or secondary radiation, variations in the geometry of the counting apparatus, and variations in iodine intake, the range of normal values for the uptake at any time interval varies among laboratories and should be determined individually. In general the range of normal values is approximately 5 to 25%. Higher values indicate thyroid hyperfunction, which usually but not always reflects hormone overproduction and a thyrotoxic state. Unfortunately, as with most other procedures, clinically difficult cases with mild hyperthyroidism often display values at or just above the upper limit of the normal range. (See Table 8–6 for a classification of factors that affect the RAIU.)

States Associated with Increased RAIU

Although an increased RAIU may reflect the overproduction and ultimate release of excessive quantities of thyroid hormone, many other factors produce a similar abnormality. An increase will occur whenever the thyroid iodide clearance rate is increased relative to that of the kidney. This may reflect not hyperthyroidism but, for example, a compensatory response to factors tending to produce hypothyroidism. The following clinical states are associated with an increased RAIU.

HYPERTHYROIDISM. Except in the case of T_3 toxicosis (see later), hyperthyroidism is almost invariably associated with an increased RAIU, unless body iodide stores are increased. Such increases in uptake are evident at all times of measurement except in patients with severe thyrotoxicosis, in whom release of hormone is so rapid that the thyroid

TABLE 8–6. Factors That Influence 24-h Thyroid Iodide Uptake

Factors That Increase Uptake
Reflecting increased hormone synthesis
  Hyperthyroidism
  Response to glandular hormone depletion
    Recovery from thyroid suppression
    Recovery from subacute thyroiditis
    Antithyroid agents
  Excessive hormone losses
    Nephrosis
    Chronic diarrheal states
    Soybean ingestion
Not reflecting increased hormone synthesis
  Iodine deficiency
    Dietary supply
    Excessive loss (dehalogenase defect, pregnancy)
  Hormone biosynthetic defects

Factors That Decrease Uptake
Reflecting decreased hormone synthesis
  Primary hypofunction
    Thyroprivic hypothyroidism
    Antithyroid agents
    Some hormone biosynthetic defects
    Hashimoto disease
    Subacute thyroiditis
  Secondary hypofunction
  Exogenous thyroid hormones
Not reflecting decreased hormone synthesis
  Increased availability of iodine
    Dietary or pharmacological supply
    Cardiac or renal insufficiency
  Increased hormone release
    Very severe hyperthyroidism (rare)

content of I* has decreased to the normal range by the time the measurement is made; this is rare and is usually associated with flagrant thyrotoxicosis. Unfortunately, in cases that are clinically marginal, values of the RAIU are often within or just above the upper limit of the normal range, as would be expected.

ABERRANT HORMONE SYNTHESIS. RAIU is increased in the absence of hyperthyroidism in a number of disorders in which accumulated iodine is inefficiently or ineffectively used to synthesize and secrete active hormone. Here the impairment in iodine use leads to enhanced sensitivity to TSH, hypersecretion of TSH, or both; this in turn produces both goiter and stimulation of all steps in hormone synthesis capable of response. As a result, synthesis of normal quantities of hormone may resume; the patient will be metabolically normal but goitrous. Alternatively, secretion of hormone may remain inadequate, and the patient will display goitrous hypothyroidism. This sequence occurs as a consequence of defects in the organic binding or coupling mechanisms or in the structure of the thyroglobulin molecule. It is also a consequence of disorders in which hormonally inactive products are released from the gland in the form of iodotyrosines (dehalogenase defect) or iodoproteins, including thyroglobulin. The magnitude of the increase in uptake and the time at which the plateau is achieved vary with the nature and severity of the disorder. Differentiation of the foregoing states from hyperthyroidism is generally not difficult, because in the former, clinical evidence of hyperthyroidism will be lacking and indeed hypothyroidism may be present. Furthermore, other indices of thyroid hormone production and thyroregulatory control will be concordant with the clinical state.

IODINE DEFICIENCY. Increases in RAIU occur in response to acute or chronic iodine deficiency. Such can be demonstrated by measurement of urinary iodine excretion, values lower than 100 µg/d indicating a deficiency state. Chronic iodine deficiency is most often the result of an inadequate content of iodine in the food and water on which the patients subsist (endemic iodine deficiency). In regions of the world where iodine intake is sufficient as in the United States, deficiency of iodine may result from other than environmental factors. Patients with cardiac, renal, or hepatic disease may develop iodine deficiency if given diets severely restricted in salt, especially if diuretic agents are administered. Iodine deficiency not uncommonly occurs in patients with thyrotoxicosis treated with antithyroid drugs and may forestall recurrence of thyrotoxicity when treatment is withdrawn. Iodine deficiency also plays a role in the goitrous hypothyroidism associated with deficiency of thyroid and peripheral iodotyrosine dehalogenase, in which large quantities of iodine are lost in the urine as iodotyrosines.

In severe iodine deficiency, in addition to the quantitative adjustments in thyroid avidity for iodide that the increased RAIU reflects, a qualitative adaptation occurs in which T_3 is preferentially synthesized and secreted. As a result, the ratio of T_3 to T_4 in the plasma is increased. This mechanism has important adaptive value, because for each atom of iodine secreted the calorigenic impact is approximately four times as great when the iodine is affixed to T_3 as when it is part of T_4.

RESPONSE TO THYROID HORMONE DEPLETION. Withdrawal of factors that lead to thyroid hormone depletion is associated with a rebound increase in thyroid hormone synthesis without an associated increase in hormone release. If hormone depletion has been produced by factors that lead to decreased hormone supply to the tissues, such as antithyroid drugs, the rebound response may reflect in part enhanced TSH stimulation and in part an autoregulatory response to depletion of thyroid hormone stores. In other instances, only the latter mechanism appears to be responsible. Rebound increases in RAIU are seen after withdrawal of antithyroid therapy, after subsidence of transient or subacute thyroiditis, and after prolonged suppression of thyroid function by exogenous hormone. A striking increase in uptake is evident in patients with iodide-induced myxedema after cessation of iodide administration. The duration of the rebound is variable and probably depends on the time required to replenish thyroid hormone stores. Generally it is no longer than several weeks, but after withdrawal of prolonged thyroid suppression, high uptake may persist for many weeks. Differentiation from thyrotoxicosis is evident from the history and from differences in the values of other indices of thyroid function.

EXCESSIVE HORMONE LOSSES. Instances in which excessive losses of thyroid hormone occur may be associated with a compensatory increase in hormone synthesis that is evident in an increased RAIU. In nephrosis excessive losses of hormone occur in the urine in association with urinary loss of binding protein. In addition, diminished binding of T_4 in the plasma in nephrosis may lead to excessive loss of hormone via the feces. A similar sequence may occur when losses of hormone via the gastrointestinal tract are abnormal, as in chronic diarrheal states or during ingestion of agents, such as soybean protein and cholestyramine, that bind the hormone in the gut.

States Associated with Decreased RAIU

As indicated earlier, in the United States the RAIU has largely lost its value in the diagnosis of the most common varieties of hypothyroidism. A general increase in iodine intake has made values of the RAIU in these disorders indistinguishable from those at the lower end of the normal range.

Ironically, therefore, the major indication for measuring the RAIU is to establish the diagnosis of the causes of thyrotoxicosis that are associated with decreased values of the RAIU. As discussed subsequently, these are disorders in which the source of the excess thyroid hormone either is outside the thyroid gland or is a leakage of hormone from a gland that is not actively synthesizing hormone. In addition, the RAIU is subnormal in true hyperthyroidism associated with or actually caused by excessive iodine intake (jodbasedow phenomenon). The value of measurements of urinary stable iodine excretion in differentiating excess iodine from other causes of subnormal RAIU cannot be overemphasized.

HYPOTHYROIDISM. The technical problem involved in utilizing the RAIU as an aid to the diagnosis of hypothyroidism needs no further discussion. A special variety of thyroid failure is that which occurs when destruction of thyroid tissue by chronic inflammation or ablative treatment (surgery or ^{131}I) is incomplete. In this syndrome, often interchangeably termed *decreased thyroid reserve* or *subclinical hypothyroidism*, mild symptoms of hypothyroidism may or may not be present. The RAIU values are often normal but fail to increase after administration of exogenous TSH. The main diagnostic features of this syndrome are, however, evidence of predisposing causes and the presence of mild or moderate elevations of the serum TSH concentration.

EXOGENOUS THYROID HORMONE: THYROTOXICOSIS FACTITIA. Except in disorders in which homeostatic control is disrupted or overridden (e.g., Graves disease or autonomously functioning thyroid nodules), administration of exogenous thyroid hormone will suppress the TSH secretory mechanism and reduce the RAIU, usually to values below 5%. Suppression of uptake can be effected by adequate quantities of any thyroactive material. Suppression of the RAIU by physiological quantities of hormone is, of course, the basis for the normal response in the thyroid suppression test (discussed later in this section). In the same way, lowering of the RAIU level is often used as an index of the adequacy of suppressive therapy in nontoxic goiter. Failure of the RAIU to be suppressed nearly completely when adequate doses of exogenous hormone are administered to patients with nontoxic goiter suggests the presence of foci whose function does not depend on TSH stimulation. This should be confirmed by performance of a thyroid scintiscan while exogenous hormone therapy is continued (suppression scan).

Low values of the RAIU in a patient who is clinically thyrotoxic may indicate the presence of thyrotoxicosis factitia, the syndrome produced by the ingestion, often surreptitious, of excess quantities of thyroid hormone. A nonpalpable thyroid is often another clue. If the offending agent is levothyroxine (T_4) or thyroid extract, values for both the total and free T_4 and T_3 concentrations in serum will be increased. On the other hand, if liothyronine (T_3) is the hormone being consumed in excess, the serum total and free T_4 concentrations will be decreased and the serum T_3 concentration will be increased. The serum TSH concentration is subnormal in either instance. Unmeasurably low levels of thyroglobulin in serum serve to differentiate thyrotoxicosis factitia from other causes of thyrotoxicosis with decreased RAIU. In the latter, which include disorders of hormone storage, serum thyroglobulin concentrations are increased.[134]

DISORDERS OF HORMONE STORAGE. Values of the RAIU are usually low in the early phase of subacute thyroiditis and in the syndrome of chronic thyroiditis with transient hyperthyroidism. Here inflammatory disease leads to follicular disruption, loss of the normal storage function of the gland, and leakage of hormone into the blood. In the early stage of subacute thyroiditis, leakage of hormone accompanied by hormonally inactive iodoproteins is usually sufficient to suppress TSH secretion and decrease the RAIU greatly and is often sufficient to produce thyrotoxicosis. Damage to the follicular epithelium also plays a role in some cases, because the RAIU may not respond well to exogenous TSH. In the syndrome of chronic thyroiditis with transient hyperthyroidism, thyrotoxicosis is present, by definition, and TSH secretion is suppressed. In both disorders the thyrotoxic phase is transient and should not be treated by the measures employed for patients who are hyperthyroid, in whom ongoing overproduction of hormone is present. Transient hypothyroidism often occurs late in both diseases, presumably when stores of preformed hormone are depleted; the RAIU may return to normal or increased values at that time. Clinical features of these diseases are discussed more fully in the section on thyrotoxicosis.

EXPOSURE TO EXCESSIVE IODINE. Exposure to excessive iodine and expansion of body iodide stores are probably the most common cause of a subnormal RAIU. Such decreases are spurious in the clinical sense because they do not indicate decreased absolute iodine uptake or decreased hormone production. They are not spurious in the physiological sense, however, because they reflect a desirable homeostatic response to overavailability of the iodide substrate.

The decreased fractional uptake of iodide is the consequence of an autoregulatory inhibition of the iodide transport mechanism as a result of the increase in the glandular stores of organic iodine. In addition, when plasma iodide concentrations are sufficiently high, dilution of the administered isotope by stable iodide would lead to a decreased percentage accumulation of the isotope. As indicated earlier, the compensatory response to excessive iodine stores is not perfect, and total iodine accumulation during continued overabundance of iodide exceeds normal values. Nevertheless, the excess iodine is not incorporated into active hormone but is organified and then lost from the gland, largely as iodide itself.

A decreased RAIU can be produced by the introduction of excessive quantities of iodine into the body in any form—inorganic, organic, or elemental. Special offenders in this regard are organic iodinated dyes used as x-ray contrast media. The duration of suppression of the uptake varies from individual to individual and with the compound administered, depending on its rapidity of excretion or deiodination. In general, dyes used for pyelography are cleared relatively rapidly, whereas those used in cholecystography persist longer and may influence the uptake for several months. Inorganic iodide may be ingested directly, usually as an expectorant, and after a single large dose a decreased uptake may persist for several days. Chronic ingestion of iodide may depress the uptake for many weeks. Lugol solution or saturated solution of potassium iodide (SSKI) in the dosage usually given (five drops three times per day) delivers up to about 500 mg of iodine daily, as opposed to the customary intake of 500 μg/d in the United States. In addition to iodide per se and iodinated dyes, excessive quantities of iodine may be encountered in a variety of vitamins and mineral preparations, vaginal or rectal suppositories, and iodinated antiseptics such as povidone. Because of its storage in fat, the highly iodinated antiarrhythmic agent amiodarone may serve as a source of excess iodine while it is being used and for many months thereafter. Some preparations of barium sulfate used in x-ray diagnosis may contain substantial quantities of iodine. Large quantities of iodine are ingested in the form of kelp by dietary faddists. Inhibition of uptake resulting from excess stable iodine is of shorter duration in hyperthyroid than in normal individuals.

The measurement of urinary iodine excretion is an invaluable means of establishing or excluding the existence of excessive body iodide stores. When this is desired, a spot urine sample can be obtained and the 24-h iodine excretion extrapolated from the iodine/creatinine ratio. Values in excess of several milligrams daily are sufficient in themselves to explain a low RAIU value, whereas values less than 1 mg daily strongly suggest that a low RAIU value is due to one of the other disorders discussed in this section.

Tests Related to Concentration and Binding of Thyroid Hormones in Blood

Measurements of the concentration of thyroid hormones in serum, together with tests that assess the extent of their association with thyroid hormone–binding proteins, are the most commonly employed laboratory aids for differentiating hypothyroid, euthyroid, and thyrotoxic states. Such tests, when combined with a suggestive clinical picture and measurements of serum TSH levels, are sufficient to establish an accurate functional diagnosis in well over 90% of the cases. Because of their general use and importance, their physiological interest, and the large number of factors that influence their interpretation, these tests will be discussed in considerable detail.

General Considerations

Sensitive and specific radioimmunoassays are widely available for measuring the serum concentrations of the thyroid hormones that are of major clinical importance: T_4, T_3, and in rare instances rT_3. Moreover, the manner in which the concentration of these hormones is influenced by changes in the thyroid hormone–binding proteins, especially TBG, is generally well understood. What emerges from these considerations is that the metabolic state correlates more closely with the free hormone concentration in serum than with the total hormone concentration. Hence the physician must take account of this fact, at least in the initial evaluation of the patient, by obtaining some datum that provides evidence of the free hormone concentration. This can be a measurement of the free hormone concentration itself, an estimate thereof as in a free hormone index, or perhaps a measurement of the concentration of the major binding protein, TBG. A profusion of tests exists by which any or all of these can be assessed.

Nonetheless, some problems persist. First, the degree of abnormality in the tests employed is generally well correlated with the severity of the functional disturbance. Consequently, in patients with mild hypothyroidism or mild thyrotoxicosis, concentrations of the thyroid hormones in the serum, both total and free, may not be clearly different from normal values, and other types of diagnostic tests will be required. Further, many factors other than the supply or production of T_4 and T_3 and the concentration of TBG in plasma can influence the concentration of the two hormones, either singly or together. Acute and chronic illness, starvation, and a variety of drugs decrease the peripheral conversion of T_4 to T_3 (see Table 8–3) and thereby decrease the serum T_3 concentration but leave the serum T_4 level unchanged, slightly increased, or decreased. Further, increased concentrations of T_4 or T_3, but not both, can be caused by the presence in plasma of increased concentrations of protein binding sites that bind one or another of the hormones with greater selectivity than TBG does. For example, serum T_4 concentrations well above the normal range, unaccompanied by abnormal serum T_3 concentrations, are seen in patients with increased TBPA levels and in those with the syndrome of familial dysalbuminemic hyperthyroxinemia. Finally, some patients develop circulating antibodies against T_4 or T_3. These endogenous antibodies interfere with radioimmunoassays for their specific antigens, causing spurious values that are either too high or too low, depending on the method employed.

In the section that follows, the thyroid and nonthyroid disorders that alter serum T_4 and T_3 concentrations, either together or separately, will be defined and discussed. Because of the diverse combinations of change that can be seen and the many factors that produce them, no classification that is both comprehensive and completely consistent can be devised. Therefore, to assist the reader in locating a topic of interest, Table 8–7 contains an outline of the topics discussed and the major heading under which they will be found.

Measurements of Hormone Concentrations

For the thyroid hormones that are of principal clinical interest, T_4, T_3, and rT_3, total concentrations in the blood are almost always measured in whole serum by radioimmunoassays, but nonisotopic immunoassays, some of which are subject to automation, are receiving increasing attention. The quantities of serum required are small (10 to 100 μL). Apart from the usual errors to which any measurement is susceptible, errors peculiar to tests for the thyroid hormones result from competition for the labeled antigen between the specific antibody and other binding proteins. This can occur if binding of the hormone-antigen to plasma proteins is not adequately inhibited by the agents used for this purpose, or if the patient's serum contains an endogenous antibody to the hormone that is being measured.

SERUM T_4 CONCENTRATION. Measurement of the serum T_4 concentration, preferably with some means of

TABLE 8–7. Common Causes of Concordant and Divergent Abnormalities in Serum T₄ and T₃ Concentrations in Untreated Patients*

T₄ Increased, T₃ Increased
All varieties of thyrotoxicosis (see Table 8–11)
Increased TBG (see Table 8–4)
T₄ Increased, T₃ Normal or Low
T₄ toxicosis (thyrotoxicosis with decreased T₄-to-T₃ conversion; see Table 8–3)
Euthyroid sick patient (?)
Familial isolated hyperthyroxinemia
Increased TBPA
Oral cholecystographic agents
Amiodarone
T₄ Normal, T₃ Increased
T₃ toxicosis
Thyrotoxicosis factitia related to liothyronine (T₄ usually decreased)
Iodine deficiency
T₄ Normal, T₃ Decreased
Most patients with decreased T₄-to-T₃ conversion (see Table 8–3)
T₄ Decreased, T₃ Normal
Mild or moderate thyroid failure
Iodine deficiency
Phenytoin, carbamazepine
T₄ Decreased, T₃ Decreased
Severe hypothyroidism
Severe systemic illness (euthyroid patient)
Decreased TBG
Salicylates in high doses (>2.0 g/d)

*See also Table 8–8.

evaluating the state of thyroid hormone binding, is the test usually employed first in the diagnosis of hypothyroidism or thyrotoxicosis. The normal range in healthy, euthyroid adults lies between approximately 64 and 142 nmol/L (5 and 11 μg/dL), but small variations in the normal range among different laboratories should be taken into account. Serum T_4 concentrations at birth are higher than values in the normal adult because of the higher concentration of TBG in neonatal plasma; free T_4 concentrations are about the same as in normal adults. Values rise abruptly within a few hours after birth, peak at about 24 h, and then gradually decrease but, until the age of about 5, remain somewhat higher than those present later in life. They then remain unchanged through the remainder of life.

SERUM T_3 CONCENTRATION. Measurements of the serum T_3 concentration are valuable in diagnosing hyperthyroidism and in following the course of this disorder. They may be useful adjuncts in avoiding overtreatment in patients with hypothyroidism being given synthetic T_4 (levothyroxine). In this respect they may supplement measurements of the serum T_4 and TSH concentrations.

Normal values of the serum T_3 concentration are 1.1 to 2.9 nmol/L (70 to 190 ng/dL). Serum T_3 concentrations display age-related variations. At birth, concentrations are below those found in normal adults. Within a few hours, however, the serum T_3 concentration rises abruptly, peaking at about 24 h at values well into the thyrotoxic range for adults.[5] These gradually decrease during the next few weeks but are somewhat higher through early adolescence (by about 25%) than those in normal adults (see Fig. 8–15). As noted earlier, some reports describe a slight decline in serum T_3 values with age, but others do not. The infirmities of old age, rather than old age itself, may produce the age-related decrease in serum T_3 concentration that has been observed. This problem bears heavily on the question of the levels of the serum T_3 concentration that are diagnostic of thyrotoxicosis in elderly patients. Values at the upper end of the usual normal range in elderly patients should be considered suggestive of this condition.

SERUM rT_3 CONCENTRATION. Measurements of the serum rT_3 concentration are not widely available because they have value only in highly selected clinical circumstances.

The rT_3 in serum is present almost entirely as a result of its generation from T_4 in the peripheral tissues. Consequently the quantity of T_4 available is an important determinant of the serum rT_3 concentration, so that it rises in thyrotoxicosis and declines in hypothyroidism. A second determinant of serum rT_3 concentration is the rate of its catabolism, which proceeds mainly by 5'-monodeiodination to yield 3,3'-T_2. As a result, serum rT_3 concentrations are almost always elevated in euthyroid individuals subjected to those factors that inhibit the conversion of T_4 to T_3, a process that also involves 5'-monodeiodination (see Fig. 8–4, Fig. 8–16, and Table 8–3).

The concentration of rT_3 in serum is much lower than that of T_3 because of the faster metabolic clearance of rT_3. Serum rT_3 concentrations are elevated at birth but decrease to stable values by about the fifth day of life. Values in the elderly tend to increase somewhat, possibly in accord with a concomitant decrease in the serum T_3 level, but uncertainties regarding the frequency and cause of any such increase are analogous to those already described in relation to the serum T_3 concentration.

SERUM PROTEIN-BOUND IODINE (PBI). Although the mainstay of thyroid diagnosis for many years, measurements of PBI are now infrequently performed. The serum PBI measures iodine in T_4, the exceedingly small quantity of iodine in other iodothyronines, a great variety of iodinated materials of exogenous origin that are bound to protein, and endogenous iodoproteins, in which iodine is covalently bound within the peptide sequence of the protein molecule. Hence, when exogenous contaminants are absent, the difference between the PBI and the T_4-iodine is an index of the iodine contained in iodoproteins. Such iodoproteins are commonly found in the sera of patients with Hashimoto disease and subacute thyroiditis and may also be present in the sera of patients with nontoxic goiter and thyroid neoplasms. Here, measurement of the PBI–T_4-iodine difference may be of some diagnostic value.

Measurements of Hormone Binding

As indicated earlier, tests that reflect hormone binding in serum afford the most convenient means of determining whether a change in the total concentration of hormone is due to a change in its binding or a change in its production rate. To put it somewhat differently, they provide clues to free hormone concentration in serum. They assume critical importance, therefore, in interpreting measurements of the serum T_4 and T_3 concentrations to differentiate hyperthyroidism and hypothyroidism from the euthyroid state.

PROPORTION AND CONCENTRATION OF FREE T_4 AND T_3. The absolute concentrations of free T_4 and free T_3 in serum are low and difficult to measure directly. Such measurements are commonly performed by difficult and cumbersome dialysis or ultracentrifugation techniques, particularly the former. Serum is enriched with a tracer concentration of the labeled hormone of interest. This quickly distributes between free and bound forms to match the distribution of the endogenous hormone. The fraction of hormone that dialyzes or ultrafilters through a semipermeable membrane is then measured. The absolute concentration of free hormone can then be calculated as the product of the total hormone concentration and the fraction that is dialyzable or ultrafiltrable. Alternatively, the concentration of T_3 or T_4 can be measured directly in the dialysate. The normal value for the proportion of free T_4 is about 2×10^{-4} (0.02%). Because of the lower affinity of T_3 for TBG, the proportion of free T_3 is normally about 15 times that of T_4, i.e., 3×10^{-3} (0.3%) Normal values for the free hormone concentrations are given in Table 8–2.

Several commercially developed radioimmunoassay methods for estimating the free T_4 level have been used in view of the cumbersome and time-consuming dialysis method used in some laboratories. Two general approaches are used. In the first, the so-called two-step method, serum diluted in buffer is allowed to interact briefly with anti-T_4 antibodies coated on the inner surface of a plastic tube. During this incubation, free T_4 in the serum is extracted and bound by the antibody so that some of its binding sites become occupied. After thorough removal of the dilute serum, a solution containing ^{125}I-labeled T_4 is added to the tube and a second incubation is carried out. This solution is then removed, and the tube is washed and counted. The quantity of labeled T_4 bound to the antibody during the second incubation is inversely related to the number of occupied binding sites on the tube surface and hence to the free T_4 level of the test specimen. Results obtained with this method agree well with those obtained by dialysis across a wide range of clinical disorders.[39]

The other approach to the direct measurement of free T_4 is the so-called one-step or tracer analogue technique. Here, dilute serum and an ^{125}I-labeled analogue of T_4 are placed in tubes coated with anti-T_4 antibodies. Although capable of binding to the anti-T_4 antibody, the analogue is predicated not to be bound significantly by any serum protein; it should, therefore, be totally available to the anti-T_4 antibody. Free, unlabeled T_4 in the serum is bound by the antibody. This decreases the availability of antibody binding sites so that the quantity of labeled analogue bound by the antibody at the end of the incubation is inversely related to the amount of free T_4 in the test specimen. Although methods of this type are theoretically sound and yield values comparable to those obtained with dialysis techniques in patients with hyperthyroidism or hypothyroidism, specious values are seen in other disorders because the tracer analogue does indeed bind to serum albumin and perhaps other proteins. As a consequence, low values are obtained in nonthyroidal illness or hypoalbuminemic states including pregnancy, and high values may be seen in patients with familial dysalbuminemic hyperthyroxinemia or endogenous anti-T_4 antibodies.

The lack of a simultaneous measurement of total T_4 concentration and the free T_4 fraction is a major disadvantage of many of the one- or two-step kits that are used to estimate the free T_4. Such tests often provide only a single value. If this value deviates from the clinical expectation it is not possible for the physician to analyze whether the deviation from normal is due to an unexpectedly altered total T_4 concentration or an unusual value for the free fraction.

IN VITRO UPTAKE TEST: THE THYROID HORMONE–BINDING RATIO. The traditional means of circumventing the technical difficulties inherent in measuring free T_4 by dialysis and direct radioimmunoassay techniques has been the in vitro T_3 or T_4 uptake test. Such tests are performed by enriching the patient's serum with a tracer quantity of I^*-labeled T_4 or T_3 and incubating the serum with a solid-phase matrix, usually a resin particle, or a tube coated with T_3 or T_4 antibody, capable of binding the hormone and competing with the binding proteins of the serum phase. After a standard interval, the proportion of labeled T_4 or T_3 bound by the solid phase is measured. This, like the proportion of free T_4 measured directly by dialysis, varies inversely with the overall concentration of unoccupied binding sites in the serum. As a consequence, this value is proportional to the free fraction of T_3 and T_4 in the original serum. Because of its less intense binding by serum proteins, which leads to higher uptake values and thereby reduces both counting time and error, labeled T_3 is used more often

than is labeled T_4 in the performance of in vitro uptake tests. Because of this it has been customary to refer to such determinations as T_3 uptake or T_3 resin uptake tests. This practice has led to much confusion since T_3 radioimmunoassays have become available. Such terminology is discouraged because it engenders confusion.[135] In addition, when tracer T_3 is used, its distribution among the proteins is determined largely by the concentration of T_4, not of T_3, because T_4 is present in roughly 50- to 60-fold higher concentrations than is T_3, has a higher affinity for the proteins, and occupies virtually the same binding sites.

To obviate this potential source of confusion and to improve the understanding of results obtained in different laboratories, the American Thyroid Association has recommended that the results of such tests be compared with the results obtained for standard control sera from a euthyroid patient with normal quantities of thyroid hormone–binding proteins.[135] This is generally done by dividing the result for the unknown serum by that obtained for the control serum in the same assay. This approach corrects for individual technical variations and for results obtained using different kits for the assays. The quotient of these results has been termed the thyroid hormone binding ratio (THBR) and has a value of 0.85 to 1.10.[135] This number relates the fraction of the tracer free in the patient's serum to that present in normal sera. A value of 1.0 indicates that the two values are identical. Because the THBR value is also proportional to the free fraction of the endogenous thyroid hormone in the serum, it can be multiplied by the total hormone concentration to obtain an estimate of the free thyroid hormone concentration, termed the *free T_4 index* or *free T_3 index*. As discussed earlier under binding protein analyses, the principal binding protein in human serum is TBG. The degree of saturation of this protein with T_4 determines the free fraction of both T_3 and T_4 in virtually all patients. A schematic demonstration of the relationships between total and free T_4, occupied and unoccupied TBG binding sites, and the THBR is shown in Figure 8–17 for normal individuals and those with acquired or congenital alterations in TBG and in Figure 8–18 for subjects with alterations in thyroid function. One advantage of the THBR normalization is that the normal range for the FT_4I is numerically the same as is the total T_4 or T_3.

From Figure 8–17 one can appreciate the utility of the FT_4I calculation. Estrogen, pregnancy, and severe illness are

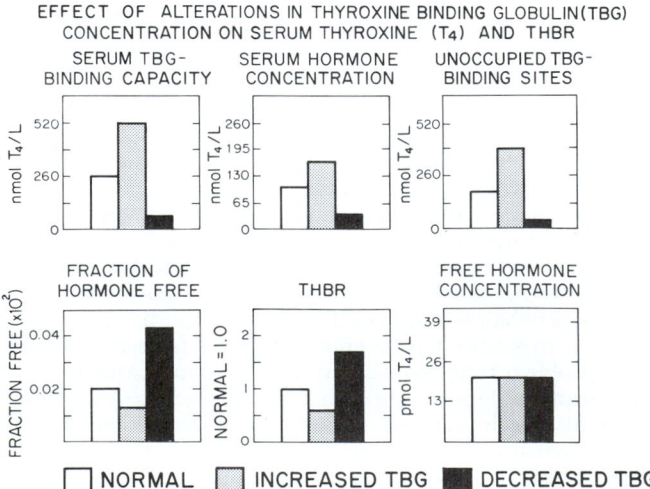

EFFECT OF ALTERATIONS IN THYROXINE BINDING GLOBULIN (TBG) CONCENTRATION ON SERUM THYROXINE (T_4) AND THBR

Figure 8–17. Pattern of changes in the total serum hormone concentration and THBR in euthyroid patients with alterations in the circulating concentration of TBG.

EFFECT OF ALTERATIONS IN THYROID HORMONE PRODUCTION ON
SERUM THYROXINE (T₄) AND THBR

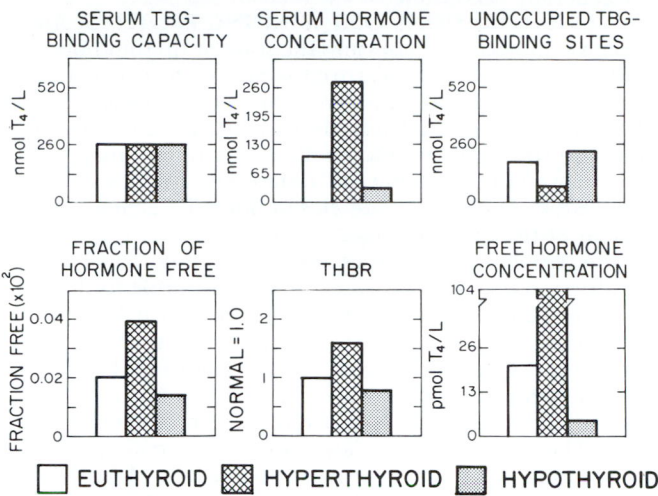

Figure 8–18. Pattern of changes in total serum hormone concentration and THBR in patients with hyperthyroidism or hypothyroidism with normal circulating TBG concentrations.

more common causes of changes in TBG concentration than are hyper- and hypothyroid states (Table 8–4). Therefore, an estimate of the binding ratio or a true estimate of free hormones must be obtained to ascertain the levels of active hormone in serum. Under normal circumstances only about one third of the available binding sites on TBG are occupied by T_4. Thus the concentration of unoccupied TBG binding sites is about 160 nmol/L. Given its intrinsic binding association constant, this leads to a free fraction of T_4 of 2×10^{-4}. During pregnancy, for example, the TBG binding capacity is doubled, the serum T_4 level is also doubled and the level of unoccupied binding sites is increased by the same factor. This increase leads to a reduction of about the same degree in the free fraction, which is reflected in the THBR. If the reduced THBR or free fraction is multiplied by the increased serum hormone concentration, an accurate reflection of the free hormone concentration is obtained. The opposite occurs in patients with reductions in TBG binding capacity. When the serum hormone concentration is reduced the concentration of unoccupied binding sites is reduced to an even greater extent and a substantial increase in free fraction or THBR occurs. Thus free hormone concentrations and the FT_4I remain in the normal range. Under ideal circumstances the THBR is linearly related to the free fraction of thyroid hormones, but this is unfortunately not the case at the extremes of the free fraction range. Thus it is not possible for the THBR to be reduced as much as the free fraction in patients with TBG excess, nor can the degree of increase in the free fraction with TBG deficiency be accurately estimated using the THBR test. Therefore, it is important not only to examine the calculated FT_4I but also to inspect the patterns of the deviations of total hormone measurements and THBR from normal to derive the maximal information from these results. As shown in the two center panels of Figure 8–17, when levels of binding proteins are increased the deviation of total T_4 measurements from normal is in the opposite direction from that of the THBR. If these tests are altered in this fashion, one should be very suspicious that it is an alteration in binding protein concentration that is responsible for the abnormality in the total thyroid hormone measurements rather than an alteration in thyroid hormone production. As discussed later, the opposite pattern occurs when hormone production changes; that

is, the deviations from normal in total hormone level and THBR are in the same direction.

When thyroid hormone production is changed (see Fig. 8–18), the TBG binding capacity is not significantly altered, so the change in unoccupied binding sites is due to the increased quantity of circulating T_4. When the T_4 level is elevated, the concentration of unoccupied TBG binding sites is reduced and both the free fraction and the THBR are increased. Therefore, the free hormone concentration and index are increased to an even greater extent than would be suspected from the change in the total hormone level. The changes in hypothyroidism are generally in the opposite direction. However, because the concentration of unoccupied TBG binding sites does not change greatly when T_4 decreases from a normal mean of 100 nmol/L to a typically hypothyroid value of 30 nmol/L, the change in the free fraction of T_4 is not large, nor is the change in the THBR. Thus although the calculated level of free hormone is markedly reduced, this is not due so much to a reduction of the free fraction as to a reduction in total hormone concentration. In hypothyroidism a typical pattern is a reduction in serum T_4 level and a low normal THBR. From the two central panels in Figure 8–18 it is immediately apparent that when thyroid hormone production is altered the deviations in these two tests away from normal occur in the same direction, whereas the opposite is the case when the abnormality in serum thyroid hormone concentration is the consequence of an altered quantity of circulating TBG. All the analyses just described apply equally well to serum T_3 and T_4.

Simultaneous abnormalities in both TBG and thyroid hormone production can occur. One should be suspicious of hyperthyroidism in a pregnant patient with an extremely high total hormone concentration if the THBR is not subnormal. Likewise, a serum T_4 level in the normal range for a nonpregnant individual accompanied by a severe reduction in THBR should lead to the consideration of hypothyroidism in the pregnant woman. An appreciation of these relationships is critically important for the proper interpretation of thyroid function tests and will remain so until simple, readily available, and reliable techniques are developed for direct assessment of free T_4 and T_3 levels.

Despite the general accuracy of these tests, several caveats should be kept in mind in their interpretation. Theoretically, one should employ radioactive T_4 to estimate the free rT_4 level, but for technical reasons radioactive T_3 is generally used. This can produce difficulties in three situations. One of these is the previously mentioned familial dysalbuminemic hyperthyroxinemia (FDH), an inherited disorder in which a usually minor component of serum albumin is increased (Fig. 8–19). This albumin binds T_4 with increased affinity, but its binding affinity for T_3 is not comparably increased.[136, 137] In sera of such patients total T_4 concentrations may be increased 1.5 to 2-fold, and although the free fraction of T_4 is appropriately reduced, the free fraction of T_3 is not. Thus if one uses tracer T_3 to estimate the free fraction, the THBR is normal and the FT_4I is increased. Before this condition was recognized, such patients were sometimes treated for hyperthyroidism because of the abnormal values even when symptoms of thyrotoxicosis were not clear-cut. Possible artifacts in thyroid function testing should always be considered when the results of the clinical assessment do not agree with the laboratory finding. As will be discussed subsequently, patients with this syndrome should have normal serum T_3 concentrations. This feature can be used to differentiate them from patients with true hyperthyroidism. In addition the serum TSH level is normal, not suppressed as in a patient with true hyperthyroidism. A similar high-affinity T_4-binding TBPA has been described.

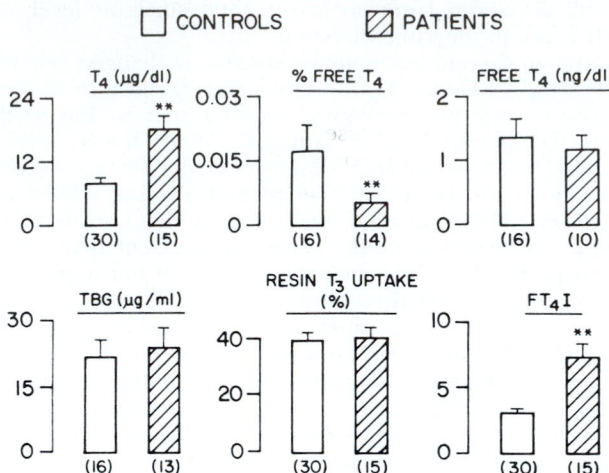

Figure 8–19. Indices of thyroid function in serum of patients with FDH and of euthyroid controls. Increased intensity of overall T₄ binding is evident in the decrease in the percentage of free T₄, but the resin uptake of T₃ is unchanged because the overall intensity of T₃ binding is little affected. As a result, the calculated FT₄I is greatly increased and no longer reflects the true free T₄, which is normal. (From Ruiz M, Rajatanavin R, Young RA, et al. Familial dysalbuminemic hyperthyroxinemia, a syndrome that can be confused with thyrotoxicosis. Reprinted, by permission of The New England Journal of Medicine, 306; 635–639, 1982.)

A second rare problem is due to the presence of endogenous antibodies directed against either T_4 or T_3. If the antibodies are directed against T_3, a THBR based on tracer T_3 will be markedly reduced even though the free fraction of T_4 is normal. Such patients have normal total serum T_4 concentrations, but serum T_3 concentrations may be altered artifactually by the antibody depending on the techniques used to assay it. If an immobilized antibody method is used, the T_3 level appears to be elevated because the endogenous antibody reduces the amount of tracer T_3 bound to the immobilized anti-T_3 antibody. On the other hand, if a charcoal separation of bound and free tracer T_3 is used, an inappropriately low result is obtained. In patients with a circulating anti-T_4 antibody, the total T_4 level is usually elevated but the free T_4 level is unchanged. As in FDH, the free fraction estimated using tracer T_3 is not altered.

A third situation in which the FT₄I may be unreliable is in patients who are ill, as already discussed. There is disagreement in the literature about the true free hormone level under these circumstances. As data from more carefully assayed samples accumulate, it is seen that the free T_4 level is rarely reduced in euthyroid patients regardless of the severity of illness.[126, 127] Why does the THBR based on T_3 not reflect the true increase in the free fraction of T_4 under these circumstances? One possibility is that a substance in the serum of these individuals competes with T_4 for binding to TBG but is diluted during the in vitro assessment so that it does not compete effectively under those circumstances. Such a substance would be not unlike salicylate or phenytoin.[102] Another possible cause may be the generation of a significant quantity of free fatty acid that competes with T_4 for TBG binding. This occurs after heparin administration.[138] Another possibility is that as a concomitant of the complex changes in serum thyroid hormone–binding proteins during illness, TBG with altered binding properties accumulates in the serum. Such TBG might not bind T_4 and T_3 with the same relative affinities as the normal protein. Accumulation of a deglycosylated TBG that has these properties has been suggested to explain the inappropriately normal free T_3 fraction in the sera of ill patients. Many of these problems could be corrected by the use of tracer T_4

(as opposed to T_3) in the uptake determination, but this has not generally been done.

CONCENTRATIONS OF T₄-BINDING PROTEINS. An alternative approach to assessing the state of thyroid hormone binding in serum is to measure the activity or concentration of the T_4-binding proteins. With the aid of labeled T_4 and of filter paper electrophoresis to separate the individual binding proteins from one another, saturation analysis can be employed to determine the T_4-binding capacities of TBG and TBPA. These correlate closely with the actual concentrations of the two proteins.

Electrophoretic analysis of T_4-binding capacities is mainly a research tool because an important role for binding of T_4 by TBPA has not been demonstrable, at least in the static sense, and satisfactory radioimmunoassays for TBG have been developed. Normal concentrations of TBG measured by radioimmunoassay are about 260 nmol/L (1.0 to 1.5 mg/dL) and tend to be slightly higher in women than in men. The disorders associated with abnormalities in the concentration of TBG are shown in Table 8–4. Measurement of the serum TBG concentration can be employed in diagnosing hypothyroidism or thyrotoxicosis in one of two ways. First, calculation of a T_4/TBG or a T_3/TBG ratio yields values that correlate well with the FT₄I or FT₃I. Second, on the assumption that TBG is the major determinant of the overall intensity of T_4 binding, a calculated value of the free T_4 can be derived from the concentrations of TBG and total T_4 and the association constant for the interaction between the two. In most instances, values calculated in this manner correlate very well with free T_4 values directly determined.

States Associated with Abnormal Hormone Concentrations in Blood

As indicated earlier, the concentrations of T_4 and T_3 in the blood are a function of two factors. The first is their rate of production or supply. Unless T_4 is being ingested, its supply is a reflection only of its rate of secretion from the thyroid, but the supply of T_3 reflects both secretion from the gland and production from T_4 in the peripheral tissues. The second factor is the rate of clearance of T_4 and T_3 from the blood, and this is a function largely of the intensity of their binding by serum proteins. In view of the many pathophysiological factors and pharmacological agents that affect one or another aspect of thyroid hormone economy-thyroregulatory mechanisms, the thyroid gland itself, and the peripheral transport and metabolism of the thyroid hormones—it is not surprising that in addition to the characteristic increases or decreases in serum thyroid hormone concentrations seen in thyrotoxicosis and hypothyroidism, respectively, one finds aberrations in serum T_4 and T_3 concentrations, and even in free T_4 and free T_3 values, in many conditions in which the patient's thyroid function is intrinsically normal, i.e., in which there is no definite thyroid disease. This section discusses the conditions in which values of the serum T_4 concentration or serum T_3 concentration or both are abnormal and seeks to differentiate those associated with intrinsic thyroid disease from those in which thyroid function is intrinsically normal. Unfortunately, disorders that cause changes in serum hormone concentrations are so diverse that no classification of them is satisfactory. In earlier editions of this book an effort was made to classify disorders in relation to whether they produced concordant or discordant changes in the serum total T_4 and T_3 concentrations. In the present edition this mode of classification is retained in Table 8–7. The table makes evident, however, the great heterogeneity of the disorders within each major category. Consequently, the discussion of disorders that alter serum T_4 and T_3 concentrations is organized primarily according to the type of disorder, rather than the nature of the change in hormone concentrations. Consideration of the table and the text will provide a vertical and horizontal view of the topic.

Disorders Associated with Thyrotoxicosis

Thyrotoxicosis is the syndrome that reflects the response of the peripheral tissues to an excess of thyroid hormone. The disorders that lead to thyrotoxicosis can be divided into two categories: those that are associated with true hyperthyroidism (e.g., ongoing overproduction of hormone by the thyroid gland) and those that are not. In the latter category the excess hormone either is extrathyroidal in origin or leaks from an inflamed, hypofunctioning thyroid gland. Classification of the causes of thyrotoxicosis into these two categories is useful because their modes of treatment are different.

INCREASED SERUM T_4 AND T_3 CONCENTRATIONS. An increase in both the serum T_4 and T_3 concentrations is the usual pattern in patients with hyperthyroidism, regardless of whether this is caused by Graves disease, toxic multinodular goiter, toxic adenoma, or the unusual varieties of thyroid hyperfunction caused by ectopic or inappropriate thyroid stimulators (molar pregnancy, choriocarcinoma in the uterus or testis, hypothalamic-pituitary dysfunction, or pituitary tumor leading to hypersecretion of TSH). Serum T_4 concentrations range from values that are only slightly elevated in patients with mild disease to values in excess of 320 nmol/L (25 μg/dL) in the most severe cases. Concentrations of T_3 are almost invariably increased, sometimes to many times the mean normal value. Usually the increase in T_3 concentration is proportionately greater than the increase in serum T_4 level, so the T_3/T_4 ratio in serum is almost always elevated.[59] This stems from the fact that in hyperthyroidism the serum T_3 reflects not only peripheral generation from T_4 but also hypersecretion from the thyroid gland of a product with a high T_3/T_4 ratio. The thyroglobulin from the Graves disease patient has a T_3/T_4 ratio about twice that of normal thyroglobulin.[18] As a consequence the serum T_3 concentration may be elevated when the serum T_4 concentration is not. Hence, the diagnosis of hyperthyroidism should never be abandoned on the basis of measurements involving T_4 alone.

Increased values of both the serum T_4 and T_3 concentrations are usual in thyrotoxic states that are not associated with true hyperthyroidism: thyrotoxicosis factitia related to ingestion of large quantities of levothyroxine or thyroid extract, overproduction of hormone by ectopic thyroid tissue, and leakage of hormone from the gland in the early phase of subacute thyroiditis or in the syndrome of chronic thyroiditis with transient thyrotoxicosis. T_3/T_4 concentration ratios in serum are usually not as high as those seen in true hyperthyroidism. In these nonhyperthyroid varieties of thyrotoxicosis there is no abnormal thyroid stimulator, no excess of TSH, and no focus of autonomous function within the gland. Consequently, suppression of TSH secretion by the excess of hormone in the blood is reflected in subnormal values of the RAIU. Thyrotoxicosis in the presence of a decreased RAIU should also suggest the possibility of iodine-induced hyperthyroidism (jodbasedow). This can be confirmed or excluded by measurement of the urinary iodine excretion.

In all the foregoing disorders, owing to the increase in serum T_4 concentration and frequently to a modest decrease in the concentration of TBG, the concentration of unoccupied binding sites on TBG is reduced and the proportions of free T_4 and free T_3 and the THBR are increased. Hence, values of the free T_4 and free T_3, as well as their corresponding indices, are increased even more markedly (see Fig. 8–18).

T_3 TOXICOSIS. Thyrotoxicosis associated with an increased serum T_3 concentration but a normal or occasionally low serum T_4 concentration is the entity termed T_3 *toxicosis*. It can occur in the course of any disorder that causes hyperthyroidism. Except for thyrotoxicosis factitia related to ingestion of liothyronine (T_3), it is unlikely to occur in thyrotoxic disorders that are not associated with true hyperthyroidism. The prevalence of T_3 toxicosis among patients initially diagnosed as being thyrotoxic is uncertain but may be as high as 5%, or even higher in areas of iodine deficiency.

T_3 toxicosis almost certainly reflects a predominant hypersecretion of T_3 by the thyroid, rather than an increase in the peripheral conversion of T_4 to T_3. Some patients with T_3 toxicosis, if left untreated, develop the usual variety of hyperthyroidism in which the serum T_4 and T_3 concentrations are both increased. Similarly, in patients with Graves disease who have been in remission following prior therapy, an increase in the serum T_3 concentration may herald recurrence of a thyrotoxic state.

The proportion of free T_4 and the THBR values are generally *normal* in patients with T_3 toxicosis, as are values for the free T_4 and FT_4I. This is due to the fact that the excess T_3 occupies a negligible fraction of the TBG binding sites. Values for free T_3 and FT_3I would, of course, be increased.

T_4 TOXICOSIS. Thyrotoxicosis in association with an elevated serum T_4 concentration and a normal or slightly decreased serum T_3 level is termed T_4 *toxicosis*. It is seen in patients with intercurrent illness, the elderly, and patients who have recently been exposed to large quantities of iodine, as in x-ray contrast studies.[131–133] The pathogenesis of T_4 toxicosis is not clear, but the relatively low serum T_3 concentration may result from loss of that component contributed by peripheral conversion of T_4 to T_3 owing to inhibition of this process by intercurrent illness or by agents that inhibit the conversion of T_4 to T_3, such as oral cholecystographic agents or amiodarone.[75–77] Excess iodine may also cause the thyroid secretory product to have a lowered T_3/T_4 ratio.

Euthyroid Hyperthyroxinemia: Increased Serum Thyroxine Level Associated with Intrinsically Normal Thyroid Function

Many disorders are characterized by an elevation of the serum T_4 concentration in patients whose thyroid function is intrinsically normal and who have no definable thyroid disease. These disorders, which cover a broad spectrum of abnormal states, have been categorized as states of euthyroid hyperthyroxinemia, a topic that has been extensively reviewed.[33] The causes of euthyroid hyperthyroxinemia can be subdivided into four major categories: increased T_4 binding by serum protein, peripheral resistance to thyroid hormones, the effects of certain drugs and hormones, and the effects of certain illnesses. The major laboratory features of the various disorders associated with euthyroid hyperthyroxinemia are indicated in Table 8–8. It is only in the category of increased T_4 binding that the free T_4 level is normal. In conditions associated with increased T_4 binding, the basal serum TSH concentration is also normal, providing additional evidence of a euthyroid state. In all the remaining varieties of euthyroid hyperthyroxinemia, in contrast, the free T_4 level is elevated, and in some the serum T_3 concentration is increased in addition, sometimes in association with abnormalities in the serum TSH concentration. Thus in some of the disorders to be considered, thyroid function and the supply of active hormone to the peripheral tissues

TABLE 8–8. Causes of Euthyroid Hyperthyroxinemia

Cause	FT$_4$I	FT$_4$	T$_3$	TSH
Alteration in T$_4$ binding in serum				
Increased TBG concentration	N*	N	I	N
Familial dysalbuminemic	I	N†	N	N
hyperthyroxinemia	I	N	N	N
Increased T$_4$ binding to TBPA and	I	N‡	N	N
anti-T$_4$ antibodies				
Generalized peripheral tissue and	I	I	I	N or I
pituitary resistance to thyroid hormone				
Nonthyroidal illness				
Sick euthyroid syndrome	I or N	I or N	D	N, D, or I
Acute psychiatric illness	I	I	N or I	N or D
Hyperemesis gravidarum	I	—	N	D
Drugs				
Oral cholecystographic agents	I	I	D	I
Amiodarone	I	I	D	I§
Amphetamines	I	I	N	I
Heparin (in vitro artifact)	I	I	N	—
Propranolol (>200 mg/d)	I	I	D	N
Exogenous T$_4$ administration				
Levothyroxine administration	I	I	N	D
Dextrothyroxine administration	I	I	I	D
High altitude	I	I	I	N or I

*I, increased; D, decreased; N, normal.

†Free T$_4$ is increased when assessed by radioimmunoassay methods that employ ^{125}I-labeled T$_4$ analogues.

‡Free T$_4$ is increased when assessed by radioimmunoassay methods that employ ^{125}I-labeled analogues. Free T$_4$ (equilibrium dialysis) is increased when serum total T$_4$ is measured by double-antibody or solid-phase methods in unextracted serum and decreased when serum T$_4$ is measured by methods that employ polyethylene glycol, dextran-coated charcoal, or ammonium sulfate.

§Observed during during first 3 mo of treatment.

Modified from Rajatanavin R, Braverman LE. Euthyroid hyperthyroxinemia. J Endocrinol Invest 1983; 6:493–505.

may be abnormal. Nonetheless, these disorders are classified as euthyroid hyperthyroxinemia because the abnormalities are transitory, disappearing when the causative factor is withdrawn and leaving the patient with normal thyroid function and no identifiable thyroid disease.

INCREASED T$_4$ BINDING. An increase in the serum T$_4$ concentration secondary to increased binding of T$_4$ by serum proteins is a common variant of euthyroid hyperthyroxinemia. As revealed in Table 8–8, the true free T$_4$ value is normal in all patients with euthyroid hyperthyroxinemia caused by increased T$_4$ binding, but the FT$_4$I level, as usually calculated from the THBR, is normal only when increased T$_4$ binding is due to an increase in the serum TBG concentration. As discussed earlier, the use of radioactive T$_3$ to estimate the free T$_4$ fraction is not valid when some serum protein other than TBG binds T$_3$ little if at all but contributes substantially to the binding of T$_4$. The physician should be alerted to the possible presence of an abnormal T$_4$-binding protein if, in the face of marked elevation of the serum T$_4$ value, the serum T$_3$ and THBR results are normal.

An increased serum TBG concentration is the commonest cause of concurrent elevations of the serum T$_4$ and T$_3$ concentrations. This occurs in a variety of clinical states (see Table 8–4), and in these situations a number of secondary consequences occur (see Fig. 8–6). Most important clinically are secondary increases in the serum T$_4$ and T$_3$ concentrations, coupled with both decreases in the percentages of free T$_4$ and free T$_3$ and lowered values of the THBR (see Fig. 8–17). The extent of increase in the serum T$_4$ and T$_3$ concentrations varies with the increase in TBG; in pregnancy the concentration of TBG is approximately doubled. The free T$_4$ and FT$_4$I values remain normal. The increase in serum T$_3$ concentration is less, with the result that values for the free T$_3$, although within the normal range, aggregate toward its lower end. Kinetically, decreases in the metabolic clearance rate of T$_4$ and T$_3$ are counterbalanced by the increase in serum concentrations, so that calculated production rates for the two hormones are normal and the patients remain euthyroid.

The most common causes of an increase in the concentration of TBG in plasma are those associated with hyperestrogenemia, notably pregnancy and the taking of contraceptive steroids. This phenomenon is due to an estrogen-induced increase of the sialic acid content of TBG.[27] This change prolongs the half-life of the molecule in the circulation, resulting in a higher plasma concentration with no change in the rate of TBG synthesis. Increased TBG values are also seen in women taking natural or synthetic estrogens for the treatment of menopausal symptoms, in some patients using topical estrogens, and in some with estrogen-producing tumors. The serum TBG level is also increased by the estrogen antagonist tamoxifen, which functions as a weak estrogen agonist.

The increase in TBG during normal pregnancy is detectable at about the third week after impregnation, is clearly evident several weeks thereafter, and persists throughout the remainder of gestation. Levels of TBG begin to decline immediately post partum and return to normal 4 to 6 wk later. A similar course follows the administration and withdrawal of exogenous estrogens. As a result of abnormalities in the conceptus, likely accompanied by a subnormal secretion of estrogens, the increase in TBG level in gravid patients who undergo spontaneous abortion by the 10th or 12th week of pregnancy is absent or subnormal.

An increase in TBG concentration is found in some patients with acute intermittent porphyria, especially women. The reason for this finding is unknown. Several diseases of the liver are associated with an increased concentration of TBG in the plasma. Among them are acute hepatitis, chronic active hepatitis, and biliary cirrhosis. In the latter two disorders, the free T$_4$ and FT$_4$I values may be subnormal, indicating some degree of associated thyroid failure, possibly with an autoimmune basis. Chronic abusers of heroin and methadone also display an increase in TBG level, probably because of associated liver disease.

Rarely, increased TBG concentration is the result of a familial disorder that is usually transmitted as an X chromosome–linked trait. This abnormality can be discovered during neonatal screening programs or in the screening of families of propositi known to have elevated TBG values. More commonly it is recognized after the chance finding of an elevated serum T$_4$ concentration, with the consequence that some patients have been treated mistakenly for hyperthyroidism. The familial variety is not associated with hyperestrogenemia, and, unlike the increase in TBG level induced by estrogen, it is not accompanied by an increase in the serum concentration of other estrogen-sensitive transport proteins, such as ceruloplasmin and corticosteroid-binding globulin. The presence of a familial elevation in TBG does not exclude the possibility of associated thyroid disease. In such patients, the sialylation of TBG is normal, as it its metabolic clearance.[27, 28]

Serum T$_4$ concentrations are also increased (usually two to three times normal) in patients with FDH (see Fig. 8–19). The syndrome is due to the appearance in serum of significant amounts of albumin(s) with an unusually high affinity for T$_4$, similar to that of TBPA.[136, 137] Because these albumins bind T$_3$ only weakly, they contribute little to the overall net binding affinity for T$_3$. As a consequence, both the serum T$_3$ concentration and the THBR remain in the normal range in patients with FDH, but FT$_4$I calculated from the THBR is high because of the increase in T$_4$. Further, serum TBG and TBPA concentrations are normal and, accordingly, the T$_4$/TBG ratio is elevated. For reasons discussed earlier, one-step analogue estimates of free T$_4$ are artifactually elevated in this syndrome because the abnormal albumin binds the analogue. Although the foregoing tests suggest the presence of thyrotoxicosis, patients with FDH are euthyroid, and both directly measured free T$_4$ values and serum TSH levels are normal. FDH is transmitted as an autosomal dominant trait and is expressed equally in males and females. Its prevalence is uncertain.

Two syndromes of euthyroid hyperthyroxinemia are due to increased binding of T$_4$ by TBPA. The first is caused by a pronounced increase in the serum TBPA concentration and has been described in two patients, both with a glucagon-secreting tumor of the pancreatic islet cells. The first patient had a serum T$_4$ concentration approximately twice normal and a three- to fourfold elevation of the serum concentration of TBPA.[139] TBPA was demonstrated both in tumor cells and in alpha cells of normal human pancreatic islets by immunofluorescence, suggesting that TBPA can be synthesized in these cells. The second syndrome in this category has been described in several members of a single family.[140] Here the abnormality is apparently an increase in the binding affinity of TBPA, because both the concentration and T$_4$-binding capacity of TBPA are normal. As would be expected from the negligible T$_3$-binding activity of TBPA, serum T$_3$ concentrations and the THBR results remain normal, and as a result values of the FT$_4$I calculated in the usual manner are increased, mistakenly suggesting that the patient is thyrotoxic.

Because all patients with euthyroid hyperthyroxinemia are euthyroid, measurements of serum TSH can be used to confirm that the thyroid hormone concentrations are artifactually elevated and that hyperthyroidism is not present.

PERIPHERAL RESISTANCE TO THYROID HORMONES. Patients have been reported whose peripheral tissues appear to be at least partially resistant to the actions of thyroid hormone. In such patients serum total and free T$_4$ and T$_3$ concentrations are elevated, although clinical features of thyrotoxicosis are lacking, and both basal serum TSH concentrations and the response to TRH are normal or increased. Clinical features vary widely. Some patients have goiters; others do not. None has had the full-blown clinical picture of hypothyroidism associated with thyroid failure, and some appear euthyroid. Others display selected features of thyroid hormone lack, such as growth retardation, stippled epiphyses, delayed bone maturation, and deaf-mutism. Some degree of resistance to thyroid hormones at the pituitary level is evident in the combination of laboratory findings already described, but the ease of suppression of TSH secretion by exogenous hormone is variable. Theoretically the syndrome may be related to that in which excessive secretion of TSH leads to frank hyperthyroidism, but, if so, the latter would appear to reflect resistance to thyroid hormone action mainly or solely at the level of the pituitary gland. In some clinically euthyroid patients with thyroid hormone resistance the disorder appears to be sporadic, but in others it is familial, although its mode of inheritance is unclear. The molecular mechanisms responsible for resistance to the actions of thyroid hormone are uncertain and may vary among different patients.[141–144]

NONTHYROIDAL ILLNESS. Almost any illness or physiological stress of sufficient severity is capable of inducing changes in one or more aspects of thyroid hormone metabolism. These responses constitute what is commonly termed the *low-T$_3$ syndrome* (see Table 8–2). Other responses seem more specifically related to the type of illness from which they arise. Notable among them are acute psychiatric illness[145] and hyperemesis gravidarum.[112] Hyperthyroxinemia may occur in these disorders, but the mechanisms responsible are doubtless different and have been addressed

under the section on the thyroid pathophysiology during illness and pregnancy. The single exception to the pattern of illness-related alterations in thyroid function is found in patients with human immunodeficiency virus (HIV) infection resulting in acquired immunodeficiency syndrome (AIDS) (Table 8–9). At all levels of illness the composite laboratory profile is dominated by an elevation in the TBG level. The explanation for this elevation is not known.[146]

Acute psychiatric illness is also associated with a number of perplexing alterations in results of various thyroid function tests, among which are increases in the serum T$_4$ concentration. Approximately one third of the patients who are hospitalized display this abnormality, and in most the free T$_4$ and FT$_4$I values are increased as well. Serum T$_3$ concentrations are normal or increased. These abnormalities are not a function of the nature of the psychiatric illness, although they are more common in patients with schizophrenia. They are also unrelated to medications the patients may have been taking and disappear without specific treatment within a few weeks. A puzzling aspect of this pattern is that responses to TRH in patients with hyperthyroxinemia are normal or flat and are poorly correlated with the initial serum T$_4$, free T$_4$, or FT$_4$I value. Further, after the serum T$_4$ and FT$_4$I values return to normal, the abnormal response to TRH stimulation may or may not persist.[145]

DRUGS. Drugs can lead to elevations of the serum T$_4$ concentration by different mechanisms. Some act by inhibiting the conversion of T$_4$ to T$_3$, others by interfering with the tissue binding of T$_4$, and still others, apparently, by an effect on central thyroregulatory mechanisms.[147]

Among the agents that inhibit peripheral T$_3$ production are certain oral cholecystographic agents, including iopanoic acid, sodium ipodate, tryopanoate, and iobenzamic acid (see Table 8–3). After administration of these agents, the serum T$_3$ concentration decreases and the serum rT$_3$ concentration increases. The accompanying hyperthyroxinemia presumably results from stimulation of the thyroid, because modest increases in the serum TSH value and its responsiveness to TRH are also seen.[77] This, in turn, is probably the result of both decreased delivery of T$_3$ to the pituitary from the circulation and inhibition of local T$_3$ formation by the contrast agents.[86] Agents of this type also discharge T$_4$ from its intrahepatic binding sites, but the extent to which this contributes to hyperthyroxinemia is uncertain. Amiodarone, a heavily iodinated antiarrhythmic agent, is also a potent inhibitor of the 5'-monodeiodinase for T$_4$ and produces effects on thyroid-related hormones similar to those produced by the contrast agents.[75, 76] After relatively short-term administration, effects may persist for as long as 6 wk because of storage of the drug in fat, but effects of the drug on the serum TSH level tend to regress after several months despite continued treatment. Amiodarone is also apt to induce either hyperthyroidism or hypothyroidism, probably as a result of the iodine released as the drug is metabolized.[148]

TABLE 8–9. Thyroid Function Studies in Patients with HIV Infection

Group	T$_4$ (nmol/L)	THBR	T$_3$ (nmol/L)	rT$_3$ (nmol/L)	TBG (nmol/L)
Reference value	95	1.00	2.3	0.28	288
Patients with AIDS-related complex	112	0.87	2.2	0.21	419
Patients with AIDS	99	0.88	2.1	.17	423
Patients with *Pneumocystis carinii* infection					
Survivors	110	0.92	1.3	0.28	476
Nonsurvivors	83	1.02	0.56	0.35	379

Data from LoPresti JS, Fried JC, Spencer CA, et al. Unique alterations of thyroid hormone indices in the acquired immunodeficiency syndrome (AIDS). Ann Intern Med 1989; 110:970–975.

That amiodarone could be a T_3 antagonist[149] seems unlikely given the fact that serum T_3 and TSH concentrations are normal in most patients receiving this drug.[150] Propranolol is also capable of inhibiting peripheral 5'-monodeiodinases and, as a consequence, lowers the serum T_3 concentration and elevates the rT_3 concentration. Serum TSH concentrations and responses to TRH are generally unchanged.[151]

The capacity of L-propranolol to inhibit conversion of T_4 to T_3 is apparently related not to its beta-adrenergic blocking activity but to its membrane-stabilizing effect, because it is reproduced by D-propranolol, which is not an effective beta-blocker. Other beta-adrenergic agonists, such as atenolol and sotalol, which lack a membrane-stabilizing effect, do not inhibit T_3 neogenesis.[152] The effect of heparin to increase the free T_4 level is now thought to be an artifact consequent to the generation of free fatty acids in vitro during the estimate of the free fraction.[138]

An effect on hypothalamic or pituitary function may explain the elevations in the serum T_4, free T_4, and FT_4I levels observed in patients taking large doses of amphetamines. Despite this, the TSH-secretory response to TRH is enhanced, possibly because serum T_3 concentrations remain normal.[153] The latter finding makes it difficult to ascribe the rise in the serum T_4 value to a stimulation of thyroid function, which would be expected to increase secretion of both T_4 and T_3.

THYROID-RELATED HORMONES. The serum T_4 concentration in patients receiving replacement or suppressive therapy with levothyroxine varies with the dose. In most patients receiving physiological replacement doses (approximately 1.6 μg/kg of body weight daily) the serum free T_4 level and FT_4I are high normal or slightly elevated. These patients are clinically euthyroid, presumably because the serum free T_3 concentrations are normal. Nonetheless, the serum TSH concentration may be suppressed because of the intracellular production of T_3 within the pituitary or central nervous system, as previously discussed under the topic of feedback regulation of thyroid function.[86] The serum T_3/T_4 ratio is always subnormal in the athyreotic patient receiving levothyroxine because thyroidal secretion of T_3 is absent. In addition, if the serum T_4 level is high normal, the conversion of T_4 to T_3 may be less efficient than when the serum T_4 level is reduced. Whatever the mechanism, in otherwise healthy patients receiving levothyroxine therapy the serum T_3 concentration is likely to be a better indication of metabolic status than is the serum T_4 level.

Because of the cross-reactivity between L-T_4 and D-T_4 in most radioimmunoassays for T_4, patients receiving dextrothyroxine (D-T_4), an agent used for the treatment of hypercholesterolemia, display elevations of the serum T_4 concentration. Serum T_3 concentrations are increased for a similar reason, because D-T_4 is converted to D-T_3. Values of free T_4, FT_4I, and FT_3I are increased as well, and the TSH level is reduced.[154]

Disorders Associated with Hypothyroidism

Hypothyroidism follows on an inadequate supply of active thyroid hormone to the peripheral tissues. The term implies failure of adequate production of hormone within the thyroid gland. However, in euthyroid individuals the active thyroid hormone, T_3, is mainly generated in the peripheral tissues, and this process is inhibited in many abnormal situations generically designated as the low-T_3 syndrome. In circumstances such as these the supply of active thyroid hormone to the tissues is inadequate and thyroid hormone-dependent functions are decreased despite the absence of disease within the hypothalamic-pituitary-thyroid axis. Although many causes of the low-T_3 syndrome

are known, it is uncertain whether they are associated with metabolic abnormalities directly related to thyroid hormone deficiency. This paradox has already been discussed in the section on effects of illness on thyroid economy.

The manifestations of thyroid hormone lack are conditioned by both severity and duration. Functional changes antecede structural changes, such as the integumentary changes, which are very slow to appear. In the discussion of hypothyroid states that follows, several of the disorders are associated with thyroid hypofunction that is mild or of short duration, or both. In these conditions, evidence of hypothyroidism is largely biochemical, rather than clinical.

DECREASED SERUM T_4 AND T_3 VALUES. In the absence of deficiency of TBG or of severe systemic illness, subnormal concentrations of T_4 and T_3 in serum denote the presence of thyroid hypofunction. Severe thyroid failure is characteristically associated with decreases in both serum T_4 and T_3 concentrations, but in less severe hypothyroidism the reduction in the serum T_3 concentration is less dramatic than that in the serum T_4 concentration. This is because the thyroid that has not totally failed and that is being stimulated by high concentrations of TSH secretes a product with a high T_3/T_4 ratio. Thus in mild or moderate primary (thyroprivic) hypothyroidism, low levels of the serum T_4 may be accompanied by an increased serum TSH concentration and by concentrations of T_3 that are near normal, normal, or even elevated (see Table 8–7). Maintenance of the serum T_3 concentration in this manner does not occur in hypothyroidism secondary to decreased secretion of TSH (trophoprivic hypothyroidism).

When the serum T_4 concentration is low as a result of thyroid failure, the proportion of free T_4 and free T_3, as well as in vitro uptake tests, would be expected to be subnormal. As discussed earlier and shown in Figure 8–18, the free fraction of the thyroid hormones is not reduced to as great an extent as during pregnancy because the increment in unoccupied TBG binding sites is more modest in this circumstance. Absolute values of the free T_4 level and FT_4I are subnormal because of the decrease in the serum total T_4 concentration.

Decreased serum T_4 and T_3 concentrations occur during the late phase of subacute thyroiditis and in some patients with chronic thyroiditis, especially post partum. In both disorders, decreased secretion of T_4 and T_3 is presumed to result from depletion of glandular hormone owing to earlier leakage of preformed hormone stores. This is consonant with the fact that the hypothyroid phase in these disorders is often anteceded by a transient phase of thyrotoxicosis.

After the withdrawal of suppressive thyroid hormone therapy in euthyroid patients, serum thyroid hormone concentrations decrease to subnormal levels, where they may remain for several weeks before returning to normal. During this period, basal serum TSH concentrations remain low and responses to exogenous TRH are absent or diminished. This clearly indicates that suppression of TSH secretion can be followed by a period of decreased TSH reserve and secondary hypothyroidism.[155] The duration of this period varies with the length and completeness of previous suppression and seems shorter when caused by T_3 than by T_4. Not surprisingly, a similar period of decrease in serum thyroid hormone concentrations and in responsiveness to TRH, sometimes of several months' duration, also follows relief of hyperthyroidism or treatment of autonomously functioning thyroid nodules. This transient phenomenon may account for some cases of hypothyroidism that appear soon after ablative therapy for hyperthyroidism. When it is uncertain whether postablative hypothyroidism is likely to be transient or permanent, the physician can either withhold treatment and observe the patient or, preferably, treat the patient with liothyronine or a subreplacement quantity of levothyroxine while monitoring the serum TSH level.

T_3 EUTHYROIDISM. As indicated earlier, the thyroid gland that is hyperstimulated, whether by the stimulator of Graves disease leading to hyperthyroidism or by TSH in an effort to compensate for failing thyroid function, secretes a product with a high T_3/T_4 ratio. As a result there are some patients with partial thyroid failure in whom serum T_4 concentrations are low but serum T_3 concentrations are normal or even slightly increased (Table 8–10). Most often this occurs in patients with Hashimoto disease or patients whose hyperthyroidism has been treated surgically or with ^{131}I. They usually appear euthyroid from the clinical standpoint and may be properly included among patients designated as having *subclinical hypothyroidism*. Presumably their normal or near-normal metabolic state is maintained by the normal quantity of T_3 in the circulation. Nonetheless, serum TSH concentrations in such patients display a better inverse correlation with the serum T_4 concentration than with the serum T_3 concentration. This gives credence to the view that the intrapituitary conversion of T_4 to T_3 plays a major role in the regulation of TSH secretion.[86]

A special example of T_3 euthyroidism is seen in patients with severe iodine deficiency. The relative or absolute hypersecretion of T_3 that this reflects constitutes an efficient mechanism for the defense of their metabolic status, because the calorigenic yield of an iodine atom secreted in T_3 is approximately four times that of an iodine atom secreted in T_4.

Euthyroid Hypothyroxinemia: Decreased Serum Thyroxine Level Associated with Intrinsically Normal Thyroid Function

Just as an increase in the serum T_4 concentration does not necessarily denote the presence of thyrotoxicosis, a decreased serum T_4 concentration does not necessarily indicate the presence of thyroid hormone insufficiency. Hypothyroxinemia may result, instead, from a decrease in the concentration of T_4-binding proteins, from the action of drugs that alter T_4 binding or peripheral hormone metabolism, or from the consequences of severe systemic illness. The reduction in the serum T_4 concentration that is compensated for by an increase in the secretion of T_3, such as occurs in mild or moderate thyroid failure or in dietary iodine deficiency, has been discussed.

DECREASED T_4 BINDING: DECREASED TBG CONCENTRATION. In view of the predominant role of TBG in the extracellular binding of both T_4 and T_3, it is not surprising that significant decreases in the concentrations of TBPA and albumin do not materially influence the concentrations of the hormones with which they can associate. Decreases in the rate of synthesis and plasma concentration of TBPA that

accompany acute and chronic illness are not responsible for the lowering of the serum T_4 concentration seen in these circumstances. Further, although a decrease in the serum T_4 concentration may occur in association with severe hypoalbuminemia, this probably reflects an associated loss of TBG, as in nephrosis, or other effects of illness. In two patients with hereditary analbuminemia studied by one of the authors, serum T_4 concentrations were not decreased.

The consequences of a decrease in the concentration of TBG are the direct antithesis of those associated with increased TBG (see Fig. 8–6 and Table 8–4). The majority of patients are metabolically normal, although the serum T_4 and T_3 concentrations are in the hypothyroid range. The proportions of free T_4 and T_3 are increased, as are values of the THBR (see Fig. 8–17). The free T_4 and free T_3 concentrations are normal. The fractional rate of T_4 turnover and the T_4 clearance rate are increased, but daily T_4 disposal is normal. Similar kinetic changes occur in the case of T_3.

Pharmacological doses of testosterone and several of its derivatives decrease the TBG concentration greatly, usually to values one half or one third of normal. Values of the serum T_4 concentration decrease pari passu but rarely into the hypothyroid range. These agents also increase the binding capacity of TBPA. This may account for the failure of the serum T_4 concentration to decrease more markedly, because binding of T_4 by TBPA becomes more important when the TBG level is decreased.

Very high doses of ACTH or glucocorticoids decrease the TBG level and increase the TBPA level. Values of the serum T_4 concentration often decrease but do not reflect sustained thyroid hypofunction. Similar changes in TBG, TBPA, and serum T_4 concentration are seen in some patients with Cushing syndrome. Serum TBG concentrations are also decreased in patients with acute lymphatic leukemia treated with asparaginase.[30]

Decreases in TBG concentration are seen in some patients with active acromegaly. As in the case of glucocorticoid excess, the mechanism of this change is unknown. Urinary loss of TBG (and TBPA) occurs in nephrotic states; here the decrease in serum hormone concentrations may also reflect some direct loss of hormone into the urine. Losses of TBG may also occur in patients with protein-losing enteropathy. Patients with hepatic cirrhosis may have a low concentration of TBG in the serum, and some decrease in serum TBG concentration is common in patients with other acute or chronic systemic illness, as discussed later.

Occasionally a decreased concentration of TBG in serum occurs as an X chromosome–linked heritable trait. The cloning of the cDNA for this protein and studies of isoelectric focusing pattern have revealed heritable abnormalities in both quantity and quality of protein.[26, 29, 32] The abnormality is more severe in males than in females. Findings in the blood with respect to the thyroid hormones are similar to those in other states associated with a decrease in TBG concentration, and patients are usually discovered by the demonstration of an anomalously low serum T_4 concentration. Data from neonatal screening programs indicate that inherited abnormalities in TBG occur in 1 of about every 2000 people, deficiency of TBG being much more common than excess.[156]

DRUGS. Many pharmacological agents lower the serum T_4 concentration by interfering with the binding of T_4 to one or more plasma proteins, accelerating the metabolism of T_4 intracellularly, or both.[147]

Phenytoin is a drug with complex effects on endocrine and metabolic systems, including the metabolism of thyroid hormones. Therapeutic doses of phenytoin lower the serum T_4 concentration, sometimes into the hypothyroid range.

TABLE 8–10. Serum Hormone Concentrations in Patients with Primary Hypothyroidism of Increasing Severity

Group*	T_4 (nmol/L)	T_3 (nmol/L)	TSH (mU/L)
Control	64–154	1.1–2.9	0.5–5.0
I	>77	1.8 ± 0.6†	5.3 ± 2.3†
II	52–77	1.6 ± 0.3	13 ± 10
III	26–52	1.6 ± 0.5	63 ± 56
IV	<26	0.7 ± 0.4	149 ± 144

*I→IV, worsening thyroid failure.
†Mean ± SD.
Data from Bigos ST, Ridgway EC, Kourides IA, et al. Spectrum of pituitary alterations with mild and severe thyroid impairment. J Clin Endocrinol Metab 1978; 46:317–325.

Although high concentrations are capable of inhibiting the binding of T_4 and T_3 by TBG, this effect probably cannot explain the lowering of the serum T_4, because free T_4 concentrations are also depressed.[72] Rather, an effect of the drug on the activity of intracellular enzymes for T_4 degradation and disposal appears to be responsible. The majority of data indicate that the serum total and free T_3 concentrations, as well as the serum TSH level, are essentially unchanged despite the reduction in serum T_4.[157] This may reflect an action of phenytoin to enhance the conversion of T_4 to T_3, possibly within the liver. Serum rT_3 concentrations are decreased in proportion to the lowering of the serum T_4 concentration. Either maintenance of the normal total and free T_3 concentrations or a direct effect on the pituitary may explain the normality of the serum TSH level despite reduced concentrations of total and free T_4.

Phenobarbital can interfere with the binding of T_4 by serum proteins when added in vitro but does not exert this effect in therapeutic doses. Phenobarbital enhances hepatic disposal of T_4 in rats, however, and probably in humans as well. Although some reports indicate no clear effect of therapeutic doses on serum T_4 and T_3 concentrations in euthyroid subjects, other data indicate that phenobarbital increases the rate of metabolic clearance of T_4; enhances its fecal excretion; and decreases serum T_4, free T_4, and T_3 concentrations modestly when given to patients with hyperthyroidism or to subjects with hypothyroidism receiving replacement doses of levothyroxine. In patients of this type, in contrast to euthyroid individuals, compensatory responses to the decreased circulating hormone concentrations are not possible and the levothyroxine dose must be increased. Carbamazepine and rifampin have similar effects.[158, 159]

Like phenytoin and phenobarbital, salicylates are capable of inhibiting the binding of T_4 and T_3 by serum proteins in vitro. In contrast to the former agents, however, they have a comparable effect in vivo when given in high doses. Initially, serum free T_4 and free T_3 concentrations are increased, but the increased metabolic clearance rates of the hormones associated with their decreased binding lead to the establishment of a new equilibrium in which the serum total T_4 and T_3 values are decreased, while the free T_4 and free T_3 values are restored to normal.[102]

Marked lowering of the serum T_4 concentration and moderate decreases in the serum T_3 concentration are seen in patients receiving another nonsteroidal anti-inflammatory agent, fenclofenac. Despite the decrease in serum total T_4 concentration, the free T_4 value remains in the normal range. Patients are clinically euthyroid and serum TSH concentrations are normal.[160]

Miscellaneous States

NUTRITIONAL ABNORMALITIES. Both acute and chronic alterations in nutritional state greatly influence the pathways of peripheral iodothyronine metabolism and, with them, the concentrations of the major initial metabolites of T_4, namely, T_3 and rT_3. (See earlier under Nutritional Influences in the section Factors That Influence Hormone Economy.)

ENDOGENOUS ANTIBODIES AGAINST T_4 AND T_3. The effects of anti-T_3 or anti-T_4 antibodies on quantitation of T_4 and T_3 and on estimation of the free fraction of these hormones have already been discussed in the section on hormone assays.[161] Because endogenous antibodies against T_4 and T_3 appear to occur almost entirely in patients with underlying thyroid disease, the distortions of serum T_4 and T_3 concentrations are likely to be ascribed to the disease itself. Their presence should be suspected, however, when the serum T_4 or T_3 values are discordant with the clinical

state. Inordinately low values for the THBR should also arouse suspicion because they reflect the capacity of the endogenous antibody to withhold its labeled antigen from the absorbing particle.

SYSTEMIC ILLNESS: SICK EUTHYROID SYNDROME. This subject has already been discussed under the categories of thyroid hormone metabolism and thyroid hormone economy.[74, 124] From the laboratory standpoint, the uniform finding in the syndrome is a decrease in the serum T_3 concentration consequent to a decrease in the conversion of T_4 to T_3 in peripheral tissues, at least in the tissues (including liver and kidney) whose T_3 neogenesis is responsible for maintenance of the serum T_3 concentration. One exception to the typical pattern of illness-induced changes in results of thyroid function tests occurs in patients with HIV infection (Table 8–9).[146] These patients have an increased TBG level and a very slight decrease in serum T_3 concentration (considering the increased TBG). rT_3 and the rT_3/T_4 ratio are subnormal except in patients with fatal *Pneumocystis* infection. The etiology of this unusual response to severe illness is not known. As noted under the topic of the in vitro estimates of hormone binding, there is a growing consensus that the free T_4 level, when measured accurately, is normal in all but a small fraction of sick patients.[126, 127]

Although a reduced free T_4 level is rare, there is suppression of the hypothalamic-pituitary axis because there is no compensatory response to the decrease in serum T_3 concentration. This is the typical pattern, but serum TSH concentrations may be reduced, normal, or even elevated in patients who appear undistinguishable in regard of the type and severity of illness and the degree of suppression in thyroid hormone levels.[129] The pathophysiology of these changes is reminiscent of that of the changes induced by starvation or malnutrition and has already been discussed. The hypothalamic-pituitary-thyroid response to severe illness is incompletely understood. In the clinical setting this group of findings can present a difficult diagnostic problem, because patients with underlying hypopituitarism can obviously develop severe systemic illness. Measurements of the plasma cortisol concentration and a search for evidence of long-standing and continuing overall pituitary insufficiency may serve to establish or exclude this diagnosis. A judicious trial of levothyroxine and cortisol replacement may be in order in such patients until the clinical situation permits conclusive evaluation.

Tests That Assess Metabolic Impact of Thyroid Hormones

Abnormalities in the supply of hormone to the peripheral tissues are associated with alterations in a number of metabolic processes. Some of these alterations are susceptible to measurement in a clinical setting and provide, in theory, a means of determining whether the supply of hormone to the tissues falls short of or exceeds normal requirements. Results of such measurements, often referred to as *metabolic indices*, were for many years the only ones available for use in the diagnosis of thyroid disease, and they remain the sole means of evaluating the metabolic impact of thyroid hormones within the peripheral tissues. Measurements of metabolic indices have virtually no place among current diagnostic tools, having been supplanted by tests of generally greater sensitivity, specificity, and diagnostic accuracy. However, some metabolic indices are of historical interest; others are of value in special circumstances, mainly for physiological exploration; and others are important because they can be confused with metabolic changes that occur in other diseases. For example, inhibition of T_4-to-T_3 conversion by an oral cholecystographic agent causes a reduction in oxygen consumption when the serum T_3 concentration is reduced despite the increase in serum T_4 concentration.[77] For these reasons, certain metabolic indices will be discussed briefly.

The negative view of metabolic indices reflects the reality of the indices that are currently known, not the substantial extent to which there remains an important role for test procedures that are clinically practical and specifically and sensitively reflect the metabolic impact of thyroid hormone within the tissues. There are several reasons why such a need exists. First, mild degrees of hormone excess or insufficiency are difficult to detect and are usually unaccompanied by clear-cut changes in the total and free T_4 and T_3 concentrations in the serum. Because the normal concentration ranges are broad, values within the normal range may represent a significant abnormality for the individual patient. Further, a great many conditions are associated with divergent changes in serum T_4 and T_3 concentrations, and, in the light of current knowledge, reliable inferences cannot be drawn from them concerning the supply of active hormone to the tissues. Examples are disorders in which the serum T_3 concentration is low and the serum T_4 normal, as in the sick euthyroid syndrome, and those in which the serum T_4 concentration is low and the serum T_3 normal, as in some patients with a failing thyroid gland. In addition, recognition of the role of T_3 neogenesis from T_4 within the pituitary as an important determinant of TSH secretion makes apparent the possibility that in some circumstances, as in starvation or the sick euthyroid syndrome, the serum TSH concentration may not accurately reflect an insufficiency of thyroid hormone in the other peripheral tissues. Finally, as judged from some patients with autonomous thyroid nodules or Graves disease who appear euthyroid in all respects, feedback inhibition of the TSH-secretory mechanism is so finely poised that a subnormal TSH value may not reflect a significant degree of thyroid hormone excess. Admittedly the latter patients may have a mild degree of thyrotoxicosis, but by current techniques there is no way to make certain that this is the case.

In these and other circumstances, availability of a thyroid hormone–specific metabolic index would contribute immensely to clinical diagnosis and physiological understanding. It may be unrealistic to hope, however, that such an index can be discovered. Few metabolic processes are under the control of a single hormone or are unaffected by changes in regional blood flow or influences from the nervous system. Moreover, even if an entirely specific and clinically measurable response to thyroid hormone were found, it likely would (and should) reflect the severity of thyroid hormone excess or insufficiency and might, therefore, have limited value in the diagnosis of mild thyrotoxicosis and hypothyroidism.

Basal Metabolic Rate

Thyroid hormones exert a calorigenic effect, increasing energy expenditure and heat production; this is manifest in the weight loss, increased caloric requirement, and heat intolerance of the thyrotoxic patient. The test that reflects this effect is the measurement of the BMR. Because it is impractical to measure heat production directly, the test measures oxygen consumption under specified basal conditions of fasting, rest, and tranquil surroundings. Under these conditions, the energy equivalent of 1 L of oxygen (at standard temperature and pressure) is equivalent to 4.83 kcal, corresponding to a respiratory quotient of 0.82.

Under basal conditions approximately 25% of oxygen consumption represents energy expenditure in visceral organs, including liver, kidney, and heart; 10% in brain; 10% in respiratory activity; and the remainder in skeletal mus-

culature. Because energy expenditure is related to functioning tissue mass, the measured oxygen consumption is related to some index thereof, most often body surface area. Calculated in this way, basal oxygen consumption is higher in men than in women. It declines rapidly from infancy to the third decade and more slowly thereafter. Values in patients, after normalization for surface area, are consequently calculated as a percentage of established normal means for sex and age. Normal values range between -15 and $+5\%$. In severely hypothyroid patients values may be as low as -40%. In thyrotoxic patients even greater deviations in excess of the norm can be seen. Abnormal, usually elevated, values are seen in burn patients and may be produced by a variety of technical factors and by a number of systemic disorders, notably febrile illnesses, pheochromocytoma, myeloproliferative disorders, anxiety, and disorders associated with involuntary muscular activity.

Achilles Reflex Time

The duration of the deep tendon reflexes is prolonged in hypothyroidism and shortened in thyrotoxicosis. These differences are due not to differences in the neural component of the arc but to differences in the speed of both muscular contraction and relaxation, particularly the latter. In about 90% of the patients with moderate to severe hypothyroidism, this delay is readily apparent. Several types of apparatus make it possible to quantify the Achilles tendon reflex. They are not now used as primary diagnostic tools, even in hypothyroidism, because of extensive overlap of the values with those in normal individuals. Adding to the problem is the delay in reflex relaxation that occurs in nonthyroidal disorders, including diabetes mellitus, pernicious anemia, anorexia nervosa, edematous states, peripheral vascular disease, and, most important, in hypothermia of any cause. Several drugs, including morphine, propranolol, quinidine, and procainamide, also prolong the relaxation time.[162]

Delay in the relaxation of the deep tendon reflexes is a valuable clinical sign in hypothyroidism, but there appears to be little merit in attempts to quantify the measurement.

Enzymes and Metabolites in Blood

The concentrations in serum of several enzymes that apparently originate in skeletal muscle are usually elevated in hypothyroidism. The enzymes principally affected are the MM variant of creatine phosphokinase and less often lactate dehydrogenase and serum glutamic transaminase.[163] Concentrations of these enzymes may be slightly depressed in patients with thyrotoxicosis. Such alterations are of negligible value in the diagnosis of thyroid dysfunction but are important to recognize so that they are not confused with those due to other diseases. Activities of a variety of erythrocyte enzymes are altered in the presence of thyroid dysfunction, but these changes are also not of diagnostic value.

The serum cholesterol concentration is frequently elevated in patients with hypothyroidism and tends to be lowered in patients with thyrotoxicosis. The former acts through a combination of increased low-density lipoprotein (LDL) production and decreased degradation. Cholesterol measurements are of no value diagnostically, although they may have some value in following the response to therapy in hypothyroidism.

Although basal plasma cyclic AMP concentrations are not consistently affected by thyroid status, the increase in concentration that follows the administration of glucagon is greater than normal in patients with thyrotoxicosis and subnormal in those with hypothyroidism. Studies of urinary cyclic AMP excretion, either measured alone or in relation to creatinine excretion, have yielded variable results, but the increase in cyclic AMP excretion after administration of epinephrine appears to be greater than normal in patients with thyrotoxicosis.[164]

Noninvasive techniques for estimating thyroid hormone effects on myocardial contractility have been devised. The interval between the initiation of the QRS complex and the arrival of the pulse wave at the brachial artery at diastolic pressure (QKd), which is normally in the range of 200 ms, is shortened in thyrotoxicosis and lengthened in hypothyroidism. The degree of abnormality appears to correlate with the extent of thyroid dysfunction. However, values of the interval are also decreased in high-output states, in conditions associated with increased adrenergic tone, and because of arterial inelasticity in old age. Prolongation of the interval occurs in aortic stenosis, during beta-adrenergic blockade, and in the presence of ventricular conduction defects. If extrathyroidal factors such as these can be excluded, the QKd interval may be a reasonable means of evaluating the impact of thyroid hormone on a particularly critical organ, the heart. A related index of myocardial contractility, the pre-ejection period (PEP), is shortened in patients with thyrotoxicosis, owing mainly to a decrease in the period of isovolumetric systole; lengthening of the PEP may occur in hypothyroidism. As with QKd, extrathyroidal factors affect the measurement; the PEP is shortened in patients with aortic stenosis or insufficiency or by the administration of epinephrine.[165] Measurements of systolic time intervals, as determined from these indices, have been used in evaluating the time course and magnitude of peripheral tissue responses to thyroid hormone replacement in patients with hypothyroidism.[166]

Tests That Assess Mechanisms for Regulating Thyroid Function

Tests that provide information concerning the state of thyroregulatory control, i.e., whether the TSH-secretory mechanism is functioning normally, is enhanced, or is inhibited, play a critical role in the diagnosis of thyrotoxicosis and hypothyroidism. This can be readily understood from a consideration of the role of thyroregulatory mechanisms in the causation of or response to thyroid hormone excess or insufficiency. Thyrotoxicosis can arise from a multiplicity of causes. In rare cases thyroid hyperfunction follows hypersecretion of TSH because of the presence of TSH-secreting pituitary tumor or because the feedback mechanism for control of TSH secretion is insensitive to thyroid hormones. More commonly, thyroid hormone excess results from one of the following: an abnormal thyroid stimulator whose secretion is not homeostatically regulated, as in patients with Graves disease or trophoblastic tumor; one or more foci of autonomous hyperfunction within the thyroid gland; or entry into the blood of excess hormone owing to leakage from an inflamed gland, synthesis by autonomous ectopic thyroid tissue, or ingestion of exogenous hormone. In the latter varieties of thyrotoxicosis, the TSH-secretory mechanism is shut down, a response that is entirely appropriate to the prevailing excess of thyroid hormone. The relationships that pertain in hypothyroid states are analogous, but converse, to those in thyrotoxicosis. In trophoprivic hypothyroidism, primary disease in the hypothalamus or pituitary leads to insufficient production of biologically active TSH, with consequent thyroid atrophy and hypofunction. More commonly, insufficient hormone production arises at the level of the thyroid itself (thyroprivic hypothyroidism), re-

flecting destruction of thyroid tissue, iodine deficiency, abnormalities in the pathways of hormone synthesis and storage, or the action of exogenous goitrogenic agents. Here the TSH-secretory mechanism is activated, a response that is again appropriate to the deficiency of thyroid hormone.

These considerations lead to a rule to which there are as yet no known exceptions—that all varieties of thyrotoxicosis or hypothyroidism are associated with changes in thyroregulatory function that represent either the primary cause of or an appropriate response to thyroid hormone excess or insufficiency. These changes in thyroregulatory function can invariably be demonstrated if appropriately sought, and consequently the tests by which they are demonstrated have great diagnostic value. These are measurements of basal serum TSH concentration supplemented in selected patients by assessment of the TSH-secretory response to exogenous TRH.

Serum TSH Concentration

Measurements of the serum TSH concentration are valuable in the diagnosis and management of hypothyroidism and thyrotoxicosis and in the differentiation between hypothyroidism of thyroid origin and that due to disease in the pituitary or hypothalamus.[88] The application of immunometric assay technology to the measurement of human serum TSH level is a substantive advance. With this technique it is possible to define both the upper and lower limits of the normal excursion for serum TSH, permitting the clinician to interpret the full range of the hypothalamic-pituitary-thyroid feedback loop. It is thus possible to ascertain not only when thyroid function is inadequate but also when the hormone supply is excessive. This test has nearly obviated the need for TRH infusion tests and thyroid suppression tests. Most kits for this assay use monoclonal antibody technology. The principle of the technique is to allow the TSH molecule to be the link between one antibody bound to an inert surface and a second antibody directed against one TSH epitope labeled with a detectable marker (^{125}I or an enzyme or chemiluminescent reagent) linked to an antibody to a second TSH epitope. Accordingly, the signal generated is proportional to the amount of TSH in the serum. Because it does not depend on displacement technology, the basis of radioimmunoassays, this technique is more sensitive and rapid. The use of monoclonal antibodies directed against unique TSH epitopes makes it extremely specific. The normal range of the TSH concentration for this test is 0.5 to 5 mU/L. Patients with primary hypothyroidism have serum TSH concentrations greater than 5 mU/L (Fig. 8–20). Individuals with hyperthyroidism have concentrations less than 0.1 mU/L. The zone between 0.5 and 0.1 mU/L indicates intermediate degrees of suppression of the normal hypothalamic-pituitary axis. Patients with such values usually have variable degrees of autonomous function or receive slightly excessive quantities of exogenous hormone.[167]

These immunometric TSH assays have been called "sensitive" or "supersensitive" by various manufacturers. These terms are relative, and it is not clear whether all available commercial assays perform equally well.[135] It is important for each clinician to develop experience with the assay employed so that a particular result can be interpreted in the context of the clinical picture. An assay of this type should be able to measure concentrations of TSH as low as 0.1 mU/L with confidence. The correlation between the basal serum TSH concentration and the response of TSH to TRH is linear, e.g., if the basal TSH concentration is suppressed, TRH-induced TSH release is also impaired.

There is one major caution, an artifactually elevated result may be obtained for serum from a patient with heterologous antibodies against mouse immunoglobulin G (IgG).[168] Such antibodies may serve as the bridge between the first and second antibodies thus acting in the same way as the TSH molecule. Most manufacturers have added mouse serum or IgG to the assay matrix to obviate this problem, but the quantity present may be insufficient for an individual with a large amount of antibody. In general, results for such patients are elevated out of proportion to the clinical state or to the levels of the serum T_4 and are readily recognized as artifactual. Occasionally, however, more modest elevations may cause difficulties in interpretation. For example, a modest TSH elevation in a patient with mild hyperthyroidism suggests the possibility of a TSH-induced form of this disease. In these situations one may assay the serum by a different technique, such as radioimmunoassay, or use a kit produced by another manufacturer. Alternatively, a TRH test may prove useful. In such a situation an increase in TSH level following TRH administration would point to a hypothalamic-pituitary cause for the hyperthyroidism. The absence of a change in TSH response would suggest an artifactual elevation or fixed production of TSH from a TSH-producing tumor.

As shown in Figure 8–20, patients with primary hypothyroidism have elevated serum TSH concentrations that can range from minimally elevated to values as high as 1000 mU/L. In general, there is a correlation between the degree of TSH elevation and the clinical symptoms. Patients with serum TSH values in the range of 6 to 15 mU/L have few if any symptoms. When such patients are given hormone replacement it is difficult to demonstrate objective clinical improvement. In patients with serum TSH values in this range the serum free T_4 level may be low normal or even slightly reduced, but serum T_3 concentrations are virtually always normal. Such findings are usually indicative of early thyroidal decompensation associated with a compensatory increase in TSH secretion.

Two groups of patients with subnormal TSH values can generally be demarcated: those with values between 0.5 and 0.1 mU/L and those with values less than 0.1 mU/L. Individuals in the latter category almost invariably have symptoms of hyperthyroidism and significant elevations in free T_3 and T_4 levels. Individuals in the former group often have high normal serum free T_4 values and may have elevations in free T_3 level. Patients with hypothalamic or pituitary hypothyroidism generally have normal values for serum TSH, although rarely the TSH level may be slightly elevated.[169, 170] In some of these patients the circulating TSH is not biologically active by cytochemical bioassay.

Among patients with TSH-induced hyperthyroidism, those with primary tumors have disproportionate increases in the concentration of alpha, but not beta, subunits in the serum relative to the concentration of TSH, and their serum TSH or subunit concentration fails to increase after they receive TRH. In those lacking a pituitary tumor, the concentration of subunits relative to that of TSH is not high, and both TSH and subunit concentrations increase after administration of TRH.[171–173]

Although enhanced secretion of TSH is commonly implicated in its pathogenesis, simple or nontoxic goiter is not usually associated with an increased serum TSH concentration. However, when the pathogenetic factors that lead to simple goiter are sufficiently severe to produce hypothyroidism (goitrous hypothyroidism), increased serum TSH concentrations are seen. In endemic goiter associated with severe iodine deficiency, serum TSH concentrations are often high and may be in part responsible for the hypersecretion of T_3 that occurs in these circumstances. In areas of less severe iodine deficiency, endemic goiter is associated with normal serum TSH concentrations, much as it is in sporadic nontoxic goiter already discussed. In the human neonate, the serum TSH concentration increases greatly during the first few hours after parturition and returns to normal values during the first day post partum. This response is thought to be due to the entry of the neonate into the relatively cool extrauterine environment.[5] Cold exposure in the adult, however, has no apparent effect.

Except when massive doses of hormone are administered initially, the treatment of patients with hypothyroidism progressively lowers the elevated serum TSH concentration, but normal levels are not attained for several weeks. Early in the course of replacement therapy, a paradoxical and unexplained increase in the basal serum TSH concentration and, more often, in the peak response to TRH may occur.[174] After withdrawal of replacement liothyronine in patients with hypothyroidism, a progressive increase in the serum TSH concentration begins within a few days. By contrast, when patients have been treated for long periods with levothyroxine, a return of the serum TSH concentration to elevated values may require a few weeks, even though the serum T_4 and T_3 concentrations have fallen to subnormal values in the interim.

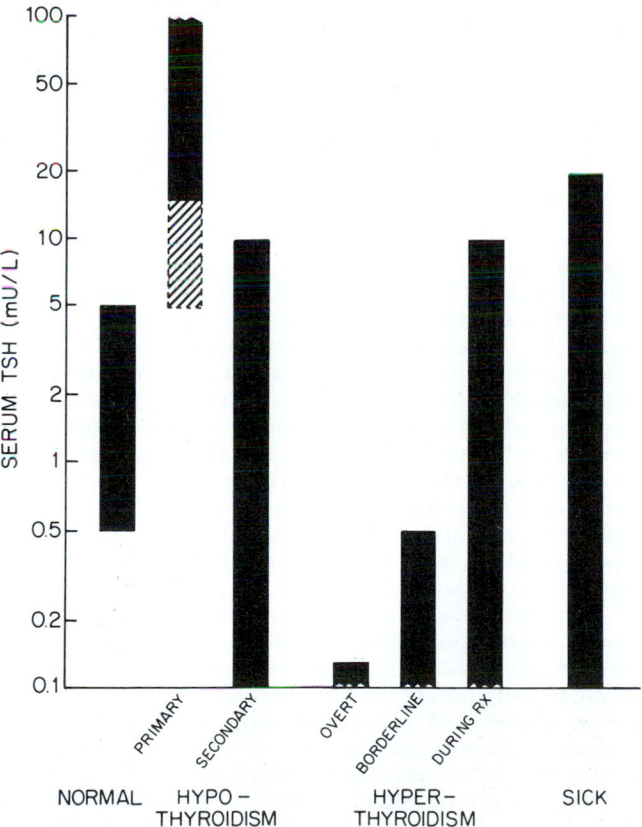

Figure 8–20. Typical serum TSH concentrations in individuals with various disorders of thyroid-pituitary function or with nonspecific illness. These results are typical of those expected using immunometric assay technology. It should be noted that in primary hypothyroidism serum TSH concentrations can exceed 100 mU/L and that TSH values between 5 and 15 mU/L are not generally associated with symptoms of thyroid hormone deficiency. In secondary hypothyroidism serum TSH levels may range from undetectable to slightly elevated. The presence of overt hyperthyroidism is associated with a reduction in the TSH concentration below the lower limit of normal of 0.1 mU/L, and individuals who are euthyroid but have autonomous thyroid function may have values between 0.1 and 0.5 mU/mL. During therapy, hyperthyroid patients may continue to have undetectable TSH, depending on the duration of therapy and the degree of suppression of thyroid function by antithyroid drugs. In illness, TSH can range from undetectable to modestly elevated levels.

Accurate measurement of both elevated and suppressed TSH concentrations has led to the proposal that an *immunometric TSH* assay could be used in screening individuals for thyroid disease. Such a strategy would have the advantage of immediate identification of patients with hypofunction or hyperfunction and elimination of patients without thyroid disease. There are several drawbacks to this approach. First, a number of significantly ill individuals who have elevated TSH levels do not have primary hypothyroidism.[128–130] Second, in hospitalized patients, especially those receiving dopamine or glucocorticoids, the TSH level may be suppressed in the absence of hyperthyroidism. It thus seems unlikely that such a screening approach would be cost effective in this population.[129] This screening strategy might be more useful for outpatients, in whom nonthyroidal causes of abnormal TSH secretion are less common. However, in neither population would this test be reliable in eliminating the possibility of hypothalamic or hypopituitary hypothyroidism, in which the serum TSH concentration may be normal. However, the method is effective in situations in which measurements of the free hormone index give ambivalent results. One example is in patients receiving amiodarone, in whom a compensatory increase in the FT_4I is found because of impaired T_4-to-T_3 conversion.[75, 76] In some of these individuals, hyperthyroidism may develop because of the large iodide load.[148] These individuals can be distinguished from those with compensatory elevations in FT_4I by measurement of the TSH concentration.[150] If the TSH concentration is reduced, autonomous thyroid hyperfunction is present; if it is normal or elevated, the elevated FT_4I is a compensatory response.

TRH Stimulation Test

In some laboratories, a reliable immunometric TSH assay may not be available, and there may still be a need for TRH testing. By providing a standard supraphysiological challenge to the TSH-secretory mechanism within the thyrotropic cell, exogenous TRH makes it possible to determine the intrinsic TSH-secretory reserve and the extent to which the mechanism is inhibited by thyroid hormones or other factors. Over a broad range, the extent of increase in the serum TSH concentration induced by TRH is closely correlated with the basal serum TSH concentration. Hence, in most circumstances, exogenous TRH acts as an amplifier to exaggerate any abnormality in the rate of TSH secretion and hence in the plasma TSH concentration. In view of the improved sensitivity of the current TSH immunoassays, this strategy is no longer necessary.

TRH is effective in activating TSH secretion, whether given orally, intramuscularly, or intravenously; however, the intravenous route is by far the most commonly used. A dose of 400 μg, which produces a maximal response, is administered as a single bolus (Fig. 8–21). In normal individuals, the serum TSH concentration rises rapidly, reaches a peak in 20 to 30 min, and then decreases more slowly, returning to basal values in 2 or 3 h. In clinical practice, specimens for TSH analysis need be drawn only just before and 30 min after TRH administration. Unfortunately, the normal increment in the serum TSH concentration varies among subjects and varies in the same subject from time to time. In general, normal increments range between 5 and 30 mU/L and average about 15 mU/L. Responses in premenopausal women are slightly greater during the preovulatory phase of the menstrual cycle and are, in general, slightly greater than in men. These differences are not clinically significant, except in elderly men, in whom responsiveness to TRH declines. Responses to TRH are decreased by pharmacological doses of glucocorticoids and by somatostatin. Increased

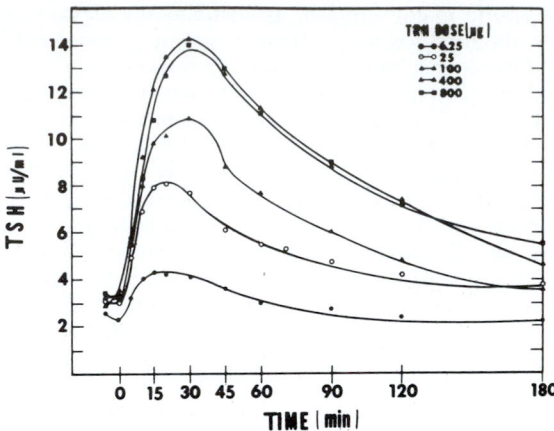

Figure 8–21. Response of serum TSH concentration to intravenous TRH in normal subjects. (From Snyder PJ, Utiger RD. Response to thyrotropin releasing hormone [TRH] in normal man. J Clin Endocrinol Metab 1972; 34:380–385. © 1972, The Endocrine Society.)

endogenous levels somatostatin may account for the lessened response to TRH seen in patients receiving growth hormone. Diminished responses are also seen in patients receiving levodopa, dopamine, and bromocriptine, whereas responses are augmented by the dopaminergic antagonists metoclopramide and domperidone.

The poise of the negative feedback inhibition of TSH secretion and of TRH responsiveness is extremely fine, so that very small doses of exogenous hormone, insufficient to increase the serum T_4 and T_3 concentrations appreciably and insufficient to bring them above the normal range, promptly and markedly decrease the response to TRH. Conversely, small decreases in serum T_4 and T_3 concentration, such as those produced by large doses of iodides, are associated with increased basal serum TSH concentrations and an increased response to TRH (see Fig. 8–11). Indeed, in the clinical sense, the feedback mechanism may be too finely poised, because the response characteristic of thyrotoxicosis may be seen in patients with autonomously functioning nodules or in patients receiving replacement or suppressive doses of thyroid hormone, even though they are clinically euthyroid by all other criteria. This may account for the lack of response to TRH in some patients with euthyroid Graves disease and ophthalmopathy, some patients who are apparently euthyroid after treatment of hyperthyroidism, and some apparently euthyroid relatives of patients with Graves disease.[175]

As would be expected, in hypothyroidism of primary thyroid origin, the response to TRH is accentuated; peak increments in serum TSH concentration are increased, often greatly so. An appreciably increased serum TSH concentration in a setting of proven or suspected hypothyroidism makes a TRH test unnecessary. When hypothyroidism is present without an increase in basal serum TSH concentration, the TRH test should serve to distinguish between hypothyroidism of pituitary origin and that of hypothalamic origin, but this approach is far from infallible.[170, 176] Typically the patient whose disease arises in the pituitary displays a subnormal response or no response to TRH, whereas the patient with hypothalamic hypothyroidism displays a normal, but retarded, response, so that peak serum concentrations of TSH are not achieved until about 60 min after TRH administration. Quite frequently, however, a pattern contrary to that expected is seen, possibly because a lesion in the one site interferes anatomically or physiologically with the other. Some hypothyroid patients with disease in the hypothalamic-pituitary area have serum TSH concentrations, as measured by radioimmunoassay, that are slightly elevated and display an exaggerated response to TRH. This apparent paradox evidently results from the secretion of a TSH that has a low ratio of biological activity to immunoreactivity. This may be due to abnormalities in the glycosylation of the peptide skeleton of TSH, a process that appears to be under the control of TRH.[93, 95] In patients with the rare syndrome of isolated TSH deficiency, TRH fails to elicit an increase in the serum TSH concentration, but the increase in serum prolactin concentration induced by TRH is normal.

By far the most frequent and most important use of the TRH test is its application to the diagnosis of thyrotoxicosis when the clinical findings are suggestive, the serum total and free T_4 and T_3 concentrations are equivocal, and an immunometric TSH assay is not available. Because of the extreme sensitivity of the TSH-secretory mechanism to feedback inhibition, a normal response excludes the possibility that the patient has thyrotoxicosis. A subnormal or flat response may be suggestive or conclusive if the clinical picture is unequivocal. However, subnormal or flat responses to TRH in association with a seeming euthyroid state are observed in most patients with hyperfunctioning thyroid adenomas, about 50% of patients with the ophthalmopathy of Graves disease, many patients with treated hyperthyroidism in Graves disease and some of their relatives, 20% or more of patients with multinodular goiter, and many patients receiving replacement or suppressive therapy with exogenous thyroid hormone. Hence, a subnormal response to TRH is not pathognomonic of thyrotoxicosis. Admittedly, patients of the types described may be experiencing a slight excess of thyroid hormone, insufficient to produce clinical manifestations or to bring the serum T_4 and T_3 concentrations out of the normal range. Hence, in patients with suspected thyrotoxicosis, the ultimate decision about whether treatment should be instituted is a matter of clinical judgment.

Apart from their use in the diagnosis of thyrotoxicosis, TRH tests may be valuable in establishing that Graves disease is the cause of ophthalmopathy in a euthyroid patient. In this use, as opposed to its use in the diagnosis of thyrotoxicosis, an abnormal response provides strong evidence that the ophthalmopathy is related to Graves disease rather than an intracranial or intraorbital lesion. A negative test, in contrast, does not exclude the possibility that Graves disease is the cause of ophthalmopathy, and in such patients differentiation between so-called endocrine and nonendocrine ophthalmopathy is best accomplished by ultrasonography or computed tomographic scans of the orbits. In patients with treated hyperthyroidism, persistence of an abnormal response to TRH is said to increase the likelihood of later recurrence. However, caution should be exercised in interpreting the results of TRH tests soon after restoration of a euthyroid state, because the TSH-secretory mechanism that has been suppressed for long periods of time by either replacement doses of exogenous hormone or excessive quantities of endogenous hormone may be hyporesponsive to TRH for a few weeks or a few months, respectively.

Thyroid Suppression Test

When normal individuals are given thyroid hormone in quantities adequate to meet peripheral requirements, suppression of endogenous thyroid function occurs. Such suppression, which is the result of decreased secretion of TSH, is associated with both a decrease in the rate of hormone secretion and a decrease in the RAIU. This principle forms the basis for the thyroid suppression test, which has been of exceptional value in diagnosing suspected thyrotoxicosis and in establishing the presence of Graves dis-

ease. This test is rarely useful now because either a suppressed basal TSH level or an absent TSH response to TRH provides the same information.

Miscellaneous Tests

TSH Stimulation Test

The TSH stimulation test formerly played a prominent role in the diagnosis of thyroid hypofunction. Currently, however, it need be applied in only a few conditions. The test depends on the fact that normal or potentially normal thyroid tissue can respond to an increase in TSH stimulation by increasing its rate of iodine accumulation and hormone release. On the other hand, a thyroid that is failing or has failed because of intrinsic disease should already be maximally stimulated by endogenous TSH, provided the TSH-secretory mechanism is intact. Thus the TSH test was used mainly to differentiate between thyroprivic and trophoprivic hypothyroidism and to demonstrate the presence of so-called decreased thyroid reserve. This term is used to denote the condition in which the maximal functional capacity of a failing thyroid gland has been evoked by an increased secretion of TSH, sufficient to yield a normal or nearly normal rate of hormone secretion. These uses of the TSH stimulation test have been almost entirely supplanted, however, by measurements of the basal serum TSH concentration and the response to TRH.

The TSH stimulation test retains its utility in three major circumstances. The test can be used to determine whether the potential for thyroid function exists in a patient taking full replacement doses of thyroid hormone. Here it may serve to establish or exclude a diagnosis of thyroprivic hypothyroidism without the need to withdraw hormone therapy. Stimulation by exogenous TSH can also be employed to determine whether areas of the thyroid that are not functioning, as indicated by scanning techniques, are capable of function. Scintiscans obtained after TSH administration can be employed to determine whether absence of I* accumulation in one lobe of the thyroid is due to hemiagenesis or to demonstrate, before therapy, whether the extranodular thyroid tissue of a patient with a hyperfunctioning thyroid adenoma will be able to resume function after ablation of the nodule.

Significant untoward reactions to bovine TSH are uncommon. Virtually all patients experience some discomfort at the site of injection. Less common reactions include nausea and vomiting, pain and tenderness in the thyroid or salivary glands, fever, urticaria, symptoms of thyrotoxicosis, dysrhythmias, and angina. In rare instances, anaphylactoid reactions have led to death. For this reason, the authors recommend intracutaneous tests for sensitivity to the bovine protein before the full intramuscular doses are administered.[177]

Assessment of Organic Binding of Iodide

In normally functioning or generally hyperfunctioning thyroids, oxidation of iodide and organic binding are sufficiently rapid that relatively little free iodide is present in the thyroid at any time. Consequently little loss of iodide from the normal thyroid can be demonstrated after the administration of agents, such as perchlorate, that inhibit iodide transport and thereby discharge accumulated iodide. When organic binding is incomplete, however, substantial accumulation of iodide occurs, and significant discharge follows inhibition of iodide transport. Two tests of the integrity of the organic binding mechanism have been devised, the standard perchlorate discharge test and the iodide-perchlorate discharge test. In the former, a dose of radioiodine is allowed to accumulate in the thyroid, and after measurement of the thyroid I* content, a blocking dose of perchlorate is administered. A significant decrease in epithyroid radioactivity within 1 h constitutes a positive response and indicates a defect in organic binding when the plasma stable iodide, and hence the intrathyroid iodide, concentration is normal or nearly normal. The iodide-perchlorate discharge test affords a more severe challenge to the organic binding mechanism, because an initial load of stable iodine is administered with the radioiodine. As a result the concentration of intrathyroid iodide is greatly increased, and even a mild impairment of organic binding will leave a significant portion of thyroid radioiodine unbound and susceptible to discharge. Hence, subtle defects can be demonstrated by means of this test. However, the interpretation of the iodide-perchlorate discharge test is more complex than is that of the standard test. When normal individuals are given sufficient quantities of stable iodide, an acute inhibition of organic binding (acute Wolff-Chaikoff effect) ensues and a variable proportion of thyroid iodide becomes dischargeable. Although the dose of stable iodide used in the iodide-perchlorate discharge test is less than that required to induce an inhibition of organic binding in the normal gland, it may be sufficient to do so in the stimulated gland in which iodide transport activity is increased. This probably explains the positive test results that are seen in some patients with hyperthyroidism and in some normal individuals who have been given TSH.[178]

A positive response to the standard test is seen in patients with a genetically determined defect in organic binding, in some patients with Hashimoto disease, and in patients with diffuse toxic goiter shortly after treatment with radioiodine. A positive response to the iodide-perchlorate discharge test is seen more commonly or more strikingly in all the foregoing disorders, as well as in some patients with untreated hyperthyroidism and those previously treated surgically or with radioiodine or antithyroid drugs. A positive response to the iodide-perchlorate discharge test is thought to be a forerunner of thyroid failure and a likely indication that the patient is prone to the development of hypothyroidism if iodides are given for a prolonged period.

Tests for Antithyroid Antibodies

As discussed more extensively later, Graves disease, Hashimoto disease, and primary thyroprivic hypothyroidism compose a triad of interrelated autoimmune thyroid disorders. Among the several lines of evidence that support the role of autoimmunity in their pathogenesis is the frequency with which antibodies against one or another thyroid antigen can be demonstrated in the blood of patients with these diseases. Four types of antithyroid antibody have been demonstrated:

1. An antithyroglobulin antibody that is detectable by the agar gel diffusion precipitin technique, by the tanned red cell agglutination technique, by the fluorescent antibody technique using fixed sections of thyroid tissue, or by radioimmunoassay.

2. An antibody directed against a component of thyroid microsomes that is demonstrable by complement fixation, by the fluorescent antibody technique using unfixed tissue, by radioimmunoassay, and by tanned red cell agglutination. Thyroid peroxidase is the major component of the microsomal antigen.[13]

3. An antibody directed against a colloid antigen distinct from thyroglobulin, demonstrable by the fluorescent antibody technique using fixed tissue.

4. An antibody that reacts with a nuclear component of thyroid cells, detectable by the fluorescent antibody technique using unfixed sections of thyroid tissue.

These autoantibodies are immunoglobulins and, except for the antinuclear antibody, are organ specific. Only the antithyroglobulin and antimicrosomal antibodies have been used as diagnostic tools to any extent, because the tests for their detection in serum are more readily available.

Although radioimmunoassay techniques are the most sensitive tests for antithyroid antibodies available, antithyroglobulin and antimicrosomal antibodies are most often measured by determining the highest dilution of the test serum capable of agglutinating sheep red blood cells that have been treated with tannic acid and coated with the appropriate antigen. The tests are simple and specific, and commercial kits with which they can be performed are available. Of the two tests, that for the antimicrosomal antibody is the more useful, because it is more frequently positive and usually in higher titer. This is particularly the case in patients younger than age 20 y. Among young patients, positive tests for antithyroglobulin antibody are obtained for only about 50% of the patients with other evidence of Hashimoto thyroiditis, and titers are usually low, but the antimicrosomal antibody test result is usually positive. Among adult patients with Hashimoto disease, antimicrosomal antibodies are found in nearly all and antithyroglobulin antibodies are present in about 85% (Fig. 8–22). Among patients with Graves disease, the corresponding values are about 80 and 30%, respectively. A somewhat lower frequency of antithyroid antibodies is found in patients with primary hypothyroidism.

The sera of approximately 10% of seemingly normal individuals contain antimicrosomal or antithyroglobulin antibodies, or both, usually in low titer. The frequency increases with age, particularly in women. Antibody titers correlate with the presence of foci of lymphocytic infiltration within the thyroid, and positive tests within a normal population probably reflect the presence of chronic thyroiditis. The frequency of antithyroid antibodies in the sera of patients with diseases other than Hashimoto disease, Graves disease, or primary myxedema is apparently no greater than that in an unselected population.

Tests for antithyroid antibodies have diagnostic value in several clinical situations. High titers are indicative of chronic thyroiditis, in a generic sense; with the appropriate clinical picture, they confirm the diagnosis of Hashimoto disease. Antibodies in moderate titer appear transiently in patients with subacute thyroiditis and may be present in patients with the syndrome of chronic thyroiditis associated with transient thyrotoxicosis (also referred to as hyperthyroiditis or painless thyroiditis). Demonstration of antithyroid antibodies may help to distinguish these disorders, in their thyrotoxic phase, from other disorders associated with a decreased RAIU, notably thyrotoxicosis factitia. Demonstrable antibodies also suggest that hypothyroidism is thyroid, rather than suprathyroid, in origin and that ophthalmopathy in the absence of hyperthyroidism is related to Graves disease, rather than to an intraorbital or intracranial lesion.

Titers of antimicrosomal and antithyroglobulin antibodies in the sera of women with Hashimoto disease or Graves disease decrease progressively during pregnancy and increase transiently thereafter, reaching their peak at 3 to 4 mo post partum. This may explain the appearance of transient thyrotoxicosis or hypothyroidism in patients with chronic thyroiditis during the first several months after delivery.[179]

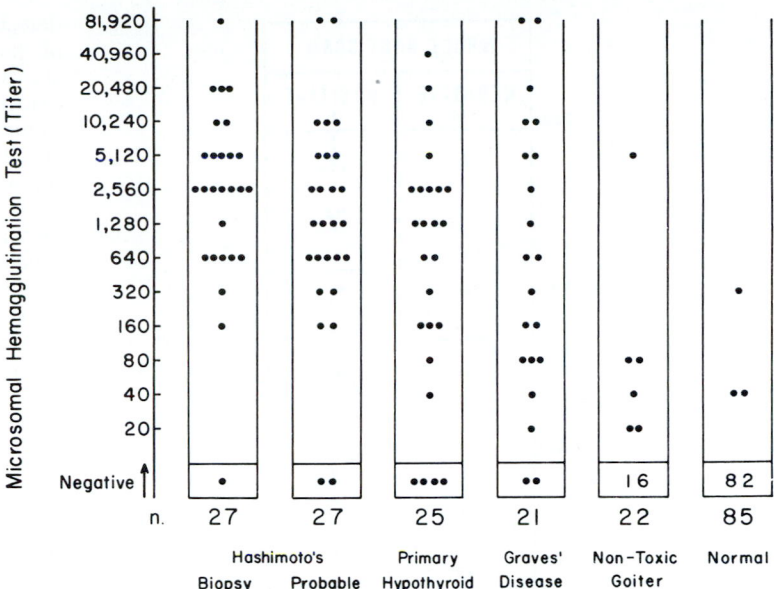

Figure 8–22. Titers of antimicrosomal antibodies in normal subjects and patients with various thyroid diseases. (From Abreau CM, Vagenakis AG, Roti E, et al. Clinical evaluation of a hemagglutination method for microsomal and thyroglobulin antibodies in autoimmune thyroid disease. Ann Clin Lab Sci 1977; 7:73–78.)

Thyroglobulin

Thyroglobulin is present in the sera of virtually all normal individuals. Concentrations are low, ranging up to 30 pmol/L (20 ng/mL); mean normal values vary with the assay used but are on the order of 15 pmol/L (10 ng/mL). Concentrations tend to be somewhat higher in women than in men and are moderately (several-fold) elevated in pregnant women and in the newborn. Distinctly elevated values are present mainly in three types of thyroid disorder: goiter and thyroid hyperfunction, inflammatory or physical injury to the thyroid, and differentiated thyroid tumors. Values are elevated in both endemic and sporadic nontoxic goiter, and the degree of elevation varies in general with the thyroid size. Increased levels are also present in the sera of patients with hyperthyroidism. In Graves disease, values tend to be lower when the disease is in remission but not with sufficient frequency to afford a reliable prognostic index. Administration of exogenous TSH and the surge of TSH secretion that follows administration of TRH are followed by transient increases in the serum thyroglobulin concentration. Transient elevations of the serum thyroglobulin concentration also occur in patients with subacute thyroiditis and as a result of trauma to the gland during thyroid surgery. Subnormal or undetectable concentrations are found in patients with thyrotoxicosis factitia and aid in differentiating this disorder from other causes of thyrotoxicosis associated with a low RAIU.[134] Even low concentrations of antithyroglobulin antibodies interfere with measurements of the serum thyroglobulin concentration as they are commonly carried out. Consequently there are few data concerning the concentration of free thyroglobulin in the serum of patients with Hashimoto disease.[180]

The major clinical value of measurements of the serum thyroglobulin concentration is in the management, but not the diagnosis, of differentiated thyroid carcinoma. Serum thyroglobulin concentrations are increased in patients with both benign and differentiated malignant tumors of the thyroid in situ and do not serve to distinguish between the two. After removal of the tumors, values decrease into the normal range and remain normal if metastatic disease is not present. Almost all patients who have undergone excision of a thyroid cancer are given suppressive doses of thyroid hormone to prevent TSH-dependent growth of the tumor.

Elevations of the serum thyroglobulin level while suppressive therapy is being taken suggest the presence of residual local or metastatic cancer. Evidently, in a small proportion of cancers, secretion of thyroglobulin is TSH dependent, so that elevated values of the serum thyroglobulin level do not develop until suppressive therapy is withdrawn. Such elevations, however, may bespeak the presence of functioning thyroid remnants rather than tumor. The most desirable finding is a low serum thyroglobulin concentration in the absence of suppressive therapy, but even among patients with this finding, a few have positive ^{131}I scans for metastatic disease. In some, elevation of the serum thyroglobulin concentration indicates the presence of metastatic disease although ^{131}I scans are negative (Fig. 8–23). Whether sequential measurements of the serum thyroglobulin level should be used with, or can replace, ^{131}I scans is uncertain.[181, 182]

Tests for Immunoglobulins Related to Graves Disease

Thyroid hyperfunction in Graves disease results from the action on the gland of abnormal immunoglobulins that bind to the thyroid plasma membrane; activate adenylate cyclase therein; and induce thyroid growth, increased vascularity, and an increased rate of hormone production and secretion. Because the responsible immunoglobulins cannot at present be differentiated by chemical or immunological means, demonstration of their presence is based on tests of their bioactivity.[183]

At present, two types of tests are most often employed. The first assesses the capacity of IgG to inhibit the binding of ^{125}I-labeled TSH to its receptors in human thyroid membrane preparations (TSH-displacing antibody, TDA; TSH-binding inhibitory immunoglobulin, TBII). The frequency of positive responses in patients with active disease is on the order of 60 to 90%. The second test assesses the capacity of IgG to stimulate adenylate cyclase or increase the concentration of cyclic AMP in human thyroid slices or membrane preparations (thyroid-stimulatory immunoglobulin, TSI). Tests of this type are positive in 80% or more of the patients with active Graves disease. Because of the proliferation of acronyms describing such antibodies, we will designate them *TSH receptor antibodies* (TRAb) with a phrase "measured by——assay" to denote the bioassay used where this is relevant.[135]

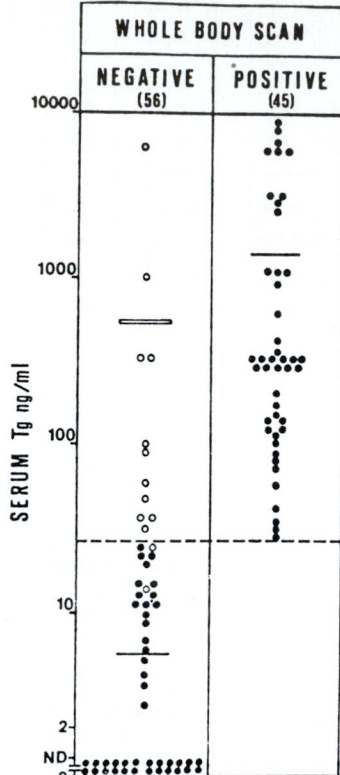

Figure 8–23. Serum thyroglobulin concentrations in patients with differentiated thyroid carcinoma after surgical and ^{131}I ablation of residual thyroid tissue; results classified according to the findings on whole body scan. Note the log scale. In the left column, filled circles indicate values in patients with no detectable metastatic tissue; open circles indicate those with detectable but nonfunctioning metastases. Dashed line, upper limit of normal value; horizontal bar, mean for each group. (From Baschieri L, Giani C, Taddei P, et al. Serum thyroglobulin as a marker of thyroid carcinoma. In: Andreoli M, Monaco F, Robbins J, eds. Advances in Thyroid Neoplasia 1981. Rome: Field Education Italia, 1981: 187–199.)

These tests are now available on a commercial basis, and there are special circumstances in which efforts should be made to have them performed. Demonstration of TRAb may be of diagnostic value in the euthyroid patient with ophthalmopathy, especially when it is unilateral and the serum TSH concentration is normal. High TRAb titers in the pregnant woman with Graves disease indicate the possibility that neonatal thyrotoxicosis will be present in her offspring. The greatest potential utility of such tests, however, would be as prognostic indicators in patients with diffuse toxic goiter who have been given a course of treatment with antithyroid agents, as some data suggest. This possibility requires further evaluation, however.[184, 185]

Imaging Techniques

External Scintiscanning

Localization of functioning or nonfunctioning thyroid tissue in the area of the thyroid gland or elsewhere is sometimes of value in the diagnosis or management of the patient with thyroid disease and is made possible by techniques of external scintiscanning. The general principle that underlies these techniques is that isotopically labeled materials that are differentially accumulated by thyroid tissue can be detected and quantified in situ and the data transformed into a visual display. Two types of apparatus are available.

The first, a rectilinear scanner, comprises a mechanical device that moves a highly collimated (focused) scintillation detector back and forth across the area of study in a series of parallel tracks moving progressively downward from above. A printing device that moves in concert with the detector is activated to record a mark whenever a predetermined number of counts have been received. In this way, a visual representation of the localization of radioactivity in the area being scanned is obtained, areas of greater radioactivity corresponding to areas of greater density in the scan. Other modifications make use of a light source that moves synchronously with the detector and whose intensity is proportional to the counting rate. The light exposes a sheet of x-ray film, and the degree of darkening of the final image corresponds roughly to the counting rate at the appropriate site in the thyroid photo scan.

The second type of apparatus is a stationary scintillation camera equipped with a pinhole collimator that views the entire field of interest and translates the counting rates from specific areas of the field into photographic images or images on a fluorescent screen that can be viewed directly or photographed. Electronic and recording instruments permit the quantification of radioactivity in specific areas or the subtraction of extrathyroid radioactivity. The information can be recorded on tape for later study.

Several types of radioisotopes are employed in thyroid imaging. ^{99m}Tc-pertechnetate (TcO_4^-) is a monovalent anion that, like iodide, is actively concentrated by the thyroid gland but, unlike iodide, undergoes negligible organic binding. Thus it is free to diffuse out of the thyroid as its concentration in the plasma decreases. The short physical half-life of ^{99m}Tc (6 h), together with its transient stay within the thyroid, makes the radiation delivered to the thyroid by a standard dose very low. Consequently large doses (>37 MBq[1 m Ci]) can be administered, permitting high counting rates and often an adequate image of the thyroid when the fractional uptake is too low to permit scintiscanning with radioiodine. Pertechnetate is usually given as a single intravenous bolus, and imaging is performed about 30 min later. With the scintillation camera, imaging can be begun almost immediately after administration of the tracer and serial images can be obtained thereafter. This makes possible studies of the dynamics of thyroid blood flow and isotope accumulation.

Three radioactive isotopes of iodine have been or are used in thyroid imaging, ^{131}I, ^{125}I, and ^{123}I. ^{131}I was commonly used in the past, and it retains utility, particularly when functioning metastases of thyroid carcinoma are being sought. The physical half-life of ^{125}I (60 d) is longer than that of ^{131}I (8 d), but its lower radiation energy results in a radiation dose to the thyroid per unit of radioactivity administered that is only about two thirds that delivered by ^{131}I. The third isotope, ^{123}I, is in many respects ideal. Its short half-life and the absence of beta radiation result in a radiation dose to the thyroid that is about 1% of that delivered by a comparable dose of ^{131}I. All three isotopes of iodine provide satisfactory images of the thyroid in its normal location.

Imaging of thyroid tissue is performed for a variety of indications. The technique can be used to provide some, although not accurate, evidence of overall thyroid size. Its most important use is to define areas of increased or decreased function ("hot" or "cold" areas, respectively) relative to function of the remainder of the gland, provided these are 1 cm or more in diameter (Fig. 8–24). Small cold nodules may be obscured by overlying functioning tissue, but superior discrimination can be achieved if the gland is scanned in the lateral or oblique, in addition to the anterior-posterior, projection. Although the majority of nonfunctioning nodules are not malignant, lack of function increases the likelihood of malignant disease, particularly if only one nodule is present. Conversely, functioning nodules, particularly if they

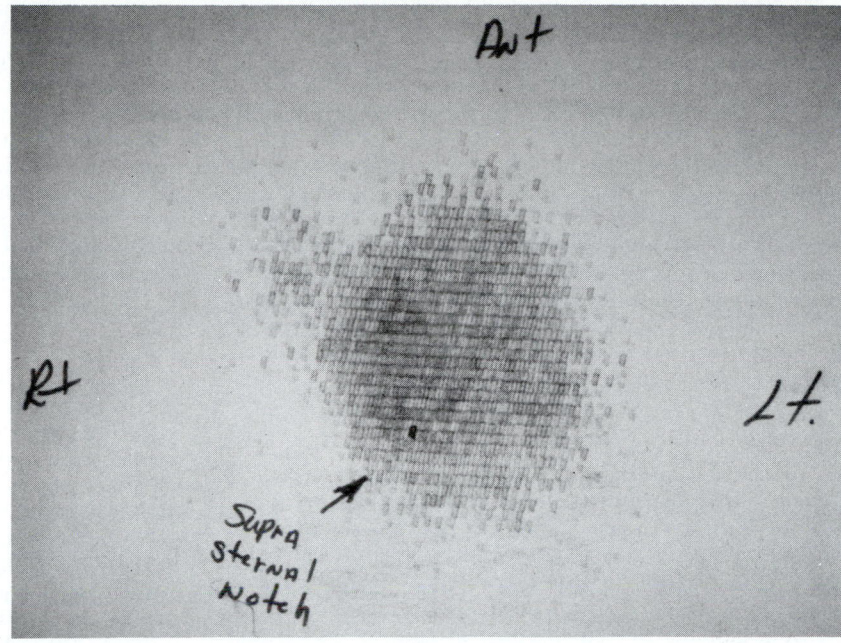

A

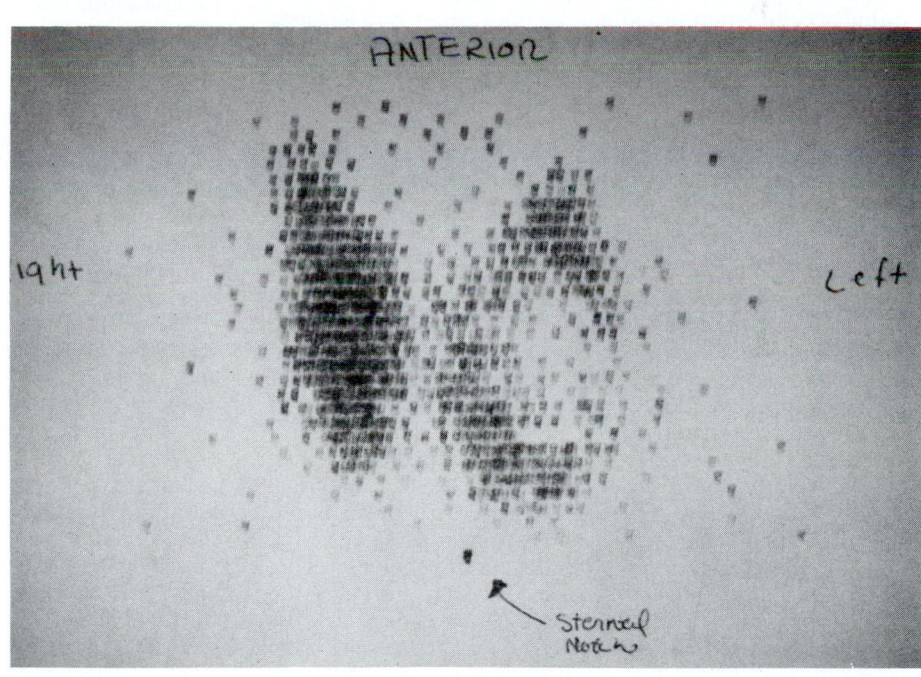

B

Figure 8–24. Scans of hyperfunctioning and non-functioning thyroid nodules. *A*, Scan of hyperfunctioning follicular adenoma arising at the junction of the isthmus and left lateral lobe. Function of the extranodular tissue is almost completely suppressed. *B*, Scan of nonfunctioning thyroid nodule in the corpus of the lateral left lobe. At operation, the lesion was a papillary carcinoma.

are either more active than surrounding tissue or the sole functioning tissue ("hot nodule"), are virtually never malignant. Occasionally irregularities in thyroid images occur in the absence of palpable abnormalities. Irregularity of the image of the lateral margin of the thyroid is suggestive of tumor, but images must be interpreted judiciously, lest unnecessary surgery be performed.

Scintiscans obtained after administration of exogenous TSH may be useful in demonstrating the presence of hemiagenesis of the thyroid and in documenting the intrinsic functional capability of suppressed thyroid tissue. Conversely, scans performed after a period of exogenous thyroid hormone administration (suppression scans) can reveal areas of autonomous function that may not have been detectable in baseline studies. Scintiscanning can also be used to dem-

onstrate that substernal or intrathoracic masses represent thyroid tissue, and they are useful in detecting ectopic thyroid tissue in the tongue or ovary. They are also useful in detecting functioning metastases of thyroid carcinoma.

Choice of the scanning agent depends on many factors. Pertechnetate is readily available in isotope laboratories, and because imaging is performed soon after administration of the scanning agent, the entire procedure requires only a single visit to the laboratory. Another advantage is the very low radiation dose delivered to the thyroid. On the other hand, pertechnetate provides information only about the iodide transport function of thyroid tissue and not about organic binding or retention. It may therefore be used in patients receiving propylthiouracil or methimazole. Some tumors of the thyroid appear to be functioning when examined with pertechnetate but not with radioiodine. Because pertechnetate imaging is done early, radiation from intravascular sources or from salivary tissue may obscure or confuse the findings. For the same reason, pertechnetate is an inappropriate agent for scans of substernal or intrathoracic goiter.

All three isotopes of iodine provide satisfactory thyroid scans, but many believe that superior scans are obtained with [123]I. The short half-life, which limits the radiation dose delivered to the thyroid, precludes its use in the search for functioning thyroid metastases. In the case of ^{125}I, its low energy emissions preclude scanning from deep sources, such as substernal goiter or distant metastases, so that either ^{123}I or ^{131}I should be used in the former and ^{131}I should be used in the latter.

Fluorescent Scans

Fluorescent scanning provides information concerning the content of stable iodine within the gland and its topological distribution. In this technique, discrete zones of the thyroid are subjected to gamma radiation from a source of radioactive americium ([241]Am). Upon encountering [127]I, this induces the emission of a fluorescent x-ray, which is appreciated by a suitable detector. Thus, in contrast to gamma scintillation imaging, which localizes and quantifies the continuing accumulation of iodine, the fluorescent scan localizes and quantifies iodine stored within the gland. The technique has interesting research applications, but its clinical utility is limited. Nonfunctioning nodules generally have a low iodine content and are, therefore, "cold" on fluorescent scan. The technique may provide useful information in conditions in which isotopic scanning is either unsuccessful or contraindicated, as in iodine overload or during pregnancy.[186]

Ultrasonography

The technique of ultrasonography has been applied successfully to the thyroid gland for the purpose of revealing several aspects of its pathological anatomy.[187] Highly focused sound waves of extremely high frequency (greater than 1 MHz) produced by a piezoelectric transducer are directed internally perpendicular to the skin surface. Echoes generated at interphases of differing acoustic impedance return to the apparatus and are detected and processed for visual display. A-mode scans are single-point recordings displayed in a linear format, in which echoes appear as spikes. The height of the spikes varies with the intensity of the echo, and the distance between spikes accurately indicates the distance between echoic interphases. In B-mode scans, the transducer is moved linearly across the neck in the horizontal plane and the data are processed to yield a transverse sonic laminogram. In gray-scale scans, the data are displayed in shades of gray across the spectrum from black to white in proportion to the intensity of the echoes generated. At the frequencies employed, ultrasonograms produce no known tissue damage; they can presumably be used, therefore, repeatedly and with impunity in children and pregnant women.

The normal thyroid produces a pattern of sparse, fine echoes in the paratracheal region. Ultrasonograms are capable of revealing diffuse or localized enlargements of the gland and provide an objective means of assessing changes in their size, as in the response to suppressive therapy. Ultrasonograms may also reveal the presence of thyroid nodules that are difficult or impossible to palpate and may, therefore, indicate that what seems a solitary nodule is in fact part of a multinodular process. The major value of ultrasonography is, however, in the differentiation of cystic from solid lesions of the gland. Purely cystic lesions are sonolucent, creating echoes only at their anterior and posterior walls. Solid lesions, in contrast, create multiple echoes, and they are often surrounded by a sonolucent halo. Mixed solid and cystic lesions are often encountered, and many lesions that are predominantly solid have small cystic areas, representing zones of focal degeneration. The demonstration that a nodule is purely cystic reduces, but does not eliminate, the likelihood that the lesion is malignant. Mixed lesions have the same significance as solid lesions, but benign and malignant lesions cannot be differentiated by ultrasonography alone.

Thyroid Biopsy

Biopsy of the thyroid, particularly closed percutaneous needle biopsy, is employed to obtain an anatomical diagnosis in certain types of thyroid disease. Although biopsy can be applied to the diagnosis of a variety of thyroid disorders, such as subacute thyroiditis in atypical cases, Hashimoto disease, or multinodular goiter, the major rationale for thyroid biopsy is to differentiate between benign and malignant thyroid nodules. Initially, open biopsy, a surgical procedure performed under general or local anesthesia, was the sole type of biopsy performed. In diseases involving the thyroid diffusely, a specimen was taken for histological examination, but nodular lesions were usually removed in toto; hence, the procedure was often therapeutic as well as diagnostic.

Subsequently, closed percutaneous biopsies intended to obtain a core of tissue for histological diagnosis were introduced. In these office procedures, after local anesthesia, a large Vim-Silverman or Tru-cut needle (about 15 gauge) is introduced through a small nick in the skin, and one or more specimens for histological examination are obtained. In experienced hands, cutting needle biopsies are safe, and a diagnostic accuracy of about 90% is obtained.[188] In less experienced hands, however, such complications as hemorrhage, tracheal puncture, laryngoparalysis, and transient injury to the recurrent laryngeal nerve are less infrequent, and specimens are more often insufficient for histological diagnosis.

The major reasons for the growth of interest in and use of thyroid biopsy are a lessening fear of disseminating malignant cells and the introduction of the fine-needle aspiration biopsy coupled with cytological examination.[189] In this technique, which is simple and quite safe, the patient is placed in a supine position with the neck extended; local anesthesia is rarely required. The nodule is then penetrated with a fine (21 to 25 gauge) needle attached to a 10-mL syringe with a nozzle tip, and suction is applied manually. The contents of the needle are spread on a glass slide, dried or fixed, and stained.

Both large- and fine-needle biopsies have limitations. In both techniques, only a limited amount of tissue is obtained, and that may not be representative of the entire lesion. Neither technique is reliable in the diagnosis of differentiated follicular carcinoma, in which evidence of capsular or blood vessel invasion is required for diagnosis, and neither can reliably distinguish between Hashimoto disease and lymphoma of the thyroid on pure cytological grounds. In the case of fine-needle biopsy, the strongest caveat, however, is that slides be read by an experienced thyroid cytologist. Papillary carcinoma is the most readily diagnosed malignancy. Differentiation of follicular adenoma from carcinoma is more difficult. False-positive results vary depending on the criteria used, but in general 30 to 40% of patients are referred for surgery on the basis of the cytological features. About 10 to 15% of these have a malignancy. The false-negative rate is generally less than 3%.[189]

Thyroid biopsy of any type should not be performed as an isolated diagnostic procedure but rather should be integrated into a systematic approach to the management of the thyroid nodule that includes, in addition, careful clinical examination, scintiscanning, and ultrasonography.

EFFECTS OF THYROID HORMONES ON METABOLIC PROCESSES

The thyroid hormones play upon a great multiplicity of metabolic processes, influencing the concentration and activity of numerous enzymes; the metabolism of substrates, vitamins, and minerals; the secretion and degradation rates of virtually all other hormones; and the response of their target tissues to them. It can truly be said that no tissue or organ system escapes the adverse effects of thyroid hormone excess or insufficiency.

Effects on Calorigenesis

Thyroid hormones stimulate calorigenesis. This is reflected in increased oxygen consumption in the whole animal or in isolated tissues in vitro. This response occurs after a latent period of several hours or days and is evident in most tissues, the spleen, brain, and testis being notable exceptions. T_3 causes a more prompt but somewhat shorter-lived effect than does T_4.

The precise mechanism of the calorigenic effect of the thyroid hormones remains uncertain. Direct effects of the hormone on mitochondrial metabolism have been and remain a topic of interest, and thyroid hormone–induced thermogenesis may represent the energy expenditure of increased transport of sodium and potassium across the cell membrane by the enzyme Na^+,K^+-ATPase. This concept has been challenged because tissue slices, used in early studies of this topic, have artificially high Na^+,K^+-ATPase levels due to leakage of Na^+ and K^+ into the medium. Studies of intact hepatic cells have given conflicting results,[190] and studies of perfused liver do not substantiate the high sensitivity of oxygen consumption to inhibition of ATPase by ouabain. Thyroid hormone does cause a two- to threefold increase in mRNA for alpha and beta subunits of Na^+,K^+-ATPase in rat liver and kidney, and the change in cell membrane K^+ permeability appears to be the initial step by which thyroid hormone increases ATPase activity.[191, 192] Other explanations for the thyroid hormone–induced calorigenesis include the stimulation of futile cycles involving either carbohydrate or lipid synthesis and breakdown, for which there is considerable experimental support.

The increase in oxygen consumption of the whole animal requires an increased exchange of ADP and ATP across the mitochondrial membrane. This increase is not due to a primary effect of thyroid hormone on adenine nucleotide translocase, although the function of this carrier protein is clearly increased.[193] Thus no differences were observed in either the mRNA or the protein itself between hypothyroid and hyperthyroid heart, liver, or kidney.[193] Several investigators have explored the possibility that there is a specific low-capacity, high-affinity T_3-binding protein in the inner mitochondrial membrane, but it has not been possible to demonstrate convincing relationships between effects on oxygen consumption and the occupancy of this putative receptor by T_3.[194]

Effects on Protein Metabolism

The effects that thyroid hormones exert on protein metabolism may be fundamental to the metabolic actions of the hormones. Stimulation of protein synthesis may be responsible for a portion of their calorigenic effect, and enhanced synthesis of specific enzymes may result in other metabolic sequelae. For example, thyroid hormones enhance the synthesis of lysozymal enzymes in muscle and are necessary for the catabolic response to a variety of stimuli in this tissue.

The effect of thyroid hormones on protein metabolism depends on the metabolic state of the recipient organism and the size of the administered dose. In thyroidectomized rats, moderate doses of T_4 increase protein synthesis and decrease nitrogen excretion. Larger doses inhibit protein synthesis and increase the concentration of free amino acids in plasma, liver, and muscle. A similar biphasic response of protein synthesis has been noted in rabbit bone marrow slices incubated in varying concentrations of T_4 in vitro. In rats, optimal doses of thyroid hormone are necessary for the elicitation of the full growth response to growth hormone; the nature of the interaction of these hormones is uncertain. Synthesis and secretion of normal quantities of growth hormone require adequate thyroid hormone supplies. Not all proteins are affected in a similar way by thyroid hormone. For example, the half-life of several thyroid hormone–dependent liver enzymes is not influenced by thyroid function.[195]

Variations in the overall growth rate are probably the most general reflection of the effects of thyroid hormones on protein synthesis, and here too the effects are biphasic. In immature animals and people, growth is retarded by hypothyroidism, is restored by replacement doses, and is inhibited by excessive doses of hormones. In the thyrotoxic state, nitrogen excretion is increased, but it is not clear whether the catabolic response to thyroid hormones is an obligatory effect or is due to negative caloric balance. In adults with hypothyroidism, studies with ^{15}N-labeled glycine indicate a decreased rate of protein synthesis, and observations with I*-labeled serum albumin indicate that the synthesis and degradation of this protein are retarded. These functions in the hypothyroid patient are restored to normal by replacement doses of thyroid hormone.

Effects on Carbohydrate Metabolism

Thyroid hormones affect virtually all aspects of carbohydrate metabolism. Many effects are dependent on or modified by other hormones, in particular catecholamines and insulin. Thyroid hormones appear to regulate the magnitude of the glycogenolytic and hyperglycemic actions of epinephrine, possibly by enhancing responsiveness of the adenylate cyclase–cyclic AMP system, and to potentiate the effects of insulin on glycogen synthesis and glucose utilization. Some of the effects of thyroid hormones depend on the dose, and as a result biphasic actions have been observed. For example, in rats, small doses of T_4 increase glycogen synthesis in the presence of insulin, whereas large doses increase hepatic glycogenolysis, causing glycogen depletion. This biphasic action of T_4 modifies the subsequent glycogenolytic response to epinephrine, small doses of T_4 enhancing and large doses depressing the response. Large doses of T_4 enhance gluconeogenesis by increasing the availability of precursors, such as lactate and glycerol. Thyroid hormones enhance the rate of intestinal absorption of glucose and galactose. They also increase the rate of uptake of glucose by adipose tissue and muscle and potentiate the effect of insulin in this respect. Insulin degradation appears to be increased by thyroid hormones. Increased insulin degradation may account for the diminished sensitivity to exogenous insulin and consequent worsening of the clinical status of type I diabetes mellitus sometimes seen when thyrotoxicosis develops. The converse occurs in hypothyroidism.

By increasing the activity of the mitochondrial enzyme α-glycerophosphate dehydrogenase, thyroid hormone enhances the synthesis of oxaloacetic acid and subsequently malate from pyruvate. Activities of a number of important enzymes involved in carbohydrate synthesis and breakdown are increased by thyroid hormone in the liver, including pyruvate carboxylase, phosphoenolpyruvate carboxykinase, and glucose-6-phosphatase. This could explain the increased gluconeogenesis characteristic of the hyperthyroid liver.[196]

Effects on Lipid Metabolism

Thyroid hormones appear to stimulate virtually all aspects of lipid metabolism, including synthesis, mobilization, and degradation. In general, degradation is affected more than synthesis, the net effect in states of hormone excess being a decrease in the stores of most lipids and usually their concentrations in plasma. This is true for triglycerides, phospholipids, and cholesterol. Converse changes are seen in states of thyroid hormone deficiency. The metabolism of various apolipoproteins is also affected.[197]

Most closely related to the changes in energy metabolism that accompany states of thyroid hormone excess or deficiency are changes in the metabolism of fatty acids at their sites of storage and degradation. Thyroid hormones increase lipolysis in adipose tissue both by a direct effect through the adenylate cyclase–cyclic AMP system and by sensitizing the tissue to other lipolytic agents, such as catecholamines, growth hormone, glucocorticoids, and glucagon. In the case of glucagon, an increase in receptor number induced by thyroid hormone may be responsible. Oxidation of free fatty acids is also increased, and this may account for some of the calorigenic action of thyroid hormones.[198]

Hepatic synthesis of triglycerides is increased, probably as a result of the increased availability of free fatty acids and glycerol mobilized from adipose tissue. Concomitantly, removal of triglycerides from plasma is accelerated, possibly because of an increase in lipoprotein lipase concentration.

Thyroid hormones lower the concentration of cholesterol in plasma, probably through a variety of actions.[199] Synthesis of cholesterol is enhanced at the stage of conversion of β-hydroxy-β-methylglutaryl-coenzyme A to mevalonate, probably by increasing the activity of the enzyme concerned. Thyroid hormone action on the elimination of cholesterol is effected by an increase in both the excretion of cholesterol and its conversion to bile acids. The lowering of the plasma cholesterol level is presumed to occur because cholesterol excretion or degradation is enhanced more than cholesterol synthesis. A further effect of the thyroid hormones is to enhance the turnover of LDL to which cholesterol and phospholipids are bound. These effects may result from stimulation of the synthesis of LDL receptors and of LDL degradation.[200]

Effects on Vitamin Metabolism

Thyroid hormones increase the demand for coenzymes and the vitamins from which they are derived. In hyperthyroidism, the requirements for water-soluble vitamins, such as thiamine, riboflavin, vitamin B_{12}, and vitamin C, are increased and their tissue concentrations are reduced. The conversion of some water-soluble vitamins to the coenzyme form may be impaired, possibly as a result of defective energy transfers. For example, phosphorylation of pyridoxine to pyridoxal-5-phosphate (codecarboxylase) and synthesis of pyridine nucleotides (NAD and NADP) from nicotinamide appear to be defective in tissues of hyperthyroid animals. On the other hand, the synthesis of some coenzymes from vitamins requires thyroid hormones. For example, the synthesis of flavin mononucleotide and flavin adenine dinucleotide from riboflavin requires the stimulatory effect of thyroid hormones on the enzyme flavokinase.

The metabolism of fat-soluble vitamins is also influenced by thyroid hormones. They are required for the synthesis of vitamin A from carotene and for the conversion of vitamin A to retinal, the pigment required for dark adaptation. In hypothyroidism, the serum carotene concentration is increased and may give the skin a yellow tint, and clinical manifestations of vitamin A deficiency may occur. In hyperthyroidism, the requirement for vitamin A is increased and the tissue concentration is reduced. Vitamins D and E appear to be deficient in hyperthyroid animals.

Interactions with the Sympathetic Nervous System

Many of the manifestations of thyrotoxicosis and of sympathetic nervous system activation are similar. As judged from the plasma concentrations of epinephrine and norepinephrine, as well as their urinary excretion and that of their metabolites, the activity of the sympathetic nervous system is not increased in patients or animals with thyrotoxicosis. Another possibility is that thyroid hormones exert effects separate from, but similar and additive to, those of the catecholamines. A careful examination of the relationship between catecholamines and thyroid hormone excess and deficiency reveals the futility of attempting a generalization in this area.[201] The reduction in heart rate and in some clinical manifestations of hyperthyroidism induced by beta-blockade in patients with this condition has led to the concept that there is increased sympathetic tone or increased cardiac sensitivity to the sympathetic nervous system. Careful studies have shown that this is clearly not the case in terms of the heart.[202, 203] Adequate beta-adrenergic blockade changes the basal level of cardiac output, but the slope of the dose-response curve to epinephrine is not altered in hyperthyroidism.

In other tissues, the situation may be even more complex, and species differences may exist. In the rat, thyroid status does not affect the number of beta-adrenergic receptors on rat adipocytes; however, in hypothyroid rats adenylate cyclase activity in white fat cells is reduced in response to beta-adrenergic stimuli, and cyclic AMP accumulation is impaired in both white and brown fat cells. Although there is decreased sensitivity of lipolysis to beta-agonists, the magnitude of the maximal response is not changed. In hyperthyroid rats, white fat cells have a normal number of beta-adrenergic receptors but show increased sensitivity and maximal cyclic AMP responses to such agents.[201] Thus these changes must occur at steps distal to receptor-agonist interaction. In rat liver, on the other hand, beta-adrenergic receptor number is increased in hypothyroidism and decreased in hyperthyroidism. This produces the expected changes in the sensitivity of glycogen phosphorylase, which is increased in hypothyroidism and decreased in hyperthyroidism. Myocardial beta-adrenergic receptor number is slightly increased in rats given pharmacological doses of thyroid hormone, but the significance of such observations for clinical hyperthyroidism is not clear.

Several recent studies have dealt with these issues in humans. In hyperthyroid individuals there are no alterations in beta-adrenergic receptor number on lymphocytes and no changes in lymphocyte beta-adrenergic responsiveness. In normal subjects receiving 100 μg of liothyronine for 10 d the beta-adrenergic receptor number in fat and skeletal muscle increased 60 and 30%, respectively. Despite this change, metabolic and hemodynamic sensitivity to infused epinephrine in vivo was not altered.[204] There was no evidence of increased glycemic, lipolytic, glycogenolytic, or ketogenic sensitivity to catecholamines. It was speculated that this might be due to a concomitant increase in endogenous insulin secretion that compensated for these changes.

In another study, the accelerated basal energy expenditure and body protein catabolism caused by 150 μg of liothyronine were unaffected by propranolol infusion.[205] The dose of beta-antagonist used completely blocked the stimulatory effect of epinephrine infusion on these parameters. These results indicate that the calorigenic stimulation by thyroid hormone is independent of catecholamines. On the other hand, because the basal energy expenditure was increased by liothyronine, the absolute increment in energy expenditure during epinephrine infusion was also greater in the thyrotoxic subjects. Thus propranolol blockade of epinephrine-induced increases in energy expenditure had a greater effect in the thyrotoxic subjects than in normal individuals. This would justify the use of beta-adrenergic blockade in thyrotoxic subjects in states characterized by sympathetic activation, such as thyroid storm, or during emergency surgery.

THEORIES CONCERNING MECHANISM OF ACTION OF THYROID HORMONES

There is an appealing parsimony in the concept that the manifold physiological and biochemical effects of the thyroid hormones reflect a single action, or perhaps a few basic actions, at the cellular or molecular level. That this may be the case is suggested by the very diversity of hormonal effects, because it is unlikely that a distinct mechanism is responsible for each. More likely, many of the effects observed are secondary consequences of one or more fundamental actions. Furthermore, most actions of the thyroid hormones are demonstrable only after a latent period, suggesting that they are preceded by some more proximal event.[206] It is not surprising, therefore, that considerable effort has been directed at uncovering "*the* mechanism of action" of the thyroid hormones. Patterns of investigation have conformed to concepts standard in modern cell biology and applicable to studies of the mechanisms of action of other hormones. These involve a search for specific cellular receptors for hormone, for the signal(s) generated by binding of the hormone to its receptor, and for the manner in which generation of the signal results in diverse, yet specific, manifestations of hormone action. Progress in this field includes the identification of two genes coding for human thyroid hormone receptors[207-218] and recognition that the thyroid hormone receptor proteins are part of a superfamily of genes coded for by v-*erb* A oncogene–related mRNAs.

Shown in Figure 8–25 are schematic diagrams of the v-*erb* A protein and the thyroid hormone receptors. In humans, rats, and mice there are two thyroid hormone receptor proteins termed alpha and beta c-*erb* A (c = cellular).[207-217] These will be referred to as TRα and TRβ. Alternate splicing of the mRNAs can lead to several different proteins coded by the same gene,[211, 212, 214-216] and these are denoted by subscripts. The deduced protein of the human $TR\beta_1$ is 456 amino acids in length with a predicted molecular size of 52 kd. The human TRβ gene has been localized to chromosome 3. The $TR\alpha_1$ protein is slightly smaller, 408 to 410 amino acids in length (45 kd), and its gene is found on chromosome 17. There is considerable homology between the TRα and TRβ proteins and between the receptors of rat, mouse, and human. Translation of these cDNAs in vitro has demonstrated that the proteins bind T_3 with high affinity (the K_d for rat TRβ is 1.8×10^{-10} M), and triac has about a 3-fold

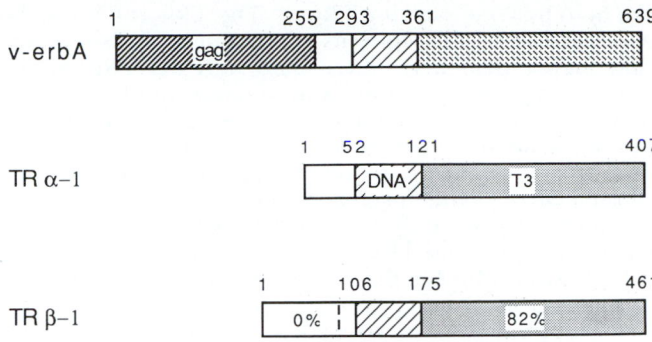

Figure 8–25. Diagrams of the viral *erb* A protein (v-*erb* A) and the thyroid hormone receptors $TR\alpha_1$ and $TR\beta_1$. The numbers indicate amino acids deduced from the cDNA sequence. Putative DNA and ligand binding domains are indicated by shading. The percent figures in the $TR\beta_1$ protein show the degree of amino acid homology to the $TR\alpha_1$ receptor. GAG denotes the portion of the v-*erb* A mRNA that codes for a structural protein of the virus particle. The v-*erb* A protein does not bind thyroid hormone but can compete with the TR proteins for DNA binding.

higher, T_4 about a 10-fold lower, and rT_3 about a 300-fold lower binding affinity than T_3 (Fig. 8–26). Similar information has been reported for $TR\alpha_1$. These receptors are expressed in all tissues shown to have high-affinity nuclear T_3-binding proteins and are less well expressed or absent in testes and spleen. In addition to binding thyroid hormone with high affinity, cDNAs coding for these proteins confer thyroid hormone responsiveness to cells that do not possess receptors in their native state, thus establishing that they function as true hormone receptors.[210, 212] The presence of two genes coding for thyroid hormone receptors was unanticipated, and the physiological significance of these two proteins has not yet been clarified. Both TRα and TRβ are expressed in many tissues, although some, particularly the liver, have high ratios of β to α.[213] A further unanticipated development was recognition that both α and β forms of the receptor have a number of different mRNAs derived from alternate splicing. Most notable is a splice variant of the α receptor referred to as $TR\alpha_2$, initially identified in a human testes cDNA library.[214, 215] This protein is identical to $TR\alpha_1$ until amino acid 370, at which point a different exon is inserted that continues for a further 120 amino acids. The mRNA coding for $TR\alpha_2$ is 2.4 kb in length, as opposed to

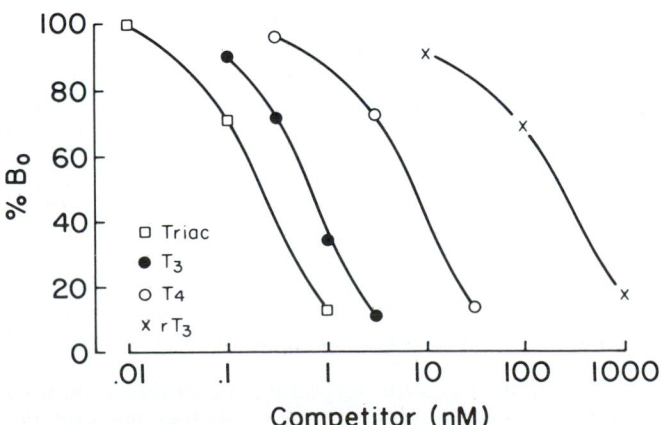

Figure 8–26. Binding isotherms for T_3 and several analogues for the protein translated in vitro from a cDNA coding for the rat TRβ. These analogues compete with T_3 for binding to rat $TR\beta_1$ with the same relative affinities as they do with native T_3 receptor or whole nuclei. (From Koenig RJ, Warne RL, Brent GA, et al. Isolation of a cDNA clone encoding a biologically active thyroid hormone receptor. Proc Natl Acad Sci USA 1988; 85:5031–5035.)

the 5- to 6-kb message for $TR\alpha_1$.[215] The $TR\alpha_2$ mRNA is also expressed in brain, where its concentration is five- or six-fold higher than that of the $TR\alpha_1$ mRNA. $TR\alpha_2$ is also found in significant quantities in pituitary and kidney. The $TR\alpha_2$ variant does not bind T_3,[215] and this raised the intriguing possibility that it could act as an antagonist of the $TR\alpha_1$ and $TR\beta_1$ forms of the receptor, a prediction that has been substantiated.[217] This antagonism could occur either through the formation of nonfunctional heterodimers between the normal receptor and $TR\alpha_2$ or through competition of $TR\alpha_2$ with $TR\alpha$ or $TR\beta$ for the T_3 response elements of thyroid hormone–responsive genes.

The complexity of regulation of thyroid hormone receptor protein expression is only beginning to be unraveled. There is homology in the DNA binding domains of a number of hormonal ligands. For example, there is considerable homology between the DNA binding domains of the thyroid hormone receptors and those for the vitamin D, estrogen, and retinoic acid receptors.[218–224] Less closely related are the DNA-binding sequences of glucocorticoid, mineralocorticoid, progesterone, and androgen receptors. The sequence of the DNA binding domain of the receptor contains two amino acid loops, the so-called zinc finger structure common to the family of thyroid/steroid hormone receptors.[218, 219] These finger domains constitute the DNA recognition portion of the molecule, and their sequence provides a significant portion of the specificity for the respective sequences of DNA in the genes regulated by the cognate hormones (see later). These results indicate that the receptors function as hormone-dependent transcriptional regulatory proteins. It seems likely that the T_3-receptor complex is bound to specific sequences on DNA and can alter the rate of transcription of these genes, presumably by making such sequences more or less attractive to RNA polymerase II and other nuclear factors required for mRNA synthesis. The receptors probably bind in a dimeric form to produce a stable, transcriptionally active unit.

The recognition sites for thyroid hormone receptor on DNA of thyroid hormone–responsive genes have now been defined in considerable detail. A major model for this type of study is the rat growth hormone gene, of which transcription is increased by thyroid hormone.[220–222] Analysis of the 5′-flanking region of this gene has revealed a hexameric motif, AGGTC(or A)A, that is repeated with varying fidelity in three segments of the gene spaced about 10 nucleotides (or one helical turn) apart.[223] Similar sequences are present in the cardiac α-myosin heavy chain gene, another thyroid hormone–inducible gene.[212] This hexanucleotide motif is referred to as a putative T_3 response element (T_3RE) and is thought to be a site for the binding of one member of the two receptor homo- or heterodimers.[224] Two such elements are required for a functional site, and a palindromic arrangement is preferred to confer a maximal T_3 response. As shown in Figure 8–27, the T_3RE is similar to the response element for estrogen, and the thyroid hormone receptor will bind to sequences in the vitellogenin estrogen response element although the capacity of T_3 to cause hormone-dependent activation of this gene is weak.[224] It is thought that the different nucleotide spacings of the two hexamers along the gene allow the estrogen receptor, but not the thyroid hormone receptor, to bind in a transcriptionally active fashion.

The human growth hormone gene (unlike that in the rat or cow) is not induced by T_3 and does not contain a putative T_3RE.[225] This is consistent with the finding of significant quantities of human growth hormone in the sera of hypothyroid children.[226–228]

The findings just described provide strong evidence that the primary action of thyroid hormones is exerted at the

HALF-SITE CONSENSUS SEQUENCES FOR THYROID AND STEROID HORMONES

$$T_3RE \qquad AGGT\!\!\begin{smallmatrix}C\\A\end{smallmatrix}\!\!A$$

$$ERE \qquad NGGTCA$$

$$GRE \qquad \begin{smallmatrix}A\\\ \\G\end{smallmatrix}GNACA$$

Figure 8–27. Putative DNA-binding sequences for thyroid and steroid hormones. These sequences provide a relatively high-affinity binding site for the nuclear proteins that have been characterized as receptors for thyroid and steroid hormones. These sequences are thought to constitute a half-site to which one receptor molecule could bind. To function optimally, the two half-sites are present in a palindromic arrangement. It is thought that receptors bind as homodimers to these half-sites. Shown are sequences currently thought to be specific for the thyroid hormone response element (T_3RE), estrogen response element (ERE), and glucocorticoid response element (GRE). Differentiation between the T_3RE and ERE may be conferred by the number of nucleotides separating the two half-sites.

nuclear level to alter gene transcription. Furthermore, nuclear occupancy by T_3 is correlated with metabolic response. There is, in general, a good concordance between the biological potency of various thyroid hormone analogues and their binding to nuclear receptors. Some tissues that fail to respond to thyroid hormones with an increase in oxygen consumption display a relatively low concentration of nuclear receptors for T_3.[206] These results, as well as the important role played by the deiodinase in activating the prohormone, T_4, are summarized in Figure 8–28.

An unresolved issue is whether any physiological effects of thyroid hormones are mediated by non-nuclear mechanisms. There are a few examples in which a non-nuclear mechanism appears possible. Uncoupling of oxidative phosphorylation is not the mechanism by which thyroid hormones increase oxygen consumption, as originally thought. Other mitochondrial effects of the thyroid hormones have been observed. In vivo, T_4 induces an increase in the number and size of mitochondria and in the number of mitochondrial cristae. It induces swelling of mitochondria in vitro with loss of mitochondrial constituents, an effect seen in T_4-responsive tissues but not in tissues whose oxygen consumption fails to increase in response to T_4, such as brain, testis, and spleen. In hypothyroid animals, T_4 promptly stimulates mitochondrial respiration in the absence of added ADP (state 4 respiration), and later it stimulates ADP-dependent respiration (state 3) as well. The stimulation of state 4 respiration may reflect the action of a specific mitochondrial protein whose synthesis is induced by thyroid hormones. T_4 and T_3, both in vitro and in vivo, promptly stimulate mitochondrial protein synthesis, and both, after several days, increase the carrier-mediated uptake of ADP by rat liver mitochondria, an effect thought to mediate enhanced ATP generation. It is not known whether or how the foregoing effects are interrelated, but their net result would presumably be an enhanced rate of oxygen consumption, an increased number of respiratory units, and an increased availability of high-energy phosphate (energy charge) within the cell.

Thyroid hormones may also exert a primary effect at the level of the cell membrane. High-affinity, limited-capacity binding sites for T_3 are present in highly purified plasma membrane fractions derived from rat liver and rat thymocytes. Thyroid hormones enhance the accumulation of exogenous free amino acids by rat muscle and brain in vivo

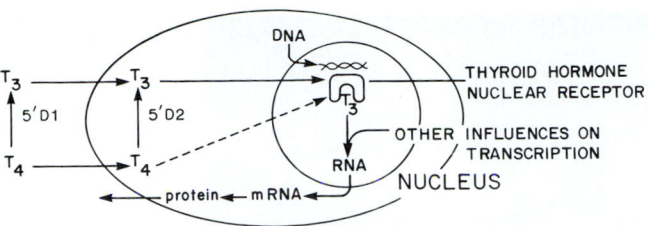

Figure 8–28. Current theory of the mechanism of thyroid hormone action. The prohormone T_4 is deiodinated to T_3 either by the propylthiouracil-sensitive iodothyronine 5'-deiodinase (5'D1) or the propylthiouracil-resistant deiodinase (5'D2). The T_3 formed enters the cell and/or is produced within it and is then transported into the nucleus, where it binds to specific high-affinity nuclear proteins, the thyroid hormone nuclear receptors. At least two active thyroid hormone receptors are coded for by different genes. The interaction of the ligand T_3 with the unoccupied receptor changes the rate of transcription of mRNA from genes that contain specific T_3 receptor–binding DNA sequences. Thyroid hormone may also influence the stability of the mRNA. Depending on the gene in question, the transcription rate may be enhanced or repressed by the T_3 receptor–DNA complex. The changes in the quantities of these thyroid hormone–dependent proteins are responsible for the characteristic pattern of biochemical changes that occur when thyroid function is altered.

and increase amino acid accumulation in vivo in chick embryo cartilage and rat thymocytes. Inward transport of 2-deoxyglucose (2-DG) is enhanced by T_3 in vitro in cultured myocardial cells of the chick embryo and in freshly isolated rat thymocytes. The latter response is the one best characterized in this area of study. The effect of T_3 on 2-DG accumulation by the thymocyte is prompt in onset, is calcium dependent, does not require new protein synthesis, and is elicited by physiological concentrations of T_3. The effect is apparently mediated by a T_3-induced increase in cellular cyclic AMP concentration, because T_3 increases cellular cyclic AMP within a few minutes, well before its effect on 2-DG uptake. The effect of T_3 is mimicked by the addition of dibutyryl cyclic AMP, and manipulations that block the cyclic AMP response to T_3, such as the omission of calcium from the incubation medium or the addition of alprenolol, also block the effect of T_3 on 2-DG uptake. T_3 and epinephrine act synergistically in respect to cyclic AMP concentration and 2-DG uptake. T_3 stimulates adenylate cyclase activity in thymocyte plasma membrane preparations, increasing the likelihood that T_3 is producing its effects at the level of the plasma membrane. Additional evidence of a direct action of thyroid hormones at the cell membrane is the capacity of T_4 and T_3, in physiological concentrations, to increase promptly the activity of Ca^{2+}-ATPase in human erythrocytes and rabbit myocardial sarcolemma. In addition, the down-regulation of type 2 deiodinase by thyroid hormones in various tissues does not require protein synthesis.[229] In this process rT_3 and T_4 are much more potent than T_3 itself, which argues for a non-nuclear event.

On the basis of foregoing evidence, although it cannot be concluded unequivocally that all thyroid hormone–dependent processes are initiated by the interaction of thyroid hormone with the nuclear receptor, the nuclear mechanism is the most important one for regulating protein synthesis in thyroid hormone–responsive cells.

APPROACH TO CLINICAL DIAGNOSIS OF THYROID DISEASE

Diseases of the thyroid gland almost always manifest themselves through symptoms resulting from excessive or insufficient production of thyroid hormone, through local symptoms in the neck, principally goiter (but occasionally pain or compression of adjacent structures), or, in the case of Graves disease, through ophthalmopathy or dermopathy. Although attention is directed initially at the major clinical evidence, the physician seeks ultimately to establish both a functional and an anatomical diagnosis, i.e., to define the metabolic state and to ascertain the nature of the underlying disorder. These two aspects of the diagnosis are not arrived at independently, because the functional state delimits the possible specific diagnoses and vice versa.

A functional diagnosis of thyroid disease is based on a carefully taken history, a thorough search for the physical signs of hypothyroidism or thyrotoxicosis, and an appraisal of the results of laboratory tests. Characteristic alterations in these aspects will be found in the discussions of the various disease states. Although conditioned by the functional diagnosis, the anatomical diagnosis depends largely on the examination of the thyroid gland itself (Fig. 8–29).

Local examination of the neck is best accomplished with the patient seated in a good light with the neck moderately extended. The patient should be provided with a glass of water to facilitate swallowing. The physician should first inspect the neck from the front and sides. The presence of old surgical scars, distended veins, and redness or fixation of the overlying skin should be noted. If a mass is present, attention should be directed to its location and to whether it moves on swallowing. The position of the trachea should be documented. Movement on swallowing is a characteristic of the thyroid gland and occurs because the gland is ensheathed by the pretracheal fascia; this feature distinguishes a goiter from most other masses arising in the neck. However, if a goiter is so large that it occupies all the available space in the neck, or if the thyroid gland is the seat of an invasive carcinoma or Riedel thyroiditis that has led to fixation to adjacent structures, movement on swallowing may be lost. The physician should also inspect the dorsum of the tongue, which is the origin of the thyroglossal duct and occasionally the seat of a goiter (lingual goiter).

Palpation of the neck may be accomplished by standing behind the seated patient and palpating with the fingertips of both hands. The position of the cricoid cartilage is first determined; this is an important landmark, because the superior border of the isthmus lies just below it. The isthmus is a band of tissue crossing the front of the trachea and joining the two lateral lobes on either side of the trachea. The examiner then attempts to outline the thyroid gland and to determine the limits of the lower borders of the lateral lobes, while the patient swallows sips of water at appropriate intervals. A normal thyroid gland can usually be palpated. An alternative approach is to stand facing the patient using the thumb to locate the thyroid isthmus. The right thumb is then moved laterally to compress the right lobe of the thyroid against the trachea as the patient swallows. A similar strategy with the left thumb is used for the left lobe. This technique may be especially useful for evaluating small nodules that might not be easily appreciated using the posterior approach. The examiner should note the shape of the gland, its size in relation to normal, and its consistency. The normal gland feels rubbery. A literal rule of thumb is that the normal thyroid lobe has approximately the same size in frontal projection as the terminal phalanx of the thumb. Whereas the diffuse colloid goiter and the hyperplastic gland of Graves disease tend to be softer than normal, the gland of Hashimoto disease tends to be firm, and the gland that is the seat of carcinoma or Riedel thyroiditis may be "stony" hard. Irregularities of the surface, variations in consistency, and tender areas should be noted. If nodules are palpated, their shape, size, position, and consistency in relation to the surrounding tissue should be

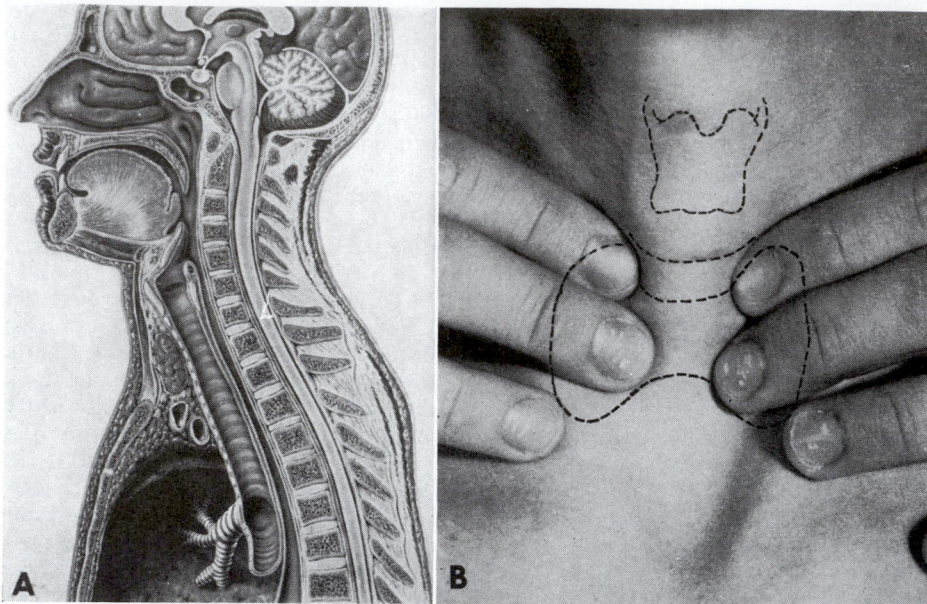

Figure 8–29. *A,* This sagittal section demonstrates the relations of the isthmus of the normal thyroid gland. The superior border is inferior to the cricoid cartilage. The inferior thyroid border is essentially at the level of the superior surface of the manubrium. The inferior portions of the lateral lobes (not shown) extend more inferiorly than the isthmus.

B, The cricoid cartilage is regarded as an important landmark. Especially when the thyroid gland is thought to be essentially normal or subnormal in size, the cricoid should be located. This is easily accomplished. The index fingers are then inserted so that their superior portion rests against the inferior portion of the cricoid, while the inferior portion of these fingers is over the superior portion of the thyroid. The second and third fingers are rotated over other portions of the gland, evaluating its size, contour, consistency, possible adherence to surrounding structures, and other features. Because there is marked variation among different subjects in the length and thickness of the neck and in the length of the trachea superior to the level of the manubrium, there is variation in the relative position of the thyroid. In some cases, essentially all of the thyroid rests posterior to the sternum. In most instances, however, by having the patient extend the neck maximally (short of markedly tightening the neck muscles) and swallow repeatedly, it is possible to palpate most or all of the gland. In spite of marked variations in neck-chest relations, thyroid tissue, when present, is found within 1 cm of the cricoid. By concentrating the palpation meticulously in the area where the thyroid is normally found, with rare exceptions it is possible to outline small as well as enlarged glands.

determined. A search should be made for the pyramidal lobe; this is a band of tissue extending upward from the isthmus to the right or left of the midline. The pyramidal lobe may be mistaken for the pretracheal or "delphian" lymph node that sometimes accompanies thyroid carcinoma or thyroiditis. Another midline mass that may lead to confusion is a thyroglossal cyst, but because this often remains attached to the base of the tongue by the obliterated thyroglossal duct, it moves upward when the tongue is protruded. During palpation a vascular thrill may be felt and, in the absence of cardiac disease, is suggestive of hyperthyroidism. Finally, palpation should always include examination of the regional lymph nodes.

Auscultation of the neck should be performed, because it gives some indication of the vascularity of the gland. A systolic or continuous bruit is commonly heard over a hyperplastic gland. Care should be taken to distinguish a thyroid bruit from a murmur transmitted from the base of the heart or from a venous hum that can be obliterated by compression of the external jugular vein or by turning the head.

Two useful clinical maneuvers that are often neglected are transillumination and the arm-raising test. Transillumination is readily performed with a penlight and serves to distinguish between cystic and solid masses in the thyroid. Because the normal tissues of the neck transilluminate to some extent, the transillumination in the lesion should be compared with that in an indifferent area. The arm-raising test is useful when a retrosternal goiter is suspected. The basis for this maneuver is that if the size of the thoracic inlet is already reduced by a retrosternal goiter, raising both arms until they touch the sides of the head will further narrow the thoracic inlet and cause congestion of the face and respiratory distress (Pemberton sign).

In addition to examination of the thyroid gland and regional lymph nodes, evidence of compression or displacement of adjacent structures should be sought. Hoarseness may indicate compression of the recurrent laryngeal nerve, usually by a malignant thyroid neoplasm, and this should be confirmed by laryngoscopy. Displacement of the trachea may be evident, and inspiratory stridor may indicate compression of the trachea. Radiological examination may reveal retrosternal extension of a goiter, displacement or narrowing of the trachea, and, during a barium swallow, displacement of the esophagus. Calcification in the thyroid gland may also be seen and, by its nature, aid in distinguishing between benign and malignant lesions.

THYROTOXICOSIS

The term thyrotoxicosis refers to the biochemical and physiological complex that results when the tissues are presented with excessive quantities of the thyroid hormones. The authors prefer the general term *thyrotoxicosis* rather than hyperthyroidism to describe this syndrome, because the disorder need not originate in the thyroid gland. The term *hyperthyroidism* is best reserved for disorders in which thyrotoxicosis results from overproduction of hormone by the thyroid itself, Graves disease being the most common. The various causes of thyrotoxicosis are listed in Table 8–11. The manifestations of thyrotoxicosis depend on the severity of the syndrome, the age of the patient, and the presence or absence of disease in other organ systems. Additional clinical features are conditioned by the specific disorder producing the thyrotoxicosis.

TABLE 8–11. Varieties of Thyrotoxicosis

Associated with Sustained Hormone Overproduction (Hyperthyroidism)*
Graves disease
Toxic multinodular goiter
Toxic adenoma
Iodine-induced (jodbasedow)
Trophoblastic tumor
Increased TSH secretion
Not Associated with Hyperthyroidism†
Thyrotoxicosis factitia
Subacute thyroiditis
Chronic thyroiditis with transient thyrotoxicosis (painless thyroiditis, hyperthyroiditis, silent thyroiditis)
Ectopic thyroid tissue (struma ovarii, functioning metastatic thyroid cancer)

*Except for iodine-induced hyperthyroidism, associated with increased values of RAIU.

†Associated with decreased values of RAIU.

Peripheral Manifestations of Thyrotoxicosis

Skin and Appendages

Thyrotoxicosis leads to a variety of changes in the skin and its appendages. Most characteristic is the warm moist feel of the skin that results from cutaneous vasodilation and excessive sweating as part of the hyperdynamic circulatory state. The hands are usually warm and moist, but the texture of the skin in this area is often altered by occupational or environmental factors; hence, texture is best assessed on the inner aspect of the arm or thigh or over the thorax. The elbows are typically smooth and pink. The complexion is rosy and the patient blushes readily. Palmar erythema, indistinguishable from "liver palms," is common, and there may be some telangiectasia. Increased diffuse pigmentation is found occasionally and may resemble that in Addison disease, but buccal pigmentation does not occur in uncomplicated thyrotoxicosis. Patchy vitiligo may also occur. Increased pigmentation may result from hypersecretion of ACTH secondary to accelerated turnover of cortisol.

The hair is fine and friable and does not retain a wave; some may fall out. A history of early graying in the patient or in relatives is common in Graves disease. The nails are often soft and friable. A characteristic finding is Plummer nails, a term applied to separation of the distal margin of the nail from the nail bed with irregular recession of the junction (onycholysis). Dirt often accumulates under the nail. Usually these changes are best seen in the fourth finger and are frequently accompanied by a thin, shiny appearance of the skin surrounding the nail.

Eyes

Retraction of the upper eyelid, evident as the presence of a rim of sclera between the lid and the limbus, is a frequent manifestation of all forms of thyrotoxicosis, regardless of the underlying cause. It is responsible for the bright-eyed "stare" of the patient with thyrotoxicosis. Accompanying lid retraction are the phenomena of lid lag, in which the upper lid lags behind the globe when the patient is asked to gaze slowly downward, and globe lag, in which the globe lags behind the upper lid when the patient gazes slowly upward. The movements of the lids are jerky and spasmodic, and a fine tremor of the lightly closed lids can often be observed. These ocular manifestations appear to be the result of increased adrenergic activity. It is important to differentiate these ocular manifestations, which occur in all forms of thyrotoxicosis, from those of infiltrative ophthalmopathy, which are characteristic of Graves disease.

Cardiovascular System

Alterations in cardiovascular function are among the most prominent manifestations of thyrotoxicosis. Increased circulatory demands result from both the hypermetabolism and the need to dissipate the excess heat produced. At rest, peripheral vascular resistance is decreased, and cardiac output is increased as a result of an increase in both stroke volume and heart rate. Thyroid hormones in excess have a direct cardiostimulatory action, possibly mediated by alterations in the state of contractile proteins or in the function of sarcoplasmic reticulum.

Tachycardia is almost always present, even at rest. Tachycardia during sleep (pulse rate greater than 90 beats/min) serves to distinguish tachycardia of thyrotoxic origin from that of psychogenic origin. The pulse pressure is widened as a result of both an increase in systolic pressure and a decrease in diastolic pressure. The increased force of cardiac contraction is often felt by the patient as palpitation and is evident on inspection or palpation of the precordium. Because of the diffuse and forceful nature of the apex beat, the heart often seems enlarged, but x-ray study generally does not confirm this impression. Heart sounds are loud and ringing, and a systolic or even a late diastolic or presystolic murmur may be present at the apex. A scratchy systolic sound along the left sternal border, resembling a pericardial friction rub, may also be heard. Mitral valve prolapse may be seen in echocardiograms, probably as a result of papillary muscle dysfunction. These manifestations abate when a normal metabolic state is restored.

Cardiac arrhythmias are common with thyrotoxicosis and are almost invariably supraventricular. Approximately 10% of the patients with thyrotoxicosis manifest atrial fibrillation, and a similar percentage of patients with otherwise unexplained atrial fibrillation prove to be thyrotoxic. Paroxysmal supraventricular tachycardia may be demonstrable or may be suggested by the history. Systolic time intervals are altered in thyrotoxicosis; the pulse wave propagation is accelerated; the pre-ejection period is distinctly shortened; and the ratio of pre-ejection period to left ventricular ejection time is decreased.

The adequacy of the circulation is a question of importance in the patient with thyrotoxicosis. The arteriovenous oxygen difference is generally normal, but the significance of this is obscured because, for purposes of heat loss, a considerable proportion of the cardiac output may be directed to the skin, in which relatively little oxygen consumption occurs. Although the cardiovascular cost of a standard workload or metabolic challenge is increased, this is adequately met if the patient is not or has not previously been in heart failure. Thus, in most patients without underlying heart disease, cardiac competence is maintained. Mild edema not uncommonly occurs in the absence of heart failure. Thyrotoxicosis may lead to congestive heart failure, but even so the circulation time may remain shortened. Heart failure usually occurs in patients with pre-existing heart disease, but it may not be possible to determine whether underlying heart disease is present until after thyrotoxicosis is relieved. There is little doubt that pure thyrocardiac disease does occur, but it occurs uncommonly and usually in association with atrial fibrillation. Because the latter decreases the efficiency of the cardiac response to any increased circulatory demand, it may play a role in bringing about cardiac failure. Attempts to convert atrial fibrillation to sinus rhythm are usually of no avail while thyrotoxicosis is present. Regardless of the type of rhythm, the response to digitalis is decreased, possibly because of accelerated metabolism of the drug, and large quantities may be required to produce a clinical effect. Resistance to digitalis, as well as failure of cardiac decompensation to respond to a usually adequate regimen, should suggest the possibility of thyrotoxicosis.

The frequency of coronary artery disease in patients with thyrotoxicosis is uncertain. Myocardial infarction is uncommon; however, when angina pectoris is present, it is aggravated by thyrotoxicosis and relieved by treatment.

Respiratory System

Dyspnea is a common symptom and need not be due to heart failure. Several factors may contribute to this symptom. Vital capacity is commonly reduced; this appears to result mainly from weakness of the respiratory muscles, but decreased pulmonary compliance may also play a role. During exercise, ventilation is increased out of proportion to the increase in oxygen uptake; the diffusing capacity of the lung is normal, however. Pulmonary function returns to normal when a normal metabolic state is restored.

Alimentary System

An increase in appetite, both at mealtimes and between meals, is a common symptom, but the mechanism whereby this occurs is unknown. Except in unusual cases, increased intake of food is inadequate to meet the increased caloric requirements, and weight is lost at a variable rate. In the occasional, usually younger, patient with mild disease, weight gain may occur instead. Anorexia, rather than hyperphagia, sometimes accompanies severe thyrotoxicosis. It occurs in about one third of elderly thyrotoxic patients and contributes to the picture of "masked" thyrotoxicosis.

The commonest symptoms referable to the alimentary tract are those related to bowel function. Diarrhea is rare; more often stools are less well formed, and the frequency of bowel movements is increased. In the authors' experience, patients may display intolerance to milk products while thyrotoxic. When constipation has anteceded the development of thyrotoxicosis, bowel function may return to normal. Anorexia, nausea, and vomiting are uncommon but may occur in patients with severe disease. These symptoms, as well as abdominal pain, may be forerunners of thyroid storm. Gastric emptying and intestinal motility are increased in thyrotoxicosis, and this appears to be responsible for slight malabsorption of fat. The mechanism underlying the gastrointestinal hypermotility has not been elucidated, but the hypermotility disappears when a normal metabolic state is restored. Gluten enteropathy and Graves disease may coexist more frequently than can be accounted for by chance. A high proportion of patients display gastric achlorhydria. In the majority, acid secretion returns after relief of the thyrotoxicosis, but in some it does not. Circulating autoantibodies against gastric parietal cells are found in approximately one third of the patients with Graves disease, and approximately 3% have been reported to have pernicious anemia. It is commonly thought that intestinal absorption is accelerated in thyrotoxicosis, but evidence for this is sparse. It is also stated that the oral glucose tolerance curve displays a high early peak in patients with thyrotoxicosis, but in fact the glycemic peak is frequently delayed.

Hepatic dysfunction occurs in thyrotoxicosis, particularly when the disease is severe; hypoproteinemia and increases in serum transaminase and alkaline phosphatase levels may be present. In the most severe cases, hepatomegaly and jaundice may be found. Gynecomastia is present in about 5% of affected men. In thyrotoxicosis, splanchnic oxygen consumption is increased while splanchnic blood flow is essentially unchanged. As a result, the arteriovenous oxygen difference across the splanchnic bed is increased; hence, hypoxia may contribute to hepatic dysfunction.[230]

Hypoxia, together with the state of relative caloric deprivation, may partly account for the depletion of hepatic glycogen that is evident both in the response to glycogenolytic agents and on direct analysis. In the absence of severe thyrotoxicosis or congestive heart failure, the liver may appear normal on light microscopic examination. In severe cases, centrilobular fatty infiltration may occur, together with patchy portal fibrosis, lymphocytic infiltration, and proliferation of bile ducts. Ultramicroscopic examination of the liver reveals enlarged mitochondria and hypertrophic smooth endoplasmic reticulum. Graves disease and chronic active hepatitis occur together more often than can be explained by chance.

Nervous System

Alterations in the function of the nervous system are an almost invariable accompaniment of thyrotoxicosis and are commonly manifested by nervousness, emotional lability, and hyperkinesia. The nervousness of the thyrotoxic patient is not that of the patient who is chronically anxious but rather is characterized by restlessness, shortness of attention span, and a compulsion to be moving around, despite a feeling of fatigue. Unlike the patient with neurocirculatory asthenia, the thyrotoxic patient wishes to be active but is hampered by fatigability and is tired from the neck down, rather than from the top of the head down. Fatigue may be a manifestation of muscle weakness and the insomnia of which patients with thyrotoxicosis commonly complain. In some patients, asthenia and fatigue are so severe that the overall activity is decreased.

Emotional lability is also prominent. Patients lose their tempers easily and have episodes of crying without apparent reason. Crying may be evoked by merely questioning the patient about the symptom. In rare cases, severe psychic disturbance may occur; manic-depressive, schizoid, or paranoid reactions may emerge during the illness.

The hyperkinesia of the thyrotoxic patient is characteristic. During the interview the patient cannot sit still, drums on the table, taps a foot, or shifts positions frequently. Movements are quick, jerky, exaggerated, and often purposeless. In children, in whom such manifestations tend to be more severe, Sydenham chorea may be suggested. Examination also reveals a fine rhythmic tremor of the hands, tongue, or lightly closed eyelids. With the aid of a magnifying glass, a tremor of the eyeballs may be seen. The tremor may sometimes mimic that of parkinsonism, and a pre-existing parkinsonian tremor is accentuated during thyrotoxicosis. In patients with convulsive disorders, the frequency of seizures is increased. The electroencephalogram reveals an increase in fast-wave activity, and in experimental animals the convulsive threshold is decreased.

The physiological basis of the findings referable to the nervous system is not well understood. In part, they may reflect increased adrenergic activity because some improvement occurs during treatment with adrenergic antagonists. Although the cerebral blood flow is increased, the arteriovenous oxygen difference is diminished and oxygen extraction is unchanged. This correlates well with the apparent inability of thyroid hormones to increase the oxygen consumption of brain tissue in animals. Nevertheless, failure of overall oxygen consumption to increase does not exclude the likelihood that other alterations in cerebral metabolism are induced by thyroid hormone.

Muscle

Weakness and fatigability are frequent. In most instances these are not accompanied by objective evidence of local disease of muscle save for the generalized wasting associated with loss of weight. Often the weakness is most prominent in the proximal muscles of the limbs, with the result that the patient experiences difficulty in climbing stairs or in maintaining the leg in an extended position. The latter maneuver can be employed to assess the degree of muscle weakness. In occasional cases, involvement of muscles is associated with wasting that again tends to be proximal and is out of proportion to the overall loss of weight (thyrotoxic myopathy). In the extreme form, the patient may be unable to rise from a sitting or lying position and may be virtually unable to walk. This disorder may resemble progressive muscular atrophy or polymyositis, but fasciculation is absent and, on biopsy, little if any inflammatory change is evident. Instead atrophy of muscle and infiltration of fat cells and lymphocytes are present. Electron microscopy reveals abnormal mitochondria and focal dilations of the transverse tubular system. Electromyograms reveal a decreased duration of mean action potentials and an increased percentage of polyphasic potentials. The biochemical basis of the muscular weakness is uncertain but may be related to the impaired ability of thyrotoxic muscle to phosphorylate creatine. Creatinuria is present and creatine tolerance is diminished.

Myopathy affects men with thyrotoxicosis more commonly than women and may overshadow the other manifestations of the syndrome. In the most severe forms, the myopathy may involve the more distal muscles of the extremities as well as muscles of the trunk and face. Although involvement of ocular muscles is unusual, the disorder may mimic myasthenia gravis. In uncomplicated thyrotoxic myopathy, some improvement of muscular strength may follow the administration of edrophonium, but, unlike that in myasthenia, the response is incomplete. Muscular strength returns to normal when a normal metabolic state has been restored, but muscle mass takes longer to recover.

Graves disease occurs in about 3 to 5% of the patients with myasthenia gravis, and about 1% of the patients with Graves disease develop myasthenia gravis. These associations are of interest in view of the frequent association of thymic enlargement with Graves disease.[231] Further, antibodies against specific receptors, i.e., the TSH receptor and the acetylcholine receptor, are involved in the pathogenesis of the two diseases. Unlike thyrotoxic myopathy, the association of myasthenia gravis with Graves disease has a distinct female sex preponderance. The effect of both thyrotoxicosis and its alleviation on the course of myasthenia gravis is variable, but in the majority of instances, myasthenia is accentuated during the thyrotoxic state and improves when a normal metabolic state is restored.

Periodic paralysis of the hypokalemic type may occur together with thyrotoxicosis, and its severity is accentuated by the latter disorder. The coincidence of the two disorders is particularly common in Japanese and Chinese patients, in whom the incidence of periodic paralysis has been reported to be as high as 13% in men and 0.4% in women with thyrotoxicosis.[232]

Skeletal System: Calcium and Phosphorus Metabolism

Thyrotoxicosis is generally associated with increased excretion of calcium and phosphorus in urine and stool. Excessive loss of mineral is sometimes associated with radiologically demonstrable demineralization of bone and occasionally with pathological fractures, especially in elderly women. In such instances the histological appearance of bone is variable, suggesting osteitis fibrosa, osteomalacia, or osteoporosis. Osteoporosis has been traditionally ascribed to loss of protein matrix, but severely negative calcium balance has been found in some patients who are in virtual nitrogen equilibrium, making this explanation unlikely. Urinary excretion of hydroxyproline is increased in thyrotoxicosis, indicating increased turnover of collagen. Kinetic studies indicate an increase in the exchangeable calcium pool and acceleration of both bone resorption and accretion, the former especially so.

Hypercalcemia occurs in a significant proportion of patients with thyrotoxicosis. The total serum calcium concentration is reportedly increased in as many as 27% of the patients and the ionized serum calcium level in 47% is elevated.[233] The concentrations of heat-labile serum alkaline phosphatase and osteocalcin are also frequently increased.[234-236] These findings are reminiscent of those of primary hyperparathyroidism, but the concentration of immunoreactive parathyroid hormone in serum is decreased in most thyrotoxic patients with hypercalcemia. True primary hyperparathyroidism and thyrotoxicosis may sometimes coexist. Hypercalcemia may be sufficient to induce anorexia, nausea, vomiting, polyuria, or even impairment of renal function. The alterations in calcium metabolism in thyrotoxicosis may be due to a direct effect of thyroid hormones in stimulating bone resorption and are reversed when the eumetabolic state is restored.

The impact of thyroid hormone excess on vitamin D metabolism is still uncertain. Plasma 25-hydroxycholecalciferol concentrations are decreased in thyrotoxic patients, and this alteration could contribute to the decreased intestinal absorption of calcium and osteomalacia noted in some patients.

The average height is above normal in thyrotoxic children. Maturation of bone may be stimulated so that bone age is advanced, but usually this is not of marked degree.

Renal Function: Water and Electrolyte Metabolism

In the absence of hypercalcemia or diabetes mellitus, thyrotoxicosis produces no symptoms referable to the urinary tract save for mild polyuria. Nevertheless, rates of renal blood flow and glomerular filtration as well as tubular reabsorptive and secretory maxima are increased. Total amounts of body water and exchangeable potassium are decreased, possibly because of a decrease in lean body mass, but the amount of exchangeable sodium tends to be increased. Serum sodium, potassium, and chloride concentrations are normal, however. In thyrotoxicosis the level of exchangeable magnesium is normal but the serum magnesium concentration is often decreased and urinary magnesium excretion is increased.

Hematopoietic System

In most patients with thyrotoxicosis, the red blood cells are normal as judged by the usual indices, but the red blood cell mass is increased. The increase in erythropoiesis appears to be due both to the direct effect of thyroid hormones on the erythroid marrow and to increased production of erythropoietin. A parallel increase in plasma volume also occurs, with the result that the hematocrit value remains normal. Other red blood cell abnormalities in thyrotoxicosis include a reduced content of zinc and carbonic anhydrase 1 and an increased content of sodium, probably because activity of Na^+,K^+-ATPase is impaired (in contrast to the increased Na^+,K^+-ATPase activity that may be seen in other tissues).

Approximately 3% of the patients with Graves disease have pernicious anemia, and a further 3% have intrinsic factor autoantibodies with normal absorption of vitamin B_{12}.

Circulating autoantibodies against gastric parietal cells occur in about one third of the patients with Graves disease. In thyrotoxicosis the requirements for vitamin B_{12} and folic acid appear to be increased. Rarely thyrotoxicosis is associated with a mild hypochromic anemia that is characterized by adequate stores of iron in the marrow and a response to large doses of pyridoxine.

The total white blood cell count is often low because of a decrease in number of neutrophils. The absolute lymphocyte count is normal or increased, leading to a relative lymphocytosis. Numbers of monocytes and eosinophils may also be increased. Splenic enlargement occurs in about 10% of the patients, and thymic and lymph node enlargement is common.[231] It is not known whether these abnormalities are a reflection of the autoimmune aspects of Graves disease, but this is unlikely because comparable alterations do not occur in Hashimoto disease. Alternatively, these alterations may result from a direct effect of thyroid hormone on lymphoid tissue.

Blood platelets and the intrinsic clotting mechanism are normal. However, the concentration of factor VIII is often increased, and it returns to normal when the thyrotoxicosis is treated.[237] Despite this increase, the hyperthyroid patient has an increased sensitivity to anticoagulants of the coumarin series because of the accelerated metabolic clearance of the vitamin K–dependent clotting factors. Somewhat paradoxically then, the dosage of such anticoagulants should be reduced in thyrotoxic patients whereas the requirement for anticoagulants is sometimes increased in the hypothyroid patient.[238]

Pituitary and Adrenocortical Function

In some respects the thyrotoxic state imposes a challenge on pituitary and particularly adrenocortical function. The metabolic transformations leading to the inactivation of cortisol are accelerated. These include reduction of the A ring, which is rapidly followed by conjugation, and oxidation of the 11-hydroxy group to a keto group as a result of an increase in 11β-hydroxysteroid dehydrogenase activity; the 11-keto compounds are less active than their 11-hydroxy precursors. As a result of these changes the disposal of cortisol is accelerated, but its rate of secretion is also increased so that the plasma cortisol concentration remains normal. The concentration of corticosteroid-binding globulin in plasma is normal. The urinary excretion of 17-hydroxycorticosteroids (17-OHCS) is normal or slightly increased, whereas the urinary excretion of 17-ketosteroids (17-KS) may be moderately reduced.

The foregoing alterations require that some degree of adrenocortical hyperfunction be sustained in thyrotoxic patients, but proof of increased secretion of ACTH is lacking. Pituitary-adrenal function is adequate for basal demands, as indicated by normal plasma cortisol concentrations, and the response to an acute challenge, such as that imposed by insulin-induced hypoglycemia, is generally adequate.

The rate of turnover of aldosterone is increased, but its plasma concentration is normal. Plasma renin activity is increased, and sensitivity to angiotensin II is reduced.[239]

The response of plasma growth hormone concentration to insulin-induced hypoglycemia is subnormal, particularly in those with severe disease. This observation need not indicate deficient growth hormone production but may reflect depletion of pituitary stores from prolonged caloric inadequacy or accelerated removal of growth hormone from plasma. Incomplete suppression of plasma growth hormone concentration by induced hyperglycemia may also reflect prolonged caloric deprivation.

Reproductive Function

Thyrotoxicosis in early life may be associated with delayed sexual maturation, although general physical development is normal and skeletal growth is often accelerated. Thyrotoxicosis after puberty also influences reproductive function, especially in women. An increase in libido sometimes occurs in both sexes, and menstrual function is usually disturbed in women. The intermenstrual interval may be either prolonged or shortened, and menstrual flow at first is diminished and ultimately ceases altogether. Fertility may be reduced, and if conception takes place, abortion may result.

In some patients, cycles are predominantly anovulatory, but in most ovulation occurs, as indicated by a secretory endometrium. In the former, a subnormal midcycle surge of LH may be responsible, but the cause of the menstrual abnormalities in the latter group is unclear. In premenopausal women with thyrotoxicosis, basal plasma concentrations of LH and FSH are reportedly normal and display normal responsiveness to luteinizing hormone–releasing hormone (LHRH).

Both quantitative and qualitative alterations occur in the metabolism of gonadal steroids. With respect to the quantitative alterations, thyrotoxicosis, whether spontaneous or induced by T_3, is accompanied by a great increase in the concentration of testosterone-binding globulin (TeBG) in plasma. As a result the plasma concentrations of testosterone, dihydrotestosterone, and estradiol are increased, but their unbound fractions are decreased. The increased binding in plasma is responsible for the decreased metabolic clearance rate of testosterone and dihydrotestosterone. In the case of estradiol, however, the metabolic clearance rate is normal, suggesting that tissue metabolism of the hormone is increased. Conversion rates of androstenedione to testosterone, estrone, and estradiol, and of testosterone to dihydrotestosterone are increased. The increased rate of conversion of androgens to estrogens has been invoked as a mechanism for gynecomastia in some thyrotoxic men.

With respect to the qualitative alterations, thyrotoxicosis favors metabolism of estradiol and estrone via 2-oxygenation over that via 16α-hydroxylation, with the result that formation of 2-hydroxyestrone and its derivative, 2-methoxyestrone, is increased while formation of estriol is decreased. In the case of androgens, thyrotoxicosis favors metabolism of testosterone to androsterone over that to etiocholanolone. These alterations occur in both spontaneous thyrotoxicosis and that induced by T_3, whereas the converse alterations occur in hypothyroidism. The physiological significance of these alterations is uncertain.[239]

Catecholamines and Serotonin

Many of the effects induced by excessive quantities of the thyroid hormones are reminiscent of those induced by epinephrine, including tachycardia, increased cardiac output, and enhanced glycogenolysis, lipolysis, and calorigenesis. Moreover, some of the clinical manifestations of thyrotoxicosis, among them eyelid retraction, tremor, excessive sweating, and tachycardia, are at least partly alleviated by adrenergic antagonists that either deplete tissue stores or block the action of catecholamines. These observations have been interpreted as indicating that a state of increased adrenergic activity exists in the thyrotoxic organism. However, as discussed earlier, this apparent adrenergic hyperactivity appears to be a consequence of a direct effect of thyroid hormones on these tissues because a number of careful studies have failed to provide evidence for increased cardiac sensitivity to catecholamines in hyperthyroid subjects.[201–203, 205] The secretion rates of both epinephrine and norepinephrine, as well as their plasma concentrations, are normal.[240, 241]

Some manifestations of thyrotoxicosis, such as flushing, sweating, tachycardia, and gastrointestinal hypermotility, are reminiscent of those of the carcinoid syndrome. However, the plasma serotonin concentration, urinary 5-hydroxyindoleacetic acid excretion, and platelet monoamine oxidase activity are normal.

Energy Metabolism: Protein, Carbohydrate, and Lipid Metabolism

The stimulation of energy metabolism and heat production is reflected in the increased BMR, increased appetite, and heat intolerance and in the slightly elevated basal body temperature of the patient with thyrotoxicosis. Despite the increased food intake, a state of chronic caloric and nutritional inadequacy almost always ensues.

Both synthesis and degradation of protein are increased, the latter to a greater extent than the former, with the result that there is net degradation of tissue protein. This is evident in negative nitrogen balance, loss of weight, muscle wasting, weakness, and mild hypoalbuminemia.

The oral glucose tolerance curve is often abnormal and varies from one in which the peak glycemia is increased and somewhat delayed to one that is frankly diabetic in form. Plasma insulin concentrations, however, are increased, suggesting the existence of insulin antagonism. The pathogenesis of these alterations remains to be defined. Pre-existing diabetes mellitus is aggravated by thyrotoxicosis, perhaps as a result of increased degradation of insulin.

Both synthesis and degradation of triglycerides and of cholesterol are increased, but the net effect is one of lipid degradation. This is reflected in an increase in the plasma concentration of free fatty acids and glycerol and a decrease in the serum cholesterol level; serum triglyceride levels are usually slightly decreased. Postheparin lipolytic activity has been reported as being decreased in some studies and increased in others. The mobilization and oxidation of free fatty acids in response to fasting, catecholamines, and growth hormone are enhanced. These alterations, which appear to be due to activation of adenylate cyclase, result in a tendency to ketosis and to fatty infiltration of the liver, depending on the degree of caloric inadequacy.

Composite Clinical Picture and Laboratory Tests in Thyrotoxic States

The effects of an excess of thyroid hormones on the major organ systems are common to thyrotoxic states regardless of their underlying etiology. Their frequency and intensity as well as the other findings with which they are associated are influenced by the nature of the underlying disorder. To a large extent, the same may be said of laboratory tests. Consequently it is propitious to consider the clinical picture, characteristic laboratory findings, and differential diagnosis of thyrotoxic states in relation to each of the specific etiologies.

Graves Disease

The disorder known as Graves disease in the English-speaking world and as Basedow disease on the continent of Europe is the most enigmatic and, in areas of iodine abundance, the most important of all thyroid diseases.

Graves disease is characterized by diffuse goiter, thyrotoxicosis, infiltrative ophthalmopathy, and occasionally infiltrative dermopathy. In the individual patient, the thyroid disease and the infiltrative phenomena may occur singly or together and run courses that are largely independent of one another. The thyroid component is closely related to that of two other thyroid diseases that are probably of autoimmune origin, primary thyroid atrophy and Hashimoto disease. Together, they form a triad of autoimmune thyroid disorders that are related in certain aspects of their pathogenesis and clinical course. In Graves disease, hyperthyroidism occurs in the presence of some degree of chronic thyroiditis and may ultimately be replaced by thyroid hypofunction. Conversely, hyperthyroidism may supervene in patients with pre-existing Hashimoto disease and rarely can arise in a patient with pre-existing primary myxedema.[184, 242]

Evidence for the existence of humoral autoimmunity, i.e., for the presence of thyroid-sensitive B lymphocytes, in the three diseases is the regular occurrence in the serum of antibodies against thyroid peroxidase (a microsomal enzyme) and often against thyroglobulin.[243] Titers tend to be highest in Hashimoto disease and lowest in primary thyroid atrophy at the time it is diagnosed. All share evidence of cell-mediated immunity against thyroid antigen and evidence of sensitized T lymphocytes, as judged from a variety of criteria, including the ability of the lymphocytes to elaborate various lymphokines and to exhibit a mitogenic response when exposed to thyroid antigens. All three are characterized by lymphocytic infiltration of the thyroid gland or remnant thyroid bed, and they share, in patients or their relatives, the frequent clinical or serological evidence of other disorders of autoimmune origin, such as insulin-dependent diabetes mellitus, pernicious anemia, myasthenia gravis, idiopathic adrenal atrophy, Sjögren syndrome, lupus erythematosus, rheumatoid arthritis, and idiopathic thrombocytopenic purpura.

More nearly specific to Graves disease are circulating immunoglobulins that appear to be antibodies to components of the thyroid cell membrane.[183] These antibodies are capable of inhibiting the binding of TSH to its specific receptor site in the cell membrane and are able to activate adenylate cyclase therein. But factors of this type are sometimes found in the serum of patients who, by conventional criteria, appear to have Hashimoto disease.

Prevalence

The prevalence of Graves disease is uncertain, but it has been estimated to occur in 0.4% of the population of the United States. An epidemiological survey in Wickham, England (population about 2800) indicated an incidence of 2.7%, past and present, in women and about one tenth as much in men. Overall, the incidence was estimated to be 1 or 2 cases per 1000 per year.[244] Graves disease is the most common cause of spontaneous hyperthyroidism in patients younger than age 40 and, except perhaps in the elderly, is several times more common than primary thyroprivic hypothyroidism, approaching Hashimoto disease in frequency. Indeed, the overall prevalence of autoimmune thyroid disease, comprising Graves disease, Hashimoto thyroiditis, and primary hypothyroidism, approaches or exceeds that of diabetes mellitus.

Pathogenesis

There is almost universal agreement that the thyroid abnormalities characteristic of Graves disease result from the action on the gland of immunoglobulins of the IgG class that may be antibodies against components or regions of the thyroid plasma membrane, possibly regions that include the receptor for TSH itself. These immunoglobulins are thought to bind to their complementary antigenic regions on the plasma membrane and activate adenylate cyclase, thereby initiating a chain of reactions that leads to thyroid growth, increased vascularity, and hypersecretion of hormone. In view of the complexities to be described later, this view is an oversimplification but nevertheless is an accurate generalization overall.

Diverse procedures have been developed to demonstrate the presence of Graves disease–related IgG in the blood. All assay procedures are of a biological nature and detect an activity, not necessarily a specific compound or class of specific compounds. The terminology used in describing these assays is confusing, owing in some cases to the application of misnomers or to the application of different names to the same activity. For many years, the common procedure for testing serum for Graves-related IgG was to administer IgG to a mouse whose thyroid had been prelabeled with radioactive I and to seek evidence of subsequent enhancement in thyroid hormone secretion into blood. Unlike the stimulation produced by TSH, which peaks at about 2h, that of Graves IgG peaks later, around 16 h. The IgG responsible for this activity was designated long-acting thyroid stimulator or LATS. LATS, which is demonstrable in the serum of about 50% of patients with active Graves disease, has the ability to stimulate the mouse thyroid gland (hence the suggestion that it be renamed the mouse thyroid stimulator). Whether all Graves-related IgGs are capable of stimulating the thyroids of mice and other species, but with less potency than the human thyroid, or whether they exhibit true species specificity is debatable. An alternative assay derives from the observation that when IgG preparations containing LATS are incubated with a human thyroid particulate fraction (containing plasma membranes), LATS activity can be reversibly absorbed from IgG. Sera of a large percentage (approximately 90%) of patients with active Graves disease, although they contain IgG that lacks LATS activity, are capable of preventing the absorption of LATS by the particulate fraction. The IgGs responsible for this activity have been designated LATS-protector or LATS-p. Although sensitive, this assay is difficult and cumbersome and has been undertaken in few laboratories. IgGs from the sera of many patients with Graves disease are capable of stimulating colloid droplet formation when incubated with slices of human thyroid gland. The active factor(s) in this assay has been given the generic name human thyroid stimulator, but this assay is also technically difficult and has not been broadly used.

The two types of assay most widely employed derive from knowledge related to the mechanism of action of peptide hormones on their target organs. In the first, radioreceptor techniques are employed to demonstrate that IgG is capable of inhibiting the binding of ^{125}I-labeled bovine TSH to specific binding sites in human or porcine thyroid membranes (TBII, Fig. 8–30). This is thought to result from competitive binding of IgG at or near the TSH receptor so as to preclude the receptor's binding of TSH. The responsible factor(s) may act elsewhere on the membrane and, in so doing, induce a conformational change in the TSH receptor that prevents the binding of TSH, but studies with a purified radioiodinated Graves IgG have revealed saturable, disease-specific binding that is inhibited by TSH.[245] Although some have referred to the IgGs that possess this activity as thyroid-stimulating immunoglobulins (TSIs), the term is inappropriate because the test does not evaluate the ability of the IgG to induce a functional stimulation. A preferable nomenclature is to refer to these proteins as TSH receptor antibodies (TRAb) and indicate the bioassay employed in parentheses.[135] TRAb are present in more than 90% of patients with active Graves disease (Fig. 8–31).

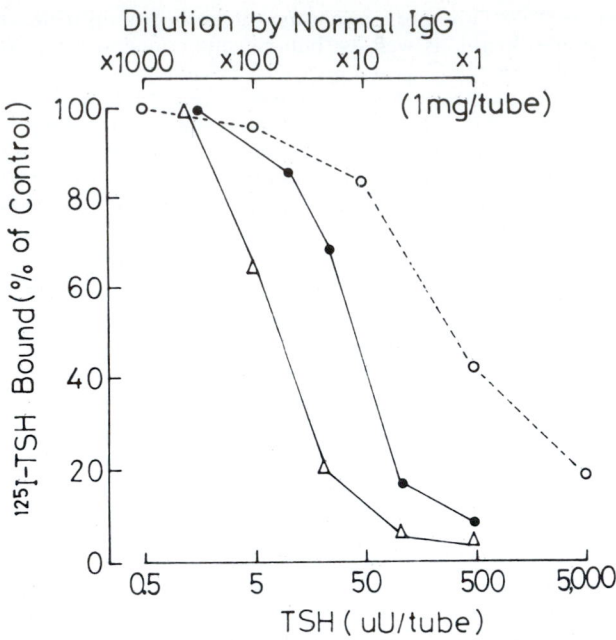

Figure 8–30. Inhibition of the binding of ^{125}I-labeled TSH to receptors in human thyroid membranes by increasing concentrations of bovine TSH (o---o) and by increasing concentrations of IgG containing TSH-binding inhibitory immunoglobulin (TBII) activity (●—● and △—△). (From Endo K, Kashagi K, Konishi J, et al. Detection and properties of TSH-binding inhibitor immunoglobulins in patients with Graves' disease and Hashimoto's thyroiditis. J Clin Endocrinol Metab 1978; 46:734–739. © 1978, The Endocrine Society.)

In another assay, IgG is tested for its ability to stimulate adenylate cyclase activity in human thyroid slices, isolated cells, or particulate preparations. Active TRAb have been designated human thyroid adenylate cyclase stimulators or, more simply, TSIs. TSI activity is present in approximately 80% of patients with active Graves disease (Fig. 8–32). Less common assays include stimulation of iodine accumulation or hormone release in thyroids of various species in vitro and stimulation of either cyclic AMP or iodine accumulation in a line of rat thyroid cells (FRTL) that are particularly sensitive.[246]

A distressing finding is that the TBII and TSI activities in IgG from patients with Graves disease do not correlate well with one another. Some sera potent in TBII activity

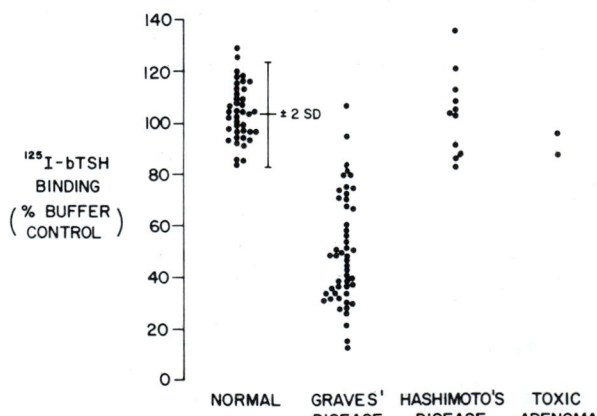

Figure 8–31. Results of TSH-binding inhibition (TBI) assays in patients with various thyroid diseases. (From Borges M, Ingbar JC, Endo K, et al. A new method for assessing the thyrotropin binding inhibitory activity in the immunoglobulins and whole serum of patients with Graves' disease. J Clin Endocrinol Metab 1982; 54:552–558. © 1982, The Endocrine Society.)

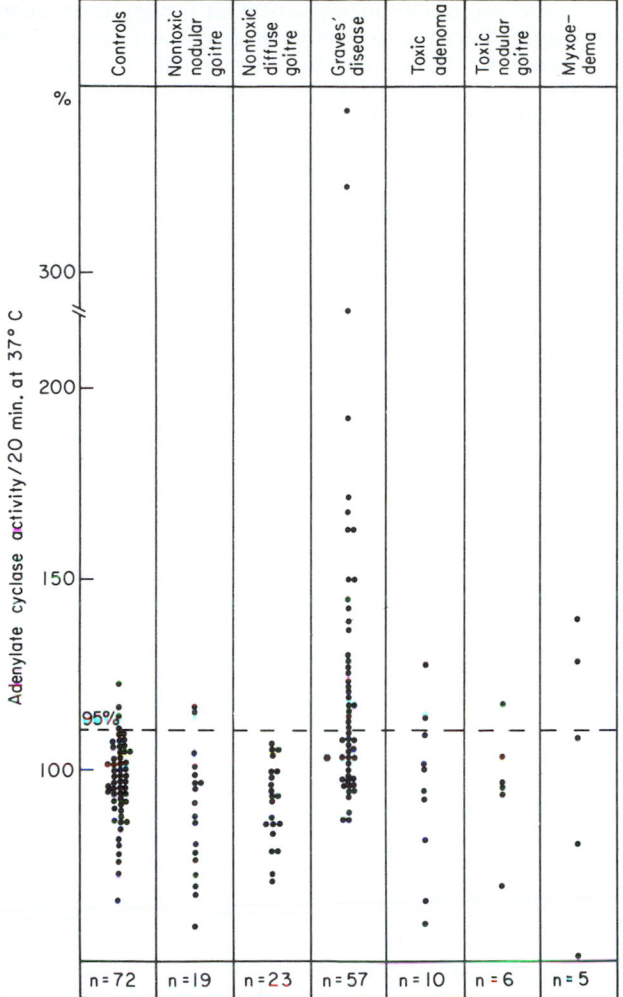

Figure 8–32. Stimulation of adenylate cyclase activity in human thyroid membranes by preparations of IgG from the serum of normal control subjects and patients with various thyroid diseases. (From Bech K, Nistrup Madsen SN. Thyroid adenylate cyclase stimulating immunoglobulins in thyroid disease. Clin Endocrinol 1979; 11:47–58.)

display no TSI activity, and apparently the reverse is also the case. On the other hand, a good correlation exists between one or another of these factors, usually TBII, and nonsuppressibility of thyroid function, the degree of thyroid hyperfunction, and relapse following withdrawal of antithyroid drug therapy.[247–249] TBIIs are also detectable in approximately one half of patients with euthyroid Graves ophthalmopathy and occasionally in patients with Hashimoto thyroiditis and in euthyroid relatives of patients with Graves disease. The absence of hyperthyroidism in these circumstances has been attributed either to limitation of thyroid responsiveness to stimulation or to dissociation between thyroid-stimulating and TSH-displacing activities. Indeed, in some patients with hypothyroidism and adult-onset primary nongoitrous myxedema, thyroid hypofunction results from the action of a class of IgGs that interact with the thyroid membrane but do not stimulate adenylate cyclase. Instead they inhibit stimulatory responses to TSH in vitro and presumably in vivo also. They also inhibit the response to stimulatory IgGs from other patients and perhaps to any that may be present in the patient's own blood. Surprisingly, not all preparations of inhibitory IgGs possess TBI activity, and some are devoid of typical antithyroid antibodies.[250] Transplacental passage of inhibitory IgGs of this type has

been strongly implicated in the pathogenesis of transient hypothyroidism in the neonate,[251] a syndrome that appears to be analogous, but functionally opposite, to neonatal Graves disease.

The concept that some Graves-related IgGs are primarily antagonists, and others agonists, with respect to thyroid stimulation is supported by studies with monoclonal antibodies, including those raised against human thyroid membranes and others derived from fusion of lymphocytes from patients with Graves disease with mouse myeloma cells. Among both types of antibodies, some inhibit the binding of TSH but do not stimulate, some have the reverse activity, and some do both. From these observations and studies related to the TSH receptor itself, it has been proposed that the TSH receptor contains two domains. One, a glycoprotein, is concerned with the binding of TSH but not directly with adenylate cyclase activation; the other, a moiety that contains ganglioside, is concerned with and required for adenylate cyclase activation. Within this construct, predominant binding of Graves IgG to one or another of these sites may determine the nature of its biological activity.[252] This hypothesis concerning the nature and function of the TSH receptor has been disputed.[253]

In any event, the thyroid-related IgGs in autoimmune thyroid disease are a heterogeneous group of antibodies directed at various sites within the thyroid cell membrane. Certain of them may be responsible for cellular damage (cytotoxicity) that causes thyroid function in all of the three diseases to fail with variable degrees of rapidity. Others are capable of eliciting functional stimulation and the clinical entity of diffuse toxic goiter. Even within the latter group there is heterogeneity, so that some are capable of stimulating the thyroids of other species, some interfere with binding of TSH to its receptor in the plasma membrane, some are agonists of the adenylate cyclase system, and some are antagonists to the agonistic action of other stimulators.

Cell-mediated immunity has also been invoked as a possible pathogenetic factor in the hyperthyroidism of Graves disease. This would require that sensitized T lymphocytes infiltrate the thyroid and elaborate stimulatory lymphokines, but evidence that this occurs is lacking. On the other hand, cooperativity between cell-mediated and humoral autoimmunity is suggested by the observation that the mitogen phytohemagglutinin stimulates the lymphocytes from patients with Graves disease to elaborate thyroid-stimulating IgG.

The final link in the pathogenetic chain of autoimmune thyroid diseases would explain why these autoimmune responses arise and, more important, persist. Both cell-mediated and humoral thyroid autoimmunity are evident during the course of subacute thyroiditis but abate when the disease becomes inactive. In chronic autoimmune thyroid disease, a sustained, genetically determined disorder of immune surveillance permits the persistence of clones of thyroid-sensitized immunocytes. This is likely the result of abnormalities in suppressor T cell function.[254]

A further question that is central to the pathogenesis of autoimmune thyroid diseases is why clones of thyroid-sensitized lymphocytes arise in the first instance. It has commonly been accepted that they reflect the occurrence of random mutations, but a variety of evidence links autoimmune thyroid disease to infection with the gram-negative enteric pathogen *Yersinia enterocolitica*. The demonstration that this organism, as well as *E. coli* and other gram-negative organisms, contains a TSH binding site that also binds Graves-related IgG raises the possibility that the initiating event is infection with an organism that gives rise to antibodies that cross-react with components of the human thyroid membrane. In an individual with the predetermined abnormality in immune surveillance, these antibodies would persist and give rise to clinical thyroid disease.[255]

The pathogenesis of the ophthalmopathy of Graves disease is even more enigmatic. One hypothesis holds that an abnormal IgG acting in concert with an exophthalmos-producing factor composed in part of the beta subunit of TSH induces mucopolysaccharide synthesis and edema formation in retro-orbital tissues. Such a mechanism is difficult to reconcile, however, with the absence of measureable quantities of beta subunit in the sera of patients with ophthalmopathy. There is no convincing evidence that antibodies against orbital tissue contents, such as fat or muscle, play a primary pathogenic role, and conclusions concerning the pathogenesis of the ophthalmopathy of Graves disease must be delayed.[256] There has been no evident progress toward elucidation of the pathogenesis of the dermopathy of Graves disease.

Constitutional Factors

Whatever its basic etiology, both the emergence of clinically evident Graves disease and its subsequent course are modified by such factors as heredity, gender, and perhaps emotions. The role of heredity is manifest in several ways. Population studies reveal an increased frequency of haplotypes HLA-B8 in whites, HLA-BW46 in Chinese, and HLA-BW35 in Japanese patients with Graves disease. Of particular importance in whites is the HLA-DR3, which increases the risk of Graves disease and may affect its response to treatment.[257] A further complexity is introduced by the finding that among families in which two or more members have Graves disease, virtually all affected members share the same HLA and Gm haplotypes, indicating that two genes may be associated with the development of this disorder.[258] In addition, a higher concordance rate of Graves disease has been noted in monozygotic than in dizygotic twins. Studies by one of the authors revealed a high incidence of abnormalities in iodine metabolism in euthyroid relatives, some of whom were goitrous. Thyroid ^{131}I uptakes were increased in approximately 20% of the relatives studied, especially in sisters and daughters of the propositi. An increase in the fractional rate of peripheral turnover of T_4 was similar to that observed in clinically overt Graves disease. IgG in the serum of some euthyroid relatives of patients with Graves disease may contain LATS-p or TBII activity, as well as antimicrosomal and antithyroglobulin antibodies. Function studies reveal nonsuppressible thyroid function in some, hyporesponsiveness to TRH in some, hyper-responsiveness in others, and occasional elevations of serum T_3 concentration.

The hereditary factor in Graves disease also appears to involve its autoimmune aspects. This is suggested by the increased incidence in patients with Graves disease or in members of their families of other autoimmune disorders, such as Hashimoto disease or pernicious anemia, and of autoantibodies against thyroid tissue components, gastric parietal cells, and intrinsic factor.

A relationship also exists between gender and the frequency and clinical manifestations of Graves disease. Overall, the disorder is more common in women than in men (7 to 10:1). Furthermore, it tends to become manifest during puberty, pregnancy, and the menopause. In men the disease tends to occur at a later age, to be more severe, and more often to be accompanied by significant ophthalmopathy. It is not known whether the influence of gender in Graves disease is a direct result of genetic determinants or of physiological factors related to reproductive function. The female preponderance is consonant with the autoimmune aspects, because most disorders of an autoimmune nature occur more commonly in women. The foregoing evidence for the operation of autoimmune and genetic factors has led to a concept that Graves disease is the result of a genetically determined immunological defect. This unifying concept does not explain the greater frequency of almost all other thyroid diseases in women than in men.

From the earliest descriptions of Graves disease, a possible role of emotional factors in its emergence has been suggested. Those who see the disease frequently are repeatedly impressed by instances in which Graves disease becomes evident either after severe emotional stress, such as the actual or threatened separation from an individual upon whom the patient is emotionally dependent, or after an acute fright, such as an automobile accident. This could reflect an effect of stress on the function of the immune system. It has also been suggested that patients with Graves disease may be drawn from a population with a characteristic pattern of personality, but some data do not support this hypothesis. Controlled studies in this field are needed if conclusions concerning the role of emotional factors in the pathogenesis of Graves disease are to be drawn.

Natural History and Course

The course of the thyrotoxic component of untreated Graves disease is variable and often erratic. In some patients the thyrotoxic component is persistent although it may vary in severity; in others it may be cyclic, exhibiting exacerbations of varying frequency, intensity, and duration. This cyclic feature has an important bearing on the treatment of the disorder and must also be encompassed by any comprehensive theory of its pathogenesis. With the passage of time, which may be months or years, the thyrotoxic component tends to "burn itself out." Approximately one third of patients treated at least 20 y earlier with antithyroid agents became hypothyroid.[259]

The ophthalmopathy of Graves disease may or may not commence together with the thyrotoxic component. Thus, thyrotoxic patients may be initially free of ophthalmopathy but may develop this manifestation months or years later or not at all. Conversely, the disease may begin with ophthalmopathy and only later, if at all, be associated with thyrotoxicosis. In patients with "euthyroid Graves disease," a small proportion show no evidence of thyroid abnormality, as judged from tests for LATS-p, thyroid suppressibility, or response to exogenous TRH. Others variously display thyroid nonsuppressibility and subnormal or elevated responses to exogenous TRH. Some become hypothyroid within a few years of initial observation, some become hyperthyroid, and still others remain euthyroid but have altered responses to exogenous T_3 or TRH. Many have evidence of chronic thyroiditis.[260] The important element that emerges is that most patients with euthyroid Graves disease display some abnormality of thyroregulatory control, evidence of thyroid autoimmunity, or both. These considerations are important in establishing a positive diagnosis of thyroid-related eye disease. Of further importance is recognition that the functional status of the thyroid in these patients is unstable.

Histopathology

A convenient designation for the thyroid gland of Graves disease during the period of active thyrotoxicosis is the term *diffuse toxic goiter*, which denotes that the gland is both enlarged and uniformly affected. Diffuse toxic goiters vary in consistency from softer than normal to firm and rubbery. The outer surface is usually smooth but may be somewhat lobular; rarely, if ever, is it grossly nodular in the early stages of the disease before treatment. The cut surface is red and glistening. Microscopically, the follicles are small, are lined by hyperplastic columnar epithelium, and contain scant colloid that displays much marginal scalloping and vacuolization (Fig. 8–33). The nuclei are vesicular, are basally situated, and exhibit mitoses. Papillary projections of the hyperplastic epithelium extend into the lumina of the follicles. Vascularity is increased, and there is infiltration to a varying degree by lymphocytes and plasma cells. These cells collect in aggregates, forming lymphoid follicles. When the patient is treated with iodine, the thyroid undergoes *involution*, in which the hyperplasia and increased vascularity abate, the papillary projections recede, and the follicles enlarge and become filled with colloid. No characteristic alterations have been described in the pituitary in Graves disease.

In patients with *infiltrative ophthalmopathy*, the volume of orbital contents is increased because of both an increase in retrobulbar connective tissue and an increase in mass of the extraocular muscles. Some of the increase in connective tissue is due to edema resulting from the increased content in the ground substance of hyaluronic acid, which is hydrophilic. The extraocular muscles are swollen, and the fibers display loss of striation, fragmentation, and lymphocytic infiltration. The lacrimal glands may also be involved. Ultimately, fibrosis of the tissues occurs.

In infiltrative dermopathy, the content of hyaluronic acid in the dermis is increased with resulting edema; the collagen fibers are separated and fragmented, and there is lymphocytic infiltration.

Pathophysiology

All aspects of thyroid hormone economy are abnormal in patients with diffuse toxic goiter. Thus, there occur disruptions of normal regulatory control of thyroid function; alterations in thyroid function itself; changes in the concentration, binding, and metabolism of thyroid hormones; and manifestations of thyroid hormone excess in the peripheral tissues. Abnormalities in all these aspects also occur in other disorders associated with thyrotoxicosis but may differ in kind or amount.

An abnormality or override of normal regulatory control is inherent in all forms of thyrotoxicosis. In Graves disease, normal regulatory mechanisms are overridden by the action of abnormal stimulatory immunoglobulins. The resulting hyperfunction of the thyroid leads to an appropriate suppression of secretion of TSH that is reflected in an undetectable serum TSH level and no TSH response to TRH. A reduced basal TSH and reduced TRH response can also be noted in patients with euthyroid Graves disease, relatives of patients with Graves disease, or patients with diffuse toxic goiter in remission, indicating that an overriding of normal regulatory control is not necessarily associated with clinical thyrotoxicosis. Evidence of the intrinsic normality of regulatory control in almost all disorders associated with thyrotoxicosis is the re-emergence of TSH secretion when thyrotoxicosis is relieved.

Within this context, the term "functional autonomy" is often misused when the intent is to imply that thyroid

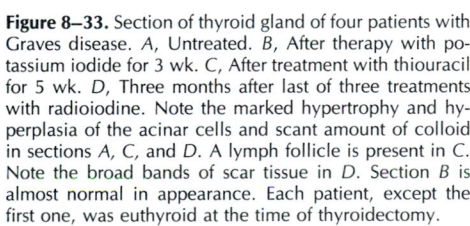

Figure 8–33. Section of thyroid gland of four patients with Graves disease. *A,* Untreated. *B,* After therapy with potassium iodide for 3 wk. *C,* After treatment with thiouracil for 5 wk. *D,* Three months after last of three treatments with radioiodine. Note the marked hypertrophy and hyperplasia of the acinar cells and scant amount of colloid in sections *A, C,* and *D.* A lymph follicle is present in *C.* Note the broad bands of scar tissue in *D.* Section *B* is almost normal in appearance. Each patient, except the first one, was euthyroid at the time of thyroidectomy.

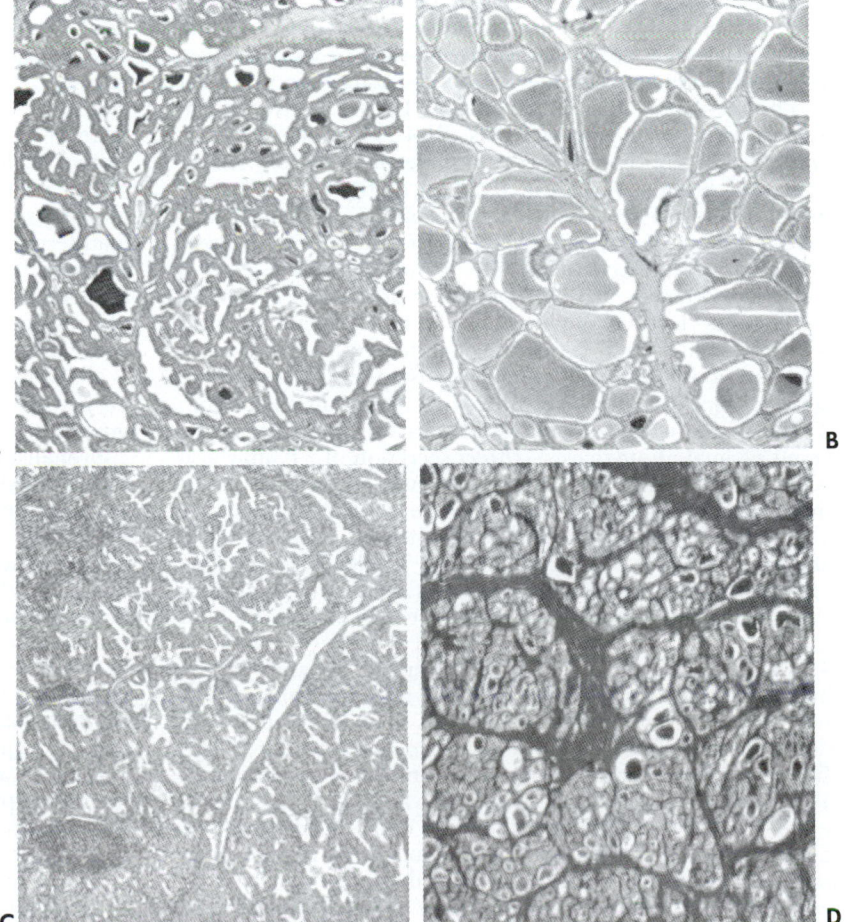

function is independent of TSH stimulation. Rather, true functional autonomy is present when thyroid function is capable of proceeding at a normal or increased pace in the absence of stimulation not only by TSH but also by any other circulating thyroid stimulator. Defined in this way, functional autonomy is characteristic of toxic multinodular goiter and toxic adenoma, but not of Graves disease. In Graves, the thyroid is not intrinsically autonomous but is merely responding to an abnormal stimulator (as in molar pregnancy). When that stimulator is withdrawn, i.e., when the disease enters remission, hyperfunction subsides and the nonautonomous nature of thyroid function becomes evident in the re-emergence of normal thyroid suppression test results. Functional autonomy also does not necessarily imply unresponsiveness to TSH stimulation. Thyroid tissue may be capable of functioning in the absence of external stimulation but may still retain the capacity to respond to TSH.

With respect to thyroid function per se, the disturbance in Graves disease is one that ultimately leads to hypersecretion of the thyroid hormones. Thyroid avidity for iodine is increased, so that thyroid iodide clearance rate is increased from its normal range of approximately 6 to 7 mL/min to values that may approach 2 L/min in the most severe cases. As a result, both RAIU and absolute uptake of iodine are enhanced. The increase in iodide clearance rate must reflect enhanced thyroid blood flow, even if extraction of iodine is assumed to be complete. Hypervascularity of the thyroid in turn may be due to humoral or neurogenic mechanisms but is almost certainly due in part to the increased rate of energy metabolism in the gland itself. The enhanced thyroid iodide clearance rate is usually the result of an increase in both the overall glandular mass and its unit functional activity. Iodide transport and probably organic binding are accelerated. The increase in iodide transport is partly responsible for the enhanced susceptibility of the thyroid gland of Graves disease to the inhibitory effects of iodide on organic binding reactions. As judged from the normal ratio of iodotyrosines to iodothyronines, the rate of the coupling reaction must also be increased. The molar ratio of T_3 to T_4 in thyroglobulin is about twice normal. This disproportionate increase in T_3 production cannot be ascribed to intrathyroid iodine deficiency because the iodine content of thyroglobulin and the number of T_4 residues per molecule are normal. It may reflect chronic hyperstimulation of the thyroid.[18] The rate of turnover and release of the glandular iodine pool is increased, often greatly so. The major product of glandular secretion is T_4, but the ratio of T_3 to T_4 in the thyroid secretion is increased several-fold, reflecting disproportionate overproduction of T_3. In some instances, T_3 appears to be the major secretory product, with the result that serum T_3 concentration alone is increased, serum T_4 concentration being normal (T_3 toxicosis). Direct secretion of rT_3 may also occur, augmenting the increase in serum rT_3 concentration that reflects enhanced peripheral generation from T_4.

Thyroid hormone–protein interactions in the plasma are disturbed, the proportion of total T_4 and T_3 in the free or unbound state being increased (see Fig. 8–18). This change results from a slight decrease in concentration of TBG, as well as from the increase in the concentration of T_4. The fractional rates of turnover of T_4 and T_3 are increased, and this, together with the increased amounts of hormone in the peripheral pool, leads to an increase in total daily disposal of T_4 and T_3. In severe cases, values of this function may increase from the normal of approximately 100 nmol T_4 and 50 nmol T_3 daily to values in excess of 600 nmol/d for both hormones. The total daily disposal of T_3 is disproportionately increased relative to that of T_4, indicating that the production rate of T_3 is disproportionately increased. Whether this results solely from a preferential increase in thyroid secretion of T_3 or whether there is also an increase in the peripheral conversion of T_4 to T_3 is uncertain. The proportionate disposal of T_4 and T_3 by deiodination relative to fecal excretion is not altered.

The abnormalities in hormone turnover in thyrotoxicosis irrespective of the underlying cause are probably the result of several factors, including a disturbance in hormone binding and hypermetabolism. In addition, in Graves disease an intrinsic abnormality may exist in the peripheral metabolism of T_4. For example, an acceleration of the fractional rate of turnover of T_4 has been found in some patients long after thyrotoxicosis had been relieved and also has been noted in some euthyroid relatives of patients with Graves disease. Persistent acceleration of the fractional rate of turnover of T_3 continues in patients with Graves disease after a normal metabolic state has been restored with treatment. The relationship of this abnormality to the other physiopathological alterations in Graves disease is unclear.

Clinical Picture

Graves disease is most commonly manifest in patients in the third and fourth decades of life. The disease is rare before the age of 10 y, and, although unusual, it does occur in the elderly. Like other diseases of the thyroid, it displays a striking preponderance in women of approximately 7 to 10:1. The syndrome comprises diffuse goiter, thyrotoxicosis, infiltrative ophthalmopathy, and occasionally infiltrative dermopathy. Because the infiltrative ophthalmopathy and dermopathy may occur independently of the former two manifestations, they will be discussed separately.

DIFFUSE TOXIC GOITER. The term diffuse toxic goiter is a convenient nosological entity that connotes the presence of thyrotoxicosis resulting specifically from Graves disease. Actual thyroid enlargement is its most common manifestation, by definition, but is absent in a small percentage of cases. The symptoms of diffuse toxic goiter usually begin gradually, the patient noting nervousness, irritability, palpitation, fatigue, heat intolerance, weight loss, or change in menstrual pattern. Any one of these symptoms may predominate (Table 8–12). Enlargement of the thyroid may be noted as a fullness in the neck or rarely may produce obstructive symptoms. In about one third of cases, ocular manifestations begin coincidentally with the onset of thyrotoxicosis. Symptoms may remain mild or progress to a florid state characterized by aggravation of the foregoing complaints together with weakness, insomnia, voracious appetite, and excessive sweating.

Several features merit further consideration. Nervousness, which is probably the most common symptom, may manifest itself in various ways, notably as a feeling of apprehension and inability to concentrate. Emotional lability and irritability may lead to difficulty in interpersonal relationships and to inappropriate spells of crying or euphoria. Fatigability frustrates the desire of the patient to be continuously active. Weakness is noted particularly on climbing stairs, and this activity, as well as others, is prone to produce breathlessness. Heat intolerance, associated with increased sweating, is also a prominent symptom and may be a cause of familial discord. The patient prefers a cooler environment than do others and may lower the thermostat, open the windows, sleep with fewer blankets, or kick off the covers while asleep. The patient usually prefers winter to summer and often finds hot weather intolerable. The change in menstrual pattern usually takes the form of oligomenorrhea with a variable intermenstrual period, occasionally progressing to amenorrhea. Frank diarrhea is uncommon, but increase in the frequency of bowel movements and softening of the stools are often noted. Palpitation may be continuous

TABLE 8–12. Incidence of Symptoms and Signs in 247 Patients with Thyrotoxicosis

Symptom	%	Symptom	%
Nervousness	99	Increased appetite	65
Increased sweating	91	Eye complaints	54
Hypersensitivity to heat	89	Swelling of legs	35
Palpitation	89	Hyperdefecation (without diarrhea)	33
Fatigue	88	Diarrhea	23
Weight loss	85	Anorexia	9
Tachycardia	82	Constipation	4
Dyspnea	75	Weight gain	2
Weakness	70		

Sign	%	Sign	%
Tachycardia*	100	Eye signs	71
Goiter†	100	Atrial fibrillation	10
Skin changes	97	Splenomegaly	10
Tremor	97	Gynecomastia	10
Bruit over thyroid	77	Liver palms	8

*In other studies, thyrotoxic patients with normal pulse rate have been observed.

†Data in this table from Williams RH. Thiouracil treatment of thyrotoxicosis. J Clin Endocrinol 1946; 6:1–22. In the experience of the present authors, enlargement of the thyroid is lacking in approximately 3% of patients with thyrotoxicosis.

or episodic, suggesting paroxysmal dysrhythmia. Although weight loss despite increase in appetite is common, the occasional patient notes a gain in weight, and in more severe cases the appetite may be decreased. Women may complain of excessive fineness of the hair and of its inability to hold a wave. The skin may become more pigmented. In some patients the skin may itch; others are prone to urticaria, sometimes on exposure to the sun. The authors have seen several patients who report urticarial rash on exposure to the sun only when they are taking propylthiouracil. The ocular manifestations of thyrotoxicosis per se are due to spasm and retraction of the eyelids and are noted as a bright-eyed, staring appearance.

Although this symptom complex may develop over a period of months or even years before the patient is first seen, the disease is sometimes fulminant in its emergence, the florid clinical picture developing within a few weeks or less. In such patients, emotional stress may be a forerunner. In some patients with pre-existing heart disease, mild or moderate thyrotoxicosis may precipitate heart failure, which then dominates the clinical picture. In others, severe weakness and wasting of muscles may be the major manifestations. The last two forms are often designated "masked" hyperthyroidism. This term implies that the characteristic manifestations of thyrotoxicosis are absent, but a careful history and examination will usually reveal that this is not the case.

The characteristic physical signs are manifold. Apart from the goiter and exophthalmos, which in themselves may suffice to establish a clinical diagnosis, other aspects of appearance and behavior may be virtually pathognomonic of thyrotoxicosis. The patient usually displays an exaggerated alertness, fidgets, responds quickly to questions or commands, is bright eyed, may appear flushed, and often looks younger than would be expected from the chronological age.

The thyroid is enlarged in most, but not all, patients; thyrotoxicosis in Graves disease may occur in association with a gland of normal size in approximately 3% of patients, and in the elderly goiter may be absent in as many as 20%. The thyroid gland is most commonly two to three times normal size, but it may be massively enlarged (Fig. 8–34). Its consistency varies from somewhat softer than normal to firm and rubbery. The enlargement is usually symmetrical, but sometimes the right lateral lobe is larger than the left. The surface of the gland is generally smooth but may feel lobular. In more severe cases, a thrill may be felt, usually over the upper poles, and a bruit may be audible. The bruit is usually continuous but is sometimes heard only in systole and is most readily detected at the upper or lower poles. It should not be confused with a venous hum or murmur arising from the base of the heart. A thrill or bruit is highly suggestive but not pathognomonic of hyperthyroidism.

Spasm and retraction of the eyelids lead to widening of the palpebral fissure, with the result that sclera is exposed

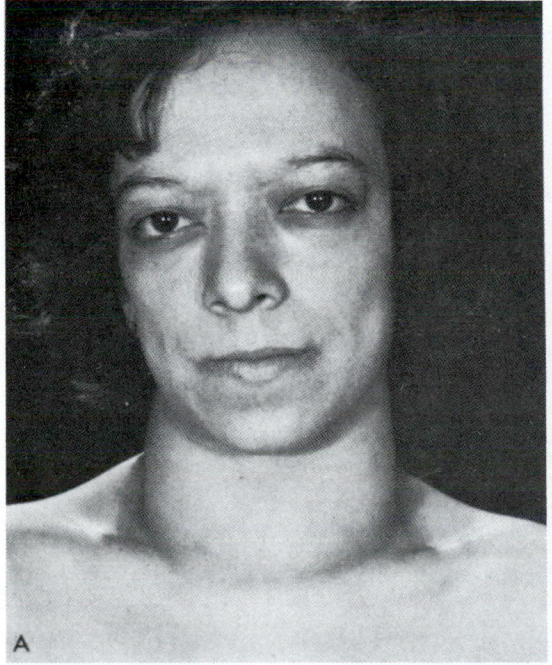
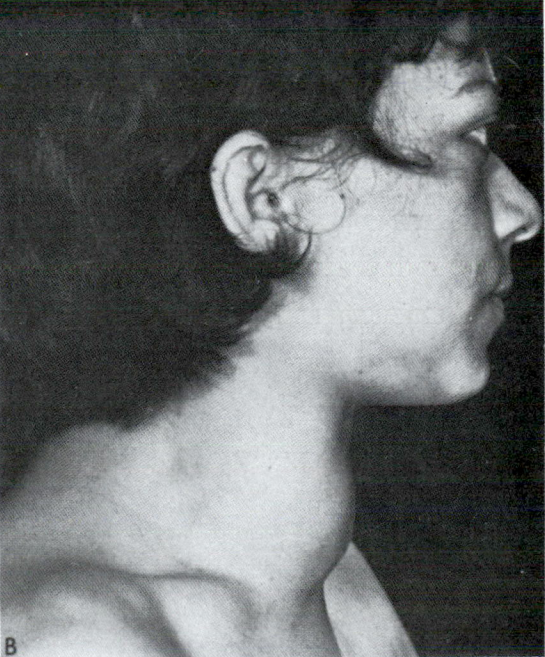

Figure 8–34. Massive thyroid enlargement related to diffuse toxic goiter. Note the sulcus between the thyroid and the lateral aspect of the neck in *B*, as well as the dilated veins overlying the thyroid gland. The patient was severely thyrotoxic and maintained a PBI of 40 μg/100 mL while receiving 1200 mg of propylthiouracil daily. The only ocular abnormality was slight widening of the right palpebral fissure, without true exophthalmos.

above the superior margin of the limbus. The retraction may be asymmetrical. When the patient looks downward, the upper lid lags behind the globe, exposing more of the sclera, and when the patient gazes upward the globe often lags behind the lid (lid lag and globe lag). The movements of the lids are jerky and spasmodic, and a tremor of the lightly closed lids can often be elicited.

The remaining peripheral manifestations of thyrotoxicosis were discussed according to the individual organ systems in a previous section. Among these are the warm, smooth, moist texture of the skin; Plummer nails; physical signs of a hyperdynamic circulation; tremor of the hands and tongue; muscular wasting; and a rapid reflex response.

In general, men tend to develop the disease at a somewhat older age than women, and although the degree of thyroid hyperfunction is often more severe in men, the severity of the symptoms is often less. Men also seem prone to develop myopathy as well as the more severe forms of ophthalmopathy. In older patients the circulatory manifestations may predominate, while the nervous manifestations are lacking. Ophthalmopathy is less common in elderly patients, who are also more likely to display muscular weakness, prostration, and anorexia (apathetic hyperthyroidism).

Infiltrative Ophthalmopathy and Dermopathy

Ophthalmic changes are a major manifestation of Graves disease. As has been suggested, it is important to differentiate between the ocular changes that result from thyrotoxicosis per se and those that not only are more proximately related to the disease process but also may pose serious problems in treatment and prognosis. The latter form has been designated *infiltrative ophthalmopathy*. The thyrotoxic ocular manifestations have already been described. If present alone, these usually abate when the thyrotoxicosis is relieved. Infiltrative ophthalmopathy, on the other hand, follows a course that may be independent of the thyrotoxic aspect and is to a large extent uninfluenced by its treatment (Fig. 8–35). Infiltrative ophthalmopathy is clinically evident in about 50% of patients. However, B-mode ultrasonographic examination of the orbits reveals changes, such as swelling of extraocular muscles and increased retro-orbital fat, in virtually all patients with Graves disease, including those in whom the clinical changes are minimal or absent.[261, 262] Occasionally, infiltrative ophthalmopathy occurs in the absence of diffuse toxic goiter, an entity that is termed euthyroid ophthalmic Graves disease.

The symptoms associated with infiltrative ophthalmopathy are diverse and may appear in varying combinations. Early symptoms often include a sense of irritation in the eyes, resembling that caused by a foreign body, and excessive tearing that is often made worse by exposure to cold air or wind, especially if exophthalmos is present. The conjunctivae may be injected. Exophthalmos, which is frequently asymmetrical, may be accompanied by a feeling of pressure behind the globes. When exophthalmos is pronounced, the patient may sleep with the eyes partly open, a condition termed *lagophthalmos*. Exophthalmos may be masked by periorbital edema, which is a common accompaniment and source of complaint. Patients frequently report that their vision is blurred and that their eyes tire easily. Double vision may occur, either in combination with the foregoing symptoms or alone. In severe cases, visual acuity may be decreased or lost, and corneal ulceration or infection may develop.

The ocular findings are variable (Fig. 8–36). Exophthalmos is probably the most common manifestation. This is usually bilateral and is often asymmetrical. True unilateral exophthalmos is rare and usually occurs in the absence of thyrotoxicosis; most often the other eye is eventually affected. In following the course of the disease, objective measurements of the degree of exophthalmos must be made with the aid of either the Hertel or the Luedde exophthalmometer. These instruments permit measurement of the distance between the lateral angle of the bony orbit and imaginary perpendicular tangent to the most anterior part of the cornea. Generally this distance does not exceed 16 mm, and 20 mm is the upper limit of normal. In severe exophthalmos, readings may be as high as 30 mm. A rough estimate of the degree of exophthalmos may be obtained by standing behind the seated patient and looking downward from above to ascertain the extent to which the eyes protrude beyond the plane of the forehead.

The lids are often reddened, and enlarged lacrimal glands may cause a bulging of their surface. The extent to which the upper and lower lids can be completely apposed should be determined, because failure of apposition promotes drying and ulceration of the cornea. Injection of the bulbar conjunctiva is common and may be accompanied by edema or frank chemosis, in which the edematous conjunctiva bulges from under the lids and around the corneal limbus.

Weakness of the extraocular muscles is most commonly evident in an inability to achieve or maintain convergence. Limitation of upward gaze and especially of superolateral gaze may be present. Occasionally there is paralysis of upward gaze; in such cases, a characteristic position of the head is assumed in which the neck is extended to make possible a field of vision above the horizontal. Rarely, downward or inward gaze is impaired. Ophthalmoplegic manifestations usually are noted in association with other signs of infiltrative ophthalmopathy but may occur alone. In some cases, only a single muscle is affected (Fig. 8–37).

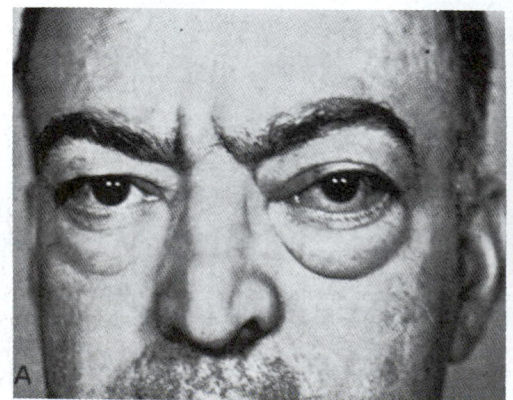

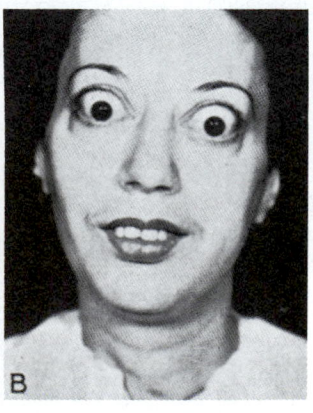

Figure 8–35. Patient *A* was euthyroid and had marked orbital swelling, exophthalmos, conjunctival injection, and chemosis. The proptosis, limitation of extraocular movements, edema, and other manifestations of infiltrative ophthalmopathy are much more marked in *A* than in *B*, who had mild hyperthyroidism, with slight diffuse enlargement of the thyroid, marked widening of the palpebral fissures, with marked stare and proptosis.

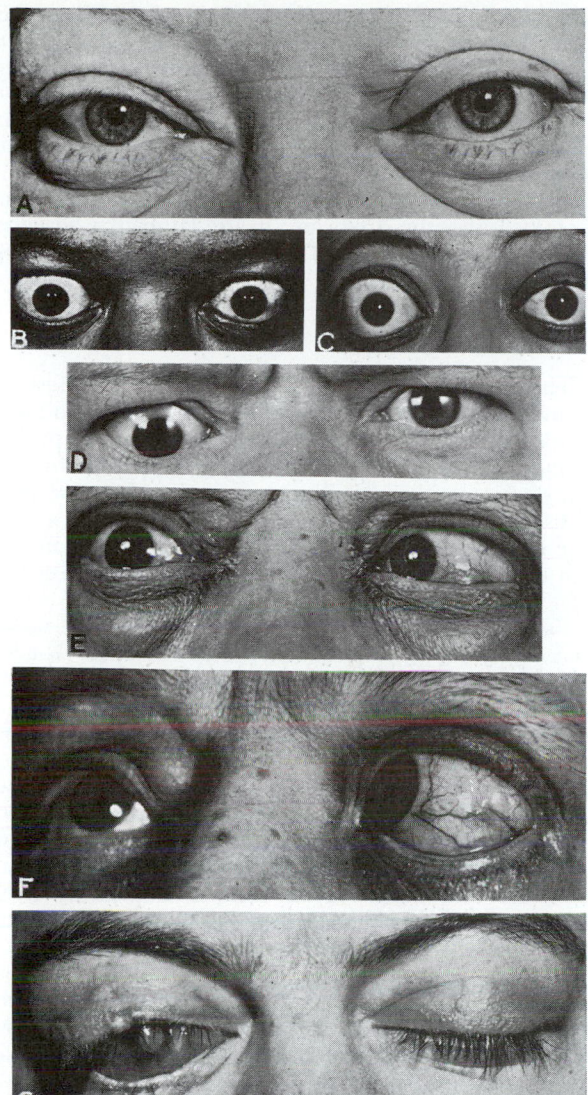

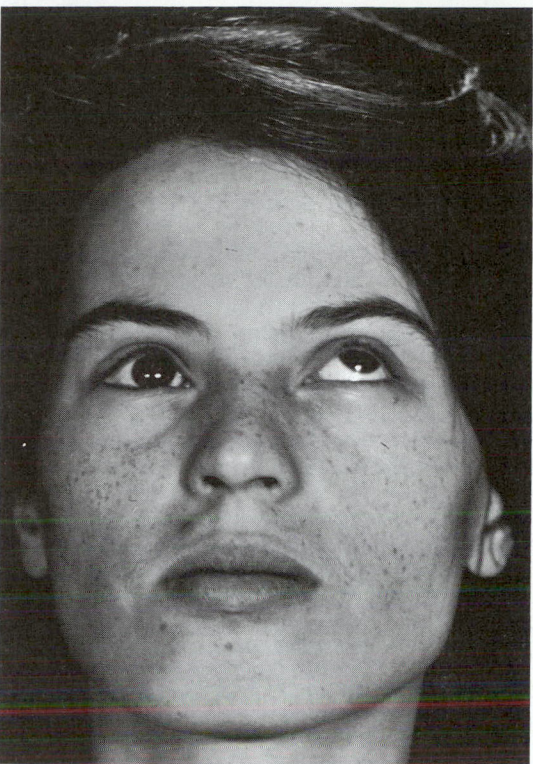

Figure 8–37. Ophthalmoplegia in Graves disease. The patient was severely hyperthyroid. Other than slight conjunctival injection, the only ocular abnormality was paralysis of upward gaze on right.

Figure 8–36. Infiltrative ophthalmopathy. *A,* Palpebral edema. This patient's eyeballs protruded anteriorly 1 cm more than normal, but there is no "pop-eye" appearance, owing to edema of the surrounding structures. *B,* Marked widening of palpebral fissures; slight palpebral swelling. *C,* Unequal degrees of ophthalmopathy. *D,* Unilateral lid retraction. *E,* Palpebral swelling, presumably because of fat pads and edema; paralysis of right external rectus muscle. *F,* Marked conjunctival injection and chemosis, together with ophthalmoplegia. *G,* Failure to close lids on right because of marked exophthalmos, corneal scarring, and panophthalmitis; the eye had to be enucleated.

Some indication of the severity of the infiltrative process in the orbit is provided by an assessment of intraorbital tension. An instrument for this purpose has been devised (orbitonometer), but clinical assessment can be accomplished by having the patient close the eyes lightly and determining the ease with which the globe can be displaced posteriorly by pressure from the thumb.

The manifestations of the extreme forms of ophthalmopathy may be catastrophic. These include subluxation of the globe and ulceration or infection of the cornea secondary to incomplete apposition of the lids. This may lead to panophthalmitis and destruction of one or both eyes. Ophthalmoscopic examination may reveal venous congestion and papilledema; these may be accompanied by visual field defects.

A classification of the eye changes of Graves disease has been developed by the American Thyroid Association. As shown in Table 8–13, the first letters of each category constitute the mnemonic NO SPECS. NO connotes the absent or mild degree of involvement; SPECS, the more serious degrees of involvement.

Infiltrative dermopathy occurs in about 5 to 10% of cases and is almost always accompanied by infiltrative ophthalmopathy, usually of severe degree. This lesion appears as a violaceous induration of the skin over the pretibial area (pretibial myxedema) and over the dorsa of the feet, usually in the form of individual plaques but occasionally becoming confluent. Rarely it is seen on the face or dorsa of the hands. Clubbing of the digits and osteoarthropathy are occasionally associated manifestations (thyroid acropachy).

Laboratory Tests

In moderate or severe diffuse toxic goiter, results of laboratory tests are abnormal and are consonant with the pathophysiology of this disorder. Serum T_4, T_3, and THBR levels are increased, and the serum TSH level is subnormal. The free T_4 and free T_3 indices are increased to a greater degree than are the respective total hormone concentrations.

TABLE 8–13. American Thyroid Association Abridged Classification of Eye Changes of Graves Disease

Class	Definition
0	No physical signs or symptoms
1	Only signs, no symptoms (signs limited to upper lid retraction, stare, lid lag, and proptosis to 22 mm)
2	Soft tissue involvement (symptoms and signs)
3	Proptosis > 22 mm
4	Extraocular muscle involvement
5	Corneal involvement
6	Sight loss (optic nerve involvement)

The serum T_3 concentration is typically more elevated than the serum T_4 concentration. The increase in thyroid iodide clearance rate is reflected in the increased RAIU. In patients with severe accompanying illness, decreased T_4- to- T_3 conversion may permit serum T_3 concentration, but usually not free T_3 or FT_3I, to return to normal (T_4 toxicosis), and a similar effect on the relation between serum T_4 and T_3 concentrations is often seen in patients with diffuse toxic goiter who have been exposed to iodine. Occasionally, this discrepancy is exaggerated, the serum T_4 concentration being normal and the serum T_3 concentration alone being elevated (T_3 toxicosis); in this circumstance, the RAIU may also be within the normal range. Metabolic indices, such as the BMR and serum cholesterol concentration, reflect the action of excessive amounts of thyroid hormone on the peripheral tissues.

An extensive discussion of the physiological basis of these tests and the manner in which they are affected by factors other than thyroid disease has been presented earlier. Some practical aspects of the use of the tests in the diagnosis of diffuse toxic goiter deserve emphasis. It is neither desirable nor feasible that all the major laboratory tests be used to assist in the diagnosis. Measurement of serum T_4 concentration alone will establish or exclude the diagnosis in the great majority of cases. To exclude the possibility that the increase in serum T_4 concentration is the result of an increase in hormone binding in the blood, concomitant measurement of either the free T_4 concentration or FT_4I should be made. If the last two functions are increased, a diagnosis of thyrotoxicosis is virtually assured. In the unusual instance in which values for serum total or free T_4 concentrations are not increased, measurement of serum T_3 concentration should be performed.

Measurement of serum T_3 concentration, together with the free T_3, FT_3I, or some indicator of hormone binding, will establish or exclude the diagnosis of hyperthyroidism in an even greater proportion of patients than will values of serum total T_4 and free T_4 concentrations and might therefore be regarded as the best initial approach, were it not for the occurrence of T_4 toxicosis or iodine-induced hyperthyroidism (jodbasedow phenomenon).

The diagnostic accuracy of the RAIU in hyperthyroidism may approach that of the serum T_4 concentration alone but does not approach that of the free T_4 or FT_4I or serum T_3 concentration. Therefore, measurement of RAIU is not necessary as a diagnostic test in patients with straightforward clinical Graves disease. Measurement of the RAIU is the most useful test for excluding thyrotoxicosis that is not due to active overproduction of hormone by the thyroid where a question exists as to the etiology of the thyrotoxicosis. Very low values of the RAIU in association with thyrotoxicosis signal the presence of thyrotoxicosis factitia, ectopic thyroid tissue, subacute thyroiditis, or the syndrome of chronic thyroiditis with transient thyrotoxicosis (hyperthyroiditis). A low value may also alert one to unsuspected iodine-induced hyperthyroidism, in which, of course, production of hormone by the thyroid gland is indeed increased.

It is in the borderline case of thyrotoxicosis that the laboratory tests are most greatly needed. In this circumstance, values are likely to be only slightly abnormal, if at all. It is here that the tests of thyroregulatory mechanisms, namely an immunometric TSH assay or the TRH stimulation test, have their greatest utility. A TSH concentration less than 0.1 mU/L is virtually pathognomonic of an excessive thyroid hormone supply. A value between 0.1 and 0.5 mU/L suggests a supranormal exposure but not a condition likely to be associated with significant clinical manifestations. The serum TSH level should be measured before initiation of treatment in all patients to eliminate the possibility of TSH-induced hyperthyroidism (see later).

The presence of TRAb in the serum strongly suggests Graves disease but does not always correlate with the presence of thyrotoxicosis. Measurement of these factors may have some utility in the pregnant patient and in the patient completing a course of antithyroid drug therapy. In the former, high levels of TRAb raise the likelihood of neonatal thyrotoxicosis in the offspring; in the latter, the absence of these factors may augur well for a long-term remission after withdrawal of therapy.

Differential Diagnosis

The patient who displays all the major manifestations of Graves disease, namely thyrotoxicosis, goiter, and infiltrative ophthalmopathy, does not pose a diagnostic problem. In some patients, however, one of the major manifestations either dominates the clinical picture or is present alone, and the disorder may mimic some other disease. Because the major manifestations are so different, the conditions from which they require differentiation will be considered separately.

Various disorders have features that resemble those of thyrotoxicosis in a general way. The disorder that most frequently simulates thyrotoxicosis is an anxiety state characterized by fatigue, palpitation, nervous irritability, and insomnia. Fatigue is pronounced and differs from that in thyrotoxicosis in that it is not accompanied by a desire to be active. The patient is listless and often feels tired on awakening. Tachycardia is common during examination but, in contrast to thyrotoxicosis, the sleeping pulse rate is normal. The palms are characteristically cool and clammy, rather than warm and moist. Hyper-reflexia is present in both disorders. In neurasthenia, goiter is absent and laboratory indices of thyroid function are normal. *Chronic obstructive pulmonary disease* may require differentiation from thyrotoxicosis. Here, retention of carbon dioxide may lead to a warm, flushed skin, tremulousness, and a bounding pulse. Mild exophthalmos may also be present. The BMR is increased by respiratory insufficiency.

Pheochromocytoma may closely resemble thyrotoxicosis in that tachycardia and hypermetabolism are common to both. Similarities include nervous irritability, eyelid retraction, tremulousness, and excessive sweating. The patient may have weight loss despite a good appetite and may have hyperglycemia with glucosuria. However, in the patient with pheochromocytoma, diastolic hypertension is often present (as opposed to reduced diastolic pressure in thyrotoxicosis) and urinary excretion of vanillylmandelic acid, metanephrine, and catecholamines is increased, features that are lacking in thyrotoxicosis. In the patient with pheochromocytoma, goiter is absent, and with very rare exceptions the laboratory indices of thyroid function are normal.

In *diabetes mellitus*, weight loss despite a good appetite, muscle wasting, and occasionally diarrhea may suggest thyrotoxicosis. Moreover, the incidence of goiter in patients with diabetes mellitus may be higher than in the general population. However, other features of thyrotoxicosis are usually lacking.

Myeloproliferative disorders may be accompanied by hypermetabolism, manifested by increased sweating, weight loss, and tachycardia, especially if anemia is present. Goiter is absent and laboratory indices of thyroid function are normal.

Cirrhosis of the liver may require differentiation from thyrotoxicosis because patients with cirrhosis often display weight loss, excessive sweating, a bounding pulse, and occasionally mild exophthalmos. Furthermore, the RAIU may be increased in cirrhosis as a result of iodine deficiency secondary to an inadequate diet. However, serum T_4 concentration is normal, serum T_3 concentration is often low, and goiter is generally absent. The RAIU returns to normal when a nutritious diet is given.

One rare disorder that simulates thyrotoxicosis is of theoretical interest. A single case has been reported of a woman who displayed severe hypermetabolism (in the range of $+200\%$), weight loss despite good appetite, profuse sweating, and progressive asthenia associated with myopathy. These symptoms had been present since childhood. Goiter was absent, and the RAIU was normal. The disorder was ascribed to structural abnormalities in the mitochondria leading to loosening of respiratory control.[263]

Thyrotoxic myopathy may require differentiation from progressive muscular atrophy or polymyositis. In *progressive muscular atrophy*, fasciculation is present and the deep tendon jerks are diminished or absent. *Polymyositis* may resemble thyrotoxic myopathy, but muscle biopsy discloses inflammatory and degenerative changes. In both progressive muscular atrophy and polymyositis, other features of thyrotoxicosis are lacking and laboratory indices of thyroid function are normal.

The diffuse goiter of Graves disease may rarely be confused with that of other thyroid diseases if thyrotoxicosis is present. Exceptions include the unusual case of Hashimoto disease in which there is concurrent hyperthyroidism, the early stage of subacute thyroiditis, and the syndrome of painless thyroiditis. In subacute thyroiditis, asymmetry of the gland, tenderness, and systemic evidence of inflammation assist in the diagnosis. The subnormal RAIU aids in distinguishing this disease, as well as painless thyroiditis, from Graves disease. When Graves disease is in a latent or inactive phase and thyrotoxicosis is absent, the diffuse goiter usually persists and may require exclusion of Hashimoto thyroiditis or simple nontoxic goiter as possible diagnoses. The goiter of Hashimoto disease tends to be somewhat lobulated and firmer than that of Graves disease. Antithyroid antibodies are present more commonly in the serum in Hashimoto disease, and the titers are generally higher but are not helpful in distinguishing Graves disease and Hashimoto disease in the individual patient. In the absence of thyrotoxicosis, the diffuse goiter of Graves disease cannot be distinguished from nontoxic goiter. An abnormal serum TSH concentration or the presence of TRAb indicates underlying Graves disease, but their absence does not exclude the diagnosis.

The ophthalmopathy of Graves disease, if bilateral and associated with the thyrotoxicosis past or present, does not require differentiation from exophthalmos of other origin. However, unilateral exophthalmos, even when associated with thyrotoxicosis, should alert the physician to the possibility of a local cause. When exophthalmos occurs in the patient who has not been thyrotoxic, other diseases that may produce either unilateral or bilateral exophthalmos must be actively excluded. These include orbital neoplasms, caroticocavernous fistulae, cavernous sinus thrombosis, infiltrative disorders affecting the orbit, and pseudotumor cerebri. Mild bilateral exophthalmos, generally without infiltrative signs, is occasionally present on a familial basis and also sometimes occurs in patients with Cushing syndrome, cirrhosis, uremia, chronic obstructive pulmonary disease, and the superior vena cava syndrome. Ophthalmoplegia as the sole manifestation of the ophthalmopathy of Graves disease requires exclusion of diabetes mellitus and other disorders affecting the brain stem and its connections. The demonstration of swelling of the extraocular muscles by orbital ultrasonog-raphy or computed tomography[261, 262] strongly suggests that the ophthalmopathy is a manifestation of Graves disease, as does the detection of TSI or TBII in serum or the demonstration of an abnormal TSH or TRH test.

Treatment of Hyperthyroidism

Although considerable progress has been made toward an understanding of the pathogenesis of Graves disease, it has not yet led to the development of therapeutic measures aimed at the basic pathogenetic factors in the disease. Existing therapies for both the thyrotoxic and the ophthalmopathic manifestations are merely palliative in that they may relieve but do not cure the disease. The lack of general agreement as to which of the several therapies is the best reflects the fact that none is ideal. Because the therapeutic problems posed by the thyrotoxicosis and the ophthalmopathy differ so widely and because they run independent courses, their treatments will be discussed separately.

The thyrotoxicosis of Graves disease is due to an abnormal rate of hormone synthesis and release, and thus all major forms of treatment impose restraints on the rate of hormone secretion. This is accomplished either by means of chemical agents that inhibit one or more stages in hormone synthesis or release or by so reducing the quantity of thyroid tissue that overproduction of hormone is no longer possible.

ANTITHYROID AGENTS. The first stage in hormone biosynthesis susceptible to chemotherapeutic inhibition is the iodide transport mechanism. Both thiocyanate and perchlorate inhibit thyroid iodide transport. However, theoretical and practical disadvantages attend their use. The ameliorative effect of these agents depends on their ability to decrease the net flux of iodide into the thyroid, thereby limiting the quantity of substrate available for hormone biosynthesis. Such treatment leaves the patient at the mercy of iodine intake, because if plasma inorganic iodide concentration is increased, sufficient iodide can enter the thyroid by diffusion to permit re-establishment of an excessive rate of hormone formation. Furthermore, this consideration makes it impossible to use iodine together with these agents in the preparation of the patient for subtotal thyroidectomy. Serious adverse reactions, such as irreversible aplastic anemia, have led to abandonment of their use.

The major agents employed in chemotherapy for thyrotoxicosis are drugs of the thionamide class having the chemical structure shown in Figure 8–14. The agents most commonly employed are propylthiouracil, methimazole, and carbimazole.[264] These agents probably exert their antithyroid action by inhibiting the oxidation and organic binding of thyroid iodide. They therefore produce a state of intrathyroidal iodine deficiency that further increases the ratio of T_3 to T_4 in thyroid secretion. This is reflected in the high T_3/T_4 ratio in the serum during chronic treatment with these agents. In addition to inhibiting hormone synthesis, propylthiouracil, but not methimazole, impairs the conversion of T_4 to T_3 in the peripheral tissues (Fig. 8–38). Because of this additional action, propylthiouracil is generally used in preference to methimazole when rapid alleviation of severe thyrotoxicosis is sought.[59, 265-267]

Data concerning the distribution and metabolism of these agents are somewhat limited. The half-life in plasma of methimazole is about 6 h, whereas that of propylthiouracil is about 1½ h. However, the plasma concentration of drug may have little bearing on the duration of antithyroid action. Both drugs are accumulated by the thyroid, and a single 30-mg dose of methimazole may exert an antithyroid effect for longer than 24 h. This provides a rational basis for the single daily dose regimen of methimazole in the patient with

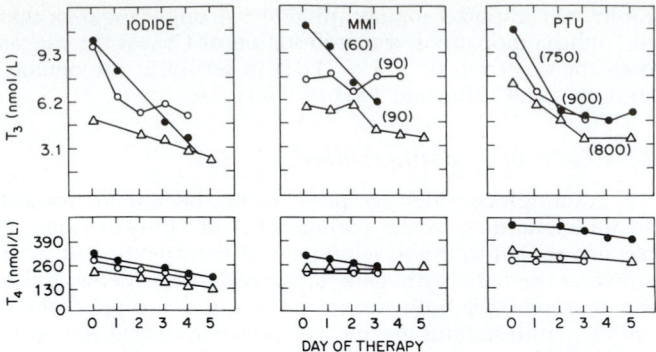

Figure 8–38. Effects of various antithyroid agents on the serum levels of T_3 and T_4 in patients with Graves disease. In the first panel are shown the effects of potassium iodide (SSKI, five drops every 8 h). A rapid reduction in T_3 concentration in all patients and a decrease in T_4 concentration are seen over the first 5 d of therapy. Methimazole, given at the indicated doses, has a variable effect on T_3 concentrations. In one patient the serum T_3 level falls rapidly over the first 3 d, whereas in the other two individuals, receiving an even larger daily dosage, there is no change. Serum T_4 concentration does not change significantly over this time interval. The effects of propylthiouracil (PTU) are shown in the right-hand panel. In all patients, administration of high-dose propylthiouracil causes a marked decrease in serum T_3 concentrations to about one third to one half of those found initially. This decrease is due to the propylthiouracil-induced inhibition of type 1 iodothyronine 5'-deiodinase. (Data from Abuid J, Larsen PR. Triiodothyronine and thyroxine in thyrotoxicosis: acute response to therapy with anti-thyroid agents. J Clin Invest 1974; 39:263–268.)

mild or moderate thyrotoxicosis.[268] There is a good correlation between the propylthiouracil concentration in serum and the extent of blockade of organic binding of iodine within the thyroid.[264]

These drugs cross the placenta and are capable, therefore, of inhibiting thyroid function in the fetus. Methimazole may cross the placenta more readily than propylthiouracil (see later under Hyperthyroidism and Thyrotoxicosis in Pregnancy).

The initial dose of propylthiouracil most commonly employed is 200 to 300 mg given orally at intervals of 8 to 12 h. An equivalent dose of methimazole is 10 to 20 mg every 12 h. Carbimazole is converted to methimazole in vivo and is equivalent in potency. It is not used in the United States.

These doses are effective in most patients, but in some no therapeutic response is seen. It is unlikely, however, that a true state of complete resistance to these agents ever occurs, although in some patients doses of up to 1200 mg propylthiouracil or an equivalent amount of methimazole daily may be required. This relative lack of effect usually occurs in patients with severe thyroid hyperfunction and large thyroid glands, possibly because of more rapid degradation of the drug either within the gland or extrathyroidally. When large doses are required, it is often advantageous to increase the frequency of administration to intervals of 4 to 6 h. The response to effective antithyroid therapy invariably occurs only after a latent period. This follows from the fact that these agents inhibit the synthesis but not the release of hormone, and hence a reduction in the supply of hormone to the tissues must await depletion of glandular hormone stores (see Fig. 8–38). Although propylthiouracil differs from methimazole in additionally inhibiting the peripheral generation of T_3 from T_4, there appears to be little difference in the duration of the latent period when either of these agents is employed alone in the usual dosage. The extrathyroidal effect of propylthiouracil on T_4-to-T_3 conversion is dose related and is more apparent at dosages greater than 600 mg/d. This effect may be an advantage in the acute treatment of severe hyperthyroidism (see Fig. 8–38).[59, 265–267]

Several factors influence the duration of the latent period. Among these are the quantity of hormone initially present in the thyroid, its inherent rate of release, and the degree of blockade of new hormone synthesis that is achieved. In the thyroid rich in iodine, such as occurs when the patient has received medications containing iodine, the clinical response to antithyroid agents may be delayed for long periods, even months. As would be expected, the latent period is shortened by administration of large doses (more than 600 mg daily of propylthiouracil), and such should be used when a more rapid therapeutic response is required. Generally, some improvement occurs within the first 2 wk; the patient may note a decrease in nervousness and palpitations, an increase in strength, and a gain in weight. Usually, a normal metabolic state can be restored within about 6 wk. At this time, the dosage can often be reduced by approximately one half and a normal metabolic state thereafter maintained.

During treatment, the size of the thyroid decreases in one third to one half of the patients. In others it may remain unchanged, while in the remainder it enlarges. The latter change signals either an intensification of the disease process, which often requires that the dosage of drug be increased, or the production of hypothyroidism as a result of excessive dosage. It is important to differentiate between these extremes. Clinical criteria should be the main guidelines by which the adequacy of treatment is judged, but confirmation may be sought in the serum T_4, T_3, and TSH concentrations. Mild thyrotoxicosis may persist despite a serum T_4 concentration in the normal range, because the peripheral turnover of T_4 may remain accelerated for some time and the serum T_3 concentration may still be increased. The latter phenomenon may also account for maintenance of a normal metabolic state in the face of a subnormal serum T_4 concentration. The serum TSH concentration or the response to TRH may remain subnormal, sometimes for months.

The antithyroid agents have the potential of inducing hypothyroidism if given in excessive quantities over prolonged periods. When this occurs, the patient often complains of excessive gain in weight, sluggishness, and fatigue. Signs of mild hypothyroidism may be present, especially a delay in the relaxation phase of the deep tendon jerks. Important signs of incipient hypothyroidism are enlargement of the thyroid gland and the appearance or accentuation of a bruit. These result from hypersecretion of TSH, together with hypothyroidism, and can be reversed either by reducing the dosage of the antithyroid drug or by administering supplemental thyroid hormone. To forestall this development, which may have adverse effects on preexisting ophthalmopathy, some physicians employ supplemental thyroid hormone routinely. The authors do not regularly prescribe this regimen.

A central question in the long-term use of antithyroid drugs is the appropriate duration of treatment. No arbitrary answer can be given, but the problem is best understood in the light of the pathophysiology of the disorder. There is no reason to believe that antithyroid therapy alters the course of the underlying disease process, and persistence of remission after withdrawal of treatment will occur only if the disorder through its natural evolution has entered a latent or inactive phase. This latter transition is more likely to occur the longer the course of treatment. This reasoning is the basis for the traditional practice of continuing antithyroid treatment for 12 mo or longer. One study has suggested that the frequency of remission is as good when the antithyroid agent is withdrawn on attainment of a eumetabolic state as when the agent is continued for 12 mo or longer.[269] Another study indicates, however, that this is not the case.[270] Certain features may serve to indicate the likelihood of long-

TABLE 8–14. Factors Favoring Long-Term Remission After Antithyroid Therapy for Diffuse Toxic Goiter

T_3 toxicosis
Small goiter
Decrease in goiter size during therapy
Normal thyroid function tests
Normal TRH stimulation test or serum TSH
Negative tests for immunoglobulins of Graves disease

term remission after withdrawal of therapy (Table 8–14). The presence initially of T_3 toxicosis or of a small thyroid (less than twice normal) augurs well for a long-term remission. In addition, a decrease in size of the thyroid and return of the TSH concentration to normal during treatment are favorable indicators. Several studies suggest that disappearance of circulating TRAb during treatment of Graves disease also portends a long-term remission after withdrawal of antithyroid drugs.[248, 249]

Treatment is often continued for about 12 mo and then withdrawn gradually. This permits an immediate exacerbation to be detected while some antithyroid effect is still maintained. Of the patients who relapse, about three quarters do so in the first 3 mo after withdrawal of therapy and the bulk of the remainder relapse during the subsequent 6 mo. Elevation of serum T_3 concentration, despite maintenance of a normal serum T_4 level, may signal exacerbation of the disease.

There is uncertainty as to the frequency with which long-term remission occurs after withdrawal of antithyroid therapy. For many years, there was nearly universal agreement that about one half of patients with diffuse toxic goiter would experience a long-term remission. Several subsequent analyses have indicated a decreasing overall remission rate over the past 30 y, however.[269, 271] This phenomenon does not appear to be due to the recent general increase in dietary iodine intake, as had been suggested, because it also occurred in a geographic region where iodine intake has remained constant and relatively low for the past 30 y. The foregoing has led to some disenchantment with antithyroid agents as the therapy of choice for thyrotoxicosis in Graves disease. Nevertheless, about one third of patients experience a lasting remission. Thus a significant place for antithyroid agents as sole therapy in the treatment of thyrotoxicosis continues to exist.

Adverse reactions occur in a small percentage of patients taking antithyroid drugs of the thionamide class (Table 8–15). The most significant is agranulocytosis, which is seen in a fraction of 1% of the patients. Agranulocytosis, like the other adverse reactions, generally occurs within the first few weeks or months of treatment. It is accompanied by fever and sore throat, and when therapy is begun the patient should be instructed to discontinue the drug and notify the physician immediately should these symptoms develop. This precaution is more important than the frequent measurement of leukocyte counts, because agranulocytosis may develop within a day or two. If agranulocytosis occurs, the drug should be discontinued immediately and the patient treated with antibiotics as indicated. Recovery almost invar-

iably takes place. Lymphocytes of patients who have developed agranulocytosis while taking propylthiouracil undergo blast transformation when exposed in vitro to propylthiouracil or methimazole.[272] Consequently, such patients should not usually be given a thionamide drug again.

Granulocytopenia may also occur during antithyroid therapy and is sometimes a forerunner of agranulocytosis. On the other hand, mild granulocytopenia may be merely a manifestation of thyrotoxicosis. For this reason, a total white blood cell count and differential should always be obtained prior to the initiation of treatment with thionamide drugs. Granulocytopenia detected during the first few weeks of therapy may present the physician with a difficult decision—whether or not treatment should be continued. In this circumstance, serial measurements of the leukocyte count should be made, and if these display a downward trend, the antithyroid drugs should be discontinued. Usually, however, serial measurements reveal a return of the white blood cell count to normal, and treatment need not be interrupted. A rash, which may take many forms, is common and in the authors' experience occurs more frequently with methimazole than with propylthiouracil.

Other reactions occur less frequently. These include arthralgia, myalgia, neuritis, hepatitis with evidence of cholestasis, thrombocytopenia, loss of or abnormal pigmentation of the hair, loss of taste sensation, enlargement of lymph nodes or salivary glands, edema, a lupus-like syndrome, and toxic psychoses. The nature of the pathological disturbances underlying these reactions is not known, although some may disappear despite continuance of treatment. Nonetheless, it is the authors' view that appearance of any of these manifestations is an indication for abandonment of antithyroid therapy and recourse to surgery or [131]I.

IODINE AND IODINE-CONTAINING AGENTS. Iodine, which until 1943 was the major chemotherapeutic agent for thyrotoxicosis, is now rarely used as sole therapy. The mechanism of action of iodine in relieving thyrotoxicosis differs from that of the thionamides. Although quantities of iodine in excess of several milligrams are capable of inducing an acute inhibition of organic binding (acute Wolff-Chaikoff effect), this is a transient phenomenon that in all likelihood does not contribute to the therapeutic action of iodine. Rather, the major action of iodine is to inhibit hormone release.

First, administration of iodine is associated with an increase in glandular organic iodine stores. Second, the beneficial effect of iodine is evident more quickly than is the effect of even large doses of agents that inhibit hormone synthesis. Finally, in patients with diffuse toxic goiter, iodine acutely retards the rate of secretion of T_4; this effect is rapidly lost when iodine is withdrawn. These features of its action provide both the disadvantages and advantages of iodine therapy. The enrichment of glandular organic iodine stores that occurs when this agent is given alone may retard the clinical response to subsequently administered thionamide, and furthermore the decrease in RAIU that iodine produces will prevent the use of radioiodine as treatment for a period of weeks or more. In addition, if iodine is withdrawn, resumption of a rapid rate of release from an enriched glandular hormone pool may produce an exacerbation of thyrotoxicosis. Still another reason for not using iodine alone is that in some patients the therapeutic response is either incomplete or lacking, and even if initially effective, iodine may lose its effect with time. (This phenomenon, which has been termed *iodine escape*, should not be confused with the escape from the acute Wolff-Chaikoff effect; see earlier under Thyroid Autoregulation.) On the other hand, the rapid slowing of hormone release that iodine induces makes it a more effective agent than the thionamide drugs

TABLE 8–15. Percent Incidence of Toxic Reactions with Antithyroid Drugs

Drug	All Reactions	Agranulocytosis
Methimazole	7.1	0.1
Carbimazole	1.9	0.8
Propylthiouracil	3.3	0.4
Methylthiouracil	13.8	0.5

when prompt relief of thyrotoxicosis is mandatory (see Fig. 8–38). Therefore, aside from its use in preparation for subtotal thyroidectomy, iodine is mainly useful for patients with actual or impending thyrotoxic crisis, severe thyrocardiac disease, or acute surgical emergencies—all conditions in which thyrotoxicosis is life-threatening.

If iodine is used in these circumstances, it should be administered with large doses of a thionamide, as the severity of the thyrotoxicosis would itself indicate. The dose of iodine required for control of thyrotoxicosis has been estimated to be approximately 6 mg daily, a quantity less than that usually given. Six milligrams of iodine would be contained in approximately one eighth of a drop of saturated solution of potassium iodide (SSKI) or eight tenths of a drop of Lugol solution; many physicians, however, prescribe 5 to 10 drops of one of these agents three times daily. Although it is advisable to administer amounts larger than the suggested minimal effective dose, huge quantities of iodine are disadvantageous in that they are more likely to produce adverse reactions, including iodide myxedema. The authors recommend the use of three drops of SSKI three times daily. In patients who are so ill that medications cannot be taken by mouth, antithyroid agents can be triturated and administered by stomach tube; iodine can be given by the same route. When use of a stomach tube is contraindicated, thionamide drugs cannot be administered because preparations for parenteral use are not available. Here, the disadvantages attendant upon administration of iodine may be accepted if the clinical situation is sufficiently serious, and a preparation of sodium iodide is available for intravenous use. The dosage is the same as for the oral preparations. Adverse reactions to iodine are unusual and, although varied, are generally not serious.[273, 274] These include rash, which may be acneiform; drug fever; sialadenitis; conjunctivitis and rhinitis; vasculitis; and a leukemoid eosinophilic granulocytosis. Sialadenitis may respond to reduction of dosage; in the case of the other reactions, iodine should be withdrawn. As discussed later, iodine appears to be particularly effective when given after administration of a therapeutic dose of ^{131}I. This combination may be very useful when rapid alleviation of thyrotoxicosis is required.

The iodine-containing cholecystographic contrast agent sodium ipodate (or iopanoate) is effective in bringing about a prompt decrease in serum T_4, and especially serum T_3, concentration in patients with hyperthyroidism when given in doses of 1 g daily.[275] These effects are doubtless the result of the conjoint release of iodine and the ability of the agent to inhibit peripheral T_3 neogenesis, a combination that could be highly useful in the seriously ill patient. However, as with iodine itself, withdrawal of the drug carries the risk of an exacerbation. Hence, in the authors' view, if the patient is sufficiently ill to warrant treatment with ipodate, concomitant administration of large doses of antithyroid agents is also indicated.

Lithium carbonate also inhibits thyroid hormone secretion, but experience with this agent is limited. Unlike iodine, it has the advantage that it does not interfere with the accumulation of a subsequently administered dose of radioiodine. Lithium is employed only to provide temporary control of thyrotoxicosis in patients who are allergic to both thionamide and iodide.

DEXAMETHASONE. This drug has become an important therapeutic adjunct when rapid alleviation of thyrotoxicosis is desired. Dexamethasone in a dosage of 2 mg every 6 h inhibits both the glandular secretion of hormone and the peripheral conversion of T_4 to T_3.[118] With respect to the latter action, the inhibitory effect of dexamethasone is additive to that of propylthiouracil, suggesting different mechanisms of action. Concurrent administration of propyl-

thiouracil, SSKI, and dexamethasone to the patient with severe thyrotoxicosis effects a rapid reduction in serum T_3 concentration, often to within the normal range in 24 to 48 h.[276] Addition of ipodate to this regimen, or substitution of ipodate for SSKI, may prove even more effective.

ADRENERGIC ANTAGONISTS. Agents that either deplete tissues of their catecholamine content (reserpine or guanethidine) or block the response to catecholamines at the receptor site (propranolol) are capable of antagonizing to a variable extent some of the manifestations of thyrotoxicosis. Hence, they are sometimes used as adjuncts in the management of patients with this disorder. Tremulousness, palpitation, excessive sweating, eyelid retraction, and heart rate decrease. When administered in sufficient dosage, these agents have effects that are rapidly manifest and appear to be mediated largely through the adrenergic nervous system, although propranolol may also impair to some extent the conversion of T_4 to T_3.

Adrenergic antagonists have their greatest use in patients with severe thyrotoxicosis, such as those with impending or actual thyrotoxic crisis (see later under Special Aspects of Thyrotoxicosis). They are of more limited value, however, in patients with less severe disease. Adrenergic antagonists are especially useful in patients with thyrocardiac disease in whom tachycardia of either sinus or ectopic origin is contributing to cardiac insufficiency. Beta-adrenergic blockers usually reduce cardiac output without altering oxygen consumption. This may have adverse effects in some organs, such as the liver, where the arteriovenous oxygen difference is already elevated in the hyperthyroid state.[230] Moreover, because thyroid hormone has a direct effect on the myocardium independent of the adrenergic nervous system, the adrenergic antagonists reduce the heart rate by an independent mechanism (see earlier discussion of catecholamine/thyroid interrelationships). Adrenergic antagonists should be considered as adjunctive rather than primary tools in the treatment of thyrotoxicosis. They are most useful in the interval during which the response to thionamide or radioiodine therapy is being awaited.

Of the agents available, propranolol is the drug of choice, as it is relatively free of adverse effects. It can be given orally in a dose of 40 to 80 mg every 6 or 8 h. For intravenous use, a shorter-acting agent may be preferable (see treatment of thyroid storm). Propranolol is contraindicated in patients with asthma or chronic obstructive pulmonary disease because it aggravates bronchospasm. Because of its myocardial depressant action, it is also contraindicated in patients with heart block and in patients with congestive failure, unless severe tachycardia is a contributory factor. Whether propranolol should be given chronically to pregnant women with hyperthyroidism is a matter of debate. Although some studies indicate that no significant complications attend its use,[277, 278] other authors report an association with small size of the fetus, low Apgar scores, and postnatal bradycardia and hypoglycemia.

SURGERY. As mentioned earlier, there is no reason to believe that antithyroid therapy with a thionamide drug has any direct effect on the thyroid that persists after treatment is discontinued. By contrast, the other major types of therapy, i.e., surgery and radioiodine, exert their effects through permanent removal or destruction of thyroid tissue, rendering the gland incapable of producing excessive quantities of hormone. Antithyroid therapy and ablative therapy are diametrically different, and their opposite properties may be considered advantageous or disadvantageous, depending on one's point of view.

The impermanence of antithyroid therapy leads to a relatively frequent recurrence of thyrotoxicosis, whereas with ablative therapy recurrence is uncommon. On the other hand, antithyroid therapy never produces permanent hypothyroidism, whereas with ablative therapy the frequency of permanent hypothyroidism may be unacceptably high. The effectiveness of surgery in relieving hyperthyroidism is unquestioned. In most series, the frequency of recurrent hyperthyroidism after subtotal thyroidectomy in adults is less than 10%. On the other hand, the combined prevalence of postoperative hypothyroidism and other surgical complications is relatively high, rendering surgery less than ideal as a form of treatment.

Table 8–16 is taken from a report that summarizes the results of surgery for hyperthyroidism in eight series.[279] The major postoperative complication is permanent hypothyroidism, which ranged in frequency between 4% and approximately 30%. The highest frequency of permanent postoperative hypothyroidism was reported from clinics in which internists did the follow-ups on the patients. In a study conducted by internists, a mean frequency of 28% was found in patients followed for 1 to 16 y and the frequency in patients followed for 10 y was 43%.

Although it has been assumed that hypothyroidism will usually develop within 1 y after operation if it is to occur at all, long-term studies indicate a progressive increase in the cumulative incidence with time similar to that produced by radioiodine but of lesser magnitude. It may be presumed that the overall frequency of some impairment of thyroid function is even higher than that of frank hypothyroidism because subtotal thyroidectomy is one important cause of decreased thyroid reserve. The increasing frequency of hypothyroidism with time may result from progressive restriction of blood supply or from autoimmune destruction of the thyroid remnant. If eventual thyroid failure is a frequent consequence of the Graves disease process itself, the large increase in cumulative frequency of hypothyroidism with time that follows both surgery and radioiodine therapy is both expected and unavoidable. Treatment that destroys thyroid tissue would accelerate the emergence of hypothyroidism resulting from the disease process itself.

An inverse relationship obtains between the frequency of recurrence and that of hypothyroidism, and the relative frequency of the two partly depends on the quantity of thyroid tissue left in place. What is more remarkable is that among patients whose thyroid glands vary greatly in size and degree of hyperfunction, and who are operated on by surgeons whose techniques must vary to a considerable extent, a normal metabolic state is restored, at least for long periods, in most patients. This favorable outcome may result because the amount of tissue remaining after operation is alone insufficient to sustain a normal metabolic state and hence becomes stimulated by the necessary quantity of endogenous TSH. In this way, the patient's homeostatic mechanism provides the adjustment in thyroid function that surgery, quite naturally, could not. This hypothesis is supported by the return of TSH to the sera of patients restored to a normal metabolic state by surgery.

Bleeding into the operative site is the most serious postoperative complication, because it can rapidly produce

death by asphyxia. This complication requires immediate evacuation of the hematoma and ligation of the bleeding vessel. Damage to the recurrent laryngeal nerve is also a major complication. If unilateral, it results in dysphonia that usually improves in a few weeks but may leave the patient slightly hoarse. If damage is bilateral, obstruction of the airway usually occurs within a few hours, producing severe stridor; tracheostomy is then required, and at this time the nature of the damage to the nerves should be explored.

Hypoparathyroidism may be either transient or permanent. Transient hypoparathyroidism results from two factors: inadvertent removal of some parathyroids and impairment of blood supply to those that remain. Depending on the severity of these insults, symptoms and signs of hypocalcemia appear, usually within 1 to 7 d after operation. The earliest indication of hypoparathyroidism may be anxiety and mental depression, followed by paresthesia and evidence of heightened neuromuscular excitability, such as Chvostek and Trousseau signs and carpopedal spasm. The serum calcium level is subnormal, and the serum inorganic phosphate level is increased. When hypoparathyroidism is severe, it should be treated initially with intravenous calcium gluconate. Milder cases can be treated with oral calcium carbonate in a dose of 1 g three times daily. It is impossible at the onset to ascertain whether the hypoparathyroidism will be permanent or will regress within a few weeks, as usually occurs.

The hypocalcemia that occurs in the thyrotoxic patient in the immediate postoperative period may not be due to transient hypoparathyroidism, because it occurs more frequently here than after surgery for other thyroid disorders. Rather, it has been ascribed to retention of calcium by bone in the thyrotoxic patient but what initiates this phenomenon has not been determined.[280] It is well recognized that hyperthyroidism leads to bone demineralization.[234–236] This process is rapidly reversed after cure of the hyperthyroid state and could possibly contribute to the modest elevation in alkaline phosphatase during recovery. The frequency of permanent hypoparathyroidism varies in a general way with the proportion of the thyroid removed and hence with the frequency of postoperative hypothyroidism. The frequency of mild hypoparathyroidism (or diminished parathyroid reserve) detectable years after operation is probably greater than is generally supposed. The treatment of permanent hypoparathyroidism is discussed in Chapter 27.

The hazards of subtotal thyroidectomy are inversely related to the experience and skill of the surgical team. Consequently, as surgery is less frequently performed, the hazards attendant on it increase. For these reasons, it is impossible to generalize about the frequency of complications, and statistics drawn from the former era in which surgery was commonly undertaken are probably no longer applicable. Unless circumstances are otherwise compelling, thyroidectomy should not be performed by surgeons who carry out this operative procedure only occasionally.

Preoperative use of antithyroid agents has greatly decreased the morbidity and mortality rates of surgery for diffuse toxic goiter because of the ability of these drugs to deplete glandular hormone stores and secondarily to restore the patient to an entirely normal metabolic state before operation. On the other hand, these agents do not have the favorable influence on the hyperplasia and hypervascularity of the gland that is exerted by iodine. Iodine induces involution characterized by a decrease in height of the follicular cells, enlargement of follicles with retention of colloid, and last, but most important, reduction of hypervascularity. Hence, the aim of preoperative management is to restore a normal metabolic state with antithyroid agents and then to bring about involution of the gland with iodine.

TABLE 8–16. Range of Results of Surgery for Hyperthyroidism, as Reported from Eight Clinics

Result	%
Mortality	0.0–3.1
Recurrent hyperthyroidism	0.6–17.9
Vocal cord paralysis	0.0–4.4
Permanent hypoparathyroidism	0.0–3.6
Permanent hypothyroidism	4.0–29.7

From Hershman JM. The treatment of hyperthyroidism. Ann Intern Med 1966; 64:1306–1314.

Achievement of these objectives makes the patient a better operative and postoperative risk in all respects. Patients who are to undergo subtotal thyroidectomy are first given antithyroid therapy in the manner described earlier. Often, relatively large doses are given, either to hasten the clinical response or because the patients for whom surgery is recommended are frequently those with severe disease or very large goiters. After a normal metabolic state has been restored, SSKI is given as three drops three times daily for a further 7 to 10 d. During this period, a pre-existing bruit or thrill may decrease in intensity or disappear entirely; the gland usually becomes firmer and may appear to have enlarged.

Within this general approach, several specific guidelines should be followed. First, no definite date for surgery should be set until the patient has been restored to a normal metabolic state. Much too often, the operation is planned well in advance and the patient is given a standardized regimen largely independent of his or her clinical progress. Second, therapy with iodine should not be started until metabolic control has been produced by the antithyroid drug; iodine should not be relied on to complete an as yet incomplete response to antithyroid therapy. This is true because if the antithyroid drug is not entirely effective the additional iodine will enrich glandular hormone stores. Finally, antithyroid agents should not be withdrawn when iodine therapy is begun.

Propranolol may be a useful adjunct in controlling some symptoms (see earlier) while the patient is being prepared for surgery. It has also been advocated that it be used alone in preoperative preparation of the patient in whom surgery is to be undertaken.[281] This mode of therapy is probably safe and effective in many patients, but thyroid storm has been reported to occur in patients already receiving propranolol. The authors believe, therefore, that unless there is some compelling indication for use of propranolol alone, restoration of the patient to a eumetabolic state, as outlined earlier, is desirable before the patient is subjected to the stress of general anesthesia and surgery.

RADIOIODINE. Radioiodine is a simple and economical means of treating thyrotoxicosis.[282] It produces the ablative effects of surgery without the immediate operative and postoperative complications of the latter. The principal disadvantage of the use of radioiodine is the high frequency of late hypothyroidism. Previously, there was concern that this form of therapy might also produce thyroid carcinoma, leukemia, or transmissible genetic damage. However, during the years in which radioiodine has been in use, no increased prevalence of thyroid carcinoma in patients so treated has been noted. Indeed, the prevalence may be lower than that in the general population, presumably because the radiation dose usually delivered to the thyroid interferes with cell replication. This phenomenon is to be contrasted with the increased prevalence of thyroid carcinoma in patients treated with lower doses of radiation in childhood or adolescence. The prevalence of leukemia is also no greater in patients treated with radioiodine. Finally, the frequency of genetic damage in the offspring of patients treated earlier with radioiodine does not appear to be increased. Indeed, the conventional dose of radioiodine employed in the treatment of thyrotoxicosis delivers to the gonads a radiation dose approximately equivalent to that delivered by a barium enema examination or intravenous urogram. In view of the lack of evidence for significant carcinogenic, leukemogenic, or teratogenic effects of radioiodine in doses generally employed for treating hyperthyroidism, the age limit for the use of radioiodine has been lowered progressively from the initial limit of 40, so that in some clinics it is now employed in children and adolescents.

During the early years of radioiodine therapy, attempts were made to standardize the radiation delivered to the thyroid gland by varying the dose of radioiodine according to the size of the gland, the uptake of ^{131}I, and its subsequent rate of release. However, such calculations do not provide uniform results, probably because of variations in individual sensitivity. Hence, the authors, and many clinics, have settled on an arbitrary dose calculated to result in 185 to 222 MBq (5 to 6 mCi of ^{131}I) in the thyroid gland 24 h after administration.

Until the early 1960s most reports indicated that the frequency of postradioiodine hypothyroidism after doses of this magnitude was approximately 7 to 12%, most of this occurring during the first year or two after treatment. Although an occasional patient developed hypothyroidism later, this was considered uncommon. In 1961, however, there appeared the first of several reports that by now have completely altered this view. Not only is the incidence of hypothyroidism higher during the first year or two after treatment than was originally thought, but also it continues to increase at a rate of approximately 3%/y thereafter. Thus the incidence of postradioiodine hypothyroidism at 5 y is approximately 30% and at 10 y approximately 40%, although values as high as 70% have been reported (Fig. 8–39).

There is little doubt that the early beneficial effect of radioiodine and the early induction of hypothyroidism both depend on radiation-induced destruction of thyroid parenchyma. Within the first few weeks after treatment, there occur epithelial swelling and necrosis, disruption of follicular architecture, edema, and infiltration with leukocytes (radiation thyroiditis). Resolution of the acute inflammation is followed by fibrosis, vascular narrowing, and lymphocytic infiltration. These structural changes account for the early response to radioiodine, be it favorable or excessive. In themselves, however, they do not appear sufficient to account for the increasing incidence of hypothyroidism with time, and more subtle factors appear to be operative. In some studies, the likelihood of hypothyroidism is increased by the presence of high titers of antithyroid antibodies at the time of treatment and by increasing age of the patient. The two predisposing factors may be related to one another.

Defective organic binding of thyroid iodide follows apparently successful therapy; this is evident in the enhanced susceptibility to iodide-induced hypothyroidism. This phenomenon may be only one of several abnormalities that

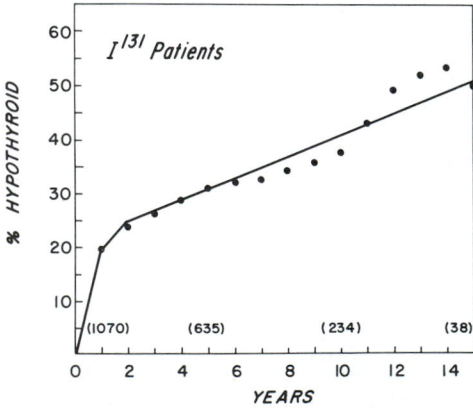

Figure 8–39. Incidence of postradioiodine hypothyroidism in relation to the duration of follow-up. The total number of patients followed for each of the indicated time periods is shown in parentheses. (From Dunn JT, Chapman EM. Rising incidence of hypothyroidism after radioactive-iodine therapy in thyrotoxicosis. Reprinted, by permission of The New England Journal of Medicine, 271; 1037–1042, 1964.)

eventually produce thyroid failure. Among these may be damage to the nucleus of the follicular cell, leading to failure of normal replication, progressive autoimmune destruction, or progressive restriction of blood supply. Such factors could interact with factors related to the disease process itself that lead to eventual thyroid failure.

In view of the foregoing, it is unlikely that the early ablative effects can be obtained free of subsequent late effects. If this is true, doses of radioiodine sufficient to exert an early therapeutic action would inevitably be associated with a high frequency of delayed hypothyroidism.

This statement summarizes the therapeutic dilemma with respect to radioiodine therapy. From various clinics, several approaches to this dilemma have emerged. Some continue to administer the conventional dose because of its relatively rapid and high effectiveness and because hypothyroidism, when it eventually occurs, is readily treated. A disadvantage of such an approach is that the onset and progression of hypothyroidism may be insidious, that prolonged follow-up of patients may not be possible, and that patients may not associate symptoms arising as a complication of therapy long past with the therapy. A rebuttal in favor of using this approach would be that the dangers of persistent or recurrent thyrotoxicosis in patients lacking follow-up exceed those of hypothyroidism, especially in the elderly.

Other approaches have been undertaken in an attempt to minimize the frequency of hypothyroidism. One is to administer a dose per gram of estimated weight that is larger the greater the gland size. In this way, the larger than usual thyroids are treated with disproportionately large doses, and the converse is true for thyroids that are particularly small. It appears, however, that a regimen of this type does not improve the ability to eliminate hyperthyroidism in the short run while forestalling the development of hypothyroidism years later. Another approach involved the use of ^{125}I, rather than ^{131}I, on the basis that the lower energy and shorter path length of the beta emission might permit irradiation of the apical portion of the thyroid cell with resulting impairment of hormone biosynthesis, while sparing the more distantly situated nucleus and its replicative machinery. However, follow-up of patients treated with ^{125}I has revealed a frequency of hypothyroidism similar to that following ^{131}I. Consequently, ^{125}I offers no advantages over ^{131}I.

Another approach employs smaller than usual doses of radioiodine, the rationale being that the small dose may be sufficient to prevent both the high incidence of delayed hypothyroidism and the late recurrence of thyrotoxicosis. Although such small doses are likely insufficient to control thyrotoxicosis acutely, such control can be achieved by administration of antithyroid drugs or stable iodine after radioiodine has been given.

The efficacy of this last approach is not yet certain. Retrospective analysis indicates that the frequency of hypothyroidism varies directly with the magnitude of the dose used.[279] Moreover, in a controlled prospective study, the effects of a single conventional dose of approximately 5.2 MBq/g (140 µCi/g) of estimated glandular weight were compared with the effects of half the dose.[283] Although the therapeutic effect of radioiodine appeared more slowly in patients receiving the half-dose, and a greater proportion required antithyroid drug therapy until this effect became apparent, the frequency of remission after 2 y was the same as that in patients receiving the conventional dose and recurrence of thyrotoxicosis was no more common. Of great importance was the finding that in the full-dose group the incidence of hypothyroidism was 8% at 1 y and 29% at 5 y, whereas in the half-dose group the corresponding values were 4 and 7%. However, although the use of low doses of

^{131}I reduces the incidence of hypothyroidism during the first few years, thereafter the cumulative frequency with time is similar to that observed with conventional doses.[284] Further observations of this type are required.

Several additional hazards may attend the use of radioiodine, particularly large doses. The parathyroids are exposed to radiation in patients treated with radioiodine, but the appearance of clinically overt hypoparathyroidism is rare. Parathyroid reserve may be diminished in some patients. The effect of radioiodine on other tissues that concentrate iodide, such as the salivary and gastric glands, has received little attention. Another potential hazard of radioiodine therapy, namely radiation thyroiditis, may influence the therapeutic regimen. This complication may lead to an exacerbation of thyrotoxicosis about 10 to 14 d after the radioiodine is administered. Serious consequences occasionally have occurred in patients with severe thyrotoxicosis or thyrocardiac disease; these include precipitation of thyrotoxic crisis and aggravation of cardiac insufficiency. In cases of this type, therefore, it is advisable to administer antithyroid drugs for several weeks before radioiodine is given, to deplete glandular hormone stores. This prevents an outpouring of hormone should severe radiation thyroiditis occur. The antithyroid agent is withdrawn about 5 d before administration of the radioiodine and, if the clinical condition warrants, can be given again 7 d later.

Because ^{131}I administration is contraindicated during pregnancy, a pregnancy test should be carried out in women of childbearing age before they are given ^{131}I therapy if there is any possibility of pregnancy.

GENERAL MEASURES. Several general measures may contribute to the well-being of the thyrotoxic patient. Bed rest is an excellent treatment. Help with family responsibilities by spouses and avoidance of physical exertion are also important. In addition, a dietary regimen rich in protein, calories, and vitamins serves to repair the general and specific nutritional deficiencies that thyrotoxic patients frequently develop.

CHOICE OF THERAPY. The choice of therapy for thyrotoxicosis is often difficult because a variety of factors interplay with the disease to modify the therapeutic decision. Among these are emotional attitudes, economic considerations, and factors within the family and home.

The authors' choice of therapy in diffuse toxic goiter accommodates factors related to the natural history of the disease, the advantages and disadvantages of the several therapeutic modalities discussed above, and the factors pertinent to the population group in which the patient falls. Surgery is recommended only in patients for whom shortcomings of other modes of therapy have special importance. This conclusion leaves to surgery a minimal role in the treatment of diffuse toxic goiter.

Considerations peculiar to the treatment of thyrotoxicosis in children and adolescents are discussed in a later section dealing with special aspects of thyrotoxicosis. The remainder of this section is confined to the choice of therapy in adults. One approach is to initiate therapy with antithyroid drugs in all patients to produce a euthyroid state before reaching a final decision regarding a definitive therapeutic strategy. This allows the patient to return to a euthyroid status as rapidly as possible and provides an estimate of the antithyroid drug dose requirement. The magnitude of the drug requirement and the size of the thyroid gland are factors considered in the evaluation of the patient with regard to the likelihood of a remission. The three options for treatment are explained to the patient during these first months of contact, and individual recommendations are then formulated. This time period also allows the establishment of a suitable physician-patient relationship, which is especially important in addressing anxieties regarding potential adverse effects of radioiodine. Such concerns lead many patients, especially those under the age of 50, to elect a trial of antithyroid drugs before definitive therapy with [131]I. Individuals with large thyroid glands or a high maintenance thionamide dose requirement (>400 mg propythiouracil/d) are advised that the chance of spontaneous remission is less than 30%. Therapeutic trials are generally pursued for 1 y if long-term thionamide therapy is selected. When a decision in favor of ^{131}I is made, it is prescribed at a dose designed to result in 186 to 222 MBq (5 to 6 mCi) [131]I retained in the thyroid gland at 24 h. This estimate is based on a ^{123}I uptake test performed immediately before treatment and at least 5 d after stopping the thionamide. Because ^{131}I is given when the patient is euthyroid and this is a relatively large dose, no additional therapy is required immediately after treatment except for patients in whom a recurrence of hyperthyroidism poses a medical risk, e.g., patients with coronary artery disease or congestive heart failure. Patients are seen at 4-wk intervals after ^{131}I administration, and hypothyroidism is treated when it appears, generally within 3 mo.

Women planning to become pregnant are advised to wait for an arbitrary period of 6 mo after ^{131}I therapy to allow for resolution of any transient effects of gonadal radiation exposure. If, after a period of 6 to 8 mo, hyperthyroidism is still present and the patient is symptomatic, the treatment is repeated, generally using about 1.5 times the initial dose of [131]I.

HYPOTHYROIDISM IN THE RECENTLY HYPERTHYROID PATIENT. Distinct symptoms may occur when the onset of hypothyroidism occurs rapidly in the previously thyrotoxic patient, as after ^{131}I or surgical treatment or even after high doses of thionamide drugs. Such patients may experience severe muscle cramps, often in large muscle groups such as the trapezius or latissimus dorsi or the proximal muscles of the extremities. Such cramps can occur even when the serum hormone levels are still only low normal or slightly decreased and before the TSH level has risen. It is possible to mistake these symptoms, such as back pain, for an unrelated illness unless the patient is warned in advance.

In the occasional young adult, it becomes necessary to remove a diffuse toxic goiter because of obstructive symptoms or cosmetic disfigurement. Although the foregoing reflects the authors' general approach to therapy, it is important to be aware of the great extent to which opinions of thyroidologists differ.[285] In view of the several approaches to treatment available, each with its advantages and disadvantages, it is incumbent upon the physician to explain these factors thoroughly, to indicate his or her preference and the reasons for it, and to allow the final choice to rest with the patient.

Treatment of Infiltrative Ophthalmopathy and Infiltrative Dermopathy

Infiltrative ophthalmopathy varies in severity from a mild form, which is common, to a severe form that may threaten the vision and even the life of the patient. Fortunately the latter is rare, because it presents difficult problems of treatment. The variety of treatments proposed and the continuing, often heated, discussion of their relative efficiency bespeak the general inadequacy of all, the most effective being merely palliative. The natural course of the disorder, which is variable and characterized by exacerbations and remissions, makes conclusions about the efficacy of most treatments dubious. This is all the more the case because the number of patients afflicted with the severe form is relatively small and controlled studies are difficult to perform. A further source of confusion is the variable terminology for describing the manifestations of ophthalmopathy and the lack of rigid criteria for defining their severity. General use of the American Thyroid Association classification that defines these variables is therefore strongly recommended (see Table 8–13).

The first question that arises is whether various forms of treatment for thyrotoxicosis affect the course of the ophthalmopathy. Subtotal thyroidectomy, radioiodine therapy, or antithyroid therapy in themselves do not influence ophthalmopathy except insofar as they may lead to the development of hypothyroidism.[286] Hypothyroidism has an adverse effect on the disorder and should be avoided; when it occurs it should be treated fully, but exogenous thyroid hormone in the absence of hypothyroidism does not favorably influence the ophthalmopathy. Similarly, no evidence exists for a favorable action of iodine, once widely used. Indeed, this agent may actually induce a hypothyroid state (iodide myxedema).

The measures used in treatment can be divided into those that are largely symptomatic (useful mainly in the mild form) and those that attempt to arrest or reverse the progression of the disorder, either by an attack on its presumed pathogenesis or by mechanical means. In milder forms of the disorder, little treatment is required.[287] The patient who experiences photophobia and sensitivity to wind or cold air is benefited by wearing dark glasses, which also afford protection from foreign bodies. Elevation of the head of the bed at night and instillation of lubricants, such as 1% methylcellulose, may benefit the patient whose lids do not appose completely during sleep. Artificial tears can be used during the day. Because the ophthalmic manifestations tend to be self-limited and the progression to a more severe form is uncommon, such measures usually suffice to tide the patient over until the disorder regresses spontaneously.

The appearance of increasing proptosis, with inability to appose the lids, or of severe infiltrative manifestations such as chemosis, indicates progression of the disorder and warrants the use of more vigorous therapeutic measures. When the condition is serious but not desperate, several methods of treatment have been proposed. Changes of this type, even when severe, may respond favorably and rapidly to massive doses of prednisone (120 to 140 mg/d). If improvement occurs, the daily dose is decreased to the lowest level at which improvement is maintained. The latter is still likely to be large, but it is hoped that a halt to the progression or actual regression of the disease will occur before untoward effects make withdrawal of the drug necessary. To circumvent the inevitable side effects of large doses of glucocorticoids given systemically, periodic injection of depot preparations of glucocorticoids given subconjunctivally or into the retro-orbital space has been advocated. Such treatment may have a dramatic effect on irritative symptoms as well as on diplopia, but its efficacy varies, and mild systemic effects of the glucocorticoids are sometimes seen. Moreover, this treatment entails the risk of puncture of the globe or a retro-orbital hematoma.

As an alternative to glucocorticoid therapy, external radiation to the orbits has been employed. The value of such treatment is not established because reported results have been variable. Highly collimated supervoltage radiation of the retro-orbital space has been applied, with seemingly rapid and beneficial effects on infiltrative and inflammatory manifestations, but usually exophthalmos and ophthalmoparesis are little affected.[288]

There appears to be no merit to the suggestion that infiltrative ophthalmopathy is benefited or its progression retarded by total ablation of the thyroid, whether performed surgically or by radioiodine, or by a combination of the two.

In view of the foregoing considerations, the authors

recommend a trial of oral glucocorticoid therapy for patients with severe or progressive ophthalmopathy. If effective doses cannot be tolerated, a course of external radiation may be attempted. Local measures should be employed, along with these major forms of treatment. Ulceration and infection of the cornea should be treated with antibiotics, lubricants, and protective shields. An attempt to appose the lids by means of sutures (tarsorrhaphy) should be performed only by an experienced ophthalmologist, as the sutures may tear out and scarring result.

If glucocorticoid therapy and external radiation fail to halt progression of the disease, and if loss of vision is threatened either by ulceration or infection of the cornea or by changes in the retina or optic nerve, orbital decompression is performed. This usually involves removal of either the lateral wall or the roof of the orbit, or resection of the lateral wall of the ethmoid sinus and the roof of the maxillary sinus.[289]

The management of severe ophthalmopathy should never be undertaken by the internist or endocrinologist or by the ophthalmologist acting alone. Close and coordinated observation of the effects of medical therapy and the progress of the disease is necessary to determine whether and when the surgical approach to treatment, which almost invariably halts the progress of the disease and preserves vision if performed in time, should be employed.

Treatment of infiltrative dermopathy is seldom necessary. However, if this manifestation is severe, a topical glucocorticoid preparation along with an occlusive dressing will produce regression of the lesion.

Toxic Multinodular Goiter

Toxic multinodular goiter is a disorder in which hyperthyroidism arises in a multinodular goiter, usually of long standing. It is uncertain whether it represents one disease or is the clinical expression of one of several pathogenetic factors. It is important to avoid the term toxic nodular goiter because this encompasses both toxic multinodular goiter, as here described, and toxic adenoma of the thyroid gland, which will be discussed in a succeeding section.

Pathogenesis, Histopathology, and Pathophysiology

The pathogenesis of toxic multinodular goiter cannot be considered apart from that of its invariable forerunner, nontoxic multinodular goiter, from which it emerges slowly and surreptitiously. Two hallmarks of the disorder, structural and functional heterogeneity and functional autonomy, develop over time; the steady increase in the extent of autonomous function causes the disease to move from the nontoxic to the toxic phase. Sometimes, hyperthyroidism appears abruptly, but this almost always results from exposure to increased quantities of iodine, which permits autonomous foci to increase their rate of hormone secretion to truly excessive levels (iodine-induced hyperthyroidism, jodbasedow).

The patterns of function displayed by toxic multinodular goiters are consonant with the two hallmarks of the disease and are evident in scintiscans and in autoradiographs of excised tissue.[290] In general, two patterns are seen. The first is a diffuse but somewhat uneven ("patchy") distribution of radioisotope that is altered little, if at all, by administration of exogenous thyroid hormone. Histopathological examination reveals multiple aggregates of small follicles with hyperplastic epithelium, interspersed with variably sized nodules that appear as if they should be inactive. However, the correlation between histological appearance and func-

tion, as judged from radioiodine accumulation, is poor. Very likely at least some, and possibly many, of the nonfunctioning areas are capable of functioning but are inactive because TSH secretion is suppressed by the hyperfunction in autonomous areas.

The second type of toxic multinodular goiter is also distinguished by its functional pattern. Here, radioiodine becomes localized in one or more discrete nodules, while iodine accumulation in the remainder of the gland is suppressed. No further suppression is produced by exogenous thyroid hormone, but TSH stimulates accumulation of iodine in the areas previously inactive. Histopathologically, the functioning areas resemble adenomas in being reasonably well demarcated from surrounding tissue. They generally consist of large follicles, sometimes with hyperplastic epithelium, but here too the correlation of architecture with functional state is not good. The remaining tissue appears inactive, and zones of degeneration are present in both functioning and nonfunctioning areas. These findings suggest that areas that are functioning can do so without TSH and may therefore be termed areas of adenomatous hyperfunction. The remaining areas, in contrast, retain their dependence on TSH, their function being suppressed as a consequence of hyperfunction in the autonomous zones. It is unlikely that function in this type of gland is sustained by an external stimulator of normal or abnormal origin. Hence, from the pathophysiological standpoint, this disorder resembles the normal thyroid that harbors a solitary hyperfunctioning adenoma. Whether the hyperfunctioning areas represent adenomas in a biological sense is unknown.

The extent of overproduction of thyroid hormone in toxic multinodular goiter is usually mild compared with that in Graves disease. First, the clinical manifestations of thyrotoxicosis are rarely flagrant. Second, the serum T_4 and T_3 concentrations are often only marginally increased. Finally, the RAIU is not greatly increased and may even be within the normal range. The relative mildness of the hyperthyroidism is consistent with either of its presumed pathogenetic origins. The effectiveness of any stimulus to hyperfunction may well be blunted in a thyroid that is the seat of a preexisting nontoxic goiter, because the latter disorder results from an impairment in the efficiency of the gland with respect to hormone synthesis; this explanation is of course speculative.

Clinical Picture

Toxic multinodular goiter is a common complication of its nontoxic precursor, but its precise incidence in the latter disorder is unknown. It usually occurs after the age of 50 in patients who have had multinodular goiter for many years. Like its forerunner, it is many times more common in women than in men. Toxic multinodular goiter is almost never accompanied by infiltrative ophthalmopathy, but when it is, it represents the emergence of Graves disease.

The clinical manifestations tend to differ from those in diffuse toxic goiter. Cardiovascular manifestations tend to predominate, possibly because of the age of the patient. These may include atrial fibrillation or tachycardia, with or without heart failure. Frequently, a decreased response to digitalis first alerts the physician to the presence of thyrotoxicosis. Weakness and wasting of muscles are common. The nervous manifestations are less prominent than in the younger patient with thyrotoxicosis, but emotional lability may be pronounced. Because of the physical characteristics of the thyroid gland as well as its frequent retrosternal extension, obstructive symptoms are more common than in diffuse toxic goiter. On palpation, the characteristics of the goiter are the same as those of the more common nontoxic multinodular goiter discussed later. In as many as 20% of elderly patients with thyrotoxicosis, the thyroid gland is firm and irregular but not distinctly enlarged.

Laboratory Tests and Differential Diagnosis

The main clinical problem is to determine whether the patient with a multinodular goiter is thyrotoxic. Laboratory tests will generally resolve this issue. The most important results are the FT_4I and the TSH concentration. If the FT_4I is elevated and the TSH level suppressed, hyperthyroidism is confirmed. In some patients only the serum FT_3I is increased, but the serum TSH must be below 0.1 mU/L to establish the diagnosis of hyperthyroidism related to Graves disease. Levels intermediate between this and the 0.5 mU/L lower limit of normal are not usually associated with significant symptoms. Such patients have thyroid autonomy but are not frankly thyrotoxic. The pituitary-hypothalamic axis provides the most sensitive indicator of an excess supply of thyroid hormone that is specifically relevant to the individual patient. Monitoring the concentration of serum TSH takes advantage of this sensitivity and is one of the most useful ways of establishing the existence of autonomous thyroid function. The RAIU may be of little help because thyrotoxicosis may exist in association with values that are normal or only slightly increased.

Treatment

Radioiodine appears to be the treatment of choice for most patients with toxic multinodular goiter, despite considerable disagreement concerning the magnitude and number of doses required to achieve a therapeutic response. In general, experience along the eastern seaboard of the United States indicates that the responsiveness to radioiodine of toxic multinodular goiter differs little from that of diffuse toxic goiter. On the other hand, in areas where goiter was formerly endemic, such as the Great Lakes area of the United States, toxic multinodular goiter is said to be resistant to radioiodine. Although no correlative studies necessary to support this hypothesis have been reported, the type that readily responds to radioiodine may resemble diffuse toxic goiter in displaying a relatively diffuse accumulation of iodine. The more resistant variety, on the other hand, may be associated with adenomatous hyperfunction, in which focal accumulation of radioiodine occurs; here, tissue previously suppressed may regain function and ultimately achieve autonomy after the hyperactive tissue has been destroyed.

Because of the age of the patient and variations in sensitivity to radioiodine, conventional doses should be administered. In any event, these are likely to be larger than those used in diffuse toxic goiter, because the percentage uptake of ^{131}I tends to be lower and the size of the gland greater. Many patients with this disorder have underlying heart disease. Therefore, the administration of radioiodine should be preceded by a course of antithyroid therapy until a eumetabolic state is achieved. Medication is then discontinued for 3 to 5 d before radioiodine is administered. Seven days thereafter, the antithyroid drug is reinstituted so that control of thyrotoxicosis is maintained until radioiodine exerts its effect. After 6 to 8 wk the antithyroid drug is gradually withdrawn, and if thyrotoxicosis recurs, a second course of therapy should be given. Surgical therapy is recommended after adequate preoperative preparation in patients in whom obstructive manifestations are present or in whom it is feared that such manifestations may result from the temporary thyroid enlargement that radioiodine sometimes produces.

Toxic Adenoma

A third and far less common form of hyperthyroidism is that sometimes produced by one or more autonomous adenomas of the thyroid gland. As herein employed, the term refers to adenomas present in a thyroid that is otherwise intrinsically normal, differentiating this lesion from areas of adenomatous hyperfunction within a toxic multinodular goiter. The disorder is usually caused by a single adenoma that is palpable as a solitary nodule and hence is sometimes referred to as *hyperfunctioning solitary nodule* or *toxic nodule*. Occasionally, two or three adenomas of similar character are present.

Pathogenesis, Histopathology, and Pathophysiology

Toxic adenomas are true follicular adenomas of the thyroid gland (for histopathological characteristics, see under Thyroid Neoplasms); hence, their basic pathogenesis is unknown.

By definition, the adenoma is capable of functioning without stimulation by TSH, and no abnormal thyroid stimulators are present in the blood. The natural course is one of slow, progressive growth and increasing function over many years. At first it may be present as a small nodule or may be impalpable, but in either case it may be detectable in the scintiscan as a localized area of increased radioiodine accumulation. On administration of exogenous thyroid hormone, the function of the remainder of the gland is suppressed, but function in the adenoma persists. Later, with further growth, a progressively increasing share of glandular function is assumed by the adenoma, with the result that the remaining tissue is increasingly suppressed. Ultimately, atrophy and complete suppression of the remainder of the gland occur, and the scintiscan reveals function only in the adenoma (hot nodule) (see Fig. 8–24). Although continued growth of the adenoma is associated with secretion of excessive quantities of hormone, some time may pass before overt thyrotoxicosis is manifest. The extranodular tissue generally retains its capacity to function if TSH is provided, either by exogenous administration or as a result of ablation of the nodule. Some adenomas of this type secrete T_3 predominantly, and some, in addition to the normal thyroid hormones, secrete an iodinated protein that is measurable as PBI, leading to a disproportionate elevation of the latter relative to T_4 iodine.

Clinical Picture

Toxic adenoma occurs in a younger age group than does toxic multinodular goiter, often in patients in their 30s or 40s. Frequently, there is a history of a long-standing, slowly growing lump in the neck. Rarely does the lesion develop sufficient function to produce thyrotoxicosis until it has achieved a diameter of 2.5 to 3 cm. The adenoma may undergo central necrosis and hemorrhage; as a result, the thyrotoxicosis may be relieved, the remainder of the thyroid may resume its function, and the adenoma may appear on the scintiscan as a cold area, suggesting a thyroid carcinoma. Calcification in the area of hemorrhage may take place and be evident on x-ray examination. Such calcification is usually gross and irregular and does not resemble the finely stippled calcification of the psammoma bodies seen in papillary cancers.

The peripheral manifestations of toxic adenoma are generally milder than those of diffuse toxic goiter and are notable for the absence of infiltrative ophthalmopathy and myopathy; cardiovascular manifestations, however, may be prominent. The nodule is usually felt as a smooth, well-defined, round or ovoid mass that is firm and moves freely on swallowing. Often, the remainder of the gland is not palpable. A bruit is never present.

Laboratory Tests

The results of laboratory tests depend on the stage of the disorder. At first serum thyroid hormone concentrations may be normal except for borderline suppression of the serum TSH. Later a thyroid scintiscan (see Fig. 8–24) may show localization of radioisotope to the palpated nodule. This does not occur until TSH secretion is suppressed. If the nodule continues to grow, frank hyperthyroidism may supervene with elevation of serum thyroid hormone concentrations and metabolic indices. When the nodule is small, the RAIU is normal but cannot be suppressed completely by exogenous thyroid hormone. However, TSH and, therefore, function in the extranodular tissue will be suppressed by exogenous hormone, allowing identification of the autonomous nature of the nodular lesion by scanning even before the lesion has become sufficiently large to suppress serum TSH. Occasionally, values for serum T_4 concentration are normal and serum T_3 concentration alone is increased (T_3 toxicosis). Relative to its overall rate of occurrence, toxic adenoma is the most frequent cause of T_3 toxicosis. If there is any question about the presence of the suppressed lobe, exogenous TSH may be administered before scintiscanning to demonstrate uptake in this tissue. However, with the availability of a sensitive TSH assay this should rarely be necessary. Incidental thyroid carcinoma may coexist with a hyperfunctioning adenoma, although a malignant nodule causing functional hyperthyroidism has not, to the authors' knowledge, been documented.

Treatment

Although many hyperfunctioning adenomas eventually cause hyperthyroidism, some do so slowly and others not at all. Therefore, treatment of asymptomatic patients with functional adenomas is decided on an individual basis. The degree of TSH suppression may be used to monitor the progression of thyroid hormone production by the adenoma. Suppression below the lower limits of normal indicates that hyperthyroidism is present, as defined by this sensitive index, and that therapy should be given except in unusual situations. Two treatment modalities are available: radioiodine and surgery. Large nodules with concomitant physical symptoms are most readily treated by surgical excision. Surgical excision is also used in patients under age 20, for whom the radiation from ^{131}I to the perinodular normal thyroid tissue could theoretically predispose to the risk of future development of radiation-related thyroid neoplasia.[291]

In terms of the specificity of treatment, functioning thyroid nodules are ideal candidates for radioiodine therapy. The radiation is directed almost exclusively to the diseased tissue; because TSH is suppressed, the normal thyroid tissue surrounding the nodule does not take up radioiodine. For the patient older than the age of 20 with a nodule 5 cm and less in diameter, ^{131}I is the treatment of choice. In general, doses of radioiodine similar to those given in Graves disease are successful, 185 to 222 MBq (~5 to 6 mCi) deposited at 24 h.[292] Because of the potential for delayed hypothyroidism with higher ^{131}I doses, prolonged follow-up is mandatory.[293]

The thyroid that is the seat of a toxic adenoma is not diffusely hypervascular and hence preoperative preparation with iodine is not required, but in the patient with overt thyrotoxicosis, restoration to a normal metabolic state with an antithyroid drug before surgery is desirable.

Hyperthyroidism in Trophoblastic Disease

Thyroid hyperfunction often accompanies hydatidiform mole, choriocarcinoma, or metastatic embryonal carcinoma of the testis. Such neoplasms, particularly hydatidiform mole, elaborate a thyroid stimulator that is distinct from pituitary TSH and and may be native hCG or a protein closely related to it.[109–111] Some patients present with clinically overt thyrotoxicosis, but in the majority clinical manifestations are not prominent and goiter is absent, despite frequent laboratory evidence of a hyperthyroid state.[294] Free T_4 and/or free T_3 concentrations are increased and TSH values are suppressed. The reason for this discordance between the clinical and laboratory indices is not known but may be the relatively short duration of the thyroid hormone excess.

The possibility of a molar pregnancy should always be considered in a young woman with thyrotoxicosis, because appropriate therapy would be evacuation of the uterus.

Hypersecretion of TSH

Rarely, hyperthyroidism results from hypersecretion of TSH because of either of two causative factors: a TSH-secreting pituitary adenoma or inappropriate hypersecretion of TSH secondary to (1) localized pituitary resistance to thyroid hormones, (2) increased secretion of TRH, or (3) an elevated threshold for feedback control, possibly the result of the first or second cause. All varieties are associated with a diffuse hyperfunctioning goiter. Features of autoimmune thyroid disease are absent in the patient and in the patient's family. This is the only hyperthyroid condition in which serum TSH concentrations are not suppressed at a time when serum free T_4 and/or T_3 concentrations are elevated.[173] In the adenomatous variety, a mass lesion in the region of the pituitary may be present. The concentration of free alpha subunits of TSH in serum is elevated, and serum TSH concentrations fail to increase after TRH administration. In patients with nonadenomatous TSH hypersecretion, in contrast, alpha subunits are not present in the blood in high concentrations and the response to TRH is usually normal.[171–173] Such patients present a difficult therapeutic problem. In some cases, TSH secretion can be suppressed if very large doses of thyroid hormone are administered, but this results in worsening of the thyrotoxicosis. Hyperthyroidism can be controlled, of course, by thyroid ablation, but the serum TSH level then increases still further and concern arises as to whether a TSH-producing adenoma may ultimately develop. Bromocriptine, a dopamine agonist, may be effective in depressing TSH secretion and alleviating the hyperthyroidism in this disorder.[295] Somatostatin analogues have also been employed. But TSH-producing tumors usually require surgical resection.[296, 297] Successful treatment with 3,5,3′-triiodothyroacetic acid has also been reported.[298]

The occurrence of TSH-induced hyperthyroidism raises the question of whether serum TSH concentration should be measured as part of the initial work-up of every patient who is hyperthyroid and has a diffuse goiter. The authors do not recommend this when other stigmata of Graves disease or of an autoimmune diathesis are evident. When these are lacking, however, measurement of the serum TSH concentration along with a serum FT_4I is indicated. The remote possibility that a patient with Graves disease might have an artifactual elevation of TSH concentration because of a heterophilic antibody cross-reacting with mouse immunoglobulin (see discussion of TSH assay) must be kept in mind.[168] For some sera, the use of a different assay kit may confirm the elevated level. A standard TSH radioimmunoassay may be sufficient to resolve the issue because these assays are not subject to such artifacts. Alternatively, mouse serum may be added to the assay tube to absorb the heterophilic antibody.

Iodine-Induced Hyperthyroidism

Administration of supplemental iodine to subjects with endemic iodine-deficiency goiter can result in overproduction of thyroid hormone. This response, termed iodine-induced hyperthyroidism or jodbasedow, occurs in only a small fraction of individuals at risk. The best studied experience has been in Tasmania, where a temporary increase in thyrotoxicosis occurred shortly after the addition of small quantities of iodine to bread as a means of correcting iodine deficiency. Studies revealed two major patterns of underlying thyroid disorder. In the first, especially common in older individuals, nodular goiter with areas of autonomous function were present and abnormal thyroid stimulators akin to those found in Graves disease were not detectable in the blood. The second pattern typically occurred in younger individuals with diffuse goiter, and here thyroid-stimulating immunoglobulins were often present. These findings indicate that jodbasedow occurs only in thyroid glands in which function is independent of TSH stimulation. The occurrence of jodbasedow should not be construed as a reason for failing to treat endemic iodine deficiency. Apart from the many other benefits that accrue from the treatment and prophylaxis, over the long run the frequency of spontaneous hyperthyroidism associated with the development of autonomous nodules is diminished.

Iodine-induced hyperthyroidism is an important disorder in areas of the world in which dietary iodine intake is sufficient.[274] In regions in which iodine intake is marginal but overt iodine deficiency is absent, moderate increments in iodine intake may induce hyperthyroidism in patients with autonomous thyroid nodules, and large pharmacological doses of iodine, such as are employed in the treatment of pulmonary disease, can do so in geographic areas in which the iodine intake is more than adequate. Consequently, the physician must be alert to the possibility of inducing hyperthyroidism when administering to patients with nodular goiter large quantities of iodine in the form of expectorants, x-ray contrast media, medications containing iodine, or any other form. Because nodular goiter is generally a disease of the older population, induction of the jodbasedow phenomenon may have serious consequences, particularly because enrichment of the thyroid with iodine forestalls administration of ^{131}I and delays the response to antithyroid agents.

In these patients, serum T_3 concentration is sometimes normal, although total and free T_4 concentrations are increased. Confirmation that the patient has been exposed to large quantities of iodine can be obtained by demonstrating that the RAIU is low and urinary iodine excretion greatly increased (more than several milligrams per day).

Although physiological reasoning dictates that the jodbasedow phenomenon can occur only when the thyroid is free of normal regulatory control, a number of patients with iodine-induced hyperthyroidism have been reported in whom thyroid function was normal, and normally suppressible, after iodine was withdrawn and a euthyroid state restored. The mechanism by which iodine induces thyrotoxicosis in such instances is unknown. The treatment of these individuals may be difficult. Even after discontinuation of exogenous iodide, the uptake of ^{131}I by the thyroid gland may remain low, not adequate for conventional doses of radioiodine. The elevated thyroid hormone content also makes thionamide drugs less effective. In some cases it may be necessary to treat such individuals for prolonged periods (6 to 9 mo) before the use of radioiodine therapy. On the other hand, if detectable uptake is present, larger doses of radioiodine may be administered to cause destruction of thyroid tissue.

Thyrotoxicosis Without Hyperthyroidism

Several disorders are associated with thyrotoxicosis, but without hyperthyroidism, i.e., ongoing overproduction of thyroid hormone. These disorders fall into two general categories: those in which the excess of hormone originates outside the thyroid gland, as in thyrotoxicosis factitia and in ectopic hyperfunctioning thyroid tissue, and those in which inflammatory disease of the thyroid leads to loss of storage function and leakage of hormone into the blood, as in subacute thyroiditis and painless or silent thyroiditis. These disorders are recognized in part by the presence of low values of the RAIU, owing to suppression of TSH secretion, inflammatory injury to the gland, or a combination of the two.

Recognition of these forms of thyrotoxicosis is important because their treatment differs from that of true thyroid hyperfunction.

Thyrotoxicosis Factitia

This term designates thyrotoxicosis that arises from the ingestion, usually chronic, of excessive quantities of thyroid hormone. The disorder usually occurs in women with a background of underlying psychiatric disease, especially in paramedical personnel who have access to thyroid hormone or in patients for whom thyroid hormone medication has been prescribed in the past.[299] Generally, the patient is aware of taking thyroid hormone but may adamantly deny it. In other instances, large doses of thyroid hormone or other thyroactive material, such as iodocasein, may be given without the knowledge of the patient, usually as part of a regimen for weight reduction.

Symptoms are typical of thyrotoxicosis and may be severe. In the absence of pre-existing disease of the thyroid, diagnosis is made from the combination of typical thyrotoxic manifestations, together with thyroid atrophy and hypofunction. Infiltrative ophthalmopathy never occurs, but lid lag, stare, and other "thyrotoxic" eye signs may be present. Hypofunction of the thyroid gland is evidenced by subnormal values of the RAIU, which can be increased by administration of TSH. Serum T_4 concentrations are increased unless the patient is taking T_3, in which case they will be subnormal. Serum T_3 concentrations are increased in either case. Low, rather than elevated, values of serum thyroglobulin concentration suggest that thyrotoxicosis results from exogenous hormone, rather than thyroid hyperfunction.[134]

This disorder may be confused with other varieties of thyrotoxicosis associated with a subnormal RAIU and absence of goiter. These include the syndrome of chronic thyroiditis with transient thyrotoxicosis; ectopic thyroid tissue; and hyperfunctioning metastatic follicular carcinoma. Evidence for the two latter disorders can be obtained by demonstration of low values for the sum of thyroid and urinary ^{131}I after a tracer dose and by localization of the ectopic focus or foci by external scintiscanning. Differentiation from painless thyroiditis may be difficult. The presence of circulating antithyroid antibodies points to painless chronic thyroiditis, whereas a firm thyroid and brief history suggest the painless variant of subacute thyroiditis.

Treatment of thyrotoxicosis factitia consists of withdrawing the offending medication. Psychotherapy will usually be necessary.

HAMBURGER THYROTOXICOSIS. An unusual form of exogenous thyrotoxicosis occurred in the midwestern por-

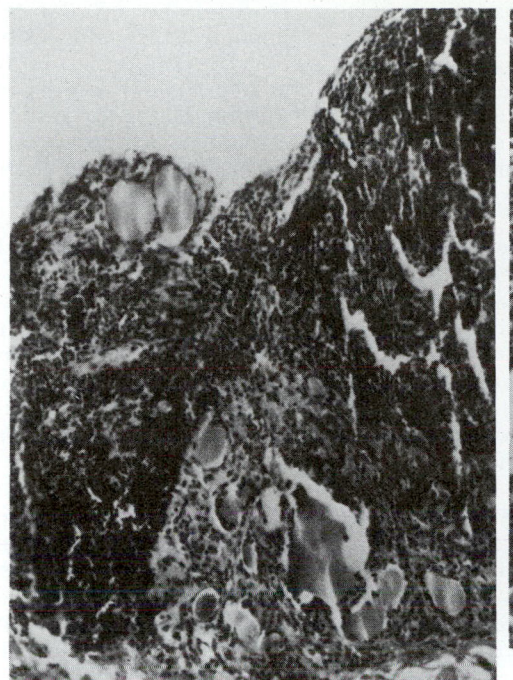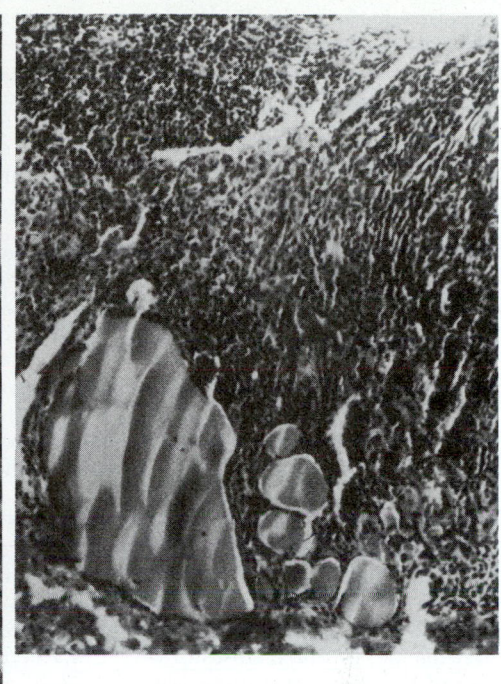

Figure 8–40. High- and low-power magnification views of open biopsy of thyroid gland during hypothyroid phase of "silent thyroiditis." Note extensive lymphocytic infiltration and patchy distribution of poorly preserved follicles. (From Woolf PD. Transient painless thyroiditis with hyperthyroidism: a variant of lymphocytic thyroiditis? Endocr Rev 1980; 1:411–420. © 1980, The Endocrine Society.)

tion of the United States in 1984 and 1985. The source was the inclusion of large quantities of bovine thyroid in ground beef preparations.[300] When the slaughtering practices were changed, this condition disappeared. Such a possibility, however remote, should be considered, especially if confronted with epidemic exogenous thyrotoxicosis.

Ectopic Thyroid Tissue

Thyroid tissue may be present in teratomas, especially in the ovary (struma ovarii), and such foci may produce thyrotoxicosis. Rarely, hyperfunctioning metastases of follicular carcinoma can produce thyrotoxicosis. The distinguishing features of such lesions were discussed earlier under Thyrotoxicosis Factitia.

Silent or Painless Thyroiditis, and Postpartum Thyroiditis Syndrome

Thyrotoxicosis is associated with the early phase of subacute or giant cell thyroiditis, in both its painful and its painless variants. Thyrotoxicosis can also occur with a painless form of thyroiditis in which biopsy of the thyroid reveals the histopathological changes of lymphocytic thyroiditis rather than those of subacute thyroiditis (Fig. 8–40).[301] This syndrome has variously been alluded to as silent or painless thyroiditis with thyrotoxicosis or as "hyperthyroiditis." This terminology is unfortunate because it does not clearly distinguish the syndrome from the painless variant of subacute thyroiditis. A better name for the syndrome might be chronic thyroiditis with transient thyrotoxicosis.

The cardinal features are thyrotoxicosis associated with greatly depressed values of the RAIU in the absence of excess body iodide stores, lack of pain or tenderness in the thyroid area, and spontaneous resolution of the thyrotoxic phase of the disease. Additional features include a tendency to pass through a transient euthyroid and then a hypothyroid phase before a long-term return to euthyroidism and a tendency for the syndrome to recur (Fig. 8–41). The thyroid gland is enlarged in only about 50% of cases, and enlarge-

ment is usually mild and unaccompanied by nodularity. Thyrotoxicosis is rarely severe, and this is reflected in the extent of elevation of serum T_4 and T_3 concentrations. Although antithyroid microsomal antibodies can be detected in almost all patients by sensitive assays, conventional assays reveal antithyroid antibodies in only about one half of the patients. Systemic manifestations of inflammation are lacking, and unlike the situation in subacute thyroiditis, the erythrocyte sedimentation rate is normal or near normal.

Several aspects of the pathophysiology of this disorder are instructive. Reduction in the RAIU cannot be explained by iodine excess, as it is in the jodbasedow phenomenon. Thus, as in subacute thyroiditis, the rate of ongoing synthesis of thyroid hormones is negligible, justifying the classification of this disorder among those that lead to thyrotoxicosis without hyperthyroidism. Decreased values of the RAIU are due partly to suppression of TSH secretion by the excess of circulating hormones, because the serum TSH level is suppressed, but function of the thyroid follicular cell is also

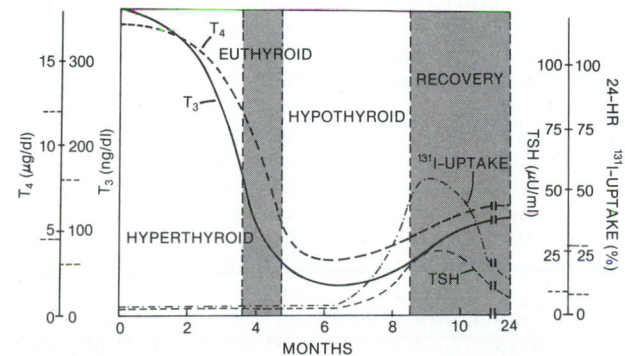

Figure 8–41. Schematic of the typical course in patients with silent thyroiditis syndrome (chronic thyroiditis with transient thyrotoxicosis). The duration of each phase may vary, and some patients do not experience a discernible hyperthyroid or hypothyroid phase. (From Woolf PD. Transient painless thyroiditis with hyperthyroidism: a variant of lymphocytic thyroiditis? Endocr Rev 1980; 1:411–420. © 1980, The Endocrine Society.)

impaired because the RAIU does not increase after administration of TSH. Although not grossly excessive, urinary iodine excretion is at the upper limit, or slightly in excess, of normal. This can readily be explained by the subnormal RAIU. Finally, the tendency of the disorder to pass through a hypothyroid phase is not surprising in view of the extensive depletion of glandular hormone stores that must occur while hormone is leaking from the gland and new hormone synthesis is reduced.

The duration of the thyrotoxic phase averages about 2 mo. About one half of the patients return to a euthyroid phase and remain well, at least for some time. In the remaining half, a hypothyroid phase that varies in duration from about 2 to 9 mo may follow. This, in turn, gives way to a restoration of euthyroidism, but a small proportion, approximately 5%, develop permanent hypothyroidism years later.[302] About one third retain a goiter, usually with persistence of antithyroid antibodies in the serum. The opposite sequela, recurrence of thyrotoxicosis, may occur months or years after restoration of a euthyroid state, and some patients experience multiple recurrences.

Treatment of the thyrotoxic phase of this disorder consists of alleviation of its peripheral manifestations through the use of propranolol or sedatives. Reportedly, prednisone, in initial doses of 50 mg/d, decreases the duration of the thyrotoxic phase without risk of relapse upon its withdrawal.[303] If mild and brief, the hypothyroid phase may not require treatment. When treatment is required, it should be undertaken with the understanding that it will be withdrawn approximately 1 y later, as the hypothyroidism is unlikely to be permanent.

The underlying nature of this disorder remains mysterious. It has many features that suggest an autoimmune basis. Extensive lymphocytic infiltration and presence of plasma cells within the thyroid are reminiscent of, although not identical to, those in Hashimoto thyroiditis, as are the circulating antithyroid antibodies. The latter, however, may merely reflect a response to inflammatory release of antigens. The occurrence of the syndrome in patients known to have Graves disease, which the authors and others have observed, and the later emergence of hypothyroidism or Hashimoto disease are also consonant with an autoimmune etiology. On the other hand, the absence of high titers of circulating antithyroid antibodies and the permanent resolution in most would argue against this.

Similar in presentation, course, and pathophysiology is the postpartum thyroiditis syndrome.[304] Transient thyrotoxicosis with low RAIU may occur some time within a few months after delivery and often is followed by a period of hypothyroidism of several months' duration, with eventual return to a euthyroid state. In some patients, only a hypothyroid phase may be evident. Postpartum hypothyroidism may occur in as many as 10% of women with positive antimicrosomal antibodies.[305, 306] This argues for prenatal assessment for the presence of antimicrosomal antibodies and postpartum assessment of thyroid function at 2 and 4 mo in women with significant antimicrosomal antibody titers. As in the similar syndrome not temporally related to pregnancy, recurrences are common after subsequent pregnancies and may also take place between pregnancies. Very likely, the postpartum thyroiditis syndrome has an autoimmune basis. Most patients have a small goiter and positive tests for antimicrosomal antibodies, although titers are low. The syndrome has been observed post partum in patients known to have Graves disease. There is a strong association with the HLA-DR3 and HLA-DR5 haplotypes,[306] which are also associated with the atrophic and goitrous varieties, respectively, of Hashimoto disease. The postpartum occur-

rence of the disorder is probably due to a rebound of immune activity after its suppression during pregnancy.[307]

The nonpostpartum syndrome may account for as many as 15% of new-onset thyrotoxicosis, although it has not been this common in the authors' experience. Most remarkable is a report from Japan that among more than 500 pregnant women studied post partum, approximately 5% displayed evidence of the postpartum thyroiditis syndrome, about 50% had transient thyrotoxicosis alone, 25% had transient hypothyroidism alone, and the remainder had both phases of the disease.[308] This high frequency has apparently been confirmed in other centers. An even more surprising finding in the same study was the nearly 4:1 ratio of females to males among babies born to women with the syndrome. Tentative conclusions of potential import can be drawn from the data. Surveillance of thyroid function with measurements of serum T_4 and T_3 concentrations should be carried out, if not in all women in the postpartum period, certainly in those who have symptoms suggestive of thyroid dysfunction, some of which may have been ascribed to psychological factors or other disease in the past. Further, patients who have experienced one episode of the postpartum thyroiditis syndrome should be considered at risk for recurrence of the syndrome both after and between pregnancies. By the same token, women of childbearing age who have experienced an episode of transient thyrotoxicosis unrelated to pregnancy should be considered at risk for development of the postpartum syndrome after any subsequent pregnancy.

Special Aspects of Thyrotoxicosis

T_3 Toxicosis

Concurrent measurements of T_4 and T_3 production rates have revealed a disproportionate increase in T_3 production in most patients with spontaneous hyperthyroidism.[75] Whether this phenomenon results solely from the preferential increase in thyroid secretion of T_3 or whether there is in addition a disproportionate increase in peripheral conversion of T_4 to T_3 is uncertain, but the former factor is likely responsible in the majority.[18] In the extreme case, the production rate of T_3 alone is increased; the thyrotoxic state resulting therefrom has been designated T_3 toxicosis. In some patients, T_3 toxicosis may be the forerunner of the usual form of thyrotoxicosis in which production of both T_3 and T_4 is increased, whereas in other patients it may persist as such. T_3 toxicosis may occur in association with Graves disease, toxic multinodular goiter, or toxic adenoma. Its true prevalence is not known but it appears to be more common, relative to the conventional laboratory presentation of hyperthyroidism, in areas of iodine deficiency. In the authors' experience, it tends to be more frequent in the elderly population; consequently, in this age group especially, reliance should not be placed solely on measurement of the serum T_4 concentration to exclude the presence of thyrotoxicosis.

The diagnosis of T_3 toxicosis should be suspected in a patient with clinical manifestations of thyrotoxicosis in whom the serum T_4 concentration and free T_4 concentration or index are normal or decreased while the serum TSH concentration is suppressed, and elevation of the FT_3I confirms the diagnosis. Palpable goiter and normal or increased RAIU exclude the presence of thyrotoxicosis factitia induced by ingestion of T_3. Preliminary experience suggests that patients with T_3 toxicosis are more likely to enjoy a long-term remission after withdrawal of antithyroid drug therapy than patients with the usual form of thyrotoxicosis, in which production of both T_4 and T_3 is increased.

T_4 Toxicosis

T_4 toxicosis refers to thyrotoxicosis with an increased serum T_4 concentration and free T_4 concentration or index, but with a normal or decreased serum T_3 concentration. This phenomenon occurs in two circumstances. One is that of iodine-induced thyrotoxicosis, discussed earlier.[274] Here, as many as one third of the patients display a normal serum T_3 concentration and the remainder display proportionate elevations of the serum T_3 and T_4 concentrations.[309] The presumption is that the availability to autonomous foci of abundant quantities of iodide leads to increased production of both T_4 and T_3 but in the proportions in which they are normally synthesized. The second circumstance is that of thyrotoxicosis accompanied by severe intercurrent illness.[131,132] Here, that component of the serum T_3 usually contributed by peripheral T_3 neogenesis is decreased or lacking so that the serum T_3 concentration, now sustained mainly or entirely by direct thyroid secretion, is normal or low although the serum T_4 concentration is high. Concomitantly, the serum rT_3 concentration is increased, often very markedly, owing to inhibition of its 5'-monodeiodination. With recovery from the intercurrent illness, serum rT_3 concentration declines and serum T_3 concentration increases into the thyrotoxic range.[310] T_4 toxicosis of this type is to be differentiated from the elevation of serum T_4 concentration, with a low serum T_3 concentration, that occasionally occurs in the course of intercurrent illness in patients who are intrinsically euthyroid.[133] A reduced serum TSH level will distinguish patients who are hyperthyroid from those who are not.

Thyrotoxicosis in Children and Adolescents

Thyrotoxicosis in childhood and adolescence is almost always the result of Graves disease. Thyrotoxicosis in this age group is worthy of special consideration because treatment is less satisfactory than in adults; hence, there is more uncertainty and greater disagreement concerning its management.[311] Several factors weigh against the use of radioiodine in children. First, the enhanced carcinogenic potential of radiation in the thyroid gland of the infant or child is evidenced by the correlation between childhood thyroid carcinoma and a history of x-ray therapy to the neck or chest in childhood.[312] Second, among all patients with thyrotoxicosis, those treated in childhood or adolescence are feared to be at greatest risk of transmitting genetic damage, although available data suggest that this may not be likely.[313] Finally, postradioiodine hypothyroidism is a particularly undesirable complication in young children because inadequate or interrupted therapy can have profound effects on growth and development and on scholastic performance. For these reasons, radioiodine is not commonly used in the treatment of childhood thyrotoxicosis.

The choice between surgical and antithyroid therapy is a difficult one. The data indicate a lower frequency of long-term remission after antithyroid therapy than is the case in adults, although some believe that thyrotoxicosis often undergoes remission after adolescence. On the other hand, most surgical series reveal a relatively high frequency of postoperative hypothyroidism, which is no more desirable after surgery than after radioiodine administration. Recurrences are also more frequent, presumably as a result of attempts to avoid hypothyroidism. Furthermore, the occasional operative death seems more tragic in a child than in an adult, and such complications as hypoparathyroidism and recurrent laryngeal nerve damage must be borne over a longer life span. On the basis of these considerations, a course of 1 to 2 y of antithyroid therapy seems most reasonable. In contrast to the recommendation for young adults, a second course of antithyroid therapy is regularly employed if recrudescence or relapse occurs after the first course. If sustained remission does not follow a second course of therapy and, particularly, if the patient has passed through adolescence during this period, radioiodine or surgery may be considered.

Hyperthyroidism and Thyrotoxicosis in Pregnancy

As discussed in the section on painless thyroiditis, transient thyrotoxicosis without true hyperthyroidism, often followed by transient hypothyroidism, may occur with some frequency (approximately 5%) during the postpartum period. When thyrotoxicosis is present during pregnancy, it is usually associated with hyperthyroidism, and this in turn is usually due to Graves disease. Difficulty in conception and fetal wastage are increased in women with Graves disease. Nonetheless, an occasional patient becomes pregnant despite antecedent untreated hyperthyroidism. More commonly, a woman under treatment for hyperthyroidism becomes pregnant, or hyperthyroidism develops after pregnancy is under way. Whatever the response, pregnancy complicates the diagnosis and treatment of hyperthyroidism in Graves disease and also influences its severity and near-term course.[314]

Pregnancy and hyperthyroidism have many features in common. Both are accompanied by thyroid enlargement, manifestations of a hyperdynamic circulation, and hypermetabolism. Amenorrhea may occur in thyrotoxicosis not associated with pregnancy. In the two conditions, the total serum T_4 and T_3 concentrations are increased. Laboratory tests useful in this differentiation are measurements of the proportion of free T_4 or T_3 in serum (THBR) and of the TSH level. The former tests demonstrate whether a decrease is present in the free fraction of thyroid hormone consequent to the pregnancy-associated increase in TBG. TSH is suppressed in hyperthyroidism during pregnancy just as it is in the nonpregnant individual. However, there is sometimes a modest suppression of TSH (between 0.1 and 0.5 mU/L) during the 8th to 14th week of normal pregnancy because of hCG stimulation of the thyroid during this interval.[108-111] A TSH level of 0.1 mU/L together with an elevated FT_4I and/or FT_3I strongly suggest coexistent hyperthyroidism.

An even greater problem is posed by the management of hyperthyroidism during pregnancy. Surgery during the last trimester and probably during the first trimester as well is not desirable because of the possible induction of premature labor. Although surgery may be successful during the middle trimester, it is best to avoid any major surgical procedure during pregnancy if possible. Because antithyroid drug treatment poses no greater risk to the mother or fetus than does surgery and possibly involves less risk, medical therapy is the method of choice. Furthermore, pregnancy appears to have an attenuating influence on the hyperthyroid state. This may be a reflection of the general immunosuppression associated with pregnancy, manifested here by a decrease in titers of associated antithyroid antibodies.[307] Although titers of TRAb also decrease during pregnancy, they may not correlate with the clinical disease under these conditions.[315-317] Whatever the cause, the consequence is that the dosage of antithyroid drug required to control the disease in the latter phases of pregnancy is generally less than that required in the same patient when not pregnant.

Certain aspects of placental permeability should be borne in mind when antithyroid drugs are used. First, propylthiouracil and methimazole readily cross the placenta,[318] are concentrated in the fetal thyroid, and, if present in sufficient quantity, can produce goitrous hypothyroidism in the fetus. The administration of as little as 100 to 300 mg propylthiouracil/d to the mother can cause a slight reduction in serum T_4 concentration and an elevated TSH concentration in neonates.[319, 320] There is no known long-term complication of this mild hypothyroidism, but the possibility must be kept in mind. Although maternal T_4 crosses the placenta (at least in infants with congenital hypothyroidism), this is not an efficient process.[7] For these reasons, the flux of antithyroid agent to the fetus should be limited by giving the mother the smallest dosage of antithyroid agent that maintains the state consistent with normal pregnancy. The serum free T_4 concentrations should be maintained in the upper normal range. However, the concentration of hormone per se is not as critical as the clinical status of the patient. A modest tachycardia is a physiological response to the increased metabolic demands of pregnancy, and pulse rates of 90 to 100 are well tolerated without evidence of myocardial decompensation during delivery. The daily maintenance dose of propylthiouracil should in most cases be 200 mg or less, although doses up to 450 mg may rarely be required. Propylthiouracil is preferred to methimazole because of the greater transplacental passage of the latter drug.[318] In a compliant patient, a dose requirement in excess of 400 mg propylthiouracil/d would be a reasonable threshold for considering subtotal thyroidectomy, preferably in the second trimester. All pregnant patients with significant Graves disease should be managed in close cooperation with obstetricians experienced with modern techniques for monitoring the fetus for intrauterine thyroid dysfunction. These techniques normally include fetal heart rate monitoring and ultrasound assessment of fetal growth rate. With advanced ultrasound it may even be possible to examine the fetus for the presence of goiter. Convincing evidence of fetal hyperthyroidism would be a strong indication to switch the mother to large doses of methimazole (~60 to 120 mg/d) to attempt in utero treatment of the fetus.[315] Levothyroxine supplementation of the mother would be required in these rare situations. The earlier fears of a congenital defect, *cutis aplasia*, in infants of mothers receiving methimazole or carbimazole have been allayed.[321] However, experience with the effects of high doses (>30 mg/d) is still limited.

Iodine should not be used as adjunctive or sole therapy for any length of time in the pregnant woman, because it readily crosses the placenta and is capable of inducing in the fetus a very large goiter that may cause airway obstruction and even death. Whether propranolol should be used in the pregnant woman with hyperthyroidism is a matter of debate. In the experience of some, it may lead to intrauterine growth retardation, as well as neonatal hypoglycemia or depression, but other studies suggest that it can be employed with safety.[277,278]

Assays for TRAb in the serum of pregnant women with Graves disease may be of value in selected cases.[315] Because transplacental passage of maternal immunoglobulins occurs, there may be a rough correlation between the maternal level of stimulatory immunoglobulin and the possibility of fetal thyrotoxicosis. However, fetal thyrotoxicosis occurs in only 1% of infants of mothers with Graves disease. Thus it is difficult to justify routine screening. Two general points can be made. One should be suspicious of the development of fetal hyperthyroidism in patients with high circulating titers of TRAb. Such patients would include more severely hyperthyroid pregnant patients or those with significant Graves eye disease or pretibial myxedema. Second, the prior ablative treatment of the mother with either surgery or radioiodine may not be accompanied by a reduction in TRAb. Thus, the fetus of a treated patient with Graves disease is still at risk of developing neonatal thyrotoxicosis and might require in utero treatment as described earlier.

Pregnancy and the postpartum state apparently influence the course of hyperthyroidism in Graves disease. Patients in clinical remission during pregnancy appear to be prone to postpartum relapse.[316,317] Prospective studies have revealed several most interesting relationships. In 41 pregnancies in 35 patients in remission, 78% were followed by development of thyrotoxicosis during the postpartum period. Patients with Graves disease and postpartum thyrotoxicosis could be classified into three categories. Some developed persistent recurrent hyperthyroidism with an elevated RAIU; this outcome was associated with an increase in the FT_4I early in pregnancy. Others developed a transient disorder associated with a normal or elevated RAIU, and still others, those with the highest titers of antimicrosomal antibodies, developed a transient thyrotoxicosis with a decreased RAIU, similar to that in the postpartum thyroiditis syndrome.

A special problem related to hyperthyroidism and pregnancy is presented by the patient who either is early in a remission after a course of antithyroid treatment or is being treated with antithyroid agents and wants to become pregnant in the near future. Management with antithyroid agents can be continued through pregnancy, or reinstituted should hyperthyroidism recur, but in such instances definitive therapy (radioiodine or surgery) should be considered so that the complexities of managing hyperthyroidism during pregnancy are forestalled. As with the therapy of Graves disease in general, such decisions must involve education of the patient so that the risks and benefits of the various alternatives are clearly appreciated.

Significant amounts of methimazole, but probably not propylthiouracil, appear in breast milk of women receiving this drug.[322] Women who take antithyroid drugs should be advised not to nurse their infants.

Thyrotoxic Crisis

Thyrotoxic crisis or thyroid storm is an extreme accentuation of thyrotoxicosis. It is an uncommon but serious complication, usually occurring in association with Graves disease but sometimes with toxic multinodular goiter. Before the availability of adequate means for achieving full preoperative control, crisis frequently followed subtotal thyroidectomy ("surgical crisis"); currently "medical crisis" is the more common. Thyrotoxic crisis is almost always of abrupt onset and occurs in patients in whom pre-existing thyrotoxicosis has been treated either incompletely or not at all. Crisis is almost always evoked by a precipitating factor, such as infection, trauma, surgical emergencies, or operations. Less common precipitating factors include radiation thyroiditis, diabetic ketoacidosis, toxemia of pregnancy, and parturition. The mechanism whereby such factors lead to an accentuation of thyrotoxicosis has not been ascertained. The serum thyroid hormone concentrations in crisis are not appreciably greater than those seen in uncomplicated thyrotoxicosis. The clinical picture is dominated by manifestations of severe hypermetabolism. Fever is almost invariably present and may be extreme; profuse sweating occurs. Marked tachycardia of sinus or ectopic origin may be accompanied by pulmonary edema or congestive heart failure. Early, tremulousness and restlessness are invariably present; delirium or frank psychosis occasionally occurs. Nausea, vomiting, and abdominal pain are common early manifestations. As the disorder progresses, apathy, stupor, and coma may supervene, and the blood pressure, which initially is well maintained, may fall to hypotensive levels. If the condition goes unrecognized, it is invariably fatal. This clinical picture in a patient with a history of pre-existing thyrotoxicosis, or with goiter or exophthalmos or both, is sufficient to establish the diagnosis, and treatment, which is urgently required, should not await laboratory confirmation.

There are no foolproof criteria by which severe thyrotoxicosis complicated by some other serious disease can be distinguished from thyrotoxic crisis induced by that disease. In any event, the differentiation between these alternatives is of no great significance, because treatment of the two is the same. Treatment of thyrotoxic crisis aims to correct both the severe thyrotoxicosis and the precipitating illness and to provide general supportive therapy. The therapy of crisis per se consists of efforts to inhibit both hormone synthesis and release and to antagonize the adrenergically mediated aspects of peripheral thyroid hormone action. Large doses of an antithyroid agent (300 to 400 mg of propylthiouracil every 4 h) are given by mouth or stomach tube. Propylthiouracil is used in preference to methimazole since it has the additional action of inhibiting the peripheral generation of T_3 from T_4.[59, 267] Immediate administration of propylthiouracil serves to initiate therapy for the postcrisis period and to prevent enrichment of glandular hormone stores by the iodine, whose administration is of more immediate importance. The latter agent, administered either as SSKI (five drops every 6 h) or as sodium iodide intravenously (0.250 g/6 h), is intended to retard acutely the release of hormone from the thyroid. In theory, it is desirable to administer propylthiouracil before iodine to inhibit completely the synthesis of additional thyroid hormones therefrom. Nonetheless, because iodine is the only agent that blocks release of preformed thyroid hormones from the thyroid gland, its administration should not be delayed or omitted in the severely toxic patient because propylthiouracil (or methimazole) is not immediately available. The latter agents may be given by intragastric infusion if necessary. Large doses of dexamethasone (2 mg orally every 6 h) are also given because, in addition to providing glucocorticoid support, dexamethasone inhibits both the release of hormone from the thyroid and the peripheral generation of T_3 from T_4, synergizing with iodide and propylthiouracil, respectively, in these actions. Indeed, the combined use of propylthiouracil, iodide, and dexamethasone restores serum T_3 concentration to within the normal range in 24 to 48 h,[276] and substitution of sodium ipodate or iopanoate for iodide may be even more effective.[275] In the absence of significant cardiac insufficiency, a beta-adrenergic blocking agent should be given to ameliorate some of the physiological manifestations of thyrotoxicosis. Most experience has been with propranolol given at a dose of 40 to 80 mg orally every 6 h or 2 mg intravenously, but a short-acting beta-adrenergic blocker such as labetalol may be safer than propranolol in this situation. Patients with severe thyrotoxicosis may develop high-output congestive heart failure, and a beta-adrenergic antagonist may further reduce cardiac output. The patient suspected of having thyroid storm should be monitored in a medical intensive care unit during the initial phases of therapy. Supportive measures include correction of the inevitable dehydration and possible hypernatremia. Glucose should be administered together with large amounts of vitamins of the B complex. A vigorous attack on the hyperpyrexia should be made. In milder cases, acetaminophen may suffice, but more often wet packs, fans, or ice packs may be required. Salicylates should be avoided because they compete with T_3 and T_4 for binding to TBG and TBPA and therefore increase the free hormone concentrations.[102] In addition, in large doses salicylates increase the metabolic rate. If heart failure or pulmonary congestion is present, digitalis and diuretics are indicated. Digitalis derivatives should be used in patients with atrial fibrillation and a rapid ventricular response to block atrioventricular node conduction.

Regimens similar to the foregoing have reduced the mortality rate in this disorder to approximately 20%, a figure that is still disturbingly high. When treatment is successful, improvement is usually manifest within 1 or 2 d and recovery occurs within a week. At this time, iodide and dexamethasone are gradually withdrawn and plans for long-term management are made.

THYROID HORMONE DEFICIENCY

Many structural or functional abnormalities can lead to deficient production of thyroid hormones. The clinical state resulting therefrom is termed hypothyroidism. A convenient classification of the causes of hypothyroidism is presented in Table 8–17 and divides the causes into three principal categories: (1) loss or atrophy of thyroid tissue (thyroprivic hypothyroidism), (2) insufficient stimulation of an intrinsically normal gland as a result of hypothalamic or pituitary disease (trophoprivic hypothyroidism), and (3) compensatory goitrogenesis as a result of defective hormone biosynthesis (goitrous hypothyroidism). Of the three categories, thyroprivic and goitrous hypothyroidism together account for approximately 95% of cases, only 5% or less being trophoprivic in origin.

In neonatal screening programs in many areas of the world hypothyroidism is present in one of every 4000 to 5000 newborns. Although screening programs are moderately costly (approximately $5000 per patient with hypothyroidism), the benefit/cost ratio of early diagnosis and treatment, in terms of prevention of later institutional care and of suffering, is enormous.[323]

Peripheral Manifestations of Thyroid Hormone Deficiency

The clinical state of hypothyroidism is manifest in all organ systems. These manifestations are to a large extent independent of the underlying disorder in the thyroid gland and are closely related to the degree of hormone deficiency.

Skin and Appendages

In the dermis as well as other tissues, an accumulation of hyaluronic acid alters the composition of the ground substance. This material binds water, producing the mucinous edema that is responsible for the thickened features and puffy appearance (termed *myxedema*) of the patient with full-

TABLE 8–17. Classification of Causes of Hypothyroidism

Thyroprivic
Postablative hypothyroidism
Primary idiopathic hypothyroidism
Sporadic athyreotic cretinism (thyroid aplasia or dysplasia)
Trophoprivic
Sheehan syndrome
Infiltrative disorders of pituitary or hypothalamus
Goitrous
Hashimoto thyroiditis
Endemic iodine deficiency
Antithyroid agents (para-aminosalicylic acid, phenylbutazone, resorcinol, lithium; cruciferous plants; cassava)
Iodide goiter and hypothyroidism
Heritable defects in hormone biosynthesis and action
Peripheral resistance to thyroid hormone (may be nongoitrous)

blown hypothyroidism. Myxedema is characteristically boggy and nonpitting and is most apparent around the eyes, on the dorsa of the hands and feet, and in the supraclavicular fossae. It causes enlargement of the tongue and thickening of the pharyngeal and laryngeal mucous membranes. A histologically similar deposit may occur in patients with Graves disease, usually over the pretibial area (infiltrative dermopathy or pretibial myxedema). In addition to having a puffy appearance, the skin is pale and cool as a result of cutaneous vasoconstriction. Anemia commonly contributes to the pallor; hypercarotenemia gives the skin a yellow tint. The secretions of the sweat glands and sebaceous glands are reduced, leading to dryness and coarseness of the skin, which in extreme cases may resemble ichthyosis.

Wounds of the skin tend to heal slowly. A bruising tendency results from an increase in capillary fragility.

Head and body hair is dry and brittle, lacks luster, and tends to fall out. Loss of hair from the temporal aspects of the eyebrows is common. Growth of hair is retarded so that haircuts and shaves are required less often. The nails are brittle and grow slowly.

In pituitary hypothyroidism, the changes in the skin and its appendages are less striking than in thyroprivic hypothyroidism. Although the skin is pale and cool, it tends to be thinner and finely wrinkled, and myxedematous infiltration of the tissues is less prominent. Depigmentation of areas that are normally pigmented, such as the areolae, frequently occurs in pituitary but not thyroprivic hypothyroidism.

Histopathological examination of the skin reveals hyperkeratosis with plugging of hair follicles and sweat glands. The dermis is edematous, and the connective tissue fibers are separated by an increase in the normal amount of metachromatically staining, PAS-positive mucinous material. This material consists of protein complexed with two mucopolysaccharides, hyaluronic acid and chondroitin sulfate B, especially the former. It is mobilized early during treatment with thyroid hormone, leading to an increase in urinary excretion of nitrogen and hexosamines.

Cardiovascular System

The cardiac output at rest is decreased because of a reduction in both stroke volume and heart rate, reflecting loss of the inotropic and chronotropic effects of thyroid hormones. Peripheral vascular resistance at rest is increased, and blood volume is reduced. These hemodynamic alterations result in narrowing of pulse pressure, prolongation of circulation time, and decrease in blood flow to the tissues. The decrease in cutaneous circulation is responsible for the coolness and pallor of the skin and the sensitivity to cold. In most tissues, the decrease in blood flow is proportional to the decrease in oxygen consumption, so that the mixed arteriovenous oxygen difference remains essentially normal. The hemodynamic alterations at rest resemble those of congestive heart failure, but cardiac output increases normally and peripheral vascular resistance decreases normally in response to exercise.

In thyroprivic hypothyroidism, the heart is enlarged (Fig. 8–42) and the heart sounds are diminished in intensity. These findings are due largely to effusion into the pericardial sac of fluid rich in protein and mucopolysaccharides, but dilation of a "flabby" myocardium may also be a factor. Pericardial effusion is rarely of a degree sufficient to cause tamponade. In pituitary hypothyroidism, the heart is frequently small.

Angina pectoris is uncommon in hypothyroidism and occasionally disappears when the eumetabolic state is restored. More commonly, angina either appears or is worsened during treatment of the hypothyroid state with thyroid hormone. There has been much discussion as to whether the hypercholesterolemia that accompanies primary hypothyroidism accelerates the development of coronary atherosclerosis. Necropsy data suggest that the hypercholesterolemia of hypothyroidism predisposes to coronary atherosclerosis only in the presence of hypertension; in normotensive hypothyroid patients, the degree of coronary atherosclerosis appears to be no greater than that in age- and sex-matched normotensive control subjects.[324]

Electrocardiographic (ECG) changes include sinus bradycardia, prolongation of the PR interval, low amplitude of the P wave and QRS complex, alterations of the ST segment, and flattened or inverted T waves. Pericardial effusion is probably responsible in part for ECG changes. Rarely, complete heart block may be present, but this disappears when hypothyroidism is treated.[325] Systolic time intervals are altered; the pre-ejection period is prolonged, and the ratio of pre-ejection period to left ventricular ejec-

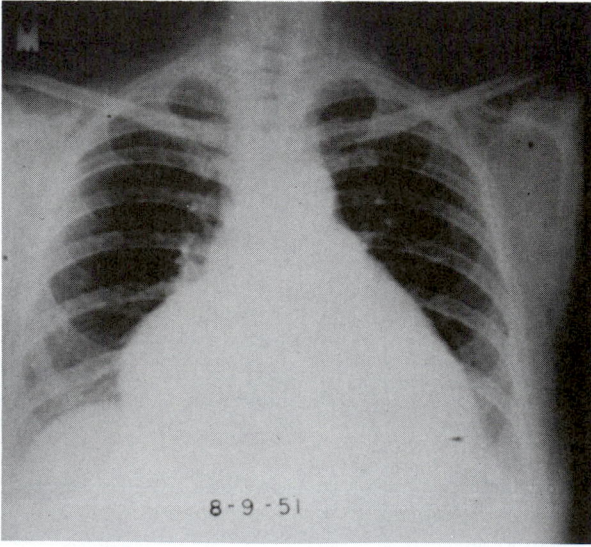
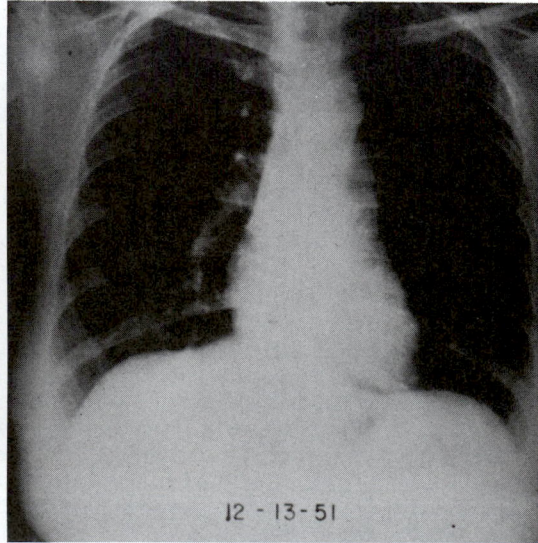

Figure 8–42. Chest roentgenograms in a patient with myxedema heart disease. The patient had signs of severe congestive heart failure and was treated with thyroid hormone alone. Within 4 mo, the heart had returned to normal size and there was no evidence of underlying heart disease.

tion time is increased. Echocardiographic studies have revealed a high frequency of asymmetrical septal hypertrophy and apparent obstruction of the left ventricular outflow tract, suggesting idiopathic hypertrophic subaortic stenosis. These findings disappear when myxedema is treated, and their hemodynamic significance is uncertain.[326]

The concentrations in serum of such enzymes as creatine kinase, glutamic-oxalacetic transaminase, and lactate dehydrogenase may be increased. Furthermore, the isoenzyme patterns sometimes suggest that the source of the increased creatine kinase and lactate dehydrogenase is cardiac muscle.

The large heart, together with the hemodynamic and ECG alterations and the serum enzyme changes, has been termed *myxedema heart*. There has been considerable discussion as to whether myxedema heart ever is the sole cause of heart failure. If it is, this must be quite rare, because in hypothyroidism the usual hemodynamic response to exercise is normal. Furthermore, the response of pulse pressure to the acute reduction in filling pressure induced by the Valsalva maneuver differs from that in heart failure. In the patient with hypothyroidism, as in the normal individual, the Valsalva maneuver leads to a decrease in pulse pressure, whereas in the patient with heart failure the pulse pressure does not decrease but displays a so-called square-wave response. In the absence of coexisting organic heart disease, treatment with thyroid hormone corrects the hemodynamic, ECG, and serum enzyme alterations of myxedema heart and restores heart size to normal (see Fig. 8–42).

On pathological examination, the pericardial sac contains fluid rich in protein and mucopolysaccharides. The heart is dilated and the myocardium is pale and flabby. Coronary atherosclerosis is commonly present. Histopathological examination of the myocardium reveals interstitial edema and swelling of the muscle fibers, with loss of striations.

Respiratory System

Pleural effusions are common. These usually are evident only on radiological examination but rarely may be sufficient to cause dyspnea. Lung volumes are usually normal, but maximal breathing capacity and diffusing capacity are reduced. In severe hypothyroidism, myxedematous involvement of respiratory muscles as well as depression of both the hypoxic and hypercapnic ventilatory drive may lead to alveolar hypoventilation and carbon dioxide retention, which in turn may contribute to the development of myxedema coma.[327] Obstructive sleep apnea, reversible with restoration of a euthyroid state, occurs with increased frequency.[328]

Alimentary System

Although most patients show a modest gain in weight, the appetite is characteristically reduced. Gross obesity is never a feature of hypothyroidism per se. Such weight gain as occurs is due largely to retention of fluid by the hydrophilic mucopolysaccharide deposits in the tissues. Peristaltic activity is decreased and, together with the decreased food intake, is responsible for the frequent complaint of constipation. The latter may be extreme, leading to fecal impaction (myxedema megacolon). Gaseous distention of the abdomen may occur (myxedema ileus) and, if accompanied by colicky pain and vomiting, may mimic mechanical ileus. Elevations in the serum concentration of carcinoembryonic antigen, which may occur on the basis of hypothyroidism alone,[329] add to the impression that an organic obstructing lesion is present. Clinically discernible ascites in the absence of other cause is unusual in hypothyroidism, but it may occur, usually in association with pleural and pericardial effusions. Like effusions into the other serous cavities, the ascitic fluid is rich in protein and mucopolysaccharides.

Achlorhydria after maximal histamine stimulation is present in about one half of patients with primary hypothyroidism. Even in the absence of overt anemia, many of these patients absorb vitamin B_{12} poorly and have low concentrations of vitamin B_{12} in serum. The impaired absorption of vitamin B_{12} is corrected by ingesting intrinsic factor. Circulating antibodies against gastric parietal cells have been found in about one third of patients with primary hypothyroidism and probably reflect the presence of an atrophic gastric mucosa. Overt pernicious anemia is reported in about 12% of patients with primary hypothyroidism. The coexistence of pernicious anemia and other presumed autoimmune diseases with primary hypothyroidism supports the view that autoimmunity plays a primary role in the pathogenesis of primary hypothyroidism.

The effects of hypothyroidism on intestinal absorption are complex. Although the rates of absorption of many substances are decreased, the total amount eventually absorbed may be normal or even increased because the decreased motility of the bowel may allow more time for absorption to take place. Overt malabsorption occasionally occurs.

Liver function tests are usually normal but mild elevations of transaminases occur, probably because of impaired clearance. Cholecystography often reveals a distended gallbladder that contracts sluggishly, but whether these changes predipose to the development of gallstones is unknown. Radiological examination of the abdomen may reveal a greatly distended colon (myxedema megacolon).

Histopathological examination frequently reveals atrophy of the gastric and intestinal mucosa and myxedematous infiltration of the bowel wall. The colon may be greatly distended. The volume of fluid in the peritoneal cavity is usually increased. The liver and pancreas are normal.

Nervous System

Thyroid hormone is essential for the development of the central nervous system. Deficiency in fetal life or at birth results in retention of the infantile characteristics of the brain, hypoplasia of cortical neurons with poor development of cellular processes, retarded myelination, and reduced vascularity.[330] If the deficiency is not corrected in early postnatal life, irreversible damage results. Deficiency of thyroid hormone beginning in adult life causes manifestations of lesser severity that usually respond to treatment with thyroid hormone. The cerebral circulation shares in the hemodynamic alterations of hypothyroidism in that cerebral blood flow is reduced. Cerebral oxygen consumption, however, may be normal; this is in accord with the observation that the oxygen consumption in vitro of isolated brain tissue, unlike that of most other tissues, is not stimulated by administration of thyroid hormones. In severe cases the decrease in cerebral blood flow may lead to cerebral hypoxia.

One of the characteristic features is a general slowing of all intellectual functions, including speech. There is loss of initiative. Slow-wittedness and memory defects are common. Lethargy and somnolence are prominent. Dementia may occur and in the elderly patient may be mistaken for senile dementia. Psychiatric reactions are not uncommon and are usually of the paranoid or depressive type, but agitated states have also been described (myxedema madness). Headache occurs quite frequently. Cerebral hypoxia resulting from the circulatory alterations may predispose to confusional attacks and syncope. Syncope may be prolonged, leading to stupor or coma. Other factors predisposing to coma in hypothyroidism include exposure to severe cold, infection, trauma, hypoventilation with carbon dioxide retention, and depressant drugs. Epileptic seizures have been reported and are especially liable to occur in myxedema coma. Night blindness is due to deficient synthesis of the pigment required for dark adaptation. Hearing loss of the perceptive type is frequent. Perceptive deafness may also occur in association with a defect in the organic binding of thyroidal iodide (Pendred syndrome) or with endemic creatinism, but in these instances it is not due to hypothyroidism per se. Thick, slurred speech and hoarseness are common and are due to myxedematous infiltration of the tongue and larynx, respectively. Movements are slow and clumsy, and pronounced ataxia of cerebellar type may occur. Numbness and tingling of the extremities are frequent; in the fingers, these symptoms are often due to compression by mucinous deposits in and around the median nerve in the carpal tunnel (carpal tunnel syndrome). The tendon jerks are slow, especially during the relaxation phase, producing the characteristic "hung-up reflexes"; this phenomenon appears to result from a decrease in the rate of muscle contraction and relaxation, rather than from a delay in nerve conduction. The presence of extensor plantar responses or diminished vibration sense should alert the physician to the possibility of coexisting pernicious anemia with combined system disease.

Electroencephalographic changes include slow alpha wave activity and general loss of amplitude. The concentration of protein in cerebrospinal fluid is often increased, but pressure is normal.

On histopathological examination, the nervous system is edematous, with mucinous deposits in and around nerve fibers. In patients with cerebellar ataxia, neural myxedematous bodies, comprising deposition of glycogen and mucinous material, are found in the cerebellum. There may be foci of degeneration and an increase in glial tissue. The cerebral vessels commonly show atherosclerosis.[331]

Muscular System

Stiffness and aching of muscles are common complaints. Delayed muscle contraction and relaxation are responsible for the slowness of movement and delayed tendon jerks. These changes are aggravated by cold. Muscle strength is usually normal. Muscle mass may be slightly increased and the muscles tend to be firmer than normal. Rarely, a great increase in muscle mass accompanied by slowness of muscular activity may be the predominant manifestation (the Kocher-Debré-Sémélaigne or Hoffmann syndrome). Myoclonus may be present. The electromyogram may be normal or may reveal disordered discharge, hyperirritability, and polyphasic action potentials.

Urinary excretion of creatine is reduced and creatine tolerance is increased, but these changes are generally not of a magnitude sufficient to afford a clear separation from normal values. The concentrations in serum of some enzymes of muscular origin, such as creatine kinase and glutamic-oxalacetic transaminase, are increased.

On histopathological examination, the muscles appear pale and swollen. The muscle fibers may show swelling, loss of normal striations, and separation by mucinous deposits. Type I muscle fibers tend to predominate.[332]

Skeletal System: Calcium and Phosphorus Metabolism

Thyroid hormone is essential for normal growth and maturation of the skeleton. The effect on growth appears to be due to a stimulation of protein synthesis as well as to a potentiation of the action of growth hormone. Before puberty, thyroid hormone is the major prerequisite for normal maturation of bone. Deficiency of thyroid hormone beginning in early life leads to both a delay in the development of and an abnormal, stippled appearance of the epiphyseal centers of ossification (epiphyseal dysgenesis). Linear growth is severely impaired, leading to dwarfism in which the limbs are disproportionately short in relation to the trunk.[226-228] Bone age is always retarded in relation to chronological age.

Data concerning the effects of hypothyroidism on calcium and phosphorus metabolism are scant. In general, urinary excretion of calcium is decreased, whereas fecal excretion of calcium and urinary and fecal excretion of phosphorus are variable. Calcium balance is also variable, and the changes reported are slight. The exchangeable pool of calcium and its rate of turnover are consistently reduced. These changes reflect decreases in the rates of bone formation and resorption. Because levels of parathyroid hormone are often increased, some degree of resistance to its action may be present; levels of 1,25-dihydroxycholecalciferol are also increased.[333] Aching and stiffness of the joints are not uncommon complaints, and joint effusions are occasionally seen.

Concentrations of calcium and phosphorus in serum are usually normal, but the alkaline phosphatase level is characteristically low in infantile and juvenile hypothyroidism. Bone density may be increased on radiological examination. The radiological appearances of the skeleton in cretinism and juvenile hypothyroidism are discussed subsequently.

Renal Function: Water and Electrolyte Metabolism

As part of the hemodynamic alterations that accompany hypothyroidism, renal blood flow and glomerular filtration rate are decreased and tubular reabsorptive and secretory maxima are reduced. Blood urea nitrogen and serum creatinine levels, however, are normal. Urine flow is reduced, and the excretion of a water load may be delayed, resulting in a reversal of the normal diurnal pattern of urine excretion. The delay in water excretion appears to be due to decreased volume delivery to the distal diluting segment of the nephron as a result of the diminished renal perfusion as well as to disordered regulation of arginine vasopressin secretion.[334] It is reversed by treatment with thyroid hormone. The ability to concentrate urine may be slightly impaired. Proteinuria of mild degree may occur.

The impaired renal excretion of water along with retention of water by the hydrophilic deposits in the tissues results in an increase in total body water, even though plasma volume is reduced. This increase accounts for the hyponatremia commonly noted, because the level of exchangeable Na^+ is increased in hypothyroidsm. Exchangeable K^+ concentration is usually normal in relation to lean body mass. Serum Mg^{2+} concentration may be increased, but exchangeable Mg^{2+} concentration and urinary Mg^{2+} excretion are decreased.

Hematopoietic System

Several hematological abnormalities may occur. In response to the diminished oxygen requirements and decreased production of erythropoietin, the red blood cell mass is decreased; this is evident in the mild normocytic, normochromic anemia that often occurs. Less commonly, the anemia is macrocytic, and usually this results from deficiency of vitamin B_{12}. Reference has already been made to the high incidence of pernicious anemia (and of achlorhydria and vitamin B_{12} deficiency without overt anemia) in patients with primary hypothyroidism. The defective absorption of vitamin B_{12} in primary hypothyroidism cannot be ascribed to lack of thyroid hormone per se because it is not found to the same extent in the hypothyroid state that follows radioiodine treatment of thyrotoxicosis and is not corrected by treatment with thyroid hormone. In fact, defective absorption of vitamin B_{12} may develop or progress during treatment of hypothyroidism. Because this abnormality appears to be corrected by intrinsic factor, the macrocytic anemia sometimes seen in patients with primary hypothyroidism is more likely to be the result of deficiency of vitamin B_{12} than of thyroid hormone per se. Nevertheless, thyroid hormone may be required for an optimal hematological response to vitamin B_{12}. Conversely, in patients with pernicious anemia, disordered thyroid function is common. Overt and subclinical hypothyroidism were present in 11.7 and 14.7% of patients, respectively.[335] (Overt hyperthyroidism was present in 8.6% and TSH values were low in 6.3%.) Folate deficiency resulting from malabsorption or dietary inadequacy may also be responsible for a macrocytic anemia. Both the frequent menorrhagia and the defective absorption of iron resulting from achlorhydria may lead to a microcytic, hypochromic anemia.

The total and differential white blood cell count is usually normal, and platelets are adequate in hypothyroidism although platelet adhesiveness is frequently depressed. An aspirate of bone marrow often has a gelatinous consistency, and the bone marrow may be hypocellular. If pernicious anemia or significant folate deficiency is present, the characteristic changes in peripheral blood and bone marrow will be found. The intrinsic clotting mechanism may be defective because of decreased concentrations in plasma of factors VIII and IX, and this, together with an increase in capillary fragility and the decrease in platelet adhesiveness, may account for the bleeding tendency that sometimes occurs.[336]

Pituitary and Adrenocortical Function

In long-standing hypothyroidism of thyroid origin, the pituitary gland is frequently enlarged, and this can be detected radiologically as an increase in volume of the pituitary fossa.[337, 338] Rarely, such hypertrophy and hyperplasia of the thyrotropes may be of such a degree that the function of other pituitary cells is compromised, resulting in pituitary insufficiency. Many patients with hypothyroidism display an increase in serum prolactin concentration that correlates with the increase in serum TSH concentration, and some patients develop galactorrhea.[339] Treatment with thyroid hormone results in a decrease in serum prolactin, as well as TSH, concentration and in disappearance of galactorrhea, if present. The mechanism underlying the hyperprolactinemia in hypothyroidism is uncertain, but it may be an enhanced sensitivity of the lactotropes to TRH. In thyroprivic hypothyroidism, the responsiveness of growth hormone to provocative stimuli, such as insulin-induced hypoglycemia, is usually subnormal.

The rate of turnover of cortisol is decreased. (See also Chapter 9.) As a result of the decreased rate of turnover of cortisol, the 24-h urinary excretion of 17-OHCS and 17-KS is decreased, but the plasma cortisol concentration is usually normal. The response of urinary 17-OHCS to exogenous ACTH and metyrapone are usually normal in thyroprivic hypothyroidism but may be decreased. The response of plasma cortisol to insulin-induced hypoglycemia may be impaired in some patients. In severe, long-standing, thyroprivic hypothyroidism, secondary depression of pituitary and adrenal function may occur, and adrenal insufficiency may

be precipitated by stress or by rapid replacement therapy with thyroid hormone.

The rate of turnover of aldosterone is decreased, but the plasma concentration is normal. Plasma renin activity is decreased and sensitivity to angiotensin II is increased.

On histopathological examination, the pituitary in thyroprivic hypothyroidism shows an increase in the number of actively secreting thyrotropes. The adrenals are usually normal but occasionally show cortical atrophy.[239]

Reproductive Function

In both sexes, thyroid hormone influences sexual development and reproductive function. Thyroprivic hypothyroidism from infancy, if untreated, leads to sexual immaturity, and hypothyroidism beginning before puberty causes a delay in onset of puberty followed by anovulatory cycles. Paradoxically, thyroprivic hypothyroidism has also been reported in association with precocious sexual development and galactorrhea.

In adult women, hypothyroidism is commonly associated with diminished libido and failure of ovulation. Secretion of progesterone fails and endometrial proliferation persists, resulting in excessive and irregular menstrual bleeding. These changes may be due to deficient secretion of LH. In severe, long-standing, thyroprivic hypothyroidism, secondary depression of pituitary function may occur, leading to ovarian atrophy and amenorrhea. Fertility is reduced, and if conception does take place, abortion may result, although many pregnancies are successful.[340] In men, hypothyroidism may be accompanied by diminished libido, impotence, and oligospermia.

Values for plasma gonadotropins are usually in the normal range in thyroprivic hypothyroidism. In postmenopausal women with this disorder, these values are usually somewhat lower than in euthyroid women of the same age, but they are nevertheless increased. This provides a valuable means of differentiating thyroprivic from pituitary hypothyroidism.

The metabolism of both androgens and estrogens is altered in hypothyroidism. Secretion of androgens is decreased, and the metabolic transformation of testosterone is shifted toward etiocholanolone rather than androsterone. With respect to estradiol and estrone, hypothyroidism favors metabolism of these steroids via 16α-hydroxylation over that via 2-oxygenation, with the result that formation of estriol is increased at the expense of 2-hydroxyestrone and its derivative, 2-methoxyestrone. The binding activity of TeBG in plasma is decreased, with the result that the plasma concentrations of both testosterone and estradiol are decreased but their unbound fractions are increased. The alterations in steroid metabolism disappear when the euthyroid state is restored.[239]

Histopathological examination of the ovaries and testes may reveal degenerative changes, especially if hypothyroidism began before puberty. In long-standing postpubertal hypothyroidism, the ovaries may be atrophied.

Catecholamines and Serotonin

The plasma cyclic AMP response to epinephrine is depressed, lending support to the view that a state of decreased adrenergic activity accompanies thyroid hormone deficiency. In addition, the responses of cyclic AMP to glucagon and parathyroid hormone are depressed, suggesting a general modulating influence of thyroid hormones on cyclic AMP–mediated effects. The mechanism underlying the decreased adrenergic responsiveness is uncertain. The secretion rate and plasma concentration of epinephrine are normal, but the corresponding functions in the case of norepinephrine are increased.[240, 241] Plasma serotonin concentration, urinary 5-hydroxyindoleacetic acid excretion, and platelet monoamine oxidase activity are normal.

Energy Metabolism: Protein, Carbohydrate, and Lipid Metabolism

The effects of thyroid hormone on intermediary metabolism are clinically evident in the patient with hypothyroidism.

The decrease in energy metabolism and heat production is reflected in the low BMR, decreased appetite, cold intolerance, and slightly low basal body temperature.

Both the synthesis and degradation of protein are decreased, the latter especially so, with the result that nitrogen balance is usually slightly positive. The decrease in protein synthesis is reflected in retardation of both skeletal and soft tissue growth. In addition, thyroid hormone deficiency is accompanied by both a decrease in secretion and a lessened effectiveness of growth hormone, perhaps related to impaired formation of insulin-like growth factor I (IGF I, also called somatomedin-C).[227–229]

Permeability of capillaries to protein is increased, accounting for the high concentration of protein in effusions and perhaps in cerebrospinal fluid. In addition, the total exchangeable albumin pool is increased, as a result of the relatively greater decrease in albumin degradation than in albumin synthesis. A greater than normal proportion and quantity of exchangeable albumin is localized in the extravascular space. The total concentration of serum proteins may be increased.

The oral glucose tolerance curve is characteristically flat and the insulin response is delayed. These alterations may be due to a decreased rate of absorption of glucose from the gut. The disappearance from plasma of an intravenous load of glucose is delayed, reflecting the slow rate of uptake of glucose by the tissues. Degradation of insulin is slower than normal, with the result that there may be an increased sensitivity to exogenous insulin. This, as well as the decrease in appetite, presumably accounts for the diminished insulin requirement that occurs when hypothyroidism supervenes in a patient with pre-existing diabetes mellitus.

Both the synthesis and degradation of lipid are depressed, the latter especially so, the net effect being one of lipid accumulation. The decrease in lipid degradation may reflect a decrease in postheparin lipolytic activity, as well as a decreased delivery of lipid to degradative sites. Although an increase in serum cholesterol is the most commonly recognized abnormality of lipid metabolism in thyroprivic (but not pituitary) hypothyroidism, serum phospholipid phosphorus and serum triglycerides are also increased, and the concentration of LDL in serum is increased. Concentrations of high-density lipoprotein cholesterol are decreased.[341] Plasma free fatty acid levels are decreased and the mobilization of free fatty acids in response to fasting, catecholamines, and growth hormone is impaired.

Composite Clinical Picture of Hypothyroidism

Adult Hypothyroidism

The onset of hypothyroidism is usually so insidious that the classic clinical manifestations may take months or years to appear and frequently go unnoticed by persons well acquainted with the patient. The gradual development of the hypothyroid state is due to a slow progression both of

TABLE 8–18. Symptoms of Myxedema
(77 Cases: 64 Women, 13 Men)

Symptom	% of Cases	Symptom	% of Cases
Weakness	99	Constipation	61
Dry skin	97	Gain in weight	59
Coarse skin	97	Loss of hair	57
Lethargy	91	Pallor of lips	57
Slow speech	91	Dyspnea	55
Edema of eyelids	90	Peripheral edema	55
Sensation of cold	89	Hoarseness or aphonia	52
Decreased sweating	89	Anorexia	45
Cold skin	83	Nervousness	35
Thick tongue	82	Menorrhagia	32
Edema of face	79	Palpitation	31
Coarseness of hair	76	Deafness	30
Pallor of skin	67	Precordial pain	25
Memory impairment	66		

Data from Means JH. The Thyroid and Its Diseases. 2nd ed. Philadelphia: J. B. Lippincott, 1948: 233.

thyroid hypofunction and of the clinical manifestations after thyroid failure is complete. This course is in contrast to the more rapid development of the hypothyroid state that occurs when replacement therapy is discontinued in a patient with treated thyroprivic hypothyroidism or when the thyroid gland of a normal subject is surgically removed. In these circumstances the overall metabolic effect of thyroid hormone withdrawal can be judged from measurements of BMR and compared with the emergence of the classic clinical picture. The BMR decreases to about −20% and symptoms of mild hypothyroidism appear within 3 wk. After 6 wk, the BMR has decreased to −30% and manifestations of frank hypothyroidism are present; by 3 mo, full-blown myxedema is usually evident.

The early symptoms of hypothyroidism are variable and nonspecific (Table 8–18). Tiredness and lethargy are common and lead to difficulty in performing a full day's work. Constipation may develop or, if present, become worse. Sensitivity to cold may be an early manifestation; its presence is often suggested by the use of more blankets on the bed or a preference for warm weather. Women may complain of menstrual disturbance, especially menorrhagia, or difficulty in conceiving because of anovulatory cycles. Loss of libido occasionally occurs in both men and women. At this stage of the disease the BMR is moderately decreased. With progression of the disease the BMR falls to its minimal value, usually between −35 and −45%, but the clinical picture continues to evolve slowly. Drowsiness and slowing of intellectual and motor activity appear. The patient becomes apathetic and listless and loses interest in work and environment. Women frequently complain of hair loss, brittle nails, and dry skin (Fig. 8–43). Despite a reduction in appetite, modest weight gain often occurs. The voice becomes husky, which may be attributed to laryngitis. Periorbital puffiness may be present (Fig. 8–44). Mucus collects in the eyes, and the lids are often stuck together when the patient awakens in the morning. Stiffness and aching of muscles are sometimes prominent and may be attributed to "rheumatism." Numbness and tingling of the fingers may occur. Progressive deafness may lead the patient to seek medical advice. Eventually, the picture of full-blown myxedema results, with thickened features, enlarged tongue, hoarseness, nonpitting edema, and extreme mental and physical lethargy. Mild hypothermia may call the physician's attention to the diagnosis. Many structural and functional manifestations become evident, but occasionally those arising in a particular organ predominate. The patient, if untreated, may remain in this state for years, finally developing myxedema coma or succumbing to an intercurrent infection or a vascular occlusion.

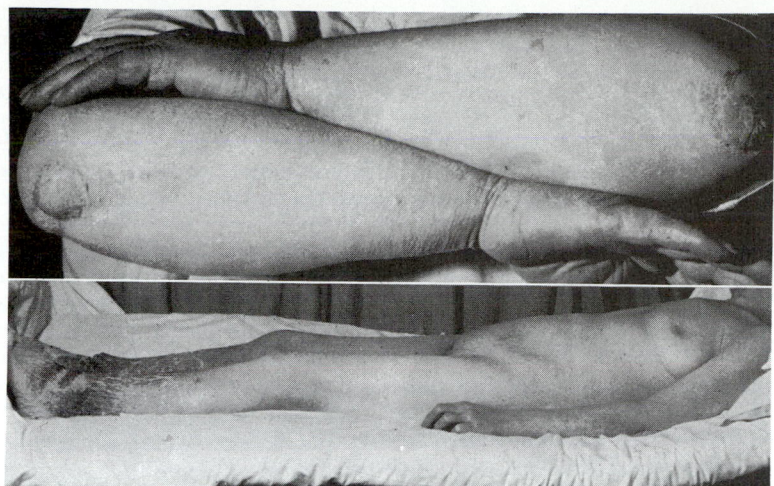

Figure 8–43. Dry, scaly skin with marked hyperkeratosis over elbows and legs.

The unusual syndrome of acute hypothyroidism in the previously hyperthyroid patient has been discussed earlier, in the section on radioiodine treatment of Graves disease.

Infantile Hypothyroidism and Cretinism

Even severe hypothyroidism is seldom apparent at birth.[342] The age at which symptoms appear depends on the degree of impairment of thyroid function. Severe hypothyroidism in infancy is termed cretinism. As the age of onset increases, the clinical picture of cretinism merges imperceptibly with that of juvenile hypothyroidism. Retardation of mental development and growth is the hallmark of cretinism. Because these changes become manifest only in later infancy and are by then largely irreversible, early recognition is crucial and can be achieved by routinely measuring serum T_4 or TSH concentrations in the neonate. During the first few months of life, symptoms of hypothyroidism include feeding problems, failure to thrive, constipation, a hoarse cry, and somnolence. In succeeding months, especially in severe cases, protuberance of the abdomen, dry skin, poor growth of hair and nails, and delayed eruption of the deciduous teeth become evident. Retardation of mental and physical development is manifested by delay in reaching the normal milestones of development, such as holding up the head, sitting, walking, and talking.

Linear growth is severely impaired, resulting in dwarfism, with the limbs disproportionately short in relation to the trunk. Closure of the fontanelles is delayed, leading to a head that is large in relation to the body. The naso-orbital configuration of the infant is retained. Maldevelopment of the femoral epiphyses results in a waddling gait. The teeth are malformed and readily become carious. The appearance is characteristic, with broad flat nose, widely set eyes, periorbital puffiness, large protruding tongue, sparse hair, rough skin, short neck, and protuberant abdomen with an umbilical hernia. Mental deficiency is usually severe.

Radiological examination of the skeleton is diagnostic. The skull shows a poorly developed base, delayed closure of the fontanelles, widely set orbits, and a short flat nasal bone. The pituitary fossa may be enlarged. Shedding of deciduous teeth and eruption of permanent teeth are delayed. A radiological feature that is virtually pathognomonic of hypothyroidism in infancy and childhood is epiphyseal dysgenesis. This abnormality may affect any center of endochondral ossification, depending on the age of onset of the hypothyroid state, but is usually best seen in larger centers, such as the femoral and humeral heads and the navicular bone of the foot. The center of ossification appears late, with the result that bone age is retarded in relation to chronological age. When the center eventually appears, instead of a single center, multiple small centers are scattered through a misshapen epiphysis. These small centers of ossification eventually coalesce, forming a single center that has an irregular outline and a stippled appearance (stippled epiphysis). Epiphyseal dysgenesis is evident only in centers that would

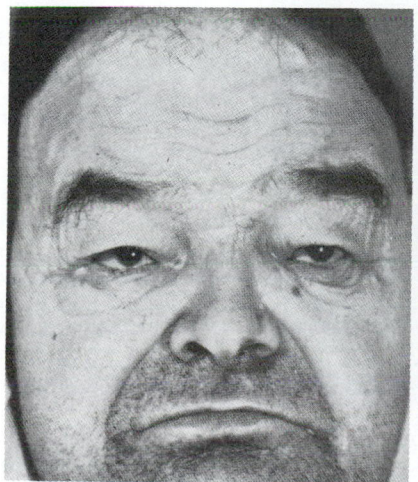
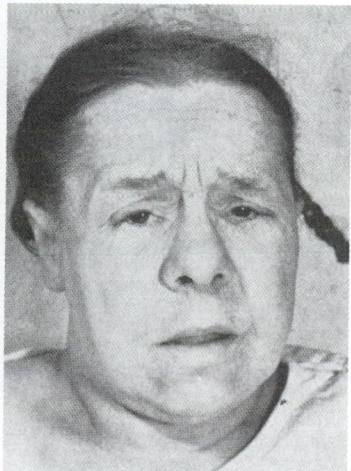

Figure 8–44. Typical facial appearance of myxedematous patients.

normally undergo ossification at a time after onset of the hypothyroidism. After a normal metabolic state has been restored by treatment, development of the centers destined to ossify at a later age proceeds normally.

Hypothyroidism beginning in childhood is termed *juvenile hypothyroidism*. The clinical manifestations of this state are intermediate between those of infantile and adult hypothyroidism, in that the developmental retardation is not as severe as that of cretinism and the manifestations of full-blown adult myxedema are rarely seen. Growth and sexual development are predominantly affected. Linear growth is severely retarded. The rate of linear growth is characteristically less than that of weight gain. Maturation of the facial bones is impaired, so that the naso-orbital configuration of the infant or young child is retained. Eruption of permanent teeth is delayed. Sexual maturation is retarded and the onset of puberty is delayed. The result is a child who appears much younger than his or her chronological age (Fig. 8–45). Rarely, precocious puberty and galactorrhea occur. Intellectual performance is distinctly poor, but the severe mental deficiency that characterizes cretinism is not found. The clinical manifestations of adult hypothyroidism are present to a varying, but usually milder, degree. On radiological examination, epiphyseal dysgenesis may be present, and epiphyseal union is always delayed, resulting in a bone age that is retarded in relation to chronological age.

Laboratory Tests

A decrease in secretion of the thyroid hormones is common to all varieties of hypothyroidism, irrespective of underlying etiology. The decrease in feedback inhibition of TSH secretion results in an increase in basal serum TSH

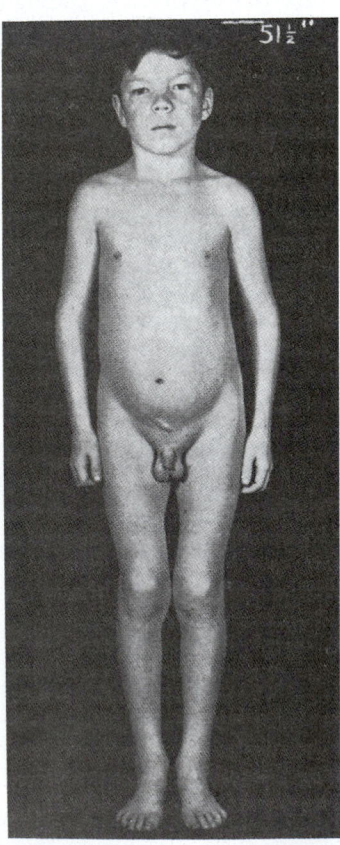

Figure 8–45. Juvenile hypothyroidism in a boy aged 17. Dwarfism and delayed sexual development are apparent. The trunk is longer than legs. Appearance is youthful.

concentration (see Fig. 8–20) and increased serum TSH response to exogenous TRH. This is the earliest laboratory abnormality in patients with intrinsic disease of the thyroid. With the passage of time, serum T_4 and T_3 concentrations progressively approach subnormal values, the former more rapidly than the latter. This is due to preferential synthesis and secretion of T_3 by residual functioning thyroid tissue under the influence of greatly increased plasma TSH concentrations. An additional factor may be that the efficiency of T_4-to-T_3 conversion is increased as serum T_4 level falls.[343] Accordingly, serum T_3 concentration may be within the normal range at a time when serum T_4 concentration is depressed (see Table 8–10). On the other hand, serum T_3 concentration is frequently decreased in euthyroid patients with severe systemic illness. For these reasons, serum T_3 concentration is less specific than serum T_4 concentration in the diagnosis of hypothyroidism.

The decrease in circulating hormone concentrations, as well as a slight increase in the concentration of TBG, results in low-normal values for the THBR or the proportions of free T_4 and T_3 (see Fig. 8–18). Calculated values for the FT_4I and sometimes the serum FT_3I are low, reflecting decreased free hormone concentration.

The BMR is decreased in all varieties of hypothyroidism. Serum cholesterol concentration may be increased to values in excess of 300 mg/dL, but in pituitary hypothyroidism the levels may be normal or low. In cretinism, hypercholesterolemia may not appear until late infancy. Other manifestations of the hypothyroid state include increased serum concentrations of creatine kinase, serum glutamic-oxalo-acetic transaminase, lactate dehydrogenase, and carcinoembryonic antigen. In infantile and juvenile hypothyroidism, the serum alkaline phosphatase concentration does not display the usual increase seen during the period of active growth.

Tests that employ radioiodine and assess the function of the thyroid gland per se display a variable pattern, depending on the underlying thyroid disorder. When the amount of thyroid tissue is reduced (thyroprivic hypothyroidism), the RAIU is subnormal. However, the diagnostic value of this finding is minimized by the decrease in the range of normal values that has resulted from the increase in dietary iodine intake. On the other hand, in disorders in which hypothyroidism results primarily from biochemical rather than anatomical failure and in which compensatory goitrogenesis usually occurs, the RAIU may be normal or increased. Specific functional patterns are discussed later in relation to the several causes of hypothyroidism.

The differentiation of hypothyroidism related to intrinsic thyroid failure (thyroprivic and goitrous hypothyroidism) from that related to diminished TSH secretion as a result of hypothalamic or pituitary disease (trophoprivic hypothyroidism) is important, because failure to recognize the latter may have serious consequences for the patient when thyroid replacement is instituted. The measurement of serum TSH concentration is the most discriminating, because it is invariably increased in intrinsic thyroid failure, regardless of underlying etiology, but may be normal, decreased, or only slightly increased in trophoprivic hypothyroidism. In some patients with pituitary tumor, the basal serum TSH concentration and its response to TRH may be elevated, but the TSH may have reduced biological potency even though it is immunologically reactive.[94] On occasion, patients with severe illnesses may have modest elevations in serum TSH levels. This is particularly common during the recovery phase.[128–130] In such patients the elevated serum TSH concentrations are rarely in excess of 20 mU/L and usually return to normal as serum thyroid hormone concentrations return to normal.

In summary, laboratory confirmation of hypothyroidism is best achieved through measurement of the FT_4I and TSH concentration. The serum TSH concentration is required to establish whether the hypothyroidism is due to intrinsic disease of the thyroid or whether it is secondary to hypothalamic or pituitary disease.

Differential Diagnosis

The clinical picture of fully developed myxedema is usually characteristic enough to leave the diagnosis in little doubt. In its milder forms, hypothyroidism may require differentiation from several other states. The fact that these disorders, like hypothyroidism, tend to occur in elderly patients is partly responsible for diagnostic uncertainty. In some elderly patients, slowing of mental and physical activity, dry skin, and loss of hair, especially from the lateral third of the eyebrows, may mimic similar findings in hypothyroidism. Furthermore, the elderly often become hypothermic on exposure to cold. In elderly patients the results of conventional laboratory tests, such as the RAIU and serum T_4 concentration, are not significantly different from those in younger individuals, but the overall turnover of thyroid hormone is slowed. The features may reflect, therefore, a diminished flux of hormone to the tissues. In patients with chronic renal insufficiency, anorexia, torpor, periorbital puffiness, sallow complexion, and anemia may suggest hypothyroidism. However, retinopathy, azotemia, an abnormal urinalysis, and hypertension provide a clear differentiation between the diseases. The differentiation of nephrotic states from hypothyroidism is more difficult. Here, waxy pallor, edema, hypercholesterolemia, and hypometabolism may suggest hypothyroidism. In addition, a decrease in serum T_4 concentration may occur if there is significant loss of TBG in the urine, but the FT_4I will be normal or increased. Serum T_3 concentration is frequently decreased, suggesting impaired T_3 neogenesis from T_4, but serum TSH concentration is not increased. In pernicious anemia, psychiatric abnormalities, a lemon-yellow tint of the skin, and numbness and tingling of the extremities may mimic similar findings in hypothyroidism. On the other hand, histamine-fast achlorhydria and mild macrocytosis in hypothyroidism may suggest pernicious anemia. Although there is a clinical and immunological overlap between primary hypothyroidism and pernicious anemia, this association is not invariable, and when pernicious anemia occurs alone it is not accompanied by stigmata and laboratory evidence of thyroid hypofunction.

The presence of hypothyroidism is often suspected in patients who are severely ill, especially if they are elderly. In the ill patient, serum T_3 concentration is almost invariably decreased, because of decreased peripheral generation of T_3 from T_4. This should pose no problem, because measurements of serum T_3 concentration should not be employed in the diagnosis of hypothyroidism. In more severely ill patients, however, the serum T_4 concentration is also decreased, often markedly so, but the free T_4 level is generally normal.[126, 127] This, together with the absence of elevation of serum TSH concentration, serves to differentiate the severely ill but intrinsically euthyroid patient from the patient with thyroprivic hypothyroidism.

Down syndrome resembles cretinism in that both are accompanied by retardation of mental development and shortness of stature. The differentiation of these two diseases is not difficult and can usually be made on clinical grounds alone, but subclinical or frank hypothyroidism and evidence of thyroid autoimmunity may be present in as many as 30% of patients with Down syndrome.[344] The infant with Down syndrome is more active, lacks the dry skin of the cretin, and displays specific stigmata, such as obliquely set eyes, epicanthal folds, white flecks in the iris (Brushfield spots), inward-curving fifth fingers, and abnormal palmar and plantar creases. In addition, analysis of the chromosomes usually reveals either trisomy-21 or 15/21 translocation. Epiphyseal dysgenesis and laboratory evidence of thyroid hypofunction are lacking in Down syndrome. Dwarfism resulting from cretinism or juvenile hypothyroidism differs from dwarfism of other causes, such as hypopituitarism, rickets, and achondroplasia, in that it is usually accompanied by mental retardation, retarded bone age, and epiphyseal dysgenesis. Replacement therapy with thyroid hormone restores growth in hypothyroid dwarfism but is ineffective in dwarfism with other causes. The dysgenesis of the femoral epiphysis resembles that of Legg-Perthes disease, but evidence of thyroid hypofunction is lacking in the latter disorder.

Thyroprivic Hypothyroidism

Disorders characterized by loss or atrophy of thyroid tissue result in decreased production of thyroid hormone despite stimulation of the thyroid remnant by TSH. The disorders in this category include primary thyroid atrophy, the hypothyroid state that follows therapeutic ablation of the thyroid gland by surgery or radioiodine (postablative hypothyroidism), and sporadic athyreotic cretinism.

Primary Hypothyroidism

Primary hypothyroidism is, after postablative hypothyroidism, the most common cause of thyroid failure in the adult. It is more common in women than in men and occurs most often between the ages of 40 and 60. The cause is unknown. The presence of circulating thyroid autoantibodies in up to 80% of the patients and the clinical and immunological overlap with autoimmune diseases suggest, however, that it represents the end stage of an autoimmune thyroiditis in which goiter either was absent or had gone unnoticed. Although most cases probably reflect autoimmune destruction of the thyroid parenchyma, an indeterminate proportion of cases of nongoitrous hypothyroidism arise through the influence of antibodies that block the response to endogenous TSH.[250, 345] In others, thyroid atrophy may reflect the action of antibodies that specifically inhibit thyroid growth. Primary hypothyroidism may occur as part of an autoimmune syndrome of polyglandular failure in association with one or more of the following: idiopathic adrenal atrophy, idiopathic hypoparathyroidism, idiopathic hypogonadism, insulin-dependent diabetes mellitus, and pernicious anemia (see Chapter 31). Primary thyroid failure also occurs in patients with Hodgkin disease who have been treated with mantle irradiation[346] or after high-dose neck radiation for other forms of lymphoma or carcinoma.[347]

On histopathological examination, the small thyroid remnant consists largely of fibrous tissue, with an occasional thyroid follicle and focus of lymphocytic infiltration.

The clinical manifestations have been discussed. The thyroid is usually impalpable, normal in size or even somewhat enlarged. Typical laboratory indices include a low serum T_4 and a high serum TSH concentration. Values for the THBR are often subnormal but may be in the normal range. Autoantibodies to thyroid microsomal antigen or to thyroglobulin are detectable in the serum in up to 80% of patients but may be absent in long-standing disease. Serum cholesterol concentration is usually increased.

In addition to spontaneous hypothyroidism, both surgical and radioiodine therapy may lead to a functional state of "subclinical hypothyroidism," which represents a phase in the evolution of thyroid failure. During this phase, the patient is eumetabolic with an increased serum TSH concentration, normal serum T_3 concentration, and normal or moderately decreased serum T_4 concentration (see Table 8–10).

Postablative Hypothyroidism

Postablative hypothyroidism is a common cause of thyroid failure in the adult. One type follows thyroidectomy. Although functioning remnants may be present, as indicated by foci of radioiodine accumulation, hypothyroidism invariably develops after total thyroidectomy. This procedure, which is associated with a high frequency of recurrent laryngeal nerve palsy and postoperative hypoparathyroidism, is often performed in patients with thyroid carcinoma.

The most common type of postoperative hypothyroidism follows subtotal resection of the diffuse goiter in Graves disease. Its frequency is influenced by the amount of tissue removed. In addition, autoimmune destruction of the thyroid remnant may sometimes be a factor, because some studies suggest a correlation between the presence of circulating thyroid autoantibodies in thyrotoxicosis and the development of hypothyroidism after surgery.[348] Hypothyroidism often becomes manifest during the first year after surgery, but, as in the case of postradioiodine hypothyroidism, there is a rising incidence with time. The frequency may approach 30% or more.[280] In some patients, mild hypothyroidism appears during the early postoperative period and then goes into remission, as is also the case after treatment with radioiodine. In adults, therefore, it may be justified to withhold replacement therapy for 1 or 2 mo, provided that close observation is maintained. Alternatively, replacement therapy can be administered and withdrawn later to ascertain whether thyroid function has recovered. In children, treatment should be instituted whenever hypothyroidism supervenes.

Hypothyroidism after destruction of thyroid tissue with radioiodine is common and is the only verified disadvantage of this form of treatment for hyperthyroidism. Its frequency is determined in large part by the dose of radiation delivered to the thyroid, but it is also influenced by variations in individual susceptibility that are conditioned by other factors, including autoimmune phenomena.[348] The incidence of postradioiodine hypothyroidism increases progressively with time. The data currently available indicate an incidence at 10 y of approximately 40%, although values as high as 70% have been reported.

Sporadic Cretinism

Developmental defects of the thyroid are responsible for most hypothyroidism in the newborn, that is, in 1 in every 4000 to 5000 births. These defects may take the form of complete absence of thyroid tissue or failure of the thyroid to descend properly during embryological development. Thyroid tissue may then be found anywhere along its route of descent from the foramen cecum at the junction of the anterior two thirds and posterior third of the tongue (lingual thyroid) to the normal site or below. Absence of thyroid tissue or its ectopic location, if present, can be ascertained by scintiscanning after administration of TcO_4^-. In a small percentage of patients, neonatal hypothyroidism results from biosynthetic defects in the thyroid or from pituitary or hypothalamic failure. Hypothyroidism has also been described in one family with a mutation in the gene coding for the TSH beta subunit.[349]

Hypothyroidism is difficult to detect by clinical examination at birth or shortly thereafter. Suggestive signs are a high birth weight owing to postmaturity, enlargement of the posterior fontanelle, delay in the passage of meconium, persistence of neonatal jaundice, and hypothermia. When several of these signs are present, the diagnosis of hypothyroidism should be sought promptly in measurements of serum T_4 and TSH concentrations. Problems in recognition of this condition have been largely eliminated by neonatal screening.

Failure to institute therapy in patients with neonatal hypothyroidism results in development of full-blown cretinism. If treatment is initiated after the clinical signs of hypothyroidism appear, the somatic manifestations of this condition may be forestalled, but psychomotor development can be permanently impaired. A similar outcome may occur if adequate treatment (suppression of TSH and elevation of the T_4 concentration to greater than 130 nmol/L [10 μg/dL]) is not maintained throughout the first 3 to 4 y of life.[350, 351] This consideration highlights the urgency of routine screening of newborns for hypothyroidism, which is accomplished by routine measurements of serum T_4 or TSH concentrations, or both, in cord blood or in blood spots dried in filter paper, as in routine screening for phenylketonuria. In some cases, neonatal hypothyroidism is transient and permanent hormone replacement therapy is not required. Rather than temporize, however, it is better to initiate treatment early, during the critical period of central nervous system development, and to withdraw treatment some months later to see if continued therapy is needed.[323]

Trophoprivic Hypothyroidism

A discussion of pituitary insufficiency is presented in Chapter 6. This section will deal mainly with the features that differentiate hypothyroidism of primary thyroid origin from that arising from disease in higher centers. When the intrinsically normal thyroid gland is deprived of TSH stimulation as a result of hypothalamic or pituitary disease, partial atrophy of the thyroid and decreased production of thyroid hormones occur. In most cases, hyposecretion of TSH is accompanied by decreased secretion of other pituitary hormones, with the result that evidence of gonadal and adrenocortical insufficiency is also present. Instances in which hyposecretion of TSH is the sole demonstrable abnormality (unitropic deficiency) are rare. Hypothyroidism resulting from pituitary insufficiency varies in severity, from instances in which it is mild and overshadowed by features of gonadal and adrenocortical failure to instances in which the features of the hypothyroid state are predominant.

The differentiation of pituitary from thyroprivic hypothyroidism is important because, in the former, treatment with thyroid hormone alone fails to correct the associated endocrine abnormalities and indeed, by precipitating acute adrenocortical insufficiency, may be dangerous. Three major aspects serve to differentiate pituitary from thyroprivic hypothyroidism: (1) features arising from the cause of the pituitary insufficiency itself, (2) differences in clinical manifestations, and (3) differences in laboratory indices.

In most cases, pituitary hypothyroidism results either from postpartum pituitary necrosis (Sheehan syndrome) or from tumors of the pituitary or adjacent structures. The tumors most commonly responsible are chromophobe adenomas of the pituitary or craniopharyngiomas (suprasellar cysts). Postpartum pituitary necrosis is suggested by a history of bleeding or shock after delivery necessitating blood transfusion, followed by deficient lactation, persistent amenorrhea, and loss of libido and of pubic and axillary hair. Symptoms of hypothyroidism may appear rapidly, in contrast to their usual slow evolution in thyroprivic hypothyroidism. Although these are the usual manifestations of Sheehan syndrome, many years may elapse before symptoms of pituitary insufficiency appear. The presence of a tumor in the region of the pituitary is suggested by headache (especially if retro-orbital in location), by visual field defects, and by enlargement of the pituitary fossa. Intracranial pressure may be increased, and diverse neurological manifestations may occur if the tumor extends beyond the pituitary fossa. Radiological examination of the skull usually reveals enlargement of the pituitary fossa and erosion of the clinoid processes. Computed tomography with contrast material and magnetic resonance imaging are helpful in defining sellar architecture and sometimes in defining extrasellar localization of a soft tissue mass. Rarely, hyperplasia and hypertrophy of the thyrotropic cells as a result of long-standing thyroprivic disease may lead to enlargement of the pituitary fossa. A craniopharyngioma or germinoma is suggested by suprasellar calcification. Cerebral angiograms may help to demonstrate a tumor or an aneurysm of the internal carotid artery, which in rare instances may cause pituitary insufficiency.

The clinical manifestations of pituitary hypothyroidism tend to differ in certain respects from those of thyroprivic hypothyroidism as described earlier. Changes in skin, hair, and tongue are less prominent. Differentiating features of pituitary insufficiency may result from inadequate secretion of other pituitary hormones, notably gonadotropins and corticotropin. In women of premenopausal age, amenorrhea rather than menorrhagia occurs and the breasts are atrophic. As regards manifestations of adrenocortical hypofunction, some similarities may exist. Loss of axillary and pubic hair is common in women with either disease. In pituitary hypothyroidism, however, the heart is usually small and blood pressure is low. Furthermore, manifestations of hypoglycemia may occur in pituitary hypothyroidism but are rare in thyroprivic hypothyroidism.

Conclusive differentiation of pituitary from thyroprivic hypothyroidism depends on the results of laboratory tests. Indices of thyroid function tend to differ in the extent to which they are abnormal. In pituitary insufficiency, serum T_4 concentration is usually not as low as in thyroprivic hypothyroidism, values at or near the lower limit of the normal range commonly being found. Because of the lack of increased TSH drive, the T_3/T_4 ratio in serum may not be increased in trophoprivic hypothyroidism as it is in primary hypothyroidism. Values of the RAIU are usually not as low as they are in primary hypothyroidism, but for reasons discussed earlier the test has little diagnostic value. Serum cholesterol concentration, usually increased in thyroprivic hypothyroidism, is low in pituitary hypothyroidism. Positive tests for circulating antithyroid antibodies suggest the presence of autoimmune thyroid disease rather than hypothalamic-pituitary failure.

Measurement of serum TSH concentration by radioimmunoassay provides the most direct means of differentiating between pituitary and thyroprivic hypothyroidism. In pituitary hypothyroidism, serum TSH is usually undetectable or within the normal range, whereas in thyroprivic hypothyroidism the serum TSH concentration is invariably increased, often greatly so (see Fig. 8–20). Measurements of the response of the serum TSH concentration to exogenous TRH are rarely required to confirm the diagnosis of thyroprivic hypothyroidism but may provide useful information in patients with pituitary or hypothalamic disease. Subnormal responses would be expected in the former and normal, but perhaps delayed, responses in the latter. Frequently, however, the pattern is not that expected, and overall the TRH test has not been particularly helpful in differentiating between the two.[176] Sometimes, in patients with pituitary or hypothalamic disease, basal serum TSH concentrations are increased and responses to TRH are augmented. These unexpected findings have been ascribed to secretion of a form of TSH that is immunoreactive but has little or no bioactivity.[94, 169]

Measurement of plasma concentration of gonadotropins can provide a means of differentiating pituitary from thyroprivic hypothyroidism. In postmenopausal women with thyroprivic hypothyroidism, the values may be somewhat lower than those found normally at the same age, but they remain elevated nevertheless. In women of premenopausal age the values are less discriminatory because they are normally much lower. In pituitary hypothyroidism, gonadotropins are often absent from plasma.

Tests of the pituitary-adrenal axis are generally less useful. Although values for the basal 24-h urinary excretion of 17-OHCS and 17-KS are characteristically reduced in hypopituitarism, subnormal values are also usually encountered in thyroprivic hypothyroidism. The latter results, at least in large part, from decreased metabolic disposal of cortisol, with the result that the plasma cortisol concentration is usually normal despite a decreased rate of cortisol secretion. In pituitary hypothyroidism, the plasma cortisol concentration is usually low. Further evidence may be obtained by assessing the response of urinary 17-OHCS to metyrapone. In thyroprivic hypothyroidism, the response is usually normal, the maximal increase in 17-OHCS occurring the day after administration of metyrapone. In some cases of thyroprivic hypothyroidism, however, the response is either subnormal or delayed, the maximal increase in 17-OHCS occurring 2 or 3 d after administration of metyrapone. By contrast, in pituitary hypothyroidism, the response to metyrapone is usually subnormal, reflecting the diminished reserve of ACTH.[352]

In pituitary insufficiency, the increases in plasma growth hormone and cortisol concentrations that normally occur in response to insulin-induced hypoglycemia either are blunted or fail to occur. Subnormal responses are also usually seen in thyroprivic hypothyroidism, so this test does not provide a useful means of differentiating between these two varieties of hypothyroidism.

Goitrous Hypothyroidism

This section will deal with a variety of disorders characterized by a relatively or absolutely impaired ability to synthesize thyroid hormone, either because of some extrinsic factor or because of an intrinsic, usually heritable, defect in hormone biosynthesis. Inadequate synthesis of hormone leads to hypersecretion of TSH, which in turn produces both goiter and stimulation of all steps in hormone biosynthesis capable of response. This compensatory response may be inadequate, and goiter with hypothyroidism or cretinism results. In many instances, however, the compensatory response overcomes the impairment in hormone biosynthesis and the patient is eumetabolic but goitrous. The latter condition, termed simple or nontoxic goiter, will be discussed in a later section. Although Hashimoto disease is the most common cause of goitrous hypothyroidism in areas of iodine sufficiency, it is discussed in the section dealing with thyroiditis.

Endemic Goiter

The term *endemic goiter* denotes any goiter occurring in a region where goiter is prevalent. Endemic goiter usually occurs in areas of environmental iodine deficiency and has been ascribed to this pathogenic factor; however, other factors may also be operative. This disease is one of vast public health significance and has been estimated to afflict more than 200 million people throughout the world. Except perhaps in North America, it is prevalent on all continents and is most common in mountainous areas such as the Alps, Himalayas, and Andes. In the United States, goiter was formerly common in the region around the Great Lakes, but here, as in other areas of endemic disease, its incidence has been greatly reduced by the use of iodized salt. The belief that iodine deficiency plays a major role in the genesis of endemic goiter is supported by an inverse correlation between the iodine content of soil and water and the incidence of goiter, the kinetics of iodine metabolism in patients with this disorder, and a decrease in incidence with iodine prophylaxis. Both the isolated geographic locale and the cultural patterns of some populations in areas of severe endemic incidence favor inbreeding, with the result that genetically determined abnormalities in hormonal biosynthesis may also play a role. The frequent occurrence of deaf-mutism, mental retardation, and motor defects in the populations of such areas supports this view. Furthermore, severe iodine deficiency and its associated abnormalities in the kinetics of iodine metabolism may occur in the absence of goiter. Endemic goiter may display a spotty incidence, even within an area of known iodine deficiency; the role of dietary minerals or naturally occurring goitrogens and of pollution of water supplies has been questioned in instances of this type. Indeed, in the Cauca Valley of Colombia, water-borne goitrogens have been implicated. In many areas of endemic iodine deficiency, consumption of cassava meal, which gives rise to thiocyanate, aggravates the iodine-deficient state by inhibiting thyroid iodide transport.[353]

Various abnormalities in iodine metabolism occur in patients with endemic goiter. Most are consistent with the expected effects of iodine deficiency. Others, such as those indicating the existence of heterogeneous pools of thyroidal iodine and the secretion of butanol-insoluble iodinated products, are probably mere exaggerations of processes occurring in the normal gland but made more prominent by prolonged hyperfunction. To date, no abnormality related to a primary defect in iodine metabolism has been described in endemic goiter. Thyroid iodide clearance rates and RAIU are increased inversely with the decrease in urinary stable iodine excretion. The absolute iodine uptake is normal or low. The thyroid hyperfunction can be suppressed by exogenous hormone, indicating that it represents a homeostatic compensatory response. In areas of only moderate iodine deficiency, the serum T_4 concentration is usually in the lower range of normal; in areas of severe deficiency, however, values may be decreased. Nevertheless, most patients in these areas do not appear to be hypothyroid, a discrepancy that is due to an increase in synthesis of the calorigenically more efficient hormone, T_3, at the expense of T_4.[354]

The severity of goiter is also not uniform among all inhabitants of an area of endemic incidence. As a group, goitrous inhabitants display lower serum T_4 concentrations and higher serum TSH concentrations than do nongoitrous inhabitants, indicating a less efficient adaptation to the iodine deficiency, but the reason for this difference in adaptive response is unclear.[354]

The gross and histopathological appearance of endemic goiter depends on the duration of the goiter and the severity of the pathogenetic insult. In the initial stages, the stimulus of iodine deficiency leads to hypertrophy and hyperplasia of the epithelial cells lining the follicles. The cells increase in height and number and may protrude into the follicular lumen, forming papillary projections. The amount of colloid in the follicles decreases. The hyperplasia is accompanied by an increase in vascularity. This is the diffuse hyperplastic goiter usually seen in children in endemic areas. If the iodine intake is increased, the hypertrophy and hyperplasia of the epithelial cells disappear and colloid reaccumulates in the follicles. This process of involution leads to a return of the gland to normal size if the hyperplasia is of relatively short duration but probably results in a diffuse colloid goiter if the hyperplastic phase has been present for years. In long-standing goiter, repeated cycles of hyperplasia and involution eventually lead to formation of nodules of involuted tissue, and a multinodular goiter results. Localized hyperplasia with the formation of encapsulated adenomas (adenomatous hyperplasia) is a less common cause of nodularity in endemic goiter; it may be difficult to distinguish this lesion from true neoplasia. Nodules often undergo hemorrhagic or cystic degeneration and may become calcified or ossified.

The incidence and severity of endemic goiter, as well as the metabolic state of the goitrous patient, depend mainly on the degree of iodine deficiency. In the absence of hypothyroidism, the effects of the goiter are mainly disfiguring. When the goiter has become nodular, however, hemorrhage into a nodule may cause acute pain and swelling, mimicking subacute thyroiditis or neoplasia. Occasionally, a goiter may cause symptoms by compressing adjacent structures, such as the trachea, esophagus, and recurrent laryngeal nerves.

The development of hyperthyroidism is unusual in patients with endemic goiter. This is in contrast to the tendency of multinodular goiter in nonendemic regions to produce hyperthyroidism in later life. It seems likely that iodine deficiency protects some patients with endemic goiter from developing hyperthyroidism. The incidence of thyrotoxicosis in an endemic goiter region increases after the introduction of measures to increase iodine intake. The incidence of thyroid carcinoma in endemic goiter is probably not increased.

The incidence of endemic goiter has been greatly reduced in many areas by the introduction of iodized salt. In the United States, table salt is enriched with potassium iodide to a concentration of 0.01%, which, if the intake of salt is average, would provide an iodine intake of approximately 500 µg/d, the desired amount in an adult. In areas where the salt is crude and moist, iodine added as potassium iodide may be lost by sublimation; in this instance, potassium iodate is preferable because it is more stable. In primitive communities, an annual injection of iodized oil is an effective means of administering iodine, and endemic goiter can be treated by the introduction of iodine into communal drinking water.

Administration of iodine has little if any effect on a colloid or multinodular goiter, but it will cause the early hyperplastic goiter to regress. Similarly, thyroid hormone usually has no effect on goiters of long standing or on established mental or skeletal changes, but it should be given in full replacement doses if there is evidence of hypothyroidism; this is of paramount importance in pregnant women. Surgical treatment is indicated if the adjacent structures are compressed or if the goiter is either very large or enlarging rapidly.

Endemic Cretinism

Endemic cretinism is a specific developmental disorder that occurs in regions of severe endemic goiter. Both parents of an endemic cretin are usually goitrous. In addition to, or instead of, the classic features of hypothyroid cretinism described earlier, endemic cretins often display deaf-mutism, spasticity, and motor dysfunction. Thus, one can distinguish three types of cretins: hypothyroid cretins, neurological cretins, and those with combined features of the two. The pathogenesis of neurological cretinism is obscure, but it may represent severe thyroid hormone deficiency during a critical phase of central nervous system development, with remission later.

Some cretins are goitrous, but often the thyroid is

atrophic. This has been ascribed either to exhaustion atrophy, resulting from continuous overstimulation, or to a requirement for iodine in normal thyroid growth. Neither explanation seems wholly satisfactory, however.

Although the role of iodine deficiency in the pathogenesis of endemic cretinism has been questioned, there can be no doubt that it is somehow implicated, because cretinism appears to have been eradicated when maternal iodine supplementation has been undertaken. Of major public health import are observations indicating that some degree of hypothyroidism, later associated with psychomotor retardation, is common in noncretinous children born in areas of severe iodine deficiency and that this can also be eliminated or alleviated by maternal iodine supplementation.[355]

Goiter Related to Antithyroid Agents

The ingestion of compounds with antithyroid actions is an occasional cause of goiter with or without hypothyroidism. Apart from the agents commonly used in the treatment of thyrotoxicosis, antithyroid agents may be encountered either as drugs used in the treatment of disorders unrelated to the thyroid gland or as agents occurring naturally in foodstuffs.

Of the drugs with potential goitrogenic action lithium is the most important. Goiter with or without hypothyroidism is sometimes encountered in patients receiving lithium as treatment for a psychiatric disorder. Lithium, like iodide, decreases thyroid hormone synthesis. Lithium-induced hypothyroidism appears to be largely confined to women, particularly those older than 40, of whom as many as one third will be hypothyroid. Many such women display evidence of thyroid autoimmunity, suggesting that autoimmune thyroid disease is a predisposing factor.

Other drugs that occasionally produce goitrous hypothyroidism include para-aminosalicylic acid, phenylbutazone, topically applied resorcinol, and ethionamide.[103] Like the commonly used antithyroid agents, these drugs exert their effect by interfering with both the organic binding of iodine and the later steps in hormone biosynthesis.

Antithyroid agents occur naturally in certain plants, particularly those of the family Cruciferae. Some of these are eaten by humans; among them, rutabaga and white turnip appear to be richest in goitrogen. It is uncertain, however, whether goitrogenic quantities of such foods are ever directly ingested. Rather, such foods may accentuate the effects of dietary iodine deficiency, as is almost certainly the case with cassava meal.

Although soybean is not an antithyroid agent, soybean products in feeding formulas formerly led to goiter in infants by enhancing fecal loss of hormone, which, together with the low iodine content of soybean products, produced a state of iodine deficiency. Feeding formulas containing soybean products are now enriched with iodine.

Both the goiter and the hypothyroidism usually subside after the antithyroid agent is withdrawn, but if continued administration of pharmacological goitrogens is required, replacement therapy with thyroid hormone will cause the disorder to regress.

Iodide Goiter and Hypothyroidism

Goiter and hypothyroidism, either alone or in combination, are sometimes induced by chronic administration of large doses of iodine in either organic or inorganic form. This is seen most commonly in patients with chronic respiratory disease, who are often given potassium iodide as an expectorant. Iodide goiter develops in only a small proportion of patients given iodine. The development of iodide goiter has also been reported to follow a single administration of radiographic contrast medium from which iodide is released slowly over a long period. Iodide goiter without hypothyroidism occurs endemically on the island of Hokkaido, Japan, where seaweed is consumed in large quantity.

From an analysis of reported cases and from the fact that only a small percentage of patients who receive iodides chronically develop goiter, it is clear that the disorder develops on a background of underlying thyroid dysfunction. Several categories of susceptible patients have been identified, including those with Hashimoto disease; those with Graves disease, especially after treatment with radioiodine; and those with cystic fibrosis. Among these groups, many but not all patients display a positive iodide-perchlorate discharge test, indicating a defect in the thyroid organic binding mechanism. However, intrinsic thyroid disease need not be present, because a propensity to develop iodide goiter and hypothyroidism has also been demonstrated in patients who have undergone hemithyroidectomy for a solitary thyroid nodule and in whom the remaining lobe was histologically normal. In these patients, as in those with Hashimoto disease or Graves disease studied prospectively, individuals with the highest basal serum TSH concentrations, even within the normal range, were those who developed iodide goiter.

Goiter and hypothyroidism commonly occur in newborn infants of women given iodine during pregnancy, and death from neonatal asphyxia has been reported (Fig. 8–46). In such cases, the mother is usually free of goiter. Pregnant women should not be given large doses of iodine. It is not known whether iodide goiter in newborns results from an inherent hypersensitivity of the fetal thyroid or from the fact that the placenta concentrates iodide several-fold.

As discussed earlier, large doses of iodine cause an acute inhibition of organic binding that in the normal individual abates, despite continued iodine administration (acute Wolff-Chaikoff effect and escape). Iodide goiter appears to result

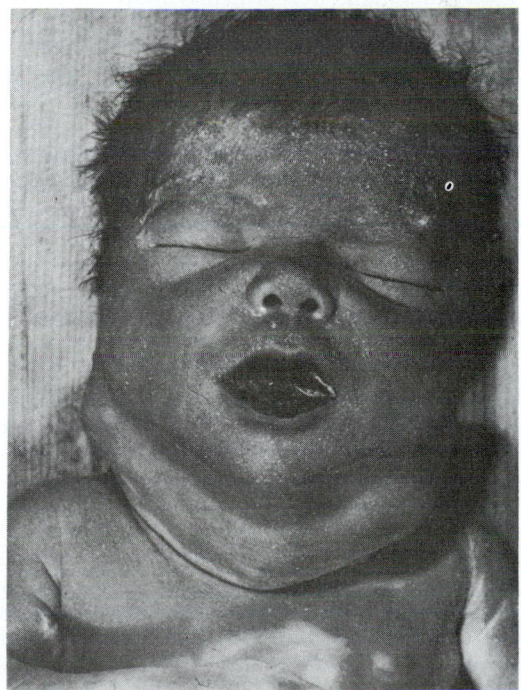

Figure 8–46. Large goiter in newborn that caused death by asphyxiation. The mother had received an iodine-containing medication for asthma during pregnancy. (From Galina MP, Avnet NL, Einhorn A. Iodides during pregnancy. An apparent cause of neonatal death. Reprinted, by permission of The New England Journal of Medicine, 267; 1124–1127, 1962.)

from a more pronounced inhibition of organic binding and a failure of escape. As a consequence of decreased hormone synthesis, iodide transport is enhanced. Because inhibition of organic binding is a function of the intrathyroidal concentration of iodide, a cycle, augmented by an increase in serum TSH concentration, is set in motion.

The disorder usually appears as a goiter with or without hypothyroidism; rarely, iodine may produce hypothyroidism unaccompanied by goiter. The thyroid is firm and diffusely enlarged, often greatly so. Histopathological examination reveals hyperplasia that is often intense.

The laboratory indices in patients with iodide goiter are consistent with the physiopathology of this disorder. While iodine is being administered, the RAIU within the first few hours after radioiodine administration is often high, reflecting both the large size of the thyroid and the hyperactive iodide transport mechanism. Because organic binding is inhibited, however, inorganic radioiodine is not retained and the thyroid uptake at 24 h is subnormal. Serum TSH concentration is increased, while serum T_4 level is normal or subnormal, in accord with the metabolic state of the patient. The 24-h urinary iodine excretion and the serum inorganic iodide concentration are greatly increased.

The disorder regresses after iodine is withdrawn. Thyroid hormone may also be given to hasten regression.

Defects in Hormone Biosynthesis

Genetically determined defects in hormone biosynthesis are rare causes of goitrous hypothyroidism.[1-4] Several members of a family are usually affected. In most instances, the defect appears to be transmitted as an autosomal recessive trait. Individuals with goitrous hypothyroidism are presumably homozygous for the abnormal gene, whereas euthyroid relatives with slightly enlarged thyroids are presumably heterozygous. In the latter, appropriate functional testing may disclose a milder abnormality of the same biosynthetic step that is defective in the homozygous individual. In contrast to nontoxic goiter, which is more common in females than in males, these defects as a group affect females only slightly more commonly than males.

Although goiter may be present at birth, it more often does not appear until several years later. Therefore, the absence of goiter in a child with functioning thyroid tissue does not exclude the presence of hypothyroidism. Initially, the goiter is diffusely hyperplastic, often intensely so, suggesting papillary carcinoma; eventually, it becomes nodular. In general, the more severe the biosynthetic defect, the earlier the goiter appears, the larger it is likely to be, and the greater is the likelihood of early emergence of manifestations of hypothyroidism. In severe cases, cretinism results.

Five specific defects in the pathways of hormone synthesis have been identified.

IODIDE TRANSPORT DEFECT. This defect, which is rare, is characterized by nonfunction of the iodide transport mechanism and is reflected in a low RAIU. Impaired iodide transport is also demonstrable in other tissues, such as salivary gland and gastric mucosa, that share a similar embryological origin with the thyroid and normally also transport iodide actively. Administration of iodine, by raising the plasma concentration, increases the intrathyroidal concentration of iodide sufficiently to permit the production of normal quantities of hormone and thereby causes regression of both goiter and hypothyroidism.[11]

ORGANIFICATION DEFECT. This is a heterogeneous group of disorders all of which impair the ability of the thyroid to carry out organic iodination. The various categories of deficiency have been defined in only a few cases and include either quantitative or qualitative abnormalities of the thyroid peroxidase enzyme, an abnormality of hydrogen peroxide generation, alterations of the amino acid sequences that serve as the iodine acceptors in thyroglobulin, and the most common of these forms, a mild defect in organification accompanied by sensory nerve deafness (Pendred syndrome). The common characteristic of these conditions is a goiter associated with an enhancement of iodide transport manifested by a high uptake of ^{123}I or TcO_4^-. The ^{123}I can be discharged almost completely by subsequent administration of 500 mg of perchlorate, which competes with the circulating iodide for reuptake by the thyroidal trapping mechanism. The deafness associated with Pendred syndrome may be present at birth or develop during early childhood, but it is not due to hypothyroidism per se because most patients with this syndrome, although goitrous, are euthyroid. The fact that infants with complete thyroid peroxidase deficiency, whose thyroid glands are unable to form T_4, have cord serum T_4 concentrations about one third to one half of normal provides clear evidence of the transplacental passage of maternal T_4.[7]

IODOTYROSINE-COUPLING DEFECT. In this defect, there appears to be an inability to couple iodotyrosines to form iodothyronines. The thyroid accumulation of I^* is rapid, approaching 100% of the administered dose within the first 2 h. Kinetic analysis reveals very rapid turnover and recycling of thyroid iodine. Analysis of thyroid tissue in this disorder reveals little or no T_4 and T_3, most of the organic iodine being in the form of MIT and DIT. Of the several defects in hormone biosynthesis, this is the least well characterized, and indeed some question has been raised whether the postulated abnormality truly exists.

IODOTYROSINE DEHALOGENASE DEFECT. The pathogenesis of goiter and hypothyroidism in this defect is complex. The major abnormality is an impairment of both intrathyroidal and peripheral deiodination of iodotyrosines, presumably because the enzyme is absent in these tissues. As a consequence of both intense thyroid stimulation and lack of intrathyroidal recycling of iodide derived from dehalogenation, I^* is rapidly accumulated by the thyroid gland and rapidly released; labeled MIT and DIT are found in the blood and, together with their deaminated derivatives, in the urine. Hypothyroidism is presumed to result from an intense stimulation of the thyroid release mechanism, leading to the loss of large quantities of MIT and DIT. Iodine deficiency is secondary to the loss of these iodotyrosines in the urine. The goiter and hypothyroidism are relieved by administration of large doses of iodine. The most specific test for the presence of this defect is the appearance in the urine of a large proportion of unchanged MIT or DIT after their systemic administration. A milder defect of similar type is seen in some patients with nontoxic goiter and in nongoitrous relatives of patients with the severe defect.

ABNORMAL SECRETION OF IODOPROTEINS. Release of abnormal iodinated proteins or polypeptides occurs in a variety of thyroid diseases, including Hashimoto disease, benign adenomas, diffuse toxic goiter, thyroid carcinoma, and endemic goiter. In addition, release of similar compounds appears to be the sole or major physiopathological abnormality leading to goiter with or without hypothyroidism. Goiter presumably develops because these calorigenically inactive compounds make up a major proportion of the products of hormone biosynthesis. They are collectively measured as PBI, but not as T_4, resulting in an abnormally large difference between the value for the PBI and the calculated value of the T_4 iodine; this discrepancy is the laboratory hallmark of the disorder. Reflecting the diversion of iodine into hormonally inactive iodoproteins, the RAIU is increased. A small quantity of similar iodoproteins is present in the serum of normal individuals. Hence, the abnormality in the goitrous group appears to be quantitative rather than qualitative. In their physical properties, these compounds usually resemble serum albumin, but an iodoprotein resembling prealbumin is present in some. A more extensive discussion of the nature of these iodoproteins and their relation to intrathyroidal proteins other than thyroglobulin appears in the section dealing with thyroid iodoproteins. Formation and release of these compounds are under the control of TSH, because exogenous TSH increases and exogenous thyroid hormone decreases their concentration in serum. The severity of the defect ranges from cretinism to nontoxic goiter in the adult. The frequency with which the disorder is familial has not been established.

CONGENITAL HYPOTHYROIDISM NOT ASSOCIATED WITH GOITER. In addition to thyroid gland aplasia or dysgenesis, several individuals have been described with what appears to be either a mutation in the TSH molecule leading to its ineffectiveness as a thyroid stimulator[349] or a defect in the capacity of the thyroid gland to respond to TSH.[356] Such patients present with congenital hypothyroidism of a moderate or severe degree, depending on the nature of the biochemical abnormality, but respond to exogenous TSH (in the case of a defect in TSH synthesis) or not (if the defect is in the thyroid gland per se). Decreased responsiveness to TSH has also been observed in familial type I pseudohypoparathyroidism (Chapter 27). Transplacental passage of thyrotropin receptor–blocking antibodies may also cause transient neonatal hypothyroidism without goiter.[357]

HORMONE RESISTANCE SYNDROMES. Resistance of the peripheral tissues to the action of thyroid hormones is a heterogeneous group of disorders. The syndrome in its most severe form includes deaf-mutism, skeletal anomalies, goiter, and a euthyroid clinical state.[142, 143] The serum total and free T_4 and T_3 concentrations are increased in the presence of a detectable serum TSH concentration. Administration of large quantities of exogenous T_4 or T_3 results in only incomplete suppression of thyroid function, suggesting that the thyrotropic cells also share in the resistance to the action of thyroid hormones. The molecular mechanisms responsible for peripheral resistance to the action of thyroid hormone are under intensive investigation. In many families, studies of restriction fragment length polymorphism suggest that this disorder segregates with the gene coding for the beta form of the thyroid hormone receptor (chromosome 3). At least two different amino acid substitutions have been observed in the ligand binding domain of the encoded receptor. (See earlier under Theories Concerning Mechanism of Action of Thyroid Hormones.) Because the defect is heterozygous in all patients studied so far, it remains to be explained how a single copy of a defective gene can lead to resistance to thyroid hormone. The abnormal response may be due to the formation of nonfunctional heterodimers of normal and abnormal receptor or to competition of the abnormal receptor for the specific DNA binding sites on responsive genes. Such an inhibitory effect has been observed with the non–T_3-binding splicing variant of the TRα receptor (TRα$_2$).

In general, patients with thyroid hormone resistance can be classified into two groups: those with generalized resistance to thyroid hormone and those with pituitary resistance.[142, 143] The latter group present with hyperthyroidism and varying degrees of inappropriate TSH elevation and have already been discussed. The former group in general show heterogeneous defects of thyroid response in peripheral tissues, which may involve any of the various body systems dependent on thyroid hormone. They may present with congenital hypothyroidism or be clinically euthyroid. There is only a single well-documented case in which the hormone resistance is confined to peripheral tissues and pituitary sensitivity is normal.[144]

Treatment of Hypothyroidism

Adults

Hypothyroidism in the adult is one of the most gratifying diseases to treat because of the ease and completeness with which it responds to administration of thyroid hormone. Treatment is carried out with one of two general types of preparations, either synthetic hormone or thyroprotein derived from animal thyroid glands. In the former category, levothyroxine sodium, liothyronine sodium, or a combination of the two (liotrix) has been employed. In the second category, thyroid extract, USP, is most commonly used. This preparation is a powder derived from dried, defatted thyroid glands that is now standardized with respect to its T_4 and T_3 content. The specific quantities are 38 μg of T_4 and 9 μg of T_3 for each 65-mg (1 grain) thyroid tablet. Thyroglobulin tablets have a slightly higher T_3/T_4 ratio and are stipulated to contain 36 μg of T_4 and 12 μg of T_3. The latter is generally prepared from porcine thyroid, whereas thyroid USP is generally prepared from mixtures of beef and pork thyroid. These requirements should eliminate much of the biological variation in the tablet preparations of different manufacturers.[358] However, even with the improved standardization, the ratio of T_3 to T_4 in desiccated thyroid preparations is higher than in human thyroid secretion. Furthermore, the 70 to 80% intestinal absorption of T_4 and virtually 100% absorption of T_3 make the effective T_3/T_4 ratio from these preparations even higher. Accordingly, in individuals given desiccated thyroid, the serum free T_4 concentration is invariably lower than normal. The serum T_3 concentration depends on the elapsed time between administration of the tablet and serum sampling. Peak serum T_3 values are reached 2 to 4 after administration. In contrast, in patients who are given replacement doses of levothyroxine the ratio of serum T_4 to serum T_3 concentration is higher than normal. There are no data demonstrating superior clinical results obtained with one type of replacement preparation or the other. There are theoretical advantages and disadvantages of each. A disadvantage of thyroid USP (or products containing chemically synthesized hormones in similar quantities) is the rapid rise and fall in serum T_3 level, which in a few patients results in subjective symptoms of hyperthyroidism or palpitations during the time when T_3 concentrations are supraphysiological. Another disadvantage is that it is difficult to educate physicians about the fact that serum T_4 concentrations should be low normal in patients receiving complete replacement with these agents, and there is, therefore, a tendency to over-replace the deficit. The average replacement dose for thyroid extract, which should provide normal quantities of T_3 to a 70-kg individual, is approximately 1.5 to 2 grains (120 mg), as opposed to 112 to 150 μg of levothyroxine. An analysis of the sources of T_3 in a hypothetical patient given either 150 μg of levothyroxine or 2 grains of thyroid USP is shown in Table 8–19. About 50% of the T_3 produced per day derives directly from the desiccated-thyroid tablet. With levothyroxine, the estimated T_3 production is the same even though the serum T_4 concentration in such patients would be about twice that during treatment with desiccated thyroid. Note also that the T_4 absorbed per day is about 1.5 times that in an individual with an intact thyroid.

A primary advantage of levothyroxine is that the body has a greater opportunity to regulate the amount of T_3 generated by normal physiological mechanisms. For exam-

TABLE 8–19. Comparison of the Sources of T_3 in an Individual Receiving Levothyroxine (150 μg) or Thyroid USP (120 mg)

Drug	Tablet Content (μg)		Quantity Absorbed* (μg/d)		Quantity Absorbed* (nmol/d)		T_3 from T_4* (nmol/d)	Total T_3 Produced (nmol/d)	Normal Production Rates for 70-kg Individual (nmol/d)	
	T_4	T_3	T_4	T_3	T_4	T_3			T_4	T_3
Levothyroxine	150	0	119	0	154	0	62	62		
									100	50
Thyroid USP	78	18	62	18	80	28	32	59		

*Assumes 80% absorption of T_4 and 40% deiodination of T_4 to T_3.

ple, the brain may derive over 80% of its T_3 from T_4 in situ (see Fig. 8–8). It is still not established whether the impairment of T_4-to-T_3 conversion during illness or fasting is physiologically beneficial. Nonetheless, if one accepts that replicating the natural state is the general goal of hormone replacement, it is logical to provide the prohormone T_4 and allow the tissues to activate it by physiologically regulated mechanisms. On the other hand, because T_4 is converted to T_3 intracellularly in the pituitary and therefore will suppress TSH by this route in addition to that occurring via circulating T_3,[86] serum TSH concentrations tend to be somewhat lower for T_3 produced from T_4 than would be the case if the same quantity of T_3 were provided directly (see Table 8–19). Because the current assays permit adjustment of the dose of thyroid hormone to return TSH levels to normal, it is critical to establish the optimal TSH concentration for a patient receiving levothyroxine replacement. Unfortunately, the serum TSH concentration is the most sensitive measure for assessing thyroid status and there is no equally sensitive physiological response variable that can be used to assess its correlation with metabolic status. This is important because one would predict that if the serum T_4 concentration were normalized by administration of levothyroxine, serum T_3 concentrations would be only about 80% of those present in normal individuals even though the TSH level might well be in the normal range.

The modestly lower bone density in women receiving excessive doses of thyroid hormone makes the approach to replacement of thyroid hormone an important practical issue.[359–361] Thyroid disease occurs five to eight times more commonly in women than in men, whether it is a consequence of Hashimoto disease or of radioiodine or surgical ablation for Graves disease. Hypothyroidism occurs in as many as 2 to 3% of women who also have an intrinsically high risk of postmenopausal osteoporosis. In the absence of definitive data, the authors believe that levothyroxine is the agent of choice for maintenance therapy in hypothyroidism. For most patients in whom replacement (as opposed to TSH suppression) is the goal of therapy, a dose of levothyroxine of about 1.6 to 1.7 μg/kg ideal body weight (about 0.7 to 0.8 μg T_4/lb) should result in adequate therapy for most patients. Typically this dose results in a serum FT_4I that is high normal, a serum FT_3I slightly below the normal mean, and a normal serum TSH concentration. Some patients require slightly higher or lower doses, presumably because of individual variations in absorption. This estimated dose is about 20 to 30% lower than that previously recommended.[362, 363] The higher estimates in earlier years were based on dose titrations using a brand of levothyroxine that was subsequently found to be subpotent based on specific assays for T_4 as opposed to the earlier USP standard of hormonal iodine.[362–364] It may be necessary to increase the dose of thyroxine in some patients during pregnancy, when, because of either increases in metabolic clearance or decreases in absorption, the quantity of oral levothyroxine required may

increase about 20 to 50%. After delivery the dose should be reduced.

When first diagnosed, hypothyroidism is usually of long standing and seldom requires prompt reversal. Consequently, the restoration of a normal metabolic state should be undertaken gradually. The initial dose of levothyroxine recommended depends on the degree of hypothyroidism and the age and general health of the patient. At one extreme, the young individual with no associated medical abnormalities can be started on a complete replacement dose without fear of adverse effects. The gradual increase in serum T_4 concentration that occurs with treatment is sufficiently delayed that patients do not experience an immediate impact. At the other extreme, the elderly patient with heart disease, particularly angina, must be given extremely small initial doses of thyroid hormone (12.5 or 25 μg levothyroxine/d). When subreplacement doses are given, dose adjustments are made at 4- to 6-wk intervals after clinical and biochemical evaluation of the response. Adverse effects of therapy are rare in younger patients. One exception, pseudotumor cerebri, has been reported occasionally in juveniles between the ages of 8 and 12 with profound hypothyroidism who were given modest initial replacement doses. This appeared 1 to 10 mo after initiation of treatment and responded to standard treatment with acetazolamide and dexamethasone.[365] In addition, a few reports suggest the possibility of a manic-affective disorder in adults given rapid thyroid hormone replacement. In both situations, levothyroxine dosage should be decreased temporarily until the symptoms resolve.

Because thyroid status influences the metabolic clearance of thyroid hormone, the adequacy of replacement should be reassessed after 6 mo to determine whether a further increase in dosage is required.[366] Also, because the metabolic clearance of T_4 decreases with increasing age, the dose of levothyroxine given to patients over age 70 should be reduced about 20% (Fig. 8–47).[116, 367] In patients with trophoprivic hypothyroidism, serum TSH concentrations cannot be used as an end point. Dependence must be on the serum FT_4I in these patients.

The interval between initiation of treatment and appearance of the first evidence of improvement depends on the size of dose given. Early clinical evidence of response is the occurrence of diuresis, and this is accompanied by loss of weight and some regression of puffiness. Even earlier, the serum Na^+ level increases if hyponatremia was present initially. Thereafter, pulse rate and pulse pressure increase, appetite improves, and constipation may disappear. Psychomotor activity increases, and the delay in the deep tendon jerks disappears. Hoarseness abates slowly, and changes in skin and hair generally require several months to disappear.

Besides myxedema coma, which is discussed later, there are a few instances in which it seems mandatory to alleviate hypothyroidism rapidly. Patients with severe hypothyroidism withstand acute infections poorly and may descend rapidly

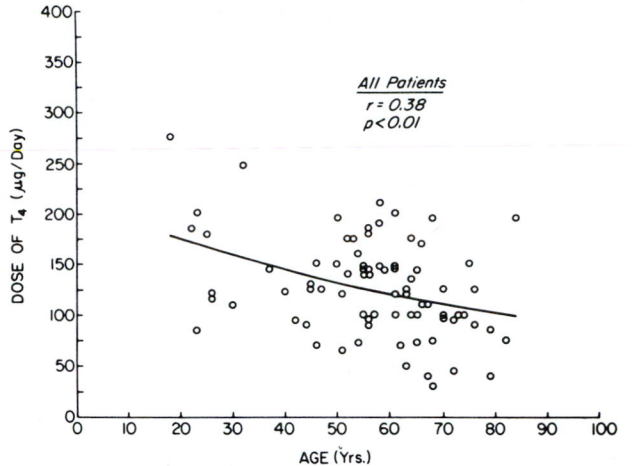

Figure 8–47. Relationship of daily maintenance dose of levothyroxine to age in male and female patients with hypothyroidism. Maintenance dose is that required to lower the serum TSH concentration into the normal range. (From Sawin C, Herman T, Molitch ME, et al. Aging and the thyroid. Decreased requirement for thyroid hormone in older hypothyroid patients. Am J Med 1983; 75:206–209.)

into myxedema coma as a result. In these circumstances, rapid repletion of the peripheral hormone pool is necessary. This can be accomplished by a single intravenous dose of 500 μg of levothyroxine in the average adult. Alternatively, by virtue of its rapid onset of action, liothyronine (25 μg orally every 8 h) can be used if the patient is able to take medication by mouth, as an intravenous preparation is not available. With both regimens, the initial effect is achieved within several hours. Oral therapy with levothyroxine is instituted as soon as possible, as outlined earlier. Because of the possibility that acute increases in metabolic rate will overtax existing pituitary-adrenocortical reserve, supplemental glucocorticoid should be administered. Finally, in view of the tendency of hypothyroid patients to retain water, intravenous fluids should be given with caution.

When hypothyroidism results from administration of iodine or drugs with antithyroid activity, withdrawal of the offending agent usually suffices to relieve both the hypothyroidism and the accompanying goiter.

Infants and Children

In the cretin the critical factor determining eventual intellectual attainment is the age at which adequate treatment with thyroid hormone was begun. The initiation of treatment for infants with congenital hypothyroidism should consist of raising the serum T_4 level to greater than 130 nmol/L (10 μg/dL) as rapidly as possible and maintaining it there for the first 3 to 4 y of life. This is usually accomplished by administering an initial levothyroxine dose of 50 μg/d,[115] which is considerably higher than the adult dose on a weight basis and accords with the higher metabolic clearance of the hormone in the infant. The serum TSH concentration may not normalize completely on this high dose because of an apparent residual reset of the pituitary feedback mechanism.[366] After age 1 to 2, a TSH result in the normal range may be used as an index of optimal therapy in infants and in children, as it is in adults.

Special Aspects of Hypothyroidism

SUBCLINICAL HYPOTHYROIDISM. The term *subclinical hypothyroidism* designates a situation in which an asymptomatic patient has normal free thyroid hormone indices but a slightly elevated TSH level. Other synonyms for this common condition are *mild hypothyroidism, preclinical hypothyroidism, biochemical hypothyroidism,* and *decreased thyroid reserve.* There is a modest elevation of the TSH level in such patients between 5.5 and 15 mU/L. This syndrome is most often seen in patients with Hashimoto disease or with Graves disease after treatment with surgery or radioactive iodine. It is also observed in patients with no evidence of autoimmune thyroid disease other than circulating antithyroid antibodies.[368] Patients with type I diabetes mellitus,[369] primary biliary cirrhosis,[370] and vitiligo[371] are prone to develop subclinical or frank hypothyroidism, as are patients with pernicious anemia[235] and progressive systemic sclerosis.[372]

A number of studies have evaluated the utility of thyroid hormone treatment in such patients. Physiological end points used to judge its effects include measurements of various serum enzymes, systolic time intervals, and psychometric testing, and the effects have been variable. In the most carefully controlled studies, one or another of the physiological or psychological parameters has responded in a positive fashion in about 25% of such patients.[373-375] In one study that employed a double-blind crossover approach, the 4 of 17 women who improved could be differentiated only by a somewhat lower serum free T_3 concentration at the start of the study.[375] Thus, when confronted with this clinical situation, there is no clearly correct approach. It is of interest vis-à-vis the issue of the relative roles of T_4 and T_3 in the regulation of TSH in humans that in virtually all such studies, levothyroxine treatment causes an increase in the free T_4 level, the serum free T_3 level remains constant, and the serum TSH level is suppressed to normal. This is consistent with expectations based on animal studies discussed earlier and on studies of human iodine deficiency and hypothyroidism (see Table 8–10).[65, 86] In the authors' opinion, one factor favoring institution of levothyroxine therapy is the presence of antithyroid microsomal antibodies in significant titers ($>^1/_{1600}$) or the presence of goiter. There is a risk of progression of thyroid dysfunction in patients with Hashimoto disease and, depending on the clinical circumstances, this premonitory sign of thyroid failure may be sufficient justification for initiation of therapy. To be weighed against this are the expense and bother of daily medication, not acceptable to many patients, as well as the possibility that overdosage with levothyroxine may aggravate osteoporosis. If a therapeutic trial is performed, the TSH concentration should be monitored carefully and not be permitted to fall below normal. If no therapy is given, patients should be monitored at intervals of 6 to 12 mo.

METABOLIC INSUFFICIENCY. It is apparent that many of the symptoms of true hypothyroidism are nonspecific. These include mild lassitude, fatigue, slight anemia, constipation, apathy, cold intolerance, menstrual irregularities, loss of hair, and weight gain. For this reason many patients with such complaints have been treated with thyroid hormone. Adequate laboratory documentation of thyroid hormone deficiency is lacking. The response to thyroid hormone therapy is sometimes gratifying, at least initially, but often symptomatic improvement disappears after a time unless the dose is increased. In this way, the total dosage increases progressively until the amounts given exceed those required for complete hormone replacement in frank myxedema. Eventually, even such large doses may fail to alleviate the symptoms. This alone suggests that the symptoms do not arise from deficiency of thyroid hormone. Some patients report that omission of a single dose of thyroid hormone results in a rapid emergence (often within hours) of the previous symptoms and that these are equally rapidly relieved by a single dose. These responses are inconsistent with the time of onset and duration of action of thyroid hormones. Thus thyroid hormone therapy should be avoided in all patients for whom there is no biochemical documentation of impaired thyroid function. Furthermore, even in patients with preclinical or subclinical hypothyroidism shown by biochemical tests, symptoms may be far out of proportion to these abnormalities. It is unwise to raise the patient's expectations regarding the relief of severe symptoms by treatment of mild biochemical abnormalities.

WITHDRAWAL OF THYROID HORMONE THERAPY. Physicians are frequently confronted with patients in whom the diagnosis of hypothyroidism, often mild, has already been made, and replacement therapy has been given. In this circumstance, it is impossible to determine from clinical or laboratory findings whether thyroid hormone replacement is truly required, because a normal thyroid would have been suppressed. Often, a strong indication that the patient is not truly hypothyroid can be obtained from the nature of the initial complaints or from peculiarities in the response to treatment, as already described. The best way to assess whether levothyroxine therapy is required in such patients is to reduce the levothyroxine dose to 50% of the replacement value (about 50 μg) and re-evaluate thyroid function after 6 to 8 wk. If there has been no significant increase in TSH concentration during that period, levothyroxine is completely withdrawn and blood tests are repeated 4 and 8 wk later. After withdrawal of prolonged replacement therapy, patients with an intrinsically normal hypothalamic-pituitary-thyroid axis have a return of thyroid function to normal over a 6-wk interval. If levothyroxine is completely withdrawn from such patients, the TSH level is reduced for the first 2 to 3 wk despite a decrease in the FT_4I to borderline low values. As time progresses, TSH becomes detectable and serum T_4 and T_3 concentrations rise to normal. This pattern of recovery suggests that prolonged replacement results in depletion of pituitary TSH that is reversible when therapy is withdrawn. On the other hand, in patients with a true but modest impairment of thyroid reserve, a transient period of elevated TSH production may follow the discontinuation of thyroid hormone.

EMERGENT SURGERY IN THE HYPOTHYROID PATIENT. The perioperative course of patients with untreated hypothyroidism has been compared with that of euthyroid individuals in several studies. In general, such patients were not recognized to be hypothyroid at the time of surgery or had significant illnesses requiring surgery despite the presence of clinically significant hypothyroidism. Most of these patients have had remarkably few complications. In one series[376] there were higher frequencies of perioperative hypotension, ileus, and central nervous system disturbances in hypothyroid patients, and patients with significant infections were less frequently febrile than were euthyroid controls.[377] Other complications possibly related to hypothyroidism were delayed recovery from anesthesia and abnormal hemostasis, possibly the consequence of an acquired form of von Willebrand disease that has been described in some patients with hypothyroidism.[336] This condition was reversible after administration of thyroid hormone. One may conclude from these studies that emergent surgery should not be postponed in hypothyroid patients, although one should monitor such patients more rigorously for evidence of carbon dioxide retention, bleeding, and infection as well as for water retention because of the recognized pathophysiological changes that occur in this condition. These results are also relevant to the issue of the treatment of individuals with symptomatic coronary artery disease in hypothyroidism. Considering the lack of significant increase in perioperative complications in the hypothyroid patient, the option of surgery for remediable coronary artery lesions is open to hypothyroid individuals without the risk of a myocardial infarction in association with restitution of the euthyroid state (see later).

ANGINA AND HYPOTHYROIDISM. Patients with hypothyroidism and angina or other symptoms of coronary artery insufficiency present a special problem in terms of therapy. Replacement of thyroid hormone in such patients may cause improvement or worsening of coronary symptoms, and it is difficult to predict which will occur in a particular patient. Some decades ago, it was noted that the deliberate induction of hypothyroidism caused relief of symptoms of angina in patients who were otherwise incapacitated with these symptoms. However, this relief was at the expense of the symptomatic hypothyroidism that ensued. Accordingly, the clinician confronted with the combination of angina and hypothyroidism must consider the possibility that coronary artery blood flow is already severely restricted. For this reason, it has been advocated that such patients have angiographic evaluation of the coronary circulation even before levothyroxine replacement is attempted. This view is supported by the fact that in several retrospective series, patients with surgically remediable coronary artery obstruction survived the operative procedure despite hypothyroidism. The coronary revascularization permitted the subsequent administration of physiological replacement doses and the reinstitution of normal thyroid status.[378, 379] Such an approach is especially appropriate for patients who cannot receive full thyroid hormone replacement or in whom thyroid replacement leads to an exacerbation of symptoms of coronary insufficiency. Medical management of such patients can be extremely difficult.

Myxedema Coma

Myxedema coma is the ultimate stage of severe long-standing hypothyroidism. This state, which invariably affects the elderly patient, occurs most commonly during the winter months and is associated with a high mortality rate. It is usually, but not always, accompanied by a subnormal temperature, values as low as 23.3°C having been recorded. Because the ordinary clinical thermometer is graduated only to 32.4 or 34.5°C, the true depth of hypothermia may not be appreciated. The external manifestations of severe myxedema, as well as bradycardia and severe hypotension, are invariably present. The characteristic delay in deep tendon reflexes may be lacking because the patient is often areflexic. Epileptic seizures may accompany the comatose state.

Although the pathogenesis of myxedema coma is not known, several factors predispose to its development: exposure to cold, infection, trauma, and central nervous system depressants. Alveolar hypoventilation, leading to carbon dioxide retention and narcosis, and dilutional hyponatremia resembling that seen during inappropriate secretion of antidiuretic hormone are common accompaniments and may contribute to the clinical state.

From the foregoing, it appears that the diagnosis of myxedema coma should be obvious. This is not the case. Elderly patients may resemble patients with myxedema, and after a brain stem infarction they may be both comatose and hypothermic. In addition, hypothermia of any cause, most commonly exposure to cold and renal insufficiency, may induce physiological alterations suggestive of myxedema, including a delay in relaxation of deep tendon reflexes. The importance of difficulty in diagnosing myxedema coma is that a delay in therapy worsens the prognosis. Consequently the diagnosis should be made on clinical grounds, and therapy should be initiated without awaiting the results of confirmatory tests, such as the serum T_4 concentration.

Treatment consists of administration of thyroid hormone and of attempts to correct the associated physiological disturbances. Because of the sluggish circulation and severe hypometabolism, absorption of therapeutic agents from the gut or from subcutaneous or intramuscular sites is unpredictable; hence, medications should be administered intravenously if possible. Thyroid hormone is best given as single intravenous dose of 500 µg of levothyroxine. This serves to replete the peripheral hormone pool and is often followed by some improvement within several hours. Daily doses of 100 µg intravenously are given there after. Hydrocortisone (100 mg daily) should also be administered because of the possibility of associated adrenocortical insufficiency, especially as the metabolic rate increases. Hypotonic fluids should not be given because of the danger of water intoxication in syndrome of inappropriate antidiuretic hormone (SIADH) and reduced renal perfusion. Hypertonic saline and glucose may be required to alleviate severe dilutional hyponatremia and the occasional hypoglycemia. A critical element in therapy is support of respiratory function by means of assisted ventilation and controlled oxygen administration. External warming should be avoided because it may lead to vascular collapse, but further heat loss should be prevented by blankets. An increase in temperature is seen within 24 h in response to levothyroxine. General measures applicable to the comatose patient should be undertaken, such as frequent turning, prevention of aspiration, and attention to fecal impaction and urinary retention. Finally, the physician should be alert to the presence of coexisting disease, such as infection and cardiac or cerebrovascular disease. It should be recalled that myxedematous patients are often afebrile despite a significant infection. Ideally, management should be undertaken in an intensive care unit. As soon as the patient is able to take medication by mouth, treatment with oral levothyroxine should be instituted.

Although myxedema coma carries a poor prognosis, survivals have been achieved with the therapeutic regimen just outlined.[380]

SIMPLE OR NONTOXIC GOITER: DIFFUSE AND MULTINODULAR

Simple or nontoxic goiter may be defined as any thyroid enlargement that is not associated with hyper- or hypothyroidism and that does not result from an inflammatory or neoplastic process. The term is usually restricted to the form that occurs sporadically, i.e., in regions that are not the locus of endemic goiter. Although useful to connote the presence of the characteristics just noted, the term simple goiter may itself be too simplistic because the disorder can be a result of different underlying abnormalities.

Pathogenesis and Pathophysiology

Any comprehensive theory concerning the pathogenesis of simple goiter must take into account the possibility that the cause may differ from one patient to another and must also explain its natural history. Diffuse symmetrical goiters tend to progress in size but may regress when TSH is suppressed. Multinodular goiters are structurally and functionally heterogeneous and tend to develop areas of functional autonomy.

The traditionally held theory concerning the pathogenesis of simple goiter suggests that it represents a response to any of several factors that impair the efficiency of the thyroid in manufacturing adequate quantities of hormone. When such factors are operative, hypersecretion of TSH leads to stimulation of thyroid growth and increase in the activity of the processes concerned with hormone biosynthesis that are

capable of response. As a consequence of the increase in thyroid mass and unit functional activity, a normal rate of hormone secretion is restored and the patient is eumetabolic but goitrous. Thus the disorder differs from goitrous hypothyroidism only in degree and is presumed to result from the same etiological factors as those discussed in the previous section. This sequence is evident in some patients with iodine deficiency and in others who develop goiter in response to specific agents. For example, some patients develop goiter, with or without hypothyroidism, when given lithium. Goiter regresses when iodine is administered (if iodine deficiency is the cause), when lithium or another offending agent is withdrawn, or if suppressive doses of exogenous thyroid hormone are administered. In most patients with nontoxic goiter, however, no extrinsic goitrogenic factor can be identified. As a consequence, it has been generally thought that the cause is some intrinsic, probably inborn, abnormality in thyroid hormone synthesis akin to one of those that produce goitrous hypothyroidism. In some cases, moderately severe defects of this type can be detected, as by the perchlorate discharge test, but more often no abnormality can be demonstrated. In such instances, it has been presumed that the abnormality is too mild to be detected by the relatively insensitive in vivo techniques available.

This concept of the pathogenesis of nontoxic goiter is inconsistent with the demonstration that the serum TSH concentration is not increased in most patients with nontoxic goiter.[381] Nonetheless, a participatory role of TSH in the maintenance of goiter is indicated by the regression of goiter that sometimes follows administration of suppressive doses of thyroid hormone. Several possible mechanisms may accommodate these seemingly divergent findings. The one with the greatest experimental support derives from the observation that in hypophysectomized rats the response of thyroid weight to standard doses of TSH is augmented by previous thyroid iodine depletion.[382] Hence, any factor that impairs normal iodine usage may lead to gradual development of goiter in response to normal concentrations of TSH. A second possibility is that the increase in serum TSH concentration is small and therefore not readily detected by the radioimmunoassay methods generally available. Finally, the primary goitrogenic stimulus may no longer be present at the time of study, and the residual normal TSH concentration may maintain but not initiate the goiter.

An alternative concept that would explain thyroid growth in nontoxic goiter has been proposed. In some patients there may exist a class of "thyroid growth immunoglobulins" (TGIs) that, like TSH, stimulate growth but do not appreciably stimulate thyroid adenylate cyclase activity, as do TSH and Graves IgG; this might explain why the thyroid is not hyperfunctioning. Differences in TGIs might also account for differences in thyroid size among patients with Graves disease and explain atrophy of the thyroid in nongoitrous hypothyroidism. TGIs and their inhibitory counterparts are detected by one or another index of growth, such as incorporation of labeled thymidine, increase in DNA content, or increase in cell number in cultured thyroid cell systems. Patients in whom "autoimmune nontoxic goiter" is thought most likely are those in whom other autoimmune phenomena are present in themselves or their families and those in whom goiter recurs after subtotal thyroidectomy. The observations in support of this concept are few, however, and more study is required.[383, 384]

Neither TSH nor TGI would explain why long-standing nontoxic goiter becomes nodular and why it is characterized by anatomical and functional heterogeneity and by functional autonomy. These characteristics have been assumed to result either from prolonged hyperstimulation by TSH or from repeated cycles of hyperstimulation and involution.

Hyperstimulation or cycles of hyperstimulation and involution could lead to the emergence of areas of hyperplasia, possibly associated with functional autonomy, coupled with areas of involution (exhaustion atrophy), the whole made more heterogeneous by localized hemorrhage, fibrosis, and sometimes calcification. Another concept has been introduced, largely on the basis of autoradiographic and clinical studies of normal, nontoxic, and toxic multinodular goiters.[290] Early in the disorder, areas of microheterogeneity of structure and function are intermixed and include areas of functional autonomy and small areas of focal hemorrhage. Indeed, as judged from the presence of scattered foci of persistent radioiodine uptake in the thyroids of patients given suppressive doses of thyroid hormone before surgery, some cells with functional autonomy are present in normal thyroid gland. Thus, in addition to the role of variations in the thyroid microcirculation, heterogeneity may result from clonal differences among the cells that give rise to thyroid follicles, some being more and some less responsive to external stimulation by TSH and some being autonomous at the outset. Individual responses to TSH might also vary from clone to clone in respect to iodine accumulation, exocytosis of thyroglobulin, or resorption of colloid. This concept implies that the basis of anatomical and functional heterogeneity exists within the thyroid at the outset of the disease and is exaggerated by prolonged stimulation.

Evidently, with the passage of time, the quantity of functionally autonomous tissue is sufficient to suppress the TSH-secretory mechanism. Initially this has been manifested by subnormal responses to TRH or lack of thyroid suppression during administration of exogenous hormone.[381] Presumably such abnormalities would now be recognizable by a suppression of the basal TSH concentration to less than 0.5 mU/L. Ultimately, autonomous hyperfunction may be sufficient to produce thyrotoxicosis, or thyrotoxicosis may supervene only when the patient is exposed to an iodine load. For this reason, patients with nontoxic multinodular goiter should not be given medications that contain iodine and should be observed after radiological procedures that involve administration of iodinated contrast media. Some investigators advocate administering antithyroid agents to patients with nodular goiter who are to receive agents containing iodine; this seems a reasonable suggestion, especially in areas of iodine deficiency, where jodbasedow is especially prone to occur.

Nontoxic goiter has a female preponderance (7 to 9:1) and seems to occur more commonly during adolescence or pregnancy. The pathogenetic relationship of these events to the development of goiter is unknown. In some patients, the goiter that appears at these times later regresses; in others, it persists. Patients often have the impression that their thyroid enlarges during times of emotional stress or during the menses, but this is not well documented. During prolonged follow-up of a group of patients with nontoxic adolescent goiter, one of the authors observed that diffuse toxic goiter supervened with high frequency, in some cases even when suppressive doses of thyroid hormone were being administered. This suggests that some varieties of nontoxic diffuse goiter may be precursors of Graves disease. Heredity appears to play a role in the genesis of nontoxic goiter; this is evident in statistical studies and in particular families.

Histopathology

The histopathological picture of nontoxic goiter from its initial diffuse form to its late multinodular stage is similar to that described for endemic goiter in the preceding section (Fig. 8–48).

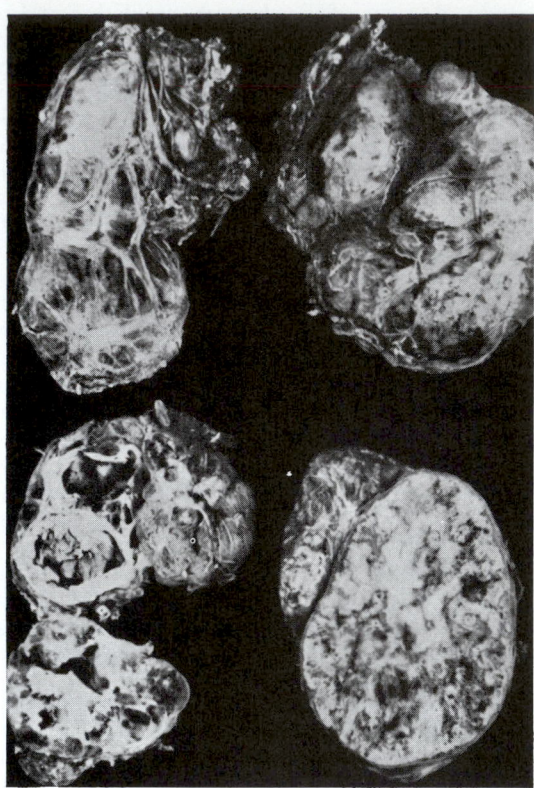

Figure 8–48. Outer and cut surface of a nontoxic nodular goiter observed by patient for 15 y. Note variations in size and structure of the nodules; there are thick areas of fibrous tissue, flecks of calcium, scattered areas of thyroid tissue, cysts, and small hemorrhages.

Clinical Picture

The clinical features of nontoxic goiter are those that result from thyroid enlargement. Most commonly, the effect either is merely disfiguring or is felt as a tightening of garments worn about the neck. With larger goiters, displacement or compression of the esophagus or trachea may occur, leading to dysphagia, a choking sensation, and inspiratory stridor. Narrowing of the thoracic inlet may compromise the venous return from the head, neck, and upper limbs sufficiently to produce venous engorgement. This obstruction is accentuated when the patient's arms are raised (Pemberton sign); dizziness and even syncope may result. Compression of the recurrent laryngeal nerve leading to hoarseness suggests carcinoma rather than nontoxic goiter. Hemorrhage into a nodule or cyst produces acute, painful enlargement locally and, if appropriately situated, can enhance or induce obstructive symptoms.

Laboratory Tests

In patients with nontoxic goiter, serum T_4 and T_3 concentrations are within the normal range, but the T_3/T_4 ratio is often increased, perhaps reflecting defective iodination of thyroglobulin. Serum thyroglobulin concentrations are increased in the majority.[385] The RAIU is usually normal but may be increased, because of either mild iodine deficiency or a biosynthetic defect. In patients with long-standing multinodular goiter, functional autonomy may be reflected in diminished or absent responsiveness of the serum TSH concentration to TRH or a reduced basal TSH concentration.

Differential Diagnosis

The differential diagnosis of nontoxic goiter can be considered from both functional and anatomical aspects. As indicated earlier, the same factors that lead to goitrous hypothyroidism can, if less severe, cause nontoxic goiter, consequently, some patients with nontoxic goiter prove to be slightly hypothyroid. On the other hand, when multinodularity has developed, foci of autonomous function may appear. Thus in multinodular goiter, the spectrum of function can range from clinical euthyroidism with intact regulatory control, through euthyroidism with some degree of functional autonomy, to thyrotoxicosis (toxic multinodular goiter).

From the anatomical standpoint, the diffuse stage of nontoxic goiter resembles the thyroid of either Graves or Hashimoto disease. If the Graves disease is not in an actively thyrotoxic phase and if the ocular manifestations are lacking, there is no way to differentiate the two disorders except to demonstrate the presence of TRAb in the serum. Diffuse nontoxic goiter is sometimes difficult to differentiate from Hashimoto disease. Functional patterns in the two may be similar. The thyroid of Hashimoto disease is usually more firm and more irregular. Demonstration of high titers of antithyroid antibodies would indicate Hashimoto disease.

In its multinodular stage, nontoxic goiter may suggest thyroid carcinoma. The approach to differentiating between the two is discussed in the section dealing with thyroid neoplasms.

Treatment

The treatment of nontoxic goiter depends on its cause and stage of development. If a pharmacological goitrogen such as phenylbutazone or lithium is being given, its removal will suffice. If this is not possible, levothyroxine may be administered in replacement doses to interrupt the endogenous thyroid stimulation. Because iodine deficiency is not a common cause, at least in the United States, administration of iodine is generally ineffective, and its use is to be deplored in view of its capacity to induce thyrotoxicosis. As the etiology of goiter is usually obscure, the most useful therapy is thyroid hormone administration, which will be successful only if TSH secretion is still present. Therefore an accurate assessment of basal TSH must be made before initiation of treatment. In younger patients with a diffuse goiter, the serum TSH level is often normal or somewhat increased, and therefore a trial with replacement doses of thyroid hormone as described earlier is indicated. However, nontoxic goiter, particularly of the nodular form, usually presents in women over the age of 50. The multinodular goiter common in this age group is often associated with a TSH concentration less than 0.5 mU/L even though serum thyroid hormone levels may still be in the normal range. In such individuals further suppression of TSH is ineffective and may lead to thyrotoxicosis resulting from a combination of exogenous and endogenous thyroid hormone. Before instituting treatment, one must determine that the serum TSH level is greater than 0.5 mU/L. If an appropriate TSH assay is not available, a TRH test should be done to demonstrate that releasable TSH is still present in the pituitary gland and, by inference, basal TSH secretion is normal or nearly so. Furthermore, measurement of the basal TSH level is useful because a reduced level may be the first sign of impending hyperthyroidism related to autonomous function of one or more nodules. In such patients, depending on the configuration of the goiter, amelioration of local symptoms can be achieved by radioactive iodine therapy. Because such problems most commonly occur in the elderly, radiation-related acute thyroid hormone discharge from the gland must be considered as a rare but possible complication of treatment. If transient hyperthyroidism is unacceptable, as in a patient with coronary artery disease, pretreatment with antithyroid drugs should be carried out. The thyroid uptake should be determined and a scan should be performed to assess the intrathyroidal localization of function. Because of the heterogeneity of thyroidal iodine uptake, the dose of radioiodine required for treatment of the multinodular goiter is generally about twice that required for Graves disease. Thus administration of a dose designed to result in about 370 to 444 MBq (10 to 12 mCi) in the thyroid gland at 24 h is usually prescribed. The 24-h radioiodine uptake in such glands is often lower than in Graves disease, and outpatient administration may be proscribed because the Nuclear Regulatory Commission does not permit amounts greater than 1.1 GBq (30 mCi) to be given to outpatients. Because there is rarely a need for rapid treatment, administration of the radioiodine in divided doses is acceptable for most patients.

If a therapeutic trial with thyroid hormone replacement is undertaken in patients with nontoxic goiter and normal TSH concentrations, the quantity of the thyroid hormone administered should be such that TSH concentrations are not reduced to those consistent with thyrotoxicosis. In the elderly patient, a dose of 50 μg of thyroxine may be sufficient to achieve an acceptable degree of TSH suppression (0.2 to 0.5 mU/L). In addition, the possible exacerbation of osteoporosis with excessive thyroid hormone therapy must be kept in mind at all times. On balance, medical therapy of nontoxic goiter in the patient whose TSH level is not greater than 1 mU/L is usually unsuccessful, and the risk/benefit ratio is generally too high to justify an aggressive approach.

Surgery for simple nontoxic goiter is physiologically unsound because it further restricts the ability of the thyroid to meet hormone requirements. Nevertheless, surgery may become necessary because of persistence of obstructive symptoms despite a trial of exogenous thyroid hormone. Surgery is sometimes indicated because a carcinoma is thought to be present in a multinodular goiter. It should never be performed for prophylaxis of carcinoma, however. Surgery should always be followed by full replacement therapy with thyroid hormone to inhibit regrowth of the goiter.

THYROID NEOPLASMS

The subject of thyroid neoplasms has received attention far beyond its importance as a cause of morbidity in the general population. In the 1970s the incidence of thyroid cancer was about 36 new cases per million population per year, and the death rate was about 9 per million per year. There are, however, several reasons why diagnosis and management have been a focus for much concern. To begin with, thyroid cancer usually presents as an asymptomatic thyroid nodule in a euthyroid patient, and nontoxic nodular goiter is a common disorder among the adult population of the United States, especially women. Estimates place its prevalence, as judged from clinical examination, at about 4%.[386] This, too, would pose no problem were it not for the fact that nodularity of the thyroid is a nonspecific manifestation of a variety of thyroid diseases with differing implications for the patient's ultimate well-being. Further, in the absence of a histological specimen, there is no means of differentiating benign from malignant nodules, and, until the widespread acceptance of needle biopsy, this usually required excisional biopsy. Nonetheless, clinical criteria for the suspicion of malignancy have been sufficiently good, and selection of patients for surgery sufficiently reliable, that surgical series have been biased to reveal a frequency of thyroid cancer in patients operated on that is apparently higher than that present in the entire population of patients with nodular thyroids. Finally, the frequency of thyroid cancer has increased, probably by about 50% in 25, because of the emergence of thyroid cancer after a long latent period from previous radiation of the head and neck areas for a variety of reasons.

The proper diagnosis and management of thyroid cancer have also been controversial (and remain so) because of variations in the biological behavior of the tumors, some being nonaggressive; because excisional biopsy, although required for diagnosis, was inherently a therapeutic measure; and because there was not a sufficiently large series of patients with various thyroid tumors treated in different ways to permit an analysis of the optimal mode of therapy for each. Thus the literature on this subject reflected considerable ignorance. Fortunately, many of the problems cited above are being resolved and the topic is less vexing than formerly. The authors' approach to diagnosis and management of the nodular thyroid gland is presented later in this section. First, it is necessary to consider the characteristics of that variety of thyroid nodule of greatest concern, the thyroid neoplasm.

Benign Neoplasms

Benign neoplasms of the thyroid are termed *adenomas*. The problem of their etiology and the biological properties that cause their behavior to differ from that of normal tissue, on the one hand, or of malignant neoplasms, on the other, are unknown. Nevertheless, adenomas have the properties of being well encapsulated, of not invading adjacent tissues or metastasizing to noncontiguous areas, of displaying few mitoses, and, in the case of endocrine adenomas, of being at least relatively free of the usual homeostatic restraints on growth and function. The most clear-cut lesions of the thyroid that display these properties are those arising in glands that are otherwise entirely normal. Much of the confusion concerning thyroid nodules stems from the fact that lesions that are anatomically similar or identical (differing architecturally from surrounding tissue and separated therefrom by fibrous tissue) are found in the late stage of nontoxic multinodular goiter. Because of this similarity, they are often termed adenomas, and the disorder itself is termed *adenomatous goiter*. In most instances, it is not known whether these are true adenomas in the basic biological sense and whether they arise de novo or as a consequence of the hyperplastic stimulus that is thought to underlie the pathogenesis of nontoxic goiter. Lacking such basic biological criteria, the term adenoma, in relation to a normal or an otherwise diseased gland, should be applied to lesions that display the anatomical properties just described, together with evidence of some degree of autonomy of growth and function. A further source of confusion is that, in the case of thyroid neoplasms, the architectures of benign and malignant lesions may be so similar that even careful histopathological examination fails to reveal local evidence of malignancy, although the tumor displays evidence of malignancy by its clinical course. Finally, as with neoplasms in other organs, it is uncertain whether benign neoplasms of the thyroid gland ever undergo malignant transformation.

The clearly defined benign neoplasms of the thyroid can be classified according to their histopathological characteristics.

Histopathology

Typical examples of the following tumors are illustrated in Figure 8–49.

EMBRYONAL ADENOMA. Here, the histopathological appearance resembles that of the embryonic thyroid before the development of follicles in that the cells are closely packed, forming a cordlike or trabecular pattern. For this reason, the lesion is sometimes termed a *trabecular adenoma*.

FETAL ADENOMA. This lesion is characterized by an architecture that resembles the fetal thyroid in its stage of early follicle formation. The cells are arranged in a tubular pattern, but colloid is scant or absent.

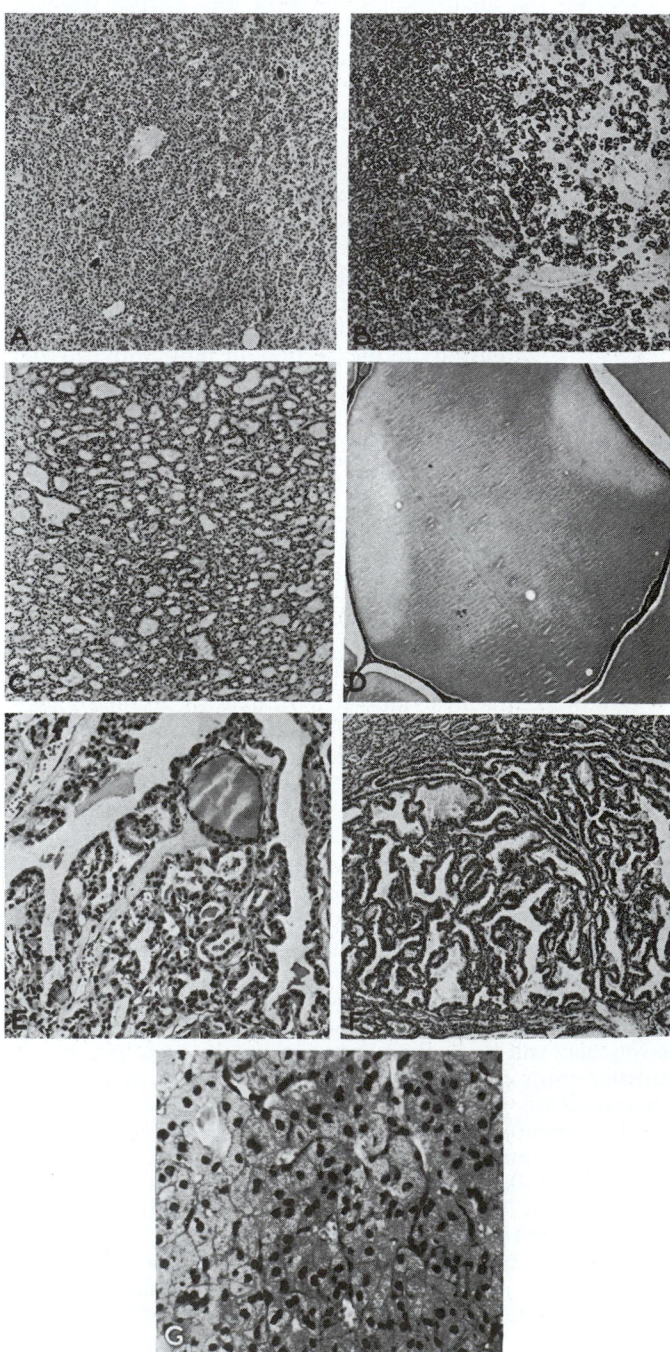

Figure 8–49. Thyroid adenomas. *A,* Embryonal (×80). *B,* Fetal (×80). *C,* Microfollicular (×80). *D,* Macrofollicular (×60). *E* and *F,* Papillary cystadenomas (×40). *G,* Hürthle cell (×450).

MICROFOLLICULAR ADENOMA. This lesion is composed of small, closely packed follicles lined by a cuboidal epithelium and containing little colloid.

MACROFOLLICULAR ADENOMA. Here well-formed follicles are present. These are usually large, well filled with colloid, and lined by a flat epithelium. Small follicles and areas of epithelial hyperplasia are often present. Another term applied to this lesion is *colloid adenoma*.

PAPILLARY CYSTADENOMA. This lesion, although classified as an adenoma, is typically unencapsulated, merges into the adjacent tissue, and often cannot be distinguished on histopathologic grounds from low-grade papillary carcinoma. It is composed of columnar epithelium that is thrown into folds, forming papillary projection with connective tissue stalks and cyst-like cavities. Follicular elements may be present to a varying degree.

HÜRTHLE CELL ADENOMA. This rare lesion is composed of large, pale, acidophilic cells that are usually arranged in a trabecular pattern. The granular appearance of these cells derives from the large numbers of mitochondria present within the cytoplasm.

The foregoing classification suggests that adenomas are uniform in structure, but in fact their architecture is often variegated; macrofollicular, microfollicular, and fetal elements are often found in the same lesion. In addition, multiple adenomas of different histopathological types are frequently present in the same gland, often in opposite lobes.

Clinical Picture and Laboratory Tests

The chief importance of thyroid adenomas lies in the need to differentiate them from carcinoma and in their ability in some instances to produce sufficient hormone to suppress the remaining thyroid tissue and induce a thyrotoxic state. Some other features merit consideration. Most thyroid adenomas are predominantly follicular in type and are unable to accumulate and retain radioactive iodine. Studies of benign nodular tissue have indicated that this defect is a consequence of loss of the trapping mechanism in cells that are in every other respect capable of responding as normal tissue.[387] If a thyroid scintiscan is performed, about 95% of such benign tumors do not concentrate TcO_4^- or radioiodine sufficiently well to be visualized. They are therefore referred to as "cold," and this test does not differentiate them from malignant tumors. The rare adenomas that concentrate radioiodine and organify it to form T_4 usually present as an area of increased uptake, but the degree of suppression of the surrounding thyroid tissue depends on the size and function of the nodule. In the earliest stages, the serum thyroid hormone and TSH levels are normal and the functioning adenoma is visible as an area of increased uptake on the scan. As the nodule enlarges, increase in T_4 and T_3 secretion and suppression of TSH are accompanied by loss of function in the surrounding normal tissue on a thyroid scan. With further enlargement of the nodule, usually to 4 cm or more in diameter, serum thyroid hormone concentrations become elevated and the patient develops clinical signs.[388] At this stage the lesion may properly be referred to as a "hot" nodule, as opposed to the earlier situation in which the nodule is "warm" and has not as yet caused thyrotoxicosis. As discussed earlier under Thyrotoxicosis, the choice of treatment for the toxic adenoma is influenced by the age of the patient, but radioiodine is generally used (see earlier).

Therapy of the nonfunctioning adenoma consists of suppression of TSH, because the tumor cells do synthesize TSH receptors and respond to TSH by elevation in adenylate cyclase activity.[387] A dose of levothyroxine is given that reduces TSH to about 0.2 to 0.5 mU/L. The patient is followed at 4- to 6-mo intervals, and if a reduction in size occurs therapy is maintained for several years. These individuals are followed at 6-mo intervals with documentation of TSH suppression and clinical evaluation of the nodule and of potential systemic symptoms. The size of these nodules can be monitored by palpation or by ultrasound if palpation is difficult. The proportion of nodules that will be reduced in size over 6 mo of levothyroxine therapy varies from series to series.[389, 390] Most have documented that decreases will occur in some patients and a therapeutic trial seems to be the logical approach to such patients. The diagnosis of follicular adenoma is usually made by fine-needle aspiration cytology, which is described later.

Malignant Neoplasms

Virtually all malignant neoplasms of the thyroid are epithelial in origin and hence are carcinomas. Two general types occur, those arising from follicular epithelium and those arising from parafollicular (C cell) elements. Rarely, the thyroid is the seat of a metastatic deposit or of a fibrosarcoma or lymphosarcoma, both of which are highly malignant. Metastases of extrathyroid cancers to the thyroid are rare but occasionally present a problem in diagnosis.

Thyroid carcinoma is the most common endocrine malignancy and yet is a rare cancer, accounting for only 1% or so of new cases of invasive cancer in a given year. The American Cancer Society estimated that in 1987 there were 10,000 to 11,000 new cases of thyroid cancer and about 1100 deaths in the United States were attributed to this condition. These estimates refer to the incidence of clinically significant thyroid cancer. Careful pathological sectioning of thyroid glands removed at autopsy shows that anywhere from 1 to 30% of apparently normal thyroid glands contain microscopic areas that meet the criteria for papillary carcinoma. Whether such lesions would ever become clinically apparent is impossible to determine. Eighty percent of patients with thyroid cancer are between the ages of 25 and 65. The prognosis for patients with thyroid cancer varies from virtually no associated morbidity to an extremely aggressive form of tumor and is related to the histological picture. Fortunately, the most aggressive tumors are the least common and occur most often in older patients.

Carcinoma of Follicular Epithelium: Histopathology and Clinical Features

Various classifications have been proposed, but the one most commonly used is that of Woolner and associates, which demarcates three categories of carcinoma of follicular origin: papillary, follicular, and anaplastic (Fig. 8–50).[391] A fourth category, that of medullary carcinoma with amyloid stroma, is discussed separately because of its parafollicular origin and distinctive manifestations.

PAPILLARY CARCINOMA. In most series, carcinoma that is either purely or predominantly papillary in structure is the most common, accounting for about 50 to 70% of all thyroid carcinomas. By definition, any carcinoma with papillary elements is included in this group even though follicular elements may dominate the microscopic appearance of the tumor or its metastasis. Papillary carcinoma may occur at any age but is seen more frequently in children and young adults than are the other types of thyroid malignancy; almost one half of the cases occur before the age of 40 (Fig. 8–51). Women are affected two to three times more commonly than men. Young patients with this disease sometimes give a history of having received x-ray therapy during childhood for cervical lymphadenitis or thymic enlargement, suggesting

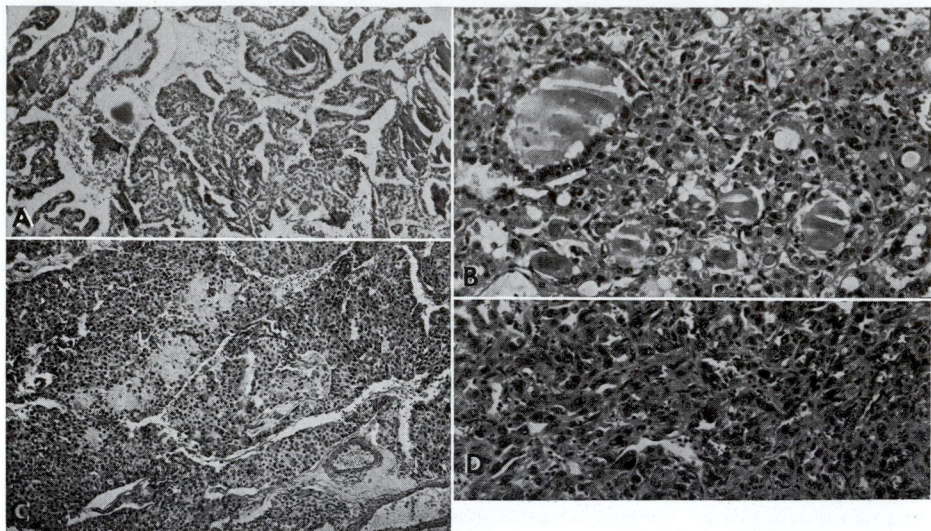

Figure 8–50. Thyroid carcinomas. *A,* Papillary carcinoma. *B,* Follicular carcinoma. *C,* Medullary carcinoma with amyloid stroma. *D,* Anaplastic carcinoma. (From Hazard JB, Hawk WA, Crile G. Medullary [solid] carcinoma of the thyroid; a clinicopathologic entity. J Clin Endocrinol Metab 1959; 19:152–161. © 1959, The Endocrine Society.)

that radiation in the vicinity of the thyroid gland may play a pathogenetic role. In general, papillary carcinoma is the slowest growing of all thyroid carcinomas, often remaining localized to the thyroid gland for many years. It tends to spread via the intraglandular lymphatics from its primary site to other parts of the thyroid and to the pericapsular and regional lymph nodes, where it may remain localized for years. Sometimes, the metastases in the cervical lymph nodes so overshadow the primary lesion that their true nature is overlooked. In the past, such lesions were thought to arise from the fourth pharyngeal pouch; these were called lateral aberrant thyroids. Hematogenous spread to distant sites such as lung is uncommon. The growth of papillary carcinoma is thought by some to depend partly on TSH stimulation,

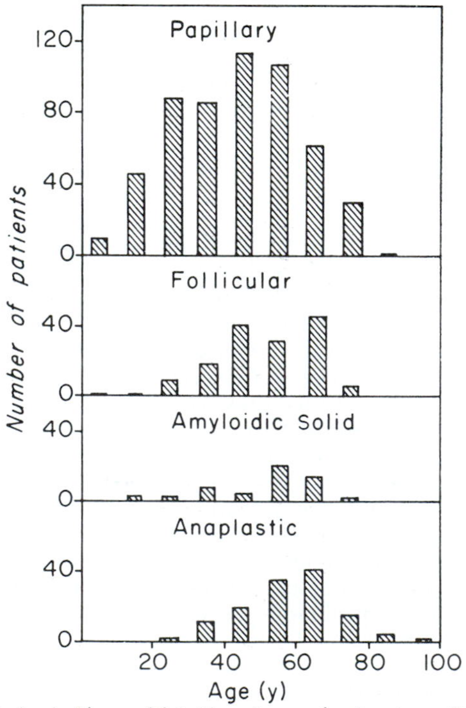

because administration of suppressive doses of thyroid hormone sometimes leads to regression of metastases from a primary lesion that was predominantly papillary in type. However, most papillary carcinomas contain follicular elements, and the metastases may be composed predominantly of the latter. In vitro studies, however, have demonstrated distinct responses of papillary carcinoma to TSH in terms of parameters such as adenylate cyclase activation or cyclic AMP formation. However, when compared with the surrounding normal tissue, the papillary carcinoma lesions are less responsive.[392] In contrast, in adenomas the TSH response of the intracellular second messengers is normal or enhanced.[387]

Papillary carcinoma has a tendency to become more malignant with advancing age; indeed, the highly malignant anaplastic carcinomas may not arise de novo but may develop from pre-existing low-grade papillary or follicular carcinomas. The age of the patient appears to be one of the most important factors in determining the prognosis of papillary carcinoma. Whereas the prognosis is excellent in young adults, in children younger than 5 y of age metastatic lymph node and pulmonary involvement is not uncommon at the time of initial presentation. Between 30 and 40% of individuals of all ages with papillary carcinoma have metastatic cervical nodes at the time of the original surgery, but the presence of positive nodes does not alter the prognosis either for recurrence or for death from thyroid cancer. In one study of 856 patients, only 6.5% died as a result of this condition over a 25-y follow-up period.[393] The factors associated with a higher risk of death are age greater than 50, male sex, a presenting lesion greater than 4 cm in diameter, extension of the primary thyroid tumor through the thyroid capsule, presence of distant metastatic lesions (outside the neck), and absence of histological evidence of Hashimoto thyroiditis in the surrounding gland. The cause of death from thyroid cancer is usually metastatic pulmonary disease, obstruction of the trachea or esophagus, or metastatic disease of the brain or spinal cord.

Grossly, the carcinoma varies in size and is usually unencapsulated. On histopathological examination, it is composed of columnar epithelium that is thrown into folds, forming papillary projections with connective tissue stalks. There is frequently a mixed papillary and follicular pattern, the former predominating. Occasionally, there are foci of large cells with well-defined nuclei and pale, acidophilic cytoplasm (Hürthle cells). Clear nuclear inclusions and grooved nuclei are typical. Concentrically layered deposits

Figure 8–51. Age incidence of thyroid carcinoma of various types. (From data of Woolner LB, Beahrs OH, Black BM, et al. Classification and prognosis of thyroid carcinoma. A study of 885 cases observed in a thirty-year period. Am J Surg 1961; 102:354–387.)

of calcium (psammoma bodies) are commonly found. There may be gross or microscopic foci of carcinoma in other parts of the glands, resulting from spread via the intraglandular lymphatics.

Clinically, papillary carcinoma usually appears either as an asymptomatic nodule in an otherwise normal thyroid or as an enlargement of the regional lymph nodes, sometimes without a palpable thyroid nodule. Invasion of adjacent structures and distant metastases are late manifestations.

Because papillary carcinoma accumulates iodine less efficiently than does the surrounding normal thyroid tissue, it will appear as a cold area in the thyroid scintiscan, provided that it is large enough to allow resolution by the scanner (>0.5 cm) and is not surrounded by a large amount of functioning tissue (see Fig. 8–24). Radiological examination of the neck may disclose the punctate calcifications of the psammoma bodies.

FOLLICULAR CARCINOMA. In most series, about 10 to 15% of all thyroid carcinomas are purely follicular in structure. Follicular carcinoma occurs in an older age group than papillary carcinoma, most cases arising after the age of 40 (Fig. 8–51). Women are affected two to three times more commonly than men. As in papillary carcinoma, there may be a history of radiotherapy to the neck area during infancy or childhood. The degree of malignancy varies but generally exceeds that of papillary carcinoma. Follicular carcinoma seldom spreads to the regional lymph nodes, but invasion of blood vessels with hematogenous spread to distant sites, particularly bone, lung, and liver, often occurs relatively early. As is the case in primary papillary carcinoma, the metastases sometimes regress under the influence of suppressive doses of thyroid hormone.

Grossly, follicular carcinoma varies in size and is typically encapsulated. The histopathological appearance of the lesion varies from area to area. In some areas it resembles normal thyroid tissue except that the follicles are smaller and contain subnormal amounts of colloid; in other areas it is composed of solid sheets of cells. The cells exhibit mitoses to a varying degree. There may be foci of Hürthle cells; rarely, these are the predominant cells and these tumors are referred to as Hürthle cell carcinomas. Invasion of blood vessels and adjacent thyroid parenchyma is often observed. The degree of invasiveness, which is greatest in the older age group of patients, largely determines the prognosis in follicular carcinoma. In minimally invasive lesions, a 10-y survival rate of 86% has been reported, whereas the comparable figure for the more invasive variety is only 44%. The metastases may display either a follicular or a mixed follicular and papillary pattern. In some cases, the histological appearance of the metastatic lesion so closely resembled that of normal thyroid tissue that the term benign metastasizing struma was applied.

The clinical features of follicular carcinoma differ in several respects from those of the usual case of papillary carcinoma. In some patients, a goiter has been present for many years. The carcinoma usually consists of a single nodule or mass and sometimes involves one whole lobe. Pain and invasion of adjacent structures are late manifestations. The regional lymph nodes are seldom enlarged. Occasionally, either a pathological fracture related to a metastatic deposit in bone or a pulmonary metastatic nodule(s) is the major manifestation.

Follicular carcinoma differs from other types of thyroid malignancy in that it may accumulate radioiodine. However, uptake is not as efficient as in normal thyroid tissue. Thus, a follicular carcinoma can present as a cold thyroid nodule by scintiscan. However, the capacity of the primary tumor and the metastatic lesions to accumulate radioiodine, especially if the TSH level is elevated, may provide a therapeutic opportunity. Rarely, function in the metastases may be sufficient to produce thyrotoxicosis, including T_3 toxicosis.

ANAPLASTIC CARCINOMA. Anaplastic carcinoma constitutes about 10% of all thyroid carcinomas. It usually occurs after the age of 50 and is slightly more common in women. It is a highly malignant lesion, rapidly invading adjacent structures and metastasizing extensively throughout the body.

Grossly, anaplastic carcinoma is unencapsulated and extends widely, distorting the shape of the thyroid. Its consistency varies, being stony hard in some areas and soft or friable in others. Evidence of invasion of adjacent structures, such as skin, muscle, nerve, blood vessels, larynx, and esophagus, is common. On histopathological examination, the lesion is composed of atypical cells that exhibit numerous mitoses and form a variety of patterns. Spindle-shaped cells and multinucleate giant cells are usually predominant. In some cases, small cells are most prominent; as a result, there may be difficulty in distinguishing the lesion from lymphosarcoma. Rarely, the lesion is composed of clear cells, resembling hypernephroma, or large epithelial cells (epidermoid carcinoma). Areas of necrosis and polymorphonuclear infiltration are frequently present. Sometimes elements of papillary or follicular carcinoma can be detected, suggesting that they may be the precursors of anaplastic carcinoma.

The usual clinical complaint is of a rapid, often painful enlargement of a mass that may have been present in the thyroid gland for many years. The mass rapidly invades adjacent structures, causing hoarseness, inspiratory stridor, and difficulty in swallowing. On examination, the overlying skin is often warm and discolored. The mass is large and tender and is often fixed to adjacent structures, with the result that it moves poorly on swallowing. It is stony hard in consistency, but some areas may be soft or fluctuant. The regional lymph nodes are enlarged, and there may be evidence of distant metastases. The patient usually succumbs within several months after diagnosis. In general, anaplastic carcinomas do not accumulate iodine. Rarely, extensive replacement of the thyroid parenchyma may produce hypothyroidism.

Carcinoma of Parafollicular Origin (Medullary Carcinoma)

This distinctive type of thyroid carcinoma makes up about 1 to 2% of the cases. It usually occurs after the age of 40 and is slightly more common in women. It is more malignant than follicular carcinoma. Medullary carcinoma readily invades the intraglandular lymphatics, spreading to other parts of the gland and to the pericapsular and regional lymph nodes. In this respect it resembles papillary carcinoma, but unlike the latter it also spreads via the bloodstream to distant sites, particularly lung, bone, and liver.

Grossly, medullary carcinoma of the thyroid is firm and usually unencapsulated. On histopathological examination, it is composed of cells that vary widely in morphological features and arrangement. Round, polyhedral, and spindle-shaped cells form a variety of patterns, but formation of papillary folds or follicles is not seen. The cells may appear undifferentiated and exhibit mitoses, but, unlike the findings in anaplastic carcinoma, necrosis and polymorphonuclear infiltration are absent. There is an abundant hyaline connective tissue stroma that gives the staining reactions for amyloid; apart from plasmacytoma, this feature is unique to solid thyroid carcinoma. Gross or microscopic foci of carcinoma are often evident in other parts of the gland. Invasion of blood vessels may be seen. The histopathological appearance of the metastases closely resembles that of the primary lesion.

Clinically, the cancer first appears either as a hard nodule or mass in the thyroid gland or as an enlargement of the regional lymph nodes. Occasionally, a metastatic lesion in a distant site is found first. Lesions are sometimes bilateral but are usually localized to the upper two thirds of the gland, which is the anatomical location of the parafollicular cells. Some medullary carcinomas present as cold nodules, but surprisingly this is often not the case.

Medullary carcinoma is an extremely interesting disease for several reasons. It arises from the parafollicular cells of the thyroid, rather than the follicular epithelium; it secretes a characteristic hormone, calcitonin; it is frequently associated with one or more paraendocrine manifestations; it may be familial; and it provides an early biochemical signal, in hypersecretion of calcitonin, that permits its early detection, treatment, and cure.[394, 395] (See also Chapters 27 and 30.)

This tumor occurs in both sporadic and familial forms, the latter making up about 20% of the total. The familial variety usually appears at a younger age, is more often bilateral, is less likely to have associated cervical metastases when diagnosed, and has a better prognosis. Most important, the familial variety is anteceded by a premalignant hyperplasia of the C cells that is curable by total thyroidectomy. Survival in both the sporadic and familial forms is mainly determined by the presence or absence of metastases and the age of the patient at the time of diagnosis, older patients generally doing much less well. Overall, long-term survival is moderate, estimated at about two thirds at 10 y.

A variety of symptoms, other than those related to mass lesions, are present in patients with medullary thyroid cancer. The carcinoid syndrome and Cushing syndrome may occur, owing to secretion of serotonin and ACTH, respectively. Prostaglandins, kinins, and vasoactive intestinal peptide may also be secreted and are variously responsible for the attacks of watery diarrhea that about one third of patients experience. In patients with the familial variety, there is often clinical or laboratory evidence of hyperparathyroidism and pheochromocytoma (Sipple syndrome; multiple endocrine neoplasia type 2A, MEN 2A). Hyperparathyroidism is most commonly due to parathyroid hyperplasia, rather than adenoma, with or without characteristic symptoms of hypercalcemia, nephrolithiasis, or nephrocalcinosis. Pheochromocytomas are often bilateral and are prone to secrete epinephrine, so that urinary total catecholamine and vanillylmandelic acid excretions are normal. Specific measurements of urinary epinephrine excretion will often reveal some elevation, however. A variant of the MEN 2A syndrome is one in which medullary thyroid cancer, pheochromocytoma, and possibly parathyroid hyperplasia are associated with ganglioneuromas, mucosal neuromas ("bumpy lip" syndrome), a marfanoid habitus, and typical facies (MEN 2A or MEN 2B [3]). (See also Chapter 30.)

In patients with the sporadic form of medullary thyroid cancer, differentiation from other types of thyroid nodule on clinical grounds alone may be difficult. In patients with a family history of thyroid cancer, hypertension, and either hyperparathyroidism or nephrolithiasis, the MEN 2A syndrome should be suspected. Measurements of basal plasma calcitonin concentrations should be made, these being elevated in about one third to two thirds of patients with medullary thyroid cancer. Infusions of pentagastrin or calcium elicit secretion of calcitonin,[395] and the response is exaggerated in patients with medullary thyroid cancer or the antecedent C cell hyperplasia. Patients are usually normocalcemic, but those suspected of having the MEN 2A syndrome should be evaluated for hyperparathyroidism and for pheochromocytoma as well.

When diagnosis has been made from calcitonin measurements or needle biopsy, total thyroidectomy with removal of regional nodes should be carried out. In patients with MEN 2A, pheochromocytomas should be treated first. First-degree relatives of patients with MEN 2A, including small children, should be screened regularly for the emergence of one or more manifestations of the syndrome (see Chapter 30).

LYMPHOMA OF THE THYROID. Thyroid lymphoma is rare but presents with manifestations that may be confused with those of anaplastic carcinoma. Differentiation of the two is important because the prognosis for lymphoma is better and the therapeutic approach is different. The histopathological evaluation of thyroid lymphoma indicates that most are diffuse histiocytic (Rappaport classification) or follicular center cell with centroblastic, centrocytic cell types (Kehoe classification). Hashimoto thyroiditis is almost always present in the surrounding thyroid. The relative risk of thyroid lymphoma is 67-fold higher in patients with Hashimoto thyroiditis than in thyroid glands with colloid nodules. Nonetheless, the disease is a rare complication of Hashimoto thyroiditis and in one series occurred in only 4 of 829 patients with this condition.[396] The typical clinical picture is that of a rapidly enlarging thyroid mass in a patient with a history of Hashimoto thyroiditis or of hypothyroidism. The lesion is nonfunctional on thyroid scintiscan, and the size suggests the need for surgical decompression. This can often be avoided by the use of radiation therapy once an appropriate diagnosis is made. Diagnostic tests of choice are either fine-needle or Vim-Silverman needle biopsy with appropriate immunohistochemical staining for monoclonal lymphocytic infiltration.[397, 398] It is especially important to make a pathological distinction between a lesion often referred to as small cell carcinoma of the thyroid and lymphoma, because lymphoma is a curable lesion, whereas undifferentiated thyroid carcinoma is fatal within a few months to a year.

Diagnosis and Management of a Thyroid Nodule

In previous editions, it was stated that benign and malignant thyroid nodules cannot be differentiated from one another with absolute certainty on clinical grounds alone and that cytopathological examination is required for this purpose. This remains the case. A reasonably accurate clinical judgment can be made as to whether a particular nodule is probably benign or malignant, so that the likelihood of either leaving a carcinoma in place or performing an excisional biopsy of a benign nodule is reduced. Nonetheless, the approach to diagnosis and management of the nodular thyroid gland has been substantially modified, and the accuracy of diagnosis increased, by the application of fine-needle aspiration or core needle biopsy. Not all authorities agree on the importance to be attached to certain findings or on how often various diagnostic procedures should be applied.

Fine-needle aspiration biopsy is an important tool for the evaluation of patients presenting with a nodular goiter. Although its use is most important in the evaluation of solitary thyroid nodules, it can also be employed with advantage to investigate any nodular lesion of the thyroid.[399] The major prerequisite is the availability of a cytopathologist experienced in the evaluation of thyroid needle aspiration specimens.[400, 401] A schematic approach to the investigation of either a solitary thyroid nodule or a dominant nodule in a multinodular gland is shown in Figure 8–52. If such expertise is not available, a less direct approach to evaluation of the solitary thyroid nodule should be taken, as shown in

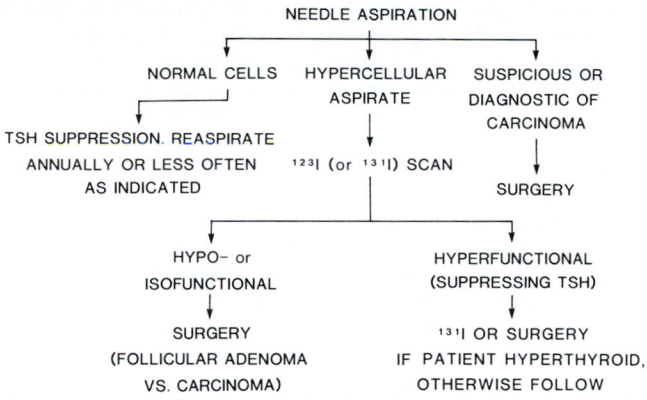

Figure 8–52. Approach to the evaluation of a solitary or dominant thyroid nodule starting with a fine-needle aspiration. (From Larsen PR. The thyroid. In: Wyngaarden JB, Smith LH Jr, eds. Cecil Textbook of Medicine. 18th ed. Philadelphia: W. B. Saunders, 1988: 1315–1340.)

Table 8–20. Initial Evaluation of Patients with Solitary or Dominant Thyroid Nodules

History
Radiation to face or neck during infancy or childhood
Familial history of tumors
Recent change in size
Hypothyroidism or Hashimoto thyroiditis
Thyrotoxicosis
Physical Examination
Thyroid status
Tracheal deviation or hoarseness
Single vs. multiple nodules
Fixation, consistency, tenderness
Lymphadenopathy
Laboratory Tests
FT$_4$I, TSH
Thyroid microsomal antibodies
Serum T$_3$, calcitonin, serum Ca^{2+} only if indicated
Needle aspiration

Figure 8–53. The prevalence of thyroid carcinoma in solitary thyroid nodules or dominant nodules in multinodular glands is about 5%. One cannot justify surgery for all such patients to find the 1 in 20 who has a malignancy, especially given the fact that thyroid malignancies rarely cause death. Accordingly, evaluation of the patient with a solitary nodule is designed to select a group of patients with a 10 to 30% risk of having a malignant lesion.

Table 8–20 lists several characteristics that increase the suspicion of thyroid malignancy in a patient. Because of the increased frequency of malignancy in patients who have received neck radiation for a benign or malignant disease in childhood, this is a critically important historical factor.[402, 403] It may be necessary for the patient to question parents regarding this possibility. Irradiated patients should have a surgical exploration even though many of these tumors are benign.[402] A familial history of tumors suggests the possibility of medullary carcinoma, and if this diagnosis is suspected, a serum calcitonin assay should be performed. In general, however, one cannot justify the expense of serum calcitonin measurements in all patients with thyroid nodules if there is no additional reason to suspect this disease. A history of a rapid growth of tumor or the enlargement of local lymph nodes suggests the possibility of malignancy. The presence of these historical factors will generally lead to surgical exploration. A needle aspiration will merely confirm a diagnosis for use in designing a surgical plan. Because benign nodules are much less common in men than in women, a solitary nodule in a man has a higher risk of malignancy than does the same lesion in a woman. In children, the presence of a thyroid nodule is sufficiently disturbing that

one should proceed directly with a thyroid scintiscan. If the nodule is not functioning, surgery is indicated, as a higher fraction of such lesions in children are malignant (~30%). A history of Hashimoto thyroiditis or hypothyroidism together with an enlarging mass suggests the possibility of lymphoma.

During the physical examination, an assessment of thyroid status should be made to exclude the possibility of either hypothyroidism or hyperthyroidism. A nodule in a hypothyroid patient may be due to a fragment of residual functioning thyroid tissue in a patient with Hashimoto thyroiditis. On the other hand, a functioning nodule greater than 4 cm in size can cause hyperthyroidism. A hyperfunctioning nodule producing excess thyroid hormone is virtually never malignant, although a small malignancy may be contained within the nodule.

Laboratory studies are used to document the presence or absence of underlying or associated thyroid disease. A serum T$_3$ determination is indicated only if hyperthyroidism is suspected, and calcitonin should be measured only if there is a high suspicion of medullary carcinoma. The possibility of a parathyroid adenoma is considered if needle aspiration reveals watery clear cystic fluid characteristic of a parathyroid cyst. In general, a parathyroid adenoma is not palpable unless it is large enough to cause significant hypercalcemia.

The pathological processes to be considered in a patient with a solitary nodule are listed in Table 8–21. More than 95% of lesions fall into one of the first five categories under primary thyroid lesions. Unless one of the historical or physical factors suggests otherwise, the simplest approach at this juncture is to proceed using the algorithm shown in Figure 8–52. The thyroid needle aspiration has been discussed extensively (see earlier under Laboratory Tests of Thyroid Hormone Economy), and several reviews are available.[398–400, 403–405] In general, the authors prefer to use a 7/8- or 1½-inch 25-gauge needle attached to a 10-mL syringe. After local anesthesia is given, the needle is introduced into

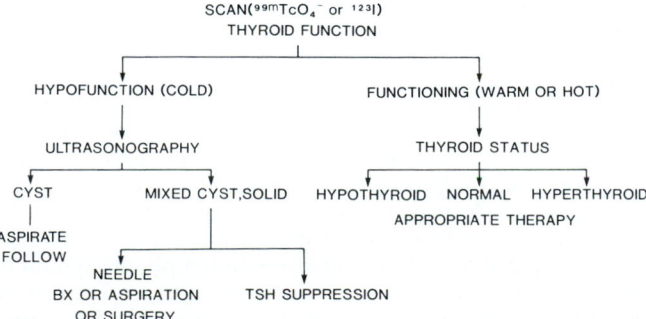

Figure 8–53. Approach to the evaluation of a solitary or dominant thyroid nodule starting with a thyroid scintiscan. (From Larsen PR. The thyroid. In: Wyngaarden JB, Smith LH Jr, eds. Cecil Textbook of Medicine. 18th ed. Philadelphia: W. B. Saunders, 1988: 1315–1340.)

Table 8–21. Differential Diagnosis of a Solitary Thyroid Nodule

Primary Thyroid Lesions	Nonthyroid Lesions
Adenoma	Lymphadenopathy
Carcinoma	Parathyroid cyst or adenoma
Cyst	Cystic hygroma
Multinodular goiter	Bronchocoele
Hashimoto thyroiditis	Laryngocoele
Thyroglossal duct cyst	Carotid aneurysm
Lymphoma	Metastasis
Prior hemithyroidectomy	
Thyroid hemiagenesis	

the nodule with the patient lying prone with a pillow supporting the shoulders, thus causing extension of the neck. When the needle tip is in the nodule, about 5 to 8 mL of suction is applied as the tip is advanced and retracted 1 or 2 mm to disrupt the cells. As soon as liquid appears in the needle hub of the syringe, suction is released and the needle withdrawn. The needle is then removed from the syringe, the barrel withdrawn, the needle replaced, and the contents of the needle and the hub deposited on a slide that is immediately sprayed or placed into alcohol for Papanicolaou (Pap) staining. Alternatively, air-dried smears can be stained with Giemsa, although the Pap smear provides better nuclear detail. The aspiration is usually repeated five times to sample different portions of the nodule. Suction is released if blood appears in the hub of the syringe, because this produces a dilute specimen. The authors also rinse the needle and syringe with an isotonic solution and concentrate and stain this material. If cystic fluid is encountered, it is unlikely that it will contain cells even though the specimen is filtered. In the case of partially cystic nodules, the needle should be directed away from the central cavity of the cyst to obtain cellular material from the wall of the nodule. A cyst that is completely removed by this procedure and is less than 4 cm in size is generally benign. However, recurrence of cystic fluid in the nodule after two aspirations raises the possibility of thyroid carcinoma and generally leads to its removal. Few complications of this procedure have been reported. Some patients experience slight tenderness in the nodule and hemorrhage may occur into cystic nodules. One should not attempt aspiration of lesions suspected to be vascular. The 25-gauge needle has been used without complications even in patients receiving anticoagulant therapy.

The necessity for an experienced cytopathologist cannot be overemphasized. In collaboration with such an individual, the clinician should determine the adequacy of sampling. One authority recommends that six or more cell clusters on at least two slides should all be benign before a diagnosis of benign lesion is accepted.[399–401] A diagnosis of papillary carcinoma, the commonest malignant lesion, is usually readily made in such samples. In the authors' clinic, an attempt is made to classify the cytological material into three general categories: benign, which consists of nodular goiters or colloid adenomas; suspicious or possibly malignant, which includes hypercellular follicular specimens or samples that consist uniformly of Hürthle cells;[406] and malignant, in which the cytological characteristics are diagnostic or nearly so. For patients with diagnoses in the latter two categories, surgical exploration is generally advocated. It is assumed that the individuals with high-risk historical or physical factors have already been referred for surgery. In the hands of experienced individuals using this approach, the specificity of a diagnosis of malignancy was 77% in a group categorized as malignant and 11% in the suspicious category.[407] About 60% of the needle aspiration diagnoses were in the benign category. Patients with apparently benign nodules are then treated with levothyroxine and followed as described for follicular adenomas. If the lesion enlarges during TSH suppression (TSH 0.2 to 0.4 mU/mL), surgery is advised if the patient is a suitable candidate. If the lesion does not enlarge, such patients may be followed at 6-mo intervals for several years. At that time, it is reasonable to withdraw levothyroxine to determine whether the nodule is TSH dependent. If it is not, annual monitoring is indicated with no TSH suppressive therapy. If the nodule enlarges, one must weigh the risk/benefit ratio of prolonged TSH suppression, particularly in women who are at risk of osteoporosis, versus that of surgery. Until the latter risk is more accurately defined, therapy must be determined on an individual basis.

As indicated in the algorithm in Figure 8–52, in the case of a hypercellular follicular cell specimen, a thyroid scintiscan should be performed using ^{123}I to determine whether the lesion is functional. Radioiodine is preferred to TcO_4^- for such studies because a few malignant lesions are capable of trapping TcO_4^- but not organifying iodine. A functioning nodule would be especially likely if the serum TSH concentration were suppressed, although this by itself would not be sufficient evidence to confirm that the lesion is responsible for the autonomous thyroid function.

The approach shown in Figure 8–53 can be employed when experienced cytopathological evaluation is not available. It is less direct than the alternative, but it has been a standard approach for many years. Its disadvantage is that because most adenomas are nonfunctioning solid tumors, the fraction of patients referred for surgery is higher than would be the case if fine-needle aspiration were used. In addition, patients with papillary carcinoma, a lesion readily recognized by fine-needle aspiration, may wait 6 mo or more before surgery if the nodule does not regress. However, considering the indolent nature of papillary carcinoma in most patients, this is not usually a significant disadvantage.

Occasional patients with malignancy of or in the thyroid present with features suggesting subacute thyroiditis, including pain, elevation of erythrocyte sedimentation rate, and decrease in the RAIU. Occasionally the tenderness is limited to the palpable nodule. In some situations this may be due to hemorrhage into a benign or malignant nodule. On the other hand, tenderness in a nodule even without hemorrhage does not eliminate the possibility of malignancy.[408]

Treatment of Thyroid Carcinoma

For individuals with suspected or established malignancy the opinions regarding the appropriate extent of surgery vary.[1–4, 409–413] Factors to be considered in this decision are the histological diagnosis, size of the original lesion, presence of distant metastasis, and age and sex of the patient. The surgeon must be experienced in procedures involving the thyroid gland. The authors recommend the following as general guidelines. In the case of papillary carcinoma, lesions less than 2.0 cm in diameter can usually be treated by lobectomy and isthmectomy with exploration of the ipsilateral lymph nodes. For larger lesions and those that have extended through the thyroid capsule into periglandular tissues, a total lobectomy on the involved side and a subtotal or nearly total thyroidectomy on the contralateral side are recommended. Such patients are likely to be considered for ^{131}I treatment, and the resection of normal tissue is indicated. The prognosis of papillary carcinoma becomes worse with increasing age, with the line drawn for men aged about 40 and for women aged about 50.[393] All patients should have exploration for, and resection of, involved lymph nodes.

For follicular lesions and Hürthle cell tumors, a total resection on the ipsilateral side and subtotal on the contralateral side are indicated because of the more aggressive nature of this lesion and the accompanying need for evaluation for radioactive iodine therapy. Medullary carcinoma is treated by total thyroidectomy and removal of involved soft tissue and nodes in the central portion of the neck and upper mediastinum. There is no therapy for medullary carcinoma other than surgery. Patients with anaplastic carcinoma generally have lesions that are too extensive for any procedure but palliative surgery. Chemotherapy and radiation are then given.[414] Individuals with lymphoma should be evaluated in collaboration with an oncologist, and appropriate therapy for the stage of lymphoma should be initiated. In some patients, the thyroid gland may be the only organ involved, and resection may be indicated. However, in most cases radiation and chemotherapy will be employed.

For individuals with malignant epithelial lesions in whom immediate surgery cannot be performed, institution of TSH-suppressive therapy with levothyroxine is indicated when the basal serum TSH concentrations are normal or elevated. This can usually be accomplished by administration of levothyroxine at approximately 1.8 to 2.0 μg/kg (about 0.9 μg/lb) of ideal body weight.

In recommending surgery, the endocrinologist should discuss the potential complications of this procedure in some detail. Unilateral lobectomy is virtually never associated with permanent hypocalcemia but can be associated with vocal cord paralysis in as many as 3% of patients. Bilateral near-total thyroidectomy causes temporary hypocalcemia in 7 to 10% of patients and permanent hypocalcemia in 0.5 to 1%; temporary vocal cord paralysis also occurs in about 1 to 2% of such patients. A true extracapsular total thyroidectomy may lead to hypoparathyroidism in as many as 30% of individuals,[393, 411] an unacceptable complication rate for most patients with indolent malignancy. In addition, vocal cord paralysis is more common after such a procedure. The experience of the surgeon is important in terms of the finer technical points of thyroidectomy such as preservation of the external branch of the recurrent laryngeal nerve, which is important in the fine regulation of voice pitch. This is especially pertinent for individuals who depend on their voice for their livelihood.

SURGERY AND FOLLOW-UP OF INDIVIDUALS WITH HISTORY OF NECK RADIATION IN CHILDHOOD. A history of radiation in childhood increases the risk of both benign and malignant thyroid nodules in later life. This risk varies with the type of radiation, the size of the radiation port, and the dose. Several issues are relevant for the thyroidologist. First, given that surgical exploration is required for patients with a history of thyroid radiation and thyroid nodules, what should be the extent of surgery and how should such patients be treated subsequently? With respect to the extent of surgery, opinions vary from near-total thyroidectomy at the time of the initial procedure to an individual assessment of the thyroid gland and the extent of surgery depending on the degree of thyroid involvement.[402, 409, 410] Individuals with bilateral nodular disease should have a near-total thyroidectomy. Because of its malignant potential, residual thyroid tissue should be ablated with radioiodine. If there is no involvement of the opposite lobe at the time of surgery, one must weigh the relative risk of complications associated with a more extensive surgical procedure against the possibility of recurrence of thyroid nodules in the residual thyroid tissue. In one radiated population, both benign and malignant nodules were recurrent in individuals who had subtotal thyroidectomy previously.[402] The risk of recurrence overall in this study was approximately 20%. As expected, it was lower in patients who had more thyroid tissue removed than in those who had less extensive procedures. Of interest is that, in this group of patients, suppression of TSH by thyroid hormone led to a reduction in recurrence from 35% to approximately 8%. Of these nodules, 20% were malignant, but TSH suppression had no influence on the prevalence of malignant nodules. Thus the recommendations for such patients must take into account the nature of the radiation exposure and the experience of the operating surgeon, and no general rule can be given. However, radiated patients who have had thyroid nodules removed should receive TSH-suppressive doses of thyroid hormone regardless of the extent of surgery. The appearance of new thyroid nodules is to be expected, and such patients should be monitored indefinitely for this possibility. A second question is whether this phenomenon could be extrapolated to suggest that all radiated patients should have TSH suppression therapy even if nodularity is not present. This cannot be determined at present because it seems likely that patients who do not have thyroid nodules may not have received sufficient exposure to have a propensity for thyroid neoplasia. Second, the risks of long-term TSH suppression in women, especially vis-à-vis osteoporosis, have not been clearly defined and may be significant.

POSTOPERATIVE MANAGEMENT. In view of the foregoing uncertainties and the different needs of individual patients, postoperative treatment of thyroid carcinoma cannot always accord with a rigid algorithm. One must consider the operative findings and the histology of the tumor, as well as the age and sex of the patient.

In a large group of patients with differentiated (papillary, papillary-follicular, or follicular) carcinoma only 9% developed distant metastasis.[415] Most of the patients had papillary carcinoma and of these 7% developed distant metastasis, as opposed to metastases in 19% of patients with follicular cancer and 34% of patients with Hürthle cell cancer. Mortality rates at 5 and 10 y after diagnosis of metastasis were 65 and 75% for all patients with distant metastasis, and nearly 80% of the deaths were due to thyroid cancer. Thus, distant metastases are an ominous development. Age was an important factor, with younger patients having a better prognosis. The prognosis was also better for individuals whose metastases concentrated radioiodine. Micronodular (diffuse) pulmonary metastases have a better prognosis than do macronodular lesions. The former tend to concentrate radioiodine better than the latter. As might be expected, multiple-organ involvement (usually bone and lung) was a worse prognostic sign than was single-site involvement. In the total group, only a small number of patients could be evaluated for the efficacy of ^{131}I therapy, and this therapy did not have a positive influence on survival. In contrast, other studies found that radioiodine prolonged life.[412, 416] A possible explanation for the lack of effect of radioiodine therapy in the study was that routine thyroid remnant ablation was not performed, nor were whole body scans routinely done, as has been recommended by some authorities.

The treatment of individuals with well-differentiated carcinoma depends to a great extent on their risk group. Small papillary carcinomas (<2.0 cm) in women between the ages of 20 and 50 and men between the ages of 20 and 40 can be followed clinically by physical examination, with levothyroxine given in quantities to suppress TSH to just above the hyperthyroid range. Patients less than 10 y of age with papillary or follicular carcinoma should generally have radioiodine studies and therapy, because pulmonary metastases are more common in this age group and may not be detectable with standard x-rays. Such patients are usually treated to ablate these lesions, although it is difficult to prove that this prolongs survival. Adults with a papillary carcinoma greater than 2 cm in diameter, especially if it extends through the thyroid capsule into the surrounding tissues, or those who have known unresectable or metastatic disease should be evaluated for radioiodine therapy. Men over the age of 40 and women over the age of 50 with papillary carcinoma should also be evaluated for ablative radioiodine therapy, as should all patients with follicular carcinoma.

RADIOIODINE TREATMENT. The use of radioiodine in the treatment of thyroid carcinoma has a sound theoretical basis.[417] Iodine organification is a thyroid-specific function and ^{131}I is an effective agent for delivering radiation to the thyroid tissue with low radiation to other portions of the body. To be useful, however, the ^{131}I must be concentrated by the tissue.[418] This is generally not the case in euthyroid patients because initially these tumors are cold. For either primary or metastatic thyroid tumors to concentrate ^{131}I, the function must be stimulated by TSH in almost every patient.

As already described, TSH is a less effective stimulator of neoplastic than of normal thyroid tissue. Therefore, not all thyroid tumors can be treated by this modality. Because human TSH is safer and more effective than bovine TSH, at present the patient must be made hypothyroid in order to stimulate endogenous TSH secretion to evaluate the potential for radioiodine treatment. This may be achieved by performing a nearly total thyroidectomy at the time of the initial operation or subsequently by the administration of radioiodine to a patient with significant residual normal thyroid tissue. Usually a dose of 2.6 GBq (70 mCi) of radioiodine is required with pretreatment studies demonstrating a significant degree of uptake in the residual gland. When sufficient normal thyroid tissue has been destroyed to cause hypothyroidism, the patient may receive a "tracer" dose of ^{131}I, usually 110 MBq (3 mCi) while hypothyroid, and dosimetric studies are performed with the help of computerized data collection systems, which are now available in most nuclear medicine departments.[418]

Despite the theoretical suitability of thyroid carcinoma for radioiodine treatment, there is considerable controversy about whether such therapy prolongs life (Fig. 8–54). Various series report either no effect[415, 419] or an effect only in a subset of patients.[416–420] However, the paucity of long-term complications and acute adverse effects leads physicians to employ this modality because it may be effective and appears to be without side effects, at least in the adult. This does not apply when the accumulated ^{131}I dose exceeds 19 GBq (0.5 Ci), at which point an increase in the incidence of leukemia occurs.

It is incumbent on the physician to demonstrate that significant quantities of the administered dose will accumulate in the residual tumor lesions before employing this treatment.[418–420] The effectiveness of radioiodine in ablation of thyroid tissue can be appreciated from the fact that the

deposition of 186 MBq (5 mCi) of ^{131}I in a typical 50-g Graves thyroid results in an average radioiodine content of approximately 3.7 MBq/g (100 μCi/g). This dose is sufficient to cause hypothyroidism in most patients and could theoretically provide the same radiation dose in a 1-g metastasis. Such an amount of ^{131}I could be accumulated in a nodule with only 0.1% uptake after administration of 3.7 GBq (100 mCi) ^{131}I. This oversimplifies the situation because the hyperthyroid gland is more homogeneous than a tumor metastasis and because the mean residence time of ^{131}I may vary considerably between the hyperthyroid and the carcinomatous follicular cell. Nonetheless, the detection system for evaluating radioiodine uptake and the dose given should be sensitive enough to quantitate radioiodine uptakes in this range.

Because this therapy is given by a specialist, the details are beyond the scope of this chapter.[417–421] However, several general guidelines should be followed. First, several months should elapse between surgery and radioiodine therapy if patients are exposed to povidone-iodine during the procedure. All contrast agents should be avoided in the 6 wk before test. If required, myelography should be performed only with water-soluble dyes because residual iodine will be present for many years after lipid-soluble agents such as lipiodol. Patients should be begun on a low-iodine diet 1 wk before administration of radioiodine and should avoid all foods (especially seafoods), medicines, and antiseptics containing iodinated dyes or iodine per se. After surgery, the patient can be maintained on replacement doses of levothyroxine. This is discontinued about 4 wk before the planned uptake study, and the patient is given liothyronine at 50 μg/d for 2 wk. At 10 d to 2 wk after stopping liothyronine, the patient is given about 111 MBq (3 mCi) ^{131}I. This approach allows controlled timing of the onset of hypothyroidism. The mean residence time of radioiodine in metas-

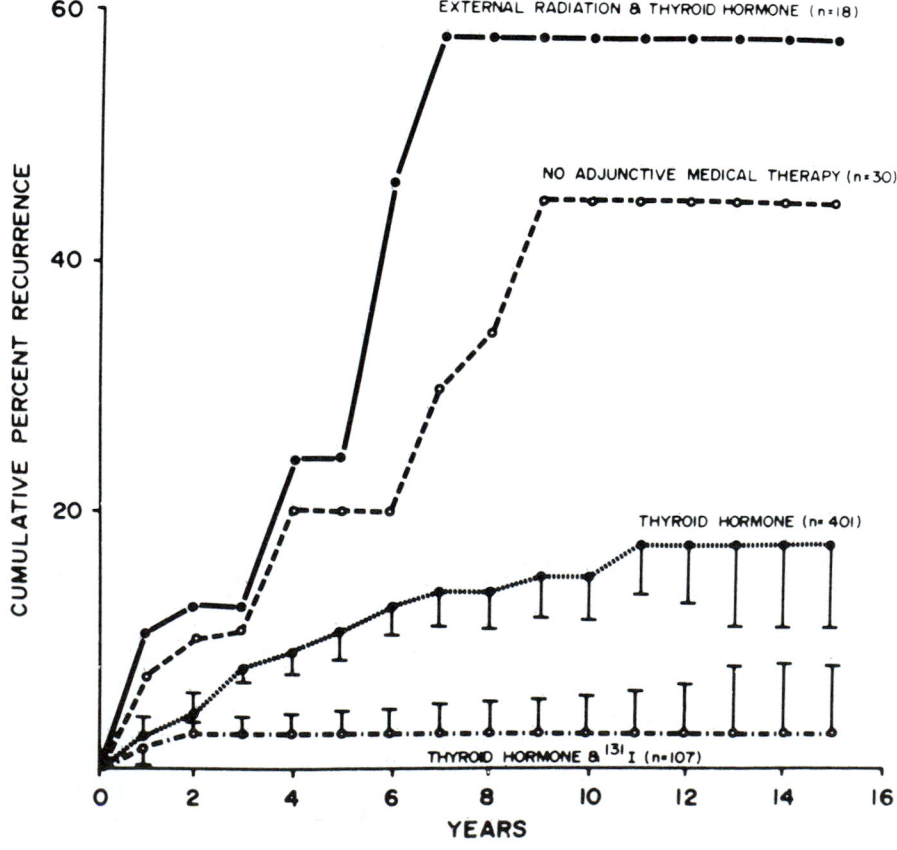

Figure 8–54. Influence of mode of therapy on the rate of postoperative recurrence in patients with papillary carcinoma of the thyroid. (From EL Mazzaferri, RL Young, JE Oertel, et al., Papillary thyroid carcinoma: the impact of therapy in 576 patients, Medicine, 56, 171–196, © by Williams & Wilkins, 1977.)

tases does not always increase with increasing TSH concentration because TSH may accelerate hormone turnover in the metastatic lesion.[422] In general, total body scans are performed 3 to 4 d after administration of radioiodine, it having been established at the time of radioiodine administration that the TSH concentration is elevated. Complete absence of uptake in the neck should lead to a determination of a urinary iodine/creatinine ratio to determine whether unsuspected iodine in the body is saturating iodine uptake in tumor tissue. Doses of radioiodine greater than 7.4 GBq (200 mCi) are rarely given outside specialized centers, and the calculated uptake in a metastasis should be sufficient to allow accumulation of a significant amount of radioiodine in the tumor tissue after administration of this amount or less. On the other hand, the upper limits of radioiodine deposition should not be exceeded. Because of the possibility of radiation fibrosis and pneumonitis, less than 3 GBq (80 mCi) should be retained in the lungs at 48 h when diffuse metastases are present. The total body retention should be less than 4.5 GBq (120 mCi) at 48 h, and less than 2 Gy (200 rad) should be delivered to whole blood by the radioiodine dose given.[420] In adults, such limitations are rarely an issue, but in children appropriate adjustments in the administered dosage should be made.

In general, radioiodine is more useful in the treatment of soft tissue metastases than of bone metastases, which are generally treated by 20 Gy (2000 rad) of external radiation. Anaplastic carcinoma rarely concentrates ^{131}I, and this modality also is not useful for patients with medullary carcinoma or lymphoma. After ablation of the thyroid gland and radioiodine therapy, patients should be followed with serum thyroglobulin and serum TSH determinations. The presence of thyroglobulin in the serum of the patient without residual normal thyroid tissue (i.e., after radioiodine ablation) indicates the presence of metastatic tissue and should lead to further evaluation for possible treatable metastases (see Fig. 8–23). On the other hand, undetectable serum thyroglobulin during TSH suppression therapy does not indicate that tumor tissue is absent. The most sensitive use of the serum thyroglobulin determination is when the patient is no longer receiving thyroid hormone and the TSH level is elevated (see Fig. 8–23). Under these circumstances, the absence of serum thyroglobulin indicates that little functioning tumor tissue is present, although poorly differentiated thyroid carcinoma may not synthesize this protein.

Should repeated ^{131}I treatments of asymptomatic patients with residual thyroid metastases be performed? There is no conclusive evidence that such an approach prolongs life. An initial treatment with ^{131}I can be justified as an attempt to destroy small residual deposits of tumor, but it is more difficult to demonstrate that periodic radioiodine therapy is either effective or, when the total dose accumulates beyond 19 GBq (500 mCi), not harmful. Because TSH may stimulate thyroid tumor cells, repeated exposure of the tumor to TSH is undesirable. However, if the patient is symptomatic because of nonresectable lesions, radioiodine therapy may be beneficial. The first author prefers to employ ^{131}I in symptomatic patients, recognizing that there are alternative opinions. For symptomatic lesions (e.g., bone or soft tissue) that do not concentrate ^{131}I, palliative external radiation should be considered.

LONG-TERM FOLLOW-UP OF THE THYROID CARCINOMA PATIENT. Patients with papillary and follicular carcinoma are followed on TSH suppression at 3-mo and then 6-mo intervals for the first 2 y after their initial surgical/radioiodine treatment. If no abnormality appears, they are then followed on an annual basis. In the absence of specific indications, chest x-rays are performed each year, and the serum FT_4I and TSH and thyroglobulin concentra-

tions are measured. Periodic estimates of bone density should be obtained in women. Solitary recurrences in lymph nodes or in the neck can be dealt with most easily by the surgeon. Depending on the individual situation, such a recurrence may indicate the need for re-evaluation for radioiodine treatment after resection of the lesion. The appearance of pulmonary nodules, particularly in a miliary pattern, should lead to an evaluation for ^{131}I treatment. Without such indications, the authors do not obtain regular ^{131}I scans or bone x-rays. Because over 80% of the recurrences of papillary carcinoma appear in the first 10 y after treatment, this is the earliest time interval at which one may begin to feel secure about the success of the initial surgery. One may consider a reduction in levothyroxine at that time, particularly if bone density is decreasing in female patients. The incidence of death from papillary thyroid cancer in one large series was 6.5% at 30 y,[415] and 73% of those who died did so within 10 y of the diagnosis. Only 1% of the patients with positive lymph nodes but no other metastatic lesion at the time of initial presentation died of thyroid cancer, again emphasizing the lack of correlation of lymph node metastases with prognosis. The presence of a distant metastasis is an alarming sign and is an indication for more aggressive therapy with radioiodine, although only 30 to 60% of such tumors concentrate sufficient ^{131}I to allow this. An unfortunate combination of thyroid diseases is that of Graves disease and thyroid cancer. The TRAb in such patients can apparently promote tumor growth.[423] Patients with medullary carcinoma can be followed with determinations of calcitonin, which is an excellent tumor marker for this condition (see Chapters 27 and 30).

THYROIDITIS

Hashimoto Disease (Lymphocytic Thyroiditis, Struma Lymphomatosa)

Until the demonstration of circulating antithyroid antibodies, Hashimoto disease could be diagnosed with certainty only by biopsy of the thyroid. Demonstration of high titers of circulating antibodies in most patients with Hashimoto disease and evidence of cell-mediated immunity to thyroid antigens have led to the use of the term *autoimmune thyroiditis* to describe this disorder.

Although its true prevalence is uncertain, Hashimoto disease is common and may be increasing in frequency. It affects women more often than men and occurs most often between the ages of 30 and 50, although no age is exempt. It is the most common cause of goitrous hypothyroidism in areas of iodine sufficiency. There is often a family history of Hashimoto disease, goiter, hypothyroidism, or Graves disease, and circulating antithyroid antibodies may be detected in relatives without overt thyroid disease. Other diseases with autoimmune components, such as pernicious anemia, diabetes mellitus, idiopathic adrenal atrophy, rheumatoid arthritis, chronic active hepatitis, vitiligo, early graying of the hair, biliary cirrhosis, and Sjögren syndrome, may occur in patients with Hashimoto disease and in their relatives more often than can be accounted for by chance (see Chapter 31). An association between Hashimoto disease and angioimmunoblastic lymphadenopathy has also been noted.

Pathogenesis

The presence of lymphocytic infiltration of the thyroid, of circulating antithyroid antibodies, and of a clinical or immunological overlap with other diseases with autoimmune components provides compelling evidence that immunological factors are involved in the pathogenesis of Hashimoto disease. Indeed, it is generally agreed that Hashimoto disease is one of the triad of autoimmune thyroid disorders that also includes Graves disease and primary thyroid atrophy. What is unclear, however, is the manner in which immunological factors bring about thyroid damage. A humorally mediated autoimmune mechanism has been suggested by the observation that antimicrosomal antibodies are cytotoxic to thyroid tissue in vitro. On the other hand, the extensive lymphocytic infiltration of the thyroid as well as the observation that lymphocytes from patients with Hashimoto disease elaborate various lymphokines and undergo blast transformation when exposed to thyroid tissue in vitro has led to the suggestion that cell-mediated autoimmune mechanisms are pathogenetically involved. A third mechanism for which there is some experimental support accommodates both of the foregoing by invoking lymphocyte-mediated cytotoxicity that is targeted and initiated by the antithyroid antibodies.

These manifestations of autoimmunity in Hashimoto disease, as in other autoimmune thyroid disorders, may reflect a genetically determined deficiency of suppressor cells that allows persistence of a forbidden clone of immunocytes directed against thyroid antigens.[254] The observation that infusion of interleukin 2 and lymphokine-activated killer cells causes progression or the appearance of hypothyroidism in patients with detectable antimicrosomal antibodies confirms the autoimmune nature of this disease.[424]

Constitutional Factors

Reference has already been made to the preponderance in women and to the familial predisposition to thyroid disease in Hashimoto disease. A significant association also exists between Hashimoto disease and the human leukocyte antigen HLA-DR3 in patients with atrophic thyroiditis[425] and between Hashimoto disease and HLA-DR5 in those with goitrous thyroiditis.[426] Both are also associated with the HLA-B8 haplotype. Hashimoto disease occurs with unexpected frequency in patients with Down syndrome and probably also in those with Turner syndrome. The fact that thyroid cells can express HLA-DR antigens, at least as a secondary phenomenon, indicates the potential role of these cells in perpetuating the immune response and may be related to the relative specificity of autoimmune disease for certain HLA-DR subgroups.[427]

Histopathology

The glandular tissue is pale and firm. The histopathological changes vary in type and extent but in general consist of diffuse lymphocytic infiltration, obliteration of thyroid follicles, and fibrosis (Fig. 8–55). In most cases, there is destruction of epithelial cells and degeneration and fragmentation of the follicular basement membrane. The remaining epithelial cells may be larger and show oxyphilic changes in the cytoplasm; these so-called Askanazy cells are virtually pathognomonic. In some cases epithelial hyperplasia may be prominent. Colloid is sparse. The interstitial tissue is infiltrated with lymphocytes that may form typical lymphoid follicles with germinal centers. Plasma cells may be prominent. Fibrosis is generally present, especially in the older lesions, but not to the extent seen in Riedel thyroiditis. Histologically, two variants can often be distinguished. The more common oxyphilic variant displays more oxyphilic change, less fibrosis, and more prominent infiltration with lymphocytes forming germinal centers. The fibrous variant is infiltrated mainly with plasma cells and displays more fibrosis. Clinical differences between the two are described later.

Lymphocytic infiltration of a focal or diffuse nature may be found in the thyroid gland in Graves disease, in thyroid neoplasms, and in simple or nontoxic goiter. In the past, a diagnosis of coexisting Hashimoto disease was not made unless Askanazy cells or lymphoid follicles were present. Because the lymphocytic infiltration in these other diseases is usually associated with circulating antithyroid antibodies, the pathogenetic mechanisms leading to lymphocytic infiltration in these disorders may be similar. In Graves disease, lymphocytic infiltration and associated antibodies may favor the development of hypothyroidism after partial thyroidectomy or radioiodine therapy.

Pathophysiology

Abnormalities in hormone biosynthesis include a defect in organic binding of thyroid iodide, as evidenced by a positive perchlorate discharge test, and accelerated turnover of a depleted organic iodine pool. In addition, abnormal release of iodoproteins occurs; in their physical properties, these may resemble either thyroglobulin or the albumin-like iodoprotein found in the sera of patients with other thyroid disorders. The foregoing abnormalities in hormone biosynthesis may occur in clinically normal individuals who either are relatives of patients with Hashimoto disease or have circulating antithyroid antibodies.

Because of the faulty synthesis of hormone, hypersecretion of TSH causes thyroid hyperactivity without thyrotoxicosis. Maximal stimulation by endogenous TSH may take place, with the result that no further stimulation is brought about by exogenous TSH (decreased thyroid reserve).

A high proportion of patients with Hashimoto disease develop iodide myxedema when iodide is taken chronically.

Clinical Picture

Goiter is the outstanding clinical feature of Hashimoto disease. It usually appears gradually and is often found during examination for some other complaint. In occasional instances, however, the thyroid enlarges rapidly, and when accompanied by pain and tenderness the disorder may mimic de Quervain or subacute thyroiditis. A moderate proportion of patients, especially those with the fibrous variant, are hypothyroid when first seen. The goiter is generally moderate in size and firm in consistency and moves freely when the patient swallows. Its surface is either smooth or scalloped, but well-defined nodules are unusual. Both lobes are enlarged, but one is often larger than the other. Enlargement of the pyramidal lobe is common. Compression of adjacent structures, such as trachea, esophagus, and recurrent laryngeal nerves, occurs rarely. Enlargement of regional lymph nodes may be present but is unusual.

Although primary (thyroprivic) hypothyroidism is thought to be the end result of autoimmune destruction of the thyroid, the progression of Hashimoto disease to classic thyroprivic hypothyroidism has not been observed in the individual patient. Indeed, the histopathological picture tends to remain rather static, except for some increase in fibrous tissue. Clinically, the goiter tends either to remain unchanged or to enlarge gradually over many years if left untreated. The clinical features of hypothyroidism commonly develop over several years in patients who are euthyroid when first seen. Although some studies suggest an increased prevalence of thyroid carcinoma in the thyroid in

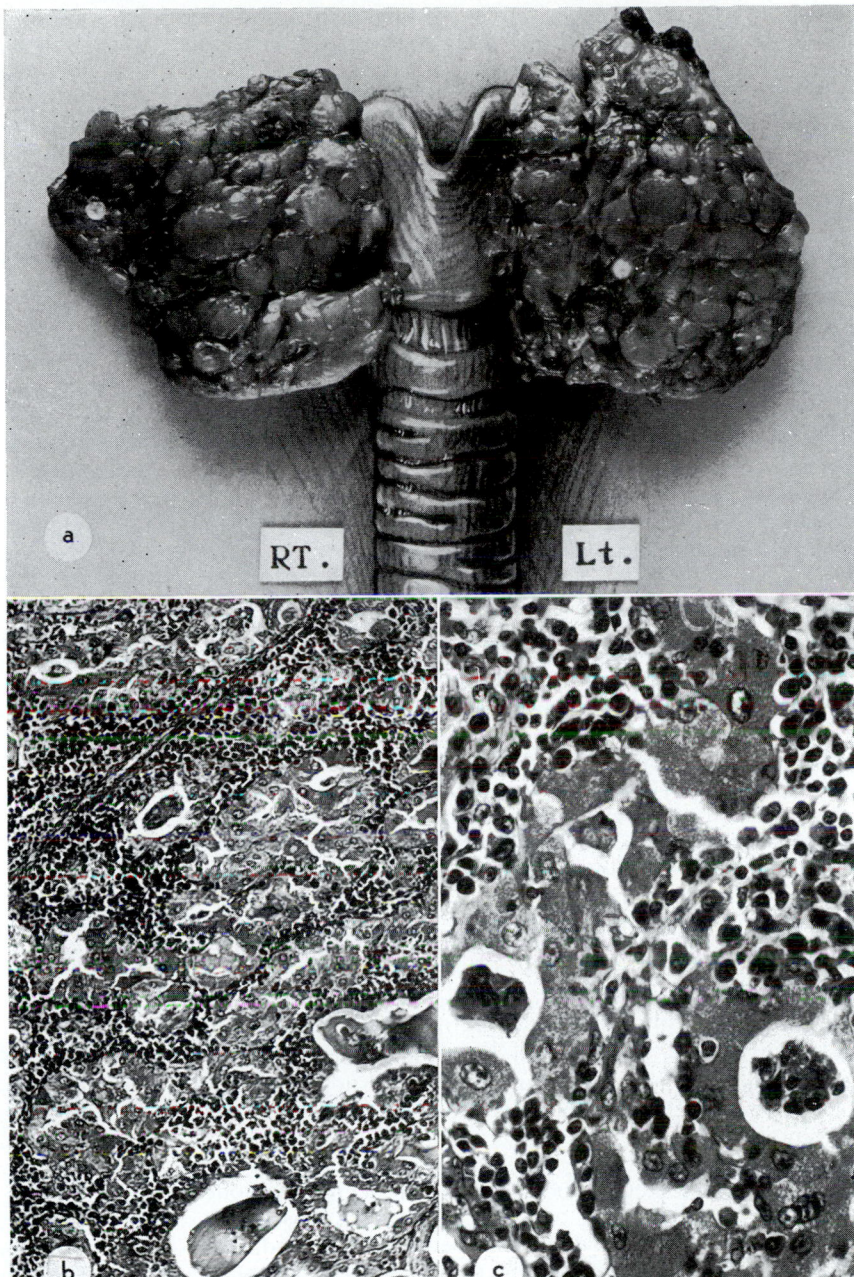

Figure 8–55. Hashimoto disease. *A,* Note the exaggeration of the normal lobular pattern. *B,* Interfollicular infiltration by lymphocytes and plasma cells. C, Granular, oxyphilic changes in the cytoplasm of the follicular epithelium (Askanazy cells). (From Woolner LB, McConahey WM, Beahrs OH. Struma lymphomatosa [Hashimoto's thyroiditis] and related thyroidal disorders. J Clin Endocrinol Metab 1959; 19:53–83. © 1959, The Endocrine Society.)

Hashimoto disease, other observations do not support this association.[428] As mentioned earlier, the presence of coexistent Hashimoto disease is a favorable prognostic factor in patients with papillary carcinoma.

Patients with Hashimoto disease may rarely develop manifestations of Graves disease, including hyperthyroidism with evidence of ongoing thyroid hyperfunction. Other patients with chronic thyroiditis develop transitory thyrotoxicosis (painless thyroiditis with thyrotoxicosis; see under Thyrotoxicosis). Here, evidence of ongoing thyroid hyperfunction is lacking because the thyroid RAIU is depressed. A phase of transient hypothyroidism beginning several weeks post partum occurs in 10 to 15% of women with chronic thyroiditis.[304-308] Often, there is a history suggesting mild thyrotoxicosis some time earlier. (See earlier discussion of postpartum thyroiditis syndromes.)

Laboratory Tests

The results of the common tests of thyroid function are variable, depending on the stage of the disease. At first, the tests indicate the presence of thyroid hyperfunction, but without overproduction of active hormone. At this time, the serum TSH concentration and RAIU are often increased, but serum T_4 and T_3 concentrations are normal. At this stage, the patient is eumetabolic, indicating that the glandular response to TSH is adequate to compensate for the abnormalities in hormone biosynthesis. With the passage of time, the ability of the thyroid to respond to TSH diminishes, and the RAIU and serum T_4 concentration progressively approach subnormal values. The serum T_3 concentration, however, may be slightly increased, reflecting in all likelihood maximal stimulation of the failing thyroid by the increased serum TSH concentration. The foregoing sequence in the evolution of complete thyroid failure reflects the development of what has been termed *diminished thyroid reserve* or *subclinical hypothyroidism*. Ultimately, the serum T_3 concentration also decreases to subnormal values, and the clinical state of the patient is that of frank hypothyroidism.

The diagnosis of Hashimoto disease is confirmed by the finding of antithyroid antibodies, usually of high titer, in the serum. Antimicrosomal (peroxidase) antibodies are more commonly detected, and in higher titer. Although circulating antibody titers tend to be higher in patients with the fibrous variant than in those with the oxyphilic type, almost all patients display elevated titers of antithyroid or antimicrosomal antibodies, or both. In young patients, however, the presence of low antibody titers does not exclude the diagnosis.

Because the diagnosis of Hashimoto disease in most patients can readily be confirmed by tests for antithyroid antibodies, needle biopsy is no longer an important adjunct in diagnosis. When a neoplastic lesion is suspected, fine-needle aspiration biopsy can be undertaken.

Differential Diagnosis

Differentiation of Hashimoto disease from other uncomplicated disorders of the thyroid has been facilitated by the demonstration that high titers of antithyroid antibodies occur commonly in Hashimoto disease but less frequently in other thyroid disorders. The frequent coexistence of hypothyroidism with Hashimoto disease also serves to distinguish this disease from others, such as nontoxic goiter and thyroid neoplasm, from which it must be differentiated. Differentiation of Hashimoto disease from diffuse nontoxic goiter is often difficult on clinical grounds, although the goiter in the latter disorder tends to be softer than that of Hashimoto disease. In adolescent patients differentiation from a diffuse nontoxic goiter is even more difficult because in this age group Hashimoto disease may not be accompanied by the high titers of antithyroid antibodies found in adult patients. Biopsy of the thyroid gland will then be necessary to establish the diagnosis. The presence of well-defined nodules generally serves to distinguish nontoxic multinodular goiter from Hashimoto disease.

Differentiation between Hashimoto disease and thyroid carcinoma can sometimes be made on clinical grounds alone. A goiter that is the seat of a thyroid carcinoma is usually nodular and firm or hard and may become fixed to adjacent structures. Compression of the recurrent laryngeal nerve with consequent hoarseness is virtually pathognomonic of thyroid carcinoma. A history of a recent enlargement of the goiter is more frequent in thyroid carcinoma than in Hashimoto disease. Enlargement of regional lymph nodes is common in thyroid carcinoma but unusual in Hashimoto disease. Finally, in thyroid carcinoma, scintiscanning of the thyroid may reveal isolated areas of nonfunction, whereas in Hashimoto disease activity is usually present throughout.

Treatment

In many patients, no treatment is required because the goiter is small and the disease asymptomatic. In others, treatment with thyroid hormone is directed at alleviating goiter or hypothyroidism, or both. Treatment is indicated in patients in whom the goiter is pressing on adjacent structures or is unsightly. This is most likely to be effective in the goiter of recent onset. In long-standing goiter, treatment with thyroid hormone is often ineffective, possibly because the gland is fibrotic. Glucocorticoids cause regression of the goiter and decrease antibody titers, but in view of

their untoward side effects and the fact that the activity of the disease returns after treatment is withdrawn, these agents are not recommended in the usual case. Full replacement doses of thyroid hormone should be given when hypothyroidism supervenes or when subclinical hypothyroidism has been demonstrated. Although surgery is a popular form of treatment in some centers, it is justified only if pressure symptoms or unsightly enlargement persists after a trial of suppressive therapy. Administration of hormone should be continued after surgery, because hypothyroidism inevitably results.

Subacute Thyroiditis

Subacute thyroiditis has been termed granulomatous, giant cell, or de Quervain thyroiditis. It is caused by a viral infection of the thyroid gland and often follows an upper respiratory illness. A tendency to a seasonal and geographic aggregation of cases has been noted. The mumps virus has been implicated in some cases and coxsackievirus, influenza virus, echoviruses and adenoviruses may also be etiological agents.[429] Although evidence of thyroid autoimmunity is often present during the active phase of the disease,[430] this is usually transitory, except perhaps in the rare patient in whom the disease progresses to hypothyroidism.

This disease is uncommon, but mild cases may be mistakenly diagnosed as pharyngitis. Women are more frequently affected than men, and the maximal incidence is in the fourth and fifth decades.

Histopathology

The histopathological changes are distinctive (Fig. 8–56) and different from those in Hashimoto disease. The lesions are patchy in distribution and vary in their stage of development from area to area. In affected areas, follicles

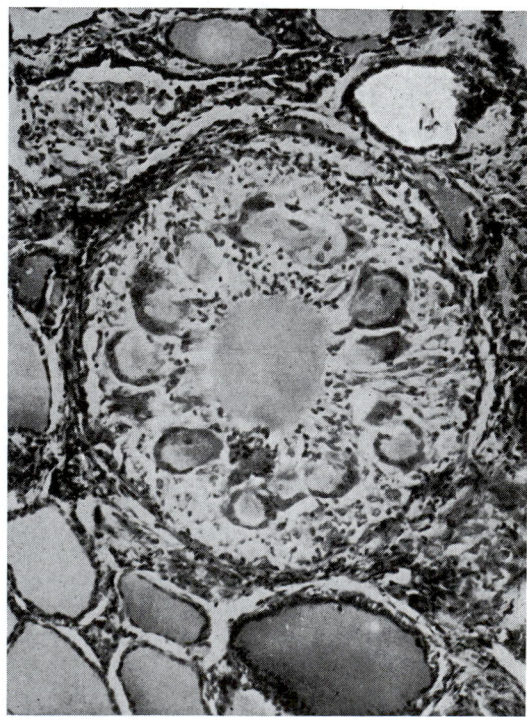

Figure 8–56. Subacute thyroiditis. Intrafollicular giant cell surrounding a central core of colloid. (From Meachim G, Young MH, De Quervain's subacute granulomatous thyroiditis: histological identification and incidence. J Clin Pathol 1963; 16:189–199.)

are infiltrated with cells predominantly of the mononuclear type. These infiltrated follicles show disruption of epithelium, partial or complete loss of colloid, and fragmentation and duplication of the basement membrane. To this extent, the histopathological appearance may resemble that in Hashimoto disease. A characteristic feature is the well-developed follicular lesion that consists of a central core of colloid surrounded by the multinucleate giant cells, from which stems the designation "giant cell" thyroiditis. Colloid may be found in the interstitium or within the giant cells (colloidophagy). The follicular changes progress to form granulomas. Interfollicular fibrosis and an interstitial inflammatory reaction are present to varying degrees. When the disease has subsided, an essentially normal histological appearance is restored.

Pathophysiology

Destruction of follicular epithelium and loss of follicular integrity are the primary events in the pathophysiology of subacute thyroiditis. Preformed hormone is released, along with abnormal iodinated materials, often in quantities sufficient to elevate the serum T_4 and T_3 concentrations, produce clinical thyrotoxicosis, and suppress TSH secretion. As a result of the latter, thyroid function is decreased, the RAIU decreases to low levels, and new hormone synthesis is interrupted. Destruction of the follicular epithelium contributes to lowering of the RAIU and disruption of hormone synthesis, because TSH may fail to increase the RAIU appreciably. Later in the disease, when stores of preformed hormone are depleted, serum T_4 and T_3 concentrations decrease, sometimes into the hypothyroid range, and the serum TSH concentration rises, often to elevated values. As the disease becomes inactive, the RAIU may be greater than normal for a time, as granular hormone stores are repleted. Ultimately, as hormone secretion resumes, serum T_4 and T_3 concentrations rise and serum TSH concentration decreases to normal values.

Clinical Picture

The characteristic feature is the gradual or sudden appearance of pain in the region of the thyroid gland accompanied in severe cases by fever. The pain, which is aggravated by turning the head or swallowing, characteristically radiates to the ear, jaw, or occiput and may mimic disorders arising in these areas. Absence of pain does not exclude the diagnosis, because biopsy-proven painless subacute thyroiditis has been reported.[431] Hoarseness and dysphagia may be present. Patients frequently complain of palpitation, nervousness, and lassitude; lassitude is often extreme, considering the local nature of the disease. Although severe cases may have acute manifestations, in milder cases, which are often wrongly diagnosed, symptoms may have been present for months. On palpation, at least part of the thyroid is slightly to moderately enlarged, firm, often nodular, and usually exquisitely tender, one lobe generally being more severely affected than the other. The overlying skin may be warm and red. Occasionally, the locus of maximal involvement migrates over the course of a few weeks to other parts of the gland. The disease usually subsides within a few months, leaving no residual deficiency of thyroid function, but often passes through an earlier transient phase of hypothyroidism, resembling the syndrome of chronic thyroiditis with transient thyrotoxicosis (silent thyroiditis) in this respect (see Fig. 8–41). In rare cases, the disease may smolder with repeated exacerbations over many months, hypothyroidism being the result.

Laboratory Tests

The laboratory findings in patients with subacute thyroiditis vary with the phase of the disease. During the active phase, the erythrocyte sedimentation rate is increased, often to a remarkable extent. Indeed, a diagnosis of active subacute thyroiditis is hardly tenable when the sedimentation rate is normal. The leukocyte count is normal or, at most, moderately increased.

Subacute thyroiditis is one of several causes of "low-uptake thyrotoxicosis," the others being so-called silent thyroiditis (see earlier), thyrotoxicosis factitia, and iodine-induced hyperthyroidism. For reasons described earlier, the RAIU is subnormal, despite the presence of normal, or often elevated, values of serum T_4 and T_3 concentrations. At this point in the course, basal serum TSH is suppressed. In the typical patient, antibodies directed against thyroid peroxidase or thyroglobulin are either not detectable or present in low titer. Subnormal values of the RAIU are found, even when only one portion of the gland seems involved clinically. Occasionally, especially in milder cases, some uptake of radioiodine may persist in unaffected portions of the gland, as revealed by scintiscan, but this is unusual, and a diagnosis of active subacute thyroiditis should be viewed with suspicion if the RAIU is normal.

In the hypothyroid phase of the disease, serum T_4 and T_3 concentrations are low and the serum TSH concentration is appropriately elevated. With recovery, the RAIU returns to normal or high values, and normal values for serum T_4 and T_3 concentrations are restored.

Differential Diagnosis

Subacute thyroiditis must be differentiated mainly from acute hemorrhagic degeneration in a pre-existing thyroid nodule, from Hashimoto disease of acute onset, from silent or painless thyroiditis, and from acute pyogenic thyroiditis. Differentiation from hemorrhage into a nodule presents no difficulty when this occurs in a multinodular goiter, because other nontender nodules will be felt. Decision is more difficult when there is hemorrhage into a solitary nodule. In both varieties of hemorrhage, however, function in the remainder of the gland persists, and marked elevation of the sedimentation rate is rarely present. Hashimoto disease of acute onset may be accompanied by pain and tenderness in the thyroid gland, but the gland usually is diffusely affected. Painless thyroiditis with thyrotoxicosis and a decreased RAIU, but with a histological picture of chronic thyroiditis and no giant cells, often termed *hyperthyroiditis*, may be difficult to distinguish from painless subacute thyroiditis. Lack of elevation of the erythrocyte sedimentation rate and high titers of antithyroid antibodies strongly suggest the former. Acute pyogenic thyroiditis is distinguished by the presence of a septic focus elsewhere, by a greater inflammatory reaction in the tissues adjacent to the thyroid, and by much greater leukocytic and febrile responses. The RAIU is usually preserved in acute pyogenic thyroiditis. Rarely, extensively infiltrating cancer of the thyroid can present with a clinical and laboratory picture almost indistinguishable from that of subacute thyroiditis.[408]

Treatment

Many forms of treatment have been recommended for subacute thyroiditis, including thionamide drugs, TSH, and suppressive doses of thyroid hormone. The evidence that these agents influence the course of the disease is unconvincing. In mild cases, aspirin is generally adequate to control the symptoms. In more severe cases, glucocorticoids (e.g., prednisone up to 40 mg/d) rapidly alleviate the clinical manifestations but do not influence the underlying disease process. Hence, the symptoms may be exacerbated if treatment is withdrawn too early but will again respond if treatment is reinstituted. It has been suggested that a relapse can be avoided if glucocorticoid therapy is continued at a dose that maintains the patient in an asymptomatic state until the RAIU has returned to normal.[432]

Riedel Thyroiditis

Riedel thyroiditis is rare and is observed chiefly in middle-aged women.[433, 434] The etiology is unknown. In the past, Riedel thyroiditis was considered to be an advanced state of Hashimoto disease, but it is now generally considered to be a separate disease entity. It is characterized by extensive fibrosis of the thyroid gland and adjacent structures and may be associated with fibrosis elsewhere, especially in the retroperitoneal area.[433]

Symptoms develop insidiously and are related chiefly to compression of adjacent structures, in particular the trachea, esophagus, and recurrent laryngeal nerves. Constitutional symptoms of inflammation are uncommon. The thyroid gland is moderately enlarged and stony hard. The enlargement is usually asymmetrical. The stony hard consistency of the gland and the invasion of adjacent structures suggest carcinoma, but there is no enlargement of regional lymph nodes. Temperature, pulse, and leukocyte count are normal. Hypothyroidism occurs occasionally.

The RAIU may be normal or low. Some patients have circulating antithyroid antibodies, but much less frequently and in lower titer than is usually seen in Hashimoto disease.

In general, surgical treatment is required to preserve tracheal and esophageal function. There may be extensive involvement of perithyroid tissues, and resection of the isthmus may relieve some of the symptoms. Treatment with thyroid hormone relieves the hypothyroidism but has no effect on the primary process.

Miscellaneous Types of Thyroiditis

Acute pyogenic thyroiditis is a rare disorder that is due to an infection of the thyroid by pyogenic organisms, usually as a result of dissemination from a septic focus elsewhere or a pyriform sinus fistula.[435] It is characterized by severe pain and tenderness in the region of the thyroid, dysphagia, fever, and malaise. There are signs of acute inflammation in the gland and in the surrounding tissues. Needle biopsy of the thyroid should be performed so that the infecting organism can be identified and treatment with the appropriate antibiotic can be instituted. Surgical drainage is indicated when fluctuation is present.

Rarely, the thyroid gland is the seat of tuberculosis or coccidioidal infection disseminated from some other focus.

REFERENCES

1. Burrow GN, Oppenheimer JH, Volpe R. Thyroid Function and Disease. Philadelphia: W. B. Saunders, 1990.
2. DeGroot LJ, Larsen PR, Refetoff S, et al. The Thyroid and Its Diseases. 5th ed. New York: John Wiley & Sons, 1984.
3. Van Middlesworth L, ed. The Thyroid Gland: A Practical Clinical Treatise. Chicago: Year Book Medical, 1986.
4. Ingbar SH, Braverman LE, eds. Werner's The Thyroid: A Fundamental and Clinical Text. 5th ed. Philadelphia: J. B. Lippincott, 1986.
5. Fisher DA, Klein AH. Thyroid development and disorders of thyroid function in the newborn. N Engl J Med 1981; 304:702–712.
6. Roti E, Gnudi A, Braverman LE, et al. Human cord blood concentrations of thyrotropin, thyroglobulin, and iodothyronines after maternal administration of thyrotropin-releasing hormone. J Clin Endocrinol Metab 1981; 53:813–817.
7. Vulsma T, Gons MH, de Vijlder JJM. Maternal-fetal transfer of thyroxine in congenital hypothyroidism due to a total organification defect or thyroid agenesis. N Engl J Med 1989; 321:13–16.
8. Ericson LE. Exocytosis and endocytosis in the thyroid follicle cell. Mol Cell Endocrinol 1981; 22:1–24.
9. Sobrinho-Simoes M, Johannessen JV. Surface features in human thyroid disorders. A scanning electron microscopic study of 95 cases. J Submicrosc Cytol 1982; 14:187–202.
10. Berkowitz M, Daughtridge D, Sherwin JR. Autoregulation of thyroid iodide transport: possible mediation by modification in sodium cotransport. Am J Physiol 1981; 240:E37–E42.
11. Gershengorn MC, Wolff J, Larsen, PR. Thyroid-pituitary feedback during iodine repletion. J Clin Endocrinol Metab 1976; 43:601–605.
12. Magnusson RP, Chazenbalk GD, Gestautas J, et al. Molecular cloning of the complementary deoxyribonucleic acid for human thyroid peroxidase. Mol Endocrinol 1987; 1:856–861.
13. Portmann L, Fitch FW, Havran W, et al. Characterization of the thyroid microsomal antigen, and its relationship to thyroid peroxidase, using monoclonal antibodies. J Clin Invest 1988; 81:1217–1224.
14. Magnusson RP, Taurog A, Dorris ML. Mechanisms of thyroid peroxidase- and lactoperoxidase-catalyzed reactions involving iodide. J Biol Chem 1984; 259:13783–13790.
15. Björkman U, Ekholm R, Denef JF. Cytochemical localization of hydrogen peroxide in isolated thyroid follicles. J Ultrastruct Res 1981; 74:105–115.
16. Vassart G, Brocas H, Cabrer B, et al. Structure and expression of the thyroglobulin gene. In: Eggo MC, Burrow GN, eds. Thyroglobulin—The Prothyroid Hormone. Vol 2. New York: Raven, 1985: 55–68.
17. Dunn JT, Anderson PC, Fox JW, et al. The sites of thyroid hormone formation in rabbit thyroglobulin. J Biol Chem 1987; 262:16948–16952.
18. Izumi M, Larsen PR. Triiodothyronine, thyroxine and iodine in purified thyroglobulin from patients with Graves' disease. J Clin Invest 1977; 59:1105–1112.
19. Erickson VJ, Cavalieri RR, Rosenberg LL. Thyroxine-5'-deiodinase of rat thyroid, but not that of liver, is dependent on thyrotropin. Endocrinology 1982; 111:434–440.
20. Ishii H, Inada M, Tanaka K, et al. Induction of outer and inner ring monodeiodinases in human thyroid gland by thyrotropin. J Clin Endocrinol Metab 1983; 57:500–505.
21. Laurberg P. Mechanisms governing the relative proportions of thyroxine and 3,5,3'-triiodothyronine in thyroid secretion. Metabolism 1984; 33:379–392.
22. Izumi M, Larsen PR. Correlation of sequential changes in serum thyroglobulin, triiodothyronine, and thyroxine in patients with Graves' disease and subacute thyroiditis. Metabolism 1978; 27:449–460.
23. Burger AG, Engler D, Buergi U, et al. Ether link cleavage is the major pathway of iodothyronine metabolism in the phagocytosing human leukocyte and also occurs in vivo in the rat. J Clin Invest 1983; 71:935–949.
24. Balsam A, Sexton F, Borges M, et al. Formation of diiodotyrosine from thyroxine. Ether-link cleavage, an alternate pathway of thyroxine metabolism. J Clin Invest 1983; 72:1234–1245.
25. Robbins J, Cheng S-Y, Gershengorn MC, et al. Thyroxine transport proteins of plasma. Molecular properties and biosynthesis. Recent Prog Horm Res 1978; 34:477–519.
26. Flink IL, Bailey TJ, Gustafson TA, et al. Complete amino acid sequence of human thyroxine-binding globulin deduced from cloned DNA: close homology to the serine antiproteases. Biochemistry 1986; 83:7708–7712.
27. Ain KB, Mori Y, Refetoff S. Reduced clearance rate of thyroxine-binding globulin (TBG) with increased sialylation: a mechanism for estrogen-induced elevation of serum TBG concentration. J Clin Endocrinol Metab 1987; 65:689–696.
28. Ain KB, Refetoff S. Relationship of oligosaccharide modification to the cause of serum thyroxine-binding globulin excess. J Clin Endocrinol Metab 1988; 66:1037–1043.
29. Murata Y, Takamatsu J, Refetoff S. Inherited abnormality of thyroxine-binding globulin with no demonstrable thyroxine-binding activity and high serum levels of denatured thyroxine-binding globulin. N Engl J Med 1986; 314:694–699.
30. Garnick MB, Larsen PR. Acute deficiency of thyroxine-binding globulin during L-asparginase therapy. N Engl J Med 1979; 301:251–253.
31. Bartalena L, Martino E, Antonelli A, et al. Effect of the antileukemic agent L-asparaginase on thyroxine-binding globulin and albumin synthesis in cultured human hepatoma (HEP G2) cells. Endocrinology 1986; 119:1185–1188.
32. Mori Y, Refetoff S, Flink IL, et al. Detection of the thyroxine-binding globulin (TBG) gene in six unrelated families with complete TBG deficiency. J Clin Endocrinol Metab 1988; 67:727–733.
33. Cody V. Thyroid hormone interactions: molecular conformation, protein binding and hormone action. Endocr Rev 1980; 1:140–166.
34. Dickson PW, Howlett GJ, Schreiber G. Rat transthyretin (prealbumin). Molecular cloning, nucleotide sequence, and gene expression in liver and brain. J Biol Chem 1985; 260:8214–8219.
35. Dickson PW, Aldred AR, Menting JGT, et al. Thyroxine transport in choroid plexus. J Biol Chem 1987; 262:13907–13915.

36. Refetoff S, Dwulet FE, Benson MD. Reduced affinity for thyroxine in two of three structural thyroxine-binding prealbumin variants associated with familial amyloidotic polyneuropathy. J Clin Endocrinol Metab 1986; 63:1432–1437.

37. Skiest D, Braverman LE, Emerson CH. Concentration of free thyroxin in serum of a patient with euthyroid hyperthyroxinemia secondary to increased thyroxin-binding prealbumin: results by various methods compared. Clin Chem 1986; 32:687–689.

38. Benvenga S. The 27-kilodalton thyroxine (T$_4$)-binding protein is human apolipoprotein A-I: identification of a 68-kilodalton high density lipoprotein that binds T$_4$. Endocrinology 1989; 124:1265–1269.

39. Bayer MF, McDougall IR. Radioimmunoassay of free thyroxine in serum: comparison with clinical findings and results of conventional thyroid-function tests. Clin Chem 1980; 26:1186–1192.

40. Mendel CM. The free hormone hypothesis: a physiologically based mathematical model. Endocr Rev 1989; 10:232–274.

41. Pardridge WM. Plasma protein-mediated transport of steroid and thyroid hormones. Am J Physiol 1987; 252:E157–E164.

42. Mendel CM, Weisiger RA, Jones AL, et al. Thyroid hormone-binding proteins in plasma facilitate uniform distribution of thyroxine within tissues: a perfused rat liver study. Endocrinology 1987; 120:1742–1749.

43. Mendel CM, Cavalieri RR, Gavin LA, et al. Thyroxine transport and distribution in Nagase analbuminemic rats. J Clin Invest 1989; 83:143–148.

44. Mendel CM, Weisiger RA, Cavalieri RR. Uptake of 3,5,3'-triiodothyronine by the perfused rat liver: return to the free hormone hypothesis. Endocrinology 1988; 123:1817–1824.

45. Krenning EP, Docter R, Visser TJ, et al. Plasma membrane transport of thyroid hormone: its possible pathophysiological significance. J Endocrinol Invest 1983; 6:59–66.

46. Hennemann G, Krenning EP, Polhuys M, et al. Carrier-mediated transport of thyroid hormone into rat hepatocytes is rate-limiting in total cellular uptake and metabolism. Endocrinology 1986; 119:1870–1872.

47. Blondeau JP, Osty J, Francon J. Characterization of the thyroid hormone transport system of isolated hepatocytes. J Biol Chem 1988; 263:2685–2692.

48. Pontecorvi A, Robbins J. Energy-dependent uptake of 3,5,3'-triiodo-L-thyronine in rat skeletal muscle. Endocrinology 1986; 119:2755–2761.

49. Docter R, Krenning EP, Bernard HF, et al. Active transport of iodothyronines into human cultured fibroblasts. J Clin Endocrinol Metab 1987; 65:624–628.

50. Centanni M, Robbins J. Role of sodium in thyroid hormone uptake by rat skeletal muscle. J Clin Invest 1987; 80:1068–1072.

51. Pontecorvi A, Lakshmanan M, Robbins J. Different intracellular and intranuclear transport of triiodothyronine enantiomers in rat skeletal myoblasts. Endocrinology 1988; 123:2922–2929.

52. Goncalves E, Lakshmanan M, Robbins J. Triiodothyronine transport into differentiated and undifferentiated mouse neuroblastoma cells (NB41A3). Endocrinology 1989; 124:293–300.

53. Movius EG, Phyillaier MM, Robbins J. Phloretin inhibits cellular uptake and nuclear receptor binding of triiodothyronine in human hep G2 hepatocarcinoma cells. Endocrinology 1989; 124:1988–1997.

54. van der Heyden, JTM, Docter R, van Toor H, et al. Effects of caloric deprivation on thyroid hormone tissue uptake and generation of low-T$_3$ syndrome. Am J Physiol 1986; 251:E156–E163.

55. Oppenheimer JH, Schwartz HL. Stereospecific transport of triiodothyronine from plasma to cytosol and from cytosol to nucleus in rat liver, kidney, brain, and heart. J Clin Invest 1985; 75:147–154.

56. Braverman LE, Ingbar SH, Sterling K. Conversion of thyroxine (T$_4$) to triiodothyronine (T$_3$) in athyreotic human subjects. J Clin Invest 1970; 49:855–864.

57. Hennemann G, ed. Thyroid Hormone Metabolism. New York: Marcel Dekker, 1986.

58. Visser TJ, Kaptein E, Terpstra OT, et al. Deiodination of thyroid hormone by human liver. J Clin Endocrinol Metab 1988; 67:17–24.

59. Abuid J, Larsen PR. Triiodothyronine and thyroxine in thyrotoxicosis: acute response to therapy with anti-thyroid agents. J Clin Invest 1974; 54:201–208.

60. Otten MH, Mol JA, Visser TJ. Sulfation preceding deiodination of iodothyronines in rat hepatocytes. Science 1983; 221:81–83.

61. Rooda SJE, van Loon MAC, Visser TJ. Metabolism of reverse triiodothyronine by isolated rat hepatocytes. J Clin Invest 1987; 79:1740–1748.

62. Rutgers M, Bonthuis F, de Herder WW, et al. Accumulation of plasma triiodothyronine sulfate in rats treated with propylthiouracil. J Clin Invest 1987; 80:758–762.

63. LoPresti JS, Eigen A, Kaptein E, et al. Alterations in 3,3',5'-triiodothyronine metabolism in response to propylthiouracil, dexamethasone, and thyroxine administration in man. J Clin Invest 1989; 84:1650–1656.

64. Visser TJ, Leonard JL, Kaplan MM, et al. Kinetic evidence suggesting two mechanisms for iodothyronine 5'-deiodination in rat cerebral cortex. Proc Natl Acad Sci USA 1982; 79:5080–5084.

65. Larsen PR, Silva JE, Kaplan MM. Relationships between circulating and intracellular thyroid hormones: physiological and clinical implications. Endocr Rev 1981; 2:87–102.

66. Leonard JL, Kaplan MM, Visser TJ, et al. Cerebral cortex responds rapidly to thyroid hormones. Science 1981; 214:571–573.

67. Visser TJ, Kaplan MM, Leonard JL, et al. Evidence for two pathways of iodothyronine 5'-deiodination in rat pituitary that differ in kinetics, propylthiouracil sensitivity, and response to hypothyroidism. J Clin Invest 1983; 71:992–1002.

68. Silva JE, Larsen PR. Pituitary nuclear 3,5,3'-triiodothyronine and thyrotropin secretion: an explanation for the effect of thyroxine. Science 1977; 198:617–619.

69. Larsen PR, Dick TE, Markovitz MM, et al. Inhibition of intrapituitary thyroxine to 3,5,3'-triiodothyronine conversion prevents the acute suppression of thyrotropin release by thyroxine in hypothyroid rats. J Clin Invest 1979; 64:117–128.

70. Riesco G, Taurog A, Larsen PR, et al. Acute and chronic responses to iodine deficiency in rats. Endocrinology 1977; 100:303–313.

71. Gardner DF, Kaplan MM, Stanley CA, et al. Effect of triiodothyronine replacement on the metabolic and pituitary responses to starvation. N Engl J Med 1979; 300:579–584.

72. Larsen PR, Atkinson AJ Jr, Wellman HN, et al. The effect of diphenylhydantoin on thyroxine metabolism in man. J Clin Invest 1970; 49:1266–1279.

73. Smith PJ, Surks MI. 5,5'-Diphenylhydantoin (Dilantin) decreases cytosol and specific nuclear 3,5,3'-triiodothyronine binding in rat anterior pituitary in vivo and in cultured GC cells. Endocrinology 1984; 115:283–290.

74. Wartofsky L, Burman KD. Alterations in thyroid function in patients with systemic illness: the "euthyroid sick syndrome." Endocr Rev 1982; 3:164–217.

75. Wiersinga WM, Trip MD. Amiodarone and thyroid hormone metabolism. Postgrad Med J 1986; 62:909–914.

76. Borowski GD, Garofano CD, Rose LI, et al. Effect of long-term amiodarone therapy on thyroid hormone levels and thyroid function. Am J Med 1985; 78:443–450.

77. Lim VS, Zavala DC, Flanigan MJ, et al. Basal oxygen uptake: a new technique for an old test. J Clin Endocrinol Metab 1986; 62:863–868.

78. Brent GA, Hershman JM. Thyroxine therapy in patients with severe nonthyroidal illnesses and low serum thyroxine concentration. J Clin Endocrinol Metab 1986; 63:1–8.

79. Becker RA, Vaughan GM, Ziegler MG, et al. Hypermetabolic low triiodothyronine syndrome of burn injury. Crit Care Med 1982; 10:870–875.

80. Borges M, Labourene J. Changes in hepatic iodothyronine metabolism during ontogeny in the chick embryo. Endocrinology 1980; 107:1751–1761.

81. Segerson TP, Kauer J, Wolfe HC, et al. Thyroid hormone regulates TRH biosynthesis in the paraventricular nucleus of the rat hypothalamus. Science 1987; 238:78–80.

82. Zoeller RT, Wolff RS, Koller KJ. Thyroid hormone regulation of messenger ribonucleic acid encoding thyrotropin (TSH)-releasing hormone is independent of the pituitary gland and TSH. Mol Endocrinol 1988; 2:248–252.

83. Dyess EM, Segerson TP, Liposits Z, et al. Triiodothyronine exerts direct cell-specific regulation of thyrotropin-releasing hormone gene expression in the hypothalamic paraventricular nucleus. Endocrinology 1988; 123:2291–2297.

84. Brenner-Gati L, Gershengorn MC. Effects of thyrotropin-releasing hormone on phosphoinositides and cytoplasmic free calcium in thyrotropic pituitary cells. Endocrinology 1986; 118:163–169.

85. Kolesnick RN, Gershengorn MC. Thyrotropin-releasing hormone and the pituitary. Am J Med 1985; 79:729–739.

86. Larsen PR. Feedback regulation of thyrotropin secretion by thyroid hormones. Thyroid-pituitary interaction. N Engl J Med 1982; 306:23–32.

87. Gershengorn MC. Bihormonal regulation of the thyrotropin-releasing hormone receptor in mouse pituitary thyrotropic tumor cells in culture. J Clin Invest 1978; 62:937–943.

88. Morley JE. Endocrine control of thyrotropin secretion. Endocr Rev 1981; 2:396–436.

89. Pierce JG, Parsons TF. Glycoprotein hormones: structure and function. Annu Rev Biochem 1981; 50:465–495.

90. Shupnik MA, Chin WW, Habener JF, et al. Transcriptional regulation of the thyrotropin subunit genes by thyroid hormone. J Biol Chem 1985; 260:2900–2903.

91. Shupnik MA, Ardisson LJ, Meskell MJ, et al. Triiodothyronine (T$_3$) regulation of thyrotropin subunit gene transcription is proportional to T$_3$ nuclear receptor occupancy. Endocrinology 1986; 118:367–371.

92. Shupnik MA, Greenspan SL, Ridgway EC. Transcriptional regulation of thyrotropin subunit genes by thyrotropin-releasing hormone and dopamine in pituitary cell culture. J Biol Chem 1986; 261:12675–12679.

93. Joshi LR, Weintraub BD. Naturally occurring forms of thyrotropin with low bioactivity and altered carbohydrate content act as competitive antagonists to more bioactive forms. Endocrinology 1983; 113:2145–2154.

94. Beck-Peccoz P, Amr S, Menezes-Ferreira MM, et al. Decreased receptor binding of biologically inactive thyrotropin in central hypothyroidism. N Engl J Med 1985; 312:1085–1090.

95. Menezes-Ferreira MM, Petrick PA, Weintraub BD. Regulation of thyrotropin (TSH) bioactivity by TSH-releasing hormone and thyroid hormone. Endocrinology 1986; 118:2125–2130.

96. Kourides IA, Re RN, Weintraub BD. Metabolic clearance and secretion

rates of subunits of human thyrotropin. J Clin Invest 1977; 59:508–516.

97. Silva JE. Effects of iodine and iodine-containing compounds on thyroid function. Med Clin North Am 1985; 69:881–898.

98. Wolff J. Physiological aspects of iodide excess in relation to radiation protection. J Mol Med 1980; 4:151–165.

99. Uchimura H, Chiu SC, Kuzaya N, et al. Effect of iodine enrichment in vitro on the adenylate-cyclase adenosine, 3′,5′-monophosphate system in thyroid glands from normal subjects and patients with Graves' disease. J Clin Endocrinol Metab 1980; 50:1066–1070.

100. Michalkiewicz M, Huffman LJ, Connors JM. Alterations in thyroid blood flow induced by varying levels of iodine intake in the rat. Endocrinology 1989; 125:54–60.

101. Ahren B, Alumets J, Ericsson M, et al. VIP appears in thyroidal nerves and stimulates thyroid hormone secretion. Nature 1980; 287:343–345.

102. Larsen PR. Salicylate-induced increases in free-triiodothyronine (T_3) in human serum: evidence of inhibition of T_3 binding to thyroxine-binding globulin and thyroxine-binding prealbumin. J Clin Invest 1972; 51:1125–1134.

103. Drucker D, Eggo MC, Salit IE, et al. Ethionamide-induced goitrous hypothyroidism. Ann Intern Med 1984; 100:837–839.

104. Jubiz W, Nolan G. The effects of 6-mercaptopurine (6-MP) on the thyroid gland. Endocrinology 1974; 94:1583–1586.

105. Transbol I, Christiansen C, Baastrup PC, et al. Endocrine effects of lithium. 1. Hypothyroidism, its prevalence in long-term patients. Acta Endocrinol 1978; 87:759–767.

106. Ermans AM. Goitrogens of vegetable origin as possible aetiological factors in endemic goiter. Ann Endocrinol 1981; 42:435–438.

107. Meyer JD, Gaitan E, Merino H, et al. Geologic implications in the distribution of endemic goiter in Colombia, South America. Int J Epidemiol 1978; 7:25–30.

108. Guillaume J, Schussler GC, Goldman J. Components of the total serum thyroid hormone concentrations during pregnancy: high free thyroxine and blunted thyrotropin (TSH) response to TSH-releasing hormone in the first trimester. J Clin Endocrinol Metab 1985; 60:678–684.

109. Pekonen F, Alfthan H, Stenman U, et al. Human chorionic gonadotropin (hCG) and thyroid function in early human pregnancy: circadian variation and evidence for intrinsic thyrotropic activity in hCG. J Clin Endocrinol Metab 1988; 66:853–856.

110. Hershman JM, Lee H, Sugawara M, et al. Human chorionic gonadotropin stimulates iodide uptake, adenylate cyclase, and deoxyribonucleic acid synthesis in cultured rat thyroid cells. J Clin Endocrinol Metab 1988; 67:74–79.

111. Yoshikawa N, Nishikawa M, Horimoto M, et al. Thyroid-stimulating activity in sera of normal pregnant women. J Clin Endocrinol Metab 1989; 69:891–895.

112. Bouillon R, Naesens M, van Assche FA, et al. Thyroid function in patients with hyperemesis gravidarum. Am J Obstet Gynecol 1982; 143:922.

113. Dowling JT, Appleton WG, Nicoloff JT. Thyroxine turnover during human pregnancy. J Clin Endocrinol Metab 1964; 27:1749–1750.

114. Silva JE, Larsen PR. Potential of brown adipose tissue type II thyroxine 5′-deiodinase as a local and systemic source of triiodothyronine in rats. J Clin Invest 1985; 76:2296–2305.

115. Fisher DA, Foley BL. Early treatment of congenital hypothyroidism. Pediatrics 1989; 83:785–789.

116. Ingbar SH. The influence of aging on human thyroid hormone economy. In: Greenblatt R, ed. Geriatric Endocrinology. New York: Raven, 1978: 13–32.

117. Visser TJ, Lambert SWJ. Regulation of TSH secretion and thyroid function in Cushing's disease. Acta Endocrinol 1981; 96:480–483.

118. Williams DE, Chopra IJ, Orgiazzi J, et al. Acute effects of corticosteroids on thyroid activity in Graves' disease. J Clin Endocrinol Metab 1975; 41:354–361.

119. Gharib H, Hodgson SF, Gastineau CF, et al. Reversible hypothyroidism in Addison's disease. Lancet 1972; 2:734–736.

120. Smals AG, Ross HA, Kloppenborg PWC. Seasonal variation in serum T_3 and T_4 levels in man. J Clin Endocrinol Metab 1977; 44:998–1001.

121. Schussler GC, Orlando J. Fasting decreases triiodothyronine receptor capacity. Science 1978; 189:686–688.

122. Danforth E Jr, Horton ES, O'Connell M, et al. Dietary-induced alterations in thyroid hormone metabolism during overnutrition. J Clin Invest 1979; 64:1336–1347.

123. Kaplan MM, Larsen PR, Crantz FR, et al. Prevalence of abnormal thyroid function test results in patients with acute medical illnesses. Am J Med 1982; 72:9–16.

124. Brent GA, Hershman JM. Effects of nonthyroidal illness on thyroid function tests. In: Van Middlesworth L, ed. The Thyroid Gland: A Practical Treatise. Chicago: Year Book Medical, 1986: 83–110.

125. Nelson JC, Weiss RM. The effect of serum dilution on free thyroxine (T_4) concentrations in the low T_4 syndrome of nonthyroidal illness. J Clin Endocrinol Metab 1985; 61:239–246.

126. Surks MI, Hupart KH, Pan C, et al. Normal free thyroxine in critical nonthyroidal illnesses measured by ultrafiltration of undiluted serum and equilibrium dialysis. J Clin Endocrinol Metab 1988; 67:1031–1039.

127. Faber J, Kirkegaard C, Rasmussen B, et al. Pituitary-thyroid axis in critical illness. J Clin Endocrinol Metab 1987; 65:315–320.

128. Brent GA, Hershman JM, Braunstein GD. Patients with severe nonthyroidal illness and serum thyrotropin concentrations in the hypothyroid range. Am J Med 1986; 81:463–466.

129. Spencer C, Eigen A, Shen D, et al. Specificity of sensitive assays of thyrotropin (TSH) used to screen for thyroid disease in hospitalized patients. Clin Chem 1987; 33:1391–1396.

130. Bacci V, Schussler GC, Kaplan TB. The relationship between serum triiodothyronine and thyrotropin during systemic illness. J Clin Endocrinol Metab 1982; 54:1229–1235.

131. Gavin LA, Rosenthal M, Cavalieri RR. The diagnostic dilemma of isolated hyperthyroxinemia in acute illness. JAMA 1979; 242:251–253.

132. Birkhauser M, Burer T, Busset R, et al. Diagnosis of hyperthyroidism when serum thyroxine alone is raised. Lancet 1977; 2:53–56.

133. Burman KD, Borst GC, Eil C. Euthyroid hyperthyroxinemia. Ann Intern Med 1983; 98:366–378.

134. Mariotti S, Martino E, Cupini C, et al. Low serum thyroglobulin as a clue to the diagnosis of thyrotoxicosis factitia. N Engl J Med 1982; 307:410–412.

135. Larsen PR, Alexander NM, Chopra IJ, et al. Revised nomenclature for tests of thyroid hormones and thyroid-related proteins in serum. J Clin Endocrinol Metab 1987; 64:1089–1092.

136. Docter R, Bos G, Krenning EP, et al. Inherited thyroxine excess: a serum abnormality due to an increased affinity for modified albumin. Clin Endocrinol 1981; 15:363–371.

137. Ruiz M, Rajatanavin R, Young RA, et al. Familial dysalbuminemic hyperthyroxinemia, a syndrome that can be confused with thyrotoxicosis. N Engl J Med 1982; 306:635–639.

138. Mendel CM, Frost PH, Kunitake ST, et al. Mechanism of the heparin-induced increase in the concentrations of free thyroxine in plasma. J Clin Endocrinol Metab 1987; 65:1259–1264.

139. Jacobsson B, Pettersson T, Sandstedt B, et al. Prealbumin in the islets of Langerhans. IRCS Med Sci 1979; 7:590–591.

140. Moses AC, Lawlor J, Haddow J, et al. Familial euthyroid hyperthyroxinemia resulting from increased thyroxine binding to thyroxine binding prealbumin. N Engl J Med 1982; 306:966–969.

141. Pagliara AS, Caplan RH, Gundersen CB, et al. Peripheral resistance to thyroid hormone in a family: heterogeneity of clinical presentation. J Pediatr 1983; 103:228–232.

142. Refetoff S. Syndromes of thyroid hormone resistance. Am J Physiol 1982; 243:E88–E98.

143. Smallridge RC, Parker RA, Wiggs EA, et al. Thyroid hormone resistance in a large kindred: physiologic, biochemical, pharmacologic, and neuropsychologic studies. Am J Med 1989; 86:289–296.

144. Kaplan MM, Swartz SL, Larsen PR. Partial peripheral resistance to thyroid hormone. Am J Med 1981; 70:1115–1121.

145. Spratt DI, Pont A, Miller MB, et al. Hyperthyroxinemia in patients with acute psychiatric disorders. Am J Med 1982; 73:41–48.

146. LoPresti JS, Fried JC, Spencer CA, et al. Unique alterations of thyroid hormone indices in the acquired immunodeficiency syndrome (AIDS). Ann Intern Med 1989; 110:970–975.

147. Cavalieri R, Pitt-Rivers R. The effect of drugs on the distribution and metabolism of thyroid hormones. Pharmacol Rev 1981; 33:55–80.

148. Martino E, Safran M, Aghini-Lombardi F, et al. Environmental iodine intake and thyroid dysfunction during chronic amiodarone therapy. Ann Intern Med 1984; 101:28–34.

149. Norman MF, Lavin TN. Antagonism of thyroid hormone action by amiodarone in rat pituitary tumor cells. J Clin Invest 1989; 83:306–313.

150. Wiersinga WM, Endert E, Trip MD, et al. Immunoradiometric assay of thyrotropin in plasma: its value in predicting response to thyroliberin stimulation and assessing thyroid function in amiodarone-treated patients. Clin Chem 1986; 32:433–436.

151. Cooper DS, Daniels GH, Ladenson PW, et al. Hyperthyroxinemia in patients treated with high-dose propranolol. Am J Med 1982; 73:867–871.

152. Perrild H, Molhom Hansen J, Skovsted L, et al. Different effects of propranolol, alprenolol, sotalol, atenolol, and metoprolol on serum T_3 and serum rT_3 in hyperthyroidism. Clin Endocrinol 1983; 18:139–142.

153. Morley JE, Shafer RB, Elson MK. Amphetamine-induced hyperthyroxinemia. Ann Intern Med 1980; 93:707–709.

154. Bantle JP, Oppenheimer JH, Schwartz HL, et al. TSH response to TRH in euthyroid, hypercholesterolemic patients treated with graded doses of dextrothyroxine. Metabolism 1981; 30:63–66.

155. Vagenakis AG, Braverman LE, Azizi F, et al. Recovery of pituitary thyrotropic function after withdrawal of prolonged thyroid-suppression therapy. N Engl J Med 1975; 293:681–684.

156. Fisher DA, Burrow GN, Dussault JH, et al. Recommendations for screening programs for congenital hypothyroidism. J Pediatr 1976; 89:692–694.

157. Evans PJ, Woodhead JS, Weeks I, et al. Circulating TSH levels measured with an immunochemiluminometric assay in patients taking drugs interfering with biochemical thyroid status. Clin Endocrinol 1987; 26:717–721.

158. DeLuca F, Arrigo T, Pandullo E, et al. Changes in thyroid function tests induced by 2 month carbamazepine treatment in L-thyroxine-substituted hypothyroid children. Eur J Pediatr 1986; 145:77–79.

159. Isley WL. Effect of rifampin therapy on thyroid function tests in a hypothyroid patient on replacement L-thyroxine. Ann Intern Med 1987; 107:517–518.

160. Ratcliffe WA, Hazelton RA, Thomson JA, et al. The effect of fenclofenac on thyroid function tests in vivo and in vitro. Clin Endocrinol 1980; 13:569–575.

161. Konishi J, Iida Y, Kousaka T, et al. Effect of antithyroxine antibodies on radioimmunoassay of free thyroxine in serum. Clin Chem 1982; 28:1389–1391.

162. Waal-Manning HJ. Effect of propranolol on the duration of the Achilles tendon reflex. Clin Pharmacol Ther 1969; 10:199–206.

163. Jenkins DJ. An investigation into creatine kinase and other plasma enzymes in thyroid disorders. Clin Chim Acta 1978; 85:197–204.

164. Peracchi M, Bamonti-Catena F, Lombardi L, et al. Plasma and urine cyclic nucleotide levels in patients with hyperthyroidism and hypothyroidism. J Endocrinol Invest 1983; 6:173–177.

165. Parisi AF, Hamilton BP. The short cardiac pre-ejection period. An index to thyrotoxicosis. Circulation 1974; 49:900–904.

166. Landenson PW, Goldenheim PD, Ridgway EC. Rapid pituitary and peripheral tissue responses to intravenous L-triiodothyronine in hypothyroidism. J Clin Endocrinol Metab 1983; 56:1252–1259.

167. Spencer CA, Lai-Rosenfeld AO, Guttler RB, et al. Thyrotropin secretion in thyrotoxic and thyroxine-treated patients: assessment by a sensitive immunoenzymometric assay. J Clin Endocrinol Metab 1986; 63:349–355.

168. Kahn BB, Weintraub BD, Csako G, et al. Factitious elevation of thyrotropin in a new ultrasensitive assay: implications for the use of monoclonal antibodies in "sandwich" immunoassay. J Clin Endocrinol Metab 1988; 66:526–533.

169. Faglia G, Beck-Peccoz P, Ballabio M, et al. Excess of β-subunit of thyrotropin (TSH) in patients with idiopathic central hypothyroidism due to the secretion of TSH with reduced biological activity. J Clin Endocrinol Metab 1983; 56:908–914.

170. Blunt S, Woods CA, Joplin GF, et al. The role of a highly sensitive amplified enzyme immunoassay for thyrotrophin in the evaluation of thyrotroph function in hypopituitary patients. Clin Endocrinol 1988; 29:387–393.

171. Kourides IA, Ridgway EC, Weintraub BD, et al. Thyrotropin-induced hyperthyroidism: use of alpha and beta subunit levels to identify patients with pituitary tumors. J Clin Endocrinol Metab 1977; 45:534–543.

172. Faglia G, Beck-Peccoz P, Piscitelli G, et al. Inappropriate secretion of thyrotropin by the pituitary. Horm Res 1987; 26:79–99.

173. Smallridge RC. Thyrotropin-secreting pituitary tumors. Endocrinol Metab Clin North Am 1987; 16:765–792.

174. Ridgway EC, Kourides IA, Chin WW, et al. Augmentation of pituitary thyrotropin response to thyrotropin releasing hormone during subphysiological triiodothyronine therapy in hypothyroidism. Clin Endocrinol 1979; 10:343–353.

175. Tamai H, Suematsu H, Ikemi Y, et al. Responses to TRH and T₃ suppression tests in euthyroid subjects with a family history of Graves' disease. J Clin Endocrinol Metab 1978; 47:475–479.

176. Snyder PJ, Jacobs LS, Rabello MM, et al. Diagnostic value of thyrotrophin-releasing hormone in pituitary and hypothalamic disease. Ann Intern Med 1974; 81:751–757.

177. Uller RP, Van Herle A, Chopra IJ. Comparison of alterations in circulating thyroglobulin, triiodothyronine and thyroxine in response to exogenous (bovine) and endogenous (human) thyrotropin. J Clin Endocrinol Metab 1973; 37:741–745.

178. Suzuki H, Mashimo K. Significance of the iodide-perchlorate discharge test in patients with ¹³¹I-treated and untreated hyperthyroidism. J Clin Endocrinol Metab 1972; 34:332–338.

179. Amino N. Postpartum autoimmune endocrine syndromes. In: Davies TF, ed. Autoimmune Endocrine Disease. New York: John Wiley & Sons, 1983: 247–272.

180. Schneider AB, Ikekubo K. Measurement of thyroglobulin in the circulation: clinical and technical considerations. Ann Clin Lab Sci 1979; 9:230–235.

181. Schneider AB, Line BR, Goldman JM, et al. Sequential serum thyroglobulin determinations, ¹³¹I scans, and ¹³¹I uptakes after triiodothyronine withdrawal in patients with thyroid cancer. J Clin Endocrinol Metab 1981; 53:1199–1206.

182. Colacchio TA, LoGerfo P, Colacchio DA, et al. Radioiodine total body scan versus serum thyroglobulin levels in follow-up of patients with thyroid cancer. Surgery 1982; 91:42–45.

183. Smith BR, McLachlan SM, Furmaniak J. Autoantibodies to the thyrotropin receptor. Endocr Rev 1988; 9:106–121.

184. Zakarija M, McKenzie JM, Banovac K. Clinical significance of assay of thyroid-stimulating antibody in Graves' disease. Ann Intern Med 1980; 93:28–32.

185. Kidd A, Okita N, Row VV, et al. Immunologic aspects of Graves' and Hashimoto's diseases. Metabolism 1980; 29:80–99.

186. Rapoport B, Block MB, Hoffer PB, et al. Depletion of thyroid iodine during subacute thyroiditis. J Clin Endocrinol Metab 1973; 36:610–611.

187. Rosen IB, Walfish PG, Miskin M. The ultrasound of thyroid masses. Surg Clin North Am 1979; 59:19–33.

188. Wang C, Vickery Al Jr, Maloof F. Needle biopsy of the thyroid. Surg Gynecol Obstet 1976; 143:365–368.

189. Hamburger JI, Hamburger SW. Fine needle biopsy of thyroid nodules: avoiding the pitfalls. NY State J Med 1986; 86:241–249.

190. Clark DG, Brinkman M, Filsell OH, et al. No major thermogenic role for (Na⁺, K⁺) dependent adenosine triphosphatase apparent in hepatocytes from hyperthyroid rats. Biochem J 1982; 202:661–665.

191. Gick GG, Ismail-Beigi F, Edelman IS. Thyroidal regulation of rat renal and hepatic Na,K-ATPase gene expression. J Biol Chem 1988; 263:16610–16618.

192. Haber RS, Loeb JN. Early enhancement of passive potassium efflux from rat liver by thyroid hormone: relation to induction of Na,K-ATPase. Endocrinology 1984; 115:291–297.

193. Hoppner W, Rasmussen UB, Abuerreish G, et al. Thyroid hormone effect on gene expression of the adenine nucleotide translocase in different rat tissues. Mol Endocrinol 1988; 2:1127–1131.

194. Sterling K. Thyroid hormone action at the cell level. N Engl J Med 1979; 300:117–121.

195. Oppenheimer JH, Silva E, Schwartz HL, et al. Stimulation of hepatic mitochondrial alpha-glycerophosphate dehydrogenase and malic enzyme by L-triiodothyronine. I. Characteristics of the response with specific nuclear thyroid hormone binding sites fully saturated. J Clin Invest 1977; 59:517–527.

196. Sestoft L. Metabolic aspects of the calorigenic effect of thyroid hormone in mammals. Clin Endocrinol 1980; 13:489–506.

197. Muls E, Blaton V, Rosseneu M, et al. Serum lipids and apolipoproteins A-I, A-II, and B in hyperthyroidism before and after treatment. J Clin Endocrinol Metab 1982; 55:459–464.

198. Stakkestad JA, Bremer J. The outer carnitine palmitoyltransferase and regulation of fatty acid metabolism in rat liver in different thyroid states. Biochim Biophys Acta 1983; 750:244–252.

199. Abrams JJ, Grundy SM. Cholesterol metabolism in hypothyroidism and hyperthyroidism in man. J Lipid Res 1981; 22:323–338.

200. Chait A, Bierman EL, Albers JJ. Regulatory role of triiodothyronine in the degradation of low density lipoprotein by cultured human skin fibroblasts. J Clin Endocrinol Metab 1979; 48:887–889.

201. Bilezekian JP, Loeb JN. The influence of hyperthyroidism and hypothyroidism on the α- and β-adrenergic receptor system and adrenergic responsiveness. Endocr Rev 1983; 4:378–388.

202. Aoki VS, Wilson WR, Theilen EO, et al. The effects of triiodothyronine on hemodynamic responses to epinephrine and norepinephrine in man. J Pharmacol Exp Ther 1967; 157:62–68.

203. Landsberg L. Catecholamines and hyperthyroidism. Clin Endocrinol Metab 1977; 6:697–718.

204. Liggett SB, Shah SD, Cryer PE. Increased fat and skeletal muscle β-adrenergic receptors but unaltered metabolic and hemodynamic sensitivity to epinephrine in vivo in experimental human thyrotoxicosis. J Clin Invest 1989; 83:803–809.

205. Gelfand RA, Hutchinson-Williams KA, Bonde AA, et al. Catabolic effects of thyroid hormone excess: the contribution of adrenergic activity to hypermetabolism and protein breakdown. Metabolism 1987; 36:562–569.

206. Oppenheimer JH. Thyroid hormone action at the cellular level. Science 1979; 203:971–979.

207. Sap J, Munoz A, Damm K, et al. The c-erb-A protein is a high-affinity receptor for thyroid hormone. Nature 1986; 324:635–640.

208. Weinberger C, Thompson CC, Ong ES, et al. The c-erb-A gene encodes a thyroid hormone receptor. Nature 1986; 324:641–646.

209. Thompson CC, Weinberger C, Lebo R, et al. Identification of a novel thyroid hormone receptor expressed in the mammalian central nervous system. Science 1987; 237:1610–1614.

210. Koenig RJ, Warne RL, Brent GA, et al. Isolation of a cDNA clone encoding a biologically active thyroid hormone receptor. Proc Natl Acad Sci USA 1988; 85:5031–5035.

211. Sakurai A, Nakai A, DeGroot LJ. Expression of three forms of thyroid hormone receptor in human tissues. Mol Endocrinol 1989; 3:392–399.

212. Izumo S, Mahdavi V. Thyroid hormone receptor α isoforms generated by alternative splicing differentially activate myosin HC gene transcription. Nature 1988; 334:539–542.

213. Murray MB, Zilz ND, McCreary NL, et al. Isolation and characterization of rat cDNA clones for two distinct thyroid hormone receptors. J Biol Chem 1988; 264:12770–12777.

214. Benbrook D, Pfahl M. A novel thyroid hormone receptor encoded by a cDNA clone from a human testis library. Science 1987; 238:788–791.

215. Mitsuhashi T, Tennyson GE, Nikodem VM. Alternative splicing generates messages encoding rat c-erbA proteins that do not bind thyroid hormone. Proc Natl Acad Sci USA 1988; 85:5804–5808.

216. Prost E, Koenig RJ, Moore DD, et al. Multiple sequences encoding potential thyroid hormone receptors from mouse skeletal muscle cDNA libraries. Nucleic Acids Res 1988; 16:6248.

217. Koenig RJ, Lazar MA, Hodin RA, et al. Inhibition of thyroid hormone action by a non-hormone binding c-erbA protein generated by alternative mRNA splicing. Nature 1989; 337:659–661.
218. Evans RM. The steroid and thyroid hormone receptor superfamily. Science 1988; 240:889–895.
219. Umesono K, Evans RM. Determinants of target gene specificity for steroid/thyroid hormone receptors. Cell 1989; 57:1139–1146.
220. Koenig RJ, Brent GA, Warne RL, et al. Thyroid hormone receptor binds to a site in the rat growth hormone promoter required for induction by thyroid hormone. Proc Natl Acad Sci USA 1987; 84:5670–5674.
221. Glass CK, Franco R, Weinberger C, et al. A c-erb-A binding site in rat growth hormone gene mediates trans-activation by thyroid hormone. Nature 1987; 329:738–741.
222. Samuels HH, Forman BM, Horowitz ZD, et al. Regulation of gene expression by thyroid hormone. J Clin Invest 1988; 81:957–967.
223. Brent GA, Harney JW, Chen Y, et al. Mutations of the rat growth hormone promoter which increase response to thyroid hormone and strengthen thyroid hormone receptor binding: a consensus thyroid hormone response element. Mol Endocrinol 1989; 3:1996–2004.
224. Glass CK, Holloway JM, Devary OV, et al. The thyroid hormone receptor binds with opposite transcriptional effects to a common sequence motif in thyroid hormone and estrogen response elements. Cell 1988; 54:313–323.
225. Brent GA, Harney JW, Moore DD, et al. Multihormonal regulation of the human, rat, and bovine growth hormone promoters: differential effects of 3′,5′-cyclic adenosine monophosphate, thyroid hormone, and glucocorticoids. Mol Endocrinol 1988; 2:792–798.
226. Chernausek SD, Underwood LE, Utiger RD, et al. Growth hormone secretion and plasma somatomedin-C in primary hypothyroidism. Clin Endocrinol 1983; 19:337–344.
227. Valcavi R, Jordon V, Kieguez C, et al. Growth hormone responses to GRF 1–29 in patients with primary hypothyroidism before and during replacement therapy with thyroxine. Clin Endocrinol 1986; 24:693–696.
228. Cavaliere H, Knobel M, Medeiros-Neto G. Effect of thyroid hormone therapy on plasma insulin-like growth factor I levels in normal subjects, hypothyroid patients and endemic cretins. Horm Res 1987; 25:132–139.
229. Obregon MJ, Larsen PR, Silva JE. The role of 3,3′,5′-triiodothyronine in the regulation of type II iodothyronine 5′-deiodinase in the rat cerebral cortex. Endocrinology 1986; 119:2186–2192.
230. Myers JD, Brannon ES, Holland BC. A correlative study of the cardiac output and the hepatic circulation in hyperthyroidism. J Clin Invest 1950; 29:1069–1077.
231. Bergman TA, Mariash CN, Oppenheimer JH. Anterior mediastinal mass in a patient with Graves' disease. J Clin Endocrinol Metab 1982; 55:587–588.
232. Engel AG. Neuromuscular manifestations of Graves' disease. Mayo Clin Proc 1972; 47:919–925.
233. Burman RD, Monchik JM, Earll JM, et al. Ionized and total serum calcium and parathyroid hormone in hyperthyroidism. Ann Intern Med 1976; 84:668–671.
234. Garrel DR, Delmas PD, Malaval L, et al. Serum bone Gla protein: a marker of bone turnover in hyperthyroidism. J Clin Endocrinol Metab 1986; 62:1052–1055.
235. Eriksen EF, Mosekilde L, Melsen F. Trabecular bone remodeling and bone balance in hyperthyroidism. Bone 1985; 6:421–428.
236. Rhone DP, Berlinger FG, White FM. Tissue sources of elevated serum alkaline phosphatase activity in hyperthyroid patients. Am J Clin Pathol 1980; 74:381–386.
237. Rogers JS, Shane SR, Jencks FS. Factor VIII activity and thyroid function. Ann Intern Med 1982; 97:713–716.
238. Self TH, Straughn AB, Weisburst MR. Effect of hyperthyroidism on hypoprothrombinemic response to warfarin. Am J Hosp Pharm 1976; 33:387–389.
239. Gordon GG, Southren AL. Thyroid-hormone effects on steroid-hormone metabolism. Bull NY Acad Med 1977; 53:241–259.
240. Coulombe P, Dussault JH, Walker P. Plasma catecholamine concentrations in hyperthyroidism and hypothyroidism. Metabolism 1976; 25:973–979.
241. Coulombe P, Dussault JH, Walker P. Catecholamine metabolism in thyroid disease. II. Norepinephrine secretion rate in hyperthyroidism and hypothyroidism. J Clin Endocrinol Metab 1977; 44:1185–1189.
242. Kohut WD, Gharib H, Anderson MW. Triiodothyronine thyrotoxicosis complicating primary hypothyroidism in a patient with autoimmune thyroiditis. Am J Med 1982; 72:843–846.
243. Salvi M, Fukazawa H, Bernard N, et al. Role of autoantibodies in the pathogenesis and association of endocrine autoimmune disorders. Endocr Rev 1988; 9:450–466.
244. Tunbridge WMG, Evered DE, Hall R, et al. The spectrum of thyroid disease in a community: the Wickham Survey. Clin Endocrinol 1977; 7:481–493.
245. Endo K, Borges M, Amir S, et al. Preparation of 125I-labeled receptor-purified Graves' immunoglobulins: properties of their binding to human thyroid membranes. J Clin Endocrinol Metab 1982; 55:566–576.
246. Carayon P, Adler G, Roulier R, et al. Heterogeneity of the Graves' immunoglobulins directed toward the thyrotropin receptor–adenylate cyclase system. J Clin Endocrinol Metab 1983; 56:1202–1208.
247. Endo K, Kasagi K, Konishi J, et al. Detection and properties of TSH-binding inhibitor immunoglobulins in patients with Graves' disease and Hashimoto's thyroiditis. J Clin Endocrinol Metab 1978; 46:734.
248. O'Donnell J, Trokoudes K, Silverberg J, et al. Thyrotropin displacement activity of serum immunoglobulins from patients with Graves' disease. J Clin Endocrinol Metab 1978; 46:770–777.
249. Bliddal H, Kirkegaard C, Siersback-Nielsen K, et al. Prognostic value of thyrotropin binding inhibiting immunoglobulins (TBII) in long term antithyroid treatment, 131I therapy given in combination with carbimazole and in euthyroid ophthalmopathy. Acta Endocrinol 1981; 98:364–369.
250. Konishi J, Iida Y, Endo K, et al. Inhibition of thyrotropin-induced adenosine 3′,5′-monophosphate increase by immunoglobulins from patients with primary myxedema. J Clin Endocrinol Metab 1983; 57:544–549.
251. Matsuura N, Yamada Y, Nohara Y, et al. Familial neonatal transient hypothyroidism due to maternal TSH-binding inhibitor immunoglobulins. N Engl J Med 1980; 303:738–741.
252. Ealey PA, Kohn LD, Ekins RP, et al. Characterization of monoclonal antibodies derived from lymphocytes from Graves' disease patients in a cytochemical bioassay for thyroid stimulators. J Clin Endocrinol Metab 1984; 58:909–914.
253. Beckner SK, Brady RO, Fishman PH, et al. Reevaluation of the role of gangliosides in the binding and action of thyrotropin. Proc Natl Acad Sci USA 1981; 78:4848–4852.
254. Volpe R. Immunoregulation in autoimmune thyroid disease. N Engl J Med 1987; 316:44–46.
255. Weiss M, Ingbar SH, Winblad S, et al. Demonstration of a saturable binding site for thyrotropin in Yersinia enterocolitica. Science 1983; 219:1331–1333.
256. Wall JR, Henderson J, Strakosch CR, et al. Graves' ophthalmopathy. Can Med Assoc J 1981; 124:855–866.
257. Dahlberg PA, Holmlund G, Karlsson FA, et al. HLA-A, -B, -C and -DR antigens in patients with Graves' disease and their correlation with signs and clinical course. Acta Endocrinol 1981; 97:42–47.
258. Uno H, Sasazuki T, Tamai H, et al. Two major genes, linked to HLA and Gm, control susceptibility to Graves' disease. Nature 1981; 292:768–770.
259. Wood LC, Ingbar SH. Hypothyroidism as a late sequela in patients with Graves' disease treated with antithyroid agents. J Clin Invest 1979; 64:1429–1436.
260. Solomon DH, Chopra IJ, Chopra U, et al. Identification of subgroups of euthyroid Graves' ophthalmopathy. N Engl J Med 1977; 296:181–186.
261. Forrester JV, Sutherland GR, McDougall IR. Dysthyroid ophthalmopathy: orbital evaluation with beta-scan ultrasonography. J Clin Endocrinol Metab 1977; 45:221–224.
262. Dallow RH, Momose KJ, Weber AL, et al. Comparison of ultrasonography, computerized tomography (EMI scan) and radiographic techniques in evaluation of exophthalmos. Trans Am Acad Ophthalmol Otolaryngol 1976; 81:305–322.
263. Luft R, Ikkos D, Palmieri G, et al. A case of severe hypermetabolism of nonthyroid origin with a defect in the maintenance of mitochondrial respiratory control: a correlated clinical, biochemical, and morphological study. J Clin Invest 1962; 41:1776–1804.
264. Cooper DS. Antithyroid drugs. N Engl J Med 1984; 311:1353–1362.
265. Geffner DL, Azukizawa M, Hershman JM. Propylthiouracil blocks extrathyroidal conversion of thyroxine to triiodothyronine and augments thyrotropin secretion in man. J Clin Invest 1975; 55:224–229.
266. Saberi M, Sterling FH, Utiger RD. Reduction in extrathyroidal triiodothyronine production by propylthiouracil in man. J Clin Invest 1975; 55:218–223.
267. Laurberg P, Weeke J. Dynamics of inhibition of iodothyronine deiodination during propylthiouracil treatment of thyrotoxicosis. Horm Metab Res 1981; 13:289–292.
268. Jansson R, Dahlberg PA, Johansson H, et al. Intrathyroid concentrations of methimazole in patients with Graves' disease. J Clin Endocrinol Metab 1983; 57:129–132.
269. Greer MA, Kammer H, Bouma DJ. Short-term antithyroid drug therapy for the thyrotoxicosis of Graves' disease. N Engl J Med 1977; 297:173–176.
270. Tamai H, Nakagawa T, Fukino O, et al. Thionamide therapy in Graves' disease: relation of relapse rate to duration of therapy. Ann Intern Med 1980; 92:488–490.
271. Solomon BL, Evaul JE, Burman KD, et al. Remission rates with antithyroid drug therapy: continuing influence of iodine intake? Ann Intern Med 1987; 107:510–512.
272. Wall JR, Fang SL, Kuroki T, et al. In vitro immunoreactivity to propylthiouracil, methimazole, and carbimazole in patients with Graves' disease: a possible cause of antithyroid drug-induced agranulocytosis. J Clin Endocrinol Metab 1984; 58:868–872.
273. Becker DV, Braverman LE, Dunn JT, et al. The use of iodine as a thyroidal blocking agent in the event of a reactor accident. JAMA 1984; 252:659–661.

274. Fradkin JE, Wolff J. Iodide-induced thyrotoxicosis. Medicine (Baltimore) 1983; 62:1–20.

275. Wu S-Y, Shyh T-P, Chopra I, et al. Comparison of sodium ipodate (Orografin) and propylthiouracil in early treatment of hyperthyroidism. J Clin Endocrinol Metab 1982; 54:630–634.

276. Croxson MS, Hall TD, Nicoloff JT. Combination drug therapy for treatment of hyperthyroid Graves' disease. J Clin Endocrinol Metab 1977; 45:623–630.

277. Rubin PC. Beta-blockers in pregnancy. N Engl J Med 1981; 305:1323–1326.

278. Gladstone R, Hordf A, Gersony WM. Propranolol administration during pregnancy: effects on the fetus. J Pediatr 1975; 86:962–964.

279. Hershman JM. The treatment of hyperthyroidism. Ann Intern Med 1966; 64:1306–1314.

280. Michie W, Stowers JM, Duncan T, et al. Mechanism of hypocalcemia after thyroidectomy for thyrotoxicosis. Lancet 1971; 1:508–514.

281. Toft AD, Irvine WJ, McIntosh D, et al. Propranolol in the treatment of thyrotoxicosis by subtotal thyroidectomy. J Clin Endocrinol Metab 1976; 43:1312–1316.

282. Hennemann G, Krenning EP, Sankaranarayanan K. Place of radioactive iodine in treatment of thyrotoxicosis. Lancet 1986; 1:1369–1372.

283. Smith RN, Wilson GM. Clinical trial of different doses of I^{131} in treatment of thyrotoxicosis. Br Med J 1967; 1:129–132.

284. Malone JF, Cutten MJ. Hypothyroidism after ^{125}I therapy. Ann Intern Med 1977; 86:823–824.

285. Dunn JT. Choice of therapy in young adults with hyperthyroidism of Graves' disease. Ann Intern Med 1984; 100:891–893.

286. Sridama V, DeGroot LJ. Treatment of Graves' disease and the course of ophthalmopathy. Am J Med 1989; 87:70–73.

287. Jacobson DH, Gorman CA. Endocrine ophthalmopathy: current ideas concerning etiology, pathogenesis, and treatment. Endocr Rev 1984; 5:200–220.

288. Teng CS, Crombie AL, Hall R, et al. An evaluation of supervoltage orbital irradiation for Graves' ophthalmopathy. Clin Endocrinol 1980; 13:545–551.

289. Ogura J, Wessler S, Avioli LV, et al. Surgical approach to the ophthalmopathy of Graves' disease. JAMA 1971; 216:1627–1631.

290. Studer H, Ramelli F. Simple goiter and its variants: euthyroid and hyperthyroid multinodular goiters. Endocr Rev 1982; 3:40–61.

291. Gorman CA, Robertson JS. Radiation dose in the selection of ^{131}I or surgical treatment for toxic thyroid adenoma. Ann Intern Med 1978; 89:85–90.

292. Ross DS, Ridgway EC, Daniels GH. Successful treatment of solitary toxic thyroid nodules with relatively low-dose iodine-131, with low prevalence of hypothyroidism. Ann Intern Med 1984; 101:488–490.

293. Goldstein R, Hart IA. Follow-up of solitary autonomous thyroid nodules treated with ^{131}I. N Engl J Med 1983; 309:1473–1476.

294. Nagataki S, Mizuno M, Sakamoto S, et al. Thyroid function in molar pregnancy. J Clin Endocrinol Metab 1977; 44:254–263.

295. Kourides IA. A patient with thyroid-stimulating hormone (TSH) hypersecretion. Med Grand Rounds 1983; 2:222–228.

296. Wemeau JL, Dewailly D, Leroy R, et al. Long term treatment with the somatostatin analog SMS 201-995 in a patient with a thyrotropin- and growth hormone–secreting pituitary adenoma. J Clin Endocrinol Metab 1988; 66:636–639.

297. Oppenheim DS, Klibanski A. Medical therapy of glycoprotein hormone-secreting pituitary tumors. Endocrinol Metab Clin North Am 1989; 18:339–358.

298. Beck-Peccoz P, Piscitelli G, Cattaneo MG, et al. Successful treatment of hyperthyroidism due to nonneoplastic pituitary TSH secretion with 3,5,3'-triiodothyroacetic acid (TRIAC). J Endocrinol Invest 1983; 6:217–223.

299. Cohen JH, Ingbar SH, Braverman LE. Thyrotoxicosis due to ingestion of excess thyroid hormone. Endocr Rev 1989; 10:113–124.

300. Hedberg CW, Fishbein DB, Janssen RS, et al. An outbreak of thyrotoxicosis caused by the consumption of bovine thyroid gland in ground beef. N Engl J Med 1987; 316:993–998.

301. Woolf PD. Transient painless thyroiditis with hyperthyroidism: a variant of lymphocytic thyroiditis? Endocr Rev 1980; 1:411–420.

302. Nikolai TF, Coombs GJ, McKenzie AK. Lymphocytic thyroiditis with spontaneously resolving hyperthyroidism and subacute thyroiditis. Long-term follow-up. Arch Intern Med 1981; 141:1455–1458.

303. Nikolai TF, Coombs GJ, McKenzie AK, et al. Treatment of lymphocytic thyroiditis with spontaneously resolving hyperthyroidism (silent thyroiditis). Arch Intern Med 1982; 142:2281–2283.

304. Jansson R, Bernander S, Karlsson A, et al. Autoimmune thyroid dysfunction in the postpartum period. J Clin Endocrinol Metab 1984; 58:681–687.

305. Freeman R, Rosen H, Thysen B. Incidence of thyroid dysfunction in an unselected postpartum population. Arch Intern Med 1986; 146:1361–1364.

306. Tachi J, Amino N, Tamaki H, et al. Long term follow-up and HLA association in patients with postpartum hypothyroidism. J Clin Endocrinol Metab 1986; 66:480–484.

307. Amino N, Kuro R, Tanizawa O, et al. Changes of serum antithyroid antibodies during and after pregnancy in autoimmune thyroid diseases. Clin Exp Immunol 1978; 31:30–37.

308. Amino N, Mori H, Iwatuni Y, et al. High prevalence of transient postpartum thyrotoxicosis and hypothyroidism. N Engl J Med 1982; 306:849–852.

309. Sobrinho LG, Limbert ES, Santos MA. Thyroxine toxicosis in patients with iodine induced thyrotoxicosis. J Clin Endocrinol Metab 1977; 45:25–29.

310. Engler D, Donaldson EB, Stockigt JR, et al. Hyperthyroidism without triiodothyronine excess: an effect of severe non-thyroidal illness. J Clin Endocrinol Metab 1978; 46:77–82.

311. Hayles AB. Problem of childhood Graves' disease. Mayo Clin Proc 1972; 47:850–853.

312. Favus MJ, Schneider AB, Stachura ME, et al. Thyroid cancer occurring as a late consequence of head-and-neck irradiation. N Engl J Med 1976; 294:1019–1025.

313. Safa AM, Schumacher OP, Rodriguez AA. Long term follow-up results in children and adolescents treated with radioactive iodine (^{131}I) for hyperthyroidism. N Engl J Med 1975; 292:167–171.

314. Davis LE, Lucas MJ, Hankins GDV, et al. Thyrotoxicosis complicating pregnancy. Am J Obstet Gynecol 1989; 160:63–70.

315. Zakarija M, McKenzie JM, Hoffman WH. Prediction and therapy of intrauterine and late-onset neonatal hyperthyroidism. J Clin Endocrinol Metab 1986; 62:368–371.

316. Yabu Y, Amino N, Mori H, et al. Postpartum recurrence of hyperthyroidism and changes of thyroid-stimulating immunoglobulins in Graves' disease. J Clin Endocrinol Metab 1980; 51:1454–1458.

317. Amino N, Tanizawa D, Mori H, et al. Aggravation of thyrotoxicosis in early pregnancy and after delivery in Graves' disease. J Clin Endocrinol Metab 1982; 55:108–112.

318. Marchant B, Brownlie BEW, Hart DM, et al. The placental transfer of propylthiouracil, methimazole and carbimazole. J Clin Endocrinol Metab 1977; 45:1187–1193.

319. Cheron RG, Kaplan MM, Larsen PR, et al. Neonatal thyroid function after propylthiouracil therapy for maternal Graves' disease. N Engl J Med 1981; 304:525–528.

320. Momotani N, Noh J, Oyanagi H, et al. Antithyroid drug therapy for Graves' disease during pregnancy. N Engl J Med 1986; 315:24–28.

321. van Dijke CP, Heydendael RJ, de Kleine MJ. Methimazole, carbimazole, and congenital skin defects. Ann Intern Med 1987; 106:60–61.

322. Low LCK, Lang J, Alexander WD. Excretion of carbimazole and propylthiouracil in breast milk. Lancet 1979; 2:1011.

323. Fisher DA, Dussault J, Foley TP, et al. Screening for congenital hypothyroidism: results of screening one million North American infants. J Pediatr 1979; 94:700–705.

324. Steinberg AD. Myxedema and coronary artery disease—a comparative autopsy study. Ann Intern Med 1968; 68:338–344.

325. Lee JK, Lewis JA. Myxoedema with complete A-V block and Adams-Stokes disease abolished with thyroid medication. Br Heart J 1962; 24:253–256.

326. Santos AD, Miller RP, Puthenpurakal KM, et al. Echocardiographic characterization of the reversible cardiomyopathy of hypothyroidism. Am J Med 1980; 68:675–682.

327. Zwillich CW, Pierson DJ, Hofeldt FD, et al. Ventilatory control in myxedema and hypothyroidism. N Engl J Med 1975; 292:662–665.

328. Orr WC, Males JL, Imes NK. Myxedema and obstructive sleep apnea. Am J Med 1981; 70:1061–1066.

329. Amino N, Kuro R, Yabu Y, et al. Elevated levels of circulating carcinoembryonic antigen in hypothyroidism. J Clin Endocrinol Metab 1981; 52:457–462.

330. Rosman NP. Neurological and muscular aspects of thyroid dysfunction in childhood. Pediatr Clin North Am 1976; 23:575–594.

331. Sanders V. Neurologic manifestations of myxedema. N Engl J Med 1962; 266:547–552, 599–603.

332. Khaleeli AA, Griffith DG, Edwards RHT. The clinical presentation of hypothyroid myopathy. Clin Endocrinol 1983; 19:365–376.

333. Bouillon R, Muls E, De Moor P. Influence of thyroid function on the serum concentration of 1,25-dihydroxyvitamin D_3. J Clin Endocrinol Metab 1980; 51:793–797.

334. Skowsky WR, Kikuchi TA. The role of vasopressin in the impaired water excretion of myxedema. Am J Med 1978; 64:613–621.

335. Carmel A, Spencer CA. Clinical and subclinical thyroid disorders associated with pernicious anemia. Arch Intern Med 1982; 142:1465–1469.

336. Dalton RG, Dewar MS, Savidge GF, et al. Hypothyroidism as a cause of acquired von Willebrand's disease. Lancet 1987; 1:1007–1009.

337. Yamada T, Tsukui T, Ikejiri K, et al. Volume of sella turcica in normal subjects and in patients with primary hypothyroidism and hyperthyroidism. J Clin Endocrinol Metab 1976; 42:817–822.

338. Lecky BRF, Williams TDM, Lightman SL, et al. Myxoedema presenting with chiasmal compression: resolution after thyroxine replacement. Lancet 1987; 1:1347–1350.

339. Onishi T, Miyai K, Aono T, et al. Primary hypothyroidism and galactorrhea. Am J Med 1977; 63:373–378.

340. Montoro M, Collea JV, Frasier SD, et al. Successful outcome of pregnancy in women with hypothyroidism. Ann Intern Med 1981; 94:31–34.

341. Agdeppa D, Macaron C, Mallik T, et al. Plasma high density lipoprotein cholesterol in thyroid disease. J Clin Endocrinol Metab 1979; 49:726–729.

342. LaFranchi SH. Hypothyroidism. Pediatr Clin North Am 1979; 26:33–51.

343. Lum SM, Nicoloff JT, Spencer CA, et al. Peripheral tissue mechanism for maintenance of serum triiodothyronine values in a thyroxine-deficient state in man. J Clin Invest 1984; 73:570–575.

344. Lobo E DeH, Khan M, Tew J. Community study of hypothyroidism in Down's syndrome. Br Med J 1980; 280:1253.

345. Konishi J, Yasuhiro I, Kasagi K, et al. Primary myxedema with thyrotrophin-binding inhibitor immunoglobulins. Ann Intern Med 1985; 103:26–31.

346. Smith RE Jr, Adler RA, Clark P, et al. Thyroid function after mantle irradiation in Hodgkin's disease. JAMA 1981; 245:46–49.

347. Kaplan MM, Garnick MB, Gelber R, et al. Risk factors for thyroid abnormalities after neck irradiation for childhood cancer. Am J Med 1983; 74:272–280.

348. Green M, Wilson GM. Thyrotoxicosis treated by surgery or iodine-131. With special reference to development of hypothyroidism. Br Med J 1964; 1:1005–1010.

349. Hayashizaki Y, Hiraoka Y, Endo Y, et al. Thyroid-stimulating hormone (TSH) deficiency caused by a single base substitution in the CAGYC region of the β-subunit. EMBO J 1989; 8:2291–2296.

350. New England Congenital Hypothyroidism Collaborative. Characteristics of infantile hypothyroidism discovered on neonatal screening. J Pediatr 1984; 104:539–544.

351. Larsen PR. Maternal thyroxine and congenital hypothyroidism. N Engl J Med 1989; 321:44–46.

352. Bigos ST, Ridgway EC, Kourides JA, et al. Spectrum of pituitary alterations with mild and severe thyroid impairment. J Clin Endocrinol Metab 1978; 46:317–325.

353. Delange F, Iteke FB, Ermans AM, eds. Nutritional Factors Involved in the Goitrogenic Action of Cassava. Ottawa: International Development Research Center, 1982.

354. Goslings BM, Djokomoeljanto R, Docter R, et al. Hypothyroidism in an area of endemic goiter and cretinism in Central Java, Indonesia. J Clin Endocrinol Metab 1977; 44:481–490.

355. Thilly CH, Delange F, Lagasse R, et al. Fetal hypothyroidism and maternal thyroid status in severe endemic goiter. J Clin Endocrinol Metab 1978; 47:354–360.

356. Codaccioni JL, Carayon P, Michel-Bechet M, et al. Congenital hypothyroidism associated with thyrotropin unresponsiveness and thyroid cell membrane alterations. J Clin Endocrinol Metab 1980; 50:932–937.

357. Takasu N, Mori T, Koizumi Y, et al. Transient neonatal hypothyroidism due to maternal immunoglobulins that inhibit thyrotropin-binding and post-receptor processes. J Clin Endocrinol Metab 1984; 59:142–146.

358. Rees-Jones RW, Larsen PR. Triiodothyronine and thyroxine content of desiccated thyroid tablets. Metabolism 1977; 26:1213–1218.

359. Coindre JM, David JP, Riviere L, et al. Bone loss in hypothyroidism with hormone replacement. Arch Intern Med 1986; 146:48–53.

360. Ross DS, Neer RM, Ridgway EC, et al. Subclinical hyperthyroidism and reduced bone density as a possible result of prolonged suppression of the pituitary-thyroid axis with L-thyroxine. Am J Med 1987; 82:1167–1170.

361. Paul TL, Kerrigan J, Kelly AM, et al. Long-term L-thyroxine therapy is associated with decreased hip bone density in premenopausal women. JAMA 1988; 259:3137–3141.

362. Hennessey JV, Evaul JE, Tseng YC, et al. L-Thyroxine dosage: a reevaluation of therapy with contemporary preparations. Ann Intern Med 1986; 105:11–15.

363. Fish LH, Schwartz HL, Cavanaugh J, et al. Replacement dose, metabolism, and bioavailability of levothyroxine in the treatment of hypothyroidism. N Engl J Med 1987; 316:764–770.

364. Sawin CT, Surks MI, London M, et al. Oral thyroxine: variation in biologic action and tablet content. Ann Intern Med 1984; 100:641–645.

365. van Dop C, Conte FA, Koch TK, et al. Pseudotumor cerebri associated with initiation of levothyroxine therapy for juvenile hypothyroidism. N Engl J Med 1983; 308:1076–1080.

366. Sato T, Suzuki Y, Taketani T, et al. Age-related change in pituitary threshold for TSH release during thyroxine replacement therapy for cretinism. J Clin Endocrinol Metab 1977; 44:553–559.

367. Sawin C, Herman T, Molitch ME, et al. Aging and the thyroid. Decreased requirement for thyroid hormone in older hypothyroid patients. Am J Med 1983; 75:206–209.

368. Bastenie PA, Bonnyns M, Van Haelst L. Grades of subclinical hypothyroidism in asymptomatic autoimmune thyroiditis revealed by the thyrotropin-releasing test. J Clin Endocrinol Metab 1980; 51:163–166.

369. Gray RS, Borsey DQ, Seth J, et al. Prevalence of subclinical thyroid failure in insulin-dependent diabetes. J Clin Endocrinol Metab 1980; 50:1034–1037.

370. Crowe JP, Christensen E, Butler J, et al. Primary biliary cirrhosis: the prevalence of hypothyroidism and its relationship to thyroid antibodies and sicca syndrome. Gastroenterology 1980; 78:1437–1441.

371. Pal SK, Ghosh KK, Banerjee PK. Thyroid function in vitiligo. Clin Chim Acta 1980; 106:331–332.

372. Gordon MB, Klein I, Dekker A, et al. Thyroid disease in progressive systemic sclerosis: increased frequency of glandular fibrosis and hypothyroidism. Ann Intern Med 1981; 95:431–435.

373. Cooper DS, Halper R, Wood LC, et al. L-Thyroxine therapy in subclinical hypothyroidism. Ann Intern Med 1984; 101:18–24.

374. Bell GM, Todd WTA, Forfar JC, et al. End-organ responses to thyroxine therapy in subclinical hypothyroidism. Clin Endocrinol 1985; 22:83–89.

375. Nystrom E, Caidahl K, Fager G, et al. A double-blind cross-over 12-month study of L-thyroxine treatment of women with 'subclinical' hypothyroidism. Clin Endocrinol 1988; 29:63–76.

376. Weinberg AD, Brennan MD, Gorman CA, et al. Outcome of anesthesia and surgery in hypothyroid patients. Arch Intern Med 1983; 143:893–897.

377. Becker C. Hypothyroidism and atherosclerotic heart disease: pathogenesis, medical management, and the role of coronary artery bypass surgery. Endocr Rev 1985; 6:432–440.

378. Hay ID, Duick DS, Vlietstra RE, et al. Thyroxine therapy in hypothyroid patients undergoing coronary revascularization: a retrospective analysis. Ann Intern Med 1981; 95:456–457.

379. Drucker DJ, Burrow GN. Cardiovascular surgery in the hypothyroid patient. Arch Intern Med 1985; 145:1585–1587.

380. Nicoloff JT. Thyroid storm and myxedema coma. Med Clin North Am 1985; 69:1005–1007.

381. Dige-Petersen H, Hummer L. Serum thyrotropin concentrations under basal conditions and after stimulation with thyrotropin-releasing hormone in idiopathic non-toxic goiter. J Clin Endocrinol Metab 1977; 44:1115–1120.

382. Bray GA. Increased sensitivity of the thyroid in iodine-depleted rats to the goitrogenic effect of thyrotropin. J Clin Invest 1968; 47:1640–1647.

383. Valente WA, Vitti P, Rotella CM, et al. Antibodies that promote thyroid growth. A distinct population of thyroid-stimulating autoantibodies. N Engl J Med 1983; 309:1028–1034.

384. Pezzino V, Vigneri R, Squatrito S, et al. Increased serum thyroglobulin levels in patients with nontoxic goiter. J Clin Endocrinol Metab 1978; 46:653–657.

385. Vander JB, Gaston EA, Dawber TR. The significance of non-toxic thyroid nodules. Final report of a 15-year study of the incidence of thyroid malignancy. Ann Intern Med 1968; 69:537–540.

386. Shimaoka K, Badillo J, Sokal JE, et al. Clinical differentiation between thyroid cancer and benign goiter. JAMA 1962; 181:179–185.

387. Field JB, Larsen PR, Yamashita K, et al. Demonstration of iodide transport defect but normal iodide organification in non-functioning nodules of human thyroid glands. J Clin Invest 1973; 52:2404.

388. Hamburger JI. The autonomously functioning thyroid nodule: Goetsch's disease. Endocr Rev 1987; 8:439–447.

389. Gharib H, James EM, Charboneau JW, et al. Suppressive therapy with levothyroxine for solitary thyroid nodules. N Engl J Med 1987; 317:70–75.

390. Morita T, Tamai H, Ohshima A, et al. Changes in serum thyroid hormone, thyrotropin and thyroglobulin concentrations during thyroxine therapy in patients with solitary thyroid nodules. J Clin Endocrinol Metab 1989; 69:227–230.

391. Woolner LB, Beahrs OH, Black BM, et al. Classification and prognosis of thyroid carcinoma. A study of 885 cases observed in a thirty-year period. Am J Surg 1961; 102:354–387.

392. Field JB, Bloom G, Chou MCY, et al. Effects of thyroid-stimulating hormone on human thyroid carcinoma and adjacent normal tissue. J Clin Endocrinol Metab 1978; 47:1052–1058.

393. McConahey WM, Hay ID, Woolner LB, et al. Papillary thyroid cancer treated at the Mayo Clinic, 1946 through 1970: initial manifestations, pathologic findings, therapy, and outcome. Mayo Clin Proc 1986; 61:978–996.

394. Stepanas AV, Samaan NA, Hill CS, et al. Medullary thyroid carcinoma. Cancer 1979; 43:825–837.

395. McLean GW, Rabin D, Moore L, et al. Evaluation of provocative tests in suspected medullary carcinoma of the thyroid: heterogeneity of calcitonin responses to calcium and pentagastrin. Metabolism 1984; 33:790–796.

396. Holm LE, Blomgren H, Lowhagen T. Cancer risks in patients with chronic lymphocytic thyroiditis. N Engl J Med 1985; 312:601–604.

397. Hamburger JI, Miller JM, Kini SR. Lymphoma of the thyroid. Ann Intern Med 1983; 99:685–693.

398. Larsen, PR. Case records of the Massachusetts General Hospital Case 15-1987. N Engl J Med 1987; 316:931–938.

399. Miller JM, Hamburger JI, Kini S. Diagnosis of thyroid nodules. Use of fine-needle aspiration and needle biopsy. JAMA 1979; 241:481–484.

400. Kini SR. Guides to Clinical Aspiration Biopsy: Thyroid. New York: Igaku-Shoin Medical, 1987.

401. Lowhagen T. Cytological diagnosis of thyroid disease. Ann Chir Gynaecol 1983; 72:90–95.

402. Fogelfeld L, Wiviott MBT, Shore-Freedman E, et al. Recurrence of

thyroid nodules after surgical removal in patients irradiated in childhood for benign conditions. N Engl J Med 1989; 320:835–840.

403. Van Herle AJ, Rich P, Ljung BE, et al. The thyroid nodule. Ann Intern Med 1982; 96:221–232.

404. Ramacciotti CE, Pretorius HT, Chu EW, et al. Diagnostic accuracy and use of aspiration biopsy in the management of thyroid nodules. Arch Intern Med 1984; 144:1169–1173.

405. Gharib H, Goellner JR, Zinsmeister AR, et al. Fine-needle aspiration biopsy of the thyroid: the problem of suspicious cytologic findings. Ann Intern Med 1984; 101:25–28.

406. Gosain AK, Clark OH. Hürthle cell neoplasms: malignant potential. Arch Surg 1984; 119:515–519.

407. Hamburger JI, Husain M, Nishiyama R, et al. Increasing the accuracy of fine-needle biopsy for thyroid nodules. Arch Pathol Lab Med 1989; 113:1035–1041.

408. Rosen IB, Strawbridge HG, Walfish PG, et al. Malignant pseudothyroiditis: a new clinical entity. Am J Surg 1978; 136:445–449.

409. Segal RL, Cobin RH, Futterweit W, et al. Thyroid nodules in irradiated patients: an indication for total thyroidectomy. J Surg Oncol 1986; 28:126–130.

410. Scanlon EF, Berk RW, Khandekar JD. Postirradiation neoplasia: a symposium. Curr Probl Cancer 1978; 3:1–45.

411. Rossi RL, Nieroda C, Cady B, et al. Malignancies of the thyroid gland. The Lahey experience. Surg Clin North Am 1985; 65:211–230.

412. Mazzaferri EL, Young RL. Papillary thyroid carcinoma: a 10 year follow-up report of the impact of therapy in 576 patients. Am J Med 1981; 70:511–518.

413. Samaan NA, Maheshwari YK, Nader S, et al. Impact of therapy for differentiated carcinoma of the thyroid: an analysis of 706 cases. J Clin Endocrinol Metab 1983; 56:1131–1138.

414. Kim JH, Leeper RD. Treatment of anaplastic giant and spindle cell carcinoma of the thyroid gland with combination Adriamycin and radiation therapy. Cancer 1983; 52:954–957.

415. Reugemer JJ, Hay ID, Bergstralh EJ, et al. Distant metastases in differentiated thyroid carcinoma: a multivariate analysis of prognostic variables. J Clin Endocrinol Metab 1988; 67:501–508.

416. Schlumberger M, Tubiana M, de Vathaire F, et al. Long-term results of treatment of 283 patients with lung and bone metastases from differentiated thyroid carcinoma. J Clin Endocrinol Metab 1986; 63:960–967.

417. Beierwaltes WH. The treatment of thyroid carcinoma with radioactive iodine. Semin Nucl Med 1979; 8(1):79–94.

418. Maxon HR, Thomas SR, Hertzberg VS, et al. Relation between effective radiation dose and outcome of radioiodine therapy for thyroid cancer. J Engl J Med 1983; 309:937–941.

419. Leeper RD. The effect of ^{131}I therapy on survival of patients with metastatic papillary or follicular thyroid carcinoma. J Clin Endocrinol Metab 1973; 36:1143–1152.

420. Leeper RD. Thyroid cancer. Med Clin North Am 1985; 69:1079–1096.

421. Samaan NA, Schultz PN, Haynie TP, et al. Pulmonary metastasis of differentiated thyroid carcinoma: treatment results in 101 patients. J Clin Endocrinol Metab 1985; 65:376–380.

422. Goldman JM, Line BR, Aamodt RL, et al. Influence of triiodothyronine withdrawal time on ^{131}I uptake postthyroidectomy for thyroid cancer. J Clin Endocrinol Metab 1980; 50:734–739.

423. Filetti S, Belfiore A, Amir SM, et al. The role of thyroid-stimulating antibodies of Graves' disease in differentiated thyroid cancer. N Engl J Med 1988; 318:753–759.

424. Atkins MB, Mier JW, Parkinson DR, et al. Hypothyroidism after treatment with interleukin-2 and lymphokine-activated killer cells. N Engl J Med 1988; 318:1557–1563.

425. Moens H, Farid NR. Hashimoto's thyroiditis is associated with HLA-DRW3. N Engl J Med 1978; 299:133–135.

426. Farid NR, Sampson L, Moens H, et al. The association of goitrous autoimmune thyroiditis with HLA-DR5. Tissue Antigens 1981; 17:265–268.

427. Bottazzo GF, Pujol-Borrell R, Hanafusa T, et al. Role of aberrant HLA-DR expression and antigen presentation in induction of endocrine autoimmunity. Lancet 1983; 2:1115–1119.

428. Crile G Jr. Struma lymphomatosa and carcinoma of the thyroid. Surg Gynecol Obstet 1978; 147:350–352.

429. Stancek D, Stancekova-Gressnerova M, Janotka M, et al. Isolation and some serological and epidemiological data on the viruses recovered from patients with subacute thyroiditis de Quervain. Med Microbiol Immunol (Berl) 1975; 161:133–144.

430. Wall JR, Fang SL, Ingbar SH, et al. Lymphocytic transformation in response to human thyroid extract in patients with subacute thyroiditis. J Clin Endocrinol Metab 1976: 43:587–590.

431. Papapetrou PD, Jackson IMD. Thyrotoxicosis due to "silent" thyroiditis. Lancet 1975; 1:361–363.

432. Vagenakis AG, Abreau CM, Braverman LE. Prevention of recurrence in acute thyroiditis following corticosteroid withdrawal. J Clin Endocrinol Metab 1970; 31:705–708.

433. Bartholomew LG, Cain JC, Woolner LB, et al. Sclerosing cholangitis: its possible association with Riedel's struma and fibrous retroperitonitis: report of two cases. N Engl J Med 1963; 269:8–13.

434. Chopra D, Wool MS, Grossen A, et al. Riedel's struma associated with subacute thyroiditis, hypothyroidism and hypoparathyroidism. J Clin Endocrinol Metab 1978; 46:869–871.

435. Miyauchi A, Matsuzuka F, Kuma K, et al. Pyriform sinus fistula: an underlying abnormality common in patients with acute suppurative thyroiditis. World J Surg 1990; 14:400–405.

THE ADRENAL CORTEX

David N. Orth, William J. Kovacs, and C. Rowan DeBold

THE NORMAL ADRENAL CORTEX

History

The anatomy of the adrenal glands appears to have been described first in 1563 by Bartholomeo Eustachius as the "glandulae renis incumbentes" in his *Tabulae Anatomicae* (Fig. 9–1), edited and published in 1774 by Lancisius[1] (cited in Gaunt,[2] Medvei,[3] and Page and co-workers[4]). Emil Huschke (1797–1858) first differentiated the cortex from the medulla anatomically[5] (cited in Medvei[3]). Edme F. A. Vulpian[6] demonstrated the differential staining of the two, and Rudolph Albert von Kölliker[7] described the formation of the fetal adrenal cortex and its subsequent invasion by the neural precursors of the medulla, which were called "chromaffin" cells because they stained selectively with potassium dichromate.[8] J. Arnold[9] described the three concentric zones of the cortex and gave them their current designations: zonae glomerulosa, fasciculata, and reticularis.

Ideas about the function of the adrenal glands lagged behind their initial description. Thomas Bartholin[10] proposed that these "capsulae atrabilariae" purified black bile that subsequently drained into the renal veins. In 1716 the Académie des Sciences de Bordeaux offered a prize for the answer to the question, "What is the purpose of the supra-renal glands?" Charles de Montesquieu, judging the responses, found the essays so unsatisfactory that he was unable to award the prize, concluding that "Perhaps some

day chance will reveal what all of this work was unable to do" (cited in ref. 2). As early as 1659, Walter Charleton distinguished glands with ducts from those without them. John Ranby showed in 1725 that the adrenal "ducts" are arteries, and Théophile de Bordeu[11] first espoused the theory of internal secretion by such glands. William B. Carpenter[12] wrote in 1852 that the "vascular glands," among them the adrenals, produced substances that, "instead of being carried out of the body, are destined to be restored to the circulating current, apparently in a state of more complete adaptiveness to the wants of the nutritive function." Claude Bernard[13] popularized the concept and introduced the term "sécrétion interne," by which he meant glucose, however, not the hormones, which were yet to be discovered. Forty years later the physiologist Edward A. Schäfer[14] elevated Bernard's concept of internal secretions to the status of full-fledged theory.

Evidence for a physiological role for the adrenal glands came from clinical observation. On March 15, 1849 Thomas Addison[15] presented a paper to the South London Medical Society entitled "On anaemia: disease of the supra-renal capsules," a result of his interest in idiopathic, or pernicious, anemia. Three of the patients he described had adrenal disease at autopsy, and it was the only abnormality identified in two of them. However, 6 years passed before he was persuaded to publish his classic monograph, On the Constitutional and Local Effects of Disease of the Supra-Renal Capsules,[16] describing the "anaemia, general languor and

489

debility, remarkable feebleness of the heart's action, irritability of the stomach, and a peculiar change of colour of the skin" he observed in 11 patients with the disease that has since borne his name.[17] The following year, Charles E. Brown-Séquard[18] provided experimental confirmation of Addison's theory that the adrenal glands are essential to life by performing adrenalectomies in several species of animals, although his operative technique and conclusions were chal-

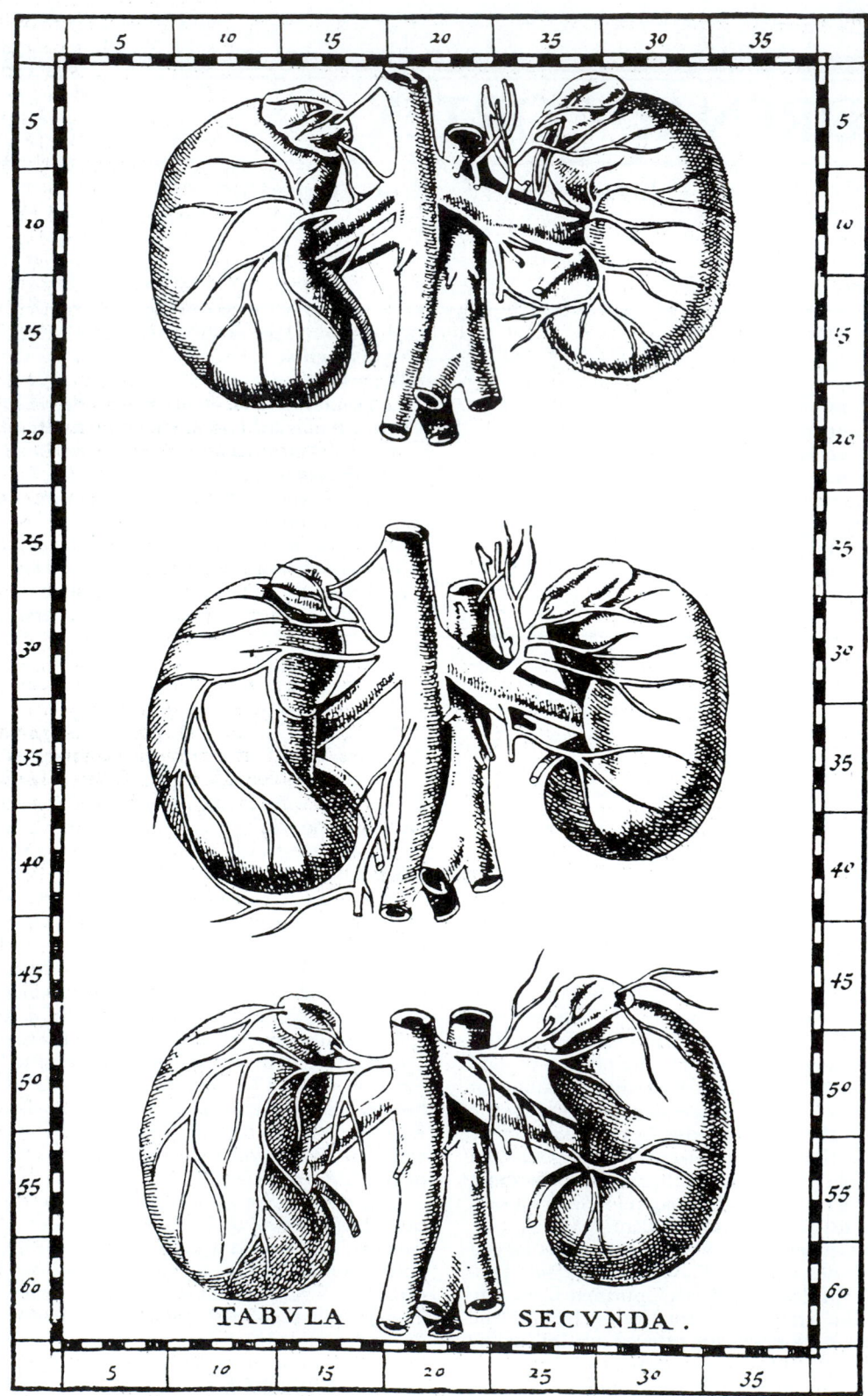

Figure 9–1. Anatomy of the adrenal gland by Eustachius.[1] (Courtesy of the Vanderbilt University History of Medicine Collection.)

lenged. Neither Brown-Séquard's nor Addison's conclusions were quickly or universally accepted.

The importance of the adrenal cortex relative to the medulla was a matter of debate well into the 20th century. George Oliver and Schäfer described a vasopressor agent in extracts of the adrenal medulla in 1894, and epinephrine was subsequently characterized[19, 20] and purified.[21] The issue was settled for most scientists by the demonstration that removal of one adrenal and half of the other and cauterization of the medulla in the remaining half adrenal were compatible with healthy survival in dogs,[22] a result corroborated by Bernardo A. Houssay and Juan T. Lewis.[23] Nonetheless, some persisted in considering epinephrine the vital adrenal principle on into the 1920s.

Early studies of the physiological role of adrenal corticosteroids were complicated because their actions appeared almost ubiquitous, adrenocortical extracts were usually contaminated with catecholamines, and the chemical nature of what was assumed to be a single active cortical principle was unknown. The turning point came in 1930, when it was found that lipid extracts of adrenal cortex had high potency for maintaining normal health and growth of adrenalectomized cats.[24-26] The extracts were immediately and successfully applied to treating humans with Addison's disease.[27] The isolation, identification, and synthesis of the adrenal steroids then began in earnest. Deoxycorticosterone (DOC), synthesized by M. von Steiger and Tadeus Reichstein[28] in 1937, had weak mineralocorticoid and negligible glucocorticoid activity, but it established the steroidal nature of the adrenocortical hormones. Cortisone was identified at about the same time, yet it was not until 1949 that cortisone acetate was synthesized in quantities sufficient for therapeutic use. The possible existence of a salt-retaining principle had been suggested in 1916 by evidence of decreased plasma volume in adrenalectomized cats[29] and the subsequent observation of hyponatremia, hypomagnesemia, and hyperkalemia in adrenalectomized dogs, the lives of which were prolonged by administration of sodium salts.[30] However, aldosterone was the most elusive of the steroids to isolate and characterize and by far the most difficult to synthesize, a feat not accomplished until 1955.[31, 32]

The mechanisms by which adrenocortical function is regulated have been elucidated in the 20th century. The work of Philip E. Smith[33] revealed the existence of a functional pituitary-adrenal axis, and D. J. Ingle and Edward C. Kendall[34] showed in 1937 that an adrenocortical extract inhibited the adrenocorticotropic effect of the pituitary, establishing the presence of a homeostatic negative feedback mechanism characteristic of most endocrine regulatory systems. They also observed the existence of other control mechanisms, such as the one mediating the response to stressful stimuli. The development of bioassays for adrenocortical hormones—reduction in numbers of circulating eosinophils, depletion of adrenal cholesterol, and depletion of adrenal ascorbic acid—facilitated the identification of corticotropin (ACTH, adrenocorticotropin), the structure of which was determined in the decade beginning in 1956.[35] Geoffrey W. Harris[36] predicted the existence of a hypothalamic factor that is secreted into the hypothalamic-hypophyseal portal blood and stimulates ACTH release from the anterior pituitary. This factor, corticotropin-releasing hormone (CRH), was characterized and synthesized by Wylie W. Vale and his co-workers[37] in 1981; aspects of its physiological effects are still being investigated.

Until the late 1940s, the only clinical use of adrenal steroids was as replacement therapy in patients with adrenal insufficiency. However, it had been observed that the inflammation of rheumatoid arthritis is often mitigated in patients who are jaundiced or pregnant. Philip S. Hench, reasoning that the effect must be mediated by an endogenous factor that is unusually abundant in those conditions, eliminated a number of other possible factors before deciding to test glucocorticoids in 1941. It was not until 1949, however, that sufficient cortisone was available, and Hench and co-workers[38] found that both it and ACTH were effective in improving "certain clinical and biochemical features of rheumatoid arthritis" but that, when "use of them was discontinued, symptoms and signs of rheumatoid arthritis usually, but not always, returned or increased promptly." The effect was entirely unexpected. Glucocorticoids have since been used with enormous benefit as anti-inflammatory agents, but their adverse side effects and inappropriate use have also resulted in enormous harm.

Knowledge of the function of the adrenal gland and its products has increased rapidly since 1949. The advances include the synthesis of potent steroids such as prednisone, prednisolone, dexamethasone, triamcinolone, and fludrocortisone; elucidation of steroid structure-function relationships; and diagnostic, therapeutic, and experimental application of these compounds. Development of inhibitors of steroid biosynthesis such as metyrapone, aminoglutethimide, and ketoconazole; inhibitors of steroid action such as cyproterone and mifepristone (RU-486); and the cytotoxic drug for the adrenal cortex mitotane has provided important diagnostic and therapeutic agents and investigative tools. There have been advances in knowledge of the structure and physiology of hypothalamic factors such as CRH, arginine vasopressin (AVP, also called antidiuretic hormone, ADH), and catecholamines that regulate pituitary ACTH secretion. The structures of pro-opiomelanocortin (POMC), its messenger RNA (mRNA), and its gene have all been described. The normal levels and metabolic fate of ACTH and other POMC-derived peptides in plasma have been defined. The pulsatile nature and circadian pattern of release of these peptides and their intracellular mechanisms of action are now known in considerable detail. Many aspects of steroid biosynthesis, including the intracellular location and structure of the steroidogenic cytochrome P-450 enzymes and the genes that encode them, have been revealed. The discovery of cytoplasmic receptors for steroids and elucidation of their structures and those of the genes that encode them have provided insight into the mechanisms by which the steroid-receptor complex interacts with specific DNA response elements to regulate the transcription of target genes. Finally, proteins, such as the lipocortins, that may be involved in steroid hormone action have been identified. Despite these advances, however, one need not probe deeply to discover the limits of present knowledge.

Anatomy

Embryology

Each adrenal consists of two functionally distinct endocrine glands within a single capsule. The cortex derives from mesenchymal cells attached to the coelomic cavity lining adjacent to the urogenital ridge. The fetal adrenal is recognizable by 2 mo of gestation, when it is invaded by neuroectodermal cells that will form the medulla. It becomes quite vascular and increases rapidly in size, to become larger than the kidney at midgestation.[39] By the second trimester, the thin outer "definitive" zone that will form the adult cortex is distinct; the inner "fetal" zone makes up most of the adrenal mass and still represents three quarters of the cortex at birth. The fetal zone degenerates rapidly after birth, accounts for only one quarter of the cortical mass at age 2 mo, and has vanished by 1 y. The definitive zone, which has distinct zonae glomerulosa and fasciculata at birth, proliferates, but total adrenal weight decreases until age 2 to 3 mo. Adrenal growth thereafter parallels somatic growth. The zona reticularis develops during the first year of life.[40]

Gross Anatomy

Each adult adrenal is a roughly pyramidal structure, 2 to 3 cm wide, 4 to 6 cm long, and about 1 cm thick, lying above or posteromedial to and occasionally attached to the upper pole of the kidney but usually surrounded by perirenal fat. Each gland is encased in a thin layer of loose areolar connective tissue and a thick fibrous capsule. The right adrenal usually lies lower and slightly more lateral than the left. Each normally weighs about 4 g, regardless of age, weight, or sex, but may weigh as much as 22 g at autopsy, apparently because of the stress of terminal illness.[41] About 10% of the adrenal weight is medulla.[4] Up to 3% of normal adults may have macroscopic nodules in the adrenal gland.[42] Micronodular changes are seen in two thirds of normal adults.[43] Most of these nodules are variants of normal structure but on occasion must be distinguished functionally from those that arise under conditions of abnormal stimulation or that secrete steroids autonomously (see later).

Ectopic Adrenal Tissue

Adrenal tissue can develop in ectopic sites. Except when situated medial to the gland's normal location, it consists only of cortical cells. Ectopic adrenals can be located in the retroperitoneal celiac plexus; in the hilum of the spleen; adjacent to the ovaries; in the broad ligaments; in the scrotum adjacent to the epididymis or spermatic cord; rarely within the liver; and even more rarely in the wall of the gallbladder, within the ovary itself, or adjacent to the brain.[4]

Vascular Supply

The adrenals are supplied with blood by an average of 11 or 12 small arteries branching from the aorta and the inferior phrenic, renal, often intercostal, and occasionally left ovarian or left internal spermatic arteries.[44] Sixty or more small branches form a subcapsular arteriolar plexus that drains into a rich array of radial capillaries, some of which anastomose as they penetrate the deeper zona fasciculata. These vessels then create a dense sinusoidal plexus around the cells of the zona reticularis and form veins that traverse the medulla to empty into the central vein (Fig. 9–2). There is no direct arterial blood supply to the zonae fasciculata and reticularis.[45] A separate medullary capillary sinusoidal network is supplied by medullary arteries that penetrate the cortex; the network also drains into the central vein.[46] Thus only a minority of chromaffin cells (those that lie adjacent to the smaller radicles of the central vein) are exposed to cortical venous blood. The central vein has two to four conspicuous longitudinal smooth muscle bundles, the function of which is unknown, but which presumably constrict outflow from the gland and may thereby increase the exposure of cortical cells to systemic factors, such as ACTH, and the exposure of medullary cells to cortisol.[47] In humans the central vein and its main branches are surrounded by a cuff of cortical tissue that invaginates at the head and fuses with the cortex in the tail.[48] The right adrenal vein is short and drains into the inferior vena cava, and the longer left adrenal vein usually drains into the left renal vein directly or after being joined by the left inferior phrenic vein. Smaller emissary veins may drain into the inferior phrenic, renal, or rarely the hepatic portal veins.[49, 50]

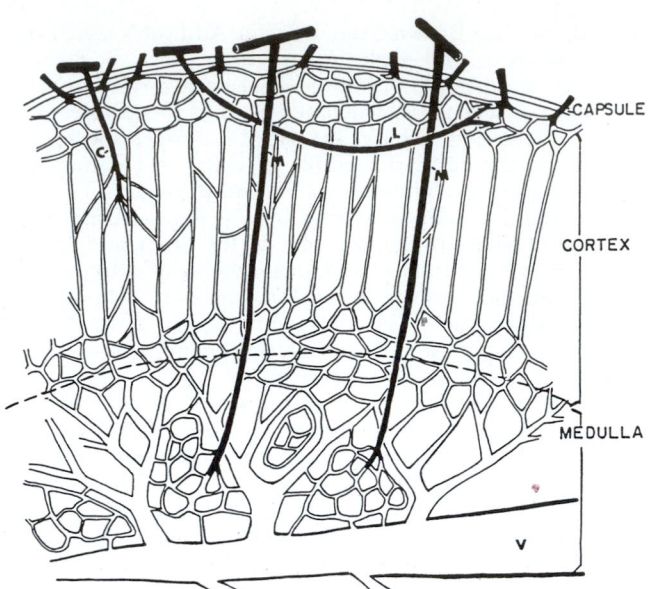

Figure 9–2. Vasculature of the mammalian adrenal gland. Arterial supply is indicated in black, venous drainage in white. C, cortical artery; L, looped artery; M, medullary arteries; V, central vein. (From Coupland RE. Blood supply of the adrenal gland. In: Greep RO, Astwood EB, eds. Handbook of Physiology. Sect 7: Endocrinology. Vol VI. Adrenal Gland. Washington, DC: American Physiological Society, 1975: 283–294.)

Nerve Supply

Efferent sympathetic axons from lower thoracic and upper lumbar plexus preganglionic neurons and efferent parasympathetic axons from the celiac branch of the posterior vagal trunk form a plexus medial to the adrenal, enter with the arterioles, and traverse the cortex to end in the medulla. Sympathetic axons also innervate the subcapsular arteriolar plexus and regulate adrenal blood flow.[51] Nerves that end on glomerulosa cells contain catecholamines and neuropeptide Y. Zona glomerulosa cells and the subcapsular plexus are also innervated by axons containing vasoactive intestinal peptide, but most, if not all, of these axons arise and radiate outward from adrenomedullary cells that are under splanchnic regulation.[52] In addition, chromaffin cells may be scattered throughout all three zones of the cortex.[53] The function of these nerves is unknown, but beta-adrenergic agonists and vasoactive intestinal peptide may influence aldosterone and cortisol secretion.[53, 54] An afferent pathway is postulated to exist between the adrenal and hypothalamus and may modulate stress-induced secretion of ACTH.[55]

Light Microscopic Structure

Arnold's division of the cortex into three concentric zones[9] was based primarily on differences in vascular and connective tissue structure that are most evident in species, like the human, whose adrenocortical cells contain abundant cytoplasmic lipid inclusions (Fig. 9–3). The zona glomerulosa constitutes about 15% of the cortex and consists of a poorly demarcated layer of U-shaped or spherical nests, several cells in diameter, lying just under the capsule. The zona glomerulosa may be penetrated by extensions of the zona fasciculata that may reach the capsule. The glomerulosa cells are small and have a lower cytoplasmic/nuclear ratio, an intermediate number of lipid inclusions, and smaller nuclei containing more condensed chromatin than the other two layers. The fasciculata constitutes about 75% of the cortex, is not demarcated from the glomerulosa, and consists of

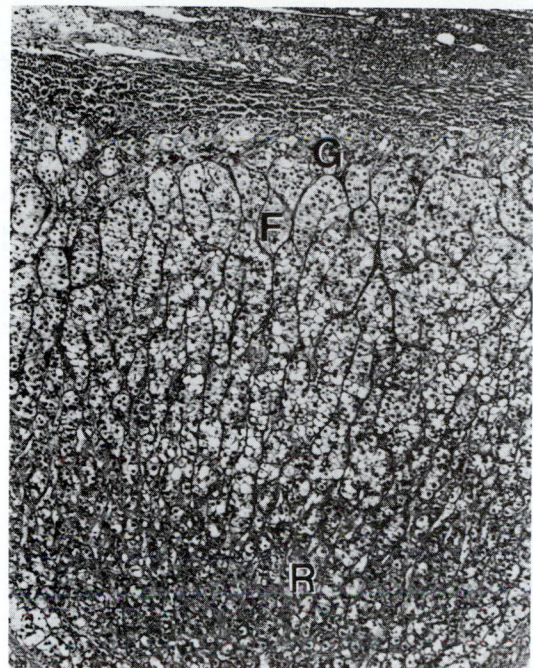

Figure 9–3. Light microscopic section of the human adrenal cortex from an unstressed individual who died of a gunshot wound. The narrow zona glomerulosa (G) lies just within the capsule, shown at the top. The broad lipid-filled zona fasciculata (F) lies between the zona glomerulosa and the dense compact cells of the zona reticularis (R). The medulla, which lies below the zona reticularis at the bottom, is not shown. (From Page DL, DeLellis RA, Hough AJ Jr. Tumors of the adrenal. In: Hartmann WH, Sobin LE, eds. Atlas of Tumor Pathology. 2nd ser. Fasc 23. Washington, DC: Armed Forces Institute of Pathology, 1986.)

radial cords of cells lying between delicate fibrovascular trabeculae. Its large cells have a high cytoplasmic/nuclear ratio and a foamy, vacuolated, "clear" cytoplasm because of the many lipid inclusions. The innermost zona reticularis is sharply demarcated from both the fasciculata and medulla and consists of irregular anastomosing cords of cells separated by thin-walled sinusoids. The cytoplasmic/nuclear ratio is intermediate, and the "compact" cytoplasm is lipid poor and, in the adult, contains numerous lipofuscin granules. The cortical cuff around the central vein resembles zona glomerulosa centrally and fasciculata peripherally.[4]

As discussed later, the zona glomerulosa cells produce the mineralocorticoid aldosterone, whereas the zonae fasciculata and reticularis secrete the glucocorticoid cortisol and the weak adrenal androgen dehydroepiandrosterone (DHEA), which is sulfated almost exclusively in the zona reticularis. However, these functional differences do not provide an adequate explanation for the different arrangements and morphologies of the cells in the three cortical zones.

Ultrastructure

The ultrastructure of adrenocortical cells is similar to that of other steroid-secreting cells (Fig. 9–4). Zona glomerulosa cells have small, elongated mitochondria with lamelliform cristae, scant finely vesiculated smooth endoplasmic reticulum, occasional lipid inclusions, and few lysosomes, lipofuscin granules, or microvilli. These gradually blend into typical fasciculata cells that contain small, spherical to ovoid mitochondria with vesicular cristae, abundant smooth and occasional rough endoplasmic reticulum arrayed as large vesicles in a honeycomb pattern, abundant lipid inclusions, increased numbers of lipofuscin granules, and prominent

microvilli. Zona reticularis cells possess small, mostly ovoid mitochondria with tubulovesicular cristae, densely packed smooth endoplasmic reticulum, rare lipid inclusions, abundant lipofuscin granules in the adult, and numerous microvilli.[4, 45]

Growth, Regeneration, and Hypertrophy

The factors that regulate adrenal growth in the fetus and maintain adrenal size in the adult are only partially understood. Because the adrenal gland of the anencephalic fetus develops normally for about 15 wk,[56] growth during this phase is presumed to be independent of fetal pituitary ACTH stimulation. The role of placental ACTH,[57] if any, is unknown, and there is no direct evidence that chorionic gonadotropin or other placental factors are involved. ACTH is required but may not be sufficient for later growth and maturation of the fetal gland. Factors that may regulate adrenal weight in the adult[58] include the NH_2-terminal fragment of POMC,[59, 60] epidermal growth factor, fibroblast growth factor, and insulin-like growth factor I (IGF I, also known as somatomedin-C).[61]

Maintenance of normal adrenal size and function may involve cell division in the zona glomerulosa, subsequent centripetal cell migration and differentiation in the fasciculata, and eventual senescence and death in the reticularis. Although the adult adrenal zonae fasciculata and reticularis clearly have the ability to regenerate from subcapsular remnants,[62] even in ectopic locations,[63] it is less clear whether this capability is utilized in the maintenance of normal

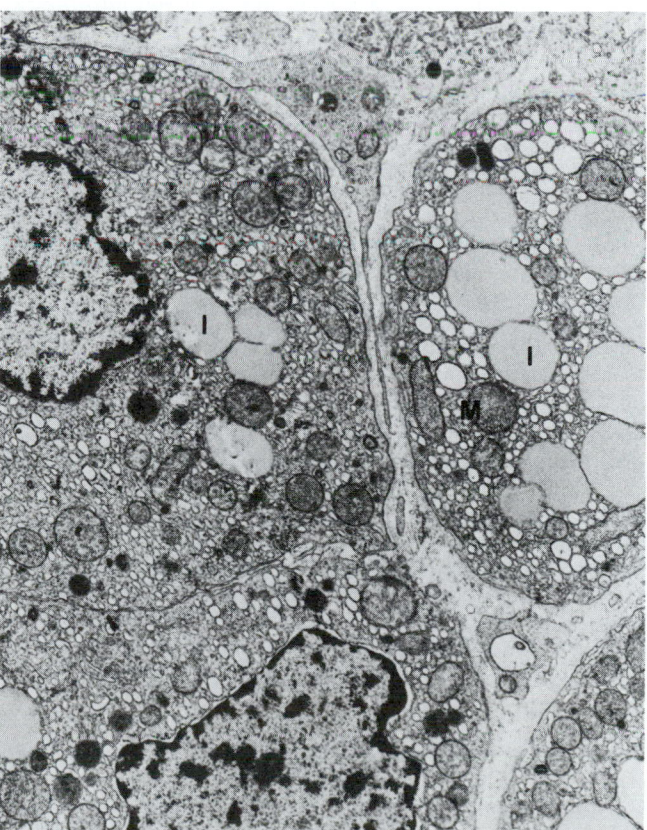

Figure 9–4. Ultrastructure of the human adrenal cortex. Cells from the inner zona fasciculata containing prominent lipid droplets (L), numerous ovoid mitochondria (M), and abundant smooth endoplasmic reticulum, which fills the cytoplasm. Uranyl acetate–lead citrate. (From Page DL, DeLellis RA, Hough AJ Jr. Tumors of the adrenal. In: Hartmann WH, Sobin LE, eds. Atlas of Tumor Pathology. 2nd ser. Fasc 23. Washington, DC: Armed Forces Institute of Pathology, 1986.)

adrenal anatomy.[64] Chronic labeling experiments with [³H]thymidine provide evidence for centripetal cell movement.[65] Furthermore, chronic ACTH stimulation and the consequent exposure to increased ambient glucocorticoid concentrations change the phenotype of glomerulosa cells to that of fasciculata cells structurally and in terms of the stimuli to which they respond and the steroids they produce.[45, 66, 67] Chronic ACTH stimulation has the further effects of converting the innermost fasciculata cells to the reticularis phenotype, a process that extends outward until the reticularis may completely replace the zona fasciculata, and of initially causing cell hypertrophy and, later, cortical hyperplasia that is reversible when ACTH is withdrawn.[43, 68]

Cells divide mainly within the zona glomerulosa, but the mechanisms that regulate the rate of division and the differentiation of some, but not all, glomerulosa-type cells into the fasciculata phenotype are poorly understood. The glomerulosa phenotype of some cells persists without obligate conversion to the fasciculata phenotype. Chronic administration of angiotensin II[69] or its physiological equivalent, dietary salt restriction, causes hypertrophy of the zona glomerulosa and increased aldosterone secretion without increasing fasciculata size or function. Furthermore, adequate secretion of aldosterone can persist during years of ACTH and consequently cortisol deficiency.[1] Finally, some patients who are "medically adrenalectomized" with mitotane, a cytotoxic drug that preferentially destroys zona fasciculata cells, maintain normal aldosterone secretion without recovery of normal cortisol secretion.[70] On the basis of these observations, it appears either (1) that the glomerulosa and fasciculata/reticularis cells arise from two different stem cells or, possibly, (2) that some (presumably local) factors stimulate the differentiation of a common stem cell into the two major types of adrenocortical cells.

After the removal of one adrenal gland, the remaining gland can undergo compensatory hypertrophy. Such hypertrophy does not occur in the absence of the pituitary gland.[2] ACTH appears to be the most important pituitary factor, but other hormones, such as growth hormone and the NH₂-terminal fragment of POMC, which may be processed locally to a bioactive product,[59, 60] may also be involved. Release from chronic beta-adrenergic inhibition[52, 54] and, possibly, other neurally mediated factors may also be involved.[71]

Steroid Biochemistry

The steroid hormones produced by the adrenal cortex are members of a large family of compounds derived from the cyclopentanoperhydrophenanthrene ring structure, which consists of three cyclohexane rings and one cyclopentane ring (Fig. 9–5). These compounds are widely distributed in the plant and animal kingdoms. They have a remarkable diversity of biological effects that depend on the nature of the chemical modifications of the basic steroid nucleus. The modifications include unsaturation of the carbon-carbon bonds in the rings and the attachment of hydroxyl, ketone, or other groups to specific carbon atoms.

Nomenclature

Steroid nomenclature follows either the chemical system established by the International Union of Pure and Applied Chemistry (IUPAC) or the collection of trivial names based in part on the compounds' biological properties (Table 9–1).[72, 73]

IUPAC NOMENCLATURE. The rings are referred to by letter and the individual carbon atoms by number (see Fig. 9–5). Parent structures have unique names. The unsaturated 17-carbon ring structure is termed *gonane*. Steroids with 18

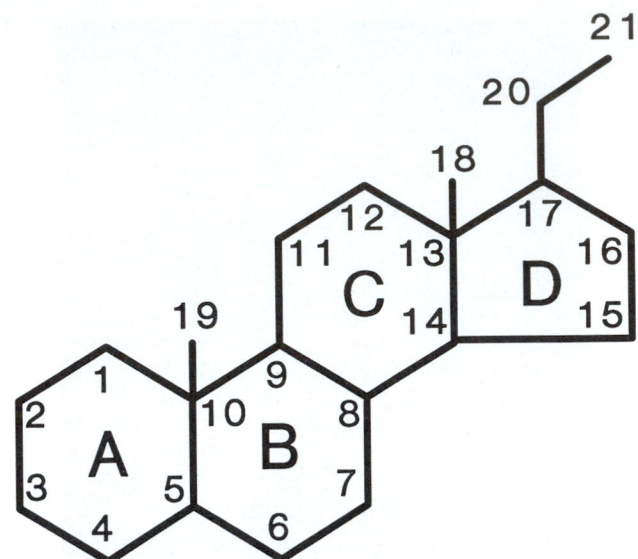

Figure 9–5. Basic steroid ring structure. The four rings are identified by letters. Individual carbon atoms of the steroid ring are numbered as shown. Substituent groups in derivative steroid molecules are designated by the number of the carbon atom to which they are attached. Double bonds in the ring structure are identified by the lower-numbered of the two carbon atoms they bind.

carbons (C_{18}-steroids) derived from this molecule by addition of a methyl group at C-13 are *estranes*. A C_{19}-steroid formed by the addition of another methyl at C-10 is an *androstane*. Further addition of an ethyl group at C-17 (a C_{21}-steroid) produces a *pregnane*. A double bond is indicated by adding "-ene" to the name of the parent compound, its position designated by the lower-numbered carbon to which it is attached. The position of a group is indicated by the number of the carbon to which it is attached. The stereochemistry of modifying groups is designated by alpha for those projecting behind the plane of the steroid ring, beta for those in front. In structural formulas the alpha configuration is denoted by a dashed line, the beta configuration by a solid line.

TRIVIAL NOMENCLATURE. The IUPAC system is too cumbersome for clinical application, and trivial names for most steroid hormones are generally used. Table 9–1 lists both systematic and trivial names for some commonly en-

TABLE 9–1. IUPAC and Trivial Names of Several Natural and Synthetic Steroids

Trivial Name	IUPAC Name
Aldosterone	4-Pregnen-11β,21-diol-3,18,20-trione
Androstenedione	4-Androsten-3,17-dione
Cortisol	4-Pregnen-11β,17α,21-triol-3,20-dione
Cortisone	4-Pregnen-17α,21-diol-3,11,20-trione
Dehydroepiandrosterone	5-Androsten-3β-ol-17-one
Deoxycorticosterone	4-Pregnen-21-ol-3,20-dione
Dexamethasone	1,4-Pregnadien-9α-fluoro-16α-methyl-11β,17α,21-triol-3,20-dione
Dihydrotestosterone	5α-Androstan-17β-ol-3-one
Estradiol	1,3,5(10)-Estratrien-3,17β-diol
Fludrocortisone	4-Pregnen-9α-fluoro-11β,17α,21-triol-3,20-dione
17-Hydroxyprogesterone	4-Pregnen-17α-ol-3,20-dione
Methylprednisolone	1,4-Pregnadien-6α-methyl-11β,17α,21-triol-3,20-dione
Prednisolone	1,4-Pregnadien-11β,17α,21-triol-3,20-dione
Prednisone	1,4-Pregnadien-17α,21-diol-3,11,20-trione
Pregnenolone	5-Pregnen-3β-ol-20-one
Progesterone	4-Pregnen-3,20-dione
Testosterone	4-Androsten-17β-ol-3-one
Triamcinolone	1,4-Pregnadien-9α-fluoro-11β,16α,17α,21-tetrol-3,20-dione

countered steroid hormones. Estrogens are C_{18}-steroids with an aromatized (fully unsaturated) A ring, androgens are C_{19}-steroids, and progestogens and glucocorticoids are C_{21} derivatives. The symbol Δ indicates an unsaturated bond; its superscript number indicates the lower-numbered carbon to which it is attached.

Steroid Hormone Biosynthesis

SOURCES OF CHOLESTEROL FOR ADRENAL STEROIDOGENESIS. All human steroid hormones are derived from cholesterol. The cells of steroidogenic tissues can synthesize cholesterol de novo from acetate, mobilize intracellular cholesteryl ester pools, or import lipoprotein cholesterol from plasma. About 80% of the cholesterol is usually provided by circulating plasma lipoproteins.[74-76] Adrenal tissue in vitro utilizes low-density lipoprotein (LDL) cholesterol via a specific receptor-mediated pathway.[77-79] Such receptors are present in mouse adrenocortical tumor cells[77, 80] and normal adrenal tissue from a variety of species.[81-87] Specific cell-surface receptors for LDL, localized to structures called *coated pits*, bind circulating LDL and internalize it by receptor-mediated endocytosis.[88] The coated pit invaginates to form a coated vesicle containing receptor-bound LDL. The coated vesicles fuse with lysosomes, where cholesteryl esters are hydrolyzed to liberate free cholesterol for use as steroidogenic substrate.

Adrenal glands of animals other than rat and mouse do not have specific binding sites for high-density lipoprotein (HDL),[78, 89, 90] and most species apparently do not use HDL cholesterol for adrenal steroid biosynthesis.[76, 77]

The adrenal cortex can also synthesize cholesterol de novo from acetyl coenzyme A. Under normal conditions about 20% of steroidogenic capacity[74-76] depends on intracellular cholesterol biosynthesis. In disorders that impair delivery of exogenous cholesterol, basal adrenal steroidogenesis is normal. Abetalipoproteinemia is a hereditary deficiency of apolipoprotein B production in which LDL is absent from plasma. Patients with this disorder have normal basal adrenal steroid hormone production.[91, 92] Patients with familial hypercholesterolemia have defective LDL receptors but have normal basal steroidogenesis, possibly because elevated plasma LDL levels promote LDL cholesterol uptake by nonspecific pathways. However, even though basal steroidogenesis is unimpaired by defects in extracellular cholesterol delivery, increased steroidogenesis stimulated by prolonged ACTH administration cannot be sustained by de novo synthesis of cholesterol alone.[91, 93]

The amount of free intracellular cholesterol available for adrenal steroidogenesis is metabolically regulated, and negative feedback is exerted via the LDL pathway to control the amount of free intracellular cholesterol in adrenocortical cells. LDL uptake suppresses cellular cholesterol synthesis by reducing the activity of hydroxymethylglutaryl–coenzyme A (HMG-CoA) reductase, the rate-limiting enzyme in cholesterol biosynthesis. Esterification of imported cholesterol is stimulated, and cell-surface LDL receptor number is down-regulated as a consequence of LDL cholesterol uptake by receptor-mediated endocytosis.[84] ACTH increases the number of LDL receptors on the cell surface, the activity of the cholesterol esterase that liberates free cholesterol from cholesteryl esters delivered by LDL or stored in lipid droplets, and, as a consequence, the amount of free intracellular cholesterol.[94, 95] ACTH does not stimulate HMG-CoA reductase activity or alter the ability of LDL to suppress it.[94, 95]

BIOSYNTHETIC PATHWAYS

Glucocorticoid Biosynthesis. **General Features.** Four cytochrome P-450 enzymes are involved in adrenal corticosteroid biosynthesis. Cytochromes P-450 are a large family of oxidative enzymes that have a characteristic 450-nm absorbance maximum when reduced with carbon monoxide. They serve a variety of biological functions[96] involving transfer of electrons from NADPH, provided by an electron transport protein intermediary, to molecular oxygen with concomitant oxygenation of substrates. The substrates of the steroidogenic cytochromes P-450 are various ring carbons of cholesterol. For example, P-450$_{scc}$ (side-chain cleavage enzyme), an adrenal mitochondrial enzyme, cleaves the side chain from C-21 of cholesterol. A second mitochondrial enzyme, P-450$_{c11}$ (11β-hydroxylase), catalyzes the beta-hydroxylation at C-11. Two enzymes of the smooth endoplasmic reticulum, P-450$_{c17}$ (17α-hydroxylase) and P-450$_{c21}$ (21-hydroxylase), catalyze hydroxylations at C-17 and C-21, respectively.[96] A fifth enzyme required for adrenal steroidogenesis, 3β-hydroxysteroid dehydrogenase, is thought not to be a P-450 enzyme, is associated with the smooth endoplasmic reticulum, and catalyzes the conversion of pregnenolone to progesterone. The biosynthetic pathways for adrenal steroidogenesis are shown in Figure 9–6 and described in the following subsections.

Pregnenolone Synthesis by P-450$_{scc}$. Each enzymatic step in cortisol biosynthesis is compartmentalized within the cell by virtue of the subcellular localization of the enzyme involved. Free cholesterol must be transported through the cytosol to the inner mitochondrial membrane, the site of the enzyme that catalyzes the first and rate-limiting step in steroidogenesis. A number of peptide factors play a role in the regulation of cholesterol access to the inner mitochondrial membrane,[97] including a 13.5-kd sterol carrier protein 2,[98, 99] a 3.2-kd steroidogenesis activator peptide,[100, 101] and an 8.2-kd protein.[102] These proteins are thought to have the capacity to enhance cholesterol transfer to the inner membrane of isolated mitochondria and consequently to stimulate the first step in steroidogenesis. The precise physiological roles of these proteins are poorly understood.[97]

Within the mitochondrion, pregnenolone is derived from cholesterol by removal of the side chain at C-20. Cleavage of the cholesterol side chain to yield pregnenolone was originally thought to proceed via the generation of several intermediates—20-hydroxycholesterol, 22-hydroxycholesterol, and 20,22-dihydroxycholesterol[103-107]—and three distinct enzymes were thought to be involved. However, a single protein catalyzes the complete reaction.[108-111] Full-length cDNAs for bovine[112] and human[113] P-450$_{scc}$ were used to show that a single mRNA species codes for the enzyme in steroidogenic tissues. A single P-450$_{scc}$ gene exists on human chromosome 15.[113] Thus the enzyme is the same in all steroidogenic tissues.

The electrons are transferred by P-450$_{scc}$ during side-chain cleavage through an electron transport system composed of adrenodoxin, a nonheme iron–binding protein that exists in soluble form in the mitochondrial matrix, and adrenodoxin reductase, a mitochondrial membrane–bound flavoprotein. Adrenodoxin reductase accepts electrons from NADPH and transfers them to adrenodoxin, which serves as a shuttle to deliver reducing equivalents to various cytochromes P-450[114] (Fig. 9–7). Humans have a single expressed gene for adrenodoxin, two adrenodoxin pseudogenes,[115] and a single gene for adrenodoxin reductase, although alternative splicing produces two forms of adrenodoxin reductase mRNA.[116] The functional significance of the two forms of adrenodoxin reductase is unknown.[117]

Conversion of Pregnenolone to Progesterone by 3β-Hydroxysteroid Dehydrogenase/$\Delta^{4,5}$-Isomerase. The newly synthesized pregnenolone is returned to the cytosolic compartment, where a series of microsomal enzymes convert it to 11-deoxycortisol. First, it is converted to progesterone by dehydrogenation of the 3-hydroxyl group of pregnenolone

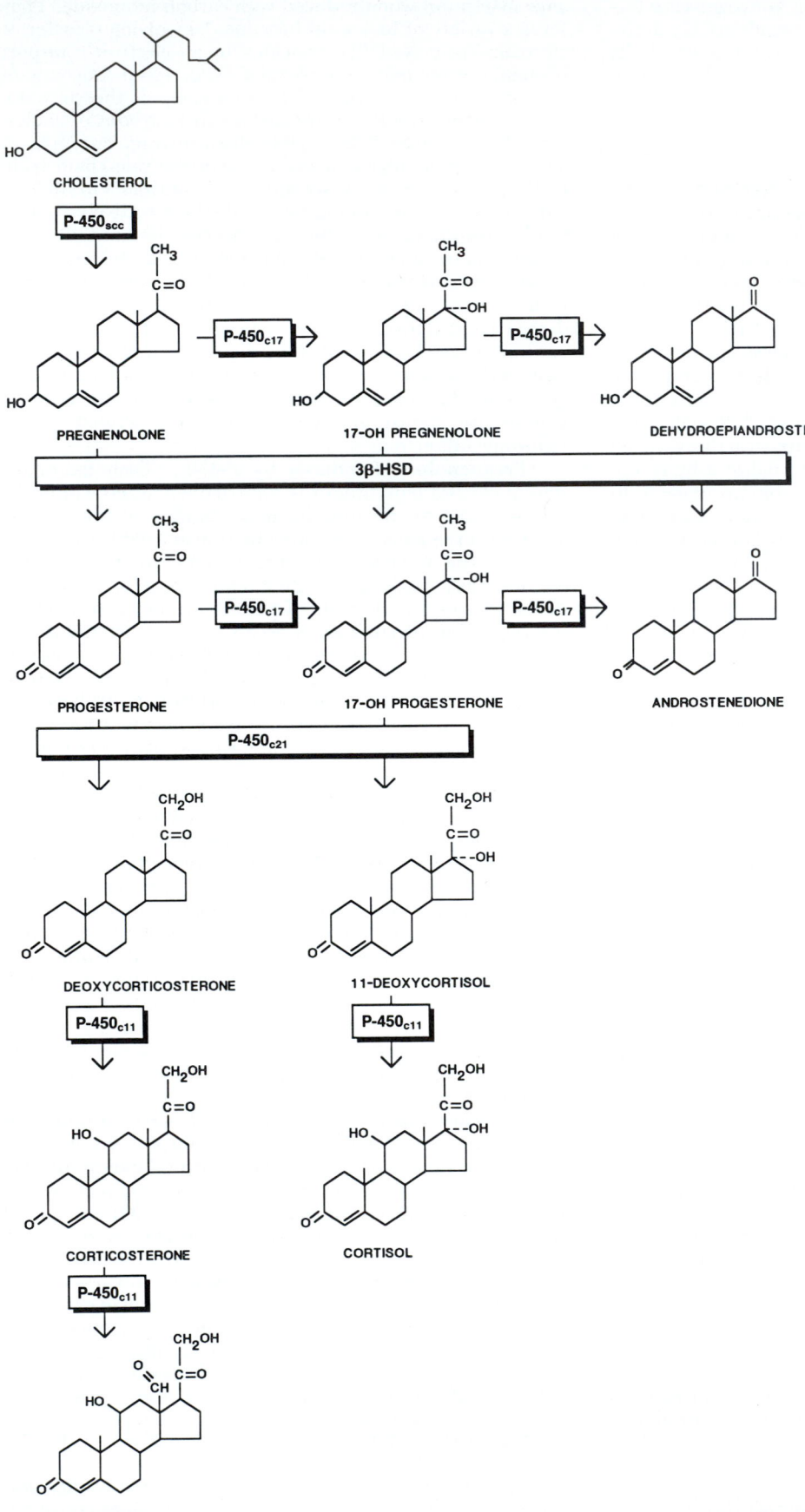

Figure 9–6. Steroid biosynthetic pathways in the adrenal cortex. The branching pathways for glucocorticoids, mineralocorticoids, and adrenal androgens and the structures of these steroids and their biosynthetic precursors are shown. The biosynthetic enzymes are represented by the boxes. 3β-HSD, 3β-hydroxysteroid dehydrogenase.

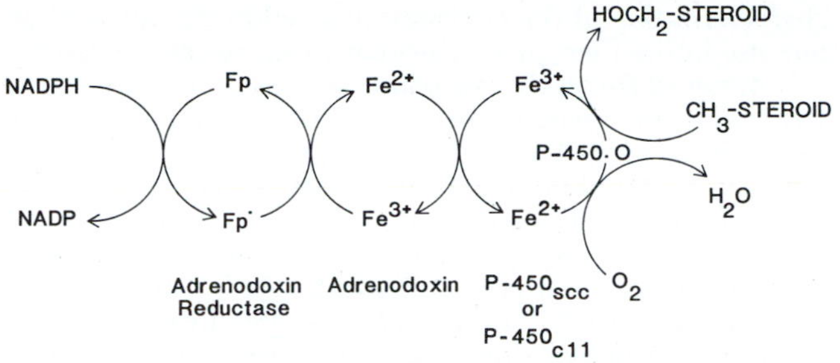

Figure 9–7. Electron shuttle system for the mitochondrial enzymes, P-450$_{scc}$ and P-450$_{c11}$. Adrenodoxin reductase receives electrons from NADPH and reduces adrenodoxin, which transfers reducing equivalents to the P-450 enzyme. The enzyme then transfers it, by way of oxygen, to the steroid. Fp, flavoprotein; Fp', reduced form of flavoprotein.

and isomerization of the double bond at C-5. The enzymatic processes responsible are poorly understood. A single form of the dehydrogenase is thought to exist in all steroidogenic tissues,[118] but various substrate-specific isomerase isoenzymes have been characterized.[119]

Conversion of Progesterone to 17α-Hydroxyprogesterone by P-450$_{c17}$. P-450$_{c17}$ is a microsomal enzyme that catalyzes both hydroxylation of C-17 of progesterone or pregnenolone (17α-hydroxylase activity) and cleavage of the residual two-carbon side chain at C-17 (17,20-lyase activity).[120–123] This dual function allows the enzyme to direct steroid precursors along several different pathways: 17α-hydroxylated substrates with the side chain intact are glucocorticoid precursors, whereas generation of C$_{19}$-steroids by both 17α-hydroxylase and 17,20-lyase activities directs substrate toward androgen and estrogen synthesis. In the zona glomerulosa, which lacks both P-450$_{c17}$ activities, pregnenolone is converted into mineralocorticoids. Whether a given steroid molecule undergoes both 17α-hydroxylation and lysis of the 17,20 bond appears to depend on the supply of electrons to P-450$_{c17}$ from a flavoprotein distinct from mitochondrial adrenodoxin. This protein, P-450 reductase, also supplies electrons to P-450$_{c21}$, the other microsomal P-450 enzyme.[124] P-450 reductase transfers two electrons sequentially from NADPH to P-450$_{c17}$. Cytochrome b_5 may also donate the second electron (Fig. 9–8). Because P-450$_{c17}$, with both 17α-hydroxylase and 17,20-lyase activities, and P-450$_{c21}$ are present in large molar excess over the reductase, they compete for the same pool of electrons.[96, 125–127] With a sufficient flux of electrons from P-450 reductase and/or cytochrome b_5, both 17α-hydroxylation and C-21 side-chain cleavage occur.

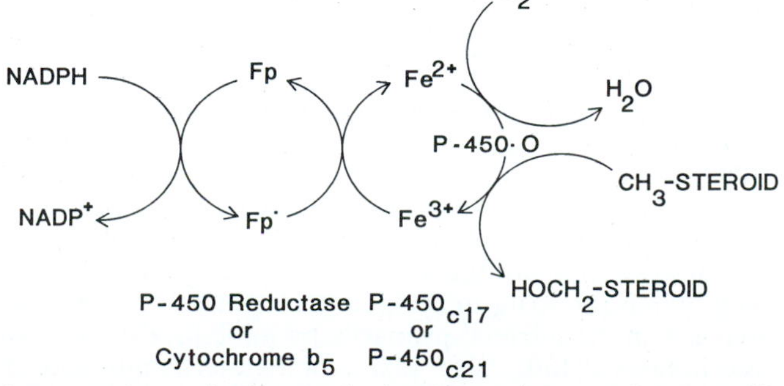

Figure 9–8. Electron shuttle system for the microsomal enzymes, P-450$_{c17}$ and P-450$_{c21}$. P-450 reductase, a flavoprotein, accepts electrons from NADPH and transfers them to the P-450 enzyme. The enzyme then transfers electrons, by way of oxygen, to the steroid. A second reducing equivalent may be supplied to P-450$_{c17}$ by P-450 reductase or cytochrome b_5.

Conversion of 17α-Hydroxyprogesterone to 11-Deoxycortisol by P-450$_{c21}$. Both progesterone and its 17α-hydroxylated derivative undergo 21-hydroxylation by a single P-450$_{c21}$ enzyme in the smooth endoplasmic reticulum.[124] There are two genes for P-450$_{c21}$,[128–132] but only one is actively transcribed in humans.[133]

Conversion of 11-Deoxycortisol to Cortisol by P-450$_{c11}$. The last step in cortisol biosynthesis is the 11β-hydroxylation of 11-deoxycortisol, catalyzed by the mitochondrial enzyme P-450$_{c11}$. Like P-450$_{scc}$, the other P-450 enzyme of the inner mitochondrial membrane, P-450$_{c11}$ receives electrons from NADPH via adrenodoxin reductase and adrenodoxin.[134, 135] This enzyme also catalyzes the 18-hydroxylation step in mineralocorticoid biosynthesis (see later). The gene product is more closely related to P-450$_{scc}$ than to the microsomal cytochromes P-450.[136–138]

Mineralocorticoid Biosynthesis. Progesterone is also the substrate for mineralocorticoid synthesis (see Fig. 9–6). In the zona glomerulosa progesterone is hydroxylated at C-21 by P-450$_{c21}$ to yield DOC. All three terminal steps in the conversion of this intermediate to aldosterone (11β-hydroxylation, 18-hydroxylation, and 18-methyl oxidation) are catalyzed by a single mitochondrial P-450$_{c11}$ enzyme.[139] Because P-450$_{c11}$ activity is also present in the zona fasciculata, it was not clear how aldosterone synthesis could be restricted to the zona glomerulosa. Studies with antibodies prepared against purified bovine P-450$_{c11}$ have revealed two different forms of the enzyme, a salt-regulated 49-kd protein restricted to the zona glomerulosa and a 51-kd form found in both zona glomerulosa and zona fasciculata.[140–142] Although the two are immunologically related, their NH$_2$-terminal amino acid sequences reveal that they are distinct proteins.[136, 137] Molecular cloning suggests the existence of two genes for P-450$_{c11}$, but the relationship of these genes to the 51- and 49-kd enzymes is unclear.[136, 137]

Adrenal Androgen Biosynthesis. Steroids with 19 carbon atoms that serve as weak androgens or androgen precursors are synthesized by the adrenal (see Fig. 9–6). In fact, DHEA and its sulfate, DHEAS, are the most abundant products of the adrenal glands. They are formed from 17α-hydroxypregnenolone by the 17,20-lyase activity of P-450$_{c17}$. Androstenedione, another 19-carbon steroid (Table 9–2), is produced by side-chain cleavage of 17α-hydroxyprogesterone by P-450$_{c17}$ and is subsequently converted to testosterone by 17-ketosteroid reductase mainly in peripheral tissues; synthesis of testosterone in the adrenal is minimal.

Adrenal Estrogen Biosynthesis. Estrogens are produced from C$_{19}$ androgens by the microsomal enzyme P-450 aromatase,[96, 143] whose net effect is to remove carbon 19 and create a conjugated double bond system (aromatization) in the A ring with a hydroxyl group in position 3. Only small amounts of estrogen are synthesized by the normal adrenal, but DHEA, DHEAS, and androstenedione are substrates for estrogen production by peripheral tissues such as adipose tissue, which contain considerable aromatase activity[144] (see Chapters 12 and 13).

Fetal Adrenal Steroid Biosynthesis. A morphologically and functionally distinct fetal zone exists in the human fetal

TABLE 9–2. Relative Androgenic Activity of Adrenal Androgens

Steroid	Activity
Dihydrotestosterone	300
Testosterone	100
Androstenedione	10
DHEA, DHEAS	5

Adapted from Nelson DH. The Adrenal Cortex: Physiological Function and Disease. Philadelphia: W. B. Saunders, 1980:102–112.

adrenal gland until birth, after which it rapidly involutes.[145] Under ACTH stimulation, the fetal zone both imports LDL cholesterol[146–148] and synthesizes cholesterol de novo[149] to produce mainly pregnenolone sulfate and DHEAS,[150–152] beginning at about 25 wk of gestation.[153] Predominant secretion of Δ^5-steroids such as DHEAS apparently is due to low activity of the 3β-hydroxysteroid dehydrogenase/$\Delta^{4,5}$-isomerase required to convert 17α-hydroxypregnenolone to 17α-hydroxyprogesterone.[154] DHEAS is converted to 16α-hydroxy-DHEAS in peripheral fetal tissues[155] and serves as substrate for placental estrogen synthesis. Estrogen, in turn, inhibits 3β-hydroxysteroid dehydrogenase activity in the fetal adrenal, thus perpetuating production of its DHEAS precursor.[156]

FUNCTIONAL ANATOMY. The structural zonation of the adrenal cortex roughly correlates with the biosynthesis of different steroids. As already noted, the fetal zone of the fetal adrenal is deficient in 3β-hydroxysteroid dehydrogenase and therefore produces little cortisol but prodigious amounts of DHEAS. The definitive zone of the fetal adrenal produces mainly cortisol, the major glucocorticoid in humans. In the mature gland, the zona glomerulosa and the outermost fasciculata synthesize the major mineralocorticoid aldosterone. The fasciculata and, less importantly, the reticularis synthesize cortisol. In addition to DOC and 18-hydroxy-DOC, which are mainly products of the zona glomerulosa, DHEA and other adrenal androgens and estrogens are also synthesized by the fasciculata and reticularis,[157–160] sulfation occurring exclusively in the reticularis.[161] DHEAS is still the major steroid product of the mature adrenal in terms of quantity but is physiologically not the most important one.

INHIBITORS OF STEROIDOGENESIS. A number of compounds (Fig. 9–9) can inhibit adrenal steroidogenesis by interfering with one or more of the enzymatic processes just described. These compounds have been useful not only for

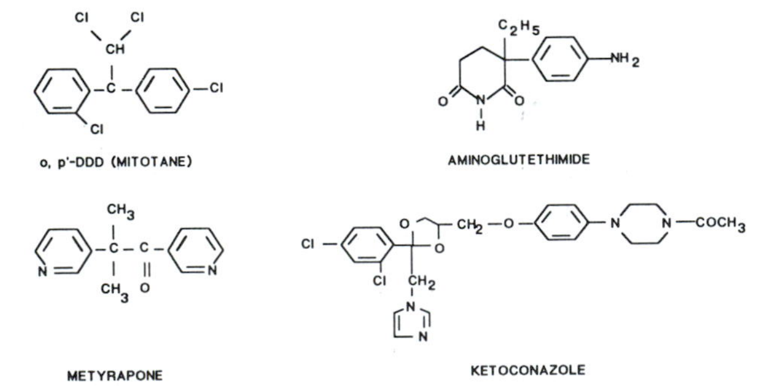

Figure 9–9. Structures of inhibitors of steroid synthesis or action. Mitotane is an adrenocorticolytic drug. Aminoglutethimide, metyrapone, cyanoketone, ketoconazole, trilostane, and etomidate are inhibitors of steroidogenesis. Mifepristone (RU-486) is a competitive antagonist of glucocorticoid binding to its receptor in target cells and is an even more potent antagonist of progesterone binding to its receptor.

characterization of the enzymes involved in steroid synthesis but also in the therapy of glucocorticoid excess (see later).

Adrenocorticolysis: Mitotane. In 1949 the insecticide DDT was first recognized to produce adrenocortical deficiency in dogs.[162] The active component was shown to be 2,2-bis(2-chlorophenyl-4-chlorophenyl)-1,1-dichloroethane or *o,p'*-DDD, usually called mitotane.[163] Brief administration of mitotane to dogs caused necrosis and hemorrhage in the zonae fasciculata and reticularis, with relative sparing of the zona glomerulosa.[164] There is considerable intraspecies variation in sensitivity to the drug, but normal and neoplastic human adrenal glands are sensitive to the cytotoxic effect. Mitotane is used to produce a "medical adrenalectomy" under certain circumstances (see later).[165–167] Mitotane also alters the peripheral metabolism of cortisol.[168] Ordinarily, cortisol is metabolized to compounds measurable in urine as 17-hydoxycorticosteroids (17-OHCS) (see later). Mitotane causes a 50 to 80% reduction in these metabolites by diverting metabolism toward formation of a more polar compound, 6β-hydroxycortisol, that is not measured in the assay.[168]

P-450$_{scc}$ Inhibition: Aminoglutethimide. Aminoglutethimide was used as an anticonvulsant for several years before discovery of its antisteroidogenic activity in vitro.[169] A principal action is to inhibit P-450$_{scc}$, which converts cholesterol to Δ^5-pregnenolone,[170] resulting in hypocortisolemia and a compensatory increase in pituitary ACTH secretion,[171] which tends to override the drug-induced blockade. Because an early step in steroidogenesis is inhibited, mineralocorticoid biosynthesis is also decreased. Although there is a compensatory increase in plasma renin activity, it cannot completely overcome the blockade, and individuals treated with the compound have decreased aldosterone secretion.[171] Aminoglutethimide is useful for controlling hypercortisolism in patients with Cushing's syndrome resulting from autonomous secretion of cortisol or ACTH (see later).

P-450$_{c11}$ Inhibition: Metyrapone. One of the earliest and clinically most useful inhibitors of steroidogenesis, metyrapone, is mainly an inhibitor of P-450$_{c11}$, which catalyzes the final step in cortisol biosynthesis, conversion of 11-deoxycortisol to cortisol.[172–174] Because P-450$_{c11}$ also catalyzes the terminal steps in aldosterone synthesis, metyrapone also inhibits aldosterone secretion,[175] but its effect on electrolyte metabolism is mitigated by increased DOC production. Production of adrenal androgen precursors is also increased. Metyrapone is useful for diagnostic testing of hypothalamic-pituitary-adrenal axis function and for controlling hypercortisolism in patients with Cushing's syndrome associated with autonomous secretion of cortisol or ACTH (see later).

3β-Hydroxysteroid Dehydrogenase Inhibition: Cyanoketone. Cyanoketone (2α-cyano-4,4,17α-trimethylandrost-5-ene-17β-ol-3-one) is a C_{19}-steroid analogue that inhibits 3β-hydroxysteroid dehydrogenase activity in rats.[176] It inhibits the enzyme in all steroidogenic tissues and thereby reduces production of both gonadal and adrenal steroids. It has not been used clinically.

Multiple Enzyme Inhibition: Ketoconazole and Etomidate. In the early 1980s a new class of imidazole-derived antifungal drugs were found to have antisteroidogenic actions in humans. These compounds exert their fungicidal effects by inhibiting a fungal P-450 enzyme system.[177] Effects on human testosterone production were first recognized[178] because men taking the drug developed gynecomastia.[179] Ketoconazole acts in the adrenal primarily by inhibiting P-450$_{c11}$ and also inhibits P-450$_{scc}$.[180, 181] Like aminoglutethimide and metyrapone, it is useful in treating some patients with Cushing's syndrome (see later).

Etomidate, another imidazole derivative, is a parenteral anesthetic used to sedate patients on mechanical ventilators in intensive care units. Like ketoconazole, etomidate's major effect is inhibition of 11β-hydroxylation,[182–186] but higher doses also inhibit P-450$_{scc}$.[182, 187] It can be used to control cortisol secretion in hospitalized Cushing's patients[188] (see later).

Blockade of Cortisol Action: Mifepristone. Mifepristone (RU-486) does not inhibit steroidogenesis, but it antagonizes the peripheral actions of glucocorticoids and progestogens because it is a competitive inhibitor of binding to their cytosolic receptor proteins.[189, 190] It is an effective abortifacient and has been used in patients with Cushing's syndrome (see later).

Regulation of Glucocorticoid Secretion

The Hypothalamic-Pituitary-Adrenal Axis

Glucocorticoid secretion is regulated by hormonal interactions among the hypothalamus, the pituitary, and the adrenal glands and by neural and other stimuli (Fig. 9–10).[191–193] Neural stimuli from the brain, as in the response to stress, cause the release into the hypothalamic-hypophyseal portal blood of CRH, AVP, and other agents from hypothalamic neurons. They are carried to the pituitary, where they stimulate ACTH secretion into the systemic blood. ACTH acts on the adrenal cortex to cause secretion of cortisol and other steroids. The negative feedback loop is completed by the inhibitory effect of glucocorticoids on CRH, AVP, and ACTH synthesis and secretion.

Pro-opiomelanocortin

STRUCTURE, SYNTHESIS, AND PROCESSING. *The POMC Gene.* ACTH is synthesized as part of a large precursor (241 amino acids in humans), POMC, which also contains the sequences for other peptides, including the lipotropins (LPHs), melanocyte-stimulating hormones (MSHs), and β-endorphin (β-END) (Fig. 9–11).[194–196] The human POMC gene is located on chromosome 2[197] and consists of three exons separated by two large introns (see

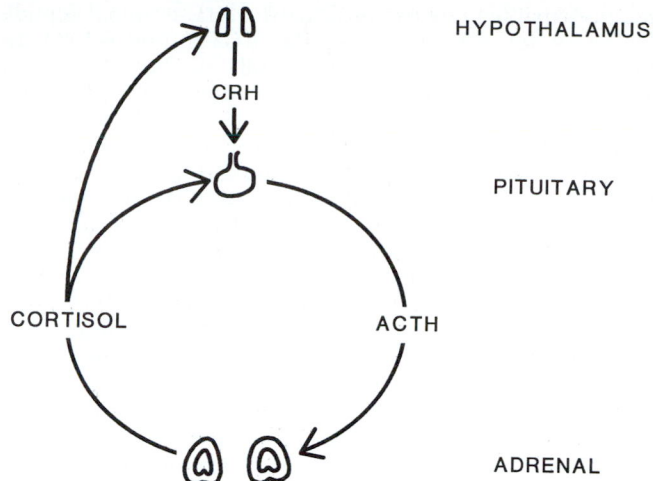

Figure 9–10. Normal regulation of adrenal glucocorticoid secretion. Secretion of CRH and other hypothalamic releasing factors, such as AVP, is regulated by central nervous system afferents mediating the circadian rhythm and responses to stress. ACTH and other POMC-derived peptides are released in equimolar amounts from anterior pituitary corticotropes. ACTH stimulates the cells of the inner two zones of the adrenal cortex to produce cortisol, which inhibits the synthesis and release of CRH and the action of CRH, AVP, and other secretagogues on the pituitary corticotrope.

Fig. 9–11).[194–196] The gene structure is the same in different species, and there is considerable sequence homology. Exon 3 codes for most of the translated sequence, and exon 2 codes for the signal peptide and the 18 NH$_2$-terminal amino acids of POMC.

Post-Translational Processing. POMC undergoes extensive post-translational processing, including cleavage, glycosylation, phosphorylation, sulfation, and NH$_2$-terminal acetylation and COOH-terminal amidation of certain cleaved peptides (see Fig. 9–11).[198–200] Multiple peptides are produced from the POMC precursor by enzymatic cleavage. The cleavage pattern is tissue specific. In the anterior lobe,

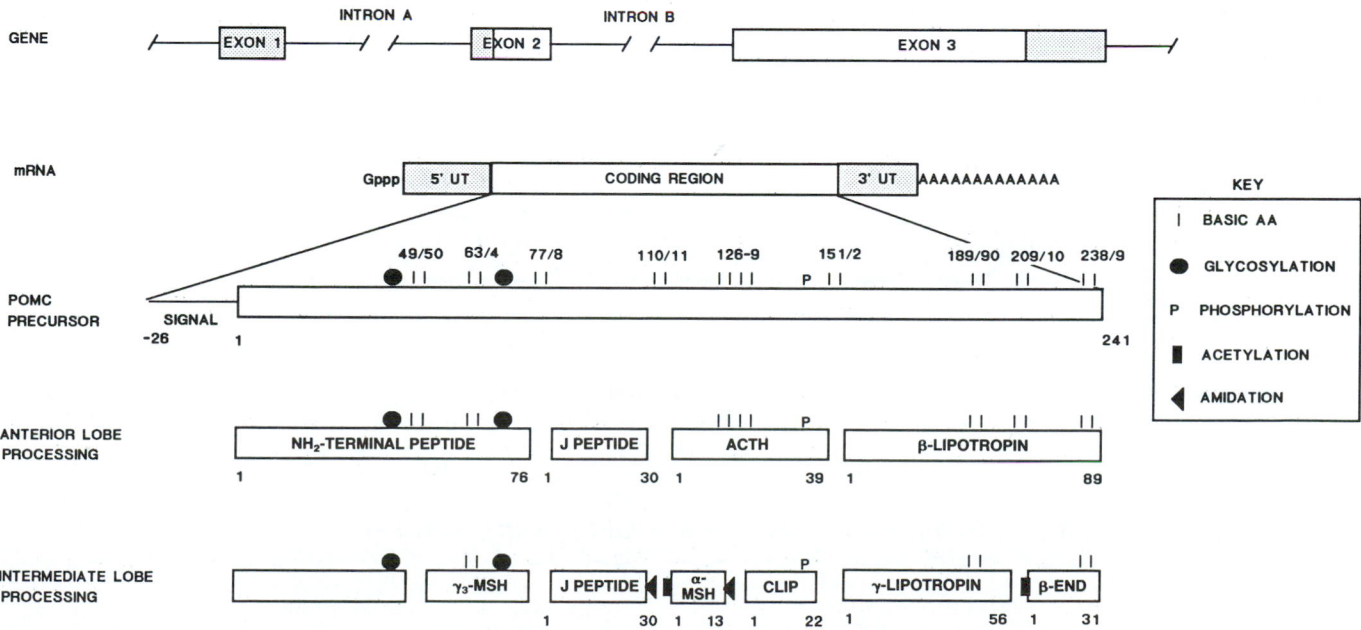

Figure 9–11. Structures of the human POMC gene, its mRNA, prePOMC with its 26-amino-acid signal sequence, and the mature peptides produced from POMC by cleavage at basic dipeptides in the anterior lobe and, in the fetus and pregnant woman, the intermediate-lobe–like corticotropes. UT, flanking untranslated region; J PEPTIDE, joining peptide; CLIP, corticotropin-like intermediate-lobe peptide.

the principal peptide products are the NH$_2$-terminal peptide (NT peptide), the joining peptide, ACTH, and β-LPH. In the intermediate lobe, which is fully developed in most subprimates but is active in humans only during fetal life and during pregnancy, ACTH is cleaved into ACTH(1–14) (the precursor of α-MSH) and corticotropin-like intermediate-lobe peptide (ACTH(18–39) or CLIP), β-LPH is completely processed into γ-LPH and β-END, and the NT peptide is cleaved to yield γ$_3$-MSH. Glycosylation can occur at Thr-45 and Asn-65 of the NT peptide.[201] ACTH is glycosylated in rodents but not in humans. The joining peptide and ACTH(1–14) are further modified by cleavage of the COOH-terminal glycine and amidation of the adjacent amino acid.[202] β-END and ACTH(1–13) amide (desacetyl-α-MSH) can be modified by the addition of one or two acetyl groups to the NH$_2$ termini, yielding acetyl–β-END and α-MSH (acetyl-ACTH(1–13) amide) or diacetyl–α-MSH.[203] In the anterior lobe, less than 1% of ACTH and β-LPH undergoes similar cleavage, and the products are not acetylated[204] because the necessary enzyme is not present. In the testis and other nonpituitary tissues, four or five amino acids can be cleaved from the COOH-terminal end of β-END to produce γ-END (β-END(1–27)) or α-END (β-END(1–26)).[205] About a third of ACTH in the human pituitary is phosphorylated at Ser-31,[206] and the carbohydrate side chains of POMC peptides may be sulfated,[207] but the significance of these modifications is unknown. Although the sequence for met-enkephalin is present in the NH$_2$ terminus of β-END, this peptide arises from a different precursor protein.

PLASMA POMC-DERIVED PEPTIDES AND THEIR ACTIONS. *Anterior-Lobe Peptides.* ACTH is a 39-amino-acid peptide that stimulates secretion of glucocorticoids, androgenic steroids, and, to a lesser extent, mineralocorticoids from the adrenal cortex (Fig. 9–12). The first 24 NH$_2$-terminal amino acids of ACTH are the same in all species studied, but there are minor species differences in the COOH-terminal portion of the molecule. The half-life of circulating ACTH depends on how it is measured. Bioactivity disappears from the circulation with a half-life of 4 to 8 min, whereas immunoreactivity may disappear more or less rapidly, depending on which part of the molecule is recognized by antibody.[208–210] There is minimal urinary excretion of ACTH. The biologically active portion of ACTH is the first 18 NH$_2$-terminal amino acids. Because of rapid metabolic degradation of this molecule, synthetic ACTH(1–24) or, in

countries other than the United States, synthetic ACTH(1–18) amide is used for clinical purposes.

ACTH, β-LPH, joining peptide, and NT peptide arise from the same precursor protein, so they are secreted in approximately equimolar amounts, resulting in similar plasma levels basally and after stimulation by low plasma cortisol levels (e.g., during metyrapone administration), hypoglycemia, CRH, or AVP.[211–214] However, the longer half-life of circulating β-LPH compared with ACTH results in a much slower decline in the plasma level of β-LPH and an elevated plasma β-LPH/ACTH ratio after a secretory episode or during prolonged hypersecretion. The ratio is also elevated in patients undergoing chronic hemodialysis.[215] These observations imply that β-LPH has no direct or indirect feedback effect on POMC synthesis. The physiological function of β-LPH, an 89-amino-acid peptide in humans, is unknown, although it has weak steroidogenic and lipolytic activities[216] and may have potent melanotropic activity.[217] The NT peptide and its NH$_2$-terminal fragments may be adrenal growth factors[59, 60, 218] and may potentiate the action of ACTH on steroidogenesis.[219]

There are three MSH regions in the POMC precursor, alpha, beta, and gamma, consisting of identical 6-amino-acid core sequences and similar flanking regions. The MSHs stimulate melanin synthesis by melanocytes, resulting in darkening of the skin. Although they are flanked by basic dipeptides that are sites of post-translational cleavage, the MSHs are not produced in appreciable amounts in humans. Thus the hyperpigmentation that occurs in Addison's disease and Nelson's syndrome is presumably due to the much weaker melanotropic activity of the elevated plasma ACTH and, possibly, β-LPH levels. Reported effects of α-MSH include stimulation of aldosterone secretion in hypophysectomized rats,[220] enhancement of growth of the adrenal zona glomerulosa,[221] and gonadotropin-releasing activity.[222] α-MSH may also potentiate the acute stimulatory effect of ACTH on aldosterone secretion, but plasma α-MSH levels are too low to exert these effects in humans.

Intermediate-Lobe Peptides. The intermediate-lobe peptides are not present in significant amounts in normal human plasma but may be secreted by some pituitary and nonpituitary tumors. α-MSH and diacetyl–α-MSH are potent melanotropins, β-MSH has moderate melanotropic activity, and corticotropin-like intermediate-lobe peptide is a weak insulin secretagogue[223] and may stimulate pancreatic exocrine func-

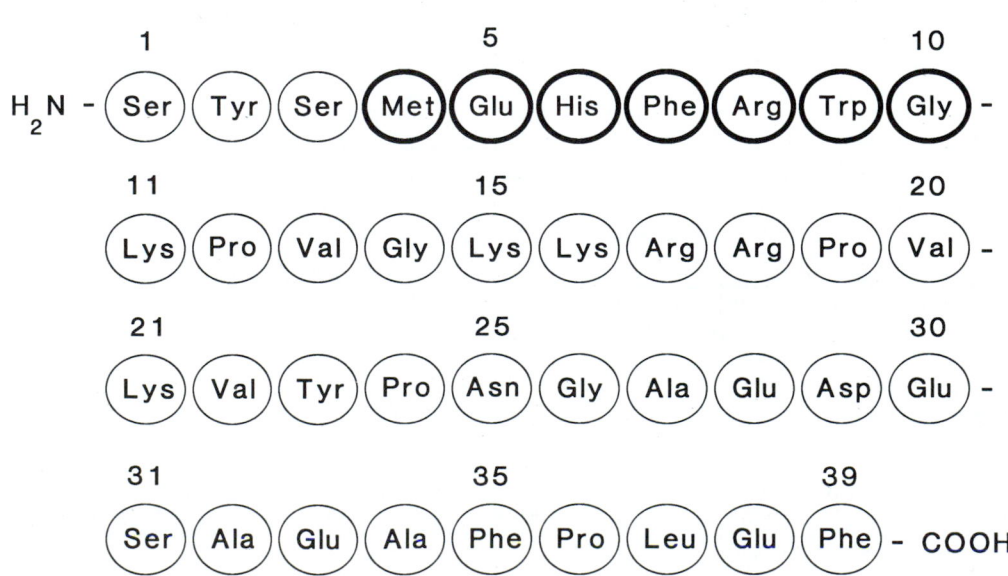

Figure 9–12. Amino acid sequence of human ACTH. The heptapeptide core sequence common to ACTH, α-MSH, β-MSH, and, with slight modification, γ-MSH is indicated by the heavy circles.

tion.[224] β-END has potent opioid activity in the central nervous system, but its function in peripheral plasma is unknown. Acetyl–β-END is devoid of opioid activity.

Nonpituitary Production of ACTH and POMC-Related Peptides. It was originally thought that the POMC gene is expressed only in the pituitary. However, detection of multiple POMC peptides, a POMC-like precursor protein, and POMC-like mRNA in many nonpituitary tissues indicates that this gene is widely expressed.[200, 225–229] These tissues include the brain, hypothalamus, liver, kidney, gastrointestinal and reproductive tissues, placenta, lymphocytes, and monocytes. Except perhaps in the placenta, the peptide levels are so low that it is unlikely they contribute significantly to circulating levels. The POMC-like mRNA in all tissues except the hypothalamus is shorter than in the pituitary and lacks exons 1 and 2 and part of exon 3.[230] Consequently, it may not be translated efficiently[228] and, because the product lacks a signal peptide, may not be secreted. The POMC peptide levels in nonpituitary tissues are not altered by dexamethasone treatment,[226] but gonadal POMC peptide and POMC-like mRNA levels are increased by gonadotropins and lowered by androgen treatment.[231, 232] The function of these peptides in nonpituitary tissues is uncertain, but they may have paracrine or autocrine actions.

ACTIONS OF ACTH ON THE ADRENAL CORTEX. Steroidogenesis. The primary action of ACTH on the adrenal cortex is to increase cortisol secretion by increasing its synthesis; intra-adrenal cortisol storage is minimal.[233, 234] ACTH depletes adrenal cholesterol content,[235] which correlates with enhanced steroid synthesis.[236]

ACTH acts by binding to specific cell-surface receptors.[237, 238] There is a single class of high-affinity receptors with an apparent dissociation constant (K_d) of 1.6 nmol/L. About 3600 sites are present on each adrenocortical cell. Extracellular calcium is required for optimal ACTH binding[237] but not for ACTH-induced steroidogenesis. Release of intracellular calcium may play a role in steps subsequent to ACTH binding.[234, 238] ACTH binding promotes adenylate cyclase activation, which increases cyclic AMP (cAMP) concentration, which in turn activates cAMP-dependent protein kinase (protein kinase A) and phosphorylation of a number of proteins.[239] Most, if not all, of the actions of ACTH appear to be mediated through cAMP.[240–242]

The effects of ACTH on steroidogenesis can be divided into acute effects, which occur within minutes, and chronic effects, which require hours or days.[243, 244] The acute effect of ACTH is to increase conversion of cholesterol to Δ^5-pregnenolone, the initial and rate-limiting step in cortisol biosynthesis.[234, 243, 244] As discussed earlier, this effect is mediated by activation of existing side-chain cleavage enzyme P-450$_{scc}$. In contrast, the chronic effects of ACTH involve increased synthesis of most of the enzymes of the steroidogenic pathway and more general actions on adrenocortical cell protein, RNA and DNA synthesis, and cell growth.[234, 243, 244] When ACTH levels are low, such as after hypophysectomy or during glucocorticoid administration, steroid biosynthesis declines and there is a dramatic decrease in the levels of all steroidogenic P-450 enzymes[243] and in protein and RNA synthesis.[239, 244] With prolonged ACTH deficiency or suppression, the adrenal glands become small and atrophic. These changes are reversed by ACTH administration, although steroidogenesis may take several days to return to normal and return of adrenal size to normal takes even longer. ACTH is essential for normal steroidogenesis, and it is required but is not sufficient, by itself, to maintain normal adrenal size.[58, 245]

In bovine adrenocortical cells, ACTH increases the rate of synthesis of all steroidogenic cytochrome P-450 enzymes, including P-450$_{scc}$,[246] P-450$_{c17}$,[247] P-450$_{c21}$,[248] and P-450$_{c11}$[249]

plus the electron transport protein adrenodoxin[250] and adrenodoxin reductase.[244] The maximal rate of protein synthesis occurs 24 to 36 h after stimulation.[244] The levels of mRNAs coding for all of these enzymes increase, some within 4 h of exposure to ACTH.[244] The increased mRNA levels are due to increased rates of gene transcription rather than to changes in the rates of mRNA turnover.[244, 251] These effects, like the acute effects of ACTH, are reproduced by cAMP analogues, indicating that they are mediated by cAMP.[244, 252] The exact mechanism by which cAMP increases adrenocortical P-450 enzyme gene transcription is not known. Cycloheximide, which inhibits protein synthesis at the level of translation, blocks the ACTH-induced increase in the P-450 mRNA levels, suggesting that the mechanism involves a rapidly turning over trans-acting nuclear protein.[251]

ACTH also increases the synthesis of other proteins required for steroidogenesis, such as the LDL receptor, which is required for uptake of circulating cholesterol; adrenodoxin,[250] which is needed for transfer of reducing equivalents; sterol carrier protein 2,[145, 253] which is required for transport of cholesterol from intracellular lipid stores to mitochondria; and, in fetal but not adult adrenals, HMG-CoA reductase,[254] which catalyzes the rate-limiting step in de novo cholesterol biosynthesis. The increase in HMG-CoA reductase synthesis and part of the increase in LDL receptor synthesis are thought to be secondary to cholesterol depletion rather than to a direct action of ACTH or cAMP.[145, 254] Because the major source of cholesterol for steroid synthesis is uptake of circulating LDL,[79] the supply of LDL cholesterol may under some circumstances be the rate-limiting factor in steroid biosynthesis.[77, 145, 244]

Maintenance of Adrenal Weight. In addition to stimulating steroidogenesis, ACTH stimulates adrenal growth. Supraphysiological plasma ACTH concentrations stimulate adrenocortical hypertrophy and hyperplasia, and adrenal atrophy results from absence of ACTH.[255] An early effect of ACTH is increased adrenal blood flow.[256] Longer exposure to ACTH increases total RNA and protein synthesis and, later, DNA content and adrenal weight.[255] Removal of one adrenal gland in rats causes compensatory growth of the remaining adrenal that occurs mainly by cell proliferation. The role of ACTH in this process is in some doubt because administration of ACTH antibodies that decrease steroidogenesis does not alter adrenal growth.[257] However, physiological concentrations of ACTH inhibit compensatory hypertrophy of the remaining adrenal[258] and inhibit proliferation of cultured adrenal cells.[259, 260] Therefore, it is likely that other factors participate in maintaining normal adrenal weight. One candidate, a peptide consisting of the 28 NH$_2$-terminal amino acids of POMC, has mitogenic effects on adrenal cells in vivo and in vitro and partially prevents adrenal atrophy after hypophysectomy.[59, 60] Neural stimuli that originate from the site of the removed adrenal gland, ascend through the spinal cord to the medial basal hypothalamus, and descend to the remaining adrenal gland may also play a role in stimulating compensatory hypertrophy.[261, 262]

EXTRA-ADRENAL ACTIONS OF ACTH. Large doses of ACTH increase glucose and amino acid transport into muscle cells,[263] increase hepatic protein synthesis,[264] and increase cAMP concentration and stimulate lipolysis in adipocytes.[265] Physiological levels of ACTH do not cause these effects, but markedly elevated plasma ACTH concentrations, such as those observed in some patients with Nelson's syndrome or untreated Addison's disease, may be sufficient. ACTH has weak melanotropic activity and, alone or together with β-LPH, may be the major cause of hyperpigmentation when plasma POMC peptide levels are elevated.

Corticotropin-Releasing Hormone

STRUCTURE AND SYNTHESIS. In 1955 two groups demonstrated independently that a hypothalamic factor increases ACTH release from pituitary cells.[266, 267] More than 25 years later, ovine CRH was isolated and sequenced.[37, 268] Subsequently, the CRHs of other species were characterized.[269–271] CRH is a 41-amino-acid peptide that appears to be the major physiological ACTH secretagogue (Fig. 9–13).[272–274] There is considerable sequence homology among species, particularly in the NH_2-terminal region, which is required for biological activity. Rat and human CRHs are identical. CRH belongs to a family of peptides that includes sauvagine from frog skin and urotensin 1 from teleost fish, both of which have ACTH-releasing and hypotensive activities like those of CRH.[268, 275, 276] Analysis of ovine[277] and rat[278] CRH cDNAs and human[279] and rat[280] genomic DNAs indicates that CRH is synthesized as a larger precursor (191 amino acids in humans) from which it is cleaved at flanking basic amino acid pairs. The single human CRH gene is located on chromosome 8.[281]

BIOSYNTHESIS. CRH is synthesized by neurons of the parvicellular division of the hypothalamic paraventricular nucleus.[282–284] Their axons project to the median eminence, where CRH is secreted into the hypophyseal portal blood. These neurons, particularly after adrenalectomy, may also contain other ACTH secretagogues, such as AVP[285, 286] and cholecystokinin;[287] opioid peptides, such as met-enkephalin[288] and dynorphin(1–8);[289] and the 27-amino-acid peptide (P) having NH_2-terminal histidine (H) and COOH-terminal isoleucine (I) amide (PHI-27), a prolactin secretagogue.[288] In addition, CRH is present in a subpopulation of oxytocin-containing neurons in the magnicellular division of the paraventricular nucleus that project to the posterior pituitary.[290] CRH is also widely distributed throughout the brain and spinal cord[282, 283] and in peripheral tissues, such as the adrenal medulla,[291] testis,[292] gastrointestinal tract,[293, 294] pancreas,[294, 295] and placenta.[296, 297] The presence of CRH and its receptor[298, 299] in the brain suggests that CRH functions as a neurotransmitter. In other tissues, CRH may exert local regulatory effects. For instance, CRH inhibits human chorionic gonadotropin–stimulated androgen production by the testis.[300]

MECHANISM OF ACTION. CRH acts on the anterior pituitary corticotrope by binding to cell-surface receptors[301, 302] and activating adenylate cyclase, thereby increasing intracellular cAMP levels and activating cAMP-dependent protein kinase A.[303] This results within a few seconds in secretion of ACTH and other POMC-related peptides and subsequently in increased POMC gene transcription and increased POMC mRNA biosynthesis and concentration.[196, 304, 305] Chronic CRH stimulation causes corticotrope hyperplasia.[306] The ACTH response may be modulated by corticotrope CRH receptor number, which is reduced in the anterior pituitary, but not in the brain, by immobilization stress, adrenalectomy, and administration of CRH, AVP, or glucocorticoid.[302, 307–310] CRH also stimulates intermediate-lobe melanotropes to synthesize POMC mRNA[305] and secrete α-MSH.[311]

PLASMA LEVELS. There is disagreement about whether peripheral plasma CRH levels reflect hypothalamic secretion in nonpregnant individuals. Some reports suggest that patients with Addison's disease[312] and normal subjects during metyrapone administration[312] or insulin-induced hypoglycemia[312a, 313] have increased plasma CRH levels and that patients with hypothalamic hypopituitarism or Cushing's syndrome with hypercortisolism associated with pituitary or adrenal adenomas have low CRH levels.[312, 312a] A diurnal rhythm in plasma CRH concentration has also been reported,[314] but this finding, too, has yet to be confirmed.[315, 316] The disagreements may be due to methodological differences but more likely indicate that peripheral plasma CRH

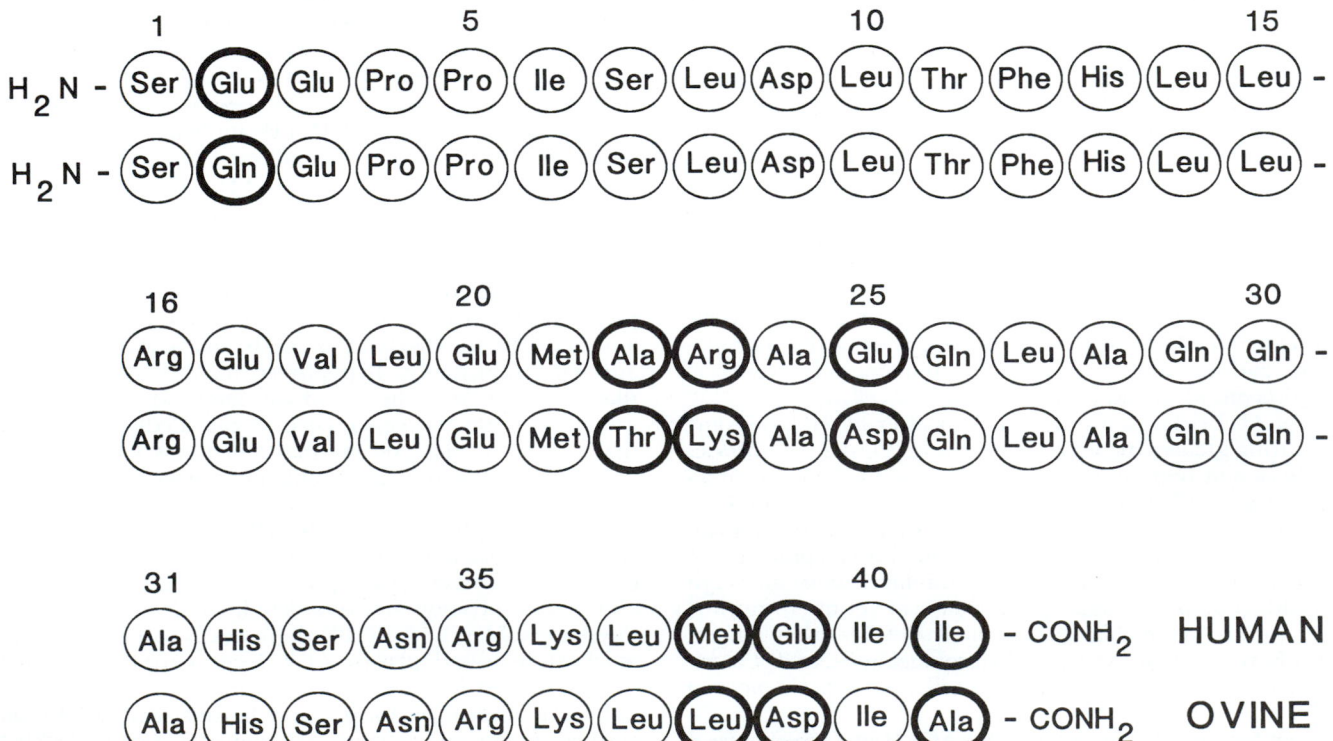

Figure 9–13. Amino acid sequences of human and ovine CRH. The latter is used in most diagnostic testing and is equipotent with and longer-acting than human CRH. Differences between the two sequences are indicated by the heavy circles.

levels reflect nonhypothalamic secretion of CRH.[312a, 317, 318] Plasma CRH levels increase markedly in third-trimester pregnancy because the placenta secretes CRH.[297, 319] In human plasma, CRH circulates bound to a high-affinity binding protein,[320] in which state its bioactivity is reduced,[321] which probably explains why the high concentrations of CRH in pregnancy do not cause increased ACTH secretion. A similar binding protein has not been found in other species.[320] Despite the binding to this protein, the half-life of circulating CRH in humans is only 4 min.[322] Ovine CRH is used for most clinical studies because, although it does not bind to the binding protein,[320] it has a half-life of 55 min and consequently a prolonged duration of action.[323, 324]

EFFECTS ON PITUITARY ACTH SECRETION. Human and ovine CRHs cause a rapid, dose-dependent increase in plasma ACTH concentration without affecting the plasma levels of other anterior pituitary hormones, AVP, or catecholamines.[322, 325, 326] Human CRH is equipotent to ovine CRH but, because of its shorter circulating half-life, the duration of plasma ACTH elevation is shorter and less total ACTH is secreted.[322] The ACTH released by CRH stimulates secretion of cortisol and other adrenal steroids, such as aldosterone and DHEA.[326, 327] There is no sex- or age-related difference in the plasma ACTH or cortisol response to CRH,[327–329] but the DHEA response is reduced in elderly men and the cortisol response is blunted in obese subjects.[327, 330] The time of day has little effect on the plasma ACTH response to CRH, but the increment in plasma cortisol is much greater in late afternoon or evening than in the morning.[331] A major factor influencing the magnitude of the plasma ACTH response to CRH is the circulating glucocorticoid concentration. For example, the plasma response to CRH varies inversely with the basal plasma cortisol concentration.[331] Thus both CRH and ACTH levels are increased during metyrapone-induced hypocortisolemia[332] and reduced by glucocorticoid administration.[332, 333]

EXTRAPITUITARY EFFECTS. CRH has a variety of peripheral and central effects. Systemic administration causes mesenteric vasodilation, which at high doses can result in hypotension and tachycardia,[325, 334] and stimulates respiration through a central effect.[335] Intracerebroventricular injection activates the autonomic nervous system,[336] resulting in increased plasma catecholamine, glucagon, and glucose concentrations; elevated blood pressure and heart rate; decreased gastric acid secretion;[337] and behavioral changes in animals.[338] CRH may modulate reproductive function because it reduces the sexual receptivity of female rats,[339] lowers luteinizing hormone (LH) levels by inhibiting LH-releasing hormone (LHRH, also called gonadotropin-releasing hormone, GnRH) secretion,[340] and inhibits human chorionic gonadotropin–stimulated testosterone production by cultured Leydig cells.[300]

Multihormonal Control of ACTH Secretion

ACTH secretion is regulated by multiple hormones. CRH and AVP are physiologically the most important, but catecholamines, angiotensin II, serotonin, oxytocin, atrial natriuretic factor (ANF), cholecystokinin, vasoactive intestinal peptide, PHI-27 (a gastrointestinal and hypothalamic peptide), and gastrin-releasing peptide have been implicated.[191–193]

CRH is probably the most important ACTH secretagogue.[37] AVP is a weak stimulator of ACTH secretion, but it potentiates the action of CRH in vivo or in vitro.[341, 342] AVP alone does not increase cAMP levels, but it augments CRH-induced cAMP levels. AVP exerts its effect by binding to a novel V_1 pressor-like receptor, thereby activating phospholipase C–mediated hydrolysis of phosphatidylinositol 4,5-

bisphosphate (PIP_2) to produce inositol 1,4,5-trisphosphate (IP_3), which mobilizes intracellular calcium stores, and diacylglycerol, which activates phospholipid/calcium-dependent protein kinase C.[343–345] Oxytocin probably acts via the AVP receptor and postreceptor pathway,[346] but the postreceptor mechanisms used by angiotensin II and cholecystokinin are not fully understood. Moreover, angiotensin II and cholecystokinin may act in vivo mainly via central mechanisms to stimulate CRH release.[347] The role of oxytocin is controversial, because in vivo studies in humans have shown either no effect or an inhibitory effect on ACTH secretion.[348] It is not clear how vasoactive intestinal peptide or PHI-27 stimulates ACTH secretion. ANF(1–28) has been detected in hypothalamic neurons and is reported to inhibit CRH-induced ACTH release from cultured anterior pituitary cells.[349] Opioid peptides inhibit ACTH secretion in humans,[350, 351] perhaps by binding to delta or kappa receptors. In contrast, opioid agonists stimulate ACTH secretion in rats via central mu or kappa receptors.[352] The role of catecholamines remains controversial.[353] Circulating plasma catecholamines have no role in regulating CRH or ACTH secretion in humans, but activation of central alpha-1–adrenergic receptors appears to be an important stimulus for CRH and thus ACTH secretion; central beta-adrenergic receptor activation has minimal effect.

Interactions with the Immune System

Interactions occur between the immune system and the hypothalamic-pituitary-adrenal axis.[354] Interleukin 1 and interleukin 6 are cytokines secreted by monocytes in response to an antigenic challenge. These cytokines increase ACTH secretion by stimulating hypothalamic CRH release. Cachectin (also known as tumor necrosis factor), released by macrophages in response to infection, directly stimulates pituitary ACTH secretion.[355] Interleukin 2, secreted by T lymphocytes, also stimulates ACTH secretion by indirect and, possibly, direct pituitary actions. Lymphocytes, like many other tissues, have very low levels of POMC mRNA and may or may not release very small amounts of ACTH and other POMC-derived peptides.[356–359] However, there is no convincing evidence that immune cells secrete sufficient ACTH or other POMC-derived peptides to influence the hypothalamic-pituitary-adrenal axis.[360, 361]

Regulation of Intermediate-Lobe POMC Peptide Secretion

Regulation of secretion of α-MSH, β-END, and other POMC peptides from the pituitary intermediate lobe differs from that in the anterior lobe. Secretion is mainly under tonic inhibitory control by hypothalamic dopamine.[362] Glucocorticoids do not inhibit secretion. CRH and beta-adrenergic agonists stimulate α-MSH secretion through a cAMP-mediated mechanism, which is inhibited by dopamine. γ-Aminobutyric acid, a neurotransmitter, also inhibits secretion.[363] As already noted, a functional intermediate lobe exists only during fetal life and in late pregnancy in humans.

Normal Patterns of ACTH and Cortisol Secretion

PULSATILE SECRETION. ACTH is secreted in brief episodic bursts, which cause sharp rises in plasma cortisol concentrations, followed by slower declines because of cortisol's prolonged clearance from plasma (Fig. 9–14). The normal diurnal rhythm results from ACTH-secretory episodes of greater amplitude.[364–366] The secretory episodes increase in amplitude (Fig. 9–15)—but not in frequency, as

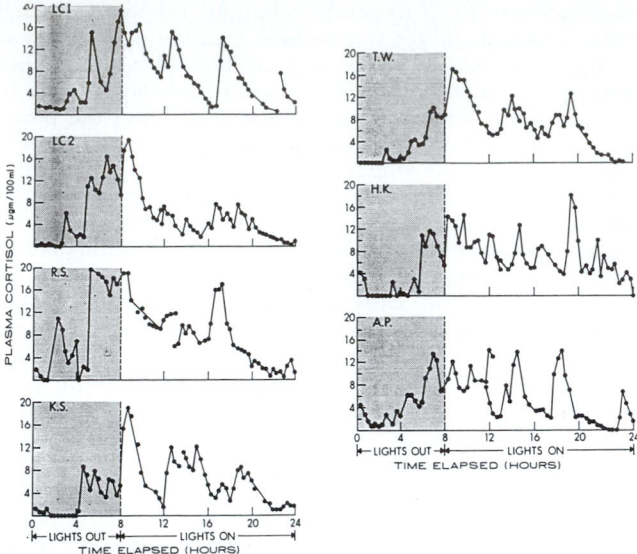

Figure 9–14. Circadian rhythm in plasma cortisol concentrations in seven normal subjects. Samples were drawn every 20 to 30 min. (From ED Weitzman, DK Fukushima, C Nogeire, et al., Twenty-four hour pattern of the episodic secretion of cortisol in normal subjects, J Clin Endocrinol Metab 33, 14–22, 1971, © by The Endocrine Society.)

bright light after such a change may speed the readjustment and perhaps lessen the symptoms of jet lag.[378, 379]

Little is known about the mechanism responsible for the circadian rhythm, except that neurons in or fibers passing through the suprachiasmatic nucleus of the ventral hypothalamus are essential.[380] CRH is the most potent ACTH secretagogue, but its role in producing the ACTH circadian rhythm is unclear. Thus, in the rat, either a peak[381] or a nadir[382] in hypothalamic CRH immunoreactivity has been observed before peak ACTH secretion. A diurnal rhythm in plasma CRH in humans, with the highest levels at 6 AM, has been reported by some investigators[314] but not others.[315, 316] When CRH is infused continuously in humans, the plasma ACTH circadian rhythm persists,[383] suggesting that factors other than CRH must be involved in generating the circadian ACTH rhythm.

Factors independent of ACTH release regulate adrenal responsiveness to ACTH in some animals but probably not in humans.[381, 384–386] In normal rats the plasma corticosterone rhythm persists even though endogenous ACTH secretion is suppressed with dexamethasone, and in hypophysectomized rats, plasma corticosterone levels show a diurnal pattern during continuous exogenous ACTH administration.[384] Adrenal innervation may be responsible for these

was once thought—after 3 to 5 h of sleep, reach a maximum during the last few hours before and the hour after awakening, and then decline throughout the morning and are minimal in the evening.[366] Consequently, plasma ACTH and cortisol levels are highest at about the time of waking in the morning, are low in the late afternoon and evening, and reach a nadir an hour or two after sleep begins. Additional secretory episodes frequently coincide with lunch and sometimes with dinner and are dependent on the protein content of the meal.[367, 368]

CIRCADIAN RHYTHM. In humans, as in other organisms, there is an endogenous pacemaker, presumably located in the suprachiasmatic nucleus of the hypothalamus, that generates a circadian ("about a day") rhythm in a variety of physiological processes. The activity of the hypothalamic-pituitary-adrenal axis is among those processes in humans. The timing of the circadian rhythm is synchronized with the solar day by dark-light shifts, which normally are a reflection of the habitual sleep-wake pattern.[369–371] As long as it is thus synchronized, it is a diurnal rhythm. In totally blind subjects (i.e., individuals without a dark-light synchronizer), the diurnal rhythm reverts to a free-running circadian rhythm with a periodicity of 24.5 to 25 h.[370] In the chronic absence of external time cues, both plasma cortisol levels and sleep-wake cycles gradually revert to a similar, synchronized circadian rhythm.[371]

The normal diurnal rhythm is said to become apparent only after age 1 y and to become well established only after 3 y.[372, 373] However, 24-h sampling has not been performed in individual children. The rhythm probably establishes itself at different ages in different individuals, possibly related to development of adult sleep-wake patterns. In the elderly the rhythm shifts about 3 h earlier.[374] It is not clear if this shift is due to the earlier time of awakening in the elderly, if the earlier time of awakening is dictated by the shift in cortisol rhythm, or if both are the consequence of some other factor. The cortisol-secretory pattern is resistant to acute change. Prolonged bed rest, continuous feeding, 5 d of fasting,[375] or 2 to 3 d of sleep deprivation does not alter the rhythm.[376] After a major time shift, as after long-distance jet travel, it takes 1 to 2 wk for the rhythm to readjust.[377] Exposure to

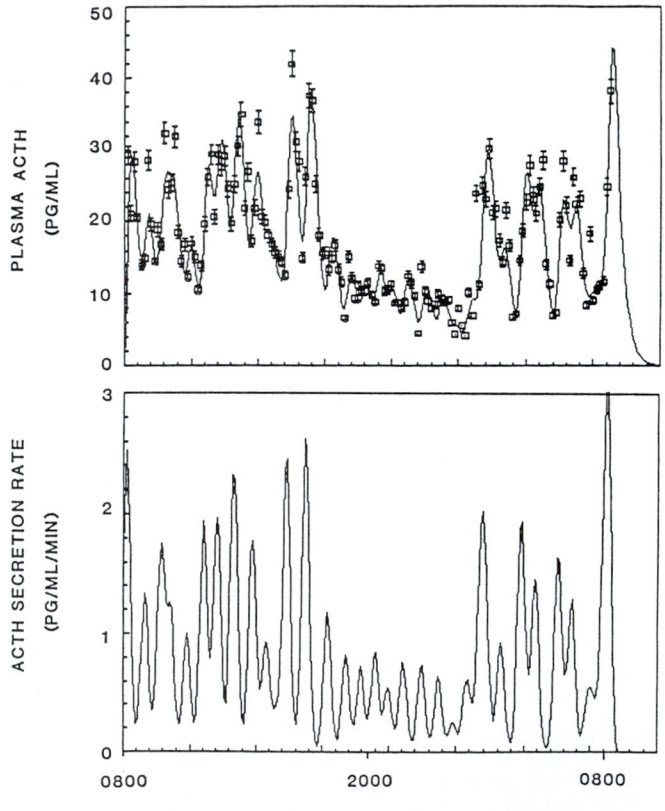

CLOCKTIME

Figure 9–15. Pulse analysis of plasma ACTH sampled at 10-min intervals for 24 h. The upper panel shows (boxes) the measured serial plasma ACTH concentrations, (brackets) the concentration-dependent standard deviation of the assay, and (solid line) the ACTH concentrations predicted by the deconvolution program. The lower panel shows the computer-calculated ACTH secretion rate plotted as a function of time. To convert picograms per milliliter to picomoles per liter, multiply by 0.22. Variation in the amplitude, not the frequency, of the pulses is responsible for the circadian rhythmicity of plasma ACTH concentration. (From JD Veldhuis, A Iranmanesh, ML Johnson, et al., Amplitude, but not frequency, modulation of adrenocorticotropin secretory bursts gives rise to the nyctohemeral rhythm of the corticotropic axis in man, J Clin Endocrinol Metab 71, 452–463, 1990, © by The Endocrine Society.)

changes in adrenal sensitivity, because the rhythm is lost with spinal cord transection at T-7 but not at L-1.[387] Cutting the splanchnic nerves reduces sensitivity to ACTH in lambs.[388] Adrenal autotransplantation abolishes the rhythm in some studies[389] but not others.[390] The mechanism of this neural influence on adrenal sensitivity may be related to changes in adrenal blood flow.[391]

EFFECT OF STRESS. Acute physical or psychological stress activates the hypothalamic-pituitary-adrenal axis, resulting in increased plasma ACTH and cortisol levels. Stress is a poorly defined term. It cannot usually be quantified, nor are the mechanisms by which it elicits a response completely understood. Physical stresses include severe trauma, burns or illness, major surgery, hypoglycemia, fever, hypotension, exercise, cold exposure, and cigarette smoking.[392–396] Surgery is one of the most potent activators of the hypothalamic-pituitary-adrenal axis. Plasma ACTH levels may increase at the time of incision and during the surgery, but the greatest ACTH secretion occurs during reversal of anesthesia, extubation, and the immediate postoperative recovery period.[395, 397] This response can be reduced by use of morphine-like analgesics,[397, 398] which blunt the pituitary ACTH response to CRH but may also act centrally to inhibit secretion of ACTH secretagogues.[397, 399] The ACTH and cortisol response to surgery can be abolished by interrupting the neural connections from the operative site, such as by sectioning the spinal cord[400] or with epidural anesthesia,[401] indicating that afferent nerve impulses mediate the response. Pretreatment with glucocorticoids will block the pituitary-adrenal response to minor stress but may not alter the response to major stress.[397, 402, 403] The pituitary-adrenal response is proportional to the extent of a burn[392] or intensity of exercise.[396]

Acute psychological stress also causes ACTH and cortisol secretion. Its degree may appear to be relatively mild, as in anticipation of athletic competition[404] or surgery[405] or performing mental tasks.[406] Chronic anxiety and schizophrenia are not usually associated with increased adrenal activity, but hypercortisolemia is a common feature of depression, in which the nocturnal quiescent period is shortened, the morning rise occurs early,[407] and the overall cortisol level is increased.[407–409] The abnormality disappears after spontaneous recovery from or successful treatment of the depression.

Stress exerts its effects via as-yet unknown central pathways that stimulate the hypothalamus to release multiple ACTH secretagogues, CRH and AVP being the most important.[193] Hypoglycemia exerts a direct effect on the medial basal hypothalamus[410] and stimulates CRH release from isolated rat hypothalami[411] but has no direct effect on pituitary ACTH secretion. Hypoglycemia also increases plasma CRH, AVP, epinephrine, and norepinephrine levels.[313] AVP probably plays a role in the pituitary response to hypoglycemia, but peripheral catecholamines are not involved.[353, 412] Fever, caused by systemic infection or induced by pyrogen administration, stimulates ACTH and cortisol secretion.[413] Infection or exposure of mononuclear leukocytes to bacterial endotoxin causes release of interleukins 1 and 6, which stimulate hypothalamic CRH secretion; interleukin 2, which causes ACTH secretion by indirect and, possibly, direct actions on the pituitary; and cachectin, which directly stimulates pituitary ACTH release.[354, 355]

GLUCOCORTICOID NEGATIVE FEEDBACK. This feedback occurs at both pituitary and hypothalamic levels. In the anterior pituitary, glucocorticoids inhibit both ACTH secretion and POMC gene transcription, resulting in greatly reduced POMC mRNA levels and POMC synthesis.[196] To a lesser extent, glucocorticoids also decrease CRH and AVP mRNA and peptide levels in the hypothalamic paraventric-

ular nuclei.[414–416] In addition, glucocorticoids block the stimulatory effect of CRH on POMC gene transcription[417] and acute ACTH release.[418] As a consequence of these actions of glucocorticoids, plasma ACTH levels are elevated in untreated Addison's disease and are suppressed in patients with Cushing's syndrome associated with a cortisol-secreting adrenal tumor or exogenous steroid administration.

Glucocorticoid feedback inhibition of ACTH secretion in rats involves at least two phases.[419] Fast feedback occurs within seconds to minutes and is proportional to the rate of increase in plasma glucocorticoid concentration rather than the absolute level. It is thought to represent a membrane-stabilizing effect, although there is no direct evidence for such an action, and we have been unable to demonstrate a rapid effect in dispersed rat anterior pituitary cells in vitro (unpublished observations, D.N. Orth and W.E. Nicholson). Delayed feedback occurs in hours to days and is proportional to the glucocorticoid dose, potency, duration of administration,[419] and, therefore, plasma levels. It presumably is mediated through the glucocorticoid receptor. Initially, the secretion but not the synthesis of ACTH and CRH is inhibited. Later, POMC and CRH gene transcription is decreased, leading to decreased hormone synthesis.[417]

Data on the mechanisms of glucocorticoid negative feedback in humans are limited. Any glucocorticoid can suppress ACTH secretion, but the degree of suppression depends on the dose, potency, and duration of action of the steroid and the duration and time of its administration. The shorter the interval before the normal early morning peak of ACTH secretion, the greater the suppressive effect. The longer the duration of action and the greater the dose administered, the greater the interval after which it has the same suppresive effect. After withdrawal of chronic administration of pharmacological doses of glucocorticoid, the hypothalamic-pituitary-adrenal axis may remain suppressed for weeks to months (see later).

The possibility of short-loop glucocorticoid negative feedback has been suggested by evidence for a direct inhibitory effect on adrenal steroidogenesis in cultured adrenal cells.[420] This effect must be minimal in vivo, however, because dexamethasone administration does not inhibit ACTH-stimulated cortisol production.[421, 422]

Regulation of Mineralocorticoid Secretion

The major circulating mineralocorticoid is aldosterone, which is synthesized exclusively in the zona glomerulosa. Its precursors, 18-hydroxycorticosterone, corticosterone, and DOC, also have weak mineralocorticoid activity. The three precursors are synthesized in all three zones of the adrenal cortex, but 18-hydroxycorticosterone is produced predominantly in the zona glomerulosa, so its secretion correlates with that of aldosterone. Much more corticosterone and DOC are produced in the zona fasciculata than in the zona glomerulosa. Their secretion correlates with that of cortisol and is ACTH dependent.[423, 424] Cortisol also has modest mineralocorticoid activity, which becomes significant during the hypercortisolemia of Cushing's syndrome. Secretion of 18-oxygenated cortisol derivatives, which have weak mineralocorticoid activity and are implicated in the hypertension of glucocorticoid-suppressible aldosteronism, is also ACTH dependent.[425] 19-Nor-DOC is a potent mineralocorticoid that is produced by extraglandular conversion of 19-oxygenated DOC precursors and may be involved in the pathogenesis of some forms of hypertension.[426] The factors regulating its secretion are not clear, although acute ACTH administration increases the plasma concentration.[426]

Aldosterone secretion, unlike that of cortisol, is governed by multiple factors that have complex regulatory interactions (Fig. 9–16).[427, 428] The renin-angiotensin system and potassium ion are the major regulators; ACTH and other POMC-derived peptides, sodium ion, and other agents such as AVP, dopamine, ANF, beta-adrenergic agents, serotonin, and somatostatin are minor modulators. These factors regulate aldosterone secretion by modulating one or more biosynthetic steps. The early step is the conversion of cholesterol to pregnenolone, and the late step is the conversion of corticosterone to aldosterone (corticosterone 18-hydroxylase/corticosterone 18-methyl oxidase [CMO I/CMO II] reaction, sometimes referred to as the 18-hydroxylase/isomerase reaction)[427] catalyzed by a single mitochondrial enzyme, cytochrome P-450$_{c11}$.[139]

The Renin-Angiotensin System

Renin is an enzyme that cleaves angiotensinogen (renin substrate), an alpha-2–globulin (about 60 kd) synthesized by the liver, to produce the decapeptide angiotensin I (Fig. 9–17).[429] Angiotensin I is rapidly cleaved by angiotensin-converting enzyme in the lungs and other tissues to form the octapeptide angiotensin II. Cleavage of the NH$_2$-terminal Asp residue of angiotensin II produces the heptapeptide angiotensin III, which is present in the circulation at a level of 20% of that of angiotensin II. Angiotensin I has no known biological action. Angiotensins II and III are equipotent in stimulating aldosterone secretion, but angiotensin II is a more potent vasopressor agent.[429, 430] Neither stimulates cortisol production. The angiotensins are inactivated within minutes by tissue and plasma peptidases.

The level of circulating renin is the rate-limiting factor in this process.[428] Renin is synthesized by the juxtaglomerular cells in the renal cortex. Its secretion is controlled mainly by renal arteriolar blood pressure, the sodium concentration of tubular fluid sensed by the macula densa, and renal sympathetic nerve activity.[431] Factors that decrease renal blood flow, such as hemorrhage, dehydration, salt restriction, upright posture, or renal artery narrowing, increase plasma renin levels. Factors that increase blood pressure, such as high salt intake, peripheral vasoconstrictors, or supine posture, decrease renin secretion. Acute infusions of norepinephrine stimulate renin release. Beta-adrenergic blockers and central alpha-1–adrenergic blockers, such as clonidine,

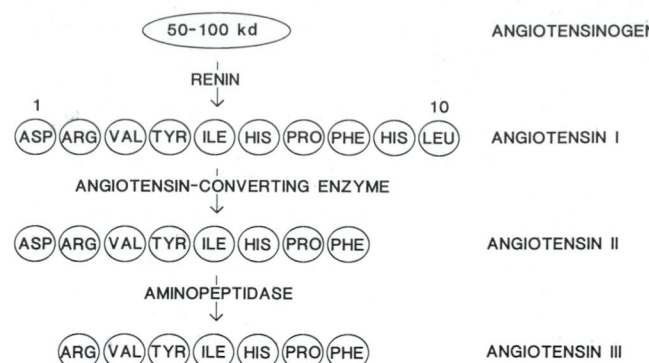

Figure 9–17. Amino acid sequences of angiotensins I, II, and III and the sequence of their production from angiotensinogen (renin substrate).

inhibit renin release, whereas peripheral alpha-blockers are without effect. In addition, angiotensin II inhibits renin secretion by direct short-loop feedback.[428] Aldosterone administration reduces renin activity indirectly through increased sodium reabsorption and plasma volume expansion. Hypokalemia increases and hyperkalemia decreases renin release.[428] Prostaglandins may play a role in renin release because infusion of prostaglandin A$_1$ increases and because inhibition of prostaglandin biosynthesis by indomethacin reduces basal and stimulated renin release.[432] An additional complexity of uncertain physiological importance is the ability of the adrenal zona glomerulosa itself to synthesize both angiotensinogen and renin and generate angiotensin II.[433]

The action of angiotensins II and III on the adrenal glomerulosa is mediated by high-affinity cell-surface receptors, which may be coupled to one or more GTP-binding proteins.[427] (Also see Chapter 4.) The primary intracellular signal transduction mechanism is activation of phospholipase C, which hydrolyzes PIP$_2$ to IP$_3$, which in turn releases intracellular calcium ions, and 1,2-diacylglycerol, which activates protein kinase C and thereby causes influx of extracellular calcium.[427] These events lead to stimulation of both conversion of cholesterol to pregnenolone and conversion of corticosterone to aldosterone.[434–436] Angiotensin II does not stimulate adenylate cyclase activity.[437] The mechanism of the increased cholesterol conversion to pregnenolone is similar to that mediating the acute effect of ACTH on cortisol biosynthesis in the zona fasciculata.[244] A series of steps are initiated that transfer cholesterol to the inner mitochondrial membrane for P-450$_{ssc}$ action.[436] However, unlike the case of cortisol biosynthesis, there is no effect on cholesterol ester synthesis or hydrolysis, and protein synthesis is apparently not required for this transfer. Protein synthesis is required, however, to activate 18-hydroxylation by P-450$_{c11}$.[436] There is little evidence that prostaglandins regulate aldosterone secretion, but lipoxygenase pathway products of arachidonic acid, such as 12-hydroxyeicosatetraenoic acid, may influence angiotensin II–mediated aldosterone production.[438] Sodium intake and potassium intake affect the response to angiotensin II (see later).

Potassium

There is a reciprocal relation between serum potassium and aldosterone concentrations. Potassium directly increases aldosterone secretion by the adrenal cortex, and aldosterone lowers the serum potassium concentration by stimulating potassium excretion by the kidney. Small changes in serum potassium concentration within the physiological range af-

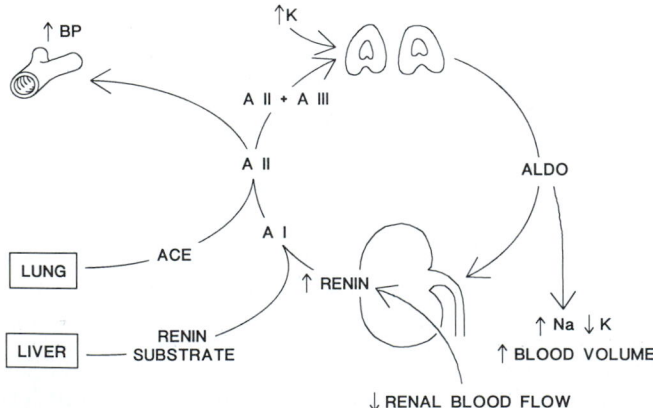

Figure 9–16. The normal renin-angiotensin-aldosterone regulatory system. Renin, secreted by the kidney, cleaves angiotensin I from renin substrate (angiotensinogen), an alpha-2–globulin produced by the liver. Angiotensin I is converted into biologically active angiotensin II by angiotensin-converting enzyme (ACE), mainly in the lung. Angiotensin II increases peripheral vascular resistance, and it and angiotensin III stimulate aldosterone secretion, which results in sodium retention and increases plasma volume.

fect aldosterone secretion. For instance, an increase in serum potassium level of as little as 0.1 mmol/L increases the aldosterone level by 35%, and a decrease in serum potassium of only 0.3 mmol/L reduces the aldosterone level by 46%.[439] High dietary potassium intake increases the plasma aldosterone concentration and enhances the aldosterone response to a subsequent potassium or angiotensin II infusion, whereas reduced potassium intake results in decreased responsiveness.[427, 440, 441]

The initial signal transduction mechanism by which potassium stimulates aldosterone secretion is different from that of the other aldosterone secretagogues. The primary action of potassium is to depolarize the plasma membrane, which activates voltage-dependent calcium channels, permitting influx of extracellular calcium.[427, 442] Potassium may also cause some release of calcium from intracellular stores. In addition, there is a small increase in cAMP levels after exposure to potassium.[427, 442] The cytosolic calcium, which increases in concentration, stimulates the same two steps in aldosterone biosynthesis as angiotensin II.[434, 435] Cortisol production is not influenced by serum potassium concentrations.

Pituitary Factors

POMC PEPTIDES. ACTH, other POMC-derived peptides, and possibly additional pituitary hormones influence aldosterone secretion. CRH administration or stresses that cause ACTH secretion increase circulating aldosterone levels,[326, 428] an effect that is blocked by hypophysectomy.[428] However, the role of ACTH in aldosterone secretion is minor. Aldosterone secretion usually remains normal after hypophysectomy because the renin-angiotensin system and potassium are the major regulators. ACTH acutely increases aldosterone secretion in humans, but, in contrast to the effect of angiotensin II, this effect lasts less than 24 h despite continued ACTH administration.[443] The lack of a prolonged response to ACTH appears to be due to a direct effect on the glomerulosa cells, such as down-regulation of ACTH receptors or the postreceptor signal transduction mechanism, rather than an indirect effect, such as suppression of renin or lowering of the serum potassium level caused by the mineralocorticoid action of cortisol.[444] Other POMC peptides, such as NT peptide, α-MSH, β-MSH, β-LPH, and β-END, stimulate aldosterone secretion,[220, 445–449] and γ-MSH potentiates ACTH-induced aldosterone secretion.[449] However, pharmacological peptide concentrations were often used in such studies. The weak effect of β-LPH is probably due to contamination with ACTH,[450] and β-END has no effect on rat glomerulosa cells in vitro.[446] POMC peptides are produced by the adrenal medulla but because of centripetal blood flow presumably do not reach the cortex.

ACTH increases aldosterone secretion by binding to specific glomerulosa cell-surface receptors, activating adenylate cyclase, and increasing intracellular cAMP levels,[437, 451] just as it increases cortisol production by fasciculata cells. The response is dependent on extracellular calcium influx[427] and can be partially blocked by calmodulin inhibitors.[452] Like other agents, ACTH stimulates the same two early and late steps of aldosterone biosynthesis.[435]

VASOPRESSIN. AVP has a modest, transient stimulatory effect on aldosterone secretion from zona granulosa cells in vitro.[453] This effect is probably mediated by binding to V_2-type receptors and activating phospholipase C to generate IP_3 and diacylglycerol.[427, 453]

Sodium

Sodium intake influences aldosterone secretion by indirect effects through changes in renin secretion and to a minor extent by direct effects on zona glomerulosa responsiveness to angiotensin II. High sodium intake increases vascular volume, which suppresses renin secretion and angiotensin II generation, whereas sodium deprivation leads to increased renin secretion. A low-sodium diet increases and a high-sodium diet decreases the sensitivity and magnitude of the aldosterone response to angiotensin II in vivo and in vitro.[454, 455]

Other Stimulatory Agents

Ammonium chloride administration induces a metabolic acidosis that stimulates aldosterone secretion without changes in serum potassium, renin, angiotensin II, or cortisol concentrations, which suggests a direct effect of hydrogen ion concentration.[456] Beta-adrenergic agonists,[457] neuropeptide Y,[67] vasoactive intestinal peptide,[458] leu-enkephalin,[459] calcitonin gene–related peptide,[460] and serotonin[427] affect aldosterone secretion, but the physiological importance is not clear.

Inhibitory Agents

DOPAMINE. Dopamine has a direct inhibitory effect on aldosterone secretion in humans that is independent of effects on prolactin, ACTH, electrolytes, and the renin-angiotensin system.[461, 462] The adrenals must be under maximal tonic dopaminergic inhibition, because dopamine infusion does not lower basal, angiotensin II–stimulated, or ACTH-stimulated aldosterone levels, but dopaminergic blockade with metoclopramide increases aldosterone secretion.[462] The mechanism of the inhibitory dopamine effect may involve binding to D_2 receptors on glomerulosa cells.[463] There are conflicting reports of the effect of dopamine on cAMP levels.[427]

ATRIAL NATRIURETIC FACTOR. ANF directly inhibits aldosterone secretion and blocks the stimulatory effects of angiotensin II, potassium, and ACTH, partly by interfering with extracellular calcium influx.[464, 465] ANF may inhibit zona glomerulosa growth because chronic infusion in the setting of constant ACTH and renin stimulation induces glomerulosa atrophy.[465]

SOMATOSTATIN. Somatostatin inhibits angiotensin II–stimulated aldosterone production in vitro. The mechanism is not clear, but high-affinity binding sites are present on glomerulosa cells.[427]

Regulation of Adrenal Androgen and Estrogen Secretion

Adrenal Androgens

The major androgens secreted by the adrenal cortex are DHEA, DHEAS, and androstenedione.[466, 467] They are not themselves effective androgens (see Table 9–2), but they can be converted to the potent androgens testosterone and 5α-dihydrotestosterone in peripheral tissues. Peripheral conversion contributes significantly to circulating testosterone levels in women (Fig. 9–18) but not in men, in whom testosterone is produced predominantly by the testis. Peripheral tissues also interconvert DHEA and DHEAS. During the follicular phase of the menstrual cycle, the adrenal glands of women secrete 3 to 4 mg of DHEA, 7 to 14 mg of DHEAS, 1 to 1.5 mg of androstenedione, and 50 μg of testosterone per day.[466] This accounts for about 50%, more than 90%, and about 50% of circulating DHEA, DHEAS, and androstenedione, respectively. An additional 30% of circulating DHEA arises from peripheral conversion of DHEAS. In women, about 67 and 50% of the plasma

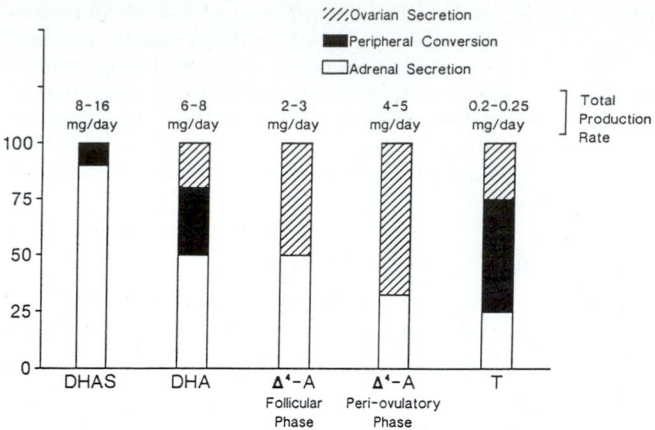

Figure 9–18. Percent contributions to total androgen production in women of adrenal secretion, conversion in peripheral tissues, and ovarian secretion. DHA, dehydroepiandrosterone (DHEA); DHAS, DHEAS; Δ⁴-A, Δ⁴-androstenedione; T, testosterone. Total daily production is shown at the top. To convert to micromoles per day, multiply DHAS values by 2.721, DHA by 3.467, Δ⁴-A by 3.491, and T by 3.467. (From Longcope C. Adrenal and gonadal androgen secretion in normal females. Clin Endocrinol Metab 1986; 15:213–228.)

testosterone and 5α-dihydrotestosterone, respectively, come from androstenedione (see Fig. 9–18).[466, 468] The ovaries produce the remainder. Androstenedione and testosterone levels rise at midcycle because of increased ovarian secretion. Adrenal secretion of androgens in men is similar to that in women during the follicular phase.

POSSIBLE STIMULATORS OF ADRENAL ANDROGEN SECRETION. ACTH. Control of adrenal androgen secretion is less well understood than that of glucocorticoids and mineralocorticoids. ACTH clearly plays a role. Plasma DHEA, androstenedione, and testosterone concentrations closely parallel the circadian rhythm in plasma cortisol level (Fig. 9–19).[469, 470] Plasma DHEAS does not exhibit a circadian rhythm because of its longer half-life in the circulation.[467] Similarly, ACTH acutely increases circulating DHEA and androstenedione levels, but 1 or 2 d of treatment is needed before an increase in DHEAS level can be detected.[466, 471] Dexamethasone administration lowers plasma adrenal androgen levels.[466, 471]

Cortical Androgen-Stimulating Hormone. Factors other than ACTH also appear to be involved, because the ACTH-induced increase in androgen levels is relatively small compared with the cortisol response. Furthermore, chronic dexamethasone administration, which suppresses cortisol production, fails to reduce androgen levels below 20% of baseline in castrated subjects.[471] Most important, adrenal androgen secretion diverges from that of ACTH and cortisol in a number of circumstances. For example, plasma levels of adrenal androgen begin to increase during adrenarche at age 6 to 8, reach adult levels during puberty,[471] and decrease during fasting[471] and aging[472] and in anorexia nervosa[473, 474] and severe illness[471, 475] without concomitant changes in ACTH and cortisol levels. In addition, adrenal androgen secretion is suppressed more readily than cortisol secretion with low doses of dexamethasone[476] and recovers more slowly after glucocorticoid withdrawal,[471] despite the incomplete suppression with high-dose dexamethasone mentioned earlier.

Evidence for a non-ACTH pituitary factor that stimulates adrenal androgen secretion was provided by a study of hypophysectomized chimpanzees in which ACTH replacement produced normal secretion of cortisol but not of DHEA and DHEAS.[477] A 60-kd glycopeptide[478] and an 18-amino-acid peptide corresponding to the NH₂-terminal region of the joining peptide of POMC,[479] both isolated from human

pituitary extracts, have been proposed as possible cortical androgen-stimulating hormones. Other studies have not confirmed an androgen-stimulating activity of the POMC derivative.[479a, 479b]

Other Possible Factors. Prolactin has been suggested as an androgen-stimulating hormone because of the increase in circulating adrenal androgen levels in some patients with hyperprolactinemia[466, 471] and subsequent fall during bromocriptine treatment.[480, 481] Synergism between prolactin and ACTH in stimulation of DHEA and DHEAS, but not cortisol or androstenedione, secretion by human adrenal cells in vitro was reported by one group[481] but not by others.[471, 482] It seems unlikely that prolactin has a physiologically important

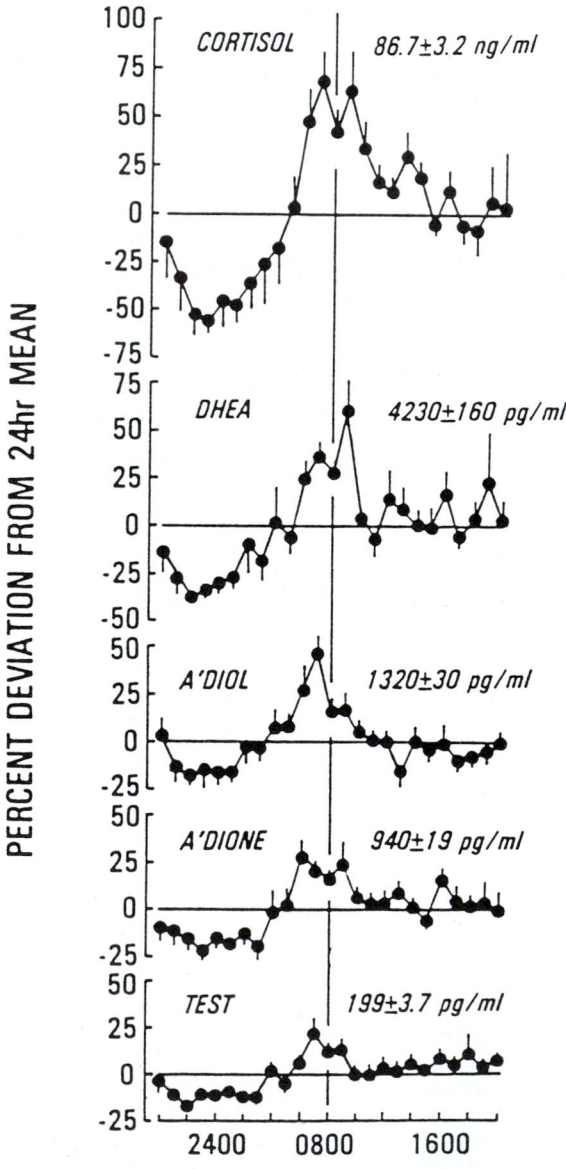

Figure 9–19. Circadian rhythm in plasma concentrations of adrenal androgens and cortisol. A'DIOL, androstenediol; A'DIONE, Δ⁴-androstenedione; TEST, testosterone. The mean (± SEM) 24-h secretion values are shown at the right. To convert to nanomoles per liter, multiply cortisol values by 2.759, DHEA by 0.003467, A'DIOL by 0.003443, A'DIONE by 0.003491, and TEST by 0.003467. (From GCL Lachelin, M Barnett, BR Hopper, et al., Adrenal function in normal women and women with the polycystic ovarian syndrome, J Clin Endocrinol Metab 49, 892–898, 1979, © by The Endocrine Society.)

effect on adrenal androgen secretion, but an extra-adrenal effect on androgen metabolism has not been excluded.

IGF I has been proposed as an adrenal androgen stimulator because an increase in its plasma levels precedes that of androgens during weight gain in anorexia nervosa.[474] Growth hormone (GH) and gonadotropins appear to have no direct effect on adrenal androgen secretion.[471]

Adrenal Estrogens

The adrenal cortex secretes estrone and estradiol, but the amounts are minimal compared with those secreted by the ovary. Most adrenal estrogens are derived indirectly from peripheral conversion of androstenedione, mainly in adipose tissue and muscle.[483]

Steroids in Circulating Plasma

Circulating steroid hormones are largely bound to plasma proteins. The major binding proteins are corticosteroid-binding globulin (CBG, or transcortin), testosterone-binding globulin (TeBG, also called sex hormone–binding globulin), and albumin.[484–487] The binding globulins have high affinity but low capacity for steroid binding, whereas albumin has low affinity and high capacity. In physiological concentrations, 90 to 97% of circulating cortisol is protein bound, most to CBG and the rest to albumin (Table 9–3). The adrenal androgens DHEA, DHEAS, and androstenedione are also largely bound to plasma proteins, about 90% to albumin and 3% to TeBG.[484] Testosterone is transported almost equally by TeBG and albumin; estrogens are bound more to albumin than to TeBG. Except for prednisone and its active metabolite, prednisolone, most synthetic steroids, including dexamethasone and fludrocortisone, are not bound to protein.[488] Aldosterone is weakly associated with CBG (20%) and albumin (40%),[484, 485] and most of the rest is thought to be non–protein bound, or free. However, a specific high-affinity aldosterone-binding protein has been reported.[489] Most circulating DOC is bound by plasma proteins, 36% by CBG and 60% by albumin.[484] In addition to binding to circulating proteins, cortisol and other steroids are associated with red blood cells.[490, 491] Erythrocyte-associated cortisol is a major component of total blood cortisol, exceeding that which is albumin bound or free.[491]

Steroid-Binding Plasma Proteins

CORTICOSTEROID-BINDING GLOBULIN. CBG is a glycosylated 383-amino-acid alpha-2–globulin with a molecular mass of 59 kd[492] that binds cortisol with an association constant of 760 nmol/L.[484] The sequence is highly conserved between rat and human CBGs,[492, 493] and there is similarity to the amino acid sequence[492] and gene structure[494] of members of the serine protease inhibitor superfamily, which includes serine protease inhibitors, thyroxine-binding globulin, angiotensinogen (renin substrate), and egg white proteins.[486] They exhibit no significant similarity to TeBG or the intracellular glucocorticoid receptor. CBG is produced primarily in the liver, but low levels of CBG mRNA in lung, kidney, and testis indicate that it is also synthesized in other tissues.[492, 493] CBG is also present in human milk.[495] The presence of a protein with CBG-like steroid-binding characteristics and immunoreactivity in other glucocorticoid-responsive tissues, such as brain, pituitary, uterus, and lymphocytes,[487] and of specific, high-affinity binding sites for CBG on cell membranes[487, 496] suggests that there may be a transport mechanism to deliver CBG-bound steroids into target cells, as there is, for example, for iron bound to transferrin.

CBG can bind other endogenous steroids[484] (Table 9–4). The Δ^4-3-ketone structure of the A ring and the 20-ketone group are essential for binding. Hydroxylation at the 11β, 17α, and 21 positions increases binding affinity. CBG has minimal or no binding affinity for the tetrahydro metabolites of endogenous steroids or for most synthetic glucocorticoids, except for prednisone and prednisolone, for which it has affinities of 5 and 59%, respectively, relative to that of cortisol.[488, 497] In normal plasma, CBG's binding capacity is limited to about 690 nmol/L (25 µg/dL) of cortisol.[497] Consequently, as the total cortisol level rises above this, the proportion of free cortisol (Fig. 9–20) and other steroids (e.g., aldosterone and DOC) that are bound by CBG and that bind to the same site as cortisol increases relative to that of the bound steroids.[483] Thus high plasma cortisol concentrations displace aldosterone from CBG, leading to an increase in the free fraction, erythrocyte binding, and plasma metabolic clearance rate of aldosterone.[483, 498, 499] Likewise, therapeutic levels of prednisolone decrease the amount of CBG-bound cortisol by about 32%, resulting transiently in increased levels of free cortisol.[488]

The level of CBG in normal plasma is about 700 nmol/L (35 to 40 mg/L), and its circulating half-life is about 5 d.[497] CBG levels in newborns are about half of those in adults, which favors fetal-to-maternal transplacental passage of glucocorticoids.[497] Prepubertal children have slightly higher CBG levels and the elderly have lower levels than young adults.[497] There is no diurnal variation, difference between

---

TABLE 9–3. Transport of Natural Steroids in Plasma of Normal Humans

Steroid	Total Concentration* (nmol/L)	% Unbound	% Bound to CBG	% Bound to Albumin	% Bound to TeBG
Cortisol	400	3.9	89.5	6.6	0.1
Cortisone	72	16.2	38.0	45.3	0.5
Corticosterone	12	3.4	77.5	19.0	0.1
11-Deoxycortisol	1.4	3.4	77.1	18.9	0.7
17-Hydroxyprogesterone	5.4	2.5	41.3	55.9	0.3
Progesterone	0.57	2.4	17.2	80.1	0.3
Deoxycorticosterone	0.2	2.7	36.4	60.1	0.8
Aldosterone	0.35	37.1	21.2	41.6	0.1
DHEA	24	4.1	<0.1	92.4	3.4
Androstenedione	4.1	7.9	1.4	88.0	2.8
Testosterone	23	2.2	3.6	49.9	44.3
Dihydrotestosterone	1.7	0.9	0.2	39.2	59.7
Estrone	0.08	4.0	<0.1	88.6	7.4
Estradiol	0.08	2.3	<0.1	78.0	19.6
Estriol	0.04	8.2	<0.2	91.3	0.4

*Physiological concentrations.

Modified from JF Dunn, BC Nisula, D Rodbard, Transport of steroid hormones: binding of 21 endogenous steroids to both testosterone-binding globulin and corticosteroid-binding globulin in human plasma, J Clin Endocrinol Metab 53, 58–68, 1981, © by The Endocrine Society.

TABLE 9–4. Relative Binding Affinity and Association Constant of Natural and Synthetic Steroids for Corticosteroid-Binding Globulin

Steroid	Relative Binding*	Association Constant†
Cortisol	100	76
Cortisone	12	7.8
Corticosterone	100	76
11-Deoxycortisol	100	76
17-Hydroxyprogesterone	76	55
Progesterone	36	24
Deoxycorticosterone (DOC)	63	45
Aldosterone	2.9	1.9
DHEA	<0.1	<0.1
Androstenedione	0.9	0.58
Testosterone	8.3	5.3
Dihydrotestosterone	1.3	0.8
Dexamethasone	<0.1	<0.1
Fludrocortisone	0.7	0.5
Prednisolone	59	41
Prednisone	5	3.2
Spironolactone	<0.1	<0.1

*Percent binding relative to cortisol. Relative binding of DHEA, DHEAS, androstenedione, estrogens, and most synthetic steroids except prednisolone and prednisone is less than 1%.
†In µmol/L (M × 10⁶).
  Data for endogenous steroids are from Dunn et al.,[484] and those for synthetic steroids are from Pugeat et al.[488]

sexes, or change during the menstrual cycle.[497, 500] However, CBG levels increase two- to threefold with estrogen administration to either sex and during pregnancy, particularly during the third trimester.[497, 500, 501] The estrogen effect on CBG level is dose dependent, is demonstrable within 2 to 4 d, reaches a maximum by 14 d that continues during therapy, and returns to normal 7 to 10 d after discontinuation of therapy.[497, 501] Decreased CBG concentrations occur with cirrhosis, hyperthyroidism, nephrosis, and other protein-losing conditions.[497, 500] Increased CBG levels can occur during chronic active hepatitis[502] and during treatment with anticonvulsant drugs.[500] Inherited abnormalities of CBG are less frequent than those of thyroxine-binding globulin. Only two families have been described with partial CBG deficiency, one with total CBG deficiency, one with a variant CBG that bound cortisol with decreased affinity, and one with abnormally high CBG concentrations.[503, 504] In states of altered plasma CBG concentration, free plasma cortisol levels remain within the normal range despite changes in total cortisol content. The exception is during third-trimester

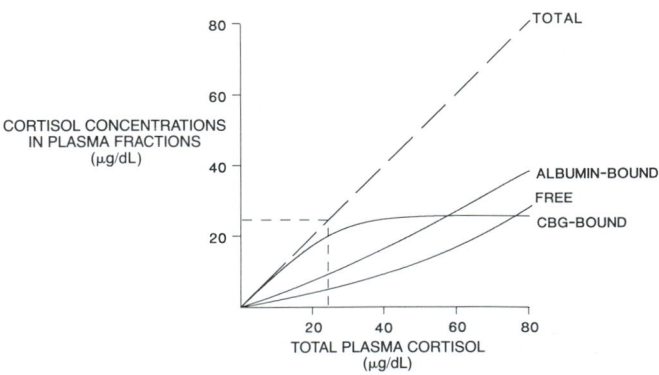

Figure 9–20. Distribution of plasma cortisol between bound and free fractions at various total cortisol concentrations. The square indicates the binding capacity of CBG and the approximate upper limit of normal plasma cortisol concentration. The sum of free, CBG-bound, and albumin-bound plasma cortisol is total plasma cortisol *(dashed line)*. To convert cortisol values to nanomoles per liter, multiply by 27.59. (Adapted from Ballard PL. Delivery and transport of glucocorticoids to target cells. In: Baxter JD, Rousseau GG, eds. Glucocorticoid Hormone Action. New York: Springer-Verlag, 1979: 25–48.)

pregnancy, when the serum free cortisol level is slightly increased.[497, 500] There is no effect of short-term pharmacological doses of glucocorticoids or ACTH on CBG levels, although levels are decreased in Cushing's syndrome.[497, 500] CBG levels are normal in adrenal insufficiency.[497, 500]

OTHER STEROID-BINDING PROTEINS. Albumin. Albumin has a greater binding capacity for cortisol than does CBG, because the circulating level of about 550 µmol/L (38 g/L) is almost 800 times greater than that of CBG. However, albumin binding is much weaker, with an association constant of 1 mmol/L, about 1300-fold lower than that of CBG. Synthetic steroids bind to albumin with an affinity similar to or slightly greater than that of cortisol.

Testosterone-Binding Globulin. TeBG is produced by the liver and binds testosterone, dihydrotestosterone, and estradiol (see Table 9–3). It is a 90-kd glycoprotein composed of two identical 373-amino-acid subunits.[505, 506] It is structurally related to cytoplasmic androgen-binding protein, which is synthesized in Sertoli cells. In fact, these proteins may arise from the same gene by alternate splicing of exons.[486] Plasma TeBG levels are increased by estrogens and pregnancy and decreased by testosterone administration, suggesting that estrogens and androgens regulate hepatic TeBG production.[487, 507, 508] However, these may represent pharmacological effects on liver metabolism, because physiological changes in gonadal steroid levels do not always correlate with changes in TeBG levels.[508] For instance, TeBG levels do not vary during the menstrual cycle, are only slightly greater in women than in men, are greater in children than in adults, and decrease in both boys and girls during puberty.[508] TeBG levels are also increased with thyrotoxicosis, cirrhosis, hypogonadism, and fasting and are decreased in hypothyroidism, acromegaly, and obesity.[487, 507, 508] Estrogens and thyroxine stimulate TeBG production by cultured hepatoma cells, whereas insulin and prolactin decrease it.[487, 509] Androgens decrease circulating TeBG levels in vivo but increase its synthesis and secretion in vitro.[487]

Orosomucoid. Orosomucoid, or alpha-1 acid glycoprotein, is a 41-kd plasma protein that plays a minor role in binding progesterone and other steroids. It has an association constant for cortisol of 200 µmol/L.[510] It is an acute-phase reactant that is involved in the binding of many drugs.[511]

Role of Steroid-Binding Plasma Proteins

FREE HORMONE HYPOTHESIS. According to the widely held free hormone hypothesis, the intracellular concentration of a hormone, and thus its biological activity, is proportional to the concentration of free hormone in plasma, not to the concentration of plasma protein–bound hormone.[512] This hypothesis is not valid for every hormone (e.g., progesterone) in every tissue because other factors, such as blood flow and rates of dissociation from plasma binding proteins, influx into cells, and intracellular degradation, may play a rate-limiting role in net hormone uptake. Evidence supporting this hypothesis for cortisol is that (1) addition of CBG inactivates the suppressive effect of cortisol on mononuclear cell DNA synthesis in vitro,[513] (2) CBG-bound cortisol is partially protected from metabolic degradation, (3) regulation of cortisol production correlates with free plasma cortisol rather than with total cortisol level, and (4) plasma free cortisol concentration and urinary free cortisol excretion are usually normal in subjects with abnormal CBG levels.[512]

FREE HORMONE TRANSPORT HYPOTHESIS. The free hormone hypothesis should be distinguished from the free hormone transport hypothesis, according to which a hormone enters tissues exclusively from the pool of free hormone after spontaneous dissociation from its binding protein in the circulating blood during its passage through a tissue.[512] Protein binding presumably inhibits diffusion of the hormone into a tissue. However, hepatic uptake of cortisol is several times greater than the amount of free cortisol in plasma. It is possible that albumin-bound or even CBG-bound cortisol can be transported into some tissues,[485, 514] but the apparent paradox is probably explained by the fact that the half-time of dissociation of cortisol from CBG (<1 s) is brief compared with its transit time in blood through the hepatic capillary/sinusoidal system (9 s).[514] Thus protein-bound hormone may be available for intracellular transport in tissues, such as liver, in which the circulation time is slow compared with the rate of dissociation. In fact, the rate of uptake of cortisol and other steroids from protein-free solutions by perfused rat liver is high enough to account fully for the observed hepatic uptake of the steroids from serum.[515] Thus all of the cortisol taken up from plasma can be accounted for by the pool of free cortisol, which is rapidly replenished by cortisol dissociating from binding proteins. Dissociation may be enhanced by a transient conformational change of the binding protein or by receptor-mediated uptake.[516]

PHYSIOLOGICAL ROLE. The physiological role of plasma protein binding of steroid hormones is not fully understood. Binding is not necessary for steroid hormone transport because steroids are sufficiently water soluble at physiological concentrations. The traditional explanation is that hormone-binding proteins serve as reservoirs to lessen the rapid swings in free steroid hormone levels that would occur with cortisol, for example, because of episodic ACTH secretion.[483, 497, 512] When radiolabeled thyroxine is perfused through the portal vein in a solution containing thyroxine-binding globulin, it is uniformly distributed, but in the absence of the globulin, virtually all of the hormone is taken up by the first cells it encounters.[517] Thus the principal function of hormone-binding proteins may be to ensure uniform hormone distribution among all the cells of its target tissues.[516]

Steroid Metabolism

The processes that terminate the physiological actions of steroids in target tissues are not completely known. However, catabolism of the biologically active hormone to inactive forms is one mechanism by which this could be achieved. The complex processes by which corticosteroids are inactivated are understood in some detail. The relative abundances of various urinary metabolites are shown in Table 9–5.

Hepatic Metabolism of Glucocorticoids
(Fig. 9–21)

REDUCTION. The Δ^4 double bond, usually in conjugation with a 3-ketone, is a structural feature of many steroid hormones, including cortisol and its precursors. Most of these steroids are inactivated by reducing this unsaturated ketone system. Reduction of the double bond results in an asymmetrical carbon at position 5, with two possible isomers. The liver, principal site of this modification, contains two stereospecific enzymes that catalyze the process.[518] 5α-Reductase produces the isomer with the hydrogen atom below, and 5β-reductase the isomer with the hydrogen atom above, the plane of the steroid ring. In rat liver, 5α-reductase activity is in the endoplasmic reticulum and 5β-reductase is a cytosolic enzyme.[519]

Reduction of the Δ^4 double bond apparently is the rate-limiting step in cortisol metabolism.[518] Various hepatic 5α-

TABLE 9–5. Relative Amounts of Various Metabolites of Cortisol in Urine

Steroid	Approximate % of Total*
Tetrahydrocortisols	20
Tetrahydrocortisones	20
Cortolones	20
Cortols	10
Cortolic and cortolonic acids	10
11-Hydroxyetiocholanolone	5
6β-Hydroxycortisol	1
11-Hydroxyandrostenedione	1
Cortisol	1

*These figures are approximations drawn from reviews of cortisol metabolism by Peterson[518] and Monder and Bradlow.[1626]

reductases were thought to exist, each of which metabolized a separate class of steroids,[520] but the fact that humans with single-gene defects in androgen 5α-reductase have concomitant defects in glucocorticoid 5α-reduction suggests that a single enzyme metabolizes different classes of steroids.[521] Similarly, several substrate-specific 5β-reductases are thought to exist, but an electrophoretically pure preparation of rat liver 5β-reductase is capable of reducing a variety of steroids.[522] The 5β-reduction of cortisol predominates in humans,[523] and 5β-dihydrocortisol is produced in considerable excess over the 5α isomer.[519]

The 3-keto group of 5α- and 5β-dihydrocortisol can be reduced by 3α-hydroxysteroid dehydrogenase to yield tetrahydrocortisols. Only trace amounts of 3β-hydroxytetrahydrocortisols are formed.[523] Thus the major tetrahydrocortisol excreted in urine is 3α,5β-tetrahydrocortisol (THF).

Cortisol, cortisone, and their tetrahydro derivatives may also be reduced by 20α- and 20β-hydroxysteroid dehydrogenases to yield cortols and cortolones.

OXIDATION. Three types of oxidative reactions involving cortisol and its metabolites occur in the liver. Oxidative removal of the C-20–C-21 side chain yields a C_{19}-steroid with a 17-ketone group.[524] These compounds mostly have the 5β configuration. A second reaction is conversion of the 11β-hydroxyl group to a ketone, as in the reversible conversion of cortisol to cortisone.[525] The third is conversion of the C-21 hydroxyl to a carboxylic acid. The products are called cortolic acids if they are cortisol derivatives (11β-hydroxyl) and cortolonic acids if they are derived from cortisone (11-ketone).

HYDROXYLATION. 6β-Hydroxylation of cortisol occurs in the liver, normally only to a minor extent. The product is highly soluble in water. When plasma cortisol levels are elevated, as in Cushing's syndrome, the normal pathways apparently become saturated and disproportionately large amounts of 6β-hydroxycortisol are produced and are excreted in the urine.[526]

CONJUGATION. The C_{19} and C_{21} metabolites of cortisol are rendered more water soluble by conjugation with glucuronic acid or sulfate. Glucuronidation predominates and is catalyzed by one of the family of uridine diphosphate (UDP) glucuronosyltransferases. These enzymes catalyze the glucuronidation of xenobiotics, bilirubin, and steroids in the hepatic endoplasmic reticulum.[527] Distinct isoenzymes catalyze the glucuronidation of different substrates, even among the steroid hormones.[528, 529] Glucuronide may be conjugated to any hydroxyl group, but the 3α-hydroxyl is preferred. Most 3α,5β-tetrahydro derivatives of cortisol are excreted as glucuronides. Sulfation, catalyzed by cytosolic sulfotransferases, accounts for only a minor fraction of conjugates of the 3α-hydroxysteroids but for most of those of the 3β-hydroxysteroids (both C_{19} and C_{21}).

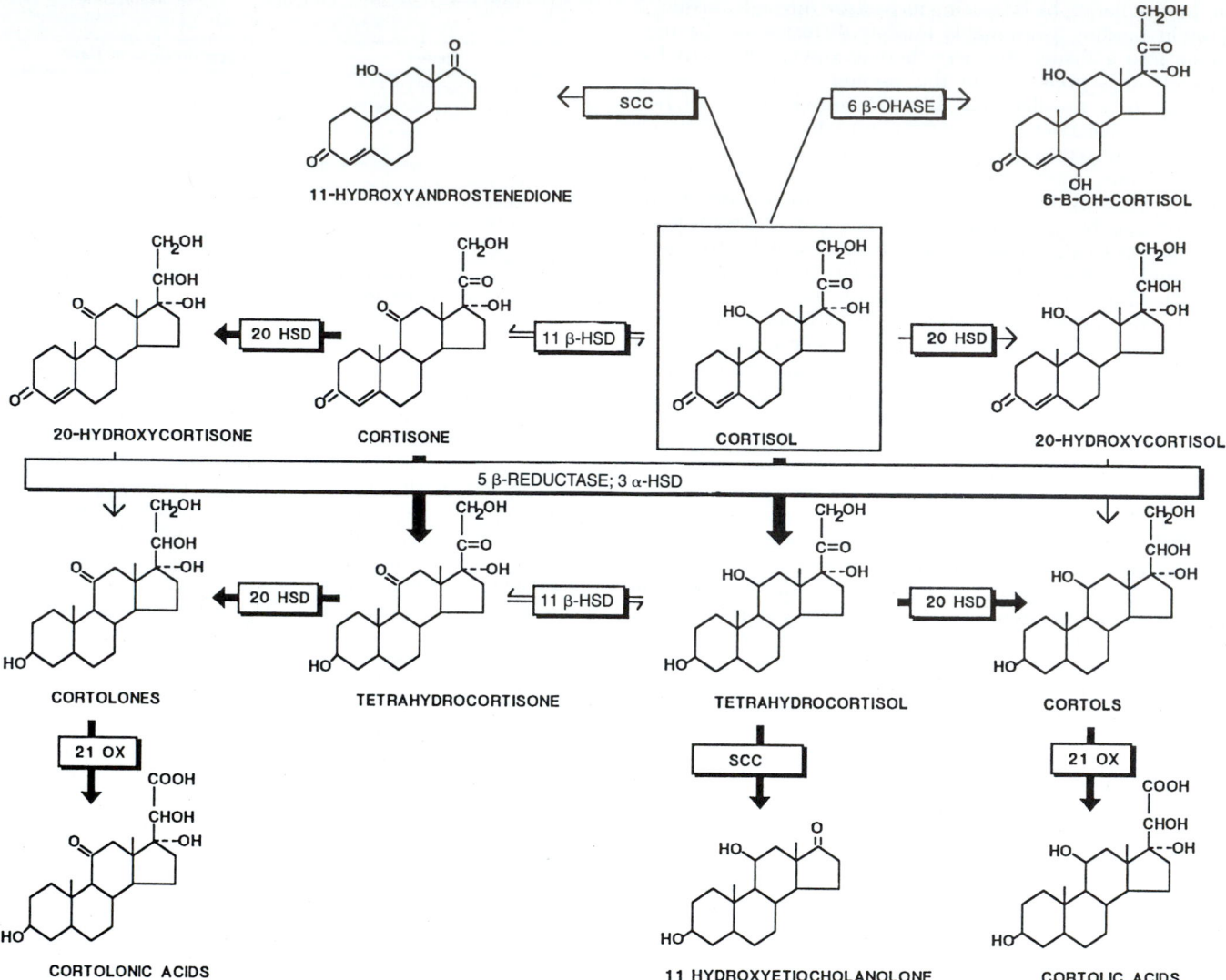

Figure 9–21. Cortisol metabolism in vivo. The relative importance of the pathways under normal conditions is indicated by the width of the arrows. Both 5α- and 5β-reduction occur, but the 5β pathway predominates. Enzymes are indicated by the boxes. SCC, side-chain cleavage activity; 6β-OHASE, 6β-hydroxylase; 20 HSD, 20α-hydroxysteroid dehydrogenase; 11β-HSD, 11β-hydroxysteroid dehydrogenase; 3α-HSD, 3α-hydroxysteroid dehydrogenase; 21 OX, 21-oxidase.

ALTERATIONS IN HEPATIC METABOLISM OF CORTISOL. A number of factors may alter the usual hepatic metabolism of cortisol. These include hormonal factors, age, intercurrent disease states, obesity, and drug-induced changes in hepatic function.

Hormonal Factors. Thyroid hormone affects cortisol metabolism. In hyperthyroid states, the removal of infused cortisol is accelerated but plasma cortisol levels remain normal.[530] In hypothyroid states, the metabolic turnover of cortisol is slowed. Plasma cortisol levels remain normal, but urinary excretion of cortisol metabolites is decreased. The effect of thyroxine is largely due to regulation of the hepatic Δ^4-5α- and Δ^4-5β-reductase activity.[531] There are few data for humans, but hepatic steroid-metabolizing hormones are sexually dimorphic in the rat. 5β-Reductase is apparently androgen induced because its activity is two- to threefold greater in males than in females.[532] Glucocorticoids in high concentrations (as from exogenous steroid therapy or endogenous production in some forms of Cushing's syndrome) also affect cortisol metabolism. Diminished proportional excretion of cortols and cortolones, tetrahydrocortisone (THE), and 5α-THF has been observed in states of glucocorticoid excess.[518]

Age and Disease. Urinary excretion of 17-OHCS (THF, THE) diminishes with age,[533] but plasma cortisol levels remain unchanged. Enzymatic metabolism of cortisol usually is unaffected by renal impairment, but clearance of glucuronides is diminished and these inactive compounds may accumulate in plasma.[518] Significant hepatic disease does affect the metabolism of cortisol. In cirrhosis of the liver there is selective loss of Δ^4-5α- and -5β-reductase activities, but 3α-hydroxysteroid dehydrogenase and glucuronosyltransferase activities remain normal.[534]

Obesity. Obese persons excrete more cortisol metabolites than do lean individuals. This difference persists even when the data are normalized for body surface area.[535] The cortisol production rate is also accelerated in obese subjects, however, so that plasma cortisol levels remain normal.[535]

Drugs. Hepatic metabolism of cortisol is altered by a number of drugs. As discussed earlier, the adrenocorticolytic drug mitotane alters the flux of cortisol metabolites from the usual pathway (tetrahydro metabolites) to the pathway of direct 6β-hydroxylation. Phenytoin and phenobarbital exert similar effects.[536, 537] The antituberculous drug rifampin accelerates the metabolism of both synthetic steroids (including fludrocortisone) and cortisol.[538–540] The responsible enzyme is not known. However, increased quantities of 6β-hydroxycortisol are found in the urine of rifampin-treated patients[541] and induction of 6β-hydroxylase is thought to be the underlying mechanism. The effect may be quantitatively more significant in the case of synthetic steroids. Although cimetidine inhibits several hepatic cytochrome P-450 enzymes, it has no significant effect on prednisolone metabolism.[542]

Glucocorticoids. As already noted, steroids affect their own metabolism and, when their plasma levels are elevated, may alter the flux through individual pathways.[526]

Extrahepatic Metabolism of Cortisol

Cortisol is converted to cortisone by 11β-hydroxysteroid dehydrogenase, which can also catalyze the reverse reaction.[543] The reaction presumably occurs in part in the liver, but the major site of conversion is the kidney,[544] where the enzyme protects the type I glucocorticoid receptor (i.e., the mineralocorticoid receptor) from cortisol (see later), thereby allowing aldosterone to regulate salt metabolism.[545, 546] The enzyme appears to reside mainly in the proximal convoluted tube and pars recta.[546] Plasma cortisone concentration[544] and, presumably, the urinary excretion of cortisone metabolites (THE, cortolones, and cortolonic acids) progressively decrease with increasing renal impairment. This conversion also takes place in fetal lung, where it is thought to involve two separate enzymes, 11β-hydroxysteroid dehydrogenase and 11-oxosteroid reductase.[547]

Hepatic Metabolism of Aldosterone
(Fig. 9–22)

REDUCTION. Like cortisol, aldosterone is reduced predominantly by a Δ⁴-3-ketosteroid reductase and a 3α-hydroxysteroid dehydrogenase. The principal Δ⁴-reductase is a cytosolic 5β-reductase, so the product is 3α,5β-tetrahydroaldosterone. This metabolite accounts for 35 to 40% of the metabolites of aldosterone detectable in urine.[548] A 21-deoxy form of tetrahydroaldosterone[549] is further reduced to the 20α-hydroxy form. The 20α-hydroxyl can then condense with the hydroxyl of the C_{18}-hemiacetal to form a unique aldosterone metabolite with bicyclic acetal rings.[550]

CONJUGATION. Tetrahydroaldosterone is conjugated in the liver to glucuronide at the 3-oxo position. This is the major urinary metabolite of aldosterone.[551] Another conjugate, aldosterone-18-glucuronide, is produced by direct conjugation of unreduced aldosterone. Thus unaltered aldosterone can be recovered from urine by acid hydrolysis followed by nonpolar solvent extraction[552] and accounts for approximately 10% of the aldosterone metabolites excreted in urine.

ALTERATIONS IN THE METABOLISM OF ALDOSTERONE. In patients with cirrhosis of the liver and ascites, the production rate and plasma levels of aldosterone are frequently elevated.[534] The liver apparently has reduced ability to metabolize the aldosterone in plasma, so greater amounts are metabolized extrahepatically.[553, 554] Patients with severe congestive heart failure and hypoperfusion of the liver also exhibit decreased aldosterone clearance.[555]

Metabolism of Adrenal Androgens (Fig. 9–23)

The steroid produced in greatest quantity by the adrenal and the major C_{19} androgenic steroid is DHEA, including DHEAS. Most of the unconjugated steroid is converted to androstenedione by oxidation of the 3β-hydroxyl and isomerization of the Δ⁵ double bond to the Δ⁴ position. Androstenedione is sequentially 5α- or 5β-reduced and the 3-ketone is reduced to yield androsterone and etiocholanolone,

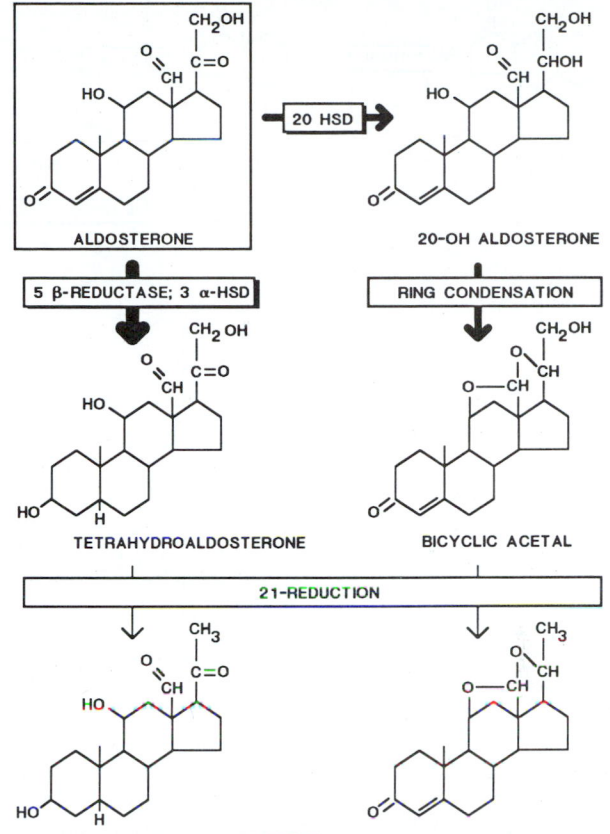

Figure 9–22. Aldosterone metabolism in vivo. The relative importance of the pathways under normal conditions is indicated by the width of the arrows. Enzymes are indicated by the boxes. 20 HSD, 20α-hydroxysteroid dehydrogenase; 3α-HSD, 3α-hydroxysteroid dehydrogenase. Ring condensation proceeds after reduction at C-20.

respectively, which are 17β-reduced to yield the respective diol derivatives, conjugated, and excreted.[518] DHEAS can be directly excreted in the urine; the sulfate group can be hydrolyzed to yield free DHEA, which is metabolized as just described; or the intact ester can be metabolized by 16- and/or 7-hydroxylation or by reversible 17β-reduction to yield androstenediol sulfate.[556] DHEAS and its metabolites are cleared more slowly from plasma by the kidney than their nonsulfated analogues.[556] Fecal excretion of DHEA and its metabolites is quantitatively more significant than that of other adrenal steroids. Of the radiolabeled metabolites of an intravenous dose of radioactive DHEAS, 30 to 45% may appear in the feces.[518] Biliary excretion of DHEA and DHEAS metabolites accounts for several percent of the metabolites of these steroids.[518]

Molecular Mechanisms of Adrenal Steroid Action*

Glucocorticoids

Glucocorticoids exert their effects on every system of the body, although their name derives from their effects on carbohydrate metabolism. Because so many physiological processes are affected, it is difficult to formulate a unifying definition of glucocorticoid action.[557] Presumably all physiological actions of glucocorticoids are mediated by binding to a specific intracellular protein receptor molecule, however,

---

*Also see Chapter 3.

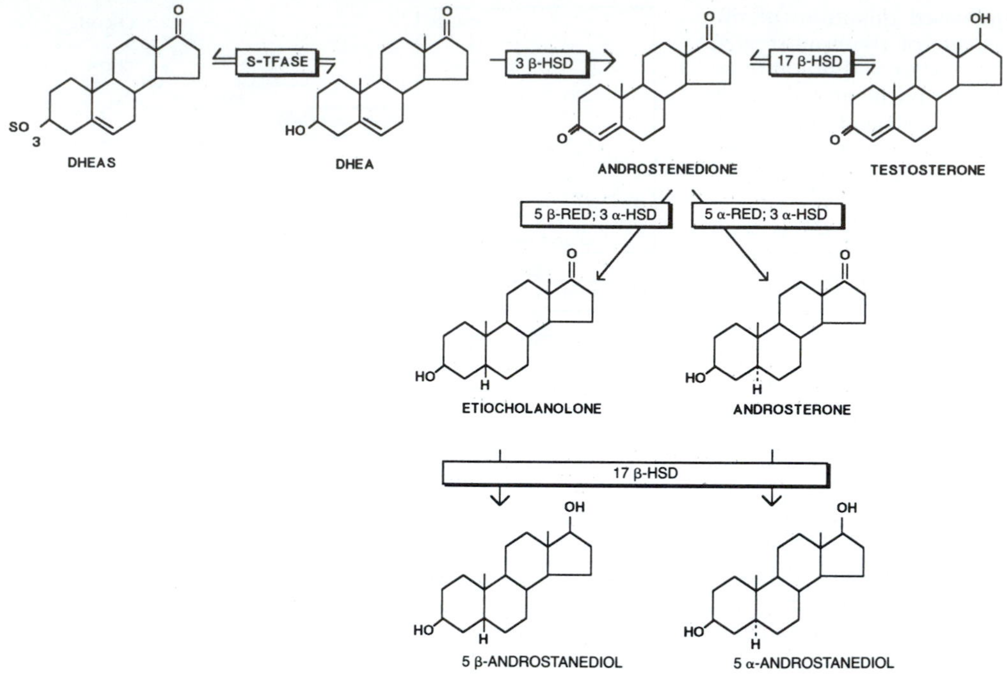

Figure 9–23. Adrenal androgen metabolism in vivo. The relative importance of the pathways under normal conditions is indicated by the width of the arrows. Enzymes are indicated by the boxes. S-TFASE, sulfotransferase; 3 β-HSD, 3β-hydroxysteroid dehydrogenase; 17 β-HSD, 17β-hydroxysteroid dehydrogenase; 5 β-RED, 5β-reductase; 5 α-RED, 5α-reductase.

and this mediation could serve as a functional definition of a "glucocorticoid effect."

The naturally occurring glucocorticoids are C_{21}-steroids with a Δ^4 configuration and 11β- and 21-hydroxyl and 3- and 20-ketone groups (Fig. 9–24). These structural features appear to be necessary for high-affinity binding to the glucocorticoid receptor.

MOLECULAR AND CELLULAR MECHANISMS OF ACTION

The Glucocorticoid Receptor. **Biochemistry and Physiology.** Glucocorticoids, like all steroid hormones, exert their effects on target cells by interacting with soluble intracellular receptor proteins[558] (Fig. 9–25). The steroid is thought to enter the cell by passive diffusion, although other transport mechanisms have been proposed.[559–561] Once inside the cell, the steroid is bound to the specific glucocorticoid receptor.

Receptor purification[562, 563] and affinity labeling[564–567] studies have shown that the receptor is a single chain polypeptide of about 94 kd. It binds glucocorticoids with high affinity and in a saturable and specific manner. In the presence of sodium molybdate, the receptor can be extracted from cells complexed with other proteins that do not have steroid-binding capacity. The molecular mass of the complex is 270 to 320 kd.[568, 569] One component of this complex is a 90-kd heat shock phosphoprotein (hsp90).[570–576]

Once the steroid is bound, the hormone-receptor complex acquires the capacity to bind to DNA.[577] The nature of this activation process is not precisely known, but it involves dissociation of the hsp90 moiety from the steroid-binding subunit of the receptor.[566, 568] Transformation of the complex to a DNA-binding form can be achieved in vitro by increasing temperature or ionic strength. Cell fractionation experiments indicate that the unoccupied receptor resides in the cytoplasm and, after binding, the steroid-receptor complex translocates to the nucleus and binds to DNA.[578] Most immunocytochemical studies support this concept,[579–581] but

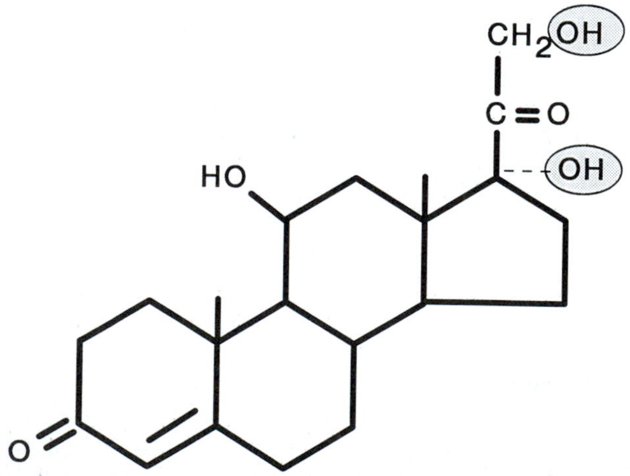

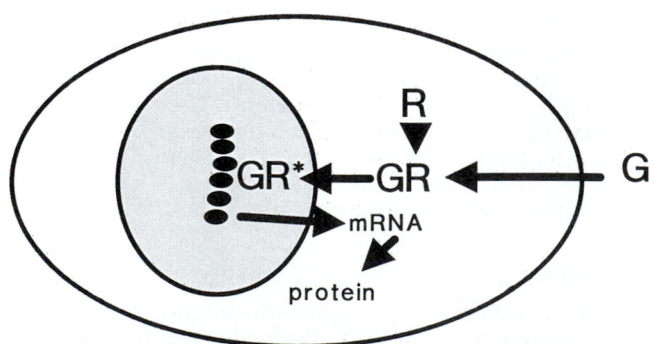

Figure 9–24. Basic structure of a glucocorticoid. The features that are essential for glucocorticoid activity are shown with heavy lines and letters. Those that are not required for basic activity, but that enhance glucocorticoid potency, are shown in the shaded areas. (Adapted from Liddle GW. The adrenals. In: Williams RW, ed. Textbook of Endocrinology. 6th ed. Philadelphia: W. B. Saunders, 1981: 242–292.)

Figure 9–25. Glucocorticoid action in target cells. Like other steroids, glucocorticoids (G) are thought to enter cells by a passive process. They bind to a cytoplasmic glucocorticoid receptor protein (R) to form a glucocorticoid-receptor complex (GR) capable of activating transcription of target genes. The mRNA is translated into new proteins that express the biological activity of the glucocorticoid. GR*, transformed complex.

others have suggested that the receptor resides in the nuclear compartment under both occupied and unoccupied conditions.[582]

Domain Structure. Specific domains of the glucocorticoid receptor molecule are responsible for steroid- and DNA-binding functions. The steroid binding site is at the COOH-terminal region of the protein.[583] Studies with covalently reactive ligands suggest that specific residues are involved in steroid binding. Whether they are also critical for binding natural ligands is not known. The region of DNA binding is located in midmolecule.[584] Most antibodies against purified receptor protein react with a third, NH₂-terminal "immunogenic" domain.[585–589]

The structural features of rat, human, and mouse glucocorticoid receptors have been defined by molecular cloning methods.[590–593] The human glucocorticoid receptor cDNA sequence predicts two forms of the receptor protein, a more abundant 777-residue alpha form and a 742-amino-acid beta form. Their sequences are identical up to residue 727 and diverge thereafter.[592] The glucocorticoid receptor is one of a family of DNA-binding proteins that act as regulators of gene transcription. This family includes receptors for all classes of steroid hormones, thyroid hormone (v-*erb* A), and retinoic acid[594] (Fig. 9–26). The hormone binding domains of these proteins are relatively conserved, but the most distinctive feature is the highly conserved "zinc finger" structure[594] in the central DNA binding domain (Fig. 9–27). A similar structure in the DNA-binding protein *Xenopus* transcription factor IIIA (TFIIIA) forms a finger-like loop structure of 12 amino acids anchored at the base by a zinc ion chelated between two pairs of cysteine and histidine residues.[595] Similar finger-like structures are assumed to exist in the glucocorticoid and other receptors of this class and presumably interact with the coils of the DNA double helix.

Steroid binding is at the COOH terminus.[596–598] Mutant human receptors transcribed in vitro lose dexamethasone-binding ability when small three- to four-codon segments are inserted into the genomic DNA past the codon for amino acid 527, whereas insertions before the codon for amino acid 500 have no affect on hormone binding.[596] Deletion mutations in the same region also impair steroid binding, whereas deletions in other parts of the coding sequence do not.[597] The DNA-binding zinc finger domain of the human

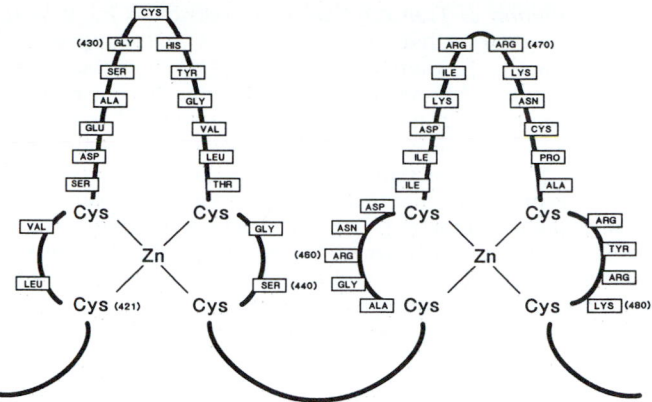

Figure 9–27. Putative "zinc finger" structures in the DNA binding domain of the glucocorticoid receptor. The eight highly conserved cysteine residues are thought to chelate Zn^{2+} to form the finger structure observed in other trans-acting transcriptional regulatory factors.

glucocorticoid receptor lies between amino acids 421 and 481.[599] Mutant human receptors with deletions in this region do not bind to DNA.[597] Studies of naturally occurring mutations of the glucocorticoid receptor in murine S49 lymphoma cells yield similar conclusions.[593] Other regions of the glucocorticoid receptor are required for its nuclear translocation[600] and its effects on gene transcription.

MECHANISMS OF GENE REGULATION BY GLUCOCORTICOIDS

Induction of Transcription. Glucocorticoid-receptor complexes regulate gene expression by interacting with specific regulatory DNA sequences, termed *glucocorticoid response elements* (GREs), which are usually located near the promoter region of target genes.[601, 602] Studies of a number of glucocorticoid-inducible genes have produced a consensus sequence for one such GRE,[601, 603–606] although not all functional GREs share this sequence.[607] The GRE is a partially palindromic structure with the sequence GGTACAnnnTGTTCT. Dimerization of the steroid-receptor complex appears to be necessary for it to bind to the GRE and exert its regulatory effect. Other steroid hormone–receptor complexes can bind to this GRE, although some (e.g., complexes with the estrogen receptor) apparently cannot induce transcription of the target gene.[608] Some specificity for induction appears to be conferred by the first zinc finger, because a chimeric estrogen receptor whose first zinc finger is replaced with the first finger of the glucocorticoid receptor is capable of inducing transcription from a GRE.[609]

The unoccupied steroid binding domain of the glucocorticoid receptor appears to have a tonic inhibitory influence on the transcriptional activation function of the receptor. Mutant receptors missing the steroid binding domain are constitutive (i.e., no longer hormone dependent) activators of target gene transcription.[599, 610, 611]

Exactly how binding of the hormone-receptor complex to the hormone response element affects gene transcription is the subject of intense investigation. Sequences in the receptor's NH₂-terminal region, the DNA binding domain, and the COOH-terminal half of the molecule all appear to be required for full transcriptional activation.[596, 610, 612, 613] The quantitative contributions of the individual domains to the total trans-activation effect are not clear.[601] Transcriptional activation may depend not only on interaction of the DNA binding and activation domains with the GRE but also on the interaction of other transcription factors. In vitro, binding sites for other trans-acting factors, as well as the presence of additional GREs, can augment the effect of a single GRE on an adjacent promoter.[614]

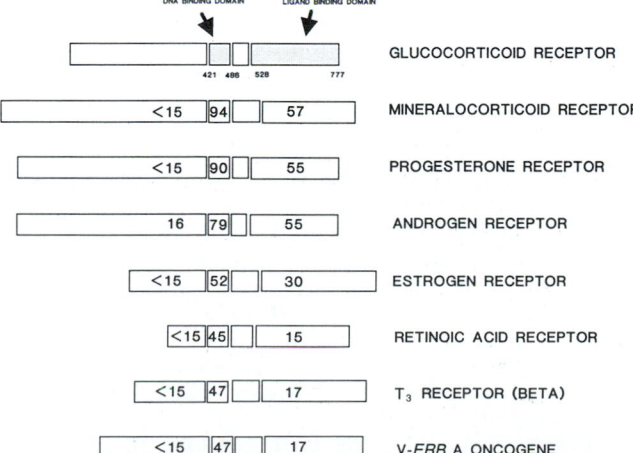

Figure 9–26. Domain structure of the glucocorticoid receptor protein and its homology with other steroid receptors, the retinoic acid receptor, the thyroid hormone (T₃) receptor, and the v-*erb* A oncogene. The 777-amino-acid alpha form of the receptor contains DNA binding (residues 421 to 486) and ligand binding (residues 528 to 777) domains. The DNA binding region is highly conserved among the various receptors (figures indicate the percent homology in each domain).

Inhibition of Transcription. Glucocorticoids increase the transcriptional activity of many genes but suppress the transcription of others, such as the POMC, prolactin, and glycoprotein hormone alpha subunit genes. No clear consensus sequence for a negative response element has emerged from studies of these genes.[601] Proposed mechanisms for the inhibitory effects of glucocorticoids in these systems include interference with other transcription factors by direct protein-protein interaction,[615a] interference with binding of another transcription factor to its own response element near the negative GRE,[616, 617] and direct action by binding of the receptor to negative response elements that alter the receptor structure in a manner that prevents transcriptional activation.[618]

Mineralocorticoids

Mineralocorticoids are named for the ability to regulate electrolyte transport across epithelial surfaces. The principal physiological mineralocorticoid is aldosterone. Its major target tissues, which include the kidney, colon, and salivary glands,[619, 620] have high-affinity type I glucocorticoid (i.e., mineralocorticoid) receptors that bind aldosterone.[621–623] Type I receptors are also present in liver, brain (particularly hippocampus), pituitary, and peripheral blood mononuclear cells.[624–627] Aldosterone promotes active sodium absorption and excretion of potassium in its major target tissues. These effects are presumably mediated via transcriptional activation mechanisms similar to those for all other members of the steroid–thyroid hormone–retinoic acid receptor family.[601]

MOLECULAR AND CELLULAR MECHANISMS OF ACTION

Mineralocorticoid Receptor. **Structure.** The mineralocorticoid receptor has been studied at the protein biochemical level by examining the binding of radiolabeled aldosterone to soluble extracts of target cells or tissues. Aldosterone binds to at least two different proteins in kidney cytosol preparations: high-affinity type I binding sites and more abundant low-affinity type II binding sites.[628, 629] The type I site is thought to be the receptor that mediates aldosterone's action. The type II site is the glucocorticoid receptor. The type I receptor displays a curious lack of specificity.[630] Radiolabeled aldosterone can be displaced from the receptor by approximately equimolar concentrations of glucocorticoids. Thus it was not clear how these receptors specifically recognized mineralocorticoids in the presence of physiological concentrations of glucocorticoids.

Molecular cloning of human mineralocorticoid receptor cDNA was achieved with a cDNA probe directed at the highly conserved DNA binding domain shared by all steroid receptor molecules.[631] The predicted 984-amino-acid protein (107 kd) is similar to but distinct from the human glucocorticoid receptor. Their NH_2 termini are unrelated. The central, cysteine-rich, DNA-binding zinc finger domain that is characteristic of this gene family is highly conserved.[595] This 65-amino-acid sequence has 94% homology with the corresponding portion of the glucocorticoid receptor. The COOH-terminal, steroid binding domain is about 50% homologous with the glucocorticoid and progesterone receptors.[631] When expressed in mammalian cells, the recombinant receptor, like the native receptor, cannot distinguish between mineralocorticoids and glucocorticoids.[631]

Basis of Specificity of Response. The aldosterone receptor cannot distinguish between glucocorticoids and mineralocorticoids in vitro, but administered radiolabeled aldosterone accumulates in type I sites in mineralocorticoid target cells in vivo. It was proposed that mineralocorticoid target tissues might be rich in extravascular CBG, which could sequester glucocorticoids and prevent them from binding to the mineralocorticoid receptor.[632] However, this did not prove to be the case.[633] Rather, specificity is conferred by the $P-450_{c11}$ enzyme system that converts cortisol to cortisone, which has low affinity for the mineralocorticoid type I receptor.[544, 545] Aldosterone-responsive tissues express $P-450_{c11}$ activity at higher levels than nonresponsive tissues.[545, 546] In some tissues in which the 11β-hydroxysteroid dehydrogenase function is lacking, such as the hippocampus and heart, type I receptors bind glucocorticoids and glucocorticoids express their biological effects via type I receptor binding. In fetal lung, $P-450_{c11}$ activity appears to require two independent enzymes, an 11β-hydroxysteroid dehydrogenase and an 11-oxosteroid reductase.[547] In other target tissues, it is not clear whether the activities reside in a single enzyme or in two enzymes. There are both inherited and acquired states of 11β-hydroxysteroid dehydrogenase deficiency (see later).

Effects of Glucocorticoids

Effects on Metabolism

GLYCOGEN METABOLISM. It was known by the mid-19th century that the adrenal glands are essential for life, but their role in intermediary metabolism was not established until 1927 when it was noted that adrenalectomized animals cannot maintain hepatic glycogen stores.[634] Replacement of adrenocortical steroids reversed both glycogen depletion and hypoglycemia in fasting adrenalectomized animals.[635] Glucocorticoids both activate glycogen synthase[636, 637] and inactivate the glycogen-mobilizing enzyme glycogen phosphorylase.[637] The total amount of glycogen synthase remains unchanged, but the enzyme is activated by dephosphorylation. It is not known whether glucocorticoids achieve this effect directly by activating a hepatic phosphatase or indirectly by inactivating glycogen phosphorylase, a phosphatase inhibitor.

GLUCONEOGENESIS. Glucocorticoids increase hepatic glucose production in part by increasing substrate availability and stimulating release of glucogenic amino acids from peripheral tissues, such as skeletal muscle[638] (Fig. 9–28). The effect is most apparent when a physiological replacement dose is administered to adrenalectomized animals.[635] Glucocorticoids also directly activate key hepatic gluconeogenic enzymes, such as glucose-6-phosphatase and phosphoenolpyruvate carboxykinase (PEPCK).[638] The increased PEPCK activity results from glucocorticoid-induced activation of PEPCK gene transcription,[639, 640] mediated by interaction of the glucocorticoid–type II receptor complex with a specific GRE located in the 5'-flanking region of the PEPCK gene.[607, 640]

Other gluconeogenic hormones, such as glucagon and epinephrine, are ineffective without the permissive effect of glucocorticoids.[638, 641] Glucocorticoids enhance the sensitivity of lipolysis to catecholamines in target tissues.[638] The glycerol released during lipolysis provides a substrate for glucose production, and released fatty acids provide an energy source for the process. Glucocorticoids also enhance the sensitivity of lactate production to catecholamine stimulation in muscle. Increased sensitivity also underlies the permissive effect of glucocorticoids on glucagon action, but the mechanism is unknown.[638]

PERIPHERAL GLUCOSE UTILIZATION. In addition to mobilizing substrate for hepatic gluconeogenesis, glucocorticoids inhibit glucose uptake and utilization by peripheral tissues,[642–645] in part by direct inhibition of glucose transport into the cells[646, 647] (see Fig. 9–28). The number of glucose transporters in adipocytes is decreased by glucocorticoids because transporter mRNA levels are decreased.[648]

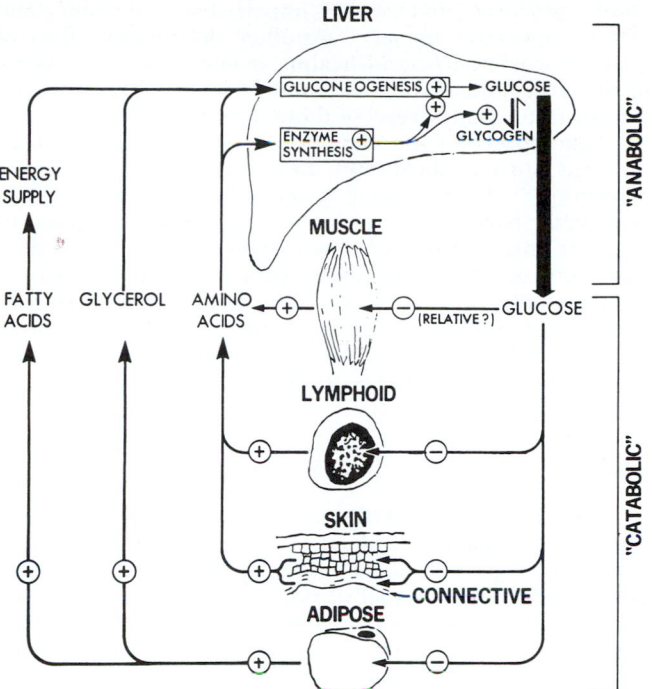

Figure 9–28. Glucocorticoid effects on hepatic glucose metabolism and peripheral tissue metabolism of protein and fat. Stimulation is indicated by plus signs, inhibition by minus signs. (From Baxter JD, Rousseau GG. Glucocorticoid hormone action: an overview. In: Baxter JD, Rousseau GG, eds. Glucocorticoid Hormone Action. New York: Springer-Verlag, 1979: 1–24.)

LIPID METABOLISM. Glucocorticoids acutely activate lipolysis in adipose tissue[645] (see Fig. 9–28). Lipolytic activity and, consequently, plasma free fatty acid levels are reduced in adrenalectomized animals and return to normal within 2 h after glucocorticoid administration.[649, 650] This permissive effect may be mediated by altered sensitivity to other lipolytic hormones, such as catecholamines and GH,[649–651] but the molecular mechanisms are not known.

Glucocorticoids also exert chronic effects on lipid metabolism. One of the most striking in humans is the redistribution of body fat after chronic glucocorticoid excess. There is relative sparing of the extremities, whereas the dorsocervical and supraclavicular regions, the trunk, and the anterior mediastinum and mesentery are sites of marked fat deposition. Animals exposed to excess glucocorticoids generally do not exhibit similar fat redistribution and may lose weight, although protein loss exceeds that of fat.[652] Hyperinsulinemia resulting from glucocorticoid effects on glucose metabolism may underlie the lipogenic effect,[653] but the reason for the central predisposition for fat deposition is unknown.

Effects on Immunological Function and Inflammatory Processes

Endogenous glucocorticoid excess suppresses immunological responses,[654] and reactivation of latent infections, such as tuberculosis, may result from administration of pharmacological doses of glucocorticoids. Various effects on components of the immunological and inflammatory responses have been described in vitro, but their relevance to a physiological role for glucocorticoids in normal immunomodulation is not clear. Immune cells have high-affinity glucocorticoid receptors, but in vitro results have usually been characterized at supraphysiological hormone concentrations. Moreover, the clinical immunosuppressive and anti-inflammatory properties of glucocorticoids are, in general, observed only when pharmacological amounts of the hormones are administered.

TRAFFIC OF CELLS OF THE IMMUNE SYSTEM. One of the principal glucocorticoid effects on immune cells is on their traffic to and from the peripheral circulation. Glucocorticoids produce a marked decrease in human peripheral lymphocyte numbers within about 4 h. Thymus-derived lymphocytes (T cells) are depleted more completely than marrow-derived lymphocytes (B cells). The effect is due to redistribution of lymphocytes from the intravascular compartment to the spleen, lymph nodes, thoracic duct, and bone marrow.[655, 656] Glucocorticoids also cause a similar redistribution of monocytes, but the opposite effect is exerted on granulocytes, which leave the bone marrow and enter the circulating blood. At the same time, glucocorticoids inhibit the accumulation of neutrophils at sites of inflammation.[657] These effects are manifested clinically by increased numbers of circulating neutrophils and suppression of local inflammatory responses.

T CELL FUNCTION. Lymphocytes have long been recognized to be targets for glucocorticoid action.[658] In fact, the effects of glucocorticoids on glucose uptake and amino acid incorporation were first defined in these cells.[659, 660] Glucocorticoids also elicit specific responses that affect immune function in lymphoid cells. In certain species, particularly rat and mouse, they induce lysis of normal and neoplastic T cells and thymocytes,[661, 662] a process that may involve induction of a specific nuclease that degrades their DNA.[663] Mature human T cells and immature human thymocytes contain specific high-affinity glucocorticoid receptors,[664] but they are relatively insensitive to glucocorticoid-induced lysis. Thus the acute effects of glucocorticoids on human lymphocyte numbers are the result of vascular redistribution, not cell lysis. Nevertheless, glucocorticoids exert immunosuppressive effects on human T cells in vitro, such as inhibition of proliferation[665] and inhibition of transcription of the gene for interleukin 2, a potent T cell growth factor.[666]

B CELL FUNCTION. Glucocorticoid modulation of B cell function may be both direct and mediated by effects on monocytes and T cell subpopulations. Resting B cells presumably first undergo an activation process, then proliferate in response to T cell–derived growth factors, such as interleukin 4, and terminally differentiate to produce immunoglobulins.[667] Glucocorticoids appear to modulate this process. Early events, such as B cell activation and proliferation, are inhibited.[668] Accessory mononuclear cells may play a role under certain conditions. Terminal B cell differentiation is much less sensitive to glucocorticoid inhibition.[668] In fact, glucocorticoids may enhance immunoglobulin production under some in vitro conditions.[667, 669–671]

MONOCYTE AND MACROPHAGE FUNCTION. Glucocorticoids inhibit the proliferative response of monocytes to colony-stimulating factor[672] and their differentiation into macrophages.[673] They also inhibit the phagocytic and cytotoxic functions of macrophages.[674]

MEDIATORS OF INFLAMMATION. Glucocorticoids inhibit the movement of cells and fluid from the intravascular compartment that characterizes the local inflammatory response.[675] They also inhibit the action of histamine, a potent vasoactive agent,[676] by an unknown mechanism. Prostaglandins are probable mediators of the inflammatory response[677] and glucocorticoids inhibit prostaglandin synthesis,[678–681] possibly by inducing increased levels of one of the lipocortins, a family of Ca^{2+}/phospholipid-dependent proteins that inhibit phospholipase A_2 activation and thus synthesis of prostaglandins and other arachidonic acid derivatives.[682–684] Lipocortin I, which is also called calpactin II and is the 35-kd substrate of epidermal growth factor receptor tyrosine kinase activity,[685] may be the inhibitor of phospholipase A_2.[686] However, lipocortin I does not have anti-inflammatory activity, and, although it inhibits phospholipase A_2 in vitro, it does not inhibit arachidonate release from macrophages.[687] Furthermore, steady-state lipocortin I mRNA levels are not regulated by glucocorticoids in several in vitro cell systems.[688] Finally, lipocortin I appears to be an intracellular protein, whereas only secreted proteins that inhibit phospholipase A_2 appear to be regulated by glucocorticoids. The specific glucocorticoid-induced phospholipase A_2-inhibitory protein has not been identified. Another possible mechanism of glucocorticoid anti-inflammatory action involves inhibition of plasminogen activators (PAs),[689–691] serine proteases that convert plasminogen into active plasmin. Plasmin cleaves the plasma globulin, kininogen, into potent kinins that cause the vasodilatation and increased capillary permeability characteristic of inflammation. Specific PA-inhibitory proteins exist, so it is unclear whether glucocorticoids regulate PA biosynthesis, PA inhibitor synthesis, or both. Although the net effect is decreased PA activity, glucocorticoids may actually increase transcription of some PA genes, the increase being offset by induction of PA inhibitor gene expression.[692]

Effects on Musculoskeletal and Connective Tissues

BONE AND MINERAL METABOLISM. The fact that chronic glucocorticoid excess causes osteopenia suggests possible direct steroid effects on bone cells. Glucocorticoids inhibit osteoblast function, decreasing new bone formation.[693–695] Steroid-induced osteopenia is associated with increased osteoclast numbers,[695] and glucocorticoids enhance the ability of osteoclasts to bind to bone surfaces as a consequence of altered expression of N-acetylglucosamine and N-acetylgalactosamine on the cell surface.[696] Whether osteoclast-mediated bone resorption is stimulated or suppressed remains controversial.[697, 698]

Glucocorticoids also exert indirect effects on bone by decreasing intestinal calcium absorption,[695, 699–701] which appears not to be due to decreased serum 25-hydroxycholecalciferol or 1,25-dihydroxycholecalciferol concentrations[695, 702, 703] or, at least in vitro, decreased intestinal epithelial sensitivity to vitamin D.[704]

A secondary effect of glucocorticoids is increased serum parathyroid hormone (PTH) concentration,[695, 705] presumably resulting from impaired intestinal calcium absorption. The increase is reversed by vitamin D and calcium administration. Glucocorticoids may also have a direct effect on the parathyroid glands. Serum PTH concentration rapidly increases without a measurable change in intestinal calcium absorption in hyperparathyroid patients given glucocorticoids.[706] Glucocorticoids also stimulate PTH release from rat parathyroid glands in vitro.[707]

Glucocorticoids increase urinary calcium excretion by decreasing renal reabsorption.[708, 709] In hyperparathyroidism, glucocorticoids, together with the PTH-induced increased filtered calcium load, produce marked hypercalciuria.[706]

SKELETAL MUSCLE. Glucocorticoid effects on intermediary metabolism (see earlier) involve skeletal muscle, a major source of amino acid substrate for gluconeogenesis. Their catabolic effect on muscle protein is the basis for the profound myopathy that sometimes results from glucocorticoid excess.

CONNECTIVE TISSUE. Glucocorticoids modulate fibroblast proliferation and a number of differentiated functions of fibroblasts. Most effects are inhibitory, such as suppression of fibroblast DNA, RNA, and protein synthesis.[710] They also suppress synthesis of the extracellular matrix components, collagen[711–715] and hyaluronidate.[716, 717] The clinical result of chronic glucocorticoid excess is impaired wound healing and friable connective tissues.[718] Another deleterious effect of glucocorticoids on wound healing is impairment of macrophage recruitment to the wound site.[718] Transforming growth factor β may reverse these defects.[719]

Glucocorticoids stimulate production of some fibroblast products, such as fibronectin, an extracellular matrix glycoprotein.[720–722] Transforming growth factor β also induces fibronectin biosynthesis and is synergistic with glucocorticoids in this regard. Glucocorticoids appear to stabilize fibronectin mRNA, whereas transforming growth factor β stimulates fibronectin mRNA transcription.[722] The level of elastin, a product of fibroblasts that have differentiated into ligament cells, is also increased by glucocorticoids.[723] This increase may also be due to mRNA stabilization rather than to transcriptional regulation.

Effects on Fluid and Electrolyte Homeostasis

MINERALOCORTICOID ACTIVITY. Evidence of glucocorticoid modulation of blood pressure comes largely from patients with glucocorticoid excess or deficiency. Those with glucocorticoid excess usually have hypertension, which often occurs without elevated plasma mineralocorticoid concentrations or evidence of functional mineralocorticoid excess, such as hypokalemia or suppressed plasma renin activity.[724, 725] The principal endogenous glucocorticoids in humans and rodents, cortisol and corticosterone, respectively, have weak mineralocorticoid activity under ordinary physiological conditions. Furthermore, studies in a rat model of glucocorticoid-induced hypertension suggest that the hypertension is not due to supraphysiological concentrations of glucocorticoids acting on type I mineralocorticoid receptors.[726] Thus, although it is generally assumed that excessive concentrations of glucocorticoids exert a direct mineralocorticoid effect on target tissues, the evidence for this is not convincing. Other glucocorticoid effects have been implicated. Glucocorticoids induce hepatic production of angiotensinogen (renin substrate), but the mechanism is unclear, as is the issue of whether increased circulating levels of angiotensinogen result in increased angiotensin II generation. Enhanced vascular sensitivity to the pressor effects of infused angiotensin II and norepinephrine is observed in patients with Cushing's syndrome,[725] but its mechanism, too, is unknown. Finally, decreased levels of the vasodilators prostaglandin E_2 and kallikrein are found in the urine of animals and humans with glucocorticoid excess.[725, 727] In summary, the basis for the hypertension in patients with glucocorticoid excess is not understood.

Patients with glucocorticoid deficiency may be hypotensive and refractory to the effects of pressor agents, in part because of the resulting renin substrate deficiency.[728] Loss of glucocorticoid inhibition of production of prostaglandin I_2, a potent vasodilator, may result in decreased peripheral vascular tone.[728]

VASOPRESSIN. A defect in free water clearance in patients with glucocorticoid deficiency[729, 730] is associated with increased plasma AVP concentrations.[731] Glucocorticoid deficiency increases AVP mRNA levels in the paraventricular nucleus but not in the supraoptic or suprachiasmatic nucleus of the rat.[414] It is not known whether this and the increased plasma AVP concentrations are direct effects of loss of glucocorticoid negative feedback on AVP gene expression or secondary to changes in intravascular volume and plasma osmolarity. However, glucocorticoid receptors are present in AVP-producing cells of the parvicellular division of the paraventricular nucleus.[732] Increased circulating AVP levels may play a role in maintaining blood pressure in adrenal insufficiency.[733]

ATRIAL NATRIURETIC FACTOR. Animals subjected to adrenal enucleation (removal of the adrenals, with the capsules and adherent zona glomerulosa cells left in situ) are unable to excrete a salt load.[734, 735] Glucocorticoid replacement results in a natriuresis that was thought to be due to a glucocorticoid-induced increase in glomerular filtration rate[736] but that now appears to involve ANF. The regulatory regions of both human and rat ANF genes contain putative GREs,[737-739] and glucocorticoids induce increased plasma ANF levels in intact[740] and adrenalectomized animals.[741] They stimulate increased ANF mRNA content[741] and ANF synthesis and secretion by cardiac myocytes in vitro.[742, 743] Glucocorticoids also increase processing of the ANF(1-126) precursor into mature ANF(99-126) by cultured rat atrial myocytes.[744]

Neuropsychiatric and Behavioral Effects

MOOD. Glucocorticoids have multiple effects on human behavior, including modulation of sleep patterns, mood, cognition, and reception of sensory input.[745] The duration of rapid eye movement sleep is decreased in patients with Cushing's syndrome[746] and in normal subjects given pharmacological doses of exogenous glucocorticoid[747] or in whom excessive production of endogenous cortisol is stimulated by ACTH.[748] Evidence for steroid-induced alterations of mood and cognitive function comes largely from clinical observation. About half of patients with either spontaneous or iatrogenic Cushing's syndrome have psychological disturbances, depression being the most common.[749-753] Patients with exogenous Cushing's syndrome may have euphoria more often than those with spontaneous Cushing's syndrome. Varying degrees of manic behavior and even overt psychosis can occur. Patients with adrenal insufficiency also may suffer from psychiatric disturbances, mainly depression, apathy, and lethargy. The mechanisms that mediate these behavioral effects of glucocorticoids are unknown.

CENTRAL NERVOUS SYSTEM. At the cellular level, glucocorticoids exert a number of effects on the nervous system. Cells in several parts of the central nervous system contain glucocorticoid receptors, but neurons exhibit responses that seem too rapid to be mediated by transcriptional activation of target genes by glucocorticoid-receptor complexes. These responses include changes in electrical activity, such as hyperpolarization of the cell membrane[754] or suppression of spontaneous electrical activity.[755, 756] They occur so rapidly (i.e., within 2 min of exposure to the hormone) that a direct membrane effect is likely. Hyperpolarization is blocked by antiglucocorticoids, suggesting involvement of a receptor-like molecule.[755] Effects of more chronic exposure include inhibition of the regenerative axon sprouting that follows deafferentation of hippocampal neurons[757, 758] and reduction in their number.[759] Central nervous system glial cells also appear to be targets for glucocorticoids, which induce glutamine synthetase activity in cultured astrocytes[760-762] and glycerol-3-phosphate dehydrogenase activity in cultured oligodendrocytes.[763, 764] These effects appear to be exerted at the transcriptional level.[765]

Gastrointestinal Effects

ION TRANSPORT. Glucocorticoids have direct effects on ion transport in the colon.[766] Although the colon contains mineralocorticoid receptors that might mediate such effects (see later), two lines of evidence suggest that glucocorticoid-induced sodium transport is a true glucocorticoid receptor–mediated effect. First, the use of steroid analogues specific for glucocorticoid receptors reveals a saturable effect on sodium transport.[767] Second, blockade of mineralocorticoid

receptors with spironolactone does not diminish the response of sodium transport to low doses of dexamethasone.[768]

ULCER FORMATION. Chronic administration of pharmacological doses of glucocorticoids is thought to increase the risk of peptic ulcer formation in the upper gastrointestinal tract.[769] The mechanism of ulcer induction may involve inhibition of healing of ulceration caused by other factors. Acute administration of pharmacological doses of glucocorticoids is not associated with increased ulcer formation.

Developmental Effects

LINEAR GROWTH. Supraphysiological concentrations of endogenous or exogenous glucocorticoids inhibit linear skeletal growth in children.[770, 771] The mechanism is unknown. GH may be suppressed[772] but is usually not markedly so in children, and serum IGF I levels are not decreased.[773] Furthermore, GH gene transcription is activated by glucocorticoids in vitro.[774] Therefore, growth arrest is presumably due to direct inhibitory effects on bone and connective tissue (see earlier). In addition, circulating inhibitors of IGF I action are induced by glucocorticoids,[775] but their significance is unknown.

LUNG. Glucocorticoids stimulate differentiation of many cell types.[776] In the lung, for example, glucocorticoid induces surfactant production by type II pneumocytes, a normal developmental process that is accelerated by pharmacological amounts of exogenous glucocorticoid.[777] Glucocorticoids also cause morphological changes in type II cells,[778, 779] induce enzymes involved in phospholipid biosynthesis, and regulate transcription of the gene for the major surfactant protein (SP-A or SP28-36).[779, 780] The effect on surfactant mRNA levels is biphasic: lower concentrations are stimulatory, but higher levels are inhibitory.[780]

NERVOUS SYSTEM AND ADRENAL MEDULLA. In the nervous system glucocorticoids regulate the differentiation of neural crest epithelial cells into chromaffin cells. Neural crest cells are precursors of a variety of more differentiated cell types, including autonomic ganglion cells and adrenomedullary cells. Cells all along the neural crest apparently are pluripotential, hormonal environment playing a major role in determining developmental fate.[781] Under the influence of nerve growth factor, for example, sympathetic ganglion cells enlarge, develop neuronal processes and synaptic vesicles, and produce a variety of neuron-specific proteins, such as SCG-10, GAP-43 (thought to be involved in neuronal growth and plasticity), and NF-68 (a neurofilament component).[782-786] Under the influence of glucocorticoids, neural crest precursor cells that invade the embryonic adrenal gland cease to express "neuron-specific" gene products, such as neurofilaments, and acquire the characteristic morphology of adrenomedullary chromaffin cells.[786] They also lose their neural processes and begin to produce catecholamine-synthesizing enzymes, such as phenylethanolamine N-methyltransferase. The mechanism by which glucocorticoids induce this differentiation is not known.

Dissociation of Biological Effects

There is an obvious attraction to finding synthetic glucocorticoids that have desirable therapeutic effects and lack undesirable side effects. The synthesis of fludrocortisone, which has salt-retaining activity out of proportion to its glucocorticoid activity, was such an accomplishment. However, the fact that a natural steroid, aldosterone, demonstrated similar dissociation of activity foretold the possibility of success, and we now know that the type I glucocorticoid (i.e., mineralocorticoid) receptor and the P-450$_{c11}$ present in the kidney mediate the mineralocorticoid response. The search for synthetic glucocorticoids that exert anti-inflammatory effects but are devoid of effects on intermediary metabolism or calcium metabolism has been generally unsuccessful. However, a new synthetic steroid, deflazacort, has been reported in preliminary studies to possess such characteristics.[787, 788] These claims are based on imprecise indices of anti-inflammatory effect, however, and because all glucocorticoid effects are thought to be mediated via the same type II receptor, it is difficult to conceive how such a dissociation might occur. In view of the discovery of the role of $P-450_{c11}$ in mediating mineralocorticoid action, however, it is possible that non–receptor-mediated mechanisms might influence steroid hormone action in other tissues.

DISEASES OF THE ADRENAL CORTEX

Hypofunction

Adrenal insufficiency results from inadequate adrenocortical function, which may be due to destruction of the adrenal cortex (primary adrenal insufficiency, Addison's disease), deficient pituitary ACTH secretion (secondary adrenal insufficiency), or deficient hypothalamic secretion of CRH or other ACTH secretagogues (tertiary adrenal insufficiency). (Also see Chapter 6.) In 1855 Thomas Addison described the clinical features, natural history, and autopsy findings of the disease that now bears his name.[16] Its incidence is only about 40 to 60 cases per million adults,[789, 790] but it causes morbidity and frequent mortality. It can be reliably diagnosed and easily treated. Its symptoms of weakness, fatigue, weight loss, and gastrointestinal complaints are common to many disorders, so it must be considered in their differential diagnosis. Secondary adrenal insufficiency related to natural causes is also uncommon, but iatrogenic tertiary adrenal insufficiency caused by suppression of hypothalamic-pituitary-adrenal function by glucocorticoid administration is common.

Pathophysiology

Adrenal insufficiency is primary, secondary, or tertiary (Fig. 9–29). Primary adrenal insufficiency results from adrenal gland destruction or dysfunction caused by a local lesion or disease process. Secondary adrenal insufficiency is due to insufficient pituitary ACTH secretion and subsequent insufficient adrenal cortisol secretion. Tertiary adrenal insufficiency results from insufficient secretion of CRH or other hypothalamic ACTH secretagogues and secondary pituitary ACTH hyposecretion.

PRIMARY ADRENAL INSUFFICIENCY. In primary adrenal insufficiency, all three zones of the adrenal cortex are usually involved by a destructive process. The process can be local or, more commonly, a manifestation of systemic disorders. These disorders include autoimmune disease, either isolated or part of the polyglandular autoimmune syndrome; granulomatous diseases such as histoplasmosis and tuberculosis; metastatic malignancies such as lung and breast carcinoma; hemorrhage associated with anticoagulant therapy or meningococcemia; and rare hereditary diseases. The result is inadequate glucocorticoid, mineralocorticoid, and androgen secretion (see Fig. 9–29). Clinical signs and symptoms do not become manifest until at least 90% of the adrenocortical tissue is destroyed.[791, 792] Thus the onset of manifestations is usually gradual, going first through a stage of partial glucocorticoid deficiency that results only in inadequate cortisol increase in response to stress and rarely,

because of deficiencies of both glucocorticoid and epinephrine, mild postprandial hypoglycemia. Partial mineralocorticoid deficiency may be manifest only as mild transient postural hypotension. Complete glucocorticoid deficiency causes a variety of effects, including a decreased sense of well-being, gastrointestinal disturbances, and problems with glucose metabolism. Mineralocorticoid deficiency results in reduced renal potassium and hydrogen ion excretion and decreased sodium retention, the latter leading to decreased intravascular volume, hypotension, and dehydration. This is compounded by reduced peripheral vascular adrenergic tone because of glucocorticoid deficiency and can lead to vascular collapse and shock. Potassium retention leads to high serum potassium concentrations that can cause cardiac arrhythmias and death. A mild acidosis occurs, which contributes to the hyperkalemia by permitting potassium to shift from the intracellular to the extracellular space. Adrenal androgen deficiency is evident in women only as decreased pubic and axillary hair and decreased libido; men derive most androgens from the testes. Loss of adrenal epinephrine secretion may contribute to postprandial hypoglycemia.

The lack of cortisol negative feedback increases hypothalamic CRH synthesis and secretion, which stimulates increased synthesis and secretion of pituitary ACTH and other POMC-related peptides (see Fig. 9–29). These peptides are responsible for hyperpigmentation of the skin and mucous membranes. CRH and possibly other growth factors cause corticotrope hyperplasia, which, in the absence of adequate glucocorticoid replacement therapy, is occasionally evident on a pituitary computed tomographic (CT) scan[793, 794] and rarely can lead to an autonomous corticotrope adenoma.[795] However, ACTH secretion, although increased, usually retains a normal circadian rhythm[796] and is normally suppressed by glucocorticoid administration.

SECONDARY AND TERTIARY ADRENAL INSUFFICIENCY. In secondary adrenal insufficiency, cortisol production is inadequate because of inadequate pituitary ACTH secretion (see Fig. 9–29). As a result of decreased cortisol negative feedback inhibition, hypothalamic CRH synthesis and secretion and plasma CRH concentrations are increased.[229] In tertiary adrenal insufficiency, the defect is a lack of normal CRH secretion (see Fig. 9–29). The intrinsically normal pituitary can secrete ACTH in response to exogenous CRH.[797–799] In secondary and tertiary adrenal insufficiency, the clinical presentation is one of pure glucocorticoid deficiency and, in women, loss of adrenal androgen secretion. Because ACTH secretion is decreased rather than increased, patients are not hyperpigmented. Mineralocorticoid secretion usually remains normal because it is regulated by the renin-angiotensin system. Hence, hypotension, dehydration, and shock are seldom encountered, and adrenal crisis is a rarity. As with primary adrenal insufficiency, the process is usually gradual, going first through a stage of partial ACTH deficiency that results only in inadequate ACTH and cortisol responses to stress. With prolonged and more profound ACTH deficiency, the adrenal fasciculata and reticularis atrophy and lose their ability to respond acutely to ACTH. However, the adrenal cortex can recover the ability to produce cortisol in response to continuous maximal ACTH stimulation over a period of a few days to a week.

Clinical Presentation

The signs and symptoms depend on the rate and degree of loss of adrenal function, whether mineralocorticoid production is preserved, as it usually is in secondary and tertiary adrenal insufficiency, and the degree of physiological stress. Adrenal insufficiency is often insidious in onset and may go

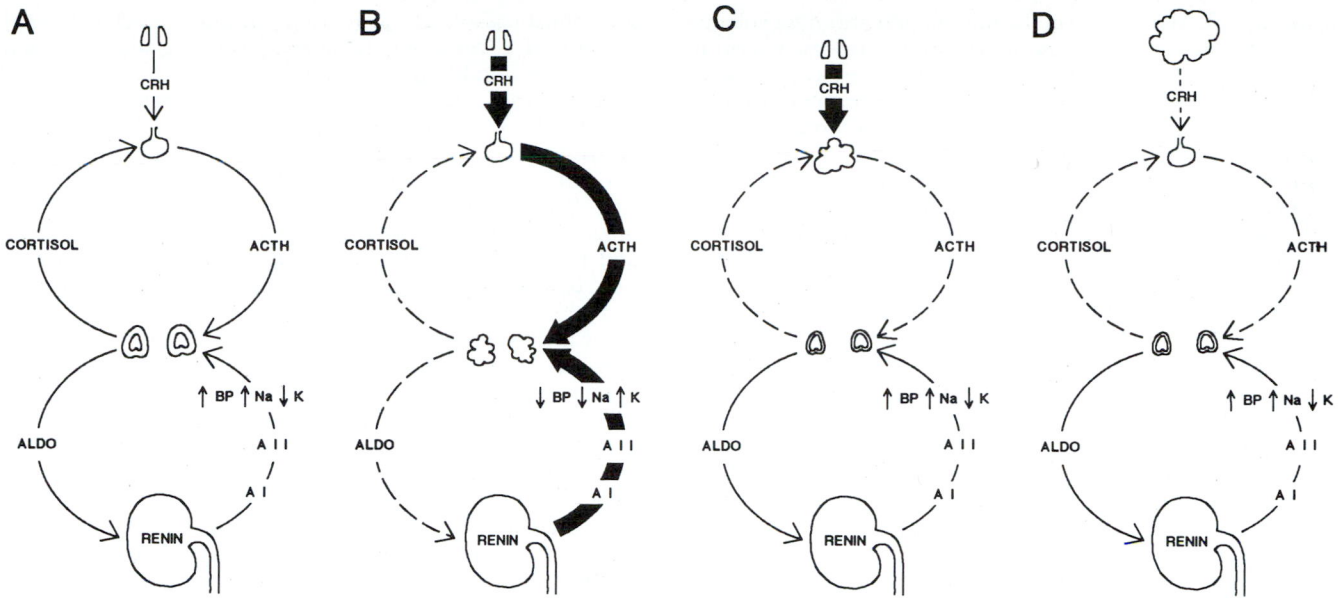

Figure 9–29. Hypothalamic-pituitary-adrenal and renin-angiotensin-aldosterone regulatory system function in (A) normal individuals and patients with (B) primary, (C) secondary, and (D) tertiary hypoadrenocorticism.

undetected until an intercurrent illness or stress precipitates a crisis.

ADRENAL CRISIS: ACUTE ADRENAL INSUFFICIENCY.
Primary Adrenal Insufficiency. Acute adrenal insufficiency, or adrenal crisis, usually presents as shock in a previously undiagnosed patient with primary adrenal insufficiency who has been subjected to a major physiological stress or in a patient with established adrenal insufficiency who does not increase glucocorticoid replacement during a bacterial infection or other major illness or cannot retain medication because of persistent vomiting resulting from viral gastroenteritis or other causes. In addition to shock, patients often have other nonspecific symptoms, such as anorexia, nausea, vomiting, abdominal pain, weakness, fatigue, lethargy, confusion, or coma (Table 9–6). Abdominal tenderness on deep palpation without localizing signs is due to an unknown cause. Fever is often present, is usually due to a precipitating infection, and may be exaggerated because of the hypocortisolemia. The abdominal pain and fever may lead to incorrect diagnosis of an acute surgical abdomen and potentially catastrophic surgical exploration without steroid replacement. Hypoglycemia rarely may be the presenting manifestation. Patients with long-standing adrenal insufficiency who are seen in crisis may be hyperpigmented and have weight loss and other symptoms of chronic adrenal insufficiency (see Table 9–6).[800]

It is important to recognize that the major pathophysi-

ology precipitating adrenal crisis is mineralocorticoid, not glucocorticoid, deficiency. In fact, adrenal crisis can occur in patients who are receiving physiological or even pharmacological dosages of synthetic glucocorticoids, if mineralocorticoid requirements are not met.[801] However, glucocorticoid deficiency can contribute to the hypotension, perhaps resulting from decreased sensitivity to angiotensin II and norepinephrine,[725] decreased synthesis of renin substrate,[728] and increased prostaglandin I_2 production.[728]

Adrenal crisis may also occur as a result of sudden, bilateral adrenal infarction associated with hemorrhage, embolus, or sepsis or, very rarely, adrenal vein thrombosis after a back injury.[802, 803] These patients do not have evidence of pre-existing adrenal insufficiency. Until the development of the CT scan, the diagnosis of adrenal hemorrhage was usually made at autopsy.[803] Presenting signs and symptoms are hypotension or shock (>90%); abdominal, flank, back, or lower chest pain (86%); fever (66%); anorexia, nausea, or vomiting (47%); neuropsychiatric manifestations such as confusion or disorientation (42%); and abdominal rigidity or rebound (22%).[802] Surprisingly, hypotension is observed in only about half of the patients before shock develops. Evidence of occult hemorrhage, such as a sudden fall in hemoglobin and hematocrit values, and progressive hyperkalemia, hyponatremia, and volume contraction should suggest the diagnosis. Major risk factors include anticoagulant therapy or coagulopathy, thromboembolic disease such as recurrent intravascular thrombosis, and the postoperative state. In patients treated with anticoagulants, clotting indices are usually within the therapeutic range and spontaneous bleeding elsewhere may not be evident.[802] This condition is difficult to recognize and must be considered whenever these symptoms develop in a patient with one or more risk factors. Without appropriate therapy, shock progresses to coma and death. Adrenal hemorrhage and often death have been associated with meningococcemia (Waterhouse-Friderichsen syndrome),[804] but *Pseudomonas aeruginosa* was the most common pathogen in 51 children dying of sepsis and bilateral adrenal hemorrhage.[805]

Chronic Secondary/Tertiary Adrenal Insufficiency. Adrenal crisis is uncommon in patients with secondary or tertiary adrenal insufficiency, because normal renin-angiotensin-al-

TABLE 9–6. Clinical and Laboratory Features Suggesting Adrenal Crisis in a Patient with Chronic Primary Adrenal Insufficiency

Dehydration, hypotension, or shock out of proportion to severity of current illness
Nausea and vomiting with a history of weight loss and anorexia
Abdominal pain, so-called acute abdomen
Unexplained hypoglycemia
Unexplained fever
Hyponatremia, hyperkalemia, azotemia, hypercalcemia, or eosinophilia
Hyperpigmentation or vitiligo
Other autoimmune endocrine deficiencies, such as hypothyroidism or gonadal failure

Adapted from Burke CW. Adrenocortical insufficiency. Clin Endocrinol Metab 1985; 14:947–976.

dosterone physiology is usually maintained and hypovolemia is rare. Hypoglycemia is the more common presentation in these patients, who often also have signs and symptoms of deficiency of other anterior pituitary hormones. Patients with pituitary apoplexy resulting from infarction of a large tumor usually complain of severe headache and may have acute visual loss or reduction in visual fields (see Chapter 6). Because glucocorticoids have a role in maintaining peripheral vascular adrenergic tone, sudden loss of ACTH secretion, particularly in conjunction with other serious illness, can lead to hypotension and shock.

CHRONIC ADRENAL INSUFFICIENCY. Patients with chronic primary adrenal insufficiency have manifestations of glucocorticoid, mineralocorticoid, and androgen deficiency. Patients with secondary or tertiary adrenal insufficiency generally maintain adequate mineralocorticoid function. The diagnosis is usually obvious in patients with the full-blown syndrome of adrenal insufficiency. However, the onset is often insidious, with gradual development of signs and symptoms, each of which, alone, is nonspecific. In the early stage, therefore, the disease presents a difficult differential diagnosis.

Primary Adrenal Insufficiency. The most common clinical features of chronic primary adrenal insufficiency are listed in Table 9–7.[790, 800, 806–808] Regardless of the immediate complaint, patients with adrenal insufficiency consistently have chronic weakness, fatigability, general malaise, lassitude, weight loss, and anorexia. The weakness is generalized, rather than being limited to particular muscle groups. The fatigue is worsened by exertion and improved with bed rest. Weight loss, which is due mostly to anorexia but partly to dehydration, may vary from 2 to as much as 15 kg but may not become evident until adrenal failure is well advanced.[806] Patients may exhibit extreme sensitivity to drugs, such as narcotics or anesthetics, and may recover slowly from illnesses or operations that do not themselves precipitate an adrenal crisis.

Gastrointestinal complaints, usually nausea, occasionally vomiting, abdominal pain, or diarrhea that may alternate

with constipation, are also common and correlate with the severity of adrenal insufficiency. Vomiting and abdominal pain often herald an adrenal crisis (see earlier). The mechanism of these gastrointestinal disorders has not been systematically investigated. Esophagogastroduodenoscopy and gastrointestinal radiographs are usually normal,[809] but gastric emptying time may be delayed.[810] Peptic ulcer disease is rare.[811] Steatorrhea, responsive to glucocorticoid replacement, has occasionally been reported in Addison's disease and has been studied in adrenalectomized rats, in which it may be due to decreased intestinal mucosal enzyme activity.[811, 812]

Cardiovascular symptoms include postural dizziness or syncope. In most patients the blood pressure is low, but initially only postural hypotension may be evident. Blood pressure control improves in patients with pre-existing hypertension. Thus the presence of systolic hypertension is strong evidence against a diagnosis of adrenal insufficiency.[806–808] Salt craving, sometimes with massive salt ingestion, is a distinctive feature in some patients.[808] Salt is often "chased" with lemon juice. Increased thirst for iced liquids is common.

The loss of the gluconeogenic effects of cortisol may appear, in adult patients, as hypoglycemia after prolonged fasting or, rarely, several hours after a high-carbohydrate meal.[806–808, 813] It is infrequent in adults in the absence of infection, fever, or alcohol ingestion. In contrast, hypoglycemia is common in infants and children with primary adrenal insufficiency[814] (see later) and in patients with secondary adrenal insufficiency associated with isolated ACTH deficiency.[800, 815] Hypoglycemia is thought to be due to increased peripheral glucose utilization associated with increased sensitivity to insulin[816] and impairment of gluconeogenesis, hepatic glucose production, and glycogen synthesis.[800] In addition, patients with adrenal insufficiency may tolerate greater degrees of hypoglycemia without developing symptoms.[813] Presumably other symptoms develop in patients with primary adrenal insufficiency or panhypopituitarism before symptomatic hypoglycemia occurs.

Patients are often aware of darkening of the skin. Hyperpigmentation, which is evident in most but not all[817] patients with primary adrenal insufficiency (see Table 9–7), is one of the characteristic physical findings (Fig. 9–30). It is caused by an increased content of melanin in the skin, which is thought to be due to the melanocyte-stimulating activity of the increased circulating POMC peptide levels, although it is not clear whether ACTH, β-LPH, or the combination of the two is responsible. In amphibians, α-MSH is the most potent melanotropin, but in reptiles β-LPH or any combination of the heptapeptide core common to all melanotropins plus the tetrapeptide COOH terminus of β-LPH or β-END is more potent.[217] Skin darkening in both of these species reflects acute dispersion of intracellular melanin granules within stellate cells called melanophores. In humans, hyperpigmentation is a more chronic process involving synthesis of melanin by epidermal melanocytes lying just subjacent to the basal cells. The melanin is packaged in secretory granules called melanosomes, which are phagocytosed by the basal cells of the epidermis.[818] The hormone primarily responsible for regulating this process in humans has not been established. The resulting brown hyperpigmentation is generalized but is most conspicuous in areas exposed to light, such as the face, neck, and backs of hands, and areas exposed to chronic mild trauma, friction, or pressure, such as the elbows, knees, spine, knuckles, waist (belt), midriff (girdle), and shoulders (brassiere straps). Patchy buccal pigmentation occurs on the inner surface of lips and the buccal mucosa along the line of dental occlusion, the site of repeated trauma (see Fig. 9–30). It may also occur

TABLE 9–7. Major Symptoms, Signs, and Laboratory Findings in Patients with Chronic Primary Adrenal Insufficiency

Symptom, Sign, or Laboratory Finding	Frequency (%)
Symptom	
Weakness, tiredness, fatigue	100
Anorexia	100
Gastrointestinal symptoms	92
Nausea	86
Vomiting	75
Constipation	33
Abdominal pain	31
Diarrhea	16
Salt craving	16
Postural dizziness	12
Muscle or joint pains	6–13
Sign	
Weight loss	100
Hyperpigmentation	94
Hypotension (systolic blood pressure <110 mm Hg)	88–94
Vitiligo	10–20
Auricular calcification	5
Laboratory Finding	
Electrolyte disturbances	92
Hyponatremia	88
Hyperkalemia	64
Hypercalcemia	6
Azotemia	55
Anemia	40
Eosinophilia	17

Compiled from Thorn,[808] Irvine and Barnes,[807] Nerup,[790] Jarvis et al.,[809] Dunlop,[806] and Burke.[800]

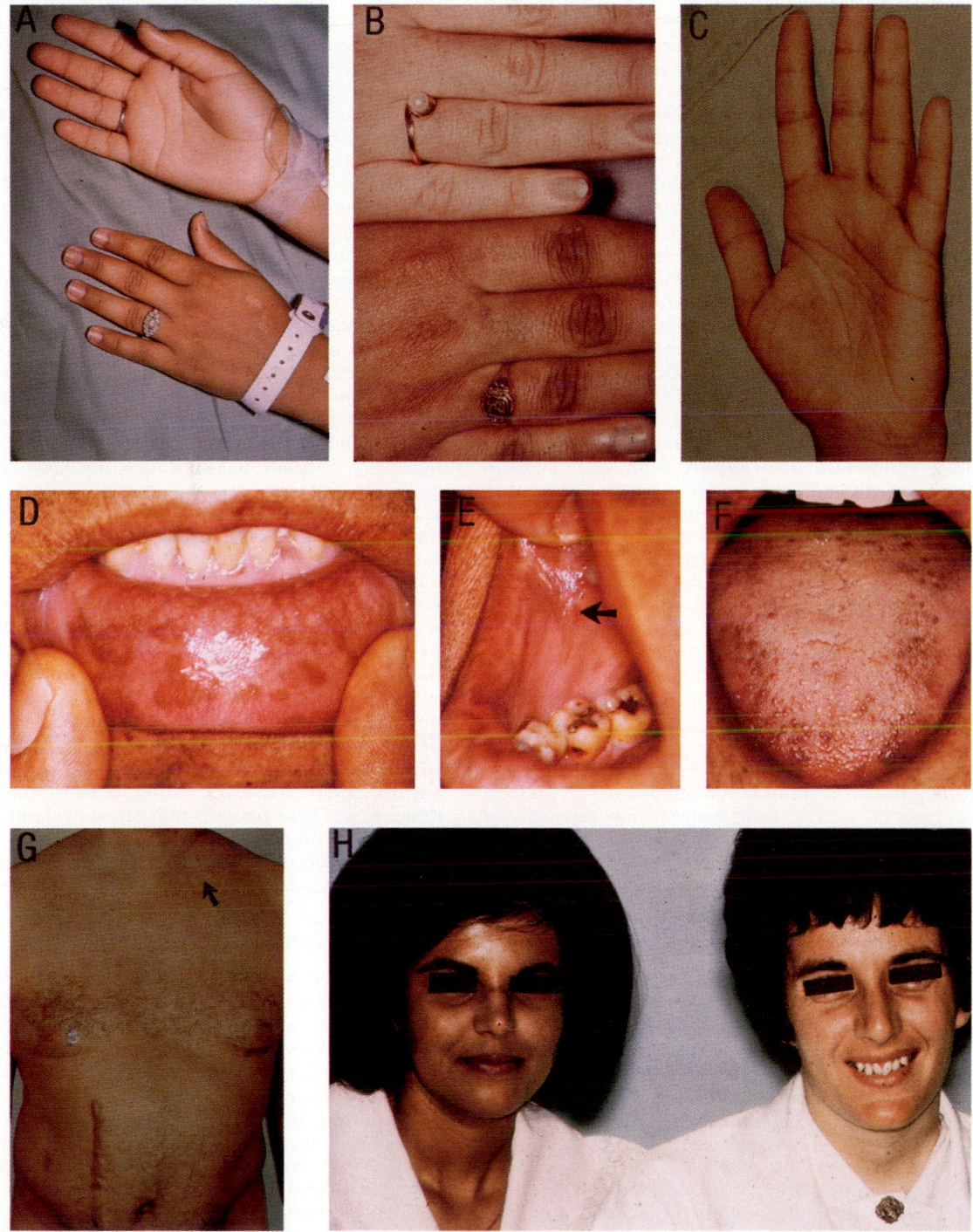

Figure 9–30. Cutaneous hyperpigmentation related to POMC-derived peptide hypersecretion. *A*, Hands of an 18-y-old girl with polyglandular autoimmune syndrome and Addison's disease. Note vitiligo above the left thumb. *B*, Hand of a 16-y-old girl with Nelson's syndrome 2 y after bilateral adrenalectomy for Cushing's disease, compared with a normal girl's hand. Note deep pigmentation of the knuckles. *C*, Hand of the same girl as in *B* at age 24. Note deep pigmentation of the palmar creases. *D*, Buccal pigmentation in 32-y-old man with tuberculous Addison's disease. Note clustering along the line of dental occlusion on the lower lip and inflammatory periodontal disease on the gums. *E*, Same as man in *D*. Note pigmentation in the cheek mucosa along the line of dental occlusion *(arrow)*. *F*, Pigmentation of the tongue in a 20-y-old girl with Nelson's syndrome 1 y after bilateral adrenalectomy for Cushing's disease. *G*, Pigmented scar from a right adrenalectomy in a 47-y-old man with Cushing's disease. The linear traumatic scar above the left medial clavicle that was formed before the onset of Cushing's disease *(arrow)* is nonpigmented. *H*, Generalized deep pigmentation in a 19-y-old white woman with Nelson's syndrome 5 y after bilateral adrenalectomy for Cushing's disease *(left)*, as contrasted with a normally pigmented woman *(right)*. (*B, C, F,* and *H* courtesy of Dr. H. Patrick Higgins.)

under the tongue, along the gingival border in patients with chronic periodontal disease, and on the hard palate. Generalized buccal, vaginal, and anal mucosal membrane hyperpigmentation may occur, but it is usually seen only in patients whose skin is normally pigmented, such as black persons and American Indians. Pigmentation is also prominent in the palmar creases, where it escapes being worn away by friction, and in areas that are normally pigmented, such as the areolae, axillae, perineum, and umbilicus[806–808] (see Fig. 9–30). Existing freckles (lentigines) become darker, and numerous new brown or black freckles may appear. Hyperpigmentation is less noticeable in black persons but a generalized darkening may be evident. Scars acquired during untreated primary adrenal insufficiency are permanently pigmented; those acquired before the onset of adrenal failure remain unpigmented, and those acquired after treatment do not become pigmented (see Fig. 9–30). The hair and nails may become darker, the nails showing longitudinal bands of darkening. The cutaneous hyperpigmentation begins to fade within several days and disappears after several weeks to a few months of adequate adrenal hormone replacement; fading on hair and nails takes longer, and scars never fade.

Patchy, often bilaterally symmetrical areas of depigmented skin, vitiligo, occur on the trunk or extremities in 10 to 20% of patients with autoimmune but not with other varieties of adrenal insufficiency (see Fig. 9–30).[807, 808]

Decreased axillary and pubic hair and loss of libido occur frequently in women but not in men because androgen production in women is principally from the adrenal glands.[807] Amenorrhea occurs in about 25% of women and may be due to the effects of chronic illness, weight loss, or autoimmune-mediated primary gonadal failure.[807]

Diffuse myalgias and arthralgias are common (see Table 9–7). Occasionally a patient may have predominantly musculoskeletal complaints and rarely flexion contractures of the lower extremities.[819, 820] Muscle enzymes and biopsy and electromyographic results are usually normal. Relief occurs rapidly with glucocorticoid and mineralocorticoid replacement, but reversal of the contractures may take several months and require orthopedic measures. Hyperkalemic neuromyopathy with symmetrical, ascending flaccid quadriplegia has been reported in a few patients with adrenal insufficiency.[821]

Calcification of the auricular cartilages may occur in long-standing primary or secondary adrenal insufficiency.[809, 822] A high incidence of multiple dental caries has been reported.[809]

Splenomegaly and lymphoid tissue hyperplasia, particularly of the tonsils, may occur.[800, 808] Patients with polyglandular autoimmune syndrome type I often have chronic moniliasis of the vagina, mouth, and, sometimes, nails that does not respond to replacement hormone therapy; antifungal agents afford only temporary relief.

Psychiatric symptoms are present in most patients with severe or long-standing adrenal insufficiency.[823] These may include (1) mild to moderate organic brain syndrome in 5 to 20%, usually impairment of memory that can progress to confusion, delirium, and stupor; (2) depression in 20 to 40%, manifested by apathy, poverty of thought, and lack of initiative; and (3) psychosis in 20 to 40%, manifested by social withdrawal, irritability, negativism, poor judgment, agitation, hallucinations, paranoid delusions, and bizarre or catatonic posturing. Perceptual disturbances, with enhanced sensitivity but impaired recognition and interpretation of auditory, tactile, gustatory, and olfactory stimuli, may also occur. These psychiatric manifestations occur early in the disease and may predate other physical findings, making the diagnosis of their etiology difficult. Most of these symptoms

disappear within a few days after adequate glucocorticoid therapy is initiated. However, the psychosis may persist for several months. Improvement does not correlate with correction of electrolyte imbalance except, on occasion, in patients with severe hyponatremia and organic brain syndrome.

In children the clinical presentation is similar to that of adults, except that weight loss is not as prominent.[824] They are usually short, ranging between the 3rd and 25th percentiles for their ages. Those with polyglandular autoimmune syndrome type I often have antecedent moniliasis of the mouth and nails and hypocalcemia associated with hypoparathyroidism,[825] whereas those with adrenoleukodystrophy or adrenomyeloneuropathy may initially have neurological symptoms.[826, 827] Neonates with primary adrenal insufficiency, which is usually due to congenital adrenal hypoplasia or adrenoleukodystrophy, are particularly susceptible to hypoglycemia.[814]

Secondary Adrenal Insufficiency. The clinical features of secondary adrenal insufficiency are similar to those of primary adrenal insufficiency with two major exceptions. First, hyperpigmentation is not present because plasma ACTH and other POMC peptide levels are not elevated. Second, dehydration is not present, and hypotension is less prominent.[800, 815] Weakness, fatigability, myalgias, arthralgias, and psychiatric changes are as common as in primary adrenal insufficiency, indicating that most of these symptoms are due to glucocorticoid rather than mineralocorticoid deficiency. However, gastrointestinal symptoms are less common,[800] suggesting that electrolyte disturbances may be involved in their etiology. Hypoglycemia is more common in secondary adrenal insufficiency.[800] This difference is not simply due to concomitant loss of GH secretion because hypoglycemia is the presenting feature in over a third of the cases with isolated ACTH deficiency.[800, 815] Perhaps hypoglycemia occurs frequently because, in the absence of dehydration and severe hypotension, these patients tolerate their illness longer and present with symptoms of chronic glucocorticoid deficiency rather than of mineralocorticoid deficiency. These patients may show evidence of a pituitary or hypothalamic tumor, such as signs and symptoms of hypersecretion or hyposecretion of other anterior pituitary hormones, headaches, or visual field defects (see Chapter 6).

Laboratory Findings

PRIMARY ADRENAL INSUFFICIENCY. *Hormonal Findings.* Cortisol secretion is low and does not increase normally with acute or chronic ACTH stimulation. Levels of plasma ACTH and other POMC-derived peptides, such as β-LPH and β-END, are elevated but still exhibit a normal diurnal rhythm.[796] Secretion of aldosterone, DHEA, DHEAS, and androsterone is low.[828, 829] The serum testosterone level is normal in men, because it is produced largely by the testes, but is low in women, in whom it is derived almost entirely from peripheral conversion of adrenal androgens.

An increased basal plasma AVP level is due partly to a decreased circulating volume and partly to a lower osmotic threshold for AVP secretion.[830] The increased AVP level results in impaired free water clearance, which is one of the causes of the hyponatremia. It also plays an important role in maintaining blood pressure in these patients, as demonstrated by the acute hypotensive effect of an AVP antagonist in adrenalectomized dogs.[733] Plasma ANF concentration is appropriately low.[831]

The volume depletion resulting from aldosterone deficiency causes increased plasma renin concentration and activity.[728] Glucocorticoid deficiency reduces angiotensinogen (renin substrate) levels,[728] but plasma concentrations of angiotensin II are increased[832] and, because of a direct peripheral vasoconstrictor effect, play an important role in maintaining blood pressure in Addison's disease.[833] Serum angiotensin-converting enzyme levels are also elevated.[834]

Serum thyroxine concentration is normal or low, and thyrotropin (TSH) concentration is often elevated. The levels of both may return to normal after several months of steroid replacement.[835] These changes may reflect associated autoimmune thyroiditis or be a direct effect of glucocorticoid deficiency.[800] The diagnosis of primary hypothyroidism cannot be established definitively at presentation, so the decision to begin thyroid hormone replacement must be based on clinical findings and the serum thyroxine level. Thyroid function must be re-evaluated after the adrenal insufficiency has been corrected. Modest hyperprolactinemia (up to 50 ng/L), with hyper-responsiveness to thyrotropin-releasing hormone, may be observed[800] and usually returns to normal after steroid replacement.

Other Findings. Electrolyte abnormalities are the rule[790, 800, 807] (see Table 9–7). Hyponatremia and hyperkalemia are present at diagnosis in 88 and 64%, respectively, of patients.[790] The hyperkalemia is due to aldosterone deficiency. The hyponatremia, which occurs mostly with glucocorticoid deficiency, is caused by elevated AVP levels and the resulting increased free water retention,[830] decreased sodium pump activity and the resulting shift of extracellular sodium into cells,[836] and decreased delivery of filtrate to diluting segments of the nephron as a result of decreased glomerular filtration rate.[837] Mild hyperchloremic acidosis and increased blood urea nitrogen/creatinine ratio are a result of prerenal azotemia associated with dehydration and decreased cardiac output.[800, 807] Mild to moderate hypercalcemia has been reported in up to 6% of patients.[838] Elevated levels of calcium-binding proteins resulting from hemoconcentration are a factor, but volume repletion with saline does not restore the calcium concentration to normal, for which glucocorticoid replacement therapy is required.[839]

Serum levels of hepatic aspartate transaminase may be elevated but fall to normal after a few days of glucocorticoid replacement.[800] The fasting blood glucose value is usually in the low-normal range, but occasionally fasting or, rarely, postprandial hypoglycemia may occur.

Mild to moderate eosinophilia, relative lymphocytosis, and anemia are common. The normocytic, normochromic anemia, which may initially be masked by hemoconcentration, is probably a direct effect of glucocorticoid deficiency.[800] A macrocytic anemia may occur in patients with polyglandular autoimmune syndrome and associated pernicious anemia. Some patients also have neutropenia, which presumably is caused by increased sequestration of neutrophils in the marginal pool.[800]

Electrocardiographic abnormalities are frequently seen in adrenal insufficiency. Hyperkalemia is responsible for peaked T waves, low P waves, and wide QRS complexes and, in the extreme case, atrial asystole, intraventricular block, and, ultimately, ventricular asystole.[820] Other abnormalities, including flattened or inverted T waves, prolonged Q-T$_c$ interval, and low QRS voltage, are due to glucocorticoid deficiency because they occur when the electrolyte levels are normal and are reversed by glucocorticoid replacement.[800, 840]

SECONDARY ADRENAL INSUFFICIENCY. The laboratory findings in secondary adrenal insufficiency are the same as those in primary adrenal insufficiency, except that (1) plasma ACTH levels are not elevated, (2) hyperkalemia does not occur and azotemia is less common in the unstressed patient because of continued mineralocorticoid secretion, (3) hypoglycemia is more common,[800, 815] and (4) hypercalcemia is less common.[800] Hyponatremia does occur in secondary adrenal insufficiency, largely because of increased AVP levels.[800]

Radiological Findings

PRIMARY ADRENAL INSUFFICIENCY. Adrenal enlargement associated with tuberculosis or other granulomatous diseases, metastatic cancer, or hemorrhage may be seen on abdominal CT scans[802, 841] but not in patients with autoimmune adrenal destruction (Fig. 9–31).[809] Chest x-ray films frequently reveal a small heart.[790, 809] In chronic untreated or inadequately treated primary adrenal insufficiency, the sella turcica may be enlarged on skull x-ray films[809, 842] and CT scan may reveal pituitary enlargement that is reversible with steroid treatment.[793] This is usually due to corticotrope hyperplasia,[794] but rarely an ACTH-secreting adenoma can develop.[795]

SECONDARY AND TERTIARY ADRENAL INSUFFICIENCY. Adrenal atrophy cannot reliably be demonstrated by CT or magnetic resonance imaging (MRI) scan. Primary or metastatic mass lesions in the hypothalamus, median eminence, or pituitary fossa can usually be detected by CT or MRI scan (see Chapter 6).

Pathogenesis

PRIMARY ADRENAL INSUFFICIENCY. When Addison first described the clinical manifestations and autopsy findings in primary adrenal insufficiency,[16] bilateral adrenal destruction by tuberculosis was the most common cause and remained so until the advent of effective treatment for tuberculosis. Today, tuberculosis causes only about 20% of cases, autoimmune destruction accounts for about 75%, and the remainder are due to other granulomatous or fungal diseases, replacement by metastatic cancer, or adrenal hemorrhage.[806, 807, 843] However, disseminated tuberculosis and fungal infections are still major causes of adrenal insufficiency in populations that have a high prevalence of these diseases.[844, 845] Similarly, bilateral metastatic disease is probably the most common cause on oncology services.

Autoimmune Adrenalitis. What previously was known as idiopathic primary adrenal insufficiency appears to be the result of an autoimmune process that destroys the adrenal cortex. Evidence of both humoral and cell-mediated immune mechanisms directed at the adrenal cortex, including lymphocytic infiltration of the adrenal glands, is found in association with autoimmune destruction of other endocrine glands and a genetic predisposition manifested by familial aggregation and increased prevalence of certain human leukocyte antigen (HLA) subtypes. (Also see Chapter 31.)

Patients with autoimmune adrenal insufficiency associated with polyglandular autoimmune syndrome at all ages are predominantly female (70%). In contrast, patients with isolated autoimmune adrenal insufficiency are predominantly male (71%) in the first two decades of life, equally male and female in the third decade, and predominantly female (81%) thereafter.[846] The explanation for these sex-related differences is unknown.

Humoral Immunity. Antibodies that react with all three zones of the adrenal cortex have been identified by complement fixation or immunofluorescence techniques. They are found in the serum of 60 to 70% of patients with idiopathic primary adrenal insufficiency but rarely in serum from patients with other causes of adrenal insufficiency, from first-degree relatives of patients with idiopathic primary adrenal insufficiency who themselves have no autoimmune endocrine disease, or from normal subjects.[807, 838, 847-849] Antibodies are more common in women, particularly those with polyglandular autoimmune syndrome. After onset of overt

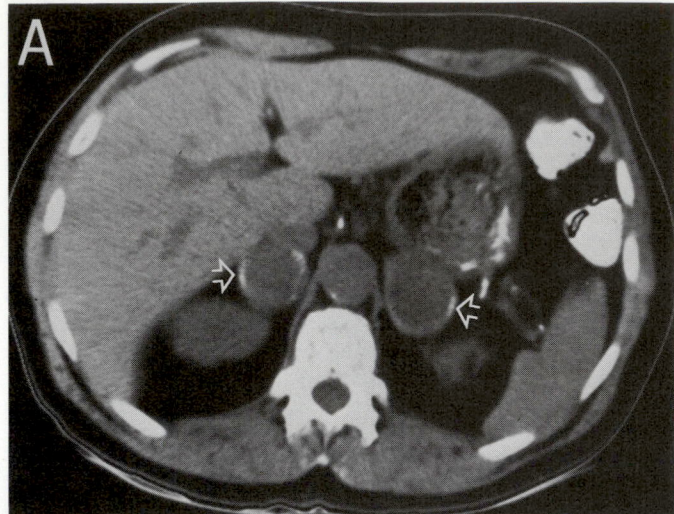

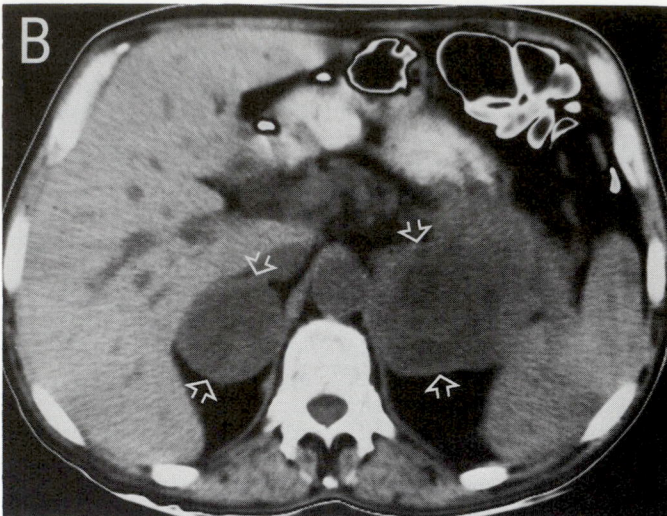

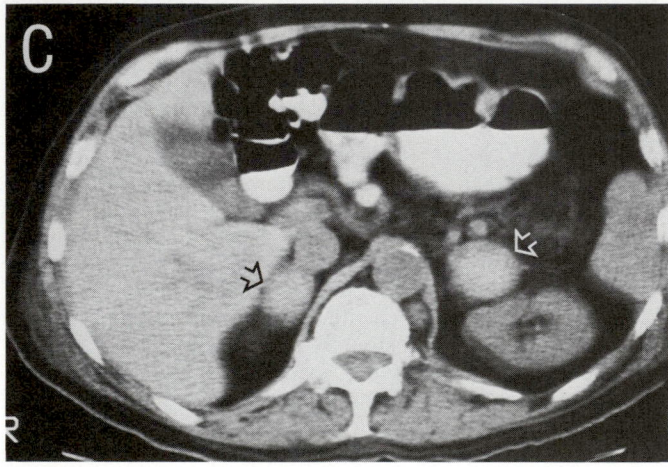

Figure 9–31. CT scans of patients with primary adrenal insufficiency. The affected adrenal glands are indicated by arrows. *A,* CT scan of a 59-y-old man with histoplasmosis. Note the subcapsular calcium in both glands. *B,* CT scan of a 59-y-old man with metastatic melanoma. *C,* CT scan of an 80-y-old man with bilateral adrenal hemorrhage resulting from anticoagulation for pulmonary emboli. (*A* and *B* courtesy of Dr. William D. Salmon; *C* courtesy of Dr. Craig R. Sussman.)

adrenal insufficiency, the titers progressively decrease and sometimes disappear completely. Some patients with other autoimmune endocrine diseases but without adrenal insufficiency also have antiadrenal antibodies (Table 9–8). The presence of antiadrenal antibodies seems to precede the development of adrenal insufficiency by several years.[850, 851] Not all patients who have antiadrenal antibodies have adrenal insufficiency, but as a group subjects with antiadrenal antibodies develop adrenal insufficiency at a rate of up to 19% per year.[851] The first sign of adrenal insufficiency is an increase in plasma renin activity in association with a normal or low serum aldosterone level, which suggests that the zona glomerulosa is affected initially.[851, 852] After several months to years, zona fasciculata dysfunction becomes evident, first by a decreased plasma cortisol response to ACTH, later by

an increased basal plasma ACTH level, and finally by a decreased plasma cortisol level and overt symptoms.[850, 851]

The nature of the antigens with which the antiadrenal antibodies react is unknown, but they are located in adrenal microsomes and/or plasma membranes.[853] Some antiadrenal antibodies are directed at an adrenal-specific 55-kd microsomal protein.[854] Immunoglobulins from most patients with autoimmune adrenal insufficiency block the stimulatory effect of ACTH on adrenal cortisol production and DNA synthesis in vitro.[855] They may bind to the ACTH receptor or interfere with ACTH binding to the receptor, as proposed for TSH receptor–blocking antibodies in atrophic thyroiditis.[856]

Cell-Mediated Immunity. Cell-mediated immune processes may also be important in the development of adrenal insufficiency. Decreased suppressor T lymphocyte function[857] and increased levels of circulating Ia-positive T lymphocytes[858] have been described in patients with idiopathic adrenal insufficiency. Human adrenal homogenates inhibited the in vitro migration of leukocytes from 14 of 30 patients with idiopathic adrenal insufficiency but from only 1 of 7 patients with tuberculous adrenal insufficiency,[859] and activated mouse macrophages blocked ACTH-induced steroidogenesis in cultured rabbit adrenocortical cells.[860] Evidence of lymphocytic infiltration of the adrenal glands further supports this concept.[861]

Associated Endocrine Autoimmunity. Antibodies against other endocrine glands are common in patients with autoimmune adrenal insufficiency but rare in control pop-

TABLE 9–8. Incidence of Antiadrenal Antibodies in Patients with Nonadrenal Autoimmune Endocrine Diseases

Autoimmune Endocrine Disease	Incidence of Antiadrenal Antibodies (%)
Hypoparathyroidism	16
Hashimoto's thyroiditis	1.9
Diabetes mellitus	1.2
Thyrotoxicosis	1.9
Atrophic hypothyroidism	1.7
Pernicious anemia	<1

Compiled from Irvine and Barnes,[807] Ketchum et al.,[864] Blizzard et al.,[862] Scherbaum and Berg,[865] Betterle et al.,[851] and Nerup.[790]

TABLE 9–9. Incidence of Autoantibodies in Patients with Autoimmune Adrenal Insufficiency

Tissue	Incidence of Antibodies (%)
Adrenal	60–70
Thyroid microsomal	50
Parathyroid	26
Islet cell	8
Gonad	
Ovary	22
Testes	5
Stomach	
Parietal cell	30
Intrinsic factor	9

Compiled from Irvine et al.,[849] Blizzard et al.,[847] McHardy-Young et al.,[863] Irvine and Barnes,[807] and Blizzard et al.[862]

ulations (Table 9–9).[807, 847, 849, 862, 863] Thyroid microsomal antibodies are present in about 50% of the patients. Of this group, half have overt hypothyroidism and most of the others have subclinical hypothyroidism (i.e., increased serum TSH levels, normal serum thyroxine levels, and exaggerated responses to thyrotropin-releasing hormone) and are at risk for later development of overt hypothyroidism.[847, 849, 863] The increased incidence of gastric parietal cell and intrinsic factor antibodies correlates with atrophic gastritis and pernicious anemia, respectively. The presence of antigonadal antibodies correlates with premature ovarian failure in women. Antigonadal antibodies are less common in men, as is the incidence of gonadal failure. The incidence of antiadrenal antibodies in serum from patients with other autoimmune endocrine diseases but not adrenal insufficiency is low (<2%) except in subjects with hypoparathyroidism (16%) (see Table 9–8).[807, 851, 862, 864, 865]

Associated Disorders: Polyglandular Autoimmune Syndromes. About 50% of the patients with autoimmune adrenal insufficiency have one or more other autoimmune or endocrine disorders (Table 9–10).[790, 807, 847, 863] On the other hand, patients with the more common autoimmune endocrine disorders, such as insulin-dependent diabetes mellitus or thyroid diseases, rarely develop adrenal insufficiency. The disorders associated with autoimmune adrenal insufficiency are referred to as polyglandular autoimmune syndrome types I and II and by many other names.[825, 866–868] A third type of polyglandular autoimmune syndrome is not associated with adrenal insufficiency and will not be discussed further here (see Chapter 31).

Polyglandular autoimmune syndrome type I is a rare syndrome, inherited in an autosomal recessive pattern, in which females are affected slightly more frequently (0.8 to 1.7 times) than males.[825, 846, 866–868] Hypoparathyroidism or mucocutaneous candidiasis is usually the first manifestation and characteristically appears during childhood or early

adolescence, always by the early 20s (Table 9–11).[825, 846, 866–868] The candidiasis is chronic or recurrent, relatively resistant to conventional therapy, almost always involves the mouth,[866] but may involve just the nail beds or may be widespread. Adrenal insufficiency usually develops later, at a mean age of 12 to 13. About half of patients develop all three of these features, if followed carefully.[866] Diabetes mellitus is relatively infrequent. Autoimmune thyroid disease is uncommon: atrophic thyroiditis and Hashimoto's thyroiditis are seen with equal frequency, and Graves' disease is not associated with this syndrome. Other endocrine and nonendocrine autoimmune disorders are even less common (see Table 9–11). In a series of 68 Finnish patients,[866] the incidence of various manifestations was different from that reported in smaller series and in reviews of the literature, diabetes mellitus being 12 times more prevalent, for example. Furthermore, manifestations of ectodermal dysplasia, including dental enamel hypoplasia, pitted dystrophy of the nails, keratopathy, and calcified plaques on the tympanic membranes, were present in one third to two thirds of the patients. These differences may reflect a peculiar variant of the disorder or represent a more complete description of the several components of the syndrome.

In the more common polyglandular autoimmune syndrome type II, primary adrenal insufficiency is the principal manifestation.[825, 867, 868] Autoimmune thyroid disease, usually Hashimoto's or atrophic thyroiditis but occasionally Graves' disease, and insulin-dependent diabetes mellitus are common (see Table 9–11). Patients with autoimmune thyroid disease or diabetes mellitus who have adrenal autoantibodies but do not yet have adrenal insufficiency and relatives who have one or more components of the syndrome should also be included. About half of the cases are familial, but various modes of inheritance have been reported.[825, 846, 867] Women are affected 1.8 times more frequently than men.[825, 867] Onset

TABLE 9–10. Incidence of Other Endocrine and Autoimmune Diseases in Patients with Autoimmune Adrenal Insufficiency*

Disease	Incidence (%)
Thyroid disease	
Hypothyroidism	8
Nontoxic goiter	7
Thyrotoxicosis	7
Gonadal failure	
Ovarian	20
Testicular	2
Insulin-dependent diabetes mellitus	11
Hypoparathyroidism	10
Pernicious anemia	5
None	53

*Total number = 365.
Compiled from Irvine and Barnes,[807] Blizzard et al.,[847] and Nerup.[790]

TABLE 9–11. Clinical Manifestations of Polyglandular Autoimmune Syndromes Associated with Adrenal Insufficiency

Disorder	Prevalence (%)
Type I	
ENDOCRINE	
Hypoparathyroidism	89
Chronic mucocutaneous candidiasis	75
Adrenal insufficiency	60
Gonadal failure	45
Hypothyroidism	12
Insulin-dependent diabetes mellitus	1
Hypopituitarism	<1
Diabetes insipidus	<1
NONENDOCRINE	
Malabsorption syndromes	25
Alopecia totalis or areata	20
Pernicious anemia	16
Chronic active hepatitis	9
Vitiligo	4
Type II	
ENDOCRINE	
Adrenal insufficiency	100
Autoimmune thyroid disease	70
Insulin-dependent diabetes mellitus	50
Gonadal failure	5–50
Diabetes insipidus	<1
NONENDOCRINE	
Vitiligo	4
Alopecia, pernicious anemia, myasthenia gravis, immune thrombocytopenic purpura, Sjögren's syndrome, rheumatoid arthritis	<1

Modified from Leshin M. Polyglandular autoimmune syndromes. Am J Med Sci 1985; 290:77–88; and Neufeld M, Maclaren NK, Blizzard RM. Two types of autoimmune Addison's disease associated with different polyglandular autoimmune (PGA) syndromes. Medicine 1981; 60:355–362.

ranges from childhood to late adulthood, most cases occurring between ages 20 and 40.[790, 825, 846] Adrenal insufficiency is the initial manifestation in about 50% of patients, occurs simultaneously with thyroiditis or diabetes mellitus in about 20%, and follows their development in about 30%.[790, 846, 867] Hypogonadism may occur first and, as in type I syndrome, ovarian failure is more frequent than testicular failure.[790, 825, 867] Hypoparathyroidism is not seen in this syndrome, and alopecia and pernicious anemia occur much less frequently than in type I syndrome. Other nonendocrine autoimmune disorders, such as vitiligo, myasthenia gravis, thrombocytopenic purpura, Sjögren's syndrome, rheumatoid arthritis, and primary antiphospholipid syndrome (recurrent deep vein thrombosis with antibodies to cardiolipin), are occasionally associated.[825, 867, 869] Serositis with pericardial and/or pleural involvement has been reported.[870]

Genetics. Autoimmune adrenal insufficiency may be familial or nonfamilial. It is less likely to be familial when it occurs alone: about one third of such patients have affected family members, whereas about one half of patients with adrenal insufficiency as part of polyglandular autoimmune syndrome type I or II have positive family histories.[790, 825, 846, 867] Polyglandular autoimmune syndrome type I is inherited as an autosomal recessive trait, whereas pedigrees compatible with autosomal recessive, autosomal dominant, or polygenic inheritance have been reported for polyglandular autoimmune syndrome type II.[825, 846, 867, 871]

Genetic susceptibility to autoimmune adrenal insufficiency is strongly linked with HLA-B8, HLA-DR3, and HLA-DR4 alleles, except when adrenal insufficiency occurs as part of polyglandular autoimmune syndrome type I, in which no HLA association has been found.[825, 872, 873] Similar HLA associations are seen in patients with insulin-dependent diabetes mellitus, which implies a common pathogenesis. However, some families with polyglandular autoimmune syndrome type II do not have a demonstrated HLA linkage.[871, 872] Furthermore, Hashimoto's thyroiditis, pernicious anemia, and premature primary gonadal failure, all components of polyglandular autoimmune syndrome type II, do not have a strong HLA linkage.[872, 873] These observations suggest that a gene or genes linked to certain HLA antigens convey susceptibility to autoimmune adrenal insufficiency and diabetes mellitus and that different non–HLA-associated genes are involved in thyroid and gastric autoimmune disease and in polyglandular autoimmune syndrome type I.

Pathology. In long-standing disease, the adrenal glands are small and sometimes difficult to locate. The capsule is thickened and fibrotic. The cortex is completely destroyed, although a few small clusters of residual adrenocortical cells may be surrounded by lymphocytes. The medulla is relatively spared. In early stages, the glands may be enlarged, with extensive lymphocytic infiltration.[848, 861, 874] Adrenal insufficiency becomes clinically manifest only when at least 90% of the cortex is destroyed.[791, 792] Patients with other associated autoimmune endocrine diseases have lymphocytic infiltration and varying degrees of destruction and fibrosis of the involved glands.[848]

Infectious Adrenalitis. Tuberculosis can destroy the adrenal glands. The incidence of tuberculous primary adrenal insufficiency in most countries has decreased in the past few decades from about 80 to 20% because of effective prevention and drug treatment of tuberculosis.[806, 807, 843] Tuberculous adrenalitis results from hematogenous spread from active infection elsewhere in the body.[874] Extra-adrenal tuberculosis usually is evident but may be clinically latent.[841, 874] Adrenal destruction is gradual. The medulla is more frequently destroyed than the cortex for unknown reasons.[874] The adrenal glands are usually enlarged in the early stage of the disease, often enough to be demonstrable on CT scans,[841]

and become completely replaced by caseous nodules and fibrosis.[874] After about 2 y of adrenal insufficiency, the adrenals become normal or small in size.[841] Calcifications can be seen radiographically in 50% of cases[809, 841] (see Fig. 9–31). However, absence of enlarged or calcified adrenal glands does not exclude tuberculosis as the cause of adrenal insufficiency.

Disseminated fungal infections can involve the adrenal glands and cause adrenal insufficiency. Histoplasmosis[875] and paracoccidioidomycosis (South American blastomycosis)[844, 876] have a predilection for the adrenal glands and are important causes of adrenal insufficiency in endemic areas. In contrast, cryptococcosis,[877] coccidioidomycosis,[878] and North American blastomycosis[879] are rare causes. The adrenal glands are enlarged and may become calcified. Recovery of adrenal function after prolonged antifungal treatment has been reported.[880, 881]

Syphilis causes adrenal insufficiency rarely. The adrenals are sclerotic, with gumma formation and demonstrable spirochetes.[874]

Metastatic Replacement. Infiltration of the adrenal glands by metastatic cancer is common, probably because of the ample sinusoidal blood supply. Most autopsy series find adrenal metastases in 40 to 60% of patients with disseminated lung or breast cancer, 30% with melanoma (see Fig. 9–31), and 14 to 20% with stomach or colon cancer, but clinically recognized adrenal insufficiency is uncommon.[792, 882–884] Lymphoma often involves the adrenals but rarely causes adrenal insufficiency.[885] The incidence of clinical adrenal insufficiency may be low partly because most of the adrenal cortex must be destroyed before hypofunction becomes evident[791, 792] and partly because the symptoms may mistakenly be attributed to cancer. In fact, two small studies have suggested that a fifth to a third of patients with bilateral adrenal metastases have partial adrenal insufficiency and benefit from glucocorticoid treatment.[883, 884]

Miscellaneous Causes. **Acquired Immunodeficiency Syndrome.** Endocrine abnormalities are common in asymptomatic patients who are positive for human immunodeficiency virus (HIV) and those with acquired immunodeficiency syndrome (AIDS), but the adrenocortical abnormalities are of most clinical significance.[886] The adrenal glands often show a necrotizing adrenalitis associated with cytomegalovirus infection, but infections with *Mycobacterium avium-intracellulare* or *Cryptococcus* and involvement with metastatic Kaposi's sarcoma also occur.[887] Adrenal insufficiency has been reported in patients with AIDS.[888] Frank adrenal insufficiency is uncommon and basal cortisol levels are often elevated. However, decreased cortisol responses to the short ACTH stimulation test occur in 8 to 14% of AIDS patients, and most AIDS patients have decreased adrenal reserve as measured by the cortisol response to prolonged (3-d) ACTH stimulation.[889, 890] In addition, there is a defect in 17-deoxysteroid production by the zona fasciculata.[890] Even patients with AIDS-related complex may have a subnormal cortisol response to ACTH administration.[890] Thus all HIV-infected patients are at risk for developing overt adrenal insufficiency.

Some drugs used to treat the opportunistic infections in AIDS, such as ketoconazole, which inhibits cortisol synthesis,[891] and rifampin, which increases cortisol metabolism,[540, 892] may precipitate adrenal crisis in patients with unsuspected partial adrenal insufficiency.[893]

Adrenoleukodystrophy and Adrenomyeloneuropathy. These inherited disorders are characterized by progressive neurological dysfunction and primary adrenal insufficiency. These disorders are caused by abnormal fatty acid metabolism that leads to accumulation of very-long-chain saturated fatty acids as cholesterol esters and gangliosides in the brain, adrenal cortex, and other organs.[827] Adrenoleukodystrophy begins in childhood and progresses rapidly to dementia, blindness, and quadriparesis. Adrenomyeloneuropathy begins in adolescence and early adulthood with weakness, spasticity, and distal polyneuropathy as the initial complaints. It is milder and more slowly progressive.[826, 827] Both disorders are transmitted as X-linked recessive traits, so most affected individuals are males. It was thought that the neurological symptoms of both disorders developed before adrenal insufficiency, but five of eight boys with idiopathic adrenal insufficiency were found to have adrenomyeloneuropathy.[894] Thus adrenomyeloneuropathy should be considered in any boy presenting with adrenal insufficiency. Therapy with dietary oleic acid may be of benefit.[895]

Congenital Adrenal Hypoplasia. In this rare familial condition the adult adrenal cortex does not develop normally. The disorder is seen at birth with any of four forms of primary adrenal insufficiency: (1) a sporadic form associated with pituitary hypoplasia, (2) an autosomal recessive form, (3) an X-linked cytomegalic form associated with hypogonadotropic hypogonadism, and (4) an X-linked form associated with glycerol kinase deficiency, psychomotor retardation, and, in most cases, muscular dystrophy.[896]

Familial Glucocorticoid Deficiency. In this rare disorder the secretion of glucocorticoid and androgen is deficient and unresponsive to ACTH stimulation. Mineralocorticoid secretion is normal or only partially deficient and responds to postural stimuli and volume depletion.[897] The disorder is usually seen in childhood with hyperpigmentation, muscle weakness, hypoglycemia, and seizures and may be associated with achalasia and alacrima.[897, 898] Its etiology is not known, but a defect at the level of the ACTH receptor has been proposed.

Defective Cholesterol Metabolism. Most cortisol is synthesized from cholesterol provided to the adrenals by circulating LDL.[79] Therefore, patients with no LDL, such as those with abetalipoproteinemia,[91, 92] or with no LDL receptors, such as those with homozygous familial hypercholesterolemia,[93] have a moderately impaired cortisol response to ACTH, although they maintain normal basal cortisol production and do not have clinically significant adrenal insufficiency. The hypocholesterolemic drug lovastatin, which inhibits cholesterol biosynthesis at the HMG-CoA reductase step, does not further impair adrenal function in patients with familial hypercholesterolemia.[899]

Drugs. A number of drugs may cause adrenal insufficiency by inhibiting cortisol biosynthesis, such as the antiepileptic aminoglutethimide,[171, 900] the anesthetic etomidate,[182] the antimycotic ketoconazole,[891] the glucocorticoid biosynthesis–inhibiting metyrapone,[172] and the antiparasitic suramin.[901, 902] These agents usually do not produce clinical adrenal insufficiency in subjects with normal hypothalamic-pituitary-adrenal function, because enzyme inhibition is incomplete and increased ACTH secretion overrides the blockade. However, patients with limited pituitary or adrenal reserve may develop symptomatic adrenal insufficiency. Other drugs accelerate the metabolism of cortisol and of most synthetic steroids by inducing hepatic mixed-function oxygenase enzymes. Such agents include phenytoin,[892, 903] barbiturates,[892] and rifampin.[540, 892] These agents can provoke adrenal insufficiency in patients with limited pituitary or adrenal reserve and those with adrenal insufficiency who are receiving replacement steroids.

SECONDARY ADRENAL INSUFFICIENCY. *Panhypopituitarism.* Any process that involves the pituitary and interferes with the ability to secrete ACTH will cause secondary adrenal insufficiency. Large pituitary tumors or craniopharyngiomas, infectious diseases such as tuberculosis or histoplasmosis, infiltrative diseases, lymphocytic hypophysitis, head trauma, and large intracranial artery aneurysms can destroy the normal pituitary tissue. Pituitary metastases are frequent (about 5%) in patients with disseminated cancer at autopsy but rarely disrupt hormone secretion.[904] Pituitary infarction may occur at the time of delivery if excessive blood is lost and if hypotension occurs (Sheehan's syndrome) or with hemorrhage into a pituitary tumor (pituitary apoplexy). These patients usually have evidence of other pituitary hormone deficiencies.

Isolated ACTH Deficiency. Isolated ACTH deficiency is rare.[815] The defect probably is at the pituitary level because there is no ACTH-secretory response to CRH, as usually occurs in hypothalamic disorders.[905] The disorder has multiple causes, but its frequent association with other autoimmune endocrine disorders, the fact that lymphocytic hypophysitis and selective corticotrope absence are a common accompaniment,[906] the finding of antipituitary antibodies in the serum of 10 of 21 patients in one series,[907] and the description of anticorticotrope antibodies in the serum of one patient[908] suggest that most occurrences are due to an autoimmune process.

TERTIARY ADRENAL INSUFFICIENCY. *Chronic Pharmacological Administration of Glucocorticoids*. Suppression of hypothalamic-pituitary-adrenal function by chronic administration of pharmacological dosages of glucocorticoids is the most common cause of adrenal insufficiency. It decreases CRH synthesis by and secretion from the hypothalamus and blocks its tropic and secretagogue actions on the pituitary corticotropes. This results in decreased synthesis of ACTH by the anterior pituitary corticotropes, which decrease in size and in the amount of stored ACTH. Eventually, the number of identifiable corticotropes decreases.[909] In the absence of ACTH stimulation, the adrenal zonae fasciculata and reticularis atrophy and can no longer secrete cortisol. However, cortisol production can be restored after prolonged ACTH administration, a feature that is used to distinguish primary from secondary adrenal insufficiency. Another important difference is that the adrenals retain nearly normal mineralocorticoid secretion because this function depends mostly on the renin-angiotensin system rather than on ACTH. This condition is treated in greater detail later in this chapter.

After Cure of Cushing's Syndrome. Tertiary adrenal insufficiency also occurs in patients who are cured of Cushing's syndrome by removal of a pituitary or nonpituitary ACTH-secreting or adrenal cortisol-secreting tumor. The chronic endogenous hypercortisolemia suppresses the hypothalamic-pituitary-adrenal axis in the same manner as exogenous glucocorticoids.

Other Causes. Any process that involves the hypothalamus and interferes with CRH secretion can cause tertiary adrenal insufficiency. Such processes include tumors, infiltrative diseases such as sarcoidosis, and cranial radiation. The CRH test can be used to distinguish between secondary and tertiary adrenal insufficiency. In patients with a pituitary defect, the ACTH-secretory response to CRH is inappropriately low or absent, whereas in those with a hypothalamic defect, this response is usually exaggerated and prolonged.[191, 910]

Diagnosis

DIFFERENTIAL DIAGNOSIS. When classic signs and symptoms of advanced disease are present, the diagnosis of adrenal insufficiency is obvious. However, the diagnosis often is not immediately apparent, because the early symptoms, such as fatigue and lassitude, are nonspecific. Consequently, the diagnosis is sometimes overlooked while other possibilities are pursued. The weight loss and gastrointestinal complaints often raise suspicion of gastric carcinoma. Even the hyperpigmentation is not always reliable, because primary adrenal insufficiency can occur without hyperpigmentation[817] and because hyperpigmentation can be caused by antineoplastic, antimalarial, and other drugs, such as tetracyclines, phenothiazines, and zidovudine,[911] and by heavy metals.[912] The pigmentation of hemochromatosis is similar except that it seldom involves the mucous membranes. Nail pigment abnormalities may also occur in Peutz-Jeghers syndrome and with pregnancy or radiotherapy.[913] Even when the diagnosis appears obvious, endocrine evaluation should be conducted to confirm the diagnosis and determine the type of adrenal insufficiency and its cause before initiating lifelong therapy.

LABORATORY DIAGNOSIS

Adrenal Insufficiency. **Basal Cortisol Secretion.** A scheme for establishing the diagnosis of adrenal insufficiency and determining its cause is shown in Figure 9–32. The basis of the diagnosis of adrenal insufficiency depends on demonstration of inadequate cortisol production. Plasma cortisol concentration is normally high in the early morning (i.e., before 8 AM) and increases with stress. Therefore, a low plasma cortisol level (i.e., <140 nmol/L [<5 μg/dL]) in these situations provides presumptive evidence of adrenal insufficiency, and a value of <275 nmol/L (<10 μg/dL) strongly suggests the diagnosis. Conversely, a level of 550 nmol/L (20 μg/dL) or greater precludes the diagnosis. An intermediate plasma cortisol level is not diagnostic. Plasma cortisol level is normally low in the late afternoon and evening, so its determination in a sample drawn at these times is of no value. Although a basal morning plasma cortisol level of more than 275 nmol/dL (>10 μg/dL) predicts a normal cortisol response to insulin-induced hypoglycemia in most patients,[914, 914a] patients with partial adrenal insufficiency may have normal basal cortisol levels but an inadequate adrenal response to stress. As with basal serum cortisol levels, basal urinary free cortisol and 17-OHCS levels are low in patients with severe adrenal insufficiency, but they may be low normal in patients with partial adrenal insufficiency.

Response to Acute ACTH Stimulation. A short ACTH stimulation test should be performed for virtually all patients in whom the diagnosis is being considered. The details of the test are discussed later in this chapter. A normal response is a rise in plasma cortisol level by 60 min to a peak of 550 nmol/L (20 μg/dL) or more.[915] An impaired response confirms adrenal insufficiency, but further studies are necessary to establish its type and cause. A normal response in the short ACTH stimulation test excludes primary adrenal insufficiency but does not eliminate secondary adrenal insufficiency of recent onset (e.g., within a week or two after pituitary surgery); in the latter setting only an insulin-induced hypoglycemia or metyrapone test is reliable.[916, 917] The overnight metyrapone test is as reliable as and quicker than the standard 3-d metyrapone test.[918] Neither should be performed for an outpatient in whom adrenal insufficiency is considered a possibility.

Treatment of patients who present in possible adrenal crisis should not be delayed while diagnostic tests are performed. Blood for plasma cortisol and electrolyte determinations should be drawn, and therapy should be initiated immediately with intravenous saline and dexamethasone, as discussed later in this chapter. The short ACTH stimulation test can be performed after initiation of glucocorticoid treatment provided that (1) glucocorticoid therapy has not been given for more than a few days, after which it can suppress the hypothalamic-pituitary-adrenal axis and compromise the adrenal response, and (2) neither hydrocortisone (cortisol) nor cortisone (which is converted to cortisol) is used for glucocorticoid therapy, because both are measured in cortisol radioimmunoassays. Dexamethasone is the drug of choice in this circumstance.

Primary vs. Secondary or Tertiary Adrenal Insufficiency. **Basal Plasma ACTH.** In primary adrenal insufficiency, basal 8 AM plasma ACTH concentrations are elevated, sometimes as high as 880 pmol/L (4000 pg/mL) and occasionally even higher (see Fig. 9–29). In secondary or tertiary adrenal insufficiency, plasma ACTH levels are low or low normal. The ACTH level must be measured in a sample drawn before initiating glucocorticoid therapy or at least 24 h after the last dose of a short-acting glucocorticoid, such as hydrocortisone. Otherwise, the ACTH level may be suppressed by glucocorticoid negative feedback. If the patient has been on replacement glucocorticoids, the steroid must be replaced with hydrocortisone for several days before measuring morning plasma ACTH. If the sample is drawn in the proper setting and the ACTH assay is reliable, this measurement by itself is sufficient to establish whether the adrenal insufficiency is primary.

Response to Prolonged ACTH Stimulation. Prolonged ACTH stimulation will also distinguish between primary and secondary or tertiary adrenal insufficiency, because the atrophic adrenal glands in secondary and tertiary adrenal insufficiency recover cortisol-secretory capacity if chronically exposed to ACTH, whereas the adrenal glands in primary adrenal insufficiency are partially or completely destroyed, are already exposed to maximally stimulating levels of endogenous ACTH, and do not respond to further ACTH stimulation (Fig. 9–33). This test is performed by administering ACTH as a continuous infusion for 48 h[919] or as daily 8-h infusions or twice-daily intramuscular injections for 4 to 5 d, while measuring daily urinary 17-OHCS or free cortisol excretion and plasma cortisol concentrations (see section on testing in this chapter). Glucocorticoid replacement should be given as dexamethasone 0.5 to 1 mg daily for at least 24 h before and during the test, because dexamethasone does not significantly interfere at this dosage with either plasma or urinary steroid measurements. There is a progressive increase in cortisol secretion in secondary or tertiary adrenal insufficiency, but little or no response in primary adrenal insufficiency. The 48-h ACTH infusion is preferred because

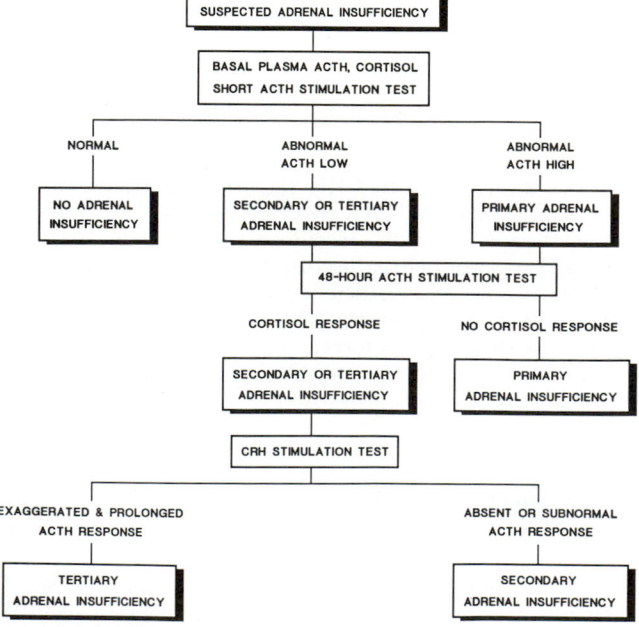

Figure 9–32. Diagnostic laboratory approach to confirming the diagnosis of adrenal insufficiency and determining whether it is primary, secondary, or tertiary.

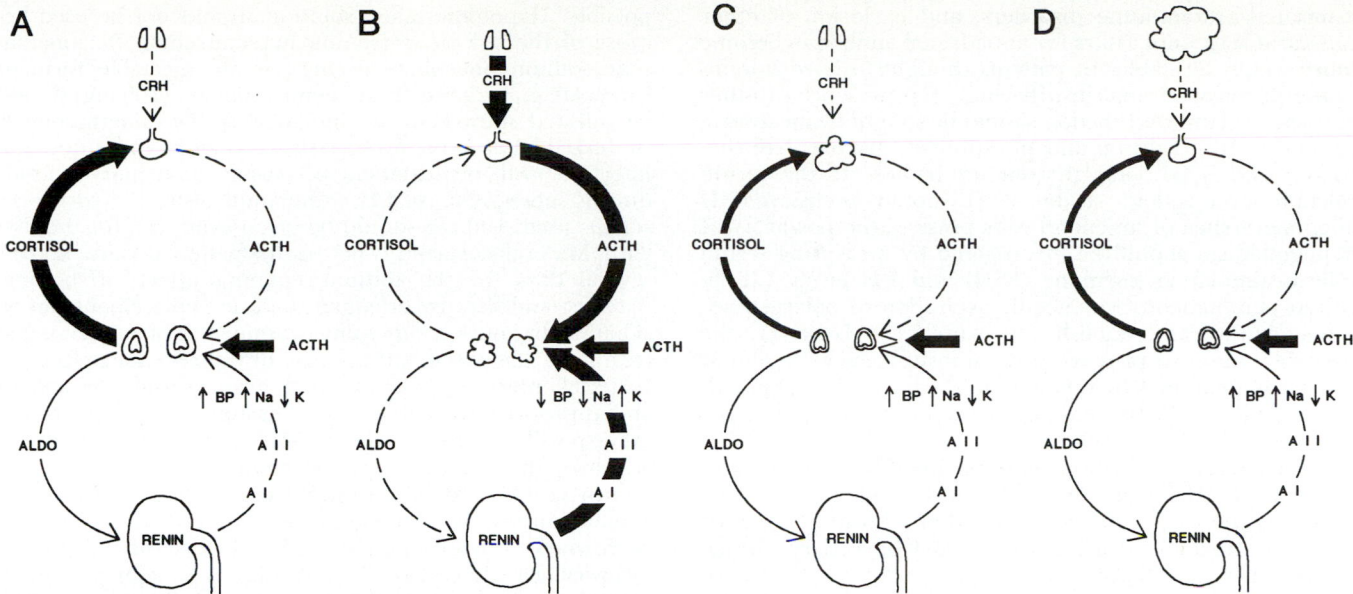

Figure 9–33. Response of (A) a normal individual and those of patients with (B) primary, (C) secondary, and (D) tertiary adrenal insufficiency to prolonged (48-h) stimulation with maximal dosage of ACTH.

it reliably separates primary from secondary or tertiary adrenal insufficiency in the shortest time.

Secondary vs. Tertiary Adrenal Insufficiency. ACTH Response to Corticotropin-Releasing Hormone. The differentiation between secondary and tertiary adrenal insufficiency can be made with a CRH test (Fig. 9–34), although from a therapeutic standpoint this distinction is rarely important. There is little or no ACTH response in patients with secondary adrenal insufficiency, whereas patients with tertiary adrenal insufficiency usually have an exaggerated and prolonged ACTH response.[191, 910]

Cause of Adrenal Insufficiency. Primary Adrenal Insufficiency. It is important to determine the cause of the adrenal insufficiency because it may be due to a disease that has other clinical ramifications, such as tuberculosis in primary adrenal insufficiency or a pituitary tumor in secondary

adrenal insufficiency. In primary adrenal insufficiency, the age of the patient, the clinical setting (i.e., anticoagulation), and the presence of other autoimmune-mediated endocrine disorders are important. An abdominal CT scan provides useful information because enlarged adrenal glands or the presence of calcium eliminates an autoimmune process and suggests an infectious, hemorrhagic, or metastatic cause.[841] (See Fig. 9–31.) However, absence of enlarged or calcified adrenal glands does not exclude tuberculosis as the cause. Patients who present initially with tuberculous adrenal insufficiency usually have active tuberculosis elsewhere.[841, 874] Chest x-ray, urine culture for *Mycobacterium tuberculosis*, and tuberculin skin testing should be done if the diagnosis is suspected. Complement fixation titers for histoplasmosis should be obtained. The diagnosis of autoimmune adrenal insufficiency is based on circumstantial evidence, such as

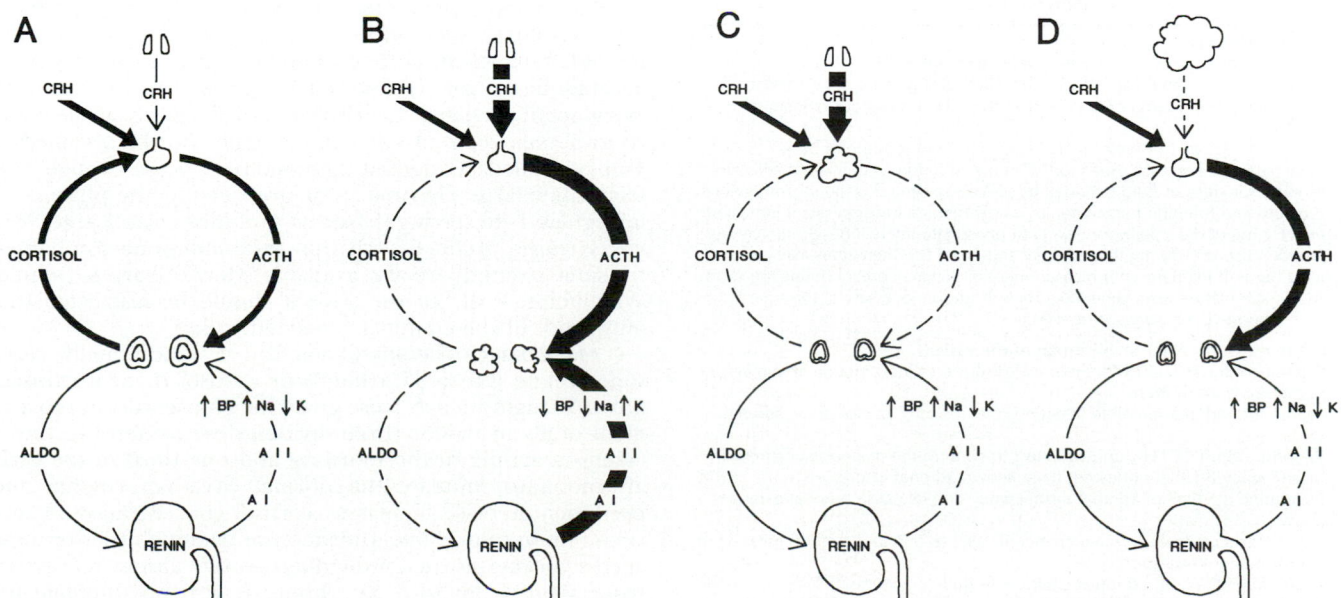

Figure 9–34. Response of (A) a normal individual and those of patients with (B) primary, (C) secondary, and (D) tertiary adrenal insufficiency to CRH stimulation.

associated autoimmune disorders, and exclusion of other causes, at least until assays for antiadrenal antibodies become more widely available. In patients thought to have autoimmune primary adrenal insufficiency, the presence of other endocrine gland dysfunction should be sought by measuring serum levels of calcium and phosphorus, glucose, free thyroxine and TSH, and thyroid antibodies. If the serum calcium level is low, serum PTH should be assayed. If oligomenorrhea or amenorrhea is present, the possibility of hypogonadism should be investigated by measuring serum follicle-stimulating hormone (FSH) and LH levels. CT-directed percutaneous fine-needle aspiration of enlarged adrenal glands can establish the cause.[877, 920] However, the treatable causes of primary adrenal insufficiency can almost always be identified by other, noninvasive means, although it may establish the presence of metastases from a previously unsuspected malignancy.

Secondary or Tertiary Adrenal Insufficiency. A pituitary CT or MRI scan should be performed to exclude a tumor as the cause. A variety of other disorders, some of which are treatable, can cause secondary or tertiary adrenal insufficiency (see Chapter 6).

Treatment

The introduction of adrenocortical extracts by Swingle and Pfiffner in 1931[26] and the use of large doses of salt in the 1930s[30] improved the treatment of adrenal insufficiency slightly, and the synthesis of DOC by von Steiger and Reichstein in 1937[28] helped further, but it was not until synthetic cortisone became available for therapeutic use in 1949[38, 921] that it was possible to treat adrenal insufficiency easily and successfully.[806]

ACUTE ADRENAL INSUFFICIENCY: ADRENAL CRISIS. Adrenal crisis is a life-threatening emergency that requires immediate and appropriate treatment (Table 9–12). When there is strong clinical suspicion of the diagnosis, therapy should not be delayed to perform diagnostic studies or await laboratory results. The initial goal of therapy is reversal of the hypotension and electrolyte abnormalities. Large volumes (i.e., 2 to 3 L) of 0.9% saline solution or 5% dextrose in saline should be infused intravenously as quickly as possible. Hypotonic saline solution should not be used because of the risk of worsening hyponatremia. Dexamethasone sodium phosphate (4 mg) or an injectable form of cortisol (e.g., hydrocortisone hemisuccinate) (100 mg) should be injected intravenously immediately. Dexamethasone is preferred because the effect lasts 12 to 24 h, and it does not interfere with measurement of plasma or urinary steroids during subsequent ACTH stimulation tests. If hydrocortisone is used, 100 mg should be given every 6 h for the first 24 h. Mineralocorticoid is not useful acutely because it takes several days for the sodium-retaining effects to become manifest and because adequate sodium replacement can be achieved by intravenous saline administration. After initial treatment, the precipitating cause of the adrenal crisis (e.g., bacterial infection, viral gastroenteritis) should be sought and appropriately treated. Consideration should be given to other possible causes of shock. After the patient's condition is stable, the diagnosis can be confirmed in patients not known to have adrenal insufficiency with a short ACTH stimulation test (see section on testing), and studies can be performed to determine the type and cause of the adrenal insufficiency (see earlier). Unless there is a major precipitating or complicating illness, glucocorticoid therapy can be tapered over 1 to 3 d to an oral maintenance dose. Most patients who present with adrenal crisis have primary adrenal insufficiency and therefore require lifelong mineralocorticoid replacement as well. Fludrocortisone (0.1 mg/d is the usual dosage) can be started when the saline infusion is stopped and the patient is taking food and fluids by mouth.

CHRONIC PRIMARY ADRENAL INSUFFICIENCY. *Education of the Patient and Emergency Precautions.* Education of the patient is the key to successful treatment of this disease. The patient must be taught that an active and vigorous life of normal length can be led as long as the prescribed medication regimen and a few commonsense precautions are observed. The patient and responsible family members should be instructed about (1) the nature of the hormonal deficit and the rationale for replacement therapy, (2) maintenance medications, (3) changes in medications during minor illnesses, (4) when to consult a physician, and (5) when and how to inject dexamethasone for emergencies.

Every patient should at all times wear a medical alert (Medic Alert) bracelet or necklace and carry the Emergency Medical Information Card that is supplied with it. Both should indicate the diagnosis and daily medications. Every patient should have at least three 1-mL syringes prefilled with dexamethasone sodium phosphate 4 mg/mL in 154 mmol/L NaCl solution: one at home, one at work or school, and one in the car. In addition, it is wise for the patient to carry such a syringe at all times, particularly while away from home, work, or car. The syringes can be obtained as 1-mL prefilled syringes (Organon, Inc., West Orange, NJ) from some large pharmacies or prepared by the pharmacist in regular 1-mL syringes from a multidose vial. Larger 2.5-mL syringes prefilled with the dexamethasone solution of the same strength are also available (Merck Sharp & Dohme, West Point, PA), but the patient should be instructed that only 1 mL of the contents is needed.

Maintenance Therapy (Table 9–13). Traditionally, cortisone acetate (25 to 37.5 mg/d) or cortisol (hydrocortisone) (20 to 30 mg/d) tablets were given for glucocorticoid replacement orally in two or three divided doses, often two thirds taken on arising in the morning and one third in the early afternoon to simulate the normal circadian rhythm and postlunch increase in plasma cortisol concentration. There is no reason to give late afternoon or evening doses of these agents because normal individuals secrete almost no cortisol from about 6 PM to 3 AM. There is also no rationale for using cortisone acetate under any circumstances. It is not

---

TABLE 9–12. Treatment of Suspected Acute Adrenal Insufficiency (Adrenal Crisis)

Emergency Measures
1. Establish intravenous access with a large-gauge needle.
2. Draw blood for immediate serum electrolyte and glucose assays and routine measurement of plasma cortisol and ACTH. Do not wait for laboratory results.
3. Infuse 2 to 3 L of 154 mmol/L NaCl (0.9% saline) solution or 50 g/L (5%) dextrose in 154 mmol/L NaCl (0.9% saline) solution as quickly as possible. Monitor for signs of fluid overload by following central or peripheral venous pressure and listening for pulmonary rales. Reduce infusion rate if indicated.
4. Inject 4 mg of dexamethasone sodium phosphate intravenously. Intravenous hydrocortisone (100 mg immediately and every 6 h thereafter) may also be used but will interfere with measurement of plasma cortisol during the short ACTH stimulation test. Mineralocorticoids are unnecessary at this time.
5. Use supportive measures as needed.

Subacute Measures After Stabilization of the Patient
1. Continue intravenous 154 mmol/L NaCl (0.9% saline) solution at a lower rate for next 24 to 48 h.
2. Search for and treat possible infectious precipitating causes of the adrenal crisis.
3. Perform a short ACTH stimulation test to confirm the diagnosis of adrenal insufficiency if patient does not have known adrenal insufficiency.
4. Determine the type of adrenal insufficiency and its cause if not already known.
5. Taper glucocorticoids to maintenance dosage over 1 to 3 d if precipitating or complicating illness permits.
6. Begin mineralocorticoid replacement with fludrocortisone (0.1 mg by mouth daily) when saline infusion is stopped.

TABLE 9–13. Treatment of Chronic Primary Adrenal Insufficiency

Maintenance Therapy

Glucocorticoid Replacement
1. Dexamethasone 0.5 (0.25–0.75) mg or prednisone 5 (2.5–7.5) mg orally at bedtime. Supplement with hydrocortisone 5–10 mg orally in midafternoon if indicated.
2. Alternative therapy is with hydrocortisone 15–20 mg on awakening and 5–10 mg in early afternoon.
3. Monitor clinical symptoms and morning plasma ACTH level.

Mineralocorticoid Replacement
1. Fludrocortisone 0.1 (0.05–0.2) mg orally.
2. Liberal salt intake
3. Monitor blood pressure and pulse taken in lying down and standing positions, edema, serum potassium concentration, and plasma renin activity.

Educate patient about the disease, how to manage minor illnesses and major stresses, and how to inject dexamethasone intramuscularly.

Obtain a medical alert bracelet or necklace, an emergency medical information card, and prefilled syringes containing dexamethasone 4 mg in 1 mL saline.

Treatment of Minor Febrile Illness or Stress

Increase glucocorticoid dose two- to threefold for the few days of illness. Do not change mineralocorticoid dose.

Contact physician if illness worsens or persists for more than 3 d.

No extra supplementation is needed for most uncomplicated, outpatient dental procedures done with local anesthesia. General anesthesia or intravenous sedation should not be used in the office.

Emergency Treatment of Severe Stress or Trauma

Inject contents of prefilled dexamethasone (4 mg) syringe intramuscularly.

Get to physician as quickly as possible.

Steroid Coverage for Illness or Surgery in Hospital

For moderate illness give hydrocortisone 50 mg twice a day orally or intravenously. Taper rapidly to maintenance dose as partient recovers.

For severe illness give hydrocortisone 100 mg intravenously every 8 h. Taper dose to maintenance level by decreasing in half every day. Adjust dose according to course of illness.

For minor procedures under local anesthesia and most radiological studies, no extra supplementation is needed.

For moderately stressful procedures, such as barium enema, endoscopy, or arteriography, give a single 100-mg IV dose of hydrocortisone just before the procedure.

For major surgery, give hydrocortisone 100 mg IV just before induction of anesthesia and continue every 8 h for first 24 h. Taper dose rapidly, decreasing by half per day, to maintenance level.

---

biologically active and must undergo hepatic metabolism to cortisol, over which it holds no advantage. Furthermore, when given intramuscularly, it is either largely unabsorbed or not metabolized.[922] Unfortunately, the administration of cortisone acetate or hydrocortisone by mouth does not achieve the desired goal of mimicking the normal daily rhythm, because the plasma cortisol concentration increases rapidly in the 30 min or so after ingestion, quickly exceeds the CBG binding capacity of about 690 nmol/L (25 µg/dL), reaches much higher than normal levels, and then rapidly declines to 690 nmol/L before slowing to a disappearance half-time of about 80 min. This results in high, transient cortisol concentrations followed by low levels before the next dose.[923] In addition, by the time the patient takes the morning cortisol dose, plasma cortisol levels would normally already be at or near the peak. This transient adrenal insufficiency probably accounts for the symptoms of fatigue, lassitude, mild nausea, or headache of which many patients complain on awakening and that are relieved within 30 to 60 min of taking their glucocorticoid. Furthermore, plasma ACTH levels are much higher than normal for several hours in the early morning and for about 3 h after the cortisol is taken.[923, 924] The elevated plasma levels of ACTH and other POMC-derived peptides account for the persistent hyperpigmentation frequently seen in patients treated with this regimen. Moreover, because the enhanced ACTH secretion is chronically inadequately inhibited by glucocorticoid negative feedback, ACTH secretion may become relatively nonsuppressible[793, 794, 925] and pituitary hyperplasia[795, 842] or, rarely, corticotrope adenomas may develop.[842]

Therefore, replacement therapy with a long-acting synthetic glucocorticoid, dexamethasone or prednisone, is preferred to that with short-acting cortisol or cortisone acetate, because the longer duration of action provides a smoother physiological effect and avoids the extremes of plasma glucocorticoid level that occur even when multiple daily doses of shorter-acting steroids are given. The usual oral daily replacement dosages are 0.5 mg and 5 mg for dexamethasone and prednisone, respectively. Occasional patients require dosage adjustments ranging from 0.25 to 0.75 mg for dexamethasone and from 2.5 to 7.5 mg for prednisone. A larger dosage may be required for very large patients or for those who metabolize the steroid more rapidly than normal, and a smaller dosage is appropriate for children or small adults and for those who metabolize the steroid less rapidly. The dosage must be increased for patients taking drugs that accelerate hepatic steroid metabolism, such as phenytoin,[892] barbiturates,[892] rifampin,[540, 892] mitotane,[926] and aminoglutethimide.[927] The dosage can be adjusted based on relief of clinical symptoms of adrenal insufficiency, decreased hyperpigmentation, and return of morning plasma ACTH concentration to less than 18 pmol/L (80 pg/mL). Excessive weight gain, facial plethora, or other signs and symptoms of Cushing's syndrome and a suppressed morning plasma ACTH concentration (i.e., <4 pmol/L [<20 pg/mL]) suggest excessive glucocorticoid replacement.

The ideal time to administer the glucocorticoid would be at 3 or 4 AM, just as circadian ACTH secretion begins to increase. Because a timed-release preparation is not available, the next best option is to give the dexamethasone or prednisone at bedtime. This lowers morning plasma ACTH levels into the normal range and provides adequate circulating glucocorticoid activity when the patient awakens. It can be given upon awakening for the rare patient in whom the bedtime dose causes insomnia. A 5- to 10-mg dose of hydrocortisone may be given in early to middle afternoon for the occasional patient who seems to require more glucocorticoid in the late afternoon. Steroid is virtually never required later in the day.

Mineralocorticoid replacement is required for all patients with primary adrenal insufficiency to prevent sodium loss, intravascular volume depletion, and hyperkalemia. The natural mineralocorticoids, aldosterone and DOC, are not used because of rapid hepatic degradation after oral ingestion and the high cost of aldosterone. DOC, which is available in a long-acting, oil-based preparation for intramuscular injection, was used extensively in the 1940s but is little used at present. Fludrocortisone (9α-fluorohydrocortisone), a potent synthetic mineralocorticoid, is given orally in a usual dose of 0.1 mg daily. Some patients require up to 0.2 mg daily.[832, 928] Patients receiving hydrocortisone, which has some mineralocorticoid activity, may require a lower dose, such as 0.05 mg daily. Adequacy of mineralocorticoid replacement can be monitored by inquiring for symptoms of postural hypotension and measuring supine and upright blood pressure and pulse, serum potassium concentration, and plasma renin activity. The dose may have to be doubled during the summer, when salt loss in perspiration increases, especially if the patient is routinely exposed to temperatures above about 29°C (85°F). Salt intake should be liberal, especially when exercising. Hypertension, edema, and hypokalemia are signs of excessive mineralocorticoid replacement.

Essential hypertension in patients with adrenal insufficiency should be treated with restriction of dietary sodium and reduced mineralocorticoid replacement, rather than with sodium-wasting diuretics.[929] Mineralocorticoid therapy usually cannot be discontinued without risking sodium depletion. Antihypertensive agents other than sodium-wasting diuretics or spironolactone should be used.

Treatment During Illness or Surgery. Cortisol secretion normally increases with the stress of illness and surgery. Recommendations for increased glucocorticoid treatment during minor or major illnesses, minor procedures, and major surgery are given in Table 9–13. Despite evidence from studies in monkeys that supraphysiological glucocorticoid doses may not be required for survival of major surgery,[930] the usual approach is to provide high doses of glucocorticoid to all patients with proven or suspected adrenal insufficiency, starting before induction of anesthesia.

Pregnancy in Addison's Disease. Before glucocorticoid replacement therapy became available, pregnancy in patients with Addison's disease was associated with maternal mortality rates as high as 35 to 45%.[931] Now most patients with adrenal insufficiency experience pregnancy, labor, and delivery without difficulty. The usual glucocorticoid and mineralocorticoid replacement dosages are continued.[807, 932] An occasional patient may require slightly more glucocorticoid in the third trimester. During labor, adequate saline hydration and 25 mg of intravenous cortisol (hydrocortisone hemisuccinate) every 6 h should be administered. At the time of delivery or if labor is prolonged, high-dosage parenteral hydrocortisone should be administered as 100 mg every 6 h or as a continuous infusion. After delivery, the dosage can be tapered rapidly to maintenance within 3 d.[932] An occasional patient with severe nausea and vomiting in the first trimester may require intramuscular dexamethasone at a slightly increased dosage (i.e., 1 mg daily). If the patient cannot take medicines by mouth, 1 to 2 mg/d of desoxycorticosterone acetate in sesame oil may be administered intramuscularly.

CHRONIC SECONDARY AND TERTIARY ADRENAL INSUFFICIENCY. Treatment of chronic secondary or tertiary adrenal insufficiency is identical to that of chronic primary adrenal insufficiency (see Table 9–13), except that mineralocorticoid replacement is rarely required and replacement of other pituitary hormones may be necessary. Treatment of adrenal insufficiency caused by pharmacological administration of glucocorticoids and withdrawal of the steroids is discussed later in this chapter.

Prognosis and Survival

The prognosis in Addison's disease was grim before the availability of glucocorticoids in the 1950s; more than 80% of patients died within 2 y after diagnosis.[806] Today, a patient with autoimmune Addison's disease should have a normal life span and can lead a fully active life, including vigorous exercise.[806, 807] The prognosis for patients with other causes of adrenal insufficiency depends mostly on the underlying disease. However, heart failure has been reported in 7 of 22 patients with long-standing primary adrenal insufficiency receiving appropriate treatment after a mean of 26 y;[929] the causal relationship, if any, is unclear. Essential hypertension occasionally occurs in patients with Addison's disease[929] and must be treated. Linear growth and pubertal development proceed normally in correctly (i.e., adequately but not overly) treated children with adrenal insufficiency.[824, 829]

Isolated Mineralocorticoid Deficiency

Deficient aldosterone production occurs in conditions other than Addison's disease. Isolated mineralocorticoid deficiency states include acquired secondary aldosterone deficiency (hyporeninemic hypoaldosteronism), acquired primary aldosterone deficiency, and inherited enzymatic defects in aldosterone biosynthesis.

HYPORENINEMIC HYPOALDOSTERONISM. The most common form of isolated hypoaldosteronism is attributed to impaired renin release from the kidney. The syndrome was first described in 1957,[933] and the hyporeninemia was first recognized in 1972.[934, 935] The typical patient is 50 to 70 y old and has unexplained, chronic, asymptomatic hyperkalemia and mild to moderate renal insufficiency (creatinine clearance greater than 15 mL/min).[936] A minority of patients present with muscle weakness or cardiac arrhythmias. About half have diabetes mellitus.[936] Other associated disease states include systemic lupus erythematosus, multiple myeloma, renal amyloidosis, cirrhosis, sickle cell anemia, and AIDS.[937–942]

Pathophysiology. **Aldosterone Deficiency**. Urinary aldosterone excretion, an index of aldosterone production, is low under basal conditions and fails to increase after sodium restriction.[934] Plasma renin activity is also low and does not increase appropriately during sodium restriction, periods of prolonged upright posture, or diuretic administration.[934] It has been postulated that interstitial renal disease and consequent damage to the juxtaglomerular apparatus result in a primary defect in renin generation or release and secondary deficiency of aldosterone secretion.[934] However, no specific anatomical lesion to explain the deficient renin production has been identified. Aldosterone-secretory capacity appears to respond to administration of angiotensin II in some patients,[943–945] whereas in others the response is absent[946] or blunted.[936] Failure to respond could indicate a coexisting primary defect in aldosterone secretion or reflect atrophy of the zona glomerulosa caused by chronic renin deficiency. Instances of frankly elevated[947] or inappropriately high basal levels and normal responsiveness of plasma 18-hydroxycorticosterone to angiotensin II infusion[948] suggest a defective terminal enzymatic step in aldosterone biosynthesis. However, it is not known whether this defect is primary or a consequence of chronic renin deficiency.

Renin Deficiency. Various mechanisms have been invoked to explain the hyporeninemia. One explanation is physiological suppression of renin secretion by hypervolemia. In hypertensive patients (up to 50% of patients with hyporeninemic hypoaldosteronism have elevated blood pressure), expanded extracellular fluid volume might suppress renin. Prolonged sodium restriction and diuretic administration result in a rise in plasma renin activity in these patients,[949] but the increments in plasma renin activity and aldosterone concentration are less than those in normal subjects. A second possible mechanism is autonomic insufficiency, particularly in patients with diabetic neuropathy, in whom a deficient norepinephrine response to postural change is thought to contribute to deficient renin release. Furthermore, these patients exhibit decreased sensitivity to administered beta-agonists, so there appear to be defects in both catecholamine production and action.[950] A third proposed mechanism is secretion of abnormal forms of renin. A defect in the conversion of prorenin to renin may exist in some patients.[947, 951, 952] Kallikrein, a neutral serine protease produced in the macula densa, activates prorenin, and some patients with hyporeninemic hypoaldosteronism have low kallikrein levels.[952] However, the suppression of kallikrein may be a secondary phenomenon, because mineralocorticoid replacement may restore kallikrein levels to normal.[953] Prostaglandin deficiency is a fourth possibility, because vasodilatory prostaglandins, particularly prostaglandin I$_2$, mediate renin release.[954] Furthermore, cyclooxygenase inhibitors, such as indomethacin, produce a reversible defect in renin production.[955] The finding of deficient prostaglandin E$_2$ in hyporeninemic hypoaldosteronism[955] has not been confirmed,[956, 957] but prostaglandin I$_2$ (prostacyclin) production, as assessed by measurement of the stable urinary metabolite 6-keto prostaglandin F$_{1\alpha}$, apparently is diminished in these patients.[958] Furthermore, the prostaglandin I$_2$ was unresponsive to the potent stimulators norepinephrine and calcium. Prostaglandin I$_2$ deficiency might cause hyporeninemic hypoaldosteronism by inhibiting conversion of prorenin to renin[959, 960] and renin release.

Hyperkalemia. The pathogenesis of hyperkalemia is probably multifactorial. Several factors interact to regulate ion transport processes in the distal nephron. They include rates of tubular flow and sodium reabsorption, transepithelial voltage gradients, dietary potassium intake, systemic pH, and mineralocorticoid action. Aldosterone has an acute effect on epithelial potassium transport in isolated renal tubules in vitro.[961, 962] However, chronic exposure to mineralocorticoids does appear to increase the potassium-secretory capacity of the tubule, presumably by indirect means. An additional factor in diabetic patients is the decreased insulin effect on internal potassium balance.[963]

Acidosis. Patients with hyporeninemic hypoaldosteronism have a unique form of renal tubular acidosis, termed type IV to distinguish it from other forms of this disorder.[964] The acidosis apparently is a consequence of decreased renal ammoniagenesis, reduced hydrogen ion–secretory capacity in the distal nephron, and mild reduction in the proximal tubular threshold for bicarbonate reabsorption. The impaired ammoniagenesis is not directly attributable to aldosterone deficiency but is the consequence of hyperkalemia. Correction of hyperkalemia by means other than mineralocorticoid replacement improves urinary ammonium excretion and sometimes results in correction of the urinary acidification defect.[965] Mineralocorticoid replacement also corrects the hyperkalemia and thereby increases urinary ammonium excretion, but net acid excretion also increases, implying that mineralocorticoid has an additional effect on hydrogen ion–secretory capacity.[964] Aldosterone acutely increases sodium-independent hydrogen ion secretion in the medullary collecting duct in vitro.[966]

Clinical Diagnosis. The diagnosis of hypoaldosteronism must be considered in any patient with unexplained chronic hyperkalemia. Spurious serum potassium values associated with in vitro hemolysis, thrombocytosis, or leukocytosis must be excluded. Dietary or medicinal sources of excess potassium should be sought, but they usually do not cause sustained hyperkalemia if renal function is normal. Renal function should be evaluated, and drugs that impair renal tubular potassium excretion should be withdrawn.

The clinical diagnosis is confirmed by finding low plasma renin activity and low plasma aldosterone concentration or low urinary aldosterone excretion under conditions that ordinarily activate the renin-angiotensin-aldosterone axis. The standard methods for achieving this are maintaining upright posture for 3 or 4 h and administering furosemide (see Chapter 11 for further details).

Treatment. The therapeutic approach must take into consideration the age of the patient and other associated disorders. If the hyperkalemia is moderate and no electrocardiographic changes are evident, periodic measurement of serum potassium concentration should suffice. Drugs that tend to promote hyperkalemia, such as beta-adrenergic antagonists, cyclooxygenase inhibitors, angiotensin-converting enzyme inhibitors, heparin, and potassium-sparing diuretics, should be avoided. Dietary potassium intake should be reduced, if possible. Diuretic therapy should be the initial treatment for patients who have coexisting diseases associated with sodium retention, such as hypertension and congestive heart failure. Mineralocorticoid replacement with fludrocortisone is reserved for patients who have more severe hyperkalemia and no hypertension or congestive heart failure. The usual starting dose is 0.1 mg of fludrocortisone per day, but some patients require higher doses.

PRIMARY HYPOALDOSTERONISM. P-450$_{c11}$ (Corticosterone 18-Methyl Oxidase II) Deficiency. Congenital hypoaldosteronism is a rare inherited disorder transmitted as an autosomal recessive trait. The clinical presentation is typical of aldosterone deficiency. The defect is in the activity of one of the terminal enzymes in the aldosterone biosynthetic pathway. Corticosterone 18-methyl oxidase I (CMO I) refers to the enzymatic activity responsible for hydroxylation of corticosterone at C-18. CMO II (sometimes called isomerase) activity converts the 18-hydroxyl group to an aldehyde.[967] CMO I deficiency would be expected to produce low plasma levels of products derived from corticosterone (18-hydroxycorticosterone and aldosterone) and low urinary excretion of their metabolites,[968] whereas CMO II deficiency should be associated with high plasma 18-hydroxycorticosterone levels and low plasma aldosterone levels.[969] Urinary excretion of tetrahydro-18-hydroxy-11-dehydrocorticosterone, the major metabolite of 18-hydroxycorticosterone, is increased, but urinary excretion of tetrahydroaldosterone is decreased.[968]

Thus far, all reported patients with inherited isolated defects in aldosterone biosynthesis apparently have had deficient CMO II activity. Reanalysis of the original reports of CMO I defects[970, 971] indicates that the subjects actually had CMO II deficiency.[968, 969, 972] Because a single gene product, mitochondrial P-450$_{c11}$, catalyzes all steps in the conversion of deoxycorticosterone to aldosterone,[139] the P-450$_{c11}$ gene presumably is the site of mutations causing these disorders. CMO II deficiency is associated with a restriction fragment length polymorphism involving the P-450$_{c11}$ gene, suggesting a mutation in or near the gene.[973] The syndrome is treated by replacing mineralocorticoid with the usual dosage of fludrocortisone.

Acquired Forms of Primary Hypoaldosteronism. Several conditions may be associated with aldosterone biosynthetic defects. Heparin therapy causes natriuresis, with or without frank hyperkalemia, in certain patients,[974–976] some of whom may have diabetes mellitus. Heparin suppresses aldosterone synthesis, leading to a compensatory rise in plasma renin activity, which in most subjects is sufficient to prevent aldosterone deficiency.[976] The compensatory mechanism apparently is insufficient in some individuals because of an impaired renin-angiotensin system, as might exist in diabetes mellitus.[976] Persistently hypotensive, critically ill patients also have inappropriately low plasma aldosterone concentrations relative to the activity of the renin-angiotensin system. The defect is at the level of the adrenal but is not associated with any particular disease state or therapy;[977] the mechanism is unknown.

PSEUDOHYPOALDOSTERONISM. This is a rare salt-wasting syndrome of infancy first described in 1958[978] and postulated to be due to renal tubular insensitivity to mineralocorticoids. Its clinical hallmarks are those of aldosterone deficiency: hyponatremia, hyperkalemia, hyper-reninemia, and renal salt wasting. However, plasma aldosterone levels and urinary excretion are elevated.[979] Hypothalamic-pituitary-adrenal function is normal. Autosomal recessive transmission has been observed in some kindreds.[979] In other instances the disorder seems to be due to obstructive uropathy[980] or prematurity[981] or follows renal transplantation.[982] Neither the clinical nor the biochemical abnormalities respond to mineralocorticoid treatment; sodium supplementation and potassium-binding resins are usually successful. One study documented spontaneous improvement in electrolyte balance with increasing age, although plasma renin activity and aldosterone concentrations remained elevated.[983]

Pseudohypoaldosteronism may be caused by an abnormal mineralocorticoid receptor. Mineralocorticoid receptors are expressed in circulating blood mononuclear cells,[984] so one can assess receptor status in patients suspected of having this disorder without having to take biopsy samples of classic target tissues, such as kidney. Patients may have absent or greatly reduced numbers of mineralocorticoid receptors.[985]

Hyperfunction

Glucocorticoids: Hypercortisolism (Cushing's Syndrome)

HISTORY. Cushing's syndrome is the constellation of clinical signs and symptoms resulting from chronic glucocorticoid excess. Harvey Cushing described a 23-y-old woman with "painful obesity, hypertrichosis and amenorrhea" in 1912[986] and postulated 20 y later that the "polyglandular syndrome" was due to primary pituitary dysfunction ("pituitary basophilism") (Fig. 9–35).[987] At that time a pituitary factor was thought to regulate the adrenal cortex,[33, 34] but neither ACTH nor adrenal steroids had yet been identified. Adrenal tumors were known to cause the syndrome in some patients.[988] A patient with Cushing's syndrome and a nonendocrine tumor was described in 1928,[989] but ectopic ACTH production was not demonstrated until 1962.[990]

CLINICAL PRESENTATION. The more common features of Cushing's syndrome are listed in Table 9–14. None is pathognomonic, but initial development or increasing severity of several of these features should arouse suspicion. The manifestations depend on both the degree and duration of

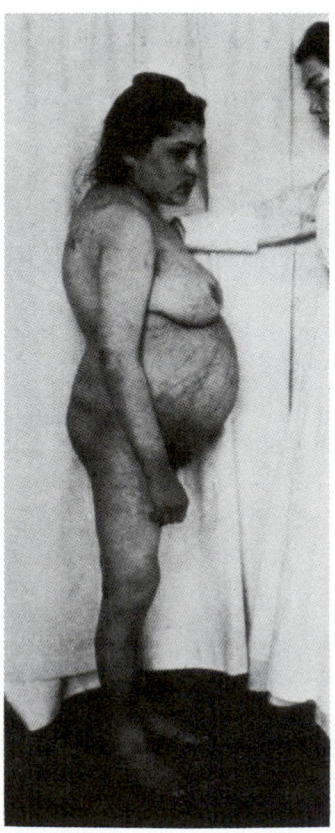

Figure 9–35. Minnie G., Cushing's index patient, at age 23 y. (From Cushing H. The basophil adenomas of the pituitary body and their clinical manifestations [pituitary basophilism]. Bull Johns Hopkins Hosp 1932; 50:137–195.)

TABLE 9–14. Signs and Symptoms of Cushing's Syndrome

Sign or Symptom	Reported Incidence (%)
Centripetal obesity	79–97
Facial plethora	50–94
Glucose intolerance	39–90
Weakness, proximal myopathy	29–90
Hypertension	74–87
Psychological changes	31–86
Easy bruisability	23–84
Hirsutism	64–81
Oligomenorrhea or amenorrhea	55–80
Impotence	55–80
Acne, oily skin	26–80
Abdominal striae	51–71
Ankle edema	28–60
Backache, vertebral collapse, fracture	40–50
Polydipsia, polyuria	25–44
Renal calculi	15–19
Hyperpigmentation	4–16
Headache	0–47
Exophthalmos	0–33
Tinea versicolor infection	0–30
Abdominal pain	0–21

Adapted from a table in Howlett et al.[1228] summarizing data from Cushing,[987] Plotz et al.,[992] Ross et al.,[993] Gold,[1627] Jeffcoate et al.,[749] Cohen,[750] Liddle,[1122] Urbanic and George,[997] and Ross and Linch.[991]

hypercortisolism, the presence or absence of androgen excess (pure hypercortisolism does not cause hirsutism or seborrhea), and additional tumor-related effects in the case of adrenal carcinoma or ectopic ACTH syndrome. These clinical manifestations are now usually less severe than in Cushing's day[987] because of earlier diagnosis.

Progressive obesity is the most common sign. It is usually central (centripetal), involving the face, neck, trunk, and abdomen, with the extremities spared or even wasted (Fig. 9–36A). Some authors report generalized obesity in a majority of patients,[991] but in our experience a minority of adults develop generalized obesity. In contrast, generalized obesity is almost the rule in children, in whom linear growth is slowed or arrested, often as the first indication of glucocorticoid excess. A child whose weight begins to rise across the percentiles as height declines across the percentiles (Fig. 9–37) should be considered to have Cushing's syndrome until proved otherwise. Facial fat accumulation can produce a moon face, often accompanied by plethora over the cheeks, anterior neck, and sun-exposed chest (see Fig. 9–36C). The neck is thick and appears shortened. There is usually a dorsocervical fat pad, or buffalo hump, consistent with the degree of obesity. Enlarged fat pads characteristically fill the supraclavicular fossae (see Fig. 9–36C). They are less common in exogenous obesity. Patients who diet and exercise rigorously may have little or no weight gain, facial rounding, or central weight redistribution (see Fig. 9–36L to O). Exophthalmos is present in about 6% of patients,[992] probably the result of retro-orbital fat deposition. It has no inflammatory component.

Weakness is usually associated with proximal muscle wasting, including the gluteus maximus. Most patients cannot rise from a squatting position without assistance, and those with severe disease may be unable to climb stairs or get up from a deep chair. In patients with extreme hypercortisolemia or those receiving thiazide diuretics, hypokalemia may aggravate the weakness.

Cardiovascular complications are a major cause of morbidity and death in untreated Cushing's syndrome.[992] Moderate hypertension (diastolic blood pressure >100 mm Hg) is common.[993] Dependent edema is another sign of mineralocorticoid excess, one of several causes of hypertension in Cushing's syndrome.[725, 994] Congestive heart failure was present in almost half of patients older than 40 in one series[993]

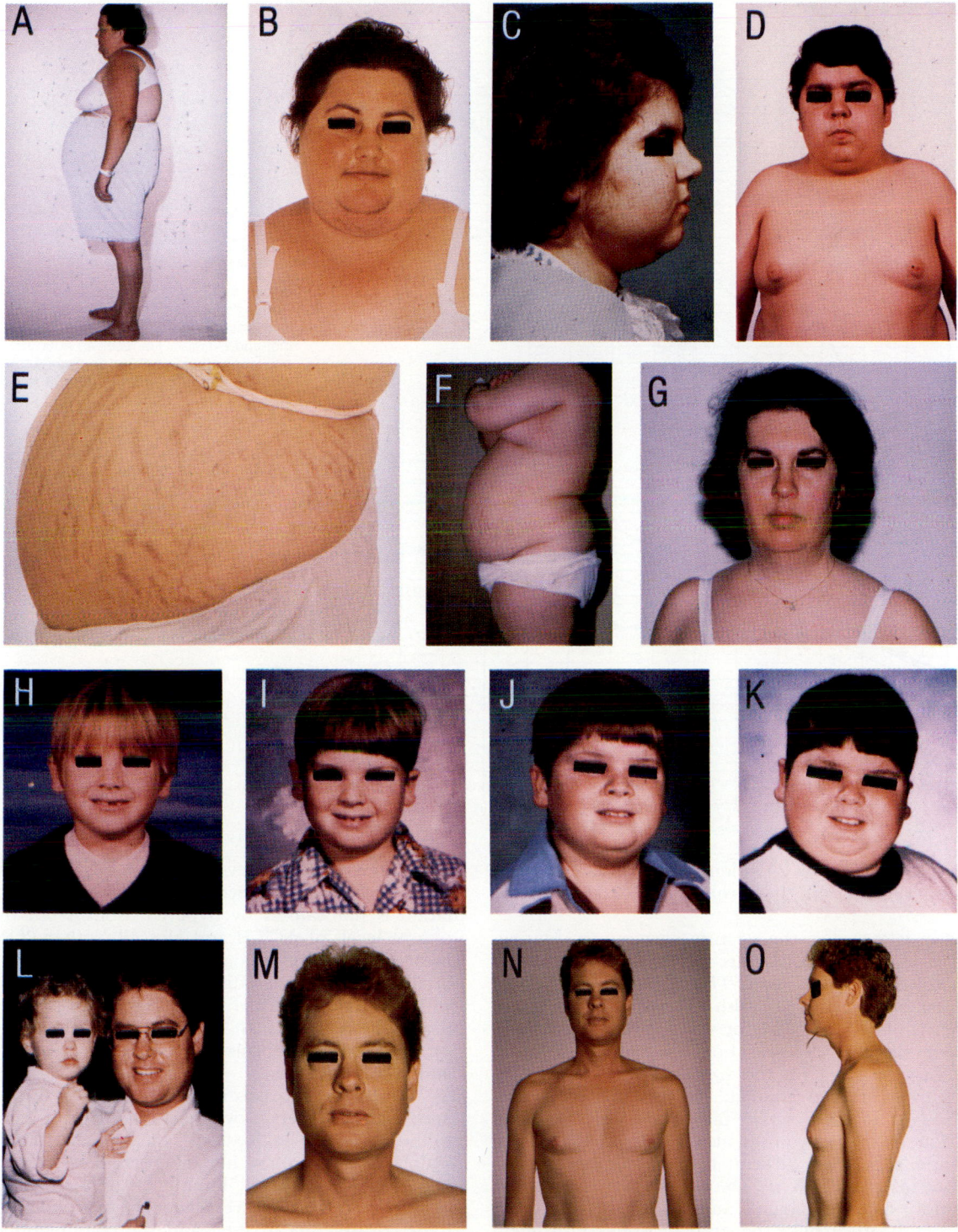

Figure 9–36. Physical appearance of patients with Cushing's syndrome. *A*, Centripetal and some generalized obesity and dorsal kyphosis in a 30-y-old woman with Cushing's disease. *B*, Same woman as in *A*, showing moon facies, plethora, hirsutism, and enlarged supraclavicular fat pads. *C*, Facial rounding, hirsutism, and acne in a 14-y-old girl with Cushing's disease. *D*, Central and generalized obesity and moon facies in a 14-y-old boy with Cushing's disease. *E*, Abdominal striae in the 30-y-old patient shown in *A*. *F*, Striae on the breast, abdomen, and thigh of a 9-y-old girl with generalized obesity and Cushing's disease. *G*, Facial plethora, mild hirsutism, and increased supraclavicular fat pads in a 42-y-old woman with a centripetal shift in weight distribution without weight gain. *H to K*, Development of childhood Cushing's disease from normal at age 7, early Cushing's disease at age 8, to progressive Cushing's disease at ages 9 and 11. *L to O*, Effects of diet and exercise on Cushing's syndrome. The patient at age 37 with a 2-y history of Cushing's disease before and after 8 mo of self-imposed diet and vigorous exercise; minimal central fat distribution and mild residual loss of proximal muscle mass are seen. (*C* courtesy of Dr. H. Patrick Higgins.)

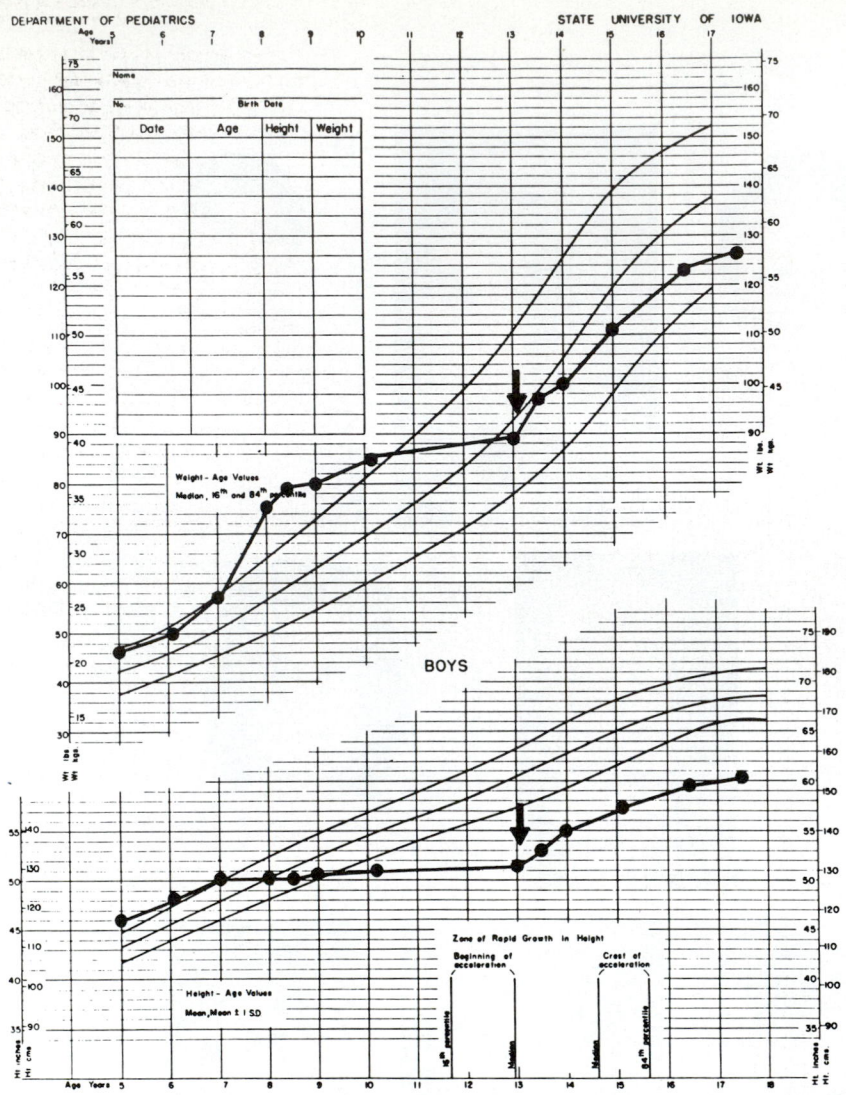

DEPARTMENT OF PEDIATRICS   STATE UNIVERSITY OF IOWA

Figure 9–37. Growth chart of a boy with childhood Cushing's syndrome beginning at about age 7. Weight gain was minimized from age 8½ to age 13 by rigorous diet and exercise. He received 4000 rad of megavoltage pituitary radiation at age 13 *(arrows)*. Note the lack of catch-up linear growth. At age 25, the height was unchanged, the weight was 70 kg, and pituitary function was normal.

but is less frequent in our experience. Like other features, it presumably reflects both the chronicity and severity of the disease.

The skin is atrophic, the stratum corneum is thinned, and there is loss of subcutaneous fat,[995] allowing subcutaneous blood vessels to be seen. The skin becomes fragile and, in extreme cases, peels off with adhesive tape like damp tissue paper (Liddle's sign). Minor wounds heal slowly, and surgical wounds may dehisce. Loss of connective tissue results in easy bruising on the forearms and shins after minimal, unremembered trauma; patients are sometimes initially thought to have senile purpura[996] or a bleeding diathesis. Extensive ecchymoses at venipuncture sites are common, and it is often difficult to maintain intravenous lines without infiltrating fluid. The fragile skin is stretched by the rapidly enlarging trunk and abdomen, producing striae (see Fig. 9–36). Unlike the striae of pregnant women, they appear purplish or reddish because the thin, transparent skin reveals the color of venous blood in the dermis. The striae are also more numerous and often more than 1 cm wide. Such striae are most frequent on the lower flanks and abdomen but can be found on the breasts, hips, buttocks, upper abdomen, shoulders, and upper thighs and in the axillae. They occur more frequently in younger patients (see Fig. 9–36).[997] Cutaneous fungal infections, especially tinea versicolor, are often found on the chest. Oral candidiasis is encountered only in severe hypercortisolism. Fungal infections of the nails are occasionally observed. Hyperpigmentation is not caused by hypercortisolism but by increased plasma levels of ACTH and, possibly, other POMC-derived melanotropins. As a consequence, hyperpigmentation may occur with Cushing's disease and, much more frequently, with the ectopic ACTH syndrome but not with adrenocortical tumors. It has an addisonian distribution but is less pronounced. Acanthosis nigricans may occur in the axillae and around the neck.

Androgen excess is manifested by oily facial skin, acne, and mild hirsutism in women. Hirsutism is usually limited to the face (see Fig. 9–36) but can be generalized. Thinning scalp hair is common, but temporal balding is rare. Oligomenorrhea in women, impotence in men, and decreased libido in both sexes are frequent, presumably because of hypercortisolemia in men and the combination of cortisol and androgen excess in women.

Low-back pain is common. Back pain, vertebral compression fractures, pathological rib fractures, and, less commonly, long bone fractures result from osteoporosis, which can be demonstrated even in most young patients with dual-energy photon absorptiometry or CT scan densitometry of the lumbosacral vertebrae. Up to 20% of patients have radiologically demonstrable vertebral compression fractures.[993, 998] We have encountered several patients with aseptic necrosis of the femoral and, in one instance, the humeral heads (Fig. 9–38), a condition known to be associated with chronic administration of potent synthetic glucocorticoids. Because of increased bone resorption, hypercalciuria and renal calculi may be present. Hypercalcemia is unusual, and, when it is encountered, coexisting primary hyperparathyroidism must be excluded.

Polydipsia and polyuria are usually seen in patients with hypercalciuria or glycosuria. Glucose intolerance and hyperinsulinemia are common because of the effect of cortisol on gluconeogenesis, but true diabetes mellitus occurs in only 10 to 15% of patients, usually those with a family history. Ketoacidosis is rare and indicates unsuspected insulinopenic diabetes that has been exacerbated by the hypercortisolism.

Psychiatric complications occur in over half of patients with Cushing's syndrome of all etiologies[749, 992] and are, therefore, presumably due to hypercortisolemia. Emotional lability, agitated depression, loss of energy and libido, irritability, anxiety, panic attacks, and mild paranoia are most common. Most patients have increased appetite and weight gain, but anorexia may rarely predominate.[999] Occasional patients may be suicidal.[992] One must be alert to this possibility and take precautions to protect the patient. Some patients appear euphoric or manic, particularly during the early course of the disease. Children tend to be tireless overachievers, often ranking near the top of their classes. Some patients with psychiatric complications have underlying personality disorders that were present before the hypercortisolism occurred[1000] and persist after it is cured. Insomnia is often an early symptom and is presumably caused by high cortisol levels during sleep.[1001]

Phlebothrombosis and thromboembolic events are said to be increased in frequency,[991, 1002] presumably because of increased plasma clotting factor and prothrombin levels,[1003] but others dispute this claim.[1004]

Glucocorticoids suppress immune function, but infection with organisms of low pathogenicity occurs only with severe hypercortisolemia.[654] Inflammatory and febrile responses to bacterial infection are suppressed, masking its presence. Thus asymptomatic urinary tract infection is common and may become apparent only after cure of the disease.

Intraocular pressure is increased in about one quarter of patients[1005] and aggravates pre-existing glaucoma.

Chronic hypercortisolism results in a number of nonspecific abnormalities in laboratory screening tests. Packed red blood cell volume and hemoglobin concentration tend to be high normal, but a true increase in red blood cell mass is unusual.[993] The total leukocyte count is usually normal but may be elevated. There is relative or absolute lymphopenia in half of all patients.[993] Total eosinophil numbers are usually low and are less than 10/mm³ in one third of patients. Hypercalciuria occurs in almost half of the patients,[993] but serum calcium and phosphorus levels are normal. Electrolyte levels are normal except in extreme hypercortisolism, mild fasting hyperglycemia occurs in about 15% of patients, and serum cholesterol and triglyceride concentrations are often elevated because of increased very-low-density lipoprotein (VLDL), LDL, and HDL concentrations.[1006] Levels of clotting factors V and VIII and prothrombin may be elevated.[1003]

PATHOPHYSIOLOGY. Cushing's syndrome may be either ACTH dependent or ACTH independent. The ACTH-dependent varieties are Cushing's disease (primary pituitary ACTH hypersecretion), the ectopic ACTH syndrome (inappropriate secretion of ACTH by nonpituitary tumors), and the ectopic CRH syndrome (inappropriate secretion of CRH by nonhypothalamic tumors causing pituitary hypersecretion of ACTH). Iatrogenic or factitious Cushing's syndrome associated with administration of exogenous ACTH is rare. These conditions all cause bilateral adrenocortical hyperplasia and cortisol hypersecretion. The ACTH-independent varieties of Cushing's syndrome are primary adrenocortical adenoma or carcinoma, the much more rare bilateral micronodular dysplasia,[1007–1011] and the even more rare bilateral ACTH-independent macronodular hyperplasia.[1012] Iatrogenic or factitious Cushing's syndrome is also ACTH independent and is caused by administration of potent synthetic glucocorticoids, usually for their anti-inflammatory effect.

Normal hypothalamic-pituitary-adrenal physiological

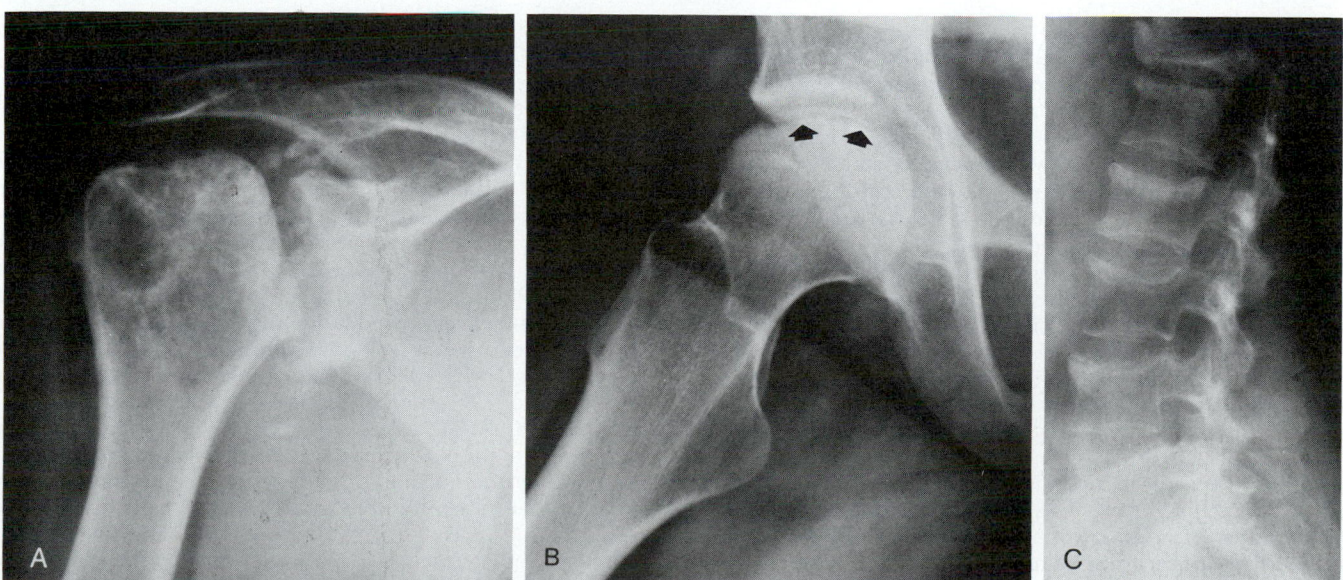

Figure 9–38. Aseptic necrosis of bone in Cushing's disease. *A,* Aseptic necrosis of the right humeral head of a 43-y-old woman with Cushing's disease of about 8 mo duration. *B,* Aseptic necrosis of the right femoral head in a 24-y-old woman with Cushing's disease of about 4½ y duration. The arrows indicate the crescent subchondral radiolucency best seen in this lateral view. *C,* Diffuse osteoporosis, vertebral collapse, and subchondral sclerosis in the patient whose shoulder is shown in *A.* (From Phillips KA, Nance EP Jr, Rodriguez RM, et al. Avascular necrosis of bone: a manifestation of Cushing's disease. Reprinted by permission from the Southern Medical Journal [79:825–829, 1986].)

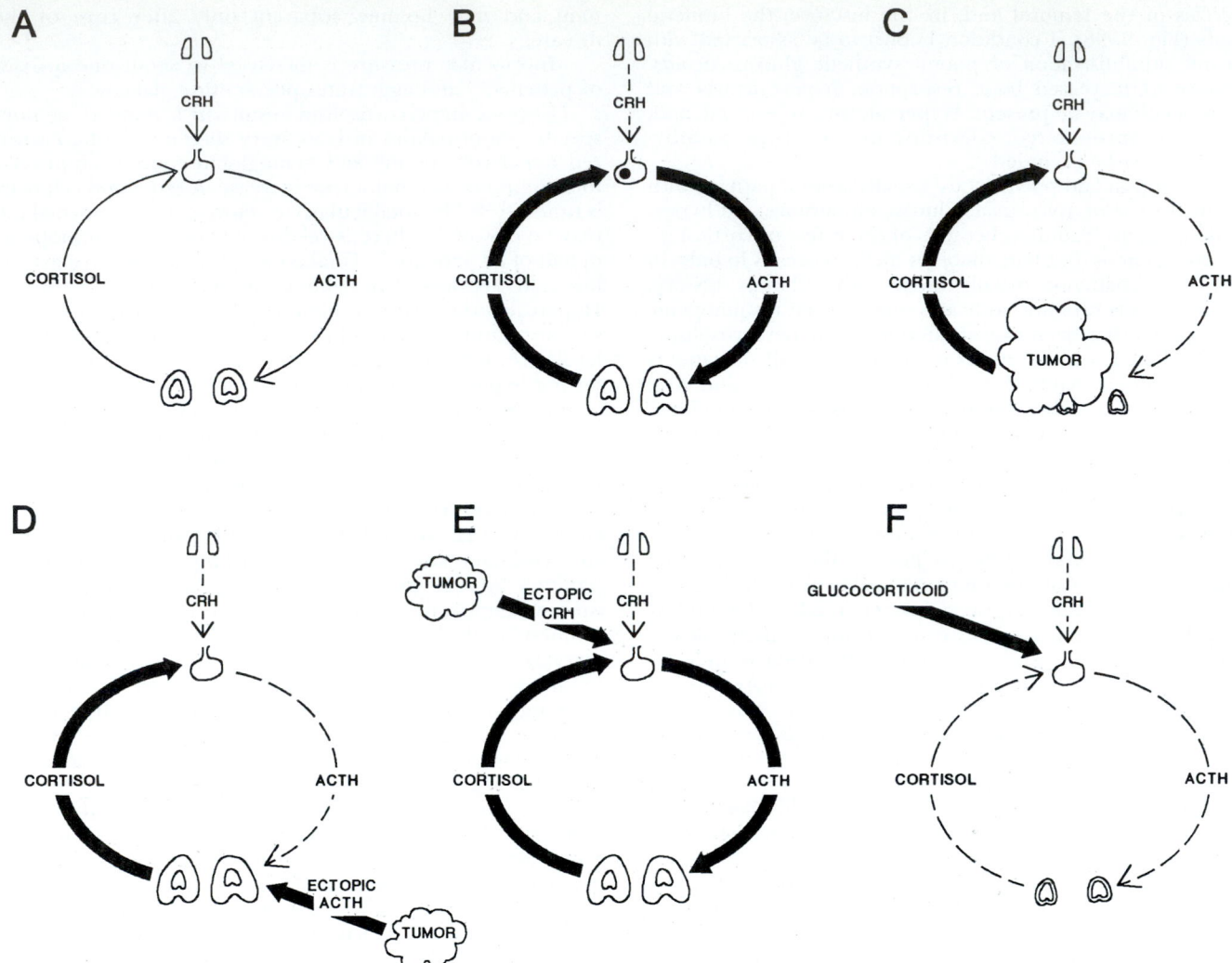

Figure 9–39. Hypothalamic-pituitary-adrenal function in (A) normal individuals and the pathophysiological aberrations in (B) pituitary ACTH-dependent Cushing's disease, (C) primary adrenocortical disease (i.e., cortisol-secreting adrenal tumor, bilateral micronodular dysplasia, and bilateral ACTH-independent macronodular hyperplasia), (D) ectopic ACTH syndrome, (E) ectopic CRH syndrome, and (F) iatrogenic Cushing's syndrome resulting from pharmacological dosage of glucocorticoids.

relationships and the pathophysiological aberrations in Cushing's syndrome of different etiologies are diagrammed in Figure 9–39.

Normal Relationships. CRH and other hypothalamic factors are released into hypophyseal portal blood in the median eminence and carried to the anterior pituitary, where they stimulate synthesis and release of ACTH and other POMC-derived peptides (see Fig. 9–39A). The increased plasma ACTH concentrations stimulate increased adrenocortical cortisol secretion. Increased plasma cortisol concentration inhibits hypothalamic CRH synthesis and secretion, blocks the action of CRH and other secretagogues on pituitary corticotropes, and inhibits synthesis of POMC and release of ACTH and other POMC-derived peptides. Falling plasma ACTH levels reduce the stimulus for cortisol production, and the system returns to the basal state. The circadian rhythm in ACTH secretion results in highest secretion rates at about the time of awakening and lowest rates about an hour after beginning sleep. Plasma ACTH and cortisol concentrations reflect this changing rate. Finally, various stressful stimuli increase ACTH and, consequently, cortisol secretion. Plasma free cortisol is filtered into saliva and urine, its metabolites are excreted in the urine as 17-OHCS, and some of its precursors are excreted in the form of 17-ketosteroids (17-KS).

ACTH-Dependent Cushing's Syndrome. **Cushing's Disease.** In Cushing's disease, the amplitude but not the number of ACTH-secretory episodes is increased[1013–1016] and the normal ACTH circadian rhythm is lost (Fig. 9–40). The increased plasma level of ACTH, alone or with other growth factors,[59, 1017] stimulates the development of bilateral adrenocortical hyperplasia and the hypersecretion of cortisol (see Fig. 9–39B). The normal circadian rhythm in cortisol secretion is lost. Morning plasma ACTH and cortisol levels may be normal, but late evening concentrations are elevated (Figs. 9–40 and 9–41). Increased daily cortisol secretion is reflected by increased urinary free cortisol and 17-OHCS excretion. Because the cortisol biosynthetic enzymes are normal, production and excretion of cortisol and its precursors are proportionately increased. The chronic hypercortisolemia suppresses hypothalamic CRH secretion and inhibits ACTH secretion by the normal, nonadenomatous pituitary corticotropes, which atrophy. The adenomatous cells do respond to decreased plasma cortisol levels by increasing ACTH secretion and to increased plasma glucocorticoid concentration by decreasing ACTH secretion, but the hallmark of the disorder is the relative resistance of ACTH secretion to glucocorticoid negative feedback inhibition. In effect, the adenoma functions at a higher than normal set point for cortisol feedback.[1018] As the adrenals become hyperplastic,

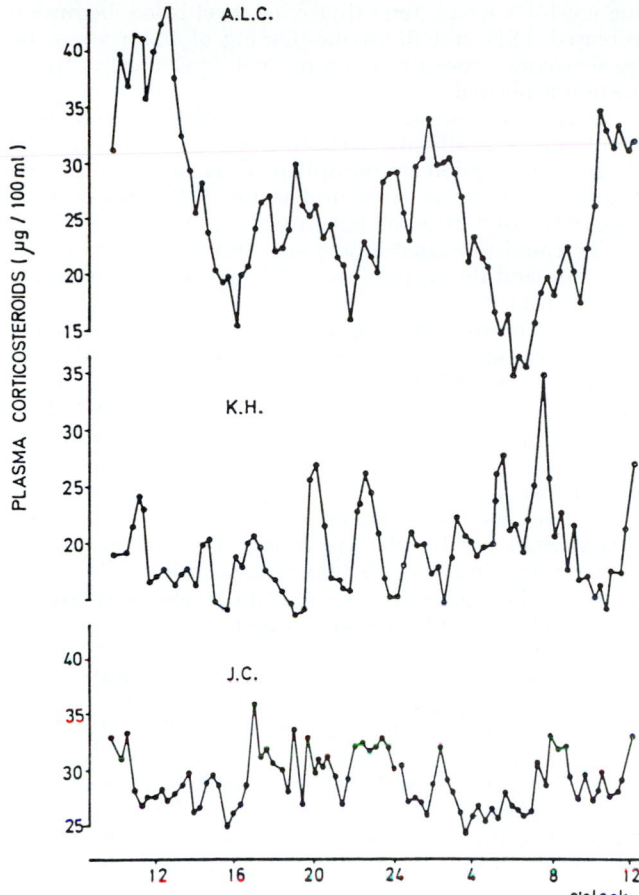

Figure 9–40. Abnormal circadian rhythm in plasma cortisol in Cushing's disease. Samples were drawn every 20 min. To convert to nanomoles per liter, multiply by 27.59. Note that the ordinate scales do not extend to zero and compare with Figure 9–14. (From P Sederberg-Olsen, C Binder, H Kehlet, et al., Episodic variation in plasma corticosteroids in subjects with Cushing's syndrome of differing etiology, J Clin Endocrinol Metab 36, 906–910, 1973, © by The Endocrine Society.)

they secrete proportionately more cortisol in response to a given increment in plasma ACTH, levels of which fall as the result of "autosuppression." This phenomenon is especially pronounced in patients with severe bilateral macronodular hyperplasia,[4, 45, 994, 1019–1022] in whom the plasma ACTH level may not exceed 3 pmol/L (15 pg/mL) (unpublished data, D. N. Orth). Such cases may be interpreted erroneously as ACTH independent.[1023] No case of Cushing's disease that progressed to ACTH-independent adrenocortical Cushing's syndrome has been documented.

Ectopic ACTH Syndrome. In the ectopic ACTH syndrome,[1024] the nonpituitary tumor secretes ACTH, which stimulates bilateral adrenal hyperplasia and hyperfunction (see Fig. 9–39D). Increased plasma cortisol concentration suppresses hypothalamic CRH synthesis and secretion and blocks CRH action on the normal pituitary corticotropes, suppressing pituitary ACTH secretion. With rare exceptions,[1025] tumor ACTH secretion is not regulated by plasma glucocorticoid concentrations. As in Cushing's disease, urinary excretion of cortisol and its precursors is increased proportionately.

Ectopic Corticotropin-Releasing Hormone Syndrome. The ectopic CRH syndrome[1026] is similar to the ectopic ACTH syndrome, except that CRH secreted by the nonhypothalamic tumor stimulates hyperplasia of anterior pituitary corticotropes[1026] and hypersecretion of ACTH (see Fig. 9–39E). The ACTH stimulates bilateral adrenocortical hy-

perplasia and hypersecretion of cortisol,[1027] which presumably suppresses hypothalamic CRH secretion. Somewhat surprisingly, ACTH secretion is usually not suppressed by high glucocorticoid concentrations.[1026, 1027] This may be because most of these tumors also produce ACTH[1028–1030] and because in those cases the hypercortisolism is actually caused by ectopic ACTH, not CRH, production. When CRH alone is produced, dosages of dexamethasone higher than 8 mg/d may be required to suppress ACTH secretion.

An interesting variant of this syndrome was produced by a CRH-secreting gangliocytoma composed of hypothalamic-like neurons that was located within the sella turcica adjacent to the pituitary gland.[1031] There appeared to be partial (i.e., 40%) suppression with low-dose dexamethasone; the high-dose test was not performed. However, there was a fourfold increase in urinary 17-OHCS levels in response to metyrapone, further indicating that ACTH secretion responded to glucocorticoid negative feedback. The corticotropes were hyperplastic, and the patient recovered normal hypothalamic-pituitary-adrenal function after the tumor was removed.[1031]

ACTH-Independent Cushing's Syndrome. Primary Adrenocortical Hyperfunction. In Cushing's syndrome associated with primary adrenocortical disease (i.e., adrenocortical tumor, micronodular dysplasia, or ACTH-independent macronodular hyperplasia), increased cortisol secretion sup-

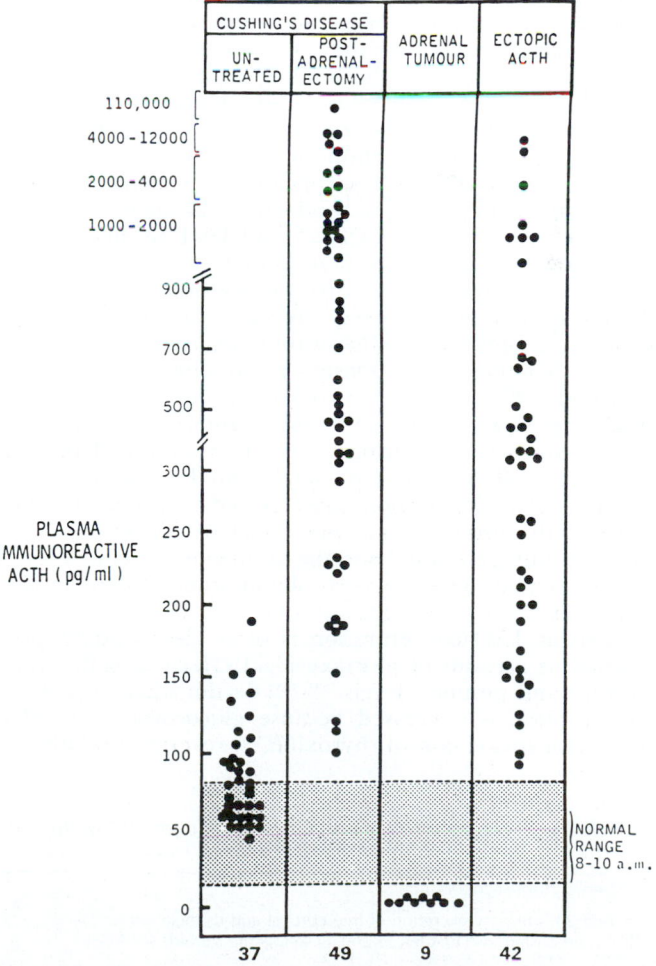

Figure 9–41. Plasma ACTH concentrations in patients with Cushing's disease and Cushing's syndrome associated with adrenocortical tumors and ectopic ACTH syndrome. To convert to picomoles per liter, multiply by 0.2202. (From Besser GM, Edwards CRW. Cushing's syndrome. Clin Endocrinol Metab 1972; 1:451–490.)

presses CRH synthesis, release, and action, thereby suppressing POMC synthesis and ACTH secretion (see Fig. 9–39*C*). Pituitary corticotropes atrophy, as does the normal adrenal cortex. Adrenal carcinomas produce excessive amounts of steroid hormones only because of their size; they are usually inefficient per unit weight in converting cholesterol to cortisol, and production of cortisol precursors is disproportionately high. In contrast, adrenal adenomas can exhibit efficient steroidogenesis, and urinary excretion of DHEAS and 17-KS is often low relative to that of 17-OHCS or free cortisol and may even be normal.

Iatrogenic Cushing's Syndrome. This syndrome is usually caused by administration of excessive amounts of potent synthetic glucocorticoids, rarely by ACTH administration. The steroid inhibits hypothalamic synthesis and secretion of CRH, suppresses pituitary ACTH synthesis and secretion (see Fig. 9–39*F*), and results in bilateral adrenocortical atrophy. Plasma ACTH and (usually) cortisol concentrations are low.

ENDOCRINE LABORATORY FINDINGS. The laboratory findings in endogenous Cushing's syndrome of any cause (Table 9–15) reflect increased synthesis and secretion of cortisol. Early morning plasma cortisol levels may be normal, but the normal circadian rhythm is lost, late evening plasma cortisol level is elevated, and mean plasma cortisol concentration is increased. This leads to increased salivary excretion of free cortisol[1032] and urinary excretion of free cortisol and 17-OHCS. Urinary and salivary free cortisol levels reflect plasma free cortisol concentration and are more sensitive indicators of increased cortisol secretion than is urinary 17-OHCS excretion because they increase more rapidly after plasma cortisol exceeds the binding capacity of transcortin (CBG) at about 690 nmol/L (25 μg/dL). Similarly, the normal hepatic metabolic pathway becomes saturated at high plasma cortisol concentrations, shunting metabolism toward 6β-hydroxycortisol, which is disproportionately increased in the urine.[526] Cortisol precursor production also increases, as do plasma concentrations of DHEA and DHEAS and urinary 17-KS and DHEAS excretion. Plasma concentrations of deoxycorticosterone, 18-hydroxydeoxycorticosterone, and corticosterone, all 17-deoxy steroids, are elevated, but levels of 18-hydroxycorticosterone and aldosterone are normal or decreased.[424] Plasma renin substrate levels are increased[725, 1033] as a result of cortisol's action on the liver,[1033] plasma renin activity[724, 725, 1033] and aldosterone levels[1034] are usually normal, and urinary excretion of the depressor substances kallikrein and prostaglandin E$_2$ is decreased.[725] Plasma ANF concentrations are elevated,[1035] presumably because of the direct stimulatory effect of cortisol on ANF synthesis and secretion[743] and the indirect effect of increased plasma volume caused by cortisol and other weak mineralocorticoids.

Serum TSH concentration is often decreased,[1036] presumably as a result of glucocorticoid effects at both hypothalamic and pituitary levels.[1037, 1038] Serum triiodothyronine concentration is decreased because glucocorticoids inhibit peripheral conversion of thyroxine,[1039] reverse triiodothyro-

nine level is normal, total thyroxine level is low because of decreased TSH and thyroxine-binding globulin levels, but free thyroxine concentration is normal.[1036] Clinically, thyroid function is normal.

Serum concentrations of PTH, 25-hydroxycholecalciferol, and 1,25-dihydroxycholecalciferol are normal, but tubular reabsorption of phosphate increases, serum phosphorus concentration rises, and serum 1,25-dihydroxycholecalciferol concentration falls after cure.[703] The causes of the decreased intestinal absorption and renal reabsorption of calcium and the severe loss of calcium from bone may be multifactorial.[1040]

Serum testosterone concentrations are low in men,[1041] in part because of direct glucocorticoid action on the Leydig cell.[1042] Serum LH concentration, however, is low normal,[1041, 1043] and LH and FSH responses to LHRH are inhibited, indicative of a reversible hypogonadotropic hypogonadism,[1043] which is clinically mild in adults but may be profound in children.

Serum insulin and glucagon levels are higher than can be accounted for by obesity alone.[1044–1046] The hyperinsulinemia may contribute to hypertriglyceridemia.[1046] Serum GH and IGF I concentrations tend to be low, and levels of IGF I–binding protein are suppressed.[1046, 1047]

INCIDENCE. Estimates of the incidence of Cushing's syndrome are imprecise. All series grossly underestimate the incidence of iatrogenic Cushing's syndrome and the ectopic ACTH syndrome.[1048] With perhaps 10 million Americans receiving pharmacological doses of glucocorticoids each year, iatrogenic Cushing's syndrome must be more common than any other form, but it is seldom reported. Ectopic ACTH syndrome is probably the second most common form of Cushing's syndrome but is often not diagnosed. Because (1) about 1% of patients with small cell lung cancer have ectopic ACTH syndrome, (2) small cell lung carcinoma causes half of all cases of the syndrome,[1024] and (3) the incidence of small cell lung carcinoma is about 33,000 per million population per year,[1049] the incidence of ectopic ACTH syndrome can be estimated to be about 660 per million per year. Adrenal carcinoma is somewhat more common than adenoma, but each causes a similar number of cases of Cushing's syndrome. The incidence of adrenal carcinoma is unknown[1050] but is estimated by the National Cancer Institute to be 2 per million per year.[1051] Cushing's disease is five to six times more common than Cushing's syndrome associated with benign and malignant adrenal tumors combined.[1048] Thus the incidence of Cushing's disease may be 5 to 25 per million per year. All other causes of Cushing's syndrome are extremely rare.

The sex-related distribution of Cushing's syndrome varies with the cause. Men had a three times greater incidence of ectopic ACTH syndrome two decades ago, but the increasing incidence of lung cancer in cigarette-smoking women has narrowed that margin. Women are three to eight times more likely to develop Cushing's disease.[1048] Women are about three times more likely than men to have either benign or malignant adrenal tumors and about four to five times more likely to have Cushing's syndrome associated with an adrenal tumor.[1048, 1052–1054] The reasons for this female preponderance are unknown.

The age at which ectopic ACTH syndrome develops parallels the development of lung carcinoma, which increases rapidly after age 50. Ectopic ACTH secretion associated with carcinoid tumors can occur at earlier ages, but is uncommon in children. Cushing's disease occurs mainly in women aged 25 to 45. It is unusual in children but still accounts for about one third of childhood Cushing's syndrome, occurring mostly after puberty. Boys and girls are about equally affected. Adrenal tumors have a bimodal age distribution,

---

TABLE 9–15. Endocrine Abnormalities in Endogenous Cushing's Syndrome of All Etiologies

Increased cortisol-secretory rate

Increased 24-h urinary excretion of free cortisol and its metabolites: 17-hydroxycorticosteroids (17-OHCS) and 17-ketogenic steroids (17-KGS)

Loss of normal diurnal rhythm in plasma cortisol concentration with increased late evening and mean daily plasma cortisol concentrations

Relative or absolute resistance to glucocorticoid negative feedback suppression of cortisol secretion

with small peaks in the first decade of life for both adenomas and carcinomas and major peaks at about 52 y for adenomas and 39 y for carcinomas.[1053, 1054] About one quarter of adrenal tumors occur in children. Adrenal carcinoma is the cause of one half of all cases of childhood Cushing's syndrome, and adenoma accounts for another one sixth.[1055] Girls are affected slightly more frequently than boys.

COMMON CAUSES OF CUSHING'S SYNDROME

ACTH-Dependent Cushing's Syndrome

Cushing's Disease. *Distinctive Clinical Features.* Cushing's disease is usually characterized by chronic, moderate hypersecretion of ACTH and other POMC-derived peptides. Consequently, its clinical features are usually those of chronic, moderate cortisol excess of gradual onset. Central obesity, moon facies, striae, muscle wasting, easy bruising, menstrual abnormalities, low-back pain, depression, decreased libido, and impotence are the predominant features. Hirsutism is usually mild because, although secretion of DHEA, a weak adrenal androgen, is increased, testosterone secretion is normal or low.[1041, 1043] Virilization is rare. Hyperpigmentation is uncommon and mild because the levels of plasma melanotropins are usually not very high. Patients frequently are moderately hypertensive and have mild to moderate glucose intolerance. Most have symptoms for 3 to 6 y before diagnosis.

Pathogenesis. Most patients have ACTH-secreting anterior pituitary corticotrope microadenomas, but a small minority have diffuse corticotrope hyperplasia.[1056–1058] Some patients have "intermediate-lobe–like" microadenomas that tend to be multifocal, poorly suppressed with dexamethasone, but responsive to the dopaminergic agonist bromocriptine.[1059] These tumors have not been encountered by others, including the authors, and their distinctive pathology has been challenged.[1060, 1061] If they occur, they are quite infrequent. Rarely, a corticotrope adenocarcinoma may cause Cushing's disease.[1062] Cushing's disease has twice been reported to arise from a previously nonfunctioning pituitary tumor.[1063, 1064]

The nature of the basic defect in Cushing's disease is unclear. The hypothalamic hypothesis proposes that hypersecretion of CRH (or other hypothalamic factors) causes corticotrope hyperplasia and that the hyperplastic corticotropes subsequently undergo adenomatous change, growing and secreting ACTH independently of stimulation by CRH,[1065, 1066] which is suppressed by the resulting hypercortisolemia (Fig. 9–42A).[229] The pituitary hypothesis proposes that the corticotrope adenoma develops as the result of loss of normal restraints on cell growth and secretes excessive amounts of ACTH and that the resulting chronic hypercortisolemia suppresses CRH secretion (Fig. 9–42B). Neither hypothesis offers an explanation for the CRH hypersecretion on the one hand or the autonomous growth of the corticotropes on the other.

Several types of evidence suggest that Cushing's disease is a primary disorder of the pituitary. The prolonged period of ACTH and cortisol deficiency[1067] and subsequent recovery of normal plasma ACTH circadian rhythm, dexamethasone suppressibility, and response to CRH after successful microadenomectomy[1015, 1068–1072] support the pituitary hypothesis. Abnormalities in secretion of GH,[1073–1075] prolactin,[1076–1079] TSH,[1076] and gonadotropin[1041, 1043] invoked as evidence of a hypothalamic disorder,[1066] resolve after cure.[1015, 1067, 1070, 1071, 1080] Responses to neurotransmitter drugs are probably mediated by direct actions on the pituitary.[1081–1086] CRH physiology has not been carefully studied after cure, but there is no evidence of CRH hypersecretion. Soon after cure, patients respond suboptimally to exogenous CRH.[1072] If a hypothalamic abnormality were present, one might expect to see recurrent disease after successful microadenomectomy. Cushing's disease recurs in only 0 to 2% of patients as long as 8 y after documented cure.[1087, 1088] Recurrence may represent development of a new tumor or growth of residual tumor cells. However, corticotrope adenomas appear to be monoclonal,[1089] arguing against, although not disproving, a role for hypothalamic hyperstimulation. Somatic mutation in the gene encoding the alpha subunit of the G_s protein that regulates adenylate cyclase activity, rendering adenylate cyclase constitutively active, has been reported to be the cause of some tumors causing acromegaly,[1090] but this mutation was not found in any of seven corticotrope tumors.[1091]

Perhaps there are two kinds of Cushing's disease, one of which may have a hypothalamic component,[1092, 1093] but most microadenomas causing Cushing's disease probably arise as a primary pituitary disorder.

Laboratory Findings. Early morning plasma ACTH and cortisol concentrations are often normal, but late evening levels are elevated (see Figs. 9–40 and 9–41). Other POMC-derived peptides parallel ACTH.[1094] Plasma concentration and urinary excretion of cortisol precursors (e.g., DHEA, DHEAS, and 17-KS) are usually increased in proportion to those of cortisol. Mild hyperprolactinemia is present in perhaps 25% of patients with Cushing's disease but not in those with adrenocortical tumors.[1095] Prolactin responses to thyrotropin-releasing hormone and hypoglycemia are normal or only slightly blunted.[1079, 1095] The tumors themselves contain prolactin-secreting cells.[1095] Hypokalemia occurs in fewer than 2% of patients who are not receiving diuretics.[1048]

Radiographic/Nuclear Medicine Findings. The tumors are usually microadenomas (<10 mm in diameter), most of which are not visible in conventional x-ray views of the sella turcica. Even high-resolution, contrast-enhanced, thin-section CT scans detect only about one third of adenomas,[1048, 1096–1098] which appear hypodense with contrast medium or reveal themselves only by displacing the diaphragm of the sella upward or by local bone resorption (Fig. 9–43). CT scans define bony structures, however, and are useful to the neurosurgeon. Coronal projections of high-resolution MRI scans at 1.5 T are reported in some studies to be able to localize microadenomas in a majority of patients.[1099] These results may or may not improve in individual patients with gadolinium–diethylenetriaminepentaacetic acid MRI enhancement[1100] (Fig. 9–44). False-positive CT or MRI scans can be obtained in patients with "nonfunctioning" microadenomas, and false-negative scans can be reported when an adenoma is present in an empty sella.[1101]

The adrenal glands may be normal in size on high-resolution, thin-section CT or MRI scans or show bilateral diffuse enlargement or unilateral or bilateral macronodular enlargement (Fig. 9–45A and B). Nodules less than 1 cm in diameter may be detected on occasion.[1102] Scintiscans with ^{131}I-labeled cholesterol and adrenal arteriograms, veno-

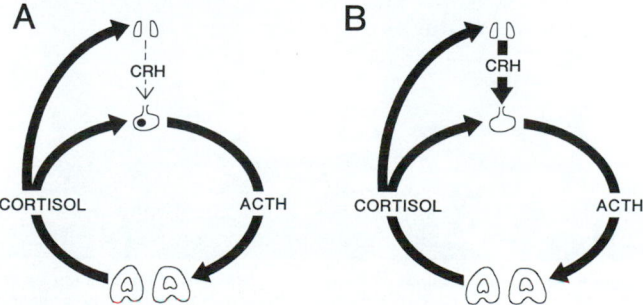

Figure 9–42. Hypothalamic-pituitary-adrenal relationships in (A) the hypothalamic and (B) the pituitary hypotheses about the pathogenesis of Cushing's disease.

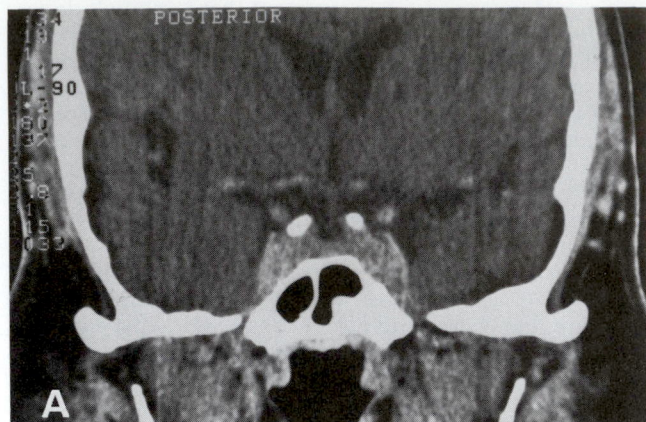

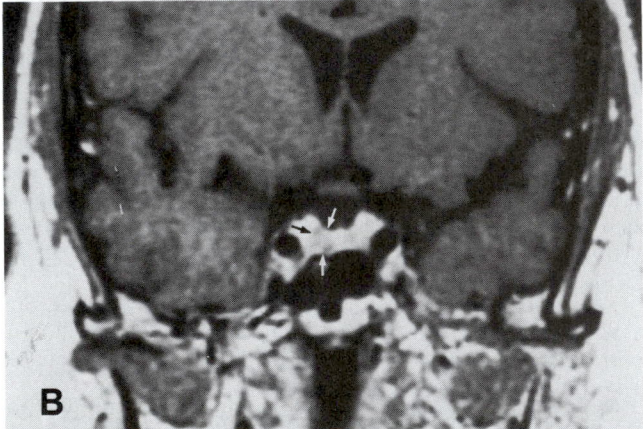

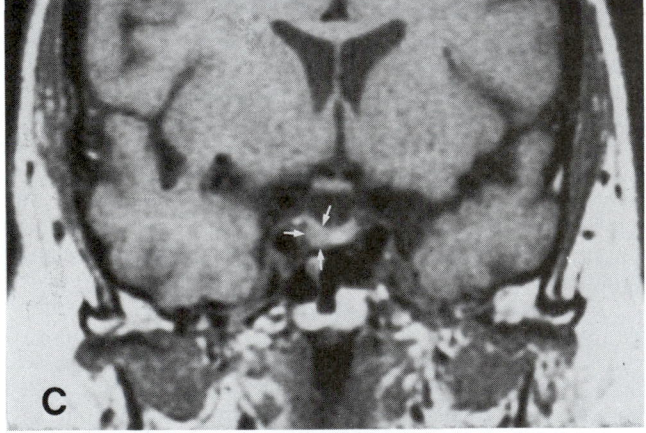

Figure 9–43. Coronal sections of CT and T1-weighted MRI scans of the sella turcica of a 59-y-old man with Cushing's disease of about 2 y duration. The CT scan *(A)* is normal; the gadolinium-enhanced MRI scan *(B)* reveals a 5- to 6-mm microadenoma *(arrows)* in the right side of the pituitary gland that is visible as an area of decreased signal in the nonenhanced scan *(C)*. *(B* and *C* courtesy of Dr. Jorge A. Pino.)

grams, or venous cortisol sampling are rarely indicated, and ultrasonography is not useful.

Osteopenia may be observed on plain films or documented by dual-energy photon absorptiometry or CT bone densitometry in most patients.[992, 1103] Cerebral cortical atrophy, without an apparent functional deficit, is an incidental finding.[1104] The anterior mediastinal fat pad is often enlarged and can be confused with a pulmonary or thymic tumor.

Laboratory Diagnosis. A scheme for confirming the clinical diagnosis of Cushing's syndrome is shown in Figure 9–46.[1105] The diagnosis of Cushing's disease involves dem-

onstrating (1) increased basal cortisol production, (2) dependence of cortisol secretion on ACTH stimulation, (3) relative resistance to glucocorticoid negative feedback,[1018] (4) ACTH response to falling plasma cortisol levels, (5) ACTH response to CRH and/or AVP, (6) cortisol response to exogenous ACTH stimulation, and (7) a pituitary source of the ACTH. Details of all these tests are provided at the end of this chapter. Schematic diagrams of the responses of normal subjects and patients with Cushing's disease to all of these tests are presented in Figures 9–47 and 9–48.

Various authors have compared the value of one test versus another for demonstrating and defining the cause of Cushing's syndrome (e.g., refs. 1106, 1107). In the end, the dexamethasone suppression tests remain the sine qua non of diagnosis, but all of the tests are useful, sometimes essential, adjuncts.[1108] Performing most of the tests in most patients and insisting that all of the results be consistent with a single diagnosis before recommending therapy entail additional time and expense but sometimes help to prevent costly therapeutic errors. Most physicians proceed only to the third step (i.e., the high-dose dexamethasone suppression test), some only to the second, before recommending therapy. If the laboratory is reliable and the results are unequivocal, this may be sufficient. However, we would rarely be willing to proceed to therapy without the results of at least one additional test, either the metyrapone or the CRH test.

INCREASED BASAL CORTISOL PRODUCTION: BASAL PLASMA CONCENTRATIONS AND URINARY EXCRETION OF

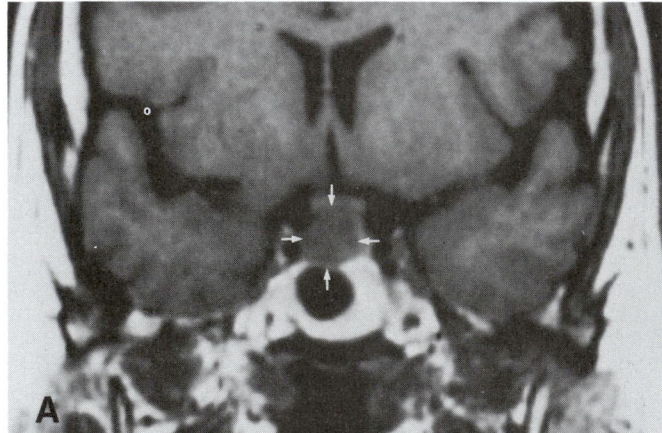

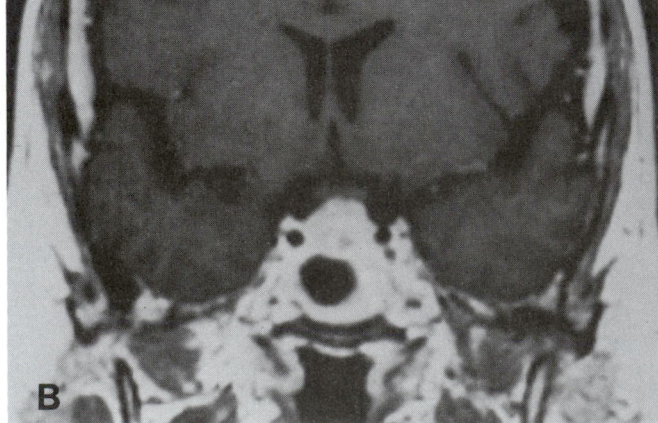

Figure 9–44. Coronal sections of T1-weighted MRI scans of the sella turcica of a 37-y-old woman with Cushing's disease of 10 y duration caused by a pituitary macroadenoma (14 × 11 × 9 mm) *(arrows)* *(A)* before and *(B)* after gadolinium enhancement.

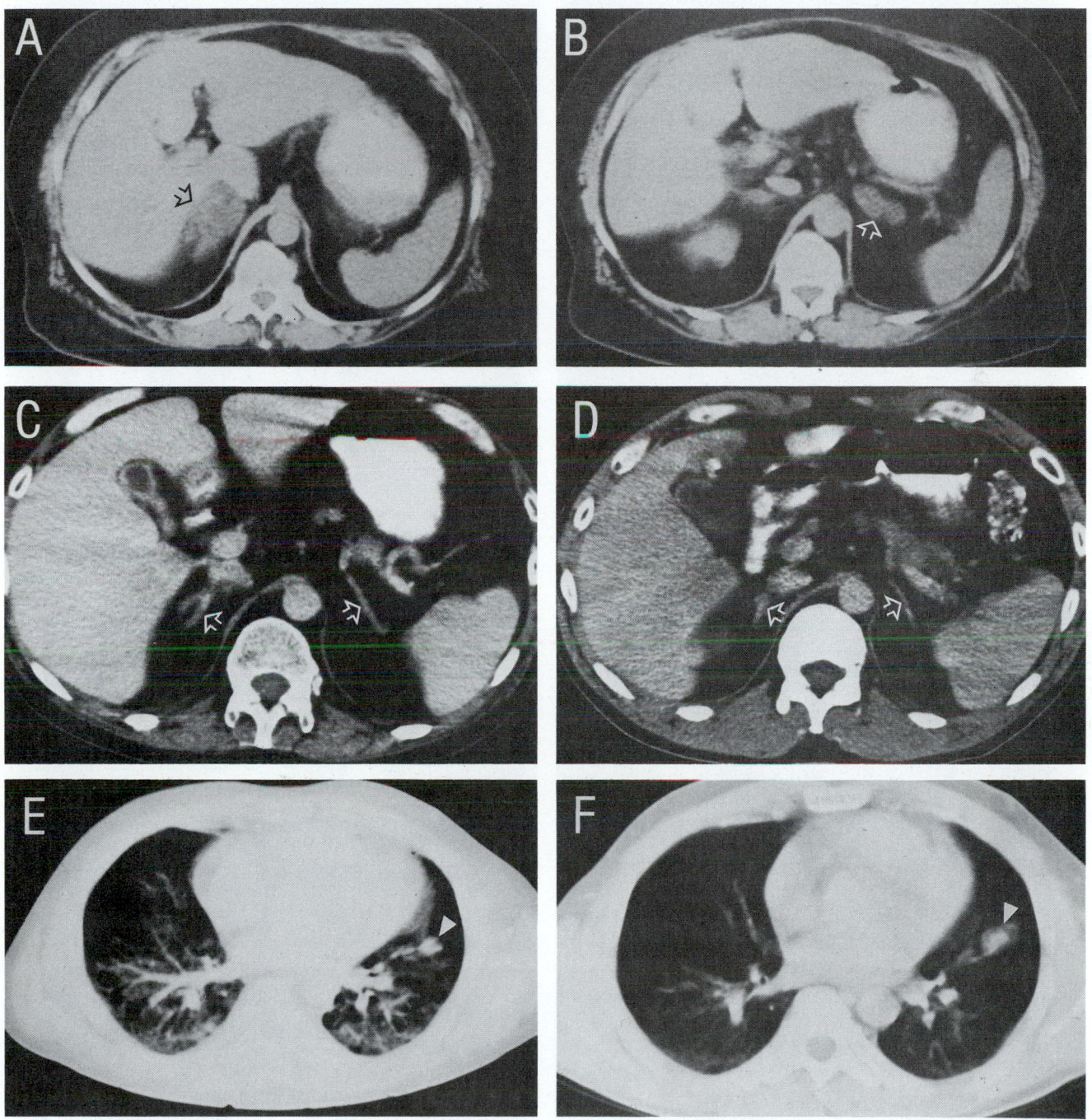

Figure 9–45. CT and MRI scans of the adrenal glands in Cushing's syndrome. The adrenals or other objects of interest are indicated by the *arrows. A, B,* CT scans of a 57-y-old woman with a 2-y history of Cushing's syndrome demonstrating bilateral macronodular hyperplasia. CT scans of *(C)* the adrenal glands and *(E)* chest of a 32-y-old man with a 2-y history of Cushing's syndrome. He has diffuse bilateral adrenal hyperplasia and a left lung lesion thought to represent old granulomatous disease. *D, F,* The same patient as in *C* 3 y later, during which time hypercortisolism was controlled with the use of adrenal enzyme inhibitors, showing no change in the adrenal glands but an increase in the size of the lung lesion, an ACTH-secreting bronchial carcinoid tumor.

Illustration continued on following page

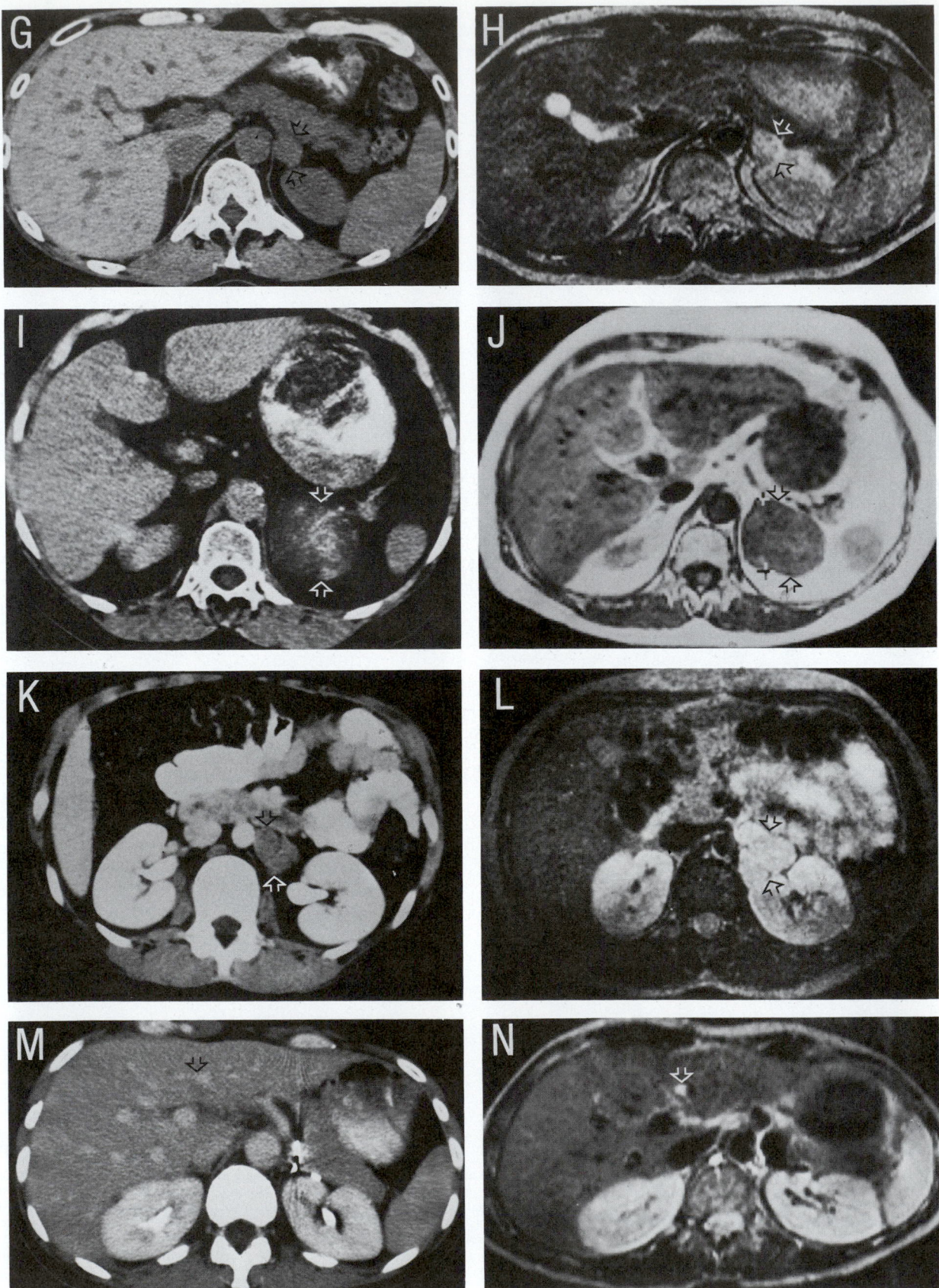

Figure 9–45 *Continued G, H,* CT and MRI scans of an adrenal adenoma causing Cushing's syndrome in a 38-y-old man. *I, J,* CT and MRI scans of a left adrenal adenoma causing Cushing's syndrome in a 59-y-old woman. The nonhomogeneity of the images, which could lead to the diagnosis of malignancy, was due to hemorrhage. *K, L,* CT and MRI scans of 13-y-old boy with left adrenal carcinoma. *M, N,* CT and T2-weighted MRI scans of one of three metastases in the liver of a 50-y-old woman. The sections are virtually identical, as shown by the relative positions of the intrahepatic veins (light on the CT scan, dark on the MRI scan). The lesion, which is visible on the MRI but not the CT scan, was surgically resected. (*L* and *M* courtesy of Dr. Kenneth Lee Jones.)

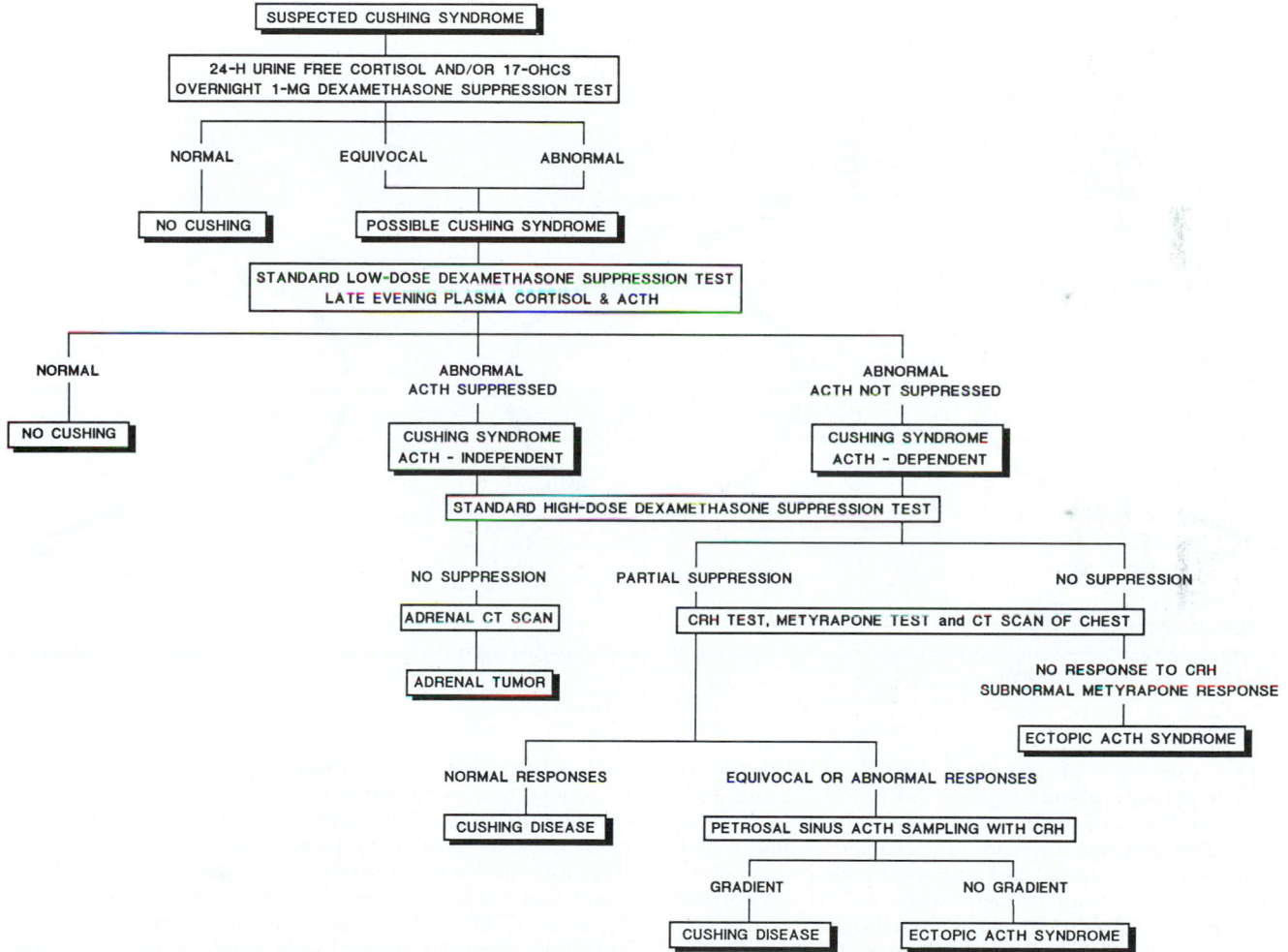

Figure 9–46. A diagnostic laboratory approach to confirming the existence of Cushing's syndrome and determining its cause.

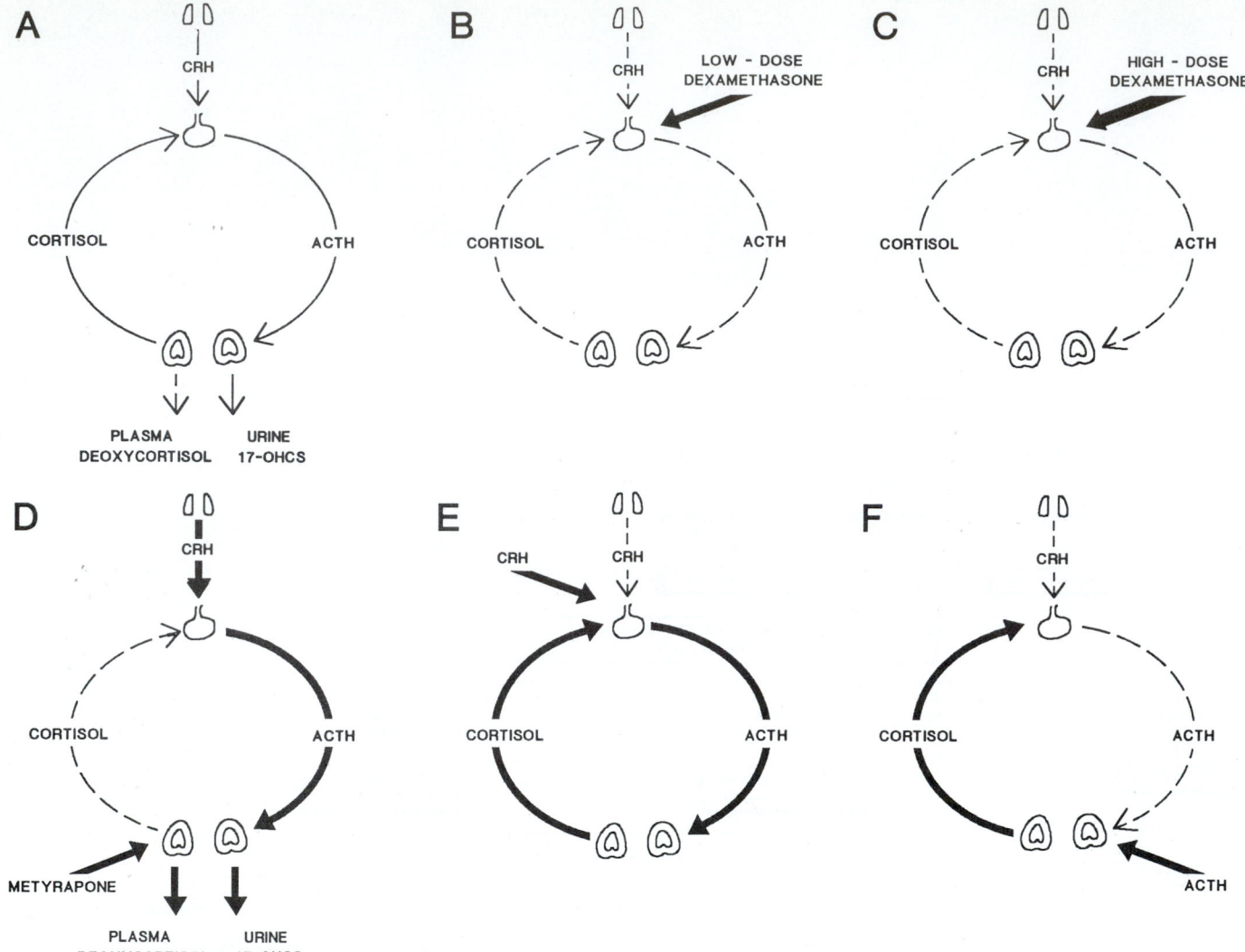

Figure 9–47. Hypothalamic-pituitary-adrenal responses of a normal individual *(A)* to the *(B)* low-dose and *(C)* high-dose dexamethasone suppression, *(D)* metyrapone, *(E)* CRH, and *(F)* ACTH stimulation tests.

CORTISOL AND/OR ITS METABOLITES (see Figs. 9–47*A* and 9–48*A*). Late evening plasma cortisol concentrations and 24-h urinary excretion of free cortisol and 17-OHCS are increased. The greatest disparity between the plasma values in normal control subjects and Cushing's patients is at about 1 h after the usual hour of sleep, when ACTH and cortisol levels normally reach their nadirs; morning plasma cortisol levels are usually within the normal range. In practice, the sample can be drawn at 1 AM regardless of the patient's sleep status that evening. To avoid a false-positive result caused by stress, (1) the sample should not be obtained the first night in hospital, (2) the patient should not be told a sample will be collected, and (3) an intravenous access line should be established in advance. Normal 1-h postsleep cortisol concentrations should be near or below the limit of detection (<140 nmol/L [<5 μg/dL]). Cortisol secretion is episodic in Cushing's disease, so it is advisable to obtain a sample on two consecutive nights to confirm the result.

Two consecutive basal 24-h urine specimens should be collected because hormone secretion may vary from day to day, especially from adrenal[1053] or ectopic ACTH-secreting tumors[1109] but also in some Cushing's disease patients.[1110–1112] One must be aware of this possibility if one is to interpret correctly the results of subsequent diagnostic tests. Cooper-

ative subjects can collect urine as outpatients. Creatinine excretion must be measured to assess adequacy of collection. In addition, expressing steroid excretion as a function of creatinine excretion in complete collections corrects for lean body mass and renal function and brings the values of most obese non-Cushing's patients within the normal range.[1113] Steroids, ACTH, CRH, or adrenal enzyme inhibitors should not be administered during baseline collections, and all other unnecessary medications should be discontinued.

DEPENDENCE OF CORTISOL SECRETION ON ACTH STIMULATION: BASAL PLASMA ACTH CONCENTRATIONS (see Figs. 9–47*A* and 9–48*A*). If cortisol secretion is dependent on ACTH secretion, as in Cushing's disease and ectopic ACTH or CRH syndrome, plasma ACTH concentrations will be inappropriately high (i.e., within or above the normal range), whereas if cortisol secretion is independent of ACTH secretion, as in adrenal tumor or other primary adrenal causes of Cushing's syndrome, these concentrations will be suppressed. Samples for plasma ACTH measurements are drawn at the same time as those for plasma cortisol. Normal 1-h postsleep plasma ACTH concentration should be low, usually less than 2 pmol/L (10 pg/mL). Because ACTH secretion is episodic and the circulating half-life of ACTH is brief, sampling on two consecutive evenings is essential.

RELATIVE RESISTANCE TO GLUCOCORTICOID NEGATIVE FEEDBACK INHIBITION: THE LOW-DOSE DEXAMETHASONE SUPPRESSION TEST (see Figs. 9–47*B* and 9–48*B*). The low-dose dexamethasone suppression test differentiates patients with Cushing's syndrome of any cause from those who do not have hypercortisolism. Its principle is that dexamethasone suppresses pituitary ACTH secretion, has no direct effect on the adrenal cortex, and is many times more potent than cortisol so that much less steroid is required to achieve the same effect. It does not cross-react in most radioimmunoassays for serum or urinary free cortisol. It is a 17-OHCS, but because so little is administered its contribution to urinary 17-OHCS concentrations is negligible.

The test can be performed either as the standard 2-d test[1018] or as an overnight screening test.[1114] Both can be performed safely on an outpatient basis if the patient is capable of cooperating. The overnight test is faster, but the standard test produces fewer false-positive results. Failure to take the drug, episodic ACTH secretion, and rapid metabolism of dexamethasone[1115, 1116] are some causes for the 10 to 15% false-positive results in the overnight test. Rare false-negative results may be due to slow metabolism of dexamethasone[1117] or, in the standard 2-d test, dexamethasone-induced increase in glomerular filtration rate.[1118] Measuring serum dexamethasone, as well as cortisol, at the completion of the tests avoids false interpretation. Urinary 17-OHCS and free cortisol levels on the second day of the test should be suppressed to less than 6.9 μmol (2.5 mg) and less than 55 nmol (20 μg) per day, respectively, regardless of body weight. Plasma cortisol and ACTH levels 6 h after the last 0.5-mg dose should be suppressed to less than 140 nmol/L (5 μg/dL) and less than 4.4 pmol/L (20 pg/mL), respectively, and serum dexamethasone concentration at that time should be 5 to 15 nmol/L (200 to 600 ng/dL) with a mean of 9.4 nmol/L (370 ng/dL),[1115] essentially the same as that 8 h after 1 mg dexamethasone in the overnight test. In the overnight screening test, plasma cortisol values of less than 140 nmol/L (5 μg/dL) are normal, but values of 140 to 275 nmol/L (5 to 10 μg/dL) are equivocal and mandate performing the standard suppression test. In fact, we would perform the standard test on any patient with a value higher than 140 nmol/L (5 μg/dL), unless basal plasma and urine steroid values are unequivocally increased.

If the results, including the plasma dexamethasone concentration, are normal, no further evaluation is required. If they are abnormal, the patient has Cushing's syndrome or, rarely, pseudo-Cushing's syndrome associated with acute alcoholism or severe depression.[1119, 1120] One must next determine the cause of the hypercortisolism.

RELATIVE VS. ABSOLUTE RESISTANCE TO GLUCOCORTICOID NEGATIVE FEEDBACK: THE HIGH-DOSE DEXAMETHASONE SUPPRESSION TEST (see Figs. 9–47*C* and 9–48*C*). There

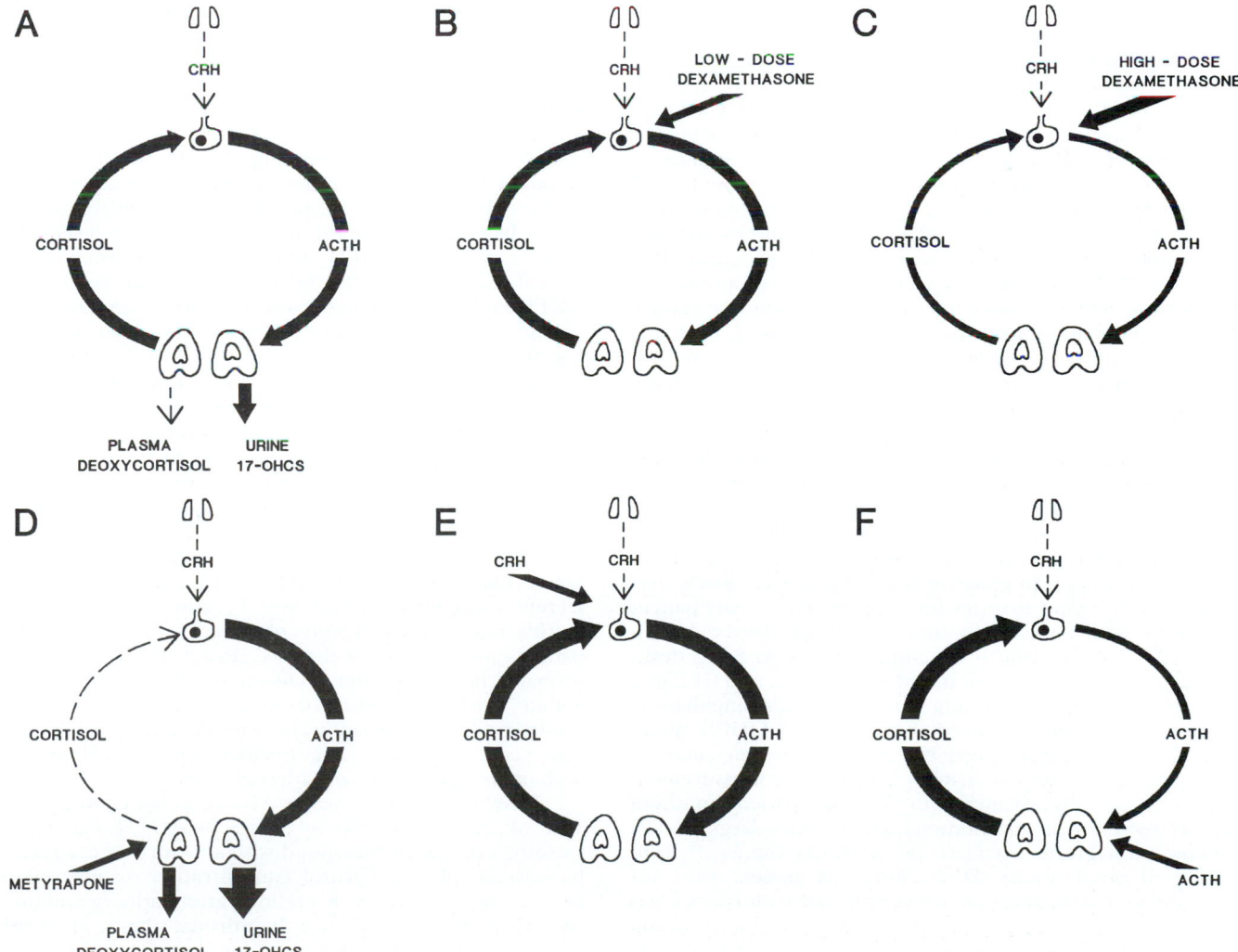

Figure 9–48. Responses of a patient with Cushing's disease *(A)* to the *(B)* low-dose and *(C)* high-dose dexamethasone suppression, *(D)* metyrapone, *(E)* CRH, and *(F)* ACTH stimulation tests.

are standard 2-d[1018] and overnight[1121] high-dose tests. Laboratory results are not available immediately, so it is efficient and cost effective to perform the high-dose test immediately after the low-dose test. If this is not done, the high-dose test must be preceded by at least 1 d of baseline urine collection. The principle of the high-dose test is that ACTH secretion in patients with Cushing's disease will be suppressed partially by this large dose of glucocorticoid (see Fig. 9–48C), whereas in patients with adrenal tumor, in whom pituitary ACTH secretion is already suppressed (see later, Fig. 9–53C), and in those with ectopic ACTH syndrome, in whom pituitary ACTH secretion is suppressed and ectopic ACTH secretion, with rare exceptions,[1025] is unresponsive to glucocorticoid regulation (see later, Fig. 9–50C), dexamethasone has no effect. The dexamethasone dose in the standard high-dose test is 16 times the usual 0.5-mg daily replacement dosage for addisonian patients. If a patient has mild Cushing's disease, with the negative feedback set point only twice normal (i.e., mean plasma cortisol level of 440 nmol/L [16 μg/dL] and urinary free cortisol excretion of 410 nmol/d [150 μg/d]), ACTH secretion will be partially suppressed even with low-dose dexamethasone (four times the replacement dosage) and profoundly suppressed with high-dose dexamethasone. However, ACTH secretion may not be suppressed significantly even by high-dose dexamethasone in a patient with Cushing's disease who has severe hypercortisolism (e.g., mean plasma cortisol level of 2.5 μmol/L [90 μg/dL] and urinary free cortisol excretion of 16.5 μmol/d [6 mg/d]). In general, the degree of suppression is inversely proportional to basal steroid production.

The criterion for deciding whether this test is positive is widely misquoted and frequently improperly applied. Urinary 17-OHCS excretion in most patients with Cushing's disease is suppressed by more than 50% from baseline,[1018] but some "have been known merely to exhibit decreases to 70–80% of their control values" after the high-dose test.[1122] *Any* degree of suppression, as long as it is *significant* (i.e., greater than daily variation and assay error) and *reproducible*, is indicative of Cushing's disease. If one recognizes that pituitary ACTH secretion, which is already suppressed in Cushing's syndrome associated with adrenal tumor or ectopic ACTH syndrome, cannot be further suppressed, then it is clear that one is seeking evidence of *any* degree of suppressibility in Cushing's disease, and most of the up to 12% false-negative results reported in some large series[1020, 1087] will be eliminated. A similar criterion can be applied to urinary free cortisol excretion. Using the criterion of reproducibility, the phenomenon of "paradoxical" response to dexamethasone also usually yields to rational explanation, such as variable day-to-day or true cyclic hormone secretion.[1109–1112, 1123]

Patients whose basal steroid production is high, reflecting great resistance to glucocorticoid negative feedback, may require even higher dosages for suppression.[1124] Any patient who otherwise appears to have Cushing's disease but in whom ACTH secretion is not suppressed with 8 mg dexamethasone a day should be tested with 16, 32, and 64 mg/d, remembering that increasing amounts of dexamethasone metabolites will be measured in urine as 17-OHCS: about 5.6, 11, and 22 mg, respectively. At these high dexamethasone dosages, therefore, urinary free cortisol measurement becomes especially advantageous. The rare patients in whom ACTH secretion is autonomous usually have large, locally invasive, low-grade corticotrope adenocarcinomas[1125] (unpublished observations, D. N. Orth). A patient who was resistant to dexamethasone but suppressed with cortisol has been reported.[1126] However, evidence of cortisol suppression consisted of measuring plasma ACTH during one 2-h cortisol infusion. Because ACTH secretion is episodic in Cushing's disease,[1016] the demonstration was inadequate. Furthermore, the mechanism for such selective glucocorticoid recognition is obscure.

Plasma dexamethasone concentration should be 18 to 51 nmol/L (700 to 2000 ng/dL) with a mean of 35 nmol/L (1350 ng/dL)[1115] 6 h after the last 2-mg dose in the standard test; values after the 8-mg overnight test have not been published but should be greater.

Macronodular adrenal hyperplasia, like diffuse hyperplasia, is ACTH dependent. The confusion in the literature, in which as many as two thirds of patients are reported to be resistant to high-dose dexamethasone,[1020] results from inappropriate criteria for suppression, poor documentation that urine collections are complete, usually no supporting plasma cortisol or ACTH data, and incorrect pathological diagnosis. If the intervening cortex is not hyperplastic, the patient does not have ACTH-dependent nodular adrenal hyperplasia. As a group, these patients are somewhat more resistant on average to dexamethasone suppression,[1022] probably simply because of the large, efficient, cortisol-producing cell mass, which requires little ACTH to secrete relatively large amounts of steroid.

If steroid production is partially or completely suppressed by high-dose dexamethasone, the diagnosis of Cushing's disease is secure. However, a CT scan of the chest should be obtained to detect ACTH-secreting bronchial[1025, 1127–1129] or thymic carcinoid tumors, about half of which may be suppressed with dexamethasone, thereby mimicking Cushing's disease. These tumors tend to be small and can be missed even on high-resolution, thin-section CT scan.

RESPONSE TO FALLING CORTISOL CONCENTRATION: THE METYRAPONE TEST (see Figs. 9–47D and 9–48D). The metyrapone test was designed as a test of pituitary ACTH-secretory reserve.[1130] As plasma cortisol levels fall, the normal (or, in patients with Cushing's disease, adenomatous) corticotropes respond by increasing ACTH production. This response can be assessed by measuring increased urinary levels of 17-OHCS, which include the tetrahydro metabolite of 11-deoxycortisol, or the increase in plasma levels of 11-deoxycortisol and ACTH. The response is normal in Cushing's disease because the microadenoma can secrete more ACTH and the hyperplastic adrenal cortex can secrete more steroid in response to increased plasma levels of ACTH (see Fig. 9–48D).

RESPONSE TO CRH AND/OR AVP: THE CRH AND AVP TESTS (see Figs. 9–47E and 9–48E). CRH and AVP are physiological ACTH secretagogues, and the microadenomas of most, but not all, patients respond to them.[797–799, 1131–1134] CRH is the more potent, together they exert an additive or synergistic effect, and both release more ACTH when endogenous cortisol production is blocked with metyrapone.[1135] The combination of CRH and AVP, with or without metyrapone, may be the most reliable means of stimulating ACTH secretion in Cushing's disease[1135] because it eliminates the 8 to 10% false-negative results observed with the CRH test in patients with Cushing's disease. However, the combination probably has no greater ability than CRH alone to differentiate Cushing's disease from other causes of Cushing's syndrome (i.e., eliminating the 3 to 5% false-positive results observed with CRH in patients with ectopic ACTH syndrome and, occasionally, primary adrenal disease).

RESPONSE TO INCREASED ACTH STIMULATION: INJECTION OR INFUSION OF COSYNTROPIN OR ACTH. Patients with Cushing's disease will respond with a normal or exaggerated increase in plasma cortisol concentration or urinary free cortisol or 17-OHCS excretion after administration of ACTH, demonstrating that the adrenal glands are neither maximally stimulated nor autonomously functioning. This test is rarely necessary.

PITUITARY SOURCE OF ACTH SECRETION: INFERIOR

PETROSAL SINUS VENOUS SAMPLING. This test was developed to demonstrate pituitary microadenomas undetected by CT or MRI scans[1136] and to lateralize the tumor within the gland.[1137] Because of the episodic nature of ACTH secretion in Cushing's disease, it is a matter of chance whether samples are drawn at the time of a spontaneous secretory episode. Thus this procedure is of questionable value unless peripheral intravenous injection of CRH is used to stimulate a secretory episode.[1138] A simultaneous peripheral venous sample must be obtained for each central sample. CRH releases prolactin from most microadenomas, which may provide a useful complement to ACTH measurements.[1139] The test appears to be reliable in experienced hands.[1138] Its limitations include the technical difficulty in simultaneously catheterizing both inferior petrosal veins, anatomical variations in venous drainage,[1140–1144] the reliability of plasma ACTH assays, potential thrombotic and hemorrhagic complications, and expense. It can be helpful in unusual patients in whom the distinction between Cushing's disease and ectopic ACTH syndrome is equivocal or in those thought to have Cushing's disease who are not cured by subtotal or total hypophysectomy. It is unlikely that its routine use may obviate the need for other diagnostic tests, as some have proposed.[1144] Some have used the data from this test to perform successful hemihypophysectomy in patients whose microadenomas could not be identified at surgery,[1138] whereas others,[1144] like the authors, have found the test of little value in predicting tumor location. More experience is required to assess the value of this procedure.

Radiographic/Nuclear Medicine Procedures. In addition to the pituitary-adrenal function tests discussed earlier, a chest CT or MRI scan should be obtained in all patients with apparent Cushing's disease who have not had petrosal venous sampling to exclude the presence of a bronchial or thymic carcinoid tumor that is mimicking Cushing's disease. MRI scans obtained both with and without gadolinium enhancement are useful for identifying the location of more than half of the pituitary microadenomas, and the CT scan provides the neurosurgeon with information about the structure of the sphenoid sinus and sella. Adrenal CT or MRI scans are not necessary but may reveal the existence of macronodular hyperplasia.

Pathology. A solitary adenoma, usually centrally located,[1145] is found in the anterior pituitary of 80 to 90% of patients. Of the adenomas, 80 to 90% are microadenomas (<10 mm in diameter) that do not enlarge the sella,[1145–1148] over half are less than 5 mm in diameter, and the average size is 5.6 mm.[1148] The larger tumors often extend beyond the sella and are locally invasive, but malignancy is rare[1149, 1150] and systemic metastases are even rarer.[1062] Those that extend beyond the sella may[1151] or may not[1152] cause increased levels of ACTH in the cerebrospinal fluid. Occasional patients have diffuse corticotrope hyperplasia.[987, 1148]

The adenomas are usually nonencapsulated and basophilic, occasionally chromophobic (i.e., sparsely granulated). Sheets of cells are arranged in a sinusoidal pattern. ACTH and other POMC-derived peptides can be demonstrated in tumor extracts[1094] or by immunocytochemical staining.[1153, 1154] Alterations in post-translational processing of POMC may result in abnormal ratios of final peptide products.[1066] Most adenomas contain cells that produce desacetyl-α-MSH, as do scattered corticotropes in normal anterior pituitaries.[1155] The microadenomas may also have a second cell subpopulation that produces prolactin.[1156] As in normal corticotropes, the secretory granules vary from 200 to 700 nm in diameter and tend to cluster below the cell membrane.[1153] Crooke's hyaline change results from chronic exposure of corticotropes to glucocorticoids and consists of an array of microfilaments surrounding the nucleus.[1153] In Cushing's disease

the hyaline change is prominent in the adenomatous corticotropes. Corticotropes in the nonadenomatous pituitary are sparse and contain relatively small amounts of POMC-derived peptides,[1153] but hyperplastic corticotropes have occasionally been reported.[1157, 1158] A few patients have diffuse corticotrope hyperplasia.[987, 1057] In some instances, no pathological changes can be found.[1056]

Bilateral diffuse adrenocortical hyperplasia is characteristic. The glands typically weigh 1.5 to 2 times normal (12 to 16 g), occasionally 3 times normal (24 g). The cut surface reveals inner brown and outer yellow cortical layers of equal thickness.[4] On microscopic examination, the widened inner zone of compact cells is sharply demarcated from an outer zone of clear cells.[4] The smooth endoplasmic reticulum is prominent, lipid droplets are decreased in size, and mitochondrial structure is altered. Multiple small nodules (< 0.25 cm in diameter), consisting predominantly of clear cells, are often seen. The zona glomerulosa is normal.

Unilateral or bilateral macronodular hyperplasia is found in 20% of patients, particularly in children[1055] and older patients with long-standing Cushing's disease.[43, 1022] The nodules are almost always bilateral, although disparate in size, ranging in diameter from 0.25 to 5 cm and more,[1020] and may be incorrectly identified as adenomas.[1159] They consist mainly of clear cells arranged in acini and cords. They compress the surrounding cortex, which is, without exception, hyperplastic. It is this last histopathological feature, more than any other, that distinguishes them functionally from the nodules in ACTH-independent bilateral micronodular dysplasia.[4, 1007, 1009, 1010, 1160, 1161] The reason for this difference is functional: if the nodules function autonomously, the cortisol they secrete suppresses ACTH secretion and the remainder of the cortex atrophies; in contrast, when the nodules are the result of ACTH hyperstimulation, the remaining cortex is also hyperplastic. The hyperplastic nodules themselves cannot be distinguished pathologically from adenomas, a feature that has led to confusion in the literature. Whether there is ever progression to true autonomy[1023] is still uncertain but unlikely, as previously discussed. There are two cases that seem to demonstrate some features of both ACTH-dependent and ACTH-independent macronodular hyperplasia.[1162, 1163] In addition, in the rare condition ACTH-independent bilateral macronodular hyperplasia,[1012, 1164] the cortex between the large nodules appears hyperplastic and contains micronodules that are indistinguishable from those found in ACTH-dependent diffuse hyperplasia, despite the fact that ACTH is suppressed and cortisol secretion is, therefore, resistant to dexamethasone suppression. The pathophysiology in these conditions is unclear.

Treatment. Ideal treatment of Cushing's disease, as of other causes of Cushing's syndrome, includes the following goals: (1) to cure the syndrome by reducing cortisol secretion to normal, (2) to eradicate any tumor threatening the health of the patient, (3) to avoid permanent dependence on medications, and (4) to avoid permanent hormone deficiency.[1105] One or more of the last three goals may have to be sacrificed to achieve the first one. The progressive stages of treatment that may be required to cure a patient of Cushing's disease are shown in Figure 9–49. Each stage provides the maximal probability of cure with the least chance of permanent endocrine deficiency.

Treatment is aimed first at the anterior pituitary gland, the apparent site of the primary cause of Cushing's disease. This is equally true for patients with ACTH-dependent macronodular hyperplasia, with or without "autosuppression" of ACTH secretion. Transsphenoidal microadenomectomy is the most rational treatment for Cushing's disease because the patient is cured and left with normal hypotha-

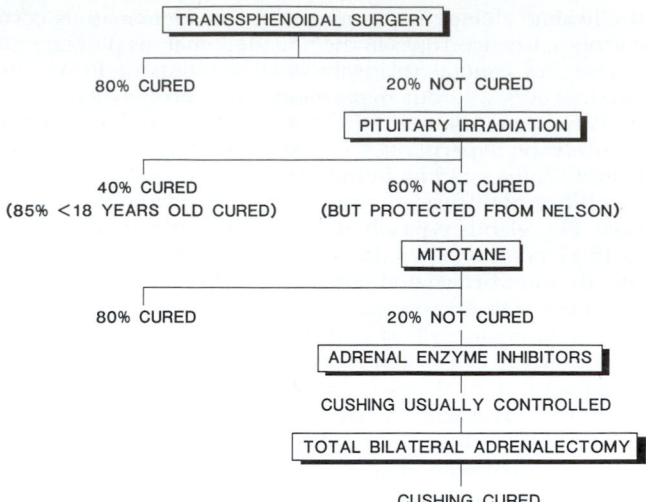

Figure 9–49. Treatment of Cushing's disease, showing the sequence of treatments that may be required for cure.

lamic-pituitary-adrenal function. In adult patients in whom a microadenoma cannot be identified and for whom fertility is not an issue, 80 to 90% of the pituitary should be resected, leaving a small island attached to the stalk. A neurosurgeon experienced with Cushing's patients can achieve a cure rate of 80 to 90% with microadenomas[1069, 1070, 1087, 1145–1148, 1165, 1166] but less than 50% with macroadenomas.[1167] In less experienced hands, the cure rate can fall to zero.[1168] Other than inexperience, the reasons for failure are unclear. Not all of the sella can be directly visualized at surgery, so adenoma tissue may be missed. Diffuse corticotrope hyperplasia may be responsible for other failures.[1148] Rarely, adenomatous ectopic pituitary tissue may be the cause.[1169] Intraoperative measurement of ACTH levels in peripituitary venous blood may be useful in localizing the adenoma and ensuring that the resection is adequate.[1170]

Patients should be given higher than normal glucocorticoid replacement intraoperatively and postoperatively to avoid acute steroid withdrawal: 200 mg of hydrocortisone by constant infusion or in divided doses over the first 24 h after induction of anesthesia and 100 mg, 75 mg, 50 mg, and maintenance hydrocortisone (10 to 25 mg each morning) on successive days thereafter. Occasional patients become anorexic and have generalized malaise and postural hypotension 3 or 4 d after surgery. These problems often respond to increasing glucocorticoid replacement for another day or two. Transient diabetes insipidus is common, but permanent AVP deficiency occurs in only a few percent, even of patients who have subtotal resection of the gland.

To assess cure, an early morning serum cortisol value can be obtained 24 h after the first maintenance dose of hydrocortisone. It is always less than 140 nmol/L (5 μg/dL) and usually less than 28 nmol/L (1 μg/dL) in cured patients; plasma ACTH is always lower than 2 pmol/L (10 pg/mL) and is usually undetectable (<1 pmol/L [<5 pg/mL]). Occasionally, morning plasma ACTH and cortisol values decrease over a few days, possibly indicating progressive necrosis of remaining ischemic cells. A persistent normal morning cortisol level, even if it represents a major decrease from preoperative levels, always indicates incomplete resection and almost certain recurrence. The ACTH response to CRH is blunted.[1171]

In patients who are not cured, three options remain: (1) reoperate on the pituitary gland, (2) radiate the pituitary gland, or (3) perform a medical or surgical adrenalectomy.

Reoperation has a lower success rate than initial surgery. It can usually be avoided by performing the most extensive resection warranted during the first operation.

Pituitary radiation is the rational next choice—and may be initial therapy in pediatric patients[1172]—because it has a reasonable probability of success, is a benign procedure rarely associated with untoward side effects, and may decrease the incidence of Nelson's syndrome (enlarging, locally invasive pituitary corticotrope tumors causing hyperpigmentation)[1173, 1174] in patients who are not cured and must undergo medical or surgical adrenalectomy. About 80% of children are cured,[1172] whereas the cure rate in adults is only about 15%.[1105] Another 25 to 30% of adults are sufficiently improved, however, to require no additional therapy or modest doses of adrenal enzyme inhibitors.[1105] The percent responding may be somewhat higher after failed transsphenoidal surgery.[1048] A total of 42 to 45 Gy (4200 to 4500 rad) of conventional megavoltage radiation is delivered to the pituitary gland at a rate of 1.8 to 2 Gy/d (180 to 200 rad/d) via opposed temporal or other multiple collimated ports with a ^{60}Co source or linear accelerator. It may require 12 to 18 mo to achieve maximal benefit, and occasional "improved" patients may be cured several years after treatment. Pediatric patients generally respond much more rapidly, often within 3 mo.[1172] During and after treatment, while awaiting full benefit of radiation, hypercortisolism can be ameliorated or controlled by use of adrenal enzyme inhibitors.[1105]

With this treatment schedule, we have encountered no serious side effects in either adult or pediatric patients, some of whom have been followed for 30 y (unpublished observations, D. N. Orth). Less than 5% of the patients have developed clinical GH or TSH deficiency months to years after radiation. With provocative testing, some degree of pituitary deficiency may be detected in a majority of patients who receive two to three times the dose we have employed.[1175] Others[1176] have corroborated our experience. Higher cure rates can be attained by delivering up to 110 Gy (11,000 rad) of alpha particle or proton beam external radiation over a few days[1177, 1178] or [198]Au or ^{90}Y interstitial radiation,[1179, 1180] but with a higher incidence of side effects, especially hypopituitarism. Stereotactic radiation with the ^{60}Co gamma knife[1181] or the linear accelerator photon knife[1182] is now available. These instruments can deliver over 100 Gy (10,000 rad) of radiation in one treatment with great precision. There are as yet no reliable data on the efficacy in Cushing's disease, but one can anticipate that it will be as good as that of Bragg's peak proton beam radiation and may be accompanied by fewer untoward side effects.

Mitotane (see Fig. 9–9) is an adrenocorticolytic drug that can be used to achieve a medical adrenalectomy during or after pituitary radiation.[70, 1183, 1184] It is more difficult to achieve control of adrenocortical function in patients who are not radiated. The drug can be started as a 0.5-g dose given at bedtime and adding single 0.5-g doses at mealtimes every few days to increase the dose to 4 g/d, with half of the daily dosage taken at bedtime to reduce nausea.

The goal is total ablation of cortisol secretion, not attainment of normal adrenal function, because, as with subtotal surgical adrenalectomy, incomplete ablation with mitotane does not permanently cure the hypercortisolism, which recurs. For instance, Schteingart and co-workers[1184] initially reported a cure rate of 80%, a minority of whom were hypocortisolemic. They have now treated 46 patients and followed them from 5 to 15 y. Eight eventually had pituitary surgery, and nine had bilateral surgical adrenalectomy; the sustained cure rate was 59% (personal communication, D. E. Schteingart), similar to that of Luton and colleagues,[1183] who used higher doses of mitotane without radiation. Four of Schteingart's 46 patients (personal communication, D. E. Schteingart) and none of Luton's 46 nonradiated patients[1183] developed Nelson's syndrome. These are lower than the incidence after surgical adrenalectomy, perhaps because mitotane acts in some manner on the pituitary as well.[1185] Our experience is limited to five patients, all of whom have been cured and remained hypocortisolemic for up to 3 y (unpublished observations, D. N. Orth). The usual duration of mitotane therapy is 6 to 9 mo.

One cannot easily predict when a patient will become hypocortisolemic, so replacement glucocorticoid, usually 0.5 mg dexamethasone each day, is begun when mitotane is started. Mitotane increases the metabolism of dexamethasone[926] and fludrocortisone and, perhaps, cortisol and other steroids. Therefore, it may be necessary to increase the dosage of these drugs to three to seven times the usual dose, using amelioration of symptoms of hypocortisolism or serum dexamethasone levels for guidance. Mitotane is taken up by fatty tissues and persists in plasma long after the drug is discontinued.[1186] Thus one may have to taper the dosage of glucocorticoid over a period of several weeks to months after mitotane is stopped until the usual maintenance dose is attained.

Efficacy during treatment must be assessed by measuring plasma or salivary cortisol or urinary free cortisol. Mitotane shifts the extra-adrenal metabolism of cortisol toward 6β-hydroxycortisol, which is not measured as a 17-OHCS, so urinary 17-OHCS levels are low.

Mitotane is expensive and not an easy drug to use. Acceptance of the drug by patients is variable, but most can tolerate 4 g/d. Major complaints are nausea, vomiting, and anorexia, but rash, diarrhea, ataxia, gynecomastia, arthralgias, and leukopenia also occur. The reward for this effort is avoidance of a major surgical procedure in most patients and the probability of retaining normal aldosterone secretion.[926, 1105, 1186] When aldosterone secretion is retained, the patient is at less risk for developing stress-related adrenal crisis; clinically, the situation is more like isolated ACTH deficiency. Despite these potential benefits, surgical adrenalectomy may be preferred to the intensive care required for 6 to 9 mo or more for mitotane therapy.

In patients in whom rapid cure of hypercortisolism is necessary or in whom all other therapies have failed, bilateral total surgical adrenalectomy is the definitive treatment.[1105, 1187, 1188] Unilateral or subtotal adrenalectomy[1184] is virtually never successful unless the patient has been improved but not cured by prior pituitary radiation (i.e., ACTH secretion is partially inhibited) or the adrenalectomy is inadvertently total because of subsequent infarction of the remnant. This is because the adrenal remnant, under continued stimulation by elevated levels of ACTH, eventually becomes hyperplastic. For the same reason, total adrenalectomy with subcutaneous autotransplantation is likely to fail; three of eight patients were reported to have developed recurrent Cushing's syndrome.[1189]

Transabdominal adrenalectomy causes major morbidity. When possible, the bilateral flank approach should be used.[1190] The glands must be removed en bloc, and care must be taken to ensure that the fragile capsule is not broken,[1190] because cells spilled locally can cause recurrent disease. An unusual cause of failure is the existence of ectopic adrenal tissue,[1191] which can sometimes be located by scintiscan with ^{131}I-labeled cholesterol.[1192] Cure should be confirmed by measuring plasma cortisol or urinary steroid levels. Steroid coverage is similar to that for transsphenoidal surgery, except that lifelong mineralocorticoid replacement therapy with fludrocortisone must be begun as soon as intravenous saline is discontinued.

We have performed medical or surgical adrenalectomy on 53 patients with Cushing's disease, all but 3 of whom had pituitary radiation before or shortly after adrenalectomy. Only one has developed Nelson's syndrome, one of the three who was not radiated. Nelson's syndrome occurs in about 20% of adults and over 50% of children who are adrenalectomized for Cushing's disease without pituitary radiation.[1193–1196] Consequently, we have concluded that radiation tends to prevent later development of Nelson's syndrome and do not recommend adrenalectomy for a patient who has not been radiated. However, radiation does not guarantee that Nelson's syndrome will not develop in some patients.[1187, 1197, 1198]

Other therapies include the administration of centrally active drugs, adrenal enzyme inhibitors, antiglucocorticoid agents, and a long-acting somatostatin analogue. Bromocriptine, cyproheptadine, and valproate are centrally active drugs that have been advocated as treatment by some investigators.[1065, 1199–1202] Although occasional successes have been reported, the results have generally been disappointing,[1203] the drugs do not provide permanent cure, and effective treatment is delayed.

The adrenal enzyme inhibitors aminoglutethimide, ketoconazole, metyrapone, trilostane, and etomidate (see Fig. 9–9) have been used as treatment.[188, 1204–1206] If the pharmacological blockade is incomplete, ACTH levels increase and override the blockade, as in incomplete congenital enzyme deficiencies. Aminoglutethimide, an anticonvulsant, blocks mainly the first step in cortisol biosynthesis and is used at a dosage of 250 mg two or three times a day. Most patients develop a transient, generalized, pruritic rash that can usually be treated symptomatically with diphenhydramine hydrochloride (Benadryl) for a few days without stopping the aminoglutethimide. Metyrapone inhibits mainly the final step in cortisol biosynthesis and may also inhibit ACTH secretion directly at high dosages.[1207] In dosages of about 4 g/d, metyrapone decreases but usually does not return cortisol secretion to normal in patients with untreated Cushing's disease.[1204] Thus, like the other adrenal enzyme inhibitors, this agent is useful mainly as adjunctive therapy in patients with mild disease or after pituitary radiation,[1105, 1204, 1208] in whom further increase in ACTH secretion is inhibited.[1209] For this purpose, dosages of 500 to 750 mg three or four times a day are usually required. Ketoconazole, which acts mainly on the first step in cortisol biosynthesis but also inhibits the conversion of 11-deoxycortisol to cortisol, may be the most effective of the three drugs because it also inhibits ACTH secretion[1210] at therapeutic dosage (200 to 400 mg two or three times a day) by impairing corticotrope adenylate cyclase activation.[1210] Unfortunately, it also is a rare cause of significant reversible hepatotoxicity[1211] and commonly causes nausea and vomiting in our experience. Trilostane, the least well studied of this group of drugs, is effective in some patients.[1212] Etomidate, a substituted imidazole anesthetic that blocks 11β-hydroxylation of deoxycortisol, may be useful in hospitalized patients when infused intravenously in a low, nonhypnotic dosage of 0.3 mg/kg/h.[188] It lowers the plasma cortisol level to the mean normal range (i.e., 275 nmol/L [10 μg/dL]) within about 10 h.[188] The plasma ACTH level remains within the normal range after 5 h of infusion in normal subjects, but ACTH concentration might increase and overcome the etomidate blockade after more chronic administration in Cushing's disease patients.

Other side effects include, with aminoglutethimide, somnolence at daily dosages of 1 g or more, especially in adults, headache, goiter, hypothyroidism, and, rarely, cholestasis and bone marrow suppression; with ketoconazole, headache, sedation, gynecomastia, decreased libido, and impotence; with metyrapone, nausea, headache, sedation, and rash; with trilostane, diarrhea, abdominal pain, nausea, burning mucous membranes, flushing, headache, rhinorrhea, decreased libido, and impotence; and with etomidate, tiredness. With combinations of these drugs, additive or synergistic therapeutic effects can be achieved at lower individual dosages and thus side effects are minimized. Aminoglutethimide increases the metabolism of dexamethasone but not of cortisol.[1213] Therefore, cortisol or cortisone acetate may be the glucocorticoid therapy of choice with this drug. Aminoglutethimide, which may cause aldosterone deficiency without a compensatory increase in DOC level, may occasionally necessitate fludrocortisone replacement. In addition to their other limitations as long-term treatment, the enzyme inhibitors are expensive. A therapeutic dosage of aminoglutethimide is by far the least expensive of the four.

Mifepristone (RU-486) (see Fig. 9–9) is an antiprogestational drug that, at much higher dosages, competes with glucocorticoids for binding to the receptor and thus blocks their action. This drug has been used acutely in several patients with Cushing's disease.[1214] Plasma cortisol levels increase about twofold. It appears to be effective, but it also blocks exogenous glucocorticoids. Thus it is difficult to assess and treat systemic glucocorticoid deficiency induced by mifepristone. At present, it is an investigational drug.

The long-acting somatostatin analogue octreotide appears to have little role in treating Cushing's disease. It may act at the level of the adrenal gland, not the pituitary.[1215]

Prognosis. Cushing's syndrome is often fatal, the result of cardiovascular, thromboembolic, or hypertensive complications or inability to respond to bacterial infection. There was once a 50% mortality 5 y after development of symptoms.[992] For Cushing's disease the prognosis is certainly not that ominous today. Cushing's disease is virtually always curable, although rarely patients may die of perioperative or other complications. Rare exceptions are patients with large, locally invasive, or metastatic tumors, who can succumb to effects of the tumor itself. No patient should die from persistent hypercortisolism, because hypercortisolism can virtually always be controlled by adrenal enzyme inhibitors, mitotane, or surgical adrenalectomy.

Signs and symptoms of Cushing's syndrome disappear gradually over a period of 2 to 12 mo. Hypertension and glucose intolerance improve but may not be cured. Unlike other forms of osteoporosis, the osteopenia of Cushing's syndrome regresses rapidly after hypercortisolemia is cured.[1216] Unfortunately, vertebral compression fractures and aseptic necrosis of proximal long bones cause permanent deformity and are a major reason for the importance of early cure of Cushing's syndrome.

Patients are hypocortisolemic for up to 12 mo after microadenomectomy and require glucocorticoid replacement therapy, which must be supplemented during stress. The rationale and methods for ensuring rapid, safe recovery are discussed later in this chapter.

The incidence of recurrence after cure by transsphenoidal microadenomectomy is not known, but one center has performed over 200 operations and reports that the recurrence rate is about 2% and that recurrences can occur as long as 8 y after operation.[1087] The rate may be higher in children.[1148] Patients with recurrent Cushing's syndrome should be studied and treated as if they had developed the disorder for the first time.

Patients who have been adrenalectomized, particularly those who have not had pituitary radiation, may develop Nelson's syndrome, in which an enlarging pituitary tumor is associated with progressive hyperpigmentation. Plasma ACTH levels range from as low as about 175 pmol/L (800 pg/mL) to as high as 5500 pmol/L (25,000 pg/mL) and more. The syndrome appears several months to many years after adrenalectomy, but the average is about 3 y. The pathogen-

esis of these tumors is uncertain. Presumably they represent the growth of pre-existing microadenomas, but it is not clear why some but not all of these tumors continue to grow in size. There are no predictive clinical or laboratory indices, except that the plasma ACTH level in those who subsequently develop tumors increases much more (1) during prolonged preadrenalectomy treatment with mitotane (but not during acute suppression of cortisol biosynthesis with metyrapone) and (2) during the first year after adrenalectomy while taking equivalent steroid replacement therapy (500 vs. 77 pmol/L, or 2300 vs. 350 pg/mL) (personal communication, J.-P. Luton, H. Escourelle, X. Y. Bertagna, and B. Guilhaume). Because this appears to be a chronic rather than an acute response to decreased glucocorticoid negative feedback, it presumably reflects the tendency of these tumors to grow and produce more ACTH-secreting cells when the effect of glucocorticoids is reduced. Once the tumors become large enough to expand the sella, they are locally invasive and are difficult to cure. Therefore, adrenalectomized patients should be followed indefinitely with periodic CT or MRI scans of the pituitary and measurements of basal and dexamethasone-suppressed plasma ACTH levels.[1193, 1217] Transsphenoidal surgery or radiation should be performed before the tumor becomes a macroadenoma. Proton beam radiation may be more successful than conventional radiation, although satisfactory results can usually be achieved with the latter.[1176] Stereotactic ^{60}Co gamma knife[1181] or photon knife[1182] radiation may prove useful, but there are as yet few reported results.[1218] Sustained remission after a course of cyproheptadine therapy has been reported,[1219] but this is an isolated instance and may represent spontaneous infarction of the tumor.

Ectopic ACTH Syndrome. *Distinctive Clinical Features.* The majority of patients with ectopic ACTH syndrome have malignant tumors, half of them small cell lung carcinoma.[1024] Plasma ACTH concentrations are often very high and may be associated with hyperpigmentation. The metabolic manifestations are those of the acute salt-retaining and gluconeogenic effects of extreme hypercortisolemia, i.e., hypertension, edema, hypokalemia, weakness, and glucose intolerance,[990, 1024] which appear suddenly and progress rapidly. The typical Cushing's habitus is often absent. Hirsutism is unusual. The findings may be complicated by secretion of other ectopic hormones, such as AVP.[1024] Anorexia, weight loss, and anemia are frequent, unrelated manifestations of the malignancy causing the hypercortisolism. About 20% of patients have more indolent tumors, such as bronchial, thymic, and pancreatic carcinoid tumors or medullary carcinoma of the thyroid. The clinical presentation in subjects with the more indolent tumors may be indistinguishable from that of patients with Cushing's disease, and the tumors, in contrast to those in the usual patient with ectopic ACTH syndrome, may not be apparent even after careful investigation.

Pathogenesis. A wide variety of tumors, most of them carcinomas, have been reported to secrete ACTH and other POMC-derived peptides ectopically.[1024] Trace amounts of POMC-like mRNA and peptides can be found in many normal tissues and tumors not associated with ectopic ACTH syndrome.[1220] As discussed earlier, the mRNA in most normal tissues is smaller than in the pituitary,[1221] whereas the mRNA in tumors tends to be larger, suggesting that alternative initiation sites are responsible for the transcription of the gene in normal and neoplastic tissues.[1221, 1222] Thus it is not clear whether ectopic hormone secretion is merely inappropriate secretion of a normal product (see Chapter 34) or is truly ectopic.[1024] Possibly, examples of both phenomena exist. With rare exceptions,[1025] ACTH production by these tumors is not regulated by glucocorticoid negative feedback, either because of absent glucocorticoid receptors[1223] or because of some other defect in steroid action.[1224]

Laboratory Findings. Hypokalemic hyponatremic alkalosis is due to the mineralocorticoid effect of the high steroid concentrations in these patients. Plasma ACTH levels usually exceed the normal range (i.e., about 20 pmol/L [90 pg/mL]) and may be 175 pmol/L (800 pg/mL) and higher but overlap with those in Cushing's disease and may occasionally be only 9 pmol/L (40 pg/mL) (see Fig. 9–41). Other POMC-derived peptides are similarly elevated. Plasma cortisol concentration reflects the increased ACTH level and ranges from 550 to more than 5500 nmol/L (20 to >200 µg/dL). Typically, plasma ACTH and cortisol concentrations are two to four times normal morning values. The NH_2-terminal 22-kd intermediate of POMC (31 kd) is found in plasma of some but not in that of most patients with pituitary tumors.[1125] Similarly, one finds more evidence of production of 18-amino-acid β-melanocyte-stimulating hormone (β-MSH), corticotropin-like intermediate-lobe peptide, and high amounts of γ-lipotropin (γ-LPH) by POMC-producing non-pituitary tumors than by pituitary tumors,[1225–1227] which suggests altered post-translational processing by these tumors. There is no circadian rhythm in plasma ACTH or cortisol levels. Urinary steroid excretion is increased in proportion to the increase in plasma steroids. The enzymatic machinery for cortisol biosynthesis is normal, so levels of androgenic precursors (DHEA, DHEAS, 17-KS) are increased in proportion to those of cortisol and 17-OHCS.

Radiographic/Nuclear Medicine Findings. The tumors are often obvious, and about half are found on routine x-ray film or CT scan of the chest. Usually both adrenal glands are diffusely enlarged. Macronodular hyperplasia is unusual, presumably because the duration of ACTH hypersecretion is usually brief. Bronchial carcinoid tumors are usually quite small and may be difficult or impossible to identify, even with high-resolution, thin-section CT scans. Hyperplasia of the anterior mediastinal fat may be mistaken for a bronchial or thymic tumor. Pituitary CT and MRI scans are normal.

Laboratory Diagnosis. The diagnosis of ectopic ACTH syndrome (see Fig. 9–46) requires demonstrating (1) increased basal cortisol production, (2) dependence of cortisol secretion on ACTH stimulation, (3) absolute resistance to glucocorticoid negative feedback, (4) reduced ACTH response to falling plasma cortisol levels, (5) lack of response to CRH and/or AVP, and (6) cortisol response to exogenous ACTH stimulation. Details of these tests are provided at the end of this chapter.

INCREASED BASAL CORTISOL PRODUCTION: BASAL PLASMA CONCENTRATIONS AND URINARY EXCRETION OF CORTISOL AND/OR ITS METABOLITES (Fig. 9–50A). The means of demonstrating increased basal cortisol production by measuring plasma cortisol concentrations and urinary excretion of cortisol and cortisol metabolites are discussed in the section on Cushing's disease. There is more likely to be day-to-day variation in hormone secretion in ectopic ACTH syndrome, and occasional patients have cyclic or episodic secretion,[1109] making interpretation of results more difficult.

DEPENDENCE OF CORTISOL SECRETION ON ACTH STIM-

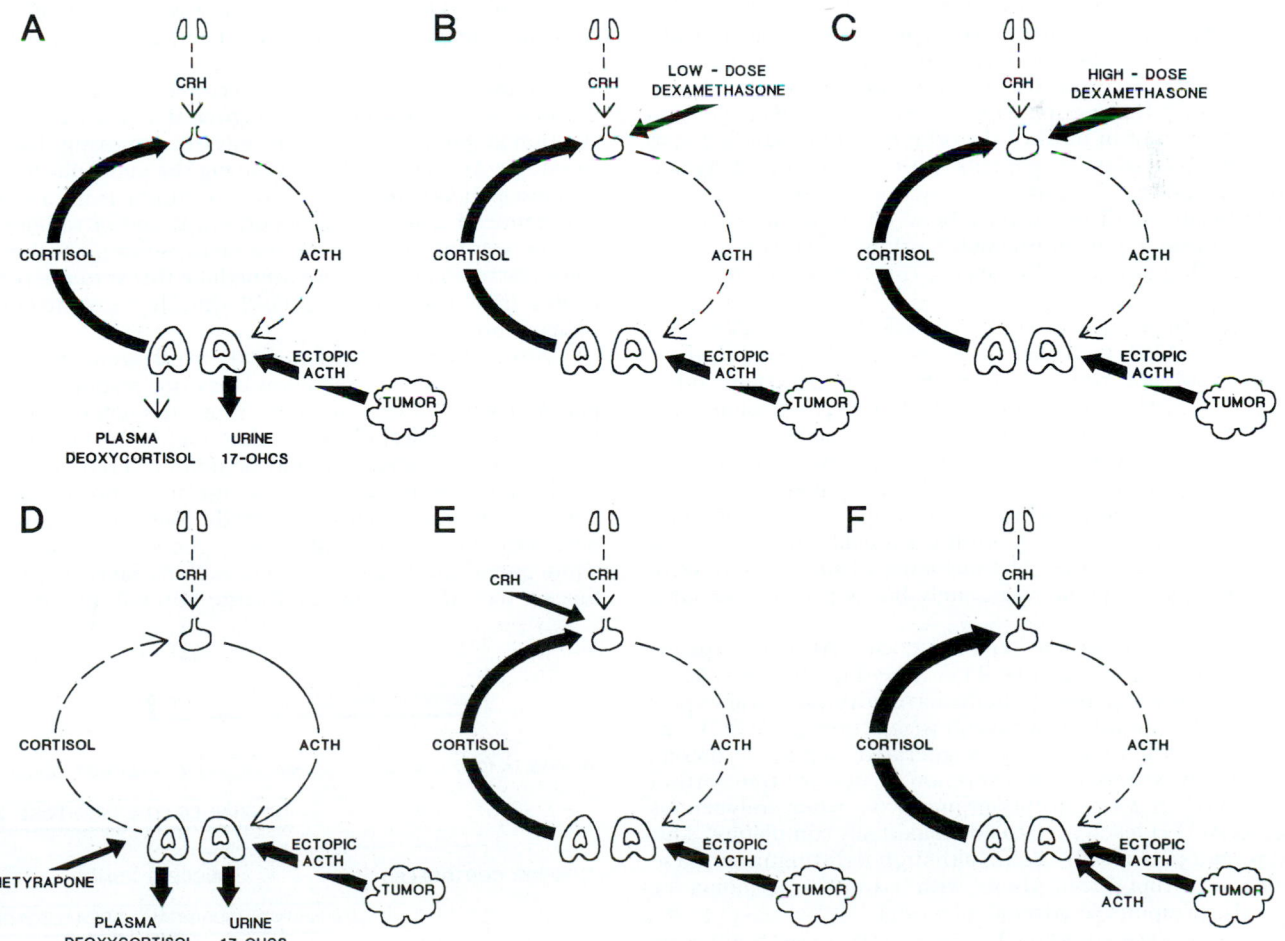

Figure 9–50. Responses of a patient with ectopic ACTH syndrome (A) to the (B) low-dose and (C) high-dose dexamethasone suppression, (D) metyrapone, (E) CRH, and (F) ACTH stimulation tests.

ULATION: BASAL PLASMA ACTH CONCENTRATIONS (see Fig. 9–50A). Plasma ACTH concentrations are measured in the same blood specimens as cortisol. Plasma ACTH concentrations tend to be higher in ectopic ACTH syndrome but overlap with levels in patients with Cushing's disease. Although, as mentioned earlier, there is abnormal processing of POMC,[1125, 1225–1229] no specific peptides in plasma distinguish these tumors from pituitary tumors.

ABSOLUTE RESISTANCE TO GLUCOCORTICOID NEGATIVE FEEDBACK: THE HIGH-DOSE DEXAMETHASONE SUPPRESSION TEST (see Fig. 9–50B and C). Unless basal steroid production is unequivocally increased, the patient should first have a low-dose dexamethasone suppression test to confirm the diagnosis of Cushing's syndrome. In patients with ACTH-dependent hypercortisolism, the high-dose test differentiates those with Cushing's disease with relative resistance to glucocorticoid negative feedback inhibition from those with ectopic ACTH syndrome, the vast majority of whom demonstrate absolute resistance. Suppression is reported in about half of the 5% of patients with ectopic ACTH syndrome associated with bronchial carcinoid tumors[1025, 1127, 1230] and occasional patients with thymic carcinoid.[1024] No more than about 3% of all patients with ectopic ACTH syndrome fall in this category. A chest CT or MRI scan in all patients who appear to have Cushing's disease will identify some of them.

REDUCED ACTH RESPONSE TO FALLING PLASMA CORTISOL LEVELS: THE METYRAPONE TEST (see Fig. 9–50D). ACTH-secreting nonpituitary tumors do not respond to falling plasma cortisol levels by increasing ACTH secretion. However, patients with acute ectopic ACTH syndrome, usually caused by small cell lung carcinoma, do not have prolonged or profound suppression of pituitary ACTH secretion. Moreover, they have hyperplastic adrenal glands capable of responding to increased ACTH stimulation. Urinary 17-OHCS levels rise in response to metyrapone in about half of these patients, albeit subnormally,[1227] and remain constant in most of the others, rather than falling as they do invariably in patients with benign or malignant adrenal tumors.[1053] Thus the metyrapone test provides another means of distinguishing between these two forms of dexamethasone-nonsuppressible Cushing's syndrome. If one has reliable plasma ACTH assays, this test is seldom necessary.

LACK OF TUMOR RESPONSE TO CRH AND/OR AVP: THE CRH AND AVP TESTS (see Fig. 9–50E). In general, these patients do not respond to CRH or, presumably, other normal ACTH secretagogues.[1134] However, occasional patients do respond normally, and at least some responders are those with bronchial carcinoid tumors who are difficult to differentiate from Cushing's disease patients.[1230] It has not been determined whether the tumor or the pituitary responds in these patients, but it is probably the pituitary in some, if not most, cases. The incidence of such false-positive CRH tests is not known accurately but is probably about 5 to 8%.

CORTISOL RESPONSE TO EXOGENOUS ACTH STIMULATION: THE SHORT ACTH TEST (see Fig. 9–50F). As in Cushing's disease, these patients have adrenocortical hyperplasia and respond to intravenous injection of ACTH (cosyntropin) with a normal or exaggerated increase in plasma cortisol concentration and excretion of urinary free cortisol and 17-OHCS. Rare exceptions may occur when endogenous plasma ACTH levels are already maximally stimulating. This test is seldom clinically useful, although it distinguishes these patients further from those with adrenal carcinoma or ACTH-unresponsive adrenal adenoma.

OTHER PROCEDURES: DEMONSTRATING THE SOURCE OF ACTH SECRETION—VENOUS ACTH SAMPLING AND PERCUTANEOUS BIOPSY. Occasionally it is possible to localize the tumor by measuring plasma ACTH levels in central and peripheral samples obtained simultaneously by venous catheterization.[1228, 1231] Unfortunately, the majority of these tumors are located in the pulmonary or splanchnic vascular beds, where the veins directly draining the tumor are inaccessible by procedures other than trans–left ventricular pulmonary vein or transhepatic portal vein catheterization. Thus the yield from venous sampling is low. Percutaneous aspiration biopsy of bronchial or thymic carcinoid tumors with a 22-gauge Chiba needle under CT or ultrasound guidance may provide sufficient tissue for ACTH measurement and thus confirm the source of ACTH.[1232] Measurement of ACTH levels in lavage fluid obtained during bronchoscopy is not helpful.[1233]

Pathology. The nonpituitary tumors are distinguished from others of the same histological type only by the fact that they contain ACTH, which can be demonstrated in tumor extracts or by immunocytochemical techniques.[1225, 1234, 1235] Secretory granules can usually be found by electron microscopy; they tend to be relatively numerous in tumors such as bronchial carcinoids and scarce in small cell carcinoma, and the number does not correspond closely with the concentration of ACTH in the tumor.[1236] These tumors also contain neuroendocrine cell markers, such as neuron-specific enolase and carcinoembryonic antigen.[1237, 1238]

The adrenal glands are markedly and diffusely enlarged, weighing 12 to 30 g each. The cut surface reveals a greatly thickened, regular, uniformly brown cortex without nodules. The cortex consists almost exclusively of straight columns of compact cells. There are few clear cells, and compact cells often penetrate the zona glomerulosa to reach the capsule.[4] The typical appearance is distinct from that in Cushing's disease and reflects relatively acute stimulation by very high concentrations of ACTH.

Treatment. The therapy for ectopic ACTH syndrome is outlined diagrammatically in Figure 9–51. When possible, the tumor should be surgically excised, removing the source of ectopic ACTH and thereby curing the metabolic disorder. In most patients, unfortunately, the tumor is nonresectable at the time of diagnosis. Chemotherapy and/or radiotherapy may be helpful. In any case, hypercortisolism, which may in some instances pose a more immediate threat to the patient's health than the tumor, should quickly be controlled by pharmacological means.

Adrenal enzyme inhibitors are ideal agents in this situation. Tumor ACTH secretion does not respond to falling plasma cortisol levels, so there is no tendency to override the pharmacological blockade. Aminoglutethimide, ketoconazole, and metyrapone should be administered, alone or in combination. Etomidate may be useful in hospitalized patients.[1239] Hypercortisolism is usually controlled within a few days with one or two of these agents (e.g., 250 mg of aminoglutethimide and/or 250 to 500 mg metyrapone three times a day) (Fig. 9–52), and acute adrenal insufficiency is

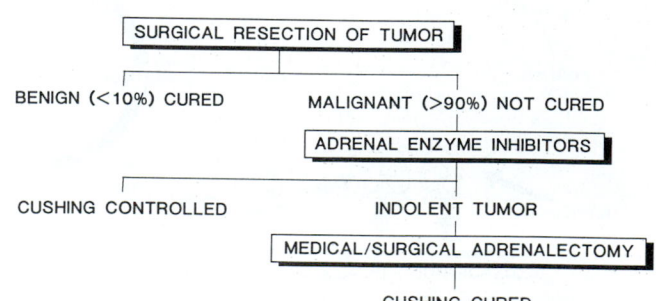

Figure 9–51. Treatment of patients with ectopic ACTH syndrome.

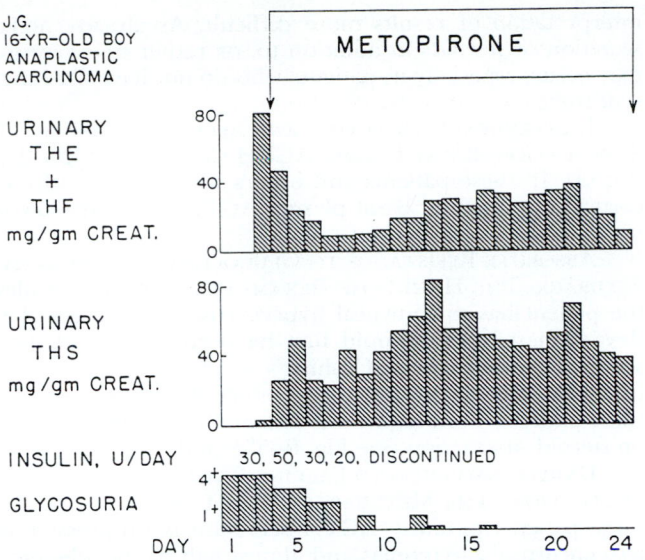

J.G.
16-YR-OLD BOY
ANAPLASTIC
CARCINOMA

Figure 9–52. Changes in urinary steroid excretion, serum K+ concentration, and insulin requirements in an adolescent patient with severe hypercortisolemia resulting from ectopic ACTH secretion after treatment with metyrapone (metopirone). Metabolites of cortisol (tetrahydrocortisol, THF, its major renal metabolite) and cortisone (tetrahydrocortisone, THE) rapidly decrease in concentration and are replaced with the tetrahydro metabolite of 11-deoxycortisol (THS), the biologically inactive immediate precursor of cortisol. This is reflected by the normalization of serum K+ concentration (not shown) and reduction in and elimination of the insulin requirement. The patient, who was moribund on arrival at hospital, returned to a fully active life before succumbing suddenly to intracranial metastatic disease. (From Liddle GW, Nicholson WE, Island DP, et al. Clinical and laboratory studies of ectopic humoral syndromes. Recent Prog Horm Res 1969; 25:283–314.)

possible. Because it is difficult to adjust the dose of inhibitor to achieve normal adrenal function, a replacement dosage of glucocorticoid should be started at the same time as the enzyme inhibitor. Aminoglutethimide induces increased hepatic clearance of steroids, so a higher than normal glucocorticoid dosage may be required.

Patients sometimes escape suddenly from enzymatic blockade, even though the peripheral venous ACTH concentrations remain constant. Metastases to the adrenal are common, particularly with small cell carcinoma.[4] This produces extremely high local concentrations of ACTH, resulting in increased steroidogenesis. Escape can usually be overcome by increasing the dosage of the drug(s). In the rare patients in whom it cannot, addition of small daily doses (1 to 3 g) of mitotane will induce adrenal insufficiency within a few days.

In patients in whom a tumor cannot be identified, enzyme inhibitors can be maintained and the patient can be re-examined periodically with CT or MRI scans for several years, if necessary, until the tumor can be diagnosed and treated. In patients with indolent tumors and a long life expectancy who cannot be cured surgically, mitotane can be used, as already described for the treatment of Cushing's disease, to achieve a medical adrenalectomy; pituitary radiation is unnecessary, of course. In appropriate patients, bilateral surgical adrenalectomy may be an alternative to mitotane.

The glucocorticoid antagonist mifepristone has been used successfully for 9 wk in one patient.[1240] It has the limitations already discussed. Octreotide, a long-acting analogue of somatostatin, can rapidly reduce ectopic ACTH secretion by some nonpituitary tumors[1241, 1242] but has no effect on tumor size. The drug must be injected twice daily and is expensive. It has little value in treating ectopic ACTH syndrome.

Prognosis. The prognosis is determined by the nature

of the tumor and is usually poor. Most patients succumb to the malignant disease within a year, whereas patients with indolent tumors may survive for over a decade. None of these patients should have persistent hypercortisolism, which can readily be controlled.

ACTH-Independent Cushing's Syndrome

Adrenocortical Tumors. *Distinctive Clinical Features*. Patients with adrenal adenoma usually have gradual onset of signs of hypercortisolism. Hirsutism and other androgenic effects are absent, as is hyperpigmentation. In contrast, patients with adrenocortical carcinoma tend to have a more acute and progressive course, and hyperandrogenic effects may predominate.[1053] The carcinoma may be palpable or the left kidney may be displaced downward, making the lower pole readily palpable. Abdominal, back, and flank pain and other tumor-related symptoms may be present.

Although most adrenal tumors cause Cushing's syndrome, with or without accompanying hypertension or virilization, adrenal adenomas may cause only virilization[1243, 1244] and adrenal carcinomas may cause only hypertension, virilization, or feminization or produce no endocrine syndrome.[1053, 1054, 1245] In patients with Cushing's disease caused by adrenocortical tumors, DOC, testosterone, estradiol, estrone, or no steroid levels may be elevated; basal plasma ACTH and cortisol concentrations may be normal; and basal cortisol production by the normal adrenal cortex may be normal and suppressible with low-dose dexamethasone. The reported incidence of nonfunctional carcinomas varies considerably, depending in part on how rigorously autonomous steroid secretion was excluded. The true incidence probably does not exceed 20%.[1053, 1054]

Pathogenesis. The cause of these tumors is not known. There are isolated instances in which adenomas[1246] or carcinomas[1247] occur in a setting of chronic ACTH excess and nodular hyperplasia, but there is no compelling evidence that either excessive stimulation by or sensitivity to ACTH plays a role in development.

Laboratory Findings. Plasma cortisol concentration may be normal in the morning but is inappropriately high in late evening. Plasma ACTH is suppressed and is often undetectable (<1 pmol/L [<5 pg/mL]) even in the morning. Urinary 17-OHCS and free cortisol levels are elevated to a similar degree in patients with benign or malignant tumors causing Cushing's syndrome. In patients with adenoma, plasma DHEAS and urinary DHEAS and 17-KS levels are often either normal or increased in proportion to cortisol and 17-OHCS levels; urinary 17-KS levels are usually less than 20 mg/d. In carcinoma the precursors tend to be disproportionately elevated, and urinary 17-KS levels are usually higher than 20 mg/d and sometimes extremely elevated.[1053] In some "nonfunctioning" carcinomas, measuring steroid precursors such as pregnenolone[1248] may establish the diagnosis.

Radiographic/Nuclear Medicine Findings. Adenomas and carcinomas are almost always visible on either high-resolution, thin-section CT or MRI scans (see Fig. 9–45G to N). Adrenal arteriograms may be of value to the surgeon but are usually unnecessary for diagnosis. Intravenous pyelograms are seldom indicated except to define renal involvement, and sonography can define large adrenal cysts but generally provides little additional useful information. Vena-caval contrast studies are useful in patients with carcinoma to define external compression, invasion, or thrombus formation by the tumor. CT or MRI scans are superior to and less time-consuming and expensive than ^{131}I-labeled cholesterol scans,[1249, 1250] which may miss relatively large adenomas causing Cushing's syndrome (unpublished observations, D. N. Orth). Most carcinomas do not take up the labeled cholesterol efficiently, although even some nonfunctioning tumors may take up the agent.[1251] Furthermore, T2-weighted

MRI images may differentiate adrenal adenomas from carcinomas.[1252]

Imaging techniques provide anatomical information only; they do not define function. They cannot, for example, differentiate between a nonfunctioning adenoma ("incidentaloma") (see Chapter 11) and one causing hypercortisolism. When the results of endocrine function studies disagree with the radiographic results, the latter should always be questioned first.

Laboratory Diagnosis. The basis for establishing the diagnosis of Cushing's syndrome caused by adrenal tumor (see Fig. 9–46) involves demonstrating (1) increased basal cortisol production, (2) cortisol secretion independent of ACTH stimulation, (3) absolute resistance to glucocorticoid negative feedback, (4) lack of response to falling plasma cortisol levels, (5) unresponsiveness to CRH and/or AVP, and (6) responsiveness, or lack thereof, to exogenous ACTH stimulation, which may help distinguish malignant from benign tumors.

INCREASED BASAL CORTISOL PRODUCTION: BASAL PLASMA CONCENTRATIONS AND URINARY EXCRETION OF CORTISOL AND/OR ITS METABOLITES. The procedure for establishing the presence of hypercortisolism has been described in the section on Cushing's disease. As in ectopic ACTH syndrome, day-to-day hormone secretion by adrenal tumors, especially carcinomas, may be variable. This renders interpretation of results more difficult. As already noted, secretion of steroids in addition to, or rather than, cortisol may occur, especially in patients who do not have Cushing's syndrome.

INDEPENDENCE OF CORTISOL SECRETION OF ACTH STIMULATION: BASAL PLASMA ACTH CONCENTRATION (Fig. 9–53A). In these patients and others with primary adrenocortical dysfunction, basal plasma ACTH levels are low or undetectable at all times of the day.

ABSOLUTE RESISTANCE TO GLUCOCORTICOID NEGATIVE FEEDBACK: THE HIGH-DOSE DEXAMETHASONE TEST. Unless the patient has unequivocal hypercortisolism, the low-dose dexamethasone test should first be performed to demonstrate the existence of Cushing's syndrome. Because the hypercortisolemia suppresses pituitary ACTH secretion in these patients, even high-dose dexamethasone has no effect on steroid production (see Fig. 9–53B and C).

UNRESPONSIVENESS TO FALLING PLASMA CORTISOL CONCENTRATION: THE METYRAPONE TEST (see Fig. 9–53D). In these patients pituitary ACTH secretion is suppressed, all adrenocortical carcinomas and almost half of the adenomas are nonresponsive to ACTH, and the remaining normal adrenal cortex is atrophic. Furthermore, metyrapone blocks not only conversion of deoxycortisol to cortisol but also conversion of cholesterol to pregnenolone. Thus even though plasma ACTH level may rise in some patients whose

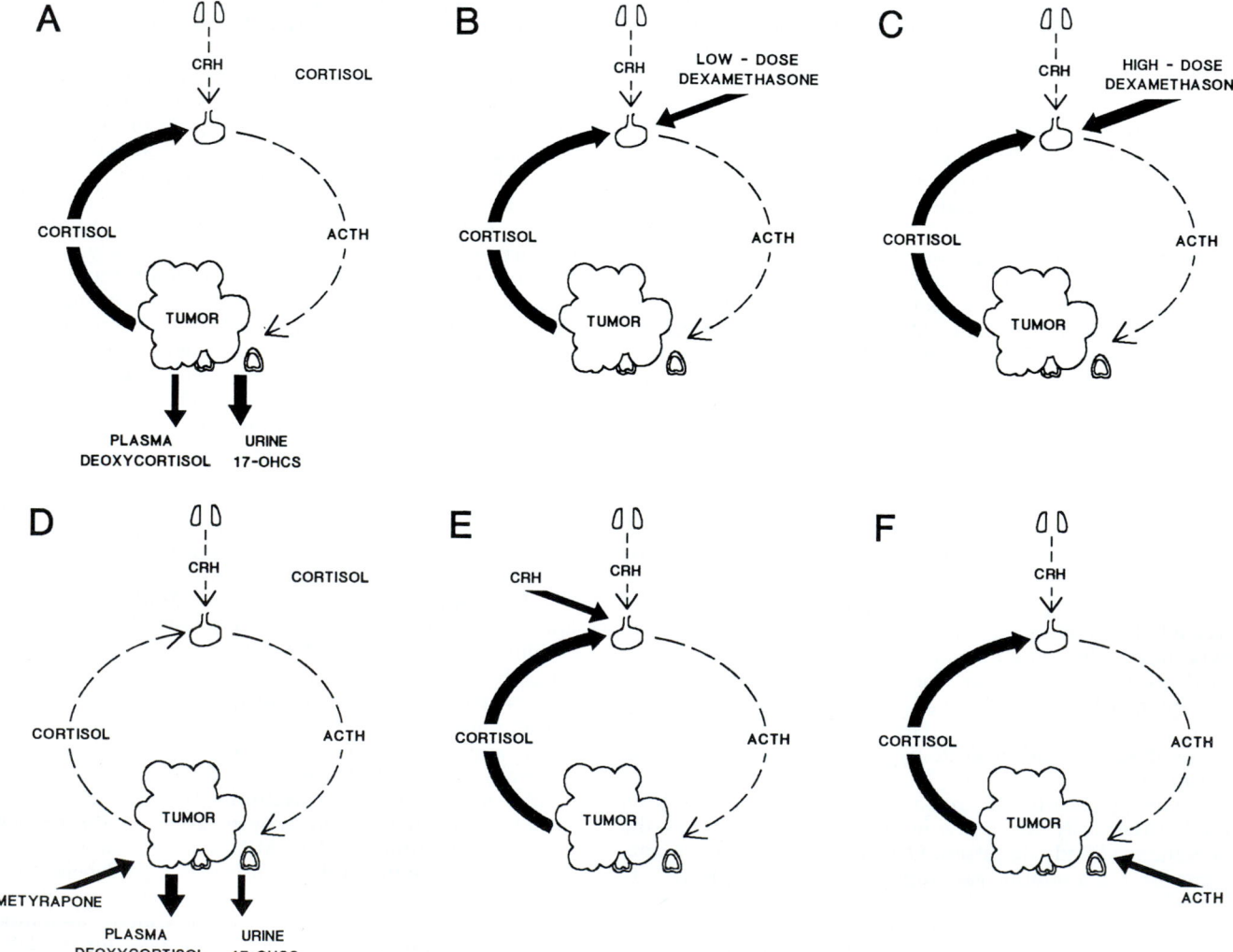

Figure 9–53. Responses of a patient with Cushing's syndrome caused by adrenocortical tumor *(A)* to *(B)* low-dose and *(C)* high-dose dexamethasone suppression, *(D)* metyrapone, *(E)* CRH, and *(F)* ACTH stimulation tests.

pituitary function is not profoundly suppressed, the serum 11-deoxycortisol level does not rise normally and urinary 17-OHCS excretion uniformly falls.[1053]

Unresponsiveness to CRH and/or AVP: The CRH and AVP Tests (see Fig. 9–53E). Because pituitary ACTH secretion is suppressed and the high plasma cortisol level blocks the action of CRH and AVP, most patients with adrenal tumors do not respond to CRH[1134] or, presumably, AVP or the combination of CRH plus AVP. However, occasional patients whose cortisol level is not markedly elevated at the time of the test and, presumably, whose disease is of such short duration that the pituitary is not profoundly suppressed do respond (unpublished observations, D. N. Orth and C. R. DeBold).

Responsiveness, or Lack Thereof, to ACTH Stimulation: The ACTH Stimulation Test (see Fig. 9–53F). Although, by definition, no adrenocortical tumor that causes Cushing's syndrome is dependent on ACTH secretion, about 60% of adenomas are responsive to maximal ACTH stimulation and, because of their large size, may sometimes produce exaggerated steroid responses.[1053] The remaining adenomas and virtually all carcinomas are unresponsive.[1053]

Pathology. True adenomas of the adrenal are rare, if incidental adrenocortical nodules are discounted.[4] The left and right adrenal glands are about equally affected. Bilateral adenomas are rare, as are familial adenomas.[1253] On occasion ectopic adenomas are found in the scrotum, broad ligaments, ovary, perirenal area, or body of the pancreas or liver.[1254] The cut surface of the adenoma is usually yellow, mottled with brown, but rarely they are filled with lipofuscin pigment and are black. They average 4 cm in diameter and are encapsulated, and the remaining cortex is atrophied because pituitary ACTH secretion is suppressed. Characteristically, the adenoma is composed of mixtures of compact, zona reticularis–type cells and clear, zona fasciculata–type cells. Clear cells predominate in the adenomas that respond to ACTH. Necrosis and nuclear pleomorphism are unusual, but myelolipomatous foci are common.[4] Atrophic normal cortex shows decreased or absent reticularis cells or thinning of both inner zones. The zona fasciculata is intact, and the capsule appears thickened.[4] The ultrastructure resembles that of normal cortex, with some variation in mitochondrial morphology.[4]

Adrenocortical carcinoma affects the left and right adrenal glands with equal frequency. Bilateral tumors and ectopic sites are uncommon. Tumors can weigh more than 5 kg (>20 cm in diameter); carcinomas weighing less than 100 g (<5.5 cm in diameter) are rare. They are usually encapsulated, soft, pink, gray, brown, or yellow masses with areas of hemorrhage and necrosis. Larger tumors may be cystic and vascular. Local tissue invasion is common. It is often difficult to find the normal adrenal remnant. The histological appearance of carcinomas varies among tumors and from one area to another within a tumor. Clear and compact cell types are mixed. Nuclear pleomorphism is usually prominent, even when the cells look uniform under low power. Mitotic figures and vascular invasion are uncommon but are indicative of malignancy, as are large areas of necrosis and broad fibrous connective tissue bands traversing the tumor.[4] There is not a perfect correlation between histology and biological behavior,[1255] but, when combined with certain clinical criteria, histological features can be highly predictive of metastatic potential.[1256] The ultrastructure is more abnormal than that of adenomas in terms of mitochondrial number and morphology, increased numbers of microvilli, and, characteristically, loss of integrity of the basement membrane surrounding alveolar groups of cells.[4] The normal cortex is atrophic. Rarely, carcinomas arise in ectopic adrenocortical tissue in the kidney, liver, para-aortic

region, and gonads. Needle aspiration biopsy has been used for the diagnosis of adrenal tumors,[1257, 1258] but we rarely find that it is useful.

Treatment. The treatment of adrenal tumors is outlined in Figure 9–54. When possible, the tumor should be removed surgically, thereby correcting the steroid excess and curing the syndrome, as well as removing a neoplasm that may threaten the health of the patient. The cure rate with surgical removal of adrenal adenoma is virtually 100%.[1053, 1259] These patients generally have rather profound suppression of the hypothalamic-pituitary-adrenal axis and require glucocorticoid replacement for several months after tumor resection. The principles are identical to those for patients cured of Cushing's disease by microadenomectomy (see earlier).

Results in adrenal carcinoma, in contrast, are dismal and are unrelated to the size of the tumor or the duration of symptoms but do correlate with tumor stage.[1054] It is impossible to resect completely the vast majority of malignant adrenocortical tumors.[1053, 1054, 1260] Even when the surgeon believes that the entire tumor has been resected and there is no radiological or hormonal evidence of residual tumor, one must assume that micrometastases are present in the liver, lungs, or other sites (see Fig. 9–45M and N) and will become clinically apparent within a period of months. Median survival after diagnosis in adults is 14.5 mo[1054] to 3 y;[1053] without treatment, survival averages 3 mo.[1260] Children may have somewhat less aggressive tumors,[1261] and patients aged 40 or younger survive longer than older patients.[1054] Reoperation to resect abdominal recurrences or distant metastases may prolong survival in some patients.[1262, 1263]

Mitotane has been used for nonresectable or recurrent disease.[1052, 1053, 1264, 1265] It is usually given to tolerance (10 to 20 g/d) to produce serum levels of at least 44 to 78 μg/mL).[1266] It has been reported to produce a hormonal response in up to 75% of patients and reduction in tumor size in up to 30%,[1052, 1267] but these results have not been confirmed by others.[1053, 1264, 1265] Tumor regression with mitotane is transient;[1054] treatment is never curative. In the most optimistic series, median survival was only 6.5 mo after beginning the drug,[1052, 1267] and there is no evidence that mitotane prolongs life.[1054, 1268] Even those who have an objective response are often incapacitated by the side effects of large dosages of mitotane,[1269] although a preparation available outside the United States is better tolerated.[1054, 1260]

There is preliminary evidence that the administration of mitotane in the absence of metastatic disease may delay or prevent recurrent disease.[1262, 1268, 1270] Mitotane is begun immediately after removal of the primary tumor and continued indefinitely. Two of four patients in one series remained free of metastases, and mean survival (75 ± 33 mo) was longer than in those who received no mitotane (10 ± 8.7 mo).[1262] Four of another 11 patients survived for 4 to 15.5 y

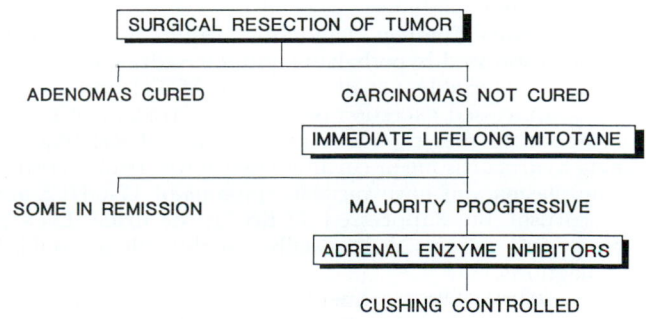

Figure 9–54. Treatment of patients with adrenocortical tumors that cause Cushing's syndrome.

without recurrent tumor.[1270] Other patients develop recurrent local or metastatic disease despite taking mitotane. The optimal dosage and duration of treatment are not established. Nevertheless, this disease is so uniformly fatal that it is rational to treat every patient, beginning immediately after tumor resection, with 4 g of mitotane per day, or the maximal dose the patient can tolerate, half of it at bedtime to minimize nausea, and to maintain treatment indefinitely. Efficacy can be assessed periodically by CT or MRI scan of the chest and upper abdomen and by measuring 24-h urinary free cortisol excretion. As mentioned previously, mitotane increases the rate of metabolism of dexamethasone, fludrocortisone, and, presumably, other steroids. Some symptoms ascribed to mitotane may be due to adrenocortical insufficiency, and dosages of up to seven times the usual maintenance level of these steroids may be required to cure the symptoms and maintain normal serum electrolytes and blood pressure.

Various other chemotherapeutic drugs have been tested in adrenal carcinoma, alone and in combination with mitotane. None of them has been shown to have greater efficacy than mitotane.[1271]

It is generally agreed that radiotherapy is not useful in this disease, but one study reported a 10-y survival for three of nine patients.[1272] However, two of the three died of other malignancies.

Excess steroid production can usually be controlled by use of adrenal enzyme inhibitors in these patients, and none should suffer from persistent Cushing's syndrome. The adrenal enzyme inhibitors already mentioned, administered alone or in combination, should be used so as to render the patient hypoadrenal, because it is too difficult to achieve and maintain normal serum cortisol levels. Replacement steroid therapy should be given. There is no advantage to using antiglucocorticoids, such as mifepristone, because enzyme inhibitors are less expensive, easily available, and less difficult to manage.

Prognosis. As already noted, the prognosis with adrenal adenoma is excellent because surgery is virtually always curative. The prognosis with adrenal carcinoma is poor because most have distant micrometastases at diagnosis and because there is no effective therapy for metastatic or recurrent disease. The symptoms of steroid excess, however, can easily be controlled.

Iatrogenic, Factitious, or Exogenous Cushing's Syndrome. *Distinctive Clinical Features.* These patients usually have signs of pure glucocorticoid excess because most have received potent synthetic steroids, such as dexamethasone or prednisone, which have little or no mineralocorticoid activity and no androgenic activity. Hirsutism is absent, and hypertension occurs only if the patient has incidental hypertension or is taking hydrocortisone or cortisone. A careful medical history is necessary because some patients take medications that, unbeknownst to them, contain steroids or have received depot injections of steroids weeks or more before seeking assistance.

Laboratory Findings. Laboratory results are characteristic of suppressed hypothalamic-pituitary-adrenal function: low or undetectable morning plasma ACTH and cortisol levels; suppressed excretion of urinary steroids; and failure to respond to metyrapone, cosyntropin, or CRH. Patients taking hydrocortisone or cortisone may have residual cortisol in the plasma and have variable amounts of 17-OHCS and free cortisol, but suppressed 17-KS, in the urine. Even in malingering patients, it is usually not difficult to establish the diagnosis.

Treatment. The treatment is to stop the steroid. Most patients who have taken enough steroid long enough to cause Cushing's syndrome will have a period of hypotha-

lamic-pituitary-adrenal insufficiency when steroids are discontinued, so gradual steroid withdrawal is necessary.

UNCOMMON CAUSES OF CUSHING'S SYNDROME
ACTH-Dependent Cushing's Syndrome
Pseudo-Cushing's Syndromes. *Depression.* Patients with depression severe enough to warrant hospitalization can have all of the hormonal abnormalities of patients with Cushing's disease, including the responses to most of the standard pituitary-adrenal function tests.[1273] Circadian rhythmicity of ACTH and cortisol secretion is maintained, but ACTH pulse frequency may be increased and resulting cortisol pulses are of greater amplitude and duration.[1274] In general, depressed patients do not have the physical signs of Cushing's syndrome and are thus not difficult to distinguish from patients with Cushing's disease. However, depression is common in Cushing's syndrome, and depressed patients can be obese, hypertensive, and diabetic. There are two ways to differentiate them from patients with Cushing's disease: (1) they have blunted responses to CRH,[1275] presumably because the hypercortisolemia, like that of acutely stressed patients,[325] blocks the effect of CRH on the intrinsically normal corticotropes, and (2) all of the hormonal abnormalities disappear as soon as the depression is corrected, spontaneously, by psychotherapy, or by antidepressant drug therapy. The pathogenesis of the hormonal disorder and its role in the manifestations of depression are unknown. Therapy is directed solely at the psychiatric disorder. Transient hypothalamic-pituitary-adrenal insufficiency does not occur after cure.

Alcoholism. A few cases of alcoholic pseudo-Cushing's syndrome have been reported.[1276, 1277] These patients may have round, plethoric faces, centripetal obesity, thin extremities, and other features of Cushing's syndrome, although whether they are due to hypercortisolism or other causes is uncertain. A careful history and laboratory evidence of abnormal liver function are the keys to correct diagnosis. These patients all have significant alcoholic liver disease, with elevated hepatic enzymes in the serum. The pathogenesis is unknown, but altered hepatic metabolism of cortisol alone cannot explain the abnormality. An alcohol-induced central nervous system disorder may be a major factor. The treatment is abstinence from alcohol.

Ectopic Corticotropin-Releasing Hormone Syndrome.
Distinctive Clinical Features. A handful of cases of ectopic CRH secretion have been reported.[1024] No clinical features distinguish this disorder from the ectopic ACTH syndrome. The patients have had a variety of tumors, mostly carcinoids.

Laboratory Findings. Material that appears immunologically, biologically, and physicochemically identical to human CRH has been extracted from normal and neoplastic non-hypothalamic tissues.[291] Plasma ACTH and cortisol levels and urinary steroid excretion are increased, as in ectopic ACTH syndrome. Plasma CRH levels, when measured, are elevated.[1026, 1028, 1030] Responses to pituitary-adrenal function tests are characteristic of those in ectopic ACTH syndrome.

It is curious, as noted earlier, that steroid production in about half of these patients is resistant to high-dose dexamethasone suppression, because one would assume that the action of endogenous ectopic CRH could be blocked by glucocorticoids, as can that of exogenous CRH.[332] In fact, steroid hypersecretion caused by an intrasellar gangliocytoma producing CRH was partially suppressed by low-dose dexamethasone.[1031] However, most[1029, 1030, 1278] but not all[1026, 1027] of the reported CRH-producing tumors also contain ACTH, suggesting that the adrenal glands in at least some of these patients are stimulated by ectopic ACTH, secretion of which is not dexamethasone suppressible. It is unlikely that the cosecreted ectopic CRH stimulates pituitary

ACTH secretion in the presence of the resulting ACTH-induced hypercortisolemia. Thus, whereas tumors may synthesize and secrete CRH, patients whose tumors also secrete ACTH and display resistance to dexamethasone suppression should be considered to be examples of the ectopic ACTH syndrome until proved otherwise. The proof should include inferior petrosal sinus sampling for ACTH before and after stimulation with exogenous CRH. There should be a central-to-peripheral ACTH gradient if ectopic CRH is involved. Furthermore, intraoperative sampling of CRH in the tumor venous drainage and a peripheral vein should reveal a central-to-peripheral CRH gradient.

Pathology. The pituitary corticotropes may be hyperplastic,[1026] but CT scan of the pituitary is normal, the adrenal glands are both increased in size, and the tumor may or may not be detected by CT or MRI scans. The histopathology of the tumors is unremarkable, except that they stain for CRH and, in most cases, ACTH. The two hormones may be contained in the same or different populations of cells. There has been one instance of an intrasellar, extrapituitary, CRH-secreting gangliocytoma consisting of hypothalamic-like neurons.[1031] The corticotropes were hyperplastic.

Treatment. Therapy is the same as that for the ectopic ACTH syndrome. The prognosis is also similar: the Cushing's syndrome can easily be controlled, but the ultimate prognosis depends on the malignancy of the tumor and whether it can be completely resected.

Ectopic Gastrin-Releasing Peptide Secretion. There is a report that a medullary carcinoma of the thyroid secreted gastrin-releasing peptide, the mammalian homologue of bombesin, which acted together with hypothalamic CRH to cause Cushing's syndrome.[1279] However, there is disagreement whether gastrin-releasing peptide has any effect on ACTH secretion.[1280, 1281]

Factitious Cushing's Syndrome Related to ACTH Administration. These rare patients can appear in all ways similar to those with endogenous ACTH hypersecretion. If a careful history and a search for injection sites do not reveal the cause and the patient wishes to deceive, it can be difficult to diagnose these patients. Neither pituitary nor ectopic sources of ACTH will be identified, of course, but neither will they be found in a significant fraction of patients with endogenous Cushing's syndrome. Commercial ACTH prepared from animal sources is contaminated with α-MSH derived from the intermediate lobe. Because α-MSH concentration is increased minimally, if at all[1155] (unpublished data, D. N. Orth), in endogenous Cushing's syndrome, measurement of plasma α-MSH concentration can be helpful. Many patients receiving ACTH develop anti-ACTH antibodies,[1282] which can also be measured. If the patient can be isolated from the source of ACTH, hypothalamic-pituitary-adrenal insufficiency will develop in a matter of several days, just as in the patient with Cushing's disease after microadenomectomy.

ACTH-Independent Cushing's Syndrome
Bilateral Micronodular Dysplasia. *Distinctive Clinical Features.* About half of the patients with this disorder have no distinctive clinical presentation other than being young, always less than age 30, half aged 15 or less, and some infants.[1007] Median duration of symptoms before diagnosis is 1 y, although intervals of up to 18 y have been reported.[1011] The other half of patients have a familial form of the disorder that is inherited as a dominant trait and accompanied by pigmented lentigines and blue nevi on the face, neck, and trunk, including the lips, conjunctiva, or sclera. These patients may also have cutaneous, mammary, and atrial myxomas, testicular tumors, pituitary somatotrope adenomas, and other tumors.[1010] Only about 20% of the patients have Cushing's syndrome, and none has all features

of the syndrome. Two siblings presented in infancy with hypertelorism, profuse dark hair, heavy eyebrows, large fontanelles, and marked hypotonia; the girl had clitoral enlargement, the boy, severe hypertension.[1009]

Pathogenesis. The pathogenesis is unknown, but a circulating immunoglobulin that stimulates steroidogenesis[1283] and adrenal cell growth[1284] may be involved. However, it is unclear why the cells that form the nodules, but not the intervening cells, should be susceptible to stimulation by these autoantibodies.[1285] Other autoimmune disorders are not common in these patients or in their families.

Laboratory Findings. Plasma cortisol concentration is usually moderately elevated and exhibits no diurnal rhythm. Cortisol precursors have not often been measured but appear to be proportionately elevated.[1009] Plasma ACTH concentration is low or undetectable. Steroid production may be irregular[1160] or frankly cyclic.[1161]

Radiographic/Nuclear Medicine Findings. The adrenal glands are normal or slightly enlarged and may or may not have discernible nodules on CT or MRI scans.[1286] Scans with ^{131}I-labeled cholesterol reveal bilateral symmetrical uptake. The pituitary appears normal. A high percentage of patients have marked osteopenia that is out of proportion to other manifestations of hypercortisolism and presumably occurs in both the sporadic[1007, 1160] and familial[1010, 1161] forms of the disease.

Laboratory Diagnosis. As with adrenal tumor, the other example of primary adrenal hypercortisolism, ACTH secretion is suppressed, so steroid production is not suppressed by either low- or high-dose dexamethasone. Urinary 17-OHCS levels fall, but plasma 11-deoxycortisol concentration does not rise normally during metyrapone administration.[1007, 1160] The cells forming the dysplastic nodules do not respond to ACTH;[1160] the occasional responses are subnormal and are probably due to either variable daily steroid production or the response of the atrophic adrenocortical cells. There is no ACTH response to CRH (unpublished observation, D. N. Orth) or, presumably, to vasopressin.

Pathology. The adrenals are either normal or slightly enlarged. Both glands contain many nodules ranging from microscopic to 5 mm in diameter and from yellow-brown to bluish black, most often brown or black. The nodules consist of large cells with eosinophilic cytoplasm containing brown lipofuscin pigment. Nuclei are enlarged and somewhat pleomorphic. The ultrastructure of the cells resembles that of fasciculata cells. The intervening non-nodular cortex consists of small cells with clear cytoplasm characteristic of adrenal atrophy.[4]

Treatment. Surgical bilateral adrenalectomy by the flank approach is the treatment of choice. The pituitary is intrinsically normal, so pituitary surgery or radiation is not helpful, nor is subtotal adrenalectomy.[1011]

Prognosis. Results of treatment are excellent. The surgery produces permanent adrenal insufficiency. Nelson's syndrome has not been described in patients adrenalectomized for this disorder. One infant died of refractory hypertension and heart failure a month after subtotal adrenalectomy.[1009]

Bilateral ACTH-Independent Macronodular Hyperplasia. There are only one or two reported cases of this syndrome.[1012, 1164] One was a 47-y-old man with gradual onset of Cushing's syndrome, impotence, and gynecomastia,[1012] the other a 62-y-old man with gradual onset of Cushing's syndrome, impotence, and dementia.[1164] Plasma and urinary steroids were two to three times increased and appeared to vary from day to day. Plasma ACTH was undetectable basally or after metyrapone or CRH. Steroid production was suppressed minimally, if at all, during high-dose dexamethasone administration. The response to metyrapone was low in the first patient,[1012] paradoxically normal in the second.[1164] Plasma cortisol and, in the first patient, elevated basal serum estrone concentrations increased after cosyntropin administration. Pituitary CT scans were normal. The adrenal glands weighed 62 and 24 g and 260 and 500 g, respectively, and contained multiple macroscopic nonpigmented nodules more than 5 mm in diameter. The nodules consisted of two populations of clear cells that differed in size in the first patient and were typical of benign adrenal nodules in the second. The internodular cortex appeared hypertrophic; atrophic cells were not observed. Bilateral adrenalectomy cured the hypercortisolemia in both patients. The pathogenesis of this disorder is unknown, but there is no evidence that ACTH hypersecretion is involved.

Cortisol Hyper-reactive Syndrome. One 54-y-old man was reported[1287] with centripetal obesity, moon facies, and non–insulin-dependent diabetes mellitus but normal blood pressure and no striae. He had low cortisol production, undetectable plasma ACTH (i.e., <2 pmol/L [<9 pg/mL]), normal CBG concentration, markedly decreased responses to rapid administration of cosyntropin, insulin-induced hypoglycemia and repeated CRH-plus-lysine vasopressin tests, and an absent response to metyrapone. However, the plasma cortisol concentration increased to about 660 nmol/L (24 μg/dL), urinary 17-OHCS excretion to 64 μmol/d (23 mg/d), and urinary free cortisol excretion to 1800 nmol/d (650 μg/d) after 2 d of intramuscular depot cosyntropin administration. CT scans of the pituitary and adrenal glands were normal. Prolonged observation in hospital and low glucocorticoid radioreceptor activity of the patient's serum excluded surreptitious self-medication with glucocorticoids. Aromatase activity in cultured skin fibroblasts was 1.5- to 1.8-fold greater than normal, and [³H]thymidine incorporation was inhibited about 33 to 44% more than normal. In vitro studies of his receptors did not fully explain the greater glucocorticoid sensitivity. The authors concluded that the patient's Cushing's syndrome was due to hyper-reactivity to cortisol. It is unclear, however, why the patient developed Cushing's syndrome, given his extremely low basal cortisol production and suppressed ACTH secretion, or why he developed it only in his sixth decade. This cause of Cushing's syndrome, if it exists, requires further explanation.

Mineralocorticoid: Hyperaldosteronism

PRIMARY ALDOSTERONISM. Inappropriate hypersecretion of aldosterone is an uncommon cause of hypertension, accounting for less than 1% of cases of the disorder. The initial patient in whom such a syndrome was described had asymptomatic hypertension, hypokalemia, and a single adrenal adenoma.[1288]

Clinical Presentation. The diagnosis should be considered in an asymptomatic patient with hypertension and spontaneous hypokalemia. Early reports described a higher incidence of physical symptoms than has subsequently been observed.[8] Some patients may have frontal headaches, muscular weakness, or flaccid paralysis associated with hypokalemia[1289] or polyuria. The peak incidence occurs between ages 30 and 50, and most patients are women. The hypertension may be severe. Malignant hypertension is rare.[1290, 1291]

Pathophysiology. Primary aldosteronism is usually caused by solitary unilateral adrenal adenomas, which were thought to account for 80 to 90% of all cases of hyperaldosteronism.[1292] The remaining 10 to 20% of cases are caused by bilateral adrenal hyperplasia, so-called idiopathic hyperaldosteronism. However, bilateral adrenal hyperplasia is now reported to account for almost 50% of cases in some referral

centers.[1293] The apparent shift is probably due to more careful evaluation of hypertensive patients. Adrenal carcinoma is a rare cause of primary hyperaldosteronism.[1294] Unilateral adrenal hyperplasia is an even rarer cause.[1295]

Adrenal Adenoma. The pathogenesis of aldosterone-secreting adrenocortical adenomas is unknown. The clinical features of primary hyperaldosteronism of all etiologies are the consequences of aldosterone excess. Renal distal tubular sodium reabsorption increases and, consequently, so does total body sodium content. Water is also retained, so serum sodium concentration remains normal. Continued renal exposure to excess mineralocorticoid results in an "escape" phenomenon, possibly mediated by a compensatory increase in ANF secretion.[1296–1299] For this and other reasons, the hypertension in hyperaldosteronism may not be due solely to volume expansion. Peripheral vascular resistance may also be elevated.[1300–1302] In animal models of mineralocorticoid-induced hypertension, intracellular vascular smooth muscle cell sodium content is increased, presumably causing vasoconstriction and increased peripheral vascular resistance.[1303, 1304]

Aldosterone also causes potassium loss in the distal renal tubule, resulting in hypokalemia. The electrochemical gradient generated by avid sodium retention also causes hydrogen ion loss in the distal tubule. As hypokalemia increases, so does renal ammoniagenesis, contributing to the alkalosis. Renal concentrating capacity diminishes, causing polyuria. Inappropriate urinary potassium excretion continues despite hypokalemia. Plasma renin activity is suppressed and is unresponsive to maneuvers that deplete intravascular volume.[1292, 1305, 1306]

Bilateral Adrenocortical Hyperplasia. The pathogenesis of zona glomerulosa hyperplasia is unknown. The possibilities include the action of normal intermediate-lobe POMC products, such as β-MSH,[446, 1307] γ-MSH,[1308, 1309] and β-END.[1310, 1311] Putative aldosterone-stimulating pituitary factors unrelated to POMC have also been reported but not structurally characterized.[1312, 1313] Indirect evidence for possible intermediate-lobe involvement is the serotoninergic control of aldosterone secretion observed in these patients.[1314, 1315] However, the intermediate lobe normally is functional only in the fetus and during pregnancy in humans, and there is no evidence that any of its POMC products circulates in sufficient concentration to stimulate glomerulosa cell function.

The biochemical abnormality observed in zona glomerulosa hyperplasia is usually less severe than in patients with adenomas: aldosterone levels are not as high, and the hypokalemia and renin suppression are not as profound. Consequently, some authorities do not consider this syndrome to be clinically distinct from low-renin essential hypertension.[1316]

There are two rare types of bilateral adrenal hyperplasia. The first is dexamethasone-suppressible hyperaldosteronism, which is found predominantly in young men and may in some cases be a genetically transmitted autosomal dominant disorder.[1317–1319] Aldosterone levels fall after glucocorticoid administration and remain suppressed during chronic therapy, indicating the dependence of aldosterone secretion on ACTH stimulation. The pathophysiology may be failure of normal differentiation of transitional zone cells to zona fasciculata cells, which should lose P-450$_{c11}$ (i.e., 11β-hydroxylase, 18-hydroxylase, and 18-methyl oxidase) activity as they migrate from the transitional zone between the zonae glomerulosa and fasciculata. The postulated defect results in ACTH-responsive cells that retain the ability to synthesize aldosterone and 18-hydroxylated corticosteroids.[1320, 1321] In one patient, however, glucocorticoids no longer suppressed aldosterone secretion after 7 y.[1322] The second rare type of bilateral adrenal hyperplasia has been described as primary hyperplasia because subtotal (75%) adrenalectomy apparently results in permanent cure.[1323] Its pathogenesis, too, is unknown.

Unilateral Adrenocortical Hyperplasia. In rare instances the adrenal hyperplasia may be unilateral,[1295, 1324] and hyperaldosteronism may be cured by resecting the affected adrenal. The pathogenesis is unknown.

Laboratory Diagnosis. The diagnostic approach consists of two phases. In the first, primary hyperaldosteronism is distinguished from other causes of hypertension by demonstrating hyperaldosteronemia and suppressed plasma renin activity. In the second, various dynamic tests and imaging procedures are used to distinguish between surgically remediable forms of hyperaldosteronism and those that respond to medical management.

The criterion for deciding which hypertensive patients to evaluate is the presence of hypokalemia.[1325] Diuretics should be discontinued 2 to 4 wk before evaluation, and dietary sodium intake should be at least 100 mmol/d. As many as 12% of patients with adrenal adenoma and 50% of those with bilateral hyperplasia have serum potassium levels above 3.5 mmol/L.[1306] A serum potassium level of less than 4.0 mmol/L increases the sensitivity to 100%, but the specificity falls to 64%.[1326, 1327] Urinary potassium excretion is inappropriately high in aldosteronism. A rate of less than 30 mmol/d is unusual.[1327] Adequate dietary sodium (i.e., urinary excretion of at least 100 mmol of sodium per day) is required for renal sodium-potassium exchange to demonstrate the kaliuresis.

Increased Basal Aldosterone Secretion, Suppressed Plasma Renin Activity. Screening aldosterone measurements can be made on plasma or 24-h urine collections. Measuring plasma aldosterone levels after 3 h of upright posture is most widely used. Plasma renin activity should be measured in the same sample. Elevated plasma aldosterone concentration in the presence of unequivocally suppressed plasma renin activity is suggestive of the diagnosis. The ratio of plasma aldosterone concentration (in nanograms per deciliter) to plasma renin activity (in nanograms per milliliter per hour) best discriminates between patients with essential hypertension and those with primary hyperaldosteronism. A plasma aldosterone/plasma renin activity ratio greater than 20 to 25 indicates the need for further study.[1293, 1328]

Failure of Aldosterone Secretion to Be Suppressed Normally. In the hypertensive patient with hypokalemia and/or kaliuresis or with an elevated plasma aldosterone/renin ratio, the diagnosis of hyperaldosteronism is confirmed by demonstrating failure of plasma aldosterone concentration to be suppressed normally. The saline suppression test[1329] is most widely used. Medications that affect the renin-angiotensin-aldosterone system must be discontinued, preferably for several weeks before testing, and potassium deficits must be corrected.[1293] Isotonic saline is infused intravenously at a rate of 300 to 500 mL/h for 4 h, after which plasma aldosterone concentration and renin activity are measured. Aldosterone levels normally fall to less than 0.28 mmol/L (10 ng/dL), and renin activity is suppressed. Failure of normal suppression usually identifies patients with aldosterone-producing adenomas.[1325] Normal subjects and most patients with secondary forms of hyperaldosteronism have normal suppression. False-negative results (i.e., suppressibility) are most frequent in patients with bilateral hyperplasia.[1330-1332]

An alternative test uses the angiotensin-converting enzyme inhibitor captopril to inhibit angiotensin II generation pharmacologically. This has the same net effect on plasma angiotensin concentration as suppressing renin secretion with saline infusion. The captopril test is recommended for patients in whom the risks from volume overload preclude performance of the saline infusion test. Plasma aldosterone is measured 2 h after oral administration of 25 mg of captopril. Plasma aldosterone concentration is normally suppressed to less than 0.42 nmol/L (15 ng/dL).[1333-1335] The test may not always be diagnostic but is a useful alternative when saline suppression cannot be performed.[1336, 1337]

Adenoma vs. Bilateral Hyperplasia. After the diagnosis of primary hyperaldosteronism is established, one must distinguish between aldosterone-producing adrenal adenoma and bilateral adrenal hyperplasia. The hypertension caused by adenomas can be cured by surgical therapy, whereas the hypertension associated with bilateral hyperplasia is often not cured even by total bilateral adrenalectomy. Adenomas tend to produce more severe hyperaldosteronism, with consequent more severe hypertension, more profound hypokalemia, and more complete renin suppression,[1292] but these features do not reliably distinguish them from hyperplasia. One widely used test for this distinction is based on the less complete suppression of renin activity generally observed in hyperaldosteronism caused by bilateral hyperplasia. Plasma renin activity rises slightly and aldosterone concentration increases significantly after 2 to 4 h of upright posture, presumably because the hyperplastic glands are sensitive to small increments in plasma renin activity. In contrast, renin activity remains suppressed and aldosterone concentration does not rise in patients with adenomas,[1338] in whom a paradoxical fall in plasma aldosterone level is often observed.[1339] A diagnostic accuracy of 85% was reported in a review of 246 cases,[1340] although others have not found the test as reliable.[1341] Measuring the plasma concentration of 18-hydroxycorticosterone, a late precursor in the aldosterone biosynthetic pathway, may be useful. It is elevated in most patients with aldosterone-producing adenomas but not in those with bilateral adrenal hyperplasia.[1325, 1342]

Patients with glucocorticoid-suppressible hyperaldosteronism, like those with adenomas, may have an anomalous postural decrease in plasma aldosterone concentration.[1343] If the patient's CT or MRI scan has no evidence of an adenoma, particularly if there is a family history of hypertension associated with hypokalemia, the diagnosis should be excluded by administering dexamethasone 2 mg/d for 3 to 4 wk. Plasma concentration and urinary excretion of aldosterone should remain suppressed; they may be transiently suppressed in patients with adenomas or the common form of bilateral adrenal hyperplasia.[1343] Primary adrenal hyperplasia produces dynamic test results similar to those in adrenal adenoma but is not lateralized by CT, MRI, or [6β-[131I]iodomethyl-19-norcholesterol (NP-59) imaging or adrenal venous sampling.[1323, 1325] Aldosterone-secreting adrenal carcinomas are usually remarkable for the severity of hypertension and hypokalemia they produce but may be similar to adenomas with respect to all dynamic tests. However, a large adrenal mass is usually found by imaging procedures, whereas adenomas are typically quite small.[1294, 1344-1347]

Lateralization of Aldosterone Secretion. If all else fails, including the imaging procedures described later, adrenal venous sampling is reliable in experienced hands.[1348] Catheterizing the right adrenal vein is a technically difficult procedure, unsuccessful about 25% of the time,[1293] but adenomas may be localized despite failure to catheterize the vein.[1349] ACTH (5 IU cosyntropin per hour) is administered continuously during the test to minimize episodic adrenocortical steroid secretion resulting from stress-induced release of endogenous ACTH.[1306] Ideally, both adrenal veins should be catheterized, and aldosterone and cortisol should be measured in plasma obtained simultaneously from both veins and a peripheral site. Criteria for lateralization have not been validated, but adrenal vein aldosterone concentration on the side of the tumor is usually at least 10 times that of the nontumorous, presumably suppressed adrenal gland.[1325] Only enough contrast material to show proper catheter placement is used because of the risk of adrenal hemorrhage.

Radiographic/Nuclear Medicine Findings. Imaging procedures can assist in differentiating causes of hyperaldosteronism, as well as in lateralizing adenomas. CT scanning of the adrenals is usually done first. About 1% of upper abdominal CT scans performed for other reasons reveal incidental adrenal masses, most of which are not associated with abnormal hormone secretion.[1350] The clinical significance of such nonfunctioning incidentalomas is unclear. High-resolution CT scanners can detect adrenal tumors as small as 7 to 8 mm in diameter.[1325, 1351, 1352] The diagnostic accuracy is only about 70% for aldosterone-producing adenomas, in part because of the incidence of nonfunctioning adrenal adenomas.[1293, 1350] Aldosterone-producing adenomas usually have attenuation values lower than those of cortisol-secreting adenomas or pheochromocytomas but similar to those of some incidental adenomas.[1353] MRI is no better than CT scanning in differentiating aldosterone-secreting from other adrenal tumors.[1354] Scintigraphic imaging with ^{131}I-labeled cholesterol derivatives during dexamethasone suppression provides an image based on functional properties of the adrenal. NP-59 is useful for this purpose.[1355, 1356] Dexamethasone and stable iodide treatment are necessary to suppress ACTH secretion and prevent thyroidal uptake of the tracer. Asymmetrical uptake after 48 h indicates an adenoma, whereas symmetrical uptake after 72 h indicates bilateral hyperplasia. Diagnostic accuracy in 308 reported cases was 72%.[1293] However, if the adrenal CT scan is normal, iodocholesterol scanning is unlikely to be helpful.[1249] This procedure is generally used only when other data are contradictory. Adrenal venography is associated with risk of adrenal hemorrhage and has been abandoned as a diagnostic technique.

Treatment. Total unilateral surgical adrenalectomy is the treatment of choice for adrenal adenoma if the patient does not face unacceptable operative risk. Cure rates as high as 90% are reported, but the long-term cure rate in a review of 694 cases was 69%.[1293] The patient should be prepared for surgery with spironolactone (200 to 400 mg/d) for several weeks to control blood pressure and restore normal potassium balance. The dosage may be reduced after control is achieved. Electrolyte imbalances disappear promptly after successful surgery, but return of blood pressure to normal may require months. Some patients with primary bilateral hyperplasia may be cured by subtotal adrenalectomy,[1323, 1325] but there is no reliable method for identifying such patients preoperatively. Ease of control of blood pressure and serum potassium with spironolactone before surgery may be a favorable prognostic sign.[1323]

Medical therapy is indicated for patients with bilateral adrenal hyperplasia and for those with adenomas who are not surgical candidates. Spironolactone (200 to 400 mg/d) usually controls the hypokalemia, but additional antihypertensive therapy is often needed, especially in patients with hyperplasia. Side effects of spironolactone, which include menstrual disturbances in women and gynecomastia, impotence, and decreased libido in men, are mainly due to its inhibition of steroid biosynthetic P-450 enzymes and its action as an antiandrogen. Amiloride, an inhibitor of distal tubular sodium transport, has been used in hyperaldosteronism[1357] but rarely controls blood pressure in subjects with hyperplasia. Some consider it the drug of choice for men with hyperaldosteronism who are not cured by surgery.[1293] Calcium channel blockers have also been used because increased cytoplasmic free calcium stimulates aldoste-

rone synthesis. Calcium channel blockers also inhibit vascular smooth muscle contraction and lower peripheral vascular resistance. Although they initially appeared to decrease plasma aldosterone concentration and blood pressure,[1358, 1359] more recent studies demonstrated no effect on aldosterone and incomplete blood pressure control.[1360, 1361]

11β-HYDROXYSTEROID DEHYDROGENASE DEFICIENCY. There are both inherited and acquired states of 11β-hydroxysteroid dehydrogenase deficiency, both of which cause syndromes of mineralocorticoid excess.

Hereditary 11β-Hydroxysteroid Dehydrogenase Deficiency. The inherited defect causes low-renin hypertension and hypokalemia not accompanied by increased plasma aldosterone levels, yet responds to spironolactone therapy.[1362] Although some of these patients were known to have abnormal cortisol metabolism, they were initially thought to provide evidence for the existence of "cryptic" mineralocorticoids.[1363] These individuals excrete metabolites of cortisol, but not cortisone, whereas normal humans excrete more tetrahydro metabolites of cortisone than of cortisol.[1364] Furthermore, sodium retention, potassium wastage, and renin suppression are corrected by suppressing endogenous cortisol production with dexamethasone administration, and exogenous hydrocortisone, administered with the dexamethasone, re-creates the syndrome.[1362] Thus cortisol acts as a mineralocorticoid in the kidney if the 11β-hydroxysteroid dehydrogenase system fails to "protect" the relatively nonspecific mineralocorticoid type I receptor from exposure to it.

Acquired 11β-Hydroxysteroid Dehydrogenase Deficiency. Additional evidence for the protection hypothesis comes from studies of patients with licorice-induced hypokalemia. Chronic excessive ingestion of glycyrrhizic acid, the active principle in licorice, suppresses the renin-aldosterone system and causes kaliuresis. One possibility was that glycyrrhizic acid inhibits hepatic 5α-reductase activity, decreasing the metabolic clearance of aldosterone and prolonging its action. However, it was not clear how such a mechanism could affect the steady-state level of aldosterone. Another possibility was that glycyrrhizic acid or its hydrolytic product, glycyrrhetinic acid, or both bind to the type I receptor and exert a mineralocorticoid effect.[1365–1367] However, the affinity of glycyrrhetinic acid for the receptor is only about 0.01% that of aldosterone, and a mineralocorticoid effect of glycyrrhetinic acid cannot consistently be demonstrated in vitro.[1367] Furthermore, the adrenal glands must be present for licorice to have a mineralocorticoid effect in animals,[1368] and licorice is an effective mineralocorticoid replacement in human primary adrenal insufficiency only if given with hydrocortisone.[1369, 1370] The explanation for all of these observations is that glycyrrhizic acid produces a pharmacological 11β-hydroxysteroid dehydrogenase deficiency state[1371] that allows glucocorticoids to exert effects via the mineralocorticoid receptor.

BARTTER'S SYNDROME. A rare syndrome of hyperreninemia, hyperaldosteronism, hypokalemia, and alkalosis without hypertension or edema was described in 1962 by Bartter and associates.[1372] Renal juxtaglomerular cell hyperplasia and increased urinary prostaglandin E_2 excretion are observed.[1373] The disorder usually begins in childhood and presents with muscle weakness, cramps, urinary frequency, or developmental impairment. A number of primary defects have been proposed to account for Bartter's syndrome, but the cause is unknown. A chloride reabsorption defect may be present in the thick ascending limb of loop of Henle of the renal tubule, but similar defects have been found at other sites in the nephron, and one patient developed the tubular defect after exhibiting other features of the syndrome.[1374–1376] The hyperaldosteronism presumably is not the cause of the hypokalemia because bilateral adrenalectomy does not correct the kaliuresis.[1377]

SECONDARY HYPERALDOSTERONISM. Plasma aldosterone concentrations may be elevated in a number of disease states associated with formation of peripheral edema. These states include congestive heart failure, cirrhosis, and nephrotic syndrome. In none of these situations is aldosterone excess the primary abnormality. Aldosterone secretion increases physiologically in response to a decrease in effective circulating blood volume caused by diminished cardiac output or transudation of intravascular volume into extravascular sites. In addition, decreased hepatic metabolism of aldosterone occurs in patients with liver disease. In cirrhosis, the sodium-retaining effect of aldosterone persists because the usual mechanisms of escape are not activated. Other secondary forms of hyperaldosteronism include renin-secreting tumors, renal artery stenosis, and salt-wasting nephropathies.

Congenital Adrenal Hyperplasia*

The term congenital adrenal hyperplasia refers to syndromes caused by inherited enzymatic defects in cortisol biosynthesis. Any of the enzymes can be affected, but the common feature is decreased negative feedback inhibition of cortisol on pituitary ACTH secretion. The clinical manifestations are consequences both of deficient synthesis of cortisol and, in some types, aldosterone and of excessive secretion of precursor steroids that are synthesized before the defective enzyme step.

A syndrome now recognized to be a form of congenital adrenal hyperplasia was first described in 1865.[1378] The patient had apparent male external genitalia but first-degree hypospadias and absent palpable external gonads. Internally, a uterus, fallopian tubes, and ovaries were present, as were enlarged adrenals.[1379] The nature of the disorder, presumably P-450$_{c21}$ deficiency, remained obscure until the mid-20th century. It was then observed that urinary 17-KS excretion is increased and urinary 17-OHCS levels are diminished in some individuals with ambiguous genitalia,[1380] apparently as the result of defective cortisol biosynthesis.[1381] Rapid advances have since been made in understanding the biochemical pathophysiology of these disorders.

Deficiency of P-450$_{c21}$ (21-Hydroxylase Deficiency)

The common form of congenital adrenal hyperplasia, P-450$_{c21}$ deficiency, accounts for more than 90% of cases.[1382, 1383] Incidence of the classic disorder, based on neonatal screening studies, varies from approximately 1 in 5000 to 15,000 live births in most white populations[1384] to 1 in 300 to 700 in Alaskan Yupik Eskimos.[1385, 1386]

CLINICAL PRESENTATION. *Classic Forms.* P-450$_{c21}$ deficiency manifests itself in several syndromes. Two of these syndromes, simple virilizing and salt-wasting congenital adrenal hyperplasia, are recognized in neonates. Female infants exhibit pseudohermaphroditism, whereas affected males usually have normal sexual development. Androgen excess results from loss of cortisol negative feedback regulation of ACTH secretion. Adrenal androgen production is unimpaired by the enzymatic defect, and chronic excess ACTH stimulation results in increased flow of cortisol precursors into the androgen biosynthetic pathway. Female fetuses may be virilized in utero. Clitoral enlargement, labial fusion, and formation of a urogenital sinus result from androgen effects on development of the external genitalia. Genital ambiguity may be so profound that inappropriate sex assignment may be made at birth. Patients with signs only of androgen excess are said to have the simple virilizing form of P-450$_{c21}$ deficiency. About two thirds of patients also have mineralocorticoid deficiency. The salt-wasting variety results in hyponatremia, hyperkalemia, volume depletion, and increased plasma renin activity characteristic of hypoaldosteronism and is usually apparent within the first 2 wk of life.[1379, 1382, 1383]

When the diagnosis is not made during the neonatal period, a syndrome of androgen excess may appear in early infancy: sexual precocity in boys and further clitoral enlargement and growth of pubic hair in girls. The excess androgens accelerate both linear growth and epiphyseal closure, so despite the early accelerated growth velocity, bone age advances rapidly and ultimate adult height is diminished.[1387, 1388]

Reproductive function is impaired in adult women with untreated P-450$_{c21}$ deficiency. Establishing fertility depends on two factors.[1388] Labial fusion resulting from fetal androgenization may leave the vaginal introitus inadequate for successful coitus; surgical correction may be necessary. In addition, high circulating levels of progestogens and androgens may suppress normal hypothalamic-pituitary-gonadal function, preventing cyclic ovulatory function. Strict adherence to glucocorticoid replacement therapy is necessary to correct this defect.[1388-1390] In contrast, untreated males with P-450$_{c21}$ deficiency may be fertile,[1387] although some may have a reversible form of azoospermia that responds to glucocorticoid replacement.[1391]

Nonclassic Forms. Some individuals with P-450$_{c21}$ deficiency do not manifest any developmental abnormalities or salt-wasting tendencies but present in childhood or at the time of puberty with evidence of androgen excess.[1392-1399] The clinical syndrome may be indistinguishable from polycystic ovary disease.[1400] Relatives of patients with this attenuated form of the disorder may have identical biochemical abnormalities (see later) but no signs of androgen excess. The latter form is called cryptic P-450$_{c21}$ deficiency.[1401, 1402] Males usually are asymptomatic, but men rarely may have testicular adrenal rest "tumors" (i.e., hyperplasia) that regress after glucocorticoid suppression of ACTH secretion.[1403, 1404]

PATHOPHYSIOLOGY. *Biochemistry.* P-450$_{c21}$ is a microsomal enzyme responsible for conversion of 17α-hydroxyprogesterone to 11-deoxycortisol. Defects in enzyme quantity or activity decrease adrenocortical capacity for cortisol biosynthesis and result in accumulation of cortisol precursors, which are converted to adrenal androgens (Fig. 9–55). Because of deficient cortisol secretion, pituitary ACTH secretion is uninhibited, and cortisol precursors and adrenal androgens are produced in excess. Basal plasma concentrations of 17α-hydroxyprogesterone, the substrate for P-450$_{c21}$, may be increased several hundredfold above normal.[1382, 1383] There is an exaggerated 17α-hydroxyprogesterone response to ACTH stimulation in persons either homozygous or heterozygous for the abnormal gene. Increased quantities of precursor metabolities, notably pregnanetriol and 17-KS, are excreted in the urine. Pregnanetriol is the chief metabolite of 17α-hydroxyprogesterone, and 17-KS are metabolites of adrenal androgens. Untreated patients with the salt-wasting form may be hyponatremic and hyperkalemic. One cannot distinguish simple virilizing from salt-wasting classic P-450$_{c21}$ deficiency on the basis of plasma 17α-hydroxyprogesterone levels.[1382, 1383, 1405]

Genetics. P-450$_{c21}$ deficiency is transmitted as a single-gene autosomal recessive trait linked to the major histocompatibility complex locus on the short arm of human chromosome 6 (Fig. 9–56).[1406, 1407] Linkage disequilibrium

---

*Also see Chapter 14.

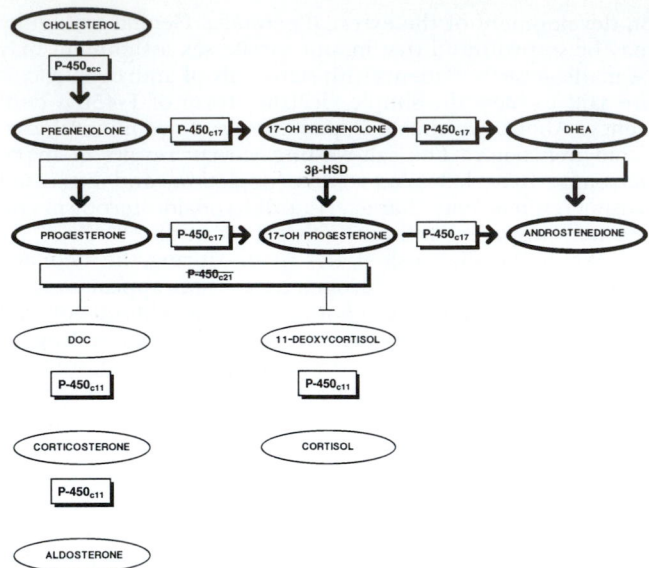

Figure 9–55. Biosynthetic defect in classic salt-wasting cytochrome P-450$_{c21}$ enzyme (21-hydroxylase) deficiency and resulting aberrations in adrenal steroidogenesis. Relative concentrations of steroids in plasma are shown by the width of the ovals. Simple virilizing and late-onset forms of P-450$_{c21}$ deficiency are associated with less impairment of cortisol and mineralocorticoid biosynthesis.

(nonrandom association) has been reported to exist between P-450$_{c21}$ deficiency and specific HLA alleles, including B14, B35, Bw47, B51, and Bw60.[1408–1412] The specific HLA types with which it is associated vary among populations. Bw47, a very rare allele, is strongly associated with classic forms of P-450$_{c21}$ deficiency in northern Europe[1410, 1411, 1413] but is absent in affected Italians.[1414] HLA associations with various clinical forms of P-450$_{c21}$ deficiency are fairly distinct: HLA-Bw47 and HLA-DR7 are associated with both classic forms of the disease, particularly the salt-wasting variant, and the simple virilizing form is associated with HLA-B51 (or HLA-B5, which has more narrow specificity).[1413] The nonclassic forms of the disorder are associated with HLA-B14.[1413, 1415, 1416] Possessing the Bw47 allele carries with it a 50-fold greater risk of classic P-450$_{c21}$ deficiency carrier status than not having this allele. This risk of carrier status for nonclassic P-450$_{c21}$ deficiency is increased 250-fold in persons with the HLA-B14 allele.[1413]

The human genome contains two P-450$_{c21}$ genes, designated A and B, both located in a 50-kb stretch of the short arm of human chromosome 6 within the major histocompatibility locus[1417, 1418] (see Fig. 9–56). The more 3' P-450$_{c21B}$ gene codes for the functioning human enzyme.[1418–1420] The P-450$_{c21A}$ gene does not code for a functional enzyme because it contains, among other differences from the P-450$_{c21B}$ gene, a deletion of eight of the nine bases constituting codons 110 to 112, changing the reading frame and producing a stop codon 18 codons downstream.[1419, 1420]

Digestion of genomic DNA with the restriction endonuclease *Taq*I results in a 3.2-kb band specific for the P-450$_{c21A}$ gene and a 3.7-kb band specific for the P-450$_{c21B}$ gene. This provides the basis for restriction fragment length polymorphism analysis of DNA from patients with P-450$_{c21}$ deficiency. Those with classic forms of the disorder may have gene deletions, gene conversion events, or point mutations underlying the inherited abnormality of the enzyme. Loss of the 3.7-kb band in patients with clinical P-450$_{c21}$ deficiency[1421–1423] suggested that the P-450$_{c21B}$ gene is deleted in up to 25% of the non–HLA-Bw47-bearing group.[1382, 1383] It now appears that a phenomenon called gene conversion, rather than actual physical loss of the gene, accounts for

many cases of P-450$_{c21}$ deficiency.[1424] Gene conversion refers to any of a number of processes by which two closely related genes become identical; in this instance the normal functional gene has acquired the properties of the nearby pseudogene.[1425] The relative frequency of conversion and deletional events has not been established, but both are causes of P-450$_{c21}$ deficiency.[1426–1431] The rare HLA haplotype A3, Bw47, DR7 appears always to be associated with deletion of the P-450$_{c21B}$ and adjacent serum complement C4B genes.[133] P-450$_{c21B}$ point mutations generally produce P-450$_{c21A}$ gene sequences and probably represent gene conversion events.[1427, 1428, 1432, 1433]

Patients who have nonclassic late-onset P-450$_{c21}$ deficiency and carry the HLA-B14 and HLA-DR1 antigens have a Val-to-Leu change at position 281 resulting from a single base change. It does not appear to be a normal polymorphism and is not found in other patients with late-onset P-450$_{c21}$ deficiency.[1434]

DIAGNOSIS. P-450$_{c21}$ deficiency should be considered in any newborn infant with genital ambiguity, salt wasting, or hypotension. Infants and children with less severe salt-wasting congenital adrenal hyperplasia may be discovered as the result of routine serum chemistry screening. Later in life, the diagnosis is usually considered because of apparent androgen excess. Adrenal androgen (DHEAS and androstenedione) and cortisol precursor (progesterone and 17α-hydroxyprogesterone) concentrations in plasma are elevated. Current laboratory diagnosis depends mostly on demonstrating increased basal or ACTH-stimulated plasma 17α-hydroxyprogesterone concentration, which has largely supplanted measurement of urinary excretion of metabolites of adrenal androgens (17-KS) or 17α-hydroxyprogesterone (pregnanetriol). Nomograms have been developed relating basal and ACTH-stimulated 17α-hydroxyprogesterone levels in classic and nonclassic forms of P-450$_{c21}$ deficiency and their carrier states[1382, 1383, 1405] (see later Fig. 9–66). Plasma aldosterone concentration may be low or normal in patients with salt wasting, depending on the severity of the enzyme deficiency, but plasma renin activity is virtually always increased.

Prenatal diagnosis would be desirable if there were a safe and effective prenatal treatment to prevent severe masculinization of female fetuses. Measurement of amniotic fluid 17α-hydroxyprogesterone levels, HLA typing of fetal

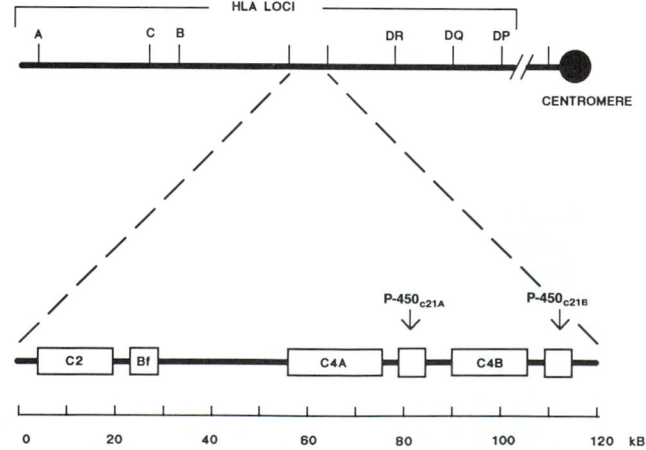

Figure 9–56. Map of the short arm of human chromosome 6 (*upper bar*), showing the relative positions of the genes encoding the major histocompatibility proteins A, C, B, DR, DQ, and DP. The detail (*lower bar*) shows the approximately 120-kb region containing the genes for complement component C2, properdin factor B (Bf), and the duplicated complement C4 gene (C4A and C4B). The pseudogene P-450$_{c21A}$ and the functional gene P-450$_{c21B}$ are in tandem array with the two C4 genes.

cells both serologically and by DNA hybridization, and restriction fragment length polymorphism analysis of fetal genomic DNA have all been proposed as screening methods.[1435–1439] Genotyping fetal cells obtained by chorionic villus sampling with P-450$_{c21}$ cDNA probes appears to be a promising approach.[1439]

TREATMENT. Therapy of P-450$_{c21}$ deficiency is directed toward the replacement of glucocorticoids and mineralocorticoids and the suppression of ACTH secretion and the consequent hyperandrogenemia so as to permit normal growth and skeletal maturation. These goals of optimal therapy are frequently difficult to achieve. The usual doses of hydrocortisone used are in the range of 20 to 25 mg/m^2 of body surface area given as two doses during the day.[1440] Because the results of therapy are frequently suboptimal in terms of eventual adult height and fertility[1387–1389, 1441–1442] and because the consequences of excessive glucocorticoid therapy are also deleterious, a number of alternative therapeutic tactics have been evaluated. A long-acting glucocorticoid such as dexamethasone, given at bedtime, suppresses early morning ACTH secretion more effectively than daytime doses of a short-acting glucocorticoid like hydrocortisone, and there is no a priori reason why such treatment should produce more side effects if the dosage is properly adjusted. Nevertheless, its use has largely been restricted to adults or adolescents who have completed linear growth.[1443, 1444] It has also been suggested that single daily doses of hydrocortisone are as effective as the traditional divided dose and even that alternate-day therapy with pharmacological doses of glucocorticoid can be successful.[1445, 1446]

Response to therapy is assessed by measuring growth velocity and rate of skeletal maturation, as well as plasma 17α-hydroxyprogesterone and adrenal androgen or testosterone levels.[1447, 1448] The biochemical markers serve as indicators of the adequacy of current treatment and the patient's compliance and are the basis for adjustments in the treatment regimen. Measurements of bone age and growth rate reflect long-term control. Ideally, treatment should be modified well before there is evidence of reduced growth rate or advanced bone age.[1449] Patients with salt wasting are given mineralocorticoid, usually fludrocortisone, in a dosage sufficient to lower plasma renin activity to normal without inducing hypertension. Occasionally, daily dosage greater than 0.1 to 0.2 mg is required; it can be titrated upward as long as blood pressure remains normal.[1448] Plasma renin activity is elevated in patients with the simple virilizing form of P-450$_{c21}$ deficiency even in the absence of overt salt wasting,[1450] and the addition of mineralocorticoid therapy may improve linear growth in non–salt-wasting patients.[1451, 1452]

In addition to medical therapy, reconstructive surgery, usually clitoral recession and vaginoplasty, is required in females with genital ambiguity.[1453]

The administration of dexamethasone to the pregnant woman suppresses both maternal and fetal pituitary ACTH secretion and should minimize or prevent virilization of female infants.[1454, 1455] The virilizing effects of androgens on genital tract development can begin as early as 6 wk of gestation, so treatment must be initiated before the onset of phenotypic sexual development or diagnosis of congenital adrenal hyperplasia via second-trimester amniocentesis or even chorionic villus biopsy at 8 to 10 wk. Consequently, treatment in most cases is initiated too late and is, therefore, unwarranted.[1456] Furthermore, the effect of maternally administered dexamethasone on genital development of affected females has been variable.[1457–1459] These facts and the potential risks of the diagnostic procedures and the steroid treatment to mother and fetus need to be considered before beginning in utero preventive therapy.

Deficiency of P-450$_{c11}$ (11β-Hydroxylase Deficiency)

INCIDENCE. P-450$_{c11}$ deficiency is the second most common cause of congenital adrenal hyperplasia, with an incidence of 1 in 100,000 live births, and it accounts for about 5% of adrenal steroidogenic defects.[1382, 1383] In Israel, it is thought to be more common among Jews of Moroccan or Iranian ancestry.[1460, 1461]

CLINICAL PRESENTATION. Classic Forms. P-450$_{c11}$ deficiency results in impaired conversion of 11-deoxycortisol and 11-DOC to cortisol and corticosterone, respectively. Decreased cortisol production results in increased ACTH secretion, which stimulates excessive production of non–11β-hydroxylated steroid precursors and adrenal androgens. The excess androgens cause female fetal virilization, which can be relatively mild or as severe as that of P-450$_{c21}$ deficiency. In a series of 25 patients,[1461] about half had relatively severe genital ambiguity or hyperandrogenism. Milder cases presented in childhood as early puberty in boys or hyperandrogenism in girls. Others were seen in young adulthood because of acne in men or menstrual irregularities and hirsutism in women.[1461]

What distinguishes P-450$_{c11}$ deficiency from P-450$_{c21}$ deficiency is hypertension. It is thought to be due to increased circulating concentrations of 11-DOC, despite lack of good correlation between DOC levels and blood pressure.[1461] Hypertension does not always occur in P-450$_{c11}$ deficiency, and salt wasting may occur in some patients.[1461, 1462] The reasons for this heterogeneity are not known. Hypokalemia may be present, presumably as a result of mineralocorticoid excess.

Nonclassic Forms. The milder late-onset form of P-450$_{c11}$ deficiency, with symptoms of androgen excess, is analogous to nonclassic P-450$_{c21}$ deficiency. However, the variable clinical severity of the disorder precludes sharp distinction between classic and nonclassic forms. There is no genetic evidence as yet that adult-onset patients inherit an allelic variant of a P-450$_{c11}$ gene distinct from that responsible for more severe childhood disease.

PATHOPHYSIOLOGY. Biochemistry. P-450$_{c11}$ catalyzes the terminal hydroxylation step in cortisol biosynthesis. Because 11-deoxycortisol and its precursors have virtually no biological glucocorticoid activity, deficiency of the enzyme results in loss of glucocorticoid negative feedback control of pituitary ACTH secretion. As in P-450$_{c21}$ deficiency, chronic ACTH hyperstimulation results in excess production of cortisol precursor steroids. Increased substrate flow through the androgen biosynthetic pathway results in excess adrenal androgen secretion (Fig. 9–57). The plasma concentrations of adrenal androgens and cortisol precursors, especially 11-deoxycortisol and DOC, increase, as does urinary excretion of their tetrahydro metabolites, which are normally excreted in only trace quantities.[1463] The androgens contribute to urinary 17-KS. It should be remembered that 11-deoxycortisol is measured as a 17-OHCS.

The hypertension observed in some patients with P-450$_{c11}$ deficiency presumably is due to a volume-expanded state induced by excess secretion of DOC, a weak mineralocorticoid.[1439] Increased plasma DOC levels suggest that the same P-450$_{c11}$ enzyme is involved in cortisol and aldosterone biosynthesis in the zonae fasciculata and glomerulosa, respectively. However, some investigators think that at least two types of P-450$_{c11}$ deficiency exist, one affecting only the cortisol pathway and the other affecting both the cortisol and aldosterone pathways. After one patient was given dexamethasone to suppress ACTH, plasma DOC levels fell and plasma renin activity rose to normal, but aldosterone levels actually increased, implying that aldosterone synthesis

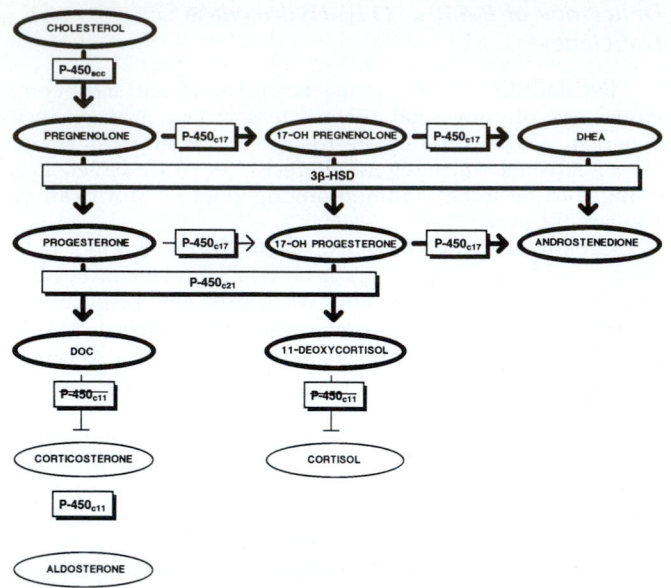

Figure 9–57. Biosynthetic defect in cytochrome P-450$_{c11}$ enzyme (11β-hydroxylase) deficiency and resulting aberrations in adrenal steroidogenesis. Relative concentrations of steroids in plasma are indicated by the width of the ovals. Elevated DOC levels produce a state of mineralocorticoid excess despite defects in the terminal steps of aldosterone synthesis.

depends on a distinct P-450$_{c11}$.[1464] There are two forms of the enzyme in the rat, one specific to the zona glomerulosa and one distributed in both glomerulosa and fasciculata.[140–142] There are also two distinct P-450$_{c11}$ mRNA species in the bovine adrenal cortex.[1465] Presumably, humans also have two P-450$_{c11}$ enzymes. How defects in these specific genes might be related to different clinical syndromes of P-450$_{c11}$ deficiency is unknown.

Genetics. P-450$_{c11}$ deficiency is inherited as an autosomal recessive disorder without evidence of linkage to the HLA locus.[1466] At least one P-450$_{c11}$ gene is located on human chromosome 8.[137]

DIAGNOSIS. P-450$_{c11}$ deficiency should be considered whenever there is apparent androgen excess in newborn infants (i.e., ambiguous genitalia), children, or adults, particularly when it is associated with hypertension. However, the rarity of this disorder and the frequency of other conditions that cause hyperandrogenism and hypertension, particularly in adults, should be borne in mind.

The diagnosis rests on the biochemical demonstration of impaired cortisol biosynthesis, with excess production of precursor steroids proximal to the 11β-hydroxylation step. Basal or ACTH-stimulated plasma 11-deoxycortisol concentration and urinary excretion of tetrahydro-11-deoxycortisol (THS), which is measured as a 17-OHCS, are increased. Adrenal androgen (DHEAS, androstenedione, and testosterone) levels in plasma are increased, as is urinary excretion of adrenal androgens and their metabolites, some of which are measured as 17-KS. In classic forms of the disorder, measurement of basal plasma 11-deoxycortisol levels and urinary excretion of THS usually establishes the diagnosis.[1382, 1383] In milder adult cases, ACTH stimulation is often necessary to reveal the defect.[1467, 1468] Unlike subjects heterozygous for P-450$_{c21}$ deficiency, P-450$_{c11}$ carriers exhibit no abnormal plasma precursor steroid elevation after ACTH stimulation.[1469] P-450$_{c11}$ deficiency can be diagnosed prenatally by measuring THS levels in amniotic fluid.[1470]

TREATMENT. P-450$_{c11}$ deficiency is treated by replacement of physiological amounts of glucocorticoid. As in P-450$_{c21}$ deficiency, therapy must be adjusted in individual cases. The usual hydrocortisone dosage is about 20 mg/m^2 divided in two doses during the day. Useful biochemical parameters in monitoring therapy are plasma 11-deoxycortisol, androgens, and renin activity. Steroid precursor and androgen levels fall with adequate therapy, and the suppressed plasma renin activity rises into the detectable range. As in P-450$_{c21}$ deficiency, linear growth rates and skeletal maturation indices are monitored to assess long-term adequacy of treatment. Hypertension may persist after suppression of mineralocorticoid (DOC) excess and require additional therapy. Aldosterone deficiency may become apparent in some infants and children, particularly those on low-salt diets, after DOC secretion is suppressed with glucocorticoid. Mineralocorticoid replacement therapy may be necessary. As in P-450$_{c21}$ deficiency, genital malformations in affected females must be corrected surgically.

Deficiency of 17α-hydroxylase activity is a rare form of congenital adrenal hyperplasia; fewer than 25 patients have been reported. The enzymatic defect was first described in a woman with sexual infantilism and hypertension,[1471] but it can also cause male pseudohermaphroditism.[1472] Because of the rarity of the disorder, its clinical presentations and course are not as well characterized as those of more common forms of adrenal steroidogenic defects.

CLINICAL PRESENTATION. Females have primary amenorrhea and absent secondary sexual characteristics. Not all patients in early reports had karyotypic analysis to establish genotypic sex, however. Male (46,XY) patients usually have complete male pseudohermaphroditism with female external genitalia, a blind-ended vagina, and absent uterus and fallopian tubes. The testes are usually intra-abdominal and exhibit Leydig cell hyperplasia on microscopic examination.[1472]

Most patients with P-450$_{c17}$ deficiency are hypertensive, including the first three women described with the disorder.[1471, 1473, 1474] However, the first male described with the syndrome was not hypertensive,[1472] and the age of development of hypertension is variable. Hypokalemia accompanies the hypertension in some patients but may be mild.

P-450$_{c17}$ deficiency usually does not cause adrenal insufficiency. Patients tolerate general anesthesia and surgery without glucocorticoid replacement. Frequent respiratory infections have been reported, but the relationship between them and the steroidogenic defect is unclear.

PATHOPHYSIOLOGY. *Biochemistry.* The P-450$_{c17}$ gene encodes an enzyme with both 17α-hydroxylase and 17,20-lyase (desmolase, or side-chain cleavage) activities. Hydroxylation of C-17 of progesterone is required to synthesize cortisol, androgens, and estrogens. Lyase activity is required to produce all androgenic C$_{19}$-steroids (DHEA, androstenedione, and testosterone) and their derivatives, the estrogenic C$_{18}$-steroids. A single enzyme possesses both activities in vitro, yet human P-450$_{c17}$ deficiency includes patients who apparently lack only 17,20-lyase activity and others who have the combined defect.[1475, 1476] In patients with the combined defect, production of glucocorticoids, androgens, and estrogens is impaired[1477] (Fig. 9–58). Plasma concentrations of progesterone, the substrate for P-450$_{c17}$, are increased. Plasma levels of cortisol, 11-deoxycortisol, and 17α-hydroxyprogesterone are low, and ACTH levels are increased. Testosterone, estradiol, and DHEAS, production of which depends on P-450$_{c17}$ activity, are also low. Because gonadal steroidogenesis is impaired, FSH and LH concentrations are elevated.

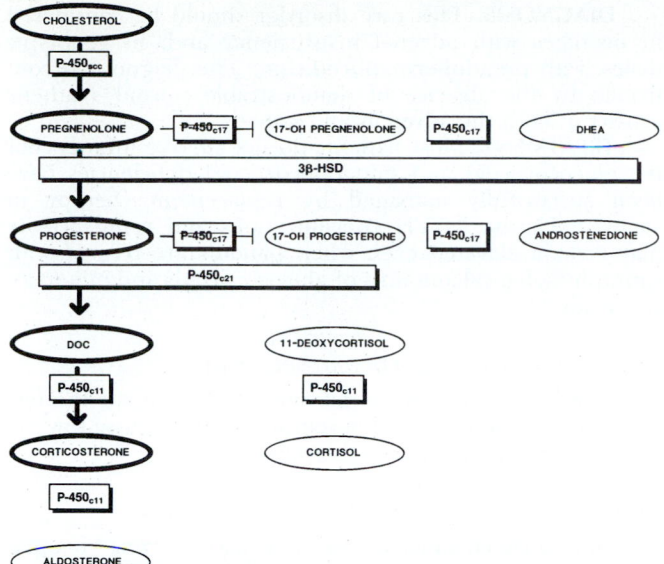

Figure 9–58. Biosynthetic defect in cytochrome P-450$_{c17}$ enzyme (17α-hydroxylase) deficiency and resulting aberrations in adrenal steroidogenesis. Relative concentrations of steroids in plasma are indicated by the width of the ovals. Enzymatic capacity for aldosterone biosynthesis is intact, but the renin-angiotensin system is suppressed by the excessive synthesis of DOC.

Mineralocorticoid biosynthesis, on the other hand, does not depend on P-450$_{c17}$ activity. Increased substrate flux along this pathway results in increased production and plasma levels of DOC and corticosterone. Plasma renin activity is suppressed, and plasma aldosterone concentrations are low.[1478] Thus P-450$_{c17}$ deficiency appears to cause a state of mineralocorticoid excess induced by DOC, 18-hydroxycorticosterone, 18-hydroxy-DOC, 19-nor-DOC, or some combination of these mineralocorticoids, all of which are increased in concentration,[1479, 1480] and secondary hypoaldosteronism.[1481] One patient apparently had deficiencies of both P-450$_{c21}$ and P-450$_{c17}$.[1482]

Genetics. Like other forms of congenital adrenal hyperplasia, P-450$_{c17}$ deficiency is inherited as an autosomal recessive trait. Several reported patients are the offspring of consanguineous marriages, and obligate heterozygotes have mild defects in P-450$_{c17}$ activity that can be revealed by ACTH stimulation.[1477, 1478, 1483]

A 46,XY patient with male pseudohermaphroditism, hypertension, and deficiency of both 17α-hydroxylase and 17,20-lyase activities had a duplicated four-base sequence in exon 8 of the P-450$_{c17}$ gene.[1484] As a result of the reading frameshift, the sequence after amino acid 479 was different from that of the normal protein and was three residues shorter because there was a new stop codon 26 codons downstream. The affected sequence is thought to be involved in the interaction of the enzyme with NADPH–cytochrome P-450 reductase. The same mutation has been observed in two Mennonite families.[1484] Another 46,XX patient had a mutation at codon 17 that changed the reading frame and produced a stop codon in exon 1 so that no functional protein was synthesized.[1485]

DIAGNOSIS. The diagnosis of P-450$_{c17}$ deficiency relies on demonstration of increased serum concentrations of steroid precursors proximal to the P-450$_{c17}$ step; decreased concentrations of cortisol, adrenal androgens, and C$_{19}$ and C$_{18}$ gonadal steroids; and increased plasma levels of DOC and corticosterone. Prenatal diagnosis has not been reported.

TREATMENT. Treatment is based on glucocorticoid administration to suppress ACTH and the consequent precur-

sor steroid excess and on gonadal steroid replacement at the time of expected puberty. Because experience with the disorder is limited, few data are available on therapeutic results. Suppression of the renin-angiotensin-aldosterone axis can be reversed by glucocorticoid administration in some patients[1481] but persists for years despite glucocorticoid therapy in others.[1479] Most patients are reared as females, regardless of genotypic sex.

Deficiency of 3β-Hydroxysteroid Dehydrogenase

3β-Hydroxysteroid dehydrogenase (sometimes referred to as 3β-ol) deficiency is a rare form of congenital adrenal hyperplasia in which synthesis of all steroid hormone classes is impaired. Excessive amounts of steroid precursors with the Δ^5-3-hydroxy configuration (i.e., Δ^5-pregnenolone, 17α-hydroxypregnenolone, and DHEA) are produced, but synthesis of progesterone and, consequently, of glucocorticoids, mineralocorticoids, androgens, and estrogens is decreased.[1379]

CLINICAL PRESENTATION. The classic disorder presents in early infancy,[1439] usually with adrenal insufficiency. Females have a mild degree of virilization of the external genitalia, presumably because of increased ACTH-stimulated secretion of DHEA, a small fraction of which is converted peripherally to testosterone. Males have varying degrees of failure of normal genital development, ranging from hypospadias to nearly normal female external genitalia. A few patients appear to have severe 3β-hydroxysteroid dehydrogenase deficiency without evidence of mineralocorticoid deficiency.[1486] The nature of the defect in these patients is not clear.

An attenuated or late-onset form has also been described that typically presents in peripubertal or adult women as hirsutism and/or oligomenorrhea.[1487, 1488] The incidence of late-onset 3β-hydroxysteroid dehydrogenase deficiency is not known.

PATHOPHYSIOLOGY. Biochemistry. Inability to convert any of the Δ^5-3-hydroxysteroids (i.e., Δ^5-pregnenolone, 17α-hydroxypregnenolone, and DHEA) into the respective Δ^4-3-ketosteroids (i.e., progesterone, 17α-hydroxyprogesterone, Δ^4-androstenedione) is the hallmark of this disorder (Fig. 9–59). Nevertheless, 17α-hydroxyprogesterone levels may be increased in the classic form of this syndrome, presumably because of extra-adrenal conversion of 17α-hydroxypregnenolone.[1489] The different clinical syndromes suggest not only that there are different degrees of enzyme deficiency but also that specific pathways may be affected or spared in different patients. However, the human enzyme has not been purified; whether specific isoforms exist is not known. Neither the cDNA nor the gene for 3β-hydroxysteroid dehydrogenase has been cloned.

Genetics. The disorder is thought to be transmitted as an autosomal recessive trait. There have been no molecular genetic studies of the mutation. Whether the late-onset form is an allelic variant of the classic form is not known.

DIAGNOSIS. The diagnosis is usually established by demonstrating a greatly increased ratio of Δ^5- to Δ^4-steroids in plasma or urine. ACTH stimulation may be required to reveal the abnormality in attenuated forms of the disorder.[1487]

TREATMENT. Therapy of the disorder is directed at replacing deficient hormones, which in the classic form may include cortisol, aldosterone, and gonadal steroids. The principles of therapy in 3β-hydroxysteroid dehydrogenase deficiency are similar to those in the treatment of P-450$_{c21}$ deficiency. Adequate cortisol replacement is given to suppress any ACTH-stimulated androgen (DHEAS) overpro-

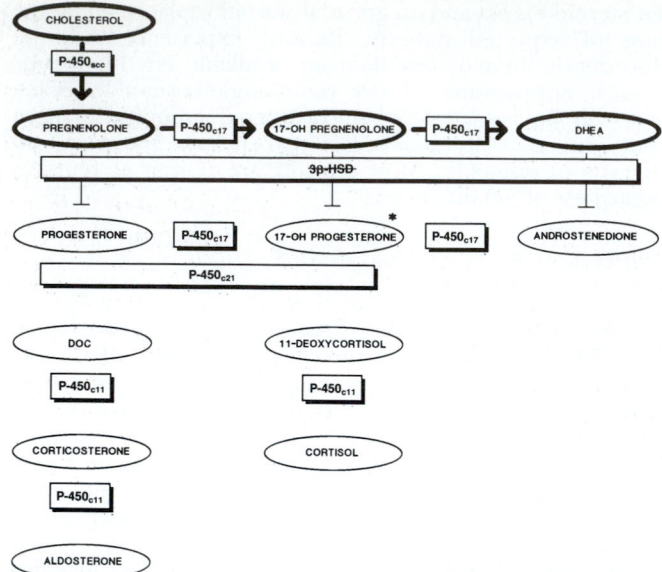

Figure 9–59. Biosynthetic defect in 3β-hydroxysteroid dehydrogenase deficiency and resulting aberrations in adrenal steroidogenesis. Relative concentrations of steroids in plasma are indicated by the width of the ovals. 17α-Hydroxyprogesterone levels *(asterisk)* may be elevated in plasma despite the adrenal enzyme deficiency because of extra-adrenal conversion of 17α-hydroxypregnenolone.

duction along with adequate mineralocorticoid. The dosages of such replacements would be similar to those described earlier. In addition, gonadal steroid replacement is needed at the time of expected puberty. Female infants who have been virilized in utero may require surgical correction of genital anomalies. In the late-onset form of the disorder, a long-acting glucocorticoid such as dexamethasone is administered to suppress ACTH and reduce adrenal DHEA hypersecretion.

Deficiency of Cholesterol Side-Chain Cleavage Enzyme (P-450$_{scc}$)

Apparent deficiency of the enzyme activity responsible for cholesterol side-chain cleavage, the rate-limiting step in adrenal and gonadal steroidogenesis, is a rare autosomal recessive trait. P-450$_{scc}$ deficiency has proved fatal in infancy in about two thirds of 34 patients reported.[1490]

CLINICAL PRESENTATION. Severe adrenal insufficiency presents during the neonatal period, with failure to thrive, vomiting, diarrhea, hyponatremia, and hypokalemia. 46,XY infants usually have female external genitalia because of lack of testicular androgen production.

PATHOPHYSIOLOGY. *Biochemistry.* Because P-450$_{scc}$ is the rate-limiting step in steroidogenesis, patients with deficiency of the enzyme have immeasurably low cortisol and aldosterone secretion rates[1490] (Fig. 9–60). Production of gonadal steroids is also impaired, and plasma levels of ACTH, FSH, LH, and renin activity are all increased. Increased ACTH stimulation is thought to cause the massive adrenal hyperplasia and cholesterol ester deposition characteristic of the disorder.

Genetics. Like other varieties of congenital adrenal hyperplasia, P-450$_{scc}$ deficiency is transmitted as an autosomal recessive trait. No deletions or other gene abnormalities have yet been detected using specific human P-450$_{scc}$ cDNA probes.[1491] The defect may be small, perhaps a point mutation. Alternatively, abnormalities of adrenodoxin or adrenodoxin reductase may account for some cases of apparent P-450$_{scc}$ deficiency.

DIAGNOSIS. This rare disorder should be considered in neonates with adrenal insufficiency and, in genotypic males, with pseudohermaphroditism. The diagnosis is confirmed by the absence of demonstrable steroid synthetic activity in both the adrenals and gonads.

TREATMENT. Most patients do not survive infancy, but the glucocorticoid and mineralocorticoid deficiencies have been successfully managed by replacement therapy in some.[1490] Plasma ACTH concentrations and renin activity may remain elevated even when patients are treated with supraphysiological amounts of glucocorticoids and mineralocorticoids.[1490]

Defects in Mineralocorticoid Biosynthesis

The inherited enzyme deficiencies that impair the terminal steps of aldosterone biosynthesis are discussed in the section on isolated hypoaldosteronism.

Pharmacological Use of Glucocorticoids

Since adrenal steroids were first used to treat rheumatoid arthritis,[38, 921] natural and synthetic glucocorticoids have been used to manage a wide variety of conditions (Table 9–16). In most disorders, the intent is not merely to replace deficient adrenal secretion of these hormones, but to achieve pharmacological effects not necessarily related to normal physiological roles. In general, the desired effect is suppression of immune reactivity or the inflammatory process. In some conditions (e.g., septic shock or cerebral edema) the exact nature of the pathophysiological processes targeted by steroid therapy is not known. Specific indications for glucocorticoid therapy in these diverse disorders will not be listed here. Rather, the pharmacological properties of natural and synthetic glucocorticoids, general guidelines for their use, and descriptions of the side effects of chronic pharmacological glucocorticoid therapy will be discussed.

Structure-Function Relationships

STRUCTURES OF COMMON SYNTHETIC STEROIDS. *Modification of Biological Activity.* Empirical chemical mod-

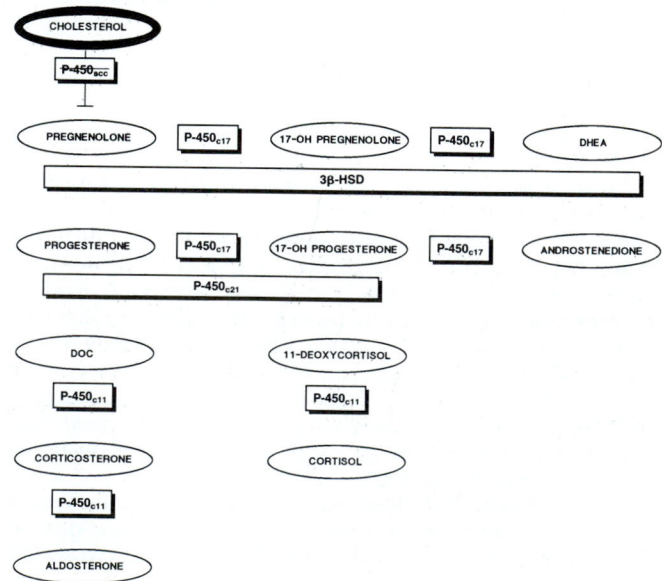

Figure 9–60. Biosynthetic defect in cytochrome P-450$_{scc}$ enzyme deficiency and resulting aberrations in adrenal steroidogenesis. Relative concentrations of steroids in plasma are indicated by the width of the ovals. Synthesis of all classes of steroid hormones, gonadal as well as adrenal, is impaired by the defect in the initial step in steroid biosynthesis.

TABLE 9–16. Examples of Nonendocrine Disorders Treated with Glucocorticoids

Allergic Diseases
Asthma, atopic dermatitis, anaphylactic shock
Autoimmune Diseases
Systemic lupus erythematosus, rheumatoid arthritis, systemic vasculitis, polymyalgia rheumatica, temporal arteritis, Graves' ophthalmopathy, autoimmune hemolysis, myasthenia gravis
Inflammatory Disorders
Crohn's disease, ulcerative colitis
Neoplastic Diseases
Lymphomas
Graft Rejection
Kidney, heart, lung, liver, and other tissue transplantation
Miscellaneous
Sarcoidosis, vitamin D intoxication, thyroid storm, septic shock, cerebral edema, altitude sickness, chronic bronchitis, emphysema

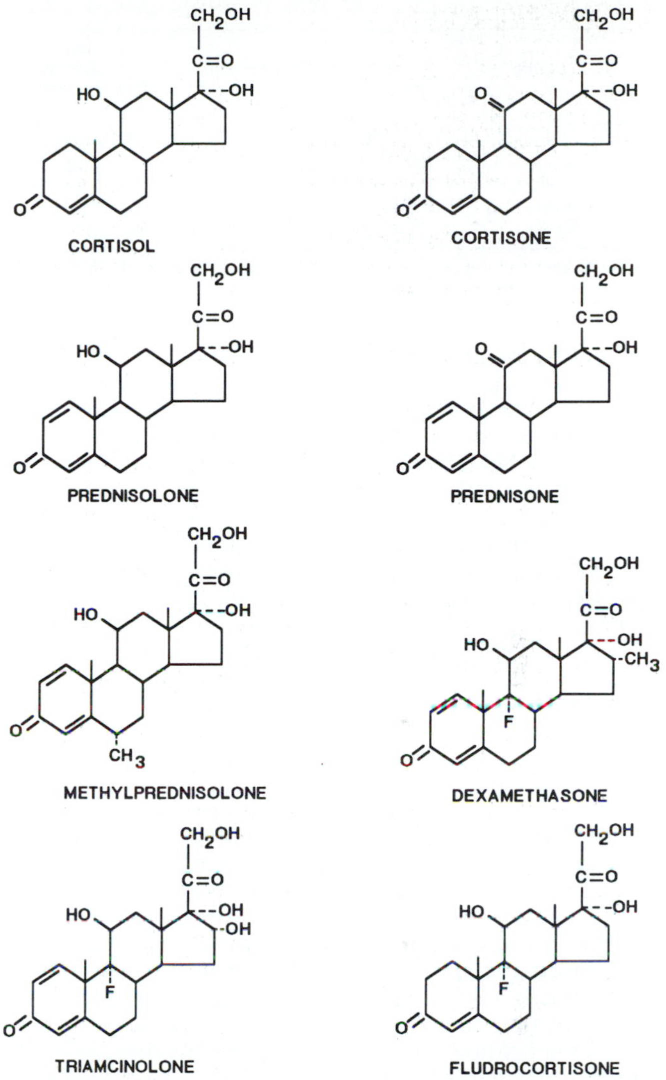

Figure 9–62. Structures of the natural glucocorticoid cortisol, some of the more commonly prescribed synthetic glucocorticoids, and the mineralocorticoid fludrocortisone. Note that triamcinolone is identical to dexamethasone except that a 16α-hydroxyl group is substituted for the 16α-methyl group. Betamethasone, another widely used glucocorticoid, has a 16β-methyl group.

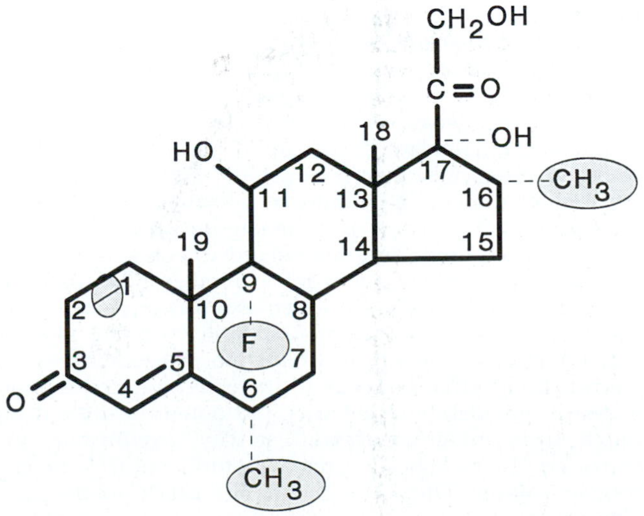

ifications of the natural steroids achieved in the 1950s revealed a number of structural features essential to their biological activities. The Δ^4-3-keto-11β,17α,21-trihydroxyl configuration (Figs. 9–5 and 9–61) is essential for glucocorticoid activity and is present, therefore, in all synthetic glucocorticoids.[1492, 1493] The addition of a 1,2-unsaturated (Δ^1) bond to hydrocortisone (cortisol) yields prednisolone (Δ^1-hydrocortisone), a compound with three- to fourfold greater glucocorticoid activity than cortisol (Fig. 9–62, Table 9–17).[1494, 1495] Prednisone, a widely used oral synthetic steroid, is prednisolone with an 11-keto group (see Fig. 9–62) and must be converted to prednisolone to become biologically active.[1496] Addition of a 6α-methyl group to prednisolone yields methylprednisolone (see Fig. 9–62), which has about five- to sixfold greater activity than cortisol.[1497] Addition of a 9α-fluoro atom to hydrocortisone (to produce fludrocortisone; see Fig. 9–62) increases its glucocorticoid and mineralocorticoid potencies by about 12-fold and 125-fold, respectively.[1498] Because aldosterone, the naturally occurring mineralocorticoid, is difficult to synthesize, fludrocortisone is used to replace the salt-retaining effect of aldosterone in patients with primary adrenal insufficiency. Combining the Δ^1 and 9α-fluoro modifications produces Δ^1-9α-fluorohydrocortisone (Δ^1-fludrocortisone, once called Δ^1FF), which has about 30-fold greater glucocorticoid activity than hydrocortisone but also has almost twice the mineralocorticoid activity of fludrocortisone (see Table 9–17). This limited its useful-

ness as a glucocorticoid, and it is no longer available. However, adding a 16α-methyl group to Δ^1-fludrocortisone produces dexamethasone (see Fig. 9–62), which retains the glucocorticoid potency of Δ^1-fludrocortisone but has almost no mineralocorticoid activity.[1492] Dexamethasone is widely used for both diagnostic and therapeutic purposes. Betamethasone, the same steroid with a 16β-methyl group, is equipotent with dexamethasone. It is used in nasal aerosol sprays and in other formulations. Triamcinolone has a 16α-hydroxyl group, rather than a methyl group (see Fig. 9–62). It has less glucocorticoid activity than dexamethasone, about the same glucocorticoid activity as methylprednisolone, and negligible salt-retaining activity. It is widely used in topical preparations.

Formulations. Steroids are essentially insoluble in water. Consequently, except when prepared in extremely dilute solution, they are formulated as organic esters (e.g., acetates, butyrates, dipropionates, valerates), which have very limited solubility, or as salts (e.g., hydrochlorides, sodium phosphates, sodium succinates), which are freely soluble. Except for the salts, many steroids are so insoluble that even at concentrations of 3% or less they form suspensions and are

Figure 9–61. The basic glucocorticoid structure and chemical modifications *(circled areas)* that can be introduced to enhance glucocorticoid or mineralocorticoid activity.

TABLE 9–17. Relative Biological Potencies of Synthetic Steroids in Bioassay Systems

Steroid	Eosinophil Suppression	Liver Glycogen	Anti-inflammatory	Hypothalamic-Pituitary Axis Suppression	Salt Retention
Cortisol	1[a]	1[b]	1[b]	1[g]	1[a]
Prednisolone	4[a]	3[b]	3[b]	4[g]	0.75[a]
Methylprednisolone	4.8[a]	10[b]	6.2[b]	4[g]	0.5[a]
Fludrocortisone	9.2[a]	12[c]	12[c]	12[g]	125[a]
Δ¹-Fludrocortisone	31.2[a]	50[d]	14[e]		225[a]
Triamcinolone		5[b]	5[c]	4	0[c]
Dexamethasone			26[f]	17[g]	0[f]

Data are from [a]Liddle,[1628] [b]Dulin et al.,[1632] [c]Soffer and Orr,[1630] [d]Stafford et al.,[1495] [e]Dulin,[1629] [f]Slater et al.,[1631] and [g]Meikle and Tyler.[1510]

unsuitable for intravenous use, although they can be used in topical creams and for intramuscular and intra-articular injection. The insoluble free alcohols, on the other hand, can be prepared as tablets for oral administration.

PHARMACOKINETICS. *Binding to Corticosteroid-Binding Globulin and Other Plasma Proteins.* Most of the cortisol circulating in human plasma is bound to protein, chiefly CBG and albumin; much of the biologically available cortisol may be bound to erythrocytes.[1499] However, most synthetic glucocorticoids bind poorly, if at all, to CBG.[1500] Their affinity for erythrocytes has not been investigated but is presumably of little importance. Prednisolone has about half of cortisol's affinity for CBG, whereas methylprednisolone, dexamethasone, betamethasone, and triamcinolone have less than 1% of its affinity.[1500] Lacking significant binding to CBG, synthetic steroids other than hydrocortisone and prednisolone circulate in two forms: about two thirds bound weakly to albumin and one third as free steroid.[1501] Although it might appear that CBG binding would affect bioavailability of a steroid, there is little evidence that CBG binding plays a major role in determining the relative potencies. CBG binding prolongs the plasma half-lives of steroids, but it is not the major factor in determining their plasma half-lives.

Plasma Disappearance Half-Life. The half-lives of synthetic glucocorticoids are generally longer than that of cortisol, which is about 80 min when its concentration remains within the binding capacity of CBG, i.e., less than about 690 nmol/L (25 μg/dL).[1502, 1503] Half-lives range from about 1 h for prednisolone to over 4 h for dexamethasone, with considerable interindividual variation.[1503, 1504] Patients who metabolize the steroid more slowly may be more likely to develop side effects;[1505] whether this is a distinct population is not clear. Clearly, binding to CBG is not the major determinant of the plasma half-life of most glucocorticoids. In addition to genetic variability, a variety of drugs can influence the rate of disappearance of steroids from plasma (see later).

BINDING TO THE CYTOSOL GLUCOCORTICOID RECEPTOR. In contrast to their weak affinities for CBG, synthetic glucocorticoids have higher affinities than cortisol for the intracellular type II glucocorticoid receptor. The affinities of prednisolone and triamcinolone are approximately 2-fold higher than that of cortisol, that of betamethasone is 5-fold higher, that of dexamethasone is 7-fold higher, and that of methylprednisolone is 11-fold higher.[1500] Prednisone has low affinity for the glucocorticoid receptor and, consequently, has negligible glucocorticoid bioactivity. Like cortisone, which must be converted to cortisol by hepatic 11β-hydroxysteroid dehydrogenase, prednisone must be converted to prednisolone to exert glucocorticoid effects.[1496] Cortisone acetate was the first glucocorticoid available for clinical use, and, although it is a relatively weak glucocorticoid and has significant mineralocorticoid activity, it is still used by some physicians. In contrast, the type I (mineralocorticoid) receptor–mediated activities of potent glucocorticoids such as prednisolone, methylprednisolone, dexameth-

asone, and triamcinolone are negligible compared with their glucocorticoid activities.

BIOLOGICAL POTENCIES AND DURATION OF ACTION. The affinity of a steroid for the glucocorticoid receptor and its pharmacokinetics do not entirely accurately predict biological potency. The magnitude and duration of the response to a steroid also depend on a number of other factors, including the efficiency and rate of its absorption into the systemic circulation and the rate of metabolism.

Absorption. Orally administered steroids are absorbed almost quantitatively within about 30 min.[1506] Absorption of topically administered steroid varies depending on the area of the body (e.g., intertriginous areas >> forehead > scalp > face > forearm) on which it is placed,[1507] whether the vehicle contains urea, dimethyl sulfoxide, or other agents (such as salicylic acid) that enhance absorption, and whether the area is covered with an occlusive dressing, which may enhance absorption 10-fold.[1508] Infants, whose stratum corneum is thinner than that of an adult, absorb topical steroids more readily.[1509] Injected steroids vary considerably in the rate of their absorption. Hydrocortisone salts are rapidly absorbed from an intramuscular injection site, and less soluble hydrocortisone esters are absorbed within an hour. Cortisone acetate is more slowly absorbed, and triamcinolone salts and esters may be absorbed for 3 to 6 wk. Absorption from intra-articular sites can be variable.

Metabolism. The metabolism of endogenous steroids is discussed earlier in this chapter. Exogenous steroids are subject to the same reduction, oxidation, hydroxylation, and conjugation reactions. The effects of drugs (phenobarbital, phenytoin, rifampin, mitotane) on these reactions, particularly by inducing increased 6β-hydroxylase activity,[168, 536, 537, 541] have also been discussed. The potential effects of these drugs must be considered in any patient who is receiving steroids.

Assays of Biological Activity. The potencies of synthetic glucocorticoids have been assessed in systems that are usually not influenced by variable absorption and metabolism of the steroid. Classic bioassays test the ability of the steroid to suppress the circulating eosinophil count in peripheral blood, to enhance hepatic glycogen deposition, or to inhibit the accumulation of an oil-induced inflammatory exudate in rats. The last two assays presumably measure directly the "glucocorticoid" and "anti-inflammatory" potency of the test steroid, respectively. Data from a number of sources are summarized in Table 9–17, which also lists estimates of the ability of the steroids to inhibit sodium excretion in adrenalectomized rats, an index of mineralocorticoid activity. All glucocorticoid effects appear to increase or decrease more or less in parallel, but glucocorticoid potency can be dissociated from mineralocorticoid activity. Prednisone, like cortisone, is biologically inactive and requires hepatic transformation. The active metabolite prednisolone has a glucocorticoid potency four- to fivefold greater than that of cortisol. Methylprednisolone and triamcinolone have similar potencies and dexamethasone has about 30-fold greater potency than cortisol in these assay systems. However, most of these estimates do not take into account differences in plasma clearance rates. Thus dexamethasone has a higher potency than its traditional estimate, depending on how long after administration bioactivity is assessed.[1510] Consequently, the values listed in Table 9–17 must be considered as estimates only.

Endocrinological Uses of Glucocorticoids

Endocrinological uses of corticosteroids constitute only a minute fraction of their total application in medical practice. The diagnostic use in detecting Cushing's syndrome and in differentiating its cause and the therapeutic use in adrenal insufficiency and congenital adrenal steroidogenic defects are discussed elsewhere in this chapter.

Nonendocrinological Uses of Glucocorticoids

Glucocorticoids are widely used as pharmacological agents for a variety of allergic, autoimmune, inflammatory, and neoplastic disorders. They are given to treat certain hypercalcemic states, manage thyroid storm, and prevent immune rejection of transplanted organs. They have been used in an attempt to reduce cerebral edema associated with intracranial masses, treat septic shock, and prevent altitude sickness (see Table 9–16). This broad array of applications is based on effects that range from inhibiting cell-mediated immune function to altering metabolic conversion of non-steroidal hormones from inactive to active forms.[1511–1513] However, many of the uses are empirical; the clinical efficacy and the mechanism underlying a number of applications of glucocorticoid therapy have not been rigorously established. Indeed, when subjected to controlled, double-blind, placebo crossover trials, glucocorticoids often produce no beneficial effect in conditions for which they are widely prescribed.

CRITERIA FOR INITIATING USE. The decision to initiate steroid therapy for a nonendocrinological illness may arise in an emergency, such as sudden anaphylactic shock, during a less acute but potentially life-threatening illness, such as lupus nephritis, or in the setting of a poorly controlled chronic illness, such as rheumatoid arthritis. The criteria for initiating therapy depend on the clinical setting.

Medical Emergencies. Even high doses of glucocorticoids can be administered for a few days with little risk. Therefore, it may be warranted to use them empirically in emergencies or in novel situations in which therapeutic benefit is not demonstrated but might be anticipated. However, because of the potentially serious side effects, they should never be administered for more than a few days for diseases for which therapeutic benefit is not established. Even in a medical emergency, their use must never replace or delay more specific primary therapies, such as antibiotics in septic shock or epinephrine and antihistamines in anaphylaxis.[1493]

Chronic Therapy. In less urgent circumstances, more careful consideration must be given to the evidence for efficacy of glucocorticoids in the disease process; the particular steroid preparation to be used and its dosage, frequency, and route of administration; and the disease indices to be monitored to assess therapeutic efficacy.

The criteria to be fulfilled before embarking on a course of chronic glucocorticoid therapy are listed in Table 9–18 and should be kept in mind during therapy. The importance of objective criteria of response deserves special emphasis. In addition to the possible placebo effect of any therapy, glucocorticoids make almost all patients feel better acutely. Therefore, a sense of well-being is not a useful criterion of response. Rather, the forced expiratory volume in 1 s (FEV$_1$) in asthma, liver enzyme levels in chronic active hepatitis,

TABLE 9–18. Guidelines for Pharmacological Glucocorticoid Administration

Initiate only if published data establish objective therapeutic benefit.
Use only after other specific therapies fail.
Identify a specific therapeutic objective.
Use objective criteria of response.
Administer sufficient steroid for a sufficient time to achieve the desired response.
Administer no more steroid for no longer than is necessary to achieve the desired response.
Terminate if objective therapeutic benefit is not observed when expected, if complications arise, or if maximal benefit has been achieved.

and similar quantifiable indices in other diseases should be used in deciding whether glucocorticoids are achieving their desired effect.

DOSAGE REGIMENS. Dosage and route of administration depend on the disorder being treated. Parenteral administration of high doses may be warranted in emergencies, such as septic shock and severe acute asthma. Intravenous boluses of gram doses of methylprednisolone have been used in transplant rejection and in some autoimmune diseases,[1514–1516] although the efficacy and mechanism of action of massive doses of steroid remain to be established. Oral preparations are generally used for chronic therapy. When possible, other forms of nonsystemic glucocorticoid therapy should be administered. Intra-articular injection for joint inflammation,[1517] inhalation of aerosolized steroids for asthma, and topical application for inflammatory dermatological disorders are examples. This makes it possible to deliver higher concentrations of steroid to the involved tissue with fewer systemic effects. However, all topical steroids are absorbed to some extent and, therefore, have potential systemic effects.

In patients whose condition warrants systemic, high-dose glucocorticoid, high concentrations of the steroid presumably should be present in plasma most of the time. Although the duration of biological activity of the glucocorticoids exceeds the relatively short plasma half-lives, multiple doses of oral steroids should be given each day for maximal efficacy. Injected steroids can be administered at longer intervals.

Glucocorticoid therapy usually involves giving supraphysiological dosages of glucocorticoid. However, in some diseases, such as mild rheumatoid arthritis, chronic control may be achieved with dosages equivalent to or even less than normal daily adrenal production.[467, 1518] This phenomenon has not been studied carefully, but presumably the exogenous steroid, usually given as a single dose early in the day, does not suppress the next morning's circadian peak in endogenous cortisol secretion. Thus the patient is exposed to the sum of the exogenous steroid plus normal or near-normal endogenous cortisol production. The potential advantage of such a regimen, when chronic low-dose therapy is required, is maintenance of normal hypothalamic-pituitary-adrenal function.

Alternate-day regimens were devised to alleviate the undesirable side effects of chronic high-dose glucocorticoid therapy.[1519, 1520] Approximately twice the usual daily steroid dose is given on alternate days, the rationale being that the patient is not exposed to high steroid levels every other day and has less chance of developing Cushing's syndrome. Furthermore, because the hypothalamic-pituitary-adrenal axis is exposed to high concentrations of exogenous steroid only on alternate days, suppression of the axis should be less of a problem. Adjunctive therapy, such as bronchodilators in asthma, must be applied optimally during the non-steroid days to prevent exacerbation of the disease process.

Regrettably, this approach is unsuccessful in virtually all patients who require high doses of glucocorticoid. In fact, one can argue that a patient who does not require any steroid on alternate days requires no steroid at all. This dosage regimen has not withstood rigorous examination in patients with disorders in which objective indices of response were monitored, and, despite initial enthusiasm, it is now used infrequently.

COMPLICATIONS OF CHRONIC ADMINISTRATION. The goal of glucocorticoid therapy, as with any therapy, is to obtain maximal benefit with minimal adverse side effects. The potent synthetic glucocorticoids are virtually devoid of mineralocorticoid, androgenic, or estrogenic activity, so the systemic side effects are those of suppression of hypothalamic-pituitary-adrenal axis function and Cushing's syndrome.

Hypothalamic-Pituitary-Adrenal Axis Suppression. The mechanisms by which endogenous and exogenous glucocorticoids exert negative feedback on the hypothalamic-pituitary-adrenal axis are described earlier. The net effect is suppression of hypothalamic CRH production and pituitary ACTH secretion, with resulting atrophy of the adrenal zonae fasciculata and reticularis and loss of cortisol-secretory capability. Although suspected adrenal insufficiency after steroid withdrawal was reported soon after steroids became available,[1504] the first well-documented case was reported in 1961.[1521]

The time required to achieve significant suppression depends on the dosage and varies among individuals, probably because of differences in rates of steroid metabolism. Any patient who has received any dose of steroid for less than 3 wk can be assumed not to be suppressed. Likewise, anyone who has taken less than 10 mg of prednisone or its equivalent per day—provided that it is not taken as a single bedtime dose[1522]—for any length of time can safely be considered not to be suppressed.[1523, 1524] Although it may be possible to demonstrate inadequate responses to metyrapone, hypoglycemia, or exogenous ACTH for brief intervals after stopping the steroid,[1525, 1526] clinical adrenal insufficiency in this setting is exceedingly rare.[1493, 1504, 1527] Chronic alternate-day glucocorticoid therapy rarely suppresses hypothalamic-pituitary-adrenal function.[1519, 1520, 1528] On the other hand, anyone who has received more than 20 mg of prednisone a day for more than 3 wk should be considered to have functional suppression of the hypothalamic-pituitary-adrenal axis.[1529] Any patient who develops Cushing's syndrome is certainly suppressed. In practical terms, this means that the patient should be treated like any patient with adrenal insufficiency (i.e., chronic ACTH deficiency), including wearing a medical alert bracelet or necklace, carrying an emergency medical information card in the wallet or purse, and, arguably, carrying a preloaded 1-mL syringe containing 4 mg dexamethasone phosphate to inject in emergencies. These precautions are discussed in detail elsewhere in this chapter.

Cushing's Syndrome. Like hypothalamic-pituitary-adrenal suppression, development of Cushing's syndrome depends on the dosage and duration of glucocorticoid administration and varies among individuals. With high-dose steroid therapy, however, signs of Cushing's syndrome can be observed within a month.

Certain features are much more common in exogenous Cushing's syndrome.[751, 1504] They include aggravation of glaucoma, formation of posterior subcapsular cataracts, and occurrence of benign intracranial hypertension, aseptic necrosis of the femoral and humeral heads, pancreatitis, and panniculitis. These features appear to reflect the severity and the chronicity of the glucocorticoid excess. In contrast, hypertension, hirsutism, acne, menstrual disturbances, and impotence are rare. Osteoporosis is perhaps the most common serious complication. Loss of muscle mass, weakness, worsening of diabetes mellitus, increased susceptibility to infection, poor wound healing, excessive weight gain, activation of latent tuberculosis or histoplasmosis, arrest of linear growth in children, and psychiatric disturbances may also occur. Herpetic keratitis may take an accelerated course, leading to blindness. These conditions warrant careful consideration before starting glucocorticoids. Any of them may require reducing or discontinuing the steroid, and some, like herpetic keratitis and acute psychosis, demand immediate withdrawal.

Certain measures may ameliorate the effects of glucocorticoids. Appropriate exercise programs may reduce the risk of myopathy. Exercise, calcium and vitamin D supplementation, and, in postmenopausal women, estrogen replacement may minimize steroid-induced skeletal calcium loss.[1530] The efficacy of these interventions during long-term glucocorticoid administration has not been evaluated, but they are the best that is available at present.

Steroid Withdrawal

Two factors limit the process of steroid withdrawal. The first is the activity of the underlying disease process. For example, allergic reactions treated with glucocorticoids are unlikely to worsen after cessation of therapy, yet very minor reductions in steroid dosage may result in exacerbation of autoimmune diseases such as systemic lupus erythematosus. In general, disease activity limits the rate of reduction to physiological doses of glucocorticoid. The second limiting factor is the recovery of normal function of the hypothalamic-pituitary-adrenal axis. This limits the ability to withdraw physiological glucocorticoid support.

DYNAMICS OF GLUCOCORTICOID WITHDRAWAL. Recovery of hypothalamic-pituitary-adrenal function appears to recapitulate its suppression. Hypothalamic CRH synthesis and secretion presumably recover first. Apparently, a period of several weeks is required after CRH recovery for corticotrope proliferation and POMC synthesis to restore normal ACTH secretion. The remainder of the process is known.[1531] Morning plasma ACTH secretion gradually reaches normal levels, but adrenal steroidogenesis remains low for several weeks. Morning plasma ACTH concentration continues to rise, actually reaching above-normal levels, as adrenal steroidogenesis begins to recover. As morning plasma cortisol concentration and daily urinary steroid excretion approach normal, ACTH—and, presumably, CRH—secretion returns to the normal range.[1531] Basal cortisol production returns to normal before responsiveness to stresses such as insulin-induced hypoglycemia recovers.[1527, 1532] The entire process may require 6 to 9 mo to complete[1531] (Fig. 9–63).

SYNDROMES OF GLUCOCORTICOID WITHDRAWAL. Other than exacerbation of the illness being treated, the symptoms and signs of steroid withdrawal are anorexia, mild nausea, weight loss, arthralgias, myalgias, lethargy, and mild postural hypotension or tachycardia. Some patients have low-grade fever, but it is uncertain to what extent the underlying inflammatory illness contributes to it. These patients have deficient basal cortisol secretion and fail to respond normally to acute ACTH stimulation.[1529] Some authors describe a similar syndrome, associated with fine desquamation of the skin, that occurs even in the presence of normal basal and stress-induced cortisol production. This syndrome is considered a form of physical dependence on physiological doses of glucocorticoids[1533, 1534] and appears to occur most often in patients who have been on relatively low doses of glucocorticoids for long periods. The incidence and pathophysiology are unknown, but it must be relatively

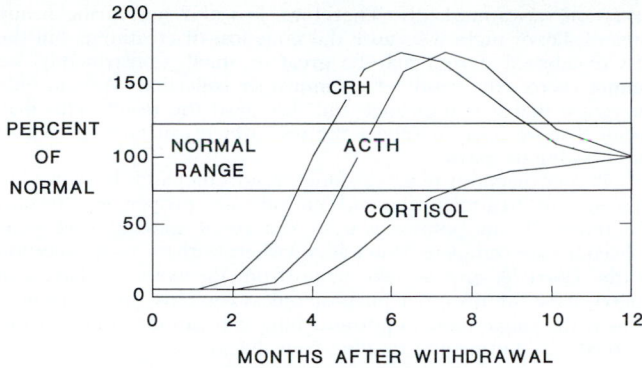

Figure 9–63. Recovery of the hypothalamic-pituitary-adrenal axis whose function has been chronically and profoundly suppressed in a patient who has had chronic endogenous hypercortisolemia (Cushing's syndrome) or has received chronic pharmacological dosages of synthetic glucocorticoids. The ACTH and cortisol curves are schematized from the data of Graber and colleagues.[1531] The CRH data are hypothetical. However, it appears that CRH secretion recovers before recovery of ACTH secretion, which in turn recovers several weeks before adrenal cortisol secretion returns to normal. The actual rate of recovery depends in part on how chronically and profoundly the hypothalamic-pituitary-adrenal axis has been suppressed.

uncommon because we have not encountered it. These patients respond normally to stress, so there is no apparent compelling reason for weaning them from maintenance steroid dosage.

PROTOCOL FOR WITHDRAWAL. The standard protocol for steroid withdrawal[1532a] is based on studies of the natural history of recovery (see Fig. 9–63). The first stage of withdrawal consists of weaning the patient from a pharmacological steroid dosage. The steroid dosage is tapered gradually, while observing the patient for objective evidence of exacerbation of the disease. Symptoms at this stage are not due to steroid insufficiency or dependence. If the disease flares, the steroid dosage must be increased temporarily. Once the disease is quiescent, tapering can resume. This stage usually takes several weeks, often several months. When one has reached a physiological dose of steroid, therapy should be changed to the short-acting glucocorticoid hydrocortisone. The usual maintenance dose is 20 mg orally each morning. Some patients may require an additional 5-mg dose at 2 to 3 PM. Long-acting steroids and large doses of short-acting steroids should be avoided in late evening. They are unnecessary and may delay recovery by suppressing the morning circadian increase in hypothalamic-pituitary activity. In the second stage of withdrawal, the patient recovers normal basal steroid-secretory activity. The daily hydrocortisone dosage should be tapered by 2.5 mg every week, or as rapidly as can be tolerated, to 10 mg in the morning. The syndromes of glucocorticoid insufficiency and dependence are seen during this stage, which typically takes a month or more to complete. The patient still requires supplemental steroid for stress and should continue to wear medical alert identification and carry a dexamethasone syringe. After 2 to 3 mo, an early morning plasma cortisol value should be obtained 24 h after the last dose of hydrocortisone. If it is 275 nmol/L (10 μg/dL) or more, maintenance hydrocortisone can be stopped, but steroid supplementation should be given during stress. If it is less than 275 nmol/L, the hydrocortisone is continued and the morning plasma cortisol value is measured after a similar interval. When the morning plasma cortisol concentration is 275 nmol/L and maintenance hydrocortisone is not required, the patient begins the third stage of withdrawal, recovery of response to stress. An acute ACTH (cosyntropin) test is performed. If it is normal (30- or 60-min plasma cortisol level is 550 nmol/L [20 μg/dL] or

more), hypothalamic-pituitary-adrenal function is normal, steroid supplementation is no longer required during stress, and the patient can discard bracelet, card, and syringe. If it is abnormal, the cosyntropin test should be repeated at intervals of 2 to 3 mo until it becomes normal. One can sometimes complete the process a few months earlier by testing more often, thereby detecting recovery earlier. In general, this is neither necessary nor cost effective.

EVALUATION OF ADRENOCORTICAL FUNCTION

Introduction

The adrenal cortex consists of three functional entities: (1) the glomerulosa, which secretes aldosterone and is primarily under the control of the renin-angiotensin system; (2) the fasciculata, which secretes cortisol and is regulated by the CRH-ACTH system; and (3) the fasciculata/reticularis, which secretes DHEA, DHEAS, and small amounts of testosterone and other 19-carbon steroids and is under the control of ACTH and, perhaps, other POMC-derived peptides.[243, 244] Consequently, evaluation of function requires measurement of the relevant adrenal hormones and their metabolites and of the secretagogues that regulate their secretion.

The normal values in this section and in the endpapers of this volume are intended only as general guidelines. Each laboratory has different normal ranges. Normal ranges should, in general, be viewed with some skepticism with regard to how they were established, particularly if they deviate significantly from those listed herein.

Laboratory Errors

IMPORTANCE OF A RELIABLE REFERENCE LABORATORY. An endocrinologist is only as good as the reference laboratory. Because the symptoms and signs of adrenocortical disorders are often subtle and nonspecific, assessment of basal, stimulated, and suppressed hormone secretion is usually essential to establish the clinical diagnosis. Even the most reliable laboratory is capable of occasional error. Regrettably, some reference laboratories consistently provide erroneous results for one or more of assays required for evaluation of the hypothalamic-pituitary-adrenal axis. The assays most subject to error are the plasma ACTH radioimmunoassay and the urinary 17-OHCS colorimetric assay.

DETECTING INCONSISTENCIES IN THE LABORATORY DATA. One cannot detect all laboratory errors, but there are some useful principles for evaluating results. Most important is awareness that any result may be incorrect, particularly when it conflicts with a body of otherwise consistent data. For example, 24-h urinary steroid excretion reflects integrated 24-h plasma steroid concentration. Mean plasma cortisol concentration during a 24-h day is about 220 nmol/L (8 μg/dL). Average daily urinary free cortisol and 17-OHCS excretions are about 150 nmol (55 μg) and 15 μmol (5.5 mg), respectively. Thus multiplying mean plasma cortisol (in nmol/L) by 0.7 and 0.07, respectively, approximates 24-h urinary excretion of free cortisol (in nmol) and 17-OHCS (in μmol), respectively. Multiplying mean plasma cortisol (in μg/dL) by 7 and 0.7, respectively, approximates 24-h urinary free cortisol (in μg) and 17-OHCS (in mg), respectively. Urinary free cortisol excretion becomes disproportionately greater, however, as plasma cortisol exceeds the normal binding capacity of transcortin of about 690 nmol/L (25 μg/dL). Thus if a patient suspected of having secondary adrenal insufficiency has a morning plasma cortisol level of 83 nmol/L (3 μg/dL) and a late evening plasma cortisol level of less than 28 nmol/L (1 μg/dL) (i.e., a mean daily plasma cortisol level of 47 nmol/L [1.7 μg/dL]), urinary free cortisol and 17-OHCS excretions should be no more than 33 nmol (12 μg) and 3.3 μmol (1.2 mg) per day, respectively. Conversely, if a patient with Cushing's syndrome has plasma cortisol levels of 550 to 690 nmol/L (20 to 25 μg/dL), the 24-h urinary free cortisol and 17-OHCS excretions should be around 440 μmol (160 μg) and 44 μmol (16 mg), respectively. If the results are significantly different from these, one measurement probably is incorrect. In the case of these three assays, plasma cortisol is most likely to be correct and urinary 17-OHCS is most likely to be incorrect. Conflicting results should be checked and repeated in the same or another laboratory. Diagnosis should not be made in the face of inconsistent laboratory data.

Patients' Errors

There are three major sources of patients' errors: (1) failure to take prescribed medications or to take them on the proper schedule; (2) failure to inform the physician of other medications that may interfere with the diagnostic tests, the hormonal assays, or both; and (3) failure to collect 24-h urine specimens properly. The first two must be dealt with by diligence on the part of both physician and patient, particularly when tests are more and more being conducted on an ambulatory basis. It is essential that the patient inform the physician when a collection error is made so that the sample can be discarded and the test repeated, if necessary.

HOW TO COLLECT A 24-HOUR URINE SPECIMEN. Improper 24-h urine collections can be minimized by explaining to the patient in detail how they should be obtained, emphasizing how important they are to the diagnosis, and making the patient—either in or out of hospital—responsible for their accuracy. The following is a complete, detailed explanation to a patient on how to collect a proper 24-h urine specimen.

I want you to collect every drop of your urine during each 24-h period. I do not care what the volume of the urine is, as long as it represents every drop that you pass during that 24-h period. If you need to have a bowel movement, you may separate the urine in time or space, but I want every drop.

Begin the collection at [usually 8:00 AM in hospital] o'clock tomorrow. At that time, pass your urine, flush it down the toilet, and note the exact time. Now you will have an empty bladder and an empty bottle. That starts the collection. Collect every drop all during the day and night until exactly the same time the next morning, when you should pass your urine and add it to the bottle. I want you to pass your urine at exactly the same time each morning, varying by no more than 5 or 10 min. If you have to go an hour before the appointed time, drink a full glass of water or more so that you can go again in an hour. If you have to go 20 min before, hold it until the proper time. This is essential to the proper interpretation of the test results. Now you will have an empty bladder, a full first bottle, and an empty second bottle. This completes your first 24-h collection and starts the second one. For your second 24-h collection, add the urine that you pass during that day and the next night, completing the collection by passing your urine at exactly the same time the next day and adding it to the second bottle. That completes the second collection and begins the third.

The bottle(s) may be kept at room temperature. It contains a weak acid. If you get acid or urine from the bottle on your skin or clothing, rinse your skin or clothing immediately with plenty of cold water, and you will have no problem.

We will measure a substance, called creatinine, in your urine. It will tell us whether each urine collection is complete. Unfortunately, that is all that it can tell us, because it is excreted more or less constantly during the day, whereas the rate of adrenal steroid excretion varies markedly. Therefore, loss of 2 h of urine at any time of day or night will cause the same loss of creatinine, but the loss of adrenal steroid may be great or small. Consequently, we cannot correct the result of an improper collection. We can only recognize that it is improper and disregard the result. This may mean that we have to repeat the test, which can take as long as three additional days.

Proper diagnosis (e.g., Cushing's syndrome) and decision as to appropriate treatment depend entirely on proper test results. Therefore, I am putting you in charge of making sure your collections are complete. Don't go anywhere without your collection bottle. Don't let anyone take urine from the bottle or have you collect urine for any other purpose unless you have my permission. This is the single most important thing you can do to assist us in correctly diagnosing and treating your illness.

The patient should then be requested to repeat exactly how the urine is to be collected to be certain that the instructions are understood. It is helpful to have printed instructions to which the patient can refer.

Measurement of Plasma Peptide and Steroid Hormone Concentrations

Hypothalamic Peptides

Peripheral plasma concentrations of hypothalamic releasing factors are lower than those in hypothalamic-hypophyseal portal plasma, and a strong correlation between peripheral and portal plasma levels has not been demonstrated. Hypothalamic peptide levels are rarely measured for clinical endocrinological evaluation.

CORTICOTROPIN-RELEASING HORMONE. Like other peptide hormones, CRH is measured by radioimmunoassay.[323] Human CRH is largely bound to a plasma CRH-binding protein.[320, 1535] It must be extracted by immunoaffinity chromatography[229] or methanol[326] before assay. Peripheral plasma CRH concentration ranges from about 0.2 to 2.2 pmol/L (1 to 10 pg/mL) and increases progressively during pregnancy to as high as 585 pmol/L (2700 pg/ml).[297, 319] According to some investigators, plasma CRH levels are increased in adrenal insufficiency, after metyrapone administration, and during insulin-induced hypoglycemia but are suppressed in all forms of Cushing's syndrome[229] except, presumably, ectopic CRH syndrome.[1026] Most investigators do not find that peripheral plasma CRH correlates with plasma ACTH or cortisol levels.

ARGININE VASOPRESSIN, OXYTOCIN, ANGIOTENSIN II, AND OTHER HYPOTHALAMIC PEPTIDES. Assays are available for AVP, oxytocin, angiotensin II, catecholamines, and other hypothalamic factors, but the relation of their peripheral plasma concentrations to ACTH secretion, if any, is uncertain.

ACTH and Other Anterior Pituitary POMC-Derived Peptides

There is disagreement about the degree to which POMC is normally processed in the anterior pituitary,[1536, 1537] and differential processing may take place in different subpopulations of anterior pituitary corticotropes. Therefore, POMC-derived peptides may not necessarily be released in equimolar concentrations into circulating blood. Furthermore, they appear to be metabolized at different rates, so that some may persist longer than others in the circulation. They are released in concert, however, so that when the concentration of one of them increases or decreases, so do those of the others.[211] Thus peripheral plasma concentrations provide a direct index of pituitary secretion.

ACTH. *Assay.* This peptide can be measured accurately and with adequate sensitivity by radioimmunoassay[1538] or two-site immunoradiometric assay.[1539, 1540] Nevertheless, results provided by some reference laboratories and by some commercial kits are unreliable.

Normal Values. Plasma ACTH concentrations are usually between 4.5 and 18 pmol/L (20 and 80 pg/mL) at 8 AM. Levels fall during the waking hours and are usually less than 4.5 pmol/L (20 pg/mL) at 4 PM and less than 2.2 pmol/L (10 pg/mL), often less than 1.1 pmol/L (5 pg/mL), 1 h after the usual time of sleep.

Interpretation. Plasma ACTH concentration is best interpreted together with a simultaneous plasma cortisol determination. Early morning plasma ACTH level is elevated, and cortisol level is low, in primary adrenal insufficiency (see Fig. 9–1), whereas both are low in hypothalamic CRH deficiency or pituitary ACTH deficiency (i.e., hypopituitarism). In congenital adrenal hyperplasia, early morning ACTH level tends to be elevated, whereas plasma cortisol level may be normal or low, depending on the severity of the disease. Late evening plasma ACTH and cortisol levels are of little value in diagnosing adrenal insufficiency or congenital adrenal hyperplasia, although evening plasma ACTH levels tend to be somewhat elevated. In Cushing's disease, late evening plasma ACTH and cortisol values are helpful. Whereas morning values may be within the normal range, there is loss of the normal circadian rhythm in secretion and late evening concentrations are elevated. In patients with adrenocortical tumors, bilateral micronodular dysplasia, or other primary adrenocortical disorders (i.e., ACTH-independent Cushing's syndrome), plasma ACTH is suppressed, usually to undetectable levels, but cortisol concentrations are elevated. In contrast, patients with Cushing's disease or ectopic ACTH syndrome (i.e., ACTH-dependent Cushing's syndrome) have increased ACTH and cortisol concentrations in plasma in late evening. Both ACTH and cortisol levels tend to be higher in the ectopic ACTH syndrome than in Cushing's disease, but there is considerable overlap.

Several factors may influence plasma ACTH assay results. ACTH is unstable in blood at room temperature, is cleaved by enzymes in blood cells and platelets, and adheres to glass and some plastic surfaces.[209] Therefore, how blood is collected and plasma is prepared and stored may affect apparent ACTH concentration, and this phenomenon varies with the antibody used in the assay.[208] The normal circadian rhythmicity of ACTH concentration reflects variation in the amplitude of secretory episodes during the day.[366] Because the plasma disappearance half-time is measured in minutes, a single plasma ACTH value, particularly if obtained between about 4 and 10 AM, may not be representative of average secretory activity. ACTH secretion remains episodic in primary adrenal insufficiency, congenital adrenal hyperplasia, and ACTH-dependent Cushing's syndrome, so the same caveat obtains. Normal subjects and patients with these disorders respond rapidly to stress with increased ACTH secretion. For this reason, it is best not to obtain postsleep values the first night in hospital. Ideally, all samples should be obtained with indwelling needles or catheters. Levels in samples that require more than 2 or 3 min to obtain by venipuncture must be interpreted with caution, if elevated. The definition of stress, as it pertains to hypothalamic-pituitary-adrenal function, is imprecise. Chronic stress usually does not increase plasma ACTH concentrations, but high fever, pain, trauma, and terminal illness can all increase ACTH secretion. Patients with major depressive disorders may also have elevated plasma ACTH concentrations.[409] One must also be certain that the patient is not taking, or has not recently taken, glucocorticoids, which may acutely or chronically suppress hypothalamic-pituitary-adrenal function.

Two-site "sandwich" immunoassays for ACTH use two different monoclonal or affinity-purified polyclonal antibodies, are sufficiently sensitive for clinical use, and are theoretically more specific than one-site immunoassays. However, they may not react with POMC or forms intermediate between POMC and ACTH.[1541] This specificity may be a disadvantage in diagnosing the ectopic ACTH syndrome, in which a large percentage of circulating immunoreactive ACTH may represent incompletely processed or unprocessed POMC. Excessive concentrations of ACTH fragments, such as ACTH(1–24), can compete for binding to one or the other of the two antibodies, preventing intact ACTH from coupling the two antibodies and yielding factitiously low ACTH concentrations.[1542] This is unlikely to be a problem in measuring endogenous ACTH levels. These assays represent a significant improvement over those previously available.

OTHER POMC-DERIVED PEPTIDES. Radioimmunoassays have been developed for other POMC-derived peptides, including α-MSH, γ-MSH, β-LPH, γ-LPH, β-END, the NT peptide of POMC, and the joining peptide between the NT peptide and ACTH.[215, 1536, 1543–1546] None appears to have a significant advantage over the ACTH assay for confirming the diagnosis of Cushing's syndrome and defining the cause. Most are not commercially available. Plasma β-LPH concentration, which usually also measures γ-LPH and β-END concentration to some degree, tends to be higher in the ectopic ACTH syndrome than in pituitary Cushing's disease.[1547] The reason for this is unclear, but it may reflect differential processing of POMC by pituitary and nonpituitary tumor cells.

Peptides of the Renin-Angiotensin-Aldosterone System

RENIN ACTIVITY. *Assay.* Renin is measured in terms of its enzymatic activity, not its mass. As the assay for plasma renin activity is usually performed, the plasma is incubated at 37°C without adding angiotensinogen (renin substrate), relying instead on endogenous angiotensinogen in the plasma specimen.[1548] Renin cleaves angiotensinogen to produce a decapeptide, angiotensin I, which can be measured by radioimmunoassay.[1549] If the radioimmunoassay is sufficiently sensitive, incubation time can be 30 min or less, during which the rate of angiotensin I generation is linear. Less sensitive assays require that more angiotensin I accumulate over a longer interval, and because of the limited amount of endogenous angiotensinogen, the relationship of renin activity to angiotensin I generation may become nonlinear. Plasma renin activity is expressed as the amount of angiotensin I generated per unit of time, subtracting the amount of preformed angiotensin I in a control aliquot incubated at 4°C.

Normal Values. Plasma renin activity ranges from about 0.77 to 4.6 nmol/L/h (1 to 6 ng/mL/h) but is dependent on sodium intake and posture.[1550]

Interpretation. Plasma renin activity is usually normal in secondary adrenal insufficiency (i.e, hypopituitarism or isolated ACTH deficiency), elevated in primary adrenal insufficiency, and normal or suppressed in Cushing's syndrome, depending on the degree of hypercortisolism and the secretion of other mineralocorticoids, such as deoxycorticosterone, which may occur especially in adrenal carcinoma. Plasma renin activity is increased in salt-losing P-450$_{c21}$ deficiency[1450] and is suppressed in hypertensive P-450$_{c11}$ or P-450$_{c17}$ deficiency.[1461, 1478] Plasma renin activity increases somewhat in the luteal phase of the menstrual cycle and during pregnancy,[1551, 1552] perhaps in part because of the mineralocorticoid antagonist activity of progesterone.[1553] Plasma renin activity is discussed further in Chapter 11.

ANGIOTENSINS I AND II. These peptides are measured by radioimmunoassay. They both tend to reflect plasma renin activity because the conversion of angiotensin I to angiotensin II, an octapeptide, by angiotensin I–converting enzyme is virtually complete in a single pass through the pulmonary circulation. Because of this and the fact that sensitive and specific radioimmunoassays are not widely available, these peptides are rarely measured in the evaluation of adrenal dysfunction.

Glucocorticoids

CORTISOL. Assay. Cortisol can be measured in plasma or serum (we use plasma to refer to both here) by a variety of methods, beginning with the assay of Porter-Silber chromogens (17,21-dihydroxy-20-ketosteroids, referred to as 17-hydroxycorticosteroids, or 17-OHCS)[1554] (see later), as modified for plasma.[1555] Plasma 17-OHCS are no longer measured, but this and other historically important assays are described to permit one to interpret the older literature.

Competitive protein-binding assay uses competition of endogenous cortisol with ³H-labeled cortisol tracer for a limited number of binding sites on CBG (transcortin) to quantify the steroid.[1556, 1557] The advantage is absence of drug interference; the disadvantage is that many steroids (e.g., progesterone, 17α-hydroxyprogesterone, DOC, corticosterone, 11β-deoxycortisol, and aldosterone) bind to CBG and, therefore, interfere in the assay. Normally present in concentrations too small to matter, these steroids may be increased in pregnancy, adrenal carcinoma, and congenital adrenal hyperplasia and after administration of adrenal enzyme inhibitors, such as metyrapone. Prednisolone, the active metabolite of prednisone, and its 16α-hydroxy derivative also bind to CBG and interfere in this assay. Interfering steroids can be removed before assay by solvent partition or thin-layer chromatography. This assay is now seldom used.

Fluorometric assay exploits the fluorescence of Δ⁴-11β,21-dihydroxy-3,20-ketosteroids (11-hydroxycorticosteroids, or 11-OHCS) in sulfuric acid and alcohol.[1558] Cortisol and corticosterone are the major steroids detected by this assay, whereas potent synthetic glucocorticoids are not. The major advantage is its simplicity and relative specificity for cortisol. The main disadvantage is drug interference by spironolactone, quinine, quinidine, niacin, and the benzoyl alcohol preservative in some intravenous solutions. Normal steroid-free plasma produces a blank of about 55 nmol/L (2 μg/dL), a level that is exaggerated in patients with hepatic or renal failure. This assay has been replaced by radioimmunoassays.

High-performance liquid chromatography separates cortisol from other steroids and steroid metabolites; cortisol can then be measured fluorometrically or spectrophotometrically.[1559] The advantages are specificity and freedom from drug interference, but the technique is slow and labor intensive and is not, therefore, widely used.

Radioreceptor assay uses the type II glucocorticoid receptor as cortisol-binding agent.[1560] This assay is specific for bioactive steroids, including synthetic glucocorticoids. The disadvantage is the limited supply and instability of the cytosol receptor. As a result, this assay is not generally available.

Radioimmunoassay is the assay method of choice. Polyclonal or monoclonal antibodies are raised to a steroid analogue that has been conjugated to a protein carrier. Each antibody is characterized in terms of its affinity and its cross-reactivity with other steroids found in plasma. Antibody, ¹³¹I- or ³H-labeled steroid tracer, and steroid standard are used to perform the assay. Both liquid-phase and solid-phase assays of requisite sensitivity and specificity are widely available in reference laboratories and in kit form. Total plasma cortisol concentration is measured.

Normal Values. Plasma cortisol concentration normally reflects that of ACTH and demonstrates circadian rhythmicity. Highest concentrations range from 275 to 550 nmol/L (10 to 20 μg/dL) and are seen in the early morning, within an hour of the usual time of awakening. Plasma cortisol concentration ranges from 85 to 275 nmol/L (3 to 10 μg/dL) at 4 PM, and lowest levels, less than 140 nmol/L (5 μg/dL), are observed an hour after the usual time of sleep.

Interpretation. Patients with primary or secondary adrenal insufficiency have low early morning plasma cortisol concentrations, and those with congenital adrenal hyperplasia may have low or normal values (corresponding to simple virilizing and "late-onset" P-450$_{c21}$ deficiency types). Most patients with Cushing's syndrome have early morning plasma cortisol concentrations within or slightly above the normal range. In contrast, cortisol concentrations an hour after sleep are almost always elevated and are often equal to the early morning values (i.e., they have an abnormal or absent circadian rhythm). Because normal hour-after-sleep plasma cortisol is often undetectable, measurement at that time does not identify patients with adrenal insufficiency or congenital adrenal hyperplasia. Thus the time at which a sample should be drawn depends on the suspected endocrine dysfunction.

Several factors must be considered in interpreting plasma cortisol results. Normal values vary with the particular assay: those we have given are representative of an average radioimmunoassay, those obtained by competitive protein-binding assay would be similar, and fluorometric assay results are about 85 nmol/L (3 μg/dL) higher.[1561] Cortisol secretion normally reflects ACTH secretion, so the same caveats concerning circadian rhythmicity, stress, and glucocorticoid administration also pertain to it, except that recent hydrocortisone (cortisol) or cortisone administration may produce elevated plasma cortisol levels. The longer disappearance half-time of cortisol than of ACTH (about 80 vs. 8 min) and the several-minute lag in its secretion after ACTH stimulation both tend to damp its excursions relative to those of ACTH. Hepatic CBG synthesis is increased by estrogens,[497, 500, 501] and early morning plasma cortisol concentrations of 1400 nmol/L (50 μg/dL) and more are not unusual during pregnancy or oral contraceptive use.[1562, 1563] Cortisol dissociates rapidly from CBG, so hour-after-sleep values are usually normal. Even relatively severe hepatic dysfunction has little effect on plasma cortisol levels.[502, 1564] Renal failure also has little effect on plasma cortisol levels, although retained cortisol metabolites may interfere in some radioimmunoassays.[1565] Thyroid hormone regulates the rate of cortisol metabolism, but hypothalamic-pituitary feedback mechanisms are intact and plasma cortisol levels are normal in hypo- and hyperthyroidism. Body weight has no appreciable effect on plasma cortisol levels, but severe malnutrition apparently has a greater inhibitory effect on cortisol metabolism than on cortisol production, resulting in increased plasma cortisol concentrations.[1566] It requires a year or more for infants to establish an adult sleep-wake cycle, entrain circadian rhythms, and establish an adult plasma ACTH and cortisol pattern.[372] Except for this phenomenon and the fact that for the first several days of life the normal infant produces more cortisone than cortisol and has low plasma cortisol concentrations,[1567] age has no effect on plasma cortisol levels. Major depressive disorders can produce plasma cortisol dynamics similar to those of Cushing's disease.[408, 409, 1568]

A number of drugs induce hepatic cytochrome P-450 enzymes that metabolize steroids. Barbiturates, phenytoin, rifampin, aminoglutethimide, and mitotane increase the metabolic clearance of steroids and of metyrapone. They may have a preferential effect on synthetic 9α-fluoro steroids (e.g., dexamethasone, fludrocortisone, triamcinolone, and betamethasone) over natural steroids. These drugs do not alter plasma cortisol levels in normal subjects, but they can interfere with dexamethasone suppression and metyrapone stimulation tests and necessitate increased steroid replacement dosage in patients with adrenal insufficiency. Alcohol abuse sufficient to increase serum hepatic enzyme levels, especially that of γ-glutamyltransferase, can cause pseudo-Cushing's syndrome and elevated plasma cortisol levels.[1569]

The biologically active fraction of total plasma cortisol is free cortisol. Although various methods have been developed for estimating plasma free cortisol concentration,[1500, 1560, 1570, 1571] these technically demanding and expensive assays are not in general use.

CORTISOL PRECURSORS. Assay. A number of biosynthetic precursors of cortisol, including pregnenolone, 17α-hydroxypregnenolone, progesterone, 17α-hydroxyprogesterone, and 11β-deoxycortisol, can be measured by radioimmunoassay directly or after solvent partition and/or chromatography.[1570, 1572]

Normal Values. Plasma 11-deoxycortisol concentration is normally undetectable by current assays (i.e., <30 nmol/L [<1 μg/dL] at 8 AM). Early morning 17α-hydroxyprogesterone concentration ranges from 1.8 to 9 nmol/L (60 to 300 ng/dL) in men, 0.6 to 3 nmol/L (20 to 100 ng/dL) in women during the follicular phase of the menstrual cycle, 1.5 to 10.6 nmol/L (50 to 350 ng/dL) during the luteal phase, and 18 nmol/L (600 ng/dL) and more by the end of pregnancy.

Interpretation. These assays are not commonly used for assessment of hypothalamic-pituitary-adrenal function, but some of them do have specific applications. Plasma 17α-hydroxyprogesterone can be measured before and after administration of cosyntropin in the diagnosis of the P-450$_{c21}$ deficiency variant of congenital adrenal hyperplasia,[1382, 1405] for example, and return of early morning plasma 17α-hydroxypregnenolone or 17α-hydroxyprogesterone concentration to normal can be used as an index of adequacy of treatment in this disorder.[1573] Plasma 11-deoxycortisol can be measured in tests of pituitary ACTH-secretory reserve using metyrapone.[1574] Levels of one or more of these cortisol precursors may be increased in the plasma of patients with adrenal carcinoma.[1053, 1248]

Mineralocorticoids

ALDOSTERONE. Assay. Aldosterone is measured by radioimmunoassay in the same manner as other adrenal corticosteroids. It requires a high-affinity antibody because plasma aldosterone concentration is only about 1% of that of cortisol.

Normal Values. Plasma aldosterone concentration ranges from 36 to 830 pmol/L (1.3 to 30 ng/dL), with a mean of about 215 pmol/L (7.7 ng/dL),[1575] in normal subjects with normal salt intakes.

Interpretation. There is a diurnal variation in plasma aldosterone concentration, with highest levels at about the time of awakening and lowest concentrations shortly after sleep, like those of cortisol, but levels are unrelated to ACTH secretion.[1576] Plasma aldosterone levels are increased by upright posture to 140 to 560 pmol/L (5 to 20 ng/dL), by dietary sodium restriction or sodium diuresis to 270 to 560 pmol/L (9.7 to 20 ng/dL), and by the combination of sodium restriction or diuresis and upright posture to 415 to 1720 pmol/L (15 to 62 ng/dL).[1577] Plasma levels are suppressed by saline infusion to less than 240 pmol/L (8.5 ng/dL). Aldosterone values are usually normal in secondary adrenal insufficiency and are decreased in primary adrenal insufficiency.

Plasma aldosterone concentration is normal or suppressed in Cushing's syndrome, depending on the rate of secretion of cortisol and other mineralocorticoids. It is low in salt-losing congenital adrenal hyperplasia and is low normal or suppressed in hypertensive P-450$_{c11}$ deficiency. Levels tend to be increased modestly in the luteal phase of the menstrual cycle and are increased up to 10 times normal by the third trimester of pregnancy.[1551, 1552] Plasma aldosterone and its role in hypertension are discussed further in Chapter 11.

DEOXYCORTICOSTERONE. DOC is measured by radioimmunoassay. Normal early morning levels range from 0.12 to 0.36 nmol/L (40 to 120 pg/mL). Plasma DOC levels may be increased in some patients with adrenal carcinoma; indeed, a DOC-secreting carcinoma has been described.[1053] DOC concentration is increased in congenital adrenal hyperplasia resulting from P-450$_{c11}$ or P-450$_{c17}$ deficiency, the degree of elevation corresponding to the degree of biosynthetic blockade.

Adrenal Androgens

DEHYDROEPIANDROSTERONE SULFATE. Assay. DHEAS, the major adrenal 19-carbon steroid, is measured by radioimmunoassay.[1578] DHEA is by far the major steroid product of the adrenal cortex, and over 99% of DHEA is sulfated before secretion.

Normal Values. DHEA concentrations range from 7 to 31 nmol/L (2 to 9 μg/L), whereas DHEAS levels range from about 2 to 10 μmol/L (0.75 to 3.7 μg/L) in men and about 3 to 127 μmol/L (1.1 to 4.7 μg/L) in women. DHEA levels increase about twofold and DHEAS levels fall by about 75% by the end of pregnancy.[1579]

Interpretation. DHEA concentration exhibits a circadian rhythm that reflects the secretion of ACTH and also varies during the menstrual cycle. DHEAS levels do not exhibit a circadian rhythm because of the longer circulating half-life. DHEA and DHEAS are derived from 17α-hydroxypregnenolone and 17α-hydroxyprogesterone and their levels are, therefore, increased in conditions in which concentrations of these steroids are elevated. The levels also tend to be elevated in all varieties of Cushing's syndrome. However, they are highest in Cushing's syndrome associated with adrenal carcinoma and lowest in adrenal adenoma, especially when expressed as a function of cortisol secretion. These differences reflect the relative inefficiency and efficiency of carcinomas and adenomas, respectively, in converting cholesterol to cortisol. DHEA and DHEAS levels are often markedly increased in patients with virilizing adrenal carcinoma without Cushing's syndrome. They are increased in the congenital adrenal hyperplasias resulting from P-450$_{c11}$, P-450$_{c21}$, and 3β-hydroxysteroid dehydrogenase deficiency; normal in the type I and type II corticosterone methyl oxidase (CMO) deficiency varieties; and low or undetectable in the P-450$_{c17}$ and P-450$_{scc}$ deficiency forms, the degree of deviation from normal being dependent in part on the degree of enzyme deficiency.

TESTOSTERONE AND ANDROSTENEDIONE. Normal Values. Plasma testosterone concentrations, which are measured by radioimmunoassay, range from 0.17 to 0.7 nmol/L (0.05 to 0.2 ng/mL) in prepubertal children, increase rapidly during puberty in boys to reach adult male levels of 10 to 35 nmol/L (3 to 10 ng/mL), and remain 0.7 to 2.6 nmol/L (0.2 to 0.7 ng/mL) in women. Androstenedione levels range from 5.6 to 7 nmol/L (1.6 to 2 ng/mL) in women and 3.2 to 4.7 nmol/L (0.9 to 1.4 ng/mL) in men.

Interpretation. Testosterone is of little value in assessing adrenal function in men because virtually all of it is produced by the testis. In women, in contrast, two thirds of plasma testosterone derives from the adrenal cortex, mostly via peripheral formation from DHEA and androstenedione. Testosterone concentration tends to be increased in the P-450_{c11} and P-450_{c21} deficiency forms of congenital adrenal hyperplasia, normal in CMO I/CMO II deficiency, and low or undetectable in the 3β-hydroxysteroid dehydrogenase and P-450_{c17} deficiency forms. In the latter two disorders, testosterone concentration is low or undetectable in males as well, because the enzymes are also missing from the testes. Testosterone levels tend to be increased in Cushing's syndrome, least in adrenal adenomas and most in adrenal carcinomas; in rare adrenal carcinomas the major product is testosterone.[1580] Conversely, testosterone levels are low in prepubertal children and women with primary or secondary adrenal insufficiency. Androstenedione is a product of 17α-hydroxyprogesterone and DHEA and is the immediate precursor of testosterone. Consequently, changes in its levels tend to mirror those of testosterone. Dihydrotestosterone is a target tissue product of testosterone and has no special value in assessing hypothalamic-pituitary-adrenocortical function. The androgens are discussed further in Chapter 13.

Measurement of Salivary Steroid Concentration

Cortisol

ASSAY. Saliva (2.5 mL) is obtained after rinsing the mouth, either by unstimulated flow or after chewing uncoated gum, is stored frozen and is assayed by competitive protein-binding assay[1556, 1581] or radioimmunoassay.[1582]

NORMAL VALUES. With the competitive protein-binding assay, normal values at 8 AM are 16 ± 8.2 nmol/L (5.8 ± 0.30 ng/mL) (range, 6.4 to 32.2 nmol/L [2.3 to 12 ng/mL]) for men and 9.8 ± 3.1 nmol/L (3.5 ± 1.1 ng/mL) (range, 4.8 to 18.2 nmol/L [1.7 to 6.6 ng/mL]) for women; the values at 8 PM for men and women are 3.9 ± 0.2 nmol/L (1.4 ± 0.7 ng/mL) (range, 2.2 to 4.2 nmol/L [0.80 to 1.5 ng/mL]).[1581]

INTERPRETATION. Plasma free cortisol diffuses freely into saliva. Therefore, salivary cortisol concentration more accurately reflects plasma free cortisol than total plasma cortisol and is independent of salivary flow rate. Morning salivary cortisol concentration is decreased in adrenal insufficiency, whereas late evening salivary cortisol concentration is increased in Cushing's syndrome. Both the competitive protein-binding assay and cortisol radioimmunoassays cross-react with other steroids. The competitive protein-binding assay cross-reacts with 17α-hydroxyprogesterone and 11-deoxycortisol, for example, so cortisol levels may appear artifactually increased in patients with congenital adrenal hyperplasia and adrenal carcinoma and after metyrapone administration. Cortisol can be chromatographically separated from other steroids before assay in these situations.[1581] Salivary cortisol concentration is especially useful in assessing cortisol secretion serially in ambulatory patients, who can collect multiple samples and store them in a freezer between clinic visits.

Measurement of Daily Urinary Steroid Excretion

Cortisol and Cortisol Metabolites

17-HYDROXYCORTICOSTEROIDS. *Assay.* Steroids with the 17,21-dihydroxy-20-ketosteroid configuration react with phenylhydrazine in acid to form yellow compounds (Porter-Silber chromogens) that can be measured colorimetrically.[1554] The specimen is first reacted with β-glucuronidase to convert glucuronide metabolites to the free steroids; an alkali wash removes the keto acids, which also react; and the steroids are extracted by organic solvent partition. In normal urine, the assay measures mostly the tetrahydro metabolites of cortisol and cortisone (THF and THE), which together constitute about one third of the total urinary metabolites of cortisol. The assay also measures THS, the tetrahydro metabolite of 11-deoxycortisol.

Normal Values. Urinary excretion of 17-OHCS in adults ranges from 8.2 to 22 μmol (3 to 8 mg) per 24 h except in extreme obesity, in which it can reach 28 μmol (10 mg) per 24 h. The effects of body weight can be corrected by expressing 17-OHCS excretion as a function of creatinine excretion.[1113] In these terms, normal excretion ranges from 5.5 to 18 μmol (2 to 6.5 mg) per gram of creatinine, independent of body weight, per 24 h.[1113]

It should be noted that, although concentrations of 17-OHCS, 17-KS, and 17-ketogenic steroids (17-KGS) can be reported in SI units, these assays measure mixtures of steroids and various steroid metabolites, the ratios of which vary depending on a variety of circumstances.

Interpretation. Urinary 17-OHCS concentrations are increased in all forms of Cushing's syndrome and decreased in primary and secondary adrenal insufficiency. They are normal in both forms of CMO deficiency and mild to moderate deficiency of P-450_{c21} and are low normal to undetectable in most other forms of congenital adrenal hyperplasia, depending on the degree of enzyme deficiency. The exception is P-450_{c11} deficiency, in which 17-OHCS excretion is elevated, the degree depending on the degree of enzyme deficiency, because THS is a Porter-Silber chromogen. For the same reason, 17-OHCS excretion increases after pharmacological blockade of 11β-hydroxylase action with metyrapone.

Urinary 17-OHCS excretion was the standard means of assessing glucocorticoid production for almost four decades. When performed correctly, which is not done in many reference laboratories, the assay is reliable. Measuring daily urinary steroid excretion has the advantage of providing an integrated index of steroid production over a period of 24 h, whereas measurement of plasma cortisol concentration provides information only about an instant in time. Certain factors must be kept in mind when interpreting the results, however, many of which were introduced during the discussion of plasma cortisol assay. In addition, steroid production can vary markedly from day to day in patients with Cushing's syndrome, particularly those with adrenal carcinoma or ectopic ACTH syndrome. The importance of complete urine collections has been stressed. A 17-OHCS value without a corresponding creatinine value is generally useless. The creatinine value provides reliable information about the reproducibility of a series of collections but little information about the completeness of an isolated collection, unless it is extremely high or low. A person who weighs 70 kg (154 lb) excretes about 1 g of creatinine per day.

Various drugs interfere in the 17-OHCS assay, among them antihypertensives (spironolactone) and tranquilizers (chlordiazepoxide, hydroxyzine, methaqualone). Their color spectra are not identical with those of THF and THE, so spectrophotometric readings at three different wavelengths can detect the presence of interfering substances. These drugs can usually be removed by solvent partition and/or chromatography. In addition, various drugs induce hepatic cytochrome P-450 enzymes, thereby enhancing the metabolism of cortisol to derivatives, mainly 6β-hydroxycortisol and 6β-cortisone, that do not form Porter-Silber chromogens. These drugs include aminoglutethimide, mitotane, phenobarbital, phenytoin, primidone, and rifampin. When possible, these drugs should be discontinued at least a week, and preferably longer, before collecting the urine specimen.

Because of these problems, urinary 17-OHCS assay has largely been supplanted by 24-h urinary free cortisol measurement.

17-KETOGENIC STEROIDS. *Assay.* The 17-KGS assay measures 17-KS[1583] after the 17,20-dihydroxycorticosteroids (which include 17-OHCS, cortols, and cortolones, the major urinary metabolites of cortisol) and pregnanetriol are oxidized to 17-KS with periodate. Before oxidation, the preformed 17-KS are reduced with borohydride, eliminating them from the assay, and THE and THF are converted to 17,20-dihydroxysteroids that can be oxidized and measured. Thus the 17-KGS assay measures more of the metabolic products of cortisol than the 17-OHCS assay. Unfortunately, it also measures 21-deoxysteroids, such as pregnanetriol, which are not cortisol metabolites.

Normal Values. Urinary 17-KGS excretion ranges from 21 to 69 µmol (6 to 20 mg) per 24 h in both men and women. Excretion is increased in extreme obesity but can be expressed as a function of creatinine excretion.

Interpretation. Despite the apparent benefit of measuring additional cortisol metabolites, 17-KGS determination has no practical advantage over 17-OHCS assay. Changes in 17-KGS concentrations mimic those of 17-OHCS, except in congenital adrenal hyperplasia resulting from P-450$_{c11}$ and P-450$_{c21}$ deficiency, in which increased 17-KGS values reflect increased excretion of pregnanetriol and other 21-deoxycorticosteroids. Furthermore, a number of drugs interfere in this assay, penicillin increasing the values and glucose, meprobamate, and radiopaque dyes (meglumine iodipamide and iothalamate) decreasing them. Although these effects usually can be minimized, the availability of the 17-OHCS and free cortisol assays has rendered the 17-KGS assay of little value in current practice.

URINARY FREE CORTISOL. *Assay.* Unconjugated cortisol concentration was measured originally by competitive protein-binding assay[1584] and is now measured by radioimmunoassay. With the development of high-affinity antisera that react specifically with the D ring of cortisol, sensitivity has been improved and interference by other steroids has been minimized.

Normal Values. Urinary free cortisol excretion ranges from 55 to 250 nmol/L (20 to 90 µg) per 24 h.

Interpretation. Although urinary free cortisol excretion represents less than 1% of the cortisol secreted each day, it provides a valid index of glucocorticoid secretion. Urinary free cortisol excretion results from glomerular filtration of plasma free cortisol and is therefore an index of integrated 24-h plasma free cortisol. As total plasma cortisol levels exceed the binding capacity of CBG at about 690 nmol/L (25 µg/dL), plasma free cortisol concentration increases more rapidly, as reflected by a more rapid increase in urinary free cortisol excretion. Urinary 17-OHCS excretion, on the other hand, continues to rise at a nearly constant rate. Thus increased urinary free cortisol excretion is a more sensitive indicator of endogenous hypercortisolism. Urinary free cortisol excretion decreases in primary and secondary hypoadrenocorticism and in congenital adrenal hyperplasia.

Urinary free cortisol concentration is not a good indicator of the adequacy of cortisol or cortisone replacement. The same daily replacement dosage of cortisol (e.g., 25 mg), given as a single oral dose, produces a greater 24-h urinary free cortisol value than when the same amount is given in multiple divided doses. The single dose is absorbed within 20 to 30 min, plasma cortisol level temporarily exceeds the binding capacity of CBG, and plasma free cortisol level is temporarily high. This free cortisol is filtered into the urine until total plasma cortisol concentration, falling rapidly, reaches the binding capacity of CBG. However, the same amount of steroid, given in multiple doses, may never exceed

the binding capacity of CBG, plasma free cortisol level does not rise to an exaggerated peak, and 24-h urinary free cortisol excretion is lower and more representative of the integrated free cortisol levels to which the patient's cells have been exposed. Disproportionately high urinary free cortisol excretion is also observed after major episodes of endogenous cortisol secretion, such as during ACTH and CRH stimulation tests. Urinary 17-OHCS levels provide a somewhat better indicator of the adequacy of cortisol replacement because they more closely reflect the total effective amount of cortisol to which tissues are exposed during 24 h. However, they, too, can be misleading, tending to underestimate effective replacement.

OTHER STEROIDS. A variety of other cortisol precursors and metabolites can be measured. THS can be extracted by solvent partition and chromatography and measured as a 17-OHCS or by specific radioimmunoassay. It is normally less than 5% of total urinary 17-OHCS, but its concentration is increased in P-450$_{c11}$ deficiency, with some adrenal carcinomas, and after metyrapone administration. Pregnanetriol can be measured after β-glucuronidase treatment, solvent extraction, and alumina column purification by colorimetric measurement of its sulfuric acid chromogen.[1585] Its excretion is normally less than 6.3 nmol/d (2 mg/d) in adults and less than 1.6 nmol/d (0.5 mg/d) in children. Its concentration is elevated in the P-450$_{c11}$ and P-450$_{c21}$ deficiency forms of congenital adrenal hyperplasia.

Urinary Androgens

17-KETOSTEROIDS. *Assay.* This assay exploits the formation of a pinkish-purple derivative of urinary 17-KS with *m*-dinitrobenzene in the presence of alkali.[1583] The 17-KS consist of 19-carbon steroids, mainly DHEA and DHEAS; their metabolites, including Δ^4-androstenedione, etiocholanolone, and estrone glucuronides; and etiocholanolone sulfate. Testosterone and dihydrotestosterone, the only potent androgens, constitute less than 1% of the total urinary 17-KS.[1586]

Normal Values. Urinary 17-KS excretion ranges from about 17 to 52 µmol (5 to 15 mg) per 24 h in women and 34 to 69 µmol (10 to 20 mg) per 24 h in men.

Interpretation. Urinary 17-KS levels are not as accurate an index of cortisol production as is urinary 17-OHCS or free cortisol excretion or as useful a measure of androgen production as are measurements of plasma testosterone, dihydrotestosterone, DHEA, DHEAS, and androstenedione. They have three major uses, however. First, they are often markedly and disproportionately increased, with respect to 17-OHCS, in patients with adrenal carcinoma, with or without Cushing's syndrome, reflecting high plasma DHEAS concentrations.[1587] They tend to be lower and may be normal in patients with adrenal adenoma.[1053] Second, they are elevated in patients with congenital P-450$_{c11}$ and P-450$_{c21}$ deficiency and can be used, in conjunction with plasma 17α-hydroxyprogesterone, to monitor the efficacy of glucocorticoid replacement therapy. Third, they lend support to the less reliable 17-OHCS results obtained in some reference laboratories. In normal subjects and patients with ACTH-dependent Cushing's syndrome, 17-KS excretion is 1.5 to 2 times that of 17-OHCS. 17-KS excretion changes more slowly than that of 17-OHCS in response to pharmacological manipulation.

Various drugs interfere in the 17-KS assay, several of which also interfere in the 17-OHCS assay. These include agents that produce falsely elevated values (e.g., chlorpromazine, ethinamate, meprobamate, nalidixic acid, penicillin, phenaglycodol, and spironolactone) and those that factitiously depress 17-KS values (e.g., chlordiazepoxide, progestational agents, propoxyphene, and reserpine). As in the 17-OHCS assay, these drugs can be detected and can often be eliminated by solvent partition or chromatography. However, because of these problems and the development of more specific assays for plasma and urinary androgens, 17-KS levels are assayed only rarely.

OTHER URINARY ANDROGENS. DHEA, DHEAS, and testosterone levels can all be measured in urine, as they can in plasma, by radioimmunoassay, but this is seldom performed. Rather, urinary 17-KS levels are measured. DHEAS is the most abundant androgen in urine and the major component of the 17-KS. Conversely, testosterone, the most potent androgen, constitutes but a tiny fraction of total 17-KS. It is sometimes useful to measure excretion of these steroids, but determining their plasma levels usually provides the necessary clinically relevant information.

Urinary Mineralocorticoids

ALDOSTERONE. Aldosterone, in the form of its 18-glucuronide, is measured by radioimmunoassay.[1588] Its excretion varies from about 14 to 53 nmol (5 to 19 μg) per 24 h. The excretion of tetrahydroaldosterone-18-glucuronide, a more abundant metabolite, ranges from about 33 to 178 nmol (12 to 65 μg) per 24 h. Because aldosterone secretion is regulated by renal perfusion and, therefore, by intravascular volume, spironolactone (an aldosterone antagonist) should be withheld for at least 6 wk, other diuretics should be discontinued for at least 4 wk, and antiadrenergic antihypertensive medications should be withheld for at least 1 wk before urinary aldosterone is measured. The patient should follow a diet with a liberal (greater than 120 mmol/d) sodium intake. Urinary aldosterone excretion is low or undetectable in primary hypoadrenocorticism, is usually normal in secondary adrenal insufficiency (ACTH deficiency), and may be low in patients with chronic panhypopituitarism. Urinary aldosterone excretion is usually normal or slightly low in Cushing's syndrome, the extent of suppression depending on the degree of hypersecretion of cortisol and other salt-retaining steroids. It is low or undetectable in P-450$_{scc}$, 3β-hydroxysteroid dehydrogenase, and CMO deficiencies. It ranges from normal in the mild form to undetectable in the severe forms of P-450$_{c21}$ deficiency because of the variable degree of the defect. It is normal or suppressed in the P-450$_{c11}$ and P-450$_{c17}$ deficiency forms of the disorder because of increased secretion of DOC and, in the latter, possibly of corticosterone. Aldosterone excretion is high in most patients with primary or secondary hyperaldosteronism and low or undetectable in those with isolated (hyperreninemic) or secondary (hyporeninemic) hypoaldosteronism. Rare instances of aldosterone-secreting adrenal carcinomas have been reported. The role of aldosterone in hypertension is further discussed in Chapter 11.

Measurement of Steroid Secretion Rates

Assay

Steroid secretion or production rates can be measured by isotopic dilution methods.[1589, 1590] The steroid, labeled at an appropriate position with a radioactive or nonradioactive isotope, is injected intravenously. Either a series of blood samples or a 24-h urine collection is then obtained. The extent of dilution of labeled by endogenous unlabeled steroid (i.e., the decrease in specific activity) is determined and can be used to calculate the amount of endogenous steroid secreted during the interval. The use of 24-h urinary excretion assumes that the metabolic clearance rate for the steroid is constant during the time of collection and that there is a unique steroid metabolite (i.e., one derived only from the steroid in question) that can be measured.

Normal Values

Cortisol secretion ranges from 22 to 69 μmol (8 to 25 mg) per 24 h. The mean is probably about 25 μmol (9.2 mg) per 24 h,[1590] about half of what was previously estimated. Aldosterone secretion ranges from about 139 to 694 nmol (50 to 250 μg) per 24 h. Secretion rates of other adrenal steroids are not of clinical importance.

Interpretation

The rate of cortisol secretion is increased in Cushing's syndrome of all causes except administration of pharmacological dosage of glucocorticoids, is decreased in primary and secondary adrenal insufficiency, and is normal or decreased in all types of congenital adrenal hyperplasia. It also tends to be increased in obesity,[1591] hyperthyroidism,[1592] and pregnancy[1562] and is decreased in malnutrition[1566] and hypothyroidism. Secretion rates in obese patients can be corrected by expressing them as a function of creatinine excretion.[1113] Aldosterone secretion rate is increased in primary and secondary hyperaldosteronism, is low in primary adrenal insufficiency and in primary and secondary hypoaldosteronism, and is normal in most cases of secondary adrenal insufficiency. It is increased in normal pregnancy.[1593]

These measurements theoretically provide precise indices of adrenocortical function, but their interpretation is not without problems. There is no unique urinary metabolite for cortisol, for example, and secretion rates differ with the use of different metabolites.[1594] Secretion rates calculated from blood dilution differ from those calculated from urinary dilution, perhaps because the metabolic clearance rate for steroids varies during the day.[1595] A study with a nonradioactive isotope resulted in an estimate of daily cortisol secretion lower than most previous estimates.[1590] For these reasons and because these assays are technically demanding, time-consuming, and expensive and the infomation required for clinical decisions can usually be obtained by other means, steroid secretion rates are rarely calculated.

Dynamic Tests of Hypothalamic-Pituitary-Adrenal Function

Analysis of basal hormone secretion is useful but provides limited information about the status of hypothalamic-pituitary-adrenal axis interactions. For example, an individual with a pituitary lesion may maintain normal basal cortisol secretion but be unable to respond to hypocortisolemia or stress by increasing ACTH secretion. Conversely, a patient with an adrenal tumor may not produce excessive amounts of cortisol each day, yet most or all of the daily cortisol production may be autonomous, the hypothalamic-pituitary axis may be partially suppressed, and the remaining normal adrenal cortex may be atrophic. The purpose of dynamic tests of hypothalamic-pituitary-adrenal function is to define abnormalities in the functional relationships between the elements of the axis that may not be reflected in altered basal secretion.

Tests For Evaluating Primary and Secondary Adrenal Insufficiency

Hypocortisolism can result from (1) a primary adrenal disorder resulting in failure to produce cortisol (primary adrenal insufficiency), (2) a primary pituitary disorder resulting in lack of ACTH secretion (secondary adrenal insufficiency), or (3) a primary hypothalamic disorder resulting in lack of CRH secretion and secondarily in lack of ACTH secretion ("tertiary" adrenal insufficiency). Measurement of basal plasma ACTH and cortisol concentrations and urinary steroid excretion and the responses of the anterior pituitary gland and adrenal cortex to a variety of stimuli will define the site at which the defect exists.

A major problem with relying on observations of unstimulated plasma hormone levels as the basis for the diagnosis is that hormone secretion is episodic. A single plasma level, if it falls within the range of normal, is inconclusive. Furthermore, the normal ranges are broad, and an individual can have pituitary or adrenal insufficiency but maintain ACTH and/or cortisol secretion within the range of the normal population. For these reasons, dynamic function tests should be performed when there is reasonable doubt about the hypothalamic-pituitary-adrenal status.

Nevertheless, a basal early morning plasma cortisol value can be very helpful in excluding adrenal hypo- or hyperfunction. If the level is greater than 300 nmol/L (11 μg/dL) it is unlikely that the patient has clinically important hypothalamic-pituitary-adrenal insufficiency, whereas if it is less than about 80 nmol/L (3 μg/dL) the probability of adrenal insufficiency is high.[914, 1596] Conversely, a patient whose plasma cortisol level 1 h after sleep is less than 140 nmol/L (5 μg/dL) has virtually no probability of having Cushing's syndrome. Similarly, patients whose salivary cortisol level at 8 AM is greater than 16 nmol/L (5.8 ng/mL) are highly unlikely to have adrenal insufficiency, whereas if the level is less than about 5 nmol/L (1.8 ng/mL) the probability of adrenal insufficiency is high. A patient whose late evening salivary cortisol level is less than 4 nmol/L (1.4 ng/mL) is unlikely to have Cushing's syndrome, whereas if it is greater than 16 nmol/L (5.8 ng/mL) the probability is high. Patients whose basal plasma or salivary cortisol concentrations do not meet these criteria are the major candidates for dynamic function testing.

ACTH TEST: ADRENOCORTICAL RESPONSE TO EXOGENOUS ACTH. *Rationale.* If the primary disorder is hypopituitarism with deficient ACTH secretion and secondary adrenal insufficiency, the intrinsically normal adrenal gland should respond to maximally stimulating concentrations of exogenous ACTH (see Fig. 9–33C and D). Conversely, in primary adrenal insufficiency, endogenous ACTH levels are already elevated and there should be no adrenal response to exogenous ACTH (see Fig. 9–33B).

Procedure. **One-Hour ACTH Stimulation Test.** Plasma cortisol measurements are made immediately before and 30 and 60 min after intravenous (IV) injection of cosyntropin (synthetic ACTH(1–24) (250 μg [85 nmol, or 25 IU]). Plasma ACTH can also be measured in the basal sample. This dose of cosyntropin produces pharmacological concentrations of plasma ACTH for the 60-min duration of the test. The test can be performed on an outpatient basis. There are no untoward side effects. Allergic reactions, which were rare with purified animal ACTH, are almost unheard of with cosyntropin.

Eight-Hour ACTH Stimulation Test. This test is performed by infusing 250 μg (56 nmol, 25 IU) cosyntropin or 40 IU purified bovine ACTH continuously over 8 h in 500 mL of physiological saline solution. A 24-h urine specimen is collected the day before and the day of the infusion for 17-OHCS and creatinine determination, and plasma cortisol concentration is determined at the end of the infusion. Plasma ACTH levels are maintained at supraphysiological levels for the duration of the infusion. The infusion solution must contain isotonic saline (154 mmol/L [9 g/L] NaCl) because addisonian patients, who may already be hyponatremic and lack salt-retaining aldosterone, can become severely hyponatremic if infused with hypotonic solutions. This is a particular problem when purified bovine ACTH, which is contaminated with variable amounts of AVP, is used; the AVP causes renal free water retention, aggravating hyponatremia. Cosyntropin is also preferable to bovine ACTH because of rare instances of allergic reactions to contaminating proteins in purified ACTH preparations. In countries where it is available, 1 mg (444 nmol) of a long-acting cosyntropin preparation (ACTH(1–18)-NH₂) can be injected intramuscularly. The 8-h ACTH infusion test is now rarely performed.

Two-Day ACTH Infusion Test. The 2-d ACTH infusion test[919] is similar to the 8-h infusion test, except that the same dose of ACTH is infused every 8 h. Alternatively, 40 IU of a depot formulation of purified bovine ACTH in gelatin is injected intramuscularly every 12 h for 48 h. Daily 444 nmol (1 mg) intramuscular injections of long-acting ACTH(1–18)-NH₂ can be used outside the United States. The same precautions should be observed as during the 8-h test. This test is the most widely used prolonged ACTH stimulation test.

Three- to Five-Day ACTH Infusion Tests. The 3- to 5-d ACTH stimulation tests are generally conducted in the same way as the 2-d test but are prolonged an additional 1 to 3 d.

Normal Values. **One-Hour ACTH Stimulation Test.** Using radioimmunoassay to determine plasma cortisol, a value of 550 nmol/L (20 μg/dL) or more at any time during the test, including before injection, is indicative of normal adrenal function.[915] Earlier criteria that included a minimal increment in plasma cortisol[1597] are invalid because patients who have a high basal plasma cortisol level, because of either normal circadian rhythmicity or acute stress, may be nearly maximally stimulated and unable to increase cortisol secretion further. Salivary cortisol increases to 52 ± 2.2 nmol/L (19 ± 0.8 ng/mL) (range, 24 to 99 nmol/L [8.7 to 36 ng/mL]) 1 h after injection.[1581]

Eight-Hour ACTH Stimulation Test. The 24-h urinary excretion of 17-OHCS should increase three- to fivefold over the baseline value on the day of ACTH infusion. If measured, plasma cortisol concentration should reach 550 nmol/L (20 μg/dL) 30 to 60 min after and exceed 690 nmol/L (25 μg/dL) 6 to 8 h after the infusion is begun.

Two-Day ACTH Stimulation Test. Urinary excretion of 17-OHCS should exceed 74 nmol (27 mg) during the first 24 h of infusion and 130 nmol (47 mg) during the second 48 h. If measured, plasma cortisol concentration should reach 550 nmol/L (20 μg/dL) 30 to 60 min after and exceed 690 nmol/L (25 μg/dL) 6 to 8 h after the infusion is begun. Both plasma and urinary steroid levels increase progressively thereafter, but ranges of normal are not standardized.

Three- to Five-Day ACTH Stimulation Test. Urinary 17-OHCS concentration should increase three- to fivefold over the baseline value on the first day of ACTH infusion. If measured, plasma cortisol concentration should reach 550 nmol/L (20 μg/dL) 30 to 60 min after and exceed 690 nmol/L (25 μg/dL) 6 to 8 h after the infusion is begun. Both plasma and urinary steroid levels will increase progressively thereafter, but ranges of normal are not standardized.

Interpretation. A subnormal response to the 1-h ACTH stimulation test is diagnostic of primary or secondary adrenal insufficiency, and a normal response excludes both disorders.[1598] The test does not distinguish between the primary and secondary forms of adrenal insufficiency. However, if the response is inadequate, one can measure the plasma ACTH concentration in the basal sample. If it is higher than normal, the patient has primary adrenal insufficiency; if it is low, the diagnosis is secondary adrenal insufficiency. In primary insufficiency, prolonged stimulation with exogenous ACTH for 1 to 5 d will result in little, if any, increase in cortisol production. In secondary insufficiency, on the other hand, the adrenal gland is intrinsically normal but is atrophic because of chronic ACTH deficiency. In most of these patients, stimulation for 1 d (8 h) is too brief to exert a major effect. Continuous infusion of ACTH for 2 d results in an increase in 24-h urinary 17-OHCS excretion to 25 nmol (9 mg) or more during the second day of infusion in most patients with hypopituitarism. Occasional patients may require 3 to 5 d of stimulation. However, even after 5 d, plasma cortisol levels may not attain those observed after 1 to 8 h of ACTH stimulation in normal individuals[1599] and 24-h urinary 17-OHCS levels may increase only threefold over baseline.[1600] In practice the prolonged ACTH stimulation test is seldom used because sensitive assays of plasma ACTH, used in conjunction with the 1-h test, have supplanted it.

An area in which there continues to be controversy is whether the 1-h ACTH test accurately predicts the ability to respond adequately to stress, such as major surgery. This is because occasional patients have normal responses to cosyntropin but subnormal responses to insulin-induced hypoglycemia,[917, 1601] although the hypoglycemia has not always been adequate.[1597] Rarely, patients who respond normally to the 1-h ACTH test have a subnormal cortisol response to surgery,[1597] but these patients, in fact, tolerate surgery normally.[1601a] Furthermore, the plasma cortisol responses of most individuals to the 1-h ACTH test and to insulin-induced hypoglycemia, a standard stress, are virtually identical.[1601] Presumably, the reason is that the endogenous plasma ACTH levels elicited in response to insulin-induced hypoglycemia are maximally stimulating during the hour or less that the test lasts, as are the plasma levels of exogenous ACTH achieved during the 1-h ACTH stimulation test. In both tests, a normal response is predicated on the fact that the adrenal gland has been stimulated daily with sufficient endogenous ACTH to prevent adrenal atrophy and maintain the required basal activity of the steroidogenic cytochrome P-450 enzymes. The reason why patients do well during major surgery, even though their cortisol levels may not rise normally, may be that one does not require more than basal daily cortisol secretion to survive surgery.[930]

With one exception, the patient who responds normally to the 1-h ACTH test does not require glucocorticoid supplementation for stress, surgical or otherwise. The exception is the patient with acute ACTH deficiency, such as a patient who has just had a hypophysectomy.[1601] During the several days after cessation of ACTH secretion, the adrenocortical zonae fasciculata and reticularis undergo functional and anatomical atrophy. However, during part of that interval the adrenals may respond normally to pharmacological doses of exogenous ACTH, whereas the pituitary gland is unable to release ACTH in response to stress. These patients respond normally to the 1-h ACTH test but fail to respond to insulin-induced hypoglycemia and require steroid supplementation during surgical or other stresses.

Because the 1-h ACTH test gives results identical to those of the insulin-induced hypoglycemia test, can be performed in an outpatient setting without a physician being present and without risk, and is less expensive to perform, it has supplanted the insulin-induced hypoglycemia test in standard clinical endocrinological practice except in patients with suspected recent loss of ACTH-secretory capacity.

INSULIN-INDUCED HYPOGLYCEMIA TEST: THE HYPOTHALAMIC-PITUITARY RESPONSE TO HYPOGLYCEMIC STRESS. *Rationale.* Stress is difficult to define, let alone to reproduce. However, hypoglycemia produces a major stress response, with increases in plasma ACTH, cortisol, GH, and prolactin and activation of the adrenergic system.[1602] Furthermore, (1) the degree of hypoglycemia can easily be quantified, (2) the test is safe, if a physician is present, in patients without a history of seizures or cardiovascular or cerebrovascular disease, and (3) the hypoglycemia can be corrected within seconds by IV infusion of hypertonic glucose solution. The magnitude of the response depends on the degree of hypoglycemia. Criteria (i.e., rate and degree of fall in plasma glucose) that are adequate to elicit a maximal GH response are inadequate to ensure a maximal ACTH response. Because the purpose of the test is to define the magnitude of a maximal stress response, more stringent criteria of adequate hypoglycemia must be applied. In a patient with a morning plasma cortisol level of less than 140 nmol/L (5 μg/dL) and 24-h urinary free cortisol excretion of less than 55 nmol (20 μg), there is rarely any indication for this test.

Procedure. The patient fasts for at least 8 h before and must remain supine during the procedure. A physician must be present during the entire procedure. A 30-mL syringe containing 50% glucose solution should be at bedside. An IV line is established, and insulin (0.15 U/kg body weight) is injected IV. The insulin dose is decreased to 0.1 U/kg body weight for patients thought to have hypopituitarism or primary adrenal insufficiency and is increased, because of insulin resistance, to 0.25 U/kg for obese patients or those with diabetes mellitus or suspected acromegaly or Cushing's syndrome. Blood is obtained for plasma glucose and cortisol assays immediately before insulin is injected and 30 and 45 min thereafter. All patients in whom adequate hypoglycemia is achieved (1.9 mmol/L [35 mg/dL] or less) will develop a profuse cold sweat. In fact, if the patient does not have a sweat, irrespective of plasma glucose level, the adequacy of stress stimulus must remain suspect. Most patients also have a hyperactive precordium (but not tachycardia or hypotension, because they are supine) and feelings of hunger, drowsiness, detachment, or anxiety. The last is common and sometimes severe, and many patients find this an unpleasant experience. Hypoglycemia is usually achieved 30 to 45 min after insulin injection. If adequate hypoglycemia is not achieved, a second identical dose of regular insulin should be injected IV. Adequate hypoglycemia should be achieved within 30 to 45 min. Ideally, an automated glucose oxidase analyzer should be available at the bedside. Unfortunately, most glucose oxidase strips are inaccurate at low plasma glucose levels and tend to underestimate the plasma glucose concentration, leading to premature abortion of the test. The final, definitive blood sample should be obtained 5 to 10 min after the patient develops a profuse sweat or, if it can reliably be measured, when plasma glucose level falls below 1.9 mmol/L. Patients with primary or secondary adrenal insufficiency or long-standing diabetes mellitus have an impaired compensatory response to hypoglycemia. Therefore, it is prudent to terminate the test, after achieving a plasma glucose concentration of 1.9 mmol/L, by infusing 10% glucose solution or giving sweetened orange juice or cola by mouth. A 50% glucose solution should be infused over a period of 1 min or so (because of its hypertonicity) if seizure, chest pain, confusion, disorientation, or other potentially serious complications occur; the latter will produce hyperglycemia within 30 s.

Normal Values. Plasma cortisol level is measured by radioimmunoassay and should reach 550 nmol/L (20 μg/dL) at some point during the test. If it does, it is unimportant whether hypoglycemia was adequate. Failure to reach this level, however, indicates an inadequate response only if plasma glucose level fell to 1.9 mmol/L (35 mg/dL) or less. Otherwise, the stimulus was inadequate and the test must be repeated. The increment in plasma cortisol is irrelevant, as discussed in relation to the 1-h ACTH stimulation test. Plasma ACTH level can also be measured. The response has not been carefully standardized, but the value should exceed 33 pmol/L (150 pg/mL).[213, 1603–1606] Finally, as discussed in greater detail in Chapter 6, plasma GH levels should also increase; their measurement provides another index of anterior pituitary function.

Interpretation. An inadequate response can be due to hypopituitarism of any etiology, including hypothalamic CRH deficiency, isolated ACTH deficiency, partial or panhypopituitarism, and acute or chronic ingestion of synthetic glucocorticoids. Because adrenocortical secretion of cortisol is used as a bioassay of ACTH secretion, primary, as well as secondary, adrenal insufficiency can also cause an abnormal cortisol response. Hypoglycemia is a stronger stimulus for ACTH secretion than is hypocortisolemia. Consequently, patients may have a normal response to hypoglycemia but an inadequate response to metyrapone administration. The reverse is almost never true.

Although the response to insulin-induced hypoglycemia is a valid, and perhaps the most rational, test of hypothalamic-pituitary-adrenal response to stress, the 1-h ACTH test provides the same information, is less difficult and expensive to perform, and can be performed without risk in any patient. Consequently, there is little, if any, reason for performing the insulin-induced hypoglycemia test in clinical practice except in patients with suspected recent ACTH deficiency.[1601] The test is discussed further in Chapter 6.

METYRAPONE TEST: THE PITUITARY RESPONSE TO HYPOCORTISOLEMIA. *Rationale.* The metyrapone test (see Fig. 9–47D) is based on the fact that ACTH secretion is inhibited by plasma cortisol. Metyrapone blocks the conversion of 11β-deoxycortisol to cortisol by P-450$_{c11}$, the last step in the biosynthetic pathway from cholesterol to cortisol (see Fig. 9–6). 11-Deoxycortisol is essentially devoid of glucocorticoid bioactivity and does not inhibit ACTH secretion. As plasma cortisol concentration falls, therefore, ACTH secretion increases, adrenal steroidogenesis is stimulated, and the secretion of cortisol precursors, especially 11-deoxycortisol, the substrate of P-450$_{c11}$ (see Fig. 9–6), increases rapidly (see Fig. 9–47D). The 11-deoxycortisol can be measured either in blood by protein-binding radioassay[1607, 1608] or radioimmunoassay or in urine as a 17-OHCS,[1130] providing an index of the increase in ACTH secretion.

Procedure. **Standard Three-Day Metyrapone Test.** This test[1130] is performed by obtaining a baseline 8 AM to 8 AM 24-h urine collection. Immediately after completing this collection, the patient begins taking metyrapone (750 mg every 4 h for six doses) by mouth with a glass of milk or a small snack to minimize gastrointestinal symptoms. The 24-h urine specimens are collected throughout the day of and the day after metyrapone administration for measurement of urinary 17-OHCS and creatinine excretion. Plasma 11-deoxycortisol, cortisol, and ACTH can also be measured 4 h after the last dose of metyrapone.[1607, 1608] Obviously, the metyrapone test cannot be performed on a patient who is taking any glucocorticoid.

Overnight Single-Dose Metyrapone Test. This test[1608] is performed by oral administration of metyrapone (30 mg/kg body weight, or 2 g for <70 kg, 2.5 kg for 70 to 90 kg, and 3 g for >90 kg body weight) at midnight with a small snack. Plasma 11-deoxycortisol and cortisol concentrations are measured by radioimmunoassay in an 8 AM blood sample. Plasma ACTH concentration can also be measured.[1609–1611]

These tests can result in hypotension, nausea, and vomiting in patients with primary or secondary adrenal insufficiency and should not be performed outside the hospital, certainly not in patients suspected of having these disorders. If symptoms of adrenal insufficiency occur, the patient should be infused with physiological saline solution and the test should be continued. Saline can usually be stopped a few hours after the last dose of metyrapone.

Normal Values. A normal response to the standard 3-d test is a two- to threefold increase above the baseline 24-h urinary 17-OHCS excretion on either the day of or, more often, the day after metyrapone administration.[1130] A normal response to the overnight single-dose test is an 8 AM plasma 11-deoxycortisol concentration of 210 to 660 nmol/L (7 to 22 μg/dL) or more.[1607, 1608] Plasma ACTH concentrations should exceed 17 pmol/L (75 pg/mL), with a mean of about 44 pmol/L (200 pg/mL), at 8 AM after the overnight dose[1611, 1612] and, presumably, 4 h after the last dose in the 3-d test.

Interpretation. The metyrapone test is the most sensitive test of pituitary ACTH-secretory reserve. It depends on the release of pituitary ACTH secretion from negative feedback inhibition by cortisol, which is a much less powerful stimulus to increased ACTH secretion than hypoglycemia or other stresses. Thus a patient with partial hypopituitarism may maintain normal daily ACTH and cortisol secretion and respond to insulin-induced hypoglycemia or other stresses with a normal increase in ACTH and cortisol secretion, yet be unable to increase ACTH secretion normally when cortisol biosynthesis is blocked by metyrapone. Conversely, a patient who responds normally to metyrapone essentially always responds normally to hypoglycemia and other stresses.

An individual who responds normally to either metyrapone test has an intact hypothalamic-pituitary-adrenal axis and requires no further investigation. An abnormal test can result from several causes. Because adrenal steroid secretion is used as the assay of ACTH activity, primary adrenal insufficiency can be the cause. This can be determined by finding either a high ACTH concentration in the basal plasma specimen or an inadequate plasma ACTH response to metyrapone[1611–1613] and can be confirmed, if necessary, by lack of a normal plasma cortisol response to cosyntropin. Acute or chronic ingestion of synthetic glucocorticoids can also result in a subnormal response. Any of the drugs that interfere in the assay of 17-OHCS can interfere with interpretation of the standard 3-d test results.

One of the more common causes of a factitious abnormal result is unusually rapid clearance of metyrapone from plasma, resulting in inadequate blockade of cortisol biosynthesis. This is manifested by a plasma cortisol level greater than 210 nmol/L (7.5 μg/dL) in the sample drawn at 8 AM in the overnight test,[1607] by a plasma cortisol level greater than 140 nmol/L (5 μg/dL) 4 h after the last dose of metyrapone, or by urinary free cortisol excretion greater than 55 nmol (20 μg) per 24 h the day metyrapone was administered in the standard 2-d test. Rapid clearance occurs in about 4% of the normal population.[1610, 1612] Metyrapone is metabolized by hepatic cytochrome P-450 enzymes that are induced by many of the same agents that increase steroid metabolism (e.g., phenobarbital, phenytoin, rifampin, mitotane, and glucocorticoids), so these drugs should be stopped well before the metyrapone test is performed. An alternative is to perform the 3-d test with twice the dosage of metyrapone (750 mg every 2 h for 12 doses; presumably, 1.5 g every 4 h for 6 doses would be equally effective). A normal response is said to be indicated by a plasma 11-deoxycortisol level greater than 300 nmol/L (10 μg/dL) 2 h after the last dose or urinary 17-OHCS excretion of more than 16 nmol (6 mg) per 24 h on the day of metyrapone administration.[1613] However, because the double dosage of metyrapone is given to overcome the increased metabolic clearance, it is not clear why the criterion for a normal response should be different from that in the standard 3-d test. Consequently, one can reasonably assume that a two- to threefold increase above the baseline 24-h 17-OHCS excretion during the day of or the day after metyrapone administration is indicative of normal ACTH-secretory reserve. Furthermore, if baseline 17-OHCS excretion is 16 nmol (6 mg) per 24 h, a similar value on the day of metyrapone administration indicates a lack of response.

CORTICOTROPIN-RELEASING HORMONE TEST: THE PITUITARY RESPONSE TO CORTICOTROPIN-RELEASING HORMONE. *Rationale.* The conceptual basis of the CRH test is the use of a maximally stimulating dose of exogenous CRH to stimulate ACTH secretion by anterior pituitary corticotropes. If the defect in hypothalamic-pituitary-adrenal function is at the hypothalamic level, CRH administration should cause release of ACTH, whereas if the primary defect is in the pituitary, ACTH secretion should be subnormal or absent even after maximal CRH stimulation. Synthetic ovine CRH is equipotent to human CRH and has a more prolonged duration of action than human CRH,[322-324] which makes it useful for clinical testing.[1614]

Procedure. The patient usually fasts for 4 h or more, after which an IV access line is established and synthetic ovine CRH (1 μg/kg body weight) is injected as an IV bolus. Blood samples for plasma ACTH and cortisol assays are drawn 15 and 0 min before and 5, 10, 15, 30, 45, 60, 90, and 120 min after CRH injection. If one measures only the plasma cortisol response, the samples at 0, 45, and 60 min are sufficient. Some patients experience mild, brief facial flushing immediately after injection, but there are no other side effects at this dose level.[325] Allergic reactions have not been reported.

Normal Values. The normal range of the ACTH response to ovine CRH is not well characterized. Absolute increments in plasma ACTH concentration are variable among individuals and from one time to another in the same individual (unpublished data, D. R. Davis and D. N. Orth). The cause of this variability is unknown, but it cannot be accounted for simply by inhibition by variable basal plasma cortisol concentrations (unpublished data, D. R. Davis and D. N. Orth). However, basal ACTH concentration increases two- to fourfold in 95% of normal subjects, in our experience, and reaches a peak of 4.4 to 22 pmol/L (20 to 100 pg/mL) 10 or 15 min after CRH injection, and plasma cortisol level usually increases to 550 to 690 nmol/L (20 to 25 μg/dL), reaching a peak 30 to 60 min after CRH injection.[324, 325, 328, 1134] Whereas the increment in ACTH is the same in the morning and evening, the peak ACTH value is higher in the morning, when basal ACTH is higher. In contrast, the peak cortisol value is similar at both times of day but the increment is smaller in the morning, when the basal cortisol level is higher.[331]

Interpretation. Patients with primary pituitary ACTH deficiency (secondary adrenal insufficiency) have decreased plasma ACTH and cortisol responses to CRH. Patients with hypothalamic disease (i.e., CRH deficiency), in general, have exaggerated and prolonged plasma ACTH responses; plasma cortisol responses are subnormal. Patients with primary adrenal deficiency have high basal plasma ACTH concentrations and greatly exaggerated responses to CRH, and plasma cortisol concentrations are low before and after CRH injection. However, the CRH test is not recommended for differentiating primary from secondary adrenal deficiency.

This test can be performed as part of a combined anterior pituitary function test in which CRH, GH-releasing hormone, LHRH, and thyrotropin-releasing hormone are administered simultaneously and plasma concentrations of all of the anterior pituitary hormones are measured.[328] The function test is useful in evaluating the site (i.e., hypothalamic vs. pituitary) and extent (i.e., partial vs. panhypopituitarism) of deficiency in patients with suspected pituitary dysfunction and in evaluating residual pituitary function after pituitary surgery and radiation. This test is discussed further in Chapter 6.

UPRIGHT PLASMA RENIN ACTIVITY/ALDOSTERONE TEST: THE RENAL-ADRENAL RESPONSE TO UPRIGHT POSTURE. *Rationale.* Renin secretion is regulated by effective renal perfusion, so anything that decreases renal blood flow will increase plasma renin levels. If the adrenal is intact, the increased plasma renin concentration will stimulate increased aldosterone secretion. Patients with primary adrenal insufficiency also lack aldosterone secretion, whereas those with secondary adrenal insufficiency generally do not (see Fig. 9–29). Although it is not necessary to document this fact to establish the diagnosis, it is sometimes important to assess the status of the renin-angiotensin-aldosterone system in a patient with primary adrenal insufficiency in whom electrolyte disturbances are mild or absent.

Procedure. Salt should not be restricted without careful monitoring in a patient with primary adrenal insufficiency, and diuretics are dangerous. On the other hand, the patient should not be overly hydrated with saline solution. In these patients, upright posture alone will suffice to stimulate increased renin secretion. The patient maintains an upright posture, preferably standing, sitting when necessary, but never lying down, for 3 h. Blood pressure should be monitored. If the patient becomes hypotensive, the test can be terminated after a blood sample is obtained. Otherwise, blood is obtained before and at the end of the 3-h period for assay of plasma renin activity and aldosterone concentration.

Normal Values. Normal upright plasma renin activity is 0.5 to 2.6 nmol/L/h (0.7 to 3.3 ng/mL/h). Normal upright plasma aldosterone concentrations range from 140 to 560 pmol/L (5 to 20 ng/dL).

Interpretation. Patients with primary adrenal insufficiency have a low plasma aldosterone level and increased plasma renin activity in response to upright posture. Patients with secondary adrenal insufficiency (hypopituitarism) usually have a normal response, although some patients with chronic ACTH deficiency may develop aldosterone deficiency.[1588, 1615] Tests of renin-angiotensin-aldosterone axis function are discussed in Chapter 11.

OTHER TESTS. The blood eosinophil response[1616] and water-loading tests[1617] no longer have a role in the evaluation of pituitary insufficiency.

Tests for Evaluating Adrenocortical Hypersecretion: Cushing's Syndrome

DEXAMETHASONE SUPPRESSION TESTS: THE PITUITARY RESPONSE TO GLUCOCORTICOID NEGATIVE FEEDBACK INHIBITION OF ACTH SECRETION. Dexamethasone (see Fig. 9–62) is a potent glucocorticoid, about 40 times more potent than cortisol (see Table 9–17). Thus the average daily maintenance dosage of dexamethasone for an addisonian patient is 0.5 mg, whereas the average daily dosage of cortisol is 20 mg. Dexamethasone and its tetrahydro metabolite both form Porter-Silber chromogens and are measured in urine as 17-OHCS. As in the case of cortisol, only about one third of the urinary metabolites of dexamethasone are detected as 17-OHCS. Because so little dexamethasone is required to suppress pituitary ACTH secretion, its contribution to total urinary 17-OHCS level is relatively small, about 0.7 mg/d in the standard 2-d low-dose dexamethasone suppression test and about 2.4 mg/d in the 2-d high-dose test. Furthermore, current antibodies used in cortisol radioimmunoassay are directed toward the D ring of the molecule and react very poorly with dexamethasone, which has a 16α-methyl modification of the D ring. Thus measurements of plasma cortisol and urinary free cortisol levels are unaffected by the presence of dexamethasone.

Low-Dose Dexamethasone Suppression Tests. Rationale. The purpose of the low-dose dexamethasone suppression test is to differentiate patients with Cushing's syndrome of any etiology (see Figs. 9–48*B*, 9–50*B*, and 9–53*B*) from patients with normal hypothalamic-pituitary-adrenal function (see Fig. 9–47*B*). Glucocorticoid receptors in the adrenal cortex bind dexamethasone, and dexamethasone apparently directly inhibits steroidogenesis to a degree in rat adrenals.[1618] However, dexamethasone has no inhibitory effect on steroid production when exogenous ACTH is infused in humans; if anything, it augments the effect.[1619] Therefore, for the purpose of this test, one can assume that the only action of dexamethasone is to suppress pituitary ACTH secretion (see Fig. 9–47*B*). If the hypothalamic-pituitary axis is intrinsically normal, the excess dosage of dexamethasone is sufficient to suppress most of pituitary ACTH secretion. Consequently, adrenal cortisol secretion falls, and the plasma concentration and urinary excretion of cortisol and cortisol metabolites also decrease.

Procedure. *Standard Two-Day Test.* At least one basal 24-h urine specimen is collected, usually beginning at 8 AM, for 17-OHCS, free cortisol, and creatinine assays. Immediately after the basal urine collection is completed, the patient begins taking 0.5 mg dexamethasone orally every 6 h for a total of eight doses, and urine collection is continued. The dose can be modified in children who weigh less than about 45 kg (100 lb).[1113] Six hours after the last dose of dexamethasone, the last urine collection is completed and blood can be drawn for assay of cortisol, ACTH, and dexamethasone.

Overnight Screening Test. Dexamethasone (1 mg) is taken orally between 11 PM and midnight, and a single blood sample is drawn at 8 AM the next morning for assay of cortisol and, if one wishes, ACTH and dexamethasone. A dose of 0.3 mg/m² surface area can be used in children.[1620]

No special precautions are required, untoward side effects are virtually absent, and either test can be conducted on an outpatient basis by an intelligent and compliant patient. Obviously, the test is invalid in a patient who is receiving exogenous ACTH or glucocorticoids.

Normal Values. *Standard Two-Day Test.* Urinary 17-OHCS concentration should fall to 6.9 μmol (2.5 mg) or less per 24 h, irrespective of creatinine excretion (i.e., lean body weight), and urinary free cortisol concentration should decrease to less than 55 nmol (20 μg) per 24 h on the second day of dexamethasone administration. Although the test does not require it, confirmatory data are provided by a plasma cortisol value of less than 140 nmol/L (5 μg/dL), a plasma ACTH value of less than 4.4 pmol/L (20 pg/mL), and a plasma dexamethasone value of 7.7 to 10 nmol/L (3 to 4 ng/mL).[1116]

Overnight Test. The 8 AM plasma cortisol level should be less than 140 nmol/L (5 μg/dL), plasma ACTH should be less than 4.4 pmol/L (20 pg/mL), and plasma dexamethasone should be from 2.6 to 7.7 nmol/L (1 to 3 ng/mL). Salivary cortisol concentration at 8 AM is 2.1 ± 1.1 nmol/L (0.8 ± 0.4 ng/mL) (range, 1.7 to 3 nmol/L [0.6 to 1.1 ng/mL]).[1581]

Interpretation. The overnight test is a quick and reliable screening test for Cushing's syndrome (12 to 15% false-positive results[1621]). If the morning plasma cortisol level is less than 140 nmol/L (5 μg/dL), the syndrome is essentially excluded. Between 140 and 275 nmol/L (5 and 10 μg/dL), the test is equivocal, and the standard 2-d test should be performed. If the 8 AM plasma cortisol level is greater than 275 nmol/L (10 μg/dL), the patient has a high probability of

having Cushing's syndrome, and further diagnostic tests must be performed to confirm the diagnosis and determine its etiology.

Measurement of plasma cortisol concentration at the end of the standard 2-d test provides reassurance that the urinary steroid values are correct. Measurement of plasma ACTH concentration, if either of the tests is positive, gives an indication of the etiology of the hypercortisolism; it will usually be high normal or elevated in ectopic ACTH syndrome, within the normal range in Cushing's disease, and undetectable in adrenal tumor.

Measuring plasma dexamethasone concentration is recommended for all dexamethasone suppression tests. It provides verification that the drug was taken and indicates whether the plasma concentration is within the limits expected in an individual who metabolizes the drug normally. Nomograms are available that relate plasma dexamethasone levels to plasma cortisol concentrations in normal subjects and in some patients with Cushing's disease,[1115, 1116] but these are not widely applied. However, finding an abnormally high or low dexamethasone level allows one to interpret the cause of an unusual cortisol response and to repeat the test, if necessary, with the same or another dexamethasone dosage.

Two forms of pseudo-Cushing's syndrome in which results of the low-dose dexamethasone suppression tests may be abnormal are major depressive disorders and alcoholism. These disorders are considered earlier in this chapter.

High-Dose Dexamethasone Suppression Tests. Rationale. The basis for the high-dose suppression tests is the fact that ACTH secretion in Cushing's disease is not completely, but only relatively, resistant to glucocorticoid negative feedback inhibition.[1018, 1122] Therefore, by increasing the dosage of dexamethasone four- to eightfold (i.e., 16 times the usual daily maintenance dosage), ACTH secretion can almost always be suppressed (see Fig. 9–48*C*). In contrast, most nonpituitary tumors that produce ectopic ACTH are not responsive to glucocorticoid negative feedback, and adrenal tumors that cause Cushing's syndrome are not dependent on ACTH secretion. In both of these varieties of Cushing's syndrome, pituitary ACTH secretion is already suppressed (see Figs. 9–50*A* and 9–53*A*). Therefore, dexamethasone cannot suppress ACTH secretion further and has no effect on cortisol secretion at any dosage (see Figs. 9–50*C* and 9–53*C*).

Procedure. *Standard Two-Day Test.* The patient collects at least one baseline 24-h urine specimen, usually beginning at 8 AM. After the baseline collection is completed, the patient begins taking 2 mg dexamethasone orally every 6 h for a total of 8 doses, and the urine collections are continued. In practice, this test is often performed immediately after completing the low-dose dexamethasone suppression test and no intervening baseline urine collection is obtained. The urine collections are assayed for 17-OHCS, free cortisol, and creatinine levels. In addition, a blood specimen can be collected 6 h after the last dose of dexamethasone for cortisol, dexamethasone, and ACTH radioimmunoassays.

Overnight Test. Dexamethasone (8 mg) is taken orally between 11 PM and midnight, and a single blood sample is drawn at 8 AM the next morning for assay of plasma cortisol and, if one wishes, ACTH and dexamethasone.

Normal Values. *Standard Two-Day Test.* Urinary 17-OHCS levels are suppressed to less than 6.9 μmol (2.5 mg) per 24 h, most of which consists of dexamethasone metabolites. Urinary free cortisol excretion is less than 28 nmol/d (10 μg/d), and plasma cortisol and ACTH concentrations are low and usually undetectable. Plasma dexamethasone concentrations range from about 31 to 41 nmol/L (12 to 16 ng/mL).

Overnight Test. The 8 AM plasma cortisol level is less than 140 nmol/L (5 μg/dL) and is usually undetectable. Plasma ACTH level is also low and often undetectable. Plasma dexamethasone concentrations range from about 20 to 61 nmol/L (8 to 24 ng/mL).

Interpretation. Patients with Cushing's disease demonstrate significant suppression (i.e., greater than day-to-day baseline variation) of urinary 17-OHCS and free cortisol levels, most showing suppression of 50% or more.[1018] However, reproducible suppression of any degree is diagnostic of Cushing's disease. Excretion of 17-OHCS in patients with Cushing's syndrome associated with primary adrenocortical disease is not suppressed. This is also true of the vast majority of patients with ectopic ACTH syndrome. However, about half of patients with hypercortisolism associated with bronchial carcinoid tumors are reported to respond with decreased tumor secretion of ACTH and reduced urinary steroid excretion.[1025] This may rarely be true of other ectopic ACTH-secreting tumors, such as thymic carcinoid tumors and hepatomas.[1024] Taken together, these patients represent less than 5% of all patients with ectopic ACTH syndrome. As in the low-dose tests, plasma cortisol concentration responds similarly and reinforces the 17-OHCS results. Plasma ACTH levels provide a more definitive indication of etiology, because they should be significantly suppressed in Cushing's disease, and plasma dexamethasone concentrations provide information about compliance and steroid metabolism.

There are five common sources of error in the dexamethasone suppression tests: (1) improper urine collection; (2) day-to-day variation in hormone secretion by tumors, particularly by malignant pituitary and nonpituitary ACTH-secreting and cortisol-secreting adrenocortical tumors; (3) failure of the patient to take the dexamethasone; (4) abnormal metabolism of dexamethasone; and (5) application of improper criteria for normal suppression. The first of these errors can be detected by measuring creatinine excretion, the second can be detected only by serial baseline urine collections,[1109, 1110, 1622] and the third and fourth can be detected by measuring dexamethasone levels in blood a few hours after the last dose. The drugs that influence the metabolism of dexamethasone have already been discussed. Because cortisol may be less affected than fluorinated steroids such as dexamethasone, it has been suggested that a cortisol suppression test be substituted; in this case the index of suppression would be plasma corticosterone levels measured by radioimmunoassay, because exogenous cortisol cannot be distinguished from endogenous cortisol in the urinary 17-OHCS and free cortisol assays or the plasma cortisol assay.[1623] Like most other variations on the original dexamethasone suppression tests, this has not been widely applied.

As discussed earlier in this chapter, the last error is the result of misapplication of the original criteria for suppression in the high-dose dexamethasone suppression test.[1018] Although the urinary 17-OHCS and free cortisol excretion of most patients with Cushing's disease is suppressed by more than 50%, the higher the baseline ACTH and cortisol secretion, in general, the greater the resistance to suppression. In less than 5% of patients with Cushing's disease, higher dosages of dexamethasone (16 to 100 mg/d) are required to produce significant suppression. These patients tend to have large tumors. There are also rare reports of paradoxical responses to dexamethasone (i.e., cortisol secretion that increases, rather than decreases, in response to dexamethasone administration[1624]), but most of these are poorly documented in terms of reproducibility of the response. In only one well-documented case has the cause (spontaneous variation in tumor ACTH secretion) been defined.[1110] As in the other three cases with which we have

been acquainted (unpublished observations, D.N. Orth), this patient had a malignant pituitary tumor.

METYRAPONE TEST: THE RESPONSE TO HYPOCORTISOLEMIA. Rationale and Procedure. The rationale for the metyrapone test and the procedure for performing it have already been described. Although it was designed as a sensitive test of pituitary ACTH-secretory reserve, it can also be applied in the diagnosis of Cushing's syndrome.

Interpretation. Patients with Cushing's disease usually have a normal two- to fourfold increase in urinary 17-OHCS excretion and a large increase in plasma 11-deoxycortisol concentration. The rate of steroid production may be very high because it starts from a much greater baseline than normal. The reason for the increase is that (1) the microadenoma responds to hypocortisolemia with increased ACTH secretion and (2) the hyperplastic adrenal cortex is able to respond with still greater steroid production to increased ACTH stimulation (see Fig. 9–48D).

Patients with adrenal tumors and, presumably, other forms of primary adrenal hypersecretion almost always show a fall in urinary 17-OHCS excretion[1053] (see Fig. 9–53D). The decrease occurs because (1) the chronic hypercortisolemia has suppressed hypothalamic CRH and pituitary ACTH synthesis and secretion, (2) little ACTH is, therefore, released in response to hypocortisolemia, (3) adrenal carcinomas and about half of adenomas are unable to respond even to maximal ACTH stimulation, (4) the normal adrenal cortices are atrophic because of prolonged ACTH deficiency and are unable to respond acutely, and (5) metyrapone also blocks earlier steps in cortisol biosynthesis, so that total 17-OHCS excretion (THE, THF, and THS) is decreased.

Patients with ectopic ACTH syndrome are intermediate in their responses (see Fig. 9–50D). Although the tumors do not respond to hypocortisolemia with increased ACTH secretion, the hypercortisolemia is usually of short duration, hypothalamic-pituitary suppression is, therefore, incomplete so that the pituitary is able to secrete some ACTH, and the hyperplastic adrenals respond to even a small increment in plasma ACTH with increased cortisol secretion. These patients tend to have a less than normal response to metyrapone, but urinary 17-OHCS secretion rarely falls. Little has been published on patients with chronic ectopic ACTH syndrome associated with relatively indolent tumors, but in our experience these patients do not respond to metyrapone, presumably because the hypothalamic-pituitary axis is chronically and profoundly suppressed.

Thus in patients with dexamethasone-nonsuppressible Cushing's syndrome the metyrapone test tends to differentiate ACTH-dependent (ectopic ACTH syndrome) from ACTH-independent (primary adrenocortical disease) etiologies, with the exception of patients with chronic ectopic ACTH syndrome.

CORTICOTROPIN-RELEASING HORMONE STIMULATION TEST: THE PITUITARY RESPONSE TO CORTICOTROPIN-RELEASING HORMONE. Rationale. The concept underlying this test is that pituitary tumors that cause Cushing's disease respond to CRH[1131] (see Fig. 9–48E), whereas ectopic ACTH-secreting tumors do not respond (see Fig. 9–50E), and in these patients and those with adrenal tumors the suppressed pituitary gland is unable to respond (see Fig. 9–53E). Thus a normal response should differentiate Cushing's disease from all other causes of Cushing's syndrome.

Procedure. The procedure, which involves injecting synthetic ovine CRH (1 μg/kg body weight) IV, has already been described.

Interpretation. Most patients with Cushing's disease respond with a normal two- to fourfold increase in plasma ACTH levels 10 to 15 min after CRH injection.[797, 798, 1131–1134] The plasma cortisol response is more variable. The absolute

ACTH response tends to be exaggerated, although the percent increase above the elevated baseline is not much different from that in normal subjects (unpublished observations, D.N. Orth). Most patients with Cushing's syndrome related to adrenal tumors and most patients with ectopic ACTH syndrome do not respond to CRH.[797, 798, 1132–1134] There are, however, exceptions to these generalizations. About 5% of patients with Cushing's disease do not respond to CRH, but most of these patients respond to vasopressin (10 pressor units, intramuscular).[1135] Simultaneous administration of both agents elicits a plasma ACTH response in virtually all patients, and the response is synergistic. However, not enough patients with adrenal tumor or ectopic ACTH syndrome have been tested to assess the ability of the combined test to differentiate among the three common causes of Cushing's syndrome. Occasional patients with ectopic ACTH syndrome or primary adrenal disease respond, presumably because the hypothalamic-pituitary axis is not completely suppressed.

For these reasons and because it is a relatively expensive procedure, the CRH test should be considered an adjunct to the dexamethasone suppression tests and measurements of plasma ACTH and probably should be reserved to differentiate difficult cases of Cushing's disease and chronic ectopic ACTH syndrome.

INFERIOR PETROSAL VENOUS SAMPLING AFTER CRH STIMULATION: LOCALIZATION OF ACTH SECRETION. *Rationale.*

In most patients, pituitary venous blood drains into the cavernous sinuses and thence into the inferior petrosal veins (Fig. 9–64). Therefore, Cushing's disease patients, who have a pituitary source of excessive ACTH secretion, should demonstrate a central-to-peripheral gradient in ACTH concentration. Spontaneous ACTH secretion in Cushing's disease is pulsatile, reducing the probability of demonstrating a gradient, but one should be able to induce a secretory pulse in most patients by administering CRH. Furthermore, the drainage of the pituitary tends to lateralize,[1140, 1142] so it is sometimes possible to determine the side on which the microadenoma lies[1137, 1138, 1144] (Fig. 9–65).

Procedure. Catheters are inserted via the femoral vein into both inferior petrosal veins. It is important that each catheter be in the petrosal vein, not in the jugular bulb or vein, because of the tremendous dilution factor by blood returning from other areas of the cranium. A third IV access is placed in a peripheral vein. Before and 2, 5, 10, and 15 min after peripheral IV injection of ovine CRH (1 μg/kg body weight), blood samples are drawn simultaneously from all three sites for plasma ACTH radioimmunoassay. Some groups anticoagulate patients with heparin before the procedure and give protamine afterward to minimize the possibility of inferior petrosal and/or cavernous sinus venous thrombosis, but most do not think this is necessary.

Interpretation. A central-to-peripheral ACTH gradient of twofold or more is probably significant, although the gradient is usually greater (see Fig. 9–65). The gradient is usually greatest within 10 min of injecting CRH because of the progressive accumulation of ACTH in the peripheral circulation. Although one group finds strong lateralization of secretion that predicts tumor location,[1138] we and others[1144] have not found such a strong predictive value.

One must, for the present, retain some reservations about this test. In the 5 to 10% of Cushing's patients who do not respond to CRH, the test presumably will be negative unless one happens to encounter a spontaneous secretory episode. This problem may be circumvented by the simultaneous administration of 10 pressor units of vasopressin together with CRH. In the occasional patients with ectopic ACTH syndrome and adrenal tumors who respond to CRH, one must assume that the ACTH is coming from the pituitary. Therefore, one would anticipate false-positive results in a catheterization study. In fact, one might predict that any patient with ectopic ACTH syndrome who responded to metyrapone with increased steroid production would respond to CRH and have a false-positive catheterization result. With respect to lateralization, most corticotrope adenomas are said to lie near the midline.[1145] Thus it is surprising that venous drainage predicts location so accurately.[1138] Because there is a 50% chance of correctly predicting the location without the aid of any anatomical data, this expensive, invasive, and potentially dangerous procedure cannot be justified on this basis alone.

This test probably should be reserved for the differential diagnosis of difficult cases of Cushing's disease versus ectopic ACTH syndrome. Another candidate is the patient with results diagnostic of Cushing's disease who has undergone subtotal or total hypophysectomy without any effect on ACTH secretion.

ACTH STIMULATION TEST: THE ADRENOCORTICAL RESPONSE TO ACTH.

Patients with Cushing's disease or ectopic ACTH syndrome respond briskly to exogenous ACTH (see Figs. 9–48F and 9–50F) because there is bilateral adrenocortical hyperplasia in both conditions. Patients with Cushing's syndrome caused by adrenal carcinoma virtually never have a normal response to ACTH (see Fig. 9–53F) because the tumors do not respond and the normal adrenal cortices are atrophic.[1053] However, patients with adrenal carcinoma who do not have hypercortisolism may have an intact hypothalamic-pituitary-adrenal axis, and the normal adrenal cortex may, therefore, respond normally. A little over half of adrenal adenomas that cause Cushing's syndrome will respond, sometimes dramatically, to ACTH.[1053] This test has little or no place in the evaluation of the Cushing's patient.

INSULIN-INDUCED HYPOGLYCEMIA TEST.

It was once claimed[1073] that the failure of the pituitary to respond to hypoglycemia with increased secretion of GH and ACTH (cortisol) was a unique feature of Cushing's disease. In fact, this response is characteristic of chronic hypercortisolemia of all etiologies.[1080] Presumably, for the same reason, severely depressed patients, who have mild hypercortisolemia of relatively short duration, were thought to respond normally

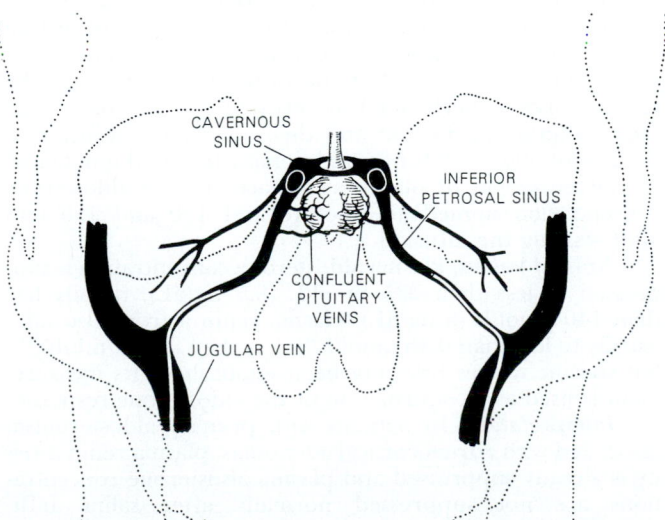

Figure 9–64. Anatomy of the venous drainage of the pituitary gland via the inferior petrosal venous sinuses. (From Oldfield EH, Chrousos GP, Schulte HM, et al. Preoperative lateralization of ACTH-secreting pituitary microadenomas by bilateral and simultaneous inferior petrosal venous sinus sampling. Reprinted, by permission of The New England Journal of Medicine, 312; 100–103, 1985.)

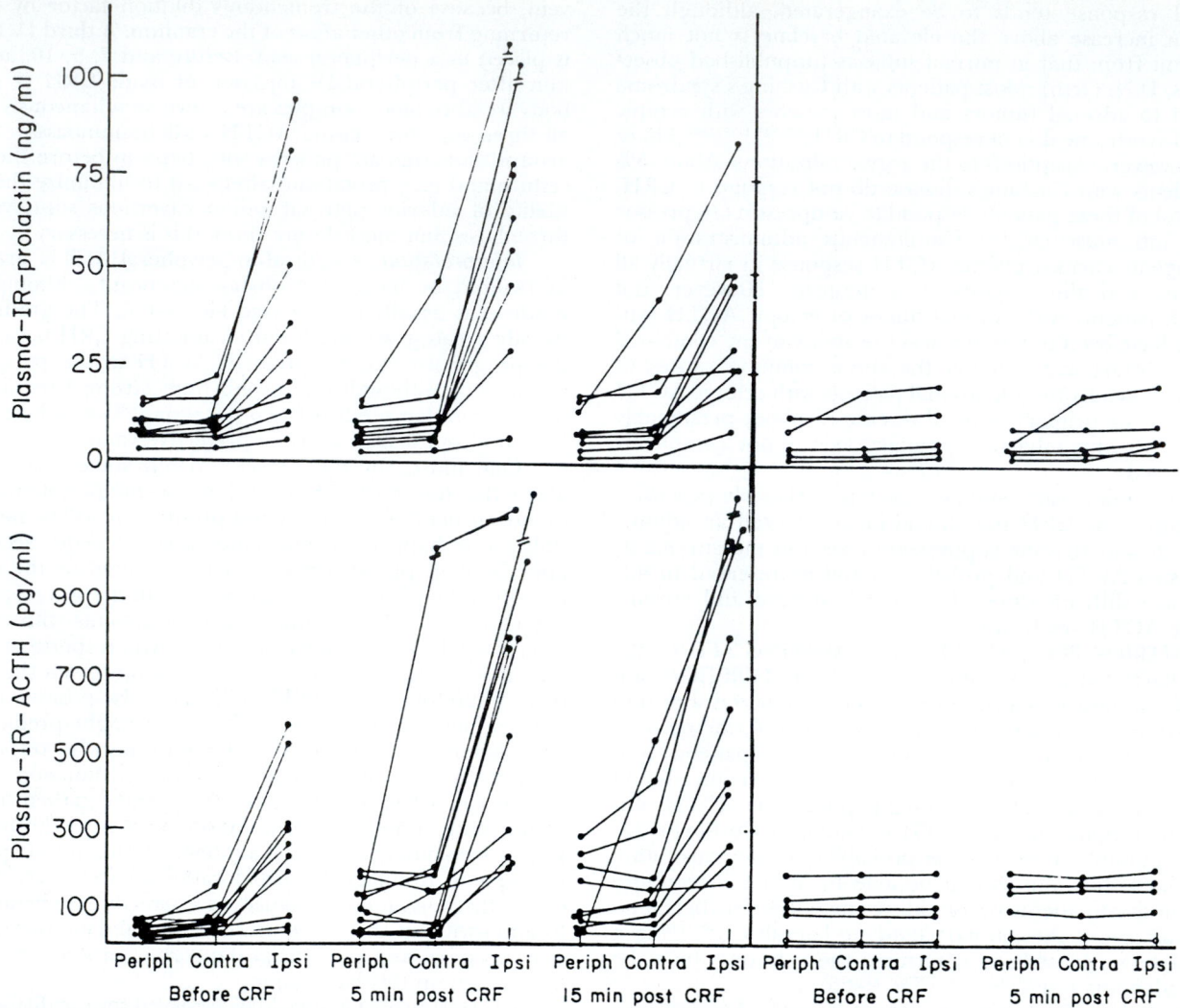

Figure 9–65. Lateralization of a microadenoma causing Cushing's disease by simultaneous inferior petrosal venous sampling for ACTH and prolactin before and after stimulation with CRH (CRF). (From Schulte HM, Allolio B, Günther RW, et al. Selective bilateral and simultaneous catheterization of the inferior petrosal sinus: CRF stimulates prolactin secretion from ACTH-producing microadenomas in Cushing's disease. Clin Endocrinol 1988; 28:289–295.)

to hypoglycemia, although a blunted GH response is now known to occur in many, at least in depressed postmenopausal women.[1624a] The response is also blunted in alcoholics.[1625] The test is nonspecific and has no place in the evaluation of patients with suspected Cushing's syndrome of any cause.

Tests for Evaluating Adrenocortical Hypersecretion: Hyperaldosteronism

SALINE SUPPRESSION TEST. *Rationale.* In the normal individual and in patients with essential hypertension, supine posture and acute expansion of the plasma volume increase renal perfusion and suppress release of renin, decrease conversion of angiotensinogen to angiotensin I, and, because of decreased generation of angiotensin II, decrease secretion of aldosterone (see Fig. 9–16). In patients with autonomously functioning aldosterone-secreting tumors, however, normal suppression is not observed.

Procedure. There are two accepted procedures for performing this test. Both are started before 9 AM in patients who have had no more than a light breakfast and who have normal serum potassium concentrations. In the preferred

test, normal saline solution is infused IV at a rate of 500 mL/h for 4 h. Blood is obtained for determination of plasma renin activity and aldosterone concentration immediately before and 2 and 4 h after the infusion is begun.[1329] The test can also be performed by infusing 500 mL of normal saline solution in 30 min and then continuing infusion at the rate of 500 mL/h for an additional 2 h. Blood is obtained for measurement of plasma renin activity and aldosterone concentration immediately before and 120 and 150 min after starting the infusion.

Normal Values. Plasma aldosterone concentration is suppressed to less than 235 pmol/L (8.5 ng/dL), usually less than 140 pmol/L (5 ng/dL). Plasma renin activity also falls, usually to less than 0.46 nmol/L/h (less than 0.6 ng/mL/h),[1331] but specific ranges have not been established. Its measurement is used as a confirmation of the aldosterone response.

Interpretation. In patients with primary aldosteronism associated with adrenocortical adenomas, plasma renin activity is already suppressed and plasma alsosterone concentrations are not suppressed normally after saline infusion.[1306, 1329] Hypokalemia can decrease aldosterone secretion in these patients.

The evaluation of endocrine hypertension is discussed in detail in Chapter 11.

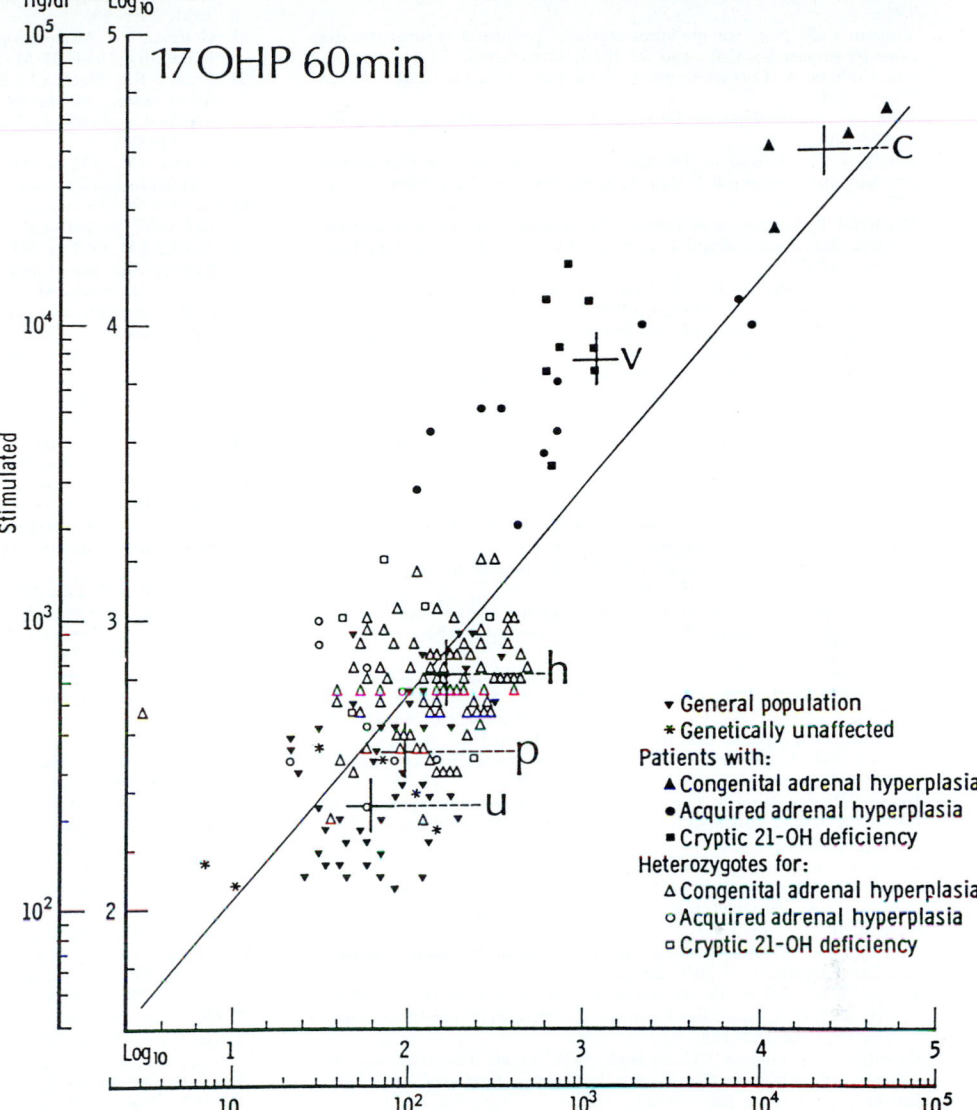

Figure 9–66. Basal and stimulated plasma 17α-hydroxyprogesterone (17 OHP) concentrations in patients with P-450_{c21} enzyme (21-hydroxylase) deficiency. To convert to nanomoles per liter, multiply by 0.0303. The mean for each group is indicated by a large cross and the adjacent letter: h, heterozygotes for all forms of P-450_{c21} deficiency; p, general population; u, known unaffected persons (e.g., siblings of patients with P-450_{c21} deficiency who carry neither affected parental haplotype as determined by HLA typing). (From White PC, New MI, Dupont B. Congenital adrenal hyperplasia. Part 1. Reprinted, by permission of The New England Journal of Medicine, 316; 1519–1524, 1987.)

Tests for the Diagnosis of Adrenocortical Hypersecretion: Hyperandrogenism

The effects of the several varieties of congenital adrenal hyperplasia on basal adrenocortical secretion have already been discussed.

ONE-HOUR ACTH STIMULATION TEST. *Rationale.* In the evaluation of hirsutism, the possibility of mild P-450_{c21} deficiency must be considered,[1382, 1383] although its incidence in the general population is low compared with that in unique groups such as Ashkenazi Jews[1398] and Eskimos.[1385, 1386] In some such patients, basal adrenal androgen levels are within the normal range, but the defect can be unmasked by acutely stimulating the adrenal cortex with pharmacological amounts of ACTH and measuring the abnormal production of the cortisol precursor 17α-hydroxy-progesterone.

Procedure. The test is conducted exactly like the 1-h ACTH (cosyntropin) test described earlier, except that blood is sampled immediately before and 30 to 60 min after the injection of cosyntropin for measurement of 17α-hydroxy-progesterone.

Interpretation. Basal and stimulated 17α-hydroxyprogesterone concentrations are compared with those of normal subjects (Fig. 9–66). Patients whose concentrations exceed normal limits may be considered to have mild "adult-onset" P-450_{c21} deficiency. According to some investigators, its incidence may be as high as 12% in hirsute women,[1418] but this appears to reflect experience with an ethnic subset. In our experience and that of others, the incidence appears to be lower. It should also be noted that there is a linear relationship between basal and stimulated plasma 17α-hydroxyprogesterone concentrations. Theoretically, therefore, basal levels should be as useful as stimulated ones for establishing this diagnosis.

The evaluation of virilizing syndromes is discussed in detail in Chapters 12 and 14.

REFERENCES

1. Eustachius B. Tabulae Anatomicae. Lancisius B, ed. Amsterdam, 1774.
2. Gaunt R. History of the adrenal cortex. In: Greep RO, Astwood EB, eds. Handbook of Physiology. Sect 7: Endocrinology. Vol VI. Adrenal Gland. Washington, DC: American Physiological Society, 1975: 1–12.
3. Medvei VC. A History of Endocrinology. Bath: Pitman, 1982.
4. Page DL, DeLellis RA, Hough AJ Jr. Tumors of the adrenal. In: Hartmann WH, Sobin LH, eds. Atlas of Tumor Pathology. 2nd ser. Fasc 23. Washington, DC: Armed Forces Institute of Pathology, 1986.
5. Schoenwetter HP. Zur Vorgeschichte der Endokrinologie. Zürcher

medizingeschichtliche Abhandlungen, Neue Reihe Nr 61. Juris Druck, 1968.

6. Vulpian EFA. Note sur quelques réactions propres à la substance des capsules surrenales. C R Acad Sci 1856; 43:663–665.

7. von Kölliker A. Entwicklungsgeschichte des Menschen und hoheren Thiere. 1861.

8. Kohn A. Das chromaffine Gewebe. Z Anat Entwicklungsgesch 1902; 12:253–348.

9. Arnold J. Ein Beitrag zu der feineren Structur und dem Chemismus der Nebennieren. Arch Pathol Anat Physiol Klin Med 1866; 35:64–107.

10. Bartholin T. Anatomica ex Caspari Bartholini Parentis Institutionibus. Lugdini Batavorum: Apud Fraciseum Hackium, 1651. London: John Streeter, 1668.

11. de Bordeu T. Recherches Anatomiques sur la Position des Glandes et sur Leur Action. Paris: Quillau, 1752.

12. Carpenter WB. Cyclopaedia of Anatomy and Physiology. Todd RB, ed. Vol IV. London, 1852.

13. Bernard C. Remarques sur la sécrétion du sucre dans le foie faites à l'occasion de la communication de M. Lehmann. C R Acad Sci 1855; 40:589–592.

14. Schäfer EA. Address in physiology on internal secretions. Lancet 1895; 2:321–324.

15. Addison T. On anaemia: disease of the supra-renal capsules. Lond Med Gaz 1849; 517–518.

16. Addison T. On the Constitutional and Local Effects of Disease of the Supra-Renal Capsules. London: Highley, 1855.

17. Trousseau A. Capsules surrenales, maladie bronze d'Addison. Arch Gen Med 1856; Ser 5, No 8:478–481.

18. Brown-Sequard CE. Recherches expérimentales sur la physiologie et la pathologie des capsules surrenales. Arch Gen Med 1856; Ser 5, No 8:385–401.

19. Szymonowicz L. Die Function der Nebenniere. Pflugers Arch Gesamte Physiol Menschen Tiere 1896; 64:97–164.

20. Abel JJ, Crawford AC. On the blood-pressure-raising constituent of the suprarenal capsule. Bull Johns Hopkins Hosp 1897; 8:151–157.

21. Aldrich TB. A preliminary report on the active principle of the suprarenal gland. Am J Physiol 1919; 5:457–461.

22. Wheeler TD, Vincent S. The question as to the relative importance to life of the cortex and medulla of the adrenal bodies. Trans Soc Can 1917; 11:125–127.

23. Houssay BA, Lewis JT. The relative importance to life of cortex and medulla of the adrenal glands. Am J Physiol 1923; 64:513–521.

24. Hartman FA, Brownell KA. The hormone of the adrenal cortex. Science 1930; 72:76.

25. Hartman FA, Thorn GW. A biological method for the assay of cortin. Proc Soc Exp Biol Med 1930; 28:94–95.

26. Swingle WW, Pfiffner JJ. Studies on the adrenal cortex. I. The effect of a lipid fraction upon the life-span of adrenalectomized cats. Am J Physiol 1931; 96:153–163.

27. Rowntree LG, Greene CH, Swingle WW, et al. The treatment of patients with Addison's disease with the "cortical hormone" of Swingle and Pfiffner. Science 1930; 72:482–483.

28. von Steiger M, Reichstein T. Desoxy-cortico-steron (21-oxyproges-teron) aus Δ5-3-oxy-atiocholensaure. Helv Chim Acta 1937; 20:1164–1179.

29. Marshall EK, Davis DM. The influence of adrenals on the kidneys. J Pharmacol Exp Ther 1916; 8:525–550.

30. Marine D, Baumann EJ. Duration of life after suprarenalectomy in cats and attempts to prolong it by injections of solutions containing sodium salts, glucose and glycerol. Am J Physiol 1927; 81:86–100.

31. Simpson SA, Tait JF. Recent progress in methods of isolation, chemistry, and physiology of aldosterone. Recent Prog Horm Res 1955; 11:183–210.

32. Schmidlin J, Anner G, Billeter JR, et al. Uber Synthesen in der aldosteron-reihe. I. Total Syntheses des racemischen Aldosterons. Experientia 1955; 11:365–368.

33. Smith PE. Hypophysectomy and a replacement therapy in the rat. Am J Anat 1930; 45:205–273.

34. Ingle DJ, Kendall EC. Atrophy of the adrenal cortex of the rat produced by the administration of large amounts of cortin. Science 1937; 86:245.

35. Graf L, Bajusz S, Patthy A, et al. Revised amide location for porcine and human adrenocorticotropic hormone. Acta Biochim Biophys Acad Sci Hung 1971; 6:415–418.

36. Harris GW. Neural control of the pituitary gland. Physiol Rev 1948; 28:139–179.

37. Vale W, Spiess J, Rivier C, et al. Characterization of a 41-residue ovine hypothalamic peptide that stimulates secretion of corticotropin and beta-endorphin. Science 1981; 213:1394–1397.

38. Hench PS, Kendall EC, Slocumb CH, et al. The effect of a hormone of the adrenal cortex (17-hydroxy-11-dehydrocorticosterone; compound E) and of pituitary adrenocorticotropic hormone on rheumatoid arthritis. Mayo Clin Proc 1949; 24:181–197.

39. Russell RP, Masi AT, Richter ED. Adrenal cortical adenomas and hypertension. Medicine 1972; 51:211–225.

40. Tähkä H. On the weight and structure of the adrenal glands and the factors affecting them in children of 0–2 years. Acta Paediatr Scand 1951; 40:1–95.

41. Gelfman NA. Morphologic changes of adrenal cortex in disease. Yale J Biol Med 1964; 37:31–54.

42. Russell RP, Masi AT, Richter ED. Adrenal cortical adenomas and hypertension. A clinical and pathologic analysis of 690 cases with matched controls and a review of the literature. Medicine 1972; 51:211–225.

43. Neville AM, O'Hare MJ. Histopathology of the human adrenal cortex. Clin Endocrinol Metab 1985; 14:791–820.

44. Gagnon R. The arterial supply of the human adrenal gland. Rev Can Biol 1957; 16:421–433.

45. Neville AM, O'Hare MJ. The Human Adrenal Cortex. Pathology and Biology—An Integrated Approach. Berlin: Springer-Verlag, 1982.

46. Hamaji M, Miyata M, Kawashima Y. A study of the vascular arrangement of the rat adrenal gland using non-radioactive microspheres. Cell Tissue Res 1985; 240:277–280.

47. Coupland RE, Dobbie JW, Symington T. Blood supply of the adrenal gland. In: Greep RO, Astwood EB, eds. Handbook of Physiology. Sect 7: Endocrinology. Vol VI. Adrenal Gland. Washington, DC: American Physiological Society, 1975: 283–294.

48. Dobbie JW, Symington T. The human adrenal gland with special reference to the vasculature. J Endocrinol 1966; 34:479–489.

49. Gagnon R. The venous drainage of the human adrenal gland. Rev Can Biol 1956; 14:350–359.

50. Monkhouse WS, Khalique A. The adrenal and renal veins of man and their connections with azygos and lumbar veins. J Anat 1986; 146:105–115.

51. Engeland WE, Lilly MP, Gann DS. Sympathetic adrenal denervation decreases adrenal blood flow without altering the cortisol response to hemorrhage. Endocrinology 1985; 117:1000–1010.

52. Holzwarth MA. The distribution of vasoactive intestinal peptide in the rat adrenal cortex and medulla. J Auton Nerv Syst 1984; 11:269–283.

53. Bornstein SR, Ehrhart-Bornstein M, Scherbaum WA, et al. Effects of splanchnic nerve stimulation on the adrenal cortex may be mediated by chromaffin cells in a paracrine manner. Endocrinology 1990; 127:900–906.

54. Holzwarth MA, Cunningham LA, Kleitman N. The role of adrenal nerves in the regulation of adrenocortical functions. Ann NY Acad Sci 1987; 512:449–464.

55. Dallman MF. Adrenal feedback on stress-induced corticoliberin (CRF) and corticotropin (ACTH) secretion. In: Jones MT, Gillham B, Dallman MF, et al., eds. Interaction Within the Brain-Pituitary-Adrenocortical System. New York: Academic, 1979: 149–162.

56. Carr BR, Parker CR Jr, Porter JC, et al. Regulation of steroid secretion by adrenal tissue of a human anencephalic fetus. J Clin Endocrinol Metab 1980; 50:870–873.

57. Odagiri E, Sherrell BJ, Mount CD, et al. Human placental immuno-reactive corticotropin, lipotropin and β-endorphin: evidence for a common precursor. Proc Natl Acad Sci USA 1979; 76:2027–2031.

58. Liddle GW, Island D, Rinfret AP, et al. Factors enhancing the response of the human adrenal to corticotropin: is there an adrenal growth factor? J Clin Endocrinol Metab 1954; 14:839–858.

59. Estivariz FE, Morano MI, Carino M, et al. Adrenal regeneration in the rat is mediated by mitogenic N-terminal pro-opiomelanocortin peptides generated by changes in precursor processing in the anterior pituitary. J Endocrinol 1988; 116:207–216.

60. Estivariz FE, Iturriza F, McLean C, et al. Stimulation of adrenal mitogenesis by N-terminal proopiocortin peptides. Nature 1982; 297:419–422.

61. Hornsby PJ, Sturek M, Harris SE, et al. Serum and growth factor requirements for proliferation of human adrenocortical cells in culture: comparison with bovine adrenocortical cells. In Vitro 1983; 19:863–869.

62. Skelton FR. Adrenal regeneration and adrenal regeneration hypertension. Physiol Rev 1959; 39:162–182.

63. Belloni AS, Neri G, Musajo FG, et al. Investigations on the morphology and function of adrenocortical tissue regenerated from gland capsular fragments autotransplanted in the musculus gracilis of the rat. Endocrinology 1990; 126:3251–3262.

64. Long JA. Zonation of the mammalian adrenal cortex. In: Greep RO, Astwood EB, eds. Handbook of Physiology. Sect 7: Endocrinology. Vol VI. Adrenal Gland. Washington, DC: American Physiological Society, 1975: 13–24.

65. Zajicek G, Ariel I, Arber N. The streaming adrenal cortex: direct evidence of centripetal migration of adrenocytes by estimation of cell turnover rate. J Endocrinol 1986; 111:477–482.

66. Hornsby PJ. Physiological and pathological effects of steroids on the function of the adrenal cortex. J Steroid Biochem 1987; 27:1161–1171.

67. Mazzocchi G, Nussdorfer GG. Neuropeptide-Y acutely stimulates rat zona glomerulosa in vivo. Neuropeptides 1987; 9:257–262.

68. Gill GN. ACTH regulation of the adrenal cortex. In: Gill GN, ed. Pharmacology of Adrenal Cortical Hormones. New York: Pergamon, 1979: 35.

69. Riondel AM, Rebuffat P, Mazzochi G, et al. Long-term effects of

ACTH combined with angiotensin II on steroidogenesis and adrenal zona glomerulosa morphology in the rat. Acta Endocrinol 1987; 114:47–54.

70. Temple TE Jr, Jones DJ Jr, Liddle GW, et al. Treatment of Cushing's disease. Correction of hypercortisolism by o,p'DDD without induction of aldosterone deficiency. N Engl J Med 1969; 281:801–805.

71. Dallman MF. Control of adrenocortical growth in vivo. Endocr Res 1984; 10:213–242.

72. IUPAC. Definitive rules for the nomenclature of steroids. J Am Chem Soc 1960; 82:5577–5581.

73. IUPAC. Definitive rules for the nomenclature of steroids. Pure Appl Chem 1972; 31:285–322.

74. Borkowski AJ, Levin S, Delcroix C, et al. Blood cholesterol and hydrocortisone production in man: quantitative aspects of the utilization of circulating cholesterol by the adrenals at rest and under adrenocorticotropin stimulation. J Clin Invest 1967; 46:797–811.

75. Bolt E, Coudert S, Lefebvre Y. Steroid production from plasma cholesterol. II. In vivo conversion of plasma cholesterol to ovarian progesterone and adrenal C_{19} and C_{21} steroids in humans. J Clin Endocrinol Metab 1967; 38:394–400.

76. Gwynne JT, Strauss JF. The role of lipoprotein in steroidogenesis and cholesterol metabolism in steroidogenic glands. Endocr Rev 1982; 3:299–329.

77. Faust JR, Goldstein JL, Brown MS. Receptor-mediated uptake of low density lipoprotein and utilization of its cholesterol for steroid synthesis in cultured mouse adrenal cells. J Biol Chem 1977; 252:4861–4871.

78. Kovanen PT, Schneider WJ, Hillman GM, et al. Separate mechanisms for the uptake of high and low density lipoproteins by the mouse adrenal in vivo. J Biol Chem 1979; 254:5498–5505.

79. Brown MS, Kovanen PT, Goldstein JL. Receptor-mediated uptake of lipoprotein-cholesterol and its utilization for steroid synthesis in the adrenal cortex. Recent Prog Horm Res 1979; 35:215–257.

80. Kita T, Beiseigel U, Goldstein JL, et al. Antibody against low density lipoprotein receptor blocks uptake of low density lipoprotein (but not high density lipoprotein) by the adrenal gland of the mouse in vivo. J Biol Chem 1981; 256:4701–4703.

81. Kovanen PT, Brown MS, Goldstein JL. Increased binding of low density lipoprotein to liver membranes from rats treated with 17α-ethinyl estradiol. J Biol Chem 1979; 254:11367–11373.

82. Windler EET, Kovanen PT, Chao YS, et al. The estradiol-stimulated lipoprotein receptor of rat liver. A binding site that mediates the uptake of rat lipoproteins containing apoproteins B and E. J Biol Chem 1980; 255:10464–10471.

83. Kovanen PT, Goldstein JL, Chappel DA, et al. Regulation of low density lipoprotein receptors by adrenocorticotropin in the adrenal glands of mice and rats in vivo. J Biol Chem 1980; 255:5591–5598.

84. Kovanen PT, Faust JR, Brown MS, et al. Low density lipoprotein receptors in bovine adrenal cortex. I. Receptor-mediated uptake of low density lipoprotein and utilization of its cholesterol for steroid synthesis in cultured adrenocortical cells. Endocrinology 1979; 104:599–609.

85. Kovanen PT, Basu S, Goldstein JL, et al. Low density lipoprotein receptors in bovine adrenal cortex. II. Low density lipoprotein binding to membranes prepared from fresh tissue. Endocrinology 1979; 104:610–616.

86. Kovanen PT, Bilheimer DW, Goldstein JL, et al. Regulatory role for hepatic low density lipoprotein in the dog. Proc Natl Acad Sci USA 1981; 78:1194–1198.

87. Kita T, Brown MS, Watanabe Y, et al. Deficiency of low density lipoprotein receptors in liver and adrenal gland of the WHHL rabbit, an animal model of familial hypercholesterolemia. Proc Natl Acad Sci USA 1981; 78:2268–2272.

88. Goldstein JL, Anderson RGW, Brown MS. Coated pits, coated vesicles, and receptor-mediated endocytosis. Nature 1979; 279:679–685.

89. Gwynne JT, Hess B. The role of high density lipoproteins in rat adrenal cholesterol metabolism and steroidogenesis. J Biol Chem 1980; 255:10875–10883.

90. Gwynne JT, Hess B. Binding and degradation of human ^{125}I HDL by rat adrenal cortical cells. Metabolism 1978; 27:1593–1600.

91. Illingworth DR, Kenny TA, Orwoll ES. Adrenal function in heterozygous and homozygous hypobetalipoproteinemia. J Clin Endocrinol Metab 1982; 54:27–33.

92. Illingworth DR, Orwoll ES, Connor WE. Impaired cortisol secretion in abetalipoproteinemia. J Clin Endocrinol Metab 1980; 50:977–979.

93. Illingworth DR, Lees AM, Lees RS. Adrenal cortical function in homozygous familial hypercholesterolemia. Metabolism 1983; 32:1045–1052.

94. Shima S, Mitsunaga M, Nakao T. Effect of ACTH on cholesterol dynamics in rat adrenal tissue. Endocrinology 1972; 98:808–814.

95. Beins DM, Vining R, Balasubramanian S. Regulation of neutral cholesterol esterase and acyl-CoA: cholesterol acyltransferase in the rat adrenal gland. Biochem J 1982; 202:631–637.

96. Miller W. Molecular biology of steroid hormone biosynthesis. Endocr Rev 1988; 9:295–318.

97. Strott CA. The search for the elusive adrenal steroidogenic "regulatory" protein. Trends Endocrinol Metab 1990; 1:312–314.

98. Noland BJ, Arebalo RE, Hansbury E, et al. Purification and properties of sterol carrier protein. J Biol Chem 1980; 255:4282–4289.

99. Chanderbhan R, Tanaka T, Strauss JF, et al. Evidence for sterol-carrier protein 2–like activity in hepatic, adrenal and ovarian cytosol. Biochem Biophys Res Commun 1983; 117:702–709.

100. Pedersen RC, Brownie AC. Cholesterol side-chain cleavage in the rat adrenal cortex: isolation of a cycloheximide-sensitive activator peptide. Proc Natl Acad Sci USA 1983; 80:1882–1886.

101. Pedersen RC, Brownie AC. Steroidogenesis-activator polypeptide isolated from a rat Leydig cell tumor. Science 1987; 236:188–190.

102. Yanagibashi K, Ohno Y, Kawamura M, et al. The regulation of intracellular transport of cholesterol in bovine adrenal cells: purification of a novel protein. Endocrinology 1988; 123:2075–2082.

103. Roberts KD, Bandy L, Lieberman S. The occurrence and metabolism of 20α-hydroxycholesterol in bovine adrenal preparations. Biochemistry 1969; 8:1259–1270.

104. Dixon R, Furutachi T, Lieberman S. The isolation of crystalline 22R-hydroxycholesterol and 20α, 22R-dihydroxycholesterol from bovine adrenals. Biochem Biophys Res Commun 1970; 40:161–166.

105. Hume T, Boyd GS. Cholesterol metabolism and steroid hormone production. Biochem Soc Trans 1978; 6:893–898.

106. Larroque C, Rousseau J, Van Lier JE. Enzyme-bound sterols of bovine adrenocortical cytochrome P-450scc. Biochemistry 1981; 20:925–929.

107. Lieberman S, Greenfield NJ, Wolfson A. A heuristic proposal for understanding steroidogenic processes. Endocr Rev 1984; 5:128–148.

108. Shikita M, Hall PF. Cytochrome P-450 from bovine adrenocortical mitochondria: an enzyme for the side chain cleavage of cholesterol. II. Subunit structure. J Biol Chem 1973; 248:5598–5604.

109. Takemori S, Suhara K, Hashimoto S, et al. Purification of cytochrome P450 from bovine adrenocortical mitochondria by an "aniline-Sepharose" and the properties. Biochem Biophys Res Commun 1975; 63:588–593.

110. Wang HP, Kimura T. Purification and characterization of the adrenal cortex mitochondrial cytochrome P450 specific for cholesterol side-chain cleavage activity. J Biol Chem 1976; 251:6068–6074.

111. Tilley BE, Watanuki M, Hall PF. Preparation and properties of side-chain cleavage cytochrome P-450 from bovine adrenal cortex by affinity chromatography with pregnenolone as ligand. Biochim Biophys Acta 1977; 493:260–271.

112. John ME, John MC, Ashley P, et al. Identification and characterization of cDNA clones specific for cholesterol side-chain cleavage cytochrome P-450. Proc Natl Acad Sci USA 1984; 81:5628–5632.

113. Chung B, Matteson KJ, Voutilainen R, et al. Human cholesterol side-chain cleavage enzyme, P450scc: cDNA cloning, assignment of the gene to chromosome 15, and expression in the placenta. Proc Natl Acad Sci USA 1986; 83:8962–8966.

114. Kimura T, Suzuki K. Components of the electron transport system in adrenal steroid hydroxylase. Isolation and properties of non-heme iron protein (adrenodoxin). J Biol Chem 1967; 242:485–491.

115. Morel Y, Picardo-Leonard J, Wu DA, et al. Assignment of the functional gene for adrenodoxin to chromosome 11q1.3–qterm and two adrenodoxin pseudogenes to chromosome 20cent–q13.1. Am J Hum Genet 1988; 43:52–59.

116. Solish SB, Picardo-Leonard J, Morel Y, et al. Human adrenodoxin reductase: two mRNAs encoded by a single gene on chromosome 17cen–q25 are expressed in steroidogenic tissues. Proc Natl Acad Sci USA 1988; 85:7104–7108.

117. Suhara K, Nakayama K, Takikawa O, et al. Two forms of adrenodoxin reductase from mitochondria of bovine adrenal cortex. Eur J Biochem 1982; 125:659–664.

118. Ishi-Ohba H, Juano H, Tamaoki B. Purification and properties of testicular 3β-hydroxy-5-ene steroid dehydrogenase and 5-ene–4-ene isomerase. J Steroid Biochem 1986; 25:555–560.

119. Ewald W, Werbin H, Chaikoff IL. Evidence for two substrate-specific delta⁵-3-ketosteroid isomerases in beef adrenal glands, and their separation from 3β-hydroxysteroid dehydrogenase. Biochim Biophys Acta 1964; 81:199–201.

120. Nakajin S, Hall PF. Microsomal cytochrome P450 from neonatal pig testis. J Biol Chem 1981; 256:3871–3896.

121. Nakajin S, Hall PF, Onoda M. Testicular microsomal cytochrome P450 for C_{21} steroid side chain cleavage. J Biol Chem 1981; 256:6134–6139.

122. Nakajin S, Shively JE, Yuan P, et al. Microsomal cytochrome P450 from the neonatal pig testis: two enzymatic activities (17α-hydroxylase and C17,20 lyase) associated with one protein. Biochemistry 1981; 20:4037–4042.

123. Zuber MX, Simpson ER, Waterman MR. Expression of bovine 17α-hydroxylase cytochrome P-450 cDNA in nonsteroidogenic (COS-1) cells. Science 1986; 234:1258–1261.

124. Kominami S, Ochi H, Koboyashi T, et al. Studies on the steroid hydroxylation system in adrenal cortex microsomes: purification and characterization of the cytochrome P450 specific for steroid 21 hydroxylation. J Biol Chem 1980; 255:3386–3394.

125. Estabrook RW, Franklin MR, Cohen B. Influence of hepatic microsomal mixed function oxidation reactions on cellular metabolic control. Metabolism 1971; 20:187–199.

126. Onoda M, Hall PF. Cytochrome b_5 stimulates purified testicular micro-

somal cytochrome P450 (C_{21} side-chain cleavage). Biochem Biophys Res Commun 1982; 108:454–460.

127. Yanigabashi K, Hall PF. Role of electron transport in the regulation of lyase activity of C_{21} side-chain cleavage P450 from porcine adrenal and testicular microsomes. J Biol Chem 1986; 261:8429–8433.

128. Chung B, Matteson KJ, Miller WL. Cloning and characterization of the bovine gene for steroid 21-hydroxylase (P450$_{c21}$). DNA 1985; 4:211–219.

129. White PC, New MI, Dupont B. Cloning and expression of cDNA encoding a bovine adrenal cytochrome P450 specific for steroid 21-hydroxylation. Proc Natl Acad Sci USA 1984; 81:1986–1990.

130. White PC, Chaplin DD, Weis JH, et al. Two steroid 21-hydroxylase genes are located in the murine S region. Nature 1984; 312:465–467.

131. Amor M, Tosi M, Duponchel C, et al. Liver cDNA probes disclose two cytochrome P450 genes duplicated in tandem with the complement C4 loci of the mouse H2-S region. Proc Natl Acad Sci USA 1985; 82:4453–4457.

132. Yoshioka H, Morohashi K, Sogawa K, et al. Structural analysis of cloned cDNA for mRNA of microsomal cytochrome P450 (C_{21}) which catalyzes steroid 21-hydroxylation in bovine adrenal cortex. J Biol Chem 1986; 261:4106–4109.

133. White PC, New MI, Dupont B. HLA-linked congenital adrenal hyperplasia results from a defective gene encoding a cytochrome P450 specific for steroid 21-hydroxylation. Proc Natl Acad Sci USA 1984; 81:7505–7509.

134. Chu JW, Kimura T. Molecular and catalytic properties of adrenodoxin reductase (a flavoprotein). J Biol Chem 1973; 248:2089–2094.

135. Suhara K, Kamayama K, Takemori S, et al. Bovine adrenal steroid hydroxylase system. III. Reconstitution of adrenal iron-sulfur protein. Biochim Biophys Acta 1974; 336:309–317.

136. John ME, John MC, Simpson ER, et al. Regulation of cytochrome P-450–11β gene expression by adrenocorticotropin. J Biol Chem 1985; 260:5760–5767.

137. Chua SC, Szabo P, Vitek A, et al. Cloning of cDNA encoding steroid 11β-hydroxylase P450c11. Proc Natl Acad Sci USA 1987; 84:7193–7197.

138. Morohashi K, Yoshioka H, Gotoh O, et al. Molecular cloning and nucleotide sequencing of DNA of mitochondrial P450 (11β) of bovine adrenal cortex. J Biochem (Tokyo) 1987; 102:559–568.

139. Yanigabashi K, Haniu M, Shively JE, et al. The synthesis of aldosterone by the adrenal cortex. Two zones (fasciculata and glomerulosa) possess one enzyme for 11β-, 18-hydroxylation, and aldehyde synthesis. J Biol Chem 1986; 261:3556–3562.

140. Lauber M, Sugano S, Ohnishi T, et al. Aldosterone biosynthesis and cytochrome P450 11β: evidence for two different forms of the enzyme in rats. J Steroid Biochem 1987; 26:693–698.

141. Ohnishi T, Wada A, Lauber M, et al. Aldosterone biosynthesis in mitochondria of isolated zones of adrenal cortex. J Steroid Biochem 1988; 31:73–81.

142. Ogishima T, Mitani F, Ishimura Y. Isolation of aldosterone synthase cytochrome P450 from zona glomerulosa mitochondria of rat adrenal cortex. J Biol Chem 1989; 264:10935–10938.

143. McPhaul MJ, Noble JF, Simpson ER, et al. The expression of a functional cDNA encoding the chicken cytochrome P450$_{arom}$ (aromatase) that catalyzes the formation of estrogen from androgen. J Biol Chem 1988; 263:16358–16363.

144. Nimrod A, Ryan KJ. Aromatization of androgens by human abdominal and breast fat tissue. J Clin Endocrinol Metab 1975; 40:367–372.

145. Carr BR, Simpson ER. Lipoprotein utilization and cholesterol synthesis by the human fetal adrenal gland. Endocr Rev 1981; 2:306–326.

146. Simpson ER, Carr BR, Parker CR, et al. The role of serum lipoproteins in steroidogenesis by the human fetal adrenal cortex. J Clin Endocrinol Metab 1979; 49:146–148.

147. Carr BR, Parker CR, Milewich L, et al. The role of low density, high density, and very low density lipoproteins in steroidogenesis by the human fetal adrenal gland. Endocrinology 1980; 106:1854–1860.

148. Carr BR, Porter JC, MacDonald PC, et al. Metabolism of low density lipoprotein by human fetal adrenal tissue. Endocrinology 1980; 107:1034–1040.

149. Carr BR, Simpson ER. De novo synthesis of cholesterol by the human fetal adrenal gland. Endocrinology 1981; 108:2154–2162.

150. Chang RJ, Buster JE, Blakely JL, et al. Simultaneous comparison of Δ^5-3β-hydroxysteroid levels in the fetoplacental circulation of normal pregnancy in labor and not in labor. J Clin Endocrinol Metab 1976; 42:744–751.

151. Huhttaniemi I. Studies on steroidogenesis and its regulation in human fetal adrenals and testis. J Steroid Biochem 1977; 8:491–497.

152. Carr BR, Parker CR, Milewich L, et al. Steroid secretion by ACTH-stimulated human fetal adrenal tissue during the first week in organ culture. Steroids 1980; 36:563–574.

153. Branchaud CL, Goodyer CG, Shore P, et al. Functional zonation of the midgestation human fetal adrenal cortex: fetal versus definitive zone use of progesterone for cortisol synthesis. Am J Obstet Gynecol 1985; 151:271–277.

154. Goldman AS, Yackovas WC, Bongiovanni AM. Development of activity of 3β-hydroxysteroid dehydrogenase in human fetal tissues and in two anencephalic newborns. J Clin Endocrinol Metab 1966; 26:14–22.

155. Siiteri PK, MacDonald PC. The utilization of dehydroisoandrosterone sulphate for estrogen synthesis during human pregnancy. Steroids 1963; 2:713–730.

156. Fujieda K, Faiman C, Feyes FI, et al. The control of steroidogenesis by human fetal adrenal cells in tissue culture. IV. The effects of exposure to placental steroids. J Clin Endocrinol Metab 1982; 54:89–94.

157. Brooks RV. Biosynthesis and metabolism of adrenocortical steroids. In: James VHT, ed. The Adrenal Gland. New York: Raven, 1979: 67–92.

158. Neville AM, O'Hare MJ. Aspects of structure, function and pathology. In: James VHT, ed. The Adrenal Gland. New York: Raven, 1979: 1–65.

159. O'Hare MJ, Nice EC, Neville AM. The regulation of androgen secretion and sulfoconjugation in the adult human adrenal cortex: studies with primary monolayer cultured cells. In: Genazzani AR, Thijssen JHH, Siiteri PK, eds. Adrenal Androgens. New York: Raven, 1980: 7–25.

160. Hyatt PJ, Bhatt K, Tait JF. Steroid biosynthesis by zona fasciculata and zona reticularis cells purified from the mammalian adrenal cortex. J Steroid Biochem 1983; 19:953–959.

161. Kennerson AR, McDonald DA, Adams JB. Dehydroepiandrosterone sulfotransferase localization in human adrenal glands: a light and electron microscopic study. J Clin Endocrinol Metab 1983; 56:786–790.

162. Nelson AA, Woodward G. Severe adrenal cortical atrophy produced by feeding DDD. Arch Pathol 1949; 48:387–390.

163. Cueto C, Brown JH. Biological studies on an adrenocorticolytic agent and the isolation of the active components. Endocrinology 1958; 62:334–339.

164. Vilar O, Tullner WW. Effects of o,p'DDD on histology and 17-hydroxycorticosteroid output of the dog adrenal cortex. Endocrinology 1959; 65:80–86.

165. Bergenstal DM, Hertz R, Lipsett MB, et al. Chemotherapy of adrenocortical cancer with o,p'DDD. Ann Intern Med 1960; 53:672–682.

166. Hutter AM Jr, Kayhoe DE. Adrenal cortical carcinoma. Results of treatment with o,p'DDD in 138 patients. Am J Med 1966; 41:581–592.

167. Southren AL, Tochimoto S, Strom L, et al. Remission in Cushing's syndrome with o,p'DDD. J Clin Endocrinol Metab 1966; 26:268–278.

168. Bledsoe T, Island DP, Ney RL, et al. An effect of o,p'-DDD on the extra-adrenal metabolism of cortisol in man. J Clin Endocrinol Metab 1964; 24:1303–1311.

169. Kahnt FW, Neher R. Uber die adrenale Steroid-Biosythese in vitro. III. Selektive Hemmung der Nebennierenrinden-Funktion. Helv Chim Acta 1966; 49:725–732.

170. Dexter RN, Fishman LM, Ney RL, et al. Inhibition of adrenal corticosteroid synthesis by aminoglutethimide: studies of the mechanism of action. J Clin Endocrinol Metab 1967; 27:473–480.

171. Fishman LM, Liddle GW, Island DP, et al. Effects of amino-glutethimide on adrenal function in man. J Clin Endocrinol Metab 1967; 27:481–490.

172. Liddle GW, Island D, Lance EM, et al. Alterations of adrenal steroid patterns in man resulting from treatment with a chemical inhibitor of 11β-hydroxylation. J Clin Endocrinol Metab 1958; 18:906–912.

173. Jenkins JS, Meakin JW, Nelson DH, et al. Inhibition of adrenal steroid 11-oxygenation in the dog. Science 1958; 128:478–480.

174. Chart JJ, Sheppard H, Allen MJ, et al. New amphenone analogs as adrenocortical inhibitors. Experientia 1958; 14:151–152.

175. Coppage WS, Island DP, Smith M, et al. Inhibition of aldosterone secretion and modification of electrolyte excretion in man by a chemical inhibitor of 11β-hydroxylation. J Clin Invest 1959; 38:2101–2109.

176. Goldman AS. Experimental congenital adrenocortical hyperplasia: persistent postnatal deficiency in activity of 3β-hydroxysteroid dehydrogenase produced in utero. J Clin Endocrinol Metab 1967; 27:1041–1049.

177. Feldman D. Ketoconazole and other imidazole derivatives as inhibitors of steroidogenesis. Endocr Rev 1986; 7:409–420.

178. Pont A, Williams PL, Azhar S, et al. Ketoconazole blocks testosterone synthesis. Arch Intern Med 1982; 142:2137–2140.

179. DeFelice R, Johnson DG, Galgoani JN. Gynecomastia with ketoconazole. Antimicrob Agents Chemother 1981; 19:1073–1074.

180. Loose DS, Kan PB, Hirst MA, et al. Ketoconazole blocks adrenal steroidogenesis by inhibiting cytochrome P450 dependent enzymes. J Clin Invest 1983; 71:1495–1499.

181. Engelhardt D, Dorr G, Jaspers C, et al. Ketoconazole blocks cortisol secretion in man by inhibition of adrenal 11β-hydroxylase. Klin Wochenschr 1985; 1:607–612.

182. Wagner RL, White PF, Kan PB, et al. Inhibition of adrenal steroidogenesis by the anesthetic etomidate. N Engl J Med 1984; 310:1415–1421.

183. Fellows IW, Bastow MD, Byrne AJ. Adrenocortical suppression in multiply injured patients: a complication of etomidate treatment. Br Med J 1983; 287:1835–1837.

184. Wagner RL, White PF. Etomidate inhibits adrenocortical function in surgical patients. Anesthesiology 1984; 61:647–651.

185. Fry DE, Griffiths H. The inhibition by etomidate of the 11β-hydroxylation of cortisol. Clin Endocrinol 1984; 20:625–629.

186. deJong FH, Mallois C, Jansen C, et al. Etomidate suppresses adrenocortical function by inhibition of 11β-hydroxylation. J Clin Endocrinol Metab 1984; 59:1143–1147.

187. Fraser R, Watt I, Gray CE, et al. The effect of etomidate on adrenocortical function in dogs before and during hemorrhagic shock. Endocrinology 1984; 115:2266–2270.

188. Schulte HM, Benker G, Reinwein D, et al. Infusion of low dose etomidate: correction of hypercortisolemia in patients with Cushing's syndrome and dose-response relationship in normal subjects. J Clin Endocrinol Metab 1990; 70:1426–1430.

189. Gaillard RC, Poffet D, Riondel AM, et al. RU 486 inhibits peripheral effects of glucocorticoids in humans. J Clin Endocrinol Metab 1985; 61:1009–1011.

190. Bertagna X, Basin C, Picard F, et al. Peripheral antiglucocorticoid action of RU 486 in man. Clin Endocrinol 1988; 28:537–541.

191. Taylor AL, Fishman LM. Corticotropin-releasing hormone. N Engl J Med 1988; 319:213–222.

192. Jones MT, Gillham B. Factors involved in the regulation of adrenocorticotropic hormone/β-lipotropic hormone. Physiol Rev 1988; 68:743–818.

193. Antoni FA. Hypothalamic control of adrenocorticotropin secretion: advances since the discovery of 41-residue corticotropin-releasing factor. Endocr Rev 1986; 7:351–378.

194. Takahasi I, Teranishi Y, Nakanishi S, et al. Isolation and structural organization of the human corticotropin–β-lipotropin precursor gene. FEBS Lett 1981; 135:97–102.

195. Whitfeld PL, Seeburg PH, Shine J. The human pro-opiomelanocortin gene: organization, sequence, and interspersion with repetitive DNA. DNA 1982; 1:133–143.

196. Lundblad JR, Roberts JL. Regulation of proopiomelanocortin gene expression in pituitary. Endocr Rev 1988; 9:135–158.

197. Owerbach D, Rutter WJ, Roberts JL, et al. The proopiocortin (adrenocorticotropin/β-lipotropin) gene is located on chromosome 2 in humans. Somat Cell Genet 1981; 7:359–369.

198. Eipper BA, Mains RE. Structure and biosynthesis of pro-adrenocorticotropin/endorphin and related peptides. Endocr Rev 1980; 1:1–27.

199. Douglass J, Civelli O, Herbert E. Polyprotein gene expression: generation of diversity of neuroendocrine peptides. Annu Rev Biochem 1984; 53:665–715.

200. Smith IA, Funder JW. Proopiomelanocortin processing in the pituitary, central nervous system, and peripheral tissues. Endocr Rev 1988; 9:159–179.

201. Seidah NG, Chrétien M. Complete amino acid sequence of a human pituitary glycopeptide: an important maturation product of pro-opiomelanocortin. Proc Natl Acad Sci USA 1981; 78:4236–4240.

202. Seidah NG, Rochemont J, Hamelin J, et al. The missing fragment of the pro- sequence of human proopiomelanocortin: sequence and evidence for C-terminal amidation. Biochem Biophys Res Commun 1981; 102:710–716.

203. Seizinger BR, Höllt V. In vitro biosynthesis and N-acetylation of β-endorphin in pars intermedia of the rat pituitary. Biochem Biophys Res Commun 1980; 96:535–543.

204. Coates PJ, Doniach I, Holly JMP, et al. Demonstration of desacetyl α-melanocyte–stimulating hormone in fetal and adult human anterior pituitary corticotrophs. J Endocrinol 1989; 120:525–530.

205. Lebouille JLM, Burbach JPH, De Kloet ER, et al. γ-Endorphin–generating endopeptidase: distribution in body tissues and cellular localization in rat testis. Endocrinology 1986; 118:372–376.

206. Mains RE, Eipper BA. Phosphorylation of rat and human adrenocorticotropin-related peptides: physiological regulation and studies of secretion. Endocrinology 1983; 112:1986–1995.

207. Hoshina H, Hortin G, Boime I. Rat pro-opiomelanocortin contains sulfate. Science 1982; 217:63–64.

208. Besser GM, Orth DN, Nicholson WE, et al. Dissociation of the disappearance of bioactive and radioimmunoreactive ACTH from plasma in man. J Clin Endocrinol Metab 1971; 32:595–603.

209. Orth DN. Adrenocorticotropic hormone (ACTH). In: Jaffe BM, Behrman HR, eds. Methods of Hormone Radioimmunoassay. 2nd ed. New York: Academic, 1979: 245–284.

210. Donald RA. ACTH and related peptides. Clin Endocrinol 1980; 12:491–524.

211. Jackson RV, DeCherney GS, DeBold CR, et al. Synthetic ovine corticotropin-releasing hormone: simultaneous release of proopiolipomelanocortin peptides in man. J Clin Endocrinol Metab 1984; 58:740–743.

212. Gilkes JJH, Bloomfield GA, Scott AP, et al. Development and validation of a radioimmunoassay for peptides related to β-melanocyte–stimulating hormone in human plasma: lipotropins. J Clin Endocrinol Metab 1975; 40:450–457.

213. Krieger DT, Liotta AS, Suda T, et al. Human plasma immunoreactive lipotropin and adrenocorticotropin in normal subjects and in patients with pituitary-adrenal disease. J Clin Endocrinol Metab 1979; 48:566–571.

214. Yamaguchi H, Liotta AS, Krieger DT. Simultaneous determination of human plasma immunoreactive β-lipotropin, γ-lipotropin, and β-endorphin using immuno-affinity chromatography. J Clin Endocrinol Metab 1980; 51:1002–1008.

215. Bertagna XY, Stone WJ, Nicholson WE, et al. Simultaneous assay of immunoreactive β-lipotropin, γ-lipotropin, and β-endorphin in plasma of normal human subjects, patients with ACTH/lipotropin hypersecretory syndromes, and patients undergoing chronic hemodialysis. J Clin Invest 1981; 67:124–133.

216. Richter WO, Schwandt P. Physiologic concentrations of β-lipotropin stimulate lipolysis in rabbit adipocytes. Metabolism 1985; 34:539–543.

217. Carter RJ, Shuster S, Morley JS. Melanotropin potentiating factor is the C-terminal tetrapeptide of human β-lipotropin. Nature 1979; 279:74–75.

218. Lowry PJ, Silas L, McLean C, et al. Pro-γ-melanocyte–stimulating hormone cleavage in adrenal gland undergoing compensatory growth. Nature 1983; 306:70–73.

219. Al-Dujaili EAS, Hope J, Estivariz FE, et al. Circulating human pituitary pro-γ-melanotropin enhances the adrenal response to ACTH. Nature 1981; 291:156–159.

220. Shenker Y, Villareal JZ, Sider RS, et al. α-Melanocyte–stimulating hormone stimulation of aldosterone secretion in hypophysectomized rats. Endocrinology 1985; 116:138–141.

221. Robba C, Rebuffat P, Mazzocchi G, et al. Long-term trophic action of α-melanocyte–stimulating hormone on the zona glomerulosa of the rat adrenal cortex. Acta Endocrinol 1986; 112:404–408.

222. Reid RL, Ling N, Yen SSC. Gonadotropin-releasing activity of α-melanocyte–stimulating hormone in normal subjects and in subjects with hypothalamic-pituitary dysfunction. J Clin Endocrinol Metab 1984; 58:773–777.

223. Beloff-Chain A, Morton J, Dunmore S, et al. Evidence that the insulin secretagogue, β-cell–tropin, is ACTH 22–39. Nature 1983; 301:255–258.

224. Marshall JB, Kapcala LP, Manning LD, et al. Effect of corticotropin-like intermediate lobe peptide on pancreatic exocrine function in isolated rat pancreatic lobules. J Clin Invest 1984; 74:1886–1889.

225. Tsong SD, Phillips D, Halmi N, et al. ACTH and β-endorphin–related peptides are present in multiples sites in the reproductive tract of the male rat. Endocrinology 1982; 110:2204–2206.

226. Saito E, Iwasa S, Odell WD. Widespread presence of large molecular weight adrenocorticotropin-like substances in normal rat extrapituitary tissues. Endocrinology 1983; 113:1010–1019.

227. Bardin CW, Chen CLC, Morris PL, et al. Proopiomelanocortin-derived peptides in testis, ovary, and tissues of reproduction. Recent Prog Horm Res 1987; 43:1–28.

228. DeBold CR, Nicholson WE, Orth DN. Immunoreactive proopiomelanocortin (POMC) peptides and POMC-like messenger ribonucleic acid are present in many rat nonpituitary tissues. Endocrinology 1988; 122:2648–2657.

229. DeBold CR, Menefee KJ, Nicholson WE, et al. Proopiomelanocortin gene is expressed in many normal human tissues and in tumors not associated with ectopic ACTH syndrome. Mol Endocrinol 1988; 2:862–870.

230. Lacaze-Masmonteil T, de Keyzer Y, Luton JP, et al. Characterization of proopiomelanocortin transcripts in human nonpituitary tissues. Proc Natl Acad Sci USA 1987; 84:7261–7265.

231. Melner MH, Young SL, Czerwiec FS, et al. The regulation of granulosa cell proopiomelanocortin messenger ribonucleic acid by androgens and gonadotropins. Endocrinology 1986; 119:2082–2088.

232. Chen CLC, Madigan MB. Regulation of testicular proopiomelanocortin gene expression. Endocrinology 1987; 121:590–596.

233. Dickerman Z, Grant DR, Faiman C, et al. Intraadrenal steroid concentrations in man: zonal differences and developmental changes. J Clin Endocrinol Metab 1984; 59:1031–1036.

234. Hall PF. Trophic stimulation of steroidogenesis: in search of the elusive trigger. Recent Prog Horm Res 1985; 41:1–31.

235. Long CNH. Relations of cholesterol and ascorbic acid to secretion of adrenal cortex. Recent Prog Horm Res 1945; 1:99–122.

236. Péron FG, Koritz SB. On the location of the stimulation in vitro by Ca++ and freezing of corticoid production by rat adrenal homogenates. J Biol Chem 1960; 235:1625–1628.

237. Catalano RD, Stuve L, Ramachandran J. Characterization of corticotropin receptors in human adrenocortical cells. J Clin Endocrinol Metab 1986; 62:300–304.

238. Ramachandran J, Tsubokawa M, Gohil K. Corticotropin receptors. Ann NY Acad Sci 1987; 512:415–425.

239. Gill GN. ACTH regulation of the adrenal cortex. Pharmacol Ther [B] 1976; 2:313–338.

240. Sala GB, Hayashi K, Catt KJ, et al. Adrenocorticotropin action in isolated adrenal cells. J Biol Chem 1979; 254:3861–3865.

241. Rae PA, Gutmann NS, Tsao J, et al. Mutations in cyclic AMP–dependent protein kinase and corticotropin (ACTH)-sensitive adenylate cyclase affect adrenal steroidogenesis. Proc Natl Acad Sci USA 1979; 76:1896–1900.

242. Schimmer BP. Cyclic nucleotides in hormonal regulation of adrenocortical function. Adv Cyclic Nucleotide Res 1980; 13:181–214.

243. Simpson ER, Waterman MR. Regulation by ACTH of steroid hormone

biosynthesis in the adrenal cortex. Can J Biochem Cell Biol 1983; 61:692–707.

244. Simpson ER, Waterman MR. Regulation of the synthesis of steroidogenic enzymes in adrenal cortical cells by ACTH. Annu Rev Physiol 1988; 50:427–440.

245. Colby HD, Caffrey JL, Kitay JI. Interaction of growth hormone and ACTH in the regulation of adrenocortical secretion in rats. Endocrinology 1973; 93:188–192.

246. DuBois RN, Simpson ER, Kramer RE, et al. Induction of synthesis of cholesterol side chain cleavage cytochrome P-450 by adrenocorticotropin in cultured bovine adrenocortical cells. J Biol Chem 1981; 256:7000–7005.

247. Zuber MX, Simpson ER, Hall PF, et al. Effects of adrenocorticotropin on 17α-hydroxylase activity and cytochrome P-450$_{17α}$ synthesis in bovine adrenocortical cells. J Biol Chem 1985; 260:1842–1848.

248. Funkenstein B, McCarthy JL, Dus KM, et al. Effect of adrenocorticotropin on steroid 21-hydroxylase synthesis and activity in cultured bovine adrenocortical cells. J Biol Chem 1983; 258:9398–9405.

249. Kramer RE, Simpson ER, Waterman MR. Induction of 11β-hydroxylase by corticotropin in primary cultures of bovine adrenocortical cells. J Biol Chem 1983; 258:3000–3005.

250. Kramer RE, Anderson CM, Peterson JA, et al. Adrenodoxin biosynthesis by bovine adrenal cells in monolayer culture. J Biol Chem 1982; 257:14921–14925.

251. John ME, John MC, Boggaram V, et al. Transcriptional regulation of steroid hydroxylase genes by corticotropin. Proc Natl Acad Sci USA 1986; 83:4715–4719.

252. Kramer RE, Rainey WE, Funkenstein B, et al. Induction of synthesis of mitochondrial steroidogenic enzymes of bovine adrenocortical cells by analogs of cyclic AMP. J Biol Chem 1984; 259:707–713.

253. Trzeciak WH, Simpson ER, Scallen TJ, et al. Studies on the synthesis of sterol carrier protein-2 in rat adrenocortical cells in monolayer culture. J Biol Chem 1987; 262:3713–3717.

254. Rainey WE, Shay JW, Mason JI. ACTH induction of 3-hydroxy-3-methylglutaryl coenzyme A reductase, cholesterol biosynthesis, and steroidogenesis in primary cultures of bovine adrenocortical cells. J Biol Chem 1986; 261:7322–7326.

255. Gill GN. Progress in endocrinology and metabolism: mechanism of ACTH action. Metabolism 1972; 21:571–588.

256. Maier R, Staehelin M. Adrenal responses to corticotrophin in the presence of an inhibitor of protein synthesis. Acta Endocrinol 1968; 58:619–629.

257. Rao AJ, Long JA, Ramachandran J. Effects of antiserum to adrenocorticotropin on adrenal growth and function. Endocrinology 1978; 102:371–378.

258. Dallman MF, Engeland WC, Holzwarth MA, et al. Adrenocorticotropin inhibits compensatory adrenal growth after unilateral adrenalectomy. Endocrinology 1980; 107:1397–1404.

259. Ramachandran J, Suyama AT. Inhibition of replication of normal adrenocortical cells in culture by adrenocorticotropin. Proc Natl Acad Sci USA 1975; 72:113–117.

260. Hornsby PJ, Gill GN. Hormonal control of adrenocortical cell proliferation: desensitization to ACTH and interaction between ACTH and fibroblast growth factor in bovine adrenocortical cell cultures. J Clin Invest 1977; 60:342–352.

261. Dallman MF, Engeland WC, Shinsako J. Compensatory adrenal growth: a neurally mediated reflex. Am J Physiol 1976; 231:408–414.

262. Engeland WC, Dallman MF. Compensatory adrenal growth is neurally mediated. Neuroendocrinology 1975; 19:352–362.

263. Lebovitz HE, Bryant K, Frohman LA. Acute effects of corticotropin and related peptides on carbohydrate and lipid metabolism. Ann NY Acad Sci 1965; 131:274–287.

264. Lando D, Secchi J, Roche J, et al. Adrenocorticotropin analogs and glucocorticoids in the hypophysectomized rat. I. Effects on liver polyribosomes and rough endoplasmic reticulum. Endocrinology 1980; 107:2055–2062.

265. Grunfeld C, Hagman J, Sabin EA, et al. Characterization of adrenocorticotropin receptors that appear when 3T3-L1 cells differentiate into adipocytes. Endocrinology 1985; 116:113–117.

266. Guillemin R, Rosenberg B. Humoral hypothalamic control of anterior pituitary: study with combined tissue cultures. Endocrinology 1955; 57:599–607.

267. Saffran M, Schally AV. Release of corticotrophin by anterior pituitary tissue in vitro. Can J Biochem Physiol 1955; 33:408–415.

268. Spiess J, Rivier J, Rivier C, et al. Primary structure of corticotropin-releasing factor from ovine hypothalamus. Proc Natl Acad Sci USA 1981; 78:6517–6521.

269. Rivier J, Spiess J, Vale W. Characterization of rat hypothalamic corticotropin-releasing factor. Proc Natl Acad Sci USA 1983; 80:4851–4855.

270. Esch F, Ling N, Bohlen P, et al. Isolation and characterization of the bovine hypothalamic corticotropin-releasing factor. Biochem Biophys Res Commun 1984; 122:899–905.

271. Patthy M, Horvath J, Mason-Garcia M, et al. Isolation and amino acid sequence of corticotropin-releasing factor from pig hypothalami. Proc Natl Acad Sci USA 1985; 82:8762–8766.

272. Rivier C, Brownstein M, Spiess J, et al. In vivo corticotropin-releasing factor–induced secretion of adrenocorticotropin, β-endorphin and corticosterone. Endocrinology 1982; 110:272–278.

273. Rivier C, Rivier J, Vale W. Inhibition of adrenocorticotropic hormone secretion in the rat by immunoneutralization of corticotropin-releasing factor. Science 1982; 218:377–379.

274. Vale W, Rivier C, Brown MR, et al. Chemical and biological characterization of corticotropin releasing factor. Recent Prog Horm Res 1983; 39:245–270.

275. Rivier C, Rivier J, Lederis K, et al. In vitro and in vivo ACTH-releasing activity of ovine CRF, sauvagine and urotensin I. Regul Pep 1983; 5:139–143.

276. Lederis K. Non-mammalian corticotropin release–stimulating peptides. Ann NY Acad Sci 1987; 512:129–138.

277. Furutani Y, Morimoto Y, Shibahara S, et al. Cloning and sequence analysis of cDNA for ovine corticotropin releasing factor precursor. Nature 1983; 301:537–540.

278. Jingami H, Mizuno N, Takahashi H, et al. Cloning and sequence analysis of cDNA for rat corticotropin releasing factor precursor. FEBS Lett 1985; 191:63–65.

279. Shibahara S, Morimoto Y, Furutani Y, et al. Isolation and sequence analysis of the human corticotropin-releasing factor precursor gene. EMBO J 1983; 2:775–779.

280. Thompson RC, Seasholtz AF, Herbert E. Rat corticotropin-releasing hormone gene: sequence and tissue-specific expression. Mol Endocrinol 1987; 1:363–370.

281. Arbiser JL, Morton CC, Bruns GAP, et al. Human corticotropin releasing hormone gene is located on the long arm of chromosome 8. Cytogenet Cell Genet 1988; 47:113–116.

282. Olschowka JA, O'Donohue TL, Mueller GP, et al. Hypothalamic and extrahypothalamic distribution of CRF-like immunoreactive neurons in the rat brain. Neuroendocrinology 1982; 35:305–308.

283. Swanson LW, Sawchenko PE, Rivier J, et al. Organization of ovine corticotropin-releasing factor immunoreactive cells and fibers in the rat brain: an immunohistochemical study. Neuroendocrinology 1983; 36:165–168.

284. Bloom FE, Battenberg ELF, Rivier J, et al. Corticotropin releasing factor (CRF): immunoreactive neurons and fibers in rat hypothalamus. Regul Pep 1982; 4:43–48.

285. Kiss JZ, Mezey E, Skirboll L. Corticotropin-releasing factor–immunoreactive neurons of the paraventricular nucleus become vasopressin positive after adrenalectomy. Proc Natl Acad Sci USA 1984; 81:1854–1858.

286. Sawchenko PE, Swanson LW, Vale WW. Co-expression of corticotropin-releasing factor and vasopressin immunoreactivity in parvocellular neurosecretory neurons of the adrenalectomized rat. Proc Natl Acad Sci USA 1984; 81:1883–1887.

287. Mezey E, Reisine TD, Skirboll L, et al. Role of cholecystokinin in corticotropin release: coexistence with vasopressin and corticotropin-releasing factor in cells of the rat hypothalamic paraventricular nucleus. Proc Natl Acad Sci USA 1986; 83:3510–3512.

288. Hökfelt T, Fahrenkrug J, Tatemoto K, et al. The PHI (PHI-27)/corticotropin-releasing factor/enkephalin immunoreactive hypothalamic neuron: possible morphological basis for integrated control of prolactin, corticotropin, and growth hormone secretion. Proc Natl Acad Sci USA 1983; 80:895–898.

289. Roth KA, Weber E, Barchas JD, et al. Immunoreactive dynorphin-(1–8) and corticotropin-releasing factor in subpopulation of hypothalamic neurons. Science 1983; 219:189–191.

290. Sawchenko PE, Swanson LW, Vale WW. Corticotropin-releasing factor: co-expression within distinct subsets of oxytocin-, vasopressin-, and neurotensin-immunoreactive neurons in the hypothalamus of the male rat. J Neurosci 1984; 4:1118–1129.

291. Nicholson WE, DeCherney GS, Jackson RV, et al. Pituitary and hypothalamic hormones in normal and neoplastic adrenal medullae: biologically active corticotropin-releasing hormone and corticotropin. Regul Pep 1987; 18:173–188.

292. Yoon DJ, Sklar C, David R. Presence of immunoreactive corticotropin-releasing factor in rat testis. Endocrinology 1988; 122:759–761.

293. Nieuwenhuijsen Kruseman AC, Linton EA, Ackland J, et al. Heterogeneous immunocytochemical reactivities of oCRH-41–like material in the human hypothalamus, pituitary and gastrointestinal tract. Neuroendocrinology 1984; 38:212–216.

294. Suda T, Tomori N, Tozawa F, et al. Distribution and characterization of immunoreactive corticotropin-releasing factor in human tissues. J Clin Endocrinol Metab 1984; 59:861–866.

295. Petrusz P, Merchenthaler I, Maderdrut JL, et al. Corticotropin-releasing factor (CRF)–like immunoreactivity in the vertebrate endocrine pancreas. Proc Natl Acad Sci USA 1983; 80:1721–1725.

296. Grino M, Chrousos GP, Margioris AN. The corticotropin releasing hormone gene is expressed in human placenta. Biochem Biophys Res Commun 1987; 148:1208–1214.

297. Sasaki A, Shinkawa O, Margioris A, et al. Immunoreactive corticotropin-releasing hormone in human plasma during pregnancy, labor, and delivery. J Clin Endocrinol Metab 1987; 64:224–229.

298. De Souza EB, Perrin MH, Insel TR, et al. Corticotropin-releasing

factor receptors in rat forebrain: autoradiographic identification. Science 1984; 224:1449–1450.

299. De Souza EB. Corticotropin-releasing factor receptors in the rat central nervous system: characterization and regional distribution. J Neurosci 1987; 7:88–100.

300. Ulisse S, Fabbri A, Dufau ML. Corticotropin-releasing factor receptors and actions in rat Leydig cells. J Biol Chem 1989; 264:2156–2163.

301. Millan MA, Abou Samra AB, Wynn PC, et al. Receptors and action of corticotropin-releasing hormone in the primate pituitary gland. J Clin Endocrinol Metab 1987; 64:1036–1041.

302. Wynn PC, Harwood JP, Catt KJ, et al. Regulation of corticotropin-releasing factor (CRF) receptors in the rat pituitary gland: effect of adrenalectomy on CRF receptors and corticotropin responses. Endocrinology 1985; 116:1653–1659.

303. Giguère V, Labrie F, Côt J, et al. Stimulation of cyclic AMP accumulation and corticotropin release by ovine corticotropin-releasing factor in rat anterior pituitary cells: site of glucocorticoid action. Proc Natl Acad Sci USA 1982; 79:3466–3469.

304. Bruhn TO, Sutton RE, Rivier CL, et al. Corticotropin-releasing factor regulates proopiomelanocortin messenger ribonucleic acid levels in vivo. Neuroendocrinology 1984; 39:170–175.

305. Loeffler JP, Kley N, Pittius CW, et al. Corticotropin-releasing factor and forskolin increase proopiomelanocortin messenger RNA levels in rat anterior and intermediate cells in vitro. Neurosci Lett 1985; 62:383–387.

306. Gertz BJ, Contreras LN, McComb DJ, et al. Chronic administration of corticotropin-releasing factor increases pituitary corticotroph number. Endocrinology 1987; 120:381–388.

307. Hauger RL, Millan MA, Catt KJ, et al. Differential regulation of brain and pituitary corticotropin-releasing factor receptors by corticosterone. Endocrinology 1987; 120:1527–1533.

308. Holmes MC, Catt KJ, Aguilera G. Involvement of vasopressin in the down-regulation of pituitary corticotropin-releasing factor receptors after adrenalectomy. Endocrinology 1987; 121:2093–2098.

309. Wynn PC, Harwood JP, Catt KJ, et al. Corticotropin-releasing factor (CRF) induces desensitization of the rat pituitary CRF receptor–adenylate cyclase complex. Endocrinology 1988; 122:351–358.

310. Hauger RL, Millan MA, Lorang M, et al. Corticotropin-releasing factor receptors and pituitary adrenal responses during immobilization stress. Endocrinology 1988; 123:396–405.

311. Proulx-Ferland L, Labrie F, Dumont D, et al. Corticotropin-releasing factor stimulates secretion of melanocyte-stimulating hormone from the rat pituitary. Science 1982; 217:62–63.

312. Suda T, Tomori N, Yajima F, et al. Immunoreactive corticotropin-releasing factor in human plasma. J Clin Invest 1985; 76:2026–2029.

312a. Sasaki A, Sato S, Murakami O, et al. Immunoreactive corticotropin-releasing hormone present in human plasma may be derived from both hypothalamic and extrahypothalamic sources. J Clin Endocrinol Metab 1987; 65:176–182.

313. Watabe T, Tanaka K, Kumagae M, et al. Hormonal responses to insulin-induced hypoglycemia in man. J Clin Endocrinol Metab 1987; 65:1187–1191.

314. Watabe T, Tanaka K, Kumagae M, et al. Diurnal rhythm of plasma immunoreactive corticotropin-releasing factor in normal subjects. Life Sci 1987; 40:1651–1655.

315. Linton EA, McLean C, Niewenhuyzen-Kruseman AC, et al. Direct measurement of human plasma corticotropin-releasing hormone by "two-site" immunoradiometric assay. J Clin Endocrinol Metab 1987; 64:1047–1053.

316. Cunnah D, Jessop DS, Besser GM, et al. Measurement of circulating corticotropin-releasing factor in man. J Endocrinol 1987; 113:123–131.

317. Bruhn TO, Engeland WC, Anthony ELP, et al. Corticotropin-releasing factor in the dog adrenal medulla is secreted in response to hemorrhage. Endocrinology 1987; 120:25–33.

318. Edwards AV, Jones CT. Secretion of corticotropin releasing factor from the adrenal during splanchnic nerve stimulation in conscious calves. J Physiol (Lond) 1988; 400:89–100.

319. Campbell EA, Linton EA, Wolfe CDA, et al. Plasma corticotropin-releasing hormone during pregnancy and parturition. J Clin Endocrinol Metab 1987; 64:1054–1059.

320. Orth DN, Mount CD. Specific high-affinity binding protein for human corticotropin-releasing hormone in normal human plasma. Biochem Biophys Res Commun 1987; 143:411–417.

321. Linton EA, Wolfe CDA, Behan DP, et al. A specific carrier substance for human corticotropin releasing factor in late gestational maternal plasma which could mask the ACTH-releasing activity. Clin Endocrinol 1988; 28:315–324.

322. Schürmeyer TH, Avgerinos PC, Gold PW, et al. Human corticotropin-releasing factor in man: pharmacokinetic properties and dose-response of plasma adrenocorticotropin and cortisol secretion. J Clin Endocrinol Metab 1984; 59:1103–1108.

323. Nicholson WE, DeCherney GS, Jackson RV, et al. Plasma distribution, disappearance half-time, metabolic clearance rate, and degradation of synthetic ovine corticotropin-releasing factor in man. J Clin Endocrinol Metab 1983; 57:1263–1269.

324. DeBold CR, DeCherney GS, Jackson RV, et al. Effect of synthetic ovine corticotropin-releasing factor: prolonged duration of action and biphasic response of plasma adrenocorticotropin and cortisol. J Clin Endocrinol Metab 1983; 57:294–298.

325. Orth DN, Jackson RV, DeCherney GS, et al. Effect of synthetic ovine corticotropin-releasing factor: dose response of plasma adrenocorticotropin and cortisol. J Clin Invest 1983; 71:587–595.

326. Conaglen JV, Donald RA, Espiner EA, et al. The effect of ovine corticotropin-releasing factor on catecholamine, vasopressin, and aldosterone secretion in normal man. J Clin Endocrinol Metab 1984; 58:463–466.

327. Pavlov EP, Harman SM, Chrousos GP, et al. Responses of plasma adrenocorticotropin, cortisol, and dehydroepiandrosterone to ovine corticotropin-releasing hormone in healthy aging men. J Clin Endocrinol Metab 1986; 62:767–772.

328. Sheldon WR, DeBold CR, Evans WS, et al. Rapid sequential intravenous administration of four hypothalamic releasing hormones as a combined anterior pituitary function test in normal subjects. J Clin Endocrinol Metab 1985; 60:623–630.

329. Ross JL, Schulte HM, Gallucci WT, et al. Ovine corticotropin-releasing hormone stimulation test in normal children. J Clin Endocrinol Metab 1986; 62:390–392.

330. Kopelman PG, Grossman A, Lavender P, et al. The cortisol response to corticotropin-releasing factor is blunted in obesity. Clin Endocrinol 1988; 28:15–18.

331. DeCherney GS, DeBold CR, Jackson RV, et al. Diurnal variation in the response of plasma adrenocorticotropin and cortisol to intravenous ovine corticotropin-releasing hormone. J Clin Endocrinol Metab 1985; 61:273–279.

332. DeBold CR, Jackson RV, Kamilaris TC, et al. Effects of ovine corticotropin-releasing hormone on adrenocorticotropin secretion in the absence of glucocorticoid negative feedback inhibition in man. J Clin Endocrinol Metab 1989; 68:431–437.

333. Won JGS, Jap TS, Chang SC, et al. Evidence for a delayed, integral, and proportional phase of glucocorticoid feedback on ACTH secretion in normal human volunteers. Metabolism 1986; 35:254–259.

334. Hermus ARMM, Pieters GFFM, Willemsen JJ, et al. Hypotensive effects of ovine and human corticotropin-releasing factors in man. Eur J Pharmacol 1987; 31:531–534.

335. Oppermann D, Huber I, Nink M, et al. Human corticotropin-releasing hormone in man: dose-response of minute ventilation and end-tidal partial pressures of carbon dioxide and oxygen. J Clin Endocrinol Metab 1987; 64:292–296.

336. Brown MR, Fisher LA, Spiess J, et al. Corticotropin-releasing factor: actions on the sympathetic nervous system and metabolism. Endocrinology 1982; 111:928–931.

337. Lenz HJ, Hester SE, Brown MR. Corticotropin-releasing factor: mechanisms to inhibit gastric acid secretion in conscious dogs. J Clin Invest 1985; 75:889–895.

338. Sutton RE, Koob GF, LeMoal M, et al. Corticotropin releasing factor produces behavioral activation in rats. Nature 1982; 297:331–333.

339. Sirinathsinghji DJS, Rees LH, Rivier J, et al. Corticotropin-releasing factor is a potent inhibitor of sexual receptivity in the female rat. Nature 1983; 305:232–235.

340. Petraglia F, Sutton S, Vale W, et al. Corticotropin-releasing factor decreases plasma luteinizing hormone levels in female rats by inhibiting gonadotropin-releasing hormone release into hypophysial-portal circulation. Endocrinology 1987; 120:1083–1088.

341. Vale W, Vaughan J, Smith M, et al. Effects of synthetic ovine corticotropin-releasing factor, glucocorticoids, catecholamines, neurohypophysial peptides, and other substances on cultured corticotropin cells. Endocrinology 1983; 113:1121–1131.

342. DeBold CR, Sheldon WR, DeCherney GS, et al. Arginine vasopressin potentiates adrenocorticotropin release induced by ovine corticotropin-releasing factor. J Clin Invest 1984; 73:533–538.

343. Bilezikjian LM, Blount AL, Vale WW. The cellular actions of vasopressin on corticotrophs of the anterior pituitary: resistance to glucocorticoid action. Mol Endocrinol 1987; 1:451–458.

344. Won JGS, Oki Y, Orth DN. Roles of intracellular and extracellular calcium in the kinetic profile of adrenocorticotropin secretion by perifused rat anterior pituitary cells. II. Arginine vasopressin, oxytocin, and angiotensin-II stimulation. Endocrinology 1990; 126:858–868.

345. Oki Y, Nicholson WE, Orth DN. Role of protein kinase C in the adrenocorticotropin secretory response to arginine vasopressin (AVP) and the synergistic response to AVP and corticotropin-releasing factor by perifused rat anterior pituitary cells. Endocrinology 1990; 127:350–357.

346. Watanabe T, Oki Y, Orth DN. Kinetic actions and interactions of arginine vasopressin, angiotensin-II, and oxytocin on adrenocorticotropin secretion by rat anterior pituitary cells in the microperifusion system. Endocrinology 1989; 125:1921–1931.

347. Rivier C, Vale W. Effect of angiotensin II on ACTH release in vivo: role of corticotropin-releasing factor. Regul Pep 1983; 7:253–258.

348. Lewis DA, Sherman BM. Oxytocin does not influence adrenocorticotropin secretion in man. J Clin Endocrinol Metab 1985; 60:53–56.

349. King MS, Baertschi AJ. Physiologic concentrations of atrial natriuretic

factors with intact N-terminal sequences inhibit corticotropin-releasing factor–stimulated adrenocorticotropin secretion from cultured anterior pituitary cells. Endocrinology 1989; 124:286–292.

350. Allolio B, Deuss U, Kaulen D, et al. FK 33–824, a met-enkephalin analog, blocks corticotropin-releasing hormone–induced adrenocorticotropin secretion in normal subjects but not in patients with Cushing's disease. J Clin Endocrinol Metab 1986; 63:1427–1431.

351. Taylor T, Dluhy RG, Williams GH. β-Endorphin suppresses adrenocorticotropin and cortisol levels in normal human subjects. J Clin Endocrinol Metab 1983; 57:592–596.

352. Pfeiffer A, Herz A, Loriaux DL, et al. Central kappa- and mu-opiate receptors mediate ACTH-release in rats. Endocrinology 1985; 116:2688–2690.

353. Al-Damluji S. Adrenergic mechanisms in the control of corticotrophin secretion. J Endocrinol 1988; 119:5–14.

354. Bateman A, Singh A, Kral T, et al. The immune-hypothalamic-pituitary-adrenal axis. Endocr Rev 1989; 10:92–112.

355. Milenkovic L, Rettori V, Snyder GD, et al. Cachectin alters anterior pituitary hormone release by a direct action in vitro. Proc Natl Acad Sci USA 1989; 86:2418–2422.

356. Buzzetti R, McLouglin L, Lavender PM, et al. Expression of pro-opiomelanocortin gene and quantification of adrenocorticotropic hormone–like immunoreactivity in human normal peripheral mononuclear cells and lymphoid and myeloid malignancies. J Clin Invest 1989; 83:733–737.

357. Lolait SJ, Clements JA, Markwick AJ, et al. Pro-opiomelanocortin messenger ribonucleic acid and posttranslational processing of beta endorphin in spleen macrophages. J Clin Invest 1986; 77:1776–1779.

358. Oates EL, Allaway GP, Armstrong GR, et al. Human lymphocytes produce pro-opiomelanocortin gene–related transcripts. J Biol Chem 1988; 263:10041–10044.

359. Bohme MWJ, Becker K, Scherbaum WA, et al. No expression of IR-ACTH on stimulated peripheral blood leukocytes. Horm Metab Res 1987; 19:670–671.

360. Smith EM, Meyer WJ, Blalock JE. Virus-induced corticosterone in hypophysectomized mice: a possible lymphoid adrenal axis. Science 1982; 218:1311–1312.

361. Dunn AJ, Powell ML, Gaskin JM. Virus-induced increases in plasma corticosterone. Science 1987; 238:1423–1424.

362. Munemura M, Eskay RL, Kebabian JW. Release of α-melanocyte–stimulating hormone from dispersed cells of the intermediate lobe of the rat pituitary gland: involvement of catecholamines and adenosine 3′,5′-monophosphate. Endocrinology 1980; 106:1795–1803.

363. Tomiko SA, Taraskevich PS, Douglas WW. GABA acts directly on cells of pituitary pars intermedia to alter hormone output. Nature 1983; 301:706–707.

364. Krieger DT, Allen W, Rizzo F, et al. Characterization of the normal temporal pattern of plasma corticosteroid levels. J Clin Endocrinol Metab 1971; 32:266–284.

365. Weitzman ED, Fukushima DK, Nogeire C, et al. Twenty-four hour pattern of the episodic secretion of cortisol in normal subjects. J Clin Endocrinol Metab 1971; 33:14–22.

366. Veldhuis JD, Iranmanesh A, Johnson ML, et al. Amplitude, but not frequency, modulation of adrenocorticotropin secretory bursts gives rise to the nyctohemeral rhythm of the corticotropic axis in man. J Clin Endocrinol Metab 1990; 71:452–463.

367. Quigley ME, Yen SSC. A mid-day surge in cortisol levels. J Clin Endocrinol Metab 1979; 49:945–947.

368. Slag MF, Ahmed M, Gannon MC, et al. Meal stimulation of cortisol secretion: a protein induced effect. Metabolism 1981; 30:1104–1108.

369. Orth DN, Island DP. Light synchronization of the circadian rhythm in plasma cortisol (17-OHCS) concentration in man. J Clin Endocrinol Metab 1969; 29:479–486.

370. Orth DN, Besser GM, King PH, et al. Free-running circadian plasma cortisol rhythm in a blind human subject. Clin Endocrinol 1979; 10:603–617.

371. Moore-Ede MC, Czeisler CA, Richardson GS. Circadian timekeeping in health and disease. Part 1. N Engl J Med 1983; 309:469–476.

372. Franks RC. Diurnal variation of plasma 17-hydroxycorticosteroids in children. J Clin Endocrinol Metab 1967; 27:75–78.

373. Krieger DT. Rhythms of ACTH and corticosteroid secretion in health and disease, and their experimental modification. J Steroid Biochem 1975; 6:785–791.

374. Sherman B, Wysham C, Pfohl B. Age-related changes in the circadian rhythm of plasma cortisol in man. J Clin Endocrinol Metab 1985; 61:439–443.

375. Vance ML, Thorner MO. Fasting alters pulsatile and rhythmic cortisol release in normal man. J Clin Endocrinol Metab 1989; 68:1013–1018.

376. Krieger DT. Rhythms in CRF, ACTH, and corticosteroids. In: Krieger DT, ed. Endocrine Rhythms. New York: Raven, 1979: 123–142.

377. Dèsir D, Van Cauter E, Fang VS, et al. Effects of "jet lag" on hormonal patterns. I. Procedures, variations in total plasma proteins, and disruption of adrenocorticotropin-cortisol periodicity. J Clin Endocrinol Metab 1981; 52:628–641.

378. Czeisler CA, Kronauer RE, Allan JS, et al. Bright light induction of strong (type 0) resetting of the human circadian pacemaker. Science 1989; 244:1328–1333.

379. Czeisler CA, Johnson MP, Duffy JF, et al. Exposure to bright light and darkness to treat physiologic maladaptation to night work. N Engl J Med 1990; 322:1253–1259.

380. Szafarczyk A, Ixart G, Malaval F, et al. Effects of lesions of the suprachiasmatic nuclei and of p-chlorophenylalanine on the circadian rhythms of adrenocorticotrophic hormone and corticosterone in the plasma, and on locomotor activity of rats. J Endocrinol 1979; 83:1–16.

381. Nicholson S, Lin JH, Mahmoud S, et al. Diurnal variations in responsiveness of the hypothalamo-pituitary-adrenocortical axis of the rat. Neuroendocrinology 1985; 40:217–224.

382. Moldow RL, Fischman AJ. Circadian rhythm of corticotropin releasing factor–like immunoreactivity in rat hypothalamus. Peptides 1984; 5:1213–1215.

383. Schulte HM, Chrousos GP, Gold PW, et al. Continuous administration of synthetic ovine corticotropin-releasing factor in man. J Clin Invest 1985; 75:1781–1785.

384. Dallman MF, Engeland WC, Rose JC, et al. Nycthemeral rhythm in adrenal responsiveness to ACTH. Am J Physiol 1978; 235:R210–R218.

385. Engeland WC, Byrnes GJ, Presnell K, et al. Adrenocortical sensitivity to adrenocorticotropin (ACTH) in awake dogs changes as a function of the time of observation and after hemorrhage independently of changes in ACTH. Endocrinology 1981; 108:2149–2153.

386. Kaneko M, Kaneko K, Shinsako J, et al. Adrenal sensitivity to adrenocorticotropin varies diurnally. Endocrinology 1981; 109:70–75.

387. Ottenweller JE, Meier AH. Adrenal innervation may be an extrapituitary mechanism able to regulate adrenocortical rhythmicity in rats. Endocrinology 1982; 111:1334–1338.

388. Edwards AV, Jones CT, Bloom SR. Reduced adrenal cortical sensitivity to ACTH in lambs with cut splanchnic nerve. J Endocrinol 1986; 110:81–85.

389. Ottenweller JE, Meier AH, Ferrell BR, et al. Extrapituitary regulation of the circadian rhythm of plasma corticosteroid concentration in rats. Endocrinology 1978; 103:1875–1879.

390. Wilkinson CW, Shinsako J, Dallman MF. Return of pituitary-adrenal function after adrenal enucleation or transplantation: diurnal rhythms and responses to ether. Endocrinology 1981; 109:162–169.

391. Wood CE, Shinsako J, Dallman MF. Comparison of canine corticosteroid responses to mean and phasic increases in ACTH. Am J Physiol 1982; 242:E102–E108.

392. Vaughan GM, Becker RA, Allen JP, et al. Cortisol and corticotropin in burned patients. J Trauma 1982; 22:263–272.

393. Gossain VV, Sherma NK, Srivastava L, et al. Hormonal effects of smoking—II: effects on plasma cortisol, growth hormone, and prolactin. Am J Med Sci 1986; 291:325–327.

394. Fish HR, Chernow B, O'Brian JT. Endocrine and neurophysiologic responses of the pituitary to insulin-induced hypoglycemia: a review. Metabolism 1986; 35:763–780.

395. Udelsman R, Norton JA, Jelenich SE, et al. Responses of the hypothalamic-pituitary-adrenal and renin-angiotensin axes and the sympathetic system during controlled surgical and anesthetic stress. J Clin Endocrinol Metab 1987; 64:986–994.

396. Luger A, Deuster PA, Kyle SB, et al. Acute hypothalamic-pituitary-adrenal responses to the stress of treadmill exercise. N Engl J Med 1987; 316:1309–1315.

397. Raff H, Norton AJ, Flemma RJ, et al. Inhibition of the adrenocorticotropin response to surgery in humans: interaction between dexamethasone and fentanyl. J Clin Endocrinol Metab 1987; 65:295–298.

398. George JM, Reier CE, Lanese RR, et al. Morphine anesthesia blocks cortisol and growth hormone response to surgical stress in humans. J Clin Endocrinol Metab 1974; 38:736–741.

399. Rittmaster RS, Cutler GB Jr, Sobel DO, et al. Morphine inhibits the pituitary-adrenal response to ovine corticotropin-releasing hormone in normal subjects. J Clin Endocrinol Metab 1985; 60:891–895.

400. Redgate ES. Spinal cord and ACTH release in adrenalectomized rats following electrical stimulation. Endocrinology 1962; 70:263–266.

401. Brandt M, Kehlet H, Binder C, et al. Effect of epidural analgesia on the glycoregulatory endocrine response to surgery. Clin Endocrinol 1976; 5:107–114.

402. Estep HL, Island DP, Ney RL, et al. Pituitary-adrenal dynamics during surgical stress. J Clin Endocrinol Metab 1963; 23:419–425.

403. Copinschi G, L'Hermite M, Leclercq R, et al. Effects of glucocorticoids on pituitary hormonal responses to hypoglycemia. Inhibition of prolactin release. J Clin Endocrinol Metab 1975; 40:442–449.

404. Sutton JR, Casey JH. The adrenocortical response to competitive athletics in veteran athletes. J Clin Endocrinol Metab 1975; 40:135–138.

405. Czeisler CA, Ede MCM, Regestein QR, et al. Episodic 24-hour cortisol secretory patterns in patients awaiting elective cardiac surgery. J Clin Endocrinol Metab 1976; 42:273–283.

406. Brandenberger G, Follénius M, Wittersheim G, et al. Plasma catecholamines and pituitary adrenal hormones related to mental task demand under quiet and noise conditions. Biol Psychol 1980; 20:239–252.

407. Linkowski P, Mendlewicz J, Kerkhofs M, et al. 24-Hour profiles of adrenocorticotropin, cortisol, and growth hormone in major depressive

illness: effect of antidepressant treatment. J Clin Endocrinol Metab 1987; 65:141–152.

408. Pfohl B, Sherman B, Schlechte J, et al. Pituitary-adrenal axis rhythm disturbances in psychiatric depression. Arch Gen Psychiatry 1985; 42:897–903.

409. Pfohl B, Sherman B, Schlechte J, et al. Differences in plasma ACTH and cortisol between depressed patients and normal controls. Biol Psychiatry 1985; 20:1055–1072.

410. Aizawa T, Yasuda N, Greer MA. Hypoglycemia stimulates ACTH secretion through a direct effect on the basal hypothalamus. Metabolism 1981; 30:996–1000.

411. Widmaier EP, Plotsky PM, Sutton SW, et al. Regulation of corticotropin-releasing factor secretion in vitro by glucose. Am J Physiol 1988; 255:E287–E292.

412. Jezová D, Kvetnansky R, Kovács K, et al. Insulin-induced hypoglycemia activates the release of adrenocorticotropin predominantly via central and propranolol insensitive mechanisms. Endocrinology 1987; 120:409–415.

413. Streeten DHP, Anderson GH Jr, Dalakos TG, et al. Normal and abnormal function of the hypothalamic-pituitary-adrenocortical system in man. Endocr Rev 1984; 5:371–394.

414. Davis LG, Arentzen R, Reid JM, et al. Glucocorticoid sensitivity of vasopressin mRNA levels in the paraventricular nucleus of the rat. Proc Natl Acad Sci USA 1986; 83:1145–1149.

415. Itoi K, Mouri T, Takahashi K, et al. Suppression by glucocorticoid of the immunoreactivity of corticotropin-releasing factor and vasopressin in the paraventricular nucleus of rat hypothalamus. Neurosci Lett 1987; 73:231–236.

416. Beyer HS, Matta SG, Sharp BM. Regulation of the messenger ribonucleic acid for corticotropin-releasing factor in the paraventricular nucleus and other brain sites of the rat. Endocrinology 1988; 123:2117–2123.

417. Eberwine JH, Jonassen JA, Evinger MJQ, et al. Complex transcriptional regulation by glucocorticoids and corticotropin-releasing hormone of proopiomelanocortion gene expression in rat pituitary cultures. DNA 1987; 6:483–492.

418. Oki Y, Peatman TW, Qu Z-C, et al. Effects of intracellular Ca²⁺ depletion and glucocorticoid on stimulated adrenocorticotropin release by rat anterior pituitary cells in a microperifusion system. Endocrinology 1991; 128:1589–1596.

419. Keller-Wood ME, Dallman MF. Corticosteroid inhibition of ACTH secretion. Endocr Rev 1984; 5:1–24.

420. Saito E, Mukai M, Muraki T, et al. Inhibitory effects of corticosterone on cell proliferation and steroidogenesis in the mouse adrenal tumor cell line Y-1. Endocrinology 1979; 104:487–492.

421. Rosenfield RL, Helke J, Lucky AW. Dexamethasone preparation does not alter corticoid and androgen responses to adrenocorticotropin. J Clin Endocrinol Metab 1985; 60:585–589.

422. Graybeal ML, Fang VS, Landau RL. Enhancement of adrenal cortisol secretion after intravenous high dose dexamethasone. J Clin Endocrinol Metab 1985; 61:607–611.

423. Tan SY, Mulrow PJ. The contribution of the zona fasciculata and glomerulosa to plasma 11-deoxycorticosterone levels in man. J Clin Endocrinol Metab 1975; 41:126–130.

424. Kater CE, Biglieri EG, Brust N, et al. Stimulation and suppression of the mineralocorticoid hormones in normal subjects and adrenocortical disorders. Endocr Rev 1989; 10:149–164.

425. Gomez-Sanchez CE, Montgomery M, Ganguly A, et al. Elevated urinary excretion of 18-oxocortisol in glucocorticoid-suppressible aldosteronism. J Clin Endocrinol Metab 1984; 59:1022–1024.

426. Griffing GT, Dale SL, Holbrook MM, et al. The regulation of urinary free 19-nor-deoxycorticosterone and its relation to systemic arterial pressure in normotensive and hypertensive subjects. J Clin Endocrinol Metab 1983; 56:99–103.

427. Quinn SJ, Williams GH. Regulation of aldosterone secretion. Annu Rev Physiol 1988; 50:409–426.

428. Williams GH, Dluhy RG. Control of aldosterone secretion. In: Genest J, Küchel O, Hamet P, et al., eds. Hypertension: Physiopathology and Treatment. 2nd ed. New York: McGraw-Hill, 1983: 320–337.

429. Goodfriend TL, Gibbons GH, Dzau VJ, et al. Interaction of signals influencing renin release. Annu Rev Physiol 1984; 46:291–308.

430. Blair-West JR, Coghlan JP, Denton DA, et al. A dose-response comparison of the actions of angiotensin II and angiotensin III in sheep. J Endocrinol 1980; 87:409–417.

431. Gibbons GH, Dzau VJ, Farhl ER, et al. Interaction of signals influencing renin release. Annu Rev Physiol 1984; 46:291–308.

432. Speckart P, Zia P, Zipser R, et al. Effect of sodium restriction and prostaglandin inhibition on the renin-angiotensin system in man. J Clin Endocrinol Metab 1977; 44:832–837.

433. Campbell DJ. Circulating and tissue angiotensin systems. J Clin Invest 1987; 79:1–6.

434. McKenna TJ, Island DP, Nicholson WE, et al. The effects of potassium on early and late steps in aldosterone biosynthesis in cells of the zona glomerulosa. Endocrinology 1978; 103:1411–1416.

435. Aguilera G, Catt KJ. Loci of action of regulators of aldosterone

436. Kramer RE, Gallant S, Brownie AC. Actions of angiotensin II on aldosterone biosynthesis in the rat adrenal cortex. J Biol Chem 1980; 255:3442–3447.

437. Fujita K, Aguilera G, Catt KJ. The role of cyclic AMP in aldosterone production by isolated zona glomerulosa cells. J Biol Chem 1979; 254:8567–8574.

438. Natarajan R, Stern N, Hsueh W, et al. Role of the lipoxygenase pathway in angiotensin II–mediated aldosterone biosynthesis in human adrenal glomerulosa cells. J Clin Endocrinol Metab 1988; 67:584–591.

439. Himathongkam T, Dluhy RG, Williams GH. Potassium-aldosterone-renin interrelationships. J Clin Endocrinol Metab 1975; 41:153–159.

440. Hollenberg NK, Williams G, Burger B, et al. The influence of potassium on the renal vasculature and the adrenal, and their responsiveness to angiotensin II in normal man. Clin Sci Mol Med 1975; 49:527–534.

441. Dluhy RG, Axelrod L, Underwood RH, et al. Studies of the control of plasma aldosterone concentration in normal man: effect of dietary potassium and acute potassium infusion. J Clin Invest 1972; 51:1950–1957.

442. Kojima I, Kojima K, Rasmussen H. Intracellular calcium and adenosine 3′,5′-cyclic monophosphate as mediators of potassium-induced aldosterone secretion. Biochem J 1985; 228:69–76.

443. Rayfield EJ, Rose LI, Dluhy RG, et al. Aldosterone secretory and glucocorticoid excretory responses to alpha 1–24 ACTH (Cortrosyn) in sodium-depleted normal man. J Clin Endocrinol Metab 1973; 36:30–35.

444. Abayasekara DRE, Vazir H, Whitehouse BJ, et al. Studies on the mechanisms of ACTH-induced inhibition of aldosterone biosynthesis in the rat adrenal cortex. J Endocrinol 1989; 122:625–632.

445. Seidah NG, Rochemont J, Hamelin J, et al. Primary structure of the major human pituitary pro-opiomelanocortin NH₂-terminal glycopeptide: evidence for an aldosterone-stimulating activity. J Biol Chem 1981; 256:7977–7984.

446. Matsuoka H, Mulrow PJ, Franco-Saenz R. Effects of β-lipotropin and β-lipotropin–derived peptides on aldosterone production in the rat adrenal gland. J Clin Invest 1981; 68:752–759.

447. Güllner HG, Gill JR Jr. Beta-endorphin selectively stimulates aldosterone secretion in hypophysectomized, nephrectomized dogs. J Clin Invest 1983; 71:124–128.

448. Vinson GP, Whitehouse BJ, Batemen A, et al. The actions of N-terminal fragments of corticotropin on steroidogenesis in dispersed rat adrenal cells in vitro. J Endocrinol 1986; 109:275–278.

449. Pedersen RC, Brownie AC, Ling N. Pro-adrenocorticotropin/endorphin–derived peptides: coordinate action on adrenal steroidogenesis. Science 1980; 208:1044–1045.

450. Washburn DD, Kem DC, Orth DN, et al. Effect of β-lipotropin on aldosterone production in the isolated rat adrenal cell preparation. J Clin Endocrinol Metab 1982; 54:613–618.

451. Kojima I, Kojima K, Rasmussen H. Role of calcium and cAMP in the action of adrenocorticotropin on aldosterone secretion. J Biol Chem 1985; 260:4248–4256.

452. Aguilera G, Catt KJ. Participation of voltage-dependent calcium channels in the regulation of adrenal glomerulosa function by angiotensin II and potassium. Endocrinology 1986; 118:112–118.

453. Woodcock EA, McLeod JK, Johnston CI. Vasopressin stimulates phosphatidylinositol turnover and aldosterone synthesis in rat adrenal glomerulosa cells: comparison with angiotensin II. Endocrinology 1986; 118:2432–2436.

454. Hollenberg NK, Chenitz WR, Adams DF, et al. Reciprocal influence of salt intake on adrenal glomerulosa and renal vascular response to angiotensin II in normal man. J Clin Invest 1974; 54:34–42.

455. Williams GH, Braley LM. Effects of dietary sodium and potassium intake and acute stimulation on aldosterone output by isolated human adrenal cells. J Clin Endocrinol Metab 1977; 45:55–64.

456. Schambelan M, Sebastian A, Katuna BA, et al. Adrenocortical hormone secretory response to chronic NH₄Cl-induced metabolic acidosis. Am J Physiol 1987; 252:E454–E460.

457. Pratt JH, Turner DA, McAteer JA, et al. β-Adrenergic stimulation of aldosterone production by rat adrenal capsular explants. Endocrinology 1985; 117:1189–1194.

458. Cunningham LA, Holzwarth MA. Vasoactive intestinal peptide simulates adrenal aldosterone and corticosterone secretion. Endocrinology 1988; 122:2090–2097.

459. Bruzzone ME, Marusic ET. Effects of opioid peptides on aldosterone production: stimulatory effects of leu-enkephalin. Endocrinology 1988; 122:402–406.

460. Murakami M, Suzuki H, Nakajima S, et al. Calcitonin gene–related peptide is an inhibitor of aldosterone secretion. Endocrinology 1989; 125:2227–2229.

461. Sowers JR, Brinkman AS, Sowers DK, et al. Dopaminergic modulation of aldosterone secretion in man is unaffected by glucocorticoids and angiotensin blockade. J Clin Endocrinol Metab 1981; 52:1078–1084.

462. Carey RM. Acute dopaminergic inhibition of aldosterone secretion is

independent of angiotensin II and adrenocorticotropin. J Clin Endocrinol Metab 1982; 54:463–469.

463. Missale C, Liberini P, Memo M, et al. Characterization of dopamine receptors associated with aldosterone secretion in rat adrenal glomerulosa. Endocrinology 1986; 119:2227–2232.

464. Chartier L, Schiffrin EL. Role of calcium in effects of atrial natriuretic peptide on aldosterone production in adrenal glomerulosa cells. Am J Physiol 1987; 252:E485–E491.

465. Rebuffat P, Mazzocchi G, Gottardo G, et al. Further investigations on the atrial natriuretic factor (ANF)–induced inhibition of the growth and steroidogenic capacity of rat adrenal zona glomerulosa in vivo. J Steroid Biochem 1988; 29:605–609.

466. Longcope C. Adrenal and gonadal androgen secretion in normal females. Clin Endocrinol Metab 1986; 15:213–228.

467. Nelson DH. The Adrenal Cortex: Physiological Function and Disease. Philadelphia: W. B. Saunders, 1980.

468. Abraham GE. Ovarian and adrenal contribution to peripheral androgens during the menstrual cycle. J Clin Endocrinol Metab 1974; 39:340–346.

469. Lachelin GCL, Barnett M, Hopper BR, et al. Adrenal function in normal women and women with the polycystic ovarian syndrome. J Clin Endocrinol Metab 1979; 49:892–898.

470. Rosenfeld RS, Rosenberg BJ, Fukushima DK, et al. 24-Hour secretory pattern of dehydroisoandrosterone and dehydroisoandrosterone sulfate. J Clin Endocrinol Metab 1975; 40:850–855.

471. Parker LN, Odell WD. Control of adrenal androgen secretion. Endocr Rev 1980; 1:392–410.

472. Orentreich N, Brind JL, Rizer RL, et al. Age changes and sex differences in serum dehydroepiandrosterone sulfate concentrations throughout adulthood. J Clin Endocrinol Metab 1984; 59:551–555.

473. Zumoff B, Walsh BT, Katz JL, et al. Subnormal plasma dehydroisoandrosterone to cortisol ratio in anorexia nervosa: a second hormonal parameter of ontogenic regression. J Clin Endocrinol Metab 1983; 56:668–672.

474. Winterer J, Gwirtsman HE, George DT, et al. Adrenocorticotropin-stimulated adrenal androgen secretion in anorexia nervosa: impaired secretion at low weight with normalization after long-term weight recovery. J Clin Endocrinol Metab 1985; 61:693–697.

475. Parker LN, Levin ER, Lifrak ET. Evidence for adrenocortical adaptation to severe illness. J Clin Endocrinol Metab 1985; 60:947–952.

476. Rittmaster RS, Loriaux DL, Cutler GB Jr. Sensitivity of cortisol and adrenal androgens to dexamethasone suppression in hirsute women. J Clin Endocrinol Metab 1985; 61:462–466.

477. Albertson BD, Hobson WC, Burnett BS, et al. Dissociation of cortisol and adrenal androgen secretion in the hypophysectomized, adrenocorticotropin-replaced chimpanzee. J Clin Endocrinol Metab 1984; 59:13–18.

478. Parker LN, Lifrak ET, Odell WD. A 60,000 molecular weight human pituitary glycopeptide stimulates adrenal androgen secretion. Endocrinology 1983; 113:2092–2096.

479. Parker L, Lifrak E, Shively J, et al. Human adrenal gland cortical androgen–stimulating hormone (CASH) is identical with a portion of the joining peptide of pituitary pro-opiomelanocortin (POMC). Endocr Soc Abstr 1989: 97.

479a. Mellon SH, Shively JE, Miller WL. Human proopiomelanocortin-(79–96), a proposed androgen stimulatory hormone, does not affect steroidogenesis in cultured human fetal adrenal cells. J Clin Endocrinol Metab 1991; 72:19–22.

479b. Penchoat A, Sanchez P, Jaillard C, et al. Human proopiomelanocortin-(79–96), a proposed cortical androgen-stimulating hormone, does not affect steroidogenesis in cultured human adult adrenal cells. J Clin Endocrinol Metab 1991; 72:23–26.

480. Lobo RA, Kletzky OA, Kaptein EM, et al. Prolactin modulation of dehydroepiandrosterone sulfate secretion. Am J Obstet Gynecol 1980; 138:632–636.

481. Higuchi K, Nawata H, Maki T, et al. Prolactin has a direct effect on adrenal androgen secretion. J Clin Endocrinol Metab 1984; 59:714–718.

482. Feher T, Szalay KS, Szilagyi G. Effect of ACTH and prolactin on dehydroepiandrosterone, its sulfate ester and cortisol production by normal and tumorous human adrenocortical cells. J Steroid Biochem 1985; 23:153–157.

483. James VHT, Few JD. Adrenocorticosteroids: chemistry, synthesis and disturbances in diseases. Clin Endocrinol Metab 1985; 14:867–892.

484. Dunn JF, Nisula BC, Rodbard D. Transport of steroid hormones: binding of 21 endogenous steroids to both testosterone-binding globulin and corticosteroid-binding globulin in human plasma. J Clin Endocrinol Metab 1981; 53:58–68.

485. Pardridge WM. Transport of protein-bound hormones into tissues in vivo. Endocr Rev 1981; 2:103–123.

486. Hammond GL. Molecular properties of corticosteroid binding globulin and the sex steroid binding proteins. Endocr Rev 1990; 11:65–79.

487. Rosner W. The function of corticosteroid binding globulin and sex hormone–binding globulin: recent advances. Endocr Rev 1990; 11:80–91.

488. Pugeat MM, Dunn JF, Nisula BC. Transport of steroid hormones:

interaction of 70 drugs with testosterone-binding globulin and corticosteroid-binding globulin in human plasma. J Clin Endocrinol Metab 1981; 53:69–75.

489. Katayama S, Yamaji T. A binding-protein for aldosterone in human plasma. J Steroid Biochem 1982; 16:185–192.

490. Chavarri M, Luetscher JA, Dowdy AJ, et al. The effects of temperature and plasma cortisol on distribution of aldosterone between plasma and red blood cells: influence on metabolic clearance rate and on hepatic and renal extraction of aldosterone. J Clin Endocrinol Metab 1977; 44:752–759.

491. Hiramatsu R, Nisula BC. Erythrocyte-associated cortisol: measurement, kinetics of dissociation, and potential physiological significance. J Clin Endocrinol Metab 1987; 64:1224–1232.

492. Hammond GL, Smith CL, Goping IS, et al. Primary structure of human corticosteroid binding globulin, deduced from hepatic and pulmonary cDNAs, exhibits homology with serine protease inhibitors. Proc Natl Acad Sci USA 1987; 84:5153–5157.

493. Smith CL, Hammond GL. Rat corticosteroid binding globulin: primary structure and messenger ribonucleic acid levels in the liver under different physiological conditions. Mol Endocrinol 1989; 3:420–426.

494. Underhill DA, Hammond GL. Organization of the human corticosteroid binding globulin gene and analysis of its 5′-flanking region. Mol Endocrinol 1989; 3:1448–1454.

495. Rosner W, Beers PC, Awan T, et al. Identification of corticosteroid-binding globulin in human milk: measurement with a filter disk assay. J Clin Endocrinol Metab 1976; 42:1064–1073.

496. Singer CJ, Khan MS, Rosner W. Characteristics of the binding of corticosteroid-binding globulin to rat cell membranes. Endocrinology 1988; 122:89–96.

497. Brien TG. Human corticosteroid binding globulin. Clin Endocrinol 1981; 14:193–212.

498. Zager PG, Burtis WJ, Luetscher JA, et al. Increased plasma protein binding and lower metabolic clearance rate of aldosterone in plasma of low cortisol concentration. J Clin Endocrinol Metab 1976; 42:207–214.

499. Zipser RD, Speckart PF, Zia PK, et al. The effect of ACTH and cortisol on aldosterone and cortisol clearance and distribution of plasma and whole blood. J Clin Endocrinol Metab 1976; 43:1101–1109.

500. Coolens JL, Van Baelen H, Heyns W. Clinical use of unbound plasma cortisol as calculated from total cortisol and corticosteroid-binding globulin. J Steroid Biochem 1987; 26:197–202.

501. Musa BU, Seal US, Doe RP. Elevation of certain plasma proteins in man following estrogen administration: a dose-response relationship. J Clin Endocrinol Metab 1965; 25:1163–1166.

502. Orbach O. Increased serum cortisol binding in chronic active hepatitis. Am J Med 1989; 86:39–42.

503. Coolens JL, Heyns W. Marked elevation and cyclic variation of corticosteroid-binding globulin: an inherited abnormality. J Clin Endocrinol Metab 1989; 68:492–494.

504. Roitman A, Bruchis S, Bauman B, et al. Total deficiency of corticosteroid-binding globulin. Clin Endocrinol 1984; 21:541–548.

505. Walsh KA, Titani K, Takio K, et al. Amino acid sequence of the sex steroid binding protein of human plasma. Biochemistry 1986; 25:7584–7590.

506. Danzo BJ, Bell BW, Black JH. Human testosterone-binding globulin is a dimer composed of two identical protomers that are differentially glycosylated. Endocrinology 1989; 124:2809–2817.

507. Plymate SR, Leonard JM, Paulsen CA, et al. Sex hormone–binding globulin changes with androgen replacement. J Clin Endocrinol Metab 1983; 57:645–648.

508. von Schoultz B, Carlsröm K. General review: on the regulation of sex-hormone-binding globulin—challenge of an old dogma and outlines of an alternative mechanism. J Steroid Biochem 1989; 32:327–334.

509. Plymate SR, Matej LA, Jones RE, et al. Inhibition of sex hormone–binding globulin production in the human hepatoma (Hep G2) cell line by insulin and prolactin. J Clin Endocrinol Metab 1988; 67:460–464.

510. Westphal U. Steroid-Protein Interactions. New York: Springer-Verlag, 1971; 375–433.

511. Routledge PA. Clinical relevance of alpha 1 acid glycoprotein in health and disease. Prog Clin Biol Res 1989; 300:185–198.

512. Mendel CM. The free hormone hypothesis: a physiologically based mathematical model. Endocr Rev 1989; 10:232–274.

513. Ogawa K, Sueda K, Matsui N. The effect of cortisol, progesterone, and transcortin on phytohemagglutinin-stimulated human blood mononuclear cells and their interplay. J Clin Endocrinol Metab 1983; 56:121–126.

514. Pardridge WM, Sakiyama R, Judd HL. Protein-bound corticosteroid in human serum is selectively transported into rat brain and liver in vivo. J Clin Endocrinol Metab 1983; 57:160–165.

515. Mendel CM, Kuhn RW, Weisiger RA, et al. Uptake of cortisol by the perfused rat liver: validity of the free hormone hypothesis applied to cortisol. Endocrinology 1989; 124:468–476.

516. Pardridge WM. Plasma protein–mediated transport of steroid and thyroid hormones. Am J Physiol 1987; 252:E157–E164.

517. Mendel CM, Weisiger RA, Jones AL, et al. Thyroid hormone–binding

proteins in plasma facilitate uniform distribution of thyroxine within tissues: a perfused rat liver study. Endocrinology 1987; 120:1742–1749.

518. Peterson RE. Metabolism of adrenal cortical steroids. In: Christy NP, ed. The Human Adrenal Cortex. New York: Harper & Row, 1971: 87–189.

519. Clark AF. Steroid delta-4 reductases: their physiologic role and significance. In: Hobkirk R, ed. Steroid Biochemistry. Boca Raton, FL: CRC Press, 1979: 1–27.

520. McGuire JS, Tomkins GM. The heterogeneity of delta⁴ 3-ketosteroid reductases (5α). J Biol Chem 1960; 235:1634–1638.

521. Fisher LK, Kogut MD, Moore RJ, et al. Clinical, endocrinological, and enzymatic characterization of two patients with 5α-reductase deficiency: evidence that a single enzyme is responsible for the 5α-reduction of cortisol and testosterone. J Clin Endocrinol Metab 1978; 47:653–664.

522. Okuda A, Okuda K. Purification and characterization of delta⁴-3-ketosteroid 5β-reductase. J Biol Chem 1984; 259:7519–7524.

523. Fukushima DK, Bradlow HL, Hellman L, et al. Metabolic transformation of hydrocortisone ¹⁴C in man. J Biol Chem 1960; 235:2246–2252.

524. Sandberg AA, Chang E, Slaunwhite WR Jr. The conversion of 4-C¹⁴ cortisol to C¹⁴-17-ketosteroids. J Clin Endocrinol Metab 1957; 17:437–440.

525. Peterson RE, Wyngaarden JB, Guerra SL, et al. The physiological disposition and metabolic fate of hydrocortisone in man. J Clin Invest 1955; 34:1779–1794.

526. Voccia E, Saenger P, Peterson RE, et al. 6β-Hydroxycortisol excretion in hypercortisolemic states. J Clin Endocrinol Metab 1979; 48:467–471.

527. Siest G, Antoine B, Fournel S, et al. The glucuronosyl transferases: what progress can pharmacologists expect from molecular biology and cellular enzymology? Biochem Pharmacol 1987; 36:983–989.

528. Falany CN, Green M, Tephly TR. The enzymatic mechanism of glucuronidation catalyzed by two purified rat liver steroid UDP-glucuronosyltransferases. J Biol Chem 1987; 262:1218–1222.

529. Falany CN, Green M, Swain E, et al. Substrate specificity and characterization of rat liver p-nitrophenol, 3α-hydroxysteroid and 17β-hydroxysteroid UDP-glucuronosyltransferases. Biochem J 1986; 238:65–73.

530. Peterson RE. The influence of the thyroid on adrenocortical function. J Clin Invest 1958; 37:736–743.

531. McGuire JS, Tomkins GM. The effects of thyroxine administration on the enzymic reduction of delta⁴ 3-ketosteroids. J Biol Chem 1959; 234:791–794.

532. Mode A, Rafter I. The sexually differentiated delta⁴-3-ketosteroid-5β-reductase of rat liver. Purification, characterization, and quantitation. J Biol Chem 1985; 260:7137–7141.

533. West CD, Brown H, Simon EL, et al. Adrenocortical function and cortisol metabolism in old age. J Clin Endocrinol Metab 1961; 21:1197–1207.

534. Peterson RE. Adrenocortical steroid metabolism and adrenocortical function in liver disease. J Clin Invest 1960; 39:320–331.

535. Migeon CJ, Green OC, Eckert JP. Study of adrenocortical function in obesity. J Clin Endocrinol Metab 1963; 12:718–739.

536. Werk EE Jr, MacGee J, Sholiton LJ. Effect of diphenylhydantoin on cortisol metabolism in man. J Clin Invest 1964; 43:1824–1835.

537. Burstein S, Klaiber EL. Phenobarbital induced increase in 6β-hydroxycortisol excretion: clue to its significance in human urine. J Clin Endocrinol Metab 1965; 25:293–296.

538. Edwards OM, Courtenay-Evans RJ, Galley JM, et al. Changes in cortisol metabolism following rifampicin therapy. Lancet 1974; 2:549–551.

539. Baciewicz AM, Self TH, Bekemeyer WB. Update on rifampin drug interactions. Arch Intern Med 1987; 147:565–568.

540. Kyriazopoulou V, Parparousi O, Vagenakis AG. Rifampicin-induced adrenal crisis in addisonian patients receiving corticosteroid replacement therapy. J Clin Endocrinol Metab 1984; 59:1204–1206.

541. Yamada S, Iwai K. Induction of hepatic cortisol-6-hydroxylase by rifampicin. Lancet 1976; 2:366–367.

542. Sirgo MA, Rocci ML Jr, Ferguson RK, et al. Effects of cimetidine and ranitidine on the conversion of prednisone to prednisolone. Clin Pharmacol Ther 1985; 37:534–538.

543. Monder C, Shackleton CHL. 11β-Hydroxysteroid dehydrogenase: fact or fancy? Steroids 1984; 44:383–417.

544. Whitworth JA, Stewart PM, Burt D, et al. The kidney is the major site of cortisone production in man. Clin Endocrinol 1989; 31:355–361.

545. Funder JW, Pearce PT, Smith R, et al. Mineralocorticoid action: target tissue specificity is enzyme, not receptor, mediated. Science 1988; 242:583–585.

546. Edwards CRW, Stewart PM, Burt D, et al. Localisation of 11β-hydroxysteroid dehydrogenase–tissue specific protector of the mineralocorticoid receptor. Lancet 1988; 2:986–989.

547. Abramovitz M, Branchaud CL, Murphy BEP. Cortisol-cortisone interconversion in human fetal lung: contrasting results using explants and monolayer cultures suggest that 11β-hydroxysteroid dehydrogenase (E.C. 1.1.1.146) comprises two enzymes. J Clin Endocrinol Metab 1982; 54:563–568.

548. Melby JC. Intermediary metabolism of aldosterone. In: Page IH, Bumpus FN, eds. Handbook of Experimental Pharmacology. Vol 37. New York: Springer-Verlag, 1973: 298–321.

549. Kelly WG, Bandy L, Lieberman SL, et al. Isolation and characterization of human urinary metabolites of aldosterone. V. Dehydroaldosterone and 21-deoxytetrahydroaldosterone. Biochemistry 1963; 2:1249–1254.

550. Kelly WG, Bandy L, Lieberman SL. Isolation and characterization of human urinary metabolites of aldosterone. IV. The synthesis and stereochemistry of two bicyclic acetal metabolites. Biochemistry 1963; 2:1243–1248.

551. Ulick S, Laragh S, Lieberman SL. The isolation of a urinary metabolite of aldosterone and its use to measure the rate of secretion of aldosterone by the adrenal cortex of man. Trans Assoc Am Physicians 1958; 71:225–235.

552. Axelrad BJ, Cates JE, Johnson BB, et al. Aldosterone in urine of normal men and of patients with oedema: its increased recovery after hydrolysis with acid and with β-glucuronidase. Br J Med 1955; 1:196–199.

553. Coppage WS, Island DP, Cooner AE, et al. The metabolism of aldosterone in normal subjects and in patients with hepatic cirrhosis. J Clin Invest 1962; 41:1672–1680.

554. Bledsoe T, Liddle GW, Riondel A, et al. Comparative fates of intravenously and orally administered aldosterone: evidence for extrahepatic formation of acid-hydrolyzable conjugate in man. J Clin Invest 1966; 45:264–269.

555. Tait JF, Little B, Tait SA. Splanchnic extraction and clearance of aldosterone in subjects with minimal and marked cardiac dysfunction. J Clin Endocrinol Metab 1965; 25:219–228.

556. Baulieu EE, Corpechot C, Dray F. An adrenal secreted androgen: dehydroisoandrosterone sulfate. Its metabolism and a tentative generalization on the metabolism of other steroid conjugates in man. Recent Prog Horm Res 1965; 21:411–500.

557. Cahill G. Action of adrenal cortical steroids on carbohydrate metabolism. In: Christy NP, ed. The Human Adrenal Cortex. New York: Harper & Row, 1973: 205–239.

558. Gustafsson JA, Carlstedt-Duke J, Poellinger L, et al. Biochemistry, molecular biology, and physiology of the glucocorticoid receptor. Endocr Rev 1987; 8:185–234.

559. Harrison RW, Fairfield S, Orth DN. Evidence for glucocorticoid transport through the target cell membrane. Biochem Biophys Res Commun 1974; 61:1262–1267.

560. Rao GS, Schultze-Hagen K, Rao ML, et al. Kinetics of steroid transport through cell membranes: comparison of the uptake of cortisol by isolated rat liver cells with the binding of cortisol to rat liver cytosol. J Steroid Biochem 1976; 7:1123–1129.

561. Rao ML, Rao GS, Eckel J, et al. Factors involved in the uptake of corticosterone by rat liver cells. Biochim Biophys Acta 1977; 500:322–332.

562. Wrange O, Carlstedt-Duke J, Gustafsson JA. Purification of the glucocorticoid receptor from rat liver cytosol. J Biol Chem 1979; 254:9284–9290.

563. Govindan MV, Manz B. Three-step purification of glucocorticoid receptors from rat liver. Eur J Biochem 1980; 108:47–53.

564. Eisen HJ, Schleenbaker RE, Simons S. Affinity labeling of the rat liver glucocorticoid receptor with dexamethasone 21-mesylate. Identification of the covalently labeled receptor by immunochemical methods. J Biol Chem 1981; 256:12920–12925.

565. Nordeen SK, Lan NC, Showers MO, et al. Photoaffinity labeling of glucocorticoid receptors. J Biol Chem 1981; 256:10503–10508.

566. Simons SS, Thompson EB. Dexamethasone 21-mesylate: an affinity label of glucocorticoid receptors from rat hepatoma tissue. Proc Natl Acad Sci USA 1981; 78:3541–3545.

567. Dellweg HG, Hotz A, Mugele K, et al. Active domains in wild-type and mutant glucocorticoid receptors. EMBO J 1982; 1:285–289.

568. Vedeckis W. Subunit dissociation as a possible mechanism of glucocorticoid receptor activation. Biochemistry 1983; 22:1983–1989.

569. Okret S, Wikstrom AC, Gustafsson JA. Molybdate-stabilized glucocorticoid receptor: evidence for a receptor heterodimer. Biochemistry 1985; 24:6581–6586.

570. Housley PR, Pratt WB. Direct demonstration of glucocorticoid receptor phosphorylation by intact L-cells. J Biol Chem 1983; 258:4630–4635.

571. Housley PR, Sanchez ER, Westphal HM, et al. The molybdate-stabilized L-cell glucocorticoid receptor isolated by affinity chromatography or with a monoclonal antibody is associated with a 90–92 kDa nonsteroid-binding protein. J Biol Chem 1985; 260:13810–13817.

572. Catelli MG, Binart N, Jung-Testas I, et al. The common 90-kd protein component of non-transformed "8S" steroid receptors is a heat shock protein. EMBO J 1985; 4:3131–3135.

573. Sanchez ER, Toft DO, Schlesinger MJ, et al. Evidence that the 90 kDa phosphoprotein associated with the untransformed L-cell glucocorticoid receptor is a murine heat-shock protein. J Biol Chem 1985; 260:12398–12401.

574. Sanchez ER, Meschinchi S, Tienrungroj W, et al. Relationship of the 90-kDa murine heat shock protein to the untransformed and transformed states of the L cell glucocorticoid receptor. J Biol Chem 1987; 262:6986–6991.

575. Mendel DB, Bodwell JE, Gametchu B, et al. Molybdate-stabilized glucocorticoid-receptor complexes contain a 90 kDa non–steroid-binding phosphoprotein that is lost on activation. J Biol Chem 1986; 261:3758–3763.

576. Denis M, Wikstrom AC, Gustafsson JA. The molybdate-stabilized nonactivated glucocorticoid receptor contains a dimer of M_r 90,000 non–hormone-binding protein. J Biol Chem 1987; 262:11803–11806.

577. Schmidt TJ, Litwack G. Activation of the glucocorticoid-receptor complex. Physiol Rev 1982; 62:1131–1192.

578. Rousseau GG, Baxter JD, Higgins SJ, et al. Steroid-induced nuclear binding of glucocorticoid receptors in intact hepatoma cells. J Mol Biol 1973; 79:539–554.

579. Govindan MV. Immunofluorescence microscopy of the intracellular translocation of glucocorticoid-receptor complexes in rat hepatoma (HTC) cells. Exp Cell Res 1980; 127:293–297.

580. Papamichail M, Tsokos G, Tsawdaroglou N, et al. Immunocytochemical demonstration of glucocorticoid receptors in different cell types and their translocation from cytoplasm to the cell nucleus in the presence of dexamethasone. Exp Cell Res 1980; 125:490–493.

581. Wikstrom AC, Bakke O, Okret S, et al. Intracellular localization of the glucocorticoid receptor: evidence for cytoplasmic and nuclear localization. Endocrinology 1987; 120:1232–1242.

582. Welshons WV, Krummel BM, Gorski J. Nuclear localization of unoccupied receptors for glucocorticoids, estrogens, and progesterone in GH_3 cells. Endocrinology 1985; 117:2140–2147.

583. Carlstedt-Duke J, Stronstedt PE, Wrange O, et al. Domain structure of the glucocorticoid receptor protein. Proc Natl Acad Sci USA 1987; 84:4437–4440.

584. Wrange O, Gustafsson JA. Separation of the hormone- and DNA-binding sites of the hepatic glucocorticoid receptor by means of proteolysis. J Biol Chem 1978; 253:856–865.

585. Govindan MV. Purification of glucocorticoid receptors from rat liver cytosol. Preparation of antibodies against the major receptor proteins and application of immunologic techniques to study activation and translocation. J Steroid Biochem 1979; 11:323–332.

586. Okret S, Carlstedt-Duke J, Wrange O, et al. Characterization of an antiserum against the glucocorticoid receptor. Biochim Biophys Acta 1981; 677:205–219.

587. Westphal HM, Moldenhauer G, Beato M. Monoclonal antibodies to rat liver glucocorticoid receptors. EMBO J 1982; 1:1467–1471.

588. Okret S, Wikstrom AC, Wrange O, et al. Monoclonal antibodies against the rat liver glucocorticoid receptor. Proc Natl Acad Sci USA 1984; 81:1609–1613.

589. Gametchu B, Harrison RW. Characterization of a monoclonal antibody to the rat liver glucocorticoid receptor. Endocrinology 1984; 114:274–279.

590. Miesfield R, Okret S, Wikstrom AC, et al. Characterization of a steroid hormone receptor gene and mRNA in wild-type and mutant cells. Nature 1984; 312:779–781.

591. Weinberger C, Hollenberg SM, Ong ES, et al. Identification of human glucocorticoid receptor complementary DNA clones by epitope selection. Science 1985; 228:740–742.

592. Hollenberg SM, Weinberger C, Ong ES, et al. Primary structure and expression of a functional human glucocorticoid receptor cDNA. Nature 1985; 318:635–641.

593. Danielsen M, Northrup JP, Ringold GM. The mouse glucocorticoid receptor: mapping of functional domains by cloning, sequencing, and expression of wild-type and mutant receptor proteins. EMBO J 1986; 5:2513–2522.

594. Evans RM. The steroid and thyroid hormone receptor superfamily. Science 1988; 240:889–895.

595. Evans RM, Hollenberg SM. Zinc fingers: guilt by association. Cell 1988; 52:1–3.

596. Giguere V, Hollenberg SM, Rosenfeld MG, et al. Functional domains of the glucocorticoid receptor. Cell 1986; 46:645–652.

597. Hollenberg SM, Giguere V, Segui P, et al. Colocalization of DNA-binding and transcriptional activation functions in the human glucocorticoid receptor. Cell 1987; 49:39–46.

598. Rusconi S, Yamamoto KR. Functional dissection of the hormone and DNA binding activities of the glucocorticoid receptor. EMBO J 1987; 6:1309–1315.

599. Weinberger C, Hollenberg SM, Rosenfeld MG, et al. Domain structure of the human glucocorticoid receptor and its relationship to the v-erb-A oncogene product. Nature 1985; 318:670–672.

600. Picard D, Yamamoto KR. Two signals mediate hormone-dependent nuclear localization of the glucocorticoid receptor. EMBO J 1987; 6:3333–3340.

601. Beato M. Gene regulation by steroid hormones. Cell 1989; 56:335–344.

602. Yamamoto KR. Steroid receptor regulated transcription of specific genes and gene networks. Annu Rev Genet 1985; 19:209–215.

603. Scheidereit C, Geisse S, Westphal HM, et al. The glucocorticoid receptor binds to defined nucleotide sequences near the promoter of the mouse mammary tumor virus. Nature 1983; 304:749–752.

604. Scheidereit C, Beato M. Contacts between the receptor and DNA double helix within a glucocorticoid regulatory element of mouse mammary tumor virus. Proc Natl Acad Sci USA 1984; 81:3029–3033.

605. Scheidereit C, Westphal HM, Carlson C, et al. Molecular model of the interaction between the glucocorticoid receptor and the regulatory elements of inducible genes. DNA 1986; 5:383–391.

606. Strahle U, Klock G, Shutz G. A DNA sequence of 15 base pairs is sufficient to mediate both glucocorticoid and progesterone induction of gene expression. Proc Natl Acad Sci USA 1987; 84:7871–7875.

607. Petersen DD, Magnuson MA, Granner DK. Location and characterization of two widely separated glucocorticoid response elements in the phosphoenolpyruvate carboxykinase gene. Mol Cell Biol 1988; 8:96–104.

608. Otten AD, Sanders MM, McKnight GS. The MMTV LTR promoter is induced by progesterone and dihydrotestosterone but not by estrogen. Mol Endocrinol 1988; 2:143–147.

609. Green S, Kumar V, Thenlaz I, et al. The N-terminal DNA binding zinc finger of the oestrogen and glucocorticoid receptors determines target gene specificity. EMBO J 1988; 7:3037–3044.

610. Godowski PJ, Rusconi S, Miesfield R, et al. Glucocorticoid receptor mutants that are constitutive activators of transcriptional enhancement. Nature 1987; 325:365–368.

611. Miesfield R, Godowski PJ, Maler BA, et al. Glucocorticoid receptor mutants that define a small region sufficient for enhancer activation. Science 1987; 236:423–427.

612. Hollenberg SM, Evans RM. Multiple and cooperative trans-activation domains of the human glucocorticoid receptor. Cell 1988; 55:899–906.

613. Webster NJG, Green S, Rui JI, et al. The hormone binding domains of the estrogen and glucocorticoid receptors contain inducible transcription activation function. Cell 1988; 54:199–207.

614. Schule R, Muller M, Otsuka-Murakami H, et al. Cooperativity of the glucocorticoid receptor and the CACCC-box binding factor. Nature 1988; 332:87–90.

615. Adler S, Waterman MI, He X, et al. Steroid receptor–mediated inhibition of rat prolactin gene expression does not require the receptor DNA-binding domain. Cell 1988; 52:685–695.

615a. Jonat C, Rahmsdorf HJ, Park KK, et al. Antitumor promotion and antiinflammation: down modulation of AP-1 (fos/jun) activity by glucocorticoid hormone. Cell 1990; 62:1189–1204.

615b. Yang-Yen H-F, Chambard J-C, Sun Y-L, et al. Transcriptional interference between c-jun and the glucocorticoid receptor: mutual inhibition of DNA binding due to protein-protein interaction. Cell 1990; 62:1205–1215.

615c. Schule R, Rangarajan P, Kliewer S, et al. Functional antagonism between oncoprotein c-jun and the glucocorticoid receptor. Cell 1990; 62:1217–1226.

616. Drouin J, Charron J, Gagner JP, et al. The pro-opiomelanocortin gene: a model for negative regulation of transcription by glucocorticoids. J Cell Biochem 1987; 35:293–304.

617. Akerblom IE, Slater EP, Beato M, et al. Negative regulation by glucocorticoids through interference with a cAMP responsive element. Science 1988; 241:350–353.

618. Sakai DD, Helms S, Carlstedt-Duke J, et al. Hormone-mediated repression: a negative glucocorticoid response element for the bovine prolactin gene. Genes Dev 1988; 2:1144–1154.

619. August JT, Nelson DH, Thorn GW. Response of normal subjects to large amounts of aldosterone. J Clin Invest 1958; 37:1549–1555.

620. Morris DJ. The metabolism and mechanism of action of aldosterone. Endocr Rev 1981; 2:234–247.

621. Funder JW, Feldman D, Edelman IS. Specific aldosterone binding in rat kidney and parotid. J Steroid Biochem 1972; 3:209–213.

622. Marver D, Goodman D, Edelman IS. Relationships between renal cytoplasmic and nuclear aldosterone receptors. Kidney Int 1972; 1:210–223.

623. Pressley W, Funder JW. Glucocorticoid and mineralocorticoid receptors in gut mucosa. Endocrinology 1975; 97:588–596.

624. McEwen BS, Weiss JM, Schwartz LS. Selective retention of corticosterone by limbic structures in rat brain. Nature 1968; 220:911–912.

625. McEwen BS, Weiss JM, Schwartz LS. Uptake of corticosterone by the brain and its concentration by certain limbic structures. Brain Res 1969; 16:227–241.

626. Moguilewsky M, Raynaud JP. Evidence for a specific mineralocorticoid receptor in rat pituitary and brain. J Steroid Biochem 1980; 12:309–314.

627. Armanini D, Strasser T, Weber PC. Characterization of mineralocorticoid receptors in human mononuclear leukocytes. Am J Physiol 1985; 248:E338–E390.

628. Rousseau G, Baxter JD, Funder JW, et al. Glucocorticoid and mineralocorticoid receptors for aldosterone. J Steroid Biochem 1972; 3:219–227.

629. Funder JW, Feldman D, Edelman IS. The roles of plasma binding and receptor specificity in the mineralocorticoid action of aldosterone. Endocrinology 1973; 92:994–1004.

630. Krozowski ZS, Funder JW. Renal mineralocorticoid receptors and hippocampal corticosterone-binding species have identical intrinsic steroid specificity. Proc Natl Acad Sci USA 1983; 80:6056–6060.

631. Arriza JL, Weinberger C, Cerelli G, et al. Cloning of human mineralo-corticoid receptor complementary DNA: structural and functional kinship with the glucocorticoid receptor. Science 1987; 237:268–275.

632. Stephenson G, Krozowski Z, Funder JW. Extravascular CBG-like sites in rat kidney and mineralocorticoid specificity. Am J Physiol 1984; 246:F227–F233.

633. Sheppard K, Funder JW. Mineralocorticoid specificity of renal type I receptors: in vivo binding studies. Am J Physiol 1987; 252:E224–E229.

634. Cori CF, Cori GT. Fate of sugar in animal body: carbohydrate metabolism of adrenalectomized rats and mice. J Biol Chem 1927; 74:473–494.

635. Long CNH, Katzin B, Fry EG. The adrenal cortex and carbohydrate metabolism. Endocrinology 1940; 26:309–344.

636. Hornbrook KR, Burch HB, Lowry OH. The effects of adrenalectomy and hydrocortisone on rat liver metabolites and glycogen synthetase activity. Mol Pharmacol 1966; 2:106–116.

637. Stalmans W, Laloux M. Glucocorticoids and hepatic glycogen metabolism. In: Baxter JD, Rousseau GG, eds. Glucocorticoid Hormone Action. New York: Springer-Verlag, 1979: 518–533.

638. Exton JH. Regulation of gluconeogenesis by glucocorticoids. In: Baxter JD, Rousseau GG, eds. Glucocorticoid Hormone Action. New York: Springer-Verlag, 1979: 535–546.

639. Yoo-Warren H, Cimbala MA, Felz K, et al. Identification of a DNA clone to phosphoenolpyruvate carboxykinase (GTP) from rat cytosol. Alterations in phosphoenolpyruvate carboxykinase RNA levels detectable by hybridization. J Biol Chem 1981; 256:10224–10227.

640. Magnuson MA, Quinn PG, Granner DK. Multihormonal regulation of phosphoenolpyruvate carboxykinase–chloramphenicol acetyltransferase fusion genes. Insulin's effects oppose those of cAMP and dexamethasone. J Biol Chem 1987; 262:14917–14920.

641. Friedmann N, Exton JH, Park CR. Interaction of adrenal steroids and glucagon on gluconeogenesis in perfused rat liver. Biochem Biophys Res Commun 1967; 29:113–119.

642. Munck A. Studies on the mode of action of glucocorticoids in rats. II. The effects in vivo and in vitro on net glucose uptake by isolated adipose tissue. Biochim Biophys Acta 1962; 57:318–326.

643. LeBoeuf B, Renold AE, Cahill GF. Studies on rat adipose tissue in vitro. IX. Further effects of cortisol on glucose metabolism. J Biol Chem 1962; 237:988–991.

644. Fain JN, Scow RO, Chernick SS. Effects of glucocorticoids on metabolism of adipose tissue in vitro. J Biol Chem 1963; 238:54–58.

645. Fain JH. Inhibition of glucose transport in fat cells and activation of lipolysis by glucocorticoids. In: Baxter JD, Rousseau GG, eds. Glucocorticoid Hormone Action. New York: Springer-Verlag, 1979: 547–560.

646. Olefsky JM. Effect of dexamethasone on insulin binding, glucose transport, and glucose oxidation of isolated rat adipocytes. J Clin Invest 1975; 56:1499–1508.

647. Livingston JN, Lockwood DH. Effect of glucocorticoids on the glucose transport system of isolated fat cells. J Biol Chem 1975; 250:8353–8360.

648. Garvey WT, Huecksteadt TP, Lima FB, et al. Expression of a glucose transporter gene cloned from brain in cellular models of insulin resistance: dexamethasone decreases transporter mRNA in primary cultured adipocytes. Mol Endocrinol 1989; 3:1132–1141.

649. Goodman HM, Knobil E. Some endocrine factors in regulation of fatty acid mobilization during fasting. Am J Physiol 1961; 201:1–3.

650. Fain JH. Effects of dexamethasone and growth hormone on fatty acid mobilization and glucose utilization in adrenalectomized rats. Endocrinology 1962; 71:633–635.

651. Havel R. Transport and metabolism of chylomicrons. Am J Clin Nutr 1958; 6:662–668.

652. Rudman D, Di Girolamo M. Effects of adrenal cortical steroids on lipid metabolism. In: Christy NP, ed. The Human Adrenal Cortex. New York: Harper & Row, 1971: 241–255.

653. Hausberger FX. Influence of insulin and cortisone on hepatic and adipose tissue metabolism of rats. Endocrinology 1958; 63:14–19.

654. Graham BS, Tucker WS Jr. Opportunistic infections in endogenous Cushing's syndrome. Ann Intern Med 1984; 101:334–338.

655. Fauci AS, Dale DC. The effect of in vivo hydrocortisone on subpopulations of human lymphocytes. J Clin Invest 1974; 53:240–246.

656. Yu DTY, Clements PJ, Paulus HE, et al. Human lymphocyte subpopulations. Effect of corticosteroids. J Clin Invest 1974; 53:565–571.

657. Dale DC, Fauci AS, Guerry D, et al. Comparison of agents producing a neutrophilic leucocytosis in man: hydrocortisone, prednisone, endotoxin, and etiocholanolone. J Clin Invest 1975; 56:808–813.

658. Munck A, Crabtree GR, Smith KA. Glucocorticoid receptors and actions in rat thymocytes and immunologically stimulated human peripheral lymphocytes. In: Baxter JD, Rousseau GG, eds. Glucocorticoid Hormone Action. New York: Springer-Verlag, 1979: 341–355.

659. Morita Y, Munck A. Effect of glucocorticoids in vivo and in vitro on net glucose uptake and amino acid incorporation by rat thymus cells. Biochim Biophys Acta 1964; 93:150–157.

660. Makman MH, Dvorkin B, White A. Alterations in protein and nucleic acid metabolism of thymocytes produced by adrenal steroids in vitro. J Biol Chem 1966; 241:1646–1648.

661. Horibata K, Harris AW. Mouse myelomas and lymphomas in culture. Exp Cell Res 1970; 60:61–77.

662. Sibley CH, Yamamoto KR. Mouse lymphoma cells: mechanisms of resistance to glucocorticoids. In: Baxter JD, Rousseau GG, eds. Glucocorticoid Hormone Action. New York: Springer-Verlag, 1979: 357–376.

663. Compton MM, Cidlowski JA. Identification of a glucocorticoid induced nuclease in thymocytes. A potential "lysis gene" product. J Biol Chem 1987; 262:8288–8292.

664. Lipmann ME, Barr RD. Glucocorticoid receptors in purified subpopulations of human peripheral blood lymphocytes. J Immunol 1977; 118:1977–1981.

665. Gillis S, Crabtree GR, Smith KA. Glucocorticoid-induced inhibition of T cell growth factor production. I. The effect on mitogen-induced lymphocyte proliferation. J Immunol 1979; 123:1624–1631.

666. Arya SK, Wong-Staal F, Gallo RC. Dexamethasone-mediated inhibition of human T cell growth factor and gamma interferon messenger RNA. J Immunol 1984; 133:273–276.

667. Fauci AS, Pratt KR, Whalen G. Activation of human B lymphocytes. IV. Regulating effects of corticosteroids on the triggering signal in the plaque-forming response of human peripheral B lymphocytes to polyclonal activation. J Immunol 1977; 119:598–603.

668. Cupps TR, Gerrard TL, Falko JM, et al. Effects of in vitro corticosteroids on B cell activation, proliferation, and differentiation. J Clin Invest 1985; 75:754–761.

669. Smith RW, Sherman WA, Middleton E Jr. Effect of hydrocortisone on immunoglobulin synthesis and secretion by human peripheral lymphocytes in vitro. Int Arch Allergy Appl Immunol 1972; 43:859–870.

670. Cooper DA, Duckett M, Petts V, et al. Corticosteroid enhancement of immunoglobulin synthesis by pokeweed mitogen–stimulated human lymphocytes. Clin Exp Immunol 1979; 37:145–151.

671. Grayson J, Dooley NJ, Koski IR, et al. Immunoglobulin production induced in vitro by glucocorticoid hormones. T cell–dependent stimulation of immunoglobulin production without B cell proliferation in cultures of human peripheral blood. J Clin Invest 1981; 68:1539–1547.

672. Ishii Y, Shinoda M, Shikita M. Specificity of the suppressive action of glucocorticoids on the proliferation of monocyte/macrophages in the CSF-stimulated cultures of mouse bone marrow. Exp Hematol [Copenh] 1983; 11:178–186.

673. Rinehart JJ, Wuest D, Ackerman GA. Corticosteroid alteration of human monocyte to macrophage differentiation. J Immunol 1982; 129:1436–1440.

674. Rinehart JJ, Sagone AL, Balcerzak SP, et al. Effects of corticosteroid therapy on human monocyte function. N Engl J Med 1975; 292:236–241.

675. Zweifach BW, Schorr E, Black MM. The influence of the adrenal cortex on the terminal vascular bed. Ann NY Acad Sci 1953; 56:626–633.

676. Fauci AS. Immunosuppressive and antiinflammatory effects of glucocorticoids. In: Baxter JD, Rousseau GG, eds. Glucocorticoid Hormone Action. New York: Springer-Verlag, 1979: 449–465.

677. Vane JR. Prostaglandins as mediators of inflammation. Adv Prostaglandin Thromboxane Res 1979; 2:791–801.

678. Kantrowitz F, Robinson DR, McGuire MB, et al. Corticosteroids inhibit prostaglandin production by rheumatoid synovia. Nature 1975; 258:737–739.

679. Tashjian AH Jr, Voelkel EF, McDonough J, et al. Hydrocortisone inhibits prostaglandin production by mouse fibrosarcoma cells. Nature 1975; 258:739–741.

680. Hong SC, Levine L. Inhibition of arachidonic acid release from cells as a biochemical action of anti-inflammatory steroids. Proc Natl Acad Sci USA 1976; 73:1730–1734.

681. Russo-Marie F, Paing M, Duval D. Involvement of glucocorticoid receptors in steroid-induced inhibition of prostaglandin secretion. J Biol Chem 1979; 254:8498–8504.

682. Flower RJ, Blackwell GJ. Anti-inflammatory steroids induce biosynthesis of a phospholipase A_2 inhibitor which prevents prostaglandin generation. Nature 1979; 278:456–459.

683. Flower RJ, Wood JN, Parente L. Macrocortin and the mechanism of action of glucocorticoids. Adv Inflammation Res 1984; 7:61–69.

684. Flower RJ. Background and discovery of lipocortins. Agents Actions 1985; 17:255–262.

685. Fava RA, Cohen S. Isolation of a calcium-dependent 35-kilodalton substrate for the epidermal growth factor receptor/kinase from A-431 cells. J Biol Chem 1984; 259:2636–2645.

686. Wallner BP, Mattaliano RJ, Hession C, et al. Cloning and expression of human lipocortin, a phospholipase A_2 inhibitor with potent antiinflammatory activity. Nature 1986; 320:77–81.

687. Northrup JK, Valentine-Braun KA, Johnson LK, et al. Evaluation of the antiinflammatory and phospholipase-inhibitory activity of calpactin II/lipocortin I. J Clin Invest 1988; 82:1347–1352.

688. Bronnegard M, Andersson O, Edwall D, et al. Human calpactin II (lipocortin I) messenger ribonucleic acid is not induced by glucocorticoids. Mol Endocrinol 1988; 2:732–739.

689. Werb Z. Biochemical actions of glucocorticoids on macrophages in

culture. Specific inhibition of elastase, collagenase and plasminogen activator secretion and effects on other metabolic functions. J Exp Med 1978; 147:1695–1712.

690. Hamilton JA, Bootes A, Phillips PE, et al. Human synovial fibroblast plasminogen activator. Modulation of enzyme activity by antiinflammatory steroids. Arthritis Rheum 1981; 24:1296–1302.

691. Vassalli JD, Hamilton J, Reich E. Macrophage plasminogen activator: modulation of enzyme production by anti-inflammatory steroids, mitotic inhibitors, and cyclic nucleotides. Cell 1976; 8:271–281.

692. Medcalf RL, Van den Berg E, Schleuning WD. Glucocorticoid-modulated gene expression of tissue and urinary-type plasminogen activator and plasminogen activator inhibitor 1 and 2. J Cell Biol 1988; 106:971–978.

693. Frost HM, Villanueva AR. Human osteoblastic activity. III. The effect of cortisone on lamellar osteoblastic activity. Henry Ford Hosp Med Bull 1961; 9:97–99.

694. Jowsey J, Riggs BL. Bone formation in hypercortisolism. Acta Endocrinol 1970; 63:21–28.

695. Hahn TJ, Halstead LR, Teitelbaum SL, et al. Altered mineral metabolism in glucocorticoid-induced osteopenia. Effect of 25-hydroxyvitamin D administration. J Clin Invest 1979; 64:655–665.

696. Bar-Shavit Z, Kahn AJ, Pegg LE, et al. Glucocorticoids modulate macrophage surface oligosaccharides and their bone binding activity. J Clin Invest 1984; 73:1277–1283.

697. Raisz LG, Trummel CL, Wener JA, et al. Effect of glucocorticoids on bone resorption in tissue culture. Endocrinology 1972; 90:961–967.

698. Teitelbaum SL, Malone JD, Kahn AJ. Glucocorticoid enhancement of bone resorption by rat peritoneal macrophages in vitro. Endocrinology 1981; 108:795–799.

699. Wajchenberg BL, Pereira VG, Kieffer J, et al. Effect of dexamethasone on calcium metabolism and ^{47}Ca kinetics in normal subjects. Acta Endocrinol 1969; 61:173–192.

700. Lukert BP, Adams JS. Calcium and phosphorus homeostasis in man: effects of corticosteroids. Arch Intern Med 1976; 136:1249–1253.

701. Klein RG, Arnaud SB, Gallagher JC, et al. Intestinal calcium absorption in exogenous hypercortisolism: role of 25-hydroxyvitamin D and corticosteroid dose. J Clin Invest 1977; 60:253–259.

702. Hahn TJ, Halstead LR, Baran DT. Effects of short term glucocorticoid administration on intestinal calcium absorption and circulating vitamin D metabolite concentrations in man. J Clin Endocrinol Metab 1981; 52:111–115.

703. Findling JW, Adams ND, Lemann J Jr, et al. Vitamin D metabolites and parathyroid hormone in Cushing's syndrome: relationship to calcium and phosphorus homeostasis. J Clin Endocrinol Metab 1982; 54:1039–1044.

704. Lee DB. Unanticipated stimulatory activity of glucocorticoids on epithelial calcium absorption. J Clin Invest 1983; 71:322–328.

705. Fucik RF, Kukreja SC, Hargis GK. Effect of glucocorticoids on the function of the parathyroid glands in man. J Clin Endocrinol Metab 1975; 40:152–155.

706. Breslau NA, Zerwekh JE, Nicar MJ, et al. Effects of short term glucocorticoid administration in primary hyperparathyroidism: comparison to sarcoidosis. J Clin Endocrinol Metab 1982; 54:824–830.

707. Au WYW. Cortisol stimulation of parathyroid hormone secretion by rat parathyroid glands in organ culture. Science 1976; 193:1015–1017.

708. Jackson WPU, Duncaster C. A consideration of the hypercalciuria in sarcoidosis, idiopathic hypercalciuria, and that caused by vitamin D. A new suggestion regarding calcium metabolism. J Clin Endocrinol Metab 1959; 19:658–680.

709. Laake H. The action of corticosteroids on the renal absorption of calcium. Acta Endocrinol 1960; 34:60–64.

710. Pratt WB, Aronow L. The effect of glucocorticoids on protein and nucleic acid synthesis in mouse fibroblasts growing in vitro. J Biol Chem 1966; 241:5244–5250.

711. Ehrlich HP, Tarver H, Hunt TK. Effects of vitamin A and glucocorticoids upon inflammation and collagen synthesis. Ann Surg 1973; 177:222–227.

712. Ponec M, Hasper I, Vianden GDNE, et al. Effects of glucocorticosteroids on primary human skin fibroblasts. II. Effects on total protein and collagen synthesis by confluent cell cultures. Arch Dermatol Res 1977; 259:125–134.

713. Sterling KM, Harris MJ, Mitchell JJ, et al. Dexamethasone decreases the amounts of type I procollagen mRNAs in vivo and in fibroblast cell cultures. J Biol Chem 1983; 258:7644–7647.

714. Shull S, Cutroneo KR. Glucocorticoids coordinately regulate procollagens type I and type III synthesis. J Biol Chem 1983; 258:3364–3369.

715. Raghow R, Gossage D, Kang AH. Pretranslational regulation of type I collagen, fibronectin, and a 50-kilodalton noncollagenous extracellular protein by dexamethasone in rat fibroblasts. J Biol Chem 1986; 261:4677–4684.

716. Mapleson JL, Buchwald M. Effect of cycloheximide and dexamethasone phosphate on hyaluronic acid synthesis and secretion in cultured human skin fibroblasts. J Cell Physiol 1981; 109:215–222.

717. Smith TJ. Dexamethasone regulation of glycosaminoglycan synthesis in cultured human skin fibroblasts. Similar effects of glucocorticoid and thyroid hormones. J Clin Invest 1984; 74:2157–2163.

718. Leibovich SJ, Ross R. The role of the macrophage in wound repair. A study with hydrocortisone and antimacrophage serum. Am J Pathol 1975; 78:71–100.

719. Pierce GF, Mustoe TA, Lingelbach J, et al. Transforming growth factor β reverses the glucocorticoid-induced wound healing deficit in rats: possible regulation in macrophages by platelet-derived growth factor. Proc Natl Acad Sci USA 1989; 86:2229–2233.

720. Furcht LT, Mosher DF, Wendelshafer-Crabb G, et al. Dexamethasone-induced accumulation of a fibronectin and collagen extracellular matrix in transformed human cells. Nature 1979; 277:393–395.

721. Oliver N, Newby RF, Furcht L, et al. Regulation of fibronectin biosynthesis by glucocorticoids in human fibrosarcoma cells and normal fibroblasts. Cell 1983; 33:267–296.

722. Dean DC, Newby RF, Bougeois S. Regulation of fibronectin biosynthesis by dexamethasone, transforming growth factor β, and cAMP in human cell lines. J Cell Biol 1988; 106:2159–2170.

723. Mecham RP, Morris SL, Levy BD, et al. Glucocorticoids stimulate elastin production in differentiated bovine ligament fibroblasts but do not induce elastin synthesis in undifferentiated cells. J Biol Chem 1984; 259:12414–12418.

724. Krakoff L, Nicolis G, Amsel B. Pathogenesis of hypertension in Cushing's syndrome. Am J Med 1975; 58:216–220.

725. Saruta T, Suzuki H, Handa M, et al. Multiple factors contribute to the pathogenesis of hypertension in Cushing's syndrome. J Clin Endocrinol Metab 1986; 62:275–279.

726. Grunfeld JP. Effects of antiglucocorticoids on glucocorticoid hypertension in the rat. Hypertension 1985; 7:292–299.

727. Handa M, Kondo K, Suzuki H, et al. Urinary prostaglandin E_2 and kallikrein excretion in glucocorticoid hypertension in rats. Clin Sci 1983; 65:37–42.

728. Stockigt JR, Hewett MJ, Topliss DJ, et al. Renin and renin substrate in primary adrenal insufficiency: contrasting effects of glucocorticoid and mineralocorticoid deficiency. Am J Med 1979; 66:915–922.

729. Slessor A. Studies concerning the mechanism of water retention in Addison's disease and in hypopituitarism. J Clin Endocrinol Metab 1951; 11:700–723.

730. Garrod O, Burston RA. The diuretic response to ingested water in Addison's disease and panhypopituitarism and the effect of cortisone thereon. Clin Soc Lond 1952; 11:113–128.

731. Raff H. Glucocorticoid inhibition of neurohypophysial vasopressin secretion. Am J Physiol 1987; 21:R635–R644.

732. Uht RM, McKelvy JF, Harrison RW, et al. Demonstration of glucocorticoid receptor–like immunoreactivity in glucocorticoid-sensitive vasopressin and corticotropin-releasing factor neurons in the hypothalamic paraventricular nucleus. J Neurosci Res 1988; 19:405–411.

733. Schwartz J, Keil LC, Maselli J, et al. Role of vasopressin in blood pressure regulation during adrenal insufficiency. Endocrinology 1983; 112:234–238.

734. Gaunt R, Renzie AA, Gisoldi E, et al. A sodium retaining influence of enucleate rat adrenal glands. Endocrinology 1967; 81:1331–1337.

735. Gaunt R, Gisoldi E, Herkner J, et al. Sodium retention after adrenal enucleation: drug and salt appetite studies. Endocrinology 1968; 83:927–932.

736. Bengele HH, McNamara ER, Alexander EA. Natriuresis after adrenal enucleation: effect of spironolactone and dexamethasone. Am J Physiol 1977; 231:F8–F12.

737. Greenberg BD, Bencen GH, Seilhamer JJ, et al. Nucleotide sequence of the gene encoding human atrial natriuretic factor precursor. Nature 1984; 312:656–658.

738. Seidman CE, Bloch KD, Klein KA, et al. Nucleotide sequences of the human and mouse atrial natriuretic factor genes. Science 1984; 226:1206–1209.

739. Argentin S, Nemer M, Drouin J, et al. The gene for rat atrial natriuretic factor. J Biol Chem 1985; 260:4568–4571.

740. Gardner DG, Hane S, Trachewsky D, et al. Atrial natriuretic peptide mRNA is regulated by glucocorticoids in vivo. Biochem Biophys Res Commun 1986; 139:1047–1054.

741. Garcia R, Debinski W, Gutkowska J, et al. Gluco- and mineralocorticoids may regulate the natriuretic effect and the synthesis and release of atrial natriuretic factor by the rat atria in vivo. Biochem Biophys Res Commun 1985; 131:806–814.

742. Matsubara H, Hirata Y, Yoshimi H, et al. Effects of steroid and thyroid hormones on the synthesis of atrial natriuretic peptide by cultured atrial myocytes of rat. Biochem Biophys Res Commun 1987; 145:336–343.

743. Shields PP, Glembotski CC. The post-translational processing of rat pro–atrial natriuretic factor by primary atrial myocyte cultures. J Biol Chem 1988; 263:8091–8098.

744. Shields PP, Dixon JE, Glembotski CC. The secretion of atrial natriuretic factor-(99–126) by cultured cardiac myocytes is regulated by glucocorticoids. J Biol Chem 1988; 263:12619–12628.

745. McEwen BS. Influences of adrenocortical hormones on pituitary and brain function. In: Baxter JD, Rousseau GG, eds. Glucocorticoid Hormone Action. New York: Springer-Verlag, 1979: 467–492.

746. Kreiger DT. The central nervous system and Cushing's disease. Mt Sinai J Med (NY) 1972; 39:416–442.

747. Gillin JC, Jacobs LS, Fram DH, et al. Acute effect of glucocorticoid on human sleep. Nature 1972; 237:398–399.

748. Gillin JC, Jacobs LS, Snyder F, et al. Effects of ACTH on the sleep of normal subjects and patients with Addison's disease. Neuroendocrinology 1974; 15:21–31.

749. Jeffcoate WJ, Silverstone JT, Edwards CRW, et al. Psychiatric manifestations of Cushing's syndrome: response to lowering of plasma cortisol. Q J Med 1979; 48:465–472.

750. Cohen SI. Cushing's syndrome: a psychiatric study of 29 patients. Br J Psychiatry 1980; 136:120–124.

751. Christy NP. Iatrogenic Cushing's syndrome. In: Christy NP, ed. The Human Adrenal Cortex. New York: Harper & Row, 1979: 395–425.

752. Starkman MN, Schteingart DE, Schork MA. Cushing's syndrome after treatment: changes in cortisol and ACTH levels, and amelioration of the depressive syndrome. Psychiatry Res 1986; 19:177–188.

753. Loosen PT, Chambliss B, DeBold CR, et al. Psychiatric phenomenology in Cushing's disease. Arch Gen Psychiatry (in press).

754. Hua SY, Chen YZ. Membrane receptor–mediated electrophysiological effects of glucocorticoid on mammalian neurons. Endocrinology 1989; 124:687–691.

755. Ruf K, Steiner FA. Steroid-sensitive single neurons in rat hypothalamus and midbrain: identification by microelectrophoresis. Science 1967; 156:667–668.

756. Mandelbrod I, Feldman S, Werman R. Inhibition of firing is the primary effect of microelectrophoresis of cortisol to units in the rat tuberal hypothalamus. Brain Res 1974; 80:303–315.

757. Scheff SW, Benardo LS, Cotman CW. Hydrocortisone administration retards axon sprouting in the rat dentate gyrus. Exp Neurol 1980; 68:195–201.

758. Scheff SW, Cotman CW. Chronic glucocorticoid therapy alters axon sprouting in the hippocampal dentate gyrus. Exp Neurol 1982; 76:644–654.

759. Sapolsky RM, Krey LC, McEwen BS. Prolonged glucocorticoid exposure reduces hippocampal neuron number: implications for aging. J Neurosci 1985; 5:1222–1227.

760. Juurlink GHJ, Schousboe A, Jorgensen OS, et al. Induction by hydrocortisone of glutamine synthetase in mouse primary astrocyte cultures. J Neurochem 1981; 36:136–142.

761. Hallermayer K, Harmening C, Hamprecht B. Cellular localization and regulation of glutamine synthetase in primary cultures of brain cells from newborn mice. J Neurochem 1981; 37:43–52.

762. Patel AJ, Hunt A. Observations on cell growth and regulation of glutamine synthetase by dexamethasone in primary cultures of forebrain and cerebellar astrocytes. Dev Brain Res 1985; 18:175–184.

763. McCarthy KD, deVellis J. Preparation of separate astroglial and oligodendral glial cell cultures from rat cerebral tissue. J Cell Biol 1980; 85:890–902.

764. Cammer WD, Snyder S, Zimmerman TR, et al. Glycerol phosphate dehydrogenase, glucose-6-phosphate dehydrogenase, and lactate dehydrogenase: activities in oligodendrocytes, neurons, astrocytes, and myelin isolated from developing rat brains. J Neurochem 1982; 38:360–367.

765. Kumar S, Holmes E, Scully S, et al. The hormonal regulation of gene expression of glial markers: glutamine synthetase and glycerol phosphate dehydrogenase in primary cultures of rat brain and in C6 cell line. J Neurosci Res 1986; 16:251–264.

766. Sandle GI, McGlone F. Acute effects of dexamethasone on cationic transport in colonic epithelium. Gut 1987; 28:701–706.

767. Bastl CP. Regulation of cation transport by low doses of glucocorticoids in in vivo adrenalectomized rat colon. J Clin Invest 1987; 80:348–356.

768. Bastl CP. Effect of spironolactone on glucocorticoid-induced colonic cation transport. Am J Physiol 1988; 255:F1235–F1242.

769. Messer J, Reitman D, Sacks HS, et al. Association of adrenocorticosteroid therapy and peptic-ulcer disease. N Engl J Med 1983; 309:21–24.

770. Blodget FM, Burgin L, Iezzou D, et al. Effects of prolonged cortisone therapy on the statural growth, skeletal maturation, and metabolic status of children. N Engl J Med 1956; 254:636–641.

771. Martial JA, Seeburg PH, Matulich DT, et al. Regulation of growth hormone messenger RNA. In: Baxter JD, Rousseau GG, eds. Glucocorticoid Hormone Action. New York: Springer-Verlag, 1979: 279–289.

772. Frantz AG, Rabkin MT. Human growth hormone. Clinical measurements, response to hypoglycemia, and suppression by corticosteroids. N Engl J Med 1964; 271:1375–1381.

773. Strickland AL, Underwood LE, Voina SJ. Growth retardation in Cushing's syndrome. Am J Dis Child 1972; 123:207–213.

774. Martial JA, Baxter JD, Goodman HM, et al. Regulation of growth hormone messenger RNA by thyroid and glucocorticoid hormones. Proc Natl Acad Sci USA 1977; 74:1816–1820.

775. Unterman TG, Phillips LS. Glucocorticoid effects on somatomedins and somatomedin inhibitors. J Clin Endocrinol Metab 1985; 61:618–626.

776. Ballard PL. Glucocorticoids and differentiation. In: Baxter JD, Rousseau GG, eds. Glucocorticoid Hormone Action. New York: Springer-Verlag, 1979: 493–515.

777. Ballard PL. Glucocorticoid regulation of lung maturation. Mead Johnson Symp Perinat Dev Med 1987; 22–27.

778. Liley HG, Hawgood S, Wellenstein GA, et al. Surfactant protein of molecular weight 28,000–36,000 in cultured human fetal lung: cellular localization and effect of dexamethasone. Mol Endocrinol 1987; 1:205–215.

779. Odom MJ, Snyder JM, Boggaram V, et al. Glucocorticoid regulation of the major surfactant associated protein (SP-A) and its messenger nucleic acid and of morphological development of human fetal lung in vitro. Endocrinology 1988; 123:1712–1720.

780. Boggaram V, Mendelson CR. Transcriptional regulation of the gene encoding the major surfactant protein (SP-A) in rabbit fetal lung. J Biol Chem 1988; 263:19060–19065.

781. LeDouarin NM. Cell line segregation during peripheral nervous system ontogeny. Science 1986; 231:1515–1522.

782. Levi-Montalcini R, Angeletti PU. Nerve growth factor. Physiol Rev 1968; 48:534–569.

783. Thoenen H, Barde YA. Physiology of nerve growth factor. Physiol Rev 1980; 60:1285–1335.

784. Anderson DJ, Axel R. Molecular probes for the development and plasticity of neural crest derivatives. Cell 1985; 42:649–662.

785. Anderson DJ, Axel R. A bipotential neuroendocrine precursor whose choice of fate is determined by NGF and glucocorticoids. Cell 1986; 47:1079–1090.

786. Federoff HJ, Grabczyk E, Fishman MC. Dual regulation of GAP-43 gene expression by nerve growth factor and glucocorticoids. J Biol Chem 1988; 263:19290–19295.

787. Balsan S, Steru D, Bourdeau A, et al. Effects of long-term maintenance therapy with a new glucocorticoid, deflazacort, on mineral metabolism and statural growth. Calcif Tissue Int 1987; 40:303–309.

788. Papagano G, Bruno A, Cavallo-Perin P, et al. Glucose intolerance after short-term administration of corticosteroids in healthy subjects. Prednisone, deflazacort, and betamethasone. Arch Intern Med 1989; 149:1098–1101.

789. Mason AS, Meade TW, Lee JAH, et al. Epidemiological and clinical picture of Addison's disease. Lancet 1968; 2:744–747.

790. Nerup J. Addison's disease. Clinical studies. A report of 108 cases. Acta Endocrinol 1974; 76:127–141.

791. Barker NW. The pathologic anatomy in twenty-eight cases of Addison's disease. Arch Pathol 1929; 8:432–450.

792. Cedermark BJ, Sjöberg HE. The clinical significance of metastases to the adrenal glands. Surg Gynecol Obstet 1981; 152:607–610.

793. Mineura K, Goto T, Yoneya M, et al. Case report: pituitary enlargement associated with Addison's disease. Clin Radiol 1987; 38:435–437.

794. Scheithauer BW, Kovacs K, Randall RV. The pituitary gland in untreated Addison's disease. Arch Pathol Lab Med 1983; 107:484–487.

795. Krautli B, Müller J, Landolt AM, et al. ACTH-producing pituitary adenomas in Addison's disease: two cases treated by transsphenoidal microsurgery. Acta Endocrinol 1982; 99:357–363.

796. Sekiya K, Nawata H, Kato KI, et al. Diurnal rhythms of proopiomelanocortin-derived N-terminal peptide, β-lipotropin, β-endorphin and adrenocorticotropin in normal subjects and in patients with Addison's disease and Cushing's disease. Endocrinol Jpn 1986; 33:713–719.

797. Nakahara M, Shibasaki T, Shizume K, et al. Corticotropin-releasing factor test in normal subjects and patients with hypothalamic-pituitary-adrenal disorders. J Clin Endocrinol Metab 1983; 57:963–968.

798. Lytras N, Grossman A, Perry L, et al. Corticotrophin releasing factor: responses in normal subjects and patients with disorders of the hypothalamus and pituitary. Clin Endocrinol 1984; 20:71–84.

799. Fukata J, Nakai Y, Imura H, et al. Human corticotropin-releasing hormone test in normal subjects and patients with hypothalamic, pituitary or adrenocortical disorders. Endocrinol Jpn 1988; 35:491–502.

800. Burke CW. Adrenocortical insufficiency. Clin Endocrinol Metab 1985; 14:947–976.

801. Jacobs TP, Whitlock RT, Edsall J, et al. Addisonian crisis while taking high-dose glucocorticoids. JAMA 1988; 260:2082–2084.

802. Rao RH, Vagnucci AH, Amico JA. Bilateral massive adrenal hemorrhage: early recognition and treatment. Ann Intern Med 1989; 110:227–235.

803. Xarli VP, Steele AA, Davis PJ, et al. Adrenal hemorrhage in the adult. Medicine 1978; 57:211–221.

804. Migeon CJ, Kenny FM, Hung W, et al. Study of adrenal function in children with meningitis. Pediatrics 1967; 40:163–183.

805. Margaretten W, Nakai H, Landing BH. Septicemic adrenal hemorrhage. Am J Dis Child 1963; 105:346–351.

806. Dunlop D. Eighty-six cases of Addison's disease. Br Med J 1963; 2:887–891.

807. Irvine WJ, Barnes EW. Adrenocortical insufficiency. Clin Endocrinol Metab 1972; 1:549–594.

808. Thorn GW. The Diagnosis and Treatment of Adrenal Insufficiency. Springfield, IL: Charles C Thomas, 1949.

809. Jarvis JL, Jenkins D, Sosman MC, et al. Roentgenologic observations in Addison's disease. A review of 120 cases. Radiology 1954; 62:16–29.

810. Valenzuela GA, Smalley WE, Schain DC, et al. Reversibility of gastric dysmotility in cortisol deficiency. Am J Gastroenterol 1987; 82:1066–1068.
811. Tobin MV, Aldridge SA, Morris AI, et al. Gastrointestinal manifestations of Addison's disease. Am J Gastroenterol 1989; 84:1302–1305.
812. McBrien DJ, Jones RV, Creamer B. Steatorrhoea in Addison's disease. Lancet 1963; 1:25–26.
813. Thorn GW, Koepf GF, Lewis RA, et al. Carbohydrate metabolism in Addison's disease. J Clin Invest 1940; 19:813–832.
814. Artavia-Loria E, Chaussain JL, Bougnères PF, et al. Frequency of hypoglycemia in children with adrenal insufficiency. Acta Endocrinol 1986; 279:275–278.
815. Stacpoole PW, Interlandi JW, Nicholson WE, et al. Isolated ACTH deficiency: a heterogenous disorder. Critical review and report of four new cases. Medicine 1982; 61:13–24.
816. Takeda N, Yasuda K, Kitabchi AE, et al. Increased insulin binding of erythrocytes and insulin sensitivity in adrenal insufficiency. Metabolism 1987; 36:1063–1066.
817. Barnett AH, Espiner EA, Donald RA. Patients presenting with Addison's disease need not be pigmented. Postgrad Med J 1982; 58:690–692.
818. Quevedo WC Jr. The control of color in mammals. Am Zool 1969; 9:531–540.
819. Ebinger G, Six R, Bruyland M, et al. Flexion contractures: a forgotten symptom in Addison's disease and hypopituitarism. Lancet 1986; 2:858 (letter).
820. Shapiro MS, Trebich C, Shilo L, et al. Myalgias and muscle contractures as the presenting signs of Addison's disease. Postgrad Med J 1988; 64:222–223.
821. Pollen RH, Williams RH. Hyperkalemic neuromyopathy in Addison's disease. N Engl J Med 1960; 263:273–278.
822. Barkan A, Glantz I. Calcification of auricular cartilages in patients with hypopituitarism. J Clin Endocrinol Metab 1982; 55:354–357.
823. Leigh H, Kramer SI. The psychiatric manifestations of endocrine disease. Adv Intern Med 1984; 29:413–445.
824. Grant DB, Barnes ND, Moncrieff MW, et al. Clinical presentation, growth, and pubertal development in Addison's disease. Arch Dis Child 1985; 60:925–928.
825. Neufeld M, Maclaren NK, Blizzard RM. Two types of autoimmune Addison's disease associated with different polyglandular autoimmune (PGA) syndromes. Medicine 1981; 60:355–362.
826. Griffin JW, Goren E, Schaumburg H, et al. Adrenomyeloneuropathy: a probable variant of adrenoleukodystrophy. I. Clinical and endocrinologic aspects. Neurology 1977; 27:1107–1113.
827. Moser HW, Moser AE, Singh I, et al. Adrenoleukodystrophy: survey of 303 cases: biochemistry, diagnosis, and therapy. Ann Neurol 1984; 16:628–641.
828. Cutler GB Jr, Davis SE, Johnsonbaugh RE, et al. Dissociation of cortisol and adrenal androgen secretion in patients with secondary adrenal insufficiency. J Clin Endocrinol Metab 1979; 49:604–609.
829. Urban MD, Lee PA, Gutai JP, et al. Androgens in pubertal males with Addison's disease. J Clin Endocrinol Metab 1980; 51:925–929.
830. Laczi F, Janáky T, Iványi T, et al. Osmoregulation of arginine-8-vasopressin secretion in primary hypothyroidism and in Addison's disease. Acta Endocrinol 1987; 114:389–395.
831. Gordon RD, Tunny TJ, Klemm SA, et al. Elevated levels of plasma atrial natriuretic peptide in Bartter's syndrome fall to normal with indomethacin: implications for atrial natriuretic peptide regulation in man. J Hypertens [Suppl] 1986; 4:S555–S558.
832. Oelkers W, L'Age M. Control of mineralocorticoid substitution in Addison's disease by plasma renin measurement. Klin Wochenschr 1976; 54:607–612.
833. Ogihara T, Hata T, Nakamaru M, et al. Decreased blood pressure in response to an angiotensin II antagonist in Addison's disease. Clin Endocrinol 1979; 10:377–381.
834. Falezza G, Santonastaso CL, Parisi T, et al. High serum levels of angiotensin-converting enzyme in untreated Addison's disease. J Clin Endocrinol Metab 1985; 61:496–498.
835. Topliss DJ, White EL, Stockigt JR. Significance of thyrotropin excess in untreated primary adrenal insufficiency. J Clin Endocrinol Metab 1980; 50:52–55.
836. Ng LL, Evans DJ, Burke CW. The human leucocyte sodium pump in adrenocortical insufficiency. Clin Endocrinol 1987; 27:235–243.
837. Spital A. Hyponatremia in adrenal insufficiency: review of pathogenic mechanisms. South Med J 1982; 75:581–585.
838. Nerup J. Addison's disease—serological studies. Acta Endocrinol 1974; 76:142–158.
839. Muls E, Bouillon R, Boelaert J, et al. Etiology of hypercalcemia in a patient with Addison's disease. Calcif Tissue Int 1982; 34:523–526.
840. Hartog M, Joplin GF. Effects of cortisol deficiency on the electrocardiogram. Br Med J 1968; 2:275–277.
841. Vita JA, Silverberg SJ, Goland RS, et al. Clinical clues to the cause of Addison's disease. Am J Med 1985; 78:461–466.
842. Himsworth RL, Lewis JG, Rees LH. A possible ACTH secreting tumour of the pituitary developing in a conventionally treated case of Addison's disease. Clin Endocrinol 1978; 9:131–139.
843. Irvine WJ, Toft AD, Feek CM. Addison's disease. In: James VHT, ed. The Adrenal Gland. New York: Raven, 1979: 131–164.
844. Del Negro G, Melo EHL, Rodbard D, et al. Limited adrenal reserve in paracoccidiomycosis: cortisol and aldosterone responses to 1–24 ACTH. Clin Endocrinol 1980; 13:553–559.
845. Eason RJ, Croxson MS, Perry MC, et al. Addison's disease, adrenal autoantibodies and computerized adrenal tomography. NZ Med J 1982; 95:569–573.
846. Spinner MW, Blizzard RM, Childs B. Clinical and genetic heterogeneity in idiopathic Addison's disease and hypoparathyroidism. J Clin Endocrinol Metab 1968; 28:795–804.
847. Blizzard RM, Chee D, Davis W. The incidence of adrenal and other antibodies in the sera of patients with idiopathic adrenal insufficiency (Addison's disease). Clin Exp Immunol 1967; 2:19–30.
848. Irvine WJ, Barnes EW. Addison's disease, ovarian failure and hypoparathyroidism. Clin Endocrinol Metab 1975; 4:379–434.
849. Irvine WJ, Stewart AG, Scarth L. A clinical and immunological study of adrenocortical insufficiency (Addison's disease). Clin Exp Immunol 1967; 2:31–70.
850. Ahohen P, Miettinen A, Perheentupa J. Adrenal and steroidal cell antibodies in patients with autoimmune polyglandular disease type I and risk of adrenocortical and ovarian failure. J Clin Endocrinol Metab 1987; 64:494–500.
851. Betterle C, Scalici C, Presotto F, et al. The natural history of adrenal function in autoimmune patients with adrenal autoantibodies. J Endocrinol 1988; 117:467–475.
852. Saenger P, Levine LS, Irvine WJ, et al. Progressive adrenal failure in polyglandular autoimmune disease. J Clin Endocrinol Metab 1982; 54:863–868.
853. Bright GM, Singh I. Adrenal autoantibodies bind to adrenal subcellular fractions enriched in cytochrome-c reductase and 5'-nucleotidase. J Clin Endocrinol Metab 1990; 70:95–99.
854. Furmaniak J, Talbot D, Reinwein D, et al. Immunoprecipitation of human adrenal microsomal antigen. FEBS Lett 1988; 231:25–28.
855. Wulffraat NM, Drexhage HA, Bottazzo GF, et al. Immunoglobulins of patients with idiopathic Addison's disease block the in vitro action of adrenocorticotropin. J Clin Endocrinol Metab 1989; 69:231–238.
856. Arikawa K, Ichikawa Y, Yoshida T, et al. Blocking type antithyrotropin receptor antibody in patients with nongoitrous hypothyroidism: its incidence and characteristics of action. J Clin Endocrinol Metab 1985; 60:953–959.
857. Fairchild RS, Schimke RN, Abdou NI. Immunoregulation abnormalities in familial Addison's disease. J Clin Endocrinol Metab 1980; 51:1074–1077.
858. Rabinowe SL, Jackson RA, Dluhy RG, et al. Ia-positive T lymphocytes in recently diagnosed idiopathic Addison's disease. Am J Med 1984; 77:597–601.
859. Nerup J, Bendixen G. Anti-adrenal cellular hypersensitivity in Addison's disease. II. Correlation with clinical and serological findings. Clin Exp Immunol 1969; 5:341–353.
860. Mathison JC, Schreiber RD, La Forest AC, et al. Suppression of ACTH-induced steroidogenesis by supernatants from LPS-treated peritoneal exudate macrophages. J Immunol 1983; 130:2757–2762.
861. Neville AM, Mackay AM. The structure of the human adrenal cortex in health and disease. Clin Endocrinol Metab 1972; 1:361–395.
862. Blizzard RM, Chee D, Davis W. The incidence of parathyroid and other antibodies in the sera of patients with idiopathic hypoparathyroidism. Clin Exp Immunol 1966; 1:119–128.
863. McHardy-Young S, Lessof MH, Maisey MN. Serum TSH and thyroid antibody studies in Addison's disease. Clin Endocrinol 1972; 1:45–56.
864. Ketchum CH, Riley WJ, Maclaren NK. Adrenal dysfunction in asymptomatic patients with adrenocortical autoantibodies. J Clin Endocrinol Metab 1984; 58:1166–1170.
865. Scherbaum WA, Berg PA. Development of adrenocortical failure in non-addisonian patients with antibodies to adrenal cortex. Clin Endocrinol 1982; 16:345–352.
866. Ahonen P, Myllärniemi S, Sipilä I, et al. Clinical variation of autoimmune endocrinopathy–candidiasis–ectodermal dystrophy (APECED) in a series of 68 patients. N Engl J Med 1990; 322:1829–1836.
867. Leshin M. Polyglandular autoimmune syndromes. Am J Med Sci 1985; 290:77–88.
868. Trence DL, Morley JE, Handwerger BS. Polyglandular autoimmune syndromes. Am J Med 1984; 77:107–116.
869. Asherson RA, Hughes GRV. Recurrent deep vein thrombosis and Addison's disease in "primary" antiphospholipid syndrome. J Rheumatol 1989; 16:378–380.
870. Tucker WS Jr, Niblack GD, McLean RH, et al. Serositis with autoimmune endocrinopathy: clinical and immunogenetic features. Medicine 1987; 66:138–147.
871. Butler MG, Hodes ME, Conneally PM, et al. Linkage analysis in a large kindred with autosomal dominant transmission of polyglandular autoimmune disease type II (Schmidt syndrome). Am J Med Genet 1984; 18:61–65.
872. Farid NR, Bear JC. The human major histocompatibility complex and endocrine disease. Endocr Rev 1981; 2:50–86.

873. Maclaren NK, Riley WJ. Thyroid, gastric, and adrenal autoimmunities and insulin-dependent diabetes mellitus. Diabetes Care 1985; 8:34–38.

874. Guttman PH. Addison's disease. A statistical analysis of five hundred and sixty-six cases and a study of the pathology. Arch Pathol 1930; 10:742–785.

875. Sarosi GA, Voth DW, Dahl BA, et al. Disseminated histoplasmosis: results of long-term follow-up. Ann Intern Med 1971; 75:511–516.

876. Abad A, Gomez I, Velez P, et al. Adrenal function in paracoccidioidomycosis: a prospective study in patients before and after ketoconazole therapy. Infection 1986; 14:22–26.

877. Walker BF, Gunthel CJ, Bryan JA, et al. Disseminated cryptococcosis in an apparently normal host presenting as primary adrenal insufficiency: diagnosis by fine needle aspiration. Am J Med 1989; 86:715–717.

878. Maloney PJ. Addison's disease due to chronic disseminated coccidioidomycosis. Arch Intern Med 1952; 90:869–878.

879. Abernathy RS, Melby JC. Addison's disease in North American blastomycosis. N Engl J Med 1962; 266:552–554.

880. Osa SR, Peterson RE, Roberts RB. Recovery of adrenal reserve following treatment of disseminated South American blastomycosis. Am J Med 1981; 71:298–301.

881. Washburn RG, Bennett JE. Reversal of adrenal glucocorticoid dysfunction in a patient with disseminated histoplasmosis. Ann Intern Med 1989; 110:86–87.

882. Cedermark BJ, Blumenson LE, Pickren JW, et al. The significance of metastases to the adrenal glands in adenocarcinoma of the colon and rectum. Surg Gynecol Obstet 1977; 144:537–546.

883. Redman BG, Pazdur R, Zingas AP, et al. Prospective evaluation of adrenal insufficiency in patients with adrenal metastasis. Cancer 1987; 60:103–107.

884. Seidenwurm DJ, Elmer EB, Kaplan LM, et al. Metastases to the adrenal glands and the development of Addison's disease. Cancer 1984; 54:552–557.

885. Huminer D, Garty M, Lapidot M, et al. Lymphoma presenting with adrenal insufficiency: adrenal enlargement on computed tomographic scanning as a clue to diagnosis. Am J Med 1988; 84:169–172.

886. Dluhy RG. The growing spectrum of HIV-related endocrine abnormalities. J Clin Endocrinol Metab 1990; 70:563–565.

887. Glasgow BJ, Steinsapir KD, Anders K, et al. Adrenal pathology in the acquired immune deficiency syndrome. Am J Clin Pathol 1985; 84:594–597.

888. Greene LW, Cole W, Greene JB, et al. Adrenal insufficiency as a complication of the acquired immunodeficiency syndrome. Ann Intern Med 1984; 101:497–498.

889. Dobs AS, Dempsey MA, Ladenson PW, et al. Endocrine disorders in men infected with human immunodeficiency virus. Am J Med 1988; 84:611–616.

890. Membreno L, Irony I, Dere W, et al. Adrenocortical function in acquired immunodeficiency syndrome. J Clin Endocrinol Metab 1987; 65:482–487.

891. Sonino N. The use of ketoconazole as an inhibitor of steroid production. N Engl J Med 1987; 317:812–818.

892. Elias AN, Gwinup G. Effects of some clinically encountered drugs on steroid synthesis and degradation. Metabolism 1980; 29:582–594.

893. Ediger SK, Isley WL. Rifampicin-induced adrenal insufficiency in the acquired immunodeficiency syndrome: difficulties in diagnosis and treatment. Postgrad Med J 1988; 64:405–406.

894. Sadeghi-Nejad A, Senior B. Adrenomyeloneuropathy presenting as Addison's disease in childhood. N Engl J Med 1990; 322:13–16.

895. Moser AE, Borel J, Odone A, et al. A new dietary therapy for adrenoleukodystrophy: biochemical and preliminary clinical results in 36 patients. Ann Neurol 1987; 21:240–249.

896. Wise JE, Matalon R, Morgan AM, et al. Phenotypic features of patients with congenital adrenal hypoplasia and glycerol kinase deficiency. Am J Dis Child 1987; 141:744–747.

897. Spark RF, Etzkorn JR. Absent aldosterone response to ACTH in familial glucocorticoid deficiency. N Engl J Med 1977; 297:917–920.

898. Stuckey BG, Mastaglia FL, Reed WD, et al. Glucocorticoid insufficiency, achalasia, alacrima with autonomic and motor neuropathy. Ann Intern Med 1987; 106:62–64.

899. Laue L, Hoeg JM, Barnes K, et al. The effect of mevinolin on steroidogenesis in patients with defects in the low density lipoprotein receptor pathway. J Clin Endocrinol Metab 1987; 64:531–535.

900. Vermeulen A, Paridaens R, Heuson JC. Effects of aminoglutethimide on adrenal steroid secretion. Clin Endocrinol 1983; 19:673–682.

901. Ashby H, DiMattina M, Linehan WM, et al. The inhibition of human adrenal steroidogenic enzyme activities by suramin. J Clin Endocrinol Metab 1989; 68:505–508.

902. Stein CA, Saville W, Yarchoan R, et al. Suramin and function of the adrenal cortex. Ann Intern Med 1986; 104:286–287.

903. Keilholz U, Guthrie GP Jr. Adverse effect of phenytoin on mineralocorticoid replacement with fludrocortisone in adrenal insufficiency. Am J Med Sci 1986; 291:280–283.

904. Modhi G, Bauman W, Nicolis G. Adrenal failure associated with hypothalamic and adrenal metastases. Cancer 1981; 47:2098–2101.

905. Koide Y, Kimura S, Inoue S, et al. Responsiveness of hypophyseal-adrenocortical axis to repetitive administration of synthetic ovine corticotropin-releasing hormone in patients with isolated adrenocorticotropin deficiency. J Clin Endocrinol Metab 1986; 63:329–335.

906. Jensen MD, Handwerger BS, Scheithauer BW, et al. Lymphocytic hypophysitis with isolated corticotropin deficiency. Ann Intern Med 1986; 105:200–203.

907. Sugiura M, Hashimoto A, Shizawa M, et al. Heterogeneity of anterior pituitary cell antibodies detected in insulin-dependent diabetes mellitus and adrenocorticotropic hormone deficiency. Diabetes Res 1986; 3:111–114.

908. Sauter NP, Toni R, McLaughlin CD, et al. Isolated adrenocorticotropin deficiency associated with an autoantibody to a corticotroph antigen that is not adrenocorticotropin or other proopiomelanocortin-derived peptides. J Clin Endocrinol Metab 1990; 70:1391–1397.

909. Phifer RF, Spicer SS, Orth DN. Specific demonstration of the human hypophyseal cells which produce adrenocorticotropic hormone. J Clin Endocrinol Metab 1970; 31:347–361.

910. Schulte HM, Chrousos GP, Avgerinos P, et al. The corticotropin-releasing hormone stimulation test: a possible aid in the evaluation of patients with adrenal insufficiency. J Clin Endocrinol Metab 1984; 58:1064–1067.

911. Merenich JA, Hannon RN, Gentry RH, et al. Azidothymidine-induced hyperpigmentation mimicking primary adrenal insufficiency. Am J Med 1989; 86:469–470.

912. Granstein RD, Sober AJ. Drug- and heavy metal–induced hyperpigmentation. J Am Acad Dermatol 1981; 5:1–18.

913. Daniel CR. Nail pigmentation abnormalities. Dermatol Clin 1985; 3:431–433.

914. Hägg E, Asplund K, Lithner F. Value of basal plasma cortisol assays in the assessment of pituitary-adrenal insufficiency. Clin Endocrinol 1987; 26:221–226.

914a. Watts NB, Tindall GT. Rapid assessment of corticotropin reserve after pituitary surgery. JAMA 1988; 259:708–711.

915. May ME, Carey RM. Rapid adrenocorticotropic hormone test in practice. Am J Med 1985; 79:679–684.

916. Cunningham SK, Moore A, McKenna TJ. Normal cortisol response to corticotropin in patients with secondary adrenal failure. Arch Intern Med 1983; 143:2276–2279.

917. Lindholm J, Kehlet H. Re-evaluation of the clinical value of the 30 minute ACTH test in assessing the hypothalamic-pituitary-adrenocortical function. Clin Endocrinol 1987; 26:53–59.

918. Spiger M, Jubiz W, Meikle AW, et al. Single-dose metyrapone test: review of a four-year experience. Arch Intern Med 1975; 135:698–700.

919. Rose LI, Williams GH, Jagger PI, et al. The 48-hour adrenocorticotrophin infusion test for adrenocortical insufficiency. Ann Intern Med 1970; 73:49–54.

920. Pagani JJ. Non–small cell lung carcinoma adrenal metastases: computed tomography and percutaneous needle biopsy in their diagnosis. Cancer 1984; 53:1058–1060.

921. Hench PS, Kendall EC, Slocumb CH, et al. Effects of cortisone acetate and pituitary ACTH on rheumatoid arthritis, rheumatic fever, and certain other conditions: a study in clinical physiology. Arch Intern Med 1950; 85:545–666.

922. Fariss BL, Hane S, Shinsako J, et al. Comparison of absorption of cortisone acetate and hydrocortisone hemisuccinate. J Clin Endocrinol Metab 1978; 47:1137–1140.

923. Scott RS, Donald RA, Espiner EA. Plasma ACTH and cortisol profiles in addisonian patients receiving conventional substitution therapy. Clin Endocrinol 1978; 9:571–576.

924. Feek CM, Ratcliffe JG, Seth J, et al. Patterns of plasma cortisol and ACTH concentrations in patients with Addison's disease treated with conventional corticosteroid replacement. Clin Endocrinol 1981; 14:451–458.

925. Dexter RN, Orth DN, Abe K, et al. Cushing's disease without hypercortisolism. J Clin Endocrinol Metab 1970; 30:573–579.

926. Robinson BG, Hales IB, Henniker AJ, et al. The effect of o,p'-DDD on adrenal steroid replacement therapy requirements. Clin Endocrinol 1987; 27:437–444.

927. Santen RJ, Lipton A, Kendall J. Successful medical adrenalectomy with amino-glutethimide. Role of altered drug metabolism. JAMA 1974; 230:1661–1665.

928. Smith SJ, Markandu ND, Banks RA, et al. Evidence that patients with Addison's disease are undertreated with fludrocortisone. Lancet 1984; 1:11–14.

929. Knowlton AI, Baer L. Cardiac failure in Addison's disease. Am J Med 1983; 74:829–836.

930. Udelsman R, Ramp J, Gallucci WT, et al. Adaptation during surgical stress: a reevaluation of the role of glucocorticoids. J Clin Invest 1986; 77:1377–1381.

931. Brent F. Addison's disease and pregnancy. Am J Surg 1950; 79:645–652.

932. Burrow GN, Ferris TF. Medical Complications During Pregnancy. Philadelphia: W. B. Saunders, 1988.

933. Hudson JB, Chobanian AV, Relman AS. Hypoaldosteronism. A clinical study of a patient with isolated mineralocorticoid deficiency, resulting

in hypokalemia and Stokes-Adams attacks. N Engl J Med 1957; 257:529–536.

934. Schambelan M, Stockigt JR, Biglieri EG. Isolated hypoaldosteronism in adults. A renin-deficiency syndrome. N Engl J Med 1972; 287:573–578.

935. Perez G, Siegel L, Schreiner GE. Selective hypoaldosteronism with hyperkalemia. Ann Intern Med 1972; 76:757–763.

936. DeFronzo R. Hyperkalemia and hyporeninemic hypoaldosteronism. Kidney Int 1980; 17:118–134.

937. Kiley J, Zager P. Hyporeninemic hypoaldosteronism in two patients with systemic lupus erythematosus. Am J Kidney Dis 1984; 4:39–43.

938. Kozeny GA, Hurley RM, Fresco R, et al. Systemic lupus erythematosus presenting with hyporeninemic hypoaldosteronism in a 10 year old girl. Am J Nephrol 1986; 6:321–324.

939. Rai Mehta B, Cavallo T, Remmers AR, et al. Hyporeninemic hypoaldosteronism in a patient with multiple myeloma. Am J Kidney Dis 1984; 4:175–178.

940. Escarce JJ. Hyporeninemic hypoaldosteronism in a patient with cirrhosis and ascites. Arch Intern Med 1986; 146:2407–2408.

941. Yoshimo M, Amerian R, Brautbar N. Hyporeninemic hypoaldosteronism in sickle cell disease. Nephron 1982; 31:242–244.

942. Kalin MF, Poretsky L, Seres DS, et al. Hyporeninemic hypoaldosteronism associated with acquired immune deficiency syndrome. Am J Med 1987; 82:1035–1038.

943. Weidmann PR, Reinhart R, Maxwell MH, et al. Syndrome of hyporeninemic hypoaldosteronism and hyperkalemia in renal disease. J Clin Endocrinol Metab 1973; 36:965–977.

944. Brown JJ, Chinn RH, Fraser R, et al. Recurrent hyperkalemia due to selective aldosterone deficiency: correction by angiotensin infusion. Br Med J 1973; 1:650–654.

945. Schambelan M. Hyporeninemic hypoaldosteronism. Adv Intern Med 1979; 24:385–405.

946. Sunderlin FS, Anderson GH, Streeten DHP, et al. The renin-angiotensin-aldosterone system in diabetic patients with hyperkalemia. Diabetes 1981; 30:335–340.

947. DeLeiva A, Christlieb AR, Melby JC, et al. Big renin and biosynthetic defect of aldosterone in diabetes mellitus. N Engl J Med 1976; 295:639–643.

948. Tuck ML, Mayes DM. Mineralocorticoid biosynthesis in patients with hyporeninemic hypoaldosteronism. J Clin Endocrinol Metab 1980; 50:341–347.

949. Perez GO, Lespier LE, Oster JR, et al. Effect of alterations of sodium intake in patients with hyporeninemic hypoaldosteronism. Nephron 1977; 18:259–265.

950. Tuck ML, Sambhi MP, Levin L. Hyporeninemic hypoaldosteronism in diabetes mellitus. Studies of the autonomic nervous system's control of renin release. Diabetes 1979; 28:237–241.

951. Tan SY, Antonpillai I, Mulrow PJ. Inactive renin and prostaglandin E_2 production in hyporeninemic hypoaldosteronism. J Clin Endocrinol Metab 1980; 51:849–853.

952. Hahn JA, Zipser RD, Brag A, et al. Studies of the renal vasoactive systems in hyporeninemic hypoaldosteronism. Prostaglandins Med 1981; 6:549–556.

953. Kaufman JS, Peck M, Hamburger RJF. Isolated hypoaldosteronism and abnormalities in renin, kallikrein, and prostaglandin. Nephron 1986; 43:203–210.

954. Oates JA, Whorton AR, Gerkens JF, et al. The participation of prostaglandins in the control of renin release. Fed Proc 1979; 38:72–74.

955. Tan SY, Shapiro R, Franco R, et al. Indomethacin-induced prostaglandin inhibition with hyperkalemia: a reversible cause of hyporeninemic hypoaldosteronism. Ann Intern Med 1979; 90:783–785.

956. Hahn J, Zipser R, Zia P, et al. Induction of renin release by exogenous prostaglandins in hyporeninemic hypoaldosteronism. Prostaglandins 1980; 20:15–23.

957. Farese RV, Rodriguez-Colomé M, O'Malley BC. Urinary prostaglandins following frusemide treatment and salt depletion in normal subjects and subjects with diabetic hyporeninaemic hypoaldosteronism. Clin Endocrinol 1980; 13:447–453.

958. Nadler JL, Lee FO, Hsueh W, et al. Evidence of prostacyclin deficiency in the syndrome of hyporeninemic hypoaldosteronism. N Engl J Med 1986; 314:1015–1020.

959. Fitzgerald GA, Hossman V, Hummerich W, et al. The renin-kallikrein-prostaglandin system: plasma active and inactive renin and urinary kallikrein during prostacyclin infusion in man. Prostaglandins Med 1980; 5:445–456.

960. Ohde H, Ogihara T, Nakamaru M, et al. Effect of prostacyclin infusion on active and inactive renin release in the isolated perfused kidney. Life Sci 1982; 31:3031–3035.

961. Kokko J. Primary acquired hypoaldosteronism. Kidney Int 1985; 27:690–702.

962. Wingo CS, Kokko J, Jacobson HR. Effects of in vitro aldosterone on the rabbit cortical collecting duct. Kidney Int 1985; 28:51–57.

963. Cox M, Sterns RH, Singer I. The defense against hyperkalemia: the roles of insulin and aldosterone. N Engl J Med 1978; 299:525–532.

964. Sebastian A, Schambelan M, Lindenfeld S, et al. Amelioration of

metabolic acidosis with fludrocortisone therapy in hyporeninemic hypoaldosteronism. N Engl J Med 1977; 297:576–583.

965. Szylman P, Better O, Chaimowitz C, et al. Role of hyperkalemia in the metabolic acidosis of isolated hypoaldosteronism. N Engl J Med 1976; 294:361–365.

966. Stone DK, Seldin DW, Kokko JP, et al. Mineralocorticoid modulation of rabbit medullary collecting acidification: a sodium-independent effect. J Clin Invest 1983; 72:77–83.

967. Ulick S. Diagnosis and nomenclature of the disorders of the terminal portion of the aldosterone biosynthetic pathway. J Clin Endocrinol Metab 1976; 43:92–96.

968. Veldhuis JD, Melby JC. Isolated aldosterone deficiency in man: acquired and inborn errors in the biosynthesis or action of aldosterone. Endocr Rev 1986; 2:495–517.

969. Lee PDK, Patterson BD, Hintz RL, et al. Biochemical diagnosis and management of corticosterone methyl oxidase type II deficiency. J Clin Endocrinol Metab 1986; 62:225–229.

970. Visser HKA, Cost WS. A new hereditary defect in the biosynthesis of aldosterone: urinary C21 corticosteroid pattern in three related patients with a salt-losing syndrome, suggesting an 18-oxidation defect. Acta Endocrinol 1964; 47:589–612.

971. Degenhart HJ, Frankena L, Visser HKA, et al. Further investigations of a new hereditary defect in the biosynthesis of aldosterone: evidence for a defect in 18-hydroxylation of corticosterone. Acta Physiol Pharmacol Neerl 1966; 14:88–93.

972. Veldhuis JD, Kulin HE, Wilson TE. Detection of isolated aldosterone deficiency in the neonate. J Pediatr 1983; 102:83–85.

973. Globerman H, Rosler A, Theodor R, et al. An inherited defect in aldosterone biosynthesis caused by a mutation in or near the gene for steroid 11-hydroxylase. N Engl J Med 1988; 319:1193–1197.

974. Wilson ID, Goetz FC. Selective hypoaldosteronism after prolonged heparin administration. Am J Med 1964; 36:635–640.

975. Conn JW, Rovner OE, Cohen EL, et al. Inhibition by heparinoid of aldosterone biosynthesis in man. J Clin Endocrinol Metab 1966; 26:527–532.

976. O'Kelly R, Magee F, McKenna TJ. Routine heparin therapy inhibits adrenal aldosterone production. J Clin Endocrinol Metab 1983; 56:108–112.

977. Zipser RD, Davenport MW, Martin KL, et al. Hyperreninemic hypoaldosteronism in the critically ill: a new entity. J Clin Endocrinol Metab 1981; 53:867–872.

978. Cheek DB, Perry JW. A salt wasting syndrome in infancy. Arch Dis Child 1958; 33:252–256.

979. Speiser PW, Stoner E, New MI. Pseudohypoaldosteronism: a review and report of two new cases. Adv Exp Med Biol 1986; 196:173–195.

980. Rodriguez-Soriano J, Vallo A, Oliveros R, et al. Transient pseudohypoaldosteronism secondary to obstructive uropathy in infancy. J Pediatr 1983; 103:375–380.

981. Keszler M, Sivasubramanian KN. Pseudohypoaldosteronism: fulminant presentation in a premature infant. Am J Dis Child 1983; 137:738–740.

982. Uribarri J, Oh MS, Butt KMH, et al. Pseudohypoaldosteronism following kidney transplantation. Nephron 1982; 31:368–370.

983. Rosler A. The natural history of salt-wasting disorders of adrenal and renal origin. J Clin Endocrinol Metab 1984; 59:689–700.

984. Armanini D, Strasser T, Weber C. Characterization of aldosterone binding sites in circulating human mononuclear leukocytes. Am J Physiol 1985; 248:E388–E390.

985. Armanini D, Kuhnle U, Strasser T, et al. Aldosterone receptor deficiency in pseudohypoaldosteronism. N Engl J Med 1985; 313:1178–1181.

986. Cushing HW. The Pituitary Body and Its Disorders. Philadelphia: J. B. Lippincott, 1912.

987. Cushing H. The basophil adenomas of the pituitary body and their clinical manifestations (pituitary basophilism). Bull Johns Hopkins Hosp 1932; 50:137–195.

988. Walters W, Wilder RM, Kepler EJ. The suprarenal cortical syndrome with presentation of ten cases. Ann Surg 1934; 100:670–688.

989. Brown WH. A case of pluriglandular syndrome. "Diabetes of bearded women." Lancet 1928; 2:1022–1023.

990. Meador CK, Liddle GW, Island DP, et al. Cause of Cushing's syndrome in patients with tumors arising from "nonendocrine" tissue. J Clin Endocrinol Metab 1962; 22:693–703.

991. Ross EJ, Linch DC. Cushing's syndrome—killing disease: discriminatory value of signs and symptoms aiding early diagnosis. Lancet 1982; 2:646–649.

992. Plotz CM, Knowlton AI, Ragan C. The natural history of Cushing's syndrome. Am J Med 1952; 13:597–614.

993. Ross EJ, Marshall-Jones P, Friedman M. Cushing's syndrome: diagnostic criteria. Q J Med 1966; 35:149–192.

994. Kaplan NM. Other forms of secondary hypertension. In: Kaplan NM, ed. Clinical Hypertension. Baltimore: Williams & Wilkins, 1982: 390–410.

995. Ferguson JK, Donald RA, Weston TS, et al. Skin thickness in patients with acromegaly and Cushing's syndrome and response to treatment. Clin Endocrinol 1983; 18:347–353.

996. Rosenberg EM, Hahn TJ, Tanaka D, et al. ACTH-secreting medullary carcinoma of the thyroid presenting as severe idiopathic osteoporosis and senile purpura: report of a case and review of the literature. J Clin Endocrinol Metab 1978; 47:255–262.

997. Urbanic RC, George JM. Cushing's disease—18 years' experience. Medicine 1981; 60:14–24.

998. Soffer LJ, Iannaccone A, Gabrilove JL. Cushing's syndrome: a study of fifty patients. Am J Med 1961; 30:129–146.

999. Black MM, Hall R, Kay DWK, et al. Anorexia nervosa in Cushing's syndrome. J Clin Endocrinol Metab 1965; 25:1030–1034.

1000. Hudson JI, Hudson MS, Griffing GT, et al. Phenomenology and family history of affective disorder in Cushing's disease. Am J Psychiatry 1987; 216:171–175.

1001. Born J, Späth-Schwalbe E, Schwakenhofer H, et al. Influences of corticotropin-releasing hormone, adrenocorticotropin, and cortisol on sleep in normal man. J Clin Endocrinol Metab 1989; 68:904–911.

1002. Welbourn RB, Manolas KJ. The role of adrenalectomy in the management of Cushing's syndrome. In: Johnston IDA, Thompson NW, eds. Endocrine Surgery. London: Butterworths, 1983: 53–75.

1003. Sjöberg HE, Blombäck M, Granberg PO. Thromboembolic complications, heparin treatment and increase in coagulation factors in Cushing's syndrome. Acta Med Scand 1976; 199:95–98.

1004. Small M, Lowe GDO, Forbes CD, et al. Thromboembolic complications in Cushing's syndrome. Clin Endocrinol 1983; 19:503–511.

1005. Sayegh F, Weigelin E. Intraocular pressure in Cushing's syndrome. Ophthalmic Res 1975; 7:390–394.

1006. Taskinen MR, Nikkilä EA, Pelkonen R, et al. Plasma lipoproteins, lipolytic enzymes, and very low density lipoprotein triglyceride turnover in Cushing's syndrome. J Clin Endocrinol Metab 1983; 57:619–626.

1007. Meador CK, Bowdoin B, Owen WC Jr, et al. Primary adrenocortical nodular dysplasia: a rare cause of Cushing's syndrome. J Clin Endocrinol Metab 1967; 27:1255–1263.

1008. Schweizer-Cagianut M, Froesch ER, Hedinger C. Familial Cushing's syndrome with primary adrenocortical microadenomatosis (primary adrenocortical nodular dysplasia). Acta Endocrinol 1980; 94:529–535.

1009. Donaldson MDC, Grant DB, O'Hare MJ, et al. Familial congenital Cushing's syndrome due to bilateral nodular adrenal hyperplasia. Clin Endocrinol 1981; 14:519–526.

1010. Carney JA, Gordon H, Carpenter PC, et al. The complex of myxomas, spotty pigmentation, and endocrine overactivity. Medicine 1985; 64:270–283.

1011. Larsen JL, Cathey WJ, Odell WD. Primary adrenocortical nodular dysplasia, a distinct subtype of Cushing's syndrome. Case report and review of the literature. Am J Med 1986; 80:976–984.

1012. Malchoff CD, Rosa J, DeBold CR, et al. Adrenocorticotropin-independent bilateral macronodular adrenal hyperplasia: an unusual cause of Cushing's syndrome. J Clin Endocrinol Metab 1989; 68:855–860.

1013. Hellman L, Weitzman ED, Roffwarg H, et al. Cortisol is secreted episodically in Cushing's syndrome. J Clin Endocrinol Metab 1970; 30:686–689.

1014. Sederberg-Olsen P, Binder C, Kehlet H, et al. Episodic variation in plasma corticosteroids in subjects with Cushing's syndrome of differing etiology. J Clin Endocrinol Metab 1973; 36:906–910.

1015. Boyar RM, Witkin M, Carruth A, et al. Circadian cortisol secretory rhythms in Cushing's disease. J Clin Endocrinol Metab 1979; 48:760–765.

1016. Liu JH, Kazer RR, Rasmussen DD. Characterization of the twenty-four hour secretion patterns of adrenocorticotropin and cortisol in normal women and patients with Cushing's disease. J Clin Endocrinol Metab 1987; 64:1027–1035.

1017. Segal DM, Drucker WD, Benovitz H, et al. Further studies of adrenal weight-maintaining activity in the plasma of patients with Cushing's disease. Am J Med 1970; 49:34–41.

1018. Liddle GW. Tests of pituitary-adrenal suppressibility in the diagnosis of Cushing's syndrome. J Clin Endocrinol Metab 1960; 20:1539–1560.

1019. Choi Y, Werk EE Jr, Sholiton LJ. Cushing's syndrome with dual pituitary-adrenal control. Arch Intern Med 1970; 125:1045–1049.

1019a. Burke CW. Disorders of cortisol production: diagnostic and therapeutic progress. Recent Adv Endocr Metab 1978; 1:61–90.

1020. Aron DC, Findling JW, Fitzgerald PA, et al. Pituitary ACTH dependency of nodular adrenal hyperplasia in Cushing's syndrome. Report of two cases and review of the literature. Am J Med 1981; 71:302–306.

1021. Symington T. The adrenal cortex. In: Bloodworth JMB Jr, ed. Endocrine Pathology. 2nd ed. Baltimore: Williams & Wilkins, 1982: 419–471.

1022. Smals AGH, Pieters GFFM, van Haelst UJG, et al. Macronodular adrenocortical hyperplasia in long-standing Cushing's disease. J Clin Endocrinol Metab 1984; 58:25–31.

1023. Hermus AR, Pieters GF, Smals AG, et al. Transition from pituitary-dependent to adrenal-dependent Cushing's syndrome. N Engl J Med 1988; 318:966–970.

1024. Orth DN. Ectopic hormone production. In: Felig P, Baxter JD, Broadus AE, et al., eds. Endocrinology and Metabolism. New York: McGraw-Hill, 1987: 1692–1735.

1025. Strott CA, Nugent CA, Tyler FH. Cushing's syndrome caused by bronchial adenomas. Am J Med 1968; 44:97–104.

1026. Carey RM, Varma SK, Drake DR Jr, et al. Ectopic secretion of corticotropin-releasing factor as a cause of Cushing's syndrome. Clinical, morphologic, and biochemical study. N Engl J Med 1984; 311:13–20.

1027. Belsky JL, Cuello B, Swanson LW, et al. Cushing's syndrome due to ectopic production of corticotropin-releasing factor. J Clin Endocrinol Metab 1985; 60:496–500.

1028. Schteingart DE, Lloyd RV, Akil H, et al. Cushing's syndrome secondary to ectopic corticotropin-releasing hormone–adrenocorticotropin secretion. J Clin Endocrinol Metab 1986; 63:770–775.

1029. Zárate A, Kovacs K, Flores M, et al. ACTH and CRF-producing bronchial carcinoid associated with Cushing's syndrome. Clin Endocrinol 1986; 24:523–529.

1030. Jessop DS, Cunnah D, Millar JGB, et al. A phaeochromocytoma presenting with Cushing's syndrome associated with increased concentrations of circulating corticotrophin-releasing factor. J Endocrinol 1987; 113:133–138.

1031. Asa SL, Kovacs K, Tindall GT, et al. Cushing's disease associated with an intrasellar gangliocytoma producing corticotrophin-releasing factor. Ann Intern Med 1984; 101:789–793.

1032. Evans PJ, Peters JR, Dyas J, et al. Salivary cortisol levels in true and apparent hypercortisolism. Clin Endocrinol 1984; 20:709–715.

1033. Krakoff LR. Measurement of plasma renin substrate by radioimmunoassay of angiotensin I: concentration in syndromes with steroid excess. J Clin Endocrinol Metab 1973; 37:110–117.

1034. Biglieri EG, Hane S, Slaton PE Jr, et al. In vivo and in vitro studies of adrenal secretions in Cushing's syndrome and primary aldosteronism. J Clin Invest 1963; 42:516–524.

1035. Yamaji T, Ishibashi M, Yamada A, et al. Plasma levels of atrial natriuretic hormone in Cushing's syndrome. J Clin Endocrinol Metab 1988; 67:348–352.

1036. Duick DS, Wahner HW. Thyroid axis in patients with Cushing's syndrome. Arch Intern Med 1979; 139:767–772.

1037. Wilber JF, Utiger RD. The effect of glucocorticoids on thyrotropin secretion. J Clin Invest 1969; 48:2096–2103.

1038. Otsuki M, Dakoda M, Baba S. Influence of glucocorticoids on TRF-induced TSH response in man. J Clin Endocrinol Metab 1973; 36:95–102.

1039. Duick DS, Warren DW, Nicoloff JT, et al. Effect of single dose dexamethasone on the concentration of serum triiodothyronine in man. J Clin Endocrinol Metab 1974; 39:1151–1154.

1040. Reid IR. Pathogenesis and treatment of steroid osteoporosis. Clin Endocrinol 1989; 30:83–103.

1041. Smals AGH, Kloppenborg PWC, Benraad TJ. Plasma testosterone profiles in Cushing's syndrome. J Clin Endocrinol Metab 1977; 45:240–245.

1042. Doerr P, Pirke KM. Cortisol-induced suppression of plasma testosterone in normal adult males. J Clin Endocrinol Metab 1976; 43:622–629.

1043. Luton J-P, Thieblot P, Valcke J-C, et al. Reversible gonadotropin deficiency in male Cushing's disease. J Clin Endocrinol Metab 1977; 45:488–495.

1044. Marco J, Calle C, Román D, et al. Hyperglucagonism induced by glucocorticoid treatment in man. N Engl J Med 1973; 288:128–131.

1045. Olefsky JM, Kimmerling G. Effects of glucocorticoids on carbohydrate metabolism. Am J Med Sci 1976; 271:202–210.

1046. Johnston DG, Alberti KGMM, Nattrass M, et al. Hormonal and metabolic rhythms in Cushing's syndrome. Metabolism 1980; 29:1046–1052.

1047. Gourmelen M, Girard F, Binoux M. Serum somatomedin/insulin-like growth factor (IGF) and IGF carrier levels in patients with Cushing's syndrome or receiving glucocorticoid therapy. J Clin Endocrinol Metab 1982; 54:885–892.

1048. Carpenter PC. Diagnostic evaluation of Cushing's syndrome. Endocrinol Metab Clin North Am 1988; 17:445–472.

1049. Parkin DM, Läärä E, Muir OS. Estimates of the worldwide frequency of sixteen major cancers in 1980. Int J Cancer 1988; 41:184–197.

1050. Brennan MF. Adrenocortical carcinoma. CA 1987; 37:348–365.

1051. Cutler SJ, Young JL. Third National Cancer Survey: Incidence Data. National Cancer Institute Monograph 41. DHEW Publication No. 287. Washington, DC: Government Printing Office, 1975.

1052. Hutter AM Jr, Kayhoe DE. Adrenal cortical carcinoma: clinical features of 138 patients. Am J Med 1966; 41:572–580.

1053. Bertagna C, Orth DN. Clinical and laboratory findings and results of therapy in 58 patients with adrenocortical tumors admitted to a single medical center (1951–1978). Am J Med 1981; 71:855–875.

1054. Luton JP, Cerdas S, Billaud L, et al. Clinical features of adrenocortical carcinoma, prognostic factors, and the effect of mitotane therapy. N Engl J Med 1990; 322:1195–1201.

1055. Neville AM, Symington TS. Bilateral adrenocortical hyperplasia in children with Cushing's syndrome. J Pathol 1972; 107:95–106.

1056. Schnall AM, Kovacs K, Brodkey JS, et al. Pituitary Cushing's disease without adenoma. Acta Endocrinol 1980; 94:297–303.

1057. McKeever PE, Koppelman MCS, Metcalf D, et al. Refractory Cushing's disease caused by multinodular ACTH-cell hyperplasia. J Neuropathol Exp Neurol 1982; 41:490–499.

1058. Young WF Jr, Scheithauer BW, Gharib H, et al. Cushing's syndrome due to primary multinodular corticotrope hyperplasia. Mayo Clin Proc 1988; 63:256–262.

1059. Lamberts SWJ, de Lange SA, Stefanko SZ. Adrenocorticotropin-secreting pituitary adenomas originate from the anterior or the intermediate lobe in Cushing's disease: differences in the regulation of hormone secretion. J Clin Endocrinol Metab 1982; 54:286–291.

1060. McNicol AM, Teasdale GM, Beastall GH. A study of corticotroph adenomas in Cushing's disease: no evidence of intermediate lobe origin. Clin Endocrinol 1986; 24:715–722.

1061. Raffel C, Boggan JE, Eng LF, et al. Pituitary adenomas in Cushing's disease: do they arise from the intermediate lobe? Surg Neurol 1988; 30:125–130.

1062. Kaiser FE, Orth DN, Mukai K, et al. A pituitary parasellar tumor with extracranial metastases and high, partially suppressible levels of adrenocorticotropin and related peptides. J Clin Endocrinol Metab 1983; 57:649–653.

1063. Gogel EL, Salber PR, Tyrrell JB, et al. Cushing's disease in a patient with a "nonfunctioning" pituitary tumor. Arch Intern Med 1983; 143:1040–1042.

1064. Vaughan NJA, Laroche CM, Goodman I, et al. Pituitary Cushing's disease arising from a previously non-functional corticotrophic chromophobe adenoma. Clin Endocrinol 1985; 22:147–153.

1065. Krieger DT, Amorosa L, Linick F. Cyproheptadine-induced remission of Cushing's disease. N Engl J Med 1975; 293:893–896.

1066. Krieger DT. Physiopathology of Cushing's disease. Endocr Rev 1983; 4:22–43.

1067. Schnall AM, Brodkey JS, Kaufman B, et al. Pituitary function after removal of pituitary microadenomas in Cushing's disease. J Clin Endocrinol Metab 1978; 47:410–417.

1068. Tyrrell JB, Brooks RM, Fitzgerald PA, et al. Cushing's disease. Selective transsphenoidal resection of pituitary microadenomas. N Engl J Med 1978; 298:753–758.

1069. Salassa RM, Laws ER Jr, Carpenter PC, et al. Transsphenoidal removal of pituitary microadenoma in Cushing's disease. Mayo Clin Proc 1978; 53:24–28.

1070. Bigos ST, Somma M, Rasio E, et al. Cushing's disease: management by transsphenoidal pituitary microsurgery. J Clin Endocrinol Metab 1980; 50:348–354.

1071. Fitzgerald PA, Aron DC, Findling JW, et al. Cushing's disease: transient secondary adrenal insufficiency after selective removal of pituitary tumors; evidence for a pituitary origin. J Clin Endocrinol Metab 1982; 54:413–422.

1072. Avgerinos PC, Nieman LK, Oldfield EH, et al. The effect of pulsatile human corticotropin-releasing hormone administration on the adrenal insufficiency that follows cure of Cushing's disease. J Clin Endocrinol Metab 1989; 68:912–916.

1073. James VHT, Landon J, Wynn V, et al. A fundamental defect of adrenocortical control in Cushing's disease. J Endocrinol 1968; 40:15–28.

1074. Morrow LB, Mellinger RC, Prendergast JJ, et al. Growth hormone in hypersecretory diseases of the adrenal gland. J Clin Endocrinol Metab 1969; 29:1364–1368.

1075. Krieger DT, Glick SM. Growth hormone and cortisol responsiveness in Cushing's syndrome. Relation to a possible central nervous system etiology. Am J Med 1972; 52:25–40.

1076. Kuku SF, Child DF, Nader S, et al. Thyrotrophin and prolactin responsiveness to thyrotrophin releasing hormone in Cushing's disease. Clin Endocrinol 1975; 4:437–442.

1077. Salassa RM, Laws ER Jr, Carpenter PC, et al. Prolactin secretion in Cushing's disease. J Clin Endocrinol Metab 1981; 53:843–846.

1078. Caufriez A, Désir D, Szyper M, et al. Prolactin secretion in Cushing's disease. J Clin Endocrinol Metab 1981; 53:843–846.

1079. Lamberts SWJ, de Quijada M, Visser TJ. Regulation of prolactin secretion in patients with Cushing's disease. A comparative study on the effects of dexamethasone, lysine vasopressin and ACTH on prolactin secretion by the rat pituitary gland in vitro. Neuroendocrinology 1981; 32:150–154.

1080. Tyrrell JB, Wiener-Kronish J, Lorenzi M, et al. Cushing's disease: growth hormone response to hypoglycemia after correction of hypercortisolism. J Clin Endocrinol Metab 1977; 44:218–221.

1081. Adams EF, Ashby MJ, Brown SM, et al. Bromocriptine suppresses ACTH secretion from human pituitary tumour cells in culture by a dopaminergic mechanism. Clin Endocrinol 1981; 15:479–484.

1082. Ishibashi M, Yamaji T. Direct effects of thyrotropin-releasing hormone, cyproheptadine, and dopamine on adrenocorticotropin secretion from human corticotroph adenoma cells in vitro. J Clin Invest 1981; 68:1018–1027.

1083. Shibasaki T, Masui H. Effects of various neuropeptides on the secretion of proopiomelanocortin-derived peptides by a cultured pituitary adenoma causing Nelson's syndrome. Clin Endocrinol Metab 1982; 55:872–876.

1084. Lamberts SWJ, Verleun T, Bons EG, et al. Effect of cyproheptadine, desmethylcyproheptadine, τ-amino-butyric acid and sodium valproate on adrenocorticotrophin secretion by cultured pituitary tumour cells from three patients with Nelson's syndrome. J Endocrinol 1983; 96:401–406.

1085. Tucci JR, Nowakowski KJ, Jackson IMD. Cyproheptadine may act at the pituitary in Cushing's disease: evidence from CRF stimulation. J Endocrinol Invest 1989; 12:197–200.

1086. Whitehead HM, Beacom R, Sheridan B, et al. The effect of cyproheptadine and/or bromocriptine on plasma ACTH levels in patients cured of Cushing's disease by bilateral adrenalectomy. Clin Endocrinol 1990; 32:193–201.

1087. Carpenter PC. Cushing's syndrome: update of diagnosis and management. Mayo Clin Proc 1986; 61:49–58.

1088. Tagliaferri M, Berselli ME, Loli P. Transsphenoidal microsurgery for Cushing's disease. Acta Endocrinol 1986; 113:5–11.

1089. Schulte HM, Oldfield EH, Allolio B, et al. Clonal composition of corticotroph adenomas in patients with Cushing's disease: determination by X-chromosome inactivation analysis. Endocr Soc Abstr 1990; 221.

1090. Landis CA, Masters SB, Spada A, et al. GTPase inhibiting mutations activate the alpha chain of G_s and stimulate adenylyl cyclase in human pituitary tumours. Nature 1989; 340:692–696.

1091. Lyons J, Landis CA, Harsh G, et al. Two G proteins in human endocrine tumors. Science 1990; 249:655–659.

1092. Pieters GFFM, Smals AGH, Goverde HJM, et al. Adrenocorticotropin and cortisol responsiveness to thyrotropin-releasing hormone and luteinizing hormone–releasing hormone discloses two subsets of patients with Cushing's disease. J Clin Endocrinol Metab 1982; 55:1188–1197.

1093. Van Cauter E, Refetoff S. Evidence for two subtypes of Cushing's disease based on the analysis of episodic cortisol secretion. N Engl J Med 1985; 312:1343–1349.

1094. Suda T, Demura H, Demura R, et al. Anterior pituitary hormones in plasma and pituitaries from patients with Cushing's disease. J Clin Endocrinol Metab 1980; 51:1048–1053.

1095. Yamaji T, Ishibashi M, Teramoto A, et al. Hyperprolactinemia in Cushing's disease and Nelson's syndrome. J Clin Endocrinol Metab 1984; 58:790–795.

1096. Aron DC, Findling JW, Tyrrell JB. Cushing's disease. Endocrinol Metab Clin North Am 1987; 16:705–730.

1097. Marcovitz S, Wee R, Chan J, et al. The diagnostic accuracy of preoperative CT scanning in the evaluation of pituitary ACTH-secreting adenomas. AJR 1987; 149:803–806.

1098. Saris SC, Patronas NJ, Doppman JL, et al. Cushing syndrome: pituitary CT scanning. Radiology 1987; 162:775–777.

1099. Peck WW, Dillon WP, Norman D, et al. High-resolution MR imaging of pituitary microadenomas at 1.5 T: experience with Cushing disease. AJR 1989; 152:145–151.

1100. Dwyer AJ, Frank JA, Doppman JL, et al. Pituitary adenomas in patients with Cushing disease: initial experience with Gd-DTPA–enhanced MR imaging. Radiology 1987; 163:421–426.

1101. Lipkin EW, Fujimoto WY. Cushing's syndrome in a patient with suppressible hypercortisolism and an empty sella. West J Med 1984; 140:613–615.

1102. White FE, White MC, Drury PL, et al. Value of computed tomography of the abdomen and chest in investigation of Cushing's syndrome. Br Med J 1982; 284:9–12.

1103. Howland WJ Jr, Pugh DG, Sprague RG. Roentgenologic changes of the skeletal system in Cushing's syndrome. Radiology 1958; 71:69–78.

1104. Momose KJ, Kjellberg RN, Kliman B. High incidence of cortical atrophy of the cerebral and cerebellar hemispheres in Cushing's disease. Radiology 1971; 99:341–348.

1105. Orth DN, Liddle GW. Results of treatment in 108 patients with Cushing's syndrome. N Engl J Med 1971; 285:243–247.

1106. Hankin ME, Theile HM, Steinbeck AW. An evaluation of laboratory tests for the detection and differential diagnosis of Cushing's syndrome. Clin Endocrinol 1977; 6:185–196.

1107. Sindler BH, Griffing GT, Melby JC. The superiority of the metyrapone test versus the high-dose dexamethasone test in the differential diagnosis of Cushing's syndrome. Am J Med 1983; 74:657–662.

1108. Orth DN. The old and the new in Cushing's syndrome. N Engl J Med 1984; 310:649–651 (editorial).

1109. Bailey RE. Periodic hormonogenesis—a new phenomenon. Periodicity in function of a hormone-producing tumor in man. J Clin Endocrinol Metab 1971; 32:317–327.

1110. Brown RD, Van Loon GR, Orth DN, et al. Cushing's disease with periodic hormonogenesis: one explanation for paradoxical response to dexamethasone. J Clin Endocrinol Metab 1973; 36:445–451.

1111. Jordan RM, Ramos-Gabatin A, Kendall JW, et al. Dynamics of adrenocorticotropin (ACTH) secretion in cyclic Cushing's syndrome: evidence for more than one abnormal ACTH biorhythm. J Clin Endocrinol Metab 1982; 55:531–537.

1112. Kuchel O, Bolté E, Chrétien M, et al. Cyclical edema and hypokalemia due to occult episodic hypercorticism. J Clin Endocrinol Metab 1987; 64:170–174.

1113. Streeten DHP, Stephenson CT, Dalakos TG, et al. The diagnosis of hypercortisolism: biochemical criteria differentiating patients from lean and obese normal subjects and from females on oral contraceptives. J Clin Endocrinol Metab 1969; 29:1191–1211.

1114. Nugent CA, Nichols T, Tyler FH. Diagnosis of Cushing's syndrome: single dose dexamethasone test. Arch Intern Med 1965; 116:172–176.

1115. Meikle AW, Lagerquist LG, Tyler FH. Apparently normal pituitary-adrenal suppressibility in Cushing's syndrome: dexamethasone metabolism and plasma levels. J Lab Clin Med 1975; 86:472–478.

1116. Meikle AW. Dexamethasone suppression tests; usefulness of simultaneous measurement of plasma cortisol and dexamethasone. Clin Endocrinol 1982; 16:401–408.

1117. Meikle AW, Clarke DH, Tyler FH. Cushing syndrome from low doses of dexamethasone. A result of slow plasma clearance. JAMA 1976; 235:1592–1593.

1118. Haigh SE, Tevaarwerk GJM. A rise in the glomerular filtration rate as the cause of a "paradoxical" increase in urinary free cortisol during dexamethasone suppression in a patient with an adrenal adenoma: a case report. Clin Endocrinol 1981; 15:53–56.

1119. Noth RH, Walter RM Jr. The effects of alcohol on the endocrine system. Med Clin North Am 1984; 68:133–146.

1120. Carroll BJ, Feinberg M, Greden JF, et al. A specific laboratory test for the diagnosis of melancholia. Standardization, validation, and clinical utility. Arch Gen Psychiatry 1981; 38:15–22.

1121. Tyrrell JB, Findling JW, Aron DC, et al. An overnight high-dose dexamethasone suppression test for rapid differential diagnosis of Cushing's syndrome. Ann Intern Med 1986; 104:180–186.

1122. Liddle GW. The adrenals. In: Williams RW, ed. Textbook of Endocrinology. 6th ed. Philadelphia: W. B. Saunders, 1981: 242–292.

1123. Atkinson AB, Kennedy AL, Carson DJ, et al. Five cases of cyclical Cushing's syndrome. Br Med J [Clin Res] 1985; 291:1453–1457.

1124. Linn JE Jr, Bowdoin B, Farmer TA, et al. Observations and comments on failure of dexamethasone suppression. N Engl J Med 1967; 277:403–405.

1125. Hale AC, Millar JBG, Ratter SJ, et al. A case of pituitary dependent Cushing's disease with clinical and biochemical features of the ectopic ACTH syndrome. Clin Endocrinol 1985; 22:479–488.

1126. Carey RM. Suppression of ACTH by cortisol in dexamethasone-nonsuppressible Cushing's disease. N Engl J Med 1980; 302:275–279.

1127. Mason AMS, Ratcliffe JG, Buckel RM, et al. ACTH secretion by bronchial carcinoid tumours. Clin Endocrinol 1972; 1:3–25.

1128. Komor J, Laeng RH, Heitz PU, et al. Cushing-Syndrome bei Bronchuskarzinoid: supprimierbare ektopische ACTH-Sekretion. Schweiz Med Wochenschr 1982; 112:1507–1514.

1129. Ward PS, Mott MG, Smith J, et al. Cushing's syndrome and bronchial carcinoid tumour. Arch Dis Child 1984; 59:375–377.

1130. Liddle GW, Estep HL, Kendall JW Jr, et al. Clinical application of a new test of pituitary reserve. J Clin Endocrinol Metab 1959; 19:875–894.

1131. Orth DN, DeBold CR, DeCherney GS, et al. Pituitary microadenomas causing Cushing's disease respond to corticotropin-releasing factor. J Clin Endocrinol Metab 1982; 55:1017–1019.

1132. Müller OA, Stalla GK, von Werder K. Corticotropin releasing factor: a new tool for the differential diagnosis of Cushing's syndrome. J Clin Endocrinol Metab 1983; 57:227–229.

1133. Pieters GFFM, Hermus ARMM, Smals AGH, et al. Responsiveness of the hypophyseal-adrenocortical axis to corticotropin-releasing factor in pituitary-dependent Cushing's disease. J Clin Endocrinol Metab 1983; 57:513–516.

1134. Chrousos GP, Schulte HM, Oldfield EH, et al. The corticotropin-releasing factor stimulation test. An aid in the evaluation of patients with Cushing's syndrome. N Engl J Med 1984; 310:622–626.

1135. DeBold CR, Dickstein G, Orth DN. Plasma ACTH and cortisol responses to ovine corticotropin-releasing hormone (CRH), arginine vasopressin (AVP), CRH plus AVP and CRH plus metyrapone in patients with Cushing's disease. Endocr Soc Abstr 1989; 460.

1136. Findling JW, Aron DC, Tyrrell JB, et al. Selective venous sampling for ACTH in Cushing's syndrome. Differentiation between Cushing's disease and the ectopic ACTH syndrome. Ann Intern Med 1981; 94:647–652.

1137. Manni A, Latshaw RF, Page R, et al. Simultaneous bilateral venous sampling for adrenocorticotropin in pituitary-dependent Cushing's disease: evidence for lateralization of pituitary venous drainage. J Clin Endocrinol Metab 1983; 57:1070–1073.

1138. Oldfield EH, Chrousos GP, Schulte HM, et al. Preoperative lateralization of ACTH-secreting pituitary microadenomas by bilateral and simultaneous inferior petrosal venous sinus sampling. N Engl J Med 1985; 312:100–103.

1139. Schulte HM, Allolio B, Günther RW, et al. Selective bilateral and simultaneous catheterization of the inferior petrosal sinus: CRF stimulates prolactin secretion from ACTH-producing microadenomas in Cushing's disease. Clin Endocrinol 1988; 28:289–295.

1140. Doppman JL, Oldfield E, Krudy AG, et al. Petrosal sinus sampling for Cushing syndrome: anatomical and technical considerations. Radiology 1984; 150:99–103.

1141. Oldfield EH, Girton ME, Doppman JL. Absence of intercavernous venous mixing: evidence supporting lateralization of pituitary microad-

enomas by venous sampling. J Clin Endocrinol Metab 1985; 61:644–647.

1142. Doppman JL, Krudy AG, Girton ME, et al. Basilar venous plexus of the posterior fossa: a potential source of error in petrosal sinus sampling. Radiology 1985; 155:375–378.

1143. Zovickian J, Oldfield EH, Doppman JL, et al. Usefulness of inferior petrosal sinus venous endocrine markers in Cushing's disease. J Neurosurg 1988; 68:205–210.

1144. McCance DR, McIlrath E, McNeill A, et al. Bilateral inferior petrosal sinus sampling as a routine procedure in ACTH-dependent Cushing's syndrome. Clin Endocrinol 1989; 30:157–166.

1145. Hardy J. Cushing's disease: 50 years later. Can J Neurol Sci 1982; 9:375–380.

1146. Fahlbusch R, Buchfelder M, Müller OA. Transsphenoidal surgery for Cushing's disease. J R Soc Med 1986; 79:262–269.

1147. Chandler WF, Schteingart DE, Lloyd RV, et al. Surgical treatment of Cushing's disease. J Neurosurg 1987; 66:204–212.

1148. Mampalam TJ, Tyrrell JB, Wilson CB. Transsphenoidal microsurgery for Cushing disease. A report of 216 cases. Ann Intern Med 1988; 109:487–493.

1149. Rovitt RL, Duane TD. Cushing's syndrome and pituitary tumors. Pathophysiology and ocular manifestations of ACTH-secreting pituitary adenomas. Am J Med 1969; 46:416–427.

1150. Gabrilove JL, Anderson PJ, Halmi NS. Pituitary pro-opiomelanocortin–cell carcinoma occurring in conjunction with a glioblastoma in a patient with Cushing's disease and subsequent Nelson's syndrome. Clin Endocrinol 1986; 25:117–126.

1151. Lenhard L, Deftos LJ. Adenohypophyseal hormones in the CSF. Neuroendocrinology 1982; 34:303–308.

1152. Nakao N, Oki S, Tanaka I, et al. Immunoreactive β-endorphin and adrenocorticotropin in human cerebrospinal fluid. J Clin Invest 1980; 66:1383–1390.

1153. Robert F, Pelletier G, Hardy J. Pituitary adenomas in Cushing's disease. A histologic, ultrastructural, and immunocytochemical study. Arch Pathol Lab Med 1978; 102:448–455.

1154. Olivier L, Vila-Porcile E, Dubois MP. Localisations cellulaires des peptides dérivés de la pro-opiocortine dans l'adénohypophyse humaine normale et dans les tumeurs de la maladie de Cushing. Horm Res 1980; 13:211–229.

1155. Coates PJ, Doniach I, Wells C, et al. Peptides related to α-melanocyte–stimulating hormone are commonly produced by human pituitary corticotroph adenomas: no relationship with pars intermedia origin. J Endocrinol 1989; 120:531–536.

1156. Sherry SH, Guay AT, Lee AK, et al. Concurrent production of adrenocorticotropin and prolactin from two distinct cell lines in a single pituitary adenoma: a detailed immunohistochemical analysis. J Clin Endocrinol Metab 1982; 55:947–955.

1157. Peillon F, Racadot J, Oliver L, et al. Microadenomas: structure and function. In: Faglia G, Giovanelli MA, MacLeod RM, eds. Microadenomas. London: Academic, 1980: 91.

1158. Lamberts SWJ, Stefanko SZ, de Lange SA, et al. Failure of clinical remission after transsphenoidal removal of a microadenoma in a patient with Cushing's disease: multiple hyperplastic and adenomatous cell nests in surrounding pituitary tissue. J Clin Endocrinol Metab 1980; 50:793–795.

1159. Schteingart DE, Tsao HS. Coexistence of pituitary adrenocorticotropin-dependent Cushing's syndrome with a solitary adrenal adenoma. J Clin Endocrinol Metab 1980; 50:961–966.

1160. Ruder JH, Loriaux DL, Lipsett MB. Severe osteopenia in young adults associated with Cushing's syndrome due to micronodular adrenal disease. J Clin Endocrinol Metab 1974; 39:1138–1147.

1161. Carson DJ, Sloan JM, Cleland J, et al. Cyclical Cushing's syndrome presenting as short stature in a boy with recurrent atrial myxomas and freckled skin pigmentation. Clin Endocrinol 1988; 28:173–180.

1162. Hashimoto K, Kawada Y, Murakami K, et al. Cortisol responsiveness to insulin-induced hypoglycemia in Cushing's syndrome with huge nodular adrenocortical hyperplasia. Endocrinol Jpn 1986; 33:479–487.

1163. Makino S, Hashimoto K, Sugiyama M, et al. Cushing's syndrome due to huge nodular adrenocortical hyperplasia with fluctuation of urinary 17-OHCS excretion. Endocrinol Jpn 1989; 36:655–663.

1164. Cheitlin RA, Westphal M, Cabrera CM, et al. Cushing's syndrome due to bilateral adrenal macronodular hyperplasia with undetectable ACTH: cell culture of adenoma cells on extracellular matrix. Horm Res 1988; 29:162–167.

1165. Laws ER, Ebersold MJ, Peipgras DG, et al. The results of transsphenoidal surgery in specific clinical entities. In: Laws ER, ed. Management of Pituitary Adenomas and Related Lesions with Emphasis on Transsphenoidal Microsurgery. New York: Appleton-Century-Crofts, 1982: 277–305.

1166. Styne DM, Grumbach MM, Kaplan SL, et al. Treatment of Cushing's disease in childhood and adolescence by transsphenoidal microadenomectomy. N Engl J Med 1984; 310:889–893.

1167. Aron DC, Findling JW, Fitzgerald PA, et al. Cushing's syndrome: problems in management. Endocr Rev 1982; 3:229–244.

1168. Burch W. A survey of results with transsphenoidal surgery in Cushing's disease. N Engl J Med 1983; 308:103–104 (letter).

1169. Kammer H, George R. Cushing's disease in a patient with an ectopic pituitary adenoma. JAMA 1981; 246:2722–2724.

1170. Lüdecke DK. Intraoperative measurement of adrenocorticotropic hormone in peripituitary blood in Cushing's disease. Neurosurgery 1989; 24:201–205.

1171. Hotta MN, Shibasaki T, Suda T, et al. The use of the corticotropin-releasing hormone test to monitor the recovery of patients with Cushing's disease or Cushing's syndrome due to an adrenal adenoma after adenomectomy. Endocrinol Jpn 1985; 32:113–125.

1172. Jennings AS, Liddle GW, Orth DN. Results of treating childhood Cushing's disease with pituitary irradiation. N Engl J Med 1977; 297:957–962.

1173. Salassa RM, Kearns TP, Kernohan JW, et al. Pituitary tumors in patients with Cushing's syndrome. J Clin Endocrinol Metab 1959; 19:1523–1539.

1174. Nelson DH, Meakin JW, Thorn GW. ACTH-producing pituitary tumors following adrenalectomy for Cushing's syndrome. Ann Intern Med 1960; 52:560–569.

1175. Sharpe GF, Kendall-Taylor P, Prescott RWG, et al. Pituitary function following megavoltage therapy for Cushing's disease: long term follow up. Clin Endocrinol 1985; 22:169–177.

1176. Howlett TA, Plowman PN, Wass JAH, et al. Megavoltage pituitary irradiation in the management of Cushing's disease and Nelson's syndrome: long-term follow-up. Clin Endocrinol 1989; 31:309–323.

1177. Linfoot JA. Heavy ion therapy: alpha particle therapy of pituitary tumors. In: Linfoot JA, ed. Recent Advances in Diagnosis and Treatment of Pituitary Tumors. New York: Raven, 1979: 245–267.

1178. Kjellberg RN, Kliman B, Swisher B, et al. Proton beam therapy of Cushing's disease and Nelson's syndrome. In: Black PM et al., eds. Secretory Tumors of the Pituitary Gland. New York: Raven, 1984: 295–307.

1179. Burke CW, Doyle FH, Joplin GF, et al. Cushing's disease. Treatment by pituitary implantation of radioactive gold or yttrium seeds. Q J Med 1973; 42:175–204.

1180. Cassar J, Doyle FH, Mashiter K, et al. Treatment of Cushing's disease in juveniles with interstitial pituitary irradiation. Clin Endocrinol 1979; 11:313–321.

1181. Lunsford LD, Flickinger J, Lindner G, et al. Stereotactic radiosurgery of the brain using the first United States 201 cobalt-60 source gamma knife. Neurosurgery 1989; 24:151–159.

1182. Friedman WA, Bova FJ. The University of Florida radiosurgery system. Surg Neurol 1989; 32:334–342.

1183. Luton JP, Mahoudeau JA, Bouchard P, et al. Treatment of Cushing's disease by o,p' DDD. Survey of 62 cases. N Engl J Med 1979; 300:459–464.

1184. Schteingart DE, Tsao HS, Taylor CI, et al. Sustained remission of Cushing's disease with mitotane and pituitary irradiation. Ann Intern Med 1980; 92:613–619.

1185. Takamatsu J, Kitazawa A, Nakata K, et al. Does mitotane reduce endogenous ACTH secretion? N Engl J Med 1981; 305:957 (letter).

1186. Hogan TF, Citrin DL, Johnson BM, et al. o,p'-DDD (mitotane) therapy of adrenal cortical carcinoma. Observations on drug dosage, toxicity, and steroid replacement. Cancer 1978; 42:2177–2181.

1187. Moore TJ, Dluhy RG, Williams GH, et al. Nelson's syndrome: frequency, prognosis, and effect of prior pituitary irradiation. Ann Intern Med 1976; 85:731–734.

1188. Kelly WF, MacFarlane IA, Longson D, et al. Cushing's disease treated by total adrenalectomy: long-term observations of 43 patients. Q J Med 1983; 52:224–231.

1189. Hardy JD. Surgical management of Cushing's syndrome with emphasis on adrenal autotransplantation. Ann Surg 1978; 188:290–307.

1190. Scott HW Jr, Orth DN. Hypercortisolism (Cushing's syndrome). In: Scott HW Jr, ed. Surgery of the Adrenal Glands. Philadelphia: J. B. Lippincott, 1990: 115–151.

1191. Chalmers RA, Mashiter K, Joplin GF. Residual adrenocortical function after bilateral "total" adrenalectomy for Cushing's disease. Lancet 1981; 2:1196–1199.

1192. Herwig KR, Schteingart DE. Successful removal of an adrenal remnant localized by 131I-19-iodocholesterol. J Urol 1974; 111:713–714.

1193. Hopwood NJ, Kenny FM. Incidence of Nelson's syndrome after adrenalectomy for Cushing's disease in children. Results of a nationwide survey. Am J Dis Child 1977; 131:1353–1356.

1194. Cohen KL, Noth RH, Pechinski T. Incidence of pituitary tumors following adrenalectomy. A long-term follow-up study of patients treated for Cushing's disease. Arch Intern Med 1978; 138:575–579.

1195. McArthur RG, Hayles AB, Salassa RM. Childhood Cushing disease: results of bilateral adrenalectomy. J Pediatr 1979; 95:214–219.

1196. Wilson CB, Tyrrell JB, Fitzgerald PA, et al. Cushing's disease and Nelson's syndrome. Clin Neurosurg 1979; 24:19–30.

1197. Wild W, Nicolis GL, Gabrilove JL. Appearance of Nelson's syndrome despite pituitary irradiation prior to bilateral adrenalectomy for Cushing's syndrome. Mt Sinai J Med 1973; 40:68–71.

1198. Barnett AH, Livesey JH, Friday K, et al. Comparison of preoperative and postoperative ACTH concentrations after bilateral adrenalectomy in Cushing's disease. Clin Endocrinol 1983; 18:301–305.

1199. Lamberts SWJ, Birkenhäger JC. Effect of bromocriptine in pituitary-dependent Cushing's syndrome. J Endocrinol 1976; 70:315–316.

1200. Jones MT, Gillham B, Beckford U, et al. Effect of treatment with sodium valproate and diazepam on plasma corticotropin in Nelson's syndrome. Lancet 1981; 1:1179–1181.

1201. Elias AN, Gwinup G, Valenta LJ. Effects of valproic acid, naloxone and hydrocortisone in Nelson's syndrome and Cushing's disease. Clin Endocrinol 1981; 15:151–154.

1202. Dornhorst A, Jenkins JS, Lamberts SWJ, et al. The evaluation of sodium valproate in the treatment of Nelson's syndrome. J Clin Endocrinol Metab 1983; 56:985–991.

1203. Koppeschaar HPF, Croughs RJM, Thijssen JHH, et al. Response to neurotransmitter modulating drugs in patients with Cushing's disease. Clin Endocrinol 1986; 25:661–667.

1204. Jeffcoate WJ, Rees LH, Tomlin S, et al. Metyrapone in long-term management of Cushing's disease. Br Med J 1977; 2:215–217.

1205. Komanicky P, Spark RF, Melby JC. Treatment of Cushing's syndrome with trilostane (WIN 24,540), an inhibitor of adrenal steroid biosynthesis. J Clin Endocrinol Metab 1978; 47:1042–1051.

1206. Loli P, Berselli ME, Tagliaferri M. Use of ketoconazole in the treatment of Cushing's syndrome. J Clin Endocrinol Metab 1986; 63:1365–1371.

1207. Schöneshöfer M, Fenner A, Claus M. Suppressive effect of metyrapone on plasma corticotrophin immunoreactivity in normal man. Clin Endocrinol 1983; 18:363–370.

1208. Child DF, Burke CW, Burley DM, et al. Drug control of Cushing's syndrome. Combined aminoglutethimide and metyrapone therapy. Acta Endocrinol 1976; 82:330–341.

1209. Orth DN. Metyrapone is useful only as adjunctive therapy in Cushing's disease. Ann Intern Med 1978; 89:128–130 (editorial).

1210. Stalla GK, Stalla J, Huber M, et al. Ketoconazole inhibits corticotropic cell function in vitro. Endocrinology 1988; 122:618–623.

1211. McCance DR, Hadden DR, Kennedy L, et al. Clinical experience with ketoconazole as a therapy for patients with Cushing's syndrome. Clin Endocrinol 1987; 27:593–599.

1212. Semple CG, Beastall GH, Gray CE, et al. Trilostane in the management of Cushing's syndrome. Acta Endocrinol 1983; 102:107–110.

1213. Santen RJ, Wells SA, Runic S, et al. Adrenal suppression with aminoglutethimide. I. Differential effects of aminoglutethimide on glucocorticoid metabolism as a rationale for use of hydrocortisone. J Clin Endocrinol Metab 1977; 45:469–479.

1214. Bertagna X, Bertagna C, Laudat MH, et al. Pituitary-adrenal response to the antiglucocorticoid action of RU 486 in Cushing's syndrome. J Clin Endocrinol Metab 1986; 63:639–643.

1215. Invitti C, de Martin M, Brunani A, et al. Treatment of Cushing's syndrome with the long-acting somatostatin analogue SMS 201-995 (Sandostatin). Clin Endocrinol 1990; 32:275–281.

1216. Lufkin EG, Wahner HW, Bergstralh EJ. Reversibility of steroid-induced osteoporosis. Am J Med 1988; 85:887–888.

1217. Kasperlik-Zaluska AA, Nielubowicz J, Wisawski J, et al. Nelson's syndrome: incidence and prognosis. Clin Endocrinol 1983; 19:693–698.

1218. Rahn T, Thoren M, Hall K, et al. Stereotactic radiosurgery in the treatment of MB Cushing. In: Szikla G, ed. Sterotactic Cerebral Irradiation. INSERM Symposium No. 12. Amsterdam: Elsevier/North-Holland, 1979: 207–212.

1219. Aronin N, Krieger DT. Sustained remission of Nelson's syndrome after stopping cyproheptadine treatment. N Engl J Med 1980; 302:453–455.

1220. DeBold CR, Menefee JK, Nicholson WE, et al. Proopiomelanocortin gene is expressed in many normal human tissues and in tumors not associated with ectopic adrenocorticotropin syndrome. Mol Endocrinol 1988; 2:862–870.

1221. DeBold CR, Mufson EE, Menefee JK, et al. Prioopiomelanocortin gene expression in a pheochromocytoma using upstream transcription initiation sites. Biochem Biophys Res Commun 1988; 155:895–900.

1222. de Keyzer Y, Bertagna X, Lenne F, et al. Altered proopiomelanocortin gene expression in adrenocorticotropin-producing nonpituitary tumors. J Clin Invest 1985; 76:1892–1898.

1223. Garroway NW, Orth DN, Harrison RW. Binding of cytosol receptor–glucocorticoid complexes by isolated nuclei of glucocorticoid-responsive and nonresponsive cultured cells. Endocrinology 1976; 98:1092–1100.

1224. Clark AJL, Stewart MF, Lavender PM, et al. Defective glucocorticoid regulation of proopiomelanocortin gene expression and peptide secretion in a small cell lung cancer cell line. Clin Endocrinol Metab 1990; 70:485–490.

1225. Orth DN, Nicholson WE, Mitchell WM, et al. Biologic and immunologic characterization and physical separation of ACTH and ACTH fragments in the ectopic ACTH syndrome. J Clin Invest 1973; 52:1756–1769.

1226. Bertagna X, Lenne F, Comar D, et al. Human β-melanocyte stimulating hormone revisited. Proc Natl Acad Sci USA 1986; 83:9719–9723.

1227. Howlett TA, Drury PL, Perry L, et al. Diagnosis and management of ACTH-dependent Cushing's syndrome: comparison of the features in ectopic and pituitary ACTH production. Clin Endocrinol 1986; 24:699–713.

1228. Howlett TA, Rees LH, Besser GM. Cushing's syndrome. Clin Endocrinol Metab 1985; 14:911–945.

1229. Vieau D, Massias JF, Girard F, et al. Corticotrophin-like intermediary lobe peptide as a marker of alternate pro-opiomelanocortin processing in ACTH-producing non-pituitary tumours. Clin Endocrinol 1989; 31:691–700.

1230. Malchoff CD, Orth DN, Abboud C, et al. Ectopic ACTH syndrome caused by a bronchial carcinoid tumor responsive to dexamethasone, metyrapone and corticotropin-releasing factor. Am J Med 1989; 84:760–764.

1231. Schteingart DE, Conn JW, Orth DN, et al. Secretion of ACTH and β-MSH by an adrenal medullary paraganglioma. J Clin Endocrinol Metab 1972; 34:676–683.

1232. Doppman JL, Loughlin T, Miller DL, et al. Identification of ACTH-producing intrathoracic tumors by measuring ACTH levels in aspirated specimens. Radiology 1987; 163:501–503.

1233. Doppman JL, Pass HI, Nieman L, et al. Failure of bronchial lavage to detect elevated levels of adrenocorticotropin (ACTH) in patients with ACTH-producing bronchial carcinoids. J Clin Endocrinol Metab 1989; 69:1032–1034.

1234. Kameya T, Shimosato Y, Kodama T, et al. Peptide hormone production by adenocarcinomas of the lung: its morphologic basis and histogenetic considerations. Virchows Arch [A] 1983; 400:245–257.

1235. Tanaka K, Nicholson WE, Orth DN. The nature of the immunoreactive lipotropins in human plasma and tissue extracts. J Clin Invest 1978; 62:94–104.

1236. Sorenson GD, Pettengill OS, Brinck-Johnsen T, et al. Hormone production by cultures of small-cell carcinoma of the lung. Cancer 1981; 47:1289–1296.

1237. Johnson DH, Marangos PJ, Forbes JT, et al. Potential utility of serum neuron-specific enolase levels in small cell carcinoma of the lung. Cancer Res 1984; 44:5409–5414.

1238. Waalkes TP, Abeloff MD, Woo KB, et al. Carcinoembryonic antigen for monitoring patients with small cell carcinoma of the lung during treatment. Cancer Res 1980; 40:4420–4427.

1239. Gärtner R, Albrecht M, Müller OA. Effect of etomidate on hypercortisolism due to ectopic ACTH production. Lancet 1986; 1:275.

1240. Nieman LK, Chrousos GP, Kellner C, et al. Successful treatment of Cushing's syndrome with the glucocorticoid antagonist RU 486. J Clin Endocrinol Metab 1985; 61:536–540.

1241. Hearn PR, Reynolds CL, Johansen K, et al. Lung carcinoid with Cushing's syndrome: control of serum ACTH and cortisol levels using SMS 201-995 (Sandostatin). Clin Endocrinol 1988; 28:181–185.

1242. Bertagna X, Favrod-Coune C, Escourolle H, et al. Suppression of ectopic adrenocorticotropin secretion by the long-acting somatostatin analog octreotide. J Clin Endocrinol Metab 1989; 68:988–991.

1243. Imperato-McGinley J, Young IS, Huang T, et al. Testosterone-secreting adrenal cortical adenomas. Int J Gynaecol Obstet 1981; 19:421–428.

1244. Gabrilove JL, Seman AT, Sabet R, et al. Virilizing adrenal adenoma with studies on the steroid content of the adrenal venous effluent and a review of the literature. Endocr Rev 1981; 2:462–470.

1245. Mersey JH, Ceballos L, Levin P, et al. Estrogen-secreting adrenal tumor responsive to ACTH: localization by adrenal venous sampling. South Med J 1988; 81:275–278.

1246. van Seters AP, van Aalderen W, Moolenaar AJ, et al. Adrenocortical tumour in untreated congenital adrenocortical hyperplasia associated with inadequate ACTH suppressibility. Clin Endocrinol 1981; 14:325–334.

1247. Anderson DC, Child DF, Sutcliffe CH, et al. Cushing's syndrome, nodular adrenal hyperplasia and virilizing carcinoma. Clin Endocrinol 1973; 9:1–14.

1248. McKenna TJ, Miller RB, Liddle GW. Plasma pregnenolone and 17-OH-pregnenolone in patients with adrenal tumors, ACTH excess, or idiopathic hirsutism. J Clin Endocrinol Metab 1977; 44:231–236.

1249. Guerin CK, Wahner HW, Gorman CA, et al. Computed tomographic scanning versus radioisotope imaging in adrenocortical diagnosis. Am J Med 1983; 75:653–657.

1250. Fig LM, Gross MD, Shapiro B, et al. Adrenal localization in the adrenocorticotropic hormone–independent Cushing syndrome. Ann Intern Med 1988; 109:547–553.

1251. Miles HM, Wahner HW, Carpenter PC, et al. Adrenal scintiscanning with NP-59, a new radioiodinated cholesterol agent. Mayo Clin Proc 1979; 54:321–327.

1252. Doppman JL, Reinig JW, Dwyer AJ, et al. Differentiation of adrenal masses by magnetic resonance imaging. Surgery 1987; 102:1018–1026.

1253. Fraumeni JF Jr, Miller RW. Adrenocortical neoplasms with hemihypertrophy, brain tumors, and other disorders. J Pediatr 1967; 70:129–138.

1254. Marieb NJ, Spangler S, Kashgarian M, et al. Cushing's syndrome secondary to ectopic cortisol production by an ovarian carcinoma. J Clin Endocrinol Metab 1983; 57:737–740.

1255. Weiss LM. Comparative histologic study of 43 metastasizing adrenocortical tumors. Am J Surg Pathol 1984; 8:103–109.

1256. Hough AJ, Hollifield JW, Page DL, et al. Prognostic factors in adrenal cortical tumors. A mathematical analysis of clinical and morphologic data. Am J Clin Pathol 1979; 72:390–399.

1257. Levin NP. Fine needle aspiration and histology of adrenal cortical carcinoma. Acta Cytol 1981; 25:421–424.

1258. Nosher JL, Amorosa JK, Seiman S, et al. Fine needle aspiration of the kidney and adrenal gland. J Urol 1982; 128:895–899.

1259. Välimäki M, Pelkonen R, Porkka L, et al. Long-term results of adrenal surgery in patients with Cushing's syndrome due to adrenocortical adenoma. Clin Endocrinol 1984; 20:229–236.

1260. Macfarlane DA. Cancer of the adrenal cortex. The natural history, prognosis and treatment in a study of fifty-five cases. Ann R Coll Surg 1958; 23:155–186.

1261. Stewart DR, Morris Jones PH, Jolleys A. Carcinoma of the adrenal gland in children. J Pediatr Surg 1974; 9:59–67.

1262. Schteingart DE, Motazedi A, Noonan RA, et al. Treatment of adrenal carcinomas. Arch Surg 1982; 117:1142–1146.

1263. Cohn K, Gottesman L, Brennan M. Adrenocortical carcinoma. Surgery 1986; 100:1170–1177.

1264. Henley DJ, van Heerden JA, Grant CS, et al. Adrenal cortical carcinoma—a continuing challenge. Surgery 1983; 94:926–931.

1265. Nader S, Hickey RC, Sellin RV, et al. Adrenal cortical carcinoma. A study of 77 cases. Cancer 1983; 52:707–711.

1266. van Slooten H, Moolenaar AJ, van Seters AP, et al. The treatment of adrenocortical carcinoma with o,p'-DDD: prognostic implications of serum level monitoring. Eur J Cancer Clin Oncol 1984; 20:47–53.

1267. Lubitz JA, Freeman L, Okun R. Mitotane use in inoperable adrenal cortical carcinoma. JAMA 1973; 223:1109–1112.

1268. Bodie B, Novick AC, Pontes JE, et al. The Cleveland Clinic experience with adrenal cortical carcinoma. J Urol 1989; 141:257–260.

1269. Hoffman DL, Mattox VR. Treatment of adrenocortical carcinoma with o,p'-DDD. Med Clin North Am 1972; 56:999–1012.

1270. Schumacher OP. Adrenocortical tumors. In: Santen RJ, Manni A, eds. Diagnosis and Management of Endocrine-Related Tumors. Boston: Martinus Nijhoff, 1984: 219–234.

1271. Kvols LK, Buck M. Chemotherapy of endocrine malignancies: a review. Semin Oncol 1987; 14:343–353.

1272. Magee BJ, Gattamaneni HR, Pearson D. Adrenal cortical carcinoma: survival after radiotherapy. Clin Radiol 1987; 38:587–588.

1273. Carroll BJ, Curtis GC, Mendels J. Neuroendocrine regulation in depression. II. Discrimination from depressed and nondepressed patients. Arch Gen Psychiatry 1976; 33:1051–1058.

1274. Mortola JF, Liu JH, Gillin JC, et al. Pulsatile rhythms of adrenocorticotropin (ACTH) and cortisol in women with endogenous depression: evidence for increased ACTH pulse frequency. J Clin Endocrinol Metab 1987; 65:962–968.

1275. Gold PW, Loriaux DL, Roy A, et al. Responses to corticotropin releasing hormone in the hypercortisolism of depression and Cushing's disease: pathophysiologic and diagnostic implications. N Engl J Med 1986; 314:1329–1335.

1276. Smals AG, Klopoenborg PW, Njo KT, et al. Alcoholic pseudo-Cushing's. Br Med J 1976; 2:1298.

1277. Rees LH, Besser GM, Jeffcoate WJ, et al. Alcoholic pseudo-Cushing's. Lancet 1977; 1:726.

1278. Cobb CF, Van Thiel DH. Mechanism of ethanol-induced adrenal stimulation. Alcohol Clin Exp Res 1982; 6:202–206.

1279. Howlett TA, Price J, Hale AC, et al. Pituitary ACTH dependent Cushing's syndrome due to ectopic production of a bombesin-like peptide by a medullary carcinoma of the thyroid. Clin Endocrinol 1985; 22:91–101.

1280. Hale AC, Price J, Ackland JF, et al. Corticotrophin-releasing factor–mediated adrenocorticotrophin release from rat anterior pituitary cells is potentiated by C-terminal gastrin-releasing peptide. J Endocrinol 1984; 102:R1–R3.

1281. Watanabe T, Orth DN. Effects of several in vitro systems on the potencies of putative adrenocorticotropin secretagogues on rat anterior pituitary cells. Endocrinology 1988; 122:2299–2308.

1282. Fleischer N, Abe K, Liddle GW, et al. ACTH antibodies in patients receiving depot porcine ACTH to hasten recovery from pituitary-adrenal suppression. J Clin Invest 1967; 46:196–204.

1283. Wulffraat NM, Drexhage HA, Wiersinga WM, et al. Immunoglobulins of patients with Cushing's syndrome due to pigmented adrenocortical micronodular dysplasia stimulate in vitro steroidogenesis. J Clin Endocrinol Metab 1988; 66:301–307.

1284. Van Berkhout FT, Croughs RJM, Kater L, et al. Familial Cushing's syndrome due to nodular adrenocortical dysplasia. A putative receptor-antibody disease? Clin Endocrinol 1986; 24:299–310.

1285. Young WR Jr, Carney JA, Musa BU, et al. Familial Cushing's syndrome due to primary pigmented nodular adrenocortical disease. Reinvestigation 50 years later. N Engl J Med 1989; 321:1659–1664.

1286. Doppman JL, Travis WD, Nieman L, et al. Cushing syndrome due to primary pigmented nodular adrenocortical disease: findings at CT and MR imaging. Radiology 1989; 172:415–420.

1287. Iida S, Nakamura Y, Fujii H, et al. A patient with hypocortisolism and Cushing's syndrome–like manifestations: cortisol hyperreactive syndrome. J Clin Endocrinol Metab 1990; 70:729–737.

1288. Conn JW. Primary aldosteronism, a new clinical entity. J Lab Clin Med 1955; 45:6–17.
1289. Atsumi T, Ishikawa S, Miyatake T, et al. Myopathy and primary aldosteronism. Electron microscopy study. Neurology 1979; 29:1348–1353.
1290. Kaplan NM. Primary aldosteronism with malignant hypertension. N Engl J Med 1963; 269:1282–1286.
1291. Iwaoka T, Umeda T, Sato T, et al. High plasma renin activities in primary aldosteronism with malignant hypertension. Jpn Heart J 1980; 21:423–428.
1292. Ferris JB, Beevres DG, Brown JJ, et al. Low renin ("primary") hyperaldosteronism—differential diagnosis and distinction of sub-groups within the syndrome. Am Heart J 1978; 95:641–658.
1293. Young WF, Hogan MJ, Klee GG, et al. Primary aldosteronism: diagnosis and treatment. Mayo Clin Proc 1990; 65:96–110.
1294. Arteaga E, Biglieri EG, Kater CE, et al. Aldosterone-producing adrenocortical carcinoma. Ann Intern Med 1984; 101:316–321.
1295. Dye NV, Litton NJ, Varma M, et al. Unilateral adrenal hyperplasia as a cause of primary aldosteronism. South Med J 1989; 82:82–86.
1296. Yamaji T, Ishibashi M, Sekihara H, et al. Plasma levels of atrial natriuretic peptide in primary aldosteronism and essential hypertension. J Clin Endocrinol Metab 1986; 63:815–818.
1297. Tunny TJ, Higgins BA, Gordon RD. Plasma levels of atrial natriuretic peptide in man in primary aldosteronism and in Bartter's syndrome. Clin Exp Pharmacol Physiol 1986; 13:341–345.
1298. Nakamura T, Ichikawa S, Sakamaki T, et al. Role of atrial natriuretic peptide in mineralocorticoid escape phenomenon in patients with primary aldosteronism. Proc Soc Exp Biol Med 1987; 185:448–454.
1299. Kelly TM, Nelson DH. Sodium excretion and atrial natriuretic peptide levels during mineralocorticoid administration. A mechanism for the escape from hyperaldosteronism. Endocr Res 1987; 13:363–383.
1300. Tarazi RC, Ibrahim MM, Bravo EL, et al. Hemodynamic characteristics of primary aldosteronism. N Engl J Med 1973; 289:1330–1335.
1301. Brock TA, Fleming BP, Diana JN. Pre- and post-capillary vascular response to sympathetic nerve stimulation in DOCA-hypertensive dogs. Hypertension 1981; 3:471–478.
1302. Yamakado M, Nagano M, Umezu M, et al. Extrarenal role of aldosterone in the regulation of blood pressure. Am J Hypertens 1988; 1:276–279.
1303. Jones AW, Hart RG. Altered ion transport in aortic smooth muscle during deoxycorticosterone hypertension in the rat. Circ Res 1975; 37:333–341.
1304. Moreland RS, Lamb FS, Webb RC, et al. Functional evidence for increased sodium permeability in aortae from DOCA hypertensive rats. Hypertension 1984; 6(Suppl 1):88–94.
1305. Jose A, Kaplan NM. Plasma renin activity in the diagnosis of primary aldosteronism: failure to distinguish primary aldosteronism from essential hypertension. Arch Intern Med 1969; 123:141–146.
1306. Weinberger MH, Grim CE, Hollifield JW, et al. Primary aldosteronism. Diagnosis, localization, and treatment. Ann Intern Med 1979; 90:386–395.
1307. Matsuoka H, Mulrow PJ, Franco-Saenz R, et al. Stimulation of aldosterone production by β-melanotropin. Nature 1981; 291:155–156.
1308. Griffing GT, Berelowitz B, Hudson M, et al. Plasma immunoreactive γ-melanotropin in patients with idiopathic hyperaldosteronism, aldosterone-producing adenomas, and essential hypertension. J Clin Invest 1985; 76:163–169.
1309. Schiffrin EL, Chretien M, Seidah NG, et al. Response of human aldosteronoma cells in culture to the N-terminal glycopeptide of proopiomelanocortin and gamma$_3$-MSH. Horm Metab Res 1983; 15:181–184.
1310. Gullner HG, Gill JR. Beta endorphin selectively stimulates aldosterone secretion in hypophysectomized, nephrectomized dogs. J Clin Invest 1983; 71:124–128.
1311. Raibinowe SL, Taylor T, Dluhy RG, et al. β-Endorphin stimulates plasma renin and aldosterone release in normal human subjects. J Clin Endocrinol Metab 1985; 60:485–490.
1312. Sen S, Valenzuela R, Smeby R, et al. Localization, purification, and biological activity of a new aldosterone-stimulating factor. Hypertension 1981; 3(Suppl 1):81–86.
1313. Carey RM, Sen S, Dolan LM, et al. Idiopathic hyperaldosteronism: a possible role for aldosterone-stimulating factor. N Engl J Med 1984; 311:94–100.
1314. Gross MD, Grekin RJ, Gniadek TC, et al. Suppression of aldosterone by cyproheptadine in idiopathic hyperaldosteronism. N Engl J Med 1981; 305:181–185.
1315. Franco-Saenz R, Mulrow PJ, Kitai K. Idiopathic aldosteronism: a possible disease of the intermediate lobe of the pituitary. JAMA 1984; 251:2555–2558.
1316. McAreavy D, Murray GD, Lever AF. Similarity of idiopathic hyperaldosteronism and essential hypertension. Hypertension 1983; 5:116–121.
1317. Sutherland DJA, Ruse JL, Laidlaw JC. Hypertension, increased aldosterone secretion and low plasma renin activity relieved by dexamethasone. Can Med Assoc J 1966; 95:1109–1119.
1318. Giebink GS, Gotlin RW, Biglieri EG, et al. A kindred with familial
1319. glucocorticoid-suppressible aldosteronism. J Clin Endocrinol Metab 1973; 36:715–723.
1319. Fallo F, Sonino N, Boscaro M, et al. Dexamethasone-suppressible hyperaldosteronism: pathophysiology, clinical aspects, and new insights into the pathogenesis. Klin Wochenschr 1987; 65:437–444.
1320. Connell JM, Kenyon CJ, Corrie JE, et al. Dexamethasone-suppressible hyperaldosteronism. Adrenal transition cell hyperplasia? Hypertension 1986; 8:669–676.
1321. Gomez-Sanchez CE, Gill JR, Ganguly A, et al. Glucocorticoid-suppressible aldosteronism: a disorder of the adrenal transition zone. J Clin Endocrinol Metab 1988; 67:444–448.
1322. Stockigt JR, Scoggins BA. Long term evolution of glucocorticoid-suppressible hyperaldosteronism. J Clin Endocrinol Metab 1987; 64:22–26.
1323. Banks WA, Kastin AJ, Biglieri EG, et al. Primary adrenal hyperplasia: a new subset of primary aldosteronism. J Clin Endocrinol Metab 1984; 58:783–785.
1324. Ganguly A, Zager PG, Luetscher JA. Primary aldosteronism due to unilateral adrenal hyperplasia. J Clin Endocrinol Metab 1980; 51:1190–1194.
1325. Noth RH, Biglieri EG. Primary hyperaldosteronism. Med Clin North Am 1988; 72:1117–1131.
1326. Weinberger MH, Grim CE. Sensitivity and specificity of screening procedures for primary aldosteronism. JAMA 1980; 244:331–332.
1327. Kaplan NM. Hypokalemia in the hypertensive patient: with observations on the incidence of primary aldosteronism. Ann Intern Med 1967; 66:1079–1090.
1328. Hamlet SM, Tunny TJ, Woodland E, et al. Is aldosterone/renin ratio useful to screen a hypertensive population for primary aldosteronism? Clin Exp Pharmacol Physiol 1985; 12:249–252.
1329. Kem DC, Weinberger MH, Mayes DM, et al. Saline suppression of plasma aldosterone in hypertension. Arch Intern Med 1971; 128:380–386.
1330. Streeten DHP, Tomycz N, Anderson GH. Reliability of the screening methods for the diagnosis of primary aldosteronism. Am J Med 1979; 67:403–413.
1331. Holland OB, Brown H, Kuhnert LV, et al. Further evaluation of the saline infusion test for primary aldosteronism. Hypertension 1984; 6:717–723.
1332. Arteaga E, Klein R, Biglieri EG. Use of the saline infusion test to diagnose the cause of primary aldosteronism. Am J Med 1985; 79:722–728.
1333. Thibonnier M, Sassano P, Dufloux MA, et al. Teste diagnostique simple de l'hyperaldosteronisme primaire. Presse Med 1983; 12:1461–1466.
1334. Lyons DF, Kem DC, Brown RD, et al. Single dose captopril as a diagnostic test for primary aldosteronism. J Clin Endocrinol Metab 1983; 57:892–896.
1335. Naomi S, Iwaoka T, Umeda T, et al. Clinical evaluation of the captopril screening test for primary aldosteronism. Jpn Heart J 1985; 26:549–556.
1336. Muratani H, Abe I, Tomita Y, et al. Single oral administration of captopril may not bring an improvement in screening of primary aldosteronism. Clin Exp Hypertens [A] 1987; 9:611–614.
1337. Muratani H, Abe I, Tomita Y, et al. Is single oral administration of captopril beneficial in screening for primary hyperaldosteronism? Am Heart J 1986; 112:361–367.
1338. Slaton PE, Schambelan M, Biglieri EG. Stimulation and suppression of aldosterone secretion in patients with an aldosterone-producing adenoma. J Clin Endocrinol Metab 1969; 29:239–250.
1339. Ganguly A, Dowdy AJ, Luetscher JA, et al. Anomalous postural response of plasma aldosterone concentration in patients with aldosterone-producing adrenal adenomas. J Clin Endocrinol Metab 1973; 36:401–404.
1340. Young WF, Klee GG. Primary aldosteronism. Diagnostic evaluation. Endocrinol Metab Clin North Am 1988; 17:367–395.
1341. Bravo EL, Tarazi RC, Dustan HP, et al. The changing clinical spectrum of primary aldosteronism. Am J Med 1983; 74:641–651.
1342. Kem DC, Tang K, Hanson CS, et al. The prediction of anatomical morphology of primary aldosteronism using serum 18-hydroxycorticosterone levels. J Clin Endocrinol Metab 1985; 60:67–73.
1343. Ganguly A, Grim CE, Weinberger MH. Anomalous postural aldosterone response in glucocorticoid-suppressible hyperaldosteronism. N Engl J Med 1981; 305:991–993.
1344. Greathouse DJ, McDermott MT, Kidd GS, et al. Pure primary hyperaldosteronism due to adrenal cortical carcinoma. Am J Med 1984; 76:1132–1136.
1345. Scott HW, Sussman CR, Page DL, et al. Primary hyperaldosteronism caused by adrenocortical carcinoma. World J Surg 1986; 10:646–653.
1346. Farge D, Chatellier G, Pagny JY, et al. Isolated clinical syndrome of primary aldosteronism in four patients with adrenocortical carcinoma. Am J Med 1987; 83:635–640.
1347. White EA, Schambelan M, Rost CR, et al. Use of computed tomography in diagnosing the cause of primary aldosteronism. N Engl J Med 1980; 303:1503–1507.
1348. Melby JC, Spark RF, Dale SL, et al. Diagnosis and localization of

aldosterone-producing adenomas by adrenal-vein catheterization. N Engl J Med 1967; 277:1050–1056.

1349. Gordon RD, Hamlet SM, Tunny TJ, et al. Distinguishing aldosterone-producing adenoma from other forms of hyperaldosteronism and lateralizing the tumor preoperatively. Clin Exp Pharmacol Physiol 1986; 13:325–328.

1350. Copeland PM. The incidentally discovered adrenal mass. Ann Intern Med 1983; 98:940–945.

1351. Johnson CM, Sheedy PF, Welch TJ, et al. CT of the adrenal cortex. Semin Ultrasound CT MR 1985; 6:241–260.

1352. Ma JT, Wang C, Lam KS, et al. Fifty cases of primary hyperaldosteronism in Hong Kong Chinese with a high frequency of periodic paralysis. Evaluation of techniques for tumor localization. Q J Med 1986; 61:1021–1037.

1353. Miyake H, Maeda H, Tashiro M, et al. CT of adrenal tumors: frequency and clinical significance of low-attenuation lesions. AJR 1989; 152:1005–1007.

1354. Ikeda DM, Francis IR, Glazer GM, et al. The detection of adrenal tumors and hyperplasia in patients with primary aldosteronism: comparison of scintigraphy, CT, and MR imaging. AJR 1989; 153:301–306.

1355. Sarkar SD, Cohen EL, Beierwaltes WH, et al. A new and superior adrenal imaging reagent, ^{131}I–6β-iodomethyl-19-nor-cholesterol (NP-59): evaluation in humans. J Clin Endocrinol Metab 1977; 45:353–362.

1356. Miles JM, Wahner HW, Carpenter PC, et al. Adrenal scintiscanning with NP-59, a new radioiodinated cholesterol agent. Mayo Clin Proc 1979; 54:321–327.

1357. Kremer D, Boddy K, Brown JJ, et al. Amiloride in the treatment of primary hyperaldosteronism and essential hypertension. Clin Endocrinol 1977; 7:151–157.

1358. Bravo EL, Fouad FM, Tarazi RC. Calcium channel blockade with nifedipine in primary aldosteronism. Hypertension 1986; 8:191–194.

1359. Nadler JL, Hsueh W, Horton R. Therapeutic effect of calcium channel blockade in primary aldosteronism. J Clin Endocrinol Metab 1986; 60:896–899.

1360. Bursztyn M, Grossman E, Rosenthal T. The absence of long-term therapeutic effect of calcium channel blockade in the primary aldosteronism of adrenal adenomas. Am J Hypertens 1988; 1:88S–90S.

1361. Stimple M, Ivens K, Wambach G, et al. Are calcium antagonists helpful in the management of primary aldosteronism? J Cardiovasc Pharmacol 1988; 12(Suppl 6):S131–S134.

1362. Stewart PM, Corrie JET, Shackelton CHL, et al. Syndrome of apparent mineralocorticoid excess. A defect in the cortisol-cortisone shuttle. J Clin Invest 1988; 82:340–349.

1363. New MI, Levine LS, Biglieri EG, et al. Evidence for an unidentified steroid in a child with apparent mineralocorticoid hypertension. J Clin Endocrinol Metab 1977; 44:924–933.

1364. Ulick S, Levine LS, Gunczler P, et al. A syndrome of apparent mineralocorticoid excess associated with defects in the peripheral metabolism of cortisol. J Clin Endocrinol Metab 1979; 49:757–764.

1365. Ulmann A, Menard J, Corvol P. Binding of glycerrhetinic acid to kidney mineralocorticoid and glucocorticoid receptors. Endocrinology 1975; 97:46–51.

1366. Armanini D, Karbowiak I, Funder JW. Affinity of liquorice derivatives for mineralocorticoid and glucocorticoid receptors. Clin Endocrinol 1983; 19:609–612.

1367. Takeda R, Miyamori I, Soma R, et al. Glycyrrhizic acid and its hydrolysate as mineralocorticoid agonist. J Steroid Biochem 1987; 27:845–849.

1368. Girerd RJ, Rassaert CL, DiPasquale G, et al. Endocrine involvement in liquorice hypertension. Am J Physiol 1960; 198:718–720.

1369. Borst JGG, Ten Holt SP, De Vries LA, et al. Synergistic action of liquorice and cortisone in Addison's disease and Simmonds's disease. Lancet 1953; 1:657–663.

1370. Elmadjian F, Hope JM, Pincus GM. The action of mono-ammonium glycyrrhizinate on adrenalectomized subjects and its synergism with hydrocortisone. J Clin Endocrinol Metab 1956; 16:338–349.

1371. Stewart PM, Wallace AM, Valentino R, et al. Mineralocorticoid activity of liquorice: 11β-hydroxysteroid dehydrogenase deficiency comes of age. Lancet 1987; 2:821–824.

1372. Bartter FC, Pronove J, Gill JR, et al. Hyperplasia of the juxtaglomerular complex with hyperaldosteronism and hypokalemic alkalosis. Am J Med 1962; 33:811–828.

1373. Gill Jr JR, Frolich JC, Bowden RE, et al. Bartter's syndrome: a disorder characterized by high urinary prostaglandins and a dependence of hyperreninemia on prostaglandin synthesis. Am J Med 1976; 61:43–51.

1374. Puschett JB, Greenberg A, Mitro R, et al. Variant of Bartter's syndrome with a distal tubular rather than loop of Henle defect. Nephron 1988; 50:205–211.

1375. Soupart A, Unger J, Debieve MF, et al. Bartter's syndrome with a salt reabsorption defect in the cortical part of Henle's loop. Am J Nephrol 1988; 8:309–315.

1376. Milani L, Pessina AC, Macca F, et al. Does defective chloride reabsorption at the loop of Henle play a major role in the pathogenesis of Bartter's syndrome? Am J Nephrol 1987; 7:65–68.

1377. Trygstad CW, Mangos JA, Bloodworth MD Jr, et al. A sibship with Bartter's syndrome: failure of total adrenalectomy to correct the potassium wastage. Pediatrics 1969; 44:234–242.

1378. De Chrecchio L. Sopra un caso di apparenze virili in una donna. Morgagni 1865; 7:151–183.

1379. Bongiovanni AM, Root AW. The adrenogenital syndrome. N Engl J Med 1963; 268:1283–1289, 1342–1351, 1391–1399.

1380. Lewis RA, Wilkins L. The effect of adrenocorticotropic hormone in congenital adrenal hyperplasia with virilism and in Cushing's syndrome treated with methyltestosterone. J Clin Invest 1949; 28:394–400.

1381. Miller AM, Dorfman RI. Metabolism of steroid hormones: isolation of 13 steroid metabolites from a patient with (probable) adrenal hyperplasia. Endocrinology 1950; 46:514–525.

1382. White PC, New MI, Dupont B. Congenital adrenal hyperplasia. Part 1. N Engl J Med 1987; 316:1519–1524.

1383. White PC, New MI, Dupont B. Congenital adrenal hyperplasia. Part 2. N Engl J Med 1987; 316:1580–1586.

1384. Cacciari E, Balsamo A, Cassio A, et al. Neonatal screening for congenital adrenal hyperplasia. Arch Dis Child 1983; 58:803–806.

1385. Hirschfeld AJ, Fleshman JK. An unusually high incidence of salt-losing congenital adrenal hyperplasia in the Alaskan Eskimo. J Pediatr 1969; 75:492–494.

1386. Pang S, Murphey W, Levine LS, et al. A pilot newborn screening for congenital adrenal hyperplasia in Alaska. J Clin Endocrinol Metab 1982; 55:413–420.

1387. Urban MD, Lee PA, Migeon CJ. Adult height and fertility in men with congenital adrenal hyperplasia. N Engl J Med 1978; 299:1392–1396.

1388. Mulaikal RM, Migeon CJ, Rock JA. Fertility rates in female patients with congenital adrenal hyperplasia due to 21-hydroxylase deficiency. N Engl J Med 1987; 316:178–182.

1389. Klingensmith GJ, Garcia SC, Jones HW, et al. Glucocorticoid treatment of girls with congenital adrenal hyperplasia: effects on height, sexual maturation, and fertility. J Pediatr 1977; 90:996–1004.

1390. Richards GE, Grumbach MM, Kaplan SL, et al. The effect of long acting glucocorticoids on menstrual abnormalities in patients with virilizing congenital adrenal hyperplasia. J Clin Endocrinol Metab 1978; 47:1208–1215.

1391. Wischusen J, Baker HWG, Hudson B. Reversible male infertility due to congenital adrenal hyperplasia. Clin Endocrinol 1981; 14:571–577.

1392. Lipsett MB, Riter BD. Urinary steroids in post-natal adrenal hyperplasia with virilism. Acta Endocrinol 1961; 38:481–489.

1393. Mahesh VB, Greenblatt RB, Coniff RF. Adrenal hyperplasia—a case report of delayed onset of the congenital form or an acquired form. J Clin Endocrinol Metab 1968; 28:619–623.

1394. Santilli J, Martin MM. Virilizing adrenal hyperplasia presenting in a prepubertal female. J Clin Endocrinol Metab 1972; 34:427–429.

1395. Rosenwaks Z, Lee PA, Jones GS, et al. An attenuated form of congenital virilizing adrenal hyperplasia. J Clin Endocrinol Metab 1979; 49:335–339.

1396. Laron Z, Pollack MS, Zamir R, et al. Late onset 21-hydroxylase deficiency and HLA in the Ashkenazi population: a new allele at the 21-hydroxylase locus. Hum Immunol 1980; 1:55–60.

1397. Kohn B, Levine LS, Pollack MS, et al. Late onset steroid 21-hydroxylase deficiency: a variant of classical congenital adrenal hyperplasia. J Clin Endocrinol Metab 1982; 55:817–827.

1398. Speiser PW, Dupont B, Rubinstein P, et al. High frequency of nonclassical steroid 21-hydroxylase deficiency. Am J Hum Genet 1985; 37:650–667.

1399. Birnbaum MD, Rose LI. Late onset adrenocortical hydroxylase deficiencies associated with menstrual dysfunction. Obstet Gynecol 1984; 63:445–451.

1400. Chrousos GP, Loriaux DL, Mann DL, et al. Late onset 21-hydroxylase deficiency mimicking idiopathic hirsutism or polycystic ovarian disease. An allelic variant of congenital virilizing adrenal hyperplasia. Ann Intern Med 1982; 96:143–148.

1401. Levine LS, Dupont B, Lorenzen F, et al. Cryptic 21-hydroxylase deficiency in families of patients with classical congenital adrenal hyperplasia. J Clin Endocrinol Metab 1980; 51:1316–1324.

1402. Levine LS, Dupont B, Lorenzen F, et al. Genetic and hormonal characterization of cryptic 21-hydroxylase deficiency. J Clin Endocrinol Metab 1981; 53:1193–1198.

1403. Chrousos GP, Loriaux DL, Sherins RJ, et al. Unilateral testicular enlargement resulting from inapparent 21-hydroxylase deficiency. J Urol 1981; 126:127–128.

1404. Rutgers JL, Young RH, Scully RE. The testicular "tumor" of the adrenogenital syndrome. A report of six cases and review of the literature on testicular masses in patients with adrenocortical disorders. Am J Surg Pathol 1988; 12:503–513.

1405. New MI, Lorenzen F, Lerner AJ, et al. Genotyping steroid 21-hydroxylase deficiency: hormonal reference data. J Clin Endocrinol Metab 1983; 57:320–326.

1406. Dupont B, Oberfield SE, Smithwick EM, et al. Close genetic linkage between HLA and congenital adrenal hyperplasia (21-hydroxylase deficiency). Lancet 1977; 2:1309–1311.

1407. Levine LS, Zachmann M, New MI, et al. Genetic mapping of the 21-hydroxylase deficiency gene within the HLA linkage group. N Engl J Med 1978; 299:911–915.

1408. Zappacosta S, DeFelice M, Minnozi M, et al. HLA and congenital adrenal hyperplasia. Lancet 1978; 2:524 (letter).

1409. Grosse-Wilde H, Weil J, Albert E, et al. Genetic linkage studies between congenital adrenal hyperplasia and the HLA blood group system. Immunogenetics 1979; 8:41–50.

1410. Klouda PT, Harris R, Price DA. HLA and congenital adrenal hyperplasia. Lancet 1978; 2:1046–1047 (letter).

1411. Pucholt V, Fitzsimmons JS, Gelsthorpe K, et al. HLA and congenital adrenal hyperplasia. Lancet 1978; 2:1047 (letter).

1412. White PC, New MI, Dupont B. Adrenal 21-hydroxylase cytochrome P-450 genes within the MHC class III region. Immunol Rev 1985; 87:123–150.

1413. Holler W, Scholz S, Knorr D, et al. Genetic differences between the salt-wasting, simple virilizing, and nonclassical types of congenital adrenal hyperplasia. J Clin Endocrinol Metab 1985; 60:757–763.

1414. Abral M, Cuccia Belvidere M, Livieri C, et al. Italian extended HLA haplotypes in congenital adrenal hyperplasia. Tissue Antigens 1988; 32:17–23.

1415. Dupont B, Virdis R, Lerner AJ, et al. Distinct HLA-B antigen associations for the salt-wasting and simple virilizing forms of congenital adrenal hyperplasia due to 21-hydroxylase deficiency. In: Albert ED, Baur MP, Mayr WR, eds. Histocompatibility Testing. Berlin: Springer-Verlag, 1984: 660–661.

1416. Scholz S, Holler W, Knorr D. Three different HLA associations in the three types of 21-hydroxylase congenital adrenal hyperplasia. In: Albert ED, Baur MP, Mayr WR, eds. Histocompatibility Testing. Berlin: Springer-Verlag, 1984: 658–659.

1417. Carroll MC, Campbell RD, Porter RR. Mapping of the steroid 21-hydroxylase genes adjacent to complement component C4 genes in HLA, the major histocompatibility locus in man. Proc Natl Acad Sci USA 1985; 82:521–525.

1418. White PC, Grossberger D, Onufer B, et al. Two genes encoding steroid 21-hydroxylase are located near the genes encoding the fourth component of complement in man. Proc Natl Acad Sci USA 1985; 82:1089–1093.

1419. White PC, New MI, Dupont B. Structure of the steroid 21-hydroxylase genes. Proc Natl Acad Sci USA 1986; 83:5111–5115.

1420. Higashi Y, Yoshioka H, Yamane M, et al. Complete nucleotide sequence of two steroid 21-hydroxylase genes tandemly arranged in human chromosome: a pseudogene and a genuine gene. Proc Natl Acad Sci USA 1986; 83:2841–2845.

1421. Schneider PM, Carroll MC, Alper CA, et al. Polymorphism of the human complement C4 and steroid 21-hydroxylase genes. Restriction fragment length polymorphisms revealing structural deletions, homo-duplications, and size variants. J Clin Invest 1986; 78:650–657.

1422. Werkmeister JW, New MI, Dupont B, et al. Frequent deletion and duplication of the steroid 21-hydroxylase genes. Am J Hum Genet 1986; 39:461–469.

1423. Rumsby G, Carroll MC, Porter RR, et al. Deletion of the steroid 21-hydroxylase and complement C4 genes in congenital adrenal hyperplasia. J Med Genet 1986; 23:204–209.

1424. Matteson KJ, Phillips JA, Miller WL, et al. P450XXI (steroid 21-hydroxylase) gene deletions are not found in family studies of congenital adrenal hyperplasia. Proc Natl Acad Sci USA 1987; 84:5858–5862.

1425. Miller WL. Gene conversions, deletions, and polymorphisms in congenital adrenal hyperplasia. Am J Hum Genet 1988; 42:4–7.

1426. Harada F, Kimura A, Iwanaga T, et al. Gene conversion–like events cause steroid 21-hydroxylase deficiency in congenital adrenal hyperplasia. Proc Natl Acad Sci USA 1987; 84:8091–8094.

1427. Amor M, Parker KL, Globerman H, et al. Mutation in the CYP21B gene (Ile-172—Asn) causes steroid 21-hydroxylase deficiency. Proc Natl Acad Sci USA 1988; 85:1600–1604.

1428. Higashi Y, Tanae A, Inoue H, et al. Aberrant splicing and missense mutations cause steroid 21-hydroxylase [P-450(C21)] deficiency in humans: possible gene conversion products. Proc Natl Acad Sci USA 1988; 85:7486–7490.

1429. Morel Y, Andre J, Uring-Lambert B, et al. Rearrangements and point mutations of P450c21 genes are distinguished by five restriction endonuclease haplotypes identified by a new probing strategy in 57 families with congenital adrenal hyperplasia. J Clin Invest 1989; 83:527–536.

1430. White PC, Vitek A, Dupont B, et al. Characterization of frequent deletions causing steroid 21-hydroxylase deficiency. Proc Natl Acad Sci USA 1988; 85:4436–4440.

1431. Rumsby G, Fielder AHL, Hague WM, et al. Heterogeneity in the gene locus for steroid 21-hydroxylase deficiency. J Med Genet 1988; 25:596–599.

1432. Rodrigues NR, Dunham I, Yu CY, et al. Molecular characterization of the HLA-linked steroid 21-hydroxylase B gene from an individual with congenital adrenal hyperplasia. EMBO J 1987; 6:1653–1661.

1433. Globerman H, Amor M, Parker KL. Nonsense mutation causing steroid 21-hydroxylase deficiency. J Clin Invest 1988; 82:139–144.

1434. Speiser PW, New MI, White PC. Molecular genetic analysis of nonclassic steroid 21-hydroxylase deficiency associated with HLA-B14, DR1. N Engl J Med 1988; 319:19–23.

1435. Gueux B, Fiet J, Couillin P, et al. Prenatal diagnosis of 21-hydroxylase deficiency congenital adrenal hyperplasia by simultaneous radioimmunoassay of 21-deoxycortisol and 17-hydroxyprogesterone in amniotic fluid. J Clin Endocrinol Metab 1988; 66:534–553.

1436. Reindollar RH, Lewis JB, White PC, et al. Prenatal diagnosis of 21-hydroxylase deficiency by the complementary deoxyribonucleic acid probe for cytochrome P-450C-21OH. Am J Obstet Gynecol 1988; 158:545–547.

1437. Couillin P, Nicolas H, Boue J, et al. HLA typing of amniotic fluid cells applied to the prenatal diagnosis of congenital adrenal hyperplasia. Lancet 1979; 1:1976–1977.

1438. Mornet E, Boue J, Raux-Demay M, et al. First trimester prenatal diagnosis of 21-hydroxylase deficiency by linkage analysis to HLA-DNA probes and by 17-hydroxyprogesterone determination. Hum Genet 1986; 73:358–364.

1439. Miller WL, Levine LS. Molecular and clinical advances in congenital adrenal hyperplasia. J Pediatr 1987; 111:1–17.

1440. Brook CGD, Zachmann M, Prader A, et al. Experience with long-term therapy in congenital adrenal hyperplasia. J Pediatr 1974; 85:12–19.

1441. Dimartino-Nardi J, Stoner E, O'Connell A, et al. The effect of treatment on final height in classical congenital adrenal hyperplasia. Acta Endocrinol 1986; 279:305–313.

1442. Young MC, Ribeiro J, Hughes IA. Growth and body proportions in congenital adrenal hyperplasia. Arch Dis Child 1989; 64:1554–1558.

1443. Horrocks PM, London DR. Effects of long term dexamethasone treatment in adult patients with congenital adrenal hyperplasia. Clin Endocrinol 1987; 27:635–642.

1444. Young MC, Hughes IA. Dexamethasone treatment for congenital adrenal hyperplasia. Arch Dis Child 1990; 65:312–314.

1445. Winterer J, Chrousos GP, Loriaux DL, et al. Effect of hydrocortisone dose schedule on adrenal steroid secretion in congenital adrenal hyperplasia. J Pediatr 1985; 106:137–142.

1446. Linder B, Feuillan P, Chrousos GP. Alternate day prednisone therapy in congenital adrenal hyperplasia: adrenal steroid suppression and normal growth. J Clin Endocrinol Metab 1989; 69:191–195.

1447. Appan S, Hindmarsh PC, Brook CGD. Monitoring treatment in congenital adrenal hyperplasia. Arch Dis Child 1989; 64:1235–1239.

1448. Hughes IA. Management of congenital adrenal hyperplasia. Arch Dis Child 1988; 63:1399–1404.

1449. Hughes IA. Monitoring treatment in congenital adrenal hyperplasia. Arch Dis Child 1990; 65:333 (editorial).

1450. Simopoulous AP, Marshall JR, Delea CS, et al. Studies on the deficiency of 21-hydroxylation in patients with congenital adrenal hyperplasia. J Clin Endocrinol Metab 1971; 32:438–443.

1451. Rösler A, Levine LS, Schneider B, et al. The interrelationship of sodium balance, plasma renin activity, and ACTH in congenital adrenal hyperplasia. J Clin Endocrinol Metab 1977; 45:500–512.

1452. Jansen M, Wit JM, van den Brande JL. Reinstitution of mineralocorticoid therapy in congenital adrenal hyperplasia. Effects on control and growth. Acta Paediatr Scand 1981; 70:229–233.

1453. Hendren WH, Donohoe PK. Correction of congenital abnormalities of the vagina and perineum. J Pediatr Surg 1980; 15:751–763.

1454. Evans MI, Chrousos GP, Mann DW, et al. Pharmacologic suppression of the fetal adrenal gland in utero. Attempted prevention of abnormal external genital masculinization in suspected congenital adrenal hyperplasia. JAMA 1985; 253:1015–1020.

1455. David M, Forest MG. Prenatal treatment of congenital adrenal hyperplasia resulting from 21-hydroxylase deficiency. J Pediatr 1984; 105:799–803.

1456. Migeon CJ. Comments about the need for prenatal treatment of congenital adrenal hyperplasia due to 21-hydroxylase deficiency. J Clin Endocrinol Metab 1990; 70:836–837 (editorial).

1457. Forest MG, Betuel H, David M. Prenatal treatment in congenital adrenal hyperplasia due to 21-hydroxylase deficiency: update 88 of the French multicentric study. Endocr Res 1989; 15:277–301.

1458. Pang S, Pollack MS, Marshall RN, et al. Prenatal treatment of congenital adrenal hyperplasia due to 21-hydroxylase deficiency. N Engl J Med 1919; 322:111–115.

1459. Speiser PW, Laforgia N, Kato K, et al. First trimester prenatal treatment and molecular genetic diagnosis of congenital adrenal hyperplasia (21-hydroxylase deficiency). J Clin Endocrinol Metab 1990; 70:838–848.

1460. Rösler A, Leiberman E. Enzymatic defects of steroidogenesis: 11β-hydroxylase deficiency congenital adrenal hyperplasia. In: New MI, Levine LS, eds. Pediatric and Adolescent Endocrinology. Vol 13. Adrenal Diseases in Childhood. Basel: S. Karger, 1983: 47–71.

1461. Zachmann M, Tassinari D, Prader A. Clinical and biochemical variability of congenital adrenal hyperplasia due to 11β-hydroxylase deficiency. A study of 25 patients. J Clin Endocrinol Metab 1983; 56:222–229.

1462. Holcombe JH, Keenan BS, Nichols BL, et al. Neonatal salt loss in the hypertensive form of congenital adrenal hyperplasia. Pediatrics 1980; 65:777–781.

1463. Green OC, Migeon CJ, Wilkins L. Urinary steroids in the hypertensive form of congenital adrenal hyperplasia. J Clin Endocrinol Metab 1960; 20:929–946.

1464. Sizonenko PC, Riondel AM, Kohlberg IJ, et al. 11β-Hydroxylase deficiency: steroid response to sodium restriction and ACTH stimulation. J Clin Endocrinol Metab 1972; 35:281–287.

1465. Kirita S, Morohashi K, Hashimoto T, et al. Expression of two kinds of cytochrome P-450 (11β) mRNA in bovine adrenal cortex. J Biochem (Tokyo) 1988; 104:683–686.

1466. Brautbar C, Rösler A, Landau H, et al. No linkage between HLA and congenital adrenal hyperplasia due to 11β-hydroxylase deficiency. N Engl J Med 1979; 300:205–206.

1467. Dryenfurth I, Sybulski S, Notchev V, et al. Urinary corticosteroid excretion patterns in patients with adrenocortical dysfunction. J Clin Endocrinol Metab 1958; 18:391–408.

1468. Gabrilove JL, Sharma DC, Dorfman RI. Adrenocortical 11β-hydroxylase deficiency and virilism first manifest in an adult woman. N Engl J Med 1965; 272:1189–1194.

1469. Pang S, Levine LS, Lorenzen F, et al. Hormonal studies in obligate heterozygotes and siblings of patients with 11β-hydroxylase deficiency congenital adrenal hyperplasia. J Clin Endocrinol Metab 1980; 50:586–589.

1470. Rösler A, Leiberman E, Rosenmann A, et al. Prenatal diagnosis of 11β-hydroxylase deficiency congenital adrenal hyperplasia. J Clin Endocrinol Metab 1979; 49:546–551.

1471. Biglieri EG, Herron MA, Brust N. 17-Hydroxylation deficiency in man. J Clin Invest 1966; 45:1946–1954.

1472. New MI. Male pseudohermaphroditism due to 17α-hydroxylase deficiency. J Clin Invest 1970; 49:1930–1941.

1473. Goldsmith O, Solomon DH, Horton R. Hypogonadism and mineralocorticoid excess: the 17-hydroxylase deficiency syndrome. N Engl J Med 1967; 277:673–677.

1474. Malin SR. Congenital adrenal hyperplasia secondary to 17-hydroxylase deficiency: two sisters with amenorrhea, hypokalemia, hypertension, and cystic ovaries. Ann Intern Med 1969; 70:69–75.

1475. Zachmann M, Werder EA, Prader A. Two types of male pseudohermaphroditism due to 17,20-desmolase deficiency. J Clin Endocrinol Metab 1982; 55:487–490.

1476. Zachmann M, Voellmin JA, Hamilton W, et al. Steroid 17,20-desmolase deficiency, a new cause of male pseudohermaphroditism. Clin Endocrinol 1972; 1:369–385.

1477. Winter JSD, Couch RM, Muller J, et al. Combined 17-hydroxylase and 17,20-desmolase deficiencies: evidence for synthesis of a defective cytochrome P450c17. J Clin Endocrinol Metab 1989; 68:309–316.

1478. D'Armiento M, Reda G, Kater C, et al. 17α-Hydroxylase deficiency: mineralocorticoid hormone profiles in an affected family. J Clin Endocrinol Metab 1983; 56:697–701.

1479. Kater CE, Biglieri EG, Brust N, et al. The unique patterns of plasma aldosterone and 18-hydroxycorticosterone concentrations in the 17α-hydroxylase deficiency syndrome. J Clin Endocrinol Metab 1982; 55:295–302.

1480. Griffing GT, Wilson TE, Holbrook MM, et al. Plasma and urinary 19-nor-deoxycorticosterone in 17α-hydroxylase deficiency syndrome. J Clin Endocrinol Metab 1984; 59:1011–1015.

1481. Rovner DR, Conn JW, Cohen EL, et al. 17Alpha-hydroxylase deficiency. A combination of hydroxylation defect and reversible blockade in aldosterone biosynthesis. Acta Endocrinol 1979; 90:490–504.

1482. Peterson RE, Imperato-McGinley J, Gautier T, et al. Male pseudohermaphroditism due to multiple defects in steroid-biosynthetic microsomal mixed-function oxidases. A new variant of congenital adrenal hyperplasia. N Engl J Med 1985; 313:1182–1191.

1483. Wit JM, Van Roermund HPC, Oostdijk W, et al. Heterozygotes for 17α-hydroxylase deficiency can be detected with a short ACTH test. Clin Endocrinol 1988; 28:657–664.

1484. Kagimoto M, Winter JSD, Kagimoto K, et al. Structural characterization of normal and mutant human steroid 17α-hydroxylase genes: molecular basis of one example of combined 17α-hydroxylase/17,20-lyase deficiency. Mol Endocrinol 1988; 2:564–570.

1485. Yanase T, Kagimoto M, Matsui N, et al. Combined 17α-hydroxylase/17,20-lyase deficiency due to a stop codon in the N-terminal region of the 17α-hydroxylase cytochrome P-450. Mol Cell Endocrinol 1988; 59:249–253.

1486. Pang S, Levine LS, Stoner E, et al. Nonsalt-losing congenital adrenal hyperplasia due to 3β-hydroxysteroid dehydrogenase deficiency with normal glomerulosa function. J Clin Endocrinol Metab 1983; 56:808–818.

1487. Lobo RA, Goebelsmann U. Evidence for reduced 3β-ol-hydroxysteroid dehydrogenase activity in some hirsute women thought to have polycystic ovary syndrome. J Clin Endocrinol Metab 1981; 53:394–400.

1488. Pang S, Lerner AJ, Stoner E. Late-onset adrenal steroid 3β-hydroxysteroid dehydrogenase deficiency. I. A cause of hirsutism in pubertal and postpubertal women. J Clin Endocrinol Metab 1985; 60:428–439.

1489. Cara JF, Moshang T, Bongiovanni AM, et al. Elevated 17-hydroxyprogesterone and testosterone in a newborn with 3β-hydroxysteroid dehydrogenase deficiency. N Engl J Med 1985; 313:618–621.

1490. Haufa BP, Miller WL, Grumbach MM, et al. Congenital adrenal hyperplasia due to deficient cholesterol side-chain cleavage activity

1491. Matteson KJ, Chung B-C, Urdea MS, et al. Study of cholesterol side-chain cleavage (20,22-desmolase) deficiency causing congenital lipoid adrenal hyperplasia using bovine-sequence P450scc oligodeoxyribonucleotide probes. Endocrinology 1986; 118:1296–1305.

1492. Dluhy RG, Newmark SR, Lauler DP, et al. Pharmacology and chemistry of adrenal glucocorticoids. In: Azarnoff DL, ed. Steroid Therapy. Philadelphia: W. B. Saunders, 1975: 1–14.

1493. Christy NP. Principles of systemic corticosteroid therapy in nonendocrine disease. In: Bardin CW, ed. Current Therapy in Endocrinology and Metabolism. 3rd ed. Philadelphia: B. C. Decker, 1988: 104–111.

1494. Herzog HL, Nobile A, Tolksdorf S, et al. New anti-arthritic steroids. Science 1955; 121:176.

1495. Stafford RO, Barnes LE, Bowman BJ, et al. Glucocorticoid and mineralocorticoid activities of delta-1 fluorohydrocortisone. Proc Soc Exp Biol Med 1955; 89:371–374.

1496. Meikle AW, Weed JA, Tyler FH. Kinetics and interconversion of prednisolone and prednisone studied with new radioimmunoassays. J Clin Endocrinol Metab 1975; 41:717–721.

1497. Spero GB, Thompson JL, Magerlein BJ, et al. Adrenal hormones and related compounds. IV. 6-Methyl steroids. J Am Chem Soc 1956; 78:6213–6214.

1498. Fried J, Sabo EF. Synthesis of 17α-hydroxycortisone and its 9α-halo derivatives from 11-epi-17α-hydroxycorticosterone. J Am Chem Soc 1953; 75:2273–2274.

1499. Migeon CJ, Lawrence B, Bertrand J, et al. In vivo distribution of some 17-hydroxycorticoids between the plasma and red blood cells of man. J Clin Endocrinol Metab 1959; 19:1411–1419.

1500. Ballard PL, Carter JP, Graham BS, et al. A radioreceptor assay for evaluation of the plasma glucocorticoid activity of natural and synthetic steroids in man. J Clin Endocrinol Metab 1975; 41:290–304.

1501. Ballard PL. Delivery and transport of glucocorticoids to target cells. In: Baxter JD, Rousseau GG, eds. Glucocorticoid Hormone Action. Berlin: Springer-Verlag, 1979: 25–48.

1502. Nugent CA, Eik-Nes K, Samuels LT, et al. Changes in plasma levels of 17-hydroxycorticosteroids during the intravenous administration of adrenocorticotropin (ACTH). IV. Response to prolonged infusion of small amounts of ACTH. J Clin Endocrinol Metab 1959; 19:334–343.

1503. Peterson RE. Metabolism of adrenocortical hormones. Ann NY Acad Sci 1959; 82:846–853.

1504. Axelrod L. Glucocorticoid therapy. Medicine 1976; 55:39–65.

1505. Kozower M, Veatch L, Kaplan MM. Decreased clearance of prednisolone, a factor in the development of corticosteroid side effects. J Clin Endocrinol Metab 1974; 38:407–412.

1506. Kehlet H, Binder C, Blicher-Toft M. Glucocorticoid maintenance therapy following adrenalectomy: assessment of dosage and preparation. Clin Endocrinol 1976; 5:37–41.

1507. McKensie AW, Stoughton RB. Method for comparing cutaneous absorption of steroids. Arch Dermatol 1962; 86:608–610.

1508. Feldman RJ, Maibach HI. Penetration of 14C-hydrocortisone through normal skin: the effect of stripping and occlusion. Arch Dermatol 1965; 91:661–666.

1509. Feiwel M, James V, Barnett ES. Effect of potent topical steroids on plasma cortisol levels of infants and children with eczema. Lancet 1969; 1:485–487.

1510. Meikle AW, Tyler FH. Potency and duration of action of glucocorticoids. Effects of hydrocortisone, prednisone, and dexamethasone on human pituitary-adrenal function. Am J Med 1977; 63:200–207.

1511. Williams DE, Chopra IJ, Orgiazzi J, et al. Acute effects of corticosteroids on thyroid activity in Graves' disease. J Clin Endocrinol Metab 1975; 41:354–361.

1512. Croxson MS, Hall TD, Nicoloff JT. Combination drug therapy for treatment of hyperthyroid Graves' disease. J Clin Endocrinol Metab 1977; 45:623–660.

1513. Zerwekh JE, Pak CYC, Kaplan RA, et al. Pathogenetic role of 1α,25-dihydroxyvitamin D in sarcoidosis and absorptive hypercalciuria: different response to prednisolone therapy. J Clin Endocrinol Metab 1980; 51:381–386.

1514. Woods JE, Anderson CF, DeWeerd JH, et al. High-dosage intravenously administered methylprednisolone in renal transplantation: a preliminary report. JAMA 1973; 223:896–899.

1515. Cathcart ES, Scheinberg MA, Idelson BA, et al. Beneficial effects of methylprednisolone "pulse" therapy in diffuse proliferative lupus nephritis. Lancet 1976; 1:163–166.

1516. Liebling MR, Lieb E, McLaughlin K, et al. Pulse methylprednisolone in rheumatoid arthritis: a double-blind cross-over trial. Ann Intern Med 1981; 94:21–26.

1517. Gifford RH. Corticosteroid therapy for rheumatoid arthritis. In: Azarnoff DL, ed. Steroid Therapy. Philadelphia: W. B. Saunders, 1974: 78–95.

1518. Garber EK, Fan PT, Bluestone R. Realistic guidelines in corticosteroid therapy of rheumatic disease. Semin Arthritis Rheum 1981; 11:231–256.

1519. Harter JG, Reddy WJ, Thorn GW. Studies on an intermittent corticosteroid dosage regimen. N Engl J Med 1963; 269:591–596.

1520. Fauci AS. Alternate-day corticosteroid therapy. Am J Med 1978; 64:729–731.

1521. Sampson PA, Brooke BN, Winstone NE. Biochemical confirmation of collapse due to adrenal failure. Lancet 1961; 1:1377.

1522. Nichols T, Nugent CA, Tyler FH. Diurnal variation in suppression of adrenal function by glucocorticoids. J Clin Endocrinol Metab 1965; 25:343–349.

1523. Danowski TS, Bonessi JV, Sabeh G, et al. Probabilities of pituitary-adrenal responsiveness after steroid therapy. Ann Intern Med 1964; 61:11–26.

1524. Myles AB, Bacon PA, Daly JR. Single daily dose corticosteroid treatment: effect on adrenal function and therapeutic efficacy in various diseases. Ann Rheum Dis 1971; 30:149–153.

1525. Streck WP, Lockwood DH. Pituitary adrenal recovery following short-term suppression with corticosteroids. Am J Med 1979; 66:910–914.

1526. Spiegel RJ, Vigersky RA, Oliff AI, et al. Adrenal suppression after short-term corticosteroid therapy. Lancet 1979; 1:630–633.

1527. Livanou T, Ferriman D, James VHT. Recovery of hypothalamopituitary function after corticosteroid therapy. Lancet 1967; 2:856–859.

1528. Ackerman GL, Nolan CM. Adrenocortical responsiveness after alternate-day corticosteroid therapy. N Engl J Med 1968; 278:405–409.

1529. Christy NP. Corticosteroid withdrawal. In: Bardin CW, ed. Current Therapy in Endocrinology and Metabolism. 4th ed. Philadelphia: B. C. Decker, 1988: 116–124.

1530. Lukert BP, Raisz LG. Glucocorticoid-induced osteoporosis: pathogenesis and management. Ann Intern Med 1990; 112:352–364.

1531. Graber AL, Ney RL, Nicholson WE, et al. Natural history of pituitary-adrenal recovery following long-term suppression with corticosteroids. J Clin Endocrinol Metab 1965; 25:11–16.

1532. Donald RA, Espiner EA. The plasma cortisol and corticotropin response to hypoglycemia following adrenal steroid and ACTH administration. J Clin Endocrinol Metab 1975; 41:1–6.

1532a. Byyny RL. Withdrawal from glucocorticoid therapy. N Engl J Med 1976; 295:30–32.

1533. Amatruda TT, Hurst MM, D'Esopo ND. Certain endocrine and metabolic facets of the steroid withdrawal syndrome. J Clin Endocrinol Metab 1965; 25:1207–1217.

1534. Dixon RB, Christy NP. On the various forms of the corticosteroid withdrawal syndrome. Am J Med 1980; 68:224–230.

1535. Behan DP, Linton EA, Lowry PJ. Isolation of the human corticotrophin-releasing factor–binding protein. J Endocrinol 1989; 122:23–31.

1536. Wilson RE, Orth DN, Nicholson WE, et al. Human γ-lipotropin radioimmunoassay: identification of immunoreactive γ-lipotropin in human plasma and tissue. J Clin Endocrinol Metab 1981; 53:1–9.

1537. Liotta AS, Suda T, Krieger DT. β-Lipotropin is the major opioid-like peptide of the human pituitary and rat pars distalis: lack of significant β-endorphin. Proc Natl Acad Sci USA 1978; 75:2950–2954.

1538. Nicholson WE, Davis DR, Sherrell BS, et al. Rapid radioimmunoassay for corticotropin in unextracted human plasma. Clin Chem 1984; 30:259–265.

1539. Raff H, Findling JW. New immunoradiometric assay of corticotropin evaluated in normal subjects and patients with Cushing's syndrome. Clin Chem 1989; 35:596–600.

1540. Hodgkinson SC, Allolio B, Landon J, et al. Development of a non-extracted "two-site" immunoradiometric assay for corticotropin utilizing extreme amino- and carboxy-terminally directed antibodies. Biochem J 1984; 218:703–711.

1541. Fukata J, Naitoh Y, Usui T, et al. Two-site immunoradiometric assay for adrenocorticotropin: a cautionary study about the reactivity to its precursor molecules. Endocrinol Jpn 1989; 36:155–161.

1542. Raff H, Findling JW, Wong J. Short loop adrenocorticotropin (ACTH) feedback after ACTH-(1–24) injection in man is an artifact of the immunoradiometric assay. J Clin Endocrinol Metab 1989; 69:678–680.

1543. Usategui R, Oliver C, Vaudry H, et al. Immunoreactive α-MSH and ACTH levels in rat plasma and pituitary. Endocrinology 1976; 98:189–202.

1544. Hale AC, Ratter SJ, Tomlin SJ, et al. Measurement of immunoreactive γ-MSH in human plasma. Clin Endocrinol 1984; 21:139–148.

1545. Pettibone DJ, Mueller GP. Clonidine releases immunoreactive β-endorphin from rat pars distalis. Brain Res 1981; 221:409–414.

1546. Chan JSD, Seidah NG, Chrétien M. Measurement of N-terminal (1–76) of human proopiomelanocortin in human plasma: correlation with adrenocorticotropin. J Clin Endocrinol Metab 1983; 56:791–796.

1547. Kuhn JM, Proeschel MF, Seurin DJ, et al. Comparative assessment of ACTH and lipotropin plasma levels in the diagnosis and follow-up of patients with Cushing's syndrome: a study of 210 cases. Am J Med 1989; 86:678–684.

1548. Haber E, Koerner T, Page LB, et al. Application of a radioimmunoassay for angiotensin I to the physiologic measurements of plasma renin activity in normal human subjects. J Clin Endocrinol Metab 1969; 29:1349–1355.

1549. Workman RJ, Sussman CR, Burkitt DW, et al. Circulating levels of angiotensin I measured by radioimmunoassay in hypertensive subjects. J Lab Clin Med 1979; 93:847–856.

1550. Laragh JH, Sealey J, Brunner HR. The control of aldosterone secretion in normal and hypertensive man: abnormal renin-aldosterone patterns in low renin hypertension. Am J Med 1972; 53:649–663.

1551. Michelakis AM, Yoshida H, Dormois JC. Plasma renin activity and plasma aldosterone during the normal menstrual cycle. Am J Obstet Gynecol 1975; 123:724–726.

1552. Weinberger MH, Kramer NJ, Grim CE, et al. The effect of posture and saline loading on plasma renin activity and aldosterone concentration in pregnant, non-pregnant and estrogen-treated women. J Clin Endocrinol Metab 1977; 44:69–77.

1553. Sebastian A, Hernandez RE, Schambelan M. Disorders of renal handling of potassium. In: Brenner BM, Rector FC Jr (eds). The Kidney. 3rd ed. Philadelphia: WB Saunders, 1986: 519–549.

1554. Porter CC, Silber RH. A quantitative color reaction for cortisone and related 17,21-dihydroxy-20-ketosteroids. J Biol Chem 1958; 185:201–207.

1555. Nelson DH, Samuels LT. A method for the determination of 17-hydroxycorticosteroids in blood: 17-hydroxycorticosterone in the peripheral circulation. J Clin Endocrinol Metab 1952; 12:519–526.

1556. Murphy BEP. Some studies of the protein-binding of steroids and their application to the routine micro and ultramicro measurement of various steroids in body fluids by competitive protein-binding radioassay. J Clin Endocrinol Metab 1967; 27:973–990.

1557. Murphy BEP. Non-chromatographic radiotransinassay for cortisol: application to human adult serum, umbilical cord serum, and amniotic fluid. J Clin Endocrinol Metab 1971; 41:1050–1057.

1558. Mattingly D. A simple fluorimetric method for the estimation of free 11-hydroxycorticoids in human plasma. J Clin Pathol 1962; 15:374–379.

1559. Gotelli GR, Wall JH, Kabra PM, et al. Fluorometric liquid-chromatographic determination of serum cortisol. Clin Chem 1981; 27:441–443.

1560. Ballard PL, Carter JP, Graham BS, et al. A radioreceptor assay for evaluation of the plasma glucocorticoid activity of natural and synthetic steroids in man. J Clin Endocrinol Metab 1975; 41:290–304.

1561. Gore M, Lester E. Comparison of a fluorometric method and a competitive protein binding assay kit for the determination of plasma hydroxycorticosteroids. Ann Clin Biochem 1975; 12:160–162.

1562. Peterson RE, Nokes G, Chen PS Jr, et al. Estrogens and adrenocortical function in man. J Clin Endocrinol Metab 1960; 20:495–514.

1563. Aron DC, Tyrrell JB, Fitzgerald PA, et al. Cushing's syndrome: problems in diagnosis. Medicine 1981; 60:25–35.

1564. McCann VJ, Fulton TT. Cortisol metabolism in chronic liver disease. J Clin Endocrinol Metab 1975; 40:1038–1044.

1565. Ramirez G, Gomez-Sanchez C, Meikle AW, et al. Evaluation of the hypothalamic hypophyseal adrenal axis in patients receiving long-term hemodialysis. Arch Intern Med 1982; 142:1448–1452.

1566. Smith SR, Bledsoe T, Chhetri MK. Cortisol metabolism and the pituitary-adrenal axis in adults with protein-calorie malnutrition. J Clin Endocrinol Metab 1975; 40:43–52.

1567. Hillman DA, Giroud CJP. Plasma cortisone and cortisol levels at birth and during the neonatal period. J Clin Endocrinol Metab 1965; 25:243–248.

1568. Schlechte JA, Coffman T. Plasma free cortisol in depressive illness—a review of findings and clinical implications. Psychiatr Med 1985; 3:23–31.

1569. Fink RS, Short F, Marjot DH, et al. Abnormal suppression of plasma cortisol during the intravenous infusion of dexamethasone to alcoholic patients. Clin Endocrinol 1981; 15:97–102.

1570. Newsome HH Jr, Clements AS, Borum EA. The simultaneous assay of cortisol, corticosterone, 11-deoxycortisol, and cortisone in human plasma. J Clin Endocrinol Metab 1972; 34:473–483.

1571. Robin P, Predine J, Milgrom E. Assay of unbound cortisol in plasma. J Clin Endocrinol Metab 1977; 46:277–283.

1572. Anderson DC, Hopper BR, Lasley BL, et al. A simple method for the assay of eight steroids in small volumes of plasma. Steroids 1976; 28:179–196.

1573. McKenna TJ, Moore G, Orth DN, et al. The biosynthesis of androgens in 21-hydroxylase deficiency. In: Genazzani AR, et al., eds. Adrenal Androgens. New York: Raven, 1980: 135–139.

1574. Meikle AW, West SC, Weed JA, et al. Single dose metyrapone test: 11β-hydroxylase inhibition by metyrapone and reduced metyrapone assayed by radioimmunoassay. J Clin Endocrinol Metab 1975; 40:290–295.

1575. Al-Dujaili EAS, Edwards CRW. The development and application of a direct radioimmunoassay for plasma aldosterone using ^{125}I-labeled ligand—comparison of three methods. J Clin Endocrinol Metab 1978; 46:105–113.

1576. Kowarski A, de Lacerda L, Migeon CJ. Integrated concentration of plasma aldosterone in normal subjects: correlation with cortisol. J Clin Endocrinol Metab 1975; 40:205–210.

1577. Katz FH, Romfh P, Smith JA. Diurnal variation of plasma aldosterone, cortisol and renin activity in supine man. J Clin Endocrinol Metab 1975; 40:125–134.

1578. Yamaji T, Ishibashi M, Takaku F, et al. Serum dehydroepiandrosterone sulfate concentrations in secondary adrenal insufficiency. J Clin Endocrinol Metab 1987; 65:448–451.

1579. Tulchinsky D, Simmer HH. Sources of plasma 17α-hydroxyprogesterone in human pregnancy. J Clin Endocrinol Metab 1972; 35:799–808.

1580. Burr IM, Sullivan J, Graham T, et al. A testosterone-secreting tumour of the adrenal producing virilisation in a female infant. Lancet 1973; 2:643–644.

1581. Laudat MH, Cerdas S, Fournier C, et al. Salivary cortisol measurement: a practical approach to assess pituitary-adrenal function. J Clin Endocrinol Metab 1988; 66:343–348.

1582. Allolio B, Hoffmann J, Linton EA, et al. Diurnal salivary cortisol patterns during pregnancy and after delivery: relationship to plasma corticotrophin-releasing-hormone. Clin Endocrinol 1990; 33:279–289.

1583. Zimmerman W. Eine Farbreaktion der Sexualhormone und ihre Anwendung zur quantitativen colorimetrischen Bestimmung. Hoppe-Seyler's Z Physiol Chem 1935; 233:257–264.

1584. Murphy BEP. Clinical evaluation of urinary cortisol determinations by competitive protein-binding radioassay. J Clin Endocrinol Metab 1968; 28:343–348.

1585. Bongiovanni A, Eberlein WR. Critical analysis of methods for measurement of 5β-pregnane-3α,17α,20α-triol in human urine. Anal Chem 1958; 30:388–393.

1586. Maroulis GB, Manlimos FS, Abraham GE. Comparison between urinary 17-ketosteroids and serum androgens in hirsute patients. Obstet Gynecol 1977; 49:454–458.

1587. Yamaji T, Ishibashi M, Sekihara H, et al. Serum dehydroepiandrosterone sulfate in Cushing's syndrome. J Clin Endocrinol Metab 1984; 59:1164–1168.

1588. Birkhäuser M, Riondel AM, Gaillard R, et al. Plasma aldosterone response to acute stimulation in panhypopituitarism. Acta Endocrinol 1981; 97:514–521.

1589. Tait JF. Review: the use of isotopic steroids for the measurement of production rates. J Clin Endocrinol Metab 1963; 23:1285–1297.

1590. Esteban NV, Yergey AL, Liberato DJ, et al. Stable isotope dilution method using thermospray liquid chromatography/mass spectrometry for quantification of daily cortisol production in humans. Biomed Environ Mass Spectrom 1988; 15:603–608.

1591. Garces LY, Kenny FM, Drash A, et al. Cortisol secretion rate during fasting of obese adolescent subjects. J Clin Endocrinol Metab 1968; 23:1843–1847.

1592. Hellman L, Bradlow HL, Zumoff B, et al. The influence of thyroid hormone on hydrocortisone production and metabolism. J Clin Endocrinol Metab 1961; 21:1231–1247.

1593. Christy NP, Shaver JC. Estrogens and the kidney. Kidney Int 1974; 6:366–376.

1594. Gallagher TF, Fukushima DK, Hellman L. Clarification of discrepancies in cortisol secretion rate. J Clin Endocrinol Metab 1970; 31:625–631.

1595. de Lacerda L, Kowarski A, Migeon CJ. Diurnal variation of the metabolic clearance rate of cortisol. Effect on measurement of cortisol production rate. J Clin Endocrinol Metab 1973; 36:1043–1049.

1596. Jenkins D, Forsham PH, Laidlaw JC, et al. Use of ACTH in the diagnosis of adrenal cortical insufficiency. Am J Med 1955; 18:3–14.

1597. Kehlet H, Binder C. Value of an ACTH test in assessing hypothalamic-pituitary-adrenocortical function in glucocorticoid-treated patients. Br Med J 1973; 2:147–149.

1598. Speckart PF, Nicoloff JT, Bethune JE. Screening for adrenocortical insufficiency with cosyntropin (synthetic ACTH). Arch Intern Med 1971; 128:761–763.

1599. Cope CC. Adrenal Steroid and Disease. London: Pitman Medical, 1972: 275.

1600. Thorn GW. Adrenal cortical insufficiency. In: Conn HF, Clohecy R, Conn RB, eds. Current Diagnosis. Philadelphia: W. B. Saunders, 1966: 445.

1601. Borst GC, Michenfelder HJ, O'Brian JT. Discordant cortisol response to exogenous ACTH and insulin-induced hypoglycemia in patients with pituitary disease. N Engl J Med 1982; 306:1462–1464.

1601a. Jasani MK, Freeman PA, Boyle JA, et al. Studies of the rise in plasma 11-hydroxycorticosteroids (11-OHCS) in corticosteroid-treated patients with rheumatoid arthritis during surgery: correlations with the functional integrity of the hypothalamo-pituitary-adrenal axis. Q J Med 1968; 37:407–421.

1602. Landon J, Greenwood FC, Stamp TCB, et al. The plasma sugar, free fatty acid, cortisol, and growth hormone response to insulin, and the comparison of this procedure with other tests of pituitary and adrenal function. II. In patients with hypothalamic or pituitary dysfunction or anorexia nervosa. J Clin Invest 1966; 45:437–449.

1603. Staub JJ, Jenkins JS, Ratcliffe JG, et al. Comparison of corticotrophin and corticosteroid response to lysine vasopressin, insulin, and pyrogen in man. Br Med J 1973; 1:267–269.

1604. Fleisher MR, Glass D, Bitensky L, et al. Plasma corticotrophin levels during insulin-hypoglycaemia: comparison of radioimmunoassay and cytochemical bioassay. Clin Endocrinol 1974; 3:203–208.

1605. Donald RA. Plasma immunoreactive corticotrophin and cortisol response to insulin hypoglycemia in normal subjects and patients with pituitary disease. J Clin Endocrinol Metab 1971; 32:225–231.

1606. DeCherney GS, DeBold CR, Jackson RV, et al. Effect of ovine corticotropin-releasing hormone administered during insulin-induced hypoglycemia on plasma adrenocorticotropin and cortisol. J Clin Endocrinol Metab 1987; 64:1211–1218.

1607. Jubiz W, Matsukura S, Meikle AW, et al. Plasma metyrapone, adrenocorticotropic hormone, cortisol, and deoxycortisol levels. Sequential changes during oral and intravenous metyrapone administration. Arch Intern Med 1970; 125:468–471.

1608. Jubiz W, Meikle AW, West CD, et al. Single-dose metyrapone test. Arch Intern Med 1970; 125:472–474.

1609. Staub JJ, Noelpp B, Girard J, et al. The short metyrapone test: comparison of the plasma ACTH response to metyrapone and insulin-induced hypoglycaemia. Clin Endocrinol 1979; 10:595–601.

1610. Feek CM, Bevan JS, Ratcliffe JG, et al. The short metyrapone test: comparison of the plasma ACTH response to metyrapone with the cortisol response to insulin-induced hypoglycaemia in patients with pituitary disease. Clin Endocrinol 1981; 15:75–80.

1611. Dolman LI, Nolan G, Jubiz W. Metyrapone test with adrenocorticotrophic levels. Separating primary from secondary adrenal insufficiency. JAMA 1979; 241:1251–1253.

1612. Mahajan DK, Wahlen JD, Tyler FH, et al. Plasma 11-deoxycortisol radioimmunoassay for metyrapone tests. Steroids 1972; 20:609–620.

1613. Meikle AW, Jubiz W, Matsukura S, et al. Effect of diphenylhydantoin on the metabolism of metyrapone and release of ACTH in man. J Clin Endocrinol Metab 1969; 29:1553–1558.

1614. Nieman LK, Cutler GB Jr, Oldfield EH, et al. The ovine corticotropin-releasing hormone (CRH) stimulation test is superior to the human CRH stimulation test for the diagnosis of Cushing's disease. J Clin Endocrinol Metab 1989; 69:165–169.

1615. Merriam GR, Baer L. Adrenocorticotropin deficiency: correction of hyponatremia and hypoaldosteronism with chronic glucocorticoid therapy. J Clin Endocrinol Metab 1980; 50:10–14.

1616. Thorn GW, Jenkins D, Arons WL, et al. Use of desoxycorticosterone trimethyl-acetate in the treatment of Addison's disease. J Clin Endocrinol Metab 1953; 13:957–973.

1617. Soffer LJ, Gabrilove JL. A simplified water-loading test for the diagnosis of Addison's disease. Metabolism 1952; 1:504–510.

1618. Loose DS, Do YS, Chen TL, et al. Demonstration of glucocorticoid receptors in the adrenal cortex: evidence for a direct dexamethasone suppressive effect on the rat adrenal gland. Endocrinology 1980; 107:137–146.

1619. Tuck ML, Sowers JR, Asp ND, et al. Mineralocorticoid response to low dose adrenocorticotropin infusion. J Clin Endocrinol Metab 1981; 52:440–446.

1620. Hindmarsh PC, Brook CGD. Single dose dexamethasone suppression test in children: dose relationship to body size. Clin Endocrinol 1985; 23:67–70.

1621. Cronin C, Igoe D, Duffy MJ, et al. The overnight dexamethasone test is a worthwhile screening procedure. Clin Endocrinol 1990; 33:27–33.

1622. Scott RS, Espiner EA, Donald RA. Intermittent Cushing's disease with spontaneous remission. Clin Endocrinol 1979; 11:561–566.

1623. Meikle AW, Stanchfield JB, West CD, et al. Hydrocortisone suppression test for Cushing syndrome. Arch Intern Med 1974; 134:1068–1071.

1624. Fehm HL, Voigt KH, Lang RE, et al. Paradoxical ACTH response to glucocorticoids in Cushing's disease. N Engl J Med 1977; 297:904–907.

1624a. Gruen PH, Sachar EJ, Altman N, et al. Growth hormone responses to hypoglycemia in postmenopausal depressed women. Arch Gen Psychiatry 1975; 32:31–33.

1625. Berman JD, Cook DM, Buchman M, et al. Diminished adrenocorticotropin response to insulin-induced hypoglycemia in nondepressed, actively drinking male alcoholics. J Clin Endocrinol Metab 1990; 71:712–717.

1626. Monder C, Bradlow LH. Cortoic acids: explorations at the frontier of corticosteroid metabolism. Recent Prog Horm Res 1980; 36:345–400.

1627. Gold EM. The Cushing syndromes: changing views of diagnosis and treatment. Ann Intern Med 1979; 90:829–844.

1628. Liddle GW. Studies of structure-function relationships of steroids. II. The 6α-methylcorticosteroids. Metabolism 1958; 7:405–415.

1629. Dulin WE. Anti-inflammatory activity of Δ¹-9α-fluorohydrocortisone acetate. Proc Soc Exp Biol Med 1955; 90:115–117.

1630. Soffer LJ, Orr RH. Newer hydrocortisone analogs. Metabolism 1958; 7:383–386 (editorial).

1631. Slater JD, Hefflon PF, Vernet A, et al. Clinical and metabolic effects of dexamethasone. Lancet 1959; 1:173–177.

1632. Dulin WE, Barnes LE, Glenn EM. Biologic activities of some C_{21} steroids and some 6α-methyl C_{21} steroids. Metabolism 1958; 7:398–404.

10

CATECHOLAMINES AND THE ADRENAL MEDULLA

Lewis Landsberg and James B. Young

Epinephrine is the predominant catecholamine of the mammalian adrenal medulla (Fig. 10–1). It is synthesized and stored in the adrenal medulla and is released into the bloodstream to influence tissues throughout the body. Epinephrine is also a neurotransmitter in certain selected regions of the central nervous system (CNS). Norepinephrine (NE) is the peripheral adrenergic neurotransmitter. It is synthesized and stored in sympathetic nerve endings and is released in the innervated tissues; it exerts its physiological effects locally. NE is also a neurotransmitter in the CNS. Dopamine (DA), the other naturally occurring, biologically important catecholamine, is a CNS neurotransmitter. A role for DA outside the CNS is likely, but the peripheral dopaminergic system has not been well characterized.

Catecholamines resemble glucocorticoids and thyroid hormones in that they affect most tissues and influence most body processes. They resemble the peptide hormones in that they initiate physiological responses by interacting with specific receptors on the cell membranes of effector cells. There are, however, important differences between catecholamines and the other components of the endocrine system. Catecholamine release at the sympathetic nerve endings and adrenal medulla is under the direct and exclusive control of the CNS. Functionally, catecholamines are neurochemical transducers that convert electrical neural activity into physiological response. The effects of catecholamines are induced rapidly and dissipate quickly, unlike the slower, more prolonged effects of most hormones.

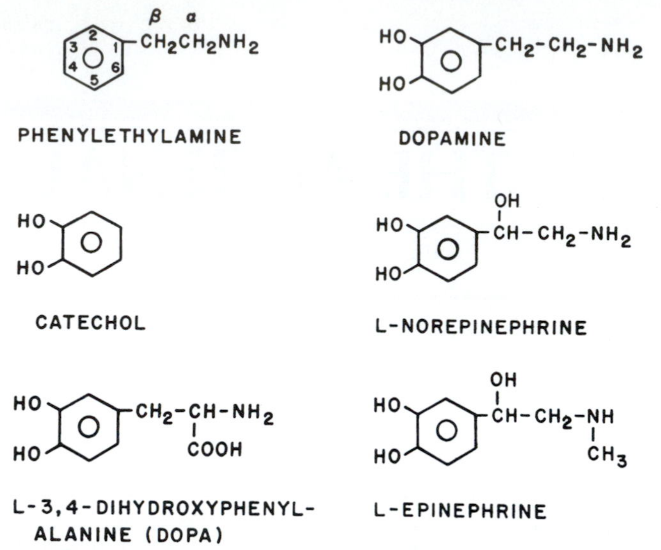

Figure 10–1. Structures of naturally occurring catecholamines and related compounds. The conventional numbering system for ring and side chain substituents is shown for phenylethylamine, which may be considered the parent compound of many sympathomimetic amines. Catecholamines are hydroxylated at positions 3 and 4 on the ring. (From Landsberg L, Young JB. Catecholamines and the adrenal medulla. In: Bondy PK, Rosenberg LE, eds. Metabolic Control and Disease. 8th ed. Philadelphia: W. B. Saunders, 1980: 1621–1693.)

STRUCTURE OF SYMPATHOADRENAL SYSTEM

Organization

The adrenal medulla and the sympathetic nervous system make up an anatomical and physiological unit that is often referred to as the *sympathoadrenal system* (Fig. 10–2). The central neural connections involved in regulating sympathoadrenal outflow are complex and only partially characterized;[1] studies with horseradish peroxidase and autoradiographic techniques demonstrate a complexity far beyond the previous concept of a single medullary "vasomotor" center.[2] The preganglionic neurons in the intermediolateral cell column of the spinal cord (see Fig. 10–2), which ultimately innervate the postganglionic sympathetic neurons in the paravertebral and preaortic sympathetic ganglia, receive neuronal inputs directly from several regions of the CNS, including specific centers within the medulla (reticular formation, raphe nuclei), pons, and hypothalamus, particularly the paraventricular nucleus. The various brain stem centers that innervate the intermediolateral cell column are, furthermore, interconnected. The neurotransmitters that are involved in regulation of the preganglionic neurons include epinephrine, DA, and NE, the last-named being particularly prominent and important, as well as serotonin (5-HT) (raphe nuclei)[3] and oxytocin (paraventricular nucleus).[2, 4] The precise anatomical pathways involved and the functional role of the various brain stem centers and neurotransmitters have not been elucidated. Spinal inputs also connect directly to the intermediolateral cell column.[2]

The axons of preganglionic neurons, which orginate between T-1 and L-2,[5] synapse with postganglionic sympathetic neurons in the paravertebral sympathetic ganglia[5] or pass through the ganglia of T-5 through L-2 and form the splanchnic nerves that innervate the adrenal medulla (see Fig. 10–2), or they synapse with postganglionic sympathetic neurons in the preaortic plexuses such as the celiac and superior mesenteric (Fig. 10–3). The preganglionic sympathetic neurons are cholinergic; the receptors on the postganglionic sympathetic neurons are predominantly nicotinic. A

system of inhibitory catecholamine-containing interneurons is present within the sympathetic ganglia. Most of these cells store DA predominantly, but in some epinephrine is the principal amine;[6] because of their fluorescent histochemical properties they are known as *small, intensely fluorescent,* or SIF, *cells*. The functional role of SIF cells is not established, but they may be interneurons in the regulation of ganglionic transmission.[6–8]

Topographic dispersion of sympathetic outflow occurs at the level of the paravertebral ganglia because each preganglionic nerve innervates several postganglionic neurons, including neurons above and below the level of the preganglionic cell. The postganglionic sympathetic fibers are distributed widely to blood vessels and viscera (see Fig. 10–3). The central nuclei that initiate descending impulse traffic are subject to regulatory influences by pathways from centers in the hypothalamus, limbic system, and cortex, as well as from a vast array of afferent impulses that initiate reflex changes in sympathetic outflow at the level of the brain stem. The composition of the extracellular fluid, including tonicity and the concentration of various substrates, hormones, and ions, also influences sympathoadrenal outflow via effects on the regulatory brain stem nuclei.

Chromaffin Cell

The endocrine cell of the adrenal medulla is commonly referred to as the *chromaffin cell*. Although most chromaffin cells are within the adrenal, some are in other sites. The term *chromaffin* is derived from histopathology and denotes an affinity for chromium salts. The characteristic chromaffin reaction is darkening of the tissue on exposure to aqueous solutions of potassium dichromate; this reaction depends on

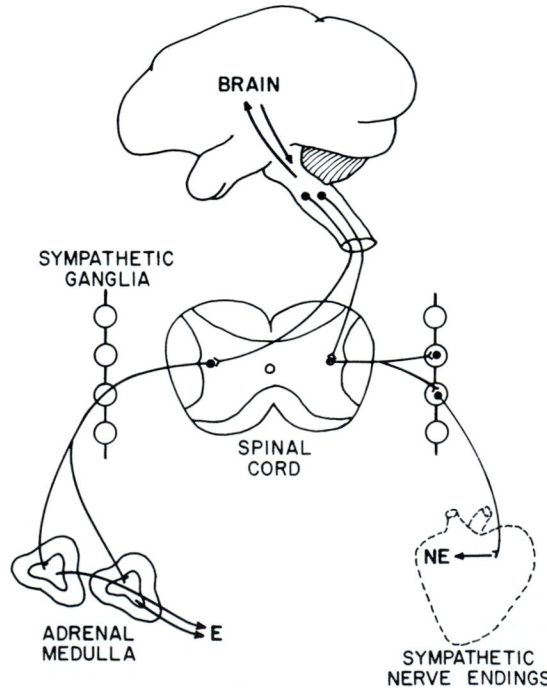

Figure 10–2. Organization of the sympathoadrenal system. Descending tracks from the medulla, pons, and hypothalamus synapse with preganglionic sympathetic neurons in the spinal cord. Preganglionic neurons, in turn, innervate the adrenal medulla directly or synapse in paravertebral ganglia with postganglionic sympathetic neurons. The latter give rise to sympathetic nerves, which are distributed widely to viscera and blood vessels. Release of epinephrine or NE at the adrenal medulla or sympathetic nerve endings occurs in response to a downward flow of nerve impulses from regulatory centers in the brain. (From Landsberg L, Young JB. Catecholamines and the adrenal medulla. In: Bondy PK, Rosenberg LE, eds. Metabolic Control and Disease. 8th ed. Philadelphia: W. B. Saunders, 1980: 1621–1693.)

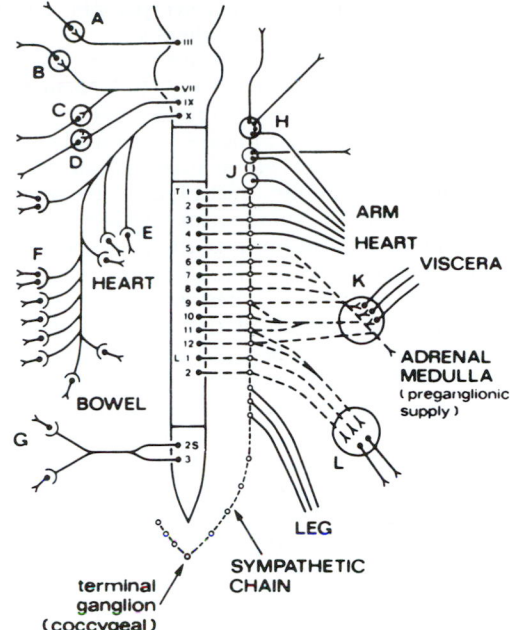

PARASYMPATHETIC   SYMPATHETIC

Parasympathetic system
from cranial nerves III, VII, IX, X
and from sacral nerves 2 and 3

Sympathetic system
from T1 to L2
preganglionic fibers ------
postganglionic fibers ———

A ciliary ganglion
B sphenopalatine (pterygopalatine)
  ganglion
C submandibular ganglion
D otic ganglion
E vagal ganglion cells in heart wall
F vagal ganglion cells in bowel wall
G pelvic ganglia

H superior cervical ganglion
J middle cervical ganglion and
  inferior cervical (stellate) ganglion
  including T1 ganglion
K coeliac and other abdominal
  ganglia
L lower abdominal sympathetic
  ganglia

Figure 10–3. Organization of the peripheral autonomic nervous system. (From Moskowitz MS. Diseases of the autonomic nervous system. Clin Endocrinol Metab 1977; 6:745–768.)

formation of colored pigments from the oxidation of catecholamines. Most workers restrict the term chromaffin to cells that, in addition to giving the characteristic chromaffin reaction, are derived from neuroectoderm; receive a preganglionic sympathetic innervation; and synthesize, store, and secrete catecholamines. This definition excludes mast cells and enterochromaffin cells, which in some circumstances give a positive chromaffin reaction, and postganglionic sympathetic neurons, which do not store catecholamines in sufficient quantity to give a positive reaction. The catecholamine-containing cells that occur in the carotid body (glomus or type I cells) and the glomus jugulare of the internal jugular vein are probably physiologically and anatomically distinct from extra-adrenal chromaffin cells, although, like the latter, these structures may give rise to catecholamine-secreting tumors.

In mature humans, most chromaffin cells are localized in the adrenal medulla. Small numbers of extra-adrenal chromaffin cells exist in and around sympathetic ganglia. In fetal and neonatal life the extra-adrenal chromaffin cells are more prominent than in later life, and clumps of cells may fuse to form encapsulated chromaffin bodies. The most prominent of these is the organ of Zuckerkandl, which lies anterior to the aorta and caudal to the inferior mesenteric artery. The function of the extra-adrenal chromaffin cells is unknown. They regress early in postnatal development, but remnants remain in the above-mentioned locations and may

be the site of subsequent tumor formation (e.g., extra-adrenal pheochromocytomas).

Development

EMBRYOLOGY. Early in embryonic development, primitive sympathetic cell precursors called *sympathogonia* appear in the region of the neural crest and neural tube. These stem cells subsequently differentiate into *neuroblasts* (sympathoblasts), which become sympathetic ganglion cells, and *pheochromoblasts,* which become pheochromocytes or mature chromaffin cells (Fig. 10–4).[9] Before differentiation, the primitive sympathetic cells migrate ventrally from the neural crest; those destined to be neuroblasts form the paravertebral and preaortic sympathetic ganglia from which the postganglionic sympathetic neurons eventually develop. Some primitive sympathetic cells remain closely associated with the developing sympathetic nervous system and give rise to the extra-adrenal chromaffin cells and chromaffin cell bodies. Other pheochromoblasts invade the developing adrenal cortex to form the primordial adrenal medulla. Most extra-adrenal chromaffin cells are, therefore, found in the abdominal preaortic sympathetic plexuses or in the paravertebral sympathetic chain, locations that are predictable on the basis of embryological development.

Extra-adrenal chromaffin cells mature earlier (9 to 11 wk of gestation in humans) in fetal and neonatal life than the sympathetic nervous system or the chromaffin cells of the adrenal medulla.[10] In the fetus, increased catecholamine secretion occurs in response to hypoxia and hypoglycemia,[10] and catecholamines contribute to the maintenance of internal homeostasis. Although extra-adrenal chromaffin cell bodies are innervated, the innervation is sparse compared with that of the adrenal medulla.[10] Postnatally, when most of the extra-adrenal chromaffin cells begin to undergo degeneration, those of the adrenal medulla complete maturation.[11] In newborn humans, primitive asympathetic cells dominate the adrenal medulla; during the first 3 y of life these cells complete maturation to chromaffin cells. Thus, the adrenal medulla develops as the extra-adrenal chromaffin bodies regress and disappear. The similar embryological origin (see Fig. 10–4) of the postganglionic sympathetic neurons and the chromaffin cells of the adrenal medulla underscores the analogy of these two cell types in terms of morphology, biochemistry, and physiology.

NERVE GROWTH FACTOR. The development of the sympathetic nervous system appears to be stimulated by nerve growth factor (NGF).[12, 13] NGF is a protein, originally isolated from rodent tumors, with the capacity to stimulate growth of the sympathetic nervous and sensory ganglia in various species. It is present in large amounts in the salivary

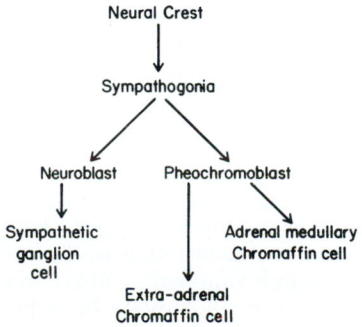

Figure 10–4. Embryological derivation of the sympathoadrenal system. (From Landsberg L, Young JB. Catecholamines and the adrenal medulla. In: Bondy PK, Rosenberg LE. Metabolic Control and Disease. 8th ed. Philadelphia: W. B. Saunders, 1980: 1621–1693.)

glands of male mice, in snake venom, and in guinea pig prostate. It has a molecular mass of 130 kd and is composed of three subunits. The biological activity resides in the beta subunit, which bears structural resemblance to proinsulin, insulin, and insulin-like growth factors. The human NGF gene, which resides on the short arm of chromosome 1, encodes a large polypeptide that is processed into a smaller, active subunit.[14] Specific antisera to NGF cause abrupt degeneration of the sympathetic nervous system when injected into newborn mice or other mammals. When administered to young animals, NGF markedly stimulates development of the sympathetic ganglia and sympathetic nerve endings; both protein and RNA synthesis are enhanced, and specific induction of tyrosine hydroxylase (TH) and dopamine β-hydroxylase (DBH), which are enzymes that are involved in catecholamine biosynthesis, is stimulated.[13] The mechanism of action of NGF is uncertain, but NGF receptors are present in sympathetic neurons, and NGF undergoes specific retrograde axonal transport, thereby establishing the potential for a target tissue to influence its innervating neuron.[13] The actions of NGF appear to be threefold:[14] (1) a tropic effect that prevents the degeneration of developing sympathetic nerve cells early in the course of growth and differentiation; (2) stimulation of neuronal differentiation manifested by enhanced neurite outgrowth and arborization; and (3) a neurotropic effect that directs neuritic growth to areas of high NGF concentration. NGF might be involved, therefore, in regulating the extent of the sympathetic innervation in different tissues.[15] Maturation of the sympathetic nervous system begins late in fetal life and proceeds to completion after gestation,[16, 17] under the influence, at least in part, of NGF.

PLASTICITY DURING EARLY DEVELOPMENT. Evidence from several laboratories[17–19] has provided insight into the differentiation of the peripheral autonomic nervous system. The neural crest cells that give rise to the peripheral components of the nervous system retain plasticity early in embryological life. Rostral portions of the neural crest ordinarily give rise to the cholinergic innervation of the gut; when these rostral portions are transplanted caudally they develop into normal adrenomedullary chromaffin cells.[18] Early in embryological life, therefore, the local environment of the autonomic cell precursors influences the subsequent differentiation of the cells in a critical way. Plasticity has also been demonstrated in the developing sympathetic neurons.[17, 19, 20] Factors derived from innervated tissues can transform an adrenergic neuron into a cholinergic one.[17, 19] Local tissue factors, hormones,[21] and, particularly, neuronal activity are all involved in establishing the neurotransmitter expressed by a given autonomic neuron. The expression of peptidergic cotransmitters in adrenergic neurons also displays plasticity.[22] Impulse traffic, for example, stimulates the expression of NE in mature rat ganglion cells while diminishing that of substance P and vice versa. The physiological implications of these developmental factors on the subsequent function of the autonomic nervous system may be considerable.

Sympathetic Nervous System

The peripheral sympathetic nerves originate from neurons in the paravertebral and preaortic ganglia (see Fig. 10–3).[23] Small, nonmyelinated postganglionic fibers arising from these ganglia are distributed widely to the viscera and blood vessels. The cranium is supplied by fibers from the superior cervical ganglion that accompany the branches of the carotid artery; the heart is innervated principally by cardiac nerves that arise from all three cervical sympathetic ganglia and the upper thoracic ganglia; the lungs are innervated by postganglionic fibers of the upper thoracic paravertebral ganglia;

the abdominal viscera are supplied by the great autonomic preaortic plexuses; and the pelvic organs receive their fibers from the sacral and coccygeal sympathetic trunks via the sacral spinal nerves and pelvic plexuses.

In sympathetically innervated tissues, the sympathetic nerve endings ramify extensively and form a plexus of terminal fibers rather than discrete nerve endings. Each sympathetic nerve fiber appears to control many effector cells, and each effector cell, in turn, is innervated by many nerve fibers. Histochemical techniques have demonstrated a nonhomogeneous distribution of neurotransmitter in the nerve endings with numerous discrete areas of high NE concentration (Fig. 10–5). These dense collections of neurotransmitter have been called *varicosities*. In some mammalian species the length of the terminal fiber of a single sympathetic neuron has been estimated at about 10 cm, and each neuron is said to contain approximately 25,000 varicosities.[24] Electron microscopic study of the sympathetic nerve endings reveals membrane-bound vesicles about 50 nm in diameter, many of which contain NE. The NE-containing granules, which have an electron-dense core, are concentrated in varicosities (Fig. 10–6).[25, 26] Each varicosity contains about 1000 granules, and each granule contains about 15,000 molecules of NE.[27]

The peripheral sympathetic nerve endings synthesize and store NE and release the stored NE in response to sympathetic nerve impulses. The nerve endings also take up catecholamines from the extracellular fluid. These processes are described later.

COTRANSMITTERS AND NEUROMODULATORS. In recent years it has become clear that central and peripheral adrenergic nerves contain chemical mediators that are stored and released along with NE.[28, 29] These substances include diverse chemical species such as peptides (neuropeptide Y, somatostatin, substance P, and enkephalins, as well as a variety of others), purines (ATP, adenosine), and amines (serotonin). These substances, when released with NE from adrenergic nerves may act as neuromodulators or cotransmitters. The term *neuromodulation* refers to effects on transmitter release (prejunctional) or modification of the response of the effector tissue (postjunctional). The term *cotransmission* implies direct stimulation of the effector tissue by interaction with a specific (nonadrenergic) receptor.[29]

Adrenal Medulla

The human adrenal medulla is enveloped within the adrenal cortex. The combined weight of the medullae from

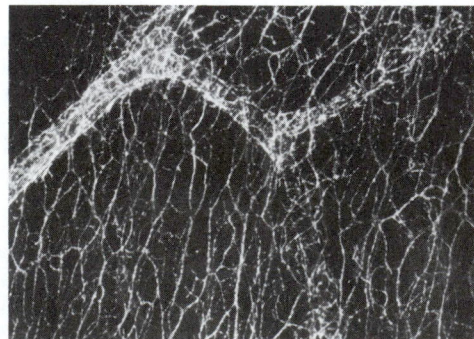

Figure 10–5. Peripheral adrenergic nerve endings demonstrated by fluorescence histochemical technique. The ground plexus of terminal sympathetic fibers is shown in a normal rat iris. The plexus is particularly dense around heavily innervated arteriole that courses through the field. Numerous discrete areas of high NE concentration (varicosities) are visible. Magnification × 160. (From Malmfors T. Studies on adrenergic nerves. Acta Physiol Scand 1965; 64[Suppl 248]:7–93.)

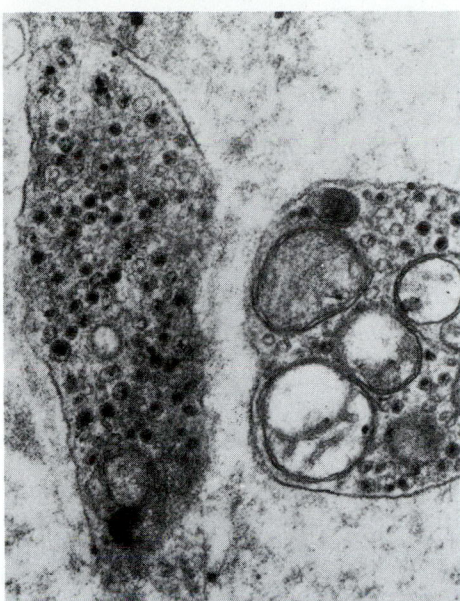

Figure 10–6. Electron photomicrograph of a sympathetic nerve ending in rat pineal gland. Note vesicles with electron-dense cores containing NE. Magnification × 45,000. (Courtesy of Dr. Floyd Bloom.)

both glands is about 1.0 g, or 10% of the total adrenal mass. The adrenal medulla is composed almost entirely of chromaffin cells. The cells are irregularly shaped polyhedrons that are organized into cords or small clumps and are surrounded by nerves, connective tissue, and blood vessels.[30] They contain numerous chromaffin granules, which are electron-dense vesicles 100 to 300 nm in diameter, that resemble the granules of the sympathetic nerve endings (Fig. 10–7).[31, 32] These granules are important in the storage and secretion of catecholamines. Individual chromaffin cells contain large amounts of either NE or epinephrine; in humans 85% of the adrenomedullary catecholamine store is epinephrine. As with the sympathetic nerve endings, a variety of potential noncatecholamine mediators have been identified in adrenomedullary chromaffin cells as well.[33]

The blood supply of the adrenal gland is derived from three adrenal arteries: the superior adrenal artery is a branch of the inferior phrenic artery; the middle adrenal artery arises directly from the aorta; and the inferior adrenal artery arises from the renal artery. The adrenal medulla has both arterial and portal venous circulations. The medullary arteries traverse the cortex and supply the medulla directly. The cortical arteries supply the cortex from the subcapsular plexus, which drains centripetally toward the medulla. In the zona reticularis the capillaries coalesce to form venous sinuses that drain into and supply the medullary tissue. The portal system contains high concentrations of steroid hormones derived from the adrenal cortex.[30] Epinephrine-secreting cells may receive a disproportionate fraction of their blood supply from the portal source. Medullary capillaries are fenestrated,[30] which may allow free diffusion of released catecholamines. These capillaries coalesce and eventually form a single adrenal vein that usually drains into the vena cava on the right and into the renal vein on the left.

The adrenal medulla is innervated by typical cholinergic preganglionic sympathetic neurons carried in the splanchnic nerves. The cell bodies of these neurons originate in the intermediolateral cell column between T-3 and L-3.[34] The major portion of the innervation is from the ipsilateral greater splanchnic nerve (T5-9). Spinal cord transections above T-3 are usually associated with deficient epinephrine

secretion, whereas transections at a lower level may not influence epinephrine output.[30]

CATECHOLAMINES

Catecholamines in Mammalian Tissues

Catecholamines have a wide distribution in the plant and animal kingdoms.[35, 36] In higher vertebrates catecholamines are localized predominantly in the sympathetic neurons, the adrenal medulla, and the CNS. In mammals epinephrine is located almost exclusively in the chromaffin cells of the adrenal medulla, where it is stored in high concentrations. The level of catecholamines in mammalian adrenal is of the order of several millimoles per kilogram (milligrams per gram) of tissue. The amounts of epinephrine in brain[37] and sympathetic ganglia[6] are small. NE, on the other hand, is widely distributed; it is found in the peripheral sympathetic nerves, the CNS, and (in very small amounts) in the extra-adrenal chromaffin cells, in addition to the adrenal medulla. Because virtually all the NE outside the CNS and the adrenal gland is located in the sympathetic nerve endings, the NE content of a particular tissue reflects the extent of its sympathetic innervation. Heavily innervated organs such as heart have NE concentrations in the range of 5 to 10 μmol/kg (1 to 2 μg/g) of tissue. The actual concentration in the nerve ending itself is much greater and has been estimated to be in the range of 5 to 50 mmol/kg (1 to 10 mg/g) of nerve cytoplasm.[38, 39] In the brain the concentration of NE is greatest in the hypothalamus, with somewhat lower levels in the brain stem and other regions.[36]

DA is also present in high concentrations in the brain, particularly in the basal ganglia and the median eminence.[40] DA outside the CNS is present in specialized interneurons in the sympathetic ganglia (SIF cells; see earlier),[41, 42] in the carotid body,[36, 43] and in some enterochromaffin cells.[44] Lower levels of DA are found in peripheral nerves of many tissues of animals.[45, 46] The extent to which these low levels of DA represent DA stored in typical sympathetic nerve endings or in distinct dopaminergic neurons is uncertain.

The regulation of physiological processes by catecholamines is mediated by both sympathetic nerves and the adrenal medulla. The concentration of catecholamines in

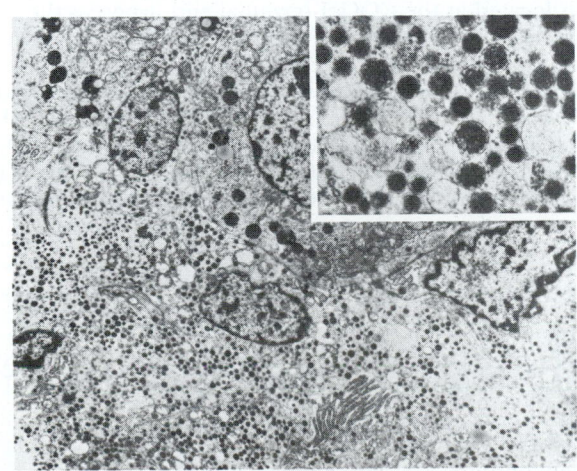

Figure 10–7. Electron photomicrograph of human adrenal medulla. Cells in the lower left containing small electron-dense particles are adrenomedullary chromaffin cells with chromaffin granules; those above are adrenocortical cells. Magnification × 7250. Inset (upper right) shows chromaffin granules with clearly defined limiting membrane under higher magnification (× 50,000). (Courtesy of Dr. James Connolly.)

the sympathoadrenal system remains relatively constant despite marked changes in the level of sympathetic activity.[47, 48] This dynamic steady state depends on a careful balance among catecholamine biosynthesis, storage, and use. Any assessment of adrenergic activity in a specific tissue must therefore take into account the rate of catecholamine turnover.[49]

Catecholamine Biosynthesis

BIOSYNTHETIC PATHWAY. The major pathway for the biosynthesis of catecholamines is shown in Figure 10–8. The sequence was predicted in 1939 after discovery of the enzyme that decarboxylates dopa and was subsequently confirmed in vitro in 1957.[30, 50] The biosynthetic pathway begins with tyrosine, which may be derived from dietary sources or synthesized from phenylalanine in the liver. It is uncertain whether specific uptake processes for tyrosine exist in adrenergic structures, but there is no evidence that tyrosine uptake is rate-limiting.[51]

Tyrosine Hydroxylase. TH (EC 1.14.16.2) catalyzes the conversion of tyrosine to dopa. Molecular oxygen and a reduced pteridine cofactor are required for activity. TH apparently causes simultaneous oxidation of tyrosine and the cofactor, with subsequent regeneration of the reduced cofactor by a pteridine reductase.[30, 50] The naturally occurring cofactor is tetrahydrobiopterin.[30] The enzyme appears to be in the cytosol of both human adrenal medulla and sympathetic nerve endings. It is found only in tissues that synthesize catecholamines and appears to be specific for L-tyrosine. At physiological tyrosine levels TH is probably saturated with regard to tyrosine but not with regard to the required cofactor tetrahydrobiopterin.[51, 52] The hydroxylation of tyrosine is the rate-limiting step in the biosynthetic pathway;[30, 50, 53] regulation of catecholamine biosynthesis involves changes in either the activity or the rate of synthesis of TH. TH is inhibited by catechols (dopa, NE, DA), which are thought to act by antagonizing activation by the reduced pteridine cofactor.[54, 55]

cDNA clones corresponding to TH messenger RNA (mRNA) have been isolated from pheochromocytoma and adrenal of humans and rats; these clones contain approximately 1900 nucleotides, show a high degree of homology, and do not appear to have large untranslated regions.[56, 57] The deduced amino acid sequence, coupled with the known biochemistry of TH action, indicates that the active catalytic site is located at the COOH-terminal end, whereas the NH$_2$-terminal domain contains sequences available for phosphorylation, which suggests a regulatory function.[58] The human TH gene has been localized to the short arm of chromosome 11.[58] Multiple TH mRNAs have been identified, which suggests that alternative splicing of pre-mRNA occurs.[58]

Aromatic-L-Amino Acid Decarboxylase. This enzyme (abbreviated AAD; EC 4.1.1.28) catalyzes the decarboxylation of dopa to DA. The enzyme, which requires pyridoxal phosphate as a cofactor, is cytosolic and is widely distributed in tissues. It is not substrate specific and decarboxylates a variety of aromatic amino acids.[59, 60] A cDNA clone of the enzyme with 2100 base pairs has been isolated from bovine adrenal medulla[61] and expressed in a mammalian cell line.

Unlike the other reactions involved in catecholamine biosynthesis, which are limited to the sympathetic nerve endings and the adrenal medulla, the decarboxylation of circulating dopa may occur in a variety of tissues, with the local production of DA. Much of the DA that is excreted in urine, for example, appears to originate from the decarboxylation of circulating dopa by the kidney.[62]

Dopamine β-Hydroxylase. DBH (EC 1.14.17.1) catalyzes the beta-hydroxylation of the DA side chain, with the formation of NE. DBH is a mixed-function oxidase that requires molecular oxygen, uses ascorbate as a hydrogen donor, and is genetically and structurally related to TH.[63] A cDNA clone that is complementary to an mRNA from rat pheochromocytoma that translates a protein functionally and structurally similar to DBH has been isolated.[63] Like TH, DBH is found only in tissues that synthesize and store catecholamines.[64, 65] The enzyme is not specific for DA and converts a variety of phenylethylamines to their beta-hydroxylated derivatives.[50] Unlike the other enzymes involved in catecholamine biosynthesis, DBH is not free in cytosol but is localized in a particulate fraction of tissue homogenates. The particulate fraction corresponds to the granulated vesicles of sympathetic nerve endings and the chromaffin granules of the adrenomedullary chromaffin cells.[30, 53, 64] DBH is present both as a structural component in the granule wall and as a soluble component inside the vesicle, which is released when the vesicle is ruptured by hypotonic lysis. DA or alternative substrates must be taken up into these storage particles before beta-hydroxylation can occur.

Phenylethanolamine N-Methyltransferase. This enzyme (abbreviated PNMT; EC 2.1.1.28) catalyzes the N-methylation of NE to epinephrine. The enzyme, which appears to be in the cytosol, is present only in epinephrine-containing cells of the adrenal medulla[34] and in small numbers of neurons in the CNS that use epinephrine as a neurotransmitter.[37] S-Adenosylmethionine is the methyl donor. PNMT is not substrate specific for NE and N-methylates a variety of phenylethanolamine derivatives.[66] Adrenomedullary PNMT appears to be inducible by high levels of glucocorticoids, a fact that has been used to explain the localization of epinephrine in the adrenal medulla, which receives steroid-rich blood from the cortex.[67] Within the adrenal, PNMT activity appears later in gestation than TH. The progressive developmental increase in PNMT activity reflects an increase in PNMT mRNA.[68] A cDNA clone of bovine PNMT has been isolated,[69] the amino acid sequence of PNMT has been deduced, and an enzymatically active protein, which is structurally similar to purified PNMT, has been produced in an

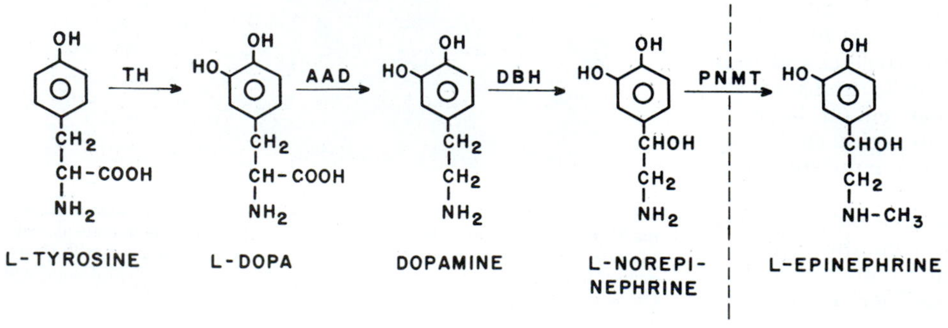

Figure 10–8. Biosynthetic pathway for catecholamines. Tyrosine hydroxylase (TH), aromatic-L-amino acid decarboxylase (AAD), and dopamine β-hydroxylase (DBH) catalyze formation of NE from tyrosine. Subsequent formation of epinephrine, catalyzed by phenylethanolamine-N-methyltransferase (PNMT), takes place in the adrenal medulla and in neurons of the CNS and peripheral ganglia that use epinephrine as a neurotransmitter. (From Landsberg L, Young JB. Catecholamines and the adrenal medulla. In: Bondy PK, Rosenberg LE, eds. Metabolic Control and Disease. 8th ed. Philadelphia: W. B. Saunders, 1980: 1621–1693.)

expression vector.[69] The enzyme has significant homology with TH, which is consistent with the previously noted immunological similarity.[69]

REGULATION OF CATECHOLAMINE BIOSYNTHESIS.

Coupling of Catecholamine Release and Biosynthesis. In vivo nerve stimulation of the adrenal medulla or of a sympathetically innervated organ such as the spleen results in release of catecholamines without much change in the catecholamine level within the tissue.[50] Similarly, catecholamine levels in the adrenal or sympathetically innervated tissues change little despite marked increases in sympathetic activity or NE turnover.[47] The stability of catecholamine levels in the face of increased sympathetic activity is the result of a simultaneous increase in catecholamine biosynthesis. (In the peripheral sympathetic nerve ending, recapture of released NE also contributes to the constancy of NE stores, as described later.) Changes in sympathoadrenal activity are coupled to catecholamine biosynthesis in two ways. In the short run, changes in the activity of TH in vivo appear to adjust the level of biosynthesis according to the rate of catecholamine release. In the long run, sustained increases in impulse traffic in the sympathoadrenal system result in induction of TH synthesis, thus creating a greater reserve of enzyme for enhanced catecholamine biosynthesis.

Activation of Tyrosine Hydroxylase. An increase in hydroxylation of tyrosine can be demonstrated rapidly after the initiation of nerve stimulation of catecholamine release.[50, 70, 71] This increase is not accompanied by an increase in TH activity assayed in vitro,[50, 72] nor does it require de novo protein synthesis.[73] Therefore, the increase in catecholamine biosynthesis after a brief period of nerve stimulation has been attributed to in vivo activation of TH. Because catechols such as dopa, DA, and NE inhibit TH activity by interacting with the reduced pteridine cofactor (see earlier),[50, 54, 55] it has been proposed that nerve stimulation reduces the concentration of catecholamines in the cytoplasm of adrenergic nerves or chromaffin cells, thereby releasing TH from end-product inhibition by freeing the pteridine cofactor.[26] Pharmacological maneuvers that increase the concentration of cytoplasmic catecholamines inhibit catecholamine synthesis,[50, 74, 75] and the inhibition is antagonized by the provision of excess pteridine cofactor.[45] There is, however, no direct evidence for the existence of a physiologically significant cytoplasmic pool of catecholamines that decreases during modest nerve stimulation. For these reasons a small, strategically located cytoplasmic pool of NE in equilibrium with the granular storage pool of TH has been postulated.[26, 70]

Release of negative feedback inhibition cannot entirely explain the increase in catecholamine biosynthesis observed with neuronal activity. Catecholamine depletion in isolated rat pheochromocytoma cells, for example, produces only a small increase in biosynthesis, and depolarization of depleted cells stimulates catecholamine biosynthesis to the same extent as in nondepleted cells.[76] Activation of TH, moreover, occurs in central noradrenergic neurons in the period after nerve stimulation in vivo[77] or depolarization in vitro,[78] which demostrates a dissociation between NE release and stimulation of biosynthesis. Acetylcholine[77, 79] and cyclic AMP (cAMP)[80–83] both increase TH activity, but cAMP, unlike depolarization, does not stimulate catecholamine secretion and does not require calcium.[81] These observations suggest two distinct mechanisms of TH activation,[81] one of which is independent of changes in catecholamine concentration. Additional evidence indicates that phosphorylation is involved in TH activation,[84] possibly mediated by a cAMP-dependent protein kinase[80–83] and/or by a calcium/calmodulin-dependent protein kinase.[85] Nicotinic stimulation in rat superior cervical ganglion appears to be associated with the latter kinase, whereas a noncholinergic mediator stimulates the cAMP kinase.[85] The situation is complicated by the presence of multiple phosphorylation sites on TH and the presence of multiple phosphorylating systems in adrenergic tissues.[85]

To summarize, the net result of nerve stimulation is induction of a conformational change in TH so that its affinity for substrate and pteridine cofactors increases and its affinity for the end-product inhibitor, NE, is diminished.[86] Both direct activation of TH and release of negative feedback inhibition are probably involved in increasing TH activity in response to nerve stimulation. Because physiologically relevant alterations in tetrahydrobiopterin may also occur,[52] changes in cofactor concentration may contribute to alterations in TH activity.

Induction of Tyrosine Hydroxylase. Prolonged stimulation of the sympathoadrenal system increases the amount of TH in the adrenal medulla and sympathetic nerves. This example of specific enzyme induction is not attributable to a general effect on protein synthesis.[50, 87, 88] Induction of TH depends on increased neuronal activity because denervation of the adrenal or decentralization of sympathetic ganglia abolishes the response. This process has been called *trans-synaptic induction.*[88] Induction of TH depends on intact transcription and protein synthesis,[50] requires a latent period of about 12 h,[87] and may involve a cAMP-dependent protein kinase.[89] cAMP has been recently shown to increase the transcription of TH[90] by interacting with the 5'-flanking region of the TH gene. Both activation and induction of TH, therefore, may be regulated by cAMP. In response to adrenomedullary stimulation, the increase in TH synthesis is preceded by an increase in the level of TH mRNA, which has been noted as early as 3 h after an appropriate stimulus.[91] Induction of TH would appear to increase the capacity of sympathetic neurons or chromaffin cells to synthesize catecholamines in response to increased physiological demand.

Catecholamine Uptake into Subcellular Storage Particles. The association of DBH with the catecholamine storage particles in adrenergic neurons and adrenal medulla means that DA must be taken up into these particles before beta-hydroxylation to NE can occur. Uptake into the storage particles is stereospecific, energy-requiring, saturable, and competitive with regard to substrate.[30, 50, 92] ATP and magnesium are required. This particle uptake process is unrelated to the axonal membrane uptake process; both of these processes are described later.

In adrenergic neurons and NE-containing chromaffin cells, the NE formed from DA is stored in the granule. In epinephrine-containing adrenomedullary chromaffin cells, the situation is more complex. Because PNMT is localized in the cytosol, it appers that the NE that is formed in the chromaffin granule must leave the granule for N-methylation to epinephrine, which in turn must enter the granule again for storage. It is possible that granular uptake protects DA from oxidative deamination by monoamine oxidase (MAO), because DA is a better substrate for MAO than NE or epinephrine and thus is more liable to enzymatic destruction.

ROLE OF ADRENAL CORTEX IN BIOSYNTHESIS OF EPINEPHRINE.

PNMT, the epinephrine-forming enzyme, is inducible by glucocorticoids.[67, 93] PNMT activity is reduced in the adrenals of hypophysectomized rats and is restored to normal by pharmacological but not physiological doses of glucocorticoids. In newborn rats, high doses of glucocorticoids can induce formation of PNMT in specialized interneurons of sympathetic ganglia if the steroid is administered within the first 5 d of life.[93] These data indicate that high levels of glucocorticoids perfusing the adrenal medulla from the cortex may be important in regulating the capacity of the adrenomedullary chromaffin cell to form epinephrine. Phylogenetically the association of adrenomedullary tissue with the adrenal cortex correlates with the capacity of the medullary tissue to form epinephrine. In human extra-adrenal chromaffin cells, only NE is found.[9] The strategic localization of the adrenal medulla within the cortex and the presence of an adrenal portal system, which results in the exposure of adrenomedullary cells to high levels of glucocorticoids, could be important in inducing the cells to form epinephrine. However, PNMT activity is not known to be rate-limiting in epinephrine biosynthesis; because epinephrine secretion is controlled by the nervous system, a direct regulatory role for glucocorticoids in epinephrine synthesis or secretion cannot be inferred. Glucocorticoids appear to confer the capacity to form epinephrine during fetal life, thus contributing to maturation of the adrenal medulla. Some forms of brain PNMT, in contrast to the adrenal enzyme, are not inducible by glucocorticoids.

Catecholamine Storage and Release

GENERAL CONSIDERATIONS. The processes of catecholamine storage and release are similar in the sympathetic nerve endings and the adrenal medulla. The adrenomedullary chromaffin cells have been better studied, and many currently held views on storage and release of catecholamines in sympathetic nerve endings are derived, by analogy, from studies of the adrenal medulla. The sympathetic nerve ending, however, by virtue of its relationship to the adrenergic synapse and the effector tissue, is subject to local regulatory influences that affect the adrenal medulla to a lesser degree.

ADRENAL MEDULLA. A pair of normal human adrenals contains about 33 μmol (6 mg) of catecholamine in the chromaffin granules.[30] There are approximately 10,000 to 30,000 chromaffin granules per chromaffin cell.[33]

Chromaffin Granules. In 1953 Hillarp and co-workers and Blaschko and Welch independently found that catecholamines are localized predominantly in a particulate fraction of adrenomedullary homogenates.[32] The particles, the chromaffin granules, were subsequently shown by electron microscopy to correspond to electron-dense membrane-bound vesicles that vary between 50 and 350 nm in diameter (see Fig. 10–7).[94] The chromaffin granules have been extensively studied[95] and contain, by dry weight, catecholamines (21%), protein (35%), lipids (22%), and ATP (15%). Ascorbic acid is present in high concentrations within the granule (20 mmol/L), predominantly (more than 90%) in the reduced form. It functions as an antioxidant, thereby preserving the catecholamine store. It is also a source of electrons for DBH in the synthesis of NE from DA.[96] Calcium is also present in high concentrations (approximately 14 mmol/L).

The protein in the granules consists of soluble and insoluble components, the soluble fraction being released on hypotonic lysis of the granules. About 75% of the protein is soluble; the remainder is associated with the limiting membrane of the chromaffin granule. DBH is one of the proteins in the chromaffin granules.[30] It is present in both the soluble and the insoluble fractions; depending on the species, between 20 and 50% of the DBH is soluble. It is interesting that the opioid peptides met- and leu-enkephalin are present in the adrenal medulla of several species including humans.[97–99] Storage is apparently within the chromaffin granule,[99, 100] with synthesis occurring from larger precursors within the adrenal.[101–105] Other neuropeptides such as neuropeptide Y[106] and galanin[107] have been identified as well. The remaining soluble granular proteins have been called *chromogranins*, a family of acidic glycoproteins. The most abundant of these proteins in bovine chromaffin granules[108] has been termed *chromogranin-A;* it accounts for almost one half of the granule matrix protein in this species.[96, 109] A

cDNA clone of chromogranin-A has been isolated from bovine adrenal medulla.[110] Chromogranins-B and -C have also been identified; these proteins are present in much lower concentrations.[111] In other species, including humans, chromogranin-B is said to predominate.[108] Chromogranin-A, or a closely related protein, has also been demonstrated in a variety of polypeptide-secreting endocrine cells that contain secretion granules, including those of the parathyroids, anterior pituitary, thyroid (parafollicular or C cells), and pancreatic islets. Chromogranin mRNA has been identified in bovine parathyroids and anterior pituitary.[110] Although the function of chromogranin-A remains unknown, its wide distribution suggests a general role in hormone storage or secretion,[109] perhaps related to the capacity of this protein to bind calcium.[110]

The chromaffin granule membrane has a low protein/lipid ratio.[96] The membrane proteins include two distinct ATPases, one of which (ATPase I) translocates protons from the cytoplasm to the interior matrix; DBH, which is accessible from the matrix side only; cytochrome *b*-561, which is capable of transmembrane electron transport; synaptin, a protein on the external membrane surface[112] that can be phosphorylated and that may be involved in secretion;[96] and structural protein elements designated chromomembrins.

Lipid is believed to be the major component of the granule membrane, with phospholipid predominating; chromaffin granule lipids are noteworthy for an unusually high concentration of lysophosphatidyl choline.[30, 95]

Uptake and Storage in Chromaffin Granules. The catecholamine store within the chromaffin granule is believed to be maintained by two processes: active uptake from the cytosol and storage in a poorly characterized intragranular complex. Several aspects of these processes have now been clarified, as summarized in Figure 10–9. A critical feature is the inwardly directed H$^+$-ATPase, which maintains a steep electrochemical proton gradient because the granule membrane has a low ionic permeability.[96, 113] The energy is derived from ATP, which translocates two protons per ATP molecule hydrolyzed. The resulting acidic internal pH (approximately 5.5) tends to trap intragranular catecholamines in a protonated form. Although this effect contributes to catecholamine storage, the proton gradient alone cannot explain amine uptake into the granules[96] because the latter process (1) is stereospecific; (2) displays structural specificity unrelated to lipophilicity; (3) is saturable; and (4) is inhibited by reserpine and related compounds. Amine uptake, therefore, depends on a specific membrane carrier protein. The specificity of the carrier favors the natural substrate DA. The amine translocator has not yet been fully characterized.

According to the chemiosmotic coupling theory the proton gradient that is established by the H$^+$ transporter and the impermeable granule membrane provides the energy for the amine carrier–mediated uptake (see Fig. 10–9). In this system the egress of H$^+$ along its concentration gradient is coupled to amine uptake against a huge concentration gradient.[96, 113]

Osmotic requirements necessitate an intragranular storage mechanism, because catecholamines within the granule at a concentration of 0.55 mol/L would cause osmotic rupture if they existed free in solution.[30, 95] Although the nature of the storage complex is not known, ATP may be involved for the following reasons: (1) ATP in the chromaffin granules is metabolically inert and is resistant to labeling with tracer radioactive phosphorus,[95] (2) the molar ratio of catecholamine to ATP is approximately 4:1,[32] and (3) ATP forms complexes with catecholamines in vitro in the presence of calcium.[30] These findings suggest that catecholamines interact with ATP in some rapidly reversible way involving

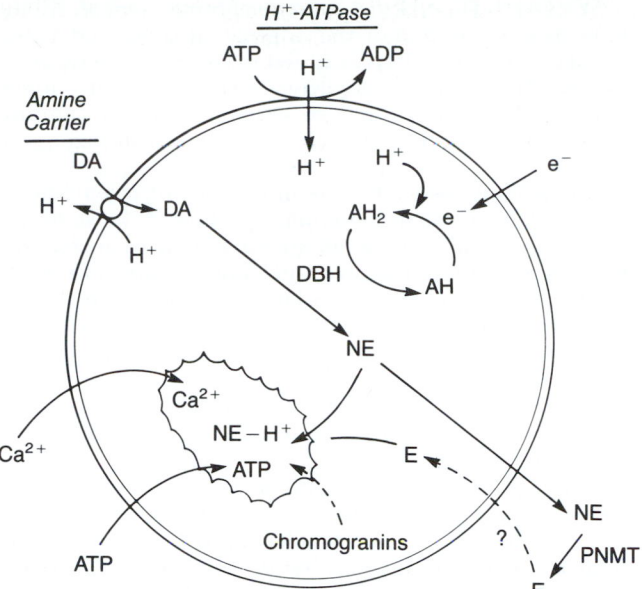

Figure 10–9. Schematic representation of a chromaffin granule. The amine carrier for DA and other catecholamines, H$^+$-ATPase, electron shuttle (e$^-$), and uptake processes for calcium and ATP are shown in the granule membrane, along with a putative process for epinephrine (E) uptake linked to NE egress. Stoichiometric relationships are not shown. AH$_2$ refers to reduced ascorbate, which is an essential cofactor for DBH that is regenerated by the electron shuttle. Calcium, ATP, catecholamines in protonated form, and chromogranins participate in a poorly understood storage complex. Synthesis of epinephrine occurs in the cytoplasm, thereby requiring translocation of NE and uptake of epinephrine for storage within the granule. Although the energetics of a linkage between NE egress (down a huge concentration gradient) and epinephrine uptake appear to be quite favorable, conclusive evidence for such a process has not appeared.

positively charged catecholamine molecules with negatively charged sites on ATP. Studies with nuclear magnetic resonance suggest, however, that ATP-catecholamine–divalent cation complexes can account for only a portion of the catecholamine store.[114] Chromogranin and other as yet undefined factors may be involved in intragranular macromolecular binding.

The chromaffin granule membrane also functions to maintain the intragranule concentration of reduced ascorbate, which is an essential cofactor for DBH;[115] reduced ascorbate is oxidized to semidehydroascorbate during the synthesis of NE from DA. Regeneration of reduced ascorbate is thought to occur via a transmembrane electron shuttle because transport of ascorbate itself across the granule membrane does not occur readily.[96, 113, 115] Cytochrome b-561, which is present in the membrane, may be involved in this transfer (see Fig. 10–9).[96, 113]

ATP and calcium levels are maintained within chromaffin granules against a high concentration gradient.[96] The transport of ATP and calcium into the granule is poorly understood.

As noted earlier, the synthesis of epinephrine requires transport of NE from the chromaffin granule into the cytosol, where PNMT is localized, with subsequent reuptake of epinephrine. The cytoplasmic synthesis of NE suggests the possibility of an exchange mechanism coupling NE efflux down its concentration gradient with epinephrine uptake. Although such a coupled mechanism is energetically favorable, supportive evidence is inconclusive.[96]

Release by Exocytosis. The physiological stimulus for catecholamine release from the adrenomedullary chromaffin cell is acetylcholine originating in the preganglionic sympathetic nerve endings. Acetylcholine, acting on nicotinic receptors, induces depolarization of the chromaffin cell by

increasing its permeability to sodium.[116] Propagated action potentials were not initially recognized in chromaffin cells after acetylcholine-induced depolarization, but they may in fact occur in adrenomedullary cells.[30] As a result of these acetylcholine-induced membrane changes, the permeability of the chromaffin cell membrane to calcium is increased, influx of calcium occurs,[116] and the intracellular calcium concentration rises. The increase in intracellular calcium level is believed to be a sufficient stimulus to trigger catecholamine secretion,[116] which involves extrusion of the soluble contents of the chromaffin granule into the extracellular space (exocytosis) (Fig. 10–10). The following evidence has been marshaled in support of this mechanism:[32] (1) the major soluble macromolecular constituents of the chromaffin granule—ATP, chromogranins, DBH, and the opioid peptides (enkephalins)[99, 117–119]—are released along with catecholamines in proportion to their concentration in the soluble fraction of the chromaffin granule; (2) cytoplasmic macromolecules are not simultaneously released; (3) the major insoluble (membrane) components of the chromaffin granules are retained in the chromaffin cell; and (4) electron photomicrographs demonstrate, for certain species, extrusion of granule contents. These observations demonstrate that the soluble contents of the granule are extruded through a temporary defect in the cell membrane, with retention of the structural granule components. Release from single chromaffin granules is probably quantal rather than partial.[120, 121] Compound, or "piggyback," exocytosis, which is the fusion of several chromaffin granules that release their contents together, seems to occur as a regular feature of the process.[113]

The molecular mechanisms that are involved in the triggering of exocytosis by calcium have received considerable attention.[113] Although a detailed, coherent picture has yet to emerge, several important components of the process have been identified. The proton gradient described earlier is not involved in exocytosis.[113] Important insights include (1) a cytosolic calcium-binding protein, synexin, that promotes aggregation of chromaffin granules has been identified. In the presence of calcium, synexin polymerizes to form rod-like hydrophobic structures that penetrate membranes and act as bridges between chromaffin granules and the cell membrane.[122] (2) Arachidonic acid is released along with catecholamines during exocytosis.[123] Arachidonic acid,

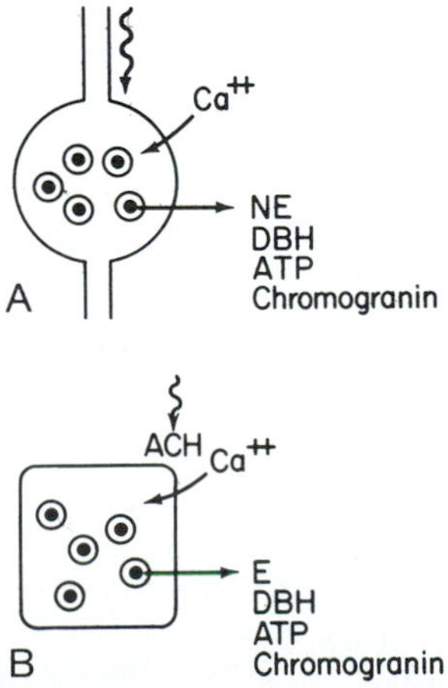

Figure 10–10. Schematic representation of catecholamine release from sympathetic nerve ending (A) and from adrenomedullary chromaffin cell (B). Catecholamines, DBH, ATP, and chromogranin, as well as enkephalins (not shown), are released in stoichiometric amounts from the storage granule in response to nerve impulses. (From Landsberg L. Catecholamines and the sympathoadrenal system. In: Ingbar SH, ed. The Year in Endocrinology. New York: Plenum, 1976: 177–231.)

which is produced from phospholipids by the action of phospholipase A$_2$, a calcium-dependent enzyme, has been shown to potentiate fusion of aggregated chromaffin granules.[113] (3) An inhibitory role for actin cytoskeletal elements in blocking chromaffin granule access to the cell membrane has been suggested.[113, 124] Nicotinic stimulation of the chromaffin cell—and perhaps an increase in calcium concentration—results in disassembly of cytoskeletal units, which potentiates chromaffin granule aggregation and docking at the cell membrane.[113, 124] (4) Phosphorylation of membrane proteins may be involved because activation of protein kinase C, which is an enzyme potentiated by calcium, has been shown to trigger secretion.[123] Calcium/calmodulin-dependent protein kinases may be involved as well.[125] Some of these relationships, although tentative, are summarized in Figure 10–11. The chromaffin granule membranes are retrieved from the plasma membrane after exocytosis and are recycled into newly formed chromaffin granules.[111]

Chromaffin cells also possess receptors for insulin[126] and insulin-like growth factor I (IGF I, also called somatomedin-C);[127] these hormones may modulate catecholamine secretion in some as yet undefined way.

Adrenomedullary Opioids. As noted earlier, the adrenal medulla of several mammalian species stores opioid peptides[97, 98, 118] within the chromaffin granule.[117, 118] Release of these peptides along with catecholamines and other constituents of the chromaffin granules occurs in response to adrenomedullary secretagogues in isolated perfused glands[117, 118] and in cultured adrenal chromaffin cells.[119] Both met- and leu-enkephalin have been identified,[118] along with related proteins, some of which may be enkephalin precursors.[100, 103, 128] In most species enkephalins are the sole opioid peptides demonstrable in the adrenal medulla; the human adrenal medulla contains, in addition, β-endorphin and other peptides derived from the pro-opiomelanocortin molecule.[129] The function of adrenomedullary opioids is uncertain, although their release has been postulated to play a role in stress-associated analgesia.[130] In addition, opioid receptors on adrenomedullary chromaffin cells may modulate nicotinic receptors in an inhibitory fashion so that stimulation of opioid receptors reduces catecholamine release in response to nicotinic agonists.[131] The opioid antagonist naloxone has been shown to increase plasma epinephrine levels in normal subjects as well as in those with pheochromocytoma.[132]

SYMPATHETIC NERVES. *Norepinephrine Content.* All the NE in tissues other than the adrenal medulla and extra-adrenal chromaffin cells is localized in the sympathetic nerve terminals. Heavily innervated tissues contain about 6 μmol/kg (1 μg of NE per gram) of tissue. As for the adrenal medulla, the NE store is largely contained in storage granules.

Storage Granules. NE in homogenates of splenic nerve is localized in a small subcellular particle.[133] Most of the storage vesicles are about 40 to 60 nm in diameter and possess an electron-dense core and a limiting membrane (see Fig. 10–6).[26, 94] There are also larger vesicles of 70 to 100 nm in diameter[26, 134] in the nerve terminal and cell bodies. These larger vesicles constitute a minority of the storage particles in the nerve ending but are the major storage particles in the cell body. The large vesicle is made in the cell body and is transported down the axon to the sympathetic nerve ending.[26, 134] Both the sympathetic nerve cell body and nerve terminal synthesize NE, but the larger vesicles are probably enriched with NE in the nerve terminals.[32] The origin of the smaller particles in the nerve terminals is not entirely clear, but they may derive from the larger vesicles.[26] Vesicles appear to be refilled with NE many times because their turnover in the sympathetic nerve endings is much slower than the turnover of NE.[26, 134, 135] As in the adrenal medulla, the large vesicles in the sympathetic nerve endings contain ATP, DBH, enkephalins,[97, 98] chromogranins,[26, 50] and, in some distributions, other neuropeptides including neuropeptide Y,[28, 111] somatostatin,[136, 137] and substance P.[138] The small vesicles contain catecholamines and nucleotides but are apparently devoid of chromogranins and neuropeptides.[111] Agranular vesicles are also found in the sympathetic nerve endings; these vesicles appear to result from either an artifact of fixation or a functional depletion of NE.[26]

Norepinephrine Storage. The storage granules of the sympathetic nerve endings accumulate amines by a process similar to that found in adrenomedullary chromaffin granules.[50, 92] This uptake process, which pumps amines from the cytosol into the storage granule, uses a proton gradient that is established by an H$^+$-ATPase. It is not specific for DA or NE; many hydroxylated phenylethylamines may be stored in the granules also.[50, 133] Uptake of amine in the storage granule is blocked by reserpine. Other drugs, such as guanethidine and sympathomimetic amines, also interfere with

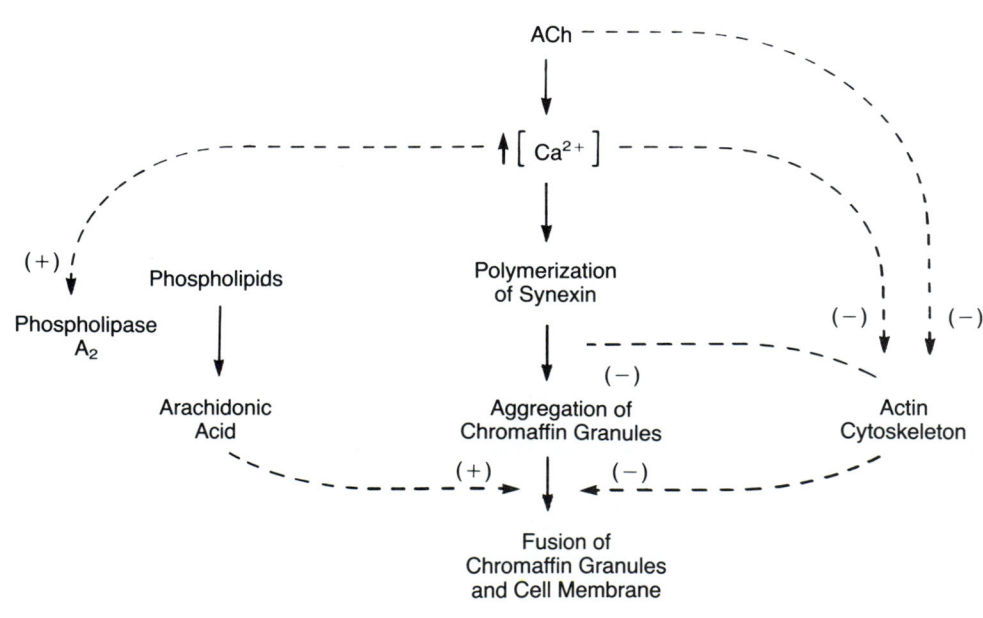

Figure 10–11. Schematic representation of the events involved in exocytosis. Note the central role of calcium. See text for details.

normal catecholamine storage.[139] The specific mechanisms that are involved in catecholamine storage are unknown, but by analogy with adrenomedullary chromaffin granules, binding to ATP and chromogranin has been implicated. Under ordinary circumstances the storage granules are not filled to capacity. Reduction in impulse traffic increases NE stores by about 25%.[133]

Role of Monoamine Oxidase in Norepinephrine Storage.
MAO is located in the mitochondria of sympathetic nerve endings; it catalyzes the oxidative deamination of NE and DA to their respective carboxylic acids.[140] NE in the granules is protected from metabolism by MAO. Cytoplasmic NE and DA are vulnerable to oxidative deamination by MAO, which suggests a competition between MAO and the storage granules for catecholamines that diffuse out of the granules, are synthesized in the cytoplasm, or are taken up from extracellular fluid (Fig. 10–12). MAO thus has an important role in regulating storage of NE in the nerve ending. When MAO is inhibited, NE stores in the cytosol (and presumably the granules) increase.[32]

False Neurotransmitters.
Under certain circumstances, compounds other than NE may be stored in the sympathetic nerve endings.[141, 142] The lack of absolute specificity of both the enzymes that are involved in catecholamine biosynthesis and the mechanisms for granular uptake and storage permits the introduction of other compounds into the neurotransmitter pool.[143] Storage of alternative transmitters may occur when MAO is inhibited or after administration of compounds that can be stored but are not substrates for MAO (such as metaraminol) or are metabolized to such compounds (such as α-methyldopa, which forms α-methyldopamine and α-methylnorepinephrine).[144] These compounds are released in response to nerve stimulation.[141, 142] Because almost all the false transmitters are less potent adrenergic agonists than NE, a sympatholytic effect is the usual result of false neurotransmitter accumulation. Under certain circumstances, epinephrine that is derived from the adrenal medulla may be stored in sympathetic nerve endings and may be released by sympathetic stimulation,[145] with modification of the physiological response.

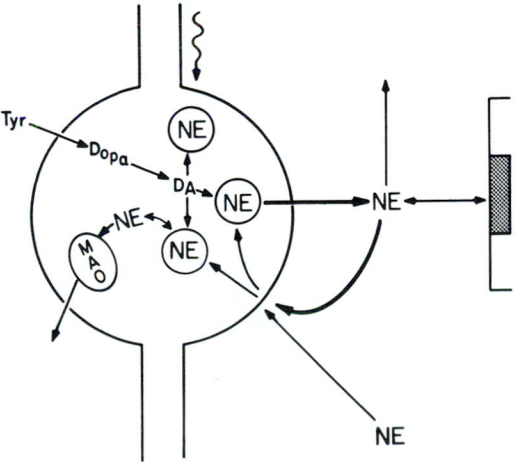

Figure 10–12. Schematic representation of sympathetic nerve ending. Tyrosine (Tyr) is taken up by the neuron and is sequentially converted to dopa and DA; after uptake into the granule, DA is converted to NE. In: response to nerve impulses, NE is released into synaptic cleft, where it may diffuse into circulation or be recaptured by a nerve. Accumulation of extragranular NE and DA is prevented by MAO. NE within the synaptic cleft also interacts with presynaptic (or prejunctional) alpha- and beta-adrenergic receptors on the axonal membrane that modulate NE release (not shown). As described in text, a variety of other mediators also affect the presynaptic membrane and modulate NE release. (From Landsberg L, Young JB. Catecholamines and the adrenal medulla. In: Bondy PK, Rosenberg LE, eds. Metabolic Control and Disease. 8th ed. Philadelphia: W. B. Saunders, 1980: 1621–1693.)

Nerve Stimulation–Induced Release by Exocytosis.
The release of NE at the sympathetic nerve ending is triggered by depolarization of the axonal membrane after a propagated action potential (see Fig. 10–10).[32] Depolarization is followed by the influx of calcium;[32, 134, 146] although the molecular role of calcium has not been established, phosphorylation of membrane proteins may be involved.[147] The final event is presumed to be exocytosis from the storage granules for the following reasons:[26, 32] (1) electrophysiological observations of effector cells are consistent with quantal release of NE; (2) cytoplasmic NE, the level of which can be markedly increased by pretreatment with an MAO inhibitor and reserpine, is not released by nerve impulses; (3) only phenylethylamine derivatives that are stored in the granules (false transmitters) are released by nerve stimulation, and the proportion of false transmitter released reflects the proportion in the granule store; (4) the soluble vesicle proteins DBH and chromogranin are released on stimulation of the sympathetic nerves, although the stoichiometry of release is less well established than is release from adrenomedullary chromaffin cells; (5) membrane-bound DBH is not released on sympathetic nerve stimulation;[134] and (6) exocytotic figures have been identified in electron photomicrographs of bovine splenic nerve.[148] Quantitative estimates of NE release are consistent with partial release of the contents of several vesicles from each varicosity every few nerve impulses.[26, 32] The process of exocytosis may explain the origin of smaller dense-core vesicles; during transport of large vesicles to the terminal varicosities, progressive depletion of the structural and functional components secondary to exocytosis might result in the formation of smaller granules. The function of the vesicles would cease when critical protein components are insufficient to support NE synthesis and storage.[26]

Dynamics of Sympathetic Nerve Ending: Summary of Role of Storage Granule in Biosynthesis, Storage, and Release of NE.
The major functions of vesicles in the peripheral sympathetic nerves include[143] (1) uptake of dopamine DA from the cytosol and formation of NE; (2) storage of NE by an active transport mechanism, with formation of an intravesicular complex involving ATP; (3) uptake and storage of NE from the cytosol after its recapture from the synapse or its uptake from the extracellular fluid; and (4) maintenance of a storage pool for NE release during nerve stimulation. During nerve stimulation, storage sites in the vesicle become available and fill with NE that has been synthesized in the cytosol and recaptured at the synapse. NE biosynthesis and recapture can proceed without interruption during NE release, because release does not require participation of cytosol or generalized changes in the axonal membrane.[143] Accumulation of cytoplasmic DA and NE during these processes is prevented by intraneuronal MAO, which deaminates amines not stored in the granules (see Fig. 10–12).

Norepinephrine Release by Sympathomimetic Amines.
Indirect-acting sympathomimetic amines, such as tyramine and metaraminol, release NE from sympathetic nerve endings. To function as sympathomimetics, amines must be substrates for the axonal membrane transport system (see later) and must release NE from the granule store (presumably by inhibiting the granule membrane amine transporter).[149] The release of stored NE, along with inhibition of NE reuptake by competition for the axonal membrane transport system, is responsible for a major portion of the sympathomimetic effects of these agents. The mechanism of release is, however, different from NE release in response to nerve impulses.[134] NE release by sympathomimetic amines does not require calcium, can occur from the cytoplasm as well as from the storage granules, and is not associated with a concomitant release of DBH. Sympathomimetic amines

thus do not release NE by exocytosis but appear to displace NE from storage sites and permit outward diffusion.[150]

Norepinephrine Storage Pools in Sympathetic Nerve Endings. The NE stores in sympathetic nerve endings are not entirely homogeneous. Newly synthesized NE is, for example, released in preference to stored NE[151] during stimulation of the sympathetic nerves. A part of the NE stores is resistant to release, even by repeated doses of tyramine.[150] The anatomical basis for the nonhomogeneity of the NE stores has not been identified. Proximity to the axonal membrane, however, may be an important factor in differential release.

PREJUNCTIONAL MODULATION OF NE RELEASE. As just described, NE release at the sympathetic nerve ending is a direct reflection of impulse traffic within the nerve. The amount of NE that is released in response to nerve impulses, however, may be influenced or modulated by a variety of systemic or local factors. A fall in pH or a decrease in temperature, for example, diminishes the amount of NE that is released when sympathetic nerves are stimulated.[152] In addition, various chemical mediators interact with the prejunctional (or presynaptic) neuronal membrane and influence the amount of NE that is released.[147, 152-154]

Prejunctional Modulation by Catecholamines. NE itself plays an important role in modulating its own release. Activation of alpha-adrenergic receptors of the alpha-2 subtype on the presynaptic neural membrane suppresses the release of NE in response to nerve stimulation. Thus NE in the synaptic cleft acts on the presynaptic nerve ending to diminish further NE release.[155, 156] Alpha-receptor–blocking agents enhance NE release by antagonizing this inhibition.[157] NE release, which is engendered by alpha-2–antagonists, is associated with the release of other constituents of the NE storage vesicles, occurs without an increase in sympathetic nerve traffic, and results in potentiated effector responses.[158] This alpha-adrenergic mechanism may also apply to neighboring nerve endings in the vicinity of the synaptic cleft; NE release at one synapse may inhibit NE release from adjacent neurons.[156] Conversely, activation of presynaptic beta-adrenergic receptors of the beta-2 subtype enhances NE release in response to nerve impulses.[159, 160] Beta-receptor–blocking agents decrease NE release.[160]

NE in the synaptic cleft thus has the potential to stimulate as well as suppress NE release.[153, 161, 162] Two hypotheses have been advanced to explain the presence of both an inhibitory and a facilitory mechanism. According to one hypothesis,[153] the concentration of NE in the synaptic cleft determines which effect predominates in vivo. Because beta-adrenergic receptors are more sensitive to low levels of agonists than are alpha-receptors, at low stimulation frequency or at the beginning of neurotransmission when the NE concentration in the synaptic cleft is low the beta-receptor mechanism may dominate and augment NE release. Conversely, at higher stimulation frequency, or late in the course of discharge when the concentration of NE in the synaptic cleft is high, the alpha mechanism may take over and inhibit release,[50, 153] because, in tissues that possess alpha- and beta-receptors, alpha-receptor effects dominate at high agonist concentrations. Such a sequence would facilitate transmission when the concentration of NE in the synaptic cleft is low and would inhibit transmission when the NE concentration at the adrenergic synapse is high. The second hypothesis relates to the fact that the beta-2–receptor is more sensitive to epinephrine than to NE.[163] Circulating epinephrine, either directly or after storage in the nerve ending and subsequent release, might facilitate transmitter release by a preferential action on the beta-2–mediated process. Such a mechanism might permit the adrenal medulla to enhance sympathetic neurotransmission. Although

the alpha-receptor–inhibitiry effect[153] is presumed to predominate in vivo, its physiological significance has been questioned.[164]

Other Prejunctional Modulators. Acetylcholine, via cholinergic receptors on the sympathetic nerve terminals, may also modulate NE release.[152, 154] Both a facilitory effect mediated by nicotinic receptors and an inhibitory effect mediated by muscarinic receptors have been identified,[154] but the muscarinic inhibitory effect appears to predominate in vivo.[154, 165, 166] Cholinergic modulation may play a regulatory role in tissues in which both cholinergic innervation and adrenergic innervation occur together; vagal stimulation, for example, decreases NE release in the heart.[166]

Prostaglandins also affect NE release from peripheral sympathetic nerve endings.[152, 154] Prostaglandins exert a predominantly inhibitory effect on NE release,[167-172] although the effect is variable in different tissues and with different prostaglandins.[152, 154, 167] Conversely, catecholamines enhance prostaglandin synthesis and release in effector tissues. The specific adrenergic receptors and second messenger systems that are involved differ in different tissues.[173] The generation of prostaglandins during the course of sympathetic stimulation provides the potential for prejunctional modulation of NE release. ATP, coreleased from sympathetic nerves with NE, is a potent stimulator of prostaglandin synthesis and release as well.

Serotonin (5-HT) exerts a prejunctional inhibitory effect on NE release that is mediated by the 5-HT_1 receptor.[174] 5-HT that is released from aggregated platelets has been shown to inhibit adrenergic neurotransmission in dog coronary arteries by a prejunctional mechanism.[175] 5-HT may also accumulate in sympathetic nerve endings and function as a false neurotransmitter,[174] thus exerting a postjunctional stimulatory effect on tissue 5-HT receptors.

Other compounds also appear to exert a prejunctional effect on NE release.[147, 152, 154] DA[176, 178] and histamine[179-181] inhibit NE release, the latter via the H_2 receptor. Purines (ATP, cAMP, and adenosine) that are released from adrenergic nerves, effector tissues, or aggregated platelets also influence adrenergic transmission and exert a predominantly inhibitory effect.[182] Angiotensin II, on the other hand, appears to facilitate adrenergic neurotransmission.[183, 184]

The physiological significance and relative importance of the various presynaptic modulators have yet to be clarified. Central sympathetic outflow is the overriding factor in the regulation of NE release, but various modulators, acting at the prejunctional membrane, may alter the relationship between impulse traffic and transmitter release. The mechanisms underlying prejunctional modulation may involve alterations in intracellular calcium and cAMP concentration.[147]

PEPTIDERGIC COTRANSMISSION AND NEUROMODULATION. Histochemical and immunohistochemical techniques have identified a variety of peptides that appear to be stored along with NE in some adrenergic nerve terminals. The peptides, which include somatostatin, enkephalins, substance P, and neuropeptide Y, occur exclusively in the large (70 to 100 nm in diameter) storage vesicles of sympathetic nerve endings.[28, 29, 136-138, 185, 186] and are released in response to nerve impulses.[111, 185] These neuropeptides may function as modulators that influence the prejunctional release or synthesis of NE, or the postjunctional effector response to NE.[29] They may serve as cotransmitters by influencing the responses of effector tissues via interaction with specific nonadrenergic receptors.[185] The peptides colocalized with NE have a specific distribution within the sympathetic outflow.[187] Neuropeptide Y, for example, is distributed principally in sympathetic fibers innervating vascular structures.

The precise distribution of other neuropeptides within the sympathetic outflow is less well defined and appears to differ among mammalian species.

An important physiological role of colocalized peptides and other mediators seems to be likely on the basis of the differential distribution and known effects of these compounds. The present state of knowledge, however, does not permit a detailed and coherent description of the role of these mediators in the elaboration of sympathetic responses in the physiological setting. The situation is complicated by the fact that these compounds have both prejunctional and postjunctional effects that may differ in their impact on a given adrenergic response. Somatostatin, for example, appears to increase TH activity in isolated ganglia;[138] the same compound inhibits NE release from hypothalamic neurons.[188] Neuropeptide Y decreases NE release prejunctionally at the same time that it potentiates the effect of NE postjunctionally and exerts a direct stimulatory effect on vascular smooth muscle.[29] Potential competing effects of different coreleased modulators from the same nerve ending further confound an attempt to define the physiological role of these compounds. It is possible that variations in impulse traffic (frequency and pattern) affect the differential release of colocalized mediators under different circumstances.

Neuropeptide Y. A 36-amino-acid peptide that is structurally related to pancreatic polypeptide, neuropeptide Y is stored and released with NE from sympathetic nerve endings that innervate the cardiovascular system.[186, 189] It is also stored in central neurons involved in the regulation of autonomic function, as well as in the adrenal medulla.[186] In peripheral sympathetic nerve endings it is found in the large dense-core vesicles of perivascular sympathetic fibers[186, 189] and in the heart,[185] but not in fibers innervating exocrine glands and other structures.[186, 189] It also occurs in nonadrenergic neurons innervating nonvascular structures. When infused exogenously, it exerts a potent pressor response which is not antagonized by adrenergic blockade.[186] It is released in response to sympathetic nerve stimulation, particularly when the stimulation frequency rate is high, and its plasma levels are increased during sympathoadrenal stimulation in humans.[186, 189] Compared with NE, the vasoconstrictor response engendered by neuropeptide Y develops more slowly and is more prolonged.[186] At the adrenergic synapse neuropeptide Y acts postjunctionally as a direct agonist and as a modulator that potentiates the effects of NE. The cerebral and coronary circulations may be particularly sensitive to the direct effects. Prejunctionally neuropeptide Y acts to decrease NE release.[186, 189] These paradoxical pre- and postjunctional effects might result in conservation of NE during periods of intense sympathetic stimulation.[186] On the basis of available evidence, therefore, it appears that neuropeptide Y participates in important ways in the cardiovascular responses that are mediated by the sympathetic nervous system.

PERIPHERAL DOPAMINERGIC SYSTEM. DA is a neurotransmitter within the CNS and is stored within the type I glomus cells of the carotid body, where it functions as an inhibitory transmitter.[190, 191] DA is also the major catecholamine of the SIF cells in sympathetic ganglia of several mammalian species.[6–8, 192–194] At this site also it functions as an inhibitory neurotransmitter, although the mechanisms involved are uncertain.[7, 194]

Several types of experimental observation suggest the presence of a peripheral dopaminergic system. A variety of physiological processes that are mediated by distinct dopaminergic receptors have been demonstrated: regulation of gut motility,[195, 196] vasodilatation in renal and mesenteric vasculature,[197–199] secretion of several hormones,[200, 201] particularly aldosterone;[202–204] regulation of renal sodium excretion[205–207] and suppression of NE release from sympathetic nerve endings by a prejunctional inhibitory mechanism.[208] The endogenous dopaminergic system that relates to these receptors, however, has not been defined. DA does not appear to be a circulating hormone because plasma levels are quite low and metabolism is rapid. DA does exist in adrenergic nerves as a biosynthetic precursor of NE but is not known to be released in sufficient quantities from these nerves to elicit distinct dopaminergic responses. Although release of DA from adrenergic nerves cannot be excluded, it seems unlikely to be a major component of the peripheral dopaminergic system. Distinct peripheral autonomic dopaminergic nerves may exist[209, 210] but have not been conclusively demonstrated. Amounts of DA in mammalian tissues[36, 211] are low, in general less than 10% of the NE concentration, which indicates sparse innervation and implies an extremely high transmitter turnover rate. DA in peripheral tissues is primarily intraneuronal because concentrations are markedly diminished by denervation.[45, 46] Thus, although a dopaminergic component of the autonomic nervous system, either as an alternative transmitter in typical sympathetic nerves or as distinct dopaminergic nerves, cannot be excluded, evidence in support of a neurally based dopaminergic system is fragmentary at best.

Renal Dopaminergic System. The best-studied peripheral dopaminergic system involves the kidney. It is generally acknowledged that most of the DA that is excreted in urine is produced by the kidney[212] for the following reasons: (1) clearance considerations show excretion far in excess of plasma flow; (2) DA levels in plasma are approximately 10% those of NE, whereas urinary levels of DA exceed those of NE by three- to fourfold; (3) plasma DA appears in the urine largely as metabolites rather than free DA.[213]

Some of the urinary DA originates from renal nerves.[214, 215] Histochemical fluorescence techniques have provided evidence in canine kidney that is consistent with the existence of specific dopaminergic nerve fibers.[216] Stimulation of specific areas of the canine brain causes renal vasodilation via specific dopaminergic receptors.[217] In some,[45, 218] but not all, studies[219] production of DA by renal nerves has been demonstrated, although only a fraction of the total DA excreted could be attributed to the nerves. In humans renal production of DA has been inferred from the fact that urinary DA excretion has a nephrogenous component; i.e., the amount of DA that is excreted in the urine exceeds the calculated renal DA clearance.[220] Renal production of DA need not, however, be confined to the renal nerves. Dopa, the precursor of DA, circulates in plasma,[221] at high levels, and renal decarboxylation of dopa could account for a substantial amount of urinary DA.[222] Current evidence indicates that the decarboxylation of circulating dopa in kidney, with the local production of DA in the renal tubule, elicits a functional dopaminergic response,[62, 223, 224] as well as contributing to urinary DA excretion.[212]

These studies suggest that an important component of the peripheral dopaminergic system in the kidney, and perhaps in other tissues as well, is the decarboxylation of circulating precursor dopa in the effector tissue with the generation of a specific response to the newly formed DA. The origin of plasma dopa is uncertain; presumably it is synthesized from tyrosine in tissues that possess TH.[225] The functional distinction between renal NE and DA, which is suggested by the observation that sodium loading increases the excretion of DA while diminishing the excretion of NE in both dogs[226] and humans[205] is consonant with such a formulation. Taken as a whole, these observations provide presumptive evidence for the existence of a renal dopaminergic system. This system may involve discrete dopaminergic nerves, the local production of DA from circulating dopa, or both. Evidence for a distinct dopaminergic system in other organs is largely inferential, but the existence of a dopaminergic mechanism of some type in regions that contain specific dopaminergic receptors seems likely.

Catecholamine Metabolism and Inactivation

The biological effects of catecholamines are terminated rapidly by uptake into the sympathetic nerve endings, by transformation to meta-*O*-methylated and deaminated metabolites, and by renal excretion.

NEURONAL UPTAKE. An important property of the sympathetic nerve ending is the capacity to take up amines from extracellular fluid.[38, 92] The axonal membrane uptake process is distinct from the uptake mechanism of the storage granules. The axonal process is energy-requiring, saturable, stereoselective (favoring the naturally occurring L isomer), sodium dependent, and competitive among a variety of naturally occurring amines and drugs.[38, 92] Neuronal uptake, which is referred to as uptake-1 to distinguish it from non-neuronal tissue uptake (uptake-2), is coupled to sodium chloride transport across the axonal membrane.[227]

Uptake-1 serves at least two important physiological functions: (1) recapture of locally released NE conserves transmitter and contributes to the constancy of the NE stores despite variation in nerve activity; and (2) uptake of circulating or locally released amines inactivates these compounds by intraneuronal storage or metabolism (by MAO) (see Fig. 10–12). When labeled catecholamines are administered to rats, the physiological effects are rapidly terminated as the catecholamines disappear from the circulation; unmetabolized catecholamines, however, can still be recovered from the tissues many hours later.[228] Chronic sympathetic denervation or drugs that block the uptake process are associated with supersensitivity to catecholamines, whereas inhibition of the metabolizing enzymes is not.[229] The isolated perfused heart inactivates twice as much catecholamine by uptake as by metabolism.[230] The relative importance of reuptake and extraneuronal metabolism varies somewhat in different tissues; in heavily innervated tissues, reuptake is more important.[50] Inactivation of locally released NE by uptake is particularly important at the postganglionic sympathetic nerve endings.[231] Uptake into nerves plays a less important role in the inactivation of circulating epinephrine.

Neuronal uptake is blocked by cocaine, sympathomimetic amines, adrenergic receptor antagonists, neuron-blocking agents, tricyclic antidepressants, and phenothiazines.[38] Because these agents compete with catecholamines and with each other for the same uptake process, the pharmacological implications are considerable. Tricyclic antidepressants or sympathomimetic amines, for example, when administered simultaneously with guanethidine, may inhibit the antihypertensive effect of that agent by blocking its uptake into the sympathetic nerve endings.[232, 233]

METABOLIC PATHWAYS. The metabolic transformations of NE and epinephrine are shown in Figure 10–13; corresponding metabolites of dopa and DA appear in Figure 10–14. The major changes include 3-*O*-methylation, oxidative deamination, and conjugation with sulfate and glucuronide.

Monoamine Oxidase. MAO (EC 1.3.2.4) catalyzes the oxidative deamination of a variety of amines with production of the corresponding aldehyde.[140] The aldehyde is immediately metabolized to the carboxylic acid or alcohol by aldehyde dehydrogenase or alcohol dehydrogenase, respectively.[234]

MAO is present in most tissues; its concentration is low in skeletal muscle and blood and high in liver, kidney, intestine, and stomach.[140] Although its properties differ in different organs and different species, some characteristics are general. MAO is a mitochondrial flavoprotein that is located in the outer mitochondrial membrane.[140] It occurs both intra- and extraneuronally. MAO oxidizes primary, secondary, and tertiary amines but requires an unsubstituted methylene group attached to the amine; alpha substituents on congeners of NE prevent metabolism by MAO.[140] Partial substrate specificity favors the naturally occurring L isomer of NE.[235, 236] More than one form of the enzyme has been identified on the basis of substrate specificity, sensitivity to different inhibitors,[237] genetic analysis,[238] and monoclonal antibodies.[239] Subtypes have been designated MAO-A and MAO-B;[240] the MAO-A subtype has a higher affinity for NE[240] and is localized in central catecholamine-containing neurons.[239] Both forms are present in liver.[241]

The action of MAO on NE or epinephrine produces the alcohol 3,4-dihydroxyphenylglycol or the acid 3,4-dihydroxymandelic acid (see Fig. 10–13). The *O*-methylated metabolites of epinephrine and NE (the metanephrines) are better substrates;[140] oxidative deamination of the metanephrines produces 3-methoxy-4-hydroxymandelic acid (vanillylmandelic acid, VMA) or the corresponding alcohol 3-methoxy-4-hydroxyphenylglycol (MOPG). The relative proportions of the glycol and the acid metabolites vary with species and tissues.[234] In humans free plasma MOPG is converted into VMA.[242] The action of MAO on DA produces 3,4-dihydroxyphenylacetic acid; the *O*-methylated metabolite of DA (3-methoxytyramine) is converted to 3-methoxy-4-hydroxyphenylacetic acid (homovanillic acid, HVA) (see Fig. 10–14).[234]

The major functions of MAO include (1) metabolism of ingested dietary amines; (2) intraneuronal metabolism of DA and NE, and hence regulation of the NE content of adrenergic neurons; and (3) metabolism of circulating catechols and their *O*-methylated metabolites.

Catechol O-Methyltransferase. This enzyme (abbreviated COMT; EC 2.1.1.6) catalyzes the meta-*O*-methylation of epinephrine, NE, and their deaminated metabolites 3,4-dihydroxyphenylglycol and 3,4-dihydroxymandelic acid (see Figs. 10–13 and 10–14). COMT was isolated originally from the soluble fraction of cells; liver and kidney have the highest levels.[243] A similar but distinct membrane-bound form of COMT with a higher affinity for catecholamines has been identified.[240] The enzyme utilizes *S*-adenosylmethionine as a methyl donor, requires a divalent cation, and is specific for the catechol group.[244] Although COMT is primarily extraneuronal, some of the enzyme may be intraneuronal.[245]

COMT functions to metabolize circulating catechols in the liver and kidney and to metabolize locally released NE in the effector tissue. The primacy of *O*-methylation, compared with deamination, in the metabolism of circulating[246] and locally released[242] catechols has been clearly demonstrated. The relative importance, at the adrenergic synapse, of local metabolism by COMT, reuptake, and diffusion into the circulation depends on local factors in the innervated tissue, the density of the adrenergic innervation, and blood flow.[50] As described earlier, neuronal recapture is of prime importance in transmitter inactivation.

The action of COMT produces normetanephrine from NE, metanephrine from epinephrine, VMA or MOPG from 3,4-dihydroxymandelic acid or 3,4-dihydroxyphenylglycol (see Fig. 10–13), 3-methoxytyramine from DA, and HVA from 3,4-dihydroxyphenylacetic acid (see Fig. 10–14).[234]

Conjugation with Sulfate or Glucuronide. The phenolic hydroxyl group of the catecholamines and catecholamine metabolites may be conjugated with sulfate or glucuronide.[234]

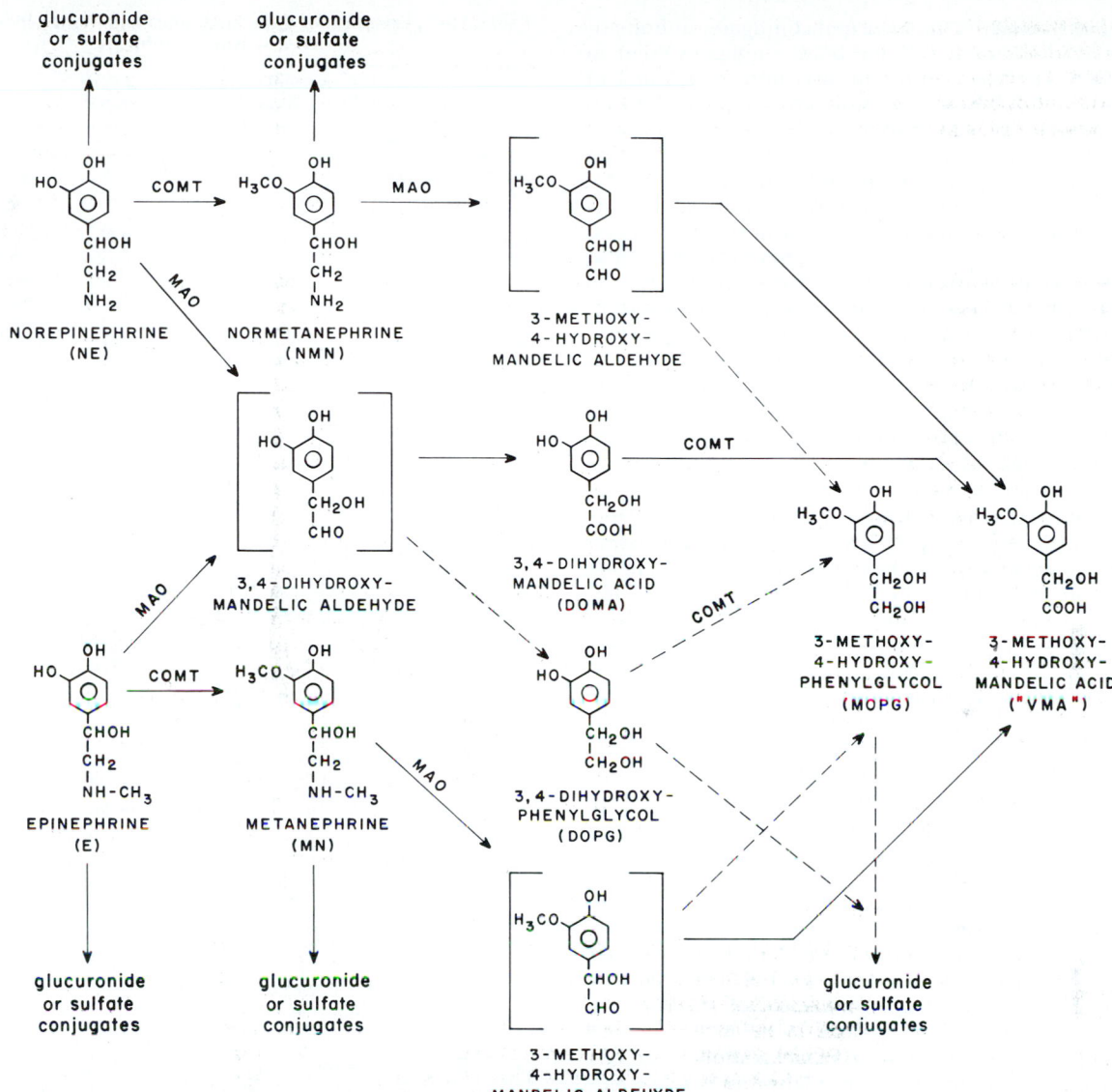

Figure 10–13. Metabolism of NE and epinephrine (E) by catechol O-methyltransferase (COMT) and MAO. The dashed lines represent the glycol pathway. Aldehyde intermediates (in brackets) exist only transiently; they are rapidly metabolized to corresponding acids and glycols by aldehyde and alcohol dehydrogenases. Conjugation of the phenolic hydroxyl group with sulfate or glucuronide also occurs. (From Landsberg L, Young JB. Catecholamines and the adrenal medulla. In: Bondy PK, Rosenberg LE, eds. Metabolic Control and Disease. 8th ed. Philadelphia: W. B. Saunders, 1980: 1621–1693.)

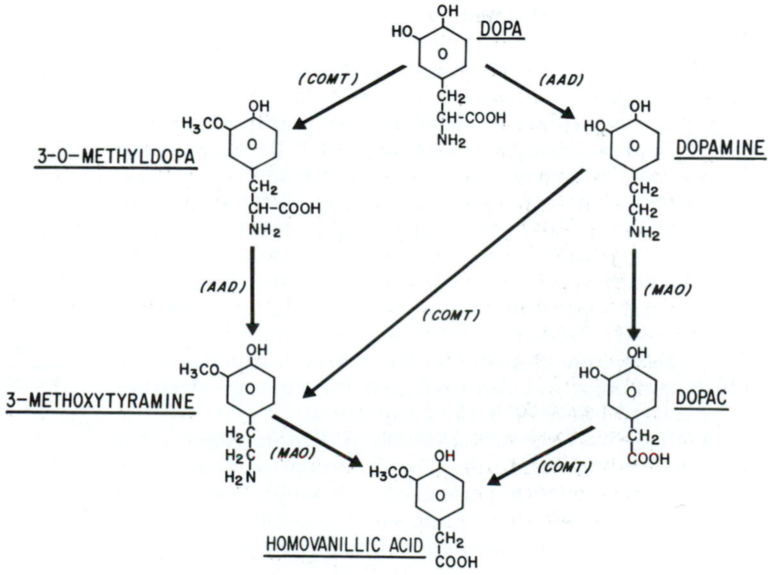

Figure 10–14. Metabolism of dopa and DA. Dopa is converted into DA by aromatic-L-amino acid decarboxylase (AAD) or 3-O-methylodpa by catechol-O-methyltransferase (COMT). The deaminated product of DA is 3,4-dihydroxyphenylacetic acid (DOPAC); the O-methylated deaminated metabolite is 3-methoxy-4-hydroxyphenylacetic acid (homovanillic acid, HVA). (Reprinted with permission from Biochemical Pharmacology, Vol 24, Landsberg L, Berardino MB, Silva R. Metabolism of ^{3}H-L-dopa by the rat gut in vivo—evidence for glucuronide conjugation. Copyright 1975, Pergamon Press, Ltd.)

In the rat glucuronide is the principal conjugate; in humans the sulfate predominates,[247, 248] but both conjugates occur in both species. The liver and gut are important sites of conjugation.[249–252] Ingested catechols are conjugated to an important degree, and catechols in the diet appear in plasma and urine principally as conjugates.[253] The enzyme that catalyzes sulfation of catechols is phenol sulfotransferase (EC 2.8.2.1).[240, 254] It occurs in two forms based on thermolability and substrate specificity and is important in the inactivation of many phenolic compounds.[254] The enzyme is present at high concentrations in platelets, brain, liver, and gut.[254]

Extraneuronal Uptake. Although catecholamines induce physiological effects by interacting with specific receptors on the plasma membrane of effector cells (see later), the formation of catecholamine metabolites in innervated tissues and systemically in liver, kidney, lung, and gut implies catecholamine uptake into a wide variety of cells. In fact, extraneuronal uptake-2 of catecholamines occurs in several organs[38, 251, 255, 256] and results in the formation of catecholamine metabolites. Locally released catecholamines are metabolized in heart and probably also in other effector tissues by COMT.[50] Circulating catecholamines and catecholamine metabolites are metabolized by COMT in kidney and liver, by MAO in liver, and by conjugation in gut.[250–252] The lung is also involved in the metabolism of circulating catecholamines, particularly NE.[257–260] The processes that are involved in extraneuronal uptake and the exact relation between uptake and metabolism are not understood.

EXCRETION OF CATECHOLAMINES AND CATECHOLAMINE METABOLITES. Catecholamines and catecholamine metabolites are excreted in the urine. The renal mechanisms that are involved in the clearance and excretion of these compounds are poorly understood. Tubular secretion of epinephrine and NE occurs in chicken[261–263] and mammalian[264–268] kidney. Mammalian kidney contains COMT and MAO,[269] metabolizes circulating catecholamines, and excretes the metabolites in urine.[268] The liver is also capable of excreting catechols and catechol metabolites in bile,[249–252] but the quantitative significance of this route is unknown.

The daily urinary excretion of catecholamines and catecholamine metabolites by normal humans is shown in Table 10–1.[270–279] Most of the catecholamines are excreted as deaminated metabolites (VMA, MOPG, HVA); a small fraction is excreted unchanged or as O-methylated amines (metanephrines). Excretion and metabolism after administration of labeled catecholamines, however, differ from the metabolism of endogenous compounds. More catecholamine is excreted unchanged or O-methylated, and less is excreted as deaminated metabolites in the tracer studies (Table 10–2).[271, 280–282] This difference reflects the fact that infused catecholamines equilibrate well with circulating catecholamines and with NE released at the adrenergic synapses, and poorly with NE in the CNS and in intraneural storage sites.[271] Because deamination is the major metabolic route for NE in the CNS and in the peripheral sympathetic nerves, deaminated metabolites constitute a lesser percentage of the catecholamine in the urine in tracer studies. Excretion of nonmetabolized catecholamines provides a better index of physiological activity of the sympathoadrenal system than excretion of catecholamine metabolites, because the latter reflect, to a considerable extent, NE that is metabolized within the nerve endings and brain and never released at adrenergic synapses in active form (see Tables 10–1 and 10–2).

INHIBITION OF MONOAMINE OXIDASE. Agents that inhibit MAO have been used for treatment of depression, angina pectoris, and hypertension. Although these drugs are not used widely at present, they are still occasionally prescribed for the management of psychiatric patients with

depression, and their use in psychiatric patients appears to be increasing. MAO inhibitors alter the storage and release of amines in the sympathetic nerve endings, thereby disrupting normal adrenergic function. The usual result of MAO inhibition is sympatholytic, which explains the use of these agents in the treatment of angina and hypertension in the past. MAO inhibitors, however, occasionally cause paroxysmal pressor crises that limit their clinical usefulness.

Sympatholytic Effects. Amines of dietary origin are ordinarily metabolized by MAO in gut and liver so that concentrations in body fluids are low. When MAO is inhibited, dietary amines reach the circulation in increased amounts, and various phenylethylamines, of which tyramine (the decarboxylation product of tyrosine) is the most important, accumulate in tissues. Because these amines are substrates for the axonal membrane uptake process, they are preferentially concentrated in the sympathetic nerve endings. Amines that are substrates for granule uptake and DBH are beta-hydroxylated and displace NE from the neurotransmitter stores. Octopamine, the beta-hydroxylated product of tyramine, accumulates in the tissues of animals that are treated with MAO inhibitors.[283] The beta-hydroxylated amines thus function as false neurotransmitters; they are released along with NE in response to sympathetic nerve impulses (Fig. 10–15A).[144, 284] Because the accumulated false

TABLE 10–1. Excretion of Catecholamines and Metabolites in Urine of Normal Human Subjects

	Amount Excreted in μmol/d (μg/d)*	% of Total from NE + E	Source†
Epinephrine (E) (free)	0.03 (5)	0.1	Adrenal medulla
Norepinephrine (NE) (free)	0.18 (30)	0.4	Sympathetic nerve endings (Adrenal medulla)
Conjugated NE + E	0.59 (100)	1.6	Dietary catecholamines (Sympathetic nerve endings) (Adrenal medulla)
Metanephrine (total)	0.33 (65)	1.0	Adrenal medulla
Normetanephrine (total)	0.55 (100)	1.6	Sympathetic nerve endings (Adrenal medulla)
Vanillylmandelic acid	20.2 (4000)	63.5	Sympathetic nerve endings Adrenal medulla CNS
3-Methoxy-4-hydroxy-phenylglycol	10.9 (2000)	31.8	Sympathetic nerve endings Adrenal medulla CNS
Dopamine (free)	1.5 (225)		Kidney
Homovanillic acid	37.9 (6900)		CNS Plasma DA

*Average values.
†Secondary sources in parentheses.

TABLE 10–2. Urinary Excretion After Infusions of Tracer Cathecholamines (% of Total Radioactivity*)

	Epinephrine		Norepinephrine	
Excreted Catecholamine	*During*	*After*	*During*	*After*
Free catecholamines	22	5	16	5
Conjugated catecholamines	—	—	8	10
Total metanephrines	37	40	18	15
Vanillylmandelic acid	28	40	34	35
3-Methoxy-4-hydroxyphenylglycol	—	7	10	15

*Average approximate figures from literature. "During" refers to distribution of catecholamines during infusion of tracer and reflects metabolism of exogenous hormone. "After" reflects metabolism of endogenous catecholamines.

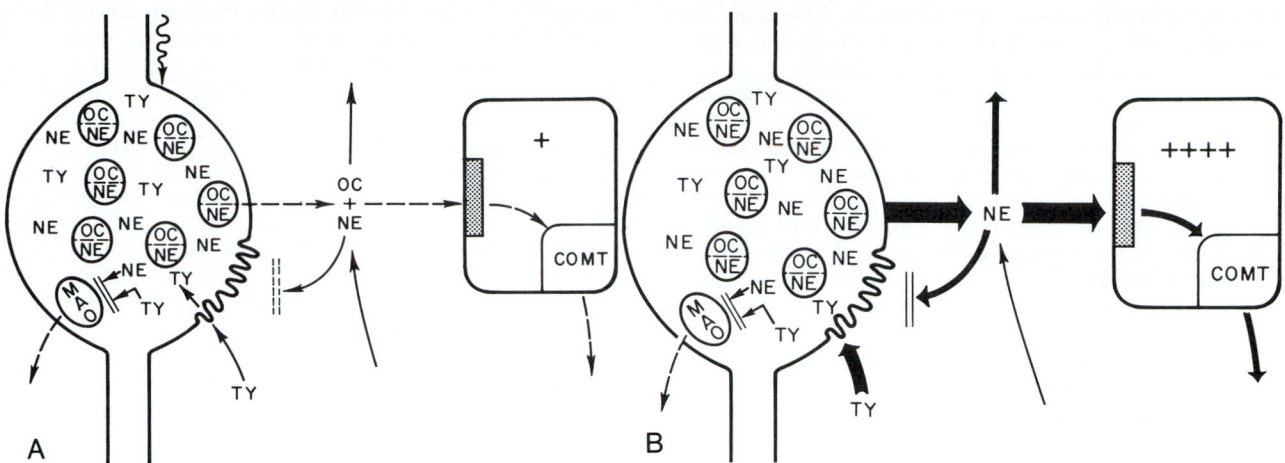

Figure 10–15. Schematic representation of a sympathetic nerve ending in the presence of MAO inhibition. *A,* When MAO is inhibited, dietary tyramine (TY) is taken up by the nerve ending and is metabolized to octopamine (OC), which displaces NE from granular storage sites. Nerve impulses release NE and octopamine by exocytosis, which results in a diminished response because NE release is diluted by octopamine, a less potent agonist. Cytoplasmic NE, which accumulates after MAO inhibition, is not released by nerve impulses. *B,* When large amounts of tyramine gain access to circulation, cytoplasmic NE is released in large amounts, which leads to an exaggerated response. This effect of high levels of tyramine does not depend on nerve impulses and does not occur by exocytosis. Although tyramine is the prototype, other amines are taken up, and false transmitters other than octopamine may be stored. Any indirect-acting sympathomimetic amine may cause release of large amounts of NE. COMT, catechol *O*-methyltransferase.

transmitters are less potent agonists than NE, dilution of the released NE with the false transmitter results in a diminished sympathetic response. Although NE increases in the nerve cytoplasm when MAO is inhibited, cytoplasmic NE is not released by nerve impulses.[134] Cytoplasmic NE can be released by indirect-acting sympathomimetic amines (of which tyramine is the prototype), but when the load of ingested amine is low, the release of NE is not appreciable and a sympathomimetic response does not occur. The low level of ingested amines, however, is sufficient to result in accumulation of false transmitters in the nerve ending.

Pressor Reactions. When a large bolus of indirect-acting sympathomimetic amine such as tyramine reaches the circulation, large amounts of NE may be released and may induce a severe hypertensive crisis. Concomitant blockade of NE reuptake into the sympathetic nerve ending by the sympathomimetic amine contributes to the pressor reaction (Fig. 10–15*B*).

A minimum of 5 to 10% of patients receiving MAO inhibitors suffer these pressor crises,[285] but many reactions may go unrecognized or unreported. Pressor reactions usually occur after several weeks of treatment with MAO inhibitors, but they may arise after only 2 d of treatment.[285]

Pressor reactions are usually precipitated by meals. Cheese (especially Cheddar) was early implicated as a precipitating agent, but other foods can produce the same effect. The tyramine content of food is the major determinant of attacks. Pickled herring, Chianti wine, and a variety of cheeses have high tyramine content,[286-288] but concentrations in foods are difficult to predict accurately because tyramine is formed from the action of bacterial decarboxylases on tyrosine, and the extent of fermentation of a particular foodstuff may be variable. Thus it is difficult to advise patients about what foods to avoid. Pressor attacks characteristically have a sudden onset 10 min to 2 h after eating. Sympathomimetic amines in drugs may also induce the syndrome.

Pressor reactions resemble the paroxysms seen in persons with pheochromocytoma. Patients suddenly feel acutely ill, and headache, sweating, palpitations, fear, anxiety, nausea, and vomiting are common. Blood pressure is increased during a paroxysm, often to alarming levels. The attack may last from 10 min to several hours. Pulmonary edema or

cardiac arrhythmias may occur. Death may result from cerebral or subarachnoid hemorrhage or from myocardial infarction.[289] The hazard is so great that the use of these agents cannot be generally recommended.

Treatment for the pressor reaction consists of the rapidly acting adrenergic blocking agent phentolamine; drugs that release NE such as reserpine, methyldopa, and guanethidine are contraindicated. Close supervision of a reliable patient by a well-informed physician is essential whenever MAO inhibitors are prescribed.

Plasma Catecholamines

METHODOLOGICAL CONSIDERATIONS. In the past, technological problems prevented accurate measurement of catecholamines in the circulation. Present techniques with radioenzymatic isotope derivative assays or high-performance liquid chromatographic (HPLC) separations with electrochemical detection are sensitive and precise enough to measure catecholamine concentrations in human plasma under basal conditions. The clinical utility of plasma catecholamine measurements is, however, limited, as described later. Interpretation in both clinical and research settings requires awareness of the limitations of these measurements in the assessment of sympathoadrenal activity.

Radioenzymatic Assays. Isotope derivative techniques that utilize partially purified enzyme preparations to transfer a labeled methyl group to the catecholamine molecule have been successfully applied to the measurement of catecholamines in plasma. In the most widely used and most useful of these assays, COMT catalyzes the transfer of a labeled methyl group from *S*-adenosylmethionine to the 3-hydroxyl position of NE, epinephrine, and DA, with the formation of labeled normetanephrine, metanephrine, and 3-methoxytyramine, respectively. The labeled products are extracted and separated chromatographically. The labeled metanephrines are then oxidized to VMA, extracted, and counted, and the catecholamine concentration in the plasma is determined from a standard curve or internal standard.[290-294]

Another radioenzymatic assay utilizes PNMT to catalyze the transfer of a labeled methyl group from *S*-adenosylmethionine to the amino group of NE in plasma.[295-297] The labeled epinephrine produced by the reaction is isolated chromatographically, eluted, and counted. This assay does not measure epinephrine or DA, and although it is simpler than the COMT assay, it is used less frequently.

HPLC-Electrochemical Detection Assays. Techniques with reverse-phase or cation-exchange HPLC in conjunction with electrochemical detection provide the requisite sensitivity for analysis of catecholamines in plasma. These techniques involve an initial purification step followed by separation of NE, epinephrine, and DA on the HPLC column and oxidation of the catecholamine at the detector with the generation of an electrical current.[298-300] As the technology improves, HPLC techniques are replacing radioenzymatic assays.

PLASMA CATECHOLAMINES IN HUMANS: SOURCE, BASAL LEVELS, AND PHYSIOLOGICAL VARIATIONS. *Protein Binding and Conjugation.*

At physiological levels 50 to 60% of catecholamines in plasma are loosely bound to albumin,[301-303] globulins, and lipoproteins.[304] A high-affinity, stereospecific, saturable site has been identified on alpha-1 acid glycoprotein.[304, 305] The significance of protein binding is unclear because water-soluble catecholamines do not require protein binding for transport. Most catecholamine assays measure both free and protein-bound catecholamines but do not measure conjugated catecholamines. Conjugated catecholamines can be determined by hydrolyzing the conjugates in the plasma sample before measurement;[248] because conjugates do not reflect acute changes in sympathetic nervous system activity,[306] they are of less interest in most circumstances. When referring to catecholamines, the designation *free* means unconjugated and does not refer to protein binding. Unless specified, reported levels of plasma catecholamines always refer to the free (or unconjugated) forms.

Sample Collection. Because catecholamine levels in plasma reflect the activity or functional state of the sympathoadrenal system, the physiological state of the subject at the time of sampling is of prime importance in interpretation. Catecholamine levels in casually collected plasma samples, without attention to the technique of phlebotomy or the physiological state of the subject, are uninterpretable and useless. Basal catecholamine levels should be obtained from a supine subject in a relaxed environment. Because pain and anxiety may transiently activate the sympathoadrenal system, samples should not be taken by direct venipuncture but rather from an indwelling intravenous line. By convention, after the intravenous line is placed, the patient remains supine for 30 min, at which time blood may be withdrawn. The blood should be collected in chilled tubes with an appropriate reducing agent to avoid oxidation of catecholamines[294] and should be placed immediately on ice; plasma should be separated promptly and stored at $-70°C$ until analysis. Drugs of different types, particularly those that affect the autonomic nervous system, may influence the circulating levels of catecholamines. Alpha- and beta-adrenergic blocking agents[307-309] and clonidine[310] are of particular concern. All medications should preferably be discontinued before plasma catecholamines are measured.

Norepinephrine. Basal plasma NE levels are generally in the range of 0.6 to 2.0 nmol/L (100 to 350 pg/mL).[292, 311, 312] NE that is released at adrenergic synapses throughout the body is subject to reuptake into sympathetic nerve endings or local metabolism within the effector tissue (see Fig. 10–12); the portion of released neurotransmitter that escapes reuptake and local metabolism diffuses into the circulation and constitutes the circulating pool.[313] Under basal conditions, venous levels of NE in the forearm exceed the arterial concentration by approximately 30%.[314] Arteriovenous differences at other sites reflect the relative contributions of metabolism, which results in NE extraction, and local release, which reflects sympathetic activity in the region being

sampled[313, 315] (Fig. 10–16). Under basal conditions the adrenomedullary contribution to the circulating pool of NE is trivial;[313] when the adrenal medulla is stimulated, however, large amounts of NE are released along with epinephrine,[316-318] and under these circumstances the adrenal medulla may contribute substantially to the plasma NE level.[319] Plasma NE turns over rapidly; the half-time of disappearance, calculated from steady-state NE infusions, is between 2.0 and 2.5 min.[320, 321] The metabolic clearance rate of plasma NE, calculated from steady-state infusions of both unlabeled and tracer NE, approximates 40 mL/min/kg.[320, 322]

Plasma NE levels are influenced by the position of the body. Orthostatic activation of the sympathetic nervous system causes a significant increase in plasma NE level; 5 min of quiet standing results in a doubling of the basal plasma NE concentration.[292, 297, 311] The predictable plasma NE response to upright posture constitutes a convenient test of sympathetic nervous system function, as described later. Aging is thought to be associated with increased plasma NE levels,[323-326] as well as enhanced NE responses to upright posture.[321] The increase in basal plasma NE in the elderly may, however, be associated with alterations in NE clearance rather than an increase in sympathetic nervous system activity.[327, 328] Men and women have similar basal plasma NE levels.[329] Cold exposure,[330] exercise,[297, 330, 331] extracellular fluid volume depletion,[332] surgery, and a variety of medical illnesses increase plasma concentrations substantially.[312, 331]

Epinephrine. Epinephrine in plasma is derived from the adrenal medulla. The basal plasma epinephrine concentration is of the order of 100 to 275 pmol/L (20 to 50 pg/mL).[292, 307, 311, 312] The metabolic clearance rate of epinephrine is higher than that of NE, approximately 90 mL/min/kg.[333] In contrast to NE, venous plasma epinephrine levels in the forearm are lower than those in the artery.[247, 308] This difference reflects significant metabolism of epinephrine by forearm tissues, principally by conjugation with sulfate,[247] and the fact that the forearm tissues do not release epinephrine into the circulation. Epinephrine levels increase minimally in response to upright posture;[292] moderately in response to cigarette smoking,[307, 334] mental stress, and exercise;[331] and markedly in response to hypoglycemia.[331] Epinephrine levels are not affected by age.[335]

Dopamine. Basal levels of free DA appear to be in the range of 165 to 330 pmol/L (25 to 50 pg/mL).[248, 336-338] Concentrations of conjugated DA are higher,[248] with the sulfate constituting about 98% of total plasma DA.[248] The

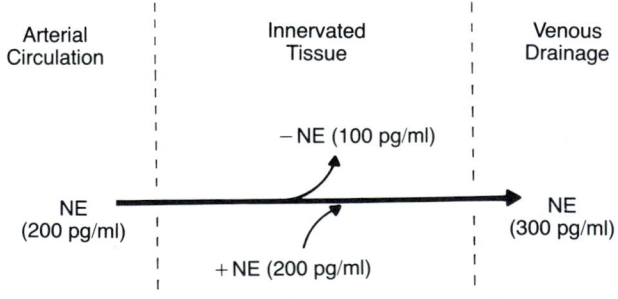

- = NE extracted (uptake in nerve endings and metabolism)
+ = NE added (release from nerve endings)

Figure 10–16. Relationship between arterial and venous NE levels. Note that the venous level depends on the amount of NE extracted as the innervated tissue is perfused with arterial blood, and on the amount of NE released from nerve endings in response to neuronal impulse traffic in the area served by the venous drainage. Only a fraction of released NE escapes reuptake and local metabolism and diffuses into the venous circulation. Both the extraction process and diffusion from the region of the synapse are influenced by blood flow. To convert NE values to nmol/L, multiply by 0.005911.

source of plasma DA is not known with certainty. In rats some DA originates from the adrenal medulla.[46] Treatments that destroy sympathetic nerves also diminish plasma DA levels, but these treatments may also affect specific dopaminergic nerves.[46] Decentralization (by spinal cord injury) has more of an effect on NE and epinephrine excretion than on the excretion of DA;[338] the significance of this observation is uncertain. Of potential interest and importance is the fact that dopa, the immediate precursor of DA, is present in substantial amounts in the plasma,[221, 222] with levels in the range of 7.6 nmol/L (1.5 ng/mL). The origin of circulating dopa is not known, but dopa may be an important source of circulating DA. The proper interpretation of plasma DA levels awaits more complete characterization of the peripheral dopaminergic system.

UTILITY OF PLASMA CATECHOLAMINE MEASUREMENTS. There are few clinical indications for the measurement of plasma catecholamines. As described later, the plasma NE level is a useful test of sympathetic nervous system function in patients with orthostatic hypotension; in patients with suspected pheochromocytoma, measurements of plasma catecholamines may be helpful, although even in this situation their usefulness is limited.

The major utility of plasma catecholamine measurements is in clinical investigation, especially in evaluation of the role of the sympathoadrenal system in the regulation of physiological and pathophysiological processes.

Assessment of Sympathoadrenal Activity

ADRENAL MEDULLA. Assessment of adrenomedullary function is relatively straightforward. Plasma levels of epinephrine accurately reflect medullary activity, although the short plasma half-time of disappearance and the technical difficulty in measuring basal levels of epinephrine, which are at the limit of sensitivity of most assays, limit clinical usefulness. Urinary epinephrine excretion provides an integrated assessment of adrenomedullary epinephrine secretion over time. An increase in plasma epinephrine level or urinary epinephrine excretion is, therefore, good evidence of adrenomedullary stimulation; the duration and intensity of such stimulation may be easily determined from urinary epinephrine excretion.

SYMPATHETIC NERVOUS SYSTEM. The assessment of sympathetic nervous system activity is more difficult. Several different strategies have been used to ascertain the functional state of the sympathetic nerves; none of these is fully satisfactory in terms of sensitivity or specificity.

Plasma and Urinary Norepinephrine Levels. NE is a neurotransmitter, not a circulating hormone. As described earlier, the plasma pool of NE is derived from the small portion of neurotransmitter that escapes reuptake and metabolism at adrenergic synapses throughout the body. This situation is reflected in the fact that, under most circumstances, plasma concentrations of NE are below the threshold for stimulation of adrenergic receptors.[320] Epinephrine, in distinction, stimulates adrenergic receptors at physiological levels,[333] as would be expected for a circulating hormone. Thus on theoretical grounds, the plasma NE level might be an insensitive index of sympathetic activity. This is indeed the case. When NE is infused, for example, the circulating level required to stimulate sympathetically mediated processes greatly exceeds the plasma NE level that occurs during physiological sympathetic stimulation of the same processes.[320, 339] Furthermore, when the sympathetic nervous system is activated, adrenergically mediated processes are stimulated before a rise in circulating NE.[307] Concomitant increases in NE clearance may accompany changes in sympathetic activity,[340] thereby lessening the impact of the change in sympathetic activity on the plasma

NE level. Thus the failure of the NE level to rise appreciably in a particular physiological setting does not exclude the possibility of significant sympathetic stimulation.

Peripheral plasma NE levels also lack specificity for two reasons. As noted earlier, the adrenal medulla secretes NE as well as epinephrine;[316–318] therefore, increases in plasma NE concentration do not always reflect the activity of the sympathetic nervous system.[319] An even greater problem is created by the fact that, as indicated in Figure 10–16, the venous NE concentration is influenced by processes in innervated tissues that result in the extraction of NE from arterial plasma and the addition of NE to the venous drainage. Extraction, which averages 30 to 50%, is highly dependent on blood flow,[315, 341, 342] whereas addition of NE is dependent on release from the sympathetic nerve endings. Because blood flow (and hence extraction)[315, 341] and sympathetic nervous system activity vary under different conditions, the venous level depends on both of these factors, as well as on the arterial level of NE perfusing the innervated tissue. The plasma NE in antecubital venous plasma is, therefore, derived principally from NE released in the tissues of the forearm (see Fig. 10–16).[343] Because the sympathetic outflow to various tissues or organ systems is not uniform,[313, 344–347] NE levels in venous plasma from the forearm may not adequately reflect changes in sympathetic activity in other organs or tissues.

Despite these limitations, antecubital venous plasma NE levels can provide a useful estimate of sympathetic activity.[348] Correspondence between sympathetic nerve impulse traffic and plasma NE concentration has been noted in humans,[349] and treatments that diminish peripheral sympathetic nerve activity reduce plasma NE concentration in animals[46, 350] and humans.[310] Furthermore, physiological manipulations that increase sympathetic nervous system activity cause increased plasma NE concentrations. The characteristic plasma NE response to upright posture is a good example (Fig. 10–17). The response indicates the functional reserve of the sympathetic nervous system; failure to increase plasma NE, if associated with a fall in blood pressure, indicates dysfunction of the sympathetic nervous system. The physiological processes that are altered reflect nerve activity and cannot be accounted for by the elevated circulating level of NE.[320]

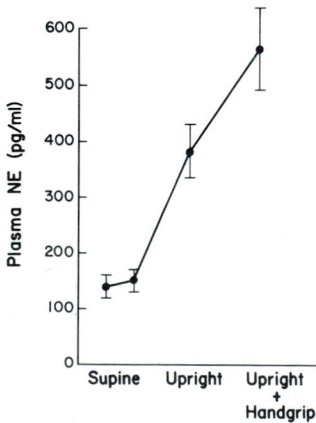

Figure 10–17. Plasma NE responses to upright posture and isometric hand grip. Mean values ± SEM are shown for eight normal male subjects; supine values represent basal plasma NE levels as defined in the text. The increase in the plasma NE concentration after 5 min of quiet upright standing reflects activation of the sympathetic nervous system in response to orthostatic stress. A further increment in plasma NE is demonstrable after 5 min more of standing upright with isometric hand grip exercise at one third maximal force. These maneuvers permit assessment of sympathetic nervous system reactivity. (From Landsberg L, Young JB. Sympathetic nervous system in hypertension. In: Brenner B, Stein JH, eds. Hypertension: Contemporary Issues in Nephrology. Vol 8. New York: Churchill Livingstone, 1981: 100–141.)

The same considerations apply to urinary NE excretion. Although a portion of NE in the urine originates from renal sympathetic nerves,[45, 218, 219, 351] the major fraction reflects the NE concentration in arterial blood.[268] Urinary NE excretion is a reasonable estimate of plasma NE concentrations integrated over time and, subject to the same limitations as the plasma NE level itself, reflects sympathetic nervous system activity.

Kinetic Techniques. In human subjects, kinetic techniques with infusion of radiolabeled NE may be more sensitive than simple plasma NE measurements in defining the overall level of sympathetic activity.[322, 340] These techniques, which permit calculation of a rate of appearance of NE in the circulation, correct for alterations in plasma NE clearance that limit changes in plasma NE levels. When coupled with venous catheterization of specific anatomical regions or organ systems, the kinetic method permits calculation of the contribution made by the various regions to the total pool of plasma NE.[352] For example, under normal circumstances the lungs contribute substantially to the circulating pool of NE.[352] In different pathophysiological states, such as hypertension, cirrhosis, or congestive heart failure, regional catheterization demonstrates a significantly increased NE release rate in heart and kidney while the total body release rate sampled at the forearm is either normal or increased to a lesser degree,[353] which is consistent with the known heterogeneity of sympathetic outflow. In an attempt to derive further information from tracer infusions by the application of kinetic modeling strategies,[354–356] various multicompartmental models are being evaluated; to date they have not provided more useful information than the noncompartmental analyses that assess the appearance rate and clearance of plasma NE. Despite their power, tracer NE infusions are too complicated for routine clinical use.

In animals, plasma catecholamine measurements are difficult to interpret because activation of the sympathoadrenal system accompanies acquisition of the plasma sample.[357, 358] Utilization of kinetic techniques in rodents, however, permits the measurement of NE turnover rate in individual sympathetically innervated tissues;[346, 359] because NE turnover rate is proportional to impulse traffic within the sympathetic nerves, such measurements provide specific, reasonably sensitive estimates of sympathetic activity independent of changes in adrenomedullary function.[360] Measurement of tissue NE turnover has not been applied to humans.

Plasma Dopamine β-Hydroxylase Activity and Chromogranin-A Levels. As described, DBH, chromogranin-A, and catecholamines are released in stoichiometric amounts during exocytosis.[361] The relatively long half-time in plasma[362] and lack of neuronal reuptake[362] raised hopes that plasma levels of DBH and chromogranin-A[363] might provide a useful measure of sympathetic activity. Although increases in plasma DBH activity and chromogranin-A levels can be demonstrated in situations that increase sympathetic activity, the changes are small in comparison with changes in plasma NE and the known degree of stimulation of the sympathetic nervous system.[363–366] These measurements are thus relatively insensitive indicators of sympathetic activity. Basal DBH levels appear to be an inherited trait[361, 367] without known physiological correlates and without major correlation with the plasma NE level. Because chromogranin-A is widely distributed in endocrine organs possessing secretory vesicles (as noted earlier), it has proved useful as an immunohistochemical marker for the identification of endocrine or neuroendocrine elements in the pathological analysis of tumor tissues. Chromogranin-A levels in plasma appear to be elevated in patients with a variety of neuroendocrine tumors,[368] which raises the possibility that these measurements

may be useful diagnostically.[109] Measurements of chromogranin-A in plasma are not generally available, however, and the clinical usefulness of these determinations has not been established.

Nerve Recordings. In both animals[344, 345] and humans,[349, 369, 370] impulse traffic from sympathetic nerves can be recorded directly. These techniques are invasive, technically demanding, and feasible only for short-term studies.

ADRENERGIC RECEPTORS

General Characteristics and Classification

The physiological changes that are induced by catecholamines are mediated via adrenergic receptors on the surface of effector cells.[371–374] Catecholamine uptake is not required for expression of the physiological effect. The interaction between catecholamine and receptor initiates events that begin in the cell membrane, progress to the cell interior, and culminate in a characteristic response. The relationship between receptor occupancy and the ultimate response of the effector tissue is at present incompletely understood (see Chapter 4), but important advances have begun to clarify the intracellular events within effector cells, as well as the molecular structure and function of the receptor itself.

Two major categories of physiological response to catecholamines or sympathetic nerve stimulation have been recognized since the early part of the 20th century. Although the different responses were originally classified as inhibitory or excitatory, their biological basis was not understood. In 1948 Ahlquist characterized the potency of a series of adrenergic agonists in eliciting various adrenergic responses.[375] On the basis of differential agonist potencies, he postulated two distinct adrenergic receptors, which he designated alpha and beta (Table 10–3). Ergot derivatives, which had been known to block many of the excitatory effects of catecholamines, appeared to block only alpha-receptor responses. The subsequent demonstration of a class of antagonists that selectively blocked beta-receptor responses provided support for the Ahlquist model.[376, 377]

Physiological responses have thus been characterized as alpha or beta on the basis of differential agonist potency and antagonism by specific alpha- or beta-receptor–blocking agents.[378, 379] The fact that many, if not all, beta-receptor responses are mediated by cAMP (see later) has provided another means of identifying beta-receptor responses; catecholamine responses that are mediated by increased intracellular cAMP are often presumed to be secondary to beta-receptor activation. Distinct subtypes of both alpha- and beta-adrenergic receptors exist.[380–382] These subtypes were defined initially on the basis of agonist potency, and the identification of relatively selective agonists and antagonists (see Table 10–3) has fortified the concept of distinct subtypes.

The application of radioligand-binding techniques to the identification of adrenergic receptors in specific tissues[371, 373, 383] also provides strong support for the existence of receptor subtypes within the alpha and beta classification. The radioligands bind to the adrenergic receptor in tissue homogenates or blood cells in vitro; the properties of the ligand binding and of its displacement in competition experiments permit characterization of the receptor.[372, 383] Radioligand techniques also provide information about receptor number and agonist affinity and have provided insight into agonist-receptor interactions and the relationship between receptor occupancy and physiological response. Ra-

TABLE 10–3. Adrenergic Receptors*

Alpha-Receptor

	Alpha-1	Alpha-2
Agonists	E, NE, PE, I	
Agonist potency	E ≥ NE > PE > I	
Antagonists	Phentolamine, phenoxybenzamine	
Subtypes	Alpha-1	Alpha-2
Selective agonists	Phenylephrine	Clonidine
	Methoxamine	α-Methyl-NE
Second messenger	Ca^{2+} ↑	cAMP ↓
	Phosphatidylinositol turnover (IP_3 ↑; DAG ↑)	
Representative responses	Vasoconstriction	Presynaptic NE release
	Intestinal relaxation	Platelet aggregation
	Uterine contraction	Vasoconstriction
	Pupillary dilation	
Selective antagonists	Prazosin	Yohimbine
	Terazosin	Rauwolscine

Beta-Receptor

	Beta-1	Beta-2
Agonist potency	I > E ≥ NE > PE	
Antagonists	Propranolol, alprenolol, nadolol, timolol	
Subtypes	Beta-1 (E = NE)	Beta-2 (E >> NE)
Selective agonists	Dobutamine	Metaproterenol
		Albuterol
		Terbutaline
		Isoetharine
		Ritodrine
Second messenger	cAMP ↑	cAMP ↑
Representative responses	Cardiac stimulation	Bronchodilation
	Lipolysis	Vasodilation
	Intestinal relaxation	Uterine relaxation
		Presynpatic NE release
Selective antagonists	Metoprolol	
	Atenolol	

*I, Isoproterenol; E, epinephrine; NE, noreprinephrine; PE, phenylephrine; IP_3, inositol 1,4,5-trisphosphate; DAG, 1,2-diacylglycerol.

dioligand techniques have also clarified some of the mechanisms that are involved in the alteration in sensitivity to catecholamines in different physiological states and as a consequence of drug treatment or disease.[372, 373, 383]

Structure-activity relationships for adrenergic agonists have been reasonably well worked out.[378, 382, 384] A three-point attachment of the catecholamine agonist to the receptor is postulated,[382] with primary interaction occurring at the amino group, the phenolic hydroxyl groups, and the benzylic hydroxyl group of the beta carbon atom on the side chain. The naturally occurring 3,4-dihydroxyphenolic groups, as well as the beta-hydroxyl group, confer maximal alpha- and beta-agonist activity; substituents on the amino group enhance beta-agonist activity, particularly of the beta-2 subtype.[384]

Dopaminergic receptors exist in certain peripheral vascular beds and visceral smooth muscle, as well as in the peripheral nervous system and the CNS, and are clearly distinct from alpha- and beta-receptors.

REGULATORY (G) PROTEINS AND SECOND MESSENGERS. The coupling of receptor occupancy with catecholamine-mediated response is now recognized to depend on specific membrane-bound regulatory proteins[385, 386] (see Chapter 4). Termed G (or N) *proteins* because they bind GTP (nucleotides), these proteins are activated by receptor-ligand interaction (Fig. 10–18). In the activated state they influence membrane-associated enzymes that alter the concentration of intracellular mediators (second messengers), thereby affecting the activity of enzymes and ion channels[385–387] that result in a tissue-specific effector response (see Fig. 10–18). Stimulatory and inhibitory G proteins that interact with adenylate cyclase have been identified and characterized.[385] The beta-adrenergic, the dopaminergic, and the alpha-2–adrenergic receptor subtypes influence effector responses by interacting with this G protein–adenylate cyclase system. The other alpha-adrenergic receptor subtype (alpha-1) also appears to interact with a G protein, as yet poorly characterized, that regulates the activity of phospholipase C (see Fig. 10–18). These membrane-associated enzymes alter the levels of cAMP, phospholipid metabolites (see later), and intracellular calcium, which act as second messengers that provoke effector responses by stimulating phosphorylation of enzymes and other intracellular proteins.

MOLECULAR STRUCTURE OF ADRENERGIC RECEPTORS. It has become clear that adrenergic receptors are membrane-associated proteins that interact with catecholamines on the extracellular side of the plasma membrane and with G proteins within the membrane. The receptor proteins, which are present in low abundance within the cell membrane, have been characterized by the application of powerful biochemical and recombinant DNA techniques.[388, 389] cDNAs for both subtypes of the alpha- and beta-adrenergic receptors have been isolated from mammalian tissues. The beta-1– and beta-2–receptors have been cloned from human placenta,[390, 391] whereas two subtypes of the human alpha-2–receptor have been cloned from platelets and kidney.[392, 393] The cDNA for the alpha-1–receptor has been cloned from cultured Syrian hamster smooth muscle cells.[394] The amino acid sequences of the various receptor proteins have been deduced from the cDNAs and have been compared. Structural analysis of these proteins reveals that the adrenergic receptors belong to a family of membrane proteins that also

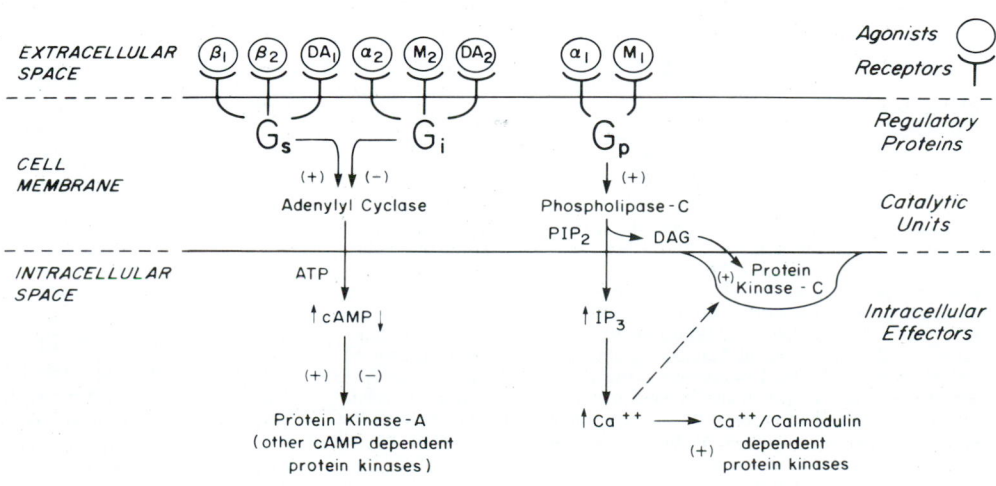

Figure 10–18. Relationships between autonomic agonists and receptors, membrane-bound regulatory proteins and enzymes, and intracellular effector systems. Adrenergic receptors are designated α and β, dopaminergic receptors DA, and muscarinic receptors M. Receptor subtypes are designated with subscripts 1 and 2. G refers to the GTP-associated regulatory protein that stimulates (s) or inhibits (i) adenylate (adenylyl) cyclase or stimulates phospholipase C (p). A (+) designates stimulation; a (−), inhibition. PIP_2, phosphatidylinositol 4,5-bisphosphate; DAG, diacylglycerol; IP_3, inositol 1,4,5-trisphosphate. See text for details. (From Landsberg L, Young JB. Physiology and pharmacology of the autonomic nervous system. In: Wilson JD, Braunwald E, Isselbacher KJ, eds. Harrison's Principles of Internal Medicine. 12th ed. New York: McGraw Hill, 1991: 380–392. Reproduced with permission of McGraw-Hill, Inc.)

includes the muscarinic acetylcholine receptors[395, 396] and the visual protein rhodopsin.[397] Distinct regions of the proteins in this family show remarkable sequence similarities; particularly well conserved are seven regions consisting of 20 to 28 hydrophobic amino acids,[397] possibly arranged as alpha helices, that form putative membrane-spanning domains. A schematic representation of the postulated topographical arrangement of this family of proteins within the cell membrane is presented in Figure 10–19.[397]

The critical structural features of this model, which appear to be common to many receptors coupled to G proteins, includes an extracellular NH₂ terminus and an intracellular COOH terminus connected by seven hydrophobic membrane-spanning domains that are connected by three extracellular and three cytoplasmic loops. Analysis of the structures of the various receptors in relation to known agonists[386, 397, 398] suggests that the membrane-spanning regions appear to be particularly important in determining ligand binding. Specificity for alpha-2– and beta-2–agonist binding apparently resides at the seventh membrane-spanning domain.[398] The size and configuration of the third cytoplasmic loop and the COOH terminus appear to be important in the relationship to specific G proteins; thus receptors coupling to G_i (see Fig. 10–18) have long third loops and short COOH termini, whereas the beta-adrenergic receptors that are coupled to G_s have relatively short third cytoplasmic loops and long COOH termini.[397] The alpha-1–receptor possesses the longest COOH terminus in the group and is most divergent in this area and in the third cytoplasmic loop.[394] In comparison, cytoplasmic loops 1 and 2 are reasonably well conserved throughout the whole group of

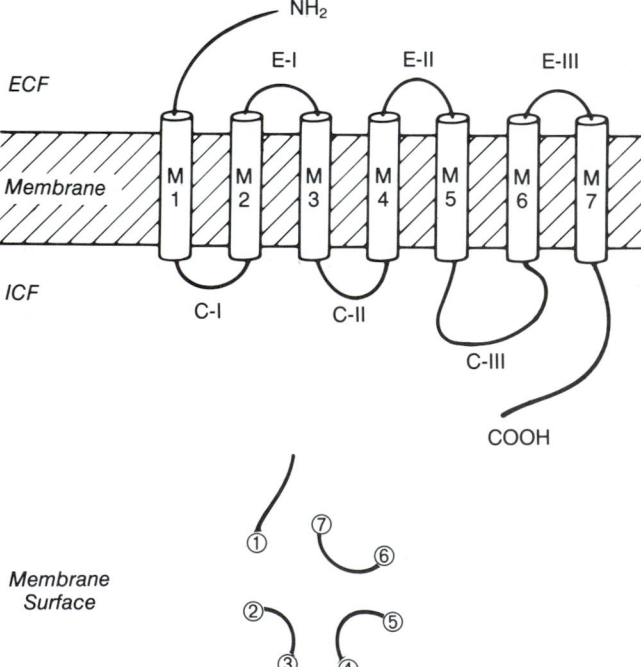

Figure 10–19. Proposed structure of prototypical adrenergic receptor as deduced from primary amino acid sequences. The receptor is composed of a single protein chain with an extracellular (ECF) hydrophilic NH₂ terminus, seven hydrophobic membrane-spanning domains (M1 to M7) connected by three extracellular loops (E-I to E-III), three cytoplasmic loops (C-I to C-III), and an intracellular (ICF) COOH terminus. The alpha- and beta-adrenergic receptors, including subtypes, appear to fit this general model. Variations in structure at the seventh membrane-spanning domain, the third cytoplasmic loop, and the COOH terminus have been shown to be important in agonist binding and in the relationship to specific G proteins as described in the text. The top portion of the figure shows the structure longitudinally; however, the three-dimensional structure within the cell membrane may be more compact, a possible arrangement of the membrane-spanning domains, extracellular loops, and NH₂ terminus as seen from the extracellular membrane surface, shown in the bottom portion of the figure.

related receptors.[386] Other structural features that are shared among the members of this family include potential sites of glycosylation near the NH₂ terminus and potential sites for phosphorylation on the cytoplasmic domains.[397]

Alpha-Adrenergic Receptors

AGONISTS AND ANTAGONISTS. Alpha-adrenergic receptors mediate a variety of responses including vasoconstriction (see Table 10–3). Epinephrine and NE are potent nonselective agonists of the alpha-receptor; phentolamine and phenoxybenzamine are nonselective alpha-receptor antagonists.[156] The alpha-1 subtype is the postsynaptic receptor that mediates a wide variety of alpha effects, most prominently involving smooth muscle. Selective alpha-1–agonists include the synthetic sympathomimetic amines phenylephrine and methoxamine.[156] At low concentrations, phenoxybenzamine is relatively selective for the alpha-1–receptor. Prazosin is a selective alpha-1–antagonist[399, 400] that is useful in the treatment of hypertension. The alpha-2–receptor is located on presynaptic sympathetic neurons,[156, 381] on cholinergic neurons within the gut,[156] on CNS neurons involved in the regulation of cardiovascular function,[4] on platelets,[401, 402] and on blood vessels. The alpha-2–receptor mediates inhibition of NE release from adrenergic neurons, inhibition of acetylcholine release from cholinergic neurons, potentiation of the baroreceptor vasodepressor response mediated via central regulatory neurons, platelet aggregation, and vasoconstriction. The relationship between the vascular effects of alpha-1– and alpha-2–receptors is considered later, along with the circulatory effects of catecholamines. Differences in selectivity between the agonist and the antagonist for alpha-1– and alpha-2–receptors may be relatively great, approaching three to four orders of magnitude.[403] This difference is considerably greater than the differences in selectivity that are noted between the subtypes of the beta-receptor. Clonidine and α-methylnorepinephrine are relatively selective alpha-2–agonists; the central inhibition of sympathetic outflow is the basis for the use of agents in the treatment of hypertension (α-methylnorepinephrine is derived in vivo from α-methyldopa). Yohimbine is a specific alpha-2–antagonist.

A variety of radioligands have been used as probes for the alpha-receptor and its subtypes.[371, 374] As with the polypeptide hormones, exposure of alpha-receptors to agonist diminishes the receptor number, thereby contributing to desensitization or tachyphylaxis.[401]

ALPHA-RECEPTOR SIGNAL TRANSDUCTION. The alpha-1– and alpha-2–receptors use different mechanisms for coupling receptor occupancy with cellular response. Both receptors relate to G proteins and regulate membrane-associated enzyme systems that lead to the generation of second messengers and ultimately to the regulation of intracellular enzyme systems and membrane channels.

The Alpha-1–Receptor. The induction of alpha-1–mediated responses in effector tissues has been recognized for some time to involve both calcium mobilization and membrane phospholipids, particularly phosphatidylinositol. Evidence has clarified considerably the relationship between alpha-1–adrenergic stimulation and these mediators, although several important aspects of this transducing system remain to be elucidated.[385, 403–409] Alpha-1–agonist binding appears to be coupled to a G protein that activates phospholipase C (see Fig. 10–18). This G protein, which awaits further characterization, has been tentatively designated G_p. Phospholipase C activation catalyzes the hydrolysis of membrane phospholipids, particularly phosphatidylinositol 4,5-bisphosphate (PIP_2), with the formation of inositol 1,4,5-trisphosphate (IP_3) and 1,2-diacylglycerol (DAG). Both IP_3

and DAG act as second messengers: IP_3 rapidly increases the cytosolic calcium concentration; DAG activates protein kinase C (see Fig. 10–18). The initial increase in cytosolic free calcium depends on mobilization of calcium from intracellular stores. The endoplasmic or sarcoplasmic reticulum appears to be the major intracellular source of calcium. The mechanisms by which IP_3 mobilizes calcium is uncertain but appears to involve a specific receptor and requires potassium.[405] In some tissues alpha-1–adrenergic responses depend, in whole or in part, on calcium influx from the extracellular fluid. Because much of the calcium that is mobilized initially in response to alpha-1–adrenergic stimulation is pumped out of the cell, uptake of calcium from the extracellular fluid is required both for support of the effector response in the presence of continued agonist stimulation and for repletion of the depleted intracellular stores. The mechanisms that are involved in coupling calcium influx with alpha-1–adrenergic stimulation remain uncertain.

DAG, the other second messenger that is produced by the action of phospholipase C on membrane phospholipids, remains associated with the plasma membrane and activates protein kinase C. Protein kinase C is also stimulated by calcium so that the two second messengers that are generated by alpha-1–agonist responses have a synergistic effect on this enzyme.[405]

The tissue-specific responses to alpha-1–adrenergic stimulation depend on the changes that are induced in regulatory enzymes and the cell membrane by changes in calcium and protein kinase C activation. Many of these responses appear to involve enzyme phosphorylation mediated by calcium/calmodulin-dependent protein kinases.[410] Phosphorylase kinase and myosin light chain kinase are examples of enzymes that are activated by calcium/calmodulin. Protein kinase C stimulates the phosphorylation of a different set of substrates that are less well characterized.[410] This enzyme may also be involved in regulating calcium influx and the hydrolysis of membrane phospholipids.[405, 410]

The Alpha-2–Receptor. Alpha-2–mediated responses in effector tissues are related, at least in part, to the inhibition of adenylate cyclase activity (see Fig. 10–18). Agonist occupancy of the alpha-2–receptor is associated with "activation" of the inhibitory G protein (G_i) in the inner plasma membrane.[385] It has also been hypothesized that subunits of G_i contribute to the inhibition of adenylate cyclase indirectly by antagonizing the activation of this enzyme by G_s.[385]

Other studies have indicated, however, that inhibition of adenylate cyclase cannot adequately account for all the intracellular effects of alpha-2–adrenergic stimulation.[411] Alpha-2–mediated effects on effector cell secretion or contraction appear to involve additional signaling mechanisms.[411] Evidence has been developed that alterations in potassium and calcium flux and acceleration of sodium-hydrogen exchange may be involved as additional cellular mediators of alpha-2–receptor stimulation.[411]

Beta-Adrenergic Receptors

AGONISTS AND ANTAGONISTS. Beta-receptors mediate cardiac stimulation, bronchodilation, and vasodilation (see Table 10–3). Subtypes of the beta-receptor are designated beta-1 and beta-2. cDNAs for beta-1– and beta-2–adrenergic receptors have been isolated from human placenta.[390, 391] Homology between the beta-1– and beta-2–adrenergic receptors is only 54%, greatest in the membrane-spanning domains and the first two cytoplasmic loops. Both receptors are products of separate genes.[390]

Epinephrine and the synthetic sympathomimetic amine isoproterenol are nonselective beta-agonists. Nonselective beta-antagonists include propranolol, alprenolol, nadolol, and timolol. NE is a potent agonist of the beta-1–receptor (equivalent to epinephrine) but is a weak agonist of the beta-2–receptor. The beta-1–receptor mediates cardiac stimulation and lipolysis; the beta-2–receptor mediates bronchodilation, vasodilation, and prejunctional stimulation of NE release from sympathetic neurons. Synthetic congeners with selective agonist or antagonist activity for the beta-1– and beta-2–receptor subtypes are given in Table 10–3. This selectivity is relative and substantially less than that for the corresponding alpha-1 and alpha-2 agents. Thus when high doses of these compounds are used therapeutically, the relative selectivity is overcome, and effects on both beta-1– and beta-2–receptors are encountered; nonetheless, at less than maximal dosages, the use of selective agonists and antagonists does have clinical utility.

Clinically Relevant Pharmacological Properties of Beta-Receptor Antagonists. Beta-blockers are widely used in clinical medicine for a variety of indications, including angina pectoris, hypertension, cardiac arrhythmias, hyperthyroidism, pheochromocytoma, hypertrophic cardiomyopathy, aortic dissection, migraine, essential tremor, and, prophylactically, after myocardial infarction. Eight beta-blocking agents are currently approved for use in the United States; although the various agents have different pharmacological properties that may be exploited to clinical advantage, the efficacy in the various indications is derived predominantly from blockade of beta-adrenergic receptors. The currently available beta-blockers are given in Table 10–4, along with a summary of distinguishing pharmacological characteristics including beta-1 selectivity, lipid and water solubility, and partial agonist activity. Some of the beta-blockers (propranolol, pindolol, acebutolol) possess membrane-stabilizing local anesthetic properties, which does not appear to contribute to efficacy or affect safety. Esmolol is rapidly metabolized because of hydrolysis of an ester linkage; it is available for intravenous use only. An additional agent, labetalol, is a combined alpha- and beta-blocking agent that is approved for the treatment of hypertension. It produces selective alpha-1–blockade and nonselective beta-blockade, with relatively greater potency on the beta-receptor.

TABLE 10–4. Pharmacology and Pharmacokinetics of Beta-Blockers

Agent	Selectivity	Lipid and Water Solubility	Partial Agonist	Half-Life (h)	Dosage Interval*
Acebutolol	Beta-1	Hydrophilic	Yes	3–4	qd
Atenolol	Beta-1	Hydrophilic	No	6–7	qd
Carteolol	Nonselective	Hydrophilic	Yes	5–6	qd
Esmolol	Beta-1	Hydrophilic	No	9 min	prn
Metoprolol	Beta-1	Lipophilic	No	3–7	qd
Nadolol	Nonselective	Hydrophilic	No	20–24	qd
Penbutolol	Nonselective	Lipophilic	Yes	5	qd
Pindolol	Nonselective	Lipophilic	Yes	3–4	bid
Propranolol	Nonselective	Lipophilic	No	4	bid
Timolol	Nonselective	Lipophilic	No	4–5	bid

*Depends on indication. Some indications may require more frequent dosing.

Pharmacological characteristics that may contribute to clinical utility include beta-1 selectivity, lipid solubility, and partial agonist activity (see Table 10–4). Beta-1–selective antagonists should theoretically produce less bronchoconstriction and vasoconstriction and have less of an impact on hepatic glucose output because bronchodilation, vasodilation, glycogenolysis, and gluconeogenesis are mediated principally by the beta-2–receptor subtype. Because selectivity between the beta-1 and beta-2 subtypes is only relative, the advantage of beta-1–selective agonists is small and may not apply at clinically relevant dosages. In recognition of these limitations, if the clinical situation dictates the need for beta-blockade in a patient with obstructive lung disease, low dosage with a beta-1–selective antagonist is a reasonable way to proceed. It is important to remember, however, that at full therapeutic doses, and perhaps even at usual therapeutic doses, selectivity is lost.[412]

The degree of lipid solubility influences the distribution and metabolism of beta-blockers. The lipophilic agents are readily absorbed from the gut, are metabolized in the liver, have large volumes of distribution, and penetrate the CNS. The hydrophilic agents are less well absorbed, are excreted in urine without extensive metabolism, and have relatively long half-lives in plasma that permit a once-daily dosage schedule. Renal failure prolongs the action of the hydrophilic group, whereas hepatic failure may prolong the half-life of the lipophilic agents, which provides a rationale for usage in the appropriate clinical setting on the basis of this property. CNS side effects may be more common in the lipophilic group, which crosses the blood-brain barrier more readily, but these side effects have been noted in the hydrophilic group as well.

Some beta-blocking agents possess partial agonist activity. These agents produce low-level stimulation of the adrenergic receptor but antagonize the effects of endogenous catecholamines.[412] As a consequence they may have less of an effect on resting heart rate than agents without agonist activity. This property may be useful when clinically significant bradycardia limits treatment in patients with low resting heart rates. Partial agonist activity may also be associated with a decrease in peripheral resistance rather than the increase that may be observed with antagonists that do not possess partial agonist activity. It has not been established that partial agonist activity avoids myocardial depression, clinically significant bronchospasm, or peripheral vascular complications.[412] Partial agonist activity may avoid the rebound increase in sensitivity to catecholamines that has been described after withdrawal of beta-blockers.[412] On theoretical grounds partial agonist activity would be undesirable in the treatment of patients with thyrotoxicosis, hypertrophic cardiomyopathy, and aortic dissection.

Selective Agonists. Dobutamine,[413, 414] an amine with modest selectivity for the beta-1–receptor, is effective in the treatment of cardiogenic shock. Similarly, agonists with selectivity for the beta-2–receptor (see Table 10–3) can cause bronchodilation at low doses with little cardiac stimulation. Other beta-2–agonists have been used in the treatment of premature labor.[415]

A variety of radioligand probes have been used in the study of the beta-receptor and its subtypes,[371, 383] which has permitted calculation of beta-receptor number and affinity. Evidence has been produced indicating a relationship between beta-adrenergic receptor density in human myocardium and that in circulating lymphocytes,[416, 417] which implies that meaningful measurements of beta-adrenergic receptors may be made with peripheral blood. Beta-2–adrenergic receptors have also been characterized in human skeletal muscle obtained by needle biopsy.[418] Exposure of beta-adrenergic receptors to agonist diminishes the receptor number on effector cells, thereby contributing to the phenomenon of desensitization.[371, 373, 383, 419–422]

BETA-RECEPTOR SIGNAL TRANSDUCTION. Beta-1– and beta-2–receptor agonists stimulate adenylate cyclase and increase intracellular cAMP, the latter serving as the second messenger (see Fig. 10–18).[423] The initial event is attachment of the agonist to the receptor. The agonist-receptor interaction induces a conformational change in the receptor that permits further interaction with the membrane-associated regulatory protein G_s.[385] Coupling of the receptor and G_s activates the catalytic portion of adenylate cyclase, which results in the formation of cAMP.[371] The increase in intracellular cAMP activates protein kinase A and other cAMP-dependent protein kinases that catalyze the phosphorylation of a variety of proteins.[372] Alterations in the functional state of these proteins generates the beta-receptor response that is characteristic of the effector tissue. Beta-receptor antagonists, on the other hand, with the exception of those with partial agonist activity, bind to the receptor but do not induce receptor interaction with the nucleotide regulatory protein[371] and therefore do not activate adenylate cyclase. As a consequence, agonist-receptor interaction is inhibited and physiological response is blocked.

Alterations in Adrenergic Receptor Number and Function

GENERAL CONSIDERATIONS: PHYSIOLOGICAL RESPONSES TO ADRENERGIC STIMULATION. The responsiveness of peripheral effector tissues to adrenergic stimulation may be modified substantially by alterations in temperature, chemical composition of the plasma, and circulating levels of various hormones. These changes in responsiveness may originate (1) at the adrenergic nerve terminals, where a variety of factors influence the amount of neurotransmitter that is released in response to nerve impulses[152] (prejunctional modulation); (2) at the adrenergic receptor, where alterations in receptor number or affinity for agonist may occur; or (3) at postreceptor sites so that the relationship between receptor occupancy and physiological response is modified. Alterations in adrenergic receptor number have been noted in various physiological and pathophysiological states.[371, 373, 383] In some of these states, a change in receptor number appears to account for the altered sensitivity to catecholamines. The term *homologous regulation* refers to alterations in the adrenergic receptor complex that are induced by adrenergic agonists; the term *heterologous regulation* designates alterations in the adrenergic receptor complex that are caused by environmental changes or other mediators that do not involve the usual agonist.[373, 419]

HOMOLOGOUS REGULATION: EFFECT OF ADRENERGIC AGONISTS. *Down-Regulation and Desensitization.* Desensitization or tachyphylaxis is the phenomenon whereby prolonged exposure of an effector tissue to an agonist results in progressive diminution in response. Homologous desensitization is agonist specific; it refers to the diminished effector response to adrenergic agonists that is engendered by prior exposure to catecholamines.[424] Responses to other agonists that affect the same intracellular effector systems are not diminished. Heterologous desensitization, in contrast, refers to a generalized attenuation of effector response.[424] Exposure of both alpha- and beta-adrenergic receptors to agonists diminishes adrenergic receptor numbers as calculated from ligand-binding experiments. Because a change in receptor number appears to correlate with the loss of physiological response, it is a reasonable presumption that agonist-induced decrease in receptor number, which is often referred to as *down-regulation*, contributes to desensitization.[383, 420] For the beta-receptor, down-regulation involves a partially reversible sequestration of the receptor[371, 419] in frog erythrocytes,[371, 425] other isolated cell systems,[419] and human monocytes.[426]

The molecular mechanisms that are involved in desensitization are complex and incompletely understood. Several different mechanisms may operate, and the importance of each may differ in different tissues. Current evidence indicates that receptor phosphorylation is associated with desensitization of adrenergic receptors.[397, 427] Structural analysis of the beta-adrenergic receptor, as noted earlier, revealed multiple potential sites of phosphorylation at the COOH terminus and the third cytoplasmic loop.[397] A specific beta-adrenergic receptor kinase has been identified and purified,[427] which is unique in catalyzing the phosphorylation of the receptor only when occupied by agonists.[427] Phosphorylation is thought to uncouple the receptor from the G protein–adenylate cyclase complex followed by sequestration of the receptor so that it is no longer available to agonists at the cell surface. The anatomical location of the sequestered receptor is uncertain and may be within the plasma membrane or the cell interior.[424] Receptors may be regenerated from the sequestered compartment by dephosphorylation and may be cycled back to functionally available sites within the plasma membrane.[427] Desensitization of the alpha-1–receptor appears to involve receptor phosphorylation and sequestration as well.[428]

Homologous desensitization, therefore, involves the receptor but is not thought to involve the regulatory G proteins or adenylate cyclase.[429] Heterologous desensitization, on the other hand, may involve the regulatory G proteins and the cyclase system itself. This difference would explain the attenuation of adrenergic responses that is induced by nonadrenergic agonists or mediators. Heterologous desensitization may involve phosphorylation of components of the effector system by protein kinase C or other cAMP-dependent protein kinases.[427] It is interesting that glucocorticoid treatment restores homologously desensitized lymphocyte beta-receptors promptly in humans.[430, 431]

An increase in adrenergic receptor numbers or increased efficacy of coupling to adenylate cyclase, along with supersensitivity to the effects of catecholamines, has been demonstrated after treatments that diminish the concentration of agonists.[373, 383] This supersensitization may be involved in the enhanced sensitivity to beta-adrenergic agonists that is noted after propranolol withdrawal.[432–434]

Physiological Significance of Alterations in Adrenergic Receptor Number: Spare Receptors. Because a maximal physiological response can be demonstrated when only a small portion of beta-receptors are occupied,[419, 435] the significance of alterations in the number of adrenergic receptors has been questioned. Interactions of agonist and receptor, however, follow the law of mass action; increased numbers of adrenergic receptors increase the likelihood of agonist-receptor interaction and thus result in a shift in dose-response relationship to the left, which indicates an increase in sensitivity.[373] Thus, the presence of "spare" receptors (or *receptor reserve*) implies that alterations in receptor number will be translated into alterations in sensitivity to agonist. In fact, an alteration in receptor number correlates with changes in sensitivity to catecholamines in a wide variety of tissues, including arteries and veins.[436] A larger question relates to the significance of alterations in receptor number in physiological as opposed to pharmacological situations. The fact that adrenergic receptor density bears an inverse relationship to catecholamine production supports the supposition that alterations in adrenergic receptor number occur under physiological as well as pharmacological conditions.[401, 420] It must be emphasized, however, that the alteration in receptor number is only one among many factors that determine sensitivity of effector tissues to catecholamines. Changes in sensitivity to the vasoconstrictor effects of NE appear to reflect, for example, alterations in the affinity of the alpha-receptor for its agonist.[437] The efficiency of coupling receptor occupancy with intracellular effector systems and the independent effect of other agonists and environmental factors on intracellular effector systems play an important role as well.

HETEROLOGOUS REGULATION: EFFECTS OF HORMONES AND OTHER MEDIATORS. Factors other than adrenergic agonists alter adrenergic receptor function and sensitivity to catecholamines. At low environmental temperatures alpha-adrenergic responses are potentiated,[438–440] an effect that may be mediated by changes in alpha-adrenergic receptor affinity for agonist.[440] Hypoxia has been shown to decrease beta-adrenergic receptor density in cultured heart cells.[441] Acute and chronic increases in cardiac afterload in guinea pigs and dogs diminishes beta-receptor number and coupling, respectively.[417, 442] Decreased adrenergic responsiveness with aging may be secondary to altered coupling of adrenergic receptor occupancy with the cellular response.[443–445]

A variety of hormones affect adrenergic responsiveness, some of which may be mediated by alterations in adrenergic receptors. Thyroid hormones potentiate beta- and diminish alpha-adrenergic responses. The mechanisms are complex but involve alterations in both receptor density and coupling (discussed in relation to hyperthyroidism later). Estrogen increases and progesterone decreases the number of alpha-receptors in rabbit uterus.[446, 447] During pregnancy in the guinea pig, myometrial alpha-receptor density increases along with uterine growth.[448] In human pregnancy the density of beta-adrenergic receptors decreases near term. This change is associated with decreased receptor coupling to adenylate cyclase.[449] These findings may explain, in part, the change in sensitivity of myometrium to catecholamines in different physiological states. Estrogens also increase the affinity of alpha-1–adrenergic receptors on rat vasculature for catecholamines;[450] the number of alpha-2–adrenergic receptors on platelets, in contrast, is reduced by estrogen treatment.[451] Glucocorticoids increase cAMP accumulation in isolated cell systems by an effect that may involve beta-receptors and G_s.[452] Autoantibodies to beta-adrenergic receptors may modify adrenergic responsiveness in patients with asthma and other allergic conditions.[453–455]

Dopaminergic Receptors

Although DA is a weak agonist for both alpha- and beta-adrenergic receptors, distinct dopaminergic receptors are present in several peripheral tissues[456, 457] and mediate specific DA responses.[458, 459] There appear to be two major types of dopaminergic receptor; subtypes within each major designation may exist as well.[460–465] By convention the CNS dopaminergic receptors have been classified D_1 and D_2 and the peripheral dopaminergic receptors have been classified DA_1 and DA_2.[461, 462] The relationship between the central and peripheral dopaminergic receptors is uncertain because agonist and antagonist potencies may differ within the CNS and on peripheral tissues.[462] Both DA_1 and D_1 appear to be coupled to adenylate cyclase via the G_s-regulatory protein, whereas many, if not all, DA_2 and D_2 responses inhibit adenylate cyclase via an interaction with G_i[461, 462] (see Fig. 10–18). DA is a potent agonist for both receptor subtypes. The DA_1 receptor mediates vasodilation in renal, mesenteric, coronary, and cerebral vascular beds. Fenoldopam is an investigational agonist that is selective for the DA_1 receptor; Sch 23390 and Sch 23982 are specific experimental DA_1 antagonists. The DA_2 receptor inhibits transmission in the sympathetic ganglia, presynaptically inhibits NE release from the sympathetic nerve endings, inhibits prolactin release from the pituitary, and evokes emesis. Selective agonists for the DA_2 receptor include bromocriptine, lergotrile, and apomorphine; selective DA_2 antagonists include butyrophenones such as haloperidol and domperidone and the benzamide sulpiride. Although DA may affect gut motility, particularly the activity of the lower esophageal sphincter, these dopaminergic responses have not been characterized with regard to receptor type.[462]

PHYSIOLOGY AND PATHOPHYSIOLOGY OF THE SYMPATHOADRENAL SYSTEM

Regulation of Sympathoadrenal Activity

CENTRAL NEURAL CONTROL. Catecholamine release at the sympathetic nerve endings and the adrenal medulla is the direct consequence of a downward flow of impulses from sympathetic centers within the CNS (see Fig. 10–2). The functional state of these centers is governed by many factors: (1) the intrinsic activity of the specific hypothalamic and brain stem nuclei that constitute the sympathetic centers and that initiate the downward flow of impulses; (2) other regions in the brain stem, hypothalamus, limbic lobe, and cortex that send projections to the sympathetic centers; (3) visceral and somatic afferents that directly (or indirectly via these other regions) relay information from the periphery to coordinate the activity of the sympathetic centers with environmental factors; and (4) the characteristics of the extracellular fluid, including the concentrations of electrolytes, substrates, and hormones, as well as temperature and tonicity, all of which may influence both the sympathetic centers and the related regions in the CNS.

Of the neural afferent pathways that are involved in regulation of sympathetic activity, only the baroreceptor reflex has been well characterized. The inhibition of sympathetic activity that follows baroreceptor stimulation by a rise in blood pressure is mediated by neurons in the nucleus of the tractus solitarius[466] and involves a central adrenergic pathway with an alpha-receptor synapse.[467] The organization of this neural response is such that sympathetic outflow is tonically inhibited by afferent impulse traffic; sympathetic activation produced by a fall in blood pressure reflects a diminished pressure signal from the baroreceptor and disinhibition of central sympathetic neurons. Similarly, afferent impulses from low-pressure volume sensors in the heart and great veins are carried by fibers in the vagus nerve and also inhibit sympathetic activity.[468, 469] Additional afferent neural signals that are potentially involved in sympathoadrenal regulation include baroreceptors in other organs (e.g., adrenal gland);[470] chemoreceptors in aortic arch, carotid body, liver, muscle, and kidney;[471–473] and cutaneous and visceral pain and temperature sensors. The participation of the sympathetic nervous system and the adrenal medulla in the control of vegetative functions undoubtedly requires a vast array of complex afferent pathways that are neither clearly identified nor well defined.

The composition of the extracellular fluid also affects sympathoadrenal activity. Low levels of metabolic fuels, such as glucose and oxygen, stimulate the sympathoadrenal system and were among the first recognized stimuli for adrenomedullary secretion. Alterations in the ionic constituents of the plasma and changes in various hormones and peptides influence the functional state of sympathetic nerves and adrenal medulla. Thus a complex series of neural reflexes and humoral feedback loops interact with central sympathetic centers to regulate sympathoadrenal outflow.

GENERALIZED VERSUS DISCRIMINANT RESPONSES. In its fully developed form, generalized or global sympathoadrenal activation results in the fight-or-flight response described by Cannon. The anatomical organization of the sympathoadrenal system is entirely consonant with the view that generalized responses represent an important aspect of sympathoadrenal function. Amplification of sympathetic outflow occurs at the level of the sympathetic ganglia where each preganglionic fiber activates several postganglionic neurons, which suggests widespread dispersion of descending nerve impulse traffic. Furthermore, the release of catecholamines from the adrenal medulla into the circulation ensures systemic distribution of the neurohumoral signal. However, the components of the sympathoadrenal system are differentially affected by a variety of physiological stimuli. Not only is sympathetic outflow distributed nonhomogeneously, but the activity of postganglionic sympathetic neurons is frequently dissociated from that of the adrenal medulla.

In animals, differential changes in impulse traffic over sympathetic nerves supplying heart, kidney, spleen, and stomach have been noted in response to baroreceptor stimulation.[344, 474] Renal and gastric sympathetic activity is affected similarly by hypoxia but not by changes in blood pressure, whereas renal and adrenal nerve activity responds similarly to changes in blood pressure but not to hypoglycemia.[345, 474, 475] In addition, after spinal cord heating and cooling, opposite changes in the rate of neuronal discharge occur in cutaneous and splenic sympathetic fibers.[476] The capacity for such discrete responses probably derives from the presence within the CNS of separate groupings of neurons for each target tissue.[1] Thus the sympathetic nervous system is capable of selectively regulating diverse vegetative functions.

RELATIONSHIP BETWEEN SYMPATHETIC NERVOUS SYSTEM AND ADRENAL MEDULLA. The relationship between the two limbs of the sympathoadrenal system is complex. The traditional view, implicit in the work of Cannon, envisages the sympathetic nervous system and the adrenal medulla working in tandem, with circulating catecholamines from the adrenal medulla supporting the effects of the sympathetic nerves. This view is consistent with the pattern of sympathoadrenal involvement in different conditions. During exposure to cold or physical exercise, for example, the initial response is predominantly one of sympathetic stimulation, but as the severity of the cold or the degree and duration of exertion increase, the secretion of adrenomedullary catecholamines progressively increases.[477, 478] A supportive role for the adrenal medulla is consistent with the fact that enhancement of adrenomedullary secretion occurs if sympathetic function is diminished by drugs, surgery, or fasting.[479–482]

In other circumstances, however, the relationship between the sympathetic nervous system and the adrenal medulla is more complex. Studies with laboratory animals in which more specific techniques were used to evaluate the sympathetic nervous system have indicated that with hypoglycemia, acute hypoxia of a moderate degree, and acute ischemia, suppression of sympathetic activity occurs in association with adrenomedullary stimulation.[483] A similar dissociation of sympathetic and adrenomedullary function occurs during fasting and after vasovagal syncope in humans.[483] One possible rationale for such a pattern of sympathoadrenal response is that the reduction in sympathetic activity lowers the rate of energy utilization, while the increase in adrenomedullary secretion sustains essential catecholamine-dependent processes at a lower net energy cost.

The relative importance of the two limbs of the sympathoadrenal system in different physiological situations in humans is difficult to assess. Most attempts to differentiate sympathetic from adrenomedullary responses have relied on measurements of NE and epinephrine in urine or plasma.[331, 484-487] Because the adrenal medulla, when stimulated, may release substantial quantities of NE, reliance on NE determinations as the sole index of sympathetic activity undoubtedly exaggerates the role of the sympathetic nervous system in some circumstances. Consequently, the precise contributions of sympathetic nerves and the adrenal medulla to the regulation of catecholamine-dependent processes are frequently not well defined.

General Features of Physiological Regulation by Sympathoadrenal System

BASAL SYMPATHOADRENAL ACTIVITY. Although the contributions of the sympathoadrenal system to physiological regulation are most often considered in relation to acute responses to internal or external stimuli such as hypoglycemia or upright posture, the chronic level of sympathoadrenal activity is also important. Unfortunately, sustained alterations in the functional level of sympathoadrenal activity are more difficult to document than those induced acutely. For example, the involvement of catecholamine release in the acute defense of blood pressure on standing or in the pressor reactions to clonidine withdrawal is readily demonstrable, whereas the potential role of a sustained elevation in sympathoadrenal activity in essential hypertension is still uncertain.

SPEED AND ANTICIPATION: IMMEDIATE RESPONSE. Because the sympathoadrenal system is an efferent limb of the nervous system, rapid onset and quick termination of the effects of released catecholamines are not surprising. Catecholamine-mediated events take place in seconds compared with the minutes, hours, or days that characterize the time course of action of other hormones. Connections between the cerebral cortex and the sympathetic centers that regulate sympathoadrenal outflow provide another measure of control. Anticipation of a particular activity, e.g., exercise, may activate the sympathoadrenal system before the exercise begins, thereby stimulating a variety of catecholamine-responsive processes in advance. Appropriate physiological adjustments can thus be initiated before alterations in the internal environment would themselves evoke a response.

DIRECT AND INDIRECT EFFECTS: INTEGRATED RESPONSE. Most catecholamine-mediated responses have both direct and indirect components. Direct effects are mediated by interaction of catecholamines and adrenergic receptors in a particular effector tissue; indirect effects involve alterations in (1) secretion of other hormones that regulate the process under study; (2) delivery of the substrate that is necessary for the process under observation; or (3) local distribution of blood flow. For example, catecholamines stimulate hepatic glucose output directly via glycogenolysis. They also inhibit insulin release and stimulate glucagon secretion, thereby activating the liver for gluconeogenesis. Finally, they may mobilize lactate and glycerol from peripheral tissues as substrates for gluconeogenesis. These indirect actions of catecholamines create the necessary hormonal and substrate milieu to favor hepatic glucose production. Circulatory adjustments that are induced by catecholamines serve to distribute the glucose that is released from the liver to tissues of greatest need. Similarly, the sympathoadrenal contribution to sodium excretion by the kidney involves not only direct stimulation of tubular sodium reabsorption, but also (1) activation of the angiotensin-aldosterone system by enhanced renin secretion and (2) sympathetically mediated redistribution of blood flow within the kidney from cortical to the more efficient juxtamedullary nephrons, changes that also foster sodium reabsorption. As a general rule, the vascular, metabolic, and hormonal effects of catecholamines reinforce one another.

Physiological Effects of Catecholamines

GENERAL CONSIDERATIONS. Catecholamines influence virtually all tissues and many functions. In most instances, however, catecholamines are not the sole or exclusive regulators; they participate with other hormonal and neuronal systems in regulation of a multitude of diverse physiological processes, thus contributing to a redundancy that ensures both a great physiological reserve and the possibility of very fine or discriminating control. Involvement of the sympathoadrenal system in regulation of multiple processes implies an important integrative role in the adjustment of organ system function in accordance with the needs of the organism as a whole.

In the following discussion, the effects of catecholamines have been arbitrarily divided into cardiovascular, visceral, and metabolic, although considerable overlap exists. In a general sense the cardiovascular effects of catecholamines serve to control cardiac output and apportion blood flow, whereas the visceral effects govern vegetative functions in organs other than the cardiovascular system. The metabolic effects involve regulation of oxygen uptake, mobilization of energy reserves from storage depots, and maintenance of the constancy of extracellular fluid.

CARDIOVASCULAR EFFECTS. The sympathetic nervous system regulates the peripheral circulation and the cardiac output[488] according to the requirements of the organism as a whole. Sympathetically mediated adjustments in peripheral resistance maintain the integrity of the circulation so as to provide adequate perfusion of vital organ systems in the face of changing circulatory and metabolic demands. Although the sympathetic nerves supplying the heart and vasculature are more important in circulatory regulation than are blood-borne catecholamines from the adrenal medulla, the latter may partially compensate for impaired or defective sympathetic responses.[479, 480]

Afferent Pathways. Stretch receptors in both low-pressure capacitance vessels and high-pressure resistance vessels continuously monitor the status of the circulation;[489] stimulation of these stretch receptors results in increased afferent neural impulses carried to the CNS in the ninth and tenth cranial nerves (Fig. 10–20). Increased stimulation from these peripheral receptors results in diminished central sympathetic outflow. The presence of receptors in both the capacitance and the resistance portions of the circulation permits the sympathetic nervous system to respond to alterations in both volume and pressure. A fall in either central venous or arterial pressure is therefore associated with an increase in sympathetic activity (see Fig. 10–20) because inhibitory input from the baroreceptors is diminished. Although the high- and low-pressure baroreceptors work in tandem to defend blood pressure and tissue perfusion, the low-pressure baroreceptors appear to be more sensitive; small decrements in venous return, such as those induced by alterations in position, stimulate the sympathetic nervous system without a fall in arterial pressure.[490]

Central Connections. The central neuronal mechanisms that are involved in the arterial baroreceptor response have been partially clarified. High-pressure baroreceptor afferents terminate in the nucleus of the tractus solitarius; increased baroreceptor afferent activity stimulates an inhibitory pathway originating in the tractus solitarius and terminating in brain stem sympathetic centers.[466] The inhibitory pathway involves an alpha-adrenergic synapse[467] of the alpha-2 subtype. Centrally acting alpha-adrenergic agonists

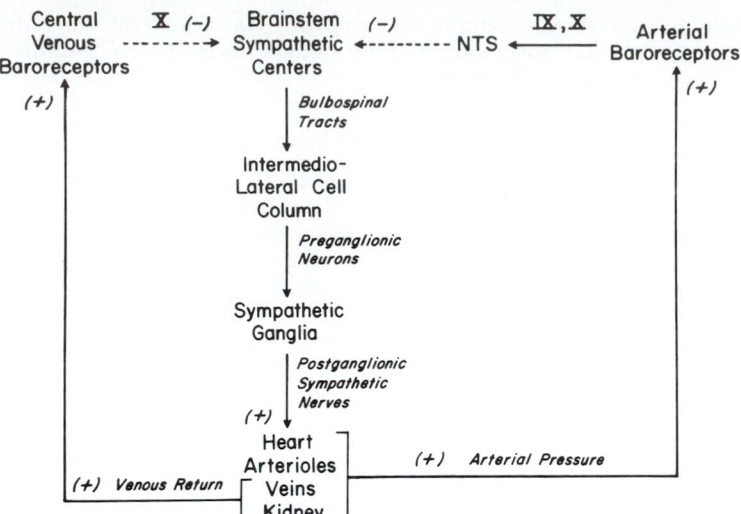

Figure 10–20. Sympathetic regulation of circulation: afferent impulses from resistance and capacitance portions of circulation. Stretch receptors in venous (low-pressure; capacitance) and arterial (high-pressure; resistance) circulations are stimulated by an increase in tension that reflects increased venous filling pressure, or increased arterial pressure. Afferent impulses from these receptors are carried to the CNS by the ninth and tenth cranial nerves. The consequence of increased afferent impulse traffic in this system is inhibition of central sympathetic outflow. Although the central connections that are involved in these circulatory reflexes are only partially clarified, the arterial baroreceptor reflex involves a relay in the nucleus tractus solitarius (NTS). When venous filling pressure or arterial blood pressure falls, impulse traffic from stretch receptors diminishes; as a consequence the tonic inhibitory effect of these circulatory afferents is diminished, with a resultant increase in central sympathetic outflow. (+) indicates stimulation; (−), inhibition. (From Landsberg L, Young JB. Physiology and pharmacology of the autonomic nervous system. In: Wilson JD, Braunwald E, Isselbacher K, et al., eds. Harrison's Principles of Internal Medicine. 12th ed. New York: McGraw-Hill, 1991: 380–392. Reproduced with permission of McGraw-Hill, Inc.)

that lower blood pressure (clonidine; α-methylnorepinephrine derived from α-methyldopa) appear to act by potentiating this baroreceptor depressor response.[1, 4, 467] The central mechanisms that are involved in the low-pressure baroreceptor response have not been clarified, although the afferent neural pathway appears to involve the vagus.[491]

Excitatory bulbospinal tracts originating in the subretrofacial region of the rostral ventrolateral medulla[492, 493] and inhibitory pathways in the caudal ventrolateral medulla[492] have been identified. The neurotransmitters that are involved in cardiovascular regulation include epinephrine, NE, and 5-HT.[494, 495] Substance P and neuropeptide Y may function as cotransmitters in some of these pathways.[494]

Efferent Cardiovascular Effects. The efferent limb of the baroreceptor reflex involves sympathetic outflow to the arterioles, heart, kidneys, and veins (Fig. 10–21). Venous return is augmented by alpha-receptor–mediated venoconstriction and, in the long run, by enhancement of sodium reabsorption (as described later). Peripheral resistance is increased by alpha-receptor–mediated vasoconstriction in the subcutaneous, mucosal, splanchnic, and renal vascular beds. Because sympathetically mediated vasoconstriction is minimal in the coronary and cerebral circulations, flow to these areas is maintained at the expense of that to the other major vascular beds. The distribution of blood flow is thus regulated by differences in sympathetically mediated arteriolar resistance in different anatomical regions.

Vascular Responses. Studies of sympathetically mediated vascular responses have demonstrated a previously unappreciated complexity. Noninnervated beta-2–receptors mediate vasodilation in response to low levels of circulating epinephrine.[496] Alpha-receptors throughout the vasculature, including lymphatics,[497] mediate vasoconstriction. Furthermore, arteries and veins in many vascular beds, including the pulmonary,[498] coronary,[499–503] and renal[504–506] circulations, are endowed with both alpha-1– and alpha-2–receptors. The physiological response in different vascular beds appears to reflect the stimulation of both alpha-receptor subtypes. On the arterial side of the circulation, alpha-receptors regulate peripheral resistance and tissue perfusion; on the venous side of the circulation, they mediate sympathetically induced changes in venous capacitance and hence plasma volume. Within the arterial circulation the alpha-1–receptor appears to be the predominant postjunctional or innervated receptor located in proximity to the sympathetic nerve endings, whereas the alpha-2–receptor is predominantly noninnervated and is therefore responsive to circulating catecholamines.[436] The situation is reversed in the venous circulation, in which the alpha-2–receptor is the innervated subtype.[436] Spare vascular alpha-1–receptors have been dem-

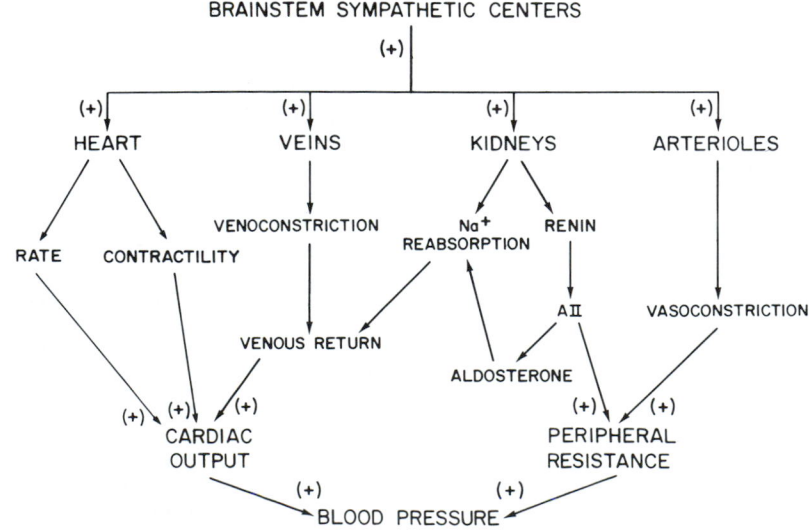

Figure 10–21. Sympathetic regulation of circulation: effects on blood pressure. Sympathetic stimulation (+) increases blood pressure by effects on the heart, veins, kidneys, and arterioles. Both cardiac output and peripheral resistance are increased by direct and indirect effects of the sympathetic nervous system. AII, angiotensin II. (From Young JB, Landsberg L. Obesity and the circulation. In: Sleight P, Jones JV, eds. Scientific Foundations of Cardiology. London: Heinemann, 1983: 201–206.)

onstrated in both the arterial and the venous systems, whereas spare alpha-2–receptors are present only in veins,[436] which implies enhanced sensitivity of venous alpha-2–receptors to the physiological agonist NE. The presence of spare alpha-2–receptors is consistent with other data indicating a more important role for the alpha-2–receptor in the regulation of venous capacitance[507, 508] than in the regulation of peripheral resistance.

In the physiological setting the vasoconstrictor response to sympathetic stimulation is modified by a variety of local factors in the innervated vascular bed. In the renal circulation, for example, prostaglandin release antagonizes the vasoconstriction that is induced by sympathetic stimulation.[509] It has also become clear that the vascular endothelium plays an important role in modulating adrenergically mediated vasoconstriction in several vascular beds,[510] including the coronary circulation.[511] Vasodilatory response engendered by the endothelium is mediated in part by endothelium-derived relaxing factor.[29, 511] NE has been shown to elicit vasodilation from isolated preparations with an intact endothelium by a mechanism that may involve the alpha-2–receptor.[511] Vasodilatory responses to epinephrine may involve the endothelium as well.[510]

In some species neurally mediated vasodilation in skeletal muscles involves sympathetic nerves that utilize acetylcholine as a neurotransmitter;[488, 496] the importance of this pathway in primates is uncertain.[488]

Cardiac Effects. The effects of catecholamines on the heart are mediated by beta-1–receptors and include increased heart rate, enhanced contractility, and augmented conduction velocity, all of which contribute to an increase in cardiac output. The increase in heart rate that is induced by catecholamines[512] is secondary to an increase in the rate of spontaneous diastolic depolarization (loss of phase 4 resting potential) in the pacemaker cells. The increase in the contractility of individual cardiac muscle fibers is expressed physiologically by a leftward shift of the ventricular function curve, which relates cardiac work to ventricular diastolic fiber length; at any initial ventricular diastolic fiber length, catecholamines increase the amount of cardiac work performed.[513] Catecholamine-induced venoconstriction also increases the force of atrial contraction, thus enhancing ventricular contractility by increasing diastolic fiber length.[513] Finally, an increase in conduction velocity in the junctional tissues causes a more synchronous ventricular contraction, thus resulting in more useful work per contraction.[513] The biological cost of catecholamine-induced cardiac stimulation is increased myocardial oxygen consumption,[514] a factor of importance in angina pectoris.[515]

VISCERAL EFFECTS. The numerous visceral effects of catecholamines are summarized in Table 10–5. All of the effects mentioned are based on experimental evidence, but the physiological importance in some cases is uncertain.

Smooth Muscle. As a general rule, catecholamines cause smooth muscle relaxation through a beta-receptor (beta-2) mechanism and smooth muscle contraction via alpha-receptor (alpha-1) stimulation.[516] Sympathetic stimulation decreases tone in intestinal and urinary bladder smooth muscle while constricting the corresponding sphincters. Dopaminergic receptors also mediate relaxation in gut and vascular smooth muscle.[195] In the intact animal the influence of catecholamines on gut smooth muscle is intimately related to the function of cholinergic parasympathetic fibers; sympathetic nerve terminals that are close to myenteric parasympathetic ganglion cells and postganglionic fibers[516, 517] have been shown to diminish acetylcholine release from the myenteric plexus[516] by an alpha-2 mechanism. The inhibition of intestinal motility that is induced by catecholamines, therefore, may represent either beta-receptor–mediated relaxa-

TABLE 10–5. Visceral Effects of Catecholamines

Smooth muscle function
  Gastrointestinal motility
  Gallbladder contraction
  Urinary bladder contraction
  Oviduct and vas deferens contractility
  Uterine contractility
  Gastrointestinal and genitourinary sphincter tone
  Bronchial smooth muscle tone
  Piloerection and activity of ciliated epithelium
  Iris and ciliary muscle function
  Milk duct contractility
  Ovarian and testicular contractility
Fluid and electrolyte transport
  Gastrointestinal tract function
    Salivary secretion
    Gastric acid secretion
    Pancreatic exocrine secretion
    Intestinal absorption
    Gallbladder reabsorption
  Epididymal duct reabsorption
  Renal tubular function
  Tracheobronchial fluid absorption
  Aqueous humor formation
  Corneal epithelium transport
  Choroid plexus secretion
  Sweat gland secretion
Protein secretion
  Gastrointestinal tract function
    Salivary secretion
    Gastric secretion of mucus
    Pancreatic exocrine secretion
  Peripheral polypeptide hormone production
  Bronchial mucin secretion
  Lacrimal secretion
Cell growth and division
  Intestinal crypts
  Erythropoiesis
  Adaptive hypertrophy
Hemostasis
Immune function

tion or alpha-2–receptor–mediated suppression of acetylcholine release. Normal regulation of intestinal motility depends on the balance between sympathetic and parasympathetic effects. Sympathetic dominance may account for several forms of paralytic ileus.[518] Neuropeptides (such as neuropeptide Y) colocalized and released with NE may affect gut motility as well.[519]

The bronchial musculature is more heavily innervated with parasympathetic than with sympathetic nerve endings,[520] and the sympathetic nervous system plays only a minor role in regulating airway resistance.[521] Circulating epinephrine may play a role in regulating bronchomotor tone by stimulating beta-2 bronchodilatory receptors.[522]

Myoepithelial cells that contain contractile elements but are not true smooth muscle cells are present in the breast (within the milk duct) and the ovary (within the wall of the graafian follicle). Catecholamines stimulate contraction of these structures, thereby contributing to lactation and ovulation.[523–526] Contractile cells are also present in the testicular capsule, and capsular contractions occur in response to NE and to nerve stimulation.[527]

Fluid and Electrolyte Transport. Catecholamines influence the movement of water and ions across membrane surfaces, including those of the intestine, gallbladder, trachea, cornea, and renal epithelium.[528–531] They likewise alter the secretion of fluid into the aqueous humor, so that both epinephrine and beta-adrenergic antagonists are useful in the treatment of glaucoma.[532] The effects of catecholamines on water and electrolyte metabolism in the kidney are discussed in subsequent sections. The effect of catecholamines on sweating deserves special comment. Apocrine sweating in the axillary and genital areas is stimulated by catecholamines, whereas eccrine sweating that is involved in temperature regulation is mediated by postganglionic sympathetic fibers that are cholinergic rather than noradrenergic.

Protein Secretion. Catecholamines stimulate the secretion of numerous peptides into tears, saliva, and pancreatic juice and also promote release of mucus from gastric mucosa and bronchial epithelium. The physiological role of catecholamines in endocrine secretion is discussed later.

Cell Growth and Division. Catecholamines stimulate cell growth and division. More than 20 years ago hypertrophy and hyperplasia of parotid tissue were observed in response to catecholamine administration or to nerve stimulation.[533] Catecholamines also modulate cell proliferation in intestinal crypts, stimulating it by an alpha-2 mechanism and inhibiting it by alpha-1 and beta mechanisms.[534] In bone marrow cells catecholamines stimulate erythroid colony formation[535] via the beta-2–receptor.[536] Proliferation of intimal smooth muscle cells may result from sympathetic innervation.[537] Catecholamines have been linked to tissue hypertrophy in several other circumstances. Ovarian hypertrophy after contralateral oophorectomy is abolished by local destruction of sympathetic nerves,[538] which implicates ovarian sympathetic activity in the hypertrophic process. Catecholamines also participate in adaptive hypertrophy in heart and in brown adipose tissue (BAT).[539–542]

Hemostasis. Epinephrine promotes platelet aggregation by an alpha-2–receptor mechanism. Administration of epinephrine also increases circulating levels of factor VIII and plasminogen activator,[543] the latter mediated by the beta-receptor.[544] Beta-adrenergic blockade attenuates the rise in factor VIII levels[545] but is without effect on plasminogen activator.

Immune Function. Catecholamines influence both humoral and cellular immunity.[546–548] The spleen and lymph nodes are heavily innervated with sympathetic fibers.[549, 550] The role played by catecholamines in immunoregulation is uncertain, but they may provide a link between the immune system and emotional state.[551]

METABOLIC EFFECTS OF CATECHOLAMINES. *Energy Metabolism: Thermogenesis.* **General Considerations: Components of Thermogenesis.** Thermogenesis means, simply, heat production. In clinical and physiological studies, oxygen consumption is a measure of thermogenesis because heat production is proportional to the rate of oxygen utilization.[552] From the rate of oxygen consumption and the respiratory quotient, the metabolic rate may be determined. The regulation of mammalian thermogenesis[553, 554] involves two major components,[555] one obligatory, the other facultative, that differ in function and regulation.

Obligatory thermogenesis refers to basal heat production in the fasting state at normal temperatures; this component includes the metabolic heat that is generated during the maintenance of homeostatis at complete rest. In normal humans under sedentary conditions, approximately 75% of total energy output falls into this category,[556] which is also known as the *basal* or the *resting metabolic rate.* Thyroid hormones are important in the regulation of obligatory thermogenesis;[555] catecholamines have only a small effect on this component.

The facultative component of thermogenesis is due to heat production in excess of that required for maintenance of the basal state. Facultative thermogenesis is said to be regulatory or adaptive when the primary goal of the increase in metabolic rate is the production of heat.[557] The heat produced by muscular exercise is facultative thermogenesis, but exercise-induced heat production is not adaptive or regulatory except in the case of shivering, in which the specific consequence of the muscular activity is the production of heat rather than work. Facultative thermogenesis also results from chemical stimulation of metabolic processes independent of muscular activity, and catecholamines are considered to be the major mediators of this process.[558]

Infusions of catecholamines increase oxygen consumption by a mechanism that is predominantly beta-receptor mediated.[557–559] The regulation of adaptive thermogenesis usually involves the sympathetic nervous system rather than the adrenal medulla because the threshold for stimulation of thermogenesis by circulating catecholamines generally exceeds normal plasma levels.[560–563] The sympathetic nervous system regulates thermogenesis in response to cold exposure (nonshivering thermogenesis) and to dietary intake (diet-induced thermogenesis).[557, 558]

Nonshivering Thermogenesis. A critical role for the sympathetic nervous system in nonshivering thermogenesis was demonstrated by Hsieh and co-workers (Fig. 10–22).[564]

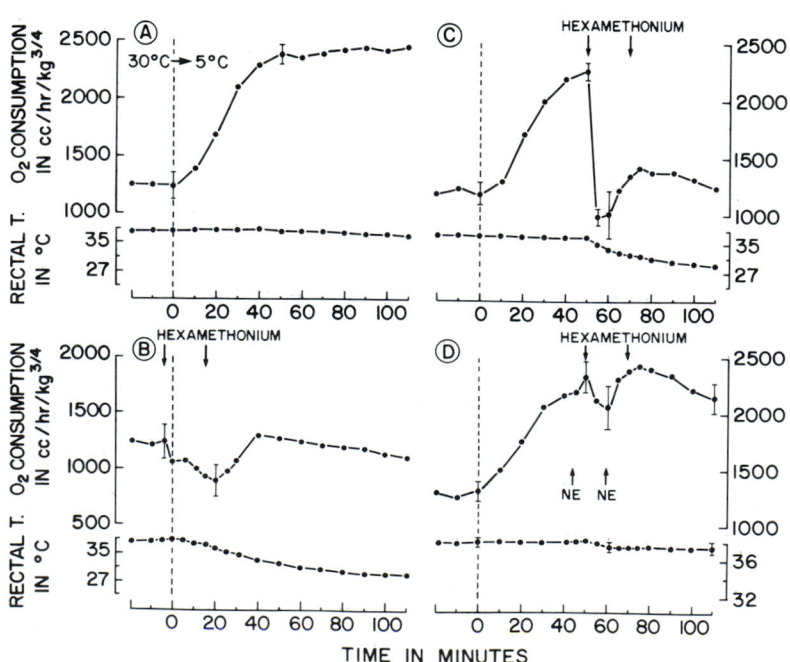

Figure 10–22. Effect of ganglionic blockade on temperature and metabolic rate in the rat during exposure to cold. Cold-acclimated curarized rats were exposed to a temperature of 5°C beginning at time 0. *A,* A normal response; oxygen consumption increases markedly and the rectal temperature is maintained when the autonomic nervous system is intact. *B,* Ganglionic blockade (hexamethonium) prevents the increase in metabolic rate, with a resultant fall in rectal temperature. The same response occurs (*C*) when ganglionic blockade is initiated after the metabolic rate has increased. *D,* Administration of NE antagonizes effect of ganglionic blockade. Because shivering was inhibited by curarization, these studies demonstrate a primary effect of the autonomic nervous system to increase the metabolic rate in response to exposure to cold (nonshivering thermogenesis). The facts that atropine had no effect on oxygen consumption in the presence of hexamethonium (not shown) and that NE was more potent than epinephrine in antagonizing the effect of ganglionic blockade indicate an important role for the sympathetic nervous system. (Modified from Hsieh ACL, Carlson LD, Gray G. Role of the sympathetic nervous system in the control of chemical regulation of heat production. Am J Physiol 1957; 190:247–251.)

These experiments demonstrated that (1) exposure to cold increases metabolic rate independent of shivering, (2) the increase in metabolic rate depends on the autonomic nervous system, and (3) the sympathetic nervous system is the portion of the autonomic nervous system that is involved.[564] NE is the major chemical mediator of nonshivering thermogenesis.[558]

Brown Adipose Tissue. BAT is the major site of metabolic heat production in the cold-acclimated rat in response to both NE[565] and cold exposure.[566] BAT also plays a major role in heat production in neonates of many mammalian species.[567, 568] Its contribution to the generation of metabolic heat in large mammals at maturity, including humans, is uncertain, although increasing evidence suggests that BAT is functional in adult humans[569–571] and other primates.[572] Catecholamine-stimulated processes in tissues other than BAT cannot convincingly explain heat production in response to cold exposure or to NE, nor can other processes conveniently account for the increased NE-induced heat production that accompanies cold acclimation.

Catecholamine-induced heat production in brown adipocytes has been the subject of considerable investigation.[573, 574] Activation of the beta-1–adrenergic receptor on the brown adipocyte cell membrane[575] stimulates the hydrolysis of triglycerides, with the intracellular liberation of free fatty acids; in conjunction with purine nucleotides the free fatty acids stimulate heat production by uncoupling oxidative phosphorylation in BAT mitochondria. This physiological uncoupling involves a unique BAT mitochondrial protein named *thermogenin* or *uncoupling protein*. According to the chemiosmotic hypothesis of mitochondrial function, the following schema operates: (1) in the normally coupled state, energy from the oxidation of fatty acid substrates by the electron transport chain is linked to the extrusion of protons from the inner mitochondrial matrix. Energy from substrate oxidation is thus stored in an electrochemical proton gradient because under normal coupled conditions the inner mitochondrial membrane is impermeable to protons and hydroxyl ions.[573] (2) ATP synthase within the mitochondrial membrane is linked to proton transport into the inner mitochondrial matrix, with the electromotive force of the proton gradient supplying the energy for the synthesis of ATP. (3) In BAT, sympathetic stimulation results in the activation of a proton conductance pathway that dissipates the proton gradient by permitting the diffusion of protons into the inner mitochondrial matrix (or the egress of hydroxyl ions).[576] Dissipation of the proton gradient is accomplished by the unique uncoupling protein that, in conjunction with purine nucleotides, renders the mitochondrial membrane permeable to protons (or hydroxyl ions). (4) The increased concentration of protons within the inner mitochondrial matrix drives the electron transport chain, which results in the oxidation of substrate that is no longer coupled to ATP synthesis because the normal proton re-entry mechanism that is coupled to ATP synthesis is bypassed.[576] Transcription of the gene that regulates the synthesis of uncoupling protein is under the direct control of NE, but it is amplified by thyroid hormone.[577]

In addition to the beta-receptor mechanism that regulates heat production in BAT, an alpha-1–receptor–mediated process exists that stimulates the deiodination of thyroxine to triiodothyronine (T_3). The BAT deiodinase has been designated type II and is distinct from the type I, propylthiouracil-responsive deiodinase that is present in liver and kidney.[578–581] The activity of this BAT deiodinase provides high local concentrations of T_3 that are essential for the full expression of the thermogenic potential of this tissue.[582, 583]

The sympathetic nerves also exert an important trophic influence on BAT growth and differentiation,[584] including a stimulatory effect on the formation of BAT mitochondria.[585] The mechanisms that are involved in this trophic stimulatory action are uncertain but may explain the increase in amount of BAT that is noted in patients with pheochromocytoma.[571] The possibilities that nonadrenergic nerves may regulate the trophic response[586] and that transmitters other than NE may be involved have also been suggested.

Diet-Induced Thermogenesis. The concept that alterations in dietary intake affect thermogenesis originated in the 19th century.[557, 558, 587] At least a portion of diet-induced thermogenesis is adaptive in nature and not solely the consequence of the energy cost that is involved in the metabolism and assimilation of nutrients.[587] The fact that dietary intake influences sympathetic activity,[557, 558] coupled with the physiological and biochemical similarity between nonshivering thermogenesis and diet-induced thermogenesis,[588, 589] suggests that the sympathetic nervous system is a principal regulator of the latter.[554, 557, 558, 590] The available evidence in humans is consistent with a role for the sympathetic nervous system in regulating the relationship between heat production and dietary intake.[591–594]

Other Situations. In several other situations, involvement of the sympathetic nervous system seems likely in increased thermogenesis. The increase in catecholamine excretion in the hypermetabolic state after trauma correlates with the elevation in oxygen consumption, and adrenergic blockade diminishes the metabolic rate.[595] The sympathetic nervous system may also participate in the alterations in thermogenesis that accompany a wide variety of physiological and pathophysiological states such as fever,[596] tetanus, and shock and in the increased metabolic rate that accompanies withdrawal from alcohol, opiates, and clonidine.

Fuel Metabolism. General Considerations. (Also see Chapters 23 and 24.) Catecholamines stimulate the breakdown of stored fuels into utilizable substrates. The liberated substrate may serve as an energy source for local metabolism, as exemplified by glycogenolysis in heart, or for systemic distribution. In fact, one of the major metabolic functions of catecholamines is the rapid mobilization of substrates from storage depots in liver, adipose tissue, and skeletal muscle (Fig. 10–23). Direct and indirect actions of catecholamines in fuel mobilization were described earlier.

Substrate mobilization depends on diverse factors including hormones, substrates, and nerves. Catecholamines, along with insulin and glucagon, participate in the regulation of these processes. The effects of catecholamines and glucagon are generally opposite to those of insulin, and the net activity of a given process reflects the interaction of these three regulators.

Liver. Catecholamines in liver promote hepatic glucose output by activating glycogenolysis and accelerating gluconeogenesis while simultaneously inhibiting glycogen synthesis. Interaction of catecholamines with the beta-adrenergic receptor activates the well-known sequence of stimulation of adenylate cyclase, generation of cAMP, and initiation of the cAMP-dependent enzymatic cascade leading to conversion of glycogen phosphorylase from the inactive to the active form.[533] This effect of epinephrine was among those reported by Rall and Sutherland in their description of adenylate cyclase.[597] Alpha-(alpha-1–)receptor stimulation also activates phosphorylase, thereby increasing glycogenolysis, and enhances gluconeogenesis in isolated hepatocytes by mechanisms that are independent of cAMP.[598–601] Amino acid uptake into liver—and perhaps lactate entry also—is augmented by alpha-agonists,[602, 603] which increases the availability of substrates for gluconeogenesis. Various factors affect the relative contributions of alpha- and beta-adrenergic receptor mechanisms to hepatic glucose production,

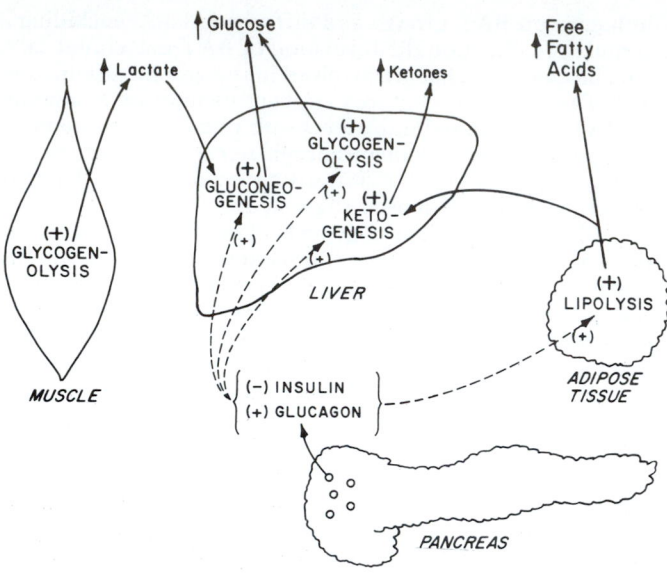

Figure 10–23. Schematic representation of catecholamine effects on fuel mobilization in liver, adipose tissue, and skeletal muscle. Direct effects are reinforced by (but do not require) catecholamine-mediated suppression of insulin and stimulation of glucagon. (+) indicates stimulation; (−), inhibition. (From Landsberg L, Young JB. Catecholamines and the adrenal medulla. In: Bondy PK, Rosenberg LE, eds. Metabolic Control and Disease. 8th ed. Philadelphia: W. B. Saunders, 1980: 1621–1693.)

including the level of extracellular glucose, gonadal steroids, glucocorticoids, endotoxin, and cholestasis.[533, 599, 604–608] Species differences also exist: alpha-adrenergic effects predominate in rats (especially males), whereas beta-adrenergic effects predominate in dogs and humans. Alpha-adrenergic stimulation, however, can enhance hepatic glucose production in humans.[609]

Catecholamines stimulate hepatic ketogenesis by increasing the delivery of free fatty acid substrate from the periphery, the rise in free fatty acids a consequence of catecholamine-stimulated lipolysis.[610, 611] Suppression of insulin and stimulation of glucagon secretion contribute to this effect.

Catecholamines, as noted previously, can also suppress insulin and stimulate glucagon secretion in the pancreas. Changes in glucagon and insulin augment the direct effects of catecholamines on hepatic glucose production. Catecholamines generally diminish hepatic blood flow,[612] and an additional effect of glucagon may be to lessen catecholamine-induced hepatic arterial vasoconstriction.[613, 614]

The relative importance of locally released NE compared with circulating epinephrine or DA in the regulation of hepatic metabolism is uncertain. Sympathetic innervation is present in the hepatic parenchyma.[615, 616] There is variation among species in the density of parenchymal innervation, human liver being among the most densely innervated and rat and mouse liver among the least.[616] The fact that increased hepatic glucose output follows electrical stimulation of hepatic sympathetic nerves emphasizes the potential importance of the neuronal contribution to regulation of hepatic metabolism.[617–620] On the other hand, circulating catecholamines, epinephrine in particular, doubtless play a major physiological role. Although early studies minimized the importance of circulating catecholamines,[621] hepatic glucose output increases during infusions of epinephrine that produce high, but physiologically attainable, arterial levels.[622] Thus both hepatic sympathetic nerves and circulating catecholamines can stimulate hepatic glucose output; the respective contributions probably differ in different physiological states.

White Adipose Tissue. Catecholamines stimulate lipolysis by activating hormone-sensitive (triacylglycerol) lipase, the enzyme that cleaves triglyceride into fatty acids and glycerol within adipose tissue.[533] The cellular processes mediating this response involve interaction of catecholamines

with the beta-1–adrenergic receptor followed by activation of adenylate cyclase and phosphorylation of the inactive lipase by a cAMP-dependent protein kinase.[623, 624] Removal of phosphate from the lipase by a phosphatase inactivates the enzyme. Catecholamines also promote triglyceride synthesis, but this effect is secondary to increased local availability of fatty acids.[533] In addition to beta-mediated lipolysis, catecholamines exert an antilipolytic effect via an alpha-2– receptor mechanism. The physiological importance of this effect is still uncertain,[623] but the effect may play a role in states that are associated with diminished catecholamine-stimulated lipolysis, such as fasting;[625, 626] in early infancy;[627] and in some discrete body regions.[628–630] It may also have sex-related function.[628] On balance, catecholamines should be considered primarily lipolytic hormones. As in liver, catecholamines stimulate glycogenolysis by activating glycogen phosphorylase and inactivating glycogen synthetase. They increase glucose uptake into adipocytes by both alpha (alpha-1) and beta mechanisms.[623, 631, 632]

Multiple factors influence the stimulation of lipolysis by catecholamines in mammalian adipose tissue. Alpha-2–adrenergic sensitivity in adipose tissue differs among species, as do lipolytic responses to catecholamines.[623, 633] Even within the same individual, fat cells from different locations exhibit different proportions of alpha- and beta-adrenergic receptors and variable rates of lipolysis in the presence of catecholamines.[629, 630, 634] In addition, numerous environmental and hormonal factors affect adipose tissue responsiveness to catecholamines, insulin being the most prominent. Insulin exerts an overriding antagonistic effect on catecholamine-mediated lipolysis; thus suppression of insulin secretion is an important component of catecholamine effects on fat mobilization. Furthermore, beta-adrenergic stimulation inhibits binding of insulin to its receptor in adipocytes.[635] Nutritional state, thyroid function, local temperature, pH, PO_2, obesity, extracellular concentrations of free fatty acids,[636] and age also influence the adipocyte response to catecholamines.[623, 637–639]

The relative importance of locally released NE versus circulating epinephrine remains uncertain. Although the vascular supply of fat is densely innervated, extensive innervation of the adipocytes has not been demonstrated, even in regions exhibiting lipolytic responses to electrical stimulation of sympathetic nerves.[640] Epinephrine that is infused at rates producing circulating levels within the physiological range increases lipolysis in humans.[641] Given the known heterogeneity among adipose tissue depots, neural stimulation of lipolysis is probably more important in some regions than in others, and the relative contribution of sympathetic nerves and circulating catecholamines in fat mobilization probably varies in different circumstances.

Blood flow to adipose tissue is controlled by sympathetic nerves. Both alpha-mediated vasoconstriction and beta-mediated vasodilation occur, but in subcutaneous adipose tissue only the alpha-adrenergic response demonstrates the phenomenon of denervation supersensitivity, which suggests that vascular alpha-receptors, but not beta-receptors, are governed by changes in sympathetic activity.[642] By inference, beta-adrenergic receptors are oriented more to circulating than to locally released catecholamines.

Brown Adipose Tissue. As noted earlier, BAT is specialized for heat production rather than for fuel storage; it contains multilobulated fat droplets and large numbers of mitochondria that give the tissue its characteristic appearance.[567] The brown fat mitochondria are uncoupled during sympathetic stimulation as described earlier. As a consequence, energy that is derived from oxidation of fuels is released as heat rather than stored as high-energy phosphate bonds. Brown adipocytes are densely innervated[643] and therefore are influenced more by changes in sympathetic nervous system activity than by fluctuations in circulating catecholamines.

Muscle. Catecholamine stimulation of glycogenolysis in muscle occurs via beta-receptor activation utilizing cAMP as the second messenger.[533] Unlike the situation in liver or adipose tissue, alpha-receptor mechanisms do not affect this process, at least in skeletal muscle.[598, 644] Because muscle lacks the enzyme glucose-6-phosphatase, the glucose-6-phosphate that is produced by glycogenolysis is metabolized to lactate before release into the circulation.[533] Catecholamines also enhance free fatty acid entry and mobilize triglyceride contained in muscle;[533] in skeletal muscle this response is beta mediated.[645] The effects of catecholamines on muscle glycogen metabolism are antagonized by insulin and require glucocorticoids.[646–648]

Although muscle protein represents a large reserve of stored fuel that is catabolized in conditions such as prolonged starvation or severe injury, the precise role of catecholamines in regulation of muscle protein metabolism is uncertain. Catecholamines, via a beta-receptor mechanism, diminish protein degradation but increase oxidation of branched chain amino acids in cardiac and skeletal muscle.[649–652] Metabolism of these amino acids elevates the ammonia content in muscle, part of which is transferred to α-ketoglutarate, with formation of glutamate and glutamine.[652–654] Both epinephrine and isoproterenol (presumably via beta-adrenergic stimulation) increase the release of glutamine and ammonia, while decreasing the release of alanine.[652, 654, 655] Because insulin antagonizes nitrogen loss from muscle,[656] suppression of insulin secretion by catecholamines may be an important component of this regulatory process.

Although in vivo studies provide firm evidence of epinephrine-induced impairment of glucose clearance from the extracellular space even when glucose and insulin levels are controlled experimentally,[657–659] the cellular mechanisms that are involved, especially in muscle, are not well defined. Epinephrine inhibits insulin-stimulated glucose accumulation in muscle in vitro by a beta-adrenergic mechanism that is independent of glucose transport.[660, 661] In the absence of insulin, epinephrine may increase glucose uptake into muscle by either alpha- or beta-receptor stimulation (as in adipose tissue), but this effect on glucose uptake is controversial.[661–663]

Because cellular events associated with muscle contraction also increase glycogenolysis and energy utilization, the separation of the effects of exercise from those of catecholamines is difficult and is confounded by the fact that catecholamines stimulate muscular contractility in skeletal, cardiac, and smooth muscle.[664] Nonetheless, catecholamines augment the effects of muscle contraction on glycogen metabolism.[665, 666] Likewise, catecholamines increase oxygen consumption in skeletal muscle beyond that induced by muscular activity or altered blood flow alone.[667, 668] Studies comparing the effects of catecholamines and those of muscle contraction on mobilization of intramuscular lipid are not available, but recruitment of this fuel source may represent a particularly important contribution of catecholamines.[669, 670]

In cardiac and smooth muscle the relative importance of sympathetic nerves and the adrenal medulla depends on the comparative levels of sympathetic and adrenomedullary activity in a given situation, as well as the degree of involvement of the beta-2–adrenergic receptor in a particular process. In skeletal muscle the balance between sympathetic and adrenomedullary influences may be affected by muscle fiber type. NE from sympathetic nerves may be of particular importance for glycogenolysis in both red and white fast twitch fibers,[665, 671] and adrenal epinephrine may play a similar role for red and intermediate muscle fibers (both fast and slow twitch).[672]

Substrate Cycling. The metabolic effects of catecholamines do not occur in isolation; in intact animals the breakdown of peripheral fuel stores increases the delivery of metabolic substrates to the liver, where they are converted into other forms, chiefly glucose, for return to peripheral tissues. As a result, studies that do not take into account the dynamic nature of intermediary metabolism may underestimate the contributions of catecholamines in a given situation. Although glucose is not the only substrate that is subject to recycling, it has been studied most extensively. Catecholamines from both sympathetic nerves and the adrenal medulla increase the rate of glucose exchange between liver and peripheral tissues. In animals epinephrine stimulates glucose-lactate exchange in the Cori cycle without substantially increasing glucose turnover.[673, 674] Comparable information in human subjects is not available, but the potential advantages of substrate cycling have been proposed in relation to human physiology.[675]

Lipoprotein Metabolism. Catecholamines exert several effects on lipoproteins, although the overall picture of sympathoadrenal regulation of lipoprotein metabolism is uncertain. Plasma levels of cholesterol increase within several hours after epinephrine administration and remain elevated with repeated injections.[676–678] Catecholamine-induced hypercholesterolemia reflects, in part, enhanced cholesterol biosynthesis. Catecholamines stimulate 3-hydroxy-3-methylglutaryl CoA reductase, the rate-limiting enzyme in cholesterol synthesis.[679–681] The mechanism of this stimulation is unknown.[677, 681–683] In rabbits catecholamines increase levels of very-low-density and low-density lipoproteins when infused over a 5-d period.[684]

The effects of catecholamines on circulating triglycerides are multiple and complex. They mobilize free fatty acids from adipose tissue, which serve as substrate for hepatic triglyceride synthesis, and inhibit triglyceride secretion from liver.[533, 685] Triglyceride levels rise during acute catecholamine infusions;[686] with more chronic administration, however, triglyceride levels are not elevated, whereas levels of both low- and high-density lipoproteins increase.[676] Treatment with prazosin, an alpha-1–receptor antagonist, reduces triglyceride levels and secretion rates in animals and humans,[682, 683] a finding that is difficult to reconcile with actions of catecholamines on free fatty acid release and on hepatic triglyceride secretion. Catecholamines also affect the activity of lipoprotein lipase in various tissues, decreasing activity in adipose tissue while increasing activity in muscle at times of fat mobilization.[687-689]

Water and Electrolyte Metabolism. General Considerations. Catecholamines play a role in the regulation of the volume and composition of the extracellular fluid. The hormonal changes that are induced by catecholamines support such a role. The interactions between the sympathoadrenal system and water and electrolyte metabolism, however, are not limited to effects of catecholamines on absorption, distribution, and excretion of water and various ions. As noted earlier, alterations in the ionic environment also elicit changes in sympathoadrenal activity and in the response of peripheral tissues to catecholamines.[152, 690]

Water. Systemic infusions of catecholamines alter renal water metabolism in humans and animals; NE increases and isoproterenol decreases free water clearance.[691-694] Although hemodynamic factors may contribute to this response, the major component is related to catecholamine effects on pituitary secretion of vasopressin. NE inhibits and isoproterenol stimulates vasopressin release via a nonpressor interaction with arterial baroreceptors.[695-697] That changes in vasopressin secretion mediate the action of infused alpha- and beta-adrenergic agonists on water excretion is clear because conditions that abolish the vasopressin response, such as acute hypophysectomy, central administration of an angiotensin II antagonist, or diabetes insipidus, block the alterations in water diuresis.[692, 693, 698-700]

The physiological role of catecholamines in regulation of water metabolism may not be mediated solely by alterations of vasopressin secretion. Alpha-adrenergic agonists inhibit vasopressin responses in cortical collecting tubules and renal papillae.[701, 702] In the absence of vasopressin[703] renal nerves may exert an antidiuretic effect. DA and levodopa also induce diuresis and an increase in free water clearance[704, 705] by a mechanism that is independent of vasopressin.[706]

Sodium. The presence of extensive adrenergic innervation in the mammalian kidney provides presumptive evidence of a role for the sympathetic nervous system in renal function. Noradrenergic fibers are found not only in relation to vascular structures but also in proximity to the juxtaglomerular apparatus (where they influence renin secretion) and the renal tubules.[707] Renal sympathetic innervation varies among species, with primate kidney displaying a greater density of fibers than rat kidney, particularly in peritubular regions.[707] DA-containing neurons are present in some species, but whether these are anatomically and functionally separate nerve fibers is uncertain.[211]

Catecholamines increase renal sodium reabsorption through vascular, hormonal, and tubular effects. The renal vascular response to strong sympathoadrenal activation is diminished glomerular filtration and increased sodium reabsorption.[708] Lesser sympathoadrenal stimulation promotes sodium reabsorption by redistributing renal blood flow from cortical to juxtamedullary nephrons, by increasing peritubular oncotic pressure, and by reducing intrarenal hydrostatic pressure.[709, 710] These changes occur in the absence of reduction in glomerular filtration. Catecholamines enhance renin release from the juxtaglomerular apparatus, thus stimulating the angiotensin-aldosterone system and inducing distal tubular sodium reabsorption. DA, on the other hand, produces renal vasodilation[711] and inhibits aldosterone secretion,[204] actions that diminish sodium reabsorption.

In addition to these vascular and hormonal effects, catecholamines directly affect renal tubular function[712] throughout the nephron.[713] Renal denervation or reflex suppression of renal sympathetic activity acutely increases sodium excretion.[714-716] Electrical or reflex stimulation of renal nerves does the reverse, both effects occurring in the absence of alterations in glomerular filtration or renal plasma flow.[715, 717-719] Fluid reabsorption in the proximal tubule is enhanced by NE and inhibited by DA.[720-722] Although earlier studies suggested that both alpha- and beta-adrenergic receptors were involved in sodium reabsorption,[708, 720, 721, 723, 724] in vivo experiments in dogs indicate that the alpha-1–receptor is principally responsible for this effect.[713]

Catecholamines also play a role in maintenance of sodium homeostasis. Alterations in sodium chloride intake affect sympathetic and dopaminergic activity. Restriction of salt intake elevates plasma and urine levels of NE and reduces urinary excretion of DA,[205, 509, 725-728] whereas salt loading increases DA excretion.[205, 207, 219] Sodium restriction increases renal sympathetic activity[509] and redistributes blood flow within the kidney in a pattern that is similar to that produced by NE infusions or sympathetic stimulation.[709, 710, 729] Pharmacological or pathological impairment in sympathetic function in human subjects interferes with renal sodium conservation.[730, 731] In various other situations, sodium retention occurs in the setting of sympathoadrenal activation.[712, 732] Oral administration of the AAD inhibitor carbidopa decreases renal DA formation and transiently reduces urinary sodium excretion.[206] Thus increased sympathetic activity may be a crucial component of the renal mechanisms for sodium conservation, with adrenomedullary catecholamines playing a subsidiary role. DA may play an important role in regulation of sodium excretion during salt loading.

Potassium. Catecholamines influence the distribution of potassium between the intracellular and the extracellular space. Epinephrine transiently elevates plasma potassium via alpha-receptor–mediated potassium efflux from liver, followed by sustained hypokalemia via beta-receptor–mediated potassium uptake into liver and skeletal muscle.[733-735] Disposal of an intravenous potassium load is also affected by the presence of adrenergic agonists or antagonists.[736, 737] Epinephrine-induced hypokalemia is a direct extrarenal effect, not dependent on changes in insulin, renin, or aldosterone concentrations,[735, 738] and is associated with diminished urinary potassium excretion.[739, 740] Beta-2–adrenergic receptor–mediated stimulation of membrane-bound Na^+,K^+-ATP-ase in muscle is also the result of a direct cellular effect of catecholamines.[741] In addition to augmenting the intracellular transfer of potassium, both epinephrine and the sympathetic nervous system protect the heart from the adverse effects of potassium toxicity.[742, 743]

Despite the effect of adrenergic agents on extrarenal potassium disposal, the physiological role of catecholamines in potassium homeostasis is uncertain. The endogenous catecholamine response to changes in plasma potassium is not clear. Although adrenal catecholamine release is induced by acute hyperkalemia in animals,[744] alterations in plasma catecholamine concentrations do not occur in humans who are infused with potassium.[737, 739] The fact that acute adrenalectomy or destruction of sympathetic nerves impairs potassium disposal in animals[744, 745] implies that the sympathoadrenal system plays at least a permissive role in maintenance of potassium homeostasis. Thus endogenous catecholamines may influence potassium disposition when the sympathoadrenal system is stimulated by other factors, such as exercise or dietary intake. In situations such as these it is possible that enhanced sympathetic tone acts as a buffer against the development of hyperkalemia.

In chronic potassium deficiency sympathetic nerves in skeletal muscle inhibit sodium-potassium exchange by an alpha-receptor mechanism that may serve to support the plasma potassium concentration by limiting intracellular storage.[746] The renal action of DA, in contrast to other catecholamines, fosters potassium excretion.[705, 747, 748] In addition, the urinary DA excretion is increased in response to oral potassium chloride.[220]

The effects of catecholamines on potassium metabolism have several clinical implications. Beta-adrenergic blockade potentiates the increase in potassium concentration during exercise or after cardiopulmonary bypass surgery.[749] This hyperkalemic effect is of therapeutic utility in treatment of hypokalemic periodic paralysis associated with thyrotoxicosis.[749, 750] The hypokalemic effect of beta-2–adrenergic agonists is of benefit in treating patients with hyperkalemic periodic paralysis,[751] but it may be a problem in situations such as the treatment of premature labor when hyperkalemia is not present.[752]

Calcium, Magnesium, and Phosphate. Catecholamines affect calcium, magnesium, and phosphate metabolism both directly and indirectly through their influence on the secretion of calcitonin and parathyroid hormone. The response of plasma calcium and magnesium to adrenergic agonists differs widely among species.[753–758] In humans the calcium level changes little, if at all, in response to acute catecholamine infusions,[759–762] whereas epinephrine infusions lower magnesium levels slightly.[763, 764] However, the hypercalcemia of pheochromocytoma and thyrotoxicosis disappears with tumor removal or beta-adrenergic blockage,[765–769] which suggests a contributory role for catecholamines in the calcium elevations. Catecholamines also stimulate urinary calcium excretion, which is an alpha-adrenergic effect independent of parathyroid function.[770] The occasional occurrence of enhanced urinary calcium excretion in patients with pheochromocytoma may be a result of this calciuric effect.[766, 770] The fact that the plasma epinephrine level increases during calcium infusion raises the possibility that adrenomedullary stimulation may participate in the defense against hypercalcemia.[761, 771]

Catecholamines exert several effects on phosphate metabolism. Epinephrine lowers serum phosphate levels in animals and humans[761, 772–776] by a beta-adrenergic receptor mechanism.[756, 776] The hypophosphatemic response to insulin-induced hypoglycemia is partially antagonized by propranolol.[776] Intrarenal infusion of NE suppresses urinary phosphate excretion,[777] whereas renal denervation enhances it.[778] DA, on the other hand, induces phosphaturia by a direct intrarenal effect.[777, 779] The low phosphate levels that are noted in situations associated with increased sympathoadrenal activity may reflect the hypophosphatemic action of catecholamines, as in the hypophosphatemia of the postoperative period[780] and after acute myocardial infarction.

Purine Metabolism. Catecholamines elevate plasma levels of uric acid; allantoin is similarly affected in species possessing uricase. Infusions of NE diminish the renal clearance of urate in human subjects;[781] in animals the administration of adrenergic agonists, electrical stimulation of the adrenal medulla, and immobilization raise plasma levels of allantoin and uric acid by a beta-receptor mechanism.[782–784] The fact that these changes occur in nephrectomized animals implies an effect on purine biosynthesis as well as clearance. Long-term beta-blockade for hypertension has been associated with elevations in serum uric acid levels in some studies,[785] although in others decreasing uric acid levels were noted as drug dosage increased.[786] Expansion of the uric acid pool after myocardial infarction may also reflect the effects of catecholamines.[787]

Effects of Catecholamines on Hormone Secretion

GENERAL CONSIDERATIONS. *Neural Control of Hormone Secretion.* Catecholamines are involved in regulating the secretion of several hormones (Table 10–6).[788] The sympathetic nerves and adrenal medulla probably provide a physiological link between the brain and the secretion of hormones not otherwise connected to the CNS. The hormones given in Table 10–6 are all regulated by specific feedback loops. Imposition of the sympathoadrenal system introduces the possibility of regulation by the CNS, an arrangement that confers advantages in the maintenance of homeostasis. Central neural control of peripheral hormone secretion implies speed, anticipation, and integration. The usual feedback loops that regulate hormone secretion operate in minutes, but catecholamine-mediated effects may occur in seconds, thereby accelerating the hormonal response to perturbations in the internal milieu. Similarly, central neural regulation allows for anticipatory changes in hormone secretion, thereby creating the proper hormonal environment for the contemplated activity and lessening the impact of the activity on the internal environment. Most important, central neural regulation provides for integration of the hormonal changes with other physiological adjustments, as well as for synchronization of changes in the secretion of several hormones. For hormones that are governed primarily by the pituitary, catecholamines may en-

TABLE 10–6. Major Effects of Catecholamines on Hormone Secretion*

Endocrine Organ	Hormone	Effect	Receptor	Usual Feedback Loop
Pancreatic islets				
Alpha cells	Glucagon	↑	Beta	Plasma substrate
Beta cells	Insulin	↓	Alpha	Plasma substrate
		↑	Beta	
Delta cells	Somatostatin	↑	Beta	?
Non-alpha, beta, delta cells	Pancreatic polypeptide	↑	Beta	?
Thyroid				
Follicles	T$_4$, T$_3$	↑	Beta	TSH
C cells	Calcitonin	↑	Beta	Plasma ionized calcium
Parathyroid	PTH	↑	Beta	Plasma ionized calcium
Gastric antrum and duodenum	Gastrin	↑	Beta	Gastric luminal pH
Kidney				
Juxtaglomerular apparatus	Renin	↑	Beta	Renal baroreceptor, distal tubular sodium
Not known	Erythropoietin	↑	Beta	Arterial P$_{O_2}$
Ovary and placenta	Progesterone	↑	Beta	LH, hCG
Testis	Testosterone	↑	Beta	LH
Pineal	Melatonin	↑	Beta	Light-dark cycle
Adrenal cortex	Aldosterone	↓	?DA	Angiotensin II, plasma potassium ACTH

*T$_4$, thyroxine; T$_3$, triiodothyronine; TSH, thyrotropin; PTH, parathyroid hormone; LH, luteinizing hormone; hCG, human chorionic gonadotropin; ACTH, corticotropin (adrenocorticotropin).

hance central regulation by altering the sensitivity of the gland to the trophic hormone. Although the sympathoadrenal system may also affect pituitary function (see earlier mention of catecholamines and vasopressin),[789] the following discussion excludes pituitary hormones, because clear distinctions cannot be made between the effects of peripheral and central (hypothalamic) catecholamines.

Effects of Catecholamines: An Overview. The effects of catecholamines on peripheral hormone secretion have common features. Beta-adrenergic receptor activation causes acute release of preformed hormone through a cAMP-dependent mechanism; this enhancement of hormone secretion is transient despite the continued presence of the agonist. Alpha-receptor effects are usually inhibitory and antagonize the principal stimulus for hormone secretion, such as glucose for insulin release and thyrotropin (thyroid-stimulating hormone, TSH) for thyroid hormone secretion, and they are frequently associated with suppression of cAMP. In addition to influencing secretion, catecholamines also affect hormone synthesis.

In some circumstances when catecholamines alone are without effect, they potentiate hormonal responses to other stimuli. Thus one role of the sympathoadrenal system may be to regulate the sensitivity of endocrine cells to stimulation by their usual secretagogues. The tonic level of sympathetic activity may be particularly important in this regard. The sympathetic nerves, moreover, contribute to ovarian and thyroid hypertrophy,[538, 790, 791] which suggests that the sympathoadrenal system may be involved in some types of glandular hypertrophy.

Sympathetic Nerves Versus Adrenal Medulla. As in other areas of metabolism, the relation between the sympathetic nerves and the adrenal medulla in regulation of hormone secretion is unclear. The presence of adrenergic fibers in proximity to the cell of origin of a particular hormone, especially synaptic contact between nerve terminal and secretory cell, provides prima facie evidence of sympathetic neuronal involvement in the secretory regulation of that hormone. Because epinephrine is a more potent agonist for the beta-2–receptor than is NE, characterization of the beta-adrenergic receptor subtype that is responsible for stimulating the release of the different hormones might, in theory, associate the beta-2–mediated responses with the adrenal medulla. Unfortunately, this pharmacological approach is not uniformly successful, in part because the receptor subtype designation is often tentative and because prejunctional beta-2–receptors that amplify sympathetic responses may be involved. In general, simultaneous catecholamine-induced alterations in the secretion of many hormones imply the global effect of adrenomedullary stimulation, whereas a selective change in one or another hormone is probably the result of the local effect of sympathetic nervous system activity.

APUD Cells and Catecholamine Effects. Many of the peptide hormones that are affected by catecholamines are secreted by cells referred to as APUD (amine precursor uptake and decarboxylation) cells.[792] As the name implies, such cells take up precursors of biogenic amines such as dopa and 5-hydroxytryptophan; decarboxylate them to DA and serotonin, respectively; and sequester them in storage granules. Among the secretory cells that are influenced by the sympathoadrenal system and are discussed in the following sections of this chapter, those responsible for the synthesis and secretion of insulin, glucagon, somatostatin, gastrin, and calcitonin are recognized members of the APUD series. An early hypothesis suggested that both APUD cells and the chromaffin cells of the adult sympathoadrenal system originated from a common progenitor in the embryonic neural crest,[792] but not all APUD cells are derived from

the neural crest.[793] An intimate association between APUD cells and catecholamines nonetheless seems likely. Because these cells possess the capacity to convert dopa into DA and because dopa circulates in plasma, local production of DA may serve an important regulatory function for APUD cells. In support of this possibility, the secretion of several of the hormones discussed later is increased after acute administration of levodopa[794–797] and DA.[200, 201, 798–800] Thus local conversion of dopa to DA may contribute to the secretory regulation of endocrine tissues.

RENIN. *Nerve Stimulation of Renin Release.* Renin is secreted by the juxtaglomerular cells of the kidney in response to changes in perfusion pressure at the afferent arteriole and in solute delivery to the distal tubule. Renal nerve stimulation or infusion of catecholamine increases renin secretion independent of changes in renal blood flow or in filtered sodium load.[788] The mammalian juxtaglomerular apparatus, exclusive of the macula densa, is innervated with sympathetic nerve endings.[801, 802] Despite the lack of direct innervation, the renin response to sympathetic stimulation depends on macula densa function.[803] Renin secretion elicited by renal nerve stimulation or administration of adrenergic agonists is mediated, in most circumstances, by beta-receptor mechanisms involving prejunctional beta-2–receptors and postjunctional beta-1–receptors.[804, 805] This response follows activation of adenylate cyclase[806] and involves the release of preformed hormone.[807, 808] The role of the alpha-receptor is less clear. Evidence is available in support of both alpha-mediated stimulation[809] and suppression[810, 811] of renin secretion; alpha-1–mediated inhibition depends on calcium.[812] Renin synthesis is enhanced in vitro in the presence of epinephrine and NE but not pure beta-agonists,[807] which suggests that an alpha-receptor mechanism, alone or in combination with beta stimulation, is responsible. In addition to these direct effects of catecholamines on renin secretion and synthesis, renal sympathetic nerves potentiate responses of renin to other stimuli.[813]

Role of Catecholamines in Physiological Regulation of Renin Release. Catecholamine stimulation of renin output is an integral part of the physiological response to volume depletion. Reflex regulation of renin release is mediated by a neural arc arising from cardiopulmonary baroreceptors; afferent impulses from these receptors travel in the vagus nerve and exert a tonic suppressive effect on renal nerve activity and renin secretion.[814] Interruption of neural afferents increases, and distention of the baroreceptors diminishes, sympathetically mediated renin secretion.[814, 815] Afferent signals from carotid baroreceptors also participate but are less potent.[816] A contribution of this reflex arc to the physiological regulation of renin secretion can be inferred from the inhibition of renin responses by beta-adrenergic blockade or renal denervation.[817–820] Deficient or discoordinated renin release in some patients with postural hypotension secondary to autonomic neuropathy demonstrates the importance of sympathetic input for postural renin responses.[821–824]

The rise in plasma renin level that accompanies chronic sodium depletion cannot, however, be attributed entirely to catecholamines. Although acute beta-adrenergic blockade lowers the elevated renin levels that are associated with sodium restriction,[825–828] chronic administration of propranolol is without effect.[825, 829–831] Patients with autonomic neuropathy have lower renin levels than control subjects, but the plasma renin level increases in response to a low-sodium diet.[731] On the other hand, surgical denervation of the canine kidney abolishes the renin response to a sodium-restricted diet.[832] Thus renal sympathetic activity, although not essential for a renin rise in the sodium-deficient state, contributes to increased renin secretion in this condition.

In other physiological and pathophysiological states in which plasma renin activity is elevated, including hemorrhage, peripheral vasodilation, exercise, respiratory acidosis, and psychological stress, the increase is mediated by the beta-adrenergic receptor.[788] With the exception of hypoglycemia, in which the increase in plasma renin level is due to adrenomedullary stimulation,[833] the sympathetic nervous system exerts a greater influence than adrenomedullary catecholamines over renin secretion. The renal sympathetic nervous system predominates in situations requiring an immediate response, such as upright posture; in the chronic situation, such as sodium restriction, additional factors participate in the renin response.

INSULIN AND GLUCAGON. *Nerve Stimulation of Insulin and Glucagon Release.* Although the secretory activity of the endocrine pancreas is governed predominantly by delivery of substrates, particularly glucose and amino acids, catecholamines influence this function. Sympathetic (and parasympathetic) nerve fibers are close to all islet cell types,[834, 835] and alterations in insulin and glucagon secretion occur in response to pancreatic nerve stimulation or administration of adrenergic agonists.[788] Beta-(beta-2)–receptor activation transiently increases secretion of both insulin and glucagon, whereas alpha-(alpha-2)–receptor stimulation suppresses insulin secretion; the effect of alpha-receptor mechanisms on glucagon secretion is uncertain. Although alpha-receptor–mediated inhibition of insulin secretion usually predominates over beta-receptor–mediated stimulation, various factors, including glucose, potassium, calcium, thyroid hormone, and properties that are intrinsic to the agonist used affect the balance between alpha- and beta-adrenergic responses.[836–839]

Studies with purified populations of alpha and beta cells indicate that catecholamine effects occur in the context of paracrine regulation of islet hormone secretion. Epinephrine and NE elicit beta-receptor–mediated stimulation of glucagon secretion from alpha cells and, in the presence of glucagon, alpha-2–receptor-mediated inhibition of insulin secretion.[840] Changes in cAMP generation parallel these secretory responses to catecholamines in both cell types.

Islet responses to nonadrenergic stimuli are also influenced by previous exposure to catecholamines. In vivo treatments that impair sympathetic function limit glucose-induced insulin and calcium-mediated glucagon secretion in vitro,[841–843] whereas exposure of islets to epinephrine or NE enhances subsequent insulin secretion in response to glucose or acetylcholine in the absence of catecholamine.[844, 845] The synergistic interaction between catecholamines and nutrient responses of beta and alpha cells may reflect catecholamine-mediated changes in cAMP formation.[846, 847] Thus catecholamines may play a role in maintenance of normal islet cell secretory responses to other stimuli.

Role of Catecholamines in Physiological Regulation of Insulin and Glucagon Release. The hormonal pattern of impaired insulin (either low insulin levels per se or normal insulin levels despite hyperglycemia) and enhanced glucagon release has suggested a role for the sympathoadrenal system in regulation of the endocrine pancreas. For pancreatic beta cells, the improvement in insulin secretion after alpha-adrenergic blockade or adrenalectomy buttresses the argument favoring active inhibition of insulin secretion by catecholamines.[788] The return of insulin responses to normal after acute adrenalectomy implicates adrenomedullary catecholamines as the primary factor. The changes in insulin secretion in other conditions, however, suggest that diminished insulin secretion may reflect not only an increase in adrenomedullary secretion but also withdrawal of the stimulatory influence of pancreatic sympathetic activity. The situation with regard to glucagon secretion is even less well

defined. Increased glucagon release is frequently coincident with sympathoadrenal activation, but whether catecholamines cause this increase is equivocal.[788]

THYROID HORMONE. A potential role for the sympathetic nervous system in the regulation of thyroid function was recognized many years ago. Nerves originating from the cervical ganglia and the vagus nerve terminate within the thyroid gland, and several lines of experimental evidence suggest that the sympathoadrenal system may influence thyroid function.

Not only is the perivascular region of the thyroid rich in sympathetic nerves, but nonvascular structures, including the thyroid follicles themselves, receive adrenergic fibers.[848] The extent of innervation varies among species and as a function of age.[849–851] Sympathetic nerve endings terminate on and even within the follicular basement membrane.[852] The morphological evidence thus suggests that sympathetic nerves are intimately involved in thyroid function.

Catecholamines influence various aspects of thyroid gland metabolism and thyroid hormone biosynthesis in vitro. Epinephrine, via an alpha-receptor mechanism, increases uptake of iodine by augmenting organification; iodine transport is not increased.[853–855] Catecholamines also stimulate iodothyronine synthesis, glucose metabolism, and protein synthesis but have no effect on degradation of iodoproteins.[855–857] Both epinephrine and NE inhibit TSH-induced and long-acting thyroid stimulator–induced thyroxine release by alpha-receptor activation.[858, 859] Thus catecholamines exert diverse effects on the thyroid.

Stimulation of the superior cervical ganglion in mammals increases,[860] whereas chemical or surgical sympathectomy reduces, thyroid hormone release.[861] Catecholamine administration after suppression of TSH increases thyroid hormone secretion by a beta-2–receptor mechanism but exerts no effect in animals with intact TSH secretion.[862, 863] Thus the physiological significance of the sympathetic nerves in regulation of thyroid function is unclear. It is conceivable, but speculative, that sympathetic stimulation enhances thyroid hormone secretion in several pathophysiological states, including acute psychiatric illness and hyperemesis gravidarum. Circulating catecholamines probably do not have a regulatory function.

PARATHYROID HORMONE AND CALCITONIN. The secretion of parathyroid hormone (PTH) and calcitonin is governed primarily by serum calcium, but catecholamines may also play a role.[788, 864] Human parathyroid tissue is innervated with nerve fibers terminating on chief cells.[865] Although sympathetic varicosities occur in interfollicular spaces,[852] synaptic contact with the calcitonin-producing C cells has not been reported. Beta-receptor stimulation increases, whereas alpha-receptor stimulation inhibits, secretion of both PTH and calcitonin in vitro.[866–873] These effects of catecholamines on PTH secretion are mediated via changes in cAMP formation.[874, 875] Similar results have been obtained in vivo with adrenergic agonists and antagonists in some[758, 759, 876, 877] but not all studies.[761, 762] Stimulation of PTH secretion by catecholamines depends, in part, on the extracellular serum calcium concentration; hypercalcemia suppresses and hypocalcemia augments the PTH response to catecholamines.[878–880]

In normal human subjects PTH and calcitonin responses to catecholamine infusions are variable,[761, 881] but catecholamine participation in PTH and calcitonin secretion can be inferred in several circumstances. In burn victims concurrent elevations in serum calcitonin and urinary NE levels may have a causal connection.[882] Likewise, in patients with chronic renal failure, which is a condition of heightened sympathetic activity,[883, 884] suppression of calcitonin and PTH levels by acute beta-blockade suggests increased sympathetic input to these secretory cells.[885] Finally, because propranolol inhibits the increase in calcitonin that occurs with feeding,[886] the sympathetic nervous system may be involved in this response. The latter observation is of interest in light of the postulated role for calcitonin in postprandial calcium homeostasis.[887]

GASTRIN. Secretion of gastrin by the G cells of the gastric antrum and proximal duodenum is governed by the interaction of intraluminal, hormonal, and neural factors that may involve catecholamines. Adrenergic nerve fibers extend into mucosal and submucosal layers of stomach and duodenum, with most fibers at the basal surface of the epithelium.[888, 889] Catecholamines increase gastrin levels acutely by a beta-adrenergic mechanism,[890–894] and the reflex increase in gastrin after denervation of the carotid baroreceptor is abolished by adrenalectomy.[895] Although beta-blockade is without effect on meal-induced gastrin secretion,[896, 897] beta-agonists potentiate the gastrin response to a meal.[898] Propranolol antagonizes arginine stimulation of gastrin.[899]

Although the overall contribution of catecholamines to physiological regulation of gastrin secretion is unknown, elevations in serum gastrin level may reflect the effects of catecholamines. The increase in gastrin after insulin-induced hypoglycemia is reduced by intravenous (but not oral) propranolol.[900–903] Likewise, beta-adrenergic blockade abolishes the rise in gastrin during respiratory acidosis.[904] The elevated gastrin levels after burns, exercise, and cigarette smoking may be related to sympathoadrenal activation, although a causal relationship has not been established.[905, 906] In patients with hyperthyroidism and duodenal ulcer, hypersecretion of gastrin has been linked to beta-adrenergic activation.[904, 907, 908]

PROGESTERONE. The sympathetic nervous system may play a role in ovarian function. In addition to participation in the regulation of compensatory ovarian hypertrophy after unilateral ovariectomy[538] and of ovarian contractility,[524] sympathetic nerves may contribute to the regulation of progesterone secretion. The extensive sympathetic nerve supply in the ovary innervates hormone-producing as well as vascular structures.[909, 910] Propranolol abolishes the rise in plasma progesterone that is associated with cervical dilation in the first trimester of pregnancy.[911] Beta-2–adrenergic activation stimulates ovarian cAMP and progesterone production.[912–915] Alpha-adrenergic stimulation has opposite effects.[916, 917] The ovarian response to catecholamines depends on gonadotropins.[909, 918–921] Catecholamines also enhance progesterone production from placenta.[922, 923] The physiological importance of catecholamine-stimulated progesterone secretion is unknown, although ovarian sympathetic activity rises at ovulation[924] and is probably increased in other regions as well during the luteal phase of the menstrual cycle and in pregnancy, when progesterone levels are also elevated.[925] Abnormalities of the ovarian sympathetic innervation have been reported in the polycystic ovary syndrome.[926]

TESTOSTERONE. Adrenergic nerves are present close to the Leydig cells in several species, including humans.[927, 928] In vitro catecholamines increase testosterone production by Leydig cells after a 24-h latent period via a beta-adrenergic mechanism involving cAMP.[929–933] Catecholamines reportedly lower circulating testosterone levels in vivo,[934–936] although beta-adrenergic stimulation raises testosterone output from perfused canine testis[937] and also increases testosterone synthesis. Alterations in plasma levels that are induced by stressful circumstances may, in part, reflect the effects of catecholamines on testicular secretion of testosterone.[938–940]

ERYTHROPOIETIN. Erythropoietin in large part determines the rate of red blood cell production in the bone marrow.[941] The release of this hormone is regulated by arterial P_{O_2}.[942] Adrenergic agonists, particularly those of the beta-2 subclass, increase plasma levels of erythropoietin.[943–945] Moreover, acute splanchnic nerve section or beta-adrenergic blockade diminishes the erythropoietin response to hypoxia and hemorrhage.[946–948] Thus the sympathetic nervous system may play a role in regulation of erythropoietin secretion.

ALDOSTERONE. In addition to angiotensin, ACTH, sodium, and potassium, DA may also regulate aldosterone secretion.[949] Plasma aldosterone levels increase after administration of the dopaminergic antagonist metoclopramide.[204, 950, 951] DA-induced suppression of aldosterone secretion is demonstrable in vivo but only if angiotensin II levels are elevated secondary to its infusion, upright posture, or dietary sodium restriction.[952–956]

The site at which DA exerts its suppressive effect is open to question. Although it inhibits aldosterone production by glomerulosa cells in vitro, high concentrations are generally required for this effect.[957–960] Delivery of DA or metoclopramide centrally is more effective in lowering or raising aldosterone levels than either systemic or intra-adrenal administration.[961, 962] The DA antagonist domperidone, which, unlike metoclopramide, does not cross the blood-brain barrier, does not affect aldosterone levels.[963, 964] Finally, the metoclopramide-induced rise in aldosterone is abolished by ganglionic blockade,[964] which implies that efferent autonomic nerves participate in this response. Thus the locus at which DA influences aldosterone secretion may reside within the CNS, although this remains unproved at present.

OTHER HORMONES. Catecholamines influence the secretion of other hormones. The regulation of melatonin secretion is reviewed elsewhere.[965] The functional state of the pineal gland is coupled to the environmental light-dark cycle by a neuronal pathway originating at the retina and reaching the pineal via adrenergic fibers from the superior cervical ganglion. Sympathetic activity—and perhaps circulating catecholamines also—influences the activities of both enzymes that are necessary to convert serotonin into melatonin, N-acetyltransferase and hydroxyindole O-methyltransferase.[966, 967]

In the pancreatic islet the secretion of somatostatin and pancreatic polypeptide is influenced by catecholamines. Beta-receptor activation stimulates, whereas alpha-receptor activation suppresses, the secretion of both hormones.[968–974] In the presence of epinephrine, however, the predominant response is inhibitory for somatostatin[969] and stimulatory for pancreatic polypeptide.[973] Because insulin, glucagon, somatostatin, and pancreatic polypeptide all manifest similar responses to pure alpha- and beta-adrenergic agonists and different responses to a mixed agonist such as epinephrine,[969] differences in alpha- and beta-adrenergic receptor sensitivity among the different endocrine cells may be involved.

Release of atrial natriuretic peptide from cardiac atria is stimulated by catecholamines both in vivo and in vitro.[975–977] Activation of alpha- and/or beta-adrenergic receptors increases atrial natriuretic peptide secretion in vitro,[976, 977] but whether these effects directly mediate the atrial natriuretic peptide response to catecholamine infusion in vivo is uncertain.[978]

Role of Sympathoadrenal System in Various Physiological and Pathophysiological States

COLD EXPOSURE. *Critical Role of Sympathoadrenal System.* An intact sympathoadrenal system is an absolute requirement for normal mammalian defense against exposure to cold. When the sympathetic nervous system and the adrenal medulla are ablated, body temperature is not maintained in a cold environment, and death from hypothermia rapidly ensues.[979, 980] Either the sympathetic nervous system or the adrenal medulla is sufficient to sustain life when the other is deficient. Under normal circumstances the sympathetic nervous system plays the dominant role.[557, 558] When the function of the sympathetic nervous system is impaired, catecholamines of adrenomedullary origin support some of the physiological functions that are normally subserved by the sympathetic nerves.[481] The sympathoadrenal response to cold is manifested by an interplay among the metabolic, cardiovascular, and hormonal effects of catecholamines.

Sympathoadrenal Activation During Cold Exposure. When a mammal is exposed to cold, a prompt increase in sympathetic nervous system activity is reflected by increased NE excretion,[981] increased plasma NE levels,[982, 983] and increased NE turnover rate.[48, 346, 984] Adrenomedullary stimulation is of a lesser degree, and the increase in adrenomedullary activity is not sustained.[981] Sympathetic stimulation during cold exposure is induced by temperature receptors in the skin and by central temperature-sensitive neurons in the hypothalamus, lower brain stem, and spinal column.[985–987] Integration of afferent neural input from these areas in the hypothalamus stimulates sympathetic outflow.[988] The increase in sympathetic activity is not distributed uniformly; sympathetic outflow to heart, pancreas, lung, spleen, skeletal muscle, and BAT is markedly increased by cold,[558] whereas submaxillary gland, liver, intestine, and kidney show little or no effect. Heat conservation is the consequence of diminished subcutaneous blood flow and, in fur-bearing mammals, of piloerection, both of which increase the insulation provided by the integument. Heat production is increased by shivering, which is regulated by the somatic motor system but is facilitated by catecholamines, and by the stimulation of nonshivering thermogenesis. The sympathoadrenal system also provides fuel for increased heat production by mobilizing substrates, and it regulates the distribution of substrates and oxygen to metabolizing tissues.

Regulation of Substrate Supply. Substrate for heat production during cold exposure is provided by the breakdown of adipose tissue triglyceride and of hepatic and skeletal muscle glycogen, and by the synthesis of glucose and ketone bodies in liver. The increase in substrate supply is regulated by the sympathoadrenal system because animals that are subjected to adrenalectomy and chemical sympathectomy fail to mobilize free fatty acids or to increase hepatic glucose output in response to cold.[989]

On exposure to a cold environment fat metabolism increases, as indicated by a decrease in respiratory quotient[990] and a rise in circulating free fatty acids,[991] which are changes that are also produced by infusions of NE.[992, 993] The sympathetic nervous system is more important than the adrenal medulla in regulating adipose tissue lipolysis in the cold because adrenal demedullation does not prevent the rise in free fatty acids that follows cold exposure.[991] Sympathetic nervous system activation may also facilitate the use of plasma triglycerides as substrate during cold exposure because both administration of NE and exposure to a cold environment increase the activity of lipoprotein lipase in BAT and heart;[687] as a consequence, plasma triglyceride and very-low-density lipoprotein levels fall,[687] although this may be due in part to catecholamine-mediated inhibition of hepatic triglyceride secretion.[685] Although increased caloric intake eventually balances the energy deficit during prolonged cold exposure, depletion of adipose stores occurs in the cold, even when access to food is unrestricted.[994]

The sympathoadrenal system is also involved in stimulation of carbohydrate metabolism during cold exposure, as demonstrated by diminution in hepatic glycogen and increased peripheral utilization of glucose.[990] Both the adrenal medulla and the sympathetic nervous system appear to be involved.[989, 995] Stimulation of glucagon[996, 997] and suppression of insulin[997–1000] occur during cold exposure, and alpha-adrenergic blockade antagonizes cold-induced suppression of insulin release.[1000, 1001] The adrenal medulla appears to be involved in suppression of insulin release, whereas the sympathetic nervous system may be involved in stimulation of glucagon.[996, 1002]

Cardiovascular Changes During Cold Exposure. Cardiovascular changes that are mediated by the sympathetic nervous system contribute both to heat conservation and to the delivery of oxygen and substrate to metabolizing tissues. Vasoconstriction in subcutaneous vascular beds diminishes heat loss through the skin by an alpha-2–receptor mechanism.[1003] Lower ambient temperatures cause enhanced vascular contractile responses to NE.[440, 1004, 1005] The superficial veins are particularly responsive, and venoconstriction shifts blood from the superficial subcutaneous veins to the deeper venae comitantes. The mechanisms that are involved in this response to cold have been well worked out and illustrate the complexity of adrenergic vascular regulation.[1006] Both superficial and deep veins in the dog are endowed with alpha-1– and alpha-2–receptors,[1006] the former predominating in the deep venous system, the latter in the superficial system. External cooling potentiates alpha-2 responses by enhancing receptor affinity but diminishes alpha-1 responses by a direct effect on the contractile process. The presence of spare alpha-1–receptors in the superficial, but not the deep, venous system maintains alpha-1 responses in the superficial system despite the lowered temperature. The resulting superficial venoconstriction shunts cooler blood to the deep system, where the direct inhibitory effect of cold decreases venous tone, thereby enhancing blood flow in the deep venous system, because deep veins have no alpha-1–receptor reserve and alpha-2–receptors are relatively sparse in this area.[1006] Increased flow in the deep veins augments the efficiency of countercurrent heat exchange in the extremities, thereby promoting the transfer of heat from arterial blood to the cooler venous blood returning to the central venous pool. The net result of increased sympathetic activity in the subcutaneous vascular beds and the enhanced sensitivity to NE that is induced by the local cold environment is conservation of heat.

Despite the vasoconstriction in the superficial vasculature, cold exposure causes a twofold increase in cardiac output in warm-acclimated human subjects,[1007] an increase that is probably attributable to the sympathetic nervous system. The increase in cardiac output correlates directly with the increase in oxygen uptake, which is consistent with a relationship between the cardiovascular changes and the delivery of oxygen and substrate to metabolizing tissues.[1007] In non–cold-acclimated primates, acute cold exposure is associated with an increase in blood pressure of about 20%.[1007–1009]

Cold Acclimation. Chronic exposure to cold, either continuous or intermittent, results in an increased capacity for metabolic heat production on re-exposure to cold,[1010] along with a decrease in the need to shiver. The hallmark of the cold-acclimated state is enhancement of the thermogenic response to NE (Fig. 10–24); the augmented response to NE provides a convenient test for the presence of cold acclimation. Cold acclimation[558, 1011] and the enhanced thermogenic response to NE[1012] occur in human subjects. In animals cold acclimation is associated with substantial hypertrophy of BAT,[1010] accompanied by an increase in both sympathetic innervation[346, 643] and the GDP-binding uncoupling protein thermogenin.[1010] The sympathetic nervous system is involved in cold acclimation because chronic administration of NE (or other beta-agonists) promotes the

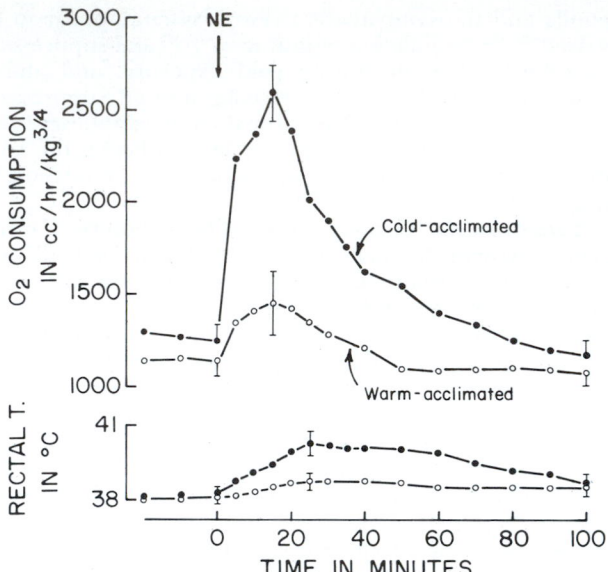

Figure 10–24. NE-stimulated thermogenesis in the rat: effect of cold acclimation. NE increases oxygen consumption (and rectal temperature) in both cold-acclimated (●) and warm-acclimated (○) curarized rats. The effect is markedly enhanced in cold-acclimated animals—the hallmark of cold acclimation. (From Hseih ACL, Carlson LD, Gray G. Role of the sympathetic nervous system in the control of chemical regulation of heat production. Am J Physiol 1957; 190:247–251.)

development of BAT[1013–1015] and enhances the thermogenic response to subsequent administration of NE.[730] However, administration of NE does not reproduce all the physiological and biochemical effects that are associated with cold acclimation.[730, 1014] Thyroid hormones do not produce the alterations associated with cold acclimation, but a permissive level of thyroid hormone is required for cold acclimation to occur.[555] It is interesting that in cold-acclimated human subjects the cardiovascular responses to both cold exposure[1009, 1016] and NE infusion[1012] are diminished in comparison with the responses noted in non–cold-acclimated subjects. In rats cold acclimation diminishes the pressor response to alpha-agonists,[1017] a finding that may explain the diminished effect of cold on blood pressure in cold-acclimated compared with warm-acclimated mammals.

HYPOGLYCEMIA. (See also Chap. 23.) *Sympathoadrenal Response to Hypoglycemia.* When the plasma glucose level is lowered, plasma and urinary levels of epinephrine promptly rise as much as 10- to 50-fold, depending on the degree and severity of the hypoglycemia (Figs. 10–25 and 10–26).[1018–1023] Small increases in plasma and urinary NE levels also occur. The latter originate in the adrenal medulla because (1) plasma NE levels do not increase when hypoglycemia is induced in adrenalectomized human subjects[319] and (2) NE levels increase in adrenal venous effluent during hypoglycemia in animals.[1024] In animals sympathetic activity is suppressed during hypoglycemia[316, 317] or 2-deoxyglucose administration[318] despite concomitant adrenomedullary stimulation. Thus during hypoglycemia the adrenal medulla is markedly stimulated while the sympathetic nervous system is suppressed.

Regulation of Adrenomedullary Response: Stimulus and Central Receptors. The plasma epinephrine concentration increases as the plasma glucose level is reduced from 5.3 to 3.3 mmol/L (95 to 60 mg/dL),[1025] which indicates that adrenomedullary stimulation occurs in response to glucose lowering within the physiological range and at glucose levels above those regarded as hypoglycemic. At about 2.8 mmol/L (50 mg/dL) a substantial further increase in adrenomedullary epinephrine secretion occurs (see Fig. 10–25), the magnitude depending on both the degree and duration of the hypoglycemia.[1026] The absolute glucose level rather than the rate of glucose fall appears to be the significant variable in triggering the adrenomedullary response.[1027–1029] In some diabetic subjects the threshold for adrenomedullary stimulation is raised.[1030]

The adrenomedullary response to hypoglycemia is elicited by glucose-sensitive neurons within the CNS. The epinephrine response to hypoglycemia is abolished by adrenal denervation, spinal cord transection,[1031] or ganglionic blockade.[1020, 1032] Neurons within the hypothalamus play a critical role in initiating the adrenomedullary response to hypoglycemia;[1033, 1034] lower centers in the caudal brain stem and upper spinal cord also possess the capacity to initiate the adrenomedullary response to hypoglycemia.[1032–1039]

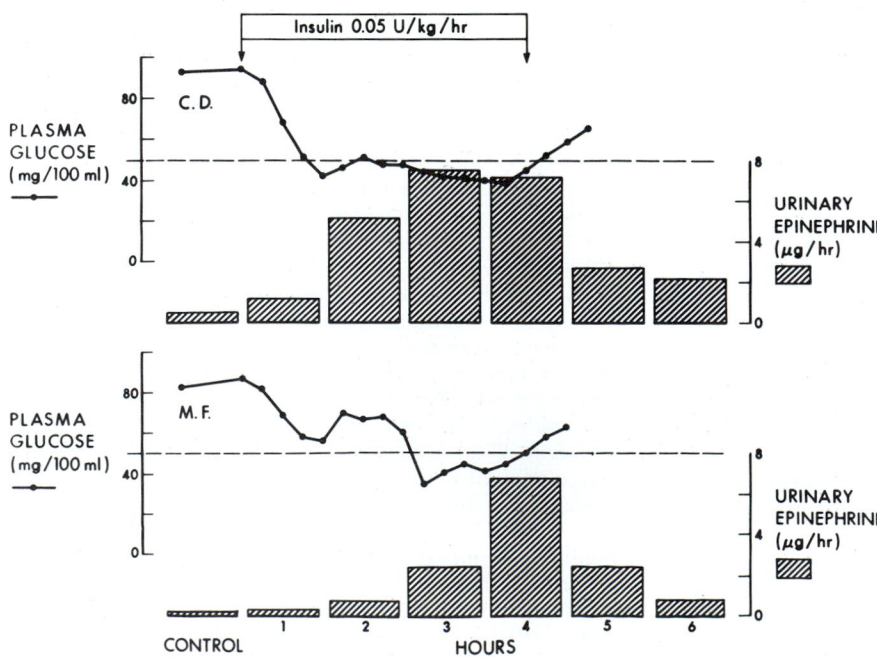

Figure 10–25. Effect of insulin-induced hypoglycemia on urinary epinephrine excretion in two normal men. Note that the urinary epinephrine excretion rises markedly when plasma glucose levels fall below 50 mg/dL. To convert glucose values to mmol/L, multiply by 0.05551. (From Landsberg L, Young JB. Catecholamines and the adrenal medulla. In: Bondy PK, Rosenberg LE, eds. Metabolic Control and Disease. 8th ed. Philadelphia: W. B. Saunders, 1980: 1621–1693.)

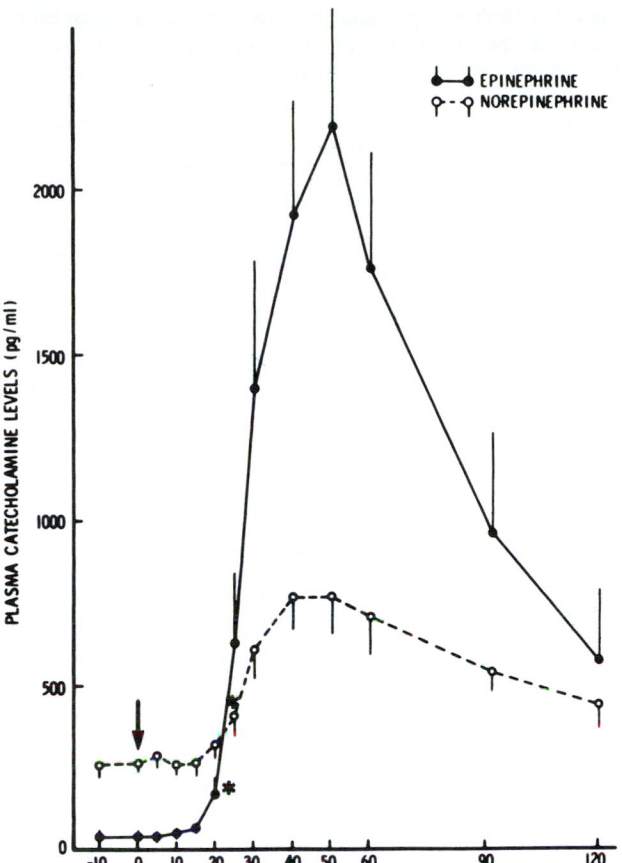

Figure 10–26. Effect of insulin-induced hypoglycemia on plasma epinephrine and NE levels. After an intravenous injection of 0.15 U/kg of regular insulin at time 0, plasma levels of epinephrine rise 50-fold in normal human subjects. To convert epinephrine values to pmol/L, multiply by 5.45. To convert norepinephrine values to nmol/L, multiply by 0.005911. (From Garber AJ, Cryer PE, Santiago JV, et al. The role of adrenergic mechanisms in the substrate and hormonal response to insulin-induced hypoglycemia in man. Reproduced from The Journal of Clinical Investigation, 1976, vol. 58, pp. 7–15 by copyright permission of The American Society for Clinical Investigation.)

Experiments with 2-deoxyglucose in both experimental animals and human subjects[1031, 1034] indicate that diminished intracellular glucose metabolism within central neurons is the proximate stimulus of the adrenomedullary response. It is interesting that the provision of alternative substrate in the form of ketones blocks the usual adrenomedullary response to hypoglycemia in dogs and rats.[1040–1042] A suppressive effect of ketone infusions on the adrenomedullary response to hypoglycemia has not been demonstrated in humans,[1043] although chronically fasted human subjects fail to increase epinephrine excretion in response to insulin-induced hypoglycemia.[1044]

Adrenal Medulla and Counterregulatory Response. The hormonal basis of glucose counterregulation after hypoglycemia is considered in Chapter 23. The redundancy of counterregulatory mechanisms, which reflects the physiological priority of continuous substrate supply for the brain, makes it difficult to document the precise role of epinephrine in mediating the various components of the counterregulatory response. Adrenalectomized, corticosteroid-replaced subjects and persons treated with adrenergic blocking agents have normal counterregulatory responses to insulin-induced hypoglycemia provided that glucagon secretion is unimpaired.[319, 1045, 1046] When glucagon secretion is blocked by somatostatin, however, epinephrine is required for normal glucose counterregulation, in response to insulin,[1047] as well as in postprandial,[1048] postabsorptive,[1049] and fasted states.[1050] These observations do not preclude the possibility that more

severe or prolonged hypoglycemia may require epinephrine for normal recovery. Because glucagon responses are deficient in most patients with insulin-dependent diabetes mellitus,[1051] this group of patients is especially dependent on epinephrine in the defense against hypoglycemia. Patients with this type of diabetes mellitus who have deficient epinephrine responses are, therefore, at particular risk for the development of hypoglycemia,[1052–1054] which limits the use of intensive insulin therapy in this group. Intensive insulin treatment lowers the epinephrine response to hypoglycemia by lowering the hypoglycemic threshold,[1055] perhaps by altering glucose transport into the CNS.

The actions of epinephrine that contribute to the counterregulatory response include (1) enhancement of hepatic glucose output (stimulation of glycogenolysis, gluconeogenesis); (2) stimulation of lipolysis in adipose tissue (provision of alternative substrate in the form of free fatty acids and glycerol); (3) inhibition of insulin-mediated glucose uptake in muscle (preservation of glucose for the CNS); and (4) suppression of endogenous insulin and stimulation of glucagon release.[1020] The cardiovascular responses to hypoglycemia—tachycardia, widened pulse pressure, and increased sweating—depend on adrenomedullary epinephrine.[1020] These signs are important for subjective recognition of hypoglycemia. Treatment with beta-adrenergic blocking agents,[1047] the presence of autonomic neuropathy,[1056–1059] or, possibly, autoimmune destruction of the adrenal medulla[1060] may increase the risk of hypoglycemia in insulin-requiring diabetic patients by altering epinephrine-dependent counterregulatory mechanisms and by impairing subjective recognition of the hypoglycemic reaction. Impaired adrenomedullary epinephrine response may contribute to the hypoglycemia that is noted in infants and children with spontaneous or ketotic hypoglycemia.[1061–1063] Decreased beta-adrenergic sensitivity has also been described in insulin-dependent diabetics who are prone to hypoglycemic episodes.[1064]

FASTING AND STARVATION. The physiological requirements of the fasted or starved state entail two major metabolic adaptations: on the one hand, energy expenditure must be reduced to conserve calories in the face of restricted intake; on the other hand, fuel stores must be mobilized to provide substrate for maintenance of vital functions. Alterations in sympathoadrenal function during fasting promote these functions.[1065]

Sympathetic Nervous System. In both animals[359, 1066, 1067] and humans,[340, 483, 1068–1071] sympathetic nervous system activity is diminished by fasting or caloric restriction. Suppression of sympathetic activity may contribute to a decrease in metabolic rate with caloric restriction.[591] Although appropriate in the setting of famine, such a mechanism decreases the efficiency of low-energy diets during dieting for weight reduction.[1065] Diminished peripheral conversion of thyroxine to T_3 with starvation exerts a synergistic effect because thyroid hormones potentiate the thermogenic effects of catecholamines. The resting metabolic rate is further diminished by fasting in hypothyroid rats, which indicates that reduced oxygen consumption with caloric restriction may be independent of changes in thyroid hormone metabolism.[1072] The mechanism appears to involve decreased insulin-mediated glucose metabolism in glucose-sensitive neurons of the hypothalamus, which stimulate an inhibitory hypothalamic pathway that suppresses central sympathetic outflow.[318, 1065, 1073]

Adrenal Medulla. The adrenal medulla, as distinct from the sympathetic nervous system, is stimulated during fasting.[483, 1074] This stimulation is modest in degree compared with that noted during frank hypoglycemia, possibly because the decrement in plasma glucose level during fasting is small.[1025] The modest increase in epinephrine secretion nonetheless may foster substrate mobilization, particularly the hydrolysis of triglyceride in adipose tissue. Lipolysis is sensitive to variations in plasma epinephrine level within the physiological range,[1075] and fasting enhances the lipolytic effect of catecholamines.[625, 626, 1076] The small increase in epinephrine secretion with fasting is unlikely to stimulate thermogenesis, because the threshold for increasing oxygen consumption in nonfasting humans is approximately 490 to 546 pmol/L (90 to 100 pg/mL) of epinephrine.[1077] The combination of sympathetic nervous system suppression and adrenomedullary stimulation may contribute to substrate mobilization with a minimal increase in energy expenditure.

FEEDING. *Adrenal Medulla.* Epinephrine secretion from the adrenal medulla serves to stabilize the postabsorptive plasma glucose level in a manner analogous to the hypoglycemic response.[1078] Plasma epinephrine levels rise 4½ to 5 h after a glucose meal, a rise that follows and may be attributable to a small decrease in plasma glucose concentration to the range of 4.2 mmol/L (75 mg/dL).[1079] When glucagon is suppressed by somatostatin, adrenergic blockade prevents stabilization of the plasma glucose level and is associated with development of frank hypoglycemia.[1078]

Sympathetic Nervous System. Dietary intake influences the sympathetic nervous system in two ways. Ingestion of a meal stimulates the sympathetic nervous system acutely, probably as a consequence of cognitive factors relating to the meal (cephalic phase) and fluid shifts with volume sequestration in the gut.[321, 1079–1083] The fact that intravenous infusions of glucose and insulin[593, 1084] also increase sympathetic activity in humans suggests that insulin-mediated glucose metabolism may be involved in sympathetic stimulation.[1085] An acute increase in sympathetic activity might be important in postprandial regulation of extracellular fluid volume, cardiac output, and distribution of blood flow.

Dietary intake also has a more prolonged influence on the sympathetic nervous system.[340, 1065] Increased sympathetic activity has been demonstrated in rats and humans chronically overfed a mixed diet.[340, 346] In the rat increments in both sucrose and fat intake increase sympathetic activity, even when total caloric intake is not increased.[359, 1067, 1086, 1087]

Involvement of the sympathetic nervous system in the chronic increase in metabolic rate that follows prolonged consumption of excessive calories is suggested by the following: (1) diet exerts an important influence on sympathetic activity in BAT in the rat (the major thermogenic organ in this species);[346] (2) beta-blockade diminishes the metabolic rate in human subjects consuming a high- but not a low-energy diet;[592] and (3) beta-blockade antagonizes a portion of the increase in metabolic rate that occurs during insulin and glucose infusions in normal subjects.[593] Because there is wide variation in the capacity for diet-induced thermogenesis,[1088, 1089] sympathetic responses to alterations in dietary intake and to the thermogenic effects of catecholamines may be involved in the pathogenesis of human obesity.[1065, 1090]

EXERCISE. *Effect of Exercise on Sympathoadrenal System.* Intense or prolonged exercise activates both sympathetic nerves and the adrenal medulla, but mild to moderate exercise principally affects the sympathetic nervous system.[478, 1091] In dogs the skeletal muscle and the cardiovascular system account for much of the increase in plasma NE during exercise.[1092] Various factors influence the relationship between exercise-induced changes in sympathetic activity and adrenomedullary secretion, including antecedent diet, environmental temperature, and inspired oxygen content.[478] The fact that plasma NE levels increase before the onset of physical activity[1093] suggests that recruitment of sympathetic activity in anticipation of need may lessen the physiological impact of the exercise. Exercise training in animals and

humans lowers sympathetic nervous system activity both at rest and in response to exertion.[1094–1099] This reduction may reflect a change in peripheral sensitivity to catecholamines because increased vascular responses to alpha-adrenergic stimulation have been noted in trained dogs compared with untrained controls.[1100] In contrast, physical training has been shown to increase plasma epinephrine responses to a variety of stimuli compared with responses in untrained human subjects.[1101]

Effects of Catecholamines During Exercise. Blood pressure and cerebral blood flow are maintained during exercise by splanchnic and renal vasoconstriction despite vasodilation in skeletal muscle and cutaneous vascular beds. These cardiovascular adjustments are consistent with the known effects of catecholamines. Adrenergic blockade, surgical denervation, or autonomic neuropathy impairs the cardiovascular responses to exercise and diminishes exercise tolerance.[480, 1102–1104]

Catecholamines contribute to the mobilization of stored fuel in support of working muscle. Stimulation of muscle glycogenolysis represents the combined effects of muscular contraction and circulating epinephrine,[666, 1105] the influence of epinephrine being most prominent in red and intermediate-type muscle fibers.[671, 672] Lipolysis in adipose tissue with exercise is mediated in part by catecholamines because beta-adrenergic blockade markedly diminishes the free fatty acid concentrations in plasma.[1106] Lipolysis within individual muscle fibers is also stimulated by catecholamines, at least in red muscle.[645] Catecholamines may also contribute to the increase in hepatic glucose output during exercise; a role for hepatic sympathetic nerves in this process seems likely. The increase in hepatic glucose output reflects physiological insulin resistance because restoration of insulin levels by insulin infusion does not suppress glucose production.[1107]

Catecholamines influence the secretion of various hormones during exercise. Beta-adrenergic mechanisms contribute to the increase in renin and pancreatic polypeptide levels,[971, 1108] whereas alpha-adrenergic stimulation suppresses insulin release.[1109] Elevations in parathyroid hormone and gastrin levels in exercising animals and humans appear to be associated with increased plasma catecholamine levels.[906, 1110] The increase in glucagon with exercise, although associated with changes in sympathoadrenal activity, is closely related to ambient glucose concentrations.[1111]

TRAUMA, CIRCULATORY FAILURE, AND HYPOXIA. *Sympathoadrenal Responses.* Alterations in sympathoadrenal activity occur in pathophysiological states that threaten the integrity of the internal environment, such as major trauma, circulatory failure, and hypoxia. Acute and chronic responses differ. The biphasic nature of metabolic responses has been most intensively studied after injury.[595] During the acute (or "ebb") phase, defense of the circulation is the chief priority and, apart from meeting that need, metabolic activity decreases. If the organism survives for hours or days, a recovery (or "flow") phase ensues that may persist for weeks to months. At this time metabolic activity increases above basal levels to a degree dependent on the extent of injury. Energy expenditure increases, and endogenous fuel stores, especially body proteins, are mobilized in support of the accelerated metabolic rate. A similar pattern of acute reduction and chronic increase in metabolic rate occurs with hypoxia and circulatory insufficiency.[1112–1114]

In experimental animals increased adrenomedullary secretion is a uniform component of the acute response to injury or illness.[1115–1118] Sympathetic nerve activity is usually not increased and under some circumstances is suppressed.[1115–1119] In vasovagal syncope, which is a transient form of circulatory insufficiency in humans that is characterized by an abrupt fall in venous return, plasma epinephrine levels increase,[486] but the frequency of sympathetic impulse traffic in superficial autonomic nerves diminishes.[1120] Thus the acute sympathoadrenal response is predominantly one of adrenomedullary activation.

In the chronic state a different pattern emerges. As the acute elevation in adrenomedullary secretion gradually abates, enhanced sympathetic nerve activity ensues after injury,[1117, 1121, 1122] hypoxia,[1118, 1123, 1124] and congestive circulatory failure.[1125, 1126] Chronic volume depletion from fluid loss or hemorrhage is similarly associated with increased sympathetic nervous system activity. As described earlier, increased renal sympathetic activity contributes to sodium conservation under these circumstances. Dehydration, with resultant hypertonicity, also increases renal sympathetic activity.[1127]

The physiological role of catecholamines in the setting of injury, hypoxia, or circulatory failure is not determined solely by changes in sympathoadrenal activity. Alteration in the sensitivity of peripheral tissues to catecholamines is the traditional explanation for hypotension in the shock state despite sympathoadrenal activation. Diminished beta-adrenergic responses have been documented in acidosis, acute and chronic hypoxia, and chronic congestive heart failure.[1128–1131]

Physiological Consequences of Sympathoadrenal Response. The sympathoadrenal response to stress has important physiological implications. The increase in mortality that is seen in acutely injured animals after sympathoadrenal ablation[1117, 1132] demonstrates the fundamental importance of catecholamines in circulatory support. Catecholamine-mediated vasoconstriction, aided by activation of the renin-angiotensin-aldosterone system, is an essential component of the defense against injury, but when prolonged the same responses can result in necrosis of vital organs and can potentiate the development of lactic acidosis from widespread tissue hypoxia. Catecholamines, in addition, may be involved in the pathogenesis of stress ulceration[1133] and paralytic ileus[518, 1134] after severe injury or surgery.

An important consequence of the sympathoadrenal response in this setting involves thermoregulation. In the reparative phase after burn injury, for example, catecholamines mediate the increase in overall energy metabolism.[1121] Increased metabolism, sweating, and a slight elevation in body temperature are also occasionally seen in patients with chronic congestive heart failure or chronic hypoxemia from pulmonary disease. The involvement of catecholamines in these phenomena, although plausible, is unproved. The role of the sympathoadrenal system in the hypometabolism of the ebb phase after injury is even less clear. Because circulating catecholamines stimulate the metabolic rate to a lesser extent than sympathetic nerves, the early predominance of adrenomedullary secretion may be protective from the standpoint of energy metabolism by sustaining catecholamine-mediated processes at a lower metabolic rate.[483]

In the acute phase after injury, plasma glucose, lactate, glycerol, and free fatty acid levels are elevated in relation to the severity of injury.[1135] Hyperglycemia in these circumstances is due to interactions of epinephrine, glucagon, and cortisol.[1136] Despite elevations in glucose level, insulin secretion is suppressed,[1137, 1138] in large measure by an alpha-adrenergic influence of adrenal catecholamines.[1138–1140] The concomitant increase in glucagon levels may also result from sympathoadrenal stimulation.[1141–1145] In the chronic state, glucose levels are nearly normal but glucose cycling is accelerated.[1137] In the later stages of injury, insulin secretion is normal despite increased sympathetic activity.[1146, 1147]

REPRODUCTION, MENSES, AND PREGNANCY. The sympathoadrenal system participates in the regulation of mammalian reproduction. Sympathetic nervous system activity increases around the time of ovulation, perhaps in association with the luteinizing hormone surge.[1148–1150] Similar changes may occur late in pregnancy.[790, 1151] Urinary epinephrine and DA excretion does not change during the menstrual cycle,[1148, 1152] but DA excretion does rise during pregnancy.[1152] Because estrogens and progestogens are capable of altering adrenergic receptors in peripheral tissues, the effects of catecholamines on reproduction may reflect changes in tissue responsiveness in addition to changes in sympathoadrenal activity, as described earlier.

Catecholamines participate in the regulation of ovulation and ejaculation.[909, 927] Myometrial tone is affected by catecholamines, and the suppression of uterine contractility by beta-2–adrenergic agonists inhibits premature labor. Catecholamines may also be involved in the control of lactation.[927]

Thyroid-Catecholamine Interrelationships

GENERAL CONSIDERATIONS: SYMPATHOMIMETIC FEATURES OF HYPERTHYROIDISM. Infusions of epinephrine produce changes that resemble those seen in thyrotoxicosis. The manifestations of pheochromocytoma are not dissimilar to those of hyperthyroidism: increased metabolic rate, sweating, heat intolerance, weight loss, tachycardia, palpitations, and nervousness. Four major areas of thyroid-catecholamine interaction will be reviewed here: (1) the effect of thyroid hormones on activity of the sympathoadrenal system; (2) the effect of catecholamines on peripheral conversion of thyroxine (T_4) to triiodothyronine (T_3); (3) the effect of thyroid hormones on the sensitivity of effector tissues to catecholamines; and (4) adrenergic blockade in hyperthyroidism. As noted earlier, thyroid follicles are innervated by sympathetic nerve endings, which may regulate thyroid hormone secretion and synethesis under some circumstances.[788]

EFFECT OF THYROID HORMONES ON FUNCTIONAL STATE OF SYMPATHOADRENAL SYSTEM. The activity of the adrenal medulla is not affected by thyroid hormones; plasma epinephrine levels, urinary epinephrine excretion, and turnover of epinephrine are not altered in hypo- or hyperthyroidism.[1153–1155] The functional state of the sympathetic nervous system is, however, significantly affected by alterations in thyroid status. Thyroid hormone excess causes a modest decrease in sympathetic activity, and thyroid hormone deficiency enhances the activity of the sympathetic nervous system. The NE turnover rate, which is a measure of sympathetic activity, is unchanged or diminished in thyroid hormone–treated animals and is markedly increased when thyroid hormone is deficient.[47, 1156] Hyperthyroid patients have either normal or diminished levels of NE in plasma and urine, whereas hypothyroid patients show significant increases.[1153, 1154, 1157–1160] Plasma NE clearance is not altered in hypo- or hyperthyroidism, but the appearance rate of NE increases in hypothyroidism.[1161] Thus the relationship between thyroid status and sympathetic activity is inverse, and the sympathomimetic features of hyperthyroidism cannot be explained by enhanced sympathetic activity.

EFFECT OF CATECHOLAMINES ON PERIPHERAL CONVERSION OF T_4 TO T_3. Catecholamines affect the rate of deiodination of T_4 in animals.[1162] Studies with humans initially failed to support such an effect.[1163, 1164] However, both hyperthyroid and hypothyroid subjects who are maintained on a fixed dose of T_4 have reduced circulating T_3 levels with beta-adrenergic blockade.[1165–1169] The magnitude of the decrease varies between 13 and 30% and is most consistently seen with propranolol as compared with other agents. In some studies the reverse T_3 level was noted to increase,[1166, 1168] which is consistent with an effect on the 5'-deiodinase. Because the selective beta-1–antagonist atenolol does not change T_3 or reverse T_3 levels[1167, 1170] in vivo, unlike the nonselective agent propranolol, the beta-adrenergic effect on T_4 deiodination has been attributed to beta-2–receptor stimulation. The situation, however, is complex and incompletely understood. The non–beta-blocking D isomer of propranolol inhibits conversion of T_4 to T_3 in vitro as effectively as the active isomer or the racemic mixture.[1171, 1172] The effect of other beta-blockers in vitro is less certain,[1171, 1172] which suggests that the membrane-stabilizing effects and the lipid solubility of propanolol may be important in blockade of deiodination. BAT, furthermore, possesses a deiodinase (type II) that is distinct from the deiodinase in kidney and liver (type I).[578–581] The BAT type II deiodinase is activated by the alpha-1–adrenergic receptor.[579] Although this BAT deiodinase has been postulated as a potential source of systemic T_3 generation in rats,[1173] the potential contribution of this mechanism in humans is uncertain. It seems likely that blockade of deiodination in particular tissues may produce effects greater than those suggested by changes in circulating levels of thyroid hormones. It should be noted that the beneficial clinical effects of beta-adrenergic blockade in patients with hyperthyroidism are similar with the beta-1–selective agent atenolol and the nonspecific beta-blocker propranolol, despite the lesser impact on peripheral thyroid hormone levels with the beta-1–selective agent.[1167, 1170]

EFFECT OF THYROID HORMONES ON SENSITIVITY OF EFFECTOR TISSUES TO CATECHOLAMINES. An effect of thyroid hormones on the sensitivity of peripheral effector tissues to catecholamines has long been suspected because the sympathomimetic features of thyroid hormone excess are blocked by adrenergic antagonists, an effect that is not explicable in terms of altered sympathoadrenal activity.[1174] Increased sensitivity is probably due to changes in the beta-adrenergic receptor–adenylate cyclase–cAMP system.

Metabolic Responses. Thyroid hormones enhance beta-receptor–mediated lipolysis, insulin secretion, thermogenesis, and cold acclimation. In rat epididymal fat pads the dose-response relationship between lipolysis and catecholamines is shifted to the right by thyroid hormone deficiency and to the left by thyroid hormone excess.[1175–1178] Human subcutaneous adipose tissue similarly demonstrates an impairment in catecholamine-stimulated lipolysis in hypothyroidism and an enhanced lipolytic response to beta-receptor agonists in hyperthyroidism.[1179, 1180] Thyroid hormone excess enhances beta-receptor stimulation of insulin secretion in both rats and humans.[838, 1181] In hypothyroid rats the responses of insulin to beta-adrenergic stimulation are diminished.[838]

The interaction between catecholamines and thyroid hormones in the regulation of thermogenesis is complex (see earlier sections on BAT and cold exposure). Thyroid hormones are the principal regulators of basal metabolic rate, which is an obligatory component of thermogenesis.[555] Catecholamines, on the other hand, regulate adaptive thermogenesis.[558] Thyroid hormones do have a permissive and synergistic function in the adaptive forms of thermogenesis. In hypothyroid rats neither exogenous catecholamines nor cold exposure stimulates metabolic heat production.[1182–1186] Sympathetically mediated thermogenesis that occurs in response to carbohydrate intake also appears to require thyroid hormones.[1183] Thyroid hormone excess enhances catecholamine-induced thermogenesis in direct relationship to the dose of thyroid hormone administered,[1015, 1182, 1186, 1187] an effect that is localized, in rats, to BAT and is mediated by uncoupling protein.[577, 582, 583]

Cardiac Effects. Thyroid hormones enhanced the effects of catecholamines on the heart in many animal studies,[1188–1197] but in others no enhancement of sensitivity to catecholamines was noted.[1198–1203] In humans, most but not all studies have demonstrated that the chronotropic response to catecholamines is increased by thyrotoxicosis.[1204–1208] The relationship between thyroid hormones and the cardiac effects of catecholamines is confounded by the fact that thyroid hormones exert direct effects on the heart[1194, 1196, 1202] and potentiate the cardiac effects of agents other than catecholamines.[1189, 1191] In general the cardiac effects of catecholamines are probably potentiated by thyroid hormones.

Miscellaneous Effects. Other beta-receptor–mediated responses that are potentiated by thyroid hormones include amino acid transport,[1209] erythropoiesis,[1210] peripheral vasodilation,[1211] and enhancement of renin[1212] and gastrin[908] secretion.

Effects of Thyroid Hormones on Beta-Adrenergic Receptor and Receptor-Linked Adenylate Cyclase–cAMP System. Thyroid hormones alter the beta-adrenergic receptor as well as the receptor-linked adenylate cyclase–cAMP system.[1213] Although variation exists among tissues and species, in general thyroid hormone excess potentiates, and thyroid hormone deficiency diminishes, sensitivity to the physiological effects of catecholamines. In rat heart, thyroid hormones increase beta-adrenergic receptor number[1195, 1213–1217] without altering receptor affinity. In contrast, beta-adrenergic receptor number is not increased by thyroid hormone excess in isolated rat adipocytes,[1177, 1178] lymphocytes, and lung[1216] or in turkey erythrocytes.[1213, 1218] Thyroid hormone deficiency diminishes beta-receptor number in rat heart[1213, 1219] and turkey erythrocytes,[1218] whereas the number of beta-receptors in rat adipose tissue is unchanged.[1213] In one study the number of beta-adrenergic receptors on circulating monocytes was unchanged in hyperthyroid humans,[1220] whereas in another, T_3 administration to normal subjects increased the beta-receptor number on monocytes.[1221] Hyperthyroidism in pigs increases beta-receptor density in myocardium; there is an associated increased sensitivity to the beta-agonist isoproteronol.[1222] In another study the number of beta-adrenergic receptors was increased in fat and skeletal muscle from human volunteers after the induction of thyrotoxicosis with T_3; despite the changes in receptor density, hemodynamic and metabolic responses to epinephrine were unaltered in vivo,[1223] which suggests a dissociation between changes in receptor number and the physiological response. The number of alpha-adrenergic receptors appears to be decreased in most tissues by both excess and deficiency of thyroid hormone.[1213]

Thyroid hormones also affect the adenylate cyclase–cAMP system.[1213] In hypothyroid patients the plasma levels of cAMP are reduced[1224] and urinary cAMP excretion is not increased by epinephrine infusion.[1225] In hyperthyroid patients the plasma levels of cAMP are increased in the untreated state and are diminished by propranolol;[1224] there is an augmented urinary cAMP response to epinephrine infusion.[1225] In some tissues, such as rat heart, changes in the cyclase system are consonant with changes in receptor number, whereas in others, such as the adipocyte, changes in cyclase activity[1176] and cAMP accumulation occur[1178, 1179] despite the fact that beta-receptor number or affinity is not altered. It thus appears that thyroid hormones may enhance the coupling of beta-receptor occupancy and cAMP generation. Some evidence suggests that thyroid hormone–induced alterations in phosphodiesterase activity may be involved,[1177, 1195, 1211, 1226] although not all data are consistent with this hypothesis.[1178]

ADRENERGIC BLOCKADE IN HYPERTHYROIDISM. Adrenergic blockade does not affect the plasma level of T_4 or the uptake of radioactive iodine in hyperthyroidism.[1174] As noted earlier, nonselective beta-receptor–blocking agents diminish the level of T_3, but this action does not account for clinical improvement because selective blockade of the beta-1–receptor produces similar clinical changes without diminishing the plasma T$_3$ level.[1167]

Clinical Effects of Adrenergic Blockade. Beta-adrenergic blockade in hyperthyroid patients has been reported to improve metabolic abnormalities.[1227–1229] The increase in metabolic rate is diminished but is not restored to normal;[1167, 1227, 1230] heat intolerance and sweating are reduced.[1178, 1231] Heart rate, cardiac output, systolic blood pressure, and pulse pressure decrease, and circulation time is increased.[1228, 1230, 1232, 1233] Cardiac contractility is frequently reduced but not to normal levels.[1233–1235] Lid lag, lid retraction, widened palpebral fissure, tremor, and hyper-reflexia are all diminished.[1231, 1236] Intestinal hypermotility is reduced,[1237] and hypercalcemia may be corrected,[1238] although urinary calcium and hydroxyproline excretion is not significantly altered.[1227]

Clinical Utility of Adrenergic Blockade. The efficacy of beta-blockade in symptomatic treatment of thyrotoxicosis is established.[1229, 1231, 1239, 1240] Although theoretical objections have been raised on the grounds that diminished cardiac output, in conjunction with increased metabolic rate, might impair vital organ function, untoward effects have rarely been noted clinically. The use of beta-blocking agents is, nonetheless, only an adjunct to conventional treatments that decrease the production of thyroid hormones. Although symptomatic improvement in the thyrotoxic state is often noted with doses as small as 40 to 80 mg of propranolol per day, higher amounts (in excess of 160 mg/d) are required in some patients with more severe disease. Because thyrotoxicosis increases propranolol metabolism,[1241–1243] the dose must be adjusted in each case depending on the clinical features and clinical response. Beta-blockade should be used only in conjunction with measures that reduce thyroid hormone production.

Beta-adrenergic blockade has been used in the preparation of thyrotoxic patients for emergency surgery; occasionally propranolol was the sole preoperative preparation.[1244–1253] The ultimate role of beta-blockade in comparison with conventional regimens involving thionamides and iodides is uncertain (see Chapter 8). Propranolol has also been used in the treatment of hyperthyroidism during pregnancy.[1254–1257] Although this agent appears to be reasonably safe,[1258] potential adverse effects on the fetus and the course of labor preclude its routine use. In emergencies, however, propranolol may be used for symptomatic management of the thyrotoxic mother.

Catecholamines and Hypertension

SYMPATHETIC NERVOUS SYSTEM EFFECTS ON BLOOD PRESSURE. *Vasoconstriction, Venoconstriction, and Cardiac Stimulation.* Sympathetic stimulation of the vasculature and the heart increases blood pressure (see Fig. 10–21). Peripheral resistance is increased by direct stimulation of arteriolar vasoconstriction and by activation of the renin-angiotensin system, with a consequent increase in production of angiotensin II. Cardiac output is increased by augmentation of myocardial contractility, as well as by an increase in venous return, the latter resulting from venoconstriction with a decrease in venous compliance and enhanced renal sodium reabsorption. The regulation of these processes has been described earlier.

Renal Sympathetic Activity. Sympathetic stimulation of the kidney enhances renal sodium reabsorption by both direct and indirect effects. The capacity of the kidney to excrete salt and water has important implications for the regulation of blood pressure.[1259, 1260] The renal response to an increase in blood pressure is an increase in salt excretion (i.e., pressure natriuresis). Factors that diminish the capability of the kidney to excrete sodium, such as increased renal sympathetic activity, increase blood pressure as a mechanism that is recruited to maintain extracellular fluid volume in the presence of a natriuretic handicap.[1261, 1262] Antinatriuretic effects would also antagonize the capacity of the kidney to compensate for an elevation in blood pressure. The importance of the renal effects of catecholamines in maintenance of an elevated blood pressure has been documented in dogs and rats.[1263, 1264] Intrarenal infusion of NE in uninephrectomized animals produces a sustained increase in blood pressure in association with a positive sodium balance; this increase is not reproduced by intravenous infusion of the same dose of NE. Renal sympathetic activity, therefore, probably plays an important role in the regulation of blood pressure.

SYMPATHOADRENAL SYSTEM AND HYPERTENSION. *Permissive Role of Sympathetic Nervous System.* The role of the sympathoadrenal system in the pathogenesis of human hypertension is complex and controversial (also see Chapter 11).[1265] Four reproducible and generally accepted observations, however, suggest that the sympathetic nervous system may be important in maintenance of the hypertensive state. First, the sympathetic nervous system is not suppressed despite elevated blood pressure in experimental or human hypertension.[1265] Urinary[1266] and plasma[1265, 1267, 1268] NE levels are normal or elevated, and plasma NE clearance is not altered.[1269] Sympathetic circulatory reflexes that defend the circulation are intact.[1270] Second, hypertensive subjects are more sensitive to the pressor effects of NE.[1269, 1271–1276] The basis of the enhanced sensitivity is uncertain but may depend on arteriolar medial hypertrophy.[1277] Third, in experimental hypertension an intact sympathoadrenal system is required for initiation and maintenance of the hypertensive state.[160, 1265, 1278–1280] In many models, increased peripheral sympathetic nervous system activity is present.[1265] Finally, sympatholytic agents lower blood pressure in hypertensive animals and human subjects. Taken as a whole, these observations suggest that the sympathetic nervous system plays at least a permissive role in maintenance of the hypertensive state.

Primary Role. Whether primary overactivity of the sympathoadrenal system is ever the proximate cause of blood pressure elevation in essential hypertension is unknown.[1265] Some patients with essential hypertension have elevated plasma levels of NE[1265, 1281] or epinephrine,[1282, 1283] or plasma NE levels that suppress poorly in response to salt loading,[1284, 1285] findings that are compatible with overactivity of the sympathoadrenal system.[1265, 1286, 1287]

A major problem in establishing a role for the sympathoadrenal system in the pathogenesis of hypertension has been the difficulty in adequately assessing sympathetic activity.[1288, 1289] Studies utilizing kinetic techniques to assess the rate of release of NE in specific sympathetically innervated regions have supported enhanced sympathoadrenal activity particularly in younger hypertensive subjects.[1290] These techniques have indicated that sympathetic outflow to the kidney, and to a lesser extent to the heart, is increased.[1290–1292]

A subgroup of "hyperadrenergic" patients with mild essential hypertension[1281, 1293] is characterized by elevated plasma renin activity when in a recumbent position and by enhanced plasma renin responsiveness to head-up tilting.[1294] This group is distinct from patients with accelerated hypertension in whom the increased plasma renin activity is attributable to renal vascular damage.[1295] The hypertension in this subgroup is not renin dependent.[1296] Rather, the increased renin activity is a marker for increased sympathetic activity, and both the hypertension and the high plasma renin activity result from increased sympathetic stimulation,[1297] as evidenced by (1) increased urinary NE excretion and plasma NE levels;[1281, 1296–1298] (2) increased sympathetic stimulation of the heart, as manifested by increased heart rate, increased cardiac output, increased cardiac contractility, and a greater negative chronotropic response to beta-adrenergic blockade;[1281, 1297–1299] (3) an enhanced blood pressure response to combined adrenergic blockade;[1281] and (4) an increased renal NE release rate, as calculated from tracer kinetics, renal venous catheterization, and estimates of renal plasma flow.[1290–1292] These findings emphasize the potentially important role of renal sympathetic activity in the pathogenesis of essential hypertension in this subgroup.[1262] It is uncertain whether this population of patients is a distinct subgroup within the larger population of patients with essential hypertension or whether it simply represents a transient stage in the development of essential hypertension.[1290] Alterations in renal alpha-adrenergic receptors have also been postulated to play a role in the pathogenesis of essential hypertension.[1300–1301]

Participation of the sympathetic nervous system in the pathogenesis of obesity-related hypertension has been suggested.[1302] Because hyperinsulinemia has been associated with hypertension in the obese patient, the possibility has been raised that insulin-mediated sympathetic stimulation may play a pathogenetic role.[1303–1305]

Role of Dopamine. Studies with patients who have salt-sensitive hypertension have raised the possibility that deficient dopaminergic stimulation in response to salt loading contributes to salt sensitivity and hypertension in this subgroup of patients.[1285, 1287, 1306] Diminished dopaminergically mediated salt excretion in this subgroup might contribute to the development of a natriuretic handicap.

DISORDERS OF SYMPATHETIC NERVOUS SYSTEM

General Considerations

ORTHOSTATIC HYPOTENSION. An orthostatic fall in blood pressure is the most prominent sign of functional or structural deficiency in the sympathetic nervous system. Under normal circumstances the assumption of erect posture is not associated with a significant decrease in blood pressure; a decrease in systolic pressure of 20 to 25 mm Hg and a diastolic fall of 10 to 15 mm Hg are abnormal,[1307, 1308] especially if associated with symptoms of lightheadedness or fainting.[1309] Maintenance of arterial pressure during postural stress depends on an adequate circulating blood volume, an unimpaired venous return, and an intact sympathetic nervous system. A postural fall in blood pressure is commonly associated with extracellular fluid volume depletion or with a loss of the sympathetic circulatory reflexes that defend arterial pressure by constricting both veins and arterioles.[1307] Disruption of the sympathetic reflexes with resultant postural hypotension (secondary orthostatic hypotension) may occur with a variety of diseases that affect the nervous system, such as tabes dorsalis, syringomyelia, diabetes mellitus, and amyloidosis. Postural hypotension also occurs in patients with adrenal insufficiency, hypopituitarism, primary hypoaldosteronism, hypokalemia, or pheochromocytoma. It is the most prominent feature of a chronic degenerative disease of the nervous system known as primary or idiopathic orthostatic hypotension. Finally, drugs that block adrenergic transmission (e.g., guanethidine), ganglionic transmission (e.g., trimethaphan and hexamethonium), or central sympathetic activity (e.g., phenothiazines and tricyclic antidepressants) commonly cause orthostatic hypotension.

TESTS OF AUTONOMIC FUNCTION. *Physiological and Pharmacological Tests.* Autonomic dysfunction can be classified and diagnosed on the basis of clinical, pharmacological, and biochemical tests.[5] Responsiveness of sympathetic reflexes can be tested by assessing the integrity of cardiovascular responses to the Valsalva maneuver, tilt table, or cold pressor test.[1310] An abnormal response to these tests indicates impaired sympathetic function but does not designate the site of the dysfunction. The integrity of the peripheral sympathetic nerve endings may be tested with an indirect-acting sympathomimetic amine such as tyramine. A normal pressor response to tyramine indicates that the peripheral sympathetic nerves and NE stores are intact; a poor response is consistent with degeneration of the peripheral sympathetic nerves.[1309, 1311] Sympathetic denervation is commonly associated with enhanced responsiveness to infusions of NE.[1309] Sudomotor and pupillary responses can be tested pharmacologically.[5, 1309]

Plasma Norepinephrine Levels. Measurement of plasma NE levels has provided a new means of diagnosis and classification of patients with orthostatic hypotension.[1310, 1312] The basal supine NE concentration is determined with blood drawn from a previously placed indwelling intravenous line after 30 min of quiet recumbency. The subject is then asked to stand for 5 min, and blood is resampled. Normally, the basal NE concentration doubles in the upright position and achieves an incremental increase of more than 0.9 nmol/L (152 pg/mL) and an absolute value in excess of 1.5 nmol/L (253 pg/mL). A blood pressure decrease on upright standing coupled with the failure to increase plasma NE indicates a disorder of the sympathetic nervous system. A normal basal plasma NE level in association with a poor increment on upright standing suggests that the peripheral sympathetic nerve endings are intact and that dysfunction of other parts of the reflex (usually within the CNS) is responsible for the inadequate sympathetic response. A low basal level with failure to respond to upright posture suggests that the peripheral sympathetic nerves are deficient.[1312] In practice the distinction between central and peripheral lesions may not always be clear on the basis of plasma NE levels alone. High levels of plasma NE with augmented postural increments indicate that volume depletion or disease of the blood vessels is a likely cause of the orthostatic hypotension.

Primary Orthostatic Hypotension

Primary involvement of the sympathetic nervous system occurs in at least two relatively distinct degenerative neurological diseases.[242, 1309, 1312, 1313] In one, the lesion occurs predominantly at the level of the postganglionic sympathetic neurons.[1311] In the other, neuronal degeneration is present at several loci within the CNS including the intermediolateral cell column, which contains the preganglionic sympathetic neurons.[1314] The latter disease, which has been termed *multiple system atrophy*, is associated with progressive evidence of CNS dysfunction. The pathogenesis of the circulatory disorder is similar in both diseases: sympathetically mediated vasoconstriction in the capacitance and resistance vessels fails to occur when venous return diminishes during upright posture.[1307, 1308] As a consequence, blood pressure falls, usually without a compensatory increase in pulse rate. In both conditions the excretion of catecholamines and catecholamine metabolites is decreased.[242]

IDIOPATHIC ORTHOSTATIC HYPOTENSION, PERIPHERAL TYPE. In this disorder, which affects middle-aged and elderly individuals, symptomatic orthostatic hypotension is the primary feature. Decreased sympathetic innervation of blood vessels has been demonstrated by histochemical fluorescence techniques.[1311] The rate of appearance of NE in the circulation is diminished,[1315] and the increment in plasma NE level after administration of tyramine is reduced.[1309] The adrenomedullary response to hypoglycemia may be normal or diminished.[1057] Constipation and urinary retention are frequent,[1309] and there is other evidence of parasympathetic dysfunction.[1316] Ptosis and nonreactive pupils are common.[1309] The basal plasma NE level is characteristically low, and the response to upright posture is minimal.[1312] Plasma renin responses may be deficient; renal sodium conservation may be subnormal.[1307] In the untreated state, spontaneous variations in supine blood pressure may occur, and occasional hypertension is noted. The alterations in blood pressure appear to reflect changes in total peripheral resistance, although the mechanisms involved are not understood.[1317] Signs of basal ganglia dysfunction are notably absent; cortical function and speech remain intact.[1309]

MULTIPLE SYSTEM ATROPHY (SHY-DRAGER SYNDROME). Multiple system atrophy, also known as the Shy-Drager syndrome, is a specific neuronal degeneration that involves the preganglionic sympathetic neurons,[1314] the basal ganglia, the cerebellum, and other regions of the CNS.[242] The disease occurs most commonly in middle-aged men. The clinical course is dominated by postural hypotension and extrapyramidal tract signs.[1318, 1319] Autonomic dysfunction includes sexual impotence, fecal and urinary incontinence, and anhidrosis. Basal plasma NE concentrations tend to be normal, but no increase occurs during upright posture.[1312] The excretion of catecholamine metabolites in urine is diminished.[242] The disease is distinguished from the peripheral type of idiopathic orthostatic hypotension by extrapyramidal dysfunction and other signs of CNS disease.

Secondary Orthostatic Hypotension: Sympathetic Dysfunction in Association with Peripheral Neuropathy

Autonomic failure may be associated with a variety of diseases that cause peripheral neuropathy, including diabetes mellitus,[1320] amyloidosis,[1321, 1322] uremia, porphyria, the Guillain-Barré syndrome, and carcinomatous neuropathy.[5] Visceral afferents or parasympathetic or sympathetic efferent neurons may be affected. Autonomic disturbance is especially common in diabetes mellitus. In most diabetic patients, autonomic dysfunction is accompanied by signs of symmetrical sensory polyneuropathy.[5] Anhidrosis, altered bladder and bowel regulation, sexual impotence, retrograde ejaculation, and abnormal pupillary responses are frequent cofeatures. Occasionally, hyperhidrosis and tachycardia may occur. Esophageal dilatation, delayed gastric emptying, nocturnal diarrhea, and fecal incontinence probably reflect a disturbance of innervation of the bowel wall.[5] Basal supine plasma NE levels in diabetics with neuropathy are low compared with those in normal control or diabetic subjects without peripheral neuropathy.[1323] The plasma NE response to upright posture is subnormal,[822, 1323, 1324] as are the increases in blood pressure and plasma NE levels that are induced by isometric hand grip.[1325] Reduction in the NE content of heart and vasculature in patients with long-standing diabetes mellitus[1326] is the result of degeneration of the peripheral sympathetic nerves.

Other Forms of Autonomic Neuropathy

ACUTE AUTONOMIC NEUROPATHY. Acute autonomic neuropathy may occur without sensory or motor deficit. Paralysis of sympathetic and parasympathetic function may be severe, with postural hypotension, bowel and bladder disturbance, impotence, poor temperature regulation, and failure of sweating and lacrimation.[1327] The defect appears to be at the level of the postganglionic autonomic neuron. Neurological function generally recovers in months to years, a feature that resembles the Guillain-Barré syndrome. An

association with infectious mononucleosis has been suggested in some cases.[5]

FAMILIAL DYSAUTONOMIA. Familial dysautonomia (the Riley-Day syndrome) is an inherited disease that results in orthostatic hypotension in addition to other disturbances in autonomic, motor, and sensory functions. The disease is found almost exclusively in children of Ashkenazi Jewish descent[1328] and is inherited as an autosomal recessive trait. It is characterized by dysphagia, absent lacrimation, vomiting, skin blotching, excessive sweating, and extreme lability of blood pressure, with both hypertensive episodes and orthostatic hypotension.[5, 1329] Hypoactive deep tendon reflexes, growth disturbance, indifference to pain, and deficient temperature regulation are also common. Fungiform papillae on the tongue are absent.[1328, 1329] Bronchopneumonia is a common complication. Children with this disease excrete more HVA, a metabolite of DA, and less VMA and MOPG than normal,[1330] which has been interpreted as reflecting inadequate synthesis of NE from DA. Hypersensitivity to infused NE is often present.[1331] Plasma NE levels are normal in the supine position, but the expected increment in response to upright posture does not occur.[365] Pathological studies reveal a loss of neurons from the sympathetic and dorsal root ganglia. The fundamental defect in this disease is unknown. A relationship between familial dysautonomia and a deficiency of nerve growth factor has been postulated.[5]

Treatment of Orthostatic Hypotension

Symptomatic orthostatic hypotension that is related to failure of the sympathetic nervous system is an indication for treatment,[1332] but if the disease is severe the results are usually disappointing. Because there is no way to restore responsiveness of the sympathetic nervous system, the major thrust of treatment is to expand the extracellular fluid volume and to enhance venous return, thereby rendering support of blood pressure in the upright position less dependent on sympathetic reflexes.[1307, 1308, 1333] An attempt to increase venous return and to prevent pooling of blood in the periphery by carefully fitted (Jobst) elastic stockings in a "pantyhose" distribution is often helpful but suffices as sole treatment in only the mildest cases.[1334] Avoidance of recumbency by sleeping partially erect may be of benefit.[1334] The potent mineralocorticoid fludrocortisone is usually the mainstay of treatment. This agent, in conjunction with a high-salt intake, expands plasma volume and enhances venous return. Mineralocorticoids may also increase the sensitivity of the vasculature to NE[1307, 1335] and thus increase peripheral resistance. Supine hypertension is a common consequence of treatment and is an additional reason for avoiding nocturnal recumbency. The goal of treatment is to increase functional status rather than to achieve arbitrary elevations in standing blood pressure.

In severe cases incapacitating orthostatic hypotension may persist despite these measures. Various other treatments have been proposed, but none has achieved general acceptance. Sympathomimetic amines such as ephedrine and newer investigational alpha-agonists[1336] have been tried but are generally not helpful when used alone; the augmented NE release that occurs when an MAO inhibitor is added may produce a beneficial response.[1337, 1338] The usefulness of this combination is limited by the possibility of uncontrolled NE release with hypertensive crises and by the fact that extremely high supine blood pressures often result before sufficient control of orthostatic symptoms can be achieved. Levodopa, with or without an MAO inhibitor, has been used in some cases, but usually without great success. Metoclopramide has been advocated as a means of blocking the vasodilatory and natriuretic effects of DA;[1339] although metoclopramide is beneficial as treatment of the gastric retention that is sometimes noted in these patients, its effects on blood pressure are usually not impressive. Indomethacin has been recommended as an antagonist of prostaglandin-mediated vasodilation;[1307] it is rarely helpful and may be associated with gastrointestinal side effects including hemorrhage. Both alpha-2–agonists (e.g., clonidine)[1340] and antagonists (e.g., yohimbine)[1341] have been advocated, the former on the basis of a postulated alpha-2 effect to constrict venous musculature, the latter to antagonize feedback inhibition of NE release. Neither has had extensive trials, and preliminary experience is not encouraging.

Two approaches seem worthy of further investigation. A closed-loop infusion pump servomechanism that delivers NE intravenously to maintain a predetermined mean arterial blood pressure level has been used in short-term experiments.[1342] Long-term use is limited by the necessity of an indwelling arterial line. A potentially useful agent appears to be a synthetic precursor of NE, 3,4-dihydroxyphenylserine, the carboxylic acid congener of NE.[1343] This agent is absorbed after oral administration and is slowly decarboxylated to NE by AAD. After a single oral dose the NE levels remain elevated for hours in association with an increase in both recumbent and upright blood pressure.[1343] This agent warrants further investigation.

PHEOCHROMOCYTOMA

Incidence and Importance

Pheochromocytoma is a catecholamine-producing tumor derived, most commonly, from adrenomedullary chromaffin cells; those tumors arising from extra-adrenal chromaffin cells are called extra-adrenal pheochromocytomas or paragangliomas. Similar clinical manifestations may occur with related tumors that secrete catecholamines, such as chemodectomas and ganglioneuromas.

Pheochromocytomas are rare; less than 0.1% of hypertensive patients harbor a chromaffin tumor as cause of increased blood pressure. The rarity of these tumors, however, should not belie their importance. Correctly diagnosed and properly treated, pheochromocytoma is curable; misdiagnosed or improperly treated, it is fatal. More than 90% of pheochromocytomas appear to be benign. They are dangerous because of their capacity to store and release catecholamines in large amounts, with subsequent production of alarming and occasionally spectacular syndromes.[1344] The potential pharmacological effects of the released catecholamines constitute a major surgical and medical therapeutic challenge. The majority of pheochromocytomas are found unexpectedly at postmortem examination;[1345, 1346] thus many potentially curable cases are undiagnosed during life. Symptoms may antedate definitive diagnosis by many years.[1347]

Pheochromocytoma is occasionally inherited as an autosomal dominant trait and may be part of a pluriglandular neoplastic syndrome. The diagnosis of pheochromocytoma may be the first clue to the presence of multiple endocrine neoplasia (MEN). Pheochromocytomas occur from infancy to old age but are rare after age 60. They are slightly more common in females than in males.

Clinical Features

GENERAL CONSIDERATIONS. *Pathogenesis.* The clinical manifestations of pheochromocytoma are largely predictable from the known physiological and pharmacological effects of catecholamines.

Presentation. Common presenting manifestations include (1) sustained hypertension, which is resistant to conventional treatment; (2) hypertensive crisis with malignant hypertension, hypertensive encephalopathy, or a constellation of signs and symptoms suggestive of aortic dissection or myocardial infarction; and (3) paroxysmal episodes or spells suggestive of seizure disorder, anxiety attacks, or hyperventilation. Less common manifestations include unexplained hypotension, shock, and severe hypertensive reactions that occur during incidental surgery or in association with trauma.

PAROXYSM. The paroxysm or crisis is the classic manifestation of pheochromocytoma.[1344, 1347, 1348] It is the physiological consequence of catecholamine release from the tumor and the subsequent stimulation of adrenergic receptors. The clinical manifestations are variable. Headache is the most common symptom and occurs in over 80% of patients (Table 10–7);[1349] it may be severe, frontal or occipital, throbbing or steady. Excessive sweating, palpitations, and apprehension are common, along with pain in the chest or abdomen, nausea, vomiting, and occasionally paresthesias. There is often a sense of impending doom. Blanching or flushing of the face is frequent during the paroxysm, with a flushed, warm feeling afterward.[1347] Blood pressure is elevated, often to alarming levels. The presence of tachycardia in the face of elevated blood pressure often suggests the diagnosis. The paroxysm may last from a few minutes to several hours; most episodes subside within 40 min. Rarely, more prolonged episodes occur.

A paroxysm may be precipitated by any movement that displaces the abdominal contents, such as lifting, straining, or bending, or by strenuous exertion of any kind. In some patients a particular stimulus reproduces an attack in a characteristic manner. In others no clearly defined precipitating event can be found, and the episodes occur in a random pattern. In contrast to anxiety states, which may be confused with pheochromocytoma, mental stress or psychological tension does not usually provoke a crisis, although anxiety may accompany the attack. A variety of therapeutic or diagnostic agents or maneuvers may provoke a crisis.

TABLE 10–7. Frequency of Symptoms in 100 Patients with Pheochromocytoma

Symptom	%	Symptom	%	Symptom	%
Headache	80	Chest pain	19	Tinnitus	3
Excessive perspiration	71	Dyspnea	19	Dysarthria	3
Palpitation (with or without tachycardia)	64	Flushing or warmth	18	Gagging	3
		Numbness or paresthesia	11	Bradycardia	3
Pallor	42	Blurring of vision	11	Back pain	3
Nausea (with or without vomiting)	42	Tightness of throat	8	Coughing	1
Tremor or trembling	31	Dizziness or faintness	8	Yawning	1
Weakness or exhaustion	28	Convulsions	5	Syncope	1
Nervousness or anxiety	22	Neck-shoulder pain	5	Unsteadiness	1
Epigastric pain	22	Extremity pain	4	Hunger	1
		Flank pain	4		

Data from Thomas JE, Rooke ED, Kvale WF. The neurologist's experience with pheochromocytoma: a review of 46 cases. J Urol 1974; 111:715–721.

Vigorous palpation of the abdomen may initiate an episode. In most patients, paroxysms occur relatively often so that over the course of 1 or 2 d it is often possible to witness an attack and measure the blood pressure.[1347] In some patients the intervals between attacks are much longer, such as weeks or months. As the disease progresses, the paroxysms tend to increase in frequency, severity, and duration.

Although pheochromocytoma is identified with the characteristic crises, paroxysmal symptoms were present in only 56% of 507 cases in one large series.[1348]

HYPERTENSION. Although the paroxysm is the most distinctive manifestation of pheochromocytoma, hypertension is the most common feature and occurs in more than 90% of patients. It is usually sustained and may be nonepisodic, resembling essential hypertension (Table 10–8).[1348] Blood pressure lability is usually present, however, and many patients with sustained hypertension also have distinct paroxysms.[1347, 1348] In 25 to 40% of patients the hypertension is truly paroxysmal, with an elevated blood pressure demonstrable only intermittently or during symptomatic episodes. The hypertension in patients with pheochromocytoma is often severe and occasionally malignant, with retinopathy, severe proteinuria, and secondary aldosteronism. Although it is generally attributed to the direct effects of high circulating levels of catecholamines, the hypertension in patients with pheochromocytoma may also depend on the sympathetic nervous system[1350] by mechanisms that remain obscure but that may be related to the increased stores of NE in sympathetic nerve endings in these patients.

The response to conventional antihypertensive treatment is usually unsatisfactory; this refractoriness may be a clue to the diagnosis. Patients with pheochromocytoma, however, respond to alpha-blocking agents that are commonly used in the treatment of essential hypertension (prazosin, terazosin, labetalol), as well as to calcium channel blockers[1351] and nitroprusside.

OTHER DISTINCTIVE FEATURES. *Orthostatic Hypotension and Shock.* Orthostatic hypotension is present in many patients.[1344, 1347] In untreated hypertensive patients, a significant postural fall in blood pressure should suggest the diagnosis. The orthostatic hypotension probably reflects the reduced plasma volume that results from high circulating levels of catecholamines. Although there has been some dispute about the cause of the orthostatic hypotension,[1347, 1352] reduced plasma volume is present in most untreated patients, particularly in those with sustained hypertension.[1344, 1353] In addition, the postural reflexes that defend upright blood pressure may lose their tone with a prolonged excess of catecholamines. Both of these factors predispose untreated patients with pheochromocytoma to develop hypotension or shock when subjected to surgery or trauma.

TABLE 10–8. Frequency of Hypertension and Crises in 507 Cases of Pheochromocytoma

Symptom	%	
Sustained hypertension	60.5	
With crises		27.0
Without crises		33.5
Paroxysmal hypertension	26.4	
Hypertension of pregnancy	3.5	
No hypertension	9.5	
Paroxysmal symptoms		2.8
Sustained symptoms		1.2
No symptoms (discovered by chance)		4.3
Local signs		1.2
Paroxysmal symptoms or crises of any kind	56.2	

Data from Hermann H, Mornex R. Human Tumors Secreting Catecholamines. New York: Macmillan, 1964: 1–14.

Cardiac Manifestations. In some cases the clinical course is dominated by signs and symptoms of cardiac disease. Chest pain, angina pectoris, and acute myocardial infarction may occur in the absence of coronary artery disease.[1344, 1354–1356] Catecholamine-induced increase in myocardial oxygen consumption and possibly coronary artery spasm may be the cause. Electrocardiographic changes are common in the absence of clinical ischemia; nonspecific ST-T wave changes and prominent U waves may be seen.[1344, 1357] Sinus tachycardia, sinus bradycardia, supraventricular tachycardias, and ventricular premature contractions[1344] have been noted and may be associated with palpitations. Conduction disturbances including right and left bundle branch block and ventricular strain sometimes occur. Clinically significant cardiomyopathy of the congestive or hypertrophic type has been noted[1344, 1358, 1359] and may be associated with congestive heart failure. Noncardiogenic pulmonary edema has also been described in patients with pheochromocytoma.[1360] Although the pathogenesis is obscure, a shift of extracellular fluid volume to the central compartment, increased pulmonary venous tone, and altered pulmonary capillary permeability may be involved.

Metabolic Alterations. The metabolic rate is increased, excessive sweating and heat intolerance are common,[1349] and fever is occasionally noted.[1361] Weight loss is usual, although obesity does not exclude the diagnosis.

Carbohydrate intolerance[1344] and elevated fasting plasma glucose concentrations may occur, most commonly during paroxysms. The elevated plasma glucose level is associated with a low plasma level of insulin, the latter reflecting alpha-receptor–mediated suppression of insulin release.[1362] Beta-receptor–mediated stimulation of hepatic glucose output may also contribute. The carbohydrate intolerance in patients with pheochromocytoma is characteristically mild but may require specific treatment, and it is reversed by removal of the tumor.

Hypercalcemia is an uncommon but well-recognized complication of pheochromocytoma.[1363] It may reflect associated hyperparathyroidism, particularly in familial cases (see later), but often occurs in the absence of parathyroid disease because it resolves after resection of the pheochromocytoma.[1364, 1365] In individual cases adrenergic stimulation of normal parathyroid glands by high circulating levels of catecholamines may be responsible.[1364, 1365] Pheochromocytomas may also produce a bone-resorbing factor that is similar to or identical with that associated with the humoral hypercalcemia of malignancy syndrome.[1363]

The watery diarrhea, hypokalemia, achlorhydria syndrome (abbreviated WHDA; also known as the Verner-Morrison syndrome) has been described in patients with pheochromocytoma[1366–1368] secondary to the ectopic production of vasoactive intestinal peptide. The syndrome resolves when the tumor is removed. Cushing syndrome secondary to ectopic production of corticotropin has also been well described in patients with pheochromocytoma.[1369, 1370]

Hematocrit. Elevation of the hematocrit is common in patients with pheochromocytoma; it is usually associated with a normal red cell mass and therefore reflects the diminished plasma volume.[1344] Erythropoietin-like activity has been demonstrated in extracts from some pheochromocytomas.[1371] The possibility of catecholamine-stimulated erythropoietin release from kidney also exists.

Adverse Drug Interactions. The clinical course of pheochromocytoma may be adversely affected by drugs or diagnostic studies that affect catecholamine metabolism in a variety of ways. Severe and even fatal crises have been induced by opiates, histamine, corticotropin,[1372] saralasin,[1373] glucagon, metoclopramide,[1374] droperidol,[1375] and pancuronium.[1376, 1377] Of these agents, the effects of opiates have been insufficiently emphasized, and patients with headache or abdominal pain may have serious paroxysms induced by administration of an opiate analgesic. Glucagon, which is used in a standard provocative test for pheochromocytoma (as described later), may precipitate crisis when administered to relax the bowel during radiological evaluations. The potent opiate agonist fentanyl may precipitate crises during induction of anesthesia in patients with unsuspected pheochromocytoma who are undergoing incidental surgery.[1375] Radiographic contrast media, when administered intra-arterially, also release catecholamines, and arteriography should be performed only in patients who have received adrenergic blocking agents. Intravenous pyelography, however, can be safely performed. Indirect-acting sympathomimetic amines, including intravenously administered methyldopa, may be associated with an unpredictable increase in blood pressure by releasing catecholamines from the augmented stores within nerve endings. Proprietary cold medicines and decongestants, which frequently contain sympathomimetic amines, are common offenders. Drugs that block the neuronal uptake of catecholamines, such as guanethidine or tricyclic antidepressants, may enhance the physiological effects of circulating catecholamines and may increase blood pressure in these patients as well. These agents should be specifically avoided in patients with known or suspected pheochromocytoma, and all medications should be administered cautiously.

Pathology

MORPHOLOGY. Pheochromocytomas are most often solitary and are located in or about the adrenal gland.[1344, 1378] In sporadic cases, about 80% are intra-adrenal and unilateral, about 10% are bilateral in the adrenals, and about 10% are extra-adrenal (Table 10–9). Sporadic, solitary lesions are more common on the right side. Familial pheochromocytomas are more often bilateral and are usually multicentric within an individual adrenal gland. Familial extra-adrenal pheochromocytomas appear to be unusual. In children the incidence of bilateral and extra-adrenal pheochromocytomas is increased compared with that in adults.

Adrenal Pheochromocytomas. Intra-adrenal pheochromocytomas are usually less than 10 cm in diameter and weigh an average of about 10 g,[1344, 1378] although tumors weighing kilograms have been reported.[1379] The cut surface often shows areas of hemorrhage and necrosis (Fig. 10–27).[1379] Microscopically the tumor is composed of large, pleomorphic chromaffin cells.[1344] Electron microscopy reveals typical dense-core chromaffin granules. Perhaps 6 to 10% of these tumors are malignant, as evidenced by either local invasion or metastases; as with other endocrine tumors, malignancy cannot be determined by microscopic appearance alone. Malignant tumors are usually slow-growing and metastasize to bone, liver, lymph nodes, and lung.[1379] Familial pheochromocytomas tend to be multinodular, which reflects their multicentric origin. The incidence of local recurrence or metastases is higher in some but not all familial cases.[1380]

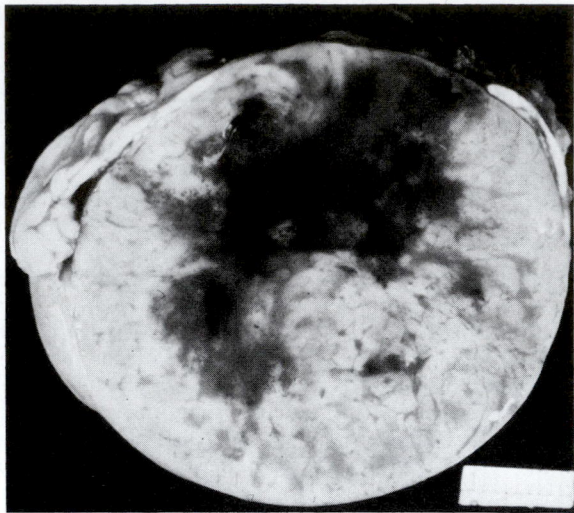

Figure 10–27. Adrenal pheochromocytoma showing cut surface. The marker is 1 cm. Note the normal adrenal surrounding the tumor, and extensive hemorrhage and necrosis. Preoperative arteriographic demonstration of this tumor is shown in Figure 10–31A. (Courtesy of Dr. Mark A. Hayes.)

Extra-Adrenal Pheochromocytomas. Extra-adrenal pheochromocytomas, or paragangliomas, make up about 10% of sporadic cases (Table 10–10). The extra-adrenal tumors are usually less than 5 cm in diameter and most often weigh between 20 and 40 g.[1344, 1348] They occur in and about the sympathetic ganglia in locations that parallel the anatomical distribution of extra-adrenal chromaffin tissue (Fig. 10–28). Most are intra-abdominal. Those in the thorax are usually located in the posterior mediastinum in close association with the sympathetic trunks, although tumors within the pericardium have been described.[1381] Rarely, tumors are in the cervical region or other locations.[1382] Extra-adrenal pheochromocytomas are usually supplied by an aberrant blood vessel of considerable size, a fact that favors their demonstration by arteriography. Malignant potential, as expressed by local recurrence or metastasis, may be greater in extra-adrenal than in intra-adrenal lesions.[1383]

Pheochromocytomas of Urinary Bladder. Pheochromocytomas within the urinary bladder produce a distinctive syndrome that is characterized by severe paroxysms occurring during or shortly after micturition.[1384, 1385] These tumors become symptomatic earlier than pheochromocytomas in other locations, an apparent consequence of their location, which subjects them to continuous changes in tension. Because symptoms can be produced when the lesions are quite small, biochemical evidence of increased catecholamine production may be less impressive than in the usual case, and the diagnosis may be more difficult to establish.[1384] Other symptoms of bladder tumor may be present; painless hematuria occurs in approximately one half of cases. Cystoscopy is usually helpful in establishing a diagnosis, the tumor being visible in most cases. It may also be visualized by

TABLE 10–9. Location of Pheochromocytomas

Location	%		
	Total*	Familial	Children
Solitary adrenal	80	<50	50
Extra-adrenal	10	<10	25
Bilateral adrenal	10	>50	25

*95% of cases are sporadic and 5% familial; 10–12% of all cases are in children.

TABLE 10–10. Location of Extra-Adrenal Pheochromocytomas*

Location	%	
Cervical	2	
Thoracic	10–20	
Intra-abdominal	70–80	
Upper abdomen		40
Organ of Zuckerkandl		30
Bladder		15

*About 10% of all pheochromocytomas are extra-adrenal.

arteriography. Localization techniques should not be undertaken before institution of adrenergic blockade.

Related Catecholamine-Secreting Tumors. Chemodectomas arising in the carotid body, glomus jugulare tumors arising from the intracranial branches of the ninth and tenth cranial nerves,[1386–1388] and ganglioneuromas arising from the postganglionic sympathetic neurons may secrete catecholamines and produce a clinical syndrome indistinguishable from that caused by extra-adrenal pheochromocytomas.[1344] From a diagnostic and therapeutic standpoint, these tumors resemble typical extra-adrenal pheochromocytomas.

BIOCHEMISTRY. *Catecholamine Storage.* Important differences in biosynthesis and storage of catecholamines have been noted[1345] in some chromaffin cell tumors compared with the normal adrenal medulla. Chromaffin granules from pheochromocytomas are morphologically and physically similar to chromaffin granules of the normal adrenal medulla. In some pheochromocytomas the catecholamine/ATP ratio is increased above the usual 4:1 relationship, which indicates a possible defect in binding or storage;[1345] in other tumors a normal ratio is observed. Similarly, for some tumors the in vitro rate of catecholamine biosynthesis is substantially greater than that in the normal adrenal medulla.[1345] This rate may be associated with an increase in the activity of TH, which is not subject to feedback inhibition by catechols.[1389, 1390] In other pheochromocytomas, TH activity is normal.[1391, 1392] The turnover rate of catecholamines may be markedly increased over the normal rate in the adrenal.[1345]

Catecholamine Release. The mechanisms of catecholamine release from pheochromocytomas are poorly understood. The role of exocytosis[1093] is unclear. Pheochromocytomas, unlike the normal adrenal medulla, are not innervated, and catecholamine release is not initiated by neural impulses.[1345] Changes in tumor blood flow, direct pressure, and a variety of chemicals and drugs may initiate catecholamine release. Pheochromocytomas, but not the normal adrenal medulla, possess receptors for glucagon.[1393]

Catecholamine Excretion. Most pheochromocytomas contain predominantly NE (unlike the normal adrenal medulla, which in humans contains 85% epinephrine). Consequently, most patients predominantly excrete increased amounts of NE in the urine.[1394] Rarely, tumors produce epinephrine exclusively; in these cases the clinical picture may be dominated by signs of excessive beta-receptor stimulation such as tachycardia and hypermetabolism.[1395] In most cases, however, it is impossible to predict the pattern of catecholamine secretion from the clinical features. Diagnosis of an epinephrine-secreting pheochromocytoma may be difficult unless epinephrine and NE are assayed selectively, because the total urinary catecholamine and catecholamine metabolite levels may be increased little, if at all.[1395] Familial pheochromocytomas are more likely to contain large amounts of epinephrine. In some familial cases, especially early in the course of the illness when the tumor is small, an increase in urinary epinephrine excretion may be the only biochemical abnormality.[1396] Because small elevations in urinary epinephrine excretion may be easily missed, pheochromocytomas in the MEN syndromes may be difficult to diagnose.

Extra-adrenal pheochromocytomas, with the occasional exception of tumors arising in the organ of Zuckerkandl (a fusion of extra-adrenal chromaffin cells caudal to the origin of the inferior mesenteric artery), typically secrete only NE. Epinephrine production by intrathoracic pheochromocytomas has, however, been reported.[1397] Epinephrine secretion increases the likelihood of tumor origin in the adrenal medulla but does not exclude an extra-adrenal site.

Excretion of DA and DA metabolites, including HVA, is usually normal in patients with benign pheochromocytoma. An increase in urinary DA or HVA excretion suggests malignancy.[1344]

Tumor Size. The size of the tumor correlates with the ratio of free catecholamines to catecholamine metabolites in the urine.[1398] Small pheochromocytomas tend to have low concentrations but high turnover rates of catecholamines and low urinary ratios of VMA to catecholamines. Conversely, large tumors tend to have high concentrations of catecholamines, low rates of turnover, and high urinary VMA/catecholamine ratios. Small tumors with high turnover rates thus appear to secrete unmetabolized catecholamines, which are physiologically active and produce clinical manifestations. Such tumors are frequently diagnosed at an early stage while still small. In contrast, tumors that store catecholamines well, or that metabolize substantial amounts of catecholamines within the tumor, secrete less catecholamines in physiologically active form and therefore attain a larger size before becoming clinically manifest.

Production of Other Substances. Pheochromocytomas contain, and presumably synthesize, opioid peptides,[97, 1399–1401] somatostatin,[1367, 1368, 1399] calcitonin,[1402, 1403] vasoactive intestinal peptide,[1366–1368] corticotropin,[1369, 1370] neuropeptide Y,[1404] and the humoral hypercalcemia of malignancy factor.[1363]

Associated Diseases

Pheochromocytoma occurs in association with hyperparathyroidism and medullary carcinoma of the thyroid in the familial MEN syndromes (MEN types 2A [2] and 2B [3]), with neurofibromas in neurofibromatosis, and with retinal and cerebellar hemangioblastomas in von Hippel-Lindau disease. As noted earlier, hypercalcemia may occur in the absence of hyperparathyroidism.[1364] For this reason hypercalcemia in a patient with pheochromocytoma should

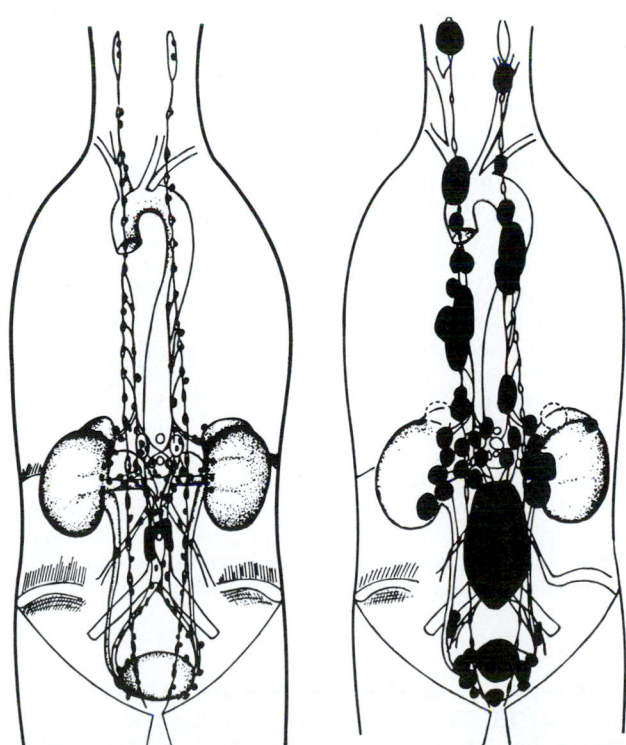

Figure 10–28. Distribution of chromaffin tissue in the newborn compared with the distribution of extra-adrenal pheochromocytomas. Extra-adrenal pheochromocytomas *(left)* occur in sites containing chromaffin tissue in the newborn *(right)*. (Modified from Coupland RE. The Natural History of the Chromaffin Cell. London: Longmans, Green, 1965: 192–194.)

be re-evaluated after the pheochromocytoma is resected because the hypercalcemia may resolve.[1364, 1365] Cholelithiasis has been reported in as many as 15 to 20% of cases.[1344] The reason for this association is obscure, but effects of catecholamines on gallbladder motility may be involved. As noted earlier, the ectopic production of corticotropin or vasoactive intestinal peptide by pheochromocytoma may be a rare cause of Cushing or WHDA syndrome.

Familial Pheochromocytoma and Multiple Endocrine Neoplasia Syndromes*

Traditionally, 5% of pheochromocytomas were considered to be inherited.[1348, 1405, 1406] The familial incidence is actually greater, however. Scores of kindreds with familial pheochromocytoma and hundreds of affected individuals have been reported.[1372, 1405–1408] In many, pheochromocytoma is part of a familial syndrome with other inherited traits. Of 29 carefully reviewed families, 11 had associated thyroid carcinoma, 2 were associated with neurocutaneous syndromes, and 16 were not associated with any other defect.[1372] Familial pheochromocytoma, alone or in combination with other familial traits, has an autosomal dominant mode of inheritance.

MEN 1. The MEN 1 syndrome (Wermer syndrome) consists of hyperparathyroidism, pituitary adenomas, and pancreatic islet cell tumors.[1409] Familial pheochromocytoma is not usually part of the MEN 1 complex.[1409] However, the familial occurrence of pheochromocytoma and islet cell tumors of the pancreas has been reported.[1410–1412] In many cases the islet cell tumors were nonfunctional.[1410] Affected kindreds with familial pheochromocytoma may display traits that are characteristic of MEN 1, MEN 2A, MEN 2B, von Recklinghausen neurofibromatosis, or von Hippel-Lindau retinocerebellar hemangioblastomatosis.[1410–1412] In one patient within an MEN 2A kindred, hypergastrinemia and the Zollinger-Ellison syndrome were present.[1413] The significance of these crossover syndromes is uncertain; although pheochromocytoma is not a regular feature of the MEN 1 syndrome, its incidence appears to be increased in any familial syndrome in which islet cell tumors are present. As usual in familial cases, pheochromocytomas in association with islet cell tumors are frequently bilateral.

MEN 2A. Also known as Sipple syndrome, MEN 2A consists of pheochromocytoma, medullary carcinoma of the thyroid, and hyperparathyroidism.[1414–1416] Pheochromocytoma occurs in about 50% of affected patients within a MEN 2A kindred and is responsible for a substantial portion of the morbidity and mortality.[1380] Pheochromocytoma in Sipple syndrome originates from adrenomedullary hyperplasia;[1380, 1417] as a result the pheochromocytomas are multicentric and frequently bilateral. Extra-adrenal pheochromocytomas are unusual. The pheochromocytomas are usually epinephrine-secreting, and early in the course of disease increased epinephrine secretion may be the only biochemical abnormality.[1418, 1419] The hypertension in MEN 2A patients with pheochromocytoma is more likely to be paroxysmal than in the usual sporadic case;[1372, 1419, 1420] less than one half of patients with pheochromocytoma within the MEN 2A complex appear to have sustained hypertension. The diagnosis of pheochromocytoma is thus more difficult than in sporadic cases.[1419, 1421] The asymptomatic normotensive patient with Sipple syndrome is at risk of dangerous and fatal paroxysms during surgery if an unsuspected pheochromocytoma is present.[1422] The incidence of malignant chromaffin tumors does not generally appear to exceed the sporadic rate in

MEN 2A, although in some kindreds local recurrence and metastases have been noted more commonly.[1380]

In MEN 2A patients with pheochromocytoma the chromaffin tumor should be removed as soon as the diagnosis is established; preoperative preparation is the same as in sporadic cases, although it may be more difficult to judge the adequacy of phenoxybenzamine treatment because a greater proportion of the patients are normotensive. Bilateral adrenalectomy is not necessary in every case; if computed tomographic (CT) scan or magnetic resonance imaging (MRI) demonstrates tumor on one side with a normal-appearing adrenal on the other, it is reasonable to leave the normal adrenal and continue observation for subsequent development of pheochromocytoma. Pheochromocytoma may develop in the remaining gland after a hiatus of many years, or not at all.[1423] After the patient has recovered from surgery for pheochromocytoma, the medullary carcinoma is treated by total thyroidectomy.

MEN 2B. Pheochromocytoma is also a part of the MEN 2B syndrome; also called the mucosal neuroma syndrome, this complex includes medullary carcinoma of the thyroid, pheochromocytoma, and multiple mucosal neuromas, often in association with a characteristic marfanoid habitus.[1424] About one half of patients show the complete syndrome. Mucosal neuromas occur in all affected subjects. Oral neuromas are most common, occurring about the lips, tongue, and buccal mucosa. Although the neuromas and the facial characteristics are often present at an early age, the disease is frequently not recognized until presentation of medullary carcinoma or pheochromocytoma later in life. The pathology, clinical behavior, and management of pheochromocytomas appear to be similar in MEN 2A and MEN 2B.

NEUROFIBROMATOSIS. The incidence of pheochromocytomas in kindreds with neurofibromatosis is uncertain, but in one large series it was present in less than 1% of the patients.[1425] About 5% of reported cases of pheochromocytomas had neurofibromatosis.[1348, 1405, 1426] Because incomplete forms of the disease are common and may be easily overlooked, the actual incidence may be higher than reported. Partial forms of neurofibromatosis include five or six café au lait spots, kyphoscoliosis, and vertebral deformity. A search for these abnormalities should be made in all patients who are suspected of having pheochromocytoma.

VON HIPPEL-LINDAU DISEASE (RETINAL CEREBELLAR HEMANGIOBLASTOMATOSIS). In a review of von Hippel-Lindau disease,[1427] pheochromocytoma was noted in 10% of patients. Four of the five cases of pheochromocytoma occurred in one family, which raises the possibility that only certain families with the trait have an increased risk of developing pheochromocytoma. Two of the five cases were bilateral. In a concomitant autopsy series,[1427] 25% of patients with von Hippel-Lindau disease had pheochromocytoma, and most of these were not diagnosed clinically. Of the seven cases in the autopsy series, two were extra-adrenal. No information is available on whether the pheochromocytomas in this disorder or in neurofibromatosis secrete predominantly epinephrine or NE. The presence of small retinal angiomata may provide a clue to incomplete von Hippel-Lindau disease and unsuspected pheochromocytoma.

Diagnosis

URINARY CATECHOLAMINES AND CATECHOLAMINE METABOLITES. The diagnosis of pheochromocytoma is established by demonstration of increased urinary excretion of catecholamines or catecholamine metabolites. The problem is to think of the diagnosis; if the possibility of pheochromocytoma is raised, the diagnosis can usually be confirmed or excluded on the basis of a single 24-h urine

---

*Also see Chapter 30.

collection, provided the patient is symptomatic or hypertensive at the time of collection.[1352, 1428, 1429]

General Considerations. Chemical determinations used in diagnosis of pheochromocytoma include VMA, total metanephrines, and unconjugated (free) catecholamines.[270, 1430, 1431] The three major determinations are probably equivalent when the assays are properly performed; the clinician should select the determination performed best by the laboratory available. Additional security is achieved when two of the three determinations are used, although this procedure is not essential as a screening in every case. The number of 24-h urine collections obtained and the number of different determinations performed on each collection depends on the clinical level of suspicion. Elevated values should always be confirmed by at least one repeat determination.

The following general considerations apply to all urinary determinations. (1) Twenty-four-hour urine collections are preferable to casual random urine samples expressed per unit of creatinine.[1428] Creatinine should be determined for each 24-h collection to assess its adequacy. (2) If possible the collection should be made with the patient at rest, while taking no medication, and without recent exposure to radiographic contrast media. When it is not feasible to discontinue all medications, those known to interfere in the assays should be avoided. Diuretics, some adrenergic blocking agents, vasodilators, calcium channel blockers, and angiotensin-converting enzyme inhibitors do not interfere appreciably. (3) The best assays are reasonably specific and dietary restrictions are minimal. (4) The urine must be acidified (pH below 3.0) and kept cold during and after collection. (5) Although most patients with pheochromocytoma, including those with paroxysmal symptoms, excrete increased amounts of catecholamines and catecholamine metabolites each day, the diagnostic yield is increased in patients with paroxysmal symptoms if a 24-h urine collection is initiated at the onset of a crisis. (6) Interfering substances depend on the specific methods that are used in the various analyses; specific questions should be referred to the clinical pathologist at the laboratory performing the assays.

Free Catecholamines. The upper limit of normal for total urinary catecholamines is generally between 591 and 890 nmol/d (100 and 150 μg/d). Most patients with pheochromocytoma have values in excess of 1500 nmol/d (250 μg/d). Specific assay of epinephrine is frequently beneficial because increased epinephrine excretion in excess of 270 nmol/d (50 μg/d) suggests an adrenal lesion and may be the only abnormality in cases that are associated with MEN. The major cause of false-positive elevations of catecholamine excretion is administration of exogenous catecholamines such as methyldopa, levodopa, or labetalol, which can elevate urine concentrations for as long as 2 wk. Excessive stimulation of the sympathoadrenal system, such as that occurring in hypoglycemia, strenuous exertion, increased intracranial pressure, and clonidine withdrawal, may also increase catecholamine excretion sufficiently to confound the diagnosis.

VMA and Total Metanephrines. In most assays the upper limit of normal for VMA excretion is in the range of 35 μmol/d (7.0 mg/d); the upper limit of normal for total metanephrines is 7 μmol/d (1.3 mg/d). Patients with pheochromocytoma almost always excrete these metabolites in excess, usually exceeding the normal range by threefold. Total metanephrine (metanephrine and normetanephrine) excretion is modestly increased by both exogenous and endogenous catecholamines and may be markedly increased by treatment with MAO inhibitors. A metabolite of propranolol also falsely elevates metanephrine excretion in one of the commonly used assays. VMA excretion is affected less by endogenous and exogenous catecholamines, but a variety of drugs may produce a spurious increase. MAO inhibitors decrease VMA excretion.

PLASMA CATECHOLAMINES. Plasma catecholamine determinations are of limited usefulness in the diagnosis of pheochromocytoma.[1429] Most patients with pheochromocytoma do have elevations in basal plasma catecholamine levels, frequently in excess of 12 nmol/L (2 ng/mL).[1428, 1432] As noted earlier, however, considerable care is required in obtaining basal catecholamine levels; casually obtained plasma levels, especially in anxious patients, frequently overlap the level in persons with pheochromocytoma.[1428] Plasma determinations should never be used as a screening test for pheochromocytoma. In an occasional problem patient in whom the clinical suspicion is high and in whom the urinary assay results are borderline, plasma catecholamine determinations may be useful. In these circumstances, basal plasma catecholamine levels higher than 12 nmol/L (2 ng/mL) support the diagnosis, whereas values lower than 3 nmol/L (0.5 ng/mL) make the diagnosis unlikely.[1428, 1432]

Suppression Tests. The usefulness of assays of plasma catecholamines may be enhanced by determining the response to agents that diminish sympathetic outflow. Administration of clonidine[1433] or the ganglionic-blocking agent pentolinium[1434] decreases plasma catecholamine levels in normal people but has a negligible effect in patients with pheochromocytoma. Prompt suppression of plasma catecholamine levels after oral clonidine is, therefore, useful at excluding the diagnosis in cases with suggestive clinical features and elevated plasma catecholamine levels. Unfortunately not all normal individuals suppress catecholamines in this test, particularly when baseline catecholamine levels are normal or low. Diuretic treatment has been shown to abort clonidine-induced suppression of plasma NE.[1435] The clonidine suppression test has also been used in suppressing overnight catecholamine excretion.[1436]

PHARMACOLOGICAL TESTS. Pharmacological tests for pheochromocytoma for the most part have been rendered obsolete by measurement of catecholamines and catecholamine metabolites in urine. The pharmacological tests were of two types: the adrenolytic test was utilized to determine catecholamine dependence in a hypertensive patient by evaluating the fall in blood pressure after administration of the rapidly acting alpha-receptor antagonist phentolamine. The provocative test was used to precipitate a crisis in normotensive patients with paroxysmal symptoms. The pharmacological tests lack sensitivity and specificity. Adrenolytic tests have a high incidence of false-positive responses, and provocative tests have a false-negative response rate of between 20 and 25%. The pharmacological tests are also potentially hazardous; fatalities have occurred from cerebral hemorrhage and myocardial infarction during provocative testing. In certain specific situations, however, modifications of the pharmacological tests may be useful. Because of the potential hazards these tests must always be carefully supervised and should never be undertaken casually.

Adrenolytic Tests. In an occasional patient presenting with malignant hypertension, the history or clinical evaluation raises the possibility of pheochromocytoma; in this setting significant blood pressure reduction by phentolamine not only suggests the diagnosis but also indicates that alpha-adrenergic blockade may be a useful form of treatment. A good response to phentolamine, however, only suggests the diagnosis; it must always be confirmed by subsequent measurement of urinary catecholamines or catecholamine metabolites.

The phentolamine test is performed with the patient in the supine position in bed and an intravenous line in place. After a stable baseline blood pressure is established and recorded, an intravenous bolus of phentolamine is administered, and blood pressure is recorded every 30 s for 3 min and then every minute for an additional 7 min or until the original values are regained. It is wise to start with a test dose of 0.5 mg; in the absence of a significant hypotensive response, the remainder of a 5-mg ampule may be administered. The test result is usually considered to be positive when the decrease in blood pressure is 35 mm Hg systolic and 25 mm Hg diastolic or greater. The response to phentolamine begins after 2 to 3 min and lasts approximately 10 min; blood pressure decreases that occur during the first 1 to 2 min after injection are nonspecific. An intravenous form of NE or phenylephrine should be immediately available for use in the event of a severe hypotensive reaction. False-positive responses are common in patients with renal failure and in those who have been treated with vasodilators.

Provocative Tests. Because of the potential hazard associated with induction of a severe paroxysm, provocative tests are almost never indicated. In the patient with paroxysmal symptoms and normal or borderline catecholamine excretion, it is preferable to document an increase in catecholamine excretion around the time of the crisis[1347] by sequential timed urine collections or, if these are not feasible, to initiate a 24-h urine collection after the onset of the paroxysm.

Previously, provocative testing used histamine, glucagon,[1437] or tyramine[1438] and assessed the blood pressure response to these agents.[1344] In addition to the danger of a severe hypertensive crisis, the false-negative rate with these agents was substantial.[1344, 1437] Glucagon releases catecholamines from pheochromocytoma[1432] but not from the normal adrenal.[1019] The sensitivity and specificity of diagnosis may be enhanced by measurement of plasma and urinary catecholamines after administration of this agent. Failure of plasma catecholamines to increase after glucagon may be helpful in excluding pheochromocytoma in difficult cases. The test must be carefully supervised by an experienced physician and requires two secure intravenous lines (one for blood sampling), close monitoring of blood pressure, and phentolamine immediately at hand. Should a severe hypertensive reaction ensue, it must be treated at once. This test should be contemplated only in extraordinary cases.

DIFFERENTIAL DIAGNOSIS. Pheochromocytoma is a rare disease with protean manifestations; as a consequence it must be considered in many patients with suggestive clinical features.

"Hyperadrenergic" Essential Hypertension. The possibility of pheochromocytoma is often suggested in patients with essential hypertension and hyperadrenergic features such as tachycardia, sweating, increased cardiac output, and anxiety.[1281, 1433] Although increased sympathetic nervous activity may contribute to the hypertension in these subjects, analysis of a 24-h urine collection is usually sufficient to exclude pheochromocytoma. Anxiety attacks resembling pheochromocytoma paroxysms may occur in these patients, and several analyses of urine collected during symptomatic episodes may be necessary before the diagnosis can be excluded with certainty.

Medications. Pressor crisis in patients who are taking MAO inhibitors, as described earlier, closely resembles pheochromocytoma paroxysms. Clonidine withdrawal[1439–1443] is also associated with pressor crises. These crises are caused by increased sympathetic nervous system activity and are frequently associated with increased urinary and plasma catecholamine levels. They can be adequately treated by alpha-adrenergic blocking agents or the reintroduction of clonidine. An accurate medication history is obviously critical for identifying the offending agents. Factitious crises produced by self-administration of sympathomimetic amines in emotionally disturbed patients should also be considered, particularly among workers in health care professions. Depending on the medication taken, urinary catecholamine excretion may be normal or abnormal. The direct addition of catecholamines to urine collections can result in a factitious diagnosis.[1444]

Intracranial Lesions. Intracranial lesions that are associated with increased intracranial pressure, particularly posterior fossa tumors[1445, 1446] or subarachnoid hemorrhage, may be confused with pheochomocytoma. Frequently these patients have experienced an obvious neurological catastrophe,[1447, 1448] and it is usually clear that the neurological disease is primary. The possibility of subarachnoid or intracranial hemorrhage secondary to pheochromocytoma, however, should not be overlooked.

Neuropsychiatric Disease. Anxiety attacks, frequently associated with hyperventilation, may suggest pheochromocytoma paroxysms. Significant blood pressure elevation during the attacks, especially when associated with tachycardia, supports the diagnosis of pheochromocytoma because in most patients anxiety attacks are not associated with hypertension. In some, however, significant elevation in both systolic and diastolic blood pressure may occur; these cases are difficult to distinguish from pheochromocytoma on clinical grounds. Several 24-h urine catecholamine or metabolite determinations may be required. Seizure disorders, especially the rare autonomic or diencephalic epilepsy, may also be confused with the paroxysms of pheochromocytoma.[1449] Modest elevations in plasma catecholamine levels have been reported during autonomic epilepsy, although urinary catecholamine excretion is usually normal. An abnormal electroencephalogram, an aura, and a beneficial response to anticonvulsant therapy usually suffice to exclude pheochromocytoma if urinary catecholamine excretion is normal.

Miscellaneous Disorders. The sympathomimetic features of thyrotoxicosis may suggest pheochromocytoma; diastolic hypertension, however, is not a feature of uncomplicated hyperthyroidism, and catecholamine excretion is normal. Some patients with angina pectoris have pressor attacks that resemble pheochromocytoma, but urinary excretion of catecholamines is normal.[1450] Patients with pheochromocytoma may present with chest pain and electrocardiographic abnormalities suggesting myocardial infarction or dissecting aortic aneurysm; the absence of pulse deficits, poor blood pressure response to conventional treatment, and the presence of tachycardia in association with a high diastolic blood pressure support the diagnosis of pheochromocytoma. Urinary catecholamine measurements usually distinguish these entities. It is best to avoid methyldopa in the initial treatment until pheochromocytoma can be excluded.

SCREENING FOR PHEOCHROMOCYTOMA. It is not feasible or necessary to screen the entire hypertensive population for pheochromocytoma. Patients with essential hypertension who have a poor response to conventional antihypertensive medications, signs of sympathetic overactivity, or paroxysms of any kind should undergo a 24-h urine collection while symptomatic. In a hypertensive patient, any of the suggestive clinical features that are given in Table 10–11 should raise the suspicion of pheochromocytoma, especially if blood pressure control is suboptimal. The personal or familial occurrence of a disease associated with pheochromocytoma is also an indication for screening. The possibility of pheochromocytoma should be considered in all members at risk in kindreds with MEN 2A, MEN 2B, neurofibromatosis, and von Hippel-Lindau disease. In the MEN kindreds, affected members should be screened yearly for pheochromocytoma, including specific estimation of epinephrine. Screening for pheochromocytoma is relatively inexpensive, harmless, and reasonably effective at establishing the diagnosis.

TABLE 10–11. Findings Suggestive of Pheochromocytoma

Clinical manifestations
  Paroxysmal attacks of any kind
  Signs of excessive adrenergic stimulation
    Tachycardia
    Excessive sweating
  Signs of hypermetabolism
    Fever
    Weight loss
  Orthostatic hypotension
  Anxiety-hyperexcitability
  Signs of cardiomyopathy
  Headaches
  Chest or abdominal pain
  Signs of neurocutaneous disease
    Five or six café au lait spots
    Neuromas or neurofibromas
    Retinal angiomas
    Vertebral abnormalities
  Unusual blood pressure response to surgery, anesthesia, or
    trauma
  Abdominal mass

Laboratory findings
  Hyperglycemia
  High hematocrit

Associated diseases
  Medullary thyroid carcinoma
  Mucosal neuroma syndrome
  Neurofibromatosis
  Retinocerebellar hemangioblastomatosis
  Hyperparathyroidism
  Islet cell tumors

Family history
  Pheochromocytoma
  Associated diseases

Management

Surgical removal is the definitive treatment of pheo-chromocytoma. Before surgery, however, a period of medical management is required to reverse the effects of excessive adrenergic stimulation. This medical treatment can be effectively achieved with adrenergic receptor blocking agents. Invasive diagnostic studies, often used in localization of pheochromocytoma (see later), should not be performed until adequate adrenergic blockade has been established.

MEDICAL ASPECTS OF TREATMENT. *Alpha-Receptor Blockade.* After the diagnosis of pheochromocytoma is established, the patient should be immediately given alpha-adrenergic blocking agents. Phenoxybenzamine is the agent of choice; it produces a stable, noncompetitive alpha-receptor blockade of long duration and is particularly suitable for preoperative management. Hypertensive crises occurring while the patient is being brought under control with phenoxybenzamine should be treated with intravenous phentolamine in doses of 1 to 5 mg. The usual initial dose of phenoxybenzamine is 10 mg every 12 h; increments of 10 mg may be added every few days until control of blood pressure is achieved and the paroxysms cease. Because of the long duration of action the therapeutic effects are cumulative and last for several days. The optimal dose, therefore, must be achieved gradually. Most patients require between 40 and 80 mg/d, although some need 200 mg/d or more. In patients without sustained hypertension, ascertainment of the appropriate dose of phenoxybenzamine is more difficult. In these individuals the dose should be titrated to the point that paroxysms cease; when postural signs and symptoms develop and persist, the dose should be stabilized. All patients who are being treated with phenoxybenzamine should have blood pressure recorded in the supine and upright positions several times each day. Dosage adjustment is best performed in a hospital setting.

Prazosin, the selective alpha-1–antagonist, has been used in preoperative management of a few patients with pheochromocytoma.[1451] Six to 10 mg/d in divided doses (every 6 h) is effective. The ultimate role of prazosin in the treatment of pheochromocytoma has not been established, but its relatively short duration of action may be a disadvantage in comparison with phenoxybenzamine.

In addition to controlling blood pressure and the paroxysms, alpha-adrenergic receptor blockade increases the blood volume. This consideration is most important for the subsequent success of surgical removal of the pheochromocytoma. Imposition of a high-salt diet augments restitution of plasma volume. Not uncommonly the hematocrit falls substantially after initiation of alpha-receptor blockade, presumably as a manifestation of volume expansion. Alpha-adrenergic blockade also improves congestive heart failure and angina pectoris, if these are present, consequent to significant afterload reduction.

All patients with pheochromocytoma (including those who are normotensive) should receive full blocking doses of phenoxybenzamine before arteriography, invasive diagnostic tests, or surgery. A 2-wk course of alpha-adrenergic blockade is the cornerstone of preoperative management.

Beta-Receptor Blockade. Propranolol is a useful adjunct in the treatment of pheochromocytoma. Although it is needed in most patients with pheochromocytoma, it should be administered only after alpha-adrenergic blockade has been introduced. When given in the absence of alpha-adrenergic blockade, propranolol may cause a paradoxical increase in blood pressure by blocking beta-receptor–mediated vasodilation in skeletal muscle. This effect is particularly prominent when the tumor secretes epinephrine. Propranolol may be introduced when tachycardia develops during institution of alpha-adrenergic blockade. Small doses are usually adequate and a reasonable starting dose is 10 mg three or four times per day, titrated as needed to control the pulse rate. Propranolol is particularly useful in controlling catecholamine-induced arrhythmias of the type that develop during administration of anesthesia. It also decreases sweating by blocking heat production and may improve angina by controlling tachycardia. If an underlying myocarditis is present caution is required because propranolol may precipitate congestive heart failure.

Inhibition of Catecholamine Biosynthesis. Metyrosine has been used to inhibit catecholamine biosynthesis by the pheochromocytoma. In doses of 0.3 to 4 g/d,[1347, 1452] 50 to 80% inhibition of catecholamine biosynthesis has been produced. This agent has been used both in preoperative preparation and in long-term treatment of inoperable patients. Usually it is not required, but it may be helpful when prolonged medical management is necessary.

LOCALIZATION OF TUMOR. Localization of the tumor or tumors facilitates surgical removal and is therefore worthwhile.[1347] CT scanning, MRI, radionuclide scanning, arteriography, and venous catheterization of the inferior vena cava, with analysis of catecholamines in the venous effluent from different levels, have all been used with more or less success. In general, localization techniques should be used after the diagnosis of pheochromocytoma is confirmed biochemically. Because the incidence of nonfunctioning "incidental" adrenal masses identifiable on CT scan is far from negligible,[1453–1455] the finding of a small nodule in the absence of catecholamine hypersecretion is problematic. Judicious use of the CT scan, nonetheless, may be helpful in the unusual difficult case in which the issue cannot be resolved by biochemical determinations. Under these circumstances the demonstration of completely normal adrenals frequently reassures both the patient and the physician that an adrenal pheochromocytoma is not responsible for the clinical picture. The demonstration of an adrenal nodule, on the other hand, frequently suggests the need for further attempts at biochemical confirmation. It should be emphasized in this context that incidentally discovered adrenal masses may be pheochromocytomas;[1456] appropriate screening is therefore indicated under these circumstances.

Adrenal Tumors. Adrenal CT scan is the major technique for demonstration of intra-adrenal pheochromocytomas (Fig. 10–29).[1457–1460] Because these tumors are usually at least 2 cm in diameter at the time of diagnosis, the lesions fall well within the resolving power of modern CT equipment. Adequate visualization of a normal-appearing adrenal is ordinarily sufficient to exclude an intra-adrenal pheochromocytoma. CT scanning has largely replaced arteriography for localization of intra-adrenal lesions. CT scanning with contrast enhancement can be performed on unblocked patients, but glucagon should not be used as an antiperistaltic agent because it may induce a severe paroxysm.[1461] Experience with MRI is still accumulating, but preliminary evidence suggests that this technique may be useful for distinguishing pheochromocytoma from adrenal cortical adenomas.[1462, 1463] Fine-needle aspiration of an adrenal mass should not be undertaken unless a pheochromocytoma is excluded, because the aspiration of an unsuspected pheochromocytoma may provoke a serious or fatal paroxysm.[1464]

Arteriography should be reserved for problem cases in which the CT scan fails to demonstrate the adrenal adequately or when an extra-adrenal pheochromocytoma is suspected. It is usually successful for demonstrating the adrenal lesion and its blood supply (Figs. 10–30 and 10–31).[1465, 1466] Although hazardous in the unblocked patient, arteriography can be safely performed after administration of alpha-adrenergic blocking agents. Because the major supply of an adrenal pheochromocytoma may be from any of the three arteries supplying the adrenal, a complete study requires demonstration of the superior, middle, and inferior adrenal arteries on each side.

Adrenal venography can identify intra-adrenal lesions (Fig. 10–32), but it is invasive, is technically demanding, and requires previous adrenergic blockade. The procedure has been rendered obsolete by the adrenal CT scan. Measurement of catecholamine levels in adrenal venous effluent is not particularly useful for identifying intra-adrenal pheochromocytomas, because a normal adrenal may secrete large amounts of catecholamines during the procedure.[1434, 1467] The

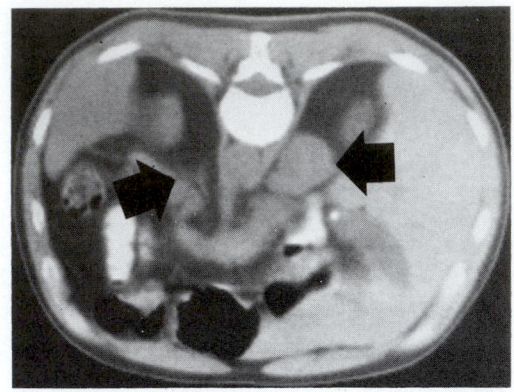

Figure 10–29. Adrenal pheochromocytoma demonstrated by CT scan. Note the normal adrenal on the left, the pheochromocytoma on the right (arrow). (From Landsberg L. Pheochromocytoma. Medical Grand Rounds 1983; 2:7–21.)

predominance of NE in the adrenal venous effluent from one side does suggest the presence of pheochromycytoma,[1434] however, because epinephrine is normally present in substantial excess.

Scintigraphic localization of pheochromocytoma using the radiopharmaceutical agent ^{131}I-meta-iodobenyzlguanidine has been described.[1468, 1469] This agent, which is a substrate for the amine uptake process, is concentrated in pheochromocytomas; if the lesion is large enough, sufficient concentration may be achieved to produce external scintigraphic images. This technique is investigational and has not been shown to demonstrate intra-adrenal pheochromocytomas in cases that could not be localized by other means. It may ultimately prove useful for localization of extra-adrenal pheochromocytomas, and may, on occasion, help to clarify the nature of a mass discovered by CT scanning or MRI when biochemical measurements are not decisive. Ultrasonography may occasionally demonstrate adrenal masses but is less sensitive than CT scanning. Pressure that is exerted by the sonogram probe has apparently provoked a paroxysm.[1461]

Extra-Adrenal Pheochromocytomas. The possibility of extra-adrenal pheochromocytoma should be considered in patients with increased catecholamine or catecholamine metabolite excretion in whom the adrenal glands appear normal on CT or MRI scan. Most extra-adrenal pheochromocytomas are located within the abdomen between the diaphragm and pelvic floor (see Table 10–10). The usefulness of CT (or

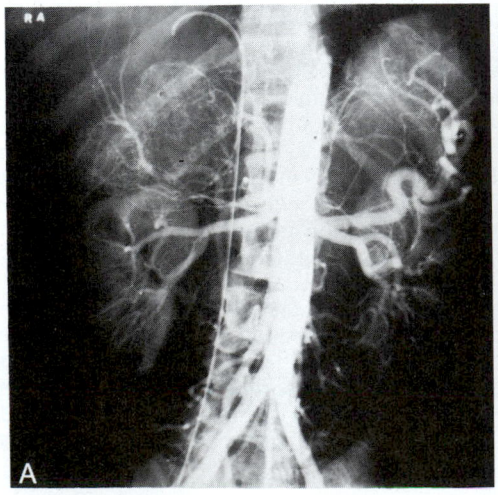 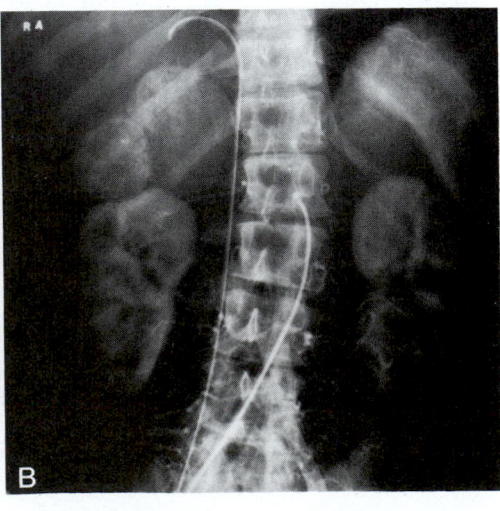

Figure 10–30. Angiographic demonstration of adrenal pheochromocytoma: abdominal aortography. Although this patient had bilateral pheochromocytomas, only the right adrenal tumor was shown clearly on arterial (A) and venous (B) phases of the study. The only suggestion of a left-sided tumor is a slight downward displacement of the splenic vein on venous-phase films. A selective injection of the left middle adrenal artery is shown in Figure 10–31B. The right-sided pheochromocytoma was bilobed at operation, which accounts for the appearance of two right suprarenal masses. (Courtesy of Dr. Harvey Eisenberg.)

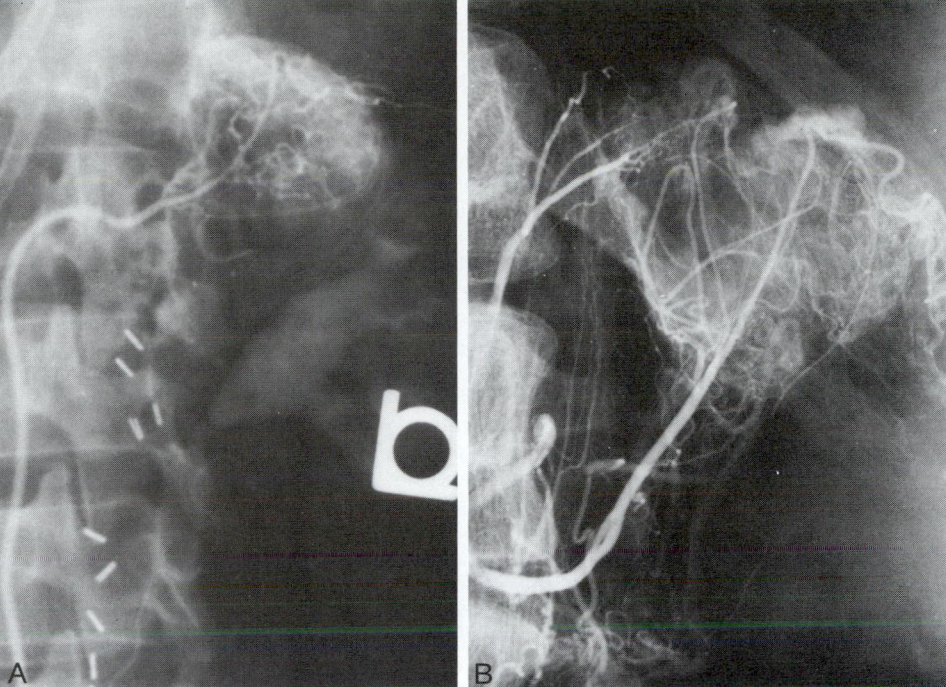

Figure 10–31. A and B, Angiographic demonstration of adrenal pheochromocytoma: selective arteriography of the middle adrenal artery. Both tumors demonstrate tumor vessels and tumor blush. The tumor in B was not visible on aortography (Fig. 10–30). (Courtesy of Drs. Dana Osborne [A] and Harvey Eisenberg [B].)

MRI) in localizing extra-adrenal pheochromocytomas has not been established, but, because these procedures are noninvasive, they are a reasonable first step in diagnosis. Abdominal aortography (after adequate blockade) should be done next because it frequently reveals extra-adrenal lesions with a blood supply derived from the aorta. The fact that extra-adrenal pheochromocytomas are often supplied by a large aberrant artery favors their demonstration by aortography.

Lesions within the thorax may be visible by chest radiography and should be obvious on CT scans. Extra-adrenal pheochromocytomas or chemodectomas in the neck may be palpable. Pressure may induce a paroxysm, but a crisis should not be intentionally provoked. If the symptoms are related to micturition, a bladder pheochromocytoma should

be sought, as described earlier. All diagnostic studies should be performed only after adrenergic blockade.

If these techniques fail to demonstrate the extra-adrenal pheochromocytoma, it is reasonable to catheterize the inferior vena cava and to obtain plasma samples for catecholamine analysis at various sites from the iliac veins to the superior vena cava. A significant step-up in catecholamine concentration that is not attributable to adrenal venous effluent may indicate the level at which the tumor drains into the vena cava.[1428, 1470] This information may allow more accurate demonstration of the tumor by arteriography or CT scanning. Scintigraphic localization of extra-adrenal pheochromocytomas may ultimately be of value, but this technique is not widely available.[1468, 1469]

SURGERY. *Preoperative Management.* Successful surgery

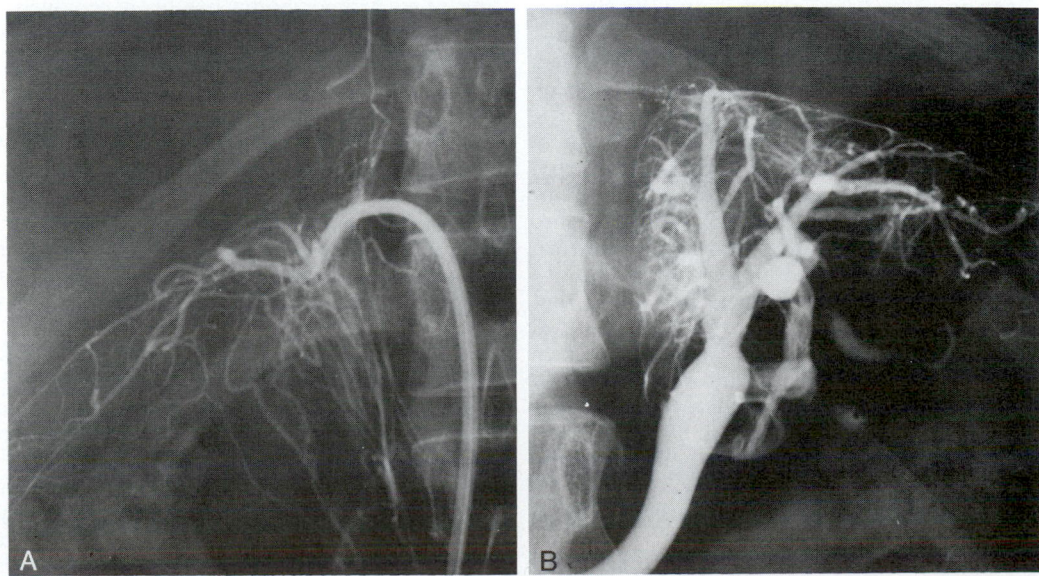

Figure 10–32. Angiographic demonstration of adrenal pheochromocytoma: selective adrenal venography. A, Normal right adrenal gland. An abnormal left adrenal venogram in the same patient (B) demonstrates a highly vascular tumor with a markedly enlarged left adrenal vein. (Courtesy of Dr. Harvey Eisenberg.)

requires the cooperation of surgeon, anesthesiologist, and endocrinologist. Surgery for pheochromocytoma is technically demanding and should not be undertaken lightly; it is preferably done in centers that have experience with this disease.

The cornerstone of successful surgery is adequate preparation, which entails a 2-wk course of alpha-adrenergic blockade with phenoxybenzamine. In conjunction with a liberal salt intake, this regimen allows restoration of plasma volume[1344, 1471] and permits recovery from the untoward effects of excessive adrenergic stimulation. There is indication for intravenous phenoxybenzamine and the rapid induction of adrenergic blockade that this produces. While adrenergic blockade is being gradually induced, a careful search can be made for a familial diathesis and associated diseases. Features suggesting MEN 2A or MEN 2B greatly increase the likelihood of bilateral tumors. Localization studies can also be performed during this period. There has been some controversy about whether phenoxybenzamine should be administered up until the day of surgery.[1352, 1471] Despite its relatively long duration of action, this agent can be continued until the time of surgery without untoward effects during the operation or in the postoperative period.[1347] Intraoperative and postoperative hypotension can be adequately controlled if sufficient time has been allowed for restoration of the extracellular fluid volume before surgery. As noted earlier, beta-blockade can be added after alpha-blockers have been started to control arrhythmias.

Anesthesia and Intraoperative Management. Scopolamine and short-acting barbiturates are satisfactory preanesthetic medications. Both pancuronium and succinylcholine have been used as muscle relaxants. The choice of anesthetic agent is controversial. A satisfactory approach utilizes a combination of nitrous oxide, thiopental, narcotics, and enflurane. All halogenated hydrocarbons (including enflurane) sensitize to the arrhythmogenic properties of catecholamines; these arrhythmias are effectively antagonized by beta-adrenergic blocking agents. Innovar, which is a combination of droperidol (a butyrophenone) and fentanyl (a narcotic), may provoke paroxysms in patients with unsuspected pheochromocytoma who are undergoing incidental surgery.[1375] The safety of this agent in blocked patients is uncertain; prudence dictates the use of other agents. Narcotics, although hazardous in unblocked patients, have been used without ill effects in blocked patients during surgery.

During the surgical procedure there should be continuous monitoring of arterial pressure (via intra-arterial catheter), central venous pressure,[1352, 1472] and electrocardiographic changes. Pulmonary wedge pressure should also be monitored in the presence of known or suspected heart disease. There should also be a careful and continuous estimation of blood loss, and particular efforts should be made to keep the rate of fluid replacement (saline, albumin, and blood) equal to the rate of loss. Hypotension generally responds better to volume replacement than to administration of vasoconstrictors. Central venous pressure or pulmonary capillary wedge pressure is a good indication of the need for volume replacement.

Hypertensive reactions and cardiac arrhythmias are most likely to occur during induction of anesthesia, intubation, and manipulation of the tumor. These effects are best controlled with intravenous administration of phentolamine and propranolol, respectively (Fig. 10–33). Phentolamine is administered as a bolus of from 1 to 5 mg intravenously, as needed. Propranolol is administered intravenously in 0.5- to 1-mg doses for tachycardia or ventricular ectopy. Lidocaine and nitroprusside may be required for treatment of arrhythmias and hypertension that are poorly responsive to propranolol and phentolamine. The need for these agents is not common in properly prepared patients. When a vasopressor agent is needed, NE or phenylephrine is satisfactory. Indirect-acting sympathomimetic amines that release catecholamines have an unpredictable effect and should be avoided.

The extent of surgical exploration depends on the results of preoperative studies that localize the tumor. When preoperative localization has not been accomplished, complete exploration of both suprarenal areas and the sympathetic chain around the abdominal aorta should be undertaken. The exploration can be limited when CT scanning, MRI, or arteriographic studies have demonstrated a pheochromocytoma in one adrenal and a normal adrenal on the contralateral side. Each pheochromocytoma should be handled as potentially malignant and should be removed with the capsule intact. Surrounding connective tissue and fat should also be removed. It is important to remove the entire adrenal gland. Patients with locally recurrent disease commonly have undergone procedures in which an attempt was made to remove the tumor but to spare the normal adrenal tissue. The malignant potential of the pheochromocytoma cannot be predicted with confidence solely on the basis of histological appearance. Malignancy is suggested by metastatic deposits or microvascular invasion.

Arterial blood pressure usually falls when the pheochromocytoma is removed (see Fig. 10–33); the failure of blood pressure to fall should raise the possibility of another tumor.

Postoperative Management. A transient episode of hypertension is not uncommon in the immediate postoperative period. This episode usually reflects fluid shifts and autonomic instability.[1347] It often responds to administration of diuretics. If there is any doubt about the hypertension being due to residual pheochromocytoma, phentolamine may be administered. A response to phentolamine suggests that all the pheochromocytoma may not have been removed. In some patients, vigorous fluid administration is required to support blood pressure in the postoperative period.

For about 1 wk the patient should be regarded as having excessive catecholamine stores in sympathetic nerve endings. Administration of catecholamine-releasing agents should be avoided during this period. Before the patient is discharged from the hospital, preferably 1 wk after removal of the tumor, assays for catecholamines and their metabolites in urine should be repeated for confirmation that all functioning pheochromocytoma has been removed. Catecholamine levels (or their metabolites) should be measured again if suggestive symptoms reappear or, if the patient remains asymptomatic, at yearly intervals thereafter for several years at least.

MALIGNANT PHEOCHROMOCYTOMA. Malignant pheochromocytoma generally recurs in the retroperitoneum or appears as metastatic deposits in bone, lung, or liver. Radiation therapy is not generally effective but may be of value for controlling symptomatic involvement of bone. Limited success has been reported with combination chemotherapy consisting of cyclophosphamide, vincristine, and dacarbazine.[1473, 1474]

LONG-TERM MEDICAL MANAGEMENT. In some patients chronic medical management is necessary because of disseminated malignancy or some other intercurrent illness that makes surgery inappropriate. Most tumors grow slowly, and the major morbidity is attributable to excessive catecholamine secretion rather than to local invasion or metastases to other organs. The disease thus may often be controlled by adrenergic blocking agents in conjunction with metyrosine, which reduces catecholamine biosynthesis by the tumor.[1452]

PREGNANCY. Pheochromocytoma complicating preg-

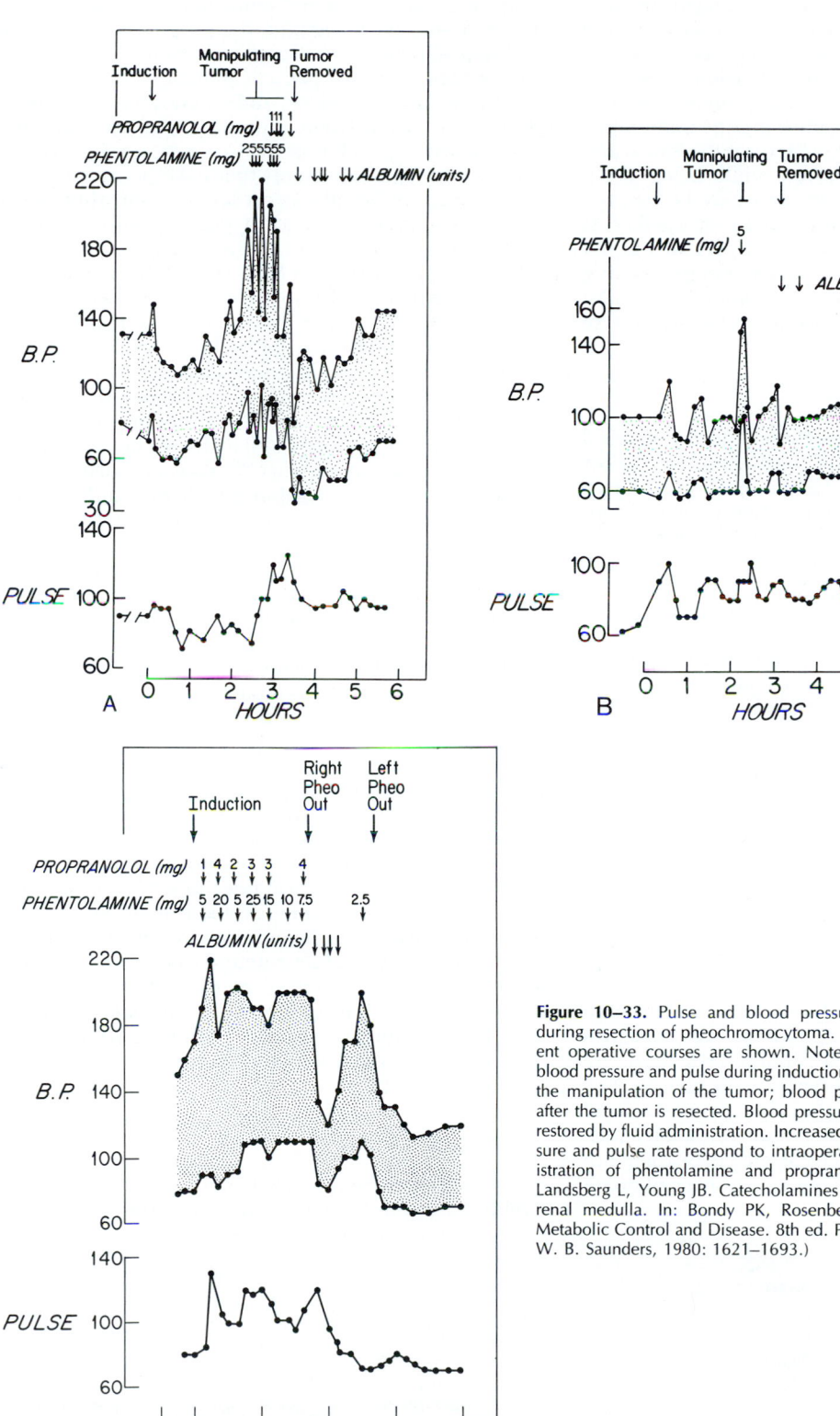

Figure 10–33. Pulse and blood pressure changes during resection of pheochromocytoma. Three different operative courses are shown. Note the rise in blood pressure and pulse during induction and during the manipulation of the tumor; blood pressure falls after the tumor is resected. Blood pressure is usually restored by fluid administration. Increased blood pressure and pulse rate respond to intraoperative administration of phentolamine and propranolol. (From Landsberg L, Young JB. Catecholamines and the adrenal medulla. In: Bondy PK, Rosenberg LE, eds. Metabolic Control and Disease. 8th ed. Philadelphia: W. B. Saunders, 1980: 1621–1693.)

nancy presents a difficult management problem. In unprepared patients, spontaneous labor with vaginal delivery is usually disastrous for mother and fetus and should therefore be avoided.[1344] After the diagnosis is established, treatment with adrenergic blocking agents should be initiated. In early or middle pregnancy, after the patient is prepared, the tumor should be removed. The pregnancy need not be terminated, but the risk of spontaneous abortion at the time of surgery is considerable. Late in the course, cesarean section followed by excision of the tumor may be undertaken if the fetus is of sufficient size.[1475] If the fetus is too immature, the patient may be closely monitored while being given adrenergic blocking drugs and operation may be delayed until fetal maturation progresses to the point of viability. If the clinical course deteriorates, however, surgery should not be postponed.[1344] Although the safety of adrenergic blocking agents during pregnancy has not been established, they have been used in several reported cases without obvious adverse effect.

Prognosis

In nonmalignant pheochromocytoma the 5-y survival rate is higher than 95%, and the recurrence rate after surgery is less than 10%.[1476, 1477] In patients with benign pheochromocytoma, the survival rate after operation approaches the age-adjusted norm. In experienced hands, surgical mortality is generally less than 2 to 3%; casually performed surgery in improperly prepared patients, on the other hand, is frequently catastrophic. In malignant pheochromocytoma the 5-y survival rate is less than 50%.[1476, 1477]

Complete resection cures the hypertension in approximately 75% of patients with pheochromocytoma; in the remaining 25%, hypertension recurs but is usually well controlled with a standard antihypertensive regimen.[1476, 1477] In this group, underlying essential hypertension or irreversible vascular damage induced by catecholamines may be involved in the persistent elevation of blood pressure.

OTHER TUMORS OF SYMPATHETIC AND ADRENOMEDULLARY ORIGIN

Neuroblastoma

GENERAL FEATURES. Neuroblastoma, ganglioneuroblastoma, and ganglioneuroma are tumors that, like pheochromocytomas, are derived from the neural crest and are located in the adrenal medulla and sympathetic ganglia (Fig. 10–34); like pheochromocytomas, they are often associated with excessive production of catecholamines and catecholamine metabolites. The pharmacological effects of their humoral products are usually minor,[5] but aggressive malignant behavior is common.

Neuroblastomas, which are the most immature and malignant of these tumors, may be considered derivatives of primitive sympathogonia or neuroblasts. Ganglioneuroblastomas are partially differentiated neuroblastomas in which mature ganglion cells and neurofibrils are present; although these tumors are malignant, the prognosis is better than that for neuroblastoma.[1478] Ganglioneuroma is a benign tumor derived from the sympathetic ganglion cells. The biology of the three tumors is poorly understood; the immature tumors appear to have a latent capacity to differentiate into more mature tissues, and this feature may account for some of the spontaneous remissions that have occurred.[5, 1478]

The excretion of catecholamines and their metabolites is almost always increased in patients with neuroblastomas and is often increased in those with ganglioneuromas.[5] NE (but not epinephrine), VMA, DA, HVA, and dopa may be excreted in increased amounts.[1448, 1479–1481] Increased excretion of DA and HVA is particularly characteristic of neuroblastomas. Compared with pheochromocytomas, the tumors themselves contain little catecholamine. Metabolism of catecholamines within the tumor may explain the absence of hypertension in most patients. Although catecholamine excretion does not correlate well with the clinical manifestations of disease in these patients,[1482] assays of urinary catecholamine excretion are useful in establishing a diagnosis[1481] and in following the results of treatment. Low ratios of VMA to HVA in the urine are correlated with a poor prognosis, perhaps because the more immature tumors have diminished DBH activity.[1483]

CLINICAL FEATURES. Neuroblastoma is one of the most common malignant tumors of children. It is characterized by rapid growth and widespread metastasis. The tumors originate either in the sympathetic chain or in the adrenal medulla; the prognosis is poorest for those of adrenomedullary origin. In younger patients the tumor is more aggressive and less likely to undergo spontaneous regression.

Neuroblastomas are more likely to undergo spontaneous regression than are any other malignant tumors in humans.[1484] A number of factors have been implicated as possibly playing a role in this spontaneous regression. One possibility is immunological rejection.[1484] Another interesting theoretical premise is the possible role of NGF,[1484] which, as described earlier, has been implicated in promoting normal maturation of sympathetic neural tissue. Such a factor might contribute to maturation of neuroblastoma cells, thus facilitating remission. The treatment of neuroblastoma is complex and involves surgery (usually partial or palliative resection of the tumor), radiation, and administration of chemotherapeutic agents.[1484–1486]

Ganglioneuroma

Ganglioneuromas are benign tumors found in both children and adults. They originate in the sympathetic chain,

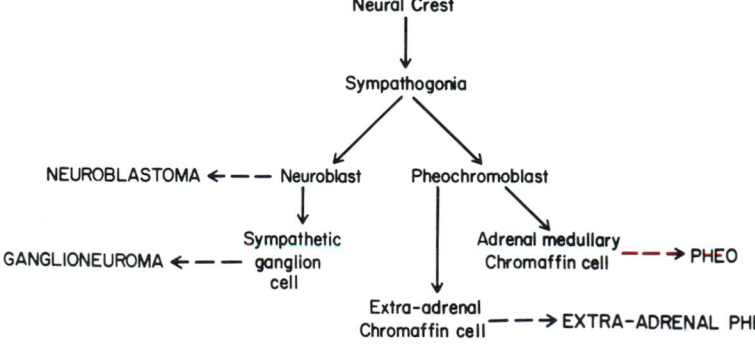

Figure 10–34. Embryological origin of sympathoadrenal tumors. (From Landsberg L, Young JB. Catecholamines and the adrenal medulla. In: Bondy PK, Rosenberg LE, eds. Metabolic Control and Disease. 8th ed. Philadelphia: W. B. Saunders, 1980: 1621–1693.)

most commonly in the posterior mediastinum. Some patients exhibit manifestations of excessive catecholamine secretion, particularly hypertension, which is more likely to occur with ganglioneuroma than with neuroblastoma.[1484] The clinical features, diagnosis, and management of NE-secreting ganglioneuromas are similar to those of extra-adrenal pheochromocytomas, as are diagnosis and management.

A syndrome of chronic diarrhea has been described in children with either ganglioneuroma or ganglioneuroblastoma.[1366, 1487] The pathogenesis of this diarrheal syndrome is obscure; it appears to be mediated by a humoral factor because it generally disappears on removal of the tumor. Vasoactive intestinal peptide secretion has been implicated in one case.[1366]

REFERENCES

1. Korner PI. Central control of blood pressure: implications in the pathophysiology of hypertension. In: Onesti G, Fernandes M, Kim KE, eds. Regulation of Blood Pressure by the Central Nervous System. New York: Grune & Stratton, 1976: 3–20.
2. Loewy AD, McKellar S. The neuroanatomical basis of central cardiovascular control. Fed Proc 1980; 39:2495–2509.
3. Cabot JB, Wild JM, Cohen DH. Raphe inhibition of sympathetic preganglionic neurons. Science 1979; 203:184–186.
4. Starke K, Endo T, Taube HD. Central noradrenergic mechanisms of neurotransmission. In: Onesti G, Fernandes M, Kim KE, eds. Regulation of Blood Pressure by the Central Nervous System. New York: Grune & Stratton, 1976: 21–34.
5. Moskowitz MS. Diseases of the autonomic nervous system. Clin Endocrinol Metab 1977; 6:745–768.
6. Heym C, Addicks K, Gerold N, et al. Catecholamines in paraganglionic cells of the rat superior cervical ganglion: functional aspects. In: Eranko O, Soinila S, Paivarinta H, eds. Histochemistry and Cell Biology of Autonomic Neurons, SIF Cells, and Paraneurons. New York: Raven, 1980: 87–94.
7. McAfee DA. Physiological evidence for cyclic AMP as a mediator of catecholamine transmission in the superior cervical sympathetic ganglion. In: Eranko O, ed. SIF Cells, Structure and Function of the Small, Intensely Fluorescent Sympathetic Cells. Fogarty International Center Proceedings No. 30. DHEW Publication No. (NIH) 76–942. Washington, DC: Government Printing Office, 1976: 132–142.
8. Libet B. The SIF cell as a functional dopamine-releasing interneuron in the rabbit superior cervical ganglion. In: Eranko O, ed. SIF Cells, Structure and Function of the Small, Intensely Fluorescent Sympathetic Cells. Fogarty International Center Proceedings No. 30. DHEW Publication No. (NIH) 76–942. Washington, DC: Government Printing Office, 1976: 163–177.
9. Coupland RE. The Natural History of the Chromaffin Cell. London: Longmans, Green, 1965.
10. Phillippe M. Fetal catecholamines. Am J Obstet Gynecol 1983; 146:840–855.
11. Stanton HC, Woo SK. Development of adrenal medullary function in swine. Am J Physiol 1978; 234:E137–E145.
12. Mobley WC, Server AC, Ishii DN, et al. Nerve growth factor. N Engl J Med 1977; 297:1096–1104, 1149–1158, 1211–1218.
13. Thoenen H, Barde Y-A. Physiology of nerve growth factor. Physiol Rev 1980; 60:1284–1335.
14. Levi-Montalcini R. The nerve growth factor 35 years later. Science 1987; 237:1154–1162.
15. Kaye MP, Wells DJ, Tyce GM. Nerve growth factor–enhanced reinnervation of surgically denervated canine heart. Am J Physiol 1979; 236:H624–H628.
16. Cochard P, Goldstein M, Black IB. Ontogenetic appearance and disappearance of tyrosine hydroxylase and catecholamines in the rat embryo. Proc Natl Acad Sci USA 1978; 75:2986–2990.
17. Bunge R, Johnson M, Ross CD. Nature and nurture in development of the autonomic neuron. Science 1978; 199:1409–1416.
18. Le Douarin NM, Smith J, Le Lievre CS. From the neural crest to the ganglia of the peripheral nervous system. Annu Rev Physiol 1981; 43:653–671.
19. Patterson PH, Potter DD, Furshpan EJ. The chemical differentiation of nerve cells. Sci Am 1978; 239:50–59.
20. Teitelman G, Baker H, Joh TH, et al. Appearance of catecholamine-synthesizing enzymes during development of rat sympathetic nervous system: possible role of tissue environment. Proc Natl Acad Sci USA 1979; 76:509–513.
21. Fukada K. Hormonal control of neurotransmitter choice in sympathetic neurone cultures. Nature 1980; 287:553–555.
22. Black IB, Adler JE, Dreyfus CF, et al. Neurotransmitter plasticity at the molecular level. Science 1984; 225:1266–1270.
23. Gabella G. Structure of the Autonomic Nervous System. London: Chapman & Hall, 1976.
24. Dahlstrom A, Haggendal J. Some quantitative studies on the noradrenaline content in the cell bodies and terminals of a sympathetic adrenergic neuron system. Acta Physiol Scand 1966; 67:271–277.
25. Potter LT. Storage of norepinephrine in sympathetic nerves. Pharmacol Rev 1966; 18:439–451.
26. Geffen LB, Livett BG. Synaptic vesicles in sympathetic neurons. Physiol Rev 1971; 51:98–157.
27. Anden NE, Carlsson A, Haggendal J. Adrenergic mechanisms. Annu Rev Pharmacol 1969; 9:119–134.
28. Millhorn DE, Hokfelt T. Chemical messengers and their coexistence in individual neurons. News Physiol Sci 1988; 3:1–5.
29. Burnstock G. Mechanisms of interaction of peptide and nonpeptide vascular neurotransmitter systems. J Cardiovasc Pharmacol 1987; 10(Suppl):S74–S81.
30. Perlman RL, Chalfie M. Catecholamine release from the adrenal medulla. Clin Endocrinol Metab 1977; 6:551–576.
31. Stjarne L. Storage particle in noradrenergic tissues. Pharmacol Rev 1966; 18:425–432.
32. Smith AD, Winkler H. Fundamental mechanisms in the release of catecholamines. In: Blaschko H, Muscholl E, eds. Catecholamines, Handbook of Experimental Pharmacology. Vol 33. Berlin: Springer-Verlag, 1972: 538–617.
33. Phillips JH, Pryde JG. The chromaffin granule: a model system for the study of hormones and neurotransmitters. Ann NY Acad Sci 1987; 493:27–41.
34. Coupland RE. The chromaffin system. In: Blaschko H, Muscholl E, eds. Catecholamines, Handbook of Experimental Pharmacology. Vol 33. Berlin: Springer-Verlag, 1972: 16–39.
35. Welsh JH. Catecholamines in the invertebrates. In: Blaschko H, Muscholl E, eds. Catecholamines, Handbook of Experimental Pharmacology. Vol 33. Berlin: Springer-Verlag, 1972: 79–105.
36. Holzbauer M, Sharman DF. The distribution of catecholamines in vertebrates. In: Blaschko H, Muscholl E, eds. Catecholamines, Handbook of Experimental Pharmacology. Vol 33. Berlin: Springer-Verlag, 1972: 110–171.
37. Saavedra JM, Grobecker H, Axelrod J. Adrenaline-forming enzyme in brainstem: elevation in genetic and experimental hypertension. Science 1975; 191:438–484.
38. Iversen LL. The Uptake and Storage of Noradrenaline in Sympathetic Nerves. Cambridge: Cambridge University Press, 1967.
39. Dahlstrom A, Haggendal J, Hokfelt T. The noradrenaline content of the varicosities of sympathetic adrenergic nerve terminals in the rat. Acta Physiol Scand 1966; 67:289–294.
40. Fuxe K, Hokfelt T. Catecholamines in the hypothalamus and the pituitary gland. In: Ganong WF, Martini L, eds. Frontiers in Neuroendocrinology. New York: Oxford University Press, 1969: 47–96.
41. Blaschko H. Catecholamine biosynthesis. Br Med Bull 1973; 29:105–109.
42. Kebabian JW, Greengard P. Dopamine-sensitive adenyl cyclase: possible role in synaptic transmission. Science 1971; 174:1346–1349.
43. Sampson SR, Aminoff MJ, Jaffe RA, et al. Analysis of inhibitory effect of dopamine on carotid body chemoreceptors in cats. Am J Physiol 1976; 230:1494–1498.
44. Hakanson R. New aspects of the formation and function of histamine, 5-hydroxytryptamine and dopamine in gastric mucosa. Acta Physiol Scand 1970; Suppl 340:1–73.
45. Stephenson RK, Sole MJ, Baines AD. Neural and extraneural catecholamine production by rat kidneys. Am J Physiol 1982; 242:F261–F266.
46. Kvetnansky R, Weise VK, Thoa NB, et al. Effects of chronic guanethidine treatment and adrenal medullectomy on plasma levels of catecholamines and corticosterone in forcibly immobilized rats. J Pharmacol Exp Ther 1979; 209:287–291.
47. Landsberg, L, Axelrod J. Influence of pituitary, thyroid, and adrenal hormones on norepinephrine turnover and metabolism in the rat heart. Circ Res 1968; 22:559–571.
48. Oliverio A, Stjarne L. Acceleration of noradrenaline turnover in the mouse heart by cold exposure. Life Sci 1965; 4:2339–2343.
49. Brodie BE, Costa E, Dlabac A, et al. Application of steady state kinetics to the estimation of synthesis rate and turnover time of tissue catecholamines. J Pharmacol Exp Ther 1966; 154:493–498.
50. Kopin IJ. Catecholamine metabolism (and the biochemical assessment of sympathetic activity). Clin Endocrinol Metab 1977; 6:525–549.
51. Vaccro KK, Liang BT, Perelle BA, et al. Tyrosine 3-monooxygenase regulates catecholamine synthesis in pheochromocytoma cells. J Biol Chem 1980; 255:6539–6541.
52. Abou-Donia MM, Viveros OH. Tetrahydrobiopterin increases in adrenal medulla and cortex: a factor in the regulation of tyrosine hydroxylase. Proc Natl Acad Sci USA 1981; 78:2703–2706.
53. Udenfriend S. Tyrosine hydroxylase. Pharmacol Rev 1966; 18:43–51.
54. Ikeda M, Fahien LA, Udenfriend S. A kinetic study of bovine adrenal tyrosine hydroxylase. J Biol Chem 1966; 241:4452–4456.
55. Udenfriend S, Zaltzman-Nirenberg P, Nagatsu T. Inhibitors of purified beef adrenal tyrosine hydroxylase. Biochem Pharmacol 1965; 14:837–845.

56. Lewis EJ, Tank AW, Weiner N, et al. Regulation of tyrosine hydroxylase mRNA by glucocorticoid and cyclic AMP in a rat pheochromocytoma cell line: isolation of a cDNA clone for tyrosine hydroxylase mRNA. J Biol Chem 1983; 258:14623–14637.

57. Lamouroux A, Faucon Biguet N, Samolyk D, et al. Identification of cDNA clones coding for rat tyrosine hydroxylase antigen. Proc Natl Acad Sci USA 1982; 79:3881–3885.

58. Mallet J, Boni C, Darmon M, et al. Molecular biology of rat and human tyrosine hydroxylase. In: Dahlstrom A, Belmaker RH, Sandler M, eds. Progress in Catecholamine Research. Part A: Basic Aspects and Peripheral Mechanisms. New York: Alan R. Liss, 1988: 21–27.

59. Lovenberg W, Weissbach H, Udenfriend S. Aromatic-L-amino acid decarboxylase. J Biol Chem 1962; 237:89–93.

60. Sourkes TL. Dopa decarboxylase: substrates, coenzymes, inhibitors. Pharmacol Rev 1966; 18:53–60.

61. Joh TH, Hwang O, Albert V, et al. Molecular biology of aromatic L-amino acid decarboxylase and dopamine beta-hydroxylase. In: Dahlstrom A, Belmaker RH, Sandler M, eds. Progress in Catecholamine Research. Part A: Basic Aspects and Peripheral Mechanisms. New York: Alan R. Liss, 1988: 29–34.

62. Williams ME, Young JB, Rosa RM, et al. Effect of protein ingestion on urinary dopamine excretion: evidence for the functional importance of renal decarboxylation of circulating 3,4-dihydroxyphenylalanine (DOPA) in man. J Clin Invest 1986; 78:1687–1693.

63. O'Malley KL, Mauron A, Raese J, et al. Genes for catecholamine biosynthesis: cloning by expression and identification of the cDNA for rat dopamine β-hydroxylase. Proc Natl Acad Sci USA 1983; 80:2161–2165.

64. Kaufman S, Friedman S. Dopamine-β-hydroxylase. Pharmacol Rev 1965; 17:71–100.

65. Kaufman S. Coenzymes and hydroxylases: ascorbate and dopamine-β-hydroxylase; tetrahydropteridines and phenylalanine and tyrosine hydroxylases. Pharmacol Rev 1966; 18:61–69.

66. Axelrod J. Methylation reactions in the formation and metabolism of catecholamines and other biogenic amines. Pharmacol Rev 1966; 18:95–113.

67. Wurtman RJ, Axelrod J. Control of enzymatic synthesis of adrenaline in the adrenal medulla by adrenal cortical steroids. J Biol Chem 1966; 241:2301–2305.

68. Sabban E, Goldstein M, Bohn MC, et al. Development of the adrenergic phenotype: increase in adrenal messenger RNA coding for phenylethanolamine-N-methyltransferase. Proc Natl Acad Sci USA 1982; 79: 4823–4827.

69. Baetge EE, Suh YH, Joh TH. Complete nucleotide and deduced amino acid sequence of bovine phenylethanolamine N-methyltransferase: partial amino acid homology with rat tyrosine hydroxylase. Proc Natl Acad Sci USA 1986; 83:5454–5458.

70. Weiner N. Regulation of norepinephrine biosynthesis. Annu Rev Pharmacol 1970; 10:273–289.

71. Weiner N, Rabadjija M. The effect of nerve stimulation on the synthesis and metabolism of norepinephrine in the isolated guinea-pig hypogastric nerve–vas deferens preparation. J Pharmacol Exp Ther 1968; 160:61–71.

72. Sedvall GC, Kopin IJ. Influence of sympathetic denervation and nerve impulse activity on tyrosine hydroxylase in the rat submaxillary gland. Biochem Pharmacol 1967; 16:39–46.

73. Weiner N, Rabadjija M. The regulation of norepinephrine synthesis: effect of puromycin on the accelerated synthesis of norepinephrine associated with nerve stimulation. J Pharmacol Exp Ther 1968; 164:103–114.

74. Vaccaro KK, Liang BT, Sheard BE, et al. Monensin inhibits catecholamine synthesis in pheochromocytoma cells. J Pharmacol Exp Ther 1982; 221:536–540.

75. Bjur RA, Weiner N. The activity of tyrosine hydroxylase in intact adrenergic neurons of the mouse vas deferens. J Pharmacol Exp Ther 1975; 193:9–26.

76. Chalfie M, Perlman RL. Regulation of catecholamine biosynthesis in a transplantable rat pheochromocytoma. J Pharmacol Exp Ther 1977; 200:588–597.

77. Salzman PM, Roth RH. Poststimulation catecholamine synthesis and tyrosine hydroxylase activation in central noradrenergic neurons. I. In vivo stimulation of the locus coeruleus. J Pharmacol Exp Ther 1980; 212:64–73.

78. Salzman PM, Roth RH. Poststimulation catecholamine synthesis and tyrosine hydroxylase activation in central noradrenergic neurons. II. Depolarized hippocampal slices. J Pharmacol Exp Ther 1980; 212:74–84.

79. Steinberg MI, Keller CE. Enhanced catecholamine synthesis in isolated rat superior cervical ganglia caused by nerve stimulation: dissociation between ganglionic transmission and catecholamine synthesis. J Pharmacol Exp Ther 1978; 204:384–399.

80. Haycock JW, Meligeni JA, Bennett WF, et al. Phosphorylation and activation of tyrosine hydroxylase mediate the acetylcholine-induced increase in catecholamine biosynthesis in adrenal chromaffin cells. J Biol Chem 1982; 257:12631–12648.

81. Chalfie M, Settipani L, Perlman RL. The role of cyclic adenosine 3':5'-monophosphate in the regulation of tyrosine 3-monooxygenase activity. Mol Pharmacol 1979; 15:263–270.

82. Meligeni JA, Haycock JW, Bennett WF, et al. Phosphorylation and activation of tyrosine hydroxylase mediate the cAMP-induced increase in catecholamine biosynthesis in adrenal chromaffin cells. J Biol Chem 1982; 257:12632–12640.

83. Vulliet PR, Langan TA, Weiner N. Tyrosine hydroxylase: a substrate of cyclic AMP–dependent protein kinase. Proc Natl Acad Sci USA 1980; 77:92–96.

84. Hoeldtke R, Kaufman S. Bovine adrenal tyrosine hydroxylase. J Biol Chem 1977; 252:3160–3169.

85. Perlman RL, Cahill AL, Horwitz J. Regulation of tyrosine hydroxylase activity in sympathetic neurons. In: Dahlstrom A, Belmaker RH, Sandler M, eds. Progress in Catecholamine Research. Part A: Basic Aspects and Peripheral Mechanisms. New York: Alan R. Liss, 1988: 53–55.

86. Morgenroth VH III, Boadle-Biber M, Roth RH. Tyrosine hydroxylase: activation by nerve stimulation. Proc Natl Acad Sci USA 1974; 71:4283–4287.

87. Mueller RA, Thoenen H, Axelrod J. Increase in tyrosine hydroxylase activity after reserpine administration. J Pharmacol Exp Ther 1969; 169:74–79.

88. Thoenen H, Mueller RA, Axelrod J. Trans-synaptic induction of adrenal tyrosine hydroxylase. J Pharmacol Exp Ther 1969; 169:249–254.

89. Kumakura K, Guidotti A, Costa E. Primary cultures of chromaffin cells: molecular mechanisms for the induction of tyrosine hydroxylase mediated by 8-Br-cyclic AMP. Mol Pharmacol 1979; 16:865–876.

90. Lewis EJ, Harrington CA, Chikaraishi DM. Transcriptional regulation of the tyrosine gene by glucocorticoid and cyclic AMP. Proc Natl Acad Sci USA 1987; 84:3550–3554.

91. Zigmond MJ, Baruchin AP, Stachowiak MK, et al. Long-term increases in tyrosine hydroxylase activity after partial injury or stress: a molecular biological analysis. In: Dahlstrom A, Belmaker RH, Sandler M, eds. Progress in Catecholamine Research. Part A: Basic Aspects and Peripheral Mechanisms. New York: Alan R. Liss, 1988: 71–74.

92. Iverson LL. Catecholamine uptake process. Br Med Bull 1973; 29:130–135.

93. Ciaranello RD. Regulation of phenylethanolamine-N-methyl-transferase. In: Usdin E, Snyder S, eds. Frontiers in Catecholamine Research. New York: Pergamon, 1973: 101–105.

94. Bloom FE. Electron microscopy of catecholamine-containing structures. In: Blaschko H, Muscholl E, eds. Catecholamines, Handbook of Experimental Pharmacology. Vol 33. Berlin: Springer-Verlag, 1972: 45–78.

95. Stjarne L. The synthesis, uptake and storage of catecholamines in the adrenal medulla: the effect of drugs. In: Blaschko H, Muscholl E, eds. Catecholamines, Handbook of Experimental Pharmacology. Vol 33. Berlin: Springer-Verlag, 1972: 231–269.

96. Johnson RG. Accumulation of biological amines into chromaffin granules: a model for hormone and neurotransmitter transport. Physiol Rev 1988; 68:232–307.

97. Yoshimasa T, Nakao K, Ohtsuki H, et al. Methionine-enkephalin and leucine-enkephalin in human sympathoadrenal system and pheochromocytoma. J Clin Invest 1982; 69:643–650.

98. North RA, Egan TM. Actions and distributions of opioid peptides in peripheral tissues. Br Med Bull 1983; 39:71–75.

99. Viveros OH, Wilson SP, Chang K-J. Regulation of synthesis and secretion of enkephalins and related peptides in adrenomedullary chromaffin cells and human pheochromocytoma. In: Costa E, Trabucchi M, eds. Regulatory Peptides: From Molecular Biology to Function. New York: Raven, 1982: 217–224.

100. Stern AS, Jones BN, Shively JE, et al. Two adrenal opioid polypeptides: proposed intermediates in the processing of proenkephalin. Proc Natl Acad Sci USA 1981; 78:1962–1966.

101. Stern AS, Lewis RV, Kimura S, et al. Isolation of the opioid heptapeptide met-enkephalin [Arg6,Phe7] from bovine adrenal medullary granules and striatum. Proc Natl Acad Sci USA 1979; 76:6680–6683.

102. Dandekar S, Sabol SL. Cell-free translation and partial characterization of mRNA coding for enkephalin-precursor protein. Proc Natl Acad Sci USA 1982; 79:1017–1021.

103. Lewis RV. Enkephalin biosynthesis in the adrenal medulla. In: Costa E, Trabucchi M, eds. Regulatory Peptides: From Molecular Biology to Function. New York: Raven, 1982: 167–174.

104. Fricker LD, Snyder SH. Enkephalin convertase: purification and characterization of a specific enkephalin-synthesizing carboxypeptidase localized to adrenal chromaffin granules. Proc Natl Acad Sci USA 1982; 79:3886–3890.

105. Wilson SP, Chang K-J, Viveros OH. Synthesis of enkephalins by adrenal medullary chromaffin cells: reserpine increases incorporation of radiolabeled amino acids. Proc Natl Acad Sci USA 1980; 77:4364–4368.

106. Majane EA, Alho H, Katokoa Y, et al. Neuropeptide Y in bovine adrenal glands: distribution and characterization. Endocrinology 1985; 117:1162–1168.

107. Bauer FE, Hacker GW, Terenghi G, et al. Localization and molecular

forms of galanin in human adrenals: elevated levels in pheochromocytomas. J Clin Endocrinol Metab 1986; 63:1372–1378.

108. Fischer-Colbrie R, Hagn C, Schober M. Chromogranins A, B, and C: widespread constituents of secretory vesicles. Ann NY Acad Sci 1987; 493:120–134.

109. Landsberg L. Chromogranin A. N Engl J Med 1984; 311:794–795.

110. Iacangelo A, Affolter H-U, Eiden LE, et al. Bovine chromogranin A sequence and distribution of its messenger RNA in endocrine tissues. Nature 1986; 323:82–86.

111. Winkler H, Sietzen M, Schober M. The life cycle of catecholamine-storing vesicles. Ann NY Acad Sci 1987; 493:3–19.

112. Bock E, Helle KB. Localization of synaptin on synaptic vesicle membranes, synaptosomal membranes and chromaffin granule membranes. FEBS Lett 1977; 82:175–178.

113. Yingst DR, Churchill PC. Cellular secretory mechanisms of the adrenal medulla. Physiologist 1985; 28:233–254.

114. Granot J, Rosenheck K. On the role of ATP and divalent metal ions in the storage of catecholamines. H NMR studies of bovine adrenal chromaffin granules. FEBS Lett 1978; 95:45–48.

115. Diliberto EJ Jr, Menniti FS, Knoth J. Co-transmitter biosynthesis in the adrenal medulla chromaffin cell: ascorbic acid availability. In: Dahlstrom A, Belmaker RH, Sandler M, eds. Progress in Catecholamine Research. Part A: Basic Aspects and Peripheral Mechanisms. New York: Alan R. Liss, 1988: 279–285.

116. Douglas WW. Stimulus-secretion coupling: the concept and clues from chromaffin and other cells. Br J Pharmacol 1968; 34:451–474.

117. Kilpatrick DL, Lewis RV, Stein S, et al. Release of enkephalins and enkephalin-containing polypeptides from perfused beef adrenal glands. Proc Natl Acad Sci USA 1980; 77:7473–7475.

118. Viveros OH, Diliberto EJ Jr, Hazum E, et al. Opiate-like materials in the adrenal medulla: evidence for storage and secretion with catecholamines. Mol Biol 1979; 16:1101–1108.

119. Livett BG, Dean DM, Whelan LG, et al. Co-release of enkephalin and catecholamines from cultured adrenal chromaffin cells. Nature 1981; 289:317–319.

120. Kirshner N, Viveros OH. Quantal aspects of the secretion of catecholamines and dopamine-β-hydroxylase from the adrenal medulla. In: Schumann HJ, Kroneberg HG, eds. New Aspects of Storage and Release Mechanisms of Catecholamines (Bayer Symposium II). Berlin: Springer-Verlag, 1970: 78–88.

121. Slotkin TA, Kirshner N. All-or-none secretion of adrenal medullary storage vesicle contents in the rat. Biochem Pharmacol 1973; 22:205–219.

122. Pollard HB, Rojas E, Burns AL. Synexin and the "hydrophobic bridge hypothesis" for membrane fusion during exocytosis. In: Dahlstrom A, Belmaker RH, Sandler M, eds. Progress in Catecholamine Research. Part A: Basic Aspects and Peripheral Mechanisms. New York: Alan R. Liss, 1988: 233–238.

123. Frye RA, Holz RW. Arachidonic acid release and catecholamine secretion from digitonin-treated chromaffin cells: effects of micromolar calcium, phorbol ester, and protein alkylating agents. J Neurochem 1985; 44:265–273.

124. Burgoyne RD, Cheek TR. Role of the chromaffin cell cytoskeleton in secretion. In: Dahlstrom A, Belmaker RH, Sandler M, eds. Progress in Catecholamine Research. Part A: Basic Aspects and Peripheral Mechanisms. New York: Alan R. Liss, 1988: 253–256.

125. Trifaro JM, Fournier S. Calmodulin and chromaffin cell secretion. In: Dahlstrom A, Belmaker RH, Sandler M, eds. Progress in Catecholamine Research. Part A: Basic Aspects and Peripheral Mechanisms. New York: Alan R. Liss, 1988: 257–262.

126. Serck-Hanssen G, Søvik O. Specific insulin binding in bovine chromaffin cells; demonstration of preferential binding to adrenalin-storing cells. Life Sci 1987; 41:2799–2806.

127. Dahmer MK, Perlman RL. Bovine chromaffin cells have insulin-like growth factor-I (IGF-I) receptors: IGF-I enhances catecholamine secretion. J Neurochem 1988; 51:321–323.

128. Lewis RV, Stern AS, Kimura S, et al. An about 50,000-dalton protein in adrenal medulla: a common precursor of (met)- and (leu)enkephalin. Science 1980; 208:1459–1461.

129. Evans CJ, Erdelyi E, Weber E, et al. Identification of pro-opiomelanocortin-derived peptides in the human adrenal medulla. Science 1983; 221:957–960.

130. Lewis JW, Tordoff MG, Sherman JE, et al. Adrenal medullary enkephalin-like peptides may mediate opioid stress analgesia. Science 1982; 217:557–559.

131. Kumakura K, Karoum F, Guidotti A, et al. Modulation of nicotinic receptors by opiate receptor agonists in cultured adrenal chromaffin cells. Nature 1980; 283:489–492.

132. Mannelli M, Maggi M, DeFeo ML, et al. Opioid modulation of normal and pathological human chromaffin tissue. J Clin Endocrinol Metab 1986; 62:577–582.

133. Von Euler US. Synthesis, uptake and storage of catecholamines in adrenergic nerves: the effect of drugs. In: Blaschko H, Muscholl E, eds. Catecholamines, Handbook of Experimental Pharmacology. Vol 33. Berlin: Springer-Verlag, 1972: 186–230.

134. Smith AD. Mechanisms involved in the release of noradrenaline from sympathetic nerves. Br Med Bull 1973; 29:123–129.

135. Dahlstrom A, Haggendal J. Studies on the transport and life-span of amine storage granules in a peripheral adrenergic neuron system. Acta Physiol Scand 1966; 67:278–288.

136. Costa M, Furness JB. Somatostatin is present in a subpopulation of noradrenergic nerve fibres supplying the intestine. Neuroscience 1984; 13:911–919.

137. Hokfelt T, Elfvin LG, Elde R, et al. Occurrence of somatostatin-like immunoreactivity in some peripheral sympathetic noradrenergic neurons. Proc Natl Acad Sci USA 1977; 74:3587–3591.

138. Kessler JA, Adler JE, Black IB. Substance P and somatostatin regulate sympathetic noradrenergic function. Science 1983; 221:1059–1061.

139. Laverty R. The mechanisms of action of some antihypertensive drugs. Br Med Bull 1973; 29:152–157.

140. Tipton KF. Biochemical aspects of monoamine oxidase. Br Med Bull 1973; 29:116–119.

141. Muscholl E. Adrenergic false transmitters. In: Blaschko H, Muscholl E, eds. Catecholamines, Handbook of Experimental Pharmacology. Vol 33. Berlin: Springer-Verlag, 1972: 618–660.

142. Kopin IJ. False adrenergic transmitters. Annu Rev Pharmacol 1968; 8:377–394.

143. Smith AD. Cellular control of the uptake, storage and release of noradrenaline in sympathetic nerves. Biochem Soc Symp 1972; 36:103–131.

144. Cohen RA, Kopin IJ, Creveling CR, et al. False neurochemical transmitters. Ann Intern Med 1966; 65:347–362.

145. Berecek KH, Brody MJ. Evidence for a neurotransmitter role for epinephrine derived from the adrenal medulla. Am J Physiol 1982; 242:H593–H601.

146. Rubin RP. The role of calcium in the release of neurotransmitter substances and hormones. Pharmacol Rev 1970; 22:389–428.

147. Weiner N. Multiple factors regulating the release of norepinephrine consequent to nerve stimulation. Fed Proc 1979; 38:2193–2202.

148. Thureson-Klein A, Klein RL, Johansson O. Catecholamine-rich cells and varicosities in bovine splenic nerve, vesicle contents and evidence for exocytosis. J Neurobiol 1979; 10:309–324.

149. Langeloh A, Bonisch H, Trendelenburg U. Mechanism of action of indirectly acting sympathomimetic amines. In: Dahlstrom A, Belmaker RH, Sandler M, eds. Progress in Catecholamine Research. Part A: Basic Aspects and Peripheral Mechanisms. New York: Alan R Liss, 1988: 155–159.

150. Trendelenburg U. Classification of sympathomimetic amines. In: Blaschko H, Muscholl E, eds. Catecholamines, Handbook of Experimental Pharmacology. Vol 33. Berlin: Springer-Verlag, 1972: 336–362.

151. Kopin IJ, Breese GR, Krauss KR, et al. Selective release of newly synthesized norepinephrine from the cat spleen during sympathetic nerve stimulation. J Pharmacol Exp Ther 1968; 161:271–278.

152. Vanhouette PM, Verbeuren TJ, Webb RC. Local modulation of adrenergic neuroeffector interaction in the blood vessel wall. Physiol Rev 1981; 61:151–247.

153. Starke K, Taube HD, Borowski E. Presynaptic receptor systems in catecholaminergic transmission. Biochem Pharmacol 1977; 26:259–268.

154. Westfall TC. Local regulation of adrenergic neurotransmission. Physiol Rev 1977; 57:659–728.

155. Enero MA, Langer SZ, Rothlin RP, et al. Role of alpha-adrenoreceptor in regulating noradrenaline overflow by nerve stimulation. Br J Pharmacol 1972; 44:672–688.

156. Vizi ES. Release-modulating adrenoceptors. In: Kunos G, ed. Adrenoceptors and Catecholamine Action. Part B. New York: John Wiley & Sons, 1983: 65–107.

157. Haggendal J. Regulation of catecholamine release. In: Usdin E, Snyder S, eds. Frontiers in Catecholamine Research. New York: Pergamon, 1973: 531–535.

158. Starke K. Presynaptic autoregulation: does it play a role? News Physiol Sci 1989; 4:1–4.

159. Alder-Graschinsky E, Langer SZ. Possible role of the β-adrenoceptor in regulation of noradrenaline release by nerve stimulation through a positive feedback mechanism. Br J Pharmacol 1975; 53:43–50.

160. deChamplain J. The sympathetic system in hypertension. Clin Endocrinol Metab 1977; 6:633–655.

161. Yamaguchi N, DeChamplain J, Nadeau RA. Regulation of norepinephrine release from cardiac sympathetic fibers in the dog by presynaptic α- and β-receptors. Circ Res 1977; 41:108–117.

162. Langer SZ. The role of α- and β-presynaptic receptors in the regulation of noradrenaline release elicited by nerve stimulation. Clin Sci Mol Med 1976; 51:423s–426s.

163. Rand MJ, Majewski H, Medgett IC, et al. Prejunctional receptors modulating autonomic neuroeffector transmission. Circ Res 1980; 46(Suppl):I70–175.

164. Angus JA, Korner PI. Evidence against presynaptic α-adrenoreceptor modulation of cardiac sympathetic transmission. Nature 1980; 286:288–291.

165. Vanhoutte PM, Verbeuren TJ. Inhibition by acetylcholine of the norepinephrine release evoked by potassium in canine saphenous veins. Circ Res 1976; 39:263–269.

166. Levy MN, Blattberg B. Effect of vagal stimulation on the overflow of norepinephrine into the coronary sinus during cardiac sympathetic nerve stimulation in the dog. Circ Res 1976; 38:81–85.

167. Hedqvist P. Activities of prostaglandins and prostaglandin endoperoxides at adrenergic neuroeffector junctions. Acta Biol Med Germ 1976; 35:1135–1139.

168. Malik K. Prostaglandin-mediated inhibition of the vasoconstrictor responses of the isolated perfused rat splenic vasculature to adrenergic stimuli. Circ Res 1978; 43:225–233.

169. Horton EW. Prostaglandins at adrenergic nerve-endings. Br Med Bull 1973; 29:148–151.

170. Hedqvist P. Modulating effect of prostaglandin E-2 on noradrenaline release from the isolated cat spleen. Acta Physiol Scand 1969; 75:511–512.

171. Hedqvist P. Control by prostaglandin E-2 of sympathetic neurotransmission in the spleen. Life Sci 1970; 9:269–278.

172. Malik KU, Ryan P, McGiff JC. Modification by prostaglandins E-1 and E-2, indomethacin, and arachidonic acid of the vasoconstrictor responses of the isolated perfused rabbit and rat mesenteric arteries to adrenergic stimuli. Circ Res 1976; 39:163–168.

173. Malik KU. Interaction of arachidonic acid metabolites and adrenergic nervous system. Am J Med Sci 1988; 295:280–286.

174. Cohen RA. Platelet 5-hydroxytryptamine and vascular adrenergic nerves. News Physiol Sci 1988; 3:185–189.

175. Cohen RA. Adenine nucleotides and 5-hydroxytryptamine released by aggregating platelets inhibit adrenergic neurotransmission in canine coronary artery. J Clin Invest 1986; 77:369–375.

176. Berkowitz BA. Dopamine and dopamine receptors as target sites for cardiovascular drug action. Fed Proc 1983; 42:3019–3021.

177. Lokhandwala MF, Buckley JP. The effect of L-dopa on peripheral sympathetic nerve function: role of presynaptic dopamine receptors. J Pharmacol Exp Ther 1978; 204:362–371.

178. Hope W, Majewski H, McCulloch MW, et al. Evidence for a modulatory role of dopamine in sympathetic transmission. Circ Res 1980; 46(Suppl):177–178.

179. Lokhandwala MF. Inhibition of sympathetic nervous system by histamine: studies with H1- and H2-receptor antagonists. J Pharmacol Exp Ther 1978; 206:115–122.

180. Powell JR. Effects of histamine on vascular sympathetic neuroeffector transmission. J Pharmacol Exp Ther 1979; 208:360–365.

181. McGrath MA, Shepherd JT. Inhibition of adrenergic neurotransmission in canine vascular smooth muscle by histamine mediation by H-2-receptors. Circ Res 1976; 39:566–573.

182. Su C. Purinergic inhibition of adrenergic transmission in rabbit blood vessels. J Pharmacol Exp Ther 1978; 204:351–361.

183. Ackerly JA, Blumberg AL, Brooker G, et al. Angiotensin II on the release of DBH and atrial cyclic AMP concentrations. Am J Physiol 1978; 235:H281–H288.

184. Zimmerman BG. Adrenergic facilitation by angiotensin: does it serve a physiological function? Clin Sci 1981; 60:343–348.

185. Archelos J, Xiang JZ, Reinecke M, et al. Regulation of release and function of neuropeptides in the heart. J Cardiovasc Pharmacol 1987; 10(Suppl 12):S45–S50.

186. Potter EK. Neuropeptide Y as an autonomic neurotransmitter. Pharmacol Ther 1988; 37:251–273.

187. Morris JL, Gibbins IL, Furness JB, et al. Chemical coding of peripheral catecholamine neurons. In: Dahlstrom A, Belmaker RH, Sandler M, eds. Progress in Catecholamine Research. Part A: Basic Aspects and Peripheral Mechanisms. New York: Alan R. Liss, 1988: 215–219.

188. Gothert M. Somatostatin selectively inhibits noradrenaline release from hypothalamic neurones. Nature 1980; 288:86–88.

189. Lundberg JM, Pernow J, Lacroix JS. Neuropeptide Y: sympathetic cotransmitter and modulator. News Physiol Sci 1989; 4:13–17.

190. Mills E, Smith PG, Slotkin TA, et al. Role of carotid body catecholamines in chemoreceptor function. Neuroscience 1978; 3:1137–1146.

191. Eyzaguirre C, Fidone SJ. Transduction mechanisms in carotid body: glomus cells, putative neurotransmitters, and nerve endings. Am J Physiol 1980; 239:C135–C152.

192. Karoum F, Garrison CK, Meff N, et al. Trans-synaptic modulation of dopamine metabolism in the rat superior cervical ganglion. J Pharmacol Exp Ther 1977; 201:654–661.

193. Neff NH, Karoum F, Hadjiconstantinou M. Dopamine-containing small intensely fluorescent cells and sympathetic ganglion function. Fed Proc 1983; 42:3009–3011.

194. Quenzer L, Yahn D, Alkadhi K, et al. Transmission blockade and stimulation of ganglionic adenylate cyclase by catecholamines. J Pharmacol Exp Ther 1979; 208:31–36.

195. Goyal RK, Rattan S. Neurohumoral, hormonal, and drug receptors for the lower esophageal sphincter. Gastroenterology 1978; 74:598–619.

196. Mukhopadhyay AK, Weisbrodt N. Effect of dopamine on esophageal motor function. Am J Physiol 1977; 232:E19–E24.

197. Yeh BK, McNay JL, Goldberg LI. Attenuation of dopamine renal and mesenteric vasodilation by haloperidol: evidence for a specific dopamine receptor. J Pharmacol Exp Ther 1969; 168:303–309.

198. Goldberg LI, Sonneville PF, McNay JL. An investigation of the structural requirements for dopamine-like renal vasodilation: phenylethylamines and apomorphine. J Pharmacol Exp Ther 1968; 163:188–197.

199. McNay JL, McDonald RH Jr, Goldberg LI. Direct renal vasodilation produced by dopamine in the dog. Circ Res 1965; 16:510–517.

200. Mizoguchi H, Dzau VJ, Siwek LE, et al. Effect of intrarenal administration of dopamine on renin release in conscious dogs. Am J Physiol 1983; 244:H39–H45.

201. Lorenzi M, Karam JH, Tsalikian E, et al. Dopamine during alpha- or beta-adrenergic blockade in man. J Clin Invest 1979; 63:310–317.

202. Sowers JR, Tuck ML, Golub MS, et al. Dopaminergic modulation of aldosterone secretion is independent of alterations in renin secretion. Endocrinology 1980; 197:937–941.

203. Whitfield L, Sowers JR, Tuck ML, et al. Dopaminergic control of plasma catecholamine and aldosterone responses to acute stimuli in normal man. J Clin Endocrinol Metab 1980; 51:724–729.

204. Carey MC, Thorner MO, Ortt EM. Effects of metoclopramide and bromocriptine on the renin-angiotensin-aldosterone system in man: dopaminergic control of aldosterone. J Clin Invest 1979; 63:727–735.

205. Alexander RW, Gill JR Jr, Yambe H, et al. Effects of dietary sodium and of acute saline infusion on the interrelationship between dopamine excretion and adrenergic activity in man. J Clin Invest 1974; 54:194–200.

206. Ball SG, Lee MR. The effect of carbidopa administration on urinary sodium excretion in man. Is dopamine an intrarenal natriuretic hormone? Br J Clin Pharmacol 1977; 4:115–119.

207. Oates NS, Ball SG, Perkins CM, et al. Plasma and urine dopamine in man given sodium chloride in the diet. Clin Sci 1979; 56:261–264.

208. Mannelli M, Pupilli C, Fabbri G, et al. Endogenous dopamine (DA) and DA2 receptors: a mechanism limiting excessive sympathetic-adrenal discharge in humans. J Clin Endocrinol Metab 1988; 66:626–631.

209. Relja M, Neff NH. Is dopamine a peripheral neurotransmitter? Introduction. Fed Proc 1983; 42:2998–2999.

210. Lackovic Z, Relja M. Evidence for a widely distributed peripheral dopaminergic system. Fed Proc 1983; 42:3000–3004.

211. Dinerstein RJ, Jones RT, Goldberg LI. Evidence for dopamine-containing renal nerves. Fed Proc 1983; 42:3005–3008.

212. Lee MR. Dopamine and the kidney. In: Lote CJ, ed. Advances in Renal Physiology. New York: Alan R. Liss, 1986: 218–246.

213. Suzuki H, Nakane H, Kawamura M, et al. Excretion and metabolism of dopa and dopamine by isolated perfused rat kidney. Am J Physiol 1984; 247:E285–E290.

214. Kopp U, Bradley T, Hjemdahl P. Renal venous outflow and urinary excretion of norepinephrine, epinephrine, and dopamine during graded renal nerve stimulation. Am J Physiol 1983; 244:E52–E60.

215. Stephenson RK, Sole MJ, Baines AD. Neural and extraneural catecholamine production by rat kidneys. Am J Physiol 1982; 242:F261–F266.

216. Dinerstein RJ, Vannice J, Henderson RC, et al. Histofluorescence techniques provide evidence for dopamine-containing neuronal elements in canine kidney. Science 1979; 205:497–499.

217. Bell C, Lang WJ. Neural dopaminergic vasodilator control in the kidney. Nature 1973; 246:25–27.

218. Baines AD. Effects of salt intake and renal denervation on catecholamine catabolism and excretion. Kidney Int 1982; 21:316–322.

219. Kopp U, Bradley T, Hjemdahl P. Renal venous outflow and urinary excretion of norepinephrine, epinephrine, and dopamine during graded renal nerve stimulation. Am J Physiol 1983; 244:E52–E60.

220. Ball AF, Oates NS, Lee MR. Urinary dopamine in man and rat: effects of inorganic salts on dopamine excretion. Clin Sci Mol Med 1978; 55:167–173.

221. Johnson GA, Gren JM, Kupiecki R. Radioenzymatic assay of DOPA (3,4-dihydroxyphenylalanine). Clin Chem 1978; 24:1927–1930.

222. Brown MJ, Collery CT. A specific radioenzymatic assay for dihydroxyphenylalanine (DOPA). Plasma dopa may be the precursor of urine free dopamine. Br J Clin Pharmacol 1981; 1:79–83.

223. Kaufman LN, Young JB, Landsberg L. Differential catecholamine responses to dietary intake: effects of macronutrients on dopamine and epinephrine excretion in the rat. Metabolism 1989; 38:91–99.

224. Baines AD, Drangova R. Neural not tubular dopamine increases glomerular filtration rate in perfused rat kidneys. Am J Physiol 1986; 250:F674–F679.

225. Eisenhofer G, Brush JE, Cannon RO III, et al. Plasma dihydroxyphenylalanine and total body and regional noradrenergic activity in humans. J Clin Endocrinol Metab 1989; 68:247–255.

226. Faucheux B, Buu NT, Kuchel O. Effects of saline and albumin on plasma and urinary catecholamines in dogs. Am J Physiol 1977; 232:F123–F127.

227. Graefe K-H. Ion dependence of neuronal amine transport. In: Dahlstrom A, Belmaker RH, Sandler M, eds. Progress in Catecholamine Research. Part A: Basic Aspects and Peripheral Mechanisms. New York: Alan R. Liss, 1988: 131–134.

228. Whitby LG, Axelrod J, Weil-Malherbe H. The fate of H^3 norepinephrine in animals. J Pharmacol Exp Ther 1961; 132:193–201.

229. Kopin IJ. Storage and metabolism of catecholamines: the role of monoamine oxidase. Pharmacol Rev 1964; 16:179–191.
230. Kopin IJ, Hertting G, Gordon EK. Fate of norepinephrine-H³ in the isolated perfused rat heart. J Pharmacol Exp Ther 1961; 138:34–40.
231. Rosell S, Kopin IJ, Axelrod J. Fate of H³-noradrenaline in skeletal muscle before and following sympathetic stimulation. Am J Physiol 1963; 205:317–321.
232. Stone CA, Porter CC, Stavorski JM, et al. Antagonism of certain effects of catecholamine-depleting agents by antidepressant and related drugs. J Pharmacol Exp Ther 1964; 144:196–204.
233. Follenfant MJ, Robison RD. The antagonism of adrenergic neurone blockade by amphetamine and dexamphetamine in the rat and guinea pig. Br J Pharmacol 1970; 38:792–801.
234. Sharman DF. The catabolism of catecholamines: recent studies. Br Med Bull 1973; 29:110–115.
235. Iversen LL, Jarrott B, Simmonds MA. Differences in the uptake, storage and metabolism of (+)- and (−)-noradrenaline. Br J Pharmacol 1971; 43:845–855.
236. Levin JA. The uptake and metabolism of ³H-L and ³H-DL-norepinephrine by intact rabbit aorta and by isolated adventitia and media. J Pharmacol Exp Ther 1974; 190:210–226.
237. Youdim MBH. Multiple forms of mitochondrial monoamine oxidase. Br Med Bull 1973; 29:120–122.
238. Hsu Y-P P, Powell JF, Chen S, et al. Molecular genetic studies of MAO genes. In: Dahlstrom A, Belmaker RH, Sandler M, eds. Progress in Catecholamine Research. Part A: Basic Aspects and Peripheral Mechanisms. New York: Alan R. Liss, 1988: 89–95.
239. Abell CW, Denney RM, Westlund KN. Localization and function of monoamine oxidases A and B. In: Dahlstrom A, Belmaker RH, Sandler M, eds. Progress in Catecholamine Research. Part A: Basic Aspects and Peripheral Mechanisms. New York: Alan R. Liss, 1988: 103–108.
240. Kopin IJ. Catecholamine metabolism: basic aspects and clinical significance. Pharmacol Rev 1985; 37:333–364.
241. Jose PA, Felder RA, Holloway RR, et al. Dopamine receptors modulate sodium excretion in denervated kidney. Am J Physiol 1986; 250:F1033–F1038.
242. Kopin IJ, Polinsky RJ, Oliver JA, et al. Urinary catecholamine metabolites distinguish different types of sympathetic neuronal dysfunction in patients with orthostatic hypotension. J Clin Endocrinol Metab 1983; 57:632–637.
243. Giachetti A. The functional state of sympathetic nerves in spontaneously diabetic mice. Diabetes 1978; 27:969–974.
244. Axelrod J, Tomchick R. Enzymatic O-methylation of epinephrine and other catechols. J Biol Chem 1958; 233:702–705.
245. Jarrott B. The cellular localization and physiological role of catechol-O-methyl transferase in the body. In: Usdin E, Snyder S, eds. Frontiers in Catecholamine Research. New York: Pergamon, 1973: 113–115.
246. Kopin IJ, Axelrod J, Gordon E. The metabolic fate of H³-epinephrine and C¹⁴-metanephrine in the rat. J Biol Chem 1961; 236:2109–2113.
247. Joyce DA, Beilin LJ, Vandongen R, et al. Epinephrine sulfation in the forearm: arteriovenous differences in free and conjugated catecholamines. Life Sci 1982; 31:2513–2517.
248. Wang P-C, Buu NT, Kuchel O, et al. Conjugation patterns of endogenous plasma catecholamines in human and rat. J Lab Clin Med 1983; 101:141–151.
249. Tyce GM. Metabolism of 3,4-dihydroxyphenylalanine by isolated perfused rat liver. Biochem Pharmacol 1971; 20:3447–3462.
250. Landsberg L, Berardino MB, Silva P. Metabolism of 3-H L-dopa by the rat gut in vivo: evidence for glucuronide conjugation. Biochem Pharmacol 1975; 24:1167–1176.
251. Landsberg L. Extraneuronal uptake and metabolism of ³H-L-norepinephrine by the rat duodenal mucosa. Biochem Pharmacol 1976; 25:729–731.
252. Landsberg L, Berardino MB, Stoff J, et al. Further studies on catechol uptake and metabolism in rat small bowel in vivo: (1) a quantitatively significant process with distinctive structural specifications; and (2) the formation of a dopamine glucuronide reservoir after chronic L-dopa feeding. Biochem Pharmacol 1978; 27:1365–1371.
253. Davidson L, Vandongen R, Beilin LJ. Effect of eating bananas on plasma free and sulfate-conjugated catecholamines. Life Sci 1981; 29:1773–1778.
254. Weinshilboum R. Phenol sulfortransferase: regulation in human tissue. In: Dahlstrom A, Belmaker RH, Sandler M, eds. Progress in Catecholamine Research. Part A: Basic Aspects and Peripheral Mechanisms. New York: Alan R. Liss, 1988: 183–189.
255. Eisenfeld AJ, Axelrod J, Krakoff L. Inhibition of the extraneuronal accumulation and metabolism of norepinephrine by adrenergic blocking agents. J Pharmacol Exp Ther 1967; 156:107–113.
256. Eisenfeld AJ, Landsberg L, Axelrod J. Effect of drugs on the accumulation and metabolism of extraneuronal norepinephrine in the rat heart. J Pharmacol Exp Ther 1967; 158:378–385.
257. Gillis CN, Greene NM, Cronau LH, et al. Pulmonary extraction of 5-hydroxytryptamine and norepinephrine before and after cardiopulmonary bypass in man. Circ Res 1972; 30:666–674.
258. Alabaster MA, Bakhle YS. The removal of noradrenaline in the pulmonary circulation of rat isolated lungs. Br J Pharmacol 1973; 47:325–331.
259. Iwasawa Y, Gillis CN. Pharmacological analysis of norepinephrine and 5-hydroxytryptamine removal from the pulmonary circulation: differentiation of uptake sites for each amine. J Pharmacol Exp Ther 1974; 188:386–393.
260. Bakhle YS, Vane JR. Pharmacokinetic function of the pulmonary circulation. Physiol Rev 1974; 54:1007–1045.
261. Rennick BR, Yoss N. Renal tubular excretion of DL-epinephrine-2-C¹⁴ in the chicken. Am J Physiol 1962; 215:347–350.
262. Quebbemann A, Rennick B. Inhibition of renal tubular transport of catecholamines by cocaine: an organic base mechanism. J Pharmacol Exp Ther 1970; 175:248–258.
263. Rennick B, Quebbemann A. Site of excretion of catechol and catecholamines: renal metabolism of catechol. Am J Physiol 1970; 218:1307–1312.
264. Jones RT. Renal excretion of L-epinephrine in the dog. Am J Physiol 1958; 215:371–374.
265. Rennick BR. Dopamine: renal tubular transport in the dog and plasma binding studies. Am J Physiol 1968; 215:532–534.
266. Hempel K, Lange HW, Kayser EF, et al. Role of O-methylation in the renal excretion of catecholamines in dogs. Naunyn-Schmiedeberg's Arch Pharmacol 1973; 277:373–386.
267. Hempel K, Carl W, Heidland A. Effect of COMT-inhibition on the renal excretion of (±)-adrenaline in dogs. Naunyn-Schmiedeberg's Arch Pharmacol 1974; 283:107–114.
268. Silva P, Landsberg L, Besarab A. Excretion and metabolism of catecholamines by the isolated perfused rat kidney. J Clin Invest 1979; 64:850–857.
269. Nagatsu T, Rust LA, DeQuattro V. The activity of tyrosine hydroxylase and related enzymes of catecholamine biosynthesis and metabolism in dog kidney—the effects of denervation. Biochem Pharmacol 1969; 18:1441–1446.
270. Crout JR. Catecholamines in urine. In: Seligson D, ed. Standard Methods of Clinical Chemistry. Vol 3. New York: Academic, 1961; 62–80.
271. Maas JW, Landis DH. The metabolism of circulating norepinephrine by human subjects. J Pharmacol Exp Ther 1971; 177:600–612.
272. von Euler US, Lishajko F. Improved technique for the fluorimetric estimation of catecholamines. Acta Physiol Scand 1961; 51:348–355.
273. Weil-Malherbe H, Smith ERB. The estimation of metanephrine, normetanephrine, and 3,4-dihydroxymandelic acid in urine. Pharmacol Rev 1966; 18:331–341.
274. Taniguchi K, Kakimoto Y, Armstrong MD. Quantitative determination of metanephrine and normetanephrine in urine. J Lab Clin Med 1964; 64:469–484.
275. Sandler M, Ruthven CRJ. The measurement of 4-hydroxy-3-methoxymandelic acid and homovanillic acid. Pharmacol Rev 1966; 18:343–351.
276. Ruthven CRJ, Sandler M. The estimation of 4-hydroxy-3-methoxyphenylglycol and total metadrenalines in human urine. Clin Chem Acta 1965; 12:318–324.
277. Maas JW, Landis DH. In vivo studies of the metabolism of norepinephrine in the central nervous system. J Pharmacol Exp Ther 1968; 163:147–162.
278. Tuchman M, Crippin PJ, Krivit W. Capillary gas-chromatographic determination of urinary homovanillic acid and vanillylmandelic acid. Clin Chem 1983; 29:828–831.
279. Moyer TP, Jiang N-S, Tyce GM, et al. Analysis for urinary catecholamines by liquid chromatography with amperometric detection: methodology and clinical interpretation of results. Clin Chem 1979; 25:256–263.
280. Goodall MC. Metabolic products of adrenaline and noradrenaline in human urine. Pharmacol Rev 1959; 11:416–425.
281. LaBrosse EH, Axelrod J, Kopin IJ, et al. Metabolism of 7-H³-epinephrine-d-barbiturate in normal young men. J Clin Invest 1961; 40:253–260.
282. Kopin IJ. Technique for the study of alternate metabolic pathways; epinephrine metabolism in man. Science 1960; 131:1372–1374.
283. Molinoff PB, Landsberg L, Axelrod J. An enzymatic assay for octopamine and other β-hydroxylated phenylethylamines. J Pharmacol Exp Ther 1969; 170:253–261.
284. Kopin IJ, Fischer JE, Musacchio JM, et al. "False neurochemical transmitters" and the mechanism of sympathetic blockade by monoamine oxidase inhibitors. J Pharmacol Exp Ther 1965; 147:186–193.
285. Blackwell B, Marley E, Price J, et al. Hypertensive interactions between monoamine oxidase inhibitors and foodstuffs. Br J Psychiatry 1967; 113:349–365.
286. Pettinger WA, Oates JA. The antihypertensive effects of MAO inhibitors. Hosp Pract 1967; 2:66–67.
287. McCabe BJ. Dietary tyramine and other pressor amines in MAO1 regimens: a review. J Am Diet Assoc 1986; 86:1059–1064.
288. Foods interacting with MAO inhibitors. Med Lett 1989; 31:11–12.
289. Liu LX, Rustigi AK. Cardiac myonecrosis in hypertensive crisis associated with monoamine oxidase inhibitor therapy. Am J Med 1987; 82:1060–1064.

290. Engelman K, Portnoy B, Lovenberg W. A sensitive and specific double-isotope derivative method for the determination of catecholamines in biological specimens. Am J Med Sci 1968; 255:259–268.
291. Passon PB, Peuler JD. A simplified radiometric assay for plasma norepinephrine and epinephrine. Anal Biochem 1973; 51:618–631.
292. Cryer PE, Santiago JV, Shah S. Measurement of norepinephrine and epinephrine in small volumes of human plasma by a single isotope derivative method: response to the upright posture. J Clin Endocrinol Metab 1974; 39:1025–1029.
293. Da Prada M, Zurcher G. Simultaneous radioenzymatic determination of plasma and tissue adrenaline, noradrenaline and dopamine within the femtomole range. Life Sci 1976; 19:1161–1174.
294. Johnson GA, Kupiecki RM, Baker CA. Single isotope derivative (radioenzymatic) methods in the measurement of catecholamines. Metabolism 1980; 29:1106–1113.
295. Saelens JK, Schoen MS, Koracsics GB. An enzyme assay for norepinephrine in brain tissue. Biochem Pharmacol 1967; 16:1043–1049.
296. Henry DP, Starman BJ, Johnson DG, et al. A sensitive radioenzymatic assay for norepinephrine in tissues and plasma. Life Sci 1975; 16:375–384.
297. Lake CR, Ziegler MG, Kopin IJ. Use of plasma norepinephrine for evaluation of sympathetic neuronal function in man. Life Sci 1976; 18:1315–1326.
298. Davis GC, Kissinger PT, Shoup RE. Strategies for determination of serum or plasma norepinephrine by reverse-phase liquid chromatography. Anal Chem 1981; 53:156–159.
299. Hjemdahl P, Daleskog M, Kahan T. Determination of plasma catecholamines by high performance liquid chromatography with electrochemical detection comparison with a radioenzymatic method. Life Sci 1979; 25:131–138.
300. Goldstein DS, Fuerstein G, Izzo JL, et al. Validity and reliability of liquid chromatography with electrochemical detection for measuring plasma levels of norepinephrine and epinephrine in man. Life Sci 1981; 28:467–475.
301. Danon A, Sapira JD. Binding of catecholamines to human serum albumin. J Pharmacol Exp Ther 1972; 182:295–302.
302. Collier JG. New dialysis technique for the continuous measurement of the concentration of vaso-active hormones. Br J Pharmacol 1972; 44:383P.
303. May P, Sanders FJ, Donabedian RK. Binding of catechol derivatives to human serum proteins. Experientia 1974; 30:304–305.
304. Sager G, Bratlid H, Little C. Binding of catecholamines to alpha-1 acid glycoprotein, albumin and lipoproteins in human serum. Biochem Pharmacol 1987; 36:3607–3612.
305. Sager G, Sandnes D, Bessen A, et al. Adrenergic ligand binding in human serum. Biochem Pharmacol 1985; 34:2812–2825.
306. Joyce DA, Beilin LJ, Vandongen R, et al. Plasma free and sulfate conjugated catecholamine levels during acute physiological stimulation in man. Life Sci 1982; 30:447–454.
307. Cryer PE, Haymond MW, Santiago JV, et al. Norepinephrine and epinephrine release and adrenergic mediation of smoking-associated hemodynamic and metabolic events. N Engl J Med 1976; 295:573–577.
308. Best JD, Halter JB. Release and clearance rates of epinephrine in man: importance of arterial measurements. J Clin Endocrinol Metab 1982; 55:263–268.
309. Hjemdahl P, Akerstedt T, Pollare T, et al. Influence of beta-adrenoreceptor blockade by metoprolol and propranolol on plasma concentrations and effects of noradrenaline and adrenaline during i.v. infusion. Acta Physiol Scand 1983; 515:45–53.
310. Metz SA, Halter JB, Porte D Jr, et al. Suppression of plasma catecholamines and flushing by clonidine in man. J Clin Endocrinol Metab 1978; 46:83–90.
311. Christensen NJ, Brandsborg O. The effect of standing and exercise on plasma catecholamines, serum insulin, and serum gastrin. Scand J Clin Lab Invest 1976; 36:591–595.
312. Halter JB, Pflug AE, Porte D Jr. Mechanism of plasma catecholamine increases during surgical stress in man. J Clin Endocrinol Metab 1977; 45:936–944.
313. Brown MJ, Jenner DA, Allison DJ, et al. Variations in individual organ release of noradrenaline measured by an improved radioenzymatic technique; limitations of peripheral venous measurements in the assessment of sympathetic nervous activity. Clin Sci 1981; 61:585–590.
314. Halter JB, Pflug AE, Tolas AG. Arterial-venous differences of plasma catecholamines in man. Metabolism 1980; 29:9–12.
315. Hjemdahl P. Measurements of plasma catecholamines by HPLC and the relation of their concentrations to sympathoadrenal activity. In: Joseph MH, Fillenz M, Macdonald IA, et al., eds. Monitoring Neurotransmitter Release During Behaviour. Chichester, England: Ellis Horwood, 1986: 17–32.
316. Young JB, Landsberg L. Sympathoadrenal activity in fasting pregnant rats: dissociation of adrenal medullary and sympathetic nervous system responses. J Clin Invest 1979; 64:109–116.
317. Landsberg L, Greff L, Gunn S, et al. Adrenergic mechanisms in the metabolic adaptation to fasting and feeding: effects of phlorizin on diet-induced changes in sympathoadrenal activity in the rat. Metabolism 1980; 29:1128–1137.
318. Rappaport EB, Young JB, Landsberg L. Effects of 2-deoxy-D-glucose on the cardiac sympathetic nerves and the adrenal medulla in the rat: further evidence for a dissociation of sympathetic nervous system and adrenal medullary responses. Endocrinology 1982; 110:650–656.
319. Gerich J, Davis J, Lorenzi M, et al. Hormonal mechanisms of recovery from insulin-induced hypoglycemia in man. Am J Physiol 1979; 236:E380–E385.
320. Silverberg AB, Shah SD, Haymond MW, et al. Norepinephrine: hormone and neurotransmitter in man. Am J Physiol 1978; 234:E252–E256.
321. Young JB, Rowe JW, Pallotta JA, et al. Enhanced plasma norepinephrine response to upright posture and glucose administration in elderly human subjects. Metabolism 1980; 29:532–539.
322. Esler M, Jackman G, Bobik A, et al. Determination of norepinephrine apparent release rate and clearance in humans. Life Sci 1979; 25:1461–1470.
323. Lake CR, Ziegler MG, Coleman MD, et al. Age-adjusted plasma norepinephrine levels are similar in normotensive and hypertensive subjects. N Engl J Med 1977; 296:208–209.
324. Saar N, Gordon RD. Variability of plasma catecholamine levels: age, duration of posture and time of day. Br J Clin Pharmacol 1979; 8:353–358.
325. de Champlain J, Cousineau D. Lack of correlation between age and circulating catecholamines in hypertensive patients. N Engl J Med 1977; 297:672.
326. Campese V, Myers MR, DeQuatro V. Plasma catecholamines and neurogenic hypertension. N Engl J Med 1977; 297:53.
327. Esler M, Skews H, Leonard P, et al. Age-dependence of noradrenaline kinetics in normal subjects. Clin Sci 1981; 60:217–219.
328. Pfeifer MA, Weinberg CR, Cook D, et al. Differential changes of autonomic nervous system function with age in man. Am J Med 1983; 75:249–258.
329. Gustafson AB, Kalkhoff RK. Influence of sex and obesity on plasma catecholamine response to isometric exercise. J Clin Endocrinol Metab 1982; 55:703–708.
330. Bergh U, Hartley H, Landsberg L, et al. Plasma norepinephrine concentration during submaximal and maximal exercise at lowered skin and core temperatures. Acta Physiol Scand 1979; 106:383–384.
331. Cryer PE. Physiology and pathophysiology of the human sympathoadrenal neuroendocrine system. N Engl J Med 1980; 303:436–444.
332. Romoff MS, Keusch G, Campese VM, et al. Effect of sodium intake on plasma catecholamines in normal subjects. J Clin Endocrinol Metab 1979; 48:26–31.
333. Clutter WE, Bier DM, Shah SD, et al. Epinephrine plasma metabolic clearance rates and physiologic thresholds for metabolic and hemodynamic actions in man. J Clin Invest 1980; 66:94–101.
334. Akerstedt T, Gillberg M, Hjemdahl P, et al. Comparison of urinary and plasma catecholamine responses to mental stress. Acta Physiol Scand 1983; 117:19–26.
335. Prinz PN, Halter J, Benedetti C, et al. Circadian variation of plasma catecholamines in young and old men: relation to rapid eye movement and slow wave sleep. J Clin Endocrinol Metab 1979; 49:300–304.
336. Van Loon GR, Sole MJ. Plasma dopamine: source, regulation, and significance. Metabolism 1980; 29:1119–1123.
337. Van Loon GR. Plasma dopamine: regulation and significance. Fed Proc 1983; 42:3012–3018.
338. Christensen NJ, Mathias CJ, Frankel HL. Plasma and urinary dopamine: studies during fasting and exercise and in tetraplegic man. Eur J Clin Invest 1976; 6:403–409.
339. Mathias CJ, Christensen NJ, Corbett JL, et al. Plasma catecholamines during paroxysmal neurogenic hypertension in quadriplegic man. Circ Res 1976; 39:204–208.
340. O'Dea K, Esler M, Leonard P, et al. Noradrenaline turnover during under- and over-eating in normal weight subjects. Metabolism 1982; 31:896–899.
341. Hjemdahl P, Freyschuss U, Juhlin-Dannfelt A, et al. Differentiated sympathetic activation during mental stress evoked by the Stroop test. Acta Physiol Scand 1984; 527(Suppl):25–29.
342. Hjemdahl P, Linde B. Influence of circulating NE and Epi on adipose tissue vascular resistance and lipolysis in humans. Am J Physiol 1983; 245:H447–H452.
343. Chang PC, Van Der Krogt JA, Vermeij P, et al. Norepinephrine removal and release in the forearm of healthy subjects. Hypertension 1986; 8:801–809.
344. Ninomiya I, Nisimaru N, Irisawa H. Sympathetic nerve activity to the spleen, kidney, and heart in response to baroceptor input. Am J Physiol 1971; 221:1346–1351.
345. Niijima A. Baroreceptor effects on renal and adrenal nerve activity. Am J Physiol 1976; 230:1733–1736.
346. Young JB, Saville E, Rothwell NJ, et al. Effect of diet and cold exposure on norepinephrine turnover in brown adipose tissue in the rat. J Clin Invest 1982; 69:1061–1071.
347. Folkow B, DiBona GF, Hjemdahl P, et al. Measurements of plasma

norepinephrine concentrations in human primary hypertension. A word of caution on their applicability for assessing neurogenic contributions. Hypertension 1983; 5:399–403.

348. Goldstein DS, McCarty R, Polinsky RJ, et al. Relationship between plasma norepinephrine and sympathetic neural activity. Hypertension 1983; 5:552–559.

349. Wallin BG, Sundlof G, Eriksson B-M, et al. Plasma noradrenaline correlates to sympathetic muscle nerve activity in normotensive man. Acta Physiol Scand 1981; 111:69–73.

350. Reid JL, Lopin IJ. The effects of ganglionic blockade, reserpine and vinblastine on plasma catecholamines and dopamine beta-hydroxylase in the rat. J Pharmacol Exp Ther 1975; 193:748–756.

351. Morgunov N, Baines AD. Renal nerves and catecholamine excretion. Am J Physiol 1981; 240:F75–F81.

352. Esler M, Jennings G, Korner P, et al. Measurement of total and organ-specific noradrenaline kinetics in humans. Am J Physiol 1984; 247:E21–E28.

353. Esler M, Jennings G, Lambert G. Regional pattern of sympathetic nervous system activation in cardiovascular disorders. In: Belmaker RH, Sandler M, Dahlstrom A, eds. Progress in Catecholamine Research. Part C: Clinical Aspects. New York: Alan R. Liss, 1988: 95–100.

354. Maas JW. A kinetic model for the study of the disposition of circulating norepinephrine. J Pharmacol Exp Ther 1970; 174:369–380.

355. Linares OA, Jacquez JA, Zech LA, et al. Norepinephrine metabolism in humans: kinetic analysis and model. J Clin Invest 1987; 80:1332–1341.

356. Linares OA, Zech LA, Jacquez JA, et al. Effect of sodium-restricted diet and posture on norepinephrine kinetics in humans. Am J Physiol 1988; 254:E222–E230.

357. Kvetnansky R, Sun CL, Lake CR, et al. Effect of handling and forced immobilization on rat plasma levels of epinephrine, norepinephrine, and dopamine-β-hydroxylase. Endocrinology 1978; 103:1868–1874.

358. Roizen MF, Moss J, Henry DP, et al. Effect of general anesthetics on handling- and decapitation-induced increases in sympathoadrenal discharge. J Pharmacol Exp Ther 1978; 204:11–18.

359. Young JB, Landsberg L. Effect of diet and cold exposure on norepinephrine turnover in pancreas and liver. Am J Physiol 1979; 236:E524–E533.

360. Landsberg L, Young JB. Assessment of sympathetic nervous activity from measurements of noradrenaline turnover in rats. In: Joseph MH, Fillenz M, Macdonald IA, et al., eds. Monitoring Neurotransmitter Release During Behaviour. Chichester, England: Ellis Horwood, 1986: 33–47.

361. Weinshilboum RM. Serum dopamine β-hydroxylase. Pharmacol Rev 1979; 30:133–166.

362. Rush RA, Geffen LB. Radioimmunoassay and clearance of circulating dopamine-beta-hydroxylase. Circ Res 1972; 31:444–452.

363. O'Connor DR, Bernstein KN. Radioimmunoassay of chromogranin A in plasma as a measure of exocytotic sympathoadrenal activity in normal subjects and patients with pheochromocytoma. N Engl J Med 1984; 311:764–770.

364. Wooten GF, Cordon PV. Plasma dopamine-beta-hydroxylase activity: elevation in man during cold pressor test and exercise. Arch Neurol 1973; 28:103–106.

365. Ziegler MG, Lake CR, Kopin IJ. Deficient sympathetic nervous response in familial dysautonomia. N Engl J Med 1976; 294:630–633.

366. Reid JL, Kopin IJ. Significance of plasma dopamine beta-hydroxylase activity as an index of sympathetic neuronal function. Proc Natl Acad Sci USA 1974; 71:4392–4394.

367. Weinshilboum RM, Schrott HG, Raymond RA, et al. Inheritance of very low serum dopamine-beta-hydroxylase activity. Am J Hum Genet 1975; 27:573–585.

368. O'Connor DT, Deftos LJ. Secretion of chromogranin A by peptide-producing endocrine neoplasms. N Engl J Med 1986; 314:1145–1151.

369. Wallin G. Intraneural recording and autonomic function in man. In: Bannister R, ed. Autonomic Failure. Oxford: Oxford University Press, 1983: 36–51.

370. Vallbo AB, Hagbarth K-E, Torebjork HE, et al. Somatosensory, proprioceptive and sympathetic activity in human peripheral nerves. Physiol Rev 1979; 59:919–957.

371. Heinsimer JA, Lefkowitz RJ. Adrenergic receptors: biochemistry, regulation, molecular mechanism, and clinical implications. J Lab Clin Med 1982; 100:641–658.

372. Pollet RJ, Levey GS. Principles of membrane receptor physiology and their application to clinical medicine. Ann Intern Med 1980; 92:663–680.

373. Lefkowitz RJ. Direct binding studies of adrenergic receptors: biochemical, physiologic and clinical implications. Ann Intern Med 1979; 91:450–458.

374. Insel PA. Identification and regulation of adrenergic receptors in target cells. Am J Physiol 1984; 247:E53–E58.

375. Ahlquist RP. A study of the adrenotropic receptors. Am J Physiol 1948; 153:586–600.

376. Moran NC, Perkins ME. Adrenergic blockade of the mammalian heart by a dichloro analogue of isoproterenol. J Pharmacol Exp Ther 1958; 124:223–237.

377. Moran NC, Perkins ME. An evaluation of adrenergic blockade of the mammalian heart. J Pharmacol Exp Ther 1961; 133:192–201.

378. Furchgott RF. The classification of adrenoceptors (adrenergic receptors): an evaluation from the standpoint of receptor theory. In: Blaschko H, Muscholl E, eds. Catecholamines, Handbook of Experimental Pharmacology. Vol 33. Berlin: Springer-Verlag, 1972:283–335.

379. Jenkinson DH. Classification and properties of peripheral adrenergic receptors. Br Med Bull 1973; 29:142–147.

380. Lands AM, Arnold A, McAuliff JP, et al. Differentiation of receptor systems activated by sympathomimetic amines. Nature 1967; 214:597–598.

381. Hoffman BB, Lefkowitz RJ. Alpha-adrenergic receptor subtypes. N Engl J Med 1980; 302:1390–1396.

382. Ruffolo RR Jr. Structure-activity relationships of alpha-adrenoceptor agonists. In: Kunos G, ed. Adrenoceptors and Catecholamine Action. Part B. New York: John Wiley & Sons, 1983; 1–50.

383. Motulsky HJ, Insel PA. Adrenergic receptors in man. Direct identification, physiologic regulation, and clinical alterations. N Engl J Med 1982; 307:18–29.

384. Weiner N. Norepinephrine, epinephrine, and the sympathomimetic amines. In: Gilman AG, Goodman LS, Gilman A, eds. The Pharmacological Basis of Therapeutics. 6th ed. New York: Macmillan, 1980; 138–175.

385. Gilman AG. G proteins: transducers of receptor-generated signals. Annu Rev Biochem 1987; 56:615–649.

386. Weiss ER, Kelleher DJ, Woon CW, et al. Receptor activation of G proteins. FASEB J 1988; 2:2841–2848.

387. Nicoll RA. The coupling of neurotransmitter receptors to ion channels in the brain. Science 1988; 241:545–551.

388. Bahouth SW, Berrios M, George ST, et al. Beta-adrenoceptors: new advances in purification and analysis. In: Dahlstrom A, Belmaker RH, Sandler M, eds. Progress in Catecholamine Research. Part A: Basic Aspects and Peripheral Mechanisms. New York: Alan R. Liss, 1988: 331–338.

389. Hoyer D, Palacios JM. Visualization of beta-adrenoceptors by autoradiography. In: Dahlstrom A, Belmaker RH, Sandler M, eds. Progress in Catecholamine Research. Part A: Basic Aspects and Peripheral Mechanisms. New York: Alan R. Liss, 1988: 339–344.

390. Frielle T, Collins S, Daniel KW, et al. Cloning of the cDNA for the human β_1-adrenergic receptor. Proc Natl Acad Sci USA 1987; 84:7920–7924.

391. Kobilka BK, Dixon RAF, Frielle T, et al. cDNA for the human β_2-adrenergic receptor: a protein with multiple membrane-spanning domains and encoded by a gene whose chromosomal location is shared with that of the receptor for platelet-derived growth factor. Proc Natl Acad Sci USA 1987; 84:46–50.

392. Kobilka BK, Matsui H, Kobilka TS, et al. Cloning, sequencing, and expression of the gene coding for the human platelet α_2-adrenergic receptor. Science 1987; 238:650–656.

393. Regan JW, Kobilka TS, Yang-Feng TL, et al. Cloning and expression of a human kidney cDNA for an α_2-adrenergic receptor subtype. Proc Natl Acad Sci USA 1988; 85:6301–6305.

394. Cotecchia S, Schwinn DA, Randall RR, et al. Molecular cloning and expression of the cDNA for the hamster α_1-adrenergic receptor. Proc Natl Acad Sci USA 1988; 85:7159–7163.

395. Peralta EG, Winslow JW, Peterson GL, et al. Primary structure and biochemical properties of an M-2 muscarinic receptor. Science 1987; 236:600–605.

396. Bonner TI, Buckley NJ, Young AC, et al. Identification of a family of muscarinic acetylcholine receptor genes. Science 1987; 237:527–532.

397. Lefkowitz RJ, Caron MG. Adrenergic receptors: models for the study of receptors coupled to guanine nucleotide regulatory proteins. J Biol Chem 1988; 263:4993–4996.

398. Kobilka BK, Kobilka TS, Daniel K, et al. Chimeric α_2, β_2-adrenergic receptors: delineation of domains involved in effector coupling and ligand binding specificity. Science 1988; 240:1310–1316.

399. Weiner N. Drugs that inhibit adrenergic nerves and block adrenergic receptors. In: Gilman AG, Goodman LS, Gilman A, eds. The Pharmacological Basis of Therapeutics. 6th ed. New York: Macmillan, 1980: 176–210.

400. Colucci WS. Alpha-adrenergic receptor blockade with prazosin. Ann Intern Med 1982; 97:67–77.

401. Hollister AS, FitzGerald GA, Nadeau JHJ. Acute reduction in human platelet α_2-adrenoreceptor affinity for agonist by endogenous and exogenous catecholamines. J Clin Invest 1983; 72:1498–1505.

402. Hsu CY, Knapp DR, Halushka PV. The effects of alpha adrenergic agents on human platelet aggregation. J Pharmacol Exp Ther 1979; 208:366–370.

403. Minneman KP. α_1-Adrenergic receptor subtypes, inositol phosphates, and sources of cell Ca^{2+}. Pharmacol Rev 1988; 40:87–119.

404. Exton JH. Mechanisms involved in alpha-adrenergic phenomena. Am J Physiol 1985; 248:E633–E647.

405. Berridge, MJ. Inositol trisphosphate and diacylglycerol: two interacting second messengers. Annu Rev Biochem 1987; 56:159–193.

406. Williamson JR. Role of inositol lipid breakdown in the generation of intracellular signals: state of the art lecture. Hypertension 1986; 8(Suppl II):II140–II156.

407. Exton JH. Mechanisms of action of calcium-mobilizing agonists: some variations on a young theme. FASEB J 1988; 2:2670–2676.

408. Fain JN, Wallace MA, Wojcikiewicz RJ. Evidence for involvement of guanine nucleotide–binding regulatory proteins in the activation of phospholipases by hormones. FASEB J 1988; 2:2569–2574.

409. Litosch I, Fain JN. Regulation of phosphoinositide breakdown by guanine nucleotides. Life Sci 1986; 39:187–194.

410. Blackshear PJ, Nairn AC, Kuo JF. Protein kinases 1988: a current perspective. FASEB J 1988; 2:2957–2969.

411. Limbird LE. Receptors linked to inhibition of adenylate cyclase: additional signaling mechanisms. FASEB J 1988; 2:2686–2695.

412. Frishman WH. Clinical significance of beta-selectivity and intrinsic sympathomimetic activity in a beta-adrenergic blocking drug. Am J Cardiol 1987; 59:33F–37F.

413. Goldberg LI, Hsieh Y-Y, Resnekov L. New catecholamines for treatment of heart failure and shock: an update on dopamine and a first look at dobutamine. Prog Cardiovasc Dis 1977; 19:327–340.

414. Sonnenblick EH, Frishman WH, LeJemtel TH. Dobutamine: a new synthetic cardioactive sympathetic amine. N Engl J Med 1979; 300:17–22.

415. Frederiksen MC. Tocolytic therapy with beta-adrenergic agonists. Ration Drug Ther 1983; 17:1–5.

416. Brodde O-E, Kretsch R, Ikezono K, et al. Human beta-adrenoceptors: relation of myocardial and lymphocyte beta-adrenoceptor density. Science 1986; 231:1584–1585.

417. Maisel AS, Ziegler MG, Carter S, et al. In vivo regulation of beta-adrenergic receptors on mononuclear leukocytes and heart. J Clin Invest 1988; 82:2038–2044.

418. Liggett SB, Shah SD, Cryer PE. Characterization of beta-adrenergic receptors of human skeletal muscle obtained by needle biopsy. Am J Physiol 1988; 254:E795–E798.

419. Harden TK. Agonist-induced desensitization of the β-adrenergic receptor–linked adenylate cyclase. Pharmacol Rev 1983; 35:5–32.

420. Fraser J, Nadeau J, Robertson D, et al. Regulation of human leukocyte beta receptors by endogenous catecholamines: relationship of leukocyte beta receptor density to the cardiac sensitivity to isoproterenol. J Clin Invest 1981; 67:1777–1784.

421. Krall JF, Connelly M, Tuck ML. Acute regulation of beta adrenergic catecholamine sensitivity in human lymphocytes. J Pharmacol Exp Ther 1980; 214:554–560.

422. Chang HY, Klein RM, Kunos G. Selective desensitization of cardiac beta adrenoceptors by prolonged in vivo infusion of catecholamines in rats. J Pharmacol Exp Ther 1982; 221:784–789.

423. Steer ML. Adrenergic receptors. Clin Endocrinol Metab 1977; 6:577–595.

424. Sibley DR, Lefkowitz RJ. Molecular mechanisms of receptor desensitization using the beta-adrenergic receptor–coupled adenylate cyclase system as a model. Nature 1985; 317:124–129.

425. Chuang D-M, Costa E. Evidence for internalization of the recognition site of beta-adrenergic receptors during receptor subsensitivity induced by (−)-isoproterenol. Proc Natl Acad Sci USA 1979; 76:3024–3028.

426. Motulsky HJ, Cunningham EMS, Deblasi A, et al. Desensitization and redistribution of beta-adrenergic receptors on human mononuclear leukocytes. Am J Physiol 1986; 250:E583–E590.

427. Sibley DR, Benovic JL, Caron MG, et al. Phosphorylation of cell surface receptors: a mechanism for regulating signal transduction pathways. Endocr Rev 1988; 9:38–56.

428. Leeb-Lundberg LMF, Cotecchia S, Lefkowitz RJ, et al. Desensitization and phosphorylation of alpha-1-adrenoceptors coupled to inositol phospholipid metabolism. In: Dahlstrom A, Belmaker RH, Sandler M, eds. Progress in Catecholamine Research. Part A: Basic Aspects and Peripheral Mechanisms. New York: Alan R. Liss, 1988: 375–382.

429. Fishman PH. Desensitization of mammalian beta-adrenoceptors. In: Dahlstrom A, Belmaker RH, Sandler M, eds. Progress in Catecholamine Research. Part A: Basic Aspects and Peripheral Mechanisms. New York: Alan R. Liss, 1988: 357–361.

430. Tashkin DP, Conolly ME, Deutsch RI, et al. Subsensitization of beta-adrenoceptors in airways and lymphocytes of healthy and asthmatic subjects. Am Rev Respir Dis 1982; 125:185–193.

431. Brodde O-E, Brinkmann M, Schemuth R, et al. Terbutaline-induced desensitization of human lymphocyte beta-2-adrenoceptors: accelerated restoration of beta-adrenoceptor responsiveness by prednisone and ketotifen. J Clin Invest 1985; 76:1096–1101.

432. Boudoulas H, Lewis RP, Kates RE, et al. Hypersensitivity to adrenergic stimulation after propranolol withdrawal in normal subjects. Ann Intern Med 1977; 87:433–436.

433. Nattel S, Rangno RE, Van Loon G. Mechanism of propranolol withdrawal phenomena. Circulation 1979; 59:1158–1164.

434. Cooper G IV, Kent RL, McGonigle P, et al. Beta adrenergic receptor blockade of feline myocardium: cardiac mechanics, energetics, and beta adrenoceptor regulation. J Clin Invest 1986; 77:441–455.

435. Kaumann AJ. On spare beta-adrenoceptors for inotropic effects of catecholamines in kitten ventricle. Arch Pharmacol 1978; 305:97–102.

436. Ruffolo RR Jr. Spare alpha adrenoceptors in the peripheral circulation: excitation-contraction coupling. Fed Proc 1986; 45:2341–2346.

437. Bevan JA, Oriowo MA, Bevan RD. Physiological variation in alpha-adrenoceptor–mediated arterial sensitivity: relation to agonist affinity. Science 1986; 234:196–197.

438. Kunos G, Szentivanyi M. Evidence favouring the existence of a single adrenergic receptor. Nature 1968; 217:1077–1078.

439. Kunos G, Yong MS, Nickerson M. Transformation of adrenergic receptors in the myocardium. Nature 1973; 241:119–120.

440. Janssens WJ, Vanhoutte PM. Instantaneous changes of alpha-adrenoceptor affinity caused by moderate cooling in canine cutaneous veins. Am J Physiol 1978; 234:H330–H337.

441. Marsh JD, Sweeney KA. Beta-adrenergic receptor regulation during hypoxia in intact cultured heart cells. Am J Physiol 1989; 256:H275–H281.

442. Vatner DE, Vatner SF, Fugii AM, et al. Loss of high affinity cardiac beta adrenergic receptors in dogs with heart failure. J Clin Invest 1985; 76:2259–2264.

443. Scarpace PJ. Decreased beta-adrenergic responsiveness during senescence. Fed Proc 1986; 45:51–54.

444. Feldman RD. Physiological and molecular correlates of age-related changes in the human beta-adrenergic receptor system. Fed Proc 1986; 45:48–50.

445. Supiano MA, Linares OA, Halter JB, et al. Functional uncoupling of the platelet alpha-2-adrenergic receptor–adenylate cyclase complex in the elderly. J Clin Endocrinol Metab 1987; 64:1160–1164.

446. Williams LT, Lefkowitz RJ. Regulation of rabbit myometrial alpha adrenergic receptors by estrogen and progesterone. J Clin Invest 1977; 60:815–818.

447. Roberts JM, Insel PA, Goldfien RD, et al. Alpha adrenoreceptors but not beta adrenoreceptors increase in rabbit uterus with oestrogen. Nature 1977; 270:624–625.

448. Arkinstall SJ, Jones CT. Myometrial alpha-1-adrenoceptors in pregnant guinea pig: their distribution and increased number. Am J Physiol 1989; 256:E215–E220.

449. Litime M-H, Pointis G, Breuiller M, et al. Disappearance of beta-adrenergic response of human myometrial adenylate cyclase at the end of pregnancy. J Clin Endocrinol Metab 1989; 69:1–6.

450. Colucci WS, Gimbrone MA Jr, McLaughlin MK, et al. Increased vascular catecholamine sensitivity and alpha-adrenergic receptor affinity in female and estrogen-treated male rats. Circ Res 1982; 50:805–811.

451. Roberts JM, Goldfien RD, Tsuchiya AM, et al. Estrogen treatment decreases alpha-adrenergic binding sites on rabbit platelets. Endocrinology 1979; 104:722–728.

452. Rodan SB, Rodan GA. Dexamethasone effects on beta-adrenergic receptors and adenylate cyclase regulatory proteins G_s and G_i in ROS 17/2.8 cells. Endocrinology 1986; 118:2510–2518.

453. Venter JC, Fraser CM, Harrison LC. Autoantibodies to beta₂-adrenergic receptors: a possible cause of adrenergic hyporesponsiveness in allergic rhinitis and asthma. Science 1980; 207:1361–1362.

454. Fraser CM, Venter JC, Kaliner M. Autonomic abnormalities and autoantibodies to beta-adrenergic receptors. N Engl J Med 1981; 305:1165–1170.

455. Parker CW. Autoantibodies and beta-adrenergic receptors. N Engl J Med 1981; 305:1212–1213.

456. Goldberg LI. The dopamine vascular receptor. Biochem Pharmacol 1975; 24:651–653.

457. DeCarle DJ, Christensen J. A dopamine receptor in esophageal smooth muscle of the opossum. Gastroenterology 1976; 70:216–219.

458. Clark BJ, Menninger K. Peripheral dopamine receptors. Circ Res 1980; 46(Suppl):I58–I62.

459. Kebabian JW, Calne DB. Multiple receptors for dopamine. Nature 1979; 277:93–96.

460. Creese I, Sibley DR, Leff SE. Agonist interactions with dopamine receptors: focus on radioligand-binding studies. Fed Proc. 1984; 43:2779–2784.

461. Felder RA, Jose PA. Dopamine₁ receptors in rat kidneys identified with ¹²⁵I-Sch 23982. Am J Physiol 1988; 255:F970–F976.

462. Willems JL, Buylaert WA, Lefebvre RA, et al. Neuronal dopamine receptors on autonomic ganglia and sympathetic nerves and dopamine receptors in the gastrointestinal system. Pharmacol Rev 1985; 37:165–216.

463. Emorine LJ, Nahmias C, Marullo S, et al. Structure of the gene for the human beta-2-adrenoceptor. In: Dahlstrom A, Belmaker RH, Sandler M, eds. Progress in Catecholamine Research. Part A: Basic Aspects and Peripheral Mechanisms. New York: Alan R. Liss, 1988: 345–349.

464. Goldberg LI. Pharmacologic basis for clinical uses of dopamine and new dopamine agonists. In: Belmaker RH, Sandler M, Dahlstrom A, eds. Progress in Catecholamine Research. Part C: Clinical Aspects. New York: Alan R. Liss, 1988: 61–64.

465. Lefebvre RA, Dupont AG, Bogaert MG. Pharmacology and clinical applications of DA-2 agonists. In: Belmaker RH, Sandler M, Dahlstrom

A, eds. Progress in Catecholamine Research. Part C: Clinical Aspects. New York: Alan R. Liss, 1988: 77–82.

466. Reis DJ, Doba N, Nathan MA. Neurogenic arterial hypertension produced by brainstem lesions. In: Onesti G, Fernandes M, Kim KE, eds. Regulation of Blood Pressure by the Central Nervous System. New York: Grune & Stratton, 1976: 35–51.

467. Haeusler G. Central adrenergic neurons in experimental hypertension. In: Onesti G, Fernandes M, Kim KE, eds. Regulation of Blood Pressure by the Central Nervous System. New York: Grune & Stratton, 1976: 53–64.

468. Thoren PN, Donald DE, Shepherd JT. Role of heart and lung receptors with nonmedullated vagal afferents in circulatory control. Circ Res 1976; 38(Suppl):II2–II9.

469. Vatner SF, McRitchie RJ. Reflex limb dilatation following norepinephrine and angiotensin II in conscious dogs. Am J Physiol 1976; 230:557–563.

470. Niijima A, Winter DL. Baroreceptors in the adrenal gland. Science 1968; 159:434–435.

471. Niijima A. Visceral afferents and metabolic function. Diabetologia 1981; 20(Suppl):325–330.

472. Liang C-S, Hood WB Jr. Afferent neural pathway in the regulation of cardiopulmonary responses to tissue hypermetabolism. Circ Res 1976; 38:209–214.

473. Recordati GM, Moss NG, Genovesi S, et al. Renal receptors in the rat sensitive to chemical alterations of their environment. Circ Res 1980; 46:395–405.

474. Nisimaru N. Comparison of gastric and renal nerve activity. Am J Physiol 1971; 220:1303–1308.

475. Niijima A. The effect of 2-deoxy-D-glucose on the efferent discharge rate of sympathetic nerves. J Physiol (Lond) 1975; 251:231–243.

476. Walther O-E, Iriki M, Simon E. Antagonistic changes of blood flow and sympathetic activity in different vascular beds following central thermal stimulation. Pflugers Arch 1970; 319:162–184.

477. Leduc J. Catecholamine production and release in exposure and acclimation to cold. Acta Physiol Scand 1961; Suppl 183:1–101.

478. Young JB, Landsberg L. The sympathoadrenal system and exercise: potential metabolic role in the trained and untrained states. In: Borer KT, Edington DW, White TP, eds. Frontiers of Exercise Biology. Champaign, IL: Human Kinetics Publishers, 1983: 152–172.

479. Ashkar E. Heart rate and blood pressure during exercise in dogs with autonomic denervation. Am J Physiol 1966; 210:950–952.

480. Ashkar E, Stevens JJ, Houssay B. Role of the sympathico-adrenal system in the hemodynamic response to exercise in dogs. Am J Physiol 1968; 214:22–27.

481. Himms-Hagen J. Role of the adrenal medulla in adaptation to cold. In: Greep RO, Astwood EB, eds. Handbook of Physiology. Sect 8: Endocrinology. Washington, DC: American Physiological Society, 1975: 637–665.

482. Young JB, Landsberg L. Effect of concomitant fasting and cold exposure on sympathoadrenal activity in rats. Am J Physiol 1981; 240:E314–E319.

483. Young JB, Rosa RM, Landsberg L. Dissociation of sympathetic nervous system and adrenal medullary responses. Am J Physiol 1984; 247:E35–E40.

484. Von Euler US. Commentary: quantitation of stress by catecholamine analysis. Clin Pharmacol Ther 1964; 5:398–404.

485. Mason JW. A review of psychoendocrine research on the sympathetic–adrenal medullary system. Psychosom Med 1968; 30:631–653.

486. Robertson D, Johnson GA, Robertson RM, et al. Comparative assessment of stimuli that release neuronal and adrenomedullary catecholamines in man. Circulation 1979; 59:637–643.

487. Christensen NJ. Biochemical methods of measuring adrenergic activity in man. Clin Physiol 1981; 1(Suppl 1):13–20.

488. Abboud FM, Heistad DD, Mark AL, et al. Reflex control of the peripheral circulation. Prog Cardiovasc Dis 1976; 18:371–403.

489. Zanchetti A, Dampney RAL, Ludbrook J, et al. Baroreceptor reflexes from different vascular areas in animals and man. Clin Sci Mol Med 1976; 51(Suppl 3):339–342.

490. Zoller RP, Mark AL, Abboud FM, et al. The role of low pressure baroreceptors in reflex vasoconstrictor responses in man. J Clin Invest 1972; 51:2967–2972.

491. Dampney RAL, Stella A, Golin R, et al. Vagal and sinoaortic reflexes in postural control of circulation and renin release. Am J Physiol 1979; 237:H146–H152.

492. Dembowsky K, Czachurski J, Seller H. Bulbospinal neurons and electrophysiology of sympathetic preganglionic neurons. In: Sandler M, Dahlstrom A, Belmaker RH, eds. Progress in Catecholamine Research. Part B: Central Aspects. New York: Alan R. Liss, 1988: 331–336.

493. McAllen RM, Dampney RAL. Functional subdivisions among subretrofacial presympathetic neurons. In: Sandler M, Dahlstrom A, Belmaker RH, eds. Progress in Catecholamine Research. Part B: Central Aspects. New York: Alan R. Liss, 1988: 337–342.

494. Chalmers JP, Minson JB, Pilowsky PM, et al. Pressor systems from ventrolateral medulla: epinephrine- and serotonin-containing neurons. In: Sandler M, Dahlstrom A, Belmaker RH, eds. Progress in Catecholamine Research. Part B: Central Aspects. New York: Alan R. Liss, 1988: 291–295.

495. Reid JL, Hamilton CA, Macrae IM, et al. Central adrenergic regulation of blood pressure: transmitter and receptor heterogeneity. In: Sandler M, Dahlstrom A, Belmaker RH, eds. Progress in Catecholamine Research. Part B: Central Aspects. New York: Alan R. Liss, 1988: 311–315.

496. Russell MP, Moran NC. Evidence for lack of innervation of beta-2 adrenoceptors in the blood vessels of the gracilis muscle of the dog. Circ Res 1980; 46:344–352.

497. Dabney JM, Buehn MJ, Dobbins DE. Constriction of lymphatics by catecholamines, carotid occlusion, or hemorrhage. Am J Physiol 1988; 255:H514–H524.

498. Hyman AL, Lippton HL, Kadowitz PJ. Nature of alpha 1 and postjunctional alpha 2 adrenoceptors in the pulmonary vascular bed. Fed Proc 1986; 45:2336–2340.

499. Young MA, Vatner DE, Knight DR, et al. Alpha-adrenergic vasoconstriction and receptor subtypes in large coronary arteries of calves. Am J Physiol 1988; 255:H1452–H1459.

500. Toda N. Alpha-adrenoceptor subtypes and diltiazem actions in isolated human coronary arteries. Am J Physiol 1986; 250:H718–H724.

501. Haws CW, Green LS, Burgess MJ, et al. Effects of cardiac sympathetic nerve stimulation on regional coronary blood flow. Am J Physiol 1987; 252:H269–H274.

502. Gwirtz PA, Overn SP, Mass HJ, et al. Alpha-1-adrenergic constriction limits coronary flow and cardiac function in running dogs. Am J Physiol 1986; 250:H1117–H1126.

503. Edwards SJ, Rattigan S, Colquhoun EQ, et al. Alpha-1-adrenergic control of contractility and coronary flow in the perfused rat heart. Am J Physiol 1989; 256:H334–H340.

504. Matherne GP, Nakamura KT, Robillard JE. Ontogeny of alpha-adrenoceptor responses in renal vascular bed of sheep. Am J Physiol 1988; 254:R277–R283.

505. Pettinger WA, Umemura S, Smyth DD, et al. Renal α_2-adrenoceptors and the adenylate cyclase–cAMP system: biochemical and physiological interactions. Am J Physiol 1987; 252:F199–F208.

506. Edwards RM, Trizna W. Characterization of alpha-adrenoceptors on isolated rabbit renal arterioles. Am J Physiol 1988; 254:F178–F183.

507. Elsner D, Stewart DJ, Sommer O, et al. Postsynaptic α_1- and α_2-adrenergic receptors in adrenergic control of capacitance vessel tone in vivo. Hypertension 1986; 8:1003–1014.

508. Appleton CP, Lee RW, Martin GV, et al. Alpha$_1$ and alpha$_2$-adrenoceptor stimulation: changes in venous capacitance in intact dogs. Am J Physiol 1986; 250:H1071–H1078.

509. Oliver JM, Pinto J, Sciacca RR, et al. Increased renal secretion of norepinephrine and prostaglandin E2 during sodium depletion in the dog. J Clin Invest 1980; 66:748–756.

510. Young MA, Vatner SF. Enhanced adrenergic constriction of iliac artery with removal of endothelium in conscious dogs. Am J Physiol 1986; 250:H892–H897.

511. Angus JA, Cocks TM, Satoh K. The alpha adrenoceptors on endothelial cells. Fed Proc 1986; 45:2355–2359.

512. Hoffman BF, Cranefield PF, Wallace AG. Physiological basis of cardiac arrhythmias (1). Mod Concepts Cardiovasc Dis 1966; 35:103–106.

513. Sarnoff SJ, Mitchell JH. The control of the function of the heart. In: Hamilton WF, Dow P, eds. Handbook of Physiology. Sect 2: Circulation. Washington, DC: American Physiological Society, 1962: 489–532.

514. Sonnenblick EH, Skelton CL. Oxygen consumption of the heart: physiological principles and clinical implication. Mod Concepts Cardiovasc Dis 1971; 38:9–16.

515. Pitt B, Ross RS. Beta adrenergic blockade in cardiovascular therapy. Mod Concepts Cardiovasc Dis 1969; 38:47–54.

516. Axelsson J. Catecholamine functions. Annu Rev Pharmacol 1971; 11:1–30.

517. Christensen J. The controls of gastrointestinal movements: some old and new views. N Engl J Med 1971; 285:85–98.

518. Catchpole BN. Ileus: use of sympathetic blocking agents in its treatment. Surgery 1969; 66:811–820.

519. Parkman HP, Reynolds JC, Ogorek CP, et al. Neuropeptide Y augments adrenergic contractions at feline lower esophageal sphincter. Am J Physiol 1989; 256:G589–G597.

520. Mathe AA, Hedqvist P. Catecholamines and pulmonary function. In: Dahlstrom A, Belmaker RH, Sandler M, eds. Progress in Catecholamine Research. Part A: Basic Aspects and Peripheral Mechanisms. New York: Alan R. Liss, 1988: 497–503.

521. Leff AR. Endogenous regulation of bronchomotor tone. Am Rev Respir Dis 1988; 137:1198–1216.

522. Sands MF, Douglas FL, Green J, et al. Homeostatic regulation of bronchomotor tone by sympathetic activation during bronchoconstriction in normal and asthmatic humans. Am Rev Respir Dis 1985; 132:992–998.

523. Lefcourt AM. Rhythmic contractions of the teat sphincter in bovines: an expulsion mechanism. Am J Physiol 1982; 242:R181–R184.

524. Walles B. Autonomic nervous control of ovarian follicular contractility. In: Polleri A, MacLeod RM, ed. Neuroendocrinology: Biological and Clinical Aspects. London: Academic, 1979: 79–96.

525. Bahr JM, Ben-Jonathan N. Elevated catecholamines in porcine follicular fluid before ovulation. Endocrinology 1985; 117:620–623.

526. Marchetti B, Cioni M, Badr M, et al. Ovarian adrenergic nerves directly participate in the control of luteinizing hormone–releasing hormone and beta-adrenergic receptors during puberty: a biochemical and autoradiographic study. Endocrinology 1987; 121:219–226.

527. Hargrove JL, MacIndoe JH, Ellis LC. Testicular contractile cells and sperm transport. Fertil Steril 1977; 28:1146–1157.

528. Bjorck S, Jansson R, Svanvik J. Adrenergic influence on concentrating function in the feline gall bladder. Gut 1982; 23:1019–1023.

529. Donowitz M, Cusolito S, Battisti L, et al. Dopamine stimulation of active Na and Cl absorption in rabbit ileum. J Clin Invest 1982; 69:1008–1016.

530. Chang EB, Field M, Miller RJ. Enterocyte alpha$_2$-adrenergic receptors: yohimbine and p-aminoclonidine binding relative to ion transport. Am J Physiol 1983; 244:G76–G82.

531. Al-Bazzaz FJ, Cheng E. Effect of catecholamines on ion transport in dog tracheal epithelium. J Appl Physiol 1979; 47:397–403.

532. Potter DE. Adrenergic pharmacology of aqueous humor dynamics. Pharmacol Rev 1981; 33:133–153.

533. Himms-Hagen J. Effects of catecholamines on metabolism. In: Blaschko H, Muscholl E, eds. Catecholamines, Handbook of Experimental Pharmacology. Vol 33. Berlin: Springer-Verlag, 1972: 363–462.

534. Kennedy MFG, Tutton PJM, Barkla DH. Adrenergic factors involved in the control of crypt cell proliferation in jejunum and descending colon of mouse. Clin Exp Pharmacol Physiol 1983; 10:577–586.

535. Kaiser G, Palm D, Quiring K, et al. The adrenergic β-receptor system of the premature erythrocyte: indication for adrenergic control of the erythron? Pharmacol Res Commun 1977; 9:93–103.

536. Brown JE, Adamson JW. Modulation of in vitro erythropoiesis. The influence of beta-adrenergic agonists on erythroid colony formation. J Clin Invest 1977; 60:70–77.

537. Bevan RD, Tsuru H. Functional and structural changes in the rabbit ear artery after sympathetic denervation. Circ Res 1981; 49:478–485.

538. Gerendai I, Marchetti B, Scapagnini U. Monaminergic peripheral regulation of compensatory ovarian hypertrophy. In: Polleri A, MacLeod RM, ed. Neuroendocrinology: Biological and Clinical Aspects. London: Academic, 1979: 103–114.

539. Ostman-Smith I. Cardiac sympathetic nerves as the final common pathway in the induction of adaptive cardiac hypertrophy. Clin Sci 1981; 61:265–272.

540. Simpson P, McGrath A. Norepinephrine-stimulated hypertrophy of cultured rat myocardial cells is an alpha$_1$ adrenergic response. J Clin Invest 1983; 72:732–738.

541. Mory G, Ricquier D, Nechad M, et al. Impairment of trophic response of brown fat to cold in guanethidine-treated rats. Am J Physiol 1982; 242:C159–C165.

542. Sundin U, Nechad M. Trophic response of rat brown fat by glucose feeding: involvement of sympathetic nervous system. Am J Physiol 1983; 244:C142–C149.

543. Hawkey CM, Britton BJ, Wood WG, et al. Changes in blood catecholamine levels and blood coagulation and fibrinolytic activity in response to graded exercise in man. Br J Haematol 1975; 29:377–384.

544. Zhu GJ, Abbadini M, Donati MB, et al. Tissue-type plasminogen activator release in response to epinephrine in perfused rat hindlegs. Am J Physiol 1989; 256:H404–H410.

545. Ingram GIC, Jones RV, Hershgold EJ, et al. Factor-VIII activity and antigen, platelet count and biochemical changes after adrenoceptor stimulation. Br J Haematol 1977; 35:81–100.

546. Bourne HR, Lichtenstein LM, Melmon KL, et al. Modulation of inflammation and immunity by cyclic AMP. Science 1974; 184:19–28.

547. Besedovsky HO, del Rey A, Sorkin E, et al. Immunoregulation mediated by the sympathetic nervous system. Cell Immunol 1979; 48:346–355.

548. Giron LT Jr, Crutcher KA, David JN. Lymph nodes—a possible site for sympathetic neuronal regulation of immune responses. Ann Neurol 1980; 8:520–525.

549. Felten DL, Felten SY, Carlson SL, et al. Development, aging, and plasticity of noradrenergic sympathetic innervation of secondary lymphoid organs: implications for neural-immune interactions. In: Dahlstrom A, Belmaker RH, Sandler M, eds. Progress in Catecholamine Research. Part A: Basic Aspects and Peripheral Mechanisms. New York: Alan R. Liss, 1988; 517–524.

550. Felten SY, Olschowka JA, Ackerman KD, et al. Catecholaminergic innervation of the spleen: are lymphocytes targets of noradrenergic nerves? In: Dahlstrom A, Belmaker RH, Sandler M, eds. Progress in Catecholamine Research. Part A: Basic Aspects and Peripheral Mechanisms. New York: Alan R. Liss, 1988; 525–531.

551. Livnat S, Eisen JN, Felten DL, et al. Behavioral and sympathetic neural modulation of immune function. In: Dahlstrom A, Belmaker RH, Sandler M, eds. Progress in Catecholamine Research. Part A: Basic Aspects and Peripheral Mechanisms. New York: Alan R. Liss, 1988: 539–545.

552. Stock M, Rothwell N. Obesity and Leanness. New York: John Wiley & Sons, 1982.

553. Girardier L, Stock MJ. Mammalian Thermogenesis. London: Chapman & Hall, 1983.

554. Rothwell NJ, Stock MJ, Stribling D. Diet-induced thermogenesis. Pharmacol Ther 1982; 17:251–268.

555. Himms-Hagen J. Thyroid hormones and thermogenesis. In: Girardier L, Stock MJ, eds. Mammalian Thermogenesis. London: Chapman & Hall, 1983: 141–177.

556. Jequier E. Energy expenditure in obesity. Clin Endocrinol Metab 1984; 13:563–580.

557. Landsberg L, Saville ME, Young JB. The sympathoadrenal system and regulation of thermogenesis. Am J Physiol 1984; 247:E181–E189.

558. Landsberg L, Young JB. Autonomic regulation of thermogenesis. In: Girardier L, Stock MJ, eds. Mammalian Thermogenesis. London: Chapman & Hall, 1983: 99–140.

559. Jung RT, Shetty PS, James WPT, et al. Reduced thermogenesis in obesity. Nature 1979; 279:322–323.

560. Girardier L. Brown fat: an energy dissipating tissue. In: Girardier L, Stock MJ, eds. Mammalian Thermogenesis. London: Chapman & Hall, 1983: 50–98.

561. Depocas F, Zaror-Behrens G, Lacelle S. Noradrenaline-induced calorigenesis in warm- or cold-acclimated rats. In vivo estimation of adrenoceptor concentration of noradrenaline effecting half-maximal response. Can J Physiol Pharmacol 1980; 58:1072–1077.

562. Depocas F, Behrens WA, Foster DO. Noradrenaline-induced calorigenesis in warm- and cold-acclimated rats: the interrelation of dose of noradrenaline, its concentration in arterial plasma, and calorigenic response. Can J Physiol Pharmacol 1978; 56:168–174.

563. Seydoux J, Girardier L. Control of brown fat thermogenesis by the sympathetic nervous system. Experientia 1977; 33:1128–1130.

564. Hsieh ACL, Carlson LD, Gray G. Role of the sympathetic nervous system in the control of chemical regulation of heat production. Am J Physiol 1957; 190:247–251.

565. Foster DO, Frydman ML. Nonshivering thermogenesis in the rat. II. Measurements of blood flow with microspheres point to brown adipose tissue as the dominant site of the calorigenesis induced by noradrenaline. Can J Physiol Pharmacol 1978; 56:110–122.

566. Foster DO, Frydman ML. Tissue distribution of cold-induced thermogenesis in conscious warm- or cold-acclimated rats reevaluated from changes in tissue blood flow: the dominant role of brown adipose tissue in the replacement of shivering by nonshivering thermogenesis. Can J Physiol Pharmacol 1979; 57:257–270.

567. Smith RE, Horwitz BA. Brown fat and thermogenesis. Physiol Rev 1969; 49:330–425.

568. Cannon B, Nedergaard J. The function and properties of brown adipose tissue in the newborn. In: Jones CT, ed. Biochemical Development of the Fetus and Neonate. New York: Elsevier Biomedical, 1982; 697–730.

569. Lean MEJ, James WPT. Brown adipose tissue in man. In: Trayhurn P, Nicholls DG, eds. Brown Adipose Tissue. London: Edward Arnold, 1986: 339–365.

570. Lean MEJ, Trayhurn P, Murgatroyd PR, et al. The case for brown adipose tissue function in humans: biochemistry, physiology and computed tomography. In: Berry EM, Blondheim SH, Eliahou HE, et al., eds. Recent Advances in Obesity Research. V: Proceedings of the 5th International Congress on Obesity. Paris: John Libbey, 1987: 109–123.

571. Lean MEJ, James WPT, Jennings G, et al. Brown adipose tissue in patients with phaeochromocytoma. Int J Obes 1986; 10:219–227.

572. Swick AG, Kemnitz JW, Houser WD, et al. Norepinephrine stimulates activity of brown adipose tissue in rhesus monkeys. Int J Obes 1986; 10:241–244.

573. Nicholls DG. Brown adipose tissue mitochondria. Biochim Biophys Acta 1979; 549:1–29.

574. Nicholls D, Locke R. Cellular mechanisms of heat dissipation. In: Girardier L, Stock MJ, eds. Mammalian Thermogenesis. London, Chapman & Hall, 1983: 8–49.

575. Bukowiecki L, Follea N, Paradis A, et al. Stereospecific stimulation of brown adipocyte respiration by catecholamines via beta-1-adrenoreceptors. Am J Physiol 1980; 238:E552–E563.

576. Selwyn MJ. Holes in mitochondrial inner membranes. Nature 1987; 330:424–425.

577. Bianco AC, Sheng X, Silva JE. Triiodothyronine amplifies norepinephrine stimulation of uncoupling protein gene transcription by a mechanism not requiring protein synthesis. J Biol Chem 1988; 263:18168–18175.

578. Leonard JL, Mellen SA, Larsen PR. Thyroxine 5'-deiodinase activity in brown adipose tissue. Endocrinology 1983; 112:1153–1155.

579. Silva JE, Larsen PR. Adrenergic activation of triiodothyronine production in brown adipose tissue. Nature 1983; 305:712–713.

580. Obregon MJ, Mills I, Silva JE, et al. Catecholamine stimulation of iodothyronine 5'-deiodinase activity in rat dispersed brown adipocytes. Endocrinology 1987; 120:1069–1072.

581. Silva JE, Mellen S, Larsen PR. Comparison of kidney and brown adipose tissue iodothyronine 5'-deiodinases. Endocrinology 1987; 121:650–656.

582. Bianco AC, Silva JE. Intracellular conversion of thyroxine to triiodo-

thyronine is required for the optimal thermogenic function of brown adipose tissue. J Clin Invest 1987; 79:295–300.

583. Bianco AC, Silva JE. Optimal response of key enzymes and uncoupling protein to cold in BAT depends on local T$_3$ generation. Am J Physiol 1987; 253:E255–E263.

584. Geloen A, Collet AJ, Guay G, et al. Beta-adrenergic stimulation of brown adipocyte proliferation. Am J Physiol 1988; 254:C175–C182.

585. Nechad M, Nedergaard J, Cannon B. Noradrenergic stimulation of mitochondriogenesis in brown adipocytes differentiating in culture. Am J Physiol 1987; 253:C889–C894.

586. Desautels M, Dulos RA. Is adrenergic innervation essential for maintenance of UCP in hamster BAT mitochondria? Am J Physiol 1988; 254:R1035–R1042.

587. Rothwell NJ, Stock MJ. Diet-induced thermogenesis. In: Girardier L, Stock MJ, eds. Mammalian Thermogenesis. London: Chapman & Hall, 1983: 208–233.

588. Rothwell NJ, Stock MJ. Similarities between cold- and diet-induced thermogenesis in the rat. Can J Physiol Pharmacol 1980; 58:842–848.

589. Rothwell NJ, Stock MJ. Influence of environmental temperature on energy balance, diet-induced thermogenesis and brown fat activity in "cafeteria"-fed rats. Br J Nutr 1986; 56:123–129.

590. Rothwell NJ, Stock MJ. Luxuskonsumption, diet-induced thermogenesis and brown fat: the case in favour. Clin Sci 1983; 64:19–23.

591. Shetty PS, Jung RT, James WPT. Effect of catecholamine replacement with levodopa on the metabolic response to semistarvation. Lancet 1979; 1:77–79.

592. Jung RT, Shetty PS, James WPT. The effect of beta-adrenergic blockade on metabolic rate and peripheral thyroid metabolism in obesity. Eur J Clin Invest 1980; 10:179–182.

593. Acheson K, Jequier E, Wahren J. Influence of beta-adrenergic blockade on glucose-induced thermogenesis in man. J Clin Invest 1983; 72:981–986.

594. Acheson KJ, Ravussin E, Wahren J, et al. Thermic effect of glucose in man. J Clin Invest 1984; 74:1572–1580.

595. Aulick LH, Wilmore DW. Hypermetabolism in trauma. In: Girardier L, Stock MJ, eds. Mammalian Thermogenesis. London: Chapman & Hall, 1983: 259–304.

596. Dascombe MJ, Rothwell NJ, Sagay BO, et al. Pyrogenic and thermogenic effects of interleukin 1-beta in the rat. Am J Physiol 1989; 256:E7–E11.

597. Rall TW, Sutherland EW. Adenyl cyclase. II. The enzymatically catalyzed formation of adenosine 3′,5′-phosphate and inorganic pyrophosphate from adenosine triphosphate. J Biol Chem 1962; 237:1228–1232.

598. Exton JH. Mechanisms involved in alpha-adrenergic phenomena: role of calcium ions in actions of catecholamines in liver and other tissues. Am J Physiol 1980; 238:E3–E12.

599. Kneer NM, Bosch AL, Clark MG, et al. Glucose inhibition of epinephrine stimulation of hepatic gluconeogenesis by blockade of the alpha-receptor function. Proc Natl Acad Sci USA 1974; 71:4523–4527.

600. Hutson NJ, Brumley FT, Assimacopoulos FD, et al. Studies on the alpha-adrenergic activation of hepatic glucose output. J Biol Chem 1976; 251:5200–5208.

601. Cherrington AD, Assimacopoulos FD, Harper SC, et al. Studies on the alpha-adrenergic activation of hepatic glucose output. J Biol Chem 1976; 251:5209–5218.

602. Exton JH, Park CR. Control of gluconeogenesis in liver. J Biol Chem 1968; 243:4189–4196.

603. Le Cam A, Freychet P. Effect of catecholamines on amino acid transport in isolated rat hepatocytes. Endocrinology 1978; 102:379–385.

604. Chan TM, Blackmore PF, Steiner KE, et al. Effects of adrenalectomy on hormone action on hepatic glucose metabolism. J Biol Chem 1979; 254:2428–2433.

605. Exton JH, Miller TB Jr, Harper SC, et al. Carbohydrate metabolism in perfused livers of adrenalectomized and steroid-replaced rats. Am J Physiol 1976; 230:163–170.

606. Aggerbeck M, Ferry N, Zafrani E-S, et al. Adrenergic regulation of glycogenolysis in rat liver after cholestasis. J Clin Invest 1983; 71:476–486.

607. Liu M-S, Ghosh S. Changes in beta-adrenergic receptors in dog livers during endotoxic shock. Am J Physiol 1983; 244:R718–R723.

608. Studer RK, Borle AB. Differences between male and female rats in the regulation of hepatic glycogenolysis. J Biol Chem 1982; 257:7987–7993.

609. Rosen SG, Clutter WE, Shah SD, et al. Direct alpha-adrenergic stimulation of hepatic glucose production in human subjects. Am J Physiol 1983; 245:E616–E626.

610. Bahnsen M, Burrin JM, Johnston DG, et al. Mechanisms of catecholamine effects on ketogenesis. Am J Physiol 1984; 247:E173–E180.

611. Beylot M, Beaufrere B, Riou JP, et al. Effect of epinephrine on the relationship between nonesterified fatty acid availability and ketone body production in postabsorptive man: evidence for a hepatic antiketogenic effect of epinephrine. J Clin Endocrinol Metab 1987; 65:914–921.

612. Hirsch LJ, Ayabe T, Glick H. Direct effects of various catecholamines on liver circulation in dogs. Am J Physiol 1976; 230:1394–1399.

613. Richardson PDI, Withrington PG. The inhibition by glucagon of the vasoconstrictor actions of noradrenaline, angiotensin and vasopressin on the hepatic arterial vascular bed of the dog. Br J Pharmacol 1976; 57:93–102.

614. Richardson PDI, Withrington PG. Glucagon inhibition of hepatic arterial responses to hepatic nerve stimulation. Am J Physiol 1977; 233:H647–H654.

615. Fuller RW, Felten SY, Perry KW, et al. Sympathetic noradrenergic innervation of guinea-pig liver; histofluorescence and pharmacological studies. J Pharmacol Exp Ther 1981; 218:282–288.

616. Moghimzadeh E, Nobin A, Rosengren E. Fluorescence microscopical and chemical characterization of the adrenergic innervation in mammalian liver tissue. Cell Tissue Res 1983; 230:605–613.

617. Seydoux J, Brunsmann MJA, Jeanrenaud B, et al. Alpha-sympathetic control of glucose output of mouse liver perfused in situ. Am J Physiol 1979; 236:E323–E327.

618. Nobin A, Falck B, Ingemansson S, et al. Organization and function of the sympathetic innervation of human liver. Acta Physiol Scand 1977; Suppl 452:103–106.

619. Nobin A, Baumgarten HG, Falck B, et al. Organization of the sympathetic innervation in liver tissue from monkey and man. Cell Tissue Res 1978; 195:371–380.

620. Jarhult J, Anderson P-O, Holst J, et al. On the sympathetic innervation to the cat's liver and its role for hepatic glucose release. Acta Physiol Scand 1980; 110:5–11.

621. Sokal JE, Sarcione EJ, Henderson AM. Relative potency of glucagon and epinephrine as hepatic glycogenolytic agents: studies with the isolated perfused rat liver. Endocrinology 1964; 74:930–938.

622. Cherrington AD, Stevenson RW, Steiner KE. Effect of epinephrine on glycogenolysis and gluconeogenesis in conscious overnight-fasted dogs. Am J Physiol 1984; 247:E137–E144.

623. Fain JN, Garcia-Sainz JA. Adrenergic regulation of adipocyte metabolism. J Lipid Res 1983; 24:945–966.

624. Belfrage P, Fredrikson G, Olsson H, et al. Control of adipose tissue lipolysis by phosphorylation/dephosphorylation of hormone-sensitive lipase. In: Angel A, Holleberg CH, Ronicari DAK, eds. The Adipocyte and Obesity: Cellular and Molecular Mechanisms. New York: Raven, 1983: 217–224.

625. Jensen MD, Haymond MW, Gerich JE, et al. Lipolysis during fasting: decreased suppression by insulin and increased stimulation by epinephrine. J Clin Invest 1987; 79:207–213.

626. Arner P, Engfeldt P. Fasting-mediated alteration studies in insulin action on lipolysis and lipogenesis in obese women. Am J Physiol 1987; 253:E193–E201.

627. Marcus C, Karpe B, Bolme P, et al. Changes in catecholamine-induced lipolysis in isolated human fat cells during the first year of life. J Clin Invest 1987; 79:1812–1818.

628. Leibel RL, Hirsch J. Site- and sex-related differences in adrenoreceptor status of human adipose tissue. J Clin Endocrinol Metab 1987; 64:1205–1210.

629. Ostman J, Arner P, Engfeldt P, et al. Regional differences in the control of lipolysis in human adipose tissue. Metabolism 1979; 28:1198–1205.

630. Kather H, Zollig K, Simon B, et al. Human fat cell adenylate cyclase: regional differences in adrenaline responsiveness. Eur J Clin Invest 1977; 7:595–597.

631. Luzio JP, Jones RC, Siddle K, et al. Dissociation of the effect of adrenalin on glucose uptake from that on adenosine cyclic 3′,5′-monophosphate levels and on lipolysis in rat-isolated fat cells. Biochim Biophys Acta 1974; 362:29–36.

632. Ludvigsen C, Jarett L, McDonald JM. The characterization of catecholamine stimulation of glucose transport by rat adipocytes and isolated plasma membranes. Endocrinology 1980; 106:786–790.

633. Péjoan C, Desbals B. Contrôle hormonal de l'activité adénylate cyclase de membranes de cellules adipeuses préparées à partir du tissu adipeux de blaireau, lapin, renard et rat. J Physiol (Paris) 1976; 72:345–358.

634. Aronovsky E, Levari R, Kornglueth W, et al. Comparison of metabolic activities of orbital fat with those of other adipose tissues. Invest Ophthalmol 1963; 2:259–264.

635. Pessin JE, Gitomer W, Oka Y, et al. Beta-adrenergic regulation of insulin and epidermal growth factor receptors in rat adipocytes. J Biol Chem 1983; 258:7386–7394.

636. Burns TW, Langley PE, Terry BE, et al. The role of free fatty acids in the regulation of lipolysis by human adipose tissue cells. Metabolism 1978; 27:1755–1762.

637. Baum D. The inhibition of norepinephrine-stimulated lipolysis by acute hypoxia. J Pharmacol Exp Ther 1969; 169:87–94.

638. Hjemdahl P, Fredholm BB. Comparison of the lipolytic activity of circulating and locally released noradrenaline during acidosis. Acta Physiol Scand 1974; 92:1–11.

639. Hjemdahl P, Sollevi A. Vascular and metabolic responses to adrenergic stimulation in isolated canine subcutaneous adipose tissue at normal and reduced temperature. J Physiol (Lond) 1978; 281:325–338.

640. Fredholm BB. Studies on the sympathetic regulation of circulation and metabolism in isolated canine subcutaneous adipose tissue. Acta Physiol Scand 1970; Suppl 354:5–37.

641. Galster AD, Clutter WE, Cryer PE, et al. Epinephrine plasma thresholds for lipolytic effects in man: measurements of fatty acid transport with [1-^{13}C] palmitic acid. J Clin Invest 1981; 67:1729–1738.

642. Rosell S, Belfrage E. Blood circulation in adipose tissue. Physiol Rev 1979; 59:1078–1104.

643. Cottle MKW, Cottle WH. Adrenergic fibers in brown fat of cold-acclimated rats. J Histochem Cytochem 1970; 18:116–119.

644. Dietz MR, Chiasson J-L, Soderling TR, et al. Epinephrine regulation of skeletal muscle glycogen metabolism. Studies utilizing the perfused rat hindlimb preparation. J Biol Chem 1980; 255:2301–2307.

645. Stankiewicz-Choroszucha B, Gorski J. Effect of beta-adrenergic blockade on intramuscular triglyceride mobilization during exercise. Experientia 1978; 34:357–358.

646. Shikama H, Chiasson J-L, Exton JH. Studies on the interactions between insulin and epinephrine in the control of skeletal muscle glycogen metabolism. J Biol Chem 1981; 256:4450–4454.

647. Foulkes JG, Cohen P, Strada SJ. Antagonistic effects of insulin and beta-adrenergic agonists on the activity of protein phosphatase inhibitor-1 in skeletal muscle of the perfused rat hemicorpus. J Biol Chem 1982; 257:12493–12496.

648. Green GA, Chenoweth M, Dunn A. Adrenal glucocorticoid permissive regulation of muscle glycogenolysis: action on protein phosphatase(s) and its inhibitors(s). Proc Natl Acad Sci USA 1980; 77:5711–5715.

649. Buse MG, Biggers JF, Drier C, et al. The effect of epinephrine, glucagon, and the nutritional state on the oxidation of branched chain amino acids and pyruvate by isolated hearts and diaphragms of the rat. J Biol Chem 1973; 248:697–706.

650. Kallfelt BJ, Hjalmarson AC, Ksaksson OG. In vitro effects of catecholamines on protein synthesis in perfused rat heart. J Mol Cell Biol 1976; 8:787–802.

651. O'Hara DS, Curfman GD, Trumbull CG, et al. The relation between reduced protein degradation and elevated adenosine 3'5'-monophosphate in isolated rat atria. Circ Res 1981; 49:609–617.

652. Li JB, Jefferson LS. Effect of isoproterenol on amino acid levels and protein turnover in skeletal muscle. Am J Physiol 1977; 232:E243–E249.

653. Goldberg AL, Chang TW. Regulation and significance of amino acid metabolism in skeletal muscle. Fed Proc 1978; 37:2301–2307.

654. Lowenstein JM, Goodman MN. The purine nucleotide cycle in skeletal muscle. Fed Proc 1978; 37:2308–2312.

655. Garber AJ, Karl IE, Kipnis DM. Alanine and glutamine synthesis and release from skeletal muscle. J Biol Chem 1976; 251:851–857.

656. Smith OLK, Huszar G, Davidson SB, et al. Effects of acute cold exposure on muscle amino acid and protein in rats. J Appl Physiol 1982; 52:1250–1256.

657. Rizza R, Haymond M, Cryer P, et al. Differential effects of epinephrine on glucose production and disposal in man. Am J Physiol 1979; 237:E356–E362.

658. Deibert DC, DeFronzo RA. Epinephrine-induced insulin resistance in man. J Clin Invest 1980; 65:717–721.

659. Bessey PQ, Brooks DC, Black PR, et al. Epinephrine acutely mediates skeletal muscle insulin resistance. Surgery 1983; 94:172–179.

660. Abramson EA, Arky RA. Role of beta-adrenergic receptors in counter-regulation to insulin-induced hypoglycemia. Diabetes 1968; 17:141–146.

661. Chiasson J-L, Shikama H, Chu DTW, et al. Inhibitory effect of epinephrine on insulin-stimulated glucose uptake by rat skeletal muscle. J Clin Invest 1981; 68:706–713.

662. Saitoh Y, Itaya K, Ui M. Adrenergic alpha-receptor–mediated stimulation of the glucose utilization by isolated rat diaphragm. Biochim Biophys Acta 1974; 343:492–499.

663. Bihler I, Sawh PC. Effect of adrenaline on sugar transport in the perifused left atrium. Can J Physiol Pharmacol 1976; 54:714–718.

664. Tomita T. Action of catecholamines on skeletal muscle. In: Greep RO, Astwood EB, eds. Handbook of Physiology. Sect 7: Endocrinology. Vol VI. Washington, DC: American Physiological Society, 1975: 537–552.

665. Nesher R, Karl IE, Kipnis DM. Epitrochlearis muscle. II. Metabolic effects of contraction and catecholamines. Am J Physiol 1980; 239:E461–E467.

666. Richter EA, Ruderman NB, Gavras H, et al. Muscle glycogenolysis during exercise: dual control by epinephrine and contractions. Am J Physiol 1982; 242:E25–E32.

667. Duran WN, Renkin EM. Influence of sympathetic nerves on oxygen uptake of resting mammalian skeletal muscle. Am J Physiol 1976; 231:529–537.

668. Nellis SH, Flaim SF, McCauley KM, et al. Alpha-stimulation protects exercise increment in skeletal muscle oxygen consumption. Am J Physiol 1980; 238:H331–H339.

669. van Hardeveld C, Kassenaar AAH. Muscle metabolism in the presence of an active and inactive nervous system. Horm Metab Res 1977; 9:136–140.

670. Masoro EJ, Rowell LB, McDonald RM, et al. Skeletal muscle lipids. II. Nonutilization of intracellular lipid esters as an energy source for contractile activity. J Biol Chem 1966; 241:2626–2634.

671. Richter EA, Galbo H, Christensen NJ. Control of exercise-induced muscular glycogenolysis by adrenal medullary hormones in rats. J Appl Physiol 1981; 50:21–26.

672. Gorski J. Exercise-induced changes of reactivity of different types of muscle on glycogenolytic effect of adrenaline. Pflugers Arch 1978; 373:1–7.

673. Kusaka M, Ui M. Activation of the Cori cycle by epinephrine. Am J Physiol 1977; 232:E145–E155.

674. Forichon J, Jomain MJ, Schellhorn J, et al. Effect of epinephrine upon irreversible disposal and recycling of glucose in dogs. Experientia 1977; 33:1171–1173.

675. Newsholme EA. A possible metabolic basis for the control of body weight. N Engl J Med 1980; 302:400–405.

676. Shafrir E, Susman KE, Steinberg D. The nature of the epinephrine-induced hyperlipidemia in dogs and its modification by glucose. J Lipid Res 1959; 1:109–117.

677. Kunihara M, Oshima T. Effects of epinephrine on plasma cholesterol levels in rats. J Lipid Res 1983; 24:639–644.

678. Dimsdale JE, Herd JA, Hartley LH. Epinephrine mediated increases in plasma cholesterol. Psychosom Med 1983; 45:227–232.

679. Edwards PA. The influence of catecholamines and cyclic AMP on 3-hydroxy-3-methylglutaryl coenzyme A reductase activity and lipid biosynthesis in isolated rat hepatocytes. Arch Biochem Biophys 1975; 170:188–203.

680. Edwards P, Lemongello D, Fogelman AM. The effect of glucagon, norepinephrine, and dibutyryl cyclic AMP on cholesterol efflux and on the activity of 3-hydroxy-3-methylglutaryl CoA reductase in rat hepatocytes. J Lipid Res 1979; 20:2–7.

681. George R, Ramasarma T. Nature of the stimulation of biogenesis of cholesterol in the liver by noradrenaline. Biochem J 1977; 162:493–499.

682. Smith U. Adrenergic control of lipid metabolism. Acta Med Scand 1983; Suppl 672:41–47.

683. Dall'Aglio E, Chang H, Reaven G. Disparate effects of prazosin and propranolol on lipid metabolism in a rat model. Metabolism 1983; 32:510–513.

684. O'Donnell L, Owens D, McGee C, et al. Effects of catecholamines on serum lipoproteins of normally fed and cholesterol-fed rabbits. Metabolism 1988; 37:910–915.

685. Chait A, Brunzell JD, Johnson DG, et al. Reduction of plasma triglyceride concentration by acute stress in man. Metabolism 1979; 28:553–561.

686. Miller HI. Plasma free fatty acid appearance in plasma triglycerides. Metabolism 1967; 16:1096–1105.

687. Radomski MW, Orme T. Response of lipoprotein lipase in various tissues to cold exposure. Am J Physiol 1971; 220:1852–1856.

688. Ashby P, Robinson DS. Effects of insulin, glucocorticoids and adrenaline on the activity of rat adipose-tissue lipoprotein lipase. Biochem J 1980; 188:185–192.

689. Lithell H, Cedermark M, Froberg J, et al. Increase of lipoprotein-lipase activity in skeletal muscle during heavy exercise. Relation to epinephrine excretion. Metabolism 1981; 30:1130–1134.

690. Tsai BS, Lefkowitz RJ. Agonist-specific effects of monovalent and divalent cations on adenylate cyclase–coupled alpha adrenergic receptors in rabbit platelets. Mol Pharmacol 1978; 14:540–548.

691. Fisher DA. Norepinephrine inhibition of vasopressin antidiuresis. J Clin Invest 1968; 47:540–547.

692. Schrier RW, Lieberman R, Ufferman RC, et al. Mechanism of antidiuretic effect of beta adrenergic stimulation. J Clin Invest 1972; 51:97–111.

693. Schrier RW, Berl T. Mechanism of effect of alpha adrenergic stimulation with norepinephrine on renal water excretion. J Clin Invest 1973; 52:502–511.

694. Levi J, Coburn J, Kleeman CR. Mechanism of the antidiuretic effect of beta-adrenergic stimulation in man. Arch Intern Med 1976; 136:25–29.

695. Shimamoto K, Miyahara M. Effect of norepinephrine infusion on plasma vasopressin levels in normal human subjects. J Clin Endocrinol Metab 1976; 43:201–204.

696. Berl T, Cadnapaphornchai P, Harbottle JA, et al. Mechanism of suppression of vasopressin during alpha-adrenergic stimulation with norepinephrine. J Clin Invest 1974; 53:219–227.

697. Berl T, Cadnapaphornchai P, Harbottle JA, et al. Mechanism of stimulation of vasopressin release during beta-adrenergic stimulation with isoproterenol. J Clin Invest 1974; 53:857–867.

698. Berl T, Harbottle JA, Schrier RW. Effect of alpha- and beta-adrenergic stimulation on renal water excretion in man. Kidney Int 1974; 6:247–253.

699. McDonald KM, Kuruvila KC, Aisenbrey GA, et al. Effect of alpha and beta adrenergic stimulation on renal water excretion and medullary tissue cyclic AMP in intact and diabetes insipidus rats. Kidney Int 1977; 12:96–103.

700. Ramsay DJ, Reid IA, Keil LC, et al. Evidence that the effects of

isoproterenol on water intake and vasopressin secretion are mediated by angiotensin. Endocrinology 1978; 103:54–59.

701. Rayson BM, Ray C, Morgan T. A study of the interaction of catecholamines and antidiuretic hormone on water permeability and the cyclic AMP system in isolated papillae of the rat. Pflugers Arch 1978; 373:99–103.

702. Krothapalli RK, Duffy WB, Senekjian HO, et al. Modulation of the hydro-osmotic effect of vasopressin on the rabbit cortical collecting tubule by adrenergic agents. J Clin Invest 1983; 72:287–294.

703. Berns AS, Anderson RJ, McDonald KM, et al. Effect of hypercapnic acidosis on renal water excretion in the dog. Kidney Int 1979; 15:116–125.

704. Abrahamsen AM, Storstein L, Westlie L, et al. Effect of dopamine on hemodynamics and renal function. Acta Med Scand 1974; 195:365–373.

705. Banasiak MF, Marshall WP, Kalkhoff RK. L-Dopa effects on renal function in obese subjects. N Engl J Med 1977; 296:1122.

706. Cadnapaphornchai P, Taher SM, McDonald FD. Mechanism of dopamine-induced diuresis in the dog. Am J Physiol 1977; 232:F524–F528.

707. Barajas L. Innervation of the renal cortex. Fed Proc 1978; 37:1192–1201.

708. Fink GD, Brody MJ. Continuous measurement of renal blood flow changes to renal nerve stimulation and intra-arterial drug administration in the rat. Am J Physiol 1978; 234:H219–H222.

709. Pomeranz BH, Birtch AG, Barger AC. Neural control of intrarenal blood flow. Am J Physiol 1968; 215:1067–1081.

710. Gotshall RW, Itskovitz HD. Redistribution of renal cortical blood flow by renal nerve stimulation and norepinephrine infusion. Proc Soc Exp Biol Med 1977; 154:60–63.

711. Breckenridge A, Orme M, Dollery CT. The effect of dopamine on renal blood flow in man. Eur J Clin Pharmacol 1971; 3:131–136.

712. Gottschalk CW. Renal nerves and sodium excretion. Annu Rev Physiol 1979; 41:229–240.

713. DiBona GF. Neural regulation of renal tubular sodium reabsorption and renin secretion. Fed Proc 1985; 44:2816–2822.

714. Bello-Reuss E, Colindres RE, Pastoriza-Munoz E, et al. Effects of acute unilateral renal denervation in the rat. J Clin Invest 1975; 56:208–217.

715. Bello-Reuss E, Pastoriza-Munoz E, Colindres RE. Acute unilateral renal denervation in rats with extracellular volume expansion. Am J Physiol 1977; 232:F26–F32.

716. Prosnitz EH, DiBona GF. Effect of decreased renal sympathetic nerve activity on renal tubular sodium reabsorption. Am J Physiol 1978; 235:F557–F563.

717. DiBona GF, Rios LL. Renal nerves in compensatory renal response to contralateral renal denervation. Am J Physiol 1980; 238:F26–F30.

718. Bello-Reuss E, Trevino DL, Gottschalk CW. Effect of renal sympathetic nerve stimulation on proximal water and sodium reabsorption. J Clin Invest 1976; 57:1104–1107.

719. DiBona GF, Sawin LL. Effect of renal nerve stimulation on NaCl and H₂O transport in Henle's loop of the rat. Am J Physiol 1982; 243:F576–F580.

720. Bello-Reuss E. Effect of catecholamines on fluid reabsorption by the isolated proximal convoluted tubule. Am J Physiol 1980; 238:F347–F352.

721. Chan YL. The role of norepinephrine in the regulation of fluid absorption in the rat proximal tubule. J Pharmacol Exp Ther 1980; 215:65–70.

722. Bello-Reuss E, Higashi Y, Kaneda Y. Dopamine decreases fluid reabsorption in straight portions of rabbit proximal tubule. Am J Physiol 1982; 242:F634–F640.

723. DiBona GF, Zambraski EJ, Aguilera AJ, et al. Neurogenic control of renal tubular sodium reabsorption in the dog. Circ Res 1977; 40(Suppl I):I127–I130.

724. Beserab A, Silva P, Landsberg L, et al. Effect of catecholamines on tubular function in the isolated perfused kidney. Am J Physiol 1977; 233:F39–F45.

725. Carey RM, Van Loon GR, Baines AD, et al. Decreased plasma and urinary dopamine during dietary sodium depletion in man. J Clin Endocrinol Metab 1981; 52:903–909.

726. Romoff MS, Keusch G, Campese VM, et al. Effect of sodium intake on plasma catecholamines in normal subjects. J Clin Endocrinol Metab 1979; 48:26–31.

727. Stene M, Panagiotis N, Tuck ML, et al. Plasma norepinephrine levels are influenced by sodium intake, glucocorticoid administration, and circadian changes in normal man. J Clin Endocrinol Metab 1980; 51:1340–1345.

728. Lilavivathana U, Campbell RG. The influence of sodium restriction on orthostatic sympathetic nervous activity. Arch Intern Med 1980; 140:1485–1489.

729. Hollenberg NK, Epstein M, Guttmann RD, et al. Effect of sodium balance on intrarenal distribution of blood flow in normal man. J Appl Physiol 1970; 28:312–317.

730. Gill JR, Bartter FC. Adrenergic nervous system in sodium metabolism. N Engl J Med 1966; 275:1466–1471.

731. Wilcox CS, Aminoff MJ, Slater JDH. Sodium homeostasis in patients with autonomic failure. Clin Sci Mol Med 1977; 53:321–328.

732. Schrier RW. Effects of adrenergic nervous system and catecholamines on systemic and renal hemodynamics, sodium and water excretion and renin secretion. Kidney Int 1974; 6:291–306.

733. Todd EP, Vick RL. Kalemotropic effect of epinephrine: analysis with adrenergic agonists and antagonists. Am J Physiol 1971; 220:1964–1969.

734. Vick RL, Todd EP, Luedke DW. Epinephrine-induced hypokalemia: relation to liver and skeletal muscle. J Pharmacol Exp Ther 1972; 181:139–146.

735. Brown MJ, Brown DC, Murphy MB. Hypokalemia from beta₂-receptor stimulation by circulating epinephrine. N Engl J Med 1983; 309:1414–1419.

736. Lockwood RH, Lum BKB. Effects of adrenergic agonists and antagonists on potassium metabolism. J Pharmacol Exp Ther 1974; 189:119–129.

737. Rosa RM, Silva P, Young JB, et al. Adrenergic modulation of extrarenal potassium disposal. N Engl J Med 1980; 302:431–434.

738. Pettit GW, Vick RL. An analysis of the contribution of the endocrine pancreas to the kalemotropic action of catecholamines. J Pharmacol Exp Ther 1974; 190:234–242.

739. DeFronzo RA, Bia M, Birkhead G. Epinephrine and potassium homeostasis. Kidney Int 1981; 20:83–91.

740. Sternheim W, Dalakos TG, Streeten DHP, et al. Action of L-epinephrine on the renin-aldosterone system and on urinary electrolyte excretion in man. Metabolism 1982; 31:979–984.

741. Clausen T. Adrenergic control of Na⁺-K⁺-homeostasis. Acta Med Scand 1983; Suppl 672:111–115.

742. Vassalle M, Greineder JK, Stuckey JH. Role of the sympathetic nervous system in the sinus node resistance to high potassium. Circ Res 1973; 32:348–355.

743. Hiatt N, Chapman LW, Davidson MB, et al. Adrenal hormones and the regulation of serum potassium in potassium-loaded adrenalectomized dogs. Endocrinology 1979; 105:215–219.

744. Lockwood RH, Lum BKB. Effects of adrenalectomy and adrenergic antagonists on potassium metabolism. J Pharmacol Exp Ther 1977; 203:103–111.

745. Silva P, Spokes K. Sympathetic system in potassium homeostasis. Am J Physiol 1981; 241:F151–F155.

746. Akaike N. Sodium pump in skeletal muscle: central nervous system–induced suppression by alpha-adrenoreceptors. Science 1981; 213:1252–1254.

747. Finlay GD, Whitsett TL, Cucinell EA, et al. Augmentation of sodium and potassium excretion, glomerular filtration rate and renal plasma flow by levodopa. N Engl J Med 1971; 284:865–870.

748. Granerus A-K, Jagenburg R, Svanborg A. Kaliuretic effect of L-dopa treatment in parkinsonian patients. Acta Med Scand 1977; 201:291–297.

749. Lundborg P. The effect of adrenergic blockade on potassium concentrations in different conditions. Acta Med Scand 1983; Suppl 672:121–125.

750. Yeung RTT, Tse TF. Thyrotoxic periodic paralysis. Am J Med 1974; 57:584–590.

751. Wang P, Clausen T. Treatment of attacks in hyperkalaemic familial periodic paralysis by inhalation of salbutamol. Lancet 1976; 1:221–223.

752. Gross TL, Sokol RJ. Severe hypokalemia and acidosis: a potential complication of beta-adrenergic treatment. Am J Obstet Gynecol 1980; 138:1225–1226.

753. Classen H-C, Marquardt P, Spath M, et al. Hypermagnesemia following exposure to acute stress. Pharmacology 1971; 5:287–294.

754. Persson J, Luthman J. The effects of insulin, glucose and catecholamines on some blood minerals in sheep. Acta Vet Scand 1974; 15:519–532.

755. Rayssiguier Y. Hypomagnesemia resulting from adrenaline infusion in ewes: its relation to lipolysis. Horm Metab Res 1977; 9:309–314.

756. Kenny AD. Effect of catecholamines on serum calcium and phosphorus levels in intact and parathyroidectomized rats. Naunyn-Schmiedebergs Arch Exp Pathol Pharmakol 1964; 248:144–152.

757. Hsu WH, Cooper CW. Hypercalcemic effect of catecholamines and its prevention by thyrocalcitonin. Calcif Tissue Res 1975; 19:125–137.

758. Fischer JA, Blum JW, Binswanger U. Acute parathyroid hormone response to epinephrine in vivo. J Clin Invest 1973; 52:2434–2440.

759. Vora NM, Williams GA, Hargis GK, et al. Comparative effect of calcium and of the adrenergic system on calcitonin secretion in man. J Clin Endocrinol Metab 1978; 46:567–571.

760. Bansal S, Woolf PD, Fischer JA, et al. Dopamine does not affect parathyroid function in man. J Clin Endocrinol Metab 1982; 54:651–652.

761. Body J-J, Cryer PE, Offord KP, et al. Epinephrine is a hypophosphatemic hormone in man. J Clin Invest 1983; 71:572–578.

762. Epstein S, Heath H III, Bell NH. Lack of influence of isoproterenol, propranolol, and dopamine on immunoreactive parathyroid hormone and calcitonin in normal man. Calcif Tissue Int 1983; 35:32–36.

763. Belz GG, Matthews JH, Longerich S, et al. Epinephrine infusion decreases magnesium plasma concentration in humans. J Cardiovasc Pharmacol 1985; 7:1205–1206.

764. Whyte KF, Addis GJ, Whitesmith R, et al. Adrenergic control of plasma magnesium in man. Clin Sci 1987; 72:135–138.

765. Swinton NW Jr, Clerkin EP, Flint LD. Hypercalcemia and familial pheochromocytoma: correction after adrenalectomy. Ann Intern Med 1972; 76:455–457.

766. Gray RS, Gillon J. Normotensive pheochromocytoma with hypercalcemia: correction after adrenalectomy. Br Med J 1976; 1:378.

767. De Plaen JF, Boemer F, De Strihou CVY. Hypercalcaemic phaeochromocytoma. Br Med J 1976; 2:734.

768. Finlayson JF, Casey JH. Hypercalcemia and multiple pheochromocytomas. Ann Intern Med 1975; 82:810–811.

769. Rude RK, Oldham SB, Singer FR, et al. Treatment of thyrotoxic hypercalcemia with propranolol. N Engl J Med 1976; 294:431–433.

770. Morey ER, Kenny AD. Effects of catecholamines on urinary calcium and phosphorus in intact and parathyroidectomized rats. Endocrinology 1964; 75:78–85.

771. Marone C, Beretta-Piccoli C, Weidmann P. Acute hypercalcemic hypertension in man: role of hemodynamics, catecholamines, and renin. Kidney Int 1980; 20:92–96.

772. Vollmer H. Die zweiphasische Wirkung des Adrenalins. Biochemische Zeitschrift 1923; 140:410–419.

773. Perlzweig WA, Latham E, Keefer CS. Inorganic phosphate in blood and urine. Proc Soc Exp Biol Med 1923; 21:33–34.

774. MacVicar R, Heller VG. Blood chloride and phosphorus content as affected by adrenalin injection. J Biol Chem 1941; 137:643–646.

775. Natelson S, Pincus JB, Rannazzisi G. Dynamic control of calcium, phosphate, citrate, and glucose levels in blood serum. Clin Chem 1963; 9:31–62.

776. Massara F, Camanni F. Propranolol block of adrenaline-induced hypophosphataemia in man. Clin Sci 1970; 38:245–250.

777. Cuche J-L, Marchand GR, Greger RF, et al. Phosphaturic effect of dopamine in dogs. J Clin Invest 1976; 58:71–76.

778. Szalay L, Bencsath P, Takacs L. Effect of splanchnicotomy on the renal excretion of inorganic phosphate in the anaesthetized dog. Pflugers Arch 1977; 367:283–286.

779. Kaneda Y, Bello-Reuss E. Effect of dopamine on phosphate reabsorption in isolated perfused rabbit proximal tubules. Miner Electrolyte Metab 1983; 9:147–150.

780. Loven L, Larsson L, Sjoberg H-E, et al. Effect of beta-blocking agents on preoperative changes in serum phosphate. Acta Chir Scand 1982; 148:339–344.

781. Ferris TF, Gorden P. Effect of angiotensin and norepinephrine upon urate clearance in man. Am J Med 1968; 44:359–365.

782. Sumi T, Umeda Y. Adrenal epinephrine in hyperuricemia induced by hypothalamic stimulation of the rat. Am J Physiol 1979; 236:E212–E215.

783. Yonetani Y, Ishii M, Ogawa Y. Stimulation by catecholamine of purine catabolism in rats and chickens. Jpn J Pharmacol 1979; 29:211–221.

784. Yonetani Y, Iwaki K. Catecholamine-induced hyperuricemia in eviscerated rats with functional hepatectomy. Jpn J Pharmacol 1981; 31:323–332.

785. Elmfeldt D, Berglund G, Wedel H, et al. Incidence and importance of metabolic side-effects during antihypertensive therapy. Acta Med Scand 1983; Suppl 672:79–83.

786. Pedersen OL, Mikkelsen E. Beta-blockers and uric-acid excretion. Lancet 1978; 2:1160.

787. Dosman JA, Crawhall JC, Klassen GA. Uric acid kinetic studies in the immediate post–myocardial-infarction period. Metabolism 1975; 24:473–480.

788. Young JB, Landsberg L. Adrenergic influence on peripheral hormone secretion. In: Kunos G, ed. Adrenoceptors and Catecholamine Action. Part B. New York: John Wiley & Sons, 1983: 157–217.

789. Tilders FJH, Berkenbosch F, Smelik PG. Adrenergic mechanisms involved in the control of pituitary-adrenal activity in the rat: a beta-adrenergic stimulatory mechanism. Endocrinology 1982; 110:114–120.

790. Young JB, Saville ME, Burgi U, et al. Sympathetic nervous system (SNS) activity in rat thyroid: evidence for a role in thyroid hypertrophy. Clin Res 1983; 31:280A.

791. Pisarev MA, Cardinali DP, Juvenal GJ, et al. Role of the sympathetic nervous system in the control of goitrogenic response in the rat. Endocrinology 1981; 109:2202–2207.

792. Pearse AGE. The APUD cell concept and its implications in pathology. Pathol Annu 1974; 9:27–42.

793. Pictet RL, Rall LB, Phelps P, et al. The neural crest and the origin of the insulin-producing and other gastrointestinal hormone-producing cells. Science 1976; 191:191–192.

794. Blair ML, Reid IA, Ganong WF. Effect of L-dopa on plasma renin activity with and without inhibition of extracerebral dopa decarboxylase in dogs. J Pharmacol Exp Ther 1977; 202:209–215.

795. Rayfield EJ, George DT, Eichner HL, et al. L-Dopa stimulation of glucagon secretion in man. N Engl J Med 1975; 293:589–591.

796. Blum JW, Schams D, Born W, et al. Effects of L-dopa on plasma levels of parathyroid hormone in calves. J Endocrinol Invest 1982; 5:311–313.

797. Ahrén B, Lundquist I. Effects of L-dopa-induced dopamine accumulation on $^{45}Ca^{2+}$ efflux and insulin secretion in isolated rat islets. Pharmacology 1985; 30:71–82.

798. Lebland H, Lachelin GCL, Abu-Fadil S, et al. The effect of dopamine infusion on insulin and glucagon secretion in man. J Clin Endocrinol Metab 1977; 44:196–198.

799. Brown EM, Carroll RJ, Aurbach GD. Dopaminergic stimulation of cyclic AMP accumulation and parathyroid hormone release from dispersed bovine parathyroid cells. Proc Natl Acad Sci USA 1977; 74:4210–4213.

800. Sowers JR, Stern N, Taylor IL. Evidence for dopaminergic modulation of pancreatic polypeptide secretion in man. Life Sci 1982; 31:2971–2975.

801. Barajas L, Muller J. The innervation of the juxtaglomerular apparatus and surrounding tubules: a quantitative analysis by serial section of electron microscopy. J Ultrastruct Res 1973; 43:107–132.

802. Wagermark J, Ungerstedt U, Ljungqvist A. Sympathetic innervation of the juxtaglomerular cells of the kidney. Circ Res 1968; 22:149–153.

803. Osborn JL, Thames MD, DiBona GF. Role of macula densa in renal nerve modulation of renin secretion. Am J Physiol 1982; 242:R367–R371.

804. Osborn JL, DiBona GF, Thames MD. Beta-1 receptor mediation of renin secretion elicited by low-frequency renal nerve stimulation. J Pharmacol Exp Ther 1981; 216:265–269.

805. Kopp UC, DiBona GF. Interaction between epinephrine and renal nerves in control of renin secretion rate. Am J Physiol 1986; 250:F999–F1007.

806. Nolly HL, Reid IA, Ganong WF. Effect of theophylline and adrenergic blocking drugs on the renin response to norepinephrine in vitro. Circ Res 1974; 35:575–579.

807. Johns EJ, Richards HK, Singer B. Effects of adrenaline, noradrenaline, isoprenaline and salbutamol on the production and release of renin by isolated renal cortical cells of the cat. Br J Pharmacol 1975; 53:67–73.

808. Katz SA, Malvin RL. Independence of beta-adrenergic stimulation of renin release on renin synthesis. Am J Physiol 1982; 243:F434–F439.

809. Blair ML. Stimulation of renin secretion by alpha-adrenoceptor agonists. Am J Physiol 1983; 7:E37–E44.

810. Vandongen R, Peart WS. The inhibition of renin secretion by alpha-adrenergic stimulation in the isolated rat kidney. Clin Sci Mol Med 1974; 47:471–479.

811. Meyer DK, Herrmann M. Inhibitory effect of tyramine-induced release of catecholamines on renin secretion. Arch Pharmacol 1978; 303:139–144.

812. Matsumura Y, Miyawaki N, Sasaki Y, et al. Inhibitory effects of norepinephrine, methoxamine and phenylephrine on renin release from rat kidney cortical slices. J Pharmacol Exp Ther 1985; 233:782–787.

813. Thames MD, DiBona GF. Renal nerves modulate the secretion of renin mediated by nonneural mechanisms. Circ Res 1979; 44:645–652.

814. Thames MD. Contribution of cardiopulmonary baroreceptors to the control of the kidney. Fed Proc 1978; 37:1209–1213.

815. Zehr JE, Hasbargen JA, Kurz KD. Reflex suppression of renin secretion during distention of cardiopulmonary receptors in dogs. Circ Res 1976; 38:232–239.

816. Thames MD, Jarecki M, Donald DE. Neural control of renin secretion in anesthetized dogs. Circ Res 1978; 42:237–245.

817. Leonetti G, Mayer G, Morganti A, et al. Hypotensive and renin-suppressing activities of propranolol in hypertensive patients. Clin Sci Mol Med 1975; 48:491–499.

818. Kiowski W, Julius S. Renin response to stimulation of cardiopulmonary mechanoreceptors in man. J Clin Invest 1978; 62:656–663.

819. Davies R, Slater JDH. Is the adrenergic control of renin release dominant in man? Lancet 1976; 2:594–596.

820. Stella A, Zanchetti A. Effects of renal denervation on renin release in response to tilting and furosemide. Am J Physiol 1977; 232:H500–H507.

821. Gordon RD, Kuchel O, Liddle GW, et al. Role of the sympathetic nervous system in regulating renin and aldosterone production in man. J Clin Invest 1967; 46:599–605.

822. Christlieb AR, Munichodoppa C, Braaten JT. Decreased response of plasma renin activity to orthostatic hypotension. Diabetes 1974; 23:835–840.

823. Rabinowitz D, Landau H, Rosler A, et al. Plasma renin activity and aldosterone in familial dysautonomia. Metabolism 1974; 23:1–5.

824. Tuck ML, Sambhi MP, Levin L. Hyporeninemic hypoaldosteronism in diabetes mellitus. Diabetes 1979; 28:237–241.

825. Bravo EL, Tarazi RC, Dustan HP. On the mechanism of suppressed plasma-renin activity during beta-adrenergic blockade with propranolol. J Lab Clin Med 1974; 83:119–128.

826. Sullivan JM, Adams DF, Hollenberg NK. Beta-adrenergic blockade in essential hypertension. Circ Res 1976; 39:532–536.

827. Yun JCH, Kelly G, Bartter FC. Suppression of renin secretion by propranolol in salt-depleted dogs. Life Sci 1977; 21:237–244.

828. Morganti A, Lopez-Ovejero JA, Pickering TG, et al. Role of the sympathetic nervous system in mediating the renin response to head-up tilt. Am J Cardiol 1979; 43:600–604.

829. Bravo EL, Tarazi RC, Dustan HP. Beta-adrenergic blockade in diuretic treated patients with essential hypertension. N Engl J Med 1975; 292:66–70.

830. Omvik P, Enger E, Eide I. Effect of sodium depletion on plasma renin concentration before and during adrenergic beta-receptor blockade with propranolol in normotensive man. Am J Med 1976; 61:608–614.

831. Sparks JC, Susic D. The effects of propranolol on plasma renin activity and renal renin concentration in rats on normal and sodium deficient diets. Pharmacol Res Commun 1977; 9:479–487.

832. Mogil RA, Itskovitz HD, Russell JH, et al. Renal innervation and renin activity in salt metabolism and hypertension. Am J Physiol 1969; 216:693–697.

833. Otsuka K, Assaykeen TA, Goldfien A, et al. Effect of hypoglycemia on plasma renin activity in dogs. Endocrinology 1970; 87:1306–1317.

834. Woods SC, Porte D Jr. Neural control of the endocrine pancreas. Physiol Rev 1974; 54:596–619.

835. Forssmann WG, Greenberg J. Innervation of the endocrine pancreas in primates. In: Coupland RE, Forssmann WG, eds. Peripheral Neuroendocrine Interaction. Berlin: Springer-Verlag, 1976: 124–133.

836. Wollheim CB, Sharp GWG. Stimulatory and inhibitory effects of epinephrine on islet Ca^{++} uptake and insulin release. Diabetologia 1978; 15:282.

837. Hiatt N, Davidson MB, Chapman LW, et al. Epinephrine enhancement of potassium-stimulated immunoreactive insulin secretion. Diabetes 1978; 27:550–553.

838. Okajima F, Ui M. Adrenergic modulation of insulin secretion in vivo dependent on thyroid states. Am J Physiol 1978; 234:E106–E111.

839. Ribes G, Blayac JP, Loubatieres-Mariani MM. Differences between the effects of adrenaline and noradrenaline on insulin secretion in the dog. Diabetologia 1983; 24:107–112.

840. Schuit FC, Pipeleers DG. Differences in adrenergic recognition by pancreatic A and B cells. Science 1986; 232:875–877.

841. Burr IM, Jackson A, Culbert S, et al. Glucose intolerance and impaired insulin release following 6-hydroxydopamine administration to intact rats. Endocrinology 1974; 94:1072–1076.

842. Lundquist I, Fanska R, Grodsky GM. Direct calcium-stimulated release of glucagon from the isolated perfused rat pancreas and the effect of chemical sympathectomy. Endocrinology 1976; 98:815–818.

843. Basabe JC, Farina JMS, Udrisar DP, et al. Effect of pancreatic adrenergic tone modifications prior to glucose-induced insulin secretion. Horm Metab Res 1977; 9:108–113.

844. Burr IM, Balant L, Stauffacher W, et al. Adrenergic modification of glucose-induced biphasic insulin release from perfused rat pancreas. Eur J Clin Invest 1971; 1:216–224.

845. Burr IM, Slonim AE, Burke V, et al. Extracellular calcium and adrenergic and cholinergic effects on islet beta-cell function. Am J Physiol 1976; 231:1246–1249.

846. Pipeleers DG, Schuit FC, Int Veld PA et al. Interplay of nutrients and hormones in the regulation of insulin release. Endocrinology 1985; 117:824–833.

847. Pipeleers DG, Schuit FC, Van Schravendijk CFH, et al. Interplay of nutrients and hormones in the regulation of glucagon release. Endocrinology 1985; 117:817–823.

848. Melander A, Sundler F, Westgren U. Intrathyroidal amines and the synthesis of thyroid hormone. Endocrinology 1973; 93:193–200.

849. Melander A, Sundler F, Westgren U. Sympathetic innervation of the thyroid: variation with species and with age. Endocrinology 1975; 96:102–106.

850. Melander A, Ljunggren JG, Norberg KA, et al. Sympathetic innervation and noradrenaline content of normal human thyroid tissue from fetal, young, and elderly subjects. J Endocrinol Invest 1978; 2:175–177.

851. Melander A, Ericson LE, Ljunggren J-B, et al. Sympathetic innervation of the normal human thyroid. J Clin Endocrinol Metab 1974; 39:713–718.

852. Tice LW, Creveling CR. Electronmicroscopic identification of adrenergic nerve endings on thyroid epithelial cells. Endocrinology 1974; 97:1123–1129.

853. Maayan ML, Ingbar SH. Epinephrine: effect on uptake of iodine by dispersed cells of calf thyroid gland. Science 1968; 162:124–125.

854. Maayan ML, Ingbar SH. Effects of epinephrine on iodine and intermediary metabolism in isolated thyroid cells. Endocrinology 1970: 87:588–595.

855. Maayan ML, Shapiro R, Ingbar SH. Epinephrine precursors: effects on the iodine and intermediary metabolism of isolated calf thyroid cells. Endocrinology 1973; 92:912–916.

856. Otten J, Dumont JE. Glucose metabolism in normal human thyroid tissue in vitro. Eur J Clin Invest 1972; 2:213–219.

857. Ahn CS, Rosenberg IN. Proteolysis in thyroid slices: effects of TSH, dibutyryl cyclic 3′5′-AMP and prostaglandin E_1. Endocrinology 1970; 86:870–873.

858. Maayan ML, Debons AF, Volpert EM, et al. Catecholamine inhibition

859. Maayan ML, Volpert EM, Debons AF. Neurotransmitter regulation of thyroid activity. Endocr Res 1987; 13:199–212.

860. Melander A, Nilsson E, Sundler F. Sympathetic activation of thyroid hormone secretion in mice. Endocrinology 1972; 90:194–199.

861. Melander A, Ericson LE, Sundler F, et al. Sympathetic innervation of the mouse thyroid and its significance in thyroid hormone secretion. Endocrinology 1974; 94:959–966.

862. Melander A, Ranklev E, Sundler F, et al. Beta₂-adrenergic stimulation of thyroid hormone secretion. Endocrinology 1975; 97:332–336.

863. Ericson LE, Melander A, Owman C, et al. Endocytosis of thyroglobulin and release of thyroid hormone in mice by catecholamines and 5-hydroxytryptamine. Endocrinology 1970; 87:915–923.

864. Heath H III. Biogenic amines and the secretion of parathyroid hormone and calcitonin. Endocr Rev 1980; 1:319–338.

865. Norberg KA, Persson B, Granberg P-O. Adrenergic innervation of the human parathyroid glands. Acta Chir Scand 1975; 141:319–322.

866. Williams GA, Hargis GK, Bowser EN, et al. Evidence for a role of adenosine 3′5′-monophosphate in parathyroid hormone release. Endocrinology 1973; 92:687–691.

867. Hanley DA, Takatsuki K, Birnbaumer ME, et al. In vitro perfusion for the study of parathyroid hormone secretion: effects of extracellular calcium concentration and beta-adrenergic regulation on bovine parathyroid hormone secretion. Calcif Tissue Int 1980; 32:19–27.

868. Brown EM, Hurwitz SH, Aurbach GD. Alpha-adrenergic inhibition of adenosine 3′5′-monophosphate accumulation and parathyroid hormone release from dispersed bovine parathyroid cells. Endocrinology 1978; 103:893–899.

869. Brown EM, Gardner DG, Windeck RA, et al. Beta-adrenergically stimulated adenosine 3′5′-monophosphate accumulation in and parathyroid hormone release from dispersed human parathyroid cells. J Clin Endocrinol Metab 1979; 48:618–626.

870. Kukreja SC, Ayala GA, Banerjee P, et al. Characterization of the beta-adrenergic receptor mediating secretion of parathyroid hormone. Horm Metab Res 1980; 12:334–338.

871. Avioli LV, Shieber W, Kipnis DM. Role of glucagon and adrenergic receptors in thyrocalcitonin release in the dog. Endocrinology 1971; 88:1337–1340.

872. Care AD, Bates RFL, Gitelman JH. A possible role for the adenyl cyclase system in calcitonin release. J Endocrinol 1970; 48:1–15.

873. Bell NH. Further studies on the regulation of calcitonin release in vitro. Horm Metab Res 1975; 7:77–83.

874. Brown EM. PTH secretion in vivo and in vitro: regulation by calcium and other secretions. Miner Electrolyte Metab 1982; 8:130–150.

875. Fitzpatrick LA, Brandi ML, Aurbach GD. Prostaglandin $F_{2\alpha}$ and alpha-adrenergic agonists regulate parathyroid cell function via the inhibitory guanine nucleotide regulatory protein. Endocrinology 1986; 118:2215–2219.

876. Kukreja SC, Hargis GK, Bowser EN, et al. Role of adrenergic stimuli in parathyroid hormone secretion in man. J Clin Endocrinol Metab 1975; 40:478–481.

877. Metz SA, Deftos LJ, Baylink DJ, et al. Neuroendocrine modulation of calcitonin and parathyroid hormone in man. J Clin Endocrinol Metab 1978; 47:151–159.

878. Kukreja SC, Johnson PA, Ayala G, et al. Role of calcium and beta-adrenergic system in control of parathyroid hormone secretion. Proc Soc Exp Biol Med 1976; 151:326–328.

879. Blum JW, Fischer JA, Hunziker WH, et al. Parathyroid hormone responses to catecholamines and to changes of extracellular calcium in cows. J Clin Invest 1978; 61:1113–1122.

880. Mayer GP, Hurst JG, Barto JA, et al. Effect of epinephrine on parathyroid hormone secretion in calves. Endocrinology 1979; 104: 1181–1187.

881. Ljunhgall S, Akerstrom G, Benson L, et al. Effects of epinephrine and norepinephrine on serum parathyroid hormone and calcium in normal subjects. Exp Clin Endocrinol 1984; 84:313–318.

882. Lennquist S, Lindell B, Nordstrom H, et al. Hypophosphatemia in severe burns. Acta Chir Scand 1979; 145:1–6.

883. McGrath BP, Ledingham JGG, Benedict CR. Catecholamines in peripheral venous plasma in patients on chronic haemodialysis. Clin Sci Mol Med 1978; 55:89–96.

884. Campese VM, Romoff MS, Levitan D, et al. Mechanisms of autonomic nervous system dysfunction in uremia. Kidney Int 1981; 20:246–253.

885. Coevoet B, Desplan C, Sebert JL, et al. Effect of propranolol and metoprolol on parathyroid hormone and calcitonin secretions in uraemic patients. Br Med J 1980; 1:1344–1346.

886. Phillippo M, Lawrence CB, Bruce JB, et al. Feeding and calcitonin secretion in sheep. J Endocrinol 1972; 53:419–424.

887. Talmage RV, Grubb SA, Norimatsu H, et al. Evidence for an important physiological role for calcitonin. Proc Natl Acad Sci USA 1980; 77:609–613.

888. Hollands BCS, Vanov S. Localization of catecholamines in visceral organs and ganglia of the rat, guinea-pig and rabbit. Br J Pharmacol 1965; 25:307–316.

of thyrotropin-induced secretion of thyroxine: mediation by an alpha-adrenergic receptor. Metabolism 1977; 26:473–475.

889. Jacobowitz D. Histochemical studies of the autonomic innervation of the gut. J Pharmacol Exp Ther 1965; 149:358–364.
890. Hayes JR, Ardill J, Kennedy TL, et al. Stimulation of gastrin release by catecholamines. Lancet 1972; 1:819–821.
891. Stadil F, Rehfeld JF. Release of gastrin by epinephrine in man. Gastroenterology 1973; 65:210–215.
892. Christensen KC, Stadil F. Effect of epinephrine and norepinephrine on gastrin release and gastric secretion of acid in man. Scand J Gastroenterol 1976; 37(Suppl):87–92.
893. DeSchryver-Kecskemeti K, Greider MH, Reiders ER, et al. In vitro gastrin secretion by rat antrum. Effects of neurotransmitter agonists, and modulators of secretion. Lab Invest 1981; 44:158–163.
894. Harty RF, Maico DG, McGuigan JE. Comparison of adrenergic and cholinergic receptor–mediated stimulation of gastrin release from rat antral fragments. Peptides 1988; 9:463–468.
895. Jarhult J, Uvnas-Wallensten K. Reflex adrenergic gastrin release evoked by unloading of carotid baroreceptors in cats. Scand J Gastroenterol 1979; 14:107–109.
896. Kronborg O. The effect of beta-adrenergic blockade upon basal and pentagastrin-stimulated gastric acid secretion and upon gastrin response to food. Scand J Gastroenterol 1975; 10:757–762.
897. Kaess H, Fanger H, Teckentrup U, et al. Serum gastrin concentration after sham feeding and feeding under the influence of propranolol in man. Digestion 1976; 14:364–367.
898. Brandsborg O, Brandsborg M, Christensen NJ. The role of the beta-adrenergic receptor in the secretion of gastrin: studies in normal subjects and in patients with duodenal ulcers. Eur J Clin Invest 1976; 6:395–401.
899. Seino S, Seino Y, Taminato T, et al. Effect of adrenergic blocking agents on plasma gastrin and secretin levels in man. Am J Gastroenterol 1980; 73:137–140.
900. Kaess H, Kuntzen O, Teckentrupp U, et al. The influence of propranolol on serum gastrin concentration and hydrochloric acid secretion in response to hypoglycemia in normal subjects. Digestion 1975; 13:193–200.
901. Christensen KC, Stadil F. On the beta-adrenergic contribution to the gastric acid and gastrin responses to hypoglycaemia in man. Scand J Gastroenterol 1976; 37(Suppl):81–86.
902. Kronborg O, Pedersen T, Stadil F, et al. The effect of beta-adrenergic blockade upon gastric acid secretion during hypoglycaemia before and after vagotomy. Scand J Gastroenterol 1974; 8:173–176.
903. Hall WH, Durkin MG, Read RC. Propranolol and serum gastrin in postvagotomy insulin tests. Digestion 1973; 9:325–331.
904. Kaess H, Utz G, Teckentrup U, et al. The effect of propranolol and phentolamine on serum gastrin concentration in response to respiratory acidosis in normal man. Eur J Clin Invest 1975; 5:401–408.
905. Orton CI, Segal AW, Bloom SR, et al. Hypersecretion of glucagon and gastrin in severely burnt patients. Br Med J 1975; 2:170–172.
906. Brandsborg O, Christensen NJ, Galbo H, et al. The effect of exercise, smoking and propranolol on serum gastrin in patients with duodenal ulcer and in vagotomized subjects. Scand J Clin Lab Invest 1978; 38:441–446.
907. Stadil F, Rehfeld JF. Effect of insulin injection on serum gastrin concentrations in duodenal ulcer patients and normal subjects. Scand J Gastroenterol 1974; 9:143–147.
908. Seino Y, Miyamoto Y, Moridera K, et al. The role of the beta-adrenergic mechanism in the hypergastrinemia of hyperthyroidism. J Clin Endocrinol Metab 1980; 50:368–370.
909. Bahr J, Kao L, Nalbandov AV. The role of catecholamines and nerves in ovulation. Biol Reprod 1974; 10:273–290.
910. Mohsin S, Pennefather JN. The sympathetic innervation of the mammalian ovary. Clin Exp Pharmacol Physiol 1979; 6:335–354.
911. Fylling P. Propranolol blockade of vasopressin induced increase in plasma progesterone in early human pregnancy. Acta Endocrinol 1971; 66:283–288.
912. Condon WA, Black DL. Catecholamine-induced stimulation of progesterone by the bovine corpus luteum in vitro. Biol Reprod 1976; 15:573–578.
913. Godkin JD, Black KL, Duby RT. Stimulation of cyclic AMP and progesterone synthesis by LH, PGE$_2$ and isoproterenol in the bovine CL in vitro. Biol Reprod 1977; 17:514–518.
914. Jordan AW III, Caffrey JL, Niswender GD. Catecholamine-induced stimulation of progesterone and adenosine 3′5′-monophosphate production by dispersed ovine luteal cells. Endocrinology 1978; 103:385–392.
915. Ratner A, Weiss GK, Sanborn CR. Stimulation by beta-2-adrenergic receptors of the production of cyclic AMP and progesterone in rat ovarian tissue. J Endocrinol 1980; 87:123–129.
916. Weiss GK, Dail WG, Ratner A. Evidence for direct neural control of ovarian steroidogenesis in rats. J Reprod Fertil 1982; 65:507–511.
917. Ratner A, Weiss GK, Sanborn CR. Alpha adrenergic mediated inhibition of progesterone and cyclic AMP production in rat ovarian tissue. Proc West Pharmacol Soc 1983; 26:25–29.
918. Ratner A, Sanborn CR, Weiss GK. Beta-adrenergic stimulation of cAMP and progesterone in rat ovarian tissue. Am J Physiol 1980; 239:E139–E143.

919. Harwood JP, Richert ND, Dufau ML, et al. Gonadotropin-induced desensitization of epinephrine action in the luteinized rat ovary. Endocrinology 1980; 107:280–288.
920. Hunziker-Dunn M. Epinephrine-sensitive adenylyl cyclase activity in rabbit ovarian tissues. Endocrinology 1982; 110:233–240.
921. Rani CSS, Nordenstrom K, Norjavaara E, et al. Development of catecholamine responsiveness in granulosa cells from preovulatory rat follicles—dependence on preovulatory luteinizing hormone surge. Biol Reprod 1983; 28:1021–1031.
922. Flint APF, Anderson ABM, Turnbull AC. Control of utero-ovarian and peripheral venous plasma progesterone by beta-sympathomimetic drugs in pregnant sheep. J Endocrinol 1974; 63:253–254.
923. Caritis SN, Hirsch RP, Zeleznik AJ. Adrenergic stimulation of placental progesterone production. J Clin Endocrinol Metab 1983; 56:969–972.
924. Wolf R, Meier-Fleitmann A, Duker E-M, et al. Intraovarian secretion of catecholamines, oxytocin, beta-endorphin, and gamma-amino-butyric-acid in freely moving rats: development of a push-pull tubing method. Biol Reprod 1986; 35:599–607.
925. Cohen WR, Galen LH, Vega-Rich M, et al. Cardiac sympathetic activity during rat pregnancy. Metabolism 1988; 37:771–777.
926. Semenova II. Adrenergic innervation of the ovaries in Stein-Leventhal syndrome. Vestn Akad Med Nauk SSSR 1969; 24:58–62.
927. Bell C. Autonomic nervous control of reproduction: circulatory and other factors. Pharmacol Rev 1972; 24:657–736.
928. Baumgarten HG, Falck B, Holstein A-F, et al. Adrenergic innervation of the human testis, epididymis, ductus deferens and prostate: a fluorescence microscopic and fluorimetric study. Z Zellforsch 1968; 90:81–95.
929. Cooke BA, Golding M, Dix CJ. Catecholamine stimulation of steroidogenesis in Leydig cells. Biochem Soc Trans 1982; 10:491–493.
930. Moger WH, Murphy PR. Beta-adrenergic agonist induced androgen production during primary culture of mouse Leydig cells. Arch Androl 1983; 10:135–142.
931. Pointis G, Latreille MT. Catecholamine-induced stimulation of testosterone production by Leydig cells from fetal mouse testis. J Reprod Fertil 1987; 80:321–326.
932. Renier G, Gaulin J, Gibb W, et al. Effect of catecholamines on porcine Sertoli and Leydig cells in primary culture. Can J Physiol Pharmacol 1987; 65:2053–2058.
933. Cooke BA, Golding M, Dix CJ, et al. Catecholamine stimulation of testosterone production via cyclic AMP in mouse Leydig cells in monolayer culture. Mol Cell Endcrinol 1982; 27:221–231.
934. Levin J, Lloyd CW, Lobotsky J, et al. The effect of epinephrine on testosterone production. Acta Endocrinol 1967; 55:184–192.
935. Damber J-E, Janson PO. The effects of LH, adrenaline and noradrenaline on testicular blood flow and plasma testosterone concentrations in anaesthetized rats. Acta Endocrinol 1978; 88:390–396.
936. Gotz F, Stahl F, Rohde W, et al. The influence of adrenaline on plasma testosterone in adult and newborn male rats. Exp Clin Endocrinol 1983; 81:239–244.
937. Eik-Nes KB. An effect of isoproterenol on rates of synthesis and secretion of testosterone. Am J Physiol 1969; 217:1764–1770.
938. Collu R, Gibb W, Ducharme JR. Role of catecholamines in the inhibitory effect of immobilization stress on testosterone secretion in rats. Biol Reprod 1984; 30:416–422.
939. Sapolsky RM. Stress-induced elevation of testosterone concentrations in high ranking baboons: role of catecholamines. Endocrinology 1986; 118: 1630–1635.
940. Woolf PD, Hamill RW, McDonald JV, et al. Transient hypogonadotropic hypogonadism after head trauma: effects on steroid precursors and correlation with sympathetic nervous system activity. Clin Endocrinol (Oxf) 1986; 25:265–274.
941. Fisher JW. Erythropoietin: pharmacology, biogenesis and control of production. Pharmacol Rev 1972; 24:459–508.
942. Rodgers GM, Fisher JW, George WJ. Renal cyclic AMP accumulation and adenylate cyclase stimulation by erythropoietic agents. Am J Physiol 1975; 229:1387–1392.
943. Fisher JW, Samuels AI, Langston J. Effects of angiotensin, norepinephrine and renal artery constriction on erythropoietin production. Ann NY Acad Sci 1968; 149:308–317.
944. Fink GD, Fisher JW. Stimulation of erythropoiesis by beta-adrenergic agonists. II. Mechanism of action. J Pharmacol Exp Ther 1977; 202:199–208.
945. Przala F, Gross DM, Beckman B, et al. Influence of albuterol on erythropoietin production and erythroid progenitor cell activation. Am J Physiol 1979; 263:H422–H426.
946. Takaku F, Hirashima K, Okinaka S. Studies on the mechanism of erythropoietin production: II. Effect of bilateral section of the splanchnic nerves. J Lab Clin Med 1962; 59:821–825.
947. Fink GD, Paulo LG, Fisher JW. Effects of beta adrenergic blocking agents on erythropoietin production in rabbits exposed to hypoxia. J Pharmacol Exp Ther 1975; 193:176–181.
948. Beynon G. The influence of the autonomic nervous system in the control of erythropoietin secretion in the hypoxic rat. J Physiol (Lond) 1977; 266:347–360.

949. Campbell DJ, Mendelsohn FAO, Adam WR, et al. Is aldosterone secretion under dopaminergic control? Circ Res 1981; 49:1217–1227.

950. Norbiato G, Bevilacqua M, Raggi U, et al. Metoclopramide increases plasma aldosterone concentration in man. J Clin Endocrinol Metab 1977; 45:1313–1316.

951. Noth RH, McCallum RW, Contino C, et al. Tonic dopaminergic suppression of plasma aldosterone. J Clin Endocrinol Metab 1980; 51:64–69.

952. Kojima I, Ogata E. Reversal by a dopamine antagonist of saline-induced attenuation of aldosterone response to angiotensin II infusion in man. Endocrinol Jpn 1982; 29:21–25.

953. Gordon MB, Moore TJ, Dluhy RG, et al. Dopaminergic modulation of aldosterone responsiveness to angiotensin II with changes in sodium intake. J Clin Endocrinol Metab 1983; 56:340–345.

954. Carey RM, Drake CR Jr. Dopamine selectively inhibits aldosterone responses to angiotensin II in humans. Hypertension 1986; 8:399–406.

955. Malchoff CD, Hughes JM, Carey RM. Effect of upright posture on the aldosterone responses to dopamine, metoclopramide, angiotensin II, and adrenocorticotropin. J Clin Endocrinol Metab 1987; 65:203–207.

956. Connell JMC, Tonolo G, Davies DL, et al. Dopamine affects angiotensin II–induced steroidogenesis by altering clearance of the peptide in man. J Endocrinol 1987; 113:139–146.

957. Zanella MT, Bravo EL. In vitro and in vivo evidence for an indirect mechanism mediating enhanced aldosterone secretion by metoclopramide. Endocrinology 1982; 111:1620–1625.

958. Braley LM, Menachery AI, Williams GH, et al. Specificity of metoclopramide in assessing the role of dopamine in regulating aldosterone secretion. Endocrinology 1983; 112:1352–1357.

959. McKenna JT, Island DP, Nicholson WE, Liddle GW. Dopamine inhibits angiotensin-stimulated aldosterone biosynthesis in bovine adrenal cells. J Clin Invest 1979; 64:287–291.

960. Sequeira SJ, McKenna TJ. Examination of the effects of epinephrine, norepinephrine, and dopamine on aldosterone response in bovine glomerulosa cells in vitro. Endocrinology 1985; 117:1947–1952.

961. Huan B-S, Malvin RL, Lee J, et al. Central dopaminergic regulation of alosterone secretion in sheep. Hypertension 1987; 10:157–163.

962. Lun S, Espiner EA, Nicholls MG, et al. Lack of direct effect of dopamine on aldosterone secretion in vivo. Endocrinology 1983; 112:60–63.

963. Sowers JR, Sharp B, McCallum RW. Effect of domperidone, an extracerebral inhibitor of dopamine receptors, on thyrotropin, prolactin, renin, aldosterone, and 18-hydroxycorticosterone secretion in man. J Clin Endocrinol Metab 1982; 54:869–871.

964. Wilson TA, Kaiser DL, Peach MJ, et al. Possible mechanism of action of metoclopramide-induced aldosterone secretion: in vivo and in vitro studies in the sheep. Endocrinology 1983; 113:887–892.

965. Cardinali DP. Melatonin. A mammalian pineal hormone. Endocr Rev 1981; 2:327–346.

966. Klein DC, Berg GR, Weller J. Melatonin synthesis: adenosine 3'5'-monophosphate and norepinephrine stimulate N-acetyltransferase. Science 1970; 168:979–980.

967. Sugden D, Klein DC. Beta-adrenergic receptor control of rat pineal hydroxyindole-O-methyltransfcrasc. Endocrinology 1983; 113:348–353.

968. Samols E, Weir GC. Adrenergic modulation of pancreatic A, B, and D cells. J Clin Invest 1979; 63:230–238.

969. Itoh M, Gerich JE. Adrenergic modulation of pancreatic somatostatin, insulin, and glucagon secretion: evidence for differential sensitivity of islet A, B, and D cells. Metabolism 1982; 31:715–720.

970. Holst JJ, Steen L, Knuhtsen JS, et al. Autonomic nervous control of pancreatic somatostatin secretion. Am J Physiol 1983; 245:E542–E548.

971. Berger D, Floyd JC Jr, Lampman RM, et al. The effect of adrenergic receptor blockade on the exercise-induced rise in pancreatic polypeptide in man. J Clin Endocrinol Metab 1980; 50:33–39.

972. Lantigua RA, Lilavivathana U, Campbell RG, et al. Adrenergic modulation of pancreatic polypeptide secretion. Metabolism 1980; 29:787–792.

973. Sive AA, Vinik I, Levitt N. Adrenergic modulation of human pancreatic polypeptide (hPP) release. Gastroenterology 1980; 79:665–672.

974. Valtysson G, Vinik AI, Glaser B, et al. Sex difference in the sensitivity of the human pancreatic polypeptide cell to autonomic nervous stimulation in man. J Clin Endocrinol Metab 1983; 56:21–25.

975. Sanfield JA, Shenker Y, Grekin RJ, et al. Epinephrine increases plasma immunoreactive atrial natriuretic hormone levels in humans. Am J Physiol 1987; 252:E740–E745.

976. Schiebinger RJ, Baker MZ, Linden J. Effect of adrenergic and muscarinic cholinergic agonists on atrial natriuretic peptide secretion by isolated rat atria. Potential role of the autonomic nervous system in modulating atrial natriuretic peptide secretion. J Clin Invest 1987; 80:1687–1691.

977. Wong NLM, Wong EFC, Au GH, et al. Effect of alpha- and beta-adrenergic stimulation on atrial natriuretic peptide release in vitro. Am J Physiol 1988; 255:E260–E264.

978. Uehlinger DE, Zaman T, Weidmann P, et al. Pressure dependence of atrial natriuretic peptide during norepinephrine infusion in humans. Hypertension 1987; 10:249–253.

979. Johnson GE. The effect of cold exposure on the catecholamine excretion of adrenalectomized rats treated with reserpine. Acta Physiol Scand 1963; 59:438–444.

980. Pouliot M. Catecholamine excretion in adreno-demedullated rats exposed to cold after chronic guanethidine treatment. Acta Physiol Scand 1966; 68:164–168.

981. Leduc J. Catecholamine production and release in exposure and acclimation to cold. Acta Physiol Scand 1961; Suppl 183:1–101.

982. Bergh U, Hartley H, Landsberg L, et al. Plasma norepinephrine concentration during submaximal and maximal exercise at lowered skin and core temperatures. Acta Physiol Scand 1979; 106:383–384.

983. Therminarias A, Chirpaz MF, Tanche M. Catecholamines in dogs during cold adaptation by repeated immersions. J Appl Physiol 1979; 46:662–668.

984. Young JB, Landsberg L. Effect of diet and cold exposure on norepinephrine turnover in pancreas and liver. Am J Physiol 1979; 236:E524–E533.

985. Boulant JA. Hypothalamic mechanisms in thermoregulation. Fed Proc 1981; 40:2843–2850.

986. Gale CC. Neuroendocrine aspects of thermoregulation. Annu Rev Physiol 1973; 35:391–430.

987. Thompson GE. Physiological effects of cold exposure. In: Robertshaw D, ed. International Review of Physiology. Environmental Physiology II. Baltimore: University Park, 1977;29–69.

988. Banet M, Hensel H, Liebermann H. The central control of shivering and non-shivering thermogenesis in the rat. J Physiol (Lond) 1978; 383:569–584.

989. Maickel RP, Matussek N, Stern DN, et al. The sympathetic nervous system as a homeostatic mechanism. I. Absolute need for sympathetic nervous function in body temperature maintenance of cold-exposed rats. J Pharmacol Exp Ther 1967; 157:103–110.

990. Depocas F. Biochemical changes in exposure and acclimation to cold environments. Br Med Bull 1961; 17:25–31.

991. Maickel R, Susman H, Yamada K, et al. Control of adipose tissue lipase activity by the sympathetic nervous system. Life Sci 1963; 3:210–214.

992. LaFrance L, Lagace G, Routhier D. Free fatty acid turnover and oxygen consumption. Effects of noradrenaline in nonfasted and non-anesthetized cold-adapted rats. Can J Physiol Pharmacol 1980; 58:797–804.

993. Maekubo H, Moriya K, Hiroshige T. Role of ketone bodies in non-shivering thermogenesis in cold-acclimated rats. J Appl Physiol 1977; 42:159–165.

994. O'Hara WJ, Allen C, Shephard RJ, et al. Fat loss in the cold—a controlled study. J Appl Physiol 1979; 46:872–877.

995. Forichon J, Jomain MJ, Patricot MC, et al. Tolerance to cold and glucose homeostasis in adrenal demedullated dogs. Experientia 1977; 33:1070–1072.

996. Seitz HJ, Krone W, Wilke W, et al. Rapid raise in plasma glucagon induced by acute cold exposure in man and rat. Pflugers Arch 1981; 389:115–120.

997. Edwards EIW, Howland RJ. Adaptive changes in insulin and glucagon secretion during cold acclimation in the rat. Am J Physiol 1986; 250:E669–E676.

998. Baum D, Dillard DH, Porte D Jr. Inhibition of insulin release in infants undergoing deep hypothermic cardiovascular surgery. N Engl J Med 1968; 279:1309–1314.

999. Blackard WG, Nelson NC, Labat JA. Insulin secretion in hypothermic dogs. Am J Physiol 1967; 212:1185–1187.

1000. Kervran AA, Gilbert M, Girard JR, et al. Effect of environmental temperature on glucose-induced insulin response in the newborn rat. Diabetes 1976; 25:1026–1030.

1001. Baum D, Porte D. Alpha-adrenergic inhibition of immunoreactive insulin release during deep hypothermia. Am J Physiol 1971; 221:303–311.

1002. Forichon J, Jomain MJ, Dallevet G, et al. Effect of cold and epinephrine on glucose kinetics in dogs. J Appl Physiol 1977; 43:230–237.

1003. Ekenvall L, Lindblad LE, Norbeck O, et al. Alpha-adrenoceptors and cold-induced vasocontriction in human finger skin. Am J Physiol 1988; 255:H1000–H1003.

1004. Millard RW, Reite OB. Peripheral vascular response to norepinephrine at temperatures from 2 to 40°C. J Appl Physiol 1975; 38:26–30.

1005. Webb-Peploe MM, Shepard JT. Responses of the superficial limb veins of the dog to changes in temperature. Circ Res 1975; 22:737–746.

1006. Vanhoutte PM, Flavahan NA. Effects of temperature on alpha adrenoceptors in limb veins: role of receptor reserve. Fed Proc 1986; 45:2347–2354.

1007. Raven PB, Niki I, Dahms TE, et al. Compensatory cardiovascular responses during an environmental cold stress, 5°C. J Appl Physiol 1970; 29:417–421.

1008. Wasserstrum N, Herd JA. Elevation of arterial blood pressure in the squirrel monkey at 10°C. Am J Physiol 1977; 232:H459–H462.

1009. Budd GM, Warhaft N. Body temperature, shivering blood pressure and heart rate during a standard cold stress in Australia and Antarctica. J Physiol (Lond) 1966; 186:216–232.

1010. Cannon B, Nedergaard J. Biochemical aspects of acclimation to cold. J Therm Biol 1983; 8:85–90.

1011. Radomski MW, Boutlier C. Hormone response of normal and intermittent cold-preadapted humans to continuous cold. J Appl Physiol 1982; 53:610–616.

1012. Joy RJT. Responses of cold-acclimatized men to infused norepinephrine. J Appl Physiol 1973; 18:1209–1212.

1013. LeBlanc J, Vallieres J, Vachon C. Beta-receptor sensitization by repeated injections of isoproterenol and by cold adaptation. Am J Physiol 1972; 222:1043–1046.

1014. Desautels M, Himms-Hagen J. Roles of noradrenaline and protein synthesis in the cold-induced increase in purine nucleotide binding by rat brown adipose tissue mitochondria. Can J Biochem 1979; 57:968–976.

1015. Leblanc J, Villemaire A. Thyroxine and noradrenaline sensitivity, cold resistance, and brown fat. Am J Physiol 1970; 218:1742–1745.

1016. LeBlanc J, Dulac S, Cote J, et al. Autonomic nervous system and adaptation to cold in man. J Appl Physiol 1975; 39:181–186.

1017. Fregly MJ, Kikta DC, Threatte RM, et al. Development of hypertension in rats during chronic exposure to cold. J Appl Physiol 1989; 66:741–749.

1018. Von Euler US, Luft R. Effect of insulin on urinary excretion of adrenaline and noradrenaline; studies in ten healthy subjects and in six cases of acromegaly. Metabolism 1952; 1:528–532.

1019. Young JB, Landsberg L, Knopp RH. Effect of intravenous glucagon on urinary catecholamine excretion. Metabolism 1976; 25:233–237.

1020. Young JB, Landsberg L. Catecholamines and intermediary metabolism. Clin Endocrinol Metab 1977; 6:599–631.

1021. Garber AJ, Cryer PE, Santiago JV, et al. The role of adrenergic mechanisms in the substrate and hormonal response to insulin-induced hypoglycemia in man. J Clin Invest 1976; 58:7–15.

1022. Christensen NJ. Plasma norepinephrine and epinephrine in untreated diabetics, during fasting and after insulin administration. Diabetes 1974; 23:1–8.

1023. Christensen NJ, Alberti KGMM, Brandsborg O. Plasma catecholamines and blood substrate concentrations: studies in insulin induced hypoglycemia and after adrenaline infusions. Eur J Clin Invest 1975; 5:415–423.

1024. Bloom SR, Edwards AV, Hardy RN, et al. Endocrine responses to insulin hypoglycemia in the young calf. J Physiol (Lond) 1975; 244:783–803.

1025. Santiago JA, Clarke WL, Shah SD, et al. Epinephrine, norepinephrine, glucagon, and growth hormone release in association with physiological decrements in the plasma glucose concentration in normal and diabetic man. J Clin Endocrinol Metab 1980; 51:877–883.

1026. Kerr D, Macdonald IA, Tattersall RB. Influence of duration of hypoglycemia on the hormonal counterregulatory response in normal subjects. J Clin Endocrinol Metab 1989; 58:1118–1122.

1027. DeFronzo RA, Tobin JD, Andres R. A test in man of the hypothesis that rate of fall in glucose concentration triggers counter-regulatory hormonal responses. Diabetes 1974; 23(Suppl 1):341.

1028. Young JB, Landsberg L, Knopp RH. Catecholamine responses to glucose lowering. Diabetes 1974; 23(Suppl 1):341.

1029. DeFronzo RA, Andres R, Bledsoe TA, et al. A test of the hypothesis that the rate of fall in glucose concentration triggers counterregulatory hormonal responses in man. Diabetes 1977; 62:445–452.

1030. DeFronzo RA, Hendler R, Christensen N. Stimulation of counterregulatory hormonal responses in diabetic man by a fall in glucose concentration. Diabetes 1980; 29:125–131.

1031. Brodows RG, Pi-Sunyer FX, Campbell RG. Neural control of counterregulatory events during glucopenia in man. J Clin Invest 1973; 52:1841–1844.

1032. Goldfien A. Effects of glucose deprivation on the sympathetic outflow to the adrenal medulla and adipose tissue. Pharmacol Rev 1966; 18:303–311.

1033. Keller-Wood M, Wade CE, Shinsako J, et al. Insulin-induced hypoglycemia in conscious dogs: effect of maintaining carotid arterial glucose levels on the adrenocorticotropin, epinephrine, and vasopressin responses. Endocrinology 1983; 112:624–632.

1034. Sun CL, Thoa NB, Kopin IJ. Comparison of the effects of 2-deoxyglucose and immobilization on plasma levels of catecholamines and corticosterone in awake rats. Endocrinology 1979; 105:306–311.

1035. Dirocco RJ. The forebrain is not essential for sympathoadrenal hyperglycemic response to glucoprivation. Science 1979; 204:1112–1114.

1036. Cantu RC, Wise BL, Goldfien A, et al. Neural pathways mediating the increase in adrenal medullary secretion produced by hypoglycemia. Proc Soc Exp Biol Med 1963; 114:10–13.

1037. Crone C. The secretion of adrenal medullary hormones during hypoglycemia in intact, decerebrate and spinal sheep. Acta Physiol Scand 1965; 63:213–224.

1038. Cane P, Artal R, Bergman RN. Putative hypothalamic glucoreceptors play no essential role in the response to moderate hypoglycemia. Diabetes 1986; 35:268–277.

1039. Biggers D, Frizzell R, Williams P, et al. Role of the central nervous system (CNS) in counterregulation during insulin induced hypoglycemia (IIH). Diabetes 1986; 35:55A.

1040. Flatt JP, Blackburn GL, Randers G, et al. Effects of ketone body infusion on hypoglycemic reaction in postabsorptive dog. Metabolism 1974; 23:151–158.

1041. Muller WA, Aoki TT, Flatt J-P, et al. Effects of beta-hydroxybutyrate, glycerol and free fatty acid infusions on glucagon and epinephrine secretion in dogs during acute hypoglycemia. Metabolism 1976; 25:1077–1086.

1042. Strickler EM, Rowland N, Saller CF. Homeostasis during hypoglycemia: central control of adrenal secretion and peripheral control of feeding. Science 1977; 196:79–81.

1043. Frolund L, Kehlet H, Christensen NJ, et al. Effect of ketone body infusion on plasma catecholamine and substrate concentrations during acute hypoglycemia in man. J Clin Endocrinol Metab 1980; 50:557–559.

1044. Drenick EJ, Alvarez LC, Tamasi GC, et al. Resistance to symptomatic insulin reactions after fasting. J Clin Invest 1972; 51:2757–2762.

1045. Clarke WL, Santiago JV, Thomas L, et al. Adrenergic mechanisms in recovery from hypoglycemia in man: adrenergic blockade. Am J Physiol 1979; 236:E147–E152.

1046. Rizza RA, Cryer PE, Gerich JE. Role of glucagon, catecholamines and growth hormone in human glucose counterregulation. J Clin Invest 1979; 64:62–71.

1047. Popp DA, Shah SD, Cryer PE. Role of epinephrine-mediated beta-adrenergic mechanisms in hypoglycemic glucose counterregulation and posthypoglycemic hyperglycemia in insulin-dependent diabetes mellitus. J Clin Invest 1982; 69:315–326.

1048. Tse TF, Clutter WE, Shah SD, et al. Mechanisms of postprandial glucose counterregulation in man: physiologic roles of glucagon and epinephrine vis-a-vis insulin in the prevention of hypoglycemia late after glucose ingestion. J Clin Invest 1983; 72:278–286.

1049. Rosen SG, Clutter WE, Berk MA, et al. Epinephrine supports the postabsorptive plasma glucose concentration and prevents hypoglycemia when glucagon secretion is deficient in man. J Clin Invest 1984; 73:405–411.

1050. Boyle PJ, Shah SD, Cryer PE. Insulin, glucagon, and catecholamines in prevention of hypoglycemia during fasting. Am J Physiol 1989; 256:E651–E661.

1051. Cryer PE, White NH, Santiago JV. The relevance of glucose counterregulatory systems to patients with insulin-dependent diabetes mellitus. Endocr Rev 1986; 7:131–139.

1052. Bolli G, de Feo P, Compagnucci P, et al. Abnormal glucose counterregulation in insulin-dependent diabetes mellitus. Interaction of anti-insulin antibodies and impaired glucagon and epinephrine secretion. Diabetes 1983; 32:134–141.

1053. Santiago JV, White NH, Skor DA, et al. Defective glucose counterregulation limits intensive therapy of diabetes mellitus. Am J Physiol 1984; 247:E215–E220.

1054. White NH, Skor DA, Cryer PE, et al. Identification of type I diabetic patients at increased risk for hypoglycemia during intensive therapy. N Engl J Med 1983; 308:485–491.

1055. Amiel SA, Tamborlane WV, Simonson DC, et al. Defective glucose counterregulation after strict glycemic control of insulin-dependent diabetes mellitus. N Engl J Med 1987; 316:1376–1383.

1056. Maher TD, Tanenberg RJ, Greenberg BZ, et al. Lack of glucagon response to hypoglycemia in diabetic autonomic neuropathy. Diabetes 1977; 26:196–200.

1057. Polinsky RJ, Kopin IJ, Ebert MH, et al. The adrenal medullary response to hypoglycemia in patients with orthostatic hypotension. J Clin Endocrinol Metab 1980; 51:1401–1406.

1058. Kennedy FP, Bolli GB, Go VLW, et al. The significance of impaired pancreatic polypeptide and epinephrine responses to hypoglycemia in patients with insulin-dependent diabetes mellitus. J Clin Endocrinol Metab 1987; 64:602–608.

1059. Hoeldtke RD, Boden G, Shuman CR, et al. Reduced epinephrine secretion and hypoglycemia unawareness in diabetic autonomic neuropathy. Ann Intern Med 1982; 96:459–462.

1060. Brown FM, Brink SJ, Freeman R, et al. Anti–sympathetic nervous system autoantibodies: diminished catecholamines with orthostasis. Diabetes (in press).

1061. Brunjes S, Hodgman J, Nowack J, et al. Adrenal medullary function in idiopathic spontaneous hypoglycemia of infancy and childhood. Am J Med 1963; 34:168–176.

1062. Christensen NJ. Hypoadrenalinemia during insulin hypoglycemia in children with ketotic hypoglycemia. J Clin Endocrinol Metab 1974; 38:107–112.

1063. Koffler H, Schubert WK, Hug G. Sporadic hypoglycemia; abnormal epinephrine response to the ketogenic diet or to insulin. J Pediatr 1971; 3:448–453.

1064. Berlin I, Grimaldi A, Landault C, et al. Lack of hypoglycemic symptoms and decreased beta-adrenergic sensitivity in insulin-dependent diabetic patients. J Clin Endocrinol Metab 1988; 66:273–278.

1065. Landsberg L, Young JB. The role of the sympathetic nervous system and catecholamines in the regulation of energy metabolism. Am J Clin Nutr 1983; 38:1018–1024.

1066. Young JB, Landsberg L. Suppression of sympathetic nervous system during fasting. Science 1977; 196:1473–1475.

1067. Rappaport EB, Young JB, Landsberg L. Initiation, duration and dissipation of diet-induced changes in sympathetic nervous system activity in the rat. Metabolism 1982; 31:143–146.

1068. Jung RT, Shetty PS, Berrand M, et al. Role of catecholamines in hypotensive response to dieting. Br Med J 1979; 1:12–13.

1069. Gross HA, Lake CR, Ebert MH, et al. Catecholamine metabolism in primary anorexia nervosa. J Clin Endocrinol Metab 1979; 49:805–809.

1070. DeHaven J, Sherwin R, Hendler R, et al. Nitrogen and sodium balance and sympathetic-nervous-system activity in obese subjects treated with a low-calorie protein or mixed diet. N Engl J Med 1980; 302:477–482.

1071. Sowers JR, Nyby M, Stern N, et al. Blood pressure and hormone changes associated with weight reduction in the obese. Hypertension 1982; 4:686–691.

1072. Wimpfheimer C, Saville E, Voirol MJ, et al. Starvation-induced decreased sensitivity of resting metabolic rate to triiodothyronine. Science 1979; 205:1272–1273.

1073. Young JB, Landsberg L. Impaired suppression of sympathetic activity during fasting in the gold thioglucose–treated mouse. J Clin Invest 1980; 65:1086–1094.

1074. Palmblad J, Levi L, Burger A, et al. Effects of total energy withdrawal (fasting) on the levels of growth hormone, thyrotropin, cortisol, adrenaline, noradrenaline, T_4, T_3, and rT_3 in healthy males. Acta Med Scand 1977; 201:15–22.

1075. Galster AD, Clutter WE, Cryer PE, et al. Epinephrine plasma thresholds for lipolytic effects in man. J Clin Invest 1981; 67:1729–1738.

1076. Arner P, Engfeldt P, Nowak J. In vivo observations on the lipolytic effect of noradrenaline during therapeutic fasting. J Clin Endocrinol Metab 1981; 53:1207–1212.

1077. Staten MA, Matthews DE, Cryer PE, et al. Physiological increments in epinephrine stimulate metabolic rate in humans. Am J Physiol 1987; 253:E322–E330.

1078. Rosen SG, Clutter WE, Berk MA, et al. Epinephrine supports the postabsorptive plasma glucose concentration, and prevents hypoglycemia, when glucagon secretion is deficient in man. J Clin Invest 1984; 73:405–411.

1079. Tse TF, Clutter WE, Shah SD, et al. Neuroendocrine responses to glucose ingestion in man: specificity, temporal relationships, and quantitative aspects. J Clin Invest 1983; 72:270–277.

1080. Antal J. Les changements dans la respiration et dans la pression du sang pendant la réception de nourriture chez les chiens. J Physiol (Paris) 1964; 56:487–488.

1081. Vatner SF, Franklin D, van Citters RL. Mesenteric vasoactivity associated with eating and digestion in the conscious dog. Am J Physiol 1970; 219:170–174.

1082. Vatner SF, Franklin D, van Citters RL. Coronary and visceral vasoactivity associated with eating and digestion in the conscious dog. Am J Physiol 1970; 219:1380–1385.

1083. Welle S, Lilavivathana U, Campbell RG. Increased plasma norepinephrine concentrations and metabolic rates following glucose ingestion in man. Metabolism 1980; 29:806–809.

1084. Rowe JW, Young JB, Minaker KL, et al. Effect of insulin and glucose infusions on sympathetic nervous system activity in normal man. Diabetes 1981; 30:219–225.

1085. Landsberg L, Young JB. Insulin-mediated glucose metabolism in the relationship between dietary intake and sympathetic nervous system activity. Int J Obes 1985; 9:63–68.

1086. Young JB, Landsberg L. Stimulation of the sympathetic nervous system during sucrose feeding. Nature 1977; 269:615–617.

1087. Schwartz JH, Young JB, Landsberg L. Effect of dietary fat on sympathetic nervous system activity in the rat. J Clin Invest 1983; 72:361–370.

1088. Sims EAH. Efficiency of gain in weight following overeating in normal subjects and in the obese. In: Bray GA, ed. Obesity in Perspective. DHEW Publication No. (NIH) 75-708. Washington, DC: Government Printing Office, 1973: 53–56.

1089. Miller DS, Mumford P. Gluttony. 1. An experimental study of overeating low- or high-protein diets. Am J Clin Nutr 1967; 20:1212–1222.

1090. Landsberg L, Young JB. Obesity and the SNS. In: Bray G, Ricquier D, Spiegelman B, eds. Obesity: Towards a Molecular Approach. UCLA Symposia on Molecular and Cellular Biology. New Series, Vol 133. New York: Alan R. Liss, 1990: 81–94.

1091. Peronnet F, Nadeau RA, de Champlain J, et al. Exercise plasma catecholamines in dogs: role of adrenals and cardiac nerve endings. Am J Physiol 1981; 241:H243–H247.

1092. Peronnet F, Beliveau L, Boudreau G, et al. Regional plasma catecholamine removal and release at rest and exercise in dogs. Am J Physiol 1988; 254:R663–R672.

1093. Mason JW, Hartley LH, Kotchen TA, et al. Plasma cortisol and norepinephrine responses in anticipation of muscular exercise. Psychosom Med 1973; 35:406–414.

1094. Hartley LH, Mason JW, Hogan RP, et al. Multiple hormonal responses to prolonged exercise in relation to physical training. J Appl Physiol 1972; 33:607–610.

1095. Hartley LH, Mason JW, Hogan RP, et al. Multiple hormonal responses to graded exercise in relation to physical training. J Appl Physiol 1972; 33:602–606.

1096. Ostman I, Sjostrand NO, Swedin G. Cardiac noradrenaline turnover and urinary catecholamine excretion in trained and untrained rats during rest and exercise. Acta Physiol Scand 1972; 86:299–308.

1097. Ostman I, Sjostrand NO. Reduced urinary noradrenaline excretion during rest, exercise and cold stress in trained rats: a comparison between physically-trained rats, cold-acclimated rats and warm-acclimated rats. Acta Physiol Scand 1975; 95:209–218.

1098. Winder WW, Hagberg JM, Hickson RC, et al. Time course of sympathoadrenal adaptation to endurance exercise training in man. J Appl Physiol 1978; 45:370–374.

1099. Jennings GL, Nelson L, Esler MD, et al. Effects of change in physical activity on blood pressure and sympathetic tone. J Hypertens 1984; 2(Suppl 3):139–141.

1100. Evans JM, Funk JN, Charles JB, et al. Endurance training in dogs increases vascular responsiveness to an α_1-agonist. J Appl Physiol 1988; 65:625–632.

1101. Kjaer M, Galbo H. Effect of physical training on the capacity to secrete epinephrine. J Appl Physiol 1988; 64:11–16.

1102. Atkins JM, Horwitz LD. Cardiac autonomic blockade in exercising dogs. J Appl Physiol 1977; 42:878–883.

1103. Hilsted J, Galbo H, Christensen NJ. Impaired cardiovascular responses to graded exercise in diabetic autonomic neuropathy. Diabetes 1979; 28:313–319.

1104. Ernst SB, Mullin WJ, Herrick RE, et al. Exercise and cardiac performance capacity in rats with partial sympathectomy. J Appl Physiol 1982; 53:242–246.

1105. Richter EA. Influence of the sympatho-adrenal system on some metabolic and hormonal responses to exercise in the rat with special reference to the effect on glycogenolysis in skeletal muscle. Acta Physiol Scand 1984; Suppl 528:1–42.

1106. Issekutz B Jr. Role of beta-adrenergic receptors in mobilization of energy sources in exercising dogs. J Appl Physiol 1978; 44:869–876.

1107. Wahren J. Glucose turnover during exercise in man. Ann NY Acad Sci 1977; 301:45–65.

1108. Lijnen PJ, Amery AK, Fagard RH, et al. The effects of beta-adrenoceptor blockade on renin, angiotensin, aldosterone and catecholamines at rest and during exercise. Br J Clin Pharmacol 1979; 7:175–181.

1109. Galbo H, Christensen NJ, Holst JJ. Catecholamines and pancreatic hormones during autonomic blockade in exercising man. Acta Physiol Scand 1977; 101:119–131.

1110. Blum JW, Bianca W, Naf F, et al. Plasma catecholamine and parathyroid hormone responses in cattle during treadmill exercise at simulated high altitude. Horm Metab Res 1979; 11:246–251.

1111. Galbo H, Christensen NJ, Holst JJ. Glucose-induced decrease in glucagon and epinephrine responses to exercise in man. J Appl Physiol 1977; 42:525–530.

1112. Braunwald E, Chidsey CA, Pool PE, et al. Congestive heart failure: biochemical and physiological considerations—combined clinical staff conference at the National Institutes of Health. Ann Intern Med 1966; 64:904–941.

1113. Gill MB, Pugh GCE. Basal metabolism and respiration in men living at 5,800 m (19,000 ft). J Appl Physiol 1964; 19:949–954.

1114. Horstman DH, Banderet LE. Hypoxia-induced metabolic and core temperature changes in the squirrel monkey. J Appl Physiol 1977; 42:273–278.

1115. Pinardi G, Talmaciu RK, Santiago E, et al. Contribution of adrenal medulla, spleen and lymph, to the plasma levels of dopamine β-hydroxylase and catecholamines induced by hemorrhagic hypotension in dogs. J Pharmacol Exp Ther 1979; 209:176–184.

1116. Chien S. Role of the sympathetic nervous system in hemorrhage. Physiol Rev 1967; 47:214–288.

1117. Young JB, Fish S, Landsberg L. Sympathetic nervous system and adrenal medullary responses to ischemic injury in mice. Am J Physiol 1983; 245:E67–E73.

1118. Johnson TS, Young JB, Landsberg L. Sympathoadrenal responses to acute and chronic hypoxia in the rat. J Clin Invest 1983; 71:1263–1272.

1119. Goldman RH, Harrison DC. The effects of hypoxia and hypercarbia on myocardial catecholamines. J Pharmacol Exp Ther 1970; 174:307–314.

1120. Wallin BG, Sundlof G. Sympathetic outflow to muscles during vasovagal syncope. J Auton Nerv Syst 1982; 6:287–291.

1121. Wilmore DW, Long JM, Mason AD Jr, et al. Catecholamines: mediator of the hypermetabolic response to thermal injury. Ann Surg 1974; 180:653–668.

1122. Jones SB, Kovarik MF, Romano FD. Cardiac and splenic norepinephrine turnover during septic peritonitis. Am J Physiol 1986; 250:R892–R897.

1123. Myles WS, Ducker AJ. The excretion of catecholamines in rats during acute and chronic exposure to altitude. Can J Physiol Pharmacol 1971; 49:721–726.

1124. Watanabe E, Ogawa K, Ban M, et al. Sympathetic nervous systems in chronic hypoxic states from pulmonary tuberculosis: a clinical study on plasma norepinephrine and cyclic AMP levels. Jpn J Med 1981; 20:180–187.

1125. Thomas JA, Marks BH. Plasma norepinephrine in congestive heart failure. Am J Cardiol 1978; 41:233–243.

1126. Francis GS, Goldsmith SR, Ziesche SM, et al. Response of plasma norepinephrine and epinephrine to dynamic exercise in patients with congestive heart failure. Am J Cardiol 1982; 49:1152–1156.

1127. Abe I, Averill DB, Ferrario CM. Activation of renal sympathetic outflow by intracisternal hypertonic NaCl in dogs. Am J Physiol 1989; 256:H411–H416.

1128. Hjemdahl P. Inhibition of the lipolytic response to nerve stimulation during acidosis. Acta Physiol Scand 1976; 98:80–84.

1129. Baum D, Oyer P. Norepinephrine-stimulated lipolysis in acute and chronic hypoxemia. Am J Physiol 1981; 241:E28–E34.

1130. Hughes MJ, Kopetzky MT, Messiha F, et al. Alterations in responses to drugs of atria from white rats acclimated to hypobaric hypoxia. J Appl Physiol 1981; 51:1607–1611.

1131. Bristow MR, Ginsburg R, Minobe W, et al. Decreased catecholamine sensitivity and beta-adrenergic-receptor density in failing human hearts. N Engl J Med 1982; 307:205–211.

1132. Ramey ER, Goldstein MS. The adrenal cortex and the sympathetic nervous system. Physiol Rev 1957; 37:155–195.

1133. Djahanguiri B, Taubin HL, Landsberg L. Increased sympathetic activity in the pathogenesis of restraint ulcer in rats. J Pharmacol Exp Ther 1973; 184:163–168.

1134. Dubois A, Kopin IJ, Pettigrew KD, et al. Chemical and histochemical studies of postoperative sympathetic activity in the digestive tract in rats. Gastroenterology 1974; 66:403–407.

1135. Stoner HB, Frayn KN, Barton RN, et al. The relationships between plasma substrates and hormones and the severity of injury in 277 recently injured patients. Clin Sci 1979; 56:563–573.

1136. Eigler N, Sacca L, Sherwin RS. Synergistic interactions of physiologic increments of glucagon, epinephrine, and cortisol in the dog. J Clin Invest 1979; 63:114–123.

1137. Wilmore DW. Carbohydrate metabolism in trauma. Clin Endocrinol Metab 1976;5:731–745.

1138. Baum D, Porte D Jr. A mechanism for regulation of insulin release in hypoxia. Am J Physiol 1972; 222:695–699.

1139. Hiebert JM, Celik Z, Soeldner JS, et al. Insulin response to hemorrhagic shock in the intact and adrenalectomized primate. Am J Surg 1973; 125:501–507.

1140. Hiebert JM, Sixt N, Soeldner JS, et al. Altered insulin and glucose metabolism produced by epinephrine during hemorrhagic shock in the adrenalectomized primate. Surgery 1973; 74:223–234.

1141. Bloom SR, Daniel PM, Johnston DI, et al. Release of glucagon, induced by stress. Q J Exp Physiol 1972; 58:99–108.

1142. Jarhult J. Role of the sympatho-adrenal system in hemorrhagic hyperglycemia. Acta Physiol Scand 1975; 93:25–33.

1143. Lindsey CA, Faloona GR, Unger RH, et al. Plasma glucagon levels during rapid exsanguination with and without adrenergic blockade. Diabetes 1975; 24:313–316.

1144. Bloom SR, Edwards AV, Hardy RN. Adrenal and pancreatic endocrine responses to hypoxia and hypercapnia in the calf. J Physiol (Lond) 1977; 269:131–154.

1145. Baum D, Porte D Jr, Ensinck J. Hyperglucagonemia and alpha-adrenergic receptor in acute hypoxia. Am J Physiol 1979; 237:E404–E408.

1146. Baum D, Griepp R, Porte D Jr. Glucose-induced insulin release during acute and chronic hypoxia. Am J Physiol 1979; 237:E45–E50.

1147. Black PR, Brooks DC, Bessey PQ, et al. Mechanisms of insulin resistance following injury. Ann Surg 1982; 196:420–425.

1148. Zuspan FP, Rao P. Thermogenic alterations in the woman. I. Interaction of amines, ovulation, and basal body temperature. Am J Obstet Gynecol 1974; 118:671–678.

1149. Rosner JM, Nagle CA, de Laborde NP, et al. Plasma levels of norepinephrine (NE) during the periovulatory period and after LH-RH stimulation in women. Am J Obstet Gynecol 1976; 124:567–572.

1150. Goldstein DS, Levinson P, Keiser HR. Plasma and urinary catecholamines during the human ovulatory cycle. Am J Obstet Gynecol 1983; 146:824–829.

1151. Young JB, Saville ME, Landsberg L. Sympathetic nervous system (SNS) activity in rat thyroid: stimulation in hypopituitarism and pregnancy. Clin Res 1982; 30:279A.

1152. Perkins CM, Hancock KW, Cope GF, et al. Urine free dopamine in normal primigravid pregnancy and women taking oral contraceptives. Clin Sci 1981; 61:423–428.

1153. Wiswell JG, Hurwitz GE, Corohno V, et al. Urinary catecholamines and their metabolites in hyperthyroidism and hypothyroidism. J Clin Endocrinol Metab 1963; 23:1102–1106.

1154. Christensen NJ. Plasma noradrenaline and adrenaline in patients with thyrotoxicosis and myxoedema. Clin Sci Mol Med 1973; 45:163–171.

1155. Coulombe P, Dussault JH, Letarte J, et al. Catecholamine metabolism in thyroid diseases. I. Epinephrine secretion rate in hyperthyroidism and hypothyroidism. J Clin Endocrinol Metab 1976; 42:125–131.

1156. Beley A, Rochette L, Bralet J. Influence de traitement par la thyroxine et le propylthiouracile sur le taux de renouvellement de la noradrenaline dans huit organes périphériques du rat. Arch Int Physiol Biochem 1973; 81:287–298.

1157. Baylis RIS, Edwards OM. Urinary excretion of free catecholamines in Graves' disease. Endocrinology 1971; 49:167–173.

1158. Christensen NJ. Increased levels of plasma noradrenaline in hypothyroidism. J Clin Endocrinol Metab 1972; 35:359–363.

1159. Coulombe P, Dussault JH, Walker P. Plasma catecholamine concentrations in hyperthyroidism and hypothyroidism. Metabolism 1976; 25:973–979.

1160. Stoffer SF, Jiang M-S, Gorman CA, et al. Plasma catecholamines in hypothyroidism and hyperthyroidism. J Clin Endocrinol Metab 1973; 36:587–589.

1161. Coulombe P, Dussault JH. Catecholamine metabolism in thyroid disease. II. Norepinephrine secretion rate in hyperthyroidism and hypothyroidism. J Clin Endocrinol Metab 1977; 44:1185–1189.

1162. Galton VA. Thyroid hormone–catecholamine interrelationships. Endocrinology 1965; 77:278–284.

1163. Hays MT, Solomon DH. Effect of epinephrine on the peripheral metabolism of thyroxine. J Clin Invest 1969; 48:1114–1123.

1164. Nicoloff JT. A new method for the measurement of acute alterations in thyroxine deiodination rate in man. J Clin Invest 1970; 49:267–273.

1165. Lumholtz IB, Siersbaek-Nielsen K, Faber J, et al. Effect of propranolol on extrathyroidal metabolism of thyroxine and 3,3′,5-triiodothyronine evaluated by noncompartmental kinetics. J Clin Endocrinol Metab 1978; 47:587–589.

1166. Kallner G, Ljunggren J-G, Tryselius M. The effect of propranolol on serum levels of T_4, T_3, and reverse-T_3 in hyperthyroidism. Acta Med Scand 1978; 204:35–37.

1167. Nilsson OR, Karlberg BE, Kagedal B, et al. Non-selective and selective β-1 adrenoceptor blocking agents in the treatment of hyperthyroidism. Acta Med Scand 1979; 206:21–25.

1168. Verhoeven RP, Visser TJ, Docter R, et al. Plasma thyroxine, 3,3′,5-triiodothyronine and 3,3′,5′-triiodothyronine during β-adrenergic blockade in hyperthyroidism. J Clin Endocrinol Metab 1977; 44:1002–1005.

1169. Wiersinga WM, Touber JL. The influence of β-adrenoceptor blocking agents on plasma thyroxine and triiodothyronine. J Clin Endocrinol Metab 1977; 45:293–298.

1170. How J, Khir ASM, Bewsher PD. The effect of atenolol on serum thyroid hormones in hyperthyroid patients. Clin Endocrinol 1980; 13:299–302.

1171. Heyma P, Larkins RG, Campbell DG. Inhibition by propranolol of 3,5,3′-triiodothyronine formation from thyroxine in isolated rat renal tubules: an effect independent of beta-adrenergic blockade. Endocrinology 1980; 106:1437–1441.

1172. Shulkin BL, Peele ME, Utiger RD. Beta-adrenergic antagonist inhibition of hepatic 3,5,3′-triiodothyronine production. Endocrinology 1984; 115:858–861.

1173. Silva JE, Larsen PR. Potential of brown adipose tissue type II thyroxine 5′-deiodinase as a local and systemic source of triiodothyronine in rats. J Clin Invest 1985; 76:2296–2305.

1174. Landsberg L. Catecholamines and hyperthyroidism. Clin Endocrinol Metab 1977; 6:697–718.

1175. Brodie BB, Davies JI, Hynie S, et al. Interrelationships of catecholamines with other endocrine systems. Pharmacol Rev 1966; 18:273–289.

1176. Krishna G, Hynie S, Brodie BB. Effects of thyroid hormones on adenyl cyclase in adipose tissue and on free fatty acid mobilization. Proc Natl Acad Sci USA 1968; 59:884–889.

1177. Goswami A, Rosenberg IN. Thyroid hormone modulation of epinephrine-induced lipolysis in rat adipocytes: a possible role of calcium. Endocrinology 1978; 103:2223–2233.

1178. Malbon CC, Moreno FJ, Cabelli RJ, et al. Fat cell adenylate cyclase and beta-adrenergic receptors in altered thyroid states. J Biol Chem 1978; 253:671–677.

1179. Arner P, Wennlund A, Ostman J. Regulation of lipolysis by human adipose tissue in hyperthyroidism. J Clin Endocrinol Metab 1979; 48:415–419.

1180. Rosenqvist U. Inhibition of noradrenaline-induced lipolysis in hypothyroid subjects by increased α-adrenergic responsiveness. Acta Med Scand 1972; 192:353–359.

1181. Wajchenberg BL, Cesar FP, Leme CE, et al. Effects of adrenergic stimulating and blocking agents on glucose-induced insulin responses in human thyrotoxicosis. Metabolism 1978; 27:1715–1720.

1182. Swanson HE. Interrelations between thyroxin and adrenalin in the regulation of oxygen consumption in the albino rat. Endocrinology 1956; 59:217–225.

1183. Rothwell NJ, Saville ME, Stock MJ. Sympathetic and thyroid influences on metabolic rate in fed, fasted, and refed rats. Am J Physiol 1982; 234:R339–R346.

1184. Hsieh ACL, Carlson LD. Role of the thyroid in metabolic response to low temperature. Am J Physiol 1957; 188:40–44.

1185. Carlson LD. Nonshivering thermogenesis and its endocrine control. Fed Proc 1960; 19(Suppl):25–30.

1186. Triandafillou J, Gwilliam C, Himms-Hagen J. Role of thyroid hormone in cold-induced changes in rat brown adipose tissue mitochondria. Can J Biochem 1982; 60:530–537.

1187. Kaciuba-Uscilko H. The effect of previous thyroxine administration on the metabolic response to adrenaline in new-born pigs. Biol Neonate 1971; 19:220–226.

1188. Brewster WR Jr, Isaacs JP, Osgood PF, et al. The hemodynamic and metabolic interrelationship in the activity of epinephrine, norepinephrine and the thyroid hormones. Circulation 1956; 13:1–20.

1189. Coville PF, Telford JM. Influence of thyroid hormones on the sensitivity of cardiac and smooth muscle to biogenic amines and other drugs. Br J Pharmacol 1970; 399:49–66.

1190. Cravey GM, Gravenstein JS. The effect of thyroxin, corticosteroids, and epinephrine on atrial rate. J Pharmacol Exp Ther 1965; 148:75–79.

1191. Field FP, Janis RA, Tribble DJ. Relationship between aortic reactivity and blood pressure of renal hypertensive, hyperthyroid, and hypothyroid rats. Can J Physiol Pharmacol 1973; 51:344–353.

1192. McDonald CH, Shepeard WL, Green MF, et al. Response of the hyperthyroid heart to epinephrine. Am J Physiol 1935; 112:227–230.

1193. Sawyer MEM, Brown MG. The effect of thyroidectomy and thyroxine on the response of the denervated heart to injected and secreted adrenine. Am J Physiol 1935; 110:620–635.

1194. Thier MD, Gravenstein JS, Hoffman RG. Thyroxin, reserpine, epinephrine and temperature on atrial rate. J Pharmacol Exp Ther 1962; 136:133–141.

1195. Tse J, Wrenn RW, Kuo JF. Thyroxine-induced changes in characteristics and activities of β-adrenergic receptors and adenosine 3′,5′-monophosphate and guanosine 3′,5′-monophosphate systems in the heart may be related to reputed catecholamine supersensitivity in hyperthyroidism. Endocrinology 1980; 107:6–16.

1196. Wildenthal K. Responses to cardioactive drugs of fetal mouse hearts maintained in organ culture. Am J Physiol 1971; 221:238–241.

1197. Wildenthal K. Studies of isolated fetal mouse hearts in organ culture: evidence for a direct effect of triiodothyronine in enhancing cardiac responsiveness to norepinephrine. J Clin Invest 1972; 51:2702–2709.

1198. Anton AH, Gravenstein JS. Studies on thyroid-catecholamine interactions in the isolated rabbit heart. Eur J Pharmacol 1970; 10:311–318.

1199. Brus R, Hess ME, Jacobwitz D. Effect of 6-hydroxydopamine and thyroxine on chronotropic response to norepinephrine. Eur J Pharmacol 1970; 10:323–326.

1200. Cairoli VJ, Crout JR. Role of the autonomic nervous system in the resting tachycardia of experimental hyperthyroidism. J Pharmacol Exp Ther 1967; 158:55–65.

1201. Margolius HS, Gaffney TE. The effects of injected norepinephrine and sympathetic nerve stimulation in hypothyroid and hyperthyroid dogs. J Pharmacol Exp Ther 1965; 149:329–335.

1202. Rutherford JD, Vatner SF, Braunwald E. Adrenergic control of myocardial contractility in conscious hyperthyroid dogs. Am J Physiol 1979; 237:H590–H596.

1203. Van Derschoot JV, Moran NC. An experimental evaluation of the reputed influence of thyroxine on the cardiovascular effects of catecholamines. J Pharmacol Exp Ther 1965; 149:336–345.

1204. Aoki VS, Wilson WR, Theilen EO. Studies of the reputed augmentation of the cardiovascular effects of catecholamines in patients with spontaneous hyperthyroidism. J Pharmacol Exp Ther 1972; 181:362–368.

1205. Goetsch E. Newer methods in the diagnosis of thyroid disorders: pathological and clinical. NY State J Med 1918; 18:259–267.

1206. Murray JF, Kelley JJ Jr. The relation of thyroidal hormone level to epinephrine response: a diagnostic test for hyperthyroidism. Ann Intern Med 1959; 51:309–321.

1207. Schneckloth RE, Kurland GS, Freedberg AS. Effect of variation in thyroid function on the pressor response to norepinephrine in man. Metabolism 1953; 2:546–555.

1208. Zwillich CW, Matthay M, Potts DE, et al. Thyrotoxicosis: comparison of effects of thyroid ablation and beta-adrenergic blockade on metabolic rate and ventilatory control. J Clin Endocrinol Metab 1978; 46:491–500.

1209. Etzkorn J, Hopkins P, Gray J, et al. Beta-adrenergic potentiation of the increased in vitro accumulation of cycloleucine by rat thymocytes induced by triiodothyronine. J Clin Invest 1979; 63:1172–1180.

1210. Popovic WJ, Brown JE, Adamson JW. The influence of thyroid hormones on in vitro erythropoiesis. J Clin Invest 1977; 60:907–913.

1211. Fregly MJ, Field FP, Ktovich MJ, et al. Catecholamine–thyroid hormone interaction in cold-acclimated rats. Fed Proc 1979; 38:2162–2169.

1212. Hauger-Klevene JH, Brown H, Zavaleta J. Plasma renin activity in hyper- and hypothyroidism: effect of adrenergic blocking agents. J Clin Endocrinol Metab 1972; 34:625–629.

1213. Bilezikian JP, Loeb JN. The influence of hyperthyroidism and hypothyroidism on alpha- and beta-adrenergic receptor systems and adrenergic responsiveness. Endocr Rev 1983; 4:378–388.

1214. Ciraldi T, Martinetti GV. Thyroxine and propylthiouracil effects in vivo on alpha and beta adrenergic receptors in rat heart. Biochem Biophys Res Commun 1977; 74:984–991.

1215. Kempson S, Marinetti GV, Shaw A. Hormone action at the membrane level. VII. Stimulation of dihydroalprenolol binding to beta-adrenergic receptors in isolated rat heart ventricle slices by triiodothyronine and thyroxine. Biochim Biophys Acta 1978; 540:320–329.

1216. Scarpace PJ, Abrass IB. Thyroid hormone regulation of rat heart, lymphocyte, and lung β-adrenergic receptors. Endocrinology 1981; 108:1276–1278.

1217. Williams LT, Lefkowitz RJ, Watanabe AM, et al. Thyroid hormone regulation of beta-adrenergic receptor number. J Biol Chem 1977; 252:2787–2789.

1218. Bilezikian JP, Loeb JN, Gammon DE. The influence of hyperthyroidism and hypothyroidism on the β-adrenergic responsiveness of the turkey erythrocyte. J Clin Invest 1979; 63:184–192.

1219. Banerjee S, Kung LS. β-Adrenergic receptors in rat heart: effects of thyroidectomy. Eur J Pharmacol 1977; 43:207–208.

1220. Williams RS, Guthrow CE, Lefkowitz RJ. β-Adrenergic receptors of human lymphocytes are unaltered by hyperthyroidism. J Clin Endocrinol Metab 1979; 48:503–505.

1221. Ginsberg AM, Clutter WE, Shah SD, et al. Triiodothyronine-induced thyrotoxicosis increases mononuclear leukocyte β-adrenergic receptor density in man. J Clin Invest 1981; 67:1785–1791.

1222. Hammond HK, White FC, Buxton ILO, et al. Increased myocardial beta-receptors and adrenergic responses in hyperthyroid pigs. Am J Physiol 1987; 252:H283–H290.

1223. Liggett SB, Shah SD, Cryer PE. Increased fat and skeletal muscle beta-adrenergic receptors but unaltered metabolic and hemodynamic sensitivity to epinephrine in vivo in experimental human thyrotoxicosis. J Clin Invest 1989; 83:803–809.

1224. Karlberg BE, Henriksson KG, Andersson RGG. Cyclic adenosine 3′,5′-monophosphate concentration in plasma, adipose tissue and skeletal muscle in normal subjects and in patients with hyper- and hypothyroidism. J Clin Endocrinol Metab 1974; 39:96–101.

1225. Guttler RG, Shaw JW, Otis CL, et al. Epinephrine-induced alterations in urinary cyclic AMP in hyper- and hypothyroidism. J Clin Endocrinol Metab 1975; 41:707–711.

1226. Van Inwegen RG, Robinson GA, Thompson WJ. Cyclic nucleotide phosphodiesterases and thyroid hormones. J Biol Chem 1975; 250:2452–2456.

1227. Georges LP, Santangelo RP, Mackin JF, et al. Metabolic effects of propranolol in thyrotoxicosis. I. Nitrogen, calcium, and hydroxyproline. Metabolism 1975; 24:11–21.

1228. Lee WY, Bronsky D, Waldstein SS. Studies of thyroid and sympathetic nervous system interrelationships. II. Effects of guanethidine on manifestations of hyperthyroidism. J Clin Endocrinol Metab 1962; 22:879–885.

1229. Mazzaferri EL, Reynolds JC, Young RL, et al. Propranolol as primary therapy for thyrotoxicosis. Arch Intern Med 1976; 136:50–56.

1230. Grossman W, Robin NI, Johnson LW, et al. The enhanced myocardial contractility of thyrotoxicosis. Role of the beta adrenergic receptor. Ann Intern Med 1971; 74:869–874.

1231. Shanks RG, Hadden DR, Lowe DC, et al. Controlled trial of propranolol in thyrotoxicosis. Lancet 1969; 1:993–994.

1232. Pietras RJ, Real MA, Poticha GS, et al. Cardiovascular response in hyperthyroidism. Arch Intern Med 1972; 129:426–429.

1233. Wiener L, Stout BD, Cox JW. Influence of beta sympathetic blockade (propranolol) on the hemodynamics of hyperthyroidism. Am J Med 1969; 46:227–233.

1234. Howitt G, Rowlands DJ, Leung DYT, et al. Myocardial contractility, and the effects of beta-adrenergic blockade in hypothyroidism and hyperthyroidism. Clin Sci 1968; 34:485–495.

1235. Lewis BS, Ehrenfeld EN, Lewis N, et al. Echocardiographic LV function in thyrotoxicosis. Am Heart J 1979; 97:460–468.

1236. Grossman W, Robin NI, Johnson L, et al. Effects of beta blockade on the peripheral manifestations of thyrotoxicosis. Ann Intern Med 1971; 74:875–879.

1237. Thomas FB, Caldwell JH, Greenberger NJ. Steatorrhea in thyrotoxicosis. Relation to hypermotility and excessive dietary fat. Ann Intern Med 1973; 78:669–675.

1238. Rude RK, Oldham SB, Singer FR, et al. Treatment of thyrotoxic hypercalcemia with propranolol. N Engl J Med 1976; 294:431–433.

1239. Mackin JF, Canary JJ, Pittman CS. Thyroid storm and its management. N Engl J Med 1974; 291:1396–1398.

1240. McLarty DG, Brownlie BEW, Alexander WD, et al. Remission of thyrotoxicosis during treatment with propranolol. Br Med J 1973; 2:333–334.

1241. Riddell JG, Neill JD, Kelly JG, et al. Effects of thyroid dysfunction on propranolol kinetics. Clin Pharmacol Ther 1980; 28:565–574.

1242. Rubenfeld S, Silverman VE, Welch KMA, et al. Variable plasma propranolol levels in thyrotoxicosis. N Engl J Med 1979; 300:353–354.

1243. Feely J, Stevenson IH, Crooks J. Increased clearance of propranolol in thyrotoxicosis. Ann Intern Med 1981; 94:472–474.

1244. Pimstone B, Joffe B. The use and abuse of beta-adrenergic blockade in the surgery of hyperthyroidism. S Afr Med J 1970; 44:1059–1061.

1245. Anderberg B, Kagedal B, Nilsson OR, et al. Propranolol and thyroid resection for hyperthyroidism. Acta Chir Scand 1979; 145:297–303.

1246. Bewsher PD, Pegg CAS, Steward DJ, et al. Propranolol in the surgical management of thyrotoxicosis. Ann Surg 1974; 181:184–192.

1247. Caswell HT, Marks AD, Channick BJ. Propranolol for the preoperative preparation of patients with thyrotoxicosis. Surg Gynecol Obstet 1978; 146:908–910.

1248. Feely J, Crooks J, Forrest AL, et al. Propranolol in the surgical treatment of hyperthyroidism, including severely thyrotoxic patients. Br J Surg 1981; 68:865–869.

1249. Michie W, Pegg CAS, Hamer-Hodges DW, et al. Beta-blockade and partial thyroidectomy for thyrotoxicosis. Lancet 1974; 1:1009–1011.

1250. Toft AD, Irvine WJ, McIntosh D, et al. Propranolol in the treatment of thyrotoxicosis by subtotal thyroidectomy. J Clin Endocrinol Metab 1976; 43:1312–1316.

1251. Toft AD, Irvine WJ, Sinclair I, et al. Thyroid function after surgical treatment of thyrotoxicosis. N Engl J Med 1978; 298:643–647.

1252. Zonszein J, Santangelo RP, Mackin JF, et al. Propranolol therapy in thyrotoxicosis. Am J Med 1979; 66:411–416.

1253. Feely J, Forrest A, Gunn A, et al. Influence of surgery on plasma propranolol levels and protein binding. Clin Pharmacol Ther 1980; 28:759–764.

1254. Bullock JL, Harris RE, Young R. Treatment of thyrotoxicosis. Am J Obstet Gynecol 1975; 121:242–245.

1255. Langer A, Hung CT, McAnulty JA, et al. Adrenergic blockade. A new approach to hyperthyroidism during pregnancy. Obstet Gynecol 1974; 44:181–186.

1256. Levy CA, Waite JH, Dickey R. Thyrotoxicosis and pregnancy. Use of preoperative propranolol for thyroidectomy. Am J Surg 1977; 133:319–321.

1257. Pruyn SC, Phelan JP, Buchanan GC. Long-term propranolol therapy in pregnancy: maternal and fetal outcome. Am J Obstet Gynecol 1979; 135:485–489.

1258. Rubin PC. Beta-blockers in pregnancy. N Engl J Med 1981; 305:1323–1326.

1259. Guyton AC, Coleman TG, Cowley AW, et al. Arterial pressure regulation. In: Laragh JH, ed. Hypertension Manual. 1st ed. New York: Yorke Medical, 1973: 111–134.

1260. Guyton AC. Personal views on mechanisms of hypertension. In: Genest J, Koiw E, Kuchel O, eds. Hypertension Physiopathology and Treatment. New York: McGraw-Hill, 1977: 566–575.

1261. Hall JE, Guyton AC, Coleman TG, et al. Regulation of arterial pressure: role of pressure natriuresis and diuresis. Fed Proc 1986; 45:2897–2903.

1262. Katholi RE. Renal nerves and hypertension: an update. Fed Proc 1985; 44:2846–2850.

1263. Katholi RE, Carey RM, Ayers CR, et al. Production of sustained hypertension by chronic intrarenal norepinephrine infusion in conscious dogs. Circ Res 1977; 40(Suppl):I118–I126.

1264. Kleinjans JCS, Smits JFM, Kasbergen CM, et al. Blood pressure response to chronic low-dose intrarenal noradrenaline infusion in conscious rats. Clin Sci 1983; 65:111–116.

1265. Landsberg L, Young JB. Sympathetic nervous system in hypertension. In: Brenner B, Stein JH, eds. Hypertension: Contemporary Issues in Nephrology. Vol 8. New York: Churchill Livingstone, 1981: 100–141.

1266. Nestel PJ, Esler MD. Patterns of catecholamine excretion in urine in hypertension. Circ Res 1970; 26–27(Suppl):II75–II81.

1267. deChamplain J, Farley L, Cousineau D, et al. Circulating catecholamine levels in human and experimental hypertension. Circ Res 1976; 38:109–114.

1268. Weidmann P. Recent pathogenic aspects in essential hypertension and hypertension associated with diabetes mellitus. Klin Wochenschr 1980; 58:1071–1089.

1269. Grimm M, Weidmann P, Keusch G, et al. Norepinephrine clearance and pressor effect in normal and hypertensive man. Klin Wochenschr 1980; 58:1175–1181.

1270. Sundlof G, Wallin BG. Muscle-nerve sympathetic activity in man. Relationship to blood pressure in resting normo- and hyper-tensive subjects. Clin Sci Mol Med 1978; 55(Suppl):387s–389s.

1271. Philipp TH, Distler A, Cordes U. Sympathetic nervous system and blood-pressure control in essential hypertension. Lancet 1978; 2:959–963.

1272. Philipp T, Distler A, Cordes U, et al. Plasma noradrenaline and the pressor action of exogenous noradrenaline in normotensive subjects and patients with essential hypertension. Clin Sci Mol Med 1978; 55(Suppl):61s–63s.

1273. Weidmann P, Keusch G, Flammer J, et al. Increased ratio between changes in blood pressure and plasma norepinephrine in essential hypertension. J Clin Endocrinol Metab 1979; 48:727–731.

1274. Weidmann P, Grimm M, Meier A, et al. Pathogenic and therapeutic significance of cardiovascular pressor reactivity as related to plasma catecholamines in borderline and established essential hypertension. Clin Exp Hypertens 1980; 2:427–449.

1275. Vlachakis ND. Blood pressure response to norepinephrine infusion in relationship to plasma catecholamines and renin activity in man. J Clin Pharmacol 1979; 19:654–661.

1276. Laurent S, Juillerat L, London GM, et al. Increased response of brachial artery diameter to norepinephrine in hypertensive patients. Am J Physiol 1988; 255:H36–H43.

1277. Bevan JA, Bevan RD, Chang PC, et al. Analysis of changes in reactivity of rabbit arteries and veins two weeks after induction of hypertension by coarctation of the abdominal aorta. Circ Res 1975; 37:183–190.

1278. Chalmers JP. Brain amines and models of experimental hypertension. Circ Res 1975; 36:469–480.

1279. Chalmers JP. Nervous system and hypertension. Clin Sci Mol Med 1978; 55(Suppl):45s–56s.

1280. Barnes KL, Brosnihan KB, Ferrario CM. Animal models, hypertension, and central nervous system mechanisms. Mayo Clin Proc 1977; 52:387–390.

1281. Esler M, Julius S, Zweifler A, et al. Mild high-renin essential hypertension: neurogenic human hypertension? N Engl J Med 1977; 296:405–411.

1282. Franco-Morselli R, Elghozi JL, Joly E, et al. Increased plasma adrenaline concentrations in benign essential hypertension. Br Med J 1977; 2:1251–1254.

1283. Franco-Morselli R, Baudouin-Legros M, Meyer P. Plasma adrenaline and noradrenaline in essential hypertension and after long-term treatment with beta-adrenoreceptor–blocking agents. Clin Sci Mol Med 1978; 55(Suppl):97s–100s.

1284. Campese VM, Romoff MS, Levitan D, et al. Abnormal relationship between sodium intake and sympathetic nervous system activity in salt-sensitive patients with essential hypertension. Kidney Int 1982; 21:371–378.

1285. Gill JR Jr, Gullner HG, Lake CR, et al. Plasma and urinary catecholamines in salt-sensitive idiopathic hypertension. Hypertension 1988; 11:312–319.

1286. Egan B, Panis R, Hinderliter A, et al. Mechanism of increased alpha adrenergic vasoconstriction in human essential hypertension. J Clin Invest 1987; 80:812–817.

1287. Tuck ML. The sympathetic nervous system in essential hypertension. Am Heart J 1986; 112:877–886.

1288. Folkow B, Di Bona GF, Hjemdahl P, et al. Measurements of plasma norepinephrine concentrations in human primary hypertension. A word of caution on their applicability for assessing neurogenic contributions. Hypertension 1983; 5:399–403.

1289. Eliasson K, Hjemdahl P, Kahan T. Circulatory and sympatho-adrenal responses to stress in borderline and established hypertension. J Hypertens 1983; 1:131–139.

1290. Esler M, Jennings G, Biviano B, et al. Mechanism of elevated plasma noradrenaline in the course of essential hypertension. J Cardiovasc Pharmacol 1986; 8(Suppl 5):S39–S43.

1291. Esler MD, Hasking GJ, Willett IR, et al. Noradrenaline release and sympathetic nervous system activity. J Hypertens 1985; 3:117–129.

1292. Esler MD, Jennings GL, Johns J, et al. Estimation of "total" renal, cardiac and splanchnic sympathetic nervous tone in essential hypertension from measurements of noradrenaline release. J Hypertens 1984; 2(Suppl 3):123–125.

1293. Hollenberg NK, Adams DF, Solomon H, et al. Renal vascular tone in essential and secondary hypertension: hemodynamic and angiographic responses to vasodilators. Medicine 1975; 54:29–44.

1294. Esler MD, Nestel PJ. Renin and sympathetic nervous system responsiveness to adrenergic stimuli in essential hypertension. Am J Cardiol 1973; 32:643–649.

1295. Hollenberg NK, Epstein M, Basch RI, et al. Renin secretion in essential and accelerated hypertension. Am J Med 1969; 47:845–859.

1296. DeQuattro V, Barbour BH, Campese V, et al. Sympathetic nerve hyperactivity in high-renin hypertension: effects of saralasin infusion. Mayo Clin Proc 1977; 52:369–373.

1297. Esler M, Zweifler A, Randall O, et al. Agreement among three different indices of sympathetic nervous system activity in essential hypertension. Mayo Clin Proc 1977; 52:379–382.

1298. Frohlich ED. Beta adrenergic blockade in the circulatory regulation of hyperkinetic states. Am J Cardiol 1971; 27:195–199.

1299. Esler MD, Julius S, Randall OS, et al. Relation of renin status to neurogenic vascular resistance in borderline hypertension. Am J Cardiol 1977; 36:708–715.

1300. DiBona GF, Sawin LL. Role of renal alpha-2-adrenergic receptors in spontaneously hypertensive rats. Hypertension 1987; 9:41–48.

1301. Michel MC, Insel PA, Brodde O-E. Renal alpha-adrenergic receptor alterations: a cause of essential hypertension? FASEB J 1989; 3:139–144.

1302. Landsberg L. Diet, obesity and hypertension: an hypothesis involving insulin, the sympathetic nervous system, and adaptive thermogenesis. Q J Med 1986; 236:1081–1090.

1303. Krieger DR, Landsberg L. Neuroendocrine mechanisms in obesity-related hypertension: the role of insulin and catecholamines. In: Laragh JH, Brenner B, Kaplan N, eds. Perspectives in Hypertension: Endocrine Mechanisms in Hypertension. New York: Raven, 1989: 105–128.

1304. Krieger DR, Landsberg L. Mechanisms in obesity-related hypertension: role of insulin and catecholamines. Am J Hypertens 1988; 1:84–90.

1305. Landsberg L, Krieger DR. Obesity, metabolism, and the sympathetic nervous system. Am J Hypertens 1989; 2:125S–132S.

1306. Shikuma R, Yoshimura M, Kambara S, et al. Dopaminergic modulation of salt sensitivity in patients with essential hypertension. Life Sci 1986; 38:915–921.

1307. Wilcox CS. Current therapy for orthostatic hypotension. J Cardiovasc Med 1983; 8:292–305.

1308. Thomas JE, Schirger A, Fealey RD, et al. Orthostatic hypotension. Mayo Clin Proc 1981; 56:117–125.

1309. Polinsky RJ, Kopin IJ, Ebert MH, et al. Pharmacologic distinction of different orthostatic hypotension syndromes. Neurology 1981; 31:1–7.

1310. Bannister R, Sever P, Gross M. Cardiovascular reflexes and biochemical responses in progressive autonomic failure. Brain 1977; 100:327–344.

1311. Kontos H, Richardson D, Norveli J. Norepinephrine depletion in idiopathic orthostatic hypotension. Ann Intern Med 1975; 82:336–341.

1312. Ziegler M, Lake R, Kopin I. The sympathetic nervous system defect in primary orthostatic hypotension. N Engl J Med 1977; 296:293–297.

1313. Hughes RC, Cartlidge WE, Milloc P. Primary neurogenic orthostatic hypotension. J Neurol Neurosurg Psychiatry 1970; 33:363–371.

1314. Johnson RH, Lee G de J, Oppenheimer DR, et al. Autonomic failure with orthostatic hypotension due to intermediolateral column degeneration: a report of two cases with autopsies. Q J Med 1966; 35:276–292.

1315. Esler M, Jackman G, Kelleher D, et al. Norepinephrine kinetics in patients with idiopathic autonomic insufficiency. Circ Res 1980; 46(Suppl):I47–I48.

1316. Polinsky RJ, Taylor IL, Chew P, et al. Pancreatic polypeptide responses to hypoglycemia in chronic autonomic failure. J Clin Endocrinol Metab 1982; 54:48–52.

1317. Niarchos AP, Magrini F, Tarazi RC, et al. Mechanism of spontaneous supine blood pressure variations in chronic autonomic insufficiency. Am J Med 1978; 65:547–552.

1318. Bannister R. Degeneration of the autonomic nervous system. Lancet 1971; 2:177–179.

1319. Shy GM, Drager GA. A neurologic syndrome associated with orthostatic hypotension. Arch Neurol 1960; 2:511–527.

1320. Hume L, Ewing DJ, Campbell IW, et al. Heart-rate response to sustained hand grip: comparison of the effects of cardiac autonomic blockade and diabetic autonomic neuropathy. Clin Sci 1979; 56:287–291.

1321. Suzuki T, Tsuge I, Higa S, et al. Catecholamine metabolism in familial amyloid polyneuropathy. Clin Genet 1979; 16:117–124.

1322. Rubenstein AE, Yahr MD, Mythilneou C, et al. Peripheral catecholamine depletion in amyloid autonomic neuropathy. Mt Sinai J Med 1978; 45:782–789.

1323. Christensen NJ. Plasma catecholamines in long-term diabetics with and without neuropathy and in hypophysectomized subjects. J Clin Invest 1972; 51:779–787.

1324. Cryer PE, Silverberg AB, Santiago JV, et al. Plasma catecholamines in diabetes. Am J Med 1978; 64:407–416.

1325. Nazar K, Taton J, Chwalbinska-Moneta J, et al. Adrenergic responses to sustained handgrip in patients with juvenile-onset–type diabetes mellitus. Clin Sci Mol Med 1975; 49:39–44.

1326. Neubauer B, Christensen NJ. Norepinephrine, epinephrine and dopamine contents of the cardiovascular system in long-term diabetics. Diabetes 1976; 25:6–10.

1327. Hopkins A, Neville B, Bannister R. Autonomic neuropathy of acute onset. Lancet 1974; 1:769–771.

1328. Brant PW, McKusick VA. Familial dysautonomia: a report of genetic and clinical studies, with a review of the literature. Medicine 1970; 49:343–374.

1329. Dancis J, Smith AA. Current concepts: familial dysautonomia. N Engl J Med 1966; 274:207–209.

1330. Smith AA, Taylor T, Wortis JB. Abnormal catecholamine metabolism in familial dysautonomia. N Engl J Med 1963; 268:705–707.

1331. Smith AA, Dancis J. Exaggerated response to infused norepinephrine in familial dysautonomia. N Engl J Med 1964; 270:704–710.

1332. Onrot J, Goldberg MR, Hollister AS, et al. Management of chronic orthostatic hypotension. Am J Med 1986; 80:454–464.

1333. Schatz IJ. Current management concepts in orthostatic hypotension. Arch Intern Med 1980; 140:1152–1154.

1334. Bannister R, Ardill L, Fentem P. An assessment of various methods of treatment of idiopathic orthostatic hypotension. Q J Med 1969; 38:377–395.

1335. Chobanian AV, Volicer L, Tifft CP, et al. Mineralocorticoid-induced hypertension in patients with orthostatic hypotension. N Engl J Med 1979; 301:68–73.

1336. Schirger A, Sheps SG, Thomas JE, et al. Midodrine: a new agent in the management of idiopathic orthostatic hypotension and Shy-Drager syndrome. Mayo Clin Proc 1981; 56:429–433.

1337. Seller RH. Idiopathic orthostatic hypotension: report of successful treatment with a new form of therapy. Am J Cardiol 1969; 23:838–844.

1338. Diamond MA, Murray RH, Schmid PG. Idiopathic postural hypotension: physiologic observations and report of a new mode of therapy. J Clin Invest 1970; 49:1341–1348.

1339. Kuchel O, Buu NT, Gutkowska J, et al. Treatment of severe orthostatic hypotension by metoclopramide. Ann Intern Med 1980; 93:841–843.

1340. Robertson D, Goldberg MR, Hollister AS, et al. Clonidine raises blood pressure in severe idiopathic orthostatic hypotension. Am J Med 1983; 74:193–200.

1341. Brodde O-E, Anlauf M, Arroyo J, et al. Hypersensitivity of adrenergic receptors and blood-pressure response to oral yohimbine in orthostatic hypotension. N Engl J Med 1983; 308:1033–1034.

1342. Polinsky RJ, Samaras GM, Kopin IJ. Sympathetic neural prosthesis for managing orthostatic hypotension. Lancet 1983; 1:901–904.

1343. Suzuki T, Higa S, Sakoda S, et al. Orthostatic hypotension in familial amyloid polyneuropathy: treatment with DL-threo-3,4-dihydroxyphenylserine. Neurology 1981; 31:1323–1326.

1344. Manger WM, Gifford RW Jr. Pheochromocytoma. New York: Springer-Verlag, 1977.

1345. Winkler H, Smith AD. Pheochromocytoma and other catecholamine producing tumors. In: Blaschko H, Muscholl E, eds. Catecholamines, Handbook of Experimental Pharmacology. Vol 33. Berlin: Springer-Verlag, 1972: 7:900–933.

1346. St John Sutton MG, Sheps SG, Lie JT. Prevalence of clinically unsuspected pheochromocytoma. Mayo Clin Proc 1981; 56:354–360.

1347. Engelman K. Pheochromocytoma. Clin Endocrinol Metab 1977; 6:769–797.

1348. Hermann H, Mornex R. Human Tumors Secreting Catecholamines. New York: Macmillan, 1964: 1–14.

1349. Thomas JE, Rooke ED, Kvale WF. The neurologist's experience with pheochromocytoma: a review of 100 cases. JAMA 1966; 197:100–104.

1350. Bravo EL, Tarazi RC, Fouad FM, et al. Blood pressure regulation in pheochromocytoma. Hypertension 1982; 4(Suppl 2):II193–II199.

1351. Mannelli M, DeFeo ML, Maggi M, et al. Effect of verapamil on catecholamine secretion by human pheochromocytoma. Hypertension 1986; 8:813–814.

1352. Sjoerdsma A, Engelman K, Waldmann TA, et al. Pheochromocytoma: current concepts of diagnosis and treatment. Ann Intern Med 1966; 65:1302–1326.

1353. Deoreo GA Jr, Stewart BH, Tarazi RC, et al. Preoperative blood transfusion in the safe surgical management of pheochromocytoma: a review of 46 cases. J Urol 1974; 111:715–721.

1354. Gupta KK. Phaeochromocytoma and myocardial infarction. Lancet 1975; 1:281–282.

1355. Radtke WE, Kazmier FJ, Rutherford BD, et al. Cardiovascular complications of pheochromocytoma crisis. Am J Cardiol 1975; 35:701–705.

1356. Short IA, Padfield PL. Malignant phaeochromocytoma with severe constipation and myocardial necrosis. Br Med J 1976; 2:793–794.

1357. Landsberg L. Pheochromocytoma. Med Grand Rounds 1983; 2:7–21.

1358. Van Vliet PD, Burchell HB, Titus JL. Focal myocarditis associated with pheochromocytoma. N Engl J Med 1966; 274:1102–1108.

1359. Northfield TC. Cardiac complications of phaeochromocytoma. Br Heart J 1967; 29:588–593.

1360. De Leeuw PW, Waltman FL, Birkenhager WH. Noncardiogenic pulmonary edema as the sole manifestation of pheochromocytoma. Hypertension 1986; 8:810–812.

1361. Fred HL, Allred DP, Garber HE, et al. Pheochromocytoma masquerading as overwhelming infection. Am Heart J 1967; 73:149–154.

1362. Colwell JA. Inhibition of insulin secretion by catecholamines in pheochromocytoma. Ann Intern Med 1969; 71:251–256.

1363. Stewart AF, Hoecker JL, Mallette LE, et al. Hypercalcemia in pheochromocytoma. Ann Intern Med 1985; 102:776–779.

1364. Kukreja SC, Hargis GK, Rosenthal IM, et al. Pheochromocytoma causing excessive parathyroid hormone production and hypercalcemia. Ann Intern Med 1973; 79:838–840.

1365. Miller SS, Sizemore GW, Sheps SG, et al. Parathyroid function in patients with pheochromocytoma. Ann Intern Med 1975; 82:372–375.

1366. Trump DL, Livingston JN, Baylin SB. Watery diarrhea syndrome in an adult with ganglioneuroma-pheochromocytoma. Identification of vasoactive intestinal peptide, calcitonin, and catecholamines and assessment of their biologic activity. Cancer 1977; 40:1526–1532.

1367. Viale G, Dell Orto P, Moro E, et al. Vasoactive intestinal polypeptide-, somatostatin-, and calcitonin-producing adreneal pheochromocytoma associated with the watery diarrhea (WDHH) syndrome: first case report with immunohistochemical findings. Cancer 1985; 55:1099–1106.

1368. Nigawara K, Suzuki T, Tazawa H, et al. A case of recurrent malignant pheochromocytoma complicated by watery diarrhea, hypokalemia, achlorhydria syndrome. J Clin Endocrinol Metab 1987; 65:1053–1056.

1369. Spark RF, Connolly PB, Gluckin DS, et al. ACTH secretion from a functioning pheochromocytoma. N Engl J Med 1979; 301:416–418.

1370. Forman BH, Marban E, Kayne RD, et al. Ectopic ACTH syndrome due to pheochromocytoma: case report and review of the literature. Yale J Biol Med 1979; 52:181–189.

1371. Shulkin BL, Shapiro B, Sisson JC. Pheochromocytoma, polycythemia, and venous thrombosis. Am J Med 1987; 83:773–776.

1372. Steiner AL, Goodman AD, Powers SR. Study of a kindred with pheochromocytoma, medullary thyroid carcinoma, hyperparathyroidism and Cushing's disease: multiple endocrine neoplasia, type 2. Medicine 1968; 47:371–409.

1373. Dunn FG, DeCarvalho JGR, Kem DC, et al. Pheochromocytoma crisis induced by saralasin; relation of angiotensin analogue to catecholamine release. N Engl J Med 1976; 295:605–607.

1374. Plouin PF, Menard J, Corvol P. Hypertensive crisis in patient with phaeochromocytoma given metoclopramide. Lancet 1976; 2:1357–1358.

1375. Bittar DA. Innovar-induced hypertensive crises in patients with pheochromocytoma. Anesthesiology 1979; 50:366–369.

1376. Fraley DS, Lemoncelli GL, Coleman A. Severe hypertension associated with pancuronium bromide. Anesth Analg 1978; 57:265–267.

1377. Jones RM, Hill AB. Severe hypertension associated with pancuronium in a patient with a phaeochromocytoma. Can Anaesth Soc J 1981; 28:394–396.

1378. Gifford RW Jr, Kvale WF, Maher FT, et al. Clinical features, diagnosis and treatment of pheochromocytoma: a review of 76 cases. Mayo Clin Proc 1964; 39:281–302.

1379. Karsner HT. Tumors of the adrenal. In: Atlas to Tumor Pathology. Sect VIII. Fascicle 29. Washington, DC: Armed Forces Institute of Pathology, 1950: 41–55.

1380. Carney JA, Sizemore GW, Sheps SG. Adrenal medullary disease in multiple endocrine neoplasia, type 2: pheochromocytoma and its precursors. Am J Clin Pathol 1976; 66:279–290.

1381. Saad MF, Frazier OH, Hickey RC, et al. Intrapericardial pheochromocytoma. Am J Med 1983; 75:371–376.

1382. Soejima H, Ogawa O, Nomura Y, et al. Pheochromocytoma of the spermatic cord: a case report. J Urol 1977; 118:495–496.

1383. Melicow MM. One hundred cases of pheochromocytoma (107 tumors) at the Columbia-Presbyterian Medical Center, 1926–1979. A clinico-pathological analysis. Cancer 1977; 40:1987–2004.

1384. Bogaert MG, Vermeulen A. Pheochromocytoma of the urinary bladder, with inconclusive chemical and pharmacologic tests. Am J Med 1972; 53:797–800.

1385. Raper AJ, Jessee EF, Texter JH Jr, et al. Pheochromocytoma of the urinary bladder: a broad clinical spectrum. Am J Cardiol 1977; 40:820–824.

1386. Rosenwasser H. Glomus jugulare tumours. Proc R Soc Med 1974; 67:259–270.

1387. Hens L, Plets C, Dom R, et al. Catecholamine secreting tumor of the glomus jugulare. Klin Wochenschr 1979; 57:741–746.

1388. Duke WW, Boshell BR, Soteres P, et al. A norepinephrine-secreting glomus jugulare tumor presenting as a pheochromocytoma. Ann Intern Med 1964; 60:1040–1047.

1389. Roth RH, Stjarne L, Levine RJ, et al. Abnormal regulation of catecholamine synthesis in pheochromocytoma. J Lab Clin Med 1968; 72:397–403.

1390. Nagatsu T, Yamamoto T, Nagatsu I. Partial separation and properties of tyrosine hydroxylase from the human pheochromocytoma: effect of norepinephrine. Biochim Biophys Acta 1970; 198:210–218.

1391. Waymire JC, Weiner N, Schneider FH, et al. Tyrosine hydroxylase in human adrenal and pheochromocytoma: localization, kinetics and catecholamine inhibition. J Clin Invest 1972; 51:1798–1804.

1392. Jarrott B, Louis WJ. Abnormalities in enzymes involved in catecholamine synthesis and catabolism in phaeochromocytoma. Clin Sci Mol Med 1977; 53:529–535.

1393. Levey GS, Weiss SR, Ruiz E. Characterization of the glucagon receptor in a pheochromocytoma. J Clin Endocrinol Metab 1975; 40:720–723.

1394. Engelman K, Sjoerdsma A. The adrenal medulla: catecholamines and pheochromocytoma. In: Clinician—I, The Adrenal Gland. New York: Medcom, 1971: 111–125.

1395. Page LB, Copeland RB. Pheochromocytoma. DM 1968; 1:1–40.

1396. Hamilton BPM, Landsberg L, Levine RJ. Sipple's syndrome: familial medullary carcinoma of the thyroid, hyperparathyroidism and epinephrine-secreting pheochromocytoma. Endocr Soc Abstr 1974; A244.

1397. Engelman K, Hammond WG. Adrenaline production by an intrathoracic phaeochromocytoma. Lancet 1968; 1:609–611.

1398. Crout JR. Pheochromocytoma. Pharmacol Rev 1966; 18:651–657.

1399. Lundberg JM, Hamberger B, Schultzberg M, et al. Enkephalin- and somatostatin-like immunoreactivities in human adrenal medulla and pheochromocytoma. Proc Natl Acad Sci USA 1979; 76:4079–4083.

1400. Yoshimasa T, Nakao K, Oki S, et al. Presence of dynorphin-like immunoreactivity in pheochromocytomas. J Clin Endocrinol Metab 1981; 53:213–214.

1401. Yanase T, Nawata H, Kato K-I, et al. Studies on adrenorphin in pheochromocytoma. J Clin Endocrinol Metab 1987; 64:692–697.

1402. O'Connor DT, Frigon RP, Deftos LJ. Immunoreactive calcitonin in catecholamine storage vesicles of human pheochromocytoma. J Clin Endocrinol Metab 1983; 56:582–585.

1403. Heath H III, Edis AJ. Pheochromocytoma associated with hypercalcemia and ectopic secretion of calcitonin. Ann Intern Med 1979; 91:208–210.

1404. Grouzmann E, Comoy E, Bohuon C. Plasma neuropeptide Y concentrations in patients with neuroendocrine tumors. J Clin Endocrinol Metab 1989; 68:808–813.

1405. Carman CT, Brashear RE. Pheochromocytoma as an inherited abnormality. N Engl J Med 1960; 263:419–423.

1406. Ljungberg O. On medullary carcinoma of the thyroid. Acta Pathol Microbiol Scand (A) 1972; Suppl 321:1–56.

1407. Melvin KEW, Tashjian AH Jr, Miller HH. Studies in familial (medullary) thyroid carcinoma. Recent Prog Horm Res 1972; 28:399–470.

1408. Hamilton BPM, Landsberg L, Levine RJ, et al. Sipple's syndrome: results of screening a large family. Clin Res 1973; 21:979A.

1409. Ballard HS, Frame B, Hartsock RJ. Familial multiple-endocrine adenoma–peptic ulcer complex. Medicine 1964; 43:481–516.

1410. Carney JA, Go VLW, Gordon H, et al. Familial pheochromocytoma and islet cell tumor of the pancreas. Am J Med 1980; 68:515–521.

1411. Janson KL, Roberts JA, Varela M. Multiple endocrine adenomatosis: in support of the common origin theories. J Urol 1978; 119:161–165.

1412. Tateishi R, Wada A, Ishiguro SM, et al. Coexistence of bilateral pheochromocytoma and pancreatic islet cell tumor. Cancer 1978; 42:2929–2934.

1413. Cameron D, Spiro HM. Zollinger-Ellison syndrome with multiple endocrine adenomatosis type II. N Engl J Med 1978; 299:152–153.

1414. Sipple JH. The association of pheochromocytoma with carcinoma of the thyroid gland. Am J Med 1961; 31:163–166.

1415. Manning PC Jr, Molnar GD, Black BM, et al. Pheochromocytoma, hyperparathyroidism and thyroid carcinoma occurring coincidentally: report of case. N Engl J Med 1963; 268:68–72.

1416. Sarosi G, Doe RP. Familial occurrence of parathyroid adenomas, pheochromocytoma and medullary carcinoma of the thyroid with amyloid stroma (Sipple's syndrome). Ann Intern Med 1968; 68:1305–1309.

1417. DeLellis RA, Wolfe HJ, Gagel RF, et al. Adrenal medullary hyperplasia: a morphometric analysis in patients with familial medullary thyroid carcinoma. Am J Pathol 1976; 83:177–196.

1418. Landsberg L. Catecholamines and the sympathoadrenal system. In: Ingbar SH, ed. The Year in Endocrinology. New York: Plenum, 1976: 177–231.

1419. Hamilton BP, Landsberg L, Levine RJ. Measurement of urinary epinephrine in screening for pheochromocytoma in multiple endocrine neoplasia type II. Am J Med 1978; 65:1027–1032.

1420. Chong GC, Beahrs OH, Sizemore GW, et al. Medullary carcinoma of the thyroid gland. Cancer 1975; 35:695–704.

1421. Siqueira-Filho AG, Sheps SG, Maher FT, et al. Glucagon-blood catecholamine test. Arch Intern Med 1975; 135:1227–1231.

1422. Cervi-Skinner SJ. Case record of the Massachusetts General Hospital. N Engl J Med 1973; 289:472–479.

1423. Gagel RF, Tashjian AH Jr, Cummings T, et al. The clinical outcome of prospective screening for multiple endocrine neoplasia type 2a. N Engl J Med 1988; 318:478–484.

1424. Khairi MRA, Dexter RN, Burzynski NJ, et al. Mucosal neuroma, pheochromocytoma and medullary thyroid carcinoma: multiple endocrine neoplasia type 3. Medicine 1975; 54:89–112.

1425. Das Gupta TK, Brasfield RD. Von Recklinghausen's disease. CA 1971; 21:174–183.

1426. Glushien AS, Mansuy MM, Littman DS. Pheochromocytoma: its relationship to the neurocutaneous syndromes. Am J Med 1953; 14:318–327.

1427. Horton WA, Wong V, Eldridge R. Von Hippel-Lindau disease: clinical and pathological manifestations in nine families with 50 affected members. Arch Intern Med 1976; 136:769–777.

1428. Jones DH, Reid JL, Hamilton CA, et al. The biochemical diagnosis, localization and follow up of phaeochromocytoma: the role of plasma and urinary catecholamine measurements. Q J Med 1980; 49:341–361.

1429. Duncan MW, Compton P, Lazarus L, et al. Measurement of norepinephrine and 3,4-dihydroxyphenylglycol in urine and plasma for the diagnosis of pheochromocytoma. N Engl J Med 1988; 319:135–142.

1430. Pisano JJ, Crout JR, Abraham D. Determination of 3-methoxy 4-hydroxy mandelic acid in urine. Clin Chim Acta 1962; 7:285–291.

1431. Pisano JJ. A simple analysis for normetanephrine and metanephrine in urine. Clin Chim Acta 1960; 5:406–414.

1432. Bravo EL, Tarazi RC, Gifford RW, et al. Circulating and urinary catecholamines in pheochromocytoma. Diagnostic and pathophysiologic implications. N Engl J Med 1979; 301:682–686.

1433. Bravo EL, Tarazi RC, Fouad RM, et al. Clonidine-suppression test: a useful aid in the diagnosis of pheochromocytoma. N Engl J Med 1981; 305:623–626.

1434. Brown MJ, Jenner DA, Allison DJ, et al. Increased sensitivity and accuracy of phaeochromocytoma diagnosis achieved by use of plasma-adrenaline estimations and a pentolinium-suppression test. Lancet 1981; 1:174–177.

1435. Hui TP, Krakoff LR, Felton K, et al. Diuretic treatment alters clonidine suppression of plasma norepinephrine. Hypertension 1986; 8:272–276.

1436. MacDougall IC, Isles CG, Stewart H, et al. Overnight clonidine suppression test in the diagnosis and exclusion of pheochromocytoma. Am J Med 1988; 84:993–1000.

1437. Sheps SG, Maher FT. Histamine and glucagon tests in diagnosis of pheochromocytoma. JAMA 1968; 205:895–899.

1438. Engelman K, Horwitz D, Ambrose IM, et al. Further evaluation of the tyramine test for pheochromocytoma. N Engl J Med 1968; 278:705–709.

1439. Hunyor SN, Hansson L, Harrison TS, et al. Effects of clonidine withdrawal: possible mechanisms and suggestions for management. Br Med J 1973; 22:209–211.

1440. Hansson L, Hunyor SN, Julius S, et al. Blood pressure crisis following withdrawal of clonidine (Catapres, Catapresan), with special reference to arterial and urinary catecholamine levels, and suggestions for acute management. Am Heart J 1973; 85:605–610.

1441. Oates HF, Stoker LM, Monaghan JC, et al. Withdrawal of clonidine: effects of varying dosage or duration of treatment on subsequent blood pressure and heart rate responses. J Pharmacol Exp Ther 1978; 206:268–273.

1442. Hunyor SN, Bailey RR. Rapid clonidine withdrawal with blood pressure overshoot exaggerated by beta-blockade. Br Med J 1973; 2:209.

1443. Cairns SA, Marshall AJ. Clonidine withdrawal. Lancet 1976; 1:368.

1444. Brandenburg RO, Gutnik LM, Nelson RL, et al. Factitial epinephrine-only secreting pheochromocytoma. Ann Intern Med 1979; 90:795–796.

1445. Cameron SJ, Doig A. Cerebellar tumors presenting with clinical features of pheochromocytoma. Lancet 1970; 1:492–494.

1446. Evans CH, Westfall V, Atuk NO. Astrocytoma mimicking the features of pheochromocytoma. N Engl J Med 1972; 286:1397–1399.

1447. Emanuele MA, Dorsch TR, Scarff TB, et al. Basilar artery aneurysm simulating pheochromocytoma. Neurology 1981; 31:1560–1561.

1448. Gitlow SE, Mendlowitz M, Bertani LM. The biochemical techniques for detecting and establishing the presence of a pheochromocytoma: a review of ten years' experience. Am J Cardiol 1970; 26:270–279.

1449. Metz SA, Halter JB, Porte D, et al. Autonomic epilepsy: clonidine blockade of paroxysmal catecholamine release and flushing. Ann Intern Med 1978; 88:189–193.

1450. Horwitz D, Sjoerdsma A. Some interrelationships between elevation of blood pressure and angina pectoris. In: Hypertension XIII. Proceedings of Council for High Blood Pressure Research. New York: American Heart Association, 1965: 39–48.

1451. Cubeddu LX, Zarate NA, Rosales CB, et al. Prazosin and propranolol in preoperative management of pheochromocytoma. Clin Pharmacol Ther 1982; 32:156–160.

1452. Fraser DG. Alpha-MPT and pheochromocytoma. Drug Intell Clin Pharm 1979; 13:597.

1453. Prinz RA, Brooks HM, Churchill R, et al. Incidental asymptomatic adrenal masses detected by computed tomographic scanning. Is operation required? JAMA 1982; 248:701–704.

1454. Mitnick JS, Bosniak MA, Megibow AJ, et al. Non-functioning adrenal adenomas discovered incidentally on computed tomography. Radiology 1983; 148:495–499.

1455. Glazer HS, Weyman PJ, Sagel SS, et al. Nonfunctioning adrenal masses: incidental discovery on computed tomography. AJR 1982; 139:81–85.

1456. Copeland PM. The incidentally discovered adrenal mass. Ann Surg 1984; 199:116–122.

1457. Stewart BH, Bravo EL, Haaga J, et al. Localization of pheochromocytoma by computed tomography. N Engl J Med 1981; 299:460–461.

1458. Laursen K, Damgaard-Pedersen K. CT for pheochromocytoma diagnosis. AJR 1980; 134:277–280.

1459. Thomas JL, Berardino ME, Samaan NA, et al. CT of pheochromocytoma. AJR 1980; 135:477–482.

1460. Hussain S, Belldegrun A, Seltzer SE, et al. Differentiation of malignant from benign adrenal masses: predictive indices on computed tomography. AJR 1985; 144:61–65.

1461. Geelhoed GW. CAT scans and catecholamines. Surgery 1980; 87:719–720.

1462. Schultz CL, Haaga JR, Fletcher BD, et al. Magnetic resonance imaging of the adrenal glands: a comparison with computed tomography. AJR 1984; 143:1235–1240.

1463. Reinig JW, Doppman JL. Magnetic resonance imaging of the adrenal. Radiologe 1986; 26:186–190.

1464. McCorkell SJ, Niles NL. Fine-needle aspiration of catecholamine-producing adrenal masses: a possibly fatal mistake. AJR 1985; 145:113–114.

1465. Rossi P, Young IS, Panke WF. Techniques, usefulness and hazards of arteriography of pheochromocytoma: review of 99 cases. JAMA 1968; 205:547–553.

1466. Boijsen E, Williams CM, Judkins MP. Angiography of pheochromocytoma. AJR 1966; 98:225–232.

1467. DeQuattro V, Margolin AH, Stocks LO. Pseudopheochromocytoma—adrenomedullary response to venography. J Clin Endocrinol Metab 1970; 30:138–140.

1468. Sisson JC, Frager MS, Valk TW, et al. Scintigraphic localization of pheochromocytoma. N Engl J Med 1981; 305:12–17.

1469. Valk TW, Frager MS, Gross MD, et al. Spectrum of pheochromocytoma in multiple endocrine neoplasia. Ann Intern Med 1981; 94:762–767.

1470. Palubinskas AJ, Roizen MR, Conte FA. Localization of functioning pheochromocytomas by venous sampling and radioenzymatic analysis. Radiology 1980; 136:495–496.

1471. Ross EJ, Prichard BNC, Kaufman L, et al. Preoperative and operative management of patients with phaeochromocytoma. Br Med J 1971; 1:191–198.

1472. Gitlow SE, Pertsemlidis D, Bertani LM. Management of patients with pheochromocytoma. Am Heart J 1971; 82:557–567.

1473. Keiser HR, Goldstein DS, Wade JL, et al. Treatment of malignant pheochromocytoma with combination chemotherapy. Hypertension 1985; 7(Suppl):I18–I24.

1474. Averbuch SD, Steakley CS, Young RC, et al. Malignant pheochromocytoma: effective treatment with a combination of cyclophosphamide, vincristine, and dacarbazine. Ann Intern Med 1988; 109:267–273.

1475. Fudge TL, McKinnon WMP, Geary WL. Current surgical management of pheochromocytoma during pregnancy. Arch Surg 1980; 115:1224–1225.

1476. Remine WH, Chong GC, Van Heerden JA, et al. Current management of pheochromocytoma. Ann Surg 1974; 179:740–748.

1477. Landsberg L. Pheochromocytoma. In: JF Fries, GE Ehrlich, eds. Prognosis. Bowie, MD: Charles Press Publishers, 1981; 413–416.

1478. Harken JL, Reed RJ. Tumors of the peripheral nervous system. In: Atlas of Tumor Pathology. 2nd Series. Fascicle 3. Washington, DC: Armed Forces Institute of Pathology, 1969: 137–151.

1479. Anton AH, Sayre DF. The distribution of dopamine and dopa in various animals and a method for their determination in diverse biological material. J Pharmacol Exp Ther 1964; 145:326–336.

1480. Voorhess ML, Gardner LI. Urinary excretion of norepinephrine, epinephrine and a 3-methoxy-4-hydroxymandelic acid by children with neuroblastoma. J Clin Endocrinol Metab 1961; 21:321–335.

1481. Gitlow SE, Bertani LM, Rausen A, et al. Diagnosis of neuroblastoma by qualitative and quantitative determination of catecholamine metabolites in urine. Cancer 1970; 25:1377–1383.

1482. Voorhess ML. The catecholamines in tumor and urine from patients with neuroblastoma, ganglioneuroblastoma and pheochromocytoma. J Pediatr Surg 1968; 3:146–155.

1483. Laug WE, Siegel ST, Shaw KNF, et al. Initial urinary catecholamine metabolite concentrations and prognosis in neuroblastoma. Pediatrics 1978; 62:77–83.

1484. Conference on the Biology of Neuroblastoma. J Pediatr Surg 1968; 3:103–193.

1485. Perez CA, Vietti TJ, Ackerman LV, et al. Treatment of malignant sympathetic tumors in children: clinicopathological correlation. Pediatrics 1968; 41:452–462.

1486. Priebe CJ, Clatworthy HW. Neuroblastoma: evaluation of the treatment of 90 children. Arch Surg 1967; 95:538–545.

1487. Hamilton JR, Radde IC, Johnson G. Diarrhea associated with adrenal ganglioneuroma. Am J Med 1968; 44:453–463.

11

ENDOCRINE HYPERTENSION

Norman M. Kaplan

INTRODUCTION

Endocrine disorders are responsible for only a small fraction of the cases of hypertension. However, because hypertension is so common, afflicting one sixth or more of adults, even small fractions represent thousands of patients. Moreover, endocrine dysfunctions may be involved, directly and indirectly, in the pathogenesis of hypertension in patients now classified as having essential or idiopathic or primary hypertension. Before considering the specific endocrine disorders responsible for secondary hypertension—almost all of which involve excessive secretion or intake of a specific hormone—general information about hypertension and the possible role of endocrine dysfunction in the primary form of the disease is presented.

Identification of Hypertension

Elevated blood pressure is one of the major risk factors for the cardiovascular diseases that cause most deaths in developed societies, and attempts have been made to identify and treat all persons with hypertension.[1] Because the disease is usually asymptomatic for 10 to 20 y (until vascular damage interferes with target organ function), it is necessary to screen the entire population. As more and more asympto-

matic people have been found to be hypertensive and treated effectively, the percentage of the U.S. population between ages 25 and 74 with unrecognized elevated blood pressure (systolic pressure 160 mm Hg or higher or diastolic pressure 95 mm Hg or higher) has diminished[2] (Fig. 11–1). The widespread control of hypertension is probably responsible in large part for the dramatic decline in mortality from strokes and heart failure since 1968.[3]

However, it is important not to label and treat inappropriately people who are not persistently hypertensive. Variability in blood pressure makes it necessary to use conservative guidelines for the diagnosis of hypertension, including measurement of blood pressure on three or more occasions.[1] In most surveys, more than one third of the people with diastolic pressures higher than 95 mm Hg at the initial screening have values lower than 90 mm Hg on re-examination.[4] Moreover, about one fifth of the patients with persistently elevated blood pressure in a physician's office have normal pressure outside of the office, i.e., "white coat hypertension."[5] In addition, "pseudohypertension," in which atherosclerotic stiffness of arteries prevents their collapse under a balloon cuff, may be a common problem in the elderly.[6]

Although it is important to prevent the inappropriate labeling of normotensive people as hypertensive—a step that

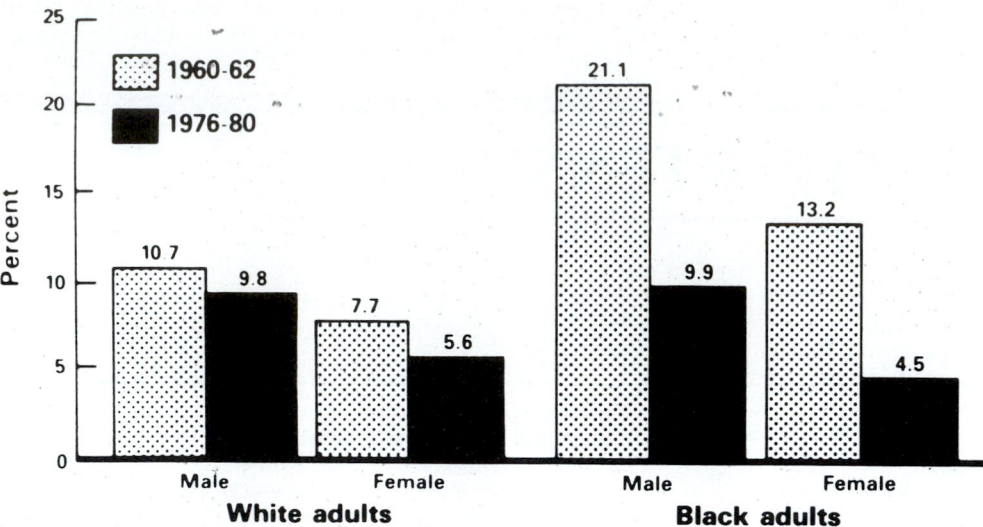

Figure 11–1. Percentage of people 18 to 74 y of age with undiagnosed hypertension, by race and sex in the United States, 1960 to 1962 and 1976 to 1980. (Data from Rowland M, Roberts J. NCHS advance data, vital and health statistics of the National Center for Health Statistics. No. 84, Oct 8, 1982. Washington, DC: U.S. Department of Health and Human Services, 1982.)

may lead to increased absenteeism from work and the worsening of overall health[7]—those who are hypertensive must be identified and directed to a healthier lifestyle and, if required, drug therapy. All people who have even transiently high blood pressure should be made aware of their readings and advised to make changes in lifestyle to reduce the likelihood of developing permanent hypertension—weight reduction for the obese, moderate sodium restriction, regular exercise, and moderation of alcohol intake.[8]

Evaluation for Endocrine Hypertension

After hypertension is diagnosed it is necessary to exclude secondary causes. The routine work-up should include a complete history and physical examination, with laboratory testing limited to a hematocrit, urinalysis, automated blood chemistry tests (including total and high-density-lipoprotein cholesterol), and an electrocardiogram. Additional laboratory testing should be obtained only if features inappropriate to uncomplicated primary or essential hypertension are noted (Table 11–1). The various secondary causes of hypertension are rare in relatively unselected populations[9–11] (Table 11–2). In contrast, secondary diseases are more frequent among patients referred to hypertension centers. Among 3520 patients evaluated in the Endocrine Section at the State University of New York Upstate Medical Center, 3% had renovascular hypertension.[12]

The low figures for secondary forms of hypertension noted in Table 11–2 could underestimate the true preva-

lence of secondary hypertension, because many patients were not adequately tested, but they are probably near the actual frequency. In fact, even these lower figures may be high for the overall hypertensive population because some of the data[10, 11] were obtained from patients with severe hypertension, in whom a higher prevalence of secondary forms is expected. Nevertheless, many patients with secondary forms of hypertension go unrecognized. During a 50-y period at the Mayo Clinic, 54 cases of pheochromocytoma were found at autopsy, only 13 of which had been correctly diagnosed during life. The unrecognized pheochromocytomas were believed to be involved in the deaths of 30 of the remaining 41 patients.[13]

Pros and Cons of Testing

Despite the relative rarity of the endocrine causes of hypertension, clinicians may perform additional tests for these disorders for several reasons.

1. Many patients have symptoms and signs suggestive of an endocrine disorder. For every patients with a pheochromocytoma, there are probably 100 with symptoms that mimic those seen in pheochromocytoma.

2. The recognition of an endocrine disorder can be curative. The management of hundreds of ordinary hyper-

---

TABLE 11–1. Features of Inappropriate Hypertension

1. Onset before age 20 or after age 50 y
2. Markedly elevated pressures (e.g., >200/120)
3. Organ damage
   a. Funduscopic findings of grade 2 or higher
   b. Serum creatinine level >0.15 mmol/L (>1.5mg/dL)
   c. Cardiomegaly (on x-ray film) or left ventricular hypertrophy (on electrocardiogram)
4. Features indicative of secondary causes
   a. Unprovoked hypokalemia
   b. Abdominal diastolic bruit
   c. Variable pressures with tachycardia, sweating, tremor
   d. Family history of renal or endocrine disease
   e. Hematuria, palpable kidneys
   f. Decreased femoral pulses
5. Poor response to usually effective therapy

From Kaplan NM. Clinical Hypertension. 5th ed. Baltimore: Williams & Wilkins, 1990. © 1990, the Williams and Wilkins Co., Baltimore.

TABLE 11–2. Frequency of Various Diagnoses in Hypertensive Subjects

Diagnosis	Percentage		
	Rudnick et al.	Danielson and Dammstrom	Sinclair et al.
Essential hypertension	94	95.3	92.1
Chronic renal disease	5	2.4	5.6
Renovascular disease	0.2	1.0	0.7
Coarctation	0.2		
Primary aldosteronism		0.1	0.3
Cushing syndrome	0.2	0.1	0.1
Pheochromocytoma		0.2	0.1
Oral contraceptive induced	0.2	0.8	1.0
Number of patients	655	1000	3783

Data from Rudnick KV, Sackett DL, Hirst S, et al. Hypertension in a family practice. Can Med Assoc J 1977; 117:492–497; Danielson M, Dammstrom B. The prevalence of secondary and curable hypertension. Acta Med Scand 1981; 209:451–458; and Sinclair AM, Isles CG, Brown I, et al. Secondary hypertension in a blood pressure clinic. Arch Intern Med 1987; 147:1289–1293.

tensives with diuretic-induced hypokalemia is lightened by the cure of even one patient with primary aldosteronism.

3. The relief of endocrine hypertension has become easier and more reliable. Transluminal renal artery dilation may relieve renovascular hypertension in patients unable to withstand major vascular surgery.

4. The search is relatively easy and relatively inexpensive. A normal spot urine metanephrine determination excludes the diagnosis of pheochromocytoma with virtual certainty.

5. Because of the difficulty of maintaining patients on lifelong antihypertensive drug therapy and because of the potential hazards of such therapy, the possibility of cure is even more attractive. Furthermore, if left untreated, curable lesions may induce vascular hypertrophy and nephrosclerosis that make the hypertension permanent even if the underlying cause is eventually removed.[14]

6. There is widespread suspicion that the endocrine causes are more common than the surveys reveal. Because adrenal tumors are now identified by abdominal computed tomographic scanning in many patients who have no obvious manifestations of adrenal dysfunction, some clinicians assume that even more detailed examinations of adrenal function should be done in more patients.

One the other hand, there are equally strong arguments to limit the search for endocrine hypertension.

1. Most endocrine disorders have symptoms and signs that are distinct from common nonspecific findings in the general population. The truncal obesity, thin skin, and muscle weakness of Cushing syndrome are distinct from the generalized obesity, postpregnancy striae, and fatigue that are common in middle-aged women with essential hypertension. Clinical judgment can usually separate the two without the need for adrenal suppression tests.

2. Because the endocrine disorders are unusual, most with a prevalence well below 1%, screening tests with relatively high sensitivity and specificity more often result in false-positive findings than in diagnoses. Even with a test such as the urine metanephrine test, which has a sensitivity approaching 100% and a specificity of 98%, the predictive value of a positive result is only 20%, assuming that the prevalence of pheochromocytoma is 0.5% of the hypertensive population (probably an overestimate). Many tests have less specificity, so that positive test results are more likely falsely positive, requiring additional tests, which are often expensive and uncomfortable and have a low predictive value.

3. The total cost of multiple screening tests done routinely in hypertensive patients would be enormous. If each test costs $40, this figure, when multiplied by 30 million patients, would result in a total cost of more than $1 billion.

4. The continued search for unlikely etiologies causes anxiety and resistance to the use of therapies designed to control hypertension.

5. The occasional oversight of a subtle endocrine hypertension usually causes no major disability. Such endocrinopathies usually become more obvious with time, during which the hypertension can usually be treated successfully with nonspecific drugs. Thus patients are usually none the worse for the delay.

6. As already stated, in most series of unselected patients these diseases are unusual. For example, in population surveys the annual incidence of primary aldosteronism is less than 1 per million people.[15]

Thus the prudent physician should limit additional tests to patients with features of inappropriate hypertension, while recognizing that even among such patients careful selection is needed and that in most patients there is no recognizable cause. This is also true for children with hypertension. More and more children are now being found to have mild, uncomplicated hypertension, and in most cases there is no secondary cause.

ENDOCRINE PARTICIPATION IN PRIMARY (ESSENTIAL) HYPERTENSION

No single, specific mechanism has been identified as the cause of the slowly rising blood pressure that occurs in most people who develop combined systolic and diastolic hypertension.

The failure to identify a specific cause for primary (combined) hypertension lends support to the mosaic concept of Irvine Page, who visualized the process as the interaction of a host of pressor and depressor mechanisms.[16] Sufficient insight has been obtained into the pathogenesis of this condition to allow the following conclusions:

Heredity is responsible for a predilection that allows environmental factors to exert their influence.[17]

Abnormalities, possibly inherited, in the structure of phospholipids in cell membranes may be markers for the predisposition to hypertension or, more important, primary defects that lead to an increase in vascular tone and thickness.[18]

Excessive amounts of short-acting pressor hormones are present relatively early in the developmental phase, including catecholamines,[19] renin-angiotensin,[20] and insulin;[21] the role of a somewhat longer-acting pressor substance, endothelin, which is derived from endothelium and works over a period ranging from minutes to hours, remains uncertain.[22]

The maintenance of sustained hypertension, however it starts, depends on increased peripheral resistance caused by hypertrophy of vessel walls.[23]

Trophic substances that can induce vascular hypertrophy include the same short-acting pressor substances previously listed, as well as additional endocrine, paracrine, and autocrine growth factors[24] (Table 11–3).

TABLE 11–3. Autocrine and Paracrine Influences on Blood Vessel Growth

Platelet derived	
Prostaglandins	Platelet-derived growth factor
Leukotrienes	Epidermal growth factor
Serotonin	Transforming growth factor β
	Thrombospondin
Endothelium derived	
Platelet-derived growth factor	Prostaglandins
Endothelial-derived growth factor	Thrombin
Interleukin 1	Fibroblast growth factor
Myocyte derived	
Platelet-derived growth factor	Prostaglandins
Insulin-like growth factor	Thrombospondin
Interleukin 1	Heparin
Neurally derived	
Norepinephrine	
Matrix	
Thrombospondin	Collagen
Fibronectin	Elastin

From Dzau VJ, Gibbons GH. Cell biology of vascular hypertrophy in systemic hypertension. Am J Cardiol 1988; 62:30G–35G.

At the same time, vasodilatory forces release an endothelium-derived relaxing factor, which may be nitric oxide.[25] This factor and other endogenous vasodilators, including atrial natriuretic factor, have been linked to elevations in the level of cyclic guanosine 3',5'-monophosphate,[26] but the method by which they induce vascular relaxation remains unknown. It is clear, however, that the normal circulation undergoes constant fine tuning by the interplay of relaxing and constricting factors, some of which arise from the endothelium itself.

Vascular Hypertrophy

Abnormalities in the functions of one or more of the relaxing and constricting factors may be involved in the development of hypertension.[27] Regardless, the perpetuation of hypertension clearly depends on the development of vascular hypertrophy. Such structural hypertrophy explains the hemodynamics of established hypertension, as shown by Folkow,[28] and is responsible for the increased tone and enhanced contractility in response to various pressor agents that are believed to play a functional role in the pathogenesis of hypertension. Small resistance vessels in subcutaneous tissue from hypertensive subjects have an average 29% increase in the ratio of media thickness to lumen diameter.[29] The in vitro response of these vessels to various pressor agents is either unchanged or depressed, which suggests that the increased contractility that is induced by pressor agents in vivo is caused by the increased muscle mass. As noted by Swales,[18] "In hypertension, there [is] no evidence for an overactive calcium second messenger system or indeed for any form of hyperresponsiveness, despite claims to the contrary over the preceding three decades. Instead, the conspicuous abnormality is hypertrophy giving rise to a generalized increase in contractility."

The search for the pathogenesis of sustained hypertension, then, must concentrate on vascular hypertrophy. The search has been further focused by recognition that multiple pressor substances serve as growth or trophic factors for vascular hypertrophy. This knowledge has come, in part, from the study of the secondary forms of endocrine hypertension, including pheochromocytoma, primary aldosteronism, and renovascular disease. Each of these causes is known to result from the direct effect of a specific pressor hormone, but, regardless of the initial hormonal action, whether it is volume retention as with primary aldosteronism or vasoconstriction as with pheochromocytoma or renovascular disease, maintenance of hypertension requires vascular hypertrophy that increases peripheral resistance, the process referred to as the "slow mechanism" by Anthony Lever in his review,[30] on which much of the following construct is based.

Lever starts with the original proposal of Folkow (Fig. 11–2), in which hypertension is initiated by a minor overactivity of a specific fast-acting pressor mechanism (A) that raises blood pressure slightly, initiating a positive feedback (BCB) that induces the vascular hypertrophy responsible for the maintenance of hypertension. The amplification (BCB) is "slowly progressive, ultimately large and probably nonspecific. Thus, different forms of chronic hypertension may resemble each other because part of the hypertension in each has the same mechanism."[30] Lever adds the action of a genetically determined hypertrophic response to pressure (D), as in the spontaneously hypertensive rat. Any inherited abnormality in the cell membrane could serve as this reinforced hypertrophic response to pressure (D). More important, one or more trophic mechanisms (E) contribute to the hypertrophy.

Lever cites renovascular hypertension as one model in which hypertension is initiated by a fast-acting pressor (an-

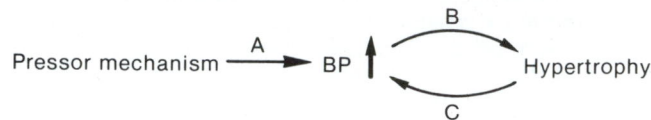

A **First hypothesis**

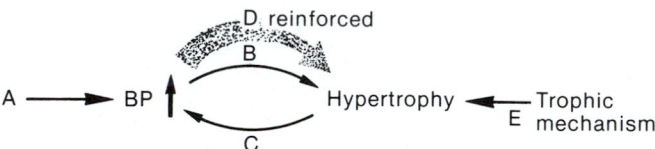

B **Second and third hypotheses**

Figure 11–2. Hypotheses for the initiation and maintenance of hypertension. *A*, Folkow's first proposal that a minor overactivity of a pressor mechanism, A, raises blood pressure slightly, initiating positive feedback (BCB) and a progressive rise of blood pressure. *B*, As in *A*, with two additional signals: D, an abnormal or "reinforced" hypertrophic response to pressure that may occur in the spontaneously hypertensive rat, and E, an increase of a humoral agent, causing hypertrophy directly. (From Lever AF. Slow pressor mechanisms in hypertension: a role for hypertrophy of resistance vessels? J Hypertens 1986; 4:515–524.)

giotensin II) and is maintained by the trophic action of the hormone to induce vascular hypertrophy. The evidence for the model derives, first, from the fact that the direct, immediate pressor actions of angiotensin II are less than the degree of chronic hypertension that occurs with equal concentrations of the hormone (Fig. 11–3), suggesting an additional contribution of a "slow mechanism." Second, lower concentrations of angiotensin II are needed to maintain hypertension than to initiate it. Third, angiotensin II is a trophin for vascular smooth muscle.

The underlying mechanisms for the immediate pressor effect, mediated by increased free intracellular calcium, and the slowly developing vascular hypertrophy are postulated to involve phosphatidylinositol metabolism in the cell membrane[31] (Fig. 11–4). The binding of angiotensin II to its receptor activates the enzyme phospholipase C, which

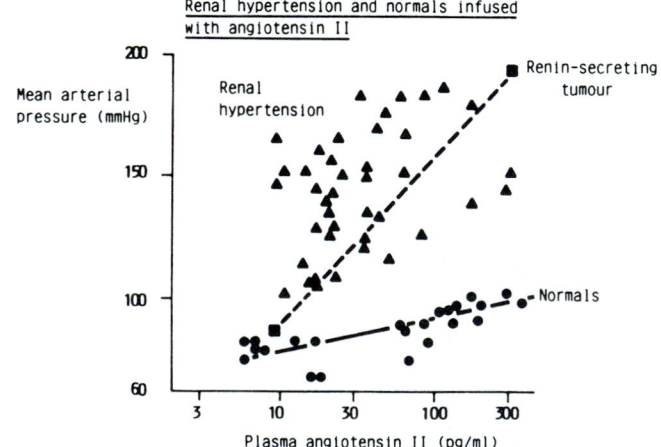

Figure 11–3. Relation of plasma angiotensin II concentration and mean arterial pressure in patients with renal hypertension (mostly caused by renal artery stenosis) (▲) compared with healthy subjects (●) before and during infusion of angiotensin II. Shown separately are values (■) from a patient with a renin-secreting tumor before and after surgery. In all of these patients the arterial pressure is higher than can be explained by the direct vasoconstrictor effect of angiotensin II as assessed by infusion of the peptide in normal subjects. (From Lever AF. Slow pressor mechanisms in hypertension: a role for hypertrophy of resistance vessels? J Hypertens 1986; 4:515–524.)

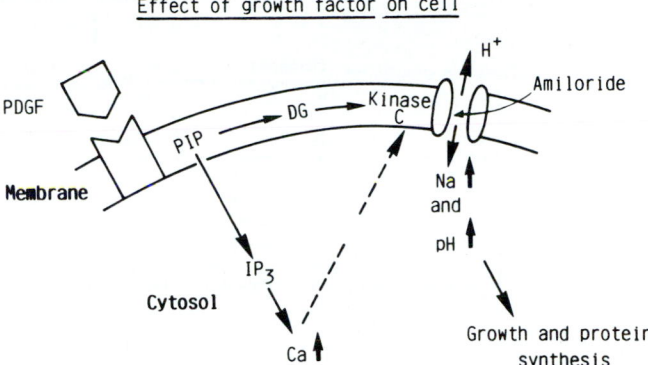

Figure 11–4. Schematic representation of the main events in a signaling system activated by growth factors. For example, platelet-derived growth factor (PDGF) occupies a membrane receptor; phosphatidylinositol 4,5-bisphosphate (PIP [PIP$_2$]) is hydrolyzed by phosphodiesterase in the membrane; inositol 1,4,5-trisphosphate (IP$_3$) is released into the cytosol and diacylglycerol (DG [DAG]) is released in the plane of the membrane. The last activates protein kinase C, linked to an amiloride-sensitive Na$^+$/H$^+$ exchanger whose activity increases. Sodium enters the cell down an electrochemical gradient, and protons are extruded. The increased intracellular pH that results promotes growth and protein synthesis. (From Lever AF. Slow pressor mechanisms in hypertension: a role for hypertrophy of resistance vessels? J Hypertens 1986; 4:515–524.)

hydrolyzes the membrane phosphatidylinositol 4,5-bisphosphate and releases inositol 1,4,5-trisphosphate into the cytosol and diacylglycerol in the plane of the membrane. The cytosolic inositol triphosphate mobilizes calcium from its intracellular stores and causes an immediate contraction. The diacylglycerol in the membrane activates protein kinase C, which increases the activity of an amiloride-sensitive Na$^+$/H$^+$ exchanger. Thereby, sodium enters the cell down an electrochemical gradient and protons are extruded so that the cell becomes more alkaline. Increased cell alkalinity is believed to initiate DNA synthesis and thereby promote cell hypertrophy.

This scheme explaining the immediate pressor action and the slow hypertrophic effect of angiotensin II is thought to be common to the action of pressor-growth promoters.[32]

When present in high concentrations over long periods, as with angiotensin II in renal artery stenosis or catecholamines in pheochromocytoma, each of these pressor-growth promoters causes hypertension. Moreover, when the source of the excess pressor-growth promoter is removed, hypertension may recede slowly, presumably reflecting the time needed to reverse vascular hypertrophy.

In the majority of hypertensive patients, no marked excess of any known pressor hormones is identifiable. Nonetheless, a lesser excess of one or more of them may have been responsible for initiation of a process sustained by the positive feedback postulated by Folkow[28] and the trophic effects emphasized by Lever.[30] This sequence encompasses a variety of specific initiating mechanisms that accentuate and maintain the hypertension by a nonspecific feedback-trophic mechanism (Fig. 11–5). If this double process is fundamental to the pathogenesis of essential hypertension, the difficulty in recognizing the initiating, causal factor is easily explained. As stated by Lever:[30]

The primary cause of hypertension will be most apparent in the early stages; in the later stages, the cause will be concealed by an increasing contribution from hypertrophy.... A particular form of hypertension may wrongly be judged to have "no known cause" because each mechanism considered is insufficiently abnormal by itself to have produced the hypertension. The cause of essential hypertension may have been considered already but rejected for this reason.

Hyperinsulinemia With or Without Obesity

Along with angiotensin and catecholamines, hyperinsulinemia may play a role in the development of hypertension.[21] This concept comes in part from the knowledge that hypertension is more common in the obese and that hyperinsulinemia is a hallmark of obesity. The associations are most striking in people with upper body obesity, who have the highest prevalence of hypertension and the most pronounced hyperinsulinemia.[33]

The high levels of insulin in people with upper body obesity arise both from increased secretion of insulin, com-

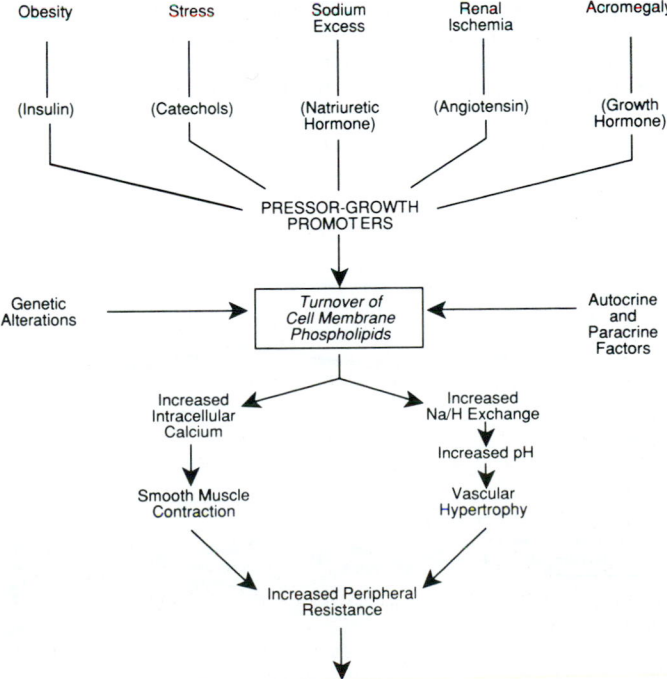

Figure 11–5. A scheme for the induction of hypertension by pressor hormones that act as vascular growth promoters.

mon to all forms of obesity, and from decreased hepatic removal and degradation of insulin, which appear to be related to the high rate of lipolysis of intra-abdominal fat[34, 35] (Fig. 11–6). The excessive amounts of free fatty acids coming from this fat are believed to be responsible for both the hyperinsulinemia and the hypertriglyceridemia common to upper body obesity.[36]

Although not ordinarily considered to be a pressor hormone, insulin can raise the blood pressure by at least two mechanisms: a rise in circulating catecholamines[37] and stimulation of renal sodium reabsorption.[38] Perhaps more important, insulin is a trophic hormone.[39] Insulin receptors are present on endothelial cells,[40] and infusion of insulin into one femoral artery of the dog causes vascular hypertrophy on that side only.[41] Insulin activates the amiloride-sensitive Na^+/H^+ exchanger[42] noted earlier to be the putative switch for protein synthesis and hypertrophy.

The presence of hyperinsulinemia in obesity and its potentially causal role in the hypertension of obesity are easily understood. Less understandable but of greater possible importance is the fact that hyperinsulinemia is also common in *nonobese* patients with primary (essential) hypertension.[21] Their hyperinsulinemia is attributable to peripheral insulin resistance,[43] but the reason for this resistance is unknown. Thus insulin is high on the list of possible pressor-growth promoters in the pathogenesis of primary hypertension both in the obese and in the nonobese.

The pathogenetic hypothesis shown in Figure 11–5 does not exclude the possibility that the environmental and genetic correlates of hypertension may be involved in other ways. However, this hypothesis serves as a reasonable way to transform a mosaic puzzle into a unified sequence.

Nonetheless, two hypotheses that do not involve the entire scheme shown in Figure 11–5 continue to receive experimental support. The first involves defects in sodium transport and the binding of calcium to cell membranes. The second implicates disturbances in the renin-angiotensin system.

Defects in Cell Transport or Binding

A causal role for sodium in the genesis of hypertension has long been assumed on the basis of circumstantial evidence (Table 11–4) that includes an increase in the level of intracellular sodium in hypertensive animals and people.[44] In addition, an increase in the intracellular calcium levels in cells from hypertensive people has been linked to the higher intracellular sodium concentration[45] (Fig. 11–7). De Wardener and MacGregor[46] proposed that an increased fluid vol-

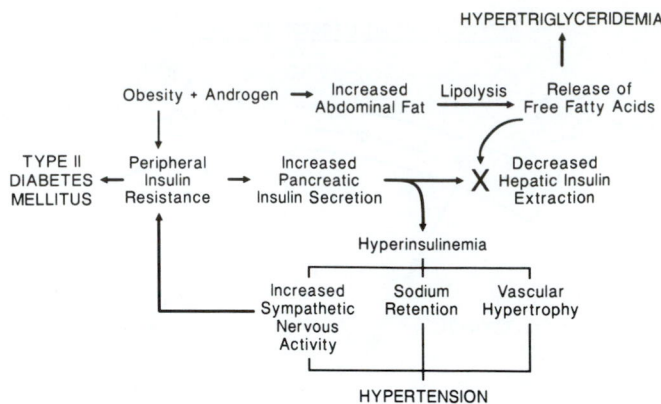

Figure 11–6. Scheme for the mechanism by which upper body obesity (via hyperinsulinemia) could promote glucose intolerance, hypertriglyceridemia, and hypertension. (From Kaplan NM. The deadly quartet. Upper-body obesity, glucose intolerance, hypertriglyceridemia and hypertension. Arch Intern Med 1989; 149:1514–1520. Copyright 1989, American Medical Association.)

ume stimulates the secretion of a digitalis-like natriuretic hormone, presumably of hypothalamic origin, that inhibits the Na^+,K^+-ATPase pump. Inhibition of the sodium pump would increase renal sodium excretion, restore vascular volume, and lead to hypertension by increasing the intracellular sodium content. A major problem with this hypothesis has been the difficulty of isolating the putative digitalis-like hormone.[47]

Although the search for the putative pressor natriuretic hormone has been unsuccessful, a natriuretic hormone from the cardiac atria has been characterized. Atrial peptide (AP, also called atrial ANF) natriuretic factor, is vasodilatory[48] and appears to be involved in the normal regulation of body fluid volume.[49] Although it appears to be released primarily in the response to acute volume expansion,[50] the concentrations may be increased in patients with established hypertension,[51] perhaps to compensate for an increased central blood volume. Lower concentrations of atrial peptide have been reported in response to high intake of sodium in normotensive sons of hypertensive parents.[52] If such a deficiency is present and persistent, it could be responsible for the initially reduced renal sodium excretion and hypervolemia (see Fig. 11–7).

Alternatively, the transport of sodium may be altered directly, for example, by an inherited defect in the structure of the cell membrane. Increased activity of the Na^+/H^+

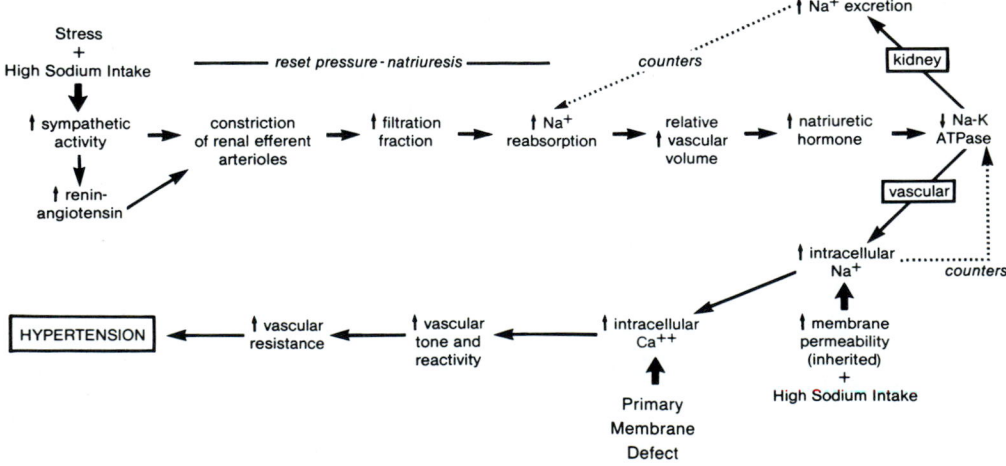

Figure 11–7. Hypothesis for the pathogenesis of primary (essential) hypertension, starting from any of three points, shown as heavy arrows. The first, at the top left, is the combination of stress and high-sodium intake, which induces an increase in the natriuretic hormone level and thereby inhibits sodium transport. The second, at the bottom right, invokes an inherited defect in sodium transport plus a high-sodium intake to induce an increase in the intracellular sodium level. The third, at the bottom middle, suggests a primary membrane defect that directly leads to an increased free intracellular calcium level. (From Kaplan NM. Systemic hypertension: mechanisms and diagnosis. In: Braunwald E, ed. Heart Disease: A Textbook of Cardiovascular Medicine. 3rd ed. Philadelphia: W. B. Saunders, 1988: 833.)

TABLE 11–4. Evidence for a Role of Sodium in Primary (Essential) Hypertension

1. In large populations the prevalence of hypertension tends to increase with increasing levels of sodium intake.
2. Multiple, scattered groups of people who consume little sodium (<50 mmol/d) have little or no hypertension. When they consume more sodium, hypertension appears.
3. Animals, if genetically predisposed, develop hypertension when given sodium loads.
4. Some people, when given large sodium loads over short periods, develop increased vascular resistance and blood pressure.
5. An increased concentration of sodium is present in the vascular tissue and blood cells of most hypertensives.
6. Sodium restriction, to a level of 60–90 mmol/d, lowers blood pressure in most people. The antihypertensive action of diuretics requires an initial natriuresis.

From Kaplan NM. Systemic hypertension: mechanisms and diagnosis. In: Braunwald E, ed. Heart Disease: A Textbook of Cardiovascular Medicine. 3rd ed. Philadelphia: W. B. Saunders, 1988.

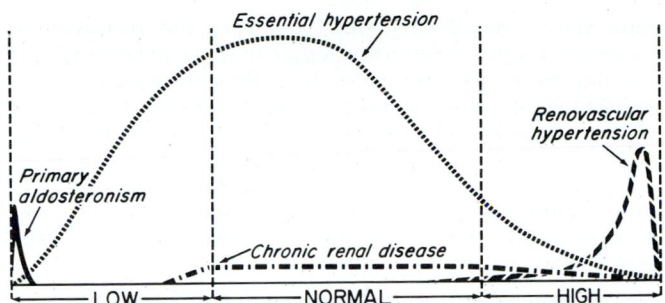

Figure 11–9. Schematic representation of plasma renin activity in various hypertensive diseases. The approximate number of patients with each type of hypertension is indicated, along with their proportion of low-, normal-, or high-renin levels. (From Kaplan NM. Renin profiles: the unfulfilled promises. JAMA 1977; 238:611–613. Copyright 1977, American Medical Association.)

antiport[44] could be involved in the amplification of the capacity of various stimuli to produce vascular smooth muscle cell contraction and hypertrophy (see Fig. 11–5).

Finally, a primary defect in calcium binding to the inner aspect of the cell membrane could increase the free cytosolic calcium concentration.[53] Defective calcium binding, in turn, could arise from alterations in the metabolism of membrane phosphoinositols.[54]

Role of the Renin-Angiotensin System

The renin-angiotensin mechanism may be involved in the pathogenesis of hypertension in various ways. All functions of renin are mediated through the synthesis of angiotensin II. As described in Chapter 9, this system is the primary stimulus for the secretion of aldosterone, and hence mediates the mineralocorticoid responses to varying sodium intakes and volume loads. When sodium intake is reduced or effective plasma volume shrinks, the increase in renin-angiotensin II stimulates aldosterone secretion, and this, in turn, is responsible for a portion of the enhanced renal retention of sodium and water (Fig. 11–8).

In addition to this primary role in the preservation of normal fluid volume, the renin-angiotensin system participates in the control of blood pressure under circumstances of sodium depletion or volume contraction. When fluid volume is normal, blockade of the renin-angiotensin system has little effect on blood pressure, but during volume contraction the increased levels of renin-angiotensin play an important role in maintaining the integrity of the circulation. When the renin-angiotensin system is blocked in normal persons with a low-sodium diet, the blood pressure may fall significantly when they stand upright.[55]

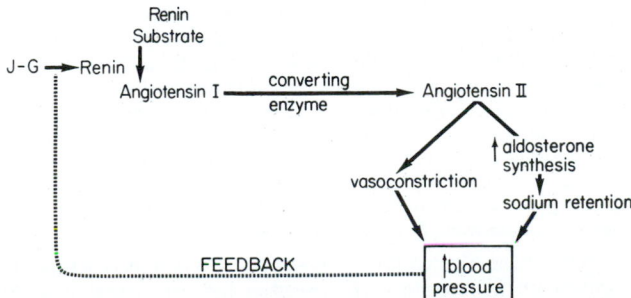

Figure 11–8. Scheme of the renin-angiotensin system. (From Kaplan NM. Clinical Hypertension. 4th ed. Baltimore: Williams & Wilkins, 1986: 96. © 1986, the Williams & Wilkins Co., Baltimore.)

As discussed later, hypertension may develop when an adrenal adenoma causes mineralocorticoid excess and suppression of renin levels or as a result of increased secretion of renin-angiotensin by a kidney made ischemic through renovascular stenosis. The fact that renin levels may be either low or high in patients with essential hypertension (Fig. 11–9) has led some to believe that an excess of mineralocorticoid activity on the one hand or a more subtle, diffuse intrarenal ischemia on the other may be involved in the pathogenesis of essential hypertension.

Low-Renin Hypertension

In keeping with current concepts (see Fig. 11–8), excess mineralocorticoid should suppress renin secretion. Nevertheless, the search for an excessively high level of mineralocorticoid among the 30% of hypertensive patients with low or suppressed levels of plasma renin activity has been largely unrewarding. Although elevated levels of deoxycorticosterone and 19-nor-deoxycorticosterone have been reported, no such elevations were found in a careful study of 46 low-renin hypertensive subjects.[56]

A syndrome of apparent mineralocorticoid excess has been identified in children[57] and in an adult.[58] Although these people exhibited flagrant evidence of mineralocorticoid excess, more subtle forms may be more widely recognized in the future. The abnormality is caused by a deficiency of 11β-hydroxysteroid dehydrogenase (11β-OHSD), which is responsible for conversion of cortisol to cortisone in the kidney. Cortisol is capable of acting as a mineralocorticoid by interacting with mineralocorticoid (type I) receptors. In the normal state, the conversion of cortisol to cortisone by 11β-OHSD prevents this from happening. In the absence of 11β-OHSD, cortisol exerts a profound mineralocorticoid effect. Of further interest, the mineralocorticoid action of licorice is the result of its inhibition of the 11β-OHSD.[59]

The absence of significant volume expansion and of hypokalemia argues against a role of mineralocorticoid excess in the pathogenesis of ordinary low-renin hypertension. People with low-renin hypertension may simply have a more normal renin mechanism than those with higher renin levels, because elevated blood pressure should diminish renin release by interaction with renal baroreceptors. Indeed, in epidemiological studies levels of plasma renin activity correlate inversely with blood pressure level.[60]

The separation of a segment of hypertensive subjects into a low-renin category is largely artifactual. The division between low and normal renin levels is arbitrary and depends on the type of analysis performed. Renin levels in essential hypertension follow a continuum, with a skewing toward low levels because a disproportionate number of hypertensive people are elderly and black, two groups whose renin levels tend to be low whether they are hypertensive or normotensive. The renin levels in these groups are lower probably because they have fewer functioning renal juxtaglomerular cells, in part the consequence of nephrosclerosis.[61]

A causal relation between a reduced number of functioning glomeruli and low-renin hypertension has been strongly supported by Brenner and co-workers.[62] They proposed that

a major renal abnormality that initiates essential hypertension is a decreased filtration surface area (FSA), due to a reduced number of nephrons and/or a decrease in FSA per glomerulus. Just as alterations in renal hemodynamics, reduced ability to excrete Na, and raised BP characterize the adaptive response to an acquired decrease in the number of functioning nephrons, inborn deficiencies may enhance susceptibility to essential hypertension. As schematized [in Fig. 11–10], this hypothesis suggests that a decrease in FSA may contribute to renal Na retention, and thus to systemic [low-renin] hypertension. Systemic hypertension then leads to glomerular capillary hypertension and eventual glomerular sclerosis, which in turn further decreases FSA, perpetuating a vicious cycle.

In keeping with the presumed role of renal sodium retention in low-renin hypertension, such patients tend to respond well to diuretics, but the better response does not necessarily reflect a greater volume component in the hypertension. By definition, low-renin patients have a renin-angiotensin-aldosterone system that is less responsive to stimuli that ordinarily increase renin levels, including diuretics. The reduced renin response to diuretic therapy enables diuretics to be more effective, because there is less compensatory rise in the angiotensin-aldosterone counter-regulatory system that limits the volume contraction and hypotensive effects of the diuretic.

Those low-renin hypertensive states in which volume expansion, usually mediated by mineralocorticoid excess, is responsible are considered in subsequent portions of this chapter.

Normal and High-Renin Hypertension

Because renin levels should be suppressed in essential hypertension, assuming that the high systemic pressure reaches the juxtaglomerular cells, the presence of normal

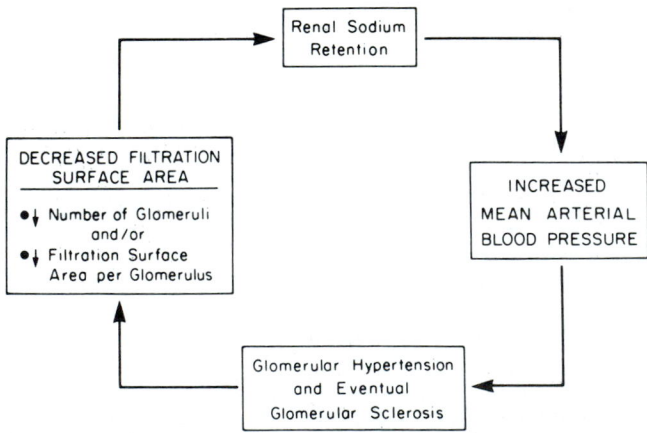

Figure 11–10. Relationship between decreased filtration surface area and mean arterial pressure. Decreased filtration surface area, caused by decreased nephron number and/or decreased filtration surface area per glomerulus, leads to renal sodium retention and thereby to increased mean arterial pressure. Systemic hypertension, in turn, promotes glomerular hypertension and eventual sclerosis, further decreasing the functioning of filtration surface area. (From Brenner BM, Garcia DL, Anderson S. Glomeruli and blood pressure: less of one, more of the other? Am J Hypertens 1988; 1:335–347.)

TABLE 11–5. The Hypothesis of Nephron Heterogeneity in Essential Hypertension

1. There are ischemic nephrons with impaired sodium excretion intermingled with adapting hyperfiltering, hypernatriuretic nephrons.
2. Renin secretion is high from ischemic nephrons and extremely low from hyperfiltering nephrons.
3. The inappropriate circulating renin-angiotensin level impairs sodium excretion because
   a. In the adapting hypernatriuretic nephrons:
      i. It increases tubular sodium reabsorption.
      ii. It enhances tubuloglomerular feedback–mediated afferent constriction.
   b. As the circulating renin level is diluted by nonparticipation of adapting nephrons, it becomes inadequate to support efferent tone in hypoperfused nephrons.
4. A loss of nephrons with age and from ischemia further impairs sodium excretion.

From Sealey JE, Blumenfeld JD, Bell GM, et al. On the renal basis for essential hypertension: nephron heterogeneity with discordant renin secretion and sodium excretion causing a hypertensive vasoconstriction-volume relationship. J Hypertens 1988; 6:763–777.

renin levels may be inappropriate and may play a role in sustaining the hypertension. Even more ominous is the presence of higher than usual levels of plasma renin activity in 10 to 20% of essential hypertensives.

A number of explanations have been offered for these inappropriately normal or high levels, beyond the proportion expected in a normal gaussian distribution curve. The concept of "nephron heterogeneity" described by Sealey and colleagues assumes a mixture of ischemic nephrons, caused by afferent arteriolar narrowing, and normal nephrons in patients with essential hypertension[20] (Table 11–5). Excess renin from the ischemic nephrons could raise the total blood renin level to varying degrees and cause some individuals to have normal or high-renin hypertension.

In support of their hypothesis, Sealey and colleagues invoke the findings of Hollenberg and Williams:[63]

These investigators have classified patients with essential hypertension as either non-modulators or modulators according to their renal hemodynamic responses to saline and angiotensin II infusions. Non-modulators have impaired plasma renin suppression, renal blood flow and natriuresis during saline infusion. The latter responses are corrected by converting enzyme inhibition therapy, suggesting that inappropriate renin secretion, perhaps from an ischemic subpopulation of nephrons, is an important contributing factor in these patients. In contrast, the modulator group of hypertensive patients responds to saline infusion with an exaggerated natriuresis, and converting enzyme inhibition does not alter the associated renal hemodynamic responses.[20]

Although "inappropriate renin secretion . . . from an ischemic subpopulation of nephrons," as suggested by Sealey and co-workers, could be involved in the pathogenesis of the nonmodulating normal renin hypertensive state, Williams and Hollenberg offer this explanation:[64]

These [nonmodulating] individuals may have either normal or high renin levels and can be characterized by a decreased adrenal responsiveness to angiotensin II on a low sodium intake and/or decreased vascular, particularly renal vascular, responsiveness to angiotensin II on a high sodium intake. While the underlying mechanisms responsible for the abnormality are unclear, it is likely that a defect in the regulation of responsiveness to angiotensin II at the tissue level and/or its receptor is a major factor. The elevated blood pressure may result either from an alteration in renal sodium handling or inappropriate increases in angiotensin II levels, depending on ambient sodium intake. Thus, the patients have either volume or angiotensin II dependent hypertension.

Whatever the explanation for the varying levels of renin-angiotensin in people with essential hypertension, it is now obvious that angiotensin II has multiple functions beyond those shown in Figure 11–8, both within the circulation and in various tissues[65] (Table 11–6).

TABLE 11–6. Diversity and Possible Functions of Tissue Renin-Angiotensin Systems

Tissue	Documented and Putative Functions
Kidney	Control of renal blood flow, glomerular filtration rate, glomerular hemodynamics, and sodium reabsorption
Blood vessel	Vascular tone, vascular hypertrophy
Heart	Myocardial metabolism, hypertrophy, and contractility
Adrenal	Aldosterone secretion, catecholamine release (?)
Brain	Thirst, behavior, blood pressure, vasopressin and catecholamine release
Pituitary	Release of corticotropin (ACTH, adrenocorticotropin), gonadotropin, and prolactin
Ovary	Ovulation (?), estrogen production (?)
Testes	Androgen production (?)
Uterus	Uteroplacental blood flow and contractility
Chorion-amnion	Unknown
Placenta	Uteroplacental blood flow, placental hormone production (?)
Gut (jejunum)	Absorption of ion and water
Salivary gland	Unknown

From Dzau VJ. Circulating versus local renin-angiotensin system in cardiovascular homeostatis. Circulation 1988; 77(Suppl I):I4–I13, by permission of the American Heart Association, Inc.

Now that the possible roles of hormones in the pathogenesis of essential (primary) hypertension have been explored, let us turn to the less common but better understood secondary forms of hypertension that have a defined endocrine connection (Table 11–7). References are provided for those forms not covered in this chapter.

RENIN-ANGIOTENSIN–MEDIATED HYPERTENSION

The prototype for renin-mediated hypertension is renovascular stenosis with resultant renal ischemia. It is likely that excess renin-angiotensin is also involved in primary hypertension (see the previous section) and in the hypertension of renal parenchymal diseases, estrogen-induced hypertension, and coarctation of the aorta. In still other conditions, renin excess may be secondary to stimulation of renin release by other primary mechanisms, including pregnancy-induced hypertension, hypercalcemic states, and pheochromocytoma. Moreover, hypertension may appear when plasma renin substrate is increased, such as in estrogen administration and glucocorticoid excess.[66]

Renovascular Hypertension

Perhaps 1% of all adults with hypertension have functionally significant renovascular stenosis (see Table 11–2). Because atherosclerotic plaques commonly develop within the renal arteries as people age, the diagnosis must be based not only on the presence of a lesion but also on proof that the kidney is ischemic.

Different types of intrinsic and extrinsic lesions may affect the renal arteries and perirenal region and thereby induce renal ischemia. Among infants, thrombosis of the renal artery after catheterization of this artery may be the most common mechanism.[67] In childhood, congenital dysplasia of the renal arteries is the usual cause. In young adults, particularly women, fibroplastic disease is most frequent, and in older adults, particularly men, atherosclerotic lesions are most common.

Two groups of patients with a high prevalence of hypertension—black persons and diabetics—have less renovascular disease than the remaining hypertensive population. Black persons develop less atherosclerosis of the main renal arteries than white persons, despite a greater degree of

intrarenal nephrosclerosis.[68] Diabetics may be protected from renovascular hypertension by their progressive loss of functioning juxtaglomerular cells, which may progress to the syndrome of hyporeninemic hypoaldosteronism.[69]

On the other hand, the prevalence of renovascular hypertension is higher among patients with accelerated-malignant hypertension. In one series of such patients, one fourth had renovascular hypertension.[70] The diagnosis should also be considered in patients with hypertension and renal insufficiency, in whom bilateral renovascular disease is relatively common.[71] In one series of such patients whose hypertension was refractory to drug therapy, one half had renovascular disease.[72] Not infrequently, such patients present with recurrent acute pulmonary edema.[73]

Pathophysiology

The sequence starts when vascular obstruction is sufficient to reduce renal perfusion pressure by at least one half, which triggers the secretion of renin. Renin levels are markedly elevated initially but, as blood pressure rises and volume retention occurs, levels tend to return toward normal. Thereafter, renin plays a continuing role, but other mechanisms, including the sympathetic nervous system, participate in the maintenance of hypertension.[74] The ischemic kidney may also release vasodepressor hormones. In rats with renal artery stenosis, blood pressure falls more if the stenosis is relieved than if the ischemic kidney is removed.[75]

In patients with long-standing renovascular hypertension, renin secretion from the affected kidney continues to be excessive. In addition, the contralateral kidney may become so damaged by nephrosclerosis that it participates in the persistence of hypertension, whereas the originally ischemic kidney's vessels are protected by the lower perfusion pressure. With repair of the stenotic kidney and removal of the contralateral kidney, the hypertension may recede.[76]

The stenosis may involve only segmental branches of one main renal artery in one tenth of patients and may involve both renal arteries in as many as one fourth.[77]

TABLE 11–7. Endocrine Causes of Hypertension

1. Primary (essential) hypertension (?)
2. Renin-angiotensin mediated
   a. Renovascular
   b. Renin-secreting tumors
   c. Renal parenchymal diseases (?)
   d. Coarctation of the aorta
   e. Estrogen induced (?)
3. Mineralocorticoid mediated
   a. Primary aldosteronism
   b. Cushing syndrome
   c. Congenital adrenal hyperplasia
   d. 11β-OHSD deficiency
   e. Exogenous: licorice, glucocorticoids, mineralocorticoids
4. Volume mediated
   a. Primary renal sodium retention (Liddle and Gordon syndromes)
   b. Acromegaly
   c. Increased intravascular volume (e.g., polycythemia)
5. Catecholamine mediated
   a. Pheochromocytoma and neuroblastoma
   b. Acute stress (e.g., postoperative, hypoglycemia, alcohol withdrawal)
   c. Neurological diseases (e.g., increased intracranial pressure, quadriplegia, porphyria)
   d. Exogenous
      i. Sympathomimetics
      ii. Monoamine oxidase inhibitors and tyramine-containing foods
6. Unknown mechanisms
   a. Hypercalcemia
      i. Hyperparathyroidism
      ii. Other hypercalcemic states
   b. Hypothyroidism
   c. Gonadal steroid therapy
   d. Gestational hypertension

Diagnosis

Renovascular hypertension should be looked for carefully in patients with certain clinical features (Table 11–8), although it may produce none of the typical features and instead may resemble the syndrome of mild essential hypertension. Nonetheless, the features listed in Table 11–8 can be used to exclude the majority of hypertensive people from additional work-up and to identify the 10% or so who should be given a more complete evaluation. As noted earlier, the routine performance of intravenous pyelography or other screening tests in all hypertensive people would result in more false-positive than true-positive results, mandating even more unnecessary work-up.

A strong case can be made for proceeding directly to renal arteriography in those patients with the suggestive clinical features listed in Table 11–8. However, in those with less suggestive features, an appropriate screening study may be adequate because, if negative, it almost certainly excludes the diagnosis.

No studies need be done if the patient is not a candidate for vascular repair; e.g., patients with long-standing, fairly mild hypertension that is easily managed by drugs, patients with extensive atherosclerosis, and in patients with coexisting contraindications to surgery. Although transluminal angioplasty may be an alternative to surgery in poor-risk subjects, it is important to remember that immediate surgery may be needed if the vessel is ruptured or severely damaged during the procedure. Angioplasty should be recommended only if a patient is capable of withstanding major surgery.

Screening Studies

Among a population with an expected prevalence of perhaps 5 to 10% (considering only those with clinical features suggestive of renovascular hypertension), an easy and safe screening procedure that gives very few false-negative results is needed. A certain number of false-positive results is expected. Considering that about 20% of all adults have primary (essential) hypertension, at least 20% of the patients with renovascular hypertension would be expected to have coexisting essential hypertension. They would thus have positive screening test results but would not be expected to be cured by repair of the stenosis and thereby would be classified as false-positives.

PERIPHERAL BLOOD RENIN ASSAYS. By themselves, unstimulated peripheral plasma renin activity (PRA) levels are of limited value in screening for renovascular hypertension. Most hypertensive patients with high levels do not have renovascular hypertension, and at least one third of the patients with proven renovascular hypertension have normal PRA levels in peripheral blood.[78]

Augmentation of peripheral blood PRA to identify renovascular hypertension has been attempted with various maneuvers and is most easily accomplished by the use of an angiotensin-converting enzyme (ACE) inhibitor. Because increased levels of renin-angiotensin II are needed to support the circulation in the stenotic kidney, the removal of this support by the action of an ACE inhibitor accentuates the ischemia, causing the release of additional renin.

In practice, blood for PRA is taken before and 1 h after a single 25- or 50-mg dose of captopril. As originally described[79] and supported,[80] the peripheral blood PRA level shows a greater relative increase (of at least 150%) and rises to much higher absolute levels (above 12 ng/mL/h) in most patients with renovascular hypertension compared with those with essential hypertension. The test has been found to be discriminatory by some[80] but not by others.[81] A review of 16 published series concluded that the data are inadequate to support the routine use of the procedure as a screening test.[82]

ISOTOPIC RENOGRAPHY. Despite the equivocal results with peripheral blood PRA, ACE inhibitors appear to be useful in accentuating the differences between ischemic and nonischemic kidneys as measured by radioisotopic renography. The procedure may use either labeled hippurate, a measure of renal blood flow, or diethylenetriamine penta-acetic acid, a measure of glomerular filtration rate. Equivocal changes before captopril use may be markedly enhanced 1 h after 25 to 50 mg of the ACE inhibitor is given[83] (Fig. 11–11).

INTRAVENOUS PYELOGRAPHY. Rapid-sequence intravenous pyelography was once the most commonly used initial screening test, but isotopic renography in conjunction with an ACE inhibitor has largely supplanted it.

Confirmatory Studies

If renovascular hypertension is suspected on the basis of either an abnormal screening test result or clinical features so suggestive that definitive testing is indicated regardless of the outcome of screening tests, confirmatory studies should be done. Some clinicians perform renal arteriography first; others measure renal vein renin concentrations. Because the patient should be taking no renin-suppressing antihypertensive drugs for several days before renal vein renin levels are measured, arteriography should be done first if the patient is taking such a drug. If the results of arteriography are negative, renal vein renin levels need not be measured. Although arteriography is a more dangerous procedure and may not be needed if the renal vein renin levels are normal, some patients with unilateral stenosis but without lateralizing renin ratios may be cured by surgery; thus arteriography appears to be the preferable confirmatory test.

MEASUREMENT OF RENAL VEIN RENIN RATIOS. In multiple series, more than 90% of the patients with a lateralizing ratio of renal vein renin concentrations, i.e., greater than 1.5 to 2.0 between the abnormal and contralateral sides, were cured or improved by surgery.[78] However, when patients with normal ratios but with other features suggestive of renovascular hypertension underwent surgery, 76% were also cured or improved. The overall sensitivity of the test is approximately 80% with 20% false-negatives, and the specificity is about 60% with 40% false-positives. The high rate of false-positives reflects the presence of an abnormal renal vein renin ratio of 1.5 or higher in one fifth of patients with essential hypertension.[84] This incidence of false-positive results in people with essential hypertension may reflect asymmetrical nephrosclerosis but probably results largely from the common practice of using a single catheter and sampling sequentially from the two renal veins. Renin secretion is episodic, and by the time the catheter is

TABLE 11–8. Clinical Clues Suggesting Renovascular Hypertension

Systolic /diastolic epigastric, subcostal, or flank bruit
Accelerated or malignant hypertension
Unilateral small kidney discovered by any clinical study
Severe hypertension in a child or young adult or after age 50 y
Sudden development or worsening of hypertension at any age
Hypertension and unexplained impairment of renal function
Sudden worsening of renal function in a hypertensive patient
Hypertension refractory to an appropriate three-drug regimen
Impairment in renal function in response to the angiotensin-converting enzyme inhibitor
Extensive occlusive disease in coronary, cerebral, and peripheral circulations
Recurrent acute pulmonary edema

From Working Group on Renovascular Hypertension. Detection, evaluation, and treatment of renovascular hypertension: final report. Arch Intern Med 1987; 147:820–829.

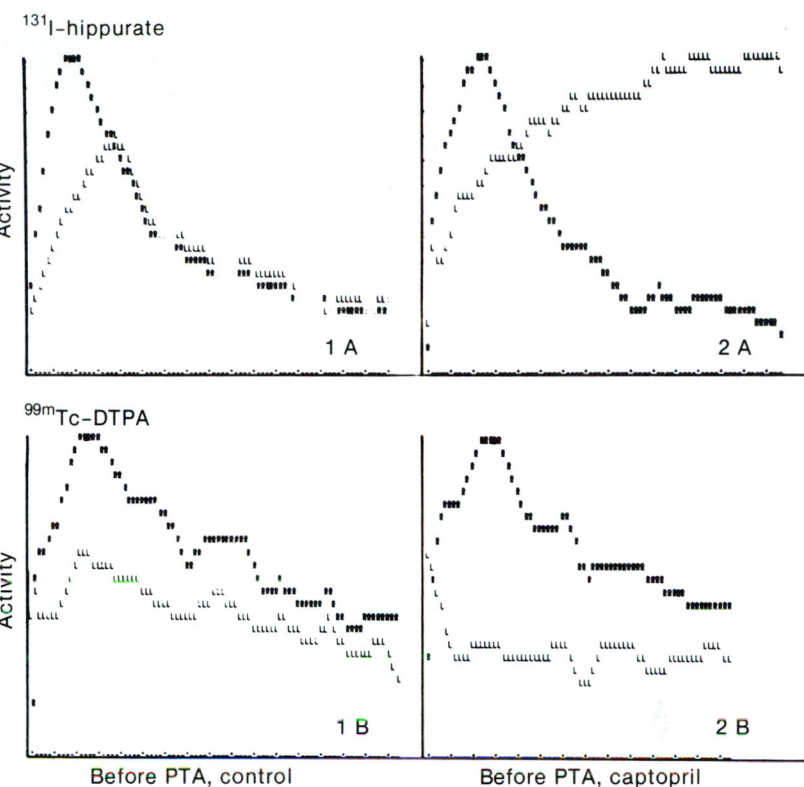

Figure 11–11. Renography in a 42-y-old man with hypertension and stenosis of the left renal artery. L indicates left kidney; R, right kidney. After percutaneous transluminal angioplasty (PTA), the hypertension was cured. The upper half of the figure shows ^{131}I-hippurate (A) and the lower half shows ^{99m}Tc-diethylenetriamine penta-acetic acid (DTPA) (B) time-activity curves in two different circumstances: (1) before PTA without any medication (control) and (2) before PTA but with 25 mg captopril taken orally 1 h before the investigation. Captopril slowed the excretion of ^{131}I-hippurate and reduced the uptake of ^{99m}Tc-DTPA only in the left kidney. (From Geyskes GG, Oei HY, Puylaert CBAJ, et al. Renovascular hypertension identified by captopril-induced changes in the renogram. Hypertension 1987; 9:451–458.)

switched, more or less renin may be coming from one renal vein than from the other.

To enhance the reliability of the procedure and to accentuate the difference between the two sides, renin secretion can be stimulated by prior volume contraction by using a low-salt diet and diuretics or a converting enzyme inhibitor. To enhance the likelihood of surgical cure in patients with suspected renovascular hypertension, it is also important to document that renin secretion from the contralateral kidney is suppressed, as evidenced by a renin level identical to that in the inferior caval blood.[85]

RENAL ARTERIOGRAPHY. Ultimately the renal vasculature must be visualized to confirm the diagnosis and to aid surgeons in deciding on the feasibility and type of repair. The transfemoral approach should be used, with selective visualization of each artery and its branches.

Although the arteriogram is necessary for the diagnosis of renovascular disease, it provides little help in predicting curability. In the Cooperative Study, neither the degree of stenosis nor the presence of poststenotic dilation nor the presence of collateral circulation was of much value in determining the success of the operation for individual patients.[86] Patients with stenosis greater than 90% may require surgery to prevent complete occlusion.

Treatment

No properly controlled study comparing medical with surgical treatment is available. Although advances in medical therapy have made it easier to control the hypertension and although the availability of transluminal angioplasty offers another curative approach, current evidence indicates that surgical repair is more likely to relieve hypertension and preserve renal function.

Surgical repair should be considered in patients with functionally significant renovascular disease if the general status and life expectancy are reasonably good. Better results

follow repair of fibroplastic disease, in part because the patients tend to be young and healthy. In various series, about 5% of the patients died during or after surgery, about 90% with fibroplastic disease were cured or improved after 1 y, and almost as many of those with atherosclerotic disease were similarly helped.[87] With newer surgical techniques, excellent results have been obtained in some patients with bilateral atherosclerotic disease and azotemia.[88]

Transluminal angioplasty has been successful in patients with all forms of renovascular disease, including some with marked renal insufficiency from stenosis of a solitary kidney or bilateral disease.[89] The procedure carries less risk than surgery and may be repeated if restenosis occurs.

The response to surgery or angioplasty may be predicted by the long-term response to ACE inhibitors,[90] which are also effective medical therapy for those unable to undergo surgery.[91] Rapid loss of renal function may occur after the administration of ACE inhibitors to patients who have renovascular hypertension in either a solitary kidney or both kidneys,[92] presumably because renal blood flow in such patients is highly dependent on the drive from high levels of angiotensin II. A calcium entry blocker such as nifedipine may provide equal control of blood pressure with less impairment of renal function in the ischemic kidney.[93]

An overall plan for the evaluation and treatment of renovascular hypertension is provided in Figure 11–12.[77]

Renin-Secreting Tumors

Renin-secreting tumors, made up of juxtaglomerular cells or hemangiopericytes, occur most commonly in young patients with severe hypertension, high renin levels both in peripheral blood and in the kidney harboring the tumor, and secondary aldosteronism manifested by hypokalemia.[94] In addition, children with Wilms tumors may have hypertension and high renin levels that revert to normal after nephrectomy.[95]

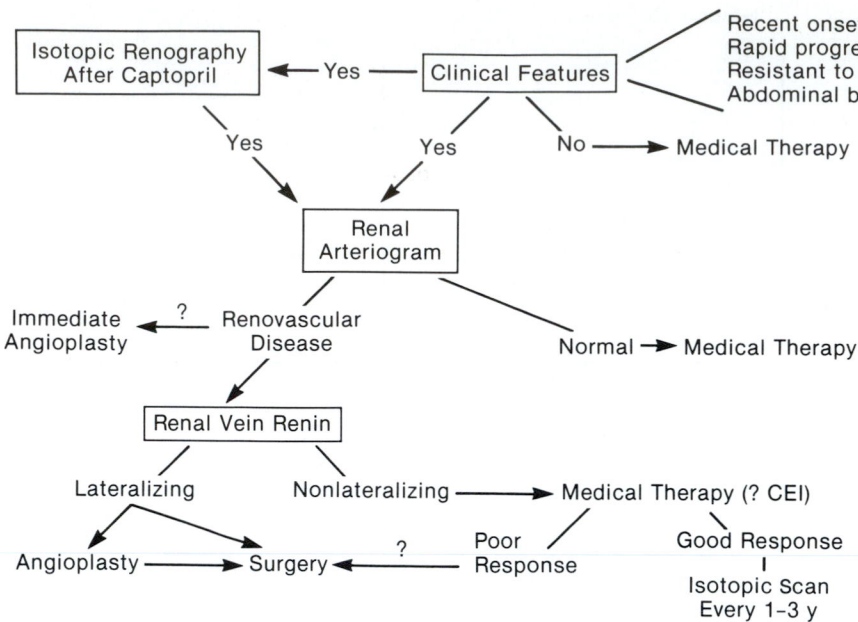

Figure 11–12. A flow diagram for the evaluation and treatment of renovascular hypertension.

Renal Parenchymal Disease

Various forms of renal injury cause progressive glomerular sclerosis, which, once it begins, sets off a vicious circle of progressive nephron loss leading to further glomerular sclerosis.[96] Elevated flow and pressure within the glomeruli are responsible for initiating the process, and various conditions associated with glomerular hypertension result in a high rate of progressive renal insufficiency.[97] Systemic hypertension and diabetes mellitus are the two leading causes, and when these conditions coexist, the progression of renal damage is particularly rapid. Hypertensive nephrosclerosis and diabetic nephropathy are, along with chronic glomerulonephritis, the leading causes of end-stage renal disease in the United States.[98]

Better understanding of the pathogenesis of progressive glomerulosclerosis has been accompanied by the availability of ACE inhibitors, which reduce glomerular hypertension by preferentially dilating renal efferent arterioles. The use of these drugs provides protection against progressive renal damage in experimental models[99] and in patients with glomerulosclerosis.[100] Although ACE inhibitors may provide a special protective effect, reduction of systemic hypertension by more traditional antihypertensive agents also slows the rate of renal damage in patients with diabetic nephropathy[101] (Fig. 11–13).

Endocrine Mechanisms

The fact that ACE inhibitors reduce the rate of progression supports the concept of a role for angiotensin II in the pathogenesis of progressive renal damage. Although peripheral renin levels are usually low in patients with chronic renal insufficiency, the high intrarenal levels immediately downstream from the juxtaglomerular cells that secrete renin are likely pathological.

As renal function worsens, the inability of the reduced renal mass to excrete salt and water becomes an increasingly important mechanism for hypertension. In addition, a deficiency of renal vasodepressor hormones may be involved in the hypertension of renal failure. Of these, renal vasodilatory prostaglandins, bradykinin,[102] and renomedullary lipids[103] may play a role.

Hyporeninemic Hypoaldosteronism

In diabetic patients the hyalinization of juxtaglomerular cells may impair renin formation to such a degree as to lead to hyporeninemic hypoaldosteronism. Although hyporeninemic hypoaldosteronism may occur in other forms of chronic renal disease as well, it is most common among diabetic patients who are unable to mobilize either the aldosterone or the insulin needed to transfer potassium from the blood to the tissues and are thus particularly vulnerable to hyperkalemia.[104]

Hypercalcemia

When the blood calcium level is higher than normal, blood pressure usually rises. Patients with chronic renal disease are particularly vulnerable to such elevation. Marked hypertensive reactions can occur when these patients are given calcium loads for any reason.[105]

Correction of Anemia

The anemia of end-stage renal disease may protect the patient against hypertension. With the use of erythropoietin, correction of the anemia may be accompanied by progressive hypertension because of volume expansion.[106]

Coarctation of the Aorta

Upper body hypertension with coarctation of the aorta may be caused by more than mechanical obstruction of the narrowed aorta. In animal models the arteriolar walls thicken in vascular beds below the coarctation where intra-arterial pressure is low.[107] Increased levels of renin-angiotensin may be involved both as a direct pressor and as a humoral growth factor.

Estrogen-Induced Hypertension

The use of estrogen-containing oral contraceptives (OCs) is likely the most common cause of secondary hypertension among women. In large surveys, about 5% of users developed a blood pressure above 140/90 in 5 y, approximately two and a half times higher than the rate of increase

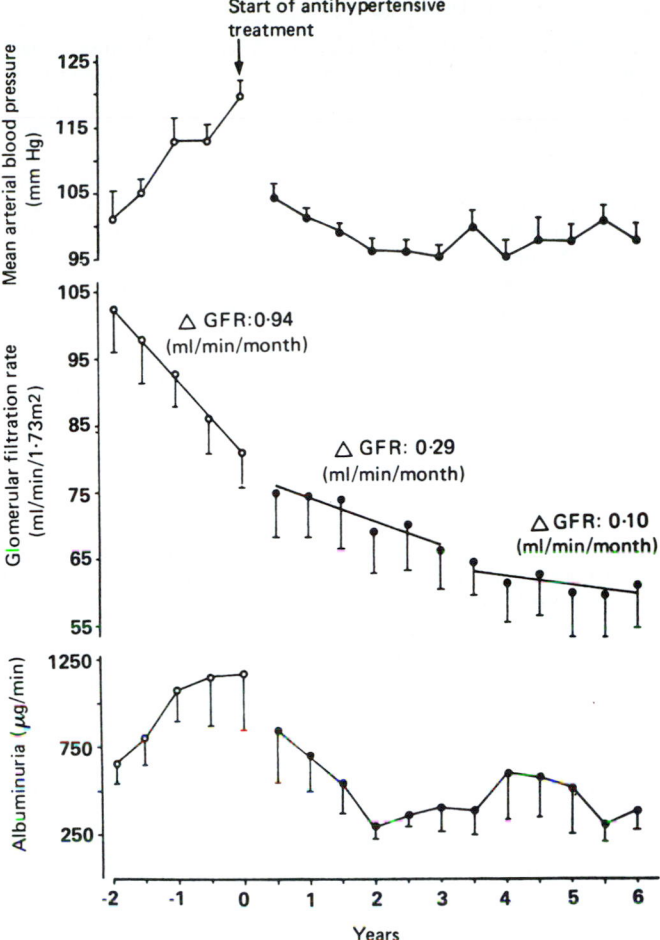

Figure 11–13. Average course of mean arterial blood pressure, glomerular filtration rate, and albuminuria before (○) and during (●) long-term effective antihypertensive treatment of nine insulin-dependent diabetic patients who had nephropathy. Therapy included furosemide, metoprolol, and hydralazine in most patients. (From Parving HH, Andersen AR, Smidt UM, et al. Effect of antihypertensive treatment on kidney function in diabetic nephropathy. Br Med J 1987; 294:1443–1447.)

in control groups.[108] Milder degrees of blood pressure elevation were even more common. The average rise in pressure after OC use noted in multiple reports was 5 mm Hg systolic and 2 mm Hg diastolic.[109]

In a prospective study of 186 women, during the first 2 y of OC use, systolic blood pressure rose in 164 and diastolic pressure increased in 150.[110] The mean rise in systolic pressure among the users was 7.7 mm Hg, whereas the mean decrease was 1.2 mm Hg in 60 women who used other types of contraception.

It is likely that the rise in blood pressure is involved in the higher mortality from cardiovascular diseases among users of OCs.[109] Most of the excess mortality occurs in women older than age 35 who smoke. Among younger, nonsmoking women, the risk is so small that the OC agent is the safest and most effective form of contraception (also see Chapter 17).

Predisposing Factors

The amounts of estrogen and progestogen in OCs may be important. Most data relating to contraceptive-induced hypertension were obtained with tablets containing either 100 or 50 μg estrogen, and it is possible that the lower doses now used in many types of OC may cause less hypertension.

In one study, eight women who were hypertensive (average blood pressure = 172/109) with a 50-μg estrogen dosage and who became normotensive when administration of the pill was stopped had a smaller increase in blood pressure when given a 30-μg estrogen pill (average blood pressure = 155/95).[110]

The amount of progestogen in the OC may also influence the development of hypertension. In some surveys,[108, 111] less hypertension developed with smaller amounts of progestogen, although others have not reported a relationship between either the type or the dose of progestogen and the development of hypertension when the dose of estrogen was kept constant.[110, 112]

As to predisposing factors in the development of hypertension among women who use OCs, the presence of obesity, a family history of hypertension, and consumption of more than 10 oz ethanol a week[115] appear to be important. Women with pre-existing hypertension or prior pregnancy-induced hypertension do not seem to have greater susceptibility.[110]

Mechanisms

Estrogens can cause both a rise in blood pressure and cardiovascular damage unrelated to hypertension. The most important estrogen effect is an increase in the hepatic synthesis of renin substrate, which leads to an increase in plasma angiotensin II levels and to aldosterone-mediated fluid retention[114] (Fig. 11–14). In addition, arterial walls have estrogen receptors that may modulate smooth muscle tone,[115] and estrogen increases the vascular sensitivity to catecholamines, apparently by increasing the affinity of alpha-adrenergic receptors for catecholamines.[116]

Clinical Management

Estrogen-containing OCs should not be used by women over age 35, particularly if they smoke and are obese. All women taking OCs should be carefully monitored. The supply should be limited initially to 3 mo and thereafter to 6 mo, and the blood pressure should be checked before an additional supply is provided. If the pressure has risen by more than 10 mm Hg, an alternative contraceptive should be offered.

If OC is the only acceptable contraceptive, the elevated blood pressure can be controlled with appropriate therapy, such as a diuretic-spironolactone combination. In those who stop taking an OC, evaluation for secondary hypertensive diseases should be postponed for at least 3 mo to allow the

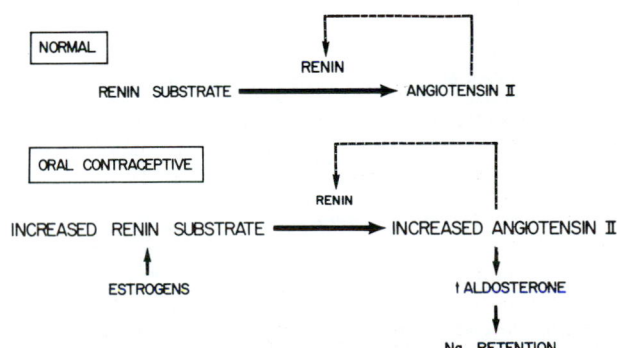

Figure 11–14. Schematic representation of changes in the renin-angiotensin system induced by OCs containing estrogen. Dotted lines show feedback suppression of renin release by angiotensin II. (From Kaplan NM. Clinical Hypertension. 4th ed. Baltimore: Williams & Wilkins, 1986: 370. © 1986, the Williams & Wilkins Co., Baltimore.)

renin-aldosterone changes to remit.[117] If the hypertension does not recede, additional work-up and therapy may be needed.

Postmenopausal Estrogen Use

The use of estrogen after menopause does not appear to induce hypertension[118] even though many hormonal and biochemical changes develop, as in younger women given OCs. The absence of a pressor effect may contribute to the apparent protection that postmenopausal estrogen use provides against both coronary disease[118] and stroke.[119]

Pregnancy-Induced Hypertension

Although the renin-aldosterone mechanism may be involved in pregnancy-induced hypertension, it now seems much more likely to be related to a prostaglandin imbalance. For this reason, it is considered under Miscellaneous Causes of Endocrine Hypertension.

MINERALOCORTICOID-INDUCED HYPERTENSION

Most of the hypertensive syndromes described in the previous section as being induced by renin-angiotensin are accompanied by a secondary increase in aldosterone synthesis. Secondary aldosteronism may aggravate the hypertension and cause significant potassium deficiency.

We now consider those hypertensive syndromes in which aldosterone or other mineralocorticoid levels are increased primarily, usually by autonomous hyperfunction of the adrenal cortex. These syndromes include two types of functional adrenal tumors.

Incidental Adrenal Tumors

Adrenal adenomas 1 mm to 4 cm in diameter were found in 9% of the 739 patients examined at autopsy in one hospital over a 6-mo interval.[120] Among the 119 patients known to have been hypertensive, adenomas were present in 12%. Although the functional state of these adenomas was not established, most were incidental or nonfunctioning tumors, well recognized and usually disregarded by pathologists. However, with the advent of computed tomographic scanning, these previously hidden masses are now diagnosed with some frequency. Unsuspected adrenal tumors can be detected in 1 to 10% of computed tomographic scans of the upper abdomen.[121, 122]

To assist in the assessment of these incidental adrenal tumors, Copeland has proposed guidelines based mainly on the size of the tumor and the results of laboratory tests[121] (Fig. 11–15). The first concern is to rule out adrenocortical cancers, which, although rare, are the major reason for surgery in those who do not have a hormonally active tumor. According to Copeland's guidelines, any solid tumor larger than 6 cm should be resected after appropriate biochemical assessment. This size was chosen because most adrenocortical cancers are larger than 6 cm and most benign tumors are smaller. However, as Belldegrun and co-workers note,[122] this approach would delay the removal of smaller cancers before they reach 6 cm; these authors propose removal of all solid, inactive masses larger than 3.5 cm. An even better approach has been offered by Gross and colleagues[123] that uses adrenal scintiscans of the uptake of the cholesterol analogue ^{131}I-6β-iodomethyl-19-norcholesterol (NP-59). In their series of 119 euadrenal patients with unilateral adrenal masses, all lesions that took up NP-59 were benign, whereas 23 of 26 with absent or markedly reduced NP-59 uptake were metastatic or primary neoplasms. Gross and colleagues propose, then, that concordance of computed tomographic and NP-59 scans

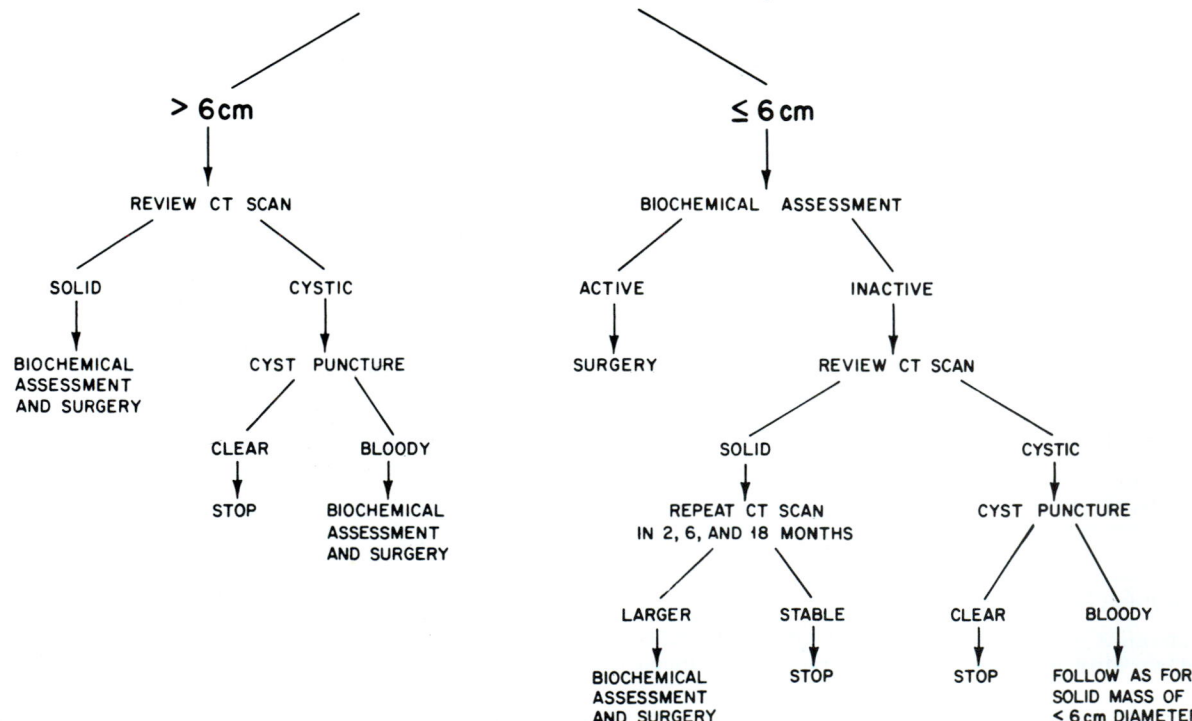

Figure 11–15. An approach to the incidentally discovered adrenal mass. The diameter of the mass can be estimated by using the radiological method by which it is detected. Biochemical assessment is described in the text. (From Copeland PM. The incidentally discovered adrenal mass. Ann Intern Med 1983; 98:940–945.)

TABLE 11–9. Evaluation of Incidental Adrenal Masses

Diagnosis	Suggestive Clinical Features	Laboratory Screening Tests
Pheochromocytoma	Paroxysmal hypertension Postural hypotension Spells of sweating, headache, palpitations	Spot urine metanephrine Normal: <5.5 nmol/mg creatinine (<1 μg/mg creatinine)
Cushing syndrome	Truncal obesity Thin skin Muscle weakness	8 AM plasma cortisol after 1 mg dexamethasone at bedtime Normal: <140 nmol/L (<5 μg/dL)
Primary aldosteronism	Hypokalemia	Urinary potassium excretion Normal: <30 mmol/24 h urine in presence of hypokalemia
Adrenocortical carcinoma	Virilization or feminization	Urinary 17-ketosteroids Normal: Women, 14–52 μmol/d (4–15 mg/d) Men, 22–88 μmol/d (7–25 mg/d)

be used to exclude the presence of a malignancy, regardless of the size of the adrenal mass.

The majority of adrenal tumors are small, and biochemical assessment is the first recommendation. As described in considerable detail in the remainder of this chapter, the assessment need not be complicated in the absence of suggestive clinical features or abnormalities in the results of routine tests. The guidelines shown in Table 11–9 should be adequate for excluding a hormonally active tumor. Tumors with suggestive clinical features or abnormal screening test results require additional testing. With these guidelines, incidentally discovered adrenal tumors can be managed appropriately.

Primary Aldosteronism*

Of the functioning adrenal tumors, those responsible for aldosterone excess tend to be smallest, but their presence is usually made obvious by the finding of unexplained, unprovoked hypokalemia in a hypertensive patient. A few patients with aldosterone-producing adenoma (APA) do not have hypokalemia,[124] and an even smaller number do not have hypertension,[125] but the combination is almost always the tip-off to the correct diagnosis.

Incidence

Solitary APAs are present in perhaps 1 of every 1000 hypertensive patients. Bilateral adrenal hyperplasia or *idiopathic hyperaldosteronism* is recognized in about one of four patients with documented primary aldosteronism and may be present in even more, because its clinical features are less distinct. In one meticulous analysis of the various features of the syndrome of hyperaldosteronism associated with bilateral adrenal hyperplasia, it was concluded that the disorder is "at the upper end of a wider-than-normal distribution of aldosterone in essential hypertension, from which it has been separated wrongly."[126] Indeed an impressive argument can be advanced that bilateral hyperplasia is not autonomous hyperaldosteronism but rather a form of essential hypertension. Because such patients should not be operated on and can usually be managed effectively with antihypertensive drugs, including aldosterone antagonists, the exclusion of this disorder from the realm of primary aldosteronism seems appropriate. This formulation is of particular importance because of the likelihood that such hyperplastic glands can be identified by abdominal computed tomographic scans and, consequently, that more cases will be recognized in the future.

Variants of primary aldosteronism include a familial glucocorticoid suppressible syndrome[127] and rare gonadal

tumors that secrete aldosterone.[128] In addition, the clinical features can be reproduced by exogenous mineralocorticoids[129] and by the action of the glycyrrhetinic acid in various forms of licorice.[59] As noted earlier, the syndrome of apparent mineralocorticoid excess that occurs with licorice ingestion is caused by inhibition of the 11β-OHSD in the kidney, thus allowing cortisol to exert its full mineralocorticoid effects.[57, 58]

Pathophysiology

In 10 patients with APAs whose disease was well controlled with the aldosterone antagonist spironolactone, administration of the drug was stopped and the syndrome was allowed to redevelop over a 6-wk interval.[130] In all, the reappearance of hypertension was initially related to volume retention with an increase in cardiac output. However, in one half, cardiac output subsequently decreased and peripheral resistance increased, a sequence that is apparently common to all forms of hypertension regardless of the initiating mechanism. Presumably other patients would have converted if the study had been conducted over a longer interval.

Contrary to what is generally believed, the hypertension can be severe and can lead to significant vascular damage; in one series of 136 patients, 4 had malignant hypertension and 31 had serious vascular complications.[131] In another series of 140 patients, 28 had mean arterial pressure higher than 120 mm Hg and were resistant to three or more antihypertensive drugs.[132]

Diagnosis

In most instances, hypokalemia in hypertensive patients is caused by loss of potassium as a result of diuretic therapy. When hypokalemia is present, the patients with diuretic-induced hypokalemia can be distinguished from the smaller group with hypokalemia caused by excessive aldosterone production by the finding of little potassium in a 24-h urine specimen collected after the administration of diuretics has been discontinued and while the patient is receiving a normal sodium intake (Fig. 11–16). Such patients should be screened first by obtaining a peripheral blood sample for aldosterone and PRA. High aldosterone and low PRA levels are strong presumptive evidence for the diagnosis.[133]

The suppression of PRA, although expected with volume-expanded hypertension, was not present in 36% of 80 patients with primary hyperaldosteronism who were studied while supine after 4 d of a 10 mmol sodium diet,[124] perhaps because many of these patients also had refractory hypertension that could have stimulated renin secretion.[132]

The most definitive diagnostic procedure is the demonstration in plasma or urine of high aldosterone levels that

*Also see Chapter 9.

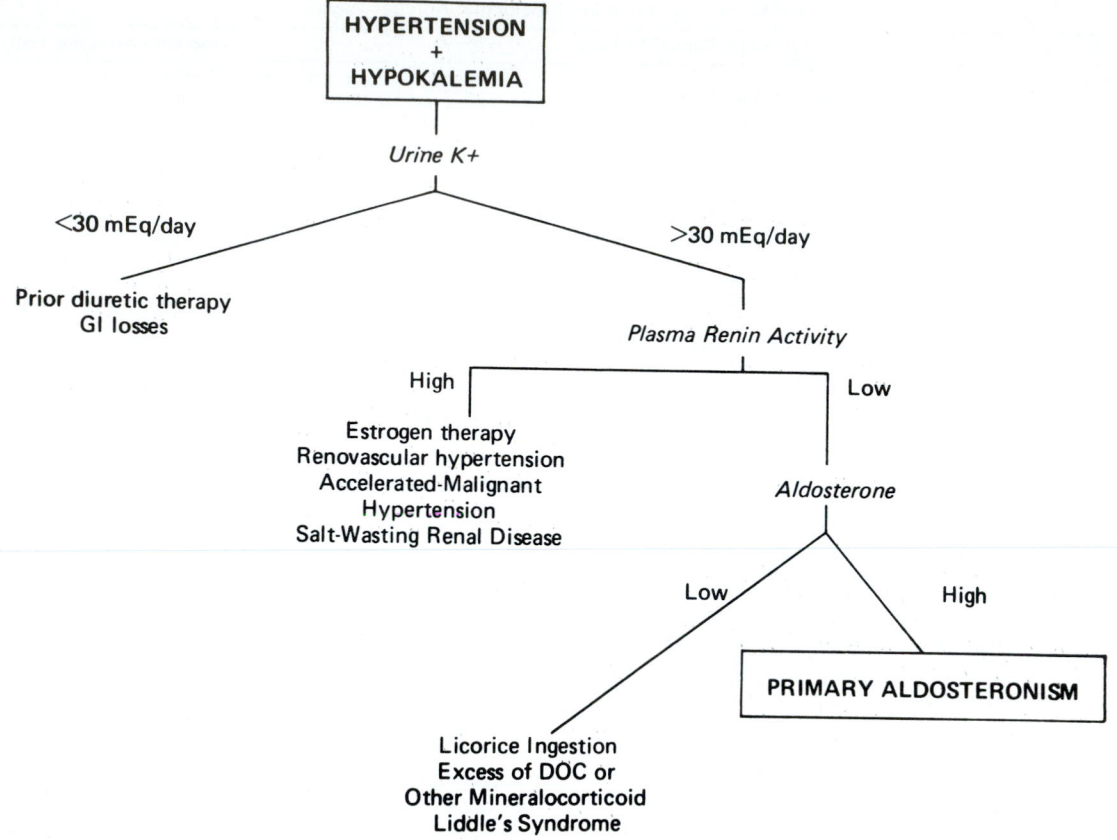

Figure 11–16. Flow diagram for the differential diagnosis of hypertension with hypokalemia. (From Kaplan NM. Clinical Hypertension. 4th ed. Baltimore: Williams & Wilkins, 1986: 413. © 1986, the Williams & Wilkins Co., Baltimore.)

do not decrease normally after volume expansion. The 4-h saline suppression test of plasma aldosterone[134] works well,[135] but some prefer longer periods of volume expansion and a demonstration of failure to suppress both plasma and urine aldosterone levels.[136]

The distinction of an APA from bilateral adrenal hyperplasia and the localization of the adenoma may be provided by a computed tomographic scan of the abdomen. If not, the diagnostic work-up shown in Figure 11–17[137] almost always makes the distinction. Rare patients with an APA may

show suppression with upright posture and saline infusion, as do patients with bilateral hyperplasia.[138]

Therapy

Surgery for APA is usually curative.[139] Patients with bilateral hyperplasia should be treated medically, usually with spironolactone, or, failing that, inhibitors of steroid synthesis.[140]

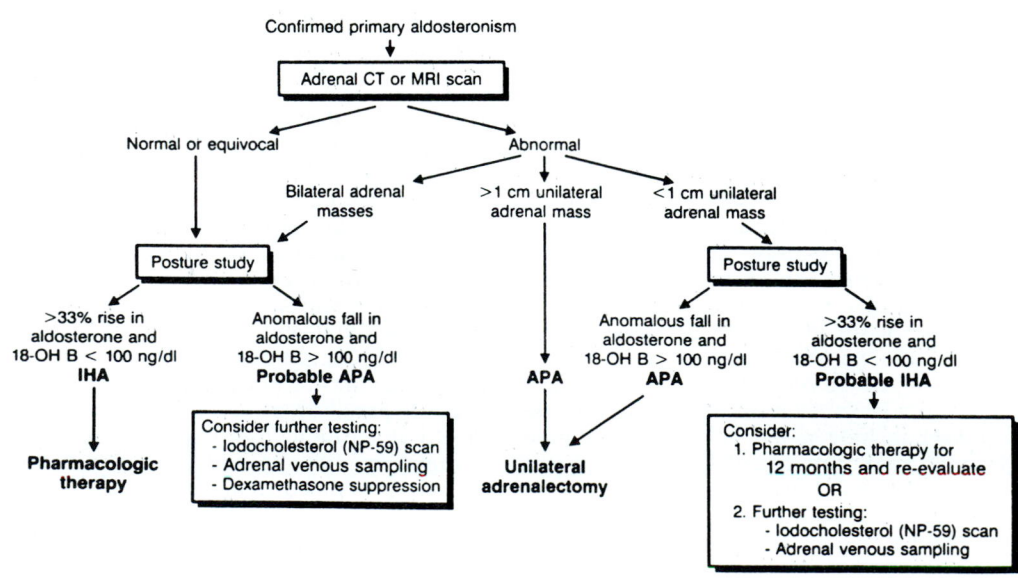

Figure 11–17. Algorithm for the diagnostic differentiation between APA and bilateral idiopathic hyperaldosteronism (IHA). The details are discussed in the text. 18-OH B, 18-hydroxycorticosterone; CT, computed tomography; MRI, magnetic resonance imaging. (From Young WF Jr, Klee GG. Primary aldosteronism. Diagnostic evaluation. Endocrinol Metab Clin North Am 1988; 17:367–395.)

Cushing Syndrome

Hypertension is present in virtually all patients with Cushing syndrome. The hypertension may be severe and may cause considerable cardiovascular damage.[141] The blood pressure may be elevated for various reasons, including high levels of renin substrate, the sodium-retaining effect of cortisol, the hypersecretion of other mineralocorticoids, and increased vascular reactivity to catecholamines.[142] The blood pressure may lose its normal circadian rhythm, apparently as a consequence of the high levels of glucocorticoids.[143]

The clinical features and the overnight dexamethasone suppression test of plasma cortisol serve as simple and accurate screening procedures to separate patients with true Cushing syndrome from those who may have cushingoid features. As described in Chapter 9, numerous additional studies may be needed to diagnose the cause of Cushing syndrome.

Congenital Adrenal Hyperplasia

A number of enzymatic defects in adrenal steroidogenesis can cause adrenal malfunction (also see Chapters 9 and 14). Hypertension is usual in the 11-hydroxylase and 17-hydroxylase defects, because the blocks in steroidogenesis occur at sites beyond those for the synthesis of deoxycorticosterone, which is therefore formed in excess. The clinical features of the hypertension in such patients are typical of other forms of mineralocorticoid-induced hypertension. The possibility exists that partial 11-hydroxylase[144] or 17-hydroxylase[145] deficiencies may be involved in a larger number of cases of less severe hypertension.

As noted earlier, the syndrome of apparent mineralocorticoid excess is now known to represent a deficiency of 11β-OHSD,[58] and the mineralocorticoid action of licorice is the result of inhibition of 11β-OHSD by glycyrrhetinic acid.[59]

VOLUME-MEDIATED HYPERTENSION

Apart from the syndromes of volume-expanded hypertension caused by an excess of a particular mineralocorticoid, rare patients have hypertension related to volume expansion that is not associated with a recognizable excess of adrenal salt-retaining hormones. An example is acromegaly,[146] in which volume expansion is associated with an endogenous digitalis-like factor in the plasma that inhibits the Na^+,K^+-ATPase pump.[147] Rare patients have primary renal retention of sodium that leads to volume expansion and hypertension.[148, 149] They may represent extremes of the subtle defect in sodium excretion described under Endocrine Participation in Primary (Essential) Hypertension.

CATECHOLAMINE-MEDIATED HYPERTENSION*

Transient hypertension is frequent during physical or emotional stress. It is likely that such rises in blood pressure reflect the combined effects of adrenomedullary secretion of epinephrine and sympathetic neuronal release of norepinephrine. With time and relaxation, blood pressure usually returns to prestress levels. Permanent hypertension, however, may be induced by an overactive sympathetic

---

*Also see Chapter 10.

nervous system, as described earlier in this chapter. Less commonly, intermittent or persistent hypertension can be caused by tumors that secrete catecholamines, mostly adrenomedullary pheochromocytomas.

Pheochromocytomas

Pheochromocytomas are responsible for 0.1 to 0.2% of hypertension, but many additional patients have suggestive symptoms. Moreover, despite the fact that symptoms and signs are usually distinctive, pheochromocytomas often remain unrecognized and cause severe hypertension and occasionally death. As cited earlier, of 54 pheochromocytomas found at autopsy at the Mayo Clinic, only 13 had been recognized before death, and in 30 cases death was directly related to the unrecognized tumor.[13]

Clinical Features

Most, but not all, pheochromocytomas cause distinctive manifestations (Table 11–10). Even when the hypertension is persistent, most patients experience superimposed paroxysms, often accompanied by orthostatic hypotension and characterized by the sudden onset of headache, sweating, palpitations, and nervousness. The presence of these "spells" should help distinguish the few who need laboratory tests to establish the diagnosis from the larger number of patients with essential hypertension, particularly those with markedly variable blood pressure. Ambulatory blood pressure monitoring is particularly useful in patients with suggestive spells who are not consistently hypertensive.[150] Most attacks that simulate those of pheochromocytomas are caused by other conditions that involve a component of excess catecholamine secretion (Table 11–11). In particular, a hyperadrenergic form of essential hypertension has been described with episodes of tachycardia and further rises in blood pressure that are triggered by emotion.[151] This form of pseudopheochromocytoma is associated with high plasma levels of dopamine sulfate.

Diagnosis

If the clinical features suggest a pheochromocytoma, a single voided urine specimen should be assayed for meta-

---

TABLE 11–10. Features Suggestive of Pheochromocytoma

Hypertension: persistent or paroxysmal
  Markedly variable blood pressure (with or without orthostatic hypotension)
  Sudden paroxysms (with or without subsequent hypertension) in relation to:
    Stress: anesthesia, angiography, parturition
    Pharmacological provocation: histamine, nicotine, caffeine, beta-blockers, saralasin, glucocorticoids, tricyclic antidepressants
    Manipulation of tumors: abdominal palpation, urination
  Rare patients persistently normotensive
  Unusual settings
    Childhood
    Pregnancy
    Familial
    Multiple endocrine neoplasia (MEN) adenomas: medullary carcinoma of thyroid (MEN 2A), mucosal neuromas (MEN 2B [3])
    Neurocutaneous lesions: neurofibromatosis

Associated symptoms
  Sudden spells with headache, sweating, palpitations, nervousness, nausea, and vomiting
  Pain in chest or abdomen

Associated signs
  Sweating, tachycardia, arrhythmia, pallor, weight loss

From Kaplan NM. Clinical Hypertension. 5th ed. Baltimore: Williams & Wilkins, 1990. © 1990, the Williams & Wilkins Co., Baltimore.

TABLE 11–11. Differential Diagnosis of Pheochromocytoma

Cardiovascular disorders
  Hyperdynamic, labile hypertension
  Paroxysmal tachycardia
  Angina, coronary insufficiency
  Acute pulmonary edema
  Eclampsia
  Hypertensive crisis during or after surgery
  Hypertensive crisis with monoamine oxidase inhibitors
  Rebound hypertension after abrupt cessation of clonidine and other
    antihypertensive drugs

Psychoneurological disorders
  Anxiety with hyperventilation
  Migraine and cluster headaches
  Brain tumor
  Stroke
  Diencephalic seizures
  Porphyria
  Lead poisoning
  Familial dysautonomia
  Acrodynia
  Autonomic hyper-reflexia, as with quadriplegia

Endocrinologic disorders
  Menopausal symptoms
  Thyrotoxicosis
  Diabetes mellitus
  Hypoglycemia
  Carcinoid
  Mastocytosis

Factitious
  Ingestion of sympathomimetic agents

From Kaplan NM. Clinical Hypertension. 5th ed. Baltimore: Williams & Wilkins, 1990. © 1990, the Williams & Wilkins Co., Baltimore.

nephrine content, expressed as micrograms per milligram of creatinine.[152] Virtually the only reason for a falsely low urine metanephrine value is the concomitant excretion of an x-ray contrast medium containing methylglucamine, which consumes the periodate used in the assay of metanephrines.[153] In the absence of this interference, a normal spot urine metanephrine test virtually excludes the disease, because most pheochromocytomas hypersecrete catechols even when the blood pressure is stable and the patient is asymptomatic. If the clinical features are highly suggestive and the spot test result is normal, or if the spot test result is elevated regardless of the clinical features, a 24-h urine specimen should be assayed for metanephrine and catecholamine levels. If the results of these more routine procedures are equivocal, greater specificity can be achieved by using a gas chromatographic–mass spectrometric analysis of free norepinephrine.[154] With all of these assays, caution is needed to exclude false-positive test results, particularly in patients who are receiving the combined alpha- and beta-blocker labetalol, a drug that is measured during the fluorometric analysis of catecholamines and the spectrophotometric analysis of metanephrines.[155]

Plasma catecholamine assays are less sensitive and specific than urine assays, likely the result of transient stimulation by stressful procedures such as venipuncture. A few patients have normal 24-h urine metanephrine levels but elevated plasma catecholamine levels,[156] an unlikely scenario unless the plasma sample was obtained during an isolated paroxysm from a tumor that is quiescent throughout the remaining time.

However, some patients have borderline urine values and suggestive symptoms, which could reflect either a hyperactive sympathetic nervous system in association with essential hypertension or an early pheochromocytoma. In such patients the measurement of plasma[156] or overnight urine[157] catecholamine levels before and after administration of a single oral 0.3-mg dose of clonidine has proved help-

ful.[158] If possible, patients should stop taking all antihypertensive medications for a few days before the collection of any specimens for catecholamine assays, particularly before suppression tests.

If urinary catechol levels are elevated and plasma catechol levels are nonsuppressible with clonidine, an abdominal computed tomographic scan should be done to localize the tumor, 80% of which arise within the adrenal glands and the remainder in chromaffin tissue outside the adrenal. Most pheochromocytomas are large enough to be diagnosed by computed tomographic scanning. Repeated venous sampling for catechols[159] or adrenal scintiscans, using an isotopically labeled guanidine derivative that localizes in adrenergic vesicles,[160] may identify tumors not found by computed tomographic scanning.

The more important clinical problem is to avoid the overdiagnosis of pheochromocytoma in hypertensive patients in whom abdominal computed tomographic scans and nonspecific catecholamine tests are performed during the hypertension work-up.[161] As noted earlier, because as many as 12% of the adrenal glands in people with essential hypertension harbor a nonfunctioning tumor at autopsy,[120] not infrequently an adrenal tumor is found by computed tomographic scanning in people with essential hypertension.[122] Because plasma catecholamine levels may be spuriously high for many reasons, the potential for diagnostic error is great. Reliance on urine assays and the proper use of suppression tests minimize the likelihood of false diagnoses. Only patients with suggestive features should be tested in the first place, and only those with unequivocal biochemical test results should undergo abdominal computed tomographic scanning.

Provocative pharmacological tests are rarely needed.[162] Such procedures should be used mainly in patients with familial multiple endocrine adenomas, who are highly likely to harbor bilateral pheochromocytomas that may be minimally symptomatic and are usually quiescent.[163] (Also see Chapters 10 and 30.)

Surgical removal should be undertaken after the institution of appropriate pharmacological blockade. With proper preoperative preparation and careful anesthesia,[164] the majority of patients are fairly easily managed. Even malignant pheochromocytoma can often be treated effectively with combination chemotherapy.[165]

Neuroblastomas

Neuroblastomas, the second most common solid tumors of childhood, may arise almost anywhere along the sympathetic nervous system chain. These poorly differentiated tumors synthesize and secrete large amounts of catecholamine precursors and metabolites, including dopa, dopamine, vanillylmandelic acid, and homovanillic acid.[166] These metabolites may also be found in patients with pheochromocytoma, but the levels tend to be higher in patients with neuroblastomas, perhaps because the storage granules for catecholamines are less well developed, exposing the catecholamines to increased breakdown by monoamine oxidase and catechol O-methyltransferase.

The increased formation and release of these inactive precursors and metabolites, rather than active catecholamines, may explain the lower frequency of hypertension in patients with neuroblastomas than in those with pheochromocytomas. In one series of 59 affected children, only one fifth had hypertension.[167] Indeed, the release by the tumors of large amounts of vasodepressor substances, dopa and dopamine, may tend to lower the blood pressure, both in children with neuroblastomas and in occasional adults with pheochromocytomas.[168] Nonetheless, hypertension, when it does occur, is often severe and poorly responsive to antihypertensive drugs, including alpha-blockers, but usually recedes after removal of the tumors.

Stress Hypertension

Stress can cause significant hypertension that recedes with the relief of the stress. Some of these stresses, such as an acute cerebrovascular accident, may stimulate central adrenergic mechanisms. Most, however, appear to induce a massive outpouring of adrenomedullary hormones, often in association with increased levels of renin-angiotensin. Examples include burns, acute pancreatitis, alcohol withdrawal, hypoglycemia, and acute myocardial infarction. A high incidence of hypertension has been noted after both cardiac[169] and carotid[170] surgery, the latter most commonly in patients with conditions that may interfere with cerebral autoregulation.

The major clinical issue is to avoid overtreatment with potent antihypertensive drugs. However, if the elevated blood pressure is an immediate threat, intravenous labetalol,[171] nitroprusside, or esmolol, a short-acting beta-blocker,[169] may be effective. Catecholamine levels should not be measured during or immediately after the stress so as to avoid the misdiagnosis of pheochromocytoma.

Neurological Diseases

Various neurological diseases may cause paroxysmal hypertension, possibly as a result of activation of the sympathetic nervous system. Examples include brain tumors, particularly in the cerebellum and brain stem, and transection of the spinal cord, in which sensory stimulation below the lesion may cause massive activation of sympathetic reflexes that are no longer held in check by central control mechanisms.[172] Acute attacks of porphyria can also cause hypertension and tachycardia, apparently as a consequence of blockade of the reuptake of catecholamines into the sympathetic neurons.[173]

Exogenous Causes

Sympathomimetic drugs that can cause severe hypertension include diet pills containing phenylpropanolamine[174] and various drugs of abuse, in particular cocaine.[175] The use of cyclosporine causes hypertension in more than one half of treated patients, and the hypertension may be severe.[176] It appears to be caused by a direct vasospastic effect of the drug, particularly on the renal arteries, and by a secondary expansion of body fluid volume.[177] Calcium entry blockers may be especially useful in this situation.[178] Patients taking monamine oxidase inhibitors may develop hypertensive crises after ingestion of certain foods (e.g., aged cheese), beverages (e.g., red wine), or drugs (e.g., levodopa) that contain large amounts of tyramine or other catecholamine precursors.

MISCELLANEOUS CAUSES OF ENDOCRINE HYPERTENSION

The coexistence of hypertension in at least 20% of patients with any other disease is expected, because few diseases protect against the development of primary (essential) hypertension. However, the frequency of hypertension is higher in some endocrine diseases, in addition to those previously described, wherein the endocrinopathy directly involves renin-angiotensin, catecholamines, or other recognized provocateurs of hypertension.

Hyperparathyroidism

The incidence of hypertension in patients with primary hyperparathyroidism varies from 10 to 60% in different series.[179] The primary diagnosis in these patients may be made only after a further sharp rise in the serum calcium level occurs with the use of thiazide diuretics to treat the hypertension.

The mechanisms of parathyroid hypertension are uncertain. There is little evidence of a direct correlation with either hypercalcemia or elevated parathyroid hormone levels[180] and a possible depressor action of phosphate depletion.[181] The hypertension may or may not remit after relief of the hyperparathyroidism.[182]

Paradox of Hypercalcemia and Calcium Intake

Hypercalcemic states other than hyperparathyroidism are often associated with hypertension. Moreover, a number of epidemiological studies have shown a positive association between total serum calcium level and high blood pressure.[183] Nevertheless, the ingestion of 1 g/d calcium reduces the blood pressure in some patients with hypertension.[184] The hypotensive effect of supplemental calcium may be limited to those hypertensives with low ionized calcium and high parathyroid hormone levels.[185] These patients may start with significant hypercalciuria as a consequence of high sodium intake and volume expansion. The hypercalciuria leads to a decrease in the plasma ionized calcium level, which stimulates release of parathyroid hormone[186] (Fig. 11–18). More data are needed to document the validity of this hypothesis and to determine the value of calcium supplements. At the least, hypertensive patients should be advised not to restrict their calcium intake, in particular by the exclusion of milk and cheese, in an attempt to moderate their dietary sodium intake.

Pseudohypoparathyroidism

Among adult patients with target organ resistance to parathyroid hormone (pseudohypoparathyroidism type I), about one half have hypertension.[187] The association may reflect the obesity commonly seen with pseudohypoparathyroidism.

Hypothyroidism

Hypothyroid patients have a higher prevalence of hypertension, mainly diastolic, which usually remits when thyroid hormone replacement therapy is adequate. In one consecutive series of 688 hypertensives, previously unrecognized hypothyroidism was found in 3.6%.[188] In addition,

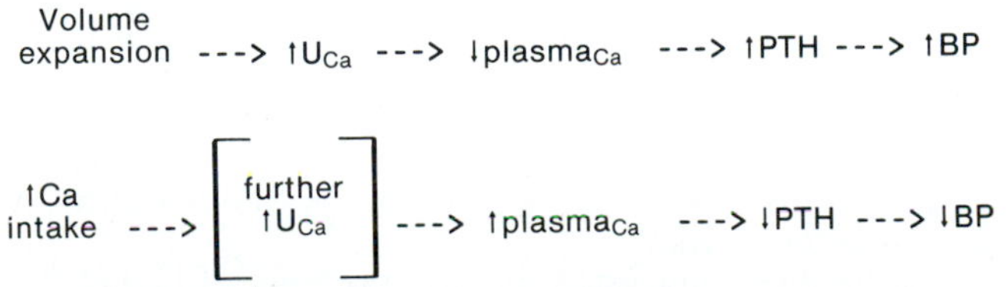

$$\text{Volume expansion} \dashrightarrow \uparrow U_{Ca} \dashrightarrow \downarrow \text{plasma}_{Ca} \dashrightarrow \uparrow PTH \dashrightarrow \uparrow BP$$

$$\uparrow Ca \text{ intake} \dashrightarrow \left[\begin{array}{c} \text{further} \\ \uparrow U_{Ca} \end{array} \right] \dashrightarrow \uparrow \text{plasma}_{Ca} \dashrightarrow \downarrow PTH \dashrightarrow \downarrow BP$$

Figure 11–18. A potential explanation for the hypotensive action of increased dietary calcium intake in patients with sodium-sensitive, low-renin hypertension who begin with a volume-expanded state that induces hypercalciuria. U_{Ca}, urine calcium excretion; PTH, parathyroid hormone; BP, blood pressure.

thyrotropin-releasing hormone may be involved in the rise in blood pressure and pulse.[189]

Hyperthyroidism

Thyrotoxic patients usually have a high cardiac output and elevated systolic blood pressure. They are often given beta-blockers to reduce tachycardia, sweating, and tremor. With the large doses of beta-blockers required to relieve these symptoms, the deiodination of thyroxine may be blocked, elevating serum free thyroxine levels and the free thyroxine index.[190] Serum triiodothyronine levels are in the low-normal range, and levels of serum reverse triiodothyronine are elevated.

Gonadal Steroid Therapy

As noted earlier, OCs containing estrogen-progestogen may induce hypertension, whereas postmenopausal replacement therapy does not. Androgens in pharmacological amounts can also induce volume expansion and hypertension.[191]

Hypertensive Disorders of Pregnancy

The onset of hypertension during the last trimester of pregnancy or immediately after delivery in a previously normotensive, nonproteinuric woman, previously called *preeclampsia* or *pregnancy-induced hypertension,* is now termed *gestational hypertension.*[192] This disorder should be distinguished from chronic hypertension and renal disease, but both may progress to eclampsia, defined as the occurrence of convulsions. The cause of gestational hypertension is unknown, but this disorder occurs more frequently in women whose mothers had the syndrome[193] and in women with trisomy-13,[194] which suggests a genetic mechanism. Immunological incompatibility between mother and fetus and racial dissimilarity of the parents may also play a role.[195] Additional predisposing factors include nulliparity, increasing age, black race, multiple gestations, concomitant heart or renal disease, and chronic hypertension.[196] In the population in which these factors were identified, diabetes mellitus did not play a significant independent role as a predisposing factor.

Making the distinction between gestational hypertension and chronic hypertension is important because their management and prognosis are different. Gestational hypertension is self-limited and rarely recurs in subsequent pregnancies, whereas chronic hypertension progresses and usually complicates all pregnancies. The separation of the two types of hypertension may be difficult because of a lack of knowledge of the prepregnancy blood pressure and because of the usual tendency for high blood pressure to fall considerably during the middle trimester, so that hypertension present before pregnancy may not be recognized.

In gestational hypertension the blood pressure rises only late in pregnancy. Among 84 patients with the onset of hypertension before 37 wk of gestation, 55 had renal disease documented by kidney biopsy 6 mo post partum, when morphological changes caused solely by gestational hypertension should have subsided.[197] Gestational hypertension was the diagnosis in only 10% of primiparas with the onset of hypertension before 37 wk, whereas it was the diagnosis in three fourths of primigravid women with onset of hypertension after 37 wk.

It has been suggested that the presence of higher than usual but not overtly elevated blood pressures in the midtrimester may make it possible to predict the development of gestational hypertension before blood pressure rises and complications occur.[198] However, Chesley and Sinai[199] noted that fewer than 10% of nulliparas who developed eclampsia had a maximal diastolic blood pressure higher than 80 mm Hg and none had pressure higher than 90 mm Hg during the second trimester. They concluded that no correlation exists between second-trimester blood pressure and the subsequent development of gestational hypertension.

Pathogenesis

The common feature of the factors that predispose to development of gestational hypertension is reduced uteroplacental perfusion. Although disturbances in the renin-angiotensin system may be involved,[200] increasing attention has been directed to the possible role of disturbed prostaglandin relationships, either as the cause or as a consequence of uteroplacental hypoperfusion.[201] Either increased activity of the lipoxygenase pathway or decreased production of prostacyclin by the fetal-placental unit can lead to the various clinical manifestations of the syndrome (Fig. 11–19). Decreased synthesis of prostacyclin may precede the appearance of hypertension.[202] Inhibition of prostacyclin production may be induced by the higher concentrations of progesterone in placentas of women with gestational hypertension.[203]

Whether or not this scheme explains the pathogenesis, small doses of aspirin, in the range of 50 to 100 mg/d, which would be expected to reduce thromboxane levels but to have little effect on prostacyclin levels, prevent development of gestational hypertension in women at high risk for the syndrome.[204, 205]

At least three other physiological abnormalities may be involved in the pathogenesis of gestational hypertension. Hyperinsulinemia is present in one half of women with hypertension during the third trimester.[206] Plasma levels of atrial natriuretic peptide are also higher in women with gestational hypertension;[207] increased amounts of this peptide may reflect a compensatory response to volume expansion, but they have the potential of increasing capillary permeability and suppressing the renin-angiotensin system.

Last, the level of a digoxin-like immunoreactive substance increases during pregnancy and could inhibit the Na^+,K^+-ATPase cellular pump, thereby inducing natriuresis and vasoconstriction. However, no difference in the level of this substance was found in pregnant patients with or without gestational hypertension.[208] Nonetheless, a reduction of the NA^+,K^+-ATPase pump in the red blood cells of pregnant women with gestational hypertension and an increase in intracellular sodium level that would be expected to accompany inhibition of the pump have been reported.[209] In brief, the pathophysiology of gestational hypertension is incompletely understood.

Treatment

Mothers with gestational hypertension and their fetuses can be protected from excessive morbidity and mortality by maneuvers that lower blood pressure without impairing uteroplacental perfusion.[210] These maneuvers include modified bed rest, a nutritious diet with normal amounts of sodium, and the use of antihypertensive agents when diastolic blood pressure higher than 100 mm Hg worsens renal function and predisposes to overt eclampsia. Low-dose aspirin is likely to be used increasingly.[205]

The traditional drug for gestational hypertension remote from term is methyldopa or, if a parenteral agent is needed closer to the time of delivery, hydralazine. Beta-blockers[211] and, if needed, the alpha-blocker prazosin are as good as or better than methyldopa.[212] The combined alpha-

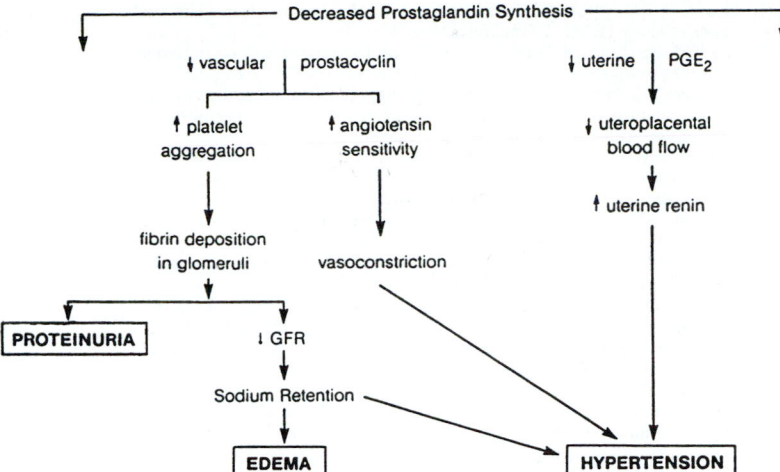

Figure 11–19. A scheme for the pathogenesis of gestational hypertension with proteinuria and edema based on decreased prostaglandin synthesis.

and beta-blocker labetalol improves the maternal and fetal outcome.[213] Caution remains necessary with the use of calcium entry blockers[214] and ACE inhibitors.[215]

Despite these generally favorable reports, caution is advised with the use of drugs for mild gestational hypertension. In one of the few controlled studies comparing modified bed rest with antihypertensive drug therapy, one half of 200 primigravidas with relatively mild hypertension at 26 to 35 wk gestation were given labetalol and the other one half were monitored while in the hospital.[216] Those given labetalol had a significant fall in blood pressure, whereas the control subjects did not, but the mothers in both groups had some worsening of renal function. However, the number of small-for-gestational age infants was higher in the labetalol group (19% vs. 9%). Thus drug treatment of maternal blood pressure did not improve the perinatal outcome and was associated with fetal growth retardation.

ENDOCRINE-METABOLIC CONSEQUENCES OF THE TREATMENT OF HYPERTENSION

A detailed review of the nondrug and drug therapies for hypertension is beyond the scope of this chapter, but

TABLE 11–12. Adverse Endocrine-Metabolic Consequences of the Treatment of Hypertension

Drug	Endocrine-Metabolic Side Effects
Diuretics	Hypokalemia
	Hyperuricemia
	Hypercholesterolemia
	Impairment of glucose tolerance
Spironolactone	Impairment of testosterone synthesis and/or action (impotence, gynecomastia)
Adrenergic inhibitors	
Reserpine	Elevation of prolactin level
Methyldopa, clonidine, guanabenz	Elevation of prolactin level, discontinuation rebound
Beta-blockers	Hypertriglyceridemia
	Decrease in high-density-lipoprotein cholesterol level
	Delayed response to insulin-induced hypoglycemia
Vasodilators	
Minoxidil	Hirsutism

mention of the endocrine and metabolic consequences of treatment seems appropriate (Table 11–12). Particular concerns have been raised about the adverse effects of diuretics and some beta-blockers on lipoproteins,[217] in part because the major trials of these agents with hypertension have failed to show protection against coronary disease.

Impotence is frequently attributed to the use of antihypertensive drugs. The problem is common in the absence of therapy and may be exacerbated by aggressive reduction of blood pressure, thereby lowering penile blood flow below the level needed to maintain an erection.[218] No one class of drug is immune to this potential problem.

Drugs may also alter the blood and urine levels of various hormones, including increases in plasma renin activity with diuretics and vasodilators and decreases in plasma renin activity with adrenergic inhibitors. In addition, modest alterations in plasma catecholamine levels may be induced by various drugs: raised by diuretics, beta-blockers, and vasodilators and lowered by centrally acting adrenergic inhibitors and alpha-blockers.

For patients taking antihypertensive drugs who require endocrine testing, the best course is to stop the administration of drugs for at least 3 or 4 d. Rebound hypertension should be avoided by gradual discontinuation. Even patients with very high blood pressure levels should not be endangered thereby, particularly if restricted to bed rest and closely observed while medications are discontinued. The possible effects of hormonal therapies—adrenal steroids, thyroxine, gonadal hormones, insulin—in inducing or aggravating hypertension should also be kept in mind. Last, patients with endocrine-metabolic disorders who are also hypertensive may have special therapeutic needs. These patients include those who are markedly obese, hyperlipidemic, or diabetic. The last type may not be controlled by traditional antihypertensive therapy[219] but may be protected by ACE inhibitors.[220]

REFERENCES

1. 1988 Joint National Committee. The 1988 report of the Joint National Committee on Detection, Evaluation, and Treatment of High Blood Pressure. Arch Intern Med 1988; 148:1023–1038.
2. Dannenberg AL, Drizd T, Horan MJ, et al. Progress in the battle against hypertension: changes in blood pressure levels in the United States from 1960 to 1980. Hypertension 1987; 10:226–233.
3. Garraway WM, Whisnant JP. The changing pattern of hypertension and the declining incidence of stroke. JAMA 1987; 258:214–217.
4. Hypertension Detection and Follow-up Program Cooperative Group. The hypertension detection and follow-up program. Circ Res 1977; 40(Suppl I):106–109.

5. Pickering TG, James GD, Boddie C, et al. How common is white coat hypertension? JAMA 1988; 259:225–228.

6. Hla KM, Feussner JR. Screening for pseudohypertension: a quantitative, noninvasive approach. Arch Intern Med 1988; 148:673–676.

7. Lefebvre RC, Hursey KG, Carleton RA. Labeling of participants in high blood pressure screening programs: implications for blood cholesterol screenings. Arch Intern Med 1988; 148:1993–1997.

8. Kaplan NM. Treatment of hypertension: nondrug therapy and the rationale for drug therapy. In: Kaplan NM, ed. Clinical Hypertension. 5th ed. Baltimore: Williams & Wilkins, 1990: 163–181.

9. Rudnick KV, Sackett DL, Hirst S, et al. Hypertension in a family practice. Can Med Assoc J 1977; 117:492–497.

10. Danielson M, Dammstroom B. The prevalence of secondary and curable hypertension. Acta Med Scand 1981; 209:451–455.

11. Sinclair AM, Isles CG, Brown I, et al. Secondary hypertension in a blood pressure clinic. Arch Intern Med 1987; 147:1289–1293.

12. Anderson GH, Blakeman N, Streeten DHP. Prediction of renovascular hypertension: comparison of clinical diagnostic indices. Am J Hypertens 1988; 1:301–304.

13. Sutton MGSJ, Sheps SG, Lie JT. Prevalence of clinically unsuspected pheochromocytoma. Mayo Clin Proc 1981; 56:354–360.

14. O'Neal LW, Kissane JM, Hartroft PM. The kidney in endocrine hypertension. Arch Surg 1970; 100:498–505.

15. Andersen GS, Totfdahl DB, Lund JO, et al. The incidence rate of pheochromocytoma and Conn's syndrome in Denmark, 1977–1981. J Hum Hypertens 1988; 2:187–189.

16. Page IH. The mosaic theory 32 years later. Hypertension 1982; 4:177.

17. Munger RG, Prineas RJ, Gomez-Marin O. Persistent elevation of blood pressure among children with a family history of hypertension: the Minneapolis children's blood pressure study. J Hypertens 1988; 6:647–653.

18. Swales JD. Blood pressure: from cells to populations: the Bradshaw lecture 1987. J R Coll Physicians Lond 1988; 22:11–15.

19. Esler M, Jennings G, Korner P, et al. Assessment of human sympathetic nervous system activity from measurements of norepinephrine turnover. Hypertension 1988; 11:3–20.

20. Sealey JE, Blumenfeld JD, Bell GM, et al. On the renal basis for essential hypertension: nephron heterogeneity with discordant renin secretion and sodium excretion causing a hypertensive vasoconstriction–volume relationship. J Hypertens 1988; 6:763–777.

21. Reaven GM, Hoffman BB. A role for insulin in the aetiology and course of hypertension? Lancet 1987; 2:435–436.

22. Yanagisawa M, Kurihara H, Kimura S, et al. A novel potent vasoconstrictor peptide produced by vascular endothelial cells. Nature 1988; 332:411–415.

23. Folkow B, Grimby G, Thulesius O. Adaptive structural changes of the vascular walls in hypertension and their relation to the control of peripheral resistance. Acta Physiol Scand 1958; 44:255–272.

24. Dzau VJ, Gibbons GH. Cell biology of vascular hypertrophy in systemic hypertension. Am J Cardiol 1988; 62:30G–35G.

25. Long CJ, Berkowitz BA. What is the relationship between the endothelium derived relaxant factor and nitric oxide? Life Sci 1989; 45:1–14.

26. Vanhoutte PM. Endothelium and responsiveness of vascular smooth muscle. J Hypertens 1987; 5(Suppl 5):S115–S120.

27. Panza JA, Quyyumi AA, Epstein SE. Impaired endothelium-dependent vascular relaxation in hypertensive patients. Circulation 1988; 78(Suppl II):II473 (abstract).

28. Folkow B. Physiology aspects of primary hypertension. Physiol Rev 1982; 62:347–504.

29. Aalkjaer C, Heagerty AM, Petersen KK, et al. Evidence for increased media thickness, increased neuronal amine uptake, and depressed excitation-contraction coupling in isolated resistance vessels from essential hypertensives. Circ Res 1987; 61:181–186.

30. Lever AF. Slow pressor mechanisms in hypertension: a role for hypertrophy of resistance vessels? J Hypertens 1986; 4:515–524.

31. Griendling KK, Berk BC, Ganz P, et al. Angiotensin II stimulation of vascular smooth muscle phosphoinositide metabolism. Hypertension 1987; 9(Suppl III):III181–III185.

32. Berridge MJ, Irvine RF. Inositol trisphosphate, a novel second messenger in cellular signal transduction. Nature 1984; 312:315–321.

33. Kaplan NM. The deadly quartet: upper body obesity, glucose intolerance, hypertriglyceridemia and hypertension. Arch Intern Med 1989; 149:1514–1519.

34. Peiris AN, Mueller RA, Smith GA, et al: Splanchnic insulin metabolism in obesity: influence of body fat distribution. J Clin Invest 1986; 78:1648–1657.

35. Stromblad G, Bjorntorp P. Reduced hepatic insulin clearance in rats with dietary-induced obesity. Metabolism 1986; 35:323–327.

36. Eckel RH, Sadur CN, Yost TJ. Deficiency of the insulin, glucose-mediated decrease in serum triglycerides in normolipidemic obese subjects. Int J Obes 1988; 12:369–376.

37. Rowe JW, Yound JB, Minaker KL, et al. Effect of insulin and glucose infusions on sympathetic nervous system activity in normal man. Diabetes 1981; 30:219–225.

38. Baum M. Insulin stimulates volume absorption in the rabbit proximal convoluted tubule. J Clin Invest 1987; 79:1104–1109.

39. Stout RW, Bierman EL, Ross R. Effect of insulin on the proliferation of cultured primate arterial smooth muscle cells. Circ Res 1975; 36:319–327.

40. Kaiser N, Tur-Sinai A, Hasin M, et al. Binding, degradation, and biological activity of insulin in vascular smooth muscle cells. Am J Physiol 1985; 249:E292–E298.

41. Cruz AB Jr, Amatuzio DS, Grande F, et al. Effect of intra-arterial insulin on tissue cholesterol and fatty acids in alloxan-diabetic dogs. Circ Res 1961; 9:39–43.

42. Rosic NK, Standaert ML, Pollet RJ. The mechanism of insulin stimulation of (Na^+,K^+)-ATPase transport activity in muscle. J Biol Chem 1985; 260:6206–6212.

43. Ferrannini E, Buzzigoli G, Bonadonna R, et al. Insulin resistance in essential hypertension. N Engl J Med 1987; 317:350–357.

44. Ng LL, Harker M, Abel ED. Mechanisms of leucocyte sodium influx in essential hypertension. Clin Sci 1988; 75:521–526.

45. Blaustein MP. Sodium ions, calcium ions, blood pressure regulation, and hypertension: a reassessment and a hypothesis. Am J Physiol 1977; 232:C165–C173.

46. de Wardener HE, MacGregor GA. Dahl's hypothesis that a saluretic substance may be responsible for a sustained rise in arterial pressure: its possible role in essential hypertension. Kidney Int 1980; 18:1–9.

47. Hamlyn JM, Harris DW, Ludens JH. A humoral digitalis-like factor in man: affinity and mechanism of inhibition. Circulation 1988; 78(Suppl II):II369 (abstract).

48. Hughes A, Thom S, Goldberg P, et al. Direct effect of alpha-human atrial natriuretic peptide on human vasculature in vivo and in vitro. Clin Sci 1988; 74:207–211.

49. Richards AM, McDonald D, Fitzpatrick MA, et al. Atrial natriuretic hormone has biological effects in man at physiological plasma concentrations. J Clin Endocrinol Metab 1988; 67:1134–1139.

50. Greenwald JE, Sakata M, Michener ML, et al. Is atriopeptin a physiological or pathophysiological substance? Studies in the autoimmune rat. J Clin Invest 1988; 81:1036–1041.

51. Saito Y, Nakao K, Sugawara A, et al. Exaggerated secretion of atrial natriuretic polypeptide during dynamic exercise in patients with essential hypertension. Am Heart J 1988; 116:1052–1057.

52. Ferrier C, Weidmann P, Hollmann R, et al. Impaired response of atrial natriuretic factor to high salt intake in persons prone to hypertension. N Engl J Med 1988; 319:1223–1224.

53. Postnov YV, Orlov SN, Shevchenko A, et al. Altered sodium permeability, calcium binding and Na-K-ATPase activity in the red blood cell membrane in essential hypertension. Pflugers Arch 1977; 371:263–269.

54. Marche P, Koutouzov S, Girard A, et al. Phosphoinositide turnover in erythrocyte membranes in human and experimental hypertension. J Hypertens 1985; 3:25–30.

55. Sancho J, Re R, Burton J, et al. The role of the renin-angiotensin-aldosterone system in cardiovascular homeostasis in normal human subjects. Circulation 1976; 53:400–405.

56. Gomez-Sanchez CE, Holland OB, Upcavage R. Urinary free 19-nor-deoxycorticosterone and deoxycorticosterone in human hypertension. J Clin Endocrinol Metab 1985; 60:234–238.

57. Ulick S, Levine LS, Gunczler P, et al. A syndrome of apparent mineralocorticoid excess associated with defects in the peripheral metabolism of cortisol. J Clin Endocrinol Metab 1979; 49:757–764.

58. Stewart PM, Corrie JET, Shackleton CHL, et al. Syndrome of apparent mineralocorticoid excess. J Clin Invest 1988; 82:340–349.

59. Stewart PM, Valentino R, Wallace AM, et al. Mineralocorticoid activity of liquorice: 11-beta-hydroxysteroid dehydrogenase deficiency comes of age. Lancet 1987; 2:821–824.

60. Meade TW, Imeson JD, Gordon D, et al. The epidemiology of plasma renin. Clin Sci 1983; 64:273–280.

61. Swales JD. Low-renin hypertension: nephrosclerosis? Lancet 1975; 1:75–77.

62. Brenner BM, Garcia DL, Anderson S. Glomeruli and blood pressure: less of one, more of the other? Am J Hypertens 1988; 1:335–347.

63. Hollenberg NK, Williams GH. Abnormal renal function, sodium-volume homeostasis, and renin-system behavior in normal-renin essential hypertension. In: Laragh JH, Brenner BM, eds. Hypertension Pathophysiology, Diagnosis, and Treatment. New York: Raven, 1990: 1349–1370.

64. Williams GH, Hollenberg NK. Abnormal adrenal and renal responses to angiotensin II in essential hypertension. In: Edwards CRW, Carey RM, eds. Essential Hypertension as an Endocrine Disease. London: Butterworth, 1985: 184–211.

65. Dzau VJ. Circulating versus local renin-angiotensin system in cardiovascular homeostasis. Circulation 1988; 77(Suppl I): I4–I13.

66. Gordon DB. The role of renin substrate in hypertension. Hypertension 1983; 5:353–362.

67. Plumer LB, Kaplan GW, Mendoza SA. Hypertension in infants—a complication of umbilical arterial catheterization. J Pediatr 1976; 5:802–805.

68. Keith TA. Renovascular hypertension in black patients. Hypertension 1982; 4:438–443.

69. Sunderlin FS Jr, Anderson GH Jr, Streeten DHP, et al. The renin-angiotensin-aldosterone system in diabetic patients with hyperkalemia. Diabetes 1981; 30:335–340.

70. Davis BA, Crook JE, Vestal RE, et al. Prevalence of renovascular hypertension in patients with grade II or IV hypertension retinopathy. N Engl J Med 1979; 23:1273–1276.

71. Jacobson HR. Ischemic renal disease: an overlooked clinical entity? Kidney Int 1988; 34:729–743.

72. Ying CY, Tifft CP, Gavras H, et al. Renal revascularization in the azotemic hypertensive patient resistant to therapy. N Engl J Med 1984; 311:1071–1075.

73. Pickering TG, Devereux RB, James GD, et al. Recurrent pulmonary oedema in hypertension due to bilateral renal artery stenosis: treatment by angioplasty or surgical revascularisation. Lancet 1988; 2:551–552.

74. Zimmerman JB, Robertson D, Jackson EK. Angiotensin II-nordrenergic interactions in renovascular hypertensive rats. J Clin Invest 1987; 80:443–457.

75. Russell GI, Bing RF, Thurston H, et al. Surgical reversal of two-kidney one clip hypertension during inhibition of the renin-angiotensin system. Hypertension 1982; 4:69–76.

76. Thal AP, Grage TB, Vernier RL. Function of the contralateral kidney in renal hypertension due to renal artery stenosis. Circulation 1963; 27:36–43.

77. Working Group on Renovascular Hypertension. Detection, evaluation and treatment of renovascular hypertension: final report. Arch Intern Med 1987; 147:820–829.

78. Rudnick MR, Maxwell MH. Limitations of renin assays. In: Narins RG, ed. Controversies in Nephrology and Hypertension. New York: Churchill Livingstone, 1984; 123–160.

79. Imai Y, Abe K, Otsuka Y, et al. Exaggerated response of renin secretion to captopril (SQ 14225) in renovascular hypertension. Jpn Heart J 1980; 21:793–802.

80. Muller FB, Sealey JE, Case DB, et al. The captopril test for identifying renovascular disease in hypertensive patients. Am J Med 1986; 80:633–644.

81. Idrissi A, Fournier A, Renaud H, et al. The captopril challenge test as a screening test for renovascular hypertension. Kidney Int 1988; 34(Suppl 25):S138–S141.

82. Gaul MK, Linn WD, Mulrow CD. Captopril stimulated renin secretion in the diagnosis of renovascular hypertension. Am J Hypertens 1988; 1:73A (abstract).

83. Geyskes GG, Oei HY, Puylaert CBAJ, et al. Renovascular hypertension identified by captopril-induced changes in the renogram. Hypertension 1987; 9:451–458.

84. Maxwell MH, Marks LS, Lupu AN, et al. Predictive value of renin determinations in renal artery stenosis. JAMA 1977; 238:2617–2620.

85. Lüscher TF, Greminger P, Kuhlmann U, et al. Renal venous renin determinations in renovascular hypertension. Diagnostic and prognostic value in unilateral renal artery stenosis treated by surgery or percutaneous transluminal angioplasty. Nephron 1986; 44(Suppl 1):17–24.

86. Bookstein JJ. Segmental renal artery stenosis in renovascular hypertension. Radiology 1968; 90:1073–1083.

87. Novick AC. Surgical management of renovascular hypertension. In: Kaplan NM, Brenner BM, Laragh JH, eds. The Kidney in Hypertension. New York: Raven, 1987; 225–237.

88. Libertino JA, Flam TA, Zinman LN, et al. Changing concepts in surgical management of renovascular hypertension. Arch Intern Med 1988; 148:357–359.

89. Schwarten DE. Percutaneous transluminal renal artery angioplasty. In: Kaplan NM, Brenner BM, Laragh JH, eds. The Kidney in Hypertension. New York: Raven, 1987; 239–250.

90. Staessen J, Wilms G, Baert A, et al. Blood pressure during long-term converting enzyme inhibition predicts the curability of renovascular hypertension by angioplasty. Am J Hypertens 1988; 1:208–214.

91. Hollenberg NK. Medical therapy for renovascular hypertension: a review. Am J Hypertens 1988; 1:338S–343S.

92. Wenting GJ, Derkx FHM, Tan-Tjiong LH, et al. Risks of angiotensin converting enzyme inhibition in renal artery stenosis. Kidney Int 1987; 31(Suppl 20):S180–S183.

93. Miyamori I, Yasuhara S, Matsubara T, et al. Comparative effects of captopril and nifedipine on split renal function in renovascular hypertension. Am J Hypertens 1988; 1:359–363.

94. Corvol P, Pinet F, Galen FX, et al. Seven lessons from seven renin secreting tumors. Kidney Int 1988; 34(Suppl 25):S38–S44.

95. Sheth KJ, Tang TT, Blaedel ME, et al. Polydipsia, polyuria, and hypertension associated with renin-secreting Wilms tumor. J Pediatr 1978; 92:921–924.

96. Klahr S, Schreiner G, Ichikawa I. The progression of renal disease. N Engl J Med 1988; 318:1657–1666.

97. Anderson S, Diamond JR, Karnovsky MJ, et al. Mechanisms underlying transition from acute glomerular injury to late glomerular sclerosis in a rat model of nephrotic syndrome. J Clin Invest 1988; 82:1757–1768.

98. Sugimoto T, Rosansky SJ. The incidence of treated end stage renal disease in the Eastern United States: 1973–1979. Am J Public Health 1984; 74:14–17.

99. Anderson S, Brenner BM. Therapeutic benefit of converting-enzyme inhibition in progressive renal disease. J Hypertens 1988; 1:380S–383S.

100. Marre M, Leblanc H, Suarez L, et al. Converting enzyme inhibition and kidney function in normotensive diabetic patients with persistent microalbuminuria. Br Med J 1987; 294:1448–1452.

101. Parving H-H, Andersen AR, Smidt UM, et al. Effect of antihypertensive treatment on kidney function in diabetic nephropathy. Br Med J 1987; 294:1443–1447.

102. Carretero OA, Scicli AG. Kinins: paracrine hormone. Kidney Int 1988; 34(Suppl 26):S52–S59.

103. Muirhead EE. The renomedullary system of blood pressure control. Am J Med Sci 1988; 295:231–233.

104. Nadler JL, Lee FO, Hsueh W, et al. Evidence of prostacyclin deficiency in the syndrome of hyporeninemic hypoaldosteronism. N Engl J Med 1986; 314:1015–1020.

105. Weidmann P, Massry SG, Coburn JW, et al. Blood pressure effects of acute hypercalcemia. Studies in patients with chronic renal failure. Ann Intern Med 1972; 76:741–748.

106. Raine AEG. Hypertension, blood viscosity, and cardiovascular morbidity in renal failure: implications of erythropoietin therapy. Lancet 1988; 1:97–99.

107. Plunkett WC, Overbeck HW. Arteriolar wall thickening in hypertensive rats unrelated to pressure or sympathoadrenergic influences. Circ Res 1988; 63:937–943.

108. Royal College of General Practitioners. Oral Contraceptives and Health. New York: Pitman, 1974: 37–42.

109. Prentice RL. On the ability of blood pressure effects to explain the relation between oral contraceptives and cardiovascular disease. Am J Epidemiol 1988; 127:213–219.

110. Weir RJ. Hypertension secondary to contraceptive agents. In: Amery A, Fagard R, Lijnen P, et al., eds. Hypertensive Cardiovascular Disease: Pathophysiology and Treatment. The Hague: Martinus Nijhoff, 1982: 612–628.

111. Khaw K, Peart WS. Blood pressure and contraceptive use. Br Med J 1983; 285:403–407.

112. Meade TW. Effects of progestogens on the cardiovascular system. Am J Obstet Gynecol 1982; 142:776–780.

113. Wallace RB, Barrett-Connor E, Criqui M, et al. Alteration in blood pressure associated with combined alcohol and oral contraceptive use—the lipid research clinics prevalence study. J Chronic Dis 1982; 35:251–257.

114. McAreavey D, Cumming AMM, Boddy K, et al. The renin-angiotensin system and total body sodium and potassium in hypertensive women taking oestrogen-progestagen oral contraceptives. Clin Endocrinol 1983; 18:111–118.

115. Horwitz KB, Horwitz LD. Canine vascular tissues are targets for androgens, estrogens, progestins, and glucocorticoids. J Clin Invest 1982; 69:750–756.

116. Colucci WS, Gimbrone MA Jr, McLaughlin MK, et al. Increased vascular catecholamine sensitivity and alpha-adrenergic receptor affinity in female and estrogen-treated male rats. Circ Res 1982; 50:805–811.

117. Hassager C, Riis BJ, Strom V, et al. The long-term effect of oral and percutaneous estradiol on plasma renin substrate and blood pressure. Circulation 1987; 76:753–758.

118. Knopp RH. The effects of postmenopausal estrogen therapy on the incidence of arteriosclerotic vascular disease. Obstet Gynecol 1988; 72:23S–30S.

119. Paganini-Hill A, Ross RK, Henderson BE. Postmenopausal oestrogen treatment and stroke: a prospective study. Br Med J 1988; 297:519–522.

120. Hedeland H, Ostberg G, Hökfelt B. On the prevalence of adrenocortical adenomas in an autopsy material in relation to hypertension and diabetes. Acta Med Scand 1968; 184:211–214.

121. Copeland PM. The incidentally discovered adrenal mass. Ann Intern Med 1983; 98:940–945.

122. Belldegrun A, Hussain S, Seltzer SE, et al. Incidentally discovered mass of the adrenal gland. Surg Gynecol Obstet 1986; 163:203–208.

123. Gross MD, Shapiro B, Gouffard JA, et al. Distinguishing benign from malignant euadrenal masses. Ann Intern Med 1988; 109:613–618.

124. Bravo EL, Tarazi RC, Dustan HP, et al. The changing clinical spectrum of primary aldosteronism. Am J Med 1983; 74:641–651.

125. Matsunaga M, Hara A, Song TS, et al. Asymptomatic normotensive primary aldosteronism. Hypertension 1983; 5:240–243.

126. McAreavey D, Murray GD, Lever AF, et al. Similarity of idiopathic aldosteronism and essential hypertension. Hypertension 1983; 5:116–121.

127. Gomez-Sanchez CE, Gill JR Jr, Ganguly A, et al. Glucocorticoid-suppressible aldosteronism: a disorder of the adrenal transitional zone. J Clin Endocrinol Metab 1988; 67:444–448.

128. Todesco S, Terribile V, Borsatti A, et al. Primary aldosteronism due to a malignant ovarian tumor. J Clin Endocrinol Metab 1975; 41:809–819.

129. Lauzurica R, Bonal J, Bonet J, et al. Rhabdomyolysis, oedema and arterial hypertension: different syndromes related to topical use of 9-alpha-fluoroprednisolone. J Hum Hypertens 1988; 2:183–186.

130. Wenting GJ, Man in't Veld AJ, Derkx FHM, et al. Recurrence of hypertension in primary aldosteronism after discontinuation of spironolactone. Time course of changes in cardiac output and body fluid volumes. Clin Exp Hypertens 1982; A4:1727–1748.

131. Beevers DG, Brown JJ, Ferriss JB, et al. Renal abnormalities and vascular complications in primary hyperaldosteronism. Evidence on tertiary hyperaldosteronism. Q J Med 1976; 45:401–410.

132. Bravo EL, Fouad-Tarazi FM, Tarazi RC, et al. Clinical implications of primary aldosteronism with resistant hypertension. Hypertension 1988; 11(Suppl I):I207–I211.

133. Hamlet SM, Tunny TJ, Woodland E, et al. Is aldosterone/renin ratio useful to screen a hypertensive population for primary aldosteronism? Clin Exp Pharmacol Physiol 1985; 12:249–252.

134. Kem DC, Weinberger MH, Mayes DM, et al. Saline suppression of plasma aldosterone in hypertension. Arch Intern Med 1971; 128:380–386.

135. Holland OB, Brown H, Kuhnert LV, et al. Further evaluation of saline infusion for the diagnosis of primary aldosteronism. Hypertension 1984; 6:717–723.

136. Stokes GS, Monaghan JC, Mennie BA. Use of an intravenous sodium load in screening for primary hyperaldosteronism. Aust NZ J Med 1984; 14:201–207.

137. Young WF Jr, Glee GG. Primary aldosteronism: diagnostic evaluation. Endocrinol Metab Clin North Am 1988; 17:367–395.

138. Gordon RD, Gomez-Sanchez CE, Hamlet SM, et al. Angiotensin-responsive aldosterone-producing adenoma masquerades as idiopathic hyperaldosteronism (IHA: adrenal hyperplasia) or low-renin essential hypertension. J Hypertens 1987; 5(Suppl 5):S103–S106.

139. Pringle SD, Macfarland PW, Isles CG, et al. Regression of electrocardiographic left ventricular hypertrophy following treatment of primary hyperaldosteronism. J Hum Hypertens 1988; 2:157–159.

140. Leal-Cerro A, Garcia-Luna PP, Villar J, et al. Ketoconazole as an inhibitor of steroid production. N Engl J Med 1988; 318:710–711 (letter).

141. Kaplan NM. Cushing's syndrome and congenital adrenal hyperplasia. In: Clinical Hypertension. 4th ed. Baltimore: Williams & Wilkins, 1986: 422–433.

142. Ritchie CM, Hadden DR, Kennedy L, et al. Pathogenesis of hypertension in Cushing's disease. J Hypertens 1987; 5(Suppl 5):S497–S499.

143. Imai Y, Abe K, Sasaki S, et al. Altered circadian blood pressure rhythm in patients with Cushing's syndrome. Hypertension 1988; 12:11–19.

144. De Simone G, Tommaselli AP, Rossi R, et al. Partial deficiency of adrenal 11-hydroxylase: a possible cause of primary hypertension. Hypertension 1985; 7:204–210.

145. Fraser R, Brown JJ, Mason PA, et al. Severe hypertension with absent secondary sex characteristics due to partial deficiency of steroid 17-alpha-hydroxylase activity. J Hum Hypertens 1987; 1:53–58.

146. Davies DL, Beastall GH, Connell JMC, et al. Body composition, blood pressure and the renin-angiotensin system in acromegaly before and after treatment. J Hypertens 1985; 3(Suppl 3):S413–S415.

147. Deray G, Rieu M, Devynck MA, et al. Evidence of an endogenous digitalis-like factor in the plasma of patients with acromegaly. N Engl J Med 1987; 316:575–580.

148. Wang C, Chan TK, Yeung RTT, et al. The effect of triamterene and sodium intake on renin, aldosterone, and erythrocyte sodium transport in Liddle's syndrome. J Clin Endocrinol Metab 1981; 52:1027–1032.

149. Tormey WP, Morgan DB. Etiological considerations in Gordon's syndrome: possible role of prostaglandins. Prostaglandins Med 1980; 4:107–112.

150. Imai Y, Abe K, Miura Y, et al. Hypertensive episodes and circadian fluctuations of blood pressure in patients with phaeochromocytoma: studies by long-term blood pressure monitoring based on a volume-oscillometric method. J Hypertens 1988; 6:9–15.

151. Kuchel O. Pseudopheochromocytoma. Hypertension 1985; 7:151–158.

152. Kaplan NM, Kramer NJ, Holland OB, et al. Single-voided urine metanephrine assays in screening for pheochromocytoma. Arch Intern Med 1977; 137:190–193.

153. Johnson LR, Reese M, Nelson DH. Interference in Pisano's urinary metanephrine assay after use of x-ray contrast media. Clin Chem 1972; 18:209–211.

154. Duncan MW, Compton P, Lazarus L, et al. Measurement of norepinephrine and 3,4-dihydroxyphenylglycol in urine and plasma for the diagnosis of pheochromocytoma. N Engl J Med 1988; 319:136–142.

155. Feldman JM. Falsely elevated urinary excretion of catecholamines and metanephrines in patients receiving labetalol therapy. J Clin Pharmacol 1987; 27:288–292.

156. Bravo EL, Gifford RW Jr. Pheochromocytoma: diagnosis, localization and management. N Engl J Med 1984; 311:1298–1303.

157. Macdougall IC, Isles CG, Stewart H, et al. Overnight clonidine suppression test in the diagnosis and exclusion of pheochromocytoma. Am J Med 1988; 84:993–1000.

158. Mannelli M, Feo ML, Maggi M, et al. Usefulness of basal catecholamine plasma levels and clonidine suppression test in the diagnosis of pheochromocytoma. J Endocrinol Invest 1987; 10:377–382.

159. Allison DJ, Brown MJ, Jones DH, et al. Role of venous sampling in locating a phaeochromocytoma. Br Med J 1983; 286:1122–1124.

160. Gross MD, Shapiro B. Scintigraphic studies in adrenal hypertension. Semin Nucl Med 1989; 19:122–143.

161. Scully RE, Mark EJ, McNeely WF, et al. Case records of the Massachu-setts General Hospital: case 46-1988: presentation of case. N Engl J Med 1988; 319:1336–1343.

162. Sheps SG, Jiang N-S, Klee GC. Diagnostic evaluation of pheochromocytoma. Endocrinol Metab Clin North Am 1988; 17:397–414.

163. Gagel RF, Tashjian AH Jr, Cummings T, et al. The clinical outcome of prospective screening for multiple endocrine neoplasia type 2a: an 18-year experience. N Engl J Med 1988; 318:478–484.

164. Pullerits J, Ein S, Balfe JW. Anaesthesia for phaeochromocytoma. Can J Anaesth 1988; 35:526–534.

165. Averbuch SD, Steakley CS, Young RC, et al. Malignant pheochromocytoma: effective treatment with a combination of cyclophosphamide, vincristine, and dacarbazine. Ann Intern Med 1988; 109:267–273.

166. Goldstein DS, Stull R, Eisenhofer G, et al. Plasma 3,4-dihydroxyphenylalanine (dopa) and catecholamines in neuroblastoma or pheochromocytoma. Ann Intern Med 1986; 105:887–888.

167. Weinblatt ME, Heisel MA, Siegel SE. Hypertension in children with neurogenic tumors. Pediatrics 1983; 71:947–951.

168. Louis WJ, Doyle AE, Heath WC, et al. Secretion of dopa in phaeochromocytoma. Br Med J 1972; 4:325–327.

169. Gray RJ, Bateman TM, Czer LSC, et al. Comparison of esmolol and nitroprusside for acute post-cardiac surgical hypertension. Am J Cardiol 1987; 59:887–891.

170. Skydell JL, Machleder HI, Baker JD, et al. Incidence and mechanism of post-carotid endarterectomy hypertension. Arch Surg 1987; 122: 1153–1155.

171. Orlowski JP, Shiesley D, Vidt DG, et al. Labetalol to control blood pressure after cerebrovascular surgery. Crit Care Med 1988; 16:765–768.

172. Naftchi NE, Demeny M, Lowman EW, et al. Hypertensive crises in quadriplegic patients. Circulation 1978; 57:336–341.

173. Beal MF, Atuk NO, Westfall TC, et al. Catecholamine uptake, accumulation, and release in acute porphyria. J Clin Invest 1977; 60:1141–1148.

174. Lake CR, Zaloga G, Clymer R, et al. A double dose of phenylpropanolamine causes transient hypertension. Am J Med 1988; 85:339–343.

175. Virmani R, Robinowitz M, Smialek JE, et al. Cardiovascular effects of cocaine: an autopsy study of 40 patients. Am Heart J 1988; 115:1068–1076.

176. Schachter M. Cyclosporine A and hypertension. J Hypertens 1988; 6:511–516.

177. Curtis JJ, Luke RG, Jones P, et al. Hypertension in cyclosporine-treated renal transplant recipients is sodium dependent. Am J Med 1988; 85:134–138.

178. Feehally J, Walls J, Mistry N, et al. Does nifedipine ameliorate cyclosporin A nephrotoxicity? Br Med J 1987; 295:310.

179. Richards AM, Espiner EA, Nicholls MG, et al. Hormone, calcium and blood pressure relationships in primary hyperparathyroidism. J Hypertens 1988; 6:747–752.

180. Lind L, Wengle B, Wide L, et al. Hypertension in primary hyperparathyroidism—reduction of blood pressure by long-term treatment with vitamin D (alphacalcidol): double-blind, placebo-controlled study. Am J Hypertens 1988; 1:397–402.

181. Cirillo M, Strazzullo P, Galletti F, et al. Development of hypertension after correction of primary hyperparathyroidism. Hypertension 1988; 11:285–287.

182. Diamond TW, Botha JR, Wing J, et al. Parathyroid hypertension: a reversible disorder. Arch Intern Med 1986; 146:1709–1712.

183. Lind L, Jakobsson S, Lithell H, et al. Relation of serum calcium concentration to metabolic risk factors for cardiovascular disease. Br Med J 1988; 297:960–963.

184. McCarron DA, Morris CD. Blood pressure response to oral calcium in persons with mild to moderate hypertension: a randomized double-blind placebo-controlled crossover trial. Ann Intern Med 1985; 103:825–831.

185. Grobbee DE, Hoffman A. Effect of calcium supplementation on diastolic blood pressure in young people with mild hypertension. Lancet 1986; 2:703–707.

186. Kaplan NM. Calcium and potassium in the treatment of essential hypertension. Semin Nephrol 1988; 8:176–184.

187. Brickman AS, Stern N, Sowers JR. Hypertension in pseudohypoparathyroidism type I. Am J Med 1988; 85:785–792.

188. Streeten DHP, Anderson GH Jr, Howland T, et al. Effects of thyroid function on blood pressure: recognition of hypothyroid hypertension. Hypertension 1988; 11:78–83.

189. Rosenthal E, Najm YC, Maisey MN, et al. Pressor effects of thyrotrophin releasing hormone during thyroid function testing. Br Med J 1987; 294:806–807.

190. Cooper DS, Daniels GH, Ladenson PW, et al. Hyperthyroxinemia in patients treated with high-dose propranolol. Am J Med 1982; 73:867–871.

191. Bretza JA, Novey HS, Vaziri ND, et al. Hypertension. A complication of danazol therapy. Arch Intern Med 1980; 140:1379–1380.

192. Davey DA, MacGillivray I. The classification and definition of the hypertensive disorders of pregnancy. Am J Obstet Gynecol 1988; 158:892–898.

193. Cooper DW, Hill JA, Chesley LC, et al. Genetic control of susceptibility to eclampsia and miscarriage. Br J Obstet Gynaecol 1988; 95:644–653.

194. Boyd P, Lindenbaum RH, Redman C. Pre-eclampsia and trisomy 13: a possible association. Lancet 1987; 2:425–427.

195. Alderman BW, Sperling RS, Daling JR. An epidemiological study of the immunogenetic aetiology of pre-eclampsia. Br Med J 1986; 292:372–374.

196. Guzick DS, Klein VR, Tyson JE, et al. Risk factors for the occurrence of pregnancy-induced hypertension. Clin Exp Hypertens 1987; B6(2):281–297.

197. Ihle BU, Long P, Oats J. Early onset pre-eclampsia: recognition of underlying renal disease. Br Med J 1987; 294:79–81.

198. Moutquin JM, Raiville C, Giroux L, et al. A prospective study of blood pressure in pregnancy: prediction of preeclampsia. Am J Obstet Gynecol 1985; 151:191–196.

199. Chesley LC, Sibai BM. Clinical significance of elevated mean arterial pressure in the second trimester. Am J Obstet Gynecol 1988; 159:275–279.

200. Symonds EM. Renin and reproduction. Am J Obstet Gynecol 1988; 158:754–761.

201. Friedman SA. Preeclampsia: a review of the role of prostaglandins. Obstet Gynecol 1988; 71:122–137.

202. Fitzgerald DJ, Entman SS, Mulloy K, et al. Decreased prostacyclin biosynthesis preceding the clinical manifestation of pregnancy-induced hypertension. Circulation 1987; 75:956–963.

203. Walsh SW. Progesterone and estradiol production by normal and preeclamptic placentas. Obstet Gynecol 1988; 71:222–226.

204. Beaufils M, Donsimoni R, Uzan S, et al. Prevention of preeclampsia by early antiplatelet therapy. Lancet 1985; 1:840.

205. Schiff E, Peleg E, Goldenberg M, et al. The use of aspirin to prevent pregnancy-induced hypertension and lower the ratio of thromboxane A₂ to prostacyclin in relatively high risk pregnancies. N Engl J Med 1989; 321:351–356.

206. Bauman WA, Maimen M, Langer O. An association between hyperinsulinemia and hypertension during the third trimester of pregnancy. Am J Obstet Gynecol 1988; 159:446–450.

207. Hirai N, Yanaihara T, Nakayama T, et al. Plasma levels of atrial natriuretic peptide during normal pregnancy and in pregnancy complicated by hypertension. Am J Obstet Gynecol 1988; 159:27–31.

208. Phelps SJ, Cochran EB, Gonzalez-Ruiz A, et al. The influence of gestational age and preeclampsia on the presence and magnitude of serum endogenous digoxin-like immunoreactive substance(s). Am J Obstet Gynecol 1988; 158:34–39.

209. Testa I, Rabini RA, Danieli G, et al. Abnormal membrane cation transport in pregnancy-induced hypertension. Scand J Clin Lab Invest 1988; 48:7–13.

210. Rasmussen K. Fetal haemodynamics before and after treatment of maternal hypertension in pregnancy. Dan Med Bull 1987; 34:170–172.

211. Frishman WH, Chesner M. Beta-adrenergic blockers in pregnancy. Am Heart J 1988; 115:147–152.

212. Lubbe WF. Hypertension in pregnancy: whom and how to treat. Br J Clin Pharmacol 1987; 24:15S–20S.

213. Plouin P-F, Breart G, Maillard F, et al. Comparison of antihypertensive efficacy and perinatal safety of labetalol and methyldopa in the treatment of hypertension in pregnancy: a randomized controlled trial. Br J Obstet Gynaecol 1988; 95:868–876.

214. Constatine G, Beevers DG, Reynolds AL, et al. Nifedipine as a second line antihypertensive drug in pregnancy. Br J Obstet Gynaecol 1987; 94:1136–1142.

215. Kreft-Jais C, Plouin P-F, Tchobroutsky C, et al. Angiotensin-converting enzyme inhibitors during pregnancy: a survey of 22 patients given captopril and nine given enalapril. Br J Obstet Gynaecol 1988; 95:420–422.

216. Sibai BM, Gonzalez AR, Mabie WC, et al. A comparison of labetalol plus hospitalization versus hospitalization alone in the management of preeclampsia remote from term. Obstet Gynecol 1987; 70:323–327.

217. Lithell H, Haglund K, Granath F, et al. Are effects of antihypertensive treatment on lipoproteins merely "side-effects"? Acta Med Scand 1988; 223:531–536.

218. Bansal S. Sexual dysfunction in hypertensive men: a critical review of the literature. Hypertension 1988; 12:1–10.

219. Kaplan NM, Rosenstock J, Raskin P. A differing view of treatment of hypertension in patients with diabetes mellitus. Arch Intern Med 1987; 147:1160–1162.

220. Parving H-H, Hommel E, Smidt UM. Protection of kidney function and decrease in albuminuria by captopril in insulin dependent diabetics with nephropathy. Br Med J 1988; 297:1086–1091.

12

DISORDERS OF THE OVARY AND FEMALE REPRODUCTIVE TRACT

Bruce R. Carr

INTRODUCTION

The ovaries are the source of ova and of the hormones that regulate female sexual life. These two functions are under precise but complex feedback control by the hypothalamic-pituitary axis. The rapid growth of a single follicle that will become dominant and release an ovum and the regularity of this process for an average of 38 y are remarkable phenomena. The complex local regulation and departmentalization in the ovary that give rise to follicular growth appear to be controlled by factors produced within the ovary itself. Estrogens, the principal hormones secreted by the ovary, promote growth and differentiation of the uterus, fallopian tubes, and vagina, as well as affect other signs of sexual maturation. Disorders of the ovary can give rise to sexual precocity, disorders of the menstrual cycle, androgen excess, and infertility. With aging, most remaining follicles undergo atresia so that by age 50 few follicles remain, estrogen levels decline, secondary sexual characteristics regress, and menopause ensues.

THE NORMAL OVARY AND OVARIAN FUNCTION

Early Development of the Ovary

Fetal Ovary

Genetic sex is determined at conception, and the development of the gonads takes place early in fetal development.

The bipotential gonadal anlagen, which give rise to either the ovaries or the testes, can be identified in human embryos by 30 d after fertilization, and the ovary can be identified histologically about day 70.[1] The ovary is composed of three principal cell types: (1) coelomic epithelial cells, which are derived from the gonadal ridge and later differentiate into granulosa cells; (2) mesenchymal cells of the gonadal ridge, which give rise to the ovarian stroma; and (3) primordial germ cells, which arise from the endoderm of the yolk sac and migrate into the gonadal ridge before differentiation into ova.

During the third week of gestation the primordial germ cells can be identified in the yolk sac at the caudal end of the ovary. The sex of the migrating primordial cells can be determined by analysis of sex chromatin. In female germ cells, one X chromosome is inactivated during migration to the gonadal ridge.[2] As formulated by Lyon,[3] X chromosome inactivation prevents the expression of more than one X chromosome in a given cell line. Primordial cell migration can be traced by cytochemical demonstration of high alkaline phosphatase activity. The mechanisms that stimulate and direct the amoeboid movement of primordial cells to the gonadal ridge are poorly understood. Fibronectin has been identified in the migratory pathway and can stimulate primordial cell movement in vitro.[4] Chemotactic substances secreted by the gonadal anlagen may also play a role in regulating the migratory process.[5] During migration the number of germ cells increases by replication. In the human embryo, 700 to 1300 germ cells are present at 5 wk, and by 8 wk 600,000 germ cells can be identified in the developing ovary.[6, 7]

Early in fetal development, the ovary is close to the mesonephros (a temporarily functioning kidney). The mesonephros influences gonadal differentiation and is essential for complete ovarian development in mammals[8] (Fig. 12–1). Whereas the ovary is not histologically distinguishable until about 10 to 11 wk of fetal life, the fetal testis can be identified by about the seventh week (see Chapter 14). After the primordial cells reach the fetal ovary, they continue to proliferate by successive mitotic division and reach the maximal number of 6 to 7 million oogonia by the 20th week of gestation[7] (Fig. 12–2). Afterward, the number of germ cells decreases (a process known as *atresia*), so that only 1 million are present at birth, 400,000 are present at menarche, and only a few remain by the menopause (Fig. 12–3). Two X chromosomes are required for normal development of the ovary. In individuals with a 45,X karyotype, ovarian development occurs and primordial germ cells appear in the gonad, but follicular development is incomplete and the rate of atresia is accelerated so that only a fibrous streak remains at birth.[9] As will be discussed later, gonadotropin is required for complete maturation of ovarian follicles. Follicular development is reduced in anencephalic human fetuses and after fetal hypophysectomy in monkeys.[10, 11]

The ovarian-mesonephros association persists during early ovarian differentiation, and the mesonephros regresses

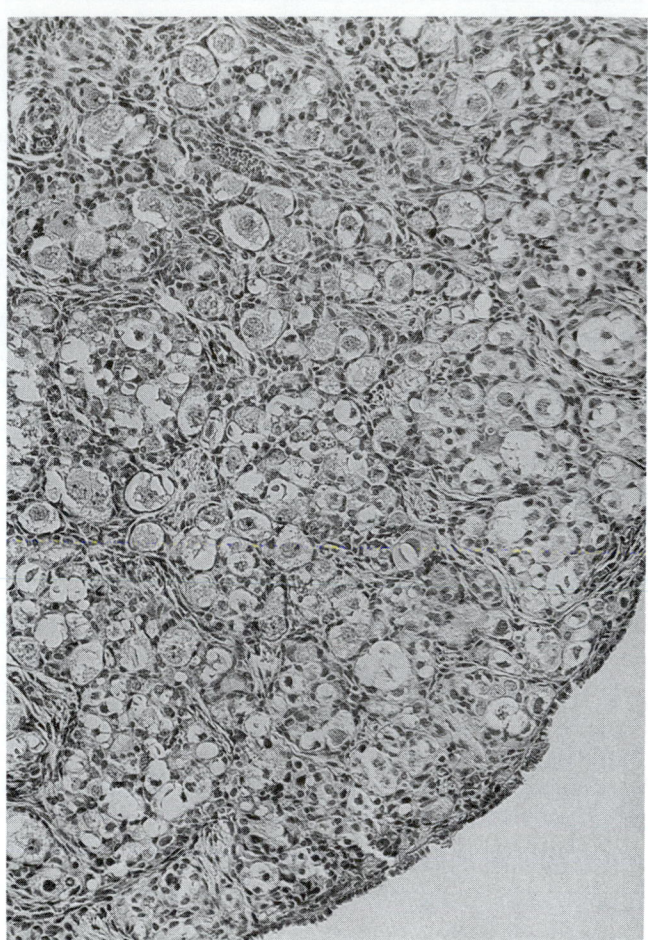

Figure 12–2. Histological section of an ovary from a 16-wk-old human fetus. (Courtesy of Dr. W. E. Rainey.)

slowly. In the human the ovary is invaded by mesonephric cells that form the medulla and force the germ cells to occupy the periphery or ovarian cortex.[12] The oogonia continue to undergo mitosis until they are converted to primary oocytes beginning as early as the 8th to the 12th week of gestation.[2, 13] The primary oocytes begin meiosis, but the process is arrested in the diplotene, or resting stage, of the first meiotic division, where the cells remain until puberty. With the onset of ovulation the first meiotic phase is completed (Fig. 12–4). The second meiotic phase occurs after ovulation and is completed after fertilization. The regulation of meiosis appears to be controlled by autocrine factors produced locally in the ovary. Meiosis-preventing substance, or oocyte maturation inhibitor, is produced by granulosa cells and arrests the oocyte in the diplotene stage. Later, meiosis is triggered by a small molecule (less than 2 kd) termed *meiosis-inducing substance*.[14, 15] When the primary oocyte is arrested at the diplotene stage it becomes surrounded by a layer of primitive granulosa cells, giving rise to the primordial follicle, the morphological marker of fetal ovarian differentiation.[10] A basement membrane separates the primordial follicle from the surrounding stromal (interstitial) tissues. The conversion of oogonia into primary oocytes and subsequent formation of primordial follicles are not completed until 6 mo after birth. Oocytes that are not incorporated into follicles undergo degeneration and account for the majority of oocytes that have disappeared by birth.[7, 16] The first primordial follicles are found at the inner part of the cortex near the medulla. Follicle formation depends on adequate numbers of mesonephric-derived

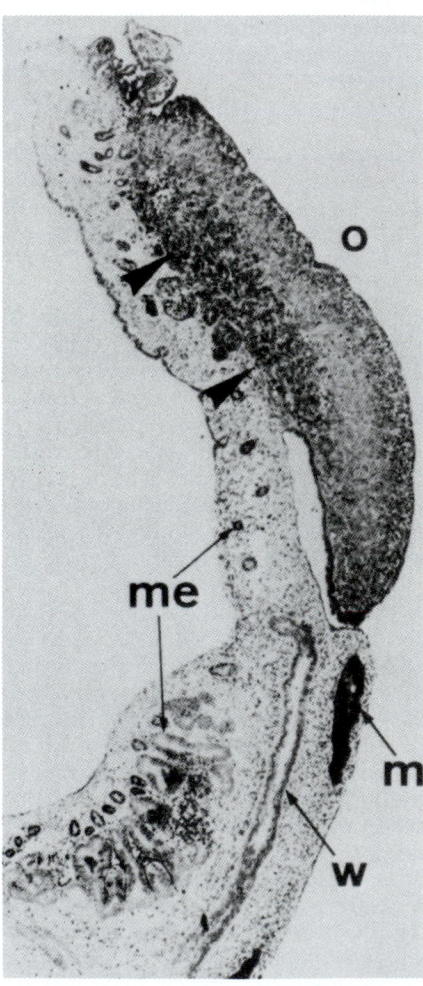

Figure 12–1. Ovary-mesonephric complex of an 11-wk-old human fetus. The ovary (o) is attached to the cranial part of the mesonephros *(arrowheads)*. Other features include the mesonephric tubules (me), wolffian duct (w), and müllerian duct (m). Magnification × 200. (From Byskov AG, Hoyer PE. Embryology of mammalian gonads. In: Knobil E, Neill J, eds. The Physiology of Reproduction. New York: Raven, 1988: 267.)

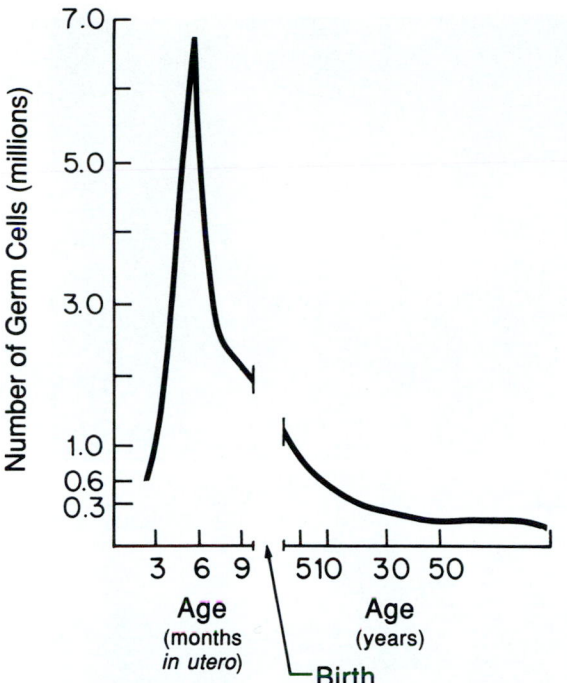

Figure 12–3. Changes in germ cell number in the human ovary with increasing age. (From Baker TG. A quantitative and cytological study of germ cells in the human ovaries. Proc R Soc Lond [Biol] 1963; 158:417–433.)

of gonadotropins (Fig. 12–5). By the seventh month of gestation, follicle maturation reaches the antrum stage.

At 8 wk of gestation the human ovary has the capacity to produce estrogens from androgens but secretes only small amounts of steroids in vitro.[17, 18] Binding sites for luteinizing hormone (LH) and human chorionic gonadotropin (hCG) are not detectable in human fetal ovaries, and LH, follicle-stimulating hormone (FSH), and hCG do not stimulate steroidogenesis in vitro, which suggests independence of gonadotropin control.[19, 20] Human fetal ovaries possess most, but not all, enzymes required for de novo synthesis of steroid hormones from cholesterol as demonstrated in vitro, but there is no convincing evidence that they secrete significant quantities of steroid hormones in vivo.[21]

The primordial genital ducts, namely the wolffian ducts (male) and the müllerian ducts (female), do not arise simultaneously. The wolffian duct develops first from the mesonephros and may participate in the formation of the müllerian ducts.[12] During normal female fetal development, the wolffian duct degenerates as a result of the lack of locally produced androgen. Degeneration of the wolffian duct begins soon after gonadal differentiation but is not completed until the beginning of the third trimester of pregnancy.[22] In the female the müllerian duct forms the fallopian tubes, the uterus, and the upper third of the vagina. At about 10 wk the uterus differentiates into an upper corpus and a lower cervix.[22] Although the cervix and corpus are initially the same length, the cervix is two thirds of the total length by the time of birth.[12] The development of the müllerian duct requires neither the gonads nor hormonal secretion because it develops normally in fetuses without gonads.[12]

granulosa cells, as discussed earlier.[12] The surface of the ovary, which is derived from coelomic epithelium and is inappropriately named the *germinal epithelium*, is not involved in the formation of germ cells or follicles.[12] At approximately 20 wk of fetal life, follicles begin to grow under the influence

Childhood and Premenarchal Ovary

After birth, the mean ovarian weight increases from about 250 mg to approximately 4000 mg by menarche.[23]

Figure 12–4. The life cycle of the oocyte. During the first trimester of fetal life the oogonium undergoes mitosis. During the second trimester meiosis I is initiated but is arrested at the diplotene stage (4n DNA). After menarche, at the time of ovulation, meiosis resumes in one ovum with the formation of the first polar body (2n DNA). Meiosis II is initiated at the time of fertilization and is completed with the formation of the second polar body (1n DNA). Fusion with the male pronucleus restores the nuclear content to 2n DNA.

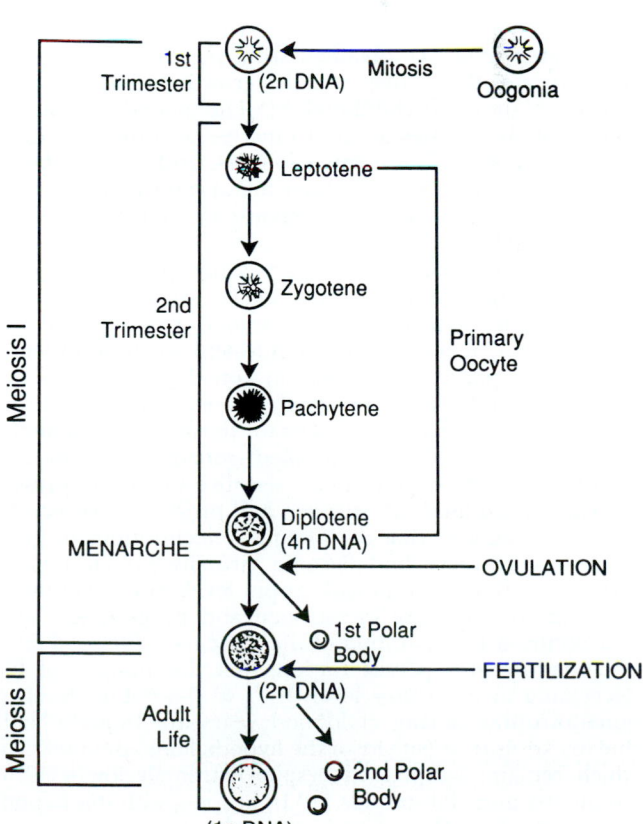

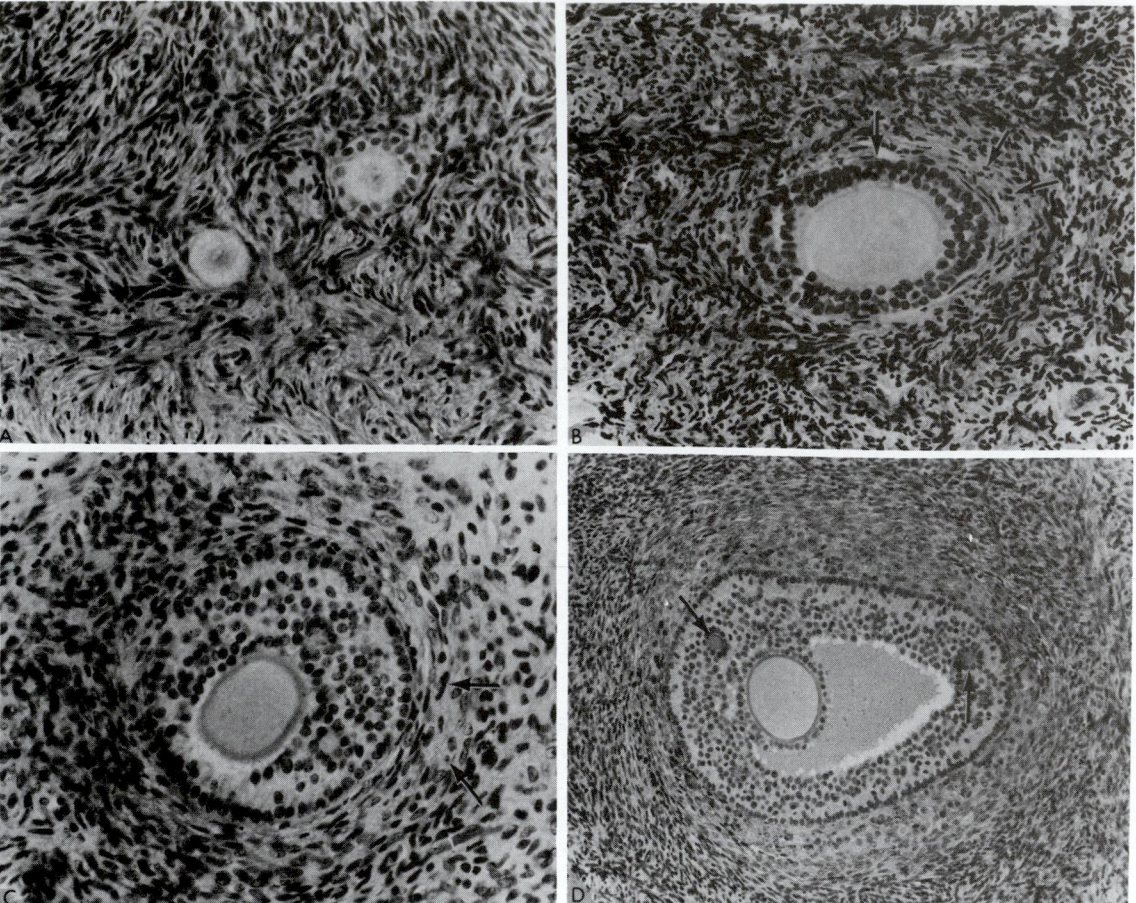

Figure 12–5. *A,* Primordial follicle *(lower left)* and primary follicle *(upper right)* in human ovary. *B,* Primary follicle with three layers of granulosa cells and incipient differentiation of theca *(arrows)* from surrounding stroma. *C,* Primary follicle with multiple layers of granulosa cells and beginning epithelioid transformation of theca *(arrows).* *D,* Graafian follicle. Note the epithelioid character of the theca cells and the Call-Exner bodies *(arrows)* among the granulosa cells.

Histological evidence obtained from postmortem examination indicates that active follicular growth and atresia occur during infancy and childhood.[16, 24] The increase in size and weight of the ovaries is due to increases in the amount of stroma, the size of individual follicles, and the number of follicles (Fig. 12–6).[16] The final maturation of the ovarian follicles at puberty occurs in response to increasing levels of FSH and LH.

Levels of gonadotropin vary significantly during the different stages of life in the female (Fig. 12–7). Plasma gonadotropins rise during the second trimester of fetal development, reaching levels equivalent to those observed in the menopause.[25] This peak in gonadotropin levels may be causally related to maximal development of follicles. During the later part of the second trimester, the hypothalamic-pituitary axis (the so-called gonadostat) undergoes maturation and becomes more sensitive to the suppressive effects of high levels of estrogen and progesterone secreted by the placenta so that the plasma concentrations of gonadotropins decrease and become virtually undetectable at birth.[26, 27] After birth, gonadotropin levels rise abruptly because of the decrease in estrogen and progestogen levels that occurs with separation of the placenta.[28] Elevated levels of gonadotropins persist for the first few months of life, decreasing again to low levels by 1 to 3 y.[28] Low levels of gonadotropins during childhood years are thought to be due to exquisite sensitivity of the hypothalamic-pituitary axis, which remains suppressed despite extremely low levels of circulating gonadal steroids.[26, 29] In keeping with this hypothesis is the fact that gonadotropin levels are elevated in

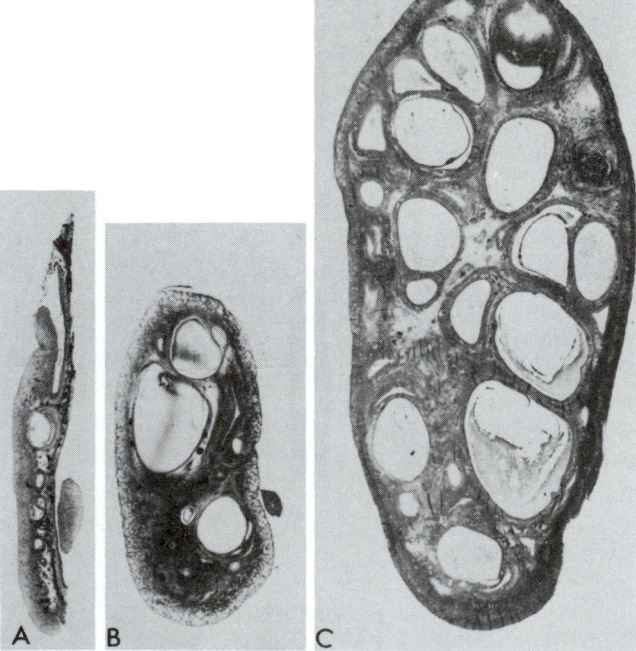

Figure 12–6. Ovaries of *(A)* a newborn, *(B)* a 10-mo-old infant, and *(C)* a 9-y-old girl. Magnification of all × 6.5. (From Peters H, Byskov AG, Grinsted J. Follicular growth in fetal and prepubertal ovaries in humans and other primates. Clin Endocrinol Metab 1978; 7:469–485.)

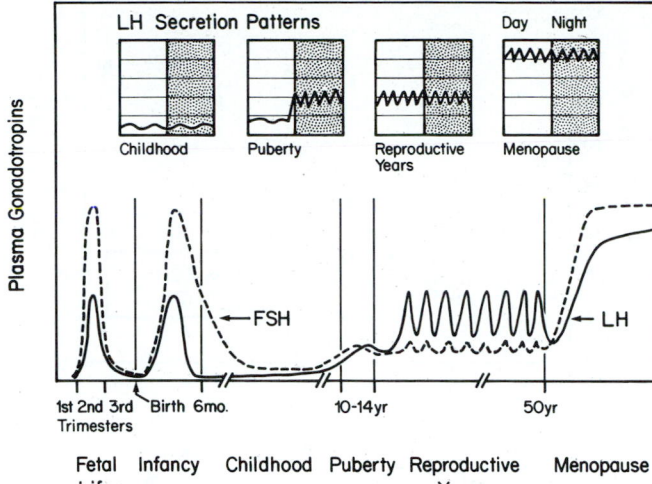

Figure 12–7. Pattern of gonadotropin secretion during different stages of life in women. The secretory patterns of LH during the waking hours (clear area) and night (stippled area) for each stage are indicated in the upper insets. (From Carr BR, Wilson JD. Disorders of the ovary and female reproductive tract. In: Braunwald E, Isselbacher KJ, Petersdorf RG, et al., eds. Harrison's Principles of Internal Medicine. 11th ed. New York: McGraw-Hill, 1987: 1818–1837. Reproduced with permission of McGraw-Hill, Inc.)

current hypothesis of hypothalamic-pituitary-gonadotropin and ovarian axis maturation is depicted in Figure 12–9.

Although basal gonadotropin secretion is low in prepubertal females, small but detectable pulses are observed at 2- to 3-h intervals, as in adults.[32] During puberty the pituitary becomes more sensitive to infusions of LHRH, and the LH and FSH responses to LHRH increase in age-dependent increments.[33] As puberty approaches, three major developments can be delineated: (1) adrenarche, the onset of adrenal androgen secretion; (2) decreased sensitivity of the gonadostat to feedback control by gonadal steroids, leading to activation or disinhibition of the LHRH neurosecretory neurons in the medial basal hypothalamus, with a consequent increase in pituitary gonadotropin release; and (3) gonadarche, the enhancement of estrogen secretion by the ovary and the onset of ovulatory cycles.

An increase in secretion of adrenal androgens occurs before maturation of gonadotropin secretion. The levels of androstenedione, dehydroepiandrosterone (DHEA), and dehydroepiandrosterone sulfate (DHEAS) increase in children beginning at approximately age 6 to 8 y. This increased secretion by the adrenal cortex is probably under the control of corticotropin (ACTH, adrenocorticotropin).[34–36] A variety of other peptide or protein hormones have been proposed as adrenal androgen-stimulating factors for the initiation of adrenarche, but evidence for the role of a hormone other than ACTH remains elusive.[36] Adrenal androgens must be converted to more potent androgens to exert androgenic effects, but they are believed to be involved in the initial spurt in skeletal growth and the development of axillary and pubic hair. Because of the close relationship between the onset of adrenarche and initiation of gonadarche, it has been proposed that the increased secretion of LHRH and gonadotropin by the hypothalamic-pituitary axis is influenced by adrenal activation. However, evidence of several types suggests that the control mechanisms for adrenarche and gonadarche are independent. Adrenarche occurs normally in both patients with Kallmann syndrome (hypogonadotropic hypogonadism) and those with gonadal dysgenesis (hypergonadotropic hypogonadism). Premature pubarche (also called premature adrenarche) with development of pubic and axillary hair before age 8 is not associated with premature gonadarche. In children with absence of adrenarche as a result of primary adrenal insufficiency, gonadarche occurs at a normal age.[37]

The factors that regulate the onset of gonadarche are thought to be initiated by a decreased sensitivity of the hypothalamic-pituitary axis to circulating levels of steroid

children with gonadal dysgenesis or in children who have been castrated during the first 4 y of life[30] (Fig. 12–8). The prepubertal hypothalamic axis (in normal children) is 6 to 15 times more sensitive to estrogen than is the adult feedback mechanism.[29] In addition to the highly sensitive gonadal steroid–dependent negative feedback system, a steroid-independent central nervous system (CNS)–inhibitory mechanism is also operative, because gonadotropin levels also fall in the absence of a gonad (see Fig. 12–8) and in children with gonadal dysgenesis between ages 5 and 11.[27] The infusion of luteinizing hormone–releasing hormone (LHRH, also called gonadotropin-releasing hormone [GnRH]) stimulates additional release of gonadotropins in agonadal children, substantiating the concept of a steroid hormone–independent mechanism of inhibition of the hypothalamic axis.[31] Although the pineal gland has been proposed to be an inhibitor of gonadotropin secretion, in the human neither the pineal gland nor melatonin has a major inhibitory effect on the hypothalamic-pituitary axis.[27] A

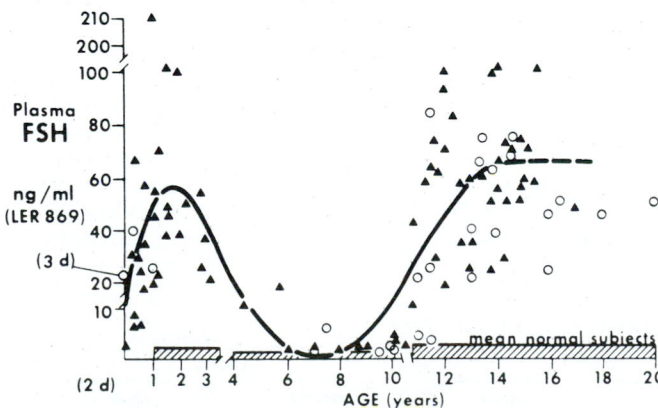

Figure 12–8. Pattern of plasma FSH in relation to age in 58 patients with gonadal dysgenesis. ▲, Patients with 45,X karyotype; ○, patients with structual abnormalities of the X chromosome and mosaics. The hatched area indicates the mean range for FSH values in normal females. To convert FSH values to international units per liter, multiply by 8.4. (From FA Conte, MM Grumbach, SL Kaplan, A diphasic pattern of gonadotropin secretion in patients with the syndrome of gonadal dysgenesis, J Clin Endocrinol Metab 40, 670–674, 1975, © by The Endocrine Society.)

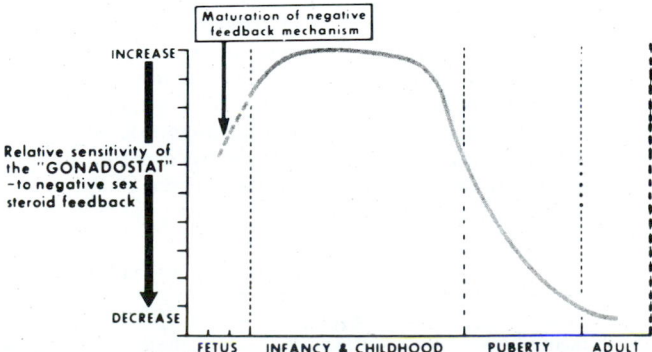

Figure 12–9. The ontogenesis of the maturation of the negative feedback system and the changes in set point of the hypothalamic gonadostat extending from the fetus through puberty to the adult. (From Styne DM, Grumbach MM. Puberty in the male and female. In: Yen SSC, Jaffe RB, eds. Reproductive Endocrinology: Physiology, Pathophysiology and Clinical Management. 2nd ed. Philadelphia: W. B. Saunders, 1986: 313–384, as modified from Grumbach MM, et al. In: Grumbach MM, Grave GD, Mayer FE, eds. Control of the Onset of Puberty. New York: John Wiley & Sons, 1974: 115–166.)

hormones. As a result, increased pulsatile secretion of FSH and LH follows. An early sign of increased pubertal gonadotropin release is a sleep-associated surge of LH release (see Fig. 12–7).[38] Similar sleep-related LH pulses also occur in children with idiopathic precocious puberty, in girls with gonadal dysgenesis after age 11, and in women during recovery from anorexia nervosa.[39] Increased secretion of ovarian estrogen enhances LH secretion (positive feedback) and leads eventually to ovulation and the menarche.

LHRH is critical for the initiation of puberty. Infantile female rhesus monkeys treated with pulsatile injections of LHRH undergo premature pubertal maturation.[40] In rhesus monkeys in which the hypothalamus has been destroyed, gonadotropin hormone levels decline. When these monkeys are treated with pulsatile LHRH given at hourly intervals, LH and FSH pulsatile secretion is re-established. Gonadotropin secretion decreases if LHRH is given continuously or if it is administered less frequently. During female puberty, frequency and amplitude of LH pulses increase. The pulsatile infusion of LHRH likewise initiates puberty in women with hypogonadotropic hypogonadism.[41] Finally, the administration of LHRH analogues causes regression of pubertal changes in girls with true isosexual precocious puberty.[42–44]

Changes in FSH and LH levels during puberty in girls are illustrated in Figure 12–10. FSH rises early, with LH following.[45] Before puberty the plasma FSH/LH ratio is greater than 1, whereas at the end of puberty the ratio is reversed. At menopause the FSH/LH ratio again becomes greater than 1. As a consequence of increased FSH, the plasma level of estradiol (more than 90% derived from the ovary) increases progressively throughout puberty.[45] The level of bioactive LH is higher during early puberty than is immunological LH. The increased ratio of bioactive to immunological LH is due to increased glycosylation of LH.[46] Serum inhibin levels increase in parallel with FSH levels during puberty in girls.[47] It is postulated that FSH stimulates granulosa cells to secrete inhibin until adult levels of inhibin are attained. Thereafter the inhibin-FSH negative feedback relationship is established (see later).

The ranges of hormone concentrations during normal puberty are presented in Table 12–1.[37] Early ovarian hormone secretion, principally estradiol, accelerates linear growth and stimulates development of female secondary characteristics (growth of breasts and maturation of the urogenital tract and femal habitus). Adrenal androgens (and, to a lesser degree, ovarian androgens) regulate axillary and pubic hair development. The age at which puberty is initiated and the rate of progression vary (Fig. 12–11). "Normal pubertal development" also varies widely among individuals. Breast development is initiated in most girls between ages 10 and 11. This is followed by the appearance of pubic and axillary hair. A growth spurt ensues, and a peak growth rate is attained at a median age of 11.4. The hormones involved include growth hormone, insulin-like growth factor I (IGF I, also called somatomedin-C), thyroid hormone, and estrogen. IGF I levels increase progressively during puberty secondary to growth hormone stimulation (see Chapter 21).

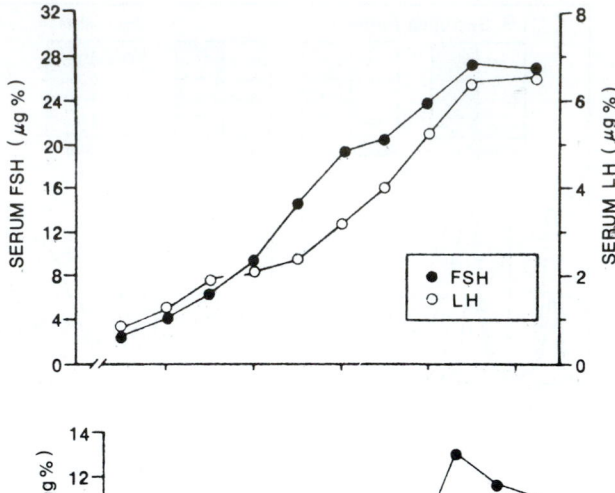

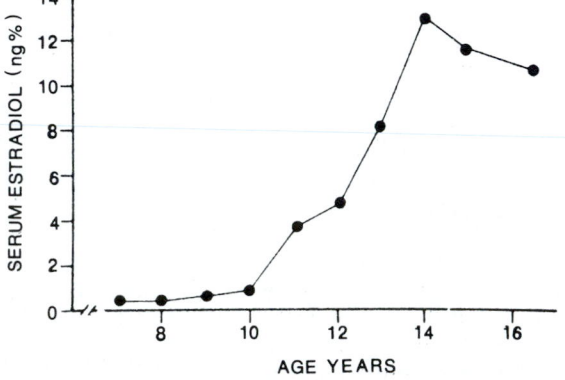

Figure 12–10. Age-related trends in blood FSH, LH, and estradiol levels before and during pubescence. To convert estradiol values to picomoles per liter, multiply by 36.7. (From Faiman C, Winter JSD. Gonadotropins and sex hormone patterns in puberty: clinical data. In: Grumbach MM, Grave GD, Mayer FE, eds. Control of the Onset of Puberty. New York: John Wiley & Sons, 1974: 32–55.)

Deficient IGF I response, as occurs in pygmies, blunts the pubertal growth spurt and results in short stature.[48] The increase in IGF I is mediated indirectly by an increase in gonadal steroids, which stimulates secretion of growth hormone.[49, 50]

It is clinically useful to classify the stages of puberty. Figures 12–12 and 12–13 depict the various stages of female puberty as formulated by Marshall and Tanner.[51] These stages are further described in Table 12–2.

Several generalizations can be made about pubertal development. Although the age of onset varies, breast development is usually the first sign. The average time between beginning breast development and the onset of menses is 4.5 y. Rates of progression from one stage to another are similar for breasts and pubic hair, averaging 0.5 to 0.9 y for each stage from stage I to stage IV. The rate of progression from stage IV to stage V is more variable. Breast changes precede the onset of the growth spurt, which becomes maximal by stage III of breast development in 75% of girls.[51]

The culmination of puberty is the onset of predictable,

TABLE 12–1. Blood Hormone Concentrations During Female Puberty

Tanner Stage	FSH (IU/L)	LH (IU/L)	Estradiol pmol/L	Estradiol pg/mL	DHEA nmol/L	DHEA ng/dL
1	0.9–5.1	1.8–9.2	<3.7	<1.0	0.6–10	19–302
2	1.4–7.0	2.0–16.6	26–136	7–37	1.6–66	45–1904
3	2.4–7.7	5.6–13.6	33–217	9–59	4.3–60	125–1730
4	1.5–11.2	7–14.4	37–573	10–156	5.3–46	153–1321
Adult: follicular	3–20	5–25	110–367	30–10	5.6–56	162–1620

Adapted from Speroff L, Glass RH, Kase NG. Clinical Gynecologic Endocrinology and Infertility. 4th ed. Baltimore: Williams & Wilkins, 1989: 417. © 1989, the Williams & Wilkins Co., Baltimore.

TABLE 12–2. Stages of Female Puberty

Stage	Breast	Pubic Hair
1	Preadolescent; only papillae are elevated.	Preadolescent; vellus hair only and hair is similar to development over anterior abdominal wall (i.e., no pubic hair).
2	Breast bud and papilla are elevated and a small mound is present; areola diameter is enlarged.	There is sparse growth of long, slightly pigmented, downy hair or only slightly curled hair, appearing along labia.
3	Further enlargement of breast mound; increased palpable glandular tissue.	Hair is darker, coarser, more curled, and spreads to the pubic junction.
4	Areola and papilla are elevated to form a second mound above the level of the rest of the breast.	Adult-type hair; area covered is less than that in most adults; there is no spread to the medial surface of thighs.
5	Adult mature breast; recession of areola to the mound of breast tissue, rounding of the breast mound, and projection of only the papilla are evident.	Adult-type hair with increased spread to medial surface of thighs; distribution is as an inverse triangle.

Adapted from Marshall WA, Tanner JM. Variations in pattern of pubertal changes in girls. Arch Dis Child 1969; 44:291–303.

cyclic, regular (and hence ovulatory) menses. The age of menarche is influenced by socioeconomic and genetic factors, general health, nutrition, geography, and altitude.[27] In the United States the median age of menarche is now 12.7 y, having decreased at a rate of 3 to 4 mo per decade over the past 100 y. The earlier onset is believed to be due primarily to improved nutrition.[52–54]

In an analysis of the growth and development of 169 girls, Frisch and McArthur observed that menarche occurs at a mean or "critical" body weight of 48 kg.[52] Additional factors that influence the onset of menarche and the maintenance of ovulatory menses include percent body fat, percent body water, ratio of lean to fat, body mass, and body "shape." Obese girls weighing 20 to 30% above the ideal experience earlier menarche than do girls of normal weight. In contrast, girls with decreased body fat as a result of participation in certain sports or ballet, malnutrition, or chronic debilitating diseases commonly have delayed menarche. Although many aspects of the theory of critical body weight are speculative and controversial, a metabolic signal related to body composition appears to be an important factor in the maturation or activation of the hypothalamic LHRH pulse generator.[27]

The Ovary of the Reproductive Years

Structural Organization of the Mature Ovary

Mature human ovaries are oval-shaped bodies with a length of 2 to 5 cm, a width of 1.5 to 3 cm, and a thickness of 0.5 to 1.5 cm. The combined weight of normal ovaries during the reproductive years is 10 to 20 g (average of 14 g). The ovaries lie in approximation with the posterior and lateral pelvic wall and are attached to the posterior surface of the broad ligament by a peritoneal fold termed the *mesovarian*. Blood vessels, nerves, and lymphatics traverse the mesovarian and enter the ovary at the hilum.[55, 56]

The ovary consists of three distinct regions: an outer cortex containing the germinal epithelium and the follicles, a central medulla consisting of stroma, and a hilum around the area of attachment of the ovary to the mesovarian. The anatomical components and function of the adult ovary are illustrated schematically in Figure 12–14.

GERMINAL EPITHELIUM. The germinal epithelium consists of coelomic-derived epithelial cells. Its function is in-

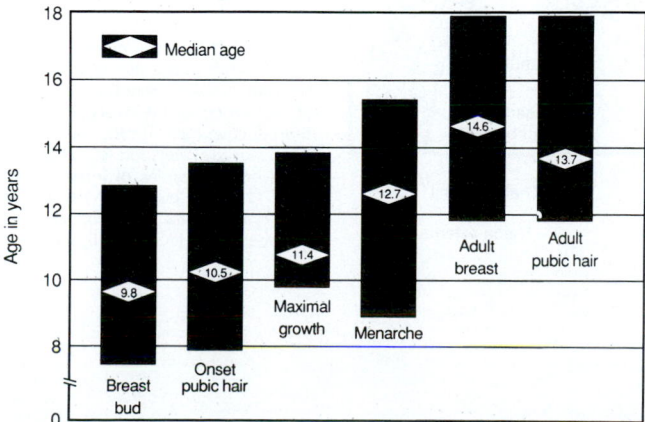

Figure 12–11. Median age and range of the signs of female sexual development during puberty. (Adapted from Speroff L, Glass RH, Kase NG. Clinical Gynecologic Endocrinology and Infertility. 4th ed. Baltimore: Williams & Wilkins, 1989: 1–688. © 1989, the Williams & Wilkins Co., Baltimore.)

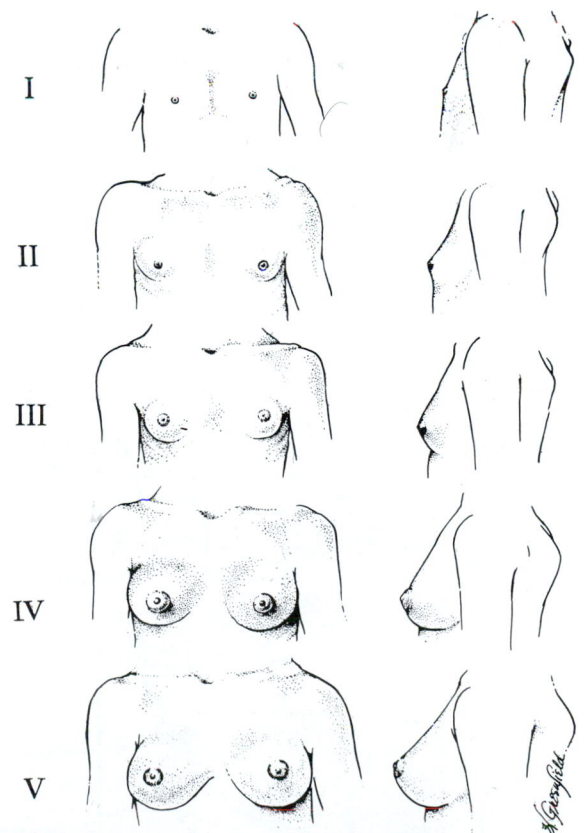

Figure 12–12. Diagrammatic representation of Tanner stages I to V of human breast maturation. (Adapted from Marshall WA, Tanner JM. Variations in patterns of pubertal changes in girls. Arch Dis Child 1969; 44:291–303.)

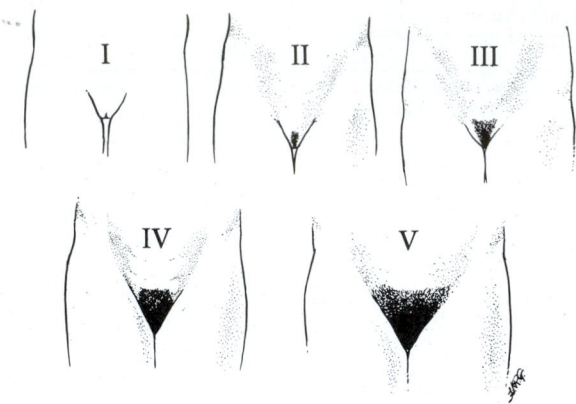

Figure 12–13. Diagrammatic representation of Tanner stages I to V for development of human pubic hair. (Adapted from Marshall WA, Tanner JM. Variations in patterns of pubertal changes in girls. Arch Dis Child 1969; 44:291–303.)

completely understood, but it is likely that germ cell number is fixed prenatally in all mammals, including humans.[57] The germinal epithelium undergoes "decidualization" in response to the hormones of pregnancy. With aging, the ovary becomes convoluted, giving rise to crypts lined with germinal epithelium. At times the continuity between the germinal epithelium in these crypts and the remaining epithelium is disrupted, giving rise to isolated rests or nests of germinal epithelium cells. After the menopause, these nests of epithelium cells can lead to the formation of inclusion cysts or solid nests of metaplastic epithelial cells.[58]

FOLLICLES. The follicles are embedded in loose connective tissue of the ovarian cortex and can be subdivided into two functional types: nongrowing, or primordial, and growing. The majority of follicles (90 to 95%) are nongrowing throughout the reproductive life (Figs. 12–5A and 12–15). Recruitment of a primordial follicle initiates dramatic

changes in growth, structure, and function. The growing follicles are divided into five stages: primary, secondary, tertiary, graafian, and atretic. The first three stages of growth can occur in the absence of the pituitary and thus appear to be controlled by intraovarian mechanisms.[59] After a follicle enters the tertiary stage, continued growth and steroidogenesis depend on the presence of gonadotropins.[60]

The primordial follicle is composed of a single layer of granulosa cells and a single immature oocyte arrested in the diplotene stage of the first meiotic division. The primordial follicle is separated from the surrounding stroma by a thin basal lamina (basement membrane). The oocyte is enclosed by a single layer of spindle-shaped cells with protoplasmic processes that reach the basal lamina, providing a route for transfer of nutrients. The oocyte and granulosa cells do not have a direct blood supply and thus exist in a microenvironment separated from contact with other cells by the basal lamina.[61]

The first sign of follicular recruitment is cuboidal differentiation in the spindle-shaped cells inside the basal lamina, which then undergo successive mitotic division to form a multilayered stratum granulosa or zona granulosa. The oocyte enlarges and secretes a glycoprotein-containing mucoid substance called the *zona pellucida* that surrounds the oocyte and separates the granulosa cells from the oocyte (see Figs. 12–5B and C and 12–15).[62, 63] This structure is a primary follicle.

The secondary follicle is formed by further proliferation of granulosa cells and by the final phase of oocyte growth, in which the oocyte reaches 120 μm in diameter. Coincident with proliferation of granulosa cells, stromal cells outside the basal lamina differentiate and become arranged in concentric perifollicular layers of cells to constitute the theca (see Figs. 12–5B and C and 12–15). The portion of the theca adjacent to the basal lamina is termed the *theca interna*. Thecal cells merging with the surrounding stroma are designated the *theca externa*. The secondary follicle acquires an independent blood supply consisting of one or more arteri-

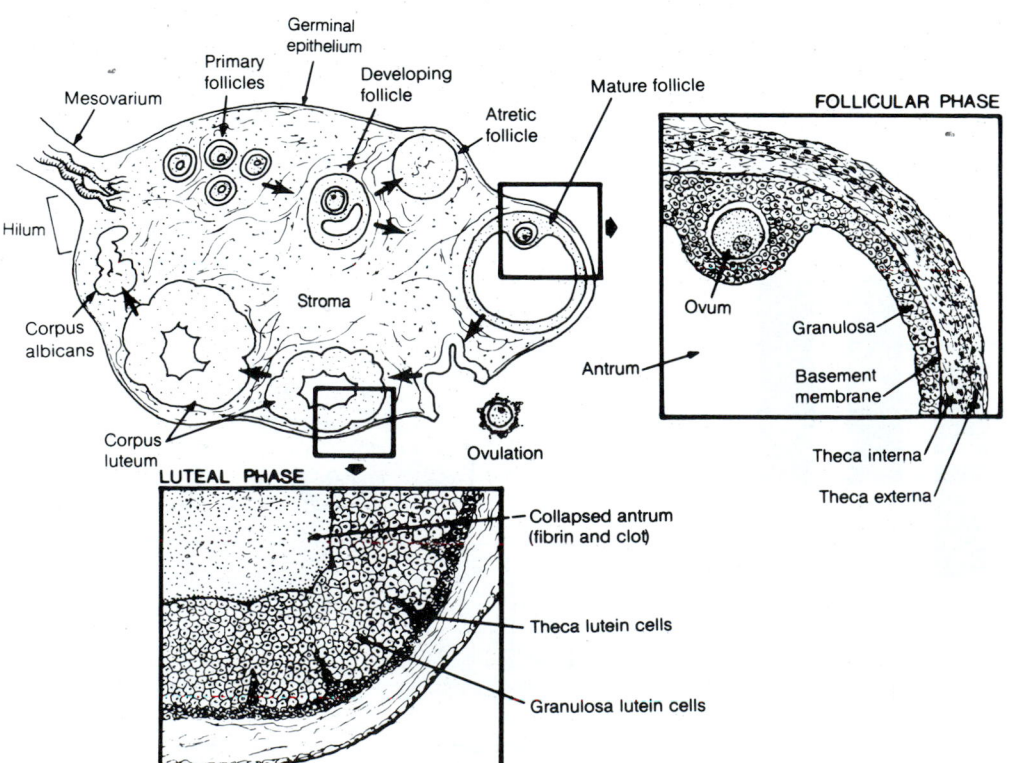

Figure 12–14. Developmental changes in the adult ovary during a complete menstrual cycle. (From Carr BR, Wilson JD. Disorders of the ovary and female reproductive tract. In: Braunwald E, Isselbacher KJ, Petersdorf RG, et al., eds. Harrison's Principles of Internal Medicine. 11th ed. New York: McGraw-Hill, 1987: 1818–1837. Reproduced with permission of McGraw-Hill, Inc.)

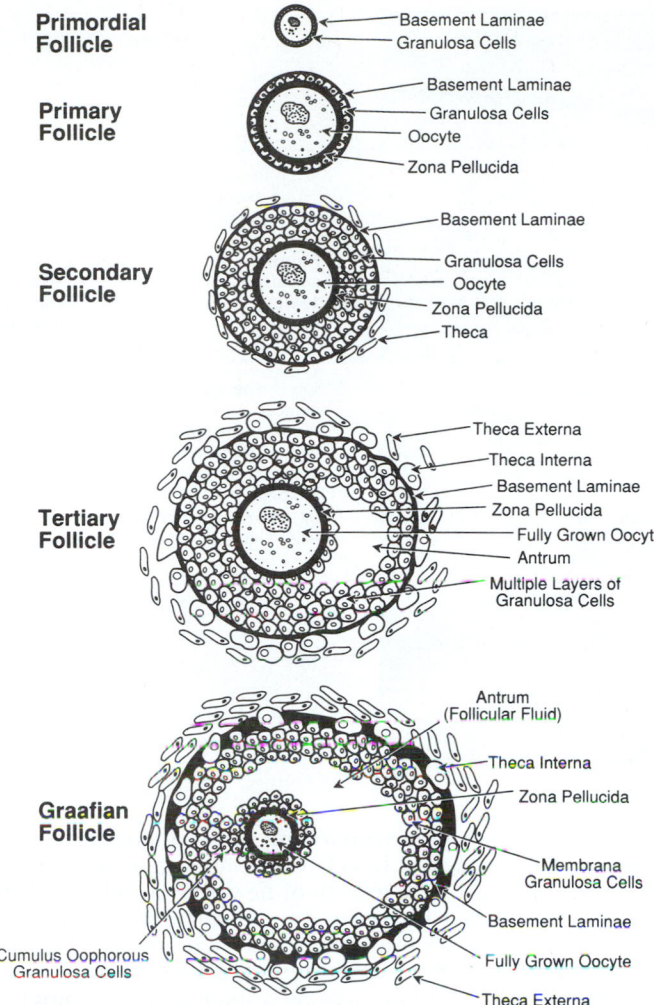

Figure 12–15. The structure and classification of the ovarian follicle during growth and development. (Adapted from GF Erickson, DA Magoffin, CA Dyer, The ovarian androgen producing cells: a review of structure/function relationships, Endocr Rev 6, 371–379, 1985, © by The Endocrine Society.)

oles that terminate in a capillary bed at the basal lamina. Capillaries do not penetrate the basement membrane, and the granulosa and oocyte remain avascular. A distinct morphological feature of the granulosa cells (termed *Call-Exner bodies*) consists of a basal lamina attached to granulosa cells associated with a cavity filled with basal lamina and a flocculent protein-like material. Call-Exner bodies appear during the development of the secondary follicle (see Fig. 12–5D). Little is known about their formation or physiological significance.

The tertiary follicle is accompanied by further hypertrophy of the theca and the appearance of a fluid-filled space among the granulosa cells named the antrum (see Figs. 12–5D and 12–15). The fluid in the antrum consists of a plasma transudate and secretory products of granulosa cells, some of which (estrogens) are found there in higher concentrations than in peripheral blood.[64] In association with the formation of the antrum, the granulosa and thecal cells develop a specialized contact between cells known as *gap junctions*.[65, 66] Gap junctions allow small molecules to pass from one cell to another, thus permitting cell-cell communication and synchronized coordination of follicular function (Fig. 12–16).

At this stage, the follicle rapidly increases in size under the influence of gonadotropins to form the mature or graafian follicle (see Fig. 12–15). During this stage the granulosa and oocyte remain encased by the basal lamina and are devoid of direct vascularization. The antral fluid increases in volume, and the oocyte, surrounded by an accumulation of granulosa cells (the cumulus oophorus), occupies a polar, eccentric position within the follicle.[67] The mature graafian follicle is ready to release the ovum by the process of ovulation (see later). Based on findings in women with natural cycles and in women with hypogonadotropic hypogonadism treated with gonadotropins, the average time for development of a primary follicle until ovulation is about 10 to 14 d.[68]

Recruited primordial follicles either develop into a dominant mature graafian follicle destined to ovulate or degenerate as a result of atresia.[64, 69] Because of atresia, the oocyte and granulosa cells within the basal laminas die and are replaced by fibrous tissue. In contrast, the thecal cells outside the basal lamina do not die but dedifferentiate and return to the pool of cells consisting of ovarian interstitial or stromal cells.[56] The process of atresia is generally thought to be secondary to the lack of hormones or growth factors formed by the mature dominant follicle through intrinsic intraovarian mechanisms.

STROMA. The ovarian stroma consists of three major cell types: connective tissue cells similar to those of other tissues, contractile cells, and several types of interstitial cells.[58] The interstitial cells are the most important in that they secrete steroid hormones (principally androgens) and undergo morphological changes in response to LH and hCG.[56] Interstitial cells are derived from mesenchymal cells of the ovarian stroma.[70] The human ovary contains four major categories of interstitial cells: primary, secondary, thecal, and hilar.

The primary interstitial cells are the first to develop and are identifiable in the fetal ovary only between 12 and 20 wk of fetal life.[71] They closely resemble early Leydig cells of the fetal testis and have the ultrastructural features of steroid-secreting cells.[71]

Secondary interstitial cells are derived from the thecal cells of atretic follicles.[70, 72] These large epithelial cells hypertrophy and maintain the active steroidogenic features of thecal interstitial cells (see later) from which they are derived. Secondary cells retain responsiveness to LH[71] but differ in that they are innervated and respond to catecholamines, which stimulate structural changes and hormone secretion.[73]

Thecal interstitial cells in tertiary follicles are the active site of androgen secretion.[74] They develop from mesenchymal cells that differentiate when secondary follicles form. Thecal interstitial cells contain LH receptors and the steroidogenic enzymes 3β-hydroxysteroid dehydrogenase (3β-HSD) and $\Delta^{4,5}$-isomerase. The transformation from stromal cells is influenced locally by the secondary follicle but appears to depend on gonadotropin stimulation.[75] These cells markedly increase in size and develop ultrastructural changes characteristic of steroid-secreting cells. Thecal interstitial cells give rise to secondary interstitial cells after follicular atresia, as stated earlier.

The hilum, where the blood vessels, lymphatics, and nerves enter the ovary, is the locus of specific interstitial cells termed *hilar cells*. These cells contain crystalloids of Reinke and are morphologically indistinguishable from Leydig cells of the testes.[56, 76] Hilar cells, which are difficult to identify before puberty, synthesize and secrete testosterone in response to LH. Occasionally, hyperplastic or neoplastic changes in hilar cells result in virilization associated with excessive testosterone secretion.[70] The physiological function of hilar cells is obscure, but because of their intimate association with nerve fibers and blood vessels they may influence ovarian function.

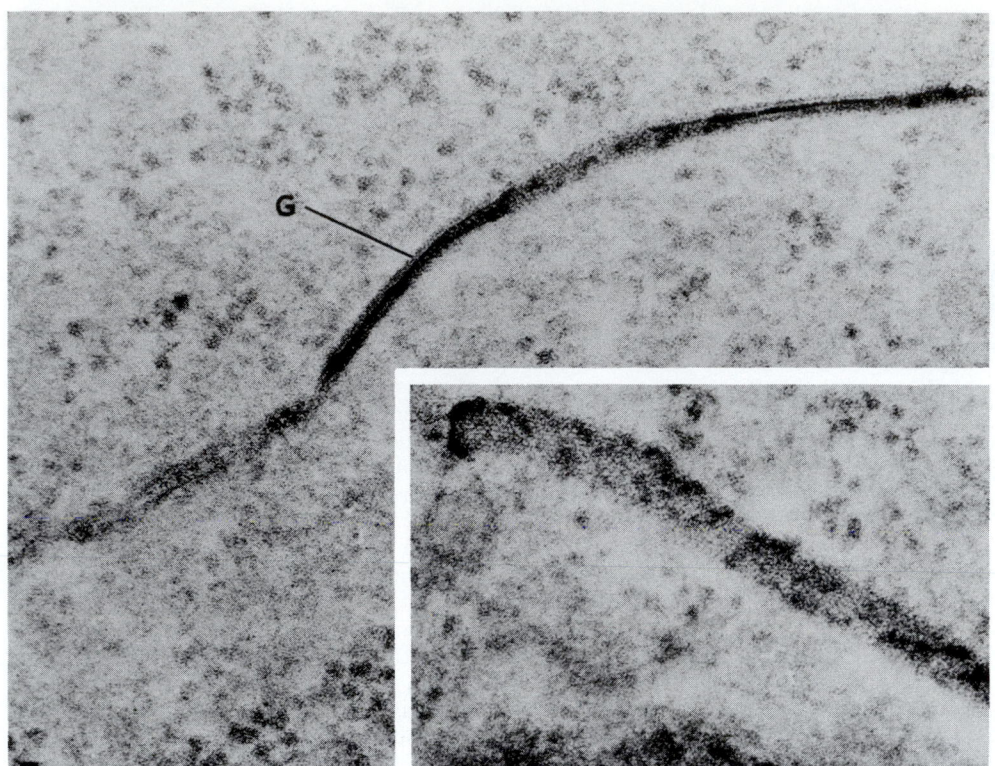

Figure 12–16. The gap junction (G) of an early antral follicle. Magnification × 139,800. Inset is an en face section of the junction revealing the quasihexagonal ordering of subunits. Magnification × 139,800. (From Albertini DF, Anderson E. The appearance and structure of intracellular connections during the ontogeny of the rabbit ovarian follicle with particular reference to gap junctions. Reproduced from the Journal of Cell Biology, 1974, vol. 63, pp. 234–250 by copyright permission of the Rockefeller University Press.)

OVUM. In the mature dominant follicle, oocyte growth occurs and meiosis is completed. During growth, the oocyte increases in diameter from 20 to 120 μm. The growth period is associated with accumulation of nutritional stores. Oocyte growth is linear until the follicle reaches the tertiary stage and thereafter ceases.[77]

The presence of granulosa cells is an absolute requirement for growth of the oocyte.[78] The oocyte is surrounded by a collection of granulosa cells termed the *corona radiata* that interact with the oocyte by gap junctions, as discussed earlier. The zona pellucida that forms between the corona radiata and the oocyte during formation of the primary follicle contains species-specific receptors for sperm, prevents polyspermy, and promotes movement of the fertilized ovum from the fallopian tube to the uterus.[79] The zona pellucida consists of three glycoproteins secreted by the growing oocyte, as noted earlier.[80]

As depicted in Figure 12–4, meiosis resumes at the time of ovulation. The role of oocyte maturation inhibitor, meiosis-inducing substance, and meiosis-preventing substance in the resumption of meiosis was discussed earlier. The resumption of meiosis occurs after the preovulatory surge of LH.[81] The oocyte of mature follicles undergoes meiosis when placed in culture, supporting the concept that an inhibitory influence suppresses meiosis before ovulation. The progression of meiosis in the mature oocyte is associated with the loss of the nuclear or germinal membrane, condensation of chromatin into bivalents, separation of homologous chromosomes, and arrest at metaphase II.[82] Meiosis is completed with the release of the second polar body at the time of fertilization. High concentrations of estradiol in follicular fluid are required for normal meiotic maturation.[83]

CORPUS LUTEUM. At the time of the preovulatory surge of LH, a series of biochemical and morphological changes occur in the cells of the granulosa and theca interna. This process is called *luteinization*. During luteinization these cells undergo hypertrophy and exhibit increased RNA and protein synthesis under the influence of LH.[84] After ovulation

the basement membrane separating the granulosa from the theca breaks down, and blood vessels and capillaries invade the granulosa cells. The growth of new vessels and invading fibroblasts is believed to be due to angiogenic factor(s) secreted by the ovary after ovulation.[85] The morphology of the developing corpus luteum (yellow body) has been well characterized.[86, 87] In brief, proliferation of the granulosa cells occurs during the day after ovulation. Capillary invasion of the granulosa cells begins on day 2 after ovulation and reaches the central cavity by day 4. Hemorrhage into the cavity can occur on any day with the formation of a fibrin clot, and fibroblasts appear in the central cavity by day 5 (Figs. 12–14 and 12–17). Maximal capillary dilation is attained by day 7 to 8, a time that corresponds to maximal progesterone secretion. The human corpus luteum secretes as much as 40 mg of progesterone per day during the midluteal phase of the ovarian cycle.[88] In view of the small size of the human corpus luteum, it is the most active steroidogenic tissue of the human. The cells that make up the corpus luteum are derived from cells that make up the follicle, namely the granulosa and the theca. The granulosa cells become granulosa-lutein cells (large cells), and the theca cells are transformed into theca-lutein cells (small cells) (see Fig. 12–17).[89] The so-called K cells, scattered throughout the corpus luteum, are believed to be macrophages.[90]

In the absence of pregnancy, the corpus luteum undergoes degeneration. This process is termed *luteolysis* and is first apparent by the eighth day after ovulation.[86] During luteolysis the granulosa-lutein cells shrink, and the thecal cells appear to be more prominent.[91] Later both types of cells undergo autolysis and necrosis. The remaining corpus luteum is composed of dense connective tissue and is termed the *corpus albicans*.

Physiology of Ovarian Function

HYPOTHALAMIC-PITUITARY-OVARIAN AXIS: AN OVERVIEW. The hypothalamus plays an important role in

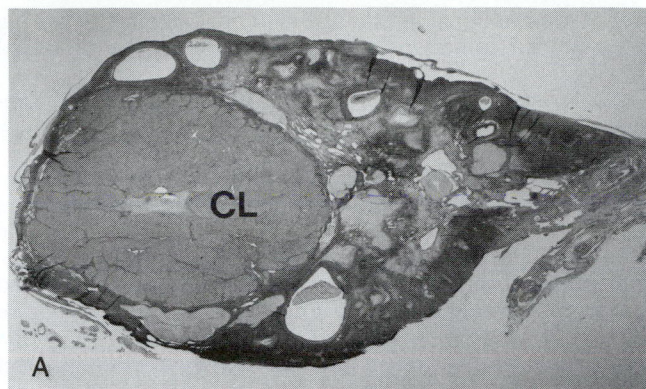

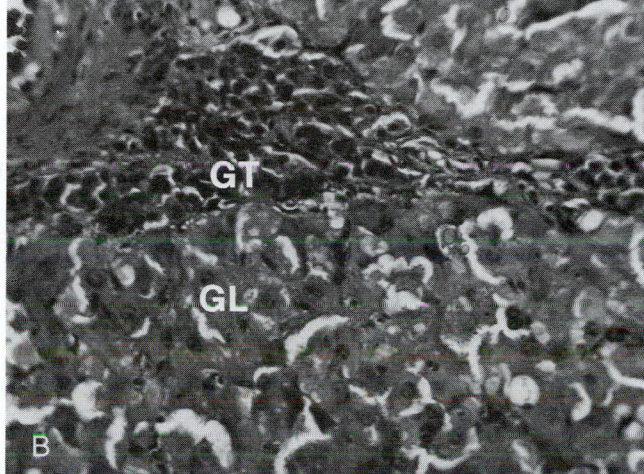

Figure 12–17. A, Photomicrograph of a human corpus luteum (CL). B, The larger pale-staining granulosa-lutein cells (GL) can readily be distinguished from the smaller, dark-staining theca-lutein cells (GT).

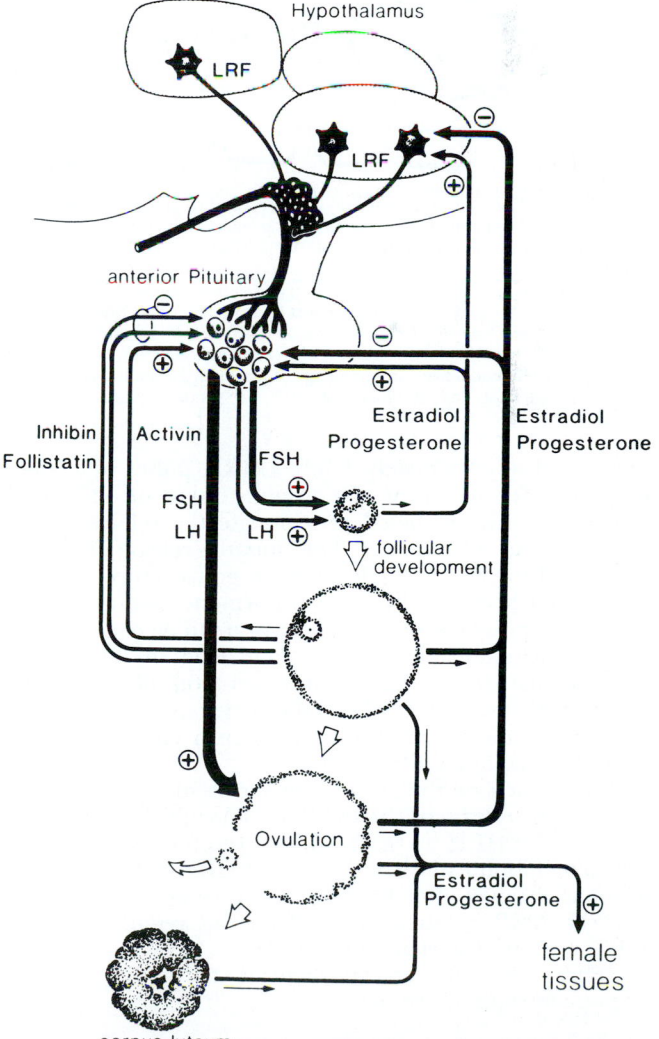

Figure 12–18. A diagrammatic representation of the hypothalamic-pituitary-ovarian axis. LRF, luteinizing-releasing factor. (From SY Ying, Inhibins, activins, and follistatins: gonadal proteins modulating the secretion of follicle-stimulating hormone, Endocr Rev 9, 267–293, 1988, © by The Endocrine Society.)

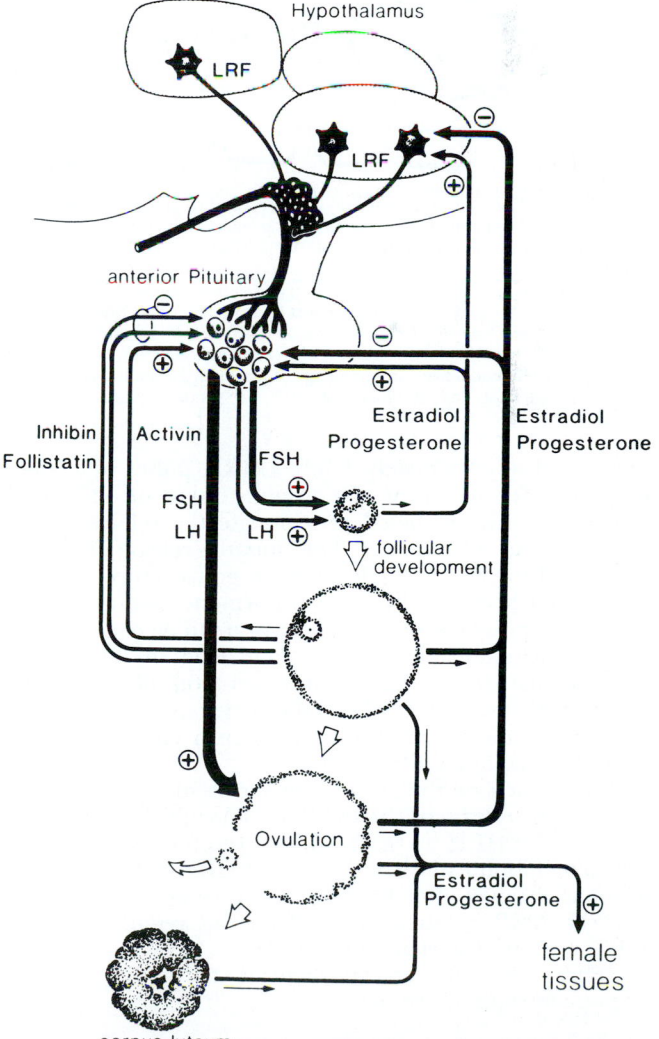

neurons from other regions of the brain whose terminals end in the arcuate nucleus. Epinephrine and norepinephrine increase LHRH release, whereas dopamine, serotonin, and endogenous opioid peptides are inhibitory (Fig. 12–19).[96] Other hormones, in particular gut-related peptide hormones, also modulate LHRH release.[96]

The half-life of LHRH is quite short (2 to 4 min), and its metabolic clearance averages approximately 800 L/d/m² body surface area.[97] The fact that LH and FSH are secreted in short pulsatile bursts led to the assumption that LHRH release is also pulsatile. This conclusion was confirmed by measurements in hypothalamic-pituitary portal venous blood from monkeys and sheep showing that LHRH is secreted in a pulsatile fashion at intervals of 70 to 90 min.[40, 98–100]

Knobil has shown in the rhesus monkey that the area of the brain responsible for the LHRH pulse generator is in the arcuate nucleus of the medial basal hypothalamus.[40] Pulsatile LHRH secretion by the arcuate nucleus is a prerequisite for normal secretion of pituitary gonadotropins.[40] This conclusion is based on studies of reactivation of gonadotropin secretion after destruction of the arcuate nucleus in the rhesus monkey in which it was shown that normal LH and FSH release requires the pulsatile infusion of LHRH at

the hormonal regulation of female reproductive function (Fig. 12–18). Understanding of the hormonal control of reproduction has progressed from the identification of ovarian steroids and pituitary gonadotropins to the discovery of hypothalamic releasing factors and the identification of a host of ovarian hormones and growth factors that modulate gonadotropin secretion and intraovarian regulation.[92] It is now believed that the follicle destined to ovulate initiates the sequence of coordinated events that control the menstrual cycle by way of the hypothalamic-pituitary system. The hypothalamus is connected to the pituitary by a portal vascular system that serves as a conduit for the transport of hormones from the brain to the pituitary. The primary direction of blood flow is from the hypothalamus to the pituitary, and interruption of this connection leads to a decline in gonadotropin levels and eventually to atrophy of the ovaries with failure of hormone secretion. Retrograde flow also occurs in the portal vessels, providing a short feedback loop from pituitary to hypothalamus.[93]

The principal hypothalamic releasing factor regulating reproductive function is LHRH, a decapeptide. Although separate releasing hormones were originally believed to exist for LH and FSH, the current predominant view is that LHRH is the only gonadotropin-releasing hormone.[92, 94] A large number of LHRH analogues have been developed. All inhibit both LH and FSH release; i.e., none selectively inhibits LH or FSH. The variations in response of LH and FSH after LHRH infusions are believed to be due to feedback effects of ovarian hormones on the hypothalamic-pituitary axis.

The hypothalamic release of LHRH is influenced by

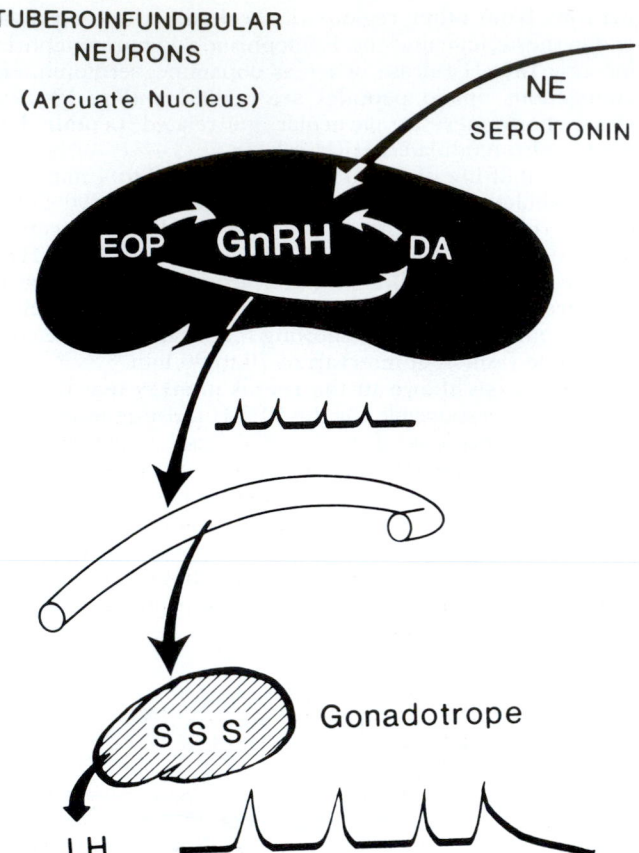

Figure 12–19. Schematic representation of the control of pituitary gonadotropin secretion by hypothalamic LHRH (also termed gonadotropin-releasing hormone, GnRH). LHRH neurons within the arcuate nucleus secrete LHRH in a pulsatile fashion that regulates the synthesis, storage, and pulsatile secretion (SSS) of LH by the pituitary gonadotropes. β-Endorphin (EOP) and dopamine (DA) within the arcuate nucleus may exert an inhibitory effect on LHRH neurons. Norepinephrine (NE) and serotonin from the midbrain may also affect LHRH neuronal release. (From Yen SSC. Neuroendocrine control of hypophyseal function. In: Yen SSC, Jaffe RB, eds. Reproductive Endocrinology: Physiology, Pathophysiology and Clinical Management. 2nd ed. Philadelphia: W. B. Saunders, 1986: 57.)

intervals of approximately 1 h.[101] LHRH pulses of a lesser or greater frequency or the administration of LHRH by continuous infusion failed to stimulate the release of LH and FSH (Fig. 12–20).[101, 102] The pulsatile release of LHRH is required for the midcycle surge of gonadotropins, which is regulated primarily by ovarian hormone feedback at the level of the pituitary, but its role appears to be permissive.[101] These observations have been confirmed in humans by showing that the pulsatile administration of LHRH to women with isolated LHRH deficiency can reproduce the hormonal changes seen during the menstrual cycle and can result in ovulation and fertility.[103]

LHRH acts on the gonadotropic cells of the pituitary to stimulate the release of LH and FSH. The initial step involves binding of LHRH to high-affinity receptor sites on the plasma membrane of these cells.[104, 105] LHRH-induced release of gonadotropins after binding to the receptor appears to be cyclic AMP independent and instead requires calcium and activation of protein kinase C.[104]

Three types of secretory patterns can be distinguished for gonadotropin in women:

1. *Trigintan* or *circatrigintan* patterns are low-frequency changes that occur approximately every 30 d during the normal menstrual cycle.[106]

2. *Diurnal* patterns are intermittent frequency changes in gonadotropin secretion that recur every 24 h. These changes are minimal in adult women but are marked during sleep at the initiation of puberty in girls, as discussed previously.[38]

3. *Circhoral* patterns are high-frequency changes in gonadotropin secretion characterized by pulses approximately every hour.[40]

LHRH regulates (1) synthesis and storage of gonadotropins, (2) activation or movement of gonadotropins from reserve to a pool ready for secretion, and (3) immediate release of gonadotropins. LH and FSH, like thyrotropin-stimulating hormone and hCG, are glycoproteins composed of two polypeptide chains designated alpha and beta. There appears to be a single gene for the expression of the alpha subunit, which is similar for all four glycoproteins and contains 92 amino acids.[107] The beta chains for the glycoprotein hormones are unique, ensuring specific biological activity for each hormone. Both subunits are required for full expression of biological activity.[108] β-hCG, the largest subunit, is similar to the beta subunit of LH except for an additional 30-amino-acid residue and a large carbohydrate moiety at the COOH end.[108] The half-life of hCG is the longest, followed by FSH and then LH, and is determined in part by the sialic content of the hormones.[109, 110]

FSH and LH are secreted in a coordinated fashion to regulate follicle growth, ovulation, and maintenance of corpus luteum (see later). As discussed previously, the release of FSH and LH requires the constant pulsatile release of LHRH from the hypothalamus. In addition, the release of LH and FSH is affected both positively and negatively by estrogen and progesterone. Whether estrogen and progesterone stimulate or inhibit gonadotropin release depends on concentration and duration of exposure to the steroids.[111] In addition to steroid hormones, at least three gonadal protein hormones modulate FSH release. Activin appears to stimulate FSH, whereas inhibin and follistatin suppress FSH (see Fig. 12–18).[92]

Negative Feedback. Estrogen exerts its inhibitory effect on both the hypothalamus and the pituitary. Negative feedback is evidenced by the increase in LH and FSH that occurs after the decrease in ovarian estrogen secretion after menopause or castration.[112] Inhibition of FSH and LH secretion occurs at low levels of estrogen but is more complete at high levels. Progesterone at high concentrations inhibits FSH and LH primarily at the level of the hypothalamus.[113] As noted, both inhibin and follistatin selectively inhibit FSH secretion.[92]

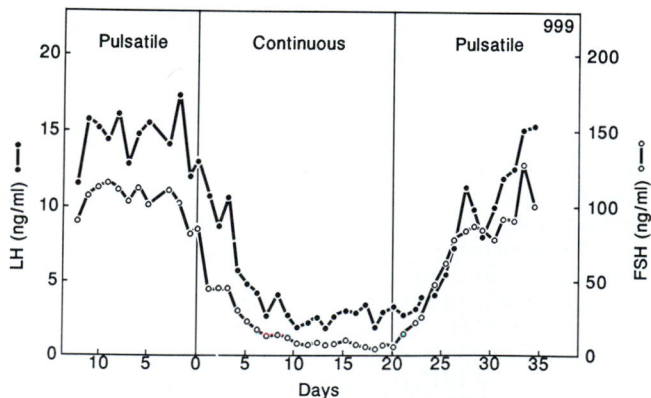

Figure 12–20. The effect of pulsatile or continuous administration of LHRH to ovariectomized monkeys rendered LHRH deficient by placement of a lesion in the hypothalamus. LH and FSH release was restored by hourly LHRH infusion, inhibited during a continuous LHRH infusion, and again restored after reinstitution of pulsatile LHRH administration. (Adapted from Belchetz PE, Plant TM, Nakai Y, et al. Hypophysial responses to continuous and intermittent delivery of hypothalamic gonadotropin-releasing hormone. Science 1978; 202:631–633. Copyright 1978 by the American Association for the Advancement of Science.)

Positive Feedback. In addition to a negative feedback, gonadal hormones exert a positive effect on gonadotropin secretion. The positive feedback is paramount in the promotion of the LH surge required to initiate ovulation and is triggered by a sharply rising plasma level of estrogen. Two features are essential for this mechanism: (1) an estradiol concentration of more than 700 pmol/L (200 pg/mL) and (2) persistence of the elevated level of estradiol for at least 48 to 50 h.[114, 115] Progesterone is reportedly responsible for the midcycle FSH surge.[116] Progesterone at low concentrations stimulates LH release but only after previous prolonged exposure of the pituitary to estrogen.[111] In addition, secretion of activin by granulosa cells serves to augment FSH release (see Fig. 12–18).[92]

OVARIAN HORMONES

Steroid Hormones

Classification. The ovarian steroids are classified on the basis of chemical structure and principal biological function and consist of three major types: estrogens, progestogens, and androgens (Fig. 12–21).[117]

Estrogens. The naturally occurring estrogens are C_{18}-steroids characterized by the presence of an aromatic A ring, a phenolic hydroxyl group at C-3, and either a hydroxyl group (estradiol) or a ketone group (estrone). The principal and most important, as well as most potent, estrogen secreted by the ovary is estradiol-17β. Although estrone is also secreted by the ovary, the principal source of estrone is from extraglandular conversion of androstenedione in peripheral tissues.[118] Estriol (16-hydroxyestradiol) is the most abundant estrogen in urine and results from the metabolism of estrone and estradiol. Obesity and hypothyroidism are associated with an increase in estriol formation.[119, 120] Catechol estrogens are formed by hydroxylation of estrogens at the C-2 or C-4 position. The physiological role of catechol estrogen, if any, is unclear. Low body weight and hyperthyroidism are associated with increased formation of catechol estrogens.[121] Estrone sulfate formed by peripheral conversion of estradiol and estrone is the most abundant estrogen in blood but is not physiologically active.[122] Estrogens promote development of the secondary sexual characteristics of women, uterine growth, thickening of the vaginal mucosa, thinning of the cervical mucus, and development of the ductal system of the breast.

Progestogens. The principal progestogens are C_{21}-steroids (see Fig. 12–21) and include pregnenolone, progesterone, and 17-hydroxyprogesterone. Pregnenolone is of primary importance in the ovary because of its key position as precursor of all steroid hormones. Progesterone is the principal secretory product of the corpus luteum and is responsible for the progestational effects (i.e., induction of secretory activity in the endometrium of the estrogen-primed uterus). Progesterone is required for implantation of the fertilized ovum and maintenance of pregnancy. It also induces decidualization of the endometrium, inhibits uterine contractions, increases the viscosity of cervical mucus, promotes glandular development of the breast, and increases body temperature (basal). However, 17-hydroxyprogesterone, also secreted by the corpus luteum, has little, if any, biological activity.[122]

Androgens. The ovary secretes a variety of C_{19}-steroids, including DHEA, androstenedione, testosterone, and dihydrotestosterone. They are produced by the thecal cells and to a lesser degree by the ovarian stroma. The major C_{19}-steroid is androstenedione (see Fig. 12–21), part of which is secreted directly into plasma, with the remainder converted to estrogen by the granulosa cells (see later). Androstenedione can be converted to estrogen or testosterone in both the ovary and extraglandular tissues. Only testosterone and dihydrotestosterone are true androgens with the capacity of interacting with the androgen receptor. Excessive production of androgens by the ovary or adrenal can cause sexual ambiguity in the newborn or hirsutism or virilization in women.[122]

Biogenesis of Steroid Hormones. All of the steroids of the ovary discussed earlier, as well as those produced by testes, adrenal, and placenta, are derived from cholesterol. Cholesterol can be obtained from three sources: (1) preformed cholesterol circulating in blood in the form of lipoproteins, (2) cholesterol synthesized de novo within the ovary from two-carbon units (acetylcoenzyme A [acetyl-CoA]), and (3) cholesterol liberated from cholesterol esters stored within lipid droplets (Fig. 12–22). The primary source of cholesterol utilized by the ovary is derived from the uptake of plasma lipoprotein cholesterol.[88, 123] In the human ovary, low-density lipoprotein (LDL) cholesterol is the principal source of cholesterol utilized for steroidogenesis.[88] In the ovary, LH stimulates the activity of adenylate cyclase, which releases cyclic AMP, which in turn serves as a second messenger to stimulate an increase in the messenger RNA (mRNA) for the LDL receptor and the binding and uptake of LDL cholesterol, as well as the formation of cholesterol esters.[123, 124] Cholesterol is then transported to the inner mitochondrial membrane by cyclic AMP–activated sterol

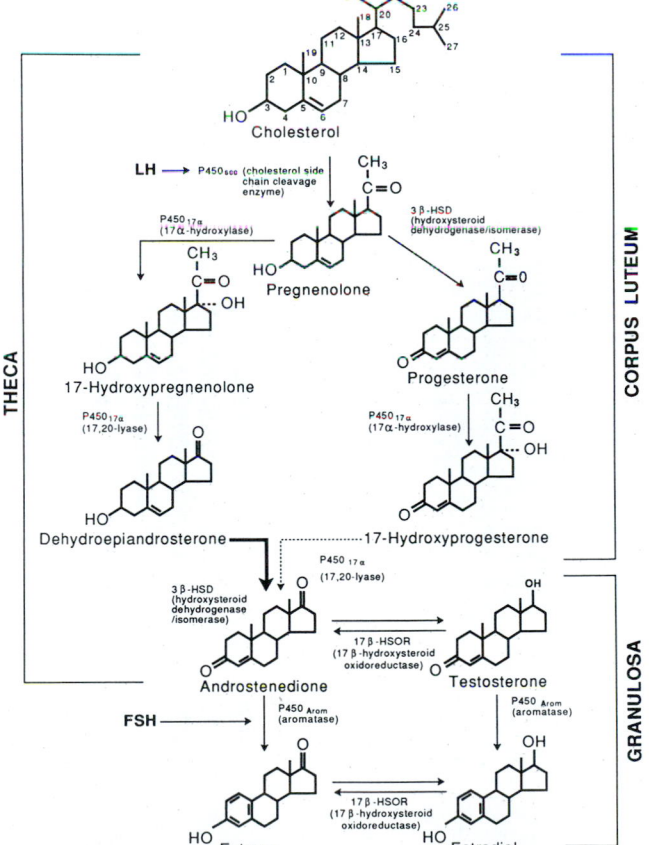

Figure 12–21. Principal pathways of steroid hormone biosynthesis in the human ovary. Although each cell type of the ovary contains the complete enzyme complement required for the formation of estradiol from cholesterol, the amounts of the various enzymes and consequently the predominant hormones formed differ among the cell types. The major enzyme complements for the corpus luteum, theca, and granulosa cells are shown in brackets; these cells produce predominantly progesterone and 17-hydroxyprogesterone (corpus luteum); androgen (theca); and estrogen (granulosa). The major sites of action of LH and FSH in mediating this pathway are shown by the horizontal arrows. The dotted line emphasizes that the metabolism of 17-hydroxyprogesterone is limited in the human ovary.

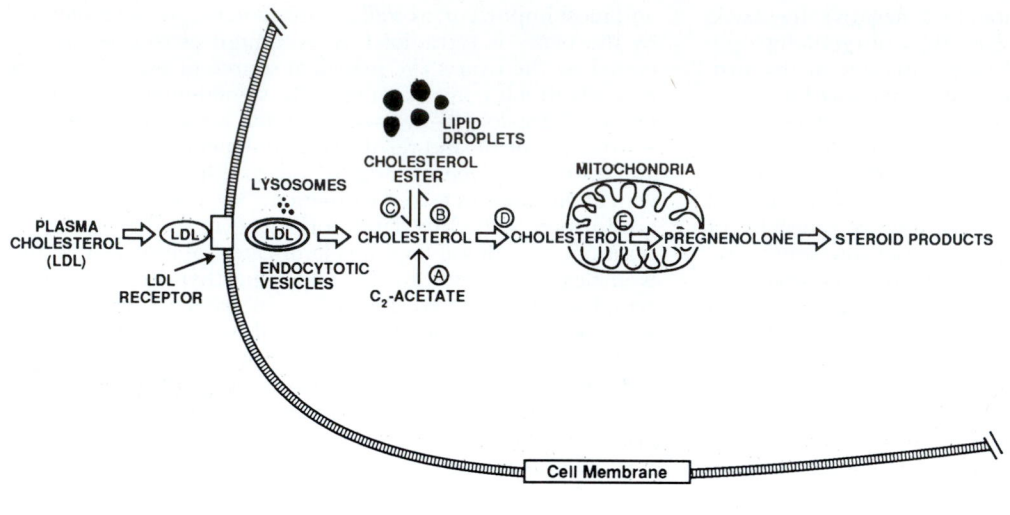

A. 3-HYDROXY-3-METHYLGLUTARYL
   COENZYME A REDUCTASE
   (HMG-CO A REDUCTASE)

B. ACYL-COENZYME A:
   CHOLESTEROL ACYL-
   TRANSFERASE (ACAT)

C. CHOLESTEROL ESTERASE

D. STEROL-CARRIER
   PROTEIN (SCP)

E. CHOLESTEROL SIDE-CHAIN
   CLEAVAGE ENZYME

Figure 12–22. Diagrammatic representation of the cellular organelles, principal sources of cholesterol, and key enzymes involved in cholesterol metabolism by the ovarian theca and corpus luteum for steroid biosynthesis. The larger arrows indicate the principal pathway. (Adapted from Hsueh AJW. Ovarian hormone synthesis, circulation and mechanism of action. In: DeGroot LJ, Besser GM, Cahill GF Jr, et al., eds. Endocrinology. 2nd ed. Philadelphia: W. B. Saunders, 1989: 1929–1939.)

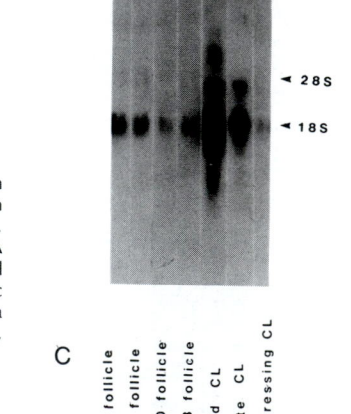

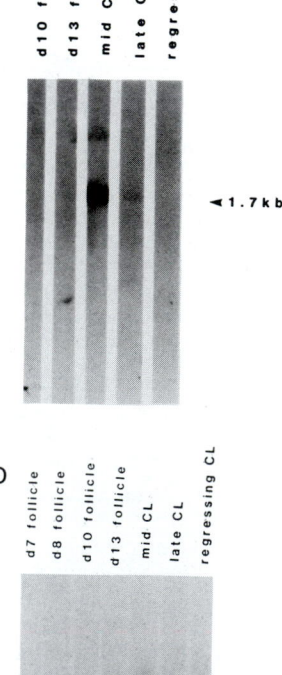

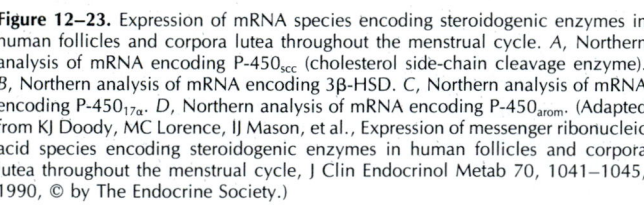

Figure 12–23. Expression of mRNA species encoding steroidogenic enzymes in human follicles and corpora lutea throughout the menstrual cycle. *A*, Northern analysis of mRNA encoding P-450$_{scc}$ (cholesterol side-chain cleavage enzyme). *B*, Northern analysis of mRNA encoding 3β-HSD. *C*, Northern analysis of mRNA encoding P-450$_{17\alpha}$. *D*, Northern analysis of mRNA encoding P-450$_{arom}$. (Adapted from KJ Doody, MC Lorence, IJ Mason, et al., Expression of messenger ribonucleic acid species encoding steroidogenic enzymes in human follicles and corpora lutea throughout the menstrual cycle, J Clin Endocrinol Metab 70, 1041–1045, 1990, © by The Endocrine Society.)

carrier protein.[123, 125] The conversion of cholesterol to pregnenolone is the rate-limiting step in ovarian steroidogenesis and is catalyzed by cholesterol side-chain cleavage enzyme complex consisting of cytochrome P-450 side-chain cleavage (P-450$_{scc}$), adrenodoxin, and flavoprotein (see Fig. 12–21).[126] The principal steroid-producing cells of the ovary, namely the granulosa, the thecal, and the corpus luteum cells, possess the complete enzymatic complement required for steroid hormone formation. The main pathway of steroid synthesis in the human corpus luteum is the Δ^4-pathway, which involves the conversion of pregnenolone to progesterone (see Fig. 12–21). In the human ovarian follicle the Δ^5-pathway is the preferred pathway for the formation of androgens and estrogens, because thecal cells of the human ovary metabolize 17-hydroxypregnenolone more efficiently than 17-hydroxyprogesterone.[127] However, the predominant steroid differs among each of these cell types so that the corpus luteum primarily forms progesterone and 17-hydroxyprogesterone, the thecal and stromal cells secrete androgen, and the granulosa cells secrete estrogen predominantly. The factors that determine which steroid is secreted by each cell type include the levels of gonadotropin and gonadotropin receptors, the expression of steroidogenic enzymes, and the availability of LDL cholesterol.

The rate of steroid production during the menstrual cycle is a function of the content of four key enzymes, P-450$_{scc}$, 3β-HSD, cytochrome P-450 17α-hydroxylase (P-450$_{17\alpha}$), and cytochrome P-450 aromatase (P-450$_{arom}$).[128–130] These important regulatory enzymes catalyze, respectively, the conversion of cholesterol to pregnenolone, pregnenolone to progesterone, pregnenolone to androgens, and androgens to estrogens (see Fig. 12–21). LH regulates the first step in steroid hormone biosynthesis by controlling the conversion of cholesterol to pregnenolone, whereas FSH controls the conversion of androgens to estrogens. The immunohistochemical localization and the expression of mRNA encoding P-450$_{scc}$, 3β-HSD, P-450$_{17\alpha}$, and P-450$_{arom}$ have been determined in human follicles and corpora lutea throughout the menstrual cycle (Fig. 12–23).[128–130] P-450$_{scc}$ mRNA is expressed in all stages of follicular development. Immunoreactive P-450$_{scc}$ is located primarily in the theca interna cells of the follicle, consistent with the requirement of this enzyme for thecal androgen biosynthesis. Expression of P-450$_{scc}$ mRNA increases in corpora lutea (see Fig. 12–23A), and immunoreactive P-450$_{scc}$ is present in both the theca-lutein and granulosa-lutein cells.[129] There is little expression of 3β-HSD mRNA in the follicle, but levels are high in corpora lutea (see Fig. 12–23B). The increases in 3β-HSD and P-450$_{scc}$ mRNAs in the corpus luteum are consistent with the enormous secretion of progesterone that occurs during the luteal phase of the cycle. The pattern of expression of P-450$_{17\alpha}$ mRNA is similar in follicles and corpora lutea (see Fig. 12–23C). Immunoreactive P-450$_{17\alpha}$ is localized histochemically only in the theca interna cells of the follicle and the theca-lutein cells of the corpus luteum and is virtually absent from granulosa and granulosa-lutein cells.[129] The studies of the steroidogenic capacities of isolated granulosa and thecal cells led to the two cell–two gonadotropin theory (Fig. 12–24), which proposed that in response to LH the thecal cells produce C$_{19}$-steroids (normally androstenedione and testosterone) and that FSH stimulates granulosa cells to aromatize those preformed C$_{19}$-steroids produced by the thecal cells to estrogens.[82, 131] The expression of P-450$_{arom}$ mRNA seen in mature follicles (see Fig. 12–23D) and immunoreactive P-450$_{arom}$ localized in granulosa cells are consistent with the marked rise in estrogen biosynthesis before ovulation. P-450$_{arom}$ mRNA is greatest in corpora lutea (see Fig. 12–23D), and immunoreactive P-450$_{arom}$ is localized in granulosa-lutein cells.[129] The amount of immunoreactive P-

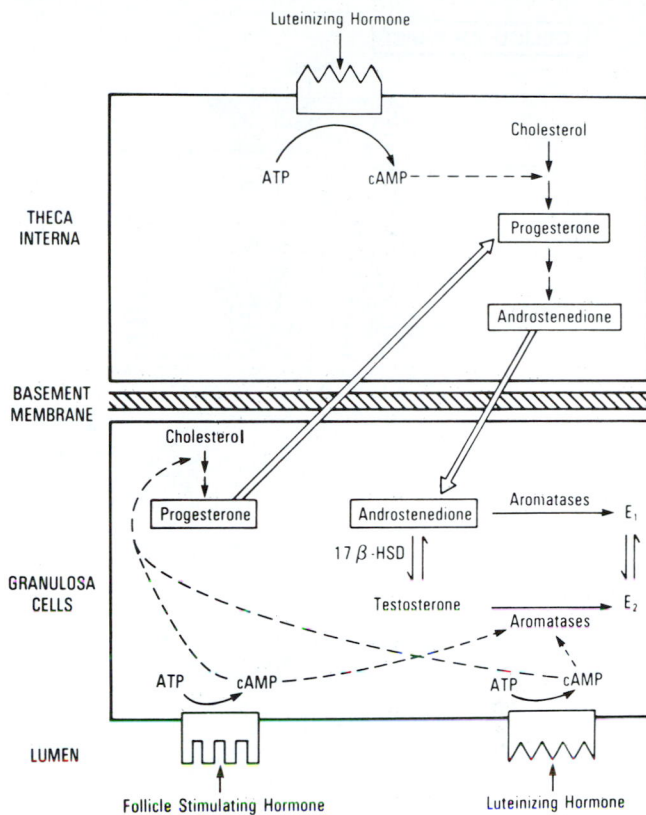

Figure 12–24. A two-cell, two-gonadotropin hypothesis of gonadotropin control of ovarian estrogen biosynthesis. (From AJW Hsueh, EY Adashi, PBC Jones, et al., Hormonal regulation of the differentiation of cultured ovarian granulosa cells, Endocr Rev 5, 76–127, 1984, © by The Endocrine Society.)

450$_{arom}$ and of P-450$_{arom}$ mRNA in human granulosa cells is enhanced by FSH.[132] In summary, studies of expression of the mRNAs encoding the various steroidogenic enzymes are consistent with the enzymatic activity of human ovaries.[130] In addition, the enzyme 17β-hydroxysteroid oxidoreductase, which converts androstenedione to testosterone and estrone to estradiol, is present in granulosa cells and in the hilus cells of the ovary (see Fig. 12–21).[133, 134] These observations explain the predominance of estrogen secreted by granulosa cells of the follicle and the corpus luteum, the secretion of androgens by the theca, and the secretion of progesterone by both types of corpus luteum cells of the human ovary.

The regulation of steroid hormone synthesis by enzymic localization is complemented by substrate availability. The granulosa cells of the follicle are avascular, as discussed previously. Thus the granulosa cells do not have ready access to LDL, and extremely low levels of LDL are found in follicular fluid bathing granulosa cells (Fig. 12–25).[135] As a result, the granulosa cells have limited ability to form progesterone. After ovulation, extensive neovascularization of the follicle takes place, providing increased amounts of cholesterol to the luteinized granulosa cells. The increased availability of LDL to the granulosa-lutein cells provides the ability for these cells to secrete increased quantities of progesterone during the luteal phase of the menstrual cycle (see later). Treatment of corpus luteum tissue in vitro with hCG and LDL increases the number of LDL receptors and enhances progesterone secretion.[135, 136] In addition, hCG also increases LDL receptor mRNA in human granulosa cells.[124] LH-hCG binding sites are maximal at midluteal phase.[137] Women with abetalipoproteinemia who have low levels of LDL cholesterol have low levels of progesterone secretion during the luteal phase.[138]

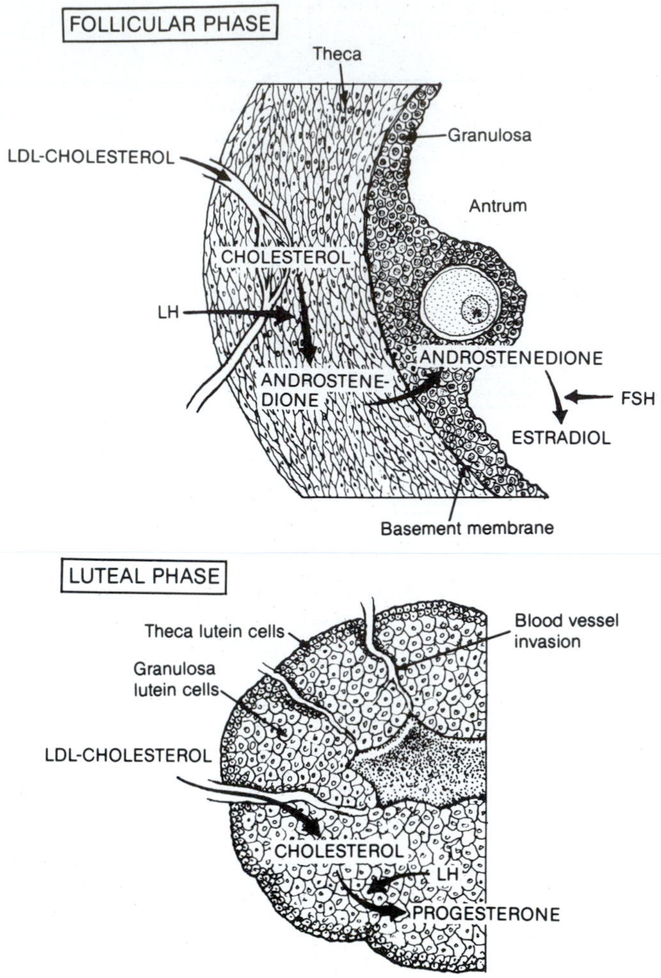

Figure 12–25. Cellular interactions in the ovary during the follicular phase *(top)* and luteal phase *(bottom)*. (From Carr BR, MacDonald PC, Simpson ER. The role of lipoproteins in the regulation of progesterone secretion by the human corpus luteum. Fertil Steril 1982; 38:303–311.)

Gonadotropin Control of Steroidogenesis. Both FSH and LH are required for estrogen synthesis, and the amount of estrogen produced depends on the relative exposure to each gonadotropin once minimal effective doses of gonadotropin have been achieved.[139] FSH is required for follicular maturation and growth, and FSH receptors are present exclusively on the granulosa cell.[140] Enhanced secretion of estradiol causes an increase in the number of estradiol receptors and further proliferation of granulosa cells and follicular growth.[140, 141] In the mature follicle, FSH in concert with estradiol causes an increase in LH receptors on granulosa cells.[140] LH acts in granulosa cells via these receptors to augment progesterone secretion, which then increases FSH release at midcycle. Taken together, these observations emphasize the important roles of autocrine and paracrine actions of steroids and validate the two cell–two gonadotropin hypothesis discussed earlier (see Fig. 12–24).

The binding of gonadotropins to their respective plasma membrane receptors stimulates adenylate cyclase (see Fig. 12–24). Deglycosylated gonadotropins can bind to receptors but do not stimulate steroidogenesis.[142] After ovulation, the number of LH receptors in the lutein cells increases, and FSH receptor number and FSH responses decrease.[140, 143] In women with the "resistant ovary" syndrome, defective ovarian response to gonadotropin occurs, and despite elevated levels of FSH and LH, these patients have immature follicles

and are thus estrogen deficient.[144] It is suspected that such patients have absent or defective gonadotropin receptors.

Extragonadal Steroidogenesis: Prohormones. The application of isotopic dilution methods made possible reliable measurements of the secretion rates of steroid hormones and provided insight into the complexity of the processes involved in secretion and metabolism of steroid hormones, particularly the role of extragonadal hormone formation in the origin of plasma estrogens (Fig. 12–26).[145, 146]

Secretion Rate. The secretory rate of hormone A is the amount of A released by the endocrine gland into the circulation per unit of time. However, hormone A may also be derived from the extraglandular or peripheral conversion of another hormone (hormone B), which may be secreted by the original or by another endocrine gland. The extraglandular conversion of androstenedione (hormone B) to estrone (hormone A) is depicted in Figure 12–26. Hormone B is the prohormone of hormone A, and this pathway of formation of A is referred to as the *prohormone pathway.*

Production Rate. The production rate of hormone A is the rate at which A enters into the circulation. In a steady state, this can also be defined as the rate by which hormone A is irreversibly removed from the circulation. If a hormone is derived exclusively via glandular secretion, the secretory and production rates are equal. However, when the hormone is formed from extraglandular conversion as well as from secretion, the production rate is greater than the secretory rate.

Metabolic Clearance Rate. The metabolic clearance rate (MCR) is the volume of blood that is irreversibly cleared of a hormone per unit of time. The blood production rate (PR) of a hormone equals the MCR multiplied by the concentration (C) of the hormone in blood: $PR = MCR \times C$.

The secretory and production rates of steroid hormones can be determined by a variety of techniques.[147, 148] The most common method involves the intravenous infusion of a radiolabeled hormone until a constant level is attained in blood. After this, the production rate or the total entry of this hormone into the circulation can be calculated from its specific activity in plasma. In the instance in which a steroid hormone is derived from more than one prohormone, infusion of each of these radiolabeled hormones makes it possible to calculate their relative contributions to the blood production rate of the hormone.[145]

The origin of plasma estrogens has been clarified by such studies. In normal women most plasma estradiol is derived by direct secretion from the ovary. There is little, if any, estradiol formed from testosterone by extraglandular conversion. On the other hand, little estrone is formed by direct ovarian secretion, and most estrone in plasma origi-

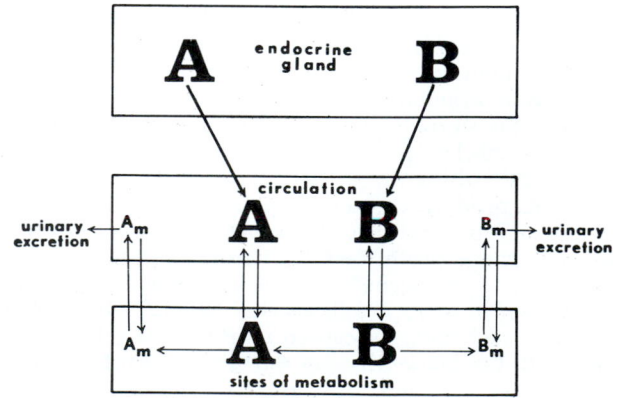

Figure 12–26. A or B may be secreted by the ovaries or adrenal. A_m and B_m represent inactive metabolites of A and B, respectively.

nates from extraglandular conversion of androstenedione and, to a minor extent, from estradiol.[146] The primary site of extraglandular aromatization of androstenedione to estrone is in adipose tissue, and the rate is influenced by age, liver function, and thyroid function.[118]

The importance of extragonadal estrogen formation is increased in a variety of clinical conditions. The formation of estrogens by the placenta depends on androgens secreted by the fetal adrenal gland and, to a lesser extent, on androgens from the maternal circulation[149] (see Chapter 16). In nonpregnant premenopausal women, estrone is formed from androstenedione secreted by the ovary and adrenal. In menopausal women the ovarian formation of androstenedione is negligible, but considerable amounts of estrone are formed by extraglandular conversion of androstenedione secreted by the adrenals. An increase in estrogen formation occurs with aging and obesity, sufficient to produce endometrial hyperplasia and bleeding in menopausal women.[118] In premenopausal women, ovarian tumors or polycystic ovarian syndrome (PCOS) can cause increased secretion of androstenedione and secondary increases in estrone formation. In such women the amount of extraglandular production of estrogen can interfere with normal feedback mechanisms and produce disturbances of the ovarian cycle.[150]

The normal ranges of plasma concentrations, production rate, metabolic clearance rate, and secretory rate of ovarian steroid hormones are presented in Table 12–3.

Transport of Ovarian Steroid Hormones in Plasma. Most steroids are bound to plasma proteins and are carried to target tissues where the hormones dissociate and pass by diffusion into cells. Transport molecules include specific globulins and albumin. For example, testosterone is largely bound to testosterone-binding globulin ([TeBG], also called sex hormone–binding globulin [SHBG]), with lesser amounts bound to albumin. The bulk of estradiol (60%) is bound to serum albumin, but 38% is bound to TeBG and 2 to 3% is free.[151] It is usually assumed that protein-bound hormone is "inactive" and that only the "free" hormone is directly available to enter target tissues, but the transport of steroid hormones may actually be more complex.[152–154]

TeBG, a beta-globulin synthesized by the liver, has a molecular mass of about 95 kd and contains 30% carbohydrate. It exhibits high-affinity (10^{-9} mol), low-capacity binding (one binding site per molecule).[155] Dihydrotestosterone has the highest binding affinity for TeBG. The affinities of

testosterone and estradiol are one third and one fifth, respectively, that of dihydrotestosterone. DHEA and progesterone have negligible affinity to TeBG.[122] The metabolic clearance rate of gonadal steroids is inversely related to the binding affinity to TeBG, and alterations in the concentration of TeBG influence gonadal steroid metabolism and target tissue action.[155] For example, women have two times the concentration of TeBG as men as a result of the fact that estrogen stimulates the formation of TeBG. The level of TeBG, and thus the level of free hormone, may be altered by a variety of clinical conditions. TeBG level is enhanced by estrogens (e.g., in pregnancy and by oral contraceptive pills) and thyroid hormones (hyperthyroidism) and is lowered by androgens, hypothyroidism, and obesity.[156]

Mechanisms of Action of Steroid Hormones (also see Chapter 3). Steroid hormones have low molecular weight and readily enter cells by diffusion, although carrier-mediated transport may occur. The affinity, specificity, and large concentration of steroid receptors in cells allow a low concentration of steroid hormones to produce biological responses. Specificity is partially determined by the number of estrogen receptors in the cells. In specific target tissues, such as the uterus, estrogens are retained, and biological action is greater and prolonged because of the large number of estrogen receptors per cell.[157] In contrast, in cells lacking estrogen receptors, estrogens are not readily retained and exit the cell.

To explain intracellular response of steroid hormones, two receptor mechanisms have been described[158] (see Chapter 3). The classic receptor or translocation model assigned a primary role to cytoplasmic receptors and required the receptor hormone complex to be translocated to the nucleus to interact with DNA. Binding of hormone was followed by transformational or conformational change of the hormone-receptor complex, which bound to DNA, leading to gene transcription and the production of mRNA. This concept was based on the observation that unoccupied receptors were found in the cytosol and that after exposure to steroid hormones, receptors were translocated to the nucleus with loss of receptors in the cytosol. Although this concept is still held by some, the finding of receptors in cytosol was based on the methods that produced artifactual results.[158]

By immunohistological techniques, it was subsequently established that most steroid receptors are localized exclusively in the nucleus.[159, 160] The steroid receptor is a nuclear

TABLE 12–3. Concentration, Metabolic Clearance Rate (MCR), Production Rate (PR), and Ovarian Secretion Rate (SR) of Steroids in Blood

Compound	MCR of Compound in Peripheral Plasma (L/d)	Phase of Menstrual Cycle	Concentration in Plasma		PR of Circulating Compound (mg/d)	SR by Both Ovaries (mg/d)
			nmol/L	µg/dL		
Estradiol	1350	Early follicular	0.2	0.006	0.081	0.07
		Late follicular	1.2–2.6	0.033–0.070	0.445–0.945	0.4–0.8
		Midluteal	0.7	0.020	0.270	0.25
Estrone	2210	Early follicular	0.18	0.005	0.110	0.08
		Late follicular	0.5–1.1	0.015–0.030	0.331–0.662	0.25–0.50
		Midluteal	0.4	0.011	0.243	0.16
Progesterone	2200	Follicular	3.0	0.095	2.1	1.5
		Luteal	36	1.13	25.0	24.0
20α-Hydroxyprogesterone	2300	Follicular	1.5	0.05	1.1	0.8
		Luteal	7.5	0.25	5.8	3.3
17-Hydroxyprogesterone	2000	Early follicular	0.9	0.03	0.6	0–0.3
		Late follicular	6	0.20	4.0	3–4
		Midluteal	6	0.02	4.0	3–4
Androstenedione	2010		5.6	0.159	3.2	0.8–1.6
Testosterone	690		1.3	0.038	0.26	
Dehydroepiandrosterone	1640		17	0.490	8.0	0.3–3

From Tagatz GE, Gurpide E. Hormone secretion by the normal human ovary. In: Greep RO, Astwood EB, eds. Handbook of Physiology. Sect 7: Endocrinology. Vol II. Female Reproductive System. Washington, DC: American Physiological Society, 1973: 603–613.

protein (occupied or unoccupied) and is immobilized by association with elements within the nucleus. In the nuclear localization model, steroid hormones diffuse across the cell membrane, enter the nucleus, and associate with a nuclear steroid receptor. The nuclear steroid receptor consists of three domains: a steroid hormone binding site (COOH terminus), a DNA binding site (middle), and a modulating domain at the NH_2 terminus.[161] Active transformation occurs after nuclear binding and involves a change in size of the receptor because of the loss of inhibiting proteins and dephosphorylation, which induces conformational changes that appear to unmask high-affinity DNA binding sites.[158] After interaction of the hormone-receptor complex with DNA, synthesis of mRNA occurs, followed by transport of mRNA to the ribosomes and finally synthesis in the cytoplasm of proteins that direct specific cellular responses.

Steroid receptors for estrogen, progesterone, glucocorticoids, and androgens have been cloned and sequenced (see Chapter 3). The unoccupied estrogen receptor is located loosely bound in the nucleus as a monomer. After exposure to estrogen, activation of the receptor involves the formation of a dimer.[162] Activation of the estrogen receptor by estrogen is followed by an increased affinity for estrogen at other sites, a process termed *positive cooperativity*. This phenomenon allows an increase in biological response with small changes in estrogen concentration. The effect is greater for estradiol-17β than for estrone.[158] Positive cooperativity allows longer duration of action as a result of increased affinity for the estrogen receptor. In some target tissues, estrogens also stimulate the formation of new estrogen receptors that are synthesized in the cytoplasm and rapidly transferred to the nucleus (receptor replenishment), which in turn further increases the biological response to a given hormone concentration. After gene activation by the estrogen-receptor complex, the receptor converts from a high-affinity site to a dissociated form with low affinity and loss of binding capacity, a phenomenon termed *receptor processing*.[158] These aspects of receptor function help to explain clinical responses to pharmacological agents and other hormones. For example, progesterone and clomiphene citrate block cooperativity and receptor replenishment, leading to a reduction in cellular biological response to estrogens.[163]

Nonsteroidal Hormones and Growth Factors of the Ovary. A variety of nonsteroidal hormones and growth factors produced by the ovary appear to modulate local steroidogenesis in the ovary by way of autocrine and paracrine mechanisms. Some of these factors may influence hypothalamic and pituitary secretion of gonadotropin via endocrine mechanisms. (For review, see refs. 164 to 166.) A list of nonsteroidal hormones and their proposed functions is presented in Table 12–4. The fact that only one follicle is destined to ovulate each month and the rest are destined to undergo atresia supports the view of a complex intraovarian regulation of growth of a single follicle and inhibition of growth of the remaining follicles. Some of these nonsteroid factors, as well as steroids produced by the dominant follicle, may play a role in local regulation of follicular growth.[164–179]

THE COORDINATION OF OVARIAN FUNCTION: THE MENSTRUAL CYCLE. The development of cyclic, predictable, regular ovulatory menstrual cycles results from regulated interactions of the hypothalamus, pituitary, ovaries, and genital tract. The menstrual cycle is usually divided into two phases: a follicular, or proliferative, phase and a luteal, or secretory, phase (Fig. 12–27).

The length of the normal menstrual cycle is defined as the time of onset of one menstrual bleeding episode until the next. The median length of the cycle in reproductive age women is 28 d, and the range is 25 to 30 d.[180–182] The greatest variability is observed at the extremes of reproductive life, menarche and menopause (Fig. 12–28). During the

TABLE 12–4. Nonsteroidal Factors Produced by the Ovary That May Regulate Endocrine-Autocrine or Paracrine Regulation of Ovarian Function

Nonsteroidal Factor	Proposed Function	Reference
Activin	Stimulates FSH release	92
Adenosine	Regulation of atresia, maintenance of corpus luteum, regulation of oocyte maturation	166
Angiogenic factors	Neovascularization of corpus luteum	168
Catecholamines	Modify steroidogenesis	166
Eicosanoids	Ovulation, corpus luteum regulation	165,167
Follicular-regulating protein	Atresia, aromatase inhibitor, inhibition of FSH action	165
Follistatin	Suppresses FSH release	92
FSH-binding inhibitor	Inhibits binding of FSH to receptor	166
γ-Aminobutyric acid	Unknown ? modulation of ovarian function	166
LHRH-like peptides	Stimulatory and inhibitory actions on FSH and LH, regulation of atresia	166,169,170
Growth factors		164–166,177
Epidermal growth factor	Mitogenic-granulosa, inhibits steroidogenesis, atresia	
Fibroblast growth factor	Mitogenic, inhibits steroidogenesis, atresia	
Insulin-like growth factors	Mitogenic, stimulate steroidogenesis	
Platelet-derived growth factor	? enhances steroidogenesis	
Transforming growth factors (TGFs)		
TGF α	Growth regulation	
TGF β	Stimulates FSH release, stimulates steroidogenesis-granulosa, inhibits steroidogenesis-theca, inhibits granulosa cell growth	
Inhibin	Inhibits FSH release	172,173
LH-binding inhibitor	Inhibits binding of LH to receptor	166
Luteinization inhibitor	Inhibits corpus luteum development and function	166
Luteinization stimulator	Stimulates corpus luteum	166
Antimüllerian hormone	Development and function unknown	174
Oocyte maturation inhibitor	Inhibits meiosis	166
Oxytocin (corpus luteum)	Modulates progesterone secretion, regulates life span of corpus luteum	166,175
Pro-opiomelanocortin-derived peptides	Unknown	166
Relaxin	Remodeling of reproductive tract, modulates corpus luteum	175,176
Renin-angiotensin	Ovulation, regulation of steroidogenesis	177
Substance P	Regulation of ovarian blood flow	166
Tissue-type plasminogen activator	Ovulation, atresia	166,178
Vasoactive intestinal peptide	Stimulates steroidogenesis	179
Vasopressin	Unknown	166

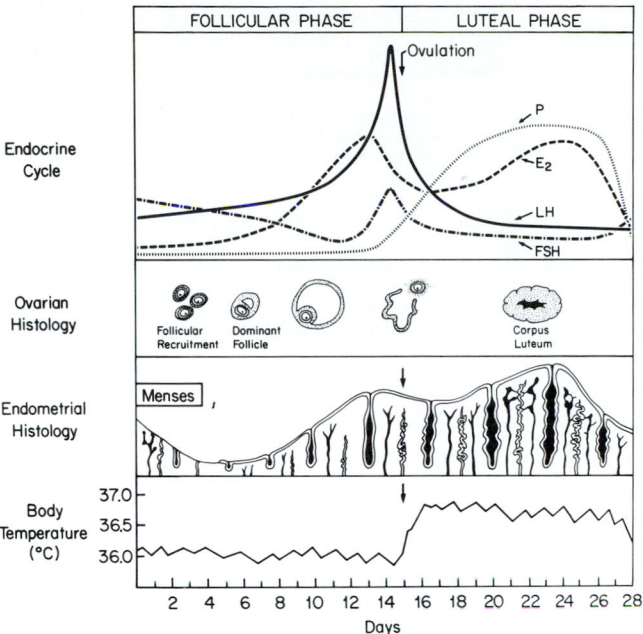

Figure 12–27. Hormonal, ovarian, endometrial, and basal body temperature changes and relationships throughout the normal menstrual cycle. (From Carr BR, Wilson JD. Disorders of the ovary and female reproductive tract. In: Braunwald E, Isselbacher KJ, Petersdorf RG, et al., eds. Harrison's Principles of Internal Medicine. 11th ed. New York: McGraw-Hill, 1987: 1818–1837. Reproduced with permission of McGraw-Hill, Inc.)

12 to 18 mo after menarche, cycle length is often prolonged and irregular as a result of inadequate follicular development and anovulatory cycles.[183, 184] A similar mechanism operates at the onset of menopause.[185] The least variability of menstrual cycle is found between ages 20 and 30. In most studies of women of reproductive age, the length of the secretory phase is remarkably constant and lasts approximately 14 d.[182] Variability in the length of the follicular phase ranging from 10 to 16 d is the cause for variation in the length of the menstrual cycle.

Follicular Phase. The initiation of follicular growth, or folliculogenesis, begins during the last few days of the luteal phase of the preceding menstrual cycle and terminates at the time of ovulation. During the last few days of the previous luteal phase, plasma progesterone and estrogen levels decline because of demise of the corpus luteum, and FSH levels rise (see Fig. 12–27).[186, 187] This rise in FSH initiates the development of follicles and the next menstrual cycle. In some primates the follicle destined to ovulate is usually in the contralateral ovary to that containing the corpus luteum.[186] However, in women ovulation probably occurs randomly during consecutive cycles, not preferentially in the contralateral ovary.[188]

After the onset of menses, follicular development continues, but FSH levels decline as a result of the negative feedback of estrogens and the effect of inhibin secreted by the developing follicle.[172, 173, 189] The decline in FSH, together with the secretion of protein hormones by the granulosa cells of the growing follicle (see Table 12–4), inhibits the development of adjacent follicles. Three stages have been described in the development of the dominant follicle (Fig. 12–29). The first stage is recruitment. From a pool of nonproliferating follicles, a cohort of follicles is recruited during days 1 to 4 of the menstrual cycle in response to FSH.[188] Once this stage is attained, the recruited follicles must either ovulate or undergo atresia.[186] The next stage is selection, in which one follicle is chosen to ovulate from those that have been recruited. This stage occurs between days 5 to 7 of the cycle. The final stage is dominance, in which the dominant follicle grows and suppresses maturation of other ovarian follicles. This stage begins between days 8 and 12 of the cycle and ends at ovulation (days 13 to 15).

During the proliferative phase, estrogen levels rise in parallel to the growth of the follicle and the number of granulosa cells (see Figs. 12–27 and 12–29). FSH receptors, as discussed previously, are exclusively located on granulosa cells. The increased levels of FSH in the late luteal phase of

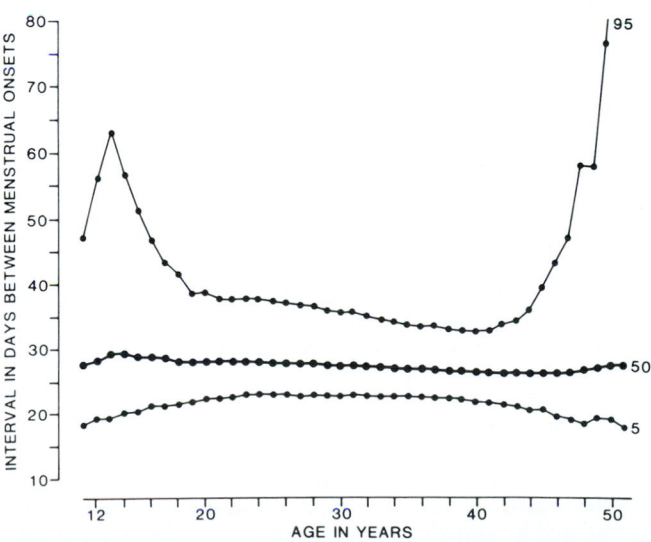

Figure 12–28. Menstrual cycle length in relation to age. The median and 5th and 95th percentiles are indicated. (Data from Treloar AE, Boynton BE, Behn BG, et al. Variations of the human menstrual cycle through reproductive life. Int J Fertil 1967; 12:77–126, as adapted by Baird DT. Amenorrhea, anovulation, and dysfunctional uterine bleeding. In: DeGroot LJ, Besser GM, Cahill GF Jr, et al., eds. Endocrinology. 2nd ed. Philadelphia: W. B. Saunders, 1989: 1950–1968.)

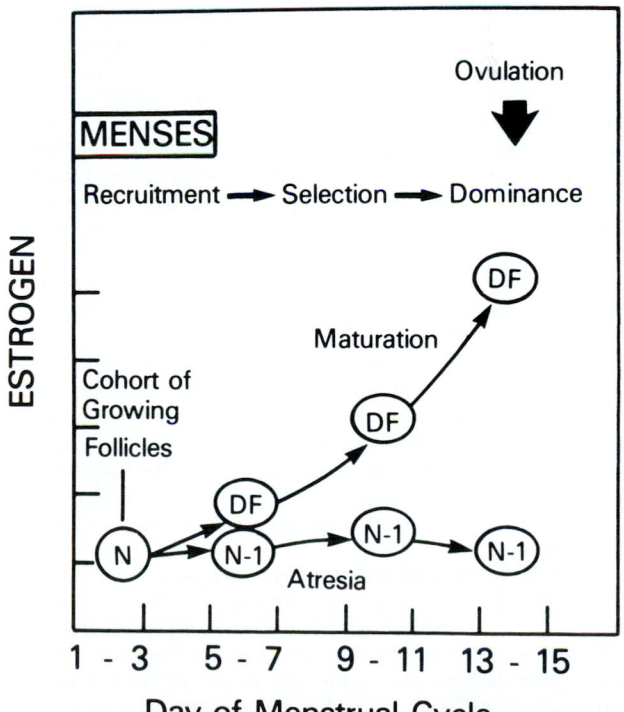

Figure 12–29. Time course for the recruitment, selection, and ovulation of the dominant ovarian follicle (DF) with onset of atresia among other follicles of the cohort (N-1). (From Hodgen GD. The dominant ovarian follicle. Fertil Steril 1982; 38:281–300.)

the previous cycle lead to an increase in the number of FSH receptors and, consequently, to an increase in estradiol secretion by granulosa cells.[190] The increase in FSH receptors appears to reflect an increase in number of granulosa cells rather than an increase in FSH receptors per cell. The granulosa cell has approximately 1500 FSH receptors per cell by the secondary stage of follicle development, and this number remains constant throughout the remainder of follicle development.[191, 192] The increase in estradiol formation appears to increase the number of estradiol receptors.[191] FSH also induces aromatase and, in the presence of estradiol, the formation of LH receptors on granulosa cells.[193, 194] After the appearance of LH receptors, the preovulatory granulosa cells begin to secrete small quantities of progesterone and 17-hydroxyprogesterone.[131] Preovulatory secretion of progesterone, although limited, may exert a positive feedback on the estrogen-primed pituitary to augment LH release, as discussed previously.[111] In addition, LH stimulates thecal cell production of androgens, which are then transferred to adjacent granulosa cells where they are aromatized to estrogen by the follicles.

During preantral and early antral follicular growth, follicles produce more androgens than estrogens.[195] This is because of the presence of the enzyme 5α-reductase, which converts testosterone to the nonaromatizable androgen dihydrotestosterone. Larger antral follicles, particularly the dominant graafian follicle with its larger quantities of aromatase, secrete more estrogens. This change in the microenvironment and the balance of androgens and estrogens of the ovary may be instrumental in the selection of the dominant follicle. The process of atresia in lesser follicles may be due to dihydrotestosterone, which inhibits aromatization.[195]

The microenvironment of the ovary and the regulation of steroidogenesis by granulosa cells are also influenced by the concentration of hormones and other substances in follicular fluid bathing the granulosa cells (Table 12–5). The concentrations of ovarian steroids in follicular fluid exceed by many-fold the concentrations in blood. Analysis of antral fluid hormone concentrations has identified two populations of antral follicles. In large follicles (>8 mm in diameter) the FSH, estrogen, and progesterone levels in follicular fluid are high. In smaller follicles the levels of androgens are higher than in large follicles. Prolactin levels also vary in follicular fluid and are reported to be high in smaller follicles and lower in larger, estrogen-progesterone–dominant follicles.[196] These observations further support the hypothesis of microenvironmental control of follicular growth by the hormones in the follicular fluid.[197–201]

Gonadotropin secretion varies during the menstrual cycle. FSH levels, which are elevated during the early part of the follicular phase, decline up until ovulation. In contrast, LH levels are low in the first part of the follicular phase. LH secretion begins to increase by the midfollicular phase as a result of the positive feedback caused by increased estrogen release. LH secretion in response to LHRH is markedly increased from the early until the late follicular phase. When two injections of LHRH are given sequentially, LH release to the second is greater, confirming the priming effect of estrogen.[202]

The frequency of spontaneous LH pulses varies during the menstrual cycle (Fig. 12–30). During the early part of the cycle, the LH pulses are of constant amplitude and occur at frequencies of 60 to 90 min. During the late follicular phase, just before the midcycle surge of LH, LH pulse frequency increases, and LH pulse amplitude may increase. In most women, LH pulse amplitude does not increase until after ovulation.[203]

Ovulation. Just before ovulation, estrogen secretion by the preovulatory follicle increases dramatically. This increase

TABLE 12–5. Substances Found in Follicular Fluid

Plasma proteins
Steroid-binding protein
Enzymes
    Side-chain cleavage enzymes
    3β-Hydroxysteroid dehydrogenase
    17α-Hydroxylase
    17,20-Lyase
    17β-Hydroxysteroid dehydrogenase
    20α-Hydroxysteroid dehydrogenase
    Aromatase
    Plasminogen (proteases)
Micropolysaccharides (proteoglycans)
    Hyaluronic acid
    Chrondroitin sulfate acid
    Heparan sulfate
Steroids
    Estrogens
    Androgens
    Progestins
Pituitary hormones
    Follicle-stimulating hormone
    Luteinizing hormone
    Prolactin
    Oxytocin
    Vasopressin
Nonsteroidal ovarian factors
    Inhibin
    Follicular protein (aromatase inhibitor)
    Oocyte meiosis inhibitor
    Luteinization inhibitor
    Luteinization stimulator

From Yen SCC. The human menstrual cycle. In: Yen SCC, Jaffe RB, eds. Reproductive Endocrinology: Physiology, Pathophysiology and Clinical Management. 2nd ed. Philadelphia: W. B. Saunders, 1986: 208.

in estrogen secretion initiates the LH surge. LH in turn initiates the process of luteinization of the granulosa cells and consequently enhances progesterone secretion, which in turn stimulates the release of the midcycle surge of FSH. The onset of the LH surge is a relatively precise predictor of the time of ovulation, occurring 34 to 36 h before release of the ovum from the follicle.[204] The peak of LH secretion occurs 10 to 12 h before ovulation.[205] The LH surge also initiates the resumption of meiosis and release of the first polar body. Luteinization of the granulosa cell increases progesterone synthesis as a result of LH-increased cyclic AMP formation.[206] Interestingly, spontaneous luteinization occurs in the absence of LH when granulosa cells are removed from the follicle and cultured. This has led to the hypothesis that oocyte maturation inhibitor or luteinization inhibitor (see Table 12–4) prevents ovulation and that the effects of these factors are overcome at the time of ovulation.[207]

Just before ovulation the follicle becomes extensively vascularized. A protrusion of the follicular wall termed the *stigma* develops and is the site at which rupture occurs with release of the oocyte-cumulus complex. The release of this complex has been photographed and appears to be explosive in nature.[208] The precise mechanism of follicular rupture is unknown. Progesterone and cyclic AMP augment or activate proteolytic enzymes such as collagenase and plasmin that digest collagen in the follicular wall, resulting in distensibility and thinning before ovum release.[209, 210] There is no evidence that an increase in follicular pressure causes follicular rupture, but measurements have not been determined at the precise instance of rupture of the follicle.[208, 209] In certain species, such as the rat, tissue plasminogen activator is stimulated by gonadotropins and increases the concentration of plasmin. Treatment of rats with antibodies to tissue plasminogen activator and α₂-antiplasmin inhibits hCG-stimulated ovulation.[211] However, in human follicular fluid, plasminogen activator does not increase in mature preovulatory follicles.[212]

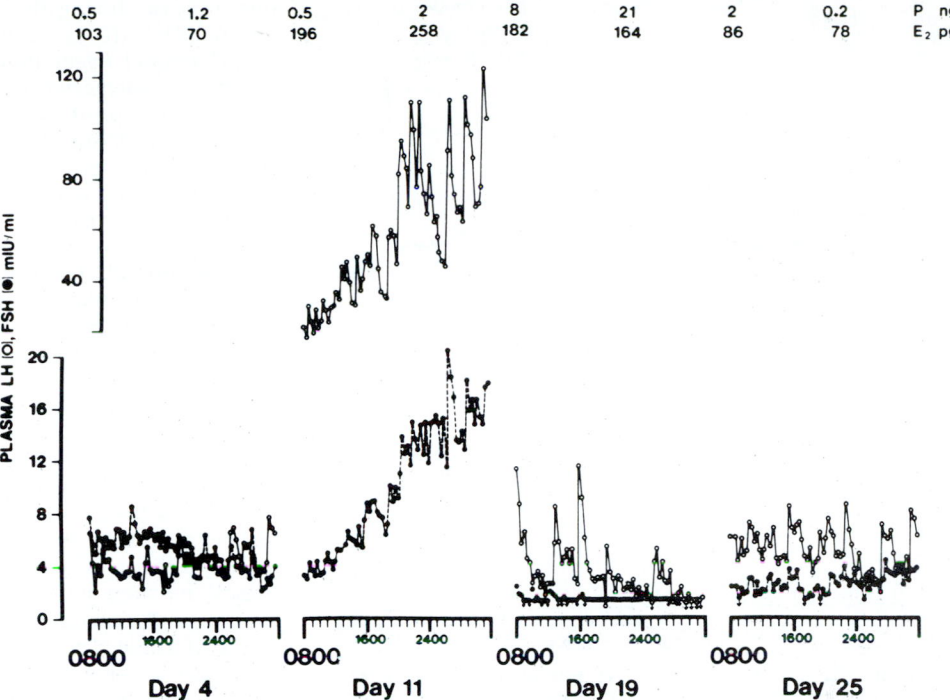

Figure 12–30. Serial measurements of plasma LH and FSH sampled every 20 min at weekly intervals where the LH surge occurred on day 11 of the menstrual cycle. *Top*, P, progesterone plasma values; E$_2$, estradiol plasma values. (Adapted from N Reame, SE Saunder, RP Kelch, et al., Pulsatile gonadotropin secretion during the menstrual cycle: evidence for altered frequency of gonadotropin-releasing hormone secretion, J Clin Endocrinol Metab 59, 328–337, 1984, © by The Endocrine Society.)

Prostaglandins of the E and F series reach a peak concentration in follicular fluid just before ovulation.[213] Prostaglandins are thought to be involved in the rupture of the follicle, possibly by stimulation of smooth muscle contraction, thereby aiding the extrusion of the oocyte-cumulus mass.[214] Occasionally, women fail to release the ovum, giving rise to the concept of the luteinized unruptured follicle syndrome.[215] However, this process appears to occur in fertile and infertile women with equal frequency.[215] Because women treated with high doses of prostaglandin synthetase inhibitors such as indomethacin develop luteinized unruptured follicles,[216, 217] infertile subjects are advised to avoid the use of such drugs before the time of expected ovulation.

Immediately before the LH peak, estradiol levels in plasma fall precipitously. This fall may be due to down-regulation of LH on LH receptors or to direct inhibition by increasing progesterone secretion (see Fig. 12–27).[218] The ovulatory peak of FSH, which is thought to be stimulated by progesterone, is believed to have a variety of functions, including stimulation of plasminogen activator and increase in granulosa cell LH receptors.[218] The postovulatory fall in LH could be due to loss of positive feedback caused by a decline in estrogen levels or by depletion of LH content of the pituitary.

Luteal Phase. After ovulation, the residual follicle undergoes dramatic changes in structure and function that result in formation of the corpus luteum. The corpus luteum is a transient endocrine organ that secretes principally progesterone for approximately 14 d. The purpose of the corpus luteum is to prepare the estrogen-primed endometrium for acceptance of the newly fertilized ovum and establishment of early pregnancy. The ingrowth of fibroblasts and the establishment of a vascular supply to the corpus luteum occurs in response to the secretion of angiogenic factors by the granulosa and thecal cells.[168] During the first few days after ovulation, the granulosa-lutein cells enlarge and are surrounded by the newly formed theca-lutein cells. At the time of peak vascularization, secretion of progesterone is maximal (see Fig. 12–27). In the absence of pregnancy the corpus luteum undergoes luteolysis and is transformed to a fibrous scar, the corpus albicans.

The pattern of secretion of hormones by corpus luteum is depicted in Figure 12–27. After ovulation, estrogen levels decrease, followed by a secondary rise at midluteal phase, followed by a second decrease at the end of the menstrual cycle. The rise of estradiol parallels the pattern of progesterone and 17-hydroxyprogesterone. Studies of ovarian venous blood indicate that the corpus luteum is the site of steroid secretion by the ovary during the luteal phase.[219]

Control of steroid secretion by the corpus luteum is not completely understood but is determined in part by (1) LH-secretory pattern and LH receptors, (2) the levels of the various enzymes regulating steroid hormone formation (see Fig. 12–23), (3) the number of granulosa cells formed by the follicle during the follicular phase, (4) the amount of cholesterol substrate (see Fig. 12–25), and (5) the secretion of other hormones by the corpus luteum (autocrine function) (see Table 12–4).

The role of LH as the primary luteotropic agent was established by studies of hypophysectomized women.[220] In these women, after induction of ovulation, the length of the luteal phase and the amount of progesterone secreted are dependent on repeated injections of LH. Administration of LH or hCG during the luteal phase can extend the functional life span of the corpus luteum and the secretion of progesterone up to two additional weeks.[221]

The secretion of progesterone during the luteal phase is episodic, and the pulses correlate with pulses of LH secretion (Fig. 12–31).[115] The fact that frequency and amplitude of LH secretion during the follicular phase regulate subsequent luteal phase function is in accord with a regulatory role for LH during the luteal phase.[222] A reduction in FSH during the follicular phase is associated with a shortened luteal phase, smaller corpora lutea, and reduced responsiveness of dispersed corpus luteum cells in vitro.[223] The continuous administration of LHRH analogues during either the follicular phase or luteal phase likewise reduces the life span of the corpus luteum.[224, 225] A reduction in LH concentration, pulse frequency, or pulse amplitude also reduces the length of the luteal phase.[226] The corpus luteum of primates, however, can recover from a transient withdrawal of LH, depending on the age of the corpus luteum.[227]

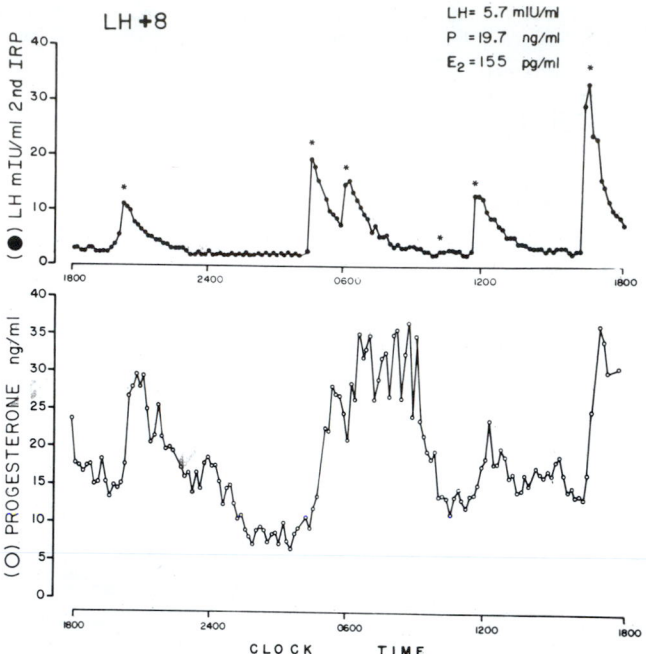

Figure 12–31. The episodic secretion of LH *(top)* and progesterone *(bottom)* during the luteal phase of a woman's cycle. P, progesterone; E_2, estradiol; LH + 8, LH surge plus 8 d. To convert progesterone values to nanomoles per liter, multiply by 3.180. To convert LH values to international units per liter, multiply by 1.0. (From Filicori M, Butler JP, Crowley WF. Neuroendocrine regulation of the corpus luteum in the human. Reproduced from the *Journal of Clinical Investigation*, 1984, vol. 73, pp. 1638–1647 by copyright permission of the American Society for Clinical Investigation.)

Progesterone secretion in the luteal phase is correlated with the number of LH/hCG receptors and their percent occupancy,[137] basal activity of adenylate cyclase, and the capacity of sodium fluoride and forskolin to enhance adenylate cyclase.

The role of other luteotropic factors in women is less clear. Prolactin does not appear to be luteotropic in women (in contrast to rats), but defective luteal function occurs when prolactin levels are either elevated or suppressed by bromocriptine.[229–331] Prostaglandin E_2 is luteotropic in isolated human corpus luteum cells and stimulates cyclic AMP and progesterone secretion.[232] The secretion of relaxin, inhibin, and oxytocin by the human corpus luteum may modulate corpus luteum function but does not appear to play a role in the maintenance of early pregnancy, because agonadal women treated with estrogen and progesterone alone have carried pregnancies to term after donor embryo transfer.[233, 234]

The function of the corpus luteum rapidly declines 9 to 11 d after ovulation, but the mechanism of luteolysis remains unclear. Both prostaglandin $F_{2\alpha}$ and exogenous estrogens appear to be luteolytic in nonhuman primates and women.[229, 235–240] On the other hand, antiestrogens and aromatase inhibitors do not decrease the length of the luteal phase or alter corpus luteum function in nonhuman primates.[241, 242] Thus the role of endogenous estrogens in luteolysis is less clear. Oxytocin and vasopressin formation within the corpus luteum may be luteolytic by modulating autocrine or paracrine mechanisms.[229, 243] Finally, LH down-regulation of its own receptor may play a role in the termination of the luteal phase.

During the normal menstrual cycle, gonadotropins, inhibin, estrogens, and progestogens undergo marked fluctuations as described. Only minimal fluctuations are seen in androgens, glucocorticoids, and pituitary hormones other than gonadotropins.[244–250] Plasma levels of deoxycorticoster-

one increase during the luteal phase as the result of extra-adrenal 21-hydroxylation of progesterone.[251, 252]

Hormonal Regulation of the Female Reproductive Tract During the Menstrual Cycle. Fluctuations in estrogen and progesterone produce striking effects on the reproductive tract. Characteristic changes occur in the endometrium during the menstrual cycle so that dating of the endometrium is possible (Fig. 12–32).[253] The proliferative phase, not as easily dated as the luteal phase, involves growth of the endometrium from 0.5 to 5 mm in depth. The glands are narrow and tubular, and mitoses and pseudostratification are present. Ovulation occurs on cycle day 14. On cycle day 16, glycogen begins to accumulate in the basal portion of the glandular epithelium, and some nuclei appear to be displaced to the midportion of the cells, resulting in the pseudostratified configuration. In formalin-fixed material, glycogen is solubilized, leaving large vacuoles in the base of the cells. This vacuolation of the glandular epithelium is evidence that a functional, progesterone-producing corpus luteum has been formed. During the luteal phase, progesterone decreases the number of estradiol receptors and increases the activity of 17β-hydroxysteroid oxidoreductase (which in turn enhances the conversion of estradiol to estrone) and the activity of estrone sulfotransferase. The net effect of these actions of progesterone is to decrease the biological action of estradiol on the endometrium during the luteal phase.[254–256] On day 17, the glands become more tortuous and dilated. By day 18, the vacuoles in the epithelium are smaller and are often located beside the nuclei. At this time, glycogen is present in the apex of the cells. On day 19, intraluminal secretion is present, and pseudostratification and vacuolation have nearly disappeared. On cycle days 21 and 22, the endometrial stroma becomes edematous. On day 23, stromal cells surrounding the spiral arterioles begin to enlarge, and stromal mitoses become apparent. Day 24 is characterized by the appearance of predecidual cells around the spiral arterioles and numerous stromal mitoses. By day 25, predecidua begins to differentiate under the surface epithelium. By day 27, the upper portion of the endometrial stroma appears as a solid sheet of well-developed decidua-like cells. Differentiation of the decidua is accompanied by a marked increase in lymphocytic infiltration. Menstruation begins on day 28.

The breakdown of the endometrium begins in the absence of conception when the decline of the corpus luteum results in a decrease of plasma estrogens and progestogens. These hormonal changes cause endometrial effects, including vascular changes, tissue death, and finally menstruation. With a reduction and shrinkage of the height of the endometrium, blood flow through the spiral vessels decreases and vasodilation ensues. The spiral vessels feeding the endometrium then undergo rhythmic vasoconstriction and vasodilation. These responses lead to disruption of the blood vessels and eventually to endometrial ischemia and cell death.[257, 258] Menstruation ensues and consists of blood and desquamated superficial endometrial tissues. The average duration of menstrual flow is 4 to 6 d, and the average amount of menstrual blood loss is 30 mL.[259] After the resumption of estrogen secretion by the ovarian follicles, endometrial healing leads to prolonged vasoconstriction and formation of a clot over the denuded endometrial vessels.[260] Necrosis of endometrium and vasospasm of the spiral vessels are thought to be due to prostaglandins. Prostaglandins are present in large amounts in secretory endometrium and menstrual blood.[261–263] Infusions of prostaglandin $F_{2\alpha}$ to women during the luteal phase induce endometrial necrosis and bleeding.[264] The release of prostaglandins is believed to be secondary to a decrease in stability of the lysosomal membranes in the endometrial cell.[265, 266] This results in the

DATING THE ENDOMETRIUM
APPROXIMATE RELATIONSHIP OF USEFUL MORPHOLOGICAL FACTORS

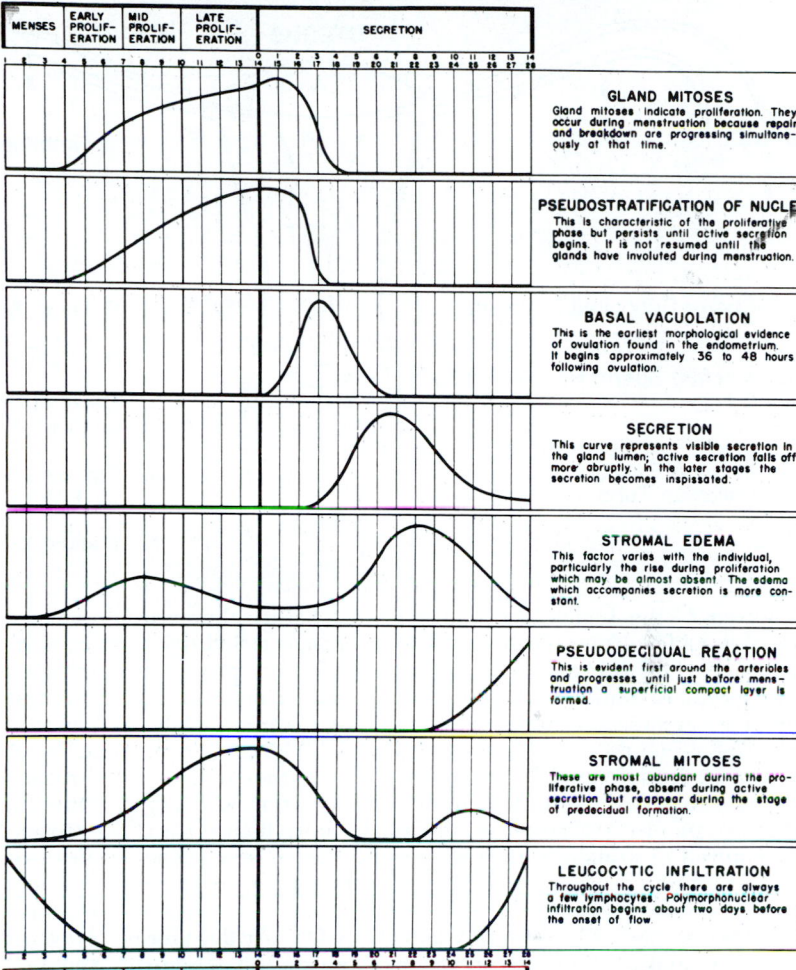

Figure 12–32. Dating the endometrium. (From Noyes RW, Hertig AW, Rock J. Dating the endometrial biopsy. Fertil Steril 1950; 1:3–25.)

liberation of phospholipids, with a subsequent synthesis of prostaglandin $F_{2\alpha}$. Prostaglandin synthetase inhibitors decrease the amount of menstrual bleeding in normal women and in women using contraceptive devices (see Chapter 18). The noncoagulability of menstrual blood may be due to the presence of fibrinolytic activity.[267]

The glands of the endocervix undergo cyclic changes more closely related to the vaginal epithelium than to the endometrium.[268] The glands of the endocervix secrete mucus. After the menses, the amount of mucus is limited and viscous. In response to increasing levels of estrogen secreted by the follicle during the later half of the follicular phase, the quantity of mucus increases up to 30-fold.[269] The mucus also changes in quality to become watery and elastic, and a fine thread can be demonstrated by stretching a drop of mucus (spinnbarkeit). In addition, a characteristic ferning or palm-leaf arborization is observed when the mucus is spread on a glass slide.[269] Progesterone reverses the effects of estrogen on the cervical mucus.

Vaginal epithelial cells are also influenced by estrogen and progesterone. During the early follicular phase, exfoliated vaginal epithelial cells are basophilic and have vesicular nuclei. In response to increasing levels of estrogen in the later half of the follicular phase, acidophilic cells with pyknotic nuclei predominate.[270] During the luteal phase, in the presence of increasing levels of progesterone, the percentage of acidophilic cells decreases and the number of leukocytes increase.[269, 270] A number of indices for characterizing vaginal cytology are available.[269]

Fertilization and Early Implantation of the Ovum

A complex and coordinated set of events leads to sperm and egg maturation, transport in the female reproductive tract, fertilization, and implantation.

SPERM TRANSPORT AND CAPACITATION. After ejaculation, sperm leave the vagina and pass through the cervix, the entire length of the uterine cavity, and the uterotubal junction to arrive at the ampullary-isthmic junction of the fallopian tube where fertilization occurs. Transport of sperm is aided by intrinsic flagellar beating, uterine contractions, and uterine and tubal cilia.[271] The process of sperm transport is rapid, and sperm have been found at the distal end of the fallopian tube 5 min after vaginal insemination.[272] However, the rate of attrition of sperm in the female reproductive tract is high. Of an estimated 250 million sperm deposited in the vagina, only 50 to 200 reach the end of the oviduct where they achieve proximity to the egg (Fig. 12–33).[273] The major loss of sperm occurs by retention in the vagina and expulsion from the introitus.

In most species sperm are required to reside in or be

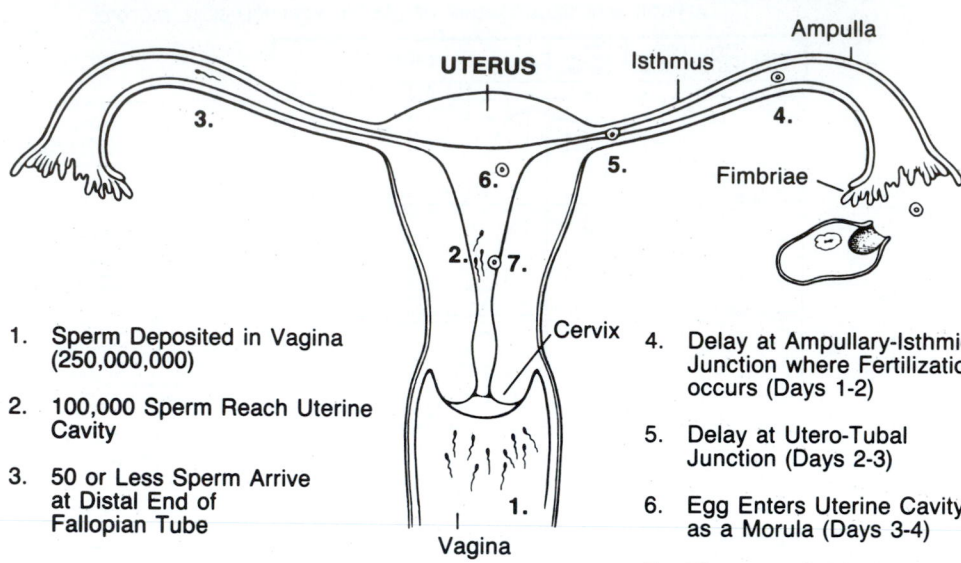

SPERM TRANSPORT

EGG TRANSPORT

1. Sperm Deposited in Vagina (250,000,000)

2. 100,000 Sperm Reach Uterine Cavity

3. 50 or Less Sperm Arrive at Distal End of Fallopian Tube

4. Delay at Ampullary-Isthmic Junction where Fertilization occurs (Days 1-2)

5. Delay at Utero-Tubal Junction (Days 2-3)

6. Egg Enters Uterine Cavity as a Morula (Days 3-4)

7. Blastocyst Implants (Day 7)

Figure 12–33. Transport of the sperm and the egg in the female reproductive tract. (From Carr BR. Fertilization, implantation and endocrinology of pregnancy. In: Griffin JE, Ojeda SR, eds. Textbook of Endocrine Physiology. New York: Oxford University Press, 1988: 186–203.)

exposed to the female reproductive tract before they are capable of fertilizing the ovum. This process is called *capacitation*.[274] This process is not well understood but prepares the sperm to undergo the acrosomal reaction involving a breakdown and merging of the plasma membrane with the acrosomal membrane of the sperm head.[271] The process of capacitation is followed by a release of enzymes that are thought to play a role in penetration of the ovum. Whether the process of capacitation in the female reproductive tract is required in women is unclear, because sperm are capable of fertilization in vitro after a short incubation in defined culture media.[275]

OVUM AND ZYGOTE TRANSPORTATION. At the time of ovulation, the fimbriated end of the fallopian tube sweeps across the surface of the ovary, and the extruded ovum and adherent granulosa cells, known as *cumulus oophorus*, are collected by the adhesive fimbriae. The transport of the egg into the tube is aided by cilial action and tubal contractions.[271] Removal of the granulosa cells before egg pickup impairs egg transport. Cells of the cumulus are able to communicate via paracrine mechanisms over a network of intracellular bridges through the zona to the perivitelline space[276] and may play a role in nutrition of the egg.

The ovum and zygote pass through the fallopian tube in three stages. The first stage encompasses the time of ovum pickup at the fimbriated end of the tube until the egg reaches the ampullary-isthmic junction, where it is retained for 1 to 2 d, during which time fertilization occurs.[271, 277] The block at the ampullary-isthmic junction is functional, because the junction is not a clearly defined anatomical entity. The second stage of transport begins soon after fertilization. The fertilized egg traverses the isthmic portion of the tube where it is again retained for 1 to 2 d at another functional block, the isthmic-utero, or uterotubal, junction. The time from ovulation until the egg enters the uterine cavity is species dependent and averages 3 to 4 d in women. The detention of the egg at these functional blocks within the fallopian tube appears to be influenced by estrogen and progesterone.[278] When the fertilized egg arrives in the uterine cavity during the final stage of transport (3 to 4 d after ovulation), it has entered the morula stage (see Fig. 12–33).[279]

FERTILIZATION. After ovulation the fertilizable life span of the human ovum is thought to be less than 24 h, and the estimated fertilizable life span for human sperm after ejac-

ulation is less than 48 h.[275, 276] The first step of fertilization involves the adherence of the sperm head to the zona pellucida surrounding the egg (Fig. 12–34). The sperm then penetrates the zona, which requires 15 to 25 min. After passage through the zona pellucida, the sperm moves rapidly across the perivitelline space, where it attaches to and penetrates the perivitelline membrane (less than 1 min).[276, 280] Once the sperm has reached this point, the male pronucleus is formed. The penetration of the vitelline membrane initiates two critical events. The first is the release of cortical granules into the perivitelline space, which blocks other sperm from penetrating the perivitelline membrane and prevents the development of polyspermia.[281] These granules contain various hydrolytic enzymes that induce the zona reaction and inactivate sperm receptors. The second event is the triggering of the final stage of meiosis of the oocyte. The second polar body is extruded from the egg and leaves a haploid complement of chromosomes in the egg pronuclei just before fertilization.[276]

The male and female pronuclei are visible about 2 to 3 h after the sperm has penetrated the vitelline membrane. By 4 h, the sperm tail is incorporated within the egg.[279] The two pronuclei move toward the center of the egg, their respective haploid chromosomes replicate, a mitotic spindle forms, and the first division occurs with the formation of two blastomeres.

The initial cleavage of the egg occurs in the fallopian tube. The rate of cleavage is remarkably constant in various mammalian species.[276] The timing in fertilized human eggs, determined from studies of in vitro fertilization, is as follows: two cells (28 h), four cells (46 to 48 h), eight cells (51 to 62 h), morula formation (111 to 135 h), and formation of a blastocyst (123 to 147 h).[282]

IMPLANTATION. In women the fertilized egg enters the uterine cavity as a morula on the third to fourth day after ovulation.[283, 284] The morula is transformed into a blastocyst by the fifth to sixth day after ovulation. At this stage of development the embryo is a hollow sphere with two cell types: the outer trophectoderm cells that will form the placenta and the inner cell mass from which the fetus will develop.[283] On the seventh day after ovulation, the blastocyst implants on the endometrial lining of the uterine cavity and penetrates the epithelium and the maternal circulation (see Fig. 12–33).[285] The blastocyst attaches to the endometrium

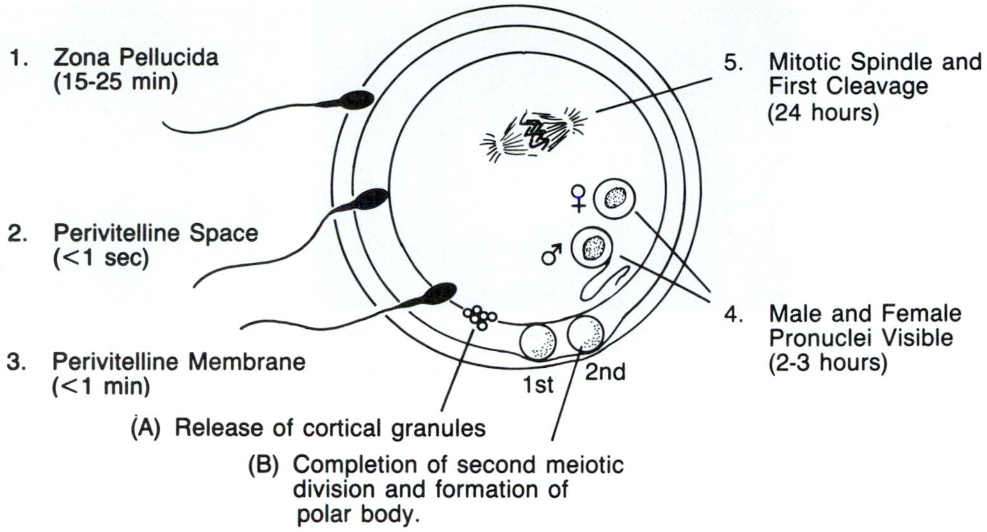

Figure 12–34. The process of fertilization of the human egg. (From Carr BR. Fertilization, implantation and endocrinology of pregnancy. In: Griffin JE, Ojeda SR, eds. Textbook of Endocrine Physiology. New York: Oxford University Press, 1988: 186–203.)

1. Zona Pellucida (15-25 min)
2. Perivitelline Space (<1 sec)
3. Perivitelline Membrane (<1 min)
    (A) Release of cortical granules
    (B) Completion of second meiotic division and formation of polar body.
4. Male and Female Pronuclei Visible (2-3 hours)
5. Mitotic Spindle and First Cleavage (24 hours)

with the embryonic pole facing the uterine cavity. The endometrium, under the influence of progesterone secreted by the corpus luteum, is transformed into a complex tissue known as *decidua*. The decidua consists of large polyhedral cells that are laden with glycogen and lipid and are often multinucleated. Continued progesterone secretion ensures the development of decidua and maintenance of pregnancy. Further decidual development appears to depend on signals from the invading embryo.[285] From studies in agonadal women provided with a fertilized donor egg after exogenous hormone treatment, it appears that the "window" for successful transfer lasts only about 3 d (days 16 to 18 of treatment).[286] After binding, endometrial cells begin to interdigitate with the microvilli of the trophectodermal cells. The layer of trophoblast cells develops into an inner cytotrophoblast layer and an outer syncytiotrophoblast layer. The syncytiotrophoblasts secrete proteolytic enzymes that erode the endometrium and allow the syncytiotrophoblast cells to invade further. The human embryo is deeply embedded and enclosed by the endometrium by the day 11 after ovulation.[285]

The biochemical events and the factors that initiate implantation are complex and involve maternal and embryonic factors, including growth factors, carbon dioxide, histamine, prostaglandins, early pregnancy factor, pregnancy-related proteins, platelet-activating factor, and others.[285, 287–291]

The Menopausal Ovary

Successive cycles of ovulation and atresia deplete the ovary of its follicles. This leads to the menopause, which is defined as the final episode of menstrual bleeding in women. The median age at menopause is 50 to 51.[292] The term *menopause* is used commonly to refer to the period of the climacteric that encompasses the transitional period between the reproductive years up to and beyond the last episode of menstrual bleeding. The basic event of the menopause is the cessation of cyclic ovarian function, and during the climacteric period women usually experience endocrine, somatic, and psychological changes. Because the average life expectancy extends 30 y after the menopause (one third of the life of women), the medical and economic impact of these changes is significant.

The average age at menopause has remained constant throughout recorded history and does not appear to be related to the age at menarche, socioeconomic conditions, race, parity, height, or weight.[293] However, menopause may occur earlier in women who smoke.[294]

As stated previously, the principal endocrine change of the menopause is a decrease in estrogen secretion as a result of the loss of ovarian follicles (Fig. 12–35). The ovary of postmenopausal women is reduced in size, weighing less than 2.5 g, and is wrinkled or prune-like in appearance. Microscopically, the cortical area is reduced because of loss of ova and follicles. Rarely, a few immature follicles undergoing maturation or atresia may be seen at the corticomedullary junction for 5 y or more after the last menses.[295] The stroma becomes hyperplastic and dominates the ovary. Interstitial and hilar cells are more readily apparent in ovaries from postmenopausal women, and virilizing syndromes secondary to hilar cell hyperplasia and neoplasia are more common after menopause.[296]

Some years before the cessation of menstruation, responsiveness of the ovary to gonadotropins begins to decrease.[185] Women who are perimenopausal but still experiencing ovulatory menstrual cycles have increased levels of FSH and LH compared with younger women, whereas the levels of estrogen and progesterone are lower. The cessation of follicular development leads to a decrease in secretion of estradiol-17β and inhibin with consequent loss of negative feedback to the hypothalamus and pituitary. The levels of gonadotropins increase, with FSH rising earlier and to a greater extent than LH (Fig. 12–36). The higher concentration of FSH may result from the decrease in inhibin levels. Intravenous infusion of LHRH to postmenopausal women elicits a release of both FSH and LH similar to that observed in women with other forms of ovarian failure.[297] The plasma levels of gonadotropins may remain elevated or decrease somewhat during the later decades of life.[297, 298] Mean plasma levels of ovarian steroids are lower in postmenopausal women (Fig. 12–36). Before the menopause, plasma androstenedione is derived equally from the adrenal and ovary; after the menopause the ovarian contribution is minimal, and plasma androstenedione levels decrease by 50%.[299]

As discussed previously, circulating estrogens in premenopausal ovulatory women are derived from two sources. Greater than 60% represents estradiol secreted directly by the ovaries, and the remainder is estrone derived from extraglandular conversion of androstenedione.[118] After the menopause, the ovarian contribution is reduced, and extraglandular formation of estrone from adrenal androstenedione secretion predominates (Fig. 12–37). Removal of the ovaries in postmenopausal women does not result in a

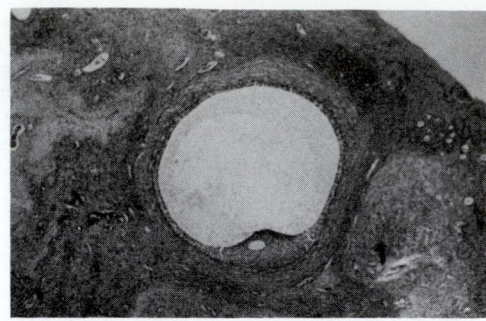
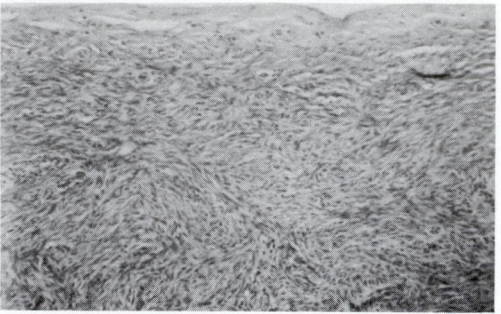

Figure 12–35. Photomicrograph of a histological section of an ovary obtained from a woman during reproductive life *(left)*. Note the large graffian follicle with a single ovum in the center of the photograph and a group of primary follicles in upper right corner. Magnification × 33. *Right,* Ovary obtained from a postmenopausal woman. Note the absence of germ cells and the prominent ovarian stroma. Magnification × 132. (From Carr BR, MacDonald PC. The menopause and beyond. In: Andres R, Bierman EL, Hazzard WR, eds. Principles of Geriatric Medicine. New York: McGraw-Hill, 1985: 325–336.)

further decline in estrogen or androstenedione levels.[299] Because a major site of extraglandular estrogen production occurs in adipose tissue, estrogen production is greater in obese than in thin postmenopausal women, and total estrogen production in the massively obese may be as great or greater than in premenopausal women.[300, 301] The predominant estrogen formed in extraglandular sites is estrone.

The fall in estrogen formation gives rise to vasomotor instability (hot flash), atrophy of the urogenital epithelium and skin, decrease in size of the reproductive organs and breasts, increased risk of cardiovascular disease, and osteoporosis.[302-307]

Hot flashes are characterized by a sensation of warmth and heat followed by profuse sweating. The frequency, duration, and intensity of vasomotor symptoms vary widely, but in the majority of women they begin to subside by 2 to 5 y after the menopause.[308] The pathogenesis of the hot flash is complex and appears to involve catecholamines, prostaglandins, endorphins, and other neuropeptides.[309]

There is a close temporal relationship between estrogen deprivation and the development of osteoporosis. Loss of both trabecular and cortical bone results in mechanical fragility and subsequent fracture (see Chapter 28). Bone loss after the menopause proceeds at a rate of 1 to 2% each year.[310] By age 80, white women have lost 50% of bone mass, and as many as 25% of women sustain a vertebral or hip fracture between the ages of 60 and 90.[311] Such fractures are a major cause of mortality and morbidity.[312] Many factors influence the development of osteoporosis, including diet, level of activity, smoking, general health, and, most important, estrogen deprivation.[313, 314]

The principal cause of death in postmenopausal women is cardiovascular disease.[315] The levels of high-density lipoprotein (HDL) cholesterol are lower and LDL cholesterol levels are higher in women who experience a natural menopause when compared with premenopausal controls, and postmenopausal women appear to be at greater risk for cardiovascular disease than matched premenopausal controls.[316] Women who undergo oophorectomy and are not treated with estrogen have an even greater risk of cardiovascular disease.[317] Abundant evidence supports the view that estrogen replacement reduces the risk of death from cardiovascular disease (discussed under Hormonal Therapy).[318, 319]

Assessment of Ovarian Function: Clinical, Laboratory, and Diagnostic Tests

The assessment of the hormonal status of women can usually be made by obtaining a thorough history and physical examination. For example, the presence of female secondary sexual characteristics such as normal breast development indicates adequate estrogen production in the past. The presence of a moist vagina and cervical mucus is evidence of current estrogen production. Regular, spontaneous, predictable, cyclic menses implies that ovulation and the secretion of gonadotropins, estrogens, progesterone, and androgens are adequate and that the female reproduction tract is intact. Thus a history and clinical examination may be more valuable and less expensive than laboratory tests in evaluating the hormonal status of a woman. However, laboratory and diagnostic tests are required in many instances to confirm a clinical diagnosis and to monitor evaluation and treatment cycles.

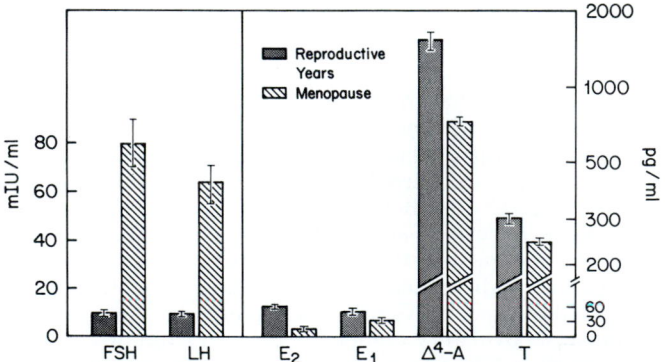

Figure 12–36. Differences in hormone concentrations in women during the reproductive years and in women during the menopause. E_2, estradiol; E_1, estrone; Δ^4-A, androstenedione; T, testosterone. (Data from Jaffe RB. The menopause and perimenopausal period. In: Yen SSC, Jaffe RB, eds. Reproductive Endocrinology: Physiology, Pathophysiology and Clinical Management. 2nd ed. Philadelphia: W. B. Saunders, 1986: 406–423; and from Carr BR, MacDonald PC. Estrogen treatment of postmenopausal women. In: Stollerman GH, ed. Advances in Internal Medicine. Vol 28. Chicago: Year Book Medical, 1983: 491–508.)

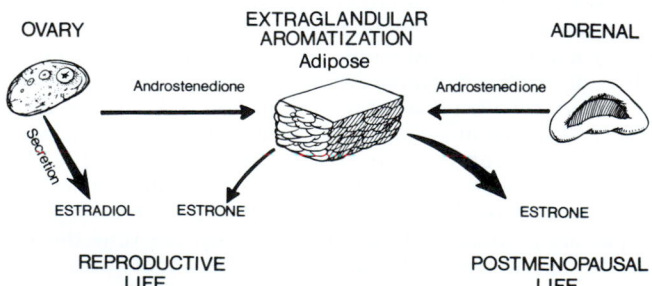

Figure 12–37. Various sources of circulating estrogens in women during reproductive and postmenopausal life. (Adapted from Carr BR, MacDonald PC. Estrogen treatment of postmenopausal women. In: Stollerman GH, ed. Advances in Internal Medicine. Vol 28. Chicago: Year Book Medical, 1983: 491–508.)

Pituitary Gonadotropins

Measurement of gonadotropins is critical in the evaluation and assessment of women with amenorrhea. For example, measurement of gonadotropins is required to determine whether amenorrhea is due to gonadal failure or to hypothalamic-pituitary failure. The most common way to evaluate gonadotropins is to measure the level in plasma or serum. The tests utilized are radioimmunoassay, fluoroimmunoassay (FIA), or enzyme-linked immunosorbent assay (ELISA). Because FSH and LH are secreted in pulses, the result obtained from a single serum sample may be difficult to interpret. Consequently, multiple samples collected at 15- to 20-min intervals may be pooled and submitted to the laboratory to obtain a mean value.[320] The value obtained depends on which reference preparation is used by the laboratory.[269] The ranges for both serum LH and FSH in normally cycling adult women are 5 to 20 IU/L.[35] However, on the day of or near ovulation, levels of FSH and LH may be two to three times normal values. Serum gonadotropin measurements are of particular usefulness in the evaluation of women with suspected ovarian failure, PCOS, or hypogonadotropic hypogonadism. A serum level of FSH greater than 40 IU/L is diagnostic of ovarian failure.[321] An elevated LH/FSH ratio in a woman with amenorrhea suggests the diagnosis of PCOS.[322] Low or undetectable levels of gonadotropins suggest hypothalamic disease or pituitary failure. The use of LHRH as a provocative test of hypothalamic-pituitary dysfunction has been described.[323] After administration of a bolus of 100 µg of LHRH, LH levels are measured at 30 to 60 min.[324] Except for a subnormal response in prepubertal children, the clinical usefulness of such testing is not established. In general the response to LHRH reflects and can be predicted by basal levels of gonadotropins.[325]

Other Pituitary Hormones

Prolactin levels are determined by radioimmunoassay, FIA, or ELISA, and the normal range in most laboratories varies from 5 to 30 µg/L.[269] In women with prolactin-secreting tumors, levels are usually greater than 100 µg/L. Amenorrhea or anovulatory bleeding can be associated with other endocrine disorders and elevated pituitary hormones. For example, primary hypothyroidism, acromegaly, and Cushing disease may be associated with disorders of ovarian function.[269]

Estrogens

Normal secondary sexual characteristics (such as breast development) imply that estrogen production was adequate in the past. Indications of the current estrogen status can be determined by the pelvic examination. The presence of a moist, rugated vagina with copious, clear, thin cervical mucus that can be stretched and exhibits arborization or ferning when spread on a slide is strong evidence of adequate estrogen production. As discussed previously, vaginal squamous epithelial cells can be graded by various techniques, and the presence of mature epithelial cells and abundant cornified squamous epithelial cells with pyknotic nuclei confirms the presence of adequate estrogen levels.[269]

The progestogen withdrawal test provides a useful functional assessment of estrogen status in women with a normal outflow tract. If menses occurs within 7 to 10 d after the end of a trial of medroxyprogesterone acetate (10 mg by mouth, once or twice daily for 5 d) or after an intramuscular injection of progesterone (100 to 200 mg), then the prior estrogen level was adequate to allow withdrawal bleeding.[326]

Plasma estradiol can also be assayed by radioimmunoassay, FIA, and ELISA, and the values fluctuate throughout the normal cycle (see Table 12–3 and Fig. 12–27). There is little indication for measuring estradiol levels in women with disorders of ovarian hormone secretion, because the clinical assessment and response to a progestogen challenge are usually adequate to indicate the status of estrogen production. However, a determination of plasma estradiol levels is helpful in monitoring anovulatory women during attempts to induce ovulation with human menopausal gonadotropins and in women undergoing in vitro fertilization. Ultrasonography is used in conjunction with this to assess adequate follicular growth.[327]

Progesterone

Spontaneous, cyclic, predictable menses imply that the patient is ovulating and that progesterone is secreted during the luteal phase. Progesterone levels in blood may be measured by radioimmunoassay, FIA, or ELISA (for normal values see Table 12–3). Progesterone measurements are used to document ovulation or adequacy of the luteal phase in infertile women and to aid in the diagnosis of women with müllerian agenesis and testicular feminization.[328, 329] The determination of 17-hydroxyprogesterone is useful in evaluation of women with adult-onset adrenal hyperplasia resulting from 21-hydroxylase deficiency.[330]

Progesterone secretion can also be assessed more simply. The simplest test is the measurement of basal body temperature throughout a cycle. Because of the thermogenic properties of progesterone, documentation of a monthly biphasic curve with an elevated temperature for approximately 13 to 14 d after ovulation indicates ovulation and suggests normal progesterone secretion during the luteal phase (see Fig. 12–27). The presence of viscous cervical mucus that does not stretch or fern, the finding of predominant intermediate cells on vaginal cytology, and the demonstration of a properly dated secretory endometrium after an endometrial biopsy during the luteal phase (see Fig. 12–27) provide additional evidence of adequate progesterone secretion.[269]

Androgen

The presence of abnormal hair growth (hirsutism) or masculinization (virilization) implies excessive androgen, principally testosterone. The woman serves as her own bioassay, and the rate of production of testosterone parallels the degree of clinical androgen excess.[331, 332] Excessive testosterone may result from increased secretion by the adrenal or ovary and increased extraglandular production from androstenedione secreted by the ovary or adrenal. Serum androgens (testosterone) and other C_{19}-steroids (DHEA, DHEAS, androstenedione) are measured by radioimmunoassay. Normal serum levels in ovulatory women are summarized in Table 12–3. Elevated urinary 17-ketosteroids (derived principally from DHEA) are sometimes useful in the diagnosis of adrenal virilizing tumors.[333]

Predicting Ovulation

Rapid urinary LH assays make it possible to predict the time of ovulation in infertile women.[334] Ultrasonography of follicles can also be used to predict the adequacy and time of ovulation.[327] These tests are widely used in evaluation and treatment of infertile women.

Specific Diagnostic Testing

IMAGING TECHNIQUES. As mentioned, ultrasonography using a vaginal probe is useful in evaluating infertility and for following follicular and endometrial growth during treatment of anovulatory women.[327] Ultrasonography or magnetic resonance imaging (MRI) can establish the presence of a uterus, uterine developmental anomaly, or a vaginal septum.[335] Hysterosalpingography, in which radiopaque dye is injected into the uterus during fluoroscopy, is helpful for delineating the uterine cavity and patency of the fallopian tubes.[336] MRI and computed tomographic (CT) scans are routinely used in the diagnosis of pituitary, hypothalamic, adrenal, uterine, and ovarian masses.[337]

CHROMOSOMAL ANALYSIS. The use of buccal smears to evaluate the chromosomal sex is not of sufficient accuracy to be clinically useful. Karyotypic analysis of peripheral blood leukocytes should be done instead.[338, 339] Cells are treated with phytohemagglutinin to stimulate cell division, which is arrested at metaphase with colchicine. The cells are then harvested, stained, and examined. The determination of a chromosomal karyotype is particularly useful in women with sexual ambiguity (see Chapter 14) and in women with ovarian failure to determine the presence of a Y chromosome.[340] To rule out mosaicism, evaluation of a large number of cells or assessment of the chromosomal complement of other tissues may be required.

OPERATIVE PROCEDURES. Diagnostic hysteroscopy is useful to evaluate the uterine cavity in women with abnormal uterine development or with infertility.[341] Diagnostic laparoscopy may be indicated in women with abnormal uterine development before a planned surgical procedure or during infertility evaluation.[342]

Diagnosis of Pregnancy

The diagnosis of pregnancy is usually suspected on the basis of the history and physical examination. For example, a woman with previous cyclic menses who develops amenorrhea accompanied by breast tenderness, malaise, lassitude, and nausea and who on physical examination exhibits a softening and enlargement of the uterus is likely pregnant. The secretion of hCG by the placenta into the maternal circulation and its excretion in urine allow the diagnosis of pregnancy before clinical signs. Modern immunoassays utilizing monoclonal antibodies directed against β-hCG improved the ability to measure small quantities of hCG in blood and urine and minimize cross-reactivity with serum LH.[343] It is now possible to detect pregnancy 8 to 10 d after ovulation and before the first missed menstrual period. β-hCG assay kits that require only 5 min can detect concentrations of 20 IU/L or greater in urine. Quantitative β-hCG immunoassays are helpful in the diagnosis of ectopic pregnancy, hydatidiform mole, and choriocarcinoma.

DISORDERS OF OVARIAN FUNCTION

Disorders of ovarian function cause different clinical presentations depending on the phase of reproductive life when the disorder is first manifest. No classification can encompass all the nuances associated with ovarian dysfunction. The developmental classification chosen here provides a rational approach to disorders of ovarian function by classifying disorders as fetal and neonatal, prepubertal, or reproductive. The menopause is not considered a disorder of ovarian function, because it is a natural process in all women. Diagnosis and classification of these disorders have improved as a result of the ability to measure small amounts of hormones in blood and the development of better imaging techniques.

Disorders During Fetal and Neonatal Life

Disturbances in female sexual differentiation during embryogenesis can arise from a variety of mechanisms and may be manifested as ambiguous genitalia at birth, delayed puberty, and/or amenorrhea. For example, gonadal dysgenesis, müllerian agenesis, and complete androgen resistance (testicular feminization) are all compatible with an apparently normal female phenotype but cause amenorrhea at the time of expected puberty. In the absence of sexual ambiguity, the majority of these disorders are in fact not diagnosed during the neonatal period unless a palpable gonad is discovered in an inguinal hernia (testicular feminization) or absence of the vagina and uterus (e.g., müllerian agenesis) is noted during the newborn physical examination; these disorders will be discussed in the section on amenorrhea. Sexual ambiguity at birth may be caused by mixed gonadal dysgenesis, true hermaphroditism, female pseudohermaphroditism, congenital adrenal hyperplasia, masculinizing syndromes in the mother, or incomplete masculinization of male infants (male pseudohermaphroditism). All may cause significant health risk and psychological trauma if not properly diagnosed. Sexual ambiguity and its management are described in Chapter 14.

During fetal life, ovarian cysts may undergo torsion and can be diagnosed by ultrasonographic studies.[344] Most of these cysts appear to be functional but regress during the neonatal period. Ovarian tumors such as embryonal cell carcinoma may also develop during infancy.

Disorders During Prepubertal Years

In girls puberty is said to be precocious when the onset of breast budding occurs before age 8 or menarche commences before age 9.[51, 345] This definition is based on statistical and practical considerations. Precocious puberty is about eight times more common in girls than in boys, and 90% of cases are idiopathic.[346] Those disorders in which the premature sexual characteristics are appropriate for the genetic and gonadal sex (i.e., feminization in girls or virilization in boys) are termed *isosexual precocity. Heterosexual precocity* occurs when sexual characteristics are inappropriate for the genetic sex (e.g., feminizing syndromes in boys or virilizing syndromes in girls). Disorders of pubertal development in boys are described in Chapter 22.

Isosexual Precocity

Isosexual precocity can be divided into three separate categories (Table 12–6). Distinction among these categories is clinically important for two reasons. First, true precocious puberty is idiopathic in most cases but is not ovarian in origin, whereas a primary ovarian disorder is often the basis for precocious pseudopuberty. Thus making this distinction helps to design appropriate therapy. Second, the cause, seriousness, and treatment of these two disorders differ. The clinical course in most girls with true precocious puberty is benign, whereas precocious pseudopuberty may be life-threatening.[27, 345–347]

The distinction among the types of isosexual precocity is complicated by the fact that the early signs are similar, and separation may be feasible only late in the course. Diagnostic procedures may also be inconclusive early, making it necessary to temporize or utilize additional diagnostic procedures. When the possibility of a life-threatening disorder can be excluded, observation is justified and is unlikely to increase the morbidity or affect prognosis adversely.

TRUE PRECOCIOUS PUBERTY, OR COMPLETE ISOSEXUAL PRECOCITY (PREMATURE ACTIVATION OF THE HY-

TABLE 12–6. Classification of Sexual Precocity

I. Isosexual precocity
   A. True precocious puberty
      1. Constitutional
      2. Organic brain disease
      3. Congenital adrenal hyperplasia (delayed treatment)
   B. Precocious pseudopuberty
      1. Ovarian tumors
      2. Adrenal tumors
      3. McCune-Albright syndrome
      4. Hypothyroidism
      5. Russel-Silver syndrome
      6. Estrogen-containing medications
   C. Isolated forms of pubertal development
      1. Premature thelarche
      2. Premature adrenarche
      3. Premature pubarche
II. Heterosexual precocity
   A. Ovarian tumors
   B. Adrenal tumors
   C. Congenital adrenal hyperplasia

POTHALAMIC-PITUITARY AXIS). True precocious puberty, also known as complete isosexual precocity, is characterized by an early but otherwise normal female pubertal development. Although puberty occurs at an early age (sometimes even in infancy), the endocrine events are normal in that the cyclic function of the hypothalamic-pituitary-ovarian axis leads to gonadotropin secretion, follicular maturation, and ovulation. Cyclic, predictable menses and ovulatory cycles are the hallmarks of true precocious puberty.[27]

Constitutional or idiopathic precocious puberty is responsible for 90% of cases. In these individuals no cause for the premature maturation of the hypothalamic-pituitary axis can be identified, and diagnosis is one of exclusion. Interestingly, about half of these individuals have abnormal electroencephalograms.[348] The basal levels of gonadotropins and gonadal steroids are increased, and the LH pulse frequency and amplitude and the response of LH to the administration of LHRH are in the normal pubertal range.[349, 350] The early appearance of secondary sexual characteristics and of ovulatory cycles with the accompanying risk of fertility may cause significant emotional disturbances. Therefore prompt diagnosis and treatment are imperative.

About 10% of girls with true precocious puberty have organic brain disease. About half of these cases are due to CNS tumors, including hamartomas, gliomas, neurofibromas, astrocytomas, ependymomas, germinomas, and, rarely, craniopharyngiomas or pinealomas.[351–357] Other CNS disorders that can give rise to true precocious puberty include encephalitis, meningitis, hydrocephalus, head injury, brain abscess, and tuberous sclerosis.[27] It is essential to separate patients with CNS causes from those with the idiopathic disorder, recognizing that some patients initially diagnosed as idiopathic may prove later to have organic brain disease. Fortunately, most patients with organic brain disease have other neurological signs and symptoms before the appearance of precocious puberty. Evaluation of patients with isosexual precocity must include imaging of the head with either CT or MRI. The location of CNS tumors that cause precocious puberty makes both surgical and radiation treatment difficult. For example, deaths have occurred after operative removal of hypothalamic hamartomas. Surgical extirpation is not recommended if the tumors are slow growing and can be monitored by imaging techniques and if precocious sexual development can be controlled by medical therapy.[27, 358]

A rare cause of isosexual precocity is virilizing adrenal hyperplasia resulting from 21-hydroxylase deficiency in girls in whom treatment is delayed until age 4 to 8. After initiation of glucocorticoid replacement, such individuals may undergo true isosexual precocious puberty.[27]

ISOSEXUAL PRECOCIOUS PSEUDOPUBERTY, OR INCOMPLETE ISOSEXUAL PRECOCITY. Isosexual precocious pseudopuberty occurs when girls feminize as a consequence of endogenous estrogen production or exogenous estrogen exposure but do not ovulate or develop cyclic menses. Ovarian cysts or tumors that secrete estrogen (granulosa or thecal cell tumors) are the most frequent cause.[359–362] The Peutz-Jeghers syndrome of intestinal polyps and mucocutaneous pigmentation is associated with ovarian tumors that secrete estrogen (or androgen that is converted to estrogen at extraglandular sites) and cause precocious pseudopuberty.[363] Most ovarian tumors can be diagnosed by rectoabdominal examination, but ultrasonography, CT, or laparoscopy may also be of help. Most tumors are unilateral and benign and can be cured by oophorectomy. Gonadotropin levels are suppressed, and the LH response to LHRH is blunted.[361] The presence of ovarian cysts can cause problems in diagnosis. The use of ultrasonography may be helpful in differentiating a benign cyst from a cystic-solid ovarian tumor, but exploratory laparotomy is ultimately necessary in the majority of cases, recognizing that unnecessary removal of a benign cyst may lead to adhesions and infertility later in life. Follicular growth of up to 3 cm may occur in patients with true precocious puberty as a consequence of increased gonadotropin secretion and is not an indication for exploration. Ovarian teratomas or choriocarcinomas that secrete pure hCG do not appear to cause precocious puberty in girls unless estrogen is secreted concomitantly by the tumor (hCG or LH in the absence of FSH does not stimulate ovarian estrogen secretion).[27, 364] Rarely, feminizing tumors of the adrenal can cause isosexual precocious puberty, either by formation of estrogen directly or by secretion of androgens that are aromatized to estrogens in extraglandular sites.[365]

Other types of isosexual precocious puberty include two disorders occasionally associated with increased gonadotropin secretion. The first is the McCune-Albright syndrome, which consists of the triad of café au lait spots, polyostotic fibrous dysplasia, and precocious puberty.[366, 367] This disorder is more common in girls, and the etiology is unknown. Although both gonadotropin-dependent and gonadotropin-independent etiologies have been suggested, most evidence supports the latter mechanism.[346, 368–371] Increased estrogen secretion by autonomous functioning cysts may spontaneously regress and recur and is not suppressed by LHRH analogues that lower plasma LH.[369] However, patients may respond to aromatase inhibitors.[371] McCune-Albright syndrome is also associated with other endocrinopathies, including excessive secretion of growth hormone, prolactin, thyroid hormone, or cortisol.[372]

The second type of incomplete isosexual precocity that may be associated with increased gonadotropin secretion is hypothyroidism. Hypothyroidism usually is associated with delayed pubertal development and amenorrhea but occasionally may present with precocious puberty, galactorrhea, and ovarian cysts.[373] In addition to increased thyrotropin-stimulating hormone levels, gonadotropin and prolactin levels are also increased; the cause for the enhanced gonadotropin secretion is unknown.[374–376] In most cases bone age is retarded, and pituitary hypersecretion and retardation of bone development respond to thyroid hormone replacement.

Another rare disease characterized by short stature, craniofacial dysostosis, and asymmetrical development of extremities is the Russell-Silver syndrome, which may be associated with precocious pseudopuberty.[377] Estrogen-containing medication, including oral contraceptives, or estrogen-contaminated meat or poultry may be a rare cause for incomplete precocious pseudopuberty.[378, 379]

ISOLATED FORMS OF PUBERTAL DEVELOPMENT. In some cases of isosexual precocity, an isolated premature pubertal event may occur such as premature breast budding (premature thelarche) or premature development of axillary or pubic hair (so-called *premature adrenarche* or *pubarche*). Premature thelarche is the development of breast budding before the age of 8 without other evidence of estrogen effect or advanced bone age.[380] This disorder is thought to be due to a transient increase in estrogen secretion or a temporary increase in end-organ sensitivity to the low levels of circulating estrogens present before puberty. It occurs most frequently by age 2 and rarely after age 4. Girls with premature thelarche exhibit increased FSH secretion after treatment with LHRH, whereas LH levels do not increase.[380] Premature thelarche is self-limited and resolves spontaneously.

Premature adrenarche (pubarche)—the appearance of axillary hair, pubic hair, or both, without other signs of pubertal development or virilization—is caused by an increased secretion of adrenal androgens, usually after age 6. Rare cases associated with transient ovarian androgen secretion resulting from ovarian cysts have also been reported.[381] In most cases of premature adrenarche (pubarche) the disorder is nonprogressive and requires no treatment. Patients enter puberty at the appropriate time.[27]

Heterosexual Precocity

Virilization in a prepubertal female is usually due to congenital adrenal hyperplasia or to testosterone secretion by an adrenal or ovarian tumor. Virilization in girls with congenital adrenal hyperplasia usually is associated with a history of sexual ambiguity at birth.

Evaluation and Treatment of Sexual Precocity*

The evaluation of sexual precocity involves a careful history and physical examination, including a rectoabdominal examination, which may often suggest the correct diagnosis. Other tests include ultrasonographic study or CT scan of ovaries and adrenals, determination of bone age, and measurement of plasma thyrotropin-stimulating hormone, gonadotropins (including hCG), and androgen and estrogen levels when appropriate. A CT or MRI scan of the head is required to rule out a CNS tumor. Treatment of CNS tumors may include surgery or radiation therapy if appropriate. Treatment of ovarian tumors is surgical.[27] LHRH analogues are the most effective treatment for most forms of gonadotropin-dependent forms of sexual precocity (idiopathic). Other agents that have been used include medroxyprogesterone acetate, danazol, and cyproterone acetate.[27] LHRH analogues are preferred, because they cause prompt regression of breast development and vaginal bleeding and cause a cessation of bone maturation.[382–384] The widest experience in the treatment of idiopathic precocious puberty has been with medroxyprogesterone acetate. It is given intramuscularly in a dose of 100 to 200 mg every 2 to 4 wk. Such a regimen is usually effective in inhibiting ovarian estrogen production and ovulation but does not consistently inhibit bone maturation or prevent premature epiphyseal closure and the resultant short stature.[385] McCune-Albright syndrome may respond to aromatase inhibitors such as testolactone.[371] Hypothyroidism is treated with thyroid hormone replacement. The diagnostic tests and treatment of sexual precocity are summarized in Table 12–7.

*Also see Chapter 22.

TABLE 12–7. Diagnostic Tests and Treatment of Sexual Precocity

Diagnostic Tests
  History and physical examination
  Bone age
  CNS imaging
  Sonography of ovaries
  CT scan of adrenal (if virilized)
  Thyroid function tests
  Estradiol
  FSH, LH, hCG
  Testosterone, DHEAS, 17-hydroxyprogesterone (if virilized)
Treatment
  Isosexual precocity
    True precocious puberty
      Constitutional
        LHRH analogues/progestogens
      Organic brain disease
        Surgery, radiation, LHRH analogues/progestogens
      Congenital adrenal hyperplasia (delayed treatment)
        LHRH analogues/progestogens
    Precocious pseudopuberty
      Ovarian tumors
        Surgery
      Adrenal tumors
        Surgery
      McCune-Albright syndrome
        Testolactone, ketoconazole
      Russel-Silver syndrome
        ? LHRH analogues/progestogens
      Estrogen-containing medications
        Discontinue it
    Isolated forms of pubertal development
      Observation
  Heterosexual precocity
    Ovarian tumors
      Surgery
    Adrenal tumors
      Surgery
    Congenital adrenal hyperplasia
      Glucocorticoids

Disorders During Reproductive Years

Disorders of the Menstrual Cycle

DYSMENORRHEA. Dysmenorrhea, or painful menstruation, is common, affecting about 50% of women at some time in life.[37] The disorder may be primary or secondary. Primary dysmenorrhea is associated with ovulatory cycles and is due to uterine smooth muscle contractions induced by prostaglandins formed in secretory endometrium.[386] Patients with primary dysmenorrhea often have additional symptoms, including nausea, diarrhea, headaches, and emotional disorders. This form of dysmenorrhea can be treated by preventing ovulation with oral contraceptives (if fertility control is desired) or with prostaglandin synthetase inhibitors. When either oral contraceptives or prostaglandin synthetase inhibitors fail to relieve symptoms after an adequate trial of therapy of 3 to 6 mo, diagnostic laparoscopy may be indicated.

Secondary dysmenorrhea is associated with a variety of conditions such as endometriosis, pelvic inflammatory disease, congenital defects in uterine development, uterine leiomyoma, and intrauterine devices. Secondary dysmenorrhea usually requires surgical or medical therapy. However, about 80% of women who experience either primary or secondary dysmenorrhea have some relief with the use of prostaglandin inhibitors.[387]

PREMENSTRUAL SYNDROME (PMS). Almost all women experience a variety of cyclic premenstrual symptoms that occur after ovulation and disappear after menstruation. These symptoms include breast tenderness, abdominal bloating, headache, weight gain, behavioral changes, and many other occasional complaints. In some women, however, the combination of symptoms, known as PMS, is more severe for unknown reasons.[388] Although the etiology is not known, prevention of ovulation by oral contraceptives or LHRH analogues is often helpful. Removal of the ovaries and uterus cures the disorder. However, castration is rarely indicated because of the sequelae of estrogen deprivation.

Short of removal of the ovaries, no single form of therapy is completely effective. Other treatments that may relieve some symptoms include bromocriptine, prostaglandin synthetase inhibitors, mild diuretics, change in lifestyle, diet, and exercise.[37, 389, 390]

ABNORMAL UTERINE BLEEDING. Between menarche and the menopause, every woman experiences one or more episodes of abnormal uterine bleeding, defined as any bleeding pattern that differs in frequency, duration, or amount from the pattern observed during a normal menstrual cycle.[37, 391, 392] A variety of descriptive terms (such as menometrorrhagia) have been used to characterize patterns of abnormal bleeding. A more logical approach is to divide abnormal bleeding patterns into those associated with ovulatory cycles and those associated with anovulatory cycles.

Abnormal Bleeding Associated with Ovulatory Cycles. Normal menstrual bleeding begins on average after the 28th day of an ovulatory cycle and is spontaneous, regular, cyclic, and predictable. The amount and duration of bleeding are also predictable, constant, and frequently associated with dysmenorrhea. The average duration of bleeding is 4 to 6 d and the average blood loss is 30 mL.[259] Regular ovulatory cycles in which the length or amount of uterine bleeding deviates from normal are often associated with pathological abnormalities of the reproductive tract or bleeding dyscrasias. For instance, regular but excessive and prolonged bleeding episodes can result from abnormalities of the uterus, including leiomyomas, adenomyosis, endometrial polyps, or coagulation defects (e.g., von Willebrand disease). Regular ovulatory cycles characterized by only spotting, light bleeding, or no bleeding at all (amenorrhea) may be due to obstructive pathological conditions of the reproductive tract, such as intrauterine adhesions (synechiae) or scarring of the cervix. Intermenstrual bleeding, or spotting between episodes of regular, ovulatory menstruation, is often due to cervical or endometrial lesions and requires surgical evaluation and treatment.

Abnormal Bleeding Associated with Anovulatory Cycles. Uterine bleeding during anovulatory cycles is unpredictable with respect to the amount, onset, and duration and is known as dysfunctional uterine bleeding (DUB). DUB is usually painless because of the absence of ovulation. This disorder is due not to primary abnormalities of the uterus but rather to interruption of the normal maturation and development of the endometrium. In the absence of ovulation and the failure of luteal progesterone support of the endometrium, bleeding is irregular and unpredictable. In contrast, the bleeding in normal ovulatory cycles is cyclic and predictable as a result of the orderly development of the endometrium induced by estrogen priming during the proliferative phase and progesterone support followed by decline of corpus luteum function during the luteal phase. In the absence of estrogen priming, as when a castrate or a postmenopausal woman is given progesterone, withdrawal bleeding usually does not occur. The exposure of endometrium to estrogen unopposed by progesterone (i.e., anovulatory bleeding, or DUB) causes a hyperplastic or proliferative endometrium.[393] Both types of endometrium have a reduced capacity to synthesize prostaglandin $F_{2\alpha}$, explaining in part the absence of painful menses.[394]

DUB occurs in normal women at the extremes of reproductive life, normally in the early postmenarcheal and late perimenopausal years.[183–185] Most causes are associated with chronic anovulation (e.g., PCOS). Anovulatory bleeding can result from several mechanisms, including estrogen breakthrough bleeding and progesterone breakthrough bleeding.

Estrogen Breakthrough Bleeding. Estrogen breakthrough bleeding occurs when continuous estrogen stimulation of the endometrium is not interrupted by cyclic progesterone exposure, as discussed earlier. This type of dysfunctional bleeding is most common and is due to anovulation associated with chronic acyclic estrogen production (PCOS). Women with this disorder have histories of irregular, unpredictable menses, oligomenorrhea, or amenorrhea (see later). Estrogen breakthrough bleeding can also occur in women with hypogonadotropic hypogonadism, in postmenopausal women given continuous estrogen therapy, and in women with estrogen-secreting tumors of the ovary or adrenal gland. In some women estrogen breakthrough bleeding may be profuse and prolonged. When bleeding is prolonged, the endometrium is typically thin and fragile, because the repair between episodes of bleeding is either incomplete or totally absent.[395]

Progesterone Breakthrough Bleeding. Progesterone breakthrough bleeding is a pharmacologically induced anovulatory bleeding that occurs in the presence of high ratios of progesterone to estrogen. This type of bleeding occurs in women treated with continuous progestogens or with continuous or cyclic low-dose oral contraceptives. In these instances the endometrium is thin and atrophic (see Chapter 18).

Diagnosis and Treatment. The approach to a patient with abnormal uterine bleeding begins with a history of menstrual patterns and prior hormonal therapy and a careful physical examination of the reproductive tract. Because not all bleeding from the urogenital tract is from the uterus, rectal and bladder sources should also be considered and evaluated. If the bleeding is from the uterus, a pregnancy-related disorder such as a threatened or incomplete abortion or ectopic pregnancy must be excluded.

The severity and frequency of bleeding dictate the extent of laboratory evaluation before therapy. If visible or palpable lesions of the reproductive tract are ruled out, then the following studies are indicated: cervical cytology, measurement of β-hCG, endometrial biopsy, and a complete blood cell count. If severe bleeding is associated with ovulatory cycles, coagulation studies are also indicated.

The diagnosis of ovulatory bleeding episodes associated with organic disease of the reproductive tract is usually established by history and physical examination, although occasionally hysteroscopy or hysterosalpingography may be required to confirm the source of uterine bleeding. In some instances, prolonged or excessive ovulatory bleeding can be reduced by half with prostaglandin synthetase inhibitors; this form of treatment can be helpful in benign types of uterine disease where future fertility is desired.[396]

The diagnosis of anovulatory bleeding is one of exclusion and is supported by the history of the bleeding episodes. Once the diagnosis of anovulatory or dysfunctional uterine bleeding is established, a rational approach to management is as follows. During a first episode of anovulatory bleeding the patient can simply be observed, provided the bleeding is not copious or the patient is not anemic. If the bleeding is moderately severe and not too prolonged, recurrent bleeding may be treated with progestogens such as medroxyprogesterone acetate (10 mg/d for 10 d). The patient should be informed that after the withdrawal of progestogen therapy she will again experience withdrawal bleeding. If this therapy is successful and the patient does not desire contraception, this form of therapy may be utilized for 10 d of each month.[37] Progestogen therapy is most often used in women in the early premenopausal or postmenopausal years. However, if symptoms of estrogen deficiency are present or if the bleeding does not respond to progestogen alone, then estrogen plus cyclic progestogen therapy is indicated (see under Hormonal Therapy).

When anovulatory bleeding is severe and prolonged, the endometrial lining of the uterus is thin and fragile and unresponsive to progestogens alone. In these instances bleeding can be controlled with a combined low-dose oral contraceptive regimen of three or four tablets per day (for a total daily dose of about 140 µg estrogen and up to 4 mg progestogen) for 1 wk, followed by tapering of the dose over 1 mo. If the bleeding is severe enough to cause anemia or hypovolemia, hospitalization and fluid and blood replacement may be required. In these instances, high doses of oral, intramuscular, or intravenous estrogens may be necessary.[397] Parenteral estrogen is no more effective than oral estrogens, but high doses of oral estrogen may induce gastrointestinal side effects such as nausea or vomiting. In either case progestogen therapy (medroxyprogesterone acetate, 10 mg/d by mouth) should be started as soon as the bleeding is controlled.

If hormone therapy does not control bleeding or if the woman is at risk for endometrial cancer (i.e., a woman approaching the age of menopause or a massively obese woman), a dilatation and curettage may be required for diagnosis and therapy. A dilatation and curettage by itself is not curative in most cases of chronic anovulatory bleeding, and dysfunctional uterine bleeding may recur. In women in the reproductive age group, long-term therapy with cyclic low-dose oral contraceptives provides adequate control of bleeding as well as effective contraception (see Chapter 18). When pregnancy is desired, contraceptive therapy is discontinued, and ovulation is stimulated (see under Infertility).

Hysterectomy or, rarely, uterine endometrial ablation by laser or cautery is the last resort for treatment of abnormal bleeding when fertility is no longer desired or significant pelvic pathological abnormality is present.

AMENORRHEA. Amenorrhea is defined as the absence or cessation of menstrual bleeding and is a manifestation of a variety of pathophysiological disorders. The criteria used to define or to determine which women require evaluation and diagnosis are not uniform. Most investigators agree that failure of menarche by age 16, regardless of the presence or absence of secondary sexual characteristics, or the absence of menstruation in a women with previous periodic menses merits evaluation. However, women who do not fulfill these criteria should be evaluated if (1) the patient or the family members are greatly concerned, (2) secondary sexual characteristics (e.g., breast enlargement) have not developed by age 14, or (3) ambiguous external genitalia or virilization is present.[398]

Women with delayed puberty by definition also have amenorrhea and need not be considered separately. Women with sexual ambiguity or virilization may also present with amenorrhea, but in these cases, the primary complaint is not

---

TABLE 12–8. Classification of Amenorrhea (Not Including Disorders of Congenital Sexual Ambiguity)

I. Anatomical defects (outflow tract)
  A. Labial agglutination/fusion
  B. Imperforate hymen
  C. Transverse vaginal septum
  D. Cervical agenesis—isolated
  E. Cervical stenosis—iatrogenic
  F. Vaginal agenesis—isolated
  G. Müllerian agenesis (Mayer-Rokitansky-Kuster-Hauser syndrome)
  H. Complete androgen resistance (testicular feminization)
  I. Endometrial hypoplasia or aplasia—congenital
  J. Asherman syndrome (uterine synechiae)
II. Ovarian failure (hypergonadotropic hypogonadism)
  A. Gonadal agenesis
  B. Gonadal dysgenesis
    1. Abnormal karyotype
      a. Turner syndrome 45,X
      b. Mosaicism
    2. Normal karyotype
      a. Pure gonadal dysgenesis
        i. 46,XX
        ii. 46,XY (Swyer syndrome)
  C. Ovarian enzymatic deficiency
    1. 17α-Hydroxylase deficiency
    2. 17,20-Lyase deficiency
  D. Premature ovarian failure
    1. Idiopathic—premature aging
    2. Injury
      a. Mumps oophoritis
      b. Radiation
      c. Chemotherapy
    3. Resistant ovary (Savage syndrome)
    4. Autoimmune disease
    5. Galactosemia
III. Chronic anovulation with estrogen present
  A. PCOS
    1. Hyperthecosis
  B. Adrenal disease
    1. Cushing syndrome
    2. Adult-onset adrenal hyperplasia
  C. Thyroid disease
    1. Hypothyroidism
    2. Hyperthyroidism
  D. Ovarian tumors
    1. Granulosa-theca cell tumors
    2. Brenner tumors
    3. Cystic teratomas
    4. Mucinous/serous cystadenomas
    5. Krukenberg tumors

IV. Chronic anovulation with estrogen absent (hypogonadotropic hypogonadism)
  A. Hypothalamic
    1. Tumors
      a. Craniopharyngioma
      b. Germinoma
      c. Hamartoma
      d. Hand-Schüller-Christian disease
      e. Teratoma
      f. Endodermal sinus tumors
      g. Metastatic carcinoma
    2. Infection and other disorders
      a. Tuberculosis
      b. Syphilis
      c. Encephalitis/meningitis
      d. Sarcoidosis
      e. Kallmann syndrome
      f. Idiopathic hypogonadotropic hypogonadism
      g. Chronic debilitating disease
    3. Functional
      a. Stress
      b. Weight loss/diet
      c. Malnutrition
      d. Psychological
        Eating disorders (anorexia nervosa, bulimia)
      e. Exercise
  B. Pituitary
    1. Tumors
      a. Prolactinomas
      b. Other hormone-secreting pituitary tumors (ACTH, thyrotropin-stimulating hormone, growth hormone)
      c. Nonfunctional tumors (craniopharyngioma)
      d. Metastatic carcinoma
    2. Space-occupying lesions
      a. Empty sella
      b. Arterial aneurysm
    3. Necrosis
      a. Sheehan syndrome
      b. Panhypopituitarism
    4. Inflammatory/infiltrative
      a. Sarcoidosis
      b. Hemachromatosis

amenorrhea. Women with sexual ambiguity should be evaluated as for a disorder of sexual differentiation, as discussed in Chapter 14. Women with hirsutism and virilization should also be evaluated differently, as discussed later in this chapter. Thus the diagnosis, evaluation, and treatment of amenorrhea are simplified.

Amenorrhea is traditionally categorized as either primary (women who have never menstruated) or secondary (women in whom menstruation is present for a variable time and then ceases). Although this distinction is useful, some disorders can cause either primary or secondary amenorrhea. For example, most women with gonadal dysgenesis have primary amenorrhea, but occasional patients have residual follicles and ovulate, so that some menstruation and rare pregnancies may occur.[399–401] Furthermore, patients with chronic anovulation (PCOS) usually have secondary amenorrhea but occasionally have primary amenorrhea.[150] For these reasons, categorization of amenorrhea into primary or secondary types is less helpful than a classification based on the underlying pathophysiological disorder: anatomical defects, ovarian failure, or chronic anovulation with current estrogen production present or absent (Table 12–8).

Anatomical Defects. A variety of anatomical defects of the female reproductive outflow tract preclude menstrual bleeding. Some may be iatrogenic or caused by infection (Fig. 12–38). Women with anatomical defects may have normal ovarian function; they ovulate and develop normal secondary sexual characteristics. Beginning at the caudal end of the female genital tract, labial agglutination secondary to infection may obstruct menstrual flow.[402] Idiopathic labial fusion may occur in the absence of other clinical findings associated with sexual ambiguity (i.e., clitoral enlargement).[403] Imperforate hymen, transverse vaginal septum, and isolated absence of the vagina or cervix can also cause amenorrhea.[404, 405] These women frequently have an accumulation of blood behind the obstruction and present with cyclic, predictable episodes of pain in the absence of menses (Fig. 12–39).[404] If undiagnosed, these disorders can lead to endometriosis, adhesions, and later infertility. More severe müllerian anomalies include müllerian agenesis (the Mayer-Rokitansky-Kuster-Hauser syndrome) and defects in lateral or vertical müllerian fusion in which the caudal portion of the müllerian duct fails to fuse normally with the urogenital sinus.[406] Defects in lateral fusion include double uterus (uterus didelphys), half uterus (uterus unicornis), partial duplication (uterus bicornis), and partial or complete uterine septum. In those patients with complete obstruction, (e.g., a

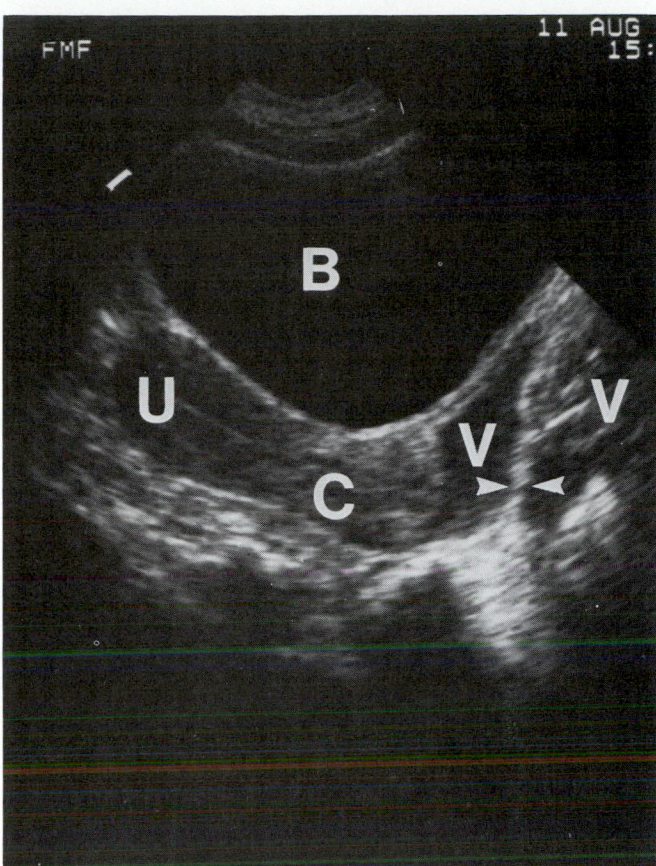

Figure 12–39. Transabdominal ultrasonographic study demonstrating a transverse vaginal septum. Arrowheads denote the location and width of the transverse septum. B, bladder; U, uterus; C, cervix; V, vagina. Menstrual blood is located between the septum and the cervix. (From Doody KM, Carr BR. Amenorrhea. Obstet Gynecol Clin North Am 1990; 17:361–387.)

blind uterine horn), amenorrhea and cyclic pain are the presenting symptoms, whereas those with communicating uterine defects characteristically present with dysmenorrhea.[406, 407]

Müllerian agenesis is the second most common cause of primary amenorrhea, after gonadal dysgenesis.[408] Women with this syndrome have a 46,XX karyotype, female secondary sexual characteristics, and normal ovarian function, including ovulation, but have absence of the vagina and either absence or severe hypoplasia of the uterus.[328] The uterus, when present, usually consists of only rudimentary bicornuate cords. If the uterus contains endometrium, cyclic abdominal pain and accumulation of blood may occur as with other disorders of vertical and lateral obstruction of the outflow tract. Women with müllerian agenesis often have associated abnormalities of the urogenital tract (15 to 40%), including unilateral absence of a kidney or a pelvic kidney.[409] About 12% have skeletal anomalies, usually involving the spine.[328] The major diagnostic problem is differentiating müllerian agenesis from complete androgen resistance (testicular feminization), in which 46,XY genetic men with testes also have female breast development, a blind-ending vaginal pouch, and an absent uterus (Table 12–9). The latter disorder is due to defects in the androgen receptor that cause profound resistance to the action of testosterone during embryogenesis and in postnatal life[329, 410, 411] (see Chapter 14). Testicular feminization is suspected if pubic and axillary hair is absent or deficient and an inguinal hernia is present. The diagnosis of testicular feminization is confirmed by

Anatomical Defects

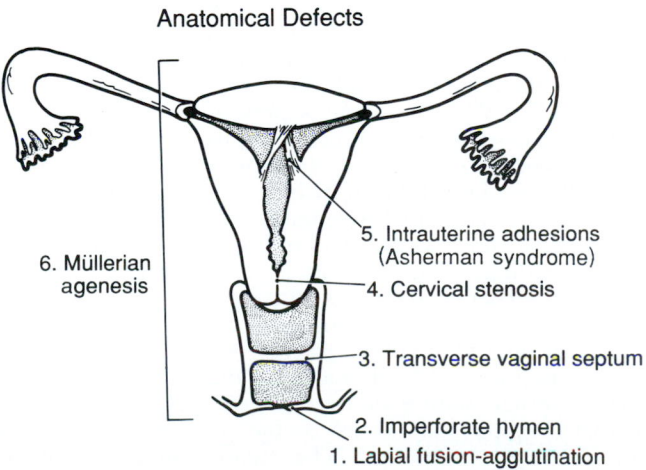

6. Müllerian agenesis

5. Intrauterine adhesions (Asherman syndrome)

4. Cervical stenosis

3. Transverse vaginal septum

2. Imperforate hymen

1. Labial fusion-agglutination

Figure 12–38. Diagrammatic representation of causes of amenorrhea resulting from disorders of the female reproductive (outflow) tract.

TABLE 12–9. Differential Diagnosis of a Phenotypic Female with Secondary Sexual Development and No Uterus

Feature	Müllerian Agenesis	Complete Androgen Resistance (Testicular Feminization)
Hereditary pattern	Sporadic	X-linked recessive
Gonad	Ovary	Testis
Chromosomes	46,XX	46,XY
Serum testosterone	Low	Male
Serum LH	Normal	Increased
Breasts	+ +	+ +
Pubic/axillary hair	+ +	—
Other anomalies	+ +	—

From Doody KM, Carr BR. Amenorrhea. Obstet Gynecol Clin North Am 1990; 17:361–387.

demonstrating a male level of serum testosterone and a 46,XY karyotype, whereas the diagnosis of müllerian agenesis can be established by documenting the presence of biphasic basal body temperatures characteristic of ovulatory women, elevated progesterone levels during the luteal phase, and a 46,XX karyotype. Subjects with testicular feminization should have the testes removed after breast development because of the risk of malignant transformation.[340]

In rare instances women lack both the uterus and female secondary characteristics but have infantile female external genitalia. In these cases a chromosomal karyotype should be obtained. Those individuals with a 46,XY karyotype have androgen deficiency, most commonly resulting from a deficiency of 17α-hydroxylase or 17,20-lyase, testicular regression syndrome, or gonadal agenesis (see Chapter 14). Those individuals with a 46,XX karyotype have müllerian agenesis along with another disorder such as ovarian failure or gonadotropin insufficiency.[412]

Other abnormalities of the uterus that cause amenorrhea include congenital absence of the cervix and obstruction of the cervix caused by scarring or stenosis. The latter is usually from dilatation and curettage or from treatment of cervical dysplasia or cervical intraepithelial neoplasia by laser, electrocautery, or cryosurgery. In rare instances amenorrhea can be due to endometrial hypoplasia or aplasia.[404] Destruction of the endometrium (Asherman syndrome) can follow vigorous curettage in association with postpartum hemorrhage, therapeutic abortion complicated by infection, or a missed abortion and is associated with endometrial adhesions or synechiae.[413] Asherman syndrome can also occur after uterine surgery such as a metroplasty, myomectomy, or cesarean section and can result from tuberculosis or schistosomiasis.[413] Women with Asherman syndrome may have amenorrhea in severe cases or scant menses at regular predictable intervals.

Diagnosis and Treatment. The diagnosis of a defect of the outflow tract is usually established by history and physical examination. In women with primary amenorrhea and no history of prior surgery of the reproductive tract, the pelvic examination may be diagnostic. Labial agglutination, labial fusion, imperforate hymen, and transverse vaginal system are easily recognizable. In cases of transverse vaginal septum, ultrasonography is helpful in determining the location and length of the septum before surgical repair (see Fig. 12–39).[414] If the vaginal opening is patent and a cervix is visualized by a speculum examination, a sound or probe can confirm the presence or absence of cervical stenosis or scarring. If a uterus is not palpated during a bimanual pelvic examination, an ultrasonographic study or MRI scan is useful in documenting whether a uterus is present and contains an endometrial cavity.[335, 336] These studies are also helpful in the diagnosis of other uterine anomalies such as double uterus or blind uterine horns. Finally hysterosalpin-

gography, hysteroscopy, and occasionally laparoscopy may be required for the diagnosis of Asherman syndrome or other abnormalities of uterine development.[336, 341, 342]

Most disorders of the outflow tract are successfully treated by surgery. Incision or excision in cases of labial fusion, imperforate hymen, or vaginal septa often leads to normal menstruation and later fertility.[415] Labial adhesions in children have been successfully treated with estrogen cream.[416] A functional vagina in women with müllerian agenesis or testicular feminization can be created either by nonsurgical dilation of a blind-ending pouch or perineal dimple or, if needed, by surgical construction using skin grafts.[417–419] Asherman syndrome is best treated by direct hysteroscopic resection.[420, 421]

Ovarian Failure. Ovarian failure, or hypergonadotropic hypogonadism, is the occurrence of amenorrhea, hypoestrogenism, and elevated gonadotropin level before age 40. Cessation of ovarian function can occur at any age, even in utero. If it occurs before puberty the presentation is as primary amenorrhea; after pubertal development and menarche the presentation is as secondary amenorrhea. Ovarian failure can result from multiple causes (see Table 12–8). Gonadal agenesis is the most severe form and is most often associated with a 46,XY karyotype and sexual infantilism. Rare cases have been associated with a 46,XX karyotype.[422] Gonadal dysgenesis results when the germ cells are lacking and the ovary is replaced by a fibrous streak[423] (see Chapter 14). Women with gonadal dysgenesis can be divided into two broad groups on the basis of karyotype. The first group has an abnormal chromosomal karyotype; deletion of genetic material in the X chromosome accounts for about two thirds of cases.[424] A 45,X karyotype is found in about half, and most of these women have somatic defects, including short stature, webbed neck, shield chest, short metacarpals, increased carrying angle of the arms, cardiovascular defects, and sexual infantilism, collectively termed *Turner syndrome* (Fig. 12–40).[425] The remainder of patients with identifiable abnormalities of the X chromosome have chromosomal mosaicism with or without structural abnormalities of the X chromosome. Short stature is seen in patients with gonadal dysgenesis who have monosomy of the short arm of the X chromosome. Genes on both the long and short arms of the X chromosome are involved in ovarian development.[426] The most common form of mosaicism in gonadal dysgenesis is 45,X/46,XX.[424] Trisomy for the X chromosome (46,XXX) is also associated with ovarian failure or premature menopause.[427]

Gonadal tumors are rare in 45,X patients, but individuals with chromosome mosaicism involving the Y chromosome have a 25% risk for the development of gonadal malignancy.[423, 428, 429] Therefore a chromosomal analysis should be obtained in all cases of ovarian failure in patients younger than age 30, and the streak gonad should be removed if a Y chromosome is present. Although patients with gonadal dysgenesis appear to have a normal complement of oocytes during early fetal development, the gonad is usually devoid of follicles by birth.[9] Thus more than 90% of women with gonadal dysgenesis resulting from deletion of genetic material in the X chromosome never have menstrual bleeding. A few individuals have sufficient residual follicles to experience menses and, rarely, fertility.[423, 424]

The second form of gonadal genesis is associated with a normal 46,XX or 46,XY karyotype and is termed *pure gonadal dysgenesis*.[399, 430] These individuals have normal or above average stature as a result of failure of estrogen-mediated epiphyseal closure in the presence of a normal chromosomal constitution. The etiology in most cases of pure gonadal dysgenesis is unknown but may be due to single-gene defects or destruction of germinal tissue in utero

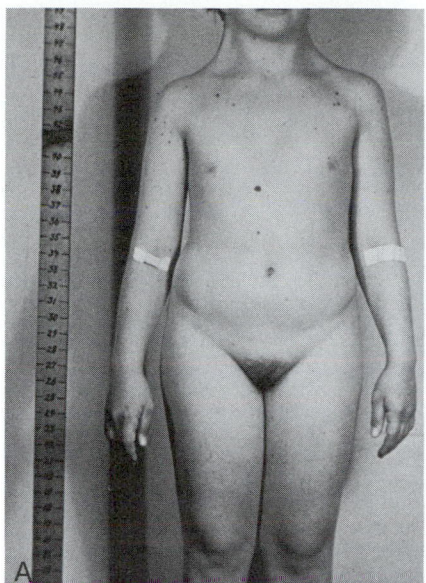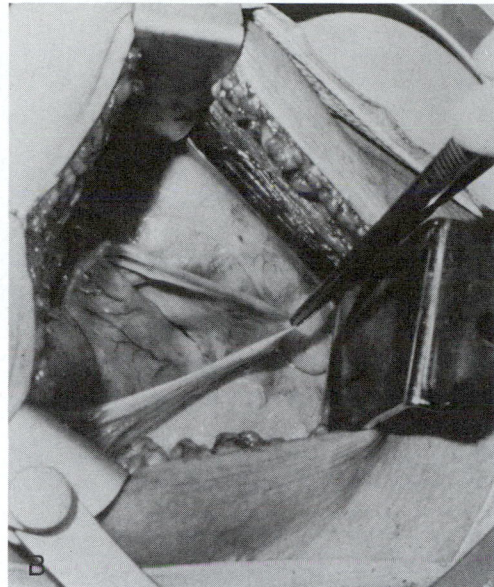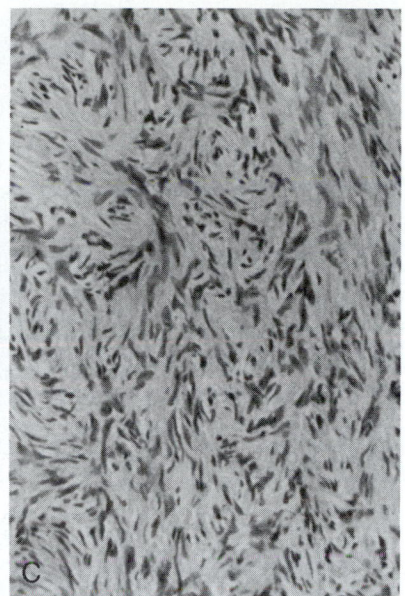

Figure 12–40. Gonadal dysgenesis. *A*, Patient with stigmata of gonadal dysgenesis, including short stature, sexual infantilism, webbed neck, and broadly spaced nipples. *B*, Streak ovary (held by forceps). *C*, Microscopic section of a streak ovary demonstrating fibrous replacement of ovarian structures and the absence of germ cells and follicles.

by environmental or infectious processes.[430] Approximately a tenth of individuals with a 46,XY karyotype develop signs of virilization, including clitorimegaly, and have an increased incidence of tumors in the gonadal streaks; as a consequence gonadal streaks should be removed prophylactically, as described previously, when a Y chromosome is present. Although signs of virilization are rare in women with 46,XX gonadal dysgenesis, the gonadal streak should be removed if the source of androgen excess is thought to be of gonadal origin.[431] Approximately two thirds of individuals with 46,XX gonadal dysgenesis experience no menses, and the remainder have one or more menstrual episodes and are occasionally fertile.[431]

Other causes of ovarian failure include deficiency of 17α-hydroxylase or 17,20-lyase, resistant ovary syndrome, galactosemia, autoimmune disorders, and physical trauma (chemotherapy and radiation therapy for malignancy or infection). 17α-Hydroxylase deficiency is characterized by primary amenorrhea, sexual infantilism, and hypertension resulting from increased production of deoxycorticosterone, whereas women with 17,20-lyase deficiency have primary amenorrhea and sexual infantilism with normal blood pressure.[432, 433] The diagnosis of these enzyme deficiencies can be established by measuring levels of progesterone and 17-hydroxyprogesterone. The resistant ovary syndrome is a rare disorder in which the ovaries contain follicles arrested in development before the antral stage, possibly because of an abnormality or deficiency of the FSH receptor.[143, 434] To differentiate this disorder from the 46,XX variety of pure gonadal dysgenesis, both of which are associated with amenorrhea and sexual infantilism, it is necessary to perform an ovarian biopsy. However, such a distinction is not clinically useful, because the treatment of infertility in both conditions is usually unsuccessful (see discussion of treatment). The ovarian failure of galactosemia is due to deficiency of galactose-containing compounds or excessive galactose-1-phosphate accumulation in the ovary.[435] Premature ovarian failure may also occur as an isolated autoimmune disorder or in association with hypothyroidism, hypoadrenalism, hypoparathyroidism, or systemic lupus erythematosus[436] (also see Chapter 31). In some of these cases antibodies to the ovary

can be identified. Because premature ovarian failure may be associated with polyglandular failure, which may be life-threatening, a thorough evaluation is indicated to rule out other endocrine failure. Ovarian failure may be due to radiation therapy and chemotherapy for treatment of malignancy.[437] A dose of more than 8 Gy (800 rad) directed to the ovary usually causes permanent ovarian failure.[438] Infection can also cause ovarian failure and infertility.[439]

Diagnosis and Treatment. The diagnosis of ovarian failure is suspected in all cases of primary amenorrhea and sexual infantilism and in women with secondary amenorrhea who develop hot flushes and other signs of estrogen deficiency. It is confirmed by documenting FSH levels in the menopausal range (i.e., >40 IU/L). In women younger than age 30, a chromosomal karyotype should be obtained, as discussed previously. If indicated, other tests may be helpful in confirming the diagnosis: progesterone, deoxycorticosterone, and 17-hydroxyprogesterone (17α-hydroxylase and 17,20-lyase deficiency); galactose-1-phosphate (galactosemia); serum levels of calcium, phosphorus, cortisol, and thyroxine; and antibodies to thyroid, adrenal, and ovary (autoimmune disorders).

Because ovarian failure is usually permanent, all patients should be treated with estrogen and progestogen replacement. Estrogen therapy promotes and maintains secondary sexual characteristics and prevents premature osteoporosis and coronary heart disease. In patients with gonadal dysgenesis and short stature, a regimen of low-dose estrogen therapy (0.3 mg/d of conjugated estrogens) has been advocated in hope of providing necessary estrogen support without hastening epiphyseal closure.[440] Growth hormone may accelerate growth if the epiphyses are not closed; whether such therapy influences final adult height is unknown (Fig. 12–41).[441, 442] In gonadal dysgenesis, estrogen is usually prescribed in a cyclic fashion with an initial dose of 0.3 mg/d of conjugated estrogens until growth ceases, at which time the daily estrogen dose is increased (to 0.625 to 1.25 mg) to augment breast development. It is necessary to initiate and continue progestogen therapy to induce regular withdrawal bleeding and reduce the risk of endometrial carcinoma. Patients with 17α-hydroxylase deficiency should

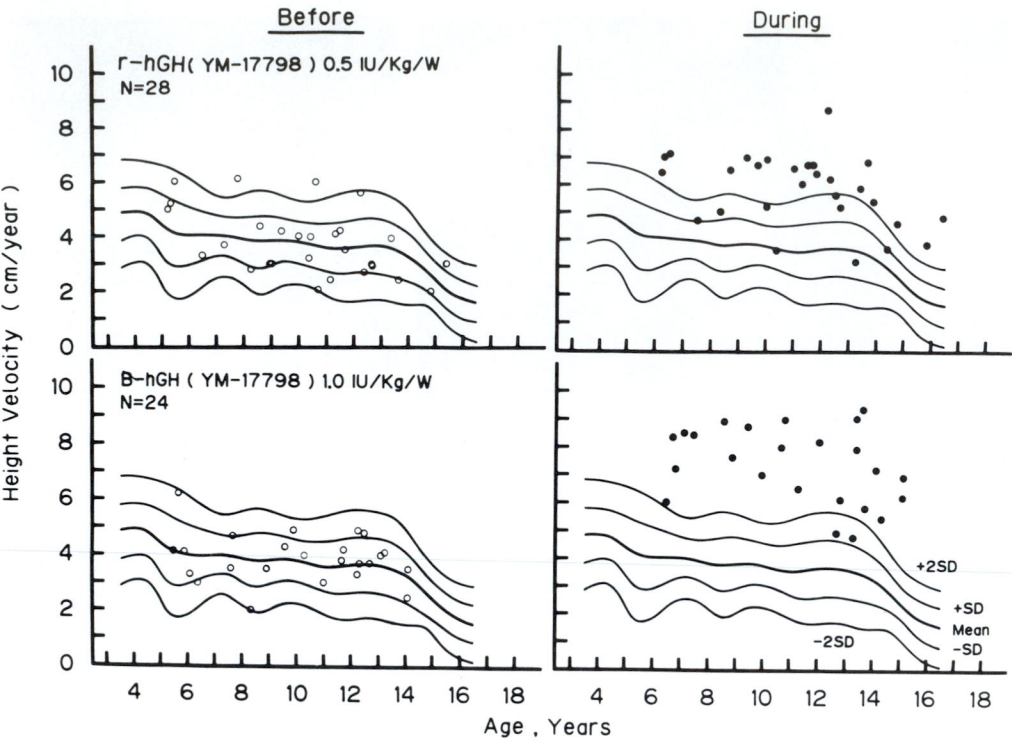

Figure 12–41. Growth rates of girls with gonadal dysgenesis before (○) and during (●) treatment with methionine-free recombinant human growth hormone plotted against the natural growth rate of girls with gonadal dysgenesis. (From Takano K, Shizume K, Hibi I, et al. Turner's syndrome: treatment of 203 patients with recombinant human growth hormone for one year. A multicentre study. Acta Endocrinol 1989; 120:559–568.)

be treated with glucocorticoids as well as estrogen and progestogen replacement. Women with autoimmune ovarian failure have been treated with short courses of glucocorticoids or plasmapheresis, with only temporary improvement in most cases.[436] Occasionally, prophylactic repositioning of the ovary (oophoropexy) may prevent ovarian failure in women who are to receive ionizing radiation.[443] Pretreatment with LHRH analogues, antiestrogens, or oral contraceptives before chemotherapy may be successful in maintaining ovarian function.[437]

In a few cases ovarian follicular depletion may not be complete, and occasional spontaneous ovulatory cycles and even pregnancy may occur.[444] Various stimulation protocols, including high-dose estrogens plus progestogens (either alone or combined with gonadotropins) or pretreatment with LHRH analogues followed by gonadotropins, have been used for women with premature menopause desiring pregnancy.[445–447] Most women with secondary ovarian failure who subsequently conceive have been treated with estrogen replacement. Estrogen is believed to suppress gonadotropins and either stimulate formation of new FSH receptors or prevent down-regulation of FSH receptors. Sporadic pregnancies have been reported with and without therapy, but because the number of reported patients is small, no definite conclusion can be drawn about the efficacy of treatment. It is difficult to predict which patients with ovarian failure will respond. An ovarian biopsy includes only a small part of the ovary, and pregnancies have occurred despite the fact that the biopsy was devoid of follicles. For this reason ovarian biopsy is not indicated. Women with small follicles demonstrated by ultrasonographic studies may be more likely to ovulate. Donor oocytes and ovum transfer combined with in vitro fertilization and cyclic exogenous estrogen and progestogen synchronization of the endometrium have also been used to achieve pregnancies (Fig. 12–42).[234]

Chronic Anovulation. The most common cause of amenorrhea is chronic anovulation. Women with chronic anovulation do not ovulate spontaneously but have ovaries with follicles and may ovulate with appropriate therapy. The ovaries of such women do not secrete estrogen in a normal cyclic pattern; it is useful to differentiate these women who produce sufficient estrogen to have withdrawal bleeding after progestogen therapy from those with hypogonadotropic hypogonadism who fail to produce enough estrogen to have withdrawal bleeding. Although this distinction is useful, some women with chronic anovulation caused by stress, weight loss, exercise, or hyperprolactinemia have reduced estrogen production but still experience withdrawal bleeding after a progestogen challenge. This result simply indicates that some estrogen is being produced.

Chronic Anovulation with Estrogen Present. Women with chronic anovulation who experience withdrawal bleeding after progesterone administration are said to be in a state of "estrus" because of the acyclic production of estrogen (largely estrone) by extraglandular aromatization of circulating androstenedione. This condition may be due to altered feedback loops. It has been proposed that the ovary is initially normal but that the hypothalamic-pituitary unit is regulated by signals that do not originate in the ovary.[150] Support for this concept is provided by animal models in which the administration of androgens to newborns before the maturation of the hypothalamic-pituitary axis permanently modifies feedback relationships. Such animals do not develop cyclic ovarian function at puberty but enter into a state of continuous estrus in which the ovaries contain many cystic follicles and overproduce androgens.[448]

The most common disorder in women resulting in chronic anovulation with estrogen present is PCOS, a complex disorder characterized by infertility, hirsutism, obesity, and various menstrual disturbances: amenorrhea, oligomenorrhea, or DUB (Table 12–10). The symptoms and features are variable even when the diagnosis is based on the presence of polycystic ovaries as determined by histological or ultrasonographic studies.[449, 450] There appears to be a strong familial component, and genetic transmission by an autosomal dominant or X-linked tract has been suggested.[451–454]

Classic PCOS, as described by Stein and Leventhal[455] in 1935, is characterized by enlarged, polycystic ovaries, but

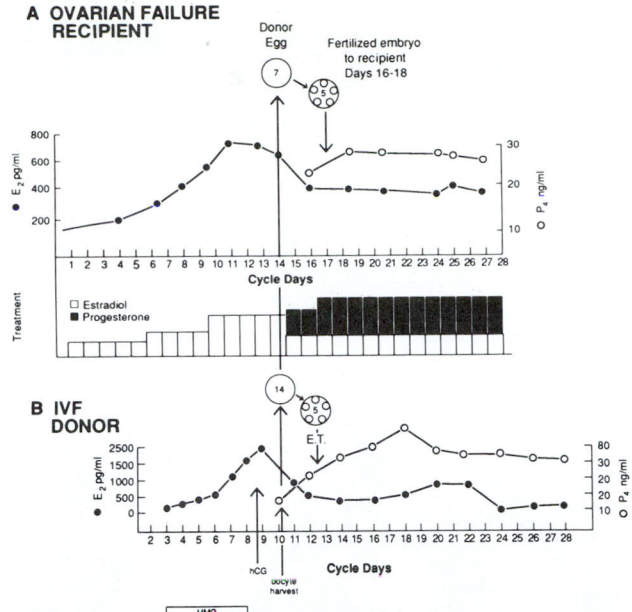

Figure 12–42. Diagrammatic representation of donation of excess oocytes by a woman undergoing in vitro fertilization (IVF) to a woman with ovarian failure treated with exogenous estrogen and progesterone. *A,* Woman with ovarian failure treated with increasing doses of estrogen during days 1 to 14 of the cycle. On day 15 exogenous progesterone was added along with estrogen until day 28 and continued if pregnancy was diagnosed. Seven donor eggs were fertilized with ovarian failure recipient husband's sperm, and five embryos were transferred to the uterus between days 16 and 18. *B,* IVF patient-donor was treated with human menopausal gonadotropin (hMG) until day 8, when hCG was given and oocytes were harvested 32 to 36 h later. Half of the eggs were donated to recipient (see earlier), and the other half were fertilized with IVF donor husband's sperm; the five fertilized eggs were transferred to the uterus of the IVF donor. E_2 (estradiol) and P_4 (progesterone) plasma levels in both women are shown. To convert estradiol values to picomoles per liter, multiply by 3.671. To convert progesterone values to nanomoles per liter, multiply by 3.180. (Adapted from Rosenwaks Z. Donor eggs: their application in modern reproductive technologies. Fertil Steril 1987; 47:895–909.)

the syndrome and its characteristic endocrine abnormalities are associated with a variety of pathological findings in the ovaries, only some of which result in their enlargement and none of which are pathognomonic.[455-459] In fact, the term *polycystic ovaries* is misleading, because the ovaries are studded with atretic follicles, not with cysts. The most common pathological finding is a white, smooth, sclerotic ovary with a thickened capsule, multiple follicles in various stages of atresia, a hyperplastic theca and stroma, and rare or absent corpora albicans (Fig. 12–43).[457-459] To lead to further confusion, polycystic ovaries as defined by ultrasonographic studies (at least 10 follicles and increased ovarian stroma) may be present in normal women with ovulatory cycles and no hirsutism.[460]

Some investigators have attempted to define PCOS in endocrine terms. Because plasma LH levels are often elevated while plasma FSH levels are normal or low, it has been suggested that an LH/FSH ratio of higher than 2 to 3 serves as a useful laboratory definition of PCOS.[461, 462] An exaggerated release of LH may occur in women with PCOS after an intravenous bolus of LHRH.[463, 464] Increases in both the pulse amplitude and the frequency of LH pulses suggest an abnormality of the LHRH pulse generator located in the hypothalamus.[465, 466] The most plausible explanation is that the increased secretion of LH occurs secondary to disturbances in steroid feedback in the hypothalamic-pituitary unit.[467] For clinical purposes, the interpretation of a single sample of gonadotropins is rarely useful for confirming the

diagnosis. Even with frequent sampling or measurement after LHRH administration, gonadotropin levels are normal in 10 to 20% of women with PCOS.[450, 463] Some have suggested that bioactive LH (as contrasted to immunoreactive LH) is elevated in these women and that this assay may help in the diagnosis.[468]

In more than half of women with PCOS, plasma androstenedione and testosterone levels (total or free levels) are elevated.[461] The principal source of androgen is the ovary. LHRH analogue treatment lowers gonadotropins and reduces androstenedione and testosterone to castrate levels, whereas levels of adrenal androgens such as DHEAS remained unchanged.[469] Although some women with PCOS have elevated plasma DHEAS levels, levels of 11β-hydroxy-androstenedione (an adrenal metabolite of androstenedione) are similar in controls and in women with PCOS.[470] About 15 to 20% of women with PCOS have mild elevations of plasma prolactin.[471, 472] Increased prolactin secretion may be due to chronic exposure to estrogen or to deficiency of hypothalamic dopamine.[467]

The diagnosis of PCOS is not based primarily on pathological changes in the ovaries or plasma hormone disturbances but is instead a clinical diagnosis based on the coexistence of chronic anovulation and varying degrees of hirsutism. In most women with PCOS, menarche occurs at the expected time, but uterine bleeding is dysfunctional and is unpredictable in onset, duration, and amount. Oligomenorrhea or amenorrhea ensues after a variable time. Five to 10% of women present with primary amenorrhea.[473] The signs of androgen excess usually become evident around the time of expected menarche. One theory suggests that this disorder originates as an exaggerated adrenarche in obese girls (Fig. 12–44).[150] The combination of elevated adrenal androgens and obesity would result in increased formation of extraglandular estrogen. In women with PCOS, levels of estrone are elevated, but so are levels of free estradiol, resulting in part from reduced levels of TeBG.[474, 475] The acyclic production of extraglandular estrogen would lead to a positive feedback on LH secretion and a negative feedback on FSH secretion, giving the characteristic LH/FSH ratio in plasma. The elevated level of LH leads to hyperplasia of the ovarian stroma and thecal cells, further increasing androgen production and in turn providing more substrate for extraglandular aromatization and perpetuation of chronic anovulation. In obese women this sequence of events is enhanced, because adipose tissue stromal cells aromatize androgens to estrogens, exaggerating inappropriate LH release.[300, 476]

Thus the fundamental defect in the PCOS is viewed as one of inappropriate signals to the hypothalamus and pitui-

TABLE 12–10. Incidence of Symptoms Associated with Polycystic Ovarian Syndrome*

Symptom	Incidence (%)		No. of Usable Cases
	Mean	Range	
Infertility	74	35–95	596
Hirsutism	69	17–83	819
Amenorrhea	51	15–77	640
Obesity	41	16–49	600
Functional bleeding	29	6–65	547
Dysmenorrhea	23		75
Corpus luteum at surgery	22	0–71	391
Virilization	21	0–28	431
Biphasic body temperature	15	12–40	288
Cyclic menses	12	7–28	395

*Tabulated from 187 references with a total of 1079 cases. The number of usable cases indicates how many of the 1079 total cases could be evaluated for the presence or absence of a particular symptom.

Adapted from Goldzieher JW, Axelrod LR. Clinical and biochemical features of polycystic ovarian disease. Fertil Steril 1963; 14:631–653.

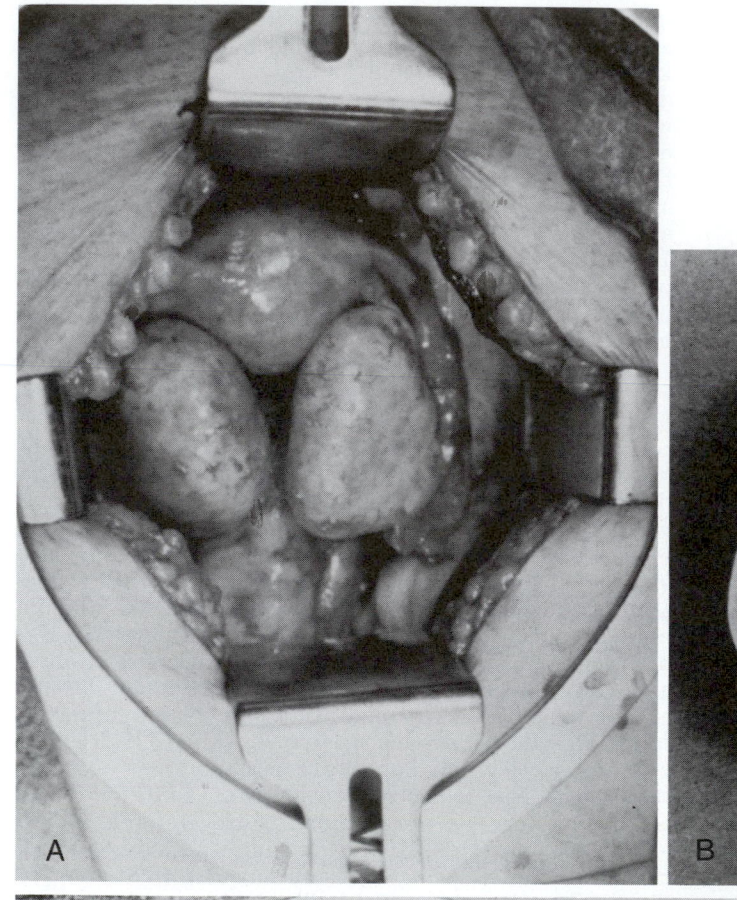

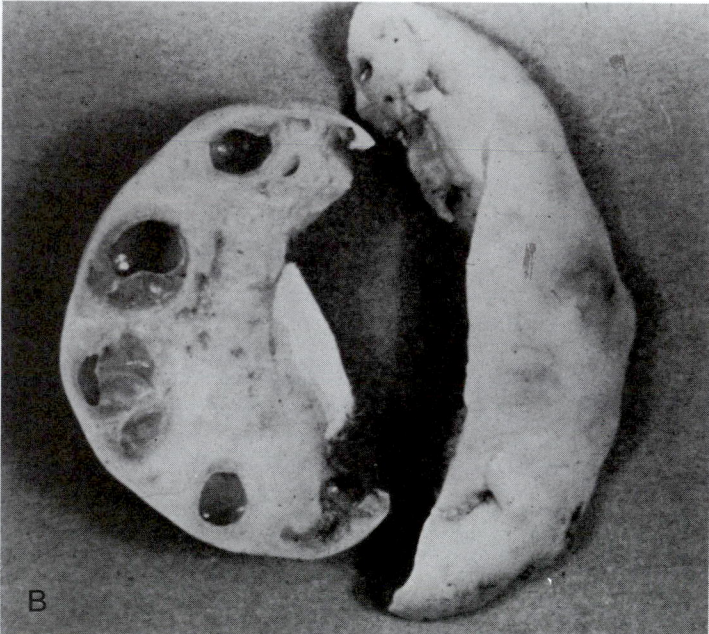

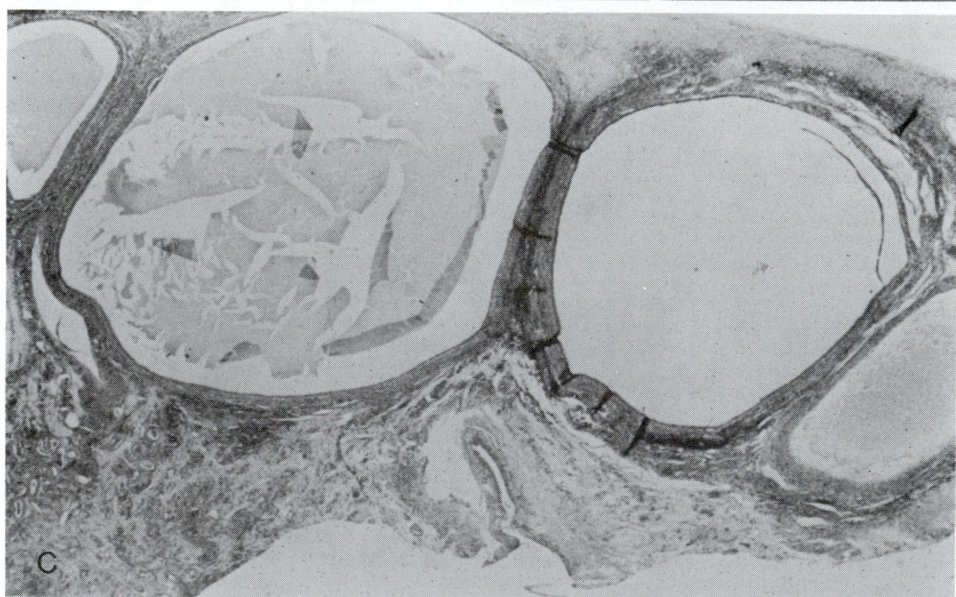

Figure 12–43. Polycystic ovaries. *A,* Operative findings of classic enlarged polycystic ovaries. The uterus is located superior to the ovaries. *B,* Sectioned polycystic ovary with numerous follicles. *C,* Histological section of polycystic ovaries demonstrating cystic follicles with reduced number of granulosa cells and increased ovarian theca and stroma. Magnification × 33.

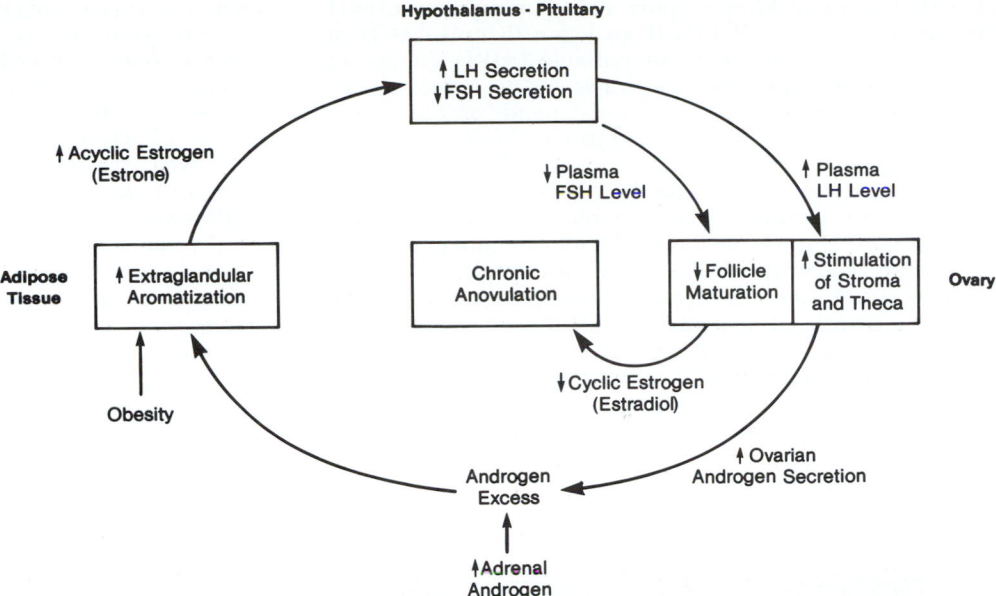

Figure 12–44. Proposed mechanism for the initiation and perpetuation of chronic anovulation in PCOS. This cycle may be entered or initiated via adrenal androgen excess or obesity, both of which result in enhanced extraglandular formation of estrogens. The therapy of this disease involves interruption of the cycle at various sites. (Adapted from Yen SSC. Chronic anovulation caused by peripheral endocrine disorders. In: Yen SSC, Jaffe RB. Reproductive Endocrinology: Physiology, Pathophysiology and Clinical Management. 2nd ed. Philadelphia: W. B. Saunders, 1986: 441–499; and from Carr BR, Wilson JD. Disorders of the ovary and female reproductive tract. In: Braunwald E, Isselbacher KJ, Petersdorf RG, et al., eds. Harrison's Principles of Internal Medicine. 11th ed. New York: McGraw-Hill, 1987: 1818–1837.)

tary. Others have proposed that a primary hypothalamic disorder independent of abnormal steroid feedback is the primary defect in PCOS.[477] However, most believe that abnormal steroid feedback signals are the primary alteration, that the hypothalamic pituitary axis responds appropriately to high levels of estrogen, and that ovulation can be induced with antiestrogens such as clomiphene citrate.[37, 450, 467] The concept that the fundamental defect is one of inappropriate signals is supported by the findings in the ovary itself. Ovarian follicles from women with PCOS have low aromatase activity, but aromatase can be induced when the follicles are treated in vitro with FSH (Fig. 12–45).[478] Also, women with PCOS can be induced to ovulate with FSH.[479, 480] In short, the anovulation does not appear to be due to an intrinsic abnormality in the ovary but rather to FSH deficiency and LH excess.

Other theories of etiology include anomalies of dopamine, endorphin, and inhibin secretion.[473, 481–483] An association of hyperandrogenemia and PCOS with insulin resistance has been documented in both obese and nonobese women.[484–486] Insulin stimulates androgen secretion in ovarian stroma in vitro,[487] and in women with PCOS plus insulin resistance, insulin may act on the ovary via IGF receptors.[488]

Chronic anovulation with estrogen present, obesity, hirsutism, and polycystic ovaries may also occur in a variety of endocrine disorders. Most such women have PCOS, but the functional abnormalities may be seen in women with Cushing syndrome, hyperthyroidism, hypothyroidism, and late-onset adrenal hyperplasia resulting from 21-hydroxylase or 11β-hydroxylase deficiency.[150, 461, 489–491] Chronic anovulation with estrogen present can also be due to tumors of the ovary, including granulosa-theca cell tumors, Brenner tumors, cystic teratomas, mucinous cystadenomas, and Krukenberg tumors (see under Hirsutism and Virilization). Such tumors can either secrete excess estrogen or produce androgens that are aromatized in extraglandular sites.[492] As a result, clinical features of PCOS are produced. Occasionally, areas of the ovary not involved with tumor demonstrate characteristic histological features of polycystic ovaries.

Treatment of PCOS is directed toward interrupting this self-perpetuating cycle and can be accomplished in several ways, including decreasing ovarian androgen secretion directly by wedge resection or indirectly by lowering LH levels (oral contraceptive pills and LHRH analogues). Other approaches include weight reduction and enhancement of FSH secretion (with clomiphene, human menopausal gonadotro-

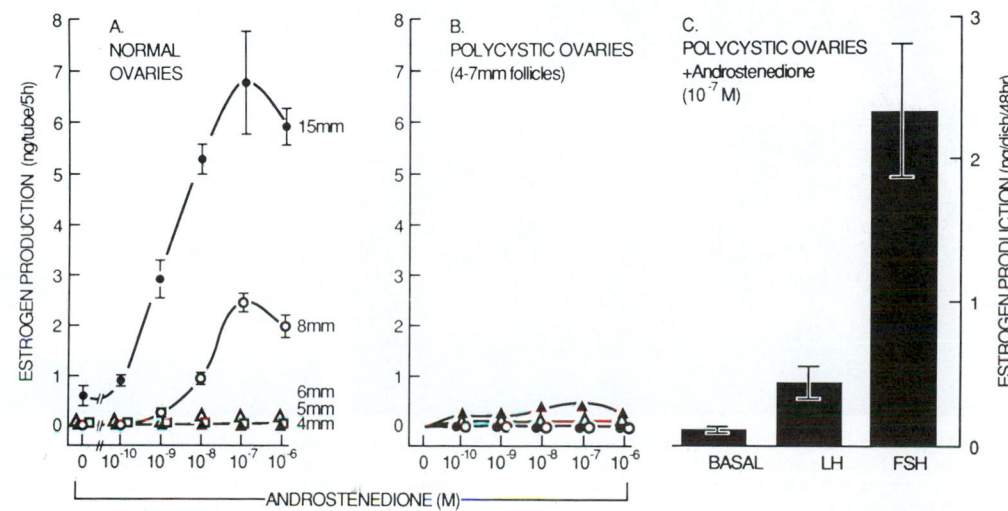

Figure 12–45. Estrogen production by granulosa cells from normal (control) and polycystic ovaries. A, Estrogen production from follicles of various sizes obtained from normal ovaries. B, Estrogen production from follicles of polycystic ovaries. C, Estrogen production from follicles of polycystic ovaries treated with adrenostenedione plus LH or FSH. (Adapted from GF Erickson, AJ Hsueh, ME Guiglen, et al., Functional studies of aromatase activity in human granulosa cells from normal and polycystic ovaries, J Clin Endocrinol Metab 49, 514–519, 1979, © by The Endocrine Society.)

pin [hMG], urofollitropin [pure FSH], or pulsatile LHRH therapy).[461, 467, 473, 493-501] LHRH analogue therapy has been combined with hMG, FSH, or pulsatile LHRH therapy in attempts to increase pregnancy rates and to reduce hyperstimulation. The choice of therapy depends on the clinical picture as well as the desires of the patient. Weight reduction is appropriate in all patients who are obese, because it reduces androgen levels and decreases insulin resistance. Weight loss may cause ovulation to return to normal in some women.[495, 501] If the woman is not hirsute and does not desire pregnancy, monthly withdrawal menses should be induced by progestogen therapy or oral contraceptives to reduce the risk of endometrial neoplasia.[502, 503] If the woman is hirsute but does not desire pregnancy, excess androgen production can be suppressed with oral contraceptives, glucocorticoids, LHRH analogues, or antiandrogens (spironolactone). Oral contraceptives are also indicated if prolonged or excessive menstrual bleeding is present. If pregnancy is desired, ovulation must be induced. The initial drug of choice is clomiphene citrate, which induces ovulation in about three fourths of patients.[473] In those women who do not ovulate or do not conceive after 6 to 12 mo of therapy, clomiphene combinations (clomiphene plus glucocorticoids, hCG, or bromocriptine), hMG, pure FSH, pulsatile LHRH by itself or pulsatile LHRH combined with an LHRH analogue, or cautery/wedge resection of the ovaries may be successful (see under Drugs to Induce Ovulation).

Chronic Anovulation with Estrogen Absent. Women with chronic anovulation and low or absent estrogen production do not experience withdrawal bleeding or have only minimal spotting after progestogen treatment. This disorder is the result of hypogonadotropic hypogonadism secondary to organic or functional disorders of the CNS-hypothalamic-pituitary axis (see Table 12–8).

A defect in the formation and migration of LHRH neurons associated with agenesis of the olfactory bulbs is known as *Kallmann syndrome*, or *isolated gonadotropin deficiency*.[504, 505] Affected women are sexually infantile with a

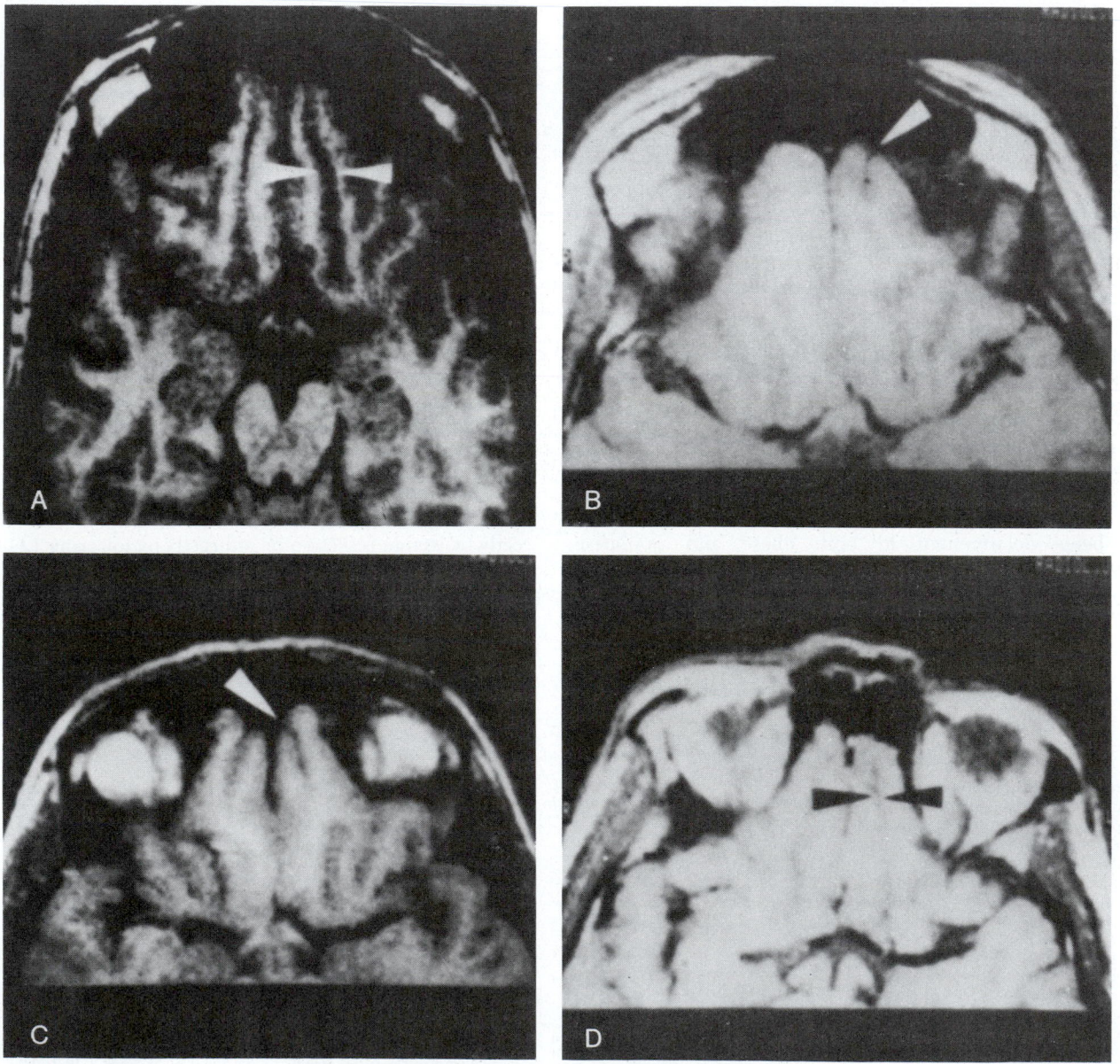

Figure 12–46. Transverse MRI images through the rhinencephalon comparing the normal anatomy of olfactory sulci (A) with the findings of three patients with Kallmann syndrome (B–D). Rudimentary sulci (B, C) or hypoplastic sulci (D) are denoted by arrowheads. (Adapted from D Klingmuller, W Dewes, T Krahe, et al., Magnetic resonance imaging of the brain in patient with anosmia and hypothalamic hypogonadism [Kallmann's syndrome], J Clin Endocrinol Metab 65, 581–584, 1987, © by The Endocrine Society.)

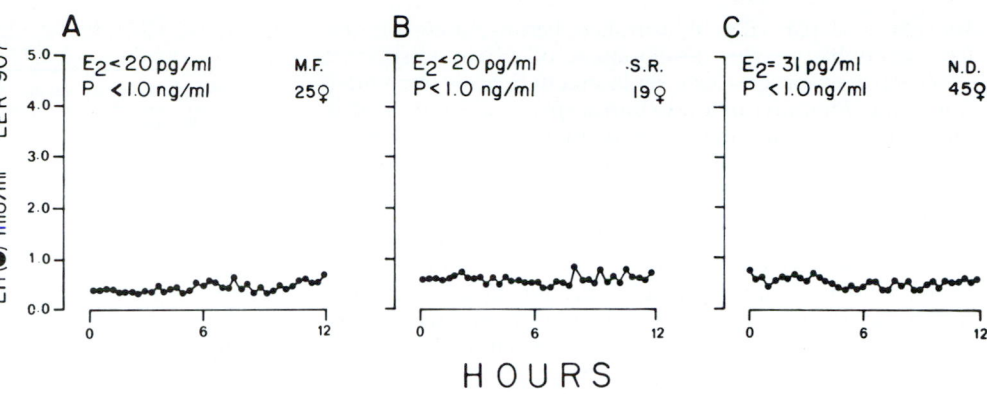

Figure 12–47. Demonstration of apulsatile secretion of LH levels in three women with hypothalamic amenorrhea. Note the complete absence of detectable LH pulses coupled with low estradiol (E₂) and progesterone (P) levels. To convert LH values to international units per liter, multiply by 1.0. To convert estradiol values to picomoles per liter, multiply by 3.671. To convert progesterone values to nanomoles per liter, multiply by 3.180. (From Crowley WF Jr, Filicori M, Spratt DI, et al. The physiology of gonadotropin-releasing hormone [GnRH] secretion in men and women. Recent Prog Horm Res 1985; 41:473–531.)

eunuchoid habitus and have low levels of gonadotropins as a result of defects in the release of LHRH. Kallmann syndrome, a familial disorder usually inherited as an autosomal dominant trait, is more commonly symptomatic in men and is frequently associated with anosmia, color blindness, and occasionally midline defects such as cleft lip and palate.[506, 507] MRI scans often demonstrate a defect in development of the olfactory bulbs and sulci of the rhincencephalon (Fig. 12–46).[508] Additional syndromes associated with hypogonadotropic hypogonadism include the Prader-Willi and the Laurence-Moon-Bardet-Biedl syndromes.[346] Rare hypothalamic lesions or developmental defects that can also impair LHRH production and cause hypogonadotropic hypogonadism include craniopharyngioma, germinoma, eosinophilic granuloma (Hand-Shuller-Christian disease), teratomas, endodermal sinus tumors, tuberculosis, syphilis, sarcoidosis, hamartomas, and metastatic tumors.[509] These disorders can usually be identified by radiographs or CT or MRI scans of the head. Trauma or radiation of the central nervous system can also cause hypothalamic amenorrhea, sometimes associated with deficiencies of other pituitary hormones.

More commonly, gonadotropin deficiency leading to chronic anovulation arises from functional disorders of the hypothalamus or higher centers in the absence of defects identifiable by MRI or CT scans. The diagnosis of a functional cause of chronic anovulation in the absence of estrogen production is one of exclusion. A history of a stressful event is frequently obtained. For example, chronic anovulation can begin suddenly in a woman who leaves home for the first time, enters college, or experiences the death of a loved one. Gonadotropin and estrogen levels are low or in the low-normal range compared with ovulatory women in the early follicular phase. In more severe cases the frequency and amplitude of LH pulses are markedly reduced (Fig. 12–47).[510] Alterations in LHRH secretion and the subsequent decreased gonadotropin levels may be due to increased dopaminergic or β-endorphin levels. Administration of naloxone, an opioid antagonist, enhances LH levels in women with functional hypogonadotropic amenorrhea.[511] In Western societies a common cause of chronic anovulation is weight loss associated with dieting.[512, 513] The extreme form is anorexia nervosa (see Chapter 25). Anorexia nervosa is characterized by the development in a young woman of weight loss with associated amenorrhea, disoriented attitudes toward eating and weight gain, self-induced vomiting, extreme emaciation, and distorted body image.[513-515] Amenorrhea in anorexia nervosa can precede, follow, or appear coincidentally with loss in body weight. Women with anorexia also exhibit disturbances of thyroid hormone and vasopressin secretion.[515] Rigorous exercises such as marathon running, ballet, or swimming can also result in weight loss and lead to chronic anovulation or amenorrhea, particu-

larly in women with a history of prior menstrual irregularity.[516-520] The etiology of amenorrhea associated with exercise is complex, because it may develop in women who exercise strenuously without weight loss or change in body composition.[521, 522] Thus other factors, including the stress of competition, fuel expenditure, and neuroendocrine disturbances, may contribute to amenorrhea.[509] Women who develop amenorrhea associated with stress, exercise, or dieting exhibit alterations that progress from the normal cycle through luteal phase dysfunction and anovulatory cycles to oligomenorrhea and, finally, amenorrhea. Withdrawal bleeding after progestogen occurs in the anovulatory phase when some estrogen is produced but does not occur when estrogen deficiency becomes severe (Fig. 12–48).[215, 520, 523] When the primary cause of amenorrhea is corrected (i.e., increase in weight, reduction in exercise or stress), a progressive reverse from amenorrhea to ovulatory menstrual cycles occurs. In addition, chronic debilitating diseases such as end-stage kidney disease, malignancy, acquired immunodeficiency syndrome, or malabsorption may lead to hypogonadotropic hypogonadism via a central mechanism.

The diagnosis of CNS-hypothalamic disorders that cause chronic anovulation with estrogen absent is suggested by the history but requires some form of imaging of the brain (CT or MRI) to rule out a tumor, because the diagnosis of functional disorders is made by exclusion. CNS imaging is especially important if amenorrhea develops suddenly or is associated with neurological signs.

Treatment of chronic anovulation resulting from CNS-hypothalamic disorders should be directed at reversal of the primary cause (i.e., reversal of stress, reduction of exercise, or correction of weight loss). Successful therapy of this

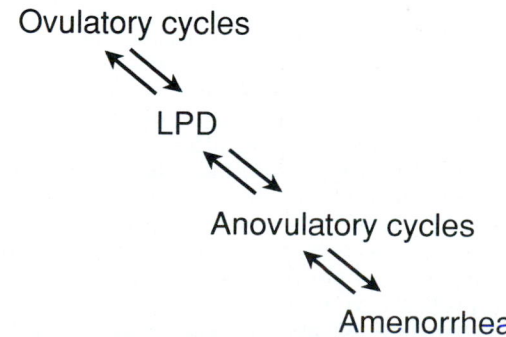

Figure 12–48. Transition from ovulatory cycles to amenorrhea that may be associated with stress, exercise, weight loss, dieting, anorexia, or hyperprolactinemia. During the development of these disorders luteal-phase defects (LPD) may occur, followed by oligoanovulatory cycles and finally amenorrhea. During the time of weight gain, the reverse may occur and amenorrhea may progress to anovulatory or luteal-phase defect cycles until normal ovulatory cycles are reestablished.

disorder is of particular importance, because these women are susceptible to the development of osteoporosis.[524-529] Cyclic estrogen-progestogen replacement therapy (see under Hormonal Therapy) or oral contraceptives are indicated if amenorrhea persists or if reversal of the primary cause is not possible; such therapy prevents further bone loss and induces or maintains normal secondary sexual characteristics. If pregnancy is desired, body weight and nutritional requirements must be returned to normal, because the risk of a low-birth-weight infant is greater in underweight women.[530] If normal body weight and nutrition are attained but amenorrhea persists, gonadotropin or pulsatile LHRH therapy is often successful in inducing ovulatory cycles.[531-533]

Several disorders of the pituitary can lead to the estrogen-deficient form of chronic anovulation: (1) space-occupying lesions that directly inhibit gonadotropin secretion by destruction of gonadotropin-producing cells or that indirectly inhibit gonadotropin release by blocking delivery or secretion of LHRH (metastatic cancer); (2) spontaneous necrosis of the pituitary (Sheehan syndrome); and (3) alterations in other CNS-hypothalamic peptides that influence LHRH neurons (prolactinomas).

Pituitary tumors make up approximately 10% of all intracranial tumors. Such tumors were previously considered to be nonfunctional, but most are now known to secrete hormones.[509] Pituitary cells of all types can be transformed into adenomatous lesions, and pituitary tumors may secrete one or more hormones, including prolactin, FSH, LH, growth hormone, ACTH, and thyrotropin-stimulating hormone (see Chapter 6). Pituitary tumors usually grow slowly; when they enlarge they may impinge on the optic chiasm, leading to blurred vision and field defects.

Prolactin-secreting adenomas are the most common pituitary tumor. Prolactinomas can be divided into microadenomas (<10 mm in diameter) and macroadenomas (>10 mm). Hyperprolactinemia is often associated with low levels of gonadotropin, and women with hyperprolactinemia commonly have amenorrhea and galactorrhea. Hyperprolactinemia from inappropriate prolactin secretion may occur in a number of disorders in addition to prolactin-secreting adenomas (Table 12–11).

Approximately a tenth of women with amenorrhea have elevated prolactin levels, and consequently serum prolactin should be measured in all cases of amenorrhea.[509] Most women with increased levels of prolactin have normal pubertal development and subsequently develop secondary amenorrhea, but prolactinomas have been reported in girls with primary amenorrhea and delayed pubertal development.[534] The most common clinical feature associated with elevated levels of prolactin is galactorrhea. However, some women with hyperprolactinemia do not exhibit galactorrhea, probably because of concomitant estrogen deficiency associated with the hypogonadotropic form of amenorrhea.[535] More than half of women with amenorrhea and galactorrhea have elevated prolactin levels. Occasionally such patients experience withdrawal bleeding after treatment with progestogens. In other women with mild elevation of prolactin, ovulatory cycles or luteal phase–deficient cycles may occur (see Fig. 12–48). Some women with hyperprolactinemia and ovulatory menses secrete high-molecular-weight forms of prolactin that are immunoreactive but lack bioactivity.[536]

Most prolactin-secreting adenomas grow slowly, and studies of their natural history suggest that the majority of women are unlikely to have significant tumor growth; indeed, many have clinical and radiographic improvement, and some experience spontaneous resolution of tumor.[537-540] The increased frequency of diagnosis of prolactin-secreting tumors during the past two decades is probably due to several factors, including increased awareness, improved

TABLE 12–11. Conditions Associated with Inappropriate Prolactin Secretion

Pharmacological Causes	Pathological Causes
Hormone therapy	Hypothalamic or pituitary lesion
Estrogen	Craniopharyngioma
Oral contraceptives	Glioma
Thyrotropin-releasing hormone	Granulomas
Anesthesia	Histocytosis
Dopamine receptor blocking agents	Sarcoid
Phenothiazines	Tuberculosis
Haloperidol	Stalk transection
Metoclopramide	Postsurgical
Domperidone	Head injury
Pimozide	Radiation damage to the
Sulpiride	hypothalamus
Dopamine reuptake blocker	Functional hypothalamic-pituitary
Nomifensine	disorders
CNS-dopamine-depleting agents	Pseudocyesis
Reserpine	Cushing disease
Methyldopa	Nelson syndrome
Monoamine oxidase inhibitor	Acromegaly
Inhibition of dopamine turnover	Prolactinoma
Opiates	Mixed growth hormone, or ACTH-
Stimulation of serotoninergic	and prolactin-secreting adenomas
system	Hypothyroidism
Amphetamines	Renal failure
Hallucinogens	Ectopic production
Histamine H_2-receptor antagonists	Bronchogenic cancer
Cimetidine	Hypernephroma

From Yen SSC. Prolactin in human reproduction. In: Yen SSC, Jaffe RB, eds. Reproductive Endocrinology: Physiology, Pathophysiology and Clinical Management. 2nd ed. Philadelphia: W. B. Saunders, 1986: 237–263.

radiographic detection methods, and availability of prolactin assays. Attempts to link the increased incidence of prolactinomas with the use of oral contraceptives have not been successful.[541] However, because prolactinomas occur more frequently in women and because exogenous estrogen use increases prolactin levels, estrogen may play a role in prolactinoma development.[542] The exact incidence of prolactinomas and hyperprolactinemia is unknown, but the prevalence of microprolactinomas in autopsy series varies from 9 to 27%.[543]

When hyperprolactinemia is present, a careful history may reveal the cause (see Table 12–11). A woman with persistent hyperprolactinemia, especially when associated with amenorrhea, should have radiographic evaluation.[544] At what level of plasma prolactin elevation radiographic investigation should be initiated in the absence of amenorrhea is not clear.[545] Some physicians recommend radiographic evaluation of all women with elevated levels of prolactin (>20 to 30 μg/L), whereas others evaluate when levels exceed a specific maximal concentration such as 50 to 100 μg/L. Women with prolactin levels greater than 50 μg/L have a 20% frequency of harboring a prolactinoma, those with 100 μg/L have a 50% frequency, and those with levels of 100 to 300 μg/L have a high frequency of at least a small macroadenoma.[544, 545] The choice of radiographic techniques with which to evaluate pituitary tumors varies in different institutions. In general, MRI is superior to CT in clarity of definition of soft tissues, optic chiasm, and vasculature. It also avoids exposure to radiation (Fig. 12–49).[546]

The management of prolactinomas includes surgery, radiation, and pharmacological therapy with dopamine analogues (see Chapter 6). Initially, transsphenoidal surgery was recommended as primary therapy for both prolactin-secreting micro- and macroadenomas. Because of the inability to achieve a complete long-term cure with a surgical approach and a high incidence of recurrence (30% for microadenomas and 90% for macroadenomas) and because of the chance of surgical complications, most physicians now recommend long-term pharmacological therapy.[545, 547, 548] Re-

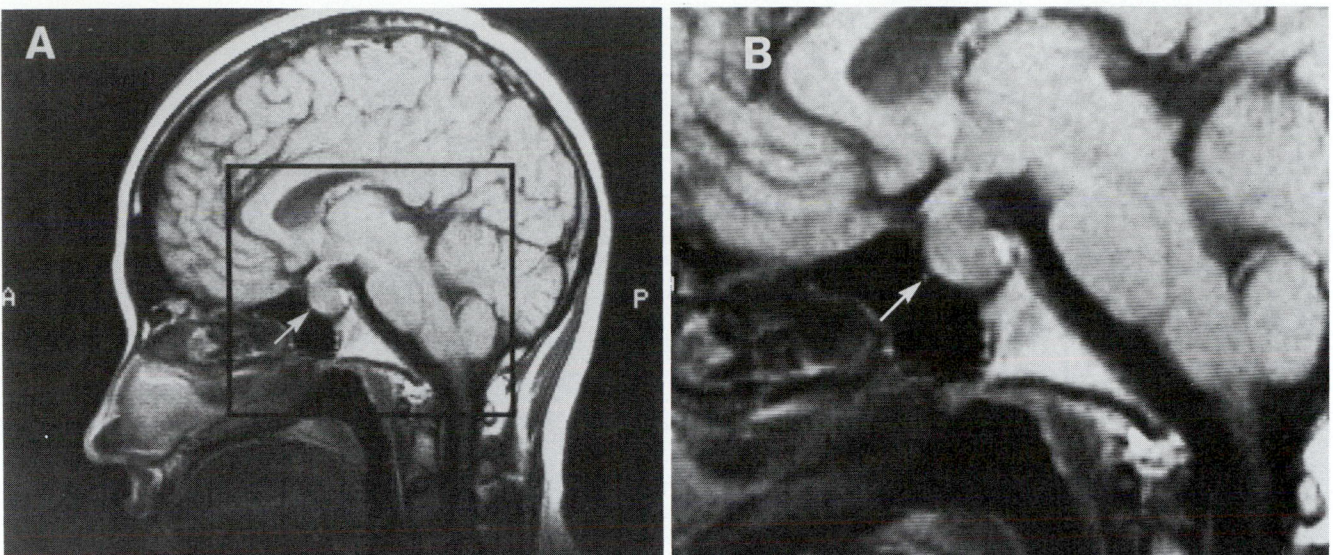

Figure 12–49. *A*, MRI scan of a woman with amenorrhea, galactorrhea, and hyperprolactinoma who had a 3 × 3 cm macroprolactinoma *(arrow)*. *B*, Enlargement of *A* demonstrating macroprolactinoma *(arrow)*. (From Doody KM, Carr BR. Amenorrhea. Obstet Gynecol Clin North Am 1990; 17:361–387.)

sults with radiation therapy are less satisfactory than those with surgical therapy, because response is slow and the incidence of panhypopituitarism is greater.[545] Microadenomas respond to bromocriptine therapy with shrinkage of tumor, and ovulatory menses resume in most women.[549–552] Bromocriptine is also successful in reducing tumor size and causing resumption of menses in women with macroadenomas, but a complete cure may require a combination of surgery and/or radiation plus bromocriptine.[545] Discontinuation of bromocriptine is usually followed by rapid regrowth of prolactin-secreting adenomas and recurrence of amenorrhea and galactorrhea so that long-term therapy is often required. Because the natural course of most microprolactinomas is benign, as previously discussed, treatment may be discontinued after a few years in some cases with resumption of spontaneous ovulatory cycles.[553] In women desiring pregnancy, the risk of tumor expansion and development of visual disturbances during pregnancy should be considered. In fact, only about 7% of women with microadenomas treated with bromocriptine to induce ovulatory cycles experience tumor growth during pregnancy.[554–556] Approximately 30% with macroadenomas develop worsening of symptoms during the course of pregnancy if bromocriptine has been discontinued.[557] If signs of visual impairment or tumor expansion occur during pregnancy, bromocriptine can be reinstituted without an effect on pregnancy or the fetus.[557–560] Some investigators have suggested that bromocriptine should be used continuously in pregnancies associated with macroadenomas, but most physicians discontinue therapy after the diagnosis of pregnancy in patients with microadenomas.

Women may develop galactorrhea and elevated prolactin levels in association with other endocrine-secreting tumors of the pituitary such as acromegaly or Cushing syndrome.[509] Craniopharyngiomas account for 30% of pituitary tumors and consist of stratified squamous epithelium containing solid and cystic components.[561] These tumors arise from remnants of the Rathke pouch and can expand to fill the pituitary sella (see Chapter 6). The degree of hypopituitarism and resultant decreased gonadotropin secretion and the degree of decreased secretion of TSH, ACTH, growth hormone, and vasopressin depend on the size of the tumor and the extent of compression of the pituitary stalk.[562]

Patients with craniopharyngiomas may present with sexual infantilism, delayed puberty, and primary amenorrhea if tumors produce symptoms before puberty, or with secondary amenorrhea if they produce symptoms after puberty. Craniopharyngiomas often calcify, and the diagnosis may be suspected by conventional skull films. Occasionally prolactin levels are elevated. In those instances in which bromocriptine fails to shrink a suspected prolactinoma, other pituitary tumors such as craniopharyngiomas need to be considered, because surgical treatment may be indicated.[563]

Panhypopituitarism may occur spontaneously, develop after surgery or radiation of pituitary adenomas, or develop after severe postpartum hemorrhage (Sheehan syndrome). Women with Sheehan syndrome exhibit characteristic manifestations, including failure to lactate or resume menses, loss of genital and axillary hair, and, in severe cases, evidence of panhypopituitarism.[509]

The empty sella syndrome is an enlargement of the pituitary sella caused by a congenital defect in the diaphragma sella, with expansion of the sella and flattening of the anterior pituitary caused by transmittal of cerebrospinal fluid pressure. Women with this disorder may develop amenorrhea or galactorrhea with elevated prolactin levels. The diagnosis is readily detected by CT or MRI scans.[564, 565]

Evaluation of Amenorrhea. A schema for the evaluation of women with amenorrhea is presented in Figure 12–50. In the physical examination, special attention should be given to three features: (1) degree of maturation of the breasts, pubic and axillary hair, and external genitalia; (2) the current estrogen status; and (3) the presence or absence of a uterus. As previously discussed, amenorrhea may coexist with disorders of sexual development, and if sexual ambiguity is present the patient should be evaluated as discussed in Chapter 14. If virilization is present, the diagnosis of a tumor of the adrenal or ovary must be considered (see discussion on evaluation of hirsutism and virilization). All reproductive-age women with amenorrhea should be assumed to be pregnant until proved otherwise. Except when pubertal development is absent (sexual infantilism), even when the history and physical examination are not suggestive, pregnancy should be excluded by urine or serum β-hCG testing. Once this is done, the cause of amenorrhea can frequently be diagnosed by history or physical exami-

EVALUATION OF AMENORRHEA

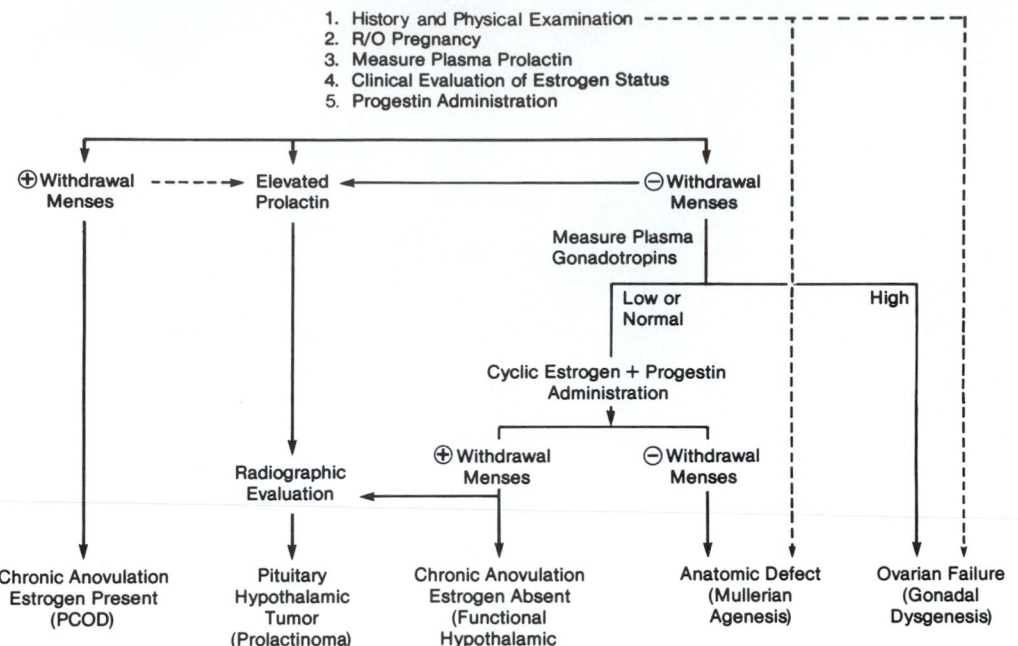

Figure 12–50. Flow diagram for the evaluation of women with amenorrhea. The most common diagnosis for each category is shown in parentheses. The dotted lines indicate that in some instances a correct diagnosis can be reached on the basis of history and physical examination alone. (From Carr BR, Wilson JD. Disorders of the ovary and female reproductive tract. In: Braunwald E, Isselbacher KJ, Petersdorf RG, et al., eds. Harrison's Principles of Internal Medicine. 11th ed. New York: McGraw-Hill, 1987: 1818–1837. Reproduced with permission of McGraw-Hill, Inc.)

nation. For example, Asherman syndrome is suggested by a history of curettage in a women who had previously menstruated; in women with primary amenorrhea, sexual infantilism, and a uterus, the differential diagnosis is between ovarian failure (most often gonadal dysgenesis) and hypogonadotropic hypogonadism. The diagnosis of gonadal dysgenesis or an anatomical defect of the outflow tract (müllerian agenesis, testicular feminization, vaginal septum, or cervical stenosis) can usually be recognized on physical examination. When a specific diagnosis is suspected, it is appropriate to proceed directly to confirmation (e.g., by obtaining a chromosomal karyotype or by measuring plasma gonadotropin levels).

After the initial examination a plasma prolactin level should be obtained. A measurement of plasma TSH can be ordered if the prolactin level is elevated or if symptoms suggest the diagnosis of hypothyroidism (see Chapter 8). Estrogen status is evaluated by determining if the vaginal mucosa is moist and rugated and if the cervical mucus can be stretched and shown to fern after drying. The woman's estrogen status can be further evaluated by a progestational challenge, most often administration of 10 mg of medroxyprogesterone acetate by mouth once or twice daily for 5 d or 100 to 200 mg of progesterone in oil intramuscularly. If estrogen levels are adequate (and the outflow tract is intact), menstrual bleeding should occur within 1 wk of ending the progestogen treatment. In women who bleed after a progestogen challenge, the plasma estradiol level is greater than 150 pmol/L (40 pg/mL), which makes a diagnosis of hypogonadotropic hypogonadism or ovarian failure unlikely.[566] The progestogen challenge test is preferable to obtaining plasma levels of estrogen for the following reasons: (1) it serves as a bioassay of current mean estrogen production, whereas estrogen levels fluctuate throughout the day and during the cycle; (2) plasma estradiol assays are expensive; and (3) the challenge test provides insight as the drug of choice to induce ovulation in women with amenorrhea (see under Drugs to Induce Ovulation). If withdrawal bleeding occurs, the diagnosis is chronic anovulation with estrogen

present (usually PCOS). If no withdrawal bleeding occurs, the subsequent work-up depends on the initial prolactin assay. If the plasma prolactin level is elevated, imaging of the pituitary by MRI or CT scan is indicated: When the plasma prolactin level is normal in women with amenorrhea and failure to bleed after a progestogen challenge, plasma gonadotropin levels should be measured. Gonadotropins should also be measured if the patient experiences minimal bleeding or spotting in the withdrawal phase or if ovarian failure is suspected. If the gonadotropin levels are elevated, the diagnosis is ovarian failure. If the gonadotropin levels are in the low or normal range, the diagnosis is either hypothalamic-pituitary disorder or an anatomical defect of the outflow tract. As discussed previously, the diagnosis of outflow tract disorders is usually established on the basis of the history and physical findings. When the physical findings are not diagnostic, it may be useful to administer cyclic estrogen plus progestogen in the form of a 1-mo package of oral contraceptives or 1.25 mg of oral conjugated estrogens daily for 4 wk plus 10 mg of medroxyprogesterone acetate for the last 10 d of treatment. If no bleeding occurs and a uterus is present, the diagnosis of Asherman syndrome is suspected and confirmed by hysterosalpingography or hysteroscopy. If withdrawal bleeding occurs after the estrogen-progestogen combination, the diagnosis of chronic anovulation with estrogen absent (functional hypothalamic amenorrhea) is suggested. Imaging of the CNS to evaluate for lesions of the pituitary or hypothalamus may be indicated, because the diagnosis of functional hypothalamic amenorrhea is one of exclusion.

Hirsutism and Virilization

Hirsutism is defined as the presence of excessive growth of hair in locations where hair growth in women is normally minimal or absent (Table 12–12). Although it may be the initial sign of a serious underlying disorder, hirsutism by itself is usually benign and is frequently associated with PCOS. In contrast, virilization is the combination of hirsu-

TABLE 12–12. Clinical Findings in Women with Hirsutism and Virilization

Hirsutism: An excessive growth of hair in women that occurs in specific androgen-sensitive areas of the body:

Face	Lower back
Chest	Buttock
Areola	Inner thigh
Linea alba	External genitalia

Virilization: The combination of hirsutism plus:
Clitoral enlargement
Deepening of voice
Temporal hair loss
Loss of female body contour

tism plus other signs of masculinization, such as clitorimegaly, deepening of voice, temporal balding, decreased breast size, and loss of female body contour (Fig. 12–51). Virilization is less common than hirsutism and is more often associated with a potentially serious disorder such as an ovarian or adrenal tumor. Hirsutism is usually associated with normal or slightly elevated levels of serum androgens, whereas virilization is associated with marked increases of ovarian and/or adrenal androgen production and with marked increases in plasma androgens. The number of hairs per unit area of skin is determined by genetic factors and is the same for both sexes of a similar ethnic background. For example, women and men of Mediterranean descent tend to have more body hairs per unit area than do Orientals.[567] Hair follicles cover the bodies of both women and men except for the lips, palms of the hands, and soles of the feet and are of two types: vellus and terminal.[568] In women, excess androgen production stimulates vellus hairs to develop into long, coarse, pigmented terminal hairs in most areas of the body except the scalp, where terminal hairs are converted to vellus hairs, eventually resulting in temporal balding.[569] Androgens stimulate, whereas estrogens inhibit, hair growth in women.[569] The primary mechanism leading to the development of hirsutism and virilization is increased secretion of androgens by the ovary or adrenal. The principal sources of circulating androgens in normal women are summarized in Figure 12–52. Under normal circumstances the circulating testosterone level in women is derived from direct secretion by the ovary and by extraglandular conversion of androstenedione secreted by the ovary and the

adrenal. Little, if any, testosterone is released by the adrenal,[570] but the adrenal is the major source of DHEA and DHEAS in the circulation.[571]

In women with isolated hirsutism, 75% of circulating testosterone is from ovarian secretion. In the presence of increased levels of testosterone, TeBG levels are reduced, leading to increased free testosterone and an increased metabolic clearance rate for testosterone.[572] In women with mild hirsutism who have ovulatory menstrual cycles and normal levels of testosterone, androstenedione, and adrenal androgens (idiopathic or simple hirsutism), the excess body hair has been explained by increased sensitivity of the pilosebaceous unit to normal plasma levels of androgen. In these women 5α-reductase activity, as well as the level of the dihydrotestosterone metabolite 5α-androstane-3α,17β-diol glucuronide and the number of androgen receptors, has been reported to be increased.[573, 574]

A classification for hirsutism is presented in Table 12–13. A frequent cause is ovarian dysfunction, and in this category the most common cause is PCOS.[575] As discussed earlier, PCOS is diagnosed on clinical grounds, and the onset of hirsutism and other symptoms associated with the syndrome usually occurs around the time of menarche. In most cases, the rate of progression of hirsutism is constant but slow. Women with PCOS may on rare occasion develop signs of virilization (e.g., clitorimegaly), usually the result of particularly high rates of testosterone secretion in women with stromal hyperthecosis,[571, 576] a condition in which islands of luteinized thecal cells are present in the ovarian stroma distant from ovarian follicles. Hyperthecosis is probably not a distinct entity from PCOS but rather an exaggerated manifestation of this disorder. Women with hyperthecosis are more likely to have an LH/FSH ratio less than 2 and to fail to ovulate after treatment with clomiphene citrate. They are also more likely to exhibit insulin resistance than those with PCOS alone.[576–578] The diagnosis is suspected from the history and the presence of bilateral enlarged ovaries. The diagnosis can be confirmed by histological section of ovaries at the time of wedge resection or oophorectomy, but only when these surgical procedures are indicated for other reasons.

The association of hyperandrogenism, insulin resistance, and acanthosis nigricans (so-called HAIR-AN syndrome) constitutes a specific subset of PCOS or hyperthe-

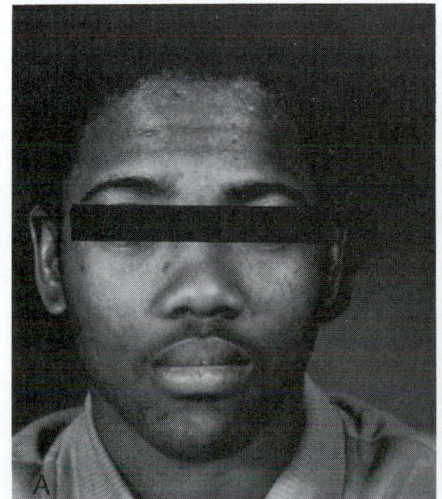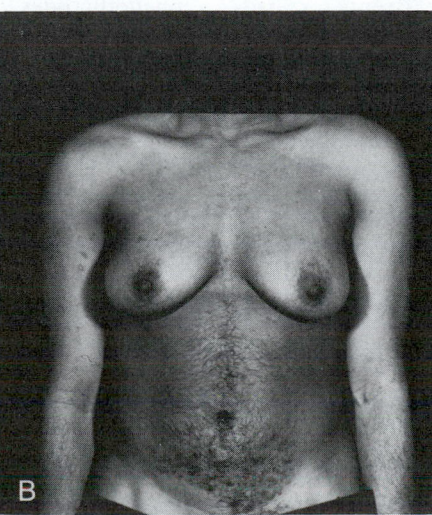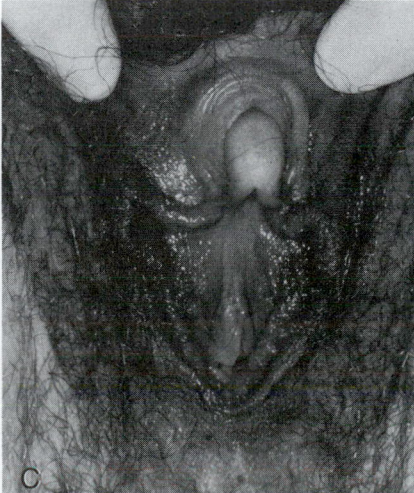

Figure 12–51. Clinical features of hirsutism and virilization in a woman with a virilizing adrenal adenoma. *A,* Photograph demonstrating facial hair and temporal balding. *B,* Photograph of the trunk and abdomen demonstrating muscle development and male escutcheon. *C,* Clitorimegaly. (Courtesy of Dr. Karen D. Bradshaw.)

TABLE 12–13. Classification of Hirsutism and Virilization

Ovarian
  PCOS
  Hyperthecosis
  Neoplasms
    Sex cord tumors
    Germ cell tumors
    Hilar cell tumors
    Adrenal rest tumors
    Mixed germ cell and gonadal tumors
    Tumors with functioning stroma
  Pregnancy associated
    Luteoma
    Hyperreactio luteinalis
Adrenal
  Congenital adrenal hyperplasia/adult-onset adrenal hyperplasia
    21-Hydroxylase deficiency
    11β-Hydroxylase deficiency
    3β-Hydroxysteroid dehydrogenase deficiency
  Neoplasms
    Adenomas
    Carcinomas
Cushing syndrome
Drugs
  Phenytoin
  Diazoxide
  Anabolic steroids
  Progestogens (19-norsteroid derivatives)
  Danazol
Idiopathic
Miscellaneous
  Hyperprolactenemia
  Acromegaly
  Menopause

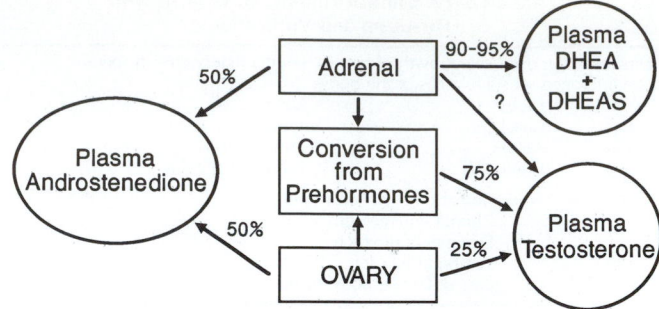

Figure 12–52. Sources of circulating androgens in normal women.

thyroid tissue (struma ovarii) may secrete thyroxine, although rarely in sufficient quantities to cause hyperthyroidism[587, 588] (see Chapter 8).

Adrenal virilization is most commonly due to congenital adrenal hyperplasia (21-hydroxylase deficiency). In women the diagnosis is usually made at birth because of sexual ambiguity[589] (see Chapter 14). Less severe forms are variously termed *late-onset, acquired, partial, attenuated, nonclassic*, or *cryptic 21-hydroxylase deficiency*.[589, 590] In women with late-onset 21-hydroxylase deficiency, hirsutism begins around the time of expected puberty. The frequency of this disorder in hirsute women has been estimated to be between 1 and 20% and probably is less than 5%.[590, 591] Women with Cushing syndrome caused by excessive production of ACTH by pituitary tumors, adrenal adenomas, or adrenal carcinomas or by ectopic secretion of ACTH may develop hirsutism, amenorrhea, and polycystic ovaries.[571] Women with acromegaly or hyperprolactinemia may also have mild hirsutism.

Virilizing adrenal tumors are a rare cause of androgen excess in women. The symptoms and clinical signs have an abrupt onset and progress rapidly, features that aid in making the diagnosis. The diagnosis is also suspected if the serum level of DHEAS is greater than 22 μmol/L (8000 ng/mL) or if urinary 17-ketosteroid levels are greater than 30 mg/d. Adrenal tumors can be readily detected by CT or MRI scan[571] (Fig. 12–54).

Iatrogenic hirsutism may result from drug therapy. One cause of hirsutism, amenorrhea, and signs of virilization is the use of androgens for the purpose of body-building or in treatment of diminished libido or menopause.[592] Other drugs that cause hirsutism include danazol, metyrapone, phenothiazides, phenytoin, diazoxide, and minoxidil.[592] Menopausal women also often complain of increased facial hirsutism, but this is physiological because of the change in the estrogen/androgen ratio.

The diagnosis and evaluation of hirsutism require a careful history and physical examination as well as laboratory testing. In terms of the history, familial occurrence, age at onset, severity, and the rate of progression are important. Hirsutism that begins at the time of expected puberty may be due to PCOS/hyperthecosis, simple hirsutism, or late-onset adrenal hyperplasia. In contrast, the sudden onset of

cosis. Three types of insulin resistance are associated with acanthosis nigricans and hirsutism (Table 12–14 and Fig. 12–53).[570] In women with type A insulin resistance resulting from intrinsic defects in the insulin receptor, the hirsutism is severe and is usually associated with hyperthecosis. The structure of the insulin receptor in women with type A insulin resistance and PCOS is abnormal.[579]

A variety of rare androgen-secreting ovarian tumors may cause virilization (Tables 12–13 and 12–15). The onset of hirsutism and virilization is more abrupt than in women with PCOS or hyperthecosis and can occur at any age. In most cases (>80%) a unilateral adnexal mass is palpable.[575] Ovarian tumors that cause virilization are derived from sex cord or stromal cells and include Sertoli-Leydig cell tumors (arrhenoblastomas), hilar cell tumors, lipoid cell tumors, and adrenal rest tumors.[580, 581] Occasionally, virilization occurs in association with other tumors of the ovary (Brenner, cystadenomas, and cystadenocarcinomas) where the tumor stimulates androgen secretion by the surrounding ovarian stroma.

Ovarian tumors may secrete a variety of hormones in addition to androgens, including estrogens, hCG, serotonin, and thyroxine (see Table 12–15). All choriocarcinomas, occasional dysgerminomas, and rare malignant ovarian teratomas secrete hCG.[582, 583] Primary ovarian carcinoids may produce serotonin in quantities sufficient to elevate 5-hydroxyindoleacetic acid excretion and produce the carcinoid syndrome[584–586] (see Chapter 35). Teratomas that contain

TABLE 12–14. Types of Insulin Resistance Associated with Hyperandrogenism and Acanthosis Nigricans

Kahn Type	Insulin Receptor Defect	Cause or Associated Disease	Hyperandrogenism
A	Defect intrinsic to insulin receptor, resulting in decreased function or decreased receptor number	Genetic or obesity	Often severe; virilization and ovarian stromal hyperthecosis common
B	Antibodies to insulin receptor	Autoimmune, collagen vascular disease	Mild to moderate
C	Receptor or postreceptor defect	Obesity	Moderate

From Barbieri RL, Smith S, Ryan KJ. The role of hyperinsulinemia in the pathogenesis of ovarian hyperandrogenism. Fertil Steril 1988; 50:197–212.

TABLE 12–15. Clinical Features of Hormone-Producing Ovarian Tumors

Tumor	Hormones Produced	Age in Years		Incidence of		Size in cm	Miscellaneous
		Peak	Range	Malignancy (%)	Bilaterality (%)		
Sex cord–stromal tumors							
Granulosa-theca cell tumors	Estrogen Androgens Progestogens	30–70	≤1–92	10–20	10–15	≤1–≥30	Most common functioning ovarian neoplasms
Androblastomas (Sertoli–Leydig cell tumors)	Androgens Estrogens	20–40	4–84	20	Rare	≥5–≤25	Most common virilizing tumors
Lipid cell tumors							
Hilar cell type	Androgens	45–75	4–86	Rare	Rare	0.5–15	
Adrenal cell type	Estrogens	20–25	6–78	20	Rare	0.5–30	Often associated with diabetes
Germ cell tumors							
Dysgerminomas Teratomas	Chorionic gonadotropin	10–30	4–76	100	5–10	3–50	
Carcinoids	Serotonin	50–70	36–79	Rare	Rare	≤1–15	Carcinoid syndrome may occur
Strumas	Thyroxine	30–60	21–69	Rare	Rare	5–20	May be clinically hyperthyroid (rare)
Mixed carcinoid and struma	Serotonin Thyroxine	40–60	21–77	Rare	None	≤1–26	
Choriocarcinomas	Chorionic gonadotropin	6–15	6–42	100	Rare		
Gonadoblastomas	Androgens Chorionic gonadotropin	10–30	6–36	50	40	≤1–≥30	Usually occur in male pseudohermaphrodites

hirsutism suggests an iatrogenic cause, or if associated with virilization, a tumor of the ovary or adrenal. The presence of acanthosis nigricans suggests the diagnosis of the HAIR-AN syndrome in association with PCOS/hyperthecosis. Clitorimegaly, as defined by a clitoral index (the product of the sagittal and transverse diameter of the glans) of greater than 35 mm², male-pattern baldness, and other virilizing signs suggest an ovarian or adrenal tumor.[593]

Useful laboratory tests in the diagnosis and management of androgen excess include measurement of serum testosterone and DHEAS levels. Serum testosterone is usually markedly elevated in ovarian causes of virilization, and DHEAS, which is derived primarily from the adrenal, is elevated in cases of virilization of adrenal origin. If mild to moderate hirsutism and normal or near-normal levels of testosterone and DHEAS are present, more extensive testing is not usually indicated if the history suggests PCOS. If there is a family history of adrenal hyperplasia or if the symptoms of hirsutism are more severe, basal 17-hydroxyprogesterone should be measured. Levels greater than 9 nmol/L (3 μg/L) suggest late-onset adrenal hyperplasia.[594] In some instances ACTH stimulation should be performed by measuring the change in levels of 17-hydroxyprogesterone before and after injection of ACTH.[571, 589, 595] A useful laboratory approach to the evaluation of androgen excess is presented in Figure 12–55.

The treatment of hirsutism is not ideal, in that cures are rarely possible. The therapeutic approach is directed first at decreasing the rate of androgen secretion or inhibiting androgen action in the pilosebaceous unit itself. Oral contraceptives are commonly used to treat ovarian causes of hirsutism. Other drugs that may be useful include LHRH analogues, antiandrogens (including spironolactone), and cyproterone acetate. Glucocorticoids are indicated if an adrenal enzyme defect such as 21-hydroxylase deficiency is present. (For a detailed discussion see under Drugs to Treat Hirsutism.)

After androgen secretion or androgen action is reduced, additional physical methods to remove hair may be instituted. These include temporary methods, such as shaving, depilatories, waxing, or tweezing, and permanent methods of hair removal (electrolysis). It should be pointed out that hormonal control requires 6 mo to 1 y to produce even partial clinical improvement in most cases. Surgical removal of the ovaries may be indicated in women with hyperthecosis

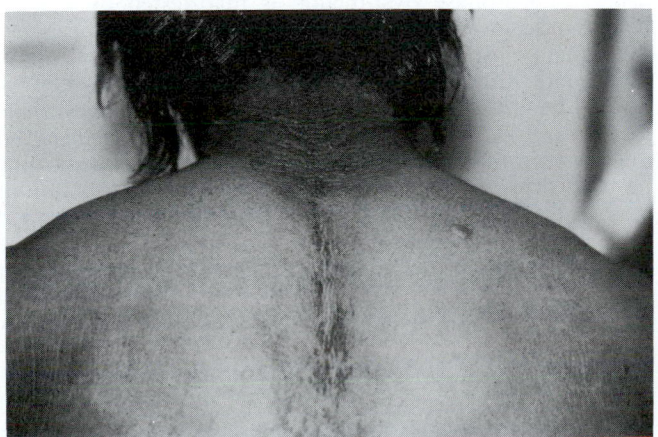

Figure 12–53. Acanthosis nigricans in a woman with insulin resistance and hyperandrogenism. Note the increased pigmentation of the neck. (Courtesy of Dr. R. Ann Word.)

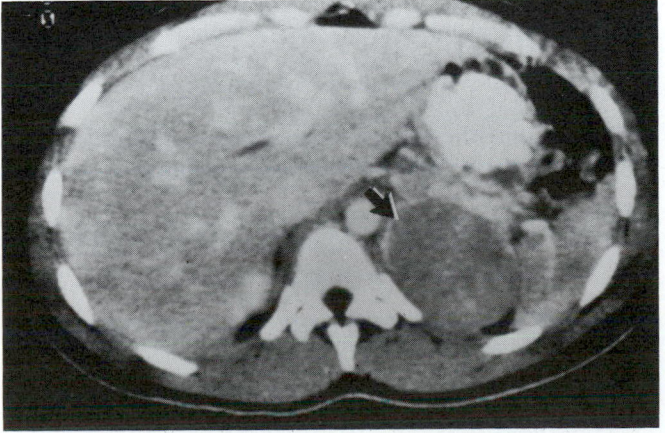

Figure 12–54. CT scan demonstrating an adrenal adenoma (arrow) of a woman with virilization. (See Fig. 12–51 for details.) (Courtesy of Dr. Karen D. Bradshaw.)

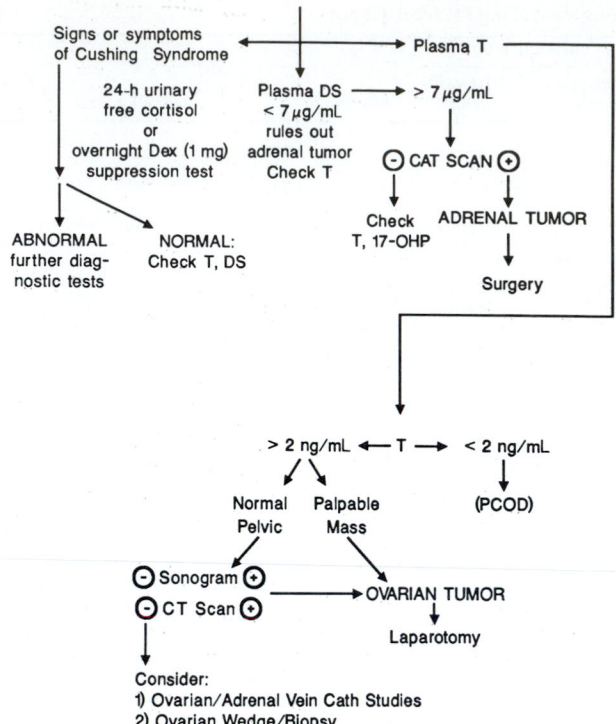

Figure 12–55. Laboratory tests and interpretations used in the evaluation of hirsutism and virilization. T, testosterone; 17-OHP, 17-hydroxyprogesterone; PCOD, polycystic ovary disease; Dex, dexamethasone; DS, dehydroepiandrosterone sulfate.

in whom childbearing is no longer desired and in whom severe hirsutism is unresponsive to standard therapy.

Infertility

Infertility, the failure to conceive after 1 y of unprotected intercourse, affects approximately 10 to 15% of couples and is one of the common complaints for which women seek gynecological care.[596] Male factors, which include decreased production and motility of spermatozoa, increased production of abnormal spermatozoa, ductal obstruction, abnormal or absent ejaculatory processes, and immunological factors, account for 40% of infertility problems (see Chapter 13). In women, ovulatory disorders account for 30%, pelvic factors (including tubal disease, uterine or cervical disease, and endometriosis) account for 50%, and immunological factors are implicated in 5% of infertility evaluations.[597] In 10 to 15% of women no etiology is found, and in about 20 to 30% of couples both male and female factors account for the infertility. The incidence of infertility increases with age, particularly in women (Table 12–16).[598]

The initial step in the evaluation of the infertile couple is to determine whether the man or the woman is the infertile partner, ordinarily by obtaining a semen analysis in the man

TABLE 12–16. The Percentage of Couples Conceiving in 12 Mo of Unprotected Intercourse Related to the Age of the Woman

Woman's Age (y)	% Conceiving in 12 Mo
20–24	86
25–29	78
30–34	63
35–39	52

Adapted from Hendershot GE, Mosher WD, Pratt WF. Infertility and age: an unresolved issue. Family Planning Perspectives. Volume 14: Number 5 (September/October 1982), p. 288. © The Alan Guttmacher Institute.

and documentation of presumed ovulation in the woman. A woman who has a history of regular, spontaneous, and cyclic menses is considered to be ovulatory. The presumptive diagnosis of ovulation is most easily and economically obtained by daily measurement of basal body temperatures throughout the month. A biphasic elevation of temperature of 0.22°C (0.4°F) during a luteal phase of at least 11 d is presumptive evidence of ovulation and a normal luteal phase. Occasionally, accurate basal body temperature records are not obtained, and other methods to evaluate ovulation are required. These methods include measurement of serum progesterone levels during the luteal phase, documentation of a secretory endometrium by biopsy, serial ultrasonographic studies to document follicular growth and subsequent rupture of a dominant follicle, and documentation of the LH surge by home urinary dipstick assay.[597]

If the infertility is associated with amenorrhea, then the work-up is the same as that described in Figure 12–50. If infertility is the result of anovulation caused by PCOS, ovulation can be induced, most commonly with clomiphene citrate. If ovulation is not induced with clomiphene citrate alone, combined treatment with clomiphene citrate and glucocorticoids (if serum androgen levels are elevated) or bromocriptine (if prolactin levels are slightly elevated) may be successful.[599, 600] Other agents to induce ovulation include hMG, urofollitropins (purified FSH), or pulsatile LHRH with or without concomitant LHRH analogues.[461, 467, 473, 496–498] Women with chronic anovulation with estrogen absent as a result of hypothalamic causes can be treated with hMG or pulsatile LHRH.[531–533] Bromocriptine is the treatment of choice to induce ovulation in women with amenorrhea and hyperprolactinemia;[545] on occasion, surgical removal or radiation therapy may be required for treatment of prolactinomas, as described previously.

Infertility may also be due to more subtle defects in folliculogenesis, including luteinized unruptured follicle syndrome, in which a mature follicle fails to rupture with entrapment of the ovum but the granulosa cells undergo luteinization.[601] This abnormality is usually diagnosed by serial ultrasonography. A spontaneous luteinized unruptured follicle may occur in as many as 10% of ovulations in normal fertile women.[216] The incidence appears to be similar in fertile and infertile women, so that at present this defect is not considered by all to be a syndrome or a cause of infertility, because most women do not exhibit repetitive luteinized unruptured follicle cycles.[601] Rupture of a follicle without release of an oocyte may also occur. Ovulation with inadequate luteinization and reduced progesterone secretion during the luteal phase has been termed *luteal-phase dysfunction*.[215] Luteal-phase dysfunction is manifested by a short luteal phase, in which the interval between the LH peak and subsequent onset of the menses is less than 10 d, or an inadequate luteal phase, in which the luteal phase is of normal length but is associated with reduced progesterone secretion.[602, 603] These types of luteal dysfunction are believed to cause infertility in about 5% of infertile women. Infertility in this disorder results from failure of implantation of fertilized ova as a result of an incompletely developed endometrium. Luteal-phase dysfunction is believed to be due to disorders of gonadotropin secretion with subsequent poor follicular development and reduced granulosa cell growth. This leads to reduced granulosa-lutein cells, low progesterone secretion, and reduced endometrial maturation during the luteal phase.[215, 222, 223] Luteal-phase dysfunction may occur sporadically in normal ovulating fertile women but is more frequent in women with hyperprolactinemia or in women who have experienced excessive exercise or weight loss and who are at the extremes of reproductive life. The diagnosis of the short luteal phase can be made by the basal body temperature chart, whereas the inadequate luteal phase is diagnosed by endometrial biopsy or measurement of serum progesterone. Although the interpretation of a single midluteal phase serum progesterone determination is fraught with difficulty, an inadequate luteal phase is rare in cycles where the value is greater than 50 nmol/L (15 µg/L).[222] Endometrial biopsy samples obtained from the uterine fundus in the late luteal phase should show results at least 2 d out of phase from those expected as determined by assessing the cycle length by the onset of the subsequent cycle or, more accurately, by the onset of the LH surge in at least two cycles.[253, 602]

Treatment of luteal-phase dysfunction varies depending on the cause and may include reduction of serum prolactin by bromocriptine, decrease in exercise, or weight gain regimens. Otherwise, follicular development may be stimulated with clomiphene citrate, gonadotropins, or progesterone replacement, usually by the administration of 25 mg of progesterone by vaginal suppositories twice daily.[215, 602]

The primary diagnostic test to evaluate tubal patency and the uterine cavity is the hysterosalpingogram.[336, 604] Further evaluation of tubal and ovarian disease can be obtained by the demonstration at diagnostic laparoscopy of dye spillage from the fimbria after transcervical injection.[342] Adhesions, filling defects, or abnormal shape of the uterus can be further evaluated and treated by operative hysteroscopy.[341] Treatment of occluded fallopian tubes or tubal ovarian adhesions by microsurgical techniques has resulted in improved pregnancy rates compared with standard macrosurgical approaches.[605, 606] If possible, adhesive disease and tubal occlusion are treated by operative laparoscopy, also called pelviscopic surgery, requiring multiple puncture sites utilizing a variety of surgical instruments, cautery, or laser.[607–610]

Endometriosis is defined by the presence and proliferation of endometrial tissue (glands and stroma) outside the endometrial cavity. The clinical manifestations are variable, but the diagnosis is often made at the time of diagnostic laparoscopy during an infertility evaluation. Although en-

dometriosis is not always associated with infertility, the fertility rate of women with moderate to severe endometriosis is reduced.[611, 612] Treatment of endometriosis associated with infertility includes operative laparoscopy with resection or ablation of endometriotic implants by cautery or laser; laparotomy with resection for more advanced disease; and temporary gonadal suppression using danazol (400 to 800 mg orally in divided doses), progestogens (medroxyprogesterone acetate, 10 to 20 mg/d by mouth), or LHRH agonists (leuprolide acetate, 3.75 mg given intramuscularly once a month, for a period usually up to 6 mo, or nafrelin acetate, 200 µg nasally twice a day).[612]

Infertility may be due to congenital anatomical defects or postsurgical scarring of the cervix. An additional problem is insufficient cervical mucus. Cervical mucus should be evaluated after coitus. The test is preferably performed at or near the time of ovulation as determined by a rise in urinary LH when the cervical mucus is thin. The aim is to evaluate penetration and survival of the sperm in the female reproductive tract. Standards of abnormality are not well defined, but a reduced number of motile sperm has been associated with a lower fertility rate in some but not all studies.[613, 614] If a cervical factor is suspected, the problem can be treated by intrauterine insemination utilizing the husband's sperm.[615, 616]

The role of antibodies to sperm in the female genital tract is controversial. Antisperm antibodies attached to sperm, as detected by immunobead testing, is associated with infertility in men. Treatment of sperm antibodies with glucocorticoids or other therapy is usually unsuccessful.[617, 618]

When standard treatment modalities for infertility caused by tubal obstructive disease, cervical factors, endometriosis, male factors, or unexplained infertility are unsuccessful, various assisted reproductive technologies including in vitro fertilization with embryo transfer (IVF-ET) have been successful.[619] Multiple follicles are stimulated by gonadotropin treatment and are subsequently aspirated at laparoscopy or under guidance by transvaginal ultrasonography (Fig. 12–56). After fertilization and cleavage in vitro, em-

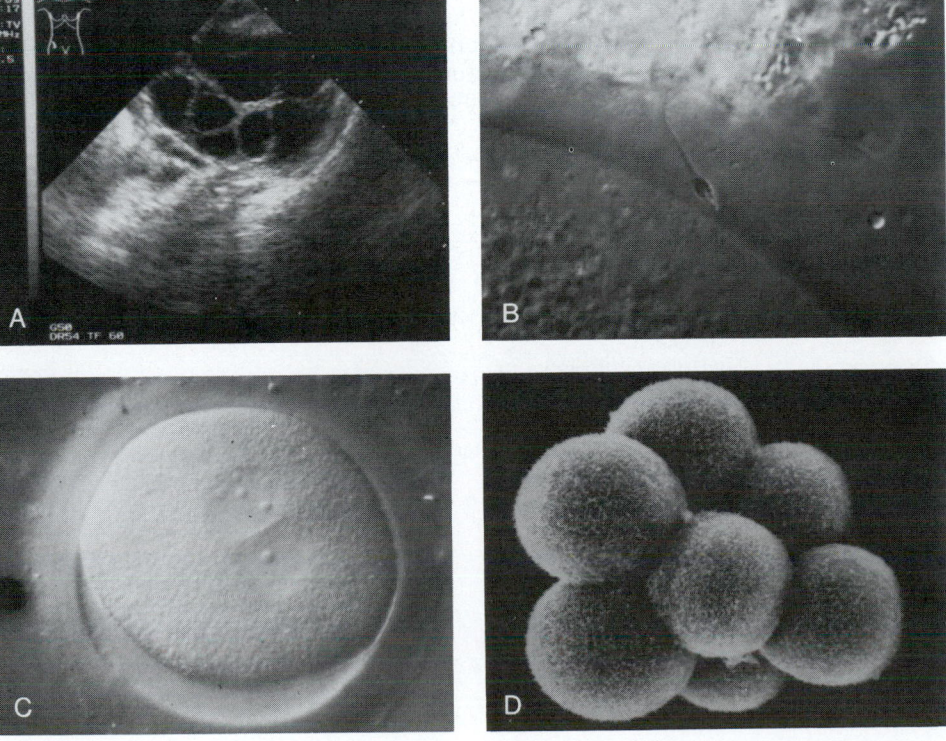

Figure 12–56. In vitro fertilization of a human oocyte. A, Ultrasonographic study of a gonadotropin-stimulated ovary demonstrating seven follicles. B, After aspiration of the follicles, ova are mixed with sperm; this figure demonstrates the attachment of sperm to the zona pellucida. C, The male and female pronuclei are present. D, A fertilized embryo ready for transfer to the uterus. (Courtesy of Dr. Karen D. Bradshaw and Dr. William Byrd.)

bryos are transferred to the uterine cavity by means of an intrauterine catheter. Although pregnancy rates vary, successful pregnancy has been reported to be as high as 30% per transfer. Term pregnancy at most centers averages 10%.[620] In women with patent fallopian tubes and infertility caused by male factors or unexplained reasons, gamete intrafallopian transfer (GIFT) or intrauterine insemination with washed sperm after stimulation with gonadotropins has resulted in pregnancy rates of 20% per cycle.[621, 622] Other technologies include zygote intrafallopian transfer (ZIFT) and pronuclear stage tubal transfer (PROST). The specific advantages of these procedures and their pregnancy rates compared with those of IVF-ET and gamete intrafallopian transfer are not known.[623, 624] Cryopreservation of embryos is now integrated into many IVF-ET programs, because often more than four to five eggs may be retrieved and fertilized. Because of the risk of multiple pregnancy no more than four to five embryos should be transferred to the uterus in one cycle. Frozen embryos can be transferred in subsequent cycles.[625] Oocyte donation using fresh or thawed embryos has been successful even in women who have ovarian failure as a result of gonadal dysgenesis or premature menopause, providing they are cycled with estrogen and progesterone before transfer.[234]

HORMONAL THERAPY

Gonadal Steroids

Progestogens

The primary use of progestogens is in conjunction with estrogen in the form of oral contraceptives (see Chapter 18). In addition, progestogens plus estrogens promote the full maturation of the endometrium in the therapy of hypogonadal premenopausal, as well as postmenopausal, women. In certain instances progestogen therapy is appropriate by itself. Indications include (1) induction of withdrawal bleeding in the diagnosis of amenorrhea, (2) fertility control (progestogen-only birth control pill), (3) inhibition of gonadotropin secretion in girls with precocious puberty or in the treatment of endometriosis, (4) treatment and prophylaxis of DUB and endometrial hyperplasia (PCOS), (5) treatment of infertility caused by luteal-phase dysfunction, and (6) palliative therapy for endometrial carcinoma.

Therapeutically useful progestogens include progesterone and synthetic progestogens. The routes of administration and doses of commonly used preparations are presented in Table 12–17. The potency of progestogens is determined from their ability to alter an estrogen-primed endometrium in animals or to induce withdrawal menstruation in women (see Chapter 18).[626] Progesterone is poorly absorbed by mouth but is well absorbed when given as a vaginal or rectal suppository (Fig. 12–57).[215] A micronized form of progesterone is absorbed orally.[627] Progesterone in oil given by injection results in higher peak plasma concentrations than those achieved by vaginal or rectal administration (see Fig. 12–57).[626]

The dosage of progestogens depends on the indication. For example, medroxyprogesterone acetate is given in a dose of 2.5 to 10 mg/d to menopausal women, 5 to 10 mg/d for a progestogen challenge, or 100 to 1000 mg/d for treatment of endometrial hyperplasia or carcinoma (see Table 12–17). Synthetic progestogens can be administered orally, intramuscularly, or transdermally.

The side effects of progestational therapy include amenorrhea, irregular bleeding or spotting, malaise, mild weight gain and edema, depression, hirsutism, acne, and adverse effects on lipoproteins (decreased HDL cholesterol and increased LDL cholesterol levels).[626] If side effects are severe, the dose may be decreased, or a different progestogen may be prescribed (see Table 12–17). Some synthetic progestogens (e.g., nortestosterone derivatives) are not recommended during pregnancy because of the potential risk of virilization of female embryos, but there is little evidence that progesterone itself is harmful.[628]

Estrogens

The primary use of estrogens in conjunction with progestogens is for fertility control in the form of oral contraceptives (see Chapter 18). Estrogens are also indicated for treatment of gonadal failure, for induction and maintenance of secondary sexual characteristics in hypogonadotropic premenopausal women, for hormone replacement therapy in postmenopausal women, for the management of DUB, for the preparation of the endometrium of hypogonadal women before donor egg and embryo transfer, and for treatment of carcinoma of the breast (see Chapter 33).

As with progestogens, therapeutically useful estrogens include naturally derived and synthetic estrogens (Table 12–

TABLE 12–17. Routes of Administration and Dosages of Commonly Used Progestogens

Progestogen	Route	Dosage* per Day (D) or Week (W)
Progesterone		
Progesterone suppositories	Vaginal	25–200 mg (D)
	Rectal	25–200 mg (D)
Progesterone in oil	Intramuscular	50–200 mg (D)
Micronized	Oral	100–300 mg (D)
17α-Hydroxy derivatives		
Medroxyprogesterone acetate	Oral	2.5–10 mg (D)
	Intramuscular	250–1000 mg (D,W)
Megestrol acetate	Oral	20–320 mg (D)
17α-Hydroxyprogesterone caproate	Intramuscular	125–250 mg (W)
19-Nortestosterone derivatives		
Ethynodiol diacetate	Oral	1 mg (D)
Norethindrone	Oral	0.35–10 mg (D)
Norethindrone acetate	Oral	1.0–10 mg (D)
Norethynodrel	Oral	2.5–5 mg (D)
Norgesterel	Oral	0.3–0.5 mg (D)
Levonorgesterel	Oral	0.075–0.5 mg (D)
Halogenated progesterone		
Cyproterone acetate	Oral	10–50 mg (D)
Retroprogesterone		
Dydrogesterone	Oral	5–20 mg (D)

*See Physicians' Desk Reference (Oradell, NJ: Medical Economics Company, 1991) for specific dose per indication.

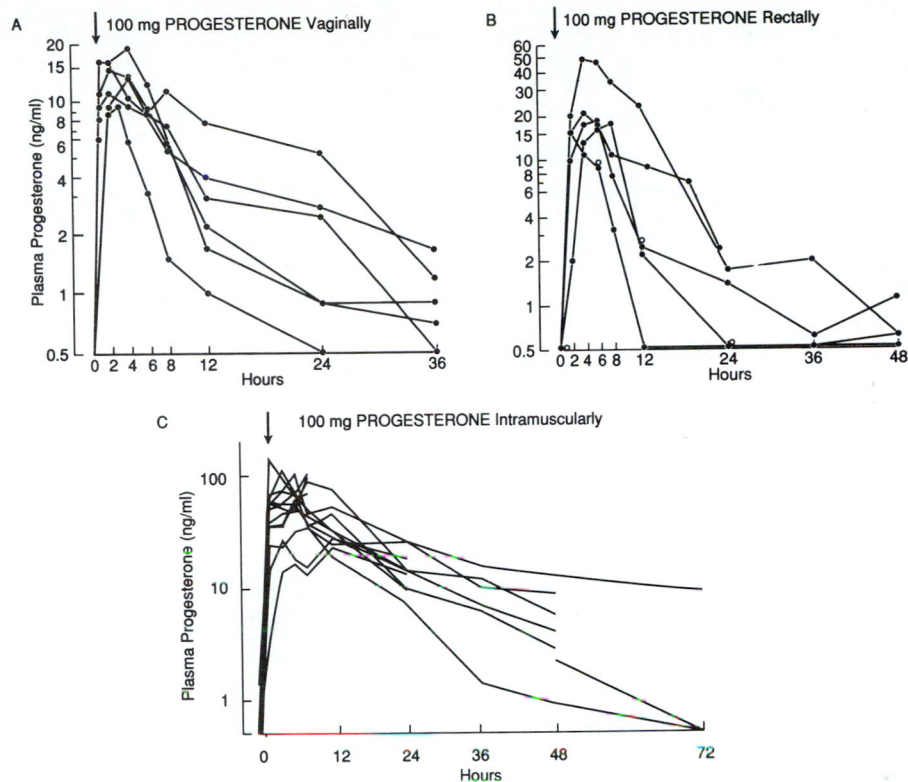

Figure 12–57. Plasma levels of progesterone after 100 mg of progesterone given by vaginal suppository (A), rectal suppository (B), or intramuscular injection in oil (C). Arrows denote time of institution of therapy by various routes. (Adapted from Nillius SJ, Johansson EDB. Plasma levels of progesterone after vaginal, rectal or intramuscular administration of progesterone. Am J Obstet Gynecol 1971; 110:470–477.)

18). Natural estrogens include estrone, estradiol, and conjugated equine estrogens. Estrogens are most often administered by mouth, but they can also be administered effectively by vaginal, intranasal, intramuscular, intravenous, and transdermal routes.[629]

When given by mouth, estrone sulfate, estradiol valerate, and micronized estradiol result in higher plasma levels of estrone than of estradiol (Fig. 12–58).[630, 631] This feature is due to the fact that estradiol is converted to estrone in the intestinal mucosa.[632] Further metabolism of estrogen occurs in the liver.[633] In contrast, the administration of estradiol vaginally or by transdermal or intramuscular injection results in higher levels in plasma of estradiol than estrone, because

the intestinal metabolism of orally administered estrogens is bypassed.[634–636] Maximal serum estrogen levels after oral ingestion are reached in 4 to 6 h.[637] Oral intake of 0.625 mg conjugated equine estrogens, 1.25 mg estrone sulfate, or 1.0 mg of micronized estradiol results in similar peak levels of estrogens (estradiol, 110 to 150 pmol/L [30 to 40 pg/mL]; estrone, 550 to 920 pmol/L [150 to 250 pg/mL]).[638] Circulating levels of estrogen after vaginal administration are about one fourth those observed with equivalent doses given by mouth.[639] Transdermal administration of estradiol with a patch applied every 3 to 4 d provides controlled and constant levels of estradiol (Fig. 12–59).[634]

The only estrogens used in contraceptives are synthetic

Table 12–18. Routes of Administration and Dosages of Commonly Used Estrogens

Estrogens	Route	Dosage* per Day (D) or Month (M)
Natural and equine estrogens		
Conjugated equine estrogens	Oral	0.3–2.5 mg (D)
	Intramuscular	25 mg (D)
	Intravenous	25 mg (D)
	Vaginal	2–4 g (D)
Piperazine estrone sulfate	Oral	0.625–2.5 mg (D)
	Vaginal	2–4 g (D)
Estradiol	Patch	0.05–0.1 mg†
	Vaginal	1–4 g (D)
Micronized, valerate	Oral	1–2 mg (D)
Valerate	Intramuscular	10 mg (M)
Cypionate	Intramuscular	1–5 mg (M)
Synthetic estrogens		
Ethinyl estradiol	Oral	20–50 μg (D)
Mestranol	Oral	50–100 μg (D)
Diethylstilbestrol	Oral	1–5 mg (D)
Quinestrol	Oral	0.1 mg (D)

*See Physicians' Desk Reference (Oradell, NJ: Medical Economics Company, 1991) for specific dose per indication.
†Every 3–4 d.

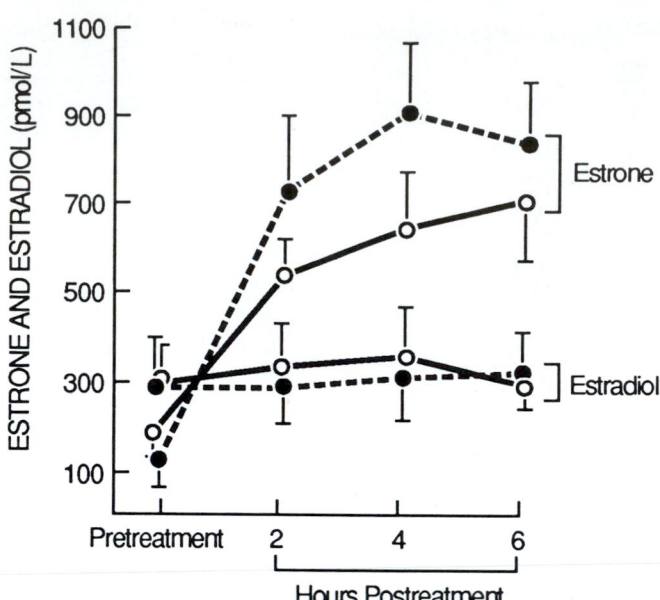

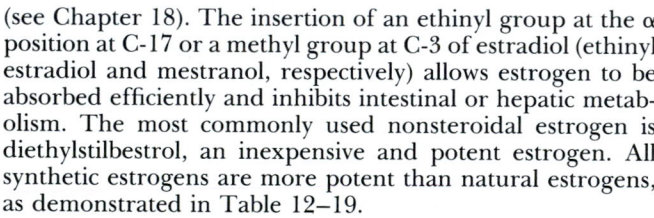

Figure 12–58. Mean serum concentrations of estradiol and estrone 2 to 6 h after oral administration of estradiol valerate (●) or piperazine estrone sulfate (○). (Adapted from Anderson ABM, Sklovsky E, Sayers L, et al. Comparison of serum oestrogen concentrations in post-menopausal women taking oestrone sulphate and oestradiol. Br Med J 1978; 1:140–142.)

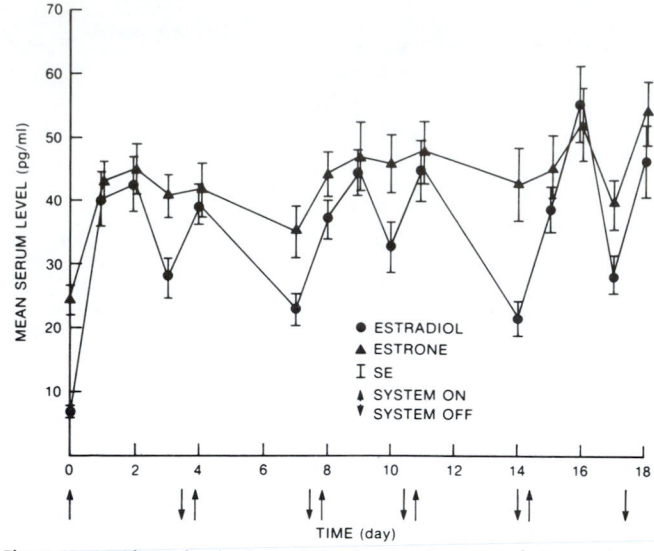

Figure 12–59. Plasma levels of estradiol and estrone in women during continuous use of an estradiol patch (0.05 mg). Arrows designate initiation and replacement of estradiol patches. To convert estrogen values to picomoles per liter, multiply by 3.671. To convert estrone values to picomoles per liter, multiply by 3.699. (From Powers MS, Schenkel L, Darley PE, et al. Pharmacokinetics and pharmacodynamics of transdermal dosage forms of 17β-estradiol: comparison with conventional oral estrogens used for hormone replacement. Am J Obstet Gynecol 1985; 152:1099–1106.)

(see Chapter 18). The insertion of an ethinyl group at the α position at C-17 or a methyl group at C-3 of estradiol (ethinyl estradiol and mestranol, respectively) allows estrogen to be absorbed efficiently and inhibits intestinal or hepatic metabolism. The most commonly used nonsteroidal estrogen is diethylstilbestrol, an inexpensive and potent estrogen. All synthetic estrogens are more potent than natural estrogens, as demonstrated in Table 12–19.

The contraindications to estrogen therapy are similar to those for oral contraceptives (see Chapter 18). Minor side effects include breast tenderness, nausea, vomiting, and mild weight gain. In these instances, the dose of estrogen may be lowered, or for gastrointestinal symptoms, alternative routes (vaginal or transdermal) may be tried.

Androgens

There are no clearly defined indications for androgen therapy in women. A few investigators have advocated androgens for treatment of menopausal symptoms and decreased libido, but in view of the side effects such as hirsutism and male-pattern baldness and the potential for increasing the risk of heart disease, such therapy is probably never indicated.

Indications for Gonadal Steroids

HYPOESTROGENEMIA. In women with decreased estrogen production, whether caused by diseases of the ovaries (gonadal dysgenesis) or by hypogonadotropic hypogonadism, treatment with cyclic estrogen plus a progestogen should be instituted at the time of expected puberty for the promotion and maintenance of female sexual characteristics, prevention of osteoporosis, and, hopefully, prevention of premature atherosclerotic heart disease.[640] The most commonly used medications are conjugated estrogens (0.625 mg to 1.25 mg/d by mouth), ethinyl estradiol (0.02 to 0.1 mg/d by mouth), micronized estradiol (1 mg/d by mouth), and transdermal estrogen (0.05 to 0.1 mg by patch every 3 to 4 d). The addition of a progestogen (medroxyprogesterone acetate, 5 to 10 mg) is recommended during the last 10 to 14 d of estrogen treatment each month to prevent development of endometrial hyperplasia. Women treated with such regimens experience withdrawal bleeding after cessation of hormone therapy at the end of each month. In women receiving these forms of hormone replacement, abnormal uterine bleeding at other times during the cycle requires histological evaluation of the endometrium. If the endometrial biopsy reveals proliferative changes or hyper-

Table 12–19. Relative Potency of Drugs According to Four Specific Measures of Estrogenicity

Estrogen Preparation	Serum FSH	Serum CBG-BC*	Serum SHBG-BC†	Serum Angiotensinogen
Piperazine estrone sulfate	1.0	1.0	1.0	1.0
Conjugated estrogens	1.4	2.5	3.2	3.5
Micronized estradiol	1.3	1.9	1.0	0.7
Diethylstilbestrol	3.8	7.9	2.8	13
Ethinyl estradiol	80–200	1000	624	232

*Corticosteroid-binding globulin–binding capacity.
†Sex hormone–binding globulin–binding capacity.
From Mashchak CA, Lobo RA, Dozono-Takano R, et al. Comparison of pharmacodynamic properties of various estrogen formulations. Am J Obstet Gynecol 1982; 144:511–518.

plasia, the dose of progestogen is increased, and the endometrium is rebiopsied in a subsequent cycle. An alternative form of therapy for treatment of hypoestrogenemia is oral contraceptives. Oral contraceptives are useful in the treatment of PCOS to control abnormal bleeding and in the treatment of hirsutism to suppress ovarian androgen secretion.

Temporary administration of estrogens in larger quantities (up to two times the usual dosage) may be necessary in pubertal girls to induce full development of secondary sexual characteristics and in older women for the control of menopausal symptoms. Occasionally, high doses of oral contraceptives or parenteral estrogens may be required for brief periods in the treatment of DUB, as discussed previously. In contrast, low doses of estrogen (100 ng/kg body weight) may stimulate bone growth in women with gonadal dysgenesis.[440]

MENOPAUSE. Estrogen replacement is successful in treating the symptoms of menopause (vasomotor symptoms and vaginal atrophy) and in reducing the risk of osteoporosis and atherosclerotic heart disease. In postmenopausal women who have undergone a hysterectomy, therapy should be with estrogen alone. The major problem is how to treat the postmenopausal woman with a uterus. The addition of a progestogen, either cyclically or continuously, to concomitant estrogen therapy reduces the risk of estrogen-induced hyperplasia or carcinoma but poses additional problems (namely, withdrawal bleeding in up to 80% of women treated with cyclic therapy or irregular spotting in women treated with continuous estrogen plus progestogen). Furthermore, progestogens appear to negate, in part, the beneficial effects of estrogen in preventing atherosclerotic heart disease (decreased HDL cholesterol, increased LDL cholesterol). Approaches to these problems and indications for endometrial biopsy are discussed later.

The menopause is not associated with a simple state of estrogen deprivation, because some estrogens continue to be produced, especially in obese women. The predominant estrogen is estrone formed by extraglandular conversion of adrenal androgens. Because estrone is a weak estrogen, most menopausal women are biologically hypoestrogenic. As is true for all estrogen therapy, treatment of the menopause, whether by replacement of estradiol or by replacement of other estrogens, does not duplicate the changes in plasma estrogen observed in the normal menstrual cycle. Estrogens recommended for replacement therapy in the postmenopausal women are the natural estrogens, including estradiol itself, conjugated equine estrogens, and estrone sulfate, which are given orally or in estrogen-containing vaginal creams or transdermal estradiol patches.[636]

The most common indication and the most proven benefit of estrogen therapy in the menopause is for the relief of vasomotor symptoms (hot flushes) and prevention or treatment of atrophy of the urogenital epithelium and skin.[304, 641] Estrogen therapy usually ameliorates these symptoms. When estrogen therapy is designed to treat hot flushes alone, such therapy should be continued only for a few years, because hot flushes tend to diminish after 2 to 5 y in untreated women.[308] Estrogen therapy of all forms is successful in treating vaginal atrophy and dryness.

Estrogen therapy is also beneficial in preventing the complications of osteoporosis, especially in high-risk women (i.e., thin white women)[305, 311–314] (see Chapter 28). This is especially true in women who have undergone premature menopause, women with gonadal dysgenesis, and those with premenopausal hypogonadotropic hypogonadism, in all of whom the incidence and complications of osteoporosis are increased. In normal menopause, estrogen therapy also prevents the loss of bone, slows the progress of osteoporosis, and reduces the risk of fractures of the hip, radius, and vertebrae.[641] To be effective for the prevention of osteoporosis, lifelong therapy is indicated. The minimal effective doses of oral estrogen that reduce the loss of bone and the incidence of fracture are 0.625 mg/d of conjugated equine estrogens, 0.625 mg/d of estrone sulfate, or 0.02 mg/d of ethinyl estradiol.[640] The effective doses of other oral estrogens, transdermal estrogen, and vaginal estrogens to prevent osteoporosis have not been clearly determined.

Estrogen replacement therapy changes the lipid profiles of older women (Table 12–20).[307, 642] The rise in HDL cholesterol and the lowering of LDL cholesterol may be beneficial in the prevention of atherosclerotic heart disease. Indeed, the risk of coronary heart disease appears to be less in estrogen-treated postmenopausal women as reported in both retrospective and prospective studies.[306, 307, 643] Unfortunately, progestogens have effects opposite to those of estrogen on the lipid profiles (see Table 12–20), and consequently progestogens should be prescribed at the lowest doses required to prevent endometrial hyperplasia. The risk of heart disease in women treated with estrogen plus progestogen is not known.

Of the potential deleterious side effects of estrogen therapy, the possibility of endometrial adenocarcinoma is the most worrisome. The relative risk of developing endometrial carcinoma in women using estrogen alone is between 6 and 8, but the actual incidence of endometrial cancer in estrogen users is low (100 to 200 per 100,000 woman-years).[644, 645] The risk is increased with duration and dosage of estrogen and is decreased in women given estrogen plus progestogen.[626] Women treated with estrogens alone who develop endometrial carcinoma have longer life expectancies than women who develop endometrial carcinoma and who never received estrogen therapy.[646]

Apprehension concerning the worsening of hypertension and thromboembolic disease appears to be due to reports associated with the use of estrogen-progestogen oral contraceptives, and such worsening does not appear to be true for estrogen use in menopausal women. There is no

Table 12–20. One-Year Prospective Study of the Effect of Estrogen and Cyclic Progestogen on Serum Lipids in Postmenopausal Women

Lipids	% Change from Pretreatment at 12 Mo			
	0.625 mg CEE,* 5 mg MPA†	0.625 mg CEE, Placebo	1.25 mg CEE, 5 mg MPA	1.25 mg CEE, Placebo
Triglycerides	↑ 39.0	↑ 34.0	↑ 42.0	↑ 19.0
Cholesterol	↓ 2.0	↑ 5.5	↓ 0.1	↓ 5.0
HDL	↑ 4.3	↑ 13.7	↑ 13.4	↑ 19.0
LDL	↓ 3.4	↓ 0.3	↓ 8.3	↓ 17.6
HDL/LDL	↑ 7.3	↑ 13.6	↑ 24.0	↑ 43.0

*Conjugated equine estrogens.
†Medroxyprogesterone acetate.
Adapted from Sherwin BB, Gelfand MM. A prospective one-year study of estrogen and progestogen in postmenopausal women: effects on clinical symptoms and lipoprotein lipids. Reprinted with permission from The American College of Obstetricians and Gynecologists (Obstetrics and Gynecology, vol. 73, 1989, pp. 759–766).

evidence that estrogen therapy in menopausal women increases the risk of hypertension; estrogen therapy can be administered to postmenopausal women with well-controlled hypertension.[647] Low-dose estrogen therapy also does not increase the incidence of thrombophlebitis, pulmonary embolism, or stroke in menopausal women. There is a slightly increased risk for the development of gallbladder disease with estrogen use during the menopause.[648]

The breast is a major target organ for estrogen, and some breast tumors are estrogen responsive (see Chapter 33). There is evidence both for and against a relationship between dose and duration of estrogen therapy and the development of breast cancer.[649–655] Based on all available data, however, long-term administration of estrogen in the doses commonly used in menopausal women does not appear to increase the risk of breast cancer substantially. Nevertheless, estrogen therapy should not be instituted if pre-existing breast disease is present and should be discontinued if malignant breast disease develops.

Whether estrogens should be given routinely in all postmenopausal women is unsettled, but evidence is accumulating that the benefits of estrogen for the prevention of complications of osteoporosis and probably for heart disease significantly outweigh the risks so that all women without contraindications to estrogen therapy should be considered to be candidates for treatment. For long-term use estrogens should be given in the minimally effective dose (0.625 mg conjugated estrogen, 0.625 mg estrone sulfate, or 1 mg of micronized estradiol). Vaginal and transdermal estrogens likely are equally effective in reducing fractures and preventing coronary heart disease, but these benefits have not been demonstrated directly. Recommended regimens of estrogen therapy include continuous daily use or cyclic replacement by prescribing estrogens for 25 d each month followed by a 5- to 6-d period of rest. For women with an intact uterus, the addition of a progestogen in cyclic fashion (medroxyprogesterone acetate, 5 to 10 mg for the last 10 to 14 d of estrogen therapy) or continuous low-dose progestogen (medroxyprogesterone acetate, 2.5 mg given daily) is usually prescribed to prevent endometrial hyperplasia. The continuous therapy has the potential benefit of reduced bleeding and amenorrhea but is occasionally complicated by breakthrough bleeding. Similar therapy is indicated in women with premature menopause. In women who have prior hysterectomy, progestogens are not recommended because they have adverse effects on serum lipids.

Each woman receiving estrogen alone or combined with progestogens must be monitored indefinitely, at a minimum at yearly intervals. Endometrial sampling is required before initiation of therapy, at yearly intervals, and when any uterine bleeding occurs in women who refuse progestogens or who experience unacceptable side effects of progestogens and are treated with estrogens alone. Sampling is also required before initiation of therapy in women treated with estrogen plus a progestogen given cyclically (10 to 14 d/mo) or if bleeding occurs at other times than expected (after cessation of the last dose of progestogen). In women treated with estrogen plus continuous progestogen, a biopsy should be obtained if irregular bleeding occurs. If no unexpected bleeding occurs in women treated with estrogen plus a progestogen given cyclically or continuously, a consensus has not been reached as to the frequency of endometrial sampling, although most advocate a biopsy at 2- to 3-y intervals.

Drugs to Induce Ovulation

The use of clomiphene citrate has replaced ovarian wedge resection as the initial therapy to induce ovulation in women with chronic anovulation and estrogen present (PCOS) who experience withdrawal menstrual bleeding after a progestogen challenge. There is little evidence to suggest that clomiphene treatment increases fertility of the infertile woman who is ovulating.

Clomiphene citrate is an antiestrogen and acts by binding to estrogen receptors and blocking estrogen action in the hypothalamus. The drug causes a rise of plasma FSH, stimulation of follicular development, and ovulation.[656] Clomiphene citrate therapy is usually initiated in a dose of 50 mg by mouth daily for 5 d commencing on the fifth day of progestogen-induced uterine bleeding. Presumptive evidence for ovulation is obtained by documenting a rise in basal body temperature, elevated progesterone levels in the luteal phase, secretory endometrium by biopsy, or ultrasonographic demonstration of collapse of a dominant follicle. If ovulation does not occur, the dose of clomiphene is serially increased by 50-mg increments up to 150 mg/d for 5 d. Some have suggested increasing the dose up to 250 mg or extending the length of therapy, but results are often unsuccessful.[656] Such therapy results in ovulation in 60 to 80% of anovulatory women and pregnancy rates of 30 to 50%.[473, 656] If ovulation does not occur on the 150-mg dose, a variety of clomiphene combinations or other treatments may be used (Table 12–21). Most women with PCOS ovulate on one or more of the regimens listed, but the percentage of women who conceive is variable. In women with PCOS who fail to ovulate with these methods, a wedge resection may be attempted, but the chance of successful ovulation or pregnancy is low. When a woman successfully ovulates but does not conceive while taking clomiphene citrate, other factors for infertility should be evaluated. Side effects of clomiphene citrate include multiple pregnancy (5 to 7%), persistant ovarian cysts, vasomotor symptoms, and occasionally visual symptoms. If these symptoms occur, the dose of clomiphene citrate should be lowered or other drugs should be used to induce ovulation.

hMG and hCG are used for women who fail to ovulate while taking clomiphene citrate and for women with hypogonadotropic hypogonadism who do not bleed after a progestogen challenge.[531, 532] Urofollitropin (FSH) may be used in place of hMG in women with PCOS.[657] The usual regimen is a schedule requiring 150 to 450 IU of hMG (1 to 3 ampules) or urofollitropin per day given intramuscularly over an 8- to 12-d period to achieve adequate follicular stimulation and growth, followed by a single injection of 5000 to 10,000 U of hCG 12 to 24 h after the last injection of hMG or urofollitropin. Ovulation is successful in 90% of hydrogonadotropic women, and pregnancy rates exceed 50 to 60%.[656] Measurement of daily estrogen levels and frequent evaluation of follicular development are required. Side effects of gonadotropin therapy include the ovarian hyperstimulation syndrome, in which excessive stimulation of ovarian follicles with resultant enlargement of the ovaries may progress to the development of ascites, hypotension,

Table 12–21. Drugs for Inducing Ovulation in Women with PCOS Who Fail to Ovulate When Given Clomiphene Citrate Alone

Clomiphene citrate combinations
  Clomiphene citrate + hCG
  Clomiphene citrate + estrogen
  Clomiphene citrate + glucocorticoids
  Clomiphene citrate + hMG + hCG
  Bromocriptine + clomiphene citrate
hMG + hCG
Gonadorelin (pulsatile LHRH)
Urofollitropin (pure FSH) + hCG
LHRH agonist + hMG, FSH, or pulsatile LHRH + hCG

and shock.[658] Gonadotropin therapy also carries a 20% risk of multiple pregnancies.[659]

Bromocriptine is a dopamine antagonist that is effective in inducing ovulation in women with elevated prolactin levels, including women with known pituitary prolactinomas. Treatment is instituted at an oral dose of 2.5 mg daily with gradual increase to 2.5 mg three times daily. Each dose should be taken with a meal. Dosage should be increased until prolactin is in the normal range. Treatment is discontinued as soon as pregnancy is diagnosed. The risk of pituitary growth during pregnancy in women with microadenomas is low, but up to 30% of women with macroadenomas develop neurological symptoms.[557] If a woman with a preexisting macroadenoma develops pituitary enlargement during pregnancy, bromocriptine therapy may be reinstituted and is often successful. Because of the high rate of development of symptoms in women with macroadenomas, some have advocated surgical or radiation treatment before attempting pregnancy or maintenance of bromocriptine treatment throughout pregnancy[554–557] (also see Chapter 6). There is no increase in complications of pregnancy or birth defects in children of women treated with bromocriptine either before or during pregnancy.[660] Long-term follow-up of children exposed to bromocriptine during pregnancy has revealed normal growth and development.[661, 662] Side effects of bromocriptine include nausea and hypotension. In women with severe nausea, bromocriptine may be given vaginally in doses of 2.5 mg three times per day.[663]

Gonadorelin (LHRH) has been used successfully to induce ovulation in hypogonadotropic women. Gonadorelin is infused subcutaneously or intravenously by a portable infusion pump that administers pulses in doses of 5 to 25 mg at 90- to 120-min intervals for 10 to 20 d. Gonadorelin promotes a "physiological" cycle in that usually only one follicle develops and the risk of multiple pregnancy is rare.[553, 664] Side effects are minimal, but inflammation or infection may occur at the site of infusion. Rates of ovulation approximate 90%, and the rate of successful pregnancy is equivalent to that observed for gonadotropins (50 to 60%).[664]

Drugs to Treat Hirsutism

Because abnormal hair growth can be caused either by excess androgen secretion or by increased sensitivity to androgens, treatment is aimed at lowering plasma levels of androgens or inhibiting androgen action in the hair follicle.

Oral Contraceptives

The most commonly used therapy for the treatment of hirsutism is the oral contraceptive pill.[499] Oral contraceptives lower androgen levels primarily by inhibiting LH release[249, 499] (see Chapter 18). They also increase TeBG levels, resulting in a disproportionate decrease in free testosterone.[665, 666] In addition, oral contraceptives suppress adrenal androgens (DHEAS), possibly by lowering plasma ACTH secretion.[249, 667–673]

High-dose oral contraceptive pills containing mestranol (75 μg) plus norethynodrel (5 mg) are effective in treating hirsutism; however, because of potential risks and side effects of this medication, this form of therapy is no longer recommended. Low-dose oral contraceptives containing norethindrone are effective in lowering testosterone (total and free) and DHEAS.[666, 670, 673] For this reason, low-dose oral contraceptives containing 35 μg or less of ethinyl estradiol are recommended in hirsutism caused by ovarian or combined ovarian/adrenal hyperandrogenism. Patients should be cautioned that therapy will need to be continued indefinitely and that 6 mo to 1 y may be required before any observable decrease in hair growth occurs.[500, 674] The goal of oral contraceptive treatment is to arrest further hair growth. Existing hairs will not disappear with hormone suppression alone, and physical methods such as electrolysis or shaving are required to remove existing hair. Treatment should be started at the earliest possible time.

Antiandrogens

The most widely used antiandrogens for the treatment of hirsutism are spironolactone (100 to 200 mg/d by mouth) and cyproterone acetate (50 to 100 mg/d by mouth). Both act primarily by blocking androgen effects at the pilosebaceous unit by competing with testosterone for the androgen receptor.[674–676] Cyproterone acetate also inhibits LH levels, whereas spironolactone inhibits P-450 enzymes involved in ovarian and adrenal steroidogenesis.[676, 677] Cyproterone acetate is not available for use in the United States but is used extensively in other countries in doses of 10 to 100 mg/d combined with low-dose oral contraceptives.[677] Side effects of spironolactone include cramping and diarrhea, drowsiness, rash, and gastritis. Side effects of cyproterone acetate include weight gain, fatigue, nausea, headaches, mastodynia, and the possibility of adrenal suppression.

Glucocorticoids

Two glucocorticoids, dexamethasone (0.25 to 0.5 mg) and prednisone (2.5 mg) given as an oral dose at bedtime, have been used for hirsutism of adrenal origin.[674] These doses are effective in women with adult-onset congenital adrenal hyperplasia, but higher doses are required in women with hirsutism typical of congenital adrenal hyperplasia. The risks of glucocorticoids include overdosage (Cushing syndrome) and adrenal suppression.

Other Treatments

LHRH analogues are potentially useful for treatment of hirsutism.[674] Routes of administration include nasal, subcutaneous, and depot forms (see later). Ketoconazole, an imidazole derivative, inhibits P-450–linked steroidogenic enzymes (principally 17α-hydroxylase) and lowers serum androgen levels in hirsute women.[678–680] A dose of 400 mg/d given orally is effective in women with PCOS, whereas 1000 mg/d may be required for those with hyperthecosis.[679, 680] Because of side effects that include gastrointestinal complaints, pruritus, and alterations in hepatic function, the widespread use of ketoconazole for the treatment of hirsute women will probably be limited.

LHRH Analogues

Inhibition of gonadotropin release to the point of hypogonadism may be produced by LHRH agonists or antagonists. The agonist gonadorelin requires continuous infusion, whereas long-acting agonists such as leuprolide acetate or antagonists can be given once daily. These agents have been used for fertility control and treatment of precocious puberty, endometriosis, leiomyomas, and hirsutism. They may be combined with gonadotropins to induce ovulation or for in vitro fertilization stimulation protocols.[681] Leuprolide can be administered subcutaneously daily or monthly in long-acting depot forms.[682] Nafrelin is an LHRH agonist available for use in a nasal spray two or three times a day.[683] Side effects of such therapy are those expected for hypogonadism, including hot flushes, vaginal dryness and atrophy, negative calcium balance with potential risk of bone loss, and possibly alteration in lipid profiles.[684] Because of these side effects, treatment is limited to a maximum of 6 mo.

REFERENCES

1. Gillman J. The development of the gonads in man, with a consideration of the whole fetal endocrines and the histogenesis of ovarian tumors. Contrib Embryol Carnegie Inst Wash 1948; 32:67–80.
2. Ohno S, Klinger HP, Atkin WB. Human oogenesis. Cytogenetics 1962; 1:42–51.
3. Lyon MF. Gene action in the X-chromosome of the mouse (Mus musculus). Nature 1961; 190:372–373.
4. Alvarez-Buylla A, Merchant-Larios H. Mouse primordial germ cells use fibronectin as a substrate for migration. Exp Cell Res 1986; 165:362–368.
5. Kuwana T, Maeda-Suga H, Fujimoto T. Attraction of chick primordial germ cells by gonadal anlage in vitro. Anat Rec 1986; 215:403–406.
6. Witschi E. Migration of the germ cells of human embryos from the yolksac to the primitive gonadal fold. Contrib Embryol 1948; 32:67–80.
7. Baker TG. A quantitative and cytological study of germ cells in the human ovaries. Proc R Soc Lond [Biol] 1963; 158:417–433.
8. Wartenberg H. Development of the early human ovary and the role of the mesonephrose in the differentiation of the cortex. Anat Embryol 1982; 165:253–280.
9. Singh RP, Carr DH. The anatomy and histology of XO human embryos and fetuses. Anat Rec 1966; 155:369–375.
10. Baker TG, Scrimgeous JB. Development of the gonad in normal and anencephalic human fetuses. J Reprod Fertil 1980; 60:193–199.
11. Guylas BJ, Hodgen GD, Tullner WW, et al. Effects of fetal and maternal hypophysectomy on endocrine organs and body weight in infant monkey (Macaca mulatta) with particular emphasis on oogenesis. Biol Reprod 1977; 16:216–227.
12. Byskov AG, Hoyer PE. Embryology of mammalian gonads and ducts. In: Knobil E, Neill JD, eds. The Physiology of Reproduction. Vol 1. New York: Raven, 1988: 265–302.
13. Baker TG, Franchi LL. The fine structure of oogonia and oocytes in human ovaries. J Cell Sci 1967; 2:213–224.
14. Byskov AG. Regulation of meiosis in mammals. Ann Biol Anim Biochim Biophys 1979; 19:1251–1261.
15. Tsafriri A, Dekel N, Bar-Ami S. The role of oocyte maturation inhibitor in follicular regulation of oocyte maturation. J Reprod Fertil 1982; 64:541–551.
16. Peters H, Byskov AG, Grinsted J. Follicular growth in fetal and prepubertal ovaries in humans and other primates. Clin Endocrinol Metab 1978; 7:469–485.
17. George FW, Wilson JD. Conversion of androgen to estrogen by the human fetal ovary. J Clin Endocrinol Metab 1978; 47:550–555.
18. Jungman RA, Schweppe JS. Biosynthesis of steroids and steroids from acetate-14C by human fetal ovaries. J Clin Endocrinol Metab 1968; 28:1599–1604.
19. Molsberry RL, Carr BR, Mendelson CR, et al. Human chorionic gonadotropin binding to human fetal testes as a function of gestational age. J Clin Endocrinol Metab 1982; 55:791–794.
20. Wilson EA, Jawad MJ. The effect of trophic agents on fetal ovarian steroidogenesis in organ culture. Fertil Steril 1979; 32:73–79.
21. Miller W. Molecular biology of steroid hormone synthesis. Endocr Rev 1988; 9:295–311.
22. O'Rahilly R. The embryology and anatomy of the uterus. In: Norris HJ, Hertig AT, Abell MR, eds. The Uterus. Baltimore: Williams & Wilkins, 1973: 17–39.
23. Wehefritz E. Systematische Gewichtsuntersuchungen am Ovarien mit Berucksichtigung anderen Drusen mit inner Sekretion. Z Gest Anat 1923; 9:161.
24. Peters H, McNatty KP. The Ovary. Berkeley: University of California Press, 1980: 12–34.
25. Faiman C, Winter JSD, Reyes FI. Patterns of gonadotropins and gonadal steroids throughout life. Clin Obstet Gynecol 1976; 3:467–483.
26. Kaplan SL, Grumbach MM, Aubert ML. The ontogenesis of pituitary hormones and hypothalamic factors in the human fetus: maturation of the central nervous system regulation of anterior pituitary function. Recent Prog Horm Res 1976; 32:161–243.
27. Styne DM, Grumbach MM. Puberty in the male and female. In: Yen SSC, Jaffe RB, eds. Reproductive Endocrinology: Physiology, Pathophysiology and Clinical Management. 2nd ed. Philadelphia: W. B. Saunders, 1986: 313–384.
28. Winter JSD, Hughes IA, Reyes FI, et al. Pituitary-gonadal steroid concentrations in man from birth to two years of age. J Clin Endocrinol Metab 1976; 42:679–686.
29. Winter JSD, Faiman C. The development of cyclic pituitary-gonadal function in adolescent females. J Clin Endocrinol Metab 1973; 37:714–718.
30. Conte FA, Grumbach MM, Kaplan SL. A diphasic pattern of gonadotropin secretion in patients with the syndrome of gonadal dysgenesis. J Clin Endocrinol Metab 1975; 40:670–674.
31. Roth JC, Kelch RP, Kaplan SL, et al. FSH and LH response to luteinizing hormone–releasing factor in prepubertal and pubertal children, adult males and patients with hypogonadotropic and hypergonadotropic hypogonadism. J Clin Endocrinol Metab 1973; 37:680–686.
32. Jakacki RI, Kelch RP, Sauder SE, et al. Pulsatile secretion of luteinizing hormone in children. J Clin Endocrinol Metab 1982; 55:453–458.
33. Grumbach MM, Roth JC, Kaplan SL, et al. Hypothalamic-pituitary regulation of puberty in man: evidence and concepts derived from clinical research. In: Grumbach MM, Grave GD, Mayer FE, eds. Control of the Onset of Puberty. New York: John Wiley & Sons, 1974: 115–166.
34. Smail PJ, Faiman C, Hobson WC, et al. Further studies on adrenarche in nonhuman primates. Endocrinology 1982; 111:844–848.
35. Kelnar CJH, Brook CGD. A mixed longitudinal study of adrenal steroid excretion in childhood and the mechanism of adrenarche. Clin Endocrinol 1983; 19:117–129.
36. Parker L, Odell WD. Control of adrenal androgen secretion. Endocr Rev 1980; 1:392–410.
37. Speroff L, Glass RH, Kase NG. Clinical Gynecologic Endocrinology and Infertility. 4th ed. Baltimore: Williams & Wilkins, 1989: 1–688.
38. Boyer RM, Rosenfeld RS, Kaplan S, et al. Simultaneous augmentation secretion of luteinizing hormone and testosterone during sleep. J Clin Invest 1974; 54:609–618.
39. Kapen S, Boyer RM, Hellman L, et al. Twenty-four-hour patterns of luteinizing hormone secretion in humans: ontogenic and sexual considerations. Prog Brain Res 1975; 42:103–113.
40. Knobil E. The neuroendocrine control of the menstrual cycle. Recent Prog Horm Res 1980; 36:53–78.
41. Crowley WF, McArthur JW. Stimulation of the normal menstrual cycle in Kallmann's syndrome by pulsatile administration of luteinizing hormone–releasing hormone (LHRH). J Clin Endocrinol Metab 1980; 51:173–175.
42. Crowley WF Jr, Comite F, Vale W, et al. Therapeutic use of pituitary desensitization with a long-acting LHRH agonist: a potential new treatment for idiopathic precocious puberty. J Clin Endocrinol Metab 1981; 53:370–372.
43. Mansfield MJ, Beardsworth DE, Loughlin JS, et al. Long-term treatment of central precocious puberty with a long-acting analogue of luteinizing hormone–releasing hormone. N Engl J Med 1983; 309:1286–1290.
44. Comite F, Cutler GB Jr, Rivier J, et al. Short-term treatment of idiopathic precocious puberty with a long-acting analogue of luteinizing hormone–releasing hormone. A preliminary report. N Engl J Med 1981; 305:1546–1550.
45. Winter JSD, Faiman C, Reyes FI, et al. Gonadotropins and steroid hormones in the blood and urine of prepubertal girls and other primates. Clin Endocrinol Metab 1978; 7:513–530.
46. Burstein S, Schoff-Blass E, Blass J, et al. Changing ratio of bioactive to immunoactive LH through puberty. J Clin Endocrinol Metab 1985; 61:508–513.
47. Burger HG, McLachlan RI, Bangah M, et al. Serum inhibin concentrations rise throughout normal male and female puberty. J Clin Endocrinol Metab 1988; 67:689–694.
48. Merimee TJ, Zapf J, Hewlett B, et al. Insulin-like growth factors in pygmies. N Engl J Med 1987; 316:906–911.
49. Mansfield MJ, Rudlin CR, Crigler JF, et al. Changes in growth and serum growth hormone and plasma somatomedin-C levels during suppression of gonadal sex steroid secretion in girls with central precocious puberty. J Clin Endocrinol Metab 1988; 66:3–9.
50. Dawson-Hughes B, Stern D, Goldman J, et al. Regulation of growth hormone and somatomedin-C secretion in postmenopausal women: effect of physiological estrogen replacement. J Clin Endocrinol Metab 1986; 63:424–432.
51. Marshall WA, Tanner JM. Variations in pattern of pubertal changes in girls. Arch Dis Child 1969; 44:291–303.
52. Frisch RE, McArthur JW. Menstrual cycles: fatness as a determinant of minimum weight for height necessary for their maintenance at onset. Science 1974; 185:949–951.
53. Frisch RE. Fatness, puberty, menstrual periodicity and fertility. In: Vaitukaitis JL, ed. Clinical Reproductive Neuroendocrinology. New York: Elsevier Biomedical, 1982: 105–135.
54. Zacharias L, Rand WM, Wurtman RJ. A prospective study of sexual development and growth in American girls: the statistics of menarche. Obstet Gynecol Surv 1976; 31:325–337.
55. Woodburne RT. Essentials of Human Anatomy. New York: Oxford University Press, 1965: 527–528.
56. Mossman HW, Duke KL. Comparative Morphology of the Mammalian Ovary. Madison, WI: University of Wisconsin Press, 1973.
57. Franchi LL, Mandl AM, Zuckerman S. The development of the ovary and the process of oogenesis. In: Zuckerman S, Mandl AM, Eckstein P, eds. The Ovary. London: Academic, 1961: 1–88.
58. Ross GT, Schreiber JR. The ovary. In: Yen SSC, Jaffe RB, eds. Reproductive Endocrinology: Physiology, Pathophysiology and Clinical Management. 2nd ed. Philadelphia: W. B. Saunders, 1986: 115–139.
59. Eshkol A, Lunenfeld B, Peters H. Ovarian development in infant mice: dependence on gonadotropic hormones. In: Butt WR, Crooke AC, Ryle M, eds. Gonadotropins and Ovarian Development. London: E and H Livingstone, 1970: 249–258.
60. Hisaw FL. Development of the graafian follicle and ovulation. Physiol Rev 1947; 27:95–119.

61. Zamboni L. Fine morphology of ovarian follicle maturation. In: Tozziniri RI, Reeves G, Pineda RL, eds. Endocrine Physiopathology of the Ovary. Amsterdam: Elsevier/North-Holland Biomedical, 1980: 63–99.

62. Greve JM, Salzman GS, Roller RS, et al. Biosynthesis of the major zona pellucida glycoprotein secreted by oocytes during mammalian oogenesis. Cell 1982; 31:749–759.

63. Dunbar BS. Morphological, biochemical and immunochemical characterization of the mammalian zona pellucida. In: Hartmann J, ed. Mechanism and Control of Animal Fertilization. London: Academic, 1983: 140–175.

64. Peters H, McNatty KP. The Ovary. Berkeley: University of California Press, 1980: 12–34.

65. Albertini DF, Anderson E. The appearance and structure of intracellular connections during the ontogeny of the rabbit ovarian follicle with particular reference to gap junctions. J Cell Biol 1974; 63:234–250.

66. Burghardt RC, Anderson E. Hormonal modulation of ovarian interstitial cells with particular reference to gap junctions. J Cell Biol 1979; 81:104–114.

67. Gougeon A. Rate of follicular growth in the human ovary. In: Rollands R, Van Hall EV, Hillier SG, et al., eds. Follicular Maturation and Ovulation. Amsterdam: Excerpta Medica, 1982: 155–162.

68. Santen RJ, Paulsen CA. Hypogonadotropic eunuchoidism. II. Gonadal responsiveness to exogenous gonadotropin. J Clin Endocrinol Metab 1973; 36:55–63.

69. Byskov AG. Follicular atresia. In: Jones RE, ed. The Vertebrate Ovary. New York: Plenum, 1978: 533–554.

70. Erickson FG, Magoffen D, Dyer CA, et al. The ovarian androgen producing cells: a review of structure/function relationships. Endocr Rev 1985; 6:371–399.

71. Gondos B, Hobel CG. Interstitial cells in the human fetal ovary. Endocrinology 1976; 93:736–739.

72. Dawson AB, McCabe M. The interstitial tissue of the ovary in infantile and juvenile rats. J Morphol 1951; 88:543–571.

73. Dyer CA, Erickson FG. Norepinephrine amplifies hCG-stimulated androgen biosynthesis by ovarian thecal-interstitial cells. Endocrinology 1985; 116:1645–1652.

74. McNatty KP, Makris A, DeGrazia C, et al. The production of progesterone, androgens and estrogens by granulosa cells, thecal tissue and stromal tissue from human ovaries in vitro. J Clin Endocrinol Metab 1979; 49:687–699.

75. Eshkal A, Lunenfeld B. Gonadotropic regulation of ovarian development in mice during infancy. In: Saxena BB, Gandy HM, Billing CG, eds. Gonadotropins. New York: John Wiley & Sons, 1972: 335–346.

76. Upadhyay S, Zamboni L. Ectopic germ cells: natural model for the study of germ cell sexual differentiation. Proc Natl Acad Sci USA 1982; 79:6584–6588.

77. Green SH, Zuckerman S. Quantitative aspects of the growth of the human ovum and follicle. J Anat 1951; 85:373–375.

78. Eppig JJ. A comparison between oocyte growth in coculture with granulosa cells and oocytes with granulosa cell–oocyte junctional contact maintained in vitro. J Exp Zool 1979; 209:345–353.

79. Austin CR. The Mammalian Egg. Springfield, IL: Charles C Thomas, 1961.

80. Bleil JD, Wassarman PM. Structure and function of the zona pellucida: identification and characterization of the proteins of the mouse oocyte's zona pellucida. Dev Biol 1980; 76:185–202.

81. Dekel N, Hillensjo T, Kraicer PF. Maturational effects of gonadotropins on the cumulus-oocyte complex of the rat. Biol Reprod 1979; 20:191–197.

82. Erickson GF. The ovary: basic principles and concepts. A. Physiology. In: Felig P, Baxter JD, Broders AG, et al., eds. Endocrinology and Metabolism. New York: McGraw-Hill, 1987: 905–950.

83. Moor RM. Role of steroids in the maturation of ovine oocytes. Ann Biol Anim Biochim Biophys 1978; 18:477–482.

84. Anderson E, Little B. The ontogeny of the rat granulosa cell. In: Toft DO, Ryan RJ, eds. Proceedings of the Fifth Ovarian Workshop. Champaign, IL: Ovarian Workshops, 1985: 203–225.

85. Koos RD, LeMaire WJ. Factors that may regulate the growth and regression of blood vessels in the ovary. Semin Reprod Endocrinol 1983; 1:295–307.

86. Corner GW Jr. Histological dating of human corpus luteum of menstruation. Am J Anat 1956; 98:377–401.

87. Crisp TM, Dessouky DA, Denys FR. The fine structure of the human corpus luteum of early pregnancy and during the progestational phase of the menstrual cycle. Am J Anat 1970; 127:37–69.

88. Carr BR, MacDonald PC, Simpson ER. The role of lipoproteins in the regulation of progesterone secretion by the human corpus luteum. Fertil Steril 1982; 38:303–311.

89. Ohara A, Mori T, Taii S, et al. Functional differentiation in steroidogenesis of two types of luteal cells isolated from mature human corpora lutea of menstrual cycle. J Clin Endocrinol Metab 1987; 65:1192–1200.

90. Gillim SW, Christensen AK, McLennon CE. Fine structure of the human menstrual corpus luteum at its stage of maximum secretory activity. Am J Anat 1970; 126:409–415.

91. Van Lennp EW, Madden LM. Electron microscopic observations on the involution of the human corpus luteum of menstruation. Z Zellforsch 1965; 66:365–380.

92. Ying SY. Inhibins, activins, and follistatins: gonadal proteins modulating the secretion of follicle-stimulating hormone. Endocr Rev 1988; 9:267–293.

93. Oliver C, Mical RS, Porter JC. Hypothalamic-pituitary vasculature: evidence for retrograde blood flow in the pituitary stalk. Endocrinology 1977; 101:598–604.

94. McCann SM, Snyder GD, Ojeda SR, et al. Roles of peptides in the control of gonadotropin secretion. In: McKerns KW, Naoro Z, eds. Hormone Control of the Hypothalamic-Pituitary-Gonadal Axis. New York: Plenum, 1984: 3–13.

95. Karten MJ, Rivier JE. Gonadotropin-releasing hormone analog design. Structure-function studies toward the development of agonists and antagonists: rationale and perspective. Endocr Rev 1986; 7:44–66.

96. Marshall JC. Regulation of gonadotropin secretion. In: DeGroot LJ, Besser GM, Cahill GF Jr, et al., eds. Endocrinology. 2nd ed. Philadelphia: W. B. Saunders, 1989: 1903–1914.

97. Huseman CA, Kelch RP. Gonadotropin response and metabolism of synthetic gonadotropin-releasing hormone (GnRH) during constant infusion of GnRH in men and boys with delayed adolescence. J Clin Endocrinol Metab 1978; 47:1325–1331.

98. Santen RJ, Bordin CW. Episodic luteinizing hormone secretion in man. J Clin Invest 1973; 52:2617–2628.

99. Carmel PW, Araki S, Ferin M. Pituitary stalk portal blood collection in rhesus monkeys: evidence of pulsatile release of gonadotropin releasing hormone (GnRH). Endocrinology 1976; 99:243–248.

100. Clarke IJ, Cummins JT. The temporal relationship between gonadotropin releasing hormone (GnRH) and luteinizing hormone (LH) secretion in ovariectomized ewes. Endocrinology 1982; 111:1737–1739.

101. Knobil E, Plan TM, Wildt TL, et al. Control of the rhesus monkey menstrual cycle: permissive role of hypothalamic gonadotropin releasing hormone. Science 1980; 207:1371–1373.

102. Belchetz PE, Plant TM, Nakai Y, et al. Hypophysial responses to continuous and intermittent delivery of hypothalamic gonadotropin-releasing hormone. Science 1978; 202:631–638.

103. Leyendecker G, Wildt L, Hansmen M. Pregnancies following chronic intermittent pulsatile administration of GnRH. J Clin Endocrinol Metab 1980; 51:1214–1216.

104. Conn PM. The molecular basis of gonadotropin-releasing hormone action. Endocr Rev 1986; 7:3–11.

105. Grant G, Vale W, Rivier J. Pituitary binding sites for H³ labeled LRF. Biochem Biophys Res Commun 1973; 50:771–776.

106. Yen SSC, Rebar RW. Endocrine rhythms in gonadotropins and ovarian steroids with reference to reproductive processes. In: Kreiger DT, ed. Endocrine Rhythms. New York: Raven, 1979: 259–298.

107. Fiddes JC, Talmadge K. Structure, expression, and evolution of the genes for human glycoprotein hormones. Recent Prog Horm Res 1984; 40:43–78.

108. Vaitukaitis JL, Ross GT, Bourstein GD, et al. Gonadotropins and their subunits: basic and clinical studies. Recent Prog Horm Res 1976; 32:289–331.

109. Kholer PO, Ross GT, Odell WD. Metabolic clearance and production rates of human luteinizing hormone in pre- and postmenopausal women. J Clin Invest 1968; 47:38–47.

110. Keller PJ. The renal clearance of follicle-stimulating and luteinizing hormone in postmenopausal women. Acta Endocrinol 1966; 53:225–233.

111. Fink G. Gonadotropin secretion and its control. In: Knobil E, Neill JD, eds. The Physiology of Reproduction. Vol 1. New York: Raven, 1988: 1349–1377.

112. Chappel SC, Resko JA, Norman RL, et al. Studies on rhesus monkeys on the site where estrogen inhibits gonadotropins: delivery of 17β-estradiol to the hypothalamus and pituitary gland. J Clin Endocrinol Metab 1981; 52:1–8.

113. Wildt L, Hutchinson JS, Marshall G, et al. On the site of action of progesterone in the blockade of the estradiol-induced gonadotropin discharge in the rhesus monkey. Endocrinology 1981; 109:1293–1294.

114. Veldius JD, Christiansen E, Evans WS, et al. Physiological profiles of episodic progesterone release during the midcycle phase of the human menstrual cycle: analysis of circadian and ultradian rhythms, discrete pulse properties, and correlations with simultaneous luteinizing hormone release. J Clin Endocrinol Metab 1988; 66:414–421.

115. Filicori M, Butler JP, Crowley WF. Neuroendocrine regulation of the corpus luteum in the human. J Clin Invest 1984; 73:1638–1647.

116. Liu JH, Yen SSC. Induction of midcycle gonadotropin surge by ovarian steroids in women: a critical evaluation. J Clin Endocrinol Metab 1983; 57:797–802.

117. Gore-Langton RE, Armstrong DT. Follicular steroidogenesis and its control. In: Knobil E, Neill JD, eds. The Physiology of Reproduction. Vol 1. New York: Raven, 1988: 331–385.

118. Siiteri PK, MacDonald PC. Role of extraglandular estrogen in human endocrinology. In: Greep RO, Astwood EB, eds. Handbook of Physiology. Sect 7: Endocrinology. Vol II. Female Reproductive System. Washington, DC: American Physiological Society, 1973: 615–630.

119. Brown JB, Matthew GD. The application of urinary estrogen methods to problems in gynecology. Recent Prog Horm Res 1962; 18:337–385.

120. Fishman J, Hellman L, Zumoff B, et al. Influence of thyroid hormone on estrogen metabolism in man. J Clin Endocrinol Metab 1962; 22:389–392.

121. Merriam GR, Lipsett MB. Catechol Estrogens. New York: Raven, 1983.

122. Lipsett M. Steroid hormones. In: Yen SSC, Jaffe RB, eds. Reproductive Endocrinology: Physiology, Pathophysiology and Clinical Management. 2nd Ed. Philadelphia: W. B. Saunders, 1986: 140–153.

123. Gwynne JT, Strauss JF. The role of lipoproteins in steroidogenesis and cholesterol metabolism in steroidogenic glands. Endocr Rev 1982; 3:299–329.

124. Golos TG, Strauss JF III, Miller WL. Regulation of low density lipoprotein receptor and cytochrome P-450$_{scc}$ mRNA levels in human granulosa cells. J Steroid Biochem 1987; 27:767–773.

125. Simpson ER. Cholesterol side-chain cleavage, cytochromic P-450, and the control of steroidogenesis. Mol Cell Endocrinol 1979; 13:213–227.

126. Waterman MR, Simpson ER. Regulation of the biosynthesis of cytochrome P-450 involved in steroid hormone synthesis. Mol Cell Endocrinol 1985; 39:81–89.

127. McAllister JM, Kerin JFP, Trant JM, et al. Regulation of cholesterol side-chain cleavage and 17α-hydroxylase/lyase activities in proliferating human theca interna cells in long term monolayer culture. Endocrinology 1989; 125:1959–1966.

128. Doody KJ, Lorence MC, Mason IJ, et al. Expression of messenger ribonucleic acid species encoding steroidogenic enzymes in human follicles and corpora lutea throughout the menstrual cycle. J Clin Endocrinol Metab 1990; 70:1041–1045.

129. Sasano H, Okamoto M, Mason JI, et al. Immunolocalization of aromatase, 17α-hydroxylase and side-chain-cleavage cytochromes P-450 in the human ovary. J Reprod Fertil 1989; 85:163–169.

130. Sano Y, Suzuki K, Arai K, et al. Changes in enzyme activities related to steroidogenesis in human ovaries during the menstrual cycle. J Clin Endocrinol Metab 1981; 52:994–1001.

131. McNatty KP, Makris A, DeGrazia C, et al. The production of progesterone, androgens, and estrogens by granulosa cells, theca tissue and stroma tissue from human ovaries in vitro. J Clin Endocrinol Metab 1979; 49:687–699.

132. Steinkampf MP, Mendelson CR, Simpson ER. Effects of epidermal growth factor and insulin-like growth factor I on the levels of mRNA encoding aromatase cytochrome P-450 of human ovarian granulosa cells. Mol Cell Endocrinol 1988; 59:93–99.

133. Corral-Gallardo J, Acevedo HA, Salazer JLP, et al. The polycystic ovary associated with PCO disease in vivo and in vitro studies. Acta Endocrinol 1966; 52:425–442.

134. Aono T, Kitamura U, Fukuda S, et al. Localization of 4-ene-5α-reductase, 17β-ol-dehydrogenase and aromatase in immature rat ovary. J Steroid Biochem 1981; 14:1369–1377.

135. Carr BR, Sadler RK, Rochelle DB, et al. Plasma lipoprotein regulation of progesterone biosynthesis by human corpus luteum tissue in organ culture. J Clin Endocrinol Metab 1981; 52:875–881.

136. Ohashi M, Carr BR, Simpson ER. Lipoprotein binding sites in human corpus luteum membrane fractions. Endocrinology 1982; 110:1477–1482.

137. Yeko TR, Shan-Dawood FS, Dawood MY. Human corpus luteum: luteinizing hormone and chorionic gonadotropin receptors during the menstrual cycle. J Clin Endocrinol Metab 1989; 68:529–534.

138. Illingworth DR, Corbin DK, Kemp ED, et al. Hormone changes during the menstrual cycle in abetalipoproteinemia: reduced luteal phase progesterone in a patient with homozygous hypobetalipoproteinemia. Proc Natl Acad Sci USA 1982; 79:6685–6689.

139. Reiter EO, Goldenberg RL, Vaitukaitis JL, et al. Evidence for a role of estrogen in the ovarian augmentation reaction. Endocrinology 1972; 91:1518–1522.

140. Hsueh AJW, Adashi EY, Jones PBC, et al. Hormonal regulation of the differentiation of culture ovarian granulosa cells. Endocr Rev 1984; 5:76–127.

141. Adashi EY, Hsueh AJW. Estrogens augment the stimulation of ovarian aromatase activity by follicle-stimulating hormone in cultured rat granulosa cells. J Biol Chem 1982; 257:6077–6083.

142. Hsueh AJW. Ovarian hormone synthesis, circulation, and mechanism of action. In: DeGroot LJ, Besser GM, Cahill GF Jr, et al., eds. Endocrinology. 2nd ed. Philadelphia: W. B. Saunders, 1989: 1929–1939.

143. Glasier AF, Baird DT, Hillier SG. FSH and the control of follicular growth. J Steroid Biochem 1989; 32:167–170.

144. Seegar-Jones G, DeMoraes-Ruehsen M. A new syndrome of amenorrhea in association with hypergonadotropism and apparently normal ovarian follicular apparatus. Am J Obstet Gynecol 1969; 104:597–600.

145. Baird DT, Horton R, Longcope C, et al. Steroid dynamics under steady state conditions. Recent Prog Horm Res 1969; 25:611–663.

146. Baird DT, Horton R, Longcope C, et al. Steroid prehormones. Perspect Biol Med 1968; 11:384–421.

147. Tait JF. Review: the use of isotopic steroids for the measurement of production rates in vivo. J Clin Endocrinol Metab 1963; 23:1285–1297.

148. Gurpide E, Gandy H. Dynamics of hormone production. In: Fuchs F, Klopper A, eds. Endocrinology of Pregnancy. New York: Harper & Row, 1971: 1–14.

149. Siiteri PK, MacDonald PC. Placental estrogen biosynthesis during human pregnancy. J Clin Endocrinol Metab 1966; 26:751–761.

150. Yen SSC. Chronic anovulation caused by peripheral endocrine disorders. In: Yen SSC, Jaffe RB, eds. Reproductive Endocrinology: Physiology, Pathophysiology and Clinical Management. 2nd ed. Philadelphia: W. B. Saunders, 1986: 441–499.

151. Wu CH, Motohashi T, Abdel-Rahman HA, et al. Free and protein-bound plasma estradiol-17β during the menstrual cycle. J Clin Endocrinol Metab 1976; 43:435–436.

152. Mendel CM. The free hormone hypothesis: a physiologically based mathematical model. Endocr Rev 1989; 10:232–274.

153. Ekins R. The free hormone concept. In: Hennemann G, ed. Thyroid Hormone Metabolism. New York: Marcel Dekker, 1986: 77–106.

154. Pardridge WM, Landaw EM. Tracer kinetic model of blood-brain barrier transport of plasma protein-bound ligands: empiric testing of the free hormone hypothesis. J Clin Invest 1984; 74:745–752.

155. Iqbal MJ, Johnson MW. Purification and characterization of human sex hormone–binding globulin. J Steroid Biochem 1979; 10:535–540.

156. Anderson DC. Sex hormone–binding globulin. Clin Endocrinol 1974; 3:69–96.

157. Barnea A, Gorsic J. Estrogen-induced protein: time course of synthesis. Biochemistry 1970; 9:1899–1904.

158. Clark JH, Markavereck BM. Actions of ovarian steroid hormones. In: Knobil E, Neill JD, eds. The Physiology of Reproduction. Vol 1. New York: Raven, 1988: 675–724.

159. Welshoun WV, Lieberman MS, Gorski J. Nuclear localization of unoccupied estrogen receptors. Nature 1984; 307:745–749.

160. Press MF, Greene GI. Localization of progesterone receptors with monoclonal antibodies to the human progestin receptor. Endocrinology 1988; 122:1165–1175.

161. Kumar V, Green S, Stack G, et al. Functional domains of the human estrogen receptor. Cell 1987; 51:941–951.

162. Scholl S, Lippman ME. The estrogen receptor in MCF-7 cells: evidence from dense amino acid labelling for rapid turnover and a dimeric model of activated nucleic acid receptor. Endocrinology 1984; 115:1295–1301.

163. DeSombre ER, Kuivanen PC. Progestin modulation of estrogen-dependent marker protein synthesis in the endometrium. Semin Oncol 1985; 12:6–11.

164. Adashi E, ed. Putative intraovarian regulators. Semin Reprod Endocrinol 1989; 7:1–100.

165. Hodgen GD, Rosenwaks Z, Spieler JM, eds. Nonsteroidal Gonadal Factors. Conrad International Workshops. Norfolk, VA: Jones Institute, 1988: 1–374.

166. Tsafriri A. Local nonsteroidal regulators of ovarian function. In: Knobil E, Neill JD, eds. The Physiology of Reproduction. Vol 1. New York: Raven, 1988: 527–565.

167. Westergaard LG. Intrafollicular factors regulating human ovarian follicular development and oocyte meiosis. Dan Med Bull 1988; 35:270–281.

168. Koos RD. Potential relevance of angiogenic factors to ovarian physiology. Semin Reprod Endocrinol 1989; 7:29–40.

169. Aten RF, Williams AT, Behrman HR. Ovarian gonadotropin-releasing hormone–like protein(s): demonstration and characterization. Endocrinology 1986; 118:961–967.

170. Li CH, Ramasharma K, Yamashiro D, et al. Gonadotropin-releasing peptide from human follicular fluid: isolation, characterization and chemical synthesis. Proc Natl Acad Sci USA 1987; 84:959–963.

171. Skinner MK, Coffey RJ Jr. Regulation of ovarian cell growth through the local production of transforming growth factor-α by theca cells. Endocrinology 1988; 123:2632–2638.

172. McNeilly AS, Tsonis CG, Baird DT. Inhibin. Hum Reprod 1988; 3:45–49.

173. Franchimont P, Hazee-Hagelstein MT, Jaspar JM, et al. Inhibin and related peptides: mechanisms of action and regulation of secretion. J Steroid Biochem 1989; 32:193–197.

174. Ueno S, Takahashi M, Manganaro TF, et al. Cellular localization of mullerian inhibiting substance in the developing rat ovary. Endocrinology 1989; 124:1000–1006.

175. Khan-Dawood FS, Goldsmith LT, Weiss G, et al. Human corpus luteum secretion of relaxin, oxytocin and progesterone. J Clin Endocrinol Metab 1989; 68:627–631.

176. Sherwood OD. Relaxin. In: Knobil E, Neill JD, eds. The Physiology of Reproduction. Vol 1. New York: Raven, 1988: 585–674.

177. Lightman A, Palumbo A, DeCherney AH, et al. The ovarian renin-angiotensin system. Semin Reprod Endocrinol 1989; 7:79–93.

178. Bicsak TA, Cajander SB, Peng XR, et al. Tissue-type plasminogen activator in rat oocytes: expression during the periovulatory period, after fertilization, and during follicular atresia. Endocrinology 1989; 124:187–194.

179. Trzeciak WH, Ahmed CE, Simpson ER, et al. Vasoactive intestinal peptide induces the synthesis of the cholesterol side-chain cleavage enzyme complex in cultured rat ovarian granulosa cells. Proc Natl Acad Sci USA 1986; 83:7490–7494.

180. Treloar AE, Boynton BE, Behn BG, et al. Variations of the human menstrual cycle through reproductive life. Int J Fertil 1967; 12:77–126.

181. Vollman RF. The Menstrual Cycle. Philadelphia: W. B. Saunders, 1977.

182. Presser HB. Temporal data relating to the human menstrual cycle. In: Ferin M, Halber F, Richart RM, et al., eds. Biorhythms and Human Reproduction. New York: John Wiley & Sons, 1974: 145–160.

183. Apter D, Raisanen I, Ylostalo P, et al. Follicular growth in relation to serum hormonal patterns in adolescence compared with adult menstrual cycles. Fertil Steril 1987; 47:82–88.

184. Fraser IS, Michie EA, Wide L, et al. Pituitary gonadotropin and ovarian function in adolescent dysfunctional uterine bleeding. J Clin Endocrinol Metab 1973; 37:407–414.

185. Sherman BM, West JH, Korenman SG. The menopausal tradition: analysis of LH, FSH, estradiol, and progesterone concentrations during menstrual cycles of older women. J Clin Endocrinol Metab 1976; 42:629–636.

186. Hodgen GD. The dominant ovarian follicle. Fertil Steril 1982; 38:281–300.

187. Goodman AL, Hodgen GD. The ovarian triad of the primate menstrual cycle. Recent Prog Horm Res 1983; 39:1–73.

188. Baird DT. A model for follicular selection and ovulation: lessons from superovulation. J Steroid Biochem 1987; 27:15–23.

189. Mais V, Cetel NS, Muse KN, et al. Hormonal dynamics during luteal-follicular transition. J Clin Endocrinol Metab 1987; 64:1109–1113.

190. Dorrington JH, Armstrong DT. Effects of FSH on gonadal functions. Recent Prog Horm Res 1979; 39:301–342.

191. Nimrod A, Erickson GF, Ryan KJ. A specific FSH receptor in rat granulosa cells: properties of binding in vitro. Endocrinology 1976; 98:56–64.

192. Amsterdam A, Rotmensch S. Structure-function relationships during granulosa cell differentiation. Endocr Rev 1987; 8:309–337.

193. Zeleznik AJ, Midgley AR Jr, Reichert LE Jr. Granulosa cell maturation in the rat: increased binding of human chorionic gonadotropin following treatment with follicle-stimulating hormone in vivo. Endocrinology 1974; 95:818–825.

194. Erickson GF, Wang C, Hsueh AJW. FSH induction of functional LH receptors in granulosa cells cultured in a chemically defined medium. Nature 1979; 279:336–338.

195. McNatty KP, Markis A, Reinhold VN, et al. Metabolism of androstene-dione by human ovarian tissue in vitro with particular reference to reductase and aromatase activity. Steroids 1979; 34:429–443.

196. Hillier SG, Van den Boogard AMJ, Reichert LE, et al. Intraovarian sex steroid hormone interactions and the regulation of follicular maturation: aromatization of androgens by human granulosa cells in vitro. J Clin Endocrinol Metab 1980; 50:640–647.

197. McNatty KP. Cyclic changes in antral fluid hormone concentrations in humans. Clin Endocrinol Metab 1978; 7:577–600.

198. McNatty KP, Smith DM, Makris A, et al. The microenvironment of the human antral follicle: interrelationships among the steroid levels in antral fluid, the population of granulosa cells, and the status of the oocyte in vivo and in vitro. J Clin Endocrinol Metab 1979; 49:851–860.

199. Sanyal MK, Berger MJ, Thompson IE, et al. Development of graafian follicles in adult human ovary. I. Correlation of estrogen and progesterone concentration in antral fluid with growth of follicles. J Clin Endocrinol Metab 1974; 38:828–835.

200. Brailly S, Gourgeon A, Milgrom E, et al. Androgens and progestins in human ovarian follicle. Differences in the evolution of preovulatory, healthy nonovulatory and atretic follicles. J Clin Endocrinol Metab 1981; 53:128–134.

201. Bomsel-Helmreich O. The preovulatory human oocyte and its microenvironment. In: Beier HM, Lindner HR, eds. Fertilization of the Human Egg In Vitro. Berlin: Springer-Verlag, 1983: 10–34.

202. Wang CF, Lasley BL, Lein A, et al. The functional changes of the pituitary gonadotropins during the menstrual cycle. J Clin Endocrinol Metab 1986; 42:718–728.

203. Ream N, Saunder SE, Kelch RP, et al. Pulsatile gonadotropin secretion during the menstrual cycle: evidence for altered frequency of gonadotropin-releasing hormone secretion. J Clin Endocrinol Metab 1984; 59:328–337.

204. Hoff JD, Quigley ME, Yen SSC. Hormonal dynamics at midcycle: a reevaluation. J Clin Endocrinol Metab 1983; 57:792–796.

205. Pauerstein CJ, Eddy CA, Croxatto HD, et al. Temporal relationships of estrogen, progesterone and luteinizing hormone levels to ovulation in women and infrahuman primates. Am J Obstet Gynecol 1978; 130:876–886.

206. Weiss TJ, Seamark RF, McIntosh JEA, et al. Cyclic AMP in sheep ovarian follicles: site of production and response to gonadotropins. J Reprod Fertil 1976; 46:347–353.

207. Channing CP, Schaerf FW, Anderson LD, et al. Ovarian follicular and luteal physiology. In: Greep RO, ed. International Review of Physiology. Vol 22. Baltimore: University Park Press, 1980: 117–201.

208. Lipner H. Mechanism of mammalian ovulation. In: Knobil E, Neill JD, eds. The Physiology of Reproduction. Vol 1. New York: Raven, 1988: 447–488.

209. Espey LL. Ovarian proteolytic enzymes and ovulation. Biol Reprod 1974; 10:216–235.

210. Beers WH. Follicular plasminogen and plasminogen activator and the effect of plasmin on ovarian follicular wall. Cell 1975; 6:379–386.

211. Tsafriri A, Bicsak TA, Cajander SB, et al. Suppression of ovulation rate by antibodies to tissue-type plasminogen activator and α_2-antiplasmin. Endocrinology 1989; 124:415–421.

212. Jones PBC, Vernon MW, Muse KN, et al. Plasminogen activator and plasminogen activator inhibitor in human preovulatory follicular fluid. J Clin Endocrinol Metab 1989; 68:1039–1047.

213. Lumsden MA, Kelly RW, Templeton AA, et al. Changes in the concentrations of prostaglandins in preovulatory human follicles after administration of hCG. J Reprod Fertil 1986; 77:119–124.

214. Yoshimura Y, Wallach EE. Studies on the mechanisms of mammalian ovulation. Fertil Steril 1987; 47:22–34.

215. Doody KJ, Carr BR. Diagnosis and treatment of luteal dysfunction. In: Hillier SG, ed. Ovarian Endocrinology. London: Blackwell Scientific, 1991: 260–318.

216. Killick S, Elstein M. Pharmacologic production of luteinized unruptured follicles by prostaglandin synthetase inhibitors. Fertil Steril 1987; 47:773–777.

217. Murdoch WJ, Cavender JL. Effect of indomethacin on the vascular architecture of preovulatory ovine follicles: possible implication in the luteinized unruptured follicle syndrome. Fertil Steril 1989; 51:153–155.

218. Yen SSC. The human menstrual cycle. In: Yen SSC, Jaffe RB, eds. Reproductive Endocrinology: Physiology, Pathophysiology and Clinical Management. 2nd ed. Philadelphia: W. B. Saunders, 1986: 200–236.

219. Niswender GD, Nett TM. The corpus luteum and its control. In: Knobil E, Neill JD, eds. The Physiology of Reproduction. Vol 1. New York: Raven, 1988: 489–525.

220. Vande Wiele RL, Bogumil J, Dyrenfurth I, et al. Mechanisms regulating the menstrual cycle in women. Recent Prog Horm Res 1970; 26:63–103.

221. Segaloff A, Sternberg WH, Gaskill CJ. Effects of luteotrophic doses of chorionic gonadotropin in women. J Clin Endocrinol Metab 1951; 11:936–944.

222. McNeely MJ, Soules MR. The diagnosis of luteal phase deficiency. Fertil Steril 1988; 50:1–15.

223. Stouffer RL, Hodgen GD. Induction of luteal phase defects in rhesus monkeys by follicular fluid administration at the onset of the menstrual cycle. J Clin Endocrinol Metab 1980; 51:669–671.

224. Sheehan KL, Casper RF, Yen SSC. Luteal phase defects induced by an agonist of luteinizing hormone releasing factor: a model for fertility control. Science 1982; 215:170–172.

225. Keyes PL, Wiltbank MC. Endocrine regulation of the corpus luteum. Annu Rev Physiol 1988; 50:465–482.

226. Cooke ID. The corpus luteum. Hum Reprod 1988; 3:153–156.

227. Hutchison JS, Zeleznik AJ. The corpus luteum of the primate menstrual cycle is capable of recovering from a transient withdrawal of pituitary gonadotropin support. Endocrinology 1985; 117:1043–1049.

228. Rojas FJ, Moretti-Rojas I, Balmaceda JP, et al. Regulation of gonadotropin-stimulable adenylyl cyclase of the primate corpus luteum. J Steroid Biochem 1989; 32:175–182.

229. Auletta FJ, Flint APF. Mechanisms controlling corpus luteum function in sheep, cows, nonhuman primates, and women especially in relation to the time of luteolysis. Endocr Rev 1988; 9:88–105.

230. Schulz KD, Geiger W, Del Poso E, et al. Pattern of sexual steroids, prolactin and gonadotropic hormones during prolactin inhibition in normally cycling women. Am J Obstet Gynecol 1978; 132:561–566.

231. Bohnet HG, McNeilly AS. Prolactin: assessment of its role in the human female. Horm Metab Res 1979; 11:533–546.

232. Hahlin M, Dennefors B, Johanson C, et al. Luteotropic effects of prostaglandin E_2 on the human corpus luteum of the menstrual cycle and early pregnancy. J Clin Endocrinol Metab 1988; 66:909–914.

233. Hodgen GD. Surrogate embryo transfer combined with estrogen-progesterone therapy in monkeys. Implantation, gestation, and delivery without ovaries. JAMA 1983; 250:2167–2171.

234. Lutjen P, Trounson A, Leeton J, et al. The establishment and maintenance of pregnancy using in vitro fertilization and embryo donation in a patient with primary ovarian failure. Nature 1984; 307:174–175.

235. Auletta FJ. The role of prostaglandin $F_2\alpha$ in human luteolysis. Contemp Obstet Gynecol 1987; 30:119–129.

236. Wentz AC, Jones GS. Transient luteolytic effect of prostaglandin $F_2\alpha$ in the human. Obstet Gynecol 1973; 42:172–181.

237. Schoonmaker JN, Bergman KS, Steiner RA, et al. Estradiol-induced luteal regression in the rhesus monkey: evidence of an extra-ovarian site of action. Endocrinology 1984; 110:1708–1715.

238. Karsch FJ, Krey LC, Weick RF, et al. Functional luteolysis in the rhesus monkey: role of estrogens. Endocrinology 1973; 92:1148–1152.

239. Johansson EDB, Gemzell C. Plasma levels of progesterone during the luteal phase in normal women treated with synthetic estrogens (RS 2874, F 6103, and ethinyloestradiol). Acta Endocrinol 1971; 68:551–560.

240. Gore BA, Caldwell BV, Speroff L. Estrogen-induced human luteolysis. J Clin Endocrinol Metab 1973; 36:615–617.

241. Westfahl PK, Resko JA. Effects of clomiphene on luteal function in the nonpregnant cynomolgus macaque. Biol Reprod 1983; 29:963–969.

242. Ellinwood WE, Resko JA. Effect on inhibition of estrogen synthesis

during the luteal phase on function of the corpus luteum in rhesus monkeys. Biol Reprod 1983; 28:636–644.

243. Khan-Dawood FS, Huang JC, Dawood MY. Baboon corpus luteum oxytocin: an intragonadal peptide modulator on luteal function. Am J Obstet Gynecol 1988; 158:882–891.

244. Givens JR, Andersen RN, Ragland JB, et al. Adrenal function in hirsutism. I. Diurnal change and response of plasma androstenedione, testosterone, 17-hydroxyprogesterone, cortisol, LH and FSH to dexamethasone and 1/2 unit of ACTH. J Clin Endocrinol Metab 1975; 40:988–1000.

245. Judd HL, Yen SSC. Serum androstenedione and testosterone levels during the menstrual cycle. J Clin Endocrinol Metab 1973; 36:475–481.

246. Abraham GE, Chakmakjian AH. Serum steroid levels during the menstrual cycle in a bilaterally adrenalectomized woman. J Clin Endocrinol Metab 1973; 37:581–587.

247. Dyrenfurth I, Jewelewica R, Warren M, et al. Temporal relationships of hormonal variables in the menstrual cycle. In: Ferin M, Halberg F, Richart RM, et al., eds. Biorhythms and Reproduction. New York: John Wiley & Sons, 1974: 171–201.

248. Genazzani AR, Lemarchand-Beraud TH, Aubert ML, et al. Pattern of plasma ACTH, hGH and cortisol during menstrual cycle. J Clin Endocrinol Metab 1975; 41:431–437.

249. Carr BR, Parker Jr CR, Madden JD, et al. Plasma levels of adrenocorticotropin (ACTH) and cortisol in women receiving oral contraceptive treatment. J Clin Endocrinol Metab 1979; 49:346–349.

250. Carr BR, Wilson JD. Disorders of the ovary and female reproductive tract. In: Braunwald E, Isselbacher KJ, Petersdorf RG, et al., eds. Harrison's Principles of Internal Medicine. 11th ed. New York: McGraw-Hill, 1987: 1818–1837.

251. Casey ML, MacDonald PC. Extraadrenal formation of a mineralocorticosteroid: deoxycorticosterone and deoxycorticosterone sulfate biosynthesis and metabolism. Endocr Rev 1982; 3:396–403.

252. Parker Jr CR, Winkel CA, Rush AJ, et al. Plasma concentrations of 11-deoxycorticosterone in women during the menstrual cycle. Obstet Gynecol 1981; 58:26–30.

253. Noyes RW, Hertig AW, Rock J. Dating the endometrial biopsy. Fertil Steril 1950; 1:3–25.

254. Tseng L, Gurpide E. Effects of progestins on estradiol receptor levels in human endometrium. J Clin Endocrinol Metab 1975; 41:402–404.

255. King RSB, Townsend PT, Whitehead MI, et al. Biochemical analysis of separated epithelium and stroma from endometria of premenopausal and postmenopausal women receiving estrogen and progestin. J Steroid Biochem 1981; 14:979–987.

256. Tseng L, Liu HC. Stimulation of arylsulfotransferase activity by progestins in human endometrium in vitro. J Clin Endocrinol Metab 1981; 53:418–421.

257. Sixma JJ, Cristiens GCML, Hospels AS. The sequence of hemostatic events in the endometrium during normal menstruation. In: Dicefalusy E, Fraser IS, Webb FTG, eds. WHO Symposium on Steroid Contraception and Endometrial Bleeding. 1980: 86.

258. Wilborn WH, Flowers CE Jr. Cellular mechanisms for endometrial conservation during menstrual bleeding. Semin Reprod Endocrinol 1984; 2:307–341.

259. Hallberg L, Hogdahl A, Nilsson L, et al. Menstrual blood loss—a population study. Acta Obstet Gynecol Scand 1966; 45:320–351.

260. Edman CD. The effects of steroids on the endometrium. Semin Reprod Endocrinol 1983; 1:79–187.

261. Pickles VR, Hall WJ, Best FA, et al. Prostaglandins in endometrium and menstrual fluid from normal and dysmenorrheic subjects. J Obstet Gynaecol Br Commonw 1965; 72:185–192.

262. Willman EA, Collins WP, Clayton SG. Studies in the involvement of prostaglandins in uterine symptomatology and pathology. Br J Obstet Gynaecol 1976; 83:337–341.

263. Schwarz BE. The production and biologic effects of uterine prostaglandins. Semin Reprod Endocrinol 1983; 1:189–195.

264. Turksoy RN, Safaii HS. Immediate effect of prostaglandin F$_2\alpha$ during the luteal phase of the menstrual cycle. Fertil Steril 1975; 26:634–637.

265. Henzl MR, Smith RE, Boost G, et al. Lysosomal concept of menstrual bleeding in humans. J Clin Endocrinol Metab 1972; 34:860–875.

266. Ferency A, Guralnick M. Endometrial microstructure: structure-function relationships throughout the menstrual cycle. Semin Reprod Endocrinol 1983; 1:205–219.

267. Todd AS. Localization of fibrinolytic activity in tissues. Br Med Bull 1964; 20:210–212.

268. Papanicolaou GN, Traut HF, Marchetti AA. The Epithelia of Women's Reproductive Organs: A Correlative Study of Cyclic Changes. New York: Commonwealth, 1948.

269. Rebar RE. Practical evaluation of hormonal status. In: Yen SSC, Jaffe RB, eds. Reproductive Endocrinology: Physiology, Pathophysiology and Clinical Management. 2nd ed. Philadelphia: W. B. Saunders, 1986: 683–733.

270. Gaudefoy M. Cytologic criteria of estrogen effect. Acta Cytol 1958; 2:347–362.

271. Harper MJK. Gamete and zygote transport. In: Knobil E, Neill JD, eds. The Physiology of Reproduction. Vol 1. New York: Raven, 1988: 103–134.

272. Settlage DSF, Motoshima M, Tredway DR. Sperm transport from the external cervical os to the fallopian tubes in women: a time and quantitation study. Fertil Steril 1973; 24:655–661.

273. Ahlgren M. Sperm transport to and survival in the human fallopian tube. Gynecol Invest 1975; 6:206–214.

274. Bedford JM. Sperm capacitation and fertilization in mammals. Biol Reprod 1970; 2(Suppl):128–158.

275. Wassarman PM. Fertilization in mammals. Sci Am 1988; 259(6):78–84.

276. Yanagimachi R. Mammalian fertilization. In: Knobil E, Neill JD, eds. The Physiology of Reproduction. Vol 1. New York: Raven, 1988: 135–185.

277. Croxatto HB, Ortiz MS. Egg transport in the fallopian tube. Gynecol Invest 1975; 6:215–225.

278. Pauerstein CJ, Eddy CA. The role of the oviduct in reproduction: our knowledge and our ignorance. J Reprod Fertil 1979; 55:223–229.

279. Blandau RJ. Gamete transport in the female mammal. In: Greep RO, Astwood EB, eds. Handbook of Physiology. Sect 7: Endocrinology. Vol II. Female Reproductive System. Washington, DC: American Physiological Society, 1973: 153–167.

280. Wassarman PM. The biology and chemistry of fertilization. Science 1987; 235:553–560.

281. Zaneveld LJD, Polakoski KL, Williams WL. Properties of a proteolytic enzyme from rabbit sperm acrosomes. Biol Reprod 1972; 6:30–39.

282. Veech LI. Atlas of the Human Oocyte and Early Conceptus. Baltimore: Williams & Wilkins, 1986: 1–331.

283. Pederson RA. Early mammalian embryogenesis. In: Knobil E, Neill JD, eds. The Physiology of Reproduction. Vol 1. New York: Raven, 1988: 187–230.

284. Hertig AT, Rock J, Adams EC, et al. Thirty-four fertilized ova, good, bad and indifferent from 210 women of known fertility. Pediatrics 1959; 23:202–211.

285. Weitauf HM. Biology of implantation. In: Knobil E, Neill JD, eds. The Physiology of Reproduction. Vol 1. New York: Raven, 1988: 231–262.

286. Chan CLK, Cameron IT, Findlay JK, et al. Oocyte donation and in vitro fertilization for hypergonadotropic hypogonadism: clinical state of the art. Obstet Gynecol Surv 1987; 42:350–362.

287. Boving BG. Implantation. Ann NY Acad Sci 1959; 75:700–725.

288. Sheleshyak MC. Inhibition of decidual cell formation in the pseudopregnant rat by histamine antagonists. Am J Physiol 1952; 170:522–527.

289. Heap RB, Flint AP, Gadsby JE. Role of embryonic signals in the establishment of pregnancy. Br Med Bull 1979; 35:129–135.

290. Kennedy TG. Evidence for a role for prostaglandins in the initiation of blastocyst implantation in the rat. Biol Reprod 1977; 16:286–291.

291. Harper MJK. Platelet-activating factor: a paracrine factor in preimplantation stages of reproduction? Biol Reprod 1989; 40:907–913.

292. A Statistical Portrait of Women in the U.S. Publication No. 58. Current Population Report, Special Studies Series. Washington, DC: U.S. Dept. of Commerce, Bureau of the Census, 1976: 23.

293. Utian WH. Menopause in Modern Perspective. New York: Appleton-Century-Crofts, 1980.

294. Linquist O, Bengtsson C. Menopausal age in relation to smoking. Acta Med Scand 1979; 205:73–77.

295. Sauramo H. Histology, histopathology and function of the senile ovary. Ann Chir Gynaecol Fenn 1952; 4(Suppl):1–66.

296. Woll EA, Hertig AT, Smith GV, et al. The ovary in endometrial carcinoma with notes on the morphological history of the aging ovary. Am J Obstet Gynecol 1948; 56:617–633.

297. Scaglia H, Medina M, Pinto-Ferriera AL, et al. Pituitary LH and FSH secretion and responsiveness in women of old age. Acta Endocrinol 1976; 81:673–679.

298. Chakravarti S, Collins WP, Forecast JD, et al. Hormonal profiles after the menopause. Br Med J 1976; 2:784–787.

299. Judd JL. Hormonal dynamics associated with the menopause. Clin Obstet Gynecol 1976; 19:775–788.

300. Edman CD, MacDonald PC. Effect of obesity on conversion of plasma androstenedione to estrone in ovulatory and anovulatory young women. Am J Obstet Gynecol 1978; 130:456–461.

301. Hemsell DL, Grodin JM, Brenner PF, et al. Plasma precursors of estrogen. II. Correlation of the extent of conversion of plasma androstenedione to estrone with age. J Clin Endocrinol Metab 1974; 38:476–479.

302. Tataryn IV, Lomax P, Bajorek JG, et al. Postmenopausal hot flushes: a disorder of thermoregulation. Maturitas 1980; 2:101–107.

303. Yen SSC. The biology of menopause. J Reprod Med 1977; 18:287–296.

304. Brincat M, Moniz CJ, Studd JW, et al. Long-term effects of the menopause and sex hormones on skin thickness. Br J Obstet Gynaecol 1985; 92:256–259.

305. Weiss NS, Ure CL, Ballard JH, et al. Decreased risk of fractures of the hip and lower forearm with postmenopausal use of estrogen. N Engl J Med 1980; 303:1195–1198.

306. Barrett-Conner E, Brown WV, Turner J, et al. Heart disease risk factors and hormone use in postmenopausal women. JAMA 1979; 241:2167–2169.

307. Ross RK, Paganini-Hill A, Mack TM, et al. Estrogen use and cardiovas-

cular disease. In: Mishell DR, ed. Menopause: Physiology and Pharmacology. Chicago: Year Book Medical, 1987: 209–223.

308. Jaszmann L, Van Lith ND, Zoat JCA. The perimenopausal symptoms. Med Gynecol Sociol 1969; 4:268–277.

309. Meldrum DR. The pathophysiology of postmenopausal symptoms. Semin Reprod Endocrinol 1983; 1:11–17.

310. Riggs BL, Wahner HW, Melton LJ III, et al. Rates of bone loss in the appendicular and axial skeletons of women. J Clin Invest 1986; 77:1487–1491.

311. Alderman BW, Weiss NS, Daling JR, et al. Reproductive history and postmenopausal risk of hip and forearm fracture. Am J Epidemiol 1986; 124:262–267.

312. Beals RK. Survival following hip fracture: long term follow-up of 607 patients. J Chronic Dis 1972; 25:235–244.

313. Nilas L, Christiansen C. Bone mass and its relationship to age and the menopause. J Clin Endocrinol Metab 1987; 65:697–702.

314. Lindsay R, Herrington BS. Estrogens and osteoporosis. Semin Reprod Endocrinol 1983; 1:55–67.

315. Henderson BE, Ross RK, Paganini-Hill A, et al. Estrogen use and cardiovascular disease. Am J Obstet Gynecol 1986; 154:1181–1186.

316. Matthews KA, Meilahn E, Kuller LH, et al. Menopause and risk factors for coronary heart disease. N Engl J Med 1989; 321:641–646.

317. Colditz GA, Willett WC, Stampfer MJ, et al. Menopause and the risk of coronary heart disease in women. N Engl J Med 1987; 316:1105–1110.

318. Bush TL, Barrett-Connor E, Cowan DK, et al. Cardiovascular mortality and noncontraceptive use of estrogen in women: results from the Lipid Research Clinics Program Follow-Up Study. Circulation 1987; 75:1102–1109.

319. Stampfer MJ, Willett WC, Colditz GA, et al. A prospective study of postmenopausal estrogen therapy and coronary heart disease. N Engl J Med 1985; 313:1044–1049.

320. Santen RJ, Bardin CW. Episodic luteinizing hormone secretion in man: pulse analysis, clinical interpretation, physiologic mechanism. J Clin Invest 1973; 52:2617–2628.

321. Goldenberg RL, Grodin JM, Rodbard D, et al. Gonadotropins in women with amenorrhea. Am J Obstet Gynecol 1973; 116:1003–1012.

322. Yen SSC, Vela P, Rankin J. Inappropriate secretion of follicle-stimulating hormone and luteinizing hormone in polycystic ovarian disease. J Clin Endocrinol Metab 1970; 30:435–442.

323. Yen SSC, VandenBerg G, Rebar R, et al. Variation of pituitary responsiveness to synthetic LRF during different phases of the menstrual cycle. J Clin Endocrinol Metab 1972; 35:931–937.

324. Rebar R, Yen SSC, VandenBerg G, et al. Gonadotropin responses to synthetic LRF: dose-response relationship in men. J Clin Endocrinol Metab 1973; 36:10–16.

325. Yen SSC, Rebar R, Vandenberg G, et al. Hypothalamic amenorrhea and hypogonadism: responses to LRF. J Clin Endocrinol Metab 1973; 36:811–816.

326. Kletzky OA, Davajan V, Nakamura RM, et al. Clinical categorization of patients with secondary amenorrhea using progesterone-induced uterine bleeding and measurement of serum gonadotropin levels. Am J Obstet Gynecol 1975; 121:695–703.

327. Ritchie WGM. Ultrasound in the evaluation of normal and induced ovulation. Fertil Steril 1985; 43:167–181.

328. Griffin JE, Edwards C, Madden JD, et al. Congenital absence of the vagina. Ann Intern Med 1976; 85:224–236.

329. Griffin JE, Wilson JD. The syndromes of androgen resistance. N Engl J Med 1980; 302:198–209.

330. New MI, Dupont B, Pang S, et al. An update of congenital adrenal hyperplasia. Recent Prog Horm Res 1981; 37:105–181.

331. Ferriman D, Gallwey JD. Clinical assessment of body hair growth in women. J Clin Endocrinol Metab 1961; 21:1440–1447.

332. Bardin CW, Lipsett MB. Testosterone and androstenedione blood production rates in normal women and women with idiopathic hirsutism or polycystic ovaries. J Clin Invest 1967; 46:891–902.

333. Lipsett MB. Clinical considerations of 17-ketosteroid and testosterone measurements. In: Sunderman FW, Sunderman Jr FW, eds. Laboratory Diagnosis of Endocrine Disease. St. Louis: Warren H. Green, 1971: 555.

334. Vermesh M, Kletzky OA, Davajan V, et al. Monitoring techniques to predict and detect ovulation. Fertil Steril 1987; 47:259–264.

335. Hricak H. MRI of the female pelvis: a review. Am J Radiol 1986; 146:1115–1122.

336. Winfield AC, Wentz AC. Diagnostic Imaging of Infertility. Baltimore: Williams & Wilkins, 1987.

337. Bradshaw JR. Magnetic resonance imaging of the CNS. Br J Hosp Med 1989; 42:472–479.

338. Tjio JH, Levan A. The chromosome number in man. Hereditas 1956; 42:1–6.

339. Seabright M. A rapid banding technique for human chromosomes. Lancet 1971; 2:971–972.

340. Manuel M, Katayama KP, Jones HW Jr. The age of occurrence of gonadal tumors in intersex patients with a Y chromosome. Am J Obstet Gynecol 1976; 124:293–300.

341. Baggish MS, Barbot J, Valle RF. Diagnostic and Operative Hysteroscopy: A Text and Atlas. Chicago: Year Book Publishers, 1989.

342. Nordenskjold F, Ahlgreen M. Laparoscopy in female infertility. Acta Obstet Gynecol Scand 1983; 62:609–615.

343. Buster JE, Simon JA. Placental hormones, hormone preparation for and control parturition, and hormonal diagnosis of pregnancy. In: DeGroot LJ, Besser GM, Cahill GF Jr, et al., eds. Endocrinology. 2nd ed. Philadelphia: W. B. Saunders, 1989: 2043–2073.

344. Gaudin J, Le Treguilly C, Parent P, et al. Neonatal ovarian cysts: twelve cysts with antenatal diagnosis. Pediatr Surg Int 1988; 3:158–164.

345. Brenner PF. Precocious puberty in the female. In: Mishell DR Jr, Davajan V, eds. Infertility, Contraception and Reproductive Endocrinology. Oradell NJ: Medical Economics Books, 1986: 223–236.

346. Dean HJ, Winter JSD. Abnormalities of pubertal development. In: Collu R, Ducharme JD, Guyda HJ, eds. Pediatric Endocrinology. 2nd ed. New York: Raven, 1989: 331–366.

347. Thamdrup E. Precocious sexual development. A clinical study of 100 children. Dan Med Bull 1961; 8:140–142.

348. Liu N, Grumbach MM, de Napoli RA, et al. Prevalence of electroencephalographic abnormalities in idiopathic precocious puberty and premature pubarche: bearing on pathogenesis and neuroendocrine regulation of puberty. J Clin Endocrinol Metab 1965; 25:1296–1308.

349. Jenner MR, Kelch RP, Kaplan SL, et al. Hormonal changes in puberty. IV. Plasma estradiol, LH and FSH in prepubertal children, pubertal females, and in precocious puberty, premature thelarche, hypogonadism, and in a child with a feminizing ovarian tumor. J Clin Endocrinol Metab 1972; 34:521–530.

350. Reiter EO, Kaplan SL, Conte FA, et al. Responsivity of pituitary gonadotropes to luteinizing hormone–releasing factor in idiopathic precocious puberty, precocious thelarche, precocious adrenarche, and in patients treated with medroxyprogesterone acetate. Pediatr Res 1975; 9:111–116.

351. Sigurjonsdottir TH, Hayles AB. Precocious puberty: a report of 96 cases. Am J Dis Child 1968; 115:309–321.

352. Saxena KM. Endocrine manifestations of neurofibromatosis in children. Am J Dis Child 1970; 120:265–271.

353. Fienman NL, Yakovac WC. Neurofibromatosis in childhood. J Pediatr 1970; 76:339–346.

354. Judge DM, Kulin HE, Page R, et al. Hypothalamic hamartoma: a source of luteinizing-hormone–releasing factor in precocious puberty. N Engl J Med 1977; 296:7–10.

355. Cabezudo JM, Perez C, Vaquera J, et al. Pubertos praecox in craniopharyngioma. J Neurosurg 1981; 55:127–131.

356. Zuniga OF, Tanner SM, Wild WO, et al. Hamartoma of CNS associated with precocious puberty. Am J Dis Child 1983; 137:127–133.

357. Kubo O, Yamasaki N, Kamijo Y, et al. Human chorionic gonadotropin produced by ectopic pinealoma in a girl with precocious puberty. J Neurosurg 1977; 47:101–105.

358. Styne DM. Precocious puberty. Compr Ther 1987; 13:14–19.

359. Towne BH, Mahour GH, Woolley MM, et al. Ovarian cysts and tumors in infancy and childhood. J Pediatr Surg 1975; 10:311–320.

360. Richards GE, Kaplan SL, Grumback MM. Sexual precocity associated with functional follicular cysts, prepubertal gonadotropins and LRF response and fluctuating estrogen levels. Pediatr Res 1977; 11:431 (abstract).

361. Thompson JP, Dockerty MB, Symonds RE, et al. Ovarian and parovarian tumors in infants and children. Am J Obstet Gynecol 1967; 97:1059–1065.

362. Eberlein WR, Bongiovanni AM, Jones IT, et al. Ovarian tumors and cysts associated with sexual precocity. J Pediatr 1960; 57:484–497.

363. Solh HM, Azoury RS, Najjar SS. Peutz-Jeghers syndrome associated with precocious puberty. J Pediatr 1983; 103:593–595.

364. Pomarede R, Finidori J, Czernichow P, et al. Germinoma in a boy with precocious puberty: evidence of hCG secretion by tumor cells. Child Brain 1984; 11:298–303.

365. Drop SLS, Bruining GJ, Visser HKA, et al. Prolonged galactorrhea in a 6-year-old girl with isosexual precocious puberty due to a feminizing adrenal tumor. Clin Endocrinol 1981; 15:37–43.

366. McCune DJ. Osteitis fibrosa cystica; the case of a nine-year-old girl who also exhibits precocious puberty, multiple pigmentation of the skin and hyperthyroidism. Am J Dis Child 1936; 52:743–747.

367. Albright F, Butler AM, Hampton AO, et al. Syndrome characterized by osteitis fibrosa disseminata, areas of pigmentation and endocrine dysfunction, with precocious puberty in females. N Engl J Med 1937; 216:726–746.

368. Lightner ES, Penny R, Frasier SD. Growth hormone excess and sexual precocity in polyostotic fibrous dysplasia (McCune-Albright syndrome): evidence for abnormal hypothalamic function. J Pediatr 1975; 87:922–927.

369. Comite F, Shawker TH, Pescovitz OH, et al. Cyclical ovarian function resistant to treatment with an analogue of luteinizing hormone releasing hormone in McCune-Albright syndrome. N Engl J Med 1984; 311:1032–1036.

370. D'Armiento RM, Camagna G, Tardella L. McCune-Albright syndrome: evidence for autonomous multiendocrine hyperfunction. J Pediatr 1983; 102:584–586.

371. Feuillan PP, Foster CM, Pescovitz OH, et al. Treatment of precocious

puberty in the McCune-Albright syndrome with the aromatase inhibitor testolactone. N Engl J Med 1986; 315:1115–1119.

372. Cuttler L, Jackson JA, uz-Zafar MS, et al. Hypersecretion of growth hormone and prolactin in McCune-Albright syndrome. J Clin Endocrinol Metab 1989; 68:1148–1154.

373. Van Wyk JJ, Grumbach MM. Syndrome of precocious menstruation and galactorrhea in juvenile hypothyroidism: an example of hormonal overlap in pituitary feedback. J Pediatr 1960; 57:416–435.

374. Pringle PJ, Stanhope R, Hindmarsh P, et al. Abnormal pubertal development in primary hypothyroidism. Clin Endocrinol 1988; 28:479–486.

375. Hemady ZS, Siler-Khodr TM, Najjar S. Precocious puberty in juvenile hypothyroidism. J Pediatr 1978; 92:55–59.

376. Castro-Magana M, Angula M, Canas A, et al. Hypothalamic-pituitary gonadal axis in boys with primary hypothyroidism and macroorchidism. J Pediatr 1988; 112:397–402.

377. Silver HK. Asymmetry, short stature and variations in sexual development: syndrome of genital malformation. Am J Dis Child 1964; 107:495–515.

378. Hertz R. Accidental ingestion of estrogens by children. Pediatrics 1958; 21:203–206.

379. Saenz de Rodriguez CA, Bongiovanni AM, Conde de Borrego L. An epidemic of precocious development in Puerto Rican children. J Pediatr 1985; 107:393–396.

380. Pescovitz OH, Hench KD, Barnes KM, et al. Premature thelarche and central precocious puberty: the relationship between clinical presentation and the gonadotropin response to luteinizing hormone–releasing hormone. J Clin Endocrinol Metab 1988; 67:474–479.

381. Muritano M, Zachmann M, Manella B, et al. Transient ovarian testosterone and androstenedione hypersecretion: a cause of virilization or premature pubarche in prepubertal girls. Horm Res 1987; 28:37–41.

382. Mansfield MJ, Beardsworth DE, Loughlin JS, et al. Long term treatment of central precocious puberty with a long acting analogue of luteinizing hormone–releasing hormone. N Engl J Med 1983; 309:1286–1290.

383. Comite F, Rescovitz OH, Rieth KG, et al. Luteinizing hormone–releasing hormone analog treatment of boys with hypothalamic hamartoma and true precocious puberty. J Clin Endocrinol Metab 1984; 59:888–892.

384. Rescovitz OH, Comite F, Hench K, et al. The NIH experience with precocious puberty: diagnostic subgroups and response to short-term luteinizing hormone releasing hormone analogue therapy. J Pediatr 1986; 108:47–54.

385. Richman RA, Underwood LE, French FS, et al. Adverse effects of large doses of medroxyprogesterone acetate (MPA) in idiopathic precocious puberty. J Pediatr 1971; 79:963–971.

386. Dawood MY, ed. Dysmenorrhea. Baltimore: Williams & Wilkins, 1981.

387. Owen PR. Prostaglandin sythetase inhibtors in the treatment of primary dysmenorrhea: outcome trials reviewed. Am J Obstet Gynecol 1984; 148:96–103.

388. Reid RL, Yen SCC. The premenstrual syndrome. Clin Obstet Gynecol 1983; 26:710–718.

389. Rubinow DR, Roy-Byrne P. Premenstrual syndromes: overview from a methodologic perspective. Am J Psychiatry 1984; 141:163–172.

390. Bancroft J, Backstrom T. Premenstrual syndrome. Clin Endocrinol 1985; 22:313–336.

391. March CM, Hoffman DI, Lobo RA. Dysfunctional uterine bleeding. In: Mishell DR Jr, Davajan V, eds. Infertility, Contraception and Reproductive Endocrinology. Oradell NJ: Medical Economics Books, 1986: 337–351.

392. Smith SK, Abel MT, Kelly RW, et al. Synthesis of prostaglandins from persistent proliferative endometrium. J Clin Endocrinol Metab 1982; 55:284–289.

393. Kurman RJ, Kaminski PT, Norris HJ. The behavior of endometrial hyperplasia. A long-term study of "untreated" hyperplasia in 170 patients. Cancer 1985; 56:403–412.

394. Van Eijkeren MA, Christiaens GCML, Sixma JJ, et al. Menorrhagia: a review. Obstet Gynecol Surv 1989; 44:421–429.

395. Ferenczy A. Studies on the cytodynamics of human endometrial regeneration: I. Scanning electron microscopy. Am J Obstet Gynecol 1976; 124:64–74.

396. Hall P, Maclachlan N, Thorn N, et al. Control of menorrhagia by the cyclo-oxygenase inhibitors naproxen sodium and mefenamic acid. Br J Obstet Gynaecol 1987; 94:554–558.

397. DeVore GR, Owens O, Kase N. Use of intravenous premarin in the treatment of dysfunctional uterine bleeding—a double-blind randomized control study. Obstet Gynecol 1982; 59:285–291.

398. Amenorrhea. American College of Obstetricians and Gynecologist Technical Bulletin No 128. 1989.

399. Simpson JL, Christakos AC, Horwith M, et al. Gonadal dysgenesis in individuals with apparently normal chromosomal complements: tabulation of cases and compilation of genetic data. Birth Defects 1971; 8:215–228.

400. Rosen GF, Kaplan B, Lobo RA. Menstrual function and hirsutism in patients with gonadal dysgenesis. Obstet Gynecol 1988; 71:677–680.

401. Hague WM, Adams J, Reeders ST, et al. 45,X Turner's syndrome in association with polycystic ovaries. Case report. Br J Obstet Gynaecol 1989; 96:613–618.

402. Capraro VJ, Greenberg H. Adhesions of the labia minora. A study of 50 patients. Obstet Gynecol 1972; 39:65–69.

403. Klein VR, Willman SP, Carr BR. Familial posterior labial fusion. Obstet Gynecol 1989; 73:500–503.

404. Soules MR. Adolescent amenorrhea. Pediatr Clin North Am 1987; 43:1083–1103.

405. Baird DT. Amenorrhea, anovulation, and dysfunctional uterine bleeding. In: DeGroot LJ, Besser GM, Cahill GF Jr, et al., eds. Endocrinology. 2nd ed. Philadelphia: W. B. Saunders, 1989: 1950–1968.

406. Rock JA. Anomalous development of the vagina. Semin Reprod Endocrinol 1986; 4:13–31.

407. Rock JA, James HW Jr. The double uterus associated with an obstructed hemivagina and ipsilateral renal agenesis. Am J Obstet Gynecol 1980; 138:339–342.

408. Reindollar RH, Byrd JR, McDonough PG. Delayed sexual development: a study of 252 patients. Am J Obstet Gynecol 1981; 140:371–380.

409. Fore SR, Hammond CB, Parker RT, et al. Urologic and genital anomalies in patients with congenital absence of the vagina. Obstet Gynecol 1975; 46:410–416.

410. Griffin JE, Wilson JD. The androgen resistance syndromes: 5α-reductase deficiency, testicular feminization, and related syndromes. In: Scriver CR, Beaudet AL, Sly WS, et al., eds. The Metabolic Basis of Inherited Disease. 6th ed. New York: McGraw-Hill, 1989: 1919–1944.

411. Perez-Palacios G, Chavez B, Mendez JP, et al. The syndromes of androgen resistance revisited. J Steroid Biochem 1987; 27:1101–1108.

412. Joshi NP, Sortrel G. Diagnostic laparoscopy in apparent uterine agenesis. J Adolesc Health Care 1988; 9:403–406.

413. Klein SM, Garcia CR. Asherman's syndrome: a critique and current review. Fertil Steril 1973; 24:722–735.

414. Rock JA, Zacur HA, Dlugi AM, et al. Pregnancy success following surgical correction of imperforate hymen and complete transverse vaginal septum. Obstet Gynecol 1982; 59:448–451.

415. Wheeless CR Jr. Excision of transverse vaginal septum. In: Wheeless CR Jr, ed. Atlas of Pelvic Surgery. 2nd ed. Philadelphia: Lea & Febiger, 1988: 74–75.

416. Aribarg A. Topical oestrogen therapy for labial adhesions in children. Br J Obstet Gynaecol 1975; 82:424–425.

417. Frank RT. The formation of an artificial vagina. Am J Obstet Gynecol 1938; 35:1053–1057.

418. Ingram, JM. The bicycle seat stool in the treatment of vaginal agenesis and stenosis: a preliminary report. Am J Obstet Gynecol 1981; 140:867–873.

419. McIndoe A. The treatment of congenital absence and obliterative conditions of the vagina. Br J Plast Surg 1950; 2:254–273.

420. Levine RU, Neuwirth RS. Simultaneous laparoscopy and hysteroscopy for intrauterine adhesions. Obstet Gynecol 1973; 42:441–445.

421. March CM, Israel R. Gestational outcome following hysteroscopic lysis of adhesions. Fertil Steril 1981; 36:455–459.

422. Levinson G, Zarate A, Guzman-Toledano R, et al. An XX female with sexual infantilism, absent gonads, and lack of mullerian ducts. J Med Genet 1976; 13:68–69.

423. Simpson JL. Gonadal dysgenesis and abnormalities of the human sex chromosomes: current status of phenotypic-karyotypic correlations. Birth Defects 1975; 11:23–59.

424. Tho PT, McDonough PG. Gonadal dysgenesis and its variants. Pediatr Clin North Am 1981; 28:309–329.

425. Turner HH. A syndrome of infantilism, congenital webbed neck, and cubitus valgus. Endocrinology 1938; 23:566–574.

426. Jaffe RB. Disorders of sexual development. In: Yen SSC, Jaffe RB, eds. Reproductive Endocrinology: Physiology, Pathophysiology and Clinical Management. 2nd ed. Philadelphia: W. B. Saunders, 1986: 283–312.

427. Michalak DP, Zacur HA, Rock JA, et al. Autoimmunity in a patient with 47,XXX karyotype. Obstet Gynecol 1983; 62:667–669.

428. Portundo JA, Neyro JL, Barral A, et al. Management of phenotypic female patients with an XY karyotype. J Reprod Med 1986; 31:611–615.

429. Simpson JL. Male pseudohermaphroditism: genetics and clinical delineation. Hum Genet 1978; 44:1–49.

430. Simpson JL. Genetic forms of gonadal dysgenesis in 46,XY individuals. Semin Reprod Endocrinol 1983; 1:93–100.

431. Carr BR, Aiman J. Steroid production in a women with gonadal dysgenesis, breast development, and clitoral hypertrophy. Obstet Gynecol 1980; 56:492–498.

432. Biglieri EG, Herron MA, Brust N. 17-Hydroxylation deficiency in man. J Clin Invest 1966; 45:1946–1954.

433. Larrea F, Lisker R, Banuelos R, et al. Hypergonadotrophic hypogonadism in an XX female subject due to 17,20 steroid desmolase deficiency. Acta Endocrinol 1983; 103:140–405.

434. Maxon WS, Wentz AC. The gonadotropin resistant ovary syndrome. Semin Reprod Endocrinol 1983; 1:147–160.

435. Kaufman FR, Xu YK, Ng WG, et al. Gonadal function and ovarian galactose metabolism in classic galactosemia. Acta Endocrinol 1989; 120:129–133.

436. LaBarbera AR, Miller MM, Ober C, et al. Autoimmune etiology in premature ovarian failure. Am J Reprod Immunol Microbiol 1988; 16:115–122.

437. Verp MS. Environmental causes of ovarian failure. Semin Reprod Endocrinol 1983; 1:101–111.

438. Ash P. The influence of radiation on fertility in man. Br J Radiol 1980; 53:271–278.

439. Morrison JC, Givens JR, Wiser WL et al. Mumps oophoritis: a cause of premature menopause. Fertil Steril 1975; 26:655–659.

440. Ross JL, Cassorla FG, Skerda MC, et al. A preliminary study of the effect of estrogen dose on growth in Turner's syndrome. N Engl J Med 1983; 309:1104–1106.

441. Raiti S. Effect of human growth hormone therapy in Turner's syndrome. Pediatr Adolesc Endocrinol 1987; 16:122–128.

442. Takano K, Shizume K, Hibi I, et al. Turner's syndrome: treatment of 203 patients with recombinant human growth hormone for one year. A multicentre study. Acta Endocrinol 1989; 120:559–568.

443. Horning SJ, Hoppe RT, Kaplan HS, et al. Female reproductive potential after treatment for Hodgkin's disease. N Engl J Med 1981; 304:1377–1382.

444. Alper MM, Jolly EE, Garner PR. Pregnancies after premature ovarian failure. Obstet Gynecol 1986; 67(Suppl):59S–62S.

445. Check JH, Wu CH, Check ML. The effect of leuprolide acetate in aiding induction of ovulation in hypergonadotropic hypogonadism: a case report. Fertil Steril 1988; 49:542–543.

446. Amos WL Jr. Pregnancy in patient with gonadotropin-resistant ovary syndrome. Am J Obstet Gynecol 1985; 153:154–155.

447. Surrey ES, Cedars MI. The effect of gonadotropin suppression on the induction of ovulation in premature ovarian failure patients. Fertil Steril 1989; 52:36–41.

448. Barraclough CA. Steroid regulation of reproductive neuroendocrine processes. In: Greep RO, Astwood EB, eds. Handbook of Physiology. Sect 7: Endocrinology. Vol II. Female Reproductive System. Washington, DC: American Physiological Society, 1973: 29–56.

449. Goldzieher JW, Axelrod LR. Clinical and biochemical features of polycystic ovarian disease. Fertil Steril 1963; 14:631–653.

450. Franks S. Polycystic ovary syndrome: a changing perspective. Clin Endocrinol 1989; 31:87–120.

451. Hauge WM, Adams J, Reeders ST, et al. Familial polycystic ovaries: a genetic disease? Clin Endocrinol 1988; 29:593–605.

452. Cooper HE, Spellacy WN, Prem KA, et al. Hereditary factors in the Stein-Leventhal syndrome. Am J Obstet Gynecol 1968; 100:371–387.

453. Wilroy RS, Givens JR, Wiser WL, et al. Hyperthecosis: an inheritable form of polycystic ovarian disease. Birth Defects 1975; 17:81–85.

454. Mandel FP, Chang RJ, Dupont B, et al. HLA genotyping in family members and patients with familial polycystic ovarian disease. J Clin Endocrinol Metab 1983; 56:862–864.

455. Stein IF, Leventhal ML. Amenorrhoea associated with bilateral polycystic ovaries. Am J Obstet Gynecol 1935; 29:181–191.

456. Smith KO, Steinberger E, Perloff WH. Polycystic ovarian disease. A report of 301 patients. Am J Obstet Gynecol 1965; 93:994–1001.

457. Shearman RP, Cox RI. The enigmatic polycystic ovary. Obstet Gynecol Surv 1966; 21:1–33.

458. Raj SG, Thompson IE, Berger MJ, et al. Clinical aspects of the polycystic ovary syndrome. Obstet Gynecol 1977; 49:552–556.

459. Seibel MM, Taymor ML. Polycystic ovarian syndrome: new insights into pathophysiology and treatment. In: Taymor ML, Nelson JH Jr, eds. Progress in Gynecology. Vol 7. New York: Grune & Stratton, 1983: 101–128.

460. Polson DW, Franks S, Reed MJ, et al. The distribution of oestradiol in plasma in relation to uterine cross-sectional area in women with polycystic or multifollicular ovaries. Clin Endocrinol 1987; 26:581–588.

461. Lobo RA. Polycystic ovary syndrome. In: Mishell DR Jr, Davajan V, eds. Infertility, Contraception and Reproductive Endocrinology. Oradell NJ: Medical Economics Books, 1986: 223–236.

462. Barnes R, Rosenfield RL. The polycystic ovary syndrome: pathogenesis and treatment. Ann Intern Med 1989; 110:386–399.

463. Rebar R, Judd HL, Yen SSC, et al. Characterization of the inappropriate gonadotropin secretion in polycystic ovary syndrome. J Clin Invest 1976; 57:1320–1329.

464. Aono T, Minagawa J, Kinugasa T, et al. The diagnostic significance of LH-releasing hormone test in patients with amenorrhea. Am J Obstet Gynecol 1974; 119:740–748.

465. Kazer RR, Kessel B, Yen SSC. Circulating luteinizing hormone pulse frequency in women with polycystic ovary syndrome. J Clin Endocrinol Metab 1987; 65:233–236.

466. Waldstreicher J, Santoro NF, Hall JE, et al. Hyperfunction of the hypothalamic-pituitary axis in women with polycystic ovarian disease: indirect evidence for partial gonadotroph desensitization. J Clin Endocrinol Metab 1988; 66:165–172.

467. McKenna TJ. Pathogenesis and treatment of polycystic ovary syndrome. N Engl J Med 1988; 318:558–562.

468. Lobo RA, Kletzky OA, Campeau JD, et al. Elevated bioactive luteinizing hormone in women with the polycystic ovary syndrome. Fertil Steril 1983; 39:674–678.

469. Chang RJ, Laufer LR, Meldrum DR, et al. Steroid secretion in polycystic ovarian disease after ovarian suppression by a long-acting gonadotropin-releasing hormone agonist. J Clin Endocrinol Metab 1983; 56:897–903.

470. Polson DW, Reed MJ, Franks S, et al. Serum 11-hydroxyandrostenedione as an indicator of the source of excess androgen production in women with polycystic ovaries. J Clin Endocrinol Metab 1988; 66:946–950.

471. Futterweit W. Pituitary tumours and polycystic ovarian disease. Obstet Gynecol 1983; 62(Suppl):S74–S79.

472. Luciano AA, Chapler FK, Sherman BM. Hyperprolactinemia in polycystic ovary syndrome. Fertil Steril 1968; 41:719–725.

473. Futterweit W. Polycystic Ovarian Disease. New York: Springer-Verlag, 1984: 1–210.

474. Lobo RA, Granger L, Goeblesmann U, et al. Elevation in unbound serum estradiol as a possible mechanism for inappropriate gonadotropin secretion in women with PCO. J Clin Endocrinol Metab 1981; 52:156–158.

475. Lobo RA, Goeblesmann U. Effect of androgen excess on inappropriate gonadotropin secretion as found in the polycystic ovary syndrome. Am J Obstet Gynecol 1982; 142:394–401.

476. Ackerman GE, Smith ME, Mendelson CR, et al. Aromatization of androstenedione by human adipose stromal cells in monolayer culture. J Clin Endocrinol Metab 1981; 53:412–417.

477. Zumoff B, Freeman R, Coupey S, et al. A chronobiologic abnormality in luteinizing hormone secretion in teenage girls with the polycystic ovary syndrome. N Engl J Med 1983; 309:1206–1209.

478. Erickson GF, Hsueh AJ, Quiglen ME, et al. Functional studies of aromatase activity in human granulosa cells from normal and polycystic ovaries. J Clin Endocrinol Metab 1979; 49:514–519.

479. Seibel MM, McArdle C, Smith D, et al. Ovulation induction in polycystic ovary syndrome with urinary follicle-stimulating hormone or human menopausal gonadotropin. Fertil Steril 1985; 43:703–708.

480. Claman P, Seibel MM, McArdle C, et al. Comparison of intermediate-dose purified urinary follicle-stimulating hormone with and without human chorionic gonadotropin for ovulation induction in polycystic ovarian disease. Fertil Steril 1986; 46:528–521.

481. Quigley ME, Rakoff JS, Yen SS. Increased luteinizing hormone sensitivity to dopamine inhibition in polycystic ovary syndrome. J Clin Endocrinol Metab 1981; 52:231–234.

482. Cumming DC, Reid RL, Quigley ME, et al. Evidence for decreased endogenous dopamine and opioid inhibitory influences on LH secretion in polycystic ovary syndrome. Clin Endocrinol 1984; 20:643–648.

483. Buckler HM, McLachlan RI, Maclachlan VB, et al. Serum inhibin levels in polycystic ovary syndrome: basal levels and response to luteinizing hormone–releasing hormone agonist and exogenous gonadotrophin administration. J Clin Endocrinol Metab 1988; 66:798–803.

484. Poretsky L, Kalin MF. The gonadotropic function of insulin. Endocr Rev 1987; 8:132–141.

485. Burghen GA, Givens JR, Kitabchi AE. Correlation of hyperandrogenism with hyperinsulinism in polycystic ovarian disease. J Clin Endocrinol Metab 1980; 50:113–116.

486. Chang RJ, Nakamura RM, Judd HL, et al. Insulin resistance in nonobese patients with polycystic ovarian disease. J Clin Endocrinol Metab 1983; 57:356–359.

487. Barbieri RL, Makris A, Randall RW, et al. Insulin stimulates androgen accumulation in incubations of ovarian stroma obtained from women with hyperandrogenism. J Clin Endocrinol Metab 1986; 62:904–910.

488. Adashi EY, Resnick CE, D'Ercole AJ, et al. Insulin-like growth factors as intraovarian regulators of granulosa cell growth and function. Endocr Rev 1985; 6:400–420.

489. Goldzieher JW, Green JA. The polycystic ovary. I. Clinical and histologic features. J Clin Endocrinol Metab 1962; 22:325–338.

490. Newmark S, Dluhy RG, Williams GH, et al. Partial 11- and 21-hydroxylase deficiencies in hirsute women. Am J Obstet Gynecol 1977; 127:594–598.

491. Cathelineau G, Brerault JL, Fiet J, et al. Adrenocortical 11β-hydroxylation defect in adult women with postmenarcheal onset of symptoms. J Clin Endocrinol Metab 1980; 51:287–291.

492. Aiman EJ, Nalick RH, Jacobs A, et al. The origin of androgen and estrogen in a virilized postmenopausal woman with bilateral benign cystic teratomas. Obstet Gynecol 1977; 49:695–704.

493. Daniell JF, Miller W. Polycystic ovaries treated by laparoscopic laser vaporization. Fertil Steril 1989; 51:232–236.

494. Dunaif A, Mandeli J, Fluhr H, et al. The impact of obesity and chronic hyperinsulinemia on gonadotropin release and gonadal steroid secretion in the polycystic ovary syndrome. J Clin Endocrinol Metab 1988; 66:131–139.

495. Pasquali R, Antenucci D, Casimirri F, et al. Clinical and hormonal characteristics of obese amenorrheic hyperandrogenic women before and after weight loss. J Clin Endocrinol Metab 1989; 68:173–179.

496. Remorgida V, Venturini PL, Anserini P, et al. Administration of pure follicle-stimulating hormone during gonadotropin-releasing hormone agonist therapy in patients with clomiphene-resistant polycystic ovarian disease: hormonal evaluations and clinical perspectives. Am J Obstet Gynecol 1989; 160:108–113.

497. Reid RL, Fretts R, Van Vugt DA. The theory and practice of ovulation induction with gonadotropin-releasing hormone. Am J Obstet Gynecol 1988; 158:176–185.

498. Eshel A, Abdulwahid NA, Armar NA, et al. Pulsatile luteinizing hormone–releasing hormone therapy in women with polycystic ovary syndrome. Fertil Steril 1988; 49:956–960.

499. Givens JR. Role of oral contraceptives in the treatment of hyperandrogenism of hirsute women. In: Mahesh VB, Greenblatt RB, eds. Hirsutism and Virilism: Pathogens, Diagnosis and Management. Boston: John Wright PSG, 1983: 351–367.

500. Gambrell RD Jr. Hormonal therapy. In: Greenblatt RB, Mahesh VB, Gambrell RD, eds. The Cause and Management of Hirsutism. Park Ridge, NJ: Parthenon, 1987: 137–146.

501. Bates GW, Whitworth NS. Effect of body weight reduction on plasma androgens in obese, infertile women. Fertil Steril 1982; 38:406–409.

502. Chamlian DL, Taylor HB. Endometrial hyperplasia in young women. Obstet Gynecol 1970; 36:659–666.

503. Jackson RL, Dockerty MB. The Stein-Leventhal syndrome: analysis of 43 cases with special reference to association with endometrial carcinoma. Am J Obstet Gynecol 1950; 73:161–173.

504. Kallmann FJ, Schoenfeld WA, Barrera SE. The genetic aspects of primary eunuchoidism. Am J Ment Defic 1944; 48:203–236.

505. Schwanzel-Fukuda M, Pfaff DW. Origin of luteinizing hormone–releasing hormone neurons. Nature 1989; 338:161–164.

506. Lieblich JM, Rogol AD, White BJ, et al. Syndrome of anosmia with hypogonadotropic hypogonadism (Kallmann syndrome). Am J Med 1982; 73:506–519.

507. Santen RJ, Paulsen CA. Hypogonadotropic eunuchoidism. I. Clinical study of the mode of inheritance. J Clin Endocrinol Metab 1973; 36:47–54.

508. Klingmuller D, Dewes W, Krahe T, et al. Magnetic resonance imaging of the brain in patients with anosmia and hypothalamic hypogonadism (Kallmann's syndrome). J Clin Endocrinol Metab 1987; 65:581–584.

509. Yen SSC. Chronic anovulation due to CNS-hypothalamic-pituitary dysfunction. In: Yen SSC, Jaffe RB, eds. Reproductive Endocrinology: Physiology, Pathophysiology and Clinical Management. 2nd ed. Philadelphia: W. B. Saunders, 1986: 500–545.

510. Santoro N, Filicori M, Crowley WF Jr. Hypogonadotropic disorders in men and women: diagnosis and therapy with pulsatile gonadotropin-releasing hormone. Endocr Rev 1986; 7:11–23.

511. Quigley ME, Sheehan KL, Casper RF, et al. Evidence for increased dopaminergic and opioid activity in patients with hypothalamic hypogonadotropic amenorrhea. J Clin Endocrinol Metab 1980; 50:949–954.

512. Vigersky RA, Anderson AE, Thompson RH, et al. Hypothalamic dysfunction in secondary amenorrhea associated with simple weight loss. N Engl J Med 1977; 297:1141–1145.

513. Gadpaille WJ, Sanborn CF, Wagner WW. Athletic amenorrhea, major affective disorders, and eating disorders. Am J Psychiatry 1987; 144:939–942.

514. Herzog DB, Coopeland PM. Eating disorders. N Engl J Med 1985; 313:295–303.

515. Warren MP, Vande Wiele RL. Clinical and metabolic features of anorexia nervosa. Am J Obstet Gynecol 1973; 117:435–449.

516. Warren MP. Effect of exercise and physical training on menarche. Semin Reprod Endocrinol 1985; 3:17–26.

517. Ronkainen H, Pakarinen A, Kirkinen P, et al. Physical exercise–induced changes and season-associated difference in the pituitary-ovarian function of runners and joggers. J Clin Endocrinol Metab 1985; 60:416–422.

518. Cumming DC, Rebar RW. Hormonal changes with acute exercise and with training in women. Semin Reprod Endocrinol 1985; 3:55–64.

519. Howlett TA, Tomlin S, Ngahfoong L, et al. Release of beta-endorphin and met-enkephalin during exercise in normal women: response to training. Br Med J 1984; 288:1950–1952.

520. Bullen BA, Skriinar GS, Beitins IZ, et al. Induction of menstrual disorders by strenuous exercise in untrained women. N Engl J Med 1985; 312:1349–1353.

521. McArthur JW, Bullen BA, Bertins IZ, et al. Hypothalamic amenorrhea in runners of normal body composition. Endocrinol Res Commun 1980; 7:13–25.

522. Abraham SF, Beumont PJV, Fraser IS, et al. Body weight, exercise and menstrual status among ballet dancers in training. Br J Obstet Gynaecol 1982; 89:507–510.

523. Shangold M, Freeman R, Thysen B, et al. The relationship between long-distance running, plasma progesterone and luteal phase length. Fertil Steril 1979; 31:130–133.

524. Drinkwater BL, Nilson K, Chestnut CH, et al. Bone mineral content of amenorrheic and eumenorrheic athletes. N Engl J Med 1984; 311:277–281.

525. Drinkwater BL, Nilson K, Ott S, et al. Bone mineral density after resumption of menses in amenorrheic athletes. JAMA 1986; 256:380–382.

526. Fisher EC, Nelson ME, Frontera WR, et al. Bone mineral content and levels of gonadotropins and estrogens in amenorrheic running women. J Clin Endocrinol Metab 1986; 62:1232–1236.

527. Lindberg JS, Fears WB, Hunt MM, et al. Exercise-induced amenorrhea and bone density. Ann Intern Med 1984; 101:647–648.

528. Marcus R, Cann CE, Madvig P, et al. Menstrual function and bone mass in elite women distance runners. Ann Intern Med 1985; 102:158–163.

529. Lloyd T, Triantafyllou SJ, Baker ER, et al. Women athletes with menstrual irregularity have increased musculoskeletal injuries. Med Sci Sports Exerc 1986; 18:374–379.

530. Van Der Spuy ZM, Steer PJ, McCusker M, et al. Outcome of pregnancy in underweight women after spontaneous and induced ovulation. Br Med J 1988; 296:962–965.

531. Gemzell C. Induction of ovulation with human gonadotropin. Recent Prog Horm Res 1965; 21:179–198.

532. Gindoff PR, Jewelewicz R. Use of gonadotropin in ovulation induction. NY State J Med 1985; 85:580–584.

533. Archer DF. Use of luteinizing hormone–releasing hormone for ovulation induction. Semin Reprod Endocrinol 1986; 4:285–291.

534. Howlett TA, Wass JAH, Grossman A, et al. Prolactinomas presenting as primary amenorrhoea and delayed or arrested puberty: response to medical therapy. Clin Endocrinol 1989; 30:131–140.

535. Schlechte J, Sherman B, Halmi N, et al. Prolactin-secreting pituitary tumors. Endocr Rev 1980; 1:295–308.

536. Jackson RD, Wortsman J, Malarkey WB. Characterization of a large molecular weight prolactin in women with idiopathic hyperprolactinemia and normal menses. J Clin Endocrinol Metab 1985; 61:258–264.

537. Schlechte J, Dolan K, Sherman B, et al. The natural history of untreated hypoprolactinemia: a prospective analysis. J Clin Endocrinol Metab 1989; 68:412–418.

538. March CM, Kletzky OA, Davajan V, et al. Longitudinal evaluation of patients with untreated prolactin-secreting pituitary adenomas. Am J Obstet Gynecol 1981; 139:835–844.

539. Sisam DA, Sheehan JP, Sheeler LR. The natural history of untreated microprolactinomas. Fertil Steril 1987; 48:67–71.

540. Martin TL, Kim M, Malarkey WB. The natural history of idiopathic hyperprolactinemia. J Clin Endocrinol Metab 1985; 60:855–858.

541. Pituitary Adenoma Study Group. Pituitary adenomas and oral contraceptives: a multicenter case-control study. Fertil Steril 1983; 39:753–760.

542. Yen SSC. Prolactin in human reproduction. In: Yen SSC, Jaffe RB, eds. Reproductive Endocrinology: Physiology, Pathophysiology and Clinical Management. 2nd ed. Philadelphia: W. B. Saunders, 1986: 237–263.

543. Burrow GN, Wortzman G, Rewcastle NB, et al. Microadenomas of the pituitary and abnormal sellar tomograms in an unselected autopsy series. N Engl J Med 1981; 304:156–158.

544. Blackwell RE, Boots LR, Goldenberg RL, et al. Assessment of pituitary function in patients with serum prolactin levels greater than 100 ng/ml. Fertil Steril 1979; 32:177–182.

545. Blackwell RE, Chang RJ, Cragen JR. Prolactin disorders in infertility. In: Seibel MM, ed. Infertility. Norwalk, CT: Appleton & Lange, 1990: 97–109.

546. Stein AL, Levenick MN, Kletzky OA. Computed tomography versus magnetic resonance imaging for the evaluation of suspected pituitary adenomas. Obstet Gynecol 1989; 73:996–999.

547. Schlechte JA, Sherman BM, Chapler FK, et al. Long term follow-up of women with surgically treated prolactin-secreting pituitary tumors. J Clin Endocrinol Metab 1986; 62:1296–1301.

548. Parl FF, Cruz VE, Cobb CA, et al. Late recurrence of surgically removed prolactinomas. Cancer 1986; 57:2422–2426.

549. Wang C, Lam KSL, Ma JTC, et al. Long-term treatment of hyperprolactinemia with bromocriptine: effect of drug withdrawal. Clin Endocrinol 1987; 27:363–371.

550. McGregor AM, Scanlon MF, Hall R, et al. Effects of bromocriptine on pituitary tumour size. Br Med J 1979; 2:700–703.

551. Molitch ME, Elton RL, Blackwell RE, et al. Bromocriptine as primary therapy for prolactin-secreting macroadenomas: results of a prospective multicenter study. J Clin Endocrinol Metab 1985; 60:698–705.

552. Thorner MO, Martin WH, Rogol AD, et al. Rapid regression of pituitary prolactinomas during bromocriptine treatment. J Clin Endocrinol Metab 1980; 51:438–445.

553. Koppelman MCS, Jaffe MJ, Rieth KG, et al. Hyperprolactinemia, amenorrhea, and galactorrhea: a retrospective assessment of twenty-five cases. Ann Intern Med 1984; 100:115–121.

554. Corenblum B. Successful outcome of ergocryptine-induced pregnancies in twenty-one women with prolactin-secreting pituitary adenomas. Fertil Steril 1979; 32:183–186.

555. Divers WA, Yen SSC: Prolactin-producing microadenomas in pregnancy. Obstet Gynecol 1983; 62:425–429.

556. Magyar DM, Marshall JR. Pituitary tumors and pregnancy. Am J Obstet Gynecol 1978; 132:739–751.

557. Molitch ME. Pregnancy and the hyperprolactinemic woman. N Engl J Med 1985; 312:1364–1370.

558. DeWit W, Coelingh Bennink HJT, Gerards LJ. Prophylactic bromocriptine treatment during pregnancy in women with macroprolactinomas: report of 13 pregnancies. Br J Obstet Gynaecol 1984; 91:1059–1069.

559. Ruiz-Velasco V, Tolis G. Pregnancy in hyperprolactinemic women. Fertil Steril 1984; 41:793–805.

560. Holmgren U, Bergstrand G, Hagenfeldt K, et al. Women with prolactinoma—effect of pregnancy and lactation on serum prolactin and on tumour growth. Acta Endocrinol 1986; 111:452–459.

561. Banna M. Craniopharyngioma: based on 160 cases. Br J Radiol 1976; 49:206–223.

562. Petito CK, DeGirolami U, Earle KM. Craniopharyngiomas, a clinical and pathological review. Cancer 1976; 37:1944–1952.

563. Bevan JS, Burke CW, Esiri MM, et al. Misinterpretation of prolactin levels leading to management errors in patients with sellar enlargement. Am J Med 1987; 82:29–32.

564. Kaufman B. The "empty" sella turcica—a manifestation of the intrasellar subarachnoid space. Radiology 1968; 90:931–941.

565. Neelon FA, Goree JA, Lebovitz HE. The primary empty sella: clinical and radiographic characteristics and endocrine function. Medicine 1973; 52:73–92.

566. Kletzky OA, Davajan V, Nakamura RM, et al. Clinical categorization of patients with secondary amenorrhea using progesterone-induced uterine bleeding and measurement of serum gonadotropin levels. Am J Obstet Gynecol 1975; 121:695–703.

567. Greenblatt RB. Hirsutism: ancestral curse on endocrinopathy. In: Greenblatt RB, Mahesh VB, Gambrell RD, eds. The Cause and Management of Hirsutism. Park Ridge, NJ: Parthenon, 1987: 17–29.

568. Hamilton JB. Effect of castration in adolescent and young males upon further changes in the proportions of bare and hairy scalp. J Clin Endocrinol Metab 1960; 20:1309–1318.

569. Uno H. Biology of hair growth. Semin Reprod Endocrinol 1986; 4:131–141.

570. Barbieri RL, Smith S, Ryan KJ. The role of hyperinsulinemia in the pathogenesis of ovarian hyperandrogenism. Fertil Steril 1988; 50:197–212.

571. Goeblesman U, Lobo RA. Androgen excess. In: Mishell DR Jr, Davajan V, eds. Infertility, Contraception and Reproductive Endocrinology. Oradell, NJ: Medical Economics Books, 1986: 303–317.

572. Chang RJ. Ovarian steroid secretion in polycystic ovarian disease. Semin Reprod Endocrinol 1984; 2:244–250.

573. Horton R, Hawks D, Lobo RA. 3α, 17β-Androstanediol glucuronide in plasma. A marker of androgen action in idiopathic hirsutism. J Clin Invest 1982; 82:1203–1207.

574. Serafini P, Ablan R, Lobo RA. 5α-Reductase activity in the genital skin of hirsute women. J Clin Endocrinol Metab 1985; 60:349–355.

575. Rebar RW. Hirsutism, hyperandrogenism, and polycystic ovarian syndrome. In: DeGroot LJ, Besser GM, Cahill GF Jr, et al., eds. Endocrinology. 2nd ed. Philadelphia: W. B. Saunders, 1989: 1982–1993.

576. Judd HL, Scully RE, Herbst AL, et al. Familial hyperthecosis: comparison of endocrinologic and histologic findings with polycystic ovarian disease. Am J Obstet Gynecol 1973; 117:976–982.

577. Nagamani M, Lingold JC, Gomez LG, et al. Clinical and hormonal studies in hyperthecosis of the ovaries. Fertil Steril 1981; 36:326–332.

578. Nagamani M, Dinh TV, Kelver ME. Hyperinsulinemia in hyperthecosis of the ovaries. Am J Obstet Gynecol 1986; 154:384–389.

579. Moller DE, Flier JS. Detection of an alteration in the insulin-receptor gene in a patient with insulin resistance, acanthosis nigricans, and the polycystic ovary syndrome (type A insulin resistance). N Engl J Med 1988; 319:1526–1529.

580. Morris M. Virilizing tumors of the ovary. Cancer Bull 1987; 39:300–303.

581. Scully RE. Ovarian tumors with endocrine manifestations. In: DeGroot LJ, Besser GM, Cahill GF Jr, et al., eds. Endocrinology. 2nd ed. Philadelphia: W. B. Saunders, 1989: 1994–2008.

582. Stone M, Bagshawe KD, Kardana A, et al. β-Human chorionic gonadotrophin and carcinoembryonic antigen in the management of ovarian carcinoma. Br J Obstet Gynaecol 1977; 84:375–379.

583. Vaitukaitis JL, Braunstein GD, Ross GT. A radioimmunoassay which specifically measures human chorionic gonadotropin in the presence of human luteinizing hormone. Am J Obstet Gynecol 1972; 113:751–758.

584. Robboy SJ, Norris HJ, Scully RE. Insular carcinoid primary in the ovary: a clinicopathologic analysis of 48 cases. Cancer 1975; 36:404–481.

585. Robboy SJ, Scully RE. Strumal carcinoid of the ovary: an analysis of 50 cases of a distinctive tumor composed of thyroid tissue and carcinoid. Cancer 1980; 46:2019–2034.

586. Brown PA, Richart RM. Functioning ovarian carcinoid tumors. Case report and review of the literature. Obstet Gynecol 1969; 24:390–395.

587. Marcus CC, Marcus SL. Struma ovarii: a report of 7 cases and a review of the subject. Am J Obstet Gynecol 1961; 81:752–762.

588. Smith FG. Pathology and physiology of struma ovarii. Arch Surg 1946; 53:603–626.

589. White PC, New MI, DuPont B. Congenital adrenal hyperplasia. N Engl J Med 1987; 316:1519–1524.

590. Brodie BL, Wentz AC. Late onset congenital adrenal hyperplasia: a gynecologist's perspective. Fertil Steril 1987; 48:175–188.

591. Kuttenn F, Couillion P, Girard F, et al. Late-onset adrenal hyperplasia in hirsutism. N Engl J Med 1985; 313:224–231.

592. Karpas AE. Iatrogenic hirsutism. In: Greenblatt RB, Mahesh VB, Gambrell RD, eds. The Cause and Management of Hirsutism. Park Ridge, NJ: Parthenon, 1987: 61–69.

593. Tagatz GE, Kopher RA, Nagel TC, et al. The clitoral index: a bioassay of androgenic stimulation. Obstet Gynecol 1979; 54:562–564.

594. Dewailly D, Vantyghem MC, Lemaire C, et al. Screening heterozygotes for 21-hydroxylase deficiency among hirsute women: lack of utility of the adrenocorticotropin hormone test. Fertil Steril 1988; 50:228–232.

595. Lobo RA, Goebelsmann U. Adult manifestation of congenital adrenal hyperplasia due to incomplete 21-hydroxylase deficiency mimicking polycystic ovarian disease. Am J Obstet Gynecol 1980; 138:720–726.

596. Mosher WD. Infertility trends among U.S. couples: 1965–1976. Fam Plann Perspect 1982; 14:22–27.

597. Seibel MM. Workup of the infertile couple. In: Seibel MM, ed. Infertility. Norwalk, CT: Appleton & Lange, 1990: 1–22.

598. Henderson GE, Mosher WD, Pratt WF. Infertility and age: an unresolved issue. Fam Plann Perspect 1982; 14:287–289.

599. Daly DC, Walters CA, Soto-Albons CE, et al. A randomized study of dexamethasone in ovulation induction with clomiphene citrate. Fertil Steril 1984; 41:844–848.

600. Seibel MM. Polycystic ovary disease. In: Seibel MM, ed. Infertility. Norwalk, CT: Appleton & Lange, 1990: 61–81.

601. Katz E. The luteinized unruptured follicle and other ovulatory dysfunctions. Fertil Steril 1988; 50:839–850.

602. Jones GS, Aksel S, Wentz AC. Serum progesterone values in the luteal phase defects. Obstet Gynecol 1974; 44:26–34.

603. Strott CA, Cargille CM, Ross GT, et al. The short luteal phase. J Clin Endocrinol 1970; 30:246–251.

604. Siegler AM. Hysterosalpingography. Fertil Steril 1983; 40:139–158.

605. Gomel V. Salpingostomy by microsurgery. Fertil Steril 1978; 29:380–387.

606. Siegler AM, Kontopoulos V. An analysis of macrosurgical and microsurgical techniques in the management of tubo-peritoneal factor in infertility. Fertil Steril 1979; 32:377–383.

607. Hunt RB. Operative laparoscopy. In: Seibel MM, ed. Infertility. Norwalk, CT: Appleton & Lange, 1990: 377–369.

608. Gomel V. Salpingo-ovariolysis by laparoscopy in infertility. Fertil Steril 1983; 40:607–611.

609. Kelly RW, Roberts DK. Experiences with the carbon dioxide laser in gynecological microsurgery. Am J Obstet Gynecol 1983; 146:585–588.

610. Keye WR, Dixon J. Photocoagulation of endometriosis by the argon laser through the laparoscope. Obstet Gynecol 1983; 62:383–386.

611. Wilson EA, ed. Endometriosis. New York: Alan R. Liss, 1987: 1–233.

612. Bayer SR, Seibel MM. Endometriosis: pathophysiology and treatment. In: Seibel MM, ed. Infertility. Norwalk, CT: Appleton & Lange, 1990: 111–128.

613. Jette NT, Glass RH. Prognostic value of the post-coital test. Fertil Steril 1972; 23:29–32.

614. Collins JA, So Y, Wilson EH, et al. The post-coital test as a prediction of pregnancy among 355 infertile couples. Fertil Steril 1984; 41:703–708.

615. Davajan V, Vargyas JM, Kletzky OA, et al. Intrauterine insemination with washed sperm to treat infertility. Fertil Steril 1983; 40:419–421.

616. Byrd W, Ackerman GE, Carr BR, et al. Treatment of refractory infertility by transcervical intrauterine insemination of washed spermatozoa. Fertil Steril 1987; 48:921–927.

617. Bronson R, Cooper RG, Rosenfeld D. Sperm antibodies: their role in infertility. Fertil Steril 1984; 42:171–183.

618. Clark GN, Elliott PJ, Smaila C. Detection of sperm antibodies in semen using the immunobead test: a survey of 813 consecutive patients. Am J Reprod Immunol Microbiol 1985; 7:118–123.

619. Seibel MM. In vitro fertilization, gamete intrafallopian transfer, and donated gametes and embryos. N Engl J Med 1988; 318:828–834.

620. Medical Research International, American Fertility Society Special Interest Group. In vitro fertilization/embryo transfer in the United States. 1985 and 1986 results from the National IVF/ET Registry. Fertil Steril 1988; 49:212–215.

621. Asch RH, Ellsworth LR, Balmaceda JP, et al. Pregnancy after translaparoscopic gamete intrafallopian tube transfer. Lancet 1984; 2:1034–1035.

622. Dodson WC, Whitesides DB, Hughes CL Jr, et al. Superovulation with intrauterine insemination in the treatment of infertility: a possible alternative to gamete intrafallopian transfer and in vitro fertilization. Fertil Steril 1987; 48:441–445.

623. Hamori M, Stuckensen JA, Rumpf D, et al. Zygote intrafallopian transfer (ZIFT): evaluation of 42 cases. Fertil Steril 1988; 50:519–521.

624. Yovick JL, Blackledge DG, Richards PA, et al. Pregnancies following pronuclear stage tubal transfer. Fertil Steril 1987; 48:851–857.

625. Van-Steirteghem AC, Van-den-Abbell E. Survey on cryopreservation. Ann NY Acad Sci 1988; 541:571–574.

626. Whitehead MI, Siddle N, Lane G, et al. The pharmacology of progestogens. In: Mishell DR Jr, ed. Menopause. Chicago: Year Book Medical, 1987: 317–334.

627. Whitehead MI, Townsend PT, Gill DK, et al. Absorption and metabolism of oral progesterone. Br Med J 1980; 280:825–827.

628. Wentz AC. Luteal phase inadequacy. In: Behrman SJ, Kistner RW, Patton GW, eds. Progress in Infertility. Boston: Little, Brown, 1988: 405–462.

629. Rigg LA, Milanes B, Villanueva B, et al. Efficacy of intravaginal and intranasal administration of micronized estradiol-17β. J Clin Endocrinol Metab 1977; 45:1261–1264.

630. Anderson ABM, Sklovsky E, Sayers L, et al. Comparison of serum oestrogen concentrations in post-menopausal women taking oestrone sulphate and oestradiol. Br Med J 1978; 1:140–142.

631. Yen SSC, Martin PL, Burnier AM, et al. Circulating estradiol, estrone

and gonadotropin levels following the administration of orally active 17β-estradiol in postmenopausal women. J Clin Endocrinol Metab 1975; 40:518–521.

632. Ryan JK, Engel LL. The interconversion of estrone and estradiol by human tissue slices. Endocrinology 1953; 52:287–291.

633. Sandberg A, Slaunwhite WR. Studies on phenolic steroids in human subjects. II. The metabolic fate and hepato-biliary-enteric circulation of C14-estrone and C14-estradiol in women. J Clin Invest 1957; 36:1266–1278.

634. Powers MS, Schenkel L, Darley PE, et al. Pharmacokinetics and pharmacodynamics of transdermal dosage forms of 17β-estradiol: comparison with conventional oral estrogens used for hormone replacement. Am J Obstet Gynecol 1985; 152:1099–1106.

635. Schiff I, Tulchinsky D, Ryan KJ. Vaginal absorption of estrone and 17β-estradiol. Fertil Steril 1977; 28:1063–1066.

636. Barnes RB, Lobo RA. Pharmacology of estrogens. In: Mishell DR Jr, ed. Menopause. Chicago: Year Book Medical, 1987: 301–315.

637. Englund DE, Johansson EDB. Plasma levels of oestrone, oestradiol and gonadotrophins in postmenopausal women after oral and vaginal administration of equine estrogens. Br J Obstet Gynaecol 1978; 85:957–964.

638. Lobo R, Mishell DR, Budoff PW. Estrogen Replacement Therapy. Symposium Proceedings, San Francisco, May 9–10, 1984. Chicago: Abbott Pharmaceuticals, 1984: 9.

639. Deutsch S, Ossowski R, Benjamin I. Comparison between degree of systemic absorption of vaginally and orally administered estrogens at different dose levels in postmenopausal women. Am J Obstet Gynecol 1981; 139:967–968.

640. Genant HK, Baylink DJ, Gallagher JC. Estrogens in the prevention of osteoporosis in postmenopausal women. Am J Obstet Gynecol 1989; 161:1842–1846.

641. Odom MJ, Carr BR, MacDonald PC. The menopause and estrogen replacement therapy. In: Andres R, Bierman E, Blass JP, eds. Principles of Geriatric Medicine and Gerontology. 2nd ed. New York: McGraw-Hill, 1990: 777–788.

642. Sherwin BB, Gelfand MM. A prospective one-year study of estrogen and progestin in postmenopausal women: effects on clinical symptoms and lipoprotein lipids. Obstet Gynecol 1989; 73:759–766.

643. Wallentin L, Larsson-Cohn U. Metabolic and hormonal effects of postmenopausal oestrogen replacement treatment. II. Plasma lipids. Acta Endocrinol 1977; 86:597–607.

644. Smith DC, Prentice R, Thompson DJ, et al. Association of exogenous estrogen and endometrial carcinoma. N Engl J Med 1975; 293:1164–1167.

645. Ziel HK, Finkle WD. Increased risk of endometrial carcinoma among users of conjugated estrogens. N Engl J Med 1975; 293:1167–1170.

646. Collins J, Allen LH, Donner A, et al. Oestrogen use and survival in endometrial cancer. Lancet 1980; 2:961–964.

647. Pfeffer RI, Kurosaki TT, Charlton SK. Estrogen use and blood pressure in later life. Am J Epidemiol 1979; 110:469–478.

648. Boston Collaborative Drug Surveillance Program. Surgically confirmed gallbladder disease, venous thromboembolism, and breast tumors in relation to postmenopausal estrogen therapy. N Engl J Med 1974; 290:15–19.

649. Ross RK, Paganini-Hill A, Gerkins VR, et al. A case-control study of menopausal estrogen therapy and breast cancer. JAMA 1980; 243:1635–1639.

650. Jick H, Walker AM, Watkins RN, et al. Replacement estrogens and breast cancer. Am J Epidemiol 1980; 112:586–594.

651. Brinton LA, Hoover RN, Szklo M, et al. Menopausal estrogen use and breast cancer. Cancer 1981; 47:2517–2522.

652. Hoover R, Glass A, Finkle WD, et al. Conjugated estrogens use and breast cancer risk. J Natl Cancer Inst 1981; 67:815–820.

653. Hiatt RA, Bawol R, Friedman GD, et al. Exogenous estrogen and breast cancer after bilateral oophorectomy. Cancer 1984; 54:139–144.

654. Kaufman DW, Miller DR, Rosenberg L, et al. Noncontraceptive estrogen use and the risk of breast cancer. JAMA 1984; 252:63–67.

655. Kelsey JL, Fischer DB, Holford TR, et al. Exogenous estrogens and other factors in the epidemiology of breast cancer. J Natl Cancer Inst 1981; 67:327–333.

656. March CM, Mishell DR Jr. Induction of ovulation. In: Mishell DR Jr, Davajan V, eds. Infertility, Contraception and Reproductive Endocrinology. Oradell, NJ: Medical Economic Books, 1986: 389–411.

657. Claman P, Seibel MM. Purified human follicle-stimulating hormone for ovulation induction. A critical review. Semin Reprod Endocrinol 1986; 4:277–283.

658. Haning RV Jr, Strawn EY, Nolten WE. Pathophysiology of the ovarian hyperstimulation syndrome. Obstet Gynecol 1985; 66:220–224.

659. March CM. Improved pregnancy rate with monitoring of gonadotropin therapy by three modalities. Am J Obstet Gynecol 1987; 156:1473–1479.

660. Weil C. The safety of bromocriptine in long-term use: a review of the literature. Curr Med Res Opin 1986; 10:25–51.

661. Turkalj I, Braun P, Krupp P. Surveillance of bromocriptine in pregnancy. JAMA 1982; 247:1589–1591.

662. Raymond JP, Goldstein E, Konopka P, et al. Follow-up of children born of bromocriptine-treated mothers. Horm Res 1985; 22:239–246.

663. Katz E, Schram HF, Adashi EY. Successful treatment of a prolactin-producing macroadenomas with intravaginal bromocriptine mesylate. A novel approach to intolerance of oral therapy. Obstet Gynecol 1989; 73:517–520.

664. Claman P, Seibel MM. Ovulation induction: GnRH. In: Seibel MM, ed. Infertility. Norwalk, CT: Appleton & Lange, 1990: 333–350.

665. Givens JR, Andersen RN, Wiser WL, et al. The effectiveness of two oral contraceptives in suppressing plasma androstenedione, testosterone, LH and FSH, and in stimulating plasma testosterone-binding capacity in hirsute women. Am J Obstet Gynecol 1979; 124:333–339.

666. Talbert LM, Sloan C. The effect of a low-dose oral contraceptive on serum testosterone levels in polycystic ovary disease. Obstet Gynecol 1979; 53:694–697.

667. Fern M, Rose DP, Fern EB. Effect of oral contraceptives on plasma androgenic steroids and their processes. Obstet Gynecol 1978; 51:541–544.

668. Madden JD, Milewich L, Parker CR Jr, et al. The effect of oral contraceptive treatment on the serum concentration of dehydroepiandrosterone sulfate. Am J Obstet Gynecol 1978; 132:380–383.

669. Wild RA, Umstot ES, Andersen RN, et al. Adrenal function in hirsutism. II. Effect of an oral contraceptive. J Clin Endocrinol Metab 1982; 54:676–681.

670. Klove KL, Roy S, Lobo RA. The effect of different contraceptive treatments on the serum concentration of dehydroepiandrosterone sulfate. Contraception 1984; 29:319–324.

671. Marynik SP, Chakmakjian ZH, McCaffree DL, et al. Androgen excess in cystic acne. N Engl J Med 1983; 308:981–986.

672. Jacobs AJ, Odom MJ, Word RA, et al. Effect of oral contraceptives on adrenocorticotropin and growth hormone secretion following CRH and GHRH administration. Contraception 1989; 40:691–699.

673. Murphy AA, Burkman RT, Cropp CS, et al. Effect of low-dose oral contraceptive on gonadotropins, androgens, and sex hormone binding globulin in nonhirsute women. Fertil Steril 1990; 53:35–39.

674. Lobo RA. Endocrine therapy of hyperandrogenism. In: Barbieri RL, Schiff I, eds. Reproductive Endocrine Therapeutics. New York: Alan R. Liss, 1988: 101–126.

675. Kuttenn F, Rigaud C, Wright F, et al. Treatment of hirsutism by oral cyproterone acetate and percutaneous estradiol. J Clin Endocrinol Metab 1980; 51:1107–1111.

676. Corvol P, Michaud A, Menard J, et al. Antiandrogenic effect of spironolactones: mechanisms of action. Endocrinology 1975; 97:52–58.

677. Hammerstein J. Cyproterone acetate. In: Greenblatt RB, Mahesh VB, Gambrell RD, eds. The Cause and Management of Hirsutism. A Practical Approach to the Control of Unwanted Hair. Park Ridge, NJ: Parthenon, 1987:147–159.

678. Sonino N. The use of ketoconazole as an inhibitor of steroid production. N Engl J Med 1987; 317:812–818.

679. Carvalho D, Pignatell D, Resende C. Ketoconazole for hirsutism. Lancet 1985; 2:560.

680. Pepper GM, Poretsky L, Gabrilove JL, et al. Ketoconazole reverse hyperandrogenism in a patient with insulin resistance and acanthosis nigricans. J Clin Endocrinol Metab 1987; 65:1047–1052.

681. Hodgen GD. Proceedings from the Symposium: current role of GnRH agonists in obstetrics and gynecology. Obstet Gynecol Surv 1989; 44(Suppl):293–296.

682. Miller JD. GnRH analog delivery systems: present and future options. Obstet Gynecol Surv 1989; 44(Suppl):326–329.

683. Friedman AJ, Barbieri RL. Leuprolide acetate: applications in gynecology. Curr Probl Obstet Gynecol Fertil 1988; 11:209–244.

684. Comite F. GnRH analogs and safety. Obstet Gynecol Surv 1989; 44(Suppl)319–325.

13

DISORDERS OF THE TESTES AND THE MALE REPRODUCTIVE TRACT

James E. Griffin and Jean D. Wilson

INTRODUCTION

The testes produce sperm and the hormones that regulate male sexual life, both functions being under complex feedback control by the hypothalamic-pituitary system. In terms of biosynthetic functions and regulatory control the testes are similar to the ovaries and the adrenals. The testes differ, however, in that the major secretory hormone, testosterone, has few direct actions; instead it serves as a circulating prohormone for two other classes of steroid hormones, 5α-reduced androgens and estrogens. These products mediate most of the cellular actions of testosterone. Testicular hormones are also responsible for the induction of male development during embryogenesis. In fulfilling this primordial function, the testes cause the differentiation of the tissues that serve as the major sites of androgen action. At puberty the testicular hormones mediate the changes of sexual maturation. As a result, abnormalities of testicular function cause different clinical consequences depending on the phase of life in which they develop, from early gestation through old age. Although these biological effects differ, the regulation of testicular hormone production and the mechanisms of hormone action are similar at all stages of life.

DEVELOPMENT OF THE TESTES

Embryogenesis

The gene or genes that control testicular differentiation are located on the Y chromosome. The Y chromosome is the third smallest human chromosome.[1] The short arm of the Y is invariable in size, whereas among normal men the long arms of the Y may differ considerably in length. Analyses of individuals with structural abnormalities of the Y chromosome indicate that the short arm of the Y carries the genes that are responsible for testicular development.[2] Additional genes on the short and/or long arms may be essential for normal spermatogenesis. The short arm of the Y chromosome is composed of two distinct regions.[3] The first region (the so-called pairing segment) is homologous to a region at the end of the short arm of the X chromosome and is responsible for pairing between the X and Y chromosomes during meiosis in the male. Pairing is essential for correct meiotic segregation of the sex chromosomes. Recombination can occur between the shared regions of the X and the Y, and genes and sequences in this region of the X chromosome fail to exhibit typical X chromosome linkage. This type of inheritance is termed *pseudoautosomal*.[1]

799

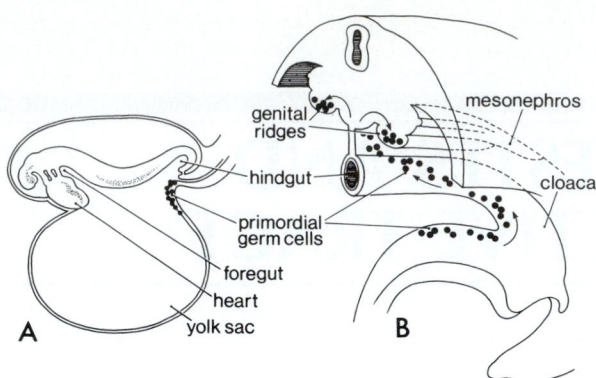

Figure 13–1. *A,* Schematic drawing of a 3-wk-old embryo showing the site of origin of germ cells in the wall of the yolk sac. *B,* Migration path of primordial germ cells along the wall of the yolk sac and along the dorsal mesentery into the genital ridge. (From George FW, Wilson JD. Embryology of the genital tract. In: Walsh PC, Gittes RF, Perlmutter AD, et al., eds. Campbell's Urology. 5th ed. Philadelphia: W. B. Saunders, 1986: 1804–1818.)

The second region of the short arm of the Y chromosome encodes genes that do not recombine with the X chromosome, including the testis-determining gene(s). The assignment of the testis-determining genes to this region was first made on the basis of studies of subjects with structural anomalies of the Y chromosome and was substantiated by the construction of detailed deletion maps of the Y chromosome.[2] Extensive analysis of the short arm of the Y chromosome between the centromere and the pseudoautosomal region has identified a gene that is believed to be responsible for testis determination; the gene is Y specific, conserved among a wide range of mammals, and encodes a testis-specific transcript.[4] This locus is distinct from the gene that encodes the H-Y antigen, a male-specific protein that was previously believed to be the testis-determining principle.[5]

The mechanism by which the testis-determining genes of the Y chromosome dictate testicular development is not known, but at a minimum three principal cell types are involved in formation of the testes: (1) germ cells that are derived from primitive ectodermal cells of the inner cell mass and that are initially identifiable in the entoderm of the yolk sac; (2) supporting cells that are derived from the coelomic epithelium of the gonadal ridge and that differentiate into the Sertoli cells in the testis (or granulosa cells in the ovary); and (3) stromal (interstitial) cells that are derived from the mesenchyme of the gonadal ridge.

The primordial germ cells, which are recognizable on the basis of size, alkaline phosphatase activity, and glycogen content, have been recognized in the 4½-d-old human blastocyst.[6, 7] Before day 23 of human gestation these cells are located in the dorsal and caudal portions of the yolk sac entoderm (Fig. 13–1A). Thereafter, they migrate by amoeboid movement from the gut endoderm through the mesentery, eventually reaching the genital ridge (Fig. 13–1B).[8] The germ cells replicate several times during this migration, so that more are found in the genital ridge than were originally present in the yolk sac.[9] The nature of the forces that control this migration is unknown. After reaching the genital ridge, the germ cells, together with adhering epithelial cells, infiltrate the underlying mesenchyme. This process is identical in male and female embryos and culminates in the formation of the genital blastema containing the three basic cell types by 5 to 6 wk of gestation. Primordial germ cells that fail to reach the genital ridge degenerate or differentiate into other cell types and may serve as the progenitors of extragonadal germ cell tumors in later life.[10]

Sexual dimorphism of the human gonad first becomes apparent with the appearance of seminiferous cords in the fetal testis between 6 and 7 wk of gestation. By contrast, histological development in the fetal ovary is not apparent until the sixth month of gestation, when granulosa cells organize around the dividing oocytes to form the primary ovarian follicle.[11] The somatic cells of the gonad can undergo partial organization into ovary or testis as specified by the genotype, even if the germ cells are prevented from migrating to the genital ridge, which implies that some determinants for gonadal development are expressed by the cells of the genital ridge.[12, 13] However, differentiation of the genital blastema into testis may also be enhanced by the germ cells themselves, probably by germ cells carrying a Y chromosome.[14]

Descent

Histological development of the testis is largely complete by the end of the third month, whereas descent of the testis from the abdominal cavity to the scrotum occurs during the latter two thirds of gestation. The forces, both chemical and physical, that regulate testicular descent are poorly understood. For didactic purposes descent can be divided into three phases: transabdominal movement, formation of the processus vaginalis, and true anatomical descent, but in reality the process constitutes a continuum.[15, 16]

At the time of endocrine differentiation of the gonad (the eighth week), the testis and mesonephros are anatomically adjacent to the kidney and are attached to the posterior abdominal wall by a broad peritoneal fold. As the mesonephros degenerates, the cranial portion of this fold disappears, but the caudal portion persists as a narrow ligament that is continuous with a band of mesenchyme extending into the genital swellings. This mesenchymal band, the gubernaculum, anchors the fetal testis to the inguinal region and may serve two functions: it probably prevents upward movement of the testis, as happens with the kidney during the rapid elongation of the trunk, and may actually pull the gonad to the edge of the anterior abdominal wall as the mesonephros degenerates with shortening of the guber-

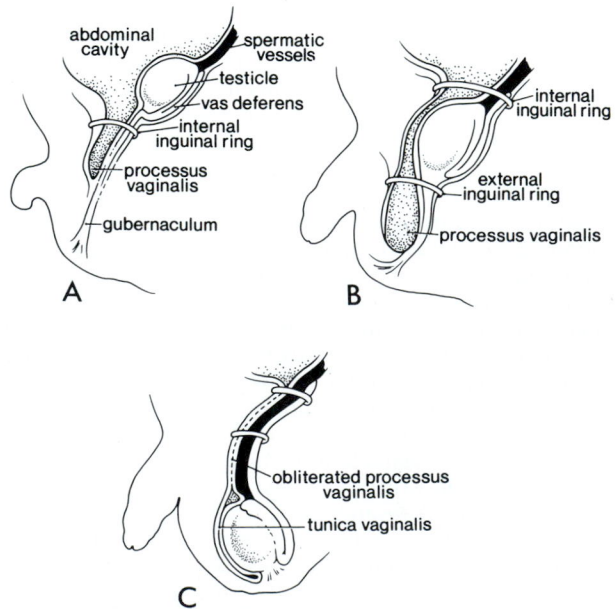

Figure 13–2. Descent of the testis. (From George FW, Wilson JD. Embryology of the genital tract. In: Walsh PC, Gittes RF, Perlmutter AD, et al., eds. Campbell's Urology. 5th ed. Philadelphia: W. B. Saunders, 1986: 1804–1818.)

naculum from about 6 to 2 mm (13 to 14 cm of crown-rump length).

During the third month of gestation, a herniation of the coelomic cavity, termed the *processus vaginalis*, forms through the ventral abdominal wall along the course of each gubernaculum (Fig. 13–2). Herniation results in part from the increase in intra-abdominal pressure that is the consequence of rapid organ development after closure of the umbilical cord. Enlargement of the processus vaginalis causes the formation of the inguinal canals. The opening through the transversalis fascia forms the deep (or internal) inguinal ring, and the opening through the aponeurosis of the external oblique muscle constitutes the superficial (or external) inguinal ring. The gubernaculum increases in thickness until the width of the inguinal canal approaches that of the testis. In the human embryo the actual movement of the testis from the abdominal cavity through the inguinal canal and into the scrotum usually occurs during the seventh month, preceded by degeneration of that portion of the gubernaculum in contact with the epididymis and testis. Continued development of the abdominal musculature causes closure of the inguinal rings, and by the time of birth the processus vaginalis has become obliterated.

A minimum of three factors are believed to participate in testicular descent: antimüllerian hormone (AMH, also called müllerian-inhibiting factor, MIF), intra-abdominal pressure, and androgen. Degeneration of the proximal portion of the peritoneal fold may be controlled by antimüllerian hormone, which is the peptide hormone formed in the seminiferous tubules; some subjects with persistent müllerian duct syndrome, which is thought to be due to deficient formation or action of antimüllerian hormone, have testes located high in the retroperitoneal space.[17, 18] Conditions that are associated with impaired development of intra-abdominal pressure, such as congenital defects in the abdominal musculature, are also commonly associated with cryptorchidism.[19–21] Finally, androgens are believed to play a role in testicular descent on the basis of two types of evidence: dihydrotestosterone promotes descent in rats,[22] and about half of subjects with severe androgen resistance, such as the testicular feminization syndrome, have intra-abdominal testes usually located near the inguinal rings.[23]

The mechanism by which androgens might promote descent is unclear, but they may promote the formation, enlargement, or degeneration of the processus vaginalis or influence the function of the gubernaculum.[24] Neurogenic factors may also be critical for testicular descent; transection of the genitofemoral nerve in the neonatal rat prevents growth of the gubernaculum and blocks transinguinal movement of the testes.[25]

In summary, testicular descent involves the disappearance of the cephalic end of the mesonephros, movement of the gut from the cord to the abdomen to cause an increase in intra-abdominal pressure, contraction of the distal end of the mesonephros, development of the processus vaginalis, passage of the testis through the inguinal canal, and closure of the exit path. In simplistic terms, the force that effects true anatomical descent appears to be intra-abdominal pressure, which causes physiological herniation of the processus vaginalis, but the factors that control the developmental and degenerative aspects of testicular descent are poorly understood.

In some normal boys the testes at birth are incompletely descended (retractile) and may be located either high in the scrotum or in the inguinal canal but will descend spontaneously by 3 mo of age.[26] Thus failure of descent cannot be identified with certainty until after 3 mo of age.

STRUCTURAL ORGANIZATION OF THE TESTES

The testes contain two functional units: a network of tubules for the production and transport of sperm to the excretory-ejaculatory ducts and a system of interstitial or Leydig cells that contain the enzymatic machinery for the production of androgenic hormones.[27–30] In functional terms, however, the structure is more complex, as illustrated in Figure 13–3. Spermatogenic tubules are composed of germ cells and Sertoli cells. Tight junctions between the Sertoli cells at a site between the spermatogonia and the primary spermatocyte form a diffusion barrier that divides the testis into two functional compartments, the basal and

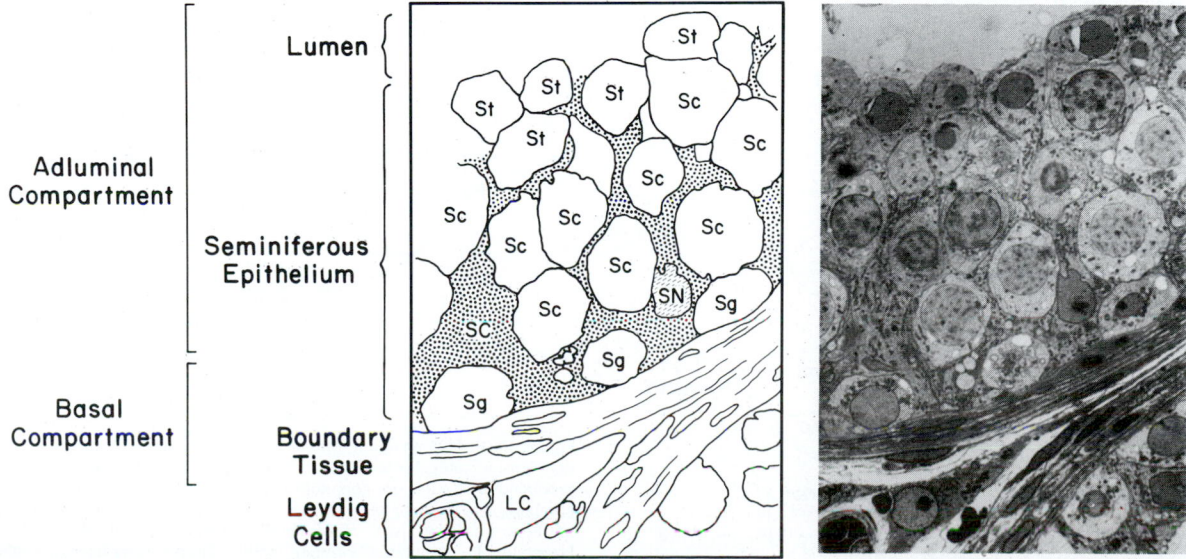

Figure 13–3. Photomicrograph, with schematic explanation, of a normal adult human testis in which proximity of the Leydig cell to the seminiferous tubule and close association of the Sertoli cell to germinal elements are demonstrated. The testis was perfused with glutaraldehyde (× 1700). SC, Sertoli cell cytoplasm; SN, Sertoli cell nucleus; Sg, spermatogonia; Sc, spermatocyte; St, spermatid; LC, Leydig cell. (Courtesy of L Johnson.)

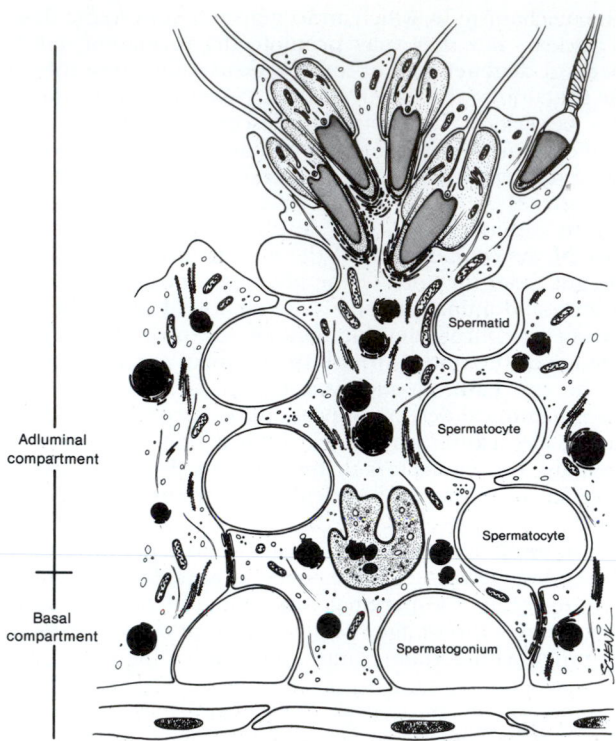

Figure 13–4. Diagram of the Sertoli cell showing the relation between Sertoli cell cytoplasm and developing spermatocytes.

the adluminal. The barrier between these two compartments has limited permeability to macromolecules, analogous to the blood-brain barrier and other epithelial barriers.[31] The basal compartment consists of the Leydig cells, the boundary tissue of the tubule, and the outer layers of the tubules containing the spermatogonia. The adluminal compartment contains the inner two thirds of the tubules, including primary spermatocytes and cells in more advanced stages of spermatogenesis.

The structure of the Sertoli cell provides insight into its function[28] (Fig. 13–4). The base of the cell is situated adjacent to the outer basement membrane of the spermatogenic tubule, whereas the inner portion consists of a progressively arborized cytoplasm containing large gaps or lacunae, analogous to the branches of a tree. The mechanism by which the spermatogonia pass through the tight junctional complexes between the Sertoli cells as they commence spermatogenesis is not known. The arborized cytoplasm of the

Sertoli cell encompasses the differentiating spermatocytes and spermatids so that spermatogenesis takes place within a network of Sertoli cell cytoplasm.

The fine structure of the Leydig cell is depicted schematically in Figure 13–5.[32] The lipid droplets that are responsible for the characteristic foamy appearance of the cytoplasm are composed mainly of esterified cholesterol, which is derived in part from circulating lipoproteins and in part from cholesterol synthesized locally within the endoplasmic reticulum of the Leydig cell. This pool of esterified cholesterol serves as a reservoir of substrate for testosterone synthesis.[33] After hydrolysis of the cholesterol ester, free cholesterol moves to mitochondria, where the rate-limiting reaction in testosterone biosynthesis takes place, namely side-chain cleavage of cholesterol to pregnenolone. Pregnenolone in turn is converted in the endoplasmic reticulum to testosterone. The amount of testosterone that is stored within the Leydig cell is small, because the newly synthesized testosterone diffuses promptly into the plasma.

PHYSIOLOGY OF TESTICULAR FUNCTION

Hypothalamic-Pituitary-Testicular Axis

HYPOTHALAMIC HORMONES. The hypothalamus is anatomically linked to the pituitary both by a portal vascular system and by neural pathways[34] (Fig. 13–6). The portal vascular system provides a mechanism for the delivery of releasing hormones from the brain to the pituitary and thus provides the major pathway by which the brain controls anterior pituitary function. Reverse flow through this hypophyseal-portal circulation may also allow pituitary hormones to reach the brain by a more direct path than through

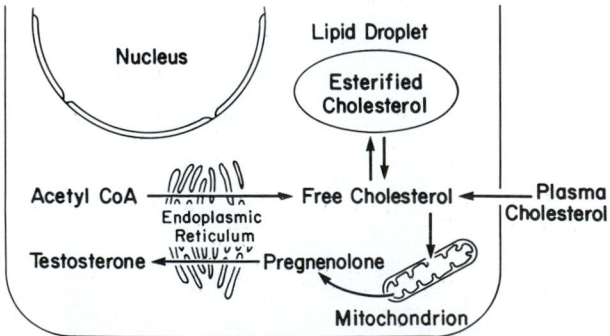

Figure 13–5. Diagram of a Leydig cell showing the origin and storage of cholesterol, the conversion of cholesterol to pregnenolone in the mitochondrion, and the conversion of pregnenolone to testosterone in the endoplasmic reticulum. Acetyl CoA, acetyl coenzyme A.

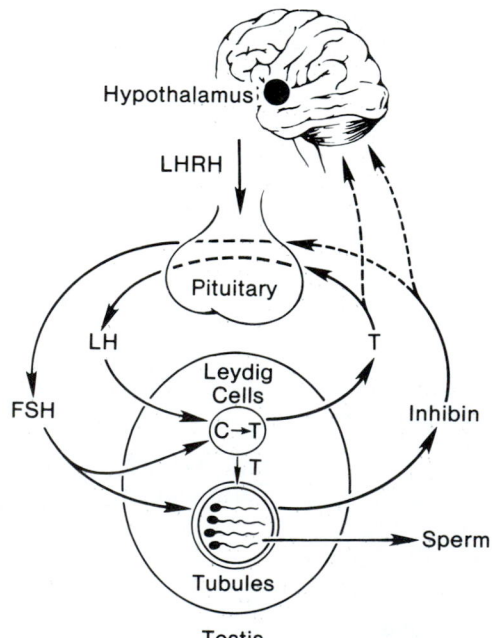

Figure 13–6. Hypothalamic-pituitary-testicular interrelationships. The schematic diagram indicates the feedback relationship of testosterone and inhibin that are produced by testes on gonadotropin secretion by the hypothalamic-pituitary complex, and the site of action of follicle-stimulating hormone and luteinizing hormone on the testis. C, cholesterol; T, testosterone; FSH, follicle-stimulating hormone; LH, luteinizing hormone; LHRH, LH-releasing hormone. (From Griffin JE, Wilson JD. The testis. In: Bondy PK, Rosenberg LE, eds. Metabolic Control and Disease. 8th ed. Philadelphia: W. B. Saunders, 1980: 1535–1578.)

the general circulation.[35] The preoptic area and the medial basal region of the hypothalamus (and particularly the arcuate nucleus) contain important centers for control of gonadotropin secretion. Peptidergic neurons in this region secrete luteinizing hormone–releasing hormone (LHRH, also called gonadotropin-releasing hormone, GnRH).[36] Neurons from other regions of the brain terminate in this area and influence LHRH synthesis and release via catecholaminergic,[37] dopaminergic,[38] and endorphin-related mechanisms.[39–41] There are excitatory noradrenergic influences, but dopamine is thought to play only a minor role. The opioid peptide involved in the endorphin-related mechanisms appears to be β-endorphin, which has an inhibitory role in the control of gonadotropin secretion.[41]

LHRH is a decapeptide that is widely distributed in the central nervous system and in other tissues as well. However, a physiological role for LHRH in sites other than the pituitary has not been established. The metabolic clearance rate of LHRH averages about 800 L/d/m² body surface area.[42] Immunoreactive metabolites of LHRH are excreted in the urine; increased urinary excretion coincides with pubertal development in boys, and in adult men the LHRH concentrations in urine correlate positively with rates of luteinizing hormone (LH) and follicle-stimulating hormone (FSH) secretion.[43]

PITUITARY HORMONES. The primary pituitary hormones that regulate the testes are LH and FSH. Both hormones were named on the basis of their function in females before their equal importance in men was recognized. LH and FSH are secreted by the same basophilic cells in the pituitary. Like thyrotropin (TSH) and human chorionic gonadotropin (hCG), LH and FSH are glycoproteins that are composed of two polypeptide chains designated alpha and beta. The alpha subunits of each of the four hormones are identical; the distinct immunological and functional characteristics of the hormones are determined by unique beta subunits.[44] Both subunits are required for full biological activity.

The structures of the beta subunits of LH and hCG are similar except that the COOH end of the beta subunit of hCG contains an additional 30 amino acids and additional carbohydrate residues.[45] The disappearance of exogenous LH from blood is described by two linear exponentials with an initial-phase half-time of 40 min and a second-phase half-time of 120 min.[46] Because of its increased glycosylation the half-life of hCG is even longer.[47] The metabolic clearance rate of LH is 25 mL/min.[48] Only a small fraction of secreted LH appears in the urine.[49] The turnover of FSH is somewhat slower, the metabolic clearance rate being 14 mL/min.[50] The disappearance of FSH from blood is also described by two exponentials with half-times of 3.9 and 70 h, respectively.[51]

MECHANISM OF ACTION OF LHRH AND GONADOTROPINS. LHRH interacts with high-affinity cell-surface receptor sites on the plasma membrane of pituitary gonadotrophs. When given in an acute fashion, it stimulates the release of both LH and FSH by a calcium-dependent mechanism that is independent of cyclic AMP (cAMP).[52] Diacylglycerols may serve as amplifiers of the calcium-mediated signal.[53] It is generally assumed that LHRH has a long-term effect on the regulation of gonadotropin synthesis as well. The amounts of LH and FSH that are released in response to LHRH depend on age and hormonal status. In monkeys the sensitivity of the gonadotrophs to LHRH reaches a peak in the first few months of life and then declines and remains low until the onset of puberty, when it again increases and attains an adult level of response.[54] Before puberty the secretion of FSH in response to LHRH is greater than that of LH.

Under certain experimental conditions it is possible to demonstrate actions of LHRH in tissues other than the pituitary.[55] For example, specific LHRH binding sites are present on Leydig cells in the rat,[56] and LHRH inhibits androgen production and causes a decrease in the number of LH receptors in rat testes.[55] However, LHRH does not appear to have a direct effect on testicular steroidogenesis in humans.[57] It is not known whether any of the extrapituitary actions of LHRH are of physiological significance.

LH interacts with specific high-affinity cell-surface receptors on the plasma membrane of Leydig cells.[58] The binding of LH to its receptor stimulates the membrane-bound adenylate cyclase that catalyzes the formation of cAMP (see Chapter 4). The release of cAMP into the cytoplasm is followed by binding of cAMP to the regulatory subunit of a protein kinase, dissociation of the regulatory subunit, and consequent activation of the catalytic subunit of the enzyme.[59] Activation of the Leydig cell protein kinase, which operates through unidentified intermediate steps, eventually results in stimulation of the conversion of cholesterol to pregnenolone. This conversion in turn enhances the synthesis of testosterone. The rate of testosterone synthesis correlates more closely with the degree of occupancy of the regulatory subunits of the protein kinase by cAMP than with the total amount of cAMP in the cells.[60] The fate of the LH-receptor complexes is not fully understood, but like other surface receptors, this complex is believed to undergo endocytosis for internalization and subsequent degradation.[61]

In the intact testis and in cultured Leydig cells the number of receptors for LH decreases after administration of LH or hCG.[62] The loss in receptor number is dose dependent, reaches a nadir 24 h after LH administration, and returns to control levels within several days.[62] This down-regulation of receptor number is associated with a decreased responsiveness (desensitization) to subsequent LH administration,[63] but the desensitization cannot be solely the result of the decrease in receptor number. Rather, the diminished steroidogenic response appears in large part to be due to inhibition of some postreceptor event, because cAMP is ineffective in reversing the desensitization phenomenon.[64] In cultured Leydig cell tumor lines the initial stimulation of steroidogenesis by LH appears to cause the subsequent desensitization, because the identical phenomenon can be induced when testosterone synthesis is stimulated by cAMP analogues under conditions that do not alter the number of LH receptors.[65] Whatever the mechanism, the diminished response of the Leydig cell to LH that follows LH administration is a critical component of an intratesticular control system for regulating testosterone production.

The epithelium of the seminiferous tubule is the primary site of action of FSH.[66] In the Sertoli cell FSH binding has been localized by autoradiography to the basal aspect of the cell.[67, 68] The initial biochemical events after the binding of FSH to its receptor are similar to those for LH. The intracellular messenger is cAMP, and adenylate cyclase activity is stimulated when seminiferous tubules are incubated with FSH in vitro.[69] In Sertoli cells the elevation in cAMP level after FSH binding activates cAMP-dependent protein kinase[70] and stimulates RNA and protein synthesis,[71] including the synthesis of androgen-binding protein[71] and the aromatase enzyme complex that converts testosterone to estradiol.[72] The precise role of FSH in the control of spermatogenesis remains uncertain and may vary with different species (see later).

FSH may play an indirect role in steroidogenesis by inducing Leydig cell maturation during development[73] or by increasing the number of LH receptors on the Leydig cell.[74, 75] Like LH and other peptide hormones, FSH regulates the number of its own receptors. After injection of a large dose of FSH the number of testicular FSH receptors de-

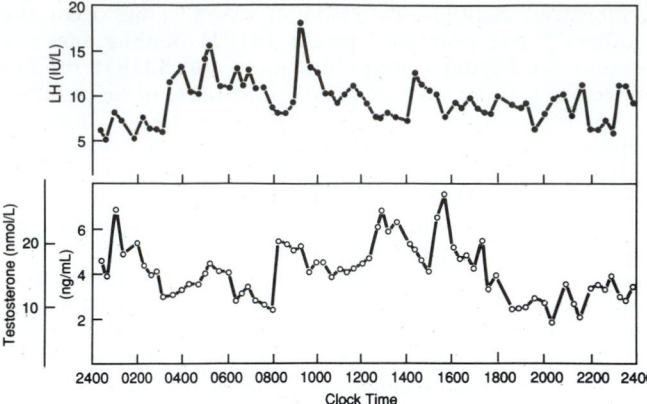

Figure 13–7. The 24-h pattern of plasma LH and testosterone levels in a 21-yr-old normal man sampled every 20 min. Variations as great as threefold were demonstrated in individual values of both LH and testosterone, depending on the time of sampling. (Courtesy of RM Boyar. From Griffin JE, Wilson JD. The testis. In: Bondy PK, Rosenberg LE, eds. Metabolic Control and Disease. 8th ed. Philadelphia: W. B. Saunders, 1980: 1535–1578.)

creases, but the physiological significance of this phenomenon is unclear.[76]

REGULATION OF SECRETION OF LHRH AND GONADOTROPINS. The secretion of LHRH into the hypophyseal-portal system is episodic,[77] and the episodic release of LHRH results, in turn, in episodic secretion of both immunoreactive and bioactive LH.[78] The secretory pulses of LH in adult men occur at a frequency of 8 to 14 pulses/24 h and vary greatly in magnitude[46] (Fig. 13–7). Pulsatile secretion of FSH is temporally coupled to that of LH but is lower in amplitude.[79]

The rate of secretion of LH is controlled by the action of gonadal steroids on the hypothalamus and the pituitary. The control of LH in men operates primarily by negative feedback because normal levels of gonadal steroids inhibit secretion (see Fig. 13–6). Both testosterone and estradiol can inhibit LH secretion. Testosterone can be converted to estradiol in the brain and the pituitary, but the two hormones are thought to act independently on the basis of studies of the effects of infusions of testosterone and estradiol in normal subjects,[80] studies of the effects of the administration of estrogen antagonists,[81, 82] and studies of patients with syndromes of androgen resistance.[82] Testosterone or its metabolites act on the central nervous system to slow the hypothalamic pulse generator and consequently decrease the frequency of LH pulsatile release.[83] Endogenous opiates have a role in the negative feedback actions of androgen and estrogen on pulsatile LH secretion in men.[84] In studies of the infusion of the nonaromatizable androgen 5α-dihydrotestosterone into normal men, selective inhibition of LH pulse frequency by the androgen was blocked by the coadministration of the opiate receptor antagonist naltrexone. Further support for a hypothalamic action of testicular steroids in the control of LH secretion comes from studies of monkeys with hypothalamic lesions that abolish endogenous LHRH release; when normal pulsatile secretion of LH is mimicked in such animals by chronic intermittent intravenous LHRH administration, bilateral orchiectomy results in only small elevations of plasma LH concentrations, whereas orchiectomy in animals with an intact hypothalamus given similar pulses of LHRH is followed by a marked rise in LH levels.[85] Acute infusions of estradiol also lower LH levels associated with an increased frequency and a decreased amplitude of the LH pulses.[80] The fact that dihydrotestosterone, which cannot be converted to estrogen, exerts a negative feedback control on LH secretion indicates that testosterone does not require aromatization to inhibit LH

secretion.[80] Testosterone also appears to have a negative feedback action on LH secretion directly at the pituitary level, because LHRH-deficient patients who are given pulsatile LHRH infusions have a decrease in mean LH levels and LH pulse amplitude when exogenous testosterone is administered.[86]

The negative feedback inhibition of testicular hormones on FSH secretion involves both gonadal peptide and steroid hormones. Serum FSH concentrations increase in proportion to the loss of germinal elements in the testis, whereas LH levels change little if at all.[87] Inhibin is a peptide inhibitor of pituitary FSH and is secreted by Sertoli cells.[88] It is also produced by the ovary. It has been purified from bovine and porcine follicular fluid and shown to be a glycoprotein consisting of two disulfide-linked subunits. The sequence of inhibin is partially homologous to transforming growth factor β and to antimüllerian hormone. An unexpected finding was that dimers of the smaller (β) subunit of inhibin stimulate FSH release from pituitary cells in vitro, whereas inhibin selectively inhibits FSH release.[88]

Inhibin is a heterodimer consisting of a 20-kd α subunit and a 15-kd β subunit. Because the β subunit can exist in two forms, there are two forms of inhibin, inhibin α and inhibin β, each 31 kd in size. FSH stimulates inhibin production by cultured rat Sertoli cells.[89, 90] One group has also reported stimulation of inhibin production in cultured Sertoli cells by androgen,[91] but this effect has not been confirmed.[89, 90] An in vivo study of the relative roles of FSH and androgen (as stimulated locally in the testes by LH) in the control of inhibin secretion in normal men concluded that both FSH and androgen are necessary for normal inhibin production.[92]

Testosterone and estradiol also have direct effects on FSH secretion.[93] In castrated rats treated with subphysiological amounts of testosterone but physiological amounts of estradiol, plasma FSH levels increase to midcastrate range, but LH concentrations are maintained at noncastrate levels. It has therefore been proposed that alterations in the testosterone/estradiol ratio might account for selective elevations in plasma FSH levels under some circumstances.[93] In addition, varying the pattern of LHRH administration to hypogonadotropic men so that the same total dose is administered with less frequent pulses results in selective increases of FSH levels.[94] Likewise, in men with isolated elevations of FSH associated with idiopathic azoospermia an increased frequency of pulsatile LHRH administration selectively decreases FSH levels.[95]

A primate model has been useful for defining the relative importance of inhibin and gonadal steroids in physiological feedback control of FSH secretion. In a hypophyseotropic clamp preparation, in which episodic gonadotropin secretion was maintained by a chronic, unchanging, intermittent LHRH infusion, neither circulating testosterone nor estradiol could account for the testicular inhibition of FSH, which implies by exclusion that inhibin must be the gonadal hormone of greatest importance for feedback control at the level of the pituitary.[96]

Androgen Physiology

TESTOSTERONE SYNTHESIS AND SECRETION. The structure of testosterone is illustrated in Figure 13–8, and the metabolic pathways by which testosterone is synthesized are summarized schematically in Figure 13–9.[97] As stated earlier, cholesterol, the precursor steroid, either can be synthesized de novo from acetyl coenzyme A or can be derived from the plasma pool by receptor-mediated endocytosis of low-density lipoprotein (LDL).[61] In the rat the cholesterol that is synthesized within the Leydig cell is the

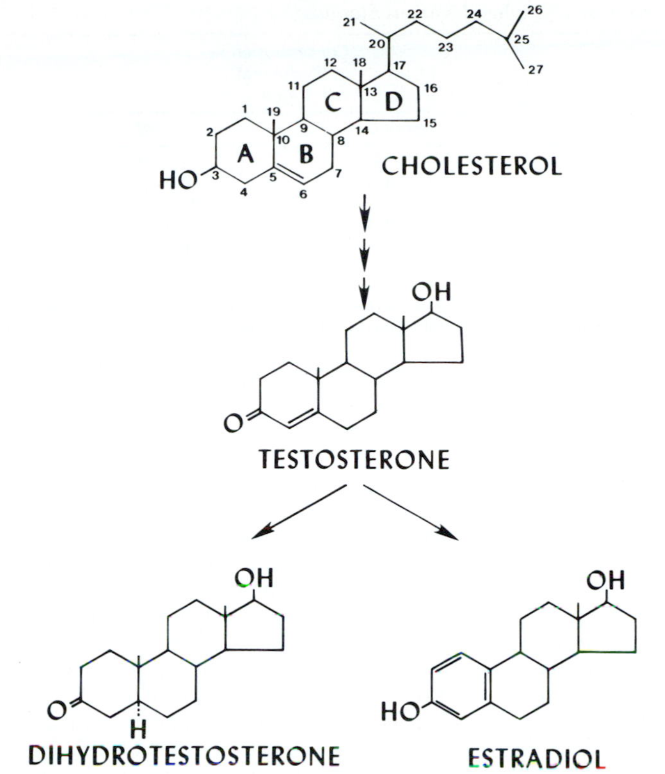

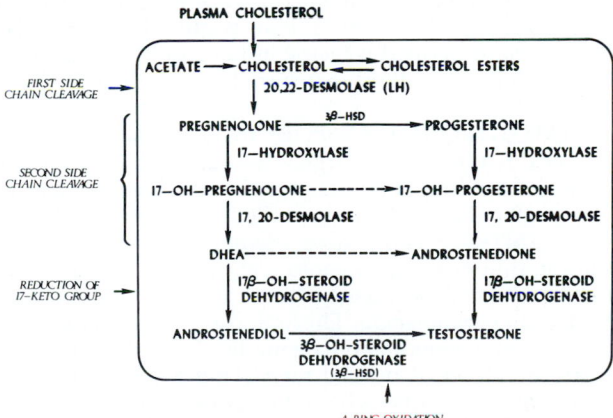

Figure 13–8. Structures of cholesterol, testosterone, and the two major active metabolites of testosterone, 5α-dihydrotestosterone and estradiol. (From Griffin JE, Wilson JD. The testis. In: Bondy PK, Rosenberg LE, eds. Metabolic Control and Disease. 8th ed. Philadelphia: W. B. Saunders, 1980 :1535–1578.)

most important source of substrate for testosterone synthesis,[98] but in the human testis both sources are quantitatively important.[99]

Five enzymatic processes are involved in the conversion of cholesterol to testosterone. As a consequence the side chain of cholesterol is cleaved in two steps to reduce the size from 27 to 19 carbons, and the A ring of the steroid is

Figure 13–9. Pathways of testosterone synthesis in human testis. The three potential sources of cholesterol for testosterone synthesis are (1) plasma cholesterol; (2) cholesterol synthesized within the cell; and (3) cholesterol stored in the form of cholesterol esters. The first side-chain cleavage of cholesterol to pregnenolone is the rate-limiting reaction in the process and is probably the process that is regulated by gonadotropins. Conversion of pregnenolone to testosterone can take place by two theoretical pathways—one in which side-chain cleavage and reduction of the 17-keto group are accomplished before A ring oxidation, and the other in which this sequence is reversed. LH, luteinizing hormone. (From Griffin JE, Wilson JD. The testis. In: Bondy PK, Rosenberg LE, eds. Metabolic Control and Disease. 8th ed. Philadelphia: W. B. Saunders, 1980: 1535–1578.)

oxidized to the Δ^4-3-keto configuration. The initial reaction in the process involves the side-chain cleavage of cholesterol by the 20,22-desmolase in mitochondria to form pregnenolone. The subsequent conversion of pregnenolone to testosterone involves, in part, a random and, in part, an ordered series of enzymatic reactions. For the second side-chain cleavage to take place, 17-hydroxylation must occur before the 17,20-desmolase reaction can be accomplished, and both reactions must take place before the reduction of the 17-ketone by 17β-hydroxysteroid dehydrogenase. In contrast, oxidation of the A ring of the steroid by the 3β-hydroxysteroid dehydrogenase–$\Delta^{4,5}$-isomerase complex can take place at any stage in the process. Thus the point in the pathway at which A ring oxidation occurs depends on the amounts and affinities of the enzymes for the various substrates and the compartmentalization of the enzymes within the endoplasmic reticulum. The predominant pathway in the human testis appears to be the Δ^5-pathway (shown on the left side of Fig. 13–9), with A ring oxidation being the terminal reaction in the sequence.[100] Although 17α-hydroxylase and 17,20-desmolase were traditionally regarded as separate enzymes, purification and in vitro reconstitution of enzyme activity indicate that both activities reside in a single cytochrome P-450 enzyme (P-450$_{c17}$).[101]

The rate-limiting reaction in testosterone synthesis is the conversion of cholesterol to pregnenolone. As mentioned earlier, LH regulates the rate of this reaction and thus controls the overall rate of testosterone synthesis.[97] When given acutely, LH may stimulate testosterone synthesis by enhancing the association between cholesterol and the cholesterol side-chain cleavage–cytochrome P-450 system in the mitochondria.[101] In the steady state, however, LH acts to stimulate steroidogenesis in the testis by enhancing formation of the side-chain cleavage enzyme.

Although testosterone is the major product, dihydrotestosterone, androsterone, androstenedione, 17-hydroxyprogesterone, progesterone, and pregnenolone are also secreted by the testis[102] (Table 13–1). The role of 5α-reduced androgens, dihydrotestosterone and androsterone, in the testis has not been established; the major sites of formation and action of dihydrotestosterone are extraglandular. Androstenedione serves as a precursor for extraglandular estrogen formation (see later). The functions of plasma progesterone and 17-hydroxyprogesterone in the male are not known.

The concentrations of testosterone in testicular lymph and testicular venous blood are similar, but the flow of testicular lymph is small compared with that of testicular blood. As a consequence the major route for steroid exit from the testis into the general circulation is via the spermatic venous blood. The mechanism of transport of testosterone and other steroids from the sites of production to blood and lymph is not completely understood. Only about 25 μg of testosterone is stored in the normal testes, so that the total hormone content turns over more than 200 times each day to provide the average of 6 mg that is secreted into plasma in normal men.[103]

GONADOTROPIN REGULATION OF TESTOSTERONE SECRETION. Rat Leydig cells have a considerable number of excess or "spare" LH receptors, i.e., a full physiological response occurs when only a fraction of the receptors are occupied by LH. These spare receptors are nevertheless coupled to cAMP generation;[104] thus maximal testosterone biosynthesis occurs at concentrations of hCG or LH that result in only 10% of maximal cAMP production.[105] Human Leydig cells contain fewer LH receptors than do rat Leydig cells, but the fact that the maximal rates of testosterone biosynthesis are similar in both cells suggests that the major difference is in the number of so-called spare receptors

TABLE 13–1. Plasma Concentration of Spermatic and Peripheral Venous Steroids*

Steroid	Concentration in Spermatic Vein		Concentration in Peripheral Vein	
	nmol/L	ng/mL	nmol/L	ng/mL
Testosterone	340–2000	100–600	8.7–35	2.5–10
Dihydrotestosterone	2–28	0.6–8.0	0.3–1.6	0.1–0.45
Androsterone	1.4–38	0.4–11	0.5–1.4	0.15–0.4
Androstenedione	3.8–42	1.1–12	1.4–3.8	0.4–1.1
17α-Hydroxyprogesterone	3–300	1.1–100	1.2–3.3	0.4–1.1
Progesterone	3.5–35	1.1–11	0.3–1.9	0.1–0.6
Pregnenolone	3.5–35	1.1–12	0.9–3.0	0.3–1.0

*Blood samples from the spermatic vein were collected, with the use of local anesthesia, from patients with carcinoma of the prostate, hernia, varicocele, or hydrocele.

Adapted from Hammond GL, Ruokonen A, Kontturi M, et al. The simultaneous radioimmunoassay of seven steroids in human spermatic and peripheral venous blood. J Clin Endocrinol Metab 1977; 45:16–24.

rather than the number of receptors that are coupled to androgen synthesis.[106]

The decreased response of target cells to LH or hCG after an initial exposure has been described earlier. Reduced LH receptor number (down-regulation) and some postreceptor binding events are involved in this phenomenon. After administration of moderate doses of hCG to rats, the 17,20-desmolase step in androgen biosynthesis is inhibited, which leads to accumulation of progesterone, 17α-hydroxyprogesterone, pregnenolone, and 17α-hydroxypregnenolone.[107] A similar inhibition of the 17,20-desmolase is produced in rat testes by the administration of estradiol, which suppresses the activity of the 17α-hydroxylase as well.[108] The possibility that hCG desensitization is mediated by a local increase in estrogen production by the testes was suggested by the findings that the testicular estradiol level is elevated within 30 min after hCG administration and that estrogen antagonists can block hCG-induced desensitization.[109] The mechanism by which estradiol produces such inhibition may involve the estrogen receptor.[110]

Testosterone itself appears to regulate its own rate of synthesis by controlling the activity of microsomal cytochrome P-450 in a cultured mouse Leydig cell system.[111, 112] Testosterone that is produced by acute stimulation with hCG binds to the active site of P-450$_{c17}$ and forms a pseudosubstrate–P-450–O$_2$ complex in the presence of oxygen. The complex breaks down, giving rise to reactive oxygen free radicals, with subsequent damage to the enzyme.[112] In contrast, during long-term stimulation by hCG in the same type of cultured mouse Leydig cells, testosterone appears to inhibit cAMP-induced synthesis of P-450$_{c17}$ by an androgen receptor–mediated mechanism.[113]

There is also evidence for temporary inhibition of steroidogenesis after hCG administration in vivo. An acute increase in plasma testosterone level occurs within 2 h after hCG administration in both rats and humans.[114] The response to hCG is biphasic; the plasma level of testosterone reaches a plateau or declines after the initial injection.[114] Plasma estradiol levels increase and peak 24 h after hCG injection, which corresponds to the nadir between the two testosterone responses.[114] The concept that the mechanism of desensitization in vivo in humans is via inhibition of the 17,20-desmolase reaction is supported by the finding of an early (24-h) increase in 17-hydroxyprogesterone after hCG and its decline while testosterone levels are rising at 48 h.[115] The administration of high doses of hCG to men for long periods results in steady-state elevations of plasma estradiol, 17-hydroxyprogesterone, and testosterone,[116] so that desensitization probably acts as a control mechanism that limits the degree of response to the hormone in the steady state. The increase in plasma testosterone levels after hCG admin-

istration is greater in the morning than in the afternoon,[117] in keeping with the normal circadian rhythm of serum testosterone concentrations.[118] The higher testosterone levels in the early morning hours in normal men do not appear to be related to sleep or to normal variations in LH or prolactin levels and may thus be the consequence of an endogenous circadian rhythm at the level of the testes.[118]

In rats prolactin receptors are present on Leydig cells,[119] and prolactin potentiates the effect of LH on Leydig cells. A possible mechanism is enhancement of lipoprotein transport into the cells, which thus increases the availability of cholesterol for steroidogenesis.[120] A role for prolactin in regulating human Leydig cell function has not been shown,[121] and there does not appear to be a prolactin receptor on human Leydig cells.[68] Atrial natriuretic peptide stimulates testosterone production in mouse Leydig cells by a mechanism that does not appear to involve cAMP.[122, 123] Arginine vasopressin and related neurohypophyseal hormones inhibit hCG-induced testosterone synthesis by inhibiting the 17α-hydroxylase reaction.[124]

Leydig cell function is also under paracrine control within the testis. Insulin-like growth factor I (IGF I, also called somatomedin-C) augments gonadotropin-stimulated testosterone production by cultured rat Leydig cells by interacting with a specific receptor on Leydig cells.[125] Likewise, heterodimers of inhibin subunits enhance rat Leydig cell testosterone production that is stimulated by LH.[126] Others have described a factor in both rat[127] and human[128] testicular interstitial fluid that stimulates Leydig cell steroidogenesis.

TESTOSTERONE TRANSPORT IN PLASMA. Testosterone circulates in the plasma largely bound to plasma proteins. The major binding molecules are albumin and testosterone-binding globulin (TeBG, also called sex hormone–binding globulin, SHBG). TeBG, a beta-globulin composed of nonidentical subunits, has a molecular mass of about 95 kd, contains about 30% carbohydrate, and has one androgen binding site per molecule. The amino acid sequence of TeBG has been determined, and its gene has been cloned.[129–131]

In the blood of normal men about 2% of testosterone is free (unbound), 44% is bound to TeBG, and 54% is bound to albumin and other proteins.[132] Albumin has about 1000-fold lower affinity for testosterone than does TeBG, but the concentration of albumin is so much higher than that of TeBG that the binding capacities of both are similar. The proportion of testosterone that is bound to TeBG in serum is proportional to the TeBG concentration. For many years the free fraction was regarded as the biologically active portion available for entry into cells and receptor interaction. It is now clear that dissociation of protein-bound testosterone can occur within a capillary bed, so that the active fraction can be larger than the free fraction measured under equilibrium conditions in vitro.[133] Interaction of binding proteins with components of the microcirculation (e.g., endothelial glycocalyx) may lead to conformational changes at the hormone binding site and result in enhanced dissociation in vivo. In studies of tissue delivery in vivo, nearly all of the albumin-bound testosterone was available for tissue uptake. Thus the bioavailable circulating testosterone in normal men is about half of the total (or equal to the free plus the albumin bound).[134]

Estradiol appears to bind differently to TeBG than does testosterone, as a consequence of which there is increased availability of TeBG-bound estradiol to tissues. The reason for these differences in testosterone and estradiol binding to what is thought to be a single competitive binding site on TeBG is thought to be the presence of multiple isoforms of TeBG in serum.[135] These isoforms are not the result of heterogeneity in the polypeptide sequence but arise from differential post-translational processing of the carbohydrate moiety of TeBG. Isoelectric focusing of concentrated glycoprotein fractions of serum indicates that testosterone is bound to the most acidic TeBG isoforms.[135]

The concentration of TeBG in plasma is regulated by several hormones. The level is increased 5- to 10-fold by estrogens, as in normal pregnancy, and is decreased 2-fold in women by testosterone administration. The level in men is one third to one half that in women, and concentrations in hypogonadal men are elevated above those of normal men.[136] Decreased TeBG levels occur in hypothyroidism, and thyroid hormone excess increases TeBG levels, possibly because of increased estrogen formation.

The physiological consequences of changes in levels of the plasma proteins that transport gonadal steroids differ, depending on the circumstances. In men who have an intact hypothalamic-pituitary-testicular axis, alterations in TeBG levels have little effect on androgen physiology in the steady state; for example, an increase in the plasma TeBG level is followed by temporary decreases in free (active) plasma testosterone and an increased rate of testosterone synthesis until the normal free (active) component is reconstituted. As a consequence, both increases and decreases in TeBG levels are compatible with normal rates of androgen synthesis and degradation and normal free hormone concentrations in plasma.

In contrast, changes in the plasma levels of binding proteins have profound consequences when the levels of the free fraction of the hormone are not so tightly regulated. Such is the case for gonadal steroids in men under two circumstances. First, in the presence of diseases of the hypothalamic-pituitary-testicular axis, the ability to regulate the free levels of the hormone is limited, and, consequently, the pharmacodynamics of androgens that are used for replacement therapy may be altered by changes in TeBG levels. Second, and more importantly, even in men with an intact hypothalamic-pituitary-testicular axis, not all plasma hormones are under such tight regulation as is testosterone. The level of plasma estradiol in men is probably determined by the amount of androgen that is available as substrate for estrogen formation and by the amount of aromatase activity in extraglandular sites and thus is not regulated directly by the usual feedback mechanisms. Because TeBG binds estradiol less avidly than testosterone or dihydrotestosterone, increases in TeBG amplify the amount of estradiol cleared by liver relative to the amount of testosterone; e.g., increases in TeBG cause decreased hepatic clearance of testosterone but have little effect on the hepatic clearance of estradiol.[137, 138] Thus even in normal men, changes in TeBG levels can cause alteration in the ratios of androgens to estrogens

that persist even when androgen levels themselves are not permanently altered.

EXTRAGLANDULAR METABOLISM OF ANDROGENS. An important feature of the metabolism of testosterone, noted earlier, is that testosterone serves as a circulating precursor, or prohormone, for the formation of two types of active metabolites, which in turn mediate many of the physiological phenomena that are involved in androgen action (see Fig. 13–8). On the one hand, testosterone can undergo irreversible reduction to 5α-reduced steroids, principally dihydrotestosterone, that are thought to mediate many of the differentiative, growth-promoting, and functional aspects of male sexual development and virilization.[139] Dihydrotestosterone, in turn, can be further metabolized to 17-ketosteroids and polar derivatives that are found in urine. Alternatively, circulating androgens can be aromatized to estrogens in the extraglandular tissues of both sexes.[140] These estrogens in some instances act in concert with androgens to influence physiological processes, but they may also exert independent effects on cellular function and even have effects opposite to those of androgens.[141, 142] Thus the physiological actions of testosterone are the result of the combined effects of testosterone itself plus those of estrogen and the active androgen metabolites of the parent molecule. In normal men small amounts of estradiol (15 to 25% of the total daily production)[143] and of dihydrotestosterone[144] are derived by direct secretion from the testis; furthermore, both can be synthesized in small amounts indirectly from adrenal androgen via the sequence androstenedione → estrone → estradiol or androstenedione → androstanedione → dihydrotestosterone.[143, 144]

The quantitative relation between circulating testosterone and the formation of estrogen in normal young men is illustrated diagrammatically in Figure 13–10. Of the average total estradiol production rate of 45 μg/d, 17 μg is derived from the aromatization of circulating testosterone, 22 μg is derived from the weak estrogen estrone, and 6 μg is secreted directly into the circulation by the testes.[143] In some instances these metabolites exert only local actions in the tissues in which they are formed, whereas in other instances the 5α-

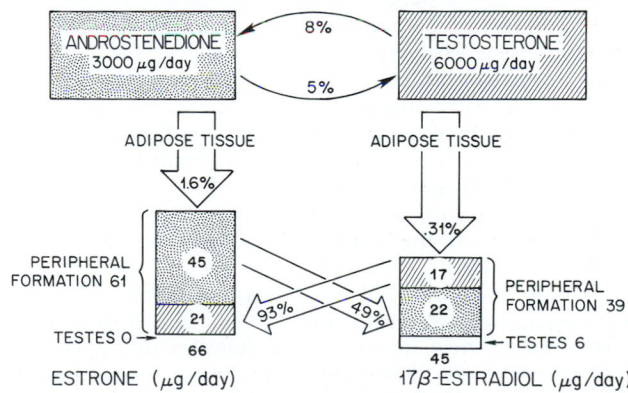

Figure 13–10. Androgen-estrogen dynamics in four normal men. The mean total production per day of estrone and estradiol is shown in lower boxes and is composed of either peripheral formation *(brace)* or direct secretion from the testes. Average amounts of androstenedione and testosterone produced per day are shown in the top boxes. Vertical arrows indicate the rate of peripheral conversion of these two prohormones to estrone and estradiol. Horizontal arrows connecting androstenedione and testosterone as well as estrone and estradiol indicate their reversible interconversion by 17β-hydroxysteroid dehydrogenase. Thus estradiol arises from plasma testosterone, from estrone derived from plasma androstenedione, and from direct secretion by testes. (From MacDonald PC, Madden JD, Brenner PF, et al. Origin of estrogen in normal men and in women with testicular feminization. J Clin Endocrinol Metab 1979; 49:905–916. © 1979, The Endocrine Society.)

reduced and estrogenic metabolites may re-enter the plasma and act as circulating hormones.[139]

The factors that regulate the metabolism of testosterone to estradiol and dihydrotestosterone are poorly understood. Circulating dihydrotestosterone is thought to be formed principally in the androgen target tissues themselves.[139] Aromatization takes place in many tissues, the most significant of which is probably adipose tissue; the overall rate of extraglandular aromatization increases with body size.[140]

The pathways of androgen catabolism were characterized before it was recognized that some testosterone derivatives are themselves active hormones rather than inactive metabolites. For example, it was known for many years that testosterone is converted in the body to a variety of 5α- and 5β-reduced isomers. Subsequently, 5α-dihydrotestosterone was shown to be the principal intracellular androgen[145] and the predominant androgen concentrated in the nucleus of androgen target tissues such as the rat prostate.[146, 147] These findings, together with the observation that dihydrotestosterone is about twice as potent as testosterone in most bioassay systems,[148] indicated that dihydrotestosterone is a cellular mediator of androgen action. The importance of dihydrotestosterone in normal androgen physiology has been confirmed both by physiological studies and by studies of human mutations in which the 5α-reductase that is responsible for dihydrotestosterone formation is defective[23, 149–152] (see Chapter 20).

5α-Reductase has a broad specificity for Δ⁴-3-ketosteroids[153] and exhibits an absolute requirement for NADPH as cofactor.[153] The reaction is not reversible under physiological conditions. 5α-Reductase has a distinct tissue localization; most activity is found in the accessory organs of reproduction, in the liver, and in the skin.[145–147, 154, 155] In human skin the highest activity is in the genital skin;[155] hair follicles from all anatomical sites contain measurable activity.[156] Fibroblasts that are cultured from human genital skin (i.e., foreskin, scrotum, and labia majora)[149–152] contain more 5α-reductase than do those cultured from other sites, such as deltoid skin. The cDNA for the gene that codes 5α-reductase has been cloned, and the amino acid sequence of the enzyme has been deduced.[157]

5α-Reductase activity varies among tissues in a given species and in the same tissue among different species. In prostate the enzyme appears to be under physiological regulation by androgens,[158] whereas in liver the enzyme is regulated by thyroid hormones.[159, 160] In humans the activity of 5α-reductase in nongenital skin is enhanced by androgens, possibly because of an androgen-mediated increase in the size and/or number of skin organelles containing the enzyme (i.e., hair follicles and sebaceous glands).[161] In normal men the production rate of dihydrotestosterone is determined predominantly by the amount of testosterone available to serve as precursor.

The conversion of C$_{19}$-steroids to estrogens in testes and in extraglandular tissues of men, principally adipose tissue, is catalyzed by the same aromatase complex that operates in placenta and ovary. Estrogen formation involves sequential hydroxylation, oxidation and removal of the carbon at position 19 of the steroid molecule, and aromatization of the A ring of the steroid. Three moles of NADPH and 3 mol of oxygen are required to convert each mole of androstenedione or testosterone to estrone or estradiol, respectively. The oxidations are of the mixed-function type involving cytochrome P-450.[162] The various enzymes involved appear to be bound in a microsomal complex that includes NADPH–cytochrome P-450 reductase, as well as cytochrome.[162] The cDNA for the human aromatase gene has been cloned, and the aromatase structure is typical for a cytochrome P-450 gene.[163]

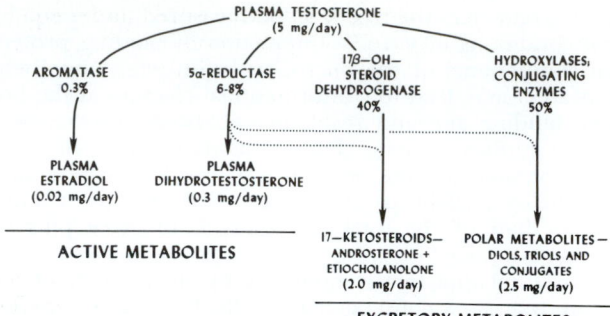

Figure 13–11. Pathways of peripheral metabolism of plasma testosterone. Testosterone can be metabolized either to active metabolites or to excretory metabolites. Active metabolites such as dihydrotestosterone may be further metabolized to excretory metabolites. (From Griffin JE, Wilson JD. The testis. In: Bondy PK, Rosenberg LE, eds. Metabolic Control and Disease. 8th ed. Philadelphia: W. B. Saunders, 1980: 1535–1578.)

Testosterone and androstenedione are the substrates for the aromatase reaction, whereas 5α-reduced steroids such as dihydrotestosterone cannot serve as estrogen precursors. Although the first part of the process, hydroxylation of C-19, can take place, prior 5α-reduction of the A ring precludes the completion of aromatization.[139]

Estrogen formation in the testis is regulated by gonadotropins (see earlier). The rate of the overall aromatase activity in nongonadal tissue is not influenced by castration or adrenalectomy but is enhanced by increasing body weight in postmenopausal women and by advancing age in men.[140] Dihydrotestosterone and 5α-androstanedione can serve as competitive inhibitors of the initial portion of the aromatization process and may serve to regulate the rate of estrogen synthesis in some tissues.

The metabolism of testosterone is schematized in Figure 13–11. The metabolites are excreted primarily in the urine (>90%), approximately half of the daily turnover being recovered as urinary 17-ketosteroids and the other half as a series of polar compounds, including diols, triols, and conjugates.[164] These various excretory metabolites are thought to be largely inactive.

ANDROGEN ACTION. Current concepts of androgen action in target cells are summarized in Figure 13–12. Major functions include regulation of gonadotropin secretion by the hypothalamic-pituitary system, initiation and maintenance of spermatogenesis, formation of the male phenotype during sexual differentiation, and promotion of sexual maturation at puberty.[139] Inside the cell, testosterone can be converted to dihydrotestosterone by 5α-reductase. The two hormones then bind to the same high-affinity androgen receptor protein. The hormone-receptor complexes interact

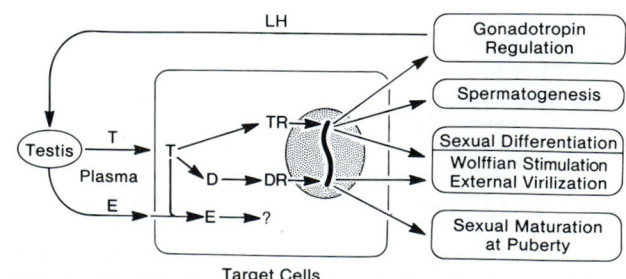

Figure 13–12. Schematic diagram of normal androgen physiology. LH, luteinizing hormone; T, testosterone; D, dihydrotestosterone; E, estradiol; R, androgen receptor. (From Griffin JE, Wilson JD. The syndromes of androgen resistance. Reprinted, by permission of The New England Journal of Medicine, 302; 198–209, 1980.)

with acceptor sites in nuclei to effect a biological response. The nature and the number of the acceptor sites within the chromosomes are unknown, but the result of the interaction is increased transcription of specific structural genes and subsequent appearance of new messenger RNA and proteins in the cytoplasm[165, 166] (see Chapter 3).

The model of androgen action shown in Figure 13–12 is based on studies of androgen metabolism in animals of various ages and on investigations of single-gene mutations that impair androgen action.[23, 139, 167] The testosterone-receptor complex regulates gonadotropin secretion and the virilization of the wolffian ducts during male sexual differentiation and is probably responsible for sexual dimorphism of muscle development. The dihydrotestosterone-receptor complex is responsible for external virilization during embryogenesis and for the development of most male secondary sex characteristics during puberty. The question of which hormone controls spermatogenesis is unresolved. On the basis of studies of androgen metabolism in rodent testis, it is generally believed that testosterone is the active hormone for this function;[168] however, dihydrotestosterone is formed in the human testis,[102] specifically in the spermatogenic tubule,[169] and spermatogenesis is impaired in subjects with 5α-reductase deficiency,[170] which suggests that dihydrotestosterone may play a role in human spermatogenesis.

As indicated in Figure 13–12 and discussed earlier, estrogens may either be secreted directly by the testis or be formed in peripheral tissues. The mechanisms by which estrogens act to augment or block androgen action are not fully understood. In the prostate, estrogens may enhance androgen action by increasing the number of androgen receptors,[141] whereas in the male breast, estrogens appear to act in opposition to androgens.[142]

Androgens and estrogens, like other steroid hormones, initiate their effects at the cellular level by interacting with high-affinity receptor proteins.[166] Androgen receptors are present in highest concentration in the accessory organs of male reproduction that depend on androgens for their growth[171] and in other major androgen target tissues.[172] Tissues such as skeletal muscle,[173] heart,[174] and placenta[175] have small amounts of receptor. In the testis the androgen receptors are present both in Sertoli cells[176] and in interstitial cells.[177] Whether the presence of androgen receptors identifies a tissue as androgen responsive is not clear.[178] The amount of receptor present in a tissue may be affected by the level of androgen or estrogen,[141, 179] by age,[180] or by single-gene mutations.[181]

A major problem in measuring the amount of androgen receptor in human tissues is to separate androgen binding to TeBG from binding to the receptor; in some species the testicular androgen-binding protein is also a potential source of confusion.[182–184] The androgen receptor appears to be the same molecule in different tissues in the rat (testis, epididymis, prostate);[171, 185–187] in these tissues an 8S to 9S form of the receptor is demonstrable in buffers of low ionic strength and is converted to a 4.5S to 5S form at salt concentrations greater than 0.1 M.[185] The androgen receptor of human prostate[180] and of fibroblasts cultured from human skin[181, 188] also sediments as an 8S to 9S species in low-salt sucrose gradients.

A single androgen receptor binds both testosterone and dihydrotestosterone, and the protein in both the mouse and the human is coded by a gene on the X chromosome.[189] The cDNA encoding the human androgen receptor has been cloned.[190–193] It predicts a protein of 917 amino acids and a molecular mass of about 99 kd.[193] Comparison with the predicted amino acid sequences of other steroid hormone receptors revealed a high degree of sequence conservation with the progesterone, glucocorticoid, and mineralocorticoid

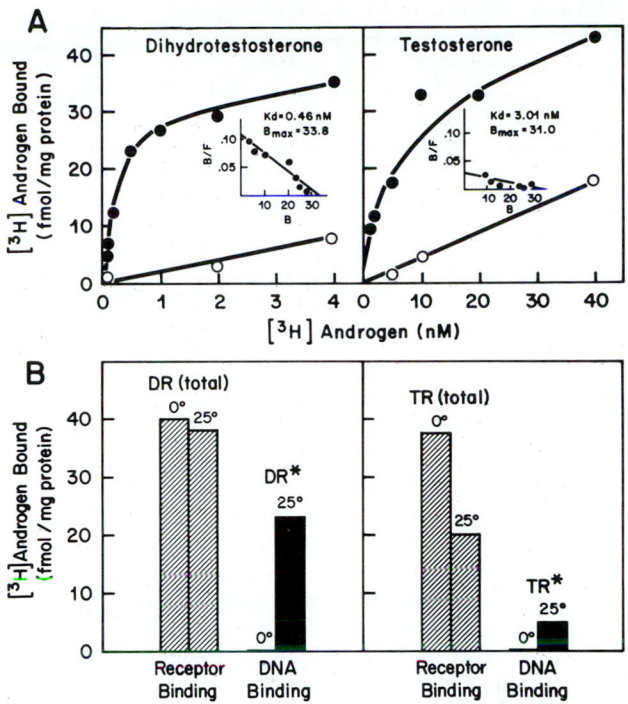

Figure 13–13. Comparison of binding of dihydrotestosterone and testosterone to human androgen receptor (A) and of the respective hormone-receptor complexes to DNA-cellulose (B). Dihydrotestosterone binds to androgen receptor with higher affinity than does testosterone, but the amount of binding (B_{max}) of the two steroids to the androgen receptor is similar (A). However, when the dihydrotestosterone-receptor complex (DR) is transformed (DR*), it binds much better to DNA than does the transformed testosterone-receptor complex (TR*) (B). (From Kovacs WR, Griffin JE, Weaver DD, et al. A mutation that causes lability of the androgen receptor under conditions that normally promote transformation to the DNA-binding state. Reproduced from The Journal of Clinical Investigation, 1984, 73, 1095–1104 by copyright permission of The American Society for Clinical Investigation.)

receptors in the putative hormone and DNA binding domains. If a single receptor mediates the action of both testosterone and dihydrotestosterone, why is dihydrotestosterone formation important for normal androgen action? A partial answer is that the affinity of the human androgen receptor for testosterone is less than that for dihydrotestosterone[182, 194–196] (Fig. 13–13A). Testosterone-receptor complexes are also less stable than dihydrotestosterone-receptor complexes[194, 195] and transform to the DNA-binding state less well (Fig. 13–13B).[196] These differences in interaction of the two steroids with the androgen receptor may serve as an amplifying mechanism for androgen action in target tissues that possess the capacity to convert testosterone to dihydrotestosterone.

Spermatogenesis and Fertilization

SPERMATOGENIC CYCLE. Spermatogenesis involves three processes: multiplication of the germ cells, reduction of the number of chromosomes from the diploid to the haploid state (meiosis), and formation of a superstructure that allows motility, generation of energy to promote motility, and protection of the chromosomal package against environmental damage.

By the second month of embryogenesis, after migration of the germ cells to the genital ridge (see Fig. 13–1), the total number of germ cells is approximately 3×10^5 per gonad. This number increases by puberty to about 6×10^8 spermatogonia per testis.[197] As a result of the hormonal events accompanying sexual maturation, a profound cellular

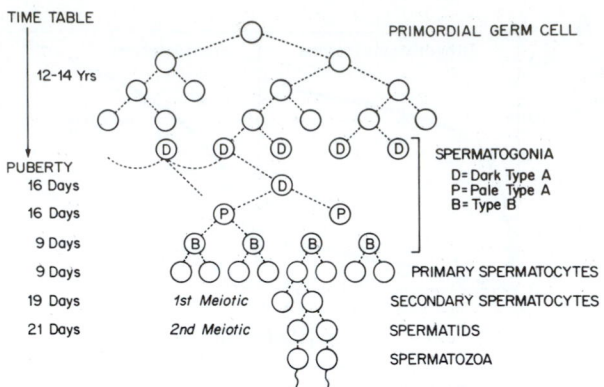

Figure 13–14. Cell divisions during spermatogenesis. The overall number of cell divisions is much higher than that in oogenesis.

proliferation ensues; the net result is the production of approximately 2×10^8 sperm each day from the completion of puberty to extreme old age, a total of more than a trillion sperm during the usual reproductive life span.

Although the process of spermatogenesis is similar among species, there are major histological differences. Indeed, spermatogenesis in the human differs in many respects from that in other primates, and certain aspects of the human system are still poorly understood. As illustrated in Figure 13–14, after puberty each spermatogonium undergoing differentiation gives rise to 16 primary spermatocytes, each of which then enters meiosis and gives rise to four spermatids and ultimately four spermatozoa. Thus 64 spermatozoa can develop from each spermatogonium. In the steady state a minimum of 1.5 million spermatogonia begin this cycle each day. Because nearly half of potential sperm production is lost during meiosis, the actual number of spermatogonia that commence this process is closer to 3 million/d.[198] On histological grounds it is clear that the commitment of spermatogonia to differentiation does not occur randomly; indeed, because clumps or groups of adjacent cells share a similar if not identical degree of histological development it is likely that contiguous groups of spermatogonia undertake the process simultaneously. Clermont identified six typical cellular associations in human seminiferous tubules;[199] thus one or two generations of spermatids at given steps of spermatogenesis are always associated with one or two generations of spermatocytes and with specific groups of spermatogonia. The succession of these six stages in any one area of tubular epithelium constitutes the cycle of the seminiferous epithelium.[199–201]

The ultrastructural features of the transformation of the human spermatocyte into a spermatozoon are illustrated diagrammatically in Figure 13–15[200, 202] and consist of a highly coordinated reorganization of nucleus and cytoplasm and development of the flagellum. The chromatin becomes progressively more dense, and the nucleus comes to occupy an eccentric position adjacent to the cranial pole of the spermatid, separated from it by an acrosomal cap. The latter begins as a cytoplasmic vacuole containing flocculent material. It is probably formed from the Golgi apparatus and is believed to be essential for the penetration of the zona pellucida of the ovum. The cilial structure that serves as the core of the sperm tail develops from a centriole near the Golgi apparatus and ultimately consists of nine outer fibers and two inner fibers. The mitochondria form a helix around the cilia from the neck to the annulus of the tail. The terminal region of the tail consists of the axial filament surrounded by the cell membrane; most of the cytoplasm is

lost as the spermatids are released from the epithelium into the lumen of the tubule.

The process of spermatogenesis takes approximately 70 d from the beginning of the differentiation of the spermatocyte to the completion of a motile sperm.[203] The transport of the sperm through the epididymis to the ejaculatory duct requires an additional 12 to 21 d;[204] the journey is probably accomplished by a combination of peristaltic movement, bulk fluid drag, and intrinsic sperm motility. When sperm leave the testes, they are relatively immature and have a poor capacity to fertilize. During passage through the epididymis, maturation is evidenced by the development of the capacity for sustained motility, modification of the structural state of the nuclear chromatin and the tail organelles, and loss of the remnant of spermatid cytoplasm (the cytoplasmic droplet).[205, 206] Final acquisition of the capacity of the sperm to fertilize is poorly understood, but completion of the process may take place in the female genital tract (see later).

The mechanism of sperm motility is not completely clear. Energy for the process is derived from the hydrolysis of ATP that is generated in the mitochondrial sheath of the middle piece of the tail (see Fig. 13–15). The axial structure of the tail contains a central pair of microtubules surrounded by nine doublet tubules and nine dense fibers; the doublets are attached to the central tubules by a series of radial spokes, to each other by dynein arms, and to the axonemal membrane by so-called Y links (Fig. 13–16). Motility is believed to involve a sliding action of the microtubules, analogous to the interaction of actin and myosin in muscles. The dynein arms contain a protein (dynein) that is a powerful ATPase.[207] Sliding is thought to be generated by interaction of the dynein arms and to be restricted by the radial spokes.[208, 209] Mutations that influence the doublet arms, the spokes, or the spoke heads can lead to the immotile cilia syndromes[210] (see later).

CONTROL OF SPERMATOGENESIS. It has been established for half a century that spermatogenesis does not occur in the hypophysectomized state; that restoration of sper-

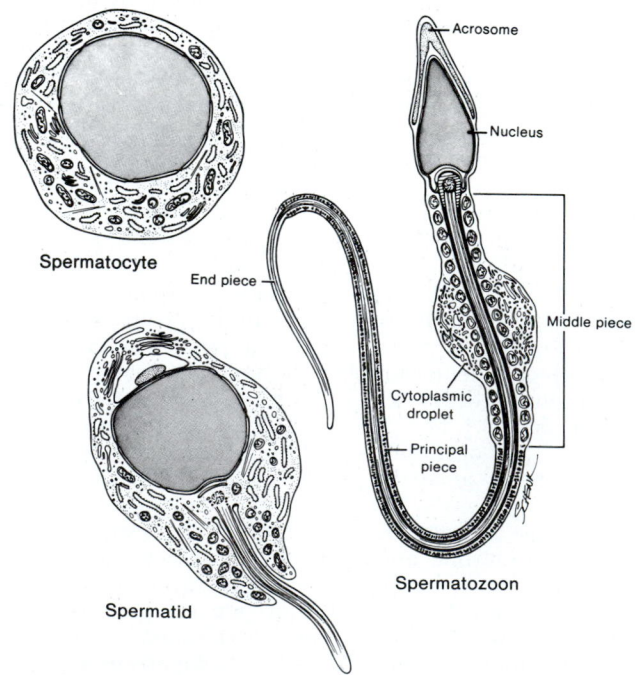

Figure 13–15. Schematic diagram illustrating conversion of spermatocyte to spermatid to spermatozoon.

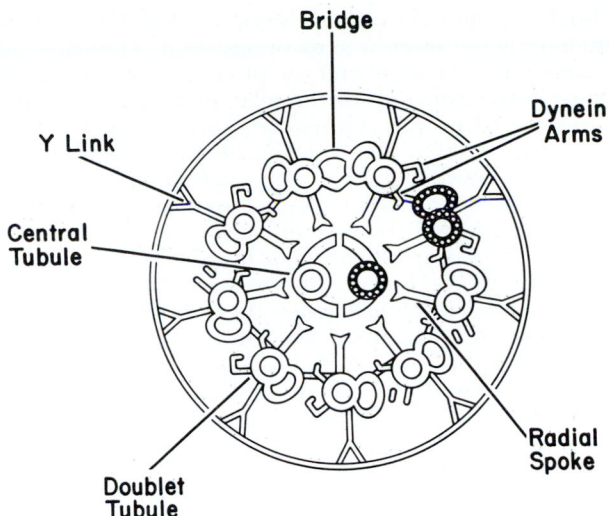

Bridge

Dynein
Arms

Y Link

Central
Tubule

Radial
Spoke

Doublet
Tubule

Figure 13–16. Schematic diagram showing a cross-section of the normal axonemal structure of human sperm.

matogenesis (or its initiation in the prepubertal state) requires LH and FSH; and that FSH appears to act directly on the spermatogenic tubule, whereas LH influences spermatogenesis indirectly by its enhancement of testosterone synthesis in the adjacent Leydig cells.[211] FSH and testosterone act in the testis by the same general mechanisms as peptide and steroid hormones in other tissues. For example, FSH binds to the surface of Sertoli cells in the spermatogenic tubule;[68, 71] this binding results in the stimulation of adenylate cyclase, an increase in intracellular cAMP concentration, the activation of protein kinases, and increased phosphorylation of a variety of proteins.[211] Likewise, the spermatogenic tubule contains high-affinity cytoplasmic and nuclear receptors for androgen;[171, 176, 212, 213] these hormone-receptor complexes act within the nuclei of cells to cause the expression of specific genes necessary for the differentiation process. Furthermore, testosterone and FSH interact by a complicated interlocking feedback system. As noted earlier, FSH may influence the sensitivity of the testis to LH (and hence the rate of testosterone biosynthesis) by regulating the number of LH receptors on the Leydig cell;[75] one function of androgen may be to control the secretion of inhibin by the Sertoli cell and hence the rate of FSH secretion.[214]

Despite these insights, major uncertainties exist at both the physiological and the molecular levels as to how spermatogenesis is controlled in the human. A portion of this problem is the consequence of differences among species. In addition, the hormonal requirements for the initiation of spermatogenesis in maturing animals differ from those required for maintenance in adults or for reinitiation after hypophysectomy. Thus extrapolations based on studies in one species and limited to one physiological situation must be made with caution.[215]

After hypophysectomy in the adult human male, no spermatocytes are formed; spermatogenesis can be restored or initiated by treatment with FSH (human menopausal gonadotropin) plus hCG.[211] After spermatogenesis is restored it can be maintained by hCG treatment alone.[211] The latter phenomenon, together with the finding that in otherwise normal subjects with suppressed FSH activity spermatogenesis can be restored by LH alone,[216] suggests that FSH may be required for initiation but not for maintenance of spermatogenesis. However, FSH appears to be necessary for quantitatively normal spermatogenesis in men.[217]

The steps in differentiation and the cellular targets on

which gonadotropins and androgens act to regulate spermatogenesis are not known with certainty. Steinberger and co-workers proposed that testosterone is necessary for meiosis and that FSH is involved in the completion of spermatid development.[215] Androgen receptors are present in Sertoli cells,[212, 213] and genetic evidence suggests that the critical action of androgens in promoting spermatogenesis takes place at this site. The primary evidence comes from studies of mouse chimeras in which sperm containing the X-linked gene for testicular feminization (and hence lacking a functional androgen receptor) can be fertile if the Sertoli cells contain an androgen receptor.[218] Because FSH receptors are also present on the Sertoli cell,[68] it is likely that both testosterone and FSH act on the Sertoli cell rather than on the spermatogonia.

A variety of biochemical effects of FSH have been characterized in immature animals both in vivo and in vitro (for reviews see refs. 71 and 219). Prominent among these effects are the increased production of androgen-binding protein, a protein that is similar to TeBG in size and binding characteristics, that appears to serve as a carrier for androgen within the tubule, and that is also present in the human testis;[220] and an increased aromatase activity in the Sertoli cell.[72, 219] However, it has not been possible to link any of these changes directly to sperm production.

In addition to the effects of FSH and androgen on seminiferous tubule function, β-endorphin production by Leydig cells may influence Sertoli cell function via a paracrine control mechanism within the testis.[221]

FERTILIZATION. Fertilization normally takes place within the fallopian tube. Spermatozoa usually require a period in the female genital tract before they can fertilize. This functional change, termed *capacitation*, is believed to consist of at least two components: (1) enhancement of the rate of flagellar beat with acceleration of sperm movement and (2) development of the capacity to undergo an acrosome reaction and consequently to allow the plasma membrane of the sperm to fuse with the ovum.[222] The time that is required for optimal capacitation of normal sperm may vary from 2 to more than 6 h.[223] Whether capacitation is an absolute requirement in the human or serves only to enhance fertilizing capabilities is not known. Because fertilization can take place in vitro when sperm and eggs are combined with no preincubation, the minimal time required for some spermatozoa to undergo capacitation must be short.[223]

The aspects of the capacitation reaction that promote motility may involve a change in the intracellular concentration or metabolism of calcium or cAMP.[224] The acrosome reaction may also involve calcium (for review see ref. 222). Neither the fallopian tube nor the egg itself appears to be essential for the acrosome reaction, which begins as a fusion between the acrosomal membrane and the overlying plasmalemma and is followed by calcium influx into the sperm down an electrochemical gradient. Subsequently fragmentation and ultimately loss of the acrosome occur. Because the acrosome is derived from lysosomes, its disintegration results in the release of hydrolytic enzymes and proteases. The fact that the acrosome reaction is followed within a few hours by a loss of sperm motility means that variability in the timing of capacitation in a sperm population relative to the moment of insemination increases the chance of a successful fertilization. Ordinarily, only about a fifth of motile spermatozoa recovered from the oviduct at variable times after insemination have undergone the reaction. The net effect of the hyperactive motility and acrosome reactions is that sperm acquire the capacity to penetrate the formidable vestments of the ovum.[222]

One consequence of this sequential acceleration of motility and initiation of the acrosome reaction is that sperm transport to the site of fertilization in the fallopian tube is a culling process. Only a small number of the millions of sperm that are ejaculated reach the site of fertilization. The characteristics of the particular spermatozoa that reach the ampulla and fertilize the egg are not known, but presumably these sperm exhibit the fastest motility and the most delayed initiation of the acrosome reaction.[225]

Understanding of the mechanism of sperm penetration is largely based on studies of fertilization of human eggs in vitro, a situation that may not be identical to the phenomenon in intact humans (for review see refs. 225 and 226). Ovulated eggs are surrounded by layers of cumulus cells embedded in a matrix of hyaluronic acid. The mechanism by which spermatozoa tunnel through the cumulus is not known. Possibly, hyaluronidase is released by the degenerating acrosome, and the mechanical agitation of the flagellum may disperse the cumulus cells.[225] Under in vitro conditions prior disposal of the cumulus with hyaluronidase is necessary to allow penetration of the zona pellucida and hence to permit fertilization by the sperm.

Phases of Normal Testicular Function

The phases of normal testicular function can be delineated in terms of the plasma testosterone concentration (Fig. 13–17). In the male embryo the production of testosterone by the testes and the concentration of plasma testosterone start to rise at the end of the second month of gestation, and shortly thereafter they attain a high value that is maintained until late in gestation when it decreases.[227, 228] At the time of birth the plasma testosterone level is only slightly higher in males than in females.[229-231] Shortly afterward the plasma testosterone level again commences to rise in the male infant and remains elevated for approximately 3 mo, falling to low levels by age 1.[229-232] The concentration then remains low, but higher in boys than in girls, until the onset of puberty when the concentration again increases in boys; it reaches adult levels by about age 17.[233, 234] Plasma concentrations remain more or less constant in the adult until late middle age and then decline somewhat during the later decades of life.[235-239] Sperm production takes place after puberty. The physiological events that take place during these various periods differ, as do the pathological consequences of derangements in testicular function that have their onset at different stages of life.

EMBRYONIC MALE SEXUAL DIFFERENTIATION. The process of sexual differentiation is described in Chapter 20.

In brief, the embryos of both sexes develop in an identical fashion until the seventh week of gestation. Thereafter, the anatomical development and the physiological development diverge, with formation of the male or female phenotype. As formulated by Jost, normal sexual development in the mammalian embryo depends on three sequential processes.[240, 241] The first involves the establishment of genetic sex, which is defined by the sex chromosome constitution that is established at the time of conception. The heterogametic sex (XY) in mammals is male, whereas the homogametic sex (XX) is female. In the second phase the sex chromosomes determine whether the indifferent gonad differentiates into a testis in the male or an ovary in the female. The third step involves the translation of gonadal sex into phenotypic sex and is the direct consequence of the type of gonad formed; i.e., during development of phenotypic sex the gonads convert indifferent internal and external genital anlagen into male or female forms.

The internal genitalia in the two sexes are derived from the wolffian and müllerian ducts that exist side by side in early embryos of both sexes.[242] The wolffian ducts serve as the excretory ducts of the mesonephric kidney and are physically attached to the indifferent gonad, whereas the müllerian duct has no continuity with the gonad. In the male the wolffian ducts give rise to the epididymis, vasa deferentia, and seminal vesicles, and the müllerian ducts disappear. In the female the fallopian tubes, uterus, and upper vagina are derived from the müllerian ducts, and the wolffian ducts disappear. The external genitalia and the urethra in the two sexes develop from common anlagen: the urogenital sinus and the genital tubercle, folds, and swelling. The urogenital sinus gives rise in the male to the prostate and prostatic urethra and in the female to the lower portion of the vagina and urethra. The genital tubercle is the origin of the glans penis in the male and the clitoris in the female. The urogenital swelling becomes the scrotum or the labia majora, and the genital folds develop into the shaft of the penis or the labia minora.

In the absence of the testis, whether in the normal female or in the male embryo castrated before the onset of phenotypic differentiation, the development of phenotypic sex proceeds along female lines.[240, 241] Thus masculinization of the fetus requires action of testicular hormones, whereas development of the female phenotype is the passive consequence of the absence of androgen. Under ordinary circumstances chromosomal sex, gonadal sex, and phenotypic sex are concordant; i.e., chromosomal sex determines gonadal sex, and gonadal sex in turn determines phenotypic sex, without deviation from the chromosomal program.

Control over the formation of the male phenotype is vested in the action of three hormones.[242] Two of the three, antimüllerian hormone and testosterone, are secretory products of the fetal testis. Antimüllerian hormone, which is a glycoprotein product of the embryonic testis, acts ipsilaterally in the male embryo to suppress the müllerian ducts and consequently to prevent development of the uterus and fallopian tubes.[243] Testosterone acts to stimulate the wolffian ducts and to induce development of the epididymis, vasa deferentia, and seminal vesicles and is also the precursor for the third fetal hormone, dihydrotestosterone.[242, 244] Dihydrotestosterone, which is formed within the urogenital sinus and lower urogenital tract from circulating testosterone, acts in the urogenital sinus to induce formation of the male urethra and prostate and in the genital tubercle, swelling, and folds to cause the midline fusion, elongation, and enlargement that eventuate in the male external genitalia.[242, 244] Thus the primary function of androgen during fetal life is to induce the formation of the accessory organs of male reproduction. Testosterone and dihydrotestosterone

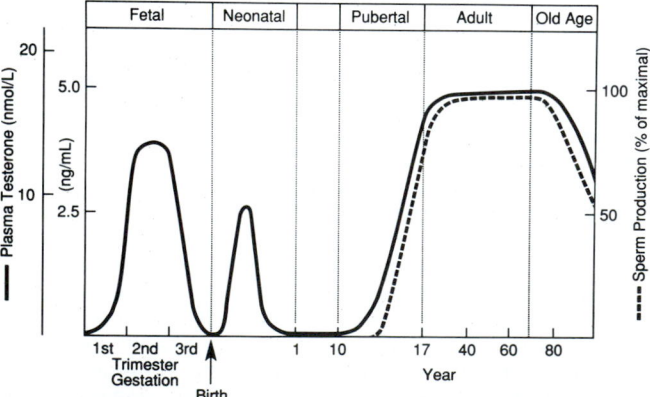

Figure 13–17. Schematic diagram of phases of male sexual function as indicated by mean plasma testosterone level and sperm production at different phases of life. (From Griffin JE, Wilson JD. The testis. In: Bondy PK, Rosenberg LE, eds. Metabolic Control and Disease. 8th ed. Philadelphia: W. B. Saunders, 1980: 1535–1578.)

act through the same receptor mechanism during embryogenesis and in the adult[245] (see Fig. 13–12). The formation of the male phenotype is largely completed by the middle of the second trimester of gestation, but at the time of completion of the male urethra the external genitalia in the two sexes do not differ in size.[242] Descent of the testes and differential growth of the external genitalia in the male take place during the second half of gestation.

The control of testosterone secretion by the embryonic testis is incompletely understood. By the 13th wk of gestation in the human, testosterone secretion appears to be regulated by LH from the fetal pituitary and/or by hCG that is present in the fetal circulation.[246] The decrease in testosterone synthesis late in gestation correlates both with a decline in the number of LH/hCG receptors in the testis[247, 248] and a decrease in the amount of hCG and LH in the fetal circulation.[246] Castration of the male rhesus monkey during late gestation results in an elevation of plasma gonadotropin and a further decrease in plasma testosterone levels.[249, 250] Anencephaly and other forms of congenital hypopituitarism result in the syndrome of microphallus.[251] Taken together, these findings indicate that testosterone production during the second half of gestation is regulated by LH, or hCG, or both and that LH production itself is under negative feedback control by testosterone.

The mechanism by which testosterone production is controlled between weeks 8 and 12 in the human embryo is not clear. In the rabbit embryo testosterone production during the analogous phase of male development appears to be independent of gonadotropins,[252] but for technical reasons this phase of embryonic development in human gestation has not been adequately examined. The fact that most male infants with anencephaly, or congenital hypopituitarism, or both have normal male urethras suggests either that androgen synthesis during early gestation is independent of gonadotropins or that chorionic gonadotropin, which is apparently not present in the rabbit, acts as a fail-safe mechanism to guarantee normal male development in the absence of LH from the fetal pituitary.[251]

In addition to their role in male phenotypic development, androgens that are secreted during fetal and/or neonatal life of some animal species exert at least two types of effects on the central nervous system: those that influence the hypothalamic-pituitary system and those that regulate diverse sexually dimorphic behavior patterns (for review see refs. 253 and 254). Androgens act in these species via the same intracellular high-affinity receptor protein in tissues as diverse as the brain and the urogenital tract. Social imprinting also plays a critical role in sex-specific behavior in some species.

The extent to which androgen action in the human central nervous system influences human sexual behavior has not been established. There is no clear-cut evidence for permanent imprinting by fetal androgens on the hypothalamic control of gonadotropin production in the human, and it is not established whether gonadal hormones have any direct effect on gender identity or gender behavior apart from their role in anatomical development of the sexual phenotype. Nevertheless, both androgens and cultural factors probably play important roles in the development of characteristic male behavior.[254] Therefore, in making clinical decisions as to sex assignment in subjects with ambiguous genitalia, it is important to undertake a thorough diagnostic evaluation and appropriate therapeutic intervention as early as possible, preferably in the newborn nursery, to ensure that the psychosocial factors are consonant with biological and anatomical development.

Male sexual development, apart from spermatogenesis, is remarkably complete during embryogenesis (see Fig. 13–17). For example, male infants have periodic erections during the later phases of gestation, which indicates that the complicated neurogenic pathways that regulate this process have developed by that time.

NEONATAL LIFE. The neonatal surge in testosterone secretion is the consequence of a rise in plasma gonadotropin levels,[250] but neither the cause for the increase in gonadotropin levels nor the precise function of the temporary increase in testosterone secretion is understood. In certain animal species neonatal testosterone is believed to be responsible for two aspects of male development: permanent virilization of the hypothalamus so that it secretes LH tonically rather than cyclically as in the female; and the priming of androgen target tissues for subsequent androgen-mediated growth and maturation in later life.[255–257] Blockade of the neonatal activation of the pituitary-testicular axis in male monkeys has been shown to result in subsequent subnormal increases in LH and testosterone and attenuated testicular enlargement at the time of puberty.[258] There is no evidence in humans that neonatal deprivation or excess of androgen has any permanent effect on hypothalamic-pituitary function.[259] Whether neonatal androgen plays a specific role in the development of human gender identity is likewise uncertain.[253, 254] However, indirect evidence suggests a role for neonatal androgen in the subsequent androgen-mediated growth of the male urogenital tract. Boys who are born with micophallus related to deficient androgen biosynthesis have inadequate androgen-mediated growth of the external genitalia if androgen replacement therapy is not started until the time of normal male puberty. However, their response may be normal if androgen is administered temporarily during infancy.[260] Such observations are consistent with the view that late fetal and/or neonatal androgen may prime the male urogenital tract by promoting early growth and by potentiating maturational effects of the hormone at puberty.

PUBERTY. In the prepubertal years the plasma levels of gonadotropins and gonadal steroids are low. The secretion of adrenal androgens, dehydroepiandrosterone, dehydroepiandrosterone sulfate, and androstenedione, starts to increase in boys as early as age 6 or 7, several years before maturation of the hypothalamic-pituitary-gonadal axis.[261] The secretion of these androgens is probably under the control of corticotropin (ACTH, adrenocorticotropin) and appears to be independent of activation of the pituitary-gonadal axis.[262] Maturation of adrenal androgen secretion is termed *adrenarche*. In part, the prepubertal growth spurt and the early development of axillary and pubic hair are mediated by these adrenal androgens, which are believed to bind to the androgen receptor only after conversion to testosterone and/or dihydrotestosterone in target tissues (see Fig. 13–12).

Before the onset of puberty, the low levels of plasma gonadotropin are under feedback control by the small amounts of androgen that are secreted by the testes,[263] as evidenced by the fact that castration at this time results in a rise in plasma gonadotropins to levels similar to those of the postpubertal castrate.[264] Gonadotropins in children, as in adults, are secreted in a pulsatile fashion, the pulses occurring at 2- to 3-h intervals.[265] These facts suggest that before puberty the negative feedback control of gonadotropin secretion is exquisitely sensitive to plasma testosterone levels.

The factors that determine the onset of puberty are poorly understood and may reside in the hypothalamic-pituitary system, the testis itself, or the adrenal, or at some undefined level (see Chapter 22). The sequence of pubertal maturation has, however, been well characterized. Its onset in boys, as well as in girls, is heralded by sleep-associated

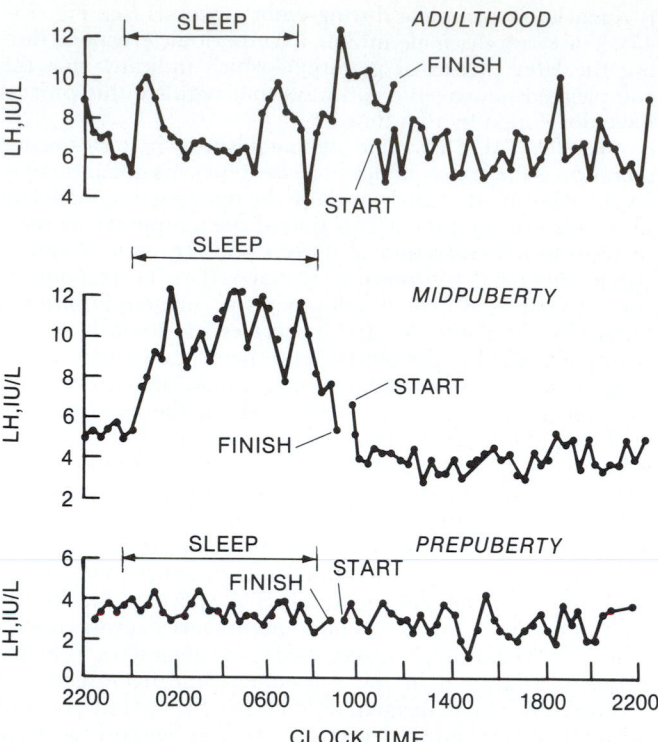

Figure 13–18. Ontogeny of LH secretion. Plasma LH concentrations were sampled every 20 min for 24 h in three normal males at different stages of development. *Top panel*, Pattern in an adult man with frequent secretory episodes throughout the 24-h period and no significant sleep-related augmentation. *Middle panel*, Secretory pattern in midpuberty in which marked secretory episodes occur during sleep. *Bottom panel*, Pattern in prepuberty in which there are no significant secretory episodes at any time throughout the sampling period. (Courtesy of RM Boyar. From Griffin JE, Wilson JD. The testis. In: Bondy PK, Rosenberg LE, eds. Metabolic Control and Disease. 8th ed. Philadelphia: W. B. Saunders, 1980: 1535–1578.)

surges in LH secretion (Fig. 13–18) and, to a lesser extent, by surges in the secretion of FSH.[266] Later in puberty the increased plasma gonadotropin levels become sustained throughout the day, as do the resulting increases in plasma testosterone and dihydrotestosterone levels.[233] The rise in gonadotropin secretion is believed to be the consequence of both an increase in LHRH secretion and an increase in sensitivity of the pituitary to LHRH.[261] Plasma levels of bioactive LH increase even more than those of the immunoreactive hormone.[267] The overall changes in gonadotropin and steroid hormone levels in plasma are compatible with the concept that with maturation, the hypothalamic-pituitary system becomes less sensitive to feedback inhibition by circulating androgens, which results in a higher mean plasma androgen concentration. As discussed earlier, endogenous opiates may be involved in the negative feedback inhibition of gonadal steroids on the hypothalamic-pituitary system.[84] Studies of prepubertal and pubertal boys suggest that there is a temporal relation between the development and/or maturation of the opioid control of LH secretion and the onset of puberty.[268, 269] How this maturational change in the hypothalamic-pituitary system is accomplished is unclear, but it appears to be triggered by the attainment of a critical body mass and/or percent body fat.[270, 271]

The changes that take place in the testes at puberty are illustrated in Figure 13–19. In prepubertal testes the interstitial cells consist of an undifferentiated mesenchyme with immature tubules. After puberty both components are fully developed; the cytoplasm of the functioning Leydig cells develops a characteristic foamy appearance, and the various stages of spermatogenesis can be delineated within the tubule. The development of spermatogenesis early in the pubertal process is associated with a rise in serum inhibin levels.[272] Assessment of the onset of sperm production in centrifuged urine samples from boys entering puberty showed that sperm production is also an early pubertal event and can occur when little or no pubic hair has developed and the testes have grown only slightly.[273]

With few exceptions, the anatomical and functional changes of puberty are the consequence of the action of gonadal steroids, principally testosterone and dihydrotestosterone. These steroids have effects on many tissues of the body, but all such actions are believed to be mediated via the same receptor machinery. Such effects have been classified as androgenic (the maturation of the male urogenital tract and spermatogenesis) and anabolic (promotion of growth in muscle and other somatic tissues), but these different effects are the result of various responses in different tissues to the same stimulus rather than the consequence of different actions of the hormone.[274] It is probable that all androgenic actions are mediated by dihydrotestosterone and/or testosterone and that other naturally occurring 19-carbon steroids can act as androgens only if they are converted to testosterone or dihydrotestosterone within peripheral tissues.[147, 274]

Multiple actions of androgen at puberty are recognized. Rugal folds appear in scrotal skin. The testes, penis, and scrotum enlarge, and the penis and scrotum become pigmented. The prostate, seminal vesicles, and epididymis increase in size during several years. The growth of the various accessory organs of reproduction accounts for about a fourth of androgen-mediated nitrogen retention of puberty.[275] One consequence of this growth and maturation process is the transformation of the cuboidal epithelia of the secretory tissues of the urogenital tract into secretory epithelia. The characteristic hair growth of male puberty involves development of the mustache and the beard; regression of the scalp line; appearance of truncal, extremity, and perianal hair; and extension of the pubic hair upward into a diamond-shaped pattern. Growth of axillary and pubic hair, which was already initiated at adrenarche, is promoted. The larynx enlarges, and the vocal cords become thickened, which results in a lowering of the pitch of the voice. Linear growth is accelerated from about 5 to about 8 cm/y and is accompanied by growth of muscle and connective tissue, which accounts for the major portion of pubertal nitrogen retention. Androgen appears to be necessary for the development of normal bone density with sexual maturation.[276] In the human the principal androgen-sensitive muscles are those of the pectoral region and the shoulder.[277] There is, in addition, an increase in the hematocrit[149] and a fall in plasma high-density lipoprotein (HDL) levels.[278] These various growth and maturation processes reach some limiting value, so that the administration even of supraphysiological amounts of exogenous androgen has little if any somatic effect after puberty is completed. The mechanism for the androgen-mediated pubertal growth spurt is thought to be the augmentation of growth hormone secretion[279] and the subsequent stimulation of increased levels of insulin-like growth factor I.[280]

A variety of behavioral and psychological changes, including development of libido and sexual potency, also take place at puberty. The extent to which the behavioral changes are the result of effects of steroids on the brain, indirect consequences of the anatomical changes at puberty, or cultural conditioning has not been defined.[254]

The events encompassing puberty vary in regard to both the time frame during which the process is initiated and completed and the sequence by which various changes take place. Because there is also extreme variability in the

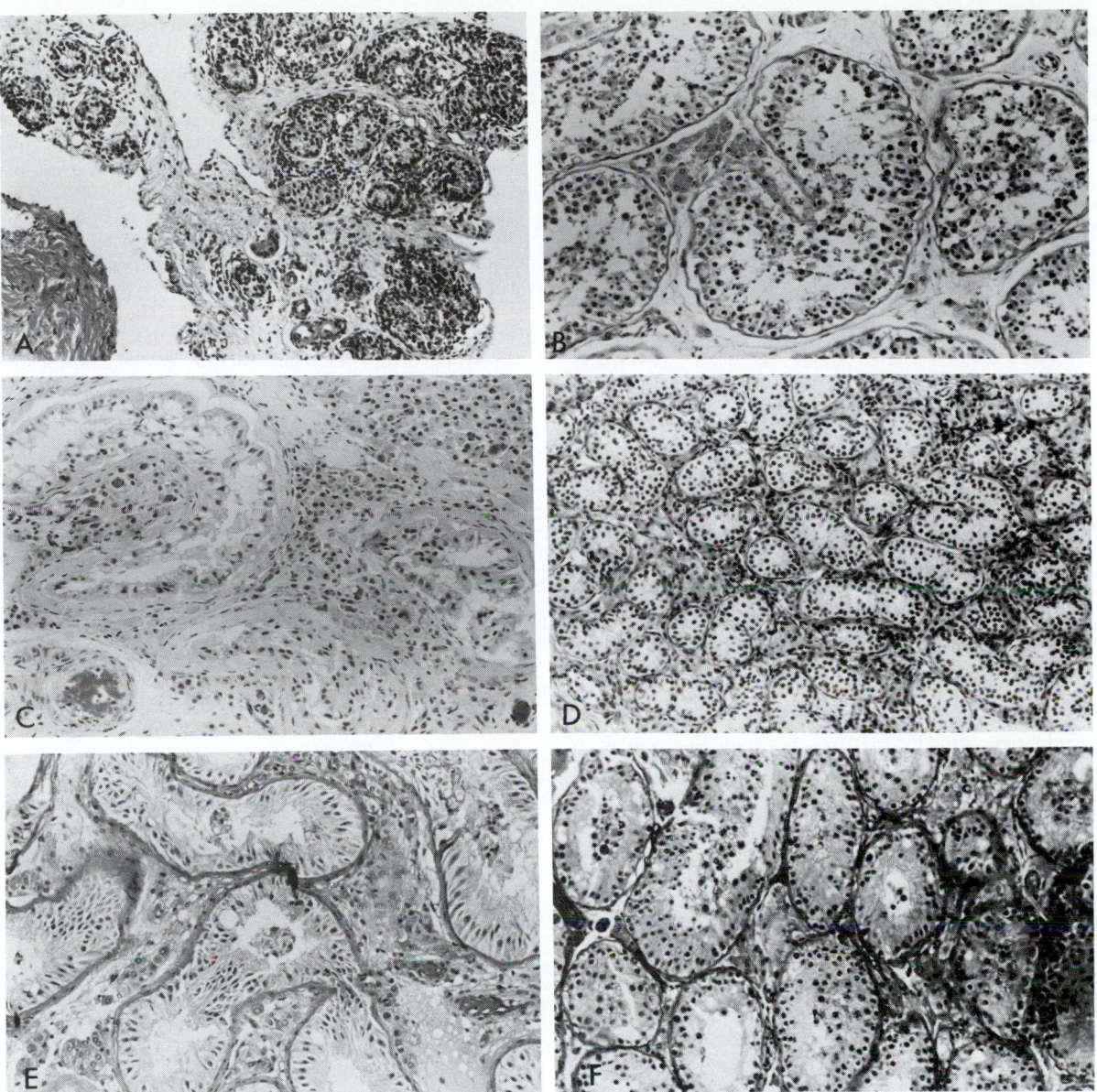

Figure 13–19. Photomicrographs (× 115) of representative testicular biopsies. *A,* Normal prepubertal boy with immature tubule development and undifferentiated interstitial (Leydig) cells; *B,* normal adult man with full spermatogenesis and mature Leydig cells; *C,* patient with Klinefelter syndrome, with marked fibrosis and hyalinization of tubules; *D,* patient with complete testicular feminization, with abundant Leydig cells and incomplete tubule maturation; *E,* patient with Sertoli cell–only syndrome (germinal cell aplasia), with normal Leydig cells and no germinal cells demonstrable within tubules; *F,* adult man with maturation arrest at spermatid stage. (Gifts of F Vellios and B Fallis. From Griffin JE, Wilson JD. The testis. In: Bondy PK, Rosenberg LE, eds. Metabolic Control and Disease. 8th ed. Philadelphia: W. B. Saunders, 1980: 1535–1578.)

end results, namely, differences in secondary sexual characteristics that depend on genetic, psychosocial, and nutritional factors, definition of the limits of normal puberty constitutes one of the most difficult and important problems of adolescent endocrinology. Several attempts have been made to establish nomograms that define the limits of normal development; however, most studies apply to only one ethnic group or nationality; such standards should be applied to other groups with caution. One system for staging pubertal development is that developed by Marshall and Tanner.[281] It is summarized in Table 13–2 and Figure 13–20. As illustrated in Table 13–3, adult male levels of plasma testosterone, LH, and FSH are usually achieved by Tanner stage 4.[282] There appears to be little doubt that under some circumstances the timing of this process is influenced by ethnic background,[283] possibly the consequence of differences in body weight among such groups.[284] However, in the United States male sexual maturation occurs on a similar time scale in black and white persons and is independent of socioeconomic status.[285]

A major problem remains in defining abnormalities of these various functions, i.e., in separating pathological delay of puberty from normal variation. For this evaluation the family history of the pattern of development (that of siblings and parents) may help. Comparisons with age-adjusted 90% confidence limits for testicular volume[283, 286] and penis size[283] are also useful in separating the normal from the abnormal. In some instances the measurement of sleep-related surges in plasma LH and/or testosterone level may provide evidence that puberty is commencing,[266] but often observation over time is required to determine whether delayed puberty is a normal variant (for the use of specific diagnostic procedures in this regard, see Chapter 22).

ADULTHOOD. On average, puberty is largely completed

TABLE 13–2. Stages of Puberty

Genital Stage	Pubic Hair Stage
Stage 1: Preadolescent. Testes, scrotum, and penis are about the same size and proportion as those in early childhood.	*Stage 1:* Preadolescent. Vellus over the pubes is no further developed than that over the abdominal wall, i.e., no pubic hair.
Stage 2: Scrotum and testes have enlarged, and there is a change in the texture of scrotal skin and some reddening of scrotal skin.	*Stage 2:* There is sparse growth of long, slightly pigmented, downy hair, straight or only slightly curled, appearing chiefly at base of penis.
Stage 3: Growth of the penis has occurred, at first mainly in length but with some increase in breadth. There has been further growth of the testes and the scrotum.	*Stage 3:* Hair is considerably darker, coarser, and more curled and spreads sparsely over junction of pubes.
Stage 4: The penis is further enlarged in length and breadth, with development of glans. The testes and the scrotum are further enlarged. There is also further darkening of scrotal skin.	*Stage 4:* Hair is now adult in type, but the area covered by it is smaller than that in most adults. There is no spread to the medial surface of the thighs.
Stage 5: Genitalia are adult in size and shape. No further enlargement takes place after stage 5 is reached.	*Stage 5:* Hair is adult in quantity and type, distributed as an inverse triangle. There is spread to the medial surface of the thighs but not up the linea alba or elsewhere above the base of the inverse triangle.

Data from Marshall WA, Tanner JM. Variations in the pattern of pubertal changes in boys. Arch Dis Child 1970; 45:13–23.

and reproductive capacity matures between the ages of 16 and 19. As indicated in Figure 13–20, most anatomical changes are also completed by this time. However, androgen-mediated hair growth is usually not maximal until the middle to late 20s.

The various physiological actions of androgen during puberty and adulthood can be separated into two general types: permanent and concurrent. Permanent effects encompass anatomical actions that are irreversible and do not regress if androgen production ceases, such as the effects on the larynx. Concurrent effects are those that require a continuing male level of the hormones, such as the enhancement of erythropoietin production and hemoglobin levels. Other physiological effects of androgen are composed of both permanent and concurrent components; e.g., beard growth slows but rarely stops in men who are castrated postpubertally. Many features of castration have been described only in anecdotal form, but two aspects have been studied in some detail. First, postpubertal castration results in a negative nitrogen balance. The source and the exact magnitude of the nitrogen loss have not been established, but probable sites of loss include the secretory tissues of the male urogenital tract and, to some extent, other androgen target tissues such as muscle. Androgen replacement to castrated men restores both nitrogen balance and the secretory capacity of the epididymis, seminal vesicles, and prostate as well.[274] Second, castration is followed by a progressive decline in male sexual drive, so that only rare castrated subjects can have intercourse after a few years. In such individuals physiological androgen replacement results in a rapid and predictable restoration of male sexual activity (reviewed in ref. 274).

At the completion of puberty the plasma testosterone levels have attained the adult male level of 10 to 35 nmol/L (3–10 ng/mL), sperm production has reached a steady level, and plasma concentrations of gonadotropins are in the adult range (5 to 20 IU/L for both LH and FSH). Thus the mature set for the feedback-regulatory system described in Figure 13–6 has been established and is sustained in a normal man for approximately 40 y. Even under the best circumstances the system can be perturbed, usually temporarily, by a variety of influences, at the level of both the testis and the hypothalamic-pituitary system. This possibility is hardly surprising considering the number of hormones and hormone receptor mechanisms and the complexity of sperm production. One of the most important of these influences is scrotal temperature; spermatogenesis is exquisitely sensitive to alterations in temperature, and temporary increases in systemic or local temperature (as in a hot bath) can be followed by temporary decreases in sperm production.[287] Spermatogenesis may also be influenced by diet, drugs, environmental agents, and a variety of psychological stresses.[288] Testosterone production is more stable than spermatogenesis but may also be impeded by some drugs.[289]

OLD AGE. The term *male climacteric* implies some analogy to the complete cessation of ovarian function that normally occurs in women. Men do not experience a relatively rapid total cessation of Leydig cell or seminiferous tubule function with old age, nor do men experience the gonadotropin-related hot flashes that are characteristic of menopause. Male sexual function does decrease with age. This decline does not appear to coincide with hormonal changes or old age as such. The rigidity of penile erection and force of expulsion of the ejaculate are greatest and the refractory period is shortest at approximately age 17. Male sexual function then begins its gradual decline.[290] The fre-

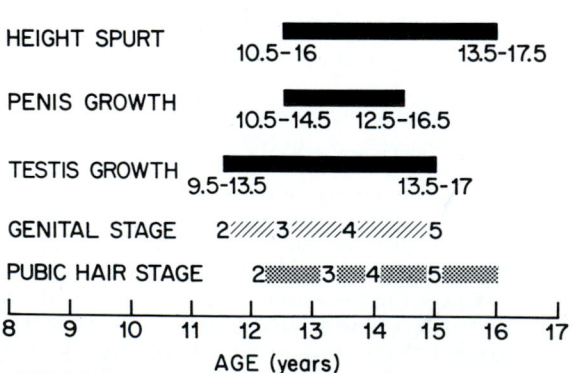

Figure 13–20. Diagram of sequence of events at puberty. The range of ages within which changes commence and terminate in normal boys is indicated by figures below each bar. (Data from Marshall WA, Tanner JM. Variations in the pattern of pubertal changes in boys. Arch Dis Child 1970; 45:13–23.)

TABLE 13–3. Comparisons of Mean Plasma Hormone Values with Stages of Puberty

Stage	Mean Testosterone Values		Mean LH Values (IU/L)	Mean FSH Values (IU/L)
	nmol/L	ng/mL		
Genital Size Staging				
1	3.0	0.9	3.3	6.1
2	8.7	2.5	4.5	7.2
3	11.7	3.4	5.3	7.6
4	18.0	5.2	6.7	8.6
5	20.0	5.7	7.9	9.8
Pubic Hair Staging				
1	1.6	0.5	3.7	6.3
2	4.6	1.4	5.0	7.3
3	11.7	3.4	5.7	7.9
4	19.4	5.6	7.4	8.8
5	21.9	6.3	8.0	9.3

Adapted from Lee PA, Jaffe RB, Midgley AR Jr. Serum gonadotropin, testosterone and prolactin concentrations throughout puberty in boys: a longitudinal study. J Clin Endocrinol Metab 1974; 39:664–672. © by The Endocrine Society.

quency of sexual activity in men appears to be established in early adulthood and maintained in the same portion of the spectrum (from relatively frequent to relatively infrequent) throughout life.[291] Male libido is separate from erectile function. Studies of serum testosterone concentrations in men with different levels of sexual activity suggest that androgen levels within the normal range are not a determinant of frequency of sexual activity.[292]

Early reports of a decline in serum testosterone levels with advanced age were flawed in that the older men being studied were either hospitalized or nursing home patients. When older men are carefully screened to exclude major health problems or medication use, some studies demonstrate no fall in serum testosterone level with age.[293] Other studies of older men with similar exclusive criteria demonstrate a clear decrease in mean serum testosterone levels with age.[294] However, almost all older men still have serum testosterone levels within the range considered to be normal for young men. Two studies have reported a loss of the normal circadian rhythmicity in serum testosterone levels with age.[238, 295] In contrast, young men have a circadian rhythm in serum testosterone, with maximal levels in the morning and minimal levels in the evening. Bioavailable testosterone, as assessed by measuring the testosterone that is not bound to TeBG, is lower, and Leydig cell reserve, as assessed by the response to gonadotropin stimulation, is decreased in older men.[296, 297] The cause of the decreased Leydig cell function with age is likely a decrease in Leydig cell number in the testes.[298] Studies of testosterone precursor concentrations in the spermatic vein or testicular tissue favor a decrease in the Δ^5-pathway of testosterone synthesis in the testes of elderly men, a pattern that is mimicked by reduced oxygen supply in in vitro incubations.[299–301]

Seminiferous tubule function also declines with age. When ejaculatory frequency is the same for selected young and old men, sperm density does not change with age, but older men have lower ejaculate volumes, decreased sperm motility, and an increased percentage of abnormal sperm.[294] However, most older men have values for these parameters that are within the range considered to be normal for young fertile men.[294] When seminiferous tubule function is quantitated by the measurement of daily sperm production on the basis of biopsy studies, there is a negative correlation of sperm production with age.[298] The decreased sperm production in older men does not correlate with Leydig cell number.[302] The hormonal function of the seminiferous tubule also declines with age, in that basal and stimulated serum inhibin levels are decreased in older men.[303]

Most studies have reported increased serum LH and FSH levels in elderly men, in keeping with some decrease in bioavailable testosterone and in sperm production.[293–295, 298, 304] Studies of pulsatile gonadotropin secretion indicate a decreased LH pulse frequency but no change in pulse amplitude with age.[305] Bioactive LH levels are increased in elderly men to a similar degree as immunoreactive LH levels, so that the LH bioactive/immunoreactive ratio is unchanged.[297] These observations suggest that the hypothalamic-pituitary responsiveness to the decreased Leydig cell function is appropriate. In one study[306] the pituitary bioactive LH reserve was found to be decreased in elderly men in response to LHRH and tamoxifen, but in another study the response to clomiphene citrate was normal.[297] Basal levels of bioactive FSH were similar in young and elderly men; immunoreactive FSH levels were higher in the elderly men.[307] Administration of clomiphene citrate increased both bioactive and immunoreactive FSH levels in serum, with similar peak levels in both assays.[307] It is unclear why the basal bioactive FSH level is not increased in elderly men in response to the decreased spermatogenesis and inhibin levels.

In summary, the decline in male sexual function with age does not appear to be endocrine mediated. However, evidence is convincing for a decrease in both Leydig cell function and seminiferous tubule function in healthy elderly men. The role of these changes in other aspects of aging is yet to be determined.

ASSESSMENT OF TESTICULAR FUNCTION

Leydig Cell Function

HISTORY AND PHYSICAL EXAMINATION. The assessment of androgen status should include inquiry about the presence of developmental abnormalities at birth (e.g., hypospadias, microphallus, and/or cryptorchidism; see later); the timing and the extent of sexual maturation at puberty; the rate of beard growth; and the current libido, sexual function, muscle strength, and energy. Inadequate Leydig cell function or androgen action during embryogenesis may manifest itself by the presence of hypospadias, cryptorchidism, or microphallus. If Leydig cell failure occurs before puberty, sexual maturation will not occur, and the individual will develop the clinical features termed *eunuchoidism*, including an infantile amount and distribution of body hair, poor development of skeletal muscles, failure of closure of the epiphyses so that the arm span is more than 5 cm greater than height and the lower body segment (heel to pubis) is more than 5 cm longer than the upper body segment (pubis to crown).

Detection of Leydig cell failure commencing after puberty requires a high index of suspicion and, usually, appropriate laboratory assessment. One reason for difficulty in detecting this failure is that the complaint of decreased sexual function is a relatively common one among adult men. In one large study of more than 1000 men in a medical outpatient clinic, about a third claimed impotence, whereas an abnormality of the hypothalamic-pituitary-testicular axis was present in only about a fifth of the impotent group.[308] The second reason is that when Leydig cell failure is severe, certain functions that require androgens for initiation continue unabated, and those functions that eventually regress may do so slowly. The frequency of shaving may not decrease for many months or even years because of the slow decline in the rate of beard growth once established.

ASSESSMENT OF PLASMA LH, ANDROGENS, AND TeBG. The plasma LH level has greater variation throughout the day than the plasma testosterone level.[309] Because the LH level must be interpreted in light of plasma testosterone, it is usually appropriate to measure both hormones by using a pool formed by combining equal quantities of blood obtained from three or four samples at 15- to 20-min intervals.[46, 309] In this way only a single pooled sample of plasma is submitted to the laboratory, and the averaging of values is accomplished before the assay. The usual assay for LH is a radioimmunoassay. The normal plasma LH values must be established for each laboratory because the antibody used in the assay may vary depending on its source. The usual normal range of plasma LH in adult men is 5 to 20 IU/L, with the National Institutes of Health Reference Standard LER-907. One microgram of LER-907 is usually equivalent to 219 mU of the Second International Reference Preparation of human menopausal gonadotropin (hMG) in the LH assay. Bioactive LH can be assessed by the rat interstitial cell assay and may be detectable at times when the immunoreactive LH is undetectable.[310]

Plasma testosterone is also measured by radioimmunoassay. Like LH, testosterone is secreted in pulsatile fashion;

the pulse height and frequency vary slightly throughout the day and at different times of the year, but these secondary variations are probably not significant in the routine clinical situation.[311] Testosterone should be measured in conjunction with plasma LH, by using a pool of samples as just described. The normal range in adult men is 10 to 35 nmol/L (3 to 10 ng/mL). The plasma testosterone level is statistically higher in prepubertal boys than in girls, the normal range in boys being 0.2 to 0.7 nmol/L (0.05 to 0.2 ng/mL). At the time of puberty, random daytime levels of plasma testosterone show a gradual increase that correlates roughly with the stages of puberty.[233] The initial rise in plasma testosterone at the start of puberty occurs as a result of sleep-related nocturnal gonadotropin surges.[266]

Dihydrotestosterone can also be measured by radioimmunoassay. In normal young men the plasma concentration averages about 10% of the testosterone value, 1 to 2.5 nmol/L (0.3 to 0.7 ng/mL; 95% confidence limits).[312] In older men with prostatic hyperplasia, plasma values are significantly higher: 1.8 to 5.2 nmol/L (0.5 to 1.5 ng/mL; 95% confidence limits).[312]

Testicular function cannot be assessed by measurement of urinary excretion of 17-ketosteroids. The androgens measured by this method are primarily of adrenal origin; testosterone and its metabolites account for only about 40% of 17-ketosteroid excretion in men.[164]

Estimation of TeBG concentration is sometimes useful for interpretation of levels of total plasma testosterone. Binding capacity of TeBG can be assessed with the use of radioactive androgen after separation of TeBG from other plasma proteins,[183] or the protein can be assayed by radioimmunoassay.

Estimates of other components of the plasma androgen pool are primarily of research interest. Free testosterone concentrations can be estimated by equilibrium dialysis, but a more accurate assessment of available testosterone in vivo can be obtained by measuring the non–TeBG-bound fraction directly. This assay can be done by removal of TeBG from plasma with concanavalin A–Sepharose.[183]

DYNAMIC TESTS OF THE HYPOTHALAMIC-PITUITARY–LEYDIG CELL AXIS. To assess Leydig cell function before puberty, it is common to measure the response of plasma testosterone to gonadotropin stimulation as an index of Leydig cell reserve.[313–315] The ability of Leydig cells to respond to gonadotropin is usually assessed after the administration of hCG in repeated doses. Normal prepubertal boys respond to 3 to 5 d of injection of 1000 to 2000 IU hCG with an increase of plasma testosterone level to about 7 nmol/L (2 ng/nL); the magnitude of the response increases with the initiation of puberty and peaks in early puberty.[313–315]

In certain circumstances the response of plasma LH to the administration of LHRH is measured to assess the functional integrity of the hypothalamic-pituitary–Leydig cell axis. The responsiveness of the pituitary to LHRH changes at the time of puberty. Before puberty the quantitative responses of LH and FSH are similar. With pubertal development the LH response to acute administration of LHRH increases, whereas the FSH response remains the same. The amount of LH released after acute administration of LHRH probably reflects the amount of stored hormone in the pituitary. When 100 μg of LHRH is given subcutaneously or intravenously to normal men, there is, on average, a four- to fivefold increase in LH, with the peak level at 30 min.[316] However, the range of response is broad, with some normal men having less than a doubling of LH levels. In general the peak LH level after a single LHRH injection correlates with the basal level.

In patients with primary testicular failure, measurement

of basal LH is usually sufficient, and measurement of the LHRH response adds little to aid the diagnosis.[317] Men who have pituitary disease or hypothalamic disease may have either a normal or an abnormal LH response to an acute dose of LHRH. Therefore, a normal response is of no value in determining the presence or absence of disease or in distinguishing hypothalamic from pituitary disease. A subnormal response is of value in determining that an abnormality exists, even though the site of the abnormality is not determined. The LHRH test is most useful for evaluation of men with secondary hypogonadism and a subnormal LH response to an acute dose of LHRH. If daily infusions of LHRH for 1 wk lead to the development of a normal LH response to an acute dose of LHRH, a hypothalamic etiology of the hypogonadism is likely.[318]

Seminiferous Tubule Function

HISTORY AND PHYSICAL EXAMINATION. Leydig cell dysfunction usually results in defective spermatogenesis. Thus men presenting with the clinical features of Leydig cell dysfunction are usually also infertile. In contrast, primary disorders of the seminiferous tubules have infertility as the sole clinical manifestation.

Examination of the testes is an essential portion of the physical examination. The seminiferous tubules account for about 60% of testicular volume. The prepubertal testis measures about 2 cm long (or 2 mL in volume, as assessed by the Prader orchidometer) and increases in size in a predictable way with puberty; the adult size is reached by about age 16. When damage to the seminiferous tubules occurs before puberty, the testes are small and firm; postpubertal damage results in characteristically small and soft testes. Considerable damage must occur before overall size is decreased below the lower limits of normal. The normal adult testis averages 4.6 cm long (range 3.5 to 5.5 cm), which corresponds to a volume of 12 to 25 mL.[319] Advanced age per se does not influence testicular size; thus the significance of small testes is the same at all ages in the adult.[319] Testis size varies among ethnic groups. Oriental men have been noted to have smaller testes than white men independent of differences in overall body size.[320] Testicular volume may be consistently overestimated with the Prader orchidometer when the actual volume is less than 20 mL.[321] Because of the frequent occurrence of varicocele among infertile men and its possible causal role in infertility, the spermatic cord should be carefully palpated with the patient in a standing position. Unilateral absence of the vas deferens is often associated with ipsilateral renal agenesis.[322]

SEMINAL FLUID EXAMINATION. Routine evaluation of the seminal fluid assesses parameters that do not necessarily reflect the functional capacity of the sperm. Although methods to measure sperm penetration of bovine cervical mucus and zona-free hamster ova have been developed, they are not sufficiently standardized for general use (see later).

Seminal fluid should be obtained by masturbation into a clean glass or plastic container. Collection in a condom or after coitus interruptus may result in incomplete samples and is not recommended. The volume of the normal ejaculate is 2 to 6 mL. Immediately after ejaculation, coagulation of the seminal fluid occurs, followed within 15 to 30 min by reliquefaction. The specimen should be analyzed within an hour.

An estimation of motility is made by examining a drop of undiluted seminal fluid and recording the percentage of motile forms. The quality of motility can be graded 1 to 3. Spermatozoa with grade 3 motility tend to move rapidly across the field, spermatozoa with grade 2 motility move aimlessly, and spermatozoa with grade 1 motility have a beating tail but do not change position. Normally 60% or more of the sperm should be motile, with an average quality of motility of grade 2.5 or more.

Sperm density may be determined by diluting seminal fluid 20-fold with an appropriate solution such as the one described in the World Health Organization laboratory manual,[323] i.e., a mixture of 75 mL glacial acetic acid; 300 mg saponin dissolved in 2 mL saline and then centrifuged for 20 min at 800 × g; 1500 mL saline; and 165 mL 5% gentian violet. After shaking of the diluted sample for 2 min, sperm density is estimated in an appropriate hemocytometer as millions per milliliter. Sperm density may also be estimated by using an electronic particle counter.[324] The normal value is usually considered to be greater than 20 million/mL, with total sperm per ejaculate higher than 60 million.

In normal men who ejaculate daily the daily sperm output is relatively constant after the first 2 d.[325] The daily sperm output is calculated from the total sperm in the ejaculate divided by the number of days since the previous ejaculation. The average daily sperm output in nine men for the third through the fifth day of daily ejaculation was 166 ± 29 million (range 47 to 579 million). Counts in the first 2 d are variable and not closely related to the output during the third through the fifth days because of differences in extragonadal sperm reserves.[325] After 6 d of sexual rest, the first ejaculate contains approximately four times as many sperm as are present in the stable daily sperm output. This change suggests either that some sperm are lost during sexual abstinence or that sperm output diminishes during sexual rest. Less than 0.1% of the daily sperm output is usually present in the urine, but a significant portion of the daily sperm output may appear in the urine after prolonged sexual rest.

In addition to the problem of variable reserves of sperm in the male excretory ducts, random sampling of sperm density is complicated by effects of factors such as hot baths, acute febrile illnesses, and use of medications. The net result is that it is difficult to define the minimally adequate ejaculate.[326] When 24 to 36 h of sexual rest was specified and ejaculates were examined at 2-wk intervals, Sherins and co-workers[326] found that average semen quality and sperm output are lower than is generally considered to be normal for fertile men. Three ejaculates are usually required to establish an inadequacy of sperm number or cytology, and as many as six estimates or more may be necessary for valid assessment if the initial ejaculates are of equivocal quality.[326]

Seminal fluid cytology is a useful index of fertility.[326] The seminal fluid smear is prepared similarly to a blood smear but with special stains.[322] Normal spermatozoa have symmetrically oval heads (3 to 5 by 2 to 3 μm), midpieces that are slightly larger at the proximal ends and that are symmetrically inserted into the head, and tails that are 7 to 15 times longer than heads. Some abnormal spermatozoa are present in all semen. The best correlations between histological abnormalities and infertility occur when a single anomaly (e.g., lack of the acrosome) is found in a large percentage of the sample. This case is not usual because variable abnormalities are more frequent. Although there is no clear delineation of the minimal structural features that are compatible with fertility, 60% or more of the spermatozoa should have normal morphological features.[326] For research purposes, the details of sperm structure can be studied by electron microscopy. Such studies are particularly useful for identifying specific abnormalities in immotile sperm (see later). However, care must be exercised in defining defects in axonemal ultrastructure because there is considerable heterogeneity among normal men.[327]

The presence of more than 2 to 3% immature sperm is thought to indicate testicular stress, which occurs within 2 to 3 wk of the onset of many illnesses, especially viral infections.[328] The upper limit of normal for the percentage of immature forms that is compatible with fertility is not known. Some leukocytes may be present in the normal ejaculate, and it may be difficult to distinguish these cells from immature sperm at times.[329]

A test for sperm penetration of cervical mucus has been developed utilizing bovine cervical mucus.[330] The cervical mucus is drawn up in flat capillary tubes and stored frozen for up to 4 wk. The capillary tube is then brought to room temperature and inserted into a semen sample for 90 min. The distance of sperm penetration is assessed microscopically. Less than 15 mm of penetration is considered to be abnormal.[330] In one report about a third of men who were evaluated for infertility had decreased penetration of bovine cervical mucus. Interestingly, the majority had normal sperm densities and motilities.[327]

Hamster eggs can be stripped of the zona pellucida and fertilized by sperm of other species, including humans.[331] The zona-free hamster egg has been used as a surrogate for a human egg in hopes that its fertilization could be used to predict the fertilizing capacities of sperm.[331] This sperm penetration test requires overnight capacitation of the sperm in vitro in a special medium, incubation of sperm and eggs together under oil for 2 to 5 h, and microscopic examination of the egg for the presence of internalized sperm heads. Sperm from fertile men usually penetrate at least 15% of the eggs, but failure to penetrate 15% of the eggs may occur in men with proven fertility.[330] Thus the sperm penetration test is expensive and is not sufficiently reliable for routine use in the evaluation of the infertile couple. It may be useful for following the efficacy of therapy in selected infertile men.[331] The bovine cervical mucus test and the sperm penetration test appear to measure different sperm properties.[332]

TESTICULAR BIOPSY. Testicular biopsy is useful in some men with oligospermia and azoospermia both as an aid in diagnosis and as a guide to treatment.[333] The most clear-cut indication for biopsy is in the group of infertile men in whom the possibility of ductal obstruction is suggested by the finding of azoospermia and normal plasma FSH levels. In such a situation, normal testicular histological findings are an indication for the performance of vasography and/or exploration of the vas deferens. Some surgeons prefer to inject the vas deferens on one side with contrast dye at the time of testicular biopsy and thus to obtain a vasogram and biopsy simultaneously. The indications for testicular biopsy in infertile men are not so clear when the plasma FSH level is elevated (implying a defect in spermatogenesis) or when some sperm are present in semen (implying that the excretory ducts are patent). However, in rare instances infertility can be associated with unilateral ductal obstruction and hence with oligospermia rather than azoospermia (see later). In most instances testicular biopsy is of little value when oligospermia is associated with infertility. The diagnosis of Klinefelter syndrome secondary to chromosomal mosaicism that is limited to the testes can be established only by tissue culture and karyotypic analysis of the biopsy material. Testicular biopsy is often followed by a transient decrease in sperm counts, but adverse effects are not permanent. The histological features of several testicular disorders are illustrated in Figure 13–19.

PLASMA FSH. Levels of plasma FSH usually correlate inversely with spermatogenesis; i.e., elevations of FSH occur in men with intact hypothalamic-pituitary axes when there is severe damage to the germinal epithelium.[334] An inverse relationship also exists between seminal plasma inhibin and serum FSH levels in men.[334] However, serum inhibin levels do not correlate with serum FSH levels or with the degree of testicular damage.[335] The failure of such a correlation raises questions as to the clinical utility of serum inhibin levels. FSH is measured by radioimmunoassay with LER-907 as the usual standard, the normal value in adult men ranging from 5 to 20 IU/L. One microgram of LER-907 is usually equivalent to 38 mU of the Second International Reference Preparation of hMG in the FSH assay. Oligospermia related to a primary defect in the testis may be associated with elevated FSH levels (see later). An FSH bioassay involving stimulation of rat granulosa cell aromatase activity has been used as an investigational tool to supplement the radioimmunoassay.[336] The role of the bioassay in the clinical evaluation of the pituitary-testicular axis is under evaluation.

CHROMOSOMAL ANALYSIS. Examination of buccal mucosal cells for the presence of chromatin clumps on the nuclear membrane (the Barr body) provides evidence for the number of X chromosomes. The Barr body, which represents the second X chromosome in XX individuals, is found in 20% or more of the nuclei of the cells of normal females and is present in less than 2% of the cells of normal males. In general there is one Barr body for every X chromosome in excess of one. If the buccal mucosal cells are stained with quinacrine or its mustard derivative and examined by fluorescence microscopy, the Y chromosome (the F body) can also be identified. This method provides a more rapid and accurate means of determining the sex chromosome complement under some circumstances, such as suspected male pseudohermaphroditism. Because the fluorescent portion of the Y chromosome is on the long arm of the Y chromosome and the male-determining factors are on the short arm, the absence of Y chromosome fluorescence must be interpreted with caution.

The analysis of chromosomal karyotype, which is the most accurate means of determining the chromosome complement, involves short-term culture of peripheral blood leukocytes or of skin or gonadal fibroblasts in medium containing an agent such as phytohemagglutinin that induces the cells to divide. A mitotic spindle poison such as colchicine, which arrests mitosis at metaphase, is added, and the cells are harvested and stained. A number of cells in metaphase are assessed to establish the number and histological characteristics of the chromosomes. This technique is valuable for establishing the exact chromosome complement, the presence of mosaicism, the presence of structural chromosome alterations, and the sex chromosome composition. The study of multiple tissues may be necessary to establish chromosome mosaicism. In a given tissue, 20 cells must be examined to exclude with 95% confidence a mosaicism of 15% or greater.

Estrogenic Function

HISTORY AND PHYSICAL EXAMINATION. Breast enlargement is the most consistent feature of feminizing states in men. Gynecomastia refers to enlargement of the male breast because of proliferation of glandular tissue. The presence of gynecomastia should be sought by examining the patient while he is in the sitting position; the fingers are used to grasp the glandular tissue. Palpation with the flat part of the hand while the patient is in a supine position may result in failure to detect early or minimal breast enlargement. In obese men it is important to try to detect the edge of the rim of glandular tissue that separates it from the adipose tissue of the chest wall. A more extensive discussion of gynecomastia is in Chapter 15.

PLASMA ESTROGENS. As discussed earlier, most of the estradiol and all of the estrone that are produced in normal men are formed by extraglandular aromatization of circulating androgens. Plasma estradiol and plasma estrone levels are measured by radioimmunoassay. The plasma estradiol level is usually less than 180 pmol/L (50 pg/mL) in normal men; the plasma estrone level is somewhat higher but usually less than 300 pmol/L (80 pg/mL).[337]

ABNORMALITIES OF TESTICULAR FUNCTION

Abnormalities of testicular function have different consequences, depending on the phase of sexual life in which they first become manifest. Although there are problems inherent in any developmental categorization, such a classification of testicular diseases has a sound physiological rationale, but it must be recognized that some aspects of the classification are arbitrary. For example, the Klinefelter syndrome is a disorder of chromosomal sex, but subjects are usually diagnosed when clinical manifestations become apparent after the time of normal puberty. Although such limitations should be remembered, the clinical disorders of the testis can be classified as abnormalities of fetal development, puberty, adult life, and senescence.

Fetal Life

ABNORMALITIES OF MALE SEXUAL DIFFERENTIATION. Disturbances in sexual differentiation can arise from a variety of mechanisms: environmental insult, as in the ingestion of a virilizing drug during pregnancy; nonfamilial aberrations of the sex chromosomes, as in 45,X/46,XY chromosomal mosaicism; developmental birth defects of multifactorial origin, as in most cases of hypospadias; or hereditary disorders resulting from single-gene mutations, as in the testicular feminization syndrome.[338]

The disorders of sexual differentiation and their management are described in Chapter 20. Because men with the Klinefelter syndrome and the XX male ordinarily present as problems of undervirilization or infertility, they will be considered later in this chapter.

CRYPTORCHIDISM. Descent of the testes is essential to normal function because spermatogenesis requires the lower temperature that is present in the scrotum. Failure of testicular descent can occur at any site in the normal pathway of descent, from high in the abdomen to the normal location in the scrotum; the clinical implications and sequelae of cryptorchidism differ, depending on the site at which descent ceases. A large portion of the clinical literature in this field is difficult to interpret because of imprecise definitions. Scorer and Farrington defined cryptorchidism as the condition of any testis that is not 4 cm or more below the pubic tubercle in an infant of normal size and subclassified the condition depending on the location of the maldescended testis, as follows:[26]

1. The intra-abdominal testis (10%) cannot be felt. Infants with bilateral intra-abdominal testes can be distinguished from female pseudohermaphrodites by assessment of the chromosomal karyotype and from boys with bilateral anorchia by demonstrating that the plasma testosterone level increases after the administration of hCG. Unilateral intra-abdominal testes should be distinguished from the syndrome of mixed gonadal dysgenesis in which a testis is present on one side and an intra-abdominal streak gonad is present on the other. Under ordinary conditions the presence and location of an intra-abdominal testis must be established by surgery; typically, it is located just above the internal inguinal ring.

2. The canalicular testis (20%) has traversed the internal inguinal ring and is present in the inguinal canal; it may be

movable and may intermittently move between the canal and the upper scrotum. Such testes are small or would not be able to pass the external inguinal ring. When the testis is in the canal, the tension of the aponeurosis of the external oblique muscle is too firm a barrier to allow palpation of the testis.

3. The high scrotal testis (40%) is further along the pathway of descent but does not reach the bottom of the scrotum. It is characteristically smaller than its normal partner and has a limited range of motion so that it can retract into the groin but not past the internal ring. Such retraction may make accurate diagnosis and classification difficult.

4. The obstructed testis (30%) is a fourth category in which failure of descent appears to be due to a physical barrier formed by a fascial cord between the inguinal pouch and the inlet of the scrotum.

On rare occasions the testis may migrate from its normal pathway of descent between the abdominal cavity and the bottom of the scrotum and become ectopic in location.[339] There are five major sites of ectopia: the perineum, the femoral canal, the superficial inguinal pouch, the suprapubic area, and the opposite scrotal compartment. Testicular ectopia is believed to be caused by abnormality of the gubernaculum, which is normally divided into five branches, one each going to the aforementioned areas.[339] The critical clinical issue is to separate this disorder from unilateral and/or bilateral anorchia.

In most situations the higher the location of the testis or the more extreme the ectopia, the more difficult surgical repair becomes. In contrast, surgical treatment of the obstructed testis is usually successful in bringing the testis into the scrotum.

About 3% of full-term male infants have at least one cryptorchid testis at birth. Completion of descent usually occurs during the first few weeks after birth, so that the incidence of cryptorchidism at 6 to 9 mo and in adult men is around 0.7 to 0.8%. In individual cases accurate diagnosis and classification require careful and, usually, repeated observations by a single observer; the factor most likely to lead to inaccurate diagnosis is retraction of a normally (or partially) descended testis into the groin. The concept that spontaneous descent can occur after a few months of age is a misconception that arose because of the failure to recognize that many normal testes are retractile in young boys. Indeed, in normal boys the testis spends much of its time in the superficial inguinal pouch, and elicitation of the cremasteric reflex can cause retraction of fully descended testes in about three fourths of boys. The frequency of retraction declines with age and rarely occurs after midpuberty.

It is important to appreciate that a testis in the superficial inguinal pouch may be a temporarily retracted normal testis, a temporarily retracted high scrotal testis, a transiently palpable canalicular testis, or an obstructed testis and that differentiation among these possibilities is not always simple.

Pathogenesis. The etiology of testicular maldescent is not well understood. As stated earlier, the cryptorchid testis functions poorly in regard to both androgen secretion and spermatogenesis, but it is not clear whether the testis functions poorly because of maldescent or fails to descend completely because it is abnormal to begin with. Discordance of testicular descent in identical twins suggests that ordinary cryptorchidism is not genetic in origin,[339] but maldescent of the testis occurs with increased frequency in more than 40 human congenital defects.[340] Such conditions include virtually all disorders that are associated with defective virilization, including hypogonadotropic hypogonadism, hereditary defects in androgen synthesis or action (a relation that supports a role for androgen in normal descent), and dis-

orders that prevent development of normal intra-abdominal pressure. In most of the congenital disorders, the relation between the defect and the failure of descent is not clear, but in some instances a clear relation exists between maldescent and malfunction of the testis. In the obstructed testis, in which a physical barrier prevents descent,[339] and in syndromes in which intra-abdominal pressure is inadequate because the abdominal muscles are absent or incomplete, such as the prune belly syndrome,[19] inadequate testicular function in later life is the consequence of impeded descent. On the other hand, in all series of patients with cryptorchidism some testes appear to have been abnormal from the first, and it is reasonable to assume that the defect in these instances plays a causal role in the maldescent.[341] Indirect evidence of several types suggests that malfunction usually precedes maldescent (reviewed in ref. 26). In one series of 29 patients with a retractile testis, assessment of the number of spermatogonia per seminiferous tubule as a marker for testicular dysgenesis suggested that an abnormality was present in more than half of cases of the retractile testis.[342]

Sequelae. About 10% of testicular tumors arise in an undescended testis, whereas cryptorchidism is present in less than 1% of adult men.[339] Thus the undescended testis is more likely to develop malignancy than a fully descended one. The greatest risk of malignancy is associated with the intra-abdominal testis. Such tumors commonly involve the germinal elements and do not differ markedly in character or course from other germ cell tumors. As in tumors arising in normally descended testes, seminomas are most common, followed by embryonal cell carcinomas.[339] Surgical correction of the cryptorchidism does not remove this risk, because malignancy may develop in a previously cryptorchid testis many years after apparently successful orchiopexy.[343] Moreover, the contralateral normal scrotal testis is the site of development of malignancy in approximately a fifth of tumors associated with unilateral cryptorchidism.[344] The frequency of malignancy in cryptorchid testes should not be exaggerated. The chance of tumor development in any individual subject with cryptorchidism is low, but lifelong follow-up is required. Each cryptorchid testis should be surgically placed in a site that allows ready examination, and if this is not possible the cryptorchid testis should be removed. Periodic examination of the testes should be a mandatory part of routine care of men with a history of cryptorchidism.[339]

In the dog[345] and the rat[346] the surgical placement of a previously descended testis into the abdomen causes a profound decrease in testosterone secretion. Likewise, androgen production declines with time in testicular feminization patients who have long-standing bilateral cryptorchidism.[143] However, in unilateral cryptorchidism, regardless of whether surgical correction has been undertaken, overall androgen production and levels are generally normal, presumably because malfunction of one testis can be compensated for by the descended testis.[347] Thus plasma testosterone and LH values are normal in adult men who had successful orchiopexy as children.[347]

Cryptorchidism is associated with defective spermatogenesis.[348, 349] Furthermore, spermatogenesis may be decreased in the normally descended testis in subjects in whom one testis is cryptorchid. For example, mean sperm density is lower in adult men after surgical repair of cryptorchid testes in childhood,[347–349] and the number of spermatogonia is less in the tubules of the undescended testis.[339] Furthermore, when unilateral vasectomy is performed on the normal side in subjects who previously had surgical correction for unilateral cryptorchidism, azoospermia frequently develops, which indicates failure of spermatogenesis in the previously cryptorchid testis.[350] Basal FSH levels and FSH responsiveness to LHRH are higher on average in such men.[347] Considered together, these types of evidence support the concept that testicular malfunction, as evidenced by impaired spermatogenesis, is fundamental to maldescent.

Additional sequelae of cryptorchidism include an increased susceptibility of the cryptorchid testis to undergo torsion, particularly after puberty,[339] and an increased incidence of herniation of intra-abdominal contents through the opening of the processus vaginalis.[339]

Neonatal Life

It is not clear whether abnormality in the neonatal surge in testosterone secretion results in pathological consequences in humans. However, as mentioned earlier, temporary inhibition of the pituitary-testicular axis in the neonatal primate is associated with impaired testicular function at puberty.[258]

Puberty

The central issue in dealing with disorders of puberty in both sexes is separating subjects with true absence or precocity of pubertal development from those at the extreme limits of normal variation. Normal puberty in the male is variable in onset, duration, and sequence of events. The spectrum of normal puberty and the disorders of sexual precocity in boys are discussed in detail in Chapter 22. (Feminizing states in prepubertal and pubertal boys can result from either absolute or relative increases in estrogen levels and are discussed in Chapter 15.) Delayed or deficient puberty in boys is also discussed in Chapter 22, but partial impairments of male sexual maturation may not be recognized until adulthood; such delayed diagnosis is common for the Klinefelter syndrome (also see Chapter 14), for some androgen resistance syndromes in phenotypic men (also see Chapter 14), and for isolated gonadotropin deficiency in men (also see Chapter 22).

Adulthood

Adult abnormalities of testicular function can be due to hypothalamic-pituitary defects, testicular disorders, or abnormalities in sperm transport (Table 13–4). Most such abnormalities are manifested by both underandrogenization and infertility, but some exhibit isolated infertility. Defective Leydig cell function usually causes infertility because spermatogenesis depends on normal androgen formation and action. Even partial decreases in testosterone production can cause infertility. Therefore, although the evaluation of the infertile man differs from that of the man who also has evidence of underandrogenization, it is essential to exclude the presence of subtle Leydig cell dysfunction in every man with infertility. Certain factors or conditions, such as hyperprolactinemia, radiation, cyclophosphamide, environmental toxins, autoimmunity, paraplegia, and androgen resistance, can cause either isolated infertility or a combined defect in testicular function (see Table 13–4).

INFERTILITY WITH UNDERANDROGENIZATION. Hypothalamic-Pituitary Disorders. Disorders of the hypothalamus and pituitary can impair secretion of gonadotropins and consequently cause decreased androgen production and defective spermatogenesis, either as an isolated defect or as part of more complex pituitary insufficiency (see Chapter 6). Thus destructive lesions of the pituitary such as infarction, pituitary macroadenomas, metastatic or suprasellar tumors, infections, or granulomatous processes can result in *panhypopituitarism* and lead to a secondary testicular defect.

TABLE 13–4. Adult Abnormalities of Testicular Function

Type of Defect	Infertility with Underandrogenization	Infertility with Normal Virilization
Hypothalamic-pituitary	Isolated gonadotropin deficiency	Isolated FSH deficiency
	Cushing syndrome	Congenital adrenal hyperplasia
	Hyperprolactinemia	Hyperprolactinemia
	Hemochromatosis	Androgen administration
Testicular	Panhypopituitarism	
	Developmental and structural defects	Developmental and structural defects
	Klinefelter syndrome	Germinal cell aplasia
	XX male syndrome	Cryptorchidism
		Varicocele
		Immotile cilia syndrome
		Other structural defects
	Acquired defects	Acquired defects
	Viral orchitis	Mycoplasmal infection
	Trauma	
	Radiation	Radiation
	Drugs (e.g., spironolactone, alcohol, ketoconazole, cyclophosphamide)	Drugs (e.g., cyclophosphamide, sulfasalazine)
	Environmental toxins	Environmental toxins
	Autoimmunity	Autoimmunity
	Granulomatous disease	
	Defects associated with systemic diseases	Defects associated with systemic diseases
	Liver disease	Febrile illness
	Renal failure	Celiac disease
	Sickle cell disease	
	Neurological disease (myotonic dystrophy, paraplegia)	Neurological disease (paraplegia)
	Androgen resistance	Androgen resistance
Sperm transport		Obstruction of epididymis or of vas deferens (cystic fibrosis, diethylstilbestrol exposure)

Primary *isolated gonadotropin deficiency* (the Kallmann syndrome) occurs in both sporadic and familial forms. The incidence of the disorder has not been established, but in most centers it is second only to the Klinefelter syndrome as a cause of hypogonadism in men. The disorder was originally described by Kallmann as a familial syndrome associated with anosmia.[351] The term *Kallmann syndrome* is now used to refer to both the sporadic and familial forms with and without anosmia, although the syndrome encompasses more than one entity.

Affected individuals can sometimes be identified in childhood because of the presence of microphallus and/or cryptorchidism.[352-355] Male urethral development is usually complete. Because major growth of the penis occurs during the later two thirds of gestation, the presence of microphallus in this disorder has been interpreted as evidence for a role of pituitary gonadotropin in regulating testosterone production only during the later portion of gestation. The growth pattern in childhood is normal, although bone age is usually retarded.

Most affected individuals are ascertained because of a failure to undergo puberty.[356] A subset of subjects, particularly familial cases, has associated congenital defects, commonly anomalies involving the midline facial and head structures, and partial deficiencies of other pituitary hormones.[357, 358] At the opposite end of the spectrum, less severely affected subjects have only partial defects in production of FSH, or LH, or both. This variant, which was originally known as the fertile eunuch syndrome, is even harder to separate from delayed puberty than is the typical disorder.[359-362] Isolated gonadotropin deficiency, of both sporadic and familial types, is less common in women than in men but is usually manifested as primary amenorrhea and sexual infantilism associated with disturbances of smell.[363-365]

The pattern of inheritance in most families is compatible either with X-linkage or with autosomal transmission with primary manifestations in males.[351, 366, 367] More than one mutant gene may be responsible for the phenotype because certain familial cases that are associated with midline abnormalities appear to be due to an autosomal recessive mutation.[357] Half or more of patients have a negative family history, which suggests that new mutations may be common. The underlying defect is at the hypothalamic level; after short-term administration of LHRH, plasma LH and FSH levels increase in about half of subjects.[368-371] After repetitive treatment for 5 d or longer, plasma gonadotropin levels rise to the normal range in most Kallmann subjects but not in individuals with panhypopituitarism.[318, 372, 373] The more severe the deficiency, the longer LHRH has to be administered to restore gonadotropin secretion.[374]

Crowley and colleagues have established that the disorder encompasses defects in the pulsatile release of LHRH, including total absence of LH secretion; defects in the amplitude and frequency of LH secretion; and altered bioactivity of the gonadotropin released.[375] Consequently, it is most appropriate to view the disorder as a spectrum of defects of LH secretion that includes the typical Kallmann syndrome, the fertile eunuch, and even less severe defects. The common defect probably involves neurogenic control mechanisms that regulate LHRH release.[376]

In the presence of olfactory disturbances, other midline defects, and/or positive family history, the diagnosis is not difficult to establish either in an infant with microphallus or an undervirilized adult. In patients with anosmia or hyposmia, defects of the rhinencephalon may be demonstrated by magnetic resonance imaging.[377] In older subjects without midline abnormalities or anosmia and with uninformative family histories, the diagnosis can be made, after the presence of a pituitary tumor is excluded, by documenting a normal acute response to LHRH administration after a week of LHRH treatment. This technique is rarely done in practice. The separation in the middle teen years of individuals with hypogonadotropic hypogonadism from those with delayed puberty may require prolonged observation (see Chapter 22).

Three forms of therapy can be used: androgen replacement to virilize, gonadotropin therapy to induce fertility, and administration of LHRH analogues to replace the deficit in the most physiological way possible. In the infant or the young child with microphallus, the administration of testosterone for limited periods (3 mo) may cause enlargement of the penis to the normal range without affecting linear growth or causing other significant virilizing signs.[260, 378] In the older child or the adult, long-acting testosterone esters are administered parenterally, as for other forms of hypogonadism.[274] Also, as in other forms of androgen deficiency, the nearer the time of onset of normal puberty that replacement therapy is begun, the more effective the promotion of normal virilization. Administration of hCG over the long term also causes serum testosterone levels to increase to normal adult male levels,[379-381] but in subjects with severe (prepubertal) hypogonadotropic hypogonadism the induction of fertility usually requires the administration of FSH in the form of human menopausal gonadotropin, in addition to administration of hCG.[382] The response to gonadotropin therapy in this disorder is not influenced by prior testosterone therapy[383] but is a function of the initial testis size, men with testes less than 4 mL in volume responding less favorably.[384] After a normal sperm count is achieved, it may be maintained by use of either hCG or, occasionally, testosterone esters.[385] In occasional patients with partial defects in gonadotropin secretion, spermatogenesis can be promoted by testosterone therapy alone.[386] The long-term administration of LHRH in a pulsatile manner to men with hypogonadotropic hypogonadism results in the achievement of normal plasma testosterone levels, normal pulsatile secretion of LH, normal mean levels of plasma LH and FSH, and, in most, mature sperm in the ejaculate.[387, 388] After the induction of spermatogenesis by such treatment, normal spermatogenesis in one study was maintained by nasal administration of LHRH.[389]

Acquired gonadotropin deficiency can be caused by factors other than pathological conditions of the hypothalamus or pituitary. For example, elevated plasma cortisol levels, as in *Cushing syndrome*, can depress LH secretion independent of a space-occupying lesion of the pituitary.[390-392] The serum LH level in these men, as in other forms of secondary testicular dysfunction, is usually in the normal range and only occasionally decreased. However, it is inappropriately low for the depressed serum testosterone level. Even when Cushing syndrome is associated with a pituitary adenoma, i.e., Cushing disease, the hypogonadotropic hypogonadism appears to be secondary to the hypercortisolism, because treatment by bilateral adrenalectomy or mitotane results in return of testosterone levels to normal.[390-391] Chronic administration of exogenous glucocorticoids can also lower testosterone levels by inhibiting LHRH secretion.[392]

Hyperprolactinemia is also a cause of secondary testicular dysfunction. Hyperprolactinemia can be produced by either microadenomas or macroadenomas of the pituitary. Macroadenomas may give rise to hyperprolactinemia either because of direct secretion by the tumor (prolactinomas) or because of interference with the delivery of normal inhibitory influences from the hypothalamus to the pituitary by the mass effect of a nonsecretory tumor. Hypogonadism can result from hyperprolactinemia itself, from diminished gonadotropin secretion because of destruction of the normal pituitary, or from a combination of these effects. Prolactin excess by itself can cause both underandrogenization and infertility and lead to impotence.[393-395] It probably causes hypogonadism by impairing LHRH release. Most men with prolactinomas respond to an injection of LHRH with a normal increase in plasma LH level.[393-395] Some patients with microadenomas respond to low doses of bromocriptine with an initial increase in plasma LH level followed by an increase in serum testosterone level.[396] Impotence that is associated with hyperprolactinemia is not always the consequence of a decreased serum testosterone level. Some hyperprolactinemic men who are given testosterone replacement do not have return of potency until the prolactin levels are corrected by the administration of bromocriptine.[395] In part because of delays in seeking evaluation, men with prolactin-secreting pituitary adenomas usually have macroadenomas at the time of diagnosis.[393-395] When a macroadenoma is present it is critical to document that deficiencies of other pituitary hormones do not coexist with the hyperprolactinemia (see Chapter 6). After surgery for macroadenomas the plasma prolactin level does not usually return to normal,[397] but it may respond to administration of bromocriptine.[398]

Idiopathic *hemochromatosis* causes iron deposition in the pituitary and testes,[399] and about half of affected men have hypogonadism, usually accompanied by testicular atrophy. The abnormalities of testicular function in this disorder may in part result from the associated liver disease,[399] but most testicular dysfunction is due to hypogonadotropic hypogonadism.[400-404] The pituitary nature of the hypogonadism was recognized because of the lack of response of LH to LHRH stimulation[401, 403, 404] and the normal response of plasma testosterone to hCG.[403, 404] However, occasional men with hemochromatosis have an elevated LH level associated with low testosterone levels, which suggests that primary testicular abnormality may also occur.[402] Acquired transfusional iron overload can cause similar abnormalities of the pituitary-testicular axis.[405] The hypogonadism that is secondary to hemochromatosis can be corrected by iron depletion therapy in some men.[406]

In several other conditions the testosterone levels may be decreased in association with normal LH levels, and the mechanism is less clear. Men with massive obesity have decreased TeBG levels and decreased levels of total and bioavailable testosterone that return toward normal with weight loss.[407] Obesity may be part of the mechanism for decreased testosterone levels in the subset of such men with pickwickian syndrome.[408] Some men with seizures of temporal lobe origin also have hormonal findings that are consistent with hypogonadotropic hypogonadism.[409] Finally, hypogonadotropic hypogonadism may occur as an apparently acquired idiopathic disorder.[410, 411]

Testicular Disorders. Abnormalities of testicular function in the adult can be grouped into several categories: developmental and structural defects of the testes, acquired testicular defects, abnormalities associated with systemic or neurological diseases, and androgen resistance.

Developmental and Structural Defects. The most common developmental defect of the testis is the *Klinefelter syndrome* (see also Chapter 14). The disorder is characterized by small, firm testes; various degrees of impaired sexual maturation; azoospermia; gynecomastia; and elevated gonadotropin levels.[412] The underlying defect is the presence of an extra X chromosome,[413-415] the common chromosomal karyotype being either 47,XXY (the classic form) or 46,XY/47,XXY (the mosaic form). The incidence is approximately 1 in 500 males.[416]

Prepubertal subjects with the Klinefelter syndrome have small testes with a decreased number of spermatogonia but are otherwise normal.[417] The diagnosis is usually made after the time of expected puberty, when the disorder is manifested by gynecomastia and/or underandrogenization, and later by infertility (Table 13–5). Damage to the seminiferous tubules and azoospermia are consistent features of the 47,XXY variety. The small, firm testes are characteristically less than 2.0 cm long and always less than 3.5 cm long (corresponding to 2 and 12 mL in volume, respectively).[418, 419] Typical histological changes in the testes include hyalinization of the tubules, absence of spermatogenesis, and apparent increase in the number of Leydig cells[420] (see Fig. 13–19C).

The increased mean body height in the disorder is the result of a longer lower body segment, a feature that is present before puberty.[421] The occurrence of this feature before puberty suggests that it is not secondary to androgen deficiency but is probably related to the underlying chromosomal abnormality. Gynecomastia occurs in about 85% of subjects;[413] it ordinarily appears during adolescence, is generally bilateral and painless, and may become disfiguring.[413] Obesity and varicose veins occur in a third to a half of subjects,[422] and mild mental deficiency and/or social maladjustment,[423, 424] subtle abnormalities of thyroid function, diabetes mellitus,[417] and restrictive pulmonary disease[426] are more common than in the general population. The risk of breast cancer is 20 times that of normal men, although the incidence is only about a fifth of that for women.[427, 428] Most individuals have a male psychosexual orientation and function sexually as men.

46,XY/47,XXY mosaicism is the cause of about 10% of cases of Klinefelter syndrome, as estimated by chromosomal karyotypes of peripheral blood leukocytes. The true prevalence may be underestimated, because chromosomal mosaicism can be present in the testes in subjects in whom the chromosomal karyotype of peripheral leukocytes is normal.[413, 414] As summarized in Table 13–5, the clinical manifestations of the mosaic form are usually less severe than are those of the 47,XXY variety, and the testes may be normal in size.[414] The endocrine abnormalities are also less severe, and gynecomastia and azoospermia are less common. Indeed, occasional patients with the mosaic form may be fertile.[429] In some individuals the diagnosis may not be suspected because of the minor degree of the associated abnormalities.

Approximately 30 additional karyotypic varieties of the Klinefelter syndrome have been described, including those with uniform cell lines (such as 48,XXYY, 48,XXXY, and 49,XXXXY) and a number of mosaicisms of the X chromosome with or without associated structural abnormalities of the X chromosome. 48,XXYY individuals have a more severe degree of mental retardation and antisocial behavior,[430] and 49,XXXXY individuals may have cryptorchidism and bone abnormalities.[431]

The 47,XXY form of Klinefelter syndrome is due to meiotic nondisjunction of the chromosomes during gametogenesis. About 40% of the responsible meiotic nondisjunctions occur in the father and 60% occur in the mother. Advanced maternal age is a predisposing factor in the latter cases.[432] The mosaic form of the disorder, in contrast, results from chromosomal mitotic nondisjunction after fertilization of the zygote and can arise either in a 46,XY zygote or a 47,XXY zygote. The latter situation (double nondisjunction, meiotic and mitotic) may be the usual cause of the mosaic form and thus explain why the mosaic form is less common than the 47,XXY disorder.[433]

Characteristic endocrine changes include elevation of plasma FSH and LH levels. FSH shows the best discrimination, and little overlap occurs with normal individuals, a consequence of the consistent damage to the seminiferous tubules.[415] In the late teen years the plasma testosterone concentration may be normal.[434, 435] By the middle 20s the plasma testosterone level averages half the normal value, but the range of values is broad and overlaps the normal range.[413, 415, 434, 435] Mean plasma estradiol levels are elevated,[436] and TeBG levels are about twice normal.[437] The reasons for the elevated plasma estradiol level (and the development of gynecomastia) are complex. In adolescence the plasma testosterone level is kept in the normal range at the expense of an elevated plasma LH value, and estradiol secretion by the testes is increased. As testicular function becomes more impaired, testicular secretion of both testosterone and estradiol decreases. Eventually, estrogen formation is almost exclusively derived from extraglandular aromatization of

TABLE 13–5. Characteristics of Patients with Classic Versus Mosaic Klinefelter Syndrome*

Characteristic	47,XXY (%)	46,XY/47,XXY (%)
Abnormal testicular histology	100	94†
Decreased length of testis	99	73†
Azoospermia	93	50†
Decreased testosterone level	79	33
Decreased facial hair	77	64
Increased gonadotropin level	75	33†
Decreased sexual function	68	56
Gynecomastia	55	33†
Decreased axillary hair	49	46
Decreased length of penis	41	21

*Table based on 519 47,XXY patients and 51 46,XY/47,XXY patients.
†Significantly different at p < .05 or better.
Data from Gordon DL, Krmpotic E, Thomas W, et al. Pathologic testicular findings in Klinefelter's syndrome. 47,XXY vs. 46,XY-47,XXY. Arch Intern Med 1972; 130:720–729.

adrenal androgen; at this point estrogen formation, although low, is high relative to that of testosterone. The net result both early and late is a variable degree of feminization and insufficient androgenization. This feminization, including the development of gynecomastia, is though to depend on the ratio of circulating estrogen to androgen (see Chapter 14). The lower the plasma testosterone and the higher the plasma estradiol levels, the more likely the development of gynecomastia. After the age of expected puberty the increase in plasma gonadotropin level after the administration of LHRH is exaggerated,[438] and the normal feedback inhibition of testosterone on pituitary LH secretion is diminished.[439] Older patients with untreated Klinefelter syndrome may have an enlarged or an abnormal sella turcica, presumably secondary to the persistent lack of gonadal steroid feedback and hyperplasia of gonadotropes.[440] It is not known whether adenoma formation takes place.

No method is available for reversing the infertility, and mastectomy is the only satisfactory treatment for gynecomastia. Some underandrogenized patients benefit from supplemental androgen,[422, 441] but such treatment may paradoxically worsen the gynecomastia, presumably by providing increased androgen substrate for the conversion to estrogens in the peripheral tissues. Androgen should be administered in the form of injections of testosterone cypionate or testosterone enanthate. After the administration of testosterone the plasma LH level returns to normal but usually only after several months.[439]

The *XX male syndrome* is a variant of the Klinefelter syndrome. The incidence of a 46,XX karyotype in phenotypic males is approximately 1 in 20,000 to 1 in 24,000 male births.[442] More than 150 XX males have been described.[443] The findings resemble those in the Klinefelter syndrome: the testes are small and firm, generally less than 2 cm long; gynecomastia is usual; the penis is normal to small in size; and azoospermia and hyalinization of the seminiferous tubules are present. Affected individuals have male psychosexual identification and an absence of female internal genitalia. The mean plasma testosterone concentration is low, whereas concentrations of plasma estradiol and gonadotropins are high.[444, 445] Affected individuals differ from typical Klinefelter patients in that the average height is less than that of normal men,[437] the incidence of mental deficiency is not increased,[437] and hypospadias is common.[446]

Four theories have been proposed to explain the pathogenesis of this disorder: (1) mosaicism in some tissues for a Y chromosome–containing cell line or early loss of a Y chromosome; (2) an autosomal gene mutation; (3) interchange of a Y chromosomal gene with the X chromosome; (4) deletion or inactivation of X chromosomal genes that normally suppress testis development.[438] Mosaicism has not been documented, and no clear-cut evidence has been adduced for an autosomal gene mutation. Forty-nine of 86 XX males whose DNA was probed with Y chromosome DNA fragments containing the testis-determining factor did have Y-related DNA.[447–450] Thus the majority of XX males appear to have the Y-linked testis-determining factor, and in this group the etiology is presumably analogous to that in the Sxr mouse, in which a critical fragment of the Y chromosome has been translocated to the X chromosome.[451] The management of XX males is similar to that described for patients with the Klinefelter syndrome.

Acquired Defects. The most common cause of acquired testicular failure in the adult is *viral orchitis*.[452] Mumps virus is most frequently responsible, although other agents act in a similar fashion, including echovirus, lymphocytic choriomeningitis virus, and group B arboviruses.[453] The orchitis is due to actual invasion of the tissue by the virus rather than to indirect effects of infection.[454] Orchitis is a common

complication of mumps; it occurs in as many as a fourth of adult men with the disease.[455] In about two thirds of cases it is unilateral. It usually develops within a few days of the onset of parotitis but occasionally precedes it. During acute orchitis the plasma LH and FSH levels are elevated, and the plasma testosterone level is decreased.[455] After the acute inflammatory phase the testis gradually decreases in size, although in some instances the swelling may persist for months. The testis may return to normal size and function or may undergo atrophy. Atrophy is due both to the direct effect of the virus on the seminiferous tubules and to ischemia that is secondary to pressure and edema within the taut tunica albuginea. The histological appearance of the atrophic testis includes progressive tubular sclerosis and hyalinization; the histological appearance is sometimes not dissimilar to that in the Klinefelter syndrome. Even when only one testis is involved clinically, degenerative changes may be seen in the other. The degree of atrophy is not necessarily proportional to the severity of the orchitis. It is usually apparent within 1 to 6 mo after the orchitis subsides, but the full extent of the damage may not be evident until 10 y later. Atrophy occurs in approximately one third of men who develop orchitis, and it is bilateral in about a tenth.[452] The hormonal changes that are associated with gynecomastia after mumps orchitis include a normal rate of extraglandular estrogen formation from adrenal androgens but a profound decrease in the production rate of testosterone.[456] The frequency with which mumps results in infertility is not known.[457] Almost half of men with unilateral mumps orchitis have sperm densities of less than 10 million/mL in the first 3 mo, but within 1 to 2 y the semen analysis returns to normal in about three fourths.[458] In contrast, semen parameters eventually return to normal in less than a third of men with bilateral orchitis.[458] The initial treatment of mumps orchitis is bed rest and scrotal support. If severe pain is present, the administration of prednisone often results in prompt defervescence and reduction of testicular swelling and pain.[459] Glucocorticoid therapy does not appear to have a significant beneficial effect on the subsequent return of the sperm count to normal.[458]

Trauma is second to viral orchitis as a cause of testicular atrophy in the adult. The exposed position of the testis in the scrotum renders it uniquely susceptible to both thermal and physical damage.

Both spermatogenesis and testosterone production are sensitive to *radiation*; the diminished secretion of testosterone appears to be a consequence of diminished testicular blood flow.[460] Although doses of radiation as low as 0.2 Gy (20 rad) result in temporary increases of both LH and FSH levels and damage to spermatogonia, a permanent decrease in testosterone production is uncommon.[461] However, a tenth of patients receiving approximately 8 Gy (800 rad) of scattered radiation to the testes during childhood[462] and most boys receiving 24 to 30 Gy (2400 to 3000 rad) of direct testicular radiation for acute lymphoblastic leukemia[463] have permanently low plasma testosterone levels. (Also see the later section on infertility with normal virilization.)

Drugs can cause underandrogenization and infertility in several ways: direct inhibition of testosterone synthesis, blockade of the peripheral actions of androgen, and enhancement of estrogen levels. Certain drugs have multiple effects. In addition, agents such as propranolol and guanethidine that affect the sympathetic nervous system can impair erectile function in men whose hypothalamic-pituitary-testicular axis is normal.[464]

Two drugs that in high doses block testosterone synthesis are spironolactone and cyproterone, both of which interfere with the late reactions in testosterone biosynthesis.[465, 466] Spironolactone appears to impair 17α-hydroxylase and

17,20-desmolase activities.[465] Plasma testosterone levels do not change appreciably, however, during usual therapeutic regimens.[465] The antifungal agent ketoconazole blocks testosterone synthesis,[289] also by inhibiting the 17,20-desmolase and the 17α-hydroxylase reactions.[467] The decrease in testosterone after a single dose of ketoconazole is transient, with the nadir occurring 4 to 8 h after administration and returning to baseline by 24 h as ketoconazole concentrations fall. However, with doses of ketoconazole greater than 400 mg/d, depression of plasma testosterone levels may be sustained.[468] The agent also inhibits the cortisol response to ACTH.[468] Tetracycline has been reported to lower testosterone levels about 20% during short-term administration.[469] Impairment of libido is common in men with epilepsy, partly as a consequence of medication.[470, 471] Enzyme-inducing antiepileptic drugs such as phenytoin and carbamazepine lower bioavailable testosterone and raise plasma LH levels. The effect is more pronounced with multiple-drug regimens.[470, 471] Valproic acid does not appear to have as severe an adverse effect in this regard.[471]

Independent of its effects on the liver, ethanol ingestion reduces testosterone levels both acutely and chronically.[472] This action is the result of inhibition of testosterone synthesis, as demonstrated both in vivo and in vitro.[473–477] In men without liver disease who are given 40% of food intake as alcohol, a 25 to 50% decrease in the plasma testosterone levels and in the testosterone production rate is demonstrable within 5 d after starting this regimen, and these effects last for as long as 3 wk.[473] In alcohol-fed rats, the decrease in plasma testosterone level is accompanied by testicular atrophy and decreased weight of androgen target tissues such as the prostate.[474] Smaller amounts of ethanol decrease only the testicular response to gonadotropin.[475] The inhibition of steroidogenesis appears to occur at the 3β-hydroxysteroid dehydrogenase reaction, as the result of a decrease in the concentration and/or availability of the pyridine nucleotide cofactors for the reaction,[476] probably mediated by the ethanol metabolite acetaldehyde.[477] The fact that the lower testosterone levels in most men given alcohol are not accompanied by appropriate elevations of plasma LH suggests that hypothalamic-pituitary function is also impaired.[472, 473] Ethanol may also interfere with the capacitation of sperm[478] and cause an increased number of morphological abnormalities in epididymal sperm.[479]

Antineoplastic and chemotherapeutic agents, especially cyclophosphamide, commonly induce infertility (see later). Combination chemotherapy for acute leukemia, Hodgkin disease, and other malignancies may also impair Leydig cell function.[480–482] In pubertal boys this effect is manifested by decreased serum testosterone levels, elevated plasma LH level, and marked gynecomastia.[480, 481] In adult men the testosterone levels do not decline, and the impaired Leydig cell function is detectable only by an exaggerated LH response to LHRH stimulation.[482] This toxic effect on the Leydig cell seems to be produced primarily by alkylating agents such as cyclophosphamide, because pubertal boys who are given other regimens for acute lymphoblastic leukemia do not develop dysfunction of Leydig cells or seminiferous tubules.[483] Treatment with alkylating agents during the prepubertal years does not interfere with testicular function in later life.[480]

Plasma testosterone levels may be low in men taking large amounts of marihuana, heroin, or methadone.[484–486] In general, elevations of plasma LH do not occur, which suggests a hypothalamic-pituitary abnormality as well as a testicular defect. Studies of the effects of marihuana on the pituitary-testicular axis in animals also suggest a dual inhibition.[487–489] Testosterone synthesis by mouse testes in vitro is reduced more than 80% by addition of the marihuana component tetrahydrocannabinol,[487] and plasma LH levels in mice decline after administration of a single oral dose of tetrahydrocannabinol.[488] In addition, marihuana may have a direct inhibitory effect on sperm motility.[490]

Elevated plasma estradiol levels and decreased plasma testosterone levels may occur in men taking digitalis preparations, the mechanism of the effect being unclear.[491] Drugs can interfere with gonadotropin production either as the result of a direct inhibition[492, 493] (as in medroxyprogesterone acetate administration) or as a secondary consequence of enhanced prolactin secretion.[494] Medroxyprogesterone acetate also seems to decrease testosterone secretion at the testicular level.[495]

Several drugs inhibit androgen action by competition at the receptor level. Although spironolactone can inhibit testosterone synthesis, in the usual dosage regimens it acts primarily by antagonizing androgen binding to the androgen receptor, which leads to gynecomastia and impotence.[465] Cyproterone also acts as an androgen antagonist.[466] The most commonly administered drug that is an androgen antagonist is cimetidine,[496–498] which binds to androgen receptors in vitro.[497] Gynecomastia can occur in men who are treated with the drug, and decreased sperm density and elevated basal testosterone levels are accompanied by a slight diminution of the LH response to LHRH.[496] Ranitidine appears to be a less potent antiandrogen.[498]

Prolonged exposure of men to lead as an *environmental toxin* appears to result in direct testicular toxicity, with an impaired pituitary response as indicated by a slight plasma LH elevation.[499] Similar hormonal changes have been documented in an animal model of lead toxicity.[500]

Testicular failure can occur as part of a generalized *autoimmune* disorder in which multiple primary endocrine deficiencies coexist and in which circulating antibodies to the basement membrane of the testes can be documented[501, 502] (see Chapter 31).

The testis can also be a site of involvement in *granulomatous disease*. Testicular atrophy occurs in 10 to 20% of men with lepromatous leprosy, as the result of direct invasion of the tissue (and in some instances the paratesticular structures as well) by the bacilli. The tubules are involved initially, followed by endarteritis and destruction of Leydig cells. The result is a decreased plasma testosterone level and elevated plasma LH and FSH levels.[503] Destruction of the testis is less common in other types of systemic granulomatous disease.

Defects Associated with Systemic Diseases. Abnormalities of the hypothalamic-pituitary-testicular axis occur in a number of systemic diseases. Given the chronic ill health and generalized wasting that may occur with these disorders, it is often difficult to distinguish effects specifically caused by the underlying condition (e.g., renal failure) from those attributable to malnutrition.

About half of men with *renal failure* who are undergoing dialysis experience decreased libido and impotence,[504] complaints that are associated with impairments in both spermatogenesis and testosterone biosynthesis. The defect in spermatogenesis varies from partial to total destruction of the germ cell population.[505, 506] The plasma testosterone level is decreased, and plasma LH and FSH levels are increased, which indicates a defect at the testicular level.[506–508] Plasma testosterone production rates are decreased,[507] and the response of plasma testosterone to hCG is subnormal.[506, 509] In Leydig cells that are isolated from uremic rats, impaired responsiveness to hCG correlates with a diminished number of LH/hCG receptors. The addition of cAMP, however, does not completely repair the defect in testosterone synthesis, which suggests an impairment distal to cAMP production as well.[510] After dialysis, plasma testosterone levels and testosterone production rates improve but usually not to the normal range.[506, 507, 509, 510] The etiology of the testicular abnormalities in renal failure is not well understood. Zinc deficiency may be a contributing factor. Uremic men have abnormal zinc metabolism and may be zinc deficient in spite of dialysis.[511] In one study oral zinc therapy led to a return of plasma testosterone level to normal, with a lowering of LH and FSH levels and an improvement in libido and potency.[512] Another potential mechanism for the testicular abnormalities in renal failure is estrogen excess. Androgen-estrogen dynamics have not been examined in detail, but the low testosterone levels coupled with normal or increased plasma estrogen levels[513] probably account for the development of gynecomastia in about half of men undergoing chronic hemodialysis. Hyperprolactinemia occurs in a fourth of men having long-term dialysis,[514] and treatment with bromocriptine to lower prolactin levels may raise testosterone levels and restore potency in some individuals.[515] There does not appear to be much difference in most parameters of testicular function before dialysis compared with men undergoing maintenance hemodialysis.[506] By contrast, successful renal transplantation is associated with a return of testosterone and prolactin levels to normal and a slight decrease in LH and FSH levels.[516, 517] Most men experience improved sexual function after transplantation, and half have sperm densities of more than 10 million/mL.[516]

The effects of *cirrhosis of the liver* on testicular function occur independent of the direct toxic effects of ethanol. Gynecomastia and testicular atrophy are present in half of men with cirrhosis, and three fourths of men with hepatic cirrhosis are impotent.[518] Histological evidence of decreased spermatogenesis and peritubular fibrosis are present in about half. The plasma estradiol level is usually elevated, and the plasma testosterone level is decreased.[518, 519] The net result is a ratio in serum of unbound estradiol to unbound testosterone of about 10 times normal.[519] Levels of the binding capacity of TeBG are about twice normal. The metabolic clearance rate and the production rate of testosterone are both decreased, and estradiol production is increased.[518] Extraglandular conversion of androgens, primarily adrenal androgens, to estradiol and estrone is increased about threefold, presumably because of decreased hepatic extraction of androgens.[520] Basal plasma levels of LH and FSH range from normal to moderately elevated.[518, 521] Dynamic testing of the pituitary-testicular axis in men with cirrhosis suggests a defect at the level of the testis. The response of plasma testosterone to hCG stimulation is diminished.[518, 521] The increase in plasma LH after the administration of LHRH is normal in most men with cirrhosis. In those with testicular atrophy, however, the response of plasma FSH is enhanced; the degree of LH responsiveness correlates inversely with the incremental response of testosterone to hCG.[522] Thus modest elevation of basal LH and FSH levels, coupled with the lack of hyper-responsiveness to LHRH, suggests that the hypothalamic-pituitary response to the diminished testosterone levels is blunted. The reason for impairment of testosterone production and of the hypothalamic-pituitary response is uncertain. Elevated estrogen levels could cause both defects. Basal prolactin levels are elevated on average fourfold in men with cirrhosis,[523] and the increased prolactin could also have an effect on the pituitary-testicular axis.

The reversibility of the gonadal changes in cirrhosis cannot be assessed as in renal failure. Testosterone therapy has been tried.[524] Although estradiol levels increased (in direct correlation with the severity of the cirrhosis) after administration of testosterone enanthate, the estrogen/androgen ratio became normal.[524] Whether such therapy is beneficial in the long term is not known, but treatment of 24 cirrhotic men for 4 wk did not cause worsening of gynecomastia or of liver function test results.[525] Men with alcoholic cirrhosis may have spontaneous recovery of sexual function when they abstain from alcohol, despite the persistence of liver abnormalities.[526] However, men with alcoholic cirrhosis and testicular atrophy are less likely to experience improvement in sexual function with abstinence from alcohol.[526]

Boys with *sickle cell anemia* have impaired skeletal and sexual maturation in adolescence.[527–529] Furthermore, in 32 adult men with sickle cell anemia, secondary sexual characteristics were abnormal in all but 2, and testicular atrophy was noted in about a third.[528] Testicular biopsy results for two men revealed maturation arrest of spermatogenesis. The defect may be either testicular[528] or hypothalamic.[529]

Abnormalities in Leydig cell function, which are frequently accompanied by decreased sperm counts, occur in a variety of chronic systemic diseases including *protein-calorie malnutrition*,[530] advanced *Hodgkin disease* and *cancer* before chemotherapy,[531, 532] *cystic fibrosis*,[533] and *amyloidosis*.[534] Except for amyloidosis, in which the abnormalities seem to be limited to the testis, all of these disorders cause a lowered plasma testosterone level coupled with normal to increased plasma LH level, which suggests combined hypothalamic-pituitary and testicular defects. The low plasma testosterone level is not the result of inhibitors that interfere with the binding to TeBG and hence is not analogous to the euthyroid sick syndrome.[535] Indeed, because the mean plasma TeBG is elevated, the decrease in available testosterone may be even greater than that indicated by the total level.[536] The above-mentioned pattern of changes in testosterone and LH may be nonspecific effects of illness, because similar changes in plasma testosterone and LH levels occur after *surgery*,[537, 538] *myocardial infarction*,[539] and severe *burns*.[540, 541]

The changes in the hypothalamic-pituitary-testicular axis in *thyrotoxicosis* may be secondary to increased estrogen levels. These changes may include decreased total sperm counts and semen volumes, increased plasma total testosterone values, and normal levels of unbound testosterone.[542] The testosterone response to hCG is blunted, in association with an increased basal LH value.[542]

Neurological disease can cause testicular abnormalities. Men with myotonic dystrophy usually have small testes, low plasma testosterone levels, and elevated plasma LH and FSH levels.[543–545] Although the effects are variable, depending on the exact nature of the defect, spinal cord lesions that result in quadriplegia or paraplegia initially cause diminished plasma testosterone levels that generally return toward normal, but defective spermatogenesis appears to persist.[546, 547] Some patients retain the capacity to obtain erections and ejaculate, depending on the extent of injury to the lumbosacral spinal cord.[548]

Men with trisomy-21 have impairment of both germinal and Leydig cell functions. Plasma FSH and LH levels are elevated.[549]

Androgen Resistance. A limited form of androgen resistance results in underandrogenization and infertility in men who have normal development of the external genitalia.[550] Some men from a family with Reifenstein syndrome were noticed to have gynecomastia and infertility without the usual hypospadias but associated with the same abnormality in the androgen receptor as more severely affected members of the same family.[181] Subsequently, men with a negative family history and apparently idiopathic infertility were found to have androgen resistance, as characterized by increased testosterone production, elevations of plasma LH levels in some, and abnormal androgen receptors in cultured genital skin fibroblasts.[550] Only one of the initial three men had gynecomastia, and underandrogenization was not present in the other two. Subsequently, in a study of unselected men with idiopathic infertility, 40% of those with idiopathic azoospermia had androgen receptor deficiency.[551] The presence of elevated testosterone and/or LH levels is not a reliable predictor of which men have a receptor defect. Testicular biopsy results for five affected men showed maturation arrests or germinal cell aplasia similar to that shown in Figure 13–19D and E.[551] An even less severe manifestation of androgen resistance related to an androgen receptor defect has been observed in men who have gynecomastia and undervirilization associated with fertility in some affected family members.[552, 533]

INFERTILITY WITH NORMAL VIRILIZATION. Some conditions lead to isolated infertility, and thus a separate group of diagnoses should be considered in the evaluation of infertile men with normal Leydig cell function. Isolated infertility can be due to defects in the hypothalamic-pituitary system, the testis, or the sperm transport system (see Table 13–4).

Hypothalamic-Pituitary Disorders. Isolated FSH deficiency has been reported in men in whom virilization, plasma LH levels, and plasma testosterone levels were normal but the plasma FSH level was persistently low.[554] Plasma FSH levels in such men increase after LHRH stimulation.[554] *Hyperprolactinemia* occasionally leads to infertility alone but more commonly also causes impotence and low testosterone levels (see earlier). In occasional patients with infertility as the sole manifestation of hyperprolactinemia, treatment with bromocriptine results in return of the sperm count to normal, in association with suppression of the hyperprolactinemia.[555] In some men with chronic untreated or undertreated *congenital adrenal hyperplasia* related to 21-hydroxylase deficiency, gonadotropin secretion is suppressed as the result of overproduction of adrenal androgens, and infertility is a consequence.[556] This diagnosis is suggested by the presence of small testes, normal to elevated levels of testosterone, and suppressed levels of gonadotropins. Diagnosis is confirmed by finding markedly elevated plasma levels of 17-hydroxyprogesterone and androstenedione[556] (see Chapters 9 and 20).

When testosterone esters, the usual form of replacement androgen, are administered intramuscularly in pharmacological doses to normal men, gonadotropins are suppressed, and about half of men develop azoospermia (see Chapter 17). Although men who present with isolated infertility are unlikely to be receiving testosterone replacement therapy, the use of *androgens* by weight-lifters and body-builders is common. Self-prescribed regimens may include parenteral testosterone esters, as well as a variety of oral and parenteral substituted androgens often termed anabolic steroids (see later). Anabolic steroids can cause reversible azoospermia in normal men.[557]

Testicular Disorders. **Developmental and Structural Defects.** *Germinal cell aplasia* is a poorly understood defect of the testis (the Sertoli cell–only syndrome). This term may encompass histological findings that can result from several etiologies. In some instances the disorder appears to be a familial syndrome related to a single gene defect. Other patients with the typical histological and clinical features have a history of viral orchitis, cryptorchidism,[558, 559] or androgen resistance.[551] The distinguishing characteristic of the testicular biopsy is complete absence of germinal elements (see Fig. 13–19E). The usual clinical findings include azoospermia in association with normal virilization, absence of gynecomastia, normal to small testes, and normal chromosomal complement. Plasma testosterone and LH values are usually normal, and plasma FSH values are high.[560] This disorder (or histological entity) apparently accounts for a tenth to a third of men with azoospermia.[559, 561]

More often the testicular biopsy of infertile men reveals either severe hypospermatogenesis or a maturation arrest, commonly at the spermatid stage, with or without sloughing of the epithelium (see Fig. 13–19F). Such a histological picture may result from several causes, including subtle abnormalities of chromosomes such as translocations or mosaicisms that affect the testis selectively.[561–563] In addition, familial male infertility with this histological pattern has been reported.[564, 565] In one family the inheritance pattern suggested X-linkage,[564] whereas in many other families parental consanguinity suggested an autosomal recessive transmission.[565] In both familial and sporadic cases, meiosis is defective because of desynapsis, lack of chiasmata, and degeneration of spermatocytes. The majority of the men with defective meiosis do not have a positive family history,[565] and in most cases the cause of this type of infertility is unknown. A variety of single-gene defects are known to influence spermatogenesis in experimental animals, and such mechanisms could operate more commonly in the human than is now recognized.[566]

Unilateral *cryptorchidism*, even when corrected before puberty, is associated with abnormal semen in many individuals (see earlier). This finding suggests that the testicular abnormality is bilateral even in unilateral cryptorchidism.

Varicocele is believed by some to be the most common treatable cause of male infertility; it may be of etiological importance in as many as a third of infertile men.[567] Varicocele is caused by retrograde flow of blood into the internal spermatic vein that eventuates in a progressive, often palpable, dilatation of the peritesticular pampiniform plexus of veins. It is thought to result from incompetence of the valve between the internal spermatic vein and the renal vein and is more common (85%) on the left (reviewed in ref. 568). The incidence of varicocele is about 10 to 15% in the general population and 20 to 40% in men with infertility. The findings on semen analysis are usually nonspecific. Decreased sperm density is often seen with medium or large varicoceles.[569, 570]

The mechanism by which varicocele leads to infertility is an enigma.[568] Clearly, not all men with varicocele are infertile, and the majority do not have any detectable abnormality of the hypothalamic-pituitary-testicular axis. The occurrence of infertility with unilateral varicocele might result from anastomoses of the venous system between the two testes, but extensive anastomoses have not been demonstrated convincingly in humans.[568] The leading theory for the adverse effect of varicocele is that it leads to an increased scrotal temperature. However, two studies have found that scrotal temperatures of infertile men are higher than those of fertile men regardless of the presence of detectable varicocele.[571, 572] Presumably an increased scrotal (and testicular) temperature would result in poor-quality semen and infertility. Studies of the effects of surgically induced unilateral varicocele in rats and dogs support the concept of obstructed venous return leading to increased testicular blood flow and increased temperature bilaterally.[573]

The preferred surgical treatment of varicocele is high spermatic vein ligation at the level of the inguinal canal. On average, semen quality improves in patients who have had varicoceles repaired. However, the effect of surgical repair on subsequent fertility is not clear. The pregnancy rate after varicocele repair is probably less than 50%. One large retrospective, uncontrolled study of almost 1000 men reported an association between subsequent fertility and preoperative sperm density.[574] Patients who had preoperative sperm densities of more than 10 million/mL (about 40% of the men in this study) had a 70% pregnancy rate after repair.[574]

The *immotile cilia syndrome* is a hereditary disorder that is characterized by immotility or poor motility of the cilia in the airways and either immotile or poorly motile spermatozoa.[210] In most instances the disorder is inherited as an autosomal recessive trait. The immotile cilia in the airways result in chronic sinusitis and bronchiectasis, and the immotile sperm cannot fertilize. Kartagener syndrome is a subcategory of the immotile cilia syndrome that is associated with situs inversus. The structural abnormality leading to impaired motility of cilia can usually be defined by electron microscopy of sperm. The specific defects known to cause the syndrome include missing or abnormally short dynein arms, short spokes with no central sheath, missing central microtubules, and displacement of one of the nine microtubule doublets (see Fig. 13–16). Cilia from epithelia and sperm tails from the same individual usually exhibit the same defects. Other less-well-understood mutations can apparently lead to immotile sperm without involvement of cilia in the lung.[575] In evaluating sperm for structural abnormalities, care should be taken to examine a number of axonemes and to confirm the structural defect, because variations in axonenemal structure occur frequently in normal functional respiratory cilia and sperm.[327] Treatment is symptomatic and is directed at the complications in the respiratory tract. There is no treatment for the infertility.

Acquired Defects. Acquired testicular causes of isolated infertility include mycoplasma infection, radiation, drugs, environmental toxins, and autoimmunity. A role for *mycoplasma (Ureaplasma urealyticum)* in infertility has been long suspected; mycoplasmal infection occurs with increased frequency in women whose infertility is associated with a "male factor," which suggests that genital tract mycoplasmal infection may cause male infertility.[576] Furthermore, when the infection is successfully eradicated the pregnancy rate is increased.[577] However, the presence of mycoplasmal infection in the male cannot be correlated with any specific alteration in sperm density or morphology.[577]

Radiation can cause isolated infertility. Spermatogonia are exquisitely sensitive to radiation, damage being demonstrable after only 0.15 Gy (15 rad).[461] With doses higher than 1.0 Gy (100 rad), extreme oligospermia or azoospermia develops. Higher doses also damage spermatids and cause more rapid decreases in sperm counts. Recovery occurs in a dose-dependent fashion. Return to preirradiation sperm densities requires 9 to 18 mo after doses of 1 Gy (100 rad) or less, 30 mo for doses of 2 to 3 Gy (200 to 300 rad), and 5 y or more for doses of 4 to 6 Gy (400 to 600 rad).[578] Fractionated radiation may have a more profound effect on the testes than single-dose radiation.[579] In a study of 27 men with variable radiation exposure to testes from scatter radiation that was associated with treatment of soft tissue sarcoma, the testicular dose varied from 0.01 to 25 Gy (1 to 2500 rad). There was a dose-dependent increase in serum FSH levels after radiation, with the maximal change at 6 mo. Only patients receiving less than 0.5 Gy (50 rad) showed complete recovery 12 mo after radiation therapy. Patients receiving greater than 2 Gy (200 rad) had significant elevations in plasma LH as well as FSH levels, and the testosterone value did not change.[579] Permanent infertility may occur after radiation treatment of malignant lymphoma of the abdomen in spite of shielding.[580] Men who are given radioactive iodine for treatment of thyroid cancer may also have impairment of spermatogenesis and elevation of plasma FSH levels. The threshold for this effect appears to be a cumulative ^{131}I dose of more than 3.7×10^3 mBq (100 mCi); recovery occurs in about 2 y.[581]

The principal *drugs* that cause isolated infertility are alkylating agents, especially cyclophosphamide. The primary histopathological lesion that is produced by the drugs studied to date is depletion of the germinal epithelium.[582] Spermatocytes and spermatogonia may disappear completely, resulting in germinal cell aplasia with only Sertoli cells lining the tubular lumen. The serum FSH level rises about fivefold in men with absent germinal epithelium and serves as a marker for germ cell loss. The serum LH and testosterone levels usually remain within normal limits in the presence of germinal cell depletion. However, in men who were treated in childhood with cyclophosphamide for nephrotic syndrome[583] and men who were treated as adults with combination chemotherapy for Hodgkin disease,[584] the serum LH level was elevated in those with severe damage to the germinal epithelium. Additional chemotherapeutic agents are associated with testicular germ cell depletion. Reversible oligospermia occurs in men receiving up to 400 mg of chlorambucil, and azoospermia and germinal aplasia may occur with cumulative doses in excess of 400 mg. Similarly, germinal aplasia is less common in patients receiving less than 6 to 10 g of cyclophosphamide. Cessation of cyclophosphamide therapy is followed by return of spermatogenesis within 3 y in about half of patients who develop azoospermia during therapy.[585] Vinblastine, doxorubicin, procarbazine, and cisplatin have all been implicated as being toxic to the germinal epithelium of animals and humans, although specific dose-toxicity relationships have not been established.

Combination-drug regimens have an even more profound impact on spermatogenesis. The combination of mechlorethamine HCl, vincristine, procarbazine, and prednisone (MOPP) causes azoospermia, germinal aplasia, testicular atrophy, and elevated FSH levels in more than 80% of men.[481, 582] Some alternative combination chemotherapy regimens for advanced Hodgkin disease may be less toxic to the germinal epithelium. The combination of doxorubicin (Adriamycin), bleomycin, vinblastine, and dacarbazine results in azoospermia only one third as often, and apparently spermatogenesis nearly always recovers in these patients.[586] Chemotherapy-induced azoospermia that follows treatment with vinblastine, bleomycin, and cisplatin for testicular cancer is usually reversible within 2 y of stopping treatment.[587] Sulfasalazine therapy may also cause infertility associated with oligospermia.[588]

Because of the potential toxic effects of many physical and chemical agents on spermatogenesis, the occupational and recreational history should be carefully evaluated in all men with infertility. Known *environmental toxins* include chemicals such as the nematocide dibromochloropropane and related compounds,[589, 590] cadmium,[591] lead,[592] microwaves,[593] and ultrasound.[594]

Although *autoimmunity* may cause combined underandrogenization and infertility, it usually results in isolated infertility. Antibodies to the basement membrane of the seminiferous tubules[595] or, more commonly, to the sperm themselves may cause a significant fraction of male infertility.[596] There is no correlation between the presence of sperm-associated antibodies and specific abnormalities in the semen analysis.[597] Not all men with antisperm antibodies are infertile, and a decrease in antibody titers is not always associated with improved fertility. Thus the exact role of antisperm antibodies in infertility is uncertain. Although immunosuppression of men with antisperm antibodies by administration of prednisone is reported to improve fertility,[598] such treatment remains investigational. The occurrence of antisperm antibodies is not always a primary phenomenon, because they have been identified in men with ductal obstruction that is either bilateral[599] or unilateral,[600] as well as after vasectomy.[601]

Defects Associated with Systemic Disease. Infertility alone may also occur in association with systemic diseases. Perhaps the most common alteration of seminiferous tubule function is the temporary decrease in semen quality, partic ularly decreased sperm density, that often follows an *acute febrile illness*. This is one of the reasons that several semen analyses must be obtained for men with suspected infertility to be confident that true basal parameters have been determined (see earlier). Men with *celiac disease* appear to have a distinct pattern of testicular dysfunction, namely, the hormonal pattern is typical of androgen resistance with elevated plasma testosterone and LH levels on average.[602–604] However, a control group of men with regional enteritis did not demonstrate this hormonal pattern, which suggests that gluten enteropathy may induce a reversible androgen resistance–like state.[602–604] As discussed earlier, the neurological disorder that results in isolated infertility is *spinal cord injury*.[546, 547]

Androgen Resistance. Androgen resistance may cause infertility without underandrogenization and may be the cause in as many as 20% of men with apparent idiopathic azoospermia (see earlier).[557, 605]

Impairment of Sperm Transport. Disorders of sperm transport may lead to infertility in as many as 6% of infertile men.[567] The abnormality may be unilateral or bilateral, congenital or acquired. In men with unilateral obstruction of sperm transport, the infertility may result from antisperm antibodies.[600] Obstructive azoospermia at the level of the epididymis also occurs in association with chronic infections of the paranasal sinuses and lungs.[606] Tuberculosis, leprosy, and gonorrhea are rare causes of acquired obstruction of the wolffian duct–derived structures. Acquired bilateral obstruction of sperm transport has also been reported in men with deep midline *müllerian duct cysts*.[607] Congenital defects of the vas deferens that result in azoospermia or oligospermia may occur as an isolated abnormality associated with the absence of seminal vesicles,[608] in patients with *cystic fibrosis*,[609] or as a portion of a more extensive anatomical disorder in sons of women who were given *diethylstilbestrol* during pregnancy.[610] Magnetic resonance imaging may be useful for visualizing the seminal vesicles in the evaluation of obstructive azoospermia.[611] In one study of the success of surgical therapy for suspected obstructive azoospermia, obstruction of the epididymis was more common than absence or obstruction of the vas deferens.[612] Vasoepididymostomy resulted in sperm densities of more than 10 million/mL in almost half and pregnancy for a fifth. Pregnancy was more likely in the absence of antisperm antibodies.[612]

Idiopathic Infertility. The preceding discussion of conditions that are associated with male infertility does not account for the problem in many men. When large series of consecutive patients are analyzed for the presence of known causal factors or associated conditions, approximately 40% of such men are classified as having *idiopathic infertility* (Table 13–6).[567, 613] Because at best only about half of the almost 40% of infertile men with a varicocele might achieve fertility after varicocele repair, it is probably more appropriate to consider that 60% of infertile men have idiopathic infertility. The actual causes of the infertility in men with a presumed idiopathic disorder are no doubt heterogeneous. Some may have androgen resistance (see earlier). Others have oligospermia or azoospermia with normal plasma LH and testosterone levels but an elevated FSH level in the absence of cryptorchidism, radiation, or drug exposure. Studies of small groups of such men indicate that the isolated FSH elevation may be associated with a decreased LHRH pulse frequency[614] and that pulsatile LHRH administration to such men may lower FSH levels.[615, 616] Whether these abnormalities are of etiological significance is not known. Another group has observed a decreased testosterone production rate in selected infertile men with isolated FSH elevations whose total serum testosterone value was within the normal range.[617]

MANAGEMENT OF INFERTILITY. The management of

TABLE 13–6. Relative Frequency of Causes and Associated Conditions in Men Who Present with Infertility

Cause or Condition	% in Study of Greenberg et al.[567] (n = 425)	% in Study of Baker et al.[613] (n = 1041)
Hypogonadotropic hypogonadism	0.9	0.6
Klinefelter syndrome	1.6	1.9
Cryptorchidism	6.1	6.4
Varicocele	37.4	40.3
Immotile sperm	0.5	0.6
Viral orchitis	1.9	1.6
Radiation/chemotherapy	—	0.5
Obstruction of epididymis or of vas deferens	6.1	4.1
Androgen resistance	—	0.1
Coital disorders	4.0	0.5
Idiopathic disorders	41.5*	43.4†

*Includes miscellaneous semen abnormalities, 10.2%, and undiagnosed primary testicular failure, 5.9%.

†Includes possible obstruction, 4.5%.

male infertility is usually unsatisfactory. Causal factors and conditions that are not amenable to therapy include azoospermia related to Klinefelter syndrome, idiopathic germinal cell aplasia, viral orchitis, trauma, radiation, androgen resistance, and totally immotile or dead sperm. However, there are also a number of potentially correctable causes of male infertility. Associated hormonal disorders and coexisting medical conditions may be treated, and offending drugs may be discontinued in appropriate circumstances. Men with hypogonadotropic hypogonadism may be given gonadotropins or LHRH (see later).

Men with infertility who do not have a specifically identifiable etiological factor and/or have a varicocele as an incidental associated condition may be considered candidates for empirical therapy. Although claims of success for several empirical therapies of infertile men with oligospermia have been made, most of these reports fail to take into account the spontaneous fertility rate in untreated men (25% in 1 y).[326] Treatment-independent pregnancy among infertile couples occurs in all forms of human infertility (male and female factors), and the possibility of its occurrence makes it necessary for all therapies to be evaluated by randomized clinical trials.[618] When several different forms of empirical therapy, including testosterone rebound, nonaromatizable androgen (mesterolone), gonadotropin, antiestrogen (clomiphene), antibiotics, bromocriptine, varicocele repair, artificial insemination, and no therapy, were evaluated and compared in one large clinical retrospective analysis of oligospermic men, no improvement in the relative pregnancy rate was demonstrated for any empirical therapy compared with no therapy.[619]

In view of the lack of efficacy of usual empirical therapy, appropriate infertile couples should be advised to consider artificial insemination with the man's semen by using newer intrauterine techniques[620] or in vitro fertilization[621] or to consider artificial insemination with donor semen (see Chapter 12). The couple may be counseled with respect to adoption or childlessness while they wait to see if fertility occurs spontaneously. Artificial insemination with donor semen has a 70% overall success rate in 1 y. Because female fertility declines with increasing age, a delay in the decision to attempt artificial insemination with donor semen may reduce the likelihood of success.

The emerging role of in vitro fertilization in management of male infertility deserves further comment. Although in vitro fertilization is less successful when poor-quality semen is used, fertility has been achieved for men with fewer than 0.5 million/mL motile sperm. Most forms of male infertility that are associated with nonspecific semen abnormalities appear amenable to therapy with in vitro fertilization; seminal inflammatory cells and low progressive motility seem to impair fertilization the most. The collection of split ejaculates and the careful preparation of the spermatozoa are important for increasing the chance of fertilization. In expert hands the pregnancy rate per treatment cycle after in vitro fertilization in couples in whom the woman is normal and the man has subnormal semen is similar to that for couples in whom in vitro fertilization is performed because of tubal disorders in women.[621]

Old Age

The decrease in total and bioavailable testosterone and the increase in estradiol that may occur in normal elderly men probably have no direct consequences for male sexual function. However, indirect evidence suggests that this changing hormonal milieu may be involved in the pathogenesis of breast enlargement in elderly men (see Chapter 14) and in the development of prostatic hyperplasia.

PROSTATIC HYPERPLASIA. Enlargement of the prostate to the extent that it produces obstruction to urethral outflow is common in elderly men.[622] The gland weighs only a few grams at birth; at puberty it undergoes androgen-mediated growth and reaches the adult size of approximately 20 g by age 20. This maturation is accompanied by transformation of the cuboidal epithelium of the acinar units of the gland to a columnar, secretory epithelium and initiation of the secretion of one component of the ejaculate. The weight and histological features of the gland remain stable for about 25 y. Commencing in the fifth decade of life, a second growth spurt occurs in the majority of men. This second growth phase, unlike the earlier growth that involves the gland diffusely, typically begins in the periurethral region as a localized proliferation involving both glandular and stromal elements. This hyperplasia may remain limited in scope, but in many men the growth continues and eventually compresses the remaining normal portion of the prostate. The progressive increase in gland size causes development of urinary tract obstruction and may cause constipation as well. Indeed, some men develop hyperplasia primarily of the periurethral region and hence experience obstruction to urine outflow in the absence of gross prostatic enlargement.

The second growth spurt, like the growth at puberty, requires a functioning testis. Dihydrotestosterone that is formed from testosterone within the prostate is the androgen that mediates the embryonic development, the pubertal growth, and the hyperplastic growth of the prostate.[623, 624] The administration to animals of an inhibitor of dihydrotestosterone formation causes involution of the gland in the face of an elevated concentration of prostatic testosterone.[625–627] Furthermore, although the plasma testosterone level declines with age, the level of dihydrotestosterone in the hyperplastic gland either remains constant or increases.[628–630]

The dog is the major species other than the human in which prostatic hyperplasia develops, and most research work on the pathogenesis of the disorder has been done in that species. The administration to the castrated dog of androgens that cause an increase in the prostatic dihydrotestosterone concentration results in prostatic enlargement that is comparable to that seen in naturally occurring canine prostatic hyperplasia.[631] Estrogen acts synergistically with dihydrotestosterone to enhance prostatic growth in the dog,[631, 632] and this interaction appears to be due to the fact that estrogen increases the amount of androgen receptor in the tissue.[141] Thus two hormones participate in the development of prostatic hyperplasia in the dog: dihydrotestosterone is responsible for prostate growth, and estradiol enhances the action of dihydrotestosterone. Whether this model applies to the endocrine role in the pathogenesis of the human disorder is unknown. The fact that estradiol levels increase with age in men[140] in the face of declining production of androgens fits with the concept that estrogen may play a role in human prostatic hyperplasia, and the fact that inhibitors of testosterone synthesis in men with prostatic hyperplasia cause a decrease in prostatic size[633, 634] indicates that continuing testosterone availability is necessary to maintain the hyperplastic state. Direct testing of the role of dihydrotestosterone formation in prostatic hyperplasia in men is now possible with the use of inhibitors of 5α-reductase.[635]

Documentation of a hormonal role in prostatic hyperplasia does not necessarily provide insight into its pathogenesis. Androgens may be involved only in a permissive sense rather than acting as true initiators of the hyperplasia, and the reason that the disorder is limited to only a few species is unclear. Even so, the possibility exists that pharmacological alteration of dihydrotestosterone levels in the gland may provide a medical means of treating the disorder in patients who are poor surgical risks.[633–637] At present the treatment is surgical.[622]

PROSTATIC CANCER. The endocrine aspects of prostatic cancer are discussed in Chapter 33.

Disorders of All Ages

TESTICULAR TUMORS. Tumors of the testes occur with an incidence of 2 to 3 per 100,000 men per year in the United States and account for about 1% of cancer deaths in men.[638–640] These tumors are the second most common malignancy (after leukemia) in men between ages 20 and 35. The frequency shows a trimodal curve, with peaks in childhood (embryonal carcinomas and teratocarcinomas), young adulthood, and old age (seminomas). The tumors are commonly bilateral (either simultaneous or sequential, e.g., a seminoma developing in one testis many years after the removal of another).[641] The incidence in black persons is a sixth or less of that in white. Reports of familial occurrence are numerous, including occasional concordance in monozygotic twins.

Several factors predispose individuals to testicular tumor development. Men with cryptorchidism have a fivefold increased risk of developing testicular tumors, intra-abdominal testes being more at risk than high inguinal testes.[642] In one series, however, only 10 of 131 men with testicular cancer had antecedent maldescent.[643] Three fourths of tumors that are associated with maldescent are seminomas, the remainder being other germ cell tumors. The effectiveness of orchiopexy in reducing the risk of developing tumors is not established, which suggests that some underlying testicular disorder may predispose individuals to both maldescent and tumor development. The incidence of gonadal malignancy may be higher in testes of patients with abnormal sexual development (i.e., 45,X/46,XY mixed gonadal dysgenesis or testicular feminization) than in patients with other forms of testicular maldescent.[644–647] Estrogen administration to pregnant women may also predispose male offspring to development of testicular tumors,[643] and men with the Klinefelter syndrome may have a higher incidence of germ cell tumors.[648]

The relation between congenital adrenal hyperplasia related to steroid 21-hydroxylase deficiency and testicular tumors is complex; most testicular tumors that occur in patients with this disorder consist of adrenal cell rests, are dependent on ACTH for growth and secretion, and develop in patients who are inadequately treated and hence have incomplete suppression of plasma ACTH concentrations.[649, 650] However, on histological grounds the tumors are difficult to separate from interstitial cell tumors.[651]

Diagnosis. Most testicular cancers produce symptoms related to the testes, but significant delay in making a diagnosis is common because of delays on the part of both physicians and patients. Most testicular cancers occur in men under age 45, and men should be educated about the need to seek prompt medical advice for any change in a previously normal testis, including the development of a mass, a feeling of heaviness, pain, swelling, or other unusual findings. To reduce delay, physicians should consider any testicular mass to be a tumor until proved otherwise. Pain occurs in half of men with testicular neoplasms and thus does not rule out cancer. If testicular symptoms or signs do not promptly regress, a surgical consultation should be obtained.[652]

Classification. The most widely used classification is that of Mostofi[653] (Table 13–7). This classification is based on the cell type from which the tumor originates, i.e., germ cells (spermatogonia), stromal cells (Leydig and Sertoli cells), and adnexal cells at the site of attachment of the testis and epididymis.

Germ cell tumors are the most common and are presumed to be derived from primordial germ cells. *Seminomas* are characterized by large cells with clear cytoplasm in a delicate fibrovascular stroma infiltrated with lymphocytes; the granulomatous reaction around the tumor can be so intense as to suggest the presence of a graft-versus-host reaction.[654] These tumors account for at least half of all testicular neoplasms and can be subdivided into spermatocytic and anaplastic varieties. Spermatocytic seminomas in older men are associated with a 90 to 95% 5-y survival, whereas the anaplastic type has a poor prognosis. *Embryonal carcinomas* are the most frequent testicular tumors in children, resemble embryonal carcinomas of the ovary, and have 5-y survivals of around 70% in infants and 25% in adults. *Choriocarcinomas* contain syncytiotrophoblastic cells and occur most commonly in the second and third decades of life; prognosis is poor. *Teratomas* contain at least two germ cell layers and may be either benign or malignant; they are second in frequency to embryonal carcinomas in childhood but occur as only a tenth of adult tumors. Tumors that contain combinations of germ cell types account for 40% of germ cell tumors; the biology of such tumors is usually determined by the least differentiated (most malignant) element. Of the *mixed tumors* that contain cells of germinal and stromal origin, perhaps the most distinctive is the *gonadoblastoma*, which consists of germ cells, sex cords, and, usually, Leydig cells. Gonadoblastomas commonly originate from dysgenetic testes containing a Y chromosome, and most synthesize androgen.[655]

Germ cell tumors of all types can originate in extragonadal sites as well as in the testes, most commonly the mediastinum[656–660] or the brain.[661–665] These extragonadal tumors are presumed to arise either from aberrant migration of germ cells early in embryogenesis or, alternatively, from some common precursor stem cell line that normally gives rise to germ cells and to cells of the thymus and the pineal.[5]

The usual presentation of a testicular germ cell tumor is a nodule or painless swelling of the testis. Occasionally the tumors are ascertained as the result of metastases or because of the peripheral manifestations of hCG secretion by the tumor. After the tumors are diagnosed, staging is performed either by surgical exploration or by computed tomographic scanning or magnetic resonance imaging. Stage I is limited to the testes, stage II involves metastases to infradiaphragmatic lymph nodes but not beyond, stage III involves supradiaphragmatic lymph nodes, and stage IV involves extralymphatic metastases.

Germinomas may secrete several distinct tumor cell markers into plasma, of which the most important is hCG, both because of its value as an indicator of relapse and because of its endocrine effects. Normal testes synthesize hCG but in such small amounts that only trace quantities reach the circulation.[666] However, hCG (or more commonly the beta chain of hCG) is secreted into the circulation in large amounts by some nonseminoma germ cell tumors (a third of teratocarcinomas and yolk sac tumors and all choriocarcinomas).[667, 668] Tumors containing yolk sac elements may also produce α-fetoprotein, and teratomas on occasion secrete carcinoembryonic antigen.[669–675] An elevated level of one of these tumor markers in plasma of a patient whose tumor has been classified as a pure seminoma usually indicates that the tumor is actually a combination tumor. These markers are particularly useful for following the response to therapy.[665, 676, 677] The secreted hCG may be endocrinologically active and cause enhanced formation of testosterone and, more importantly, of estradiol by the testes. The net result can be a feminizing syndrome, with consequent inhibition of the secretion of LH and FSH by the pituitary[678] (also see Chapter 14).

The treatment of germ cell tumors constitutes a major triumph of cancer therapy. Appropriate therapeutic strategies include debulking of the tumor mass, resection of involved lymph nodes, administration of chemotherapy (usually combinations of cisplatin, vinblastine, etoposide, and bleomycin), radiation, and the monitoring of tumor cell markers.[640, 665, 679–683] The surgical cure rates for patients with seminomas approximate 90% for stage I disease, and subjects with stage III nonseminoma tumors, which were previously uniformly lethal, now have good survival rates.[684] Because young men with germ cell tumors commonly develop infertility caused by castration, radiation, and/or chemotherapy, cryopreservation of semen before treatment has been advocated as a means of preserving fertility.[685]

Stromal tumors account for only 1 to 2% of testicular tumors. Such malignancies usually involve Leydig or Sertoli cells, and both cell types may coexist within the same tumor. Rarely, adrenal rest tumors may occur in the testes.[686] As would be expected, interstitial cell tumors commonly secrete testosterone and thus may cause virilization in prepubertal boys (precocious pseudopuberty). Leydig cell tumors are usually benign in character. Approximately a fourth of these tumors secrete estradiol as well as testosterone and thus cause mixed signs of feminization and virilization during the prepubertal years and feminizing signs in adult men. Endocrinologically active tumors cause suppression of endogenous gonadotropins, azoospermia, and decreased size of the contralateral testis. Because the tumors may be small and sometimes can be recognized only by ultrasonography, documenting that the testis is the site of increased estrogen production by selective catheterization of the testicular veins can be useful. After removal of the involved testis, gyneco-

TABLE 13–7. Classification of Testicular Tumors

    I. Germ cell tumors (95%)
       A. Single-cell–type tumors (60%)
          Seminomas
          Yolk sac tumors (embryonal cell tumors)
          Teratomas
          Choriocarcinoma
       B. Combination tumors (40%)
   II. Tumors of gonadal stroma (1–2%)
          Leydig cell
          Sertoli cell
          Primitive gonadal structures
  III. Gonadoblastomas
          Germ cell + stromal cell

Data from Mostofi FK. Pathology of germ cell tumors of testis: a progress report. Cancer 1980; 45:1735–1754.

mastia regresses, the excessive estradiol levels return to normal, and the sperm count returns to normal.[687]

Sertoli cell tumors show a bimodal age distribution, with most patients being younger than 1 y or between ages 20 and 45. The tumors are frequently bilateral, and gynecomastia occurs in about a fourth of patients. Decreased spermatogenesis and atrophy of the contralateral testis are common in the estrogen-secreting group. Leydig cell hyperplasia can occur in the area around the tumor, which implies either that the tumor is of mixed cell origin or that Sertoli cells secrete some factor or factors involved in stimulating Leydig cell differentiation.[688] The usual course is for complete cure and regression of any feminizing signs after surgical resection. The secretion of estrogen by Sertoli cell tumors, as well as Leydig cell tumors, is consistent with the current view that estrogen synthesis in the normal testis takes place in both cell types.[72] The treatment of these tumors is surgical. Approximately a tenth of stromal tumors are malignant and follow an aggressive course;[687, 688] occasionally such patients respond to mitotane.[686]

In summary, testicular tumors can cause enhanced production of estradiol and testosterone by more than one mechanism. When production of steroid hormones by the tumor is autonomous, plasma gonadotropin levels and androgen secretion by uninvolved portions of the testes are depressed, and azoospermia is common. When hCG is secreted by the tumor, the gonadotropin acts to increase estradiol and testosterone production in unaffected areas of the testes, and azoospermia is uncommon. Furthermore, occasional choriocarcinomas that cannot synthesize steroids de novo nevertheless convert circulating androgens to estrogens. When androgens, or estrogens, or both are formed directly or indirectly by the tumors, the response varies, depending on the pattern of hormones produced and the age of the subject. Some patients are clinically normal, whereas others develop feminization or virilization.

HORMONAL THERAPY

Androgen Therapy

Testosterone administered by mouth is absorbed into the portal blood and is degraded promptly by the liver so that only a small portion reaches the systemic circulation. Parenterally injected testosterone is also rapidly absorbed and degraded so that maintenance of physiological levels in plasma is difficult. As a consequence, effective androgen therapy requires either the administration in a slowly absorbed form of testosterone (dermal patches or a micronized oral preparation) or the administration of chemically modified analogues. Such chemical modifications either retard the rate of absorption or catabolism so as to maintain effective blood levels or enhance the androgenic potency of each molecule so that hormonal effects can be achieved at a lower plasma level of the drug. Three general types of modification of testosterone are clinically useful: esterification of the 17β-hydroxyl group (type A), alkylation at the 17α-position (type B), and modification of the A, B, or C rings, particularly substitutions at the 1, 2, 9, and 11 carbons (type C) (Fig. 13–21). Most agents actually contain combinations of ring structure alterations and either 17α-alkylation or esterification of the 17β-hydroxyl.

Esterification of testosterone with various carboxylic acids decreases the polarity of the steroid, makes it more soluble in the fat vehicles that are used for injection, and hence slows release of the injected steroid into the circulation.[689–691] The esters of 19-nortestosterone appear to have

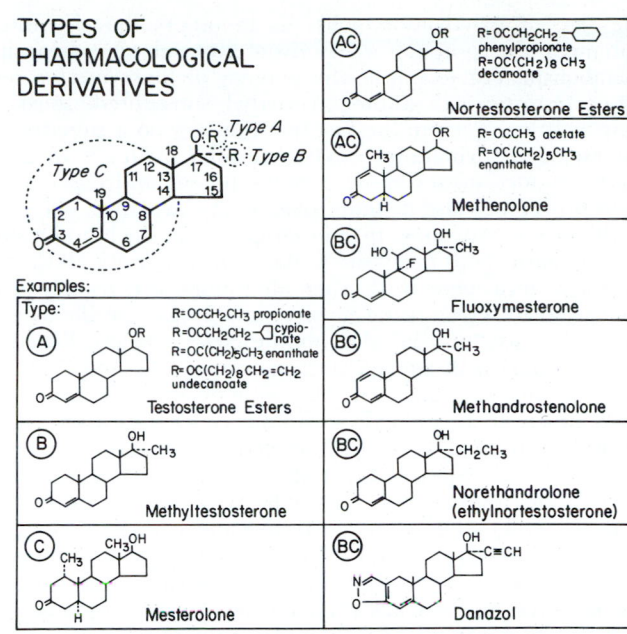

Figure 13–21. Some of the androgen preparations available for clinical use, classified into three types. Type A derivatives are esterified in the 17β-position. Type B steroids have alkyl groups in a 17α-position. Type C derivatives include a variety of additional alterations of ring structure that enhance activity, impede catabolism, or influence both functions. Most androgen preparations involve combinations of type AC or type BC changes.

particularly slow release and turnover.[557] The longer the carbon chain in the ester, the more fat soluble the steroid becomes and hence the more prolonged the action. For example, testosterone cypionate and testosterone enanthate can be administered every 2 or 3 wk, whereas testosterone propionate must be injected daily. Testosterone cypionate or enanthate is the treatment of choice for male hypogonadism.[274, 439, 692–695] Although the esters can be detected in plasma, they must be hydrolyzed before the hormone acts so that effectiveness of therapy can be monitored by assaying the plasma level of testosterone after administration. Most esters cannot be administered by mouth and must be injected. However, two esters—methenolone acetate and testosterone undecanoate—have special features that make administration by mouth possible. Testosterone undecanoate is absorbed via the lymphatic system into the systemic circulation so that physiological blood levels of testosterone can be achieved at doses of approximately 120 mg/d.[696–699] Because of rapid turnover in plasma, however, testosterone undecanoate must be administered twice daily.[700, 701] The reason for the oral effectiveness of methenolone acetate (and of mesterolone) is not entirely clear; the methyl group in the 1 position may slow the rate of hepatic inactivation and allow effective blood levels to be maintained.[702–704]

17α-Alkylated androgens, such as methyltestosterone and methandrostenolone, are effective when given by mouth because alkylated steroids are absorbed into the portal circulation but are slowly catabolized by the liver and reach the systemic circulation in effective amounts. For this reason, 17α-methyl or 17α-ethyl substitution is a common feature of most orally active androgens. Because all 17α-alkylated steroids are believed to act within the cell as such (i.e., the alkyl groups are not removed), because they may cause abnormalities of liver function, and because assays are not routinely available for monitoring blood levels, these steroids have a limited role in medicine.[705, 706]

Other alterations of the ring structure have been adopted empirically; in some instances the effect is to slow the rate of inactivation, whereas in others the alteration enhances the potency of a given molecule or alters its metabolism. For example, the potency of fluoxymesterone, 19-nortestosterone, and/or 1-methyl–substituted steroids may be due in part to the fact that they are poor precursors for estrogen formation in extraglandular tissues.[707] In contrast, 19-nortestosterone is a more potent androgen than testosterone because its more planar ring structure, like that of dihydrotestosterone, fits more tightly into the binding site of the androgen receptor.[708] As is true for 17-alkylated steroids, androgens with ring alterations are usually not converted to testosterone in vivo, and hence specific assays for each must be utilized to monitor blood levels. Because most steroids with altered ring structures also contain 17α-substitutions, they also have the same deleterious effects on liver function as methyltestosterone and thus have little clinical usefulness. One orally effective androgen, mesterolone, is neither esterified nor alkylated in the 17α-position. In addition, the molecule cannot be aromatized to estrogens in peripheral tissues, so that effective androgen replacement can be achieved by oral administration without causing abnormalities of liver function; unfortunately, the steroid has no effective feedback regulation of gonadotropin secretion and consequently is a poor agent for routine androgen replacement therapy.[702–704]

The use of a transdermal therapeutic preparation of testosterone in which a testosterone-loaded film is applied each day to scrotal skin in the form of a patch makes it possible to sustain serum testosterone levels in the normal male range.[709–711] With such preparations the serum testosterone level increases to reach a peak within 2 to 3 h and maintains a level that is 60 to 80% of the peak value throughout the day, thus avoiding the wide swings in serum testosterone values that are characteristic of therapy with parenterally administered testosterone esters.[710] This system therefore offers advantages over other modalities for administering testosterone in that it simultaneously replaces the missing molecule specifically and avoids the necessity for parenteral administration. Such therapy causes a disproportionate increase in plasma dihydrotestosterone to a level that is 30 to 40% that of testosterone, presumably because of the high level of 5α-reductase in scrotal skin.[711–713] Such increases in serum dihydrotestosterone level have also been reported after treatment with the extremely long-acting parenteral testosterone ester testosterone *trans*-4-*n*-butylcyclohexyl-carboxylate[714] and with the oral ester testosterone undecanoate.[715] As long as the total androgen level in serum is maintained within the normal range, dihydrotestosterone acts similarly to testosterone as an effective androgen and does not appear to have any deleterious side effects. Indeed, after the percutaneous administration of therapeutic preparations of dihydrotestosterone itself to men for as long as 3 mo, no change occurred in the ratio of HDL cholesterol to LDL cholesterol and no deleterious side effects were observed.[716, 717]

Other means of administering testosterone have been proposed. After subcutaneous implantation of testosterone-filled Silastic capsules, the hormone is released slowly for long periods into the plasma,[718] but this mode may not be practical in humans because of the large size of such capsules. When oral testosterone in microparticulate form is administered in large amounts (200 to 400 mg/d), physiological blood levels can be achieved, but the preparation has to be taken several times a day.[719–721] Furthermore, this dosage level of hormone induces hepatic drug-metabolizing enzymes, the long-term effects of which are uncertain.[722] Topical administration of testosterone that is suspended in creams appears to be effective insofar as the hormone can be absorbed from skin into the bloodstream and thus act systemically.[723, 724] Administration of testosterone via rectal suppository[725] or nasal drops[726] also results in only short-term elevation of plasma levels. Because of the frequency of administration that is necessary to sustain effective blood levels, none of these other techniques appear to be clinically useful.

ADMINISTRATION OF ANDROGENS TO NORMAL MEN. The administration of testosterone esters to normal men in amounts that are sufficient to replace the normal daily testicular secretion (equivalent to 5 to 10 mg/d) has little physiological effect.[439] When the plasma testosterone level is raised above the normal range, both the basal levels of LH and FSH and the peak response after LHRH administration are diminished. As a consequence the testicular volume is decreased about 20%, sperm production is uniformly decreased by 90% or more, and the volume of the ejaculate remains unchanged.[693, 727–729] The administration of comparable amounts of 17α-alkylated androgens by mouth results in decreases in the plasma testosterone level but similar changes in gonadotropin level and sperm count.[730, 731] These properties of androgens were the basis for trials of the agents as male contraceptives in hopes that sperm production could be effectively inhibited but androgen action maintained. Unfortunately, the inhibition of sperm production is not usually complete (see Chapter 17). When plasma testosterone is increased significantly above control levels, body weight increases about 3% (largely because of an increase in extracellular fluid volume), the hemoglobin level rises by about 10 g/L (1 g/dL), acne is common, and the serum estradiol concentration doubles.[727]

ADMINISTRATION OF ANDROGENS TO HYPOGONADAL MEN. The aim of androgen therapy in hypogonadal men is to restore or bring to normal male secondary sexual characteristics (beard, body hair, external genitalia) and male sexual behavior and to promote normal male somatic development (hemoglobin, voice, muscle mass, nitrogen balance, and epiphyseal closure). Because a reliable assay for plasma testosterone is widely available for monitoring therapy, the treatment of androgen deficiency is straightforward and almost universally successful. The parenteral administration of a long-acting testosterone ester such as 100 to 300 mg of testosterone enanthate at 1- to 3-wk intervals results in a sustained increase in plasma testosterone concentration to the normal male range or slightly above.[274, 439, 692, 693, 732] The usual replacement regimen is 200 mg every 2 wk.[692] Similar effects are obtained with the percutaneous administration of testosterone.[709, 713] In most subjects such regimens reduce the plasma LH level and maintain serum testosterone within the normal range.[692] If the hypogonadism is primary and of long duration (as in the Klinefelter syndrome), suppression of the plasma LH value to the normal range may not occur for many weeks, if at all.[439, 733–736] There is considerable variability in the relation between plasma testosterone and male sexual behavior, but in postpubertal testicular failure, even of many years' duration, resumption of normal sexual activity is usual after adequate replacement.[737, 738] The major effects of androgen appear to be on libido[739] and on the frequency of erections.[740] Androgen therapy does not ordinarily restore spermatogenesis to normal in hypogonadal states, but the volume of the ejaculate, which is derived largely from the prostate and seminal vesicles, and other secondary sexual characteristics return to normal. The somatic effects of endogenous androgen, including effects on hemoglobin, nitrogen balance, and skeletal development, are also reproduced.[277]

In men of all ages in whom hypogonadism develops before expected puberty (such as subjects with hypogonadotropic hypogonadism), it is appropriate to bring plasma testosterone into the adult range slowly. When therapy is

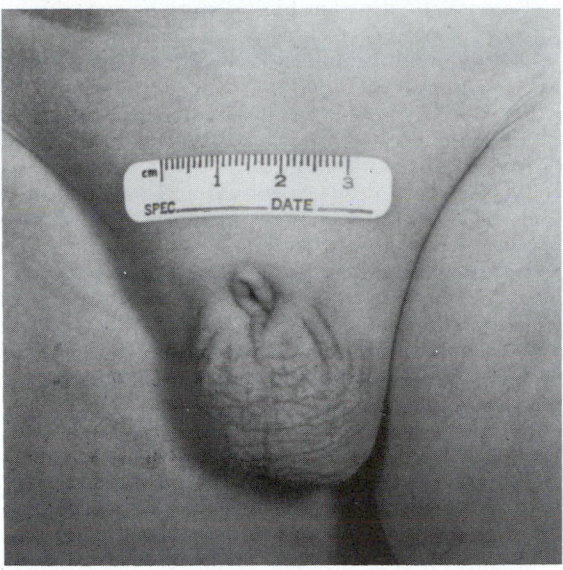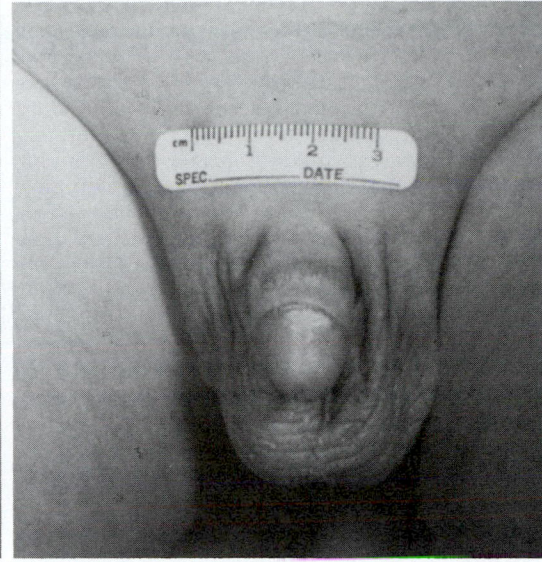

Figure 13–22. Effect of three injections of testosterone cypionate (25 mg intramuscularly at 3-wk intervals) on penis size in a 1-y-old boy with microphallus related to hypogonadotropic hypogonadism.

commenced at the time of expected puberty in such patients, the normal events of male puberty proceed in the usual fashion. If therapy is delayed until long after the time of usual puberty, the degree to which normal virilization will occur is variable. Many such patients undergo a late but relatively complete anatomical and functional male maturation. Intermittent androgen therapy is sometimes administered to prepubertal hypogonadal boys with microphallus to stimulate the growth of the external genitalia into the normal range[260, 378] (Fig. 13–22) and is useful for some boys with hypospadias and microphallus before surgical repair.[741] If patients are monitored closely and androgen is given for only short periods, such therapy probably has no adverse effects on somatic growth.

In boys of pubertal age with either isolated hypogonadotropic hypogonadism or primary testicular deficiency, the initial administration of small doses of testosterone esters followed by a gradual increase to doses of 100 to 150 mg/m^2 of body surface area per month results in the development of a normal pubertal growth spurt.[742] Penile growth, deepening of the voice, and appearance of other secondary sexual characteristics usually commence during the first year of treatment. Puberty in normal boys extends over several years, and treatment that is designed to replicate normal development cannot shorten the process greatly. The usual practice is to institute androgen therapy in hypogonadal boys between the ages of 12 and 14, depending on their subjective need for sexual development. Testosterone exerts its full action only in the presence of a balanced hormonal environment and, particularly, in the presence of adequate levels of growth hormone. Consequently, prepubertal boys with coexisting deficiency of growth hormone exhibit a diminished response to androgens in regard to both growth and the development of secondary sexual characteristics unless growth hormone is given simultaneously.[742–745] As noted earlier, testosterone may promote growth in pubertal boys by enhancing the secretion of growth hormone and insulin-like growth factor I.[279, 280, 746]

USE OF ANDROGENS FOR PURPOSES OTHER THAN REPLACEMENT THERAPY. Enhanced Nitrogen Balance and Muscle Development. Soon after the identification of testosterone as the principal androgen produced by the testis, it was recognized that the administration of the hormone to

hypogonadal or castrated men has systemic effects in addition to those on the male urogenital tract. These effects include reduction in the urinary excretion of nitrogen, sodium, potassium, and chloride and induction of a gain in weight (reviewed in ref. 274). In contrast, in normal men who are given pharmacological amounts of androgen, nitrogen retention is only about half that of hypogonadal men, and under balanced conditions in which food intake is constant, normal men gain little or no weight. In all situations other than hypogonadism, the positive nitrogen balance is short-lived (probably lasting no more than 1 to 2 mo).

A major component of androgen-induced weight gain and nitrogen retention in hypogonadal men is due to an increase in skeletal and muscle mass. In most species, including humans, the skeletal muscles that support the forelimbs, namely, the muscles of the pectoral and shoulder region, show the greatest response, but most muscles probably have some degree of response to androgen administration.[277] The enlargement of responsive muscles is due to the formation of new myofilaments along the myofibrils and to division of the enlarging myofibrils; the net consequence is an increase in the diameter of muscle fibers and fibrils.[747]

Because androgens have significant effects on muscle mass and on body weight when administered to hypogonadal men, it was initially assumed that androgens in pharmacological amounts could promote growth of muscle mass above the levels produced by the normal testicular secretion. The anabolic and androgenic actions of androgens were believed to be distinct and independent hormone actions, so a concerted effort was made to devise pure anabolic steroids with no androgenic effects. In fact, however, androgenic and anabolic effects do not result from different actions of the same hormone but represent the same action in different tissues. Krieg and Voigt showed that androgen-responsive muscle contains the same androgen receptor system that is known to mediate the action of the hormone in other androgen target tissues.[748] It is theoretically possible that a steroid might be devised that would be taken up by or retained selectively by muscle,[749] but no anabolic hormone without androgenic effects has been found.[750, 751]

All anabolic agents tested in humans so far are also androgens and in appropriate doses can be used for androgen replacement.[752–754] For example, methandrostenolone, which has a greater effect on nitrogen balance per unit weight than does methyltestosterone, is a potent androgen and can be used for replacement therapy with hypogonadal men.[752] For these reasons, because the effects of androgens on nitrogen balance are of limited magnitude and of short duration in normal men, and because no beneficial effects of androgen have been documented on muscle development in normal, postpubertal men, the likelihood of developing a specific anabolic steroid seems remote. However, androgens have been tried in a variety of clinical situations other than hypogonadism with the hope that improvement in nitrogen balance and muscle development could outweigh any deleterious side effects.

Attempts to Improve Nitrogen Balance in Catabolic States. After injury, infection, or surgery, body protein is broken down more rapidly than it is formed and as a consequence excess nitrogen is excreted in the urine. During the subsequent recovery phase, nitrogen deficits are replaced. Anabolic steroids can improve the nitrogen balance during the first few days after relatively minor operations in well-nourished subjects,[755] but the diminution in nitrogen loss is minimal and has not been shown to be of significant therapeutic benefit.[755] Likewise, any effect of androgens on weight in undernourished, debilitated, or elderly individuals is probably due to enhancement of appetite. In appropriately controlled studies, no consistent effects on weight or strength have been documented after androgen treatment.[756, 757] These negative results are probably the consequence of several factors, including the dependence of anabolic effects on adequate nutrition and health, the paucity of androgenic effects in men with normal androgen levels, and the temporary nature of any positive nitrogen balance when it does occur. In short, androgens are disappointing as therapeutic aids to promote anabolism in acute illness, continuing trauma, and protein depletion that is associated with chronic illness.

Androgens are also of no proven value in the management of nitrogen accumulation in chronic renal failure; at best they induce a transient improvement in nitrogen balance, but this effect is of doubtful benefit.[758] In acute renal failure, androgens cause a decrease in the rate of urea production and a consequent decrease in the frequency of dialysis in some patients.[759] Most of these patients do well without androgen therapy.

Androgens and Athletic Performance. The use of androgens by athletes in the belief that athletic performance will be improved constitutes a widespread form of drug abuse. Because of the secrecy surrounding their use, a great deal of the information is based on rumor and hearsay, and the amount of factual data on the subject is limited. Weightlifters and body-builders had begun to use them in the 1950s, and the usage gradually spread into football and other areas of athletics. The abuse of these substances at all levels of athletic competition from high school to professional has become widespread, despite the absence of solid evidence that such agents have a positive effect and with disregard for the adverse effects of the drugs.[760]

Whereas some observers believe that the use of androgenic steroids has been responsible for the breaking of athletic records in the recent past, the bulk of evidence indicates that the drugs do not do anything beyond the normal testicular secretion.[760] Indeed, in many appropriately controlled studies, it has not been possible to show that these agents cause an increase in muscle bulk, in strength, or in athletic ability,[760] and when effects on strength have been reported it is not clear that such effects necessarily result in improved performance. It is true, however, that published trials of efficacy involve the administration of drugs at smaller doses than are actually taken by many athletes.

Because the drugs at high dosage have multiple side effects, some of which preclude appropriate studies of efficacy in a double-blind fashion, it is not clear whether the question of efficacy can ever be resolved scientifically.[760] It should be noted that skepticism about the efficacy of the agents on athletic performance is warranted solely based on their use in adult men. Although such drugs have a positive effect on nitrogen retention in women and boys, no studies of their effects on athletic performance in these groups have been reported. The inevitable side effects of the drugs, some of which are irreversible, preclude such studies.

The question of efficacy, interesting though it may be, is independent of the question of the side effects of the drugs. Because most athletes take oral agents such as nandrolone phenpropionate (Durabolin) and stanozolol, frequently along with testosterone esters by injection, the potential toxic side effects are formidable. Nevertheless, regardless of the risk of toxicity and lack of definitive evidence for their usefulness and despite condemnation of the practice by sports organizations, abuse of androgens by athletes is widespread. The focus among organizations that sponsor athletic events has thus shifted from education and prevention to the detection of the drugs in blood and urine and to the disqualification of athletes who are shown to be using these agents.

Stimulation of Erythropoiesis. The difference in the hematocrit between men and women is the result of a positive effect of testosterone on erythropoietin formation and hence on erythropoiesis. After castration of men, there is a 10% decrease in red blood cell mass, a 36% decrease in red blood cell diameter, and an increase in osmotic fragility. Occasionally, the resulting anemia may be severe.[277] Administration of androgens to women increases erythropoiesis, and some women develop polycythemia during long-term androgen therapy, as in treatment of carcinoma of the breast. On average, the hemoglobin level increases by 43 g/L (4.3 g/dL), and the hematocrit increases by 0.11 in women who are treated with pharmacological doses of testosterone.[761] The average increase in hemoglobin is about 10 g/L (1 g/dL) in normal men who are given pharmacological doses of testosterone esters.[727] As a consequence, androgens have been used in the treatment of refractory anemia.[762] The mechanism by which androgens act to stimulate erythropoietin formation by the kidneys presumably involves the same receptor mechanism that has been documented for other androgen actions. In the human some erythropoietin is synthesized outside the kidneys, and the presence of renal tissue is not an absolute requirement for stimulation of erythropoiesis by androgens.[762, 763] The capacity to enhance erythropoiesis is shared by all active androgens. Androgen therapy has received extensive trials in the anemias associated with failure of the bone marrow and/or myelofibrosis and in the anemia of renal failure.

Occasional dramatic increases in hemoglobin level occur after the administration of androgens to subjects with bone marrow failure.[764, 765] In large numbers of unselected patients who are treated with androgens, approximately half appear to respond.[764] The improvement appears to be more consistent when the bone marrow is hypoplastic or when there is myelofibrosis than when the marrow is hypercellular.

What is uncertain, however, is the frequency with which drug administration and therapeutic response are coincidental.[766, 767] This question is a particular problem in regard to acquired anemias, in which spontaneous remission can occur during therapy. In a prospective randomized trial of androgen therapy in patients with aplastic anemia, the use of oral androgens at high dosages (1 mg/kg body weight/d) was associated with hematological improvement and increased survival in the less severe cases.[768]

Androgens may also be beneficial in the anemia of renal failure. Androgen-induced increases in erythropoietin and hemoglobin levels are less marked in the anephric state, as would be expected if the beneficial effect were due to increased erythropoietin formation.[769] In addition, the anemia of renal failure may undergo gradual improvement with time, after the institution of adequate dialysis programs and correction of other coexisting causes of anemia.[770] Nevertheless, in most studies androgen therapy results in increases in hemoglobin level (10 to 50 g/L [1 to 5 g/dL]) and in red blood cell volume (325 to 350 mL), provided dialysis is adequate and stores of iron and folate are normal.[771–776] Whether the benefits of such treatment outweigh the potential adverse effects is unclear.[777] The drugs should be discontinued after 3 mo whether or not a response has occurred, and therapy should be resumed in those who had an initial response only if the hematocrit falls to pretreatment levels after drug withdrawal.

Hereditary Angioneurotic Edema. Hereditary angioneurotic edema is an autosomal dominant disorder in which the serum inhibitor of the first component of complement is nonfunctional or absent. As a consequence there is unopposed activation of the complement cascade, which leads to the generation of factors that enhance the permeability of vessels and produce attacks of angioedema. A variety of 17α-alkylated steroids are known to increase the activity of the inhibitor in serum and to restore the complement components that are depleted secondarily in the disorder.[778–785] Orally active androgens are effective, and steroids such as danazol that are weak androgens appear to be equally or more effective than potent androgens. The response in men and women appears to be the same. Because 17α-alkylated androgens (but not testosterone or testosterone esters) cause elevations of several plasma glycoproteins, including haptoglobin, protein-bound sialic acid, plasminogen, and the inhibitor of the first component of complement,[786, 787] the beneficial effect of oral androgens in this disorder is likely the result of a side effect of 17α-alkylated steroids on liver function rather than the result of androgen action per se. No reports of the effect of testosterone esters in angioneurotic edema have been published. Therapeutic benefits of danazol have been reported for several other conditions such as endometriosis.[788–790]

Short Stature. Androgens have been used in the management of growth retardation of various causes other than pituitary insufficiency. Their administration before epiphyseal closure results in an acceleration of linear growth, and the mean advance in height age may be enhanced more profoundly than is skeletal maturation.[791–793] Such therapy, when given for short periods (6 mo or less), has no permanent effects on hypothalamic-pituitary or gonadal maturation. This acceleration of growth may be the result of an enhancement in plasma growth hormone levels.[745, 794] However, in these boys such treatment does not appear to affect the final height.[795] Furthermore, if such therapy is given to short children before the age of 9, it may actually have a deleterious effect on adult height.[792]

Carcinoma of the Breast. See Chapter 33.

Other Disorders. Androgen therapy is effective in the treatment of the osteoporosis that complicates androgen deficiency; indeed, the histological response to hormonal replacement can be dramatic.[796] A role for androgens in the treatment of osteoporosis that is unassociated with male hypogonadism has not been established.

Oral androgens cause a modest decrease in total plasma triglyceride and very-low-density lipoprotein triglyceride levels in occasional subjects with hyperlipidemia.[797] Simultaneous elevation of LDL cholesterol and reduction of HDL cholesterol also result from such therapy. Consequently, it is not clear whether androgen therapy has a net beneficial effect in hyperlipidemic patients.

SIDE EFFECTS. Some side effects of androgen therapy result from physiological actions of the hormones (via the androgen receptor) but in an inappropriate setting. For example, the virilizing actions are desirable in hypogonadal men but are undesirable in women and in young boys. In some older hypogonadal men the administration of androgens may cause previously unrecognized prostate cancer to become clinically apparent.[798] Other side effects are the results of actions of androgen metabolites, and because different androgens are metabolized differently, the side effects vary. Testosterone can be metabolized to estrogens[727] and may cause feminizing as well as virilizing effects, whereas 5α-reduced androgens such as dihydrotestosterone cannot be converted to estrogens and consequently do not feminize. Normal populations vary in the development of some side effects, just as there is variability among normal men in the degree to which they virilize at puberty. There are also striking age differences in the occurrence of some side effects. Androgens in children may cause premature closure of the epiphyses, induce gynecomastia, or produce virilization, even when used in small amounts and for relatively limited periods. The incidence of some complications may also be increased by coexisting clinical conditions. Hepatoma may occur more frequently after androgen treatment in patients with Fanconi anemia, sodium retention is worse in patients with congestive heart failure, and feminizing side effects are more prominent in patients with hepatic cirrhosis. The relation between the duration of administration or dosage and the development of side effects has never been explored systematically, and claims as to the innocuous nature of some analogues are based on studies of short duration.

Side effects of androgen therapy can also result from actions of the steroid derivatives that have no relation to the androgenic actions of these compounds. These effects constitute the true complications of androgen therapy and include the adverse effects of 17α-alkylated androgens on liver function.

Virilizing Side Effects. All androgens carry the risk of inducing virilization in women.[799, 800] Among the early manifestations are acne, coarsening of the voice, and development of hirsutism. Menstrual irregularities are common. If treatment is discontinued as soon as these effects are noticed, the manifestations may slowly subside. With prolonged treatment, male-pattern baldness, worsening of hirsutism and voice changes, and hypertrophy of the clitoris develop and are largely irreversible. There is considerable variation in the frequency and the degree to which these signs develop in women, probably because of individual differences in susceptibility, variations in steady-state blood levels of the hormones, and different durations of therapy. In general the younger the patient, the more striking the virilizing signs, but florid virilization can also occur in adult women if the plasma androgen level is raised sufficiently.

Feminizing Side Effects. The feminizing side effects of androgens are poorly understood. Testosterone can be converted (aromatized) in peripheral tissues to estradiol. Although the conversion of all androgen analogues to estrogens has not been documented, it is presumed that the majority, if not all, C_{19}-steroids with a Δ^4-3-keto configuration can be converted to estrogens and that feminization is the effect of estrogenic metabolites of the parent steroids. The administration of testosterone esters to men results in an increase in plasma estrogen levels.[727] When androgens are given to men with cirrhosis of the liver, the increase in the plasma level of estrogen is greater.[524] In contrast, 5α-reduction of the molecule precludes estrogen formation. The most common manifestation of feminization, development of gynecomastia, is unpredictable and usually occurs in adult men only after high-dose androgen treatment. However, in children who are given androgens, gynecomastia is common and correlates with an increase in urinary estrogen excretion, possibly because of a greater capacity to convert androgens to estrogens in extraglandular tissues in childhood.[801]

Toxic Side Effects. Some degree of sodium retention is a common consequence of therapy with androgens,[727] but the amount of retained sodium is usually minor. However, in patients with underlying heart disease[802] or renal failure[769] the degree of sodium retention may be sufficient to produce edema.

17α-Alkylated androgens impair liver function, as evidenced by consistent elevation of sulfobromophthalein sodium (Bromsulphalein) retention and frequent elevation of plasma alkaline phosphatase and conjugated bilirubin levels during therapy.[803–806] The predominant effect appears to be at the site of transport of metabolites from hepatocyte into bile. The clinical manifestations of abnormal liver function probably depend on the previous integrity of the liver, but jaundice can occasionally occur in the absence of pre-existing liver disease because of a hypersensitivity reaction. Among the changes in liver function that are induced by 17α-alkylated drugs are an increased level of a variety of plasma proteins[786, 787] and a decrease in the conjugation of adrenal steroids by the liver.[807]

The most serious complications of the use of oral androgens are development of peliosis hepatis (blood-filled cysts in the liver) and hepatoma. These disorders may be more common in subjects given androgens with aplastic anemia[808–811] but also occur in persons given oral androgens for other reasons, including hypogonadism.[812–819] An increased incidence of hepatocellular neoplasms may also occur in women taking oral contraceptives. Although these tumors may follow a benign course and regress after discontinuation of the drugs, in other patients the course is rapidly fatal.

Occasional hyperlipidemia has also been reported in patients treated with oral androgens;[820] the reason for this occurrence is unknown. 17α-Alkylated androgens cause striking reductions in serum HDL cholesterol levels.[821] Such unfavorable changes in the plasma lipoprotein levels were not seen in men given high-dose parenteral testosterone ester therapy.[821] Sleep apnea has been reported in occasional men given pharmacological amounts of testosterone esters,[822] possibly a consequence of an increased hematocrit.[761] Priapism was reported in one 20-y-old hypogonadal man treated with testosterone enanthate.[823]

Gonadotropin Therapy

Gonadotropin treatment can establish or restore fertility in men who have gonadotropin deficiency either as an isolated disorder or as a part of more extensive anterior pituitary failure. Because men with hypogonadotropic hypogonadism may become resistant to gonadotropins after long-term treatment (presumably as the result of the development of neutralizing antibodies), the customary strategy is to treat such subjects initially with testosterone esters as described earlier and to reserve gonadotropin therapy until fertility is desired.[824] Prior androgen therapy does not impair subsequent gonadotropin induction of spermatogenesis in subjects with hypogonadotropic hypogonadism.[825]

Two gonadotropin preparations are available: hMG and hCG. The usual preparation of hMG (menotropins), purified from the urine of postmenopausal women, contains 75 IU FSH and 75 IU LH per vial. hCG is available from several sources in vials containing 5000 to 20,000 IU. hCG is devoid of FSH activity and resembles LH in its ability to stimulate

Leydig cells. Because of the expense of hMG, treatment is usually begun with hCG alone, and hMG is added later to stimulate the FSH-dependent stages of spermatid development. A high ratio of LH to FSH activity and a long duration of treatment (3 to 6 mo) are necessary to bring about the maturation of prepubertal testes.[826] In hypophysectomized adults in whom spermatogenesis has regressed for long periods, it is not predictable whether administration of preparations with both FSH and LH activities is necessary to initiate spermatogenesis. However, after spermatogenesis has been restored in hypophysectomized patients or has been initiated in hypogonadotropic hypogonadal men by combined therapy, sperm production can usually be maintained by hCG alone.

In men with hypogonadotropic hypogonadism the dose of hCG that is required to maintain a normal plasma testosterone level varies from 1000 to 6000 IU weekly.[826] Most treatment regimens for the induction of spermatogenesis involve starting with doses of 2000 IU three times or more a week until most of the clinical parameters, including normal male plasma testosterone values, indicate an optimal effect. During initial treatment the testis volume may reach only 8 mL. Menotropins is then added, with as little as 12.5 IU of FSH and 12.5 IU LH being required three times a week to complete the development of spermatogenesis and to cause further growth of the testes. The duration of therapy for optimal spermatogenesis to be achieved may be as long as 12 mo.[826] The addition of menotropins may not be necessary in individuals with partial hypogonadotropic hypogonadism who presumably have some endogenous FSH secretion. The development of anti-hCG antibodies is common after long-term hCG treatment, but development of resistance to the action of the hormone is less common.[827]

Gonadotropin therapy in men with germ cell aplasia is ineffective in bringing about development of a germinal epithelium, but in rare azoospermic men who are not eunuchoidal (excluding those with germ cell aplasia) a combination of menotropins and hCG is said to be effective in completing maturation.[826] Men with oligospermia of unknown cause have also been treated with human gonadotropins. In uncontrolled studies of men with severe oligospermia (<10 million/mL), gonadotropin therapy leads to fertility in less than a tenth of treated cases, and in patients with moderate oligospermia (11 to 20 million/mL), fertility is said to result in about a fifth.[826] It is not clear whether the incidence of fertility in these treated patients is greater than that which would occur in appropriately matched untreated controls.

Treatment with hCG has been used to attempt to promote permanent descent of inguinal testes into the scrotum. In appropriate controlled studies only 1 of 17 cryptorchid testes actually descended into the scrotum, whereas all of 5 retractile testes descended into the scrotum.[828] These findings suggest that the wide discrepancies in apparent efficacy in previous reports of hormonal therapy in cryptorchidism may have been due to the inclusion of various proportions of patients with retractile testes. Such therapy is associated with a variety of virilizing and feminizing side effects in boys because of its enhancement of estradiol and testosterone production by the testes (see Chapter 15).

Luteinizing Hormone–Releasing Hormone Therapy

LHRH agonists can produce diametrically opposite effects, depending on the mode of administration. When administered in a pulsatile fashion that approximates the physiological secretory pattern, such therapy results in enhancement of gonadotropin secretion. In contrast, the tonic administration of the same agonist inhibits gonadotropin secretion and causes a physiological (reversible) castration. In addition, specific antagonists have been designed that have no agonist action, regardless of the mode of administration.[829]

Agonistic effects have proved to be of benefit in hypogonadotropic hypogonadism and in hypothalamic amenorrhea (see Chapter 12). Antagonist actions are useful in some subjects with precocious puberty (see Chapter 22), in women with breast cancer (see Chapter 33), and in men with prostatic cancer (see Chapter 33). LHRH analogues have also been used successfully in men with benign prostatic hyperplasia who are poor candidates for surgery.[830, 831]

As noted earlier, most patients with isolated gonadotropin deficiency are thought to have variably severe defects in the synthesis and/or release of LHRH and eventually respond to repeated stimulation by LHRH. Thus LHRH is the most "physiological" treatment for isolated gonadotropin deficiency. Induction of puberty in men with idiopathic hypogonadotropic hypogonadism can be accomplished by long-term pulsatile administration of low-dose LHRH by using a portable infusion pump; normal levels of plasma testosterone, LH, and FSH can be attained over 3 mo of therapy with 25 ng of LHRH (gonadorelin) per kilogram of body weight administered subcutaneously every 2 h.[832] However, the achievement of adult levels of spermatogenesis may require high dosages.[832] After optimal effects have been achieved by the pulsatile parenteral administration of the agonists, normal plasma androgen levels and normal sperm counts were maintained in one study with intermittent administration via the nasal route.[833] Whether pulsatile LHRH therapy will prove to have advantages over gonadotropin therapy in men with hypogonadotropic hypogonadism is uncertain. In one study LHRH therapy was more effective than gonadotropin therapy in stimulating testicular growth but not in increasing the sperm count.[834]

The administration of LHRH and its analogues by intranasal application has also been used in boys with cryptorchidism. The success (or failure) rate for descent of inguinal testes in boys so treated seems comparable to that achieved with gonadotropins.[828, 835–837]

REFERENCES

1. Vogel F, Motulsky AG. Human Genetics. Berlin: Springer-Verlag, 1979.
2. Vergnaud G, Page DC, Simmler MC, et al. A deletion map of the human Y chromosome based on DNA hybridization. Am J Hum Genet 1986; 38:109–124.
3. Burgoyne PS. Mammalian X and Y crossover. Nature 1986; 320:170–172.
4. Sinclair AH, Berta P, Palmer MS, et al. A gene from the human sex-determining region encodes a protein with homology to a conserved DNA-binding motif. Nature 1990; 346:240–244.
5. George FW, Wilson JD. Sex determination and differentiation. In: Knobil E, Neill J, eds. The Physiology of Reproduction. New York: Raven, 1988: 3–26.
6. McKay DG, Hertig AT, Adams EC, et al. Histochemical observations on the germ cells of the human embryo. Anat Rec 1953; 117:201–220.
7. Hertig AT, Adams EC, McKay DG, et al. A description of 34 human ova within the first 17 days of development. Am J Anat 1956; 98:435–493.
8. Witschi E. Migration of the germ cells of human embryos from the yolk sac to the primitive gonadal folds. Carnegie Contrib Embryol Carnegie Inst Wash 1948; 32:67–80.
9. Mintz B, Russell ES. Gene-induced embryological modification of primordial germ cells in the mouse. J Exp Zool 1957; 134:207–230.
10. Friedman NB, Van de Velde RL. Germ cell tumors in man, pleiotropic mice, and continuity of germplasm and somatoplasm. Hum Pathol 1981; 12:772–776.
11. Gillman J. The development of the gonads in man, with a consideration of the role of fetal endocrines and the histogenesis of ovarian tumors. Carnegie Contrib Embryol Carnegie Inst Wash 1948; 32:83–131.
12. Merchant H. Rat gonadal and ovarian organogenesis with and without germ cells. An ultrastructural study. Dev Biol 1975; 44:1–21.
13. McCarrey JR, Abbott UK. Chick gonad differentiation following excision of primordial germ cells. Dev Biol 1978; 66:256–265.
14. Mittwoch U. How does the Y chromosome affect gonadal differentiation? Philos Trans R Soc Lond Ser B 1970; 259:113–117.
15. Backhouse KM. The gubernaculum testis Hunteri: testicular descent and maldescent. Ann R Coll Surg Engl 1964; 35:15–33.
16. Gier HT, Marion GB. Development of mammalian testes and genital ducts. Biol Reprod 1969; 1(Suppl 1):1–22.
17. Sloan WR, Walsh PC. Familial persistent müllerian duct syndrome. J Urol 1976; 115:459–461.
18. Guerrier D, Tran D, Vanderwinden JM, et al. The persistent müllerian duct syndrome: a molecular approach. J Clin Endocrinol Metab 1989; 68:46–52.
19. Burke EC, Shin MH, Kelalis PP. Prune belly syndrome. Clinical findings and survival. Am J Dis Child 1969; 117:668–671.
20. Roberts P. Congenital absence of the abdominal muscles with associated abnormalities of the genito-urinary tract. Arch Dis Child 1965; 31:236–239.
21. Williams DI, Burkholder GV. The prune belly syndrome. J Urol 1967; 98:244–251.
22. Frey HL, Peng S, Rajfer J. Synergy of abdominal pressure and androgens in testicular descent. Biol Reprod 1983; 29:1233–1239.
23. Griffin JE, Wilson JD. The androgen resistance syndromes: 5α-reductase deficiency, testicular feminization, and related disorders. In: Scriver CR, Beaudet AL, Sly WS, et al., eds. The Metabolic Basis of Inherited Disease. 6th ed. New York: McGraw-Hill, 1989: 1919–1944.
24. George FW, Peterson KG. Partial characterization of the androgen receptor of the newborn rat gubernaculum. Biol Reprod 1988; 39:536–539.
25. Frey HL, Rajfer J. Roll of the gubernaculum and intraabdominal pressure in the process of testicular descent. J Urol 1984; 131:575–579.
26. Scorer CG, Farrington GH. Congenital Deformities of the Testis and Epididymis. New York: Appleton-Century-Crofts, 1971.
27. Burgos MH, Vitale-Calpe R, Aoki A. Fine structure of the testis and its functional significance. In: Johnson AD, Gomes WR, Vandemark NL, eds. The Testis. New York: Academic, 1970: 551–649.
28. Fawcett DW. Ultrastructure and function of the Sertoli cell. In: Greep RO, Astwood EB, eds. Handbook of Physiology. Sect 7: Endocrinology. Vol V. Male Reproductive System. Washington, DC: American Physiological Society, 1975: 21–55.
29. Steinberger E, Steinberger A. Spermatogenic function of the testis. In: Greep RO, Astwood EB, eds. Handbook of Physiology. Sect 7: Endocrinology. Vol V. Male Reproductive System. Washington, DC: American Physiological Society, 1975: 1–20.
30. de Kretser DM. Ultrastructural features of human spermiogenesis. Z Zellforsch 1969; 98:477–505.
31. Neaves WB. The blood-testis barrier. In: Johnson AD, Gomes WR, eds. The Testis. New York: Academic, 1977: 125–161.
32. Neaves WB. Leydig cells. In: Greep RO, Koblinsky MA, eds. Frontiers in Reproduction and Fertility Control. Cambridge, MA: MIT Press, 1977: 125–161.
33. Freeman DA. Cyclic AMP mediated modification of cholesterol traffic in Leydig tumor cells. J Biol Chem 1987; 262:13061–13068.
34. Green JD, Harris GW. Observation of the hypophysioportal vessels of the living rat. J Physiol (Lond) 1949; 108:359–361.
35. Oliver C, Mical RS, Porter JC. Hypothalamic-pituitary vasculature: evidence for retrograde blood flow in the pituitary stalk. Endocrinology 1977; 101:598–604.
36. Silverman AJ, Krey LC, Zimmerman EA. A comparative study of the luteinizing hormone releasing hormone (LHRH) neuronal networks in mammals. Biol Reprod 1979; 20:98–110.
37. Negro-Vilar A, Ojeda SR, McCann SM. Catecholaminergic modulation of luteinizing hormone–releasing hormone release by median eminence terminals in vitro. Endocrinology 1979; 104:1749–1757.
38. Evans WS, Rogol AD, MacLeod RM, et al. Dopaminergic mechanisms and luteinizing hormone secretion. I. Acute administration of the dopamine agonist bromocriptine does not inhibit luteinizing hormone release in hyperprolactinemic women. J Clin Endocrinol Metab 1980; 50:103–107.
39. Delitala G, Giusti M, Mazzocchi G, et al. Participation of endogenous opiates in regulation of the hypothalamic-pituitary-testicular axis in normal men. J Clin Endocrinol Metab 1983; 57:1277–1281.
40. Grossman A, Moult PJA, Gaillard RC, et al. The opioid control of LH and FSH release: effects of a met-enkephalin analogue and naloxone. Clin Endocrinol 1981; 14:41–47.
41. Veldhuis JD, Rogol AD, Johnson ML, et al. Endogenous opiates modulate the pulsatile secretion of biologically active luteinizing hormone in man. J Clin Invest 1983; 72:2031–2040.
42. Huseman CA, Kelch RP. Gonadotropin responses and metabolism of synthetic gonadotropin-releasing hormone (GnRH) during constant infusion of GnRH in men and boys with delayed adolescence. J Clin Endocrinol Metab 1978; 47:1325–1331.
43. Bourguignon J-P, Hoyoux C, Reuter A, et al. Urinary excretion of immunoreactive luteinizing hormone–releasing hormone-like material and gonadotropins at different stages of life. J Clin Endocrinol Metab 1979; 48:78–84.

44. Vaitukaitis JL, Ross GD, Braunstein GD, et al. Gonadotropins and their subunits: basic and clinical studies. Recent Prog Horm Res 1976; 32:289–331.

45. Bishop WH, Nureddin A, Ryan RJ. Pituitary luteinizing and follicle-stimulating hormones. In: Parsons JA, ed. Peptide Hormones. Baltimore: University Park Press, 1976: 273–298.

46. Santen RJ, Bardin CW. Episodic luteinizing hormone secretion in man: pulse analysis, clinical interpretation, physiologic mechanisms. J Clin Invest 1973; 52:2617–2628.

47. VanHall EV, Vaitukaitis JL, Ross GT, et al. Effects of progressive desialylation on the rate of disappearance of immunoreactive hCG from plasma in rats. Endocrinology 1971; 89:11–15.

48. Veldhuis JD, Fraioli F, Rogol AD, et al. Metabolic clearance of biologically active luteinizing hormone in man. J Clin Invest 1986; 77:1122–1128.

49. Keller PJ. The renal clearance of follicle-stimulating and luteinizing hormone in postmenopausal women. Acta Endocrinol (Kbh) 1966; 53:225–233.

50. Coble YD Jr, Kohler PO, Cargille CM, et al. Production rates and metabolic clearance rates of human follicle-stimulating hormone in premenopausal and postmenopausal women. J Clin Invest 1969; 48:359–363.

51. Yen SSC, Llerena LA, Pearson OH, et al. Disappearance rates of endogenous follicle-stimulating hormone in serum following surgical hypophysectomy in man. J Clin Endocrinol 1970; 30:325–329.

52. Conn PM, Morrell DV, Dufau ML, et al. Gonadotropin-releasing hormone action in cultured pituicytes: independence of luteinizing hormone release and adenosine 3′,5′-monophosphate production. Endocrinology 1979; 104:448–453.

53. Conn PM. The molecular basis of gonadotropin-releasing hormone action. Endocr Rev 1986; 7:3–10.

54. Huhtaniemi IT, Koritnik DR, Korenbrot CC, et al. Stimulation of pituitary-testicular function with gonadotropin-releasing hormone in fetal and infant monkeys. Endocrinology 1979; 105:109–114.

55. Hsueh AJW, Erickson GF. Extra-pituitary inhibition of testicular function by luteinizing hormone releasing hormone. Nature 1979; 281:66–67.

56. Bourne GA, Regiani S, Payne AH, et al. Testicular GnRH receptors—characterization and localization on interstitial tissue. J Clin Endocrinol Metab 1980; 51:407–409.

57. Rajfer J, Sikka SC, Swerdloff RS. Lack of a direct effect of gonadotropin hormone–releasing hormone agonist on human testicular steroidogenesis. J Clin Endocrinol Metab 1987; 64:62–67.

58. Dufau ML, Catt KJ. Gonadotropin receptors and regulation of steroidogenesis in the testis and ovary. Vitam Horm 1978; 36:461–592.

59. Podesta EJ, Dufau ML, Solano AR, et al. Hormonal activation of protein kinase in isolated Leydig cells: electrophoretic analysis of cyclic AMP receptors. J Biol Chem 1978; 253:8994–9001.

60. Catt KJ, Dufau ML. Gonadotropin receptors and regulation of interstitial cell function in the testis. Receptors Horm Action 1978; 3:291–339.

61. Goldstein JL, Anderson RGW, Brown MS. Coated pits, coated vesicles, and receptor-mediated endocytosis. Nature 1979; 279:679–685.

62. Sharpe RM. hCG-induced decrease in availability of rat testis receptors. Nature 1976; 264:644–646.

63. Saez JM, Haour F, Cathiard AM. Early hCG-induced desensitization in Leydig cells. Biochem Biophys Res Commun 1978; 81:552–558.

64. Tsuruhara T, Dufau ML, Cigorrago S, et al. Hormonal regulation of testicular luteinizing hormone receptors. J Biol Chem 1977; 252:9002–9009.

65. Freeman DA, Ascoli M. Desensitization to gonadotropins in cultured Leydig tumor cells involves loss of gonadotropin receptors and decreased capacity for steroidogenesis. Proc Natl Acad Sci USA 1981; 78:6309–6313.

66. Means AR, Vaitukaitis JL. Peptide hormone receptors: specific binding of ³H-FSH to testis. Endocrinology 1972; 90:39–46.

67. Orth J, Christensen AK. Autoradiographic localization of specifically bound ¹²⁵I-labelled follicle-stimulating hormone on spermatogonia of the rat testis. Endocrinology 1978; 103:1944–1951.

68. Wahlström T, Huhtaniemi I, Hovatta O, et al. Localization of luteinizing hormone, follicle-stimulating hormone, prolactin, and their receptors in human and rat testis using immunohistochemistry and radioreceptor assay. J Clin Endocrinol Metab 1983; 57:825–830.

69. Dorrington JH, Vernon RG, Fritz IB. The effect of gonadotropins on the 3′,5′-AMP levels of seminiferous tubules. Biochem Biophys Res Commun 1972; 46:1523–1528.

70. Fakunding JL, Means AR. Characterization and follicle-stimulating hormone activation of Sertoli cell cyclic AMP–dependent protein kinases. Endocrinology 1977; 101:1358–1368.

71. Means AR, Fakunding JL, Huckins C, et al. Follicle-stimulating hormone, the Sertoli cell, and spermatogenesis. Recent Prog Horm Res 1976; 32:477–527.

72. Dorrington JH, Armstrong DT. Follicle-stimulating hormone stimulates estradiol-17β synthesis in cultured Sertoli cells. Proc Natl Acad Sci USA 1975; 72:2677–2681.

73. Kerr JB, Sharpe RM. Follicle-stimulating hormone induction of Leydig cell maturation. Endocrinology 1985; 116:2592–2604.

74. Odell WD, Swerdloff RS, Hacobs JS, et al. FSH induction of sensitivity to LH: one cause of sexual maturation in the male rat. Endocrinology 1973; 92:160–165.

75. Ketelslegers JM, Hetzel WD, Sherins RJ, et al. Developmental changes in testicular gonadotropin receptors: plasma gonadotropins and plasma testosterone in the rat. Endocrinology 1978; 103:212–222.

76. Granaprakasam MS, Chem CJH, Sutherland JG, et al. Receptor depletion and replenishment processes: in vivo regulation of gonadotropin receptors by luteinizing hormone, follicle-stimulating hormone and ethanol in rat testes. Biol Reprod 1979; 20:991–1000.

77. Neill JD, Patton JM, Dailey RA, et al. Luteinizing hormone releasing hormone (LHRH) in pituitary stalk blood of rhesus monkeys: relationship to level of LH release. Endocrinology 1977; 101:430–434.

78. Dufau ML, Veldhuis JD, Fraioli F, et al. Mode of secretion of bioactive luteinizing hormone in man. J Clin Endocrinol Metab 1983; 57:993–1000.

79. Veldhuis JD, King JC, Urban RJ, et al. Operating characteristics of the male hypothalamo-pituitary-gonadal axis: pulsatile release of testosterone and follicle-stimulating hormone and their temporal coupling with luteinizing hormone. J Clin Endocrinol Metab 1987; 65:929–941.

80. Santen RJ. Is aromatization of testosterone to estradiol required for inhibition of luteinizing hormone secretion in men? J Clin Invest 1975; 56:1555–1563.

81. Winters SJ, Troen P. Evidence for a role of endogenous estrogen in the hypothalamic control of gonadotropin secretion in men. J Clin Endocrinol Metab 1985; 61:842–845.

82. Lacroix A, McKenna TJ, Rabinowitz D. Sex steroid modulation of gonadotropins in normal men and in androgen insensitivity syndrome. J Clin Endocrinol Metab 1979; 48:235–240.

83. Matsumoto AM, Bremner WJ. Modulation of pulsatile gonadotropin secretion by testosterone in man. J Clin Endocrinol Metab 1984; 58:609–614.

84. Veldhuis JD, Rogol AD, Samojlik E, et al. Role of endogenous opiates in the expression of negative feedback actions of androgen and estrogen on pulsatile properties of luteinizing hormone secretion in man. J Clin Invest 1984; 74:47–55.

85. Plant TM, Dubey AK. Evidence from the rhesus monkey (*Macaca mulatta*) for the view that negative feedback control of luteinizing hormone secretion by the testis is mediated by deceleration of hypothalamic gonadotropin-releasing hormone pulse frequency. Endocrinology 1984; 115:2145–2153.

86. Sheckter CB, Matsumoto AM, Bremner WJ. Testosterone administration inhibits gonadotropin secretion by an effect directly on the human pituitary. J Clin Endocrinol Metab 1989; 68:397–401.

87. Baker HWG, Bremner WJ, Burger HC, et al. Testicular control of follicle-stimulating hormone secretion. Recent Prog Horm Res 1976; 98:997–1004.

88. Robertson DM, McLachlan RI, Burger HG, et al. Inhibin-related proteins in the male. In: Burger H, de Kretser D, eds. The Testis. 2nd ed. New York: Raven, 1989: 231–254.

89. Bicsak TA, Vale W, Vaughan J, et al. Hormonal regulation of inhibin production by cultured Sertoli cells. Mol Cell Endocrinol 1987; 49:211–217.

90. Morris PL, Vale WW, Cappel S, et al. Inhibin production by primary Sertoli cell–enriched cultures: regulation by follicle-stimulating hormone, androgens, and epidermal growth factor. Endocrinology 1988; 122:717–725.

91. Verhoeven G, Franchimont P. Regulation of inhibin secretion by Sertoli cell–enriched cultures. Acta Endocrinol (Copenh) 1983; 102:136–143.

92. McLachlan RI, Matsumoto AM, Burger HG, et al. Relative roles of follicle-stimulating hormone and luteinizing hormone in the control of inhibin secretion in normal men. J Clin Invest 1988; 82:880–884.

93. Sherins RJ, Patterson AP, Brightwell D, et al. Alteration in the plasma testosterone:estradiol ratio: an alternative to the inhibin hypothesis. Ann NY Acad Sci 1982; 383:295–306.

94. Gross KM, Matsumoto AM, Bremner WJ. Differential control of luteinizing hormone and follicle-stimulating hormone secretion by luteinizing hormone–releasing hormone pulse frequency in man. J Clin Endocrinol Metab 1987; 64:675–680.

95. Gross KM, Matsumoto AM, Berger RE, et al. Increased frequency of pulsatile luteinizing hormone–releasing hormone administration selectively decreases follicle-stimulating hormone levels in men with idiopathic azoospermia. Fertil Steril 1986; 45:392–396.

96. Dubey AK, Zeleznik AJ, Plant TM. In the rhesus monkey (*Macaca mulatta*), the negative feedback regulation of follicle-stimulating hormone secretion by an action of testicular hormone directly at the level of the anterior pituitary gland cannot be accounted for by either testosterone or estradiol. Endocrinology 1987; 121:2229–2237.

97. Eik-Nes KB. Biosynthesis and secretion of testicular steroids. In: Greep RO, Astwood EB, eds. Handbook of Physiology. Sect 7: Endocrinology. Vol V. Male Reproductive System. Washington, DC: American Physiological Society, 1975: 95–116.

98. Morris MD, Chaikoff IL. The origin of cholesterol in liver, small intestine, adrenal gland, and testis of the rat: dietary versus endogenous contributions. J Biol Chem 1959; 234:1095–1097.

99. Carr BR, Parker CR Jr, Ohashi M, et al. Regulation of human fetal

testicular secretion of testosterone: low-density lipoprotein-cholesterol and cholesterol synthesized de novo as steroid precursor. Am J Obstet Gynecol 1983; 146:241–247.

100. Yanaihara T, Troen P. Studies of the human testis. I. Biosynthetic pathways for androgen formation in human testicular tissue in vitro. J Clin Endocrinol Metab 1972; 34:783–792.

101. Miller WL. Molecular biology of steroid hormone synthesis. Endocr Rev 1988; 9:295–318.

102. Hammond GL, Ruokonen A, Kontturi M, et al. The simultaneous radioimmunoassay of seven steroids in human spermatic and peripheral venous blood. J Clin Endocrinol Metab 1977; 45:16–24.

103. Morse HC, Horike N, Rowley MJ, et al. Testosterone concentrations in testes of normal men: effects of testosterone propionate administration. J Clin Endocrinol Metab 1973; 37:882–886.

104. Catt KJ, Dufau ML. Spare gonadotrophin receptors in rat testis. Nature New Biol 1973; 244:219–221.

105. Mendelson C, Dufau ML, Catt KJ. Gonadotropin binding and stimulation of cyclic adenosine 3′:5′-monophosphate and testosterone production in isolated Leydig cells. J Biol Chem 1975; 250:8818–8823.

106. Huhtaniemi I, Bolton N, Leinonen P, et al. Testicular luteinizing hormone receptor content and in vitro stimulation of cyclic adenosine 3′,5′-monophosphate and steroid production: a comparison between man and rat. J Clin Endocrinol Metab 1982; 55:882–889.

107. Cigorraga SB, Dufau ML, Catt KJ. Regulation of luteinizing hormone receptors and steroidogenesis in gonadotropin-desensitized Leydig cells. J Biol Chem 1978; 253:4297–4304.

108. Kalla NR, Nisula BC, Menard R, et al. The effect of estradiol on testicular testosterone biosynthesis. Endocrinology 1980; 106:35–39.

109. Cigorraga SB, Sorrell S, Bator J, et al. Estrogen dependence of a gonadotropin-induced steroidogenic lesion in rat testicular Leydig cells. J Clin Invest 1980; 65:699–705.

110. Nozu K, Dufau ML, Catt KJ. Estradiol receptor–mediated regulation of steroidogenesis in gonadotropin-desensitized Leydig cells. J Biol Chem 1981; 256:1915–1922.

111. Payne AH, Quinn PG, Rani CS. Regulation of microsomal cytochrome P-450 enzymes and testosterone production in Leydig cells. Recent Prog Horm Res 1985; 41:153–197.

112. Quinn PG, Payne AH. Steroid product–induced, oxygen-mediated damage of microsomal cytochrome P-450 enzymes in Leydig cell cultures. J Biol Chem 1985; 260:2092–2099.

113. Hales DB, Sha L, Payne AH. Testosterone inhibits cAMP-induced de novo synthesis of Leydig cell cytochrome P-450$_{17\alpha}$ by an androgen receptor–mediated mechanism. J Biol Chem 1987; 262:11200–11206.

114. Padron RS, Wischusen J, Hudson B, et al. Prolonged biphasic response of plasma testosterone to single intramuscular injections of human chorionic gonadotropin. J Clin Endocrinol Metab 1980; 50:1100–1104.

115. Smals AGH, Pieters GFFM, Lozekott DC, et al. Dissociated responses of plasma testosterone and 17-hydroxyprogesterone to single or repeated human chorionic gonadotropin administration in normal men. J Clin Endocrinol Metab 1980; 50:190–193.

116. Matsumoto AM, Paulsen CA, Hopper BR, et al. Human chorionic gonadotropin and testicular function: stimulation of testosterone, testosterone precursors, and sperm production despite high estradiol levels. J Clin Endocrinol Metab 1983; 56:720–728.

117. Nankin HR, Murono E, Lin T, et al. Morning and evening human Leydig cell responses to hCG. Acta Endocrinol 1980; 95:560–565.

118. Miyatake K, Morimoto Y, Oishi T, et al. Circadian rhythm of serum testosterone and its relation to sleep: comparison with the variation in serum luteinizing hormone, prolactin, and cortisol in normal men. J Clin Endocrinol Metab 1980; 51:1365–1371.

119. Davies TF, Katikineni M, Chan V, et al. Lactogenic receptor regulation in hormone-stimulated steroidogenic cells. Nature 1980; 283:863–865.

120. Bartke A. Pituitary-testis relationship: role of prolactin in the regulation of testicular function. In: Hubinont PO, ed. Progress in Reproductive Biology. Vol 1. Basel: S. Karger, 1976: 136–152.

121. Martikainen H, Vihko R. HCG-stimulation of testicular steroidogenesis during induced hyper- and hypoprolactinaemia in man. Clin Endocrinol 1982; 16:227–234.

122. Mukhopadhyay AK, Bohnet HG, Leidenberger FA. Testosterone production by mouse Leydig cells is stimulated in vitro by atrial natriuretic factor. FEBS Lett 1986; 202:111–116.

123. Pandey KN, Pavlou SN, Kovacs WJ, et al. Atrial natriuretic factor regulates steroidogenic responsiveness and cyclic nucleotide levels in mouse Leydig cells in vitro. Biochem Biophys Res Commun 1986; 138:399–404.

124. Adashi EY, Hsueh AJW. Direct inhibition of testicular androgen biosynthesis by arginine-vasopressin: mediation through pressor-selective testicular recognition sites. Endocrinology 1981; 109:1793–1795.

125. Kasson BG, Hsueh AJW. Insulin-like growth factor-I augments gonadotropin-stimulated androgen biosynthesis by cultured rat testicular cells. Mol Cell Endocrinol 1987; 52:27–34.

126. Hsueh AJW, Dahl KD, Vaughan J, et al. Heterodimers and homodimers of inhibin subunits have different paracrine action in the modulation of luteinizing hormone–stimulated androgen biosynthesis. Proc Natl Acad Sci USA 1987; 84:5082–5086.

127. Risbridger GP, Jenkin G, de Kretser DM. The interaction of hCG,

128. Verhoeven G, Cailleau J. A Leydig cell stimulatory factor produced by human testicular tubules. Mol Cell Endocrinol 1987; 49:137–147.

129. Rosner W, Smith RN. Isolation and characterization of the testosterone-estradiol–binding globulin from human plasma: use of a novel affinity column. Biochemistry 1975; 14:4813–4820.

130. Que BG, Petra PH. Characterization of cDNA coding for sex steroid–binding protein of human plasma. FEBS Lett 1987; 219:405–409.

131. Hammond GL, Underhill DA, Smith CL, et al. The cDNA-deduced primary structure of human sex hormone–binding globulin and location of its steroid-binding domain. FEBS Lett 1987; 215:100–104.

132. Dunn JF, Nisula BC, Rodbard D. Transport of steroid hormones: binding of 21 endogenous steroids to both testosterone-binding globulin and corticosteroid-binding globulin in human plasma. J Clin Endocrinol Metab 1981; 53:58–68.

133. Pardridge WM, Landaw EM. Testosterone transport in brain: primary role of plasma protein-bound hormone. Am J Physiol 1985; 249:E534–E542.

134. Pardridge WM. Serum bioavailability of sex steroid hormones. Clin Endocrinol Metab 1986; 15:259–278.

135. Terasaka T, Nowlin DM, Pardridge WM. Differential binding of testosterone and estradiol to isoforms of sex hormone–binding globulin: selective alteration of estradiol binding in cirrhosis. J Clin Endocrinol Metab 1988; 67:639–643.

136. Plymate SR, Leonard JM, Paulsen CA, et al. Sex hormone–binding globulin changes with androgen replacement. J Clin Endocrinol Metab 1983; 57:645–648.

137. Pardridge WM. Transport of protein-bound hormone into tissues in vivo. Endocr Rev 1981; 2:103–123.

138. Anderson DC. Sex-hormone–binding globulin. Clin Endocrinol Metab 1974; 3:69–96.

139. Wilson JD. Metabolism of testicular androgens. In: Greep RO, Astwood EB, eds. Handbook of Physiology. Sect 7: Endocrinology. Vol V. Male Reproductive System. Washington, DC: American Physiological Society, 1975: 491–508.

140. Siiteri PK, MacDonald PC. Role of extraglandular estrogen in human endocrinology. In: Greep RO, Astwood EB, eds. Handbook of Physiology. Sect 7: Endocrinology. Vol II. Female Reproductive System. Part I. Washington, DC: American Physiological Society, 1973: 615–629.

141. Moore RJ, Gazak JM, Wilson JD. Regulation of cytoplasmic dihydrotestosterone binding in dog prostate by 17β-estradiol. J Clin Invest 1979; 63:351–357.

142. Wilson JD, Aiman J, MacDonald PC. The pathogenesis of gynecomastia. Adv Intern Med 1980; 25:1–32.

143. MacDonald PC, Madden JD, Brenner PF, et al. Origin of estrogen in normal men and in women with testicular feminization. J Clin Endocrinol Metab 1979; 49:905–916.

144. Ito T, Horton R. The source of plasma dihydrotestosterone in man. J Clin Invest 1971; 50:1621–1627.

145. Bruchovsky N, Wilson JD. The conversion of testosterone to 5α-androstan-17β-ol-3-one by rat prostate in vivo and in vitro. J Biol Chem 1968; 243:2012–2021.

146. Anderson KM, Liao S. Selective retention of dihydrotestosterone by prostatic nuclei. Nature 1968; 219:277–279.

147. Labrie C, Belanger A, Labrie F. Androgenic activity of dehydroepiandrosterone and androstenedione in the rat ventral prostate. Endocrinology 1988; 123:1412–1417.

148. Dorfman RI, Shipley RA. Androgens: Biochemistry, Physiology, and Clinical Significance. New York: John Wiley & Sons, 1956.

149. Wilson JD. Dihydrotestosterone formation in cultured human fibroblasts. Comparison of cells from normal subjects and patients with familial incomplete male pseudohermaphroditism, type 2. J Biol Chem 1975; 250:3498–3504.

150. Moore RJ, Griffin JE, Wilson JD. Diminished 5α-reductase activity in extracts of fibroblasts cultured from patients with familial incomplete male pseudohermaphroditism, type 2. J Biol Chem 1975; 250:7168–7172.

151. Moore RJ, Wilson JD. Steroid 5α-reductase in cultured human fibroblasts: biochemical and genetic evidence for two enzyme activities. J Biol Chem 1976; 251:5895–5900.

152. Leshin M, Griffin JE, Wilson JD. Hereditary male pseudohermaphroditism associated with an unstable form of 5α-reductase. J Clin Invest 1978; 62:685–691.

153. Frederiksen DW, Wilson JD. Partial characterization of the nuclear reduced nicotinamide adenine dinucleotide phosphate: Δ⁴-3-ketosteroid 5α-oxidoreductase of rat prostate. J Biol Chem 1971; 246:2584–2593.

154. Wilson JD, Gloyna RE. The intranuclear metabolism of testosterone in the accessory organs of reproduction. Recent Prog Horm Res 1970; 26:309–336.

155. Wilson JD, Walker JD. The conversion of testosterone to 5α-androstan-17β-ol-3-one (dihydrotestosterone) by skin slices of man. J Clin Invest 1969; 48:371–379.

156. Takayasu S, Adachi K. The conversion of testosterone to 17β-hydroxy-5α-androstane-3-one (dihydrotestosterone) by human hair follicles. J Clin Endocrinol Metab 1972; 34:1098–1101.

157. Andersson S, Bishop RW, Russell DW. Expression cloning and regulation of steroid 5α-reductase, an enzyme essential for male sexual differentiation. J Biol Chem 1989; 264:16249–16255.

158. Moore RJ, Wilson JD. The effect of androgenic hormones on the reduced nicotinamide adenine dinucleotide phosphate: Δ⁴-3-ketosteroid 5α-oxidoreductase of rat ventral prostate. Endocrinology 1973; 93:581–592.

159. Kato R, Onoda K, Omori Y. Mechanism of thyroxine-induced increase in steroid Δ⁴-reductase activity in male rats. Endocrinol Jpn 1970; 17:215–219.

160. Hellman L, Bradlow HL, Zumoff B, et al. Thyroid androgen inter-relations and the hypocholesterolemic effect of androsterone. J Clin Endocrinol Metab 1959; 19:936–948.

161. Kuttenn F, Mowszowicz I, Schaison G, et al. Androgen production and skin metabolism in hirsutism. J Endocrinol 1977; 75:83–91.

162. Thompson EA, Siiteri PK. Studies on the aromatization of C-19 androgens. Ann NY Acad Sci 1973; 212:378–391.

163. Corbin CJ, Graham-Lorence S, McPhaul MJ, et al. Isolation of a full-length cDNA insert encoding human aromatase system cytochrome P-450 and its expression in nonsteroidogenic cells. Proc Natl Acad Sci 1988; 85:8948–8952.

164. Brooks RV. Androgens. Clin Endocrinol Metab 1975; 4:503–520.

165. Williams-Ashman HG. Metabolic effects of testicular androgens. In: Greep RO, Astwood EB, eds. Handbook of Physiology. Sect 7: Endocrinology. Vol V. Male Reproductive System. Washington, DC: American Physiological Society, 1975: 473–490.

166. Evans RM. The steroid and thyroid hormone receptor superfamily. Science 1988; 240:889–895.

167. George FW, Wilson JD. Sex determination and differentiation. In: Knobil E, Neill J, eds. The Physiology of Reproduction. New York: Raven, 1988: 3–26.

168. Baker HWG, Bailey DJ, Feil PD, et al. Nuclear accumulation of androgens in perfused rat accessory sex organs and testes. Endocrinology 1977; 100:709–721.

169. Payne AH, Kawano A, Jaffe RB. Formation of dihydrotestosterone and other 5α-reduced metabolites by isolated seminiferous tubules and suspensions of interstitial cells in a human testis. J Clin Endocrinol Metab 1973; 37:448–453.

170. Price P, Wass JAH, Griffin JE, et al. High dose androgen therapy in male pseudohermaphroditism due to 5α-reductase deficiency and disorders of the androgen receptor. J Clin Invest 1984; 74:1496–1508.

171. Wilson EM, French FS. Binding properties of androgen receptors: evidence for identical receptors in rat testes, epididymis, and prostate. J Biol Chem 1976; 251:5620–5629.

172. Verhoeven G. Androgen binding proteins in mouse submandibular gland. J Steroid Biochem 1979; 10:129–138.

173. Snochowski M, Dahlberg E, Gustafsson J-A. Characterization and quantification of the androgen and glucocorticoid receptors in cytosol from rat skeletal muscle. Eur J Biochem 1980; 111:603–616.

174. McGill HC Jr, Anselmo VC, Buchanan JM, et al. The heart is a target organ for androgen. Science 1980; 207:775–777.

175. McCormick PD, Razel AJ, Spelsberg TC, et al. Evidence for an androgen receptor in the human placenta. Am J Obstet Gynecol 1981; 140:8–13.

176. Tsai Y-H, Sanborn BM, Steinberger A, et al. Sertoli cell chromatin acceptor sites for androgen-receptor complexes. J Steroid Biochem 1980; 13:711–718.

177. Verhoeven G. Androgen receptor in cultured interstitial cells derived from immature rat testis. J Steroid Biochem 1980; 13:469–474.

178. Menon M, Tananis CE, Hicks LL, et al. Characterization of the binding of a potent synthetic androgen, methyltrienolone, to human tissues. J Clin Invest 1978; 61:150–162.

179. Blondeau J-P, Baulieu E-E, Robel P. Androgen-dependent regulation of androgen nuclear receptor in the rat ventral prostate. Endocrinology 1982; 110:1926–1932.

180. Rajfer J, Namkung PC, Petral PH. Identification, partial characterization and age-related changes of a cytoplasmic androgen receptor in the rat penis. J Steroid Biochem 1980; 13:1489–1492.

181. Griffin JE, Wilson JD. The syndromes of androgen resistance. N Engl J Med 1980; 302:198–209.

182. Wilbert DM, Griffin JE, Wilson JD. Characterization of the cytosol androgen receptor of the human prostate. J Clin Endocrinol Metab 1983; 56:113–120.

183. Nisula BC, Dunn JF. Measurement of the testosterone binding parameters for both testosterone-estradiol binding globulin and albumin in individual serum samples. Steroids 1979; 34:771–791.

184. Bonne C, Raynaud J-P. Methyltrienolone, a specific ligand for cellular androgen receptors. Steroids 1975; 26:227–232.

185. Wilson EM, French FS. Effects of proteases and protease inhibitors on the 4.5S and 8S androgen receptor. J Biol Chem 1979; 254:6310–6319.

186. Lea OA, Wilson EM, French FS. Characterization of different forms of the androgen receptor. Endocrinology 1979; 105:1350–1360.

187. Colvard DS, Wilson EM. Identification of an 8S androgen receptor-promoting factor that converts the 4.5S form of the androgen receptor to 8S. Endocrinology 1981; 109:496–504.

188. Griffin JE, Punyashthiti K, Wilson JD. Dihydrotestosterone binding by cultured human fibroblasts: comparison of cells from control subjects and from patients with hereditary male pseudohermaphroditism due to androgen resistance. J Clin Invest 1976; 57:1342–1351.

189. Migeon BR, Brown TR, Axelman J, et al. Studies of the locus for androgen receptor: localization on the human X chromosome and evidence for homology with the Tfm locus in the mouse. Proc Natl Acad Sci USA 1981; 78:6339–6343.

190. Lubahn DB, Joseph DR, Sullivan PM, et al. Cloning of human androgen receptor complementary DNA and localization to the X chromosome. Science 1988; 240:327–330.

191. Chang C, Kokontis CJ, Liao S. Molecular cloning of human and rat complementary DNA encoding androgen receptors. Science 1988; 240:324–326.

192. Trapman J, Klaassen P, Kuiper GGJM, et al. Cloning, structure and expression of a cDNA encoding the human androgen receptor. Biochem Biophys Res Commun 1988; 153:241–248.

193. Tilley WD, Marcelli M, Wilson JD, et al. Characterization and expression of a cDNA encoding the human androgen receptor. Proc Natl Acad Sci USA 1989; 86:327–331.

194. Maes M, Sultan C, Zerhourni N, et al. Role of testosterone binding to the androgen receptor in male sexual differentiation of patients with 5α-reductase deficiency. J Steroid Biochem 1979; 11:1385–1390.

195. Kaufman M, Pinsky L. The dissociation of testosterone- and 5α-dihydrotestosterone-receptor complexes formed within cultured human genital skin fibroblasts. J Steroid Biochem 1983; 18:121–125.

196. Kovacs WJ, Griffin JE, Weaver DD, et al. A mutation that causes lability of the androgen receptor under conditions that normally promote transformation to the DNA-binding state. J Clin Invest 1984; 73:1095–1104.

197. Vogel F, Rathenberg R. Spontaneous mutations in man. Adv Hum Genet 1975; 5:223–318.

198. Johnson L, Petty CS, Neaves WB. Further quantification of human spermatogenesis. Germ cell loss during postprophase of meiosis and its relationship to daily sperm production. Biol Reprod 1983; 29:207–215.

199. Clermont Y. The cycle of the seminiferous epithelium in man. Am J Anat 1963; 112:35–45.

200. Kerr JB, de Kretser DM. The cytology of the human testis. In: Burger H, de Kretser D, eds. The Testis. New York: Raven, 1981: 141–169.

201. Nikkanen V, Söderström K-O, Parvinen M. Identification of the spermatogenic stages in living seminiferous tubules of man. J Reprod Fertil 1978; 53:255–257.

202. Fawcett DW. The Cell. 2nd ed. Philadelphia: W. B. Saunders, 1981: 604–617.

203. Heller CG, Clermont Y. Spermatogenesis in man: an estimate of its duration. Science 1963; 140:184–186.

204. Rowley MJ, Teshima F, Heller CG. Duration of transit of spermatozoa through the human male ductular system. Fertil Steril 1970; 21:390–396.

205. Bedford JM. Maturation, transport, and fate of spermatozoa in the epididymis. In: Greep RO, Astwood EB. Handbook of Physiology. Sect 7: Endocrinology. Vol V. Male Reproductive System. Washington, DC: American Physiological Society, 1975: 303–317.

206. Hinrichsen MJ, Blaquier JA. Evidence supporting the existence of sperm maturation in the human epididymis. J Reprod Fertil 1980; 60:291–294.

207. Satir R. Basis of flagellar motility in spermatozoa: current status. In: Fawcett DW, Bedford JM, eds. The Spermatozoon. Baltimore: Urban and Schwarzenberg, 1979: 81–90.

208. Linck RW. Advances in the ultrastructural analysis of the sperm flagellar axoneme. In: Fawcett DW, Bedford JM, eds. The Spermatozoon. Baltimore: Urban and Schwarzenberg, 1979: 99–115.

209. Gibbons BH. Studies on the mechanism of flagellar movement. In: Fawcett DW, Bedford JM, eds. The Spermatozoon. Baltimore: Urban and Schwarzenberg, 1979: 91–97.

210. Afzelius BA, Mossberg B. The immotile-cilia syndrome including Kartagener's syndrome. In: Stanbury JB, Wyngaarden JB, Fredrickson DS, et al., eds. The Metabolic Basis of Inherited Disease. 5th ed. New York: McGraw-Hill, 1983: 1986–1994.

211. Setchell BP. Regulation of spermatogenesis and possible sites for contraceptive action. In: Jeffcoate SL, Sandler M, eds. Progress Towards a Male Contraceptive. New York: John Wiley & Sons, 1982: 1–18.

212. Hansson W, Weddington SC, McLean WS, et al. Regulation of seminiferous tubular function by FSH and androgen. J Reprod Fertil 1975; 44:363–375.

213. Tindall DJ, Miller DA, Means AR. Characterization of androgen receptor in Sertoli cell–enriched testis. Endocrinology 1977; 101:13–23.

214. Verhoeven G, Franchimont P. Regulation of inhibin secretion by Sertoli cell–enriched cultures. Acta Endocrinol 1983; 102:136–143.

215. Steinberger E, Steinberger A, Sanborn B. Endocrine control of spermatogenesis. Basic Life Sci 1974; 4:163–181.

216. Matsumoto AM, Paulsen CA, Bremner WJ. Stimulation of sperm production by human luteinizing hormone in gonadotropin-suppressed normal men. J Clin Endocrinol Metab 1984; 59:882–887.

217. Matsumoto AM, Karpas AE, Bremner WJ. Chronic human chorionic gonadotropin administration in normal men: evidence that follicle-stimulating hormone is necessary for the maintenance of quantitatively

normal spermatogenesis in man. J Clin Endocrinol Metab 1986; 62:1184–1192.

218. Lyon MF, Glenister PH, Lamoreux ML. Normal spermatozoa from androgen-resistant germ cells of chimeric mice and the role of androgen in spermatogenesis. Nature 1975; 258:620–622.

219. Fritz IB. Sites of action of androgens and follicle stimulating hormone on cells of the seminiferous tubule. In: Litwack G, ed. Biochemical Actions of Hormones. Vol V. New York: Academic, 1978: 249–281.

220. Cheng CY, Musto NA, Gunsalus GL, et al. There are two forms of androgen binding protein in human testes: comparison of their protomeric variants with serum testosterone-estradiol binding globulin. J Biol Chem 1985; 260:5631–5640.

221. Fabbri A, Knox G, Buczko E, et al. β-Endorphin production by the fetal Leydig cell: regulation and implications for paracrine control of Sertoli cell function. Endocrinology 1988; 122:749–755.

222. Bedford JM. Significance of the need for sperm capacitation before fertilization in eutherian mammals. Biol Reprod 1983; 28:108–120.

223. Perreault SD, Rogers BJ. Capacitation pattern of human spermatozoa. Fertil Steril 1982; 38:258–260.

224. Gorus FK, Finsy R, Pipeleers DG. Effect of temperature, nutrients, calcium, and cAMP on motility of human spermatozoa. Am J Physiol 1982; 242:C304–C311.

225. Blandau RJ. In vitro fertilization and embryo transfer. Fertil Steril 1980; 33:3–11.

226. Evans MI, Mukherjee AB, Schulman JD. Human in vitro fertilization. Obstet Gynecol Surv 1980; 35:71–81.

227. Siiteri PK, Wilson JD. Testosterone formation and metabolism during male sexual differentiation in the human embryo. J Clin Endocrinol Metab 1974; 38:113–125.

228. Reyes FI, Bordoditsky RS, Winter JSD, et al. Studies on human sexual development. II. Fetal and maternal serum gonadotropin and sex steroid concentrations. J Clin Endocrinol Metab 1974; 38:612–617.

229. Forest MG, Sizonenko PC, Cathiard AM, et al. Hypophyso-gonadal function in humans during the first year of life. I. Evidence for testicular activity in early infancy. J Clin Invest 1974; 53:819–828.

230. Forest MG, Cathiard AM. Pattern of plasma testosterone and Δ⁴-androstenedione in normal newborns: evidence for testicular activity at birth. J Clin Endocrinol Metab 1975; 41:977–984.

231. Bidlingmaier F, Dörr HG, Eisenmenger W, et al. Testosterone and androstenedione concentrations in human testis and epididymis during first two years of life. J Clin Endocrinol Metab 1983; 57:311–315.

232. Winter JSD, Hughes IA, Reyes FI, et al. Pituitary-gonadal relations in infancy. 2. Patterns of serum gonadal steroid concentrations in man from birth to two years of age. J Clin Endocrinol Metab 1976; 42:679–686.

233. Frasier SD, Gafford F, Horton R. Plasma androgens in childhood and adolescence. J Clin Endocrinol Metab 1969; 29:1404–1408.

234. August GP, Grumbach MM, Crapo L, et al. Hormonal changes in puberty. III. Correlation of plasma testosterone, LH, FSH, testicular size, and bone age with male pubertal development. J Clin Endocrinol Metab 1972; 34:319–326.

235. Vermuelen A, Reubens R, Verdonck L. Testosterone secretion and metabolism in male senescence. J Clin Endocrinol Metab 1972; 34:730–735.

236. Stearns EL, MacDonnell JA, Kaufman BJ, et al. Declining testicular function with age: hormonal and clinical correlates. Am J Med 1974; 57:761–766.

237. Pirke KM, Doerr P. Age related changes in free plasma testosterone, dihydrotestosterone and oestradiol. Acta Endocrinol 1975; 80:171–178.

238. Bremner WJ, Vitiello MV, Prinz PM. Loss of circadian rhythmicity in blood testosterone levels with aging in normal men. J Clin Endocrinol Metab 1983; 56:1278–1281.

239. Davidson JM, Chen JJ, Crapo L, et al. Hormonal changes and sexual function in aging men. J Clin Endocrinol Metab 1983; 57:71–77.

240. Jost A. The role of fetal hormones in prenatal development. Harvey Lect 1961; 55:201–226.

241. Jost A. A new look at the mechanism controlling sex differentiation in mammals. Johns Hopkins Med J 1972; 130:38–53.

242. George FW, Wilson JD. Embryology of the genital tract. In: Walsh PC, Gittes RF, Perlmutter AD, et al., eds. Campbell's Urology. 5th ed. Philadelphia: W. B. Saunders, 1986: 1804–1818.

243. Donahoe PK, Cate RL, MacLaughlin DT, et al. Mullerian inhibiting substance: gene structure and mechanism of action of a fetal regressor. Recent Prog Horm Res 1987; 43:431–468.

244. George FW, Wilson JD. Sexual differentiation. In: Beard RW, Nathanielsz PW, eds. Fetal Physiology and Medicine. The Basis of Perinatology. 2nd ed. New York: Marcel Dekker, 1984: 57–79.

245. George FW, Noble JF. Androgen receptors are similar in fetal and in adult rabbits. Endocrinology 1984; 115:1451–1458.

246. Kaplan SL, Grumbach MM. The ontogenesis of human foetal hormones. II. Luteinizing hormone (LH) and follicle stimulating hormone (FSH). Acta Endocrinol 1976; 81:808–829.

247. Molsberry RL, Carr BR, Mendelson CR, et al. Human chorionic gonadotropin binding to human fetal testis as a function of gestational age. J Clin Endocrinol Metab 1982; 55:791–794.

248. Tapanainen J, Kellokumpu-Lehtinen P, Pelliniemi L, et al. Age-related changes in endogenous steroids of human fetal testis during early and midpregnancy. J Clin Endocrinol Metab 1981; 52:98–102.

249. Reyes FI, Faiman C, Winter JSD. Development of the regulatory mechanisms of the hypothalamic-pituitary-gonadal system in the human fetus: the chorionic-hypothalamic-pituitary-gonadal axis. In: Novy MJ, Resko JA, eds. Fetal Endocrinology. New York: Academic, 1981: 283–302.

250. Ellinwood WE, Baughman WL, Resko JA. The effects of gonadectomy and testosterone treatment on luteinizing hormone secretion in fetal rhesus monkeys. Endocrinology 1982; 110:183–189.

251. Zondek LH, Zondek T. Observations on the testis in anencephaly with special reference to the Leydig cells. Biol Neonate 1965; 8:329–347.

252. George FW, Simpson ER, Milewich L, et al. Studies on the regulation of the onset of steroid hormone biosynthesis in fetal rabbit gonads. Endocrinology 1979; 105:1100–1106.

253. Reinisch JM. Effects of prenatal hormone exposure on physical and psychological development in humans and animals: with a note on the state of the field. In: Sachar EJ, ed. Hormones, Behavior, and Psychopathology. New York: Raven, 1976: 69–94.

254. Wilson JD. Gonadal hormones and sexual behavior. In: Besser GM, Martini L, eds. Clinical Neuroendocrinology. Vol II. New York: Academic, 1982: 1–29.

255. Davidson JM, Levine S. Endocrine regulation of behavior. Annu Rev Physiol 1972; 34:375–408.

256. De Moor P, Verhoeven G, Heyns W. Permanent effects of fetal and neonatal testosterone secretion on steroid metabolism and binding. Differentiation 1973; 1:241–253.

257. Gustafsson J-A, Stenberg A. Neonatal programming of androgen responsiveness of liver of adult rats. J Biol Chem 1974; 249:719–723.

258. Mann DR, Gould KG, Collins DC, et al. Blockade of neonatal activation of the pituitary-testicular axis: effect on peripubertal luteinizing hormone and testosterone secretion and on testicular development in male monkeys. J Clin Endocrinol Metab 1989; 68:600–607.

259. Reiter EO, Grumbach MM, Kaplan SL, et al. The response of pituitary gonadotropes to synthetic LRF in children with glucocorticoid-treated congenital adrenal hyperplasia: lack of effect of intrauterine and neonatal androgen excess. J Clin Endocrinol Metab 1975; 40:318–325.

260. Guthrie RD, Smith DW, Graham CB. Testosterone treatment for micropenis during early childhood. J Pediatr 1973; 83:247–252.

261. Ducharme JR, Collu R. Pubertal development: normal, precocious and delayed. Clin Endocrinol Metab 1982; 11:57–87.

262. Wierman ME, Beardsworth DE, Crawford JD, et al. Adrenarche and skeletal maturation during luteinizing hormone releasing hormone analogue suppression of gonadarche. J Clin Invest 1986; 77:121–126.

263. Forti G, Santoro S, Grisolia GA, et al. Spermatic and peripheral plasma concentrations of testosterone and androstenedione in prepubertal boys. J Clin Endocrinol Metab 1981; 53:883–886.

264. Winter JSD, Faiman C. Serum gonadotropin concentrations in agonadal children and adults. J Clin Endocrinol Metab 1972; 35:561–564.

265. Jakacki RI, Kelch RP, Sauder SE, et al. Pulsatile secretion of luteinizing hormone in children. J Clin Endocrinol Metab 1982; 55:453–458.

266. Boyar RM, Rosenfeld RS, Kapen S, et al. Human puberty: simultaneous augmented secretion of luteinizing hormone and testosterone during sleep. J Clin Invest 1974; 54:609–618.

267. Lucky AW, Rich BH, Rosenfield RL, et al. LH bioactivity increases more than immunoreactivity during puberty. J Pediatr 1980; 97:205–213.

268. Mauras N, Veldhuis JD, Rogol AD. Role of endogenous opiates in pubertal maturation: opposing actions of naltrexone in prepubertal and late pubertal boys. J Clin Endocrinol Metab 1986; 62:1256–1263.

269. Ulloa-Aguirre A, Mendez JP, Gonzalez-Castillo A, et al. Changes in the responsiveness of luteinizing hormone secretion to infusion of the opioid antagonist naloxone throughout male sexual maturation. Clin Endocrinol 1988; 29:17–28.

270. Parra A, Cervantes C, Sanchez M, et al. The relationship of plasma gonadotrophins and androgen concentrations to body growth in boys. Acta Endocrinol 1981; 98:137–147.

271. Katz SH, Hediger ML, Zemel BS, et al. Adrenal androgens, body fat and advanced skeletal age in puberty: new evidence for the relations of adrenarche and gonadarche in males. Hum Biol 1985; 57:401–413.

272. Burger HG, McLachlan RI, Bangah M, et al. Serum inhibin concentrations rise throughout normal male and female puberty. J Clin Endocrinol Metab 1988; 67:689–694.

273. Nielsen CT, Skakkebaek NE, Richardson DW, et al. Onset of the release of spermatozoa (spermarche) in boys in relation to age, testicular growth, pubic hair, and height. J Clin Endocrinol Metab 1986; 62:532–535.

274. Wilson JD, Griffin JE. The use and misuse of androgens. Metabolism 1980; 29:1278–1295.

275. Scow RO, Hagan SN. Effect of testosterone propionate on myosin, collagen and other protein fractions in striated muscle of gonadectomized rats. Endocrinology 1957; 60:273–276.

276. Finkelstein JS, Klibanski A, Neer RM, et al. Osteoporosis in men with idiopathic hypogonadotropic hypogonadism. Ann Intern Med 1987; 106:354–361.

277. Hamilton JB. The role of testicular secretions as indicated by the effects of castration in man and by studies of pathological conditions and the

short lifespan associated with maleness. Recent Prog Horm Res 1948; 3:257–322.

278. Kirkland RT, Keenan BS, Probstfield JL, et al. Decrease in plasma high-density lipoprotein cholesterol levels at puberty in boys with delayed adolescence. Correlation with plasma testosterone levels. JAMA 1987; 257:502–507.

279. Mauras N, Blizzard RM, Link K, et al. Augmentation of growth hormone secretion during puberty: evidence for a pulse amplitude-modulated phenomenon. J Clin Endocrinol Metab 1987; 64:596–601.

280. Merimee TJ, Zapf J, Hewlett B, et al. Insulin-like growth factors in pygmies. The role of puberty in determining final stature. N Engl J Med 1987; 316:906–911.

281. Marshall WA, Tanner JM. Variations in the pattern of pubertal changes in boys. Arch Dis Child 1970; 45:13–23.

282. Lee PA, Jaffe RB, Midgley AR Jr. Serum gonadotropin, testosterone and prolactin concentrations throughout puberty in boys: a longitudinal study. J Clin Endocrinol Metab 1974; 39:664–672.

283. Schonfeld WA. Primary and secondary sexual characteristics. Study of their development in males from birth through maturity, with biometric study of penis and testes. Am J Dis Child 1943; 65:535–549.

284. Takihara H, Sakatoku J, Fujii M, et al. Significance of testicular size measurement in andrology. I. A new orchiometer and its clinical application. Fertil Steril 1983; 39:836–840.

285. Harlan WR, Grillo GP, Cornoni-Huntley J, et al. Secondary sex characteristics of boys 12 to 17 years of age: the U.S. Health Examination Survey. J Pediatr 1979; 95:293–297.

286. Zachmann M, Prader A, Kind HP, et al. Testicular volume during adolescence. Cross-sectional and longitudinal studies. Helv Paediatr Acta 1974; 29:61–72.

287. Harrison RG. Effect of temperature on the mammalian testis. In: Greep RO, Astwood EB, eds. Handbook of Physiology. Sect 7: Endocrinology. Vol V. Male Reproductive System. Washington DC: American Physiological Society, 1975: 219–223.

288. Leatham JH. Nutritional influences on testicular composition and function in mammals. In: Greep RO, Astwood EB, eds. Handbook of Physiology. Sect 7: Endocrinology. Vol V. Male Reproductive System. Washington DC: American Physiological Society, 1975: 225–232.

289. Pont A, Williams PL, Azhar S, et al. Ketoconazole blocks testosterone synthesis. Arch Intern Med 1982; 142:2137–2140.

290. Masters WH, Johnson VE. Sex and the aging process. J Am Geriatr Soc 1981; 29:385–390.

291. Martin CE. Factors affecting sexual functioning in 60–79-year-old married males. Arch Sex Behav 1981; 10:399–420.

292. Tsitouras PD, Martin CE, Harman SM. Relationship of serum testosterone to sexual activity in healthy elderly men. J Gerontol 1982; 37:288–293.

293. Harman SM, Tsitouras PD. Reproductive hormones in aging men. I. Measurement of sex steroids, basal luteinizing hormone, and Leydig cell response to human chorionic gonadotropin. J Clin Endocrinol Metab 1980; 51:35–40.

294. Tsitouras PD, Hagen TC. Testosterone, LH, FSH, prolactin and sperm in aging healthy men. 7th International Congress of Endocrinology, Quebec City, Canada. 1984: 1236 (abstract).

295. Deslypere JP, Vermeulen A. Leydig cell function in normal men: effect of age, life-style, residence, diet, and activity. J Clin Endocrinol Metab 1984; 59:955–962.

296. Nankin HR, Calkins JH. Decreased bioavailable testosterone in aging normal and impotent men. J Clin Endocrinol Metab 1986; 63:1418–1420.

297. Tenover JS, Matsumoto AM, Plymate SR, et al. The effects of aging in normal men on bioavailable testosterone and luteinizing hormone secretion: response to clomiphene citrate. J Clin Endocrinol Metab 1987; 65:1118–1126.

298. Neaves WB, Johnson L, Porter JC, et al. Leydig cell numbers, daily sperm production, and serum gonadotropin levels in aging men. J Clin Endocrinol Metab 1984; 59:756–763.

299. Pirke KM, Sintermann R, Vogt HJ. Testosterone and testosterone precursors in the spermatic vein and in the testicular tissue of old men. Gerontology 1980; 26:221–230.

300. Takahashi J, Higashi Y, LaNasa JA, et al. Studies of the human testis. XVIII. Simultaneous measurement of nine intratesticular steroids: evidence for reduced mitochondrial function in testis of elderly men. J Clin Endocrinol Metab 1983; 56:1178–1187.

301. Vermeulen A, Deslypere JP. Intratesticular unconjugated steroids in elderly men. J Steroid Biochem 1986; 24:1079–1083.

302. Neaves WH, Johnson L, Petty CS. Seminiferous tubules and daily sperm production in older adult men with varied numbers of Leydig cells. Biol Reprod 1987; 36:301–308.

303. McLachlan R, Tenover J, Matsumoto A, et al. Decreased serum inhibin levels in normal elderly men: evidence for decreased Sertoli cell function with aging. Clin Res 1988; 36:125A.

304. Harman SM, Tsitouras PD, Costa PT, et al. Reproductive hormones in aging men. II. Basal pituitary gonadotropins and gonadotropin responses to luteinizing hormone–releasing hormone. J Clin Endocrinol Metab 1982; 54:547–551.

305. Deslypere JP, Kaufman JM, Vermeulen T, et al. Influence of age on

306. Urban RJ, Veldhuis JD, Blizzard RM, et al. Attenuated release of biologically active luteinizing hormone in healthy aging men. J Clin Invest 1988; 81:1020–1029.

307. Tenover JS, Dahl KD, Hsueh AJW, et al. Serum bioactive and immunoreactive follicle-stimulating hormone levels and the response to clomiphene in healthy young and elderly men. J Clin Endocrinol Metab 1987; 64:1103–1107.

308. Slag MF, Morley JE, Elson MK, et al. Impotence in medical clinic outpatients. JAMA 1983; 249:1735–1740.

309. Goldzieher JW, Dozier TS, Smith KD, et al. Improving the diagnostic reliability of rapidly fluctuating plasma hormone levels by optimized multiple-sampling techniques. J Clin Endocrinol Metab 1976; 43:824–830.

310. Rich BH, Rosenfield RL, Moll GW Jr, et al. Bioactive luteinizing hormone pituitary reserves during normal and abnormal male puberty. J Clin Endocrinol Metab 1982; 55:140–146.

311. Smals AGH, Kloppenborg PWC, Benraad TJ. Circannual cycle in plasma testosterone levels in man. J Clin Endocrinol Metab 1976; 42:979–982.

312. Horton R, Hsieh P, Barberia J, et al. Altered blood androgens in elderly men with prostate hyperplasia. J Clin Endocrinol Metab 1975; 41:793–796.

313. Toublanc JE, Canlorbe P, Job JC. Evaluation of Leydig-cell function in normal prepubertal and pubertal boys. J Steroid Biochem 1975; 6:95–99.

314. Walsh PC, Curry N, Mills RC, et al. Plasma androgen response to hCG stimulation in prepubertal boys with hypospadias and cryptorchidism. J Clin Endocrinol Metab 1976; 42:52–59.

315. Grant DB, Laurance BM, Atherden SM, et al. hCG stimulation test in children with abnormal sexual development. Arch Dis Child 1976; 51:596–601.

316. Wollesen F, Swerdloff RS, Odell WD. LH and FSH responses to luteinizing-releasing hormone in normal, adult, human males. Metabolism 1976; 28:845–863.

317. Harman SM, Tsitouras PD, Costa PT, et al. Evaluation of pituitary gonadotropic function in men: value of luteinizing hormone–releasing hormone response versus basal luteinizing hormone level for discrimination of diagnosis. J Clin Endocrinol Metab 1982; 54:196–200.

318. Synder PJ, Rudenstein RS, Gardner DF, et al. Repetitive infusion of gonadotropin-releasing hormone distinguishes hypothalamic from pituitary hypogonadism. J Clin Endocrinol Metab 1979; 48:864–868.

319. Lubs HA Jr. Testicular size in Klinefelter's syndrome in men over fifty. Report of a case with XXY/XY mosaicism. N Engl J Med 1962; 267:326–331.

320. Diamond JM. Variation in human testis size. Nature 1986; 320:488–489.

321. Rivkees SA, Hall DA, Boepple PA, et al. Accuracy and reproducibility of clinical measures of testicular volume. J Pediatr 1987; 110:914–917.

322. Donohue RE, Fauver HE. Unilateral absence of the vas deferens. A useful clinical sign. JAMA 1989; 261:1180–1182.

323. Belsey MA, Eliasson R, Callegos AH, et al., eds. Laboratory Manual for the Examination of Human Semen and Semen–Cervical Mucus Interaction. Singapore: Press Concern, 1980.

324. Gordon DL, Herrigel JE, Moore DJ, et al. Efficacy of Coulter counter in determining low sperm concentrations. Am J Clin Pathol 1967; 47:226–228.

325. Johnson L. A re-evaluation of daily sperm output of men. Fertil Steril 1982; 37:811–816.

326. Sherins RJ, Brightwell D, Sternthal PM. Longitudinal analysis of semen of fertile and infertile men. In: Troen P, Nankin HR, eds. The Testis in Normal and Infertile Men. New York: Raven, 1977: 473–488.

327. Wilton LJ, Teichtahl H, Temple-Smith PD, et al. Structural heterogeneity of the axonemes of respiratory cilia and sperm flagella in normal men. J Clin Invest 1985; 75:825–831.

328. Alexander NJ. Male evaluation and semen analysis. Clin Obstet Gynecol 1982; 25:463–482.

329. Amelar RD, Dubin L. Semen analysis. In: Amelar RD, Dubin L, Walsh PC, eds. Male Infertility. Philadelphia: W. B. Saunders, 1977: 105–140.

330. Alexander NJ. Evaluation of male infertility with an in vitro cervical mucus penetration test. Fertil Steril 1981; 36:201–208.

331. Rogers BJ. The sperm penetration assay: its usefulness reevaluated. Fertil Steril 1985; 43:821–840.

332. Takemoto FS, Rogers BJ, Wiltbank MC, et al. Comparison of the penetration ability of human spermatozoa into bovine cervical mucus and zona-free hamster eggs. J Androl 1985; 6:162–170.

333. Coburn M, Wheeler T, Lipshultz LI. Testicular biopsy. Its use and limitations. Urol Clin North Am 1987; 14:551–561.

334. Scott RS, Burger HG. An inverse relationship exists between seminal plasma inhibin and serum follicle-stimulating hormone in man. J Clin Endocrinol Metab 1981; 52:796–803.

335. deKretser DM, McLachlan RI, Robertson DM, et al. Serum inhibin levels in normal men and men with testicular disorders. J Endocrinol 1988; 120:517–523.

336. Wang C. Bioassay of follicle stimulating hormone. Endocr Rev 1988; 9:374–377.

337. Weinstein RL, Kelch RP, Jenner MR, et al. Secretion of unconjugated androgens and estrogens by the normal and abnormal human testis before and after human chorionic gonadotropin. J Clin Invest 1974; 53:1–6.

338. Wilson JD, Goldstein JL. Classification of hereditary disorders of sexual development. Birth Defects 1975; 11(4):1–16.

339. Rafjer J. Congenital anomalies of the testes. In: Walsh PH, Gittes RF, Perlmutter AD, et al., eds. Campbell's Urology. 5th ed. Philadelphia: W. B. Saunders, 1986: 1947–1968.

340. Buyse M, Feingold M. Syndromes associated with abnormal external genitalia. In: Vallet HL, Porter IH, eds. Genetic Mechanisms of Sexual Development. New York: Academic, 1979: 425–435.

341. Andersen H, Andreassen M, Quaade F. Testicular biopsies in cryptorchidism. Acta Endocrinol 1955; 18:567–569.

342. Saito S, Kumamoto Y. The number of spermatogonia in various congenital testicular disorders. J Urol 1989; 141:1166–1168.

343. Krabbe S, Berthelsen JG, Volsted P, et al. High incidence of undetected neoplasia in maldescended testes. Lancet 1979; 1:999–1000.

344. Fonger JD, Filler RM, Rider WD, et al. Testicular tumours in maldescended testes. Can J Surg 1981; 24:353–355.

345. Eik-Nes K. Secretion of testosterone by the ectopic and the cryptorchid testes in the same dog. Can J Physiol Pharmacol 1966; 44:629–633.

346. Farrer JH, Sikka SC, Xie HW, et al. Impaired testosterone biosynthesis in cryptorchidism. Fertil Steril 1985; 44:125–132.

347. Lipshultz LI, Caminos-Torres R, Greenspan CS, et al. Testicular function after orchiopexy for unilaterally undescended testis. N Engl J Med 1976; 295:15–18.

348. Scott LS. Fertility in cryptorchidism. Proc R Soc Med 1962; 55:1047–1050.

349. Hezmall HP, Lipshultz LI. Cryptorchidism and infertility. Urol Clin North Am 1982; 9:361–369.

350. Alpert PF, Klein RS. Spermatogenesis in the unilateral cryptorchid testis after orchiopexy. J Urol 1983; 129:301–302.

351. Kallmann FJ, Schoenfeld WA, Barrerra SE. The genetic aspects of primary eunuchoidism. Am J Ment Defic 1944; 48:203–236.

352. Turner RC, Bobrow M, Bobrow LB, et al. Cryptorchidism in a family with Kallmann's syndrome. Proc R Soc Med 1974; 67:33–35.

353. Walsh PC, Wilson JD, Allen TD, et al. Clinical and endocrinological evaluation of patients with congenital microphallus. J Urol 1978; 120:90–95.

354. Laron Z, Kaushanski A, Josefsberg Z. Penile size and growth in children and adolescents with isolated gonadotropin deficiency (IGnD). Clin Endocrinol 1977; 6:265–270.

355. Danish RK, Lee PA, Mazur T, et al. Micropenis. II. Hypogonadotropic hypogonadism. Johns Hopkins Med J 1980; 146:177–184.

356. Kaushanski A, Laron Z. Growth pattern of boys with isolated gonadotropin deficiency. Isr J Med Sci 1979; 15:518–521.

357. Lieblich JM, Rogol AD, White BJ, et al. Syndrome of anosmia with hypogonadotropic hypogonadism (Kallmann syndrome). Clinical and laboratory studies in 23 cases. Am J Med 1982; 73:506–519.

358. Boyar RM, Finkelstein JW, Witkin M, et al. Studies of endocrine function in "isolated" gonadotropin deficiency. J Clin Endocrinol Metab 1973; 36:64–72.

359. Faiman C, Hoffman DL, Ryan RJ, et al. The "fertile eunuch" syndrome: demonstration of isolated luteinizing hormone deficiency by radioimmunoassay technique. Mayo Clin Proc 1968; 43:661–667.

360. Del Pozo E, Bolte E, Very M. Suprasellar disturbance in the syndrome of fertile eunuchoidism: case report. Acta Endocrinol 1975; 80:165–170.

361. Boyar RM, Wu RHK, Kapen S, et al. Clinical and laboratory heterogeneity in idiopathic hypogonadotropic hypogonadism. J Clin Endocrinol Metab 1976; 43:1268–1275.

362. Smals AGH, Kloppenborg PWC, Van Haelst UJG, et al. Fertile eunuch syndrome versus classic hypogonadotrophic hypogonadism. Acta Endocrinol 1978; 87:389–399.

363. Tagatz G, Fialkow PJ, Smith D, et al. Hypogonadotropic hypogonadism associated with anosmia in the female. N Engl J Med 1970; 283:1326–1329.

364. Soules MR, Hammond CB. Female Kallmann's syndrome: evidence for a hypothalamic luteinizing hormone–releasing hormone deficiency. Fertil Steril 1980; 33:82–85.

365. Kemmann E, Conrad P, Jones JR. Cardiac abnormalities in female hypogonadotropic hypogonadism with anosmia. Am J Obstet Gynecol 1980; 136:964–966.

366. Nowakowski H, Lenz W. Genetic aspects of male hypogonadism. Recent Prog Horm Res 1961; 17:53–95.

367. Santen RJ, Paulsen CA. Hypogonadotropic eunuchoidism. I. Clinical study of the mode of inheritance. J Clin Endocrinol Metab 1973; 36:47–54.

368. Marshall JC, Harsoulis P, Anderson DC, et al. Isolated pituitary gonadotrophin deficiency: gonadotrophin secretion after synthetic luteinizing hormone and follicle stimulating hormone–releasing hormone. Br Med J 1972; 4:643–645.

369. Mortimer CH, Besser GM, McNeilly AS, et al. Luteinizing hormone and follicle stimulating hormone–releasing hormone test in patients with hypothalamic-pituitary-gonadal dysfunction. Br Med J 1973; 4:73–77.

370. Bell J, Spitz I, Slonim A, et al. Heterogeneity of gonadotropin response to LHRH in hypogonadotropic hypogonadism. J Clin Endocrinol Metab 1973; 36:791–794.

371. Oettinger M, Bruneteau DW, Psaoudakis A, et al. FSH and LH response to LHRF in Kallmann's syndrome. Obstet Gynecol 1976; 47:233–236.

372. Reitano JF, Caminos-Torres R, Snyder PJ. Serum LH and FSH responses to the repetitive administration of gonadotropin-releasing hormone in patients with idiopathic hypogonadotropic hypogonadism. J Clin Endocriol Metab 1975; 41:1035–1042.

373. Dickerman Z, Prager-Lewin R, Laron Z. The effect of repeated injections of synthetic luteinizing hormone–releasing hormone on the response of plasma luteinizing hormone and follicle-stimulating hormone in young hypogonadotropic-hypogonadal patients. Fertil Steril 1976; 27:162–166.

374. Barkan AL, Reame NE, Kelch RP, et al. Idioathic hypogonadotropin hypogonadism in men: dependence of the hormone responses to gonadotropin-releasing hormone (GnRH) on the magnitude of the endogenous GnRH secretory defect. J Clin Endocrinol Metab 1985; 61:1118–1125.

375. Santoro N, Filicori M, Crowley WF Jr. Hypogonadotropic disorders in men and women: diagnosis and therapy with pulsatile gonadotropin-releasing hormone. Endocr Rev 1976; 7:11–23.

376. Quigley ME, Sheehan KL, Casper RF, et al. Evidence for increased dopaminergic and opioid activity in patients with hypothalamic hypogonadotropic amenorrhea. J Clin Endocrinol Metab 1980; 50:949–954.

377. Klingmüller D, Dewes W, Krahe T, et al. Magnetic resonance imaging of the brain in patients with anosmia and hypothalamic hypogonadism (Kallmann's syndrome). J Clin Endocrinol Metab 1987; 65:581–584.

378. Burstein S, Grumbach MM, Kaplan SL. Early determination of androgen-responsiveness is important in the management of microphallus. Lancet 1979; 2:983–986.

379. Smals AGH, Pieters GFFM, Kloppenborg PW, et al. Lack of a biphasic steroid response to single human chorionic gonadotropin administration in patients with isolated gonadotropin deficiency. J Clin Endocrinol Metab 1980; 50:879–881.

380. Santen RJ, Paulsen CA. Hypogonadotropic eunuchoidism. II. Gonadal responsiveness to exogenous gonadotropins. J Clin Endocrinol Metab 1973; 36:55–63.

381. Wang C, Paulsen CA, Hopper BR, et al. Acute steroidogenic responsiveness to human luteinizing hormone in hypogonadotropic hypogonadism. J Clin Endocrinol Metab 1980; 51:1269–1273.

382. Finkel DM, Phillips JL, Snyder PJ. Stimulation of spermatogenesis by gonadotropins in men with hypogonadotropic hypogonadism. N Engl J Med 1985; 313:651–655.

383. Ley SB, Leonard JM. Male hypogonadotropic hypogonadism: factors influencing response to human chorionic gonadotropin and human menopausal gonadotropin, including prior exogenous androgens. J Clin Endocrinol Metab 1985; 61:746–752.

384. Burris AS, Rodbard HW, Winters SJ, et al. Gonadotropin therapy in men with isolated hypogonadotropic hypogonadism: the response to human chorionic gonadotropin is predicted by initial testicular size. J Clin Endocrinol Metab 1986; 66:1144–1151.

385. Baranetsky NG, Carlson HE. Persistence of spermatogenesis in hypogonadotropic hypogonadism treated with testosterone. Fertil Steril 1980; 34:477–482.

386. Rowe RC, Schroeder M-L, Faiman C. Testosterone-induced fertility in a patient with previously untreated Kallmann's syndrome. Fertil Steril 1983; 40:400–401.

387. Spratt DI, Finkelstein JS, Odea LSTL, et al. Long-term administration of gonadotropin-releasing hormone in men with idiopathic hypogonadotropic hypogonadism. Ann Intern Med 1986; 105:848–855.

388. Shargil AA. Treatment of idiopathic hypogonadotropic hypogonadism in men with luteinizing hormone–releasing hormone: a comparison of treatment with daily injections and with the pulsatile infusion pump. Fertil Steril 1987; 47:492–501.

389. Klingmüller D, Schweikert H-U. Maintenance of spermatogenesis by intranasal administration of gonadotropin-releasing hormone in patients with hypothalamic hypogonadism. J Clin Endocrinol Metab 1985; 61:868–872.

390. Luton J-P, Thieblot P, Valcke J-C, et al. Reversible gonadotropin deficiency in male Cushing's disease. J Clin Endocrinol Metab 1977; 45:488–495.

391. McKenna TJ, Lorber D, Lacroix A, et al. Testicular activity in Cushing's disease. Acta Endocrinol 1979; 91:501–510.

392. MacAdams MR, White RH, Chipps BE. Reduction of serum testosterone levels during chronic glucocorticoid therapy. Ann Intern Med 1986; 104:648–651.

393. Carter JN, Tyson JE, Tolis G, et al. Prolactin-secreting tumors and hypogonadism in 22 men. N Engl J Med 1978; 299:847–852.

394. Thorner MO, Besser GM. Bromocriptine treatment of hyperprolactinaemic hypogonadism. Acta Endocrinol (Suppl) 1978; 88:131–146.

395. Franks S, Jacobs HS, Marti N, et al. Hyperprolactinaemia and impotence. Clin Endocrinol 1978; 8:277–287.

396. Davis JL. Lowering prolactin level in a hyperprolactinemic man. Re-

sponses of luteinizing hormone, follicle-stimulating hormone, and testosterone. Arch Intern Med 1982; 142:146–148.

397. Randall RV, Laws ER Jr, Abboud CF, et al. Transsphenoidal microsurgical treatment of prolactin-producing pituitary adenomas. Results in 100 patients. Mayo Clin Proc 1983; 58:108–121.

398. Prescott RWG, Johnston DG, Kendall-Taylor P, et al. Hyperprolactinaemia in men—response to bromocriptine therapy. Lancet 1982; 1:245–248.

399. MacDonald RA, Mallory GK. Hemochromatosis and hemosiderosis. Study of 211 autopsied cases. Arch Intern Med 1960; 105:686–700.

400. Stocks AE, Powell LW. Pituitary function in idiopathic haemochromatosis and cirrhosis of the liver. Lancet 1972; 2:298–301.

401. Leonard JM, Milder MS. Pituitary origin of hypogonadism in idiopathic hemochromatosis (I.H.). Clin Res 1978; 26:106A.

402. Edwards CQ, Cartwright GE, Skolnick MH, et al. Homozygosity for hemochromatosis: clinical manifestations. Ann Intern Med 1980; 93:519–525.

403. Charbonnel B, Chupin M, Le Grand A, et al. Pituitary function in idiopathic haemochromatosis: hormonal study in 36 male patients. Acta Endocrinol 1981; 98:178–183.

404. Iyer R, Duckworth WC, Solomon SS. Hypogonadism in idiopathic hemochromatosis. Arch Intern Med 1981; 141:517–518.

405. Schafer AI, Cheron RG, Dluhy R, et al. Clinical consequence of acquired transfusional iron overload in adults. N Engl J Med 1981; 304:319–324.

406. Kelly TM, Edwards CQ, Meikle AW, et al. Hypogonadism in hemochromatosis: reversal with iron depletion. Ann Intern Med 1984; 101:629–632.

407. Strain GW, Zumoff B, Miller LK, et al. Effect of massive weight loss on hypothalamic-pituitary-gonadal function in obese men. J Clin Endocrinol Metab 1988; 66:1019–1023.

408. Semple PA, Graham A, Malcolm Y, et al. Hypoxia, depression of testosterone, and impotence in pickwickian syndrome reversed by weight reduction. Br Med J 1984; 29:801–802.

409. Herzog AG, Seibel MM, Schomer DL, et al. Reproductive endocrine disorders in men with partial seizures of temporal lobe origin. Arch Neurol 1986; 43:347–350.

410. Cunningham GR. Idiopathic post-pubertal LH deficiency. Clin Res 1983; 31:896A.

411. Korenman SG, Stanik-avis S, Mooradian A, et al. Evidence for a high prevalence of hypogonadotropic hypogonadism. Clin Res 1987; 35:182A.

412. Klinefelter HF Jr, Reifenstein EC Jr, Albright F. Syndrome characterized by gynecomastia, aspermatogenesis without A-Leydigism, and increased excretion of follicle-stimulating hormone. J Clin Endocrinol Metab 1942; 2:615–627.

413. Paulsen CA, Gordon DL, Carpenter KW, et al. Klinefelter's syndrome and its variants: a hormonal and chromosomal study. Recent Prog Horm Res 1968; 24:321–363.

414. Gordon DL, Krmpotic E, Thomas W, et al. Pathologic testicular findings in Klinefelter's syndrome, 47,XXY vs 46,XY/47,XXY. Arch Intern Med 1972; 130:726–729.

415. Leonard JM, Paulsen CA, Ospina LF, et al. The classification of Klinefelter's syndrome. In: Vallet HL, Porter IH, eds. Genetic Mechanisms of Sexual Development. New York: Academic, 1979: 407–423.

416. Court-Brown WM. Human Population Cytogenetics. New York: John Wiley & Sons, 1967.

417. Mikamo K, Aguercif M, Hazeghi P, et al. Chromatin-positive Klinefelter's syndrome. A quantitative analysis of spermatogonial deficiency at 3, 4, and 12 months of age. Fertil Steril 1968; 19:731–739.

418. Laron Z, Hochman IH. Small testes in prepubertal boys with Klinefelter's syndrome. J Clin Endocrinol Metab 1971; 32:671–672.

419. Caldwell PD, Smith DW. The XXY Klinefelter's syndrome in childhood: detection and treatment. J Pediatr 1972; 80:250–258.

420. Ahmad KN, Dykes JRW, Ferguson-Smith MA, et al. Leydig cell volume in chromatin-positive Klinefelter's syndrome. J Clin Endocrinol Metab 1971; 33:517–520.

421. Schibler D, Brook CGD, Kind HP, et al. Growth and body proportions in 54 boys and men with Klinefelter's syndrome. Helv Paediatr Acta 1974; 29:325–333.

422. Becker KL. Clinical and therapeutic experience with Klinefelter's syndrome. Fertil Steril 1972; 23:568–578.

423. Ratcliffe SG, Bancroft J, Axworthy D, et al. Klinefelter's syndrome in adolescence. Arch Dis Child 1982; 57:6–12.

424. Nielsen J, Pelsen B. Follow-up 20 years later of 34 Klinefelter males with karyotype 47,XXY and 16 hypogonadal males with karyotype 46,XY. Hum Genet 1987; 77:188–192.

425. Smals AGH, Kloppenborg PWC, Lequin RL, et al. The pituitary-thyroid axis in Klinefelter's syndrome. Acta Endocrinol 1977; 84:72–79.

426. Huseby JS, Petersen D. Pulmonary function in Klinefelter's syndrome. Chest 1981; 80:31–33.

427. Scheike O, Visfeldt J, Petersen B. Male breast cancer. 3. Breast carcinoma in association with the Klinefelter syndrome. Acta Pathol Microbiol Scand A 1973; 81:352–358.

428. Griesemer DA. Klinefelter syndrome and breast cancer. Johns Hopkins Med J 1976; 138:102–108.

429. Laron Z, Dickerman Z, Zamir R, et al. Paternity in Klinefelter's syndrome—a case report. Arch Androl 1982; 8:149–151.

430. Bloomgarden ZT, Delozier CD, Cohen MP, et al. Genetic and endocrine findings in a 48,XXYY male. J Clin Endocrinol Metab 1980; 50:740–743.

431. Day RW, Levinson J, Larson W, et al. An XXXXY male. J Pediatr 1963; 63:589–598.

432. Ferguson-Smith MA. Sex chromatin, Klinefelter's syndrome and mental deficiency. In: Moore KL, ed. The Sex Chromatin. Philadelphia: W. B. Saunders, 1966: 277–315.

433. Sanger R, Tippett P, Gavin J. Xg groups and sex abnormalities in people of northern European ancestry. J Med Genet 1971; 8:417–426.

434. Gabrilove JL, Freiberg EK, Thornton JC, et al. Effect of age on testicular function in patients with Klinefelter's syndrome. Clin Endocrinol 1979; 11:343–347.

435. Gabrilove JL, Freiberg EK, Nicholis GL. Testicular function in Klinefelter's syndrome. J Urol 1980; 124:825–826.

436. Wang C, Baker HWG, Burger HG, et al. Hormonal studies in Klinefelter's syndrome. Clin Endocrinol 1975; 4:399–411.

437. Wieland RG, Zorn EM, Johnson MW. Elevated testosterone-binding globulin in Klinefelter's syndrome. J Clin Endocrinol Metab 1980; 51:1199–1200.

438. de Behar BR, Mendilaharzu H, Rivarola MA, et al. Gonadotropin secretion in prepubertal and pubertal primary hypogonadism: response to LHRH. J Clin Endocrinol Metab 1975; 41:1070–1075.

439. Caminos-Torres R, Ma L, Snyder PJ. Testosterone-induced inhibition of the LH and FSH responses to gonadotropin-releasing hormone occurs slowly. J Clin Endocrinol Metab 1977; 44:1142–1153.

440. Samaan NA, Stepanas AV, Danziger J, et al. Reactive pituitary abnormalities in patients with Klinefelter's and Turner's syndromes. Arch Intern Med 1979; 139:198–201.

441. Myhre SA, Ruvalcaba RHA, Johnson HR, et al. The effects of testosterone treatment in Klinefelter's syndrome. J Pediatr 1970; 76:267–276.

442. de la Chapelle A. Analytic review: nature and origin of males with XX sex chromosomes. Am J Hum Genet 1972; 24:71–105.

443. de la Chapelle A. The etiology of maleness in XX men. Hum Genet 1981; 58:105–116.

444. Perez-Palacios G, Medina M, Ullao-Aguirre A, et al. Gonadotropin dynamics in XX males. J Clin Endocrinol Metab 1981; 53:254–257.

445. Schweikert HU, Weissbach L, Leyendecker G, et al. Clinical, endocrinological, and cytological characterization of two 46,XX males. J Clin Endocrinol Metab 1982; 54:745–752.

446. Roe TF, Alfi OS. Ambiguous genitalia in XX male children: report of two infants. Pediatrics 1977; 60:55–59.

447. Vergnaud G, Page DC, Simmler MC, et al. A deletion map of the human Y chromosome based on DNA hybridization. Am J Hum Genet 1986; 38:109–124.

448. Affara NA, Ferguson-Smith MA, Tolmie J, et al. Variable transfer of Y specific sequence in XX males. Nucleic Acids Res 1986; 14:5375–5387.

449. Muller U, Dunlon T, Schmid M, et al. Deletion mapping of the testis determining locus with DNA probes in 46,XX males and in 46,XY and 46,X,dic(Y) females. Nucleic Acids Res 1986; 14:6489–6505.

450. Seboun E, LeRoy P, Casanova M, et al. A molecular approach to the study of the human Y chromosome and anomalies of sex determination in man. Cold Spring Harbor Symp Quant Biol 1986; 51:237–248.

451. Mardon G, Mosher R, Disteche CM, et al. Duplication, deletion, and polymorphism in the sex-determining region of the mouse Y chromosome. Science 1989; 243:78–80.

452. Werner CA. Mumps orchitis and testicular atrophy. I. Occurrence. Ann Intern Med 1950; 32:1066–1074.

453. Riggs S, Sanford JP. Viral orchitis. N Engl J Med 1962; 266:990–993.

454. Bjorvatn B. Mumps virus recovered from testicles by fine-needle aspiration biopsy in cases of mumps orchitis. Scand J Infect Dis 1973; 5:3–5.

455. Adamopoulos DA, Lawrence DM, Vassilopoulos P, et al. Pituitary testicular interrelationships in mumps orchitis and other viral infections. Br Med J 1978; 1:1177–1180.

456. Aiman J, Brenner PF, MacDonald PC. Androgen and estrogen production in elderly men with gynecomastia and testicular atrophy after mumps orchitis. J Clin Endocrinol Metab 1980; 50:380–386.

457. Werner CA. Mumps orchitis and testicular atrophy. II. A factor in male sterility. Ann Intern Med 1950; 32:1075–1086.

458. Bartak V, Skalova E, Nevarilova A. Spermiogram changes in adults and youngsters after parotitic orchitis. Int J Fertil 1968; 13:226–232.

459. Petersdorf RG, Bennett IL Jr. Treatment of mumps orchitis with adrenal hormones. Report of twenty-three cases with a note on hepatic involvement in mumps. Arch Intern Med 1957; 99:222–233.

460. Wang J, Galil KAA, Setchell BP. Changes in testicular blood flow and testosterone production during aspermatogenesis after irradiation. J Endocrinol 1983; 98:35–46.

461. Oakberg EF. Effects of radiation on the testis. In: Greep RO, Astwood EB, eds. Handbook of Physiology. Sec 7: Endocrinology. Vol V. Male Reproductive System. Washington, DC: American Physiological Society, 1975: 233–243.

462. Shalet SM, Beardwell CG, Jacobs HS, et al. Testicular function following irradiation of the human prepubertal testis. Clin Endocrinol 1978; 9:483–490.

463. Brauner R, Czernichow P, Cramer P, et al. Leydig-cell function in children after direct testicular irradiation for acute lymphoblastic leukemia. N Engl J Med 1983; 309:25–28.

464. Smith CG. Drug effects on male sexual function. Clin Obstet Gynecol 1982; 25:525–531.

465. Lorioux DL, Menard R, Taylor A, et al. Spironolactone and endocrine dysfunction. Ann Intern Med 1976; 85:630–636.

466. Neumann F, van Berswordt-Wallrabe R, Elger W, et al. Aspects of androgen-dependent events as studied by antiandrogens. Recent Prog Horm Res 1970; 26:337–410.

467. Rajfer J, Sikka SC, Rivera F, et al. Mechanism of inhibition of human testicular steroidogenesis by oral ketoconazole. J Clin Endocrinol Metab 1986; 63:1193–1198.

468. Pont A, Graybill Jr, Craven PC, et al. High-dose ketoconazole therapy and adrenal and testicular function in humans. Arch Intern Med 1984; 144:2150–2153.

469. Pulkkinen MO, Mäenpää J. Decrease in serum testosterone concentration during treatment with tetracycline. Acta Endocrinol 1983; 103:269–272.

470. Rodin E, Subramanian MG, Schmalz S, et al. Testosterone levels in adult male epileptic patients. Neurology 1987; 37:706–708.

471. Macphee GJA, Larkin JG, Butler E, et al. Circulating hormones and pituitary responsiveness in young epileptic men receiving long-term antiepileptic medication. Epilepsia 1988; 29:468–475.

472. Cicero TJ. Alcohol-induced deficits in the hypothalamic-pituitary-luteinizing hormone axis in the male. Alcoholism (NY) 1982; 6:207–215.

473. Gordon GG, Altman K, Southern AL, et al. Effect of alcohol (ethanol) administration on sex-hormone metabolism in normal men. N Engl J Med 1976; 295:793–797.

474. Van Thiel DH, Gavaler JS, Lester R, et al. Alcohol-induced testicular atrophy. An experimental model for hypogonadism occurring in chronic alcoholic men. Gastroenterology 1975; 69:326–332.

475. Boyden TW, Silvert MA, Pamenter RW. Chronic ethanol feeding impairs human chorionic gonadotropin–stimulated testicular testosterone responses of dogs. Biol Reprod 1982; 27:652–657.

476. Gordon GG, Vittek J, Southern AL, et al. Effect of chronic alcohol ingestion on the biosynthesis of steroids in rat testicular homogenate in vitro. Endocrinology 1980; 106:1880–1885.

477. Van Thiel DH, Cobb CF, Herman GB, et al. An examination of various mechanisms for ethanol-induced testicular injury: studies utilizing the isolated perfused rat testes. Endocrinology 1981; 109:2009–2015.

478. Anderson RA Jr, Reddy JM, Joyce C, et al. Inhibition of mouse sperm capacitation by ethanol. Biol Reprod 1982; 27:833–840.

479. Anderson RA Jr, Willis BR, Oswald C, et al. Ethanol-induced male infertility: impairment of spermatozoa. J Pharmacol Exp Ther 1983; 225:479–486.

480. Sherins RJ, Olweny CLM, Med M, et al. Gynecomastia and gonadal dysfunction in adolescent boys treated with combination chemotherapy for Hodgkin's disease. N Engl J Med 1978; 229:12–16.

481. Whitehead E, Shalet M, Blackledge G, et al. The effects of Hodgkin's disease and combination chemotherapy on gonadal function of the adult male. Cancer 1982; 49:418–422.

482. Chapman RM, Rees LH, Sutcliff SB, et al. Cyclical combination chemotherapy and gonadal function. Lancet 1979; 1:285–289.

483. Blatt J, Poplack DG, Sherins RJ. Testicular function in boys after chemotherapy for acute lymphoblastic leukemia. N Engl J Med 1981; 304:1121–1124.

484. Kolodny RC, Masters WH, Kolodner RM, et al. Depression of plasma testosterone levels after chronic intensive marihuana use. N Engl J Med 1974; 290:872–874.

485. Wang C, Chan V, Yeung RTT. The effect of heroin addiction on pituitary-testicular function. Clin Endocrinol 1978; 9:455–461.

486. Mendelson JH, Mendelson JE, Patch VD. Plasma testosterone levels in heroin addiction and during methadone maintenance. J Pharmacol Exp Ther 1975; 192:211–217.

487. Dalterio S, Bartke A, Burstein S. Cannabinoids inhibit tetosterone secretion by mouse testes in vitro. Science 1977; 196:1472–1473.

488. Dalterio S, Bartke A, Roberson C, et al. Direct and pituitary-mediated effects of Δ^9-THC and cannabinol on the testis. Pharmacol Biochem Behav 1977; 8:673–678.

489. Tyrey L. Δ^9-Tetrahydrocannabinol: a potent inhibitor of episodic luteinizing hormone secretion. J Pharmacol Exp Ther 1980; 213:306–308.

490. Hong CY, Chaput de Saintonge DM, Turner P. Δ^9-Tetrahydrocannabinol inhibits human sperm motility. J Pharm Pharmacol 1981; 33:746–747.

491. Stoffer SS, Mynes KM, Jiang N-S, et al. Digoxin and abnormal serum hormone levels. JAMA 1973; 225:1643–1644.

492. Geller J, Fruchtman B, Meyer C, et al. Effect of progestational agents on gonadal and adrenal cortical function in patients with benign prostatic hypertrophy and carcinoma of the prostate. J Clin Endocrinol Metab 1967; 27:556–560.

493. Blumer D, Migeon C. Hormone and hormonal agents in the treatment of aggression. J Nerv Ment Dis 1975; 160:127–137.

494. Bixler EO, Santen RJ, Kales A, et al. Inverse effects of thioridazine (Mellaril) on serum prolactin and testosterone concentrations in normal men. In: Troen P, Nankin HR, eds. The Testis in Normal and Infertile Men. New York: Raven, 1977: 403–408.

495. Rosenthal SM, Grumbach MM. Gonadotropin-independent familial sexual precocity with premature Leydig and germinal cell maturation (familial testotoxicosis): effects of a potent luteinizing hormone–releasing factor agonist and medroxyprogesterone acetate therapy in four cases. J Clin Endocrinol Metab 1983; 57:571–579.

496. Van Thiel DH, Gavaler JS, Smith WI Jr, et al. Hypothalamic-pituitary-gonadal dysfunction in men using cimetidine. N Engl J Med 1979; 300:1012–1015.

497. Funder JW, Mercer JE. Cimetidine, a histamine H_2 receptor antagonist, occupies androgen receptors. J Clin Endocrinol Metab 1979; 48:189–191.

498. Peden NR, Boyd EJS, Browning MCK, et al. Effects of two histamine H_2-receptor blocking drugs on basal levels of gonadotrophins, prolactin, testosterone and oestradiol-17β during treatment of duodenal ulcer in male patients. Acta Endocrinol 1981; 96:564–568.

499. Rodamilans M, Osaba MJM, To-Figueras J, et al. Lead toxicity on endocrine testicular function in an occupationally exposed population. Hum Toxicol 1988; 7:125–128.

500. Sokol RZ, Mading CE, Swerdolff R. Lead toxicity and the hypothalamic-pituitary-testicular axis. Biol Reprod 1985; 33:722–728.

501. Murthy GG, Peress NS, Khan SA. Demonstration of antibodies to testicular basement membrane by immunofluorescence in a patient with multiple primary endocrine deficiencies. J Clin Endocrinol Metab 1976; 42:637–641.

502. Elder M, Maclaren N, Riley W. Gonadal autoantibodies in patients with hypogonadism and/or Addison's disease. J Clin Endocrinol Metab 1981; 52:1137–1142.

503. Morley JE, Distiller LA, Sagel J, et al. Hormonal changes associated with testicular atrophy and gynaecomastia in patients with leprosy. Clin Endocrinol 1977; 6:299–303.

504. Sherman FP. Impotence in patients with chronic renal failure on dialysis: its frequency and etiology. Fertil Steril 1975; 26:221–223.

505. de Kretser DM, Atkins RC, Hudson B, et al. Disordered spermatogenesis in patients with chronic renal failure undergoing maintenance haemodialysis. Aust NZ J Med 1974; 4:178–181.

506. Holdsworth S, Atkins RC, de Kretser D. The pituitary-testicular axis in men with chronic renal failure. N Engl J Med 1977; 296:1245–1249.

507. Stewart-Bentley M, Gans D, Horton R. Regulation of gonadal function in uremia. Metabolism 1974; 23:1065–1072.

508. Lim VS, Fang VS. Gonadal dysfunction in uremic men. A study of the hypothalamo-pituitary-testicular axis before and after renal transplantation. Am J Med 1975; 58:655–662.

509. Rager K, Bundschu H, Gupta D. The effect of hCG on testicular androgen production in adult men with chronic renal failure. J Reprod Fertil 1975; 42:113–120.

510. Briefel GR, Tsitouras PD, Kowatch MA, et al. Decreased in vitro testosterone production by isolated Leydig cells from uremic rats. Endocrinology 1982; 110:976–981.

511. Mahajan Sk, Prasad AS, Rabbani P, et al. Zinc metabolism in uremia. J Lab Clin Med 1979; 94:693–698.

512. Mahajan SK, Abbasi AA, Prasad AS, et al. Effect of oral zinc therapy on gonadal function in hemodialysis patients. Ann Intern Med 1982; 97:357–361.

513. Lim VS, Fang VS. Restoration of plasma testosterone levels in uremic men with clomiphene citrate. J Clin Endocrinol Metab 1976; 43:1370–1377.

514. Gomez F, de la Cueva R, Wauters J-P, et al. Endocrine abnormalities in patients undergoing long-term hemodialysis. The role of prolactin. Am J Med 1980; 68:522–530.

515. Vircburger MI, Prelevic GM, Peric LA, et al. Testosterone levels after bromocriptine treatment in patients undergoing long-term hemodialysis. J Androl 1985; 6:113–116.

516. Holdsworth SR, de Kretser DM, Atkins RC. A comparison of hemodialysis and transplantation in reversing the uremic disturbance of male reproductive function. Clin Nephrol 1978; 10:146–150.

517. Chopp RT, Mendez R. Sexual function and hormonal abnormalities in uremic men on chronic dialysis and after renal transplantation. Fertil Steril 1978; 29:661–666.

518. Baker HWG, Burger HG, de Kretser DM, et al. A study of the endocrine manifestations of hepatic cirrhosis. Q J Med 1976; 45:145–178.

519. Chopra IJ, Tulchinsky D, Greenway FL. Estrogen-androgen imbalance in hepatic cirrhosis. Studies in 13 male patients. Ann Intern Med 1973; 79:198–203.

520. Gordon GG, Olivo J, Rafii F, et al. Conversion of androgens to estrogens in cirrhosis of the liver. J Clin Endocrinol Metab 1975; 40:1018–1026.

521. Van Thiel DH, Lester R, Sherins RJ. Hypogonadism in alcoholic liver disease: evidence for a double defect. Gastroenterology 1974; 67:1188–1199.

522. Distiller LA, Sagel J, Dubowitz B, et al. Pituitary-gonadal function in men with alcoholic cirrhosis of the liver. Horm Metab Res 1976; 8:461–465.

523. Van Thiel DH, McClain CJ, Elson MK, et al. Evidence for autonomous secretion of prolactin in some alcoholic men with cirrhosis and gynecomastia. Metabolism 1978; 27:1778–1784.

524. Kley HK, Strohmeyer G, Krüskemper HL. Effect of testosterone application on hormone concentrations of androgens and estrogens in male patients with cirrhosis of the liver. Gastroenterology 1979; 76:235–241.

525. Gluud C, Bennett P, Dietrichson O, et al. Short-term parenteral and peroral testosterone administration in men with alcoholic cirrhosis. Scand J Gastroenterol 1981; 16:749–755.

526. Van Thiel DH, Gavaler JS, Sanghvi A. Recovery of sexual function in abstinent alcoholic men. Gastroenterology 1982; 84:677–682.

527. Olambiwonnu NO, Penny R, Frasier SD. Sexual maturation in subjects with sickle cell anemia: studies of serum gonadotropin concentration, height, weight, and skeletal age. J Pediatr 1975; 87:459–464.

528. Abbasi AA, Prasad AS, Ortega J, et al. Gonadal function abnormalities in sickle cell anemia. Studies in adult male patients. Ann Intern Med 1976; 85:601–605.

529. Landefeld CS, Schambelan M, Kaplan SL, et al. Clomiphene-responsive hypogonadism in sickle cell anemia. Ann Intern Med 1983; 99:480–483.

530. Smith SR, Chhetri MK, Johanson AJ, et al. The pituitary-gonadal axis in men with protein-calorie malnutrition. J Clin Endocrinol Metab 1975; 41:60–69.

531. Vigersky RA, Chapman RM, Berenberg J, et al. Testicular dysfunction in untreated Hodgkin's disease. Am J Med 1982; 73:482–486.

532. Chlebowski RT, Heber D. Hypogonadism in male patients with metastatic cancer prior to chemotherapy. Cancer Res 1982; 42:2495–2498.

533. Landon C, Rosenfeld RG. Short stature and pubertal delay in male adolescents with cystic fibrosis. Androgen treatment. Am J Dis Child 1984; 138:388–391.

534. Handelsman DJ, Yue DK, Turtle JR. Hypogonadism and massive testicular infiltration due to amyloidosis. J Urol 1983; 129:610–612.

535. Chopra IJ, Hershman JM, Pardridge WM, et al. Thyroid function in nonthyroidal illnesses. Ann Intern Med 1983; 98:946–957.

536. Goussis OS, Pardridge WM, Judd HL. Critical illness and low testosterone: effects of human serum on testosterone transport into rat brain and liver. J Clin Endocrinol Metab 1983; 56:710–714.

537. Glass AR, Smith CE, Kidd GS, et al. Response of the hypothalamic-pituitary-testicular axis to surgery. Fertil Steril 1978; 30:560–563.

538. Wang C, Chan V, Yeung RTT. Effect of surgical stress on pituitary-testicular function. Clin Endocrinol 1978; 9:255–266.

539. Wang C, Chan V, Tse TF, et al. Effect of acute myocardial infarction on pituitary-testicular function. Clin Endocrinol 1978; 9:249–253.

540. Vogel AV, Peake GT, Rada RT. Pituitary-testicular axis dysfunction in burned men. J Clin Endocrinol Metab 1985; 60:658–664.

541. Lephart ED, Baxter CR, Parker CR Jr. Effect of burn trauma on adrenal and testicular steroid hormone production. J Clin Endocrinol Metab 1987; 64:842–848.

542. Kidd GS, Glass AR, Vigersky RA. The hypothalamic-pituitary-testicular axis in thyrotoxicosis. J Clin Endocrinol Metab 1979; 48:798–802.

543. Sagel J, Distiller LA, Morley JE, et al. Myotonia dystrophica: studies on gonadal function using luteinizing hormone–releasing hormone (LRH). J Clin Endocrinol Metab 1975; 40:1110–1113.

544. Febres F, Scaglia H, Lisker R, et al. Hypothalamic-pituitary-gonadal function in patients with myotonic dystrophy. J Clin Endocrinol Metab 1975; 41:833–840.

545. Takeda R, Ueda M. Pituitary-gonadal function in male patients with myotonic dystrophy—serum luteinizing hormone, follicle stimulating hormone and testosterone levels and histological damage of the testis. Acta Endocrinol 1977; 84:382–389.

546. Claus-Walker J, Scurry M, Carter RE, et al. Steady state hormonal secretion in traumatic quadriplegia. J Clin Endocrinol Metab 1977; 44:530–535.

547. Cortes-Gallegos V, Castaneda G, Alonso R, et al. Diurnal variations of pituitary and testicular hormones in paraplegic men. Arch Androl 1982; 8:221–226.

548. Piera JB. The establishment of a prognosis for genito-sexual function in the paraplegic and tetraplegic male. Paraplegia 1973; 10:271–278.

549. Hasen J, Boyar RM, Shapiro LR. Gonadal function in trisomy 21. Horm Res 1980; 12:345–350.

550. Aiman J, Griffin JE, Gazak JM, et al. Androgen insensitivity as a cause of infertility in otherwise normal men. N Engl J Med 1979; 330:223–227.

551. Aiman J, Griffin JE. The frequency of androgen receptor deficiency in infertile men. J Clin Endocrinol Metab 1982; 54:725–732.

552. Grino PB, Griffin JE, Cushard WG, et al. A mutation of the androgen receptor associated with partial androgen resistance, familial gynecomastia, and fertility. J Clin Endocrinol Metab 1988; 66:754–761.

553. Pinsky L, Kaufman M, Killinger DW. Impaired spermatogenesis is not an obligate expression of receptor-defective androgen resistance. J Med Genet 1989; 32:100–104.

554. Mozaffarian GA, Higley M, Paulsen CA. Clinical studies in an adult male patient with "isolated follicle stimulating hormone (FSH) deficiency." J Androl 1983; 4:393–398.

555. Segal S, Polishuk WZ, Ben-David M. Hyperprolactinemic male infertility. Fertil Steril 1976; 27:1425–1427.

556. Bonaccorsi AC, Adler I, Figueiredo JG. Male infertility due to congenital adrenal hyperplasia: testicular biopsy findings, hormonal evaluation, and theapeutic results in three patients. Fertil Steril 1987; 47:664–670.

557. Schürmeyer T, Belkien L, Knuth UA, et al. Reversible azoospermia induced by the anabolic steroid 19-nortestosterone. Lancet 1984; 1:417–420.

558. Rothman CM, Sims CA, Stotts CL. Sertoli cell only syndrome 1982. Fertil Steril 1982; 38:388–390.

559. Ishida H, Isurugi K, Aso Y, et al. Endocrine studies in Sertoli-cell-only syndrome. J Urol 1976; 116:56–58.

560. Edwards JA, Bannerman RM. Familial gynecomastia. Birth Defects 1971; 7:193–195.

561. de Kretser DM, Burger HG, Fortune D, et al. Hormonal, histological and chromosomal studies in adult males with testicular disorders. J Clin Endocrinol Metab 1972; 35:392–401.

562. Jones TM, Amarose AP, Lebowitz M. Testicular chromosomal mosaicism and infertility. J Clin Endocrinol Metab 1976; 42:888–893.

563. Viguie F, Romani F, Dadoune JP. Male infertility in a case of (Y;6) balanced reciprocal translocation. Mitotic and meiotic study. Hum Genet 1982; 62:225–227.

564. Chaganti RSK, German J. Human male infertility, probably genetically determined, due to defective meiosis and spermatogenic arrest. Am J Hum Genet 1979; 31:634–641.

565. Chaganti RSK, Jhanwar SC, German J. Genetically determined asynapsis, spermatogenic degeneration, and infertility in men. Am J Hum Genet 1980; 32:833–848.

566. Reame NE, Hafez ESE. Hereditary defects affecting fertility. N Engl J Med 1975; 292:675–681.

567. Greenberg SH, Lipshultz LI, Wein AJ. Experience with 425 subfertile male patients. J Urol 1978; 119:507–510.

568. Turner TT. Varicocele: still an enigma. J Urol 1983; 129:695–699.

569. Rodriguez-Rigau LJ, Steinberger E. Varicocele and the morphology of spermatozoa. Fertil Steril 1981; 35:54–57.

570. Fariss BL, Fenner DK, Plymate SR, et al. Seminal characteristics in the presence of a varicocele as compared with those of expectant fathers and prevasectomy men. Fertil Steril 1981; 35:325–327.

571. Mieusset R, Bujan L, Mondinat C, et al. Association of scrotal hyperthermia with impaired spermatogenesis in infertile men. Fertil Steril 1987; 48:1006–1011.

572. Zorgniotti AW, Sealfon AI. Measurement of intrascrotal temperature in normal and subfertile men. J Reprod Fertil 1988; 82:563–566.

573. Saypol DC, Howards SS, Turner TT, et al. Influence of surgically induced varicocele on testicular blood flow, temperature, and histology in adult rats and dogs. J Clin Invest 1981; 68:39–45.

574. Dubin L, Amelar RD. Varicocelectomy: 986 cases in a twelve-year study. Urology 1977; 10:446–449.

575. Pedersen H, Hammen R. Ultrastructure of human spermatozoa with complete subcellular derangement. Arch Androl 1982; 9:251–259.

576. Cassell GH, Younger JB, Brown MB, et al. Microbiologic study of infertile women at the time of diagnostic laparoscopy. N Engl J Med 1983; 308:502–505.

577. Toth A, Lesser ML, Brooks C, et al. Subsequent pregnancies among 161 couples treated for T-mycoplasma genital-tract infection. N Engl J Med 1983; 308:505–507.

578. Hahn EW, Feingold SM, Nisce L. Aspermia and recovery of spermatogenesis in cancer patients following incidental gonadal irradiation during treatment: a progress report. Radiology 1976; 119:223–225.

579. Shapiro E, Kinsella TJ, Makuch RW, et al. Effects of fractionated irradiation on endocrine aspects of testicular function. J Clin Oncol 1985; 3:1232–1239.

580. Asbjornsen G, Molne K, Klepp O, et al. Testicular function after radiotherapy to inverted "Y" field for malignant lymphoma. Scand J Haematol 1976; 17:96–100.

581. Handelsman DJ, Turtle JR. Testicular damage after radioactive iodine (I-131) therapy for thyroid cancer. Clin Endocrinol 1983; 18:465–472.

582. Schilsky RL, Sherins RJ. Gonadal dysfunction. In: DeVita VT Jr, Hellman S, Rosenberg SA, eds. Cancer: Principles and Practice of Oncology. Vol 2. Philadelphia: J. B. Lippincott, 1985: 2032–2039.

583. Watson AR, Rance CP, Bain J. Long term effects of cyclophosphamide on testicular function. Br Med J 1985; 291:1457–1460.

584. Tsatsoulis A, Whitehead E, St. John J, et al. The pituitary–Leydig cell axis in men with severe damage to the germinal epithelium. Clin Endocrinol 1987; 27:683–689.

585. Buchanan JD, Fairley KF, Barrie JU. Return of spermatogenesis after stopping cyclophosphamide therapy. Lancet 1975; 2:156–157.

586. Santoro A, Viviani S, Zucali R, et al. Comparative results and toxicity of MOPP vs ABVD combined with radiotherapy in PS IIB, III Hodgkin's disease. Proc Am Soc Clin Oncol 1983; 2:223 (abstract).

587. Drasga RE, Einhorn LH, Williams SD, et al. Fertility after chemotherapy for testicular cancer. J Clin Oncol 1983; 1:179–183.

588. Birnie GG, McLeod TIF, Watkinson G. Incidence of sulphasalazine-induced male infertility. Gut 1981; 22:452–455.

589. Whorton MD. Male occupational reproductive hazards. West J Med 1982; 137:521–524.

590. Bush B, Bennett AH, Snow JT. Polychlorobiphenyl congeners, p,p'-DDE, and sperm function in humans. Arch Environ Contam Toxicol 1986; 15:334–341.

591. Dwivedi C. Cadmium-induced sterility: possible involvement of the cholinergic system. Arch Environ Contam Toxicol 1983; 12:151–156.

592. Assennato G, Paci C, Baser ME, et al. Sperm count suppression without endocrine dysfunction in lead-exposed men. Arch Environ Health 1986; 41:387–390.

593. Lancranjan I, Maicanescu M, Rafaila E, et al. Gonadic function in workmen with long-term exposure to microwaves. Health Phys 1975; 29:381–383.

594. Fahim MS, Fahim Z, Harman J, et al. Ultrasound as a new method of male contraception. Fertil Steril 1977; 28:823–831.

595. Salomon F, Saremaslani P, Jakob M, et al. Immune complex orchitis in infertile men. Immunoelectron microscopy of abnormal basement membrane structures. Lab Invest 1982; 47:555–567.

596. Bronson R, Cooper G, Rosenfeld D. Sperm antibodies: their role in infertility. Fertil Steril 1984; 42:171–183.

597. Haas GG Jr. Antibody-mediated causes of male infertility. Urol Clin North Am 1987; 14:539–550.

598. Mathur S, Baker ER, Williamson HO, et al. Clinical significance of sperm antibodies in infertility. Fertil Steril 1981; 36:486–495.

599. Phadke AM, Padukone K. Presence and significance of autoantibodies against spermatozoa in the blood of men with obstructed vas deferens. J Reprod Fertil 1964; 7:163–170.

600. Hendry WF, Parslow JM, Stedronska J, et al. The diagnosis of unilateral testicular obstruction in subfertile males. Br J Urol 1982; 54:774–779.

601. Ansbacher R. Vasectomy: sperm antibodies. Fertil Steril 1973; 24:788–792.

602. Green JRB, Goble HL, Edwards CRW, et al. Reversible insensitivity to androgens in men with untreated gluten enteropathy. Lancet 1977; 1:280–282.

603. Farthing MJG, Edwards CRW, Rees LH, et al. Male gonadal function in coeliac disease: 1. Sexual dysfunction, infertility, and semen quality. Gut 1982; 23:608–614.

604. Farthing MJG, Rees LH, Boylan LM, et al. Male gonadal function in coeliac disease: 2. Sex hormones. Gut 1983; 24:127–135.

605. Morrow AF, Gyorki S, Warne GL, et al. Variable androgen receptor levels in infertile men. J Clin Endocrinol Metab 1987; 64:1115–1121.

606. Handelsman DJ, Conway AJ, Boylan LM, et al. Young's syndrome. Obstructive azoospermia and chronic sinopulmonary infections. N Engl J Med 1984; 310:3–9.

607. Sharlip ID. Obstructive azoospermia or oligozoospermia due to müllerian duct cyst. Fertil Steril 1983; 39:435–436.

608. Sivanesaratnam V. Male infertility due to absence of vas deferens. Eur J Obstet Gynecol Reprod Biol 1982; 14:31–35.

609. Holsclaw DS, Perlmutter AD, Jockin H, et al. Genital abnormalities in male patients with cystic fibrosis. J Urol 1971; 106:568–574.

610. Gill WB, Schumacher FGB, Bibbo M. Pathological semen and anatomical abnormalities of the genital tract in human male subjects exposed to diethylstilbestrol in utero. J Urol 1977; 117:477–480.

611. McClure RD, Hricak H. Magnetic resonance imaging: its application to male infertility. Urology 1986; 27:91–98.

612. Hendry WF, Parslow JM, Stedronska J. Exploratory scrototomy in 168 azoospermic males. Br J Urol 1983; 55:785–791.

613. Baker HWG, Burger HG, de Kretser DM, et al. Relative incidence of etiological disorders in male infertility. In: Santen RJ, Swerdloff RS, eds. Male Reproductive Dysfunction: Diagnosis and Management of Hypogonadism, Infertility and Impotence. New York: Marcel Dekker, 1986: 341–372.

614. Gross KM, Matsumoto AM, Southworth MB, et al. Evidence for decreased luteinizing hormone–releasing hormone pulse frequency in men with selective elevations of follicle-stimulating hormone. J Clin Endocrinol Metab 1985; 60:197–202.

615. Gross KM, Matsumoto AM, Berger RE, et al. Increased frequency of pulsatile luteinizing hormone–releasing hormone administration selectively decreases follicle-stimulating hormone levels in men with idiopathic azoospermia. Fertil Steril 1986; 45:392–396.

616. Hönigl W, Knuth UA, Nieschlag E. Selective reduction of elevated FSH levels in infertile men by pulsatile LHRH treatment. Clin Endocrinol 1986; 24:177–182.

617. Booth JD, Merriam GR, Clark RV, et al. Evidence for Leydig cell dysfunction in infertile men with a selective increase in plasma follicle-stimulating hormone. J Clin Endocrinol Metab 1987; 64:1194–1198.

618. Collins JA, Wrixon W, Janes LB, et al. Treatment-independent pregnancy among infertile couples. N Engl J Med 1983; 309:1201–1205.

619. Baker HWG. Male infertility of undetermined etiology. In: Krieger DT, Bardin CW, eds. Current Therapy in Endocrinology 1983–1984. Philadelphia: B. C. Decker, 1983: 366–371.

620. Kerin JF, Peek J, Warnes GM, et al. Improved conception rate after intrauterine insemination of washed spermatozoa from men with poor quality semen. Lancet 1984; 1:533–535.

621. Yates CA, de Kretser DM. Male-factor infertility and in vitro fertilization. J In Vitro Fert Embryo Transfer 1987; 4:141–147.

622. Walsh PC. Benign prostatic hyperplasia. In: Walsh PC, Gittes RF, Perlmutter AD, et al., eds. Campbell's Urology. 5th ed. Philadelphia: W. B. Saunders, 1986: 1248–1265.

623. Wilson JD. The pathogenesis of benign prostatic hyperplasia. Am J Med 1980; 68:745–756.

624. Horton R. Benign prostatic hyperplasia: a disorder of androgen metabolism in the male. Am J Nephrol 1982; 2:157–163.

625. Wenderoth UK, George FW, Wilson JD. The effect of a 5α-reductase inhibitor on androgen-mediated growth of the dog prostate. Endocrinology 1983; 113:569–573.

626. Liang T, Hiss CE. Inhibition of 5α-reductase, receptor binding, and nuclear uptake of androgens in the prostate by a 4-methyl-4-aza-steroid. J Biol Chem 1981; 256:7998–8005.

627. Brooks JR, Berman C, Glitzer MS, et al. Effect of a new 5α-reductase inhibitor on size, histological characteristics and androgen concentrations of the canine prostate. Prostate 1982; 3:35–44.

628. Siiteri PK, Wilson JD. Dihydrotestosterone in prostatic hypertrophy. I. The formtion and content of dihydrotestosterone in the hypertrophic prostate of man. J Clin Invest 1970; 49:1737–1745.

629. Hammond GL. Endogenous steroid levels in the human prostate from birth to old age: a comparison of normal and diseased tissues. J Endocrinol 1978; 78:7–19.

630. Walsh PC, Hutchins GM, Ewing LL. Tissue content of dihydrotestosterone in human prostatic hyperplasia is not supranormal. J Clin Invest 1983; 72:1772–1777.

631. Walsh PC, Wilson JD. The induction of prostatic hypertrophy in the dog with androstanediol. J Clin Invest 1976; 57:1093–1097.

632. Aumüller G, Funke PJ, Hahn A, et al. Phenotypic modulation of the canine prostate after long-term treatment with androgens and estrogens. Prostate 1982; 3:361–373.

633. Peters CA, Walsh PC. The effect of nafarelin acetate, a luteinizing-hormone–releasing hormone agonist, on benign prostatic hyperplasia. N Eng J Med 1987; 317:599–604.

634. Gabrilove JL, Levine AC, Kirschenbaum A, et al. Effect of a GnRH analogue (leuprolide) on benign prostatic hypertrophy. J Clin Endocrinol Metab 1987; 64:1331–1333.

635. McConnell JD, Wilson JD, George FW, et al. An inhibitor of 5α-reductase, MK-906, suppresses prostatic dihydrotestosterone in men with benign prostatic hyperplasia. J Urol 1989; 141:239A.

636. Geller J, Albert J, Geller S. Acute therapy with megestrol acetate decreases nuclear and cytosol androgen receptors in human BPH tissue. Prostate 1982; 3:11–15.

637. Petrangeli E, Sciarra F, Di Silverio F, et al. Effects of two different medical treatments on dihydrotestosterone content and androgen receptors in human benign prostatic hyperplasia. J Steroid Biochem 1988; 30:395–399.

638. Kaplan JH, Kudish HG, Sacks SA. Testicular tumors of germ cell origin. I. Epidemiology, pathogenesis, clinical presentation, and diagnosis. Postgrad Med 1981; 70:114–121.

639. Morse MJ, Whitmore WF. Neoplasms of the testis. In: Walsh PC, Gittes RF, Perlmutter AD, et al., eds. Campbell's Urology. 5th ed. Philadelphia: W. B. Saunders, 1986: 1535–1582.

640. Hainsworth JD, Greco FA. Testicular germ cell neoplasms. Am J Med 1983; 75:817–832.

641. Lefevre RE, Levin HS, Banowsky LH, et al. Bilateral testicular tumors of germ cell origin. J Urol 1975; 114:556–559.

642. Fonger JD, Filler RM, Rider WD, et al. Testicular tumors in maldescended testes. Can J Surg 1981; 24:353–355.

643. Henderson BE, Benton B, Jing J, et al. Risk factors for cancer of the testis in young men. Int J Cancer 1979; 23:598–602.

644. Schellhas HF. Malignant potential of the dysgenetic gonad. Part I. Obstet Gynecol 1974; 44:298–309.

645. Shellhas HF. Malignant potential of the dysgenetic gonad. Part II. Obstet Gynecol 1974; 44:455–462.

646. Manuel M, Katayama KP, Jones HW Jr. The age of occurrence of gonadal tumors in intersex patients with a Y chromosome. Am J Obstet Gynecol 1976; 24:293–300.

647. Simpson JL, Photopulos G. The relationship of neoplasia to disorders of abnormal sexual differentiation. Birth Defects 1976; 12:15–50.

648. Carroll PR, Morse J, Koduru PPK, et al. Testicular germ cell tumor in patient with Klinefelter syndrome. Urology 1988; 31:72–74.

649. Kirkland RT, Kirkland JL, Keenan BS. Bilateral testicular tumors in congenital adrenal hyperplasia. J Clin Endocrinol Metab 1977; 44:369–378.

650. Kadair RG, Block MB, Katz FH, et al. "Masked" 21-hydroxylase deficiency of the adrenal presenting with gynecomastia and bilateral testicular masses. Am J Med 1977; 62:278–282.

651. Newell ME, Lippe BM, Ehrlich RM. Testis tumors associated with congenital adrenal hyperplasia: a continuing diagnostic and therapeutic dilemma. J Urol 1977; 117:256–258.

652. Bosl GJ, Vogelzang NJ, Goldman A, et al. Impact of delay in diagnosis on clinical stage of testicular cancer. Lancet 1981; 2:970–973.

653. Mostofi FK. Pathology of germ cell tumors of testis: a progress report. Cancer 1980; 45:1735–1754.

654. Marshall AHE, Dayan AD. An immune reaction in man against seminomas, dysgerminomas, pinealomas, and the mediastinal tumours of similar histological appearance? Lancet 1964; 2:1102–1104.

655. Scully RE. Gonadoblastoma: a review of 74 cases. Cancer 1970; 25:1340–1356.

656. Besznyak I, Sebesteny M, Kuchar F. Primary mediastinal seminoma. A case report and review of literature. J Thorac Cardiovasc Surg 1973; 65:930–934.

657. Luna MA, Valenzuela-Tamariz J. Germ-cell tumors of the mediastinum, postmortem findings. Am J Clin Pathol 1976; 65:450–454.

658. Bush SE, Martinez A, Bagshaw MA. Primary mediastinal seminoma. Cancer 1981; 48:1877–1882.

659. Raghavan D, Barrett A. Mediastinal seminomas. Cancer 1980; 46:1187–1191.

660. Mukai K, Adams WR. Yolk sac tumor of the anterior mediastinum. Am J Surg Pathol 1979; 3:77–83.

661. Chang CG, Kageyama N, Kobayashi T, et al. Pineal tumors: clinical diagnosis, with special emphasis on the significance of pineal calcification. Neurosurgery 1981; 8:656–668.

662. Kirshner JJ, Ginsberg SJ, Fitzpatrick AV, et al. Treatment of a primary intracranial germ cell tumor with systemic chemotherapy. Med Pediatr Oncol 1981; 9:361–365.

663. Kobayashi T, Kageyama N, Kida Y, et al. Unilateral germinomas involving the basal ganglia and thalamus. J Neurosurg 1981; 55:55–62.

664. Koide O, Iwai S. An ultrastructural study on germinoma cells. Acta Pathol Jpn 1981; 31:755–766.

665. Ellis M, Sikora K. The current management of testicular cancer. Br J Urol 1987; 59:2–9.

666. Braunstein GD, Rasor J, Wade ME. Presence in normal human testes of a chorionic-gonadotropin–like substance distinct from human luteinizing hormone. N Engl J Med 1975; 293:1339–1343.

667. Keogh B, Hreshchyshyn MM, Moore RH, et al. Urinary gonadotropins in management and prognosis of testicular tumor. Urology 1975; 5:496–503.

668. Cochran JS, Walsh PC, Porter JC, et al. The endocrinology of human chorionic gonadotropin–secreting testicular tumors: new methods in diagnosis. J Urol 1975; 114:549–555.

669. Masopust J, Kithier K, Radl J, et al. Occurence of fetoprotein in patients with neoplasms and non-neoplastic diseases. Int J Cancer 1968; 3:364–373.

670. Talerman A. Endodermal sinus (yolk sac) tumor elements in testicular germ-cell tumors in adults. Cancer 1980; 46:1213–1217.

671. Javadpour N. The role of biologic tumor markers in testicular cancer. Cancer 1980; 45:1755–1761.

672. Szymendera JJ, Zborzil J, Sikorowa L, et al. Value of five tumor markers (AFP, CEA, hCG, hPL, and SP₁) in diagnosis and staging of testicular germ cell tumors. Oncology 1981; 38:222–229.

673. Willemse PHB, Sleijfer DT, Koops HS, et al. Tumor markers in patients with non-seminomatous germ cell tumors of the testis. Oncodev Biol Med 1981; 2:117–128.

674. Willemse PHB, Sleijfer DT, Koops HS, et al. The value of AFP and hCG half-lives in predicting the efficacy of combination chemotherapy in patients with non-seminomatous germ cell tumors of the testis. Oncodev Biol Med 1981; 2:129–134.

675. Lange PH, McIntire KR, Waldmann TA, et al. Serum alpha fetoprotein and human chorionic gonadotropin in the diagnosis and management of non-seminomatous germ-cell testicular cancer. N Engl J Med 1976; 295:1237–1240.

676. Bosl GJ, Geller NL, Cirrincione C, et al. Serum tumor markers in patients with metastatic germ cell tumors of the testis. Am J Med 1983; 75:29–35.

677. Bosl GJ, Geller N, Cirrincione C, et al. Interrelationships of histopathology and other clinical variables in patients with germ cell tumors of the testis. Cancer 1983; 51:2121–2125.

678. Aiginger P, Kolbe H, Kühböck J, et al. The endocrinology of testicular germinal cell tumors. Acta Endocrinol 1981; 97:419–426.

679. Raghavan D, Vogelzang NJ, Bosl GJ, et al. Tumor classification and size in germ-cell testicular cancer. Cancer 1982; 50:1591–1595.

680. Donohue JP. Selecting initial therapy: seminoma and nonseminoma. Cancer 1987; 60:490–495.

681. Bergmann KA. Current concepts in clinical therapeutics: testicular cancer. Clin Pharm 1987; 6:693–706.

682. Bey P, Guillemin F, Malissard L, et al. Testicular seminomas: study of relapses and causes of death in a series of 86 patients. In: Khoury S, Kuss R, Murphy GP, et al., eds. Testicular Cancer. New York: Alan R. Liss, 1985: 493–498.

683. Fraley EE, Lange PH, Kennedy BJ. Germ-cell testicular cancer in adults. N Engl J Med 1979; 301:1370–1377.

684. Li FP, Connelly RR, Myers M. Improved survival rates among testis cancer patients in the United States. JAMA 1982; 247:825–826.

685. Reed E, Sanger WG, Armitage JO. Results of semen cryopreservation in young men with testicular carcinoma and lymphoma. J Clin Oncol 1986; 4:537–539.

686. Freeman DA. Steroid hormone–producing tumors in man. Endocr Rev 1986; 7:204–220.

687. Gabrilove JL, Nicolis GL, Mitty HA, et al. Feminizing interstitial cell tumor of the testis: personal observations and a review of the literature. Cancer 1975; 35:1184–1202.

688. Gabrilove JL, Freiberg EK, Leiter E, et al. Feminizing and non-feminizing Sertoli cell tumors. J Urol 1980; 124:757–767.

689. Junkmann K. Long-acting steroids in reproduction. Recent Prog Horm Res 1957; 13:389–419.

690. James KC, Nicholls PJ, Roberts M. Biological half-lives of [4-

691. Honrath WL, Wolff A, Meli A. The influence of the amount of solvent (sesame oil) on the degree and duration of action of subcutaneously administered testosterone and its propionate. Steroids 1963; 2:425–428.

692. Snyder PJ, Lawrence DA. Treatment of male hypogonadism with testosterone enanthate. J Clin Endocrinol Metab 1980; 51:1335–1339.

693. Mauss J, Borsch G, Bormacher K, et al. Effect of long-term testosterone oenanthate administration on male reproductive function: clinical evaluation, serum FSH, LH, testosterone, and seminal fluid analyses in normal men. Acta Endocrinol 1975; 78:373–384.

694. Nieschlag E. Current status of testosterone substitution therapy. Int J Androl 1982; 5:225–228.

695. Sokol RZ, Saul C, Campfield LA, et al. Testosterone enanthate kinetics: compartmental modeling. Fertil Steril 1981; 36:428 (abstract).

696. Gooren LJG. Long-term safety of the oral androgen testosterone undecanoate. Int J Androl 1986; 9:21–26.

697. Davidson DW, O'Carroll R, Bancroft J. Increasing circulating androgens with oral testosterone undecanoate in eugonadal men. J Steroid Biochem 1987; 26:713–715.

698. Nieschlag E, Mauss J, Coert A, et al. Plasma androgen levels in men after oral administration of testosterone or testosterone undecanoate. Acta Endocrinol 1975; 79:366–374.

699. Franchimont P, Kocovic PM, Mattei A, et al. Effects of oral testosterone undecanoate in hypogonadal male patients. Clin Endocrinol 1978; 9:313–320.

700. Maisey NM, Bingham J, Marks V, et al. Clinical efficacy of testosterone undecanoate in male hypogonadism. Clin Endocrinol 1981; 14:625–629.

701. Schürmeyer TH, Wickings EJ, Freischem CW, et al. Saliva and serum testosterone following oral testosterone undecanoate administration in normal and hypogonadal men. Acta Endocrinol 1983; 102:456–462.

702. Petry R, Rausch-Stroomann J-G, Hienz HA, et al. Androgen treatment without inhibiting effect on hypophysis and male gonads. Acta Endocrinol 1968; 59:497–507.

703. Aakvaag A, Stromme SB. The effect of mesterolone administration to normal men on the pituitary-testicular function. Acta Endocrinol 1974; 77:380–386.

704. Luisi M, Franchi F. Double-blind group comparative study of testosterone undecanoate and mesterolone in hypogonadal male patients. J Endocrinol Invest 1980; 3:305–308.

705. Mosbach EH, Shefer S, Abell LL. Identification of the fecal metabolites of 17α-methyltestosterone in the dog. J Lipid Res 1968; 9:93–97.

706. Alkalay D, Khemani L, Bartlett MF. Spectrophotofluorometric determination of methyltestosterone in plasma or serum. J Pharm Sci 1972; 61:1746–1749.

707. Doerr P, Pirke KM. Regulation of plasma oestrogens in normal adult males. Acta Endocrinol 1974; 75:617–624.

708. Liao S, Liang T, Fang S, et al. Steroid structure and androgenic activity. Specificity involved in the receptor binding and nuclear retention of various androgens. J Biol Chem 1973; 248:6154–6162.

709. Bals-Pratsch M, Yoon YD, Knuth UA, et al. Transdermal testosterone substitution therapy for male hypogonadism. Lancet 1986; 2:943–946.

710. Findlay JC, Place VA, Snyder PJ. Transdermal delivery of testosterone. J Clin Endocrinol Metab 1987; 64:266–268.

711. Korenman SG, Viosca S, Garza D, et al. Androgen therapy of hypogonadal men with transscrotal testosterone systems. Am J Med 1987; 83:471–478.

712. Bals-Pratsch M, Langer K, Place VA, et al. Substitution therapy of hypogonadal men with transdermal testosterone over one year. Acta Endocrinol 1988; 118:7–13.

713. Ahmed SR, Boucher AE, Manni A, et al. Transdermal testosterone therapy in the treatment of male hypogonadism. J Clin Endocrinol Metab 1988; 66:546–551.

714. Weinbauer GF, Marshall GR, Nieschlag E. New injectable testosterone ester maintains serum testosterone of castrated monkeys in the normal range for four months. Acta Endocrinol 1986; 113:128–132.

715. Gooren LJG. Long-term safety of the oral androgen testosterone undecanoate. Int J Androl 1986; 9:21–26.

716. Kuhn JM, Rieu M, Laudat MH, et al. Effects of 10 days administration of percutaneous dihydrotestosterone on the pituitary-testicular axis in normal men. J Clin Endocrinol Metab 1984; 58:231–235.

717. Vermeulen A, Deslypere JP. Long-term transdermal dihydrotestosterone therapy: effects on pituitary gonadal axis and plasma lipoproteins. Maturitas 1985; 7:281–287.

718. Marberger H. Hormonal therapy with steroid-filled Silastic rubber implants. Br J Urol 1976; 48:153–154.

719. Johnsen SG, Bennett EP, Jensen VG. Therapeutic effectiveness of oral testosterone. Lancet 1974; 2:1473–1475.

720. Daggett PR, Wheeler MJ, Nabarro JDN. Oral testosterone, a reappraisal. Horm Res 1978; 9:121–129.

721. Fogh M, Corker CS, McLean H, et al. Serum-testosterone during oral administration of testosterone in hypogonadal men and transsexual women. Acta Endocrinol 1978; 87:643–649.

¹⁴C]testosterone and some of its esters after injection into the rat. J Pharm Pharmacol 1969; 21:24–27.

722. Johnsen SG, Kampmann JP, Bennett EP, et al. Enzyme induction by oral testosterone. Clin Pharmacol Ther 1976; 20:233–237.

723. Jacobs SC, Kaplan GW, Gittes RF. Topical testosterone therapy for penile growth. Urology 1975; 6:708–710.

724. Ben-Galim E, Hillman RE, Weldon VV. Topically applied testosterone and phallic growth. Am J Dis Child 1980; 134:296–298.

725. Aakvaag A, Vogt JH. Plasma testosterone values in different forms of testosterone treatment. Acta Endocrinol 1969; 60:537–542.

726. Danner CH, Frick J. Androgen substitution with testosterone containing nasal drops. Int J Androl 1980; 3:429–435.

727. Cunningham GR, Silverman VE, Thornby J, et al. The potential for an androgen male contraceptive. J Clin Endocrinol Metab 1979; 49:520–526.

728. Swerdloff RS, Palacios A, McClure RD, et al. Male contraception: clinical assessment of chronic administration of testosterone enanthate. Int J Androl 1978; 2:731–747.

729. Palacios A, McClure RD, Campfield A, et al. Effect of testosterone enanthate on testis size. J Urol 1981; 126:46–48.

730. Vigersky RA, Easley RB, Loriaux DL. Effect of fluoxymesterone on the pituitary-gonadal axis: the role of testosterone-estradiol–binding globulin. J Clin Endocrinol Metab 1976; 43:1–9.

731. Jones TM, Fang VS, Landau RL, et al. The effect of fluoxymesterone administration on testicular function. J Clin Endocrinol Metab 1977; 44:121–129.

732. Aakvaag A, Vogt JH. Plasma testosterone values in different forms of testosterone treatment. Acta Endocrinol 1969; 60:537–542.

733. Scaglia HE, Ramirez AM, Gaytan JR, et al. Gonadotropin dynamics in Klinefelter's syndrome. Reproduction 1975; 2:7–12.

734. Smals AGH, Kloppenborg PWC, Pieters GFE, et al. Modulation of the gonadotropin response to constant luteinizing hormone–releasing hormone infusion by acute and chronic testosterone administration in Klinefelter's syndrome. J Clin Endocrinol Metab 1979; 48:148–152.

735. Fukutani K, Isurugi K, Takayasu H, et al. Effects of depot testosterone therapy on serum levels of luteinizing hormone and follicle-stimulating hormone in patients with Klinefelter's syndrome and hypogonadotropic eunuchoidism. J Clin Endocrinol Metab 1974; 39:856–864.

736. Capell PT, Paulsen CA, Derleth D, et al. The effect of short-term testosterone administration on serum FSH, LH and testosterone levels: evidence for selective abnormality in LH control in patients with Klinefelter's syndrome. J Clin Endocrinol Metab 1973; 37:752–759.

737. Davidson JM, Camargo CA, Smith ER. Effects of androgen on sexual behavior in hypogonadal men. J Clin Endocrinol Metab 1979; 48:955–958.

738. Salmimies P, Kockott G, Pirke KM, et al. Effects of testosterone replacement on sexual behavior in hypogonadal men. Arch Sex Behav 1982; 11:345–353.

739. Kwan M, Greenleaf WJ, Mann J, et al. The nature of androgen action on male sexuality: a combined laboratory–self-report study on hypogonadal men. J Clin Endocrinol Metab 1983; 57:557–562.

740. O'Carroll R, Shapiro C, Bancroft J. Androgens, behaviour and nocturnal erection in hypogonadal men: the effects of varying the replacement dose. Clin Endocrinol 1985; 23:527–538.

741. Gearhart JP, Jeffs RD. The use of parenteral testosterone therapy in genital reconstructive surgery. J Urol 1987; 138:1077–1078.

742. Zachmann M, Prader A. Anabolic and androgenic effect of testosterone in sexually immature boys and its dependency on growth hormone. J Clin Endocrinol 1970; 30:85–95.

743. Aynsley-Green A, Zachmann M, Prader A. Interrelation of the therapeutic effects of growth hormone and testosterone on growth in hypopituitarism. J Pediatr 1976; 89:992–999.

744. Tanner JM, Whitehouse RH, Hughes PCR, et al. Relative importance of growth hormone and sex steroids for the growth at puberty of trunk length, limb length, and muscle width in growth hormone–deficient children. J Pediatr 1976; 89:1000–1008.

745. Pertzelan A, Blum I, Grunebaum M, et al. The combined effect of growth hormone and methandrostenolone on the linear growth of patients with multiple pituitary hormone deficiencies. Clin Endocrinol 1977; 6:271–276.

746. Parker MW, Johanson AJ, Rogol AD, et al. Effect of testosterone on somatomedin-C concentrations in prepubertal boys. J Clin Endocrinol Metab 1984; 58:87–90.

747. Venable JH. Morphology of the cells of normal, testosterone-deprived and testosterone-stimulated levator ani muscles. Am J Anat 1966; 119:271–301.

748. Krieg M, Voigt KD. Biochemical substrate of androgenic actions at cellular levels in prostate, bulbocavernosus/levator ani and skeletal muscle. In: Symposium on Developments in Endocrinology in Honour of Dr. G. A. Overbeek. The Netherlands: Organon International Oss, 1976: 43–89.

749. Tóth M. Relative androgenic and myotropic activity plots of 19-nortestosterone. J Steroid Biochem 1981; 14:1085–1090.

750. Wynn V. The anabolic steroids. Practitioner 1968; 200:509–518.

751. Overbeek GA, van der Vies J, de Visser J. The so-called "pure" anabolic agents. J Am Med Wom Assoc 1969; 24:54–59.

752. Liddle GW, Burke HA Jr. Anabolic steroids in clinical medicine. Helv Med Acta 1960; 27:504–513.

753. Nowakowski H. Metabolic studies with anabolic steroids. Acta Endocrinol 1961; 39(Suppl 63):37–53.

754. van Wayjen RGA, Buyze G. Clinical-pharmacological evaluation of certain anabolic steroids. Acta Endocrinol 1961; 39(Suppl 63):18–36.

755. Tweedle D, Walton C, Johnston IDA. The effect of an anabolic steroid on postoperative nitrogen balance. Br J Clin Pract 1972; 27:130–132.

756. Watson RN, Bradley MH, Callahan R, et al. A six month evaluation of an anabolic drug, norethandrolone, in underweight persons. Am J Med 1959; 26:238–242.

757. Kalliomaki JL, Pirila AM, Ruikka I. A therapeutic trial with ethylestrenol in geriatric patients. Acta Endocrinol 1961; 39(Suppl 63):124–131.

758. Thaysen JH. Anabolic steroids in the treatment of renal failure. In: Gross F, ed. Protein Metabolism. Berlin: Springer-Verlag, 1962: 450–478.

759. Blagg CR, Parsons FM, Young GA. Effect of dietary glucose and protein in acute renal failure. Lancet 1962; 1:608–612.

760. Wilson JD. Androgen abuse by athletes. Endocr Rev 1988; 9:181–199.

761. Kennedy BJ, Gilbertsen AS. Increased erythropoiesis induced by androgenic-hormone therapy. N Engl J Med 1957; 256:719–726.

762. Shahidi NT. Androgens and erythropoiesis. N Engl J Med 1973; 289:72–80.

763. Evens RP, Amerson AB. Androgens and erythropoiesis. J Clin Pharmacol 1974; 14:94–101.

764. Hengstum V, Steenbergen J, Haanen C. Clinical course in 28 unselected patients with aplastic anaemia treated with anabolic steroids. Br J Haematol 1979; 41:323–333.

765. Najean Y. Long-term follow-up in patients with aplastic anemia. A study of 137 androgen-treated patients surviving more than two years. Am J Med 1981; 71:543–551.

766. Branda RF, Amsden TW, Jacob HS. Randomized study of nandrolone therapy of anemias due to bone marrow failure. Arch Intern Med 1977; 137:65–69.

767. Camitta BM, Thomas ED, Nathan DG, et al. A prospective study of androgens and bone marrow transplantation for treatment of severe aplastic anemia. Blood 1979; 53:504–514.

768. French Cooperative Group for the Study of Aplastic and Refractory Anaemias. Androgen therapy in aplastic anaemia: a comparative study of high and low doses and of 4 different androgens. Scand J Haematol 1986; 36:346–352.

769. Mirand EA, Murphy GP. Erythropoietin activity in anephric humans given prolonged androgen treatment. J Surg Oncol 1971; 3:59–65.

770. Eschbach JW, Funk D, Adamson J, et al. Erythropoiesis in patients with renal failure undergoing chronic dialysis. N Engl J Med 1967; 276:653–658.

771. Eschbach JW, Adamson JW. Improvement in the anemia of chronic renal failure with fluoxymesterone. Ann Intern Med 1973; 78:527–532.

772. Hendler ED, Goffinet JA, Ross S, et al. Controlled study of androgen therapy in anemia of patients on maintenance hemodialysis. N Engl J Med 1974; 291:1046–1051.

773. Koch KM, Patyna WD, Shaldon S, et al. Anemia of the regular hemodialysis patient and its treatment. Nephron 1974; 12:405–419.

774. Williams S, Stein JH, Ferris TF. Nandrolone decanoate therapy for patients receiving hemodialysis. Arch Intern Med 1974; 134:289–292.

775. Cattran DC, Fenton SSA, Wilson DR, et al. A controlled trial of nandrolone decanoate in the treatment of uremic anemia. Kidney Int 1977; 12:430–437.

776. von Hartitzsch B, Kerr DNS, Morley G, et al. Androgens in the anemia of chronic renal failure. Nephron 1977; 18:13–20.

777. Androgens in the anaemia of chronic renal failure. Br Med J 1977; 2:417–418 (editorial).

778. Spaulding WB. Methyltestosterone therapy for hereditary episodic edema (hereditary angioneurotic edema). Ann Intern Med 1960; 53:739–745.

779. Blohme G, Ysander L, Korsan-Bengtsen K, et al. Hereditary angioneurotic oedema in three families. Acta Med Scand 1972; 91:209–219.

780. Rosse WF, Logue GL, Silberman HR. The effect of synthetic androgens in hereditary angioneurotic edema: alteration of C1 inhibitor and C4 levels. Trans Assoc Am Physicians 1976; 89:122–132.

781. Frank MM, Gelfand JA, Atkinson JP. Hereditary angioedema: the clinical syndrome and its management. Ann Intern Med 1976; 84:580–593.

782. Gelford JA, Sherins RJ, Alling DW, et al. Treatment of hereditary angioedema with danazol. Reversal of clinical and biochemical abnormalities. N Engl J Med 1976; 295:1444–1448.

783. Sheffer AL, Fearon DT, Austen KF. Methyltestosterone therapy in hereditary angioedema. Ann Intern Med 1977; 86:306–308.

784. Saihan EM, Warin RP. Treatment of hereditary angioneurotic oedema with methandienone. Br Med J 1978; 1:367.

785. Gould DJ, Cunliffe WJ, Smiddy EG. Anabolic steroids in hereditary angioedema. Lancet 1978; 1:770–771.

786. Barbosa J, Seal US, Doe RP. Effects of anabolic steroids on haptoglobin, orosomucoid, plasminogen, fibrinogen, transferrin, ceruloplasmin, α_1-antitrypsin, β-glucuronidase and total serum proteins. J Clin Endocrinol 1971; 33:388–398.

787. Carl-Bertil L, Rannevik G. A comparison of plasma protein changes

induced by danazol, pregnancy, and estrogens. J Clin Endocrinol Metab 1979; 49:719–725.

788. Madanes AE, Farber M. Danazol. Ann Intern Med 1982; 96:625–630.

789. Gralnick HR, Rick ME. Danazol increases factor VIII and factor IX in classic hemophilia and Christmas disease. N Engl J Med 1983; 308:1393–1395.

790. Ahn YS, Harrington WJ, Simon SR, et al. Danazol for the treatment of idiopathic thrombocytopenic purpura. N Engl J Med 1983; 308:1396–1399.

791. Limbeck GA, Ruvalcaba RHA, Mahoney CP, et al. Studies on anabolic steroids. IV. The effects of oxandrolone on height and skeletal maturation in uncomplicated growth retardation. Clin Pharmacol Ther 1971; 12:798–805.

792. Bettman HK, Goldman HS, Abramowicz M, et al. Oxandrolone treatment of short stature: effect on predicted mature height. J Pediatr 1971; 79:1018–1023.

793. Moore DC, Tattoni DS, Limbeck GA, et al. Studies of anabolic steroids. V. Effect of prolonged oxandrolone administration on growth in children and adolescents with uncomplicated short stature. Pediatrics 1976; 58:412–422.

794. Clayton PE, Shalet SM, Price DA, et al. Growth and growth hormone responses to oxandrolone in boys with constitutional delay of growth and puberty (CDGP). Clin Endocrinol 1988; 29:123–130.

795. Wilson DM, Kei J, Hintz RL, et al. Effects of testosterone therapy for pubertal delay. Am J Dis Child 1988; 142:96–99.

796. Baran DT, Bergfeld MA, Teitelbaum SL, et al. Effect of testosterone therapy on bone formation in an osteoporotic hypogonadal male. Calcif Tissue Res 1978; 26:103–106.

797. Tamai T, Nakai T, Yamada S, et al. Effects of oxandrolone on plasma lipoproteins in patients with type IIa, IIb and IV hyperlipoproteinemia: occurrence of hypo–high density lipoproteinemia. Artery 1979; 5:125–143.

798. Jackson JA, Waxman J, Spiekerman, AM. Prostatic complications of testosterone replacement therapy. Arch Intern Med 1989; 149:2365–2366.

799. Kennedy BJ, Nathanson IT. Effects of intensive sex steroid hormone therapy in advanced breast cancer. JAMA 1953; 152:1135–1141.

800. Fruehan HE, Frawley TH. Current use of anabolic steroids. JAMA 1963; 184:527–532.

801. Kearns WM. Oral therapy of testicular deficiency. J Clin Endocrinol 1941; 1:126–130.

802. Laron Z. Effectiveness of fluoxymesterone on linear growth and weight in children with group retardation and underweight. Acta Endocrinol 1961; 36:541–548.

803. Foss GL, Simpson SL. Oral methyltestosterone and jaundice. Br Med J 1959; 1:259–263.

804. Kory RC, Bradley MH, Watson RN, et al. A six-month evaluation of an anabolic drug, norethandrolone, in underweight persons. II. BSP retention and liver function. Am J Med 1959; 26:243–248.

805. Arias IM. The effects of anabolic steroids on liver function. In: Gross F, ed. Protein Metabolism. Berlin: Springer-Verlag, 1962: 434–445.

806. deLorimier AA, Gordan GS, Lowe RC, et al. Methyltestosterone, related steroids, and liver function. Arch Intern Med 1965; 116:289–294.

807. Muller AF, Valatlan M, Manning EL. Effet de la 17-ethyl-19-nor-testosterone sur la sécrétion du cortisol. Helv Med Acta 1960; 27:678–682.

808. Sweeney EC, Evans DJ. Hepatic lesions in patients treated with synthetic anabolic steroids. J Clin Pathol 1976; 29:626–633.

809. Shapiro P, Ikeda RM, Ruebner BH, et al. Multiple hepatic tumors and peliosis hepatis in Fanconi's anemia treated with androgens. Am J Dis Child 1977; 131:1104–1106.

810. McDonald EC, Speicher CE. Peliosis hepatis associated with administration of oxymetholone. JAMA 1978; 240:243–244.

811. Arnold GL, Kaplan MM. Peliosis hepatis due to oxymetholone—a clinically benign disorder. Am J Gastroenterol 1979; 71:213–216.

812. Farrell GC, Uren RF, Perkins KW, et al. Androgen-induced hepatoma. Lancet 1975; 1:430–431.

813. Goldfarb S. Sex hormones and hepatic neoplasia. Cancer Res 1976; 36:2584–2588.

814. Hernandez-Nieto L, Bruguera M, Bombi JA, et al. Benign liver-cell adenoma associated with long-term administration of an androgenic-anabolic steroid (methandienone). Cancer 1977; 40:1761–1764.

815. Antunes CMF, Stolley PD. Cancer induction by exogenous hormones. Cancer 1977; 39:1896–1898.

816. Goodman MA, Laden AMJ. Hepatocellular carcinoma in association with androgen therapy. Med J Aust 1977; 1:220–221.

817. Westaby D, Paradinas FJ, Ogle SJ, et al. Liver damage from long-term methyltestosterone. Lancet 1977; 2:261–263.

818. Boyd PR, Mark GJ. Multiple hepatic adenomas and a hepatocellular carcinoma in a man on oral methyl testosterone for eleven years. Cancer 1977; 40:1765–1770.

819. Coombes GB, Reiser J, Paradinas EJ, et al. An androgen-associated hepatic adenoma in a trans-sexual. Br J Surg 1978; 65:869–870.

820. Shephard RJ, Killinger D, Fried T. Response to sustained use of anabolic steroid. Br J Sports Med 1977; 11:170–173.

821. Thompson PD, Cullinane EM, Sady SP, et al. Contrasting effects of testosterone and stanozolol on serum lipoprotein levels. JAMA 1989; 261:1165–1168.

822. Matsumoto AM, Sandblom RE, Schoene RB, et al. Testosterone replacement in hypogonadal men: effects on obstructive sleep apnea, respiratory drives, and sleep. Clin Endocrinol 1985; 22:713–721.

823. Zelissen PMJ, Stricker BHC. Severe priapism as a complication of testosterone substitution therapy. Am J Med 1988; 85:273–274.

824. Sokol RZ, McClure RD, Peterson M, et al. Gonadotropin therapy failure secondary to human chorionic gonadotropin–induced antibodies. J Clin Endocrinol Metab 1981; 52:929–933.

825. Burger HG, de Kretser DM, Hudson B, et al. Effects of preceding androgen therapy on testicular response to human pituitary gonadotropin in hypogonadotropic hypogonadism: a study of three patients. Fertil Steril 1981; 35:64–68.

826. Rosemberg E. Gonadotropin therapy of male infertility. In: Hafez ESE, ed. Human Semen and Fertility Regulation in Men. St. Louis: C. V. Mosby, 1976: 464–475.

827. Claustrat B, David L, Faure A, et al. Development of antihuman chorionic gonadotropin antibodies in patients with hypogonadotropic hypogonadism. A study of four patients. J Clin Endocrinol Metab 1983; 57:1041–1047.

828. Rajfer J, Handelsman DJ, Swerdloff RS, et al. Hormonal therapy of cryptorchidism. A randomized, double-blind study comparing human chorionic gonadotropin and gonadotropin-releasing hormone. N Engl J Med 1986; 314:466–470.

829. Vickery BH. Comparison of the potential for therapeutic utilities with gonadotropin-releasing hormone agonists and antagonists. Endocr Rev 1986; 7:115–124.

830. Gabrilove JL, George AC, Kirschenbaum A, et al. Effect of a GnRH analogue (leuprolide) on benign prostatic hypertrophy. J Clin Endocrinol Metab 1987; 64:1331–1333.

831. Peters CA, Walsh PC. The effect of nafarelin acetate, a luteinizing hormone–releasing hormone agonist, on benign prostatic hyperplasia. N Engl J Med 1987; 317:599–604.

832. Santoro N, Filicori M, Crowley WF Jr. Hypogonadotropic disorders in men and women: diagnosis and therapy with pulsatile gonadotropin-releasing hormone. Endocr Rev 1986; 7:11–23.

833. Klingmuller D, Schweirkert H-U. Maintenance of spermatogenesis by intranasal administration of gonadotropin-releasing hormone in patients with hypothalamic hypogonadism. J Clin Endocrinol Metab 1985; 61:868–872.

834. Liu L, Chaudhari N, Corle D, et al. Comparison of pulsatile subcutaneous gonadotropin-releasing hormone and exogenous gonadotropins in the treatment of men with isolated hypogonadotropic hypogonadism. Fertil Steril 1988; 49:302–308.

835. Cacciari E, Frejaville E, Becca A. Treatment of cryptorchidism by intranasal synthetic LH-RH and its analogue D-Ser(TBU)⁶-LHRH-EA¹⁰. Eur J Pediatr 1982; 139:280–284.

836. Hagberg S, Westphal O. Treatment of undescended testes with intranasal application of synthetic LH-RH. Eur J Pediatr 1982; 139:285–288.

837. Frick J. Cryptorchidism. In: Krieger DT, Bardin CW, eds. Current Therapy in Endocrinology 1983–1984. Philadelphia: B. C. Decker, 1983: 371–374.

14

DISORDERS OF SEX DIFFERENTIATION

Melvin M. Grumbach and Felix A. Conte

In our culture the distinction between male and female is considered absolute, and these terms are often used to epitomize opposites. Usually, the components of an individual's sexual make-up are indeed dominantly of one gender and conform to the chromosomal pattern established in the zygote at the time of fertilization. Most sexual characteristics, however, emerge from identical bipotential precursors in the embryo, and a spectrum of differentiation is possible at each level of sexual organization.

The remarkable accumulation of knowledge over the past three decades and new and continuing insights in the field of sex determination and differentiation represent major landmarks in biomedical science. No aspect of prenatal development is better understood. Advances in experimental embryology, steroid and molecular biochemistry, cytogenetics and genetics, endocrinology, immunology and transplantation biology, cell biology, and the behavioral sciences all have contributed to the understanding of sexual anomalies in humans and to the clinical management of these disorders. Major contributions to this understanding have stemmed from studies of patients with abnormalities of sex differentiation. Failure at any of the sequential stages of sexual development, whether the cause is genetic or environmental, can have a profound effect on the phenotype and lead to complete sex reversal, various degrees of ambisexual development, or less overt abnormalities in sexual function that first become apparent after sexual maturity. For general works on sex determination and differentiation see refs. 1 to 13.

NORMAL SEX DETERMINATION AND SEX DIFFERENTIATION

Sex determination and differentiation are sequential processes that involve successively the establishment of chromosomal (and genetic) sex in the zygote at the moment of conception, the determination of gonadal (primary) sex by the genetic sex, and the regulation by gonadal sex of the differentiation of the genital apparatus and, hence, the phenotypic sex. At puberty the development of sex-specific, secondary sexual characteristics reinforces and provides more visible phenotypic manifestations of this sexual dimorphism. Sex determination is concerned with the control of the development of the primary or gonadal sex, and sex differentiation encompasses the events subsequent to gonadal organogenesis. These processes are regulated by at least 30 different genes located on sex chromosomes or autosomes that act through a variety of mechanisms, including organizing factors, gonadal steroid and peptide hormones, and tissue receptors. Both male and female embryos possess indifferent, common primordia that have an inherent tendency to feminize unless there is active interference by masculinizing factors. The indifferent embryonic gonad develops into an ovary unless it is diverted by a testis-organizing factor regulated by the Y chromosome; female differentiation of the somatic sex structures (the internal and external genital tract) occurs independently of gonadal hormones and will take place in the absence of fetal testes

853

whether ovaries are present or not. Thus the sexual dimorphism in phenotype in placental mammals is mediated by the fetal testis and its dual hormonal secretions, and not by the ovary (Table 14–1). When testicular secretions are present, male differentiation takes place despite an environment in which the concentration of circulating estrogens and progestogens is high.

Abnormalities of sexual development can be classified into two broad categories: (1) disorders of sex determination, which most often are due to sex chromosome or gene abnormalities that affect gonadogenesis, and (2) disorders of sex differentiation, which usually are due to a genetic defect, less often to adverse intrauterine environmental factors. Before discussing the genetic control of sex determination and gonadogenesis, we shall consider aspects of cytogenetics that are important to understanding abnormalities of sex determination.

Chromosomal Sex and X and Y Chromatin

A systematized array of metaphase chromosomes from a single cell is known as a *karyotype*.[14] The meaning of this term is usually extended to imply that the chromosomal pattern in that cell typifies all the diploid cells of that individual or even of that species, although, as will be seen, this is by no means always true. When the 22 autosomes and two sex chromosomes (two X chromosomes or an X and a Y) are arranged and serially numbered according to size, the X chromosomes are identified by their resemblance to the larger autosomes in the medium-sized group with submedian centromeres (group 6–12). The Y chromosome resembles the short acrocentric autosomes in group 21–22[14] (Fig. 14–1).

Each of the pairs of chromosomes can be identified with

TABLE 14–1. Ontogeny of Sexual Characteristics

Characteristic	How Identified	Origin	Factors Determining Differentiation

Chromosomal sex	Karyotype analysis	Sex chromosomes of parental germ cell	Normal: chromosomal composition of sperm
			Abnormal:
			  Nondisjunction during meiotic divisions of parental germ cells
			  Nondisjunction or anaphase lag in early mitotic divisions of zygote
			  Structural errors due to chromosome breakage

X chromatin	Buccal smear; neutrophil spreads; smears or sections of other peripheral tissues	Late-replicating (heterochromatinized) X chromosome	Partial inactivation and heterochromatin formation of all X chromosomes in excess of one
Y body	Same as for X chromatin; also seen in sperm	Y chromosome	Distal segment of long arm of Y
Gonadal sex	Histological appearance	Testis	Testis: TDF, testes-determining gene(s) on the Y chromosome; SRY gene on the distal short arm of the Y chromosome just proximal to the pseudoautosomal boundary; downstream autosomal genes
		Ovary	Ovary: sex-determining genes on two X chromosomes
Genital ducts	Pelvic examination; pelvic exploration	Müllerian and wolffian ducts	Intrinsic tendency to feminize; müllerian involution requires antimüllerian hormone from fetal Sertoli cells; testosterone stimulates male duct development

External genitalia	Inspection; investigation of urogenital sinus by urethroscopy and/or x-ray contrast study	Genital tubercle, urethral folds, labioscrotal folds, and urogenital sinus	Intrinsic tendency to feminize; masculinization requires androgenic stimulation before 12th fetal week
			  Normal male: testosterone from fetal testes converted to dihydrotestosterone at end organ
			  Virilized female: adrenal hyperplasia (21- and 11-hydroxylase deficiency); maternal androgen
			  Incompletely differentiated male: insufficient testosterone secretion by fetal testes; 5α-reductase deficiency; end-organ androgen resistance

Hormonal sex	*Secondary sexual characteristics*
	  Male: sexual hair pattern; voice; muscularity; phallus size
	  Female: breast development; rounding of contours; growth of reproductive tract; menstruation; ovulation
	
	Hormonal patterns
	  Male: testosterone secretion from testes; tonic gonadotropin release
	  Female: cyclic secretion of gonadotropins, estrogen, and progesterone
		Hypothalamus and other neural centers; luteinizing hormone–releasing hormone
		Pituitary gonadotropin
		Secretory cells of testes, ovaries, and adrenals
			Hypothalamus and neural centers: luteinizing hormone–releasing hormone
			Pituitary: gonadotropin release governed by pulsatile secretion of hypothalamic luteinizing hormone–releasing hormone and circulating levels of gonadal steroids and inhibin
			Gonads: differentiation of secretory cells and biosynthetic enzymes; stimulation by pituitary gonadotropins
			Hormone expression may be modified by end-organ sensitivity

Gender identity	Identification of self as either male or female	Neuter at birth	Psychological environment during early years of paramount importance in establishing gender identity:
			  Attitudes of parents
			  Interactions of both sexes
			  Conformity of genitalia and secondary sexual characteristics at puberty to assigned sex
			Hormonal factors: adult sexual postures in lower species conditioned by hormonal factors in fetal and perinatal periods

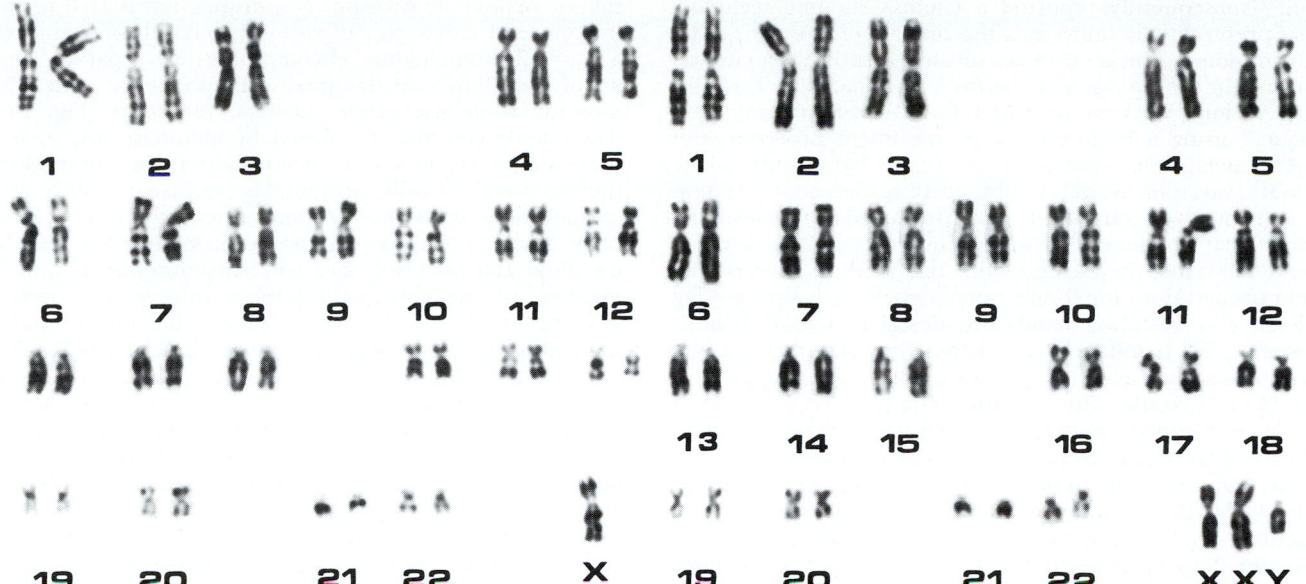

Figure 14–1. A typical G-banded karyotype of patients with abnormal gonadal differentiation. *Left,* The 45,X karyotype of a patient with streak gonads, short stature, and physical stigmata of Turner syndrome. *Right,* The 47,XXY karyotype of a phenotypic male with seminiferous tubule dysgenesis (chromatin-positive Klinefelter syndrome).

chromosome banding techniques.[14] The pattern of DNA replication in human chromosomes is disclosed by pulse labeling cell cultures with tritiated thymidine and preparing autoradiographs of the chromosomal spreads[15, 16] or by the bromodeoxyuridine dye technique.[17] One of the two X chromosomes in the female replicates late,[15, 16] and this characteristic is responsible for the distinctive X chromatin body seen in female somatic cells (see later).

Chromosome banding techniques differentially stain segments along the length of the chromosome. Caspersson and associates[18, 19] introduced fluorescent staining with substances such as quinacrine mustard or quinacrine hydrochloride. Now referred to as the Q-staining method, this staining procedure gives a distinctive fluorescent banding pattern (Q bands) for each chromosome (Fig. 14–2). The distal portion of the Y chromosome is intensely fluorescent. Pardue and

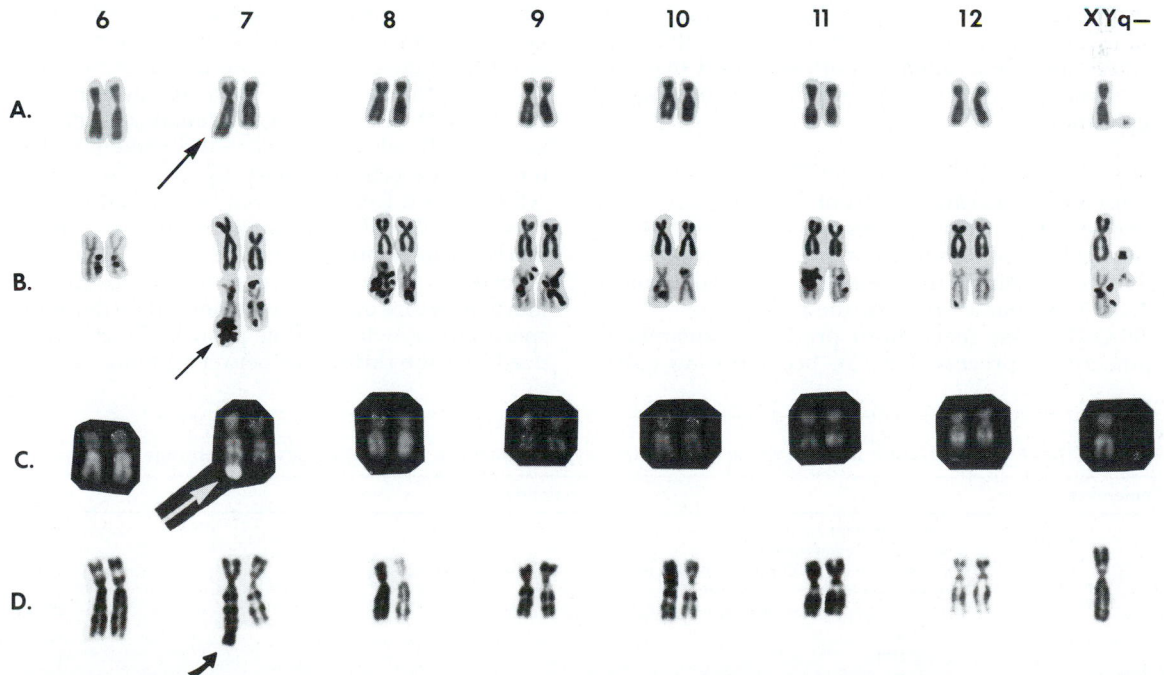

Figure 14–2. A partial karyotype of C group (chromosome numbers 6–12) and X and Y in a patient with a 46,X,t(Y;7) (q11; q36) karyotype. Standard Giemsa staining, autoradiography, fluorescent (Q), and Giemsa (G) banding techniques were used to identify the chromosome anomaly. *A,* The standard staining technique for karyotype analysis revealed an enlarged C group chromosome and a deleted G group chromosome. *B,* Autoradiography after incubation of lymphocyte culture with tritiated thymidine showed a late-labeling segment on the distal arms of the C chromosome and absence of a late-labeling segment on the deleted long arm of the presumptive Y. *C,* Quinacrine hydrochloride staining and fluorescence microscopy demonstrated a translocation of the brightly fluorescent segment of the long arm of the Y chromosome to the long arm of chromosome 7. *D,* Giemsa banding confirmed that the C group chromosome involved in the translocation was chromosome 7.

Gall[20] subsequently reported a Giemsa staining technique that preferentially stains only the centromeric regions of the chromosome. The areas of constitutive (centromeric) heterochromatin are known as C bands.[14] Stimulated by this finding, various workers modified the Giemsa staining technique,[21] using a multitude of pretreatment procedures on fixed metaphase chromosomes (e.g., hypertonic saline, NaOH, variation of pH, temperature, cation concentration, and proteolytic enzymes) that produced Giemsa-stained bands that are identical (with minor exceptions) to the Q bands described by Caspersson;[18] this method gives permanent preparations for conventional light microscopy (see Fig. 14–2). The resulting bands are designated as G bands.[14] Reverse (R) banding is a Giemsa staining method that produces a reverse pattern of chromosome banding to either the Q or G bands. The structural components of the chromosome that give rise to the banding patterns are uncertain, but the differential distribution of base composition and the state of condensation of the chromatin appear to be involved. The Q bands result from binding of quinacrine stains to adenine- and thymine-rich (A-T–rich) regions of DNA; guanine- and cytosine-rich (G-C–rich) regions of the chromosome quench the fluorescence. The G bands appear to be a consequence of differential dye binding to nonhistone protein overlying the A-T–rich regions.

In any event, high-resolution chromosome banding procedures provide precise methods for the identification of each chromosome and for the analysis of chromosome abnormalities, including complex chromosome rearrangements (see Fig. 14–2). A standard nomenclature for the identification and designation of individual chromosomes, chromosome regions and bands, and structurally altered chromosomes was embodied in the report of the 1971 Paris Conference on Standardization in Human Cytogenetics.[14] Table 14–2 summarizes the nomenclature applied to sex chromosome anomalies.

A major attempt has been made to correlate sex chromosome abnormalities with both sexual and somatic abnormalities. Anomalies in the number and structure of sex chromosomes occur with far greater frequency than suspected earlier, and these anomalies are so varied that they cannot be attributed to any single mechanism or stage of cellular replication.

Mechanisms of Chromosome Anomalies

Chromosome errors can arise from faulty replication of the germ cells during spermatogenesis or oogenesis or from faulty mitotic division of cells in the zygote after fertilization. Aneuploid cells contain a total number of chromosomes different from that characteristic of the species.

ANEUPLOIDY. One mechanism producing aneuploidy is nondisjunction, a process that can occur during either mitotic or meiotic division. Nondisjunction is characterized by failure of either pair of sister chromatids or members of a pair of homologous chromosomes to separate during anaphase. Thus one daughter cell receives an extra chromosome while the other remains one short (Fig. 14–3). Aneuploidy can also be caused by anaphase lag, in which there is a simple loss of a chromosome from one or both of the two daughter cells, presumably because of failure of one chromosome to become properly oriented at the equatorial plate during metaphase. If both chromatids are lost, both daughter cell lines will lack this chromosome. If only one member of the chromatid pair is subsequently lost, the descendant of one daughter cell will be normal and the other will be one chromosome short (see Fig. 14–3).

MOSAICISM. Mosaicism is the presence in an individual of two or more cell lines differing in chromosomal constitution but originating from a single zygote. This condition can arise only from errors in mitosis after fertilization has occurred, but embryos derived from gametes of abnormal chromosomal make-up are prone to further errors of replication.[22] Mosaicism is more common than first supposed, and many of the seeming paradoxes between genotype and phenotype are attributable to studies that lacked sufficient data to exclude this explanation. The difficulty of detecting or, especially, excluding sex chromosome mosaicism cytogenetically has been formidable in the past. However, recombinant DNA techniques offer more specific and accurate approaches to this problem.[23] Furthermore, the use of X and Y DNA probes together with the polymerase chain reaction makes it possible to detect the presence and quantity of both X and Y specific chromosome material in tissues that are not amenable to routine cytogenetic analyses. Hence, molecular analysis of sex chromosome mosaicism and structural abnormalities of sex chromosomes may make possible accurate phenotype-genotype correlations in patients with sex chromosome mosaicism and/or structural abnormalities of the X or Y chromosome.

CHIMERISM. Chimerism is the existence in an individual of two or more cell lines, each of which has a different genetic origin. In the freemartin, a common hermaphrodite in cattle, chimerism is derived by admixture of hemopoietic and primordial germ cells between biovular twins of opposite sex through anastomotic placental channels. Although it may be difficult to recognize the presence of chimerism if the separate cell lines have the same sex, the presence of cell lines of different sex will be marked by a 46,XX/46,XY karyotype. Ford[24] has discussed mechanisms by which chimerism can occur: (1) double fertilization (dispermy) of a binucleate ovum, (2) fusion of two complete zygotes or morulae before implantation, and (3) fertilization by separate sperms of an ovum and its polar body. It should be emphasized that the difference between mosaicism and chimerism

TABLE 14–2. Nomenclature for Describing Human Karyotype Pertinent to Designating Sex Chromosome Abnormalities

Paris Conference	Description	Former Nomenclature
46,XX	Normal female karyotype	XX
46,XY	Normal male karyotype	XY
47,XXY	Karyotype with 47 chromosomes including an extra X chromosome	XXY
45,X	Monosomy X	XO
45,X/46,XY	Mosaic karyotype composed of 45,X and 46,XY cell lines	XO/XY
p	Short arm	p
q	Long arm	q
46,X,del (X) (qter → p21:)	Deletion of short arm of X distal to band Xp21	Xp–
46,X,del (X) (pter → q21:)	Deletion of long arm of X distal to band Xq21	Xq–
46,X,i(Xq)	Isochromosome of long arm of X	Xqi
46,X,i(Xp)	Isochromosome of short arm of X	Xpi
46,X,r(X)	Ring X chromosome	Xr
46,X,t(Y;7) (q11; q36)	Translocation of distal fluorescent portion of Y chromosome to long arm of chromosome 7	46,XYt(Yq–,7q+)

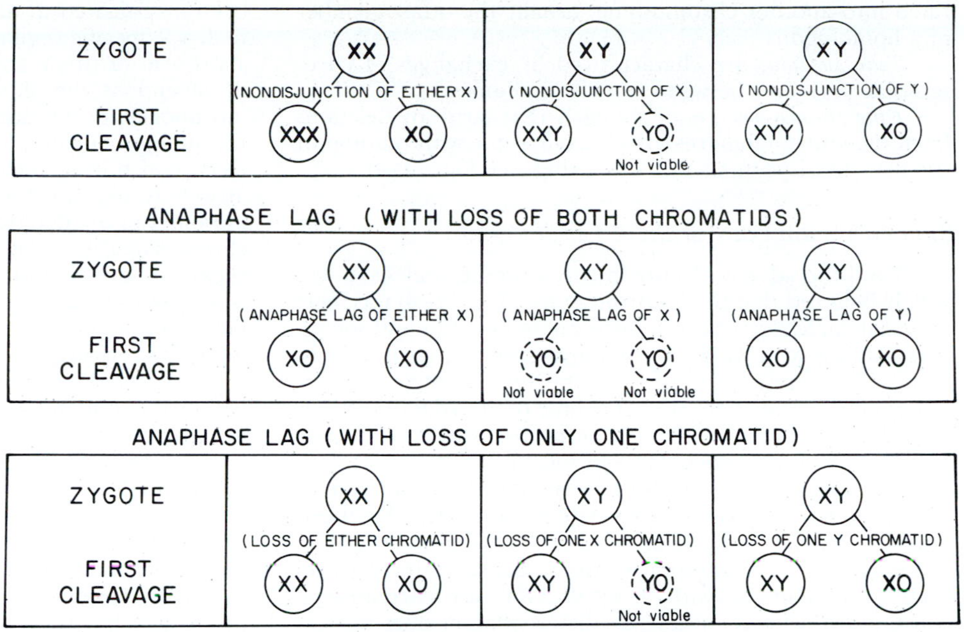

ZYGOTE	XX	XY	XY
FIRST CLEAVAGE	(NONDISJUNCTION OF EITHER X) XXX / XO	(NONDISJUNCTION OF X) XXY / YO Not viable	(NONDISJUNCTION OF Y) XYY / XO

ANAPHASE LAG (WITH LOSS OF BOTH CHROMATIDS)

ZYGOTE	XX	XY	XY
FIRST CLEAVAGE	(ANAPHASE LAG OF EITHER X) XO / XO	(ANAPHASE LAG OF X) YO / YO Not viable Not viable	(ANAPHASE LAG OF Y) XO / XO

ANAPHASE LAG (WITH LOSS OF ONLY ONE CHROMATID)

ZYGOTE	XX	XY	XY
FIRST CLEAVAGE	(LOSS OF EITHER CHROMATID) XX / XO	(LOSS OF ONE X CHROMATID) XY / YO Not viable	(LOSS OF ONE Y CHROMATID) XY / XO

Figure 14–3. Daughter cell lines can arise from mitotic nondisjunction or anaphase lag during first mitotic division in the zygote. More complex mosaicism can result if the zygote is aneuploid or if replication errors arise beyond the one-cell stage. In females, nondisjunction or anaphase lag may involve either the maternal or paternal X chromosome. Deductions regarding the origin of X chromosomes in aneuploid patients can be made by correlating sex-linked traits with those in parents and by using specific DNA probes for analysis.

depends solely on whether the different cell lines are of the same or different genetic origin.

STRUCTURAL ERRORS. With the increased ability to identify the morphological characteristics of human chromosomes by banding techniques, subtle as well as more obvious abnormalities of structure have been described. Structural errors are due to breakage or partial deletion, often followed by improper reunion of the fragments (Fig. 14–4). Most structural abnormalities that are sufficiently distinctive to be made visible by the light microscope are characterized by an abnormally long or short chromosome. Chromosome fragments lacking a centromere or containing an additional functional centromere are usually eliminated

from the cell. The following are the more common structural abnormalities (see Table 14–2).[14]

Isochromosomes are chromosomes with almost identical arms. They had been thought to arise by transverse rather than longitudinal division of the chromosome (centric fission) (Fig. 14–5). This error involves primarily the X and Y chromosomes and usually results in a chromosome consisting of two long arms (e.g., Xqi or Yqi). Isochromosomes may have either one or two centromeric bands, and some isochromosomes exhibit subtle differences in the banding pattern and size of the two arms. These observations and the limited evidence that centric fission can occur in human cells have led to the belief that isochromosomes most likely arise from deletions close to the centromere, with fusion of the sister chromatids, followed by normal division of the centromere and duplication of the entire chromatid to form an isochromosome[25] (see Fig. 14–5).

Deletion is characterized by detachment and loss of a portion of a chromosome. The notation q− refers to deletion of a portion of the long arm and p− refers to deletion of a portion of the short arm.

Duplication occurs when a deleted segment is incorpo-

PRODUCTION OF SOME STRUCTURAL ABNORMALITIES OF A CHROMOSOME

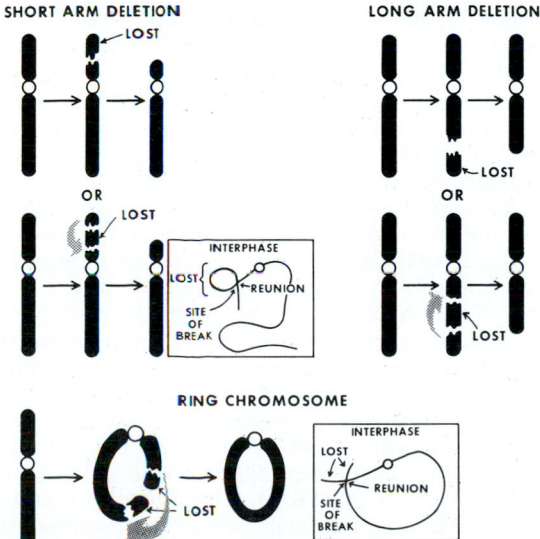

Figure 14–4. A diagram of chromosome breakage and recombination to form long and short arm deletions and ring chromosomes. Deleted segments may also be transposed to terminal portions of other chromosomes as additions, or there may be reciprocal translocations of deleted segments with those from another chromosome.

ORIGIN OF ISOCHROMOSOME

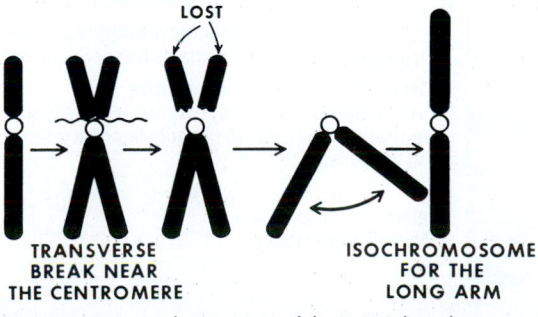

TRANSVERSE BREAK NEAR THE CENTROMERE

ISOCHROMOSOME FOR THE LONG ARM

Figure 14–5. Long arm isochromosomes of the X (Xqi) have been postulated to result from centric fission, that is, transverse rather than longitudinal division of the centromere. A more likely mechanism is shown. A deletion occurs above the centromere on the short arm. Fusion of chromatids followed by division of the centromere and duplication of entire chromatid results in an isochromosome with either one or two centromeres. The acentric fragment is lost.

rated into another chromosome, usually the other member of a homologous pair.

Translocations are characterized by exchanges of chromosome segments between two chromosomes.

Ring chromosomes, e.g., a ring X (Xr), arise by deletions from the ends (telomeres) of a chromosome with reunion of the new distal portions to form a ring (see Fig. 14–4).

Biological Functions of the Y Chromosome

Until the advent of human chromosome analysis, it was widely believed that the Y chromosome (Fig. 14–6) was inert and that male determiners were carried on the autosomes. The finding of a 47,XXY sex chromosome constitution in men with Klinefelter syndrome and only a single X chromosome in women with the syndrome of gonadal dysgenesis provided convincing evidence that the Y chromosome carries male-determining genes that can induce testicular development even in the presence of two or more X chromosomes. In subsequent work the testis-determining gene has been localized to the short arm of the Y chromosome.[26] The presence of a Y chromosome causes testicular differentiation even in individuals with a 49,XXXXY sex chromosome constitution, whereas testicular differentiation does not occur in 45,X individuals. In addition, the Y is essential to spermatogenesis.

The length of the human Y chromosome varies as much as threefold in normal men. The length and morphology of the Y are heritable, are relatively constant in male relatives, and exhibit racial variation. Most of this variation is in the length of the long arm and its distal, heterochromatic, brilliantly fluorescent segment in Q-stained preparations (see Fig. 14–6). This polymorphism in the size of the fluorescent portion and loss of part of the distal nonfluorescent portion of the long arm are consistent with normal male sex differentiation and not associated with any specific phenotypic effects; consequently, it is likely that a large segment of the long arm of the Y is not engaged in gene transcription. The long arm of the Y contains highly repetitious Y chromosome–specific and non–Y-specific sequences of DNA. The euchromatic short arm and proximal portion of the long arm of the human Y chromosome make up about 0.5% of the diploid genome (XY + 44 autosomes).

The euchromatic portion of the Y chromosome has been investigated in detail.[26] Two regions have been identified, a Y-specific region and a region at the distal end of the short arm of the Y chromosome that is homologous to the distal end of the short arm of the X chromosome. The morphogenetically distinct X and Y chromosomes pair and recombine obligately only along this small segment at the distal end during meiosis, maintaining sequence homology as well as allowing for the proper distribution of sex chromosomes to the daughter cells. This process is critical to the chromosomal basis of sex determination.[27, 28] Genes in this region of the X and Y are paired, not subject to dosage compensation (i.e., inactivation), and hence are expressed like autosomal genes rather than sex-linked genes. Accordingly, this region is designated the "pseudoautosomal" region of the X and Y chromosomes[29] (see Fig. 14–6). The homology of this region has been verified with anonymous DNA probes and by the identification in the region of the MIC2 and the GM-CSF receptor genes.[30, 31] MIC2 encodes a cell-surface molecule implicated in T cell adhesion.[30, 31] GM-CSF encodes the receptor for granulocyte-macrophage colony-stimulating factor.[32] The pseudoautosomal region is thought to extend about 2500 kb, and the boundaries are demarcated distally by the telomeres of the X and Y chromosomes and proximally by the 3′ end of the MIC2 gene and an Alu repeat sequence on the Y chromosome.[33] The pseudoautosomal regions of the X and Y chromosomes are 99% homologous distal to the Alu sequence.[33]

The second region of the euchromatic portion of the Y chromosome is the so-called sex-specific region, which extends from the proximal boundary of the pseudoautosomal region to the heterochromatic portion of the long arm of the Y chromosome. Deletion analyses of the Y chromosome in 46,XX males and 46,XY females have demonstrated that the segment just proximal to the pseudoautosomal region on the short arm of the Y chromosome has a gene(s) critical to testicular organogenesis and, hence, male sex differentiation.[26] A 35-kb region immediately adjacent to the pseudoautosomal boundary contains a gene(s) termed SRY (sex-determining region Y).[34] This gene encodes a testis-specific transcript that shows homology with two DNA-binding proteins: Mc, a mating-type protein of the fission yeast *Schizosaccharomyces pombe*, and HMG-1 and HMG-2, so-called nuclear high-mobility group proteins.[35] Proximal to SRY another gene putatively involved in sex determination has been cloned from a 230-kb portion of the short arm of the Y chromosome.[36] This gene codes for a protein that has 13 Cys-Cys/His-His zinc fingers as well as an acidic and a basic domain and has been termed ZFY (zinc finger Y).[36, 37] By analogy to other zinc finger proteins, such as *Xenopus* transcription factor IIIA, the protein is thought to bind to DNA in a sequence-specific manner and to regulate transcription.[38] Other genes localized to the euchromatic region of the long arm of the Y chromosome include the pseudogene for steroid sulfatase (STS),[39–41] a gene controlling the expression of histocompatibility Y (H-Y) antigen as assessed by the cytotoxic T cell assay,[42] and the gene for amelogenin, the major extracellular matrix enamel protein in the developing tooth bud.[43] Other genes postulated to reside on the Y chromosome but not yet cloned include genes affecting height, tooth size, and spermatogenesis,[44] as well as genes that prevent the stigmata of Turner syndrome[45] and a locus on the short arm for the control of serological H-Y antigen.[46]

Y CHROMATIN (Y BODY). The fluorescent end of the Y chromosome in human male metaphases, stained with the fluorochrome quinacrine hydrochloride or its mustard derivative, is visualized as a small, brightly fluorescent body (Y body) in a high proportion of diploid interphase nuclei of the male in tissue preparations including buccal mucosal smears, lymphocytes and polymorphonuclear leukocytes in

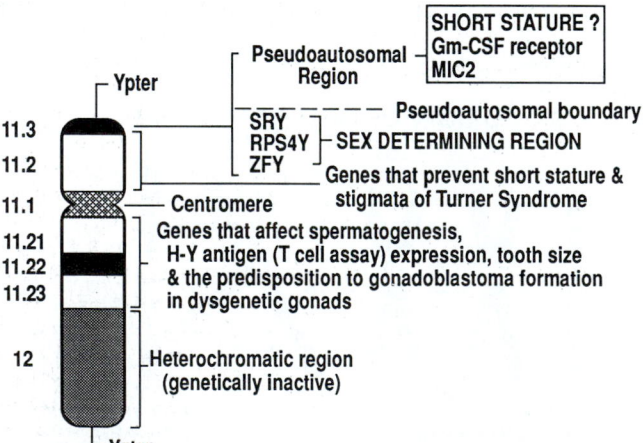

Figure 14–6. A diagrammatic representation of a G-banded Y chromosome. Y-linked genes are shown. ZFY, zinc finger Y; SRY, sex-determining region Y; GM-CSF, granulocyte-macrophage colony-stimulating factor; MIC2, gene for a cell-surface antigen recognized by monoclonal antibody 12E7; RPS4Y, ribosomal protein S4.

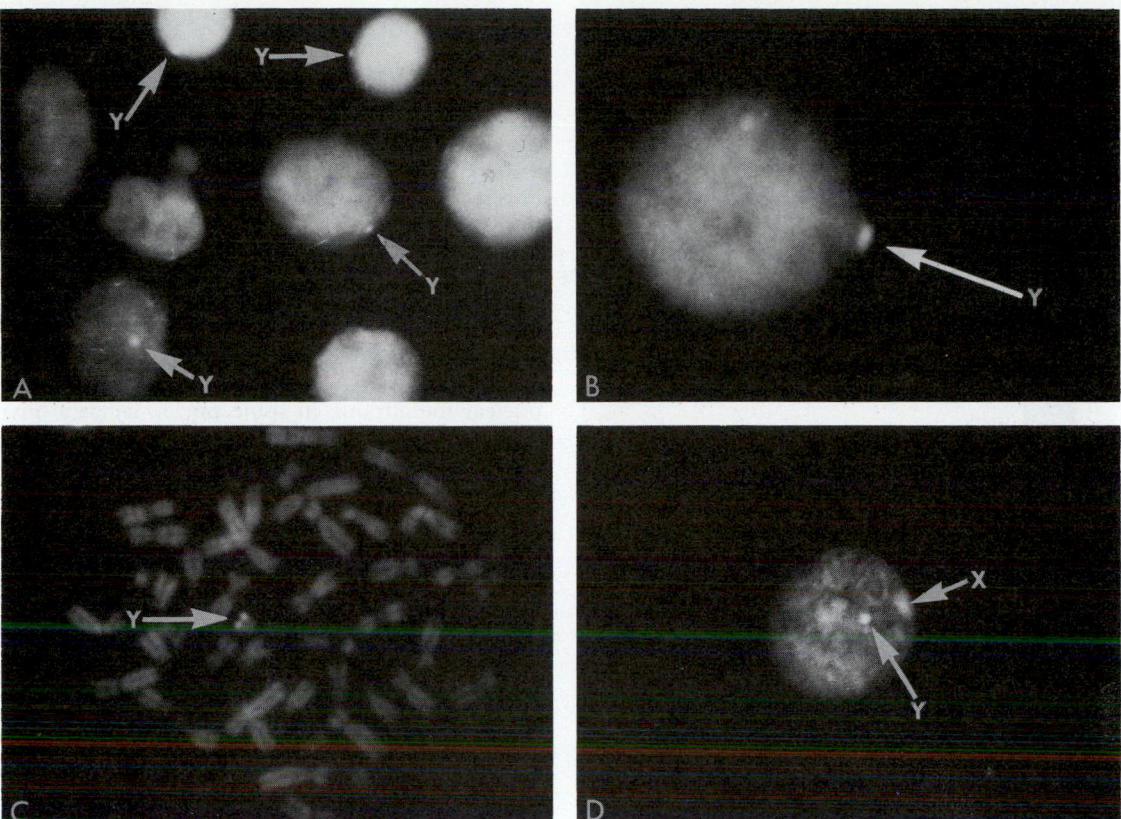

Figure 14–7. *A,* Q staining and fluorescence microscopy of interphase cells from a normal male, illustrating typical Y bodies. *B,* An enlarged photograph of one cell, showing a fluorescent Y body at the periphery of the nucleus. *C,* Metaphase chromosomes from a normal male, illustrating the brightly fluorescent distal segment of the long arm of the Y chromosome. *D,* An interphase nucleus in a buccal smear of a patient with a 47,XXY karyotype. A brightly fluorescent Y body and an X chromatin body (which exhibits much weaker fluorescence) were identified by Q staining and fluorescence microscopy.

peripheral blood smears, hair root sheath cells, and cells grown in culture.[21] In XY males, a single Y body, sometimes bipartite in structure, is present in interphase nuclei (Fig. 14–7), whereas two Y bodies are detectable in over 15% of nuclei in 47,XYY and 48,XXYY males (Table 14–3). In a small percentage of normal males (<0.05%), a small Y chromosome that lacks all or most of the distal fluorescent segment is present, and a Y body is absent in somatic nuclei. Fluorescence of Q-stained X chromatin bodies has been observed in cultured fibroblasts and certain other tissues from females, but the intensity of fluorescence of the X body is less and the size is three to five times larger than that of the Y body (see Fig. 14–7).

Biological Functions of the X Chromosome

The biological functions of the X chromosomes are more complex than those of the Y chromosome. Genes on the X have a critical influence on sex determination in both the female and male and on the differentiation of the somatic sex structures in the male. In addition, more than 130 gene loci unrelated to sex development are known to be X linked, and additional genes have been tentatively localized on the X chromosome.

The organization of the X chromosome resembles that of the Y chromosome in that it has a pseudoautosomal region on its distal short arm homologous to that on the Y (Xp22.3 → pter)[29] as well as an X-specific region (Fig. 14–8). The pseudoautosomal region of the X chromosome is the locus for two genes, MIC2 and GM-CSF, and for numerous anonymous DNA sequences.[30–32] Immediately proximal to the boundary of the pseudoautosomal region are the loci for many genes including those for the red cell antigen (XG), the gene for STS,[39, 40] the gene coding for the amelogenin enamel protein in the developing tooth bud,[43] and the locus of the zinc finger X gene (ZFX),[47] which cross-hybridizes with probes for the ZFY gene. ZFX has 13 zinc fingers with 383 of 393 amino acid residues identical to those of ZFY. Hence, it appears that both these zinc finger proteins may bind to the same nucleic acid sequences. Furthermore, ZFX is transcribed in 46,XX cell lines.[47] All genes in the area of the X chromosome immediately proximal to the pseu-

TABLE 14–3. Sex Chromosome Complement Correlated with X Chromatin and Y Bodies in Somatic Interphase Nuclei*

	Maximal Number in Diploid Somatic Nuclei	
Sex Chromosomes	**X Bodies**	**Y Bodies**
45,X	0	0
46,XX	1	0
46,XY	0	1
47,XXX	2	0
47,XXY	1	1
47,XYY	0	2
48,XXXX	3	0
48,XXXY	2	1
48,XXYY	1	2
49,XXXXX	4	0
49,XXXXY	3	1
49,XXXYY	2	2

*Maximal number of X chromatin bodies in diploid somatic nuclei is one less than the number of X's, whereas maximal number of Y fluorescent bodies is equivalent to the number of Y's in the chromosome constitution.

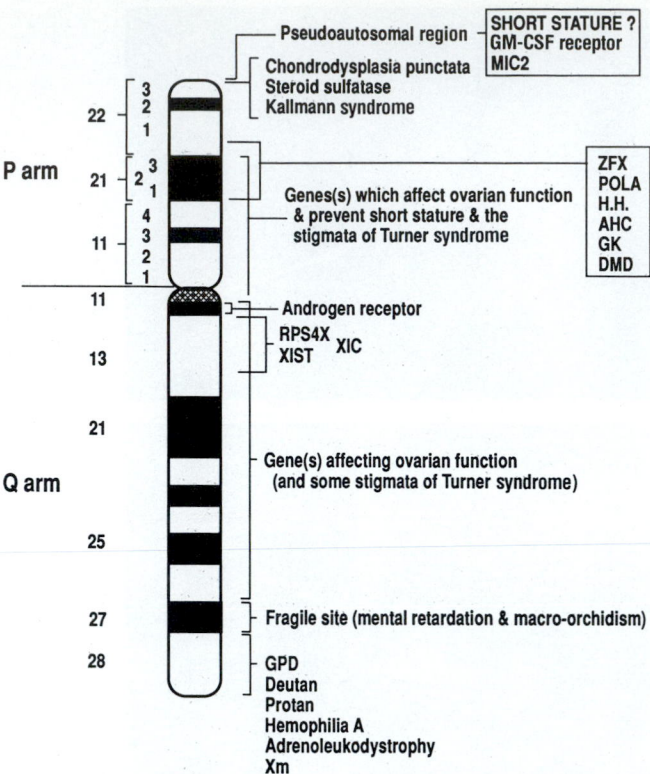

Figure 14–8. A diagrammatic representation of G-banded X chromosome. Selected X-linked genes are shown. GM-CSF, granulocyte-macrophage colony-stimulating factor; MIC2, a cell-surface antigen recognized by monoclonal antibody 12E7; ZFX, zinc finger X; POLA, RNA polymerase; HH, hypogonadotropic hypogonadism; AHC, congenital adrenal hypoplasia; GK, glycerol kinase; DMD, Duchenne muscular dystrophy; RPS4X, ribosomal protein S4; XIST, Xi-specific transcripts; XIC, X inactivation center.

doautosomal region (i.e., XG, STS, ZFX) escape X inactivation.[39, 47] Other genes postulated to reside in this region include a gene that affects the expression of H-Y antigen[46] and the gene (or genes) that prevents short stature and many of the somatic abnormalities found in the syndrome of gonadal dysgenesis.[48, 49] Proximal to this region are genes that are not represented by homologues on the Y chromosome and are subject to dosage compensation by X inactivation[50] on any X chromosome in excess of one.

Two X chromosomes are required in the human for normal ovarian differentiation and follicular maturation: 45,X individuals have bilateral streak gonads. Studies of patients with deletions of the X chromosome suggest that loci on both the short and long arms of the X chromosome are involved in ovarian differentiation and maturation.[49, 51]

The long arm of the X chromosome harbors a large number of genes subject to X inactivation and responsible for a wide variety of X-linked traits. The gene for the androgen receptor protein is located in the paracentromeric region of the long arm of the X.[52, 53] This region also contains the putative X inactivation center XIC around which the X chromosome condenses to form the Barr body and from which inactivation spreads.[54]

X CHROMATIN (X OR BARR BODY). Whereas the Y chromosome is one of the smallest human chromosomes and is mainly concerned with testis organogenesis, the X chromosome is the eighth longest and contains about 5% of the total DNA content of the haploid genome (X + 22 autosomes). Furthermore, the X chromosome contains genetic coding for functions involving every system in the body. Because females have twice as much of this genetic material in their cells as males, the biological differences between the sexes should be far greater than is the case. Theories proposed to explain this paradox are an outgrowth of Barr's pioneering observations of the X chromatin body in somatic cells of females.

In 1949 Barr and Bertram[55] described the presence of a stainable chromatin mass at the periphery of the nucleus in resting ganglion cells of female but not of male cats. This distinguishing characteristic of the female sex is present in the peripheral cells of most mammalian species and has been used as a cytological means of assessing the number of X chromosomes in humans with various errors of sex differentiation (Fig. 14–9 and Table 14–3).

The X chromatin body is usually planoconvex, with the flattened side in apposition to the inner surface of the nuclear membrane; in some nuclei, it has a bipartite structure. It is about 1 μm in diameter and stains positively for DNA. In certain tissues, such as amniotic membrane, almost every interphase nucleus is chromatin-positive. In buccal mucosal smears, the most commonly used preparation for determining the X chromatin pattern, the proportion of X chromatin–positive nuclei in females may be lower than in other somatic tissues, but in most laboratories they are detected in no less than 20% of nuclei.

In polymorphonuclear leukocytes this sexual dimorphism takes a different form; in females, 1 to 15% of neutrophils (mean 2.5%) have a drumstick-shaped, dense chromatin accessory nuclear appendage not found in normal males (Fig. 14–9D). These appendages have the same significance as X chromatin in other somatic tissues.

In patients with more than two X chromosomes, the maximal number of X chromatin bodies in any diploid nucleus is one less than the total number of X chromosomes. In 47,XXX females or 48,XXXY males, for example, at most two Barr bodies are present in diploid nuclei, whereas 46,XY and 45,X individuals are X chromatin–negative (see Table 14–3). Abnormalities in shape and size of the X chromatin body can often be correlated with structural abnormalities of the X chromosome. An abnormally small X chromatin body has been found in females with one normal X and one deleted X (46,XXp−) or with one ring X chromosome (46,XXr). A large X body is associated with a long arm isochromosome (Xqi). When a structurally abnormal X is present, it is the aberrant X chromosome that replicates late and gives rise to the X chromatin (except when the structurally abnormal X is an X-autosome translocation).

X CHROMATIN AND GENE EXPRESSION. In 1959 Ohno and co-workers[56] reported the first evidence that X chromatin arises from only one of the two X chromosomes in the interphase nuclei of female somatic cells. The staining characteristics of such nuclei arise from the fact that a portion of one X chromosome is highly condensed (heteropyknotic); the other X does not contribute to the heterochromatic material because, like the autosomes, it is extended and filamentous.[57] This difference in staining quality betokens a striking difference in the functional roles of the two X chromosomes. By studying the sequence of incorporation of [³H]thymidine into replicating chromosomes, Morishima and colleagues[15, 16] showed that the X chromosome that gives rise to X chromatin completes DNA synthesis later than does any other chromosome in the cell and that the maximal number of X chromatin bodies in a single diploid nucleus is equal to the number of late-replicating X chromosomes (Fig. 14–10). These observations and the incisive genetic studies of Lyon, Beutler, and other workers led to the concept (Lyon hypothesis) that only one X chromosome in each cell is genetically active during interphase; the other X chromosome, which retains its heterochromatic properties, is genetically inactive for many functions.[58, 59]

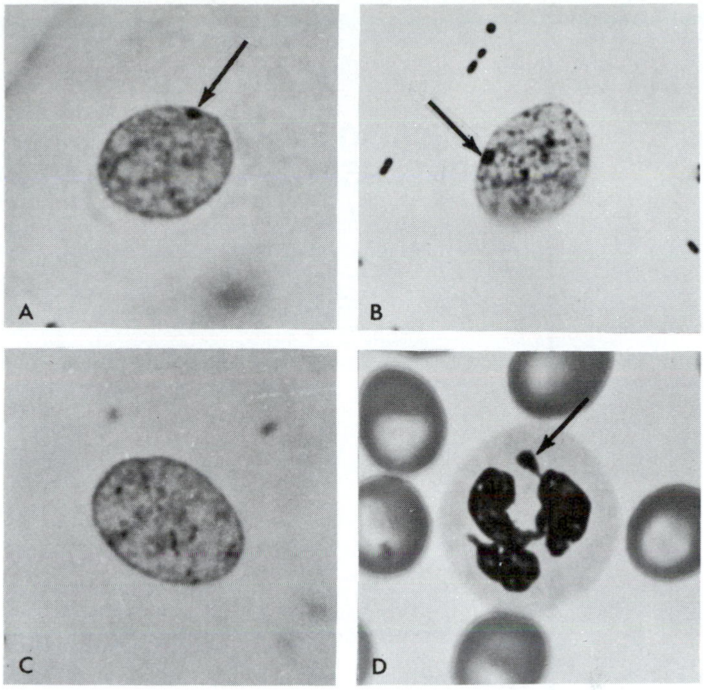

Figure 14–9. *A* and *B*, X chromatin body (Barr body) in the nucleus of buccal mucosal cells from a normal female (thionine stain, ×2000). Such cells are found in about 25% of well-preserved nuclei. *C*, A buccal mucosal cell from a normal male, illustrating absence of this body. *D*, A typical "drumstick" nuclear appendage found in a variable proportion of leukocytes of female subjects.

The change in state (heterochromatinization) of one X chromosome in each female cell occurs during the late blastocyst stage, between the 12th and the 18th day in the human embryo when cytodifferentiation begins. The female germ cells beyond the stage of oogonia are the only somatic cell lines known to be exempted from heterochromatinization, a finding in keeping with the requirement for a second X chromosome for normal ovarian differentiation. Epstein[60] has provided evidence that both X chromosomes in mouse oocytes are active and code for the X-linked genes for glucose-6-phosphate dehydrogenase and hypoxanthine-guanine phosphoribosyltransferase. This observation has been confirmed in human fetal and postnatal oocytes.[61] In all other cells, the maternally or the paternally derived X chromosome becomes inactive by random chance. Once this transformation is established, however, the inactive state of that particular X chromosome is transmitted to all descendants of that cell. This control system appears to function as a mechanism of dosage compensation by which each female somatic cell functions virtually as if it had only one active X chromosome.[59] The female, in effect, has no more active genetic material than does the male. This hypothesis is variously referred to as the inactive X theory, the Lyon hypothesis, or the fixed differentiation hypothesis of X chromosome behavior.

The implication that normal females function as genetic mosaics insofar as X-linked traits are concerned has found strong support in studies of the mouse and of X-linked traits in humans.[59] For example, Davidson and associates[62] demonstrated two populations of cells in females heterozygous for a mutant form of the X-linked gene for glucose-6-phosphate dehydrogenase, which has an electrophoretic mobility different from that of the normal form (Fig. 14–11). Heterochromatinization of all X chromosomes in excess of one also explains the relatively minor phenotypic changes in women with more than two X chromosomes, because the supernumerary X chromosomes are also heterochromatinized and therefore relatively inactive (Fig. 14–12). By contrast, trisomy for an autosome as small as chromosome 21, as in Down syndrome, is usually associated with profound effects. Biochemical analysis of DNA methylation of active and inactive X chromosomes and studies with 5-azacytidine (which impairs methylation of cytosine) suggest that DNA methylation plays an important role in the maintenance of X chromosome inactivation, late replication, and sex chromatin formation.[63] DNA methylation differs in the two X chromosomes. The double-stranded palindrome CpG dinucleotide clusters, the CpG islands, commonly found at the 5' end of genes, are methylated mainly in genes on the inactive X chromosome. The methylated cytosine residues serve to maintain the suppressed transcriptional activity and relative resistance to nuclease. The mechanism of initiation and termination of X inactivation during the meiotic cycle is not known.

In the human, in contrast to the mouse, the inactivation of an X chromosome does not involve the entire chromosome. The heteropyknotic X in the human female is only segmentally inactive in terms of transcriptional activity. Not only genes on the pseudoautosomal region of the short arm of the heterochromatic, late-replicating X chromosome, but also genes scattered along at least the short arm of the heteropyknotic X escape inactivation.[64] Individuals with a 45,X or 47,XXY constitution, for example, have abnormalities in sexual development and in somatic features unrelated to sex. Further, as noted previously, the red cell antigen XG, the STS loci, and the ZFX loci escape inactivation and are active on both X chromosomes in the female; these genes have been mapped to the distal part of the short arm of the X[39, 47] outside the pseudoautosomal region. Two genes, XIST (Xi-specific transcripts)[64a] and RPS4 (ribosomal protein S4),[64b] have been mapped to the proximal long arm of the X chromosome. Both of these genes escape inactivation on the heteropyknotic X chromosome. XIST appears to map to the region of the X chromosome inactivation center—Xq13.[64c]

Whereas the female germ cell requires two active X chromosomes to give rise to normal oocytes (in contrast to the inactivation of one X chromosome in the somatic tissues), the X chromosome must be inactivated before meiosis in male germ cells for normal spermatogenesis to occur.

USING THE DIF-
FERENTIAL BE-
HAVIOR OF THE
TWO X-CHROMO-
SOMES OF THE
HUMAN FEMALE
AS MODEL

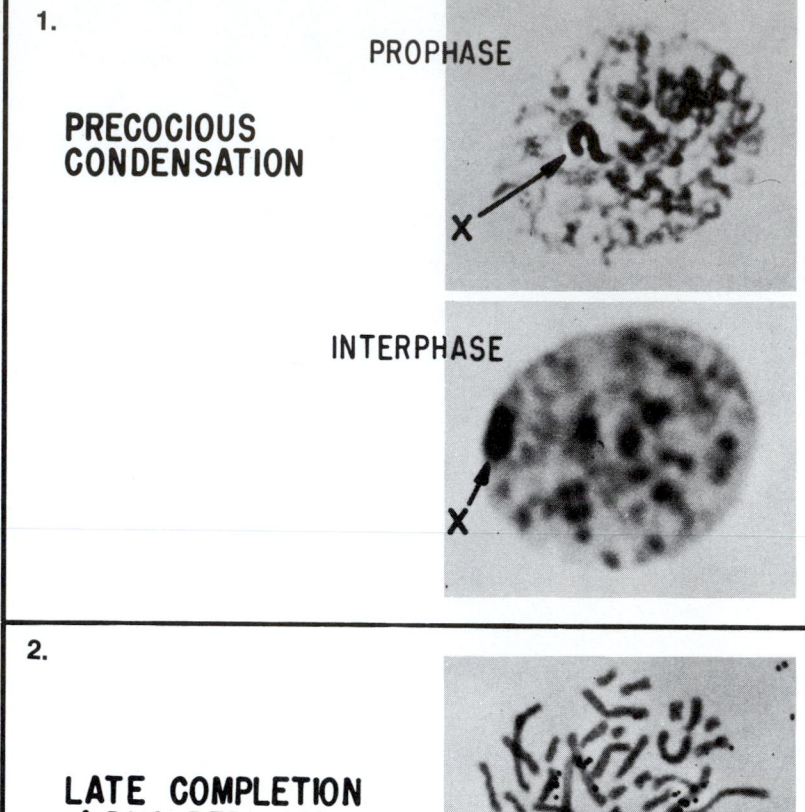

Figure 14–10. Characteristics of heterochromatin formation as exemplified by differential behavior of the two X chromosomes of the female in somatic cells. *1,* Precocious condensation of a large part of one of the two X chromosomes in prophase and formation of the X chromatin body in interphase nuclei. *2,* Delayed replication of DNA in one of the X chromosomes (arrow indicates silver grains overlying one X chromosome in the autoradiogram of metaphase chromosomes from a normal female exposed to tritiated thymidine late in the synthetic period). The gene activity on the heterochromatic late-replicating X chromosome is suppressed or modified in part. (From Grumbach MM. On the significance of sex chromatin. In: Second International Conference on Congenital Malformations. New York: International Medical Congress, 1964: 62–67.)

Genes and Testicular Organogenesis

The genetic sex of the zygote is established by the fertilization of a normal ovum by an X- or Y-bearing sperm, and the mechanisms involved in the translation of genetic sex into a testis or an ovary are understood in broad terms. From the early days of human chromosome analysis, compelling evidence was obtained for the regulation of testicular gonadogenesis by a gene (or genes) on the Y chromosome. Indeed, sex determination is essentially testis differentiation. The short arm of the Y chromosome contains a gene (or genes) that controls testis determination and, hence, maleness. The gene acts in a dominant fashion and leads to differentiation of the bipotential gonad as a testis. Several hypotheses have been proposed to explain testicular morphogenesis (Fig. 14–13). These include the H-Y antigen hypothesis, the ZFY gene as the sex-determining locus, and, most compelling, the proposal that the SRY gene is the master gene that controls male sex determination.

H-Y ANTIGEN. In 1955 Eichwald and Silmser[65] discovered in males of a highly inbred strain of mice the H-Y antigen, a male-specific cell membrane component that causes rejection by female mice of skin grafts from male donors of the same strain. Antibodies to H-Y antigen were identified serologically in male-grafted female mice by Goldberg and associates in 1971[66] and utilized by a combined absorption and sperm cytotoxicity test for measurement of H-Y antigen. Other serological assays for H-Y antigen are based on the direct or indirect detection of H-Y antibody bound to target cells.[67, 68]

After the development of the sperm cytotoxicity assay, Wachtel and co-workers[69] discovered the invariant association of serological H-Y antigen with the heterogametic sex in a wide range of vertebrates, including mammals, birds, amphibians, and bony fish. In mammals, serological H-Y antigen is expressed in the heterogametic XY male but not the homogametic XX female; in birds the female is the heterogametic sex (ZW), and H-Y (or H-W) antigen may act as an ovarian organizer in this species.[12] The conservation throughout evolution of this ubiquitous cross-reacting minor plasma membrane histocompatibility antigen, its appearance early in embryonic development (in the mouse, preimplantation male embryos at the eight-cell stage are H-Y antigen–positive[70]), and its association with the heterogametic sex led Wachtel[12] and Ohno and associates[71] to suggest that the phylogenetically conserved serological H-Y antigen is the factor responsible for inducing testicular organogenesis in humans and that it is a product of the testis-organizing gene on the Y chromosome.

Support for this hypothesis was obtained from the study of 47,XYY and 48,XXYY men who express increased amounts of serological H-Y antigen.[12] XX sex-reversed infertile human, mouse, goat, and dog males are serological H-Y antigen–positive, as are 46,XX true hermaphrodites and 46,XY women with testicular feminization.[12] Even in the absence of a discrete Y chromosome or karyotype evidence

Figure 14–11. A diagrammatic representation of the fixed differentiation or Lyon hypothesis of X chromosome behavior in somatic cells of the human female. At the late blastocyst stage (the time when X chromatin can first be identified), one of the two X chromosomes becomes heterochromatinized in each cell and gives rise to an X chromatin body; it is by chance in each cell whether this differentiation involves a maternally derived X (M) or a paternally derived X (P). Once differentiation has occurred, this characteristic is fixed in succeeding generations of somatic cells. Most of the genes on the heterochromatic portion of an X chromosome are suppressed or inactivated, thus serving as a means of "dosage compensation" for the greater number of X-linked genes in the female than in the male. This mechanism has an important bearing on expressivity and penetrance of an X-linked mutant gene in a heterozygous female. In the diagram, the maternally derived X carries a mutant gene (a) that is expressed only in cells in which this X is the isopyknotic, euchromatic active X (white X^M). Although the heterochromatinized X (black X) in this diagram is represented as wholly inactive, some loci on the heterochromatinized X do remain active and exert genetic effects. The female germ cell line beyond the oogonia stage is exempted from heterochromatinization.

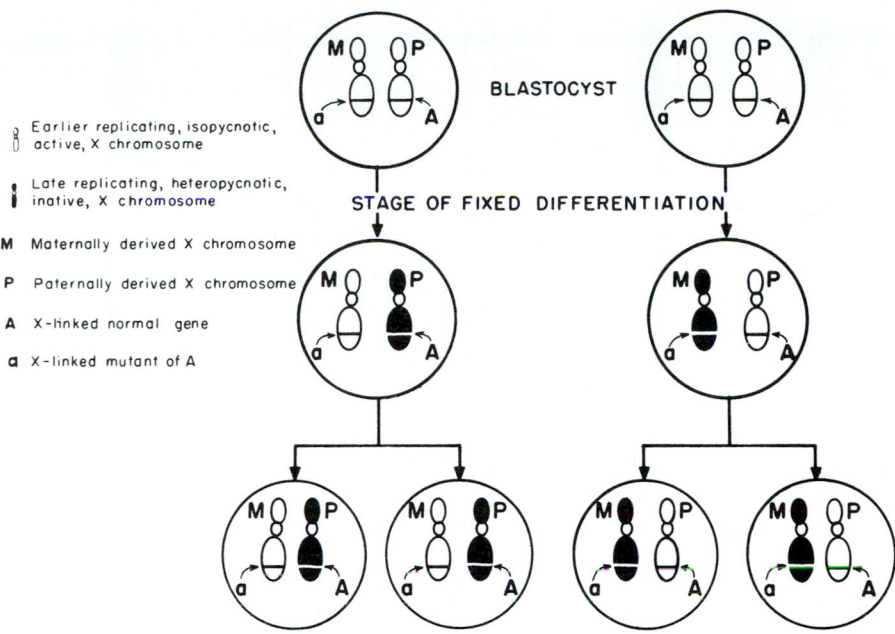

Earlier replicating, isopycnotic, active, X chromosome

Late replicating, heteropycnotic, inactive, X chromosome

M Maternally derived X chromosome

P Paternally derived X chromosome

A X-linked normal gene

a X-linked mutant of A

BLASTOCYST

STAGE OF FIXED DIFFERENTIATION

of a Y-to-X or Y-to-autosome translocation or insertion, the presence of testicular tissue was associated with a positive test for serological H-Y antigen.[12, 46, 71]

Other evidence supporting the hypothesis that H-Y antigen has a testicular organizing function came from two types of experiments: (1) transformation of dissociated XY newborn rodent testes cells into ovarian follicle-like structures by treatment with H-Y antibody[71–73] and (2) reports of induction of testicular differentiation in XX undifferentiated rat, bovine, and human gonads by exposure to H-Y antigen.[71, 74–77] Based on these observations, a hypothesis concerning the genetic control of H-Y antigen secretion and the organogenesis of the indifferent embryonic gonad was proposed by Wachtel and Ohno, namely that the short arm of the Y chromosome contains a locus (or loci) that regulates the expression of H-Y antigen. In the presence of a Y chromosome (or the Y locus that controls H-Y antigen), H-Y antigen is disseminated by cells in the gonadal blastema (possibly Sertoli cell precursors), binds to gonad-specific H-Y receptors, and induces differentiation of the primitive gonad as a testis.[46] Other genes, such as a locus on the X chromosome (Xp22.3),[46, 78] a structural gene on an autosome,[79] and genes coding for the specific H-Y antigen receptor on gonadal cells, play a role in the secretion and action of H-Y antigen.[46]

Melvold and co-authors[80] described a single XO mutant male mouse that was H-Y antigen–positive by the serological assay but H-Y antigen–negative by transplantation experiments. This finding suggested that two distinct male-specific antigenic systems exist, one recognized by transplantation assays (or assays that correlate with transplantation such as the cytotoxic T cell assay) and the other detected serologically. Studies supporting[81, 82] and refuting[83] the H-Y antigen hypothesis have been published. The discrepancies and discordant data, along with the problems of reproducibility and specificity of the H-Y antigen assay, have led to the rejection by most workers of a role for H-Y antigen in sex determination.[68]

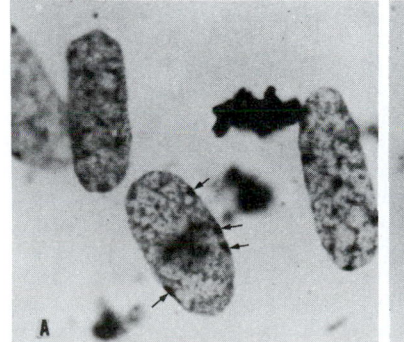
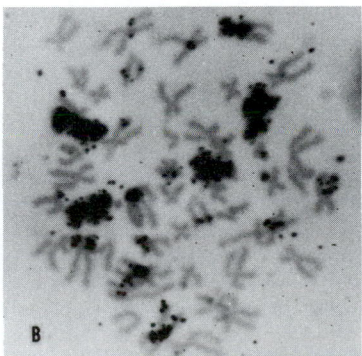
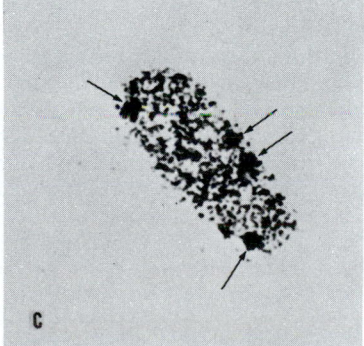

Figure 14–12. Diploid somatic cells from a girl with a 49,XXXXX karyotype. *A,* Four X chromatin bodies in an interphase nucleus from a culture of skin fibroblasts. *B,* Autoradiogram of metaphase chromosomes, illustrating four areas of high grain density overlying four of the five X chromosomes. *C,* An autoradiogram of an interphase nucleus in a culture of skin fibroblasts; four peripheral "hot" areas *(arrows)* of high grain density overlie four X chromatin bodies and provide direct evidence that each X chromatin body is derived from one late-labeling X chromosome. (Modified from Grumbach MM, Morishima A, Taylor JA. Human sex chromosome abnormalities in relation to DNA replication and heterochromatization. Proc Natl Acad Sci USA 1963; 49:581–589; and Grumbach MM. On the significance of sex chromatin. In: Second International Congress on Congenital Malformations. New York: International Medical Congress, 1964: 62–67.)

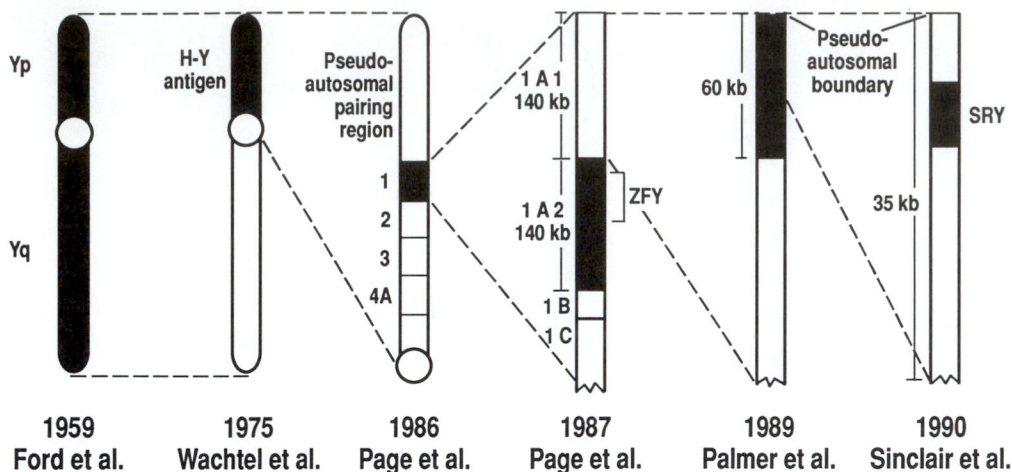

Figure 14–13. A diagrammatic representation of the historical search for the testis-determining factor (TDF). The shaded area on the Y chromosome is the region to which this factor has been localized. ZFY, zinc finger Y; SRY, sex-determining region Y; numbers 1 to 4A indicate arbitrary deletion segments on the Y chromosome. (Modified from McLaren A. What makes a man a man. Reprinted by permission from Nature vol. 346 pp. 216–217 Copyright © 1990 Macmillan Magazines Ltd.)

The genes controlling the expression of transplantation H-Y antigen and the testis-determining factor (TDF) in mice and humans are on the Y chromosome, but the genes are separate and distinct.[42, 68, 84] XX mice that inherit the Sxr (sex reversal) mutation are phenotypic males with sterile testes and are H-Y antigen–positive. Sex reversal in these mice is due to a duplication and translocation of the sex-determining region of the mouse Y chromosome to the pseudoautosomal (pairing) region. Translocation of the sex-determining region of the Y chromosome to the X chromosome occurs during meiosis, resulting in XX male mice.[85] The mouse Y chromosome carries two homologues of the zinc finger gene found in the sex-determining region of the human Y chromosome.[36, 86, 87] They have been called zinc finger Y-1 (Zfy-1) and zinc finger Y-2 (Zfy-2). A variant of Sxr has been described and termed Sxr'.[84] XX Sxr' mice are phenotypic males with testes but are H-Y antigen–negative by both cytotoxic and serological H-Y antigen assays on nongonadal cells.[68, 84] Furthermore, Sxr' mice have a deletion of the Zfy-2 locus.[86] Hence, in XX Sxr' mice, neither H-Y antigen nor Zfy-2 is necessary for testes determination.[84, 86] Furthermore, as XO Sxr' male mice lack spermatocytes and spermatids in the testes, in contrast to XO Sxr male mice, Burgoyne and associates[88] suggested that the H-Y antigen locus deleted in XO Sxr' males is either linked or related to a locus controlling spermatogenesis.

The gene(s) for H-Y antigen, as assessed by the cytotoxic T cell assay, and those for sex determination (TDF) are separate and distinct in humans.[42] Eight individuals with presumed deletions of TDF gene(s) on the Y chromosome were studied using the human leukocyte antigen (HLA)–restricted cytotoxic T cell assay for H-Y antigen. Six 46,XX men with testes were H-Y antigen–negative with this assay,[42] although all 46,XX males tested positive with the serological assay.[12, 46] As evidenced by DNA hybridization studies with Y-specific probes, these males have a small segment of the distal short arm of the Y chromosome translocated to the terminal portion of the short arm of the X chromosome. This translocation is postulated to result from anomalous recombination during meiosis between the pseudoautosomal region of the X chromosome and the sex-determining region of the Y chromosome located proximal to the pseudoautosomal region of the Y chromosome.[89, 90] Two 46,XY phenotypic females were found to be H-Y antigen–positive by the cytotoxic T cell assay[42] (other 46,XY females have serotyped both H-Y antigen–positive and –negative).[12] Hence, the gene for sex determination is located on the short arm, and the gene for H-Y antigen (cytotoxic assay) is located on the paracentromeric region of the long arm of the Y chromosome.[42]

ZFY GENE. In 1987 Page and co-workers[36] proposed that the sex-determining function of the Y chromosome is located within a 140-kb segment of the short arm of the Y chromosome. A gene in this region is conserved during evolution and encodes a protein with 13 Cys-Cys/His-His zinc fingers at the COOH-terminal end (and a basic and acidic region at the NH_2-terminal end).[91] By analogy to *Xenopus* transcription factor IIIA, it was suggested that this protein binds to DNA and/or RNA in a sequence-specific manner and regulates transcription.[36] They postulated that this zinc finger protein, termed ZFY, is the primary sex-determining signal on the Y chromosome.[36] A sequence homologous to ZFY is present on the X chromosome (ZFX) in the Xp21.2–22.1 region.[36] The latter finding initially suggested that X inactivation (dosage compensation) might play a role in sex determination.[92–94] However, ZFX escapes inactivation, so X chromosome inactivation cannot play a role in this process.[47]

SRY GENE. Convincing evidence is now available that ZFY is not the testis-determining gene. In metherian species (marsupials), sex determination is Y dependent. However, ZFY-related sequences are not located on the X and Y chromosomes of these animals but rather on autosomes.[95] Human 46,XX true hermaphrodites and 10% of 46,XX males are ZFY-negative, and Palmer and co-workers[34] reported four patients (three 46,XX males and one true hermaphrodite) who were ZFY-negative, even though all had evidence of a Y-to-X chromosome exchange. The exchange in these four patients involved Y-specific sequences distal to the ZFY locus residing within 35 kb of the pseudoautosomal boundary (Fig. 14–14). Hence, it was concluded that TDF is located in a region distal to the ZFY locus and within 35 kb of the boundary of the pseudoautosomal region of the Y. A 2.1-kb clone, pY53.3, was identified within 8 kb of the pseudoautosomal boundary. This probe detects conserved, male-specific sequences in a variety of species (Noah's ark blot) of eutherian mammals.[96] In addition, two phenotypic females with 46,XY gonadal dysgenesis have been reported in whom mutations in the SRY gene were detected.[96a, 96b] In one patient there was a conservative substitution of an isoleucine for a methionine in the putative DNA binding region of the SRY protein.[96a] In the other, a four-nucleotide deletion in the SRY gene led to a frameshift, presumably resulting in a nonfunctioning protein.[96b]

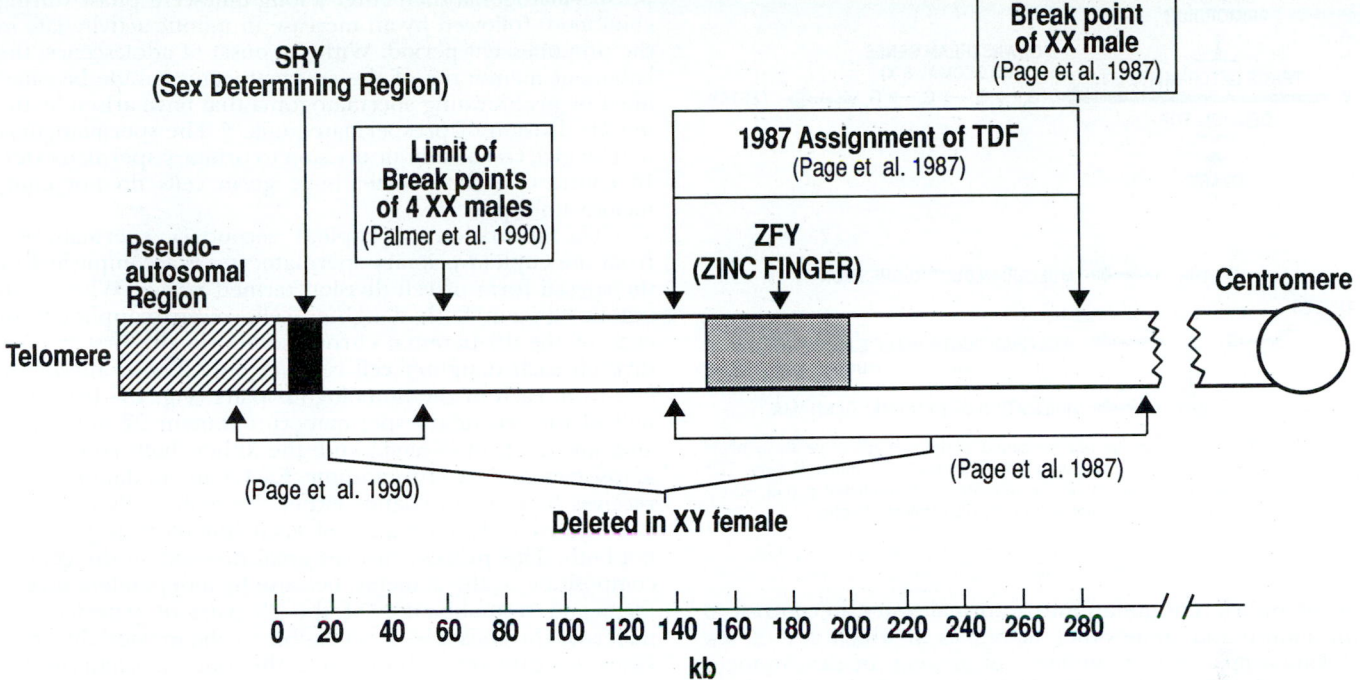

Figure 14–14. Localization of the putative sex-determining region, SRY, on the short arm of the Y chromosome (1990 putative site of TDF). The zinc finger locus ZFY is shown (the suggested site of TDF in 1987), as well as the break points observed in four 46,XX males described by Palmer and co-workers.[34] The break points of one 46,XX male and one 46,XY female studied by Page and colleagues[36] are also indicated. Note that the 46,XY female has a noncontinuous deletion that involves both ZFY and SRY.[265]

The translated nucleotide sequences of pY53.3 contain two open reading frames[96] and are homologous to a group of DNA-binding proteins, including the Mc protein encoded by the mat-3M locus of the fission yeast *S. pombe*, and to a domain in the nuclear nonhistone proteins HMG-1 and HMG-2.[96] The putative TDF is designated the SRY gene. By analogy, it appears to code for a DNA-binding protein that affects the transcription of the sex-determining gene (or genes) in a trans manner.[96]

Studies in mice support the testicular determining function of SRY. As noted earlier, mice have two zinc finger gene loci on the Y chromosome, Zfy-1 and Zfy-2.[86] Zfy-1, previously thought to be critical for sex determination, is expressed in the developing embryonic testis but not at the appropriate stage.[97] It is not expressed in the developing embryonic testis of mice homozygous for the mutation W^c/W^c, in which the testes are devoid of germ cells.[97] These findings preclude a critical role for the Zfy-1 gene in testis determination in the mouse.[97] Furthermore, fertile XY female mice have been described with a heritable mutation involving the testis-determining gene.[98, 99] Analysis of the mutant Y chromosome (designated Ȳ) did not detect a gross deletion or loss of Y-specific function except for testis determination.[99] The mutant Ȳ chromosome could be complemented by a normal Y or by Sxr', which is the smallest segment of mouse Y chromosome known to contain testis-determining genes.[100] DNA from XȲ females hybridized in Southern blots to probes for Zfy-1 and Zfy-2 but not for pY53.3 (SRY), the 2.1-kb probe cloned from the sex-determining region of the human Y chromosome.[96] However, the pY53.3 probe identified a 3.5-kb male-specific band in both XY male mice and XX Sxr' male mice. Hence, the mutation in XȲ female mice involves deletion of the gene specified for by the SRY probe pY53.3. In addition, Sry (the mouse gene analogous to human SRY) is expressed in the developing mouse gonad at 11.5 d post coitus, a stage at which the testis begins to differentiate.[99a] The mouse homologue of human pY53.3 was used to identify a family of genes including Sry on the Y chromosome and four genes on autosomes.[100]

Definitive proof that SRY is the testis-determining gene (TDF) requires the demonstration of sex reversal in XX transgenic mice carrying the Sry transcript or the production of XY females by site-directed mutagenesis of the Sry gene. Koopman and colleagues have introduced the Sry gene into mouse ova and produced XX sex-reversed transgenic mice.[100a] This is compelling evidence that SRY is TDF. Whether other genes on the short arm of the Y chromosome play a role in male sex determination and the nature and function of the "downstream" autosomal genes in the sex determination cascade remain to be determined.[101, 102]

A working scheme for sex determination suggests that the gene for SRY on the Y chromosome affects the transcription of downstream autosomal genes in a sequential fashion to induce Sertoli cell development in the bipotential primordial gonad. Differentiation of Sertoli cells evokes further testicular development including differentiation of Leydig cells. Thereafter, the fetal testis, through secretion of testosterone and antimüllerian hormone (AMH, also known as müllerian-inhibiting factor, MIF) and the actions of these hormones on specific receptors, induces male sex differentiation of the somatic sex structures (Fig. 14–15).

Genes and Ovarian Organogenesis

As early as 1958[103] it was suggested that in the human two intact X chromosomes are required for differentiation

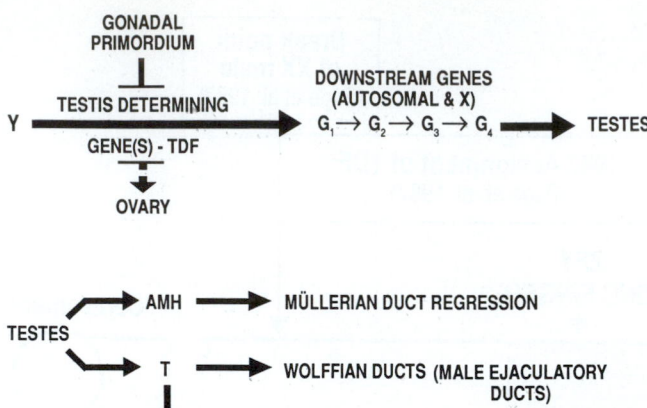

Figure 14–15. A diagrammatic representation of the cascade of genes involved in testis determination and hormones involved in male sex differentiation. TDF imposes testicular differentiation on the primordial or indifferent gonad. AMH, antimüllerian hormone; T, testosterone; DHT, dihydrotestosterone.

of the indifferent gonad into a normal ovary, in contrast to the mouse and some other mammals in which a 45,X sex chromosome constitution does not prevent the development of a fertile ovary (although it leads to accelerated atresia of ovarian follicles). In 45,X individuals, as well as those with deletions of the short arm (Xp) or long arm (Xq) of the X chromosome, ovarian development commences in utero, but oocytes usually do not survive meiosis and folliculogenesis fails to occur or is defective. This results in loss of germ cells, oocyte degeneration, and, secondarily, gonadal dysgenesis (streak gonads). Both X chromosomes appear to be active in the germ cell and oocyte from the onset of meiosis to ovulation.[104] These observations suggest that genes controlling ovarian differentiation and function are located on both arms of the X chromosome and that the viability of the germ cells and oocytes is dependent on the genetic contribution of both X chromosomes. In addition to genes on the X chromosome, the occurrence of familial 46,XX gonadal dysgenesis, which is transmitted as an autosomal recessive trait, suggests that, as in testicular development, autosomal genes, expressed through direct or indirect actions on the germ cell, are essential for ovarian organogenesis. Among the latter possibilities, a mutant autosomal gene that leads to a defect in development of the rete ovarii or in the synthesis or action of the putative meiosis-stimulating factor could result in familial 46,XX gonadal dysgenesis.

Gametogenesis

ORIGIN OF PRIMORDIAL GERM CELLS. Primordial germ cells of both sexes migrate to the undifferentiated gonads. In the 24-d embryo, germ cells are located in the dorsal endoderm of the yolk sac close to the allantoic evagination. From this site, the cells, increasing in number by mitosis, migrate during the fourth and fifth weeks to the hindgut and then through the dorsal mesentery to the primordial gonad in the urogenital ridge.[105] In the absence of primordial germ cells, the gonadal ridges in the female remain undeveloped, but germ cells are not essential for differentiation of testes.[48] Germ cells that fail to reach the gonads by the time of sex differentiation usually disappear, although persistence and teratoma formation may occur.[106]

SPERMATOGENESIS. During early testicular differentiation, the primordial germ cells become distributed throughout the primitive seminiferous tubules as progenitors of spermatogonia. A series of mitotic divisions occur, and the prespermatogonia then enter a long quiescent phase during childhood, followed by an increase in mitotic activity late in the prepubescent period. With the onset of adolescence, the basement membrane of the spermatogenic tubule becomes lined by proliferating spermatogonia that have arisen by the mitotic division of prespermatogonia.[107] The spermatogonia in turn give rise by mitotic division to primary spermatocytes. In contrast to the oocyte, male germ cells do not enter meiosis until puberty.

The formation of haploid secondary spermatocytes from the euploid primary spermatocytes is accomplished by the special form of cell division termed *meiosis*. Whereas in mitotic division both daughter cells receive duplicates of each of the 46 parental chromosomes, in the first meiotic division each daughter cell receives only 23 chromosomes, one from each of the homologous pairs (Fig. 14–16). Thus half of the secondary spermatocytes contain 22 autosomes and an X chromosome, and the other half contain 22 autosomes and a Y chromosome. Each haploid daughter cell receives by random chance either the maternally or paternally derived chromosomes of each homologous pair, but not both. This process ensures great diversity in the genetic composition of the gametes, because by independent assortment and recombination of the 23 pairs of paternal and maternal chromosomes it is possible to obtain two^{23} different kinds of gametes. This is not the only mechanism for ensuring genetic variation, however, because the special nature of the prophase during this reduction division facilitates exchanges of DNA (crossing over) between homologous chromosomes. The details of this complex process are described in standard genetics texts. Secondary spermatocytes give rise to spermatids by a second meiotic division, but this division is more analogous to mitosis than to the first meiotic division, because daughter cells are again produced by a longitudinal split of the two chromatid filaments constituting each of the unpaired chromosomes (see Fig. 14–16). Thus the haploid number is not altered.

Spermatids do not undergo further division but rather develop into spermatozoa by metamorphosis. Germ cells in the adult male are continually being renewed and undergoing maturation. Heller and Clermont[108] have shown that the complete cycle in adult males from spermatogonium to mature sperm requires about 74 ± 5 d.

OOGENESIS. Female germ cells pursue a different course. During ovarian differentiation, the primary germ cells undergo vigorous mitotic replication and successive differentiation into oogonia. When mitotic division ceases and the cells enter meiosis, they are then termed *oocytes*. Meiosis is influenced by mesonephric tissue and the secretion of a meiosis-stimulating factor. The period of oogonial proliferation results in a peak population of about 6 million to 7 million germ cells in the two ovaries at 5 mo, including oogonia, oocytes in various stages of prophase, and degenerating germ cells.[109, 110] Oocytes degenerate at different stages of meiosis. Only 5% of the peak number of germ cells in the fetal ovary reach the diplotene stage.[109] Formation of oogonia from primary germ cells ceases by the seventh month of gestation. Some oocytes remain in undifferentiated nests, whereas others form primordial follicles.[105] A follicle is formed when presumptive granulosa cells surround the diplotene oocyte and an intact basal lamina encloses this unit. If the oocyte is not enclosed in a follicle, it degenerates.[106] The number of primordial follicles in the ovary is maximal at birth, and the number then diminishes. In the germ cells that survive, the oocyte is arrested at late prophase of the first meiotic division (diplotene state) and remains in this state from before birth until ovulation occurs many years later. The arrest of the oocyte in late prophase of meiosis is thought to be due to a meiosis-preventing factor.

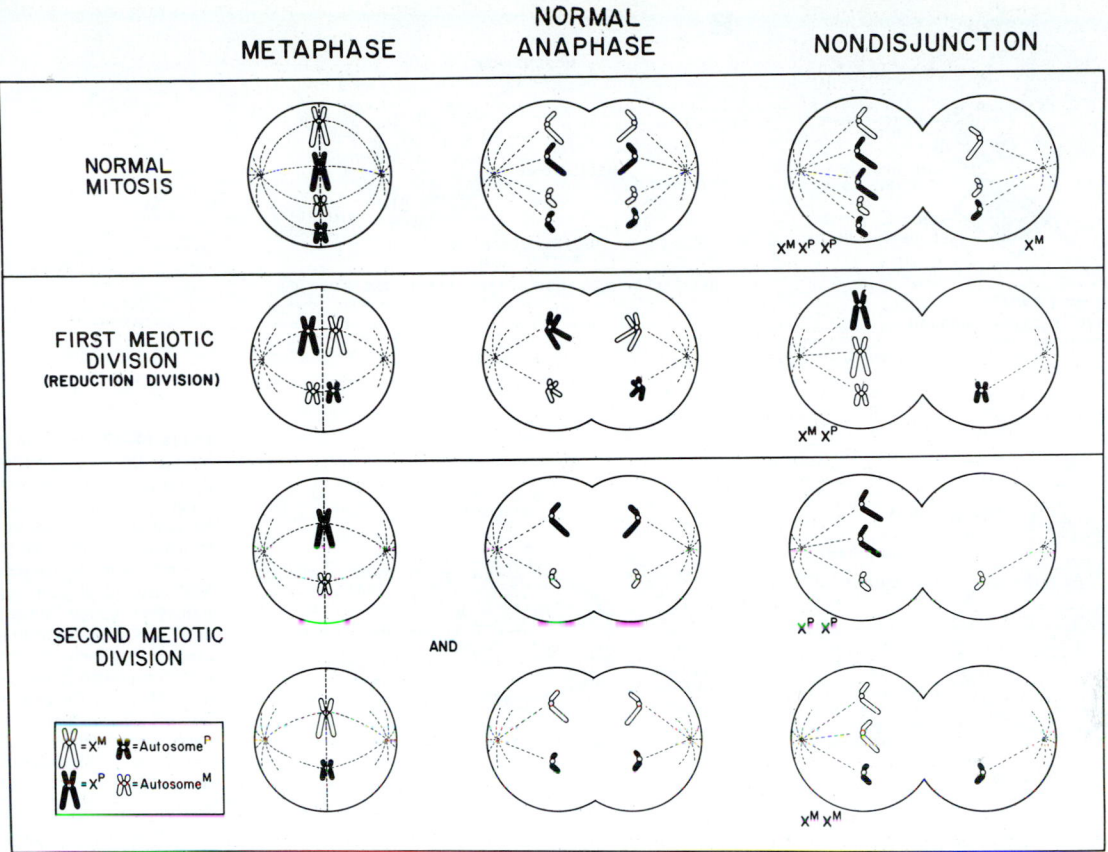

Figure 14–16. *Mitosis,* A diagram of a female somatic cell undergoing mitosis. Represented at the metaphase plate are two X chromosomes and two homologous autosomes of group 21–22. Division occurs through the centromere, giving rise to two daughter cells of identical chromosomal composition. Replication of each arm into two chromatids takes place while the chromosomes are extended and before the next metaphase. *First Meiotic Division,* This process involves pairing of homologous chromosomes. The centromere does not divide in this cell division. It is by chance whether the maternal (X^M) or paternal (X^P) member of each pair goes to the respective daughter cells. During the complex prophase of first meiotic division (not shown), multiple chiasmata are formed between the chromosomes of each pair, facilitating exchanges of chromosomal segments (crossing over) between them. *Second Meiotic Division,* During this division the centromere again divides, giving rise to daughter cells identical to the parent cell. This division more nearly resembles mitosis than the first meiotic division. Nondisjunction can take place either in mitosis or in the first or second meiotic division. Representative examples are illustrated.

The long life span of female germ cells, in contrast to that of the male, may have an important bearing on the increased prevalence of certain chromosomal anomalies with advanced maternal age.

Before ovulation, the first polar body is extruded, thus completing the first meiotic division. The haploid secondary oocyte immediately begins a second meiotic division but remains in metaphase and does not extrude the second polar body until the ovum is penetrated by a sperm cell. The triploidy found in spontaneously aborted fetuses may be due either to failure of extrusion of the second polar body (polygyny) or to double fertilization (polyspermy).

Differentiation of the Testis and the Ovary

The gonads of both sexes develop from anlagen located on the medioventral border of the urogenital ridge, adjacent to the kidney and primitive adrenal (Fig. 14–17).[4, 10, 106, 109–116] Until the 12-mm stage (approximately 42 d of gestation), the gonads of the male and female are indistinguishable on morphological grounds and could potentially differentiate either as a testis or as an ovary. The close ontogenic relationship between gonadal and adrenal cells at this early stage is noteworthy, because as differentiation proceeds nests of adrenal cells frequently separate with the gonad and are found as adrenal rests in the hilum of the mature ovary or

testis. Such rests may become a problem in patients with long-standing untreated adrenal hyperplasia. Adrenal cell rests in testes, for example, may enlarge under persistent corticotropin (ACTH, adrenocorticotropin) stimulation and be mistaken for testicular tumors or true testicular enlargement.

The primitive undifferentiated gonad is derived from proliferation of the mesodermal coelomic epithelium, the mesenchymal cell mass in the urogenital ridge, mesonephric elements,[111, 115] and the large alkaline phosphatase–containing primordial germ cells that have migrated from the posterior endoderm of the yolk sac through the mesenchyme of the mesentery to the gonad. According to Witschi, the number of migrating germ cells in the human embryo is about 700 to 1300, and by the eighth week of embryogenesis about 600,000 germ cells are present.[105, 109] These large cells later become either oogonia or spermatogonia. Lack of germ cells is incompatible with ovarian differentiation but does not completely prevent testicular morphogenesis. The role of the primordial germ cells in testis differentiation is unsettled. The precursor of the Sertoli cell of the testis and its counterpart in the ovary, the granulosa cell, are not yet firmly established. Wartenberg and co-workers[117] suggested a dual origin from both the germinal epithelium and cells of mesonephric origin. In the mouse the rete ovarii, a derivative of the mesonephric tubules, appear to give rise to the first granulosa cells.[10, 118]

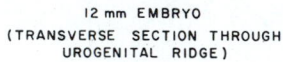

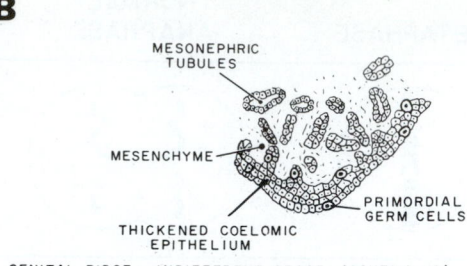

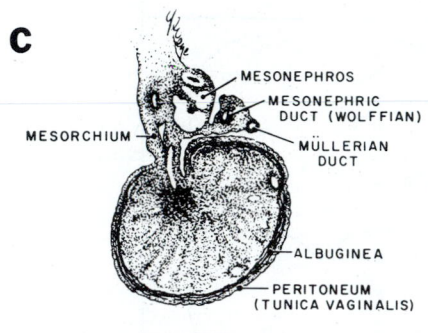

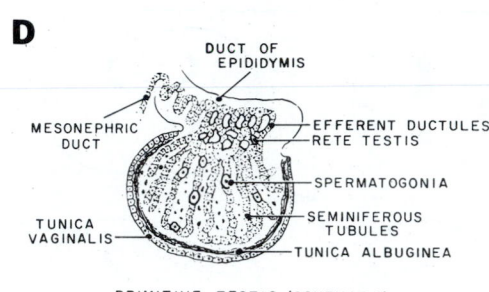

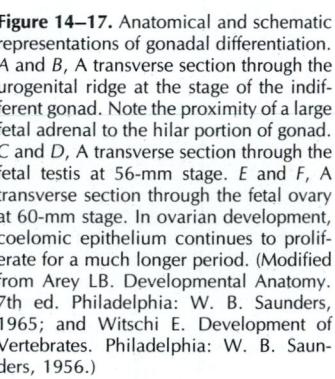

Figure 14–17. Anatomical and schematic representations of gonadal differentiation. *A* and *B*, A transverse section through the urogenital ridge at the stage of the indifferent gonad. Note the proximity of a large fetal adrenal to the hilar portion of gonad. *C* and *D*, A transverse section through the fetal testis at 56-mm stage. *E* and *F*, A transverse section through the fetal ovary at 60-mm stage. In ovarian development, coelomic epithelium continues to proliferate for a much longer period. (Modified from Arey LB. Developmental Anatomy. 7th ed. Philadelphia: W. B. Saunders, 1965; and Witschi E. Development of Vertebrates. Philadelphia: W. B. Saunders, 1956.)

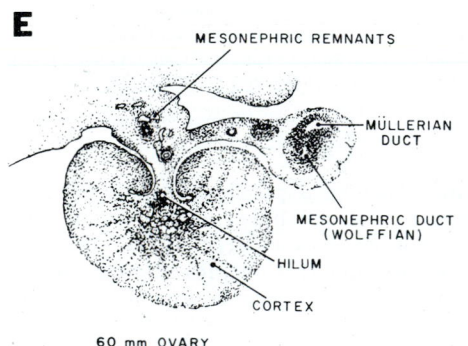

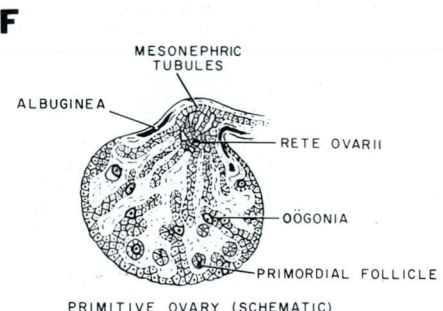

There is a striking difference between sexes in the timing of gonadal differentiation. Under the influence of the testes-determining genes, testes organization begins at about 45 d of gestation (6 to 7 wk). The ovary does not emerge from the indifferent stage until 3 mo, when the earliest sign appears—the beginning of meiosis as evidenced by the maturation of oogonia into oocytes.[4, 10, 113]

TESTIS. In the past it was widely believed that the testis is derived primarily from the medullary portion of the primitive gonad, whereas the ovary is derived from the cortical portion. According to this concept, the testis and ovary are not strictly homologous, because they differentiate from different primordial structures. Witschi and coworkers[119] suggested that in genetic males the medullary portion secretes an inductor substance that stimulates development of seminiferous tubules and inhibits cortical development; conversely, the cortex of genetic females was thought to secrete an inductor substance that inhibits testicular development and results in ovarian dominance.

Jost and co-workers,[114, 120] Jirasek,[4] and van Wagenen and Simpson,[115] among others, have called into question the histological descriptions of gonadal differentiation that served as the basis for these theories. After carefully examining early embryos, Jost[114] and Jirasek[4] concluded that it is not possible to identify primary sex cords as such before the 15-mm stage (about 45 d), when epithelial cords derived from the coelomic epithelium, the gonadal blastema, and the germ cells, antecedents of the seminiferous tubules, are apparent in the male. With the onset of testicular differentiation and the incorporation of the germ cells into the primitive seminiferous cords, proliferation of the germ cells is suppressed and differentiation is arrested at the primitive spermatogonial stage. This may be mediated by a Sertoli cell meiosis-preventing substance or by the separation of the primordial germ cell from the meiosis-inducing substance secreted by the rete testis.[106] The somatic cells of the cords are the presumptive Sertoli cells, and the germ cells are the future spermatogonia. Burgoyne and associates[121–123] have proposed from studies of XX↔XY chimeric mice that the sex-determining gene on the Y chromosome acts autonomously to induce Sertoli cell differentiation, which then mediates further testicular differentiation. Studies of mice with single-gene mutations or radiation-induced injury indicate that germ cells are not critical to testicular cord formation.[106] After testicular differentiation (43 to 50 d gestational age) occurs,[4] the male embryo can also be recognized by beginning regression of the primitive müllerian ducts (30-mm stage, about 60 d) and differentiation of male external genitalia (40-mm stage, 65 to 77 d).

An early endocrine function of the fetal testis is the secretion by the Sertoli cells of AMH, a glycoprotein that functions as a paracrine secretion and by diffusion passes to the paired müllerian ducts and induces their dissolution.[124] The versatile Sertoli cell also secretes inhibin, nurtures the germ cells, synthesizes an androgen-binding protein, and, as noted, prevents meiosis.

Leydig cells are first found in 32- to 35-mm fetuses (about 60 d) and rapidly proliferate during the third month, after differentiation of the primitive testicular cords, and during the first half of the fourth month;[4, 119, 120, 125] during this period the interstitial spaces between the seminiferous tubules are crowded with Leydig cells. The onset of testosterone biosynthesis occurs at about 9 wk[126] and the Leydig cell has human chorionic gonadotropin–luteinizing hormone (hCG-LH) cell membrane receptors by week 12 of gestation.[127, 128] The Leydig cells secrete testosterone, the regulator of male differentiation of the wolffian ducts, urogenital sinus, and external genitalia. The plasma concentration of testosterone in the male fetus correlates with the biosynthetic activity of the fetal testes.[126] Peak concentrations in the fetal circulation (7 to 21 nmol/L [2 to 6 ng/mL]) are reached by about 16 wk of gestation, comparable to values in the adult male.[129, 130] Between 16 and 20 wk the testosterone level falls to about 3.5 nmol/L (1 ng/mL); after 24 wk the concentration of testosterone is low (in the early pubertal range). Testosterone in amniotic fluid shows a similar pattern.[131] Clinical as well as biochemical data suggest that hCG secreted by the syncytiotrophoblast stimulates testosterone secretion during the critical period of male sex differentia-

tion,[127, 130] although a more recent report suggests that testosterone secretion and adenylate cyclase activity in the early fetal testis may be independent of hCG.[132] Whether hCG is required to initiate testosterone secretion in the human is not known, and this question is complicated by the detection of hCG-like material in the fetal testis.[132, 133] The pattern of testosterone secretion early in gestation follows that of hCG.[130, 134] The number of Leydig cells decreases after 18 wk, probably by dedifferentiation, and few cells show Leydig cell characteristics in the interstitium of the testis at birth. However, a low level of testosterone secretion is maintained after 15 wk of gestation under the control of fetal pituitary LH and hCG.[130, 134] Fetal pituitary gonadotropins are essential for the continued growth and function of the fetal testis after the early period of sex differentiation. Fetal pituitary LH seems necessary in concert with hCG for the normal growth of the differentiated penis and scrotum and for the descent of the testes.[134] The male fetus with anencephaly or congenital hypopituitarism often has hypoplastic male external genitalia and undescended testes containing a decreased number of Leydig cells.[130, 134]

Figure 14–18 correlates the pattern of testosterone, hCG, and fetal pituitary follicle-stimulating hormone (FSH) and LH during gestation with the histological changes in the fetal testis.

In sum, organogenesis of the testis involves successively differentiation of the seminiferous cords with primitive Sertoli cells enveloping the extragonadally derived germ cells, development of the tunica albuginea, appearance of Leydig cells, and finally differentiation of the mesonephric tubules into the ductuli efferentes, which connect the seminiferous tubules and rete network with the epididymis to provide the pathway for sperm into the ejaculatory duct system.

OVARY. In the absence of testis-determining genes, the gonadal primordium has an inherent tendency to develop as an ovary, *provided that germ cells are present and survive.* The indifferent stage persists in the female fetus weeks after testis organogenesis begins. There is, however, continued proliferation of the coelomic epithelium and primordial germ cells, which gradually enlarge and become oogonia. Despite the discordance in the histological appearance of the primordial testis and ovary, George and Wilson[135] have noted the simultaneous development at 8 wk of gestation of the capacity of the fetal testis to synthesize testosterone and

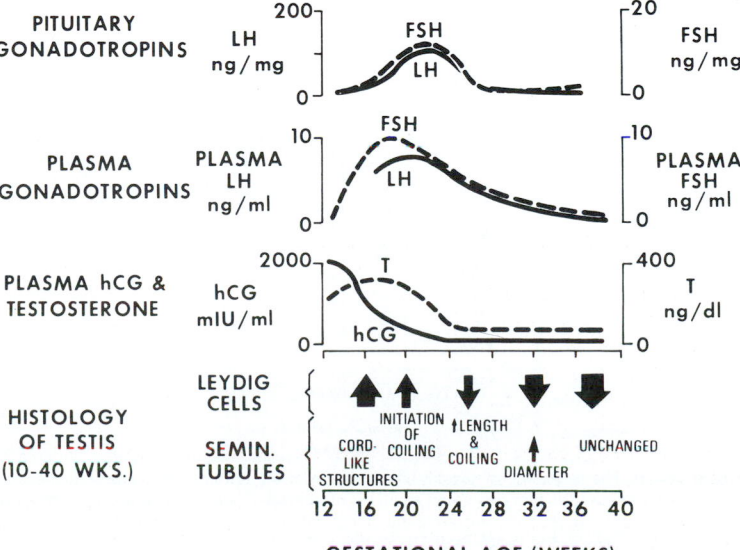

Figure 14–18. Comparison of the pattern of change of serum testosterone and hCG and serum and pituitary LH (LER-960) and FSH (LER-869) in the human male fetus during gestation with morphological changes in the fetal testis. (Adapted from Kaplan SL, Grumbach MM. Pituitary and placental gonadotropins and sex steroids in the human and subhuman primate fetus. Clin Endocrinol Metab 1978; 7:487–511.)

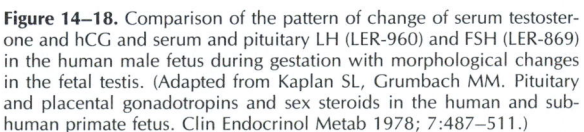

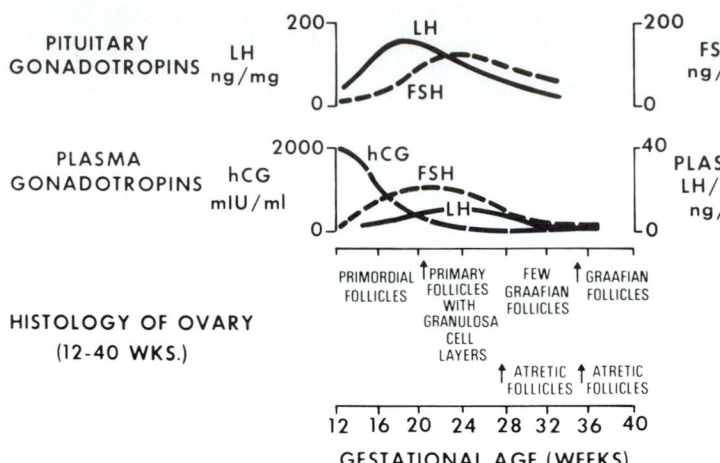

Figure 14–19. Comparison of the pattern of serum FSH, LH, and hCG and pituitary FSH and LH in the human female fetus during gestation with the developmental histology of the fetal ovary. (Adapted from Kaplan SL, Grumbach MM. Pituitary and placental gonadotropins and sex steroids in the human and sub-human primate fetus. Clin Endocrinol Metab 1978; 7:487–511.)

of the fetal "ovary" to synthesize estradiol[135] when incubated with C$_{21}$-steroid precursors. Although the gonads of both male and female fetuses have 3β-hydroxysteroid dehydrogenase (3β-HSD) activity at this stage, the activity of this enzyme is more than 50-fold greater in the fetal testis.[135] Testosterone is synthesized by the fetal Leydig cell, but the site of synthesis of estradiol in the primordial ovary is not known. However, Gondos and Hobel[136] have identified interstitial cells in the ovarian primordium at about 12 wk of gestation that have the ultrastructural characteristics of steroidogenic cells.[136] The fetus is bathed in estrogens of placental origin, and it is unlikely that the fetal ovary contributes significantly to circulating estrogens in the fetus. The ovary has no documented role in differentiation of the female genital tract.

During the ninth week the rete ovarii arise from the hilar mesonephric tubules and infiltrate the gonad as a syncytium of tubules and cords.[10] About the 11th to 12th wk (80-mm stage), long after differentiation of the testis in the male fetus, germ cells begin to enter meiotic prophase, which characterizes the transition of oogonia into oocytes and marks the onset of ovarian differentiation. The oogonia in the most central part of the ovary are the first to come in contact with the rete ovarii and the first to enter meiosis. According to Byskov,[106, 116] the rete secretes a meiosis-inducing substance. The formation of primordial follicles (in which the oocyte is enveloped by a single layer of flat granulosa cells) reaches a maximum during the 20th to the 25th wk of gestation; during this period the plasma concentration of fetal pituitary FSH attains its peak[130, 134] and the first primary follicles are formed (Fig. 14–19). Hence, by the 20th to the 25th wk, the gonad has the morphological characteristics of a definitive ovary. As discussed earlier, the maximal number of germ cells decreases from a peak of between 6 million and 7 million to 2 million at term. The last oogonia enter meiosis at 7 mo of gestation. In the anencephalic female fetus, the ovaries are small and exhibit a decreased number and hypoplasia of primary follicles,

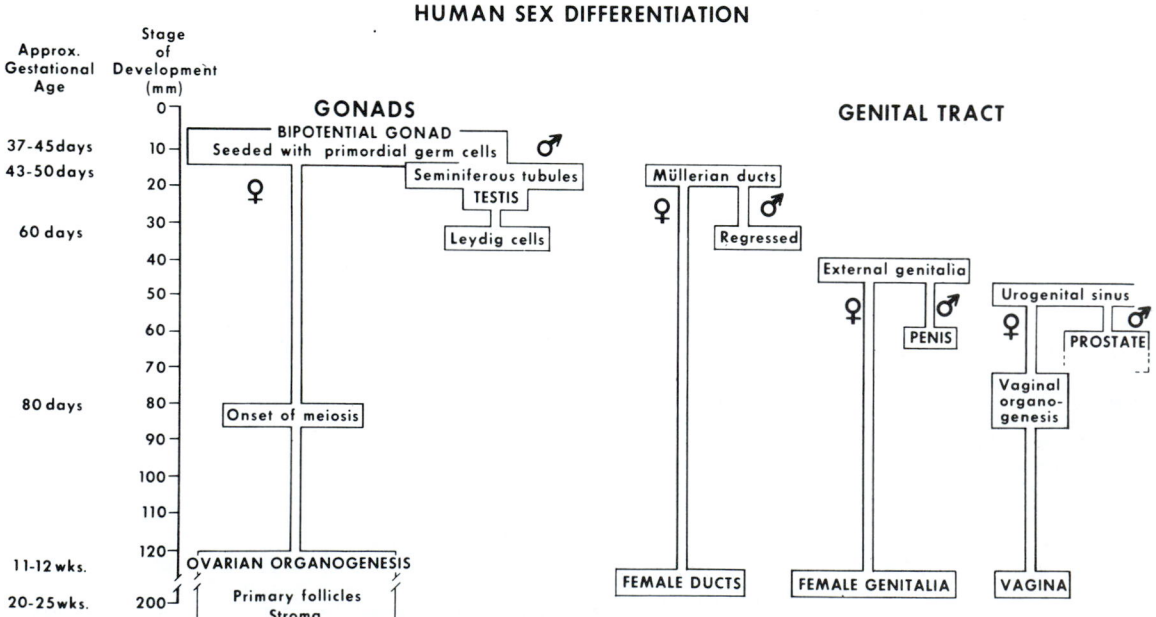

Figure 14–20. The sequence of sexual differentiation in the human fetus. The sequence as schematically depicted here emphasizes that testicular development in the male fetus precedes all other forms of sexual dimorphism. There is an inherent propensity of the gonads, genital ducts, and external genitalia to feminize, whereas masculinization requires Y chromosome–mediated differentiation of the fetal testes. (Modified from Jost A. Hormonal factors in the sex differentiation of the mammalian foetus. Philos Trans R Soc Lond [Biol] 1970; 259:119–130.)

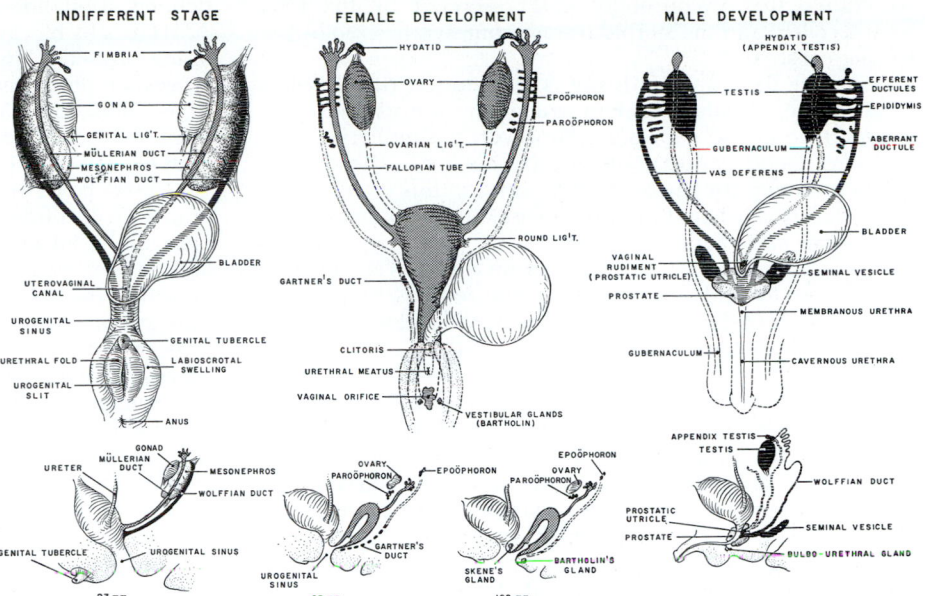

Figure 14–21. Embryonic differentiation of male and female genital ducts from wolffian and müllerian primordia. *Left,* An indifferent stage showing large mesonephric body. *Middle,* Female ducts. Remnants of mesonephros and wolffian ducts are now termed the epoophoron, paroöphoron, and Gartner duct. *Right,* Male ducts before descent into scrotum. The only müllerian remnant is the testicular appendix. Prostatic utricle (vagina masculina) is derived from urogenital sinus. (Modified from Corning HK. Lehrbuch der Entwicklungsgeschichte des Menschen. Munich: J. F. Bergmann, 192J; and Wilkins L. The Diagnosis and Treatment of Endocrine Disorders in Childhood and Adolescence. 3rd ed. 1965. Courtesy of Charles C Thomas, Publisher, Springfield, Illinois.)

whereas the hilar cells seem to be similar in anencephalic and normal fetuses, suggesting that the hilar cells differentiate independently of the effect of pituitary gonadotropins.[106, 130, 134] Whereas the meiosis-inducing factor of the rete may be essential for meiosis and the formation of primordial follicles, the growth, development, and maintenance of follicles are influenced by fetal pituitary gonadotropins, mainly FSH.

The sequence and time of events in gonadal organogenesis and the relationship to the differentiation of male and female somatic sexual characteristics are shown in Figure 14–20.

Differentiation of the Genital Ducts

At the seventh week of intrauterine life, the fetus is equipped with both male and female genital ducts derived from the mesonephros. The müllerian ducts serve as the anlagen of the uterus and fallopian tubes, whereas the mesonephric or wolffian ducts have the potential to differentiate further into the epididymis, vas deferens (the ejaculatory ducts of the male), and seminal vesicles. During the third fetal month either the müllerian or wolffian ducts complete their development, while involution occurs simultaneously in the opposite structures (Fig. 14–21).

Jost[137, 138] demonstrated that secretions from the fetal testis play a decisive role in determining the direction of genital duct development. In the presence of functional testes, the müllerian structures involute and the wolffian ducts complete their development, whereas in the absence of testes the wolffian ducts do not develop and the müllerian structures differentiate (Fig. 14–22). The retrogression of the müllerian ducts and the stabilization and differentiation of the wolffian ducts are mediated by two fetal testicular

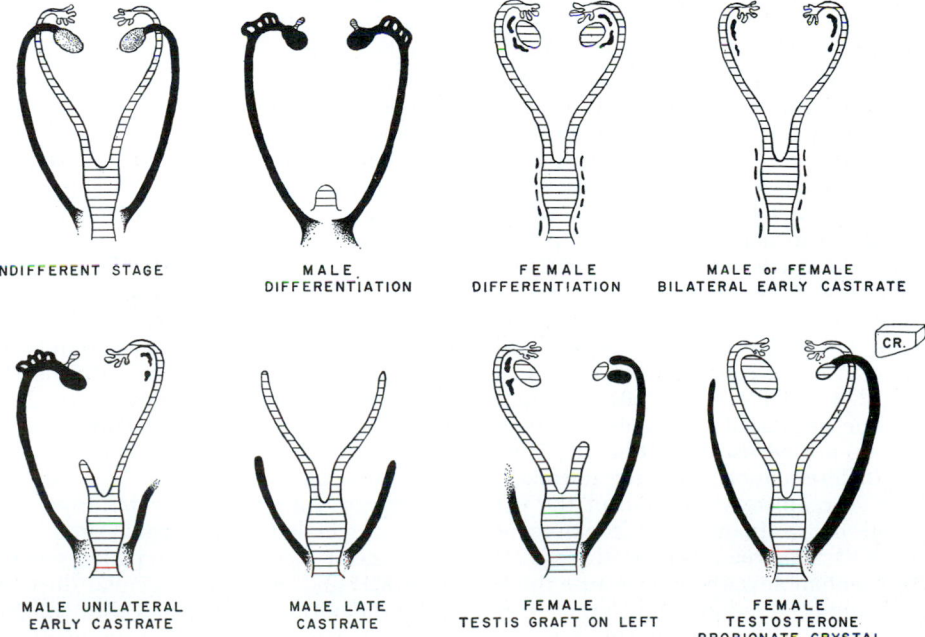

Figure 14–22. A schematic summary of Jost's experiments with rabbit embryos. The fetal testis plays a decisive role in determining the differentiation of the genital ducts. Testosterone stimulates wolffian development but fails to effect involution of müllerian structures. (Data from Jost A. Embryonic sexual differentiation [morphology, physiology, abnormalities]. In: Jones HW, Scott WW, eds. Hermaphroditism, Genital Anomalies and Related Endocrine Disorders. 2nd ed. Baltimore: Williams & Wilkins, 1971: 16.)

secretions: the glycoprotein AMH secreted by the fetal Sertoli cells[124] and the steroid testosterone synthesized by the Leydig cells.

Female development is not contingent on the presence of an ovary, because development of the uterus and tubes occurs if no gonad is present. However, the müllerian duct (paramesonephric duct) fails to differentiate in the absence of the mesonephric ducts (wolffian ducts); thus renal aplasia is commonly associated with hypoplasia of the fallopian tubes and uterus and vaginal agenesis.

The influence of the fetal testis on duct development is exerted locally and unilaterally; if one testis is removed at an early stage of development, the oviduct develops normally on that side, whereas müllerian regression occurs on the side of the intact testis.[138]

Systemic administration of androgen to an early embryo does not cause regression of müllerian structures. Even when large amounts of androgen are implanted locally in the gonadal region of female fetuses, the müllerian ducts do not atrophy, whereas the wolffian ducts become virilized.[137, 138] On the other hand, if a testis is grafted onto an ovary, müllerian regression and wolffian stimulation occur on that side (Fig. 14–22). For these reasons, Jost proposed that the fetal testis secretes a müllerian duct–inhibiting substance that is distinct from ordinary androgens.

Josso and associates[5, 124] studied the influence of the fetal testis on müllerian duct inhibition in organ culture. Direct contact between the testis and the müllerian anlage was not necessary to bring about this inhibition. By separating the testis from the müllerian ducts with dialysis membranes, they concluded that the material secreted from the testis was macromolecular and not a steroid. They also demonstrated that the human fetal testis, regardless of age, inhibits the müllerian ducts of 14.5-d-old fetal rats in similar organ culture studies and that AMH activity is present in human testes until 8 to 10 y of age.[139, 140] Using bovine fetal testes in which tubules and interstitial tissue were isolated and assayed separately, they showed that AMH actively is derived from the Sertoli cell with peak levels occurring at the time of müllerian duct regression.[124, 140] Thereafter, the levels remain high until birth, after which a steady decline occurs until the prepubertal period.[124, 140] AMH is present in the ovarian follicle and is synthesized and secreted by the granulosa cells.[141] However, both ovarian development and AMH secretion occur later in granulosa cells than in testes and after the "window" of sensitivity of the müllerian ducts to AMH. Hence, AMH secretion by the fetal and postnatal ovary does not affect the development of the fallopian tubes and the uterus. Exposure of the ovary and the müllerian structures to AMH before the refractory period occurs in the freemartin. AMH secreted by the fetal Sertoli cells of the male twin passes by placental anastomosis to the female twin. This results in müllerian regression, ovarian inhibition, tunica albuginea formation, and development of seminiferous tubule–like cords.[142, 143] Studies with transgenic female mice that persistently express the human AMH gene have produced results similar to the freemartin model.[144] The transgenic female mice lack müllerian derivatives, and at birth the ovaries have fewer germ cells than normal. During the first 2 wk of life germ cells are lost and the somatic cells become organized into seminiferous tubule–like structures that do not persist to adulthood.[144] In transgenic male mice, sex differentiation is usually normal, although some males have incomplete virilization of the external genitalia, inhibition of wolffian duct development, and undescended testes.[144] The relevance of these studies to "normal" sex differentiation is unclear because the levels of AMH and its continuous secretion are different from those in the normal mouse fetus. The mechanism of action of AMH is still to be defined. Donahoe and co-workers[145] have suggested that AMH acts by blocking phosphorylation of tyrosine on membrane proteins. Physiological roles for AMH in males after regression of the müllerian ducts and in females also are yet to be defined. AMH may play a role in testicular descent,[139, 146] and AMH may function as a meiotic inhibitor in both males[147] and females.[148]

AMH is a glycoprotein composed of identical subunits linked by disulfide bonds.[149] The monomer has a molecular mass of 72 kd and the multimer ranges from 145 to 235 kd.[124] The gene for AMH encodes a 560-amino-acid protein in which the COOH-terminal domain shows marked homology with transforming growth factor β and the β chain of porcine inhibin and activin.[149] The gene is located on the short arm of chromosome 19.[150]

Studies of humans with various forms of intersex have confirmed that AMH is the decisive factor in causing regression of the müllerian ducts. In patients with rudimentary gonads, the uterus and fallopian tubes develop normally regardless of the chromosomal sex. In true hermaphrodites who have a testis on one side and an ovary on the other, regression of the müllerian ducts is most marked on the side of the testis. Similarly, müllerian derivatives are absent in 46,XY women with the syndrome of testicular feminization, a condition characterized by unresponsiveness of tissues to the action of androgens. Conversely, early intrauterine exposure of human female fetuses to high levels of androgens (as in congenital adrenal hyperplasia) fails to hinder normal development of the uterus and fallopian tubes.

Although müllerian involution is not androgen dependent, the differentiation of primitive wolffian ducts into the epididymides, vas deferens, and seminal vesicles requires testosterone and the cytosolic androgen receptor.[151, 152] Mice, rats treated with cyproterone acetate (an agent that blocks androgen action), and androgen-resistant XY individuals show the expected regression of the müllerian ducts, but structures derived from wolffian ducts remain vestigial.[153] Jost showed that the implantation of a crystal of testosterone adjacent to the fetal rabbit ovary stimulates differentiation of male ducts on that side and to a lesser extent on the contralateral side; similar results were obtained by grafting a fetal testis adjacent to the ovary (see Fig. 14–22).

The lateralization of these effects suggests that higher local concentrations of androgen are required for male duct stimulation than for masculinization of the external genitalia and derivatives of the urogenital sinus. Unlike the masculinization of the urogenital sinus and external genitalia, in which testosterone reaches these target tissues systemically via the circulation (a classic endocrine effect), local diffusion of testosterone from the testis may be involved in stabilization and differentiation of wolffian duct derivatives. This local effect of a hormone from one cell on neighboring cells by local dissemination is referred to as a paracrine action.

During differentiation of the wolffian ducts to form the epididymides, vasa deferentia, and seminal vesicles, they lack the enzyme 5α-reductase that converts testosterone to dihydrotestosterone.[154] Thus testosterone (not dihydrotestosterone) binds to the cytosolic androgen receptor in the wolffian duct cells during the critical period of sex differentiation and induces the development of male duct derivatives. This is in striking contrast to the urogenital sinus and genital tubercle, which acquire this enzyme even before the testis has developed the capacity to synthesize testosterone.[155] It is dihydrotestosterone that mediates the masculinization of the urogenital sinus and external genitalia.

In patients with ambiguous genitalia, well-differentiated male genital ducts are seen only in those who have testes. Females with congenital adrenal hyperplasia do not display this development, even though the external genitalia may be highly virilized in utero. Patients with asymmetrical gonadal differentiation likewise have asymmetrical male duct development that correlates with the degree of testicular differentiation on that side.

If the critical role of the testis in male duct development is to provide a high local concentration of testosterone, male duct development would be expected to be deficient, even though testes are present, in patients with severe defects in steroid biosynthesis (e.g., cytochrome P-450$_{scc}$ deficiency) and in XY patients whose tissues are unresponsive to testosterone (complete syndrome of androgen resistance). The epididymides and vasa deferentia of these patients are indeed hypoplastic or rudimentary. During sex differentiation testosterone and AMH may mediate their morphogenetic actions on the underlying mesenchymal cells rather than directly affecting the epithelial cells.[156] Action of the hormone-stimulated mesenchyme on the epithelial cells appears to be a major factor in the morphogenesis of the male ducts and in retrogression of the müllerian ducts.[156]

Differentiation of External Genitalia and Urogenital Sinus

Origin of the External Genitalia

At the eighth fetal week the external genitalia of both sexes are identical and have the capacity to differentiate in either direction.[157] They consist of a urogenital slit bounded by paired urethral folds and, more laterally, by labioscrotal swellings. The urogenital slit is surmounted by a genital tubercle consisting of corpora cavernosa and glans (Fig. 14–23). The mucosa-lined urethral folds may remain separate, in which case they are called labia minora, or may fuse to form a corpus spongiosum enclosing a phallic urethra. The fleshy labioscrotal swellings may remain separate to form labia majora or fuse in the midline to form a scrotum and the ventral epidermal covering of the penis. The distinction between a clitoris and a penis is based primarily on size and whether or not the labia minora fuse to form a corpus spongiosum.

By the 50-mm crown-rump stage, male and female fetuses can be distinguished by inspection of the external genitalia; in the male, the urethral folds have fused completely in the midline to form the cavernous urethra and corpus spongiosum by 12 to 14 wk of gestation. Penile length in the male increases linearly, at about 0.7 mm/wk, from 10 wk to normal term; a 12-fold increase occurs from 0.3 cm at 10 wk to 3.5 cm at term, a rate of growth about 3.5 times that of the clitoris.[158]

Origin of the Vagina

The urogenital sinus separates from a common cloaca in early fetal life.[159] There is disagreement about the relative

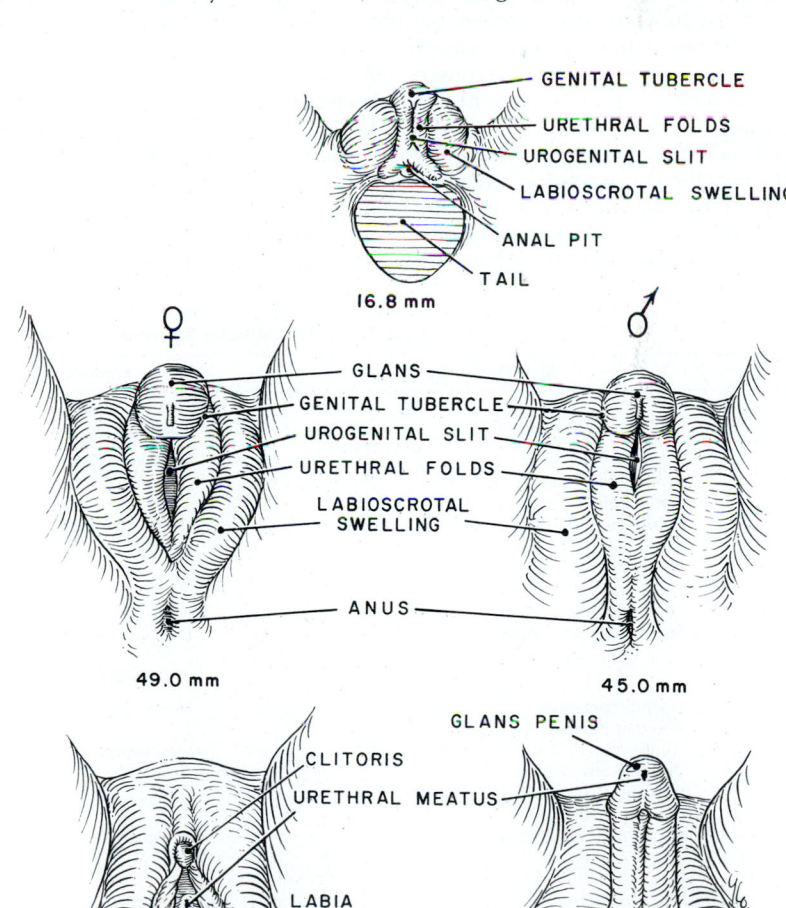

Figure 14–23. Differentiation of male and female external genitalia from indifferent primordia. Male development will occur only in the presence of androgenic stimulation during the first 12 fetal weeks. (Adapted from Spaulding MH. The development of the external genitalia in the human embryo. Contrib Embryol Carnegie Inst 1921; 13:69–88.)

contribution of the müllerian duct and the urogenital sinus to the vagina. However, the contact and interaction of the fused müllerian ducts with the urogenital sinus is essential for normal development of the vagina.[160, 161] In normal female development, proliferation of the vesicovaginal septum pushes the vaginal orifice posteriorly so that it acquires a separate external opening; thus no urogenital sinus, as such, is preserved. In male development the vaginal pouch is usually obliterated when the müllerian ducts are resorbed, although a vestigial blind vaginal pouch known as the prostatic utricle can sometimes be demonstrated.

The prostate gland and bulbourethral glands of Cowper in the male are outgrowths of the urogenital sinus; their differentiation is mediated by dihydrotestosterone and requires the presence of cytosolic androgen receptors. In the female, the paraurethral glands of Skene and the vestibular glands of Bartholin have homologous origins (Table 14–4).

Mechanism of Androgen Action

The effects of testosterone are varied and tissue specific and reflect the sum of its action and the actions of its conversion products, dihydrotestosterone and estradiol (Fig. 14–24).[162, 163] Testosterone enters the cell by diffusion. It can be 5α-reduced to dihydrotestosterone or aromatized to estradiol. Subsequently, testosterone and dihydrotestosterone bind to a high-affinity androgen receptor protein. This receptor has a twofold greater binding affinity for dihydrotestosterone than testosterone. It is encoded by a gene located between the centromere and Xq13 on the X chromosome[53] and is present in androgen-sensitive target tissues of both males and females. The androgen receptor is a member of a family of regulatory proteins that includes the specific receptors for other steroids as well as for vitamin D, thyroid hormone, and the oncogene v-*erb* A[164] (Fig. 14–25) (also see Chapter 3). These receptors have in common three domains: (1) an NH$_2$-terminal domain thought to be involved in gene transcription; (2) a DNA binding domain that contains two zinc fingers (see Fig. 14–25), of which one has information for sequence-specific binding to DNA and the other is thought to stabilize binding of the receptor to DNA (Fig. 14–26); and (3) a COOH-terminal domain that binds the ligand (androgen).[164, 165] The degree of homology between the receptors in this family is highest in the DNA binding domains and diminishes in the ligand binding domains.[164] The NH$_2$-terminal domains of these receptors show little homology.

Steroid hormone receptors, but not the vitamin D and thyroid hormone receptors, are complexed to heat shock proteins in the absence of ligand.[164] Ligand binding results in a conformational change in the receptor with dissociation from the heat shock protein and "activation" of the receptor.[162, 164] The activated steroid-receptor complex is smaller (4S or less) than the unactivated complex (8S or greater).[166] The steroid-receptor complex binds to steroid-responsive elements in genomic DNA that are upstream from CAAT and TATA boxes.[162, 164] RNA polymerase and other transcription factors are recruited to initiate transcription (messenger RNA [mRNA]) of the steroid response gene at a point 19 to 27 kb downstream of the TATA box. After transcription and processing of the mRNA, the RNA moves to the cytoplasm, where it is translated by cytoplasmic ribosomes and results in synthesis of new proteins and hence androgenic effects.

It is thought that testosterone and dihydrotestosterone have different roles. The testosterone-receptor complex modulates the secretion of LH by the hypothalamic-pituitary unit and affects the stabilization of the wolffian ducts, whereas the dihydrotestosterone-receptor complex primarily affects masculinization of the urogenital sinus and external genitalia of the fetus and pubertal maturation.[163] A defect in any of the sequential steps in the action of androgen in a male fetus results in impaired masculinization of the urogenital sinus and external genitalia (Fig. 14–27).

TABLE 14–4. Homologies Between Male and Female Sexual Structures

Male Derivative	Primordial Structure	Female Derivative
	Gonad	
	Indifferent gonad derived from	
Seminiferous tubules	Coelomic epithelium	Graafian follicles
Sertoli cells	Mesenchymal cell mass	Granulosa cells
Leydig cells	Mesonephric elements	Theca cells
		Interstitial cells
Rete testes		Rete ovarii
Septa and tunica albuginea		
Tunica vaginalis		
Spermatogonia → sperm	Primordial germ cells	Oogonia → ova
	Genital Ducts	
Ductuli efferentes	Mesonephric tubules	Epoophoron
Aberrant ductules		Paroophoron
Epididymis	Mesonephric (wolffian) ducts	Gartner ducts
Vas deferens		
Seminal vesicles		
Ejaculatory ducts		
Appendix testis (hydatid)	Müllerian ducts	Fallopian tubes
		Uterus
		Upper vagina
	External Genitalia	
Penis	Genital tubercle	Clitoris
Corpora cavernosa		Corpora cavernosa
Glans penis		Glans clitoris
Corpus spongiosum (enclosing penile urethra)	Urethral folds	Labia minora
Scrotum and ventral epidermis of penis	Labioscrotal swellings	Labia majora
Prostate	Urogenital sinus	Paraurethral glands (of Skene)
Bulbourethral glands (of Cowper)		Bartholin glands
Prostatic utricle (vagina masculina)		Vagina (lower)

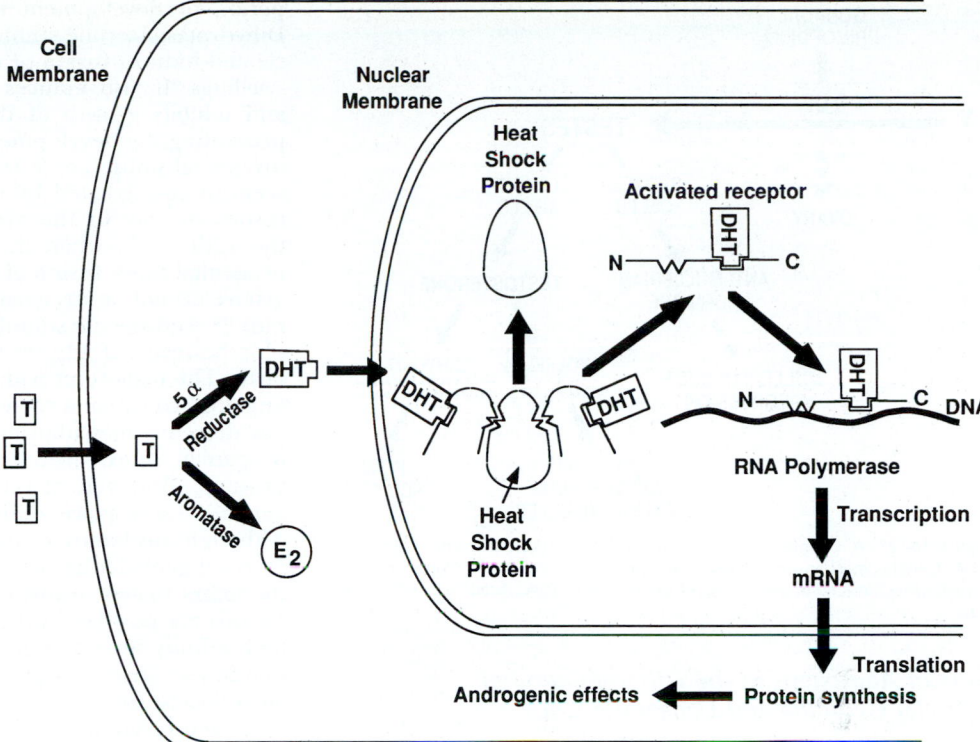

Figure 14–24. A diagrammatic representation of the putative mechanism of action of testosterone on target cells. Testosterone (T) enters the cell, where it is either 5α-reduced to dihydrotestosterone (DHT) or aromatized to estradiol. Dihydrotestosterone enters the nucleus, where it binds to the androgen receptor and "activates" it with the release of the heat shock protein. The activated androgen receptor complex then binds as a dimer (not shown) to specific hormone response elements of the DNA and initiates transcription, translation, and protein synthesis, with consequent androgenic effects.

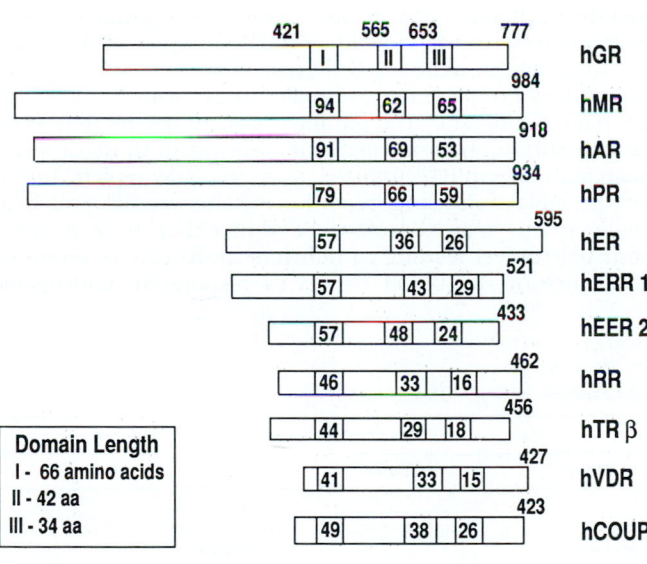

Figure 14–25. Linear representations of the steroid/thyroid hormone receptor superfamily are shown to illustrate sequence homology. hGR is the glucocorticoid receptor; hMR, the mineralocorticoid receptor; hAR, the androgen receptor; hPR, the progesterone receptor; hER, the estrogen receptor; hERR 1 and hERR 2, estrogen-related receptors; hRR, the retinoic acid receptor; hTRβ the thyroid hormone receptor; hVDR, the vitamin D receptor; and hCOUP, the chicken ovalbumin upstream promotor. The DNA binding site (region I) and the hormone binding regions (II and III) are shown. (From B O'Malley, The steroid receptor superfamily: more excitement predicted in the future, Mol Endocrinol 4, 363–369, 1990, © by The Endocrine Society.)

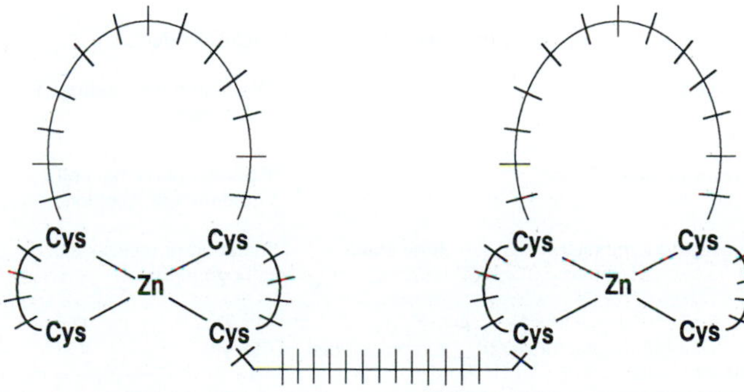

Figure 14–26. Type II zinc fingers. +++ indicates the amino acid skeleton of the zinc fingers, which specifies DNA binding in a sequence-specific manner.

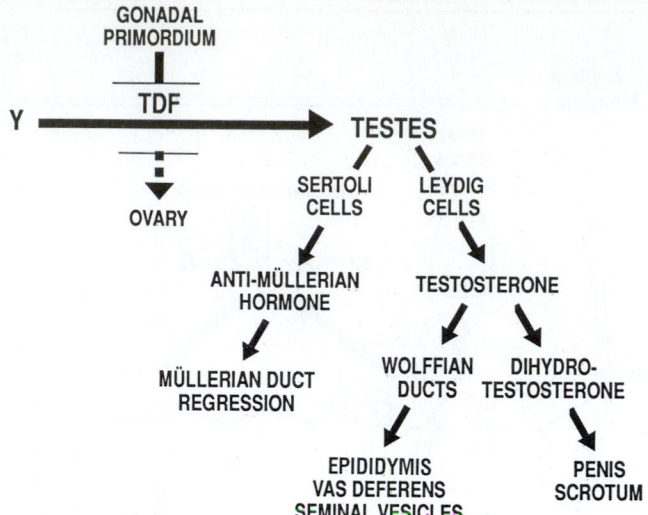

Figure 14–27. A scheme of male sex differentiation. (Modified from Grumbach MM. Genetic mechanisms of sex development. In: Vallet HL, Porter IH, eds. Genetic Mechanisms of Sexual Development. New York: Academic, 1979: 33–73.)

Role of Androgens in the Differentiation of External Genitalia and Urogenital Sinus

The induction of male differentiation of the external genitalia and urogenital sinus is effected by dihydrotestosterone, the 5α-reduced product of testosterone. Testosterone is the prohormone and is delivered via the bloodstream to these target tissues, which are rich in the enzyme 5α-reductase and can readily convert testosterone to dihydrotestosterone, even before the fetal testis secretes testosterone.[155] Dihydrotestosterone binds to the androgen receptor that is coded by an X-linked structural gene and initiates the events that lead to androgen action. As in the case of the genital ducts, there is an inherent tendency for the external genitalia and urogenital sinus to feminize in the absence of fetal gonadal secretions. Complete male differentiation of the external genitalia and urogenital sinus occurs only if the androgenic stimulus is received during the critical period of development (8 to 12 wk) early in fetal life. Dihydrotestosterone stimulates growth of the genital tubercle and induces fusion of the urethral folds and labioscrotal swellings. It also induces differentiation of the prostate[167] and inhibits growth of the vesicovaginal septum, thereby preventing the development of the vaginal derivative of the urogenital sinus. These morphogenetic effects of androgen seem to be mediated by the specific mesenchyme of these tissues and not by the overlying epithelium.[156] After about the 12th week, when the vagina has separated from the urogenital sinus, fusion of the labioscrotal folds and urethral groove cannot occur, even with an intense androgenic stimulus.[168] Androgenic stimulation can cause clitoral hypertrophy, however, at any time during fetal life as well as after birth. The male fetus with 5α-reductase deficiency and thus impaired conversion of testosterone to dihydrotestosterone has defective masculinization of the external genitalia and urogenital sinus, including absence or hypoplasia of the prostate. However, at puberty, virilization of the external genitalia takes place under the influence of testosterone. Although this failure of testosterone to masculinize the fetal external genitalia has been ascribed primarily to inability of the target tissues to form dihydrotestosterone, other explanations are possible. Although the androgen receptor has a high affinity for testosterone itself, the fetal environment is rich in estrogens and progestogens; therefore, the effect of 5α-reductase deficiency on the binding of testosterone to the androgen receptor in the male fetus and at puberty may be different.

Whereas in some species fetal pituitary gonadotropins are required to sustain the secretion of testosterone by the fetal testes, human placental hCG stimulates fetal Leydig cell development and function; human fetal pituitary gonadotropin plays a role only after differentiation of the external genitalia is already determined. This probably explains why the external genitalia of male infants with anencephaly or hypopituitarism and pituitary gonadotropin deficiency usually differentiate normally, in contrast to those of lower mammals hypophysectomized in utero. Incomplete fusion of the labial folds and retention of the vaginal pouch in male infants may therefore be due either to a primary testicular defect leading to deficient androgen secretion or to failure of the target tissues to respond to androgenic

TABLE 14–5. Paracrine and Endocrine Mechanisms in Sex Differentiation

Paracrine Mechanisms			Endocrine Mechanisms		
Agent	Source	Target	Agent	Source	Target
			TESTES		
			Chorionic gonadotropin	Syncytiotrophoblast	Leydig cell (cell membrane receptor)
Meiosis-inhibiting factor	Sertoli cell	Spermatogonia	Testosterone (dihydrotestosterone)	Leydig cell	Urogenital sinus and external genitalia (nuclear androgen receptor)
AMH	Sertoli cell	Müllerian ducts	Fetal inhibin	Sertoli cell	Pituitary gonadotrope
Testosterone	Leydig cell	Wolffian ducts (androgen receptor)			
			OVARIES		
? Ovary-inducing factor	?	Gonadal blastema (cell membrane receptors)			
Meiosis-inducing factor	Rete ovarii	Initiation of meiosis in oogonia	Fetal FSH	Fetal pituitary gonadotrope	Primordial follicle Folliculogenesis and maintenance of primary oocyte
Meiosis-inhibiting factor or (?) AMH	Granulosa cell	Oocyte	Fetal inhibin	Granulosa cell	Pituitary gonadotrope

stimulation. Conversely, if female infants are subjected in utero to androgenic stimulation from some extragonadal source, the external genitalia can exhibit any degree of masculinization, ranging from simple clitoral hypertrophy to the formation of a normal-appearing penis. Thus similar external abnormalities can be produced in the male by androgen deficiency (or failure of the target tissues to respond) and in the female by exposure to androgen from some pathological source in the fetus or mother.

Endocrine and Paracrine Control Mechanisms in Sex Differentiation

The regulation of sex differentiation by chemical messengers involves two types of control mechanisms. One is the classic endocrine mechanism: a cell, usually in a discrete endocrine gland, secretes a hormone into the bloodstream, where it is transported to a distant target tissue to regulate or induce differentiation. In this context, a striking example of an endocrine secretion is testosterone: testosterone secreted by the fetal Leydig cell is delivered via the circulation to the anlagen of the external genitalia and urogenital sinus.

Another is hCG, which is synthesized by the syncytiotrophoblast and acts on the Leydig cell to stimulate testosterone secretion.

The second type of regulation in sex differentiation is by paracrine control. This local and more primitive regulatory mechanism involves the dissemination of a hormone from its site of synthesis to its target cells by local diffusion through the extracellular space. Examples of this delivery system for chemical messengers are the action of AMH on the müllerian duct and the action of testosterone on the wolffian duct (in this instance testosterone is a paracrine secretion). Table 14–5 lists some of the chemical messengers involved in sex differentiation and classifies their effects as mediated by an endocrine or a paracrine control mechanism.

Hormonal Sex Differentiation

Sex differentiation is not complete until the secondary sexual characteristics have matured, fertility is attained, and the ultimate goal, reproduction, becomes possible (Fig. 14–28). These developments occur during puberty. In the past puberty was regarded as a de novo event because of the

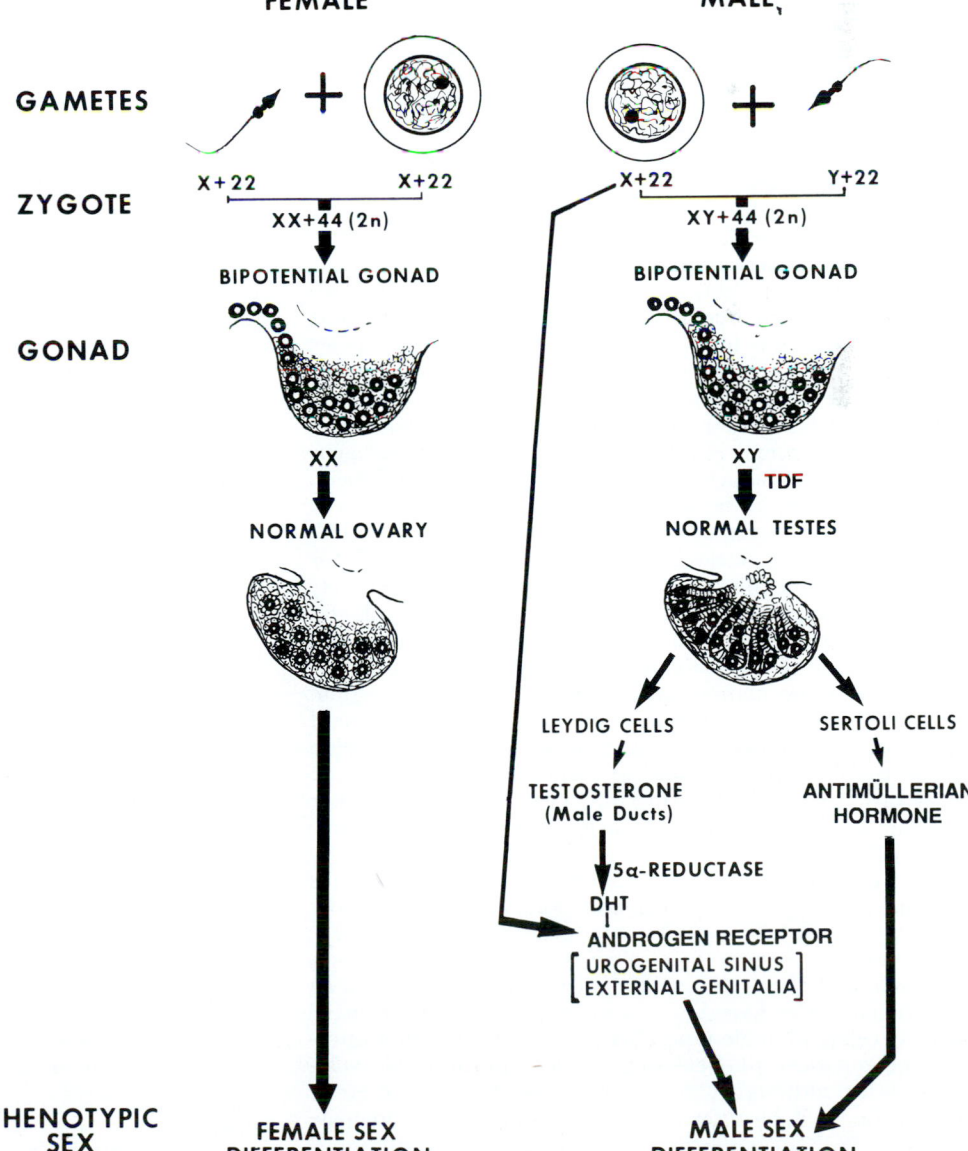

Figure 14–28. A diagrammatic representation of human sex determination and differentiation. Intrinsic or extrinsic factors adversely affecting any stage of these processes can lead to anomalies of sex.

dramatic changes brought about by the maturation of the gonads and the increased secretion of gonadal steroids. However, the development of gonadal function is actually a continuum extending from sex differentiation of the gonad and the ontogeny of the hypothalamic-pituitary-gonadal system in the fetus, through puberty, to the attainment of full sexual maturation and fertility. Puberty is not an isolated event but rather a critical stage in a sequence of complex maturational changes. The hypothalamic-pituitary gonado-tropin unit (including the pulsatile secretion of the hypotha-lamic gonadotropin-releasing factor and of FSH and LH) functions in the fetus, is suppressed to a low level of activity during childhood for about a decade, and is reactivated at the onset of puberty.[169] The hormonal changes and the neuroendocrinology of puberty, including adrenarche and gonadarche, are reviewed elsewhere in this book (see Chapter 22).

Sex Differentiation in the Hypothalamus

Although the control of gonadal function in both sexes is mediated by both FSH and LH, the secretory patterns of the gonadotropins differ in males and females. The male pituitary characteristically secretes both FSH and LH in a pulsatile but relatively constant and sustained manner—so-called tonic release—whereas in the adult female the pulsa-tile secretion of FSH and LH is cyclic and is characterized by a preovulatory gonadotropin surge that leads to ovulation.

In 1936 Pfeiffer[170] reported that during the early post-natal period the rat pituitary becomes differentiated accord-ing to the nature of the gonads. Subsequently it was shown, however, that the cyclic secretory pattern characteristic of the female pituitary is not an innate property of the pituitary itself. The pituitary of a male animal, when grafted under the hypothalamus of an adult female, is fully able to sustain the rhythm of repeated estrous cycles. When the male pituitary is grafted elsewhere in the recipient, ovulation fails to occur. Thus the hypothalamus or higher neural centers function differently in the two sexes.[171, 172] In the rat, mouse, hamster, guinea pig, and sheep there is an inherent tendency to a female neurohypophyseal pattern of gonadotropin release, and this pattern is converted to a male pattern if the newborn animal is exposed to androgens or estrogens during the neonatal period;[171, 172] in the guinea pig and sheep the androgen must be administered prenatally. Once the male pattern is imprinted on "sex centers" in the hypothal-amus (usually by testicular androgens), the potential for cyclic activity on the part of the hypophysis is irrevocably lost. In the rat, the critical period is the first 10 d of life; female rats given as little as 1 μg of testosterone during this period exhibit structural changes in the hypothalamus[173, 174] and develop permanent infertility because gonadotropin secretion at maturity is sustained rather than cyclic and ovulation does not occur. The ovaries of these rats develop multiple follicular cysts and no corpora lutea. Similarly, if male rats are castrated during the first few days of life, later ovarian implants form corpora lutea in a normal female manner.

In contrast, sex differentiation of the central nervous system mechanism mediating gonadotropin secretion does not occur even when testosterone is administered to preg-nant monkeys beginning early in gestation. Furthermore, human females with congenital virilizing adrenal hyperplasia and females who have been exposed to androgens in utero later develop a female-type FSH response to the administra-tion of gonadotropin-releasing factor[175] and normal ovula-tory cycles, although cystic ovaries have been reported in rare patients.[176] Moreover, in both castrate men and male monkeys,[177, 178] an acute rise in concentration of serum estra-diol after estrogen administration can elicit a surge in LH secretion; this suggests that in primates the potential for cyclic gonadotropin secretion is intact and that androgen-induced differentiation of the gonadotropin-regulatory mechanism described in rodents and sheep is not applicable to humans.

Psychosexual Differentiation

Sexually dimorphic human behavior may be classified into four broad categories (Table 14–6):[9, 179, 180] (1) *gender identity*, which is defined as the identification of self as either male or female; (2) *gender role*, which means the aspects of behavior in which males and females differ from one another in our culture at this time; (3) *gender orientation*, which is the choice of erotic partner, whether homosexual, heterosexual, or bisexual; and (4) *cognitive differences*.[180–184]

Studies in lower species suggest that the sexual role adopted at maturity is determined by the hormonal environ-ment in early life.[181–184] As with other aspects of sex differ-entiation, there appears to be an innate tendency to develop female sexual postures. Development of male patterns of sexual behavior in lower species is influenced to a large extent by exposure to androgens, in particular testosterone, during the prenatal and perinatal period.[176, 184, 185] This or-ganizing capacity of testosterone administered at a "critical stage" of development has been localized to specific areas of the brain.[172, 184, 185] A difference between the sexes in the volume of the sexually dimorphic nucleus in the preoptic area of the rat brain has been described, and structural differences of the brain that seem related to the sexually dimorphic nucleus of the rat are now recognized in many species including humans.[186] Moreover, current theories sug-gest that sexually dimorphic organization of target cell nuclei and behavior-related events in lower species are the result of aromatization of testosterone to estradiol in the central nervous system of these species.[184, 185] The so-called protec-tion hypothesis holds that physiological levels of estradiol cannot enter the brain and masculinize the central nervous system of the female rodent fetus because the estrogen is bound to α-fetoprotein.[185] However, in humans, α-fetopro-tein does not retard the transport of estradiol to the central nervous system, and sex steroid–binding globulin has a greater affinity for testosterone than for estradiol. Thus the protection hypothesis does not appear to be applicable to the human. Studies of human males indicate a greater prevalence of left-handedness than in females. This differ-ence has been ascribed, at least in part, to the prenatal effect of testosterone on the brain.[187] Females with congenital virilizing adrenal hyperplasia are more left biased as assessed by an index of cerebral lateralization than their normal sisters, whereas affected males do not differ in handedness from their normal brothers.[188]

Gender identity—the identification of self as either male or female—is a phenomenon applicable only to humans. The behavioral changes attributed to prenatal exposure to

TABLE 14–6. Gender-Related Behavior

Gender identity	Identification of self as male or female
Gender role	Sexually dimorphic behavior
	Energy expenditure
	Aggression
	Parenting rehearsal
	Peer and group interaction—preference of playmates by sex
	Labeling ("tomboy," "sissy")
	Grooming behavior, e.g., clothes, hair
Gender orientation	Choice of sexual partner
Cognition	Sexually dimorphic cognitive abilities

androgens and progestogens in females and to estrogens and progestogens in males are subtle, do not appear to affect gender identity, and are within the range of normal for sexually dimorphic behavior.[180, 181, 189, 190] Individuals who have been reared in a sex opposite to their chromosomal and/or gonadal sex, as well as prenatally androgenized females with congenital adrenal hyperplasia, provide strong evidence that gender identity is not coded primarily by sex chromosomes or gonadal steroids.[9, 181, 191] Gender identity is formed early in the postnatal years and is in part dependent on a process of learning.[9, 181, 191] The general rule is that gender identity agrees with the sex of assignment in the intersex patient provided that the child is raised unambiguously (free from doubt) and *appropriate surgical correction and hormone therapy* are instituted so that the child has an unambiguous male or female phenotype. Sexual identity, under these circumstances, is usually established by 18 to 30 mo.[9] Thereafter, even the development of secondary sexual characteristics of the opposite sex at puberty may not shake the conviction of gender identity if it has been firmly established in early life and if any discordant genital anatomy is corrected.[181] On the other hand, if at puberty discordant secondary sexual characteristics are allowed to mature, some individuals may develop doubts about their true gender identity. Imperato-McGinley and associates[192] have reported a geographic isolate of male pseudohermaphrodites with 5α-reductase deficiency who masculinize at puberty. In these patients, a change in gender behavior is common but not invariable.[192] These studies have cast doubt on the hypothesis that gender identity is "irreversibly fixed" by environmental factors by 2 to 3 y of age.[193] They also emphasize the effect of gonadal steroids at puberty on gender identity and behavior and attest to the plasticity of gender identity in the cultural-genetic isolate studied.[192] Another genetic isolate of patients with 5α-reductase deficiency has been reported from the Sambia tribe of New Guinea. In these patients, gender role change seemed to result from social-experiential and cultural factors rather than from an effect of hormonal imprinting.[194]

Stronger credence is now given to the role of early hormonal influences on sexually dimorphic behavior in humans. As noted, studies of patients with prenatal virilization caused by congenital virilizing adrenal hyperplasia or maternal ingestion of progestogens demonstrate no effect on gender identity in well-managed patients.[189, 195] On the other hand, gender-related behavior can be affected. Prenatally androgenized females demonstrate greater interest in outdoor play and competitive sports and are more "tomboyish."[181] As a group, they are more career oriented and tend to lack a strong interest in doll play and mothering.[181] The pattern is persistent and is not abnormal for female behavior in our culture. According to Money and associates,[196] a higher proportion of young women with congenital virilizing adrenal hyperplasia than of unaffected women rated themselves as bisexual or homosexual.

The eventual outcome of this "nature versus nurture" controversy is of practical importance. The evidence related to hypogonadal males, patients with the complete form of androgen resistance, and prenatally virilized girls supports the thesis that exposure to androgens before birth can contribute to the programming of sexually dimorphic behavior. However, these hormonal factors are rarely decisive, and more important elements in the development of gender identity are the assigned sex of rearing, the reinforcement that this assignment receives during infancy and early childhood, and appropriate gonadal steroid secretion or replacement therapy at the normal age of puberty. If this reinforcement is weak because of ambiguous attitudes of the parents and the community setting, the outlook for attaining a normal gender identity in adult life is diminished.

These interpretations are supported by experience gained from a pragmatic approach to the assignment of sex in patients with ambiguous genitalia (see later).

CLASSIFICATION OF ERRORS IN SEX DIFFERENTIATION

In the past, individuals with hermaphroditism were classified according to the gonadal morphology. In the terminology of Klebs, a true hermaphrodite is a person who possesses both ovarian and testicular tissue. A male pseudohermaphrodite is one whose gonads are exclusively testes but whose genital ducts or external genitalia, or both, exhibit the phenotype of a female or incompletely differentiated male. A female pseudohermaphrodite is a person with ovaries whose external genitalia exhibit some masculine characteristics. We have classified errors in sex differentiation by a modification and expansion of this broad framework and have attempted to blend etiological mechanisms and clinical entities into a simplified rational classification (Table 14–7). The clinical and etiological heterogeneity of syndromes with similar anatomical findings merits emphasis.

Disorders of Gonadal Differentiation and Sex Chromosome Anomalies

Not all patients with anomalies of sex chromosomes have abnormal gonads and, conversely, congenital defects in gonadal differentiation are not always due to chromosomal errors. The association is so frequent, however, that these topics are inseparable. Exceptions to this association are of special importance in defining the genetic and chromosomal determinants of gonadogenesis.

Seminiferous Tubule Dysgenesis: Klinefelter Syndrome and Its Variants

47,XXY SEMINIFEROUS TUBULE DYSGENESIS (TYPICAL KLINEFELTER SYNDROME). Seminiferous tubule dysgenesis is a common cause of primary hypogonadism and male infertility (Table 14–8). This syndrome was first defined as a clinical entity by Klinefelter and associates.[197] The characteristic features, which first become manifest during adolescence, are gynecomastia, a variable degree of eunuchoidism, small atrophic testes with hyalinization of the seminiferous tubules, aggregation of Leydig cells, aspermatogenesis, and increased urinary excretion of gonadotropin. In 1956 several groups found that a high proportion of patients with this syndrome are X chromatin–positive in contrast to their phenotypic male appearance. Soon thereafter it became evident that the syndrome is heterogeneous.

In 1959 Jacobs and Strong[198] and Ford and co-workers[199] first reported a 47,XXY sex chromosome constitution in patients with this disorder, which explained the positive sex chromatin pattern. Various other sex chromosome compositions, including mosaicism, have been described. Virtually all these variants have in common the presence of at least two X chromosomes and a Y chromosome, except for the rare group that has only a 46,XX sex chromosome complement by karyotype analysis of multiple tissues.

The differentiation of testes and lack of ovarian differentiation in patients with 47,XXY and, more strikingly, 49,XXXXY complements indicate that a single Y chromosome and the expression of testis-determining gene(s) are sufficient to bring about testicular organogenesis and male sex differentiation in the presence of as many as four X chromosomes.

TABLE 14–7. Classification of Anomalous Sexual Development

I. **Disorders of gonadal differentiation**
  A. Seminiferous tubular dysgenesis (Klinefelter syndrome)
  B. Syndrome of gonadal dysgenesis and its variants (Turner syndrome)
  C. Complete and incomplete forms of 46,XX and 46,XY gonadal dysgenesis
  D. True hermaphroditism
II. **Female pseudohermaphroditism**
  A. Congenital virilizing adrenal hyperplasia
  B. P-450 aromatase (placental) deficiency
  C. Androgens and synthetic progestogens transferred from maternal circulation
  D. Associated with malformations of intestine and urinary tract (non–androgen-induced female pseudohermaphroditism)
  E. Other teratological factors
III. **Male pseudohermaphroditism**
  A. Testicular unresponsiveness to hCG and LH (Leydig cell agenesis or hypoplasia)
  B. Inborn errors of testosterone biosynthesis
    1. Enzyme defects affecting synthesis of both corticosteroids and testosterone (variants of congenital adrenal hyperplasia)
      a. P-450$_{scc}$ (cholesterol side-chain cleavage) deficiency (congenital lipoid adrenal hyperplasia)
      b. 3β-Hydroxysteroid dehydrogenase deficiency
      c. P-450$_{c17}$ (17α-hydroxylase) deficiency
    2. Enzyme defects primarily affecting testosterone biosynthesis by testes
      a. P-450$_{c17}$ (17,20-lyase deficiency)
      b. 17β-Hydroxysteroid oxidoreductase deficiency
  C. Defects in androgen-dependent target tissues
    1. End-organ resistance to androgenic hormones (androgen receptor and postreceptor defects)
      a. Syndrome of complete androgen resistance and its variants (testicular feminization and its variant forms)
      b. Syndrome of partial androgen resistance and its variants (Reifenstein syndrome)
      c. Androgen resistance in infertile men
      d. Androgen resistance in fertile men
    2. Defects in testosterone metabolism by peripheral tissues
      a. 5α-Reductase deficiency—pseudovaginal perineoscrotal hypospadias
  D. Dysgenetic male pseudohermaphroditism
    1. X chromatin–negative variants of syndrome of gonadal dysgenesis (e.g., 45,X/46,XY, 46,XYp−)
    2. Incomplete forms of XY gonadal dysgenesis
    3. Associated with degenerative renal disease
    4. "Vanishing testes" (embryonic testicular regression syndrome; 46,XY agonadism; 46,XY gonadal agenesis; rudimentary testes; anorchia)
  E. Defects in synthesis, secretion, or response to AMH
    1. Female genital ducts in otherwise normal men—"herniae uteri inguinale"; persistent müllerian duct syndrome
  F. Maternal ingestion of progestogens
IV. **Unclassified forms of abnormal sexual development**
  A. In males
    1. Hypospadias
    2. Ambiguous external genitalia in 46,XY males with multiple congenital anomalies
  B. In females
    1. Absence or anomalous development of vagina, uterus, and fallopian tubes (Rokitansky-Küster syndrome)

Clinical Features.[200–202] In the postpubertal patient, the only constant clinical features are a male phenotype, small testes (less than 3 cm in length and often less than 1.5 cm), and azoospermia (Fig. 14–29). Gynecomastia is common. The prepubertal clinical profile indicates that children with a 47,XXY karyotype, as a group, have lower birth weights; smaller mean head circumferences; a slightly increased incidence of major and minor congenital anomalies, especially clinodactyly; height percentiles that increase with age; a lower verbal I.Q. than normal boys; and delayed emotional development and poor motor control.[202] Studies of individuals with a 47,XXY sex chromosome constitution ascertained by karyotype analyses at birth have revealed that the impairment in verbal I.Q. is slight (10 to 20 points) compared with controls and that the full-scale I.Q. is normal.[203–205, 205a] Severe retardation is uncommon.[206] There is a higher than average incidence of problems with speech development, learning problems, and social adjustment in adolescence. An increased prevalence of psychopathology, including antiso-

cial behavior and delinquency, has been reported from retrospective studies, although the true risk is uncertain because of biased ascertainment. However, several studies indicate that in spite of verbal deficits, adults with Klinefelter syndrome as a group are not significantly different from other hypogonadal males or even normal controls as far as education, employment, socioeconomic status,[205] social adjustment, and criminal behavior are concerned.[207]

Patients with a 47,XXY karyotype tend to be taller than average, mainly because of disproportionate length of the legs.[204, 208] This finding is present before clinical signs of puberty are evident and may not be accompanied by a proportional increase in arm span. The prepubertal onset of disproportionate leg length suggests that it is not related to androgen deficiency and delayed epiphyseal closure. Androgen deficiency after the age of puberty may augment the prepubertal deviation in skeletal proportions.[208]

Prepubertally, the basal plasma concentration of FSH and LH and the response to luteinizing hormone–releasing hormone (LHRH) are within the normal range.[209–211] The timing and onset of secondary sexual characteristics and puberty have been reported as normal in one study[211] and delayed in another.[212] With the onset of puberty, progressive histological changes and a decreased capacity of the Leydig cells to synthesize testosterone become apparent. Thus in postpubertal patients the concentration of testosterone[211] tends to be low, the levels of plasma estradiol are normal or increased, and gonadotropin levels are elevated. Testosterone responses to hCG appear to be normal in childhood and early adolescence, as opposed to those in adults.[211] Diminished potency is common in the adult, and Leydig cell reserve is impaired, reflected in a subnormal increase in the concentration of serum testosterone after administration of hCG and increased concentration of LH in plasma.[213] The testosterone production rate, total and free levels of testosterone, and rates of metabolic clearance of testosterone and estradiol tend to be low, while plasma estradiol levels are normal or elevated.[200, 214] Gynecomastia and signs of androgen deficiency, such as diminished facial and body hair, a female escutcheon, a small phallus, poor muscular development, and a further increase in the disproportion between leg and body length, usually become evident during puberty or postpubertally. The testicular failure in Klinefelter syndrome appears to progress with age. The gynecomastia, which occurs in about 90% of patients, is probably secondary to an increased ratio of serum estradiol to testosterone.[211] (Also see Chapter 15.)

Associated Abnormalities. Abnormalities in thyroid function include a diminished thyroid response to thyrotropin, decreased uptake of radioactive iodine, and a subnormal increase in serum thyrotropin concentration after administration of thyrotropin-releasing hormone.[215] Clinically significant thyroid disease is uncommon. An increased incidence of thyroid antibodies is not found in this disorder, in contrast to the syndrome of gonadal dysgenesis.

TABLE 14–8. Salient Features of Klinefelter Syndrome

Karyotype: 47,XXY
Inheritance: Sporadic; associated with advanced maternal age; nondisjunction during first or second meiotic division in either parent (67% maternal, 33% paternal); mitotic nondisjunction
Genitalia: Male
Wolffian duct derivatives: Normal
Müllerian duct derivatives: Absent
Gonads: Small, firm testes; seminiferous tubule dysgenesis; azoospermia; Leydig cell hyperplasia
Habitus: Poor to normal virilization at puberty: gynecomastia; disproportionately long legs
Hormone profile: Testosterone levels variable but usually ↓ ; ↑ levels of plasma LH and FSH postpubertally

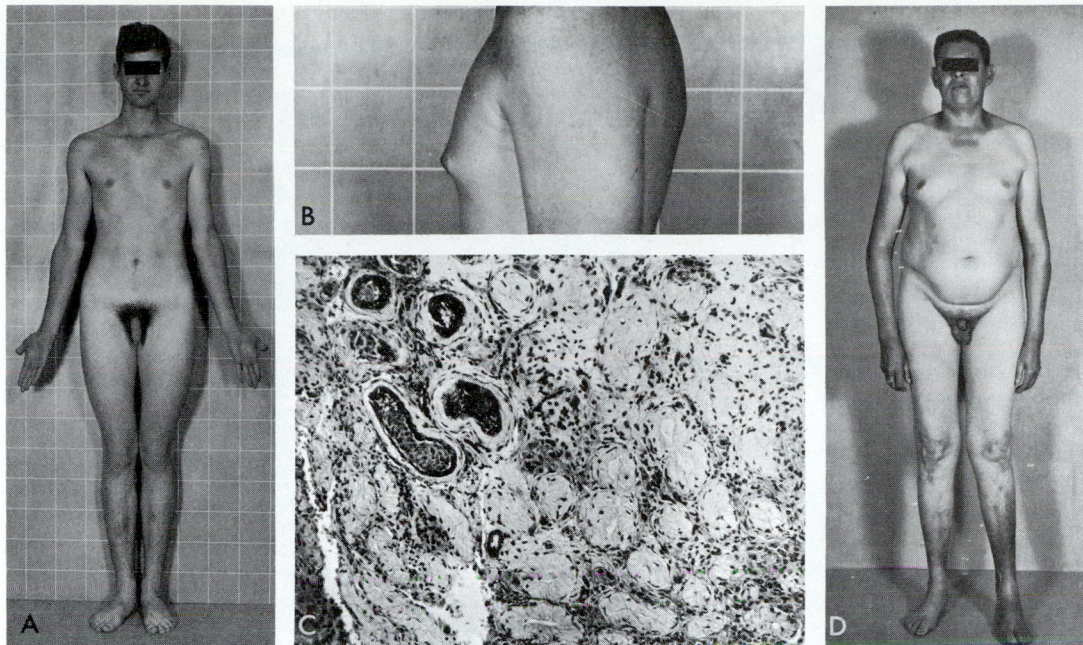

Figure 14–29. *A,* A 19-y-old phenotypic male with chromatin-positive seminiferous tubule dysgenesis (Klinefelter syndrome). The karyotype was 47,XXY, gonadotropin levels were elevated, and testosterone levels were low normal. Note normal virilization with long legs and *(B)* gynecomastia. The testes were small and firm and measured 1.8 × 0.9 cm. Testicular biopsy *(C)* revealed a severe degree of hyalinization of the seminiferous tubules and Leydig cell hypoplasia. *D,* A 48-y-old male with 47,XXY Klinefelter syndrome with severe leg varicosities.

The frequency of diabetes mellitus is increased. Nielsen[216] reported that in a group of 157 patients, 19% had impaired glucose tolerance and 8% had overt diabetes. The prevalence of diabetes mellitus was also increased in the parents. The patients with diabetes mellitus were usually under 50 y of age, and the diabetes was usually mild. Insulin resistance with secondary hyperinsulinemia has been postulated as the cause of glucose intolerance in these patients.[217]

47,XXY patients with gynecomastia have an increased predisposition to cancer of the breast. In a survey of 187 males with breast cancer, 8 patients with chromatin-positive seminiferous tubule dysgenesis were detected, about 18 times the expected prevalence.[218] Infiltrating ductal carcinoma is the most common histological pattern.[218a] Other types of neoplasia have been reported in 1.6% of 47,XXY males.[218b] Chronic pulmonary disease and varicose veins with stasis ulcers may also be more prevalent in adults with Klinefelter syndrome.[219] Sexual precocity caused by an hCG-secreting intrathoracic germ cell neoplasm has been reported in six 47,XXY boys.[220] The diagnosis was suggested by the association of small testes with sexual precocity in the absence of a virilizing adrenal disorder. Six patients with both androgen resistance and a 47,XXY karyotype have been reported.[221] These patients had female or ambiguous male genitalia and some clinical features of the 47,XXY karyotype. This combined defect is probably due to fertilization of an oocyte containing two X chromosomes, each bearing a defect in the X-linked gene coding for the androgen receptor, by a normal sperm containing a Y chromosome.

Frequency. Surveys of the prevalence of 47,XXY fetuses by karyotype analysis of unselected newborn infants indicate an incidence of about 1 per 1000 males.[222] No racial or geographic predilection has been observed.[222] Whereas 10% of clinically recognizable spontaneous abortions have a 45,X constitution, only 0.1% have a 47,XXY karyotype.

Testicular Lesions. Changes in the histological structure of the testis become more marked with age in 47,XXY individuals.[223] A limited number of studies of fetal testes have been reported, and the findings are variable. Grumbach

and associates[224] reported normal histology for the testes of a 1700-g chromatin-positive infant,[224] but examination of several other affected fetuses suggested deficient germinal epithelium and heterotopic germ cells.[225, 226] In three infants between 3 and 12 mo of age with a 47,XXY karyotype, a decrease in spermatogonia was described.[227] In later childhood, testicular biopsies have revealed small tubules with progressive reduction in spermatogonia.[228] In considering the pathogenesis of the testicular lesion, it seems that a normal or near-normal complement of germ cells is present early in fetal life. During late gestation and early infancy, a drastic loss of spermatogonia ensues. This reduction in germ cell complement in 47,XXY individuals may represent an exaggeration of the normal degeneration of spermatogonia that occurs in the neonatal period. Excessive germ cell loss could result from either defective maturation[229] or failure of the germ cells to migrate to the periphery of the tubule and align in opposition to the basement membrane.

With the approach of adolescence and even before pubertal signs are well advanced, the actions of pituitary gonadotropins on the intrinsically defective testis induce progressive hyalinization of the seminiferous tubules and pseudoadenomatous clumping of Leydig cells. Despite this clumping, the mean volume of Leydig cells is usually normal.[230] After pubescence, the testes are characterized by small dysgenetic tubules with arrested development and often early fibrosis and hyalinization. The result is testes that are small in size and firm in consistency. Peritubular elastic tissue is usually absent or diminished in the small dysgenetic tubules.[224, 228] That gonadotropin secretion plays a direct or indirect role in this change was illustrated in a 7-y-old 48,XXXY boy with precocious puberty and elevated urinary gonadotropin levels. Unlike the relatively normal architecture in most boys of this age with Klinefelter syndrome, the testes of this boy exhibited extensive hyalinization and fibrosis of the tubules and clumping of Leydig cells (Fig. 14–30). Conversely, 47,XXY patients with gonadotropin deficiency do not exhibit changes in testicular histology.

Hyalinization of the tubules is usually extensive but

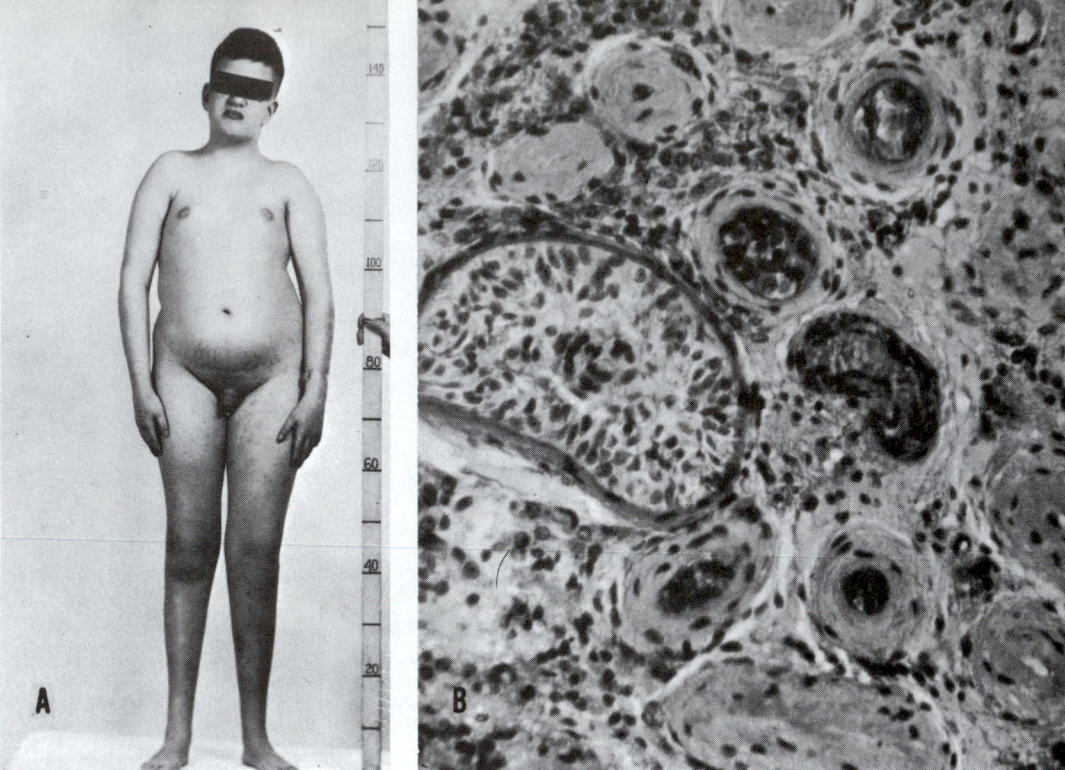

Figure 14–30. *A,* An 8½-y-old boy with a 48,XXXY chromosome constitution, mental retardation, precocious sexual development, and accelerated growth. The appearance of pubic hair was noted at age 6. By 8 y, acne, a deep voice, tall stature, and axillary hair were present. Height was 148 cm (+ 2.9 SD), weight 47.7 kg (+ 3.9 SD), span 140 cm, and upper segment/lower segment ratio 0.87. Testes measured 2.1 × 1.3 cm. Note the long legs, prognathism, small hands and feet, gynecomastia, and secondary sexual characteristics. The I.Q. was 62. The urinary 17-ketosteroid level was 3.2 mg/d and urinary gonadotropin levels were between 10 and 50 mouse units/d. Bone age was 13½. The buccal smear contained diploid nuclei with a maximum of two X chromatin bodies. Karyotype of cells derived from skin and blood was 48,XXXY. *B,* Testicular biopsy showed hyalinized tubules and clumping of Leydig cells; germ cells were absent. The findings suggest that true precocious puberty, with stimulation of juvenile testes by pituitary gonadotropin, led to premature appearance of typical histological changes of seminiferous tubule dysgenesis. (From unpublished data, M. M. Grumbach and A. Morishima.)

varies in degree from patient to patient and even between the testes of the same patient. The fibrosis tends to progress with age, and in some older patients few tubules can be identified. Conversely, in occasional patients the tubules are lined by Sertoli cells, tubular fibrosis is relatively slight, and the histological appearance resembles that of germinal cell aplasia. Rarely, spermatogenesis is found in isolated tubules. This finding could represent hidden mosaicism in the gonad or possibly mitotic nondisjunction or anaphase lag in germ cells giving rise to 46,XY cells that would then go on to spermatogenesis. There have been sporadic reports of alleged paternity; most of these cases proved to have sex chromosome mosaicism, and in others acceptable documentation of paternity was not provided. The fertile patients with 46,XY/47,XXY mosaicism often lack features that distinguish them from typical Klinefelter syndrome.

Origin of 47,XXY Constitution. 47,XXY males may develop through nondisjunction of the sex chromosomes during either the first or second meiotic division in either parent or, less commonly, mitotic nondisjunction in the zygote at the time of or after fertilization (see Figs. 14–3 and 14–16). Fertilization of a 46,XX ovum by a Y-bearing sperm or of an X ovum by a 46,XY-bearing sperm would yield a 47,XXY zygote. Mitotic nondisjunction of the sex chromosomes in a 46,XY zygote could yield a 47,XXY and a 45,Y daughter cell (Fig. 14–31). Because the 45,Y cell line is nonviable, only the 47,XXY cell line would survive.

These abnormalities of meiosis almost always occur in parents with normal sex chromosome constitution. However, Rosenkranz[231] described two 47,XXY patients whose mothers were, respectively, 47,XXX and 46,XX/47,XXX mosaic. Whether a 47,XXY karyotype is derived more frequently than previously suspected from a polysomic X constitution in the mother remains to be determined.

Family studies using X-linked markers, such as color

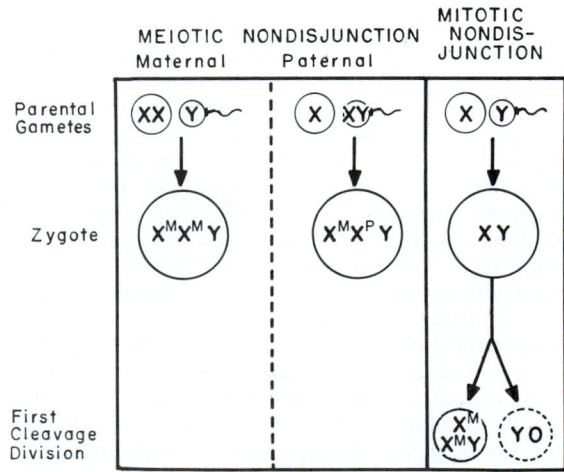

Figure 14–31. Origin of the 47,XXY karyotype. Superscripts M and P designate, respectively, maternal and paternal X chromosomes. The interrupted circle indicates a nonviable cell line. (From Grumbach MM. The testes. In: Beeson PB, McDermott W, eds. Cecil-Loeb Textbook of Medicine. 13th ed. Philadelphia: W. B. Saunders, 1971: 1804–1818.)

vision, Xg blood group, serum Xm group, and glucose-6-phosphate dehydrogenase, indicate that in informative pedigrees both X chromosomes are of maternal origin (X^MX^MY) in two thirds of cases and one X is of paternal origin (X^MX^PY) in one third.[232,233] This proportion is similar to that derived by DNA analysis.[234] Ferguson-Smith and colleagues[235] and others reported a positive association with advanced maternal age in 47,XXY patients, although this association is less marked than in trisomy-21. These various findings suggest that a high proportion of X^MX^MY cases result from nondisjunction during oogenesis rather than from mitotic nondisjunction in the first cell division of an XY zygote. Data for the X^MX^PY group indicate that paternal nondisjunction is not dependent on age,[235, 236] a finding also reminiscent of autosomal trisomies.

Rarely, Klinefelter syndrome is associated with a supernumerary X chromosome that is structurally abnormal, e.g., an X-autosome translocation or an isochromosome for the long arm of the X.

Etiological Factors. The most important factor imputed in the etiology of the 47,XXY chromosome constitution is advanced maternal age.[235, 236] As discussed earlier, the maternal age effect in chromosome abnormalities may be a consequence of the long diplotene stage of human ova. Ova remain suspended in prophase of the first meiotic division from birth to ovulation, which may not occur for many years. The defective segregation of the two X chromosomes could be caused, at least in part, by reduction of the length of the chiasma between certain chromosomes as the length of the diplotene stage increases. As in gonadal dysgenesis, the prevalence of twinning in sibships of 47,XXY individuals may be increased.

Genetic factors that predispose to nondisjunction may also be important and have been demonstrated in lower species. Although chromosome abnormalities are usually sporadic, a number of pedigrees have been reported in which leukemia and various chromosome abnormalities have occurred in siblings and relatives. In addition, patients with more than one form of trisomy seem to occur more frequently than expected by chance alone. The roles of radiation and viruses as predisposing factors are not known.

Diagnosis and Treatment. The diagnosis of Klinefelter syndrome in the postpubertal male is suggested by the typical phenotype and hormonal changes and confirmed by the finding of a 47,XXY karyotype or a variant sex chromosome complement in blood, skin, or gonads. Treatment should be directed toward androgen replacement therapy when there is evidence of androgen deficiency. In general, parenteral androgens are more effective in virilizing the patient and are safer (also see Chapters 13 and 22). Hepatic tumors and abnormalities in liver function have been associated with chronic administration of oral androgens that have substitutions at the 17α position (e.g., a methyl group). Such abnormalities are not a problem with testosterone ester preparations such as propionate or enanthate. Testosterone enanthate in oil, 200 mg intramuscularly (IM) every 2 to 3 wk, is recommended for full replacement therapy. It is wise to begin therapy at a lower dose (e.g., 50 mg IM every 4 wk) to avoid rapid virilization and bone maturation, especially in adolescent males. In general, gynecomastia, if present, does not diminish as a result of androgen replacement. Severe or psychologically disturbing gynecomastia can be corrected by reduction mammoplasty.

The diagnosis of Klinefelter syndrome should be suspected in prepubertal patients with one or more of the following: (1) long legs, (2) smaller than normal testes, (3) learning disorders, and (4) developmental delay in speech and language. Many of these features are amenable to therapy, so early detection and intervention may be beneficial to the patient. Nielsen and Pelsen[207] have suggested that prepubertally diagnosed patients with Klinefelter syndrome should be offered therapy with testosterone at 11 to 12 y of age to initiate puberty and to prevent both physical and psychological complications of hypogonadism. A regimen utilized by us primarily for patients with hypogonadotropic hypogonadism is to begin replacement testosterone therapy with 50 mg of testosterone enanthate in oil IM monthly at a bone age of 12 y.[237] After 6 mo or when the bone age has advanced to 14 y, the dose may be increased to 100 mg IM monthly. Usually, several years of treatment at this dose will result in the attainment of a height that is appropriate for genetic height potential and adequate pubertal progression. When full virilization is desired, an adult replacement dose of 200 mg every 2 wk or 300 mg every 3 wk may be given.

VARIANT FORMS OF KLINEFELTER SYNDROME.
46,XY/47,XXY Mosaicism. 46,XY/47,XXY mosaicism is the second most common karyotype in phenotypic males with X chromatin–positive patterns. The presence of a normal XY cell line in these patients can modify the clinical expression of the 47,XXY cell line. Thus, in general, these patients manifest a lesser degree of gynecomastia, androgen deficiency, and testicular pathology. As a group they are older (mean age 45 y) at the time of diagnosis than patients with 47,XXY Klinefelter syndrome. Symptoms of decreased libido and potency may not appear until the fourth or fifth decade. At the time of diagnosis, serum FSH levels are elevated and serum testosterone concentrations are often in the normal range. Secondary sexual characteristics are less impaired than those of patients with 47,XXY karyotypes, and seminiferous tubules exhibiting spermatogenesis are more common than in 47,XXY patients.[201] At least four patients with 46,XY/47,XXY mosaicism have been fertile.[201]

The diagnosis of 46,XY/47,XXY mosaicism is established by the finding of at least 5% XY cells in blood, skin, or gonads in which the second cell line is 47,XXY. 46,XY/47,XXY mosaicism may result from nondisjunction or anaphase lag in a 47,XXY zygote.

48,XXYY. Affected individuals have the typical findings of Klinefelter syndrome and often exhibit additional features. They constitute about 3% of chromatin-positive males, and most of the reported patients are mentally retarded. The 48,XXYY karyotype is usually associated with tall stature (the mean height of 26 patients was 181 cm, compared with 172 cm for 47,XXY males), disproportionately long lower extremities, gynecomastia, delinquent behavior, and unusual dermatoglyphic patterns. Peripheral vascular disease, especially varicose veins and stasis dermatitis, are common. Secondary sexual characteristics are poorly developed, and testicular histology is similar to that of 47,XXY patients. The sex chromatin pattern is indistinguishable from that of the 47,XXY groups; however, two fluorescent Y bodies are present in a high proportion of somatic nuclei.

To have two Y chromosomes, nondisjunction must occur in paternal meiosis. In two informative matings the Xg blood groups indicated that the father contributed an X as well as two Y chromosomes, which suggests that an X ovum was fertilized by an XYY sperm (arising from successive nondisjunction in the first and second meiotic divisions). The 48,XXYY karyotype in a patient whose mother was 47,XXX[238] could have arisen by the fertilization of an XX ovum by a YY sperm.

48,XXXY and 49,XXXYY. All reported patients with a 48,XXXY karyotype have been mentally retarded.[239] In addition, they have had small testes and signs of androgen deficiency. With an increase in the number of X chromosomes, the severity and frequency of somatic anomalies, such as short neck, epicanthal folds, radioulnar synostosis, and clinodactyly, also increase. Mental retardation, somatic anomalies, and small testes also occur in 49,XXXYY patients.[240]

49,XXXXY. This karyotype has been reported in more than 100 patients since the first report by Fraccaro and colleagues in 1960.[241] The diagnosis may be suspected from the clinical picture. In addition to mental deficiency, often of a severe degree, these patients have certain phenotypic similarities, including (1) skeletal abnormalities, especially radioulnar synostosis and epiphyseal dysgenesis, and (2) hypoplastic external genitalia with a small penis, underdeveloped scrotum, and very small and frequently undescended testes; the appearance of the external genitalia may be ambiguous because of hypospadias, bifid scrotum, hypoplastic phallus, and cryptorchidism.[242] In adults, gynecomastia is absent and androgen deficiency is severe. Before puberty, the testes often contain hypoplastic seminiferous tubules. Other anomalies include congenital heart disease, cleft palate, strabismus, and microcephaly. The facies not infrequently has a characteristic appearance, with a Down syndrome–like slant of the eyes, epicanthal folds, hypertelorism, strabismus, and a wide nose.[242] Sarto and co-workers[243] have suggested that the phenotypic abnormalities noted in patients with aneuploidy involving supernumerary X chromosomes result from an effect of the nonactivated genes on the X chromosomes and/or asynchronous replication of the supernumerary X chromosomes, so that more than one X chromosome is active in cells.

46,XX Males. More than 150 phenotypic males with a 46,XX karyotype have been described since 1964; this disorder occurs in about 1 per 20,000 males.[232, 244] These patients have a male phenotype and psychosocial orientation and are similar clinically and endocrinologically to individuals with "classic" Klinefelter syndrome except for minor differences.[232, 244] Postpubertally, as in Klinefelter syndrome, they have varying degrees of testosterone deficiency, gynecomastia, and small testes with azoospermia.[232, 244, 245] Testosterone production is often decreased, as is the response to hCG.[245] Both basal and LHRH-induced rises in FSH and LH levels are increased.[245] There is a 10% incidence of hypospadias in prepubertal 46,XX males that can be attributed to a deficiency of testosterone secretion by the fetal Leydig cells. 46,XX males with genital abnormalities tend to lack evidence for Y chromosomal DNA in their genome and to manifest a greater prevalence and degree of gynecomastia than their 46,XX counterparts in whom a Y-to-X translocation is present[245a] (see later). In comparison to males with a 47,XXY karyotype, 46,XX males have a lower frequency of intellectual and psychosocial problems;[232, 244] they are shorter (mean height 168 cm) than 47,XXY patients or normal males, have smaller tooth crowns (Y-linked gene) than normal males, and, in contrast to 47,XXY individuals, usually have normal skeletal proportions.[94, 244]

The histology of the testes is similar to that of 47,XXY males; seminiferous tubules are decreased in size and number, germinal cells are usually absent, and peritubular and interstitial fibrosis occurs. The Leydig cells appear hyperplastic. In some patients, the morphology of the testes is similar to that in germinal cell aplasia or intermediate between it and the morphology in seminiferous tubule dysgenesis. Unlike the case of 47,XXY patients, maternal age is not increased.[232]

The paradoxical finding of males with a 46,XX karyotype has fascinated investigators and led to an expansion of our understanding of the genes that control sex determination. Several theories were advanced to explain this type of sex reversal: (1) loss of a Y chromosome early in embryogenesis, (2) cryptic sex chromosome mosaicism in a 46,XX male with an undetected and/or circumscribed cell line containing a Y chromosome,[246] (3) translocation between a

Y and an X chromosome or autosome resulting in the presence of the testis-determining gene(s) on an X chromosome or autosome,[247] or (4) a mutation involving either an autosomal or X-linked gene in the pathway to testis differentiation.[245a, 248] Studies involving X- and Y-linked marker genes,[249] cytogenetic observations,[250, 251] and direct molecular genetic analysis[34, 89, 90, 245a, 252–262] suggest that 80 to 90% of 46,XX males result from an anomalous Y-to-X translocation during meiosis.

As discussed earlier, the X and Y chromosomes have a homologous region on the distal short arms—the pseudoautosomal region. The homology of this region and the proper segregation of sex chromosomes are maintained by an obligate crossover within the region at meiotic pairing. The sex-determining region of the Y chromosome with its candidate gene(s) (SRY) has been mapped proximal to the boundary of the pseudoautosomal region.[33, 34] 46,XX males can arise from a balanced aberrant nonhomologous interchange between Yp and Xp that includes the sex-determining locus[90, 258] (Fig. 14–32A) or from aberrant unequal nonhomologous exchange, resulting in an X chromosome that has part of its pseudoautosomal region as well as the sex-determining region of the Y and its pseudoautosomal region[259, 263] (Fig. 14–32B). Such 46,XX patients have had three copies of the pseudoautosomal gene MIC2. (The resulting Y chromosome in both the anomalous balanced and unbalanced exchanges lacks the testis-determining region of the Y chromosome and hence could give rise to a 46,XY female with pure gonadal dysgenesis[264, 265] [see Fig. 14–32].) Three patients with 47,XXX karyotypes and male sex differentiation have been reported.[262, 266] All three were Y(+). Two of the three had two maternal X chromosomes and the third had two paternal X chromosomes. These findings suggest that both anomalous Y-to-X exchange and maternal or paternal nondisjunction occurred in these patients.[266]

Three 46,XX males studied by Palmer and associates and five reported by Ferguson-Smith and colleagues[266a] were negative for all Y-specific material (including the SRY and ZFY probes). Y DNA–negative 46,XX males have occurred in rare families in which there is true hermaphroditism.[34, 258, 260, 266b] These observations are consistent with the origin of a small proportion of 46,XX males as a consequence of a mutation in a "downstream" autosomal gene(s) or an X-linked gene involved in the testis-determining cascade (see Fig. 14–15). They also suggest that 46,XX males and 46,XX true hermaphrodites may arise by similar pathogenetic mechanisms. In sum, the 46,XX male syndrome arises mainly as a result of a Y-to-X translocation; other mechanisms include an X chromosomal or autosomal abnormality as well as cryptic mosaicism that involves a Y-bearing cell line in at least the Sertoli cells.

The Syndrome of Gonadal Dysgenesis: Turner Syndrome and Its Variants

In 1938 Turner described seven phenotypic females with dwarfism, sexual infantilism, webbing of the neck, and cubitus valgus. Studies of this syndrome and its variants have made a major contribution to the evolution of current concepts of sex differentiation. (For reviews see refs. 11, 22, 267–270, 270a.)

In the early 1940s Albright and colleagues and Varney and associates found that the excretion of urinary gonadotropin was increased in affected adolescents and adults. Wilkins and Fleischmann soon thereafter described the gonads as bilateral, pale "streaks" of connective tissue situated in the mesosalpinges and devoid of any germ cells. Wilkins proposed, in the light of Jost's fetal castration experiments

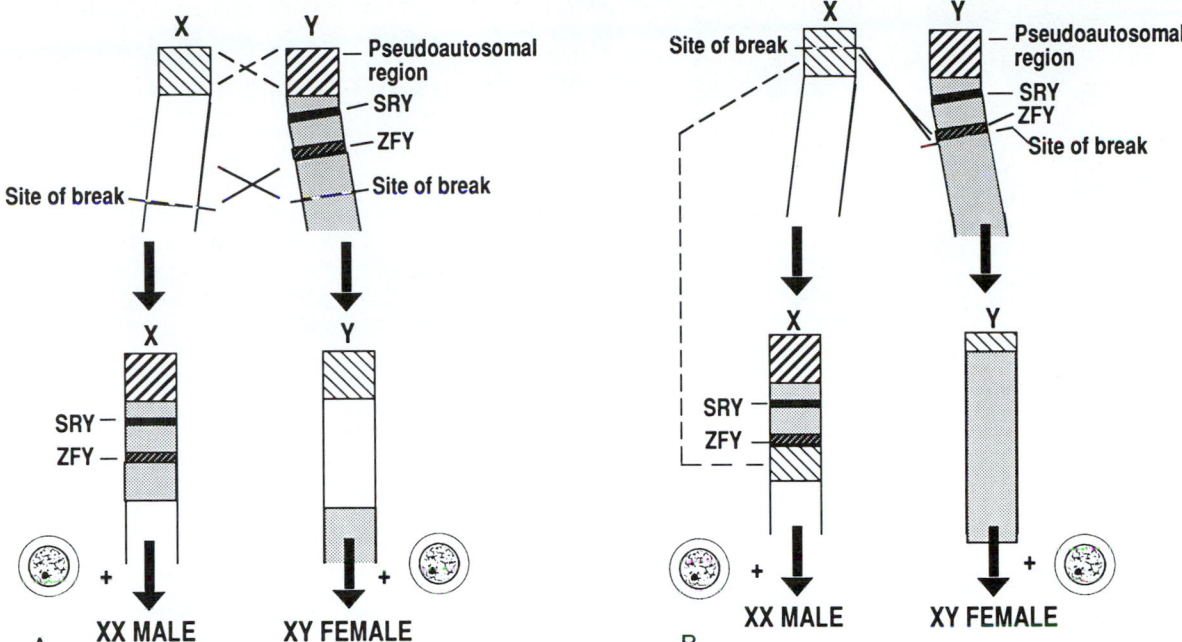

Figure 14–32. A diagrammatic representation of the short arms of the X and Y chromosomes during meiotic pairing. *A,* A crossover *(interrupted lines)* usually occurs between the pseudoautosomal regions of the X and Y chromosomes. Anomalous but equal crossovers *(solid lines)* can occur that result in an X chromosome with the sex-determining region and a Y chromosome deficient in testes-determining genes (TDF). Zygotes with these sex chromosomes will become XX males or XY females as indicated. *B,* Anomalous unequal crossovers *(solid lines)* during male meiosis can result in an X chromosome with testes-determining genes as well as the pseudoautosomal regions of both the X and Y chromosomes.

in the rabbit, that some of these functionally agonadal patients might be genetic males, because fetal castration of either sex invariably leads to a female phenotype. The discovery in 1954 that many of these patients, contrary to their phenotype, were X chromatin–negative seemed initially to confirm the hypothesis that these patients were indeed genetic males. However, soon after techniques became available to determine chromosome constitution, Ford and co-workers[271] reported that the sex chromosome constitution in a 14-y-old phenotypic female with this syndrome was 45,X rather than 46,XY. Work in many laboratories thereafter defined more precisely the chromosomal basis of this and related disorders.

The absence of a second sex chromosome (X chromosome monosomy) is associated with four cardinal features: (1) female phenotype, (2) short stature, (3) sexual infantilism owing to rudimentary gonads, and (4) a variety of associated somatic abnormalities. These features may be modified by the presence of lesser degrees of sex chromosome deficiency. It is therefore useful to consider the syndrome of gonadal dysgenesis and its variants as a continuum of features ranging from those of the typical 45,X phenotype to a normal female or male. The functional importance of chromosomal additions to the basic 45,X pattern can be deduced from the extent to which they modify toward normal, in at least some cases, the short stature, sexual infantilism, and somatic anomalies that typify the patient with complete sex chromosome monosomy.

Partial sex chromosome monosomy may be attributed to a structurally abnormal second sex chromosome (X or Y), sex chromosome mosaicism involving a 45,X cell line, or both a structural abnormality and mosaicism. Even though the modified clinical forms are almost invariably associated with partial sex chromosome monosomy, the contrary is not necessarily true; partial sex chromosome monosomies may be associated with the typical clinical picture found in 45,X patients.

TYPICAL TURNER SYNDROME (45,X GONADAL DYSGENESIS).[11, 49, 267–270]

In patients with the cardinal features of sex chromosome monosomy, the X chromatin pattern is negative in about 60 to 70%; most of these have a 45,X sex chromosome constitution (Table 14–9). Significant variability occurs in expression of the somatic anomalies associated with sex chromosome monosomy (Fig. 14–33).

Clinical Aspects. The typical patient (Fig. 14–34) is often recognizable by the distinctive facies, in which micrognathia; epicanthal folds; prominent, low-set, rotated or deformed ears or both; a fish-like mouth with a narrow, high arched palate; ptosis; and strabismus are present with varying degrees of frequency. The chest is usually square and shield-like with microthelia. The neck is short and broad with a low hairline in back. Webbing of the neck is present in 25 to 40% of the patients, and coarctation of the aorta occurs in 10 to 20%. Those with coarctation usually also have webbing of the neck. Additional anomalies include cubitus valgus, congenital lymphedema of the feet and hands (30%) (see Fig. 14–34) or puffiness of the dorsum of the fingers, short fourth metacarpal (50%), renal abnormalities (60%), high arched palate, various skeletal anomalies, increased number of pigmented nevi, tendency to keloid formation, abnormal nails, recurrent otitis media, which may result in

TABLE 14–9. Salient Features of 45,X Gonadal Dysgenesis: Turner Syndrome

Karyotype: 45,X
Inheritance: Sporadic; meiotic or mitotic nondisjunction
Genitalia: Female
Wolffian duct derivatives: Absent
Müllerian duct derivatives: Normal female
Gonads: Streak
Habitus: Short stature; sexual infantilism at puberty; somatic stigmata
Hormone profile: ↑ plasma LH and FSH concentrations; ↓ plasma estradiol levels

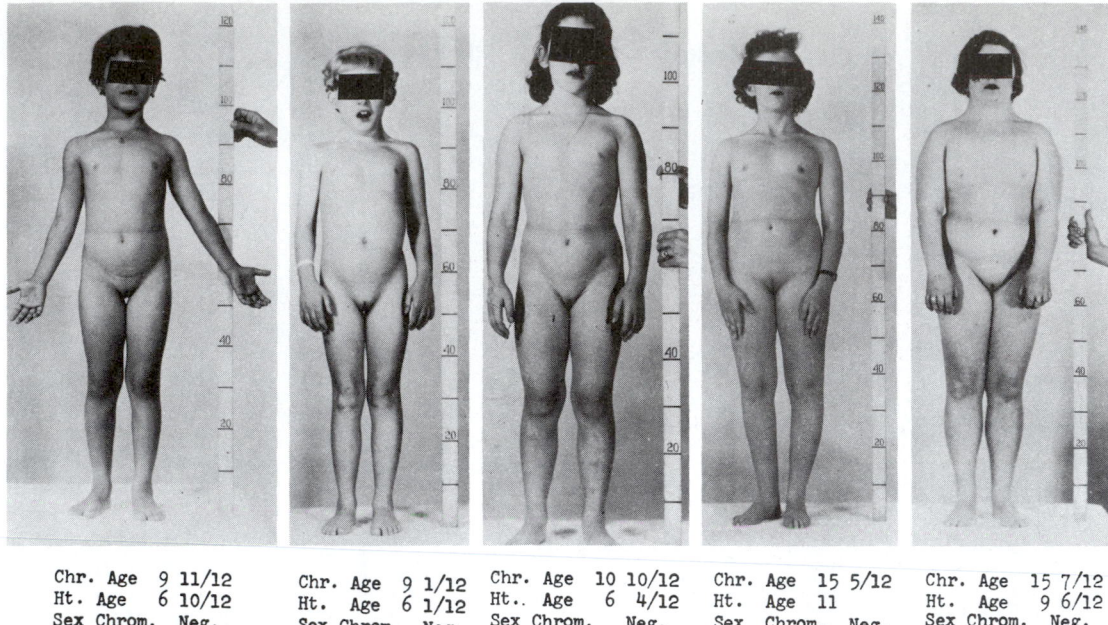

Chr. Age	9 11/12	Chr. Age	9 1/12	Chr. Age	10 10/12	Chr. Age	15 5/12	Chr. Age	15 7/12
Ht. Age	6 10/12	Ht. Age	6 1/12	Ht.. Age	6 4/12	Ht. Age	11	Ht. Age	9 6/12
Sex Chrom.	Neg.	Sex Chrom.	Neg.	Sex Chrom.	Neg.	Sex Chrom.	Neg.	Sex Chrom.	Neg.

Figure 14–33. Variation in physical appearance in five patients with the typical form of the syndrome of gonadal dysgenesis (Turner syndrome). All of these patients had a 45,X karyotype, and all had differences between height age and chronological age of 3 y or more. (Modified from Grumbach MM. Some considerations of the pathogenesis and classification of anomalies of sex in man. In: Astwood EB, ed. Clinical Endocrinology. New York: Grune & Stratton, 1960: 407–436.)

conductive hearing loss, unexplained hypertension,[272] and, rarely, gastrointestinal bleeding secondary to intestinal telangiectasia, hemangiomatoses, or dilated veins. The incidence of mental retardation is not increased over normal. Money and others have reported that impairments of directional sense and space-form recognition are common; this perceptual disability results in a lower mean performance I.Q. than in the general population, whereas verbal ability is normal.[273, 274] In general, patients with gonadal dysgenesis do not tend to differ from siblings in overall intelligence.[275, 276] Severe psychopathic manifestations are uncommon, although a small increase in anorexia nervosa has been reported.[276]

The eponym Bonnevie-Ullrich syndrome has been applied to phenotypic female infants with lymphedema of the distal extremities and loose folds of skin over the back of the neck in addition to the typical features of gonadal dysgenesis (Fig. 14–35). In the neonate, pleural effusions and ascites that clear spontaneously are not uncommon[277] and, rarely, pericardial effusion has been reported. The serous effusions and the lymphedema are attributable to hypoplasia and other defects of the lymphatic system. 45,X abortuses commonly exhibit generalized edema and a large hygroma of the neck.[278, 279] The latter abnormality results postnatally in webbing of the neck. Shephard and Fantel[280] have suggested that the severe pitting edema secondary to hypoalbuminemia and lymphatic duct hypoplasia in 45,X fetuses are responsible for many of the malformations involving the ears, hairline, neck, nipples, nails, and kidneys. The increased incidence of congenital heart disease associated with webbed neck has led to the suggestion that a pathogenetic relationship exists between the two related to lymphatic obstruction.[281, 282]

In addition to coarctation of the aorta, common cardiovascular abnormalities include bicuspid aortic valves,[283] partial anomalous venous drainage,[284] and hypoplastic left-sided heart syndrome.[285] On echocardiography, an 8 to 29% incidence of aortic root dilatation has been reported.[286, 287] In 18 patients aortic dilatation and rupture occurred.[287] Therefore,

all patients with gonadal dysgenesis should have a thorough baseline cardiac evaluation including an echocardiogram in infancy and again at adolescence. Patients with increased risk factors for dissection and rupture (e.g., those with coarctation, hypertension, and aortic root dilatation) require follow-up and therapeutic measures to decrease the risk of dissection. Patients with bicuspid aortic valves should be given prophylactic therapy to prevent bacterial endocarditis.

The most common renal abnormalities are rotation of the kidney, horseshoe kidney, duplication of the renal pelvis and ureter, and hydronephrosis secondary to ureteropelvic obstruction. Complete absence of the kidney in 4 of 141 patients and gross renal ectopia in 3 of 141 have been reported by Lippe and co-workers.[288] Abnormal differentiation of the kidneys and upper collecting system is so common in this syndrome that intravenous urography or a renal sonogram should be obtained routinely.

Skeletal maturation is normal or slightly delayed in childhood but lags in adolescence secondary to gonadal steroid deficiency. In most cases, the skeleton exhibits localized areas of rarefaction (fishnet appearance), especially of the hands, feet, elbows, and upper femurs.[289–291] Bone mineral content as assessed by single-beam photon absorptiometry can be reduced beginning as early as 8 y of age.[291] As indicated by dual-beam photon absorptiometry, lumbar bone density is also diminished, although the decrease in lumbar bone mass may develop during the pubertal years.[291] Patients not treated with estrogen often develop a severe form of the postmenopausal type of osteoporosis and may develop fractures and vertebral collapse. Osteochondrosis-like changes of the spine, vertebral hypoplasia, and scoliosis are common.[289, 290] In addition to the metacarpal sign (shortening of the fourth metacarpal), Kosowicz has described a carpal sign characterized by a more acute angular configuration of the proximal row of carpal bones. An abnormality at the wrist is the Madelung or "bayonet" deformity in about 10% of patients. Cubitus valgus (an increased carrying angle) occurs in half of patients and is a consequence of a developmental abnormality of the trochlear head. The knee may

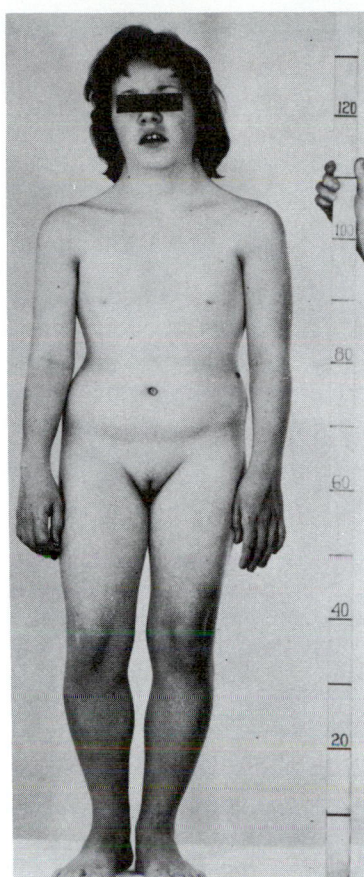

Figure 14–34. A 14^{10}/$_{12}$-y-old patient with the typical form of the syndrome of gonadal dysgenesis (Turner syndrome). The X chromatin pattern was negative and karyotype was 45,X. She was short (height 134.5 cm, height age 9^{5}/$_{12}$ y), sexually infantile except for the appearance of sparse pubic hair, and exhibited characteristic stigmata of the syndrome: a short webbed neck, shield-like chest with widely separated nipples, bilateral short fourth metacarpals, puffiness over dorsum of fingers, cubitus valgus, and an increased number of pigmented nevi. The facies were characteristic and the ears low set. The bone age was 13½ y. The urinary 17-ketosteroid level was 5.1 mg/d; plasma and urinary gonadotropin levels were elevated. Vaginal smears and urocytogram showed an immature pattern in which cornified squamous cells were absent. With estrogen therapy, female secondary sexual characteristics were induced; cyclic administration resulted in periodic estrogen-withdrawal bleeding.

between patients and normal individuals (16 cm) is close to that at maturity (20 cm).[295] Hence, there appears to be little additional loss of height relative to normal individuals after a bone age of 9 y in spite of the lack of a pubertal growth spurt (Fig. 14–36). This may be accounted for by the prolongation of growth mediated by the lack of an effect of gonadal steroids (in the untreated patient) on bone maturation.[296] Final height in untreated patients may not be achieved until late in the second decade of life. The final height correlates with birth weight[294] and midparental height.[292–294]

The short stature in this syndrome is not attributable to a deficiency of growth hormone, insulin-like growth factor I (IGF I, also called somatomedin-C), or insulin-like growth factor II (IGF II),[297] or adrenal and gonadal steroids.[298] Decreased 24-h secretion of growth hormone as manifested by decreased amplitude and frequency of growth hormone pulses has been reported in patients with the syndrome of gonadal dysgenesis after 8 y of age.[299] Likewise, IGF I levels that are normal up to 10 y of age are low thereafter;[299] however, administration of either estrogen[297] or growth hormone induces a rise in the concentration of plasma IGF I. Thus the changes in growth hormone secretory dynamics and IGF I concentrations noted after age 8 to 10 y are probably secondary to the lack of the estrogen-induced rise in plasma growth hormone concentration and consequently IGF I concentration at puberty. As yet, the etiology of the progressive growth failure has not been defined. We postulate that the abnormality resides in the response of the chondrocyte to the somatomedins.

Sexual Infantilism. The genital ducts and external genitalia in this syndrome are female in character but immature. Located in the mesosalpinges parallel to the fallopian tubes are long, attenuated, pale, fibrous streaks of connective tissue. Typically, these streak-like or spindle-shaped structures consist of fibrous stroma arranged in whorls similar to those in ovarian stroma, but they lack primordial follicles. Vestigial medullary elements and rudimentary mesonephric

show deformities of the medial tibial and femoral condyles with obliquely tipped tibial epiphyses and medial projections of the tibial metaphyses that can result in genu valgum. The pelvis tends to have a male-type inlet. Midface hypoplasia is common. An enlarged sella turcica secondary to pituitary hyperplasia may be present, especially in untreated adult patients with hypergonadotropic hypogonadism. An "empty sella" was noted on computed tomographic (CT) scan in two of our patients.

Short Stature. Short stature is an invariant feature in 45,X individuals. The mean final height of patients ranges in different series from 142 to 147 cm;[292–295, 295a] the ratio of sitting to standing height is frequently increased by late childhood and reflects the greater retardation in growth of the legs.[296] Intrauterine growth retardation is common in patients with gonadal dysgenesis, and the average birth weight (2.83 ± 0.57 kg) and length (48.2 ± 3.2 cm) are 1 standard deviation (SD) below the mean for normal infants of comparable gestational age.[294, 295]

For the first 3 y of life, growth velocity is usually within the normal range.[295] Subsequently, velocity decelerates so that by a bone age of 9 the difference in mean height

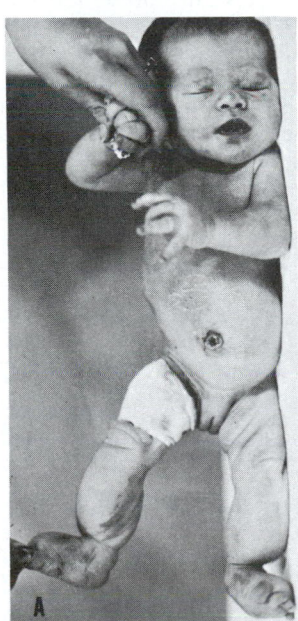
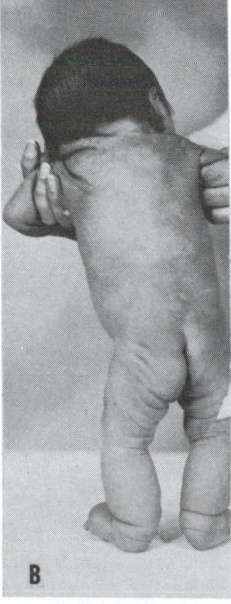

Figure 14–35. An infant with the syndrome of gonadal dysgenesis (karyotype 45,X) and associated lymphedema of extremities. The term Bonnevie-Ullrich syndrome is applied when this characteristic swelling of the feet or hands or both is associated with other features of Turner syndrome. (From Grumbach MM. Chromosomal sex and the prepubertal diagnosis of gonadal dysgenesis. Reproduced by permission of Pediatrics vol 20 page 740 Copyright 1957.)

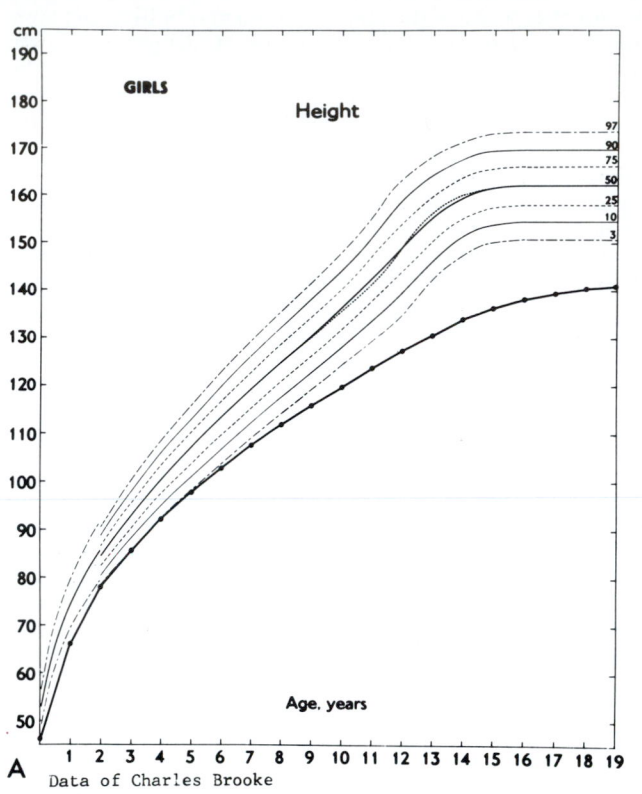

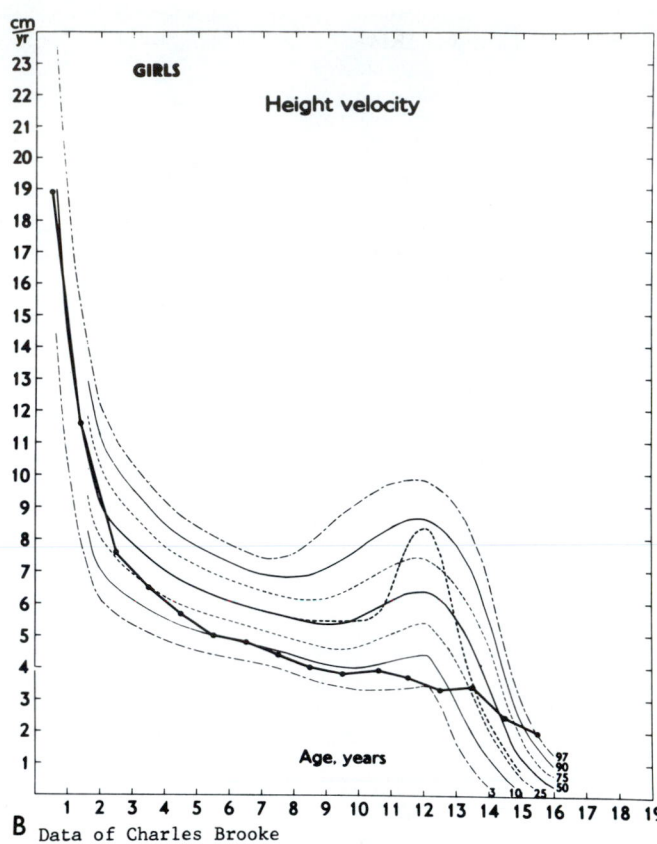

Figure 14–36. *A,* The mean height in 38 untreated patients with 45,X karyotype. *B,* Mean yearly height velocities from data on 36 untreated patients with Turner syndrome (45,X karyotype). Note the absence of a pubertal growth spurt. (From Brook CGD, Murset G, Zachmann M, et al. Growth in children with 45,X Turner's syndrome. Arch Dis Child 1974; 49:789–795.)

tubules like those found in the primitive genital ridge are common at the hilus. After puberty, aggregates of epithelioid cells resembling Leydig or hilus cells are present in variable quantity.

Singh and Carr[278] studied the gonadal ridge of eight spontaneously aborted embryos and fetuses ranging in gestational age from 5 wk to 4 mo. Primordial germ cells were observed in all eight specimens. Until the third month of gestation, no appreciable differences were noted between these gonads and those from 46,XX fetuses; after that, an increase in connective tissue stroma and impaired formation of follicles were found. These observations suggest that primordial germ cells seed the primitive gonad in 45,X individuals, many degenerate during oocyte formation and folliculogenesis, and the surviving oocytes undergo accelerated atresia.[300] Jirasek[301] has reported that in patients with a 45,X karyotype, oocytes degenerate shortly after formation of the primary follicle, possibly because the surrounding follicular cell layer is incomplete. Apparently, two active X chromosomes are required for the normal development of human oogonia and oocytes. The presence of follicles in the gonadal streaks in 45,X infants is not unusual at birth, although it is uncommon by late childhood and adolescence.

Longitudinal studies of both basal and LHRH-evoked gonadotropin secretion demonstrate a lack of feedback inhibition of the hypothalamic-pituitary axis by the dysgenetic gonad in infants and young children with gonadal dysgenesis.[302, 303] Basal levels of LH and FSH were studied in 58 patients aged 2 d to 20 y. Plasma FSH levels were elevated between 2 d and 4 y of age and decreased to high-normal values at 5 to 10 y of age (Fig. 14–37). After 10 y of age, the plasma FSH level rose again into the castrate range.[302]

Thus the pattern of plasma FSH concentration followed a diphasic curve similar to but higher than that in normal infants and children. The pattern of change in LH levels was similar, but the concentrations were one third to one tenth those of FSH. LHRH-induced LH and FSH responses exhibited a diphasic pattern with age, similar to those of basal levels.[303] In patients under 5 y of age both the mean basal levels and the rise in gonadotropin levels induced by the administration of LHRH were increased over normal

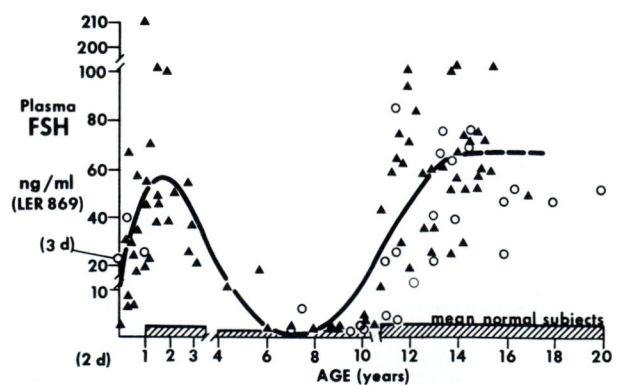

Figure 14–37. The pattern of plasma FSH concentration in relation to age in 58 patients with the syndrome of gonadal dysgenesis. ▲, patients with 45,X karyotype; ○, patients with structural abnormalities of the X chromosome and mosaics. The hatched area shows the range of FSH values in normal females. (From FA Conte, MM Grumbach, SL Kaplan, A diphasic pattern of gonadotropin secretion in patients with the syndrome of gonadal dysgenesis, J Clin Endocrinol Metab 40, 670–674, 1975, © The Endocrine Society.)

values for age. Between ages 5 and 10 y, basal concentrations of FSH and LH and LHRH-evoked responses were less than those of patients with gonadal dysgenesis under 5 y of age (see Fig. 14–37). In some patients between ages 6 and 10 y, both FSH and LH concentrations and the LHRH-induced gonadotropin responses were comparable to those in normal children. After age 11 y a striking rise in basal and readily releasable LH and FSH levels was observed. Thus between ages 5 and 10 y basal and LHRH-elicited gonadotropin responses may not reflect the functional status of the gonads in all patients with gonadal dysgenesis.

Although streak gonads are the rule in 45,X gonadal dysgenesis, exceptions have been documented. Primary follicles have been described in the ridges of some 45,X individuals at adolescence, and this correlates with the rare occurrence of menarche and a variable but attenuated period of regular menses. By means of sonography, 30% of a series of 45,X females were found to have nonstreak gonads.[304] In this study 3 of 32 patients over age 10 y had breast development but had not menstruated.[303] This number correlates with previous data suggesting that 5 to 10% of patients with gonadal dysgenesis have a sufficient number of ovarian follicles ($>10^4$) at adolescence to initiate breast development.[305] In 11 women, conceptions were documented despite extensive karyotypic studies revealing only a 45,X cell line in multiple tissues.[305–307] In addition to variability in the rate of follicular atresia, another possible explanation for the presence of oogonia in 45,X individuals is that a certain number of 45,X germ cells may undergo mitotic nondisjunction with the formation of 46,XX oogonia.[308] This process normally occurs in the female creeping vole and serves as a sex-determining mechanism in this species. Alternatively, some fertile 45,X patients may be unrecognized sex chromosome mosaics. Women with a 45,X cell line have increased fetal wastage and an increased number of chromosomally abnormal live-born infants including those with Turner and Down syndromes.[306, 307, 309–311]

Patients with gonadal dysgenesis experience adrenarche with a normal rise in adrenal androgen production in childhood and develop sparse pubic and axillary hair. Before age 10 y the plasma concentration of adrenal androgens is normal.[312] After age 15 y, levels of dehydroepiandrosterone, testosterone, and androstenedione are lower than normal, reflecting absence of the gonadal contribution.[313]

Clitoral enlargement is rare in 45,X patients. Enlargement of the clitoris may be present at birth or become manifest at puberty. Secretion of androgens by "Leydig cells" in the gonadal streak is a possible cause, as is the presence of an undetected Y cell line.

A number of males with a 45,X karyotype have been described.[314–318] Invariably, these patients have had a Y-autosome translocation involving variable segments of the euchromatic (sex-determining) region of the Y chromosome.[314–318] Translocations have been reported involving the short arm of chromosomes 5, 14, 15, and 18. The majority of reported patients have had either minor or major anomalies not usually associated with the syndrome of gonadal dysgenesis, such as the four 45,X cases with Y-5 translocations and the cri du chat syndrome. These additional anomalies are no doubt related to the autosome involved in the translocation as well as the degree of deletion involved.

Incidence in Abortuses, Newborns, and Twins.
The incidence of gonadal dysgenesis varies in newborns from 1 per 2500 to 1 per 10,000 phenotypic females.[222, 319] There is, however, a considerable loss of 45,X embryos and fetuses.[320] About 10% of all clinically recognizable spontaneous abortuses have a 45,X constitution.[221] It is estimated that the frequency of 45,X zygotes is 0.8%, probably the most common chromosome anomaly in humans, but fewer than 3%

of 45,X conceptuses survive to term.[319] Hook and Warburton[321] have analyzed chromosome genotypes in embryonic and fetal deaths and demonstrated a significant disparity between the 45,X genotype and those with mosaicism and/or an isochromosome for the long arm of the X chromosome (Xqi). They postulated a "fetoprotective" effect of more than one dose of some locus or loci on the long arm of the X chromosome.[321]

Associated Disorders.
There is an increased incidence of autoimmune disorders in patients with gonadal dysgenesis; the most prevalent is Hashimoto thyroiditis. An increased frequency of thyroid antibodies and hypothyroidism (or hyperthyroidism) occurs during childhood and adolescence.[322, 323] Early diagnosis may be facilitated by following antibody levels as well as basal and thyrotropin-releasing hormone–induced thyrotropin responses. Basal as well as thyrotropin-releasing hormone–induced prolactin concentrations may be elevated in euthyroid patients with gonadal dysgenesis. Prevalences of rheumatoid arthritis and inflammatory bowel disease are increased in patients with a 45,X karyotype.[324]

Carbohydrate intolerance and nonketotic diabetes mellitus are common, especially after age 16 y.[325, 326] During childhood, episodes of otitis media may result in conductive hearing loss.[327] Abnormalities in the growth of the temporal bone, condylar cartilage, and spheno-occipital synchrondrosis result in an abnormality in the positioning of the external auditory meatus and the relationship of the middle ear to the eustachian tube in Turner syndrome.[327] These changes, along with abnormalities in the shape of the palate, are thought to be responsible for an increased incidence of otitis media. Sensorineural deafness has also been reported in adults. In a survey of 289 patients with Turner stigmata, Wertelecki and co-workers[328] found eight patients with nongonadal tumors, suggesting a possible increased risk of malignancy.

Origin of 45,X Constitution.
A 45,X chromosome constitution may arise through a variety of chromosome errors (see Figs. 14–3 and 14–13). It may be a consequence of nondisjunction or chromosome loss during gametogenesis in either parent, resulting in a sperm or ovum lacking a sex chromosome. Although errors of mitosis in a normal zygote often lead to mosaicism, a purely 45,X constitution may arise at the first cleavage division from anaphase lag with loss of a sex chromosome or, less likely, mitotic nondisjunction with failure of the complementary 47,XXX or 47,XYY cell line to survive (see Fig. 14–3). There is indirect evidence that loss of one X or Y chromosome between fertilization and the first cleavage division may be a frequent but not the only cause of a 45,X embryo.[22]

Several lines of evidence support a mitotic error in this syndrome: (1) the lack of association with advanced maternal age, in contrast to chromatin-positive Klinefelter syndrome (indeed, an increased incidence of 45,X conceptuses occurs in teen-age pregnancies);[329] (2) the prevalence of sex chromosome mosaicism; (3) the increased frequency of twinning in sibships with a 45,X individual;[330] and (4) the occurrence of a 46,XY monozygotic co-twin of a 45,X individual.[331]

Family studies of such X-linked traits as color blindness and the Xg blood group indicate that loss of the paternally derived sex chromosome is more common than would be expected if either the maternally or paternally derived sex chromosome were lost randomly; in informative pedigrees 77% of 45,X individuals have loss of the paternal sex chromosome ($45,X^M$), and 23% have loss of the maternal X chromosome ($45,X^P$). Similar findings have been obtained using restriction fragment length polymorphisms.[332]

The underlying cause of this sex chromosome abnormality is not known. An increased frequency of thyroid autoimmunity in patients with the syndrome of gonadal dysgenesis and in their parents suggests that the genetic predisposition to develop autoantibodies in one or both parents is associated with an increased prevalence of a 45,X constitution and other chromosome abnormalities in the offspring. Of note, three patients with gonadal dysgenesis have been born after artificial insemination.[333] The familial occurrence of 45,X gonadal dysgenesis is rare.

Diagnosis and Treatment. Phenotypic females with the following features should have a karyotype analysis: (1) short stature (more than 2.5 SD below the mean height value for age), (2) somatic stigmata associated with Turner syndrome, and (3) delayed adolescence with increased plasma or urinary gonadotropin levels. In the past, X chromatin was assessed to screen for gonadal dysgenesis. Normal females have 20 to 30% sex chromatin–positive cells at all ages, including the neonatal period. 45,X patients lack an X chromatin body in interphase nuclei, and 45,X/46,XX mosaics usually have between 3 and 19% chromatin-positive cells. Although determination of the X chromatin pattern is a rapid method of screening, karyotype analysis is the definitive procedure. Levels of plasma gonadotropins, especially FSH, are useful in assessing the functional status of the gonads. It is important in patients with gonadal dysgenesis to obtain an intravenous pyelogram or ultrasonographic examination to exclude renal anomaly; to assess cardiovascular function clinically and with an echocardiogram; to test for loss of hearing periodically; to evaluate thyroid function regularly; to measure plasma glucose levels after adolescence; and to monitor bone density in late adolescence and adulthood for evidence of progressive osteopenia.

Therapy is directed toward augmenting stature, correcting somatic anomalies, and inducing secondary sexual characteristics and menses. As noted, the short stature in Turner syndrome does not seem to be related to a deficiency of growth hormone, insulin-like growth factors, thyroid hormone, or adrenal or gonadal steroids. However, data on the effect of treatment with biosynthetic growth hormone at a dose of 0.125 mg three times a week subcutaneously and oxandrolone at 0.06 mg/kg/d are encouraging.[334] Patients treated with the combination therapy had a growth velocity of 9.8 cm/y for the first year after beginning therapy, compared with 6.1 cm/y in those treated with growth hormone alone and 3.8 cm/y in control patients. Although growth velocity declined over the next 3 y of therapy, the patients treated with combined therapy had a mean increment of 8.5 cm in predicted final height. Patients treated with combined therapy for 3 to 7 y had a mean increase in height of 8 to 9 cm, and some are still growing (personal communication, R. G. Rosenfield). Daily growth hormone at the same dose per week (0.375 mg/kg/wk) appears to be as efficacious as combined therapy. This study, now in its seventh year, is still in progress. Nevertheless, the results are sufficiently encouraging to merit consideration of treatment with biosynthetic human growth hormone. Because these patients lose most of their height between ages 3 and 9, it would seem prudent to consider starting therapy early in childhood.

Estrogen therapy has commonly been deferred until age 15 or later on the assumption that treatment at an earlier age leads to rapid skeletal maturation and diminished height. This premise has been based largely on the fact that pharmacological doses of estrogens can accelerate bone maturation and lead to premature epiphyseal fusion without a proportionate increase in height. We examined the effect of early low-dose, conjugated estrogen therapy on linear growth, bone age, and the development of secondary sexual characteristics in a group of patients with gonadal dysgene-

sis.[292] Conjugated estrogens (9 μg/kg body weight/d) or ethinyl estradiol (141 ng/kg body weight/d) was given to 21 patients with gonadal dysgenesis who had a mean age of 13 and mean bone age of 10.7. A transient acceleration in growth rate occurred and declined to below the pretherapy rate after 12 mo of therapy. The final height of the patients treated with low-dose estrogen was not different from that of the control nontreated patients or that of a group of six patients with the syndrome of gonadal dysgenesis in whom normal ovarian function was documented clinically and biochemically. Hence, no increase or decrease in final height was noted in our study. The patients developed breasts within 3 mo of onset of therapy and usually experienced withdrawal bleeding within 8 mo of the start of therapy.

Serious psychological effects are frequently associated with a prolonged delay in the treatment of the sexual infantilism.[335] The institution of low-dose, conjugated estrogen or synthetic estrogen therapy at approximately 12 to 13 y of age (bone age > 11 y) elicits a growth spurt without inordinate advancement of skeletal maturation or reduction in final height and induces the development of secondary sexual characteristics at an age comparable to that of normal peers, thereby obviating the undesirable psychological consequences of a prolonged delay in sexual maturation. As yet, there are no long-term data on the effect of combination therapy with low-dose estrogen and growth hormone. However, low-dose estrogen and growth hormone in combination do not have a synergistic effect on short-term tibial growth.[336] In a 1-y study, no additional increment in growth velocity was obtained by combining growth hormone with extremely low-dose (25 ng/kg/d) ethinyl estradiol. Furthermore, breast development and an increased rate of bone maturation were noted.[336a]

A number of instances of endometrial carcinoma have been reported in patients with gonadal dysgenesis.[337] The evidence suggests that estrogens, especially when unopposed by progesterone, can produce a progression of histological changes from endometrial hyperplasia to invasive carcinoma (also see Chapter 12). To clarify the relationship between estrogen therapy and endometrial pathology in gonadal dysgenesis, Rosenwaks and colleagues[338] studied 41 patients receiving estrogen replacement therapy. Increased risk of abnormal endometrial histology correlated with (1) a lifetime dosage of conjugated estrogens of greater than 2500 mg, (2) more than 7 y of estrogen therapy, and (3) a daily dose of conjugated estrogens greater than 1.25 mg. Progestogens can modify the effect of estrogens on endometrial histology. It is therefore prudent to treat patients with gonadal dysgenesis with low-dose estrogen replacement therapy administered in a cyclic fashion, with progestogen added at the end of each cycle. Further studies will be necessary to assess the optimal dose of estrogen to reduce the risk of endometrial carcinoma and concurrently prevent osteoporosis. Rarely, patients with a 45,X karyotype and no evidence of Y chromosome material have been reported to have a gonadoblastoma;[339] however, most patients with a 45,X karyotype have little or no risk of neoplastic transformation of the streak gonads.

Replacement Therapy. We routinely initiate therapy at 12 to 13 y of age with 0.3 mg of conjugated estrogen, or ethinyl estradiol, 5 μg by mouth, for the first 21 d of the calendar month. Thereafter the dose of estrogen is gradually increased over the next 2 to 3 y to 0.6 to 1.25 mg of conjugated estrogens or 10 μg of ethinyl estradiol daily for the first 21 d of the month. The patient is maintained on the minimal dose of estrogen needed to maintain secondary sexual characteristics, to permit withdrawal bleeding, and to prevent osteopenia. Medroxyprogesterone acetate, 5 to 10 mg/d, is given from the 12th through the 21st day of the month to ensure more physiological menses and reduce the risk of endometrial carcinoma.

An important part of the management is the education of the patient and family.[340] A frank discussion of the pathophysiology of the condition with the parents is appropriate when the diagnosis is made. Thereafter, the child should be given as much information about her condition as she can comprehend to allay any false fears or anxieties. An honest assessment of reproductive function based on clinical as well as hormonal levels should be given to the patient when appropriate. Advances in in vitro fertilization and embryo transplantation have made pregnancy possible for these patients.[341] Social and psychosocial support from the parents and the physician will usually result in a normal, well-adjusted, knowledgeable, and successful adult female.[340, 342]

PARTIAL SEX CHROMOSOME MONOSOMY AND CLINICAL VARIANTS OF THE SYNDROME OF GONADAL DYSGENESIS. Partial sex chromosome monosomy may or may not modify the expression of the classic 45,X phenotype.[22, 49] Approximately 30 to 40% of patients with the typical syndrome of gonadal dysgenesis are X chromatin–positive. This group usually has a structurally abnormal X chromosome and, more commonly, sex chromosome mosaicism involving a 45,X cell line. Chromatin-positive and chromatin-negative clinical variants of gonadal dysgenesis will be discussed in relation to the more usual types of sex chromosome aberrations with which they may be associated.

A diagrammatic scheme interrelating the variable effect of partial sex chromosome monosomy on the typical features of the syndrome is shown in Figure 14–38.

In patients with sex chromosome mosaicism, the ratio in each gonad of 45,X primordial germ cells and blastemal components to those with a normal 46,XX or 46,XY constitution is probably the major determinant of whether the ultimate gonadal structure is a streak, a dysgenetic or hypoplastic ovary or testis, or a relatively normal gonad.[22, 49, 343] The weight of evidence supports the idea that, after migration into the primitive gonad, primordial germ cells that bear a 45,X constitution degenerate more rapidly than do 46,XX cells, resulting in a streak, hypoplastic, or normal ovary. Similarly, if the gonadal blastemal components, in particular the Sertoli cells, do not contain an appropriate number of 46,XY cells, testicular development will not take place[344] (Fig. 14–39).

The quantitative relation in peripheral tissues between 45,X cells and those with a 46,XX or 46,XY pattern may also be responsible for the variable effect of mosaicism on stature and associated somatic stigmata.[22]

In patients with a single cell line (euploid) containing a structurally abnormal sex chromosome, the somatic and gonadal consequences appear to be related to the nature and degree of the short or long arm deficiency of the second X or Y chromosome. Table 14–10 summarizes the correlation between structural abnormalities of the X and Y chromosomes and the clinical manifestations. The use of deletion mapping of the human sex chromosomes to clarify the

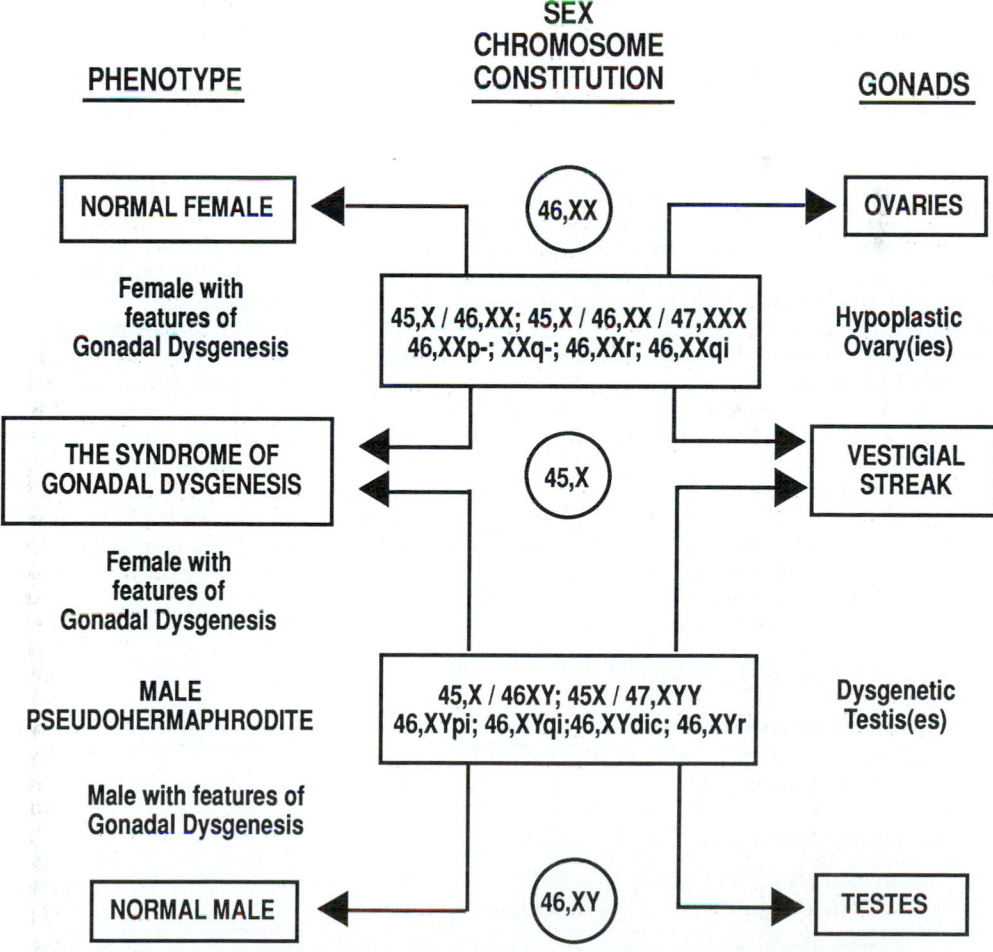

Figure 14–38. The range of phenotypic and gonadal expression in variants of the syndrome of gonadal dysgenesis and its relationship to sex chromosome constitution. Typical phenotypic and gonadal findings in monosomic 45,X gonadal dysgenesis may be modified by the presence of a mosaic chromosomal constitution or by the presence of a structurally abnormal second sex chromosome. For example, 45,X/46,XX and 45,X/47,XXX mosaicism may be associated with normal stature, minimal somatic features of Turner syndrome, and varying degrees of ovarian differentiation, or with a clinical picture indistinguishable from that of classic 45,X gonadal dysgenesis. Phenotype and gonadal differentiation apparently depend on the proportion of 45,X to 46,XX or 47,XXX cells in somatic and germ cells during differentiation. Similarly, the presence of a structurally abnormal X chromosome frequently modifies some features of the classic syndrome. When 45,X/46,XY mosaicism or a structurally abnormal Y chromosome is present, varying degrees of testicular differentiation may be found. The spectrum of clinical findings may thus extend from a phenotypic male through pseudohermaphroditism to a phenotypic female, depending on the degree of fetal testicular insufficiency. In addition, beneficial effects of a normal XY cell line or presence of some part of a Y chromosome may lead to normal stature and a modification of the somatic defects associated with 45,X monosomy. (From Jones HW Jr, Grumbach MM. Developmental disorders [females]. In: Cooke RE, ed. Biologic Basis of Pediatric Practice. New York: McGraw-Hill, 1968: 1087–1093.)

SEX CHROMOSOME CONSTITUTION

PHENOTYPE — GONADS

NORMAL FEMALE ← 46,XX → OVARIES

Female with features of Gonadal Dysgenesis

45,X / 46,XX; 45,X / 46,XX / 47,XXX
46,XXp-; XXq-; 46,XXr; 46,XXqi — Hypoplastic Ovary(ies)

THE SYNDROME OF GONADAL DYSGENESIS ← 45,X → VESTIGIAL STREAK

Female with features of Gonadal Dysgenesis

MALE PSEUDOHERMAPHRODITE

45,X / 46XY; 45X / 47,XYY
46,XYpi; 46,XYqi; 46,XYdic; 46,XYr — Dysgenetic Testis(es)

Male with features of Gonadal Dysgenesis

NORMAL MALE ← 46,XY → TESTES

-=deletion, i=isochromosome, r=ring, q=long arm, p=short arm, dic=dicentric

THE PRIMORDIAL GERM CELLS, THE SEX CHROMOSOMES AND GONADOGENESIS

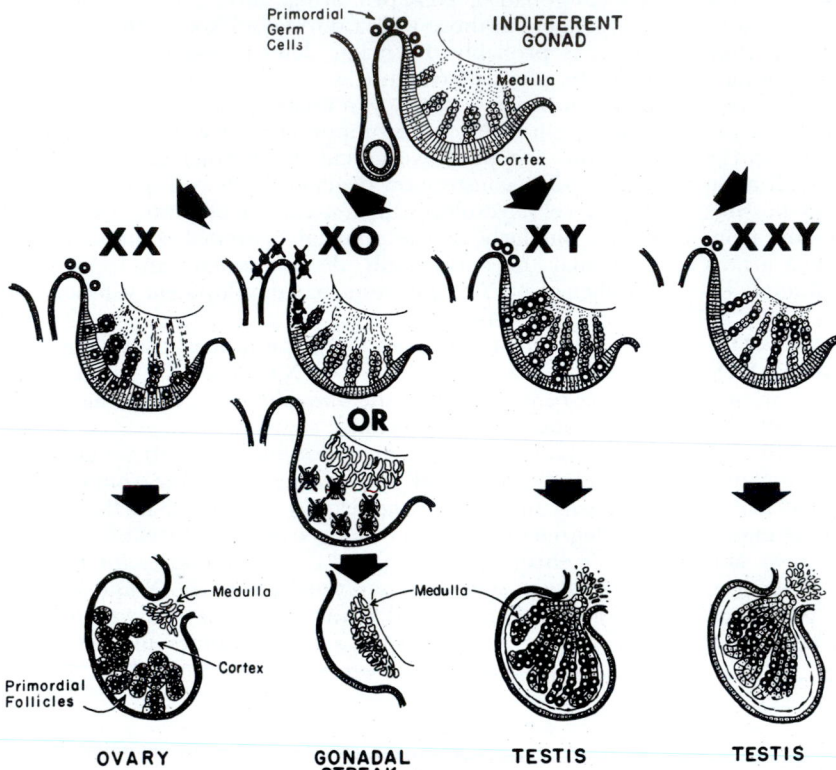

Figure 14–39. The loss of germ cells during migration to or after seeding of the indifferent gonad in a 45,X individual would give rise to a gonadal streak, as germ cells are necessary for ovarian development of the indifferent gonad; evidence suggests that loss occurs after implantation of germ cells. In the presence of 45,X/46,XX mosaicism, gonadal differentiation may vary from that of an ovary to that of a gonadal streak. Similarly, in 45,X/46,XY mosaics, depending on the sex chromosome constitution of the germ cells and gonadal blastoma, gonadal differentiation may vary from that of a testis to that of a gonadal streak. In 47,XXY individuals, germ cells become implanted in the primitive testis, but a marked loss of spermatogonia seems to occur in the perinatal period. (From Jones HW Jr, Grumbach MM. Developmental disorders [females]. In: Cooke RE, ed. Biologic Basis of Pediatric Practice. New York: McGraw-Hill, 1968: 1087–1093.)

relation of phenotype to karyotype has limitations. Structural abnormalities are often associated with mosaicism because of loss of the structurally abnormal sex chromosome from the stem cell line. Further, structural rearrangements of chromosomes are complex. However, the advent of chromosome banding and molecular genetics techniques has facilitated the analysis of structurally abnormal sex chromosomes. At present, the data suggest that (1) ovarian determiners are located on both the long and short arms of the X chromosome, and patients with short arm deletions proximal to band Xp21 or long arm deletions proximal to band Xq25 usually have streak gonads and sexual infantilism;[345–347] and (2) the short arm of the X chromosome (and to a lesser extent the long arm) contains loci that, if deleted, result in short stature and the somatic stigmata of the syndrome of gonadal dysgenesis.[346, 347] Page's group has cloned a gene from a 90-kb region of the Y chromosome

between SRY and ZFY.[64b, 64c] Its homologue on the X chromosome is in the region of the X inactivation center Xq13. This gene, RPS4, codes for a ribosomal protein. The authors suggest that this gene is implicated in the somatic stigmata of the Turner phenotype.[64b]

X CHROMATIN–POSITIVE VARIANTS OF GONADAL DYSGENESIS.[22, 49, 268] **45,X/46,XX, 45,X/47,XXX, and 45,X/46,XX/ 47,XXX Mosaicism.** 45,X/46,XX mosaicism is the most common finding in patients with chromatin-positive gonadal dysgenesis and is second in frequency only to 45,X. Patients with these forms of mosaicism usually exhibit fewer of the associated somatic anomalies, are not invariably short, and may menstruate and even be fertile. One gonad may be of the streak type, and the contralateral gonad may be either a hypoplastic or normal ovary; alternatively, both ovaries may be either normal or hypoplastic. During a family survey for a leukocyte anomaly, a normal grandmother with

TABLE 14–10. Relationship of Structural Abnormalities of X and Y to Clinical Manifestations of Gonadal Dysgenesis

Type of Sex Chromosome Abnormality	Karyotype*	Phenotype	Sexual Infantilism	Short Stature	Somatic Anomalies of Turner Syndrome
Loss of an X or Y	45,X	Female	+	+	+
Deletion of short arm of an X†	46,XXqi	Female	+ (occ. ±)	+	+
	46,XXp−	Female	+, ±, or −	+ (−)	+ (−)
Deletion of long arm of an X†	46,XXq−	Female	+	− (+)	− or +
Deletion of both arms of an X (ring X)	46,XXr	Female	− or +	+	+
Loss of short arm of Y	46,XYp−	Ambiguous	+	+	+

*Xqi, isochromosome for long arm of an X; Xp−, deletion of short arm of an X; Xq−, deletion of long arm of an X; Xr, ring chromosome derived from an X; Yp−, deletion of short arm of Y chromosome.

†In Xp− and Xq−, extent and site of deleted segment are variable.

45,X/46,XX/47,XXX mosaicism was discovered fortuitously. Some appreciation of the variable clinical features may be gleaned from nine patients with these forms of mosaicism studied by Morishima and Grumbach.[22] All had normal female external genitalia. Of seven who attained pubertal age, four showed development of some female secondary sexual characteristics and two menstruated regularly. One of the two has had three pregnancies. In some, no important somatic abnormalities were detected, and two were of normal stature. One of the 45,X/46,XX patients had a webbed neck, coarctation of the aorta, and other stigmata but was of normal stature and menstruated regularly. A 12-y-old 45,X/46,XX/47,XXX patient had primary hypothyroidism and Hashimoto thyroiditis.

46,XXqi and 45,X/46,XXqi. Patients with the Xqi structural abnormality (isochromosome for the long arm of the X) have been thought to have an X chromosome that consists primarily of two long arms (Xq) and lacks a short arm (Xp) (Fig. 14–40). Studies utilizing C and G chromosome banding techniques have demonstrated both monocentric and dicentric X isochromosomes.[348] In a review of 89 cases of Xqi, 29 of 89 were monocentric. Of these, only 5 of 17 were associated with mosaicism for a 45,X cell line.[349] In contrast, 49 of 60 patients with a dicentric isochromosome had a 45,X cell line. Dicentric X isochromosomes seem more unstable than monocentric forms and as a consequence more frequently result in sex chromosome mosaicism through loss of the heteromorphic dicentric X chromosome. Isochromosome for the long arm of the X is the most common form of structural rearrangement of the X chromosome, occurring in approximately 15% of patients with the syndrome of gonadal dysgenesis.

Patients with a long arm X isochromosome are invariably short and have streak gonads,[22, 49] although some menstruate spontaneously.[305, 350] In general, the somatic stigmata of Turner syndrome are less severe than in 45,X patients. Coarctation of the aorta and severe lymphedema of the hands and feet are conspicuously absent in 46,XXqi patients. Webbing of the neck, if present, is usually slight. The findings suggest that absence of the short arm on the second X, even in the presence of an X chromosome composed of two long arms, leads to shortness of stature, failure of ovarian development, and some somatic stigmata of Turner syndrome. The prevalence of Hashimoto thyroiditis, decreased glucose tolerance, and inflammatory bowel disease may be higher in patients with structural abnormalities of the X chromosome, especially 46,XXqi, than in 45,X individuals.

Structurally abnormal X chromosomes are usually late replicating (except in balanced X-autosome translocations) and they give rise to the X chromatin body. Thus X chromatin bodies are larger than normal in patients with a 46,XXqi constitution, but their increased size may be less evident in buccal smears than in other tissues. Karyotype analysis reveals a metacentric X chromosome with two arms of equal length whose banding pattern is similar to that of the long arm of the normal X chromosome.

46,XXpi. There is controversy about the existence of an isochromosome for the short arm of the X chromosome. Of the 11 reported cases, 3 have been revised to long arm deletions, 4 were reported as presumptive, and 2 have been questioned on cytogenetic grounds.[351] The controversy revolves around the difficulty in distinguishing Xpi from deletions of the long arm of the X chromosome because the banding pattern of Xp is quite similar to that of Xq from the centromere to Xq24. High-resolution chromosome banding and molecular genetic studies will no doubt resolve this issue.

46,XXr or 45,X/46,XXr. A ring X chromosome (Xr) usually occurs as part of 45,X/46,XXr mosaicism or a more complex karyotype (see Fig. 14–40).[11, 352] Short stature was present in the majority of patients, and most had minor stigmata of Turner syndrome; none had a webbed neck or coarctation of the aorta. Approximately one third had spontaneous menses and developed secondary sexual characteristics. A mother and daughter with 45,X/46,XXr have been described.[353]

The proportion of X chromatin–positive cells is decreased in patients with a ring X chromosome, and the X chromatin bodies tend to be small. The ring X chromosome with rare exceptions exhibits late DNA replication.[22]

The ring X chromosome arises by loss of both ends of a chromosome and union of the proximal breaks; as a consequence, a variable amount of chromatin material is lost from each arm (see Fig. 14–4). Ring chromosomes are unstable, and there is considerable variability in the size of the ring in different cells of the same subject. In relation to gonadal dysgenesis, patients with a ring X chromosome establish that loss of both terminal ends (telomere) of an X chromosome need not lead to the development of streak gonads.

Not infrequently, it is difficult to be sure of the cytoge-

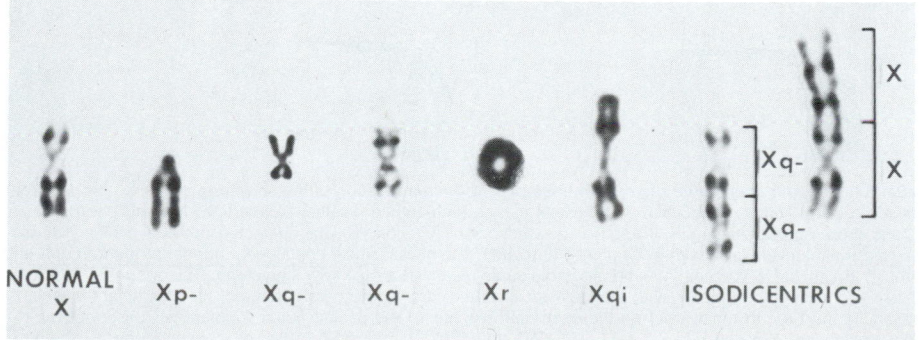

Figure 14–40. Structural anomalies of the X chromosome. The normal X at the left is G banded. A dark band on the short arm and two major dark bands on the long arm are visible. The first Xq− and the ring X chromosome (Xr) are not banded. They show late replication with tritiated thymidine. Note symmetry of the arms of the second Xq−. Even with G banding, it is difficult to distinguish this chromosome from a possible short arm isochromosome. The long arm isochromosome (Xqi) appears to be dicentric. The two chromosomes to the far right are apparent isodicentric X chromosomes. Both have two C bands but only one functional centromere. There is a mirror-like band pattern on both sides of a point between the two C bands. The first isodicentric presumably represents a break in the long arm of X at q22 with fusion of chromatids and duplication of entire chromatid. The second isodicentric appears to represent a terminal break in the short arm so that reduplication of the chromatids has produced what appears to be almost two X chromosomes.

netic origin of the ring chromosome. Its origin is critical in view of the increased risk of gonadal tumors associated with dysgenetic gonads and Y cell lines. DNA analysis with specific X and Y chromosome probes has made identification easier.[354, 355]

46,XXp− and 45,X/46,XXp−. Deletions of the short arm of the X chromosome (Xp−) are rare and frequently associated with 45,X mosaicism. Phenotypic-karyotypic analysis of 40 nonmosaic patients indicated considerable variation in somatic stigmata and gonadal function.[11, 356–360] Nevertheless, patients with a terminal deletion of the short arm of the X (distal to Xp21) can have normal ovarian function and no somatic stigmata of Turner syndrome with the possible exception of short stature.[345] Patients with deletions proximal to Xp21 usually have short stature, variable stigmata of Turner syndrome, and gonadal dysfunction (Fig. 14–41).

The abnormal X chromosome in these patients is usually the late DNA-replicating X and is the origin of the small X chromatin body in interphase nuclei in these patients. Of interest is the report of a familial group of seven patients with the syndrome of gonadal dysgenesis secondary to a deletion of the short arm of an X chromosome in which the disorder was transmitted by carriers of a balanced translocation between the X and chromosome 1.[361]

46,XXq− and 45,X/46,XXq−. Few patients have been reported with this X chromosome anomaly (Xq− designates a deletion of the long arm of the X). In general, patients with only a 46,XXq− cell line are normal in stature and exhibit few if any manifestations of Turner syndrome, but have primary amenorrhea, sexual infantilism, and streak gonads. We have studied two patients with 46,XXq− karyotypes, and the findings in one are summarized in Figure

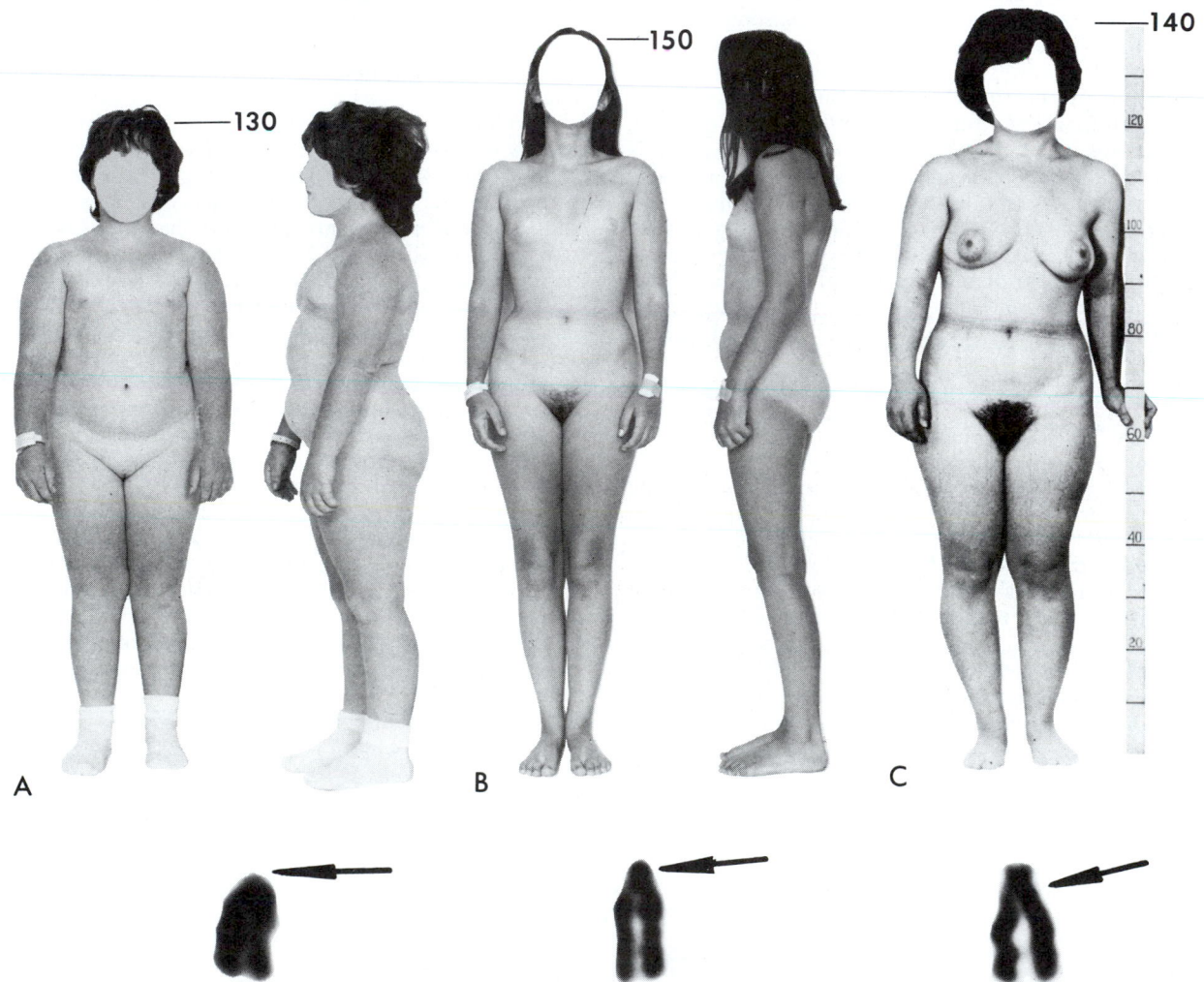

Figure 14–41. Variable gonadal function and phenotypic stigmata in three patients with a deletion of the short arm of the X chromosome (Xp−) of different degrees. *A*, A 13-y-old phenotypic female of short stature (−3.5 SD) with low-set ears, a high-arched palate, low hairline, a broad chest with wide-spaced areolae, cubitus valgus, puffy hands and feet, and short fourth metacarpals. There was no evidence of secondary sexual characteristics at age 13 y. The plasma FSH level was elevated at 26 μg/L (LER-869); the plasma estradiol level was less than 22 pmol/L (6 pg/mL). The buccal smear contained a normal proportion of X chromatin bodies in interphase nuclei, which were conspicuously small. Karyotype analysis and autoradiography revealed a 46,XXp− karyotype. The abnormal X chromosome appeared to lack the entire short arm. *B*, A 17 4/12-y-old phenotypic female with the stigmata of the syndrome of gonadal dysgenesis. Her height was 151 cm (−3 SD), and she had multiple nevi, cubitus valgus, and a short fourth metacarpal on the right hand. At age 13 the patient noted spontaneous onset of breast development, which did not progress. Plasma gonadotropin levels were elevated: LH 7.3 μg/L (LER-960) and FSH 53 μg/L (LER-869). The concentration of plasma estradiol was 70 pmol/L (19 pg/mL). On buccal smear, the cells had a normal proportion of X chromatin bodies, which appeared small. Karyotype analysis and autoradiography indicated an Xp− chromosome that had been deleted close to the centromere, but a small segment of the short arm is visible distal to the centromere. *C*, A 20-y-old phenotypic female with a chief complaint of dysfunctional uterine bleeding. She had short stature, slight puffiness of hands and feet, and short fourth metacarpals. Female secondary sexual characteristics appeared at age 11, and menarche at age 13 was followed by regular menses, which later became irregular. The buccal smear contained nuclei with a normal proportion of small sex chromatin bodies. Bilateral ovaries were identified grossly and histologically during an appendectomy. Karyotype was 46,XXp−. The extent of deletion of the short arms of the abnormal X chromosome in this patient is less than that seen in patients in *A* and *B*. A segment of the short arm is readily discernible above the centromere. It appears that, in these three patients with XXp− karyotypes, somatic and gonadal manifestations of the syndrome of gonadal dysgenesis correlated with the magnitude of deletion of the short arm of the X chromosome.

14–42. Exceptions to the rule that 46,XXq− patients lack stigmata of Turner syndrome and are of normal height were reported before chromosome banding techniques became available. Such cases may represent either hidden mosaicism or complex structural rearrangements of the X chromosome, including inversions and interstitial rather than terminal deletions. Further study with molecular genetic techniques will clarify this issue.

Isodicentric X. Isodicentric X chromosomes are large X chromosomes with two C bands. These chromosomes replicate late, form a large bipartite sex chromatin body, and apparently have one functionally suppressed centromere (see Fig. 14–40).[351] The banding pattern of isodicentric X chromosomes reveals a mirror image about a point between the two centromeres (C bands). These chromosomes are

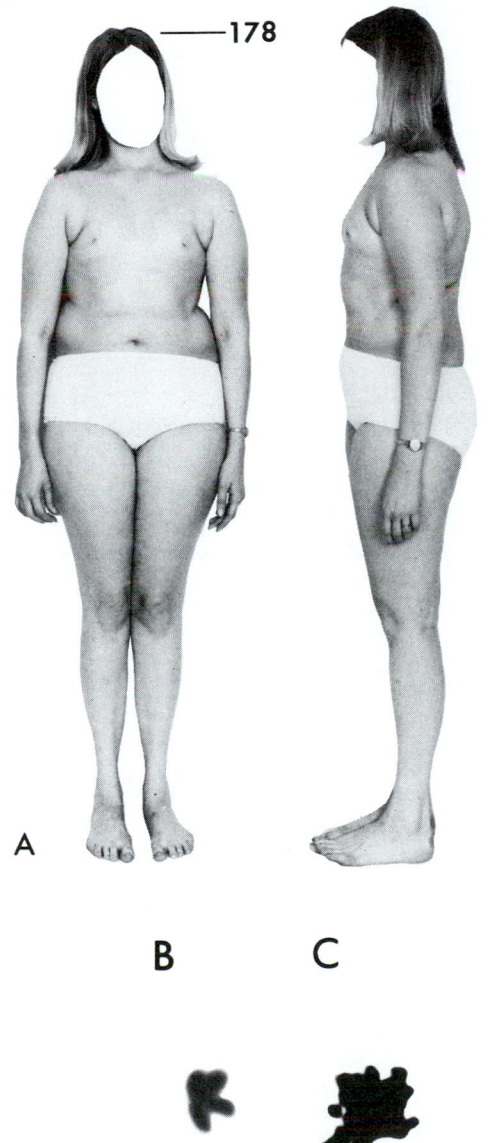

A

B   C

Figure 14–42. *A,* A 22-y-old tall female with a chief complaint of primary amenorrhea who had a deletion of the long arm of one X chromosome, Xq−. At age 12 she developed sparse pubic hair. Breast development did not occur, and she remained sexually infantile. Height was 178 cm (+2.6 SD) and weight was 70 kg (+1.2 SD). No somatic stigmata of the syndrome of gonadal dysgenesis were noted. Plasma gonadotropin levels were elevated: LH 5.6 μg/L (LER-960) and FSH 36.5 μg/L (LER-869). The buccal smear showed a normal proportion of X chromatin bodies that were slightly small. *B,* A Giemsa-stained Xq−, which exhibited the late-labeling pattern characteristic of an X chromosome (*C*).

usually associated with mosaicism for a 45,X cell line and presumably arise by chromatid break and fusion of sister chromatids. This mechanism would produce an acentric fragment that would be lost during cell division and thus result in a 45,X cell line. Phenotypic-karyotypic correlations in these patients are similar to the pattern in Xp− and Xq− patients.[362]

X-Autosome Translocations. X-autosome translocations have been reviewed.[363, 364] In general, women with a break in the X chromosome between Xp13 and Xp26 manifest infertility, confirming the belief that this region contains genes critical to gonadal differentiation and function. Male carriers of a balanced X-autosome translocation with an X chromosome break in the "critical region" Xp13 to Xp26 are usually infertile.

X CHROMATIN–NEGATIVE VARIANTS OF GONADAL DYSGENESIS. The pattern of sex chromosome mosaicism and structural abnormalities of the Y chromosome is similar to that for the X chromosome. Usually as a consequence of its effect on gonadal differentiation, a Y-bearing cell line modifies the typical female phenotype of the syndrome by causing a variable degree of masculine differentiation of the genital tract.

45,X/46,XY, 45,X/47,XYY, 45,X/46,XY/47,XYY, and Related Abnormalities (Table 14–11). A highly diverse phenotype is encountered in these forms of mosaicism.[11, 22, 365, 366] Such individuals may be phenotypic females, individuals with ambiguous external genitalia, or phenotypic males (Fig. 14–43). As in 45,X/46,XX mosaicism, short stature and the associated somatic abnormalities, although frequently present, are inconsistent features and may vary independently of each other and of gonadal differentiation. In the review by Zah and co-workers[365] of 60 patients with 45,X/46,XY mosaicism, two thirds had been reared as females.

Of nine patients with 45,X/46,XY or 45,X/46,XY/47,XYY mosaicism studied by Morishima and Grumbach,[22] one was a phenotypic female, one was a phenotypic male, and seven had ambiguous external genitalia (Table 14–12). The differentiation of the gonads varied from bilateral streaks in the phenotypic female to bilateral dysgenetic testes. In others the development was asymmetrical: one patient had a streak in one mesosalpinx and a rudimentary testis on the contralateral side (so-called mixed gonadal dysgenesis); another had a normal testis in the scrotum and a herniated streak, fallopian tube, and vestigial uterus (hernia uteri inguinale) in the contralateral inguinal region. In several cases, the streak gonad contained a few primordial follicles.

In screening a family for bone marrow transplantation donors, an adult with 45,X/46,XY mosaicism was ascertained by serendipity. Except for short stature, no stigmata of the syndrome of gonadal dysgenesis were present, and he had

TABLE 14–11. Salient Features of 45,X/46,XY Mosaicism

Karyotype: 45,X/46,XY

Genitalia: Female → ambiguous → male

Wolffian duct derivatives: / Müllerian duct derivatives: — Duct differentiation, contingent on functional integrity of homolateral fetal gonad, i.e., streak → uterus, fallopian tubes; dysgenetic testis → variable structures; testis → wolffian duct derivatives

Gonad: Streak gonads → dysgenetic testes → normal testes; Streak gonad + dygenetic testis—"mixed gonadal dysgenesis"; ↑ risk gonadal neoplasm (gonadoblastoma)

Habitus: Short, Turner stigmata; genitalia: streak gonads → female with sexual infantilism at puberty; dysgenetic testes → ambiguous genitalia; if gonadoblastoma present → gynecomastia secondary to estradiol production; testes → normal male differentiation

Hormone profile: ↑ plasma FSH and LH; ↓ testosterone concentrations

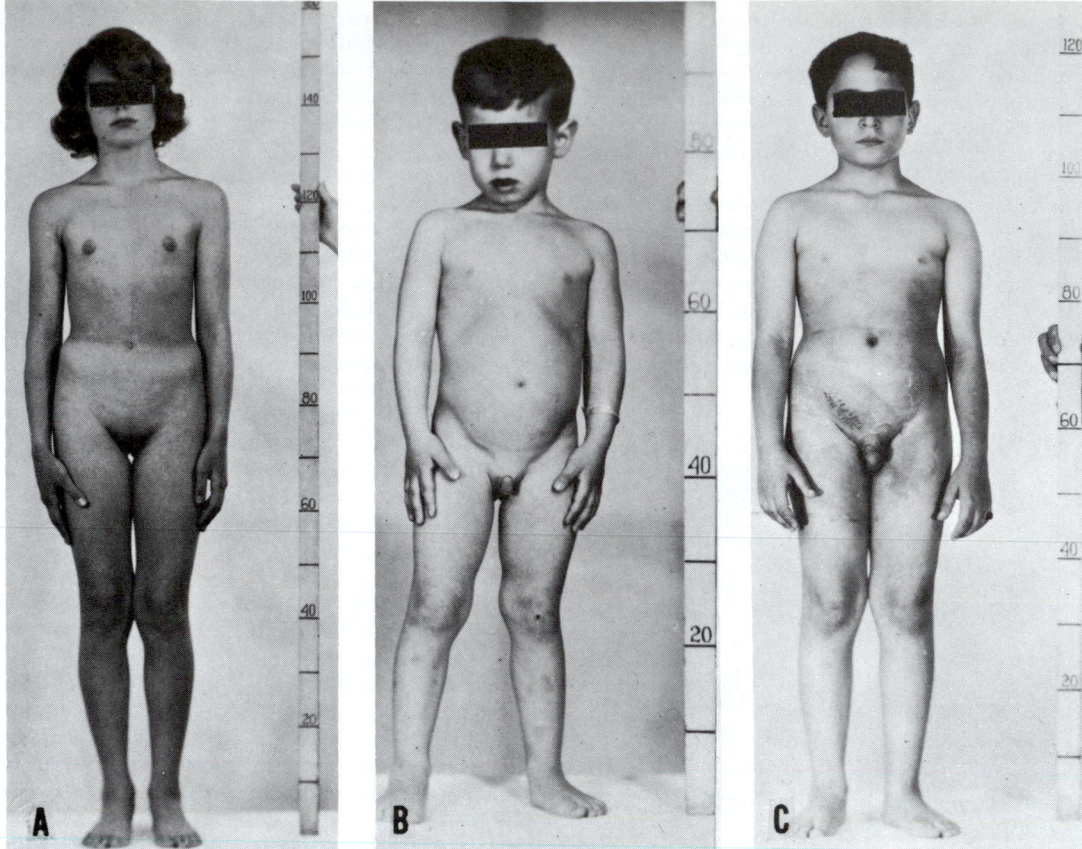

Figure 14–43. Three patients with 45,X/46,XY sex chromosome mosaicism who illustrate the highly varied phenotype in this variant of the syndrome of gonadal dysgenesis. (Numbers of the patients refer to designation in Table 14–12.) *A*, Patient 1, a phenotypic female, was 15⁴⁄₁₂ y of age. She had short stature (−3.1 SD), an increased number of pigmented nevi, puffiness over dorsum of fingers, and broad and short hands, and she was sexually infantile (breast development seen in photograph followed estrogen therapy) except for sparse pubic and axillary hair. The titer of urinary gonadotropin was greater than 80 mouse units/d. *B*, Patient 3, a 3¹⁄₁₂-y-old child, had ambiguous external genitalia, perineal hypospadias, and undescended gonads. He was of average height and had a broad chest and a duplication of the left kidney. *C*, Patient 9, an 8¹⁄₁₂-y-old phenotypic male with a penile urethra and unilateral undescended gonad, was of average height and had cubitus valgus, short fourth metacarpals, and puffiness of dorsum of fingers. By age 15, male secondary sexual characteristics were well advanced and a scrotal testis, which was normal in histological appearance, measured 4.0 × 2.4 cm.

TABLE 14–12. Genital Structures in Nine Patients with 45,X/46,XY Mosaicism

Case	External Genitalia	Urogenital Sinus	Phallus Enlargement	Gonads	Genital Ducts		
					Female		*Male*
1	Female	−	−	Rt. streak? Lt. streak?	Rt. fallopian tube? Lt. fallopian tube?	Uterus	Rt. − Lt. −
2	Ambiguous	+	+	Rt. testis Lt. streak	Rt. fallopian tube Lt. fallopian tube	Uterus	Rt. vas deferens Lt. −
3	Ambiguous	+	+	Rt. not found Lt. streak	Rt. fallopian tube Lt. fallopian tube	Uterus	Rt. − Lt. −
4	Ambiguous	+	+	Rt. dysgenetic testis Lt. dysgenetic testis	Rt. fallopian tube Lt. fallopian tube	Vestigial uterus	Rt. vas deferens Lt. −
5	Ambiguous	+	+	Rt. dysgenetic testis Lt. dysgenetic testis	Rt. fallopian tube Lt. fallopian tube	Uterus	Rt. vas deferens Lt. vas deferens
6	Ambiguous	+	+	Rt. dysgenetic testis Lt. dysgenetic testis	Rt. fallopian tube Lt. fallopian tube	Uterus	Rt. − Lt. −
7	Ambiguous	+	+	Rt. dysgenetic testis Lt. dysgenetic testis	Rt. − Lt. −		Rt. vas deferens Lt. vas deferens
8	Ambiguous	+	+	Rt. dysgenetic testis Lt. streak	Rt. fallopian tube Lt. fallopian tube	Uterus	Rt. vas deferens Lt. −
9	Male	−	Normal penis	Rt. streak Lt. testis	Rt. fallopian tube Lt. −	Vestigial uterus	Rt. − Lt. vas deferens

From Morishima A, Grumbach MM. The interrelationship of sex chromosome constitution and phenotype in the syndrome of gonadal dysgenesis and its variants. Ann NY Acad Sci 1968; 155:695–715.

normal adult male genitalia (Fig. 14–44). Plasma gonadotropin and testosterone levels both basally and in response to LHRH were within the normal range for adult men. On pelvic ultrasonography, müllerian derivatives were absent, and the testes appeared normal and homogeneous. The sperm count was 17,000,000/mL, and he demonstrated fertility both in vitro by the fertilization of hamster eggs and in vivo by the fathering of a "normal" 46,XY fetus. The finding of a short, otherwise normal fertile male with 45,X/46,XY mosaicism extends the phenotypic spectrum of this disorder.

Ascertainment bias may be responsible for the lack of well-differentiated males in reports of this disorder.[367] A review of the chromosome analyses of 58 patients in the literature ascertained because of ambiguous genitalia shows a preponderance of 45,X cells,[343] suggesting that only individuals whose abnormality occurred in the first few cell divisions are represented in this group of patients. However, 90% of the fetuses diagnosed by amniocentesis and confirmed postnatally as 45,X/46,XY mosaics have normal male genitalia.[367–369] Follow-up of these patients is limited, and hypothalamic-pituitary-gonadal function has not been characterized. However, their lack of presentation at a later date with either gonadal tumors or gonadal dysfunction suggests that, as in our patient, the majority (at least 75%) probably have normal hypothalamic-pituitary-gonadal function.

The restricted local or paracrine action of the testes on the differentiation of genital ducts is well demonstrated in patients with asymmetrical gonadal development. In such patients, development of male ducts and involution of the müllerian structures are also asymmetrical and parallel the degree of testicular development on each side. As discussed previously, local action of the testis on müllerian duct regression is mediated through AMH, whereas unilateral differentiation of male ducts is mediated by high local levels of testosterone in the wolffian ducts and their derivatives. The presence of Sertoli cells in the ipsilateral gonad correlates with the absence of müllerian structures on the same side in patients with 45,X/46,XY mosaicism.[370] This observation is consistent with the local secretion of AMH by embryonic and fetal Sertoli cells. Male differentiation of the external genitalia is, however, brought about by the systemic effects of testosterone secreted by a fetal testis. Hence, the phenotype may range from a simulant female to a completely male configuration. Although in most patients the secretion of androgenic hormones at adolescence is predictable from the degree of masculinization of the external genitalia in utero, virilization may occur at puberty in patients with a female phenotype. Breast development at or after the age of puberty occurs in about one fourth of cases and is usually associated with a gonadal neoplasm. We studied two adolescent 45,X/46,XY subjects who exhibited breast development and had pubertal levels of plasma estradiol; at laparotomy a gonadoblastoma that secreted estradiol was found (Fig. 14–45).

The propensity of patients with 45,X/46,XY mosaicism to develop gonadal tumors is high, and prophylactic removal of the streak gonads or dysgenetic undescended testes is indicated. Gonadoblastoma, a complex tumor composed of large germ cells, Sertoli cells, and stromal derivatives, is the neoplasm most often found; it can give rise to a malignant germinoma. Thus, after the removal of the gonads, serial sections should be examined for evidence of a tumor. The risk of tumor is about 20%[371] and is age related. Four 45,X/46,XY patients with incomplete virilization have been described with carcinoma in situ present in biopsies of the gonads.[372] Carcinoma in situ is though to be a premalignant lesion leading to germ cell tumors in infertile men.[372] Hence, 45,X/46,XY mosaics may have not only gonadoblastomas, roughly 30% of which are associated with germ cell tumors, but also an increased prevalence of carcinoma in situ. Thus gonadal biopsy is indicated in all individuals with a male phenotype and 45,X/46,XY mosaicism. If the testis is histologically normal and is in the scrotum or can be placed in the scrotum, it can be retained. However, careful, close follow-up is mandatory. The risk of gonadal germ cell tumors in phenotypically normal males ascertained by chance to be 45,X/46,XY mosaics has not been defined and

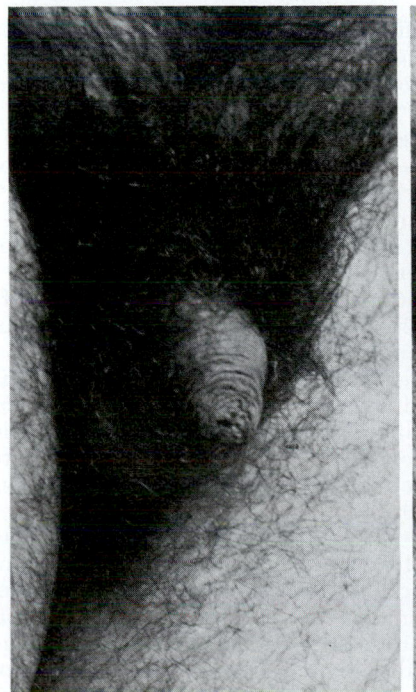
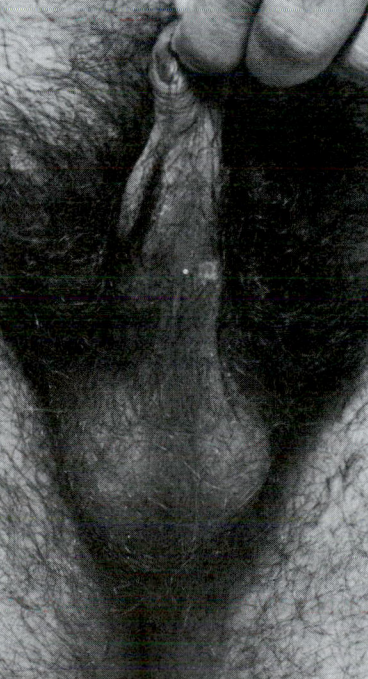

Figure 14–44. The external genitalia of a normally differentiated male with 45,X/46,XY mosaicism. Karyotype analyses revealed 16 and 68% mosaicism for a 45,X cell line in blood and skin, respectively. Gonadotropin levels, both basal and LHRH stimulated, were normal. Fertility was documented in vitro and by the conception of a normal male fetus.

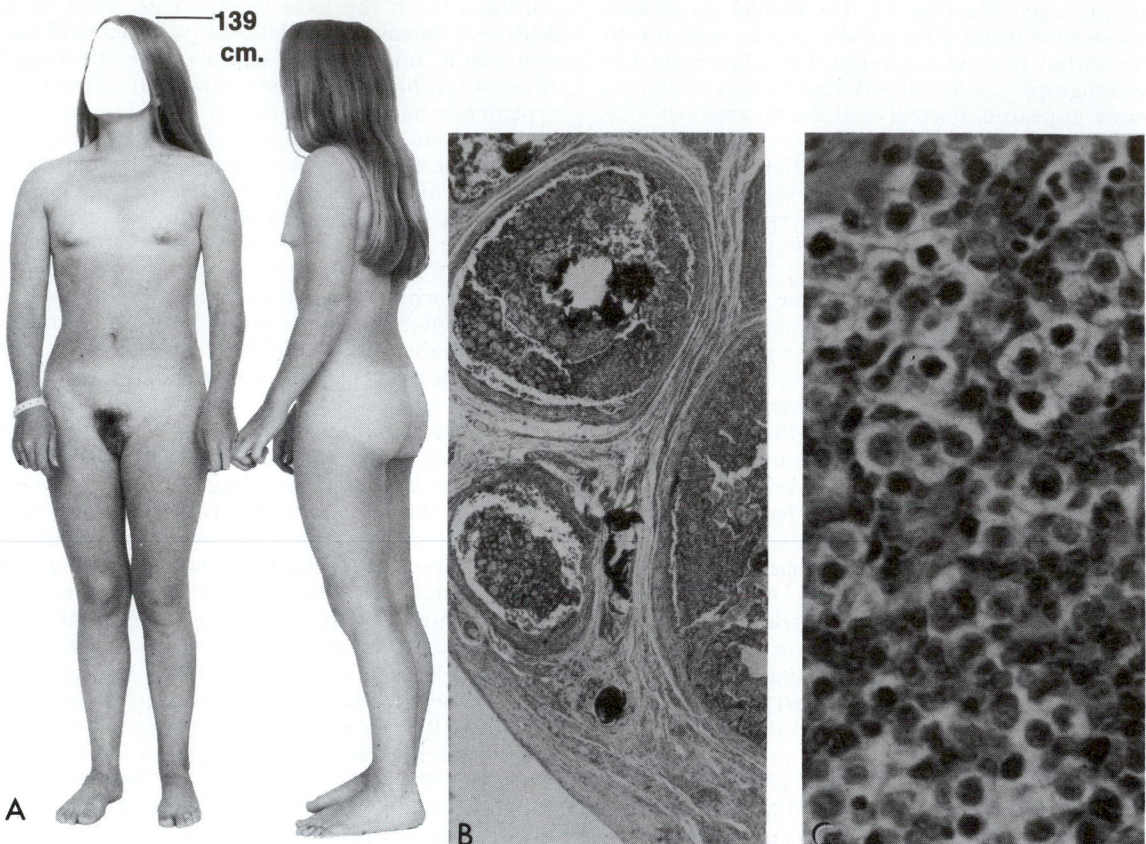

Figure 14–45. 45,X/46,XY mosaicism with a feminizing gonadoblastoma. *A*, A 20-y-old female with many stigmata of the syndrome of gonadal dysgenesis, including short stature, multiple nevi, cubitus valgus, and hyperconvex, small nails. The buccal smear was X chromatin–negative; on fluorescence microscopy, 30% of interphase nuclei had a single Y body. Karyotype was 45,X/46,XY. The patient had spontaneous development of pubic and axillary hair at age 12. At age 18, breast development was noted. Her height was 139 cm (−5.1 SD) and weight 39 kg (−2.5 SD). Bone age was 17 y; an intravenous pyelogram was normal. The concentration of plasma gonadotropins at 20 y of age was elevated; plasma LH 8 μg/L (LER-960) and FSH 50 μg/L (LER-869). A urocystogram showed a moderate estrogen effect. The concentration of plasma estradiol was 95 pmol/L (26 pg/mL) and of estrone was 117 pmol/L (32 pg/mL); plasma testosterone level was less than 0.7 nmol/L (0.2 ng/mL). On exploratory laparotomy, normal-appearing fallopian tubes and a uterus were found. The right gonad was a typical "streak," with whorls of fibrous connective tissue. *B*, The left gonad was replaced by a 1.3 × 1 × 1 cm tumor mass, which, on histological section, revealed well-defined nests and islands of Sertoli-Leydig–like cells and germ cells, as well as calcification consistent with diagnosis of gonadoblastoma. *C*, Higher magnification illustrates aggregates of germ cells and small epithelial cells resembling immature Sertoli cells, as well as cells indistinguishable from Leydig cells. After gonadectomy the concentration of plasma estradiol was prepubertal (<18 pmol/L [<5 pg/mL]).

must await further studies. Modalities such as sonography, CT, or magnetic resonance imaging (MRI) of the testes are useful noninvasive approaches to screening for gonadal neoplasms.

The presence of functional testicular elements can be detected before puberty by the rise in the concentration of serum testosterone above prepubertal values after a course of hCG (1000 to 2000 U IM, given every other day × 3).

In some patients with 45,X/46,XY or 45,X/47,XXY mosaicism the brightly fluorescent portion of the Y chromosome is absent. Caspersson and colleagues[373] noted the absence of bright fluorescence of the Y chromosome in four of seven patients. In one patient a Y-to-chromosome 2 translocation during gametogenesis was suspected. In other patients,[374, 375] no evidence of translocation or deletion of the Y was present. Fluorescence, C banding, and replication of the Y chromosome were altered compared with normal.

Magenis and Donlon[376] studied 12 structurally altered Y chromosomes with a panel of banding techniques. They concluded that the nonfluorescent Y chromosome is an isodicentric chromosome that most likely arises from a chromatid break at the heterochromatic-euchromatic junction on the long arm of the Y chromosome with sister chromatid fusion and duplication of the Y. Subsequent studies with Y-specific DNA probes have verified their interpretation but revealed variability in the break point on the Y.[377] Isodicen-

tric chromosomes are more prone to mitotic errors that result in a 45,X cell line. The relationship of nonfluorescent Y chromosomes to the risk of gonadal neoplasia is controversial.[378–380] However, in patients bearing a Y cell line who have dysgenetic gonads, gonadal extirpation is prudent. Some patients have mosaicism with a cell line containing a minute nonfluorescent chromosome fragment whose exact nature (i.e., either X or Y) is not apparent by standard chromosome banding techniques. Molecular DNA analyses should be performed in these cases to ascertain the origin of the fragment.

Mixed, asymmetrical, or atypical gonadal dysgenesis is a term that has sometimes been used to describe patients with a streak gonad on one side and a testis on the other. It is important to emphasize that, although this association is common in 45,X/46,XY mosaicism, these gonadal findings are not specific for this mosaicism and occur with a 46,XY karyotype (e.g., in familial 46,XY gonadal dysgenesis).

45,X/46,XY mosaicism probably arises mainly through anaphase lag and is frequently associated with structurally abnormal Y chromosomes.[379, 380] Thus interchromosomal rearrangements with loss of the structurally abnormal Y may be a common mechanism for the production of 45,X/46,XY mosaicism in patients who have a structurally abnormal Y chromosome.

Diagnosis and Treatment. The diagnosis is established by the demonstration of 45,X/46,XY mosaicism in blood, skin, or gonadal tissue. A Y chromosome, even one lacking the distal fluorescent portion of its long arm, can be recognized as a Y by its size, morphological appearance (parallel long arms and short, fuzzy short arms), and a segment of Giemsa 11−positive heterochromatin as well as by use of Y-specific DNA probes for the long and short arms.[354, 377] The decision as to the sex of rearing should be based on the potential for normal function of the external genitalia. In patients assigned a female gender role, the gonads should be removed and the external genitalia should be repaired by clitoral recession, vaginoplasty, and labioscrotal reduction. Estrogen therapy, initiated at the age of normal puberty, is necessary to induce female secondary sexual characteristics. In affected infants for whom a male gender assignment is selected, all gonadal tissue except that which appears functionally and histologically normal and is in the scrotum should be removed and prosthetic testes should be placed in the reconstructed scrotal sac. In these patients, removal of the müllerian duct remnants is indicated, as is repair of any hypospadias.

As discussed earlier, most 45,X/46,XY mosaic males detected by amniocentesis are born with normally differentiated male genitalia.[367–369] In these infants, it is prudent to obtain an MRI scan of the pelvis and testes to detect any müllerian structures and any inhomogeneity of the testes suggestive of dysgenesis or neoplasm. Hypothalamic-pituitary-gonadal integrity can be assessed by serial determinations of plasma gonadotropin and testosterone levels. If there is hormonal or radiological evidence of testicular dysgenesis, testicular biopsy or gonadectomy (or both) is indicated in infancy. In the absence of evidence for testicular dysgenesis, close follow-up is indicated, including a testicular biopsy at puberty to be certain of the normal structure of the testes and to ascertain malignant potential (e.g., carcinoma in situ).[372] The need for androgen replacement therapy at adolescence depends on the capacity of the testis to secrete testosterone. Because of the increased risk of neoplasm in dysgenetic testes, especially in adults, patients raised as males in whom a testis is retained must be examined regularly.

Structural Abnormalities of the Y Chromosome.[44, 379–381] Structural abnormalities of the Y chromosome that are of clinical significance are rarer than those of the X chromosome. This may be because the abnormal Y chromosome, being smaller than most structural abnormalities of the X, is more readily lost from the cell during mitosis. Some 45,X individuals may therefore occur as a consequence of a structural abnormality of the Y that is lost at an early cleavage division. Deletions of both the long and short arms of the Y chromosome, as well as rings, isochromosomes of both arms, and dicentric chromosomes, have been described, and the pseudoautosomal region of the Y chromosome with the MIC2 and GM-CSF receptor gene loci has been defined.[30, 32] Proximal to the pseudoautosomal region on the short arm of the Y chromosome are the sex-determining region and the putative sex-determining gene SRY.[34–36] Patients with deletions of the short arm of the Y lack male sex differentiation and may manifest the gonadal dysgenesis syndrome.[264, 346, 382] The findings in these patients support earlier evidence that genes responsible for the stigmata of Turner syndrome are primarily on the short arms of the X and Y chromosomes. Deletions of the long arms of the Y chromosome and, to a lesser extent, the long arms of the X chromosome do not result in these somatic stigmata.

The genes mapped to the long arm of the Y chromosome include a locus for H-Y antigen as assessed by the cytotoxic T cell assay,[42] the pseudogene for STS,[39] the gene for amelogenin,[39] and a putative locus that affects spermatogenesis.[383, 384] Page[385] has postulated that the gene for cytotoxic H-Y antigen has a role in gonadoblastoma formation in patients with dysgenetic gonads. Most patients with an isochromosome, ring, or dicentric Y chromosome are sex chromosome mosaics and have an associated 45,X cell line. The phenotypes vary from that of a normal male (depending on the presence of the sex-determining region) through individuals with ambiguous genitalia and male pseudohermaphroditism to women with infantile female external genitalia and bilateral streak gonads. The variation in phenotype is best explained by the effect of the 45,X cell line as well as the loss of genes on the Y chromosome. Several instances of apparently balanced Y-autosome translocations are known;[386] usually the distal heterochromatic region of the long arm of the Y chromosome is translocated to an autosome and male sex differentiation is normal (see Fig. 14−2).

As noted previously, Y-to-X translocations involving the sex-determining portion of the Y chromosome and a variable portion of the short arm of the X chromosome (usually the pseudoautosomal region) are found in more than 90% of XX males. Males with a 46,Y t(X:Y) karyotype have also been reported who inherited the t(X:Y) from their mothers.[387] These males have an intact Y chromosome and a deleted X chromosome. The phenotypic features are variable and correlate with the extent of the deletion of the short arm of the X chromosome. Hence, short stature, mild mental retardation, chondrodysplasia punctata, STS deficiency with ichthyosis, anosmia, and hypogonadotropic hypogonadism (Kallmann syndrome) have been variable features of this contiguous gene deletion syndrome.[39, 387] Phenotypically normal females with a 46,X t(X:Y) karyotype have been reported.[387] All females with Xp22:Yq11 translocations have been normal except for short stature. Increased fetal wastage was noted in the women with this karyotype who experienced pregnancy. In patients with Y-to-X translocation, careful cytogenetic and molecular DNA studies should be performed to define the exact break points on the X and Y chromosomes. One can assess the functional integrity of the gonads by measuring the concentration of basal as well as LHRH-evoked plasma gonadotropins and gonadal steroids. Pelvic MRI is helpful in defining the pelvic contents and gonads.

Pure Gonadal Dysgenesis

This term has been applied to phenotypic females with a 46,XX or 46,XY karotype who have rudimentary streak gonads and remain sexually infantile but are of normal or tall stature and lack the somatic stigmata of Turner syndrome. At puberty, they exhibit the usual effects of prepubertal castration and plasma and urinary gonadotropin values are increased. The X chromatin pattern may be either positive or negative. The X chromatin−negative patients occasionally have clitoral enlargement, which may be present at birth or first become manifest at puberty; clitoral enlargement is rarely present in X chromatin−positive patients. The designation *pure gonadal dysgenesis* was introduced by Harnden and Stewart in 1959 in their report of a 19-y-old phenotypic female with the described phenotype and an XY karyotype.[388] It is now known that a variety of etiological factors may lead to the development of this clinical picture. We have chosen to restrict the term pure gonadal dysgenesis to patients with XX or XY gonadal dysgenesis (see later).

FAMILIAL AND SPORADIC 46,XX GONADAL DYSGENESIS AND ITS INCOMPLETE FORMS. 46,XX gonadal dysgenesis is characterized by normal stature, sexual infantilism, bilateral streak gonads (similar in structure to those of 45,X gonadal dysgenesis), normal female internal and external genitalia, primary amenorrhea, elevated gonadotropin levels, absence of the somatic stigmata of the syndrome of gonadal dysgenesis, and a 46,XX karyotype[11, 389] (Table 14–13).

The habitus is often eunuchoid. Rare cases have had a few somatic abnormalities including cubitus valgus, but none have the typical Turner phenotype. McDonough and associates[390] reviewed the phenotypic and cytogenetic findings in 82 phenotypic female patients with primary gonadal failure. Sex chromosome anomalies were found in association with ovarian failure in 52 of 82 patients, all of whom were less than 160 cm tall. Conversely, all patients taller than 160 cm with ovarian failure had either a 46,XX or a 46,XY karyotype.[390]

Occasionally, women with clitoral enlargement, hirsutism, and other signs of virilization have serum testosterone levels above the range for normal women.[391] The streak gonads secrete testosterone, presumably from nests of hilus cells. The high concentration of gonadotropins apparently leads to hilus cell hyperplasia and a modest increase in circulating androgen levels, which, in the presence of meager estrogen production, have potent biological action.

Families may have multiple siblings affected,[11, 389] and within families the expression of the disease may vary in affected siblings. The gonads may range from bilateral streak gonads to hypoplastic ovaries with varying degrees of ovarian function. In the familial cases transmission is consistent with an autosomal recessive trait. Autosomal recessive 46,XX gonadal dysgenesis provides evidence that a mutant gene on a pair of autosomes can lead to a profound disturbance of ovarian differentiation and that an autosomal gene has an important role in the differentiation of normal ovaries. The abnormal gonadogenesis may be the consequence of the effect of a mutant gene on germ cell migration, the gonadal blastema, the rate of germ cell attrition, or a defect in the putative ovary-organizing factor or its receptor. In support of the heterogeneous nature of this syndrome, we studied a kinship in which a consanguineous mating resulted in two phenotypic female siblings, one of whom had 46,XX gonadal dysgenesis and the other 46,XY gonadal dysgenesis.

Familial 46,XX gonadal dysgenesis has been associated with sensorineural deafness.[11, 392] Genetic heterogeneity is suggested by concordance of the gonadal defect with deaf-mutism in these families and by other families in which short stature, 46,XX gonadal dysgenesis, microcephaly, and arachnodactyly occurred in affected siblings.[11] Hamet and colleagues[393] described three sisters with renal failure, adrenal hyperplasia, hypertension, sensorineural deafness, and primary hypogonadism. A kindred with cerebellar ataxia and hypergonadotropic hypogonadism and a family with mental retardation, streak gonads, myopathy, and various neurological abnormalities have been described.[394]

Sporadic cases of 46,XX gonadal dysgenesis may also

be heterogenous. For example, ovarian hypoplasia has been associated with aneuploidy, especially trisomy-13 and trisomy-18. Patients with 46,XX gonadal dysgenesis should be distinguished from those with ovarian failure secondary to infection, such as mumps in childhood or autoimmune oophoritis, and from patients with antibodies to gonadotropin receptors, biologically inactive FSH, gonadotropin-insensitive ovaries, galactosemia, or biosynthetic errors that affect estrogen formation (e.g., 17α-hydroxylase and/or 17,20-lyase deficiency [$P-450_{c17}$]).

In contrast to 46,XY gonadal dysgenesis, gonadal neoplasms are rare in 46,XX gonadal dysgenesis. The diagnosis of 46,XX gonadal dysgenesis is based on finding a normal karyotype in a sexually infantile phenotypic female with hypergonadotropic hypogonadism. In sporadic cases, it is important to confirm the presence of streak or hypoplastic gonads by sonography, pelvic MRI, or laparoscopy. Replacement therapy with estrogen is similar to that for patients with 45,X gonadal dysgenesis.

FAMILIAL AND SPORADIC 46,XY GONADAL DYSGENESIS AND ITS INCOMPLETE FORMS. 46,XY gonadal dysgenesis was first described by Swyer.[395] This syndrome in its complete form is characterized by a female phenotype, normal to tall stature, bilateral dysgenetic gonads, sexual infantilism with primary amenorrhea, eunuchoid habitus, and a 46,XY karyotype (Table 14–14). Somatic features of Turner syndrome are usually absent. The internal structures are female with bilateral tubes, a uterus, and a vagina. Clitoral enlargement is not uncommon, and the prevalence of gonadal neoplasms, especially gonadoblastoma and germinoma (seminoma, dysgerminoma), is high. In patients with the incomplete or variant form, both the internal and external genitalia may be ambiguous. Breast development after the normal age of puberty suggests the presence of an estrogen-secreting gonadal tumor, especially a gonadoblastoma.[396] Plasma and urinary gonadotropin levels are increased. In some patients the concentration of serum testosterone is higher than in adult women, presumably because of the secretion of androgens from the hilus cells of the streak gonads. A male proportion of single fluorescent Y bodies is present in interphase nuclei. In one case the Y chromosome was nonfluorescent.[397] Excluded from this syndrome are patients with variants of the syndrome of gonadal dysgenesis, such as 45,X/46,XY mosaicism and those with microscopically visible structural abnormalities of the Y chromosome.

Familial aggregates as well as sporadic cases have been described.[11, 13, 398–400] In an extensive review, Simpson[399] supported the view that 46,XY gonadal dysgenesis is a heterogeneous condition that is inherited as either an X-linked recessive or male-limited autosomal dominant trait. We obtained evidence of an autosomal recessive form. Familial

TABLE 14–13. 46,XX Gonadal Dysgenesis and Variant Form

Parameter	Complete Syndrome	Incomplete Form
Karyotype	46,XX	
Inheritance	Autosomal recessive in familial cases (sensorineural deafness in about 10%)	
Genitalia	Normal female	
Wolffian duct derivatives	Absent	
Müllerian duct derivatives	Normal female	
Gonads	Bilateral streak gonads	Hypoplastic ovary and streak or bilateral hypoplastic ovaries
Habitus	Normal stature, no somatic stigmata of Turner syndrome	
	Sexual infantilism	Incomplete puberty, premature ovarian failure
Hormone profile	↑ plasma FSH and LH concentration	Plasma estradiol variable: decreased or normal

TABLE 14–14. Salient Features of 46,XY Gonadal Dysgenesis and Variant Form

	Complete Syndrome	Incomplete Form
Karyotype	46,XY	
Inheritance	Familial cases consistent with X linked (or male-limited autosomal dominant)	
Genitalia	Female	Ambiguous
Wolffian duct derivatives	Absent	Rudimentary → hypoplastic
Müllerian duct derivatives	Normal	Variable, rudimentary → hypoplastic
Gonads	Bilateral streak gonads	Bilateral dysgenetic testes or streak gonad + dysgenetic testes (mixed gonadal dysgenesis)
	↑ risk of gonadal tumor, gonadoblastoma	
Habitus	Sexual infantilism at puberty	Variable degree of virilization at puberty
	Breast development suggests presence of gonadal tumor	
Hormone profile	↑ plasma FSH and LH and ↓ testosterone concentrations postpubertally	
	10% have deletion of TDF region of the Y chromosome; point mutation in SRY gene	

cases may vary in the appearance of the external genitalia and the development of secondary sexual characteristics. Usually the external and internal genital tracts are female and the patient is sexually infantile (complete form); however, affected siblings may have ambiguous external genitalia and ambiguous genital ducts and urogenital sinus (incomplete or variant form). The spectrum of genital ambiguity suggests variable expression of the mutant gene. In a family reported by Chemke and colleagues,[400] two siblings had 46,XY gonadal dysgenesis with bilateral streak gonads and another had the incomplete form with genital ambiguity, bilateral dysgenetic testes, and müllerian derivatives. We studied the infant born to the "normal" 46,XX sister of the Chemke propositi. This 46,XY patient had ambiguous external genitalia, bilateral dysgenetic testes, and müllerian derivatives. Inheritance in this family is consistent with an X-linked recessive or a male-limited autosomal dominant trait. Similar families have been described.[398]

Several authors who performed Y-DNA hybridization studies reported submicroscopic deletions of the sex-determining region of the short arm of the Y chromosome in approximately 10% of sporadic patients with 46,XY gonadal dysgenesis.[264, 266, 401] In general, these patients have had some of the phenotypic stigmata of Turner syndrome, except for short stature. One 46,XY patient was found to have a point mutation in the putative DNA binding region of the protein coded for by the SRY gene as noted earlier.[96a] Another had a four-nucleotide deletion resulting in a nonfunctional protein.[96b] Furthermore, four 46,XY females have been described with a duplication of an Xp segment that included the ZFX locus.[402, 403]

Of note is the association of 46,XY gonadal dysgenesis with camptomelic dwarfism, a heterogeneous, autosomal recessive form of lethal dwarfism.[404] Dysgenetic gonads resembling ovaries have been reported in affected 46,XY patients. Camptomelic dwarfism is thought to be inherited as an autosomal recessive trait. Its association with 46,XY gonadal dysgenesis suggests an autosomal mutation affecting sex determination in this syndrome. No abnormality has been noted in the gonads of 46,XX females with camptomelic dwarfism. 46,XY gonadal dysgenesis has also been associated with multiple congenital anomalies (genitopalatocardiac syndrome),[399] with Smith-Lemli-Opitz syndrome,[405] and with renal parenchymal disorders, some of which have resulted in chronic renal failure.[406, 407]

Like some 45,X patients, subjects with 46,XY gonadal dysgenesis have been reported to have follicles in the dysgenetic gonads. Cussen and MacMahon[408] described germ cells and follicles in the underdeveloped gonads of a 3-mo-old 46,XY female. Subsequent examination at age 3¹⁰/₁₂ revealed bilateral streak gonads with a gonadoblastoma in one gonad.[408] The persistence of follicles and their function at puberty have been reported in a 46,XY, serological H-Y antigen–positive phenotypic female who underwent spontaneous puberty and experienced menarche.[409] Examination of the gonads after development of secondary amenorrhea revealed only gonadal stroma and a few hilus cells.

In sum, 46,XY gonadal dysgenesis is a heterogeneous syndrome. Deletions and/or mutations involving the Y chromosome,[401] the X chromosome,[402, 403] and downstream autosomal genes involved in the testes-determining cascade have all been implicated.

There is a high prevalence of gonadal tumors, especially gonadoblastoma and germinoma, in this syndrome, and they can occur bilaterally in childhood. Bilateral prophylactic gonadectomy is indicated when the diagnosis is established.

The sex of rearing of patients with the incomplete form of 46,XY gonadal dysgenesis is determined by the extent of genital ambiguity and the age at diagnosis. Patients raised as females should be placed on estrogen replacement therapy at age 12 to 13 y and eventually be cycled monthly with estrogen and progestogen. In patients raised as males, testosterone replacement therapy is begun at the age of puberty.

"MALE TURNER SYNDROME." Many phenotypic males have been reported with short stature, webbed neck, and other somatic abnormalities associated with the syndrome of gonadal dysgenesis in whom the testes were hypoplastic and frequently undescended. The resemblance of these males to phenotypic females with 45,X gonadal dysgenesis suggested a pathogenetic parallelism or Turner syndrome in the male. However, with rare exceptions, this interrelationship is no longer tenable. A few patients with the phenotypic features of male Turner syndrome have had a sex chromosome abnormality, such as 45,X/46,XY mosaicism, and represent a variant form of Turner syndrome. In all the other karyotypic studies of these patients, the sex chromosome constitution is 46,XY. The 46,XY cases form a heterogeneous clinical group in which there may be multiple causes. Unless partial sex chromosome monosomy can be demonstrated, these patients ought not to be considered as the clinical parallel in the male of Turner syndrome. Many of the cases previously categorized as "male Turner syndrome" are examples of the syndrome of webbed neck, ptosis, hypogonadism, and short stature usually associated with congenital heart disease and mental retardation.[239]

Syndrome of Webbed Neck, Ptosis, Hypogonadism, Congenital Heart Disease, and Short Stature (46,XX and 46,XY Turner Phenotype, Pseudo-Turner Syndrome, Noonan Syndrome, Ullrich Syndrome)

Among the group of phenotypic males previously classified as having male Turner syndrome, a distinctive clinical entity was identified that led to the identification of its counterpart in the female and its distinction from the syndrome of gonadal dysgenesis.[239, 410–412] Various eponyms have been applied to this syndrome, but we prefer to exclude Turner from the designation. It is of interest that in 1938, the year Turner's paper appeared, Bizarro reported a phenotypic female with the features of this "pseudo-Turner" syndrome. Table 14–15 lists the clinical features of 2 phenotypic males and 12 phenotypic females with this entity studied by us. These patients have a characteristic facies and, frequently, a webbed neck and short stature (Fig. 14–46); in 12 of the 14 cases, congenital heart disease was present. The most common cardiac malformations have been pulmonic stenosis (approximately 50%) or atrial septal defect, or both; ventricular septal defect, patent ductus arteriosus, and ventricular hypertrophy also have been found. Coarctation of the aorta and aortic stenosis, the most common cardiovascular anomalies in the syndrome of gonadal dysgenesis, are infrequent. Pectus excavatum, cubitus valgus, and impaired mental development are often present, and lymphedema occurs in 15% of patients.[413] The chromosome constitution is normal, and gonadal differentiation is appropriate for the phenotypic and chromosomal sex. In males, cryptorchidism is common, and the testes may be hypoplastic and exhibit germinal aplasia. Androgen deficiency is not uncommon at puberty. However, some affected males have normal testicular function, including fertility. At present, we prefer to limit this diagnosis to patients with four or more of the cardinal features of the syndrome and a normal chromosome constitution. The females have functioning ovaries and, although the onset of puberty may be delayed, female secondary sexual characteristics eventually emerge.

Most cases are sporadic. Familial clusters are consistent with autosomal dominant inheritance.[413, 414] The abnormality of gonadal function and the higher incidence of congenital heart disease in males may play a part in the apparently higher maternal transmission of the mutant gene. However, we and others have studied familial cases transmitted through an affected male.

The diagnosis is based on the constellation of stigmata, the most prominent of which are short stature, webbed neck, ptosis, and right-sided congenital heart disease in a patient with a normal sex chromosome constitution. The differential diagnosis of this syndrome is extensive and includes structural abnormalities of the Y chromosome, especially those involving the short arm, 45,X/46,XY mosaicism, and dysmorphic syndromes secondary to hydantoin, primidone, and alcohol exposure during gestation.[239] At puberty, affected males may require testosterone replacement therapy.

True Hermaphroditism

The diagnosis of true hermaphroditism requires the presence of both ovarian and testicular tissue in either the same or opposite gonads.[415–417] Failure to adhere to this definition has led to considerable confusion. Gonadal stroma arranged in whorls, similar to those found in the ovary but lacking oocytes, should not be considered as sufficient evidence to designate the rudimentary gonad as an ovary. Similarly, when testicular tissue is present in the contralateral gonad, the presence of a few oocytes in a streak gonad is not considered by the authors to be adequate evidence for

TABLE 14–15. Summary of Clinical Findings in 14 Patients with the Syndrome of Webbed Neck, Ptosis, Hypogonadism, Congenital Heart Disease, and Short Stature

Clinical Characteristics	Males	Females	Clinical Characteristics	Males	Females
Short stature (>2 SD below mean)	2/2	8/12	Both PS and ASD	2/2	3/10
			Patent ductus arteriosus (PDA)	0/2	2/10
Typical facies	2/2	12/12	Undiagnosed heart disease	0/2	2/10
Triangular shape of face	2/2	7/12	Incompletely evaluated	0/2	2/12
Prominent brow	2/2	12/12			
Hypertelorism	2/2	12/12	Extremities		
Epicanthus	2/2	9/12	Cubitus valgus	2/2	9/12
Antimongoloid palpebral slant	2/2	10/12	Gracile fingers	1/2	8/12
Ptosis	2/2	12/12	Short stubby fingers	1/2	2/12
Depressed nasal bridge	1/2	2/12	Lymphedema	0/2	3/12
Broad apex nasi	2/2	11/12	Dystrophic nails	2/2	2/12
			Shortened fourth metacarpal(s)	0/2	3/12
Low-set and/or malformed ears	2/2	8/12	Clinodactyly of fifth finger(s)	1/2	2/12
			Palmar simian crease	1/2	1/12
High-arched palate	2/2	8/12			
			Undescended testes	2/2	—
Neck					
Short	2/2	10/12	Delayed puberty	1/1	3/3
Webbing	2/2	10/12			
Low hairlilne	2/2	10/12	Skeletal retardation	2/2	8/10
Chest			Mental development		
Shield-like	1/2	11/12	Retarded	2/2	4/12
Wide-spaced nipples	2/2	11/11	Borderline	0/2	5/12
Pectus excavatum	2/2	5/12	Normal	0/2	3/12
Cardiac abnormalities	2/2	11/12	Intrauterine growth retardation	1/2	4/12
Pulmonic stenosis (PS)	2/2	5/10			
PS and ventricular septal defect	0/2	1/10	Renal collecting system		
Atrial septal defect (ASD)	2/2	6/10	Normal	2/2	7/8
ASD with anomalous pulmonary venous return	0/2	1/10	Abnormal	0/2	1/8
Endocardial cushion defect (ECD)	0/2	2/10	Normal karyotype	2/2	12/12
ECD + patent ductus arteriosus and mitral insufficiency	0/2	1/10			

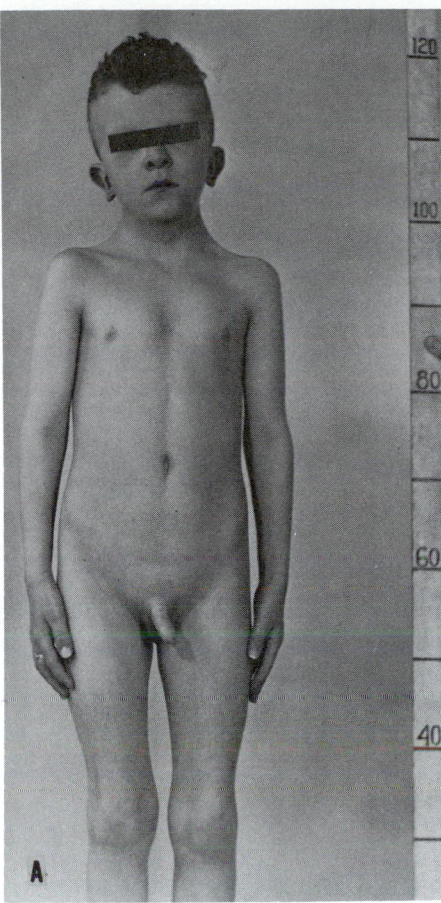
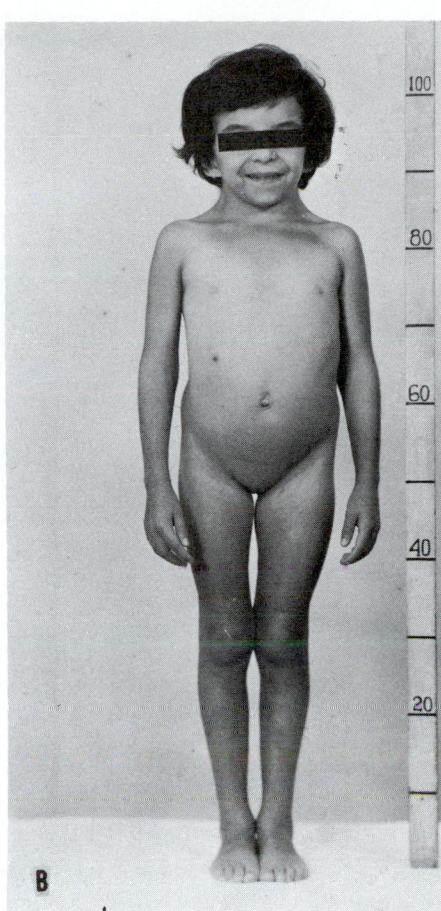

Figure 14–46. A phenotypic male and female with syndrome of webbed neck, ptosis, congenital heart disease, short stature, and hypogonadism (pseudo-Turner syndrome: Noonan syndrome). *A,* A 9⁷/₁₂-y-old boy who exhibited characteristic abnormalities: triangular facies, prominent brow, hypertelorism, ptosis, antimongoloid slant of palpebral fissures, broad apex nasi, low-set ears, webbed neck, pectus excavatum, pulmonic stenosis and atrial septal defect, short stature (−3.5 SD), bilateral undescended testes, and high-grade mental retardation. At age 18, he was 154.0 cm in height (height age 12⁵/₁₂ y); the boy had Leydig cell hypofunction. Biopsy of testes showed germinal aplasia. (From Grumbach MM, Barr ML. Cytologic tests of chromosomal sex in relation to sexual anomalies in man. Recent Prog Horm Res 1958; 14:255–334.) *B,* An 8-y-old girl with similar features. Height was 106.2 cm (height age 4⁴/₁₂ y). Pulmonic stenosis was present. 46,XX karyotype.

the diagnosis of true hermaphroditism. Because rare female-type germ cells may be found in patients with 45,X gonadal dysgenesis, it seems of little value from the clinical, cytogenetic, embryological, or nosological standpoint to classify as true hermaphrodites the 45,X/46,XY mosaics in whom a dysgenetic gonad contains rare oocytes. Similarly, the status of the internal and external genitalia, which invariably exhibit some degree of ambisexual development, should not be used as a criterion for classifying an individual as a true hermaphrodite.

CLASSIFICATION. True hermaphroditism is uncommon but has been reported in more than 350 patients.[417] Patients with this syndrome may be subclassified according to the type and location of the gonads.

Lateral. The arrangement of a testis on one side and an ovary on the other occurs in about 30% of patients. The ovary is found frequently on the left side.

Bilateral. Testicular and ovarian tissue are present bilaterally, usually as ovotestes; this disposition occurs in about 20% of patients.

Unilateral. Testicular and ovarian tissue on one side and a testis or ovary on the other occurs in slightly less than one half of cases. A testis or ovotestis may be situated along the normal pathway of descent of a testis, but an ovary is almost invariably in its normal position.

CLINICAL FEATURES. The differentiation of the genital tract and the development of secondary sexual characteristics are highly variable (Table 14–16; Fig. 14–47). The external genitalia may simulate those of either a male or a female, often they are ambiguous, and three fourths of the patients are reared as males because of the size of the phallus.[417] Almost all have hypospadias, which varies in extent from perineal to penile, with incomplete fusion of the labioscrotal

folds. In rare cases a penile urethra is present. Cryptorchidism is common, and an inguinal hernia, which may contain a gonad or uterus, is present in about one half of the cases. In virtually all cases a uterus is present. The differentiation of the genital ducts usually follows that of the gonads. The ovotestis is the most common gonad in true hermaphrodites, followed by the ovary and, least commonly, the testis.[418–421] In patients with a testis on one side and an ovary on the other, the development of the homolateral duct is usually consistent with that of the gonad, despite the varied appearance of the external genitalia. Most patients with an ovotestis have predominantly female development of the genital ducts. The relationship between gonadal structure and differentiation of the genital tract in true hermaphroditism provides added evidence for the essentially local effect of AMH secreted by the Sertoli cells of the embryonic and fetal testes.

TABLE 14–16. True Hermaphroditism

Karyotype: 46,XX (most common), 46,XX/46,XY, or 46,XY (rare)

Inheritance: Familial cases (autosomal recessive, autosomal dominant transmission) rare

Genitalia: Ambiguous; cryptorchidism frequent; ovotestis possibly located in labioscrotal fold

Wolffian duct derivatives:	Duct differentiation after that of the
Müllerian duct derivatives:	homolateral gonad

Gonad: Testis, ovary, or ovotestis

Habitus: Breast development and virilization common at puberty

Molecular studies: two of eight 46,XX cases exhibited hybridization to DNA probes for pseudoautosomal boundary region of the Y chromosome (SRY)

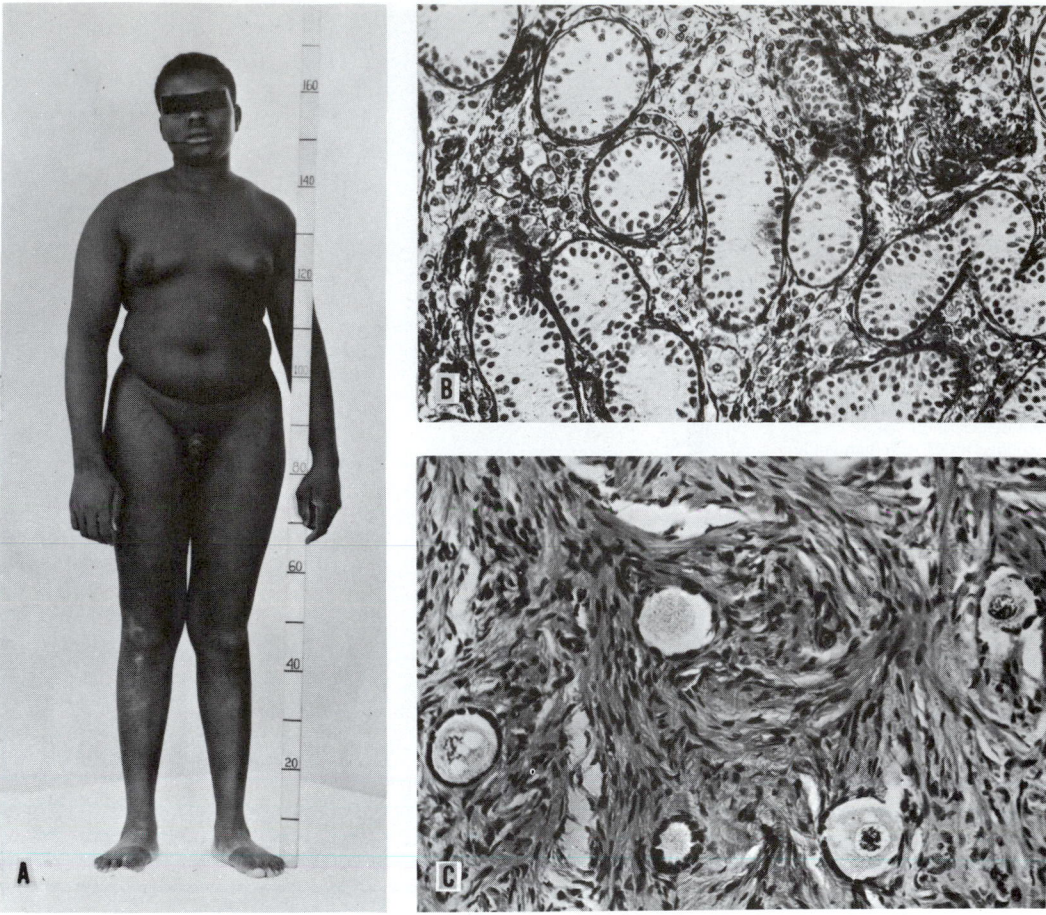

Figure 14–47. *A*, A 17-y-old true hermaphrodite with bilateral scrotal ovotestes and a 46,XX sex chromosome constitution in cultures of peripheral blood and skin, perineal hypospadias (partially repaired in photograph), moderate bilateral gynecomastia and pubic hair (recently shaved in picture), sparse axillary hair, a high-pitched voice, and absent facial hair. Height was 168 cm. Urinary 17-ketosteroid level was 1.3 mg/d; urinary gonadotropin levels were between 10 and 80 mouse units/d. A male type of urethra, bilateral scrotal fallopian tubes and ovotestes, and rudimentary bicornuate uterus and vagina attached to the posterior urethra were seen at operation. The photomicrographs show histopathology of demarcated ovarian and testicular portion of one ovotestis: *B*, immature seminiferous tubules lined with Sertoli cells and spermatogonia and Leydig cells; *C*, ova and follicles. (From Grumbach MM, Barr ML. Cytologic tests of chromosomal sex in relation to sexual anomalies in man. Recent Prog Horm Res 1958; 14:255–334.)

Breast development is frequent during puberty in true hermaphrodites, and menses occur in more than half of the patients. Periodic hematuria associated with menstruation is a late clue to the diagnosis. Spermatogenesis is rare, but ovulation is not uncommon, and pregnancy and childbirth have been reported for patients with a 46,XX karyotype.[420, 422]

Few studies of hypothalamic-pituitary-gonadal function have been carried out in true hermaphrodites. Whereas an ovary or ovarian portion of an ovotestis may function normally, with rare exceptions the testis or testicular portion of the ovotestis is abnormal.[423] A cyclic pattern of FSH and LH secretion similar to that in normal women can occur.[424] As in other men with gynecomastia, a low testosterone/estradiol ratio plays a role in the breast development that is seen frequently in postpubertal true hermaphrodites.[425]

CHROMOSOMAL FINDINGS. About 70% of true hermaphrodites are X chromatin–positive. Van Niekerk and Retief[418] analyzed the cytogenetic findings in 195 patients; 116 (60%) were 46,XX, 24 (12%) had a 46,XY karyotype, 25 (13%) were 46,XX/46,XY chimeras, and the remainder were sex chromosome mosaics.[418]

ORIGINS OF TRUE HERMAPHRODITISM. True hermaphroditism could result from sex chromosome mosaicism (apparent or cryptic), chimerism, Y-to-autosome or Y-to-X chromosome translocation,[34, 425a] or mutation of either X-linked or autosomal genes involved in sex differentiation. Studies using the ZFY probe fail to support Y-to-autosome or Y-to-X chromosome translocations in patients with true hermaphroditism.[421] However, Palmer and co-workers[34] described a "true hermaphrodite" whose sibling was a 46,XX male.[426] In this patient, a Y-to-X translocation was found involving the SRY gene. Jäger and co-workers[425a] reanalyzed seven 46,XX true hermaphrodites previously reported to be ZFY-negative. One of the seven was positive for sequences next to the Y-pseudoautosomal boundary. Thus two of eight true hermaphrodites studied with probes of Y DNA distal to ZFY have had evidence of a Y-to-X translocation.

Sex chromosome mosaicism arises from mitotic or meiotic errors. 46,XX/46,XY chimerism is usually a consequence of double fertilization or possibly fusion of two normally fertilized ova.[24, 427] Chimeric individuals have two distinct populations of cells, each of which has a different genetic origin. Study of 46,XX/46,XY chimeras provides evidence for the fertilization of a binucleate ovum by two sperms, one bearing an X and the other a Y.[428, 429] All patients with whole body chimerism do not have true hermaphroditism. One 46,XX/46,XY patient was a phenotypic male without true hermaphroditism; a likely mechanism for the chimerism in this case, based on the blood group studies and other findings, is fusion of two zygotes or fertilization of an ovum and its polar body. The experiments of

Tarkowski[430] using XX and XY blastocytes demonstrate that random fusion of two blastocytes *seldom* produces 46,XX/46,XY true hermaphroditism. Fused mouse blastocysts usually result in testicular organogenesis rather than development of ovaries or ovotestes. The presence of true 46,XX hermaphroditism in kindreds,[421, 424, 431–435] especially when the kindred includes 46,XX males,[34, 266a] suggests a common pathogenetic mechanism, either Y-to-X translocation or mutation of an X-linked or autosomal gene involved in sex determination. As previously noted, Y-DNA–negative 46,XX males have a high incidence of ambiguous genitalia and are phenotypically more similar to true hermaphrodites than are 46,XX males positive for Y DNA.[245a]

DIAGNOSIS AND THERAPY. The diagnosis of true hermaphroditism should be considered in all patients with ambiguous genitalia. A 46,XX/46,XY karyotype in a patient with ambiguous external genitalia strongly suggests the diagnosis; a 46,XX or 46,XY karyotype does not exclude the diagnosis. The finding of a gonad in the labioscrotal fold (especially on the right side) with a lobulated bipolar consistency compatible with an ovotestis is suggestive. If all other forms of pseudohermaphroditism have been ruled out, the diagnosis of true hermaphroditism should be confirmed by the histological demonstration of both ovarian and testicular tissues.

The management is contingent on the age at diagnosis and a careful assessment of the functional capacity of the internal and external genitalia. In infants in whom gender identity has not already been established, either a male or female assignment of sex can be made. If a male gender role is assigned, all müllerian and ovarian structures should be removed. The testis or testicular component of an ovotestis is usually dysgenetic, and the risk of malignant transformation is increased. Thus in 46,XX true hermaphrodites raised as males we recommend gonadectomy, the insertion of prosthetic testes, and hormone replacement at puberty. However, in 46,XX/46,XY chimeras and 46,XY true hermaphrodites, especially when a testis is present on one side and an ovary on the other and the size of the phallus is adequate, the possibility should be weighed of retaining a histologically normal-appearing testis in the scrotum and raising the patient as a male, even though the risk of malignancy may be increased. In true hermaphrodites reared as females, all testicular tissue should be removed. Normal ovarian function and, in rare instances, pregnancy have been reported in true hermaphrodites, usually of the 46,XX variety; however, it is not known whether the risk of neoplastic transformation is increased in the retained ovarian tissue in these patients.[420, 436] In older subjects gender identity is the major consideration; usually it conforms to the sex of rearing. The discordant gonad and dysgenetic gonadal tissue should be removed, and plastic repair of the external genitalia should be carried out. Appropriate gonadal hormone replacement therapy is recommended at the age of puberty.

Sex Chromosome Abnormalities Unassociated with Gonadal Defects

Five sex chromosome abnormalities are not accompanied by a typical gonadal defect but are frequently associated with mental retardation.

47,XXX. This common chromosome abnormality has the frequency of about 1 per 1000 newborn female infants.[222] The prevalence of 47,XXX individuals in institutions for the mentally retarded is 4.3 per 1000,[437] suggesting a slightly increased risk for mental retardation. Although some have delayed menarche or premature ovarian failure, most 47,XXX females have normal ovarian function. 47,XXX females can rarely give birth to 47,XXY sons. The incidence of congenital malformations is increased in the progeny of 47,XXX women.[438] Subtle clinical features in infants ascertained by karyotype analysis in the neonatal period included the following: a tendency to low birth weight, advanced mean parental age, an increased incidence of clinodactyly, normal postnatal growth patterns, an increased risk of speech and language problems, and a lower mean I.Q. than the siblings or a control group.[202, 204]

The diagnosis of 47,XXX can be confirmed by the finding of two sex chromatin bodies in interphase cells and by the demonstration of a 47,XXX karyotype by the use of appropriate banding techniques. Because of the increased risk in the offspring of a sex chromosome abnormality (47,XXY and 47,XXX) and congenital malformations, prenatal counseling and amniocentesis should be considered in 47,XXX females who become pregnant.

48,XXXX. This is a rare anomaly,[439, 440] and considerable phenotype heterogeneity exists among tetra-X individuals, making identification by clinical means difficult. The most constant feature is a variable degree of mental retardation affecting speech.[440] Ovarian function is usually normal.[440] The diagnosis is suggested by finding three sex chromatin bodies in 6 to 9% of somatic nuclei and is confirmed by karyotype analysis.

49,XXXXX.[11, 441–443] The penta-X syndrome occurs rarely. Severe prenatal and postnatal growth delay and mental retardation are invariable. Other somatic stigmata include hypertelorism, epicanthal folds, upslanted palpebral fissures, depressed nasal bridge, abnormal dentition, short neck, congenital heart disease, clinodactyly, and overlapping toes. The external genitalia are usually normal, and gonadal function is normal in some patients.[438] A proportion of interphase nuclei contain four X chromatin bodies.

47,XYY. The first subject reported by Sandberg and associates[444] was an essentially normal fertile man of average intelligence who was detected only because he had a daughter with Down syndrome. However, surveys in penal institutions suggested an increase in prevalence of this anomaly, especially in tall prisoners, and gave rise to an undeserved stereotype that has been modified by later studies.[445, 446] Among 43 XYY boys 1 to 12 y of age, ascertained by routine karyotype analysis in the newborn period, no clear-cut 47,XYY syndrome emerged in childhood.[202] No major deviations were evident that could be attributed to an extra Y chromosome, with the possible exception of a skew to the left in I.Q. scores. 47,XYY individuals have a 1% risk of exhibiting criminal behavior, as opposed to a 0.1% risk in 46,XY males.[11] 47,XYY is a common sex chromosome abnormality, occurring in 1 per 1000 male births. Among the features are tall stature, antisocial behavior, nodulocystic acne, and skeletal anomalies such as radioulnar synostosis. These individuals rarely show any abnormality in sexual development. A few reports have described hypospadias in 47,XYY patients, but this may be coincidental. The diagnosis should be suspected in tall males with nodulocystic acne who exhibit antisocial behavior and can be confirmed by demonstrating two fluorescent Y bodies in somatic interphase nuclei stained with Q or by karyotype analysis.

48,XYYY. The reported subjects with this rare karyotype have had multiple somatic abnormalities and mental retardation.[447] The diagnosis is based on finding three fluorescent Y bodies in interphase nuclei or on karyotype analysis.

Gonadal Neoplasms in Dysgenetic Gonads

The prevalence of gonadal neoplasms is increased in patients with certain types of dysgenetic gonads, in particular all those with a Y-bearing cell line.[448–454] Germinoma (dysgerminoma, seminoma), teratoma, and gonadoblastoma have been found. Cryptorchid testes, even when not associated with intersexuality, are also associated with an increased risk of malignancy. The probability that cryptorchid testes will undergo malignant degeneration is difficult to assess but is many times greater than the probability for normally descended testes.[453, 454] Approximately 7% of males with testicular neoplasms have been or are, at the time of diagnosis, cryptorchid.[454] In addition, in 33% of patients with cryptorchidism who developed carcinoma of the testis, the neoplasm occurred after orchiopexy; in patients with unilateral cryptorchidism, 25% of tumors were located in the contralateral descended testes.[453, 454] The management of cryptorchid testes has been extensively reviewed.[455]

Gonadal neoplasms are uncommon in patients with 47,XXY seminiferous tubule dysgenesis, but a small number of patients have gonadal or extragonadal germ cell tumors.[220, 454, 456] Similarly, gonadal tumors are rare in the streak gonads of 45,X patients and in 45,X mosaics with a normal or structurally abnormal X chromosome in the second cell line. Gonadoblastoma and dysgerminoma,[454, 457–459] mucinous cystadenoma,[460] and a hilus cell tumor with signs of virilization have been reported in gonadal dysgenesis.[461]

Gonadoblastomas are usually composed of three elements—large germ cells, sex cord derivatives (Sertoli-granulosa cells), and stromal elements (theca cells, Leydig cells). They are found almost exclusively in patients who have a 46,XY cell line. They may be microscopic or large, especially if overgrown by other germ cell elements, and often are calcified. A comprehensive review of gonadoblastoma has been published by Scully[452] (see Fig. 14–45). In 27 of 74 patients, a tumor was present in both gonads. Thirty patients were younger than age 15 when the tumor was diagnosed, and 10 were younger than age 10. A third of these tumors were detected incidentally on histological examination of dysgenetic gonads removed for other indications. In patients in whom chromosomal studies had been carried out, the predominant karyotypes were 45,X/46,XY and 46,XY. Although 80% of patients are reared as females, most displayed some degree of clitorimegaly or hirsutism; rarely, the tumors secrete enough estrogen to induce breast development (see Fig. 14–45). Pure gonadoblastomas can be regarded as germ cell tumors in situ and as such do not metastasize.[453] In half the cases, however, the germ cells infiltrate the stroma of the tumor to form a dysgerminoma.[462] Gonadoblastomas are also associated with more highly malignant germ cell tumors such as endodermal sinus tumors, embryonal carcinoma, and choriocarcinoma (10%).[453, 454] There is an increased risk of gonadal tumors (gonadoblastoma and/or dysgerminoma) in patients with 46,XY gonadal dysgenesis and particularly in familial cases.[454, 463] The strikingly disparate propensity for neoplastic transformation in the streak or dysgenetic gonads of patients with 46,XY gonadal dysgenesis in contrast to 46,XX gonadal dysgenesis must be emphasized.

In view of the well-documented malignant potential of dysgenetic gonads, the question of prophylactic gonadectomy merits serious attention. The neoplasms are infrequent in childhood,[464] but the risk rises appreciably in young adults.[451, 453, 454] It is possible that high gonadotropin levels play a role in their growth and that substitution therapy with gonadal steroids affords some protection. A prudent course is to advise laparotomy and removal of the dysgenetic gonads of all patients with 46,XY gonadal dysgenesis (complete and incomplete forms) and all patients with the syndrome of gonadal dysgenesis who have a cell line with a normal or a structurally abnormal Y chromosome or who have Y chromosomal material as determined by molecular biological studies. Exceptions to this rule occur in patients who are 45,X/46,XY mosaics with normal male genitalia,

histologically normal testes, and normal gonadotropin levels and in patients with 45,X/46,XY mosaicism with ambiguous genitalia who have been assigned a male gender role in whom a histologically normal gonad is located in the scrotum. However, the fact that a gonad is located in the scrotum or labial folds and is palpable does not guarantee against a disastrous result, as seminomas tend to metastasize at an early stage before a local mass is obvious. Patients with 45,X gonadal dysgenesis who have no suggestion of clitorimegaly are not at risk. The incidence of gonadal tumors in patients with other X chromosome abnormalities, such as 45,X/46,XX, 46,XXr, and 46,XXq−, is low; these patients, however, should be examined at regular intervals and followed by sonography of the pelvis for signs of gonadal or uterine neoplasm.

Female Pseudohermaphroditism

Female pseudohermaphroditism (Table 14–17) is the easiest of the sexual anomalies to comprehend, as the ovaries and müllerian derivatives are normally developed and anatomical ambisexuality is limited to the external genitalia. Because, in the absence of testes there is an inherent tendency for the external genitalia to feminize, a female fetus will be masculinized only if exposed to androgens. The degree of fetal masculinization is determined by the stage of differentiation at the time of exposure. Once the vagina has separated from the urogenital sinus (about the 12th fetal week), androgens cause only clitoral hypertrophy (Fig. 14–48). Even with severe masculinization of the external genitalia, the uterus and fallopian tubes are normal, because regression of the primordia for these structures, the müllerian duct, requires secretion of AMH by fetal testes, and this action cannot be mimicked by androgens. Although the presence of virilized genitalia usually provides prima facie evidence of an androgenic influence during gestation, ambiguous genitalia, superficially resembling those produced by androgen, are an occasional feature of other, more generalized teratological malformations.

Congenital Adrenal Hyperplasia

Congenital adrenal hyperplasia[465] accounts for most of the cases of female pseudohermaphroditism and approximately half of all patients with ambiguous external genitalia. **BIOCHEMICAL VARIANTS OF CONGENITAL ADRENAL HYPERPLASIA.** (Also see Chapter 9.) Six major biosynthetic

---

TABLE 14–17. Classification of Female Pseudohermaphroditism

I. **Androgen induced**
  A. Fetal source
    1. Congenital adrenal hyperplasia
      a. Virilism only, defective adrenal 21-hydroxylation
      b. Virilism with salt-losing syndrome, defective adrenal 21-hydroxylation
      c. Virilism with hypertension, defective adrenal 11β-hydroxylation
      d. Virilism with adrenal insufficiency, deficient 3β-HSD
    2. P-450 aromatase (placental) deficiency
  B. Maternal source
    1. Iatrogenic
      a. Testosterone and related steroids
      b. Certain synthetic oral progestogens and rarely diethylstilbestrol
    2. Virilizing ovarian or adrenal tumor
    3. Virilizing luteoma of pregnancy
    4. Congenital virilizing adrenal hyperplasia in mother
  C. Undetermined source
    1. ? virilizing luteoma of pregnancy
    2. ? placental aromatase deficiency
II. **Non–androgen-induced disturbances in differentiation of urogenital structures**

Figure 14–48. Female pseudohermaphroditism induced by prenatal exposure to androgens. Exposure after 12th fetal week leads only to clitoral hypertrophy (diagram on left). Exposure at progressively earlier stages of differentiation (depicted from left to right in drawings) leads to retention of the urogenital sinus and labioscrotal fusion. If exposure occurs sufficiently early, the labia fuse to form a penile urethra. (From Grumbach MM, Ducharme JR. The effects of androgens on fetal sexual development. Androgen-induced female pseudohermaphroditism. Fertil Steril 1960; 11:157–180. Reproduced with permission of the publisher, The American Fertility Society.)

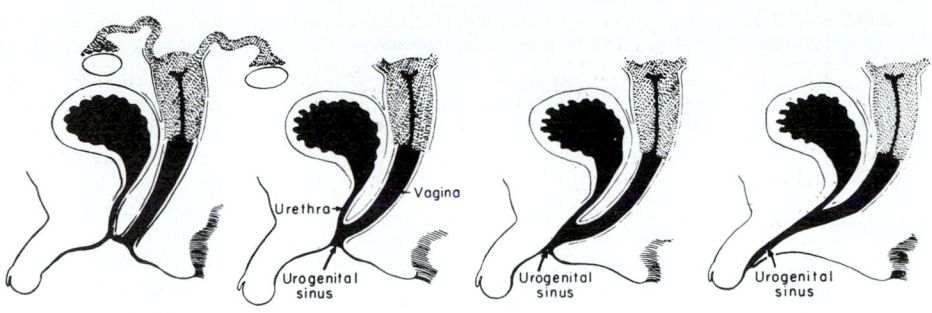

defects in steroid synthesis cause congenital hyperplasia, each with a distinctive clinical picture and specific biochemical lesion (Fig. 14–49).[465] All are transmitted as autosomal recessive traits. The common denominator in all six biochemical defects is impaired cortisol secretion, which results in hypersecretion of ACTH and consequent hyperplasia of the adrenal cortex. Only cytochrome P-450$_{c21}$ and P-450$_{c11}$ deficiencies, however, are predominantly virilizing disorders. In patients with "classic" forms of these defects, the most striking abnormality of the sexual phenotype is masculinization of the female fetus because of overproduction of adrenal androgens and androgen precursors. Affected males have no abnormalities of the genitalia. These inborn errors of steroid biosynthesis are discussed in this section as causes of female pseudohermaphroditism.

Patients with 3β-HSD, cytochrome P-450$_{c17}$, and cytochrome P-450$_{scc}$ deficiencies have in common defects in steroid hormone synthesis that not only block cortisol synthesis but also impair the production of gonadal steroids by the gonads and by the adrenal glands. Affected males exhibit varying degrees of male pseudohermaphroditism because of deficient androgen production by the fetal Leydig cells, whereas affected females may or may not exhibit virilization.

If present, virilization in females is usually less severe than in P-450$_{c21}$ and P-450$_{c11}$ deficiencies. These forms of congenital adrenal hyperplasia in the male will be discussed in the section on male pseudohermaphroditism. Administration to the pregnant rat of selective synthetic inhibitors of the enzymes involved in adrenal and testicular steroid biogenesis has produced abnormalities of sex differentiation in the offspring that are the counterparts of congenital adrenal hyperplasia in humans and served to clarify the role of steroidogenic enzymes in the control of fetal sex differentiation.[466]

P-450$_{c21}$ HYDROXYLASE DEFICIENCY (21α-HYDROXYLASE DEFICIENCY). *Simple Virilizing P-450$_{c21}$ Hydroxylase Deficiency.* P-450$_{c21}$ hydroxylase deficiency is the most common cause of ambiguous genitalia in infants. It is inherited (as are the other forms) as an autosomal recessive trait. Simple P-450$_{c21}$ hydroxylase deficiency has an incidence of about 1 per 60,000 persons (approximately 25% of subjects with P-450$_{c21}$ hydroxylase deficiency)[467] (Table 14–18).

The abnormality in adrenal biosynthesis in patients with simple P-450$_{c21}$ hydroxylase deficiency is primarily defective hydroxylation at C-21 of progesterone and 17-hydroxyprogesterone in the adrenal gland, which results in increased

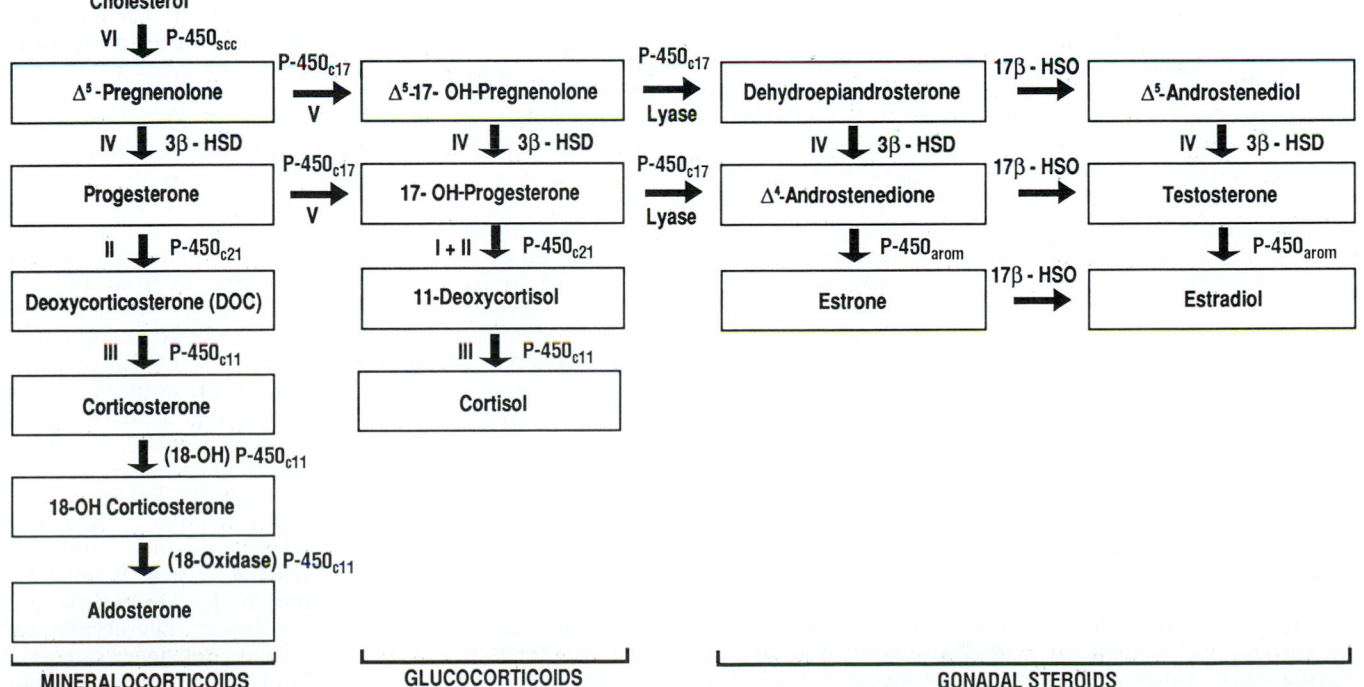

Figure 14–49. A diagrammatic representation of the steroid biosynthetic pathways. I to VI correspond to numbers for specific biosynthetic defects that result in congenital adrenal hyperplasia. P-450$_{scc}$, cholesterol side-chain cleavage; 3β-HSD, 3β-hydroxysteroid dehydrogenase/Δ^{4,5}-isomerase; P-450$_{c21}$, 21-hydroxylase; 17β-HSO, 17β-hydroxysteroid oxidoreductase; P-450$_{c11}$ catalyzes 11-hydroxylation as well as 18-hydroxylation and 18-oxidation; P-450$_{c17}$ catalyzes 17-hydroxylation and 17,20-lyase activity.

TABLE 14–18. Incidence of Classic Congenital Virilizing Adrenal Hyperplasia (P-450$_{c21}$ Deficiency) After Screening

Population	Number of Newborns Screened	Newborns Affected/Live Births	Incidence by Case Survey
Alaska	1,131	1/282	1/490
La Réunion, France	31,472	1/3,147	
Rome, Italy	22,400	1/5,600	
Lille (Lyon), France	199,624	1/11,090	1/23,000
Illinois	357,825	1/11,928	1/15,000 Wisconsin 1/40,000 USA
Sweden	370,000	1/12,758	
Portugal	100,000	1/14,285	
Emilia-Romagna, Italy	73,000	1/14,600	
Scotland	119,960	1/17,137	1/20,907
Washington	255,527	1/18,251	1/15,000 Wisconsin
New Zealand	168,965	1/18,773	
Japan	585,000	1/20,892	1/43,674

Reprinted by permission of the publisher from Newborn screening, prenatal diagnosis, and prenatal treatment of congenital adrenal hyperplasia due to 21-hydroxylase deficiency, by S Pang, A Clark, Trends Endocrinol Metab vol 1, p 302. Copyright 1990 by Elsevier Science Publishing Co., Inc.

production of progesterone and 17-hydroxyprogesterone and decreased synthesis of cortisol.[465, 468] As a consequence of defective cortisol synthesis, there is hypersecretion of ACTH with resulting hyperpigmentation; the adrenal is stimulated to produce excessive amounts of cortisol precursors, including androgens and androgen precursors, proximal to the block in the biosynthetic pathway. Hence, in affected patients the concentrations of plasma 17-hydroxyprogesterone and 21-deoxycortisol are increased, as are the plasma levels of androstenedione and testosterone. Postnatally, metabolites of these steroids are excreted as urinary 17-ketosteroids, pregnanetriol and 11-ketopregnanetriol. Prenatally, excess adrenal androgen synthesis in the female fetus results in elevated circulating testosterone levels. Before the 12th week of gestation, high fetal androgen levels lead to a varying degree of labioscrotal fusion and clitoral enlargement in the affected female fetus; exposure to androgen after 12 wk causes isolated clitorimegaly.

The genitalia of females with the virilizing forms of congenital adrenal hyperplasia (P-450$_{c21}$, P-450$_{c11}$, and 3β-HSD deficiencies) may exhibit a spectrum of masculinization from simple enlargement of the clitoris to complete labioscrotal fusion with a penile urethra (see Fig. 14–48). In severe cases the urogenital sinus is usually preserved and serves as a common outlet for both the urethra and vagina. Presumably, the hypersecretion of androgens and androgen precursors begins before the 12th week of gestation, especially in patients who manifest more than simple clitorimegaly. The uterus and fallopian tubes (müllerian structures) and the ovaries are normally formed, except in rare cases. Wolffian duct development is consistently absent regardless of the degree of virilization of the external genitalia in affected females. Thus internal genital morphogenesis corresponds to gonadal sex in affected females and males.

Postnatally, secretion of testosterone by the adrenal gland and the conversion of androstenedione to testosterone in peripheral tissues result in continued virilization of the untreated patient. In contrast to the salt-wasting form of P-450$_{c21}$ hydroxylase deficiency, the 21-hydroxylation of C$_{21}$ 17-hydroxysteroids and 17-deoxysteroids is primarily impaired.[468, 469] However, even in patients with mild late-onset P-450$_{c21}$ hydroxylase deficiency a mild defect also exists in the 21-hydroxylation of mineralocorticoids, as evidenced by elevated plasma 21-deoxycorticosterone levels after ACTH stimulation.[469] Untreated patients with simple P-450$_{c21}$ hydroxylase deficiency usually have normal plasma renin levels and normal aldosterone secretion rates,[470] although variabil-

ity has been noted. In untreated patients, increased androgen production leads to accelerated growth during childhood and to disproportionate acceleration of skeletal maturation, which results in premature closure of the epiphyses and short stature in adolescence and adulthood.[471]

P-450$_{c21}$ Hydroxylase Deficiency with Salt Loss. In patients with severe P-450$_{c21}$ hydroxylase deficiency, both virilization and salt loss can occur. This variant, which occurs in about 75% of patients with classic 21-hydroxylase deficiency (1 in 19,000 persons),[467] is due to a severe defect in adrenal 21-hydroxylation that leads to impaired cortisol (fasciculata) and aldosterone (glomerulosa) secretion[465, 469] and increased plasma renin activity. Electrolyte and fluid losses result in hyponatremia, hyperkalemia, acidosis, dehydration, and vascular collapse. About 50% of patients have their first salt-losing crisis between 6 and 14 d of age; it is infrequent before age 6 d. However, plasma potassium concentrations may be elevated before 6 d. Masculinization of the external genitalia and urogenital sinus in affected females tends to be more severe in complete P-450$_{c21}$ hydroxylase deficiency than in simple P-450$_{c21}$ hydroxylase or P-450$_{c11}$ hydroxylase deficiency. Without specific therapy, death can result from hyperkalemia, dehydration, and shock. In the affected male whose genitalia are normal, the differential diagnosis includes sepsis, pyloric stenosis, gastroenteritis, congenital heart disease, and congenital adrenal hypoplasia.

Nonclassic P-450$_{c21}$ Hydroxylase Deficiency. Studies of families affected with P-450$_{c21}$ deficiency have revealed heterogeneity in the biochemical and clinical manifestations of this condition, including asymptomatic as well as symptomatic "late-onset" P-450$_{c21}$ hydroxylase deficiency.[465, 472–474] Affected females have no genital ambiguity at birth, as opposed to those with classic P-450$_{c21}$ hydroylase deficiency, but can manifest symptoms of androgen excess, such as premature development of pubic hair in early childhood,[475] accelerated linear growth and bone maturation with resulting short stature, cystic acne, male-pattern baldness, hirsutism, and menstrual abnormalities. Symptoms and findings in women may be similar to those of polycystic ovary disease.[465]

In affected males, premature development of pubic hair, beard growth, growth spurt, and phallic maturation can all occur prepubertally as a result of the increased adrenal androgen production. Oligospermia and decreased fertility have also been attributed to late-onset P-450$_{c21}$ hydroxylase deficiency.[476]

In studies of families with classic P-450$_{c21}$ hydroxylase deficiency, individuals have been detected who manifest the hormonal criteria of this disease, i.e., elevated basal and/or ACTH-stimulated 17-hydroxyprogesterone, androstenedione, and testosterone levels, but in whom no clinical signs of androgen excess are evident.[465] These patients have been designated as having "cryptic" P-450$_{c21}$ hydroxylase deficiency. Symptoms of hyperandrogenism may wax and wane in these patients, who thus may not be truly asymptomatic over a period of time.[465]

New and co-workers,[477] using ACTH-induced rises in 17-hydroxyprogesterone and androstenedione, have defined hormone reference data in the form of a nomogram. Their studies provide a means of distinguishing patients with classic 21-hydroxylase deficiency from those with milder, variant forms, heterozygotes, and normal individuals. These hormonal data in conjunction with linkage studies with HLA typing indicate that all three variants—classic P-450$_{c21}$ hydroxylase deficiency and the cryptic and late-onset variants—result from the same biosynthetic defect. The cryptic and late-onset forms of P-450$_{c21}$ hydroxylase deficiency can occur in families with classic disease and can arise in the same patient at different times of life. The cryptic and late-onset forms are postulated to arise from allelic variants of the

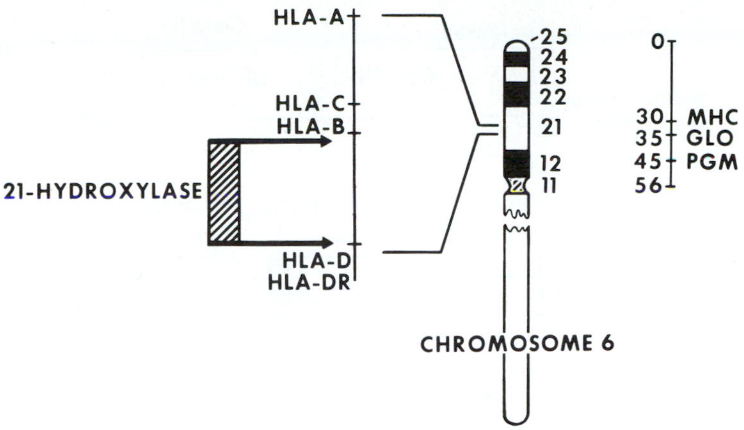

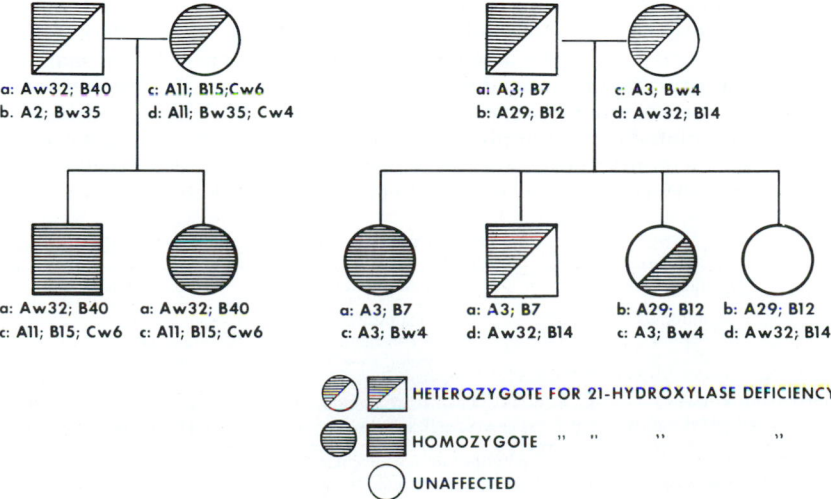

Figure 14–50. A diagrammatic representation of chromosome 6. Only the banding pattern of the short arm is shown. Numbers 11 to 25 delineate bands according to the Paris nomenclature. To right of the centromere, the sites of genes for the major histocompatibility complex (MHC), glyoxalase I (GLO), and phosphoglucomutase (PGM) are indicated on a recombinant unit scale. To left is a scheme of genes in the major histocompatibility complex. The gene for 21-hydroxylation is closely linked to HLA-B and resides between the HLA-B and HLA-D loci.

gene that causes classic 21-hydroxylase deficiency and may be either a heterozygous genetic compound in association with the classic gene or a homozygous state with two variant alleles.[465] Utilizing hormonal data and linkage studies, Speiser and co-workers[478, 479] estimated that nonclassic P-450_{c21} deficiency is the most common autosomal recessive disorder in humans, the frequency being 0.01 in all ethnic groups. The gene frequency seems to be even higher in Ashkenazi Jews, Hispanics, and Yugoslavs.[478, 479]

Molecular Genetics of P-450_{c21} Hydroxylase Deficiency.[480, 481] P-450_{c21} is a heme-containing enzyme that is bound to endoplasmic reticulum and receives electrons from NADPH by way of a flavoprotein, P-450 reductase. The gene for this enzyme is located in the major HLA complex on the short arm of chromosome 6[465] (Fig. 14–50). HLA types are codominantly inherited and can be used in informative families (those containing an affected child and the parents) to distinguish homozygotes, heterozygotes, and unaffected individuals (Fig. 14–51). Although a wide variety of HLA antigens and haplotypes is found in affected patients, disequilibrium has been found for certain specific types and haplotypes. In particular, HLA-Bw47 has a high degree of association with the salt-losing form of P-450_{c21} hydroxylase deficiency and HLA-DR1, B14 occurs more frequently in patients with the nonclassic form of the disease.[465]

Molecular genetic analysis of the 21-hydroxylase gene locus has identified two P-450_{c21} hydroxylase genes on each chromosome 6 located between HLA-B and HLA-DR[482] (Fig. 14–52). These two genes are flanked telomerically in tandem by the C4A and C4B genes, which code for the fourth component of complement.[482] The P-450_{c21} hydroxylase genes are about 3.3 kb long and have 10 exons each.[183, 184] P-450_{c21A} and P-450_{c21B} are 98% homologous; however, P-450_{c21A} is a pseudogene, i.e., does not encode an mRNA.[484] The P-450_{c21A} gene has an eight-base-pair deletion in exon 3, insertion of a thymidine residue in exon 7, and a cytosine → thymidine substitution in exon 8.[484–486] Each of these changes results in stop codons and, as a consequence, a nonfunctional gene.

It has been suggested that the tandem organization of the P-450_{c21} hydroxylase and C4 genes, as well as their sequence homology, can lead to unequal pairing of the P-450_{c21} hydroxylase–C4 genes on one chromosome 6 with the P-450_{c21}–C4 genes on its homologue (see Fig. 14–52). A crossover during meiosis of unequally paired P-450_{c21} genes can result in deletion of a P-450_{c21} + C4 gene, addition of a P-450_{c21} + C4 gene, or possibly a combined P-450_{c21A}–P-450_{c21B} gene if the recombination occurs within the paired sequences.[481, 483] Examples of all these possibilities have been reported.[481, 483] Because of methodological difficulties, differences in analyses of data, and biases in patient selection, there is controversy about estimates of the proportion of deletions, point mutations, and gene conversions in patients with P-450_{c21} hydroxylase deficiency.[481, 487] However, it appears that point mutations are more common (60 to 75%) than deletions (10 to 30%) and large gene conversions (10%)[481, 487] (Table 14–19). Gene deletions may involve all or

Figure 14–51. Pedigrees of two families with children with 21-hydroxylase deficiency. HLA haplotypes for HLA-A, HLA-B, and HLA-C are indicated for each individual. a, b (half-hatched symbol) indicates paternal haplotypes and c, d (half-hatched symbol) maternal haplotypes. Parents are heterozygotes for 21-hydroxylase deficiency. Haplotype a, c (hatched symbol) indicates patients with homozygous 21-hydroxylase deficiency. Haplotype b, d (unhatched symbol) indicates a child who has two normal genes for 21-hydroxylase activity. (Redrawn from Levine LS, Zachmann M, New MI, et al. Genetic mapping of the 21-hydroxylase deficiency gene within the HLA linkage group. Reprinted, by permission of the New England Journal of Medicine, 299; 911–915, 1978.)

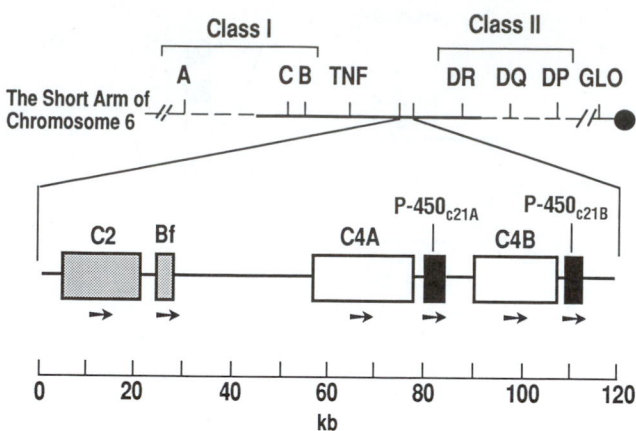

Figure 14–52. A diagrammatic representation of the two P-450$_{c21}$ hydroxylase genes, the active P-450$_{c21B}$ gene, and the inactive P-450$_{c21A}$ gene, located in tandem with the genes coding for the fourth component of complement C4A and C4B on the short arm of chromosome 6. The major histocompatibility loci are shown in the top portion of the figure. (From WL Miller, Molecular biology of steroid hormone synthesis, Endocr Rev 9, 295–318, 1988, © by The Endocrine Society.)

part of the P-450$_{c21B}$ gene. Deletions involving a portion of P-450$_{c21B}$ commonly involve a segment extending from the middle of the P-450$_{c21A}$ gene to a similar site on the P-450$_{c21B}$ gene.[487] The "fusion gene" that results is nonfunctional. A number of point mutations are associated with clinical disease, but many, if not most, appear to be "micro" gene conversions in which the base changes in the mutant P-450$_{c21B}$ gene are similar to those that occur normally in the P-450$_{c21A}$ gene.[483, 487]

Although genotype-phenotype correlations cannot be made at present, certain assumptions appear valid: classic salt-wasting 21-hydroxylase deficiency is associated with mutations, gene deletions, or conversions that abolish or severely reduce 21-hydroxylase activity, and functionally less severe mutations cause the nonclassic form of the disease. Most patients are expected to be compound heterozygotes harboring, for example, a deletion on one chromosome 6 and a point mutation or gene conversion on the other. The functionally less severe genetic defect would be the major determinant of the severity of the enzyme deficiency and thus the phenotype, i.e., classic salt-wasting or cryptic form. However, the difference between the simple salt-wasting and nonclassic variants of 21-hydroxylase deficiency may be both quantitative and qualitative. Not only the amount of enzyme produced but also its specificity may be the result of the specific combination of deletions, point mutations, and gene conversions. Indeed, individuals who are either homozygous for a P-450$_{c21B}$ gene deletion or heterozygous for a deletion and a large gene conversion of P-450$_{c21B}$ to P-450$_{c21A}$ are classic salt wasters.[488] As discussed earlier, one would expect the simple virilizing phenotypes to result from dysfunctional mutations or compound heterozygosity in which the less severe mutation dictates the phenotype. For example, eight patients with homozygosity for HLA-B14, DR1 haplotype and nonclassic P-450$_{c21}$ hydroxylase deficiency had a base

mutation involving codon 281 in which a CTG encoding valine was changed to a TTG encoding leucine.[489]

Screening for P-450$_{c21}$ Hydroxylase Deficiency. Newborn screening programs for P-450$_{c21}$ hydroxylase deficiency have been instituted in a number of regions and countries by using heel blot 17-hydroxyprogesterone levels[467] for the assessment of 21-hydroxylase deficiency. A blood heel blot specimen is obtained at 3 to 5 d of life in conjunction with screening for hypothyroidism and a variety of other inborn metabolic diseases. The 17-hydroxyprogesterone level is determined either by direct radioimmunoassay or after organic solvent extraction.[467] Variability in the "normal" levels reported from one study to another reflects differences in assay technique, antibody specificity, and thickness of the blood spot. Hence, each screening program has to establish its own diagnostic standards and take into account confounding variables such as illness and prematurity.[490]

In worldwide results from screening studies an average of 1 in 14,500 infants is homozygous for the classic (simple and salt-wasting) forms of P-450$_{c21}$ hydroxylase deficiency, and 1 in 60 is a heterozygote.[467] However, the prevalence varies from 1 in 282 among the Yupik Eskimos of southwest Alaska to 1 in 17,942 infants in the state of Washington.[467] Seventy-five percent of patients identified in such screens have the salt-losing form. Screening for 21-hydroxylase deficiency is reliable and cost effective and promises to reduce morbidity and unrecognized mortality in newborn males with severe P-450$_{c21}$ hydroxylase deficiency as well as the erroneous assignment of male sex to affected female infants.[467]

Diagnosis. The diagnosis of P-450$_{c21}$ hydroxylase deficiency should always be considered in (1) subjects with ambiguous genitalia and the features of female pseudohermaphroditism, (2) phenotypic males with bilateral cryptorchidism, (3) infants who present in shock or a severely dehydrated condition, and (4) boys and girls who virilize before puberty. The family history may reveal a previously affected sibling, an unexpected death in infancy, or a male sibling with sexual precocity. The initial evaluation of patients suspected of having P-450$_{c21}$ hydroxylase deficiency includes measurement of plasma electrolyte, 17-hydroxyprogesterone, and testosterone levels. A karyotype should be obtained. Pelvic ultrasonography is useful to determine the nature of internal structures. Increased excretion of urinary 17-ketosteroids and pregnanetriol and an elevated concentration of plasma 17-hydroxyprogesterone establish the diagnosis in affected infants and children. The concentration of plasma 17-hydroxyprogesterone is normally elevated in umbilical cord blood (mean 50 nmol/L [1640 ng/dL]) but rapidly decreases to 3 to 6 nmol/L (100 to 200 ng/dL) after 24 h of age[491] (Fig. 14–53). After 24 h of age infants with 21-hydroxylase deficiency can usually be distinguished from normal infants by measurement of 17-hydroxyprogesterone and androstenedione levels. However, "sick" unaffected infants and premature infants may have elevated androstenedione and 17-hydroxyprogesterone levels that can confound the diagnosis of 21-hydroxylase deficiency.[492–494]

TABLE 14–19. Pathological Point Mutations in P-450$_{c21B}$ Genes

Location of Mutation	Nature of Mutation	P-450$_{c21B}$ Sequence	Mutant Sequence	P-450$_{c21A}$ Sequence
Intron 2	C → G substitution	cccacctcc	cccaGctcc	cccaGctcc
Exon 4	T → A substitution	atcatctgt	atcaActgt	atcaActgt
Exon 6	3 clustered T → A substitutions	atcgtggagatg	aAcgAggagaAg	aAcgAggagaAg
Exon 7	G → T substitution	cacgtgcac	cacTtgcac	cacTtgcac
Exon 8	C → T substitution	ctgcaggag	ctgTaggag	ctgTaggag

Reprinted by permission of the publisher from Molecular genetics of congenital adrenal hyperplasia, by T Strachan, Trends Endocrinol Metab vol 1, pp 68–72. Copyright 1990 by Elsevier Science Publishing Co., Inc.

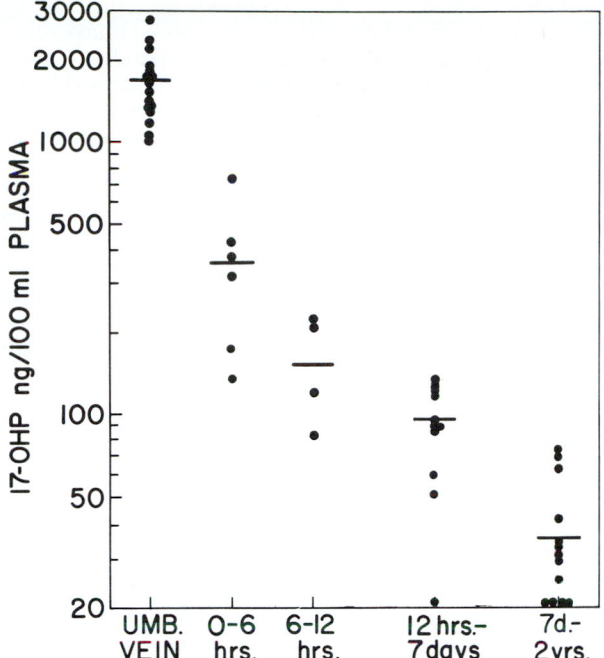

Figure 14–53. Normal plasma 17-hydroxyprogesterone levels in nonstressed infants from birth to 2 y of age. To convert 17-hydroxyprogesterone values to nanomoles per liter, multiply by 0.03026. (From Jenner MR, Grumbach MM, Kaplan SL. Plasma 17-OH progesterone in maternal and umbilical cord plasma in children, and in congenital adrenal hyperplasia [CAH]: application to neonatal diagnosis of CAH. Pediatr Res 1970; 4:380 [abstract].)

In affected patients 17-hydroxyprogesterone values usually range from 90 to 1200 nmol/L (3000 to 40,000 ng/dL), depending on age and the severity of the defect in 21-hydroxylation. Patients with nonclassic 21-hydroxylase deficiency and heterozygotes may have borderline or nondiagnostic levels of 17-hydroxyprogesterone. In these instances, determining the effect of ACTH on the increase of 17-hydroxyprogesterone, androstenedione, and 21-deoxycortisol levels will identify affected infants.[477, 495] In a kinship with an affected infant, HLA genotyping can frequently be used to distinguish between heterozygosity and a mild form of the disorder in a homozygous patient.[465]

The striking elevation in the concentration of plasma 17-hydroxyprogesterone is such a distinctive marker of 21-hydroxylase deficiency that prenatal diagnosis has been attempted by determining its concentration in amniotic fluid in pregnancies at risk.[131, 465, 496] HLA typing of cells obtained from amniotic fluid of mothers who had a previously affected offspring has also been used to identify fetuses homozygous or heterozygous for 21-hydroxylase deficiency.[497] Advances in prenatal diagnosis with amniotic fluid steroid analysis[498] and chorionic villus biopsy with restriction fragment length polymorphism analysis have led to earlier and more accurate diagnosis of infants affected with P-450$_{c21}$ hydroxylase deficiency.[499] The availability of prenatal diagnosis has led to attempts at prenatal treatment.[500] Dexamethasone crosses the placenta and suppresses the fetal adrenal gland if given in sufficient doses.[499, 500] Preliminary studies suggest that dexamethasone administration to pregnant women early in gestation (before 7 wk) can result in a decrease in virilization of the external genitalia of the affected female infant.[499–501] No significant morbidity or mortality has been reported as yet in fetuses treated to term and followed through infancy and childhood.[499–501]

In the past, diagnosis of 21-hydroxylase deficiency was based on assessment of the excretion of urinary 17-ketoste-roids and pregnanetriol. The excretion of 17-ketosteroids varies with age, and in the first few days of life in unaffected infants it can be as high as 7 to 14 μmol/d (2 to 4 mg/24 h). After 1 mo of age, urinary 17-ketosteroid levels decrease to an upper limit of approximately 1.6 μmol/d (0.5 mg per year of age) until the onset of adrenarche. Pregnanetriol, the urinary metabolite of 17-hydroxyprogesterone, is a "hallmark" of 21-hydroxylase deficiency. However, in the neonatal period the urinary pregnanetriol level may be within the normal range in affected infants. Thereafter, the levels rise and are useful diagnostically.

Infants with salt wasting usually have clinical evidence of frank or incipient adrenal insufficiency or crises after the sixth day of life and especially during the second week. Early diagnosis of the salt-losing form of congenital adrenal hyperplasia is usually based on the clinical findings of poor appetite, weight loss, vomiting, hyponatremia, hyperkalemia, and often renal acidosis. The plasma concentration and excretion of aldosterone are low, and plasma renin activity is high. Mild salt losers may have normal electrolytes under basal conditions but exhibit elevated plasma renin activity and hyponatremia, hyperkalemia, and inappropriate natriuresis with salt restriction.

Treatment. Therapy for patients with congenital adrenal hyperplasia resulting from P-450$_{c21}$ hydroxylase deficiency can be divided into two phases, acute and chronic. In acute adrenal crises in infants and children with the salt-losing form of the disorder, deficiency of both cortisol and aldosterone rapidly leads to dehydration, hypoglycemia, electrolyte imbalance, hypotension, and, consequently, vascular collapse and cardiac arrest. An intravenous infusion of 5% glucose in isotonic saline should be started immediately, and fluid and electrolyte intakes should be adequate to ensure correction of the electrolyte disorder and maintenance of normal plasma electrolyte levels and body water. In the first hour, restoration of intravascular volume is imperative.

If the patient is hypotensive, isotonic saline (20 mL/kg of body weight) may be administered by rapid infusion. (Note: If 5% glucose in isotonic saline is used, 1 g of glucose per kg of body weight will be given, and this may result in hyperglycemia.) Hydrocortisone sodium succinate (50 mg/m²) should be administered as a bolus intravenously, and another 50 to 100 mg/m² should be added to the infusion fluid over the first 24 h. When hyponatremia and hyperkalemia are present, deoxycorticosterone acetate is given (1 to 2 mg IM, depending on age) every 12 to 24 h. Alternatively, one may administer fludrocortisone at a dose of 0.1 mg in the severely hyperkalemic child. These tablets can be crushed and given in a small volume of liquid by nasogastric tube. The frequency and amount of mineralocorticoid and the amount and type of intravenous fluids are adjusted according to the serum electrolyte levels, state of hydration, body weight, and blood pressure. Excess mineralocorticoid and salt can cause hypertension, congestive heart failure, and hypertensive encephalopathy, and too little salt and mineralocorticoid will not correct the electrolyte imbalance and hypovolemia. Severe hyperkalemia may result in life-threatening cardiac arrhythmias. Under these circumstances, intravenous sodium bicarbonate and calcium and rectal cation-exchange resins are useful adjuvants for rapid correction of the serum potassium level.

After diagnosis and stabilization, maintenance therapy is begun. During the first 2 y of life, we prefer to treat infants with intramuscular cortisone acetate. This avoids the problems of regurgitation and variable absorption of oral medication. The initial suppressive dose in infants is 20 to 25 mg of cortisone acetate IM daily for 5 d. Thereafter, cortisone acetate is given every 3 d in a dose (15 to 20 mg) that approximates the daily requirement of 12 ± 3 mg/m².

With stress, febrile episodes, acute gastrointestinal disorders, and surgery, the dose is increased by giving the injection daily rather than every 3 d. This regimen of glucocorticoid replacement is usually continued until 18 to 24 mo of age.

The dose of glucocorticoids (Table 14–20) is empirical and must be adjusted for each patient by assessing bone age, linear growth, 24-h excretion of 17-ketosteroids, and clinical evidence of glucocorticoid deficiency or excess. Random measurements of plasma levels of testosterone, androstenedione, and 17-hydroxyprogesterone are no more useful than measurements of urinary 17-ketosteroid levels in assessing the adequacy of therapy in infants and children. The estimation of circadian rhythms of plasma 17-hydroxyprogesterone by measurement of salivary and heel stick levels has been reported to be efficacious in the management of patients with P-450$_{c21}$ hydroxylase deficiency.[502]

After 18 to 24 mo of intramuscular therapy, we change to oral glucocorticoids. The oral dose of cortisone acetate is approximately 22 mg/m²/d (for hydrocortisone, 18 mg/m²/d) and is divided into three equal doses.[471] These doses of cortisone acetate and hydrocortisone permit normal growth and development;[471] it is essential to readjust the dose on an individual basis, depending on the clinical findings, pattern of growth, skeletal maturation, and hormone data. Adjustment of the oral dose of the more potent and longer-acting glucocorticoids such as methylprednisolone and dexamethasone is more difficult in infants and children, and their use has resulted in overtreatment, manifested by growth suppression and development of cushingoid features. Thus we tend to avoid these long-acting glucocorticoid analogues in the treatment of infants and young children. On the other hand, such analogues are useful in postpubertal females because their long action leads to less fluctuation in adrenal suppression and may facilitate normal hypothalamic-pituitary-gonadal function and menses.[503] Many affected women, when treated appropriately, give birth to normal children. Polycystic ovaries and sterility have been reported in patients with undertreated adrenal hyperplasia, although the prevalence is not known.[176]

Patients with salt wasting require long-term therapy with both mineralocorticoid and salt. After the infant has been diagnosed and stabilized, fludrocortisone (0.05 to 0.2 mg/d) and salt supplements (1 to 3 g/d by mouth) are given to maintain normal electrolyte levels, blood pressure, and plasma renin activity.

Plasma renin activity measurements are a useful index of the adequacy of mineralocorticoid replacement therapy. Insufficient mineralocorticoid and salt therapy not only results in hypovolemia, hyperkalemia, and hyponatremia but also can lead to increased secretion of glucocorticoid precursors and adrenal androgens.[504] For optimal therapy and to ensure normal growth and development, we recommend that all salt losers and affected patients with elevated plasma renin activity be maintained on mineralocorticoid;

the dosage should be assessed periodically and especially before an increase in the maintenance dose of glucocorticoid therapy is instituted. By age 2 to 3 y, patients with salt wasting can regulate their own dietary salt intake ad libitum.

Long-term follow-up data on the effects of glucocorticoid and mineralocorticoid replacement in patients with congenital adrenal hyperplasia indicate that the mean adult height of both males and females is less than that of unaffected siblings and less than the mean value for normal adult height.[462, 505–507] Puberty and even fertility have been reported in untreated adult males with congenital adrenal hyperplasia. However, patients who have discontinued therapy or have been noncompliant are at risk for (1) hyperplasia of adrenal rests in the testes that produce tumor-like masses that usually respond to glucocorticoid suppression, (2) pituitary hyperplasia, (3) adrenal carcinoma, and (4) adrenal crises with stress. Thus we recommend that *all patients receive continuing treatment with a glucocorticoid and, if indicated, a mineralocorticoid* (Fig. 14–54).

Surgical repair of the external genitalia of female infants with ambiguous external genitalia should be inititated after the adrenal insufficiency is stabilized and before 12 mo of age. Clitoral recession or clitoroplasty is preferred to clitoridectomy.[508] Vaginoplasty should be deferred until later childhood or adolescence.[509] It is of critical importance to reassure the parents that with appropriate treatment and compliance the child will grow and develop into a normal, functional adult. Fertility in males and feminization, menstruation, and fertility in females can be expected in the adequately treated patient. Psychological guidance and support by the physician are an essential component of long-term management. As noted previously, an increased prevalence of bisexuality or homosexuality in affected females has been reported by one observer.[196]

P-450$_{c11}$ HYDROXYLASE (11β-HYDROXYLASE) DEFICIENCY (VIRILIZATION WITH HYPERTENSION).[465, 510–512] P-450$_{c11}$ hydroxylase is located on the mitochondrial inner membrane. Like other P-450 steroid enzymes, it serves as a terminal oxidase of an electron transport chain that includes adrenodoxin reductase and adrenodoxin. The enzyme is present in both the zona fasciculata and zona glomerulosa and catalyzes 11- and 18-hydroxylation in the zonae fasciculata and glomerulosa as well as 18-oxidation (corticosterone methyl oxidase II [CMO II]) in the zona glomerulosa[513, 514] (see Fig. 14–49). Two tandemly duplicated P-450$_{c11}$ genes are located on the long arm of chromosome 8; however, only one gene appears to be functional.[515, 516] Congenital adrenal hyperplasia resulting from P-450$_{c11}$ hydroxylase deficiency was first described by Eberlein and Bongiovanni.[510] In its classic form, P-450$_{c11}$ hydroxylase deficiency results in impaired conversion of 11-deoxycortisol to cortisol and of deoxycorticosterone to corticosterone in the zona fasciculata of the adrenal gland, resulting in the accumulation of the blocked metabolites.[517, 518] Cortisol defi-

TABLE 14–20. Mean Estimated Optimal Dose of Glucocorticoids for Growth in Patients with Congenital Adrenal Hyperplasia, Compared with Anti-Inflammatory Potencies

Glucocorticoid	Actual Dose in mg/m²/24 h	Equivalent Dose	Reported Potency Based on Anti-Inflammatory Effect
Dexamethasone	0.23	1	1
Methylprednisolone	2.4	10	5
Prednisone	3.7	16	7
Hydrocortisone	18.4	80	27
Cortisone acetate (IM)	13.9	60	17
Cortisone acetate (PO)	22.0	96	33

From Styne DM, Richards GE, Bell JJ, et al. Growth patterns in congenital adrenal hyperplasia. Correlation of glucocorticoid therapy with stature. In: Lee PA, Plotnick LP, Kowarski AA, et al., eds. Congenital Adrenal Hyperplasia. Baltimore: University Park Press, 1977: 247–261.

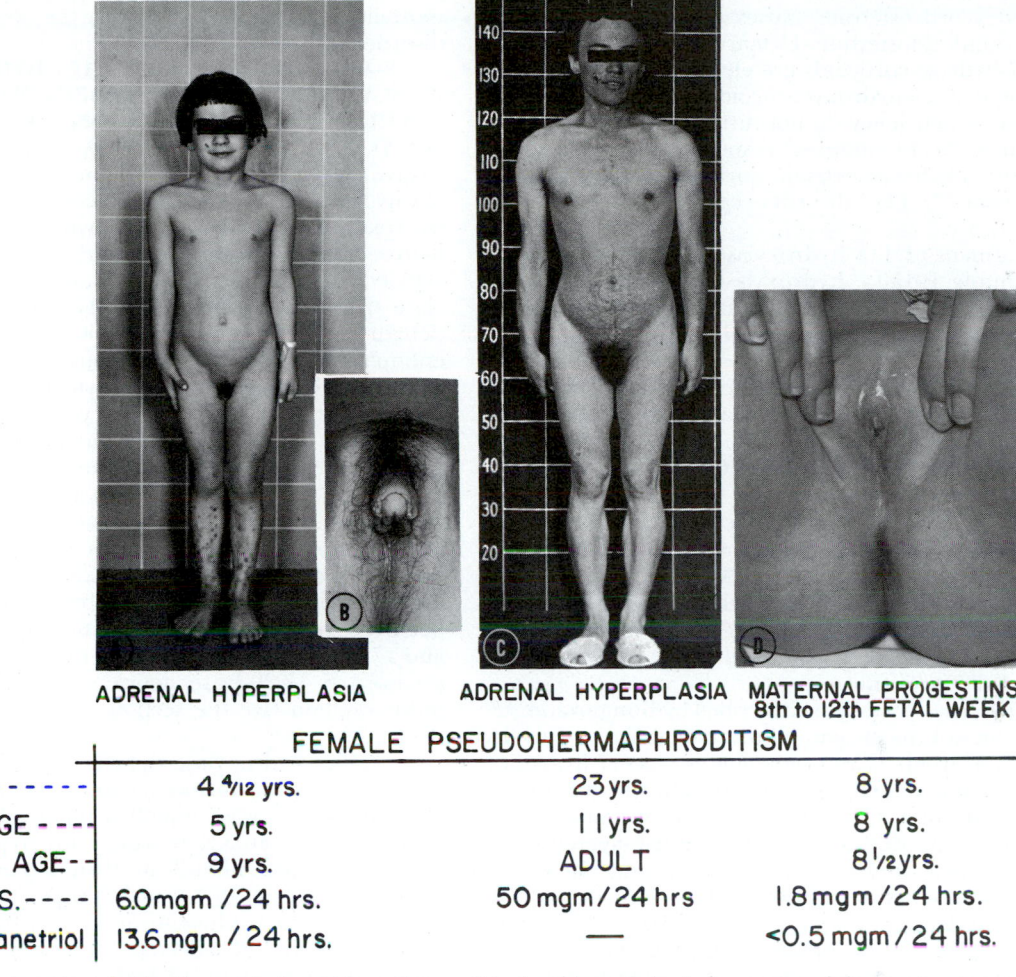

ADRENAL HYPERPLASIA   ADRENAL HYPERPLASIA   MATERNAL PROGESTINS
8th to 12th FETAL WEEK

FEMALE PSEUDOHERMAPHRODITISM

AGE	4 4/12 yrs.	23 yrs.	8 yrs.
HT. AGE	5 yrs.	11 yrs.	8 yrs.
BONE AGE	9 yrs.	ADULT	8½ yrs.
17 K.S.	6.0 mgm /24 hrs.	50 mgm/24 hrs	1.8 mgm/24 hrs.
Pregnanetriol	13.6 mgm / 24 hrs.	—	<0.5 mgm / 24 hrs.

Figure 14–54. A and B, An untreated girl with a relatively mild form of congenital adrenal hyperplasia. Androgens caused disproportionate acceleration of bone maturation compared with stature. C, Virilized adult female with adrenal hyperplasia. The patient had a deep voice, shaved daily, and wore a toupee for baldness. After treatment with cortisone, her 17-ketosteroid levels fell to normal values, her breasts enlarged, she underwent a normal menarche, and hair regrew on her head. Note short stature and short extremities. (From Wilkins L. The Diagnosis and Treatment of Endocrine Disorders in Childhood and Adolescence. 3rd ed. 1965. Courtesy of Charles C Thomas, Publisher, Springfield, Illinois.) D, Female pseudohermaphroditism caused by maternal ingestion of an oral progestational compound from 8th to 12th wk of pregnancy. Labioscrotal fusion is sufficient to obscure vaginal orifice and create a urogenital sinus. Clitoris is enlarged. There is no progressive virilizing tendency.

ciency results in increased ACTH secretion that engenders a further increase in 11-deoxycortisol, deoxycorticosterone, and androgen secretion by the adrenal gland. Excess deoxycorticosterone secretion causes salt and water retention, volume expansion, and low-renin hypertension; hypokalemia is uncommon.[512] Excess androgen secretion in utero by the fetal adrenal gland masculinizes the external genitalia of the female fetus and causes female pseudohermaphroditism. Postnatally, untreated males and females experience progressive virilization. Mild, late-onset, and even cryptic forms of P-450$_{c11}$ hydroxylase deficiency have been reported.[519, 520] Although biochemical and clinical variability is striking, patients with the more severe clinical manifestations, detected at a younger age, tend to have higher basal and ACTH-induced deoxycorticosterone and 11-deoxycortisol levels.[512, 519] Hypertension is a variable feature and is usually not present before age 2 y.[512] The presence of hypertension does not always correlate with the concentration of plasma deoxycorticosterone.[511, 512] Furthermore, salt loss has been reported in rare infants with the apparent classic 11β-hydroxylase defect.[512, 521, 521a] Prepubertal gynecomastia in untreated patients regresses with hydrocortisone replacement therapy.[512]

P-450$_{c11}$ hydroxylase deficiency is about 1/20 as frequent as 21-hydroxylase deficiency in most series of patients with congenital adrenal hyperplasia. However, this disease is more common in Middle Eastern Jews.[511] P-450$_{c11}$ hydroxylase deficiency is inherited as an autosomal recessive disorder and is not HLA linked.[465]

The 18-oxidase activity of P-450$_{c11}$ hydroxylase is apparently more sensitive to denaturation during purification than the 11- and 18-hydroxylase activities.[516] This activity can be dissociated from 11- and 18-hydroxylase activities by mutations in the P-450$_{c11}$ gene.[522] Patients with 18-oxidase deficiency, so-called CMO II deficiency, manifest salt loss alone,[523] including failure to thrive in the neonatal period and hyponatremia and hyperkalemia. Plasma cortisol levels and responses to ACTH are normal. The ratio of the concentration of serum 18-hydroxycorticosterone to aldosterone is elevated, as is plasma renin activity.[523] Sexual differentiation is normal.

The diagnosis of P-450$_{c11}$ hydroxylase deficiency can be confirmed by finding elevated plasma concentrations of 11-deoxycortisol and deoxycorticosterone, increased excretion of their metabolites in urine (mainly tetrahydro-11-deoxycortisol and tetrahydrodeoxycorticosterone), and their suppression by glucocorticoid therapy. In patients with equivocal baseline values, an ACTH stimulation test can unmask the defect. The increased secretion of the mineralocorticoid deoxycorticosterone causes low levels of plasma renin activity and aldosterone. Urinary levels of 17-ketosteroids and 17-hydroxycorticoids are elevated (tetrahydro-11-deoxycortisol is a 17-hydroxycorticoid). Heterozygotes for 11β-hydroxylase deficiency do not differ from normal individuals in their ACTH-induced responses of 17-hydroxyprogesterone, 11-deoxycortisol, cortisol, corticosterone, and aldosterone.[524] The disorder can be detected prenatally.[525, 526]

The treatment of 11β-hydroxylase deficiency is similar to that of simple P-450$_{c21}$ hydroxylase deficiency. Cortisol therapy suppresses ACTH secretion and, as a consequence, corrects the increased secretion of adrenal androgens and deoxycorticosterone. Suitable replacement therapy usually results in alleviation of the hypertension and arrest of virilization. Transient salt wasting may occur when glucocorticoid therapy is initiated.

3β-HYDROXYSTEROID DEHYDROGENASE/Δ$^{4, 5}$-ISOMERASE DEFICIENCY. 3β-HSD is not a cytochrome P-450 enzyme.[527] It requires NAD$^+$ as a cofactor and is encoded by an 8-kb gene located on the short arm of chromosome 1 at 1p11–p13.[514a]. The enzyme catalyzes 3β-hydroxysteroid dehydrogenation and isomerization of the double bond from the B ring (Δ^5-steroids) to the A ring (Δ^4-steroids) in both the adrenals and gonads.[528, 529] The deficiency is inherited as an autosomal recessive trait.

3β-HSD deficiency was first described by Bongiovanni.[530] Classic deficiency of the enzyme results in inability to convert 3β-hydroxy-Δ^5-steroids (Δ^5-pregnenolone, Δ^5-17-hydroxypregnenolone, and dehydroepiandrosterone) to 3-keto-Δ^4-steroids (progesterone, 17-hydroxyprogesterone, and Δ^4-androstenedione). The defect leads to defective synthesis of aldosterone, cortisol, and potent androgens and estrogens. In addition to adrenal insufficiency secondary to cortisol and aldosterone deficiency, severely affected females exhibit slight to moderate clitoral enlargement, whereas affected males have varying degrees of male pseudohermaphroditism. This mild virilization in affected females, which was formerly ascribed to the direct androgenic action of dehydroepiandrosterone, is more likely due to the peripheral conversion of dehydroepiandrosterone and other 3β-hydroxy C$_{19}$-steroids to testosterone by a hepatic 3β-HSD that is apparently under genetic control separate from that of the adrenal and gonadal enzyme. Heterogeneity is evident; non–salt losers have been described with classic 3β-HSD deficiency[531] as well as mild and late-onset forms of the disease.[532–534] The latter may not become apparent until late childhood or adolescence.

Diagnosis. The plasma concentrations of 17-hydroxypregnenolone, dehydroepiandrosterone and its sulfate, and other steroids with a 3β-hydroxy-Δ^5 configuration are elevated in affected patients. Plasma levels of 17-hydroxyprogesterone may be elevated as a result of peripheral conversion of 17-hydroxypregnenolone to 17-hydroxyprogesterone. However, the plasma 17-hydroxypregnenolone/17-hydroxyprogesterone ratio is strikingly elevated in patients with 3β-HSD deficiency. Levels of urinary 17-ketosteroids, especially dehydroepiandrosterone sulfate, are elevated. Bongiovanni[535] has reported that increased excretion of urinary 16-hydroxydehydroepiandrosterone and 16-hydroxypregnenolone sulfate is characteristic of 3β-HSD deficiency (except in the neonatal period, when these steroids can be present normally for the first few weeks of life).[535] In patients with partial forms of this disorder ACTH stimulation is useful in establishing the diagnosis.[475, 531–533] Suppression of the increased plasma and urinary C$_{19}$ and C$_{21}$ 3β-hydroxysteroids by glucocorticoids distinguishes 3β-HSD deficiency from virilizing adrenal tumors. Therapy is similar

to that for patients with P-450$_{c21}$ hydroxylase deficiency. The mortality is high in infants with the complete form of this disorder.

P-450$_{c17}$ HYDROXYLASE (17α-HYDROXYLASE) DEFICIENCY (MALE PSEUDOHERMAPHRODITISM, SEXUAL INFANTILISM, HYPERTENSION, AND HYPOKALEMIC ALKALOSIS). The single enzyme P-450$_{c17}$ hydroxylase catalyzes the 17-hydroxylation of both pregnenolone and progesterone (17-hydroxylase activity) and the side-chain cleavage of 17-hydroxypregnenolone and 17-hydroxyprogesterone to dehydroepiandrosterone and androstenedione (17,20-lyase activity).[536–540] Data for humans suggest that P-450$_{c17}$ hydroxylase (lyase) can convert only 17-hydroxypregnenolone to dehydroepiandrosterone.[540a] This enzyme is located in the endoplasmic reticulum and consists of a P-450$_{c17}$ and a specific flavoprotein NADPH–cytochrome P-450 reductase. Transcription of the gene is cyclic AMP dependent and appears to require a cyclohexamide-sensitive factor.[541] To function, the enzyme must interact with the microsomal membrane, and this interaction involves a specific ribonucleoprotein.[542] The gene that encodes P-450$_{c17}$ hydroxylase is approximately 13 kb long, has eight exons, and is located on chromosome 10 at 10q24–q25.[514a] Three types of enzymatic deficiency related to an abnormal P-450$_{c17}$ gene have been reported: (1) combined deficiency of 17α-hydroxylase and 17,20-lyase; (2) isolated 17α-hydroxylase deficiency; and (3) isolated 17,20-lyase deficiency. The combined form is most common (see the section on male pseudohermaphroditism).[543]

P-450$_{c17}$ hydroxylase deficiency is a rare autosomal recessive condition that occurs in approximately 1 of 50,000 individuals. It was initially reported by Biglieri and colleagues[544] in 46,XX females with hypertension, hypokalemia, and sexual infantilism.[544] Subsequently, this defect has been described in 46,XY male infants, children, and adults with pseudohermaphroditism.[545–548] A defect in 17-hydroxylation in both the adrenal cortex and gonads results in impaired synthesis of 17-hydroxyprogesterone and 17-hydroxypregnenolone and thus of cortisol, androgens, and estrogens. Decreased cortisol synthesis causes increased ACTH secretion, which results in excessive secretion of 17-deoxysteroids, including deoxycorticosterone, corticosterone, and 18-hydroxycorticosterone, by the adrenal cortex. Excess deoxycorticosterone secretion leads to hypertension, hypokalemic alkalosis, suppression of the renin-angiotensin system, and, secondarily, diminished aldosterone synthesis and secretion. Corticosterone is a weak glucocorticoid, and high plasma levels are thought to prevent the signs and symptoms of cortisol deficiency.

The phenotypic manifestations are a consequence of the biochemical defects in adrenal and gonadal steroid biosynthesis. Affected 46,XX females have normal female differentiation of the internal and external genital tract. However, their ovaries cannot secrete estrogens at puberty, and they exhibit sexual infantilism and hypogonadism with elevated plasma FSH and LH levels. In addition, the lack of adrenal and ovarian androgens can result in little or no growth of pubic and axillary hair. In affected 46,XX individuals the ovaries have a high proportion of atretic follicles. Some ovaries contain an increased number of cysts. In affected 46,XY males the testes are small, contain atrophic seminiferous tubules, and show hyperplastic Leydig cells. In males, impaired testosterone synthesis by the fetal testes can result in male pseudohermaphroditism.[545] The genitalia of affected males can vary phenotypically from female to ambiguous genitalia to hypoplastic male;[540a] female duct derivatives are usually absent, as the secretion of AMH by the fetal Sertoli cells is not impaired. In patients with less severe defects in P-450$_{c17}$ hydroxylase, significant hypertension may not be present and aldosterone secretion may be normal.[545, 547]

Winter and co-workers[548] studied six phenotypic female children with classic 17-hydroxylase deficiency. In vitro enzyme analysis indicated lack of 17-hydroxylase and 17,20-lyase activity, in spite of abundant amounts of $P-450_{c17}$ mRNA in the testes. Molecular analyses of the defective $P-450_{c17}$ hydroxylase gene from two patients revealed a four-base duplication in exon 8 of the gene that altered the reading frame and resulted in formation of a protein with a COOH-terminal amino acid sequence different from that of $P-450_{c17}$.[549] It was postulated that this mutation might interfere with the interaction of the enzyme with the specific flavoprotein NADPH–cytochrome P-450 reductase and thus result in functionally ineffective protein for 17-hydroxylase and 17,20-lyase activity.[548, 549] A variety of mutations are known.[540a] Of note is the description of a male pseudohermaphrodite with a defect in both $P-450_{c17}$ and $P-450_{c21}$ hydroxylases, which suggested a defect in the interaction of the $P-450_{c17}$ and $P-450_{c21}$ enzymes with the microsomal membrane.[550, 551] Because one affected patient had a normal microsomal electron transfer system, it remains possible that defects were present in both $P-450_{c17}$ and $P-450_{c21}$.[551a]

Diagnosis. $P-450_{c17}$ hydroxylase (17,20-lyase) deficiency should be considered in all patients with ambiguous genitalia and in phenotypic females with sexual infantilism who have hypertension with hypokalemic alkalosis. Elevated levels of 17-deoxy C_{21}-steroids such as progesterone, pregnenolone, deoxycorticosterone, and corticosterone in plasma and increased urinary excretion of their metabolites establish the diagnosis. The plasma levels of deoxycorticosterone, corticosterone, 18-hydroxycorticosterone, 18-hydroxydeoxycorticosterone, aldosterone, and cortisol and the response to ACTH challenge can be used to discriminate among homozygous, heterozygous, and nonaffected individuals.[548, 552, 553]

Glucocorticoid therapy as for $P-450_{c21}$ hydroxylase deficiency results in suppression of deoxycorticosterone and corticosterone secretion. With suppression of the excess circulating mineralocorticoids, the blood pressure and serum potassium level return to normal. At puberty, both affected males and females usually require gonadal steroid replacement.

P-450$_{scc}$ DEFICIENCY (SIDE-CHAIN CLEAVAGE DEFECT, "LIPOID ADRENAL HYPERPLASIA"): MALE PSEUDOHERMAPHRODITISM, SEXUAL INFANTILISM, AND ADRENAL INSUFFICIENCY). The first step in the synthesis of steroids in both the adrenals and the gonads is the conversion of cholesterol to pregnenolone. This step is rate-limiting and is the principal site of action of ACTH on steroid biosynthesis. 20,22-Hydroxylation of cholesterol, side-chain cleavage (scc), and conversion to pregnenolone require a complex mitochondrial mixed-function oxidase system that includes cy-

tochrome $P-450_{scc}$, flavoprotein-adrenodoxin reductase, and the iron-sulfur protein adrenodoxin.[554] The gene for $P-450_{scc}$ is at least 20 kb long, has nine exons, and is located on chromosome 15 at 15q23–q24.[514a, 555, 556] Deficiency of the enzyme, like that of all other steroid biosynthetic enzymes, is inherited in an autosomal recessive manner.

Prader first described this form of adrenal hyperplasia associated with severe glucocorticoid and mineralocorticoid deficiency in which no C_{18}-, C_{19}-, or C_{21}-steroids are elaborated by the adrenal glands or gonads. As a consequence, affected males usually have female external genitalia with a blind vaginal pouch and absent müllerian derivatives. Females with this disorder have normal internal and external genital differentiation. Clinical manifestations of adrenal insufficiency usually become apparent in the first few weeks of life. On ultrasound, CT, or MRI scans, markedly enlarged lipid-laden adrenals and downward displacement of the kidneys can be visualized. More than 30 patients with $P-450_{scc}$ deficiency have been described.[557–562] Although most have died in infancy, approximately one third have survived with replacement therapy, and we have followed one patient for 25 y.[562] The $P-450_{scc}$ enzyme was reported to be absent in the adrenals of one patient and in the testes of another; however, in these patients the coding region of the gene appeared to be intact by molecular DNA analysis.[563]

In patients with $P-450_{scc}$ deficiency, little or no C_{18}-, C_{19}-, and C_{21}-steroids are detectable in plasma or urine, even after ACTH stimulation. In 46,XX females the differential diagnosis includes congenital adrenal hypoplasia. Demonstration of the greatly enlarged adrenals in $P-450_{scc}$ deficiency by imaging techniques readily differentiates these two entities. Affected males are raised as females and require gonadectomy. Therapy requires replacement with glucocorticoids and mineralocorticoids and addition of estrogen at the time of expected puberty.

The clinical manifestations of each form of congenital adrenal hyperplasia are summarized in Table 14–21.

P-450 AROMATASE DEFICIENCY (PLACENTAL AROMATASE DEFICIENCY). Female pseudohermaphroditism related to placental aromatase deficiency has been described.[563a] Virilization of the female fetus and mother, with markedly diminished estrogen production, was noted during gestation. In vivo studies during gestation and in vitro studies post partum indicated a marked decrease in the ability of the fetoplacental unit to aromatize androgens to estrogens. Postpartum studies indicated that the aromatase deficiency appeared to be confined to the placenta.[563a] We have observed a phenotypically similar infant with pseudohermaphroditism in whom aromatase deficiency was persistent in the child. At puberty, increased androgen levels were associated with extremely low plasma estrone and estradiol levels, elevated plasma gonadotropin levels, and large follicular cysts.

TABLE 14–21. Clinical Manifestations of Various Types of Congenital Adrenal Hyperplasia

Enzymatic Defect	P-450$_{scc}$ (Cholesterol Side-Chain Cleavage) Type VI		3β-HSD Type IV		P-450$_{c17}$ (17α-Hydroxylase) Type V		P-450$_{c11}$ (11β-Hydroxylase) Type III		P-450$_{c21}$ (21α-Hydroxylase) Types II and I	
Chromosomal sex	XX	XY	XX	XY	XX	XY	XX	XY	XX	XY
External genitalia	Female	Female	Female (clitorimegaly)	Ambiguous	Female	Female or ambiguous	Ambiguous	Male	Ambiguous	Male
Postnatal virilization	− (Sexual infantilism at puberty)		±	Mild to moderate	−	+	+		+	
Addisonian crises	+		±		−		−		+ in 80% (type II)	
Hypertension	−		−		+		±		−	

Maternal Androgens and Progestogens

Masculinization of the external genitalia of female infants has been observed after maternal ingestion of testosterone or synthetic progestational agents during the first trimester of pregnancy[564-568] (see Fig. 14–54). If the exposure occurs after the 12th week of gestation, fusion of the labioscrotal folds does not occur, although there may be clitoral enlargement. Severe virilization may be caused by methyltestosterone in dosages as small as 3 mg daily, even though androgenic effects are not noticeable in the mother.

Because progesterone itself is only slightly active when administered orally, various synthetic derivatives that may be taken by mouth have been prescribed in the past for women with habitual or threatened abortion. Most of these progestogens are 19-nortestosterone derivatives, and they are intrinsically androgenic to some degree and can cause virilization of female fetuses in experimental animals. Principal among the offenders have been norethindrone and ethisterone and, less commonly, norethynodrel and medoxyprogesterone acetate.[566] Ishizuka and co-workers[568] reported some degree of masculinization of the external genitalia in 2.75% of female infants whose mothers received progestogens of various types during pregnancy. This consequence of progestogen administration to the pregnant female is mainly dose and time dependent.

Danazol, the 2,3-d-isoxazole derivative of 17α-ethinyltestosterone, is used for the treatment of endometriosis. When given to pregnant animals, danazol crosses the placenta and can cause virilization of the external genitalia of the fetus in a manner similar to other androgenic compounds.[569] There have been several reports of female pseudohermaphroditism (including one with transient 11β- and 21-hydroxylase deficiency) as a consequence of maternal ingestion of danazol.[569, 570]

In four cases of female pseudohermaphroditism, the mother received only stilbestrol in large doses.[571] The mechanism of virilization may be related to inhibition of 3β-HSD by stilbestrol or its metabolites.

Masculinization of the female fetus may rarely occur if the mother has a virilizing ovarian tumor (usually arrhenoblastoma or Krukenberg tumor) or adrenal tumor, a virilizing form of congenital adrenal hyperplasia, or virilization of some other cause during pregnancy.[168, 565, 567, 570-575] Luteoma of pregnancy, an ovarian pseudotumor composed of hyperplastic luteinized thecal cells that regress post partum, has been associated with masculinization of the external genitalia of female infants, especially when there has been maternal virilization.[576, 577] Ovarian lutein cysts in pregnancy (hyperreactio luteinalis), considered by some to be a cystic form of luteoma, are less frequently associated with maternal virilization and only rarely with fetal masculinization.[578, 579] Placental aromatization of androgens such as testosterone may protect the mother and the fetus from virilization.[567, 578, 579] Some of the rare cases of nonadrenal female pseudohermaphroditism of undetermined etiology may be a consequence of a luteoma of pregnancy that regressed spontaneously after delivery or to undiagnosed placental aromatase deficiency.[563a] In these patients a history of maternal ingestion of androgenic steroids is lacking and the postpartum course of the mother is inconsistent with a virilizing neoplasm, but the clinical features are most compatible with fetal exposure to androgens. The absence of virilism in the mother does not exclude a maternal source of androgen in these children, however, because the amounts of androgen required to masculinize the external genitalia of a female fetus may be less than those that cause overt manifestations in the mother.

Female pseudohermaphroditism arising from the transfer of androgenic steroids from the mother to the fetus is the most easily treated of all types of ambisexual development. No hormone therapy is necessary, postnatal virilism does not occur, and female secondary sexual characteristics can be expected to emerge at the usual age of adolescence. Surgical correction of the external genitalia restores feminine appearance and permits normal sexual function.

Malformations of the Intestine and the Urinary Tract (Non–Androgen-Induced Female Pseudohermaphroditism)

Genital abnormalities are frequently associated with imperforate anus, renal agenesis, and other congenital malformations of the lower intestine and urinary tract.[580, 581] Carpentier and Potter[582] reviewed the findings in such infants and suggested the term "nonspecific female pseudohermaphroditism."[582] Some, but not all, of these anomalies are incompatible with life. Renal failure, often accompanied by pyelonephritis, is frequently present and may confuse the picture with that of salt-losing congenital adrenal hyperplasia. In contrast with other forms of female pseudohermaphroditism, the internal genital ducts may also be malformed. The findings in these patients may be quite bizarre, and persistence of a primitive cloaca is not infrequent. The pathogenesis of these anomalies is different from that of other types of ambisexual development and should be considered in the context of other forms of embryonic field defects. Familial occurrence of nonadrenal female pseudohermaphroditism with multiple anomalies has been reported.[567]

Male Pseudohermaphroditism

Male pseudohermaphroditism is a heterogeneous condition in which the gonads are exclusively testes but the genital ducts and/or external genitalia are incompletely masculinized. The clinical spectrum varies from individuals with female external genitalia to those with mild forms of impaired masculinization of the external genitalia, as represented by hypospadias, cryptorchidism, and minimal ambiguity of the external genitalia.

With the advances in our knowledge of pathogenesis, systems of nomenclature based on phenotype have become less important. There are at least six major etiological categories of male pseudohermaphroditism with many subtypes, all of which are associated with incomplete masculinization of the fetal genital tract and/or incomplete regression of the müllerian ducts.

In this section, forms of male pseudohermaphroditism in 46,XY individuals with relatively normal embryonic differentiation of their testes are discussed. In such patients, defective male development must be ascribed to a more specific failure of the fetal testes to overcome the inherent tendency toward feminization of the somatic sex structures. This failure may stem either from a secretory failure of the testes during the critical period of sex differentiation or from a failure of target tissues to respond normally to androgen stimulation. Table 14–22 reflects an attempt to classify the many forms of male pseudohermaphroditism on the basis of etiology, insofar as that is known.

The ability of the testes to virilize at adolescence is frequently a recapitulation of their capacity to masculinize the external genitalia in utero. The greater the development of the phallus in an infant, the greater likelihood that male secondary sexual characteristics will emerge at the time of expected puberty. Individuals with ambiguous genitalia may remain eunuchoid, exhibit mild virilism, or develop breast enlargement and other feminine secondary sexual characteristics. Those with an external female phenotype usually either feminize or remain sexually infantile. These are only approximate guides, however, and the development of male sexual characteristics at adolescence may occur, especially in partial androgen resistance and patients with 5α-reductase deficiency.

Male pseudohermaphroditism can result from (1) testicular unresponsiveness to hCG and LH and Leydig cell hypoplasia; (2) a specific enzyme defect in testosterone biosynthesis; (3) familial end-organ resistance to androgen caused by abnormalities in the cytosolic receptor for testosterone and dihydrotestosterone and possibly postreceptor defects or by an enzyme defect in the intracellular metabolism of testosterone; (4) aberrations in testicular organogenesis (dysgenetic male pseudohermaphroditism); (5) defective synthesis, secretion, or response to AMH; and (6) administration of progestogens during pregnancy. Apart from dysgenetic male pseudohermaphroditism and the persistent müllerian duct syndrome, all other forms of male pseudohermaphroditism are characterized by the absence of müllerian duct derivatives. Except for some variants of dysgenetic male pseudohermaphroditism and the maternal ingestion of progestogens, all forms of male pseudohermaphroditism are familial and characterized by genetic heterogeneity. No doubt many subtypes will be defined and characterized by molecular, genetic, and biochemical techniques. Although we have already discussed dysgenetic male pseudohermaphroditism—the group of disorders associated with defective organogenesis of the testes—it is included under male pseudohermaphroditism because this category of intersexuality must be considered by the clinician in the differential diagnosis of male pseudohermaphroditism.

Testicular Unresponsiveness to hCG and LH (Leydig Cell Agenesis or Hypoplasia)

The production of testosterone by fetal Leydig cells is critical to male sexual differentiation of the wolffian ducts and the external genitalia. Leydig cell agenesis or hypoplasia or Leydig cell unresponsiveness to hCG-LH can result in male pseudohermaphroditism (Fig. 14–55).

This form of male pseudohermaphroditism is associated with Leydig cell agenesis or hypoplasia and unresponsiveness to hCG-LH[583–593] (Table 14–23). Phenotypically, the external genitalia vary from those of a normal-appearing female through an ambiguous appearance to hypoplastic male genitalia.[592] Müllerian derivatives are absent in all patients; wolffian derivatives have been present in some of the most severely affected patients despite the presence of female external genitalia.[584, 585] Basal FSH and LH levels as well as LHRH-evoked responses are elevated in postpubertal patients.[588] Plasma 17α-hydroxyprogesterone, androstenedione, and testosterone levels are low, and stimulation with hCG elicits little or no response. Plasma LH levels decrease after testosterone administration.[586]

On histological examination, the testes lack distinct Leydig cells in prepubertal patients. Postpubertal patients have absent or decreased numbers of Leydig cells without Reinke crystalloids,[584–586, 593] normal-appearing Sertoli cells, and seminiferous tubules with spermatogenic arrest. In the five patients who had LH receptor measurements, there was absent or diminished binding of labeled hCG and LH to the Leydig cells.[587, 588] Familial studies are consistent with autosomal recessive transmission.[593] The counterpart to this disorder described in the rat is termed the *vestigial testis syndrome* and is apparently due to an LH receptor defect.[594]

TABLE 14–22. Male Pseudohermaphroditism

I. **Testicular unresponsiveness to hCG and LH (Leydig cell agenesis or hypoplasia)**
II. **Inborn errors of testosterone biosynthesis**
    A. Enzyme defects affecting synthesis of both corticosteroids and testosterone (variants of congenital adrenal hyperplasia)
        1. P-450$_{scc}$ (cholesterol side-chain cleavage) deficiency (congenital lipoid adrenal hyperplasia)
        2. 3β-HSD deficiency
        3. P-450$_{c17}$ (17α-hydroxylase) deficiency
    B. Enzyme defects primarily affecting testosterone biosynthesis by testes
        1. P-450$_{c17}$ (17,20-lyase) deficiency
        2. 17β-Hydroxysteroid oxidoreductase deficiency
III. **Defects in androgen-dependent target tissues**
    A. End-organ resistance to androgenic hormones (androgen receptor and postreceptor defects)
        1. Syndrome of complete androgen resistance and its variants (testicular feminization and its variant forms)
        2. Syndrome of partial androgen resistance and its variants (Reifenstein syndrome)
        3. Androgen resistance in infertile men
        4. Androgen resistance in fertile men
    B. Defects in testosterone metabolism by peripheral tissues
        1. 5α-Reductase deficiency—pseudovaginal perineoscrotal hypospadias
IV. **Dysgenetic male pseudohermaphroditism**
    A. X chromatin–negative variants of syndrome of gonadal dysgenesis (e.g., 45,X/46,XY, 46,XYp−)
    B. Incomplete form of XY gonadal dysgenesis
    C. Associated with degenerative renal disease
    D. "Vanishing testes" (embryonic testicular regression syndrome: 46,XY agonadism; 46,XY gonadal agenesis; rudimentary testes; congenital anorchia)
V. **Defects in synthesis, secretion, or response to AMH: Female genital ducts in otherwise normal men—"hernia uteri inguinale"; persistent müllerian duct syndrome**
VI. **Maternal ingestion of estrogen and progestogens**

In patients with testicular unresponsiveness to hCG-LH, fetal testosterone deficiency results in poorly masculinized external genitalia, but müllerian duct regression is complete because the secretion of AMH by the fetal Sertoli cells is intact. Of interest is the paradoxical finding of wolffian derivatives, which are testosterone dependent, in some patients with minimal masculinization of the external genitalia (only posterior labial fusion). A likely explanation, supported by the variability in the virilization of the external genitalia, is that the defect in the hCG-LH receptor is of variable severity. During the early fetal period, sufficient testosterone may have been secreted *locally*, possibly autonomously,[135] to induce male duct development, but the concentration in the fetal circulation was too low to evoke male differentiation of the external genitalia and urogenital sinus. hCG is necessary to sustain Leydig cell differentiation and growth and testosterone secretion by the fetal testes, at least by about the 10th week of gestation. Variation in the magnitude of hCG-LH resistance of the undifferentiated embryonic and fetal Leydig cell would result in variable degrees of fetal testosterone deficiency and thus a variable degree of failure to develop normal male external genitalia.

In the human male fetus, deficient fetal pituitary gonadotropin secretion associated with anencephaly, hypothalamic hypopituitarism, and isolated gonadotropin deficiency (including Kallmann syndrome) is not associated with ambiguous genitalia, although undescended testes, hypoplasia of the scrotum, and microphallus are common. These clinical observations are consistent with the important role of hCG in testosterone secretion by the human fetal testis during the critical period of male sex differentiation; fetal pituitary FSH and LH are not required for differentiation of testes or male external genitalia but do play a role in their growth during the last half of gestation.

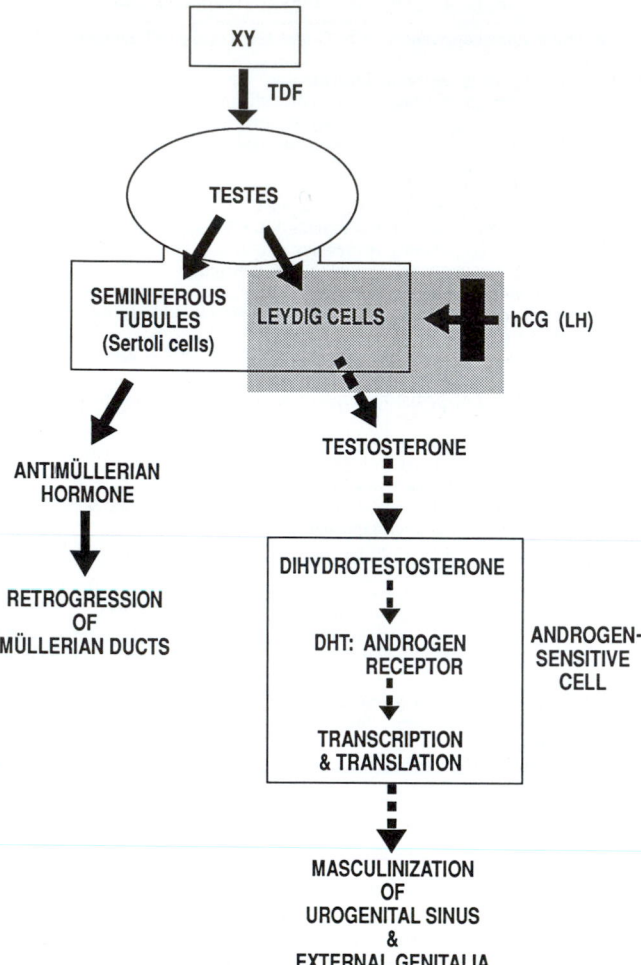

Figure 14–55. A diagrammatic scheme of male sex determination and differentiation showing a defect in Leydig cell responsiveness to hCG (LH) resulting in male pseudohermaphroditism. Solid bar delineates defect, and stippled area designates general site of defect. Interrupted lines indicate that subsequent processes may be completely or partially affected.

Enzyme Defects of Testosterone Biosynthesis Affecting Both Adrenal Steroid and Testosterone Biosynthesis (Variants of Congenital Adrenal Hyperplasia)

Five enzymatic defects in testosterone biosynthesis (Fig. 14–56) have been described, one at each of the enzymatic steps required for the conversion of cholesterol to testosterone[465, 595] (Fig. 14–57). Three of the defects (in P-450$_{scc}$, 3β-HSD, and P-450$_{c17}$ hydroxylase) involve enzymes affecting both glucocorticoid and gonadal steroid biosynthesis; these errors in steroid biosynthesis are discussed, in part, in the section on congenital adrenal hyperplasia.

P-450$_{scc}$ DEFICIENCY (CHOLESTEROL SIDE-CHAIN CLEAVAGE DEFICIENCY, LIPOID ADRENAL HYPERPLASIA). Infants with this defect (Table 14–24) present with severe adrenal insufficiency and accumulation of lipid in the cells of both the adrenal cortex and gonads. Affected males have female (or possibly ambiguous) external genitalia with a blind vaginal pouch and hypoplastic male genital ducts but no uterus or fallopian tubes; the genitalia of affected females are normal. In males, the testes may be abdominal, inguinal, or in the labia. Glucocorticoid and mineralocorticoid insufficiency is usually severe and, if untreated, usually results in death. However, three male pseudohermaphrodites survived

TABLE 14–23. Salient Features of Testicular Unresponsiveness to hCG/LH (Leydig Cell Agenesis or Hypoplasia)

Karyotype: 46,XY

Inheritance: Familial

Genitalia: Female → ambiguous male → hypoplastic male

Wolffian duct derivatives: Absent → hypoplastic

Müllerian duct derivatives: Absent

Gonads: Small undescended testes with absent or decreased number of Leydig cells

Habitus: Lack of virilization at puberty

Hormone profile: ↑ gonadotropins postpubertally, ↓ testosterone levels with ↓ or absent response to hCG stimulation, ↓ binding of hCG/LH by Leydig cell

the perinatal period without therapy and presented at 6 wk, 12 wk, and 8½ mo of age.[560–562] The patient reported by Hauffa and co-workers[562] (and in the previous editions of this chapter) is now 25 y old and well maintained with glucocorticoid and mineralocorticoid replacement therapy. Sexual hair is absent and female secondary sexual characteristics were induced by estrogen replacement. This disorder is transmitted as an autosomal recessive trait. Studies of DNA using P-450$_{scc}$ probes have not detected a gene deletion or point mutation in this patient.

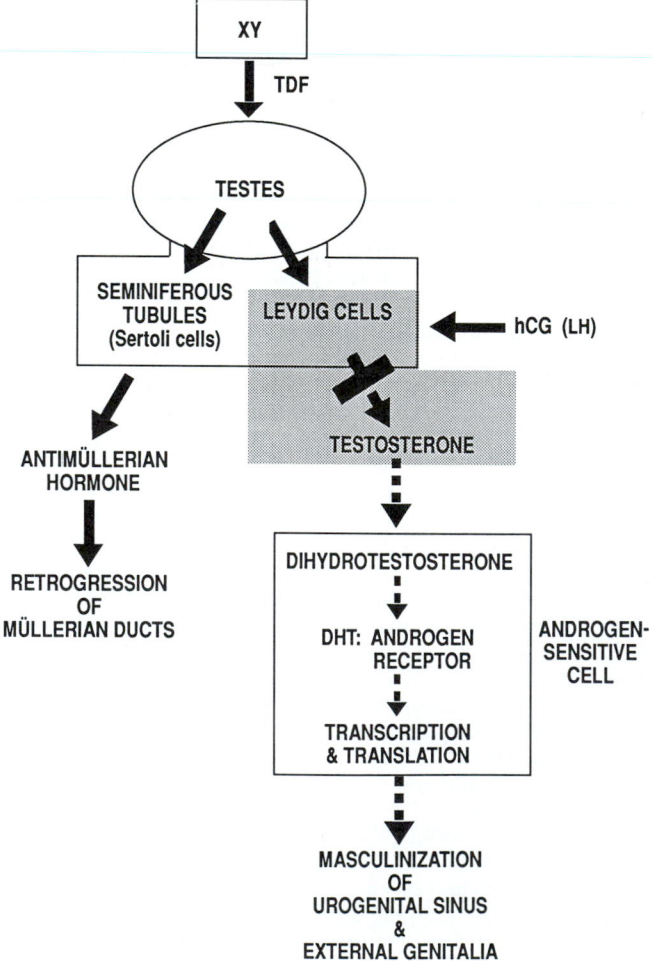

Figure 14–56. A diagrammatic scheme of male sex determination and differentiation showing consequences of an enzymatic block in biosynthesis of testosterone that results in male pseudohermaphroditism.

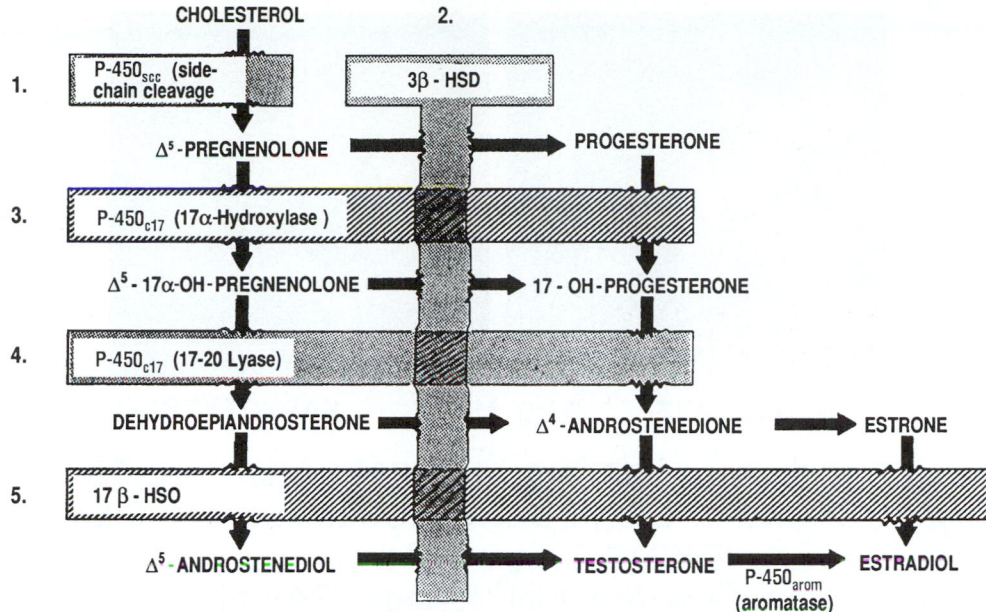

Figure 14–57. Enzymatic defects in biosynthetic pathway for testosterone. All five of the enzymatic defects cause male pseudohermaphroditism in affected males. Even though all blocks affect both gonadal and adrenocortical steroidogenesis, those at steps 1, 2, and 3 are associated with major abnormalities in biosynthesis of glucocorticoids and mineralocorticoids. P-450$_{c17}$/17,20-lyase primarily catalyzes the scission of 17-hydroxypregnenolone to dehydroepiandrosterone in humans. Therefore, synthesis of gonadal steroids is primarily through the Δ^5-pathway.

The diagnosis of P-450$_{scc}$ deficiency should be suspected in patients with male pseudohermaphroditism, including all phenotyic female infants with adrenal insufficiency. The diagnosis can be confirmed by documenting low or absent mineralocorticoids, glucocorticoids, and gonadal steroids and their metabolites in plasma and urine and an absent response to ACTH stimulation. The adrenals are large and lipid-laden on CT or MRI scans. Therapy requires glucocorticoid and mineralocorticoid replacement. All affected 46,XY males have been reared as females. Estrogen replacement therapy at puberty is indicated, as is prophylactic orchidectomy.

3β-HYDROXYSTEROID DEHYDROGENASE/$\Delta^{4,5}$-ISOMERASE DEFICIENCY. Male pseudohermaphroditism associated with adrenal insufficiency is the usual finding in affected males with 3β-HSD deficiency (Table 14–25). Because the block occurs at an early stage of steroid biosynthesis, both adrenal steroidogenesis and testosterone secretion by the fetal Leydig cells are impaired. Clinical heterogeneity in this condition may well reflect differences in the control of 3β-HSD in the adrenals, gonads, and liver as well as variability in the "severity" of the defect. Unlike affected males with the P-450$_{scc}$ defect who are uniformly phenotypic females, males with 3β-HSD deficiency exhibit partial masculinization of the external genitalia. The external genitalia of the affected male usually consist of a small phallic structure with

second- or third-degree hypospadias and partial fusion of the labioscrotal folds; a urogenital sinus and a blind vaginal pouch are present (Fig. 14–58). Wolffian duct differentiation is normal. The testes are usually in the scrotum and, as with other enzymatic blocks in testosterone biosynthesis or defects in androgen-dependent target tissues, müllerian structures are absent.

Although most of the patients reported originally died in infancy, some male pseudohermaphrodites with 3β-HSD deficiency have survived infancy and entered puberty; at least some of these patients have a partial deficiency of the enzyme, and some do not appear to be salt wasters.[596–602] All have had ambiguous external genitalia, and most develop gynecomastia at puberty.[596–601] The gynecomastia may be related to peripheral conversion of C$_{19}$-steroids to estrogen and an elevated ratio of circulating estrogen levels to androgen levels. In postpubertal 46,XY patients, low-normal concentrations of plasma testosterone, increased estrogen levels, and appearance of steroid metabolites such as pregnanetriol in the urine have been attributed by some to the maturation of hepatic and peripheral enzymes (under different genetic control than the adrenal and gonadal enzymes) with the

---

TABLE 14–24. Salient Features of P-450$_{scc}$ (Cholesterol Side-Chain Cleavage) Deficiency in 46,XY Males

Karyotype: 46,XY

Inheritance: Autosomal recessive

Genitalia: Female → ambiguous

Wolffian duct derivatives: Absent → hypoplastic

Müllerian duct derivatives: Absent

Gonads: Testes

Habitus: Severe adrenal insufficiency in infancy, little or no virilization at puberty

Hormone profile: ↓ or absent glucocorticoids, mineralocorticoids, and gonadal steroids in plasma and urine, ↑ plasma LH and FSH

TABLE 14–25. Salient Features of 3β-Hydroxysteroid Dehydrogenase Deficiency in 46,XY Males

Karyotype: 46,XY

Inheritance: Autosomal recessive

Genitalia: Hypospadiac male

Wolffian duct derivatives: Normal

Müllerian duct derivatives: Absent

Gonads: Testes

Habitus: Severe adrenal insufficiency in infancy; poor virilization at puberty with gynecomastia. Mild form: no mineralocorticoid deficiency, premature adrenarche → mild virilization

Hormone profile: ↑ concentrations of Δ^5 C$_{21}$- and C$_{19}$-steroids (e.g., 17-hydroxypregnenolone, dehydroepiandrosterone [DHEA], and their sulfates) in urine and plasma; ↑ 17-hydroxypregnenolone and DHEA response to ACTH and/or hCG; 17-hydroxypregnenolone and DHEA suppressible by dexamethasone

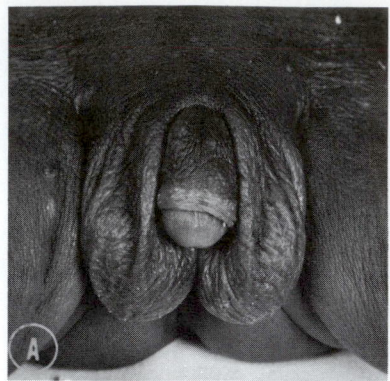 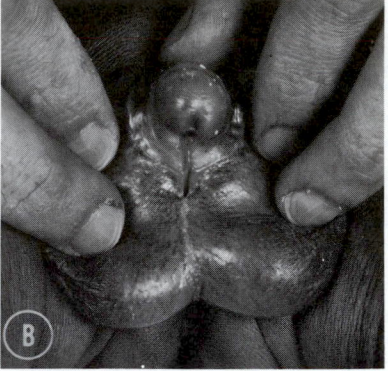

NCMH #II-74-I3   3 MO. MALE   KARYOTYPE:XY

CONGENITAL ADRENAL HYPERPLASIA DUE TO
3-β HYDROXY-STEROID DEHYDROGENASE DEFICIENCY
17 KS : 3.2 mgm / 24 hrs
"pregnanetriol": 1.4 mgm / 24 hrs.

Figure 14–58. Genitalia of male infant with congenital adrenal hyperplasia resulting from 3β-HSD deficiency. The boy was admitted at 9 d of age in a salt-losing crisis and died at 3 mo of unexplained muscular paralysis. Paresis, resembling that of Werdnig-Hoffmann syndrome, became progressively more severe even though adrenal replacement therapy was adequate and blood electrolytes were normal. Biochemical findings revealed a severe block in the conversion of Δ^5-3β-hydroxysteroids to Δ^4-3-ketosteroids.

capacity to convert C_{21} and C_{19} Δ^5-3β-hydroxysteroids to Δ^4-3-ketosteroids. However, in normal individuals the peripheral conversion of dehydroepiandrostenedione to androstenedione and testosterone is low. Alternatively, it is likely that the 3β-HSD deficiency in the testes is partial in these patients; this possibility is supported by the detection of higher testosterone concentrations in spermatic vein blood than in peripheral venous blood by de Peretti and associates.[603] Gynecomastia was absent in one postpubertal patient with 3β-HSD deficiency who did not have salt loss and who had normal spermatogenesis.[602]

The diagnosis of 3β-HSD deficiency should be suspected in all 46,XY males with ambiguous genitalia and adrenal insufficiency. The hormonal characteristics of this disorder are the increased concentrations of Δ^5-3β-hydroxy C_{21}- and C_{19}-steroids (e.g., 17-hydroxypregnenolone and dehydroepiandrosterone and their sulfates) and their metabolites in plasma and urine. However, the diagnosis in early infancy can be confounded by the elevated levels of Δ^5-3β-hydroxy C_{21}- and C_{19}-steroids that commonly occur in normal premature and full-term infants during the first few weeks of life, as well as by the peripheral conversion of Δ^5-3β-hydroxysteroids to Δ^4-3-ketosteroids. Newborn males with 3β-HSD deficiency can have elevated levels of 17-hydroxyprogesterone in infancy secondary to the peripheral conversion of 17-hydroxypregnenolone to 17-hydroxyprogesterone.[604] However, in these patients the ratio of plasma 17-hydroxypregnenolone to 17-hydroxyprogesterone is abnormally high, consistent with adrenal and gonadal deficiency of 3β-HSD. Thus in infancy it is important to interpret the increased concentrations of Δ^5-3β-hydroxysteroids in relation to normal values for age and to determine the ratios of Δ^5- to Δ^4-steroids. Therapy involves replacement of glucocorticoids and mineralocorticoids (if necessary) as in salt-wasting patients with P-450$_{c21}$ hydroxylase deficiency.

Inheritance of this disorder is consistent with an autosomal recessive trait. The clinical and biochemical variability in the severity of the enzyme defect suggests genetic heterogeneity. The gene locus is on chromosome 1. DNA probes encoding 3β-HSD have been described. Studies of affected patients have not been reported.

P-450$_{c17}$ HYDROXYLASE (17α-HYDROXYLASE) DEFICIENCY. The phenotype of 46,XY males with 17α-hydroxylase deficiency (Table 14–26), a defect that impairs both adrenal and gonadal steroidogenesis, varies from phenotypic females with normal-appearing female external genitalia and a blind vaginal pouch to (rarely) males with hypospadias and a small phallus.[545, 605] The magnitude of the impaired masculinization in the male fetus correlates with the severity of the block in 17α-hydroxylation and, hence, with the magnitude of the impairment in testosterone synthesis.[540a, 544–546, 605–611] The testes may be intra-abdominal, in the inguinal canal, or in the labioscrotal folds. Inguinal hernias are commonly present. In one affected 46,XY patient, no gonads were found at laparotomy.[612] Müllerian structures are absent, and wolffian derivatives are usually hypoplastic. The excessive secretion of deoxycorticosterone and corticosterone, the consequence of the failure to 17-hydroxylate C_{21}-steroids, usually leads to hypertension and hypokalemia. The adrenal zona fasciculata is the source of the increased plasma concentration of deoxycorticosterone, corticosterone, 18-hydroxydeoxycorticosterone, and 18-hydroxycorticosterone in these patients.[552] Salt and water retention, volume expansion, and hypertension result in suppression of renin and consequently suppression of aldosterone secretion in the classic form. This process is reversible with cortisol therapy.[546] As gonadal steroid secretion is low, severely affected patients fail to develop secondary sexual characteristics, including pubic and axillary hair. Plasma and urinary

TABLE 14–26. Salient Features of P-450$_{c17}$ (17α-Hydroxylase) Deficiency in 46,XY Males

Karyotype: 46,XY

Inheritance: Autosomal recessive

Genitalia: Female → ambiguous → hypospadiac male; blind vaginal pouch

Wolffian duct derivatives: Absent → hypoplastic

Müllerian duct derivatives: Absent

Gonads: Testes

Habitus: Absent or poor virilization at puberty, gynecomastia, hypertension with hypokalemic alkalosis

Hormone profile: ↓ plasma testosterone; ↑ plasma LH and FSH levels; ↑ plasma deoxycorticosterone, corticosterone, and progesterone concentrations; ↓ plasma renin level

FSH and LH levels are elevated. One patient with a partial deficiency of 17-hydroxylase activity manifested prominent gynecomastia and incomplete development of male secondary sexual characteristics at the time of expected puberty.[545]

The diagnosis of 17α-hydroxylase deficiency should be suspected in male pseudohermaphrodites, including 46,XY phenotypic females, with hyporeninemic hypertension and hypokalemic alkalosis. Plasma concentrations of ACTH, deoxycorticosterone, corticosterone, and progesterone are elevated, whereas the levels of aldosterone, 17-hydroxyprogesterone, cortisol, and gonadal steroids are low. Replacement therapy with physiological doses of cortisol or its analogues results in suppression of deoxycorticosterone and corticosterone secretion and the return of serum potassium levels, blood pressure, and plasma renin and aldosterone levels to normal. At puberty, appropriate gonadal steroid replacement therapy is indicated, as is gonadectomy in 46,XY patients who have been assigned a female sex of rearing.

Enzyme Defects Primarily Affecting Testosterone Biosynthesis by the Testes

P-450$_{c17}$ HYDROXYLASE/17,20-LYASE DEFICIENCY. (See Table 14–27.) The 17-hydroxylation of pregnenolone and progesterone and the conversion of the C_{21}-steroids 17-hydroxypregnenolone and 17-hydroxyprogesterone to the C_{19}-steroids dehydroepiandrosterone and androstenedione are mediated by a single enzyme encoded by the P-450$_{c17}$ gene[536–540, 540a] located on chromosome 10. In the adrenal gland, P-450$_{c17}$ catalyzes 17α-hydroxylation in the biosynthesis of glucocorticoids, and in both the adrenal and the gonad 17-hydroxylation of C_{21}-steroids and the subsequent conversion of 17-hydroxypregnenolone and 17-hydroxyprogesterone to the C_{19}-steroids dehydroepiandrosterone and androstenedione are a function of P-450$_{c17}$. Patients with mutations involving the gene encoding P-450$_{c17}$ can have both 17α-hydroxylase and 17,20-lyase deficiencies (or 17,20-lyase deficiency alone), probably as a result of different mutations or other defects in the gene (see earlier discussion of this defect). The enzyme has greater affinity for 17-hydroxypregnenolone than for 17-hydroxyprogesterone.[613]

Zachmann and colleagues[614] initially reported two first cousins and a maternal aunt with a familial form of male pseudohermaphroditism ascribed to a partial deficiency of 17,20-lyase in both the adrenals and testes. The patients had ambiguous genitalia, inguinal or intra-abdominal testes, and a 46,XY sex chromosome constitution. Both cousins had severe hypospadias with a male-type urethra and male duct

development. The aunt, who was sexually infantile, had a laparotomy and bilateral orchidectomy before the study and was reported to have a vagina and rudimentary müllerian derivatives in addition to a vas deferens and epididymis. In this study only urinary steroids were examined in vivo. A sample of testicular tissue from one cousin studied in vitro exhibited a defect in the conversion of C_{21}-steroids to testosterone (C_{19}-steroids). Subsequent studies of the cousins at ages 12 and 13 revealed a putative partial defect in the conversion of Δ^5 and Δ^4 C_{21}-steroids to C_{19}-steroids.[615] Analysis of the P-450$_{c17}$ gene in one cousin indicated compound heterozygosity with two different mutant alleles. In vitro studies indicated combined 17α-hydroxylase and 17,20-lyase deficiencies despite the clinical findings.[540a]

Three male pseudohermaphrodites have been described in a family with 17,20-lyase deficiency.[616] The two older siblings had a 46,XY karyotype, ambiguous genitalia, and normal glucocorticoid and mineralocorticoid secretion.[616] At ages 7 and 9, the older siblings had low basal levels of androstenedione, dehydroepiandrosterone, and dehydroepiandrosterone sulfate (C_{19}-steroids) that failed to rise in response to ACTH stimulation. Levels of the C_{21}-steroids 17-hydroxyprogesterone and 17-hydroxypregnenolone were elevated and rose further after both ACTH and hCG stimulation with only a minimal testosterone response.[616] In the third sibling, a small (2.5 by 1 cm) phallus, a bifid scrotum, and palpable scrotal gonads were noted at birth. Elevated levels of 17-hydroxyprogesterone and 17-hydroxypregnenolone were found in the amniotic fluid and in umbilical cord and peripheral blood at birth. As discussed in the preceding section, the disorder is transmitted as an autosomal recessive trait. In this pedigree there is strong indirect evidence of a selective defect in 17,20-lyase activity, whereas 17-hydroxylase activity is intact. Marked heterogeneity in the genetic defects has been noted.[540a]

Depending on the degree of impairment in 17,20-lyase and its effect on fetal testosterone production during gestation, the external appearance may vary from female to ambiguous to hypoplastic male.[546, 614–618] The testes may be intra-abdominal, in the inguinal region, or in the scrotum. As with other defects in testosterone synthesis, wolffian duct derivatives are either hypoplastic or normal, depending on the severity of the testosterone deficiency, and müllerian duct derivatives are absent.

In 46,XX females 17,20-lyase deficiency causes failure of pubertal development and elevated gonadotropin levels.[619]

The diagnosis of 17,20-lyase deficiency should be considered in male pseudohermaphrodites with absent müllerian derivatives and in 46,XX females who have no abnormality in glucocorticoid or mineralocorticoid synthesis but at puberty fail to develop secondary sexual characteristics and have elevated levels of FSH and LH. In prepubertal male pseudohermaphrodites 17,20-lyase deficiency must be distinguished from the partial form of androgen resistance, 5α-reductase deficiency, and 17-oxidoreductase deficiency.

Diagnosis. In the prepubertal patient both ACTH and hCG stimulation may be useful in unmasking the defect. Prenatal diagnosis is possible by the measurement of amniotic fluid C_{21}- and C_{19}-steroids.[616] The age at diagnosis and the degree of masculinization of the external genitalia are important determinants of the sex of rearing. Gonadal steroid replacement therapy is usually necessary in both sexes at puberty. Gonadectomy is recommended in 46,XY patients raised as females.

17β-HYDROXYSTEROID OXIDOREDUCTASE (17β-HYDROXYSTEROID DEHYDROGENASE, 17β-KETOSTEROID REDUCTASE DEFICIENCY). This form of male pseudohermaphroditism is caused by an enzymatic deficiency in the last step of testosterone and estradiol biosynthesis (Table

---

TABLE 14–27. Salient Features of P-450$_{c17}$/17,20-Lyase Deficiency in 46,XY Males

Karyotype: 46,XY

Inheritance: Autosomal recessive

Genitalia: Female → male with perineal hypospadias → hypoplastic male; blind vaginal pouch

Wolffian duct derivatives: Rudimentary → normal

Müllerian duct derivatives: Absent

Gonads: Testes

Habitus: Normal stature; sexual infantilism

Hormone profile: ↓ plasma testosterone, androstenedione, dehydroepiandrosterone (DHEA), and estradiol concentrations; abnormal ↑ in plasma 17-hydroxyprogesterone and 17-hydroxypregnenolone and ↑ ratio of 17-hydroxy C_{21}-deoxysteroids to C_{19}-steroids (DHEA, Δ^4-androstenedione) after hCG stimulation test; plasma LH and FSH elevated

14–28). 17β-Hydroxysteroid oxidoreductase is an NADPH-dependent microsomal enzyme that catalyzes the oxidoreduction of androstenedione to testosterone, estrone to estradiol, and dehydroepiandrosterone to Δ^5-androstenediol.[554] This is the only reversible enzyme reaction involved in steroid biosynthesis, and the enzyme is ubiquitously distributed throughout the body. Two genes in tandem that encode an enzyme that catalyzes the conversion of estrone to estradiol are located on chromosome 17 at 17q11–q12.[514a, 620] Both genes have six exons and five introns, and they show 89% homology.[621] 17β-Hydroxysteroid oxidoreductase gene 1 encodes a truncated protein of 214 amino acids because of a G→T substitution, which results in a stop codon TAA at position 218.[621] As yet, it is not known whether both genes are functional and whether they encode an enzyme that catalyzes the other functions (i.e., the reduction of androstenedione to testosterone) of this enzyme. Male pseudohermaphroditism resulting from a deficiency of this enzyme was first reported by Saez and colleagues.[622, 623] Subsequently, many patients have been described, including a large kindred with 23 affected patients who exhibit an autosomal recessive mode of inheritance.[518, 624–633]

The defect has been described mainly in genetic males and occurs primarily in the gonad. Except for a few patients with ambiguous male genitalia at birth,[631, 632] all the affected patients have had female external genitalia or subtle virilization, testes (usually located in the inguinal canal), male genital duct derivatives only, and a blind vaginal pouch. Puberty is usually characterized by progressive virilization with clitoral enlargement. In the patients described by Rosler and Kohn,[629] the phallus reached lengths of 4 to 8 cm, although it was bound down by chordee. Deepening of the voice, male body hair distribution, and an increase in muscle mass occurred. Gynecomastia has been a variable finding. Whether breast development occurs is probably related to the severity of the enzymatic defect and the relative plasma concentrations of androgens and estrogens; the estrogens (estrone) arise from direct secretion by the testes and the peripheral conversion of C_{19}-steroids from the adrenal and testes (mainly androstenedione) to estrone.

At puberty, the plasma concentrations of testosterone and dihydrotestosterone are low for a male, and plasma androstenedione and estrone levels are elevated. The testicular origin of these steroids is evident from the fact that their concentrations decrease with gonadectomy and gonadal steroid suppression of gonadotropins and are not affected by dexamethasone suppression.

In vitro studies of testicular tissue from affected patients demonstrate that the impaired conversion of androstenedione to testosterone and of dehydroepiandrosterone to Δ^5-androstenediol is more profound in prepubertal patients.[634] After puberty, the ability to synthesize testosterone appears

to be restored, as evidenced by the fact that spermatic vein testosterone levels increase to near-normal values.[634] This finding is probably the consequence of elevated plasma LH levels that result in compensatory Leydig cell hyperplasia, as the concentration of spermatic vein androstenedione remains markedly elevated.[629] Abnormal steroidogenesis is also indicated by the observation that progesterone[634] is preferentially converted to 16α-hydroxyprogesterone.

The striking virilization at puberty is in contrast to the lack of masculinization in utero. Similar to the situation in 5α-reductase deficiency, some patients have changed their gender role behavior from female to male at puberty.[628, 629] Most of these patients are from the Arab kindred studied by Rosler and Kohn.[629] We have had the opportunity to study four patients with this disorder, all of whom virilized at puberty and two of whom had gynecomastia. All had a female gender identity. Others have reported similar findings.[630]

17β-Hydroxysteroid oxidoreductase deficiency should be considered in (1) male pseudohermaphrodites who have absent müllerian derivatives and no abnormality in adrenal steroid biosynthesis and (2) male pseudohermaphrodites who virilize at puberty with or without gynecomastia. Virilization at expected puberty and development of gynecomastia occur in various subtypes of male pseudohermaphroditism. The absence of müllerian structures distinguishes patients with defective testosterone biosynthesis or androgen resistance from those with dysgenetic male pseudohermaphroditism. In the prepubertal patient or young adolescent, basal plasma androstenedione and estrone levels may be normal. However, at any age the defect in testosterone biosynthesis can be demonstrated by an hCG stimulation test. In response to hCG, there is a disproportionate rise in plasma androstenedione and estrone levels in relation to testosterone and estradiol levels.[635] We postulated in the previous edition of this text that an affected female would feminize spontaneously at puberty but might not menstruate regularly and that the biochemical hallmark of the defect, elevated androstenedione, estrone, and gonadotropin levels, would be present. A putatively affected female has been reported by Pang and co-workers.[636]

In patients reared as females (the usual case), the appropriate treatment is castration followed by estrogen substitution therapy at puberty. In the patient with ambiguous genitalia reared as a male, testosterone therapy to augment phallus size and genitoplasty are indicated in infancy. As noted previously, male pseudohermaphroditism caused by 17β-hydroxysteroid oxidoreductase deficiency is relatively common among Arabs of the Gaza Strip.[635] The natural history in this isolate is virilization at puberty; further, a change in gender role behavior is the rule. Because of this, Gross and colleagues[635] proposed that these patients should be given male gender assignment. They described seven affected 46,XY males with female external genitalia. After biochemical confirmation, each patient was treated with testosterone enanthate, 25 to 50 mg each month for 3 mo. Most patients received two or three courses of testosterone therapy, which resulted in an increase in phallic length into the normal range for age.[635] First-stage genitoplasty was then undertaken when the patients were between ages 2 and 3 y. Final results regarding the cosmetic and functional state of these patients have not yet been reported. When the patient is reared as a male, testosterone replacement therapy is indicated to achieve full masculinization and prevent, at least in some, the appearance of gynecomastia. A plausible explanation for the absence of spermatogenesis in these patients, aside from cryptorchidism, is the low concentration of testosterone in the testis. In patients raised as males with retained gonads, cryptorchidism as well as elevated gona-

---

TABLE 14–28. Salient Features of 17β-Hydroxysteroid Oxidoreductase Deficiency in 46,XY Males

Karyotype: 46,XY

Inheritance: Autosomal recessive

Genitalia: Female → ambiguous; blind vaginal pouch

Wolffian duct derivatives: Hypoplastic

Müllerian duct derivatives: Absent

Gonads: Testes

Habitus: Virilization at puberty (phallus enlargement, deepening of voice, and development of facial and body hair); gynecomastia variable

Hormone profile: ↑ plasma estrone and androstenedione; ↓ ratio of plasma testosterone/androstenedione and estradiol/estrone after hCG stimulation test; ↑ plasma FSH and LH levels

dotropin levels (postpubertally) may increase the risk for testicular neoplasm.

Defects in Androgen-Dependent Target Tissues

A defect at any step in the mechanism of action of androgens on their target cells (see Fig. 14–24)—5α-reduction of testosterone, receptor function, translocation of the steroid-receptor complex, activation of nuclear binding sites, transcription, or translation—can lead to impaired androgen action and result in male pseudohermaphroditism. Two major forms have been identified: end-organ resistance to androgenic hormones (androgen receptor defects) and errors in testosterone metabolism by peripheral tissues (5α-reductase deficiency).

END-ORGAN RESISTANCE TO ANDROGENIC HORMONES (ANDROGEN RECEPTOR DEFECTS).[637–640] Several forms of androgen resistance have been identified. The spectrum of phenotypes in 46,XY individuals with androgen resistance syndromes varies from individuals with normal female external genitalia through patients with genital ambiguity to those with a normal male phenotype who have a small phallus and are fertile. Both qualitative and quantitative defects in the cytosolic androgen receptor are known, as are receptor-positive forms. The gene for the androgen receptor has been cloned and localized to Xq11–Xq12.[641–643]

Complete Androgen Resistance and Its Variants (Testicular Feminization, Feminizing Testes). The term "testicular feminization," coined by Morris and Mahesh,[644] has been applied to a highly distinctive X-linked disorder in which affected males are phenotypic females and develop female secondary sexual characteristics at puberty but fail to menstruate (Table 14–29). That affected individuals are genetic males is shown by the 46,XY karyotype and the presence of testes. Phenotypically, these patients present with unambiguous female external genitalia; a blind vaginal pouch; absent or, rarely, vestigial müllerian structures (uterus and tubes);[645] testes

TABLE 14–29. Salient Features of Complete Androgen Resistance

Karyotype: 46,XY

Inheritance: X-linked recessive

Genitalia: Female with blind vaginal pouch

Wolffian duct derivatives: Usually absent; less commonly, rudimentary or hypoplastic

Müllerian duct derivatives: Absent

Gonads: Testes

Habitus: Scant or absent pubic and axillary hair; breast development and female habitus at puberty; primary amenorrhea ("hairless woman")

Hormone profile: ↑ plasma LH and testosterone concentration; ↑ estradiol (for men); FSH levels often normal or slightly ↑
Resistance to androgenic and metabolic effects of testosterone
Androgen receptor studies: genetic heterogeneity:
  Low or undetectable amount of normal receptor (receptor-negative)
  Unstable receptor (thermolabile, partial receptor deficiency)
  Receptor-positive form (abnormal receptor)

located in the labia or inguinal canal or intra-abdominally; and absent or vestigial wolffian derivatives (Fig. 14–59). Histologically, the testes are difficult to distinguish from normal prepubertal testes before puberty. After puberty, seminiferous tubules are small with few spermatogonia and absent spermatogenesis.[646, 647] The Leydig cells are hyperplastic and tend to form adenomatous clumps. The testes are predisposed to malignant transformation,[640, 648] although the risk of neoplasia is low before age 25,[451] after which it increases significantly. The overall risk of malignancy in patients with testicular feminization may be only slightly greater than that in otherwise normal men with cryptorchid testes.[451]

At birth and in childhood the diagnosis should be suspected in phenotypic females with an inguinal hernia and a testis-like mass in the inguinal region or in the labia. It has been estimated that 1 to 2% of phenotypic females with inguinal hernias have androgen resistance.[649] At adolescence,

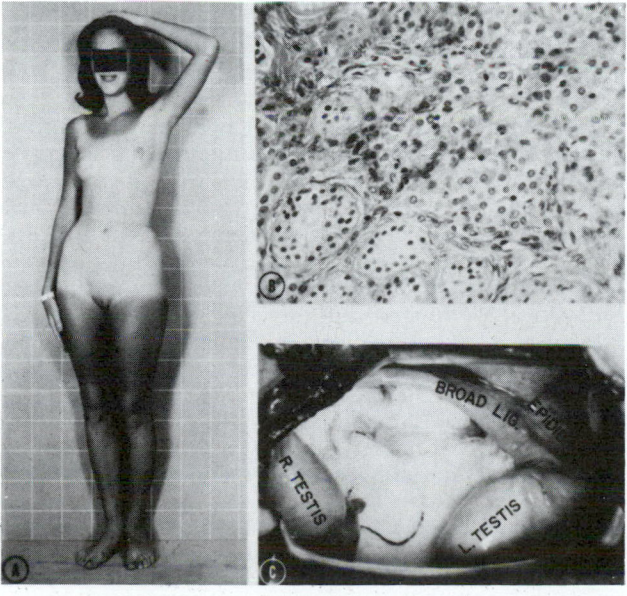

COMPLETE FORM OF SYNDROME

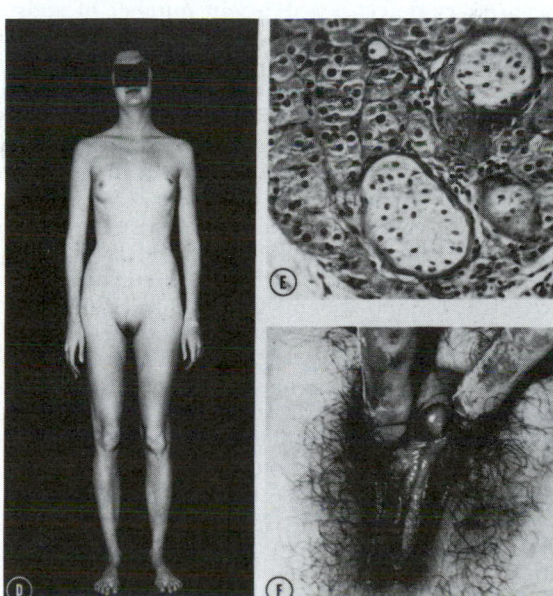

VARIANT FORM OF SYNDROME

Figure 14–59. The syndrome of complete androgen resistance and its variant form. *A,* A 17-y-old patient with the complete syndrome. This phenotypic female was chromatin-negative, had a 46,XY karyotype, and had total absence of sexual hair with female secondary sexual characteristics. A small vagina ended blindly. *B,* The testes exhibited Leydig cell hyperplasia and seminiferous tubules that lacked germinal elements. *C,* At laparotomy, abdominal testes, rudimentary wolffian structures, and no müllerian structures were found. *D,* The variant form of syndrome in a 25-y-old female. Sexual hair was present, although sparse. *E,* The testes exhibited Leydig cell hyperplasia. *F,* The clitoris was hypertrophied, but there was no labial fusion. A shallow vagina ended blindly. At laparotomy, hypoplastic wolffian structures and absent müllerian structures were noted.

female secondary sexual characteristics develop and include normal breasts and female body habitus but no menses. Pubic and axillary hair is usually sparse and is completely lacking in about one third of patients. A small amount of vulval hair is usually present. The clitoris is normal or small, the vagina is shallow and ends in a blind pouch, and the labia minora tend to be underdeveloped. Wolffian duct derivatives are absent, vestigial, or hypoplastic; vestigial müllerian structures are rarely present, presumably because of the secretion of AMH by the fetal Sertoli cells. Approximately 10% of patients have slight ambiguity of the external genitalia at birth (partial fusion of the labioscrotal folds and modest clitorimegaly). In these patients, in whom wolffian duct derivatives are hypoplastic, slight clitorimegaly and virilization often occur at puberty, as do pubic and axillary hair and feminization (breast development and a female habitus).[640, 650] We prefer to classify this condition as the variant form of complete androgen resistance rather than using the term incomplete testicular feminization.[640] Intelligence is normal, as is thyroid and adrenal function; there are no associated clinical anomalies. Gender identity is that of a normal female with strong maternal instincts. Estimates of prevalence vary from 1 in 20,000 to 1 in 64,000 male births.

Pathophysiology and Hormonal Profile. *The Androgen Receptor.* Our understanding of the pathogenesis of this syndrome has advanced rapidly over the past few years. In 1950 Wilkins first suggested that failure of androgenization of the male fetus and the development of female rather than male secondary sexual characteristics at puberty could be explained by end-organ unresponsiveness to androgen (Fig. 14–60). Studies by subsequent workers supported this contention by failing to demonstrate a clinical or metabolic response to testosterone administration in patients with the complete form of this syndrome.[651] This X-linked disorder has been described in several mammalian species, including the mouse, rat, bull, and chimpanzee.[652]

Studies in two animal models, the tfm/y mouse and rat, by Bardin and co-workers,[594] Stanley and associates,[652] Gehring and colleagues,[653] and Goldstein and Wilson[654] suggested that the primary defect is a deficient number of androgen receptors for dihydrotestosterone and testosterone. Soon thereafter, Keenan and colleagues[655] reported an undetectable or low amount of androgen receptor activity in cultured fibroblasts from the skin of karyotypic males with the syndrome. Their observations were amply confirmed by others.[656, 657] The lack of androgen binding in genital skin fibroblasts from patients with this disorder provided an explanation for the observed failure of androgen action.

Subsequent studies, mainly from the laboratories of Migeon and of Wilson, indicated that genetic heterogeneity in the defect existed in patients with androgen resistance.[640, 658–660] Initial studies of patients with complete androgen resistance revealed two groups: those with absent dihydrotestosterone binding and those with apparently normal cytosolic and nuclear binding. It was suggested that the receptor-positive patients had a subtle qualitative abnormality in the androgen receptor or an undefined postreceptor defect.[661] Additional observations of the receptor-positive patients showed that the receptor was thermolabile[662, 663] and/or unstable in the presence of molybdate.[664] Other qualitative abnormalities in androgen binding or kinetics have been described in some receptor-positive patients, including (1) an increase in the rate of dissociation of the steroid-receptor complex,[663, 665] (2) defective up-regulation of the androgen receptor,[666] (3) decreased affinity of ligand binding,[667] (4) impaired nuclear retention of the ligand,[668, 669] and (5) lability of the androgen receptor under transforming conditions.[670] In general, the severity of the defect in androgen receptor

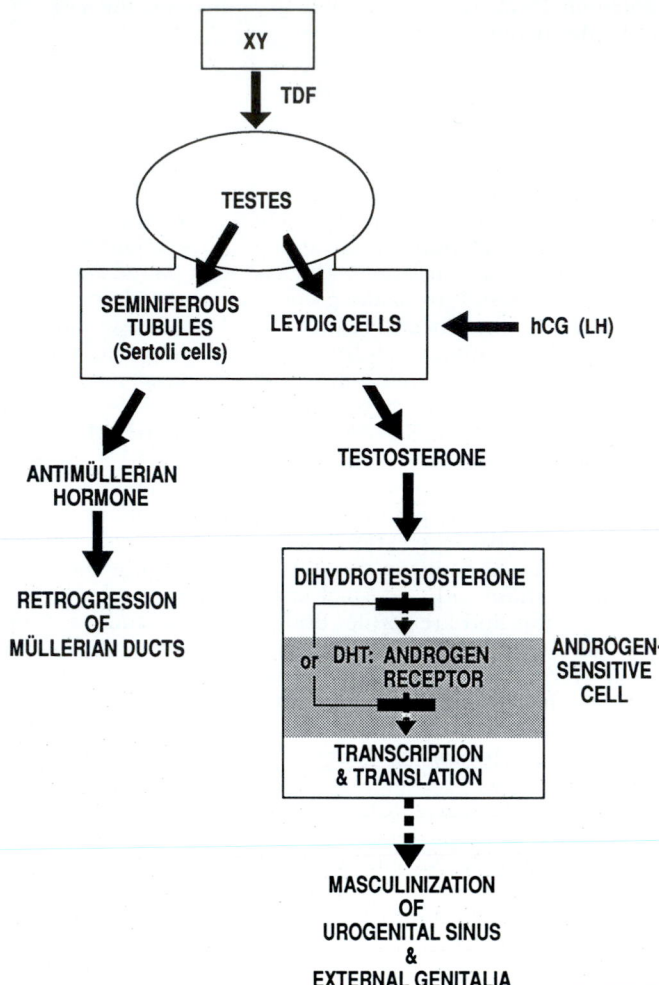

Figure 14–60. A diagrammatic scheme of male pseudohermaphroditism caused by complete or partial androgen resistance.

quantity or quality correlates with the phenotype.[640] Patients with complete androgen resistance usually have absent binding or severe qualitative abnormalities, whereas those with more virilized phenotypes, i.e., Reifenstein or infertile males, have lesser qualititative and quantitative deficits in androgen receptor activity.[640] Individuals varying in phenotype from complete testicular feminization to the infertile male syndrome have had an apparently normal receptor in qualitative and quantitative terms when assessed by steroid-binding properties.[163, 640] These patients have been termed receptor-positive. We suggest that they have a defect in the X-linked gene at sites not involved in coding of the steroid binding region of the androgen receptor.

Molecular Biology of the Androgen Receptor. The androgen receptor is one member of a family of regulatory proteins (see Chapter 3). This superfamily includes all of the steroid hormone receptors and receptors for thyroid hormone, vitamin D, and retinoic acid.[671] These receptors all contain three major regions: (1) an NH_2-terminal region thought to be involved in transcriptional activation, (2) a central cysteine-rich region with two zinc fingers that bind to specific (androgen) response elements located in genomic DNA adjacent to target genes, and (3) a COOH-terminal ligand binding domain (for dihydrotestosterone and testosterone in the case of the androgen receptor).[643, 671] The androgen receptor is encoded by a gene (Fig. 14–61) that is more than 90 kb in length; however, only 3%, represented

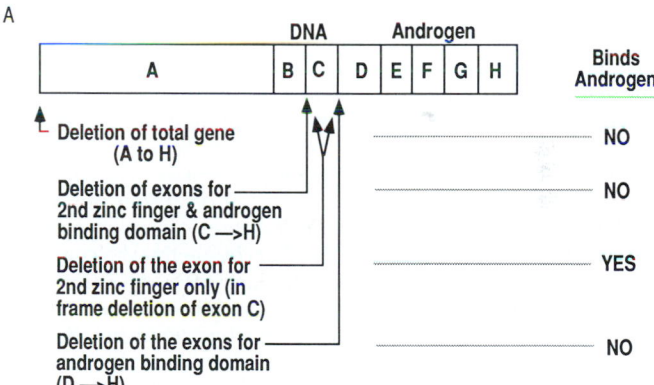

Figure 14–61. A, A diagrammatic representation of the androgen receptor gene divided into its nine exons. Exon A codes for the NH₂-terminal domain and regulates transcription. Exons B and C code for two zinc fingers. Exons D through H code for the androgen binding domain of the receptor. B, The organization of a steroid-responsive gene. Ligand binding activates the receptor, and it binds to the steroid response elements of the gene (as a dimer; not shown). Enhancers as well as a CAAT and a TATA box are present. Gene transcription begins 19 to 27 base pairs downstream of the TATA box.

by eight exons (A to H), is translated.[643, 671] Exon A codes for the NH₂-terminal domain,[672] exons B and C code for the cysteine-rich zinc finger DNA binding domain, and exons D to H code for the androgen binding region[643, 671] (see Fig. 14–61). Patients with the complete syndrome of androgen resistance have a heterogeneous group of molecular genetic defects, including lack of or decreased levels of androgen receptor mRNA caused by a deletion, insertion of a premature stop codon, or a point mutation causing a single amino acid change in exons C to H, that result in an absent or qualitatively nonfunctional androgen receptor[642, 643, 673–681] (Fig. 14–62).

Of interest are two children with receptor-positive complete androgen resistance reported by French and co-workers.[643] These patients had a twofold increase in androgen receptor level. There was no evidence of a qualitative abnormality in the receptor, that is, thermolability or defective nuclear retention. DNA analyses of these patients detected a 117-base-pair deletion involving exon C that did not disturb the translational reading frame.[643] This deletion affected the structure of the second zinc finger of the DNA binding domain, which is necessary for stabilization of the receptors to the steroid response elements of DNA.[671] A patient with receptor-positive complete testicular feminization had a G→C substitution at position 2006 within exon C, which encodes the second zinc finger.[681a] Thus in these patients receptor-positive androgen resistance was due to a defect in the region of the androgen receptor gene that encodes the DNA binding but not the steroid binding region.

Hormone Profile. In the complete form of androgen resistance, lack of effect of testosterone and dihydrotestosterone during embryogenesis blocks stabilization of the wolffian ducts and masculinization of the external genitalia. Secretion of AMH by the fetal Sertoli cells leads to regression of the müllerian ducts. The hormone profile is similar in all variants of androgen resistance but has been characterized best in those with the complete form. The hallmark is an elevated concentration of plasma LH and testosterone in the absence of virilization (or in the presence of a minimal degree of virilization). However, plasma LH and testosterone levels were normal in the first 4 mo of life in four patients with the complete form of androgen resistance (personal communication, J. L. Chaussain), in contrast to the elevated plasma levels of LH and testosterone found during the same

period in two patients with incomplete androgen resistance.[682, 683] We have found that basal plasma LH and testosterone levels are elevated after 6 mo of age in patients with the complete form, suggesting that patients with complete androgen resistance differ from those with incomplete an-

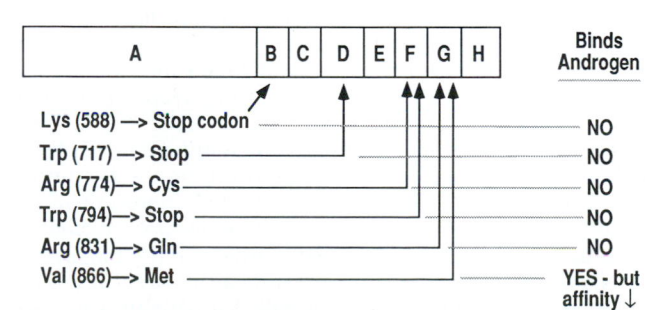

Figure 14–62. A diagrammatic representation of the androgen receptor gene divided into its nine exons. Exon A codes for the NH₂-terminal domain. Exons B and C code for two zinc fingers: the DNA binding domain. Exon D is the hinge region and in part, along with exons E and F, codes for the androgen binding domain. A, Deletions of the androgen receptor gene that have been reported in patients with complete androgen resistance. B, Point mutations and amino acid substitutions affecting the quantitative and qualitative function of the androgen receptor, which results in complete androgen resistance. (Modified from French FS, Lubahn DB, Brown TR, et al. The molecular basis of androgen insensitivity. Recent Prog Horm Res 1990; 46:1–38.)

drogen resistance with respect to the function of the hypothalamic-pituitary-gonadal axis during the first 6 mo of life. At puberty, androgen resistance at the hypothalamic-pituitary level leads to an increase in LH pulse frequency and amplitude compared with those in normal individuals.[684] This results in augmented LH secretion, which in turn stimulates an increase in testosterone secretion.[685–687] Increased testicular secretion of estradiol and peripheral conversion of androstenedione and testosterone to estradiol result in elevated plasma estradiol concentrations, which, in the presence of end-organ resistance to androgens, cause feminization.[688, 689] At puberty, these patients exhibit the type of growth spurt induced by estrogen but not by androgen, with a peak height velocity of 7.4 cm/y at a mean chronological age of 12.7 y.[690] Mean final height in five adult patients was 172 ± 4.1 cm, which is $+1.4$ SD for women and -0.6 SD for men.[690] The growth of sexual hair, normally mediated by androgens, is either absent, sparse, or normal, depending on the degree of androgen resistance. Adrenal androgen levels, including dehydroepiandrosterone sulfate, are normal. The elevated estradiol level evokes an increase in the concentration of plasma testosterone-binding globulin, which, along with the increased secretion of testosterone by the testes, results in an increase in mean plasma testosterone level.[640, 688, 689] On the other hand, the concentration of plasma dihydrotestosterone tends to be lower than normal because of a decrease in peripheral 5α-reduction of C_{19}-steroids.[689] Plasma FSH levels are variable, either normal or slightly elevated.[640] Castration results in a further elevation of plasma LH concentration and a rise in FSH concentration, which suggests that both estradiol and inhibin play a role in the negative feedback of gonadotropins in patients with androgen resistance.[640, 691]

Diagnosis. The diagnosis of complete androgen resistance (testicular feminization) can be established by clinical criteria alone after puberty and can be strongly suspected before puberty. The patients may present with an inguinal hernia or labial mass, primary amenorrhea despite female secondary sexual characteristics, and a history of an affected sister, aunt, or cousin. A phenotypic female with primary amenorrhea, breast development, scant or absent pubic and axillary hair, a shallow vagina and absent cervix on gynecological examination, and a 46,XY karyotype has the complete form of androgen resistance. Similarly, the detection of a 46,XY karyotype in a female infant or child with an inguinal hernia and/or labial mass suggests the diagnosis. A presumptive diagnosis of androgen resistance can be made in infants in whom the plasma LH and/or testosterone level is elevated despite lack of virilization;[682, 683] however, as noted previously, this may not hold true in the neonatal period for patients with the complete form of this syndrome. Absence of the uterus can be confirmed by sonography or pelvic MRI scans. Before puberty, the differential diagnosis includes defects in testosterone biosynthesis and 5α-reductase deficiency. In the prepubertal patient, the family history, phenotype, endocrine evaluation including the C_{19}- and C_{21}-steroid responses to hCG and ACTH, determination of androgen receptor activity, and, if necessary, metabolic response to testosterone are used to establish the diagnosis. As DNA analysis becomes more readily available, it will play an increasing diagnostic role, especially for patients with normal binding of dihydrotestosterone to the androgen receptor, the so-called receptor-positive form.

46,XX females heterozygous for the androgen receptor–deficient form of complete androgen insensitivity are ascertainable in some pedigrees by androgen receptor analysis of fibroblast clones derived from genital skin. Affected 46,XY fetuses may be detected by androgen receptor studies of cells from amniotic fluid or by the use of DNA probes.[643]

Treatment. Therapy includes affirmation and reinforcement of the female phenotype and gender identity. Prepubertal orchidectomy is indicated when the testes of patients with complete androgen resistance are located in the labia majora or when an inguinal hernia is present. Otherwise, we usually defer castration until late adolescence to allow the patient to undergo spontaneous feminization at puberty; the status of the intra-abdominal testes can be monitored by periodic sonography or MRI scans of the pelvis. Girls with the variant form of complete androgen resistance (with clitoromegaly and slight posterior labial fusion) may exhibit mild virilization as well as feminization at puberty; in these patients, it is prudent to remove the testes before puberty or soon after puberty begins. When the testes are removed, estrogen substitution is necessary to promote development of secondary sexual characteristics at the expected age of puberty. The vagina may be adequate in length for sexual intercourse; in patients with a short vaginal pouch, the initiation during adolescence of manual dilatation with a prosthesis is effective in increasing the size of the vagina.

We believe, as do other clinicians, that it is rarely, if ever, indicated to inform the patient directly that genetic sex and phenotypic sex do not coincide.[640] Rather, the patient must be counseled and reassured of her ability to lead a functional, normal (except for fertility) life. It is important for the patient to have an understanding of the pathophysiology of the condition. This can be explained simply, using non–sex-specific terms such as sex glands and hormones. With proper therapy and reassurance, these patients do become "normal" adult females.

Partial Syndrome of Androgen Resistance and Its Variants (Reifenstein Syndrome). A heterogenous group of 46,XY individuals have partial androgen resistance[637, 640, 692] (Table 14–30). The external genitalia are predominantly male or ambiguous. The pedigree analysis is consistent with an X-linked recessive trait. The patients described in the past by Lubs, Gilbert-Dreyfus, Reifenstein, Rosewater, Walker, and their associates quite likely had forms of partial androgen resistance.[640, 693, 694] The variable degree of masculinization of affected males within and between kinships is well illustrated by one family studied by Wilson and colleagues.[695] Eleven males were affected; two had a relatively mild defect in masculinization of the external genitalia (small penis and bifid scrotum), eight had perineal hypospadias, and one had hypospadias, a urogenital sinus with a blind vaginal pouch, and an absent vas deferens. All lacked müllerian structures. In contrast, in families with the complete form of testicular feminization there is little variability in expression of the mutant gene. The most common presentation in infancy is an apparent male with third-degree hypospadias (the ure-

TABLE 14–30. Salient Features of Partial Androgen Resistance

Karyotype: 46,XY

Inheritance: X-linked recessive

External genitalia: Ambiguous with blind vaginal pouch → hypoplastic male → normal male with infertility

Wolffian duct derivatives: Rudimentary → hypoplastic → normal

Müllerian duct derivatives: Absent

Gonads: Testes

Habitus: ↓ to normal axillary and pubic hair, beard growth, and body hair; gynecomastia common at puberty

Hormone profile: ↑ plasma LH and testosterone concentrations; ↑ estradiol (for men); FSH levels may be normal or slightly ↑

Partial resistance to androgenic and metabolic effects of testosterone

Androgen receptor studies: genetic heterogeneity:
    Partial deficiency of normal receptor
    Qualitatively abnormal receptor

thral orifice located at the base of the phallus), a small penis, and frequently cryptorchidism. Müllerian duct derivatives are absent; in some patients wolffian duct derivatives are present but usually hypoplastic. At puberty, pubic and axillary hair and gynecomastia usually appear, male secondary sexual characteristics are poorly developed, and the testes remain small and exhibit azoospermia because of germinal cell arrest beyond the primary spermatocyte stage. As in other patients with androgen insensitivity, the concentrations of plasma LH and testosterone are elevated; the high LH concentrations are resistant to suppression by exogenous androgens. Estradiol and testosterone production rates are increased. However, the degree of feminization at puberty, despite elevated estradiol secretion, is less than in the complete form of androgen resistance (Fig. 14–63).

Although a single biochemical defect had been suspected as a basis for the clinical findings in these disorders, it was not until the reports from Wilson's and Migeon's laboratories that the pathogenesis was clarified.[695, 696] Studies of dihydrotestosterone binding by cultured fibroblasts from genital skin have shown two main patterns: (1) a quantitative deficiency of the androgen receptor[697] and (2) a qualitatively abnormal androgen receptor.[637, 698–700] Some receptor-positive patients have no apparent abnormality in androgen binding.[637]

There are still fundamental gaps in our knowledge of the mechanism of androgen action. Undefined factors apart from ligand binding may influence the response of the target tissues to androgen. This is illustrated by the wide variation in phenotype in patients with partial androgen resistance, by the lack of correlation of the severity of the defect in masculinization of the external genitalia with the magnitude of the receptor abnormality in vitro, and by the variation in androgen resistance in different target tissues in the same patient (the hypothalamic-pituitary-gonadotropin complex versus the external genitalia). DNA analysis of these patients promises to advance our understanding of the molecular genetics of the androgen resistance and to provide a better correlation with the phenotype than has been the case with studies based on hormone binding by the androgen receptor.

Androgen Resistance in Infertile Men. Analysis of a large kindred with Reifenstein syndrome led to the detection of two phenotypically normal males who were infertile and lacked the clinical features of androgen resistance. These infertile males could not be distinguished endocrinologically or by androgen receptor studies from their more severely affected relatives.[637, 656, 695]

Subsequently, Aiman and co-workers[692] reported infertility in three unrelated men with uninformative family histories and a quantitative deficiency of the androgen receptor.[637] Two of the men had a normal adult male phenotype; one had slight gynecomastia, decreased body hair, and a modest reduction in testicular size. All were infertile and had severe oligospermia or azoospermia. The significant hormonal findings were normal or elevated serum concentrations of testosterone in the presence of high plasma concentrations of LH. Two of the three men had increased blood production rates for testosterone, androstenedione, and estradiol. The decreased amount of androgen receptor in genital skin fibroblasts was consistent with a quantitative deficiency of the androgen receptor. Further studies suggested the existence of both quantitative and qualitative abnormalities in the androgen receptor in infertile males.[637] To estimate the frequency of androgen receptor abnormalities in men with idiopathic infertility, Aiman and Griffin[701] studied 28 unrelated, phenotypically normal men with id-

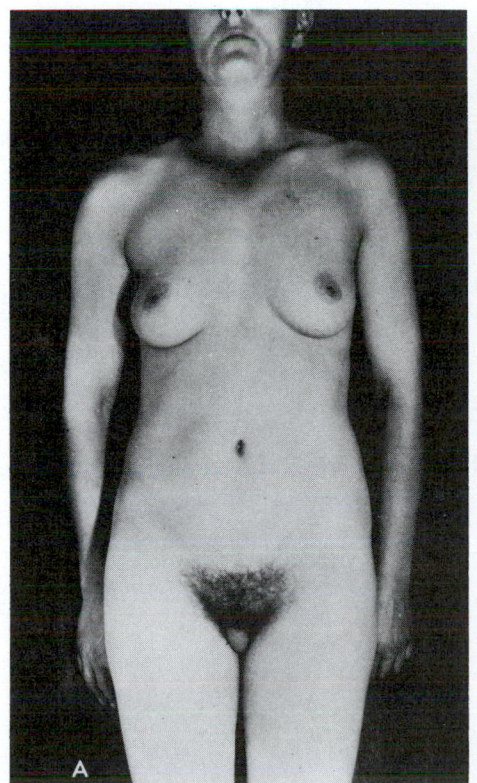
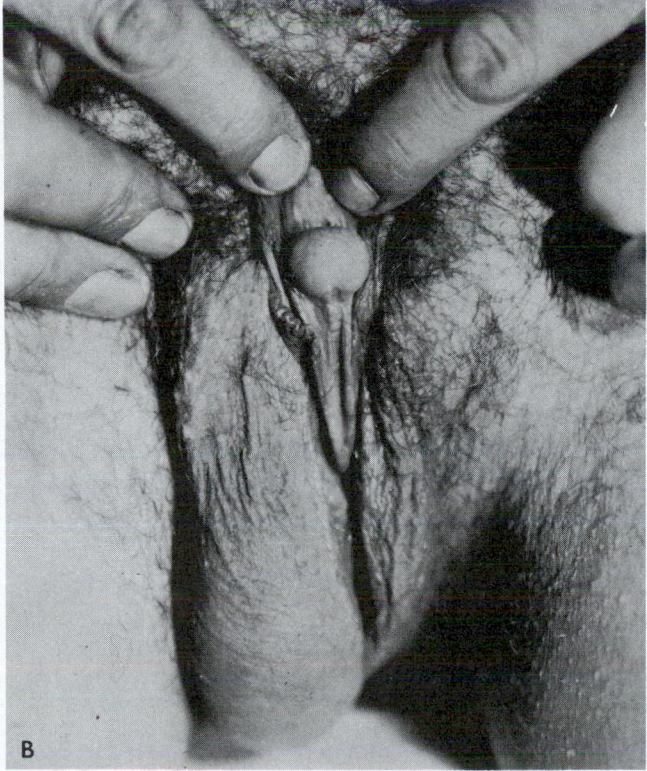

Figure 14–63. A patient with partial androgen resistance (Reifenstein syndrome). Both the patient and his brother had hypospadias, poor masculinization, and marked gynecomastia. Both had a normal 46,XY karyotype, normal wolffian duct derivatives, and no müllerian structures. (Reproduced, with permission, from Bowen P, Lee CSN, Migeon CJ, et al. Hereditary male pseudohermaphroditism with hypogonadism, hypospadias, and gynecomastia [Reifenstein's syndrome]. Ann Intern Med 1965; 62:252–270. Courtesy of Dr. E. C. Reifenstein, Jr.)

iopathic azoospermia or oligospermia. Using genital skin fibroblasts, they noted a partial deficiency of the receptor in 9 of 22 (40%) of the azoospermic or oligospermic subjects.[701] In contrast to previously studied patients with androgen resistance, plasma LH and testosterone levels were normal in six of nine infertile men, and the plasma production rate of testosterone was elevated in only two of six.[701] Other studies have detected subtle defects in the androgen receptor in some subfertile men.[703]

Androgen Insensitivity in Fertile Men. It has been postulated that infertility in otherwise normal men may be the only and most subtle clinical manifestation of quantitative and qualitative defects in the androgen receptor.[703] However, two families consisting of eight males with unambiguous male genitalia, postpubertal gynecomastia, and poor virilization in spite of elevated plasma testosterone levels have been described.[704, 705] In both cohorts, fertility was intact. Studies of androgen receptors in affected individuals revealed several qualitative abnormalities, including receptor instability, failure of up-regulation, and increased dissociation of receptor–synthetic androgen complexes.[705] Hence, gynecomastia with or without poor virilization (phallus length 5 to 6 cm in two patients) rather than infertility may represent the extreme of the phenotypic spectrum of subtle quantitative or qualitative defects in the androgen receptor.[705]

Diagnosis. The diagnosis of partial androgen resistance cannot be made from the phenotype alone. Errors in testosterone biosynthesis can cause a 46,XY patient to have a hypoplastic, hypospadiac phallus, incomplete fusion of the labioscrotal folds, blind vaginal pouch, and gynecomastia at puberty. However, the pattern of inheritance and the measurement of the levels of plasma LH and testosterone and its precursors before and after administration of hCG may distinguish patients with partial androgen resistance from those with other forms of male pseudohermaphroditism. Studies of binding of dihydrotestosterone in fibroblasts cultured from genital skin may show a qualitative and/or a quantitative defect in the androgen receptor, and molecular analysis may define an abnormality in the structure of the gene. Demonstration of a poor or absent metabolic and clinical response to testosterone can be a useful adjuvant in the diagnosis of partial androgen resistance. The finding of germinal cell aplasia (Sertoli cell–only syndrome) or spermatogenic arrest on testicular biopsy may also be a clue to androgen resistance in the otherwise normal infertile male.[701]

There is no specific therapy for partial androgen resistance; however, several patients have had at least some response to high-dose androgen therapy.[706, 707] Sex of rearing is dependent on age at diagnosis and degree of genital ambiguity. In view of the limited response to testosterone in patients with this condition and the gynecomastia at puberty, it may be prudent to raise all patients with this syndrome who have ambiguous genitalia as females. In patients assigned a female gender identity, plastic repair of the genitalia and gonadectomy are indicated before 6 mo of age. At the age of puberty, estrogen replacement therapy should be initiated.

DEFECTS IN TESTOSTERONE METABOLISM BY PERIPHERAL TISSUES: 5α-REDUCTASE DEFICIENCY; MALE PSEUDOHERMAPHRODITISM WITH NORMAL VIRILIZATION AT PUBERTY. In 1961 Nowakowski and Lenz[708] described a familial type of male pseudohermaphroditism, which they termed "pseudovaginal perineoscrotal hypospadias," that was transmitted as an autosomal recessive trait.[709] The patients resemble those with other forms of male pseudohermaphroditism by having a 46,XY karyotype, normally differentiated testes, male internal ducts, and ambiguous

external genitalia. At puberty, striking but selective signs of masculinization appear.

In 1974 Walsh and colleagues[710] and Imperato-McGinley and colleagues[711–714] reported a defect in the conversion of testosterone to its 5α-reduced metabolite dihydrotestosterone in patients with this syndrome (Fig. 14–64). Imperato-McGinley and associates described studies of a genetic isolate from villages in the southwestern part of the Dominican Republic. In 24 families, 38 male pseudohermaphrodites were identified, 24 of whom were postpubertal[711] (Table 14–31). The typical features of this form of male pseudohermaphroditism in infancy include a clitoris-like, hypospadiac phallus bound in chordee of variable degree, a bifid scrotum, and a urogenital sinus that opens on the perineum. A blind vaginal pouch opens either into the urogenital sinus or onto the perineum behind the urethral orifice. The testes are well differentiated and are located in the inguinal canal or the labioscrotal folds. No müllerian structures are present. The wolffian structures (epididymis, vas deferens, and seminal vesicle) are well differentiated; the ejaculatory ducts usually terminate in the blind vaginal pouch. If a vaginal pouch is not present, the wolffian ducts terminate on the perineum next to the urethra. The prostate is hypoplastic. At puberty, plasma testosterone levels increase into the adult male range while dihydrotestosterone levels remain disproportionately low. Affected males virilize to a variable degree without

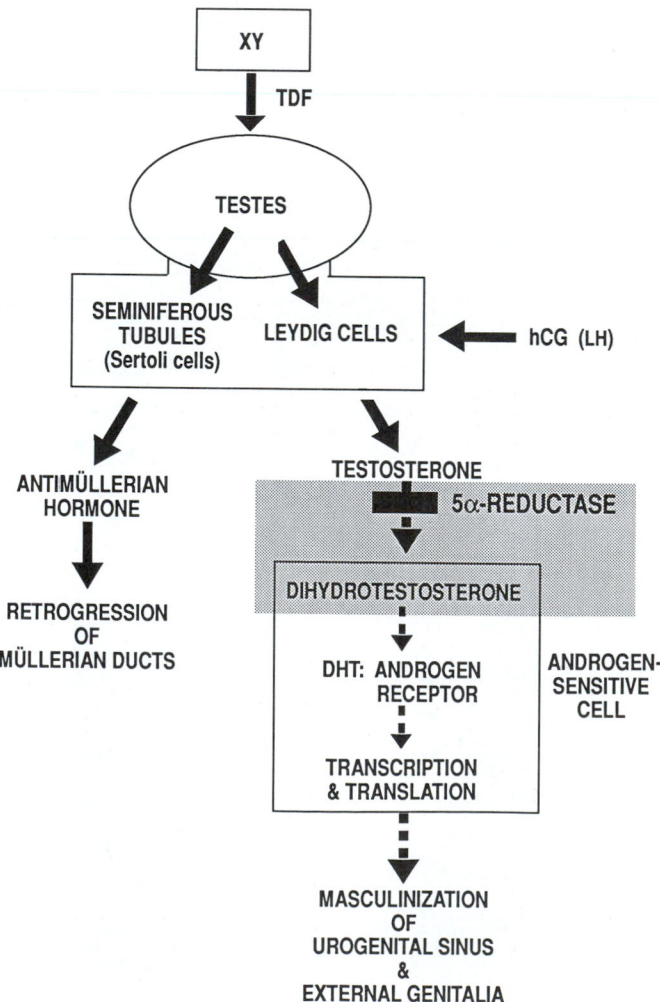

Figure 14–64. A diagrammatic scheme of male pseudohermaphroditism resulting from 5α-reductase deficiency.

TABLE 14–31. Salient Features of 5α-Reductase Deficiency

Karyotype: 46,XY

Inheritance: Autosomal recessive

Genitalia: Usually ambiguous with small, hypospadiac phallus; blind vaginal pouch

Wolffian duct derivatives: Normal

Müllerian duct derivatives: Absent

Gonads: Normal testes

Habitus: Partial virilization at puberty without gynecomastia; ↓ facial and body hair, no temporal hair recession; prostate not palpable

Hormone profile: ↓ ratio of 5α/5β C_{21}- and C_{19}-steroids in urine; ↑ plasma testosterone/dihydrotestosterone (T/DHT) ratio before and after hCG stimulation; modest ↑ plasma LH ↓ conversion of T → DHT in vivo

gynecomastia: the voice deepens, muscle mass increases, and the phallus, although bound in chordee of variable severity, enlarges to 4 to 8 cm in length. The bifid scrotum becomes rugated and pigmented, and the testes enlarge and descend into the labioscrotal folds. However, none of the postpubertal affected males had acne, more than sparse facial or body hair, temporal hair recession, or enlargement of the prostate. Histological examination of the adult testes in seven affected males demonstrates Leydig cell hyperplasia.[715] In adult patients with undescended testes, the seminiferous tubules may contain only Sertoli cells or impaired spermatogenesis may be observed.[715, 716] Patients with descended testes may have histological findings similar to those of patients with undescended testes, although spermatogenesis may be seen in some.[715, 716] Interestingly, although 18 of 38 affected male patients in this family were raised "unambiguously" as females, 17 of the 18 changed to a male gender identity and 16 changed to a male gender role after the onset of puberty[192] (Fig. 14–65A and B).

The hormonal profile in these patients is consistent with defective 5α-reduction of testosterone to dihydrotestosterone in androgen target tissues.[640, 710] After the onset of puberty, the plasma testosterone levels are normal to elevated and the dihydrotestosterone levels are decreased in affected males.[640, 713, 716] The testosterone/dihydrotestosterone concentration ratio in peripheral blood is increased to 35 to 84 in affected adults in contrast to the normal male ratio of 12 ± 3.1.[640, 717] Prepubertally, because of the low levels of plasma androgens, the testosterone/dihydrotestosterone ratio may be normal in affected males under basal conditions;[717] however, after hCG stimulation of testosterone secretion, an abnormal ratio can be readily demonstrated.[717] Postpubertally, plasma LH concentrations are minimally elevated and plasma FSH values tend to be higher than in age-matched controls. Additional features of 5α-reductase deficiency are diminished ratios of urinary 5α-reduced to 5β-reduced C_{19}- and C_{21}-steroids and deficient or abnormal 5α-reductase activity in fibroblasts cultured from genital skin (the preferred source for in vitro studies).[640, 714, 716] The androgen receptor is normal qualitatively and quantitatively. Adult females homozygous for the defect have no clinical manifestations.[716] Heterozygotes for 5α-reductase deficiency have intermediate ratios of urinary 5α-reduced to 5β-reduced C_{19}-steroids (e.g., androsterone/etiocholanolone).[640]

5α-Reductase deficiency is inherited as an autosomal recessive trait and causes abnormal sex differentiation and other clinical manifestations only in males homozygous for the trait. The enzyme defect is genetically heterogeneous. Three types of mutations that affect the 5α-reductase enzyme in this disorder have been described. In the first reports, including the families from the Dominican Republic and Dallas, enzyme studies of genital biopsy specimens and fibroblast cultures derived from genital skin indicated a very low level (deficiency) of 5α-reductase activity.[640, 718] A second type of defect, an alteration of the stability of the enzyme, was described in a family from Los Angeles.[719, 720] In this kinship, 5α-reductase activity was low in fresh biopsy specimens of genital skin but in the low-normal range in cultured

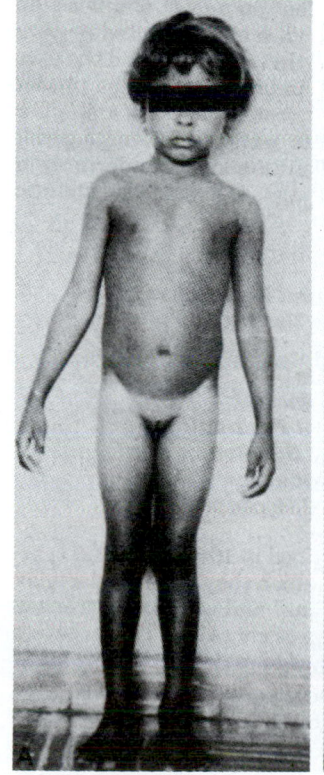
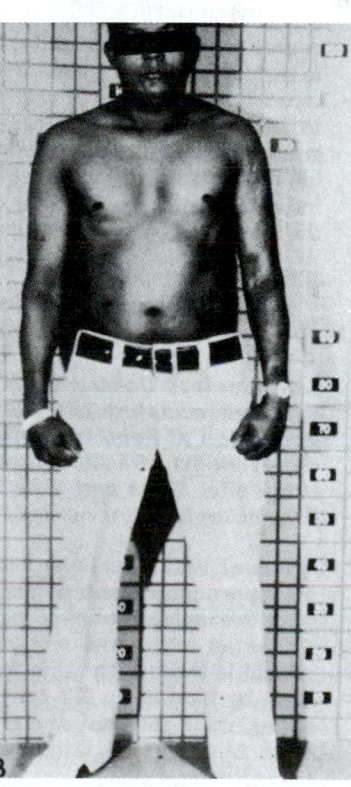

Figure 14–65. *A*, A prepubertal 46,XY child with 5α-reductase deficiency who was raised as a female. *B*, A postpubertal male with 5α-reductase deficiency who has virilized and changed gender role behavior. (From Peterson RE, Imperato-McGinley J, Gautier T, et al. Male pseudohermaphroditism due to 5α-steroid deficiency. Am J Med 1977; 62:170–191.)

fibroblasts. The enzyme bound testosterone normally but had a low affinity for the cofactor NADPH, and thus the 5α-reductase was unstable and had a rapid turnover.[720] A third variant 5α-reductase in another affected individual had intermediate activity and an intermediate turnover rate compared with those in fibroblasts in the family from Los Angeles.[721]

The phenotype of patients with 5α-reductase deficiency supports the hypothesis that testosterone induces differentiation of the male ducts and dihydrotestosterone causes male differentiation of the urogenital sinus, prostate, and external genitalia.[722] Peterson and colleagues[716] postulated that the increased muscle mass, deepening of the voice, spermatogenesis, and male sex drives seen at puberty in these patients are testosterone mediated, whereas acne, temporal hair recession, facial hair, and prostatic enlargement are dihydrotestosterone dependent. The growth of the phallus at puberty, despite the severe 5α-reductase deficiency and incomplete masculinization of the external genitalia during fetal life, is not well explained. The androgen receptor also binds testosterone, but with a lower affinity, and the sustained high levels of circulating testosterone attained at puberty may be a factor in the growth of the phallus. In addition, the enzyme defect is incomplete and at puberty the plasma concentration of dihydrotestosterone, although low, is detectable; further, the hormonal environment is different at puberty in that large quantities of steroids that compete for the androgen receptor, such as progesterone, are not present as they are in utero. Hodgins[723] suggested that 5α-reductase protects the male fetus from the antiandrogenic action of progesterone by converting it to 5α-dihydroprogesterone, which is only one fourth as effective as progesterone in displacing testosterone and dihydrotestosterone from the androgen receptor. Patients with 5α-reductase deficiency do not manifest gynecomastia at puberty because the production rate of estrogen is not increased and the testosterone/estrogen ratio is normal.[724]

The study[192] of gender identity and gender identity transformation of patients with 5α-reductase deficiency in the southwestern Dominican Republic raised questions about the relative influence and interaction of male sex hormones, sex of rearing, social conditions, and learning on psychosexual development (see section on psychosexual differentiation). Another genetic isolate of 5α-reductase–deficient patients was described from New Guinea by Herdt and Davidson.[194] As in the Dominican Republic isolate, a third category of sex was identified in this culture, the "Turnim man." However, sex reversal at puberty was not as common in this isolate and whether it occurred appeared to be a function of social and cultural pressure rather than hormonal imprinting.[194]

Diagnosis. The diagnosis of 5α-reductase deficiency should be suspected in all prepubertal male pseudohermaphrodites with perineoscrotal hypospadias with or without a blind vaginal pouch and in male pseudohermaphrodites who virilize at puberty without evidence of gynecomastia. Virilization at puberty and absence of gynecomastia in male pseudohermaphrodites are not unique to 5α-reductase deficiency. For example, 17-oxidoreductase deficiency and partial androgen insensitivity may present in this manner but can be distinguished biochemically from 5α-reductase deficiency. The diagnosis of 5α-reductase deficiency can be confirmed prepubertally as well as postpubertally by demonstrating an abnormally high testosterone/dihydrotestosterone ratio in peripheral blood before and/or after hCG administration.[717, 725–728] The testosterone/dihydrotestosterone ratio under basal conditions in postpubertal affected males is 35 to 84, whereas the ratio in normal men is 12 ± 3.1.[689, 716] In normal male infants, when

testosterone and dihydrotestosterone are detectable, the testosterone/dihydrotestosterone ratio ranges from 1.7 to 17 (mean ± SD, 4.9 ± 2.85).[717] In view of the low levels of testosterone and dihydrotestosterone in prepubertal males, it is usually necessary to administer hCG (1000 to 2000 U IM every 48 h × 3) to demonstrate the defect. Affected patients with 5α-reductase deficiency have high testosterone/dihydrotestosterone ratios after hCG administration. After a course of hCG, the ratio is 5.2 ± 1.5 in normal male infants (17 d to 6 mo) and 11 ± 4.4 in normal prepubertal males (6 mo to 14 y).[717] Similarly, the ratio of 5α to 5β metabolites of testosterone in urine is a marker both prepubertally and postpubertally of 5α-reductase deficiency.[716, 726] By using both basal and hCG-induced increases in testosterone level and urinary analyses of 5α- and 5β-steroid metabolites, Imperato-McGinley and co-workers[727] diagnosed 5α-reductase deficiency in three infants between the ages of 1 and 3 mo.[727] The plasma testosterone/dihydrotestosterone and urinary 5α/5β-steroid ratios were lower in infancy than later in life, which suggested that 5α-reductase activity decreases with age in normal as well as affected individuals.[727] Less readily available but more direct studies that can be used to confirm the diagnosis of 5α-reductase deficiency include determination of the in vitro conversion of testosterone to dihydrotestosterone by genital skin fibroblasts[640, 714, 728] and measurement of the blood production rate of dihydrotestosterone.[729] 5α-Reductase activity can be diminished in patients with other disorders, including the receptor-negative form of androgen resistance, porphyria, hypothyroidism, low-triiodothyronine syndromes (e.g., anorexia or chronic illness), and Cushing syndrome.[714]

Early diagnosis of 5α-reductase deficiency is important because of its bearing on the assignment of sex in the affected infant. The natural history of patients with this deficiency—that is, the propensity in some patients for male gender role behavior and for virilization at puberty—makes male assignment of neonatally diagnosed patients appealing. On the other hand, this decision necessitates extensive surgical repair as well as hormone therapy. Theoretically, therapy with dihydrotestosterone should increase phallus length into the normal range for age and enable repair of hypospadias. However, dihydrotestosterone has not been generally available in the past.[730] Carpenter and co-workers[731] described an infant who was diagnosed at 9 mo of age with 5α-reductase deficiency. The child had been assigned a male gender at birth. The genitalia exhibited penoscrotal hypospadias with a phallus 1.9 cm in length and bound down in chordee. The testes were normal and in the scrotum. No müllerian structures were present on pelvic sonography. Therapy was instituted with dihydrotestosterone, 25 mg/d (2% by weight in a cold cream base), applied to the patient's abdomen. The plasma dihydrotestosterone level 12 h after application was 2.0 nmol/L (58 ng/dL), which is within the normal adult male range.[731] Four months of therapy resulted in an increase of stretched phallus length from 1.8 to 3.8 cm. No advancement in bone maturation was noted. Hypospadias repair was undertaken, and a second course of dihydrotestosterone was given without consequence.[731] Our experience with males with microphallus suggests that it would be prudent to maintain the phallus length at or above the 50% range for age by using additional short courses of dihydrotestosterone until the onset of puberty and spontaneous phallus development. In adults with 5α-reductase deficiency, supraphysiological doses of testosterone have resulted in normal dihydrotestosterone levels and satisfactory virilization.[706] Hence, a short course of testosterone enanthate in oil theoretically should be effective in augmenting phallus size in infants and children with 5α-reductase deficiency. Dihydrotestosterone heptanoate would be preferable but is not yet approved by the U.S. Food and Drug Administration.[730] No experience with these regimens in affected male infants has been reported. In patients reared as females, gonadectomy before puberty, plastic repair of genitalia, and estrogen replacement at an age appropriate for puberty are indicated.

Dysgenetic Male Pseudohermaphroditism (Ambiguous Genitalia Resulting from Dysgenetic Gonads)

Ambiguous development of the genital ducts, urogenital sinus, and external genitalia occurs in patients with X chromatin–negative variants of the syndrome of gonadal dysgenesis, such as 45,X/46,XY mosaicism or certain structural abnormalities of the Y chromosome, and in patients with familial forms of 46,XY gonadal dysgenesis (see discussion of gonadal dysgenesis). These disorders are classified as abnormalities of gonadal differentiation, but patients with faulty testicular differentiation can present with the clinical syndrome of male pseudohermaphroditism[732, 733] (Fig. 14–66). Consequently, these disorders must be considered in the differential diagnosis. We have used the designation "dysgenetic male pseudohermaphroditism," a term suggested by Federman, to describe this group of patients, whose gonadal development is often asymmetrical and on either side varies from a gonadal streak to a dysgenetic testis to a normal testis. The prevalence of malignant gonadal tumors in dysgenetic male pseudohermaphroditism is increased.

MALE PSEUDOHERMAPHRODITISM ASSOCIATED WITH DEGENERATIVE RENAL DISEASE. Anomalies of the urinary tract are common in patients with abnormalities of genital differentiation.[734] Less common is the association of male pseudohermaphroditism with congenital or early-onset renal disease (diffuse mesangial sclerosis) and Wilms tumor (Drash syndrome[406, 735, 735a]) or with childhood onset of renal disease and gonadal tumors (Frasier syndrome[407]). Familial occurrence has been described. The linkage of male pseudohermaphroditism with renal disease suggests a common developmental aberration during organogenesis of the testis and kidney of undetermined origin and multifactorial etiology. Of note is the association of a deletion of band p13 on the short arm of chromosome 11 (11p−) with aniridia, mental retardation, and a high risk for developing nephroblastoma and/or gonadoblastoma in both genotypic males and females.[736] Genotypic males with this chromosomal abnormality exhibit ambiguous or hypoplastic male genitalia, including bifid scrotum, hypospadias, and cryptorchidism.

THE "VANISHING TESTES SYNDROME" (EMBRYONIC TESTICULAR REGRESSION SYNDROME; XY GONADAL DYSGENESIS→XY GONADAL AGENESIS→RUDIMENTARY TESTIS SYNDROME→CONGENITAL ANORCHIA). Various terms have been used to describe the spectrum of genital anomalies resulting from cessation of testicular function during the middle phase of male sex differentiation, from 8 to 14 wk of gestation. We first used the term vanishing testes syndrome to describe this heterogeneous group of male pseudohermaphrodites in 1957 because the genitalia in these cases suggested that the fetal testicular deficiency occurred and the testes "vanished" (for an obscure reason) at some time during the process of male sex differentiation. These patients have a 46,XY karyotype. Gonadal elements are absent, and the differentiation of the genital ducts, urogenital sinus, and external genitalia is variable. At one end of the spectrum is the group of patients with female external and internal genitalia in whom the deficiency of embryonic testicular function presumably occurred before 8 wk of

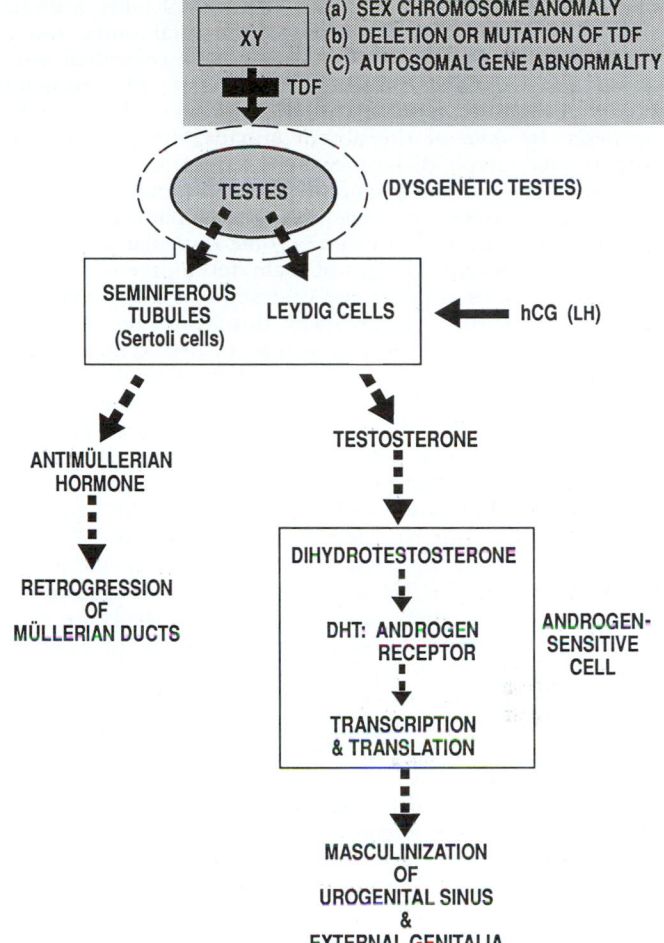

Figure 14–66. A diagrammatic representation of the pathogenesis of dysgenetic male pseudohermaphroditism. This condition can result from a sex chromosome anomaly or from a mutant gene in the male sex determination or differentiation cascade. The degree of masculinization is dependent on the functional ability of the dysgenetic gonads to produce AMH and testosterone.

gestation, that is, 46,XY gonadal dysgenesis.[737] Lack of or deficient function of the fetal testes between 8 and 10 wk of gestation would lead to ambiguous genitalia and variable development of the genital ducts, from complete absence of both müllerian and wolffian ducts to partial development of either. This form of dysgenetic male pseudohermaphroditism has been referred to by some as the "XY gonadal agenesis syndrome."[738–740] Loss of testicular function after the critical phase of male differentiation (about 12 to 14 wk) results in anorchia, a syndrome characterized by the finding of normal male differentiation both internally and externally but no gonadal tissue. Sporadic and familial forms of unilateral and bilateral anorchia, including monozygotic twins concordant and discordant for anorchia, have been described.[741–743] Fetal testicular insufficiency and incomplete regression of the fetal testes after 12 to 14 wk would be expected to produce a syndrome similar to that described by Bergada and colleagues,[744, 745] that is, small rudimentary testes with microphallus and male ejaculatory ducts.

The nature of the underlying defect, which in some cases leads to absence or regression of genital ducts as well as testes, is not known. Several sibships with multiple affected individuals have been described. Josso and Briard[746] reported two siblings, one of whom was a normally differentiated male with microphallus and anorchia. The other patient had a 46,XY karyotype but was raised as a female.

She had a normal clitoris, fused labioscrotal folds, a single perineal opening that led into a urogenital sinus, and a vagina. At laparotomy, absent gonads with coexistent müllerian and wolffian structures were found. This patient's phenotype was compatible with a diagnosis of XY gonadal agenesis. In spite of the absent gonads, the patients had marked phenotypic differences in the internal and external genitalia. The coexistence of so-called XY gonadal agenesis and anorchia in the same sibship suggests that the disorders are related and are due to embryonic testicular regression occurring at different stages of male development in utero; the familial cases support the operation of a rare, mutant gene in at least some patients with this syndrome.

The diagnosis of anorchia can be suspected in normally differentiated males with cryptorchidism and elevated gonadotropin levels. We have demonstrated a diphasic pattern of gonadotropin levels in anorchic males similar to that seen in females with gonadal dysgenesis.[747] In particular, plasma FSH levels are elevated in infancy, decrease into the normal range in midchildhood, and rise again into the agonadal range after age 9 to 10. LHRH-induced increases in gonadotropin levels are elevated throughout infancy and childhood. Hence, the LHRH test may be helpful diagnostically in midchildhood, when basal gonadotropin levels are normal.[748] It has been proposed that the finding of elevated plasma FSH levels in conjunction with lack of a plasma testosterone response to hCG (1000 to 2000 U IM every 48 h for seven doses) establishes the diagnosis of anorchia and obviates the need for laparotomy.[748] This approach has been called into question by the demonstration of testes at laparotomy in two prepubertal males in whom no testosterone response to hCG was elicited.[749] CT or MRI scans, sonography, and laparoscopy are useful procedures for evaluation of the patient with suspected anorchia.

Defects in Synthesis, Secretion, or Response to Antimüllerian Hormone

PERSISTENT MÜLLERIAN DUCT SYNDROME (FEMALE DUCTS IN OTHERWISE NORMAL MEN, HERNIA UTERI INGUINALE). More than 150 men and boys have been described who have relatively well-developed testes, male ducts, and genitalia as well as müllerian structures (Fig. 14–67).[750–754] The diagnosis is often not made until müllerian structures are encountered in patients undergoing inguinal hernia repair, orchiopexy, or abdominal surgery. Two anatomical forms exist.[755] In the more prevalent form, there is a hernia in which a partially descended testis is present. In addition, the uterus and the ipsilateral tube are in the hernia or can be brought down by traction.[755] In the other form, the uterus and tubes as well as the testes are in the pelvis. Approximately 30% of patients with this syndrome have transverse testicular ectopia.[755] The vasa deferentia are often embedded in the uterine wall, and the epididymides are contained in the mesosalpinx.

The retention of müllerian structures in otherwise normally differentiated males can be attributed to (1) failure of the testis to synthesize and secrete AMH, (2) synthesis of a structurally abnormal protein, (3) a defect in the response of the duct to the AMH, that is, a receptor defect, or (4) an abnormality in the timing of secretion of the hormone.[756] In a study of six patients, two synthesized biologically and immunologically active AMH, suggesting a receptor defect or one related to the time of onset of synthesis and release of the hormone.[755] The other four patients from a family cohort had no measurable biologically or immunologically reactive AMH. However, AMH mRNA was present in normal amounts. This study supports the genetic heterogeneity of this syndrome.

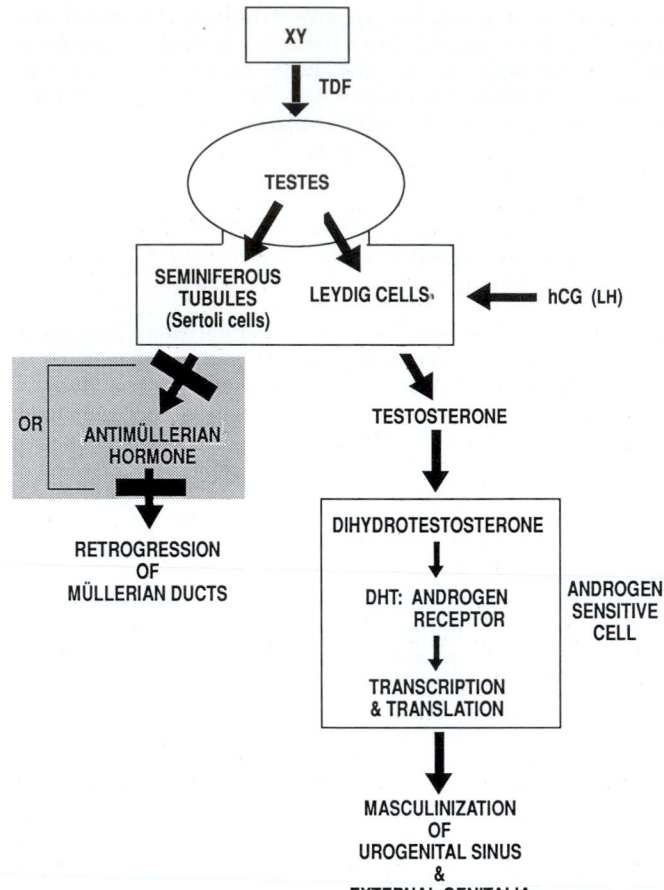

Figure 14–67. A diagrammatic representation of the pathogenesis of the persistent müllerian duct syndrome.

The gene for AMH has been cloned and mapped to chromosome 19.[757] In most familial cases, inheritance is consistent with a sex-limited, autosomal recessive trait. Care must be exercised in repair of the cryptorchidism and resection of the müllerian structures because of the proximity of the vasa deferentia and epididymides to the female duct derivative.[755] Examination of testicular biopsy specimens has revealed normal germ cell populations, and the risk of malignancy does not appear to be higher than in other patients with cryptorchidism.[755]

Maternal Ingestion of Progestogens and Estrogens

Progestogens and synthetic estrogens alone and in combination have been implicated but not proved as rare causes of male pseudohermaphroditism. Courrier and Jost[758] in 1942 were the first to demonstrate an antiandrogen effect on the male fetus induced by a synthetic progestogen, ethisterone. Neumann and colleagues[153] observed that relatively high doses of progesterone or of synthetic progestogens impaired urethral groove fusion in a low percentage of fetal male rats. Aarskog[759] reported 130 patients with hypospadias who were studied retrospectively. A history of maternal ingestion of oral progestogens in early pregnancy was obtained in 11 cases. In six the agent was administered for threatened abortion, and in five progestogen in combination with estrogens was given as a pregnancy test. Hypospadias occurred anywhere from the glans to the base of the penile shaft; the location correlated with the week of gestation in which therapy was initiated. Other studies have also suggested an association between progestogens and hypospadias.[760, 761] However, a more recent report has questioned this relationship.[762]

Aarskog postulated that maternal progestogens might inhibit testosterone synthesis by the fetal testes or impair the reduction of testosterone to dihydrotestosterone at the target tissue and thus lead to failure of urethral groove fusion and hypospadias. Some progestogens can inhibit 5α-reductase activity in vitro.[763] Inhibition of this enzymatic activity at an early fetal stage, through placental transfer of drugs given to the mother, for example, could result in impaired masculinization of the male external genitalia. Alternatively, progestogens may bind to androgen receptors and block androgen expression.[723]

Kaplan[764] described male pseudohermaphroditism in a boy whose mother received large doses of diethylstilbestrol during early pregnancy. However, no additional reports of this association have appeared. Because of the report of Herbst linking maternal diethylstilbestrol therapy during pregnancy with vaginal and cervical adenocarcinoma in daughters, abnormalities in the genital tract have been sought in males.[765] An increased incidence of meatal stenosis, epididymal cysts, hypoplastic testes, and abnormal semen has been observed, but hypospadias has not been reported.[766, 767] Thus there is no apparent relationship between the administration of large doses of estrogen during pregnancy and the occurrence of male pseudohermaphroditism.

Unclassified Forms of Abnormal Sexual Development

Significant advances in the understanding of male pseudohermaphroditism and its heterogeneity have been made since the first edition of this book. The major subgroups are now defined, including recognition of enzyme defects in testosterone biosynthesis and of disorders resulting from defective androgen action. Nonetheless, there are forms of male pseudohermaphroditism that are not readily categorized and others in which the pathogenesis is obscure.

Sexual Abnormalities of Unknown Cause in Males

HYPOSPADIAS. Hypospadias, which may be defined as incomplete fusion of the penile urethra without a urogenital sinus, is a relatively common anomaly of the lower urinary tract with an estimated incidence of 1 to 8 per 1000 male births.[760, 768–770] On theoretical grounds, deficient virilization of the external genitalia implies either subnormal Leydig cell function in utero, a mild degree of androgen insensitivity, or improper chronological correlation between hormone level and the critical time for the tissue to respond to androgen. In the past, there was little evidence for suspecting any of these mechanisms in most patients, and nonendocrine factors that impair differentiation of the primordia were assumed to be responsible for most instances of this anomaly.[768] However, more recent studies have identified a subgroup of males with simple hypospadias who appear to have an abnormality in the androgen receptor[771, 772] or a defect in the nuclear localization of androgen.[773] Further studies will be necessary to document the significance of these and other observations in the pathogenesis of simple hypospadias.[774] Approximately 40% of the cases of hypospadias have associated anomalies of the urogenital tract, most of which are mild. Hypospadias as an isolated anomaly occurs in families, has about a 10% recurrence rate, and is usually of polygenic or multifactoral origin.[768, 769, 774, 775] In addition, hypospadias is a feature of over 20 malformation syndromes.[752, 776]

Aarskog[777] has carried out a careful prospective study of 100 consecutive patients with hypospadias without other somatic anomalies, most of whom were referred from a plastic and reconstructive surgery clinic. No familial cases were encountered. One patient was a genetic female with congenital virilizing adrenal hyperplasia, five had sex chromosome abnormalities (45,X/46,XY or 46,XX/46,XY mosaicism), one had the incomplete form of 46,XY gonadal dysgenesis, and nine were from pregnancies during which the mother had taken exogenous progestational compounds during the first trimester. Hence, in 15% of these patients, a pathogenetic mechanism was found or suspected.

The mildest and most common form of hypospadias is glandular or coronal and occurs in 87% of cases. Extensive endocrine and cytogenetic evaluation of the otherwise normal male with glandular hypospadias and no somatic anomalies is probably not warranted. More severe hypospadias with or without cryptorchidism and somatic anomalies warrants complete evaluation, including karyotype analysis, gonadotropin and hCG stimulation tests, and visualization of the genitourinary tract.

CRYPTORCHIDISM. Undescended testes, the most common urogenital abnormality in malformation syndromes, is associated with more than 40 syndromes.[776] Although normal testes may fail to descend into the scrotum because of coincidental anatomical abnormalities, in many instances cryptorchidism is due to a defective testis. Fetal pituitary gonadotropin deficiency, either partial or complete, may play a role in some instances of cryptorchidism as well as microphallus.[778–780] Cryptorchidism and its management are considered in greater detail in Chapter 13 and in an extensive review.[455]

AMBIGUOUS GENITALIA IN 46,XY MALES WITH MULTIPLE ANOMALIES. Ambiguous genitalia are associated with several malformation syndromes.[249, 752, 776] In malformation syndromes such as the Aarskog and Opitz syndromes, the genital anomaly is of diagnostic significance.[776]

Other reports of rare causes of male pseudohermaphroditism include a patient with a putative "biologically inactive" but immunologically reactive LH[781] and a group of familial cases in which a defect was postulated in fetal Leydig cell maturation with inadequate fetal testosterone production and impaired differentiation of germinal elements.[782] The latter patients had ambiguous genitalia at birth but normal virilization at puberty.

Sexual Abnormalities of Unknown Cause in Females

ABSENCE OR ANOMALOUS DEVELOPMENT OF THE VAGINA ASSOCIATED WITH VARIABLE ABNORMALITIES OF THE MÜLLERIAN STRUCTURES. The association of congenital absence of the vagina with abnormal or absent müllerian structures has been recognized for more than 100 years[783–786] and is usually known as the Mayer-Rokitansky-Küster-Hauser syndrome. Congenital absence of the vagina occurs in 1 in 5000 female births.[783] It was the second most common cause of primary amenorrhea in a series of 538 patients reviewed by Ross and van de Wiele.[787] The principal features of the syndrome are primary amenorrhea in 46,XX females with well-developed female secondary sexual characteristics, an absent or hypoplastic vagina, and müllerian derivatives that vary from a normal uterus to bicornuate cords to absence of the uterus. Ovarian function is usually normal, and patients exhibit cyclic gonadotropin secretion with ovulation.[788] Renal and skeletal anomalies are usually present.[783, 786, 789] Clitorimegaly is not a feature of the Mayer-Rokitansky-Küster-Hauser syndrome, which distinguishes it from the adrenal and nonadrenal forms of female pseudohermaphroditism; the 46,XX karyotype and normal plasma gonadal steroid values differentiate this disorder from testicular feminization.

Ultrasonography and CT and MRI scans are useful for determining the presence of a uterus and its structure. Hematocolpos is a preventable complication if surgical reconstruction is begun before puberty is advanced.[790, 791] If the vagina is too small for sexual intercourse, nonsurgical or surgical correction should be undertaken at an appropriate age. Vaginal lubrication, orgasm, and marital relations have been reported to be satisfactory in adults who have had vaginal reconstruction.[792]

MANAGEMENT OF PATIENTS EXHIBITING AMBISEXUAL DEVELOPMENT

Considerations Governing Choice of Sex for Rearing

With proper assignment of sex for rearing and appropriate subsequent management, individuals with ambiguities of the genitalia should be able to lead well-adjusted lives and ultimately attain a satisfactory sex life. To obtain this favorable result, it is incumbent on the physician to make a correct diagnosis as early as possible and to reach a firm decision on the sex for rearing. We look upon the detection of genital ambiguity in a newborn infant as a neonatal psychosocial emergency. Once the sex for rearing is assigned, the gender role is thereafter reinforced by appropriate employment of whatever surgical, hormonal, and psychological measures are indicated.

Deeply ingrained in our culture is the concept that some innate biological difference between males and females is responsible for the behavioral differences between boys and girls as well as for the sexual orientation as adults. Studies of patients reared in a sex discordant with their chromosomal sex, gonadal sex, hormonal sex, and even external genital organs have clearly shown, however, that no one parameter is an infallible basis on which to assign sex for rearing. This choice should therefore be governed principally by the possibilities that exist for achieving unambiguous and sexually useful genital structures.

The hormonal sex expected at maturity and the possibilities for fertility are of secondary importance except in patients with female pseudohermaphroditism in whom the abnormality is limited to a surgically correctable ambiguity of the external genitalia. Also, in affected infants with 5α-reductase deficiency, the dramatic virilization that may take place at puberty and the consequent male gender identification make the assignment of a male sex of rearing a defensible decision.

With the exception of female pseudohermaphrodites and rare true hermaphrodites reared as females, ambiguities of the external genitalia are caused by lesions that invariably render the person infertile. Thus the major consideration in these patients should be the possibility of achieving cosmetic and functionally normal external genitalia by surgical and endocrinological means. In considering a decision to recommend a male sex of rearing, we believe that greater emphasis should be placed on the size of the shaft and glans and its potential for growth than on the degree of labioscrotal fusion. *All* phenotypic males with microphallus (penis length less than 2.5 cm at birth) should be given, after appropriate measures to exclude a sexual anomaly, a trial of testosterone enanthate in oil, 25 to 50 mg IM monthly

for three doses, to ascertain the potential of the phallus for further growth before a decision on sex of rearing is made.[779] Failure of the phallus to lengthen significantly (mean response 2.0 ± 0.6 cm [SD]) suggests that the phallus lacks the capacity for growth in later childhood and at puberty and raises for consideration a female sex assignment.[793] Principles governing the differential diagnosis and the surgical, hormonal, and psychological management of patients with genital ambiguity are treated more extensively in the following sections.

Differential Diagnosis of Ambisexual Development in Infancy (Fig. 14–68)

Abnormalities of sex differentiation should be suspected not only in infants with grossly ambiguous genitalia but also in apparent females with inguinal masses, inguinal hernias, or slight clitoral enlargement. Apparent males with cryptorchidism, hypospadias, or unusually small genitalia or gonads likewise deserve close scrutiny. Sufficient investigation should be carried out in the newborn period to permit the assignment of sex with enough firmness to preclude future uncertainty. A karyotype analysis is an imperative first step in all such newborns because the presence of a 46,XX karyotype should suggest the need for additional studies to determine whether female pseudohermaphroditism is present (see Fig. 14–68).

Infants with a 46,XX Karyotype

All infants with sexual ambiguity and a 46,XX karyotype should receive sufficient study in the neonatal period to differentiate the various forms of female pseudohermaphroditism from true hermaphroditism.

Congenital Adrenal Hyperplasia

If female pseudohermaphroditism is secondary to congenital adrenal hyperplasia (primarily $P-450_{c21}$ hydroxylase deficiency), plasma levels of 17-hydroxyprogesterone and androstenedione and excretion of urinary 17-ketosteroids should be markedly elevated. A plasma 17-hydroxyprogesterone level over 90 nmol/L (3000 ng/dL) in an infant with ambiguous genitalia who is 24 h of age or older is virtually diagnostic of $P-450_{c21}$ hydroxylase deficiency. Premature and stressed infants may have marginally elevated plasma 17-hydroprogesterone levels. The diagnosis of congenital adrenal hyperplasia is sometimes difficult in the newborn period and may require multiple steroid determinations and dynamic studies with ACTH. Any infant with ambiguous external genitalia who fails to thrive or who develops vomiting and dehydration during the first few weeks of life should be suspected of having the severe salt-losing type of congenital adrenal hyperplasia. If such an infant is found to have hyperkalemia associated with acidosis and hyponatremia, the diagnosis is virtually assured, and vigorous therapy with glucocorticoids, salt, and mineralocorticoids should be instituted on an urgent basis to prevent collapse and sudden death. Once the diagnosis of adrenal hyperplasia is established, glucocorticoid therapy should be instituted and *continued for life.*

Other Forms of Female Pseudohermaphroditism

46,XX infants may be presumed to have nonadrenal female pseudohermaphroditism if adrenal hyperplasia has been excluded and if there is a reliable history of the mother

1. History: family history, pregnancy (hormones, virilization inspection)
   Palpation of inguinal region and labioscrotal folds; rectal examination
   Karyotype analysis
   Initial studies: plasma 17-hydroxyprogesterone, androstenedione,
   dehydroepiandrosterone, testosterone, & dihydrotestosterone
   Serum electrolytes
   Sonogram or MRI of kidneys, ureters & pelvic contents
   Provisional Dx

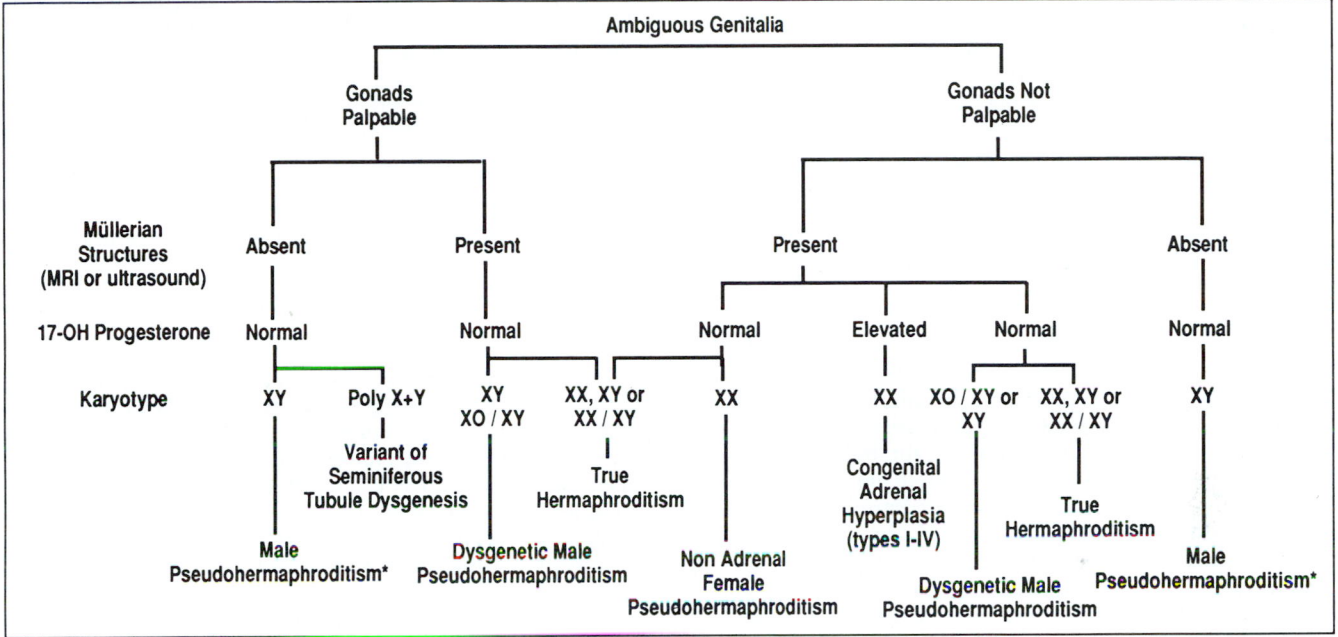

2. "Vaginogram" (urogenital sinogram): selected cases
   Endoscopy, laparotomy, gonadal biopsy: restricted to male pseudohermaphrodites, true hermaphrodites, and selected instances of nonadrenal
   female pseudohermaphroditism

   *Plasma 17-hydroxyprogesterone levels may be modestly elevated in patients with P450$_{c11}$ (Type III), 3β-hydroxysteroid dehydrogenase deficiency
   (Type IV) and are "low" in patients with P-450$_{c17}$ (Type V) and P-450$_{scc}$ deficiency (Type VI)

Figure 14–68. Steps in the diagnosis of intersexuality in infancy and childhood. Step 1 involves initial work-up and provisional diagnosis. Step 2 is utilized in selected cases.

receiving androgens or progestational hormones during pregnancy or if the mother developed some virilizing tendency during pregnancy. These children require no further hormonal medication during childhood and feminize normally at adolescence. In some of these patients nonadrenal female pseudohermaphroditism is associated with gross anomalies of the lower intestine and/or urinary tract. Such children should be studied for the presence of pyelonephritis and anomalies in other systems. Patients with female pseudohermaphroditism usually have a normal uterus and fallopian tubes with ovaries in the normal location. For this reason, the diagnosis should be viewed with suspicion if there is an inguinal hernia or if gonad-like masses are palpable in the groin. Such masses are frequently testes. The presence of a uterus can often be detected in the newborn period by digital examination via the rectum. If there is uncertainty, ultrasonography or an MRI scan of the pelvis may be useful. It is often possible to confirm the presence of endometrial tissue in the newborn infant by cytological means after expressing mucoid secretions from a urogenital sinus by bimanual manipulation of the suspected uterus. When the physiological hyperplasia of the uterus, present at birth, has regressed, the interpretation of a rectal examination may be inconclusive.

True Hermaphroditism

Most patients with true hermaphroditism have a 46,XX karyotype, and it may be difficult to distinguish some of them from the rare idiopathic cases of female pseudohermaphroditism. True hermaphrodites, however, often have gonads located in the labia or inguinal canals; a bipartite gonad is highly suggestive of ovotestes. In true hermaphrodites the assignment of sex should be deferred until the nature of the internal genital structures and gonads can be determined by sonography, MRI, urethroscopy, or radiological study with contrast media and, if necessary, pelvic exploration. The assignment of sex to a true hermaphrodite should be based on the possibilities for surgical correction of the external genitalia. Not infrequently, the heterologous gonadal tissue can be removed. It is important to emphasize the risk of malignant degeneration of the dysgenetic testicular tissue that is retained. In general, assignment of a female sex and an attempt to preserve an ovary or ovarian tissue are appropriate.

Infants with a 46,XY Karyotype

A 46,XY karyotype is found in patients with male pseudohermaphroditism. In many of these patients, the phenotype is so clearly male or female that the sex for rearing is not in question. Nonetheless, efforts should be made to establish an etiological diagnosis, because this may have an important bearing on subsequent management. A detailed family history with construction of a pedigree is important, because many sexual abnormalities are hereditary in nature and this type of historical information is not always volunteered. For example, a history of aunts who have never menstruated or of an inguinal hernia or labial mass in a phenotypic female may suggest the diagnosis of androgen resistance syndrome. The mother should also be asked about drugs or hormones that she may have received during the early part of pregnancy.

Studies during the newborn period should always include an examination of the karyotype. A sufficient number of metaphase plates should be examined to reduce the possibility of overlooking mosaicism. The morphology of the Y chromosome should be examined with the Giemsa and Q-banding techniques and, if indicated, by molecular genetic techniques.

An ultrasound or MRI scan, roentgenological studies of the urogenital sinus after injection of contrast media from a syringe with a blunt tip placed in the single perineal orifice so as to prevent leakage of dye, and fiberoptic endoscopic examination may aid in this initial evaluation. Laparotomy is usually not necessary in the neonatal period because, in choosing the sex of rearing, primary emphasis should be placed on the external genitalia and the possibilities for adequate sexual function. However, before recommending a sex assignment, the anatomical findings must be assessed in the light of karyotypic studies, the pattern of plasma gonadal steroids before and after hCG stimulation, and other measures to identify a specific type of male pseudohermaphroditism.

Urinary steroids and plasma androgens before and after ACTH and hCG (1000 to 2000 U IM every 48 h × 7) should be measured to ascertain whether the patient has a block in testosterone metabolism or 5α-reductase deficiency.[640, 794] If baseline values are available, a shorter course of hCG may be used, for example, 1000 U daily for 3 to 4 d. The testosterone response to hCG may result in significant phallus enlargement. Thus in addition to providing objective information about the functional capacity of the Leydig cells to secrete testosterone, the test may also provide evidence for the capacity of androgen-sensitive target tissues to respond to this stimulus. In the patient with male pseudohermaphroditism and no evidence of a testosterone biosynthetic error, 5α-reductase deficiency, or dysgenetic male pseudohermaphroditism, clinical or metabolic evidence of testosterone responsiveness should be documented before a sex assignment is made.

The problem of sex assignment in the male infant with a micropenis is particularly vexing. Male infants with hypopituitarism frequently have small genitalia and unilateral or bilateral cryptorchidism, and this diagnosis should be excluded by appropriate pituitary function studies before considering sex reassessment. It is our view that all male infants with microphallus should be given a trial of testosterone parenterally before concluding that the phallus lacks the capacity for growth.[779] Administration of a dose of 25 to 50 mg of testosterone enanthate IM once a month for 3 mo should provide an adequate androgen stimulus to make this assessment.[779] This treatment may cause a slight advancement of the skeletal age, but this consideration is trivial when weighed against the momentous question of deciding the future sex of rearing. It is also important to assess phallus size periodically and to repeat the course of testosterone therapy to maintain phallus size within the normal range for age. Some evidence suggests that capacity for penile growth is, at least in part, age related; that is, there is a progressive loss of growth capacity with age.[795, 796]

In most patients a precise etiological diagnosis and appropriate sex assignment can be made on the basis of the criteria just stated. In the rare patient with no evidence of defective testosterone synthesis, end-organ unresponsiveness to androgen, or testicular dysgenesis, true hermaphroditism should be considered. In these patients laparotomy and the demonstration of both ovarian and testicular tissue will establish the diagnosis.

Once the decision is made to rear the infant as a boy or girl, there should be no further indecision in the mind of the physician or the parents. Nevertheless, for most patients bearing a Y chromosome it is necessary to carry out surgical exploration to determine the structure of the internal genital ducts and gonads. Pelvic exploration can be deferred until plastic procedures on the external genitalia are undertaken.

Reassignment of Sex after the Newborn Period

Frequently, children are assigned an inappropriate sex because of errors in diagnosis or ignorance of the principles that should properly determine this choice. In such cases, the knotty decision to change the sex of rearing or to leave matters undisturbed is largely dependent on the age of the child and the degree to which the gender identity has been established. Money has shown that a change in the sex of rearing is feasible until the age of 1½ y and is sometimes successful until 2½ y,[193, 196, 793] but thereafter, in our culture, serious and sometimes calamitous psychiatric and social consequences may be encountered. Although these concepts have been challenged, change of sex after 18 mo should be undertaken only after a painstaking review of possible alternatives and only if provision has been made for close supervision and long-term counseling of the patient, parents, and siblings.

After adolescence, the patient may reach the decision that he or she has been reared in the wrong sex and may request assistance in changing his or her sex of assignment. If there are sufficient anatomical grounds for this belief, the request should be seriously considered and honored if possible. Such patients may have serious psychiatric disturbances, and both psychiatric and legal counsel should be sought.[797]

Reconstructive Surgery

Because the presence of ambiguous external genitalia is likely to reinforce doubt about the sexual identity of the infant or child, it is desirable to initiate reconstructive surgery as early as is medically and surgically feasible. Money's group has stressed the importance of both early genital operation and psychological support for the family in ensuring a successful outcome.[193, 793] Thus it is highly desirable that surgery on the external genitalia be initiated before 12 mo of age. Certainly, in patients with nonadrenal forms of female pseudohermaphroditism and in male pseudohermaphrodites assigned a female sex, genital reconstruction should be undertaken as soon as possible in the neonatal period.

The management of clitorimegaly in female pseudohermaphrodites and in male pseudohermaphrodites reared as females has been controversial. Three different operative approaches have been recommended: clitoridectomy,[798] clitoral recession,[799] and clitoroplasty.[800–802] Observations on the role of the clitoris as an erotic organ in females[803] have made it clear that clitoridectomy should be avoided. Clitoroplasty, as recommended by Spense and Allen[800] and Shaw,[801] requires excision of the shaft and corpora with retention of the glands. This procedure and modifications of it are used most widely at present. Long-term data are necessary to evaluate the efficacy of this procedure with respect to appearance and sexual function.

The extent of the initial repair of the urogenital sinus and vagina depends in large part on the skill and experience of the surgeon.[804] Even when the initial repair is done by an experienced surgeon, it is not uncommon for patients who have had vaginoplasties performed at age 1½ y or earlier to require secondary operations because of stenosis of the introitus.[805] We feel that reconstruction of a vagina in male pseudohermaphrodites reared as females and female pseudohermaphrodites can be deferred until adolescence or until requested by the patient. A small vaginal pouch can often be enlarged by daily manipulations with a suitable mold.[806] Even if the vagina remains too shallow for satisfactory sexual relations, manual dilatation makes it easier to carry out subsequent surgical correction.

A male with hypospadias usually requires multiple operations to create a phallic urethra. This is a major surgical undertaking and should not be regarded lightly. Circumcision should be avoided to preserve as much tissue as possible. Pelvic exploration can be undertaken (if necessary) simultaneously with the initial operation. It is often desirable to insert prosthetic testes to give the scrotum dependency and to improve cosmetic appearance. These may be changed to adult-sized prostheses in adolescence.

Removal of the Gonads

A high incidence of gonadal tumors in patients with certain forms of gonadal dysgenesis and various other forms of hermaphroditism makes it mandatory that an evaluation of this risk be given priority in deciding if and when the gonads should be removed. Although the incidence of gonadoblastomas and germinomas (seminoma or dysgerminoma) increases near the normal time of adolescence, some of these tumors have been discovered during the first decade. As temporizing serves no useful purpose and may expose the child to hormone secretions inappropriate to the chosen sex for rearing, it is advisable to proceed with gonadectomy concurrently with the initial repair of the external genitalia in patients who are at risk. We are evaluating the use of MRI of the pelvis every 1 to 2 y to screen for gonadal neoplasms in children at risk. Similarly, gonadectomy and removal of the uterus should be carried out as early as possible in the rare female pseudohermaphrodites who have been mistakenly reared as boys and in whom change of sex is inadvisable.

Although prevalence values of gonadal tumors as high as 9% have been reported in testicular feminization, some patients who developed tumors may have had atypical forms of gonadal dysgenesis. The prevalence of gonadal malignancy before age 25 appears to be relatively low. Although gonadectomy should ultimately be carried out in these patients, it is often desirable to leave the gonads in situ until after puberty in the hope that testicular estrogens will promote the development of normal feminine sexual characteristics. In our experience, this greatly reinforces the patient's concept of her sexual identity, and castration to prevent malignancy is often more easily explained to and readily accepted by older girls.

There is a high risk of some degree of virilization at the time of puberty in patients with the variant (incomplete) forms of androgen resistance and with other forms of male pseudohermaphroditism in which a female sex for rearing has been assigned; castration in childhood is desirable. In male pseudohermaphroditism in which a male sex for rear-

ing has been selected, at least partial development of male secondary sexual characteristics will occur with the onset of puberty. Provided the testes are not dysgenetic and are sufficiently descended to permit palpation, it is reasonable to leave the testes in situ. Such patients should be carefully examined at regular intervals for the presence of a tumor. MRI scans and examination of testicular biopsy specimens may be helpful in the early diagnosis of testicular neoplasm.[807]

Hormone substitution therapy in hypogonadal patients should be prescribed in such a way that secondary sexual characteristics emerge appropriately in both timing and sequence. The goal of therapy should be to approximate normal adolescent development as closely as possible.

In females, including patients with the syndrome of gonadal dysgenesis, hormone substitution therapy is initiated with low doses of estrogen (0.3 mg conjugated estrogens or 5 μg ethinyl estradiol) daily by mouth for the first 21 d of the month. Breast enlargement and growth of the uterus frequently occur within 3 mo. Usually, cyclic therapy with estrogen and an oral progestogen is begun after about 6 to 12 mo of estrogen therapy, or sooner if breakthrough bleeding occurs.

Better virilization is usually obtained by repository injections of testosterone than by oral preparations. Many oral androgens have the added disadvantage of predisposing to biliary stasis, jaundice, and hepatic tumors. Rapid virilization is often inadvisable, and it is preferable to bring about adolescent changes gradually over a period of many months in a manner similar to that in normal boys. It should be appreciated that the effect of gonadal steroids on skeletal maturation is dose related, whereas the effect on linear growth is less so. Thus at the inception of therapy the relation between attained stature and skeletal maturation as well as the dosage of androgen prescribed will determine the ultimate effect of this therapy on the adult height. An intial IM dose of 50 mg of testosterone enanthate or other long-acting testosterone ester may be given monthly, beginning at age 12 to 13. Thereafter the dose should be increased gradually over 3 to 4 y to the adult replacement dose of 200 mg every 2 wk, usually after a bone age of 16 y has been attained.

Psychological Management [808]

Few people are sufficiently sophisticated to accept a sex for rearing discordant with their chromosomal or gonadal sex. For this reason, it is advisable to avoid such a disclosure at the beginning and to present the issues in more readily comprehended terms. There should never be any doubt in the mind of parent or patient that a child is being reared in his or her own "true sex," although it is best initially to admit uncertainty regarding the true sex and to urge the parents not to assign a name or send out birth announcements until sufficient studies have been completed. This approach is completely honest if the physician fully recognizes that sex is not a single biological entity with one decisive parameter but rather the net expression of many morphological characteristics and functional potentialities. In the strictest sense, an infant's true sex is in fact the one to which he or she is assigned after these many factors have been thoroughly evaluated. A simple explanation of the double set of sexual organs present in early life is useful because it lays the groundwork for the concept that sex differentiation is often not complete in utero. An analogy to other congenital malformations, such as cleft lip or congenital heart disease, is accurate and easily understood. The parents should be reassured that their child does not have a "reversed sex," nor is their child "half boy and half girl." It should be clearly stated that the anatomical abnormalities in sexual development can be repaired and result in functional sexual organs.

Children reared in an atmosphere in which the sex for rearing is accepted with conviction need not have catastrophic psychological problems. With proper surgical reconstruction and hormonal substitution, most individuals with ambisexual development, although usually infertile, should reach adulthood as well-virilized men or as feminine women capable of achieving satisfactory sexual relationships.

REFERENCES

1. Austin CR, Edwards RG. Mechanisms of Sex Differentiation in Animals and Man. London: Academic, 1981.
2. Burger HM, de Kretser DM, eds. The Testis. 2nd ed. Comprehensive Endocrinology. New York: Raven, 1989.
3. Haseltine FP, McClure ME, Goldberg EH, eds. Genetic Markers of Sex Differentiation. New York: Plenum, 1987.
4. Jirasek JE. Development of the Genital System and Male Pseudohermaphroditism. Baltimore: Johns Hopkins University Press, 1971.
5. Josso N. The Intersex Child. Pediatrics, Adolescent Endocrinology. Vol 8. New York: S. Karger, 1981.
6. McKusick VA. Mendelian Inheritance in Man: Catalogs of Autosomal Dominant, Autosomal Recessive, and X-Linked Phenotypes. 7th ed. Baltimore: Johns Hopkins University Press, 1990.
7. McLaren A, Ferguson-Smith MA, eds. Sex determination in mouse and man. Philos Trans R Soc Lond [Biol] 1988; 322:1–157.
8. McLaren A. Sex determination in mammals. Trends Genet 1988; 42:153–157.
9. Money J, Ehrhardt AA. Man and Woman, Boy and Girl: The Differentiation and Dimorphism of Gender Identity from Conception to Maturity. Baltimore: Johns Hopkins University Press, 1972.
10. Peters H, McNatty KP. The Ovary: A Correlation of Structure and Function in Mammals. New York: Granada, 1980.
11. Simpson JL. Disorders of Sexual Differentiation: Etiology and Clinical Delineation. New York: Academic, 1976.
12. Wachtel SS. H-Y Antigen and the Biology of Sex Determination. New York: Grune & Stratton, 1983.
13. Goodfellow PN, Craig IW, Smith JC, et al., eds. The mammalian Y chromosome: molecular search for the sex determining factor. Development 1987; Suppl 101.
14. Hamerton JL, Jacobs PA, Klinger HP, eds. Paris Conference (1971): Standardization in Human Cytogenetics. Birth Defects: Original Article Series. Vol VIII. No 7. New York: The National Foundation, 1972; 1–46.
15. Grumbach MM, Morishima A, Taylor JH. Human sex chromosome abnormalities in relation to DNA replication and heterochromatinization. Proc Natl Acad Sci USA 1963; 49:581–589.
16. Morishima A, Grumbach MM, Taylor JH. Asynchronous duplication of human chromosomes and the origin of sex chromatin. Proc Natl Acad Sci USA 1962; 48:756–763.
17. Latt SA. Patterns of late replication in human X chromosomes. In: Vallet HL, Porter IH, eds. Genetic Mechanisms of Sexual Development. New York: Academic, 1979; 305–329.
18. Caspersson T, Zech L, Johansson C, et al. Identification of human chromosomes by DNA-binding fluorescent agents. Chromosoma 1970; 30:215–217.
19. Caspersson T, Zech L. Chromosome identification by fluorescence. Hosp Pract 1972; 7:51–62.
20. Pardue ML, Gall JG. Chromosomal localization of mouse satellite DNA. Science 1970; 168:1356–1358.
21. Pearson P. The use of new staining techniques for human chromosome identification. J Med Genet 1972; 9:264–275.
22. Morishima A, Grumbach MM. The interrelationship of sex chromosome constitution and phenotype in the syndrome of gonadal dysgenesis and its variants. Ann NY Acad Sci 1968; 155:695–715.
23. Disteche CM, Saal H, Friedman C, et al. Quantitative analysis of sex chromosome mosaicism with X-Y DNA probes. Am J Hum Genet 1986; 38:751–758.
24. Ford CE. Mosaics and chimaeras. Br Med Bull 1969; 25:104–109.
25. Harbison M, Hassold T, Kobryn C, et al. Molecular studies of the parental origin and nature of human X isochromosomes. Cytogenet Cell Genet 1988; 47:217–222.
26. Page DC. Sex reversal: deletion mapping of the male-determining function of the human Y chromosome. Cold Spring Harbor Symp Quant Biol 1986; 51:229–235.
27. Bengtsson BO, Goodfellow PN. The effect of recombination between the X and Y chromosomes of mammals. Ann Hum Genet 1987; 51:57–64.
28. Goodfellow PN, Darling SM. Genetics of sex determination in man and mouse. Development 1988; 102:251–258.
29. Burgoyne PS. Genetic homology and crossing over in the X and Y chromosomes of mammals. Hum Genet 1982; 61:85–90.
30. Goodfellow PN, Goodfellow PJ, Pym B, et al. Genes on the human Y chromosome. In: Haseltine FP, McClure ME, Goldberg EH, eds. Genetic Markers of Sex Differentiation. New York: Plenum, 1987: 99–111.
31. Goodfellow PN, Pym B, Pritchard C, et al. MIC2: a human pseudoautosomal gene. Philos Trans R Soc Lond [Biol] 1988; 322:145–154.
32. Gough N, Gearing DP, Nicola N, et al. Localization of the human GM-CSF receptor gene to the X-Y pseudoautosomal region. Nature 1990; 345:734–736.
33. Ellis NA, Goodfellow PJ, Pym B, et al. The pseudoautosomal boundary in man is defined by an Alu repeat sequence inserted on the Y chromosome. Nature 1989; 337:81–84.
34. Palmer MS, Sinclair AH, Berta P, et al. Genetic evidence that ZFY is not the testis-determining factor. Nature 1989; 342:937–939.
35. Sinclair AH, Berta P, Palmer MS, et al. A gene from the human sex determining region encodes a protein with homology to a conserved DNA-binding motif. Nature 1990; 346:240–244.
36. Page DC, Mosher R, Simpson EM, et al. The sex-determining region of the human Y chromosome encodes a finger protein. Cell 1987; 51:1091–1104.
37. Mardon G, Page DC. The sex-determining region of the mouse Y chromosome encodes a protein with a highly acidic domain and 13 zinc fingers. Cell 1989; 56:765–770.
38. Miller J, McLachlan AD, Khy A. Repetitive zinc-binding domains in the protein transcription factor IIIA from Xenopus oocytes. EMBO J 1985; 41:1609–1614.
39. Shapiro LJ. Steroid sulfatase deficiency and X-linked ichthyosis. In: Scriver CR, Beudet AL, Sly WS, et al., eds. The Metabolic Basis of Inherited Disease. 6th ed. New York: McGraw-Hill, 1989: 1945–1964.
40. Yen PH, Allen E, Marsh B, et al. Cloning and expression of steroid sulfatase cDNA and the frequent occurrence of deletions in STS deficiency: implications for X-Y interchange. Cell 1987; 49:443–454.
41. Yen PH, Marsh B, Allen E, et al. The human X-linked steroid sulfatase gene and Y-encoded pseudogene: evidence for an inversion of the Y chromosome during primate evolution. Cell 1988; 55:1123–1135.
42. Simpson E, Chandler P, Goulmy E, et al. Separation of the genetic loci for H-Y antigen and testis determination on the Y chromosome. Nature 1987; 326:876–878.
43. Lau EC, Mohandas TK, Shapiro LJ, et al. The human and mouse amelogenin loci are on the sex chromosomes. Genomics 1989; 4:162–168.
44. Buhler EM. A synopsis of the human Y chromosome. Hum Genet 1980; 55:145–175.
45. Grumbach MM. Genetic mechanisms of sex development. In: Vallet HL, Porter IH, eds. Genetic Mechanisms of Sexual Development. New York: Academic, 1979: 33–74.
46. Wolf U. Sex inversion as a model for the study of sex determination in vertebrates. Philos Trans R Soc Lond [Biol] 1988; 322:97–107.
47. Schneider-Gadicke A, Beer-Romero P, Brown LG, et al. ZFX has a gene structure similar to ZFY, the putative human sex determinant, and escapes X inactivation. Cell 1989; 57:1247–1258.
48. Grumbach MM. Male reproductive tract development, anatomy, physiology and disorders. In: Cooke RE, ed. The Biologic Basis of Pediatric Practice. New York: McGraw-Hill, 1968: 1058–1081.
49. Ferguson-Smith MA. Karyotype-phenotype correlations in gonadal dysgenesis and their bearing on the pathogenesis of malformations. J Med Genet 1965; 2:142–155.
50. McKusick V. Morbid anatomy of the human genome: a review of gene mapping in clinical medicine. Medicine 1987; 66:1–63.
51. Krauss CM, Turksoy N, Atkins L, et al. Familial premature ovarian failure due to an interstitial deletion of the long arm of the X chromosome. N Engl J Med 1987; 317:125–131.
52. Meyer WJ III, Migeon BR, Migeon CJ. Locus on human X chromosome for dihydrotestosterone receptor and androgen insensitivity. Proc Natl Acad Sci USA 1975; 72:1469–1472.
53. Lubahn DB, Joseph DR, Sullivan PM, et al. Cloning of the human androgen receptor complementary DNA and localization to the X chromosome. Science 1988; 240:327–330.
54. Therman E, Sarto GE. Inactivation center on the human X chromosome. In: Sandburg AA, ed. Cytogenetics of the Mammalian X Chromosome. Part A: Basic Mechanisms of X Chromosome Behavior. New York: Alan R. Liss, 1983: 315–325.
55. Barr ML, Bertram EG. A morphological distinction between neurones of the male and female, and the behavior of the nucleolar satellite during acceleration of nucleoprotein synthesis. Nature 1949; 163:676.
56. Ohno S, Kaplan WD, Kinosita R. Formation of the sex chromatin by a single X-chromosome in liver cells of Rattus norvegicus. Exp Cell Res 1959; 18:415–418.
57. Grumbach MM, Morishima A. Sex chromatin and the sex chromosomes: on the origin of sex chromatin from a single X chromosome. Acta Cytol 1962; 6:46–60.
58. Beutler E, Yeh M, Fairbanks VF. The normal human female as a mosaic of X-chromosome activity: studies using the gene for G-6-PD deficiency as a marker. Proc Natl Acad Sci USA 1962; 48:9–16.
59. Lyon MF. The X chromosomes and their levels of activation. In: Sandberg AA, ed. Cytogenetics of the Mammalian X Chromosome. Part

A: Basic Mechanisms of X Chromosome Behavior. New York: Alan R. Liss, 1983: 187–204.

60. Epstein CJ. Expression of the mammalian X chromosome before and after fertilization. Science 1972; 175:1467–1468.

61. Gartler SM, Andina RJ. Mammalian X-chromosome inactivation. Adv Hum Genet 1976; 7:99–140.

62. Davidson RG, Nitowsky HM, Childs B. Demonstration of two populations of cells in the human female heterozygous for glucose-6-phosphate dehydrogenase variants. Proc Natl Acad Sci USA 1963; 50:481–485.

63. Gartler SM, Dyer KA, Marshall Graves JA, et al. A two step model for mammalian X-chromosome inactivation. Prog Clin Biol Res 1985; 198:223–235.

64. Brown CJ, Willard HF. Localization of a gene that escapes inactivation to the X chromosome proximal short arm: implications for X inactivation. Am J Hum Genet 1990; 46:273–279.

64a. Brown CJ, Ballabio A, Rupert JL, et al. A gene from the region of the X inactivation center is expressed exclusively from the inactive X chromosome. Nature 1991; 349:38–44.

64b. Fisher EMC, Beer-Romero P, Brown LG, et al. Homologous ribosomal protein genes on the human X and Y chromosomes: escape from X inactivation and possible implications for Turner syndrome. Cell 1990; 61:1205–1208.

64c. Brown CJ, Lafreniere RG, Powers VE, et al. Localization of the X inactivation center in the human X chromosome in Xq13. Nature 1991; 349:82–84.

65. Eichwald EJ, Silmser CR. Untitled communication. Transplant Bull 1955; 2:148–149.

66. Goldberg EH, Boyse EA, Bennett D, et al. Serological demonstration of H-Y (male) antigen on mouse sperm. Nature 1971; 232:478–480.

67. Bradley MP, Ebensperger C, Wilberg A. Determination of the serologic H-Y antigen in birds and mammals using high-titer antisera and a sensitive urease ELISA. Hum Genet 1987; 76:352–356.

68. Goldberg E. H-Y antigen and sex determination. Philos Trans R Soc Lond [Biol] 1988; 322:72–81.

69. Wachtel SS, Koo GC, Boyse EA. Evolutionary conservation of H-Y ("male") antigen. Nature 1975; 254:270–272.

70. Krco CJ, Goldberg EH. H-Y (male) antigen: detection on eight-cell mouse embryos. Science 1976; 193:1134–1135.

71. Ohno S, Nagai Y, Ciccarese S, et al. Testis-organizing H-Y antigen and the primary sex-determining mechanism of mammals. Recent Prog Horm Res 1979; 35:449–476.

72. Ohno S, Nagai Y, Ciccarese S. Testicular cells lysostripped of H-Y antigen organize ovarian follicle–like aggregates. Cytogenet Cell Genet 1978; 20:351–364.

73. Zenzes MT, Wolf U, Gunther E, et al. Studies on the function of H-Y antigen: dissociation and reorganization experiments of rat gonadal cells. Cytogenet Cell Genet 1978; 20:365–372.

74. Zenzes MT, Wolf U, Engel W. Organization in vitro of ovarian cells into testicular structures. Hum Genet 1978; 44:333–338.

75. Nagai Y, Ciccarese S, Ohno S. The identification of human H-Y antigen and testicular transformation induced by its interaction with the receptor site of bovine fetal ovarian cells. Differentiation 1979; 13:155–164.

76. Ciccarese S, Orsini G, Massari S, et al. Free H-Y antigen induces in vitro testicular differentiation of human XX embryonic indifferent gonads. Cell Differ 1983; 12:185–190.

77. Muller U, Urban E. Reaggregation of rat gonadal cells in vitro: experiments in the function of H-Y antigen. Cytogenet Cell Genet 1981; 31:104–107.

78. Wolf U, Fraccaro M, Mayerova A, et al. A gene controlling H-Y antigen on the X chromosome. Hum Genet 1980; 54:149–154.

79. Lau Y-F, Chan K, Kan YW, et al. Male-enhanced expression and genetic conservation of a gene isolated with anti–H-Y antibody. Trans Assoc Am Physicians 1987; 100:45–53.

80. Melvold RW, Kohn HI, Yergenian G, et al. Evidence suggesting the existence of two H-Y antigens in the mouse. Immunogenetics 1977; 5:33–41.

81. Koo GC, Reidy JA, Nagamine CM. H-Y antigen in XO mice. Immunogenetics 1983; 18:37–44.

82. Simpson E, McLaren A, Chandler P. Evidence for two male antigens in mice. Immunogenetics 1982; 15:609–614.

83. Wilberg UH, Mayerova A. Serologically H-Y antigen–negative XO mice. J Immunogenet 1985; 12:55–63.

84. McLaren A, Simpson E, Tomonari K, et al. Male sexual differentiation in mice lacking H-Y antigen. Nature 1984; 312:552–555.

85. Bishop CE, Weith A, Mattei MG, et al. Molecular aspects of sex determination in mice: an alternative model for the origin of Sxr. Philos Trans R Soc Lond [Biol] 1988; 322:119–124.

86. Mardon G, Mosher R, Disteche CM, et al. Duplication, deletion and polymorphism in the sex-determining region of the mouse Y chromosome. Science 1989; 243:78–80.

87. Nagamine CM, Chan K, Kozak CA, et al. Chromosome mapping and expression of a putative testis-determining gene in mouse. Science 1989; 243:80–83.

88. Burgoyne PS, Levy ER, McLaren A. Spermatogenic failure in male mice lacking H-Y antigen. Nature 1986; 315:224–226.

89. Page DC, de la Chapelle A, Weissenbach J. Chromosome Y specific DNA in related human XX males. Nature 1985; 315:224–226.

90. Page DC, Brown LG, de la Chapelle A. Exchange of terminal portions of X and Y chromosomal short arms in human XX males. Nature 1987; 328:437–440.

91. Mardon G, Page C. The sex determining region of the mouse Y chromosome encodes a protein with a highly acidic domain and 13 zinc fingers. Cell 1989; 56:765–770.

92. Chandra HS. Is human X chromosome inactivation a sex determining device? Proc Natl Acad Sci USA 1985; 82:6947–6949.

93. German JL. Gonadal dimorphism explained as a dosage effect of a locus on the sex chromosome, the gonad-differentiation locus (GDL). Am J Hum Genet 1988; 42:414–421.

94. Ferguson-Smith MA, Affara NA. Accidental X-Y recombination and the aetiology of XX males and true hermaphroditism. Philos Trans R Soc Lond [Biol] 1988; 322:133–144.

95. Sinclair AH, Foster JW, Spenser JA, et al. Sequences homologous to ZFY, a candidate human sex determining gene, are autosomal in marsupials. Nature 1988; 336:780–782.

96. Sinclair AA, Berta P, Palmer MS, et al. A gene from the human sex-determining region encodes a conserved DNA-binding motif. Nature 1990; 346:240–244.

96a. Berta P, Ross Hawkins J, Sinclair AH, et al. Genetic evidence equating SRY and the testis determining factor. Nature 1990; 348:448–450.

96b. Jäger RJ, Anvret M, Hall K, et al. A human XY female with a frame shift mutation in the candidate testis-determining gene SRY. Nature 1990; 348:452–454.

97. Koopman P, Gubbay J, Collignon J, et al. ZFY gene expression patterns are not compatible with a primary role in mouse sex determination. Nature 1989; 342:940–942.

98. Mintz B, Russel ES. Gene-induced embryological modifications of primordial germ cells in the mouse. J Exp Zool 1957; 134:207–238.

99. Lovell-Badge R, Robertson E. XY female mice resulting from a heritable mutation in the primary testis determining gene Tdy. Development 1990; 109:635–646.

99a. Koopman P, Munsterberg A, Capel B, et al. Expression of a candidate sex determining gene during mouse testis differentiation. Nature 1990; 348:450–452.

100. Gubbay J, Collignon J, Koopman P, et al. A gene mapping to the sex-determining region of the mouse Y chromosome in a member of a novel family of embryologically expressed genes. Nature 1990; 346:245–250.

100a. Koopman P, Gubay J, Vivian N, et al. Male development of chromosomally female mice transgenic for Sry. Nature 1991; 351:117–121.

101. Eicher E. Autosomal genes involved in mammalian primary sex determination. Philos Trans R Soc Lond [Biol] 1988; 322:109–117.

102. Hodgkin J. Sex determination compared in Drosophila and Caenorhabditis. Nature 1990; 344:721–728.

103. Grumbach MM, Barr ML. Cytologic tests of chromosomal sex in relation to sexual anomalies in man. Recent Prog Horm Res 1958; 14:255–334.

104. Epstein CJ. Cellular consequences of the state of X-chromosome activity. In: Sandberg AA, ed. Cytogenetics of the Mammalian X Chromosome. Part A: Basic Mechanisms of X Chromosome Behavior. New York: Alan R. Liss, 1983: 341–353.

105. Witschi E. Embryology of the ovary. In: Grady HG, Smith DE, eds. The Ovary. Baltimore: Williams & Wilkins, 1963.

106. Byskov AG. Differentiation of mammalian embryonic gonad. Physiol Rev 1986; 66:71–117.

107. Mancini RE, Narbaitz R, Lavieri JC. Origin and development of the germinative epithelium and Sertoli cells in the human testis: cytological, cytochemical and quantitative study. Anat Rec 1960; 136:477–489.

108. Heller CG, Clermont Y. Kinetics of the germinal epithelium in man. Recent Prog Horm Res 1964; 20:545–575.

109. Baker TG. A quantitative and cytological study of germ cells in human ovaries. Proc R Soc Lond [Biol] 1963; 158:417–433.

110. Baker TG, Eastwood J. Origin and differentiation of germ cells in man. Bibl Anat 1983; 24:67–76.

111. Jost A, Vigier B, Prepin J, et al. Studies on sex differentiation in mammals. Recent Prog Horm Res 1973; 29:1–41.

112. Gondos B. Testicular development. In: Johnson AD, Gomes WR, Vandemark NL, eds. The Testis. Vol 4. New York: Academic, 1977: 1–37.

113. Gondos B. Oogonia and oocytes in mammals. In: Jones RE, ed. The Vertebrate Ovary: Comparative Biology and Evolution. New York: Plenum, 1978: 83–120.

114. Jost A. A new look at the mechanism controlling sex differentiation in mammals. Johns Hopkins Med J 1972; 130:38–53.

115. van Wagenen G, Simpson ME. Embryology of the Ovary and Testis, Homo sapiens and Macaca mulatta. New Haven: Yale University Press, 1965.

116. Byskov AG. Gonadal sex and germ cell differentiation. In: Austin CR, Edwards RG, eds. Mechanisms of Sex Differentiation in Animals and Man. London: Academic, 1981: 145–164.

117. Wartenberg H, Rodemer-Lenz E, Viebahn CH. The dual Sertoli cell system and its role in testicular development and in early germ cell differentiation (prespermatogenesis). In: Holstein AF, Voigt KD, Graes-

slin G, eds. Biologie and Klinik der Reproduction. Berlin: Diesbach, 1988.

118. Byskov AG. The anatomy and ultrastructure of the rete system of the mouse ovary. Biol Reprod 1978; 19:720–725.

119. Witschi E, Nelson WO, Segal SJ. Genetic, developmental and hormonal aspects of gonadal dysgenesis and sex inversion in man. J Clin Endocrinol Metab 1957; 17:737–753.

120. Jost A, Magre S, Agelopoulou R. Early stages of testicular differentiation in the rat. Hum Genet 1981; 58:59–63.

121. Burgoyne PS. The role of the mammalian Y chromosome in spermatogenesis. Development 1988; 101(Suppl):133–141.

122. Burgoyne PS, Buehr M, Koopman P, et al. Cell autonomous action of the testis-determining gene: Sertoli cells are exclusively XY in XX ↔ XY chimeric mouse testes. Development 1988; 102:443–450.

123. Burgoyne PS. Role of mammalian Y chromosome in sex determination. Philos Trans R Soc Lond [Biol] 1988; 322:63–72.

124. Josso N, Picard J-Y, Tran D. The antimullerian hormone. Recent Prog Horm Res 1977; 33:117–167.

125. Gondos B, Connell CJ. Cellular interrelationships in the fetal rabbit testis. Arch Androl 1978; 1:19–30.

126. Siiteri PK, Wilson JD. Testosterone formation and metabolism during male sexual differentiation in the human embryo. J Clin Endocrinol Metab 1974; 38:113–125.

127. Huhtaniemi IT, Korenbrot CC, Jaffe RB. hCG binding and stimulation of testosterone biosynthesis in the human fetal testis. J Clin Endocrinol Metab 1977; 44:963–967.

128. Molsberry RL, Cau BR, Mendelson CR, et al. Human chorionic gonadotropins binding to human fetal testis. J Clin Endocrinol Metab 1982; 55:791–794.

129. Reyes FI, Boroditsky RS, Winter JSD, et al. Studies on human sexual development. II. Fetal and maternal serum gonadotropins and sex steroid concentrations. J Clin Endocrinol Metab 1974; 38:612–617.

130. Kaplan SL, Grumbach MM. Pituitary and placental gonadotropins and sex steroids in the human and sub-human primate fetus. J Clin Endocrinol Metab 1978; 7:487–511.

131. Pang S, Levine LS, Cederqvist L, et al. Amniotic fluid concentrations of Δ^5 and Δ^4 steroids in fetuses with congenital adrenal hyperplasia due to 21-hydroxylase deficiency and in anencephalic fetuses. J Clin Endocrinol Metab 1980; 51:223–229.

132. Word RA, George FW, Wilson JD, et al. Testosterone synthesis and adenylate cyclase activity in the early human fetal testis appear to be independent of human chorionic gonadotropin. J Clin Endocrinol Metab 1989; 69:204–207.

133. Huhtaniemi IT, Korenbrot CC, Jaffe RB. Content of chorionic gonadotropin in human fetal tissues. J Clin Endocrinol Metab 1978; 46:994–997.

134. Kaplan SL, Grumbach MM, Aubert ML. The ontogenesis of pituitary hormones and hypothalamic factors in the human fetus: maturation of central nervous system regulation of anterior pituitary function. Recent Prog Horm Res 1976; 32:161–243.

135. George FW, Wilson JD. The regulation of androgen and estrogen formation in fetal gonads. Ann Biol Anim Biochim Biophys 1979; 19(4B):1297–1306.

136. Gondos B, Hobel CJ. Interstitial cells in the human fetal ovary. Endocrinology 1973; 93:736–739.

137. Jost A. Problems of fetal endocrinology: the gonadal and hypophyseal hormones. Recent Prog Horm Res 1953; 8:379–418.

138. Jost A. Embryonic sexual differentiation (morphology, physiology, abnormalities). In: Jones HW Jr, Scott WW, eds. Hermaphroditism, Genital Anomalies and Related Endocrine Disorders. Baltimore: Williams & Wilkins, 1971: 16–64.

139. Josso N. Anti müllerian hormone: new perspectives for a sexist molecule. Endocr Rev 1986; 7:421–433.

140. Josso N, Legeai L, Forest M, et al. An enzyme linked immunoassay for anti-müllerian hormone: a new tool for the evaluation of testicular function in infants and children. J Clin Endocrinol Metab 1990; 70:23–27.

141. Vigier B, Picard JY, Tran D, et al. Production of anti-müllerian hormone: another homology between Sertoli and granulosa cells. Endocrinology 1984; 114:1315–1320.

142. Vigier B, Tran D, Legeai L, et al. Origin of anti-müllerian hormone in bovine freemartin fetuses. J Reprod Fertil 1984; 70:473–479.

143. Vigier B, Watrin F, Magre S, et al. Purified bovine AMH induces a characteristic freemartin effect in fetal rat prospective ovaries exposed to it in vitro. Development 1987; 100:43–55.

144. Behringer RR, Cate RL, Froelick GJ. Abnormal sexual development in transgenic mice chronically expressing müllerian inhibiting substance. Nature 1990; 345:167–169.

145. Donahoe PK, Cate RL, MacLaughlin DT, et al. Müllerian inhibiting substance. Gene structure and mechanism of action of a fetal regressor. Recent Prog Horm Res 1987; 43:431–467.

146. Hutson JM, Donahoe PK. The control of testicular descent. Endocr Rev 1986; 7:270–284.

147. Tran D, Picard JY, Vigier B, et al. Persistence of müllerian ducts in male rabbits passively immunized against bovine anti-müllerian hormone during fetal life. Dev Biol 1986; 116:160–167.

148. Takahashi M, Hayashi M, Mangaro TE, et al. The ontogeny of müllerian inhibitory substance in granulosa cells of the mouse ovarian follicle. Biol Reprod 1986; 35:447–453.

149. Cate RL, Mattaliano RJ, Hession C, et al. Isolation of the human gene in animal cells. Cell 1986; 45:685–698.

150. Cohen-Haguenauer O, Picard JY, Mattei MG, et al. Mapping of the gene for anti müllerian hormone to the short arm of human chromosome 19. Cytogenet Cell Genet 1987; 44:2–6.

151. Wilson JD, Lasnitzki I. Dihydrotestosterone formation in fetal tissues of rabbit and rat. Endocrinology 1971; 89:659–668.

152. Wilson JD. Testosterone uptake by the urogenital tract of the rabbit embryo. Endocrinology 1973; 92:1192–1199.

153. Neumann F, von Berswordt-Wallrabe R, Elger W, et al. Aspects of androgen-dependent events as studied by antiandrogens. Recent Prog Horm Res 1970; 26:337–410.

154. Siiteri PK, Wilson JD. Testosterone formation and metabolism during male sexual differentiation in the human embryo. J Clin Endocrinol Metab 1974; 38:113–125.

155. Wilson JD, Siiteri PK. Developmental pattern of testosterone synthesis in the fetal gonad of the rabbit. Endocrinology 1973; 92:1182–1191.

156. Cunha GR, Chung LWK, Shannon JM, et al. Stromal-epithelial interactions in sex differentiation. Biol Reprod 1980; 22:19–42.

157. Wilson JD, Griffin JE, George FW, et al. The role of gonadal steroids in sexual differentiation. Recent Prog Horm Res 1981; 37:1–39.

158. Feldman KW, Smith DW. Fetal phallic growth and penile standards for newborn male infants. J Pediatr 1975; 86:395–398.

159. O'Rahilly R. The development of the vagina in the human. Birth Defects 1977; 13:123.

160. Forsberg J-G. Origin of vaginal epithelium. Obstet Gynecol 1965; 25:787–791.

161. Cunha GR. The dual origin of vaginal epithelium. Am J Anat 1975; 143:387–392.

162. Harrison RW, Lippman SS. How steroid hormones work. Hosp Pract 1989; 9:63–76.

163. Griffin JE, Wilson JD. The androgen resistance syndromes: 5α-reductase deficiency, testicular feminization, and related disorders. In: Scriver CR, Blaudet AL, Sly WS, et al., eds. The Metabolic Basis of Inherited Disease. 6th ed. New York: McGraw-Hill, 1989: 1919–1944.

164. O'Malley B. The steroid receptor superfamily: more excitement predicted in the future. Mol Endocrinol 1990; 4:363–369.

165. Liao S, Konkontis J, Tetsujun S, et al. Androgen receptors: structures, mutations, antibodies and cellular dynamics. J Steroid Biochem 1989; 34:41–51.

166. Grino PB, Griffin JE, Wilson JD. Transformation of the androgen receptor to the desoxyribonucleic acid binding state: studies in homogenates and intact cells. Endocrinology 1987; 120:1914–1920.

167. George FW, Peterson K. Dihydrotestosterone formation is necessary for embryogenesis of the rat prostate. Endocrinology 1988; 122:1159–1164.

168. Grumbach MM, Ducharme JR. The effects of androgens on fetal sexual development: androgen-induced female pseudohermaphrodism. Fertil Steril 1960; 11:157–180.

169. Grumbach MM, Kaplan SL. The neuroendocrinology of human puberty: an ontogenic perspective. In: Grumbach MM, Sizonenko PC, Aubert ML, eds. Control of the Onset of Puberty. Baltimore: Williams & Wilkins, 1990: 1–68.

170. Pfeiffer CA. Sexual differences of the hypophyses and their determination by the gonads. Am J Anat 1936; 58:195–225.

171. Harris GW. Sex hormones, brain development and brain function. Endocrinology 1964; 75:627–648.

172. Gorski RA, Jacobson CD. Sexual differentiation of the brain. In: Kogan SJ, Hafez ESE, eds. Pediatric Andrology. The Hague: Martinus Nijhoff, 1981: 109–134.

173. Raisman G, Field PM. Sexual dimorphism in the neuropil of the preoptic area of the rat and its dependence on neonatal androgen. Brain Res 1973; 54:1–29.

174. Brawer JR, Naftolin F, Martin J, et al. Effects of a single injection of estradiol valerate on the hypothalamic arcuate nucleus and on reproductive function in the female rat. Endocrinology 1978; 103:501–512.

175. Reiter EO, Grumbach MM, Kaplan SL, et al. The response of pituitary gonadotropins to synthetic LRF in children with glucocorticoid-treated congenital adrenal hyperplasia: lack of effect of intrauterine and neonatal androgen excess. J Clin Endocrinol Metab 1975; 40:318–325.

176. Sizonenko PC, Schindler AM, Kohlberg IJ, et al. Gonadotropins, testosterone and oestrogen levels in relation to ovarian morphology in 11β-hydroxylase deficiency. Acta Endocrinol 1972; 71:539–550.

177. Karsch FJ, Dierschke DJ, Knobil E. Sexual differentiation of pituitary function: apparent difference between primates and rodents. Science 1973; 179:484–486.

178. Barbarino A, De Marinis L, Lafuentl G, et al. Presence of positive feedback between oestrogen and LH in patients with Klinefelter's syndrome, and Sertoli cell–only syndrome. Clin Endocrinol 1979; 10:235–242.

179. Erhardt A. The psychobiology of gender. In: Rossi A, ed. Gender and the Life Course. New York: Aldine, 1985.

180. Baker WS. Psychosexual differentiation in the human. Biol Reprod 1980; 22:61–72.

181. Ehrhardt AA, Meyer-Bahlburg HFL. Effects of prenatal sex hormones on gender-related behavior. Science 1981; 211:1312–1318.
182. Pardridge WM, Gorski RA, Lippe BM, et al. Androgens and sexual behavior. Ann Intern Med 1982; 96:488–501.
183. Diamond M. A critical evaluation of the ontogeny of human sexual behavior. Q Rev Biol 1965; 40:147–175.
184. MacLusky NJ, Naftolin F. Sexual differentiation of the central nervous system. Science 1981; 211:1294–1303.
185. McEwen BS. Neural gonadal steroid actions. Science 1981; 211:1303–1311.
186. Allen LS, Hines M, Shryne JE, et al. Two sexually dimorphic cell groups in the human brain. J Neurosci 1989; 9:497–506.
187. Geschwind N, Galaburda AM. Cerebral lateralization. Biological mechanisms, association and pathology. II. A hypothesis and a program for research. Arch Neurol 1985; 42:521–522.
188. Nass R, Baker S, Speiser P, et al. Hormones and handedness: left handed bias in female congenital adrenal hyperplasia patients. Neurology 1987; 37:711–715.
189. Rubin RT, Reinisch JM, Haskett RF. Postnatal gonadal steroid effects on human behavior. Science 1981; 211:1318–1324.
190. Meyer-Bahlburg HFL. Hormones and psychosexual differentiation: implications for the management of intersexuality, homosexuality and transsexuality. Clin Endocrinol Metab 1982; 11:681–701.
191. Money J, Higham E. Sexual behavior and endocrinology (normal and abnormal). In: DeGroot LJ, Besser GM, Cahill GF Jr, et al., eds. Endocrinology. 2nd ed. Philadelphia: W. B. Saunders, 1989: 1848–1859.
192. Imperato-McGinley JL, Peterson MD, Gautier T, et al. Androgens and the evolution of male-gender identity among male pseudohermaphrodites with 5α-reductase deficiency. N Engl J Med 1979; 300:1233–1237.
193. Money J, Hampson JG, Hampson JL. An examination of some basic sexual concepts: the evidence of human hermaphroditism. Johns Hopkins Med J 1955; 97:301–319.
194. Herdt GH, Davidson J. The Sambia "Turnim-man": sociocultural and clinical aspects of gender formation in male pseudohermaphrodites with 5-alpha-reductase deficiency in Papua, New Guinea. Arch Sex Behav 1988; 17:33–55.
195. Ehrhardt AA, Epstein R, Money J. Fetal androgens and female gender identity in the early-treated adrenogenital syndrome. Johns Hopkins Med J 1968; 122:160–167.
196. Money J, Schwartz M, Lewis VG. Adult erotosexual status and fetal hormonal masculinization and demasculinization: 46,XX congenital virilizing adrenal hyperplasia and 46,XY androgen-insensitivity compared. Psychoneuroendocrinology 1984; 9:405–414.
197. Klinefelter HF Jr, Reifenstein EC Jr, Albright F. Syndrome characterized by gynecomastia, aspermatogenesis without a Leydigism and increased excretion of follicle-stimulating hormone. J Clin Endocrinol 1942; 2:615–627.
198. Jacobs PA, Strong JA. A case of human intersexuality having a possible XXY sex-determining mechanism. Nature 1959; 83:302–303.
199. Ford CE, Jones KW, Miller OH, et al. The chromosomes in a patient showing both mongolism and the Klinefelter syndrome. Lancet 1959; 1:709–710.
200. Hsueh WA, Hsu TH, Federman DD. Endocrine features of Klinefelter's syndrome. Medicine (Baltimore) 1978; 57:447–461.
201. Leonard JM, Paulsen CA, Ospina LF, et al. The classification of Klinefelter's syndrome. In: Vallet HL, Porter IH, eds. Genetic Mechanisms of Sexual Development. New York: Academic, 1978: 407–423.
202. Robinson A, Lubs HA, Bergsma D. Summary of clinical findings: profiles of children with 47,XXY, 47,XXX and 47,XYY karyotypes. Birth Defects 1979; 15:261–281.
203. Ratcliffe SG, Bancroft J, Axworthy D, et al. Klinefelter's syndrome in adolescence. Arch Dis Child 1982; 57:6–12.
204. Stewart DA, Netley CT, Park E. Summary of clinical findings of children with 47,XXY, 47,XYY and 47,XXX karyotypes. Birth Defects 1982; 18:1–5.
205. Porter ME, Gardner HA, De Feudis P, et al. Verbal deficits in Klinefelter (XXY) adults living in the community. Clin Genet 1988; 33:246–253.
205a. Graham JM Jr, Bashir AS, Stark RE, et al. Oral and written language abilities of XXY boys: implications for anticipatory guidance. Pediatrics 1988; 81:795–806.
206. Klinefelter syndrome. Lancet 1988; 2:1316–1317 (editorial).
207. Nielsen J, Pelsen B. Followup 20 years later of 34 Klinefelter males with karyotype 47,XXY and 16 hypogonadal males with karyotype 46,XY. Hum Genet 1987; 77:188–192.
208. Schibler D, Brook CGD, Kind HP, et al. Growth and body proportions in 54 boys and men with Klinefelter's syndrome. Helv Paediatr Acta 1974; 29:325–333.
209. Illig R, Tolkdorf M, Murset G, et al. LH and FSH responses to synthetic LH-RH in children and adolescents with Turner's and Klinefelter's syndrome. Helv Paediatr Acta 1975; 30:221–231.
210. Ratcliffe SG. The sexual development of boys with the chromosome constitution 47,XXY (Klinefelter's syndrome). Clin Endocrinol Metab 1982; 11:703–716.
211. Salenblatt JA, Bender BG, Puck MH, et al. Pituitary-gonadal function in Klinefelter syndrome before and during puberty. Pediatr Res 1985; 19:82–86.
212. Sorenson K. Klinefelter's Syndrome in Childhood, Adolescence and Youth: A Genetic, Clinical, Developmental, Psychiatric and Psychological Study. Lancaster, UK: Parthenon, 1988.
213. Smals AHG, Kloppenberg WC, Bernard TJ. Effect of short and long term human chorionic gonadotropin (hCG) administration on plasma testosterone levels in Klinefelter's syndrome. Acta Endocrinol 1974; 77:753–764.
214. Wang C, Baker HWG, Burger HG, et al. Hormonal studies in Klinefelter syndrome. Clin Endocrinol 1975; 4:399–411.
215. Smals AHG, Kloppenborg PWC, Lequin RL, et al. The pituitary-thyroid axis in Klinefelter's syndrome. Acta Endocrinol 1977; 84:72–79.
216. Nielsen J. Diabetes mellitus in patients with aneuploid chromosome aberrations and in their parents. Humangenetik 1972; 16:165–170.
217. Geffner ME, Kaplan SA, Bersche N, et al. Insulin resistance in Klinefelter syndrome. J Pediatr Endocrinol 1987; 2:173–177.
218. Harnden DG, Maclean N, Langlands AO. Carcinoma of the breast and Klinefelter's syndrome. J Med Genet 1971; 8:460–461.
218a. Sanchez AG, Villanueva AG, Redoudo C. Lobular carcinoma of the breast in a patient with Klinefelter syndrome: a case with bilateral, synchronous, histologically different breast tumors. Cancer 1986; 57:1180–1183.
218b. Kleczkowska A, Fryns JP, Van den Berghe H. X-chromosome polysomy in the male. The Leuven experience 1966–1987. Hum Genet 1988; 80:16–22.
219. Breit R. Lower leg ulcers. In: Bandmann H-J, Breit R, eds. Klinefelter's Syndrome. Berlin: Springer-Verlag, 1984: 71–79.
220. Chaussain J-L, Lemerle J, Roger M, et al. Klinefelter syndrome, tumor and sexual precocity. J Pediatr 1980; 97:607–609.
221. Eil C. Case 13-1990; case records of the Massachusetts General Hospital. N Engl J Med 1990; 322:917–925.
222. Hook EB, Hamerton JL. The frequency of chromosome abnormalities detected in consecutive newborn studies—difference between studies—results by sex and severity of phenotypic involvement. In: Hook EB, Porter IH, eds. Population Cytogenetics, Studies in Humans. New York: Academic, 1977: 63–79.
223. Rutgers JL, Scully RE. Pathology of the testis in intersex syndromes. Semin Diagn Pathol 1987; 4:275–291.
224. Grumbach MM, Blanc WA, Engle ET. Sex chromatin pattern in seminiferous tubule dysgenesis and other testicular disorders: relationship to true hermaphrodism and to Klinefelter's syndrome. J Clin Endocrinol Metab 1957; 17:703–736.
225. Citoler P, Aechter J. Histology of testis in XXY-fetuses. In: Murken J-D, Stengel-Rutkowski S, Schwinger E, eds. Prenatal Diagnosis. Proceedings of the 3rd European Conference on Prenatal Diagnosis of Genetic Disorders. Stuttgart: Ferdinand Enke, 1979: 336–337.
226. Murken J-D, Stengel-Rutkowski S, Walther J-U, et al. Klinefelter's syndrome in the fetus. Lancet 1974; 2:171 (letter).
227. Mikano K, Aguercif M, Hazeghi P, et al. Chromatin-positive Klinefelter syndrome. Fertil Steril 1968; 19:731–739.
228. Ferguson-Smith MA. The prepubertal testicular lesions in chromatin positive Klinefelter's syndrome (primarily micro-orchidism) as seen in mentally handicapped children. Lancet 1959; 1:219–222.
229. Ohno S. Control of meiotic processes. In: Troen P, Nankin HR, eds. The Testis in Normal and Infertile Men. New York: Raven, 1977: 1–33.
230. Ahmad KN, Dykes JRW, Ferguson-Smith MA, et al. Leydig cell volume in chromatin-positive Klinefelter's syndrome. J Clin Endocrinol Metab 1971; 33:517–520.
231. Rosenkranz VW. Klinefelter Syndrom bei Kindern von Frauen mit Geschlechtschromosomen-Anomalien. Helv Paediatr Acta 1965; 20:359–368.
232. de la Chapelle A. Analytic review: nature and origin of males with XX sex chromosomes. Am J Hum Genet 1972; 24:71–105.
233. Sanger R, Tippett P, Gavin J, et al. Xg groups and sex chromosome abnormalities in people of northern European ancestry: an addendum. J Med Genet 1977; 14:210–211.
234. Jacobs PA, Hassold TJ, Whittington E, et al. Klinefelter's syndrome: an analysis of the origin of the additional sex chromosome using molecular probes. Ann Hum Genet 1988; 52:147–151.
235. Ferguson-Smith MA, Mack WS, Ellis PM, et al. Parental age and the source of the X chromosomes in XXY Klinefelter's syndrome. Lancet 1964; 1:46.
236. Carothers AD, Filippi G. Klinefelter's syndrome in Sardinia and Scotland: comparative studies of parenteral age and other aetiological factors in 47,XXY. Hum Genet 1988; 81:71–75.
237. Van Dop C, Burstein S, Conte FA, et al. Isolated gonadotropin deficiency in boys: clinical characteristics and growth. J Pediatr 1987; 111:684–692.
238. Zizka J, Balicek P. XXYY son of a triple-X mother. Humangenetik 1975; 26:159–160.
239. Jones KL, ed. Smith's Recognizable Patterns of Human Malformation: Genetic, Embryologic and Clinical Aspects. 4th ed. Philadelphia: W. B. Saunders, 1988.

240. Lecluse-Van Der Bilt FA, Hagemeijer A, Smit EME, et al. An infant with an XXXYY karyotype. Clin Genet 1974; 5:263–270.
241. Fraccaro M, Kaljser K, Lindsten J. A child with 49 chromosomes. Lancet 1960; 2:899–902.
242. Borghgraeff M, Fryns JP, Smeets E, et al. The 49,XXXXY syndrome. Clinical and psychologic follow-up data. Clin Genet 1988; 33:429–434.
243. Sarto GE, Otto PG, Kuhn EM, et al. What causes the abnormal phenotype in a 49,XXXXY male? Hum Genet 1987; 76:1–4.
244. de la Chapelle A. The etiology of maleness in XX men. Hum Genet 1981; 58:105–116.
245. Perez-Palacios G, Medina M, Ullao-Aguirre, et al. Gonadotropin dynamics in XX males. J Clin Endocrinol Metab 1981; 53:254–257.
245a. Ferguson-Smith MA, Cooke A, Affara NA, et al. Genotype-phenotype correlations in XX males and their bearing on current theories of sex determination. Hum Genet 1990; 84:198–202.
246. Miro R, Cabellin MR, Marsini S, et al. Mosaicism in XX males. Hum Genet 1978; 45:103–106.
247. Ferguson-Smith MA. X-Y chromosomal interchange in the aetiology of true hermaphroditism and XX Klinefelter's syndrome. Lancet 1966; 2:475–476.
248. de la Chappelle A, Koo GC, Wachtel SS. Recessive sex-determining genes in human XX male syndrome. Cell 1978; 15:837–842.
249. de la Chapelle A, Tippett PA, Wetterstrand G, et al. Genetic evidence of X-Y interchange in a human XX male. Nature 1984; 307:170–171.
250. Evans HJ, Buckton KE, Spowart G, et al. Heteromorphic X chromosomes in 46,XX males: evidence for the involvement of X-Y interchange. Hum Genet 1979; 49:11–31.
251. Magenis RE, Webb MJ, McKeon RS, et al. Translocation (X:Y) (p22:33; p11.2) in XX males: etiology of male phenotype. Hum Genet 1982; 62:271–276.
252. Guellaen G, Casanova M, Bishop C, et al. Human XX males with Y single-copy DNA fragments. Nature 1984; 307:172–173.
253. Muller U, La Lande M, Donlon T, et al. Moderately repeated sequences for the short arm of the human Y chromosome are present in XX males and reduced in copy number in an XY female. Nucleic Acids Res 1986; 14:1325–1340.
254. Affara NA, Ferguson-Smith MA, Tolmie J, et al. Variable transfer of Y specific sequences in XX males. Nucleic Acids Res 1986; 14:5375–5387.
255. Andersson M, Page DC, de la Chapelle A. Chromosome Y–specific DNA is transferred to the short arm of X chromosome in human XX males. Science 1986; 223:786–788.
256. Buckle VJ, Boyd Y, Fraser N, et al. Localization of Y chromosome sequences in normal and XX males. J Med Genet 1987; 24:197–203.
257. Kalaitzidakis M, Therialt A, Boyd E, et al. The destination of Y specific sequences in X-Y interchange males. Development 1987; 101(Suppl):195 (abstract).
258. Petit C, de la Chapelle A, Levilliers J, et al. An abnormal X-Y interchange accounts for most but not all cases of human XX maleness. Cell 1987; 49:595–602.
259. Rouyer F, Simmler MC, Page DC, et al. A sex chromosome rearrangement in a human XX male caused by Alu-Alu recombination. Cell 1987; 51:417–425.
260. de la Chapelle A. The Y chromosome and autosomal testes-determining genes. Development 1987; 101(Suppl):33–38.
261. Magenis RE, Casanova M, Fellous M, et al. Further cytologic evidence of Xp-Yp translocation in XX males using in situ hybridization with Y-derived probe. Hum Genet 1987; 75:228–233.
262. Muller U, Latt SA, Donlon T. Y specific DNA sequences in male patients with 46,XX and 47,XXX karyotypes. Am J Med Genet 1987; 28:393–401.
263. Stalvey JRD, Durbin EJ, Erickson RP. Sex vesicle "entrapment": translocation or nonhomologous recombination of misaligned Yp and Xp as alternative mechanisms for abnormal inheritance of the sex-determining region. Am J Med Genet 1989; 32:564–572.
264. Disteche CM, Casanova M, Saal M, et al. Small deletions of the short arm of the Y chromosome in 46,XY females. Proc Natl Acad Sci USA 1986; 83:7841–7844.
265. Page DC, Fisher EMC, McGillivray B, et al. Additional deletion in sex determining region of human Y chromosome resolves paradox of X,t(Y:22) female. Nature 1990; 346:279–281.
266. Sherer G, Schempp W, Baccichetti C, et al. Analysis of two 47,XXX males reveals X-Y interchange and maternal and paternal nondisjunction. Hum Genet 1989; 81:247–251.
266a. Ferguson-Smith MA, Affara NA, Briggs H. The secret of sex. Lancet 1990; 2:809–810.
266b. Skordis NA, Stetka DG, MacGillivray MH, et al. Familial 46,XX males coexisting with familial 46,XX true hermaphrodites in same pedigree. J Pediatr 1987; 110:224–248.
267. Engel E, Forbes AP. Cytogenetic and clinical findings in 48 patients with congenitally defective or absent ovaries. Medicine 1965; 44:135–165.
268. Palmer CG, Reichman A. Chromosomal and clinical findings in 110 females with Turner syndrome. Hum Genet 1976; 35:35–49.
269. Hall JG, Sybert VP, Williamson RA, et al. Turner's syndrome. West J Med 1982; 137:32–44.
270. Rosenfeld R, Grumbach MM, eds. Turner Syndrome. New York: Marcel Dekker, 1990.
270a. Lippe BM. Primary ovarian failure. In: Kaplan SA, ed. Clinical Pediatric Endocrinology. 2nd ed. Philadelphia: W. B. Saunders, 1990: 325–366.
271. Ford CE, Jones KW, Polani PE, et al. A sex chromosome anomaly in a case of gonadal dysgenesis (Turner's syndrome). Lancet 1979;1:711–713.
272. Virdis R, Cantu MC, Ghizzoni L, et al. Blood pressure behavior and control in Turner syndrome. Clin Exp Hypertens 1986; 8:787–791.
273. Money J, Alexander D, Ehrhardt A. Visual constructional deficit in Turner's syndrome. J Pediatr 1966; 69:126–127.
274. Bender B, Puck M, Sallenblatt J, et al. Cognitive development of unselected girls with complete and partial X monosomy. Pediatrics 1984; 73:175–182.
275. Garron DC. Intelligence among persons with Turner's syndrome. Behav Genet 1977; 7:105–127.
276. Downey JI, Ehrhardt AA. The long-term behavior of patients with Turner syndrome—an update. In: Rosenfeld RG, Grumbach MM, eds. Turner Syndrome. New York: Marcel Dekker, 1990: 483–490.
277. Gordon RR, O'Neill EM. Turner's infantile phenotype. Br Med J 1969; 1:483–485.
278. Singh RF, Carr DH. The anatomy and histology of XO human embryos and fetuses. Anat Rec 1966; 155:369–384.
279. van der Putte SCJ. Lymphatic malformation in human fetuses. A study of fetuses with Turner's syndrome or status Bonnevie-Ullrich. Virchows Arch [A] 1977; 376:233–246.
280. Shephard TH, Fantel AG. Pathogenesis of congenital defects associated with Turner's syndrome: the role of hypoalbuminemia and edema. Acta Endocrinol 1986; 113(Suppl 279):440–447.
281. Clark EB. Web neck and congenital heart defects: a pathogenic association in 45XO Turner syndrome? Teratology 1984; 29:355–361.
282. Lacro RV, Jones KL, Benirschke K. Coarctation of the aorta in Turner syndrome: a pathologic study of fetuses with nuchal cystic hygromas, hydrops fetalis, and female genitalia. Pediatrics 1988; 81:445–451.
283. Miller MJ, Geffner ME, Lippe BM, et al. Echocardiography reveals a high incidence of bicuspid aortic valve in Turner syndrome. J Pediatr 1983; 102:47–50.
284. Mazzanti L, Prandstaller D, Tassinari D, et al. Heart disease in Turner's syndrome. Helv Paediatr Acta 1988; 43:25–31.
285. Van Egmond H, Orye E, Praet M, et al. Hypoplastic left heart syndrome and the 45,X karyotype. Br Heart J 1988; 60:69–71.
286. Allen DB, Hendrichs A, Levy JM. Aortic dilatation in Turner syndrome. J Pediatr 1986; 109:302–305.
287. Lin AE, Lippe BM, Geffner ME, et al. Aortic dilation, dissection, and rupture in patients with Turner syndrome. J Pediatr 1986; 109:820–826.
288. Lippe B, Geffner ME, Dietrich RB, et al. Renal malformations in patients with Turner syndrome: imaging in 141 patients. Pediatrics 1988; 82:852–856.
289. Lubin MB, Gruber HE, Rimoin DL, et al. Skeletal abnormalities in the Turner syndrome. In: Rosenfeld RG, Grumbach MM, eds. Turner Syndrome. New York: Marcel Dekker, 1989: 281–291.
290. Prager L, Steinbach HL, Moskowitz P, et al. Roentgenographic abnormalities in phenotypic females with gonadal dysgenesis. A comparison of chromatin positive patients and chromatin negative patients. Am J Roentgenol Radium Ther Nucl Med 1968; 104:899–910.
291. Ruben KR. Osteoporosis in Turner syndrome. In: Rosenfeld RG, Grumbach MM, eds. Turner Syndrome. New York: Marcel Dekker, 1990: 301–318.
292. Alexander RL, Conte FA, Kaplan SL, et al. The effect of estrogen treatment on height in patients with gonadal dysgenesis. Clin Res 1978; 26:174A.
293. Brook CGD, Murset G, Zachmann M, et al. Growth in children with 45,XO Turner's syndrome. Arch Dis Child 1974; 49:789–795.
294. Park E, Bailey JD, Cowell CA. Growth and maturation in patients with Turner's syndrome. Pediatr Res 1983; 17:1–7.
295. Ranke MB, Stubbe P, Majewski F, et al. Spontaneous growth in Turner's syndrome. Acta Paediatr Scand 1988; 343(Suppl):22–30.
295a. Lyon AJ, Preece MA, Grant DB. Growth curve for girls with Turner syndrome. Arch Dis Child 1985; 60:932–935.
296. Hughes PCR, Ribeiro J, Hughes IA. Body proportions in Turner's syndrome. Arch Dis Child; 61:506–517.
297. Cuttler L, Van Vliet G, Conte FA, et al. Somatomedin C levels in children and adolescents with gonadal dysgenesis: comparison with age related norms and effect of estrogen replacement therapy. J Clin Endocrinol Metab 1985; 60:1087–1092.
298. Sklar C, Kaplan SL, Grumbach MM. Lack of effect of oestrogens on adrenal androgen secretion in children and adolescents with a comment on oestrogens and pubic hair growth. Clin Endocrinol 1981; 14:311–320.
299. Ross JL, Long-Meyerson L, Loriaux DL, et al. Growth hormone secretory dynamics in Turner syndrome. J Pediatr 1985; 106:202–206.
300. Weiss L. Additional evidence of gradual loss of germ cells in the pathogenesis of streak ovaries in Turner's syndrome. J Med Genet 1971; 8:540–544.

301. Jirasek J. Principles of reproductive embryology. In: Simpson JL, ed. Disorders of Sexual Differentiation. Etiology and Clinical Delineation. New York: Academic, 1976: 52–110.

302. Conte FA, Grumbach MM, Kaplan SL. A diphasic pattern of gonadotropin secretion in patients with the syndrome of gonadal dysgenesis. J Clin Endocrinol Metab 1975; 40:670–674.

303. Conte FA, Grumbach MM, Kaplan SL, et al. Correlation of luteinizing hormone–releasing factor–induced luteinizing hormone and follicle-stimulating hormone release from infancy to 19 years with the changing pattern of gonadotropin secretion in agonadal patients: relation to restraint of puberty. J Clin Endocrinol Metab 1980; 50:163–168.

304. Massarano AA, Adams JA, Preece MA, et al. Ovarian ultrasound appearances in the Turner syndrome. J Pediatr 1989; 114:814–816.

305. Rosenfeld RL. Spontaneous puberty and fertility in Turner syndrome. In: Rosenfeld RG, Grumbach MM, eds. Turner Syndrome. New York: Marcel Dekker, 1990: 131–144.

306. Kohn G, Yarkoni S, Cohen MM. Two conceptions in a 45,X woman. Am J Med Genet 1980; 5:339–343.

307. King CR, Magenis E, Bennett S. Pregnancy and the Turner syndrome. Obstet Gynecol 1978; 52:617–624.

308. Speed RM. Oocyte development in XO foetuses of man and mouse: the possible role of heterologous X-chromosome pairing in germ cell survival. Chromosome 1986; 94:115–124.

309. Reyes FI, Koh KS, Faiman C. Fertility in women with gonadal dysgenesis. Am J Obstet Gynecol 1976; 126:668–670.

310. Dewhurst J. Fertility in 47,XXX and 45,X patients. J Med Genet 1978; 15:132–135.

311. Singh DN, Hara S, Foster HW, et al. Reproductive performance in women with sex chromosome mosaicism. Obst Gynecol 1980; 55:608–611.

312. Sklar CA, Kaplan SL, Grumbach MM. Evidence for dissociation between adrenarche and gonadarche. Studies in patients with idiopathic precocious puberty, gonadal dysgenesis, isolated gonadotropin deficiency, and constitutionally delayed growth and adolescence. J Clin Endocrinol Metab 1980; 51:548–556.

313. Apter D, Lenko H-L, Perheentupa J, et al. Subnormal pubertal increases of serum androgens in Turner's syndrome. Horm Res 1982: 16:164–173.

314. LoCurto F, Pucci E, Scappaticci S, et al. XO and male phenotype. Am J Dis Child 1974; 128:90–91.

315. Forabosco A, Carratu A, Assuma M, et al. Male with 45,X karyotype. Clin Genet 1977; 12:97–100.

316. de la Chapelle A, Page DC, Brown L, et al. The origin of 45,X males. Am J Hum Genet 1986; 38:330–340.

317. Gal A, Weber B, Neri G, et al. A 45,X male with Y-specific DNA translocated onto chromosome 15. Am J Hum Genet 1987; 40:477–488.

318. Munke M, Page DC, Brown LG, et al. Molecular detection of a Y/18 translocation in a 45,X holoprosencephalic male. Hum Genet 1988; 80:219–223.

319. Robinson A. Demography and prevalence of Turner syndrome. In: Rosenfeld RG, Grumbach MM, eds. Turner Syndrome. New York: Marcel Dekker, 1990: 93–99.

320. Carr DH. Chromosomes and abortion. Hum Genet 1971; 2:201–257.

321. Hook EB, Warburton D. The distribution of chromosome genotypes associated with Turner's syndrome: livebirth prevalence rates and evidence for diminished fetal mortality and severity in genotypes associated with structural X abnormalities or mosaicism. Hum Genet 1983; 64:24–27.

322. Germain EL, Plotnick LP. Age-related anti-thyroid antibodies and thyroid abnormalities. Acta Paediatr Scand 1986; 75:750–755.

323. Fleming S, Cowell C, Bailey J, et al. Hashimoto's disease in Turner's syndrome. Clin Invest Med 1988; 11:243–246.

324. Manzione NC, Kram M, Kram E, et al. Turner's syndrome and inflammatory bowel disease: a case report with immunologic studies. Am J Gastroenterol 1988; 83:1294–1297.

325. Polychronakos C, Letarte J, Collu R, et al. Carbohydrate intolerance in children and adolescents with Turner syndrome. J Pediatr 1980; 96:1009–1014.

326. Wilson DM, Frane JW, Sherman B, et al. Turner syndrome: effect of therapy with growth hormone, oxandrolone, and a combination of both. J Pediatr 1988; 112:210–217.

327. Anderson H, Fillipson R, Fluur E. Hearing impairment in Turner's syndrome. Acta Otolaryngol 1969; 247(Suppl):1.

328. Wertelecki W, Fraumeni JF Jr, Mulvihill JJ, et al.: Nongonadal neoplasia in Turner's syndrome. Cancer 1970; 26:485–488.

329. Warburton D, Kline J, Stein Z. Monosomy X: a chromosomal anomaly associated with young maternal age. Lancet 1980; 1:167–169.

330. Carothers AD, Frackiewicz A, DeMey R, et al. A collaborative study of the aetiology of Turner syndrome. Ann Hum Genet 1980; 43:355–368.

331. Al-Awadi SA, Cuschieri A, Farag TI, et al. Ullrich-Turner syndrome in monozygotic twins. Am J Med Genet 1983; 15:537–542.

332. Hassold T, Kumlin E, Takeesu N, et al. Determination of the parenteral origin of sex chromosome monosomy using restriction fragment length polymorphisms. Am J Hum Genet 1985; 37:965–972.

333. King CR, Maginis E. Turner syndrome in the offspring of artificially inseminated pregnancies. Fertil Steril 1978; 30:604–605.

334. Rosenfeld RG, Hintz RL, Johanson AJ, et al. Three year results of a randomized prospective trial of methionyl human growth hormone and oxandrolone in Turner syndrome. J Pediatr 1988; 113:393–400.

335. Ehrhardt AA. Behavioral effects of estrogen in the human female. Pediatrics 1978; 62:1166–1170.

336. Ross JL, Cassorla F, Carpenter G, et al. The effect of short term treatment with growth hormone and ethinyl estradiol on lower leg growth rate in girls with Turner's syndrome. J Clin Endocrinol Metab 1988; 67:515–518.

336a. Vanderschueren-Lodeweyckx M, Massa G, Maes M, et al. Growth promoting effect of growth hormone and low dose ethinyl estradiol in girls with Turner's syndrome. J Clin Endocrinol Metab 1990; 70:122–126.

337. Levine LS. Treatment of Turner's syndrome with estrogen. Pediatrics 1979; 62:1178–1183.

338. Rosenwaks Z, Urban MD, Wentz AC, et al. Endometrial pathology and its relation to estrogen therapy in patients with hypogonadism. Pediatrics 1979; 62:1184–1188.

339. Sinisi AA, Perrone L, Quarto C, et al. Dysgerminoma in 45,X Turner syndrome: report of a case. Clin Endocrinol 1988; 28:187–193.

340. Nielsen J. Mental aspects of Turner syndrome and the importance of information and Turner contact groups. In: Rosenfeld RG, Grumbach MM, eds. Turner Syndrome. New York: Marcel Dekker, 1990: 451–467.

341. Rosenwaks Z, Navot D. Oocyte donation in ovarian failure. In: Rosenfeld RG, Grumbach MM, eds. Turner Syndrome. New York: Marcel Dekker, 1990: 109–124.

342. McCauley E, Kay T, Ito J, et al. The Turner syndrome: cognitive deficits, affective discrimination, and behavior problems. Child Dev 1987; 58:464–473.

343. Rosenberg C, Frota-Pessoa O, Vianna-Morgante AM, et al. Phenotypic spectrum of 45,X/46,XY individuals. Am J Med Genet 1987; 27:553–559.

344. Urban E, Zenzes MT, Muller U, et al. Cell reorganization "in vitro" of heterosexual gonadal co-culture. Differentiation 1981; 18:161–168.

345. Fraccaro M, Maraschio P, Pasquali F, et al. Women heterozygous for deficiency of the (p21-pter) region of the X chromosome are fertile. Hum Genet 1977; 39:283–292.

346. Epstein CJ. Mechanisms leading to the phenotype of Turner syndrome. In: Rosenfeld RG, Grumbach MM, eds. Turner Syndrome. New York: Marcel Dekker, 1990: 13–23.

347. Therman E, Susman B. The similarity of phenotypic effects caused by Xp and Xq deletions in the human female: a hypothesis. Hum Genet 1990; 85:175–183.

348. Fujita H, Tanigawa Y, Yoshida Y, et al. Cytological findings of 10 cases of I(Xq) and one with dic(X). Hum Genet 1977; 39:147–55.

349. Otto PG, Vianna-Morgante AM, Otto PA, et al. The Turner phenotype and the different types of human X isochromosome. Hum Genet 1981; 57:159–164.

350. Stafford TM, Palmer CG, Cleary RE. Gonadal dysgenesis with isochromosome X and menstruation. Am J Obstet Gynecol 1973; 116:886.

351. Dewald GW. Isodicentric X chromosomes in humans: origin, segregation behavior, and replication band patterns. In: Sandberg AA, ed. Cytogenetics of the Mammalian X Chromosome. Part A: Basic Mechanisms of X Chromosome Behavior. New York: Alan R. Liss, 1983: 405–426.

352. Hagemeijer A, Hoovers J, Hasper-Voogt I, et al. Late-replicating ring X-chromosomes identified by R-banding after BrdU pulse. Three new examples of 45,XO/46,Xr(X). Hum Genet 1976; 34:45–52.

353. Dallapiccola B, Bruni L, Boscherini B, et al. Segregation of an X ring chromosome in two generations. J Med Genet 1980; 17:306–308.

354. Crolla JA, Llerena JC. A mosaic 45,X/46xXr(?) karyotype investigated with X and Y centromeric-specific probes using a non autoradiographic in situ hybridization technique. Hum Genet 1988; 81:81–84.

355. Disteche C. The use of DNA probes to characterize sex chromosome anomalies. In: Rosenfeld RG, Grumbach MM, eds. Turner Syndrome. New York: Marcel Dekker, 1990: 37–54.

356. Hoo JJ. A note on the Xp−. Hum Genet 1979; 50:339–40.

357. Herva R, Kaluzewski B, de la Chapelle A. Inherited interstitial del(Xp) with minimal consequences: with a note on the location of genes controlling phenotypic features. Am J Med Genet 1979; 3:43–58.

358. Kalousek D, Schiffrin A, Berguer A-M, et al. Partial short arm deletions of the X chromosome and spontaneous pubertal development in girls with short stature. J Pediatr 1979; 94:891–894.

359. Fryns JP, Petit P, Van den Berghe H. The various phenotypes in Xp deletion. Observation in eleven patients. Hum Genet 1981; 57:385–387.

360. Wilson MG, Modebe O, Towner JW, et al. Ullrich-Turner syndrome associated with interstitial deletion of Xp11.4p22.31. Am J Med Genet 1983; 14:567–576.

361. Leichtman DA, Schmickel RD, Gelehrter TD, et al. Familial Turner syndrome. Ann Intern Med 1978; 89:473–476.

362. Mirzayants GG, Baranovskaya LI. X-X translocation in a patient with gonadal dysgenesis and the problem of phenotypic-karyotypic correlations. Hum Genet 1978; 40:249–257.

363. Mattei MG, Mattei JF, Ayme S, et al. X-autosome translocations: cytogenetic characteristics and their consequences. Hum Genet 1982; 61:295–309.

364. Madan K. Balanced structural changes involving the human X: effect on sexual phenotype. Hum Genet 1983; 63:216–221.

365. Zah W, Kalderon HE, Tucci JR. Mixed gonadal dysgenesis. Acta Endocrinol 1975; 79(Suppl 197):3–39.

366. Donahoe PK, Crawford JD, Hendren WH. Mixed gonadal dysgenesis, pathogenesis and management. J Pediatr Surg 1979; 14:287–300.

367. Wheeler M, Peakman D, Robinson A, et al. 45X/46XY mosaicism: contrast of prenatal and postnatal diagnosis. Am J Med Genet 1988; 29:565–571.

368. Hsu LYF. Prenatal diagnosis of 45,X/46,XY mosaicism—a review and update. Prenatal Diagn 1989; 9:31–48.

369. Chang HJ, Clark RD, Bachman H. The phenotype of 45,X/46,XY mosaicism. An analysis of 92 prenatally diagnosed cases. Am J Med Genet 1990; 46:156–168.

370. Bonaventura L, Roth LM, Cleary RE. The Sertoli cell in mixed gonadal dysgenesis. Obstet Gynecol 1979; 53:324–329.

371. Simpson JL. Male pseudohermaphroditism: genetics and clinical delineation. Hum Genet 1978; 44:1–49.

372. Muller J, Skakkeback NE, Ritzen M, et al. Carcinoma in situ of the testis in children with 45,X/46,XY gonadal dysgenesis. J Pediatr 1985; 106:431–436.

373. Caspersson TA, Hulten M, Jonasson J, et al. Translocation causing nonfluorescent Y chromosomes in human XO/XY mosaicism. Hereditas 1971; 68:317–324.

374. Kluzewski B, Jokineu A, Hortling H, et al. A theory explaining the abnormality in 45,X/46,XY mosaicism with non-fluorescent Y chromosome. Presentation of 3 cases. Ann Genet 1978; 21:5–11.

375. Madan K, Gooren L, Shoemaker J. Three cases of sex chromosome mosaicism with a nonfluorescent Y. Hum Genet 1979; 46:295–304.

376. Magenis E, Donlon T. Non-fluorescent Y chromosomes. Cytologic evidence of origin. Hum Genet 1982; 60:133–138.

377. Ganshirt-Ahlert D, Pawlowitzki IH, Gal A. Three cases of 45,X/46,XYnf mosaicism. Hum Genet 1987; 76:153–156.

378. Lukusa T, Fryns JP, van den Berghe H. Gonadoblastoma formation and Y-chromosome fluorescence. Clin Genet 1986; 29:311–316.

379. Drummond-Borg M, Pagon RA, Bradley CM, et al. Nonfluorescent dicentric Y in males with hypospadias. J Pediatr 1988; 113:469–473.

380. Weckworth PF, Johnson HW, Pantzer JT, et al. Dicentric Y chromosome and mixed dysgenesis. J Urol 1988; 139:91–94.

381. Yanagisawa S. Structural abnormalities of the Y chromosome and abnormal external genitalia. Hum Genet 1980; 53:183–188.

382. Rosenfeld R, Luzzatti L, Hintz RL, et al. Sexual and somatic determinants of the human Y chromosome. Studies in a 46,XYp– phenotypic female. Am J Hum Genet 1979; 31:458–468.

383. Tiepolo L, Zuffardi O. Localization of factors controlling spermatogenesis in the nonfluorescent portion of the human Y chromosome long arm. Hum Genet 1976; 34:119–124.

384. Yunis E, Garcia-Conti FL, Torres de Caballero OM, et al. Yq deletion, aspermia, and short stature. Hum Genet 1977; 39:117–122.

385. Page DC. Hypothesis: a Y chromosome gene causes gonadoblastoma in dysgenetic gonads. Development 1987; 101(Suppl):151–155.

386. Kohdr G, Cadena GD, Ong TC, et al. Y-autosome translocation, gonadal dysgenesis, and gonadoblastoma. Am J Dis Child 1979; 133:277–282.

387. Bernstein R. X:Y chromosome translocations and their manifestations. In: Sandberg AA, ed. Progress and Topics in Cytogenetics, the Y Chromosome. New York: Alan R. Liss, 1985: 171–206.

388. Harnden DG, Stewart JSS. The chromosomes in a case of pure gonadal dysgenesis. Br Med J 1959; 2:1285–1287.

389. Nazareth HR de S, Farah LMS, Cunha AJB, et al. Pure gonadal dysgenesis (type XX). Report on a family with four affected sibs. Hum Genet 1977; 37:117–120.

390. McDonough PG, Byrd JR, Tho PT, et al. Phenotypic and cytogenetic findings in eighty-two patients with ovarian failure—changing trends. Fertil Steril 1977; 28:638–641.

391. Judd HL, Scully RE, Atkins L, et al. Pure gonadal dysgenesis with progressive hirsutism: demonstration of testosterone production by gonadal streaks. N Engl J Med 1970; 282:881–885.

392. Pallister PD, Opitz JM. The Perrault syndrome: autosomal recessive ovarian dysgenesis with facultative, non–sex-limited sensorineural deafness. Am J Med Genet 1979; 4:239–246.

393. Hamet P, Kuchel O, Nowaczynski W, et al. Hypertension with adrenal, genital, renal defects, and deafness. Arch Intern Med 1973; 131:563–569.

394. Skre H, Bassoe HH, Berg K, et al. Cerebellar ataxia and hypergonadotropic hypogonadism in two kindreds. Chance occurrence, pleiotropism or linkage? Clin Genet 1976; 9:234–244.

395. Swyer GIM. Male pseudohermaphrodism: a hitherto undescribed form. Br Med J 1955; 2:709–712.

396. Warner BA, Monsaert RP, Stumpf PG, et al. 46,XY gonadal dysgenesis: is oncogenesis related to H-Y antigen phenotype or breast development? Hum Genet 1985; 69:79–85.

397. Gaal M, Laszlo J, Bosze P. 46,XY pure gonadal dysgenesis with non-fluorescent Y chromosome. Clin Genet 1978; 14:83–89.

398. Simpson JL, Blagowidow N, Martin AO. XY gonadal dysgenesis: genetic heterogeneity based upon observations, H-Y antigen status and segregation analysis. Hum Genet 1981; 58:91–97.

399. Simpson JL. Genetic heterogeneity in XY sex reversal: potential pitfalls. In: Wachtel S, ed. Isolating the Testes-Determining Factor (TDF) in Evolutionary Mechanism in Sex Determination. Boca Raton, FL: CRC Press, 1989: 266–276.

400. Chemke J, Carmichael R, Stewart JM, et al. Familial XY gonadal dysgenesis. J Med Genet 1970; 7:105–111.

401. Blagowidow N, Page DC, Huff D, et al. Ullrich-Turner syndrome in an XY female fetus with deletion of the sex determining portion of the Y chromosome. Am J Med Genet 1989; 34:159–162.

402. Bernstein R, Koo GC, Wachtel SS. Abnormality of the X chromosome in human 46,XY female siblings with dysgenetic ovaries. Science 1980; 207:768–769.

403. Scherer G, Shempp W, Baccichetti C, et al. Duplication of an Xp segment that includes the ZFX locus causes sex inversion in man. Hum Genet 1989; 81:291–294.

404. Hofnagel D, Wurster-Hill DH, Dupree WB, et al. Camptomelic dwarfism associated with XY-gonadal dysgenesis and chromosome anomalies. Clin Genet 1978; 13:489–499.

405. Bialer MG, Penchaszadeh VB, Kahn E, et al. Female external genitalia and müllerian duct derivatives in a 46,XY infant with the Smith-Lemli-Opitz syndrome. Am J Med Genet 1987; 28:723–731.

406. Friedman BL, Finlay JL. The Drash syndrome revisited: diagnosis and follow-up. Am J Med Genet 1987; 3(Suppl):293–296.

407. Moorthy AV, Chesney RW, Lubinsky M. Chronic renal failure and XY gonadal dysgenesis: "Frasier" syndrome—a commentary on reported cases. Am J Med Genet 1987; 3(Suppl):297–302.

408. Cussen LJ, MacMahon RA. Germ cells and ova in dysgenetic gonads of a 46,XY female dizygotic twin. Am J Dis Child 1979; 133:373–375.

409. Russel MH, Wachtel SS, Davis BW, et al. Ovarian development in 46,XY gonadal dysgenesis. Hum Genet 1982; 60:196–199.

410. Grumbach MM, Morishima A, Liu N. A distinctive clinical entity simulating Turner's syndrome in boys and girls associated with congenital heart disease, appropriate gonadal differentiation, and a normal sex chromosome constitution. J Pediatr 1965; 67:966 (abstract).

411. Noonan J. Hypertelorism with Turner phenotype. A new syndrome with associated congenital heart disease. Am J Dis Child 1968; 116:373–380.

412. Mendez HMM, Optiz JM. Noonan syndrome: a review. Am J Med Genet 1985; 21:493–506.

413. Miller M, Motulsky AC. Noonan syndrome in an adult family presenting with chronic lymphedema. Am J Med 1978; 65:379–383.

414. Char F, Rodriquez-Fernandez HL, Scott CI Jr, et al. The Noonan syndrome—a clinical study of forty-five cases. Birth Defects 1972; 8:110–118.

415. Jones HW, Scott WW. Hermaphroditism, Genital Anomalies, and Related Endocrine Disorders. 2nd ed. Baltimore: Williams & Wilkins, 1971.

416. van Niekerk WA. True hermaphroditism: an analytic review with a report of 3 new cases. Am J Obstet Gynecol 1976; 126:890–907.

417. van Niekerk WA. True hermaphrodism. In: Josso N, ed. The Intersex Child. Pediatric and Adolescent Endocrinology. Vol 8. Basel: S. Karger, 1981: 80–99.

418. Van Niekerk WA, Retief AE. The gonads of human true hermaphrodites. Hum Genet 1981; 58:117–122.

419. McKelvie J, Jaubert F, Nezelof C. True hermaphroditism. A primary germ cell disorder. Pediatr Pathol 1987; 7:31–41.

420. Nihoul-Fekete C, Lortat-Jacob S, Cahin O, et al. Preservation of gonadal function in true hermaphroditism. J Pediatr Surg 1984; 19:50–55.

421. Ramsay M, Bernstein R, Zwane W, et al. XX true hermaphroditism in southern African blacks: an enigma of primary sexual differentiation. Am J Hum Genet 1988; 43:4–13.

422. Williamson HO, Phansey SA, Mathur RS. True hermaphroditism with term vaginal delivery and a review. Am J Obstet Gynecol 1981; 141:262–265.

423. Shannon R, Nicolaides NJ. True hermaphrodism with oogenesis and spermatogenesis. Aust NZ J Obstet Gynaecol 1973; 13:184–187.

424. Armendares S, Salamanca F, Cantu JM, et al. Familial true hermaphrodism in three siblings: clinical, cytogenetic, histologic and hormonal studies. Humangenetik 1975; 29:99–109.

425. Aiman J, Hemsell DJ, MacDonald PC. Production and origin of estrogen in two true hermaphrodites. Am J Obstet Gynecol 1978; 132:401–409.

425a. Jäger RJ, Ebensperger C, Fraccaro M, et al. A ZFY-negative 46,XX true hermaphrodite is positive for the Y pseudoautosomal boundary. Hum Genet 1990; 85:666–668.

426. Abbas NE, Toublanc JE, Boucekkine C, et al. A possible common origin of Y-negative human XX males and XX true hermaphrodites. Hum Genet 1990; 84:356–360.

427. Benirschke K, Naftolin F, Gittes R, et al. True hermaphroditism and chimerism. Am J Obstet Gynecol 1972; 113:449–458.

428. Gartler SM, Waxman SH, Giblett E. An XX/XY human hermaphrodite resulting from double fertilization. Proc Natl Acad Sci USA 1962; 48:332–335.

429. Josso N, de Grouchy J, Auvert J, et al. True hermaphroditism with

XX/XY mosaicism, probably due to double fertilization of the ovum. J Clin Endocrinol Metab 1965; 25:114–126.

430. Tarkowski AK. Mouse chimaera developed from fused eggs. Nature 1961; 190:857–860.

431. Fraccaro M, Tiepolo L, Zuffardi O, et al. Familial XX true hermaphroditism and the H-Y antigen. Hum Genet 1979; 48:45–52.

432. Clayton GW, Smith JD, Rosenberg HS. Familial true hermaphroditism in pre- and post-pubertal genetic females. Hormonal and morphological studies. J Clin Endocrinol Metab 1958; 18:1349–1358.

433. Mori Y, Mitzutami S. Familial true hermaphroditism in genetic females. Jpn J Urol 1968; 59:857–864.

434. Berger R, Abonyi D, Nodot A, et al. Hermaphrodisme vrai et "garcon XX" dans une fratrie. Rev Eur Etud Clin Biol 1970; 15:330–333.

435. Kasdan R, Nankin HR, Troen P, et al. Paternal transmission of maleness in XX human beings. N Engl J Med 1973; 288:539–545.

436. Schwartz IS, Cohen CJ, Deligdisch L. Dysgerminoma of the ovary associated with true hermaphroditism. Obstet Gynecol 1980; 56:102–106.

437. Barr ML, Sergovich FR, Carr DH, et al. The triplo-X female: an appraisal based on a study of 12 cases and a review of the literature. Can Med Assoc J 1969; 101:247–258.

438. Fryns JP, Kleczkowska A, Petit P, et al. X-chromosome polysomy in the female: personal experience and review of the literature. Clin Genet 1983; 23:341–349.

439. Nielsen J, Homma A, Christiansen F, et al. Women with tetra-X (48XXXX). Hereditas 1977; 85:151–156.

440. Collen RJ, Falk RE, Lippe BM, et al. A 48,XXXX female with absent ovaries. Am J Med Genet 1980; 6:275–278.

441. Cirillo-Silengo M, Davi GF, Franceschini P. The 49XXXXX syndrome. Report of a case with 48XXXX/49XXXXX mosaicism. Acta Paediatr Scand 1979; 68:769–771.

442. Toussi T, Halal F, Lesage R, et al. Renal hypodysplasia and unilateral ovarian agenesis in the penta-X syndrome. Am J Med Genet 1980; 6:153–162.

443. Fragoso R, Hernandez A, Plascencia ML, et al. 49,XXXXX. Ann Genet 1982; 24:145–148.

444. Sandberg AA, Koepf GF, Ishihara T, et al. An XYY human male. Lancet 1961; 2:488–489.

445. Hook EB. Extra sex chromosomes and human behavior: the nature of the evidence regarding XYY, XXY, XXYY, and XXX genotypes. In: Vallet HL, Porter IH, eds. Genetic Mechanisms of Sexual Development. New York: Academic, 1979: 437–463.

446. Owen DR. Psychological studies in XYY men. In: Vallet HL, Porter IH, eds. Genetic Mechanisms of Sexual Development. New York: Academic, 1979: 465–471.

447. Ridler MAC, Lax R, Mitchell MJ, et al. An adult male with XYYY sex chromosomes. Clin Genet 1973; 4:69–77.

448. Melicow MM, Uson AC. Dysgenetic gonadomas and other gonadal neoplasms in intersexes: report of 5 cases and review of the literature. Cancer 1959; 12:552–572.

449. Schellhas F. Malignant potential of the dysgenetic gonad. Obstet Gynecol 1974; 44:298–309 (Part I) and 455–562 (Part II).

450. Simpson JL, Photopulos G. The relationship of neoplasia to disorders of abnormal sexual differentiation. Birth Defects 1976; 12:15–50.

451. Manuel M, Katayama K, Jones HW Jr. The age of occurrence of gonadal tumors in intersex patients with a Y chromosome. Am J Obstet Gynecol 1976; 124:293–300.

452. Scully RE. Gonadoblastoma. A review of 74 cases. Cancer 1970; 25:1340–1356.

453. Scully RE. Neoplasia associated with anomalous sexual development and abnormal sex chromosomes. In: Josso N, ed. The Intersex Child. Pediatric and Adolescent Endocrinology. Vol 8. Basel: S. Karger, 1981: 203–217.

454. Verp MS, Simpson JL. Abnormal sexual differentiation and neoplasia. Cancer Genet Cytogenet 1987; 25:191–218.

455. Fonkalsrud EW, Mengel W, eds. The Undescended Testis. Chicago: Year Book Medical, 1981.

456. Sogge MR, McDonald SD, Cofold PB. The malignant potential of the dysgenetic germ cell in Klinefelter's syndrome. Am J Med 1979; 66:515–518.

457. Greenblatt RB, Byrd JR, McDonough PG, et al. The spectrum of gonadal dysgenesis: a clinical, cytogenetic and pathologic study. Am J Obstet Gynecol 1967; 98:151–172.

458. Lindsay AN, Sills IN, MacGillivray MH, et al. Dysgerminoma in a patient with the syndrome of gonadal dysgenesis with a 45,X karyotype. Am J Med Genet 1981; 10:21–24.

459. Patel SK, Prentice SA. Gonadoblastoma, distinctive ovarian tumor. Arch Pathol 1972; 94:165–170.

460. Goldberg MB, Scully AL, Solomon IL, et al. Gonadal dysgenesis in phenotypic female subjects: a review of 87 cases, with cytogenetic studies in 53. Am J Med 1968; 45:529–543.

461. Warren JC, Erkman B, Cheatum S, et al. Hilus cell adenoma in a dysgenetic gonad with XX/XO mosaicism. Lancet 1964; 1:141–143.

462. Hart WR, Burkons DM. Germ cell neoplasms arising in gonadoblastomas. Cancer 1979; 43:669–678.

463. Boczkowski K, Teter J, Sternandel Z. Sibship occurrence of XY gonadal dysgenesis with dysgerminoma. Am J Obstet Gynecol 1972; 113:952–955.

464. Isurugi K, Aso Y, Ishida H, et al. Prepubertal XY gonadal dysgenesis. Pediatrics 1977; 59:569–573.

465. New MI, White PC, Pang S, et al. The adrenal hyperplasias. In: Scriver CR, Beudet AL, Sly WS, et al., eds. The Metabolic Basis of Inherited Disease. 6th ed. New York: McGraw-Hill, 1989: 1881–1917.

466. Goldman AS. Animal models of inborn errors of steroidogenesis and steroid action. Colloq Ges Biol Chem 1970; 21:389–436.

467. Pang S, Wallace MA, Hofman L, et al. Worldwide experience in newborn screening for congenital adrenal hyperplasia due to 21 hydroxylase deficiency. Pediatrics 1988; 81:866–874.

468. Biglieri EG, Wajchenberg BL, Malerbi DA, et al. The zonal origins of the mineralocorticoid hormones in the 21-hydroxylation deficiency of congenital adrenal hyperplasia. J Clin Endocrinol Metab 1981; 53:964–969.

469. Fiet J, Gueux B, Raux-Demay M-C, et al. Increased plasma 21-deoxycorticosterone (21-DB) levels in late onset adrenal 21-hydroxylase deficiency suggest a mild defect of the mineralocorticoid pathway. J Clin Endocrinol Metab 1989; 68:542–547.

470. Kowarski A, Finkelstein JW, Spaulding JS, et al. Aldosterone secretion rate in congenital adrenal hyperplasia. A discussion of the theories on the pathogenesis of the salt-losing form of the syndrome. J Clin Invest 1965; 44:1505–1513.

471. Styne DM, Richards GE, Bell JJ, et al. Growth pattern in congenital adrenal hyperplasia: correlation of glucocorticoid therapy with stature. In: Lee PA, Plotnick LP, Kowarski AA, et al., eds. Congenital Adrenal Hyperplasia. Baltimore: University Park Press, 1977: 247–263.

472. Levine LS, Dupont B, Lorenzen F, et al. Cryptic 21-hydroxylase deficiency in families of patients with classical congenital adrenal hyperplasia. J Clin Endocrinol Metab 1980; 51:1316–1324.

473. Kohn B, Levine LS, Pollack MS, et al. Late-onset steroid 21-hydroxylase deficiency: a variant of classical congenital adrenal hyperplasia. J Clin Endocrinol Metab 1982; 55:817–827.

474. Rosenwaks Z, Lee PA, Jones GS, et al. An attenuated form of congenital virilizing adrenal hyperplasia. J Clin Endocrinol Metab 1979; 49:335–339.

475. Temeck JW, Pang S, Nelson C, et al. Genetic defects of steroidogenesis in premature pubarche. J Clin Endocrinol Metab 1987; 64:609–617.

476. Wischusen J, Bakker HWG, Hudson B. Reversible male infertility due to congenital adrenal hyperplasia. Clin Endocrinol 1981; 14:571–577.

477. New MI, Lorenzen F, Lerner AJ, et al. Genotyping steroid 21-hydroxylase deficiency: hormonal reference data. J Clin Endocrinol Metab 1983; 57:320–326.

478. New MI, Speiser PW. Genetics of adrenal steroid 21-hydroxylase deficiency. Endocr Rev 1986; 7:331–349.

479. Speiser PW, Dupont B, Rubinstein P, et al. High frequency of nonclassical steroid 21-hydroxylase deficiency. Am J Hum Genet 1985; 37:650–667.

480. Miller WL, Morel Y. The molecular genetics of 21-hydroxylase deficiency. Annu Rev Genet 1989; 23:371–393.

481. Strachan T. Molecular pathology of congenital adrenal hyperplasia. Clin Endocrinol 1990; 32:373–393.

482. White PC, Grossberger D, Onufer BJ, et al. Two genes encoding steroid 21-hydroxylase are located near the genes encoding the fourth component of complement in man. Proc Natl Acad Sci USA 1985; 82:1089–1093.

483. Strachan T. Molecular genetics of congenital adrenal hyperplasia. Trends Endocrinol Metab 1990; 1:68–72.

484. Higashi Y, Yoshioka H, Yanane M, et al. Complete nucleotide sequence of two steroid 21-hydroxylase genes tandemly arranged in human chromosome: a pseudogene and a genuine gene. Proc Natl Acad Sci USA 1986; 83:2841–2845.

485. Rodrigues NR, Dunham I, Yu C, et al. Molecular characterization of the HLA-linked steroid 21-hydroxylase B gene from an individual with congenital adrenal hyperplasia. EMBO J 1987; 6:1653–1661.

486. White PC, New MI, Dupont B. Structure of the human steroid 21-hydroxylase genes. Proc Natl Acad Sci USA 1986; 85:4436–4440.

487. Morel Y, André J, Uring-Lambert R, et al. Rearrangements and point mutations of the P450c21 genes are distinguished by five restriction endonuclease haplotypes identified by a new probing strategy in 57 families with congenital adrenal hyperplasia. J Clin Invest 1989; 83:527–536.

488. Collier S, Sinnott PJ, Dyer PA, et al. Pulsed field gel electrophoresis identifies a high degree of variability in the number of tandem 21-hydroxylase and complement C4 gene repeats in 21-hydroxylase deficiency haplotypes. EMBO J 1989; 8:1393–1402.

489. Speiser PW, New MI, White PC. Clinical and genetic characterization of nonclassic 21-hydroxylase deficiency. Endocr Res 1989; 15:257–276.

490. Thompson R, Seargeant L, Winter JSD. Screening for congenital adrenal hyperplasia: distribution of 17α-hydroxyprogesterone concentrations in neonatal blood spot specimens. J Pediatr 1989; 114:400–404.

491. Jenner MR, Grumbach MM, Kaplan SL. Plasma 17-OH progesterone in maternal and umbilical cord plasma in children, and in congenital adrenal hyperplasia (CAH): application to neonatal diagnosis of CAH. Pediatr Res 1970; 4:380 (abstract).

492. Pang S, Levine LS, Chow DM, et al. Serum androgen concentration in neonates and young infants with congenital adrenal hyperplasia due to 21 hydroxylase deficiency. Clin Endocrinol 1979; 11:575–584.

493. Godo B, Visser HKA, Degenhart JH. Plasma 17OH-progesterone in fullterm and preterm infants at birth and during the early neonatal period. Horm Res 1981; 15:65–71.

494. de Peretti E, Forest M. Pitfalls in the etiologic diagnosis of congenital adrenal hyperplasia in the early neonatal period. Horm Res 1982; 16:10–22.

495. Fiet J, Gueux B, Gourmelen M, et al. Comparison of basal and adrenocorticotropin-stimulated plasma 21-deoxycortisol and 17-hydroxyprogesterone values as biological markers of late-onset adrenal hyperplasia. J Clin Endocrinol Metab 1988; 66:659–667.

496. Frasier SD, Thorneycroft IH, Weiss BA, et al. Elevated amniotic fluid concentration of 17α-hydroxyprogesterone in congenital adrenal hyperplasia. J Pediatr 1975; 86:310–311 (letter).

497. Pollack M, Levine LS, Duchon M, et al. Prenatal diagnosis of CAH due to 21 hydroxylase deficiency by HLA typing of cultured amniotic fluid cells. Pediatr Res 1979; 13:384 (abstract).

498. Gueux B, Fiet J, Couillin P, et al. Prenatal diagnosis of 21-hydroxylase deficiency congenital adrenal hyperplasia by simultaneous radioimmunoassay of 21-deoxycortisol and 17-hydroxyprogesterone in amniotic fluid. J Clin Endocrinol Metab 1988; 66:534–537.

499. Speiser PW, Laforgia N, Kato K, et al. First trimester prenatal treatment and molecular genetic diagnosis of congenital adrenal hyperplasia (21-hydroxylase deficiency). J Clin Endocrinol Metab 1990; 70:838–848.

500. David M, Forest MG. Prenatal treatment of congenital adrenal hyperplasia resulting from 21-hydroxylase deficiency. J Pediatr 1984; 105:799–803.

501. Forest MG, Betuel H, David M. Prenatal treatment in congenital adrenal hyperplasia due to 21-hydroxylase deficiency: update 88 of the French multicentric study. Endocr Res 1989; 15:277–301.

502. Young MC, Robinson JA, Read GF. 17OH-Progesterone rhythms in congenital adrenal hyperplasia. Arch Dis Child 1988; 63:617–623.

503. Richards GE, Grumbach MM, Kaplan SL, et al. The effect of long acting glucocorticoids in menstrual abnormalities in patients with virilizing congenital adrenal hyperplasia. J Clin Endocrinol Metab 1978; 47:1208–1215.

504. Horner JM, Hintz RL, Leutscher JA. The role of renin and angiotensin in salt-losing, 21-hydroxylase–deficient congenital adrenal hyperplasia. J Clin Endocrinol Metab 1979; 48:776–783.

505. Urban MD, Lee PA, Migeon CJ. Adult height and fertility in men with congenital virilizing adrenal hyperplasia. N Engl J Med 1978; 299:1392–1396.

506. Brook CGD, Zachmann M, Prader A, et al. Experience with long-term therapy in congenital adrenal hyperplasia. J Pediatr 1974; 85:12–19.

507. Klingensmith GJ, Garcia SC, Jones HW Jr, et al. Glucocorticoid treatment of girls with congenital adrenal hyperplasia: effects on height, sexual maturation, and fertility. J Pediatr 1977; 90:996–1004.

508. Sotiropoulos A, Morishima A, Homsy Y, et al. Long-term assessment of genital reconstruction in female pseudohermaphrodites. J Urol 1976; 115:599–601.

509. Hendren WH, Donahoe PK. Correction of congenital abnormalities of the vagina and perineum. J Pediatr Surg 1980; 16:751–763.

510. Eberlein WR, Bongiovanni AM. Congenital adrenal hyperplasia with hypertension: unusual steroid pattern in blood and urine. J Clin Endocrinol Metab 1955; 15:1531–1534.

511. Rosler A, Lieberman E, Sack J, et al. Clinical variability of congenital adrenal hyperplasia due to 11β-hydroxylase deficiency. Horm Res 1982; 16:133–141.

512. Zachmann M, Tassinari D, Prader A. Clinical and biochemical variability of congenital adrenal hyperplasia due to 11β-hydroxylase deficiency. A study of 25 patients. J Clin Endocrinol Metab 1983; 56:222–229.

513. Wada A, Okamoto M, Nonaka Y, et al. Aldosterone biosynthesis by a reconstituted cytochrome P-450 11-beta system. Biochem Biophys Res Commun 1984; 119:365–371.

514. Yanagibashi K, Haniu M, Shively JE, et al. The synthesis of aldosterone by the adrenal cortex. J Biol Chem 1986; 261:3556–3562.

514a. Sparkes RS, Klisak I, Miller WL. Regional mapping of genes encoding human steroidogenic enzymes: P450scc to 15q23–q24; adrenodoxin to 11q22; adrenodoxin reductase to 17q24–q25; and P450c17 to 10q24–q25. DNA Cell Biol 10:359–366, 1991.

515. Chua SC, Szabo P, Vitek A, et al. Cloning of cDNA encoding steroid 11β-hydroxylase (P450c11). Proc Natl Acad Sci USA 1987; 84:7193–7197.

516. Miller WL. Molecular biology of steroid hormone synthesis. Endocr Rev 1988; 9:295–318.

517. Levine LS, Rauh W, Gottesdiener K, et al. New studies of the 11β-hydroxylase and 18-hydroxylase enzymes in the hypertensive form of congenital adrenal hyperplasia. J Clin Endocrinol Metab 1980; 50:258–263.

518. Rodriguez Portales JA, Arteaga E, Lopez Moreno JM, et al. Zona glomerulosa function after life-long suppression in two siblings with the hypertensive virilizing form of congenital adrenal hyperplasia. J Clin Endocrinol Metab 1988; 66:349–354.

519. Rosler A, Leiberman E. Enzymatic defects of steroidogenesis: 11β-
hydroxylase deficiency congenital adrenal hyperplasia. In: New MI, Levine LS, eds. Adrenal Diseases in Childhood. Pediatric Adolescent Endocrinology. Vol 13. Basal: S. Karger, 1984: 47–71.

520. Birnbaum MD, Rose LI. Late onset adrenocortical 11β-hydroxylase deficiency associated with menstrual dysfunction. Obstet Gynecol 1984; 63:445–451.

521. Holcombe JH, Keenan BS, Nichols BL, et al. Neonatal salt loss in the hypertensive form of congenital adrenal hyperplasia. Pediatrics 1980; 65:777–781.

521a. Hochberg Z, Benderly A, Kahana L, et al. Requirement of mineralocorticoid in congenital adrenal hyperplasia due to 11β-hydroxylase deficiency. J Clin Endocrinol Metab 1986; 63:36–40.

522. Globerman H, Rosler A, Theodur R, et al. An inherited defect in aldosterone biosynthesis is caused by a mutation in or near the gene for steroid 11-hydroxylase. N Engl J Med 1988; 319:1193–1197.

523. Lee PDK, Patterson BD, Hintz RL, et al. Biochemical diagnosis and management of corticosterone methyl oxidase type II deficiency. J Clin Endocrinol Metab 1986; 62:225–229.

524. Pang S, Levine LS, Lorenzen F, et al. Hormonal studies in obligate heterozygotes and siblings of siblings with 11β-hydroxylase deficiency congenital adrenal hyperplasia. J Clin Endocrinol Metab 1980; 50:586–589.

525. Schumert Z, Rosenmann A, Landau H, et al. 11-Deoxycortisol in amniotic fluid: prenatal diagnosis of congenital adrenal hyperplasia due to 11β-hydroxylase deficiency. Clin Endocrinol 1980; 12:257–260.

526. Rosler A, Lieberman E, Rosenmann A, et al. Prenatal diagnosis of 11β-hydroxylase deficiency congenital adrenal hyperplasia. J Clin Endocrinol Metab 1979; 49:546–551.

527. Ishi-Ohba H, Saiki N, Inano H, et al. Purification and characterization of rat adrenal 3β-hydroxysteroid dehydrogenase with steroid 5-ene-4-ene-isomerase. J Steroid Biochem 1986; 24:753–760.

528. Stalvy JRD, Meisler MA, Payne AH. Evidence that the same structural gene encodes testicular and adrenal 3β-hydroxysteroid dehydrogenase isomerase. Biochem Genet 1987; 25:181–190.

529. Luu-The V, Lachance Y, Le Blanc G, et al. Characterization of the human 3β-hydroxysteroid dehydrogenase gene. Endocr Soc Abstr 1990; 278.

530. Bongiovanni AM. The adrenogenital syndrome with deficiency of 3β-hydroxysteroid dehydrogenase. J Clin Invest 1962; 41:2086–2092.

531. Pang S, Levine LS, Stoner E, et al. Nonsalt-losing congenital adrenal hyperplasia due to 3β-hydroxysteroid dehydrogenase deficiency with normal glomerulosa function. J Clin Endocrinol Metab 1983; 56:808–818.

532. Rosenfield RL, Rich BH, Wolfsdorf JL, et al. Pubertal presentation of congenital Δ⁵-3β-hydroxysteroid dehydrogenase deficiency. J Clin Endocrinol Metab 1980; 51:345–353.

533. Bongiovanni AM. Acquired adrenal hyperplasia with special reference to 3β-hydroxysteroid dehydrogenase. Fertil Steril 1981; 35:599–608.

534. Bongiovanni AM. Congenital adrenal hyperplasia due to 3β-hydroxysteroid dehydrogenase deficiency. In: New MI, Levine LS, eds. Adrenal Diseases in Childhood. Basel: S. Karger, 1984: 72.

535. Bongiovanni AM. Urinary steroidal pattern of infants with congenital hyperplasia due to 3-beta-hydroxysteroid dehydrogenase deficiency. J Steroid Biochem 1980; 13:809–811.

536. Nakajin S, Hall PF. Microsomal cytochrome P450 from neonatal pig testis. J Biol Chem 1981; 256:3871–3876.

537. Kominami S, Shinzawa K, Takemora S. Purification and properties of cytochrome P-450 for steroid 17α-hydroxylation and C$_{17-20}$ bond cleavage from guinea pig adrenal microsomes. Biochem Biophys Res Commun 1982; 109:916–921.

538. Nakajin S, Shinoda M, Hall PF. Purification and properties of 17α-hydroxylase from pig adrenal: a second C$_{21}$ side-chain cleavage system. Biochem Biophys Res Commun 1983; 111:512–517.

539. Nakajin S, Shinoda M, Haniu M, et al. C$_{21}$ steroid side chain cleavage enzyme from porcine adrenal microsomes. Purification and characterization of the 17α-hydroxylase/C17-20 lyase cytochrome P450. J Biol Chem 1984; 259:3971–3976.

540. Chung B-C, Picardo-Leonard J, Haniu M, et al. Cytochrome P450c17 (steroid 17α-hydroxylase/17,20 lyase) cloning of the human adrenal and testes cDNAs indicate the same gene is expressed in both tissues. Proc Natl Acad Sci USA 1987; 84:407–411.

540a. Yanase T, Simpson ER, Waterman MR. 17α-Hydroxylase/17,20-lyase deficiency: from clinical investigation to molecular definition. Endocr Rev 1991; 12:91–108.

541. Rodgers RJ, Waterman MR, Simpson ER. Cytochrome P-450scc, P-450$_{17α}$, adrenodoxin, and reduced nicotinamide adenine dinucleotide phosphate–cytochrome P-450 reductase in bovine follicles and corpora lutea. Changes in specific contents during the ovarian cycle. Endocrinology 1986; 118:1366–1374.

542. Sakaguchi M, Mihara K, Sata R. Signal recognition particle is required for cotranslational insertion of cytochrome P450 into microsomal membranes. Proc Natl Acad Sci USA 1984; 81:3361–3364.

543. Matteson KJ, Picardo-Leonard J, Chung B, et al. Assignment of the gene for adrenal P450c17 (17α-hydroxylase/17,20 lyase) to human chromosome 10. J Clin Endocrinol Metab 1986; 63:789–791.

544. Biglieri EG, Herron MA, Brust N. 17-Hydroxylation deficiency in man. J Clin Invest 1966; 45:1946–1954.

545. New MI. Male pseudohermaphrodism due to a 17α-hydroxylase deficiency. J Clin Invest 1970; 49:1930–1941.

546. Peterson RE, Imperato-McGinley J. Male pseudohermaphroditism due to inherited deficiencies of testosterone biosynthesis. In: Serio M, Motta M, Zanisi M, et al., eds. Sexual Differentiation: Basic and Clinical Aspects. New York: Raven, 1984: 301–319.

547. Dean HJ, Shackelton CHL, Winter JSD. Diagnosis and natural history of 17-hydroxylase deficiency in a newborn male. J Clin Endocrinol Metab 1984; 59:513–520.

548. Winter JSD, Couch RM, Muller J, et al. Combined 17-hydroxylase and 17/20 desmolase deficiencies: evidence for synthesis of a defective cytochrome P450c17. J Clin Endocrinol Metab 1989; 68:309–316.

549. Kagimoto M, Winter JSD, Kagimoto K, et al. Structural characterization of normal and mutant human steroid 17α-hydroxylase genes: molecular basis of one example of combined 17α-hydroxylase/17,20 lyase deficiency. Mol Endocrinol 1988; 2:564–570.

550. Peterson RE, Imperato-McGinley J, Gautier T, et al. Male pseudohermaphroditism due to multiple defects in steroid-biosynthetic microsomal mixed-function oxidases. N Engl J Med 1985; 313:1182–1191.

551. Miller WL. Congenital adrenal hyperplasia. N Engl J Med 1986; 314:1321 (letter).

551a. Kagawa J, Janae A, Hashimoto N, et al. A new variant of congenital adrenal hyperplasia (CAH) with combined deficiencies of 17α-hydroxylase, 17,20-desmolase and 21-hydroxylase. Acta Pediatr Jpn 1988; 30(Suppl):239–242.

552. Kater CE, Biglieri EG, Brust N, et al. The unique patterns of plasma aldosterone and 18-hydroxycorticosterone concentrations in the 17α-hydroxylase deficiency syndrome. J Clin Endocrinol Metab 1982; 55:295–302.

553. D'Armiento M, Reda G, Kater C, et al. 17α-Hydroxylase deficiency: mineralocorticoid hormone profiles in an affected family. J Clin Endocrinol Metab 1983; 56:697–701.

554. Miller WL. Molecular biology of steroid hormone synthesis. Endocr Rev 1988; 9:295–318.

555. Morohashi K, Sogawa K, Omura T, et al. Gene structure of human cytochrome P-450(scc), cholesterol desmolase. J Biochem (Tokyo) 1987; 101:879–887.

556. Chung B, Matteson KJ, Voutilainen R, et al. Human cholesterol side-chain cleavage enzyme, P450scc: cDNA cloning, assignment of gene to chromosome 15 and expression in the placenta. Proc Natl Asad Sci USA 1986; 83:8962–8966.

557. Koizumi S, Kyoya S, Miyawaki T, et al. Cholesterol side-chain cleavage enzyme activity and cytochrome P-450 content in adrenal mitochondria of a patient with congenital lipoid adrenal hyperplasia (Prader disease). Clin Chim Acta 1977; 77:301–306.

558. Prader A, Gurtner HP. Das Syndrom des Pseudohermaphroditismus masculinus bei kongenitaler Nebennierenrinden-Hyperplasie ohne Androgenuberproduktion (adrenaler Pseudohermaphrotidismus masculinus). Helv Paediatr Acta 1955; 10:397–412.

559. Tsutsui Y, Hirabayashi N, Ito G. An autopsy case of congenital lipoid hyperplasia of the adrenal cortex. Acta Pathol Jpn 1970; 20:227–237.

560. Camacho AM, Kowarski A, Migeon CJ, et al. Congenital adrenal hyperplasia due to a deficiency of one of the enzymes involved in the biosynthesis of pregnenolone. J Clin Endocrinol Metab 1968; 28:153–161.

561. Kirkland RT, Kirkland JL, Johnson CM, et al. Congenital lipoid adrenal hyperplasia in an eight-year old phenotypic female. J Clin Endocrinol Metab 1973; 56:488–496.

562. Hauffa BP, Miller WL, Grumbach MM, et al. Congenital adrenal hyperplasia due to deficient cholesterol side-chain cleavage activity (20,22 desmolase) in a patient treated for 18 years. Clin Endocrinol 1985; 23:481–493.

563. Matteson KJ, Chung B-C, Urdea MS, et al. Study of cholesterol side chain cleavage (20,22 desmolase) deficiency causing congenital adrenal hyperplasia using bovine-sequence P450scc oligo-deoxyribonucleotide probes. Endocrinology 1986; 118:1296–1305.

563a. Shozu M, Akasofu K, Takenori T, et al. A new cause of female pseudohermaphroditism: placental aromatase deficiency. J Clin Endocrinol Metab 1991; 72:560–566.

564. Grumbach MM, Ducharme JR, Moloshok RE. On the fetal masculinizing action of certain oral progestins. J Clin Endocrinol Metab 1959; 19:1369–1380.

565. Kirk JM, Perry LA, Shard WS. Female pseudohermaphroditism due to a maternal adrenocortical tumor. J Clin Endocrinol Metab 1990; 70:1280–1284.

566. Wilkens L. Masculinization of female fetus due to use of orally given progestins. JAMA 1960; 172:1028–1032.

567. Jones HW Jr. Nonadrenal female pseudohermaphroditism. In: Josso N, ed. The Intersex Child. Pediatric and Adolescent Endocrinology. Vol 8. Basel: S. Karger, 1981: 65–79.

568. Ishizuka N, Kawashima Y, Nakanishi T, et al. Statistical observations on genital anomalies of newborns following the administration of progestins to their mothers. Obstet Gynecol Surv 1964; 19:496–497.

569. Duck SC, Katayama KP. Danazol may cause female pseudohermaphrodism. Fertil Steril 1981; 35:230–231.

570. Castro-Magana M, Cheruvanky T, Collipp PJ, et al. Transient adreno-genital syndrome due to exposure to danazol in utero. Am J Dis Child 1981; 135:1032–1034.

571. Bongiovanni AM, Di George AM, Grumbach MM. Masculinization of the female infant associated with estrogenic therapy alone during gestation: four cases. J Clin Endocrinol Metab 1959; 19:1004–1011.

572. Murset G, Zachmann M, Prader A, et al. Male external genitalia of a girl caused by a virilizing adrenal tumour in the mother. Acta Endocrinol 1970; 65:627–638.

573. Novak DJ, Lauchlan SC, McCawley JC, et al. Virilization during pregnancy. Am J Med 1970; 49:281–290.

574. Verhoeven ATM, Mastboom JL, Van Leusden HAIM, et al. Virilization in pregnancy coexisting with an (ovarian) mucinous cystadenoma: a case report and review of virilizing ovarian tumors in pregnancy. Obstet Gynecol Surv 1973; 28:597–622.

575. Kai H, Nose O, Iida Y, et al. Female pseudohermaphrodism caused by maternal congenital adrenal hyperplasia. J Pediatr 1979; 95:418–420.

576. Malinak LR, Miller GV. Bilateral multicentric ovarian luteomas of pregnancy associated with masculinization of a female infant. Am J Obstet Gynecol 1965; 91:251–259.

577. Cohen DA, Daughaday WH, Weldon VV. Fetal and maternal virilization associated with pregnancy. Am J Dis Child 1982; 136:353–356.

578. Hensleigh PA, Carter RP, Grotjan HE Jr. Fetal protection against masculinization with hyperreactio luteinalis and virilization. J Clin Endocrinol Metab 1975; 40:816–823.

579. Hensleigh PA, Woodruff JD. Differential maternal-fetal response to androgenizing luteoma or hyperreactio luteinalis. Obstet Gynecol Surv 1978; 33:262–271.

580. Park IJ, Johanson A, Jones HW, et al. Special female hermaphroditism associated with multiple disorders. Obstet Gynecol 1972; 39:100–106.

581. Gearhart JP, Rock JD. Female pseudohermaphroditism: unusual variants and their management. Adolesc Pediatr Gynecol 1989; 2:3–9.

582. Carpentier PJ, Potter EL. Nuclear sex and genital malformation in 48 cases of renal agenesis, with especial reference to nonspecific female pseudohermaphroditism. Am J Obstet Gynecol 1959; 78:235–258.

583. Perez-Palacios G, Scaglia H, Kofman-Alfaro S, et al. Inherited deficiency of gonadotropin receptor in Leydig cells: a new form of male pseudohermaphroditism. Am J Hum Genet 1975; 27:71a (abstract).

584. Berthezene F, Forest MG, Grimaud JA, et al. Leydig cell agenesis: a cause of male pseudohermaphroditism. N Engl J Med 1976; 295:969–972.

585. Brown DM, Markland C, Dehner LP. Leydig cell hypoplasia: a cause of male pseudohermaphrodism. J Clin Endocrinol Metab 1978; 46:1–7.

586. Perez-Palacios G, Scaglia H, Kofman-Alfaro S, et al. Inherited male pseudohermaphrodism due to gonadotropin unresponsiveness. Acta Endocrinol 1981; 98:148–156.

587. Schwartz M, Imperato-McGinley J, Peterson RE, et al. Male pseudohermaphroditism secondary to an abnormality in Leydig cell differentiation. J Clin Endocrinol Metab 1981; 53:123–127.

588. Perez-Palacios G, Ulloa-Aguirre A, Kofman-Alfaro S. Inherited male pseudohermaphroditism: analogies between human and rodent models. In: Serio M, Motta M, Zanisi M, et al., eds. Sexual Differentiation: Basic and Clinical Aspects. New York: Raven, 1984: 287–299.

589. Lee PA, Rock JA, Brown TR, et al. Leydig cell hypofunction resulting in male pseudohermaphroditism. Fertil Steril 1982; 37:675–679.

590. David R, Yoon D, Landin L, et al. A syndrome of gonadotropin resistance possibly due to an LH receptor defect. Endocr Soc Abstr 1983; 468:197.

591. Eil C, Austin RM, Sesterhenn I, et al. Leydig cell hypoplasia causing male pseudohermaphroditism: diagnosis 13 years after prepubertal castration. J Clin Endocrinol Metab 1984; 58:441–448.

592. Toledo SPA, Arnhold IJP, Luthold W, et al. Leydig cell hypoplasia determining familial hypergonadotrophic hypogonadism. Prog Clin Biol Res 1985; 200:311–314.

593. Saldanha PH, Arnhold IJP, Mendonca BB, et al. A clinico-genetic investigation of Leydig cell hypoplasia. Am J Med Genet 1987; 26:337–344.

594. Bardin CW, Bullock LP, Sherins RJ, et al. Androgen metabolism and mechanism of action in male pseudohermaphroditism: a study of testicular feminization. Recent Prog Horm Res 1973; 29:65–109.

595. Forest MG. Inborn errors of testosterone biosynthesis in the intersex child. In: Josso N, ed. Pediatric and Adolescent Endocrinology. Vol 8. Basel: S. Karger, 1981: 133–155.

596. Janne O, Perheentupa J, Viinikka L, et al. Plasma and urinary steroids in an eight-year old boy with 3β-hydroxysteroid dehydrogenase deficiency. J Clin Endocrinol Metab 1970; 31:162–165.

597. Aachmann M, Vollmin JA, Murset G, et al. Unusual type of congenital adrenal hyperplasia probably due to deficiency of 3β-hydroxysteroid dehydrogenase. Case report of a surviving girl and steroid studies. J Clin Endocrinol Metab 1970; 30:719–726.

598. Parks GA, Bermudez JA, Anast CS, et al. Pubertal boy with the 3β-hydroxysteroid dehydrogenase defect. J Clin Endocrinol Metab 1971; 33:269–278.

599. Kenny FM, Reynolds JW, Green OC. Partial 3-β-hydroxysteroid dehydrogenase (3-β-HSD) deficiency in a family with congenital adrenal hyperplasia: evidence for increasing 3-β-HSD activity with age. Pediatrics 1971; 48:756–765.

600. Janne O, Perheentupa J, Viinikka L. Testicular endocrine function in a pubertal boy with 3β-hydroxysteroid dehydrogenase deficiency. J Clin Endocrinol Metab 1974; 39:206–209.

601. Schneider G, Genel M, Bongiovanni AM, et al. Persistent testicular Δ5-isomerase-3β-hydroxysteroid dehydrogenase (Δ5-3β-HSD) deficiency in the Δ5-3β-HSD form of congenital adrenal hyperplasia. J Clin Invest 1975; 55:681–690.

602. Mendonca BB, Bloise W, Arnhold IJP, et al. Male pseudohermaphroditism due to non–salt losing 3β-hydroxysteroid dehydrogenase deficiency: gender role change and absence of gynecomastia at puberty. J Steroid Biochem 1987; 28:669–675.

603. de Peretti E, Forest MG, Feit JP, et al. Endocrine studies in two children with male pseudohermaphrodism due to 3β-hydroxysteroid (3βHSD) dehydrogenase defect. In: Genazzani AR, Thijssen JHH, Siiteri PK, eds. Adrenal Androgens. New York: Raven, 1980: 141–146.

604. Cara JF, Moshang T Jr, Bongiovanni AM, et al. Elevated 17-hydroxyprogesterone and testosterone in a newborn with 3-beta-hydroxysteroid dehydrogenase deficiency. N Engl J Med 1985; 313:618–621.

605. Jones HW Jr, Lee PA, Rock JA, et al. A genetic male patient with 17α-hydroxylase deficiency. Obstet Gynecol 1982; 59:254–259.

606. Mantero F, Busnardo B, Riondel A, et al. Arterial hypertension, hypokalemic alkalosis and pseudohermaphroditism caused by 17α-hydroxylase deficiency. Schweiz Med Wochenschr 1971; 101:38–43.

607. Bricaire H, Luton JP, Laudat P, et al. A new male pseudohermaphroditism associated with hypertension due to a block of 17α-hydroxylation. J Clin Endocrinol Metab 1972; 35:67–72.

608. Alvarez MN, Cloutier MD, Hayles AB. Male pseudohermaphroditism due to a 17α-hydroxylase deficiency in two siblings. Pediatr Res 1973; 7:325 (abstract).

609. Kershnar AK, Borut D, Kogut MD, et al. Studies in a phenotypic female with 17-α-hydroxylase deficiency. J Pediatr 1976; 89:395–400.

610. Tourniaire J, Audi Parera L, Loras B, et al. Male pseudohermaphroditism with hypertension due to a 17α-hydroxylation deficiency. Clin Endocrinol 1976; 5:53–61.

611. Ito S, Yamaguchi M, Miyamoto N. The 17α-hydroxylase deficiency found in genotypically female and male siblings both phenotypically female. Jpn J Hum Genet 1977; 21:247–256.

612. Tvedegaard M, Frederiksen V, Olgaard K, et al. Two cases of 17α-hydroxylase deficiency—one combined with complete gonadal agenesis. Acta Endocrinol 1981; 98:267–273.

613. Hosaka M, Oshima H, Troen P. Studies of the human testis. XIV. Properties of C17-20 lyase. Acta Endocrinol 1980; 94:389–396.

614. Zachmann M, Vollmin JA, Hamilton W, et al. Steroid 17,20-desmolase deficiency: a new cause of male pseudohermaphroditism. Clin Endocrinol 1972; 1:369–385.

615. Zachmann M, Werder EA, Prader A. Two types of male pseudohermaphroditism due to 17,20-desmolase deficiency. J Clin Endocrinol Metab 1982; 55:487–490.

616. Forest MG. Familial male pseudohermaphroditism due to 17-20 desmolase deficiency. I. In vivo endocrine studies. J Clin Endocrinol Metab 1980; 50:826–833.

617. Goebelsmann U, Zachmann M, Davajan U, et al. Male pseudohermaphroditism consistent with 17,20-desmolase deficiency. Gynecol Invest 1976; 7:138–156.

618. Kaufman FR, Costin G, Goebelsmann U, et al. Male pseudohermaphroditism due to 17,20-desmolase deficiency. J Clin Endocrinol Metab 1983; 57:32–36.

619. Larrea F, Lisker R, Banuelos R, et al. Hypergonadotropic hypogonadism in an XX female subject due to 17,20 desmolase deficiency. Acta Endocrinol 1983; 103:400–405.

620. Tremblay Y, Ringler GE, Morel Y, et al. Regulation of the gene for estrogenic 17-ketosteroid reductase lying on chromosome 17 cen → q25. J Biol Chem 1989; 264:20458–20462.

621. Van L-T, Labrie C, Simard J, et al. Structure of two in tandem human 17β-hydroxysteroid dehydrogenase genes. Mol Endocrinol 1990; 4:268–275.

622. Saez JM, de Peretti E, Morera AM, et al. Familial male pseudohermaphroditism with gynecomastia due to a testicular 17-ketosteroid reductase defect. I. In vivo studies. J Clin Endocrinol Metab 1971; 32:604–610.

623. Saez JM, Morera AM, de Peretti E, Bertand J. Further in vivo studies in male pseudohermaphroditism with gynecomastia due to a testicular 17-ketosteroid reductase defect (compared to a case of testicular feminization). J Clin Endocrinol Metab 1972; 34:598–600.

624. Givens JR, Wiser WL, Summitt RL, et al. Familial male pseudohermaphroditism without gynecomastia due to deficient testicular 17-ketosteroid reductase activity. N Engl J Med 1974; 291:938–944.

625. Goebelsmann U, Hall TD, Paul WL, et al. In vitro steroid metabolic studies in testicular 17β-reduction deficiency. J Clin Endocrinol Metab 1975; 41:1136–1143.

626. Harkness RA, Thistlethwaite D, Darling JAB, et al. 17β-Hydroxysteroid oxidoreductase deficiency causing male pseudohermaphroditism in a child. J Endocrinol 1975; 67:16P–17P.

627. Pittaway DE, Andersen RN, Givens JR. Deficient 17β-hydroxysteroid oxidoreductase activity in testes from a male pseudohermaphrodite. J Clin Endocrinol Metab 1976; 43:457–461.

628. Imperato-McGinley J, Peterson RE, Stoller R, et al. Male pseudoher-

629. Rösler A, Kohn G. Male pseudohermaphroditism due to 17β-hydroxysteroid dehydrogenase deficiency: studies on the natural history of the defect and effect of androgens on gender role. J Steroid Biochem 1983; 19:663–674.

630. Millan M, Audi L, Martinez-Mora J, et al. 17-Ketosteroid reductase deficiency in an adult patient without gynecomastia but with female psychosocial orientation. Acta Endocrinol 1983; 102:633–640.

631. Dumic M, Plavsic V, Fattorini I, et al. Absent spermatogenesis despite early bilateral orchiepexy in 17-ketoreductase deficiency. Horm Res 1985; 22:100–106.

632. Ulloa-Aguirre A, Bassol S, Poo J, et al. Endrocine and biochemical studies in a 46,XY phenotypically male infant with 17 ketosteroid reductase deficiency. J Clin Endocrinol Metab 1985; 60:639–643.

633. Wit JM, van Hooff COM, Thijssen JHH, et al. In vivo and in vitro studies in a 46,XY phenotypically female infant with 17-ketosteroid reductase deficiency. Horm Metab Res 1988; 20:367–374.

634. Eckstein B, Cohen S, Farkas A, et al. The nature of the defect in familial male pseudohermaphroditism in Arabs of Gaza. J Clin Endocrinol Metab 1989; 68:477–485.

635. Gross DJ, Landau H, Kohn G, et al. Male pseudohermaphroditism due to 17β-hydroxysteroid dehydrogenase deficiency: gender assignment in early infancy. Acta Endocrinol 1986; 112:238–246.

636. Pang S, Softness B, Sweeney WJ III, et al. Hirsutism, polycystic ovarian disease and ovarian 17-ketosteroid reductase deficiency. N Engl J Med 1987; 316:1295–1301.

637. Griffin JE, Wilson JD. The syndromes of androgen resistance. N Engl J Med 1980; 302:198–209.

638. Migeon CJ, Brown TR, Fichman KR. Androgen insensitivity syndrome. In: Josso N, ed. The Intersex Child. Pediatric and Adolescent Endocrinology. Vol 8. Basel: S. Karger, 1981: 171–202.

639. Perez-Palacios G, Ulloa-Aguirre A, Kofman-Alfaro S. Inherited male pseudohermaphroditism: analogies between the human and rodent models. In: Serio M, Motta M, Zanisi M, et al., eds. Sexual Differentiation: Basic and Clinical Aspects. New York: Raven, 1984: 287–299.

640. McPhaul MJ, Marcelli M, Tilley WD. Androgen resistance caused by mutations in the androgen receptor gene. FASEB J (in press).

641. Lubahn DB, Joseph DR, Sullivan PM, et al. Cloning of human androgen receptor complementary DNA and localization to the X chromosome. Science 1988; 240:327–330.

642. Brown CJ, Goss SJ, Lubahn DB, et al. Androgen receptor locus in the human X chromosome: regional localization to Xq11–12 and description of a DNA polymorphism. Am J Hum Genet 1989; 44:264–269.

643. French FS, Lubahn DB, Brown TR, et al. The molecular basis of androgen insensitivity. Recent Prog Horm Res 1990; 46:1–38.

644. Morris JM, Mahesh VB. Further observations on the syndrome, "testicular feminization." Am J Obstet Gynecol 1963; 87:731–734.

645. Ulloa-Aguirre A, Mendez JP, Angeles A, et al. The presence of müllerian remnants in the complete androgen insensitivity syndrome: a steroid hormone–mediated defect? Fertil Steril 1986; 45:302–305.

646. O'Leary JA. Comparative studies of the gonad in testicular feminization and cryptorchidism. Fertil Steril 1965; 16:813–819.

647. Ferenczy A, Richart RM. The fine structures of the gonads in the complete form of testicular feminization syndrome. Am J Obstet Gynecol 1972; 113:399–409.

648. O'Connell MJ, Ramsey HE, Whang-Peng J, et al. Testicular feminization syndrome in three sibs: emphasis on gonadal neoplasia. Am J Med Sci 1973; 265:321–333.

649. German J, Simpson JL, Morillo-Cucci G, et al. Testicular feminization and inguinal hernias. Lancet 1978; 1:891.

650. Madden JD, Walsh PC, MacDonald PC, et al. Clinical and endocrinologic characterization of a patient with the syndrome of incomplete testicular feminization. J Clin Endocrinol Metab 1973; 41:751–760.

651. French FS, Van Wyk JJ, Baggett B, et al. Further evidence of a target organ defect in the syndrome of testicular feminization. J Clin Endocrinol Metab 1966; 26:493–503.

652. Stanley AJ, Gumbreck LG, Allison JE. Male pseudohermaphroditism in the laboratory Norway rat. Recent Prog Horm Res 1973; 29:43–64.

653. Gehring U, Tomkins GM, Ohno S. Effect of the androgen-insensitivity mutation on a cytoplasmic receptor for dihydrotestosterone. Nature New Biol 1971; 232:106–107.

654. Goldstein JL, Wilson JD. Studies on the pathogenesis of the pseudohermaphroditism in the mouse with testicular feminization. J Clin Invest 1972; 51:1647–1658.

655. Keenan BS, Meyer WJ III, Hadjian AJ, et al. Syndrome of androgen insensitivity in man: absence of 5α-dihydrotestosterone binding protein in skin fibroblasts. J Clin Endocrinol Metab 1974; 38:1143–1146.

656. Griffin JE, Punyashthiti K, Wilson JD. Dihydrotestosterone binding by cultured fibroblasts: comparison of cells from control subjects and from patients with hereditary male pseudohermaphroditism due to androgen resistance. J Clin Invest 1976; 57:1342–1351.

657. Kaufman M, Straisfeld C, Pinsky L. Male pseudohermaphroditism presumably due to target organ unresponsiveness to androgens. Defi-

cient 5α-dihydrotestosterone binding in cultured skin fibroblasts. J Clin Invest 1976; 58:345–350.

658. Amrhein JA, Meyer WJ III, Jones HW Jr, et al. Androgen insensitivity in man: evidence for genetic heterogeneity. Proc Natl Acad Sci USA 1976; 73:891–894.

659. Kaufman M, Pinsky L, Baird PH, et al. Complete androgen insensitivity with a normal amount of 5α-dihydrotestosterone–binding activity in labium majus skin fibroblasts. Am J Med Genet 1979; 4:401–411.

660. Berkovitz GD, Brown TR, Migeon CJ. Androgen receptors. Clin Endocrinol Metab 1983; 12:155–173.

661. Migeon CJ, Amrhein JA, Keenan BS, et al. The syndrome of androgen insensitivity in man: its relation to our understanding of male sex differentiation. In: Vallet HL, Porter I, eds. Genetic Mechanisms of Sexual Development. New York: Academic, 1979; 93–128.

662. Griffin JE. Testicular feminization associated with a thermolabile androgen receptor in cultured fibroblasts. J Clin Invest 1979; 64:1624–1631.

663. Pinsky L, Kaufman M, Summitt RL. Congenital androgen insensitivity due to a qualitatively abnormal androgen receptor. Am J Med Genet 1981; 10:91–99.

664. Griffin JE, Durrant JL. Qualitative receptor defects in families with androgen resistance: failure of stabilization of the fibroblast cytosol androgen receptor. J Clin Endocrinol Metab 1982; 55:465–474.

665. Brown TR, Maes M, Rothwell SW, et al. Human complete androgen insensitivity with normal dihydrotestosterone receptor binding capacity in cultured genital skin fibroblasts: evidence for a qualitative abnormality of the receptor. J Clin Endocrinol Metab 1982; 55:61–69.

666. Kaufman M, Pinsky L, Feder-Hollander R. Defective up-regulation of the androgen receptor in human androgen insensitivity. Nature 1981; 293:735–737.

667. Pinsky L, Kaufman M, Chudley AE. Reduced affinity of the androgen receptor for 5α-dihydrotestosterone but not methyltrienolone in a form of partial androgen resistance. J Clin Invest 1985; 75:1291–1296.

668. Eil C. Familial incomplete male pseudohermaphroditism associated with impaired nuclear androgen retention. J Clin Invest 1983; 71:850–858.

669. Brown TR, Migeon CJ. Androgen binding in nuclear matrix of human genital skin fibroblasts from patients with androgen insensitivity syndrome. J Clin Endocrinol Metab 1986; 62:542–550.

670. Kovacs WJ, Griffen JE, Weaver DD, et al. A mutation that causes lability of the androgen receptor under conditions that normally promote transformation to the DNA-binding state. J Clin Invest 1984; 73:1095–1104.

671. O'Malley B. The steroid receptor superfamily: more excitement predicted for the future. Mol Endocrinol 1990; 4:363–369.

672. Faber PW, Kuiper GGJM, van Rooij HCJ, et al. The N-terminal domain of the human androgen receptor is encoded by one large exon. Mol Cell Endocrinol 1989; 61:257–262.

673. Brown TR, Lubahn DB, Wilson EM, et al. Deletion of the steroid-binding domain of the human androgen receptor gene in one family with complete androgen insensitivity syndrome: evidence for further genetic heterogeneity in this syndrome. Proc Natl Acad Sci USA 1988; 85:8151–8155.

674. Trifiro M, Prior L, Pinsky L, et al. A single transition at an exonic CpG site apparently abolishes androgen receptor (AR)–binding activity in a family with complete androgen insensitivity (CAI). Am J Hum Genet 1989; 45(Suppl):A225 (abstract).

675. Pinsky L, Trifiro M, Sabbaghian N, et al. A deletional alteration of the androgen receptor (AR) gene in a sporadic patient with complete androgen insensitivity (CAI) who is mentally retarded. Am J Hum Genet 1989; 45(Suppl):A212 (abstract).

676. Lubahn DB, Brown TR, Simenthal JA, et al. Sequences of the intron/exon junctions of the coding region of the human androgen receptor gene and identification of a point mutation in a family with complete androgen insensitivity. Proc Natl Acad Sci USA 1989; 86:9534–9538.

677. Sai T, Seino S, Chang C, et al. An exonic point mutation of the androgen receptor gene in a family with complete androgen insensitivity. Am J Hum Genet 1990; 46:1095–1100.

678. Marcelli M, Tilley WD, Wilson CM, et al. A single nucleotide substitution introduces a premature termination codon into the androgen receptor gene of a patient with receptor negative androgen resistance. J Clin Invest 1990; 85:1522–1528.

679. Marcelli M, Tilley WD, Wilson CM. Definition of the human androgen receptor gene structure permits the identification of mutations that cause androgen resistance: premature termination of the receptor protein at amino acid residue 588 causes complete androgen resistance. Mol Endocrinol 1990; 4:1105–1115.

680. Tilley WD, Marcelli M, Griffen JE. Receptor negative androgen resistance is caused by diverse abnormalities of the androgen receptor gene. Endocr Soc Abstr 792:222, 1990.

681. Brown TR, Corden JL. Point mutations in the human androgen receptor gene of subjects with the receptor negative form of complete androgen insensitivity. Endocr Soc Abstr 861:240, 1990.

681a. Marcelli M, Zoppi S, Grino PB, et al. A mutation in the DNA-binding domain of the androgen receptor gene causes complete testicular feminization in a patient with receptor-positive androgen resistance. J Clin Invest 1991; 87:1123–1126.

682. Lee PA, Brown TR, La Torre HA. Diagnosis of the partial androgen insensitivity syndrome during infancy. JAMA 1986; 25:2207–2209.

683. Nagel BA, Lippe BM, Griffen JE. Androgen resistance in the neonate: use of hormones of hypothalamic-pituitary-gonadal axis for diagnosis. J Pediatr 1986; 109:486–488.

684. Boyar RM, Moore RJ, Rosner W, et al. Studies on gonadotropin-gonadal dynamics in patients with androgen insensitivity. J Clin Endocrinol Metab 1978; 47:1116–1117.

685. Faiman C, Winter JSD. The control of gonadotropin secretion in complete testicular feminization. J Clin Endocrinol Metab 1974; 39:631–638.

686. Tremblay RR, Foley TP Jr, Corvol P, et al. Plasma concentration of testosterone, dihydrotestosterone, testosterone-oestradiol binding globulin, and pituitary gonadotropins in the syndrome of male pseudohermaphroditism with testicular feminization. Acta Endocrinol 1972; 70:331–341.

687. MacDonald PC, Madden JD, Brenner PF, et al. Origin of estrogen in normal men and in women with testicular feminization. J Clin Endocrinol Metab 1979; 49:905–916.

688. Kelch RP, Jenner MR, Weinstein R, et al. Estradiol and testosterone secretion by human, simian, and canine testes, in males with hypogonadism and in male pseudohermaphrodites with the feminizing testes syndrome. J Clin Invest 1972; 51:824–830.

689. Imperato-McGinley J, Peterson RE, Gautier T, et al. Hormonal evaluation of a large kindred with complete androgen insensitivity: evidence for secondary 5α-reductase. J Clin Endocrinol Metab 1982; 54:931–941.

690. Zachmann M, Prader A, Sokel E, et al. Pubertal growth in patients with androgen insensitivity: indirect evidence for the importance of estrogens in pubertal growth of girls. J Pediatr 1986; 108:694–697.

691. Conte FA, Grumbach MM. Bearing of abnormalities of sex differentiation on the hypothalamic-pituitary-gonadal axis at puberty. In: Serio M, Motta M, Zanisi M, et al., eds. Sexual Differentiation: Basic and Clinical Aspects. New York: Raven, 1984: 275–285.

692. Aiman J, Griffin JE, Gazak JM, et al. Androgen insensitivity as a cause of infertility in otherwise normal men. N Engl J Med 1979; 300:223–227.

693. Reifenstein EC Jr. Hereditary familial hypogonadism. Clin Res 1947; 3:86.

694. Bowen P, Lee CSN, Migeon CJ, et al. Hereditary male pseudohermaphroditism with hypogonadism, hypospadias, and gynecomastia (Reifenstein's syndrome). Ann Intern Med 1965; 62:252–270.

695. Wilson JD, Harrod MJ, Goldstein JL, et al. Familial incomplete male pseudohermaphrodism, type I. N Engl J Med 1974; 290:1097–1103.

696. Amrhein JA, Jones Klingensmith G, Walsh PC, et al. Partial androgen insensitivity: the Reifenstein syndrome revisited. N Engl J Med 1977; 297:350–356.

697. Keenan BS, Kirland JL, Kirkland RT, et al. Male pseudohermaphroditism with partial androgen insensitivity. Pediatrics 1977; 59:224–231.

698. Gyorki S, Warne GL, Khalid BAK, et al. Defective nuclear accumulation of androgen receptors in disorders of sexual differentiation. J Clin Invest 1983; 72:819–825.

699. Eil C, Blair D, Fox TD. Androgen resistance with defective nuclear androgen binding. J Cell Biochem 1982; 6(Suppl):164 (abstract).

700. Eil C. Familial incomplete male pseudohermaphroditism associated with impaired nuclear androgen retention. J Clin Invest 1982; 71:850–858.

701. Aiman J, Griffin JE. The frequency of androgen receptor deficiency in infertile men. J Clin Endocrinol Metab 1982; 54:725–732.

702. Morrow AF, Gyorki S, Warne GL, et al. Variable androgen receptor levels in infertile men. J Clin Endocrinol Metab 1987; 64:1115–1121.

703. Wilson JD, Griffin JE, Leshin M, et al. The androgen resistance syndrome: 5α-reductase deficiency, testicular feminization, and related disorders. In: Stanbury JB, Wyngaarden JB, Fredricksen DS, et al., eds. The Metabolic Basis of Inherited Disease. 5th ed. New York: McGraw-Hill, 1983: 1001–1026.

704. Larrea F, Benavides G, Scaglia H, et al. Gynecomastia as a familial incomplete male pseudohermaphroditism type 1: a limited androgen resistance syndrome. J Clin Endocrinol Metab 1978; 46:961–970.

705. Grino PB, Griffin JE, Cushard WG Jr, et al. A mutation of the androgen receptor associated with partial androgen resistance, familial gynecomastia and fertility. J Clin Endocrinol Metab 1988; 66:754–761.

706. Price P, Wass JAH, Griffin JE, et al. High dose androgen therapy in male pseudohermaphroditism due to 5α-reductase deficiency and disorders of the androgen receptor. J Clin Invest 1984; 74:1496–1508.

707. Grino PB, Isidro-Gutierrez F, Griffin JE, et al. Androgen resistance associated with a qualitative abnormality of the androgen receptor and responsive to high dose androgen therapy. J Clin Endocrinol Metab 1989; 68:578–584.

708. Nowakowski H, Lenz W. Genetic aspects in male hypogonadism. Recent Prog Horm Res 1961; 17:53–95.

709. Opitz JM, Simpson JL, Sarto GE, et al. Pseudovaginal perineoscrotal hypospadias. Clin Genet 1972; 3:1–26.

710. Walsh PC, Madden JD, Harrod MJ, et al. Familial incomplete male pseudohermaphroditism, type 2. Decreased dihydrotestosterone formation in pseudovaginal perineoscrotal hypospadias. N Engl J Med 1974; 291:944–949.

711. Imperato-McGinley JL, Guerrero L, Gautier T, et al. Steroid 5α-reductase deficiency in man: an inherited form of male pseudohermaphrodism. Science 1974; 186:1213–1215.

712. Imperato-McGinley JL, Peterson RE. Male pseudohermaphroditism: the complexities of male phenotypic development. Am J Med 1976; 61:251–272.

713. Peterson RE, Imperato-McGinley J, Gautier T, et al. Male psuedohermaphroditism due to steroid 5α-reductase deficiency. Am J Med 1977; 62:170–191.

714. Imperato-McGinley JL, Peterson RE, Gautier T. Primary and secondary 5α-reductase deficiency. In: Serio M, Motta M, Zanisi M, et al., eds. Sexual Differentiation: Basic and Clinical Aspects. New York: Raven, 1984: 233–245.

715. Johnson L, George FW, Neaves WB, et al. Characterization of the testicular abnormality in 5α-reductase deficiency. J Clin Endocrinol Metab 1986; 63:1091–1099.

716. Peterson RE, Imperato-McGinley J, Gautier T, et al. Hereditary steroid 5α-reductase deficiency: a newly recognized cause of male pseudohermaphroditism. In: Vallet HL, Porter IH, eds. Genetic Mechanisms of Sexual Development. New York: Academic, 1979: 149–173.

717. Pang S, Levine LS, Chow D, et al. Dihydrotestosterone and its relationship to testosterone in infancy and childhood. J Clin Endocrinol Metab 1979; 48:821–826.

718. Moore RJ, Griffin JE, Wilson JD. Diminished 5α-reductase activity in extracts of fibroblasts cultured from patients with familial incomplete male pseudohermaphroditism, type 2. J Biol Chem 1975; 250:7168–7172.

719. Fisher LK, Kogut MD, Moore RJ, et al. Clinical, endocrinological, and enzymatic characterization of two patients with 5α-reductase deficiency: evidence that a single enzyme is responsible for the 5α-reduction of cortisol and testosterone. J Clin Endocrinol Metab 1978; 47:653–664.

720. Leshin M, Griffin JE, Wilson JD. Hereditary male pseudohermaphroditism associated with an unstable form of 5α-reductase. J Clin Invest 1978; 62:685–691.

721. Imperato-McGinley J, Peterson RE, Leshin M, et al. Steroid 5α-reductase deficiency in a 65-year old male pseudohermaphrodite: the natural history, ultra-structure of the testes and evidence for inherited enzyme heterogeneity. J Clin Endocrinol Metab 1980; 50:15–22.

722. Wilson JD. Recent studies on the mechanism of action of testosterone. N Engl J Med 1972; 287:1284–1291.

723. Hodgins MB. Possible mechanisms of androgen resistance in 5α-reductase deficiency: implications for the physiological roles of 5α-reductase. J Steroid Biochem 1983; 19:555–559.

724. Wilson JD, Aiman J, Macdonald PC. The pathogenesis of gynecomastia. Adv Intern Med 1980; 25:1–32.

725. Saenger P, Goldman AS, Levine LS, et al. Prepubertal diagnosis of steroid 5α-reductase deficiency. J Clin Endocrinol Metab 1978; 46:627–634.

726. Greene S, Zachmann M, Manella B, et al. Comparison of two tests to recognize or exclude 5α-reductase deficiency in prepubertal children. Acta Endocrinol 1987; 114:113–117.

727. Imperato-McGinley J, Gautier T, Pichardo M, et al. The diagnosis of 5α-reductase deficiency in infancy. J Clin Endocrinol Metab 1986; 63:1313–1318.

728. Pinsky L, Kaufman M, Straidfeld C, et al. 5α-Reductase activity of genital and nongenital skin fibroblasts from patients with 5α-reductase deficiency, androgen insensitivity, or unknown forms of male pseudohermaphroditism. Am J Med Genet 1978; 1:407–416.

729. Simpson JL. Male pseudohermaphroditism: genetics and clinical delineation. Hum Genet 1978; 44:1–49.

730. Keenan BS, Eberle AJ, Sparrow JT, et al. Dihydrotestosterone heptanoate: synthesis, pharmacokinetics, and effects on hypothalamic-pituitary-testicular function. J Clin Endocrinol Metab 1987; 64:557–563.

731. Carpenter TO, Imperato-McGinley J, Boulware SD, et al. Variable expression of 5α-reductase deficiency: presentation with male phenotype in a child of Greek origin. J Clin Endocrinol Metab 1990; 71:318–322.

732. Rajfer J, Mendelsohn G, Arnheim J, et al. Dysgenetic male pseudohermaphrodism. J Urol 1978; 119:525–527.

733. Rajfer J, Walsh PC. Mixed gonadal dysgenesis—dysgenetic male pseudohermaphroditism. In: Josso N, ed. The Intersex Child. Pediatric and Adolescent Endocrinology. Vol 8. Basel: S. Karger, 1981: 105–115.

734. Curry CJR, Jensen K, Holland J, et al. The Potter sequence: a clinical analysis of 80 cases. Am J Med Genet 1984; 19:679–702.

735. Drash A, Sherman F, Hartmann WH, et al. A syndrome of pseudohermaphroditism, Wilms' tumor, hypertension and degenerative renal disease. J Pediatr 1970; 76:585–593.

735a. Habib R, Loirat C, Gubler MC, et al. The nephropathy associated with male pseudohermaphroditism and Wilms tumor (Drash syndrome): a distinctive glomerular lesion. Report of 10 cases. Clin Nephrol 1985; 6:269–278.

736. Turleau C, De Grouchy J, Dufier JL, et al. Aniridia, male pseudohermaphroditism, gonadoblastoma, mental retardation and del 11p13. Hum Genet 1981; 57:300–306.

737. Cleary RE, Caras J, Rosenfeld R, et al. Endocrine and metabolic studies in a patient with male pseudohermaphrodism and true agonadism. Am J Obstet Gynecol 1977; 128:862–867.

738. Sarto GE, Opitz JM. The XY gonadal agenesis syndrome. J Med Genet 1973; 10:288–293.

739. Edman CD, Winters A, Porter J, et al. Embryonic testicular regression. A clinical spectrum of XY agonadal individuals. Obstet Gynecol 1977; 49:208–217.

740. Coulam CB. Testicular regression syndrome. Obstet Gynecol 1979; 53:44–49.

741. Goldberg LM, Skaist LB, Morrow JM. Congenital absence of testes: anorchism and monorchism. J Urol 1974; 111:840–845.

742. Hall JG, Morgan A, Blizzard RM. Familial congenital anorchia. Birth Defects 1975; 11:115–119.

743. Aynsley-Green AA, Zachmann M, Illig R, et al. Congenital bilateral anorchia in childhood: a clinical, endocrine and therapeutic evaluation of 21 cases. Clin Endocrinol 1976; 5:381–391.

744. Bergada C, Cleveland WW, Jones HW Jr, et al. Variants of embryonic testicular dysgenesis: bilateral anorchia and the syndrome of rudimentary testes. Acta Endocrinol 1962; 40:521–536.

745. Najjar SS, Takla RJ, Nassar VH. The syndrome of rudimentary testes: occurrence in five siblings. J Pediatr 1974; 84:119–122.

746. Josso N, Briard M-L. Embryonic testicular regression syndrome: variable phenotypic expression in siblings. J Pediatr 1980; 97:200–204.

747. Lustig RH, Conte FA, Grumbach MM, et al. Ontogeny of gonadotropin secretion in congenital anorchia: sexual dimorphism versus syndrome of gonadal dysgenesis and diagnostic considerations. J Urol 1987; 138:587–591.

748. Levitt SB, Kogan SJ, Engel RM, et al. The impalpable testis: a rational approach to management. J Urol 1978; 120:515–520.

749. Bartone FF, Huseman CA, Maizels M, et al. Pitfalls in using human chorionic gonadotropin (hCG) stimulation test to diagnose anorchia. J Urol 1984; 132:563–567.

750. Brook CGD, Wagner H, Zachmann M, et al. Familial occurrence of persistent müllerian structures in otherwise normal males. Br Med J 1973; 1:771–773.

751. Weiss EB, Kiefer JH, Rowlatt UF, et al. Persistent müllerian duct syndrome in male identical twins. Pediatrics 1978; 61:797–800.

752. Summitt RL. Genetic forms of hypogonadism in the male. Prog Med Genet 1979; 3:1–72.

753. Brook CGD. Persistent müllerian duct syndrome. In: Josso N, ed. The Intersex Child. Pediatric and Adolescent Endocrinology. Vol 8. Basel: S. Karger, 1981: 100–104.

754. Josso N, Fekete C, Cachin O, et al. Persistence of müllerian ducts in male pseudohermaphroditism, and its relationship to cryptorchidism. Clin Endocrinol 1983; 19:247–258.

755. Guerrier D, Tran D, Vanderwinden JM, et al. The persistent müllerian duct syndrome: a molecular approach. J Clin Endocrinol Metab 1989; 68:46–52.

756. Taguchi O, Cunha GR, Lawrence WD, et al. Timing and irreversibility of müllerian duct inhibition in the embryonic reproductive tract of the human male. Dev Biol 1984; 106:394–398.

757. Cohen-Haguenauer O, Picard O, Mattei MG, et al. Mapping of the gene for anti-müllerian hormone to the short arm of human chromosome 19. Cytogenet Cell Genet 1987; 44:2–6.

758. Courrier R, Jost A. Intersexualité totale provoquée par la pregneninolone au cours de la grossesse. C R Soc Biol (Paris) 1942; 136:395–396.

759. Aarskog D. Maternal progestins as a possible cause of hypospadias. N Engl J Med 1979; 300:75–78.

760. Sweet RA, Schrott HG, Kurland R, et al. Study of the incidence of hypospadias in Rochester, Minnesota, 1940–1970, and a case control comparison of possible etiologic factors. Mayo Clin Proc 1974; 49:52–58.

761. Lorber CA, Cassidy SB, Engel E. Is there an embryo-fetal exogenous sex steroid exposure syndrome (EFESSES)? Fertil Steril 1979; 31:21–24.

762. Czezel A, Toth J. Correlation between the birth prevalence of hypospadias and parental subfertility. Teratology 1990; 41:167–172.

763. Voight W, Hsia SL. Further studies on testosterone 5α-reductase of human skin: structural features of steroid inhibitors. J Biol Chem 1973; 248:4280–4285.

764. Kaplan NM. Male pseudohermaphrodism: report of a case, with observations on pathogenesis. N Engl J Med 1959; 261:641–644.

765. Henderson BE, Benton B, Cosgrove M, et al. Urogenital tract abnormalities in sons of women treated with diethylstilbestrol. Pediatrics 1976; 58:505–507.

766. Driscoll SG, Taylor SH. Effects of prenatal maternal estrogen on the male urogenital system. Obstet Gynecol 1980; 56:537–542.

767. Penny R. The effect of DES on male offspring. West J Med 1982; 136:329–330.

768. Carter CO. Multifactorial genetic disease. In: McKusick VA, Claiborne R, eds. Medical Genetics. New York: HP Publishing, 1973.

769. Belman AB, Kaplan GW. Genitourinary Problems in Pediatrics. Philadelphia: W. B. Saunders, 1981.

770. Sheldon CA, Duckett JW. Hypospadias. Pediatr Clin North Am 1987; 34:1259–1272.

771. Svensson J, Snochowski M. Androgen receptor levels in preputial skin from boys with hypospadias. J Clin Endocrinol Metab 1979; 49:340–345.

772. Keenan BS, McNeel RL, Gonzales ET. Abnormality of intracellular 5α-dihydrotestosterone binding in simple hypospadias: studies on equilibrium steroid binding in sonicates of genital skin fibroblasts. Pediatr Res 1984; 18:216–220.

773. Warne GL, Gyorski S, Risibridger GP, et al. Fibroblast studies on clinical androgen insensitivity. J Steroid Biochem 1983; 18:583–586.

774. Allen T, Griffin JE. Endocrine studies in patients with advanced hypospadias. J Urol 1984; 131:310–314.

775. Bauer SB, Retik AB, Coldny AH. Genetic aspects of hypospadias. Urol Clin North Am 1981; 8:559–564.

776. Buyse M, Feingold M. Syndromes associated with abnormal external genitalia. In: Vallet HL, Porter IH, eds. Genetic Mechanisms of Sexual Development. New York: Academic, 1979: 425–435.

777. Aarskog D. Clinical and cytogenetic studies in hypospadias. Acta Paediatr Scand 1970; 203(Suppl):1–62.

778. Walsh PC, Wilson JD, Allen TD, et al. Clinical and endocrinological evaluation of patients with congenital microphallus. J Urol 1978; 120:90–95.

779. Burstein S, Grumbach MM, Kaplan SL. Early determination of androgen-responsiveness is important in the management of microphallus. Lancet 1979; 2:983–986.

780. Lovinger RD, Kaplan SL, Grumbach MM. Congenital hypopituitarism associated with neonatal hypoglycemia and microphallus: four cases secondary to hypothalamic hormone deficiencies. J Pediatr 1975; 87:1171–1181.

781. Park IJ, Burnett LS, Jones HW Jr, et al. A case of male pseudohermaphrodism associated with elevated LH, normal FSH and low testosterone possibly due to the secretion of an abnormal LH molecule. Acta Endocrinol 1976; 83:173–181.

782. Meyer WJ III, Keenan BS, De Lacerda L, et al. Familial male pseudohermaphroditism with normal Leydig cell function at puberty. J Clin Endocrinol Metab 1978; 46:593–603.

783. Griffin JE, Edwards C, Madden JD, et al. Congenital absence of the vagina. The Mayer-Rokitansky-Küster-Hauser syndrome. Ann Intern Med 1976; 85:224–236.

784. Pinsky L. A community of human malformation syndromes involving the müllerian ducts, distal extremities, urinary tract and ears. Teratology 1974; 9:65–79.

785. Michels VV, Caskey TC. Müllerian aplasia with hypoplastic thumbs: two case reports. Int J Gynaecol Obstet 1979; 17:6–10.

786. Neinstein LS, Castle G. Congenital absence of the vagina. Am J Dis Child 1983; 137:671.

787. Ross GT, van de Wiele RL. The ovaries. In: Williams RH, ed. Textbook of Endocrinology. 5th ed. Philadelphia: W. B. Saunders, 1974: 368–422.

788. Fraser ID, Baird DT, Hobson BM, et al. Cyclical ovarian function in women with congenital absence of the uterus and vagina. J Clin Endocrinol Metab 1973; 36:634–637.

789. Duncan PA, Shapiro LR, Stangel JJ, et al. The MURCS association: müllerian duct aplasia, renal aplasia, and cervicothoracic somite dysplasia. J Pediatr 1979; 95:399–402.

790. Garcia J, Jones HW. The split thickness graft technic for vaginal agenesis. Obstet Gynecol 1977; 49:328–332.

791. Haskins JL, Gysler M, Cowell CA. Anatomical amenorrhea: the problems of congenital vaginal agenesis and its surgical correction. Pediatr Clin North Am 1981; 28(2):345–354.

792. Hecker BR, McGuire LS. Psychosocial function in women treated for vaginal agenesis. Am J Obstet Gynecol 1977; 129:543–547.

793. Money J, Hampson JC, Hampson JL. Hermaphroditism: recommendations concerning assignment of sex, change of sex, and psychologic management. Johns Hopkins Med J 1955; 97:284.

794. Forest MG. Pattern of the response of testosterone and its precursors to human chorionic gonadotropin stimulation in relation to age in infants and children. J Clin Endocrinol Metab 1979; 49:132–137.

795. Kogan SJ. Micropenis: etiologic and management conditions. In: Kogan SJ, Hafez ESE, eds. Clinics in Andrology. Vol 7. Pediatric Andrology. The Hague: Martinus Nijhoff, 1981: 197–207.

796. Rajfer J, Namkung PC, Petra PH. Ontogeny of 5α-reductase and the androgen receptor in the penis. In: Kogan SJ, Hafez ESE, eds. Clinics in Andrology. Vol 7. Pediatric Andrology. The Hague: Martinus Nijhoff, 1981: 53–57.

797. Caron AM, D'Avino R. Legal implications of intersexuality. In: Josso N, ed. The Intersex Child. Pediatric and Adolescent Endocrinology. Vol 8. Basel: S. Karger, 1981: 218–227.

798. Gross RE, Randolph J, Crigler JF Jr. Clitorectomy for sexual abnormalities: indications and technique. Surgery 1966; 59:300–308.

799. Lattimer JK. Relocation and recession of the enlarged clitoris with preservation of the glans: an alternative to amputation. J Urol 1961; 86:113–116.

800. Spense HM, Allen TD. Genital reconstruction in the female with the adrenogenital syndrome. Br J Urol 1973; 45:126–130.

801. Shaw A. Subcutaneous reduction clitoroplasty. J Pediatr Surg 1977; 12:331–338.

802. Rosenfield RL, Lucky AW, Allen TD. The diagnosis and management of intersex. In: Gluck L, ed. Current Problems in Pediatrics. Vol 10. No 7. Chicago: Year Book Medical, 1980.

803. Masters HW, Johnson VE. Human Sexual Response. Boston: Little, Brown, 1966.

804. Snyder McCH III, Retik AB, Bauer SB, et al. Feminizing genitoplasty: a synthesis. J Urol 1983; 129:1024–1026.

805. Jones HW Jr, Garcia SC, Klingensmith GJ. Necessity for and the technique of secondary surgical treatment of masculinized external genitalia of patients with virilizing adrenal hyperplasia. In: Lee PA, Plotnick LP, Kowarski AA, et al., eds. Congenital Adrenal Hyperplasia, Baltimore: University Park Press, 1977: 347–353.

806. Wabrek AJ, Millard R, Wilson WB Jr, et al. Creation of a neovagina by the Frank nonoperative method. Obstet Gynecol 1971; 37:408–413.

807. Thomsen C, Jensen KE, Giwercman A, et al. Magnetic resonance: in vivo tissue characterization of the testes in patients with carcinoma in situ of the testis and healthy subjects. Int J Androl 1987; 10:191–198.

808. Baker SW. Psychological management of intersex children. In: Josso N, ed. The Intersex Child. Pediatric and Adolescent Endocrinology. Vol 8. Basel: S. Karger, 1981: 261–269.

15

ENDOCRINE DISORDERS OF THE BREAST

Andrew G. Frantz and Jean D. Wilson

NORMAL DEVELOPMENT

Fetal Life Through Adolescence

Early in fetal life epithelial cells, derived from the epidermis in the area that will later become the areola, proliferate into the underlying mesenchyme. In the human, 20 or so short cords are formed, which later develop lumina to become ducts that are connected to the nipple and open to the surface. Surrounding the ducts is a network of myoepithelial cells, destined ultimately to serve in the expulsion of milk. In the later stages of gestation the blind ends of the ducts undergo budding to form alveolar structures, and a small amount of secretory activity occurs.[1–4] This results in the formation of so-called witch's milk, which can be expressed from the breasts of most full-term infants by the fifth to seventh day after birth and which persists for 1 to 7 wk thereafter.[5, 6] Subsequently, with the decline in circulating fetal prolactin and in the absence of estrogen and progesterone of placental origin, the breast regresses to a resting stage composed of a small number of scattered ducts. Such regression may not be complete until many months post partum, however.[7] In several species there is sexual dimorphism in the embryogenesis of the excretory duct system. In the male rodent the excretory ducts regress during the later phases of embryogenesis (as a result of testicular androgen secretion), and the breast proper is left as an isolated island in the subcutaneous tissue.[8–10] However, such dimorphism has never been documented in the human embryo, and there does not appear to be any histological or functional difference between the breasts in children of the two sexes before the onset of puberty.[11] Shortly before human menarche, with increased secretion of ovarian estrogen, lengthening and branching of the ducts begin in the female breast, accompanied by budding of the terminal ends and increased formation of underlying fat and connective tissue. With the onset of menses, further growth takes place in a cyclic fashion, some regression occurring at the end of each cycle.[12–14]

Pregnancy

During pregnancy the maternal breast is exposed to high levels of estrogen, progesterone, and prolactin (also see Chapter 16). Prolactin increases in concentration steadily throughout gestation, presumably as a consequence of estrogenic stimulation. Levels of human placental lactogen also increase, particularly during the terminal phases of gestation. Under these stimuli a dramatic augmentation of breast growth takes place, characterized by increased branching of ducts and differentiation of the end buds to form alveoli; the alveoli group in clusters known as lobules. Toward the end of pregnancy, secretory vacuoles are seen within the epithelial cells, and some secretory material may be present in the ducts, although actual lactation does not occur until after parturition. The secretory material has many components, including fat, protein (casein, lactalbumin, lactoglobulin), and lactose.[15–20]

HORMONAL REGULATION OF BREAST DEVELOPMENT

Optimal development of the breast requires the coordinated action of many hormones: prolactin, estrogen, progesterone, adrenal steroids, insulin, growth hormone, and thyroid hormone.[21] In simplified terms, duct growth is promoted by estrogen, lobuloalveolar development is controlled by prolactin and progesterone, and lactation is mediated by prolactin. In spite of an enormous amount of work, however, the precise roles of each hormone have been difficult to delineate because one hormone, besides acting directly on the breast, may also regulate the secretion and activity of other hormones. In vitro findings do not always parallel those in vivo, and species differences make uncertain the application of some observations to humans, who have been less studied than other species.

Prolactin

Prolactin is critical to breast control.[22, 23] Its importance in all phases of breast development was clearly shown by the careful studies of Lyons and co-workers.[24] Using hypophysectomized, adrenalectomized, gonadectomized rats, these authors found that estrogen alone was ineffective in inducing ductal or other mammary growth. When administered together with prolactin and growth hormone, however, or if administered to animals with intact pituitaries, estrogen was an effective promoter of ductal growth. Similar ineffectiveness of estrogen in the hypophysectomized goat in the absence of pituitary hormones was reported by Cowie and colleagues.[25] Talwalker and Meites noted that large amounts of prolactin cause some ductal and lobuloalveolar growth in the triply operated rat,[26] although prolactin ordinarily requires estrogen to stimulate epithelial cell proliferation. In the presence of progesterone, prolactin fosters lobuloalveolar development. The growth-promoting properties of prolactin in various animal species have been substantiated by measurement of DNA and by microscopic observation. Prolactin also controls many steps of milk secretion, including the synthesis of the milk proteins casein and α-lactalbumin. Their measurement, along with that of other secretory products, has been used as a specific and quantitative index of prolactin activity both in vitro and in vivo.[16, 27] Prolactin receptors have been documented in mammary tissue of several species, including humans, and appear to increase in number during gestation and after parturition.[23, 28–31] They are also present in certain other tissues, e.g., rat liver, in which estrogen treatment augments the number of prolactin receptors and prolactin itself may do the same.[32] Ovine prolactin induces prolactin receptors in the rabbit mammary gland, and progesterone can block this effect.[33] Prolactin receptors in rat mammary tumors decrease after estrogen treatment.[34] Antibodies to prolactin receptors block prolactin-mediated events such as the incorporation of tritiated leucine into casein.[35] These studies indicate that binding to its receptor is an essential first step in the action of prolactin on the breast, but knowledge of subsequent stages is fragmentary. The prolactin receptor is a protein of about 600 amino acids that contains a single transmembrane domain and shares approximately 25% homology with the growth hormone receptor; the mechanism by which these receptors mediate hormone action is unknown.[36]

The chorionic hormone human placental lactogen also circulates in large amounts in maternal blood during human pregnancy. It appears to have essentially the same action as prolactin. Although of slightly lesser potency than prolactin on a weight basis,[37] human placental lactogen is present in considerably greater quantities and therefore must be regarded, along with prolactin, as a major contributor to breast growth during gestation.

Estrogen

The role of estrogen is complex. Although a highly potent mammogen, it is ineffective by itself in the absence of anterior pituitary hormones.[24, 25] Administration of estrogen to intact animals promotes the formation of lactotropic cells in the pituitary and increases the secretion of prolactin.[37] In humans estrogen also increases growth hormone secretion.[38] In the presence of these two hormones, estrogen acts on breast tissue to promote ductal development. Although estrogen prepares the breast for eventual milk formation, it inhibits lactation and in this respect acts as an antagonist to prolactin.[39] It is largely because of the high levels of circulating estrogen and progesterone that women do not lactate during pregnancy, and it is the abrupt withdrawal of these two hormones after the expulsion of the placenta that triggers the onset of lactation. As noted earlier, estrogen may act to regulate the number of prolactin receptors in breast tissue. As with actions of estrogen on other tissues, dose considerations are probably important, and differential actions of estrogen may well exist, depending on blood or tissue levels. Fat cells of breast tissue, like adipose tissue elsewhere, have the capacity to form estrogens by aromatization of the circulating androgens androstenedione and testosterone.[40–43] The relative importance of this local source of estrogen production in breast tissue is unknown.

Estrogen receptors, both cytoplasmic and nuclear, are present in normal as well as in tumorous breast tissue.[44–47] Concentrations of cytoplasmic receptor vary with the menstrual cycle[45, 47] and increase during later pregnancy and the first part of lactation. Both estrogen and progesterone are capable of stimulating estrogen receptor synthesis, but the mechanisms governing estrogen regulation are complex.[48, 49]

Progesterone

Like estrogens, progesterone has no effect on the breast in the absence of anterior pituitary hormones.[24, 25] Even in the presence of prolactin, progesterone may have little or no effect unless there is concomitant or preceding estrogen stimulation. Under these conditions progesterone acts synergistically with prolactin in promoting lobuloalveolar development.[50] Some of the actions of progesterone on the breast, like those on the uterus, appear to be antiestrogenic.[51] Like estrogen, progesterone inhibits lactation.[52, 53] Exogenously administered progesterone is less effective than estrogen in stopping lactation once the process has become established.[54] Progesterone receptors exist in breast tissue and appear to be regulated primarily by estrogens, although prolactin is probably also involved.[48, 49, 55]

Growth Hormone

Growth hormone appears to synergize with prolactin and may be able to substitute for it in promoting certain phases of breast growth such as ductal development.[24, 25] Growth hormones from different species possess varying degrees of prolactin-like activity in homologous and heterologous species. Growth hormone seems to enhance the degree of breast growth obtainable with combinations of other hormones in hypophysectomized animals, but whether it is essential for breast growth in humans is questionable. Although human and primate growth hormones have strong intrinsic prolactin-like activity, the fact that ateliotic dwarfs who lack growth hormone develop breasts and lactate normally post partum suggests that growth hormone is not required for lactation in humans.[56]

Insulin and Insulin-Like Growth Factors

Insulin is necessary for prolactin and other hormones to exert their effects on breast tissue in vitro, and insulin or insulin-like growth factors are probably necessary in vivo as well. The importance of insulin in breast function was established by the studies of Topper and colleagues.[16, 57] Insulin-like growth factor I (IGF I, also called somatomedin-C) can mimic most if not all of the effects of insulin on breast tissue, although the relative concentrations required to produce the various actions differ according to the activity being studied.[58] Receptors for IGF I, in addition to those for insulin, are present in breast tissues.[59, 60] The extent to which these two hormones act via their own receptors, as opposed to the receptor for the alternative hormone, is not wholly clear; the mitogenic action of insulin on long-term cultures of human breast cells may be mediated largely via the IGF I receptor.[59]

Other Growth Factors

Epidermal growth factor can stimulate growth of both mammary and pigeon crop-sac epithelium.[61-63] The specificity and essentiality of epidermal growth factor for breast growth are unclear. Nicoll and his colleagues have obtained evidence that prolactin acts on the liver to stimulate secretion of a substance, termed synlactin, that synergizes with prolactin in the growth of mammary epithelium and the pigeon crop sac. Synlactin activity resembles that of IGF I, but whether the two are identical is uncertain.[64, 65] A somewhat similar substance, partially mimicking the actions of prolactin, has also been found in lactating rat livers by others.[66] Newman and colleagues have found that the human pituitary contains a substance, different from prolactin, growth hormone, or other known breast stimulants, capable of promoting breast growth in both monkeys and rats.[67] There is also evidence for a number of other factors, as yet not well characterized, that appear to stimulate breast growth by local or paracrine mechanisms.[68]

Glucocorticoids

Like insulin, glucocorticoids appear to be necessary for most phases of breast growth and secretion, both in vitro and in vivo.[16] Cytoplasmic glucocorticoid receptors are present in lactating mammary tissue.[69] As with insulin, glucocorticoids probably play a permissive rather than a regulatory role.

Thyroid Hormone

Thyroid hormone does not appear to be essential for breast development or lactation, although both processes may be adversely affected in states of thyroid hormone deficiency or excess.[4]

LACTATION

Lactation begins when the maternal breast, primed by long exposure to high levels of prolactin, estrogen, and progesterone, is subjected to sudden withdrawal of the latter two placental hormones. Thereafter, lactation proceeds in an environment of relatively high (although declining) prolactin and low estrogen and progesterone. Suckling provides an essential stimulus for the release of both oxytocin and prolactin.

Oxytocin

A necessary component of effective lactation is expulsion of milk from the alveoli and ducts. This is caused by contraction of the surrounding myoepithelial cells under the influence of oxytocin. Oxytocin secretion can be caused by purely psychic factors, such as anticipation of nursing, or by sensory stimuli arising from the nipple during the act of nursing.[70] Enhanced oxytocin secretion is experienced by the mother as a sensation of milk let-down and by the appearance of milk, sometimes forcibly ejected at the nipple. Uterine cramps may also occur during nursing. Indeed, nipple stimulation in the later stages of pregnancy can be used to produce uterine contractions as part of a standardized contraction stress test.[71-74] Oxytocin secretion can be inhibited (with marked impairment of milk yield) by stress and by psychic factors, such as fright, both of which appear to involve activation of the sympathetic nervous system and release of norepinephrine and epinephrine.

Prolactin

Suckling in women post partum is a powerful stimulus for the release of prolactin. Unlike oxytocin, which is also released by nipple stimuli that are transmitted via dorsal nerve roots to the hypothalamus, prolactin does not respond to anticipatory psychic stimuli. Release of oxytocin and prolactin is independent, and one may be liberated without the other (Fig. 15–1).[70, 75, 76] In the first few weeks post partum, maternal serum prolactin levels are continuously high and undergo further elevation (5- to 10-fold) with each nursing episode. Later, somewhere between the third and seventh weeks after parturition, internursing concentrations of prolactin fall to the normal range (<20 or 25 μg/L) most of the time. Some degree of prolactin rise during each suckling episode persists in most women, however, even many months post partum (Fig. 15–2). This nursing-induced rise is probably important in maintaining the breast in an actively lactating state[75] but does not occur in all women studied many weeks post partum.[77] Thus high levels of prolactin appear to be necessary for the initiation of lactation, but once breast enzyme systems are activated lactation can continue with mean prolactin concentrations that are normal or only modestly elevated. Even at these levels, however, prolactin is essential for maintenance of lactation. If its concentration is further lowered by ergot drugs, lactation stops.

Other Hormones

The level of human growth hormone is low throughout lactation and does not rise with nursing (see Fig. 15–2), further indicating a lack of participation in this process. Thyrotropin was originally reported to be unaffected by nursing in three women studied several weeks post partum,[78] suggesting that the prolactin increase during nursing is not mediated by thyrotropin-releasing hormone. On the other hand, another study of 12 women in the early postpartum period showed major elevations of thyrotropin, oxytocin, and prolactin after nursing.[70] Because thyrotropin-releasing hormone has been shown to release oxytocin in vivo,[79] thyrotropin-releasing hormone may participate to some de-

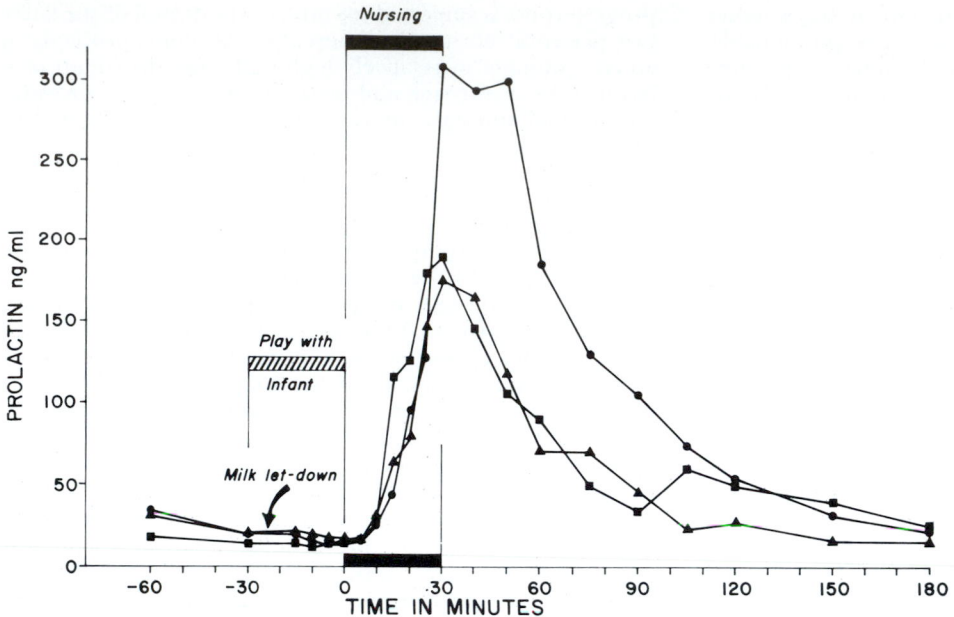

Figure 15–1. Plasma prolactin concentrations during anticipation of nursing and course of nursing in three women who were between 22 and 26 d post partum. The women played with their infants for 30 min before suckling began. Milk let-down, an oxytocin-mediated phenomenon, occurred in each case approximately 25 min before suckling. Prolactin levels did not rise until there was contact with the breast itself. (From GL Noel, HK Suh, AG Frantz, Prolactin release during nursing and breast stimulation in postpartum and nonpostpartum subjects, J Clin Endocrinol Metab, 38, 413–423, 1974, © by The Endocrine Society.)

gree in the release of all three of these pituitary hormones by nursing.

Breast Stimulation in Normal Subjects

In normally menstruating, nonpostpartum women, manual stimulation of the breast and nipple causes a twofold or greater prolactin rise in about one third[75] or more.[80] The factors that separate women who respond from those who do not are unclear. Men show no prolactin response to breast stimulation. The reflex for this type of response appears to be present in latent form in women and is somehow turned on or enhanced by the hormonal events of pregnancy and parturition.

Induction of Lactation in the Absence of Pregnancy

The attempt to induce lactation in nonpostpartum women for the purpose of breast-feeding adopted infants has received little attention in the scientific literature. Anecdotal accounts exist of women, sometimes postmenopausal and usually in primitive tribes, who were able to initiate lactation when placed in contact with an infant to be nursed. Richardson, writing in 1970, was able to find only 13 such instances documented since 1900.[81] We were unsuccessful in inducing either galactorrhea or any breast engorgement in two normal young women who underwent self-stimulation of the breast for four ½-h periods a day for 2 wk.[75] However,

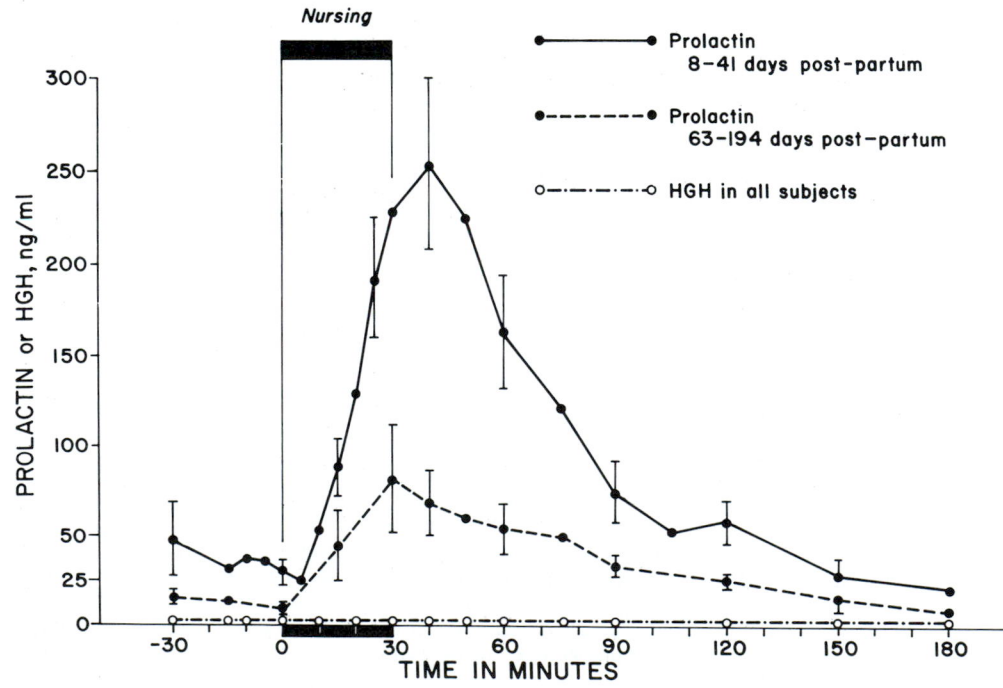

Figure 15–2. Plasma prolactin and growth hormone concentrations during nursing in postpartum women. Eight women were studied 8 to 41 d post partum and six women were studied 63 to 194 d post partum. Prenursing prolactin levels in the latter group are within the normal range. Plasma growth hormone showed no change in any of the subjects during nursing. (From GL Noel, HK Suh, AG Frantz, Prolactin release during nursing and breast stimulation in postpartum and nonpostpartum subjects, J Clin Endocrinol Metab, 38, 413–423, 1974, © by The Endocrine Society.)

a report based on answers to a questionnaire by 240 women who had tried adoptive nursing[82] suggests that successful induction of lactation may be more common than our own experience would suggest. By means of breast and nipple stimulation for several weeks beforehand, half of the women were able to induce some type and degree of breast secretion before the arrival of the infant. This secretion was milky, as opposed to clear or colostrum-like, in 43% of 102 women who had previously nursed biological offspring. In women who had not had a previous nursing episode, milky secretions were obtained in 14% of 83 who had never been pregnant and 12% of 55 who had had a previous pregnancy.[82] The amount of milk obtained after the infant began to nurse regularly was not recorded, and all but two of the women supplemented their own milk supply with external sources during part or all of the nursing period. Eleven percent of the women noted a change in menstrual cycling after initiation of breast-feeding, but only 4% reported amenorrhea. Six percent had used hormone preparations of some kind before the infant's arrival, chiefly an oxytocin nasal spray (Syntocinon) to enhance milk ejection. No hormone measurements were made.[82] Despite the many limitations of this retrospective, questionnaire-based study, the findings emphasize the importance of breast and nipple stimulation in the induction of lactation. There is little doubt that the effectiveness of such techniques in inducing lactation would be enhanced by prolonged pretreatment with estrogen and progesterone designed to simulate the hormonal conditions of pregnancy, followed by abrupt withdrawal of these agents. Few reports of such treatment have appeared in the literature.[83]

Clinical Aspects of Postpartum Lactation

SUPPRESSION OF LACTATION. If a woman does not nurse or empty the breasts post partum, lactation usually stops spontaneously in a week or two, accompanied by involution of much of the recently differentiated lobuloalveolar structure of the breast. Stasis of milk in the ducts and alveoli and a rise in intramammary pressure, leading to a degree of alveolar rupture and cell necrosis, are major factors in the cessation of lactation, but the detailed mechanisms are not altogether clear.[54] Prolactin levels revert quickly to normal, menses usually resume in 4 to 12 wk (mean 8 wk), but occasionally periods of up to 6 mo are required.[84] During the first week or two post partum in women who do not nurse, there is a variable amount of discomfort caused by breast engorgement, which can usually be treated satisfactorily by simple measures such as ice packs, a tight binder, and analgesics. To minimize discomfort in women who do not wish to nurse their babies, however, it has been common practice to prescribe drugs for the suppression of lactation. In addition to oral estrogens, which were once commonly prescribed, another effective method was the single intramuscular injection during labor of a long-acting estrogen-androgen combination (e.g., 2 or 3 mL of Deladumone, containing 4 mg of estradiol valerate and 90 mg of testosterone enanthate per mL). The hormones are less effective if administered after lactation has begun. Androgen synergizes with the estrogen in inhibiting breast secretion and minimizes the chance of later recurrence of lactation.[54] Because of growing awareness of the potential toxicities of estrogen therapy, however, as well as the availability of bromocriptine, the administration of steroids to suppress lactation has greatly declined.[85] If drug-induced suppression of lactation is deemed advisable, then bromocriptine, an ergot derivative that suppresses prolactin secretion by virtue of its long-acting dopamine agonist properties,[86] is the agent of choice. An effective dose schedule that minimizes rebound breast engorgement is 2.5 mg twice daily for 2 wk beginning after delivery, followed by 2.5 mg daily for a third week. In controlled trials the bromocriptine regimen was as effective as or more effective than steroid regimens.[86, 87] Side effects of bromocriptine, including nausea, vomiting, and postural hypotension, are less prominent in postpartum patients than in those who take the drug for other indications; the reasons for this are unclear.[87]

FAILURE OF LACTATION. The first endocrine disorder known to be associated with failure of lactation was Sheehan syndrome (also see Chapter 6). This disorder is due to infarction of the pituitary at the time of delivery and may be first manifest by lack of postpartum milk production, presumably because of low circulating prolactin. Other signs of pituitary hormone deficiency may subsequently appear: failure of menses to resume, sparse regrowth of shaved pubic hair, and development of hypothyroidism. The pattern of individual hormone deficiencies in Sheehan syndrome is variable, and rarely spontaneous amelioration may occur.[88, 89] Lymphocytic hypophysitis, a condition that may occur post partum and mimic Sheehan syndrome, may also be associated with hypoprolactinemia and failure of lactation.[90] Isolated prolactin deficiency associated with alactogenesis has also been reported.[91] Hypoprolactinemia, manifested by alactogenesis, may occasionally occur in association with other pituitary diseases. Diminished milk production, particularly in mothers of premature infants, has been successfully treated in some cases with metoclopramide, an agent that stimulates prolactin release.[92] It must be noted, however, that milk production is not a simple function of serum prolactin levels. Many instances of insufficient lactation are believed to be due to emotional factors, which could operate via noradrenergic pathways to inhibit oxytocin secretion.

LACTATION-ASSOCIATED INFERTILITY. If postpartum nursing is prolonged, amenorrhea usually continues for at least 4 to 6 mo, but menses resume in two thirds of women by 9 mo post partum despite continued lactation.[84] Lactation-associated amenorrhea is primarily due to the antigonadotropin effects of hyperprolactinemia, but other factors may also be operative, particularly in the later postpartum period when the serum prolactin level is normal much of the time. It must be emphasized that amenorrhea does not guarantee infertility, and conception can occur post partum without an intervening menstrual period. Therefore, contraception, if desired, should be begun soon after delivery, at least before the fifth week post partum, whether the mother nurses her child or not (also see Chapter 18). If oral contraceptives are used in a nursing mother, a low-dose estrogen preparation should be chosen to minimize inhibitory effects on milk yield.[84] Another possible side effect of maternal estrogen use is enlargement of the child's breast because of secretion of the steroid into the mother's milk.[93] In many species other than primates, prolonged lactation is no barrier to rapid resumption of ovulatory cycles. Insemination of domestic cows is frequently undertaken 3 mo or less post partum despite copious lactation, which proceeds, if milking continues, throughout the ensuing gestation.[4]

DISORDERS OF BREASTS IN WOMEN

Galactorrhea

Galactorrhea may be defined as any persistent discharge of milk or milk-like secretions from the breast in the absence of parturition or beyond 6 mo post partum in a non-nursing mother. Formerly regarded as rare, it is now often recognized, particularly if one includes minimal degrees of secretion that may be evident only when specifically sought by squeezing the breast. Doubt as to whether the secretion represents milk may be resolved by doing fat stains or, for greater specificity, tests for specific milk products such as α-lactalbumin, casein, or lactose. Clinically, such tests are rarely necessary. Nonmilky types of nipple discharge (serous, purulent, sanguineous) also occur, but these are rarely if ever reflective of an endocrine disturbance. In the past such discharges were thought to suggest cancer, but most non-bloody secretions are not associated with malignancy, although they may indicate that fibrocystic disease is present.[94-97] A careful search for breast nodules should nevertheless be made in patients with such discharges. True galactorrhea is not associated with an increased incidence of cancer.

CAUSES. Galactorrhea occurs in a wide variety of endocrine and nonendocrine disorders. The largest series (235 patients) reported to date is that of Kleinberg and colleagues;[98] the discussion that follows is based on this series, the findings of which are in general agreement with those of other observers.[99-101]

Galactorrhea with Pituitary Tumors. The most important diagnostic consideration in galactorrhea is pituitary tumor. Twenty percent of our patients with galactorrhea and 34% of women with associated amenorrhea had pituitary tumors. The true prevalence of tumors is undoubtedly higher because of failure to detect some small microadenomas radiologically preceding the availability of computed tomographic (CT) scans and magnetic resonance imaging (MRI). The histologic appearance is almost always that of a chromophobe adenoma, with increased lactotropes demonstrable by special stains. A minority of patients have associated acromegaly; these patients all have clinical stigmata of acromegaly as well as elevated serum growth hormone levels. As a group, patients with tumors have the highest serum prolactin values

(Fig. 15–3), and the likelihood of finding a tumor is proportional to the level of prolactin. In our experience all patients with concentrations over 300 μg/L have had tumors, and any value of more than 75 to 100 μg/L should be regarded with great suspicion. Of the few patients with tumors who had normal serum prolactin values, all but two either had acromegaly or had received treatment for acromegaly. Amenorrhea is usual (greater than 80%) in patients with galactorrhea and tumors and was the primary complaint in 10% of our patients. Menses, if present, are apt to be abnormal; only 3 of 48 patients with tumors in our series had regular periods.

Idiopathic Galactorrhea with Menses. The largest category of patients with galactorrhea consists of those with regular menses and no associated endocrine disease. Galactorrhea is often overlooked because patients may not think it worth reporting. In over half of patients the galactorrhea represents a residue of postpartum lactation that has never altogether disappeared despite resumption of menses. Most of these patients have prolactin levels within the normal range (see Fig. 15–3), and fertility is usually normal. In this group of women the abnormality probably is not primarily hormonal but rather an excessive sensitivity of the breast tissue itself—perhaps because of increased prolactin receptors—to normal levels of circulating prolactin. From a clinical standpoint, the combination of regular menses and normal serum prolactin is strong evidence against the presence of pituitary tumor. It is probably unnecessary to do MRI or CT scans in these patients, although the serum prolactin level should be redetermined on one or more occasions.

Idiopathic Galactorrhea with Amenorrhea: The Role of Hyperprolactinemia. A minority of women with galactorrhea have associated amenorrhea, no history of drug ingestion, and a normal sella turcica by conventional radiographs. Most such women have hyperprolactinemia (see Fig. 15–3). Many

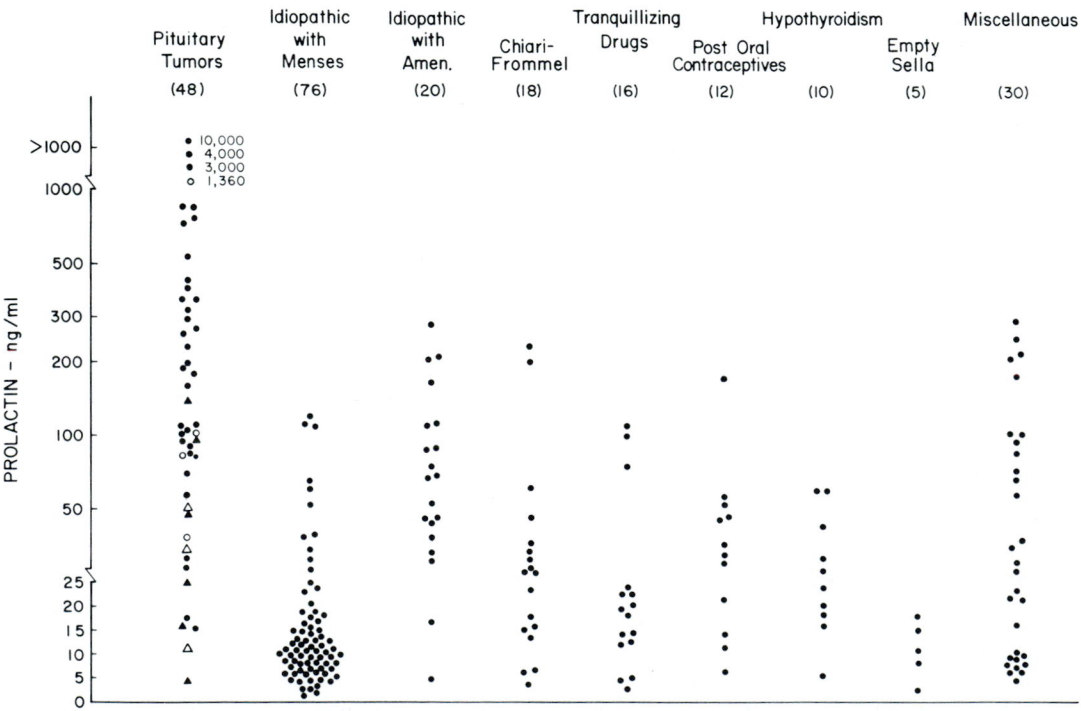

Figure 15–3. Plasma prolactin in 235 patients with galactorrhea of varying causes. Among the patients with tumor, triangles denote patients with acromegaly. Open circles or triangles denote patients studied only after radiotherapy or surgical resection. Normal female levels of prolactin are considered to be less than 25 μg/L. (From Kleinberg DL, Noel GL, Frantz AG. Galactorrhea: a study of 235 cases including 48 with pituitary tumors. Reprinted, by permission of the New England Journal of Medicine, 296; 589–600, 1977.)

have small sellar abnormalities on MRI or CT scans. In the absence of definitive radiographic changes, the likelihood of a pituitary tumor increases directly with the level of the serum prolactin. It is probable that the hyperprolactinemia, in these as in other patients with galactorrhea and amenorrhea, causes the amenorrhea, because any treatment that lowers prolactin close to or into the normal range is likely to restore menses. Possible mechanisms of amenorrhea include interference by prolactin at the hypothalamic level with the tonic or cyclic release of luteinizing hormone–releasing hormone (LHRH), alteration of pituitary sensitivity to the action of LHRH, or interference with the steroidogenic action of gonadotropins at the ovarian level. There is evidence for each of these mechanisms, but defective production of LHRH appears to be the predominant factor.[102, 103]

Chiari-Frommel Syndrome. The so-called Chiari-Frommel syndrome, defined as galactorrhea and amenorrhea persisting more than 6 mo post partum in the absence of nursing and without evident pituitary tumor, is poorly understood. Some of these patients probably harbor occult microadenomas stimulated by the hormones of pregnancy that may later become radiologically evident. In about half, menses eventually return over a period of months or years.[98] The serum prolactin level is elevated in some but not all patients (see Fig. 15–3).

Post–Oral Contraceptive Galactorrhea. Galactorrhea is less common after discontinuation of oral contraceptives than is amenorrhea, with which it is usually associated. Both sequelae are uncommon in relation to the large number of women who use oral contraceptives. As with the Chiari-Frommel syndrome, some patients eventually develop radiologically evident tumors, although most in our experience do not. In this syndrome, as in the postpartum state, milk production is triggered by the withdrawal of estrogen and progesterone after a period of stimulation by these hormones (and also in part by estrogen-enhanced prolactin secretion). Despite the lower hormone levels and shorter duration of stimulation in this disorder than in postpartum lactation, the fundamental mechanisms of the two conditions may be similar.

Hypothyroidism. Galactorrhea is a rare accompaniment of primary hypothyroidism both in children—in whom it may be associated with precocious puberty[104] (also see Chapter 22)—and in adults.[105] Among adults with primary hypothyroidism, prolactin levels may be slightly above the normal mean but are often within the normal range or only slightly elevated (see Fig. 15–3).[98, 106, 107] Enlargement of the sella turcica may occur in primary hypothyroidism, and if hyperprolactinemia is present the condition may mimic a prolactinoma.[108] Administration of thyroid hormone to restore euthyroidism lowers the prolactin somewhat and usually stops the galactorrhea. In children thyroid hormone may also cause precocious menses to stop until the normal time of menarche. The underlying mechanisms in these cases are not clear and may involve complex alterations of prolactin and gonadotropin production and degradation, as well as changes in breast tissue sensitivity. Administration of thyroid hormone to euthyroid patients with other forms of galactorrhea does not stop milk production.[109]

Thyrotoxicosis. Galactorrhea was reported in a high percentage of women with thyrotoxicosis in one report.[110] The serum prolactin level was normal in all women, and the mechanisms are obscure.

Drug Administration. Galactorrhea has been associated with a wide variety of drugs that raise serum prolactin levels,[98–100] including phenothiazines, butyrophenones, reserpine, methyldopa, tricyclic antidepressants, estrogens, opiates, metoclopramide, verapamil,[111] cimetidine,[112] and co-caine.[113] Many of these appear to act as antidopaminergic agents, decreasing dopamine-mediated inhibition of prolactin secretion at the level of the pituitary or hypothalamus, or both.

Major Surgery and Disorders of the Chest Wall. Galactorrhea occurs occasionally after major surgery such as cholecystectomy, and its likelihood may be greater after procedures that include oophorectomy.[98] Presumably, the mechanisms involve in part the acute release of prolactin[114] plus the effect of acute estrogen withdrawal in cases in which the ovaries are removed. Galactorrhea has also been reported in diseases affecting the chest wall, such as herpes zoster, or after thoracotomy.[81] This has led to speculation that increased prolactin secretion can result from stimulation of nerves originating in the breast and areola; sustained hyperprolactinemia does not occur in all patients after chest wall surgery, and it is not clear that thoracotomy is more likely to be followed by galactorrhea than are other major surgical procedures.[115]

Miscellaneous. Conditions occasionally associated with galactorrhea include various hypothalamic and pituitary diseases (sarcoidosis, Schüller-Christian disease, craniopharyngioma, Cushing disease, and head trauma), in which alteration of normal hypothalamic-pituitary connections may lead to reduced hypothalamic inhibition and consequent hyperprolactinemia. Isoniazid administration and refeeding after starvation can also cause galactorrhea.[98] Hyperprolactinemia, with or without accompanying galactorrhea, is present in some patients with renal failure[36, 116] and hepatic cirrhosis.[117] Self-manipulation of the breasts in an attempt to reduce gynecomastia has been associated with galactorrhea in adolescent boys.[118]

ROLE OF PROLACTIN IN GALACTORRHEA. Although serum prolactin concentrations are often elevated in galactorrhea, they were within the normal range in 46% of our patients. Thus galactorrhea can be present without hyperprolactinemia. Likewise, hyperprolactinemia can exist without galactorrhea. In the latter case the absence of galactorrhea may be due to inadequacy of estrogenic and progestational priming (as in most men) or lack of a suitable triggering event involving estrogen withdrawal (oophorectomy, abortion, cessation of estrogen, or oral contraceptive medication). In many cases of galactorrhea, however, no triggering event is evident from the history. In patients with galactorrhea and normal serum prolactin, an earlier transient period of hyperprolactinemia may have existed at the time of onset of the galactorrhea, analogous to the situation in nursing mothers in whom milk secretion, once established, can continue for many months with what appear to be normal prolactin levels. Galactorrhea remains prolactin dependent, however, because lowering of serum prolactin concentrations with ergot drugs usually stops the galactorrhea. In summary, although prolactin is essential for milk production, the serum levels of the hormone do not correlate with the copiousness of milk flow in all patients with galactorrhea.

CLINICAL CONSIDERATIONS IN GALACTORRHEA. *Diagnosis.* A careful history is essential with attention to menses, drug ingestion, and symptoms suggestive of pituitary or hypothalamic disease (headaches, visual disturbances, abnormalities of temperature, thirst, and appetite regulation), thyroid disease, or adrenal dysfunction. On physical examination the physician should check visual fields by confrontation; seek evidence of abnormal skin texture, pigmentation, or hirsutism; and look for signs of acromegaly, hypothyroidism, Cushing syndrome, and hyperthyroidism. The breast should be examined for nodules and gently but firmly compressed by the physician or patient to assess the degree of galactorrhea. Serum prolactin and serum gonadotropin levels should be measured in patients with amenorrhea. Thyroid function should be assessed, but other hormonal assays, e.g., for growth hormone and adrenal steroids, are not necessary in the absence of specific indications. MRI or CT scans should be performed if the serum prolactin level is even slightly elevated or if there are any other signs suggestive of a pituitary tumor; as noted earlier, such scans are not mandatory in cases of minimal galactorrhea if the serum prolactin value is within the normal range and menses are regular. At one time it was thought that prolactin stimulation and suppression tests, involving the assessment of response to such agents as levodopa, phenothiazines, thyrotropin-releasing hormone, and metoclopramide, might prove valuable in distinguishing pituitary tumors from other causes of galactorrhea or hyperprolactinemia, but such tests are too variable in their results to be useful.[119] The diagnosis of pituitary tumor rests essentially on the level of the serum prolactin and on radiographic evidence, particularly on MRI or CT scans, which have replaced polytomography.[120]

Treatment. In most cases the galactorrhea does not require treatment for its own sake. If fertility is not desired and if there is no evidence of pituitary tumor, treatment for elevated prolactin alone is not necessary, because there is no evidence that prolonged hyperprolactinemia in the absence of associated amenorrhea is deleterious. If amenorrhea accompanies hyperprolactinemia, however, as is often the case, then patients are at increased risk for the development of osteoporosis[121–123] (also see Chapters 12 and 28). Decreases in bone density appear to be greater in vertebral (trabecular) than forearm (cortical) bone.[124] Although hypoestrogenism undoubtedly accounts for some, if not most, of the increased risk of osteoporosis in such patients, hyperprolactinemia itself may contribute independently.[122] Such observations afford a rationale for treating hyperprolactinemia in amenorrheic women, but to date the effects of lowering prolactin levels on bone mineral content are not wholly clear,[122, 124] although some improvement has been reported.[125]

If MRI or CT scanning discloses the presence of a pituitary tumor but fertility is not desired, the choice of therapy depends chiefly on the size of the tumor (also see Chapter 6). If it is a microadenoma, i.e., less than 1 cm in diameter, and if the risks of osteoporosis do not appear to necessitate treatment, it may be appropriate to follow such patients without specific therapy. Although the natural history of prolactin-secreting microadenomas is not extensively documented, the majority of these tumors do not appear to progress to macroadenomas.[126–128] Furthermore, a gradual reduction of serum prolactin may take place over a period of years, and in a minority of patients this may be accompanied by spontaneous resumption of menses and cessation of galactorrhea.[127] The serum prolactin level should be assessed at 6-mo to yearly intervals, with MRI or CT scanning less frequently (e.g., at 2- to 5-y intervals). For macroadenomas some form of therapy—surgery, radiotherapy, or prolactin-lowering drugs—is usually considered advisable, to prevent further growth and to shrink the tumor if local pressure symptoms (e.g., visual field defects) are present. *Transsphenoidal surgery* in experienced hands is a safe procedure, with mortality rates averaging 0.9% for macroadenomas and 0.27% for microadenomas.[129] Return of the serum prolactin level to normal after surgery depends both on the initial level of the serum prolactin and on the size of the tumor. With initial serum prolactin values of less than 200 to 250 μg/L and with microadenomas, the immediate postoperative cure rates may be as high as 83 to 86%; with higher serum prolactin values and macroadenomas generally, the cure rate is less than 50%.[129–133] Enthusiasm for surgery as primary therapy for prolactinomas has been tempered in recent years because recurrence rates in patients originally considered cured are higher than originally anticipated.[133–137] These recurrence rates range from 17%[134] to 91%[136] several years postoperatively, but in most cases the recurrence involves only recurrence of hyperprolactinemia and not regrowth of tumor. *Radiotherapy* alone is effective in arresting tumor growth and shrinking existing tumors in most cases and it is followed by a progressive decrease in serum prolactin levels that continues over a period of many years.[138–140] Because of the slowness of the decline in prolactin levels, the availability of drug therapy, and the possibility of inducing late-developing hypopituitarism (which has ranged from 13%[140] to 100%[139] in recent series), radiotherapy is usually reserved as an adjunct to surgery with larger tumors or utilized in patients considered unacceptable risks for surgery. With either surgery or radiotherapy, restoration of menses and cessation of galactorrhea require that the serum prolactin level be lowered to within or close to the normal range.

The ergot derivatives, especially bromocriptine, are more effective than any other form of treatment in lowering serum prolactin, stopping galactorrhea, and restoring ovulatory menses in patients with hyperprolactinemia, whether related to tumor or other causes.[86, 98, 141] The usual dose of bromocriptine is 2.5 mg/d for 1 wk, increased to 2.5 mg twice or three times a day thereafter. Initial nausea is experienced by many patients but usually disappears with time. Postural hypotension and nasal stuffiness may also occur. In most cases the drug is effective only for the duration of its administration; hyperprolactinemia and the associated abnormalities recur after it is withdrawn. If ergot drugs are used to restore fertility in a patient with a prolactin-secreting macroadenoma, preliminary transsphenoidal surgery is usually performed to minimize the risk of rapid tumor growth during pregnancy. If the tumor is a microadenoma, preliminary surgery is generally not considered necessary before the use of ergot drugs to induce fertility. Under these conditions complications related to tumor growth during pregnancy are comparatively few and easily managed.[142, 143]

In addition to lowering serum prolactin levels, ergot derivatives shrink prolactin-secreting pituitary tumors. Several published series have indicated an overall shrinkage rate of approximately 73%,[144] though rates as high as 100% have been reported.[145] Tumor shrinkage can be rapid, beginning within a few days, possibly even a few hours, after bromocriptine administration. The degree of tumor shrinkage does not correlate with serum prolactin reduction. Rarely, tumor growth may occur despite continued prolactin suppression.[146] The serum prolactin level remains suppressed as long as ergot drugs are given but usually rises when they are stopped. With continued therapy (2 y or more) dose reduction may be possible in some cases,[147] and the serum prolactin level may not rise fully to its original levels on withdrawal of the drug. Some degree of tumor re-expansion must also be anticipated after withdrawal of ergot drugs but may not occur for many months when therapy has been prolonged.[145, 148, 149] Despite the need for indefinite treatment with ergot drugs, the success of these agents in lowering the serum prolactin value and shrinking tumors has led to their use in many centers as first-line therapy instead of surgery for macroadenomas.[145] A long-acting injectable form of bromocriptine may have particular advantages in achieving rapid results with tumors.[150–152] Ergot drugs may on occasion effect dramatic size reductions over a long period with some giant invasive prolactinomas.[144, 153] Short-term therapy with ergot drugs may also be useful as a preliminary to surgery by shrinking the tumor and thereby facilitating transsphenoidal resection.[154]

Hypoplasia

Hypoplasia or aplasia of the breast caused by delayed or absent sexual maturation, as in gonadal dysgenesis, usually responds to cyclic estrogen-progesterone therapy. The same is true of the breast atrophy that follows premature menopause. Occasionally, partial or total failure of breast development, sometimes only one sided,[155] occurs in a woman who is having regular menses and appears to be endocrinologically normal. Hypomastia is linked in some cases with mitral valve prolapse.[156] The problem in hypomastia may be either a deficiency of breast tissue related to a developmental defect or an insensitivity of breast tissue to normal hormonal stimulation. Estrogen or other hormone therapy should not be used to augment breast size in these patients. Estrogens are unlikely to have any significant effect in doses close to the physiological range, and the pharmacological doses that might conceivably produce slight improvement carry unacceptable risks. If treatment appears necessary for psychological reasons, mammoplasty is indicated.[155, 157]

Macromastia

Macromastia, usually defined as massive breast enlargement in women, is an uncommon but unsolved problem.[158] As is the case with breast enlargement in men, breast enlargement in women is compounded by problems of definition. To separate macromastia from cases of moderate or minimal breast enlargement, the usual practice is to limit the diagnosis to women in whom the weight bearing itself is uncomfortable or in whom stretching of the overlying skin causes ulceration. If the variant associated with extreme obesity is excluded, the disorder is most commonly classified into three types: pubertal macromastia (approximately 83%), macromastia during pregnancy (about 13%), and macromastia in adult women in whom no initiating cause is identified (about 4%).[159] In addition, the disorder may be associated with penicillamine therapy. In each of these variants the enlargement can be grossly asymmetrical and can be associated with simultaneous development of ancillary breast masses in the axillae.

Macromastia of puberty can commence before or after the onset of menses, may recur after reduction mammoplasty has reduced the size of the breasts by 3 to 8 kg of weight, and may on occasion be associated with hypothyroidism.[160-163] When associated with pregnancy, macromastia usually has its onset in the first or second trimester, may begin during the first pregnancy or after uneventful previous pregnancies, may subside minimally or completely after termination of pregnancy, and may worsen with subsequent pregnancies.[164-172] Penicillamine-induced macromastia has been reported in several women between the ages of 25 and 45 who were receiving relatively modest amounts of the drug, and it may not regress after the drug is discontinued.[173-178]

On biopsy, the histological characteristics of the breast tissue in all these various disorders are appropriate for the physiological state. Hormonal studies to date in women with macromastia are usually unremarkable, including normal levels of gonadal steroids, plasma prolactin, and placental lactogen.[176] It is assumed that the disorder results from some type of enhanced end-organ response to physiological amounts of hormone.

Reduction mammoplasty is the most common form of treatment,[179, 180] but recurrence may make total mastectomy necessary.[163, 172, 181] Various empirical therapies have been tried, including bromocriptine,[171] tamoxifen,[162, 171, 172] dydrogesterone,[158, 172] medroxyprogesterone,[162] and danazol,[176-240]

but the experience is too small to allow assessment of efficacy with any of these agents.

Mastaglia

Many women complain at times of pain in the breast.[182, 183] In the large series studied by Preece and colleagues,[182] the pain was commonly diffuse and subject to cyclic premenstrual induction or exacerbation. A smaller group had localized pain ascribed to ductal ectasia and periductal mastitis. Tietze syndrome, trauma, and cancer were diagnoses in a smaller number of cases. The response to placebo therapy among these patients tends to be so high that careful double-blind studies are necessary to document the effect of hormonal or other therapy. Evening primrose oil, a plant extract with few side effects, and bromocriptine were about equally effective, and both were more effective than placebo in relieving pain in patients with cyclic, as opposed to noncyclic, mastalgia.[184] Danazol, an antigonadotropic agent, is more effective than either of these drugs.[184, 185] In view of the menstrual irregularities, weight gain, and occasional androgenic effects that may occur with danazol, however, it seems wise to use this drug, if at all, only in severe cases when other measures have failed and then only for short periods.[186] Tamoxifen, an antiestrogen, may be as effective as danazol with fewer side effects, although its use is still experimental.[187]

DISORDERS OF BREASTS IN MEN

Gynecomastia

CLINICAL FEATURES. The consideration of gynecomastia is complicated by formidable problems of definition. The general view has been that any palpable breast tissue in men is abnormal except for three situations—the transient gynecomastia of the newborn, the breast enlargement at puberty in boys, and the gynecomastia that occasionally occurs in elderly men.[188] However, this view has been challenged by Nuttall and his colleagues, who reported that 36% of normal men between the ages of 17 and 80 have palpable breast tissue[189] and that the overall prevalence in hospitalized men is 65%.[190] In another study Ley and colleagues reported a prevalence of 34% in normal men.[191]

A confounding problem in the ascertainment of gynecomastia is that it may be difficult to distinguish true enlargement of breast tissue from lipomastia, in which the enlargement is due to adipose tissue.[192] The false-positive rate for the estimation of gynecomastia by physical examination has never been established by performing biopsies for all subjects.[193] Separating gynecomastia from lipomastia is a particular problem in overweight men, and in this regard it is important to remember that the bulk of breast tissue in normal women and in most men is in fact adipose tissue. The endocrine cause (or causes) for the local proliferation of adipose tissue in the breasts has never been defined, and most work on the endocrine control of the tissue has focused on breast tissue per se.

The available pathological data are not of much help in establishing the true prevalence of gynecomastia. In three large unselected autopsy series the incidence of active gynecomastia (epithelial hyperplasia and periductal stromal hyperplasia) was 9%,[188] 7%,[194] and 5%;[195] in these reports gynecomastia was most frequent in the young and the elderly. Evidence of inactive or burned-out gynecomastia was more common—32%[188] and 48%.[192] It is also not clear from the autopsy data what fraction of gynecomastia—active or inactive—is theoretically palpable. In summary, major uncertainties exist. On the one hand, as was previously believed, gynecomastia in contrast to lipomastia may be unusual; alternatively, gynecomastia may be so common as to be a normal variant in the absence of an obvious underlying endocrinopathy. It is also possible that an increase in the prevalence of gynecomastia may have occurred in the recent past related to some unrecognized cause.

True gynecomastia can be separated from lipomasty by mammography.[196, 197] However, most studies of mammography have been performed in men with florid breast enlargement who are being evaluated for breast cancer. Sonography may be a useful adjunct to mammography in defining gynecomastia.[198, 199]

For the purposes of this discussion, we shall assume that any palpable breast tissue in men (other than in the three so-called physiological states) may be indicative of an underlying endocrinopathy and deserves at least a limited evaluation.

HISTOPATHOLOGY AND ETIOLOGY. Gross asymmetry in the development of gynecomastia is frequent; furthermore, unilateral gynecomastia may be a temporary phenomenon in that one breast may enlarge or become painful for years or months before the other. The histological features of gynecomastia have been studied in most detail in subjects with diethylstilbestrol-induced breast enlargement, but the histology in all forms of gynecomastia correlates better with the duration rather than with the etiology, suggesting a common pathogenesis.[200-202] Initially, the disorder is characterized by proliferation of the fibroblastic stroma and of the duct system, which elongates, buds, and duplicates. In gynecomastia of longer duration (even when the stimulation is continued, as in prolonged diethylstilbestrol therapy) progressive fibrosis and hyalinization occur in association with regression of epithelial proliferation. Eventually, the ducts decrease in number. Mononuclear cell infiltration is common.

Resolution occurs by reduction in size and cell content of the ductular epithelia followed by gradual disappearance of the ducts, leaving hyaline bands that may eventually disappear. If the process is of sufficient duration, fibrosis and hyalinization may be so extensive that complete resolution never occurs even when the underlying cause is corrected.

Because estradiol is a normal male hormone, because estradiol is a growth hormone for the breast in women, and because the administration of diethylstilbestrol and other estrogens to men causes breast enlargement that is histologically indistinguishable from other forms of gynecomastia, gynecomastia has been generally viewed as a disturbance of estrogen physiology.

Lewin was apparently the first to suggest that all gynecomastia is due either to increased estrogen secretion or to a decreased androgen/estrogen ratio,[203] a formulation that has been further developed by Gabrilove[204] and has been utilized in some[205-207] but not all[208] subsequent attempts to classify the causes of gynecomastia.

ESTROGEN PRODUCTION IN MEN. A basic knowledge of androgen physiology is essential to understanding estrogen physiology in normal men (see Chapter 13). In brief, testosterone secretion by the Leydig cell of the testis is regulated largely by luteinizing hormone (LH) from the pituitary. Follicle-stimulating hormone may augment testosterone secretion, possibly by regulating the number of LH receptors on the plasma membrane of the Leydig cell. Testosterone feeds back on the pituitary to alter the sensitivity of the gland to the hypothalamic LHRH. The molecular mechanism by which testosterone regulates LH production is believed (on the basis of studies of subjects with single

gene defects that impair the function of the androgen receptor) to be identical to that by which the hormone acts in other target cells: androgen combines with a specific cytoplasmic receptor protein to form a hormone-receptor complex that activates specific genes within the nuclei of target cells.

Plasma testosterone serves as a circulating precursor or prohormone for the formation of two other types of active hormones, which in turn mediate many of the physiological processes involved in androgen action.[209] Testosterone can undergo 5α-reduction to dihydrotestosterone, which performs many of the differentiative, growth, and functional actions involved in male sexual differentiation and virilization. Alternatively, circulating androgens can be converted (aromatized) in extraglandular tissues of both sexes to estrogens. Thus the physiological consequences of testosterone represent the combined effects of testosterone plus estrogen and dihydrotestosterone. For the purposes of this discussion, it is assumed that the active androgens (testosterone and dihydrotestosterone) virilize the male and that estrogen (estradiol) acts principally in opposition to androgen to feminize.

As measured by isotope dilution techniques, urinary production rates for estrone and estradiol in normal men average about 60 and 45 μg/d (Fig. 15–4). Thus normal men produce approximately a hundred times more testosterone than estradiol. All of estrone and about 85% of estradiol production can be accounted for by formation from androstenedione and testosterone in extraglandular sites. Thus on the basis of kinetic studies in vivo it was concluded that in normal men about 6 μg of estradiol is secreted directly into the circulation by the testes each day.[210] Kelch and co-workers[211] and Weinstein and co-workers[212] reached similar conclusions in studies of arteriovenous differences of plasma estrogen content across the testes. When pharmacological amounts of human chorionic gonadotropin (hCG) are administered to normal men, however, direct secretion of estradiol by the testis increases in proportion to the enhancement of testosterone secretion.[212] This phenomenon explains why estradiol secretion by the testis is frequently elevated when the plasma LH level is increased (as in Klinefelter syndrome, testicular feminization, or chronic hCG administration). In brief, testicular secretion of estradiol is of minor significance in the normal man but may be profound in pathological states. Within the testes, estrogen is formed principally within Leydig cells but also by Sertoli cells.[213]

Estradiol exerts its growth-promoting properties in the male breast as in the female breast and other estrogen target tissues via the same high-affinity receptor protein that binds the hormone to the nuclear acceptor sites in other estrogen target tissues[214-217] (see Chapters 3 and 33).

CLASSIFICATION OF GYNECOMASTIA*

Physiological Gynecomastia. During three phases of male life, breast enlargement can be regarded as a physiological rather than a pathological event.

Gynecomastia in the Newborn. The enlargement of the neonatal breast that is present in many normal newborns probably results from the action of maternal and/or placental estrogens. The swelling may or may not be associated with witch's milk (see earlier) and ordinarily disappears in a few weeks, although it may persist longer in exceptional cases.[218]

Adolescent Gynecomastia. Transient enlargement of the breast is a normal occurrence in male adolescence. Of 1855 adolescent boys of different ages examined at one Boy Scout camp 39% had gynecomastia,[219] whereas in another

---

*See Table 15–1.

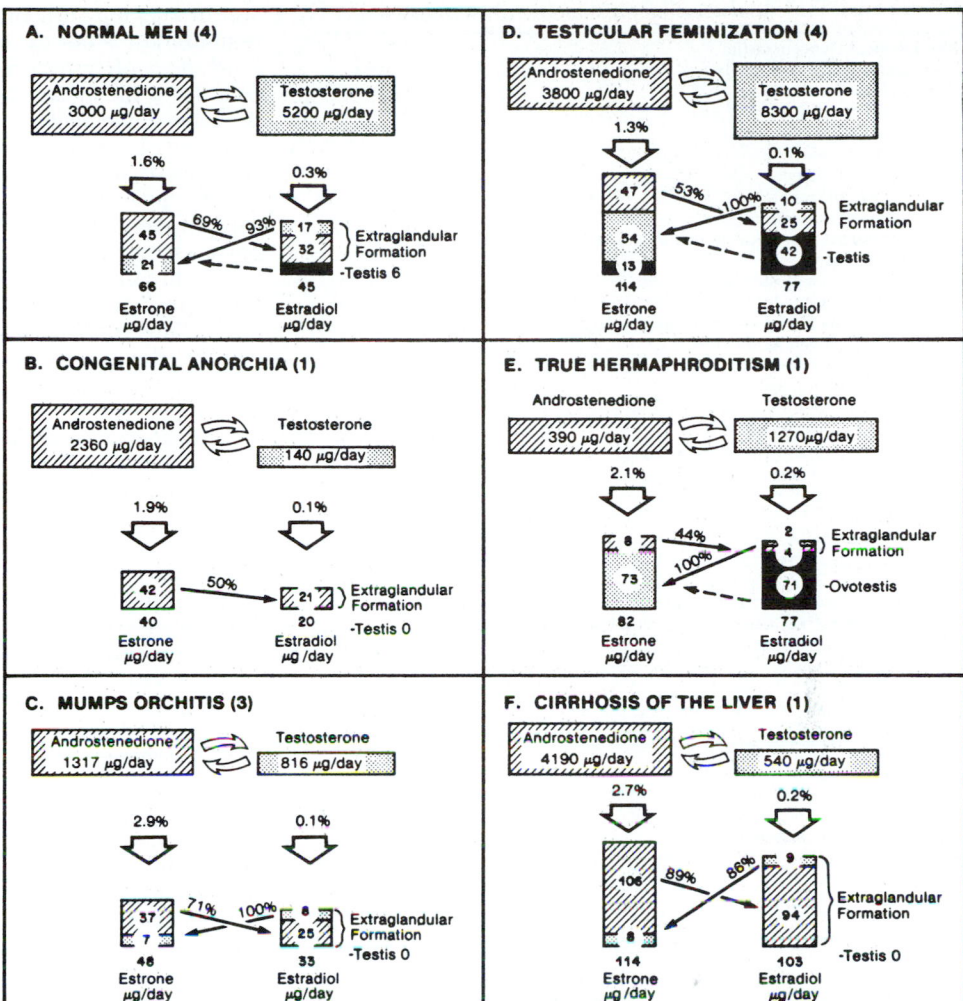

Figure 15–4. Dynamics of androgen and estrogen production in normal men and in patients with gynecomastia. Average production rates of androgen are indicated in upper boxes, and production rates of estrogen are shown at bottom of each vertical bar. The extent of conversion of plasma testosterone and androstenedione to estradiol and estrone is shown by vertical arrows, and interconversions of estradiol and estrone and of testosterone and androstenedione are indicated by horizontal arrows. Sources of estradiol and estrone are indicated by vertical bars. Black bars indicate estrogen secreted directly by the testis. Thus estradiol arises from plasma testosterone, from estrone, and from direct secretion by the testis, and estrone arises from plasma androstenedione, from estradiol, and in some instances by direct secretion from the testis. For A and D, data were taken from MacDonald et al.[241] For B, data were taken from Edman et al.[230] For C, data were taken from Aiman et al.[251] For E, data were taken from Aiman et al.[279] Data in Part F were supplied to us by Dr. C. D. Edman.

population survey the occurrence was somewhat less common.[220] The median age at onset is 14. In many boys the breasts are grossly asymmetrical and may be tender. By age 20 only a small number of men have palpable vestiges of gynecomastia in one or both breasts. The most severe form of this disorder is termed pubertal macromastia and may persist to adulthood.[221]

The exact cause of pubertal breast enlargement is uncertain. In boys the plasma estradiol value reaches the adult level before the adult level of plasma testosterone is attained.[222, 223] Furthermore, average plasma estradiol levels have been reported to be slightly higher in boys with gynecomastia.[224] As a result, in boys with pubertal gynecomastia the plasma ratios of testosterone to estradiol[225] and of adrenal androgens to estrone[226] tend to be low. This is presumably either due to the fact that the aromatase enzyme system in the Leydig and/or Sertoli cell completes maturation before androgen synthesis achieves the adult level or due to an enhanced activity of extraglandular aromatase (which can utilize adrenal androgen efficiently as a substrate for estrogen synthesis) before testosterone formation by the testes reaches its maximum so that the ratio of estrogen formed in the testes and/or extraglandular tissues to testosterone secretion by the testis is temporarily high.[210] It is also possible that local formation of estrogen within the breast itself might play a role in the gynecomastia of puberty.[227]

Gynecomastia of Aging. The fact that gynecomastia may occur in otherwise healthy elderly men has been known for many years; because gynecomastia can also be an indication of underlying pathology, the diagnosis of involutional gynecomastia is one of exclusion. What is remarkable is the frequency of this disorder; Williams reported that 40% of elderly men at autopsy have true gynecomastia,[188] and Niewoehner and Nuttall described a prevalence of 72% in hospitalized men aged 50 to 69.[190] However, many elderly patients receive other medications and have concurrent disorders of cardiovascular and liver function, and gynecomastia of aging, if it exists, may be due to the increased incidence of a variety of medical problems with age rather than to age itself.[228]

Nevertheless, changes in estrogen and androgen metabolism have been characterized in men older than age 70, including decrease in mean levels of plasma testosterone, decrease in plasma levels of bioavailable testosterone, elevation of plasma testosterone-binding globulin, increase in the rate of peripheral aromatization, decrease in the ratio of androgen to estrogen, elevation of plasma LH and follicle-stimulating hormone levels, and diminution or loss of the circadian rhythmicity of plasma testosterone levels (reviewed in Chapter 13). Such changes in elderly men might result in a sufficient alteration of the ratios of testosterone to estradiol within breast cells to feminize and thus be causal in breast enlargement in the absence of other diseases.

Pathological Gynecomastia. In pathological states gynecomastia can be caused by deficiency of testosterone formation or action, enhanced estrogen production, drugs, or unknown causes.

Deficiency of Testosterone Formation or Action. When

TABLE 15–1. Classification of Endocrine Gynecomastia

Physiological Gynecomastia
  Gynecomastia in the newborn
  Adolescent gynecomastia
  Gynecomastia of aging
Pathological Gynecomastia
  Testosterone deficiency
    Congenital defects
      Congenital anorchia
      Klinefelter syndrome
      Androgen resistance (testicular femininization and Reifenstein syndrome)
      Defects in testosterone synthesis
    Secondary testicular failure (viral orchitis, trauma, castration, neurological and granulomatous diseases, renal failure)
  Increased estrogen production
    Increased testicular estrogen secretion
      Testicular tumors
      Bronchogenic carcinoma and other tumors producing hCG
      True hermaphroditism
    Increased substrate for extraglandular aromatase
      Adrenal disease
      Liver disease
      Starvation
      Thyrotoxicosis
    Increase in extraglandular aromatase
  Drugs
    Estrogens or drugs that act like estrogens (diethylstilbestrol, estrogen-containing cosmetics, birth control bills, digitalis, estrogen-contaminated foods, phytoestrogens)
    Drugs that enhance endogenous estrogen formation (gonadotropins, clomiphene)
    Drugs that inhibit testosterone synthesis and/or action (ketoconazole, metronidazole, cimetidine, etomidate, alkylating agents, cisplatin, flutamide, spironolactone)
    Drugs that act by unknown mechanisms (busulfan, isoniazid, methyldopa, calcium channel–blocking agents, captopril, tricyclic antidepressants, penicillamine, diazepam, marijuana, heroin)
Idiopathic Gynecomastia

gynecomastia occurs as the consequence of a failure of testosterone synthesis (or action), it is generally associated with elevations of plasma gonadotropin levels and may or may not be associated with a secondary rise in testicular estrogen secretion.

Congenital Anorchia. This disorder is rare (often occurring in families); in it the testes are missing in phenotypically normal 46,XY males. Affected individuals are thought to have bilateral cryptorchidism at birth, and on surgical exploration of the abdomen no testes whatever can be located. Because testicular hormones are necessary for male phenotypic development and because penile development is normal in these boys, it is believed that testes are present and function normally until late in embryonic life and then regress for unknown reasons.

Approximately half of anorchid men develop gynecomastia. Endocrine studies have been performed in only a few such individuals. Kirschner and colleagues showed that in some anorchid men, Leydig cells are present and secrete small amounts of testosterone into the circulation even when testes cannot be found at surgery.[229] In another study two men with congenital anorchia had profound testosterone deficiency and low estradiol production; the small amounts of estradiol formed could be accounted for almost exclusively by the indirect pathway involving the aromatization of adrenal androgens in extraglandular tissues.[230] In the anorchid man with gynecomastia the plasma production of testosterone was entirely derived from extraglandular formation from androstenedione, whereas the man who did not have gynecomastia secreted small amounts of testosterone (162 μg/d), presumably from some unlocated testicular remnant.[230] These findings suggest that even small amounts of testosterone production may be sufficient to prevent gynecomastia even though not enough to virilize. The results are

also in keeping with the concept that the critical factor for feminization is not the absolute level of estrogen but rather some ratio of testosterone to estradiol. More important, it constitutes the purest example of a disturbance of ratio in the sense that smaller than normal amounts of estradiol are sufficient to feminize men unless opposed by normal amounts of androgen.

To provide insight into the meaning of the androgen/estrogen ratio, the mechanism by which androgen opposes estrogen action has been examined in detail in the mouse breast; in this tissue dihydrotestosterone competes with estradiol for binding to the cytosolic estrogen receptor.[231] Thus the antiestrogenic action of androgen in breast may be the result of effects of androgen acting via the estrogen receptor. If so, dihydrotestosterone performs one of its major actions independent of the androgen receptor.

Klinefelter Syndrome. Approximately half of nonmosaic and a third of mosaic Klinefelter men develop gynecomastia after the time of expected puberty.[232–234] Plasma and urine follicle-stimulating hormone and LH levels are high, and the average plasma testosterone level is half normal, although many such men have testosterone values within the normal range. The variability in plasma testosterone and estradiol levels may explain the variable degree of androgenization and feminization in men with this disorder.[235]

The reasons for the elevation of plasma estradiol and for the development of gynecomastia in the Klinefelter syndrome are complex.[236–238] Early in adolescence plasma testosterone may be maintained in the normal range as the result of elevated plasma LH, and as a consequence estradiol secretion by the testis is simultaneously elevated. Testis function becomes impaired with time so that after age 15 the serum testosterone levels are in the low adult range.[239] Eventually, the formation of both testosterone and estradiol by the testis declines so that the end stage resembles the situation in anorchia in which estrogen is formed predominantly by extraglandular aromatization of adrenal androgens, and estrogen formation, although low, is high relative to that of testosterone.[236] In addition, estrogen clearance may be diminished, which would result in further increase in estrogen/androgen ratios.

Androgen Resistance (Testicular Feminization and Reifenstein Syndrome). Hereditary defects in the X-linked cytoplasmic androgen receptor protein result in a spectrum of syndromes of incomplete virilization in 46,XY men who have testes and male testosterone levels but who are resistant to their own and to exogenous androgens. In the most severe form, affected individuals are phenotypic women with testicular feminization. When the impairment of receptor function is less complete, the phenotype is that of men with the Reifenstein syndrome (hypospadias and gynecomastia), lesser degrees of undervirilization, or the infertile male syndrome.[240] Detailed measurements of androgen and estrogen dynamics have been performed in six women with complete testicular feminization,[241] two men with the Reifenstein syndrome,[242] and one woman with incomplete testicular feminization.[243]

Androgen production rates are uniformly normal or elevated, and estrogen and estradiol production rates are enhanced as the result of increased secretion by the testes. Enhanced testicular secretion of estrogen and androgen is the consequence of elevated plasma gonadotropin levels, which in turn are increased because of resistance at the hypothalamic-pituitary level to the negative feedback control by testosterone. However, there is no direct relationship between the rates of estrogen secretion in these disorders and the degree of feminization that results. Two phenotypic men with the Reifenstein syndrome had average daily estradiol production rates of 212 μg and average testicular secretion rates of 160 µg of estradiol/day,[242] considerably higher than the mean daily estradiol production rates of 53 to 121 µg in patients with complete testicular feminization.[241] The estradiol production rate in a woman with incomplete testicular feminization was intermediate, 138 µg/d.[243] In contrast, testosterone production rates in the three groups overlap. Thus feminization in the androgen resistance syndromes depends on increased estradiol production after the time of puberty, but the degree of feminization must be influenced by other factors such as the severity of the androgen resistance and the variable elevation of plasma androgen levels.

Defects in Testosterone Synthesis. Five specific enzyme defects are known to result in deficient testosterone synthesis (and, usually, incomplete virilization of the male embryo during embryogenesis) (see Chapter 14). Each of the enzymes involves a critical biochemical step in the conversion of cholesterol to testosterone. There is extreme variability in the completeness of the enzyme defects and in the severity of clinical manifestations, but gynecomastia is common in two of the disorders, 3β-hydroxysteroid dehydrogenase deficiency and 17β-hydroxysteroid dehydrogenase deficiency. Androgen and estrogen dynamics have not been characterized in these disorders, but feminization could be due to normal or low levels of plasma estrogen in the face of diminished androgen production, as occurs in 3β-hydroxysteroid dehydrogenase deficiency.[244] In such a situation, development of gynecomastia is analogous to that in congenital anorchia. Alternatively, estrogen production may result from increased availability for extragonadal aromatization of steroids such as androstenedione that accumulate proximal to the enzymatic block in 17β-hydroxysteroid dehydrogenase deficiency.[245, 246]

Viral Orchitis. This disorder is the most common cause of testicular failure after puberty, and mumps is the most important etiology;[247] echovirus, lymphocytic choriomeningitis virus, and group B arboviruses may also be responsible.[248] The orchitis is due to direct effects of the virus in the testis rather than to indirect effects, because mumps virus has been isolated from the testes of affected patients.

Orchitis is the most common complication of mumps in adults and occurs in approximately a fourth of affected men. In two thirds it is unilateral, and in the remainder it is bilateral. Orchitis occurs rarely before puberty and usually develops within a few days after the onset of parotitis. After the acute phase, the testis gradually decreases in size and may either return to normal or shrink below the normal size. Testicular atrophy ensues in approximately a third of cases of viral orchitis and is bilateral in a tenth. Atrophy is believed to be the consequence either of direct action of the virus on the seminferous tubules or of ischemia secondary to pressure and edema within the tunica albuginea. The degree of atrophy is not necessarily proportional to the clinical severity of the orchitis. In a survey of 2000 adult men, Werner found atrophy of one or both testes in 2%, half of which was caused by mumps.[249] Testicular atrophy will presumably become less common because mumps is now preventable. In the acute phase, the administration of glucocorticoids is followed by rapid reduction of testicular swelling and pain, but it is not known whether this treatment influences the subsequent development of atrophy.[250]

The endocrine changes in men with bilateral testicular atrophy related to mumps orchitis have been characterized by Aiman and associates[251] and can be summarized as follows: testosterone production is about a fifth of normal, whereas production rates of estradiol and estrone are normal and can be accounted for almost entirely as arising from extraglandular sources. These findings suggest that the capacity of the Leydig cells to secrete testosterone is impaired but that total estrogen production is normal because of the increase in extraglandular aromatization that occurs with age. The net consequence of these changes is a reduction in the ratio of testosterone to estrogen, and gynecomastia commonly ensues.[251]

Trauma. The second most common cause of acquired testicular atrophy in the adult is trauma, and gynecomastia may also occur after *castration* in men.[247] Presumably, the disturbance in the ratios of androgen to estrogen in these disorders resembles that in congenital anorchia.

Neurological Disease. Testicular atrophy occurs in three fourths of cases of myotonia atrophica and is also common in men with spinal cord lesions and other neurological diseases. Biopsy of the testes reveals atrophy and hyalinization.[252–254] The nature of the endocrine abnormality is unclear but is probably similar to that in mumps orchitis.

Granulomatous Disease. Testicular atrophy, decreased plasma testosterone levels, elevated gonadotropin levels, and gynecomastia are common in leprosy.[254–256] Direct granulomatous involvement of testis and the secondary neuropathy probably both play a role in the impairment of testicular function. Liver function tests may also be deranged in men with leprosy and gynecomastia, and the correlation between the endocrine changes that have been described and the development of gynecomastia is not invariable.

Renal Failure. Gynecomastia is common in men with renal failure and is present in approximately half of men with renal failure who are undergoing hemodialysis.[251–263] The endocrine changes in renal failure are complex. In men whose creatinine (or creatine?) clearance is less than 4 mL/min, plasma LH and follicle-stimulating hormone levels are elevated (four times normal), the plasma testosterone level is depressed (30% of normal), the testes show damage to the spermatogenic tubules, the response of plasma testosterone to hCG is subnormal, and prolactin levels in plasma are elevated. The elevated plasma LH is due to both reduced metabolic clearance and increased secretion, probably the consequence of subnormal production of testosterone by the testes. The extent to which gynecomastia is due to decreased androgen production compared with increased estrogen levels is unknown. Interestingly, in one report treatment of patients on hemodialysis with bromocriptine caused a decrease in prolactin levels and a slight increase in plasma testosterone level.[263]

Increased Estrogen Production. This alteration can result from increased testicular estrogen secretion, from increased substrate for extraglandular formation, or from increased extraglandular aromatase itself.

Testicular Estrogen Secretion. TESTICULAR TUMORS. These tumors produce feminization in three ways. Some germinal cell tumors (embryonal carcinomas, choriocarcinomas, teratomas, and rarely seminomas) produce hCG or fragments of hCG, which in turn stimulate estradiol and testosterone synthesis by the uninvolved areas of the testes.[264] In contrast, stromal cell tumors (Leydig cell and Sertoli cell tumors) may secrete testosterone and estradiol autonomously; in these instances plasma gonadotropin levels are depressed, uninvolved areas of the testes are nonfunctional, and azoospermia is common.[265–270] A distinctive feature of feminizing Leydig cell tumors is that feminization can be produced before such tumors are detectable by physical examination. These small masses can frequently be identified by ultrasonography,[271, 272] and Kuhn and colleagues have concluded that a combination of a prolonged rise in plasma estradiol after administration of hCG and ultrasonographic evidence provides the best criterion for the diagnosis of feminizing testicular tumors.[273] Finally, in testicular choriocarcinomas the aromatase concentration may be high in the tumor tissue so that circulating adrenal and testicular androgens are converted to estrogen by the tumor.[274, 275]

BRONCHOGENIC CARCINOMA. This carcinoma can cause an increase in hCG levels in plasma and an increase in estrogen production as well, and the degree of gynecomastia correlates with the estrogen production. The exact mechanism of the increased estrogen production has not been elucidated, but it is likely, as in other patients with elevation of plasma hCG levels, that the elevated plasma gonadotropins result in increased secretion of estradiol by the testes.[276, 277] Indeed, hCG secretion by any tumor, such as by transitional cell tumors of the urinary tract, can cause feminizing states.[278]

TRUE HERMAPHRODITISM. In true hermaphroditism both the ovarian and the testicular components of the gonads are endocrinologically active, and at the time of expected puberty a mixed pattern of feminization and virilization takes place.[279] Gynecomastia is a consequence of gonadal estrogen secretion (admittedly this is not testicular secretion in a strict sense, because the estrogen is assumed to come from the ovarian elements of the ovotestes).[279]

Increased Substrate for Peripheral Aromatase. ADRENAL DISEASE. In adrenal disease such as feminizing adrenal carcinoma, estrogen production may reach 2 to 8 mg/d. Most feminizing adrenal cancers are associated with massive increases in the production of the adrenal androgens androstenedione and dehydroepiandrosterone; the enhanced estrogen production is usually the consequence of increased availability of these androgens to serve as substrates for extraglandular aromatization, but in rare instances the adrenal tumor itself may secrete estrogen.[280–285]

Feminization can also occur in benign forms of adrenal hyperplasia. The feminization in boys with congenital adrenal hyperplasia related to 21-hydroxylase deficiency may be complicated because it can be associated with benign testicular tumors, but in most boys with congenital adrenal hyperplasia enhanced estrogen production is believed to be the consequence of increased production of androstenedione and hence of increased availability of substrate for peripheral aromatase.[286–290] In 3β-hydroxysteroid dehydrogenase deficiency, feminization is believed to be due to a combination of decreased testosterone levels and increased availability of adrenal androgens for extraglandular aromatization.[291] As noted earlier, increased availability of adrenal androgen for extraglandular aromatization also contributes to the feminization in patients with 17β-hydroxysteroid dehydrogenase deficiency.[245, 246]

LIVER DISEASE. Liver disease (in particular cirrhosis of the liver) is a common cause of feminization. Because both plasma concentrations and urinary excretion rates of estrogens are elevated, gynecomastia is thought to be largely due to overproduction of estrogen. However, the liver is not the direct source of the estrogens. Gordon and colleagues[292] reported that the extent of extraglandular aromatization of plasma androgens to estrogen is increased in cirrhosis, and Edman and colleagues[293] showed that the increased extraglandular formation is largely the consequence of decreased hepatic extraction of androstenedione (7% of the normal rate) and a secondary increased availability of androstenedione for extrasplanchnic metabolism, including aromatization. However, the development of gynecomastia in subjects with liver disease does not correlate closely with the measurable endocrine abnormalities,[294, 295] and administration of testosterone to men with alcoholic cirrhosis causes a decreased prevalence of gynecomastia.[296] These findings imply that androgen deficiency (and possibly other factors as well) also plays a role in the gynecomastia of liver disease. In

carcinoma of the liver feminization can be the consequence of increased aromatase activity in the tumor itself.[297, 298]

STARVATION. Starvation is also associated with feminizing signs. Approximately 15% of American prisoners of war in Japanese prison camps developed gynecomastia.[299, 300] Three fourths of cases were bilateral, and most regressed within 5 to 7 mo. About a third of the cases occurred during refeeding after release, and other instances were associated with temporary improvements in the food supply during imprisonment. Infectious hepatitis and liver disease may have played a role in the pathogenesis, because some of the men affected also had spider angiomata and fatty infiltration of the liver. The exact etiology of starvation gynecomastia has never been clarified, but the pathogenesis may be similar to that of liver disease, namely, diminished hepatic clearance of androgens and consequent shunting of androgens to the extraglandular sites of aromatization.

THYROTOXICOSIS. Thyrotoxicosis causes gynecomastia in about a third of affected men, and as many as 80% may have histological evidence of gynecomastia.[301–303] Such men have elevated plasma estradiol levels,[304–307] probably the result of elevated androstenedione production rates and consequently the increased formation of estrogen in extraglandular sites (despite a normal rate constant for the reaction).[308] Thus the mechanism of increased estrogen production is probably similar to that in liver disease—increased availability of substrate for extraglandular aromatization.

Increase in Extraglandular Aromatase. Increased extraglandular estrogen production can also arise from increased activity of aromatase enzymes in peripheral tissues. Hemsell and co-workers[309] described a remarkable 8-y-old boy who developed a striking feminization syndrome; he converted half of circulating androstenedione to estrone each day for an estrogen production rate of 780 μg/d—more than 50 times the normal rate of extraglandular aromatase activity. The genetic basis of the disorder in the index case is not clear, but two brothers with a similar disorder have been described by Berkowitz and colleagues,[310] implying that it is due to a single gene mutation. A characteristic feature in the three reported cases is that the onset of the gynecomastia corresponded with the onset of adrenarche and thus occurred before the time of normal puberty. A similar trait has been characterized in the Sebright bantam chicken, in which an autosomal dominant gene causes more than a 100-fold increase in extraglandular aromatization.[311]

Drugs. Drugs can cause gynecomastia by several different mechanisms—by acting directly as estrogens, by enhancing testicular production of estrogens, by inhibiting testosterone synthesis or action, and by unknown mechanisms.

Estrogens and Drugs That Act Like Estrogens. Estrogens given to men in any form can result in severe gynecomastia. That which occurs in diethylstilbestrol-treated men[312] and transsexual men given estrogens[313] is best characterized. In some instances estrogens may be taken for other therapeutic reasons.[314] Young men and boys are particularly sensitive to estrogens and may develop gynecomastia from industrial estrogen exposure or exposure to dermal ointments containing estrogens, which are sometimes used without being unaware that the creams contain estrogens.[315–324] Unraveling the source of estrogen exposure may require a high index of suspicion, as in the cases of a barber who massaged the scalps of customers with an antibaldness nostrum containing estrogen,[319] workers in plants manufacturing oral contraceptives,[323] and children of workers in a diethylstilbestrol manufacturing plant who absorbed the drug from the clothing of their fathers.[324] Indeed, sufficient estrogen to induce gynecomastia can be absorbed by men during sexual intercourse with partners who use vaginal creams containing estrogen.[325, 326] In the United States no federal regulation governs the use of estrogens in cosmetics provided no therapeutic claims are made, and estradiol concentrations as high as 18 ng/g have been described in cosmetic creams.[327]

Furthermore, epidemics of gynecomastia among children in Bahrain and in Italy have been described in which the estrogen source was milk from estrogen-injected cows or meat from diethylstilbestrol-injected cows.[328, 329] These reports are of particular importance because they raise the possibility that long-term exposure to small amounts of estrogenic agents might be the cause of gynecomastia of unknown etiology. Such agents might be derived from meat and dairy products from animals treated with estrogenic implants other than diethylstilbestrol,[330] from endogenous estrogens in animal tissues,[331] or from fungal estrogens and phytoestrogens in foods.[332–334]

Although an association between digitalis administration and gynecomastia is well known, the pathophysiology is not well understood. About 10% of men who have been given digitalis leaf for a year develop gynecomastia,[335, 336] but LeWinn pointed out that many patients with digitalis-induced gynecomastia also have abnormal liver function.[335] The same types of preparation that cause gynecomastia also have an estrogenic effect on the squamous epithelia of the vagina in postmenopausal women.[337] The mechanism of the gynecomastia is thought to be related to the role of digitalis as an estrogen or estrogen precursor; whereas digoxin has no identifiable effect on plasma estrogens,[338] digitoxin binds to the human estrogen receptor.[339] Alternatively, Ricken has suggested that digitalis glycosides act principally to enhance the action of endogenous estrogens.[340]

Drugs That Enhance Endogenous Estrogen Formation. The administration of hCG to boys and to men may result in gynecomastia,[341] as would be predicted because it causes an increase in estradiol secretion by the testes.[211] Clomiphene citrate (both a weak estrogen and an antiestrogen) has been used to treat gynecomastia in boys, but paradoxically it can cause gynecomastia on withdrawal, presumably by increasing LH secretion and consequently increasing estradiol secretion by the testes.[342]

Drugs That Inhibit Testosterone Synthesis or Action. The antifungal drug ketoconazole blocks steroid hormone synthesis in Leydig cells (the principal step appears to be at the 17,20-desmolase reaction).[343] A similar effect occurs with other imidazole drugs including metronidazole and etomidate.[343, 344] The inhibition of synthesis by ketoconazole is transient, and plasma testosterone returns to normal when blood levels of the drug fall. Thus gynecomastia occurs only when the dosage and administration schedule are such as to cause prolonged lowering of plasma androgen levels.[345] In this situation, inhibition of testosterone synthesis presumably causes feminization by mechanisms similar to that in testicular failure, namely, by altering the ratio of estradiol to testosterone.[346, 347]

Antineoplastic agents may result in long-lasting inhibition of testosterone synthesis, presumably via toxic effects on the Leydig cell; such damage may occur when the therapy is directed either toward systemic neoplasms (alkylating agents for treatment of Hodgkin disease) or toward testicular cancers.[348–351] The precise mechanism of this phenomenon has never been elucidated, but elevation in plasma gonadotropin levels secondary to the testicular damage may play a role.[351]

Approximately half of men who receive 150 mg of spironolactone per day develop gynecomastia.[352] Spironolactone has at least two effects on androgen metabolism: it inhibits testosterone biosynthesis by inhibiting the 17,20-desmolase reaction, and it prevents the binding of androgen

to its receptor.[353–355] The incidence of gynecomastia is dose related,[356] but spironolactone may cause gynecomastia in doses as low as 50 mg/d—a dose that apparently does not have any effect on testosterone synthesis. At these dose levels the drug is believed to cause gynecomastia by inhibiting androgen binding to the receptor. At higher doses, testosterone synthesis is also inhibited, and plasma testosterone levels fall as a consequence. It is of interest that spironolactone-induced gynecomastia may disappear during treatment with the active metabolite of the drug canrenoate.[357]

Two antiandrogens that have been tried for the treatment of prostatic disease (cyproterone and flutamide) inhibit testosterone binding to the receptor, and both cause gynecomastia.[358, 359] Gynecomastia is a common side effect of cimetidine therapy.[360–364] The drug has the capacity to block the binding of androgen to the androgen receptor as well as blocking the binding of histamine to the H_2 receptor, and in addition it may inhibit the catabolism of estradiol.[365] Gynecomastia is less common in subjects receiving ranitidine than in those receiving cimetidine.[366, 367] Suggestive evidence for induction of gynecomastia by an antiandrogen has come from studies of an epidemic of temporary gynecomastia that affected about a tenth of male Haitian refugees in five detention centers set up by the U.S. government in 1981.[368] The delousing agent used in these centers has an affinity for the androgen receptor similar to that of the synthetic androgen methyltrienolone and acts as an antiandrogen in rats,[369] and it has been suggested that it might have caused the gynecomastia. From this cumulative experience it can be concluded that antiandrogens can cause gynecomastia and that unidentified antiandrogens might cause some of the cases now designated as idiopathic.

Drugs That Act by Unknown Mechanisms. A variety of drugs cause gynecomastia by unknown mechanisms. These include busulfan, methyldopa, isoniazid, tricyclic antidepressants, penicillamine, captopril, calcium channel–blocking agents, and diazepam, some of which may act by altering liver function.[370–373] Both marijuana and heroin are suspected causes of gynecomastia, but the available data make it impossible to establish a direct cause-and-effect relationship.[374–377]

Idiopathic Gynecomastia. In all published series half or more of subjects evaluated for gynecomastia do not have an underlying endocrinopathy that is diagnosable at autopsy[378, 379] or by careful endocrine work-up.[380] If one adds those instances in which the diagnosis is tenuous in all large series, the idiopathic category accounts for approximately three fourths of cases. At present we do not know whether men with gynecomastia of unknown etiology are in fact normal (as proposed by Nuttall[189]), whether they had a feminizing factor that was transient and not present at the time of work-up, whether there is widespread exposure to small amounts of one or more environmental estrogens or antiandrogens, or whether the gynecomastia is the consequence of subtle, unrecognized endocrinopathies. Endocrinopathies that are known to cause breast enlargement are associated with severe gynecomastia, and the extent to which minor endocrine disorders are not recognized with current methodologies is uncertain. The fact that gynecomastia can develop as the result of subtle environmental exposure to estrogens or to antiandrogens raises the possibility that some gynecomastia may be due to long-term, subtle exposure to unrecognized endocrine substances.[324, 328–334, 369] The problem of gynecomastia is in many ways analogous to that of the epidemiology of euthyroid goiter in that the etiology has been explained in only a fraction of cases. The critical clinical point, however, is that whatever the etiology (or etiologies) the diagnosis of idiopathic gynecomastia carries no known import as to health.

Prolactin Does Not Play a Direct Role in Gynecomastia.
Plasma prolactin levels are usually normal in men with gynecomastia of diverse etiologies, and men who have prolonged elevation in plasma prolactin secondary to psychotropic drugs do not commonly develop gynecomastia.[381-384] As a consequence, prolactin is not believed to play a direct role in the disorder; this conclusion is in keeping with the fact that prolactin is not a growth hormone for the breast. Furthermore, when gynecomastia develops in men with prolactin-secreting tumors of the pituitary and high plasma prolactin levels,[385-387] the gynecomastia is probably the consequence of secondary testicular failure as a result of either effects of the tumor mass or effects of prolactin itself on gonadotropin secretion. In other instances of gynecomastia in which the prolactin level is elevated, the elevation may be the secondary consequence of hyperestrogenemia.[388, 389]

DIAGNOSIS. The dilemma is to separate men with underlying endocrinopathies from those in the larger category of idiopathic disorders. In general, only men whose gynecomastia is symptomatic are evaluated, but if there is a serious question as to whether the gynecomastia is real the issue can probably best be solved by mammography and/or ultrasonography.[196-199]

The routine measurement of androgen and estrogen kinetics is impractical, but most of the known causes of gynecomastia can be identified by a work-up that includes (1) a careful drug history that encompasses potential environmental and indirect exposures to endocrinologically active substances; (2) detailed physical examination including the testes (the finding of small testes bilaterally suggests testicular insufficiency, and asymmetrical testes raise the possibility of testicular tumors); (3) evaluation of liver function; and (4) a limited endocrine work-up including measurement of plasma dehydroepiandrosterone or urinary 17-ketosteroids (usually elevated in adrenal feminizing states), measurement of plasma estradiol (helpful if elevated but generally normal), and measurement of plasma LH and testosterone (high LH and normal or low testosterone levels suggest testicular insufficiency; low LH and low testosterone levels suggest hypopituitarism, estrogen secretion from a tumor, or an exogenous source of estrogen; and high LH and high testosterone levels suggest androgen resistance). If these parameters are normal (as is frequently the case), the usual recourse is to follow the patient. If the symptoms persist or worsen and if the enlargement is progressive, a more extensive work-up may have to be undertaken.

TREATMENT. The difficulty in treating gynecomastia is inherent in its natural history; when the feminizing process persists for a long period the initial glandular hyperplasia is replaced by a progressive fibrosis and hyalinization that does not regress when the source of excess estrogen is corrected.[200] Consequently, surgery remains the mainstay of therapy and is frequently indicated for psychological and cosmetic reasons. Such surgery is usually accomplished through a circumareolar approach.[390-394]

Medical management is most successful when it is addressed to gynecomastia of recent onset or to prevention of its development. Testosterone administration has inconsistent effects in the Klinefelter syndrome but can cause dramatic improvement in subjects with other forms of testicular failure (anorchia or viral orchitis); the uncertain element in testosterone therapy is the result of the fact that it can serve as substrate for extraglandular estrogen formation, and under some circumstances (such as liver disease) androgen therapy can cause a disproportionate increase in plasma estrogen levels. Various drug regimens have been tried for gynecomastia with varying degrees of success, including the antiestrogens tamoxifen[395-397] and clomiphene,[398, 399] the aromatase inhibitor testolactone,[400] and danazol,[401, 402] a weak androgen that acts by inhibiting gonadotropin secretion and causing a fall in plasma testosterone. It is of interest that treatment with dihydrotestosterone (which cannot be aromatized to estrogen) is said to cause significant symptomatic improvement in gynecomastia.[403-405] Unfortunately, no suitable prospective control studies have been performed with any of these regimens, and their clinical usefulness is not established.

Perhaps the most effective form of medical therapy is prevention of its development by breast radiation before the institution of stilbestrol therapy in men who have carcinoma of the prostate.[406-408] Such therapy approaches 90% effectiveness, and the complication rate is low in the age group affected with prostatic cancer.

CONCLUSIONS. The clinical problem of gynecomastia is clouded by questions of definition and incidence. Once the diagnosis is made, the disorder must be separated into the idiopathic type (of uncertain significance as well as cause), which may account for three fourths of cases, and endocrine gynecomastia, which can arise from any of several disturbances in androgen and estrogen physiology. It is useful to consider the endocrine causes in terms of the androgen/estrogen ratio, namely, disturbances that can arise from decreases in androgen production (or action) or from increases in estrogen formation. The latter, in turn, can arise from estrogen secretion by tumors or increase in extraglandular estrogen formation. Most drugs that cause gynecomastia also act to alter the ratio of androgen to estrogen. It is rational in most instances of gynecomastia to perform only a limited endocrine work-up and to monitor the course of this disorder before undertaking more extensive diagnostic evaluation.

Galactorrhea in Men

Galactorrhea is more common in women than in men, who account for about 5% of galactorrheic patients. The relative infrequency of this disorder in men is presumably due to the fact that appropriate estrogen priming of the breast is less common in men who have elevations in plasma prolactin. When galactorrhea does occur in men it is appropriate to evaluate the patients both for feminizing syndromes and for prolactin excess. Prolactin-secreting pituitary tumors are a common cause of prolactin excess.

Carcinoma of the Male Breast

Gynecomastia is a risk factor for malignancy in that men with gynecomastia have breast cancer with a greater frequency and at a lower age than men without gynecomastia.[409-413] However, this increased risk is small, and of 228 patients with gynecomastia followed for up to 10 y none developed breast cancer.[414] When cancer is suspected mammography is helpful in establishing the diagnosis. It is puzzling that the frequency of breast cancer in men with gynecomastia is less than that of normal women.

REFERENCES

1. Ceriani RL. Hormones and other factors controlling growth in the mammary gland: a review. J Invest Dermatol 1974; 63:93–108.
2. Porter JC. Hormonal regulation of breast development and activity. J Invest Dermatol 1974; 63:85–92.
3. Salazar H, Tobon H, Josimovich JB. Developmental, gestational and postgestational modifications of the human breast. Clin Obstet Gynecol 1975; 18:113–137.
4. Cowie AT, Forsyth IA, Hart IC. Hormonal Control of Lactation. Berlin: Springer-Verlag, 1980.
5. McKiernan JF, Hull D. Breast development in the newborn. Arch Dis Child 1981; 56:525–529.
6. McKiernan JF, Hull D. Prolactin, maternal oestrogens, and breast development in the newborn. Arch Dis Child 1981; 56:770–774.

7. McKiernan J, Coyne J, Cahalane S. Histology of breast development in early life. Arch Dis Child 1988; 63:136–139.
8. Raynaud A. Morphogenesis of the mammary gland. In: Kon SK, Cowie HT, eds. Milk: The Mammary Gland and Its Secretions. Vol 1. New York: Academic, 1961: 3–46.
9. Kratochwil K. In vitro analysis of the hormonal basis for the sexual dimorphism in the embryonic development of the mouse mammary gland. J Embryol Exp Morphol 1971; 25:141–153.
10. Kratochwil K, Schwartz P. Tissue interaction in androgen response of embryonic mammary rudiment of the mouse: identification of the target tissue for testosterone. Proc Natl Acad Sci USA 1976; 73:4041–4044.
11. Pfaltz CR. Das embryonale und postnatale Verhalten den Mannlichen brustdruse beim Menschen. II. Das Mammanorgan in Kindes-, Junglings-, Mannes-, und Greisenaltern. Acta Anat 1949; 8:293–328.
12. Vogel PM, Georgiade NG, Fetter BF, et al. The correlation of histologic changes in the human breast with the menstrual cycle. Am J Pathol 1981; 104:23–34.
13. Longacre TA, Bartow SA. A correlative morphologic study of human breast and endometrium in the menstrual cycle. Am J Surg Pathol 1986; 10:382–393.
14. Going JJ, Anderson TJ, Battersby S, et al. Proliferative and secretory activity in human breast during natural and artificial menstrual cycles. Am J Pathol 1988; 130:193–204.
15. Anderson RR. Endocrinological control. In: Larson BL, Smith VR, eds. Lactation. A Comprehensive Treatise. New York: Academic, 1974: 97–140.
16. Topper YJ, Oka T. Some aspects of mammary gland development in the mature mouse. In: Larson BL, Smith VR, eds. Lactation. A Comprehensive Treatise. New York: Academic, 1974: 327–348.
17. Vorherr H. Hormonal and biochemical changes of pituitary and breast during pregnancy. Semin Perinatol 1979; 3:193–198.
18. Tucker HA. Endocrinology of lactation. Semin Perinatol 1979; 3:199–223.
19. Knight CH, Peaker M. Development of the mammary gland. J Reprod Fertil 1982; 65:521–536.
20. Battersby S, Anderson TJ. Proliferative and secretory activity in the pregnant and lactating human breast. Virchows Arch A 1988; 413:189–196.
21. Topper YJ, Freeman CS. Multiple hormone interactions in the developmental biology of the mammary gland. Physiol Rev 1980; 60:1049–1105.
22. Nicoll CS. Physiological actions of prolactin. In: Greep RO, Astwood EB, Knobil E, et al., eds. Handbook of Physiology. Sect 7: Endocrinology. Vol IV. The Pituitary Gland and Its Neuroendocrine Control. Part 2. Washington, DC: American Physiological Society, 1974: 253–292.
23. Shiu RPC, Friesen HG. Mechanism of action of prolactin in the control of mammary gland function. Annu Rev Physiol 1980; 42:83–96.
24. Lyons WR, Li CH, Johnson RE. The hormonal control of mammary growth and lactation. Recent Prog Horm Res 1958; 14:219–254.
25. Cowie AT, Tindal JS, Yokoyama A. The induction of mammary growth in the hypophysectomized goat. J Endocrinol 1966; 34:185–195.
26. Talwalker PK, Meites J. Mammary lobulo-alveolar growth induced by anterior pituitary hormones in adreno-ovariectomized and adreno-ovariectomized-hypophysectomized rats. Proc Soc Exp Biol Med 1961; 107:880–883.
27. Kleinberg DL, Todd J, Niemann W. Prolactin stimulation of α-lactalbumin in normal primate mammary gland. J Clin Endocrinol Metab 1978; 47:435–441.
28. Holdaway IM, Friesen HG. Hormone binding by human mammary carcinoma. Cancer Res 1977; 37:1946–1952.
29. Djiane J, Durand P, Kelly PA. Evolution of prolactin receptors in rabbit mammary gland during pregnancy and lactation. Endocrinology 1977; 100:1348–1356.
30. Hayden TJ, Bonney RC, Forsyth IA. Ontogeny and control of prolactin receptors in the mammary gland and liver of virgin, pregnant and lactating rats. J Endocrinol 1979; 80:259–269.
31. Dhadly MS, Walker RA. The localization of prolactin binding sites in human breast tissue. Int J Cancer 1983; 31:433–437.
32. Posner BI, Kelly PA, Friesen HG. Prolactin receptors in rat liver: possible induction by prolactin. Science 1975; 188:57–59.
33. Djiane J, Durand P. Prolactin-progesterone antagonism in self-regulation of prolactin receptors in the mammary gland. Nature 1977; 266:614–643.
34. Kledzik GS, Bradley CJ, Marshall S, et al. Effects of high doses of estrogen on prolactin-binding activity and growth of carcinogen-induced mammary cancers in rats. Cancer Res 1976; 36:3265–3268.
35. Shiu RPC, Friesen HG. Blockade of prolactin action by an antiserum to its receptors. Science 1976; 192:259–261.
36. Godowski PJ, Leung DW, Meacham LR, et al. Characterization of the human growth hormone receptor gene and demonstration of a partial gene deletion in two patients with Laron-type dwarfism. Proc Natl Acad Sci USA 1989; 86:8083–8087.
37. Frantz AG, Kleinberg DL, Noel GL. Studies on prolactin in man. Recent Prog Horm Res 1972; 28:527–590.
38. Frantz AG, Rabkin MT. Effects of estrogen and sex difference on

39. secretion of human growth hormone. J Clin Endocrinol Metab 1965; 25:1470–1480.
39. Kleinberg DL, Todd J, Babitsky G, et al. Estradiol inhibits prolactin induced α-lactalbumin production in normal primate mammary tissue in vitro. Endocrinology 1982; 110:279–281.
40. Perel E, Wilkins D, Killinger DW. The conversion of androstenedione to estrone, estradiol, and testosterone in breast tissue. J Steroid Biochem 1980; 13:89–94.
41. Perel E, Davis S, Killinger DW. Androgen metabolism in male and female breast tissue. Steroids 1981; 37:345–352.
42. Perel E, Killinger DW. The metabolism of androstenedione and testosterone to C_{19} metabolites in normal breast, breast carcinoma and benign prostatic hypertrophy tissue. J Steroid Biochem 1983; 19:1135–1139.
43. James VHT, McNeill JM, Lai LC, et al. Aromatase activity in normal breast and breast tumor tissues: in vivo and in vitro studies. Steroids 1987; 50:269–279.
44. Wagner RK, Jungblut PW. Oestradiol- and dihydrotestosterone receptors in normal and neoplastic human mammary tissue. Acta Endocrinol 1976; 82:105–120.
45. Silva JS, Georgiade GS, Dilley WG, et al. Menstrual cycle–dependent variations of breast cyst fluid proteins and sex steroid receptors in the normal human breast. Cancer 1983; 51:1297–1302.
46. Petersen OW, Hoyer PE, van Deurs B. Frequency and distribution of estrogen receptor-positive cells in normal, nonlactating human breast tissue. Cancer Res 1987; 47:5748–5751.
47. Markopoulos C, Berger U, Wilson P, et al. Oestrogen receptor content of normal breast cells and breast carcinomas throughout the menstrual cycle. Br Med J 1988; 296:1349–1351.
48. Edery M, Imagawa W, Larson L, et al. Regulation of estrogen and progesterone receptor levels in mouse mammary epithelial cells grown in serum-free collagen gel cultures. Endocrinology 1985; 116:105–112.
49. Muldoon TG. Prolactin mediation of estrogen-induced changes in mammary tissue estrogen and progesterone receptors. Endocrinology 1987; 121:141–149.
50. Freeman CS, Topper YJ. Progesterone is not essential to the differentiative potential of mammary epithelium in the male mouse. Endocrinology 1978; 103:186–192.
51. Mauvais-Jarvis P, Kuttenn F, Gompel A. Antiestrogen action of progesterone in breast tissue. Horm Res 1987; 28:212–218.
52. Davis JW, Wikman-Coffelt J, Eddington CL. The effect of progesterone on biosynthetic pathways in mammary tissue. Endocrinology 1972; 91:1011–1019.
53. Shamay A, Zeelon E, Ghez Z, et al. Inhibition of casein and fat synthesis and α-lactalbumin secretion by progesterone in explants from bovine lactating mammary glands. J Endocrinol 1987; 113:81–88.
54. Vorherr H. Suppression of lactation. In: The Breast. New York: Academic, 1974: 198–217.
55. Haslam SZ, Shyamala G. Progesterone receptors in normal mammary glands of mice: characterization and relationship to stage of development. Endocrinology 1979; 105:786–795.
56. Rimoin DL, Holzman GB, Merimee TJ, et al. Lactation in the absence of human growth hormone. J Clin Endocrinol Metab 1968; 28:1183–1188.
57. Topper YJ, Nicholas KR, Sankaran L, et al. Insulin as a developmental hormone. Prog Clin Biol Res 1984; 142:63–77.
58. Prosser CG, Sankaran L, Hennighausen L, et al. Comparison of the roles of insulin and insulin-like growth factor I in casein gene expression and in the development of α-lactalbumin and glucose transport activities in the mouse mammary epithelial cell. Endocrinology 1987; 120:1411–1416.
59. Furlanetto RW, DiCarlo JN. Somatomedin-C receptors and growth effects in human breast cells maintained in long-term tissue culture. Cancer Res 1984; 44:2122–2128.
60. Peyrat JP, Bonneterre J, Laurent JC, et al. Presence and characterization of insulin-like growth factor I receptors in human benign breast disease. Eur J Cancer Clin Oncol 1988; 24:1425–1431.
61. Tonelli QJ, Sorof S. Epidermal growth factor requirement for development of cultured mammary gland. Nature 1980; 285:250–252.
62. Imagawa W, Tomooka Y, Hamamoto S, et al. Stimulation of mammary epithelial cell growth in vitro: interaction of epidermal growth factor and mammogenic hormones. Endocrinology 1985; 116:1514–1524.
63. Anderson TR, Mayer GL, Hebert N, et al. Interactions among prolactin, epidermal growth factor, and proinsulin on the growth and morphology of the pigeon crop-sac mucosal epithelium in vivo. Endocrinology 1987; 120:1258–1264.
64. Nicoll CS, Anderson TR, Hebert NJ, et al. Comparative aspects of the growth-promoting actions of prolactin on its target organs: evidence for synergism with an insulin-like growth factor. In: MacLeod RM, Thorner MO, Scapagnini U, eds. Prolactin: Basic and Clinical Correlates. New York: Springer-Verlag, 1985: 393–410.
65. Nicoll CS, Hebert NJ, Russell SM. Lactogenic hormones stimulate the liver to secrete a factor that acts synergistically with prolactin to promote growth of the pigeon crop-sac mucosal epithelium in vivo. Endocrinology 1985; 116:1449–1453.
66. Hoeffler JP, Frawley LS. Liver tissue produces a potent lactogen that

partially mimics the actions of prolactin. Endocrinology 1987; 120:1679–1681.

67. Newman CB, Cosby H, Friesen HG, et al. Evidence for a nonprolactin, non–growth-hormone mammary mitogen in the human pituitary gland. Proc Natl Acad Sci USA 1987; 84:8110–8114.

68. Oka T, Yoshimura M. Paracrine regulation of mammary gland growth. Clin Endocrinol Metab 1986; 15:79–97.

69. Shyamala G. Specific cytoplasmic glucocorticoid hormone receptors in lactating mammary glands. Biochemistry 1973; 12:3085–3090.

70. Dawood MY, Khan-Dawood FS, Wahi RS, et al. Oxytocin release and plasma anterior pituitary and gonadal hormones in women during lactation. J Clin Endocrinol Metab 1981; 52:678–683.

71. Huddleston JF, Sutliff G, Robinson D. Contraction stress test by intermittent nipple stimulation. Obstet Gynecol 1984; 63:669–673.

72. Finley BE, Amico J, Castillo M, et al. Oxytocin and prolactin responses associated with nipple stimulation contraction stress tests. Obstet Gynecol 1986; 67:836–839.

73. Keegan KA Jr, Helm DA, Porto M, et al. A prospective evaluation of nipple stimulation techniques for contraction stress testing. Am J Obstet Gynecol 1987; 157:121–125.

74. Curtis P, Evens S, Resnick J, et al. Patterns of uterine contractions and prolonged uterine activity using three methods of breast stimulation for contraction stress tests. Obstet Gynecol 1987; 83:631–638.

75. Noel GL, Suh HK, Frantz AG. Prolactin release during nursing and breast stimulation in postpartum and nonpostpartum subjects. J Clin Endocrinol Metab 1974; 38:413–423.

76. Johnston JM, Amico JA. A prospective longitudinal study of the release of oxytocin and prolactin in response to infant suckling in long term lactation. J Clin Endocrinol Metab 1986; 62:653–657.

77. Tyson JE, Friesen HG, Anderson MS. Human lactational and ovarian response to endogenous prolactin release. Science 1972; 177:897–900.

78. Gautvik KM, Weintraub BD, Graeber CT, et al. Serum prolactin and TSH: effects of nursing and pyroGlu-His-ProNH$_2$ administration in postpartum women. J Clin Endocrinol Metab 1973; 37:135–139.

79. Weitzman RE, Firemark HM, Glatz TH, et al. Thyrotropin-releasing hormone stimulates release of arginine-vasopressin and oxytocin in vivo. Endocrinology 1979; 104:904–907.

80. Kolodny RC, Jacobs LS, Daughaday WH. Mammary stimulation causes prolactin secretion in non-lactating women. Nature 1972; 238:284–286.

81. Richardson GS. Reflex lactation (thoracotomy) and reflex ovulation (intercostal block): case report, review of the literature, and discussion of mechanisms. Obstet Gynecol Surv 1970; 25:1021–1036.

82. Auerbach KG, Avery JL. Induced lactation. Am J Dis Child 1981; 135:340–343.

83. Thearle MJ, Weissenberger R. Induced lactation in adoptive mothers. Aust NZ J Obstet Gynaecol 1984; 24:283–286.

84. Vorherr H. Lactation and reproductive function. In: The Breast. New York: Academic, 1974: 184–197.

85. Wong S, Stepp-Gilbert E. Lactation suppression. Nonpharmaceutical versus pharmaceutical method. J Obstet Gynecol Neonatal Nurs 1985; 14:302–310.

86. Vance ML, Evans WS, Thorner MO. Bromocriptine. Ann Intern Med 1984; 100:78–91.

87. Duchesne C, Leke R. Bromocriptine mesylate for prevention of postpartum lactation. Obstet Gynecol 1981; 57:464–467.

88. Sheehan HL. Atypical hypopituitarism. Proc R Soc Med 1961; 54:43–48.

89. Sheehan HL, Davis JC. Pituitary necrosis. Br Med Bull 1968; 24:59–70.

90. Cosman F, Post KD, Holub DA, et al. Lymphocytic hypophysitis. Report of 3 new cases and review of the literature. Medicine 1989; 68:240–256.

91. Kauppila A, Chatelain P, Kirkinen P, et al. Isolated prolactin deficiency in a woman with puerperal alactogenesis. J Clin Endocrinol Metab 1987; 64:309–312.

92. Ehrenkranz RA, Ackerman BA. Metoclopramide effect on faltering milk production by mothers of premature infants. Pediatrics 1986; 78:614–620.

93. Madhavapeddi R, Ramachandran P. Side effects of oral contraceptive use in lactating women—enlargement of breast in a breast-fed child. Contraception 1985; 32:437–443.

94. Rimsten A, Skoog B, Stenkvist B. On the significance of nipple discharge in the diagnosis of breast disease. Acta Chir Scand 1976; 142:513–518.

95. Urban JA, Egeli RA. Non-lactational nipple discharge. CA 1978; 28:130–140.

96. Murad TM, Contesso G, Mouriesse H. Nipple discharge from the breast. Ann Surg 1982; 195:259–264.

97. Leis HP Jr, Greene FL, Cammarata A, et al. Nipple discharge: surgical significance. South Med J 1988; 81:20–26.

98. Kleinberg DL, Noel GL, Frantz AG. Galactorrhea: a study of 235 cases, including 48 with pituitary tumors. N Engl J Med 1977; 296:589–600.

99. Tolis G, Somma M, Van Campenhout J, et al. Prolactin secretion in 65 patients with galactorrhea. Am J Obstet Gynecol 1974; 118:91–101.

100. Boyd AE III, Reichlin S, Tuskoy RN. Galactorrhea-amenorrhea syndrome: diagnosis and therapy. Ann Intern Med 1977; 87:165–175.

101. Gomez F, Reyes FI, Faiman C. Nonpuerperal galactorrhea and hyperprolactinemia: clinical findings, endocrine features, and therapeutic responses in 56 cases. Am J Med 1977; 62:648–660.

102. Evans WS, Thorner MO. Mechanisms for hypogonadism in hyperprolactinemia. Semin Reprod Endocrinol 1984; 2:9–22.

103. McNeilly AS. Prolactin and the control of gonadotrophin secretion. J Endocrinol 1987; 115:1–5.

104. Van Wyk JJ, Grumbach MM. Syndrome of precocious menstruation and galactorrhea in juvenile hypothyroidism: an example of hormonal overlap in pituitary feedback. J Pediatr 1960; 57:416–435.

105. Edwards CRW, Forsyth IA, Besser GM. Amenorrhoea, galactorrhoea, and primary hypothyroidism with high circulating levels of prolactin. Br Med J 1971; 3:462–464.

106. Bigos ST, Ridgway EC, Kourides IA, et al. Spectrum of pituitary alterations with mild and severe thyroid impairment. J Clin Endocrinol Metab 1978; 46:317–325.

107. Honbo KS, Van Herle AJ, Kellett KA. Serum prolactin levels in untreated primary hypothyroidism. Am J Med 1978; 64:782–787.

108. Grubb MR, Chakeres D, Malarkey WB. Patients with primary hypothyroidism presenting as prolactinomas. Am J Med 1987; 83:765–769.

109. Malarkey WB, Beck P. 24-hour prolactin profiles in normal and disease states: failure of thyroxine to modify prolactin secretion. J Clin Endocrinol Metab 1975; 40:708–712.

110. Kapcala LP. Galactorrhea and thyrotoxicosis. Arch Intern Med 1984; 144:2349–2350.

111. Gluskin LE, Strasberg B, Shah JH. Verapamil-induced hyperprolactinemia and galactorrhea. Ann Intern Med 1981; 95:66–67.

112. Ehrinpreis MN, Dhar R, Narula A. Cimetidine-induced galactorrhea. Am J Gatroenterol 1989; 84:563–565.

113. Mendelson JH, Mello NK, Teoh SK, et al. Cocaine effects on pulsatile secretion of anterior pituitary, gonadal, and adrenal hormones. J Clin Endocrinol Metab 1989; 69:1256–1260.

114. Noel GL, Suh HK, Stone G, et al. Human prolactin and growth hormone release during surgery and other conditions of stress. J Clin Endocrinol Metab 1972; 35:840–851.

115. MacFarlane IA, Rosin MD. Galactorrhoea following surgical procedures to the chest wall: the role of prolactin. Postgrad Med J 1980; 56:23–25.

116. Lim VS, Kathpalia SC, Frohman LA. Hyperprolactinemia and impaired pituitary response to suppression and stimulation in chronic renal failure: reversal after transplantation. J Clin Endocrinol Metab 1979; 48:101–107.

117. Van Thiel DH, McClain CJ, Elson MK, et al. Evidence for autonomous secretion of prolactin in some alcoholic men with cirrhosis and gynecomastia. Metabolism 1978; 27:1778–1784.

118. Rohn RD. Benign galactorrhea/breast discharge in adolescent males probably due to breast self-manipulation. J Adolescent Health Care 1984; 5:210–212.

119. Frantz AG. Endocrine diagnosis of prolactin secreting pituitary tumors. In: Black PM, Zervas NT, Ridgway EC, et al., eds. Secretory Tumors of the Pituitary Gland. New York: Raven, 1984: 45–52.

120. Burrow GN, Wortzman G, Rewcastle NB, et al. Microadenomas of the pituitary and abnormal sellar tomograms in an unselected autopsy series. N Engl J Med 1981; 304:156–158.

121. Klibanski A, Neer RM, Beitins IZ, et al. Decreased bone density in hyperprolactinemic women. N Engl J Med 1980; 303:1511–1514.

122. Schlechte JA, Sherman B, Martin R. Bone density in amenorrheic women with and without hyperprolactinemia. J Clin Endocrinol Metab 1983; 56:1120–1123.

123. Koppelman MCS, Kurtz DW, Morrish KA, et al. Vertebral body bone mineral content in hyperprolactinemic women. J Clin Endocrinol Metab 1984; 59:1050–1053.

124. Schlechte J, El-Khoury G, Kathol M, et al. Forearm and vertebral bone mineral in treated and untreated hyperprolactinemic amenorrhea. J Clin Endocrinol Metab 1987; 64:1021–1026.

125. Klibanski A, Greenspan SL. Increase in bone mass after treatment of hyperprolactinemic amenorrhea. N Engl J Med 1986; 315:542–546.

126. Schlechte J, Dolan K, Sherman B, et al. The natural history of untreated hyperprolactinemia: a prospective analysis. J Clin Endocrinol Metab 1989; 68:412–418.

127. Koppelman MCS, Jaffe MJ, Rieth KG, et al. Hyperprolactinemia, amenorrhea, and galactorrhea. A retrospective assessment of 25 cases. Ann Intern Med 1984; 100:115–121.

128. Sisam DA, Sheehan JP, Sheeler LR. The natural history of untreated microadenomas. Fertil Steril 1987; 48:67–71.

129. Zervas NT. Surgical results for pituitary adenomas: results of an international survey. In: Black PM, Zervas NT, Ridgway EC, et al., eds. Secretory Tumors of the Pituitary Gland. New York: Raven, 1984: 377–385.

130. Tucker HStG, Grubb SR, Wigand JP, et al. Galactorrhea-amenorrhea syndrome: follow-up of 45 patients after pituitary tumor removal. Ann Intern Med 1981; 94:302–307.

131. Faria MA Jr, Tindall GT. Transsphenoidal microsurgery for prolactin-secreting pituitary adenomas. Results in 100 women with the amenorrhea-galactorrhea syndrome. J Neurosurg 1982; 56:33–43.

132. Hardy J. Transsphenoidal microsurgery of prolactinomas. In: Black PM, Zervas NT, Ridgway EC, et al., eds. Secretory Tumors of the Pituitary Gland. New York: Raven, 1984: 73–81.

133. Laws ER Jr, Ebersold MJ, Piepgras DG, et al. The role of surgery in the management of prolactinoma. In: MacLeod PM, Thorner MO, Scapagnini U, eds. Prolactin: Basic and Clinical Correlates. New York: Springer-Verlag, 1985: 849–853.

134. Rodman EF, Molitch ME, Post KD, et al. Long-term follow-up of transsphenoidal selective adenomectomy for prolactinoma. JAMA 1984; 252:921–924.

135. Serri O, Rasio E, Beauregard H, et al. Recurrence of hyperprolactinemia after selective transsphenoidal adenomectomy in women with prolactinomas. N Engl J Med 1983; 309:280–283.

136. Parl FF, Cruz VE, Cobb CA, et al. Late recurrence of surgically removed prolactinomas. Cancer 1986; 57:2422–2426.

137. Schlechte JA, Sherman BM, Chapler FK, et al. Long term follow-up of women with surgically treated prolactin-secreting pituitary tumors. J Clin Endocrinol Metab 1986; 62:1296–1301.

138. Frantz AG, Cogen PH, Chang CH, et al. Long-term evaluation of the results of transsphenoidal surgery and radiotherapy in patients with prolactinoma. In: Crosignani PG, Rubin BL, eds. Endocrinology of Human Infertility: New Aspects. New York: Grune & Stratton, 1981: 161–170.

139. Johnston DG, Hall K, Kendall-Taylor P, et al. The long-term effects of megavoltage radiotherapy as sole or combined therapy for large prolactinomas: studies with high definition computerized tomography. Clin Endocrinol 1986; 24:675–685.

140. Mehta AE, Reyes FI, Faiman C. Primary radiotherapy of prolactinomas: eight- to 15-year follow-up. Am J Med 1987; 83:49–58.

141. Friesen HG, Tolis G. The use of bromocriptine in the galactorrhea-amenorrhea syndromes: the Canadian cooperative study. Clin Endocrinol 1977; 6(Suppl):91s–99s.

142. Gemzell C, Wang CF. Outcome of pregnancy in women with pituitary adenoma. Fertil Steril 1979; 31:363–372.

143. Molitch ME. Pregnancy and the hyperprolactinemic woman. N Engl J Med 1985; 312:1364–1370.

144. Kleinberg DL, Boyd AE III, Wardlaw S, et al. Pergolide for the treatment of pituitary tumors secreting prolactin or growth hormone. N Engl J Med 1983; 309:704–709.

145. Molitch ME, Elton RL, Blackwell RE, et al. Bromocriptine as primary therapy for prolactin-secreting macroadenomas: results of a prospective multicenter study. J Clin Endocrinol Metab 1985; 60:698–705.

146. Kupersmith MJ, Kleinberg D, Warren FA, et al. Growth of prolactinoma despite lowering of serum prolactin by bromocriptine. Neurosurgery 1989; 24:417–423.

147. Liuzzi A, Dalabonzana D, Oppizzi G, et al. Low doses of dopamine agonists in the long-term treatment of macroprolactinomas. N Engl J Med 1985; 313:656–659.

148. Johnston DG, Hall K, Kendall-Taylor P, et al. Effect of dopamine agonist withdrawal after long-term therapy in prolactinomas. Lancet 1984; 2:187–192.

149. Moriondo P, Travaglini P, Nissim M, et al. Bromocriptine treatment of microprolactinomas: evidence of stable prolactin decrease after drug withdrawal. J Clin Endocrinol Metab 1985; 60:762–772.

150. Montini M, Pagani G, Gianola D, et al. Long-lasting suppression of prolactin secretion and rapid shrinkage of prolactinomas after a long-acting, injectable form of bromocriptine. J Clin Endocrinol Metab 1986; 63:266–268.

151. Grossman A, Ross R, Wass JAH, et al. Depot-bromocriptine treatment for prolactinomas and acromegaly. Clin Endocrinol 1986; 24:231–238.

152. Benker G, Gieshoff B, Freundlieb O, et al. Parenteral bromocriptine in the treatment of hormonally active pituitary tumours. Clin Endocrinol 1986; 24:505–513.

153. Murphy FY, Vesely DL, Jordan RM, et al. Giant invasive prolactinomas. Am J Med 1987; 83:995–1002.

154. Fahlbusch R, Buchfelder M, Schrell U. Short-term preoperative treatment of macroprolactinomas by dopamine agonists. J Neurosurg 1987; 67:807–815.

155. Juri J. Mammary asymmetry: a brief classification. Aesthetic Plast Surg 1989; 13:47–53.

156. Rosenberg CA, Derman GH, Grabb WC, et al. Hypomastia and mitral-valve prolapse: evidence of a linked embryologic and mesenchymal dysplasia. N Engl J Med 1983; 309:1230–1232.

157. Pierre ML, Jouglard J-P. Treatment of unilateral congenital hypoplasia or absence of the breast. Plast Reconstr Surg 1975; 56:146–151.

158. Mayl N, Vasconez LO, Jurkiewica MJ. Treatment of macromastia in the actively enlarging breast. Plast Reconstr Surg 1974; 54:6–12.

159. Strombeck JO. Types of macromastia. Acta Chir Scand Suppl 1964; 341:37–39.

160. Fisher W, Smith JW. Macromastia during puberty. Plast Reconstr Surg 1971; 47:445–451.

161. Hollingsworth DR, Archer R. Massive virginal breast hypertrophy at puberty. Am J Dis Child 1973; 125:293–295.

162. Sperling RL, Gold JJ. Use of an anti-estrogen after a reduction mammaplasty to prevent recurrence of virginal hypertrophy of breasts. Plast Reconstr Surg 1973; 52:439–442.

163. de Castro CC. Subcutaneous mastectomy for gigantomastia in an adolescent girl. Plast Reconstr Surg 1977; 59:575–578.

164. Burslem RW, Dewhurst CJ. Massive hypertrophy of the breasts in pregnancy. J Obstet Gynaecol Br Emp 1952; 59:380–381.

165. Williams PC. Massive hypertrophy of the breasts and axillary breasts in successive pregnancies. Am J Obstet Gynecol 1957; 74:1326–1329.

166. Blaydes RM, Kinnebrew CA. Massive breast hyperplasia complicating pregnancy. Obstet Gynecol 1958; 12:601–602.

167. Lewison EF, Jones GS, Trimble FH, et al. Gigantomastia complicating pregnancy. Surg Gynecol Obstet 1960; 110:215–223.

168. Nolan JJ. Gigantomastia. Obstet Gynecol 1962; 19:526–529.

169. Greeley PW, Robertson LE, Curtin JW. Mastoplasty for massive bilateral benign breast hypertrophy associated with pregnancy. Ann Surg 1965; 162:1081–1083.

170. Miller CJ, Becker DW Jr. Management of first trimester breast enlargement with necrosis. Plast Reconstr Surg 1979; 63:383–386.

171. Lafreniere R, Temple W, Ketcham A. Gestational macromastia. Am J Surg 1984; 148:413–418.

172. Ryan RF, Pernoll ML. Virginal hypertrophy. Plast Reconstr Surg 1985; 75:737–742.

173. Desai SN. Sudden gigantism of breasts: drug induced? Br J Plast Surg 1973; 26:371–372.

174. Passas C, Weinstein A. Breast gigantism with penicillamine therapy. Arthritis Rheum 1978; 21:167–168.

175. Thew DCN, Stewart IM. D-Penicillamine and breast enlargement. Ann Rheum Dis 1980; 39:200.

176. Taylor PJ, Cumming DC, Corenblum B. Successful treatment of D-penicillamine-induced breast gigantism with danazol. Br Med J 1981; 282:362–363.

177. Rooney PJ, Cleland J. Successful treatment of D-penicillamine-induced breast gigantism with danazol. Br Med J 1981; 282:1627–1628.

178. Finer N, Emery P, Hicks BH. Mammary gigantism and D-penicillamine. Clin Endocrinol 1984; 21:219–222.

179. Versaci AD. Reduction mammaplasty for moderate macromastia. Ann Plast Surg 1981; 6:253–260.

180. Ariyan S. Reduction mammaplasty with the nipple-areola carried on a single, narrow inferior pedicle. Ann Plast Surg 1980; 5:167–177.

181. Boyce SW, Hoffman PG Jr, Mathes SJ. Recurrent macromastia after subcutaneous mastectomy. Ann Plast Surg 1984; 13:511–518.

182. Preece PE, Mansel RE, Bolton PM, et al. Clinical syndromes of mastalgia. Lancet 1976; 2:670–673.

183. Dowle CS. Breast pain: classification, aetiology and management. Aust NZ J Surg 1987; 57:423–428.

184. Pye JK, Mansel RE, Hughes LE. Clinical experience of drug treatments for mastalgia. Lancet 1985; 2:373–377.

185. Hinton CP, Bishop HM, Holliday HW, et al. A double-blind controlled trial of danazol and bromocriptine in the management of severe cyclical breast pain. Br J Clin Pract 1986; 40:326–330.

186. Mansel RE, Wisbey JR, Hughes LE. Controlled trial of the antigonadotropin danazol in painful nodular benign breast disease. Lancet 1982; 1:928–930.

187. Fentiman IS, Caleffi M, Hamed H, et al. Dosage and duration of tamoxifen treatment for mastalgia; a controlled trial. Br J Surg 1988; 75:845–846.

188. Williams MJ. Gynecomastia: its incidence, recognition and host characterization in 447 autopsy cases. Am J Med 1963; 34:103–112.

189. Nuttall FQ. Gynecomastia as a physical finding in normal men. J Clin Endocrinol Metab 1979; 48:338–340.

190. Niewoehner CB, Nuttall FQ. Gynecomastia in a hospitalized male population. Am J Med 1984; 77:633–638.

191. Ley SB, Mozaffarian GA, Leonard JM, et al. Palpable breast tissue versus gynecomastia as a normal physical finding. Clin Res 1980; 28:24A.

192. Burke CW. Gynaecomastia. Practitioner 1982; 226:1403–1410.

193. Friedman PJ. Gynecomastia in a hospitalized male population. Am J Med 1985; 78:A40–A43.

194. Andersen JA, Gram JB. Male breast at autopsy. Acta Pathol Microbiol Immunol Scand A 1982; 90:191–197.

195. Sandison AT. An autopsy study of the adult human breast. Natl Cancer Inst Monogr 1962; 8:77–80.

196. Kapdi CC, Parekh NJ. The male breast. Radiol Clin North Am 1983; 21:137–148.

197. Dershaw DD. Male mammography. AJR 1986; 146:127–131.

198. Wigley KD, Thomas JL, Bernardino ME, et al. Sonography of gynecomastia. AJR 1981; 136:927–930.

199. Jackson VP, Gilmore RL. Male breast carcinoma and gynecomastia: comparison of mammography with sonography. Radiology 1986; 149:533–536.

200. Nicolis GL, Modlinger RS, Gabrilove JL. A study of the histopathology of human gynecomastia. J Clin Endocrinol Metab 1971; 32:173–178.

201. Bannayan GA, Hajdu SI. Gynecomastia: clinicopathologic study of 351 cases. Am J Clin Pathol 1972; 57:431–437.

202. Anderson JA, Gram JB. Gynecomasty: histological aspects in a surgical material. Acta Pathol Microbiol Immunol Scand A 1982; 90:185–190.

203. Lewin ML. Gynecomastia: the hypertrophy of the male breast. J Clin Endocrinol Metab 1941; 1:511–514.

204. Gabrilove JL. Some recent advances in virilizing and feminizing syndromes and hirsutism. Mt Sinai J Med 1974; 41:636–654.

205. Wilson JD, Aiman J, MacDonald PC. The pathogenesis of gynecomastia. Adv Intern Med 1980; 25:1–32.

206. Bercovici JP, Maudelonde T. Physiologie et physiopathologie du développement mammaire chez l'homme. Ann Endocrinol 1982; 43:221–245.

207. von Werder K. Diagnostisches vorgehen bei Gynakomastie. Dtsch Med Wochenschr 1988; 113:776–778.

208. Carlson JE. Gynecomastia. N Engl J Med 1980; 303:795–799.

209. Wilson JD. Metabolism of testicular androgens. In: Greep RO, Astwood EB, eds. Handbook of Physiology. Sect. 7: Endocrinology. Vol V. Male Reproductive System. Washington, DC: American Physiological Society, 1975: 491–508.

210. Siiteri PK, MacDonald PC. Role of extraglandular estrogen in human endocrinology. In: Greep RO, Astwood EB, eds. Handbook of Physiology. Sect. 7: Endocrinology. Vol II. Female Reproductive System. Part 1. Washington, DC: American Physiological Society, 1975: 615–629.

211. Kelch RP, Jenner MR, Weinstein R, et al. Estradiol and testosterone secretion by human, simian and canine testes in males with hypogonadism and in male pseudohermaphrodites with the feminizing testis syndrome. J Clin Invest 1972; 51:824–830.

212. Weinstein RL, Kelch RP, Jenner MR, et al. Secretion of unconjugated androgens and estrogens by the normal and abnormal human testis before and after human chorionic gonadotropin. J Clin Invest 1974; 53:1–6.

213. Payne AH, Kelch RP, Musich SS, Halpern ME. Intratesticular site of aromatization in the human. J Clin Endocrinol Metab 1976; 42:1081–1087.

214. Rajendran KG, Shah PN, Bagli NP, et al. Oestradiol receptors in non-neoplastic gynaecomastic tissue of phenotypic males. Horm Res 1976; 7:193–200.

215. Poulsen HS, Hermansen C, Andersen A, et al. Gynecomasty: estrogen and androgen receptors. A clinical-pathological investigation. Acta Pathol Microbiol Immunol Scand A 1985; 93:229–233.

216. Pacheco MM, Oshima CF, Lopes MP, et al. Steroid hormone receptors in male breast diseases. Anticancer Res 1986; 6:1013–1018.

217. Andersen J, Orntoft TF, Andersen JA, et al. Gynecomastia. Immunohistochemical demonstration of estrogen receptors. Acta Pathol Microbiol Immunol Scand A 1987; 95:263–267.

218. McKiernan JF, Hudd D. Breast development in the newborn. Arch Dis Child 1981; 56:525–529.

219. Nydick M, Bustos J, Dale JD Jr, et al. Gynecomastia in adolescent boys. JAMA 1961; 178:449–454.

220. Harlan WR, Grillo GP, Cornoni-Huntley J, et al. Secondary sex characteristics of boys 12 to 17 years of age: the U.S. health examination survey. J Pediatr 1979; 95:293–297.

221. Marynick SP, Nisula BC, Pita JC Jr, et al. Persistent pubertal macromastia. J Clin Endocrinol Metab 1980; 50:128–130.

222. Bidlingmaier F, Knorr D. Plasma testosterone and estrogens in pubertal gynecomastia. Z Kinderheilkd 1973; 115:89–94.

223. Lee PA. The relationship of concentrations of serum hormones to pubertal gynecomastia. J Pediatr 1975; 86:212–215.

224. LaFranchi SH, Parlow AF, Lippe BM, et al. Pubertal gynecomastia and transient elevation of serum estradiol level. Am J Dis Child 1975; 129:927–931.

225. Eversmann T, Moito J, von Werder K. Testosteron- und Ostradiolspiegel bei der Gynäkomastie des Mannes. Klinische und endokrine Befunde bei Behandlung mit Tamoxifen. Dtsch Med Wochenschr 1984; 109:1678–1682.

226. Moore DC, Schlaepfer LV, Paunier L, et al. Hormonal changes during puberty: V. Transient pubertal gynecomastia: abnormal androgen-estrogen ratios. J Clin Endocrinol Metab 1984; 58:492–499.

227. Bulard J, Mowszkowicz I, Schaison G. Increased aromatase activity in pubic skin fibroblasts from patients with isolated gynecomastia. J Clin Endocrinol Metab 1987; 64:618–623.

228. Eversmann T, Buchner A, Bock L, et al. Diagnosis and medical treatment of gynecomastia in different endocrine and metabolic diseases. Acta Endocrinol 1983; 102:139–140.

229. Kirschner MA, Jacobs JB, Fraley EE. Bilateral anorchia with persistent testosterone production. N Engl J Med 1970; 289:240–244.

230. Edman CD, Winters AJ, Porter JC, et al. Embryonic testicular regression. A clinical spectrum of XY agonadal individuals. Obstet Gynecol 1977; 49:209–217.

231. Casey RW, Wilson JD. Antiestrogenic action of dihydrotestosterone in mouse breast. Competition with estradiol for binding to the estrogen receptor. J Clin Invest 1984; 74:2272–2278.

232. Gordon DL, Krompotic E, Thomas W, et al. Pathological testicular findings in Klinefelter's syndrome: 47,XXY vs 46,XY/47,XXY. Arch Intern Med 1972; 130:726–729.

233. Paulsen CA, Gordon DL, Carpenter RW, et al. Klinefelter's syndrome and its variants: a hormonal and chromosomal study. Recent Prog Horm Res 1968; 24:321–363.

234. Becker KL, Hoffman DL, Albert A, et al. Klinefelter's syndrome: clinical and laboratory findings in 50 patients. Arch Intern Med 1966; 118:314–321.

235. Wang C, Baker HWG, Burger HG, et al. Hormonal studies in Klinefelter's syndrome. Clin Endocrinol 1975; 4:399–411.

236. Aiman J, Hemsell DL, Brenner PF, et al. Origin of estrogen in adolescents with Klinefelter syndrome and gynecomastia. J Androl 1981; 2:6.

237. Gabrilove JL, Freiberg EK, Thornton JC, et al. Effect of age on testicular function in patients with Klinefelter's syndrome. Clin Endocrinol 1979; 11:343–347.

238. Gabrilove JL, Freiberg EK, Nicolis GL. Testicular function in Klinefelter's syndrome. J Urol 1980; 124:825–826.

239. Salbenblatt JA, Bender BG, Puck MH, et al. Pituitary-gonadal function in Klinefelter syndrome before and during puberty. Pediatr Res 1985; 19:82–86.

240. Griffin JE, Wilson JD. The androgen resistance syndromes: 5α-reductase deficiency, testicular feminization, and related disorders. In: Scriver CR, Beaudet AL, Sly WS, et al., eds. Metabolic Basis of Inherited Disease. 6th ed. New York: McGraw-Hill, 1989: 1919–1944.

241. MacDonald PC, Madden JD, Brenner PF, et al. Origin of estrogen in normal men and in women with testicular feminization. J Clin Endocrinol Metab 1979; 49:905–916.

242. Wilson JD, Harrod MJ, Goldstein JL, et al. Familial incomplete male pseudohermaphroditism, type I: evidence for androgen resistance and variable clinical manifestations in a family with the Reifenstein syndrome. N Engl J Med 1974; 290:1097–1103.

243. Madden JD, Walsh PC, MacDonald PC, et al. Clinical and endocrinologic characterization of a patient with the syndrome of incomplete testicular feminization. J Clin Endocrinol Metab 1975; 40:751–760.

244. Martin F, Perheentupa J, Adlercreutz H. Plasma and urinary androgens and oestrogens in a pubertal boy with 3β-hydroxysteroid dehydrogenase deficiency. J Steroid Biochem 1980; 13:197–201.

245. Imperato-McGinley J, Peterson RE, Stoller R, et al. Male pseudohermaphroditism secondary to 17β-hydroxysteroid dehydrogenase deficiency: gender role change with puberty. J Clin Endocrinol Metab 1979; 49:391–395.

246. Rogers DG, Chasalow FI, Blethen SL. Partial deficiency in 17-ketosteroid reductase presenting as gynecomastia. Steroids 1985; 45:195–200.

247. Werner CA. Mumps orchitis and testicular atrophy: I. Occurrence. Ann Intern Med 1950; 32:1066–1074.

248. Riggs S, Sanford JP. Viral orchitis. N Engl J Med 1962; 266:990–993.

249. Werner CA. Mumps orchitis and testicular atrophy: II. A factor in male sterility. Ann Intern Med 1950; 32:1075–1086.

250. Petersdorf RF, Bennett IL Jr. Treatment of mumps orchitis with adrenal hormones: report of twenty-three cases with a note on hepatic involvement in mumps. Arch Intern Med 1957; 99:222–233.

251. Aiman J, Brenner PF, MacDonald PC. Androgen and estrogen production in elderly men with gynecomastia and testicular atrophy after mumps orchitis. J Clin Endocrinol Metab 1980; 50:380–386.

252. Clarke BG, Shapiro S, Monroe RG. Myotonia atrophia with testicular atrophy. J Clin Endocrinol 1956; 16:1235–1244.

253. Cooper IS, Ryanson EA, Bailey AA, et al. The relation of spinal cord disease to gynecomastia and testicular atrophy. Staff Proc Mayo Clin 1950; 25:320–326.

254. Morely JE, Distiller LA, Sagel J, et al. Hormonal changes associated with testicular atrophy and gynaecomastia in patients with leprosy. Clin Endocrinol 1977; 6:299–303.

255. Rolston R, Mathews M, Taylor PM, et al. Hormone profile in lepromatous leprosy: a preliminary study. Int J Lepr 1981; 49:31–36.

256. Kannan V, Vijaya G. Endocrine testicular functions in leprosy. Horm Metab Res 1984; 16:146–150.

257. Nagel TC, Freinkel N, Bell RH, et al. Gynecomastia, prolactin, and other peptide hormones in patients undergoing chronic hemodialysis. J Clin Endocrinol Metab 1973; 36:428–432.

258. Sawin CT, Longcope C, Schmitt GW, et al. Blood levels of gonadotropins and gonadal hormones in gynecomastia associated with chronic hemodialysis. J Clin Endocrinol Metab 1973; 36:988–990.

259. Holdsworth S, Atkins RC, de Kretser DM. The pituitary testicular axis in men with chronic renal failure. N Engl J Med 1977; 296:1245–1249.

260. Schmitt GW, Shehadeh I, Sawin CT. Transient gynecomastia in chronic renal failure during chronic intermittent hemodialysis. Ann Intern Med 1968; 69:73–79.

261. Gupta D, Burdschu HD. Testosterone and its binding in the plasma of male subjects with chronic renal failure. Clin Chim Acta 1972; 36:479–484.

262. Maywood BT, Krumlowsky F, Hugh NE. Gynecomastia in the chronic renal dialysis patient: beware. Plast Reconstr Surg 1982; 69:41–44.

263. Vircburger MI, Prelevic GM, Peric LA, et al. Testosterone levels after bromocriptine treatment in patients undergoing long-term hemodialysis. J Androl 1985; 6:113–116.

264. Cochran JS, Walsh PC, Porter JC, et al. The endocrinology of human chorionic gonadotropin-secreting testicular tumors: new methods in diagnosis. J Urol 1975; 114:549–555.

265. Gabrilove JL, Nicholis GL, Mitty HA, et al. Feminizing interstitial cell tumor of the testis: personal observations and a review of the literature. Cancer 1975; 38:1184–1202.

266. Gabrilove JL, Freiberg EK, Leiter E, et al. Feminizing and non-feminizing Sertoli cell tumors. J Urol 1980; 123:757–767.

267. Perez C, Novoa J, Alcaniz J, et al. Leydig cell tumour of the testis with gynaecomastia and elevated oestrogen, progesterone and prolactin levels: case report. Clin Endocrinol 1980; 13:409–412.

268. Bercovici JP, Nahoul K, Tate D, et al. Hormonal profile of Leydig cell tumors with gynecomastia. J Clin Endocrinol Metab 1984; 59:625–630.

269. Siegel SW, Thomas AJ Jr. Gynecomastia and Leydig cell tumors in the adult. Cleve Clin Q 1984; 51:395–399.

270. Mineur P, de Cooman S, Hustin J, et al. Feminizing testicular Leydig cell tumor: hormonal profile before and after unilateral orchidectomy. J Clin Endocrinol Metab 1987; 64:686–691.

271. Hendry WS, Garvie WHH, Ah-See AK, et al. Ultrasonic detection of occult testicular neoplasms in patients with gynaecomastia. Br J Radiol 1984; 57:571–572.

272. Mellor SG, McCutchan JDS. Gynaecomastia and occult Leydig cell tumour of the testis. Br J Urol 1989; 63:420–422.

273. Kuhn JM, Mahoudeau JA, Billaud L, et al. Evaluation of diagnostic criteria for Leydig cell tumours in adult men revealed by gynaecomastia. Clin Endocrinol 1987; 26:407–416.

274. MacDonald PC, Siiteri PK. The in vivo mechanisms of origin of estrogen in subjects with trophoblastic tumors. Steroids 1966; 8:589–603.

275. Whitcomb RW, Schimke RN, Kyner JL, et al. Endocrine studies in a male patient with choriocarcinoma and gynecomastia. Am J Med 1986; 81:917–920.

276. Charles MA, Claypool R, Schaaf M, et al. Lung carcinoma associated with production of three placental proteins. Arch Intern Med 1973; 132:427–431.

277. Fairlamb D, Boesen E. Gynaecomastia associated with gonadotrophin-secreting carcinoma of the lung. Postgrad Med J 1977; 53:269–271.

278. Wurzel RS, Yamase HT, Nieh PT. Ectopic production of human chorionic gonadotropin by poorly differentiated transitional cell tumors of the urinary tract. J Urol 1987; 137:502–504.

279. Aiman J, Hemsell DL, MacDonald PC. Production and origin of estrogen in two true hermaphrodites. Am J Obstet Gynecol 1978; 132:401–409.

280. Bacon GE, Lowrey GH. Feminizing adrenal tumor in a six year old boy. J Clin Endocrinol 1965; 25:1403–1406.

281. Gabrilove JL, Nicolis GL, Hardsknecht RU, et al. Feminizing adrenocortical carcinoma in a man. Cancer 1970; 25:153–160.

282. Bhettay E, Bonnici F. Pure oestrogen-secreting feminizing adrenocortical adenoma. Arch Dis Child 1977; 52:241–243.

283. Gabrilove JL, Sharma DC, Wotiz HH, et al. Feminizing adrenocortical tumors in the male. Medicine 1965; 44:37–79.

284. Howard CP, Takahashi H, Hayles AB. Feminizing adrenal adenoma in a boy. Mayo Clin Proc 1977; 52:354–357.

285. Desai MB, Kapadia SN. Feminizing adrenocortical tumors in male patients: adenoma versus carcinoma. J Urol 1988; 139:101–103.

286. Maclaren NK, Migeon CJ, Raiti S. Gynecomastia with congenital virilizing adrenal hyperplasia (11-β-hydroxylase deficiency). J Pediatr 1975; 86:579–581.

287. Kadair RG, Block MB, Katz FH, et al. "Masked" 21-hydroxylase deficiency of the adrenal presenting with gynecomastia and bilateral testicular masses. Am J Med 1977; 62:278–282.

288. Gabrilove JL, Nicolis GL, Sohval AR. Non-tumorous feminizing adrenogenital syndrome in the male subject. J Urol 1973; 110:710–713.

289. Boyar RM, Hellman L. Syndrome of benign nodular adrenal hyperplasia associated with feminization and hyperprolactinemia. Ann Intern Med 1974; 80:389–394.

290. Durand A, Roger M, Chaussain JL, et al. L'hyperplasie congénitale virilisante des surrénales par déficit en 11 beta-hydroxylase. Semin Hop Paris 1981; 57:1392–1397.

291. Frank-Raue K, Raue F, Korth-Schutz S, et al. Clinical features and diagnosis of mild 3-beta-hydroxysteroid dehydrogenase deficiency in men. Dtsch Med Wochenschr 1989; 114:331–334.

292. Gordon GG, Olivo J, Rafii F, et al. Conversion of androgens to estrogens in cirrhosis of the liver. J Clin Endocrinol Metab 1975; 40:1018–1026.

293. Edman DC, Hemsell DL, Brenner PF, et al. Extraglandular estrogen formation in subjects with cirrhosis. Gastroenterology 1975; 69:819.

294. Bahnsen M, Gluud C, Johnsen SG, et al. Pituitary-testicular function in patients with alcoholic cirrhosis of the liver. Eur J Clin Invest 1981; 11:473–479.

295. Olivo J, Gordon GG, Rafii F, et al. Estrogen metabolism in hyperthyroidism and in cirrhosis of the liver. Steroids 1975; 26:47–56.

296. Copenhagen Study Group for Liver Diseases. Testosterone treatment of men with alcoholic cirrhosis: a double-blind study. Hepatology 1986; 6:807–813.

297. Kew MC, Kirschner MA, Abrahams GE, et al. Mechanism of feminization in primary liver cancer. N Engl J Med 1977; 296:1084–1088.

298. Aabo K, Dimitro NV. Feminization in hepatocellular carcinoma corrected by chemotherapy: a case report. Med Pediatr Oncol 1980; 8:275–280.

299. Klatskin G, Saltin WT, Humm FD. Gynecomastia due to malnutrition. Am J Med Sci 1947; 213:19–30.

300. Zurbiran S, Gomez-Mont F. Endocrine disturbances in chronic human malnutrition. Vitam Horm 1953; 11:97–132.

301. Ashkar FW, Smoak WM, Gilson AJ, et al. Gynecomastia and mastoplasia in Graves' disease. Metabolism 1970; 19:946–951.

302. Becker KL, Winnacker JL, Matthews MJ, et al. Gynecomastia and hyperthyroidism: an endocrine and histological investigation. J Clin Endocrinol 1968; 28:227–285.

303. Becker KL, Matthews MJ, Higgins GA Jr, et al. Histologic evidence of gynecomastia in hyperthyroidism. Arch Pathol 1974; 98:257–260.

304. Chopra IJ, Tulchinsky D. States of estrogen-androgen balance in hyperthyroid men with Graves' disease. J Clin Endocrinol Metab 1974; 38:269–277.

305. Chopra IJ. Gonadal steroids and gonadotropins in hyperthyroidism. Med Clin North Am 1975; 59:1109–1121.

306. Bercovici JP, Mauvais-Jarvis P. Hyperthyroidism and gynecomastia: metabolic studies. J Clin Endocrinol Metab 1972; 35:671–677.

307. Chopra IJ, Abraham GE, Chopra N, et al. Alterations in circulating estradiol-17 in male patients with Graves' disease. N Engl J Med 1972; 286:124–129.

308. Southren AL, Olivo J, Gordon GG, et al. The conversion of androgens to estrogens in hyperthyroidism. J Clin Endocrinol Metab 1974; 38:207–214.

309. Hemsell DL, Edman CD, Marks JF, et al. Massive extraglandular aromatization of plasma androstenedione resulting in feminization of a prepubertal boy. J Clin Invest 1977; 60:455–464.

310. Berkowitz GD, Gerami A, Brown TR, et al. Familial gynecomastia with increased extraglandular aromatization of plasma carbon 19-steroid. J Clin Invest 1985; 75:1763–1769.

311. Wilson JD, Leshin M, George FW. The Sebright bantam chicken and the genetic control of extraglandular aromatase. Endocr Rev 1987; 8:363–376.

312. Hendrickson DA, Anderson WR. Diethylstilbesterol therapy: gynecomastia. JAMA 1970; 213:468.

313. Orentreich N, Durr NP. Mammogenesis in transsexuals. J Invest Dermatol 1974; 63:142–146.

314. Brandt NJ, Cohn J, Hiller M. Controlled trial of oral contraceptives in haemophilia. Scand J Haematol 1973; 11:225–229.

315. Beas F, Vargas L, Spada RP, et al. Pseudoprecocious puberty in infants caused by a dermal ointment containing estrogens. J Pediatr 1969; 75:127–130.

316. Landolt R, Murset G. Premature signs of puberty as late sequelae of unintentional estrogen administration. Schweiz Med Wochenschr 1968; 98:638–641.

317. Edidin DV, Levitsky LL. Prepubertal gynecomastia associated with estrogen-containing hair cream. Am J Dis Child 1982; 136:587–588.

318. Gabrilove JL, Luria M. Persistent gynecomastia resulting from scalp inunction of estradiol. Arch Dermatol 1978; 117:1672–1673.

319. Cimorra FA, Gonzalez-Peirona E, Ferrandez A. Percutaneous oestrogen-induced gynaecomastia: a case report. Br J Plast Surg 1982; 35:209–210.

320. Halperin DK, Sizonenko PC. Prepubertal gynecomastia following topical inunction of estrogen containing ointment. Helv Paediatr Acta 1983; 38:361–366.

321. Gottswinter JM, Korth-Schutz S, Ziegler R. Gynecomastia caused by estrogen containing hair lotion. J Endocrinol Invest 1984; 7:383–386.

322. Schmidt KU, Wagner G, Mensing H. Ostrogen-induzierte gynakomastie nach anwendung ostrogenhaltiger lokaltherapeutika. Dtsch Med Wochenschr 1987; 112:926–928.

323. Harrington JM, Stein GF, Rivera RO, et al. The occupational hazards of formulating oral contraceptives—a survey of plant employees. Arch Environ Health 1978; 33:12–15.

324. Pacynski A, Budzynska A, Przylecki S. Hiperestrogenizm v pracownikow zakladow farmaceutyczach i ich dzieci jako choroba zawodowa. Endokrynol Pol 1971; 22:149–154.

325. DeRaimondo CV, Roach AC, Meador CK. Gynecomastia from exposure to vaginal estrogen cream. N Engl J Med 1980; 302:1089–1090.

326. Moore N, Paux G, Noblet C, et al. Spouse-related drug side-effects. Lancet 1988; 1:137.

327. Abramowicz M. Estrogens in cosmetics. Med Lett 1985; 27:54–55.

328. Kimball AM, Hamadeh R, Mahmood RAH, et al. Gynaecomastia among children in Bahrain. Lancet 1981; 1:671–672.

329. Fara GM, Del Vorvo G, Bernuzzi S, et al. Epidemic of breast enlargement in an Italian school. Lancet 1979; 2:295–297.

330. Sundlof SF, Strickland C. Zearalenone and zeranol: potential residue problems in livestock. Vet Hum Toxicol 1986; 28:242–250.

331. Henricks DM, Gray SL, Hoover JLB. Residue levels of endogenous estrogens in beef tissues. J Anim Sci 1983; 57:247–255.

332. Verdeal K, Ryan DS. Naturally-occurring estrogens in plant foodstuffs—a review. J Food Protect 1979; 42:577–583.

333. Katzenellenbogen BS, Katzenellenbogen JA, Fordecai D. Zearalenones: characterization of the estrogenic potencies and receptor interactions of a series of fungal β-resorcylic acid lactones. Endocrinology 1979; 105:33–40.

334. Powell-Jones W, Raeford S, Lucier GW. Binding properties of zearalenone mycotoxins to hepatic estrogen receptors. Mol Pharmacol 1981; 20:35–42.

335. LeWinn EB. Gynecomastia during digitalis therapy. N Engl J Med 1953; 248:316–320.

336. Wolfe CJ. Gynecomastia following digitalis administration. J Fla Med Assoc 1975; 62:54–55.

337. Navab A, Koss LG, LaDue JS. Estrogen-like activity of digitalis: its effect on the squamous epithelium of the female genital tract. JAMA 1965; 194:30–32.

338. Kley HK, Abendroth H, Hehrmann R, et al. Kein Einfluss von Digitalis auf Sexual- und Nebennierenrindenhormone bei gesunden Probanden und bein Patienten mit Herzinsuffizienz. Klin Wochenschr 1984; 62:65–73.

339. Rifka SM, Pita JC, Vigersky RA, et al. Interaction of digitalis and spironolactone with human sex steroid receptors. J Clin Endocrinol Metab 1977; 46:338–344.

340. Ricken K. The estrogenic potency of digitalis glycosides. Naunyn Schmiedebergs Arch Pharmacol 1975; 287(Suppl):25.

341. Maddock WO, Nelson WO. The effects of chorionic gonadotropin in adult men: increased estrogen and 17-ketosteroid excretion, gynecomastia, Leydig cell stimulation and seminiferous tubule damage. J Clin Endocrinol Metab 1952; 12:985–1014.

342. Lee PA. The occurrence of gynecomastia upon withdrawal of clomiphene citrate treatment for idiopathic oligospermia. Fertil Steril 1980; 34:285–286.

343. Feldman D. Ketoconazole and other imidazole derivatives as inhibitors of steroidogenesis. Endocr Rev 1986; 7:409–420.

344. Grosso DS, Boyden TW, Parmenter RW, et al. Ketoconazole inhibition of testicular secretion of testosterone and displacement of steroid hormones from serum transport proteins. Antimicrob Agents Chemother 1983; 23:207–212.

345. Fagan TC, Johnson DG, Grosso DS. Metronidazole-induced gynecomastia. JAMA 1985; 254:3217.

346. DeFelice R, Johnson DG, Galgiani JN. Gynecomastia with ketoconazole. Antimicrob Agents Chemother 1981; 19:1073–1074.

347. Pont A, Goldman ES, Sugar AM, et al. Ketoconazole-induced increase in estradiol-testosterone ratio. Arch Intern Med 1985; 145:1429–1431.

348. Whitehead E, Shalet SM, Blackledge G, et al. The effects of Hodgkin's disease and combination chemotherapy on gonadal function in the adult male. Cancer 1982; 49:418–422.

349. Trump DK, Pavy MD, Staal S. Gynecomastia in men following antineoplastic therapy. Arch Intern Med 1982; 142:511–513.

350. Turner AR, Morrish DW, Berry J, et al. Gynecomastia after cytotoxic therapy for metastatic testicular cancer. Arch Intern Med 1982; 142:896–897.

351. Saeter G, Fossa DK, Norman N. Gynaecomastia following cytotoxic therapy for testicular cancer. Br J Urol 1987; 59:348–352.

352. Jeunemaitre X, Chatellier G, Kreft-Jais C, et al. Efficacy and tolerance of spironolactone in essential hypertension. Am J Cardiol 1987; 60:820–825.

353. Loriaux DL, Menard R, Taylor A, et al. Spironolactone and endocrine dysfunction. Ann Intern Med 1976; 85:630–636.

354. Caminos-Torres R, Ma L, Snyder PJ. Gynecomastia and semen abnormalities induced by spironolactone in normal men. J Clin Endocrinol Metab 1977; 5:255–260.

355. Clark E. Spironolactone therapy and gynecomastia. JAMA 1965; 193:163–164.

356. De Gasparo M, Whitebread SE, Preiswerk G, et al. Antialdosterones: incidence and prevention of sexual side effects. J Steroid Biochem 1989; 32:223–227.

357. DuPont A. Disappearance of spironolactone-induced gynaecomastia during treatment with potassium canrenoate. Lancet 1985; 2:731.

358. Geller J, Vazakas G, Fruchtman B, et al. The effect of cyproterone acetate on advanced carcinoma of the prostate. Surg Gynecol Obstet 1968; 127:748–758.

359. Caine M, Perlberg S, Gordon R. The treatment of benign prostatic hypertrophy with flutamide (SCH 13521): a placebo controlled study. J Urol 1975; 114:564–568.

360. Hall WH. Breast changes in males on cimetidine. N Engl J Med 1976; 295:841.

361. Funder JW, Mercer JE. Cimetidine occupies androgen receptors. J Clin Endocrinol Metab 1979; 48:189–191.

362. Sultan C, Terraza A, Descomps B, et al. Cimetidine competition with androgens for binding to human sex skin fibroblast androgen receptors. J Steroid Biochem 1980; 13:839–840.

363. Spence RW, Celestin LR. Gynaecomastia associated with cimetidine. Gut 1979; 20:154–157.

364. Jensen RT, Collen MJ, Pandol SJ, et al. Cimetidine-induced impotence and breast changes in patients with gastric hypersecretory states. N Engl J Med 1983; 308:883–887.

365. Galbraith RA, Michnovicz JJ. The effects of cimetidine on the oxidative metabolism of estradiol. N Engl J Med 1989; 321:269–274.

366. Mignon M, Vallor TH, Mayeur S, et al. Ranitidine and cimetidine in Zollinger-Ellison syndrome. Br J Clin Pharmacol 1980; 10:173–174.

367. Allende HD, Collen MJ, Pandol SJ, et al. Cimetidine-induced impotence and gynaecomastia: reversal with ranitidine. Gastroenterology 1982; 82:1007.

368. CDC. Gynecomastia in Haitians—Puerto Rico, Florida, Texas, New York. MMWR 1982; 31:205–206.

369. Brody SA, Winters J, Down MA, et al. An epidemic of gynecomastia among Haitian refugees: possible exposure to anti-androgen. Endocr Soc Abstr 1983; 724.

370. Markusse HM, Meyboom RHB. Gynaecomastia associated with captopril. Br Med J 1988; 296:1262–1263.

371. Tanner LA, Bosco LA. Gynecomastia associated with calcium channel blocker therapy. Arch Intern Med 1988; 148:379–380.

372. Bergman D, Futterweit W, Segal R, et al. Increased oestradiol in diazepam related gynaecomastia. Lancet 1981; 1:1225–1226.

373. Reid DM, Martynoga AG, Nuki G. Reversible gynaecomastia associated with D-penicillamine in a man with rheumatoid arthritis. Br Med J 1982; 285:1083–1084.

374. Mendelson JH, Kuehnle J, Ellingboe J, et al. Plasma testosterone levels before, during and after chronic marijuana smoking. N Engl J Med 1974; 291:1051–1055.

375. Harmon JW, Aliapoulios MA. Marijuana-induced gynecomastia: clinical and laboratory experience. Surg Forum 1974; 25:423–425.

376. Cicero TJ, Bell RD, Wiest WG, et al. Function of the male sex organs in heroin and methadone users. N Engl J Med 1975; 292:882–887.

377. Mendelson JH, Mendelson JE, Patch VD. Plasma testosterone levels in heroin addiction and during methadone maintenance. J Pharmacol Exp Ther 1975; 192:211–217.

378. Sirtori C, Veronesi U. Gynecomastia: a review of 218 cases. Cancer 1957; 10:645–654.

379. Bannayan GA, Hajdu SI. Gynecomastia: clinicopathologic study of 351 cases. Am J Clin Pathol 1972; 57:431–437.

380. McFadyen IJ, Bolton AE, Camerson EHD, et al. Gonadal-pituitary hormone levels in gynaecomastia. Clin Endocrinol 1980; 13:77–86.

381. Turkington RW. Serum prolactin levels in patients with gynecomastia. J Clin Endocrinol 1972; 34:62–66.

382. Frantz AG, Kleinberg DL, Noel GL. Studies on prolactin in man. Recent Prog Horm Res 1972; 82:527–590.

383. Large DM, Anderson DC, Laing I. Twenty-four hour profiles of serum prolactin during male puberty with and without gynaecomastia. Clin Endocrinol 1980; 12:293–302.

384. Beck W. Normoprolactinemia in boys with marked gynecomastia. Eur J Pediatr 1981; 137:41–44.

385. Besser GM, Parke L, Edwards CRW, et al. Galactorrhoea: successful treatment with reduction of plasma prolactin levels by brom-ergocryptine. Br Med J 1972; 3:669–672.

386. Thorner MO, McNeilly AS, Hagan C, et al. Long-term treatment of galactorrhoea and hypogonadism with bromocriptine. Br Med J 1974; 2:419–422.

387. Scheike O. Male breast cancer. 5. Clinical manifestations in 257 cases in Denmark. Br J Cancer 1973; 28:552–561.

388. Draznin B, Maman A. Estrogen-induced galactorrhea in man. Arch Intern Med 1979; 139:1059–1060.

389. Baron SH, Sowers JR, Feinberg M. Prolactinoma in a man following industrial exposure to estrogens. West J Med 1983; 138:720–722.

390. Huang TT, Hidalgo JE, Lewis SR. A circumareolar approach in surgical management of gynecomastia. Plast Reconstr Surg 1982; 69:35–40.

391. Moss ALH, Brown GED. The surgical approach to gynecomastia. NZ Med J 1982; 95:505–506.

392. Saad MN, Kay S. The cirumareolar incision: a useful incision for gynecomastia. Ann R Coll Surg Engl 1984; 66:121–122.

393. Freiberg A, Hong C. Apple-coring technique for severe gynecomastia. Can J Surg 1987; 30:57–60.

394. Courtiss EH. Gynecomastia: analysis of 159 patients and current recommendations for treatment. Plast Reconstr Surg 1987; 79:740–753.

395. Parker LN, Gray DR, Lai MK, et al. Treatment of gynecomastia with tamoxifen: a double-blind crossover study. Metabolism 1986; 8:705–708.

396. LeRoith D, Sobel R, Glick SM. The effect of clomiphene citrate on pubertal gynaecomastia. Acta Endocrinol 1980; 95:177–180.

397. Plourde PV, Kulin HE, Santner SJ. Clomiphene in the treatment of adolescent gynecomastia. Am J Dis Child 1983; 137:1080–1082.

398. Stepanas AV, Burnet RB, Harding PE, et al. Clomiphene in the treatment of pubertal-adolescent gynecomastia: a preliminary report. J Pediatr 1977; 90:651–653.

399. LeRoith D, Sobel R, Glick SM. The effect of clomiphene citrate on pubertal gynaecomastia. Acta Endocrinol 1980; 95:177–180.

400. Zachmann M, Eiholzer U, Muritano M, et al. Treatment of pubertal gynaecomastia with testolactone. Acta Endocrinol 1986; 113:218–226.

401. Beck W, Stubbe P. Ausgeprate gynakomastie beim jungen. Monvatsschr Kinderheilkd 1984; 132:32–37.

402. Buckle R. Danazol in the treatment of gynaecomastia. Drugs 1980; 19:356–361.

403. Kuhn JM, Roca R, Laudat MH, et al. Studies on the treatment of idiopathic gynaecomastia with percutaneous dihydrotestosterone. Clin Endocrinol 1983; 19:513–520.

404. Eberle AJ, Sparrow JT, Keenan BS. Treatment of persistent pubertal gynecomastia with dihydrotestosterone heptanoate. J Pediatr 1986; 109:144–149.

405. Kuhn JM, Laudat MH, de Lignieres B, et al. Traitement androgenique percutané des hypogonadismes masculins. Efficacité comparée de la

testosterone et de la dihydrotestosterone: étude de 40 observations. Endocrinologie 1986; 14:1031–1036.

406. Gagnon JD, Moss WT, Stevens KR. Pre-estrogen breast irradiation for patients with carcinoma of the prostate: a critical review. J Urol 1979; 121:182–184.

407. Waterfall NB, Glaser MG. A study of the effects of radiation on prevention of gynaecomastia due to oestrogen therapy. Clin Oncol 1979; 5:257–260.

408. Fass D, Steinfeld A, Brown J, et al. Radiotherapeutic prophylaxis of estrogen-induced gynecomastia: a study of late sequela. Int J Radiat Oncol Biol Phys 1986; 12:407–408.

409. Scheike O, Visfeldt J. Male breast cancer. 4. Gynecomastia in patients with breast cancer. Acta Pathol Microbiol Immunol Scand A 1973; 81:359–365.

410. Scheike O. Male breast cancer. 5. Clinical manifestations in 257 cases in Denmark. Br J Cancer 1973; 28:552–561.

411. Meyskens FL, Tormey DC, Neifeld JP. Male breast cancer: a review. Cancer Treat Rev 1976; 3:83–93.

412. Langlands AO, Maclean N, Kerr GR. Carcinoma of the male breast: report of a series of 88 cases. Clin Radiol 1976; 27:21–25.

413. Mabuchi K, Bross DS, Kessler II. Risk factors for male breast cancer. J Natl Cancer Inst 1985; 74:371–375.

414. Dexter CJ. Benign enlargement of the male breast. N Engl J Med 1956; 254:996–997.

16

ENDOCRINOLOGICAL CHANGES OF PREGNANCY

M. Linette Casey, Paul C. MacDonald, and Evan R. Simpson

INTRODUCTION

The endocrine alterations that accompany pregnancy in women are among the most remarkable in mammalian physiology or pathophysiology. In pregnant women at or near term, there is a daily production of about 70 μmol (20 mg) of estradiol, 300 μmol (80 mg) of estriol, 1 mmol (300 mg) of progesterone, 3 μmol (1 mg) of aldosterone, and 30 μmol (10 mg) of deoxycorticosterone. The levels of plasma renin, angiotensinogen, and angiotensin II increase strikingly. Production of human placental lactogen (hPL, also called human chorionic somatomammotropin, hCS) is about 1 g, and large quantities of human chorionic gonadotropin (hCG) are formed. Finally, there is increased formation of human chorionic thyrotropin (hCT), chorionic corticotropin (ACTH, adrenocorticotropin), luteinizing hormone–releasing hormone (LHRH), somatostatin, possibly chorionic thyrotropin-releasing hormone (TRH), and other proteins (placental specific) that are unique to pregnancy. Thus a remarkable aspect of pregnancy is the establishment of mechanisms whereby the gravid woman and her fetus are able to adapt to this unusual endocrine milieu.

ESTROGEN FORMATION DURING PREGNANCY*

In normal pregnancy large quantities of estrogens are produced (Fig. 16–1). After the first 3 to 4 wk of human pregnancy nearly all the estrogens produced are synthesized in trophoblasts, i.e., the placenta. The mechanism by which estrogen is produced in the placenta is unique. In the human there is little or no steroid 17α-hydroxylase activity in the placenta, and consequently there is little if any conversion of C_{21}-steroids to C_{19}-steroids. Thus progesterone is not metabolized further within the placenta, except to 5α-dihydroprogesterone (in limited amounts) and to 20α-dihydroprogesterone (little of which is secreted by the placenta). Ryan[1] demonstrated in 1959 that the placenta has a remarkable capacity for the aromatization of C_{19}-steroids and that androstenedione, testosterone, and dehydroepiandrosterone are converted efficiently to estrone and estradiol by placental tissue minces and placental microsomes. At that time, how-

---

*Also see Chapter 20.

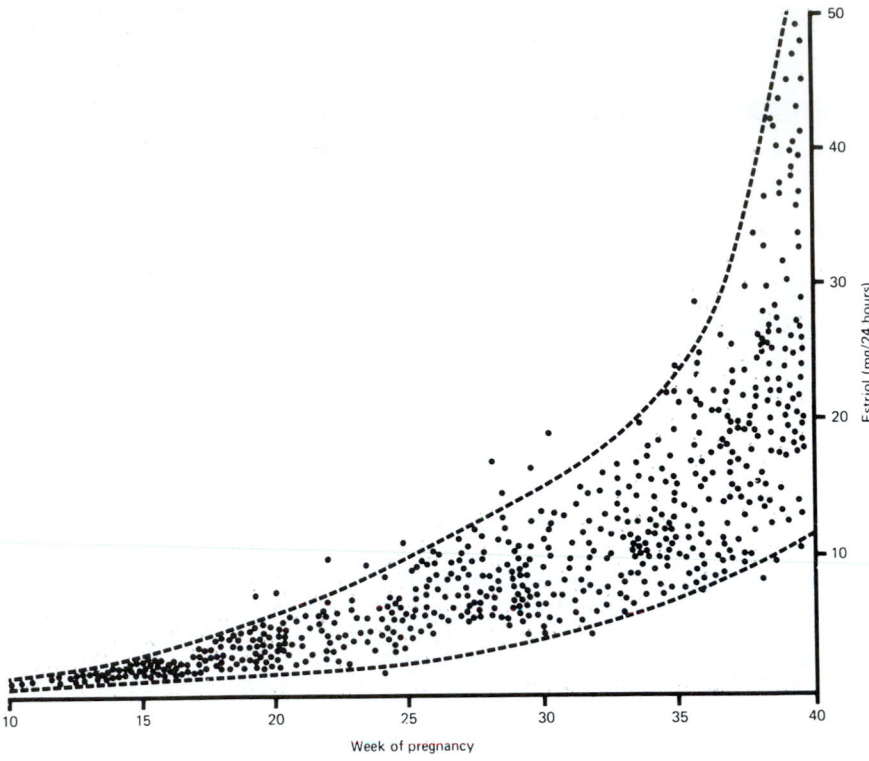

Figure 16–1. Urinary excretion of estriol-16-glucuronoside in 31 healthy pregnant women followed throughout pregnancy. Upper and lower dashed lines are the 95% confidence limits. (From Beling C. Estrogens. In: Fuchs F, Klopper A, eds. Endocrinology of Pregnancy. 2nd ed. New York: Harper & Row, 1977: 86.)

ever, another enigma existed because there also was known to be a disproportionate amount of estriol, compared with the amounts of estradiol and estrone, in the urine of pregnant women. Whereas in the urine of nonpregnant women the ratio of estriol to estrone plus estradiol is approximately 1:1, the ratio is 10:1 or more in the urine of pregnant women. This disproportionate excretion of estriol cannot be caused by an alteration in the metabolism of estrone or estradiol in the maternal compartment or to the formation of estriol from estrone or estradiol in the placenta. This conclusion follows from the fact that the fractional conversion of intravenously administered estrone and estradiol to estriol is the same in pregnant and nonpregnant women and from the observation that little or no steroid 16α-hydroxylase activity is present in placenta.

Thus two questions were posed. First, what was the source of the C_{19}-steroids used by the placenta for estrogen biosynthesis? Second, what was the mechanism by which the disproportionate amount of estriol arose in pregnant women? It seemed likely that the fetus was involved in placental estrogen biosynthesis because Frandsen and Stakeman[2] had found that urinary estrogen levels are low in women pregnant with an anencephalic fetus; in the latter, there is striking atrophy of the fetal adrenal.

PLACENTAL AROMATIZATION OF CIRCULATING C_{19}-STEROIDS. In 1963 several groups of investigators demonstrated that the human placenta depends on circulating C_{19}-steroid precursors for estrogen biosynthesis. The principal precursor of placental estradiol-17β is circulating dehydroepiandrosterone sulfate[3–5] (Fig. 16–2). Moreover, the increased amount of estriol in maternal plasma and urine is due to the secretion of estriol by the placenta. Estriol is formed in the human placenta by sequential desulfurylation and aromatization of plasma 16α-hydroxydehydroepiandrosterone sulfate.[6, 7]

Estradiol and estrone are formed in the placenta from dehydroepiandrosterone sulfate, a C_{19}-steroid that is present in both fetal and maternal plasma. Dehydroepiandrosterone sulfate is desulfurylated in placenta by steroid sulfatase. The product of the aromatization of dehydroepiandrosterone (after conversion to androstenedione) that enters the maternal compartment is principally estradiol. It is not clear whether estrone or estradiol is the primary metabolite that enters the fetal circulation. Probably both estradiol and estrone are secreted into fetal plasma, although estradiol could be converted to estrone by fetal erythrocytes or other intervillous tissues before reaching the fetus.[8] Near term, approximately half of the estradiol synthesized in the placenta is derived from precursors in the fetal circulation and half from precursors in the maternal circulation.[7] By contrast, estriol is produced principally from 16α-hydroxydehydroepiandrosterone sulfate in the fetal plasma. Dehydroepiandrosterone sulfate, secreted by the fetal adrenal cortex, is converted extensively to 16α-hydroxydehydroepiandrosterone sulfate in the fetal adrenal and liver. In any event, approximately 90% of the estriol excreted in the urine of near-term pregnant women is derived from the placental aromatization of 16α-hydroxydehydroepiandrosterone sulfate of fetal origin.[7] Steroid sulfatase activity in the placenta is great.[9, 10]

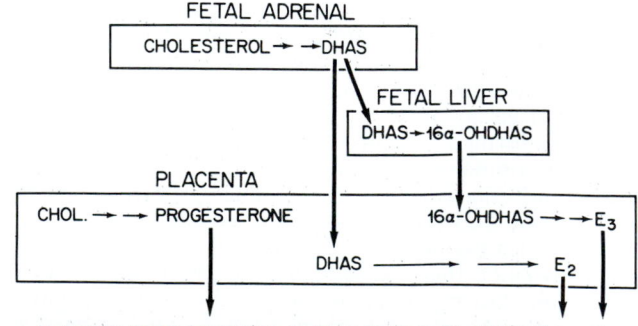

STEROID BIOSYNTHESIS IN THE FETAL-PLACENTAL UNIT

Figure 16–2. Schematic representation of steroid hormone biosynthesis in the fetal-placental unit. DHAS, dehydroepiandrosterone sulfate; E_2, estradiol; E_3, estriol; CHOL, cholesterol.

PLACENTAL SULFATASE DEFICIENCY. In placental sulfatase deficiency there is failure of hydrolysis of dehydroepiandrosterone sulfate or 16α-hydroxydehydroepiandrosterone sulfate, and thus there is a deficiency in estrogen formation by the placenta.[11] In such instances the levels of estriol in the plasma and urine of pregnant women are quite low; indeed, they may be as low as those associated with death of the fetus. The infants born of such pregnancies usually are normal at birth but develop ichthyosis later in life. All infants with placental sulfatase deficiency are male. In many pregnancies associated with placental sulfatase deficiency, there is a delay in the onset of parturition, or a refractoriness to the induction of labor by the intravenous administration of oxytocin, or both. Many women with pregnancies in which there is placental sulfatase deficiency have been hypertensive. However, placental sulfatase deficiency per se is not believed to be associated with a predisposition to pregnancy-associated hypertension. Rather, it is more likely that placental sulfatase deficiency is recognized as a consequence of the monitoring of estriol levels in hypertensive pregnant women.

ROLE OF FETAL ADRENAL IN PLACENTAL ESTROGEN BIOSYNTHESIS. The human is one of the few mammals in whom estrogens are produced in large quantities during pregnancy. The adrenals of the human fetus at term are as large as those of adults, weighing 10 g or more (Fig. 16–3).[12] Morphologically, however, the fetal adrenal differs from that of the adult. The human fetal adrenal is composed principally of an inner fetal zone that accounts for 85% of the volume of the gland. The outer zone, i.e., the neocortex, which ultimately develops into the adult adrenal cortex, makes up 15% or less of the total volume. In addition to its size, the human fetal adrenal has a remarkable capacity for steroidogenesis. Near term, the fetal adrenals secrete 100 to 200 mg steroid per day. The principal secretory products are dehydroepiandrosterone sulfate and pregnenolone sulfate.

In addition to the role of the fetal adrenal cortex in providing the precursors for placental estrogen formation, its secretions may participate in the biochemical events that lead to the initiation of parturition and to fetal lung maturation.[13, 14] Therefore the control of steroidogenesis by the human fetal adrenal is an issue of considerable importance in the endocrinology of human pregnancy. The fetal adrenal appears to be responsive to more than one trophic stimulus. First, ACTH levels in human fetal blood decline as gestation advances;[15] paradoxically, the rate of growth of the adrenals increases at a time when ACTH levels are falling. Second, the fetal adrenals secrete different steroids from those of the adult adrenals. For these reasons a trophic role has been proposed for peptides such as growth hormone, hCG, prolactin, hPL, and α-melanocyte-stimulating hormone. There is little convincing evidence, however, that any of these protein hormones serve an important role in stimulating growth or steroidogenesis directly in the fetal adrenal cortex. It is likely that a growth factor (or factors) (possibly of placental origin) stimulates growth of the adrenal without directly enhancing the synthesis of steroidogenic enzymes. The increase in the rate of steroidogenesis during gestation may be caused, at least in part, by the increase in the size of the fetal zone of the adrenal.

Attempts have also been made to define the precursors of the steroid hormones synthesized by the fetal adrenal. Some investigators have suggested that circulating progesterone and pregnenolone of placental origin could serve as precursors for fetal adrenal steroidogenesis. On the basis of the level of pregnenolone (sulfate) in umbilical venous blood, however, it can be computed that this source of steroid precursor accounts for no more than 1% of the dehydroepiandrosterone sulfate secreted by the fetal adrenal. Conceivably a portion of fetal adrenal cortisol is formed by the utilization of progesterone produced within the placenta. However, suppression of fetal ACTH secretion by dexamethasone therapy in pregnant women leads to a striking decrease in fetal plasma cortisol levels. Moreover, the fetal adrenal gland possesses the capacity for de novo synthesis of cortisol and thus likely does not require placental steroids as precursors for steroid biosynthesis in a quantitative sense.

The principal precursor for fetal adrenal steroid biosynthesis is probably cholesterol. The question then arises as to the source of cholesterol that is utilized in fetal adrenal steroidogenesis. There are two possibilities. First, cholesterol could be formed in situ in the fetal adrenal by de novo synthesis from two-carbon precursors. Second, cholesterol could be assimilated from plasma lipoproteins. Many tissues utilize cholesterol derived from circulating lipoproteins. For example, in human fibroblasts in culture, most of the cholesterol is derived from low-density lipoprotein (LDL).[16] This is also the case in mouse adrenal tumor cells in culture.[17] In addition, the adrenals of adult rats take up cholesterol from high-density lipoprotein.[18] It is important to note that the LDL cholesterol level in cord blood of newborn infants is

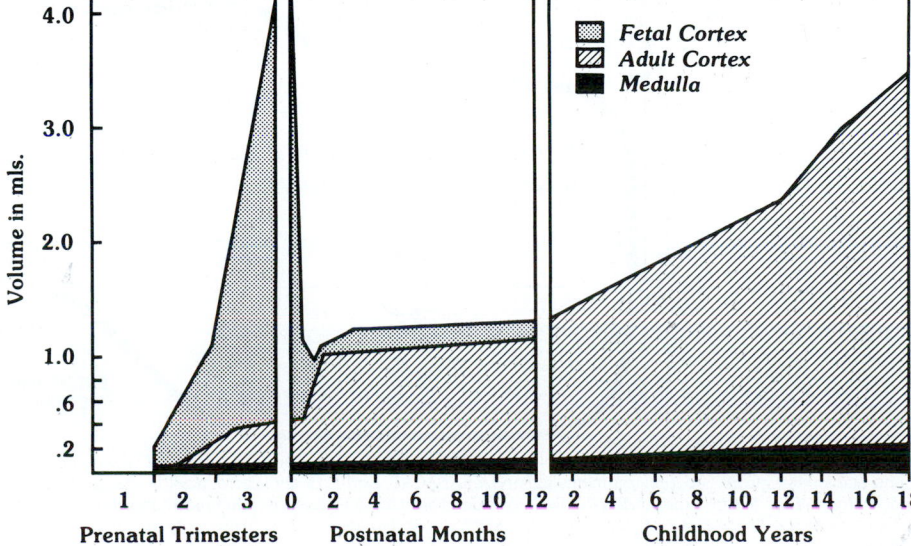

Figure 16–3. Size of adrenal gland and its component parts in utero, during infancy, and during childhood. (Adapted from Bethune JE, ed. The Adrenal Cortex, A Scope Monograph. Kalamazoo: Upjohn, 1974: 11.)

approximately 0.8 mmol/L (30 mg/dL), an amount only one fourth to one fifth of that in the plasma of normal adults.[19]

The LDL cholesterol present in the entire plasma volume of the human fetus near term is only 0.08 mmol (30 mg) of cholesterol. Thus if LDL were the principal source of cholesterol for fetal adrenal steroidogenesis, its turnover in fetal plasma must be rapid compared with that in the adult, and indeed, lipoprotein cholesterol is the form of cholesterol preferentially utilized for steroidogenesis in human fetal adrenal tissue fragments maintained in organ culture in the presence of ACTH.[20] Pregnenolone sulfate, dehydroepiandrosterone sulfate, and cortisol are the principal products. In these studies it was computed that 50 to 70% of the steroids secreted by the fetal adrenal are derived from LDL cholesterol and that the remainder is derived from cholesterol synthesized de novo in the adrenal gland.[20]

LDL is the preferred lipoprotein used for steroidogenesis by the fetal adrenal.[21] High-density lipoprotein is less effective, and very-low-density lipoprotein (VLDL) is not utilized. A scheme for the regulation of cholesterol metabolism by the human fetal adrenal is presented in Figure 16–4. It thus appears possible that the rate of fetal adrenal steroidogenesis may be regulated in part by the concentrations of LDL in the fetal plasma and hence by the rate of synthesis of lipoproteins in the fetus.

What is the source of lipoproteins in the fetus? It appears that no more than 20% of fetal cholesterol can be derived from the maternal circulation.[22] As LDL is ultimately derived from VLDL after the hydrolysis of the triacylglycerol portion of VLDL by lipoprotein lipase, it may be that the fetal lung is important in LDL formation. This obtains because there is little adipose tissue in the human fetus before the 36th wk of gestation. Lipoprotein lipase activity is present in fetal rat lung tissue, and prolactin is known to stimulate lipoprotein lipase in other tissues.[23] Thus prolactin may act to facilitate adrenal steroidogenesis through stimulation of the conversion of VLDL to LDL in fetal tissues. In keeping with this view, fetal plasma prolactin levels increase in a manner parallel to the rate of increase in the size of the fetal adrenal cortex. Thus prolactin may be an indirect trophic agent for the fetal adrenal, even though the hormone does not seem to stimulate fetal adrenal steroidogenesis directly.

SECRETION OF PLACENTAL ESTROGEN INTO MATERNAL AND FETAL COMPARTMENTS. More than 90% of the estradiol and the estriol formed in the trophoblast is secreted into the maternal compartment,[24] and 85% or more of the progesterone formed in the trophoblast enters the maternal compartment; likewise, little of the progesterone in the maternal circulation enters the fetus.[25]

PROGESTERONE FORMATION

During the last few weeks of pregnancy, the placenta secretes 0.8 mmol (250 mg) or more of progesterone per day (Fig. 16–5). Indeed, in pregnancies with multiple fetuses, up to 2 mmol (600 mg) of progesterone is formed per day. Progesterone formed by the human placenta is derived from circulating maternal cholesterol.[26, 27] Normally, the fetus does not contribute to progesterone formation by the placenta. This was shown by the finding that ligation of the umbilical cord with the placenta remaining in situ does not cause an immediate reduction in the level of progesterone in plasma or in the level of pregnanediol in maternal urine.[28] Hellig and co-workers,[27] in a study of women pregnant with an anencephalic fetus, also showed that after the administration of radiolabeled cholesterol under conditions that approximated an isotopic steady state, the specific activities of plasma progesterone and urinary pregnanediol are similar to those of maternal circulating cholesterol.

MECHANISM OF PLACENTAL PROGESTERONE FORMATION. In near-term pregnant women, the amount of progesterone formed per day is equivalent to one fourth to one third of the daily cholesterol turnover rate in nonpregnant adults. In spite of this, the rate of incorporation of [14C]acetate into cholesterol by placental tissue in the human is low, as is the activity of the rate-limiting step in cholesterol biosynthesis, 3-hydroxy-3-methylglutaryl coenzyme A reductase, in human placental microsomes. Therefore, it is also likely that the rate of de novo synthesis of cholesterol in the

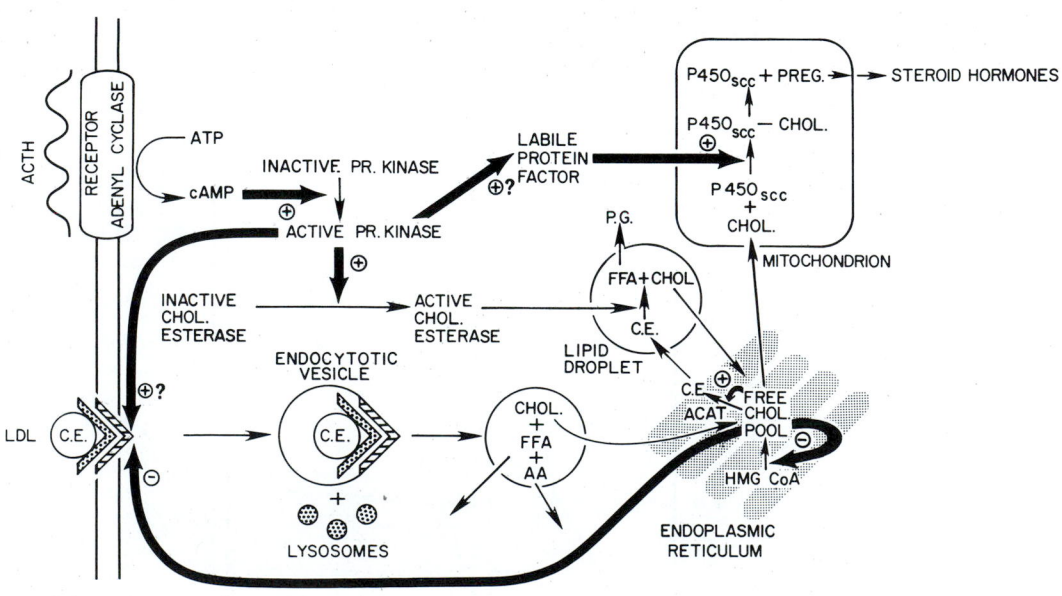

Figure 16–4. Pathways of cholesterol metabolism and its regulation in human fetal adrenal. C.E., cholesteryl esters; CHOL, cholesterol; FFA, free fatty acids; AA, amino acids; HMG CoA, 3-hydroxy-3-methylglutaryl CoA; ACAT, acyl-CoA:cholesterol acyltransferase; P.G., prostaglandins; P450scc, cholesterol side-chain cleavage cytochrome P-450. (From Simpson ER. Cholesterol side-chain cleavage, cytochrome P-450, and the control of steroidogenesis. Mol Cell Endocrinol 1979; 13:213–227.)

placenta is low. In cultured choriocarcinoma cells and human trophoblasts, lipoproteins are the principal source of cholesterol for steroidogenesis, and LDL is utilized preferentially.[29] LDL is bound to a saturable population of plasma membrane receptors on the trophoblastic cell with high affinity for LDL (also see Chapter 26). After binding of LDL to the cell-surface receptor, the lipoprotein is internalized through the process of endocytosis. The endocytotic vesicles fuse with lysosomes, and the lysosomal enzymes effect the hydrolysis of the lipoprotein. The protein moiety of LDL is broken down to amino acids, and the hydrolysis of the cholesterol esters gives rise to fatty acids and cholesterol. The liberated cholesterol is then available to serve as precursor for pregnenolone formation in mitochondria, and pregnenolone is thereafter converted to progesterone in mitochondria and in endoplasmic reticulum. The mechanism by which progesterone is believed to be synthesized from circulating LDL is illustrated diagrammatically in Figure 16–6.

Although the mechanism for progesterone biosynthesis in normal pregnancy is well established, other mechanisms may operate under certain circumstances. In a full-term pregnancy in a woman with familial homozygous hypobeta-lipoproteinemia, the plasma level of progesterone was quite low but not absent.[30] (The rate of production of progesterone by the corpus luteum during an ovulatory cycle in this woman was negligible.[31]) Estrogen levels in this pregnancy were reduced modestly, probably because of some attenuation in fetal adrenal dehydroepiandrosterone sulfate production caused by reduced levels of circulating LDL in the fetus, which is a heterozygous carrier of the mutant gene.

Ordinarily, the uptake of LDL by a tissue is associated with an increase in cholesterol ester synthesis by way of LDL stimulation of acyl-CoA:cholesterol acyltransferase (ACAT) activity.[32] Paradoxically, however, in trophoblastic tissue there are few or no cholesterol esters. The explanation for this paradox came from an investigation of the effect of progesterone on ACAT activity in placenta,[33, 34] which demonstrated that progesterone inhibits ACAT activity. Indeed, progesterone in concentrations similar to those present in trophoblastic cells inhibits ACAT activity almost completely. By preventing the sequestration of cholesterol in storage form, namely, cholesterol esters, such inhibition may ensure a continuing supply of cholesterol for progesterone biosynthesis. Amino acids derived from hydrolysis of the protein component of LDL may constitute a source of essential amino acids for the fetus; the fatty acids derived from hydrolysis of the cholesterol esters of LDL, principally linoleic acid, also may provide essential fatty acid for the fetus.

There is no evidence that any class of steroid other than

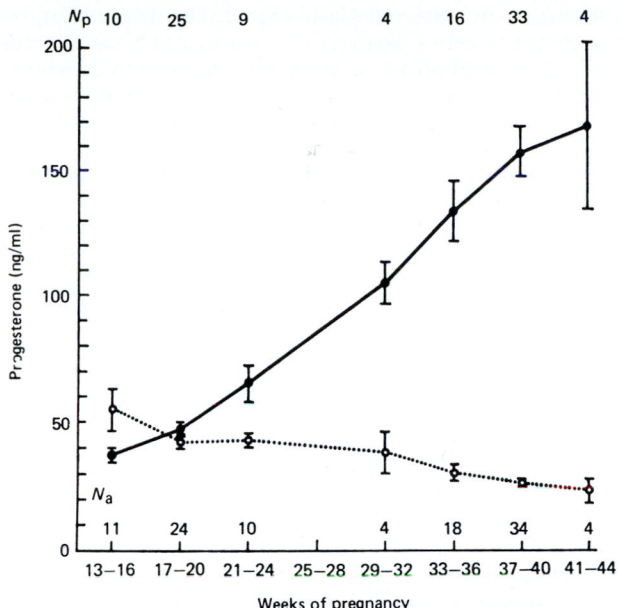

Figure 16–5. Progesterone levels in maternal plasma (—) and amniotic fluid (··········) from the same subjects. Values were grouped in 4-wk periods. N_p, number of plasma samples; N_a, number of amniotic fluid samples in each period. (From Johansson ED, Johansson LE. Progesterone levels in amniotic fluid and plasma from women. I. Levels during normal pregnancy. Acta Obstet Gynecol Scand 1971; 50:339–343.)

estrogens and progesterone is formed or secreted by the placenta. Specifically, there is no evidence for the de novo production of glucocorticoids or mineralocorticoids.

TRANSFER OF STEROID HORMONES FROM MATERNAL TO FETAL COMPARTMENTS

Little of the steroids that circulate in the maternal compartment reach the fetal compartment. Part of the reason may be that the rapid clearance of steroids from maternal plasma compared with placenta plasma flow minimizes their availability to trophoblastic cells. Perhaps more important, steroids that reach the trophoblast appear to re-enter the maternal compartment preferentially rather than to be transported into the fetal compartment. For example,

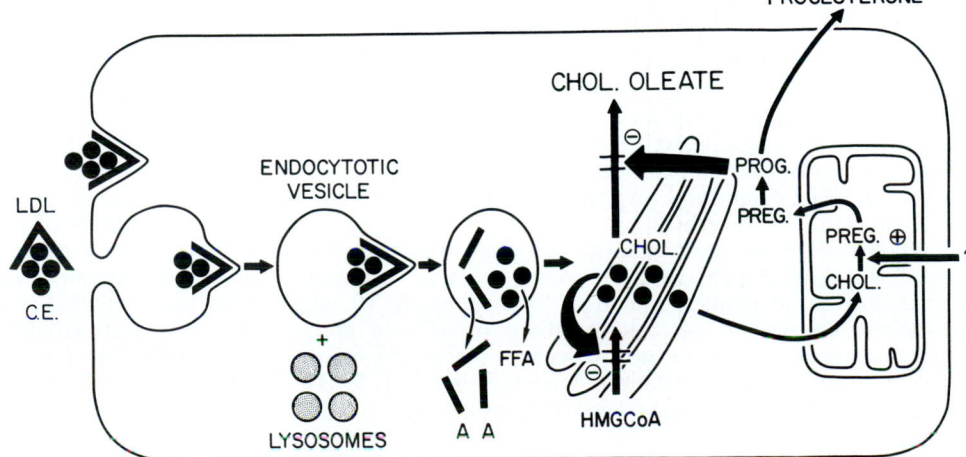

Figure 16–6. Pathways of cholesterol metabolism and its regulation in human placenta. PREG., pregnenolone; PROG., progesterone; LDL, low-density lipoprotein; C.E., cholesteryl esters; FFA, free fatty acids; AA, amino acids; CHOL., cholesterol; HMGCoA, 3-hydroxy-3-methylglutaryl CoA.

little cortisol in maternal plasma enters the trophoblast, both because the re-entry pathway dominates and because cortisol within the trophoblast is converted largely to cortisone.[35] Thus most of the cortisol molecules in the maternal compartment that enter the fetal compartment would do so in the form of cortisone.

Circulating C_{19}-steroids in the maternal compartment, namely, dehydroepiandrosterone sulfate, dehydroepiandrosterone, androstenedione, and testosterone, usually do not escape into the fetal compartment in significant quantities because of the extremely large capacity of the aromatase enzyme system of the trophoblast for the conversion of C_{19}-steroids to estrogens. Indeed, in most circumstances the aromatase system of the human trophoblast is not rate-limiting in the formation of estrogen from C_{19}-steroids in maternal plasma. This follows from the observation that the fractional conversion of circulating C_{19}-steroids to estradiol is not altered by wide fluctuations in their concentration in maternal circulation.[36] This protective mechanism prevents virilization of the female fetus of women who have or who develop androgen-secreting tumors of the ovary during pregnancy. In many women with strikingly increased rates of testosterone production, virilization of the female fetus does not occur. When virilization of the female fetus occurs as a result of excessive androgen formation in the maternal compartment, it is probably caused by C_{19}-steroids that are not estrogen prehormones, e.g., dihydrotestosterone or 5α-androstanedione. Alternatively, such fetuses may become virilized early during pregnancy at a time when the placenta may not be able to clear testosterone efficiently by aromatization.

PROTEIN HORMONES OF THE PLACENTA

Early in human pregnancy, perhaps before nidation, protein hormones begin to be produced by the human trophoblast. Among these are hCG, hPL, hCT,[37] and chorionic ACTH.[38–40] In addition, the trophoblast produces a number of hypothalamic-like releasing and inhibiting hormones, including LHRH,[41, 42] TRH,[42] corticotropin-releasing hormone,[43] inhibin,[44–45] and somatostatin.[46]

HUMAN CHORIONIC GONADOTROPIN. hCG is a glycoprotein that is composed of an alpha and a beta subunit and is secreted by the syncytiotrophoblast. Messenger RNAs (mRNAs) for both alpha and beta subunits are demonstrable in syncytial cells of the placenta, whereas the mRNA for the alpha subunit is demonstrable only in cytotrophoblasts.[47] Interestingly, however, the maximal rate of hCG secretion coincides in time with the greatest abundance of cytotrophoblasts in placenta (Fig. 16–7). As it is believed that the cytotrophoblast is the progenitor of the syncytiotrophoblast, the correlation of formation and secretion of hCG with numbers of cytotrophoblasts may simply reflect increased conversion of cytotrophoblast to syncytiotrophoblasts. Alternatively, the cytotrophoblast is the site of synthesis of LHRH; thus a paracrine mechanism may exist whereby LHRH of cytotrophoblast origin acts on syncytiotrophoblasts to stimulate the production of hCG.

The rate of secretion of hCG increases rapidly in the first few weeks of pregnancy, maximal levels in maternal blood and urine being attained at approximately 10 wk gestation. Thereafter the concentrations of hCG in both maternal serum and urine slowly decline, reaching a nadir at approximately 120 d gestation. After this time hCG levels in maternal plasma persist at a level of approximately 20,000 IU/L.

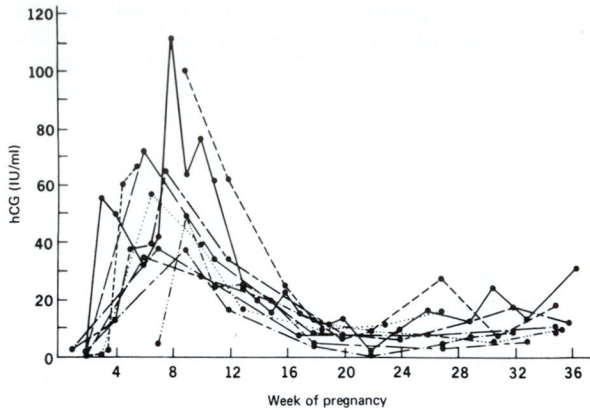

Figure 16–7. Plasma hCG levels of eight women followed longitudinally throughout gestation. Week of pregnancy is indicated, relative to time of ovulation. (From Vaitukaitis J. Human chorionic gonadotropin. In: Fuchs F, Klopper A, eds. Endocrinology of Pregnancy. 2nd ed. New York: Harper & Row, 1977: 67.)

Elevated levels of hCG are found in women with multiple fetuses and in women with hydatidiform mole or choriocarcinoma. Late in pregnancy, rising levels of hCG also may be observed in women with Rh isoimmunization and an affected fetus, and in some women with diabetes mellitus. In these latter two circumstances, cytotrophoblasts reappear in the placenta late in gestation. At approximately 10 wk gestation, when the maximal levels of hCG are attained, the mean concentration in the plasma of most pregnant women is of the order of 100,000 IU/L. Women with hydatidiform mole may have enormous levels of hCG. If hCG concentrations rise above 500,000 IU/L of plasma, the diagnosis of hydatidiform mole is virtually assured. Unfortunately, the reverse is not the case, because hCG levels below 500,000 IU/L of serum do not exclude the possibility of neoplastic trophoblastic disease. Interestingly, concentrations of hPL do not increase in women with hydatidiform mole. In fact the finding of high levels of hCG together with low levels of hPL is characteristic of this abnormality. Development of theca lutein cysts of the ovary during pregnancy usually indicates high levels of hCG. These lesions are found most often in women with hydatidiform mole but also may occur in women with multiple fetuses, diabetes mellitus, or Rh isoimmunization.

The physiological role of hCG in human pregnancy is not fully defined. It is likely that hCG acts as a luteotropin to maintain the corpus luteum and is responsible for conversion of the corpus luteum of menstruation to the corpus luteum of pregnancy via its capacity to stimulate progesterone secretion by this organ. It also is possible that hCG induces secretion of testosterone from the fetal testes before the secretion of LH by the fetal pituitary. hCG may also play a role in the provision of immunological protection to the trophoblast,[48] although others have suggested that such findings were caused by a contaminant in the hCG preparations used.[49]

Because of the biological and immunological similarity between hCG and LH, it was initially difficult to distinguish between these two gonadotropins. With the recognition that the beta subunits of the two compounds differ, antibodies were developed that are specific for the beta subunit of hCG. The measurement of hCG by specific radioimmunoassay has facilitated monitoring of the efficacy of treatment of women with hydatidiform mole and choriocarcinoma.[50]

PLACENTAL LACTOGEN. The secretion of hPL by the syncytiotrophoblast may commence on or before the day of nidation. The pattern of hPL secretion, however, differs from that of hCG (Fig. 16–8). Concentrations in maternal

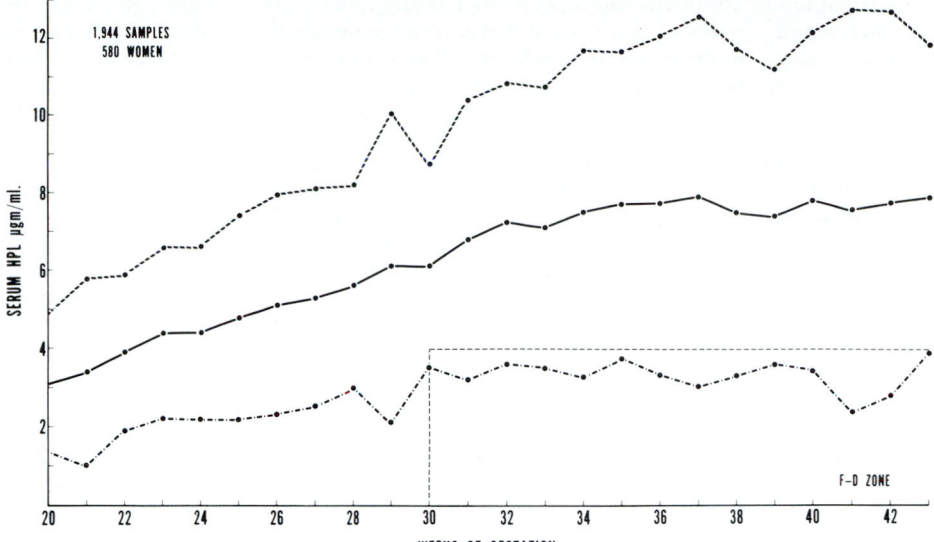

Figure 16–8. Plasma levels of hPL as a function of gestational age (± 2 SD). If, after 30 wk gestation, the level of hPL is less than 4 μg/mL, the fetus is considered to be in danger (F-D zone). (From Spellacy WN. Human placental lactogen in high-risk pregnancy. Clin Obstet Gynecol 1973; 16:298–312.)

blood increase slowly and appear to parallel the size of the placental mass. Maximal levels are attained sometime after the 32nd week of gestation and remain relatively constant after that time. The rate of hPL secretion in pregnant women is the greatest of any protein hormone in women or men, with daily production reaching 1 g or more late in normal pregnancy. Little hPL enters the fetal circulation. The hormone has both lactogenic and somatotrophic properties. Its potency in promoting growth, however, is only about 1/100 that of pituitary growth hormone. hPL is an insulin antagonist and may be responsible in part for the development of overt diabetes mellitus in pregnant women who were not known to have the disease before they became pregnant and who may not require insulin after the pregnancy is terminated (gestational diabetes). Direct evidence in support of this proposition, however, has not been obtained. Apparently normal pregnancies have been described in which no hPL could be detected in maternal blood or in placenta.[51]

HUMAN CHORIONIC THYROTROPIN. hCT has been isolated from extracts of placenta and hydatidiform molar tissue.[37] This substance is not identical to the thyroid-stimulating hormone produced by the human anterior pituitary. The role of hCT is unclear, and it is not known whether it is present in the fetal or the maternal compartment. Excessive amounts of thyroid-stimulating activity are found in neoplastic trophoblastic tissue, but it is likely that the hyperstimulation of the maternal thyroid that occurs in some women with molar pregnancy comes about largely through the action of hCG.[52]

CHORIONIC CORTICOTROPIN. An ACTH-like compound in extracts of placental tissue[38-40] appears to be biologically active and immunoreactive with antibodies prepared against human pituitary ACTH. It has not been established conclusively that the placenta produces chorionic ACTH, although the incorporation of radiolabeled amino acids into an ACTH-like compound has been reported.[39]

LUTEINIZING HORMONE– AND THYROTROPIN-RELEASING HORMONES. LHRH-like[41, 42] and TRH-like[42] substances are present in extracts of placenta. Moreover, placental tissue maintained in culture secretes LHRH.[42] It is possible that the releasing hormones control hCG and hCT production by trophoblastic tissue, but experimental support for this proposition is lacking.

INHIBIN. Inhibin is a glycoprotein with two distinct subunits (α and β) and is produced in human ovary, human testis, and human placenta.[44, 45] Inhibin of gonadal origin inhibits follicle-stimulating hormone secretion by the pitui-

tary, and placental inhibin may also prevent this secretion, thereby preventing ovulation during pregnancy. In addition, inhibin, which is produced in cytotrophoblasts, may serve a paracrine role in placenta to decrease hCG production by syncytial cells.

MEASUREMENT OF PLACENTAL HORMONES AS AN INDEX OF FETAL WELL-BEING

For decades, physicians have sought to evaluate the well-being of the fetus by monitoring the levels of various hormones that arise in the placenta or the fetal-placental unit. It was reasoned that alterations in placental function could be assessed by the measurement of such hormones, that alterations in their concentrations would reflect changes in the health of the fetus, and that information so gained would allow intervention in high-risk pregnancies to effect preterm delivery when the intrauterine environment of the fetus was deteriorating.

ESTRIOL. Determination of estriol levels in maternal plasma or urine has been, and in some institutions still is, utilized to monitor fetal well-being because estriol is formed in the placenta primarily from fetal adrenal C_{19}-steroids. Therefore a decrease in estriol level in the maternal plasma or urine could reflect a deterioration in fetal health. Moreover, after fetal death, levels of estriol in maternal plasma and urine are reduced. Indeed, the diagnosis of fetal death can be established with some reliability by the determination of estriol levels in the maternal compartment. In pregnancies in which the fetus is considered to be at risk, marked reductions in estriol levels or persistently low levels of estriol predict impending fetal demise. With such a background of information, it would seem that the measurement of estriol in the maternal compartment could give data that would constitute a reliable index of fetal well-being. Unfortunately, we do not believe this to be true. For example, in some pregnancies in which the fetus is undoubtedly at risk, there may be no reduction in estriol values. Examples of such high-risk pregnancies are those that include Rh isoimmunization with an affected fetus and those complicated by maternal diabetes mellitus. In such pregnancies, the level of estriol in maternal plasma or urine may be higher than that in normal pregnancies at the same stage of gestation.

A comment about the concept of *stress* in the fetus may be warranted. In most cases, fetal stress represents fetal hypoxia caused by decreased uteroplacental blood flow, e.g., pregnancy complicated by chronic hypertension, pregnancy-induced hypertension (preeclampsia-eclampsia), placental insufficiency (from unknown causes), fetal growth retardation (for unknown reasons), or severe diabetes mellitus. Unfortunately, fetal stress has been equated with stress as we know it in the adult, which is associated with increased ACTH secretion. If pituitary ACTH secretion were increased in the stressed fetus, one would anticipate that estriol levels in the maternal plasma or urine would increase—not decrease. This follows because the principal precursor of placental estriol is fetal 16α-hydroxydehydroepiandrosterone sulfate formed from dehydroepiandrosterone sulfate secreted by the fetal adrenal. Thus if fetal pituitary secretion of ACTH were to increase with stress, the secretion of fetal adrenal dehydroepiandrosterone sulfate should increase and result, ultimately, in an increase in the secretion of 16α-hydroxydehydroepiandrosterone sulfate, and thence, in increased levels of estriol. This is not the case. During fetal hypoxia there appears to be a decrease in the secretion of fetal pituitary ACTH, a decrease in the rate of secretion of fetal adrenal dehydroepiandrosterone sulfate, and subsequently a decrease in the rate of estriol secretion.[53, 54] Put succinctly, stress in the adult usually refers to a state in which secretion of adrenal hormones increases ("fight or flight"), whereas stress in the fetus (hypoxia) is usually associated with decreased adrenal activity.

During hypoxia there is a decrease in body[55] and thoracic[56] movements of the fetus; these findings suggest that hypoxia induces longer sleep periods for the fetus. In support of the view that fetal stress/hypoxia is accompanied by decreased adrenal activity, the levels of plasma LDL in the cord blood of newborns of mothers with chronic and pregnancy-induced hypertension are higher than those of newborns of normotensive mothers.[57] These data, together with the finding that the fetal adrenal preferentially utilizes LDL cholesterol for steroidogenesis in vitro, support the view that during fetal hypoxia utilization of circulating LDL for steroidogenesis by the fetal adrenal is reduced.

Let us return to the principal question: Does the measurement of estriol in maternal plasma or urine provide an index of fetal well-being that could allow the physician to choose the ideal timing of delivery of a fetus in whom the intrauterine environment is believed to be compromised? The choice is usually between prematurity on the one hand and a deteriorating intrauterine environment of the fetus on the other hand. It is our view that the results of measurements of estriol in maternal blood or urine do not provide meaningful information over and above that available from the clinical assessment of the pregnancy unit.[58] Clinical assessment is accomplished by measurement of the rate of fetal growth by clinical and sonographic criteria, by systematic evaluation of maternal blood pressure, and by the evaluation of renal function or the status of carbohydrate metabolism in pregnant women. It is not difficult to conclude that the fetus is at risk when maternal hypertension is worsening or in a diabetic woman in whom carbohydrate metabolism is not controlled. It is easy to recognize that the fetus is at risk when the biparietal diameter of the fetal head fails to increase at a proper rate. These considerations, together with the fact that estriol levels fluctuate widely in the same pregnant woman and from woman to woman, have led us to the view that more harm than good can come from the timing of delivery on the basis of estriol levels in the maternal compartment, without taking into account other factors. Most investigators now share this view. To date, there has been only one controlled, prospective study of the utility of estriol measurements, and in this investigation estriol values did not prove helpful in decreasing perinatal mortality or morbidity.[58]

ESTETROL. Estetrol (15α-hydroxyestriol) is formed in the fetal compartment by the action of an enzyme that effects 15α-hydroxylation of estriol or 16α-hydroxylation of 15α-hydroxylated estrogens.[24] The finding that 15α-hydroxylation occurs uniquely in the fetal compartment prompted several groups of investigators to evaluate estetrol levels in maternal plasma or urine as an index of fetal well-being. Because the placental estrogen precursors arise in the fetal adrenal cortex and because 15α-hydroxylation is unique to the fetus, it was presumed that estetrol levels might be a better index of fetal well-being than estriol. Unfortunately, this has not proved to be the case. The reservations applicable to the utility of estriol measurements in the management of complicated obstetrical problems are applicable to estetrol as well.

PLACENTAL LACTOGEN. Because hPL is secreted by the trophoblast and because the rate of its secretion generally is proportional to the placental mass, hPL has been measured in maternal plasma in attempts to evaluate placental function and, indirectly, fetal well-being. Again, the objective of such measurements was to gain insight into the health of fetuses of complicated pregnancies to determine the optimal time of delivery for a potentially adversely affected fetus. In some high-risk pregnancies, especially those complicated by hypertension, there is a reasonable correlation between the level of hPL and the outcome for the newborn.[59] Unfortunately, however, this correlation is no better than, and probably not as good as, that between the level of estriol and fetal outcome. Like estriol measurement, measurement of hPL in maternal plasma does not appear to provide information superior to that available from clinical evaluation alone.

PLACENTAL CLEARANCE OF MATERNAL PLASMA DEHYDROEPIANDROSTERONE SULFATE AND THE DEHYDROEPIANDROSTERONE LOADING TEST. Because formation of estrogen in the placenta depends on circulating C_{19}-steroids (i.e., there is no de novo estrogen synthesis), a technique has been developed for the evaluation of placental clearance of maternal plasma dehydroepiandrosterone sulfate through placental estradiol formation (PC-DSE$_2$).[60] In this test the metabolic clearance rate of maternal plasma dehydroepiandrosterone sulfate is determined together with the fractional conversion of maternal plasma dehydroepiandrosterone sulfate to estradiol. The product of these two values is the volume of maternal plasma that is cleared of dehydroepiandrosterone sulfate by the placenta through the formation of estradiol per unit time. It is believed that such measurements reflect uteroplacental blood flow.[61] This technique has been used to demonstrate that the PC-DSE$_2$ is reduced in primigravid women with pregnancy-induced hypertension and in ambulatory women with chronic hypertension (Fig. 16–9).[62] Moreover, the PC-DSE$_2$ is reduced during sodium deprivation in normal pregnant women and in women with pregnancy-induced or chronic hypertension. PC-DSE$_2$ falls even further after diuretic treatment in both normal and hypertensive pregnant women.[63] For these and other reasons, most investigators take the view that salt deprivation and diuretic treatment should not be used in most pregnant women, certainly not in women with simple edema of pregnancy or pregnancy-induced hypertension (preeclampsia) or in most pregnant women with chronic hypertension. Generally speaking, salt deprivation and diuretic administration are indicated only in pregnant women with pulmonary edema and congestive heart failure. In unusual instances of chronic hypertension, in which the woman is treated with diuretics before conception occurs, it may be reasonable to

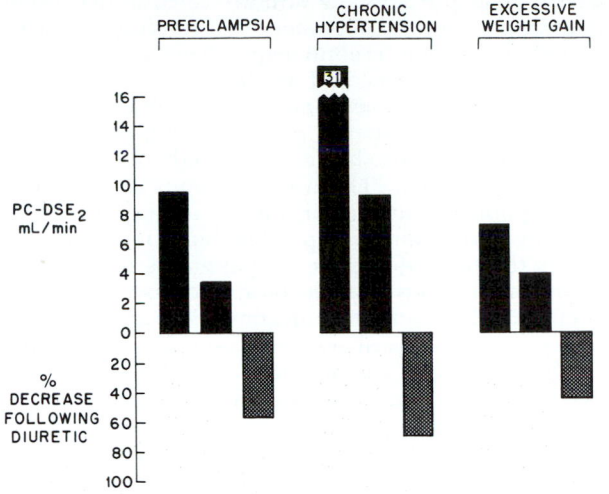

Figure 16–9. Placental clearance of dehydroepiandrosterone sulfate through estradiol formation (PC-DSE$_2$) and the effect of diuretic therapy. PC-DSE$_2$, placental clearance of dehydroepiandrosterone sulfate to estradiol.

continue diuretic therapy if the hypertension does not abate (as it commonly does) during the second trimester of pregnancy.

The determination of PC-DSE$_2$ is cumbersome and expensive and requires several weeks of laboratory analysis. For these reasons, it is not useful in the clinical management of high-risk pregnancies. Another approach has been to measure the increase in estradiol after administration of a loading dose of dehydroepiandrosterone sulfate.[64] It was reasoned that placental clearance of maternal dehydroepiandrosterone sulfate through either estradiol or estriol formation could be estimated from the change in the levels of estrogens in the maternal compartment after administration of the loading dose of the placental estrogen precursor. The results of such studies are similar to those obtained by formal determination of PC-DSE$_2$, and no prospective studies have been conducted to evaluate the utility of such measurements in determining optimal management of high-risk pregnancy.

MATERNAL ADAPTATIONS TO PREGNANCY

As stated at the beginning of this chapter, a remarkable feature of pregnancy is the successful adaptation of the woman to the enormous endocrine changes effected by steroid and protein hormones produced by the placenta. Women experience considerable blood loss at delivery. On average, 500 mL of blood is lost at the time of vaginal delivery; with cesarean section, 1000 mL; and at the time of cesarean section–hysterectomy, 1500 mL.[65] This loss is usually well tolerated because, on average, the blood volume of a woman increases from 3500 mL before pregnancy to 5000 mL by the latter part of pregnancy. In spite of the increase in blood volume, high levels of plasma renin activity, plasma angiotensin II levels, and aldosterone-secretory rates (10 to 40 times those of nonpregnant women) accompany late pregnancy. Yet systolic and diastolic blood pressures ordinarily are lower during pregnancy than before or after. This process of adaptation is not fully understood, but some of the individual components of the mechanism have been clarified.

Estrogen stimulates the hepatic synthesis of angiotensinogen, the precursor of angiotensin I that in turn is converted to angiotensin II. Estrogen and progesterone, alone or together, stimulate the secretion of renin, the enzyme that catalyzes the conversion of angiotensinogen to angiotensin I. Thus the net consequence is an enhancement in the synthesis of angiotensin II. In pregnancy, however, a dichotomy in tissue responsiveness to angiotensin II is evident. On the one hand, the zona glomerulosa of the maternal adrenal remains responsive to the trophic action of angiotensin II as aldosterone secretion increases strikingly during pregnancy. On the other hand, the maternal vasculature becomes refractory to the pressor effects of angiotensin II. These two events, acting in concert, are probably important for the expansion of blood volume that accompanies normal pregnancy. Refractoriness to the pressor effect of angiotensin II develops early in pregnancy and persists throughout gestation in women who do not develop pregnancy-induced hypertension (preeclampsia and eclampsia). In normal men and nonpregnant women, on average, the intravenous infusion of angiotensin II at a rate of 7 ng/kg body weight per minute causes a rise of 20 mm Hg in diastolic pressure. By contrast, an average of more than 16 ng of angiotensin II per kilogram of body weight per minute is required to effect a similar pressor response in pregnant women, and in some there is little pressor response even to 40 ng of angiotensin II per kilogram of body weight per minute. Prostaglandin (PG) or a PG-like substance is believed to mediate this process, because prostaglandin synthase inhibitors such as indomethacin and aspirin abolish the refractoriness of pregnant women to the pressor effects of angiotensin II.[66]

Failure of the physiological adaptations to pregnancy may be catastrophic. In a prospective study of young primigravid women who were at risk of developing pregnancy-induced hypertension, those who ultimately developed preeclampsia became refractory to the pressor effects of angiotensin II early in pregnancy.[67] Thereafter, these women began to lose refractoriness to angiotensin II—some as early as 22 wk of gestation—long before hypertension developed. This failure in the adaptive process of pregnancy is believed to be important in the pathophysiology of pregnancy-induced hypertension. After the development of hypertension, the levels of renin, angiotensin II, and aldosterone in the plasma of affected pregnant women fall, sometimes to values only slightly greater than those in nonpregnant women.

The levels in plasma of another mineralocorticoid, deoxycorticosterone (DOC), increase strikingly during pregnancy,[68, 69] principally in the last trimester, and the rate of DOC production is not controlled by the same mechanisms that modulate the secretion of aldosterone or cortisol. The administration of ACTH or dexamethasone to near-term pregnant women does not change the level of DOC in plasma,[69] and DOC secretion from the adrenal is not regulated by the action of angiotensin II. The level of DOC in umbilical cord plasma is greater than that in the maternal plasma; on the basis of the umbilical arteriovenous difference in DOC concentration,[70] however, maternal plasma DOC cannot be accounted for by transfer from the fetus. The level of DOC sulfate in the fetal circulation is even greater than that of DOC.[70] Circulating progesterone is converted to DOC in nonadrenal tissue,[71] and the fractional conversion of plasma progesterone to DOC is similar in men and in nonpregnant and pregnant women. Thus the rate of extra-adrenal DOC formation is proportional to the plasma concentration of progesterone. On the basis of these observations, extra-adrenal 21-hydroxylation of progesterone to form DOC is one of the reactions that lead to the formation of hormones from circulating precursors in extraglandular tissues. Interestingly, the fractional conversion of circulating progesterone to DOC, unlike the fractional conversion of other steroid hormones to metabolites, varies widely (i.e.,

0.002 to 0.03).[71] When progesterone secretion is high, as at the midluteal phase of the ovarian cycle (0.1 mmol/d [40 mg/d]) or during pregnancy (0.8 to 2.0 mmol/d [250 to 600 mg/d]), extraglandular formation of DOC from plasma progesterone is the principal source of DOC in plasma. The impact of DOC formation from plasma progesterone can vary widely, depending on the fractional conversion of plasma progesterone to DOC. In some pregnant women 20 μmol (7.5 mg) or more of DOC is produced each day from circulating progesterone.

The level of cortisol in the plasma of pregnant women is increased, partly because of a three- to fourfold increase in the level of corticosteroid-binding globulin.[72] The rate of secretion of cortisol by the maternal adrenal is not increased in pregnancy, but the rate of clearance is decreased so that the half-life of the hormone in plasma is prolonged. The ACTH level is suppressed in women during pregnancy,[73] presumably because of the action of estrogen and progesterone.[74] The lowest level of ACTH is found early in pregnancy, rising to a maximum between 26 wk and term.[73]

The rate of secretion of dehydroepiandrosterone sulfate by the maternal adrenal has not been studied systematically in pregnant women. Its concentration in plasma declines appreciably[75] during pregnancy because of an increase in the metabolic clearance rate of this compound through utilization by the placenta for estradiol formation and extensive 16α-hydroxylation in the maternal liver. Prolactin secretion increases steadily during pregnancy; in near-term pregnant women, the level of prolactin (of pituitary origin) in plasma ranges from 150 to 250 μg/L. The role of prolactin in adrenal function, if any, however, is not defined. Prolactin also is produced in the decidua of pregnant women and is believed to be the source of the high concentrations of the hormone in amniotic fluid. Decidual prolactin secretion does not account for that present in maternal or fetal blood. The secretion of decidual prolactin during pregnancy is not inhibited by dopamine or dopamine agonists.[76]

The physiological adaptation of the pregnant woman assures the fetus of adequate placental transfer of the nutrients required for growth and development and protects the mother from the trauma and blood loss of delivery by an expansion of blood volume without a concomitant increase in arterial blood pressure.

ENDOCRINOLOGY OF PARTURITION

Preterm birth and the attendant sequelae are the major health problems of children. Mortality in the newborn infant is related most closely to prematurity, and those premature infants who survive often incur permanent physical and mental impairment.[77–81] Indeed, a sizable proportion of persons with physical and mental impairments who require lifelong institutional or domiciliary care are disabled because of an untimely birth.[77–81] The magnitude of this problem is such that the economic, social, and health care problems of cancer, heart disease, and stroke pale by comparison. Assurance of the best possible quality of life for newborn infants, who should be expected to enjoy 70 or 80 y of good health, is a major goal for society in general and those concerned with health care in particular. Those entrusted with the health care of children and with research directed toward a solution of problems that afflict children must address prematurity as a first priority.

The major sequelae of prematurity are birth trauma and the respiratory distress syndrome.[77–80] The latter is a consequence of immaturity in the production by fetal lung of a surface-active material, surfactant. Surfactant is a lipo-protein that, after birth, reduces surface-active tension in the alveolus and prevents the alveolar collapse that would preclude oxygenation.[82] Consequences of respiratory distress in the newborn include cerebral hemorrhage, brain damage, permanent lung disorders, and death.

The mechanism or mechanisms by which labor is initiated in pregnant women are not completely understood. Several hypotheses have been formulated to explain the initiation of parturition. There are elements of plausibility for each hypothesis, but each also seems incomplete.

Human parturition is separable into three phases.[83] Phase 1 is the time of uterine preparedness for labor, in which myometrial oxytocin receptors increase in amount, the number and size of gap junctions between myometrial cells increase, and cervical softening and effacement commence. Phase 1 also is characterized commonly by uterine irritability. Phase 2 is active labor and is characterized by forceful, coordinated myometrial contractions; this phase is completed with the delivery of the newborn and the placenta. Phase 3 is that time after delivery when the uterus contracts to effect hemostasis and, thence, to return the organ to the nonpregnant state.

Uterotropins act on uterine tissues to facilitate the responsiveness of this tissue to the action of uterotonins, agents that effect uterine contractions. Uterotropins also effect the initial phase of parturition. Uterotonins, e.g., PGs, oxytocin, and other agents, can cause uterine contraction in phase 2 or 3 of parturition. The physiological uterotonin of phase 2 is not identified. Uterotonins may be produced in response to physiological or pathophysiological processes; alternatively, they may be administered pharmacologically to induce myometrial contraction, as is commonly done with oxytocin or PGs.

The fact that the infusion of oxytocin induces labor in women at or near term has led to the hypothesis that this hormone plays a physiological role in the initiation of labor, presumably being released by the neurohypophysis at the appropriate time. A careful study of the oxytocin levels in maternal, fetal, and newborn plasma, however, led Chard to conclude that a physiological role of oxytocin during early labor is unlikely.[84] He suggested that the pattern of release of oxytocin from the pituitary of pregnant women is more consistent with a permissive than an initiating function. In fact, the most important action of oxytocin may be during the expulsive phase of labor and during the postpartum period to ensure full contraction of the uterus and reduction of blood loss after the uterus is emptied of its contents. Thus the uterotonic action of oxytocin, in a physiological sense, is to facilitate phase 3 of parturition.

In 1882 Spiegelberg (as recounted by Thorburn[85]) proposed that the fetus is the origin of the signal for the initiation of human parturition, and it appears likely that a signal emanating from the fetus is important in the timing of parturition. Anomalies of the brain of the fetal calf, fetal lamb, and human fetus are associated with a delay in the timely onset of labor. If the pituitary is absent in the bovine fetus, the gestation period is prolonged by several weeks.[86] Adrenal hypoplasia in the bovine fetus also causes prolonged gestation.[87] If, early in pregnancy, the ewe eats the foliage of *Veratrum californicum,* a plant that grows wild in the northwestern United States, the fetus develops a characteristic cyclopean deformity in which there is abnormal vascularization of the pituitary from the hypothalamus in the fetus and prolonged gestation.[88] It is not certain that absence or hypoplasia of the pituitary in the human fetus causes prolonged gestation.[89]

The endocrine events of parturition have been defined most convincingly in the sheep. Whereas the sequence of events and the nature of the signal(s) that lead to the onset of parturition in the ewe appear to be different from those in women, the fundamental biochemical processes are similar in most species. In sheep the signal for the initiation of parturition emanates from the fetus; for the timely onset of labor, a properly functioning fetal hypothalamus, pituitary gland, and adrenal gland and a functional placenta are essential. The earliest known event in parturition in the sheep is an increase in the rate of cortisol production by the fetal adrenal. Fetal cortisol acts on the placenta to reduce progesterone secretion and augment estrogen formation. In consequence there is increased production of PG.[90, 91] An increase in the production of PGs in the fetal membranes or uterine decidua vera, or both, is also associated with the initiation and maintenance of labor in women. We will consider this event subsequently.

The importance of fetal brain, pituitary, and adrenal in processes that lead to the timely onset of labor is demonstrated by the observation that hypophysectomy, transection of the pituitary stalk, or adrenalectomy in the fetal sheep causes prolonged gestation.[90–94] Infusion of ACTH or a glucocorticoid into the sheep fetus causes premature parturition, whereas infusion of the same hormones into the ewe does not initiate labor.

As stated, the increased secretion of cortisol in the sheep fetus is associated with an alteration in biosynthetic processes in the placenta; ultimately, these lead to an increased rate of placental estrogen production. Cortisol acts on the sheep placenta to cause an increase in the activities of steroid 17α-hydroxylase and steroid 17,20-lyase[95] as a result of induction of mRNA and new protein synthesis.[96] An increase in the activities of these enzymes leads to increased conversion of pregnenolone to 17α-hydroxypregnenolone and thence to dehydroepiandrosterone and androstenedione, C_{19}-steroids that serve as substrates for estrogen biosynthesis (Fig. 16–10). Other factors play a role, however, because infusion of C_{19}-steroids (e.g., dehydroepiandrosterone or androstenedione) into the fetus at rates sufficient to increase the fetal plasma concentration of the C_{19}-steroid by 10-fold causes little increase in estrogen production unless the pregnancy is near term.[97] Thus in addition to an increase in the activities of steroid 17α-hydroxylase and steroid 17,20-lyase, there must be an increase in the activity of the placental or fetal aromatase system in response to cortisol,[98] as in other tissues known to respond to glucocorticoids by an increase in aromatase activity.[99]

The mechanism or mechanisms that regulate the rate of formation of PGs or related compounds before the initiation of parturition is not understood, but the previously mentioned increase in cortisol secretion by the adrenals of the lamb fetus, which leads to decreased placental secretion of progesterone and increased production of estrogen, is believed to be important in the increase in PG formation in intrauterine tissues. Of these hormones, estrogen appears to be related most closely to the increased synthesis and release of PGs within the uterus. Twenty-four hours after estrogen (diethylstilbestrol, 20 mg in oil) is administered to a pregnant ewe, the concentration of PGs in uterine venous blood increases. In women, local estradiol treatment also appears to cause cervical softening and effacement and, thereafter, increased responsiveness to oxytocin.[100]

An association between anencephaly in the human fetus and prolonged gestation was reported in 1898 by Rea.[101] In 1933 Malpas[102] extended these observations and suggested that prolonged gestation is attributable to anomalous function of the fetal brain-pituitary-adrenal system. These findings suggest that in humans, as in sheep, the fetal adrenal may serve an important role in the timely onset of labor. The adrenal glands of the anencephalic human fetus at term are small (only 5 to 10% of the weight of a normal fetal adrenal). The smallness of the gland is due largely to failure of development or early atrophy (by 20 wk of gestation) of the fetal zone—the structure that accounts for most of the mass of the human fetal adrenal.

There is another similarity between the events of parturition in humans and in sheep. In the human fetus with adrenal hypoplasia, gestation may be prolonged.[103] Hypophysectomy or adrenalectomy in the sheep fetus has the same effect.[90–93]

The endocrine events of parturition in humans and in sheep differ in regard to the role of fetal cortisol in the initiation of labor. Murphy[104] and Cawson and colleagues[105] reported that the plasma level of cortisol was higher in newborns delivered after labor than that in newborns delivered before initiation of labor by elective cesarean section. The plasma level of cortisol in babies who were delivered by cesarean section after labor commences also tended to be higher than that in newborns who were delivered by cesarean section before labor began. These investigators concluded that in the human fetus, as in the sheep fetus, a rise in the plasma cortisol level may be an important event leading to the onset of parturition. The findings of others, however, suggest an alternative conclusion. Hauth and co-workers[106] also reported that babies delivered vaginally after the spontaneous onset of labor (gestational ages of 30 to 42 wk) had a cord plasma cortisol level greater than that in newborn infants delivered before labor commenced. They found, however, that in newborn infants (gestational ages of 31 to 38 wk) delivered by cesarean section of women in spontaneous labor, the cord plasma cortisol level was similar to that in cord plasma of babies (gestational ages of 31 to 40 wk) delivered by cesarean section of women not in labor. These results may mean that the modestly elevated plasma cortisol level in newborn infants delivered vaginally is a consequence of vaginal delivery and is not related to labor per se. For example, during vaginal delivery, blood flow to the adrenals may be impaired temporarily, leading to transient hypoxia and vasodilation of the adrenal blood vessels. After delivery a reactive hyperemia could result in increased adrenal blood flow, a process known to cause increased corticosterone secretion by the rat adrenal.[107] If this were the case, the increased plasma cortisol level in newborn infants delivered vaginally is a consequence of birth rather than a cause of the initiation of parturition. Sybulski and Maughan[108] also determined the cortisol level in umbilical cord plasma and concluded that there is no surge in fetal

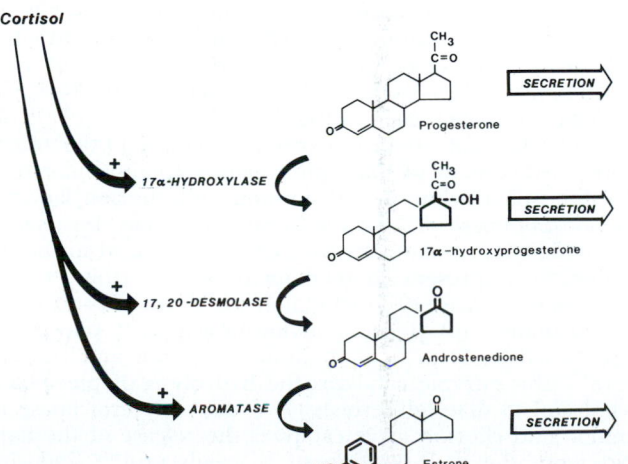

Figure 16–10. Regulation by cortisol of steroid secretion in sheep placenta. (Reprinted with permission from Pritchard JA, MacDonald PC, Gant NF. Williams Obstetrics. 17th ed. New York: Appleton-Century-Crofts, 1984: 298.)

cortisol production before the onset of spontaneous labor in the human. Moreover, Ohrlander and colleagues[109] studied the cortisol level in plasma from the fetal scalp during labor and concluded that cortisol secretion is not increased before the onset of labor. Furthermore infusion of glucocorticoids or ACTH into the human fetus does not cause premature labor, as it does in the sheep.[93, 94] Mati and associates, however, reported the induction of labor in post-term women after intra-amniotic injection of a large dose of betamethasone.[110] It is also of note that in instances in which augmented fetal cortisol production is precluded, e.g., in congenital adrenal hyperplasia, labor commences on time at term.[111–114] Thus cortisol does not appear to be as important in the initiation of parturition in the human as in the sheep. Nonetheless, the increased frequency of prolonged gestation in women with an anencephalic fetus or a fetus with adrenal hypoplasia suggests some role for the fetal adrenal in the timely onset of parturition. In accord with this view is a distinctive feature of the human fetus not found in any other species, namely, the massive enlargement of the adrenal caused by enlargement of the fetal zone of the cortex. Large quantities of C_{19}-steroids are also secreted by the human fetal adrenal, and these serve as precursors of the estrogens formed in the human placenta.

In this context, it is notable that in pregnancies in which placental sulfatase activity is absent or severely deficient, there is low estrogen production because the placenta cannot hydrolyze the sulfate ester bond of dehydroepiandrosterone sulfate. Some such women sustain prolonged gestation, and others are refractory to the action of oxytocin that is infused to induce labor.[115–117]

These three disorders, fetal adrenal hypoplasia, fetal anencephaly, and placental sulfatase deficiency, are all associated with a striking reduction in estrogen production. It would seem, therefore, that estrogen must occupy an important role in the regulation of events that lead to the timely onset of labor in women. Not all women with an anencephalic[118] or a placental sulfatase–deficient fetus have prolonged pregnancies. Nonetheless, in those who do, the prolongation of gestation may be considerable.

An understanding of the role of estrogen in human pregnancy is important for deciphering the events that lead to the onset of labor. Estrogen acts to stimulate phospholipid synthesis[119] and phospholipid turnover,[120] to increase the incorporation of arachidonic acid into glycerophospholipids,[121] to stimulate PG biosynthesis,[90] and to increase the number of lysosomes in the uterine endometrium.[122, 123]

In most mammalian species the onset of labor is preceded by a decrease in the level of progesterone in maternal plasma.[91, 124] This is not true in the monkey or in women;[125, 126] nonetheless, some form of progesterone withdrawal or deprivation may be important in the initiation of labor in these two species. In women there may be an alternative means to achieve functional progesterone withdrawal, namely, a lower capacity for progesterone binding in human myometrium at term than in myometrium from nonpregnant women.[127]

PGE_2 and $PGF_{2\alpha}$, when administered in large amounts, cause uterine contractions at any stage of pregnancy in women[128, 129] and effect cervical softening and effacement.[130] Ingestion of inhibitors of prostaglandin synthase activity by pregnant women (in large amounts) leads to prolongation of gestation.[131] Inhibitors of prostaglandin synthase (specifically, of arachidonic acid cyclooxygenase) also are alleged to be effective in arresting premature labor. PG levels in amniotic fluid and maternal plasma increase during labor.[132–137] These events are reminiscent of those at the end of the ovulatory cycle when progesterone levels are falling. In the pregnant ewe, progesterone withdrawal leads to the initiation of parturition.[138] For all these reasons, PGs are consid-

ered by some to be important in the initiation of the spontaneous onset of labor in women.

It is not clear, however, that the increase in PG production that accompanies labor commences before the onset of labor. Therefore, the role of PGs as physiological mediators of the initiation of labor is questionable. On the basis of current understanding of the biochemical events involved in the regulation of PG production, it seems possible—even highly likely—that the synthesis of PGs in increased amounts occurs as a consequence of labor. It is also likely, although not proved, that the increase in PG levels facilitates the progress of labor, i.e., cervical dilatation as well as the propagation of myometrial contractions.

A role for lipids in the initiation of parturition was suggested by the demonstration that intravenous infusion of a lipid emulsion into pregnant rabbits causes an increase in the responsiveness of the uterus to oxytocin.[139] The active component of these emulsions is phosphatidylcholine enriched with linoleic acid, a precursor of arachidonic acid.[140–142] Nathanielsz and colleagues showed that intra-aortic infusion of arachidonic acid into pregnant rabbits induces labor,[143] and Hertelendy demonstrated that the intrauterine injection of arachidonic acid induces premature oviposition in quail.[144] Arachidonic acid is the obligate precursor for the biosynthesis of PGs of the 2 series,[145, 146] and free arachidonic acid is utilized for PG formation.[147, 148]

The fetus–amniotic fluid–fetal membranes–decidua complex is a complicated unit for the transmission of a response to signals that lead to the onset of labor. The fetal membranes may be the primary site for the receipt of such signals: (1) the membranes provide a large surface area (approximately 0.6 m²) contiguous to the uterus; (2) direct communication is established between the fetus and the fetal membranes by substances that originate in the fetus and are excreted into the amniotic fluid through fetal urine, lungs, skin, and umbilical cord; (3) it would seem to be preferable to generate uterine contractions in myometrium contiguous to the fetal membranes rather than at the placental implantation site; and (4) injuries to the fetal membranes such as premature rupture with loss of amniotic fluid, stripping the chorion laeve from the contiguous decidua, infections of the membranes, or instillation of hypertonic solutions into the amniotic fluid commonly lead to the onset of uterine contractions and premature delivery of the fetus.

Additional evidence supports the concept that metabolic events in amnion and chorion laeve are crucial to the generation of PGs: (1) the specific acitivity of prostaglandin synthase in amnion is greater than that in chorion laeve, decidua vera, myometrium, or placenta;[149–151] (2) the glycerophospholipids of amnion and chorion laeve are enriched with arachidonic acid;[152] (3) as stated, the levels of free arachidonic acid, as well as those of PGE_2 and $PGF_{2\alpha}$ in amniotic fluid increase during labor;[132, 135–137, 153, 154] (4) during early labor, there is a specific decrease in the arachidonic acid content of diacylphosphatidylethanolamine and diacylphosphatidylinositol of amnion and chorion laeve;[155] (5) phospholipase A_2, with substrate specificity for diacylphosphatidylethanolamines with arachidonic acid in the sn-2 position, is present in fetal membranes[156] (this enzyme catalyzes the release of arachidonic acid from phosphatidylethanolamine); (6) phosphatidylinositol-specific phospholipase C activity is present in human amnion and chorion laeve[157] (this enzyme catalyzes the hydrolysis of phosphatidylinositol to diacylglycerols); (7) a diacylglycerol lipase in amnion and chorion laeve catalyzes the release of the fatty acid from the sn-1 position of diacylglycerol,[158] and this enzyme may be relatively specific for diacylglycerols with arachidonic acid in the sn-2 position;[158] (8) a monoacylglycerol lipase in amnion and chorion laeve catalyzes the release of the fatty acid in the *sn*-2 position of monoacylglycerols[158] (there may be relative substrate specificity of this enzyme for *sn*-2-arachidonoyl monoacylglycerols)—thus arachidonic acid is released from phosphatidylinositol in the fetal membranes by the coordinated activity of several enzymes; (9) the specific activities of phospholipases A_2 and C in human amnion increase late in gestation;[159] (10) diacylglycerols, the products of the reaction catalyzed by phosphatidylinositol-specific phospholipase C, accumulate in amnion during early labor;[160] (11) the activity of NAD^+-dependent 15-hydroxy-prostaglandin dehydrogenase, the enzyme that catalyzes the first reaction in the inactivation of PGs, is not detectable in human amnion;[149] and (12) components of amniotic fluid, such as epidermal growth factor,[161] act to stimulate de novo synthesis of prostaglandin H_2 synthase (cyclooxygenase)[162] and, thereby, prepare the amnion to produce large amounts of PGE_2 when presented with arachidonic acid.

In summary, the first events in the initiation of pregnancy appear to be hormonal, with changes occurring in the formation and release of cortisol, progesterone, and estrogen. By mechanisms still not completely understood, these changes lead to the enhanced production of PGs that accompanies labor. There are many gaps in our understanding of the involvement of PGs in human parturition. In particular, the factors that regulate PG biosynthesis and release are not understood, and the mode of action of PGs remains undefined.

Infection is commonly associated with the premature onset of labor; this is true whether the infection is localized in uterine or extrauterine maternal tissues or in the extraembryonic fetal membranes. Biochemical (endocrine and paracrine) mechanisms are involved in this process and are under investigation. Cytokines, i.e., interleukin 1β[163] and tumor necrosis factor α,[164] are produced by decidual macrophages in response to bacterial toxins that gain access to this tissue. These cytokines promote the synthesis, in uterine tissues (decidua and myometrium) and in extraembryonic fetal membranes (contiguous with decidua and myometrium), of PGs and other bioactive agents that may be instrumental in the initiation and propagation of myometrial contractions.

REFERENCES

1. Ryan KJ. Aromatization of steroids. J Biol Chem 1959; 234:268–272.
2. Frandsen VA, Stakeman G. The site of production of oestrogenic hormones in human pregnancy. Hormone excretion in pregnancy with anencephalic fetus. Acta Endocrinol 1961; 38:383–391.
3. Siiteri PK, MacDonald PC. The utilization of circulating dehydroisoandrosterone sulfate for estrogen synthesis during human pregnancy. Steroids 1963; 2:713–730.
4. Baulieu EE, Dray F. Conversion of ³H-dehydroisoandrosterone (3β-hydroxy-Δ⁵-androsten-17-one) sulfate to ³H-estrogens in normal pregnant women. J Clin Endocrinol Metab 1963; 23:1298–1301.
5. Bolte E, Mancuso S, Eriksson G, et al. Studies on the aromatization of neutral steroids in pregnant women: I. Aromatization of C-19 steroids by placentas perfused in situ. Acta Endocrinol 1964; 45:535–559.
6. Magendantz HG, Ryan KJ. Isolation of an estriol precursor, 16α-hydroxydehydroepiandrosterone, from human umbilical sera. J Clin Endocrinol Metab 1964; 24:1155–1162.
7. Siiteri PK, MacDonald PC. Placental estrogen biosynthesis during human pregnancy. J Clin Endocrinol Metab 1966; 26:751–761.
8. Gurpide E, Marks C, deZiegler D, et al. Asymmetric release of estrone and estradiol derived from labeled precursors in perfused human placentas. Am J Obstet Gynecol 1982; 144:551–555.
9. Pulkkinen MO. Arylsulphatase and the hydrolysis of some steroid sulphates in developing organism and placenta. Acta Physiol Scand 1961; 52(Suppl 180):90–92.
10. Warren JC, Timberlake CE. Steroid sulfatase in the human placenta. J Clin Endocrinol Metab 1962; 22:1148–1151.
11. Tabei T, Heinrichs WL. Diagnosis of placental sulfatase deficiency. Am J Obstet Gynecol 1976; 124:409–414.
12. Spector WS, ed. Handbook of Biological Data. Philadelphia: W. B. Saunders, 1956: 353.
13. MacDonald PC, Porter JC, Schwarz BE, et al. Initiation of parturition in the human female. Semin Perinatol 1978; 2:273–286.
14. Liggins GC. Premature delivery of foetal lambs infused with glucocorticoids. J Endocrinol 1969; 45:515–523.
15. Winters AJ, Oliver C, Colston C, et al. Plasma ACTH levels in the human fetus and neonate as related to age and parturition. J Clin Endocrinol Metab 1974; 39:269–273.
16. Goldstein JL, Brown MS. Binding and degradation of low density lipoproteins by cultured human fibroblasts. J Biol Chem 1974; 249:5153–5162.
17. Faust JR, Goldstein JL, Brown MS. Receptor-mediated uptake of low-density lipoprotein and utilization of its cholesterol for steroid synthesis in cultured mouse adrenal cells. J Biol Chem 1977; 252:4861–4871.
18. Anderson JM, Dietschy JM. Regulation of sterol synthesis in 15 tissues of rat. II. Role of rat and human high and low density plasma lipoproteins and of rat chylomicron remnants. J Biol Chem 1977; 252:3652–3659.
19. Glueck CJ, Mellies MJ, Tsang RC, et al. Low and high density lipoprotein cholesterol interrelationships in neonates with low density lipoprotein cholesterol above the 10th percentile and in neonates with high density lipoprotein cholesterol below the 90th percentile. Pediatr Res 1977; 11:957–959.
20. Simpson ER, Carr BR, Parker CR, et al. The role of serum lipoproteins in steroidogenesis by the human fetal adrenal cortex. J Clin Endocrinol Metab 1979; 49:146–148.
21. Carr BR, Parker CR, Milewich L, et al. The role of low density, high density, and very low density lipoprotein in steroidogenesis by the human fetal adrenal gland. Endocrinology 1980; 106:1854–1860.
22. Lin DS, Pitkin RM, Connor WE. Placental transfer of cholesterol into the human fetus. Am J Obstet Gynecol 1977; 128:735–739.
23. Zinder O, Hamosh M, Fleck TRC, et al. Effect of prolactin on lipoprotein lipase in mammary gland and adipose tissue of rats. Am J Physiol 1974; 226:744–748.
24. Gurpide E, Schwers J, Welch MT, et al. Fetal and maternal metabolism of estradiol during pregnancy. J Clin Endocrinol Metab 1966; 26:1355–1365.
25. Gurpide E, Tseng J, Escarcena L, et al. Fetomaternal production and transfer of progesterone and uridine in sheep. Am J Obstet Gynecol 1972; 113:21–32.
26. Bloch K. Biological conversion of cholesterol to pregnanediol. J Biol Chem 1945; 157:661–666.
27. Hellig H, Gattereau D, Lefebvre Y, et al. Steroid metabolism from plasma cholesterol. I. Conversion of plasma cholesterol to placental progesterone in humans. J Clin Endocrinol Metab 1970; 30:624–631.
28. Cassmer O. Hormone production of the isolated human placenta. Acta Endocrinol 1959; 45(Suppl):3–82.
29. Simpson ER, Bilheimer DW, MacDonald PC, et al. Uptake and degradation of plasma lipoproteins by human choriocarcinoma cells in culture. Endocrinology 1979; 104:8–16.
30. Parker CR Jr, Illingworth DR, Bissonnette J, et al. Endocrine changes during pregnancy in a patient with homozygous familial hypobetalipoproteinemia. N Engl J Med 1986; 314:557–560.
31. Illingworth DR, Corbin DK, Kemp ED, et al. Hormone changes during the menstrual cycle in abetalipoproteinemia: reduced luteal phase progesterone in a patient with homozygous hypobetalipoproteinemia. Proc Natl Acad Sci USA 1982; 79:6685–6689.
32. Brown MS, Dana SE, Goldstein JL. Cholesterol ester formation in cultured human fibroblasts. J Biol Chem 1975; 250:4025–4027.
33. Simpson ER, Burkhart MF. AcylCoA:cholesterol acyltransferase activity in human placental microsomes: inhibition by progesterone. Arch Biochem Biophys 1980; 200:79–85.
34. Simpson ER, Burkhart MF. Regulation of cholesterol metabolism by human choriocarcinoma cells in culture: effect of lipoproteins and progesterone on cholesteryl ester synthesis. Arch Biochem Biophys 1980; 200:86–92.
35. Murphy BEP, Clark SJ, Donald IR, et al. Conversion of maternal cortisol to cortisone during placental transfer to the human fetus. Am J Obstet Gynecol 1974; 118:538–541.
36. MacDonald PC, Siiteri PK. Origin of estrogen in women pregnant with an anencephalic fetus. J Clin Invest 1965; 44:465–474.
37. Osathanondh R, Tulchinsky D. Placental polypeptide hormones. In: Tulchinsky D, Ryan KJ, eds. Maternal-Fetal Endocrinology. Philadelphia: W. B. Saunders, 1980: 17–42.
38. Rees LH, Burke CW, Chard T, et al. Possible placental origin of ACTH in normal human pregnancy. Nature 1975; 254:620–622.
39. Liotta A, Osathanondtt R, Ryan KJ, et al. Presence of corticotropin in human placenta: demonstration of in vitro synthesis. Endocrinology 1977; 101:1552–1558.
40. Odagiri E, Sherrell BJ, Mount CD, et al. Human placental immunoreactive corticotropin, lipotropin and β-endorphin. Evidence for a common precursor. Proc Natl Acad Sci USA 1979; 76:2027–2031.
41. Gibbons JM, Mitnick M, Chieffo V. In vitro biosynthesis of TSH- and LH-releasing factors by human placenta. Am J Obstet Gynecol 1975; 121:127–131.
42. Khodr GS, Siler-Khodr TM. Placental luteinizing hormone-releasing factor and its synthesis. Science 1980; 207:315–317.
43. Shibasaki T, Odagiri E, Shizume K, et al. Corticotropin-releasing factor–

like activity in human placental extracts. J Clin Endocrinol Metab 1982; 117:1598–1601.

44. McLachlan RI, Healy DL, Robertson DM, et al. The human placenta: a novel source of inhibin. Biochem Biophys Res Commun 1986; 140:485–490.
45. Petraglia F, Sawchenko P, Lim AT, et al. Localization, secretion, and action of inhibin in human placenta. Science 1987; 237:187–189.
46. Lee JN, Wu P, Chard T. Identification of somatostatin in the human placenta. Acta Endocrinol 1982; 99:601–604.
47. Hoshina M, Boothby M, Hussa R, et al. Linkage of human chorionic gonadotrophin and placental lactogen biosynthesis to trophoblast differentiation and tumorigenesis. Placenta 1985; 6:163–172.
48. Adcock EW III, Teasdale F, August CS, et al. Human chorionic gonadotropin: its possible role in maternal lymphocyte suppression. Science 1973; 181:845–847.
49. Golbus MS, Siiteri PK. Effects of human chorionic gonadotropin preparations on amino acid uptake and incorporation into protein in vitro. Endocr Res Commun 1976; 3:273–279.
50. Hertz R. Choriocarcinoma and Related Gestational Tumors in Women. New York: Raven, 1978.
51. Chard T. Placental lactogen: biology and clinical applications. In: Grudzinskas JG, Teisner B, Seppälä M, eds. Pregnancy Proteins: Biology, Chemistry, and Clinical Application. New York: Academic, 1981: 101–118.
52. Kenimer JG, Hershman JM, Higgins P. The thyrotropin in hydatidiform moles is human chorionic gonadotropin. J Clin Endocrinol Metab 1975; 40:482–491.
53. Parker CR, Simpson ER, Bilheimer DW, et al. Inverse relationships between the plasma concentrations of LDL-cholesterol and the placental estrogen precursor, dehydroisoandrosterone sulfate, in the human fetus. Science 1980; 208:512–514.
54. Parker CR, Leveno K, Carr BR, et al. Umbilical cord plasma levels of dehydroisoandrosterone sulfate (DS) during human gestation. J Clin Endocrinol Metab 1982; 54:1216–1220.
55. Pearson JF, Weaver JB. Fetal activity and fetal well-being: an evaluation. Br Med J 1976; 1:1305–1307.
56. Boddy K, Mantell CD. Observations of fetal breathing movements transmitted through maternal abdominal wall. Lancet 1972; 2:1219–1220.
57. Parker CR, Hankins GDV, Carr BR, et al. The effect of hypertension in pregnant women on fetal adrenal function and fetal plasma lipoprotein-cholesterol metabolism. Am J Obstet Gynecol 1984; 150:263–269.
58. Duenhoelter JH, Whalley PJ, MacDonald PC. An analysis of the utility of plasma immunoreactive estrogen measurements in determining delivery time of gravidas with a fetus considered at high risk. Am J Obstet Gynecol 1976; 125:889–898.
59. Spellacy WN, Buhi WC, Birk SA, et al. Distribution of human placental lactogen in the last half of normal and complicated pregnancies. Am J Obstet Gynecol 1974; 120:214–223.
60. Madden JD, Siiteri PK, MacDonald PC, et al. The pattern and rates of metabolism of maternal plasma dehydroisoandrosterone sulfate in human pregnancy. Am J Obstet Gynecol 1976; 125:915–920.
61. Everett RB, Porter JC, MacDonald PC, et al. Relationship of maternal placental blood flow to the placental clearance of maternal plasma dehydroisoandrosterone sulfate through placental estradiol formation. Am J Obstet Gynecol 1980; 136:435–439.
62. Worley RJ, Everett RB, MacDonald PC, et al. Placental clearance of dehydroisoandrosterone sulfate and pregnancy outcome in three categories of hospitalized patients with pregnancy-induced hypertension. Gynecol Invest 1975; 6:28–29.
63. Worley RJ, Everett RB, Madden JD, et al. Fetal considerations: metabolic clearance rate of maternal plasma dehydroisoandrosterone sulfate. Semin Perinatol 1978; 2:15–28.
64. Pupkin MJ, Nagey DA, Schomberg DW, et al. The dehydroisoandrosterone loading test. III. A possible placental function test. Am J Obstet Gynecol 1979; 134:281–288.
65. Pritchard JA, MacDonald PC. Obstetric hemorrhage. In: Williams Obstetrics. 16th ed. New York: Appleton-Century-Crofts, 1980: 487–489.
66. Everett RB, Worley RJ, MacDonald PC, et al. Effect of prostaglandin synthetase inhibitors on pressor response to angiotensin II in human pregnancy. J Clin Endocrinol Metab 1978; 46:1007–1010.
67. Gant NF, Daley GL, Chand S, et al. A study of angiotensin II pressor response throughout primigravid pregnancy. J Clin Invest 1973; 52:2682–2689.
68. Brown RD, Strott CA, Liddle GW. Plasma deoxycorticosterone in normal and abnormal human pregnancy. J Clin Endocrinol Metab 1972; 35:736–742.
69. Nolten WE, Lindheimer MD, Oparil S, et al. Deoxycorticosterone in pregnancy. I. Sequential studies of the secretory patterns of desoxycorticosterone, aldosterone, and cortisol. Am J Obstet Gynecol 1978; 132:414–420.
70. Parker CR, Cutrer S, Casey ML, et al. Concentrations of deoxycorticosterone, deoxycorticosterone sulfate, and progesterone in maternal venous and umbilical arterial and venous sera. Am J Obstet Gynecol 1983; 145:427–432.
71. Winkel CA, Milewich L, Parker CR, et al. Conversion of plasma progesterone to deoxycorticosterone in men, nonpregnant and pregnant women, and adrenalectomized subjects: evidence for steroid 21-hydroxylase activity in non-adrenal tissues. J Clin Invest 1980; 66:803–812.
72. Doe RP, Fernandez R, Seal US. Measurement of corticosteroid-binding globulin in man. J Clin Endocrinol Metab 1964; 24:1029–1039.
73. Carr BR, Parker CR, Madden JD, et al. Maternal plasma adrenocorticotropin and cortisol relationships throughout human pregnancy. Am J Obstet Gynecol 1981; 139:416–422.
74. Vale W, Rivier C, Yang L, et al. Effects of purified hypothalamic corticotropin-releasing factor and other substances on the secretion of adrenocorticotropin and β-endorphin-like immunoreactivities in vitro. Endocrinology 1978; 103:1910–1915.
75. Milewich L, Gomez-Sanchez CE, Madden JD, et al. Dehydroisoandrosterone sulphate in peripheral blood of premenopausal, pregnant and postmenopausal women and men. J Steroid Biochem 1978; 9:1159–1164.
76. Friesen H, Forsbach G. Prolactin secretion during pregnancy. In: Jaffe RB, ed. Prolactin. New York: Elsevier, 1981: 167–180.
77. Pregnancy, birth, and the infant. NIH Publication No. 82–2304. Washington, DC: Government Printing Office, 1981.
78. Pregnancy and perinatology. NIH Publication No. 81–2347. Washington, DC: Government Printing Office, 1981.
79. Research Planning Workshop on Human Parturition. DHEW Publication No. (NIH) 76–1101. Washington, DC: Government Printing Office, 1975.
80. The advancement of knowledge of the nation's health. Public Health Service Publication No. 1649. Washington, DC: Government Printing Office, 1967: 149–152.
81. Mental retardation: past and present. DHEW Publication No. (OHD) 71–21016. Washington, DC: Government Printing Office, 1977.
82. Avery ME, Mead J. Surface properties in relation to atelectasis and hyaline membrane disease. Am J Dis Child 1959; 97:517–523.
83. Cunningham FG, MacDonald PC, Gant NF. Williams Obstetrics. 18th ed. Norwalk, CT: Appleton & Lange, 1989: 187–189.
84. Chard T. The role of the posterior pituitaries of mother and fetus in spontaneous parturition. In: Foetal and Neonatal Physiology, Proc Sir J Barcroft Centenary Symp. London: Cambridge University Press, 1973: 579–583.
85. Thorburn GD. Physiology and control of parturition: reflections on the past and ideas for the future. Anim Reprod Sci 1979; 2:1–27.
86. Kennedy PC, Kendrick JW, Stormont C. Adenohypophyseal aplasia and an inherited defect associated with abnormal gestation in Guernsey cattle. Cornell Vet 1957; 47:160–178.
87. Jasper DE. Prolonged gestation in the bovine. Cornell Vet 1950; 40:165–172.
88. Binns W, James LF, Shupe JL. Toxicosis of *Veratrum californicum* in ewes and its relationship to a congenital deformity in lambs. Ann NY Acad Sci 1964; 111:571–576.
89. Moncrief MW, Hill DS, Archer J, et al. Congenital absence of pituitary gland and adrenal hypoplasia. Arch Dis Child 1972; 47:136–137.
90. Liggins GC, Fairclough RJ, Grieves SA, et al. The mechanism of initiation of parturition in the ewe. Recent Prog Horm Res 1973; 29:111–149.
91. Thorburn GD, Challis JRG, Robinson JS. Endocrine control of parturition. In: Wynn RM, ed. Biology of the Uterus. New York: Plenum, 1977: 653–732.
92. Liggins GC, Kennedy PC, Holm LW. Failure of initiation of parturition after electrocoagulation of the pituitary of the fetal lamb. Am J Obstet Gynecol 1967; 98:1080–1086.
93. Liggins GC, Fairclough RJ, Grieves SA. Parturition in the sheep. In: Knight J, O'Connor M, eds. The Fetus and Birth. Amsterdam: Elsevier, 1977: 5–30.
94. Liggins GC. Premature parturition after infusion of corticotrophin or cortisol in foetal lambs. J Endocrinol 1968; 42:323–329.
95. Flint APF, Anderson ABM, Steele PA, et al. The mechanism by which foetal cortisol controls the onset of parturition in the sheep. Biochem Soc Trans 1975; 3:1189–1194.
96. Mason JI, France JT, Magness RR, et al. Ovine placental steroid 17 alpha-hydroxylase/C-17,20-lyase, aromatase and sulphatase in dexamethasone-induced and natural parturition. J Endocrinol 1989; 122:351–359.
97. Pierrepoint GC, Anderson ABM, Turnbull AC, et al. In vivo and in vitro studies of steroid metabolism by the sheep placenta. In: Pierrepoint GC, ed. The Endocrinology of Pregnancy and Parturition—Experimental Studies in the Sheep. Cardiff, Wales: Alpha Omega Alpha Publishing, 1973: 40–53.
98. Ricketts AP, Galil AKA, Ackland N, et al. Activation by corticosteroids of steroid metabolizing enzymes in ovine placental explants in vitro. J Endocrinol 1980; 85:457–469.
99. Simpson ER, Ackerman GE, Smith ME, et al. Estrogen formation in stromal cells of adipose tissue of women: induction by glucocorticosteroids. Proc Natl Acad Sci USA 1981; 78:5690–5694.
100. Pinto RM, Leon C, Mazzoco N, et al. Action of estradiol-17β at term and at onset of labor. Am J Obstet Gynecol 1970; 98:540–546.
101. Rea C. Prolonged gestation, acrania, monstrosity and apparent placenta praevia in one obstetrical case. JAMA 1898; 30:1166–1167.

102. Malpas P. Postmaturity and malformations of the foetus. J Obstet Gynaecol Br Commonw 1933; 40:1046–1053.

103. O'Donohue NV, Holland PDJ. Familial congenital adrenal hypoplasia. Arch Dis Child 1968; 43:717–723.

104. Murphy BEP. Does the human fetal adrenal play a role in parturition? Am J Obstet Gynecol 1973; 115:521–525.

105. Cawson JM, Anderson ABM, Turnbull AC, et al. Cortisol, cortisone, and 11-deoxycortisol levels in human umbilical and maternal plasma in relation to the onset of labour. J Obstet Gynaecol Br Commonw 1975; 81:737–745.

106. Hauth JC, Parker CR, MacDonald PC, et al. A role of fetal prolactin in lung maturation. Obstet Gynecol 1978; 51:81–88.

107. Porter JC, Klaiber MS. Corticosterone secretion in rats as a function of ACTH input and adrenal blood flow. Am J Physiol 1965; 209:811–814.

108. Sybulski S, Maughan GB. Cortisol levels in umbilical cord plasma in relation to labor and delivery. Am J Obstet Gynecol 1976; 125:236–238.

109. Ohrlander S, Gennser G, Eneroth P. Plasma cortisol levels in human fetus during parturition. Obstet Gynecol 1976; 48:381–387.

110. Mati JKG, Horrobin DF, Bramley PS. Induction of labour in sheep and in humans by single doses of corticosteroids. Br Med J 1973; 2:149–151.

111. Price HV, Cone BA, Keogh M. Length of gestation in congenital adrenal hyperplasia. J Obstet Gynaecol Br Commonw 1971; 78:430–434.

112. Kenney FM, Reynolds JW, Green OC. Partial 3β-hydroxysteroid dehydrogenase (3β-HSD) deficiency in a family with congenital adrenal hyperplasia: evidence for increasing 3β-HSD activity with age. Pediatrics 1971; 48:756–765.

113. Goldsmith O, Solomon DH, Horton R. Hypogonadism and mineralo-corticosteroid excess: the 17-hydroxylase deficiency syndrome. N Engl J Med 1967; 277:673–677.

114. New MI. Male pseudohermaphroditism due to a 17α-hydroxylase deficiency. J Clin Invest 1970; 49:1930–1941.

115. France JT, Liggins GC. Placental sulfatase deficiency. J Clin Endocrinol Metab 1969; 29:138–141.

116. France JT, Seddon RI, Liggins GC. A study of a pregnancy with low estrogen production due to placental sulfatase deficiency. J Clin Endocrinol Metab 1973; 36:1–9.

117. Bedin M, Alsat E, Tanguy G, et al. Placental sulfatase deficiency: clinical and biochemical study of 16 cases. Eur J Obstet Gynecol Reprod Biol 1980; 10:21–34.

118. Honnebier WJ, Swaab DF. The influence of anencephaly upon intra-uterine growth of fetus and placenta and upon gestation length. J Obstet Gynaecol Br Commonw 1973; 80:577–588.

119. Aizawa Y, Mueller GC. The effect in vivo and in vitro of estrogens on lipid synthesis in rat uterus. J Biol Chem 1961; 236:381–386.

120. Mueller GC. The role of RNA and protein synthesis in estrogen action. In: Karlson P, ed. Mechanisms of Hormone Action. New York: Academic, 1965: 228–239.

121. Jonsson HT Jr, Culp TW, Kaufman RH, et al. The influence of exogenous PMS and HCG on the arachidonic acid content of the immature rat ovary. Proc Soc Exp Biol Med 1975; 49:1005–1009.

122. Smith RE, Henzl MR. Role of mucopolysaccharides and lysosomal hydrolases in endometrial regression following withdrawal of estradiol and chlormadinone acetate. I. Epithelium and stroma. Endocrinology 1969; 85:50–66.

123. Henzl MR, Smith RE, Boost G, et al. Lysosomal concept of menstrual bleeding in humans. J Clin Endocrinol Metab 1972; 34:860–875.

124. Bedford CA, Challis JRG, Harrison FA, et al. The role of oestrogens and progesterone in the onset of parturition in various species. J Reprod Fertil 1972; 16(Suppl):1–23.

125. Challis JRG, Davies IJ, Benirschke K, et al. The concentrations of progesterone, estrone, estradiol-17β in the peripheral plasma of the rhesus monkey during the final third of gestation, and after the induction of abortion with PGF$_{2α}$. Endocrinology 1974; 95:547–553.

126. Batra S, Bengtsson LP, Grundsell H, et al. Levels of free protein-bound progesterone in plasma during late pregnancy. J Clin Endocrinol Metab 1976; 42:1041–1047.

127. Giannopoulos G, Tulchinsky D. Cytoplasmic and nuclear progestin receptors in human myometrium during the menstrual cycle and in pregnancy at term. J Clin Endocrinol Metab 1979; 49:100–106.

128. Embrey MP. PGE compounds for induction of labour and abortion. Ann NY Acad Sci 1971; 180:518–523.

129. Thiery J. Induction of labor with prostaglandins. In: Keirse MJNC, Anderson ABM, Bennebroek-Gravenhorst J, eds. Human Parturition. Leiden: Leiden University Press, 1979: 155–164.

130. Calder AA. Prostaglandins for pre-induction of cervical ripening. In: Karim SMM, ed. Practical Applications of Prostaglandins and Their Synthesis Inhibitors. Lancaster, England: M.T.P. Press, 1979: 301–318.

131. Zuckerman H, Karpaz-Kerpel S. Prostaglandins and their inhibitors in premature labor. In: Karim SMM, ed. Practical Applications of Prostaglandins and Their Synthesis Inhibitors. Lancaster, England: M.T.P. Press, 1979: 411–435.

132. Karim SMM. Identification of prostaglandins in human amniotic fluid. J Obstet Gynaecol Br Commonw 1966; 73:903–908.

133. Karim SMM, Devlin J. Prostaglandin content of amniotic fluid during pregnancy and labour. J Obstet Gynaecol Br Commonw 1967; 74:230–234.

134. Pattilo RA, Hussa RO, Terragno NA, et al. Absence of prostaglandin synthesis in the malignant human trophoblast in culture. Am J Obstet Gynecol 1973; 115:91–94.

135. MacDonald PC, Schultz FM, Duenhoelter JH, et al. Initiation of human parturition. I. Mechanism of action of arachidonic acid. Obstet Gynecol 1974; 44:629–636.

136. Dray F, Frydman R. Primary prostaglandin in amniotic fluid in pregnancy and spontaneous labor. Am J Obstet Gynecol 1976; 126:13–19.

137. Keirse MJNC. Endogenous prostaglandins in human parturition. In: Keirse MJNC, Anderson ABM, Bennebroek-Gravenhorst J, eds. Human Parturition. Leiden: Leiden University Press, 1979: 101–142.

138. Mitchell MD, Flint APF. Progesterone withdrawal: effects of prostaglandins and parturition. Prostaglandins 1977; 14:611–614.

139. Luukkainen TU, Csapo AI. Induction of premature labor in the rabbit after treatment with phospholipids. Fertil Steril 1963; 14:65–72.

140. Ogawa Y, Herod L, Lanman JT. Phospholipids and the onset of labor in rabbits. Gynecol Invest 1970; 1:240–248.

141. Lanman JT, Herod L, Thau R. Premature induction of labor with dilinoleyl lecithin in rabbits. Pediatr Res 1972; 6:701–704.

142. Lanman JT, Herod L, Thau R. Phospholipids and fatty acids in relation to the premature induction of labor in rabbits. Pediatr Res 1974; 8:1–4.

143. Nathanielsz PW, Abel M, Smith GW. Hormonal factors in parturition in the rabbit. In: Foetal and Neonatal Physiology, Proc Sir J Bancroft Centenary Symp. London: Cambridge University Press, 1973: 594–602.

144. Hertelendy F. Prostaglandin-induced premature oviposition in the co-turnix quail. Prostaglandins 1972; 2:269–279.

145. Van Dorp DA, Beerthuis RK, Nugteren HD, et al. The biosynthesis of prostaglandins. Biochim Biophys Acta 1964; 90:204–207.

146. Bergstrom S, Danielson H, Samuelsson B. The enzymatic formation of prostaglandin E$_2$ from arachidonic acid: prostaglandins and related factors. Biochim Biophys Acta 1964; 90:207–210.

147. Lands WEM, Samuelsson B. Phospholipid precursors of prostaglandins. Biochim Biophys Acta 1968; 164:426–429.

148. Vonkeman H, van Dorp DA: The action of prostaglandin synthetase on 2-arachidonyl-lecithin. Biochim Biophys Acta 1968; 164:430–432.

149. Okazaki T, Casey ML, Okita JR, et al. Initiation of parturition. XII. Biosynthesis and metabolism of prostaglandins in human fetal membranes and uterine decidua. Am J Obstet Gynecol 1981; 139:373–381.

150. Kinoshita K, Satoh K, Sakamoto S. Biosynthesis of prostaglandin in human decidua, amnion, chorion and villi. Endocrinol Jpn 1977; 23:343–350.

151. Mitchell MD: Prostaglandins during pregnancy and the perinatal period. J Reprod Fertil 1981; 62:305–315.

152. Schwarz BE, Schultz FM, MacDonald PC, et al. Initiation of human parturition. III. Fetal membrane content of prostaglandin E$_2$ and F$_{2α}$ precursor. Obstet Gynecol 1975; 46:564–568.

153. Keirse MJNC, Turnbull AC. E prostaglandins in amniotic fluid during pregnancy and labour. J Obstet Gynaecol Br Commonw 1973; 80:970–973.

154. Keirse MJNC, Flint APF, Turnbull AC: F prostaglandins in amniotic fluid during pregnancy and labour. J Obstet Gynaecol Br Commonw 1974; 81:131–135.

155. Okita JR, MacDonald PC, Johnston JM. Mobilization of arachidonic acid from specific glycerophospholipids of human fetal membranes during early labor. J Biol Chem 1982; 257:14029–14034.

156. Okazaki T, Okita JR, MacDonald PC, et al. Initiation of human parturition. X. Substrate specificity of phospholipase A$_2$ in human fetal membranes. Am J Obstet Gynecol 1978; 130:432–438.

157. DiRenzo GC, Johnston JM, Okazaki T, et al. Phosphatidylinositol-specific phospholipase C in fetal membranes and uterine decidua. J Clin Invest 1981; 67:847–856.

158. Okazaki T, Sagawa N, Okita JR, et al. Diacylglycerol metabolism and arachidonic acid release in human fetal membranes and decidua vera. J Biol Chem 1981; 256:7316–7321.

159. Okazaki T, Sagawa N, Bleasdale JE, et al. Initiation of human parturition. XIII. Phospholipase C, phospholipase A$_2$ and diacylglycerol lipase activities in fetal membranes and decidua vera tissues from early and late gestation. Biol Reprod 1981; 25:103–109.

160. Okita JR, MacDonald PC, Johnston JM. Initiation of human parturition. XIV. Increase in the diacylglycerol content of amnion during parturition. Am J Obstet Gynecol 1982; 142:432–435.

161. D'Souza SW, Haigh R, Micklewright L, et al. Amniotic fluid, epidermal growth factor and placental weight. Lancet 1985; 2:272–273.

162. Casey ML, Korte K, MacDonald PC. Epidermal growth factor—stimulation of prostaglandin E$_2$ biosynthesis in amnion cells: induction of PGH$_2$ synthase. J Biol Chem 1988; 263:7846–7854.

163. Romero R, Wu YK, Brody DT, et al. Human decidua: a source of interleukin-1. Obstet Gynecol 1989; 73:31–34.

164. Casey ML, Cox SM, Beutler B, et al. Cachectin/tumor necrosis factor-α formation in human decidua: potential role of cytokines in infection-induced preterm labor. J Clin Invest 1989; 83:430–436.

17

METABOLIC CHANGES IN PREGNANCY

Norbert Freinkel and Boyd E. Metzger

Pregnancy modifies fuel economy in a continuously evolving fashion. Appropriate management of disorders in the mother that may coexist with and/or be triggered by pregnancy makes it necessary to understand the changes in metabolism that occur as a function of normal gestation per se. The English obstetrician J. Matthews Duncan appreciated this fact more than a century ago when he introduced the first published description of diabetes in pregnancy with the generalization: "And it is my conviction that when our physiological knowledge is somewhat farther advanced, and when skilled observers have occupied the field, all diseases including surgical accidents will have their puerperal variations well defined and suitable therapeutics adjusted to them."[1] This chapter summarizes the metabolic realignments that characterize normal pregnancy and the implications for normal growth and development of the conceptus.

IMPLICATIONS OF PREGNANCY FOR MATERNAL METABOLISM

In the course of normal pregnancy, the average woman "eating to appetite" gains 12.5 kg of body weight.[2] The accretion is biphasic (Fig. 17–1). An accumulation of maternal body fat begins early and may be facilitated by an increased sensitivity to insulin. It achieves maximal expression during midpregnancy. In the rat this early extrauterine anabolism is manifested by increased accumulation of adipose tissue,[3] hepatic glycogen,[4] and even lean tissue.[5] In human pregnancies the increasing obesity can be documented by skinfold measurements and is typically centripetal with particular prominence over the back, upper thighs, and abdomen.[6] The increase in depot fat during the first

two trimesters has been estimated to consist of "more than 30,000 kcal" and may offset the "extra maintenance costs of late pregnancy."[7] It constitutes an anticipatory storage of nutrients that is analogous to the stockpiling that occurs in many species before physiological exercises that necessitate sustained access to endogenous reserves—e.g., hibernation in the bear, the spawning migrations of the salmon, and the migratory flights of hummingbirds. The adipogenesis of early pregnancy may have conferred survival advantages when mammalian reproductive patterns were evolving under conditions in which the availability of food was more precarious.[7] In general the increase in maternal fat accounts for about 3.5 kg of the total 12.5-kg gain in body weight. The remainder is due to the products of conception, growth of the uterus, development of the breasts, and expansion of maternal blood volume and interstitial fluids. The growth of the conceptus continues during the second half of gestation, whereas the net accretion of maternal fat occurs chiefly in the first half (see Fig. 17–1). The early *extrauterine* anabolism appears to be committed to the support of the later *intrauterine* anabolic events. These supportive functions are unmasked when food is withheld in late pregnancy. Thus adipose tissue turnover in the mother is accelerated,[3] hepatic glycogen level tends to decrease,[4] and muscle proteolysis is enhanced.[5]

The second half of pregnancy is noteworthy for the resistance to insulin action and a propensity to develop diabetes mellitus. In parallel with the growth of the conceptus, insulin requirements of diabetic mothers increase, diabetic tendencies develop in previously normal women, and the hypoglycemic potency of endogenous and exogenous insulin is diminished. Moreover, complications such as toxemia, hydramnios, and intrauterine death are more frequent in pregnant diabetics. The changes in carbohydrate and

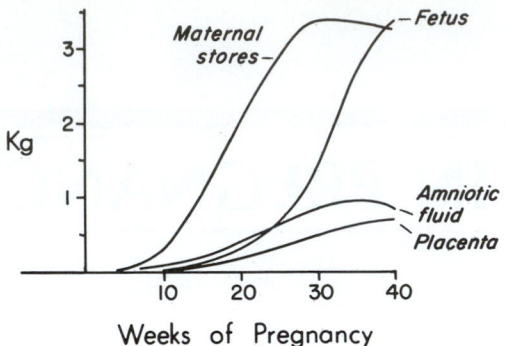

Figure 17–1. Aspects of anabolism manifested by changes in mass during pregnancy. (From Hytten FE, Leitch I. The Physiology of Human Pregnancy. 2nd ed. Oxford: Blackwell Scientific Publications, 1971.)

insulin economy are reversed in the immediate postpartum period. The temporal correlations make it likely that these phenomena are linked to some properties of the conceptus.[8, 9]

METABOLIC CONTRIBUTIONS OF THE CONCEPTUS. As a new and growing structure, the conceptus has a number of effects on maternal fuel homeostasis.[8]

Role in Maternal Endocrine Function (also see Chapter 20). The conceptus may function as a site for the removal of maternal hormones or for endocrine biosynthesis. Insulin does not cross the placenta, although some may be sequestered and bound there.[10] Insulin can be degraded in rat[11] and human[12] placentas, and this property coincides with acceleration of fractional turnover of radiolabeled insulin during late pregnancy in the rat.[9, 13] However, although insulin turnover is accelerated,[14] the extraction of maternal insulin by the placenta does not appear to be sufficient[15] to increase the fractional rate of maternal insulin turnover to a detectable degree[16–18] in monotocous species such as humans (in which the conceptus constitutes a smaller proportion of the total maternal mass).

Basal and glucose-stimulated levels of plasma insulin are increased in late human pregnancy.[19–23] The outpouring of insulin in response to oral or intravenous glucose in the last trimester of pregnancy is about 1.5 to 2.5 times greater than that under nongravid conditions.[9] By contrast, in early pregnancy, when maternal fat stores begin to expand[2] and the sensitivity to insulin is not blunted (and may be increased),[24] there is only a modest increase in insulin secretion in response to glucose.[25, 26] When the integrated secretory responses to oral glucose at different times in gestation are expressed as percentages of the values in nonpregnant subjects, the curve simulates the growth pattern of the conceptus (Fig. 17–2). The parallelism suggests that some endocrine properties of the conceptus might account for the diminished effectiveness of insulin in the mother and the enhanced secretion of insulin.

The hormonal secretions of the placenta may be implicated. The progressive increases in levels of plasma progesterone, estrogen, and the growth hormone–like human placental lactogen (hPL, also called human chorionic somatomammotropin, hCS) during pregnancy[27] parallel the curves for growth of the conceptus and the enhancement of insulin secretion (Fig. 17–3).[9] Longitudinal studies of the individual hormones indicate that the hormones change in concentration at different rates, especially in early pregnancy. For example, the elevated plasma levels of progesterone tend to remain constant between weeks 4 and 10 as the rising contributions from the placenta offset the diminishing output from the maternal corpus luteum. In contrast, the plasma estradiol level increases progressively from earliest pregnancy onward. Moreover, the relative increments with

time differ for the individual hormones.[28] Thus the concentrations of plasma progesterone at 38 wk are about seven times greater than the plateau values at 4 to 8 wk; estradiol levels increase about 130-fold between weeks 4 and 38; and prolactin values rise about 19-fold during the same interval. Plasma human chorionic gonadotropin (hCG) undergoes the most profound excursions, with a 290-fold increase during the first trimester and a further 16-fold increase above the 12-wk level during the second and third trimesters. The hCG is detectable about 6 to 8 d after conception, peaks at 10 wk of gestation, falls about 90% by week 24, and undergoes a slow but progressive increase thereafter until term.[28]

The early asynchronies and the subsequent disparities in availability of the "hormones of pregnancy" may be important in the changing patterns of maternal metabolism during early pregnancy. For example, the metabolic actions of progesterone and hCG could be dominant before new relationships supervene via the increasing levels of circulating estradiol and hPL. The endocrine elaborations of later pregnancy are more synchronized. Two aspects warrant comment. First, the changes in circulating hormone levels during the second and third trimesters for all the abovementioned hormones (except hCG) approximate straight lines when the measurements are transformed to logarithmic values.[28] Second, despite variations among women, individuals tend "to retain their rank in the spectrum of hormone values throughout the pregnancy,"[28] so that the maternal hormonal milieu for the entire pregnancy is fixed by the end of the third month of gestation. A similar relation holds for the circulating prolactin (of pituitary and decidual origin).[28]

The potential effects of the hormones of pregnancy on maternal fuel economy have been characterized with varying degrees of certitude.[24] For prolactin, the precise metabolic contributions during gestation remain to be defined. Despite conflicting reports,[29] the finding of mild reductions of glucose tolerance in the face of increased levels of plasma insulin in women with hyperprolactinemia suggests that prolactin may antagonize insulin action.[30] There are no clear-

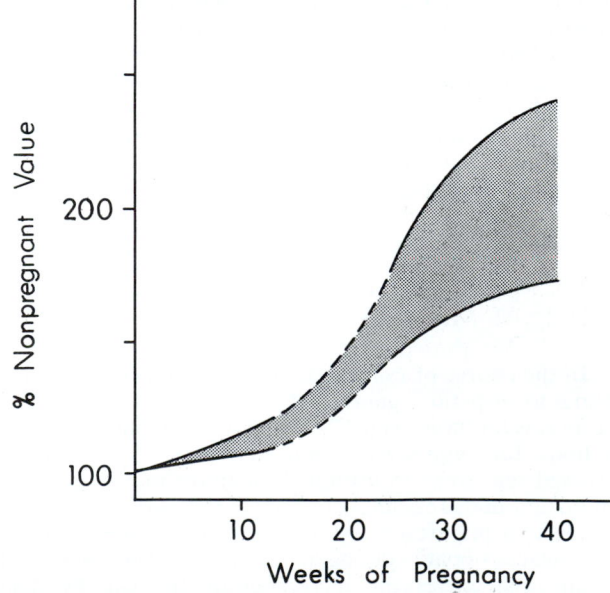

Figure 17–2. Changes in stimulated insulin secretion during normal pregnancy. Net increases in circulating insulin above basal values after glucose administration reported from many laboratories have been combined to characterize the serial secretory responses. (From Freinkel N. Banting Lecture 1980. Of pregnancy and progeny. Diabetes 1980; 29:1023–1025. Reproduced with permission from the American Diabetes Association, Inc.)

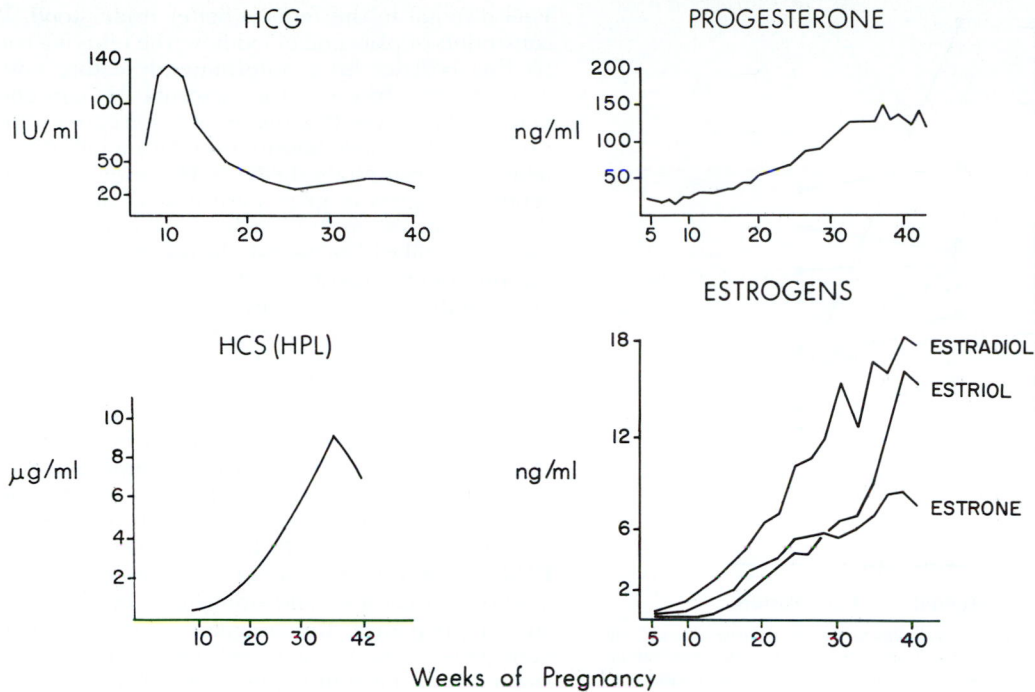

Figure 17–3. Changes in plasma levels of hormones of pregnancy during normal gestation. HCG, human chorionic gonadotropin; HCS (HPL), human placental lactogen. To convert values for hPL, progesterone, estradiol, estriol, and estrone to nanomoles per liter, multiply by 46.30, 3.180, 3.67, 3.47, and 3.70, respectively. (Adapted with permission from Pitkin RM, Spellacy WN. Physiologic adjustments in general. In: Laboratory Indices of Nutritional Status in Pregnancy, 1978. Published by National Academy Press, Washington, DC.)

cut extragonadal metabolic actions of hCG, although early studies with patients following restricted caloric diets[31] were consistent with a minor role of hCG in fat mobilization. More clear-cut metabolic actions have been demonstrated for the major placental hormones. Estrogens, progesterones, and hPL can augment islet secretory responsiveness,[24] and indeed receptors for estrogens[32] and progesterone[33] are present in pancreatic islets. hPL can exert lipolytic effects in vitro[34, 35] and can cause insulin resistance in nongravid subjects when infused overnight in amounts that are designed to replicate the plasma levels that are seen during late gestation.[36, 37] Estrogens can enhance the responsiveness of muscle to insulin action,[38, 39] whereas progesterone is a mild antagonist to insulin action in nonpregnant animals.[39] In combination, these actions of estrogen and progesterone may neutralize one another.[39] In other regards, the administration of the two hormones together may elicit responses that cannot be produced by either alone. The sequential changes in plasma glucose, alanine, and ketone levels that occur during starvation in normal subjects are not affected by treatment with either estrogens or progesterone alone, whereas the administration of both hormones enhances ketonemia, triglyceridemia, and hypoalaninemia and increases the concentration of free fatty acids (FFA) without modifying the changes in plasma glucose.[40] Similarly, brief administration of estrogen and progesterone in combination to postmenopausal women results in greater increments in total plasma ketone levels and greater reductions in alanine levels during 36-h fasts without altering plasma levels of insulin, glucose, and triglycerides beyond control values.[41] Thus placental hormones, which appear in ever-increasing amounts with increasing placental mass,[27, 28] create a metabolic state in which islet secretory performance is augmented, responsiveness to insulin is blunted, and ketogenesis is enhanced. The elaboration of these hormones by the placenta is affected minimally,[42–44] if at all,[45] by normal alimentary excursions of glucose. As a consequence, their actions are continuously operative, although expression may be influ-

enced by meal-related excursions in plasma insulin. The finding that intrinsic lipolysis and re-esterification are increased in isolated adipose tissue from pregnant rats[3] and humans,[46] even when sampling is performed in the fed state, is consistent with the known actions of the placental hormones.

Extrauterine endocrine influences may also operate. A role for glucocorticoids has been suggested.[47] Administration of corticosterone to nonpregnant rats alters the flux of glucose, alanine, and phenylalanine in muscle in a fashion that simulates the insulin-resistant pattern that is found after fasting in late pregnancy.[47] In human pregnancy the exposure of maternal tissues to glucocorticoids is increased two-fold above nongravid values,[48] and the level of circulating free cortisol is increased in the mother.[49] It seems unlikely that these increments are of fetal origin. Inappropriate adrenal biosynthesis related to autonomously functioning placental corticotropin or to placental corticotropin-releasing factor–like activity[50] also seems unlikely in view of the preservation of diurnal rhythms.[49] Thus the normally regulated hypothalamic-pituitary feedback is operative, although at a higher pituitary setting, perhaps owing to the increased availability of the gonadal steroids.

In terms of metabolic implications, none of the individual hormones of pregnancy can be discussed in isolation; they must rather be viewed in terms of interactive potentialities. Thus the absolute increments during earliest pregnancy are greatest for progesterone and hCG. Their integrated effects in association with the changes in estrogen may dominate the first trimester. Thereafter, the absolute increases in hPL (and to a lesser extent in prolactin) level may temper, if not actually condition, the subsequent metabolic responses to gonadal and adrenal steroids.

The determinants of resistance to insulin actions in the face of these complex hormonal relationships have been clarified. Insulin receptors on circulating monocytes or red blood cells are not diminished in late human pregnancy despite the increases in plasma insulin (Fig. 17–4).[51–55] In-

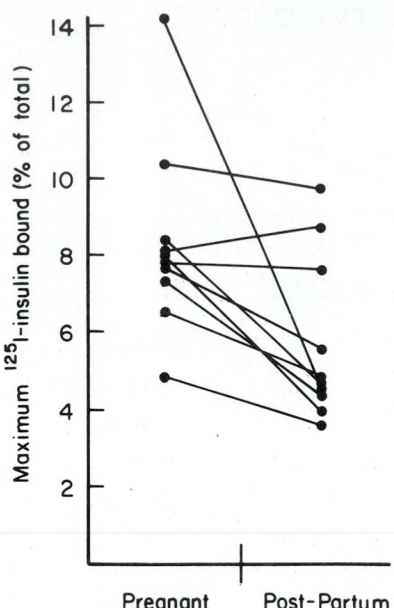

Figure 17-4. Maximal binding of ¹²⁵I-insulin to monocytes from women with normal carbohydrate metabolism and from the same women post partum. (Adapted from G Puavilai, EC Drobny, LA Domont, et al., Insulin receptors and insulin resistance in human pregnancy: evidence for a postreceptor defect in insulin action, J Clin Endocrinol Metab 54, 247–253, 1982, © by The Endocrine Society.)

deed, values for insulin binding are the same or greater than those observed in nongravid women in the luteal phase of the normal menstrual cycle.[55] There are no studies of insulin-receptor relationships in early pregnancy when the responsiveness to insulin is unchanged or increased and when the increases in circulating progesterone and estradiol are not attended by commensurate rises in hPL. However, the finding that insulin receptors on monocytes are unchanged when nongravid women are given oral contraceptives (i.e., combinations of ethinyl estradiol and norethindrone) in amounts sufficient to alter glucose tolerance and increase insulin levels[52] suggests that insulin binding is also physiologically normal in early gestation. Hence, the changes in responsiveness to insulin during pregnancy and the insulin resistance of late human pregnancy appear to reflect events distal to the binding of insulin to its receptor. These realignments could be mediated by the metabolic actions of the hormones of pregnancy, the growth of the conceptus per se, or a combination of both. Pregnancy does not appreciably alter plasma glucagon levels,[56-58] the binding of glucagon to isolated rat liver plasma membranes,[59] or the activation of adenylate cyclase by glucagon in such membranes.[59] Thus inappropriate glucagon secretion or enhanced hepatic responsiveness to glucagon need not be invoked.

Role in Maternal Fuel Disposition. The conceptus consumes considerable amounts of maternal fuels.[8] In the fed state, ingested nutrients reach the placenta and may be utilized for anabolism. Many facets of carbohydrate and lipid metabolism of the human placenta are responsive to insulin action.[8, 60] In addition, nutrients can cross the placenta and gain access to the fetus (see later).[61, 62]

For the mother, the implications of fuel disposal by the conceptus may be of particular significance in the fasted state. Increases in maternal FFA levels can cause compositional changes in the placenta,[8] and placental glycogenosis and steatosis may be induced by increased exposure to FFA and esterified fatty acids.[63-65] It is not known whether these changes are attended by alterations in placental function.

Fuel disposal in the fetus is better understood. Within the constraints of placental blood flow, the fetus is a continuously feeding boarder in an intermittently eating host. Ketones and glycerol traverse the placenta in concentration-dependent fashion so that the fetus is presented with abundant products of fat metabolism after fat mobilization and ketonemia are well established.[66-70] However, because the conceptus continues to grow even during periods of maternal dietary deprivation,[69, 71-73] other nutrients must also be employed. Uptake of maternal glucose, amino acids, and other carbon donors persists at all times, although the fetus may exert modulating influences.[69]

The needs of the human fetus include glucose utilization at the rate of approximately 0.03 mmol (6 mg)/kg body weight/min at term,[74] in contrast to glucose turnover of about 0.014 mmol (2.5 mg)/kg body weight/min in normal adults.[75] Growth of the human fetus in the third trimester also requires the net transfer of 54 mmol nitrogen/d across the placenta.[76] Furthermore, in sheep amino acids may be catabolized for oxidative energy needs of the conceptus.[77]

MODIFICATIONS OF THE FASTED STATE IN MOTHERS DURING PREGNANCY. Because of the continuous removal of glucose, lactic acid, and amino acids by the fetus, especially late in pregnancy, the pregnant mother cannot conserve endogenous fuels in the fasted state with the parsimony that characterizes the nonpregnant state. These factors prompted the suggestion more than two decades ago that pregnant women exhibit normal adaptations to dietary deprivation more rapidly in late pregnancy (accelerated starvation).[8] The more rapid shift to fat catabolism in the mother "spares" maternal glucose and amino acids for use by the fetus while minimizing the insult to maternal nitrogen and carbohydrate reserves. The persistent elaboration of placental hormones that accelerate lipolysis and antagonize insulin action might, of itself, enhance metabolism of fat and gluconeogenesis.[8] Indeed, the "increasing placental elaboration of anti-insulin factors in parallel with the growth of the fetus provides just the right temporal juxtaposition to make it all work."[73]

Substantive evidence supports the concept of accelerated starvation during the fasted state in late pregnancy.[9] More rapid mobilization of fat occurs in isolated fat pads from gravid animals[3] and in intact animals.[3, 72] Exaggerated increases in plasma and urinary ketones[72] attest to greater activation of ketogenesis.[71] The decline in plasma glucose level is enhanced in subhuman primates[78] and rodents.[71, 72] Greater intrahepatic gluconeogenic activation occurs in vivo[72, 73] and in vitro[79] and is associated with exaggerated losses of urinary nitrogen during early fasting.[72] A decrease in gluconeogenic amino acids in plasma[80, 81] results in impaired gluconeogenesis in late pregnancy; hence the hypoglycemia that occurs with fasting in late pregnancy represents a "substrate deficiency syndrome."[82] Despite the accelerated starvation, compensation for extra fuel losses is not complete, as documented by greater maternal muscle catabolism during fasting.[72, 82] Humans, like rats, display features of accelerated starvation such as enhanced ketonemia, increased urinary nitrogen excretion, and exaggerated reductions in gluconeogenic amino acids as early as midpregnancy.[81-85]

Relative Contributions of Endocrine and Metabolic Effects of the Conceptus. Replication of certain aspects of accelerated starvation by the administration of gonadal steroids to nongravid subjects (see earlier) has prompted some reservations about the degree to which these features can be ascribed to fuel removal by the conceptus. This concern has been supported by the observations that women who are not pregnant experience greater reductions in levels of plasma glucose and increases in FFA than men after prolonged fasting.[86] Is the pregnant woman behaving like a "super female" during dietary deprivation, or are effects on maternal metabolism conferred by the fuel functions of the conceptus? As outlined earlier, certain unique features devolve from the presence of the conceptus, at least in late pregnancy. For example, the exaggerated fall of plasma glucose and increases in FFA during fasting in pregnancy cannot be replicated by the administration of gonadal steroids to laboratory animals[40] or to human volunteers during dietary deprivation.[41] Moreover, the blunted responses of isolated skeletal muscle from pregnant animals to the actions of insulin in regard to glucose uptake, alanine release, and proteolysis cannot be reproduced with exogenous gonadal steroids,[39] although some inhibition is produced in the nongravid rat by the administration of glucocorticoids in amounts that approximate the levels of late pregnancy.[47] Some case reports also suggest that the metabolic realignments are due to the presence of the conceptus rather than to changes in extrauterine hormones. For example, in a woman who had been hypophysectomized during week 26 and maintained on *constant* amounts of cortisone and thyroid extract thereafter, glucose intolerance and insulin resistance occurred at week 31 of gestation, and amelioration of both alterations occurred during the early postpartum period (Fig. 17–5).[87]

Several lines of inquiry have been pursued in our laboratory to differentiate between the contributions of the hormones of pregnancy and the fuel needs of the growing conceptus in the rat. First, we have compared the responses to fasting for 48 h (during days 18 to 20 of the 22-d gestation) in sham-operated pregnant rats and in pregnant rats from whom fetuses alone or fetuses plus placentas had been excised.[78, 82] The presence of the placenta even in the absence of the fetus suffices to preserve the increases in hepatic size[72]

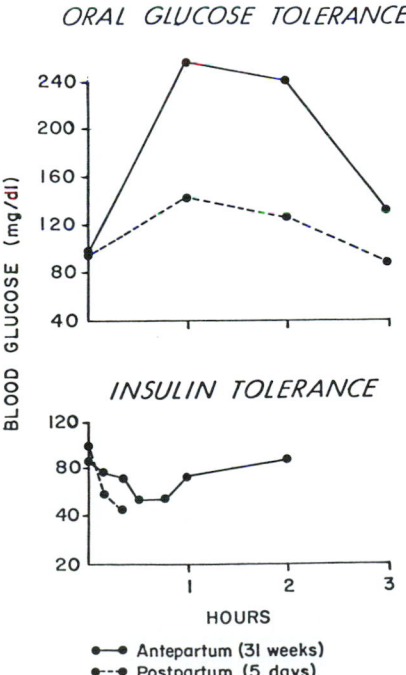

ORAL GLUCOSE TOLERANCE

INSULIN TOLERANCE

Figure 17–5. Effects of pregnancy on oral glucose tolerance and insulin tolerance in the absence of the pituitary. Total hypophysectomy was performed for breast cancer during week 26 of pregnancy, and the patient was maintained thereafter on constant replacement therapy with cortisone and thyroid extract during antepartum and postpartum studies of glucoregulation. To convert glucose units to millimoles per liter, multiply by 0.05551. (Adapted from B Little, OW Smith, AG Jessiman, et al., Hypophysectomy during pregnancy in a patient with cancer of the breast: case report with hormone studies, J Clin Endocrinol Metab 18, 425–443, 1958, © by The Endocrine Society.)

and the alterations in intrahepatic nitrogen disposition during gluconeogenesis (i.e., diminished urea synthesis and enhanced ammonia formation)[79] that occur during normal gestation. On the other hand, full replication of accelerated starvation in terms of ketonemia and hypoglycemia during fasting occurs only when fetuses as well as placentas are retained.[78, 82] These experiences with partial extirpations of the products of conception confirm earlier reports[71, 88–90] and support the proposition that the abstraction of glucose and gluconeogenic precursors by the fetus is necessary for the full expression of accelerated starvation in late gestation, although certain components of that response may be mediated by the increases in the hormones of pregnancy per se.

A similar conclusion has evolved from studies of [14C]glucose turnover during pregnancy in the rat.[91] Overall increases in maternal glucose production (to offset enhanced glucose removal by the conceptus) and exaggerated lowerings of plasma glucose with fasting are demonstrable in late pregnancy. However, identical lowerings of plasma glucose occur during fasting earlier in pregnancy before gestation-related increases in *total* glucose turnover can be demonstrated. The temporal dichotomies between the effects of pregnancy on "steady-state" fasting plasma glucose levels and rates of glucose turnover[91] suggest that at least initially the former may be mediated by the hormones of pregnancy, whereas the latter are linked to the mounting fuel needs of the conceptus.

This early resetting of steady-state plasma glucose concentrations at lower levels during fasting in pregnancy may conserve maternal glucose stores,[9] because transplacental glucose flux is proportional to ambient plasma glucose[61, 62, 92] (up to a saturable maximum).[93] This concept is strengthened by studies during late gestation in the sheep. Approximately one third of maternal glucose production in pregnant sheep is abstracted by the conceptus under conditions of normoglycemia (approximately 70% is deployed for uteroplacental metabolism, and 30% is used by the fetus).[94] These apportionments are not altered during maternal hypoglycemia, so that the absolute rate of glucose uptake by the conceptus is determined by the levels of maternal glucose.[94] However, in sheep[94] as in rat[69] pregnancy the fetus has some potential for glucose production, which may offset the fall in the delivery of glucose from the mother during maternal hypoglycemia. On the other hand, in human pregnancy at term, production of glucose by the mother is enhanced, but there is no measurable production of glucose by the fetus.[95]

Practical Significance of Accelerated Starvation. To evaluate whether accelerated starvation is significant under ordinary conditions,[96, 97] breakfast was withheld from pregnant women (at 32 to 38 wk of gestation) and from age- and weight-matched control women after a standard supper at 6 PM on the preceding evening. Blood samples were secured from indwelling venous catheters after 12, 14, 16, and 18 h of fasting (Fig. 17–6). Although the plasma glucose level was lower in pregnant women than in nonpregnant women after this 12-h fast, FFA, β-hydroxybutyrate, and alanine levels were not different.[96] Minor prolongations of the fast affect the latter fuels (see Fig. 17–6). Thus after a 16-h fast, plasma concentrations of FFA and β-hydroxybutyrate are higher, and alanine and glucose levels are lower. By 18 h of fasting, all the features of accelerated starvation are evident in pregnant subjects, whereas circulating fuels remain relatively unaffected in nonpregnant controls.[96, 97] Clearly, accelerated starvation is a real event in late pregnancy, even in pregnancies with normal carbohydrate metabolism, and the variability in the published values for fuel levels after an overnight fast in late normal pregnancy[98, 99] may be due to minor variations in the length of the fast.[96, 97] Insofar as increased ketonemia is undesirable in pregnancy (see

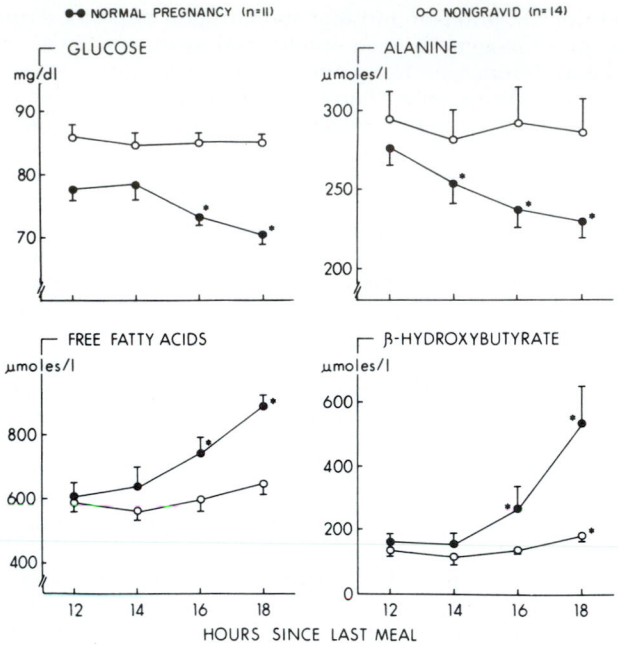

Figure 17–6. Accelerated starvation during brief dietary deprivation in late pregnancy. Dinner was administered at 6 PM to nonobese normal gravidas and to age- and weight-matched nonpregnant control subjects. Plasma samples were secured after a 12-h fast at 6 AM and at 2-h intervals thereafter. Food was withheld until lunch was served at noon (i.e., after an 18-h fast). To convert glucose values to millimoles per liter, multiply by 0.05551. (Adapted from Metzger BE, Ravnikar V, Vileisis RA, et al. "Accelerated starvation" and the skipped breakfast in late normal pregnancy. Lancet 1982; 1:588–592.)

later),[100, 101] delaying meals for medical tests should be avoided during late gestation.

MODIFICATIONS OF THE FED STATE IN MOTHERS DURING PREGNANCY. The combined contributions of the hormones of pregnancy and the fuel needs of the conceptus confer on the mother a heightened propensity for metabolism of fat in the fasted state. Significant alterations are also seen in the fed state. Administration of oral glucose (100 g) for the standard oral glucose tolerance test after a 14-h fast in late gestation provides the best example (Fig. 17–7). Such a glucose challenge elicits greater and more prolonged increases in plasma glucose than those in nonpregnant controls.[102] Concurrent increases in plasma triglyceride levels (located chiefly in the very-low-density lipoprotein [VLDL] fraction[103]) and greater decreases in plasma glucagon levels[56–58] are also evident. The sequence may facilitate anabolism.[103, 104] The exaggerated hyperglycemia after glucose ingestion causes more of the glucose to cross the placenta because of the concentration dependency of glucose transfer across the placenta (see earlier). The increased plasma triglycerides may simultaneously substitute for some of the circulating glucose as a maternal oxidative fuel, thereby sparing glucose for transplacental flux. Moreover, because triglycerides cross the placenta poorly,[105] the hypertriglyceridemia should enable some of the ingested glucose to be stored as fat for subsequent recall as glyceride-glycerol or fatty acid during lipolysis in the fasted state. Finally, the greater suppression of glucagon after glucose ingestion could facilitate anabolism, because it attenuates persistent contributions of glucagon to intrahepatic aspects of accelerated starvation such as glycogenolysis, gluconeogenesis, and ketogenesis.

A transitory fall in hPL and hCG levels during the standard oral glucose tolerance test has been observed by some[42–44] but not all[45] workers (see Fig. 17–7). Insofar as these peptides may play a moment-to-moment role in activating lipolysis, decreased concentrations in plasma could facilitate anabolism by enhancing repletion of adipose stores during glucose feeding.

The capacity of amino acids to stimulate glucagon secretion is preserved in pregnancy despite the exaggerated release of insulin from beta cells.[106] The sequence is consistent with facilitated anabolism in the fed state: increased release of insulin could blunt the gluconeogenic potential of glucagon during postprandial hyperglycemia and so spare ingested amino acids for maternal or fetal access. After disposition of the carbohydrate, the persistent hyperaminoacidemia-maintained glucagon release and a fall in insulin could re-establish gluconeogenesis and so prevent postprandial hypoglycemia and premature return to accelerated starvation.

INTEGRATED CHANGES IN MATERNAL FUELS DURING EATING OF MEALS. As a result of the changes that accompany late gestation, the diurnal patterns of maternal fuel economy are modified.[107] The resultant metabolic profiles have been characterized by collecting blood samples from

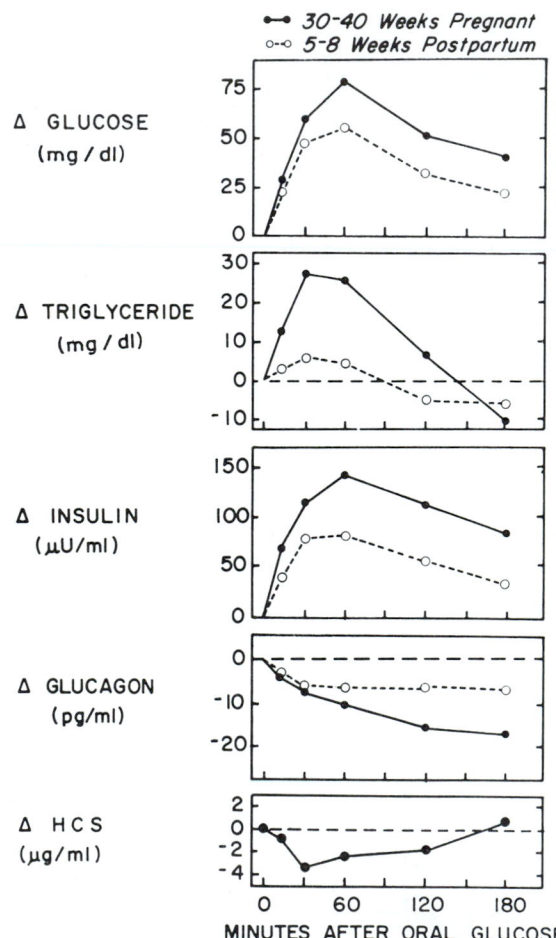

Figure 17–7. Facilitated anabolism in late pregnancy. Women with normal carbohydrate metabolism were challenged with oral glucose (100 g) after a 14-h overnight fast during late gestation, and again 5 to 8 wk post partum. Changes in levels of plasma glucose, triglycerides, immunoreactive insulin, glucagon, and hPL (HCS in figure) are expressed as absolute increments or decrements from levels that existed before glucose administration. To convert values for glucose, triglyceride, and hPL to millimoles per liter, multiply by 0.05551, 0.01129, and 46.30, respectively. To convert insulin values to picomoles per liter, multiply by 7.175. (Adapted from Freinkel N, Metzger BE, Nitzan M, et al. Facilitated anabolism in late pregnancy: some novel maternal compensations for accelerated starvation. In: Malaise WJ, Pirart J, eds. Proceedings of VIIIth Congress of International Diabetes Foundation. International Series No. 312. Amsterdam: Excerpta Medica, 1974: 474–488.)

pregnant women throughout the day under conditions of random or controlled meal eating.[99, 104, 107-117] Some results with such round-the-clock samplings[115] are summarized in Figures 17–8 and 17–9. Diurnal effects on facilitated anabolism from ingested nutrients were evaluated during the 5-h postprandial intervals after three daily meals, and sufficient time was interposed between supper and breakfast (i.e., 14 h) to allow evaluation of the accelerated starvation during an overnight fast.

Plasma glucose consistently falls to lower levels after meals and after overnight fasts in late pregnancy than in controls despite the exaggerated increases in plasma glucose with eating (see Fig. 17–8). Similarly, values for individual amino acids (with the exception of threonine) are consistently lower. The differences are not obliterated by eating; meal-induced increments for individual amino acids tend to be of lesser duration and of lower magnitude during late pregnancy.[115] FFA levels after the 14-h overnight fast differ inconsistently (Fig. 17–8 vs. Fig. 17–6) among gravid and nongravid subjects. However, the heightened propensity to fat mobilization is readily apparent from the rapid rebound of plasma FFA levels after each meal in late pregnancy even though the nocturnal spike in FFA is blunted (see Fig. 17–

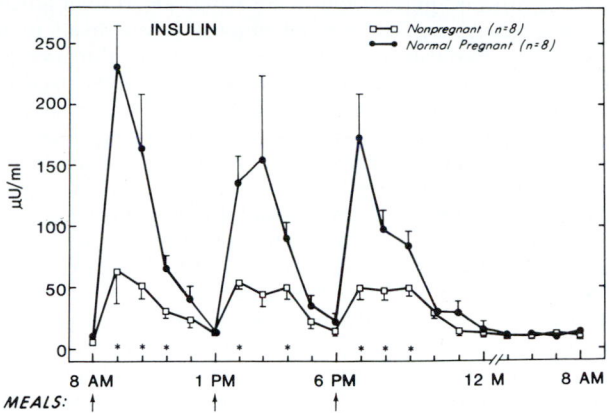

DIURNAL CHANGES IN INSULIN

Figure 17–9. Effects of late pregnancy on diurnal excursions in plasma immunoreactive insulin. The illustration summarizes insulin values for the studies shown in Figure 17–8. To convert insulin values to picomoles per liter, multiply by 7.175. (From Phelps RL, Metzger BE, Freinkel N. Carbohydrate metabolism in pregnancy. XVII. Diurnal profiles of plasma glucose, insulin, free fatty acids, triglycerides, cholesterol, and individual amino acids in late normal pregnancy. Am J Obstet Gynecol 1981; 140:730–736.)

8). Premeal levels of plasma triglycerides tend to be greater than those in controls, although exaggerated postmeal increments are difficult to demonstrate with mixed meals (see Fig. 17–8). The heightened oscillations in plasma glucose levels constitute the most striking pregnancy-related change in metabolic profiles. The greater premeal decrements and postmeal increments in circulating glucose concentrations that occur *with every meal*[115] are consistent with the patterns that are predicted on the basis of accelerated starvation and facilitated anabolism.[107]

Mean 24-h values for plasma immunoreactive insulin are increased approximately twofold in late pregnancy.[115] However, insulin secretion is more accurately reflected by the acute postprandial increases (see Fig. 17–9). Thus the plasma insulin peaks after meals are greater in late pregnancy than under nongravid conditions, and the integrated increases in plasma insulin during the 5 h after meals are enhanced approximately threefold (see Fig. 17–9). The findings support the rationale of giving some soluble insulin with each meal in insulin-dependent pregnant diabetics.[9]

Some changes in intermediary metabolism that occur during normal pregnancy are unexplained. For example, it is not known whether the blunted increases in plasma amino acid levels with meals[115] reflect gestational changes in the digestion of proteins or alterations in gastrointestinal absorption, extracellular distribution (e.g., addition of the conceptus to the distribution compartment), renal losses, or intracellular disposition of amino acids. Published assessments of the fate of amino acid after meals in pregnancy are not adequate to resolve these possibilities. Similarly, it is not known whether some of the postbinding resistance to insulin action in late gestation is linked to the altered fuel relationships. The possibility that the increased diversion to products of fat metabolism may be playing a major role (in a manner consistent with the glucose–fatty acid cycle of Randle and colleagues[118]) has served as a working hypothesis.[8, 9, 107] In this regard, Ferrannini and co-workers have obtained evidence that the glucose–fatty acid cycle operates in humans.[119] They used the hyperinsulinemic clamp technique under euglycemic and hyperglycemic conditions in nonpregnant normal subjects to demonstrate that fatty acids compete with glucose for uptake and utilization by peripheral tissues.[119] Circulating FFA were maintained at high levels

DIURNAL CHANGES IN GLUCOSE AND LIPIDS

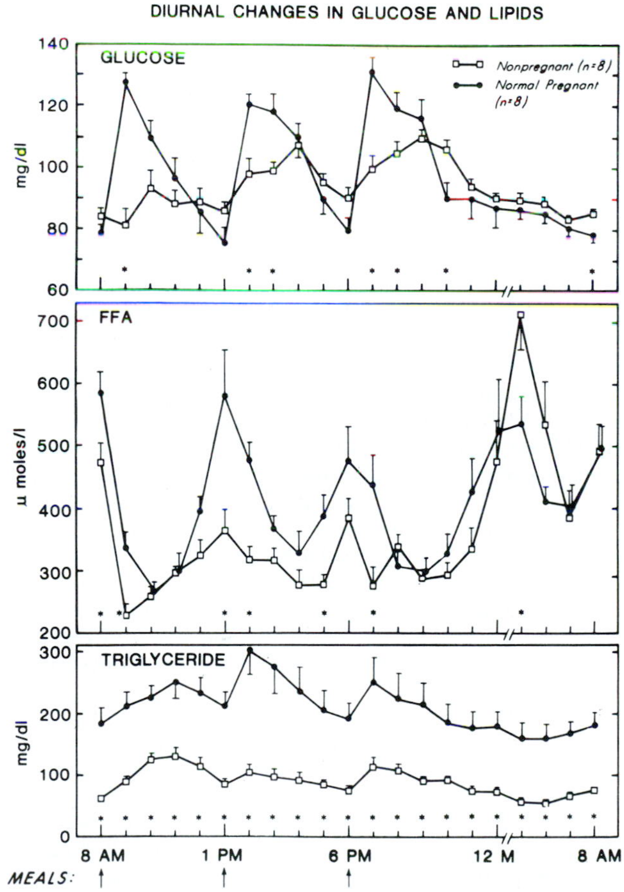

Figure 17–8. Effects of late pregnancy on diurnal excursions in plasma glucose, FFA, and triglyceride levels. Normal gravidas (weeks 33 to 39 of gestation) and age- and weight-matched, nonpregnant control subjects were given liquid formula diets (2110 kcal/d containing 275 g carbohydrate and 75 g protein) in three equal feedings at 8 AM, 1 PM, and 6 PM. Blood samples were secured from indwelling catheters at hourly intervals. Individual values are expressed as means ± SEM. Asterisks (*) denote time points at which mean values for the two groups are significantly different (p < .05). Glucose and triglyceride values can be converted to millimoles per liter as in Figure 17–7. (From Phelps RL, Metzger BE, Freinkel N. Carbohydrate metabolism in pregnancy. XVII. Diurnal profiles of plasma glucose, insulin, free fatty acids, triglycerides, cholesterol, and individual amino acids in late normal pregnancy. Am J Obstet Gynecol 1981; 140:730–736.)

by providing a triglyceride emulsion together with heparin.[120] Continued generation of FFA depressed total glucose flux at high as well as normal glucose levels, even in the presence of hyperinsulinemia; FFA activated gluconeogenesis when insulin was lacking.[119] Reaven[121] summarized evidence that such changes sustain the metabolic alterations of non–insulin-dependent diabetes mellitus. The parallelisms to late pregnancy are also striking. In pregnancy the continued and ever-increasing lipolytic input from the placental hormones may enhance generation of fatty acids from intracellular stores to compete with ambient glucose for the oxidative needs of the mother (Fig. 17–10). The exaggerated FFA concentrations of late pregnancy, which become manifest during postprandial rebounds (see Fig. 17–8) or after starvation exceeding 14 h (see Fig. 17–6), may thus reflect spillover into the circulation of these continuously generated products of intracellular lipolysis. Their release into plasma would be favored by the declines in plasma glucose and insulin levels that occur at these times and by the diminished potential for intracellular recapture by re-esterification in situ.

The correlations between basal levels of FFA[103, 104, 107] and triglycerides[104] and the exaggerated rises in plasma glucose levels after oral glucose in late normal pregnancy are consistent with the above-mentioned formulation. The normal impedance to glucose disposition after eating, despite the increased availability of insulin, may be linked to the plethora of lipids as alternative fuels. Within that framework, the correlations between maternal FFA and birth weight in the offspring of diabetic mothers[122] may be the consequence of a fatty acid–induced prolongation of postprandial hyperglycemia and a consequently increased transplacental delivery of glucose.

IMPLICATIONS OF MATERNAL METABOLISM FOR THE FETUS

Pregnancy thus modifies every facet of fuel metabolism in the mother. It follows that criteria for nongravid "normality" cannot be used to evaluate the status of metabolic regulation during pregnancy or to gauge the efficacy of measures designed to rectify maternal abnormalities. The implications for the fetus should also be considered in evaluating the metabolic realignments that occur during pregnancy. Maternal fuels are the building blocks for all fetal development. Appreciation of this relationship prompted the suggestion that the metabolic aspects of pregnancy should be viewed as a "tissue-culture experience."[104, 112] The tissue culture formulation stresses that the placenta and the fetus develop in an incubation medium that is derived

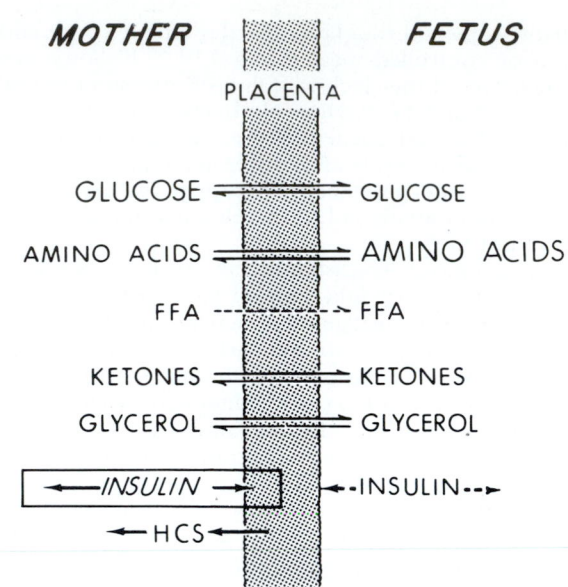

Figure 17–11. Pregnancy as a tissue culture experience. Most maternal fuels can cross the placenta in concentration-dependent fashion; maternal insulin can influence their quantitative and qualitative availability. This illustration underscores factors in maternal metabolism that may delimit the metabolic mixture (i.e., tissue culture medium) available for development of new cells in the fetus. (From Freinkel N. Banting Lecture 1980. Of pregnancy and progeny. Diabetes 1980; 29:1023–1025. Reproduced with permission from the American Diabetes Association, Inc.)

from maternal fuels. As shown schematically in Figure 17–11, maternal glucose traverses the placenta by stereospecific, carrier-mediated, facilitated diffusion,[92, 93] amino acids are transported actively in a fashion that is concentration dependent for the neutral and basic amino acids;[123] ketones and glycerol gain ready access in proportion to maternal blood levels in the rat and the human;[66–68, 70] and despite some variation in different species, FFA may be metabolized directly within the placenta[8, 64] or transported across it in sufficient amounts to provide at least the necessary essential fatty acids.[124] Derivative biotransformations may arise within the placenta (e.g., the abundant generation of lactic acid from glucose[8, 60, 125]) or the fetus (e.g., gluconeogenesis in some species[69, 94]). Additional rate-limiting determinants may also influence the incubation medium, such as uterine and/or placental blood flow,[93, 126] mechanical and/or biochemical restrictions to placental transfer, and even "genetic factors."[127] Nonetheless, in view of the parallelism between the circulating levels of nutrients in the mother and the fetus, the mother's fuels generally provide a valid sample of the tissue culture medium.[112]

All of these maternal fuels, in the fed and the fasted states, are affected quantitatively and qualitatively by maternal insulin (see Fig. 17–11). Thus although maternal insulin does not cross the placenta, it is the ultimate arbiter of the system, and pregnancy that is complicated by diabetes constitutes the optimal "experiment of nature" for demonstrating the dependence of fetal development on maternal fuel economy.[9]

OVERALL RELATIONSHIPS TO MATERNAL INSULINIZATION. Certain aspects of the tissue culture relationship warrant emphasis.

First, maternal insulin secretion is a major factor in determining the characteristics of the incubation medium. Delayed insulin release during meals results in delayed disposition of ingested nutrients (underutilization); inadequate basal insulin release in the fasted state results in excessive generation of fuels from endogenous maternal

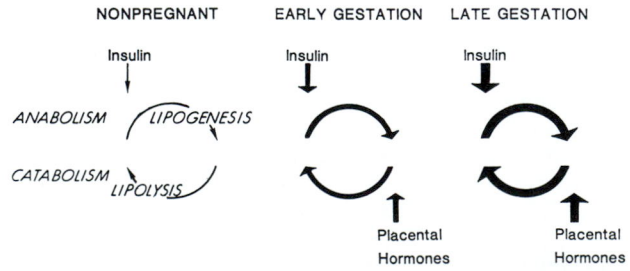

Figure 17–10. Serial changes in lipid turnover during pregnancy. As the pregnancy progresses, the ever-increasing availability of placental hormones with lipolytic potential (such as hPL) and the heightened outpouring of insulin in the fed state effect changing interactions among net lipolysis, net lipogenesis, and re-esterification in situ.

stores (overproduction). Either situation allows hyperglycemia to persist in the maternal circulation for longer periods so that increased amounts of glucose reach the fetus.

Second, maternal insulin also influences qualitative features of the incubation medium. For example, insulin affects the generation of endogenous fuels such as ketones (which also seem to cross the placenta according to maternal blood levels) (see Fig. 17–11). In the fetus, as in the adult, ketones can supplant less expendable fuels for oxidative fulfillment.[70, 128–130] However, although such "sparing" by ketones may be desirable in mature cells,[75, 131] the implications in utero may not be innocuous (see later).

Third, the interrelationships between fuels and developing fetal tissues must be considered. For example, the formation and function of beta cells in the fetal pancreas may be affected by the nutrient secretagogues in the fetal circulation.[132] Increased delivery of nutrients from the mother causes more insulin to be released by the fetus, and the "extra" fetal insulin enables more maternal nutrients to be retained by insulin-responsive tissues within the fetus.[112, 133–135] (This positive feedback has prompted efforts to use neonatal insulin secretion as a retrospective index of the integrated exposure of fetal cells to maternal fuels in utero.)[136]

This relationship between nutrients in the fetus and fetal beta cell development underscores an important aspect of the tissue culture formulation, i.e., all cells do not have equal capabilities for replication. Cells in tissues such as those in the gastrointestinal tract, liver, kidney, skin, and hematopoietic system may be renewed throughout the lifetime of the host. Other cells, such as brain cells,[137, 138] adipocytes,[139] muscle cells,[140] and perhaps even the beta cells of the pancreas,[132, 141] have more limited replicative potential; their renewal may be restricted to finite intervals (of which intrauterine life may constitute a major proportion). The consequences of altered maternal metabolism may be different for the two types of cells. In freely replicating cells with rapid rates of turnover, the characteristics of the intrauterine metabolic mixture need not have long-range implications. On the other hand, permanent changes in cell number, structure, and/or function could arise in poorly replicating, terminally differentiated cells as a consequence of the intrauterine environment. The possibility for fuel-mediated teratogenesis[9, 142] may be of significance, depending on the stage of gestation.[9, 143] Space precludes detailed consideration of the full ramifications, but a few examples will be cited.

Late Pregnancy. The latter third of pregnancy is the period of most rapid growth for adipocytes, muscle cells, and beta cells of the pancreas. The concept that these structures may be affected by fuel excess during fetal life was first advanced by Pedersen in 1954.[133] He sought to explain the macrosomia that occurs in the offspring of diabetic mothers by suggesting that maternal hyperglycemia provides more glucose for the fetus and that fetal hyperglycemia stimulates fetal insulin and causes increased deposition of fat and glycogen. This "hyperglycemia-hyperinsulinism hypothesis"[134] is supported by the demonstration of islet hyperplasia[144–146] and disparate increases in the mass of insulin-sensitive structures[146–148] in the macrosomic infants of diabetic mothers. In addition, evolving macrosomia (as judged by serial ultrasound measurements) and premature islet maturation (as judged by the insulin content of amniotic fluid) are correlated in such infants.[135] Indeed, the replicative capabilities and secretory responsiveness of fetal islet cells can be enhanced directly by the addition of supranormal amounts of glucose during prolonged tissue culture.[149–152]

One may ask whether changes in the offspring of mothers with gestational diabetes presage abnormalities in the same structures during later life. For example, are

macrosomic newborns with increased adiposity and islet responsiveness after intrauterine "stuffing" at increased risk for adult obesity, diabetes, or disturbances in appetite regulation?[9, 112, 142] Some evidence is consistent with this possibility. Aerts and Van Assche described inadequate pancreatic beta cell responses during pregnancy in the offspring of normal rats that were rendered diabetic by the administration of streptozocin.[153] Gestational beta cell limitations persisted in the second and third generations of such rats, which raises the possibility that gestational diabetes could represent an acquired disorder. Similar observations have been made in the Pima Indians—a group in whom the incidence of non–insulin-dependent diabetes mellitus is high. More obesity[154] and a higher frequency of diabetes[155] occur in the offspring (up to age 19) of Pima mothers who are diabetic during pregnancy than in the offspring of mothers who remain nondiabetic or do not become diabetic until *after* pregnancy. Development during childhood of the offspring of diabetic mothers who were enrolled between 1978 and 1983 in prospective studies of the Northwestern University Medical School Diabetes and Pregnancy Center is consistent with this fuel-mediated anthropometric teratogenesis. Follow-up through 6 y of age disclosed an increasing prevalence of obesity that is correlated with the relative degree of obesity (diabetic macrosomia) at birth,[156] antepartum maternal metabolic alterations,[156] and fetal islet function during intrauterine development.[157] All of the observations cited earlier are consistent with the concept[9, 112] that the intrauterine environment exerts long-range effects on certain poorly replicating, terminally differentiated cells, such as adipocytes and pancreatic beta cells.

Midpregnancy. The second trimester is a critical period for development of the human brain. Although oligodendroglial proliferation, myelin synthesis, synaptic connections, and neurochemical maturations take place in the third trimester and during the first 2 y of life, all the brain cells that will be present throughout life form in the second trimester.[137] The possibility that ketones may affect these processes has been an area of considerable controversy since the provocative, perhaps flawed, suggestions[100, 101] that ketonuria during pregnancy may be associated with diminished intelligence in the offspring.

Our laboratory[70, 129] and others[128, 130, 158] have shown that fetal brain cells, like those of the adult,[131] can use ketones as oxidative fuels. However, concentrations of ketones that are similar to those achieved during starvation ketosis and diabetic ketoacidosis can also reduce the formation of pyrimidines in fetal rat brain (as judged by the incorporation of bicarbonate into uridine).[159] The inhibitory effects of ketones have been localized to the steps proximal to the formation of orotic acid.[159] If these findings can be confirmed and extended and if brain cell number and intellectual performance are correlated, these observations could provide a biochemical explanation for the putative deleterious effects of maternal ketonemia on intelligence of children.[100, 101]

Early Pregnancy. The fact that metabolic disturbances during the period of organogenesis may be associated with an increased frequency of congenital lesions in diabetic pregnancies underscores the importance of fuel homeostasis during the first 2 mo of gestation.[160] Indeed, the finding that glucose regulation in the early postimplantation period may be of major significance in neural tube formation and closure provides a common mechanism through which seemingly unrelated teratogens may operate.[161] Workers in a number of laboratories have utilized whole embryo culture[162] to demonstrate that abnormal fuel mixtures per se can impair organogenesis directly. Severe hyperglycemia can cause dysmorphosis (e.g., open neural tube, faulty neural tube fusion, microcephaly, and pericardial edema);[161, 163–165] similar teratogenic insults can be elicited by high concentrations of ketones.[166, 167] Hyperglycemia and hyperketonemia interact synergistically in rodent embryo culture, and marked teratogenic effects are achieved by adding both glucose and ketones simultaneously in amounts that would be subteratogenic or minimally teratogenic if added singly.[167]

The findings have clearly established the teratogenic potentialities of aberrant fuels of maternal origin. Other fuel-related factors may also contribute. Serum from animals with experimental diabetes inhibits growth and induces malformations in rodent embryos in culture.[167, 168] Some of the inhibitory actions may be correlated with the presence of somatomedin inhibitors.[167, 169] Additional metabolic alterations that develop as a consequence of poorly controlled diabetes have also been implicated as potential teratogenic factors. The evidence regarding these various possibilities has been reviewed.[170] Finally, the relationship between diabetic control during early pregnancy and the risk of congenital malformations has been examined in several clinical reports. Taken together, these data are consistent with the hypothesis that faulty metabolism in the periconceptional period predisposes the offspring of diabetic mothers to birth defects.[171]

FUEL-MEDIATED TERATOGENESIS AND MATERNAL METABOLISM. As summarized earlier, many effects of normal pregnancy on maternal metabolism have been clarified. By contrast, the implications of maternal metabolism for the growth and development of the conceptus are only beginning to be probed. Maternal metabolism may permanently modify development in the offspring by delimiting the metabolic mixture that is available to certain tissues during critical periods in intrauterine development.[9, 112] The long-range effects of fuels (or fuel-related products) need not be restricted to cell development in early pregnancy during the period of organogenesis (i.e., "organ" teratogenesis). Equally important, albeit more subtle, expressions may arise from fuel disturbances during the period of neuronal proliferation in midgestation ("behavioral" and "intellectual" teratogenesis) or in late gestation when complex multineuronal connections are established and many minimally replicating cells undergo terminal differentiation and/or functional maturation ("anthropometric," "neuroendocrine," and "metabolic" teratogenesis).[9, 112, 142]

Models support all these possible forms of fuel-mediated teratogenesis. Knowledge of whether these models have more than heuristic merit must await results from ongoing attempts to correlate antepartum maternal metabolism with the long-range characteristics of the offspring.[9, 154–157] Insofar as offspring of diabetic mothers are at risk throughout pregnancy, they constitute the best population in which to test the possibilities of fuel-mediated teratogenesis. However, because fetal development in *all* pregnancies is influenced by maternal metabolism, the derived insights may have general relevance. Indeed, an understanding of metabolism during pregnancy may make it possible to promote the promises of nature (i.e., the genetic endowment) in optimal fashion through enlightened manipulations of nurture (i.e., the intrauterine environment).

REFERENCES

1. Duncan JM. On puerperal diabetes. Trans Obstet Soc Lond 1882; 24:256–285.
2. Hytten FE, Leitch I. The Physiology of Human Pregnancy. 2nd ed. Oxford: Blackwell Scientific, 1971.
3. Knopp RH, Herrera E, Freinkel N. Carbohydrate metabolism in pregnancy. VIII. Metabolism of adipose tissue isolated from fed and fasted pregnant rats during late gestation. J Clin Invest 1970; 49:1438–1446.
4. Paul PK. Dynamics of hepatic glycogen: oestrogen and pregnancy. Acta Endocrinol 1972; 71:385–392.
5. Naismith DJ. The foetus as a parasite. Proc Nutr Soc 1969; 28:25–31.
6. Taggart NR, Holliday RM, Billewicz WZ, et al. Changes in skinfolds during pregnancy. Br J Nutr 1967; 21:439–451.
7. Hytten FE. Nutrition in pregnancy. Postgrad Med J 1979; 55:295–302.
8. Freinkel N. Effects of the conceptus on maternal metabolism during pregnancy. In: Leibel BS, Wrenshall GA, eds. On the Nature and Treatment of Diabetes. Amsterdam: Excerpta Medica, 1965: 679–691.
9. Freinkel N. Banting Lecture 1980. Of pregnancy and progeny. Diabetes 1980; 29:1023–1025.
10. Goodner CJ, Freinkel N. Carbohydrate metabolism in pregnancy. IV. Studies on the permeability of the rat placenta to I^{131} insulin. Diabetes 1961; 10:383–392.
11. Goodner CJ, Freinkel N. Carbohydrate metabolism in pregnancy: the degradation of insulin by extracts of maternal and fetal structures in the pregnant rat. Endocrinology 1959; 65:957–967.
12. Freinkel N, Goodner CJ. Carbohydrate metabolism in pregnancy. I. The metabolism of insulin by human placental tissue. J Clin Invest 1960; 39:116–131.
13. Goodner CJ, Freinkel N. Carbohydrate metabolism in pregnancy: the turnover of I^{131} insulin in the pregnant rat. Endocrinology 1960; 67:862–872.
14. Katz AI, Lindheimer MD, Mako ME, et al. Peripheral metabolism of insulin, proinsulin, and C-peptide in the pregnant rat. J Clin Invest 1975; 56:1608–1614.
15. Metzger BE, Rodeck C, Freinkel N, et al. Transplacental arteriovenous gradients for glucose, insulin, glucagon and placental lactogen during normoglycaemia in human pregnancy at term. Placenta 1985; 6:347–354.
16. Burt RL, Davidson IWF. Insulin half-life and utilization in normal pregnancy. Obstet Gynecol 1974; 43:161–170.
17. Bellmann O, Hartmann E. Influence of pregnancy on the kinetics of insulin. Am J Obstet Gynecol 1975; 122:829–833.
18. Lind T, Bell S, Gilmore E, et al. Insulin disappearance rate in pregnant and non-pregnant women, and in non-pregnant women given GHRH. Eur J Clin Invest 1977; 7:47–51.
19. Spellacy WN, Goetz FC. Plasma insulin in normal late pregnancy. N Engl J Med 1963; 268:988–991.
20. Kalkhoff R, Schalch DS, Walker JL, et al. Diabetogenic factors associated with pregnancy. Trans Assoc Am Physicians 1964; 77:270–279.
21. Bleicher SJ, O'Sullivan JB, Freinkel N. Carbohydrate metabolism in pregnancy. V. The interrelations of glucose, insulin, and free fatty acids in late pregnancy and postpartum. N Engl J Med 1964; 271:866–872.
22. Phelps RL, Bergenstal R, Freinkel N, et al. Carbohydrate metabolism in pregnancy. XIII. Relationships between plasma insulin and proinsulin during late pregnancy in normal and diabetic subjects. J Clin Endocrinol Metab 1975; 41:1085–1091.
23. Kühl C. Serum proinsulin in normal and gestational diabetic pregnancy. Diabetologia 1976; 12:295–300.
24. Kalkhoff RK, Kissebah AH, Kim HJ. Carbohydrate and lipid metabolism during normal pregnancy: relationship to gestational hormone action. Semin Perinatol 1978; 2:291–307.
25. Lind T, Billewicz WZ, Brown G. A serial study of changes occurring in the oral glucose tolerance test during pregnancy. J Obstet Gynaecol Br Commonw 1973; 80:1033–1039.
26. Spellacy WN, Goetz FC, Greenberg BZ, et al. Plasma insulin in normal "early" pregnancy. Obstet Gynecol 1965; 25:862–865.
27. Pitkin RM, Spellacy WN. Physiologic adjustments in general. In: Laboratory Indices of Nutritional Status in Pregnancy. Washington DC: National Academy of Sciences, 1978: 1–8.
28. Aspillaga MO, Whittaker PG, Taylor A, et al. Some new aspects of the endocrinological response to pregnancy. Br J Obstet Gynaecol 1983; 90:596–603.
29. Scobie IN, Kesson CM, Ratcliffe JG, et al. The effects of prolonged bromocriptine administration on Prl secretion, GH and glycaemic control in stable insulin-dependent diabetes mellitus. Clin Endocrinol 1983; 18:179–185.
30. Landgraf R, Landgraf-Leurs MMC, Weissmann A, et al. Prolactin: a diabetogenic hormone. Diabetologia 1977; 13:99–104.
31. Asher WL, Harper HW. Effect of human chorionic gonadotropin on weight loss, hunger, and feeling of well-being. Am J Clin Nutr 1973; 26:211–218.
32. Winborn WB, Sheridan PJ, McGill HC. Estrogen receptors in the islets of Langerhans of baboons. Cell Tissue Res 1983; 230:219–223.
33. Green IC, Howell SL, El Seifi S, et al. Binding of ^{3}H-progesterone by isolated rat islets of Langerhans. Diabetologia 1978; 15:349–355.
34. Turtle JR, Kipnis DM. The lipolytic action of human placental lactogen in isolated fat cells. Biochim Biophys Acta 1967; 144:583–593.
35. Mochizuki M, Morikawa H, Ohga Y, et al. Lipolytic action of human chorionic somatomammotropin. Endocrinol Jpn 1975; 22:123–129.
36. Beck P, Daughaday WH. Human placental lactogen: studies of its acute metabolic effects and disposition in normal man. J Clin Invest 1967; 46:103–110.
37. Kalkhoff RK, Richardson BL, Beck P. Relative effects of pregnancy, human placental lactogen and prednisolone on carbohydrate tolerance in normal and subclinical diabetic subjects. Diabetes 1969; 18:153–163.
38. Shamoon H, Felig P. Effects of estrogen on glucose uptake by rat muscle. Yale J Biol Med 1974; 47:227–233.

39. Rushakoff RJ, Kalkhoff RK. Effects of pregnancy and sex steroid administration on skeletal muscle metabolism in the rat. Diabetes 1981; 30:545–550.

40. Morrow PG, Marshall WP, Kim H-J, et al. Metabolic response to starvation. I. Relative effects of pregnancy and sex steroid administration in the rat. Metabolism 1981; 30:268–273.

41. Morrow PG, Marshall WP, Kim H-J, et al. Metabolic response to starvation. II. Effects of sex steroid administration to pre- and postmenopausal women. Metabolism 1981; 30:274–278.

42. Spellacy WN, Buhi WC, Schram JD, et al. Control of human chorionic somatomammotropin levels during pregnancy. Obstet Gynecol 1971; 37:567–573.

43. Gaspard U, Sandront H, Lambotte R. Contrôle glycémique des taux sériques maternels de l'hormone chorionique somatomammotrope (HCS) au cours de la grossesse. Acta Paediatr Belg 1973; 27:218–226.

44. Surmaczynska B, Nitzan M, Metzger BE, et al. Carbohydrate metabolism in pregnancy. XII. The effect of oral glucose on plasma concentrations of human placental lactogen and chorionic gonadotropin during late pregnancy in normal subjects and gestational diabetics. Isr J Med Sci 1974; 10:1481–1486.

45. Kühl C, Gaede P, Klebe JG, et al. Human placental lactogen concentration during physiological fluctuations of serum glucose in normal pregnant and gestational diabetic women. Acta Endocrinol 1975; 80:365–373.

46. Elliot JA. The effect of pregnancy on the control of lipolysis in fat cells isolated from human adipose tissue. Eur J Clin Invest 1975; 5:159–163.

47. Rushakoff RJ, Kalkhoff RK. Relative effects of pregnancy and corticosterone administration on skeletal muscle metabolism in the rat. Endocrinology 1983; 113:43–47.

48. Burke CW, Roulet F. Increased exposure of tissues to cortisol in late pregnancy. Br Med J 1970; 1:657–659.

49. Nolten WE, Lindheimer MD, Rueckert PA, et al. Diurnal patterns and regulation of cortisol secretion in pregnancy. J Clin Endocrinol Metab 1980; 51:466–472.

50. Shibasaki T, Odagiri E, Shizume K, et al. Corticotropin-releasing factor-like activity in human placental extracts. J Clin Endocrinol Metab 1982; 55:384–386.

51. Beck-Nielsen H, Kühl C, Pedersen O, et al. Decreased insulin binding to monocytes from normal pregnant women. J clin Endocrinol Metab 1979; 49:810–814.

52. Tsibris JCM, Raynor LO, Buhi WC, et al. Insulin receptors in circulating erythrocytes and monocytes from women on oral contraceptives or pregnant women near term. J Clin Endocrinol Metab 1980; 51:711–717.

53. Moore P, Kolterman O, Weyant J, et al. Insulin binding in human pregnancy: comparisons to the postpartum, luteal, and follicular states. J Clin Endocrinol Metab 1981; 52:937–941.

54. Puavilai G, Drobny EC, Domont LA, et al. Insulin receptors and insulin resistance in human pregnancy: evidence for a postreceptor defect in insulin action. J Clin Endocrinol Metab 1982; 54:247–253.

55. Toyoda N. Insulin receptors on erythrocytes in normal and obese pregnant women: comparisons to those in nonpregnant women during the follicular and luteal phases. Am J Obstet Gynecol 1982; 144:679–682.

56. Daniel RR, Metzger BE, Freinkel N, et al. Carbohydrate metabolism in pregnancy. XI. Response of plasma glucagon to overnight fast and oral glucose during normal pregnancy and in gestational diabetes. Diabetes 1974; 23:771–776.

57. Luyckx AS, Gerard J, Gaspard U, et al. Plasma glucagon levels in normal women during pregnancy. Diabetologia 1975; 11:549–554.

58. Kühl C, Holst JJ. Plasma glucagon and the insulin:glucagon ratio in gestational diabetes. Diabetes 1976; 25:16–23.

59. Baumann G, Puavilai G, Freinkel N, et al. Hepatic insulin and glucagon receptors in pregnancy: their role in the enhanced catabolism during fasting. Endocrinology 1981; 108:1979–1986.

60. Villee CA. The metabolism of human placenta in vitro. J Biol Chem 1953; 205:113–123.

61. Cornblath M, Schwartz R. Disorders of Carbohydrate Metabolism in Infancy. 2nd ed. Philadelphia: W. B. Saunders, 1976: 29–71.

62. Pedersen J. The Pregnant Diabetic and Her Newborn. 2nd ed. Baltimore: Williams & Wilkins, 1977: 106–122.

63. Herrera E, Freinkel N. Metabolites in the liver, brain, and placenta of fed or fasted mothers and fetal rats. Horm Metab Res 1975; 7:247–249.

64. Diamant YZ, Diamant S, Freinkel N. Lipid deposition and metabolism in rat placenta during gestation. Placenta 1980; 1:319–325.

65. Diamant YZ, Metzger BE, Freinkel N, et al. Placental lipid and glycogen content in human and experimental diabetes mellitus. Am J Obstet Gynecol 1982; 144:5–11.

66. Scow RO, Chernick SS, Smith BB. Ketosis in the rat fetus. Proc Soc Exp Biol Med 1958; 98:833–835.

67. Kim YJ, Felig P. Maternal and amniotic fluid substrate levels during caloric deprivation in human pregnancy. Metabolism 1972; 21:507–512.

68. Girard JR, Cuendet GS, Marliss EB, et al. Fuels, hormones, and liver metabolism at term and during the early postnatal period in the rat. J Clin Invest 1973; 52:3190–3200.

69. Girard JR, Ferre P, Gilbert M, et al. Fetal metabolic response to maternal fasting in the rat. Am J Physiol 1977; 232:E456–E463.

70. Shambaugh GE III, Mrozak SC, Freinkel N. Fetal fuels. I. Utilization of ketones by isolated tissues at various stages of maturation and maternal nutrition during late gestation. Metabolism 1977; 26:623–636.

71. Scow RO, Chernick SS, Brinley MS. Hyperlipemia and ketosis in the pregnant rat. Am J Physiol 1964; 206:796–804.

72. Herrera E, Knopp RH, Freinkel N. Carbohydrate metabolism in pregnancy. VI. Plasma fuels, insulin, liver composition, gluconeogenesis and nitrogen metabolism during late gestation in the fed and fasted rat. J Clin Invest 1969; 48:2260–2272.

73. Freinkel N, Herrera E, Knopp RH, et al. Metabolic realignments in late pregnancy: a clue to diabetogenesis? In: Camerini-Davalos RA, Cole HS, eds. Early Diabetes. New York: Academic, 1970: 205–219.

74. Page EW. Human fetal nutrition and growth. Am J Obstet Gynecol 1969; 104:378–387.

75. Cahill GF Jr, Owen OE. Some observations on carbohydrate metabolism in man. In: Dickens F, Randle PJ, Whelan WJ, eds. Carbohydrate Metabolism and Its Disorders. New York: Academic, 1968: 497–522.

76. Young M. Placental transfer of glucose and amino acids. In: Camerini-Davalos RA, Cole HS, eds. Early Diabetes in Early Life. New York: Academic, 1975: 237–242.

77. Gresham EL, James EJ, Raye JR, et al. Production and excretion of urea by the fetal lamb. Pediatrics 1972; 50:372–379.

78. Metzger BE, Freinkel N. Regulation of maternal protein metabolism and gluconeogenesis in the fasted state. In: Camerini-Davalos RA, Cole HS, eds. Early Diabetes in Early Life. New York: Academic, 1975: 303–311.

79. Metzger BE, Agnoli F, Hare JW, et al. Carbohydrate metabolism in pregnancy. X. Metabolic disposition of alanine by the perfused liver of the fasting pregnant rat. Diabetes 1973; 22:601–608.

80. Metzger BE, Hare JW, Freinkel N. Carbohydrate metabolism in pregnancy. IX. Plasma levels of gluconeogenic fuels during fasting in the rat. J Clin Endocrinol Metab 1971; 33:869–873.

81. Felig P, Kim YJ, Lynch V, et al. Amino acid metabolism during starvation in human pregnancy. J Clin Invest 1972; 51:1195–1202.

82. Freinkel N, Metzger BE, Nitzan M, et al. "Accelerated starvation" and mechanisms for the conservation of maternal nitrogen during pregnancy. Isr J Med Sci 1972; 8:426–439.

83. Felig P, Lynch V. Starvation in human pregnancy: hypoglycemia, hypoinsulinemia, and hyperketonemia. Science 1970; 170:990–992.

84. Tyson JE, Austin KL, Farinholt JW. Prolonged nutritional deprivation in pregnancy: changes in human chorionic somatomammotropin and growth hormone secretion. Am J Obstet Gynecol 1971; 109:1080–1082.

85. Tyson JE, Austin K, Farinholt J, et al. Endocrine-metabolic response to acute starvation in human gestation. Am J Obstet Gynecol 1976; 125:1073–1084.

86. Merimee TJ, Fineberg SE. Homeostasis during fasting. II. Hormone substrate differences between men and women. J Clin Endocrinol Metab 1973; 37:698–702.

87. Little B, Smith OW, Jessiman AG, et al. Hypophysectomy during pregnancy in a patient with cancer of the breast: case report with hormone studies. J Clin Endocrinol Metab 1958; 18:425–443.

88. Campbell RM, Innes IR, Kosterlitz HW. Some dietary and hormonal effects on maternal, foetal and placental weights in the rat. J Endocrinol 1953; 9:68–75.

89. Bourdel G, Jacquot R. Role du placenta dans les facultés anabolisantes des rattes gestantes. C R Acad Sci Ser D 1956; 242:552–555.

90. Curry DM, Beaton GH. Cortisone resistance in pregnant rats. Endocrinology 1958; 63:155–161.

91. Ogata ES, Metzger BE, Freinkel N. Carbohydrate metabolism in pregnancy. XVI. Longitudinal estimates of the effects of pregnancy on D-(6^3H) glucose and D-(6-^{14}C) glucose turnovers during fasting in the rat. Metabolism 1981; 30:487–492.

92. Widdas WF. Inability of diffusion to account for placental glucose transfer in the sheep and consideration of the kinetics of a possible carrier transfer. J Physiol (Lond) 1952; 118:23–39.

93. Simmons MA, Battaglia FC, Meschia G. Placental transfer of glucose. J Dev Physiol 1979; 1:227–239.

94. Hay WW Jr, Sparks JW, Wilkening RB, et al. Partition of maternal glucose production between conceptus and maternal tissues in sheep. Am J Physiol 1983; 245:E347–E350.

95. Kalhan SC, D'Angelo LJ, Savin SM, et al. Glucose production in pregnant women at term gestation. Sources of glucose for human fetus. J Clin Invest 1979; 63:388–394.

96. Metzger BE, Ravnikar V, Vileisis RA, et al. "Accelerated starvation" and the skipped breakfast in late normal pregnancy. Lancet 1982; 1:588–592.

97. Metzger BE, Freinkel N. Accelerated starvation in pregnancy: implications for dietary treatment of obesity and gestational diabetes mellitus. Biol Neonate 1987; 51:78–85.

98. Drazancic A, Stavlenic A. Free fatty acid determinations in normal and abnormal pregnancies. Am J Obstet Gynecol 1971; 109:666–669.

99. Persson B, Lunel NO. Metabolic control in diabetic pregnancy: variations in plasma concentrations of glucose, free fatty acids, glycerol, ketone

bodies, insulin, and human chorionic somatomammotropin during the last trimester. Am J Obstet Gynecol 1975; 122:737–745.

100. Churchill JA, Berendes HW. Intelligence of children whose mothers had acetonuria during pregnancy. Pan Am Health Organ Sci Publ 1969; 185:30.

101. Stehbens JA, Baker GL, Kitchell M. Outcome at ages 1, 3, and 5 years of children born to diabetic women. Am J Obstet Gynecol 1977; 127:408–413.

102. O'Sullivan JB, Mahan CM. Criteria for the oral glucose tolerance test in pregnancy. Diabetes 1964; 13:278–285.

103. Freinkel N, Metzger BE, Nitzan M, et al. Facilitated anabolism in late pregnancy: some novel maternal compensations for accelerated starvation. In: Malaise WJ, Pirart J, eds. Proceedings of VIIIth Congress of International Diabetes Federation. International Congress Series No. 312. Amsterdam: Excerpta Medica, 1974: 474–488.

104. Freinkel N, Phelps RL, Metzger BE. Intermediary metabolism during normal pregnancy. In: Sutherland HW, Stowers JM, eds. Carbohydrate Metabolism in Pregnancy and the Newborn, 1978. New York: Springer-Verlag, 1979: 1–31.

105. Dawes GS. Foetal and Neonatal Physiology. Chicago: Year Book Medical Publishers, 1968: 210–222.

106. Metzger BE, Unger RG, Freinkel N. Carbohydrate metabolism in pregnancy. XIV. Relationships between circulating glucagon, insulin, glucose, and amino acids in response to "mixed meal" in late pregnancy. Metabolism 1977; 26:151–156.

107. Freinkel N, Metzger BE. Some considerations of fuel economy in the fed state during late human pregnancy. In: Camerini-Davalos RA, Cole HS, eds. Early Diabetes in Early Life. New York: Academic, 1975: 289–301.

108. Gillmer MDG, Beard RW, Brooke FM, et al. Carbohydrate metabolism in pregnancy. I. Diurnal glucose profile in normal and diabetic women. Br Med J 1975; 3:339–402.

109. Lewis SB, Wallin JD, Kuzuya H, et al. Circadian variation of serum glucose, C-peptide immunoreactivity and free insulin in normal and insulin-treated diabetic pregnancy subjects. Diabetologia 1976; 12:343–350.

110. Gillmer MDG, Beard RW, Oakley NW, et al. Diurnal plasma free fatty acid profiles in normal and diabetic pregnancies. Br Med J 1977; 2:670–673.

111. Jervell J, Stokke KT, Moe N, et al. Metabolic profiles in closely controlled diabetic pregnancies during the third trimester. Diabetologia 1979; 16:229–233.

112. Freinkel N, Metzger BE. Pregnancy as a tissue culture experience: the critical implications of maternal metabolism for fetal development. Ciba Found Symp 1979; 63:3–23.

113. Cousins L, Rigg L, Hollingsworth D, et al. The 24-hour excursion and diurnal rhythm of glucose, insulin, and C-peptide in normal pregnancy. Am J Obstet Gynecol 1980; 136:483–488.

114. Metzger BE, Phelps RL, Freinkel N, et al. Effects of gestational diabetes on diurnal profiles of plasma glucose, lipids, and individual amino acids. Diabetes Care 1980; 3:402–409.

115. Phelps RL, Metzger BE, Freinkel N. Carbohydrate metabolism in pregnancy. XVII. Diurnal profiles of plasma glucose, insulin, free fatty acids, triglycerides, cholesterol, and individual amino acids in late normal pregnancy. Am J Obstet Gynecol 1981; 140:730–736.

116. Potter JM, Reckless JPD, Cullen DR. Diurnal variations in blood intermediary metabolites in mild gestational diabetic patients and the effect of a carbohydrate-restricted diet. Diabetologia 1982; 22:68–72.

117. Hollingsworth DR. Alterations of maternal metabolism in normal and diabetic pregnancies: differences in insulin-dependent, non–insulin-dependent, and gestational diabetes. Am J Obstet Gynecol 1983; 146:417–429.

118. Randle PJ, Garland PB, Hales CN, et al. The glucose fatty-acid cycle. Its role in insulin sensitivity and the metabolic disturbances of diabetes mellitus. Lancet 1963; 1:785–789.

119. Ferrannini E, Barrett EJ, Bevilacqua S, et al. Effect of fatty acids on glucose production and utilization in man. J Clin Invest 1983; 72:1737–1747.

120. Schalch DS, Kipnis DM. Abnormalities in carbohydrate tolerance associated with elevated plasma nonesterified fatty acids. J Clin Nutr 1965; 44:2010–2020.

121. Reaven GM. Banting Lecture 1988. Role of insulin resistance in human disease. Diabetes 1988; 37:1595–1607.

122. Szabo AJ, Szabo O. Placental free-fatty-acid transfer and fetal adipose-tissue development: an explanation of fetal adiposity in infants of diabetic mothers. Lancet 1974; 2:498–499.

123. Holzman IR, Lemons JA, Meschia G, et al. Uterine uptake of amino acids and placental glutamine-glutamate balance in the pregnant ewe. J Dev Physiol 1979; 1:137–149.

124. Hull D, Elphick MC. Evidence for fatty acid transfer across the human placenta. Ciba Found 1979; 63:75–86.

125. Prior RL, Scott RA. Ontogeny of gluconeogenesis in the bovine fetus: influence of maternal dietary energy. Dev Biol 1977; 58:384–393.

126. Krauer G, Joyce J, Young M. The influence of high maternal plasma glucose levels and maternal blood flow on the placental transfer of glucose in the guinea pig. Diabetologia 1973; 9:453–456.

127. Burke BJ, Savage PE, Sherriff RJ, et al. Diabetic twin pregnancy: an unequal result. Lancet 1979; 1:1372–1373.

128. Adam PAJ, Räihä N, Rahiala E-L, et al. Oxidation of glucose and D-β-OH-butyrate by the early human fetal brain. Acta Paediatr Scand 1975; 64:17–24.

129. Shambaugh GE III, Koehler RA, Freinkel N. Fetal fuels. II. Contributions of selected carbon fuels to oxidative metabolism in the rat conceptus. Am J Physiol 1977; 233:E457–E461.

130. Dahlquist G, Persson U, Persson B. The activity of D-β-hydroxybutyrate dehydrogenase in fetal, infant and adult rat brain and the influence of starvation. Biol Neonate 1972; 20:40–50.

131. Owen OE, Morgan AP, Kemp HG, et al. Brain metabolism during fasting. J Clin Invest 1967; 46:1589–1595.

132. Hellerström C. Growth pattern of pancreatic islets in animals. In: Volk BW, Wellman KF, eds. The Diabetic Pancreas. New York: Plenum, 1977: 61–97.

133. Pedersen J. Weight and length at birth of infants of diabetic mothers. Acta Endocrinol 1954; 16:330–342.

134. Pedersen J. The Pregnant Diabetic and Her Newborn. Problems and Management. 2nd ed. Baltimore: Williams & Wilkins, 1977: 211–220.

135. Ogata ES, Sabbagha R, Metzger BE, et al. Serial ultrasonography to assess evolving fetal macrosomia. Studies in 23 pregnant diabetic women. JAMA 1980; 243:2405–2408.

136. Ogata ES, Freinkel N, Metzger BE, et al. Perinatal islet function in gestational diabetes: assessment by cord plasma C-peptide and amniotic fluid insulin. Diabetes Care 1980; 3:425–429.

137. Dobbing J. Prenatal nutrition and neurological development. In: Carvioto J, Hambreus L, Vahlquist B, eds. Symposia of the Swedish Nutrition Foundation XII—Early Malnutrition and Mental Development. Uppsala, Sweden: Almqvist & Wiksell, 1974: 96–110.

138. Winnick M, Morgan BLG. Nutrition and cellular growth of the brain. In: Freinkel N, ed. Contemporary Metabolism. Vol 1. New York: Plenum, 1979: 165–180.

139. Hirsch J, Faust IM, Johnson PR. What's new in obesity: current understanding of adipose tissue morphology. In: Freinkel N, ed. Contemporary Metabolism. Vol 1. New York: Plenum, 1979: 385–399.

140. Cheek DB. Muscle cell growth in normal children. In: Cheek DB, ed. Human Growth, Body Composition, Cell Growth, Energy, and Intelligence. Philadelphia: Lea & Febiger, 1968: 337–351.

141. Logothetopoulos J. Islet cell regeneration and neogenesis. In: Greep RO, Astwood EB, Steiner R, et al., eds. Handbook of Physiology. Sect 7: Endocrinology. Vol I. Endocrine Pancreas. Washington, DC: American Physiological Society, 1972: 67–76.

142. Freinkel N. Pregnant thoughts about metabolic control and diabetes. N Engl J Med 1981; 304:1357–1359 (editorial).

143. Freinkel N, Metzger BE, Cockroft D, et al. Inquiries into maternal metabolism: past, present, and future—a progress report from the Northwestern University Diabetes in Pregnancy Center. In: Mugola EN, ed. Proceedings of 11th Congress of International Diabetes Federation, Nairobi, Kenya, Nov, 1982. Amsterdam: Excerpta Medica, 1983: 423–427.

144. Dubreuil G, Anderodias J. Islets de Langerhans glands chez un nouveau-né issu de mère glycosurique. C R Soc Biol 1920; 83:1490–1493.

145. Cardell BS. The infants of diabetic mothers. A morphological study. J Obstet Gynaecol Br Commonw 1953; 60:834–853.

146. Naeye RL. Infants of diabetic mothers: a quantitative morphologic study. Pediatrics 1965; 35:980–988.

147. Osler M, Pedersen J. The body composition of newborn infants of diabetic mothers. Pediatrics 1960; 26:985–992.

148. Fee BA, Weil WB Jr. Body composition of infants of diabetic mothers by direct analysis. Ann NY Acad Sci 1963; 110:869–897.

149. Hellerström C, Lewis NJ, Borg H, et al. Method for large-scale isolation of pancreatic islets by tissue culture of fetal rat pancreas. Diabetes 1979; 28:769–776.

150. Freinkel N, Lewis NJ, Johnson R, et al. Maturation of stimulus recognition and insulin secretion during tissue culture of fetal pancreatic islets. Trans Am Clin Climatol Assoc 1979; 90:86–93.

151. Freinkel N, Lewis NJ, Johnson R, et al. Differential effects of age versus glycemic stimulation on the maturation of insulin stimulus-secretion coupling during culture of fetal rat islets. Diabetes 1984; 33:1028–1038.

152. Dudek RW, Kawabe T, Brinn JE, et al. Glucose affects in vitro maturation of fetal rat islets. Endocrinology 1984; 114:582–587.

153. Aerts L, Van Assche FA. Is gestational diabetes an acquired condition? J Dev Physiol 1979; 1:219–225.

154. Pettitt DJ, Baird HR, Aleck KA, et al. Excessive obesity in offspring of Pima Indian women with diabetes during pregnancy. N Engl J Med 1983; 308:242–245.

155. Pettitt DJ, Bennett PH, Knowler WC, et al. Gestational diabetes mellitus and impaired glucose tolerance during pregnancy. Long-term effects on obesity and glucose tolerance in the offspring. Diabetes 1985; 34(Suppl 12):119–122.

156. Green OC, Winter RJ, Depp R, et al. Fuel-mediated teratogenesis: prospective correlations between anthropometric development in childhood and antepartum maternal metabolism. Clin Res 1987; 35:657A.

157. Silverman BL, Green OC, Dooley SL, et al. Relationships between amniotic fluid insulin before birth and childhood obesity in offspring of diabetic mothers (ODM). Pediatr Res 1989; 25:203A.

158. Dierks-Ventling C. Prenatal induction of ketone-body enzymes in the rat. Biol Neonate 1971; 19:426–433.

159. Bhasin S, Shambaugh GE III. Fetal fuels. V. Ketone bodies inhibit pyrimidine biosynthesis in fetal rat brain. Am J Physiol 1982; 243:E234–E239.

160. Mills JL, Baker L, Goldman AS. Malformations in infants of diabetic mothers occur before the seventh gestational week. Implications for treatment. Diabetes 1979; 28:292–293.

161. Freinkel N, Lewis NJ, Akazawa S, et al. The honeybee syndrome—implications of the teratogenicity of mannose in rat-embryo culture. N Engl J Med 1984; 310:223–230.

162. New DAT. Whole-embryo culture and the study of mammalian embryos during organogenesis. Biol Rev 1978; 53:81–122.

163. Cockroft DL, Coppola PT. Teratogenic effects of excess glucose on head-fold rat embryos in culture. Teratology 1977; 16:141–146.

164. Sadler TW. Effects of maternal diabetes on early embryogenesis: II. Hyperglycemia-induced exencephaly. Teratology 1980; 21:349–356.

165. Garnham EA, Beck F, Clarke CA, et al. Effects of glucose on rat embryos in culture. Diabetologia 1983; 25:291–295.

166. Horton WE, Sadler TW. Effects of maternal diabetes on early embryogenesis. Alterations in morphogenesis produced by the ketone body, β-hydroxybutyrate. Diabetes 1983; 32:610–616.

167. Freinkel N, Cockroft DL, Lewis NJ, et al. The 1985 McCollum Award Lecture. Fuel-mediated teratogenesis during early organogenesis: the effects of increased concentrations of glucose, ketones or somatomedin inhibitor during rat embryo culture. Am J Clin Nutr 1986; 44:986–995.

168. Sadler TW. Effects of maternal diabetes on early embryogenesis: I. The teratogenic potential of diabetic serum. Teratology 1980; 21:339–347.

169. Sadler TW, Phillips LS, Balkan W, et al. Somatomedin inhibitors from diabetic rat serum alter growth and development of mouse embryos in culture. Diabetes 1986; 35:861–865.

170. Freinkel N. Diabetic embryopathy and fuel-mediated teratogenesis: lessons from animal models. Horm Metab Res 1988; 20:463–475.

171. Metzger BE, Buchanan TA, eds. From research to practice: diabetes and birth defects. Diabetes Spectrum 1990; 3:150–183.

18

FERTILITY CONTROL AND ITS COMPLICATIONS

Bruce R. Carr and James E. Griffin

INTRODUCTION

World population almost doubled between 1950 and 1980 and was estimated to be 4.9 billion by 1986. By the year 2000 the world population is predicted to be 7 billion, and it will increase to 10 billion by the year 2050. By the year 2050 approximately 90% of people will live in developing countries (Fig. 18–1).[1, 2] The implications of this increase and of the projected future growth of the population on food supply, energy resources, and political stability justify the present interest in fertility control. Indeed, an understanding of the methods of contraception and their application, methods of action, effectiveness, and side effects is of importance to all physicians. It must be recognized, however, that the availability of fertility control in the United States and in the rest of the world is regulated by social, religious, and political factors.

The discovery of estrogen and progesterone and their potential contraceptive effects led to an enormous amount of research on fertility regulation in women. The effectiveness and safety of oral contraceptive agents in controlling ovulation and fertility are a result of these efforts, and most research and application of fertility control techniques continue to be directed toward the control of female fertility. There is no readily reversible and effective pharmacological contraceptive for men. Some believe that this imbalance is due to prejudice as to which sex should bear the responsibility of contraception and that this has influenced investigators and granting agencies controlling monies for such research.[3] An alternative explanation is that there was not so much a lag in research in the male as a large positive stimulus for research directed toward a female contraceptive device. Thus the moral support and financial aid that the birth control advocates Margaret Sanger and Mrs. Stanley

McCormack provided for a pioneer in reproductive endocrinology, Gregory Pincus, may to a certain extent explain the rapid early development of the oral contraceptive for women.

The delay during the succeeding decades in the development of better means of fertility control in men probably has several causes. One is that it has proved to be easier to prevent the production of only one ovum per month in the female than to prevent the production of millions of sperm each day in the male. In addition, the processes of sperm migration from the vagina to the fallopian tubes, the development of the ability of sperm to fertilize an ovum, capacitation, fertilization, and implantation of the fertilized ovum all take place in women. Thus even some measures designed to affect the sperm, such as inhibition of capacitation and implantation, can be used in women but not in men.

This chapter summarizes the present status of methods

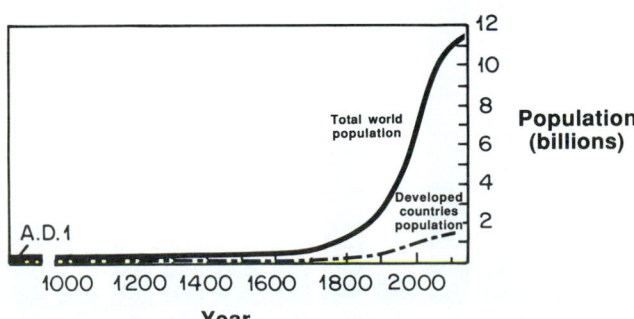

Figure 18–1. Past records and future projections of world population. (Adapted in part from Pannenborg CO. Contraception in the year 2001. Excerpta Med Int Congr Ser 1987; 759:21–44.)

TABLE 18–1. Estimated Number of Couples Using Birth Control, Worldwide, by Method, 1970, 1977, and 1984

Method	1970 Millions	1977 Millions	1984 Millions
Voluntary sterilization	20	80	137
Oral contraception	30	55	55
Condom	25	35	37
IUD	12	15	70
Other methods*	60	65	26
Total	147	250	325
Abortion (annual incidence)	40	40	—

*Barrier and natural family-planning methods.
Adapted from Hammerstein J. Contraception: an overview. Am J Obstet Gynecol 1987; 157:1020–1023.

of fertility control in women and in men and discusses areas of current investigation in contraceptive control. Some methods of fertility control that are used worldwide are given in Table 18–1. Of couples who used some form of birth control in the United States as of 1988, approximately 29% relied on surgical sterilization; 26% used oral contraceptives; 13% used condoms; 8% used intrauterine devices (IUDs) or diaphragms; and 21% used other methods[4] (Fig. 18–2).

FERTILITY CONTROL IN WOMEN

The various methods of fertility control for women and their primary targets in the body are depicted in Figure 18–3. These methods include (1) hormonal contraceptives, (2) IUDs, (3) barrier methods, (4) natural family-planning methods, (5) immunological techniques, (6) sterilization, and (7) abortion.

Hormonal Contraceptives

Steroidal Contraceptives

ORAL CONTRACEPTIVES. Background. Haberlandt was the first to provide evidence that steroids exhibit a contraceptive effect in animals by demonstrating that transplanted tissue fragments of corpus luteum produced infertility in rabbits and mice. In 1928 Fellner extended these experiments by demonstrating that estrogen extracts, which he named "feminin," were effective contraceptives in rodents.[5] Further developments utilizing steroids as contraceptive agents awaited the purification and crystallization of estrogen

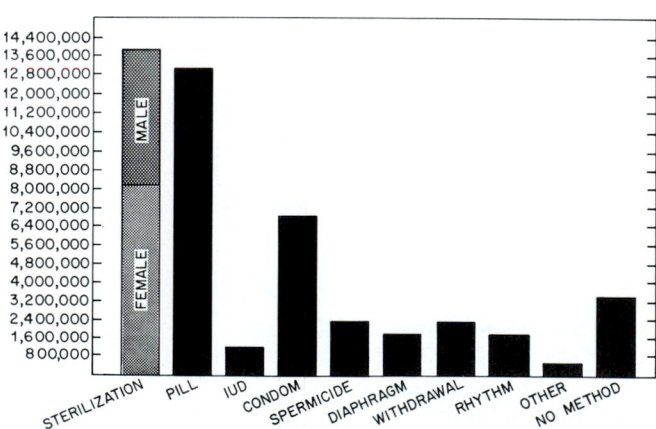

Figure 18–2. Contraceptive choices of U.S. couples aged 15 to 44 in 1988. (From Cunningham FG, Gant NF, MacDonald PC. Contraceptive choices of U.S. couples aged 15 to 44 in 1988. Williams Obstetrics. 18th ed. Norwalk, CT: Appleton & Lange, 1989: 922.)

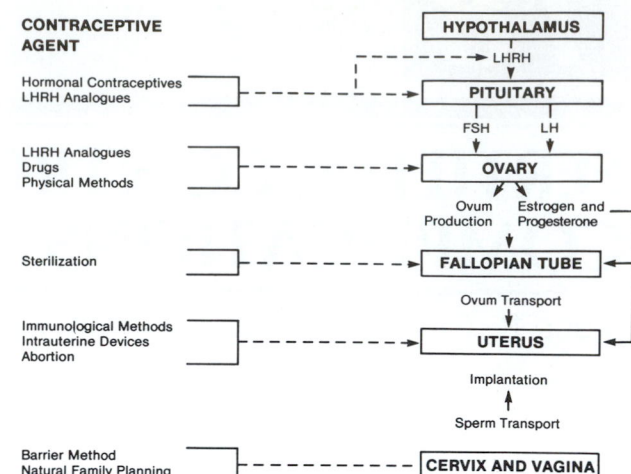

Figure 18–3. Principal sites of action of various contraceptives on the female reproductive tract.

and progesterone. Estrogens were isolated and crystallized in 1929 by Doisy and colleagues[6] and by Butenandt;[7] Butenandt and Westphal[8] isolated and subsequently synthesized progesterone.

Sturgis and Albright[9] observed that the administration of estradiol benzoate by injection caused improvement in dysmenorrhea when ovulation was inhibited. Subsequently, chemical modifications of estrogens resulted in the production of orally active estrogens—ethinyl estradiol and the 3-methyl ether of ethinyl estradiol, mestranol. In addition, it was shown that the removal of the C-19 methyl group from testosterone reduced its androgenic activity (19-nortestosterone) and that the orally active derivative containing an ethinyl group at C-17 had progestational activity. These discoveries led to the first clinical trials of oral contraceptives by Pincus and colleagues.[10]

***Pharmacology.* Structure.** The two estrogens in oral contraceptive agents are ethinyl estradiol and mestranol. In addition, five synthetic progestogens are utilized in oral contraceptives in the United States: norethindrone, norethynodrel, norethindrone acetate, ethynodiol diacetate, and norgestrel (D,L-norgestrel or D-levonorgestrel) (Fig. 18–4). Three additional progestogens (gestodene, desogestrel, and norgestimate) are available in oral contraceptives marketed in Western Europe and are undergoing investigation in the United States.[11]

Formulations. At present, four types of oral contraceptive preparations are available in the United States (Table 18–2). These include fixed-combination oral contraceptive pills in which the estrogen and progestogen composition remains constant throughout therapy; biphasic and triphasic oral contraceptive pills in which the estrogen composition remains constant or varies slightly but the progestogen composition varies markedly during the cycle; and progestogen-only contraceptive pills. The fixed-combination pills are the most widely utilized form of oral contraceptives and are the principal source of information regarding side effects. Because of potential dose-related side effects the hormonal content of oral contraceptives has declined since their introduction. At present the maximal dose of estrogen in oral contraceptives is 50 µg, and the maximal dose of progestogen is 2.5 mg. The effectiveness of all combination oral contraceptives is similar (theoretically greater than 99%) but is somewhat less for the progestogen-only (mini) pills.[12] The biphasic and triphasic oral contraceptives allow for lower doses of progestogen during the early part of the

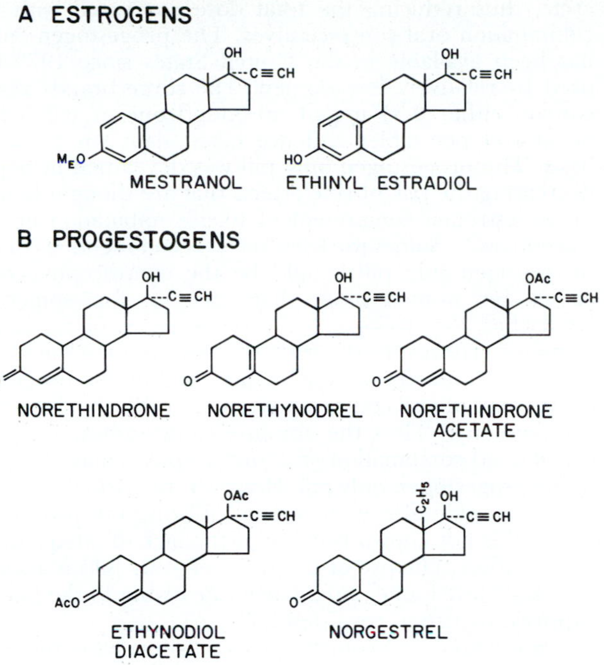

A ESTROGENS

MESTRANOL   ETHINYL ESTRADIOL

B PROGESTOGENS

NORETHINDRONE   NORETHYNODREL   NORETHINDRONE
                                    ACETATE

ETHYNODIOL   NORGESTREL
DIACETATE

Figure 18–4. Structure of estrogens (*A*) and progestogens (*B*) that are available in oral contraceptive pills.

TABLE 18–2. Composition of Oral Contraceptives

Name	Estrogen	μg	Progestogen	mg
Combination Type				
Estrogen Content = 50 μg				
Ortho-Novum 1/50	Mestranol	50	Norethindrone	1.0
Norinyl 1 + 50	Mestranol	50	Norethindrone	1.0
Ovcon-50	Ethinyl estradiol	50	Norethindrone	1.0
Ovral	Ethinyl estradiol	50	Norgestrel	0.5
Demulen	Ethinyl estradiol	50	Ethynodiol diacetate	1.0
Norlestrin 2.5/50	Ethinyl estradiol	50	Norethindrone acetate	2.5
Norlestrin 1/50	Ethinyl estradiol	50	Norethindrone acetate	1.0
Estrogen Content < 50 μg				
Ortho-Novum 1/35	Ethinyl estradiol	35	Norethindrone	1.0
Norinyl 1 + 35	Ethinyl estradiol	35	Norethindrone	1.0
Modicon	Ethinyl estradiol	35	Norethindrone	0.5
Brevicon	Ethinyl estradiol	35	Norethindrone	0.5
Ovcon-35	Ethinyl estradiol	35	Norethindrone	0.4
Demulen 1/35	Ethinyl estradiol	35	Ethynodiol diacetate	1.0
Loestrin 1.5/30	Ethinyl estradiol	30	Norethindrone acetate	1.5
Loestrin 1/20	Ethinyl estradiol	20	Norethindrone acetate	1.0
Nordette	Ethinyl estradiol	30	Levonorgestrel	0.15
Lo/Ovral	Ethinyl estradiol	30	Norgestrel	0.3
Biphasic Type				
Ortho-Novum 10/11				
First 10 d	Ethinyl estradiol	35	Norethindrone	0.5
Next 11 d	Ethinyl estradiol	35	Norethindrone	1.0
Triphasic Type				
Ortho-Novum 7/7/7				
First 7 d	Ethinyl estradiol	35	Norethindrone	0.5
Second 7 d	Ethinyl estradiol	35	Norethindrone	0.75
Third 7 d	Ethinyl estradiol	35	Norethindrone	1.0
Tri-Norinyl				
First 7 d	Ethinyl estradiol	35	Norethindrone	0.5
Next 9 d	Ethinyl estradiol	35	Norethindrone	1.0
Next 5 d	Ethinyl estradiol	35	Norethindrone	0.5
Tri-Levlen				
First 6 d	Ethinyl estradiol	30	Levonorgestrel	0.05
Next 5 d	Ethinyl estradiol	40	Levonorgestrel	0.075
Next 10 d	Ethinyl estradiol	30	Levonorgestrel	0.125
Triphasil				
First 6 d	Ethinyl estradiol	30	Levonorgestrel	0.05
Next 5 d	Ethinyl estradiol	40	Levonorgestrel	0.075
Next 10 d	Ethinyl estradiol	30	Levonorgestrel	0.125
Progestogen Only				
Micronor	None		Norethindrone	0.35
Nor-Q.D.	None		Norethindrone	0.35
Ovrette	None		Norgestrel	0.075

cycle, thus reducing the total dose compared with fixed-combination oral contraceptives. The progestogen-only pill has been available in the United States since 1973 but is used by relatively few women. The three brands available contain either 0.35 mg of norethindrone or 0.075 mg of norgestrel per tablet and are taken daily on a continual basis. The progestogen-only pill was developed in hopes of decreasing the risk of side effects that are thought to be due to the estrogen component of fixed-combination oral contraceptives.[13] Some workers have recommended that the progestogen-only pill should be the contraceptive risk of choice for women older than age 35; for women with headaches, hypertension, or varicose veins; or for lactating women.[14] However, the risk of hypertension, myocardial infarction, and stroke may be increased by the progestogen component of oral contraceptives rather than by the estrogen component. [15] Thus the absolute contraindications for the use of fixed-combination oral contraceptives may also pertain to the progestogen-only pill. However, the risk of developing significant side effects in women utilizing the progestogen-only pill is not known because of the lack of adequate long-term studies. The use of progestogen-only pills is associated with a slightly higher pregnancy rate owing to the failure to suppress ovulation consistently.[14]

Sequential oral contraceptive pills involving the administration of estrogen alone for 2 wk followed by a combination of estrogen and a progestogen for 1 wk were previously available but were banned by the Food and Drug Administration after reports of endometrial atypical hyperplasia and endometrial carcinoma in women using this form of contraception.[16] Although no definite causal relationship between endometrial carcinoma and sequential oral contraceptives could be established, the morphological changes in the endometrium associated with their use were believed to be due to the relatively low progestational activity; i.e., the progestational activity in sequential contraceptives was ineffective in protecting against the development of hyperplasia that was induced by the estrogen component. In addition, sequential contraceptives were not as effective as the other oral contraceptive agents in preventing pregnancy.[17]

Potency. The biological effects of the various synthetic estrogens and progestogens alone and in combination oral contraceptive agents have been assessed in animal as well as human subjects. Ethinyl estradiol is twice as potent as mestranol in its ability to produce vaginal keratinization in rats,[18] but in women there is little difference in potency between the two hormones.[19-21] All estrogen-containing oral contraceptive agents that contain less than 50 μg of estrogen are composed exclusively of ethinyl estradiol.

The progestogens in oral contraceptive agents do not possess all the properties of progesterone, and in addition they exhibit varying estrogenic and androgenic side effects. The most widely used means to assess progestational potency of steroids is the Clauberg test,[22] in which immature female rabbits are primed with estrogen for 6 d and receive a test compound for 5 d; the uterus is then removed and evaluated by histological grading. In this assay, norgestrel is the most potent progestogen.[23] These results, however, may not apply to humans. Attempts to assess progestational potency in women, including assessment of the delay of menses and histological analysis of the glycogen deposition in endometrial glands, are difficult to interpret because of use of various estrogens preceding progestogen administration and the failure to achieve parallel dose-response curves.[22-25]

Potency tables, which are based on delay of menses and glycogen deposition data, have been developed to try to aid in selecting the appropriate oral contraceptive pill for a particular patient.[26, 27] However, the interpretation of various tests of progestational effects is difficult,[22, 25] and there does not appear to be a good correlation between potency scales and side effects.[28] A more rational approach to drug selection takes into account data from clinical trials of the incidence of specific serious adverse side effects with specific combinations of ethinyl estradiol and progestogens.

Metabolism. Mestranol and ethinyl estradiol are absorbed efficiently in the gastrointestinal tract, and up to 60% of an oral dose is excreted in urine after 24 h.[24] Mestranol is not physiologically active until it is converted to ethinyl estradiol. The latter is metabolized principally to glucuronides and sulfates. Peak levels of ethinyl estradiol in plasma are reached 1 h after oral administration, followed by an initial rapid decline and a second slower phase of decline. Approximately 3% of ethinyl estradiol remains in plasma 24 h after administration.[29] Norethindrone, norethynodrel, and norgestrel are rapidly absorbed, peak concentrations being reached 1 to 3 h after administration; peak levels of ethynodiol diacetate and norethindrone acetate are achieved somewhat later, because they may undergo deacylation in the gastrointestinal tract before absorption. Progestogen metabolism is more complex than that of estrogens, and more than 30 metabolites have been identified.[24] Small amounts of synthetic progestogens may be metabolized to estrogens, but it is not known whether this is important clinically.[30]

Mechanism of Action. Steroid hormones in oral contraceptive pills act both within the central nervous system and in tissues of the urogenital tract to inhibit reproductive function. The principal site of action is at the level of the hypothalamus and pituitary to prevent the midcycle surge of luteinizing hormone (LH), and hence to prevent ovulation. The basal concentrations of LH and follicle-stimulating hormone (FSH) and plasma levels of estradiol and progesterone are suppressed in users of oral contraceptives, as shown in Fig. 18–5.[31] This effect on basal concentrations of plasma gonadotropins is related to dose and time.[32] The increase in plasma levels of gonadotropins after the administration of luteinizing hormone–releasing hormone (LHRH) is either normal [33, 34] or slightly decreased.[35]

Follicular growth is inhibited, although the number of primary follicles is similar to that in controls.[32] Whether

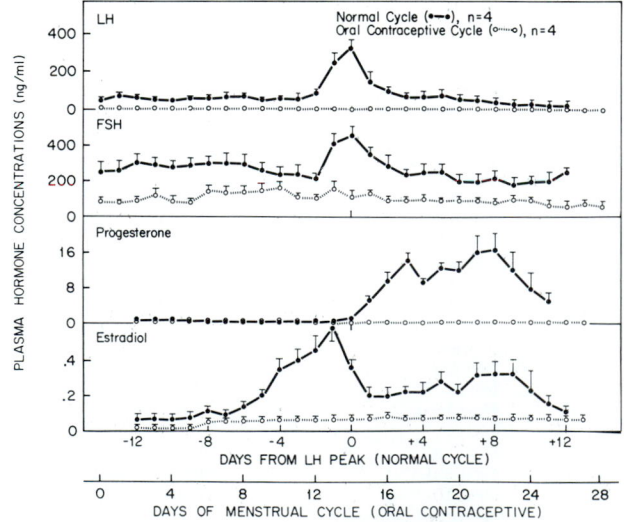

Figure 18–5. Plasma levels of gonadotropins, estradiol-17β, and progesterone during the ovarian cycles of four ovulatory women and four women treated with Norinyl 1 + 80. (Reproduced with permission from Carr BR, Parker CR Jr, Madden JD, et al. Plasma levels of adrenocorticotropin and cortisol in women receiving oral contraceptive steroid treatment. J Clin Endocrinol Metab 1979; 49:346–349. © 1979, The Endocrine Society.)

follicular atresia is increased by oral contraceptive pills is unclear, but the age at which menopause begins is not affected by previous oral contraceptive use.[32] Motility of the fallopian tubes, a process that is essential for the transport of the gametes before and after fertilization, is affected by estrogen and progestogen treatment in vitro.[36] The role of these effects on tubal motility in fertility control is unclear. Oral contraceptive agents cause glandular atrophy in uterine endometrium, induce a pseudodecidual reaction in the endometrial stroma, and cause formation of subnuclear vacuoles in the endometrial endothelium throughout the menstrual cycle.[37] The hormonal effects on the endometrium may inhibit implantation of the blastocyst. In addition, oral contraceptives cause the formation of a thick cervical mucus that inhibits sperm motility and migration.

Metabolic Effects. **Potential Risks.** No contraceptive is 100% effective and none is without risk. Oral contraceptives are usually effective, and their actions are usually reversible when treatment is stopped (Table 18–3). Furthermore, the incidence of potentially lethal side effects in oral contraceptive users (Table 18–4) may be less than the mortality risk resulting from pregnancy. The death rates from surgical procedures such as tubal sterilization (8 per 100,000 procedures) and hysterectomy (100 per 100,000 procedures) are higher than are death rates in young, nonsmoking oral contraceptive users.[38, 39]

Soon after the introduction of oral contraceptives, it was suggested that use of these agents might be associated with serious cardiovascular side effects such as ischemic heart disease (myocardial infarction), thromboembolic disease, stroke, and hypertension. This issue has been analyzed in both retrospective, case-controlled studies and prospective, cohort studies. Such data are commonly expressed either as a relative risk (the ratio of the incidence of a disease among users to that among nonusers) or attributive risk (the difference in the incidence of disease between users and nonusers).

TABLE 18–3. First-Year Failure Rates of Birth Control Methods

Method	% of Women Experiencing Accidental Pregnancy in First Year of Use		
	Lowest Expected*	Typical†	Lowest Reported‡
Chance	85	85	43
Spermicides	3	21	0
Periodic abstinence		20	—
Ovulation method	3	—	11
Symptothermal	2	—	13
Calendar	10	—	14
Postovulation	1	—	2
Withdrawal	4	18	7
Cervical cap	6	18	8
Sponge	5	18	14
Diaphragm (with spermicide)	6	18	2
Condom	2	12	4
IUD			
Medicated	2	—	2
Nonmedicated	1	—	0.5
Pill			
Combination	0.1	—	0
Progestogen only	0.5	—	1
Injectable progestogen	0.3	0.3	0
Female sterilization	0.2	0.4	0
Male sterilization	0.1	0.15	0

*Among couples who initiate use of a method and who use it perfectly, the authors' best guess of the percentage expected to experience an accidental pregnancy during the first year if they do not stop for any other reason.

†Among typical couples who initiate a method, the percentage who experience an accidental pregnancy during the first year if they do not stop use for another reason.

‡In the literature on contraceptive failure, the lowest reported percentage who experience an accidental pregnancy during the first year of use after initiation of use if they did not stop use for any other reason.

Adapted in part from Hatcher RA, Stewart F, Stewart GK, et al. Contraceptive Technology 1990–1992. New York: Irvington, 1990: 134.

TABLE 18–4. Annual Death Rates Associated with Fertility Control per 100,000 Nonsterile Women

Contraceptive Technique	Death Rate for Age Group of					
	15–19	20–24	25–29	30–34	35–39	40–44
None (birth related)	7.0	7.4	9.1	14.8	25.7	28.2
Oral contraceptives						
Smokers	2.4	3.6	6.8	13.7	51.4	117.6
Nonsmokers	0.5	0.7	1.1	2.1	14.1	32.0
IUD	1.3	1.1	1.3	1.3	1.9	2.1
Abortion	0.5	1.1	1.3	1.9	1.8	1.1
Barrier methods (birth related)	1.5	1.4	1.0	0.8	1.3	7.6

Adapted from HW Ory, Mortality associated with fertility and fertility control: 1983. Family Planning Perspectives. Volume 15: Number 2 (March/April 1983), pp 57–63. © The Alan Guttmacher Institute.

The characteristics of three major cohort studies that began in 1968 are given in Table 18–5. The mortality rates for oral contraceptive users compared with those for nonusers may have declined in recent years.[12] For example, in the Royal College of General Practitioners Oral Contraceptive Study, the relative risk of mortality in current users was 4.7 in 1977[40] and 4.0 in 1981.[41] In the Oxford study the relative risk of mortality in 140,000 woman-years of observation was 2.5, which is not statistically different from that in nonusers.[42] In the Walnut Creek study in more than 127,000 woman-years of observation, the relative risk of mortality from oral contraceptive use was 2.1, which again is not statistically significant.[43] In a prospective study by the Group Health Cooperative of Puget Sound, no deaths from cardiovascular disease were reported among oral contraceptive users between 1977 and 1988.[44] The apparent decrease in mortality rates for oral contraceptive users appears to be the consequence of (1) more observations and more exact estimates, (2) increased use of agents that contain lesser amounts of estrogens, and (3) more extensive use of other methods of birth control in women in high-risk categories.[12] In the United States, the United Kingdom, Sweden, and Taiwan the overall death rates do not appear to reflect any deleterious effects of contraceptive use.[12]

Circulatory System. ISCHEMIC HEART DISEASE (MYOCARDIAL INFARCTION). The incidence of myocardial infarction is rare in young women, increases rapidly with age, and is increased further by other risk factors such as smoking, hypertension, hypercholesterolemia, and diabetes mellitus.[45, 46] In the United States in 1976, the death rate from myocardial infarction was 1.9 per 100,000 in women aged 25 to 34 and

TABLE 18–5. Characteristics of Sample Populations of Major Cohort Studies of Oral Contraceptives

Study and Population	Number in Sample
Royal College of General Practitioners, 1968–present	
Oral contraceptive users	23,611
Never users	22,766
Oxford/Family Planning Association Study, 1968–present	
Oral contraceptive users	9,653
Diaphragm users	4,217
IUD users	3,162
Walnut Creek/Kaiser Permanente Study, 1968–1977	
Oral contraceptive users	6,107
Former users	4,217
Never users	6,503

Adapted from Lettenmaier C, Liskin L, Church CA, et al. Mothers' lives matter: maternal health in the community. Population Reports, Series L, No. 7. Baltimore: The Johns Hopkins University, Population Information Program, September 1988.

14.6 per 100,000 in women aged 35 to 44.[47] The relative risk of myocardial infarction in women who smoke varies with the number of cigarettes used. For example, the relative risk of myocardial infarction is 3.4 in women who smoke 1 to 24 cigarettes a day compared with 7.8 in women who smoke more than 25 cigarettes a day.[48]

In 1968 Inman and Vessey[49] suggested that the incidence of ischemic heart disease was increased in oral contraceptive users, and additional studies of the relationship between oral contraceptives and myocardial infarction have reported a relative risk between 2 and 6.[12] In one large cohort study Slone and colleagues[50] observed that in addition to a threefold increase in the risk of myocardial infarction in current oral contraceptive users, there is also an increased risk in previous long-term users of the agents (5 y or more). That study suggests that previous oral contraceptive use is associated with a greater risk of myocardial infarction, even when the agents have been discontinued for up to 10 y. Stampfer and colleagues[51] reported the results of a large prospective study (Nurses' Health Study Cohort) of 484,096 person-years. They observed no increase of cardiovascular risk, including coronary disease, among previous users of oral contraceptives, even with prolonged use. Several studies have demonstrated that in oral contraceptive users the risk of death from circulatory disease, principally myocardial infarction and stroke, is significantly related to age and smoking (Table 18–6).[12, 41, 51] Analysis of these data suggests that (1) smokers have a greater risk than nonsmokers regardless of age, (2) the deleterious effects of oral contraceptives and smoking increase with age, and (3) nonsmokers older than age 40 and smokers older than age 35 should not use oral contraceptives but an alternative form of fertility control. The Walnut Creek cohort study, which was somewhat small in scope, did not find an increased mortality in users of oral contraceptives who smoked compared with smokers alone.[43]

Although the mechanisms by which oral contraceptives result in an increased incidence of ischemic heart disease are not fully understood, changes in serum lipoprotein levels may be involved. The effects of oral contraceptive use on plasma lipoprotein levels and, in particular, high-density lipoprotein (HDL) cholesterol levels have been assessed because of the purported inverse relationship between the serum HDL level and the development of myocardial infarction.[46, 52] Pills containing 50 μg or more of estrogen increase levels of low-density lipoprotein and very-low-density lipoprotein, but the levels of HDL may be raised or lowered depending on the type and amount of progesto-

gen.[15, 53–57] Women using the progestogen-only or minipill have lower levels of HDL,[58, 59] and oral contraceptive pills containing a progestogen with high progestational activity,[27] such as norgestrel in combination with a low dose of estrogen, tend to produce more profound lowering of HDL levels than do other preparations.[55, 56] It is not known whether these changes are of clinical importance.

The Royal College of General Practitioners Oral Contraceptive Study noted a positive correlation and increasing rates of myocardial infarction with increasing doses of progestogens in oral contraceptive agents.[60, 61] Some progestogens may be more deleterious than others with respect to altering lipoprotein patterns and causing disease of the circulatory system.[55–57] However, the use of low-dose combination pills containing 30 to 35 μg of ethinyl estradiol does not appear to be associated with ischemic heart disease and exerts minimal effects on lipoprotein profiles.[55, 57, 60] The decline in the death rate from myocardial infarction in the recent cohort studies is believed to be due in part to the reluctance of older women and smokers to use oral contraceptive pills, as well as to the increased use of low-dose pills in the majority of women.

THROMBOEMBOLIC DISEASE. During the 1960s several retrospective studies suggested a relative risk of developing thromboembolism of 3 to 11 in users of oral contraceptives.[12] These studies were largely based on the clinical diagnosis of deep vein thrombosis, a diagnosis fraught with difficulty, and some investigators have challenged these results.[62] However, with more sophisticated techniques it now appears that the risk of developing thromboembolism, frequently subclinical, is increased in pill users.[63–65]

Three large cohort studies have observed lower relative risk rates of thromboembolism (2 to 5) than those reported in the retrospective studies.[12] The lower incidence may be due to more careful screening and elimination of women with high risk factors before oral contraceptives are prescribed. Although the incidence of thromboembolism is increased, the risk of death from venous thromboembolism is rare (5 per 450,000 woman-years).[45] Moreover, the risk of development of thromboembolism may be related to the dose of estrogen in the pill. For example, the incidence of thromboembolic disease in the Royal College study in 1974 was 112 per 100,000 woman-years with agents containing more than 50 μg estrogen, and 81 per 100,000 woman-years with lower-dose pills.[66] However, in the follow-up study by the Royal College of General Practitioners in 1978, a dose relationship could be demonstrated only for superficial thromboembolism; the incidence of deep vein thrombosis was unrelated to the dose of estrogen or to the progestogen component.[67] In Sweden, where all users were changed from high- to low-dose estrogen pills, a decrease in the incidence of thromboembolism from 25 to 9 per 100,000 woman-years occurred, unassociated with a change in mortality from thromboembolism, cardiovascular disease, or cerebrovascular accident.[68] Meade and co-workers[60] reported relatively low death rates from both arterial and venous thromboembolism with pills containing 30 μg of estrogen or less compared with those containing more than that amount. Two studies confirmed a relationship between current oral contraceptive use and venous thromboembolism but no relationship for previous use. However, the Oxford-Family Planning Association Contraceptive Study[69] observed a lower incidence with agents containing less than 50 μg of estrogen, whereas Helmrich and associates[70] reported no relation to estrogen dose. These discrepancies may be due to methodological differences.[71] The risk of developing thromboembolism in oral contraceptive users does not appear to be related to the duration of use, and any risk disappears soon after discontinuance of the pills.[45] Possible mechanisms whereby

TABLE 18–6. Circulatory Disease Mortality Rates (Deaths per 100,000 Woman-Years) and Risks by Age, Smoking Status, and Oral Contraceptive Use: Royal College of General Practitioners Oral Contraceptive Study, 1981

Age and Smoking Status	Ever Users	Never Users	Relative Risk	Excess Risk per 100,000 Woman-Years
15–24 y				
Nonsmokers	0.0	0.0	—	0.0
Smokers	10.5	0.0	—	10.5
25–34 y				
Nonsmokers	4.4	2.7	1.6	1.7
Smokers	14.2	4.2	3.4	10.0
35–44 y				
Nonsmokers	21.5	6.4	3.3	15.1
Smokers	63.4	15.2	4.2*	48.2*
≥45 y				
Nonsmokers	52.4	11.4	4.6*	40.9*
Smokers	206.7	27.9	7.4*	178.8*

*Statistically significant differences in risk (p < .05).

Adapted from Royal College of General Practitioners. Further analyses of mortality in oral-contraceptive users. Lancet 1981; 1:541–546.

oral contraceptives predispose to venous thromboembolic disease include (1) endothelial proliferation; (2) decrease in the rate of venous blood flow; and (3) increase in coagulability of blood because of changes in platelets, coagulation factors, and the fibrinolytic system.[45] In summary, with the current use of low-dose contraceptive pills the risk of developing serious thromboembolic disease is probably low.

CEREBROVASCULAR ACCIDENT. Smoking, hypertension, and age increase the risk of developing cerebrovascular accidents (stroke).[12] As with myocardial infarction, the risk of stroke is highest in older, hypertensive women who smoke. Case-control studies suggest a relative risk of 3 to 14 for development of stroke in oral contraceptive users.[12] Two cohort studies (Royal College of General Practitioners and Walnut Creek) reported higher incidences of subarachnoid hemorrhage (but not other types of stroke) in contraceptive users than in nonusers.[41, 72] Death from stroke is rare and is confined to older women. The risk increases in relation to the dose of estrogen and possibly of progestogen.[60, 73] Because of the seriousness of stroke, users of oral contraceptives who develop severe visual symptoms or headaches should discontinue the agent and use another form of fertility control.

HYPERTENSION. Most women experience small elevations in blood pressure (1 to 2 mm Hg diastolic and 5 mm Hg systolic) while taking oral contraceptives.[12] The mechanism for the development of hypertension involves the renin-angiotensin-aldosterone system and is principally due to an increase in renin substrate (angiotensinogen), with a secondary increase in angiotensin.[74] Significant hypertension, i.e., higher than 140 mm Hg systolic or 90 mm Hg diastolic, develops in a small fraction of patients; the relative risk was about 2.6 times greater in users in the Royal College study.[66] The development of hypertension appears to be related to the duration of oral contraceptive use and, in particular, to the progestogen dose.[74–76] Hypertension that develops with use of oral contraceptives usually returns to normal after discontinuation of the medication. There appears to be no significant relation between pregnancy-associated hypertension and the development of sustained hypertension with subsequent oral contraceptive use.[4] As with myocardial infarction and stroke, the risk of development of hypertension in women who use contraceptives increases with age.[46]

Carbohydrate Intolerance. Some women who take oral contraceptives develop impairment of glucose tolerance as manifested by elevated plasma glucose and elevated plasma insulin levels after a glucose load, which suggests the development of insulin resistance. These levels usually return to normal after the drug is stopped.[77] This impairment is apparently due to progestogen, because elevations in insulin levels occur in women using the progestogen-only pills.[78, 79] The use of oral contraceptives is also associated with a decrease in the number and affinity of insulin receptors on monocytes.[80, 81] The new low-dose oral contraceptives do not appear to affect insulin or glucose responses to a glucose load.[15, 82] Given the propensity to induce glucose intolerance and insulin resistance and the increased risk of cardiovascular disease in diabetics, it is probably prudent to recommend other forms of birth control in women with either insulin-dependent or non–insulin-dependent diabetes.

Neoplasia. Because some malignancies of the female reproductive tract respond to steroid hormones, a possible association with oral contraceptives and the development of neoplasia has been a major concern. No convincing evidence exists of a role for these agents in the development of cancers of the endometrium or ovary.[12, 83–86] In fact, the agents may provide beneficial, protective effects against the development of neoplasia.[83–89] The majority of the studies

suggest that the incidence of breast cancer is not increased in present or past users of oral contraceptives.[87, 90, 91] A few studies reported an increase in the incidence of breast cancer in previous users,[92] but there is no consensus regarding oral contraceptive use and the development of breast cancer.

The question of cervical cancer is also unsettled. This is due to the difficulty in controlling the risk factors for cervical neoplasia, such as sexual behavior (age at first intercourse and the number of sexual partners), and to exposure to sexually transmitted diseases. An additional problem is the difficulty in differentiating between dysplasia and invasive cancer of the cervix.[12] When sexual behavior was taken into account, a small risk factor of 1.3 to 3.4 for the development of cervical dysplasia was reported in oral contraceptive users.[87, 93]

An infrequent but serious association exists between the development of benign liver tumors (hepatocellular adenomas and peliosis hepatis) and the use of oral contraceptive agents.[12] These tumors may cause death because of spontaneous rupture and sudden massive hemorrhage. The risk apparently increases with duration of use,[94] but overall is low (1.2 per 100,000 woman-years), so that no liver tumors have been detected in the cohort studies to date.[95] However, an increased risk for the development of hepatocellular carcinoma was reported in one study.[96] Oral contraceptives should not be used by women with liver function abnormalities or by women with known acute or chronic liver disease. Oral contraceptives may induce jaundice in women predisposed to the development of recurrent jaundice of pregnancy.

In a follow-up of the Walnut Creek study a suggestion of significant increased risk of development of malignant melanomas was reported, but the study was not controlled for the effect of exposure to sunlight, which is a major risk factor in the development of this malignancy.[97] Other studies have not demonstrated any relationship between oral contraceptives and melanomas.[98, 99]

Other Potential Side Effects. Oral contraceptives produce an increase in the concentration of cholesterol in bile, which is probably the cause of the observed twofold increase in cholecystitis and cholelithiasis in women taking these agents.[100] Users are also at risk of developing pigmentation of the face (chloasma), which is augmented by exposure to sunlight. This effect appears to be related to the dose of estrogen and is unusual with the lower-dose agents currently in use.[13] Minor side effects attributed to oral contraceptives include dyspepsia, breast discomfort, weight gain, psychological changes, and changes in libido. Whether such symptoms are in fact due to contraceptive use is doubtful on the basis of double-blind crossover studies.[101]

BREAKTHROUGH BLEEDING. Women taking very-low-dose estrogen-containing combination oral contraceptives or the progestogen-only pills may develop breakthrough bleeding. If the amount of estrogen is lowered beyond some critical point, the progestogen-stimulated endometrium tends to be fragile and prone to breakdown, which results in asynchronous bleeding of two types. The initial bleed is associated with the first few months of oral contraceptive use. The recommended treatment is observation and reassurance because it usually resolves by the third month. Possible causes include incorrect use or failure to take the drug consistently, concurrent drug therapy, or poor absorption because of vomiting.[13] Late breakthrough bleeding may occur at any time after the first few months of contraceptive use and is thought to be a consequence of induction of a thin, atrophic endometrium. Originally, doubling of the pill dosage was recommended, but because this measure increases the intake of both estrogen and progestogen, the atrophic endometrium is unchanged.[13] Therefore, when the bleeding is excessive or bothersome, a pill containing a higher estrogen content may be instituted for one to two cycles, or conjugated estrogens or ethinyl estradiol may be added to the oral contraceptive in use. In most cases the latter solution appears to be sufficient because the problem is usually self-limited. When bleeding is not controlled by these methods, a thorough re-examination must be performed and other causes of bleeding (cervical, uterine, or pregnancy complications) must be excluded.

AMENORRHEA. The use of low-dose oral contraceptive agents and the progestogen-only pills may also be associated with an absence of withdrawal bleeding. The incidence of this phenomenon is unknown but is thought to be low (around 1%).[14] The mechanism for the amenorrhea is similar to that for breakthrough bleeding, i.e., atrophy of the endometrium. Such amenorrhea is reversible and hence does not result in future problems after the agents are discontinued, but it causes anxiety in the patient because of the possibility of pregnancy. A careful history and physical examination are indicated when amenorrhea occurs in oral contraceptive users, and a diagnostic test for pregnancy (such as the radioimmunoassay for the beta subunit of human chorionic gonadotropin) may be indicated. After pregnancy has been excluded, the patient can be reassured of the benign nature of the amenorrhea, and, if indicated, a pill containing a higher estrogen content can be instituted.

POSTPILL AMENORRHEA. Eighty percent of women resume normal menstrual function 3 mo after discontinuing oral contraceptives, and 95 to 98% are ovulatory within a year. The incidence of failure of the menses to resume after discontinuation of the pill is similar to that of the development of spontaneous secondary amenorrhea in the population as a whole. Thus subsequent fertility is probably not impaired by previous use of oral contraceptives, as had been suggested by some earlier studies.[102, 103]

BIRTH DEFECTS. Some, but not all, retrospective studies suggested that oral contraceptive use during pregnancy is associated with cardiovascular and limb defects in the fetus.[12, 104, 105] In most studies the incidence of birth defects is not increased after discontinuation of the pill.[12]

GALACTORRHEA/PROLACTINOMA. A slight increase in basal prolactin levels may occur, and galactorrhea may be detected in up to one tenth of women who take oral contraceptives.[106] The increased incidence of prolactinomas in men and women reported within the last decade may be due to (1) greater physician awareness, (2) availability of prolactin assays and improved radiological testing, or (3) the use of oral contraceptives. Most studies refute the oral contraceptive theory.[107–111] For example, a careful multicenter retrospective study reported no association between their use and the development of prolactinoma.[112]

EFFECT ON LABORATORY VALUES. Changes in values for a number of clinical laboratory tests occur in women taking oral contraceptive pills and need to be taken into consideration when laboratory data are evaluated (Table 18–7).

DRUG INTERACTIONS. Several drugs may interfere with the efficacy of oral contraceptives. Some act by enhancing the activity of liver enzymes and thus accelerate the clearance of estrogens by the liver.[113] Particular attention has been directed to the effect of antibiotics, in particular rifampin, because an increased incidence of pregnancy has been reported when rifampin is used concurrently with oral contraceptives.[114, 115] Individual reports have suggested that concurrent use of ampicillin, tetracycline, and chloramphenicol may also be associated with an increased risk of pregnancy.[12] Indeed, some authors recommend that women who take low-dose oral contraceptives should use additional protection during the period when simultaneous antibiotic treatment is required.

TABLE 18–7. Effects of Oral Contraceptives on Laboratory Tests

	Increased	Decreased
Hematological	Erythrocyte sedimentation rate	Prothrombin time
	Plasmin, plasminogen	Antithrombin III
	Euglobulin lysis	
	Clotting factors I, II, VII, VIII, IX, X, XII	
	Platelet count, aggregation, adhesiveness	
	Cryofibrinogen	
	Partial thromboplastin time	
	Serum iron concentration	
Liver	Alkaline phosphatase	Haptoglobin
	Bilirubin	Urobilinogen
	Glutamic-oxaloacetic transaminase, glutamic-pyruvic transaminase	
	Leucine aminopeptidase	
	Sulfobromophthalein retention	
Serum Proteins	Alpha-1, alpha-2–globulin	Immunoglobulins G, A, M
	Ceruloplasmin	Albumin
	Iron-binding capacity	
	Corticosteroid-binding globulin	
	Transferrin	
	Thyroid-binding globulin	
	Testosterone-binding globulin	
Vitamins	A	B_2, B_6, B_{12}
		C
		Folate
Hormones	Insulin	Triiodothyronine uptake (resin)
	Triiodothyronine, thyroxine, protein-bound iodine	Estradiol
	Aldosterone	Progesterone
	Angiotensinogen	Follicle-stimulating hormone, luteinizing hormone
	Angiotensin I and II	Renin
	Cortisol	Corticotropin
	Growth hormone	
	Prolactin	
	Testosterone	
Others	Glucose	Magnesium
	Cholesterol	Zinc
	Triglycerides	Calcium
	Lipoproteins	Complement-reactive protein

Selected laboratory values adapted from Hatcher RA, Stewart GK, Stewart F, et al. Contraceptive Technology, 1982–1983. New York: Irvington, 1982; and from Effects of oral contraceptives on laboratory test results. The Medical Letter 1979; 21(13):54–56.

Potential Benefits. Unanticipated benefits of contraceptive use include control of dysmenorrhea and anovulatory dysfunctional uterine bleeding, which results in a decrease in uterine blood loss.[12] Oral contraceptives have also been beneficial in preventing certain types of sexually transmitted diseases. For example, the incidence of pelvic inflammatory disease is decreased in pill users, possibly owing to changes in cervical mucus.[116] The incidence of ectopic pregnancies is also decreased.[12] In contrast to previous views, women who take oral contraceptives appear to have a reduced risk for the development of uterine leiomyomas.[117]

Oral contraceptive use may decrease the incidence of endometrial and ovarian carcinoma[83–86] and of functional ovarian cysts.[118, 119] The incidence of fibroadenomas and of fibrocystic disease of the breast is decreased.[12] Oral contraceptives may reduce the risk of development of endometriosis, and they constitute one of the treatment regimens for this disorder. Hirsutism and acne in women with polycystic ovarian disease are also effectively treated by oral contraceptive agents.[120] Contraceptive use may reduce the incidence of rheumatoid arthritis.[121]

Selection and Prescription of Oral Contraceptives: Recommendations. A thorough history and physical examination must be performed before oral contraceptive therapy is initiated. The absolute and relative contraindications to oral contraceptives should be considered before such therapy is prescribed (Table 18–8). The physical examination should include an evaluation of blood pressure, the breasts, the abdomen (with particular attention to the liver), and the pelvis, including a Papanicolaou smear. Follow-up examinations should be performed at 6 mo to 1 y. When oral contraceptives are prescribed, the woman should be told to notify her physician of the development of serious side effects, including leg swelling or pain, headache, visual disturbances, speech defects, sensory or motor impairment, and chest or abdominal pain.

The need for laboratory testing before prescribing oral contraceptives is controversial. A family history of cardiovascular disease, hormone-dependent cancer, and diabetes may suggest more frequent evaluation and at an earlier age. In women younger than age 30, screening for sexually transmitted disease, hematocrit, urinalysis, plasma lipid levels, and sickle cell testing (in black women) are sufficient. In women between age 30 and 35, a serum glucose assay and a mammogram are ordered if the history suggests diabetes or breast disease. All of these tests are recommended for women older than age 35 if oral contraceptives are to be prescribed.[122] If the plasma cholesterol level is higher than 8 mmol/L (300 mg/dL) or plasma triglyceride level is higher than 5.5 mmol/L (500 mg/dL), another form of contraception is indicated.[123]

The use of oral contraceptives by women of older reproductive age (age 35 to 50) remains controversial. Sterilization, IUDs, barrier contraceptives, and natural family planning are usually recommended for these women. However, some believe that if women of this age are healthy, without risk factors, and have negative laboratory screening test results, low-dose oral contraceptives may be safe.[120, 124]

An additional consideration when beginning oral contraceptive use is the day of the menstrual cycle on which to initiate therapy. Most commonly, the pill is started on the fifth day or the first Sunday after the beginning of menstruation. In women with chronic anovulation (such as in polycystic ovarian disease) who are amenorrheic, oral contraceptives can be started after a negative screening test result for pregnancy followed by a progestogen-induced withdrawal bleed. After a full-term pregnancy, oral contraceptives should be initiated on or after the fourth postpartum week, or 2 wk after delivery in women who are treated with bromocriptine to prevent lactation. After a spontaneous or an induced abortion, oral contraceptives are usually started within 5 d because ovulation may occur within 2 wk in these situations.[122]

TABLE 18–8. Contraindications for Oral Contraceptive Use

Absolute Contraindications

1. Known or suspected estrogen-dependent neoplasia
2. Thrombophlebitis or thromboembolic disease (or history thereof)
3. Cerebrovascular or coronary artery disease (or history thereof)
4. Active liver disease or adenoma
5. Undiagnosed vaginal bleeding
6. Known or suspected pregnancy

Relative Contraindications

1. Severe headaches or migraines
2. Hypertension
3. Diabetes mellitus
4. Gallbladder disease
5. Sickle cell disease (SS or SC)
6. Elective surgery
7. Leg injury or cast
8. Hyperlipemia

A preparation should be recommended that offers effective contraception with the greatest margin of safety and fewest side effects. Safety is probably greater with pills containing less than 50 μg of estrogen. Most physicians recommend a combination pill containing 35 μg of estrogen because doses lower than that are less effective and may produce more breakthrough bleeding.[13] Previous data regarding potency and serious side effects may not apply to the low-dose pills, which are associated with a reduced incidence of such side effects.

POSTCOITAL CONTRACEPTION (INTERCEPTION). The risk of pregnancy from unprotected midcycle intercourse ranges up to 30%, and a postcoital contraceptive or interception pill is occasionally indicated,[125] for example, after rape. Historically, women have used a variety of agents to avoid pregnancy after unprotected midcycle intercourse. Modern posthormonal interception, often called the morning-after pill, involves administration of high-dose estrogens.[126] Although these agents are effective, their use is associated with nausea and vomiting as well as menstrual disturbances. The use of 50 μg of ethinyl estradiol and 0.5 mg of norgestrel is equally effective and results in fewer side effects. The recommended dosage is two tablets within 72 h of exposure and two more tablets 12 h later.[127, 128]

LONG-ACTING CONTRACEPTIVE STEROIDS. A variety of long-acting steroid contraceptives have been developed as alternatives to oral agents. Some of these methods are being utilized extensively in developing countries. Originally, they were developed to eliminate the estrogen component of the oral contraceptives; however, agents containing only progestogen cause significant amenorrhea, breakthrough bleeding, and other deleterious side effects, as discussed earlier.

Injectable Steroids. The principal long-acting injectable contraceptives are medroxyprogesterone acetate (150 mg intramuscularly every 3 mo) and norethindrone enanthate (200 mg intramuscularly every 8 wk for 6 mo, then every 12 wk).[129] Slightly higher pregnancy rates occur with norethindrone enanthate than with medroxyprogesterone acetate, and the pregnancy rates with both treatment methods are higher shortly after the first injection.[130] The mechanism of action of long-acting progestational agents includes inhibition of ovulation; production of a thick, unfavorable cervical mucus; induction of a decidual reaction, which results in an unfavorable endometrium, and possibly delayed ovum transport. These agents are approved for contraception in more than 90 countries but have not been approved for use in the United States.[130] The Food and Drug Administration has approved medroxyprogesterone acetate for treatment of endometrial carcinoma.[131] Problems with medroxyprogesterone acetate include possible carcinogenic effects (it has induced breast tumors in dogs), increased incidence of breakthrough bleeding and amenorrhea, and diminished fertility for up to 2 y after discontinuation.[129, 131] A number of new progestogens are being tested as long-activating injectable agents in the form of microspheres or microcapsules that release hormones slowly at a constant rate and are effective for 1 to 6 mo.[129] To reduce vaginal spotting and bleeding problems with pure progestogens, monthly estrogen-progestogen formulations are used in some developing countries.[129]

Implants. Subdermal implantation of polydimethylsiloxone (Silastic) capsules or rods containing a variety of progestogens have been used for contraception.[129, 132] The capsules are implanted through a small incision on the forearm or inguinal or gluteal surfaces and must be removed after the steroid has been released. Depending on the agent used, the amount released appears to be relatively stable, and the duration of activity is from 6 mo to 5 y.[129] Although implants are effective, they require removal and are associated with breakthrough bleeding and amenorrhea similar to that seen when the agents are injected. Biodegradable implants containing progestogens that do not require removal are in the developmental phase, as are biodegradable pellets.[129]

Vaginal Rings. Steroids may also be administered in Silastic vaginal rings that are impregnated with hormone.[129, 133] Most of these rings contain a progestogen, but a few contain an estrogen and a progestogen. They are fitted as a diaphragm in the vagina, kept in place for 3 wk, removed for 1 wk to allow for withdrawal bleeding, and then reinserted. These rings are undergoing trials. Problems include vaginitis, expulsion, interference with coitus, difficulty of insertion, and occasional breakthrough bleeding.[133]

Steroid-Releasing Intrauterine Devices. The Progestasert IUD is the only hormonal IUD available in the United States (see later). Its main advantage is that its use results in decreased bleeding during menstruation (a common cause of discontinuation of the IUD) and decreased menstrual cramping.[134] The disadvantages are breakthrough bleeding and the requirement for yearly replacement. IUDs are being tested that contain norgestrel and require replacement every 3 to 5 y.

Progesterone Antagonists. The development of a synthetic competitive progesterone antagonist, mifepristone (RU 486), has opened new approaches to fertility control. Mifepristone prevents ovulation in women and induces luteolysis and premature menstruation.[135, 136] This form of medication is not associated with any major side effects and may be used in the future as a contraceptive until women reach menopause.[137] Its use as an abortifacient is described later in this chapter.

Nonsteroidal Contraceptives

A variety of LHRH analogues have been synthesized in an attempt to prolong the activity of the hormone. Paradoxically, prolonged continuous administration of LHRH and its agonists results in the lowering of gonadotropin levels.[138] Consequently, the use of LHRH as a contraceptive has been attempted in men and women. Its primary site of action is the pituitary. During long-term continuous administration of LHRH and its agonists, the rate of gonadotropin secretion increases during the first week and then decreases.[138] Potential mechanisms whereby LHRH analogues may act as contraceptives include (1) inhibition of ovulation, (2) induction of luteal-phase defects, and (3) enhancement of luteolysis.[138] Daily administration of the agonists by injection[139] or intranasally[140] inhibits ovulation and provides effective contraception. Most of the reports utilized either buserelin or nafarelin by daily intranasal administration.[140, 141] In these studies there were no pregnancies, but some women developed oligomenorrhea, irregular bleeding, or amenorrhea. To achieve regular withdrawal bleeding patterns and to prevent the possible development of endometrial hyperplasia, other investigators administered LHRH analogues for 21 d with added progestogen during days 17 to 21 and no therapy for 7 d each month.[142] This regimen results in regular withdrawal bleeding but is also associated with intermenstrual spotting. Because continous or prolonged intermittent therapy induces a pseudomenopause or low-estrogen state and increases the risk of bone loss, the use of LHRH analogues for female contraception is not an acceptable alternative at present to other forms of hormonal contraception.

The effects of smaller doses of LHRH agonists on luteal function have been investigated in hopes of preventing the low-estrogen state that accompanies the inhibition of ovulation. Administration of 50 μg of LHRH agonists by subcutaneous injection daily during the first 3 d of the menstrual cycle was followed by a significant decrease in FSH level, with prolongation of the follicular phase and shortening of the luteal phase with decreased progesterone secretion.[143] Other investigators using similar regimens found delayed ovulation but no effect on the length of the luteal phase.[138]

Attempts have also been made to induce luteolysis by injection of LHRH analogues at the time of expected ovulation,[138] and to induce luteal-phase insufficiency by administering the analogues by injection or intranasally between the fifth and eighth days of the luteal phase.[144, 145] A major problem with these alternative treatment methods is the accurate timing of ovulation.

The Intrauterine Device

Approximately 85 million women worldwide use the IUD, including more than 59 million women in the People's Republic of China.[146] The IUD was first used in antiquity, but modern use was initiated with the development of intrauterine rings. Two types of IUD are now in use: (1) unmedicated (Lippes loop, single-coil stainless steel ring) and (2) medicated, containing copper (Copper-7, TCu-200B, TCu-380A) or hormone (Progestasert). Because of economic reasons and the inability of the manufacturers to obtain liability insurance, the only devices that are currently marketed in the United States are Progestasert and a copper-containing IUD (TCu-380A). The TCu-380A contains 380 mm² of exposed copper wrapped around the vertical stem and arms of the plastic device to enhance contraceptive effectiveness.[146] Progestasert, also a T-shaped plastic device, contains 38 mg of progesterone, which is released at a daily rate of 65 μg.[134] IUDs may be inserted at any time of the menstrual cycle but are usually inserted at the time of menstrual bleeding to enhance the ease of insertion and to diminish the chance of pregnancy.

All devices now available worldwide are roughly equal in contraceptive effectiveness, with failure rates ranging from 1.4 to 4 per 100 women at 1 y after insertion.[146] The major advantages of the copper-containing IUDs are (1) a smaller increase in menstrual blood flow than with the unmedicated IUDs, (2) a lower expulsion rate, and (3) less pain after insertion. The progesterone-containing IUD is associated with a decrease in both menstrual bleeding and dysmenorrhea.[146] The drawbacks of the copper- and progesterone-containing IUDs compared with unmedicated IUDs include the necessity for frequent replacement (4 y for copper-containing IUDs and yearly for progesterone-containing IUDs) and greater cost.

The precise mechanism by which the IUD acts as a contraceptive is unclear. The devices may prevent fertilization by impairing sperm transport and by damaging sperm directly.[147, 148] Another action is thought to result from an induction of an endometrial inflammatory response, so that the endometrium is unfavorable for implantation. Plasma cells and macrophages in the inflammatory response may phagocytose spermatozoa or possibly the fertilized ovum.[149-151] Copper appears to increase the inflammatory action, and the progesterone-containing IUD interferes with the hormonal response of the endometrium.[146] Complications of IUD use include excessive bleeding, infection, and expulsion. Approximately 5 to 15% of women discontinue its use within the first year because of bleeding and pain.[146] The increased loss of blood rarely results in significant anemia, but intermittent iron replacement or use of nonsteroidal anti-inflammatory drugs may be appropriate. The increased bleeding is thought to be due to vascular disruption, increased fibrinolytic activity, or increased activity of mast cells with local release of heparin.[146, 152]

A potentially serious complication of IUD use is the development of pelvic inflammatory disease, which usually occurs soon after insertion.[146] This issue is important both because of acute morbidity and because of an increased risk of infertility related to tubal obstruction. Current IUD users are 1.6 times more likely to be hospitalized with pelvic inflammatory disease than women utilizing no forms of contraception, and 4.5 times more likely than oral contraceptive users.[153] Indeed, the incidence of pelvic inflammatory disease may actually be reduced in women using barrier contraceptives or oral contraceptives. Potential mechanisms for the increased incidence of pelvic inflammatory disease include the entry of bacteria into the endometrium at the time of or shortly after insertion, and promotion of bacterial growth by the increased volume and duration of menstrual bleeding.[146, 154] The highest rates of pelvic inflammatory disease were observed with the Dalkon Shield device. Retrospective and prospective studies suggest a lower but still significant risk of pelvic inflammatory disease in women using currently available IUDs compared with nonusers.[154] Occasionally, the infection may be so severe that it results in bilateral tubo-ovarian abscesses. Prompt recognition and treatment of pelvic inflammatory disease are critical for maintaining tubal function. Therapy includes removal of the IUD, prompt initiation of antibiotics, and hospitalization if indicated. Responsible organisms include *Neisseria gonorrhoeae, Chlamydia, Escherichia coli, Bacteroides, Peptostreptococcus,* and rarely *Actinomyces.*[155]

If pregnancy occurs, the IUD should be removed (if the string is visible) to reduce the incidence of spontaneous abortion, severe infection, and occasional maternal death that has been associated with concurrent pregnancy in IUD users.[156] If the IUD string is not visible, the choice of abortion is offered, and if abortion is not acceptable, the patient should be observed for signs of infection. Such pregnancy is more likely to be extrauterine than intrauterine, because the IUD reduces the incidence of intrauterine pregnancies more efficiently than that of ectopic pregnancies.[146]

The effects of IUD use on subsequent fertility have not been fully evaluated. Most women who discontinue IUD use conceive as rapidly as nonusers.[146] Because IUDs increase the risk of developing pelvic infection, women who have pelvic inflammatory disease may develop tubal obstruction. Until this issue is settled, women who are nulligravid should use other forms of contraception. In addition, women with a history of pelvic inflammatory disease or who have multiple sex partners run an increased risk of developing pelvic inflammatory disease and also should use an alternative form of contraception. There is no evidence that IUD users develop cancer of the reproductive tract more often than do nonusers.[157] A rare complication is perforation at the time of insertion, which is an indication for surgical removal. Absolute contraindications for IUD use include active or previous pelvic infection, abnormalities or distortion of the uterine cavity, undiagnosed genital bleeding, uterine or cervical malignancy, history of ectopic pregnancy, increased susceptibility to infection (leukemias, diabetes, valvular heart disease, acquired immunodeficiency syndrome, and long-term glucocorticoid therapy), genital actinomycosis, allergies to copper or Wilson disease (for copper-containing IUDs), and known or suspected pregnancy.[146, 158]

Barrier Methods

Barrier methods of contraception circumvent many of the potential risks that accompany the use of oral contraceptives and IUDs. These methods are among the oldest, most simple, and most widely used forms of birth control.

Originally, the term barrier implied a physical barrier that prevents the sperm from reaching the fertilizable egg. More recently, the definition has broadened to include biological, chemical, and physical means of preventing fertilization. Barrier contraceptives are often underutilized, but if they are used correctly and continuously they provide adequate contraception. In addition, they are simple to use and provide some protection against sexually transmitted diseases.[159] All barrier methods of contraception require prior planning and motivation.

The vaginal diaphragm is one of the most commonly utilized forms of female barrier contraception. The diaphragm consists of a shallow rubber cup that is stabilized by a circumscribing, rubber-covered steel spring. The three types of diaphragms (the coil spring, the flat spring, and the arching spring) are designed for various vaginal shapes. The efficacy of the diaphragm depends on selection of the appropriate type and size, proper placement, and continued usage. Proper use requires the placement of a spermicidal cream or jelly inside the dome of the diaphragm before insertion prior to intercourse. For maximal effectiveness, the diaphragm must be left in place for at least 6 h after intercourse. Failure rates vary from 2.4 to 17 per 100 women per year of usage.[14] The effectiveness, as with all forms of barrier contraception, depends primarily on continued use. Complications include occasional allergic reactions to latex or to the spermicidal agent. In addition, improperly fitted diaphragms may cause vaginal irritation or pain. A profuse, foul-smelling vaginal discharge may occur if a diaphragm is left in place too long; for this reason, it is recommended that it be removed and washed once every 24 h.[14, 159]

The cervical cap is a smaller version of the diaphragm that fits directly over the cervix and is used in conjunction with a spermicidal jelly.[159] The cervical cap requires fitting by a trained physician. Some women cannot be fitted properly because of a developmental or a surgical deformity of the cervix. The cervical cap has been approved by the Food and Drug Administration but is not widely available at present. The effectiveness and side effects of the cervical cap and the recommendations for time of insertion and removal are similar to those for the vaginal diaphragm.

Chemical or spermicidal agents can be used by themselves or as a supplement to other barrier contraceptive methods. Such agents are available in jellies, creams, suppositories, aerosol foams, film, and sponges and comprise two components: a relatively inert base that physically blocks the passage of sperm and any of several chemical spermicides.[159, 160] The active ingredients in some commonly available spermicidal agents are given in Table 18–9. The majority utilize nonoxynol 9 (nonylphenoxypolyethoxyethanol).

Toxic shock syndrome has been reported rarely in users of diaphragms and sponges.[161, 162] Women who use cervical caps may also be at risk for the development of toxic shock syndrome.

Failure rates of spermicidal agents that are used alone range from 2 to 29 pregnancies per 100 woman-years of use.[14] Like mechanical barriers, they provide some protection against sexually transmitted diseases including syphilis, gonorrhea, and disorders caused by *Chlamydia, Trichomonas, Candida,* human immunodeficiency virus, and papillomavirus.[159, 160, 163] There are relatively few complications associated with spermicidal agents other than infrequent allergic reactions or irritation.[159] In some studies a slightly increased risk of congenital abnormalities has been reported in the offspring of women who used spermicides vaginally.[164] A number of larger studies have failed to demonstrate such an association.[159, 165–167]

TABLE 18–9. Some Available Spermicidal Agents

Type	Product	Active Ingredient
Cream	Conceptrol	Nonoxynol 9 (5%)
	Ortho-Creme	Nonoxynol 9 (2%)
	Koromex II	Octoxynol (3%)
	Milex Cream	Glyceryl ricinoleate (0.36%)
Jelly	Koromex II	Octoxynol (1%)
	Ortho-Gynol	p-Diisobutylphenoxypolyethoxyethanol
	Preceptin	p-Diisobutylphenoxypolyethoxyethanol
	Ramses "10-hour"	Dodecaethylene glycol monolaurate (5%)
Suppository	Encare	Nonoxynol 9 (2.5%)
	Ortho-forms	Nonoxynol 9 (2%)
	Semicid	Nonoxynol 9 (6.6%)
	S-Positive	Nonoxynol 9 (10%)
Foam	Delfen	Nonoxynol 9 (12.5%)
	Koromex	Nonoxynol 9 (12.5%)
	Emko	Nonoxynol 9 (8%)
	Because	Nonoxynol 9 (8%)
Sponge	Today	Nonoxynol 9 (1 g)
Film	VCF	Nonoxynol 9 (72 mg)

Natural Family-Planning Methods

Natural family planning is one of the most widely used methods of fertility regulation, particularly by those who for religious, financial, or cultural reasons do not use drugs or devices for contraception. Such methods are based on periodic abstinence from sexual relations during the fertile period surrounding the time of ovulation, which usually occurs about 14 d before the next expected menstrual period. Techniques for identifying the fertile period, commonly termed rhythm methods, include the calendar method, basal body temperature method, cervical mucus method, and symptothermal method. Successful application of these techniques requires both training and motivation.[168, 169]

The calendar method is based on the work of Ogino[170] and Knaus.[171] Calculation of the fertile period rests on three assumptions: (1) ovulation occurs on day 14 before the onset of the next menses, (2) sperm remain viable for only 48 to 72 h, and (3) the unfertilized ovum survives for only 12 to 24 h.[168] This method requires the use of a menstrual calendar on which the woman records the length of her menstrual cycles for at least 6 and preferably 12 cycles. The first day of the potential fertile period is the shortest cycle minus 18 d, and the last day of the potential fertile period is the longest cycle minus 11 d. As an example, in a woman whose menstrual cycles vary from 26 to 31 d, application of the calendar method would mean a potential fertility period as follows: the first day of potential fertility, 26 − 18 = 8; the last day of potential fertility, 31 − 11 = 20. This would mean that the period of fertility would range from the 8th to the 20th days of the cycle, so that the safe days during which intercourse would be allowed, with the calendar method, would be from the first day of menstrual flow through the 7th day of the cycle and from the 20th day until the onset of the next menses. Women with grossly irregular cycles cannot use this method.

The basal body temperature method depends on identification of the rise in basal body temperature from a relatively low level during the follicular phase to the higher level during the luteal phase of the menstrual cycle in response to the thermogenic effect of progesterone.[169] The rise in temperature is small (between 0.2 and 0.5°C), occurs abruptly over a 24-h period, and is sometimes preceded by a small drop in temperature. To use this method, a woman records her basal temperature each day for 3 consecutive mo. The elevated temperatures begin 1 to 2 d after ovulation and correspond to the rising levels of progesterone. Intercourse is not permitted between the end of menses and 3 d after the temperature rise. Problems with this method include difficulty in interpreting temperature charts and the fact that abstinence is necessary for the entire preovulatory period.[168]

Changes in the character and appearance of cervical secretions occur just before ovulation in most women and are the basis of the mucus method.[168] To practice this method the woman must differentiate between sensations of dryness, moistness, and wetness of the secretions at the vaginal opening during the different phases of the menstrual cycle. The viscous mucus that is present during the pre- and postovulatory phases must be differentiated from the slippery, clear, and copious mucus that appears just before ovulation. It is necessary to identify the time at which the change in character of the mucus occurs; mucus is removed from the vagina to determine whether it possesses increased stretchiness (spinnbarkeit). By this method, abstinence must start the first day after such a change in mucus is observed and continue until the fourth day after the maximal amount of cervical mucus is observed. All other days until menstruation are considered infertile days. Care must be taken to differentiate cervical mucus from lubricants and semen.

The symptothermal method combines the previously described techniques for identifying the fertile period including changes in cervical mucus, calendar calculations to estimate the onset of the fertile period, and basal body temperature charts. In addition, symptoms such as ovulatory abdominal pain (mittelschmerz); midcycle ovulatory bleeding; self-observed changes in the position, texture, moistness, and dilation of the cervix; breast tenderness; edema; and mood changes can be used to identify the fertile period.

Natural family-planning methods can be used during the fertile days in conjunction with other forms of contraception such as condoms, diaphragms, and spermicidal agents. The major complication with all these methods is a high rate of unplanned pregnancies. The overall effectiveness is a function of the degree of patient education and dedication, and it varies from as high as 99% to an average of around 70%.[168, 169] In a prospective study, there was no difference in birth defects between the offspring of women using natural family planning and the offspring of women using other methods.[172]

The development of home urinary or blood assay kits to determine and predict precisely the time of the initial rise of estrogen before ovulation and the rise of progesterone to detect the postovulatory state is under investigation. It is hoped that these or similar methods will increase the reliability and effectiveness of natural family planning.[173, 174]

Other types of natural family planning include abstinence after pregnancy in certain societies in which intercourse is taboo during this period; coitus interruptus; or the withdrawal method. The last-named requires no devices, no chemicals, and little education; the failure rate is around 16 pregnancies per 100 women per year of usage.[14] Coitus interruptus may also be used with other natural family-planning methods during the period of expected fertility to enhance their effectiveness.

Breast-feeding has been advocated as a physiological mechanism for spacing births, but reliance on this form of birth control in certain parts of the world has probably been responsible, in part, for the exponential increase in the birth rate. The basis for this method is that breast-feeding inhibits ovulation after delivery, presumably as a consequence of the amount of prolactin that is secreted during breast stimulation. The effectiveness of this method depends on the frequency and continued use of breast-feeding, but most investigators consider it unreliable as a means of birth control.[14, 175] Even the associated amenorrhea that occurs is unreliable as an indication of a safe period of infertility, because nearly 80% of women who breast-feed ovulate unpredictably before their first menstrual period.[176] After menstruation resumes, the risk of pregnancy is similar in women who continue to breast-feed and in non–breast-feeding women. Because of the high risk of pregnancy in breast-feeding women, contraceptive counseling should begin early in the postpartum period. The preferred methods of birth control in such women include abstinence, barrier methods, and IUDs. Whereas some of the higher-dosage oral contraceptives reduce the volume of breast milk, the new low-dose estrogen and progestogen-only contraceptives have no effect or may slightly increase milk volume.[175] Small quantities of orally ingested steroid hormones are secreted in milk and are thus transmitted to the newborn infant. Because of the possible long-term effects of steroid hormones on the infant, oral contraceptives probably should not be given to nursing mothers.

Immunological Techniques

Contraceptive vaccines are under investigation as an effective method of fertility control. Hormones and proteins of the female reproductive tract or of early pregnancy are not in themselves antigenic and must be linked to other proteins such as serum albumin or tetanus toxoid to induce an antibody response.[177, 178] Anti-LHRH antibodies, anti-LH antibodies,[178] anti-FSH antibodies,[179] and antibodies against zona pellucida antigens have been used to induce infertility in experimental animals.[177–179] Anti–human chorionic gonadotropin vaccines are now being subjected to phase I clinical trials in women. No significant complications have been observed to date in women so immunized, and in most cases a variable period of temporary infertility results.[179]

Sterilization

Sterilization is now the most widely used form of birth control worldwide; by 1984 a total of 94 million women had undergone some form of sterilization procedure.[180] Between 1970 and 1980 approximately 5 million women in the United States underwent surgical sterilization procedures.[14] The increased use of such procedures during the recent past is due to improvement in surgical techniques and dissatisfaction with the complications of other contraceptive methods (Table 18–10).

Surgical

Simple ligation of the fallopian tubes through a standard abdominal or minilaparotomy incision is one of the oldest forms of tubal sterilization and one of the most common surgical procedures performed today. Other methods to interrupt fallopian tubes include ligation and crushing, simple resection, and resection of a midportion of the tube followed by insertion of the tubal stumps into the mesosalpinx or the wall of the uterus (Irving procedure). The procedure can be performed during the puerperal period, usually through a small periumbilical incision. In the non-puerperal woman, techniques for ligation and resection of the fallopian tube include a minilaparotomy incision and conventional colpotomy incision through the posterior vagina, followed by ligation and partial resection of the fallopian tubes or fimbriectomy.

Various laparoscopic techniques have been devised to reduce the duration of the hospital stay and the length of the abdominal incision. These include fulguration by hot cautery (unipolar or bipolar) and the application of clips (silicone-titanium and spring-loaded clips) or bands (Silastic rings).[180]

Surgical techniques involving the uterus include hyster-

TABLE 18–10. Methods of Sterilization of Women

Surgical
A. Fallopian tube
   1. Ligation/resection
      a. Abdominal
      b. Minilaparotomy
      c. Vaginal
   2. Laparoscopy
      a. Fulguration/division
      b. Clips
      c. Bands
B. Uterus
   1. Hysteroscopic fulguration of tubal ostia
   2. Hysterectomy

Chemical
A. Liquid installation
   1. Quinicrine
   2. Methyl-2-cyanoacrylate (MCA)
   3. Silicone polymers (Silastic)
   4. Gelatin-resorcinol-formaldehyde (GRF)
   5. Phenol (carbolic acid) compounds
B. Solid plugs
   1. Silastic
   2. Polyethylene
   3. Dacron
   4. Teflon

Data from Population Reports. Minilaparotomy and laparoscopy: safe, effective, and widely used. Series C, No. 9. Female Sterilization. Baltimore: The Johns Hopkins University, 1985.

ectomy and fulguration of tubal ostia by hysteroscopic examination. In the latter the tubal ostium is visualized through the hysteroscope, an electrode is placed in the tubal ostium, and an electrical current is applied. The principal problem is the high failure rate because of incomplete fulguration. Many clinicians prefer to introduce chemicals into the uterus to achieve tubal occlusion (see later). Hysterectomy for sterilization may be indicated if other uterine disorders or pelvic diseases are present, such as leiomyomata, menorrhagia, pelvic pain, uterine prolapse, stress urinary incontinence, or cervical intraepithelial neoplasia.

The mortality rate for tubal sterilization procedures in the United States is approximately 8 per 100,000.[39] Complications of the abdominal and minilaparotomy procedures are similar to those of other surgical procedures involving the abdomen and include anesthetic-related complications, wound infection, hemorrhage, and bowel or bladder injury. The vaginal approach is associated with an increased incidence of infection. The failure rates of the various abdominal and vaginal sterilization procedures, defined as the number of pregnancies, range between 0.2 and 0.6 per 100 procedures (Table 18–11).[181, 182]

Complications of laparoscopic procedures include perforation of the uterus by the uterine manipulator and

TABLE 18–11. Pregnancy Rates After Sterilization Procedures

Method	Pregnancy Rate (per 100 Procedures)
Ligation/resection	
Puerperal abdominal	0.2*
Interval abdominal	0.6*
Vaginal	0.3*
Laparoscopic	
Coagulation and cutting	0.8†
Spring clip	2.3†
Silastic band	0.8†
Hysteroscopic procedures	2.3*

*Adapted from Shepherd MK. Female contraceptive sterilization. Obstet Gynecol Surv 1974; 29:739.
†Adapted from Brenner WE. Evaluation of contemporary sterilization methods. J Reprod Med 1981; 26:439–453.

complications resulting from the carbon dioxide introduced into the abdomen to produce pneumoperitoneum. These complications include creation of cutaneous emphysema and the injection of carbon dioxide into the intestine or into the intravascular spaces. In addition, perforation of the intestine or vessels can occur during insertion of the trocar. These severe complications are rare; their occurrence appears to be related to the skill and experience of the surgeon.[180–183] Coagulation with a unipolar cautery, which is the original method for laparoscopic sterilization, may cause bowel burns. Bipolar cautery causes this complication less often but does not completely alleviate the danger.[180] Consequently, spring clips and Silastic band techniques were introduced. The spring clip method has a higher rate of technical failure.[184] The failure rates for the various laparoscopic methods of sterilization are summarized in Table 18–11. Although the failure rates for hysterectomy are essentially zero, the postoperative course, morbidity, and mortality are 10- to 100-fold greater than those for a tubal ligation.[38] The problems that are associated with hysteroscopic fulguration include thermal injury to the bowel and a high pregnancy rate.[180]

Chemical

Several chemical methods of sterilization are under investigation (see Table 18–10). The most extensive experience is with quinacrine, which is injected into the uterus near the tubal ostia and produces sclerosis of the tubal lumen. Complications, although relatively rare, include seizures, intrauterine adhesions, and abdominal pain; the failure rate is around 30%.[180] Adhesive substances such as Silastic (a silicone polymer), methyl-2-cyanoacrylate, and gelatin-resorcinol-formaldehyde have been instilled experimentally into the uterotubal junction to form a plug. These compounds are viscous when instilled and solidify when in place. Although morbidity is low, failure rates are significant.[180]

Various types of solid plugs have been devised that can be inserted into the uterine or fimbrial ends of the tubes. These plugs include Silastic, polyethylene, ceramic, Dacron, and Teflon devices. Preliminary results indicate that these methods of contraception are reversible when the plugs are removed.[180]

The number of women seeking sterilization continues to increase, particularly young women with relatively small families. An increasing number of these young women may later desire reversal of the sterilization procedure. As many as 1 or 2 per 1000 sterilized women may be candidates for tubal reanastomosis.[185] Before a decision is made on a reanastomosis procedure, the couple must be carefully screened for other infertility factors and coexisting medical disorders, and the woman must be evaluated for distal tubal disease and for adequacy of tubal length. Those procedures in which clips or ligation involve only a small portion of the fallopian tubes have a greater chance of successful reversal. Laparoscopic fulguration often causes severe damage to a greater length of the fallopian tube, and thus successful reversals are less frequent. Improved pregnancy rates have been reported with surgical techniques utilizing operative microscopes.[185] If the length of the remaining tubes is insufficient or the patient fails to conceive after a surgical reversal, then in vitro fertilization and embryo transfer may be offered.

Abortion

Between 30 and 50 million abortions are performed worldwide each year, primarily as a means of fertility control. In the United States a pregnant woman and her physician can make the decision to abort for fertility control through 24 to 26 wk.[186, 187] However, state governments may regulate abortions particularly during the time between the first trimester and 24 to 26 wk of gestation (now considered to be the age of fetal viability). Since abortions became legal in 1973, deaths from illegal abortions have declined markedly.[188]

The choice of method of abortion depends primarily on the stage of pregnancy, on whether associated uterine diseases are present, and on whether sterilization is desired.

Surgical

Menstrual extraction by suction can be performed in the first few weeks after a missed menstrual period. A small, flexible plastic cannula is inserted and the uterine contents are evacuated by suction applied to the cannula. The main problem with this technique is occasional failure to abort the pregnancy. The traditional dilatation and curettage procedure circumvents this difficulty but requires greater dilation of the cervix and is associated with more pain and blood loss.[4]

Suction or vacuum curettage is the most widely used method of abortion in the United States.[4] A laminaria tent, which is made from stems of the seaweed *Laminaria digitata* or *L. japonica*, is usually placed in the cervix 6 to 24 h before the procedure and slowly dilates the cervix by osmotic swelling. A small plastic cannula is then inserted into the uterus, and the contents are evacuated by utilizing an electrically powered vacuum source.

Surgical methods of abortion during the second trimester include dilation by laminaria and extraction of the products of conception by suction curettage and/or forceps. Other surgical procedures include hysterotomy (which is analogous to a small cesarean section) or hysterectomy when another clear indication for such a procedure is present. Morbidity and mortality rates after these last two procedures are high, and they are therefore used infrequently for abortion.

Chemical

Midtrimester abortions (more than 14 to 16 wk of gestational age) can be induced by the intrauterine instillation of solutions such as dinoprost (prostaglandin $F_{2\alpha}$), hypertonic saline, or hypertonic urea.[14, 189] In addition, dinoprostone (prostaglandin E_2) vaginal suppositories are available for termination of pregnancy in the second trimester in cases of fetal death in utero up to 28 wk. To shorten the abortion time and blood loss, laminaria and oxytocin are used in conjunction with these methods.

Progesterone antagonists, such as mifepristone (RU 486), have been used to induce abortions in early human gestation either alone or in combination with oral prostaglandins.[190, 191] The People's Republic of China and France have approved the use of this agent for early pregnancy termination.

Complications from chemical methods include hemorrhage, infection, retention of the products of conception, and cervical injury. The risk of death from abortions is low, but when death occurs it is more likely associated with pregnancies of more than 8 wk gestation.

FERTILITY CONTROL IN MEN

Fertility control in men involves either use of the condom or vasectomy. A major attempt has been made to

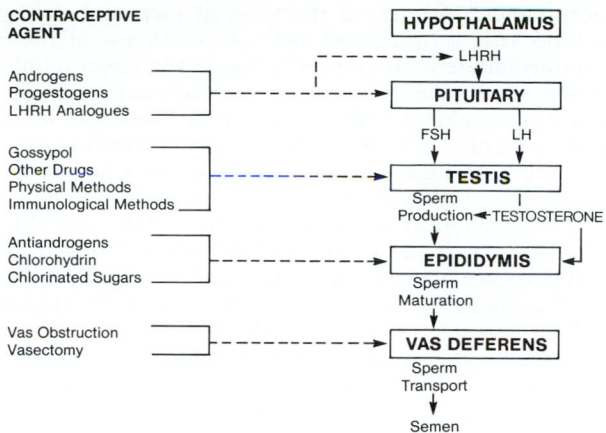

Figure 18–6. Principal sites of action of contraceptive agents on the male reproductive tract.

develop reversible contraceptives for men, but that objective still remains an unfulfilled promise. Because of the importance of such an agent, we review briefly the sites at which these agents might act: e.g., the hypothalamic-pituitary level, the testis, the epididymis, or the vas deferens (Fig. 18–6).

The Condom

The condom is the oldest form of barrier contraception, and use of the latex rubber condom is a major method of male contraception. In Japan almost 80% of couples practicing contraception rely on the condom.[192] Condoms are safe and effective; when used properly and consistently, their effectiveness is greater than 97%.[192] Like other forms of barrier contraceptives, condoms offer significant protection against sexually transmitted diseases. The only complication of condom use is a rare allergic reaction to, or irritation from, latex rubber or the lubricant used.[192]

Vasectomy

Background and Current Use

Surgical sterilization procedures have gained widespread acceptance since the 1950s.[193, 194] In the United States, almost 50% of couples choose surgical interruption of the vas deferens (vasectomy), and about 500,000 vasectomy procedures are performed each year.[195, 196] It is clear that the profile of men undergoing vasectomy has changed in that the average age, length of marriage, and number of living children were greater in 1968 to 1971 than in 1974 to 1978 (Table 18–12).[197] These figures indicate that sterilization of men has gained social acceptance in North America.

Vasectomy has also been utilized extensively as a method of fertility control in India and the People's Republic of China. In 1976 alone, three fourths of the 8 million surgical

TABLE 18–12. Characteristics of Two Groups of Vasectomy Patients in Montreal

Group	Age <35 y	No. of Children 1 or 2	Married <10 y
1968–1971	26%	31%	23%
1974–1978	55%	58%	61%
	p <.01	<.01	<.01

Adapted from Ramos-Cordero RA, Ackman CFD, Naftolin F. Changing profiles in vasectomy subjects in the past decade. Fertil Steril 1979; 31:410–412. Reproduced with permission of the publisher, The American Fertility Society.

sterilization procedures in India were performed on men.[198] Approximately 13.8 million vasectomies were performed in the People's Republic of China between 1971 and 1978.[199]

Methods, Success Rate, and Acute Complications

Bilateral partial vasectomy is a relatively simple operative procedure and is usually performed with local anesthesia. Common incisions and the surgical techniques are illustrated in Figure 18–7.[195] The dorsal lithotomy position allows the weight of the testes to elongate and stretch the vasa, which facilitates entrapment of the vas between the thumb and forefinger of the surgeon and allows infiltration of local anesthetic both in the skin and around the isolated vas. The skin is incised, the vas is separated from its surrounding sheath, and a minimum of 1 cm is excised. With all techniques for permanent closure of the remaining vasal stumps (see Fig. 18–7), the rare possibility of spontaneous recanalization is always present (see later). Usually the skin edges are only loosely approximated, and an ice pack is recommended for 12 h and scrotal support for an additional 72 h.

The Chinese have utilized a rapid "nonsurgical" method of male sterilization (less than 10 min) in which the spermatic ducts are injected with a sclerosing agent, phenol.[200] This method was reported to be successful in 91% of 50,000 men and to involve a smaller incidence of hematoma and infection than that after vasectomy.

Studies of intravasal devices aimed at producing a reversible vasectomy have been reviewed.[194] Devices used in animals include an injectable, nonocclusive chemical polymer,[201] 1.5 cm of nonocclusive copper wire,[202] and a flexible prosthetic valve device that has been implanted long-term for reversible obstruction.[203] These methods appear to be effective, but none has been tried in humans.

Common causes of failure include division or ligation of some cord-like structure other than the vas (hence the need for pathological examination of the resected tissue) and spontaneous postsurgical recanalization. In two large

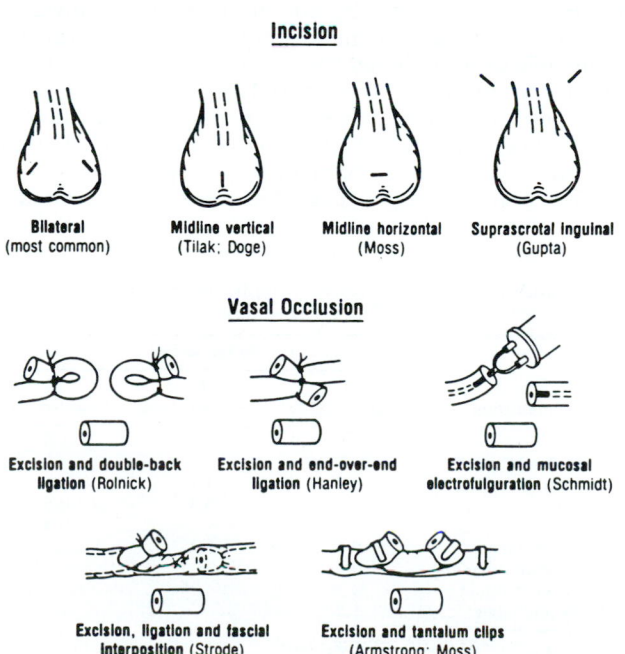

Figure 18–7. Diagram depicting common incisions for and methods of vasal occlusion. (From Lipshultz LI, Benson GS. Vasectomy—1980. Urol Clin North Am 1980; 7:89–105.)

series the failure rates related to recanalization were 0.3%[204] and 1.2%.[205] The greater the length of the vas resected, the less likely was recanalization to occur.[205]

Vasectomy is considered to be successful when sperm cannot be demonstrated in direct wet mounts of the semen on two consecutive specimens. The median time for development of azoospermia after vasectomy is 24 ejaculations, and conception caused by the presence of residual sperm has been reported 6 wk after a technically successful vasectomy.[206] Thus most patients are evaluated at 3 mo, although some physicians recommend initial examination at 1 mo with search only for motile sperm.[207] When recanalization occurs, it develops at a median time of 6 mo.[204]

The acute complications of vasectomy include swelling, hematoma formation, inflammation, and recanalization. The frequency of complications in three large series is shown in Table 18–13.[204, 208, 209] Vasitis, funiculitis, and epididymitis are not the result of infection but rather are due to extravasation of sperm into the interstitium.[208] The overall complication rate is about 6%.

Development of sperm granuloma is the most common serious postoperative complication of vasectomy.[195] It is apparently less common when a double-back ligation technique or electrofulguration is used than after simple vasal excision and ligation.[208] Immediately after vasectomy, induration and swelling develop in the stumps, probably because of compromise in the blood supply to the vas by the ligature. In most cases a scar forms and the ends of the vas become sealed off. However, necrosis of the ligated stump may occur, resulting in a leak and formation of a sperm granuloma. Sperm granulomas are painful and may initiate a spontaneous reanastomosis, thus causing the vasectomy to fail. This anastomosis is thought to occur because islands of mucosal cells in the inflammatory tissue of the granuloma can proliferate to form irregular narrow canals that finally connect the two ends.

Effects on Testicular Histology and Endocrine Function

The changes in the testis after occlusion of the vas have been extensively studied in animals.[210] They vary from species to species and with the site and type of operative vasal occlusion. Occlusion of the vas deferens in the primate is compatible with continued spermatogenesis in the testis. The sperm may be resorbed or stored in distended ducts and cysts. Testicular volume does not change after vasectomy in men.[211] The transient degeneration of the germinal epithelium that occurs in the immediate postoperative period is not demonstrable several years after vasectomy. Quantitative

TABLE 18–13. Postoperative Complications of Vasectomy in Three Large Series

Complication	% for Series*		
	A (Total No. 2711)	**B** (Total No. 1000)	**C** (Total No. 843)
Epididymitis	1.0	1.8	1.8
Abscess formation	0.7		1.5
Vasitis and funiculitis	0.4	3.2	
Hematoma	0.5	0.3	0.5
Hydrocele	0.1		0.4
Sperm granuloma	<0.1	1.2	
Vas cutaneous adhesion	0.7		
Vas cutaneous fistula	0.5		
Cellulitis and other	1.2		1.1
Recanalization	0.3	0.8	0.2
	5.5	7.3	5.5

*A, ref. 204; B, ref. 208; C, ref. 209.

morphometric studies of the testis of men undergoing vasectomy reversal disclosed increased thickness of the seminiferous tubule walls and reduction in the mean number of Sertoli cells.[212] Focal interstitial fibrosis was present in 23% and was associated with an increased likelihood of subsequent infertility in spite of a technically successful vasectomy reversal.[212] Changes in the epididymis may be permanent owing to rupture and fibrosis.[213]

Small amounts of steroid hormones are present in the seminal fluid. It has been generally believed that testicular hormones are present in the fluid that enters the epididymis and that these hormones are passed through the epididymis and the ejaculatory system to the seminal fluid. However, the content of several of these hormones in seminal fluid decreases only slightly after vasectomy, which suggests that they are derived in large part from the seminal vesicle and prostate rather than directly from the testes.[214] The fact that some (but not all) prostatic contributions to the ejaculate decrease after vasectomy suggests that prostatic function may also diminish.[215]

There appear to be no significant systemic endocrine sequelae of vasectomy. In five representative studies, levels of plasma testosterone, LH, and FSH did not change after vasectomy.[216–220] These studies include prospective trials[217, 218, 220] and follow-ups for as long as 5 y after surgery.[217, 220] In addition, Leydig cell reserve, as assessed by response to human chorionic gonadotropin, is normal 4 y after vasectomy.[220]

Antibodies and Atherosclerosis After Vasectomy

Sperm-agglutinating antibodies in the sera of vasectomized men were first reported in 1959.[221] Shortly thereafter, complement-dependent sperm-immobilizing antibodies were detected.[222] Approximately 2% of control men have sperm-agglutinating titers, whereas no immobilizing antibody can be detected in men before vasectomy.[223] Sperm antibodies are detectable beginning 7 to 11 d after vasectomy.[223] In general, 40% of men develop significant agglutinating antibody titers within a year after vasectomy, and 20% have sperm-immobilizing antibodies.[195, 223, 224] The sperm immobilization test is a sensitive and specific assay for complement-fixing antibodies to sperm.[225] All sera with agglutination titers higher than 1:80 have associated sperm-immobilizing antibodies, and sperm immobilization cannot be demonstrated in sera lacking agglutinating antibodies.[225] The immunoglobulin G fraction of postvasectomy sera possesses both sperm-agglutinating and sperm-immobilizing capacities.[226] However, these two tests probably do not measure identical antibodies because there is a greater increase in sperm-immobilizing titers after suture ligation for vasectomy than after the fulguration technique, whereas sperm-agglutinating titers are not significantly different after the two procedures.[224] Both types of antibodies persist for as long as 11 y after vasectomy.

Development of antisperm antibodies (specifically head-agglutinating antibodies) appears to be associated with the human leukocyte antigen A28.[227] Furthermore, the autoimmune antibody response to sperm surface antigens in the guinea pig is controlled by a single gene.[228]

The development of antibodies to sperm after vasectomy raised the question whether other forms of autoimmune reactions might occur in such men. In two studies involving more than 1000 vasectomized men, there was no increased incidence of antibodies directed to antigens other than sperm.[229, 230] In addition, there was no increased incidence of autoimmune disease in the vasectomized men.[230] However, in 1978 Alexander and Clarkson reported that vasectomy increases the severity of diet-induced atherosclerosis in cynomolgus monkeys.[231] It had been recognized that diet-induced atherosclerosis in rabbits could be enhanced by the induction of serum sickness (an immune complex disease).[232] In the monkey both the extent of atherosclerosis and the cholesterol content of the vessels were greater in the vasectomized group.[231] Antibodies to sperm developed in all vasectomized monkeys, and both complement and immunoglobulins were present in atherosclerotic plaques in these vasectomized animals with antibodies. In subsequent studies the occurrence and extent of atherosclerosis in rhesus monkeys fed monkey chow (devoid of cholesterol and low in fat) were more severe in vasectomized animals.[233] Almost all rhesus monkeys developed antisperm antibodies shortly after vasectomy, but by 4 to 6 mo only about half of the animals retained antisperm antibodies that were not a part of immune complexes.

It is not clear whether these findings in monkeys are relevant to humans. In a prospective study, immune complexes were sought by using sensitive enzyme-linked immunosorbent assays of sera from 35 men collected before and at timed intervals after vasectomy.[234] Less than 10% of the men ever produced sera positive for antisperm antibodies. However, sperm-related antigens were present in the sera of one fourth of the men 4 mo after vasectomy, and one fifth or more had higher circulating immune complex concentrations at various times after vasectomy. The components of the immune complexes were examined in nine patients; six contained antigen reactive with antisperm immunoglobulin G, and four contained complement components C3 and/or C1q. Thus circulating immune complexes are present in increased quantity in the sera of men after vasectomy.

The significance of the immune complexes in vasectomized men is not clear. However, studies involving several thousand subjects evaluated the incidence of nonfatal myocardial infarction, coronary artery disease, and hospitalization rates in vasectomized and control men.[235–240] No increased prevalence of atherosclerotic cardiovascular disease or its symptoms was found in the vasectomized group in any of the studies, even after 10 y or more.[235, 237, 240] It must be concluded, therefore, that there does not appear to be an association between vasectomy and atherosclerosis in men.

Psychosexual Effects

Most men who undergo vasectomy are satisfied with the procedure and would, in retrospect, have it done again.[241–243] Increased sexual enjoyment and increased frequency of intercourse are common, probably related to decreased anxiety about unwanted pregnancies. Vasectomy has no deleterious effect on potency or sexual performance, and marital harmony usually improves or remains unchanged after vasectomy.

Reversal of Vasectomy

Vasectomy should be recommended only to men who desire permanent sterilization. However, it is inevitable that some will change their minds and request reversal. Reasons for such requests include the death of children, an improved economic situation, and remarriage after divorce or death of the wife. Two vasovasostomy techniques (single-layer and double-layer microscopic closure) have been developed for such reanastomoses.[244] With both techniques the success rate for reappearance of sperm in the ejaculate is 80 to 90%. However, the associated pregnancy rate is only 30 to 50%.[245–249] A number of technical issues influence the anatomical success of the reanastomosis procedure, but the

functional success is probably determined by whether antisperm antibodies are present (Table 18–14).[250–253] In some, but not all, studies, men who are able to father a child after vasovasostomy are less likely to have antisperm antibodies than those who remain infertile.[254] The relationship is not absolute, but the antisperm antibodies presumably interfere with sperm function. Isolated immunoglobulin G and Fab antibodies from vasectomized guinea pigs inhibit fertilization in vitro.[255]

Conclusion

Vasectomy is a relatively simple procedure that is more than 99% effective in producing permanent infertility. Postoperative complications are minor. No adverse effects on the testis or its endocrine function have been detected. Although acceleration of atherosclerosis associated with immune complex formation occurs in vasectomized monkeys, there is no evidence that a similar phenomenon occurs in humans. Surgical reanastomosis can restore fertility in 30 to 50% of vasectomized men.

The Search for a Male Contraceptive

Drugs That Inhibit Hypothalamic-Pituitary Function

Because spermatogenesis requires normal gonadotropin levels, inhibition of the production of LH and FSH, either directly through an effect on the pituitary or indirectly through suppression of LHRH, will decrease sperm production.

ANDROGENS ALONE. The administration of exogenous testosterone to normal men suppresses gonadotropin secretion and inhibits spermatogenesis; it simultaneously prevents the deficiency in testosterone production that would otherwise follow gonadotropin suppression and consequently avoids the adverse effects on libido and potency. The preparations that are available for administering testosterone safely are long-acting esters, testosterone cypionate and testosterone enanthate, both of which must be given intramuscularly. The optimal replacement dose is about 200 mg every 2 wk.[256] A new testosterone ester, testosterone trans-4-n-butylcyclohexylcarboxylate, has been reported to maintain serum testosterone levels of castrated monkeys in the normal range for up to 4 mo.[257] Most oral androgen preparations have 17α-alkyl substitutions in the steroid molecule to prevent inactivation by the liver. These preparations are not safe for testosterone replacement because of the risk of their causing hepatotoxicity.[258] Nandrolone (19-nortestosterone) esters, given parenterally, were recognized to have potential contraceptive effects when abusers of anabolic steroids were noted to be infertile (see Chapter 13). When nandrolone-hexylphenylpropionate was used in a clinical study for male fertility regulation, it was of similar utility to pharmacological doses of testosterone enanthate (see later).[259]

Administration of 200 mg of testosterone enanthate every 2 wk causes azoospermia in less than one fourth of

TABLE 18–14. Percentage of Vasovasostomy Subjects with Positive Antisperm Antibody in Relation to Achieving Pregnancy

Variable	% for Series*			
	A (45 Couples)	B (51 Couples)	C (20 Couples)	D (51 Couples)
Pregnancy	48	18	8	15
No pregnancy	94	69	75	71

*A, ref. 250; B, ref 251; C, ref. 252; D, ref. 253.

men after a year, whereas a regimen of 200 mg of testosterone enanthate every 7 to 10 d causes azoospermia in about one half (Table 18–15).[260–263] This weekly regimen resulted in an average 50% increase in plasma testosterone levels above pretreatment values and suppression of plasma LH and FSH levels by 60 to 80%.[260, 262, 263]

Maximal suppression of sperm density was achieved within 8 to 10 wk, and recovery of control sperm density occurred within 20 to 28 wk after cessation of therapy.[262] The side effects of weekly 200-mg testosterone enanthate injections are minor. Libido and potency are not altered. Mild weight gain is common. Many men develop or experience a worsening of acne, but this effect is usually mild.[262, 263] Although plasma estradiol levels increase 50 to 80%,[262, 263] gynecomastia was reported in only one man in the four series summarized in Table 18–15.[261] The mean concentration of hemoglobin increased about 10 g/L (1 g/dL),[262, 263] but polycythemia did not occur. Testicular volume decreased about 20%.[264]

More extensive dose-response studies of long-term testosterone enanthate administered weekly have shown that at lower doses (25 and 50 mg) the serum LH and FSH levels are suppressed in parallel and that a dose of 300 mg is no more effective than 100 mg in suppressing LH and FSH levels and sperm density.[265] Moreover, treatment with high-dose testosterone for more than 6 mo appears to be safe, with no adverse effects. Because only about half of men who receive high-dose testosterone enanthate develop azoospermia, the same investigator evaluated whether severe oligozoospermia was associated with abnormal sperm function.[266] Penetration of zona-free hamster ova (see Chapter 13) by sperm from men with severe oligozoospermia was impaired in all and absent completely in five of six men.[266] However, the fact that some partners of men who were treated with progestational agents became pregnant (see later) suggests that azoospermia is the only absolutely reliable criterion for hormonal contraception in men.

PROGESTATIONAL AGENTS. Progestational agents inhibit pituitary gonadotropin secretion in both women and men and have been considered as a potential means of fertility control in men. Because the suppression of plasma LH results in a lowering of testosterone levels, progestogens are used in conjunction with androgens. The most extensively studied combination is 150 to 200 mg of medroxyprogesterone acetate and 200 to 500 mg of testosterone enanthate by injection,[267–269] usually on a monthly basis. Azoospermia is achieved on average in about half of the men, usually within 2 to 3 mo.[267] Escape from the suppression of spermatogenesis may occur after several months.[267] The importance of azoospermia for contraception with this drug regimen is proved by the fact that five pregnancies occurred in the partners of men receiving this regimen whose sperm densities were less than 1 million/mL.[270]

Side effects of the combination therapy include mild acne and occasional gynecomastia. Most subjects gained weight; in one study the average weight gain was 6 kg.[269] Some men reported decreased libido, possibly because the plasma testosterone value was only 10 to 30% of baseline

one month after the injection.[269] Medroxyprogesterone acetate has a longer duration of action and results in chronic gonadotropin suppression after exogenous testosterone has been depleted.[271] Depot medroxyprogesterone acetate has been combined with nandrolone esters for somewhat better suppression of spermatogenesis than with nandrolone alone.[272] However, only about two thirds of men who are treated with this regimen become azoospermic.[272]

Cyproterone acetate, a progestational agent with potent antiandrogenic properties, has been tried as an antifertility agent. In animals the drug causes both gonadotropin suppression and impairment of androgen action at the level of the testis or epididymis.[273–275] However, the drug is ineffective in lowering sperm density below the normal range in most men, and only rare men develop azoospermia.

LHRH ANALOGUES. As discussed earlier, a family of LHRH analogues (both agonists and antagonists) has been synthesized. When the LHRH agonists are modified at positions 6 and 10, they are more potent than the native hormone.[276] Prolonged administration of these agonists causes a paradoxical inhibition of gonadotropin secretion,[277] possibly because of decreases in the number of LHRH receptors and inhibiting postreceptor events involved in the secretion of gonadotropin.[278] In rats the LHRH agonists decrease testosterone production by reducing the number of LH receptors in the testis, and they inhibit steroidogenesis by partially blocking the activity of the 17-hydroxylase and 17,20-desmolase enzymes.[277] This direct inhibition of testicular function in the rat is mediated by LHRH receptors in Leydig cells.[279] LHRH agonists may also inhibit testosterone action directly, because the testosterone-induced increase in the weight of the ventral prostate and seminal vesicles is diminished in hypophysectomized-gonadectomized rats treated concurrently with the analogue and testosterone.[280]

One LHRH agonist that has been studied in humans is D-Ser(TBU)^6-EA^{10}-LHRH. The daily subcutaneous administration of 5 μg of this analogue to normal men lowers LH, FSH, and testosterone levels both acutely (1 wk)[281] and chronically (17 wk).[282] However, sperm density and potency were not significantly changed in four men treated for 17 wk, probably because the plasma hormone levels were decreased less than 50%.[282] Interestingly, when this same agent was administered to six normal men as a single intranasal dose of 500 μg, plasma LH and FSH levels temporarily increased and returned to normal within 8 to 12 h, whereas the plasma testosterone level increased and then decreased to 50% of baseline values for the subsequent 3 d.[283]

Daily administration of the agonist D-Trp^6-Pro^9-N-ethylamide-LHRH by subcutaneous injections to eight normal men resulted in a 90% decrease in plasma testosterone levels and a 50% decrease in plasma gonadotropin levels.[284] It is of interest that levels of bioactive LH decrease to a greater extent than levels of immunoreactive LH after treatment with this analogue.[285] The pulsatile pattern of LH release was diminished, and the gonadotropin response to pulsatile administration of LHRH was lost, but the Leydig cell remained responsive to exogenous human LH during treatment with the agonist.[286] Thus the locus of action of the analogue in humans appears to be at the level of the pituitary.[286] In contrast to the decreasing ratio of bioactive LH to immunoactive LH during treatment with this agonist, the ratio of bioactive to immunoactive FSH was normal.[287] Although treatment was discontinued in most men after 6 or 7 wk because of impotence, one subject developed azoospermia after 10 wk of therapy. Recovery of spermatogenesis occurred by 14 wk after cessation of therapy in all subjects.[284]

Initial trials suggested that LHRH analogues and testosterone were synergistic in inhibiting gonadotropins,[288] but

TABLE 18–15. Effect of Weekly Injections of 200 mg of Testosterone Enanthate on Sperm Density in Normal Men

Investigators	No. of Men	Duration of Treatment (wk)	% of Men with Azoospermia
Steinberger and Smith[260]	5	42	100
Paulsen et al.[261]	42	26	48
Cunningham et al.[262]	20	12	25
Swerdloff et al.[263]	17	16	59

daily injection of LHRH analogues combined with biweekly testosterone injections did not lower 24-h integrated LH concentrations and was not successful in producing azoospermia in men.[289] When the agonist was given by constant infusion and in conjunction with biweekly testosterone injections, three of seven men developed azoospermia.[290]

Because the combination of LHRH agonist and testosterone had not consistently induced azoospermia in normal men, clinical trials of LHRH antagonists have been performed. One antagonist, Nal-Glu (Ac D²NaL¹, D4Cl Phe², D3Pal³, Arg⁵, DGlu⁶ (AA) DAla¹⁰-LHRH), has been studied by several groups.[291, 292] LHRH antagonists compete with endogenous LHRH for binding to receptors in pituitary gonadotrophs and thereby inhibit gonadotropin secretion. Prolonged administration of the Nal-Glu LHRH antagonist by daily injection lowers the levels of inhibin, LH, and FSH and the ratio of bioactive to immunoactive LH and decreases the serum testosterone level by 70 to 78%.[291, 292] The combination of weekly testosterone injection plus Nal-Glu LHRH was more effective in suppressing serum LH, FSH, and inhibin levels than either Nal-Glu alone or testosterone alone.[292] Whether long-term administration of testosterone plus the LHRH antagonist will be more successful than testosterone plus agonist in inducing azoospermia remains to be demonstrated.

In summary, fertility control in men with agents aimed at pituitary inhibition does not seem promising.

Drugs and Other Agents That Affect the Testis Directly

A number of antineoplastic drugs and other relatively toxic compounds impair sperm production by direct effects on the testes. Most of these compounds produce additional unacceptable side effects. This section deals with the oral agent gossypol, reviews studies with other drugs, and describes physical and immunological attempts to inhibit spermatogenesis.

GOSSYPOL. In the late 1950s an increased frequency of infertility was noted in areas of the People's Republic of China where crude cottonseed oil was used in cooking. It was found that the antifertility agent in cottonseed oil is gossypol (Fig. 18–8), which is a naphthalphenol present in various parts of the cotton plant.

Clinical trials of gossypol as an antifertility agent in the People's Republic of China have involved almost 10,000 men for a decade.[293, 294] Gossypol affects the spermatogenic tubules predominantly, with little change in Leydig cells. The administration of 20 mg by mouth daily for 60 days (loading period) causes the sperm in the ejaculate to become immotile and to decrease in number or disappear. A sperm density of less than 4 million/mL was achieved in 99.9% of men. Because gossypol affects sperm motility as well as sperm number, the requirement for azoospermia to ensure consistent infertility may not be necessary, as in the case of drugs

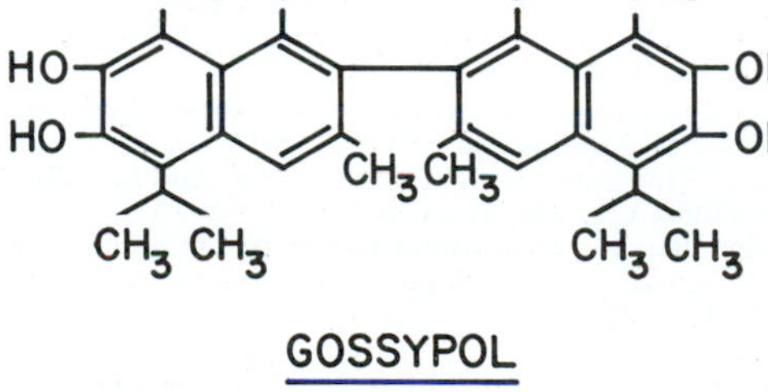

that inhibit pituitary function. The actual assessment of fertility has not been described in men receiving gossypol.[293, 294] After a low sperm count is achieved (usually 60 d), the maintenance dose is decreased to one third the original dose.

Short-term side effects included fatigue, decreased libido, and decreased appetite. During chronic therapy the incidence of symptomatic hypokalemia varied from as high as 4.7% to an undetectable amount among groups.[295] Initial fatigue and muscle cramps were followed by frank hypokalemic paralysis in a few of the hypokalemic subjects; the hypokalemia appears to be due to renal potassium wasting.[295] Attempts to decrease the dose of gossypol to prevent hypokalemia were unsuccessful.[296] Supplemental potassium salts and triamterine were also ineffective in preventing hypokalemia.[297]

The drug not only impairs spermatogenesis but also inhibits sperm maturation, with the result that motility is impaired.[294, 298] The studies of the mechanism of action and pharmacology of gossypol have been reviewed.[298] In long-term studies, male sexual function appears not to be affected after the loading period. The factor that is likely to prevent further clinical trials of gossypol is the failure of sperm density to return to normal after cessation of therapy.[294, 299] In a study at two centers, about 40% of azoospermic men at cessation of gossypol therapy did not recover normal sperm density by 2 y, and half remained azoospermic.[299]

OTHER DRUGS. Sulfasalazine is a drug that is used for the management of inflammatory bowel disease. Like gossypol, sulfasalazine appears to impair spermatogenesis and inhibit sperm motility, presumably related to effects on the epididymis.[300, 301] The incomplete inhibition of spermatogenesis and the frequency of side effects make it unacceptable as a male contraceptive.

Other drugs with antispermatogenic activity in animals include nitrofurans, thiophenes, dinitropyrroles, and bis-(dichloroacetyl)-diamines.[302] Of these, the diamines appear to be sufficiently free of severe toxic effects for human trials to be undertaken. However, the trials were abandoned when an antabuse-like effect was discovered after the use of the drugs was combined with alcohol ingestion.[302]

Indazole carboxylic acids such as tolnidamine may have potential for fertility control in men.[303] These chemicals have a selective action on the testicular germinal epithelium in rats, rabbits, and rhesus monkeys and have a paucity of side effects. Spermatogenesis returns to normal when the drug is discontinued. The site of action of tolnidamine appears to be the Sertoli cells.[303]

PHYSICAL METHODS. The suppressive effect of heat on spermatogenesis is manifested by the temporary decreases in sperm density that follow acute febrile illnesses or hot baths. The 2°C higher temperature of the abdomen than that of the scrotum is thought to account for the infertility of cryptorchidism. The thermal effect of hot water, infrared heat, microwaves, and ultrasound has been evaluated in rats as a potential antifertility therapy.[304] Electronic means of heat induction appear to be more effective than the other thermal methods in causing infertility, and ultrasound is more effective at a lower temperature than microwaves.[304]

Ultrasound as a physical means of inhibiting spermatogenesis has been investigated in several species.[304] Spermatogenesis can be suppressed in cats, dogs, and monkeys without causing histological damage to Leydig cells and without altering plasma testosterone levels. This effect is believed to be temporary. Pilot studies of ultrasound treatment in men with prostate cancer before orchiectomy demonstrated reductions in spermatogenesis without an effect on Leydig cell morphology or plasma testosterone level.[304]

IMMUNOLOGICAL METHODS. Immunological ap-

Figure 18–8. Structure of the antifertility agent gossypol.

proaches to fertility control in men have utilized the production of antibodies to hormones or the induction of autoimmune reactions to some component of the testes, sex accessory organs, or spermatozoa.[305] The ideal target hormone would appear to be FSH, which is required for the induction of spermatogenesis. When FSH is neutralized with anti-FSH antibodies in monkeys, spermatogenesis is severely impaired in mature animals. For example, in bonnet monkeys passive immunization induces reversible infertility without a reduction in plasma LH or testosterone levels.[306, 307] The effect of neutralization of FSH in humans is not known. Passive immunization with anti-FSH antibodies is impractical in the long term. Active immunization of male rhesus monkeys with purified FSH was ineffective for fertility control in a long-term study.[308]

Induction of an immunological reaction to some component of the testis may result in either the induction of an autoimmune orchitis or the elicitation of a specific antibody response to a specific sperm antigen. The injection of testicular homogenates induces allergic orchitis in at least eight mammalian species. In the guinea pig at least four different antigens have been identified in testicular homogenates when Freund complete adjuvant and repeated subcutaneous injections are used. Talwar and colleagues[309, 310] have described a technique in which intratesticular injection of bacille Calmette-Guérin vaccine alone was used to achieve aspermatogenesis. Oligospermia can be achieved within 6 wk in dogs and monkeys, whereas both basal testosterone levels and the testosterone response to human chorionic gonadotropin administration are normal.[309] These effects are reversible in some animals.[310] The effect appears to be local, no antisperm antibodies being detectable in the serum.

A specific isozyme of lactate dehydrogenase (LDH-X), which is limited to the testis and spermatozoa, is a potential candidate for induction of the immune response for fertility control in men. Immunization with this antigen does not result in aspermatogenesis or orchitis but does impair sperm motility in rabbits.[311] The resulting infertility is reversible in rabbits and in mice. The antibody to LDH-X in the seminal fluid immobilizes sperm by either mechanical impairment or metabolic inhibition. Because this antibody affects only mature spermatozoa, it is possible that immunization of women with this antigen could be used for fertility control.[311]

In summary, gossypol does not appear to be a suitable oral contraceptive for men. The risk of hypokalemia and the uncertain reversibility suggest that either a different dosage regimen or another analogue with less toxicity must be developed. The indazole carboxylic acids, other chemicals with promise, have been studied only in animals. Ultrasound may be effective and safe but is associated with an uncertain duration of effect. Most active immunization methods have an indeterminate duration of action and involve repeated injections of Freund adjuvant. Passive immunization may cause acute allergic reactions and immune complex disease.

Drugs That Affect the Epididymis

Selective inhibition of epididymal function that would cause impairment of sperm maturation would theoretically control fertility without the risk of impaired testicular function. The time required to achieve an effect on fertility with such agents should also be less than the 2 to 3 mo necessary for agents affecting the pituitary or testis.

ANTIANDROGENS. Because normal androgen action is necessary for epididymal function, antiandrogens are logical candidates to inhibit sperm maturation in the epididymis. Cyproterone acetate, an antiandrogen, does inhibit gonadotropin secretion. Both cyproterone (the free alcohol) and the nonsteroidal antiandrogen flutamide appear to be inef-

fective in inhibiting epididymal function. These agents inhibit the negative feedback of endogenous androgens and cause an increased LH and testosterone synthesis, thus overcoming any inhibitory effect of the antiandrogen in the epididymis.[312, 313]

α-CHLOROHYDRIN. α-Chlorohydrin, a monochloro derivative of glycerol (3-chloro-1,2-propanediol), is commercially available as a racemic mixture of $S(+)$ and $R(-)$ forms. The $S(+)$-3-chlorohydrin form is active in inducing infertility and has less toxicity than the mixture, whereas the $R(-)$ isomer is ineffective for fertility control.[314] These observations suggest that any antifertility properties are due to a specific metabolic action and not to their random action as alkylating agents. The compound induces temporary infertility in rats, guinea pigs, and monkeys without causing loss of libido and without alterations in ejaculation or in the morphology of ejaculated spermatozoa. α-Chlorohydrin may inhibit oxidative phosphorylation, glycolysis, and glycerol metabolism.[315] The toxicity of the agent appears to be its limiting factor. The compound causes bone marrow depression in monkeys and hepatotoxicity or nephrotoxicity in other species.[316] A better understanding of the specific mechanism of action of this drug on sperm metabolism might lead to the development of other less toxic compounds.

CHLORINATED SUGARS. The 6-chloro-6-deoxy sugars have been investigated as potential inhibitors of the glycolytic pathway in spermatozoa.[317] Like α-chlorohydrin, these compounds produce reversible infertility in male rats with a paucity of toxic side effects. No direct inhibitory effect of 6-chloro-6-deoxyglucose has been demonstrated in spermatozoa, so the compounds are probably converted to another active metabolite in the body. Rats made infertile with 6-chloro-6-deoxyglucose continue to produce normal numbers of spermatozoa and to mate with females as frequently as controls. However, spermatozoa from treated animals are unable to oxidize glucose, and they quickly become immotile after removal from the epididymis and incubation with glucose as an energy source. Unfortunately, neurotoxicity has been detected in marmoset monkeys and mice that were given high doses of 6-chloro-6-deoxyglucose.[318]

In summary, antiandrogens are ineffective. α-Chlorohydrin and chlorinated sugars are effective in animals but have significant toxicity.

REFERENCES

1. Population Reports. Migration, population growth, and development. Series M, No. 7. Baltimore: The Johns Hopkins University, 1983.
2. Pannenborg CO. Contraceptive needs in the Third World: the present paradox of a future planning–technology nexus. Excerpta Med Int Congr Ser 1987; 759:21–44.
3. Segal AJ. Contraceptive research: a male chauvinist plot? Fam Plann Perspect 1972; 4:21–25.
4. Cunningham FA, Gant NF, MacDonald PC. Williams Obstetrics. 18th ed. Norwalk, CT: Appleton & Lange, 1989: 921–943.
5. Goldzieher JW. Estrogens in oral contraceptives: historical perspectives. Johns Hopkins Med J 1982; 150:165–169.
6. Doisy EA, Veler CD, Tayer S. Folliculin from urine of pregnant women. Am J Physiol 1929; 90:329–330.
7. Butenandt A. Progynon, a crystalline female sexual hormone. Naturwissenschafen 1929; 17:879.
8. Butenandt A, Westphal V. Zur Isolierung und Charakterisierung des Corpus-Luteum-Hormons. Berl Dtsch Chem Ges 1934; 67:1440–1442.
9. Sturgis SH, Albright R. Mechanism of estrin therapy in the relief of dysmenorrhea. Endocrinology 1940; 26:68–72.
10. Pincus G, Roch J, Garcia CR. Effects of certain 19-nor steroids upon the reproductive process. Ann NY Acad Sci 1958; 71:677–690.
11. Chez RA. Three new progestins for OCs: do they offer benefits? Contemp OB/GYN 1988; 32:51–60.
12. Population Reports. Oral contraceptives in the 1980s. Series A, No. 6. Oral Contraceptives. Baltimore: The Johns Hopkins University, 1982: A190–A222.
13. Speroff L. The formulation of oral contraceptives: does the amount of estrogen make any clinical difference? Johns Hopkins Med J 1982; 150:170–176.

14. Hatcher RA, Stewart GK, Stewart F, et al. Contraceptive Technology, 1982–1983. New York: Irvington, 1982.
15. Gaspard UJ. Metabolic effects of oral contraceptives. Am J Obstet Gynecol 1987; 157:1029–1041.
16. Silverberg S, Makowski E. Endometrial carcinoma in young women taking oral contraceptive agents. Obstet Gynecol 1975; 46:503–506.
17. Liggins GC. The effect of variation in estrogen dosage on the pregnancy rate during sequential oral contraception. Fertil Steril 1967; 18:191–197.
18. Jones RC, Edgren RA. The effects of various steroids on the vaginal histology in the rat. Fertil Steril 1973; 24:284–291.
19. Goldzieher JW, Maqueo M, Chenault CB, et al. Comparative studies of the ethinyl estrogens used in oral contraceptives. I. Endometrial response. Am J Obstet Gynecol 1975; 122:615–618.
20. Goldzieher JW, de la Pena A, Chenault CB, et al. Comparative studies of the ethinyl estrogens used in oral contraceptives. II. Anovulatory potency. Am J Obstet Gynecol 1975; 122:619–624.
21. Goldzieher JW, de la Pena A, Chenault CB, et al. Comparative studies of the ethinyl estrogens used in oral contraceptives. III. Effect on plasma gonadotropins. Am J Obstet Gynecol 1975; 122:625–636.
22. Edgren RA. Relative potencies of oral contraceptives. In: Moghissi KS, ed. Controversies in Contraception. Baltimore: Williams & Wilkins, 1979:1–18.
23. Dorflinger LJ. Relative potency of progestins used in oral contraceptives. Contraception 1985; 31:557–570.
24. DeLia LE, Emery MG. Clinical pharmacology and common minor side effects of oral contraceptives. Clin Obstet Gynecol 1981; 24:879–892.
25. Edgren RA, Sturtevant FM. Potencies of oral contraceptives. Am J Obstet Gynecol 1976; 125:1029–1038.
26. Dickey RP, Stone SC. Progestational potency of oral contraceptives. Obstet Gynecol 1976; 47:106–112.
27. Dickey RP. Initial pill selection and managing the contraceptive pill patient. Int J Gynaecol Obstet 1979; 16:547–555.
28. Berger GS, Talwar PP. Oral contraceptive potencies and side effects. Obstet Gynecol 1978; 51:545–547.
29. Goldzieher JW, Dozier DT, de la Pena A. Plasma levels and pharmacokinetics of ethinyl estradiol in various populations. II. Mestranol. Contraception 1980; 21:17–22.
30. Barbieri RL, Petro Z, Canick JA, et al. Aromatization of norethindrone to ethinyl estradiol by human placental microsomes. J Clin Endocrinol Metab 1983; 57:299–303.
31. Carr BR, Parker CR Jr, Madden JD, et al. Plasma levels of adrenocorticotropin and cortisol in women receiving oral contraceptive steroid treatment. J Clin Endocrinol Metab 1979; 49:346–349.
32. Bronson RA. Oral contraception: mechanisms of action. Clin Obstet Gynecol 1981; 24:869–877.
33. Kastin AJ, Schally AV, Gual C, et al. Stimulation of LH release in men and women by LH-releasing hormone purified from porcine hypothalami. J Clin Endocrinol Metab 1969; 29:1046–1050.
34. Vandenberg G, DeVane G, Yen SSC. Effects of exogenous estrogen and oral progestin on pituitary responsiveness to synthetic luteinizing hormone–releasing factor. J Clin Invest 1974; 53:1750–1754.
35. Spellacy WN, Kalra PS, Buhi WR, et al. Pituitary and ovarian responsiveness to a graded gonadotropin releasing factor stimulation test in women using a low estrogen on a regular type of oral contraceptive. Am J Obstet Gynecol 1980; 137:109–115.
36. Greenwald GS. In vivo recording of intraluminal pressure changes in the rabbit oviduct. Fertil Steril 1963; 14:666–674.
37. Hillard GD, Norris HJ. Pathological effects of oral contraceptives. Recent Results Cancer Res 1979; 66:49–71.
38. Gray MJ, Grimes DA. Birth control, abortion and sterilization. In: Romney SC, Gray MJ, Little AB, et al., eds. Gynecology and Obstetrics: The Health Care of Women. New York: McGraw-Hill, 1981: 817–852.
39. Peterson HB, DeStefano F, Greenspan JR, et al. Mortality risk associated with tubal sterilization in United States hospitals. Am J Obstet Gynecol 1982; 143:125–129.
40. Royal College of General Practitioners Oral Contraceptive Study. Mortality among oral contraceptive users. Lancet 1977; 2:727–733.
41. Royal College of General Practitioners Oral Contraceptive Study. Further analyses of mortality in oral contraceptive users. Lancet 1981; 1:541–546.
42. Vessey MP, McPherson K, Yeates D. Mortality in oral contraceptive users. Lancet 1981; 1:549–550.
43. Ramcharan S, Pelligrin FA, Ray R, et al. Mortality. In: Ramcharan S, Pelligrin FA, Ray R, et al., eds. The Walnut Creek Contraceptive Drug Study: A Prospective Study of the Side Effects of Oral Contraceptives. Vol 3. An Interim Report—A Comparison of Disease Occurrence Leading to Hospitalization or Death in Users and Nonusers of Oral Contraceptives. Bethesda: Center for Population Research, 1981: 189–210.
44. Porter JB, Jick H, Walker AM. Mortality among oral contraceptive users. Obstet Gynecol 1987; 70:29–32.
45. Stadel BV. Oral contraceptives and cardiovascular disease (first of two parts). N Engl J Med 1981; 305:612–618.
46. Stadel BV. Oral contraceptives and cardiovascular disease (second of two parts). N Engl J Med 1981; 305:672–677.
47. World Health Organization. The world's main health problems. From WHO's sixth report on the world health situation. World Health Forum 1981; 2:264–280.
48. Shapiro S, Slone D, Rosenberg L, et al. Oral-contraceptive use in relation to myocardial infarction. Lancet 1979; 1:743–747.
49. Inman WHW, Vessey MP. Investigation of deaths from pulmonary, coronary, and cerebral thrombosis and embolism in women of child-bearing age. Br Med J 1968; 2:193–199.
50. Slone D, Shapiro S, Kaufman DW, et al. Risk of myocardial infarction in relation to current and discontinued use of oral contraceptives. N Engl J Med 1981; 305:420–424.
51. Stampfer MJ, Willett WC, Colditz GA, et al. A prospective study of past use of oral contraceptive agents and risk of cardiovascular disease. N Engl J Med 1988; 319:1313–1317.
52. Castelli WP. Cardiovascular disease in women. Am J Obstet Gynecol 1988; 158:1553–1560.
53. Wallace RB, Hoover J, Barrett-Connor E, et al. Altered plasma lipid and lipoprotein levels associated with oral contraceptive and oestrogen use: report from the Medications Working Group of the Lipid Research Clinics Program. Lancet 1979; 2:111–115.
54. Heiss G, Tamir I, Davis CE, et al. Lipoprotein-cholesterol distributions in selected North American populations: The Lipid Research Clinics Program Prevalence Study. Circulation 1980; 61:302–315.
55. La Rosa JC. The varying effects of progestins on lipid levels and cardiovascular disease. Am J Obstet Gynecol 1988; 158:1621–1629.
56. Wahl P, Walden C, Knopp R, et al. Effect of estrogen/progestin potency on lipid/lipoprotein cholesterol. N Engl J Med 1983; 308:862–867.
57. Knapp RH. Cardiovascular effects of endogenous and exogenous sex hormones over a woman's lifetime. Am J Obstet Gynecol 1988; 158:1630–1643.
58. Bradley DD, Wingerd J, Petitti DB, et al. Serum high-density-lipoprotein cholesterol in women using oral contraceptives, estrogens and progestins. N Engl J Med 1978; 299:17–20.
59. Krauss RM, Lindgren FT, Silvers A, et al. Changes in serum high density lipoproteins in women on oral contraceptive drugs. Clin Chim Acta 1977; 80:465–470.
60. Meade TW, Greenberg G, Thompson SC. Progestogens and cardiovascular reactions associated with oral contraceptives and a comparison of the safety of 50- and 30-μg oestrogen preparations. Br Med J 1980; 280:1157–1161.
61. Meade TW. Effects of progestogens on the cardiovascular system. Am J Obstet Gynecol 1982; 142:776–780.
62. Barnes RW, Krapf T, Hoak JC. Erroneous clinical diagnosis of leg vein thrombosis in women on oral contraceptives. Obstet Gynecol 1978; 51:556–558.
63. Sagar S, Stamatakis JD, Thomas DP, et al. Oral contraceptives, antithrombin-III activity, and postoperative deep-vein thrombosis. Lancet 1976; 1:509–511.
64. Stamatakis JD, Lawrence D, Kakkar VV. Surgery, venous thrombosis and anti-Xa. Br J Surg 1977; 64:709–711.
65. Alkjaersig N, Fletcher A, Burstein R. Association between oral contraceptive use and thromboembolism: a new approach to its investigation based on plasma fibrinogen chromatography. Am J Obstet Gynecol 1975; 122:199–211.
66. Royal College of General Practitioners. Oral Contraceptives and Health. New York: Pittman, 1974.
67. Royal College of General Practitioners Oral Contraceptive Study. Oral contraceptives, venous thrombosis, and varicose veins. J R Coll Gen Pract 1978; 28:393–399.
68. Bottinger LE, Boman G, Eklund G, et al. Oral contraceptives and thromboembolic disease: effects of lowering oestrogen content. Lancet 1980; 1:1097–1101.
69. Oxford-Family Planning Association Contraceptive Study. Oral contraceptives and venous thromboembolism: findings in a large prospective study. Br Med J 1986; 292:526.
70. Helmrich SP, Rosenberg L, Kaufman DW, et al. Venous thromboembolism in relation to oral contraceptive use. Obstet Gynecol 1987; 69:91–95.
71. Realini JP, Goldzieher JW. Oral contraceptives and cardiovascular disease: a critique of the epidemiologic studies. Am J Obstet Gynecol 1985; 152:729–798.
72. Ramcharan S, Pelligrin FA, Ray R, et al. Diseases of the circulatory system. In: Ramcharan S, Pelligrin FA, Ray R, et al., eds. The Walnut Creek Contraceptive Drug Study: A Prospective Study of the Side Effects of Oral Contraceptives. Vol 3. An Interim Report—A Comparison of Disease Occurrence Leading to Hospitalization or Death in Users and Nonusers of Oral Contraceptives. Bethesda: Center for Population Research, 1981:130–132.
73. Meade TW. Risks and mechanisms of cardiovascular events in users of oral contraceptives. Am J Obstet Gynecol 1988; 158:1646–1652.
74. Woods JW. Oral contraceptives and hypertension. Hypertension 1988; 11(Suppl II):II11–II15.
75. Kay CR. The happiness pill? J R Coll Gen Pract 1980; 30:8–19.
76. Royal College of General Practitioners Oral Contraceptive Study. Effect on hypertension and benign breast disease of progestogen component in combined oral contraceptives. Lancet 1977; 1:624.

77. Sondheimer S. Metabolic effects of the birth control pill. Clin Obstet Gynecol 1981; 24:927–941.

78. Spellacy WN, Buhi WC, Birk SA. The effect of the progestogen ethynodiol diacetate on glucose, insulin and growth hormone after six-month treatment. Acta Endocrinol 1972; 70:373–384.

79. Spellacy WN, Buhi WC, Birk SA. Effects of norethindrone on carbohydrate and lipid metabolism. Obstet Gynecol 1975; 46:560–563.

80. Depirro R, Forte F, Bertoli A, et al. Changes in insulin receptors during oral contraception. J Clin Endocrinol Metab 1981; 52:29–33.

81. Seed M, Godsland IF, Wyn V, et al. The effects of cyproterone acetate and ethinyl estradiol on carbohydrate metabolism. Clin Endocrinol 1984; 21:689–699.

82. der Vang NV, Kloosterboer HJ, Haspels AA. Effect of seven low-dose combined oral contraceptive preparations on carbohydrate metabolism. Am J Obstet Gynecol 1987; 156:918–922.

83. Centers for Disease Control Cancer and Steroid Hormone Study. Oral contraceptive use and the risk of ovarian cancer. JAMA 1983; 249:1596–1599.

84. Cramer DW, Hutchinson GB, Welch WR, et al. Factors affecting the association of oral contraceptives and ovarian cancer. N Engl Med J 1982; 307:1047–1051.

85. Rosenberg L, Shapiro S, Slone D, et al. Epithelial ovarian cancer and combination oral contraceptives. JAMA 1982; 247:3210–3212.

86. Centers for Disease Control Cancer and Steroid Hormone Study. Oral contraceptive use and the risk of endometrial cancer. JAMA 1983; 249:1600–1604.

87. Huggins GR, Zucker PK. Oral contraceptives and neoplasia: 1987 update. Fertil Steril 1987; 47:733–761.

88. Cancer and Steroid Hormone Study of the Centers for Disease Control and the National Institute of Child Health and Human Development. Combined oral contraceptive use and the risk of endometrial cancer. JAMA 1987; 257:796–800.

89. Cancer and Steroid Hormone Study of the Centers for Disease Control and the National Institute of Child Health and Human Development. The reduction in risk associated with oral-contraceptive use. N Engl J Med 1987; 316:650–655.

90. Centers for Disease Control Cancer and Steroid Hormone Study. Long-term oral contraceptive use and the risk of breast cancer. JAMA 1983; 249:1591–1595.

91. Schlesselman JJ, Stadel BV, Murray P, et al. Breast cancer in relation to early use of oral contraceptives. JAMA 1988; 259:1828–1833.

92. Population Reports. Oral contraceptives. Lower dose pills. Series A, No. 7. Baltimore: The Johns Hopkins University, 1988.

93. Harris RW, Brinton LA, Cowdell RH, et al. Characteristics of women with dysplasia or carcinoma in situ of the cervix uteri. Br J Cancer 1980; 42:359–369.

94. Jick H, Herman R. Oral-contraceptive–induced benign liver tumors—the magnitude of the problem. JAMA 1978; 240:828–829 (letter).

95. Rooks JB, Ory HW, Ishak KG, et al. Cooperative Liver Tumor Study Group. Epidemiology of hepatocellular adenoma: the role of oral contraceptive use. JAMA 1979; 242:644–648.

96. Neuberger J, Forman D, Doll R, et al. Oral contraceptives and hepatocellular carcinoma. Br Med J 1986; 292:1355–1357.

97. Ramcharan S, Pelligrin FA, Ray R, et al. Infective parasitic diseases: malignant neoplasms; benign neoplasms. In: Ramcharan S, Pelligrin FA, Ray R, et al., eds. The Walnut Creek Contraceptive Drug Study: A Prospective Study of the Side Effects of Oral Contraceptives. Vol 3. An Interim Report—A Comparison of Disease Occurrence Leading to Hospitalization or Death in Users and Nonusers of Oral Contraceptives. Bethesda: Center for Population Research, 1981: 43–78.

98. Adams SA, Sheaves JK, Wright NH, et al. A case-control study of the possible association between oral contraceptives and malignant melanoma. Br J Cancer 1981; 44:45–50.

99. Kay CR. Malignant melanoma and oral contraceptives. Br J Cancer 1981; 44:479 (letter).

100. Boston Collaborative Drug Surveillance Program. Oral contraceptives and venous thromboembolic disease, surgically confirmed gall-bladder disease, and breast tumours. Lancet 1973; 1:1399–1404.

101. Goldzieher JW, Moses LE, Averkin E, et al. A placebo-controlled double-blind crossover investigation of the side effects attributed to oral contraceptives. Fertil Steril 1971; 22:609–623.

102. Archer DF, Thomas RL. The fallacy of the postpill amenorrhea syndrome. Clin Obstet Gynecol 1981; 24:943–950.

103. Hull MG, Bromham DR, Savage PE, et al. Normal fertility in women with post-pill amenorrhoea. Lancet 1981; 1:1329–1332.

104. Heinonen OP, Slone D, Monson RR, et al. Cardiovascular birth defects and antenatal exposure to female sex hormones. N Engl J Med 1977; 296:67–70.

105. Janerick DT, Piper JM, Glebatis DM. Oral contraceptives and congenital limb-reduction defects. N Engl J Med 1974; 291:697–700.

106. Holtz G. Galactorrhea in oral contraceptive users. J Reprod Med 1982; 27:210–212.

107. Vaisrub S. Pituitary prolactinoma and estrogen contraceptives. JAMA 1979; 242:177–178.

108. Sherman BM, Schlechte J, Halmi NS, et al. Pathogenesis of prolactin-secreting pituitary adenomas. Lancet 1978; 2:1019–1021.

109. Coulam CB, Annegers JF, Abboud CF, et al. Pituitary adenoma and oral contraceptives: a case-control study. Fertil Steril 1979; 31:25–28.

110. Wingrave SJ, Kay CR, Vessey MP. Oral contraceptives and pituitary adenomas. Br Med J 1980; 280:685–686.

111. Shy KK, McTiernan AM, Daling JR, et al. Oral contraceptive use and the occurrence of pituitary prolactinoma. JAMA 1983; 249:2204–2207.

112. Pituitary Adenoma Study Group. Pituitary adenomas and oral contraceptives: a multicenter case-control study. Fertil Steril 1983; 39:753–760.

113. Szoka PR, Edgren RA. Drug interactions with oral contraceptives: compilation and analysis of an adverse experience report data base. Fertil Steril 1988; 49(Suppl):31S–38S.

114. Bolt HM, Bolt M, Kappus H. Interaction of rifampicin treatment with pharmacokinetics and metabolism of ethinyloestradiol in man. Acta Endocrinol 1977; 85:189–197.

115. Back DJ, Breckenridge AM, Crawford F, et al. The effect of rifampicin on norethisterone pharmacokinetics. Eur J Clin Pharmacol 1979; 15:193–197.

116. Rubin GL, Ory HW, Layde PM. Oral contraceptives and pelvic inflammatory disease. Am J Obstet Gynecol 1982; 144:630–635.

117. Ross RK, Pike MC, Vesse MP, et al. Risk factors for uterine fibroids: reduced risk associated with oral contraceptives. Br Med J 1986; 293:359–362.

118. Ory H. Functional ovarian cysts and oral contraceptives: negative association confirmed surgically. JAMA 1974; 228:68–69.

119. Vessey M, Metcalfe A, Wells C, et al. Ovarian neoplasms, functional ovarian cysts and oral contraceptives. Br Med J 1987; 294:1518–1520.

120. Speroff L, Glass RH, Kase NG. Clinical Gynecologic Endocrinology and Infertility. 3rd ed. Baltimore: Williams & Wilkins, 1983.

121. Royal College of General Practitioners Oral Contraceptive Study. Reduction in incidence of rheumatoid arthritis associated with oral contraceptives. Lancet 1978; 1:569–571.

122. Carr BR. Starting the new patient on oral contraceptives. Int J Fertil 1988; 33(Suppl):21–26.

123. Prevention and management of cardiovascular risk in women. Am J Obstet Gynecol 1988; 158(Suppl):1659–1661.

124. Mishell DR. Use of oral contraceptives in women of older reproductive age. Am J Obstet Gynecol 1988; 158:1652–1657.

125. Tietze C. Probability of pregnancy resulting from a single unprotected coitus. Fertil Steril 1960; 11:485–488.

126. Population Reports. Postcoital contraception—an appraisal. Series J, No. 9. Family Planning Programs. Washington, DC: George Washington University, 1976:J141–J156.

127. Yuzpe AA, Smith RP, Rademaker AW. A multicenter clinical investigation employing ethinyl estradiol combined with DL-norgestrel as a postcoital contraceptive agent. Fertil Steril 1982; 37:508–513.

128. Postcoital contraception. Lancet 1983; 1:855–856 (editorial).

129. Population Reports. Hormonal contraception: new long-acting methods. Series K, No. 3. Injectables and Implants. Baltimore: The Johns Hopkins University, 1987: K57–K87.

130. Goldzieher JW, Benogiano G. Long-acting injectable steroid contraceptives. In: Mishell DR, ed. Advances in Infertility Research. Vol 1. New York: Raven, 1982: 75–115.

131. Rosenfeld A, Maine D, Rochat R, et al. The Food and Drug Administration and medroxyprogesterone acetate. What are the issues? JAMA 1983; 249:2922–2928.

132. Segal SJ. Contraceptive implants. In: Mishell DR, ed. Advances in Infertility Research. Vol 1. New York: Raven, 1982:117–127.

133. Nash HA, Jackonicz TM. Vaginal rings. In: Mishell DR, ed. Advances in Infertility Research. Vol 1. New York: Raven, 1982: 129–144.

134. ALZA Corporation. The Progestasert: Progesterone Uterine Therapeutic System. Palo Alto, CA, 1976.

135. Luukkainen T, Heikinhemio O, Hasukkamaa M, et al. Inhibition of folliculogenesis and ovulation by the antiprogesterone RU 486. Fertil Steril 1988; 49:961–963.

136. Baulieu EE, Ulman A. Antiprogesterone activity of RU 486 and its contragestive and other applications. Hum Reprod 1986; 1:107–110.

137. Hodgen GD. Progesterone antagonists: useful for contraception. Contemp OB/GYN 1988; 32:65–66.

138. Andreyko JL, Marshall LA, Dumesic DA, et al. Therapeutic uses of gonadotropin-releasing hormone analogs. Obstet Gynecol Surv 1987; 42:1–21.

139. Nillius SJ, Bergquist C, Wide L. Inhibition of ovulation in women by chronic treatment with a stimulating LHRH analogue—a new approach to birth control? Contraception 1978; 17:537–545.

140. Monroe SE, Blumenfeld Z, Andreyko J, et al. Dose dependent inhibition of pituitary-ovarian function during administration of GnRH agonistic analog (nafarelin). J Clin Endocrinol Metab 1986; 63:1334–1341.

141. Bergquist C, Nillius SJ, Wide L. Peptide contraception in women. Inhibition of ovulation by chronic intranasal LRH agonist therapy. Ups J Med Sci 1984; 89:99–106.

142. Lemay A, Faure N, Labrie F, et al. Inhibition of ovulation during discontinuous intranasal luteinizing hormone–releasing hormone ago-

nist dosing in combination with gestagen. Fertil Steril 1985; 43:868–877.

143. Sheehan KL, Casper RF, Yen SSC. Luteal phase defects induced by an agonist of luteinizing hormone–releasing factor: a model for fertility control. Science 1982; 215:170–172.

144. Sheehan KL, Casper RF, Yen SSC. Induction of luteolysis by luteinizing hormone–releasing hormone factor (LRF) agonist: sensitivity, reproducibility, and reversibility. Fertil Steril 1982; 37:209–212.

145. Lemay A, Faure N, Labrie F. Sensitivity of pituitary and corpus luteum responses to single intranasal administration of (D-Ser[TBU]⁶-des-gly-NH₂¹⁰) luteinizing hormone–releasing hormone ethylamide (Buserelin) in normal women. Fertil Steril 1982; 37:193–200.

146. Population Reports. IUDs: a new look. Series B, No. 5. Intrauterine Devices. Baltimore: The Johns Hopkins University, 1988: 1–31.

147. Alvarez F, Branche V, Fernadez E, et al. New insights on the mode of action of intrauterine contraceptive devices in women. Fertil Steril 1988; 49:768–773.

148. World Health Organization. Mechanism of action, safety and efficacy of intrauterine devices. WHO Tech Rep Ser 1987; 753:12–17.

149. Gupta PK, Malkani PK, Bhasin K. Cellular responses in the uterine cavity after IUD insertion and structural changes of the IUD. Contraception 1971; 4:375–384.

150. Moyer DL, Mishell DR Jr. Reactions of human endometrium to the intrauterine foreign body. 2. Long-term effects on the endometrial histology and cytology. Am J Obstet Gynecol 1971; 111:66–80.

151. Sagiroglu N. Phagocytosis of spermatozoa in the uterine cavity of women using intrauterine device. Int J Fertil 1971; 16:1–14.

152. Toppozada T. Treatment of increased menstrual blood loss in IUD users. Contraception 1987; 36:145–157.

153. Burkman RT. The Women's Health Study. Association between intrauterine device and pelvic inflammatory disease. Obstet Gynecol 1981; 57:269–276.

154. Grimes DA. Intrauterine devices and pelvic inflammatory disease: recent developments. Contraception 1987; 36:97–109.

155. Weström L. Pelvic inflammatory disease: bacteriology and sequelae. Contraception 1987; 36:111–128.

156. Cates W Jr, Ory HW, Rochat RW, et al. The intrauterine device and deaths from spontaneous abortion. N Engl J Med 1976; 295:1155–1159.

157. Tatum HJ. A reassessment of intrauterine contraception. In: Mishell DR, ed. Advances in Infertility Research. Vol 1. New York: Raven, 1982: 47–74.

158. The intrauterine device. ACOG Technical Bulletin. No. 104. Washington, DC: American College of Obstetricians and Gynecologists, 1987.

159. Population Reports. New developments in vaginal contraception. Series H, No. 7. Barrier Devices. Baltimore: The Johns Hopkins University, 1984: H157–H190.

160. Barrier Contraceptives and Spermicides. Geneva: World Health Organization, 1987: 1–49.

161. Faich G, Pearson K, Fleming D, et al. Toxic shock syndrome and the vaginal contraceptive sponge. JAMA 1986; 255:216–218.

162. Baehler EA, Dillon WP, Cumb TJ, et al. Prolonged use of a diaphragm and toxic shock syndrome. Fertil Steril 1982; 38:248–250.

163. Feldblum PJ, Fortney JA. Condoms, spermicides, and the transmission of human immunodeficiency virus: a review of the literature. Am J Public Health 1988; 78:52–54.

164. Jick H, Walker AM, Rothman KJ, et al. Vaginal spermicides and congenital disorders. JAMA 1981; 245:1329–1332.

165. Louik C, Mitchell AA, Werler MM, et al. Maternal exposure to spermicides in relation to certain birth defects. N Engl J Med 1987; 317:474–478.

166. Warburton D, Neugut RH, Lustenberger A, et al. Lack of association between spermicide use and trisomy. N Engl J Med 1987; 317:478–482.

167. Bracken MB. Spemicidal contraceptives and poor reproductive outcomes: the epidemiologic evidence against an association. Am J Obstet Gynecol 1988; 151:552–556.

168. Population Reports. Periodic abstinence: how well do new approaches work? Series I, No. 3. Periodic Abstinence. Baltimore: The Johns Hopkins University, 1981; I34–I71.

169. Bonnar J. Natural family planning including breast feeding. In: Mishell DR, ed. Advances in Infertility Research. Vol 1. New York: Raven, 1982: 1–18.

170. Ogino K. Ovulationstermin und Konzeptionstermin. Zentralbl Gynaekol 1930; 54:464–479.

171. Knaus H. Die periodische Frucht und Unfruchtbarkeit des Weibes. Zentralbl Gynaekol 1933; 57:1393.

172. Oechsli FW. Studies of the consequences of contraceptive failure: final report. Berkeley, CA: University of California, Berkeley, Apr 8, 1976 (Contract N01-HD-5–2816): 20.

173. Brown JB, Blackwell LF, Billing JJ, et al. Natural family planning. Am J Obstet Gynecol 1987; 157:1082–1089.

174. Zinman MJ. Why you should know about natural family planning. Contemp OB/GYN 1989; 32:69–89.

175. Population Reports. Breast-feeding, fertility, and family planning. Series J, No. 24. Breast Feeding. Baltimore: The Johns Hopkins University, 1981: J526–J575.

176. Perez A. First ovulation after childbirth: the effect of breastfeeding. Am J Obstet Gynecol 1972; 114:1041–1045.

177. Talwae GP, ed. Immunologic Approaches to Contraception and Infertility. New York: Plenum, 1986.

178. Anderson DJ, Alexander NJ. A new look at antifertility vaccines. Fertil Steril 1983; 40:557–571.

179. Talwar GP, Gaur A. Recent developments in immunocontraception. Am J Obstet Gynecol 1987; 157:1075–1078.

180. Population Reports. Mini laparotomy and laparoscopy: safe, effective and widely used sterilization. Series C, No. 9. Baltimore: The Johns Hopkins University, 1985: C125–C167.

181. Shepherd MK. Female contraceptive sterilization. Obstet Gynecol Surv 1974; 29:739–787.

182. Sterilization. ACOG Technical Bulletin. No. 113. Washington, DC: American College of Obstetricians and Gynecologists, 1988.

183. Khandwala SD. Laparoscopic sterilization: a comparison of current techniques. J Reprod Med 1988; 33:463–466.

184. Brenner WE. Evaluation of contemporary female sterilization methods. J Reprod Med 1981; 26:439–453.

185. Population Reports. Reversing female sterilization. Series C, No. 8. Female Sterilization. Baltimore: The Johns Hopkins University, 1980: C97–C123.

186. Jane Roe et al. v. Henry Wade. Supreme Court of the United States. Opinion No. 70-18, Jan 22, 1973.

187. Doe et al. v. Bolton. Attorney General of Georgia et al. Supreme Court of the United States. Opinion No. 74-1151 and 74-1419, July 1, 1976.

188. Atrash HK, Mackay T, Binkin NJ, et al. Legal abortion mortality in the United States: 1972 to 1982. Am J Obstet Gynecol 1987; 156:605–612.

189. Population Reports. The use of PGs in human reproduction. Series G, No. 8. Prostaglandins. Baltimore: The Johns Hopkins University, 1980: G77–G119.

190. Grimes DA, Mishell DR, Shoupe D. Early abortion with a single dose of the antiprogestin RU 486. Am J Obstet Gynecol 1988; 158:1307–1312.

191. Cameron IT, Baird DT. Early pregnancy termination: a comparison between vacuum aspiration and medical abortion using prostaglandin (16,16 dimethyl-trans-Δ²-PGE₁ methyl ester) or the antiprogestogen RU 486. Br J Obstet Gynaecol 1988; 95:271–276.

192. Population Reports. Update on condoms—products, protection, promotion. Series H, No. 6. Barrier Methods. Baltimore: The Johns Hopkins University, 1982: H121–H155.

193. Javer PS, Ohri BB. The history of experimental and clinical work on vasectomy. J Int Coll Surg 1960; 33:482–486.

194. Hackett RE, Waterhouse K. Vasectomy—reviewed. Am J Obstet Gynecol 1973; 116:438–455.

195. Lipschultz LI, Benson GS. Vasectomy—1980. Urol Clin North Am 1980; 7:89–105.

196. Kendrick JS, Ruben GL. Vasectomies performed by private physicians, United States, 1980 to 1984. Fertil Steril 1986; 46:528–530.

197. Ramos-Cordero RA, Ackman CFD, Naftolin F. Changing profiles in vasectomy subjects in the past decade. Fertil Steril 1979; 31:410–412.

198. Population Reports. Voluntary sterilization: world's leading contraceptive method. Series M, No. 2. Washington, DC: George Washington University Medical Center, Population Information Program, 1978: 37–70.

199. Population Reports. Population and birth planning in the People's Republic of China. Series J, No. 25. Washington, DC: George Washington University Medical Center, Population Information Program, 1982: 577–618.

200. Anonymous. New method of male sterilization. Chin Med J 1980; 93:205–206.

201. Misro M, Guha SK, Singh H, et al. Injectable non-occlusive chemical contraception in the male. Contraception 1979; 20:467–473.

202. Ahsan RK, Kapur MM, Farooq A, et al. Further studies of an intravasal copper device in rats. J Reprod Fertil 1980; 59:341–345.

203. Brueschke EE, Kaleckas RA, Wingfield JR, et al. Development of a reversible vas deferens occlusion device. VII. Physical and microscopic observations after long-term implantation of flexible prosthetic devices. Fertil Steril 1980; 33:167–178.

204. Leader AJ, Axelrad SD, Frankowski R, et al. Complications of 2,711 vasectomies. J Urol 1974; 111:365–369.

205. Kaplan KA, Heuther CA. A clinical study of vasectomy failure and recanalization. J Urol 1975; 113:71–74.

206. Lo CN, Mumford SD, Atwood RJ. Postvasectomy residual sperm pregnancy. Fertil Steril 1980; 33:668–669.

207. Edwards IS. Postvasectomy testing: reducing the delay. Med J Aust 1981; 1:649.

208. Klapproth HJ, Young IS. Vasectomy, vas ligation and vas occlusion. Urology 1973; 1:292–300.

209. Penna RM, Potash J, Penna SM. Elective vasectomy: a study of 843 patients. J Fam Pract 1979; 8:857–858.

210. Neaves WB. Biological aspects of vasectomy. In: Greep RO, Astwood EB, eds. Handbook of Physiology. Sect 7. Endocrinology. Vol V. Male Reproductive System. Washington, DC: American Physiological Society, 1975: 383–404.

211. Gupta AS, Kothari LK, Dhruva A, et al. Surgical sterilization by

vasectomy and its effect on the structure and function of the testis in man. Br J Surg 1975; 62:59–63.

212. Jarow JP, Buden RE, Dym M, et al. Quantitative pathologic changes in the human testis after vasectomy: a controlled study. N Engl J Med 1985; 313:1252–1256.

213. Horan AH. When and why does occlusion of the vas deferens affect the testis? Fertil Steril 1975; 62:59–63.

214. Ying W, Hedman M, de la Torre B, et al. Effect of vasectomy on the steroid profile of human seminal plasma. Int J Androl 1983; 6:116–124.

215. Naik VK, Joshi UM, Sheth AR. Long-term effects of vasectomy on prostatic function in men. J Reprod Fertil 1980; 58:289–293.

216. Varma MM, Varma RR, Johanson AJ, et al. Long-term effects of vasectomy on pituitary-gonadal function in man. J Clin Endocrinol Metab 1975; 40:868–871.

217. Purvis K, Saksena SK, Cekan Z, et al. Endocrine effects of vasectomy. Clin Endocrinol 1976; 5:263–272.

218. Smith KD, Tcholakian K, Chowdhury M, et al. An investigation of plasma hormone levels before and after vasectomy. Fertil Steril 1976; 27:145–151.

219. Skegg DCG, Mathews JD, Guillevaud J, et al. Hormonal assessment before and after vasectomy. Br Med J 1976; 1:621–622.

220. Whitby RM, Gordon RD, Blair BR. The endocrine effects of vasectomy: a prospective five-year study. Fertil Steril 1979; 31:518–520.

221. Rumke P, Hellinga G. Autoantibodies against spermatozoa in sterile men. Am J Clin Pathol 1959; 32:357–363.

222. Ansbacher R, Keung-Yeung K, Wurster JC. Sperm antibodies in vasectomized men. Fertil Steril 1972; 23:640–643.

223. Ansbacher R. Vasectomy: sperm antibodies. Fertil Steril 1973; 24:788–792.

224. Alexander NJ, Schmidt SS, Free MJ, et al. Sperm antibodies after vasectomy with fulguration. J Urol 1976; 115:77–78.

225. Alexander JN, Wilson BJ, Patterson GD. Vasectomy: immunologic effects in rhesus monkeys and men. Fertil Steril 1974; 25:149–156.

226. Quinlivan WLG, Sullivan H, Olsher N. Circulating antispermatozoa immunoglobulin G in men after vasectomy. Fertil Steril 1975; 26:224–227.

227. Law HY, Bodmer WF, Mathews JD, et al. The immune response to vasectomy and its relation to the HLA system. Tissue Antigens 1979; 14:115–139.

228. Tung KSK, Teuscher C, Goldberg EH, et al. Genetic control of antisperm autoantibody response in vasectomized guinea pigs. J Immunol 1981; 127:835–839.

229. Mathews JD, Skegg DCG, Vessey MP, et al. Weak antibody reactions to antigens other than sperm after vasectomy. Br Med J 1976; 2:1359–1360.

230. Bullock JY, Gilmore LL, Wilson JD. Autoantibodies following vasectomy. J Urol 1977; 118:604–606.

231. Alexander NJ, Clarkson TB. Vasectomy increases the severity of diet-induced atherosclerosis in *Macaca fascicularis*. Science 1978; 201:538–541.

232. Lamberson HV Jr, Fritz KE. Immunological enhancement of atherogenesis in rabbits. Arch Pathol 1974; 98:9–16.

233. Clarkson TB, Alexander NJ. Long-time vasectomy. Effects on the occurrence and extent of atherosclerosis in rhesus monkey. J Clin Invest 1980; 65:15–25.

234. Witkin SS, Zelikovsky G, Bongiovanni AM, et al. Sperm-related antigens, antibodies, and circulating immune complexes in sera of recently vasectomized men. J Clin Invest 1982; 70:33–40.

235. Walker AM, Jick H, Hunter JR, et al. Vasectomy and non-fatal myocardial infarction. Lancet 1981; 1:13–15.

236. Wallace RB, Lee J, Gerger WL, et al. Vasectomy and coronary disease in men less than 50 years old: absence of association. J Urol 1981; 126:182–184.

237. Walker AM, Jick H, Hunter JR, et al. Hospitalization rates in vasectomized men. JAMA 1981; 245:2315–2317.

238. Goldacre MJ, Holford TR, Vessey MP. Cardiovascular disease and vasectomy: findings from two epidemiologic studies. N Engl J Med 1983; 308:805–808.

239. Massey FJ, Bernstein GN, O'Fallon WM, et al. Vasectomy and health: results from a large cohort study. JAMA 1984; 252:1023–1029.

240. Rosenberg L, Schwingl PJ, Kaufman DW, et al. The risk of myocardial infarction 10 or more years after vasectomy in men under 55 years of age. Am J Epidemiol 1986; 123:1049–1056.

241. Doty FO. Emotional aspects of vasectomy: a review. J Reprod Med 1973; 10:156–161.

242. Kohli KL, Sobrero AJ. Vasectomy: a study of psychosexual and general reactions. Soc Biol 1973; 20:298–302.

243. Vaughn RL. Behavioral response to vasectomy. Arch Gen Psychiatry 1979; 36:815–821.

244. Lipshultz LI, Benson GS. Vasectomy: an anatomical, physiologic, and surgical review. In: Cunningham GR, Schill W-B, Hafez ESE, eds. Regulation of Male Fertility. The Hague: Martinus Nijhoff, 1980: 169–186.

245. Lee HY. Observations of the results of 300 vasectomies. J Androl 1980; 1:11–15.

246. Mehrotra ML, Gupta RL, Nagar AM, et al. Fertility status of men following vaso-vasostomy. Indian J Med Res 1981; 73:33–40.

247. Martin DC. Microsurgical reversal of vasectomy. Am J Surg 1981; 142:48–50.

248. Lee HY. A 20-year experience with vasovasostomy. J Urol 1986; 136:413–415.

249. Yarbro ES, Howards SS. Vasovasostomy. Urol Clin North Am 1987; 14:515–526.

250. Sullivan MJ, Howe GE. Correlation of circulating antisperm antibodies to functional success in vasovasostomy. J Urol 1977; 117:189–191.

251. Bagshaw HA, Masters JRW, Pryor JP. Factors influencing the outcome of vasectomy reversal. Br J Urol 1980; 52:57–60.

252. Linnet L, Hjort T, Fogh-Andersen P. Association between failure to impregnate after vasovasostomy and sperm agglutinins in semen. Lancet 1981; 1:117–119.

253. Royle MG, Parslow JM, Kingscott MMB, et al. Reversal of vasectomy: the effects of sperm antibodies on subsequent fertility. Br J Urol 1981; 53:644–659.

254. Thomas AJ Jr, Pontes JE, Rose NR, et al. Microsurgical vasovasostomy: immunologic consequences and subsequent fertility. Fertil Steril 1981; 35:447–450.

255. Huang TTF Jr, Tung KSK, Yanagimachi R. Autoantibodies from vasectomized guinea pigs inhibit fertilization in vitro. Science 1981; 213:1267–1269.

256. Snyder PJ, Lawrence DA. Treatment of male hypogonadism with testosterone enanthate. J Clin Endocrinol Metab 1980; 51:1335–1339.

257. Weinbauer GF, Marshall GR, Nieschlag E. New injectable testosterone ester maintains serum testosterone of castrated monkeys in the normal range for months. Acta Endocrinol 1986; 113:128–132.

258. Wilson JD, Griffin JE. The use and misuse of androgens. Metabolism 1980; 29:1278–1295.

259. Knuth UA, Behre H, Belkien L, et al. Clinical trial of 19-nortestosterone hexylphenylprionate (Anadur) for male fertility regulation. Fertil Steril 1985; 44:814–821.

260. Steinberger E, Smith KD. Effect of chronic administration of testosterone enanthate on sperm production and plasma testosterone, follicle-stimulating hormone, and luteinizing hormone levels: a preliminary evaluation of a possible male contraceptive. Fertil Steril 1977; 28:1320–1328.

261. Paulsen CA, Leonard JM, Burgess EC, et al. Male contraceptive development: re-examination of testosterone enanthate as an effective single entity agent. In: Patanelli DJ, ed. Proceedings of Hormonal Control of Male Fertility. Washington, DC: Government Printing Office, 1978: 17–36.

262. Cunningham GR, Silverman VE, Thornby J, et al. The potential for an androgen male contraceptive. J Clin Endocrinol Metab 1979; 49:520–526.

263. Swerdloff RS, Campfield LA, Palacios A, et al. Suppression of human spermatogenesis by depot androgen: potential for male contraception. J Steroid Biochem 1979; 11:663–670.

264. Palacios A, McClure RD, Campfield A, et al. Effect of testosterone enanthate on testis size. J Urol 1981; 126:46–48.

265. Matsumoto AM. Effects of chronic testosterone administration in normal men: safety and efficacy of high dosage testosterone and parallel dose-dependent suppression of luteinizing hormone, follicle-stimulating hormone, and sperm production. J Clin Endocrinol Metab 1990; 70:282–287.

266. Matsumoto AM. Is high dosage testosterone an effective male contraceptive agent? Fertil Steril 1988; 50:324–328.

267. Alvarez-Sanchez F, Faundes A, Brache V, et al. Attainment and maintenance of azoospermia with combined monthly injections of depo medroxyprogesterone acetate and testosterone enanthate. Contraception 1977; 15:635–648.

268. Brenner PF, Mishell DR Jr, Bernstein GS, et al. Study of medroxyprogesterone acetate and testosterone enanthate as a male contraceptive. Contraception 1977; 15:679–691.

269. Faundes A, Brache V, Leon P, et al. Sperm suppression with monthly injections of medroxyprogesterone acetate combined with testosterone enanthate at a high dose (500 mg). Int J Androl 1981; 4:235–245.

270. Barfield A, Melo J, Coutinho E, et al. Pregnancies associated with sperm concentrations below 10 million/ml in clinical studies of a potential male contraceptive method, monthly depo medroxyprogesterone acetate and testosterone esters. Contraception 1979; 20:121–127.

271. Hedman M, Gottlieb C, Svanborg K, et al. Endocrine, seminal and peripheral effects of depot medroxyprogesterone acetate and testosterone enanthate in men. Int J Androl 1988; 11:265–276.

272. Knuth VA, Nieschlag E. Male contraception based on androgen/gestagen combinations. In: Cooke BA, Sharpe RM, eds. The Molecular and Cellular Endocrinology of the Testis. New York: Raven, 1988: 219–223.

273. Fogh M, Corker CS, Hunter WM, et al. The effects of low doses of cyproterone acetate on some functions of the reproduction system in normal men. Acta Endocrinol 1979; 91:545–552.

274. Wang C, Yeung KK. Use of low-dosage oral cyproterone acetate as a male contraceptive. Contraception 1980; 21:245–272.

275. Moltz L, Rommler A, Post K, et al. Medium dose cyproterone acetate

(CPA): effects on hormone secretion and on spermatogenesis in men. Contraception 1980; 21:393–413.

276. Crowley WF, Beitins IZ, Vale W, et al. The biologic activity of a potent analogue of gonadotropin-releasing hormone in normal and hypogonadotropic men. N Engl J Med 1980; 302:1052–1057.

277. Labrie F, Belanger A, Cusan L, et al. Antifertility effects of LHRH agonists in the male. J Androl 1980; 1:209–228.

278. Marchetti B, Reeves JJ, Pelletier G, et al. Modulation of pituitary luteinizing hormone–releasing hormone receptors by sex steroids and luteinizing hormone–releasing hormone in the rat. Biol Reprod 1982; 27:133–145.

279. Clayton RN, Katikineni M, Chan V, et al. Direct inhibition of testicular function by gonadotropin-releasing hormone: mediation by specific gonadotropin-releasing hormone receptors in interstitial cells. Proc Natl Acad Sci USA 1980; 77:4459–4463.

280. Sundaram K, Cao Y-Q, Qang N-G, et al. Inhibition of the action of sex steroids by gonadotropin-releasing hormone (GnRH) agonists: a new biological effect. Life Sci 1981; 28:83–88.

281. Smith R, Donald RA, Espiner EA, et al. Normal adults and subjects with hypogonadotropic hypogonadism respond differently to D-Ser(TBU)^6-LH-RH-EA^{10}. J Clin Endocrinol Metab 1979; 48:167–170.

282. Bergquist C, Nillius SV, Bergh T, et al. Inhibitory effects on gonadotropin secretion and gonadal function in men during chronic treatment with a potent stimulatory luteinizing hormone–releasing hormone analogue. Acta Endocrinol 1979; 91:601–608.

283. Belanger A, Labrie F, Lemay A, et al. Inhibitory effects of a single intranasal administration of [D-Ser-(TBU)^6, des-Gly-NH$_2$10] LHRH ethylamide, a potent LHRH agonist, on serum steroid levels in normal adult men. J Steroid Biochem 1980; 13:123–126.

284. Linde R, Doelle GC, Alexander N, et al. Reversible inhibition of testicular steroidogenesis and spermatogenesis by a potent gonadotropin-releasing hormone agonist in normal men. N Engl J Med 1981; 305:663–667.

285. Evans RM, Doelle GC, Lindner J, et al. A luteinizing hormone–releasing hormone agonist decreases biological activity and modifies chromatographic behavior of luteinizing hormone in man. J Clin Invest 1984; 73:262–266.

286. Evans RM, Doelle GC, Alexander AN, et al. Gonadotropin and steroid secretory patterns during chronic treatment with a luteinizing hormone–releasing hormone agonist analog in men. J Clin Endocrinol Metab 1984; 58:862–867.

287. Pavlou SN, Dahl KD, Wakefield G, et al. Maintenance of the ratio of bioactive to immunoactive follicle-stimulating hormone in normal men during chronic luteinizing hormone–releasing hormone agonist administration. J Clin Endocrinol Metab 1988; 66:1005–1009.

288. Bhasin S, Heber O, Steiner B, et al. Hormonal effects of GnRH agonist in the human male. II. Testosterone enhances gonadotropin suppression induced by GnRH agonist. Clin Endocrinol 1984; 20:119–128.

289. Bhasin S, Heber D, Steiner BS, et al. Hormonal effects of gonadotropin-releasing hormone (GnRH) agonist in the human male: III. Effects of long term combined treatment with GnRH agonist and androgen. J Clin Endocrinol Metab 1985; 60:998–1003.

290. Bhasin S, Yuan QX, Steiner BS, et al. Hormonal effects of gonadotropin releasing hormone (GnRH) agonist in men: effects of long term treatment with GnRH agonist infusion and androgen. J Clin Endocrinol Metab 1987; 65:568–574.

291. Pavlou SN, Wakefield G, Schlechter NL, et al. Mode of suppression of pituitary and gonadal function after acute or prolonged administration of a luteinizing hormone–releasing hormone antagonist in normal men. J Clin Endocrinol Metab 1989; 68:446–454.

292. Bagatell CJ, McLachlan RI, de Krester DM, et al. A comparison of the suppressive effect of testosterone and a potent new gonadotropin-releasing hormone antagonist on gonadotropin and inhibin levels in normal men. J Clin Endocrinol Metab 1989; 69:43–48.

293. National Coordinating Group on Male Antifertility Agents. Gossypol—a new antifertility agent for males. Chin Med J 1978; 4:417–428.

294. Liu GZ. Clinical study of gossypol as a male contraceptive. Reproduccion 1981; 5:189–193.

295. Shaozhen Q, Guangwei J, Ziaoyun W, et al. Gossypol related hypokalemia. Clinicopharmacologic studies. Chin Med J 1980; 93:477–482.

296. Liu GZ, Lyle KC, Cao J. Experiences with gossypol as a male pill. Am J Obstet Gynecol 1987; 157:1079–1082.

297. Liu GZ, Chiu-Hinton K, Cao J, et al. Effects of K salt or a potassium blocker on gossypol-related hypokalemia. Contraception 1988; 37:111–117.

298. Qian SZ, Wang Z-G. Gossypol: a potential antifertility agent for males. Annu Rev Pharmacol Toxicol 1984; 24:329–360.

299. Meng G-D, Zhu J-C, Chen Z-W, et al. Recovery of sperm production following the cessation of gossypol treatment: a two-centre study in China. Int J Androl 1988; 11:1–11.

300. Giwercman A, Skakkebaek NE. The effect of salicylazosulphapyridine (sulphasalazine) on male fertility. A review. Int J Androl 1986; 9:38–52.

301. White DR, Cuther RJ. Sulfasalazine as a male contraceptive agent. In: Zatuchini GI, Goldsmith A, Spieler JM, et al., eds. Male Contraception: Advances and Future Prospects. Philadelphia: Harper & Row, 1986: 227–236.

302. Jackson H. Antispermatogenic agents. Br Med Bull 1970; 26:79–86.

303. Spitz IM, Gunsalus GL, Mather JP, et al. The effects of the indazole carboxylic acid derivative, tolnidamine, on testicular function: I. Early changes in androgen binding protein secretion in the rat. J Androl 1985; 6:171–178.

304. Kandeel FR, Swerdloff RS. Role of temperature in regulation of spermatogenesis and the use of heating as a method for contraception. Fertil Steril 1988; 49:1–23.

305. Madhwa Raj HG, Sairam MR, Hieschlag E. Immunologic approach to regulation of fertility in the male. In: Cunningham GR, Schill W-B, Hafez ESE, eds. Regulation of Male Fertility. The Hague: Martinus Nijhoff, 1980: 209–218.

306. Sheela Rani CS, Murty GSRC, Moudgal NR. Effect of chronic neutralization of endogenous FSH on testicular function in the adult male bonnet monkey—assessment using biochemical parameters. Int J Androl 1978; 1:489–500.

307. Murty GSRC, Sheela Rani CS, Moudgal NR, et al. Effect of passive immunization with specific antiserum to FSH on the spermatogenic process and fertility of adult male bonnet monkeys. J Reprod Fertil 1979; 26:147–163.

308. Srinath BR, Wickings EJ, Witting C, et al. Active immunization with follicle-stimulating hormone for fertility control: a 4½-year study in male rhesus monkeys. Fertil Steril 1983; 40:110–117.

309. Talwar GP, Naz RK, Das C, et al. A practicable immunological approach to block spermatogenesis without loss of androgens. Proc Natl Acad Sci USA 1979; 76:5882–5885.

310. Talwar GP, Naz RK. Immunological control of male fertility. Arch Androl 1981; 7:177–185.

311. Goldberg E, Wheat TE. Induction of infertility in male rabbits by immunization with LDH-X. In: Spilman CH, Lobl TJ, Kirton KT, et al., eds. Regulatory Mechanisms of Male Reproductive Physiology. Amsterdam: Excerpta Medica, 1976: 133–139.

312. Setty BS. Regulation of epididymal function and sperm maturation—endocrine approach to fertility control in male. Endokrinologie 1979; 74:100–117.

313. Neumann F, Schenck B. Antiandrogens: basic concepts and clinical trials. In: Cunningham GR, Schill W-B, Hafez ESE, eds. Regulation of Male Fertility. The Hague: Martinus Nijhoff, 1980: 93–104.

314. Lobl TJ. α-Chlorohydrin: review of a model posttesticular antifertility agent. In: Cunningham GR, Schill W-B, Hafez ESE, eds. Regulation of Male Fertility. The Hague: Martinus Nijhoff, 1980: 109–122.

315. Ford WCL, Harrison A. Effect of α-chlorohydrin on glucose metabolism by spermatozoa from the cauda epididymis of the rhesus monkey (Macaca mulatta). J Reprod Fertil 1980; 60:59–64.

316. Morris ID, Williams LM. Some preliminary observations of the nephrotoxicity of the male antifertility drug (±)α-chlorohydrin. J Pharm Pharmacol 1980; 32:35–38.

317. Ford WCL. The contraceptive effect of 6-chloro–6-deoxysugars in the male. In: Cunningham GR, Schill W-B, Hafez ESE, eds. Regulation of Male Fertility. The Hague: Martinus Nijhoff, 1980: 123–126.

318. Jacobs JM, Ford WCL. The neurotoxicity and antifertility properties of 6-chloro-6-deoxyglucose in the mouse. Neurotoxicology 1981; 2:405–417.

19

SEXUAL DYSFUNCTION

Stanley G. Korenman

Sexual dysfunction is common in both sexes, may contribute to difficulties in relationships, and may herald the presence of serious illness.

SEXUAL DYSFUNCTION IN MEN

The study of impotence as an organic medical disorder has been accelerated by advances in technology, the availability of effective therapies, and the recognition that the behavioral model of Masters and Johnson[1] can account for only a minority of cases. This section will focus on erectile insufficiency and give some consideration to impaired libido and ejaculation. These dysfunctions are quite common, frequently of organic origin, and often amenable to therapy.

Impotence is usually defined as the inability to attain an erection of sufficient rigidity for vaginal penetration in 50% or more of attempts. Erectile insufficiency after a period of normal sexual functioning is termed *secondary impotence*. Early ejaculation often precedes development of secondary impotence. Associated sexual dysfunctions include a loss of libido and ejaculatory insufficiency. *Loss of libido* refers to a reduction in sexual interest and initiative and in the frequency and intensity of responses to external or internal erotic stimuli. Loss of libido characterizes hypogonadal men, regardless of whether the hypogonadism is due to testicular failure or to hypothalamic-pituitary failure.[2,3] Intercurrent

illness, drugs, and psychiatric problems may also be associated with reduced libido. Withdrawal from sexual activity should be construed as evidence of impotence.

Ejaculatory insufficiency refers to absent or reduced seminal emission, impaired ejaculatory contractions, and decreased or anesthetic orgasm. Ejaculatory insufficiency is most often associated with drug therapy.[4,5] A rare condition termed *ejaculatory anesthesia* refers to a lack of appropriate sensation at orgasm; its etiology is completely unknown.[6] Ejaculatory capability tends to be preserved in most cases of penile impotence.

Epidemiology

Sexual activity in men progressively declines with age, which may result in either cessation or a reduced frequency of intercourse in those remaining active. The extent to which impotence, hypogonadism, and partner unavailability contribute to this decline remains unknown.[7] A few studies have attempted to determine the age-dependent prevalence of impotence. Of these studies, only that of Kinsey dealt with men who were not identified through a medical source.[8–10] As shown in Figure 19–1, the prevalence of impotence (including an absence of sexual activity) increases rapidly after age 50. It appears to be much higher in men with diabetes mellitus, and about the same in hypertensive men and in unselected populations.[11,12] Conservative estimates of the prevalence of impotence are 10% in the sixth decade of

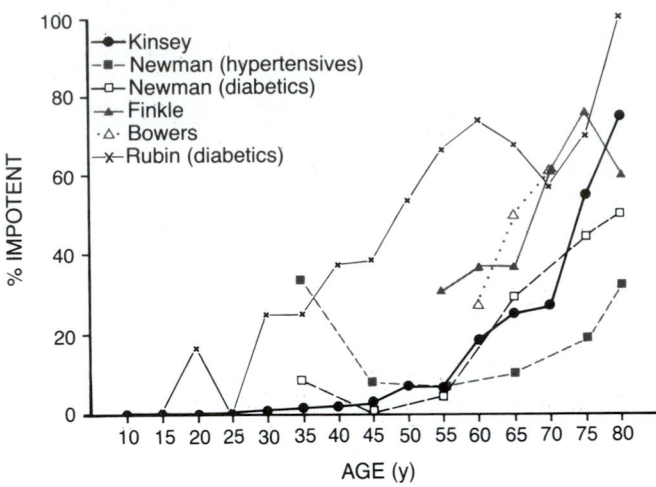

Figure 19–1. Age-dependent prevalence of impotence as derived from studies in unselected subjects,[8] veterans receiving care in Veterans Administration hospitals,[9, 10] patients with diabetes mellitus,[11] and patients with hypertension.[11]

life, 25% in the seventh, 40% in the eighth, and more than 50% in the ninth. Korenman and colleagues found that one fourth of healthy men older than age 50 (average age of 64) reported themselves as impotent.[13]

Mechanism of Erection

Penile erection results from relaxation of vascular and sinusoidal smooth muscle of the corpus cavernosum as a result of autonomic nervous system activation. The central nervous system responds to erotic stimuli by signaling the thoracolumbar and sacral erection centers that activate the nervi erigentes.[14] These parasympathetic pathways have been traced in adult human cadavers, in the monkey, and in the dog.[14, 15] In humans, fibers emerge from the intermediolateral nucleus through S2-4. They join fibers from the hypogastric nerve to form the pelvic plexus, which spreads over the lateral aspect of the rectum to innervate the rectum, bladder, seminal vesicle, and prostate, as they course mostly along blood vessels. The most caudad portion becomes the prostatic plexus as the fibers progress distally. At the distal bulbous urethra they divide. Some traverse the corpora cavernosa with the vessels, and others travel into the corpora alone and then divide to innervate the helicine arteries and central erectile tissues. Thus during pelvic surgical procedures if careful attention is not paid to the neural pathways, neurogenic impotence may be caused by transection of nerves, by an associated inflammatory response, or by ischemia.[14]

Identification of the neurotransmitters that are responsible for erection is not fully clarified. Preganglionic cholinergic neurons stimulate postganglionic neurons that activate an unknown neurotransmitter to release nitric oxide (NO), a direct vasodilator, via activation of guanylate cyclase.[16, 17] Inhibition of basal alpha-2–adrenergic contractile tone by parasympathetic preganglionic fibers also contributes to cavernosal sinusoidal and vascular smooth muscle relaxation.

As with many systems, receptors for a variety of active substances are present in corporeal tissues, so that for different species, relaxation may be produced in vitro by using nicotine, vasoactive intestinal peptide, isoproterenol, phenoxybenzamine, phentolamine, rimiterol, acetylcholine, carbachol, methacholine, prostaglandin E_1, and prostaglandin E_2. On the other hand, norepinephrine, epinephrine, dopamine, serotonin, histamine, prostaglandin $F_{2\alpha}$, brady-

kinin, vasopressin, angiotensin, substance P, ATP, phenylephrine, and prostaglandin I_2 all cause corporeal smooth muscle contraction.[18]

The hemodynamics of erection have been worked out over the last few years by Michal[19] and Wagner and Metz,[20] who used arteriography and cavernosometry, and by Lue and colleagues[18, 21–23] in studies of animals with electrodes chronically implanted in the cavernosal nerves to produce neurogenic erections.

There are five phases of erection (Fig. 19–2). In the latent phase, immediately after the onset of stimulation, there is a reduction in resistance of the penile arterioles and cavernosal sinusoids, followed promptly by a two- to three-fold increase in flow without an increase of intracavernosal pressure. At about 10 s, cavernosal pressure begins to rise to near-arterial levels. As a full erection approaches, cavernosal diastolic blood pressure remains near zero, and systolic pressure is near the systolic level, although it slowly falls as the erection persists. Cessation of the stimuli at any time leads to prompt passive detumescence. During the rigid erection phase, contraction of the ischiocavernous muscles as a result of pudendal nerve stimulation produces intracavernosal pressures much higher than the systemic pressure. This is the phase of maximal erectile strength.[18, 23] Detumescence is usually associated with alpha-2–sympathetic vasoconstrictor activity.[4]

Infusion cavernosograms document that inhibition of venous return via the cavernosal vein begins as early as 5 s after initiation of nerve stimulation, as a result of venoconstriction.[24, 25] More complete inhibition of venous flow is due to passive compression of the outflow tract of the penetrating veins by the increasing corporeal pressure and the dilated corporeal sinuses. The measurement of corporeal blood gases during up to 30 min of erection demonstrates that oxygenation and pH are preserved, which indicates that adequate tissue perfusion persists. Thus, in brief, erection is due to neurogenically controlled arterial and sinusoidal vasodilatation and simultaneous venoconstriction, but some perfusion persists in the erect penis.

Emission, Ejaculation, and Orgasm

Emission, ejaculation, and orgasm are controlled principally by sympathetic nerves and, under appropriate circumstances, may be separable from each other.[4, 26] Emission refers to the secretion of seminal fluid into the posterior

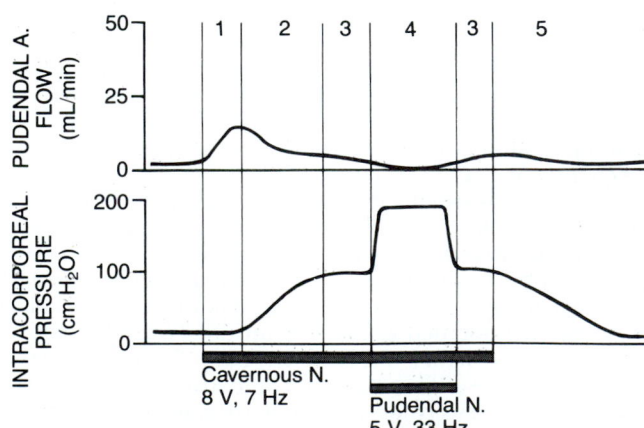

Figure 19–2. The five phases of erection, as delineated by sequential electrostimulation of the cavernosal and pudendal nerves in the monkey. 1, latent phase; 2, tumescence phase; 3, full erection phase; 4, rigid erection phase; 5, detumescence phase. (From Lue TF. The mechanism of penile erection in the monkey. Semin Urol 1986; 4:217–224.)

urethra. It is initiated by stimulation of the genitalia, which activates a specific center between T-12 and L-2, and is also under voluntary control. Emission results from peristalsis of the vas deferens and the ampulla, rhythmic contractions of the seminal vesicle, and constriction of prostatic smooth muscle. The proximal vesicle sphincter (bladder neck) and distal vesicle sphincter are both contracted, resulting in a pressure level that leads to the sensation of ejaculatory inevitability. Semen is transferred from the posterior to the bulbous urethra by intermittent relaxation of the distal vesicle sphincter. Ejaculation, which is the expulsion of semen from the urethra, is a reflex response to the entry of semen into the bulbous urethra and does not reflect cerebral input. It is due to three to seven contractions of the bulbocavernous muscle and other muscles of the pelvic floor. Normal antegrade ejaculation requires firm closure of the proximal vesicle sphincter and a functioning distal sphincter. A disordered distal sphincter will result in a seeping ejaculation. If the proximal sphincter is impaired, retrograde ejaculation occurs.

Orgasm is the subjective sensation of pleasure that is initiated at about the time of emission and continues through the ejaculatory process. Although it is associated with and enhanced by the various events of the emission and ejaculatory process, it is separable from them in that it may occur without ejaculation, as in prepubertal children, and with markedly attenuated sensation, as in anesthetic ejaculation.[6]

Ejaculate volume is androgen dependent and decreases with age. Reduced ejaculatory volume is associated with reduced sexual pleasure. Transurethral prostatectomy commonly interferes with proximal vesicle function and may result in retrograde ejaculation, which is also seen in association with some cases of autonomic nervous system neuropathy (such as in diabetes mellitus). Painful ejaculation may reflect injury to the ejaculatory ducts. A variety of surgical procedures, neurological disorders, and spinal cord injuries that interfere with the pelvic sympathetic nerves impair emission, as do drugs that impair the sympathetic nervous system, particularly alpha-2–adrenergic blockers and ganglionic blockers.[4, 5, 27]

Premature ejaculation remains an etiological puzzle, but its therapy has received a great deal of attention since Masters and Johnson reported a high cure rate[1] by use of education and simple techniques for developing voluntary control by delaying initiation of emission through desensitization to stimulatory impulses. Their success rate has not been achieved by others.[28] Reduced time to ejaculation is a common early manifestation of secondary impotence, however, and its onset should be taken seriously.

Pudendal nerve afferents stimulate nocturnal penile tumescence (NPT) and reflex erections that are maintained even with spinal cord injury. NPT occurs throughout life, primarily during rapid eye movement sleep and results, in the adult, in two to eight full erections per night that last up to 40 min each.[29] The number and quality of nocturnal erections decrease with age, in association with the decline in rapid eye movement sleep.

With aging, erotogenic stimuli must be of greater intensity to produce a response, and spontaneous pelvic swelling decreases in frequency.[1] The duration of the latent phase is increased, penile filling is slower, and there is increased venous drainage, which results in a less firm maximal erection. Paradoxically, the time to ejaculation may be prolonged, which enhances the quality of coitus. There is a lengthened absolute refractory period to the next erection. In some aging men penile sensation is decreased.

Normal sexual function depends on the interaction of libido and potency. Androgens appear to play an important role in libido and in the frequency of nonerotic or reflex

TABLE 19-1. Mechanisms Contributing to Erectile Dysfunction

Type of Condition	Disorder
Vascular	
Aortoiliac arterial obstruction	Aorto-occlusive disease
Hypogastric-penile arterial obstruction	Atherosclerosis
Arterial dysplasia	Primary impotence in young men
Veno-occlusive incompetence	Age, diabetes, Peyronie disease
Neurogenic	
Central nervous system and spinal neuronal loss	Cerebrovascular accident (stroke), multiple sclerosis, epilepsy
Peripheral autonomic neuronal loss	Surgery, Shy-Drager syndrome, diabetes
Disordered signal transmission	Drugs
Psychogenic inhibition of the erotic response	Depression (psychogenic)
Endocrine	
Deficient androgen availability	
Testicular failure	Castration, radiation, chemotherapy
Hypothalamic-pituitary disease	Age, pituitary adenoma, ethanol
Prolactin excess	Prolactinoma, uremia, drugs
Estrogen excess	Alcoholism, cirrhosis, drugs
Inhibition of androgen action	Spironolactone, cimetidine, ranitidine, flutamide, ketoconazole, ethanol
Secondary hyperparathyroidism	Uremia
Hypothyroidism and hyperthyroidism	
Local	
Peyronie disease	
Intersinusoidal fibrosis	Diabetes, aging
Penile trauma	
Pudendal nerve trauma	Bicycle rider's palsy
Penile carcinoma	

erections, including NPT.[30] Androgens are required for normal seminal fluid content and volume. They do not seem to be involved acutely in erections associated with erotic stimuli.[2]

Erectile Dysfunction

Erectile dysfunction may be due to arterial and veno-occlusive insufficiency,[19] loss of neuronal integrity, psychogenic inhibition of the erotic response, endocrinopathies,[31–33] and local cavernosal factors (Table 19–1). These mechanisms are not independent and often act together to produce erectile insufficiency.

Impotence in Medical Diseases

Patients receiving medical care who present to an impotence clinic have a wide variety of medical illnesses (Table 19–2), as reported by ourselves and others.[34–37] Patients presenting to urologists may have different characteristics.

Some etiological insight may be gained by evaluating

TABLE 19–2. Clinical Characteristics of 301 Patients Presenting to a Sexual Dysfunction Clinic*

Disorder	% of Patients with Disorder
Hypertension	45.8
Diabetes mellitus	30.0
Atherosclerosis	33.6
Myocardial infarction	16.3
Stroke	9.6
Occlusive vascular disease	7.0
Angina	9.6
Coronary bypass graft	5.3
Transurethral prostate resection	16.9
Arthritis	22.2

*Patients with active alcoholism, progressive systemic illness, psychosis, or established hypogonadism were not admitted to the study. Mean duration of impotence was 4.8 y. Ponderal index (kg/m²) was 27.3.

studies assessing the prevalence of sexual dysfunction in patients with specific conditions (Table 19–3). Although of considerable interest, these analyses used varied definitions of sexual dysfunction, had a variety of case selection biases, and often did not compare the prevalence in disease groups with that in matched controls, so that it was impossible to separate disease-related from age-related impotence.

VASCULAR DISEASE. The majority of cases of secondary impotence, particularly in older men, appear to be due to atherosclerosis.[11, 34–41] Penile arteriographic studies in a few patients with "psychogenic" impotence revealed a substantial number of obstructive or dysplastic lesions, particularly in patients older than age 35.[19] Occlusive vascular disease was associated with a 51% rate of impotence in 367 reported patients.[42–46] Impotence was associated with the most severe arterial lesions (by angiographic visualization) and the lowest penile blood pressures. Relief of major vessel obstruction did not alleviate the impotence in most cases,[44] which suggests that smaller distal arteries were involved. Impotence preceded clinical vascular symptoms half the time,[43] which

is consistent with evidence that a low penile blood pressure significantly predicts cardiovascular events[47] and an abnormal exercise stress test result.[48]

Myocardial infarction was associated with a pre-existing impotence rate of 44% and an overall sexual dysfunction rate of 64% in one large series.[49] A similar prevalence was seen in a control group under medical treatment.[50] Other studies gave comparable results.[51, 52]

DIABETES MELLITUS. Impotence in men with diabetes mellitus is common.[34] Several large series suggest a prevalence of about 50% in unselected patients[12, 53–57] (see Table 19–3), increasing steadily with age, to reach 95% in a geriatric diabetes clinic. The relation between the onset of diabetes and impotence is variable.[34, 56, 58, 59] We found that the onset of impotence is inversely related to age at diagnosis of diabetes (Fig. 19–3).

NPT is almost invariably abnormal in impotent diabetics compared with either normal subjects or potent diabetics,[60, 61] which implies an organic pathogenesis. Endocrine, neuropathic, and vascular etiologies have been proposed.

TABLE 19–3. Impotence in Patients with Different Clinical Conditions

Condition	Number of Patients	% Impotent	% with Sexual Dysfunction	Reference
Occlusive vascular disease	367	51		43–46
Myocardial infarction	229	44		49–52
At-risk controls	93	45		
Diabetes mellitus	1471	44		12, 39, 53–57
5-y follow-up	466	58		
Hypertension: active therapy	221	19		68, 70
Placebo	219	14		
No tablets	80	20		
Nonstudy patients	134	10		
Uremia	750	46		72–77
Transplanted	21	26		
Multiple sclerosis	68	63	75	88
Partial temporal lobe epilepsy	20	45		89, 90
Stroke	39	36	70	91, 92
Prostate cancer				
Pretreatment	68	25	17	100, 102
Post-treatment	68	85	79	
Nerve-sparing surgery	75	14		15, 97, 98
Pelvic cancer	55			99
Preoperative		22		
Postoperative		84		
Rectal carcinoma	103			107, 108
Abdominoperineal resection		60		
Low resection		39		
2-y operated survivors	10	80		
Chronic pain	60	23		110, 111
Obstructive pulmonary disease	20	35		112
Hypoxic pulmonary fibrosis	8	90		113
Osteoarthritis	48	2	46	116
Osteoarthritis before hip replacement	49	7	22	115
Osteoarthritis after hip replacement	49	6	12	115
Scleroderma	10	60		117, 118
Rheumatoid arthritis controls	10	0		
Depression	16	35		140
Controls	16	0		
Graves disease	7	56		33
Transurethral prostatectomy	62	26	50	105, 106
Hemachromatosis	44	25		119
Acromegaly and prolactinoma	29	76	76	120
Celiac disease	28	19		114
Alcoholism	176	47		122, 123

Hypogonadism has been suggested[53, 62] and denied[54, 55, 59, 63, 64] in the pathogenesis of diabetic impotence. A similar prevalence of primary and secondary hypogonadism was seen in men with diabetes and in nondiabetic impotent men of the same age[34] and in healthy controls[13] when both serum testosterone and bioavailable testosterone (BT) levels were measured. However, insulin-dependent diabetes mellitus is associated with infiltration of the testicular interstitial matrix with collagen-like material and abnormal seminiferous tubules.[65] Androgen therapy is generally ineffective for diabetic impotence,[54] but it may have some benefit in the small number of hypogonadal diabetic men with a normal penile blood pressure.[66]

Ellenberg's demonstration that peripheral neuropathy and bladder neuropathy are more frequent (an 80% incidence) in impotent than in potent diabetic men[54] led to the neurogenic hypothesis of diabetic impotence. That result has been difficult to confirm. Palmer and colleagues[57] evaluated both autonomic and peripheral nerves and demonstrated that slowed motor nerve conduction velocity correlates best with secondary impotence. Clinical evidence of neuropathy, age, treatment modality, or quality of control could not distinguish between impotent and potent groups. The prevalence of abnormal nerve conduction velocity reached 35% in a series of nondiabetic impotent subjects, in part because of alcohol and tobacco abuse,[36, 67] so a control group is necessary for these studies.

A major role of macro- and microvascular disease in the pathogenesis of diabetic impotence is now appreciated.[35, 40, 41] The prevalence of borderline or abnormal penile blood pressure, indicative of arterial disease, is greater in non–insulin-dependent diabetes (79%) than in insulin-dependent diabetes (47%) and is comparable to the incidence of abnormal penile blood pressure in nondiabetic impotent men (64%), which supports the importance of atherosclerosis in impotence for both groups.[34]

HYPERTENSION. Hypertension has long been thought to be associated with an increased incidence of impotence. In one large study, 20% of hypertensive men were found to be impotent before initiation of therapy, and impotence rates higher than 30% were reported in drug-treated groups.[68] However, the age-specific incidence of impotence in hypertensive men probably does not differ from that in the remainder of the general population receiving medical care.[11, 69, 70]

The onset of impotence is often attributed to initiation of antihypertensive therapy, which contributes to noncompliance of men with such drug regimens. Central and peripheral autonomic agents have been especially implicated, but all such agents including diuretics, angiotensin-converting enzyme inhibitors, and calcium channel blockers have been reported to result in impotence,[5, 27, 69] although the reports leave much to be desired.[69] None of the studies related the degree of blood pressure control to sexual dysfunction. Reduction of arterial blood pressure and reduced resistance in nonpenile vascular beds may accentuate the reduction in flow rate associated with an obstructive lesion in the hypogastric-penile arterial tree, so that adequate control of the blood pressure may result in reduced maximal penile-filling capacity.[71]

UREMIA. Uremia is associated with a prevalence of impotence of nearly 50% (see Table 19–3).[72–78] Proposed mechanisms have been reviewed.[31, 32, 79] Possible causes include elevation of prolactin level, sometimes with gynecomastia; elevation of luteinizing hormone level; and low levels of plasma testosterone.[80] There appears to be an increased secretion rate of prolactin, as well as reduced prolactin metabolic clearance.[81] Secondary hyperparathyroidism may also be implicated.[31] Zinc depletion has been proposed to contribute to the impotence of uremia,[82] as has autonomic neuropathy.[83] Vascular disease, therapy for hypertension, and volume depletion during the dialysis process may reduce the penile filling rate. The use of bromocriptine[84, 85] and clomiphene[86] has been claimed to improve sexual performance of some patients with uremia who are undergoing dialysis. Androgen therapy was of limited success. Erythropoietin has also been reported to improve sexual function, concomitant with reduction of the serum prolactin level.[87]

NEUROLOGICAL DISEASE. Multiple sclerosis,[88] temporal lobe epilepsy,[89, 90] and cerebrovascular accident (stroke)[91, 92] are associated with a high prevalence of impotence (see Table 19–3), presumably by impairing central or peripheral erectile centers or pathways. Pelvic surgery impairs erectile function by interrupting the autonomic fibers of the nervi erigentes that control the erectile process[14] or by decreasing the penile blood supply.[93]

HYPOGONADISM. Severe hypogonadism usually causes loss of libido and of erectile function and reduction in ejaculate volume,[2, 30] although there are reports of retained erectile capability in adult castrates.[94] Lesser degrees of hypogonadism are common with aging.[38, 95] Although there are reports of more severe hypogonadism in impotent men, as measured by reduced BT[96] or bioavailable luteinizing hormone[97] values, Korenman and colleagues have found that testosterone and BT levels decrease with age[38] but are identical in potent and impotent men in the presence or absence of a medical illness.[13] Because of reduced testosterone production and increased protein binding of testosterone, the bioavailable hormone level is lower in older men than in younger men, decreasing in 40% of men to values below those seen in younger men. Almost all such older

$$y = 58.844 - 0.965x \quad R = 0.75$$

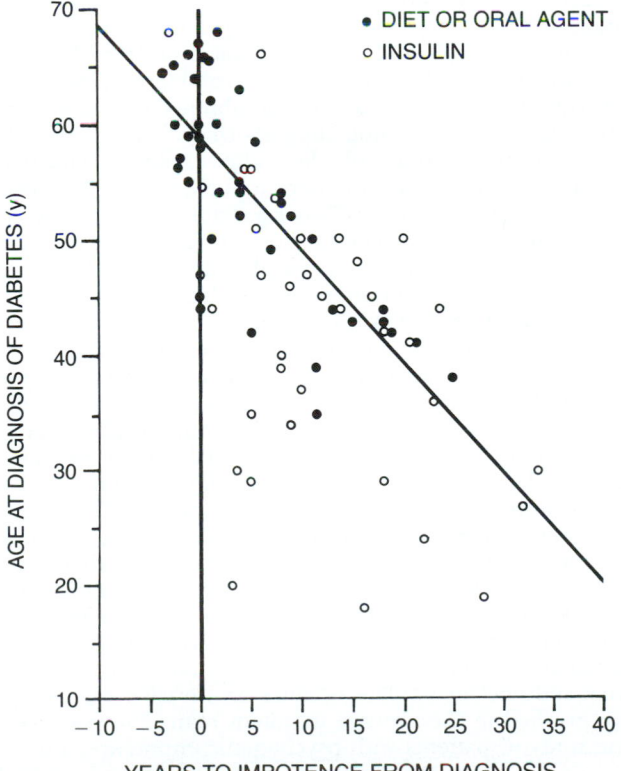

Figure 19–3. The relationship between the onset of diabetes and the onset of impotence was assessed in 64 consecutive diabetics seen in an impotence clinic.

men have values consistent with hypogonadotropic hypogonadism, and many have reduced responsiveness to luteinizing hormone–releasing hormone (LHRH, also called gonadotropin-releasing hormone, GnRH). Perhaps the more important measure is tissue availability of androgens, which is reduced with aging,[98] but levels in tissues from potent and impotent men have not been compared.

NEOPLASTIC DISEASE. Patients with cancer of a variety of types frequently have a diminution in the quality of sexual life, as well as of other parameters of life.[99, 100] With specific reference to impotence, among patients with mostly pelvic tumors, including prostatic cancer, about 20% before and 80% after surgery were impotent.[99, 101] Walsh and colleagues[15, 102, 103] developed an improved method of carrying out radical prostatectomy and cystoprostatectomy that has resulted in potency rates above 75% and acceptable recurrence rates, as confirmed by others (see Table 19–3).[104] However, it should be kept in mind that impotence and sexual dysfunction rates of about 10% have been reported even after transurethral prostatectomy.[105, 106]

Surgery for rectal cancer results in a 60 to 80% impotence rate after abdominal-perineal resection and a 40% rate after a low resection.[107, 108] Radiation therapy for such tumors also produces a high rate of impotence through changes in blood flow and fibrosis.[109] Careful attention to surgical detail and to the needs of cancer patients and their partners will help to improve the quality of their sexual life.

OTHER CHRONIC DISEASES. High rates of impotence and of loss of libido and sexual activity have been reported in men with chronic back pain,[110, 111] chronic obstructive pulmonary disease,[112] pulmonary fibrosis,[113] Graves disease,[33] celiac disease,[114] arthritis,[115, 116] scleroderma,[117, 118] hemochromatosis,[119] and acromegaly and prolactinoma[120] (see Table 19–3).

DRUG-RELATED DYSFUNCTION. Sexual dysfunction including loss of libido, impotence, and ejaculatory insufficiency is a reported complication of therapy with a wide variety of drugs, but unfortunately most studies of the phenomenon are anecdotal and uncontrolled. The reader is referred to reviews by Wein and Van Arsdale[4] and others[5, 27, 68] for discussion of individual therapeutic agents. The principal culprits are neurotransmitter agonists or antagonists that are used for the treatment of hypertension, angina, and afterload reduction or for alleviation of psychosis, anxiety, and depression. They may act by inhibiting the parasympathetic erectile mechanism, stimulating alpha-adrenergic vasoconstrictor tone, interfering with central erotic responsiveness, or influencing the reproductive endocrine system by blocking the dopaminergic inhibition of prolactin secretion. Prolactin hypersecretion both affects central nervous system control of sexual responsiveness and inhibits gonadotropin secretion. Other agents acting to reduce androgen availability or acting directly as estrogens include digitalis, cimetidine, ranitidine, spironolactone, ketoconazole, progestogens, LHRH agonists or antagonists, and estrogens themselves. The sexual effects of narcotics, cocaine,[121] and marihuana are predominantly depressive, although cocaine has a reputation for enhancing sexual pleasure.[5]

Alcoholism is associated with a high prevalence of impotence.[122, 123] Among the effects of ethanol are hypogonadism with feminization[124] (Table 19–4), neuropathy, and vascular disease associated with the smoking that commonly accompanies alcohol excess.

Alcoholics may respond to high doses of nonaromatizable androgens, which suggests that a refractory form of hypogonadism prevails in many alcoholics.[125] Entry into a rehabilitation program and abstinence are believed by some alcoholics to be associated with the onset of impotence,[121]

TABLE 19–4. Chronic Reproductive-Endocrine Consequences of Ethanol Abuse

Cell or System	Effect
Leydig cells	Increased gonadotropin receptors
	Reduced cyclic AMP concentration
	Increased sensitivity to estrogens
	Acetaldehyde toxicity
	Reduced NAD+/NADH inhibits steroidogenesis
	Reduced 3β-hydroxysteroid dehydrogenase
	Injures mitochondria
	Increased presence of testicular autoantibodies
Enhanced testosterone metabolism	Induction of 5α-reductase activity with acute or short-term exposure
Estrogen metabolism	Chronically increased aromatase activity
	Probably increased estrogen receptors in tissues (including testis and liver)
	Reduced intracellular estrogen metabolism
	Phytoestrogens in alcohol-containing beverages

particularly when antabuse is employed. Whether antabuse actually causes impotence is doubtful,[126] although NPT was reduced by antabuse in one study.[127] Long-term rehabilitation resulted in return of sexual function in only 25% of alcoholics in one study,[125] which suggests that impotence should be addressed as soon as the alcoholic is established in therapy.

Cigarette smoking has been reported as a risk factor for impotence.[35, 128] Cigarette smoking is increased in impotent men compared with age-matched controls, and there is a high prevalence of heavy smokers in the impotent group. Among impotent nonsmokers, there is frequently a history of previous smoking. Smoking is also associated with a high prevalence of abnormal penile blood pressure determinations.[129] A relationship among the use of beta-adrenergic blockers, smoking, and impotence has been proposed, and improvement has been reported after eliminating the use of the beta-adrenergic blockers.[130] In one study in dogs, electrically stimulated erections were inhibited by passive inhalation of smoke from two cigarettes per hour or by intravenous nicotine injection.[131] This inhibitory effect of nicotine was due to a reduction in corporeal blood flow and in cavernosal venoconstriction in the absence of systemic vascular effects. This finding suggests that nicotine, as well as perhaps other cigarette volatiles, either inhibits erectile nerve vasodilator activity or stimulates alpha-adrenergic vasoconstrictor activity, or both. Thus cigarette smoking may contribute to vascular impotence both by its chronic enhancement of the development of peripheral vascular disease and by acutely inhibiting neurogenic vasodilatation.

PSYCHOGENIC CAUSES. Primary psychogenic impotence is a diagnosis of exclusion. The prevalence and etiology of pure psychogenic impotence are matters of considerable debate. The results in any study of impotence depend on the sources of patients, the age distribution, the extent of the work-up, and the criteria for assignment to one or another diagnostic category. Most studies attribute less than a third of impotence to psychogenic causes.[35, 37, 132] In studies by Korenman and colleagues,[36, 38] organic etiological factors were identified in more than 90% of men older than age 50 with secondary impotence. Doubts have been raised as to the relevance of the distinction between organic and psychogenic impotence.[133, 134] Problems involved in making this distinction include the fact that vascular assessment may frequently be incomplete because an invasive evaluation is not justified in the average impotent man. For example, in one study of patients with psychogenic impotence, a degree of vascular obstruction or dysplasia was present in virtually every man older than age 35.[19] Veno-occlusive disorders have been a recognized cause of impotence for only a few years, and yet they are now reported in up to two thirds of certain subsets of impotent men with abnormal filling of penile blood during papaverine injection.[135] Furthermore, NPT is no longer accepted as a definitive means of distinguishing among causes of impotence. Patients with compromised penile blood flow related to a pelvic steal syndrome may have normal NPT.[136–138] In primary psychiatric disease, ambulatory schizophrenics do not appear to have a high prevalence of impotence.[139] Depression, on the other hand, is associated with a high prevalence of sexual dysfunction, impotence, and abnormal NPT.[140] By and large, psychometric evaluation of impotent men does not reveal the presence of significant pathological changes. Furthermore, success with sex therapy, although poorly documented, seems to be the same in organic impotence and in pure psychogenic impotence,[141] probably because such therapy is directed primarily at education and marital support.

Diagnostic Evaluation

The diagnostic evaluation for impotence requires a careful history, an appropriate physical examination, and special diagnostic procedures. The desire of the patient and his partner for corrective measures and their willingness to undergo invasive diagnostic and therapeutic interventions will determine the extent of the assessment.

The sexual history should record the extent of the dysfunction, its duration, its progression, and its characteristics. An excellent self-administered form is available for documenting such a record.[134] Appropriate questions concern current sexual activities; partner availability; the presence of spontaneous morning erections; the quality, duration, and usability of the best erections; and the ejaculatory capacity. A substantial decrease in sexual interest or responsiveness suggests the possibilities of hypogonadism, an effect of drugs, and clinical depression. The impact of self-image and interpersonal relations will help in the assessment of the urgency of diagnostic and therapeutic maneuvers.

It is essential to involve the partner early in the discussion of sexual function and of the various therapeutic alternatives. Successful therapy depends to a great degree on the availability, interest, health, and psychological status of the partner. Some women, particularly in the geriatric age group, may not be prepared for resumption of an active sex life.

A complete medical evaluation should be performed because impotence may be the presenting complaint in serious medical illness, including diabetes (see Fig. 19–2) and occlusive vascular disease.[43]

PHYSICAL EXAMINATION. The physical examination should emphasize detecting evidence of hypogonadism. Penile size and shape, the presence of Peyronie plaque or fibrous tissue, and the size, firmness, and nodularity of the prostate should also be determined. Autonomic nervous system function may be tested by evaluating for postural hypotension and assessing of heart rate responses to deep breathing.

LABORATORY TESTS. The appropriate laboratory assessment for impotence is somewhat controversial. The endocrine tests should include two morning fasting measurements of luteinizing hormone and assays for loosely bound testosterone or BT, prolactin, and ultrasensitive thyrotropin. Both hyper- and hypothyroidism may be associated with impotence and may be difficult to diagnose on clinical grounds, particularly in older men. The diagnosis of hypogonadism by hormone assay may be difficult. We consider a BT value of less than 2.2 nmol/L (70 ng/dL) to be the lower limit of normal.[13] Because a majority of older men with low BT levels have normal to low gonadotropin levels, an LHRH

responsiveness test to identify hyporesponsiveness may be appropriate. Few of these men have a pituitary adenoma, and computed tomographic scans are not routinely required. Normal prolactin and thyrotropin levels help to rule out a pituitary tumor.

SPECIAL DIAGNOSTIC TESTS. *Nocturnal Penile Tumescence.* Karacan and co-workers developed the NPT test to distinguish organic from psychogenic impotence.[29] By continuously monitoring penile diameter and sleep stage and visually assessing the rigidity of erection, it may be determined whether the reflex erectile mechanism is intact. A valid test requires at least two nights in a sleep laboratory and is thus expensive. The Rigiscan portable NPT monitor, which can be taken home by the patient, uses a mechanical constriction mechanism to measure penile rigidity and diameter and gives a record of the number and quality of erectile episodes throughout the night. The apparatus is expensive, and specialized equipment is required to process and print the report.

Simple inexpensive tests to determine whether NPT has occurred include the stamp test, in which a ring of stamps is placed around the flaccid penis at bedtime and a break indicates an episode of diameter increase, the Potentest,[137] and the Dacomed Snap Gauge,[142] which responds to three different levels of nocturnal tumescence with rupture of thin plastic strips.

Men with normal vasculature may have abnormal NPT because of disturbed sleep,[143] and normal NPT can be consistent with organic impotence associated with a pelvic steal syndrome.[138] In potent men both the frequency and the quality of NPT episodes decrease with age.[144] Thus the usefulness of measurement of NPT has come under skeptical scrutiny.[136, 138] Davis and colleagues found that more than 90% of men older than age 50 with secondary impotence had abnormal NPT.[36] We use NPT testing only rarely for patients with a normal penile blood pressure and a normal penile response to papaverine who claim to have no full erections.

Penile-Brachial Blood Pressure Index (PBPI). Development of a simple, noninvasive method of evaluating penile arterial integrity by comparing the penile and the brachial systolic pressures[145–149] was a major advance in the evaluation of impotence. The test is specific but of limited sensitivity.[150, 151] It is commonly used to demonstrate arteriogenic impotence, to predict the dose necessary for intracavernosal papaverine therapy,[152] and to determine the presence of a pelvic steal syndrome.[148] A pelvic steal syndrome occurs when obstructive lesions of the iliac or hypogastric arterial system provide adequate flow for erection at rest (or during NPT) but shunt blood to the legs during exercise.

To measure the penile blood pressure, a portable mercury manometer is connected to a 2.5-cm infant cuff. By using an inexpensive handheld 10 MHz Doppler instrument, the systolic blood pressure is listened for at 10 and 2 o'clock on the distal penile shaft to obtain right- and left-sided corporeal artery values. Brachial and penile pressure measurements are repeated after 5 min in the supine position and after performing bicycling motions in the air for up to 2 min. The PBPI is composed of the four ratios of penile to brachial pressure on each side in each position. The criteria for abnormal responses were developed mainly in men with occlusive vascular disease,[19, 45, 153] and the exercise test was described by Goldstein and colleagues.[148] For a definite abnormality

1. One of the four ratios is ≤0.6.
2. The mean of the four ratios is ≤0.65.
3. A 0.15 or more decrease in the ratio between the supine and the exercise PBPI indicates a pelvic steal syndrome.

A mean of the four determinations of 0.65 to 0.75 is suggestive of but not definitive for an obstructive arterial etiology for impotence.

Diagnostic Intracorporeal Injection. Intracorporeal injection of vasodilators is used primarily to determine erectile capability when the PBPI is not diagnostic of arterial insufficiency.[18, 154, 155] It is also employed during angiography[156] and cavernosography[157–159] to ensure adequate visualization of the penile vessels, and when performing duplex ultrasonographic assessment of arterial reactivity.[152]

Intracorporeal injection of papaverine or papaverine-phentolamine combinations diluted in normal saline using a 27-gauge needle produces an erection within 3 min and a maximal erection in 10 to 20 min in most men.[154] Before injection, a rubber band is placed on the proximal penis to impede the loss of papaverine into the systemic circulation. After 2 min the band is cut off and the patient is asked to stand to increase arterial inflow. Papaverine is not metabolized in the corpora and is thus long-acting. Patients with neurological disorders may have denervation hypersensitivity to the drugs, and those with vascular disease may require larger doses to achieve usable erections. Similar results can be attained with injections of prostaglandin E_1 (15 μg).[160] Although the last agent has the advantage of local metabolism, on occasion it causes painful erections.[161] In some studies, drug effectiveness has depended on dose.[161, 162]

Papaverine-phentolamine injections carry a risk of priapism (about 1% of injections), hematoma (3 to 10% of injections), infection (rare), local pain, and systemic hypotension (rare). We ask patients to discontinue aspirin use 5 d before each injection to minimize subcutaneous hematoma formation. The quality of the erection attained helps to determine the degree of vascular insufficiency. Cigarette smoking may inhibit the response to papaverine.[163] A strong, persistent erection excludes significant arterial or venous insufficiency as a cause of impotence, whereas a weak erection supports the diagnosis of arterial disease or impaired veno-occlusion.[155, 164] A study comparing the PBPI (with a PBPI of 0.7 at rest as the criterion for the designation abnormal) with intracorporeal papaverine injection demonstrated a poor correlation between the two.[164] Korenman and colleagues found that more than 20% of diagnostic PBPIs were due to a pelvic steal syndrome, and this situation may be one cause for such a discrepancy.

Duplex Scanning. Duplex scanning of penile arteries before and after papaverine-induced erection can determine whether corporeal arterial diameters are reduced and whether they dilate after exposure to papaverine.[18] Failure of erection after good arterial flow is diagnostic of veno-occlusive insufficiency and may render cavernosography or venography unnecessary.[152] Duplex scanning predicts whether there will be a good response to therapeutic papaverine but does not provide information as to whether a pelvic steal syndrome is present.

Penile Arteriography. Arteriography of the penile arteries and corpora cavernosa before and after papaverine-induced erection identifies arterial spasm and obstructive disease.[156, 160, 165] The induced erection dilates and extends the penile arteries, which makes it possible to visualize obstructions and collaterals consistently.[18] The most common sites of arterial disease are at the base of the penis (58%) and in the pudendal artery (31%). Asymmetrical lesions are common, and some degree of bilateral disease is necessary for erectile insufficiency.[156]

Cavernosometry and Cavernosography. Cavernosometry and cavernosography after pretreatment with vasodilators are valuable for identification of veno-occlusive incompetence[24] as well as arterial disease. Saline is injected into the corpus cavernosum to induce an erection. Cavernosal

pressure is measured on the other side. Normally, an erection occurs at about 20 mm Hg pressure. If it does not, venous insufficiency is suggested. Cavernosography with diluted contrast medium after intracorporeal administration of papaverine then localizes the venous leaks. Prevalence estimates of such leaks range from 17 to 86%,[23, 135, 166] especially in older men in the presence of atherosclerosis.[167] These procedures cause a significant incidence of local hematomas.

Electromyography. Evaluation of the neural system has been effective in demonstrating only a correlation between certain findings and impotence, not a direct causal relation, perhaps because the cavernous nerves have not been approachable. Electromyographic analysis of peripheral nerves is a time-consuming and painful means of diagnosing peripheral neuropathy, abnormal bulbocavernosus reflex latency, and defects of sacral and genitocerebral evoked potentials.[66] It provides evidence about the integrity of the neural circuits tested but not about whether those circuits play a role in the impotence. Dorsal penile nerve conduction velocity measurement is directed at the penile sensory system. Demonstration of a delay of conduction velocity to below 40 m/s indicates that a portion of the penile innervation is abnormal.[167, 168] A combination of bulbocavernosus reflex latency and somatosensory evoked potentials demonstrated abnormalities in 76 of 130 patients tested; unfortunately, no comparable potent control group was studied.[169] There is no substantiation, however, that sensory defects affect potency. Many investigators believe that a careful neurological history and physical examination suffice to determine whether neurological impairment contributes to sexual dysfunction.

Therapy

Therapeutic initiatives for impotence should follow thorough discussion of the benefits and risks of the various alternatives with the couple. Management should be based on a risk factor approach, because the presence of hypogonadism does not rule out vascular impotence, because combined arterial and veno-occlusive incompetence is common, and because psychogenic factors, when present, do not preclude other diagnoses. Age should be no barrier to therapy.

INTRACORPOREAL PHARMACOTHERAPY. Impotence of any etiology except for moderate to severe vascular disease may be treated by episodic self-administration of intracorporeal prostaglandin E_1, papaverine, or papaverine-phentolamine combinations, after appropriate education and training.[170–181] Although this approach is highly effective, it is rejected by as many as 20% of initially willing candidates during the preparation phase.[170] Only about 50% of men so treated continue long-term therapy,[171, 175, 176] but to them it may be quite satisfactory. Complications include local pain,[173] penile induration or fibrosis,[174, 182–184] prolonged erections,[171, 173, 175, 178] and systemic discomfort and dizziness in the presence of venous leaks.[180] For some men the effectiveness of the injections is reduced with time.[182] This therapy may provide a satisfactory medium-term solution to impotence for men, but the possibility of penile fibrosis engenders concern about its long-term consequences.

As an alternative method of intracavernosal therapy, Lue and Tanagho[18] and Mooradian and colleagues[185] found that a substantial proportion of men with vascular impotence who are treated with four injections of papaverine 2 wk apart have a persistent restoration of erectile function.

VASCULAR SURGERY. Vascular surgery for impotence may utilize techniques of inhibiting venous return and increasing arterial inflow. Surgical ligation of the superficial and deep dorsal veins draining the penis is a relatively simple procedure[186] that may give a 60% initially excellent or good result in restoring erectile function. Care must be taken to ensure that arterial flow is adequate before surgery so that adequate venous occlusion can take place.[152] Furthermore, in the presence of diabetes mellitus, the compliance of the corporeal sinusoids may be reduced so that venous occlusion may not be possible.

Arterialization of the dorsal penile vein by using the inferior epigastric artery has been reported to be associated with a 60% success rate.[187] Major vascular complications occurred in 6% of patients. Longer-term studies will permit assessment of the duration and quality of the therapeutic response.

PENILE PROSTHESES. Penile prostheses are devices that when inserted into the corpora cavernosa confer rigidity, either continuously as in the semirigid varieties or, on demand, as in the inflatable types. Mechanical, semirigid varieties that are more flexible than previously possible have been developed. These devices made impotence readily treatable, stimulated research in the field, and helped thousands of men. Their properties have been reviewed by Krane.[188] Penile prostheses are expensive and require surgery. Semirigid prostheses carry an overall complication rate of about 14% and are relatively easy to implant,[189] but they may produce relatively poor-quality erections. The inflatable units with a separate liquid reservoir are beset by mechanical problems; reoperation has been required in 3 to 22% of cases.[189-200] Technical advances in the device have improved those results.[190, 191, 193, 196, 199, 200] Other complications include a short-term infection rate of more than 2%,[190, 195] which may extend the duration of hospitalization and increase costs dramatically,[192] and aneurysms of the cylinders.[193, 198] Many men are not satisfied with the result[194] and complain of reduced penile size and discomfort.

None of these devices allow swelling of the glans penis, which is therefore susceptible to trauma during intercourse, and no information is available about the long-term fate of the implants. There are anecdotal reports that men with diabetes mellitus have an increased incidence of infection and externalization of the prosthesis. Krane and colleagues use prostheses only in men who are not candidates for vascular surgery or intracavernosal pharmacotherapy,[188] and we tend to reserve them for men desiring them and for men who cannot manage an external vacuum device.

EXTERNAL VACUUM TUMESCENCE DEVICES. The development of external vacuum devices dates back 80 years, but they have not been widely used in the treatment of impotence. Currently, three devices are marketed: the Erecaid, the Correctaid, and the Response. They provide assistance to the penile vascular pump and can be used regardless of the etiology of the impotence.[201-205] They produce an erection by creating a vacuum around the penis and causing increased cavernosal filling sufficient for a good erection. Venous drainage is inhibited by the use of constricting bands. After the patient learns how to use them, the devices are usually a satisfactory and cost-effective solution to the problem. Tissues are not adversely affected. The usual coital pattern may be restored (Fig. 19–4), with 2 to 10 episodes per month.[202] Erectile duration is also quite satisfactory, lasting an average of 16 min (Fig. 19–5). Some couples find the loss of spontaneity inhibiting. In patients with normal sensation, excessive negative pressure is prevented by pain. The erection is not completely normal in that the engorged penis becomes reddened and sometimes cyanotic because of the filling of the superficial penile vessels as well as the corpora. The glans penis is normally distended. The principal complications are occasional reversible hematomas, discomfort from the bands, and cold temperature of the

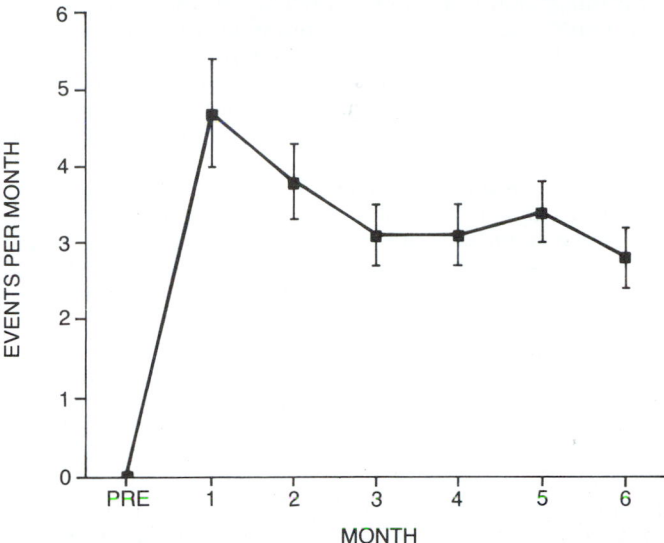

MEAN COITAL EVENTS PER MONTH OVER STUDY PERIOD

Figure 19–4. Monthly frequency of episodes of coitus in 19 impotent men screened for availability of a willing partner after initiation of the use of the Erecaid vacuum tumescence device. Before treatment, no coitus had been possible for at least 3 mo. (Reprinted with permission from the American Geriatrics Society, Use of a vacuum tumescence device in the management of impotence, by Korenman SG, Viosca SP, Kaiser FE, et al. Journal of the American Geriatrics Society, Vol 38, pp 217–220, 1990.)

erect penis, which can be treated by warming. This approach may be useful in the management of patients with an unsatisfactory result from a penile prosthesis either after its removal or with it in place. It is also effective in patients with a spinal cord injury or after major pelvic surgery.

MEDICAL THERAPIES. No medical therapy is effective for unselected patients with impotence, but some therapies may be useful in carefully selected patients.

Androgens. Androgens have long been used in the treatment of impotence. Thousands of patients were treated in the 1950s and 1960s with Afrodex, which is a combination of 5 mg of nux vomica, 5 mg of methyltestosterone, and 5 mg of yohimbine. The most careful studies of the

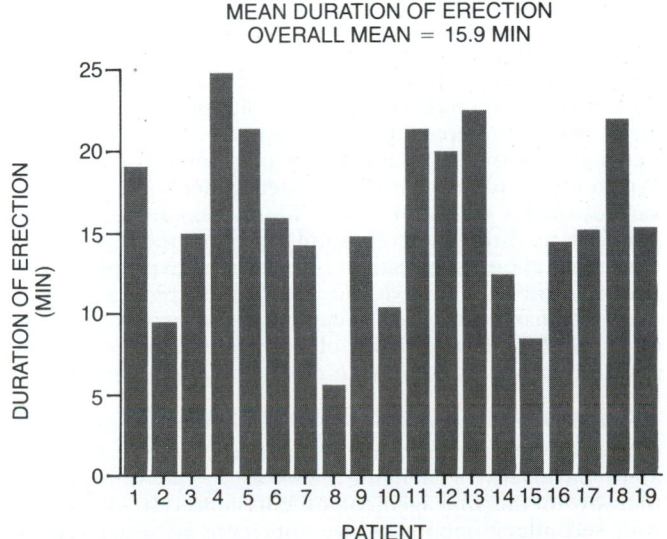

MEAN DURATION OF ERECTION
OVERALL MEAN = 15.9 MIN

Figure 19–5. Mean erectile duration reported by 19 impotent men using the Erecaid vacuum tumescence device over the course of a 6-mo study.

agent[206, 207] demonstrated a placebo effect but also a significant drug-induced improvement in both libido and erectile function;[208] however, the agent fell into disuse. Testosterone injection[209] improved sexual interest in 10 men with low interest despite normal circulating testosterone levels but had no impact on erectile problems. Oral testosterone undecanoate[210] was equally without effect, as were most of the attempts of androgen therapy for impotence in men with diabetes mellitus.[54, 55, 59, 63, 64]

Other Hormone-Directed Therapies. Bromocriptine, used because of hyperprolactinemia, seemed to be successful for some patients with impotence associated with uremia.[84, 85] Other impotent uremic men fared as well with placebo as with bromocriptine.[211] The use of clomiphene to reduce the effect of estrogen and to increase gonadotropin levels[212] caused excellent increases in testosterone and gonadotropin levels in men with uremia but only one improvement in impotence. LHRH, at a dose of 500 μg administered subcutaneously every 8 h for 4 wk, did not result in improvement in sexual function,[213] possibly because suppressive doses of the agent were given.[214] Serotonin antagonists are also ineffective.[215] In contrast, erythropoietin therapy in men with uremia may be remarkably successful, although an analysis of the changes in sexual function was incomplete.[87] The use of this agent merits further study in uremic men who do not have penile vascular insufficiency.

Other Therapies. The work of Morales and co-workers[216] resurrected the use of yohimbine, a potent alpha-2–adrenergic blocker, in the treatment of impotence by reporting a sustained improvement in erectile function in 26% of 23 impotent men. The same group subsequently reported that it is ineffective.[217]

Androgen Therapy for Hypogonadism. Hypogonadism should be treated with androgens (also see Chapter 13). In older men with a high prevalence of vascular disease, androgen therapy alone should not be expected to return erectile function to normal, even when hypogonadism is present. However, androgens in such men may improve energy, mood, and the sense of well-being. The use of the available oral preparations is not warranted because of hepatic complications. A long-acting testosterone ester such as testosterone enanthate or testosterone cypionate should be given, usually at a dose of 200 mg intramuscularly every 2 wk. Although a supraphysiological level of testosterone and BT is produced for several days and although values may fall below normal before the next injection, these preparations are the best available. In the older man the principal complication of testosterone therapy is erythremia, which sometimes requires phlebotomy (also see Chapter 13). Androgens also increase the low-density lipoprotein cholesterol level, reduce the high-density lipoprotein cholesterol level, stimulate hepatic lipoprotein lipase, and sensitize patients to the anticoagulant effects of coumarin derivatives. We routinely place androgen-treated patients on a prudent cardiovascular diet and follow lipoprotein levels and hematocrit at 3-mo intervals until the hematocrit stabilizes. Concerns about stimulation of prostatic hyperplasia and prostatic carcinoma have not been supported experimentally, nor have they been subject to rigorous scrutiny. The expected future availability of a transdermal testosterone system[218] promises to provide more physiological androgen replacement.

Sex Therapy. Changing beliefs about the pathogenesis of erectile dysfunction and the availability of effective therapies have led to changing views as to the value of sex therapy in the management of impotence. In older men with secondary impotence, we anticipate an organic cause and treat accordingly. However, depression may interfere with sexual performance. Loss of a mate often leads to depression and social isolation. Men may lose confidence in their sexual abilities, which creates anxieties that contribute greatly to their failure to initiate new relationships. The physician who sees patients for impotence may have an opportunity to identify and treat depression and to refer them for further support.

Sex therapy techniques may allow improvement of sexual attitudes and capacity in organic as well as psychogenic impotence. Sex therapy should focus on the couple. Unrealistic expectations and marital discord must be addressed, and the characteristics of a more satisfactory sex life defined. Behavioral changes that may assist in many cases include eliminating exposure to nicotine, arranging an appropriate time and environment for sexual intercourse, and encouraging intimacy, mutual pleasuring, experimentation, and communication. The effectiveness of sex therapy has never been fully evaluated. Although Zilbergeld and others proposed that an improvement in erectile function is common with sex therapy,[219, 220] the level of improvement is not satisfactory for coitus.[221]

SEXUAL DYSFUNCTION IN WOMEN

Anatomical, physiological, and psychosocial differences between women and men cause differences in patterns of sexual dysfunction, but the underlying themes are similar, just as the anatomical elements and the physiological responses to arousal are analogous. Women experience disturbances of the desire (libido), arousal (proceptivity), and orgasmic phases of the sexual response cycle, as well as painful intercourse (dyspareunia). Vaginismus, or severe contractions of the vaginal musculature that prevent penile entry, is rare.

Epidemiology

There have been few objective, population-based, detailed analyses of female sexual dysfunction, and available reports have described various diagnostic criteria. During the adult reproductive years, the principal dysfunctions reported by women in five surveys[56, 222–225] are low desire (18%), low arousal (25%), global orgasmic difficulty (9%), situational orgasmic difficulty (27%), and dyspareunia (8%) (Table 19–5). The relative consistency of the reports suggests that these average values are not far wrong. Unfortunately, there is little information on sexual dysfunction in young women.

Osborn and colleagues,[225] in a community-based study in Great Britain that evaluated the changing physiological status of women as they go through menopause, demonstrated that substantial increases in operationally defined sexual dysfunctions occur in women as they age (Table 19–6). The principal problem seems to be a decrease in sexual interest and arousability in a subset of women and an increased rate of anorgasmic episodes of coitus. These findings were related not to gynecological history or menopausal state but rather primarily to age itself. The subjects perceived themselves to be much less sexually dysfunctional than did the investigators. In this cross-sectional study, cohort effects may have an important role in sexual expectations. Only 4% of the women were interested in pursuing the "problem."

Similar findings but with a higher rate of perception of dysfunction were noted in a clinic, where 85% of patients admitted having a sexual problem and 22% of the problems were attributed to the partner.[226] A decrease in sexual activity with advancing age was considered to be normal,[227] but in a study of healthy men and women ranging in age from 80

TABLE 19–5. Sexual Dysfunction in Healthy Women with a Regular Partner

Author	Schover	Jensen	Frank et al.	Schover et al.	Osborn et al.
Reference	222	56	223	224	225
Year	1981	1981	1978	1987	1988
Number of patients	92	40	100	76	436
Mean age (y)	30	38	35	41	
Low sexual desire (%)	10	23	35	10	17
Low arousal (%)	14	24	48	10	50
Orgasmic difficulty					
Global (%)	9	7	15	4	
Situational (%)	18	30	33	26	
Total (%)	27	37	48	30	16
Dispareunia (%)	8	8		10	8

to 102, Bretschneider and McCoy[228] found considerable sexual activity in both sexes. Touching and caressing without coitus were reported by 64% of women, masturbation by 40%, and sexual intercourse by 30%. Bretschneider and McCoy comment that the principal decrease in sexual activity and enjoyment occurs during the postmenopausal years and that in healthy women, sexual interest and activity remain relatively constant after menopause, although coital opportunity and frequency decrease precipitously with age.

The Female Sexual Response Mechanism

The female response cycle consists of desire, arousal, plateau, orgasm, and resolution. The sexual response organs of the female are analogous to those of the male. Desire begins in both sexes in the brain, with perception of erotogenic stimuli. On arousal the clitoris, which is the embryonic analogue of the glans penis, becomes erect. The labia minora, which are analogous to the corpora cavernosa of the penis, become engorged. Blood flow in the entire vaginal vault triples. There is dilatation of the upper two thirds of the vagina as well as secretion of lubricant, followed by swelling and dilatation of the lower third during the orgasmic platform. The clitoris and vagina have dense somatosensory innervation and responsiveness. At orgasm, rhythmical vaginal smooth muscle and pelvic contractions occur. Women may experience multiple orgasms without a refractory period, although in some women orgasm requires intense vaginal and sometimes clitoral stimulation. Women have periodic nocturnal increases in vaginal pulse amplitude that are similar to NPT. The neurogenic elements supporting the female sexual response are similar to those for men, and some degree of dysfunction may follow pelvic or genital surgery.

Hormonal Control of Sexual Function

The role of hormones in influencing sexual function is of considerable practical as well as theoretical interest because women may receive nonphysiological amounts and proportions of estrogens and progestogens in oral contraceptives and in agents used as therapy for the postmenopausal state. They also frequently undergo surgery on fallopian tubes, uterus, and ovaries, with uncertain consequences for sexual behavior.

Estrogens, progestogens, and androgens influence sexual behavior in animals via central mechanisms. Responsiveness is a result of central nervous system–mediated autonomic nervous system signals. At least one LHRH subunit may regulate sexual behavior.[229] After somatosensory stimulation, orgasm is also an adrenergic response. Estrogens are responsible for the development and maintenance of the sexual tissues.

The menopause is associated with cessation of ovarian estrogen secretion (see Chapter 12). As a result of aromatization of adrenal precursors, many postmenopausal women continue to produce estrogen and have unchanged sexual behavior. A variable decrease in sexual behavior may characterize the perimenopausal period in other women.[225, 226] Estrogen replacement therapy appears to restore sexual desire and responsiveness in symptomatic postmenopausal women.[230]

As a result of studies with primates,[231] androgens have been proposed to be hormones of libido in women as in men. There are anecdotal reports of increased libido in women with breast cancer who are treated with large doses of androgens. However, women with the androgen excess (polycystic ovary) syndrome do not appear to have increased libido or altered sexual behavior.[232] Finally, in controlled trials, androgens do not seem to enhance the effects of estrogens in women with menopausal hyposexuality.[233, 234]

Types of Female Sexual Dysfunction

The four principal sexual dysfunctions in women are lack of interest, failure of arousal, anorgasmy, and dyspareunia. One important factor that has not been studied in "normal" populations is the effect of childhood sexual abuse and of rape on lifelong sexual behavior. With as many as 15 to 38% of girls being abused before the age of 18 and a high incidence of rape, mostly not reported,[235] such experiences could have a grave impact on lifelong sexual enjoyment. A study of 371 self-referred, previously assaulted women[236] indicated that 59% had remaining sexual problems, most of which were attributed to the assault(s). The extremely high prevalence of prior abuse in women with the

TABLE 19–6. Sexual Dysfunction in Women According to Age

Dysfunction	Ages 35–39	Ages 40–44	Ages 45–49	Ages 50–54	Ages 55–59	All Ages
			%			
Low sexual desire	4	8	6	29	28	17
Frequency of orgasm	5	8	14	22	35	16
Dyspareunia	0	1	9	17	17	8
Vaginal dryness	8	12	16	26	22	17
Any of above	14	19	32	51	48	33

unexplained pelvic pain syndrome[237] suggests that careful study of traumatic sexual experiences may shed light on the high prevalence of low desire and arousal reported for some populations (see Table 19–5). In women with regular menstrual cycles, sexuality does not seem to relate well to reproductive hormone levels,[238] and administration of either androgens or estrogens has little effect on sexuality.[239]

Relaxed vaginal outlet as a result of multiple vaginal deliveries is a common cause of reduced sexual enjoyment of both partners. The sexual symptoms are a feeling of "looseness" and a lack of feeling of penile containment. Treatment with Kegel exercises[240] designed to improve pelvic muscle tone is of dubious help.[241] In the presence of stress incontinence or uterine descensus, surgical correction may be indicated.

The impact of medical illness on sexual interest and arousal in women is difficult to assess because of the high prevalence of subjective disordered function in healthy women (see Table 19–6) and because of the difficulty of distinguishing between the effects of illness and the effects of drugs. Pelvic and breast neoplasms,[98, 242] multiple sclerosis,[243] uremia,[87] and myocardial infarction[244] cause a decrease in sexual activity. Pelvic surgery and ostomy placement also have the potential for serious impairment of sexual function,[245] but many such patients do quite well. The irritable bowel syndrome appears to be associated with more disordered sexual function than either inflammatory bowel disease or peptic ulcer disease.[246]

Diabetes mellitus in women results in far fewer sexual consequences than it does in men[247–250] and may have no effect,[56] perhaps because diabetic women have less atherosclerotic disease than diabetic men of comparable age. Arthritis[251] also has minimal sexual consequences, as does hysterectomy.[252] The consequences of hypertension and its therapy on the sexual function of women are not known.

A variety of gynecological disorders cause dyspareunia, including vaginitis resulting from infection with trichomonads, yeasts, and bacteria; pelvic infections; endometriosis; neoplasms; and postmenopausal atrophy of urogenital tissues. Other factors include infections of Skene or Bartholin glands, vulvitis, and hymenal obstruction. A similar syndrome may result from episiotomy scarring and postradiation vaginal atrophy.

There are reports of adverse effects of alpha- and beta-adrenergic inhibitors, narcotics, and mood-altering drugs on libido and orgasm in women.[27] Chronic alcoholism is associated with reduced sexual satisfaction,[253] and acute ethanol ingestion inhibits orgasmic function.[254]

Diagnostic Evaluation

A complete medical assessment should include a sensitive inquiry about sexual dysfunction. If the patient seeks help or gives a positive response to questioning, inquiry into the nature of the problem (interest, arousability, orgasm, or dyspareunia), its duration and progression, and the expectations of the patient regarding sexual activity and enjoyment should be initiated. Does the dysfunction represent a lifelong pattern or is it secondary to some event or illness? Is there general and sexual marital compatibility? Is there a history of sexual abuse? The medical evaluation should include detailing of medical illnesses and use of drugs, surgical interventions, and psychiatric background. The physical examination should include careful assessment of the pelvis, and abnormal findings must be pursued because sexual dysfunction may be a presenting complaint in serious conditions.

Endocrine diagnostic testing is unlikely to be of help in a woman with regular menstrual cycles, and all postmeno-

pausal women are hypogonadal. Perimenopausal hormone changes and abnormal or absent cycles warrant more study.

A variety of techniques have been used to measure sexual arousal in response to erotic stimuli or during sleep, including assessment of vaginal temperature or blood flow. Such techniques have not provided clinically useful information as yet because subjective arousal and objective arousal are not correlated and because the techniques have not been applied systematically to older women, in whom alterations may be expected to occur.[255]

Treatment

Treatment of sexual dysfunction in women requires evaluation of the couple and therapy for both members individually and together. Education of the couple about the basis of the problem and establishment of communication by the couple are of great help. Identified organic problems should be treated appropriately. Postmenopausal loss of desire and atrophy of urogenital tissues should be treated with estrogens and progestogens. Restoration of vaginal tissue integrity and of sexual interest may require several months and integrity may be incomplete. For women who cannot or will not take systemic estrogens, low-dose vaginal suppositories may be helpful for local symptoms. There seems to be little rationale for the use of androgens.

Sex therapy, as described earlier, may have some value for improving general sexual and marital satisfaction in women who have inhibited desire or arousal, but the results are not spectacular.[221] Ability to achieve orgasm by various means can also be helped in some women with a program of education and training in masturbation. Coital orgasm is less frequently achieved.[256]

CONCLUSION

Advances in understanding and appreciation of the importance of sexual dysfunction, insight into the pathophysiology of impotence, and development of new diagnostic tests and therapeutic alternatives have made it possible to enhance and/or restore an active sexual life for many dysfunctional couples. Alleviation of this emotionally and socially destructive problem can provide a more vital and satisfying life to couples of all ages.

REFERENCES

1. Masters WH, Johnson VE. Human Sexual Inadequacy. Boston: Little, Brown, 1970.
2. Davidson JM, Camargo CA, Smith ER. Effects of androgen on sexual behavior in hypogonadal men. J Clin Endocrinol Metab 1979; 48:955–958.
3. Salmimies P, Kockett G, Pirke KM, et al. Effects of testosterone replacement on sexual behavior in hypogonadal men. Arch Sex Behav 1982; 11:345–353.
4. Wein AJ, Van Arsdale KN. Drug-induced male sexual dysfunction. Urol Clin North Am 1988; 15:23–31.
5. Buffum J. Pharmacosexology: the effects of drugs on sexual function— a review. J Psychoactive Drugs 1982; 14:5–44.
6. Williams W. Anaesthetic ejaculation. J Sex Marital Ther 1985; 11:19–29.
7. Martin CE. Factor affecting sexual functioning in 60–79-year-old married males. Arch Sexual Behav 1981; 10:399–420.
8. Kinsey AC, Pomeroy WB, Martin CF. Sexual Behavior in the Human Male. Philadelphia: W. B. Saunders, 1948.
9. Finkle AL, Moyers TG, Tobenkin MI, et al. Sexual potency and aging males. JAMA 1959; 170:1391–1393.
10. Bowers LM, Cross RR Jr, Lloyd FA. Sexual function and urologic disease in the elderly male. J Am Geriatr Soc 1963; 11:647–652.
11. Newman HF, Marcus H. Erectile dysfunction in diabetes and hypertension. Urology 1985; 26:135–137.

12. Rubin A, Babbott D. Impotence and diabetes mellitus. JAMA 1959; 168:498–500.

13. Korenman SG, Morley JE, Mooradian AD, et al. Secondary hypogonadism in older men: its relation to impotence. J Clin Endocrinol Metab 1990; 71:963–969.

14. Lue TF, Zeinah SJ, Schmidt RA, et al. Neuroanatomy of penile erection: its relevance to iatrogenic impotence. J Urol 1984; 131:273–280.

15. Walsh P, Donker P. Impotence following radical prostatectomy: insight into etiology and prevention. J Urol 1982; 128:492–497.

16. Saenz de Tejada I, Goldstein I, Azadzoi K, et al. Impaired neurogenic and endothelium-mediated relaxation of penile smooth muscle from diabetic men with impotence. N Engl J Med 1989; 320:1025–1030.

17. Ignarro LJ, Bush PA, Buga JM, et al. Nitric oxide and cyclic GMP formation upon electric field stimulation cause relaxation of corpus cavernosum smooth muscle. Biochem Biophys Res Commun 1990; 170:843–850.

18. Lue TF, Tanagho EA. Physiology of erection and pharmacological management of impotence. J Urol 1987; 137:829–836.

19. Michal V. Arterial disease as a cause of impotence. Clin Endocrinol Metab 1982; 11:725–748.

20. Wagner G, Metz P. Arteriosclerosis and erectile failure. In: Wagner G, Green R, eds. Impotence. New York: Plenum, 1981:63–72.

21. Lue TF. The mechanism of penile erection in the monkey. Semin Urol 1986; 4:217–224.

22. Lue TF, Takamura T, Umraiya M, et al. Hemodynamics of canine corpora cavernosa during erection. Urology 1984; 24:347–352.

23. Aboseif SR, Lue TF. Hemodynamics of penile erection. Urol Clin North Am 1988; 15:1–7.

24. Lue TF, Hricak H, Schmidt RA, et al. Functional evaluation of penile veins by cavernosography in papaverine-induced erection. J Urol 1985; 134:479–482.

25. Fournier GR, Juenemann KP, Lue TF, et al. Mechanisms of venous occlusion during canine penile erection: an anatomic demonstration. J Urol 1987; 137:163–167.

26. Newman HF, Reiss H, Northrup JD. Physical basis of emission, ejaculation and orgasm in the male. Urology 1982; 19:341–350.

27. Drugs that cause sexual dysfunction. Med Lett 1987; 29:65–70.

28. Levine SB. Marital sexual dysfunction: ejaculation disturbances. Ann Intern Med 1976; 84:575–579.

29. Karacan I, Williams RL, Thornby JI, et al. Sleep-related tumescence as a function of age. Am J Psychiatry 1975; 132:932–937.

30. Kwan M, Greenleaf WJ, Mann J, et al. The nature of androgen action on male sexuality: a combined laboratory–self-report study on hypogonadal men. J Clin Endocrinol Metab 1983; 57:557–562.

31. Massry SG, Goldstein DA, Procci WR, et al. On the pathogenesis of sexual dysfunction of the uremic male. Proc Eur Dial Transplant Assoc 1980; 17:139–145.

32. Procci WR, Goldstein DA, Adelstein J, et al. Sexual dysfunction in the male patient with uremia: a reappraisal. Kidney Int 1981; 19:317–323.

33. Kidd GS, Glass AR, Vigersky RA. The hypothalamic-pituitary-testicular axis in thyrotoxicosis. J Clin Endocrinol Metab 1979; 48:798–802.

34. Kaiser FE, Korenman SG. Impotence in diabetic men. Am J Med 1988; 85:147–152.

35. Virag R, Bouilly P, Frydman D. Is impotence an arterial disorder? Lancet 1985; 1:181–184.

36. Davis SS, Viosca S, Guralnik M, et al. Evaluation of impotence in older men. West J Med 1985; 142:499–505.

37. Slag MF, Morley JE, Elson MK, et al. Impotence in medical clinic outpatients. JAMA 1983; 249:1736–1740.

38. Kaiser FE, Viosca SP, Morley JE, et al. Impotence and aging: clinical and hormonal factors. J Am Geriatr Soc 1988; 36:511–519.

39. McCulloch K, Young RJ, Prescott RJ, et al. The natural history of impotence in diabetic men. Diabetologia 1984; 26:437–440.

40. Herman A, Adar R, Rubinstein Z. Vascular lesions associated with impotence in diabetic and nondiabetic arterial occlusive disease. Diabetes 1978; 27:975–981.

41. Lehman TP, Jacobs JA. Etiology of diabetic impotence. J Urol 1983; 129:291–294.

42. Jevtich MJ, Edson M, Jarmon WD, et al. Vascular factor in erectile failure among diabetics. Urology 1982; 19:163–168.

43. Metz P. Erectile function in men with occlusive disease in the legs. Dan Med Bull 1983; 30:185–189.

44. Dewar ML, Blundell PE, Lidstone D, et al. Effects of abdominal aneurysmectomy, aortoiliac bypass grafting and angioplasty on male sexual potency: a prospective study. Can J Surg 1985; 28:154–159.

45. Forsberg L, Olsson AM, Neglen P. Erectile function before and after aortoiliac reconstruction: a comparison between measurements of Doppler acceleration ratio, blood pressure and angiography. J Urol 1982; 127:379–382.

46. Queral L, Whitehouse W, Flinn W, et al. Pelvic hemodynamics after aortoiliac reconstruction. Surgery 1979; 86:799–809.

47. Morley JE, Korenman SG, Kaiser FE, et al. Relationship of penile brachial pressure index to myocardial infarction and cerebrovascular accidents in older men. Am J Med 1988; 84:445–448.

48. Korenman SG, Udhoji V, Morley JE, et al. Cardiovascular stress test in patients with vascular impotence. Clin Res 1989; 37:519A (abstract).

49. Wabrek AJ, Burchell RC. Male sexual dysfunction associated with coronary heart disease. Arch Sex Behav 1980; 9:69–75.

50. Dhabuwala CB, Kumar A, Pierce JM. Myocardial infarction and its influence on male sexual function. Arch Sex Behav 1986; 15:499–504.

51. Bloch A, Maeder JP, Haissly JC. Sexual problems after myocardial infarction. Am Heart J 1975; 90:536–537.

52. Hellerstein HK, Friedman EH. Sexual activity and the post-coronary patient. Arch Intern Med 1970; 125:987–999.

53. Schöffling K, Federlin K, Ditschuneit H, et al. Disorders of sexual function in male diabetics. J Am Diabetes Assoc 1963; 12:519–527.

54. Ellenberg M. Impotence in diabetes: the neurological factor. Ann Intern Med 1971; 75:213–219.

55. Kolodny RC, Kahn CB, Goldstein HH, et al. Sexual dysfunction in diabetic men. Diabetes 1974; 23:306–309.

56. Jensen SB. Diabetic sexual dysfunction: a comparative study of 160 insulin treated diabetic men and women and an age-matched control group. Arch Sex Behav 1981; 10:493–504.

57. Palmer JDK, Fink S, Burger RH. Diabetic secondary impotence: neuropathic factor as measured by peripheral motor nerve conduction. Urology 1986; 28:197–200.

58. Nathan D, Singer D, Godine J, et al. Non–insulin-dependent diabetes in older patients: complications and risk factors. Am J Med 1986; 81:837–842.

59. Faerman I, Vilar O, Rivarola MA, et al. Impotence and diabetes: studies of androgenic function in diabetic impotent males. Diabetes 1972; 21:23–30.

60. Schiavi RC, Fisher C, Quadland M, et al. Nocturnal penile tumescent evaluation of erectile function in insulin-dependent diabetic men. Diabetologia 1985; 28:90–94.

61. Hosking DJ, Bennet T, Hampton JR, et al. Diabetic impotence: studies of nocturnal erections during REM sleep. Br Med J 1979; 2:1394–1396.

62. Zeidler A, Gelfand R, Tamagna E, et al. Pituitary gonadal function in diabetic male patients with and without impotence. Andrologia 1982; 14:62–68.

63. Ficher M, Zuckerman M, Fishkin R, et al. Do endocrines play an etiological role in diabetic and nondiabetic sexual dysfunctions? J Androl 1984; 5:8–16.

64. Maatman T, Montague D, Martin L. Erectile dysfunction in men with diabetes mellitus. Urology 1987; 29:589–592.

65. Cameron D, Murray F, Drylie D. Interstitial compartment pathology and spermatogenic disruption in testes from impotent diabetic men. Anat Rec 1985; 213:53–62.

66. Murray FT, Wyss HU, Thomas RG, et al. Gonadal dysfunction in diabetic men with organic impotence. J Clin Endocrinol Metab 1987; 65:127–135.

67. Mehta AJ, Viosca SP, Korenman SG, et al. Peripheral nerve conduction studies and bulbocavernosus reflex in the investigation of impotence. Arch Phys Med Rehabil 1986; 67:332–335.

68. Bulpitt CJ, Dollery CT. Side effects of hypotensive agents evaluated by a self-administered questionnaire. Br Med J 1973; 3:485–490.

69. Moss HB, Procci WR. Sexual dysfunction associated with oral antihypertensive medications: a critical survey of the literature. Gen Hosp Psychiatry 1982; 4:121–129.

70. Bauer GE, Baker J, Hunyor SN, et al. Side-effects of antihypertensive treatment: a placebo-controlled study. Clin Sci Mol Med 1978; 55:341–344.

71. Lue TF, Hricak H, Marich KW, et al. Vasculogenic impotence evaluated by high resolution ultrasonography and pulsed Doppler spectrum analysis. Radiology 1985; 155:778–782.

72. Levy NB, Wynbrandt GD. The quality of life on maintenance hemodialysis. Lancet 1975; 1:1328–1331.

73. Abram HS, Hester LR, Sheridan WF, et al. Sexual functioning in patients with chronic renal failure. J Nerv Ment Dis 1975; 160:220–226.

74. Levy NB. Sexual adjustment to maintenance hemodialysis and renal transplantation. National survey by questionnaire: preliminary report. Trans Am Soc Artif Intern Organs 1973; 19:138–143.

75. Rodger RCS, Fletcher K, Dewar J, et al. Prevalence and pathogenesis of impotence in one hundred uremic men. Uremia Invest 1984–85; 8:89–96.

76. Nghiem D, Corry R, Picon-Mendez G, et al. Factors influencing male sexual impotence after renal transplantation. Urology 1983; 21:49–52.

77. Procci WR, Martin DJ. Effect of maintenance hemodialysis on male sexual performance. J Nerv Ment Dis 1985; 173:366–372.

78. Weizman R, Weizman A, Levi J, et al. Sexual dysfunction associated with hyperprolactinemia in males and females undergoing hemodialysis. Psychosom Med 1983; 45:259–269.

79. Foulks CJ, Cushner HM. Sexual dysfunction in the male dialysis patient: pathogenesis, evaluation and therapy. Am J Kidney Dis 1986; 8:211–222.

80. Ramirez G, O'Neill WM Jr, Bloomer HA, et al. Abnormalities in the regulation of prolactin in patients with chronic renal failure. J Clin Endocrinol Metab 1977; 45:658–661.

81. Sievertsen GD, Lim VS, Nakawatase C, et al. Metabolic clearance and secretion rates of human prolactin in normal subjects and in patients with chronic renal failure. J Clin Endocrinol Metab 1980; 50:846–852.

82. Antoniou LD, Shalhoub RJ, Sudhakar T, et al. Reversal of uraemic impotence by zinc. Lancet 1977; 2:895–898.

83. Campese VM, Procci WR, Levitan D, et al. Autonomic nervous system dysfunction and impotence in uremia. Am J Nephrol 1982; 2:140–143.

84. Bommer J, Ritz E, del Pozo E, et al. Improved sexual function in male haemodialysis patients on bromocriptine. Lancet 1979; 2:496–497.

85. Muir JW, Besser GM, Edwards CRW, et al. Bromocriptine improves reduced libido and potency in men receiving maintenance hemodialysis. Clin Nephrol 1983; 20:308–314.

86. Lim VS, Fang VS. Restoration of plasma testosterone levels in uremic men with clomiphene citrate. J Clin Endocrinol Metab 1976; 43:1370–1377.

87. Schaefer RM, Kokot F, Wernze H, et al. Improved sexual function in hemodialysis patients on recombinant erythropoietin: a possible role for prolactin. Clin Nephrol 1989; 31:1–5.

88. Valleroy ML, Kraft GH. Sexual dysfunction in multiple sclerosis. Arch Phys Med Rehabil 1984; 65:125–128.

89. Herzog A, Seibel M, Schomer D, et al. Reproductive endocrine disorders in men with partial seizures of temporal lobe origin. Arch Neurol 1986; 43:347–350.

90. Hierons R, Saunders M. Impotence in patients with temporal-lobe lesions. Lancet 1966; 2:761–763.

91. Kalliomaki JL, Markkanen TK, Mustonen VA. Sexual behavior after cerebral vascular accident. Fertil Steril 1961; 12:156–158.

92. Sjogren K, Damber J-E, Liliequist B. Sexuality after stroke with hemiplegia: aspects of sexual function. Scand J Rehabil Med 1983; 15:55–61.

93. Melman A. Iatrogenic causes of erectile dysfunction. Urol Clin North Am 1988; 15:33–39.

94. Bremer J. Asexualization: A Follow-up Study of 244 Cases. Oslo, Norway: Oslo University Press, 1958.

95. Tenover JS, Matsumoto AM, Plymate SR, et al. The effects of aging in normal men on bioavailable testosterone and luteinizing hormone secretion: response to clomiphene citrate. J Clin Endocrinol Metab 1987; 65:1118–1126.

96. Nankin HR, Calkins JM. Decreased bioavailable testosterone in aging normal and impotent men. J Clin Endocrinol Metab 1986; 63:1418–1420.

97. Fabbri A, Jannini EA, Ulsse S, et al. Low serum bioactive luteinizing hormone in nonorganic male impotence: possible relationship with altered gonadotropin-releasing hormone pulsatility. J Clin Endocrinol Metab 1988; 67:867–875.

98. Deslypere JP, Vermeulen A. Influence of age on steroid concentrations in skin and striated muscle in women and in cardiac muscle and lung tissue in men. J Clin Endocrinol Metab 1985; 61:648–653.

99. Schover LR, Evans RB, von Eschenbach AC. Sexual rehabilitation in a cancer center: diagnosis and outcome in 384 consultations. Arch Sex Behav 1987; 16:445–461.

100. Anderson BL. Sexual functioning morbidity among cancer survivors. Cancer 1985; 55:1835–1842.

101. Pontes JE, Huben R, Wolf R. Sexual function after radical prostatectomy. Prostate 1986; 8:123–126.

102. Walsh PC, Mostwin JL. Radical prostatectomy and cystoprostatectomy with preservation of potency: results using a new nerve-sparing technique. Br J Urol 1984; 56:694–697.

103. Walsh PC, Schlegl PN. Radical pelvic surgery with preservation of sexual function. Ann Surg 1988; 208:391–400.

104. Surya BV, Provet S, Dalbogni G, et al. Experience with potency preservation during radical prostatectomy. Urology 1988; 32:498–501.

105. Bruskewitz RC, Larsen EH, Madsen PO, et al. 3-year followup of urinary symptoms after transurethral resection of the prostate. J Urol 1986; 136:613–615.

106. Gilling PJ, Wright WL, Gray JM. Factors associated with sexual dysfunction following transurethral resection of the prostate. NZ Med J 1988; 101:484–485.

107. Fegiz G, Trenti A, Bezzi M, et al. Sexual and bladder dysfunction following surgery for rectal carcinoma. Ital J Surg Sci 1986; 16:103–109.

108. Kinn A, Oman U. Bladder and sexual function after surgery for rectal cancer. Dis Colon Rectum 1986; 29:43–48.

109. Goldstein I, Feldman MI, Deckers PJ, et al. Radiation-associated impotence: a clinical study of its mechanism. JAMA 1984; 25:903–910.

110. Sjogren K, Fugl-Meyer AR. Chronic back pain and sexuality: sexuality and disablement. Int Rehabil Med 1981; 3:19–25.

111. Maruta T, Osborne D, Swanson DW, et al. Chronic pain patients and spouses, marital and sexual adjustment. Mayo Clin Proc 1981; 56:307–310.

112. Fletcher E, Martin R. Sexual dysfunction and erectile impotence in chronic obstructive pulmonary disease. Chest 1982; 81:413–421.

113. Semple PDA, Beastall GH, Brown TM, et al. Sex hormone suppression and sexual impotence in hypoxic pulmonary fibrosis. Thorax 1984; 39:46–51.

114. Farthing MJG, Edwards CRW, Rees L, et al. Male gonadal function in coeliac disease: sexual dysfunction, infertility, and semen quality. Gut 1982; 23:608–614.

115. Todd RC, Lightowler CDR, Harris J. Low friction arthroplasty of the hip and sexual activity. Acta Orthop Scand 1973; 44:690–693.

116. Currey HLF. Osteoarthritis of the hip joint and sexual activity. Ann Rheum Dis 1970; 29:488–493.

117. Lally E, Jimenez S. Impotence in progressive systemic sclerosis. Ann Intern Med 1981; 95:150–153.

118. Nowlin NS, Brick JE, Weaver DJ, et al. Impotence in scleroderma. Ann Intern Med 1986; 104:794–798.

119. Stremmel W, Niederau C, Berger M, et al. Abnormalities in estrogen, androgen, and insulin metabolism in idiopathic hemochromatosis. Ann NY Acad Sci 1988; 526:209–223.

120. Franks S, Jacobs HS, Martin N, et al. Hyperprolactinemia and impotence. Clin Endocrinol 1978; 8:277–287.

121. Cocores JA, Miller NS, Pottash AC, et al. Sexual dysfunction in abusers of cocaine and alcohol. Am J Drug Alcohol Abuse 1988; 14:169–173.

122. Fahrner EM. Sexual dysfunction in male alcohol addicts: prevalence and treatment. Arch Sex Behav 1987; 16:247–257.

123. Jensen SB. Sexual function and dysfunction in younger married alcoholics. Acta Psychiatr Scand 1984; 69:543–549.

124. Van Thiel DH, Gavaler JS. Hypothalamic-pituitary-gonadal function in liver disease with particular attention to the endocrine effects of chronic alcohol abuse. Prog Liver Dis 1986; 8:273–282.

125. Van Thiel DH, Gavaler JS, Sanghvi A. Recovery of sexual function in abstinent alcoholic men. Gastroenterology 1982; 84:677–682.

126. Christensen JK, Rønsted P, Vaag UH. Side effects after disulfiram. Comparison of disulfiram and placebo in a double-blind multicentre study. Acta Psychiatr Scand 1984; 69:265–273.

127. Snyder S, Karacan I, Salis PJ. Disulfiram and nocturnal penile tumescence in the chronic alcoholic. Biol Psychiatry 1981; 16:399–406.

128. Condra M, Surridge DH, Morales A, et al. Prevalence and significance of tobacco smoking in impotence. Urology 1986; 27:495–498.

129. Bornman MS, du Plessis DJ. Smoking and vascular impotence. A reason for concern. S Afr Med J 1986; 70:329–330.

130. Forsberg L, Gustavii B, Höjerback T, et al. Impotence, smoking, and β-blocking drugs. Fertil Steril 1979; 31:589–591.

131. Juenemann K, Lue TF, Luo J, et al. The effect of cigarette smoking on penile erection. J Urol 1987; 138:438–441.

132. Impotence Study Group of Western Australia. The diagnosis and treatment of impotence. Med J Aust 1988; 16:494–498.

133. Jeffcoate WJ. Impotence: science and sciencibility. Br Med J 1986; 292:783–784.

134. Schover LR, Jenson SB. Sexuality and Chronic Illness. New York: Guilford, 1988.

135. Rajfer J, Rosciszewski A, Mehringer M. Prevalence of corporeal venous leakage in impotent men. J Urol 1988; 140:69–71.

136. Condra M, Morales A, Surridge DH, et al. The unreliability of nocturnal penile tumescence as an outcome measurement in the treatment of organic impotence. J Urol 1986; 135:280–282.

137. Bertini J, Boileau MA. Evaluation of nocturnal penile tumescence with Potentest. Urology 1986; 27:492–494.

138. Marshall P, Morales A, Surridge D. Unreliability of nocturnal penile tumescence recording and MMPI profiles in assessment of impotence. Urology 1982; 17:1369.

139. Verhulst J, Schneidman B. Schizophrenia and sexual functioning. Hosp Community Psychiatry 1981; 34:259–262.

140. Matthew RJ, Weinman ML. Sexual dysfunctions in depression. Arch Sex Behav 1982; 11:323–328.

141. Finkle AL, Jackson S. Urology/sexuality clinic: results of counseling of 67 men. West J Med 1982; 137:95–98.

142. Anders EK, Bradley WE, Krane RJ. Nocturnal penile rigidity measured by the Snap Gauge band. J Urol 1983; 130:964–966.

143. Pressman MR, DiPhillipo MA, Kendrick JI, et al. Problems in the interpretation of nocturnal penile tumescence studies: disruption of sleep by occult sleep disorders. J Urol 1986; 136:595–598.

144. Schiavi RC, Schreiner-Engel P. Nocturnal penile tumescence in healthy aging men. J Gerontol 1988; 43:146–150.

145. Gaskell P. The importance of penile blood pressure in cases of impotence. Can Med Assoc 1971; 105:1047–1051.

146. Abelson D. Diagnostic value of the penile pulse and blood pressure: a Doppler study of impotence in diabetics. J Urol 1975; 113:636–639.

147. Metz P, Christensen J, Mathiesen FR, et al. Ultrasonic Doppler pulse wave analysis versus penile blood pressure measurement in the evaluation of arteriogenic impotence. Vasa 1983; 12:363–366.

148. Goldstein I, Siroky MB, Nath RL, et al. Vasculogenic impotence: role of the pelvic steal test. J Urol 1982; 128:300–306.

149. Metz P, Bengtsson J. Penile blood pressure. Scand J Urol Nephrol 1981; 15:161–164.

150. Chiu RCJ, Lidstone D, Blundell PE. Predictive power of penile/brachial index in diagnosing male sexual impotence. J Vasc Surg 1986; 4:251–256.

151. Metz P, Vestergard AS, Brunner S. Arteriographic findings and erectile function in men with occlusive arterial disease in the legs. Eur J Radiol 1982; 2:109–112.

152. Mueller SC, Lue TF. Evaluation of vasculogenic impotence. Urol Clin North Am 1988; 15:65–76.

153. Forsberg L, Olsson AM, Neglen P. Erectile function before and after aortoiliac reconstruction: a comparison between measurements of Doppler acceleration ratio, blood pressure and angiography. J Urol 1982; 127:379–382.

154. Virag R, Frydman D, Legman M, et al. Intracavernous injection of papaverine as a diagnostic and therapeutic method in erectile failure. Angiology 1984; 35:79–87.

155. Buvat J, Lemaire A, Buvat-Herbaut M, et al. Is intracavernous injection of papaverine a reliable screening test for vascular impotence? J Urol 1986; 135:476–479.

156. Bookstein JJ, Valji K, Parsons L, et al. Pharmacoarteriography in the evaluation of impotence. J Urol 1987; 137:333–337.

157. Stief CG, Diederichs W, Benard F, et al. The diagnosis of venogenic impotence: dynamic or pharmacologic cavernosometry? J Urol 1988; 140:1561–1563.

158. Jantos C, Weidner W. Pharmacocavernosography in the evaluation of erectile failure. Urol Int 1988; 43:225–230.

159. Desai KM, Gingell JC. Saline-induced artificial erection without papaverine: a potential source of error in diagnosing cavernosal venous leakage. Br J Urol 1988; 62:176–178.

160. Stackl W, Hasun R, Marberger M. Intracavernous injection of prostaglandin E_1 in impotent men. J Urol 1988; 140:66–68.

161. Waldhauser M, Schramek P. Efficiency and side effects of prostaglandin E_1 in the treatment of erectile dysfunction. J Urol 1988; 140:525–527.

162. Porst H. Value of prostaglandin E_1 in the diagnosis of erectile dysfunction in comparison with papaverine and papaverine/phentolamine in 61 patients with erectile dysfunction. Urologe [A] 1988; 27:22–26.

163. Glina S, Reichelt AC, Leao PP, et al. Impact of cigarette smoking on papaverine-induced erection. J Urol 1988; 140:523–524.

164. Abber JC, Lue TF, Orvis BR, et al. Diagnostic tests for impotence: a comparison of papaverine injection with the penile-brachial index and nocturnal penile tumescence monitoring. J Urol 1986; 135:923–925.

165. Schwartz AN, Freidenberg D, Harley JD. Nonselective angiography after intracorporeal papaverine injection: an alternative technique for evaluating penile arterial integrity. Radiology 1988; 167:249–253.

166. Stief CG, Gall H, Scherb W, et al. Erectile dysfunction due to ectopic penile vein. Urology 1988; 31:300–303.

167. Buvat J, Lemaire A, Dehaene JL, et al. Venous incompetence: critical study of the organic basis of high maintenance flow rates during artificial erection test. J Urol 1986; 135:926–928.

168. Lin JT, Bradley WE. Penile neuropathy in insulin-dependent diabetes mellitus. J Urol 1985; 133:213–215.

169. Porst H, Tackmann W, van Ahlen H. Neurophysiological investigations in potent and impotent men: assessment of bulbocavernosus reflex latencies and somatosensory evoked potentials. Br J Urol 1988; 61:445–450.

170. Zorgniotti AW, Lefleur R. Auto-injection of the corpus cavernosum with a vasoactive drug combination for vasculogenic impotence. J Urol 1985; 133:39–41.

171. Watters GR, Keogh EJ, Earle CM, et al. Experience in the management of erectile dysfunction using the intracavernosal self-injection of vasoactive drugs. J Urol 1988; 140:1417–1419.

172. Kursh ED, Bodner DR, Resnick MI, et al. Injection therapy for impotence. Urol Clin North Am 1988; 15:625–629.

173. Klinge E, Huttunen MO. Pharmacological causes of disturbances in sexual activity. Duodecim 1988; 104:1157–1168.

174. Corriere JN Jr, Fishman IJ, Benson GS, et al. Development of fibrotic penile lesions secondary to the intracorporeal injection of vasoactive agents. J Urol 1988; 140:615–617.

175. Watters GR, Keogh EJ, Carati CJ, et al. Prolonged erections following intracorporeal injection of medications to overcome impotence. Br J Urol 1988; 62:173–175.

176. Sidi AA, Reddy PK, Chen KK. Patient acceptance of and satisfaction with vasoactive intracavernous pharmacotherapy for impotence. J Urol 1988; 140:293–294.

177. Puppo P, de Rose AF, Pittaluga P, et al. Penile-brachial pressure index as a guide for the dosage of intracavernous injection of papaverine. Eur Urol 1988; 14:210–213.

178. Stief CG, Gall H, Scherb W, et al. Mid-term results of autoinjection therapy for erectile dysfunction. Urology 1988; 31:483–485.

179. Dennis RL, McDougal WS. Pharmacological treatment of erectile dysfunction after radical prostatectomy. J Urol 1988; 139:775–776.

180. Wespes E, Schulman CC. Systemic complication of intracavernous papaverine injection in patients with venous leakage. Urology 1988; 31:114–115.

181. Ami Sidi A, Lange PH. Recent advances in the diagnosis and management of impotence. Urol Clin North Am 1986; 13:489–500.

182. Girdley FM, Bruskewitz RC, Feyzi J, et al. Intracavernous self-injection for impotence: a long-term therapeutic option? Experience in 78 patients. J Urol 1988; 140:972–974.

183. Corriere JN, Fishman IJ, Benson GS, et al. Development of fibrotic penile lesions secondary to the intracorporeal injection of vasoactive agents. J Urol 1988; 140:615–617.

184. Larsen EH, Gasser TC, Bruskewitz RC. Fibrosis of corpus cavernosum after intracavernous injection of phentolamine/papaverine. J Urol 1987; 137:292–293.

185. Mooradian A, Morley JE, Kaiser FE, et al. Biweekly intracavernosal administration of papaverine for erectile dysfunction. West J Med 1989; 151:515–517.

186. Lewis RW. Venous surgery for impotence. Urol Clin North Am 1988; 15:115–121.

187. Bennett AH. Venous arterialization for erectile impotence. Urol Clin North Am 1988; 15:111–113.

188. Krane RJ. Penile prosthesis. Urol Clin North Am 1988; 15:103–109.

189. Kabalin JN, Kessler R. Five-year follow-up of the Scott inflatable penile prosthesis and comparison with semirigid penile prosthesis. J Urol 1988; 140:1428–1430.

190. Merrill DC. Clinical experience with the Mentor inflatable penile prosthesis in 301 patients. J Urol 1988; 140:1424–1427.

191. Mulcahy JJ. The Hydroflex self-contained inflatable prosthesis: experience with 100 patients. J Urol 1988; 140:1422–1423.

192. Goetz A, Yu VL, O'Donnell WF. Surgical complications related to insertion of penile prostheses with emphasis on infection and cost. Infect Control Hosp Epidemiol 1988; 9:250–254.

193. Scarzella GI. Cylinder reliability of inflatable penile prosthesis. Experience with distensible and nondistensible cylinders in 325 patients. Urology 1988; 31:486–489.

194. Pedersen B, Tiefer L, Ruiz M, et al. Evaluation of patients and partners 1 to 4 years after penile prosthesis surgery. J Urol 1988; 139:956–958.

195. Kabalin JN, Kessler R. Infectious complications of penile prosthesis surgery. J Urol 1988; 139:953–955.

196. Wilson SK, Wahman GE, Lange JL. Eleven years of experience with the inflatable penile prosthesis. J Urol 1988; 139:951–952.

197. Stanisic TH, Dean JC, Donovan JM, et al. Clinical experience with a self-contained inflatable penile implant: the Flexi-Flate. J Urol 1988; 139:947–950.

198. Furlow WL, Motley RC. The inflatable penile prosthesis: clinical experience with a new controlled expansion cylinder. J Urol 1988; 139:945–946.

199. Furlow WL, Goldwasser B, Gundian JC. Implantation of model AMS 700 penile prosthesis: long-term results. J Urol 1988; 139:741–742.

200. Brooks MB. 42 months of experience with the Mentor inflatable penile prosthesis. J Urol 1988; 139:48–49.

201. Wiles PG. Successful non-invasive management of erectile impotence in diabetic men. Br Med J 1988; 296:161–162.

202. Korenman SG, Viosca SP, Kaiser FE, et al. Use of a vacuum tumescence device in the management of impotence. J Am Geriatr Soc 1990; 38:217–220.

203. Witherington R. Suction device therapy in the management of erectile impotence. Urol Clin North Am 1988; 15:123–128.

204. Marmar JL, DeBenedictis, Praiss DE. The use of a vacuum constrictor device to augment a partial erection following an intravenous injection. J Urol 1988; 140:975–979.

205. Cooper AJ. Preliminary experience with a vacuum constriction device (VCD) as a treatment for impotence. J Psychosom Res 1987; 31:413–418.

206. Miller WW. Afrodex in the treatment of male impotence: a double-blind crossover study. Curr Ther Res 1968; 10:354–360.

207. Sobotka JJ. An evaluation of Afrodex in the management of male impotency: a double-blind crossover study. Curr Ther Res 1969; 11:87–94.

208. Roberts CD, Sloboda W. Afrodex vs placebo in the treatment of male impotence: statistical analysis of two double-blind crossover studies. Curr Ther Res 1974; 16:96–100.

209. O'Carrol R, Bancroft J. Testosterone therapy for low sexual interest and erectile dysfunction in men: a controlled study. Br J Psychiatry 1984; 145:146–151.

210. Benkert O, Witt W, Adam W, et al. Effects of testosterone undecanoate on sexual potency and the hypothalamic-pituitary-gonadal axis of impotent males. Arch Sex Behav 1979; 8:471–479.

211. Ambrosi B, Bara R, Travaglini P, et al. Study of the effects of bromocriptine on sexual impotence. Clin Endocrinol 1977; 7:417–421.

212. Cooper A, Ismail AAA, Harding T, et al. The effects of clomiphene in impotence: a clinical and endocrine study. Br J Psychiatry 1972; 120:327–330.

213. Davies T, Mountjoy C, Gomez-Pan A, et al. A double-blind cross over trial of gonadotrophin releasing hormone (LHRH) in sexually impotent men. Clin Endocrinol 1976; 5:601–607.

214. Davies T, Gomez-Pan A, Watson M, et al. Reduced gonadotropin response to releasing hormone after chronic administration to impotent men. Clin Endocrinol 1977; 6:213–218.

215. Ambrosi B, Travaglini P, Gaggini M, et al. Effects of serotonin antagonists in sexually impotent men. Andrologia 1979; 11:475–477.

216. Morales A, Surridge DHC, Marshall PG, et al. Nonhormonal pharmacological treatment of organic impotence. J Urol 1982; 128:45–47.

217. Morales A, Condra MS, Owen JE, et al. Oral and transcutaneous pharmacologic agents in the treatment of impotence. Urol Clin North Am 1988; 15:87–93.

218. Korenman SG, Viosca S, Guralnik M, et al. Androgen therapy of hypogonadal men with transscrotal testosterone systems. Am J Med 1987; 83:471–478.

219. Zilbergeld B. Alternatives to couples counseling for sex problems: group and individual therapy. J Sex Marital Ther 1980; 6:3–18.
220. LoPiccolo JL, Heiman JR, Hogan DR, et al. Effectiveness of single therapists versus cotherapy teams in sex therapy. J Consult Clin Psychol 1985; 53:287–294.
221. De Amicis LA, Goldberg DC, LoPiccolo J, et al. Three-year follow-up of couples evaluated for sexual dysfunction. J Sex Marital Ther 1984; 10:215–227.
222. Schover LR. Male and female therapists' responses to male and female client sexual material: an analogue study. Arch Sex Behav 1981; 10:477–491.
223. Frank E, Anderson C, Rubinstein D. Frequency of sexual dysfunction in "normal couples." N Engl J Med 1978; 299:111–115.
224. Schover LR, Evans RB, von Eschenbach AC. Sexual rehabilitation in a cancer center: diagnosis and outcome in 384 cases. Arch Sex Behav 1987; 16:445–461.
225. Osborn M, Hawton K, Gath D. Sexual dysfunction among middle aged women in the community. Br Med J 1988; 296:959–962.
226. Sarrell P, Whitehead MI. Sex and menopause: defining the issues. Maturitas 1985; 7:217–224.
227. Pfeiffer E, Davis GC. Determinants of sexual behavior in middle and old age. J Am Geriatr Soc 1972; 20:151–158.
228. Bretschneider JG, McCoy NL. Sexual interest and behavior in healthy 80–102 year olds. Arch Sex Behav 1988; 17:109–129.
229. Dudley CA, Moss RL. Facilitation of lordosis behavior in female rats by CNS-site specific infusions of an LH-RH fragment, Ac-LH-RH-(5-10). Brain Res 1988; 441:161–167.
230. Dennerstein L, Burrows GD, Wood C, et al. Hormones and sexuality: effect of estrogen and progestogen. Obstet Gynecol 1980; 56:316–322.
231. Herbert J. The neuroendocrine basis of sexual behavior in primates. In Money J, Musaph H, eds. Handbook of Sexology. Amsterdam: Elsevier/North-Holland, 1978: 449–457.
232. Raboch J, Kobilková J, Raboch J, et al. Sexual life of women with the Stein-Leventhal syndrome. Arch Sex Behav 1985; 14:263–270.
233. Mathews A, Whitehead A, Kellett J. Psychological and hormonal factors in the treatment of female sexual dysfunction. Psychol Med 1983; 13:83–92.
234. Dow MGT, Hart DM, Forrest CA. Hormonal treatments of sexual unresponsiveness in postmenopausal women: a comparative study. Br J Obstet Gynaecol 1983; 90:361–366.
235. Bachmann GA, Moeller TP, Benett J. Childhood sexual abuse and the consequences in adult women. Obstet Gynecol 1988; 71:631–642.
236. Becker JV, Skinner LJ, Abel GG, et al. Sexual problems of sexual assault survivors. Women Health 1984; 9:5–20.
237. Walker E, Katon W, Harrop-Griffiths J, et al. Relationship of chronic pelvic pain to psychiatric diagnoses and childhood sexual abuse. Am J Psychiatry 1988; 145:75–80.
238. Bancroft J. Hormones and human sexual behavior. J Sex Marital Ther 1984; 10:3–21.
239. Sanders D, Bancroft J. Hormones and the sexuality of women—the menstrual cycle. Clin Endocrinol Metab 1982; 11:639–657.
240. Kegel A. Sexual functions of the pubococcygeus muscle. West J Surg 1952; 60:521–524.
241. Freese MP, Levitt EE. Relationships among intravaginal pressure, orgasmic function, parity factors and urinary leakage. Arch Sex Behav 1984; 13:261–268.
242. Anderson BL, Lachenbruch PA, Anderson B, et al. Sexual dysfunction and signs of gynecologic cancer. Cancer 1986; 57:1880–1886.
243. Minderhoud JM, Leemhuis JG, Kremer J, et al. Sexual disturbances arising from multiple sclerosis. Acta Neurol Scand 1984; 70:299–306.
244. Papadopoulos C, Beaumont C, Shelley SI, et al. Myocardial infarction and sexual activity of the female patient. Arch Intern Med 1983; 143:1528–1530.
245. Neale K, Phillips R. Living with a stoma. Br Med J 1988; 297:310–311.
246. Guthrie E, Creed FH. Severe sexual dysfunction in women with the irritable bowel syndrome: comparison with inflammatory bowel disease and duodenal ulceration. Br Med J 1987; 295:577–578.
247. Kolodny RC. Sexual dysfunction in diabetic females. Diabetes 1971; 20:557–559.
248. Ellenberg M. Sexual aspects of the female diabetic. Mt Sinai J Med 1977; 44:495–500.
249. Newman AS, Bertelson AD. Sexual dysfunction in the diabetic woman. J Behav Med 1986; 9:261–270.
250. Schreiner-Engel P, Schiavi RC, Vietorisz D, et al. The differential impact of diabetes type on female sexuality. J Psychosom Res 1987; 31:23–33.
251. Blake DJ, Maisaik R, Koplan A, et al. Sexual dysfunction among subjects with arthritis. Clin Rheumatol 1988; 7:50–60.
252. Coppen A, Bishop M, Beard RJ, et al. Hysterectomy, hormones, and behaviour. A prospective study. Lancet 1981; 1:126–128.
253. Peterson JS, Hartsock N, Lawson G. Sexual dissatisfaction of female alcoholics. Psychol Rep 1984; 55:744–746.
254. Malatesta VJ, Pollack RH, Crotty TD, et al. Acute alcohol intoxication and female orgasmic response. J Sex Res 1982; 18:1–17.
255. Rogers GS, Van de Castle RL, Evans WS, et al. Vaginal pulse amplitude response patterns during erotic conditions and sleep. Arch Sex Behav 1985; 14:327–342.
256. LoPiccolo J, Stock WE. Treatment of sexual dysfunction. J Consult Clin Psychol 1986; 54:158–167.

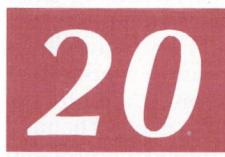

ENDOCRINOLOGY OF FETAL DEVELOPMENT

Delbert A. Fisher

INTRODUCTION

Endocrine systems are involved in virtually every aspect of pregnancy, including implantation, placentation, maternal adaptation, embryonic development, fetal growth and differentiation, parturition, and the fetal transition to extrauterine life. The pervasive role of the placenta, the parasitic aspects of fetal metabolism, the extraordinary rate of fetal growth, and the continuing fetal maturation condition an environment in which the endocrine system is vastly more complicated than that of extrauterine life. The unraveling of the complex cellular, neural, and chemical events that make up the endocrine and metabolic milieu of mammalian pregnancy represents one of the great triumphs of modern biology.

One important principle to emerge from the recent half century of study is that our understanding of endocrine system physiology derived from later stages of life can rarely be applied directly to the fetal environment (Table 20–1). Several illustrations emphasize this: (1) The placenta is a microcosm of the entire endocrine system and plays a significant role in the function of each fetal endocrine subsystem. (2) The fetus is endowed with several unique and transient endocrine organs. (3) Some endocrine glands have been adapted to special intrauterine functions and/or produce hormones that are different from those of mature glands because of changes in enzymatic processes and cell composition. (4) Hormones and especially neuropeptides may be synthesized and bioactive in many tissues of the embryo and fetus. (5) A variety of hormones and metabolites are unique or uniquely prominent in the fetus. (6) Some chemical mediators act predominantly by paracrine routes during early embryonic and fetal life and via endocrine pathways as maturation proceeds. (7) Some fetal endocrine systems are hyperactive in utero and others are suppressed relative to the extrauterine state. (8) The biological actions of selected hormones are neutralized in utero by a variety of mechanisms potentiating the anabolic milieu of the fetus. Increased insight into the complex, interlocking neural and endocrine mechanisms constituting the fetal endocrine mi-

TABLE 20–1. Features of the Fetal Endocrine Environment

Placental hormone production
   Estrogens
   Progesterone
   Polypeptide hormones
   Neuropeptides
   Growth factors
Unique fetal endocrine systems
   Fetal adrenal cortex
   Para-aortic chromaffin system
   Intermediate pituitary
Prominent fetal hormones or metabolites
   Ectopic neuropeptides
   Vasotocin
   Calcitonin
   Cortisone
   Reverse triiodothyronine
Fetal endocrine system adaptations
   Adrenal-placental interactions
   Testicular control of male differentiation
   Neuropeptides and fetal water metabolism
   Parathyroid glands and placental calcium transport
   Catecholamine and vasopressin responses to hypoxia
   Catecholamine and cortisol control of extrauterine adaptation

lieu is essential to understanding fetal growth and development, as well as postnatal endocrine systems, and is important for our continuing diagnostic and therapeutic approaches to this intrauterine endocrine frontier.

THE PLACENTA

The fetal milieu depends on a functioning placenta, which develops in parallel with the fertilized ovum.[1-3] By 6 to 7 d after conception the blastocyst consists of an outer layer of trophoblast cells and an inner cell mass destined to become the embryo. The trophoblast cells have implanted in the endometrium and by 10 d have developed two distinct layers, an inner cytotrophoblast layer and an outer, thicker layer of continuous cytoplasm, the syncytiotrophoblast, which forms the early fetal-maternal interface (Fig. 20–1). Small pockets of cytotrophoblast cells persist in the mature placenta, but their function remains unclear. They appear to serve as a reservoir of stem cells for continuing syncytiotrophoblast development. There is progressive growth of the predominantly syncytiotrophoblastic placenta throughout gestation. As the placenta develops, the chorionic villi containing the fetal capillaries extend into the maternal lakes of blood within the maternal decidua. Within the villi three layers of fetal tissue separate the fetal circulation from the maternal circulation: the trophoblast-syncytiotrophoblast layer, a layer of extraembryonic connective tissue, and the fetal capillary endothelium. The syncytiotrophoblast is the major site of diffusion between the maternal lakes of blood in the placenta and the fetal capillaries (see Fig. 20–1). The syncytiotrophoblast also manufactures large amounts of steroid and protein hormones, and after the eighth week of pregnancy it is the most active fetal or maternal endocrine organ. The steroid hormones are produced from both fetal and maternal substrates. The protein hormones are synthesized in the rough endoplasmic reticulum of the syncytiotrophoblast from amino acids of maternal origin. Secretion is predominantly into the maternal circulation, but significant amounts reach the fetal compartment.

Placental Hormone Transfer*

One important function of the placenta is to regulate maternal-fetal molecular exchange, and "thin" areas of the

*Also see Chapter 16.

syncytiotrophoblast adjacent to the fetal capillaries seem to be specialized for this function[1] (see Fig. 20–1). However, the fetal endocrine milieu is largely autonomous of maternal hormones because the placenta is impermeable to most peptide hormones. There are two major routes for the transfer of molecules across the placenta: an extracellular route via fluid-filled intercellular channels and a transcellular route. The rate of extracellular diffusion relates to the luminal diameter of the intercellular or paracellular channels and to the molecular weight (molecular radius or size) and lipid solubility or hydrophilicity of the transferred molecule. The placenta is more permeable to lipid-soluble molecules, and the permeability of both lipid-soluble and lipid-insoluble molecules decreases with increasing molecular weight.[3,4] The rate of transfer or diffusion of L-glucose is considered to be a marker for extracellular diffusion.

Table 20–2 summarizes information on placental transfer of a number of hormones that have been studied in several species.[5-27] The differences in placental structure across species appear to have a limited influence on placental hormone transfer, and data derived from some animal and primate species are included. As indicated in Table 20–2, placental transfer decreases with increasing molecular size. The threshold for transfer is the molecular mass range of 700 to 1200. Hormone molecules larger than this have little or no access to the fetal compartment.

Placental cell membranes contain a variety of receptors for polypeptide hormones and growth factors, including insulin, the insulin-like growth factors (IGFs), and epidermal growth factor (EGF).[28] These receptors bind and in some instances degrade their respective ligands but do not facilitate placental transfer.[28]

A number of hormones traverse the placenta via the transcellular route and are metabolized en route.[5,11,14,28-30] These hormones include glucocorticoids, thyroid hormones, and catecholamines. The placental cells contain an active 11β-hydroxysteroid dehydrogenase, which catalyzes the con-

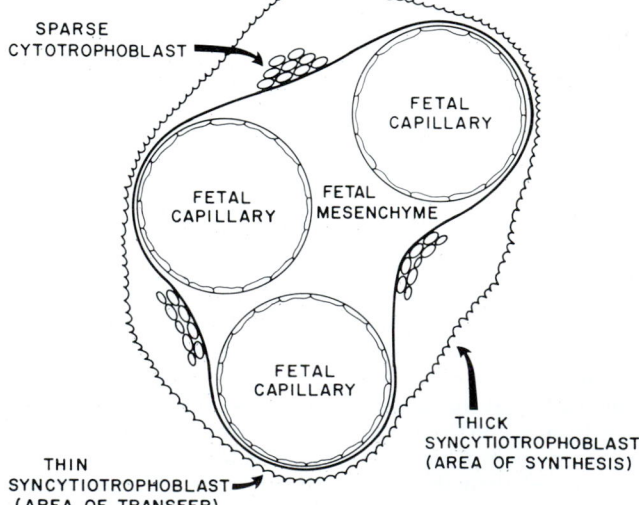

MATERNAL INTERVILLOUS SPACE

SPARSE CYTOTROPHOBLAST

FETAL CAPILLARY

FETAL CAPILLARY

FETAL MESENCHYME

FETAL CAPILLARY

THICK SYNCYTIOTROPHOBLAST (AREA OF SYNTHESIS)

THIN SYNCYTIOTROPHOBLAST (AREA OF TRANSFER)

Figure 20–1. Diagrammatic representation of a cross-section of chorionic villus extending into the maternal blood lake and showing fetal capillaries in the fetal mesenchyme. The villus is sheathed by the syncytiotrophoblast. The residual sparse areas of cytotrophoblast probably provide cells to renew and maintain the syncytiotrophoblast layer. The syncytiotrophoblast surface membrane is microvillous, which massively increases the effective surface area. The villus is surrounded by maternal blood in the maternal intervillous space. (Modified from Chard T. Proteins of the human placenta: some general concepts. In: Grudzinskas JG, Teisner B, Seppala M, eds. Pregnancy Proteins. North Ryde, Australia: Academic, 1982: 6.)

TABLE 20–2. Placental Transfer of Hormones

Hormone	Approximate Molecular Size (Daltons)	Placental Transfer
Catecholamines	180	Yes
Melatonin	230	Yes
Steroid hormones	350	Yes
Vitamin D	350	Yes
Thyrotropin-releasing hormone	360	Yes
Thyroid hormones	800	Limited
Oxytocin	1,000	No
Vasopressin	1,100	No
Luteinizing hormone–releasing hormone	1,200	Yes
Calcitonin	3,400	No
Glucagon	3,600	No
Corticotropin	4,500	No
Corticotropin-releasing hormone	4,800	No
Insulin	6,000	No
Parathyroid hormone	9,000	No
Growth hormone	22,000	No
Thyrotropin	27,000	No
Luteinizing hormone	30,000	No
Renin	40,000	No

version of most of the cortisol to inactive cortisone; measurements of cortisol/cortisone ratios in human placental tissue have shown values of much less than 1.0 near term.[11] In late gestation in the baboon, the oxidation of cortisol to cortisone by the placenta, decidua, and uterus was sevenfold higher than the reverse reaction.[28] Placental tissue also contains an iodothyronine inner ring monodeiodinase, which deiodinates most of the thyroxine (T_4) to inactive reverse triiodothyronine (rT_3) and converts active 3,5,3′-triiodothyronine (T_3) to inactive diiodothyronine.[14] In addition, catecholamine-degrading enzymes have been demonstrated in placental tissue. These enzymes include both monoamine oxidase and catechol O-methyltransferase,[14, 29, 30] and both metanephrine and dihydroxymandelic acid metabolites of catecholamines are present in placental homogenates.[14]

Placental Hormone Production*

Placental Estrogen Production

Estrogen production in nonpregnant women is less than 1 mg/d. The human placenta near term, however, secretes large amounts of estrogens, including estrone, estradiol, and estriol.[31–35] Daily excretion of these steroids approximates 2, 1, and 30 to 40 mg, respectively.[35] This production represents a combined effect of the fetal adrenal gland and the placenta, first characterized by Diczfalusy as the human fetoplacental unit.[33] Most of the estrogen is secreted into the maternal circulation, but fetal concentrations and levels in amniotic fluid are quite high. The major substrates for placental estrogen synthesis are dehydroepiandrosterone (DHEA) and androstenedione. These inactive adrenal steroids are derived from both fetal and maternal adrenal sources.[31–35] The fetal zone of the fetal adrenal cortex is deficient in an enzyme with 3β-hydroxysteroid dehydrogenase (3βHSD) and $\Delta^{4,5}$-isomerase activities, but it has high steroid sulfokinase activity.[33–35] Thus the conversion of pregnenolone to progesterone is limited, and the major product of fetal adrenal steroidogenesis is DHEA sulfate (DHEAS), which is transported to the liver for 16-hydroxylation. The placenta is deficient in 17-hydroxylase activity but sufficient in 3βHSD and sulfatase activities and contains an aromatase that converts androstenedione and testosterone to estrone

*Also see Chapter 16.

and estradiol, respectively, and 16-hydroxyandrostenedione to estriol.[35] DHEAS and 16-hydroxy-DHEAS are hydrolyzed in the placenta by the steroid sulfatase, and DHEA serves as a substrate for placental estrone and estradiol biosynthesis; 16-hydroxy-DHEA is the major substrate for placental estriol synthesis. The features of the fetoplacental unit are summarized in Figure 20–2. Placental estrogen biosynthesis is a function of placental mass and the provision of C_{19}-steroid precursors by the fetal adrenal gland.[35]

The physiological significance of the large amounts of placental estrogen produced during pregnancy remains somewhat obscure for both the mother and the fetus. Estrogens stimulate uterine and mammary growth and have other metabolic effects in the mother. Estriol is a relatively weak estrogen in many biological systems but may have a role in the maintenance of uteroplacental blood flow. However, estrogen production and circulating estrogen levels (especially estriol) may be markedly reduced in pregnancies in which the fetus (including the placenta) has an X-linked steroid sulfatase deficiency and the placenta is unable to convert DHEAS to free DHEA for estrogen biosynthesis. Only about 10% of normal estrogen biosynthesis continues in such pregnancies, with maternal DHEA and androstenedione as substrates. Although parturition may be somewhat delayed, the pregnancy proceeds normally, and the fetus seems to be otherwise normal.[32, 35]

Placental Progesterone Production

During normal pregnancy there is a marked and progressive increase in progesterone production. The maternal corpus luteum is the major source of plasma progesterone during the first 5 to 6 wk; after 12 wk the placenta is the major source.[31, 34, 35] The principal substrate for placental progesterone synthesis is circulating maternal low-density lipoprotein (LDL) cholesterol; de novo placental synthesis of cholesterol from acetate is limited.[35] Placental progester-

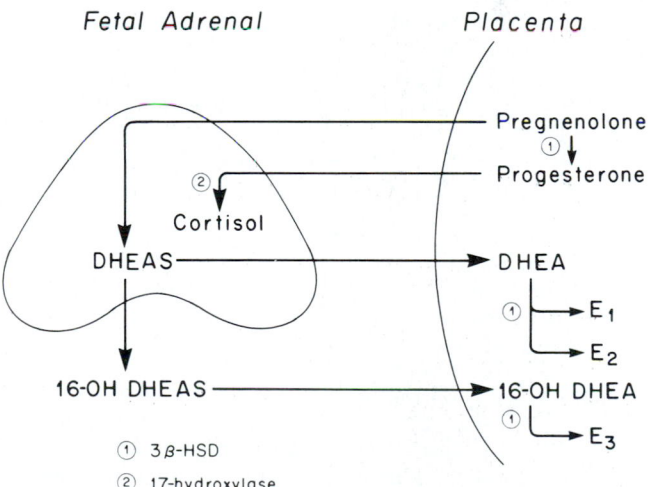

Figure 20–2. Diagrammatic representation of the fetoplacental unit composed of the fetal adrenal cortex and the placenta. The placenta is deficient in 17-hydroxylase activity and cannot synthesize estrogens from progesterone. The fetal adrenal has low 3βHSD and $\Delta^{4,5}$-isomerase activity and cannot synthesize progesterone. Sulfokinase activity is high in fetal adrenal tissue, and steroid sulfatase activity is high in placental tissue. Thus the placenta produces progesterone, which is converted by the fetal adrenal predominantly to dehydroepiandrosterone (DHEA), which can be sulfated to form DHEA sulfate (DHEAS). Part of this is 16-hydroxylated by the fetal liver, and both DHEA and DHEAS are used by the placenta as substrates for estrogen synthesis. Placental sulfatase converts DHEAS and 16-hydroxy-DHEAS to DHEA and 16-hydroxy-DHEA. DHEA serves as a substrate for estrone (E_1) and estradiol (E_2) synthesis; 16-hydroxy-DHEA is utilized for estriol (E_3) synthesis. See text and references for further details.

one production is largely independent of the maternal pituitary or adrenal glands, and fetal death in utero has little acute effect on maternal progesterone levels.[32, 35] Progesterone production is regulated by the number of LDL receptors and thus placental mass. There is evidence that estrogens may stimulate placental progesterone production via effects on the LDL receptor and the conversion of cholesterol to pregnenolone.[35] Estrogens also have a negative feedback effect on adrenal DHEA production.[35] Human chorionic gonadotropin (hCG) and the IGFs may also have a role in autoregulation of progesterone synthesis.[34, 35]

The production of progesterone approximates 200 mg daily during the third trimester, a value some 10-fold higher than that during the midluteal phase of the normal menstrual cycle, and 90% of this amount is secreted into the maternal circulation.[32, 34, 35] Progesterone acts on the uterine musculature to maintain a state of quiescence and may inhibit maternal cell-mediated immune responses to foreign (fetal) antigens. In spite of the predominant secretion of progesterone into the maternal circulation, fetal blood progesterone levels are two- to threefold higher than maternal values because of a lower metabolic clearance of progesterone in the fetus.[35] The significance of this progesterone to the fetus is not clear.

Placental Polypeptide Hormone Production

The placenta produces several pituitary-like hormones. The most abundant are hCG and human placental lactogen (hPL, also called human chorionic somatomammotropin, hCS).[2, 34] hCG is a glycoprotein of 36 to 40 kd with structural, biological, and immunological similarities to the pituitary gonadotropins and thyrotropin (TSH); hCG also has weak thyrotropic hormone–like activity. hPL is a 191-amino-acid protein with 96% homology to human pituitary growth hormone (GH).[2, 34] It has 3% or less of the growth-promoting bioactivity of GH and equivalent prolactin (PRL)–like effects. hCG is secreted predominantly during the first half of gestation, and hPL, during the second half. The control of placental synthesis and secretion of these peptide hormones is not well understood.[34] Hormone secretion is related to placental mass and continues in the absence of the fetus. Chorionic luteinizing hormone–releasing hormone (LHRH, also called gonadotropin-releasing hormone, GnRH) may have a paracrine role in modulating hCG production.[34, 36–38] In addition, glucocorticoids and cyclic AMP (cAMP) increase hCG production by placental cells in vitro; progesterone has decreased hCG production in some studies.[37, 39, 40]

The probable roles of hCG are the maintenance of the corpus luteum during the early part of pregnancy, stimulation of the fetal testes, and stimulation of placental progesterone production.[34, 41] hCG has TSH-like activity, but this activity is weak, less than 0.5 μU of TSH per unit of hCG, and hCG produces minimal changes in maternal thyroid function during normal pregnancy.[42, 43] hPL has weak GH-like and PRL-like bioactivities and has been proposed to exert an anti-insulin effect on maternal carbohydrate and lipid metabolism.[34] This effect would tend to increase maternal glucose and amino acid levels and augment maternal-to-fetal substrate flow. In addition, hPL appears to be an important stimulus of fetal growth.

Recombinant DNA studies of the glycoprotein hormone family have shown a single gene for the beta subunit expressed in the placenta for hCG and in the pituitary for production of luteinizing hormone (LH), follicle-stimulating hormone, and TSH.[44] Also, there is a single gene for the beta subunit of LH, whereas there are seven hCG beta subunit genes or pseudogenes. These hCG and LH beta genes have quite similar structures, and it seems that the

hCG gene arose from the LH beta and that the hCG beta gene family is early in the process of evolution of pseudogenes.[44] The PRL, GH, and hPL genes are also closely related.[45, 46] The PRL gene is presumed to be the ancestral gene; GH evolved nearly 400 million y ago and hPL, within the last 10 million y. The GH gene cluster includes five similar gene loci, two for GH and three for hPL; these loci have 93% messenger RNA (mRNA) homology and probably evolved by repeated duplication over time.[46, 47] Only two of the hPL sequences are expressed in the placenta and produce identical hPL molecules.[45, 46] Placental tissue also expresses pituitary PRL and one of the GH genes (GH-V), and placental GH may contribute to the maternal GH-like effects mediated by somatomedins during pregnancy.[47–49]

The placenta may also produce a separate chorionic TSH. Significant plasma levels of an antibovine TSH-like, immunoreactive material are present in pregnant women, and this hormone may be a unique placental TSH.[42] The physiological significance of this TSH, however, remains unclear; most of the thyrotropic activity in placental tissue and in maternal plasma during pregnancy is attributable to the inherent TSH bioactivity of hCG.[42, 43]

The human placenta synthesizes a pro-opiomelanocortin (POMC) and a material similar to corticotropin (ACTH, adrenocorticotropin) that is referred to as human chorionic corticotropin (hCC).[50, 51] Cleavage products of placental POMC, including β-endorphin, α-melanocyte-stimulating hormone (α-MSH), and α- and β-lipotropin, have been isolated from placental tissue.[50–53] These peptides are localized by immunohistochemical methods in the syncytiotrophoblast.[52] The control of hCC production is not understood, but corticotropin-releasing hormone (CRH) is also produced by the placenta, and CRH stimulates hCC production from perifused human placental fragments, which supports a possible paracrine role for placental CRH in modulating hCC production in the placenta.[53] Glucocorticoids have no effect on placental CRH or hCC release, and oxytocin stimulates placental POMC release, whereas it has no effect on pituitary release of ACTH.[53] Also β-endorphin and α-MSH are released from placental tissue in larger amounts than ACTH, which suggests that control of placental POMC production and processing differs from that in the anterior pituitary.[53] The significant increases in plasma levels of POMC-derived peptides in pregnant women and the resistance of maternal plasma ACTH to glucocorticoid suppression in pregnancy suggest that the placenta may be involved in regulation of the maternal pituitary-adrenal axis during pregnancy.[53, 54]

Renin activity is present in homogenates and in cultured explants of placenta and has been localized in chorionic tissue by immunohistochemical assay.[55, 56] The amino acid composition and NH₂-terminal sequence of chorionic renin are identical to those of kidney renin.[55] Renin mRNA has been demonstrated in the chorion throughout pregnancy; there was no mRNA detectable in decidua, amnion, or myometrium.[56] Placental renin mRNA concentrations at term are about 10% of kidney levels, and the total placental renin mRNA level approximates 20% of kidney content.[56] Angiotensinogen mRNA has not been detected in placenta.[56]

Functional angiotensin II receptors are present in skeletal muscle and connective tissue of the late-gestation rat embryo.[57] In fetal skin fibroblasts these receptors are coupled to membrane phospholipid turnover and mediate increases in cellular inositol phosphate and cytosolic calcium concentrations. Moreover, injection of angiotensin II into 18-d-old rat fetuses increases amino acid incorporation into skin protein.[57] These observations suggest a role for angiotensin II in fetal growth, and placental renin may play a role in the production of fetal angiotensin II.

The sheep placenta produces a parathyroid hormone (PTH)–like bioactivity that is similar in composition to the PTH-related protein produced by tumors associated with hypercalcemia.[58] Bioactivity of the partially purified sheep placental PTH-like protein is inhibited by an antiserum against synthetic human PTH-related peptide (PTHRP), whereas antiserum that neutralizes bovine PTH bioactivity has no effect on the ovine placental PTH-like bioactivity.[58] The placental PTH-like bioactivity is highest in ovine mid-gestation placentas. Similar material is present in fetal and maternal ovine parathyroid glands. Calcitonin (CT) mRNA is also present in the rat placenta, in association with a CT-like immunoreactivity.[59] The significance of these proteins is discussed later in the section describing the fetal PTH-CT system.

Placental Neuropeptide Production

The human placenta contains and produces LHRH, thyrotropin-releasing hormone (TRH), somatostatin (SRIF, somatotropin release–inhibiting factor), CRH, and growth hormone–releasing hormone (GHRH).[38, 60–78] Chorionic LHRH has not been purified and structurally characterized, but structure predicted from the cloned cDNA and human gene is identical with that of the hypothalamic peptide.[38, 62] Moreover, by high-performance liquid chromatography analysis, chorionic LHRH is similar to or identical with synthetic hypothalamic LHRH, and LHRH mRNA is present in placental tissue.[60–62] LHRH is produced in the cytotrophoblast and can bind to receptors in the syncytiotrophoblast.[63] The placental LHRH receptor has lower affinity and less selectivity for LHRH analogues than the pituitary receptor.[60] Because synthetic LHRH increases in vitro production of hCG, and perhaps progesterone, estrone, estradiol, and estriol from placental explants, endogenous chorionic LHRH may have a paracrine role in the regulation of placental hCG and steroid hormone production.[37]

The placental TRH immunoreactivity has not been completely characterized, nor has its site of production been identified.[64–66] In most studies its immunoreactivity and chromatographic characteristics are similar to those of synthetic TRH, and bioactivity has been demonstrated.[65, 66] Sheep placental TRH has immunological and chromatographic similarity to synthetic TRH, and levels vary with the thyroid status of the fetus—increasing with hypothyroidism and decreasing after administration of T_3 to the fetus.[67] These data suggest that regulation of placental TRH gene transcription resembles that of hypothalamic TRH.

Immunoreactive chorionic somatostatin, like LHRH, is localized in the cytotrophoblast.[68, 69] The observations that the somatostatin-containing cells in the placenta disappear as pregnancy progresses and that hPL production increases progressively during the second half of gestation led to the speculation that chorionic somatostatin may exert negative paracrine control on production of hPL by the syncytiotrophoblast.[69] No data for or against this hypothesis are available.

Immunoreactive CRH has been identified in human and sheep placental extracts and in third-trimester pregnancy plasma.[70, 71] It is not detected in plasma of pregnant women during the first or second trimesters, and it disappears post partum.[72–74] CRH mRNA is present in full-term human placental tissue, and immunoreactive CRH, with similar chromatographic characteristics as synthetic CRH, is produced by placental fragments in vitro.[50, 75, 76] The lack of correlation of maternal plasma ACTH or cortisol and CRH levels has suggested that placental CRH is not primarily involved in maternal pituitary ACTH regulation.[73, 74] However, CRH levels are strongly correlated with gestational age

and plasma concentrations, which suggests a relationship to placental function.[74] Moreover, studies with the baboon, which resembles the human with regard to CRH metabolism during pregnancy, have shown a blunted maternal pituitary ACTH response to CRH after CRH infusion.[77] These studies were interpreted to support a role of placental CRH in modulating maternal pituitary and adrenal function during pregnancy.[77] In contrast to the negative feedback effect of glucocorticoid on hypothalamic CRH production, glucocorticoid stimulates placental CRH mRNA and CRH production.[75, 76] This observation and the parallel increases in placental CRH and CRH mRNA concentrations during the last 5 wk of pregnancy suggest that the increase in fetal glucocorticoid production near term may stimulate placental CRH and POMC production and may further augment prenatal fetal cortisol production.

Immunoreactive GHRH and biologically active GHRH are present in rat placenta.[78] Two forms of GHRH activity were identified by high-performance liquid chromatography, one eluting identically with synthetic GHRH and one similar to the methionine sulfoxide analogue. By analogy with other placental releasing factors, chorionic GHRH may be involved in paracrine control of hPL or placental GH production. Plasma GHRH levels, like CRH concentrations, are elevated during the third trimester of human gestation, correlate with gestational age and hPL concentrations, and become undetectable 3 d post partum.[74] A relationship to placental function seems likely.

Placental Growth Factor Production

In addition to pituitary-like tropic hormones, the placenta appears to be able to produce a variety of growth factors including somatomedins. Human placental tissue contains both insulin-like growth factor I (IGF I, also called somatomedin-C) and insulin-like growth factor II (IGF II) mRNA species,[79, 80] and translation of placental RNA in vitro results in the production of a 14-kd protein that is immunoprecipitable with IGF I antiserum.[79] Term placental explants also produce a 24-kd immunoprecipitable IGF I–like protein.[79] The IGF II cDNA isolated from human placenta has a 5′-untranslated region different from that of human liver, and IGF II mRNA expression in placenta may differ from that in liver or kidney.[80] Only one IGF II gene is present in the human genome, so there may be unique tissue-specific and developmental expression of somatomedins by human placental tissue. The role of placental somatomedins and control of their production remain to be characterized. Placental cells possess IGF I receptors by the sixth week of gestation, and placental IGF I may have an autocrine or a paracrine role in placental growth.[79]

Nerve growth factor (NGF) β from human placenta has similar molecular weight, chromatographic properties, and biological (neurite-promoting) activity as mouse salivary gland NGF-β.[81, 82] Human placental NGF does not cross-react, however, with antisera to mouse NGF-β. The significance of placental NGF with regard to fetal development is not clear.

Transforming growth factor β (TGF β) has also been purified from human placenta, and precursor mRNA is present in placental tissue.[83, 84] Inhibiting effects of TGF β on DNA synthesis by human fetal fibroblasts and hepatocytes have been reported, but the significance of these effects is not clear.[85] A role for TGF β in placental growth or metabolism has not been described. EGF and transforming growth factor α (TGF α) have not been described in placental tissue. However, the placenta is richly endowed with receptors that bind both EGF and TGF α.[28, 85, 86] TGF α mRNA is localized in the maternal decidua early in gestation in the mouse, and

TGF α is present in fetal tissues.[87, 88] Moreover, EGF induces differentiation of human trophoblast to syncytiotrophoblast, and this differentiation is associated with increased production of hCG and hPL.[89] These studies have suggested that TGF α or EGF or both may have an important role in placental maturation and function.

Platelet-derived growth factor (PDGF) is probably produced by placental trophoblast cells, and PDGF receptors are present in cultured trophoblast tissue.[90] The PDGF mRNA was localized with a cDNA probe, and peptide was identified by radioreceptor assay.[90] Autocrine control of placental trophoblast cell growth by PGDF has been postulated.

ECTOPIC FETAL HORMONE PRODUCTION

Ectopic Fetal Polypeptide Hormone Production

Fetal tissues appear to be able to produce an hCG-like material. Kidney, liver, and testes from 16- to 20-wk-old human fetuses produce immunoreactive and bioactive hCG in vitro.[91, 92] Kidney tissue produces nearly half as much hCG (per milligram of protein) as placental extracts; liver activity is lower. ACTH-like immunoreactivity is present in relatively high concentrations in neonatal rat pancreas and kidney.[93] Presumably this material is derived from a POMC parent molecule.

Extraneural Fetal Neuropeptide Production

Hypothalamic neuropeptides have been demonstrated in a variety of adult tissues, particularly in the pancreas and the gut.[94–100] In the fetus, hypothalamic neuropeptides are also present in the gut and tissues derived from it. High concentrations of TRH and somatostatin immunoreactivity have been reported in neonatal rat pancreas and gastrointestinal tract tissues while hypothalamic concentrations of these immunoreactive substances are low.[101–104] These neuropeptides have immunoreactive and chromatographic properties similar to those of the synthetic hypothalamic peptides. Other peptides cleaved from pre-proTRH have been demonstrated in perinatal rat pancreas.[105] In addition, encephalectomy does not alter the circulating TRH levels in the neonatal rat, whereas significant reductions are produced by pancreatectomy.[102] TRH production by monolayer cultures of fetal rat pancreatic cells is stimulated by serotonin and is inhibited by carbachol; catecholamines, γ-aminobutyric acid, and histamine have no effect.[106] Specific neurotransmitter control has been postulated. In the sheep fetus, thyroid hormones modulate pancreatic and gut TRH concentrations, which suggests thyroid hormone control of extrahypothalamic TRH gene transcription or translation in the fetus.[67]

TRH and somatostatin are present in the human neonatal pancreas[107, 108] and in blood of the human newborn.[109–111] It seems likely for both hormones that most of the circulating peptide is derived from extrahypothalamic sources.[72, 106, 110] The presence of TRH at high concentrations in fetal ovine blood and the control of fetal pancreatic, placental, and blood TRH levels by thyroid hormones suggest a role of extrahypothalamic TRH in the control of fetal pituitary TSH secretion before the near-term maturation of hypothalamic TRH.[67] There also may be other TRH actions in the fetus: TRH infusion to the fetal sheep evokes behavioral arousal, causes increased body and eye movements, and stimulates fetal breathing.[112] The role of extraneural somatostatin in the fetus is undefined.

There is a general tendency to hypersecretion of fetal pituitary hormones in the sheep during the last half of gestation, and pituitary hormones found at high levels in cord blood in aborted human fetuses and premature human infants include GH, TSH, ACTH, β-endorphin, β-lipotropin, LH, and follicle-stimulating hormone.[113–116] Maturation of hypothalamic-pituitary control is complex, and the mechanism of fetal pituitary hyperfunction during late embryonic life is not yet clear. Immaturity of higher nervous system inhibitory input has been postulated for GH,[113] and immature negative feedback control clearly plays a role for TSH and the gonadotropins and perhaps for ACTH. Extrahypothalamic neuropeptides may play a role in regulation of fetal pituitary–target organ function, but evidence currently is limited.

FETAL ENDOCRINE SYSTEMS

The Anterior Pituitary

Development

The human fetal forebrain is identifiable by 3 wk of gestation; the diencephalon and telencephalon are distinguishable by 5 wk. Rathke pouch, the buccal precursor of the anterior pituitary gland, separates from the primitive pharyngeal stomodeum by 5 wk.[117, 118] The neural components of the transducer system—the hypothalamus, the pituitary stalk, and the posterior pituitary—are largely developed by 7 wk, and the bony floor of the sella turcica is present by this time and separates the adenohypophysis from the primitive gut.[117, 118] Capillaries develop within the proliferating anterior pituitary mesenchymal tissue about Rathke pouch and the diencephalon by 8 wk, and intact hypothalamic-pituitary portal vessels are present by 12 to 17 wk.[119] Maturation of the pituitary portal vascular system continues, and functional integrity of the system matures during the period of histological differentiation of the hypothalamus and development of the portal vascular extension into hypothalamic tissue; this maturation process extends to 30 to 35 wk of gestation.

The median eminence of the hypothalamus is evident by 9 to 10 wk, and the hypothalamic cell condensations, which represent the hypothalamic nuclei, and the interconnecting fiber tracts are demonstrable histologically by 15 to 18 wk.[120, 121] Hypothalamic cells and diencephalic fiber tracts for the hypothalamic neuropeptides somatostatin, CRH, GHRH, and LHRH are also visible by this time.[122–126] Concentrations of dopamine, TRH, LHRH, and somatostatin are significant in hypothalamic tissue by 10 to 14 wk.[127–129] Specialized anterior pituitary cell types, including lactotropes, somatotropes, corticotropes, thyrotropes, and gonadotropes, can be recognized in the anterior pituitary between 7 and 16 wk.[130, 131] Anterior pituitary hormones, including GH, PRL, TSH, LH, follicle-stimulating hormone, and ACTH, are detectable by radioimmunoassay between 10 and 17 wk.[113, 128] Thus the anatomy and biosynthetic mechanisms that make up the hypothalamic-pituitary neuroendocrine transducer appear to be functional by 12 to 17 wk of gestation in the human.

Fetal Pituitary Growth Hormone and Prolactin

The fetal pituitary can synthesize and secrete GH by 8 to 10 wk of gestation.[113, 115, 128] Pituitary GH content increases from about 1 nmol (20 ng) at 10 wk to 45 nmol (1000 ng) at 16 wk. Fetal plasma concentrations measured in cord blood samples are in the 1 to 4 nmol/L range during the first trimester and increase progressively to a mean peak of approximately 6 nmol/L at midgestation (Fig. 20–3). Plasma GH levels fall progressively during the second half of gestation to a mean value of 1.5 nmol/L at term.[113, 128] There are similar increases in pituitary GH mRNA and pituitary GH content, which generally parallel the increase in plasma GH concentration between 16 and 24 wk of gestation.[132] This pattern of ontogenesis of plasma GH reflects a progressive maturation of hypothalamic-pituitary and forebrain function. The responses of plasma GH to somatostatin and GHRH and to insulin and arginine are mature at term in human infants.[113, 115] Plasma GH levels are low in anencephalic infants.[113]

The high plasma GH concentrations at midgestation, after the development of the pituitary portal vascular system, may reflect unrestrained secretion.[113, 128] Studies of 9- to 16-wk-old human fetal pituitary cells in culture have shown a predominant response to GHRH and a limited effect of somatostatin, which suggests that the inhibitory action of somatostatin develops late in gestation.[133] This interpretation has been substantiated by in vivo studies with the sheep fetus, which have shown a failure of somatostatin to inhibit GHRH-stimulated GH release early in the third trimester and maturation of the inhibitory response to somatostatin near term.[134] Thus a predominant GHRH enhancement and limited somatostatin inhibition of GH secretion exist at midgestation, presumably associated with a limited capacity for somatomedin feedback inhibition of GH release. In addition, there may be unrestrained GH secretion at the pituitary cell level and/or immaturity of limbic and forebrain inhibitory circuitry that modulates hypothalamic function.[113, 128] Whatever the mechanisms, control of GH secretion becomes progressively mature during the last half of gestation and the early weeks of postnatal life.[113] Mature responses to sleep, glucose, and levodopa appear during the first 3 mo of postnatal life.

The pattern of ontogenesis of fetal plasma PRL differs significantly from that of GH (see Fig. 20–3); levels are low until 25 to 30 wk and increase to a mean peak value of approximately 11 nmol/L at term.[113, 115] Pituitary PRL content increases progressively from 12 to 15 wk, and in vitro fetal pituitary cells from midgestation fetuses show limited autonomous PRL secretion, although PRL release increases in response to TRH and decreases in response to dopamine.[115] It appears that maturation of brain and hypothalamic control of PRL develops late in gestation and during the first months of extrauterine life.[113, 115, 128] Estrogen stimulates PRL synthesis and release by pituitary cells, and the marked increase in fetal plasma PRL concentration in the last trimester parallels the increase in fetal plasma estrogen levels, although lagging by several weeks.[113, 115, 128] Anencephalic fetuses have plasma PRL concentrations in the normal or low-normal range.[113, 115] These data support a role for estrogen in stimulating fetal PRL release, which accounts in part for the in utero pattern of maturation of fetal plasma PRL levels. In addition, studies with the sheep, which demonstrate a similar pattern of fetal plasma PRL levels, indicate that maturation and integration of brain and hypothalamic mechanisms modulating PRL release develop late in gestation and postnatally, which accounts for the delayed postnatal fall in plasma PRL level in the neonate of this species.[113]

Control of somatomedin production in the fetus is not well understood, but GH does not appear to be involved. Postnatally, GH acts via receptors in liver and other tissues to stimulate production of IGF I and, to a lesser degree, IGF II. Prenatally, in contrast, GH does not bind to fetal liver cells and does not stimulate somatomedin production; rather, fetal tissues contain specific hPL receptors distinct from GH and PRL receptors.[135, 136] Moreover, IGF II mRNA levels are higher in fetal tissues than in adult tissues, and unique IGF II production control systems may be present in the fetus.[136] Further evidence that hPL may play a role in control of fetal growth is provided by the observations that ovine placental lactogen stimulates glycogen synthesis in fetal ovine liver and that hPL stimulates amino acid transport, DNA synthesis, and IGF I production in human fetal fibroblasts and muscle cells. GH and PRL have little activity in these tissues.[135, 136]

The Fetal Pituitary-Adrenal System

The primordium of the fetal adrenal gland can be recognized just cephalad of the developing mesonephros at 3 to 4 wk of gestation. By 6 to 8 wk an inner fetal zone of cells is surrounded by a subcapsular rim of immature cells referred to as the outer or definitive zone. The fetal adrenal gland grows rapidly and progressively in mass; the combined glandular weight approximates 8 g at term, when the fetal zone makes up about 80% of the mass of the gland.[137, 138] The large eosinophilic cells of the fetal zone are well differentiated by 9 to 12 wk and are capable of active steroidogenesis. The regulation of fetal adrenal growth appears to be complex and has been reviewed.[139] Fetal pituitary and placental factors and growth factors acting via paracrine and endocrine routes are probably involved at different times.[139]

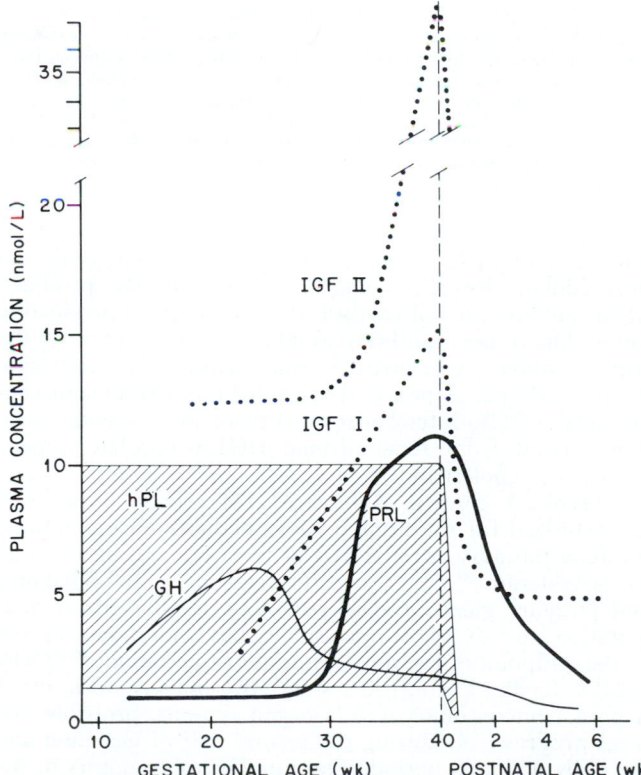

Figure 20–3. Patterns of change of average fetal plasma hPL, GH, PRL, IGF I, and IGF II during gestation and in the neonatal period. The range of fetal plasma hPL concentrations is shown as the hatched area. (Data from Bennett A, Wilson DM, Liu R, et al. Levels of insulin like growth factors I and II in human cord blood. J Clin Endocrinol Metab 1983; 57:609–612; Kaplan SL, Grumbach MM, Aubert ML. The ontogenesis of pituitary hormones and hypothalamic factors in the human fetus: maturation of central nervous system regulation of anterior pituitary function. Recent Prog Horm Res 1976; 32:161–243; and Bala RM, Lopatka J, Leung A, et al. Serum immunoreactive somatomedin levels in normal adults, pregnant women at term, children at various ages, and children with constitutionally delayed growth. J Clin Endocrinol Metab 1981; 52:508–512.)

The fetal adrenal can produce the same five steroidogenic apoenzymes as the adult gland, including the two mitochondrial cytochrome P-450 enzymes for cholesterol side-chain cleavage (P-450$_{scc}$) and hydroxylation of C-11 and C-18 of the steroid nucleus (P-450$_{c11/18}$), and the two microsomal enzymes with 17-hydroxylase and 17,20-desmolase (P-450$_{c17}$) and 21-hydroxylase (P-450$_{c21}$) activities.[138–140]. The fifth enzyme, in the smooth endoplasmic reticulum, has both 3βHSD and Δ^{4,5}-isomerase activities. Expression of these genes appears to be independent of fetal pituitary stimulation, because specific mRNA levels are similar in the adrenal tissue of normal and anencephalic fetuses.[140, 141] However, there are quantitative differences in relative enzymatic activities in the zones of the fetal adrenal that influence the pattern of steroids produced. The most important of these is a paucity of 3βHSD activity in the fetal zone.[33–35, 138, 139]

The fetal adrenal gland also manifests relatively high steroid sulfotransferase activity,[142] and because of the low 3βHSD and high sulfotransferase activities the major steroid products of the fetal adrenal are DHEA, DHEAS, pregnenolone sulfate, several Δ^5-3β-hydroxysteroids, and limited amounts of Δ^5-3-ketosteroids, including cortisol and aldosterone.[138, 139, 143] The definitive zone contributes only a small fraction of total fetal adrenal steroid output compared with the fetal zone but may produce more cortisol per cell.[138, 139] Cholesterol, which is the major substrate for fetal adrenal steroidogenesis, is derived from circulating LDL and from de novo adrenal synthesis;[138, 139, 144, 145] LDL cholesterol, largely of fetal liver and testicular origin, is estimated to contribute 70% of the total.[138, 139] The fetal zone contains more LDL binding sites and manifests a greater rate of de novo cholesterol synthesis than the definitive zone, in keeping with the greater steroidogenic activity of the fetal zone.[146]

The major stimulus to fetal adrenal function appears to be fetal pituitary ACTH. In the anencephalic fetus the fetal adrenal involutes sometime between 14 and 20 wk of gestation, and studies with the rhesus monkey show little effect of hCG, PRL, or α-MSH on fetal adrenal activity, which suggests that any role of placental factors in control of fetal ACTH is limited.[138, 139, 147, 148] Other pituitary peptides, including β-endorphin, β-lipotropin, α-MSH, and corticotropin-like intermediate peptide (CLIP), also have little adrenotropic effect.[138] Maternal levels of CRH are elevated during the last trimester of gestation and reach values of 0.5 to 1.0 nmol/L at term; normal nonpregnant values are less than 0.01 nmol/L.[149] This CRH is bioactive, and levels correlate with maternal cortisol concentrations, which suggests that CRH plays a role in stimulating maternal ACTH release.[149] Fetal plasma CRH levels at term, however, approximate 0.03 nmol/L and, relative to the presumably high levels in pituitary portal blood, probably have little role in modulating fetal ACTH release.[149] Midgestation fetal plasma ACTH concentrations average about 55 pmol/L (250 pg/mL), levels that maximally stimulate fetal adrenal steroidogenesis, and although concentrations fall near term, they are higher throughout gestation than in postnatal life (Fig. 20–4).[138, 150] The fetal ACTH secretion in the sheep fetus is approximately 1 pmol/min/kg body weight (5 ng/min/kg), compared with the adult rate of about 0.3 pmol/min/kg body weight.[151]

Thus the fetal adrenal cortex, maximally stimulated by pituitary ACTH, produces large quantities of DHEA and pregnenolone and their sulfate conjugates. Much of the DHEA is converted to 16-hydroxy-DHEAS by the fetal adrenal and fetal liver. As already discussed, DHEA serves as a substrate for placental estrone and estradiol production; 16-hydroxy-DHEA undergoes metabolism to estriol in the placenta. In the anencephalic fetus placental estrogen production is reduced to about 10% of normal.[32] An important factor in fetal adrenal function appears to be substrate

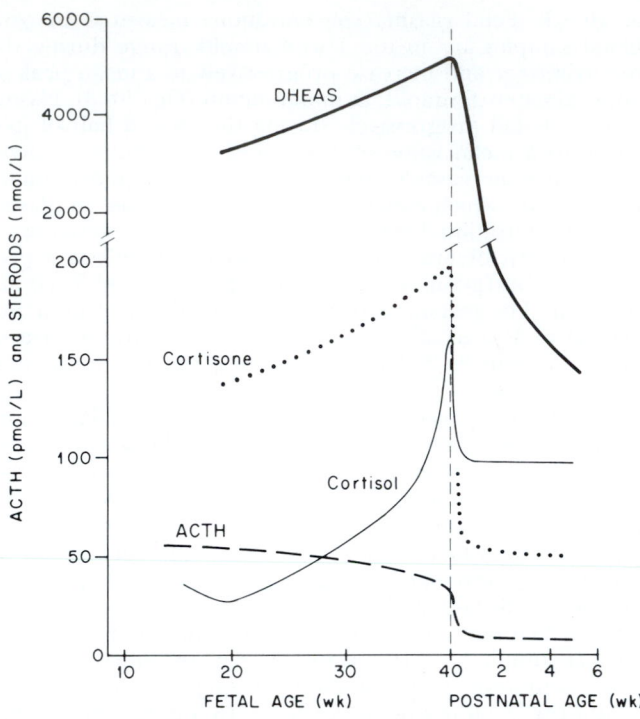

Figure 20–4. Pattern of change of fetal plasma ACTH, cortisol, cortisone, and DHEAS during gestation and in the neonatal period. The trend of average values is shown for each hormone in nanomoles per liter. Note the broken scale for DHEAS. (Data from Winters AJ, Oliver C, Colston C, et al. Plasma ACTH levels in the human fetus and neonate as related to age and parturition. J Clin Endocrinol Metab 1974; 39:269–273; Murphy BEP. Human fetal serum cortisol levels related to gestational age: evidence of a midgestational fall and a steep late gestational rise, independent of sex or mode of delivery. Am J Obstet Gynecol 1982; 144:276–282; Beitins IZ, Bayard F, Ances FIG, et al. The metabolic clearance rate, blood production, interconversion and transplacental passage of cortisol and cortisone in pregnancy near term. Pediatr Res 1973; 7:509–513; and Winter JSD. Fetal and neonatal adrenocortical physiology. In: Polin RA, Fox WW, eds. Neonatal and Fetal Medicine. Philadelphia: W. B. Saunders, 1992: 1829–1841.)

inhibition of 3βHSD activity by placental estrogens and intracellular adrenal steroids.[138, 152] The fetus also produces significant amounts of cortisol; the fetal cortisol production rate in blood, per unit body weight, is similar to that in the adult.[153] About two thirds of fetal cortisol is derived from the fetal adrenal glands, and one third is derived via placental transfer.[139] Both fetal adrenal cortisol and placental estradiol derived from fetal adrenal DHEA regulate hepatic synthesis of cholestrol.[139]

Feedback control of fetal ACTH release is not well characterized for the human. Dexamethasone can suppress the fetal pituitary-adrenal axis at term but not at 18 to 20 wk of gestation.[138, 139, 154, 155] In the fetal sheep, hypothalamic and pituitary glucocorticoid receptors are present at midgestation, and ACTH suppressibility has been demonstrated by the midpoint of the third trimester of gestation.[156, 157] The ACTH feedback control system, by analogy with other hypothalamic-pituitary–target organ systems, probably matures progressively during the second half of gestation and the early neonatal period. The number of receptors in the pituitary gland increases at term, at the time of increasing glucocorticoid levels.[157] It was suggested that this change might allow normal autoregulation of glucocorticoid receptors to be overridden at term.[157]

Fetal cortisol is metabolized rapidly to inactive cortisone via an 11β-hydroxysteroid dehydrogenase in fetal tissues, and levels of circulating cortisone in the midgestation fetus are four- to fivefold higher than cortisol concentrations (see Fig. 20–4). Teleologically, this metabolism protects the anabolic milieu of the fetus because glucorticoids can retard both placental and fetal growth and because cortisone is a relatively inactive glucocorticoid.[158] Glucocorticoid receptors are present at birth and probably are present at midgestation in most tissues, including placenta, lung, brain, liver, and gut.[157, 159, 160] As term approaches, selected fetal tissues express 11-ketosteroid reductase activity and an increasing capacity for local conversion of cortisone to cortisol; these tissues include liver and lung.[11, 34, 138] Cortisol serves as an important maturational stimulus to prepare the fetus for extrauterine survival. An increase in fetal cortisol concentration occurs during the last 10 wk of gestation, probably as a result of increased cortisol secretion and decreased fetal conversion of cortisol to cortisone[138] (see Fig. 20–3). This fetal cortisol surge has an important role in maturation of several fetal systems or functions that are critical to extrauterine survival.[138, 159, 161, 162]

The human fetal adrenal appears to be capable of aldosterone secretion near term, and fetal plasma aldosterone concentrations in infants who are born by cesarean section are three- to fourfold higher than the maternal levels.[138, 163] Vaginal delivery increases levels in both mother and infant, as does maternal salt restriction.[163] The increased aldosterone levels are due to increased secretion, which persists during the first year of extrauterine life.[164] However, there is a poor correlation between plasma renin activity (PRA) and aldosterone levels in cord blood.[165] Aldosterone secretion is quite low in the midgestation human fetal adrenal and is unresponsive to the secretagogues that are known to modulate alsoterone production in the adult.[143] In the sheep model, fetal aldosterone becomes responsive to PRA and angiotensin in the neonatal period.[166] In this species, in which late fetal aldosterone levels are also high relative to the adult, furosemide stimulates PRA during the third trimester, whereas aldosterone is not responsive until the neonatal period.[166] This situation appears to be the case also in the human fetus and neonate.[143] The mechanism for the hyperactivity of the renin-angiotensin-aldosterone system in the late fetal and early infancy periods is unclear. A role for placental renin production is possible.[55, 56] However, the persistence of relatively high PRA and aldosterone levels in the neonatal period suggests that other mechanisms are also involved.[164] Plasma atrial natriuretic factor concentrations are high in the fetus, so that the increased PRA and aldosterone levels are not accountable on the basis of relative atrial natriuretic factor deficiency.[167, 168] Relative renal salt wasting is unlikely because it probably would not induce PRA hypersecretion in the fetus. A relative resistance to the vasoconstrictive effect of angiotensin II is a possibility.

Aldosterone affects renal sodium excretion in the fetal sheep and in premature infants.[138, 163, 166] Despite the fact that the newborn human kidney is relatively unresponsive to exogenous aldosterone, signs and symptoms of mineralocorticoid deficiency in the newborn term infant can occur as a result of aldosterone deficiency or blockade of renal receptors.[138] Relatively reduced glomerular filtration in the newborn limits sodium loss, but by 1 wk of age salt loss related to aldosterone deficiency produces the characteristic manifestations of hyponatremia, hyperkalemia, and volume depletion.

The Fetal Pituitary-Thyroid System

The thyroid gland is a derivative of the primitive buccopharyngeal cavity and develops from contributions of two anlagen, a midline thickening of the pharyngeal floor (median anlage) and paired caudal extensions of the fourth pharyngobranchial pouches (lateral anlagen).[169–171] These structures are discernible by 16 to 17 d of gestation, and by 24 d the median anlage develops a thin, flask-like diverticulum extending from the floor of the buccal cavity down to the fourth branchial arch. By 50 d the median and lateral anlagen have fused and the buccal stalk has ruptured. During this period, the thyroid gland migrates caudally to its definitive location in the anterior neck, aided in part by its relationship with developing cardiac structures. By 70 d of gestation, colloid accumulations are visible histologically, and at this time thyroglobulin synthesis and iodide can be demonstrated within the gland.[170] During the final follicular phase of development, there is a further increase in the size of the colloid spaces, as well as progressive cell growth and accumulation of thyroid hormones. At 12 wk the fetal thyroid weight is approximately 80 mg; at term the gland weighs 1 to 2 g.[170]

The parathyroid glands develop between 5 and 12 wk of gestation from the third and fourth pharyngeal pouches. The third pouches encounter the migrating thyroid anlage and the parathyroid anlagen are carried caudally with the thyroid gland. They finally come to lie at the lower poles of the thyroid lobes as the inferior parathyroid glands. The fourth pouches encounter the thyroid anlage later and come to rest at the upper poles of the thyroid lobes as the superior parathyroid glands. The individual parathyroid glands increase in diameter from less than 0.1 mm at 14 wk to 1 to 2 mm at birth. The fifth pouches contribute paired ultimobranchial bodies that are incorporated into the developing thyroid gland as the parafollicular or C cells, the calcitonin-secreting cells.[172]

As indicated earlier, maternal thyroid hormones have limited access to the fetal circulation. However, some maternal-fetal transfer of T_4 and T_3 occurs.[173, 174] At term the fetal serum T_4 levels in the athyroid fetus range from 30 to 70 nmol/L (2.3 to 5.4 µg/dL).[173] Isotopic equilibrium studies with pregnant rats at term suggest that 15 to 20% of the T_4 in fetal tissues is of maternal origin.[174] Fetal serum T_4 and T_3 concentrations are low before midgestation and are largely accountable by maternal transfer, if similar maternal-fetal hormone kinetics early and late in gestation are assumed.

Pituitary and plasma TSH concentrations begin to increase during the second trimester in the human fetus, about the time that pituitary portal vascular continuity develops[175–178] (Fig. 20–5). Plasma TSH levels increase progressively during the last half of gestation (see Fig. 20–5). Plasma thyroxine-binding globulin and total T_4 concentrations increase progressively from low levels at 16 to 18 wk to plateau at 35 to 40 wk. Free T_4 levels also increase progressively as a consequence of the increase in T_4 production. The increases in plasma TSH and T_4 concentrations during the third trimester reflect a progressive maturation of hypothalamic-pituitary control of TSH and thyroid gland responsiveness to TSH (see Fig. 20–5). TSH responsiveness to TRH is present early in the third trimester. Premature infants born at 26 to 28 wk of gestation respond to exogenous TRH with an increase in plasma TSH concentration comparable to that in adults.[179] Moreover, injection of T_4 into the amniotic fluid 24 h before elective cesarean section increases fetal plasma T_4 and decreases TSH levels, which indicates negative feedback control of TSH.[175, 178] This concept is further supported by the progressive maturation of the ratios of free T_4/TSH and free T_3/TSH, which approach adult values by 2 mo of extrauterine life.[171, 176]

The thyroid follicular cell of the adult can to a large extent modify iodine transport or uptake relative to dietary iodine intake, exclusive of variations in serum TSH levels.[180] Before 36 to 40 wk the developing thyroid lacks this autoregulatory mechanism and is relatively susceptible to iodine-induced inhibition of thyroid hormone synthesis.[181, 182] The

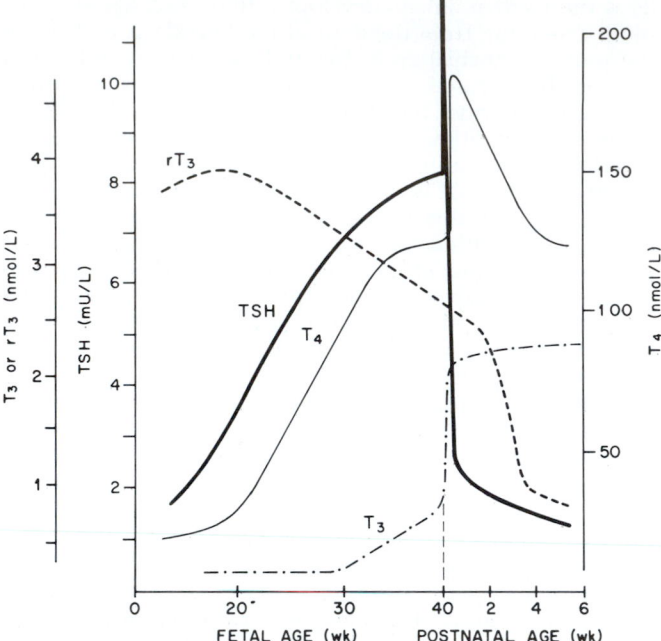

Figure 20–5. Pattern of change of average fetal plasma TSH, T_4, T_3, and rT_3 levels during gestation and in the neonatal period. (Data from Fisher DA, Klein AH. Thyroid development and disorders of thyroid function in the newborn. N Engl J Med 1981; 304:702–712.)

fetal thyroid follicular cell, when exposed to high circulating levels of iodide, is unable to reduce iodide trapping and prevent the high intracellular iodide concentrations that produce the blockade of hormone synthesis referred to as the Wolff-Chaikoff effect.[181] The membrane autoregulatory mechanism is not well characterized, but preliminary evidence suggests that the failure of the immature thyroid to exhibit autoregulation relates to the absence or reduced iodination of an 8- to 10-kd protein component of the thyroid follicular cell.[181] In addition to maturation of autoregulation, there is progressive maturation of thyroidal responsiveness to TSH.[175, 176]

These data and studies with rats, sheep, and nonhuman primates indicate that hypothalamic-pituitary-thyroid control matures during an interval corresponding to the third trimester and early neonatal period of human development.[171, 176, 178] This maturation includes coordinate maturation of hypothalamic TRH secretion, pituitary TRH sensitivity, TSH negative feedback control, and thyroid follicular cell responsiveness to TSH. The fetus progresses from a state of both primary (thyroidal) and tertiary (hypothalamic) hypothyroidism at midgestation through a state of mild tertiary hypothyroidism during the final weeks in utero to a fully mature hypothalamic-pituitary-thyroid axis by 2 mo postnatally (see Fig. 20–5).

Iodothyronine metabolism proceeds through a progressive series of monodeiodinations.[183] Several enzymes are involved, acting on the iodines in the outer (phenolic) ring or the inner (tyrosyl) iodothyronine ring. Most of the circulating, biologically active T_3 in adults is derived via outer ring monodeiodination of T_4 to T_3 in liver and other nonthyroidal tissues; biologically inactive rT_3 also derives from inner ring deiodination of T_4 in peripheral tissues. Several iodothyronine monodeiodinase (MDI) subtypes have been characterized. Type I outer ring MDI expressed in liver and kidney is a high-K_m enzyme, inhibited by propylthiouracil and stimulated by thyroid hormone. This enzyme also has

inner ring deiodinative activity and catalyzes the conversion of rT_3 to 3,3'-diiodothyronine. Type II outer ring MDI in brain, pituitary, and brown adipose tissue is a low-K_m enzyme, insensitive to propylthiouracil and inhibited by thyroid hormone.[183] Type III MDI is present in liver, heart, skin, and placenta and is responsible for inner ring deiodination of T_4 to rT_3. The type I MDI is believed to be responsible for production of T_3 that escapes from the cells into the circulation, whereas the type II enzyme is responsible for production of local T_3 in brain, pituitary, and brown adipose tissue. rT_3 apparently diffuses out of most tissues to appear in plasma.

The type III enzyme that converts T_4 to rT_3 and T_3 to diiodothyronine is present in most fetal tissues and in the placenta early in gestation and is responsible for production of the high levels of fetal plasma rT_3, which peak at midgestation in the 3 to 4 nmol/L range (200 to 300 ng/dL).[14, 175, 176] The persistence of the high plasma levels of rT_3 in the neonate for several weeks after birth indicates that production by fetal tissues, rather than by the placenta, is the major source of circulating of rT_3 (see Fig. 20–5).[175]

There is little conversion of T_4 to active circulating T_3 in the midgestation human fetus; plasma T_3 levels are low (<0.2 nmol/L [15 ng/dL]) until 30 wk, after which the mean value increases to reach 0.7 nmol/L (50 ng/dL) at term[175, 176] (see Fig. 20–5). Early in the third trimester in the fetal sheep, the daily T_4 production rate is approximately 50 nmol/kg body weight, whereas the daily T_3 production rate averages about 7 nmol/kg body weight.[184] The T_3 production rate increases progressively to term, presumably because of maturation of type I MDI activity in the liver and other tissues. In the fetal sheep, hepatic type I MDI activity increases progressively during the last trimester.[185] Type II MDI activity is present in the brain at midgestation and may be important to guarantee adequate brain T_3 in the sheep, a species in which brain maturation depends on thyroid hormone during the second half of gestation.[185] Both enzyme activities are T_4 responsive during the third trimester.[185]

Relatively high levels of nuclear T_3 receptors are present in brain tissue of the fetal sheep at midgestation; liver binding matures during the third trimester to reach adult levels at term.[186, 187] The sheep is relatively mature at birth, and the sensitivity of brain maturation to thyroid hormones begins about midgestation. Thyroid effects on skin and bone maturation are evident during the third trimester. Demonstrable thyroid hormone effects on heart, lung, kidney, and liver are delayed until the early weeks of postnatal life.[176, 187]

There is limited information on maturation of tissue iodothyronine receptors and responses to thyroid hormones in the human fetus and neonate. In the human fetus, thyroid nuclear receptors are present in lung, brain, heart, and liver at 13 to 19 wk of gestation.[188, 189] However, there are few manifestations of thyroid hormone deficiency in the infant born without thyroid tissue and with very low plasma T_4 and high TSH concentrations.[175, 176] Size, weight, appearance, behavior, biochemical parameters, extrauterine adaptation, and neonatal course are usually normal. The paucity of manifestations of hypothyroidism in the fetus may be due to the effects of maternal T_4 or to a lack of effect of thyroid hormones in the fetus. However, about 60% of hypothyroid infants do manifest a 3 to 6 wk delay in bone maturation, and there may be an abnormal set point of the TSH feedback control system so that TSH levels remain relatively high for the prevailing plasma T_4 concentration.[175, 176] During the first 6 to 8 wk of postnatal life, growth, brain development, and metabolism become thyroid dependent, and prevention of permanent sequelae of congenital hypothyroidism requires prompt replacement therapy with thyroid hormones.

The Fetal Pituitary-Gonadal Axis*

The mammalian gonad is derived from two tissue anlagen, the primordial germ cells of the yolk sac wall and somatic, stromal cells that migrate from the primitive mesonephros.[190-192] By 4 to 5 wk of gestation, the germ cells have begun their migration from the yolk sac, and the gonadal ridge has appeared as a derivative of the mesonephros. The germ cells are incorporated into the developing gonadal ridge during the sixth week, when the primitive gonad is composed of a surface epithelium, primitive gonadal cords continuous with the epithelium, and a dense cellular mass referred to as the gonadal blastema.[192] Development of the undifferentiated gonads into testes or ovaries after 6 wk of gestation is regulated largely by genetic determinants. Studies have characterized Y and X chromosome genes, which code for DNA-binding zinc finger proteins that are postulated to play a role in male gonadal differentiation.[193, 194] The interaction of the two genes is not clear; differential expression during embryonic development has been proposed.[194]

Male gonadal differentiation begins at 7 wk, with organization of the gonadal blastema into interstitium and germ cell–containing testicular cords. The primitive cords lose their connections with the epithelium, primitive Sertoli cells and spermatogonia become visible within the cords, and the epithelium differentiates to form the tunica albuginea.[192] Leydig cells derived from the undifferentiated interstitium are visible by the end of the eighth week and are capable of androgen synthesis at this time. By 14 wk these cells make up as much as 50% of the cell mass; their numbers decrease to low levels at birth. The fetal testes grow from approximately 20 mg at 14 wk to 800 mg at birth; at 5 to 6 mo they descend into the inguinal canal, in association with the epididymis and the ductus deferens.[192]

In females, differentiation of ovaries begins during the seventh week of gestation. The gonadal blastema differentiates into interstitium and medullary cords containing the primitive germ cells now referred to as oogonia. The cords degenerate, and cortical layers of surface epithelium, containing individual small oogonia, appear. By 11 to 12 wk clusters of dividing oogonia surrounded by cord cells appear within the cortex; the medulla at this time consists largely of connective tissue.[192] At 12 wk primitive granulosa cells appear and begin to replicate, and many of the large oogonia in the deepest layers of the cortex enter their first meiotic division; other oogonia degenerate. Maturation continues toward the superficial layers through the ninth month, by which time all of the surviving oogonia have undergone the first meiotic division to become primary oocytes. Primordial follicles are present by 5 mo, and during the seventh month stroma-derived theca cells develop around the primordial follicles as they mature to primary follicles. This process continues after birth, again progressing toward the superficial layers. Each fetal ovary weighs about 15 mg at 14 wk of gestation and 300 to 350 mg at birth.[192]

In the male the development of responsive Leydig cells and the high level of circulating hCG in the fetus lead to an increase in fetal testosterone production between weeks 10 and 20 (Fig. 20–6). In vitro studies with the rat have shown that hCG binding to fetal testis cells does not down-regulate LH receptors.[195] If this is true in vivo, continuous exposure of the Leydig cell to hCG would not desensitize the fetal testis and would allow the maintenance of augmented testosterone production during development. Fetal LH may contribute to fetal Leydig cell stimulation, but, quantitatively, hCG is the predominant gonadotropin (see Fig. 20–6). The

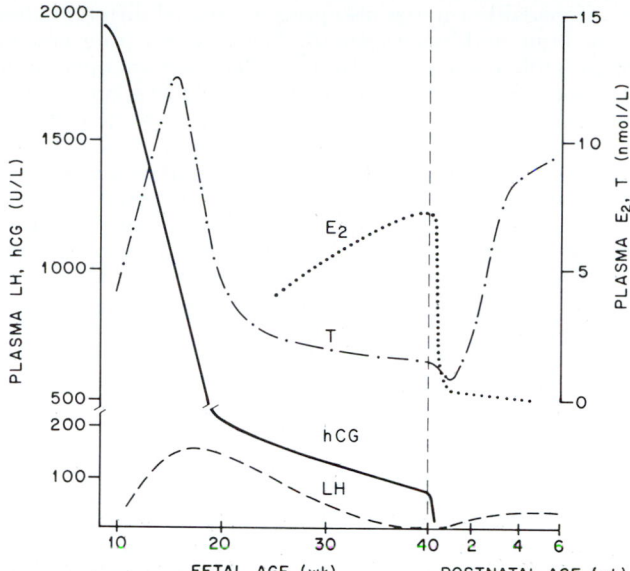

Figure 20–6. Pattern of change of average plasma levels of hCG, LH, testosterone (T), and estradiol (E₂) in a male fetus during gestation and in the neonatal period. (Data from Reyes FI, Boroditsky RS, Winter JS, et al. J Clin Endocrinol Metab 1974; 38:612–617; Kaplan SL, Grumbach MM, Aubert ML. Recent Prog Horm Res 1976; 32:161–243; Winter JS, Faiman C, Hobson WC, et al. J Clin Endocrinol Metab 1975; 40:545–551; Forest MG, Cathiard AM. J Clin Endocrinol Metab 1975; 41:977–980; and Penny R, Parlow AF, Frasier SD. Pediatrics 1979; 64:604–608.)

increased testosterone production stimulates differentiation of the primitive mesonephric ducts into bilateral ductus deferens, epididymides, seminal vesicles, and ejaculatory ducts. Testosterone also stimulates male differentiation of the urogenital sinus and external genitalia, including differentiation of the prostate, growth of the genital tubercle to form a phallus, and fusion of the urogenital folds to form the penile urethra. Whereas testosterone stimulates mesonephric ductal differentiation, conversion to dihydrotestosterone is essential for male differentiation of the urogenital sinus and external genitalia. This process requires maturation of the 5α-reductase enzyme for conversion of testosterone to dihydrotestosterone and appearance of the dihydrotestosterone receptor in the responsive tissues.

The fetal testis also produces antimüllerian hormone (AMH), which causes dedifferentiation of the müllerian duct system in the male fetus.[196-198] AMH is a glycoprotein with a monomer molecular size of approximately 72 kd and multimer sizes ranging from 145 to 235 kd.[197, 198] It is produced by testicular Sertoli cells and reaches the müllerian ducts largely by diffusion; duct regression in vitro requires a 24- to 36-h exposure to AMH.[199] AMH is synthesized by fetal testis tissue early in gestation, and production peaks at the time of müllerian duct regression. Biosynthesis in the testis continues throughout gestation and decreases after birth.[197, 198, 200] AMH mRNA levels are modulated by cAMP, but the ligand controlling fetal AMH production is not known; testosterone and hCG do not stimulate expression of the AMH gene.[197, 198, 200]

AMH may have a role in testicular descent and is present in adult granulosa cells.[197, 200] Male phenotypic differentiation is mediated by testicular testosterone and AMH and occurs between 8 and 14 wk of gestation. In the female fetus the müllerian duct system differentiates in the absence of AMH, the mesonephric ducts fail to develop in the absence of testosterone, and the undifferentiated urogenital sinus and external genitalia mature into female structures.

---

*Also see Chapter 14.

Gonadal hormones also program sexual differentiation of the brain and hypothalamus. The female is programmed for pulsatile release of LHRH and feedback modulation of gonadotropin secretion that mediate cyclic ovarian function postpubertally. Testosterone administration to neonatal female rats produces irreversible inhibition of cyclic hypothalamic control via local aromatization to estradiol and estrogen receptor binding.[201, 202] In primates and humans, estrogens per se seem to be more effective in this regard.[202–204] However, androgen receptors and aromatase activity are present at midgestation in most brain areas of both male and female monkey fetuses, and there appear to be no major tissue biochemical differences between the sexes in utero to account for sexual dimorphic behavioral or gonadotropic programming.[204] Thus the mechanisms for these effects are not yet clear in the primate and human fetus.

The Intermediate Pituitary

In the human and sheep fetus an intermediate lobe of the pituitary is prominent, in addition to the anterior and the posterior lobes.[114, 205, 206] Intermediate lobe cells begin to disappear near term and are virtually absent in the adult human pituitary, although the intermediate lobe in the adult of some lower species is anatomically and functionally distinct.[114, 205] The major secretory products of the intermediate lobe are α-MSH and β-endorphin derived from cleavage of the POMC molecule. Cleavage of POMC in the anterior lobe results predominantly in ACTH and β-lipotropin.

In rhesus monkeys and humans, the fetal pituitary, in contrast to the adult gland, contains high concentrations of compounds resembling α-MSH and CLIP;[139, 207, 208] α-MSH concentrations in the human fetus decrease progressively with increasing fetal age.[209] The circulating levels of both β-endorphin and β-lipotropin are high in the fetal lamb, and the basal ratio of β-endorphin to β-lipotropin is greater than that during hypoxic stimulation of the anterior pituitary.[114] Because hypoxia provokes ACTH release and β-lipotropin production from the anterior pituitary, these data have been interpreted to suggest intermediate lobe origin of basal β-endorphin levels in the fetus.[114] A role for α-MSH and CLIP in fetal adrenal activation has been proposed, and α-MSH may play a role in fetal growth.[34, 114, 139, 210, 211] However, these effects are probably minor; the processing of pituitary POMC in the human fetus by the end of the second trimester is similar to that in the adult,[212] but the role of these intermediate lobe peptides in the fetus remains obscure.[138, 139]

The Posterior Pituitary

The fetal neurohypophysis is well developed by 10 to 12 wk of gestation and contains both arginine vasopressin (AVP, also called antidiuretic hormone, ADH) and oxytocin.[213, 214] In addition, arginine vasotocin (AVT), the parent neurohypophyseal hormone in submammalian vertebrates, has been identified in the fetal pituitary and pineal glands and in adult pineal glands from several mammalian species, including humans.[215–217] AVT is present in the pituitary only during fetal life; it disappears in the neonatal period.[215] In adult mammals the instillation of AVT into cerebrospinal fluid inhibits anterior pituitary gonadotropin and ACTH release, stimulates PRL release, and induces sleep; however, its physiological importance in these regards remains unclear.[216] No role for AVT in the fetal pineal gland has been proposed.

Data for fetal AVP secretion have been derived largely from sheep. In this species the baseline fetal plasma AVP concentrations are similar to maternal levels after midgestation. During the last trimester of gestation, fetal hypotha-lamic and pituitary responsiveness to both volume and osmolar stimuli for AVP secretion are well developed, and an antidiuretic effect of AVP on the fetal kidney is well established.[213, 218, 219] Baseline plasma levels of AVT in fetal sheep during the last trimester approximate values for AVP and oxytocin.[217] Presumably, this AVT is derived from the posterior pituitary, but the stimuli for AVT secretion in the fetus remain to be defined.

In the fetus, AVP appears to function as a stress responsive hormone. Perhaps the major potential stress for the fetus is hypoxia, and the response of AVP to hypoxia is augmented relative to the maternal response and relative to the fetal AVP responses to osmolar stimuli.[220–222] Plasma AVP concentrations in human cord blood are elevated with intrauterine bradycardia and meconium passage.[223] The vasopressor action of AVP may be important in the maintenance of fetal circulatory homeostasis during hemorrhage and during hypoxia; AVP has a limited effect on fetoplacental blood flow.[224, 225] Fetal hypoxia is also a major stimulus for catecholamine release.[226] There is little information on interaction between AVP and catecholamines during fetal hypoxia, but both fetal hypoxia and AVP have been shown to stimulate anterior pituitary function.[114, 216, 226] A role for AVP as a CRH is established in the adult, and the ovine fetal pituitary responds separately and synergistically to AVP and CRH early in the third trimester.[227–229] The relative role of AVP in stimulating fetal ACTH release seems to decrease with gestational age.[228] Whether AVT functions as a fetal CRH is not known.

There is little information on maturation of fetal neurohypophyseal hormone receptors and their physiological effects in the fetus. Oxytocin receptors have been demonstrated in neonatal rat brain and in human fetal membranes at term; AVP receptors have been found in renal medullary membranes of newborn sheep.[230–232] Both AVP and AVT manifest antidiuretic effects in the sheep fetus during the third trimester of gestation.[233, 234] In addition, both peptides inhibit lung fluid production in fetal sheep and goats.[235–237] AVP has also been shown in vitro to stimulate contracture of aortic rings from neonatal rats and may have an effect on water transport via the amniotic membranes.[238, 239] Thus both hormones act in the fetal environment to conserve water for the fetus, by inhibiting fluid loss into amniotic fluid via the lungs and the kidneys (Fig. 20–7). Whether AVT exerts its effects via AVP receptors or separate fetal AVT receptors is not clear. The ability of the newborn human infant to respond to isotonic dextran or to hypertonic saline with appropriate alterations in kidney free water clearance indicates that both volume and osmolar control

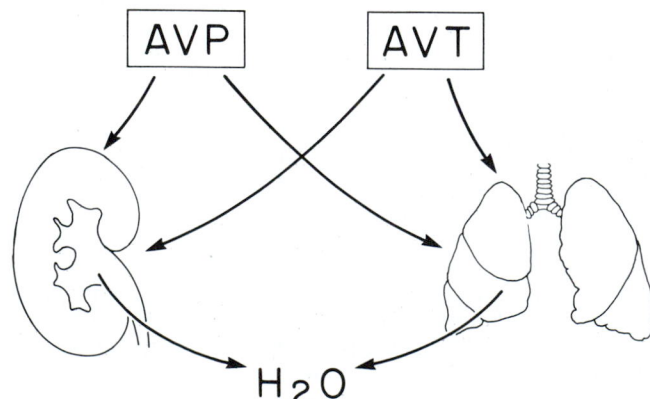

Figure 20–7. Effect of AVP and AVT on fetal water metabolism. Both peptides act to decrease output of urine and to decrease tracheal fluid outflow in the fetus. Thus both act to decrease production of amniotic fluid. See text for details.

systems for modulation of AVP secretion are mature at birth.[240] Maximal concentrating capacity by the fetal kidney is limited to about 600 mmol/L. This limitation is not due to inadequate AVP stimulation but rather to inherent immaturity of the renal tubules.[240]

The Fetal Autonomic Nervous System

In the human fetus the primordia of the sympathetic trunk ganglia are visible by 6 to 7 wk of gestation. The preaortic sympathetic primordia at this time are composed of primitive sympathetic neurons and chromaffin cells, which condense into chains of cell masses along the abdominal aorta. By 10 to 12 wk the paired adrenal masses are well developed. In addition, numerous extramedullary paraganglia (derived from preaortic condensations of sympathetic neurons and chromaffin cells) are scattered throughout the abdominal and pelvic sympathetic plexuses[241] (Fig. 20–8). Most of the chromaffin tissue in the fetus is represented by these extramedullary paraganglia, each of which may reach a maximal diameter of 2 to 3 mm by 28 to 30 wk of gestation. The largest of these paraganglia, the organs of Zuckerkandl near the origin of the inferior mesenteric arteries, enlarge to 10 to 15 mm in length at term. After birth the paraganglia gradually atrophy and completely disappear by 2 to 3 y of age. Progressive growth of the adrenal medullae, increasing catecholamine content with increasing gestational age, and a progressive maturation of adrenomedullary functional capacity occur[241, 242] (see Fig. 20–8). Histologically, the adrenal medullae are somewhat immature at birth but by the age of 1 y they resemble the adult glands.[241]

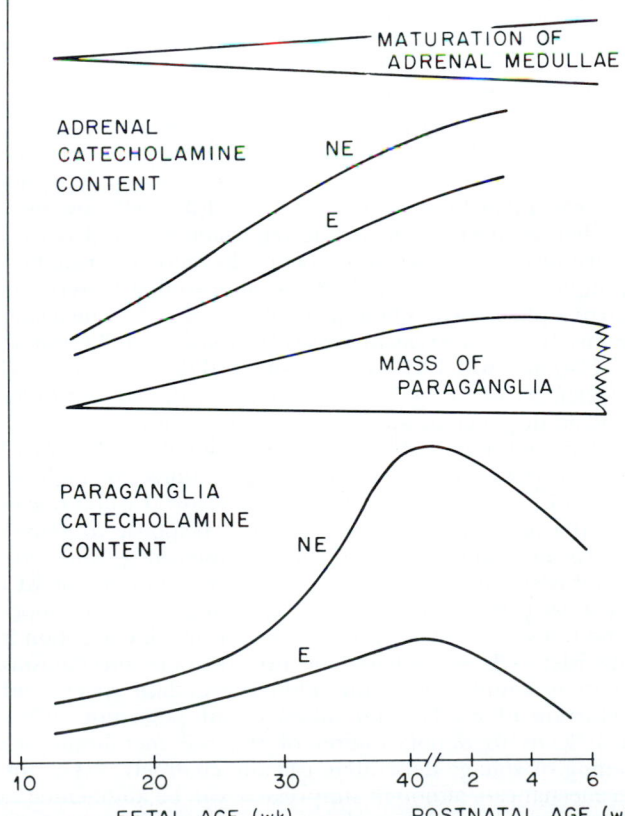

Figure 20–8. Patterns of maturation of chromaffin tissue and chromaffin tissue catecholamine concentrations in the human fetus during gestation and infancy. The general patterns of change in norepinephrine (NE) and epinephrine (E) levels in adrenomedullary and aortic paraganglial tissue are shown. (Modified from Fisher DA. Fetal endocrinology: endocrine disease and pregnancy. In DeGroot LJ, Besser GM, Cahill GF Jr, et al., eds. Endocrinology. 2nd ed. Philadelphia: W. B. Saunders, 1989: 2102–2120.)

Both chromaffin cells and sympathetic nerve cells are derived from common neuroectodermal stem cells, and both respond to NGF.[243, 244] Sympathetic nervous system development is NGF dependent, and injections of NGF antiserum into neonatal rats lead to degeneration of immature chromaffin cells, sympathetic cells, and pheochromoblasts.[244] Whether NGF and other growth factors are involved in the transient life span and function of the paraganglia in the human fetus and neonate remains to be clarified. Also, the role of placental NGF in maturation of the fetal autonomic nervous system is unclear.[81, 82]

Catecholamines are present in the para-aortic chromaffin tissue by 10 to 15 wk of gestation, and concentrations increase to term.[242] The predominant catecholamine is norepinephrine (NE), presumably because of low activity of phenylethanolamine N-methyltransferase in para-aortic chromaffin tissue. This enzyme, which catalyzes the methylation of NE to epinephrine, appears to be activated by the high concentrations of cortisol that diffuse into the adrenal medulla from the adrenal cortex; in contrast to cortisol levels in the adrenal medulla, levels in extramedullary chromaffin tissue are low.[245] Fetal hypophysectomy reduces adrenomedullary epinephrine content in rats, and ACTH restores this content.[246] In fetal mammals the chromaffin cells of the adrenal medulla can respond directly to asphyxia, long before splanchnic innervation develops, by secreting NE, and it is likely that the noninnervated para-aortic tissue responds similarly.[246, 247] In the developing rat, splanchnic innervation of the adrenal medulla develops by day 10 postnatally, and in neonatal rats acute hypoxia markedly increases adrenal catecholamine synthesis and plasma epinephrine and NE levels.[248] In the fetal sheep a similar developmental transition occurs at 120 to 135 d of the 150-d gestation.[247–250] The central nervous system responds to stimuli that evoke sympathetic nervous system responses before the adrenomedullary splanchnic innervation, but the adrenal medulla is relatively unresponsive to such stimuli. The transition is heralded by an adrenomedullary response to hypoglycemia mediated by the central nervous system.[249] This response is present in developing sheep, monkeys, and human fetuses during the third trimester of gestation.[251–253] Central and adrenal enkephalins are also involved in fetal autonomic reactivity.[249, 250] Pretreatment with naloxone potentiates and methadone inhibits the catecholamine response to hypoxia.[249, 250]

There is limited information about the source of catecholamines in the human fetus. Basal plasma catecholamine levels are easily measured during the last third of gestation in the sheep, and levels decrease progressively as term approaches; this is true for epinephrine, NE, and dopamine.[254] The metabolic clearance rate of epinephrine increases with gestational age while the production rate remains unchanged,[255] which indicates that the decreasing basal catecholamine levels with fetal age are due, at least in part, to maturation of clearance mechanisms. The fetal sheep responds to maternal exercise or hypoxia with increased catecholamine levels.[256, 257] The human neonate responds to parturition with an increase in plasma epinephrine and NE concentrations, and these responses are augmented by hypoxia and acidosis.[249, 258–260] The newborn infant also increases catecholamine secretion after cold exposure and hypoglycemia.[249, 253]

Catecholamines, like the fetal neurohypophyseal peptides, provide an important stress response system in the fetus, and both systems respond to hypoxia during fetal and neonatal life.[219–223, 249] The fetal adrenal and the para-aortic chromaffin masses provide for the rapid and effective discharge of relatively large amounts of catecholamines directly into the circulation to provide the circulatory and metabolic adjustments to defend against fetal hypoxia.[249] Moreover, the defense of hypoxia in the fetus involves catecholamine actions mediated through cardiac alpha-receptors that are unique to immature animals.[249, 261] Alpha-adrenergic receptors predominate, relative to the adult, in immature cardiac tissue, and these receptors gradually decline in number as the number of beta-adrenergic receptors increases with maturation. Catecholamine release and alpha-receptor stimulation protect the fetal heart from the conduction and metabolic sequelae of hypoxia.[249] Chromaffin tissue in the fetus is also innervated by opiate receptors and contains relatively large amounts of opiate peptides that appear to be cosecreted with the catecholamines.[249, 250] The extent to which these peptides or pituitary endorphins are involved in modulating fetal catecholamine secretion remains unclear.

The Parathyroid Hormone–Calcitonin System

As indicated earlier under The Fetal Pituitary Thyroid System, the fetal parathyroid glands and the thyroid parafollicular C cells (the CT-secreting cells) are identifiable at the end of the first trimester, and both endocrine systems are functional during the second and third trimesters. Studies conducted with fetal sheep and monkey models and measurements in human preterm and term infants indicate that during pregnancy, high concentrations of fetal calcium (averaging 2.75 to 3.0 mmol/L in the last trimester) are maintained by active placental transport from maternal blood.[262, 263] The placental transport of calcium probably occurs across the syncytiotrophoblast. This tissue contains a calcium-binding protein that buffers intracellular calcium ions as they are transported across the syncytial cell to the basement membrane. An ATP-dependent calcium pump transports the calcium across the cell membrane to the fetal circulation.[263] PTH levels in human cord blood during the last trimester are relatively low and CT concentrations are high.[262-265] 25-Hydroxycholecalciferol and 1,25-dihydroxycholecalciferol ($1,25(OH)_2D$) are transported across the placenta, and free vitamin D concentrations in the fetal circulation are similar to or higher than maternal values.[264, 266, 267] It is postulated that the high prevailing levels of total and ionized calcium maintained in fetal blood by active maternal-fetal transport tend to suppress fetal PTH and stimulate fetal CT secretion.

In the fetal sheep thyroparathyroidectomy results in a rapid decrease in fetal plasma calcium concentration and a loss of the placental calcium gradient.[268] Ovine fetal parathyroid glands contain relatively high concentrations of a PTH-like bioactivity with chemical and immunological characteristics of the PTHRP isolated from tumor tissues associated with hypercalcemia.[58] Partially purified placental PTHRP increases calcium transport in in vitro perfused placentas from thyroparathyroidectomized fetuses, whereas PTH does not.[58] Recombinant 1–84 or 1–141 PTHRP can also stimulate calcium transport.[263] These data support the hypothesis that fetal parathyroid PTHRP acts on the placenta to stimulate maternal-fetal calcium transfer.[263] Placental PTHRP may also play a role.[58, 263] Synthetic bovine PTH 1–34 has been shown to inhibit phosphate uptake by human placental brush border membranes, which suggests a role in modulating placental transport of phosphate.[269] PTH receptors are localized in both the brush border and apical plasma membranes of human placental cells, and PTH stimulates adenylate cyclase activity in these membranes.[269, 270]

Fetal nephrectomy also reduces fetal calcium concentrations, and the hypocalcemia can be prevented by administration of $1,25(OH)_2D$.[266, 268] Moreover, infusion into the sheep fetus of antibody to $1,25(OH)_2D$ reduces the placental calcium gradient.[266] Thus fetal PTHRP and PTH appear to stimulate fetal renal $1,25(OH)_2D$ production, which acts to enhance maternal-fetal transport of calcium by the placenta. The fetal kidney can synthesize $1,25(OH)_2D$, and the placenta contains specific $1,25(OH)_2D$ receptors and a vitamin D–dependent calcium-binding protein.[264, 266] In the sheep fetus the endogenous production rate of $1,25(OH)_2D$ during the last third of gestation is six times greater than that in the mother.[271] The metabolic clearance of $1,25(OH)_2D$ is also higher in the fetus than in the mother.[271] The high turnover of the hormone may be related to tissue uptake, but the significance of $1,25(OH)_2D$ in fetal mineral metabolism is not yet clear.

The fetal parathyroid-placental axis is oriented to the maintenance of maternal-fetal transfer of bone mineral and hence to fetal bone mineral accretion. The high blood levels of CT in the fetus are probably due to the chronic stimulation by fetal hypercalcemia; CT responds to calcium in the sheep and primate fetus and in the newborn infant.[262, 263, 265] A prominent effect of CT is to inhibit bone resorption, and the high fetal serum calcium concentrations coupled with high circulating CT promote bone mineral anabolism.[272] CT has been called a vestigial hormone because of its limited role in postnatal calcium regulation,[272] but it may have an important role in the fetus. Placental CT production may contribute to the high CT levels in fetal plasma,[59] but the persistence of high plasma CT levels in neonatal plasma argues for predominant fetal production.[262] $1,25(OH)_2D$ or $24,25(OH)_2D$ may play a role in fetal cartilage growth and bone mineral accretion.[273] These concepts are summarized in Figure 20–9.

The Endocrine Pancreas: Insulin and Glucagon

The fetal pancreas is identifiable by 4 wk of gestation, and alpha and beta cells can be recognized by 8 to 9 wk; insulin, glucagon, somatostatin, and pancreatic polypeptide are measurable by 8 to 10 wk.[274-278] Alpha cells are more prevalent than beta cells in the fetal pancreas and reach a relative peak at midgestation; beta cells increase in number throughout the second half of gestation so that by term the ratio of alpha to beta cells approximates 1:1.[277, 278] The insulin content of the pancreas increases from less than 3.6 pmol/g (0.5 U/g) at 7 to 10 wk to 30 pmol/g (4 U/g) at 16 to 25 wk and then 93 pmol/g (13 U/g) near term; the concentration in the adult pancreas approximates 14 pmol/g (2 U/g).[275, 277]

Although the fetal beta cell is functional by 14 to 24 wk and fetal pancreatic hormone concentrations are high, secretion of insulin by the fetal pancreas is low. Insulin release from the fetal rat pancreas in vitro in response to glucose or pyruvate is minimal, but insulin release can be stimulated in fetal islet cells by leucine, arginine, tolbutamide, or KCl, so at least parts of the secretory mechanism are developed in the fetus.[277, 279] There is evidence that insulin secretion in adult islet cells is mediated by two or more mechanisms, including stimulation of the adenylate cyclase system with production of cAMP, and inhibition of potassium efflux, which leads to depolarization of the cell membrane and opening of voltage-dependent calcium channels.[279] The former mechanism, although suppressed, can be augmented by theophylline, but calcium channel activation does not occur in fetal islets in response to initiators of insulin release that cause depolarization of adult islet cells.[279] In in vivo studies preceding hysterotomy in pregnant women, glucose or arginine failed to provoke insulin secretion at midgestation or near term, and before the onset of labor, plasma insulin

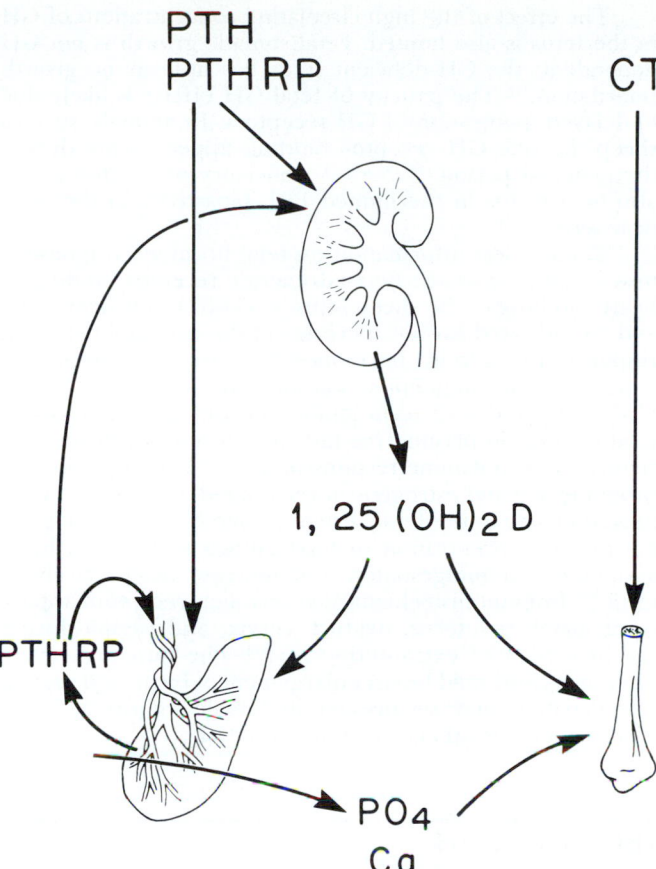

Figure 20–9. Proposed actions of PTH, PTHRP, and CT in the fetus. PTHRP and perhaps PTH from the parathyroid glands and PTHRP from the placenta act on the placenta to promote calcium (Ca) and phosphate (PO₄) transport from the maternal to the fetal circulation to maintain the relative fetal hypercalcemia and the high rate of fetal bone formation during the last half of gestation. PTHRP also acts on the kidney to promote 1-hydroxylation of 25-hydroxycholecalciferol to 1,25(OH)₂D, which augments placental calcium transport and promotes fetal bone growth. High fetal CT levels tend to promote bone accretion. See text for details.

levels in the human fetus are relatively unresponsive to high glucose concentrations.

Similar observations have been made with the fetal monkey, in vivo, near term. In this species neither glucose nor arginine stimulates insulin release, whereas glucagon evokes prompt insulin release.[277] Late in gestation in the ovine fetus, epinephrine inhibits insulin release via a receptor pathway.[277] In the anencephalic human fetus, the endocrine pancreas develops normally if maternal carbohydrate metabolism is not impaired. However, in contrast to the situation for normal fetuses, beta cell hypertrophy and hyperplasia do not occur in the anencephalic fetus or in decapitated fetal rabbits exposed to chronic hyperglycemia. This lack of beta cell response to hyperglycemia may be the result of GH deficiency because GH stimulates insulin gene expression and may exert a permissive role in beta cell hyperplasia and hypertrophy.[280]

Pancreatic glucagon concentrations are also relatively high in fetal plasma and increase progressively with fetal age. The fetal pancreatic glucagon content at midgestation is approximately 6 μg/g compared with an adult level of 2 μg/g.[276–278] As is true for insulin, the capacity for glucagon secretion is blunted in the fetus. Hyperglycemia does not suppress fetal plasma glucagon levels in rats, monkeys, and sheep, and acute hypoglycemia does not evoke glucagon secretion in the rat fetus. Amino acids, which are important

secretagogues for insulin and glucagon in the adult, probably have little role in modulating insulin and glucagon secretion in the preterm fetus.[278] However, infusion of alanine into women at term increases both maternal and cord blood glucagon levels, which indicates a fetal glucagon reponse to amino acids in the term fetus. Catecholamines also evoke glucagon release in the near-term ovine fetus.[277]

Thus, although the fetal pancreatic islet cells are histologically mature and capable of hormone synthesis and hyperplasia, they are functionally immature at birth with regard to a capacity to secrete both insulin and glucagon. The relatively rapid maturation of responsiveness to glucose in the neonatal period in both premature and mature infants suggests that this blunted state may be a secondary result of the relatively stable fetal serum glucose levels maintained by placental transfer of maternal glucose, rather than a primary, temporally fixed maturation process. The blunted capacity for insulin and glucagon secretion has been related to a deficient capacity of the fetal pancreatic islet cells to generate cAMP and/or to rapid cAMP destruction by phosphodiesterase. A two- to threefold increase in islet cell cAMP concentration occurs in newborn rats during the first 72 h after birth, in keeping with this hypothesis.[281] The metabolism of nutrient secretagogues (such as glucose) in the fetal islets fails to couple with the potassium channel to depolarize the cell membrane.[282]

Insulin and glucagon are not normally necessary for substrate metabolism in the fetus.[278, 283] Glucose is obtained by placental transfer via facilitated diffusion. The fetal respiratory quotient approximates 1.0, which suggests that glucose is the primary energy substrate for the fetus. Other substrates such as amino acids and lactate may be utilized in the human as in the sheep fetus.[283] However, at least early in gestation, hepatic metabolism and substrate utilization appear to be independent of insulin and are modulated in an autoregulatory fashion by glucose.[277] In addition, the constant supply of glucose normally precludes the necessity for endogenous gluconeogenesis, and gluconeogenic enzyme activities are low in the fetal liver.[277, 284, 285]

Glycogen storage in the fetus is modulated by fetal corticoidsteroids and probably by placental hPL. Fetal insulin plays a role near term, when insulin also has the capacity to increase fetal glucose uptake and lipogenesis.[277, 278, 286] Insulin receptors are present on most fetal cells in higher numbers than on adult cells; moreover, hyperinsulinemia fails to down-regulate fetal insulin receptors.[277, 287] Fetal hepatic glucagon receptors, in contrast, are relatively reduced in number in fetal liver cells, and fetal liver is relatively resistant to the glycemic effect of glucagon.[288] These conditions tend to potentiate the fetal anabolic milieu during the period of rapid growth in the last trimester of gestation.

NEUTRALIZATION OF HORMONE ACTIONS IN THE FETUS

Production of Inactive Metabolites

Throughout the latter part of gestation, cortisol is metabolized in fetal tissues to inactive cortisone via an 11β-hydroxysteroid dehydrogenase. The placenta is permeable to steroid hormones including cortisol. Through the period of midgestation, placental 11β-hydroxysteroid dehydrogenase activity is low and cortisol is transferred to the fetus. Placental 11β-hydroxysteroid dehydrogenase activity is progressively stimulated during the second half of pregnancy by placental estrogens, and enzyme activity near term is high.[139] Thus maternal-fetal cortisol transfer decreases progressively. In addition, although many adult tissues can convert cortisone to cortisol, fetal tissues seem devoid of this capacity during most of fetal life. Thus most of the cortisol that crosses the placenta or is produced by the fetus is inactivated to cortisone by the placenta or by fetal tissues. Levels of cortisone in fetal plasma exceed those of cortisol by three- to fourfold until after 30 wk (see Fig. 20–4). Teleologically, this would help preserve the anabolic and growth-promoting milieu of the fetus and minimize premature maturational and parturitional effects of cortisol. After 30 wk the ratio of cortisol to cortisone in fetal tissues and plasma increases as a result of both increased fetal secretion and decreased 11-ketosteroid reductase activity within fetal tissues.[11, 36, 138, 139] Cortisol has important maturational action on several fetal tissues (see later under The Transition to Extrauterine Life).

Thyroid hormones also have limited action during fetal life. The athyroid human fetus grows normally and usually without stigmata of thyroid hormone deprivation.[175, 187] Treatment with thyroid hormone early after birth makes possible continued normal physical and mental growth and maturation. Fetal thyroid hormone metabolism is characterized by conversion of T_4 to inactive rT_3 and by limited receptor and postreceptor responsiveness to thyroid hormone. The placenta contains an iodothyronine inner ring MDI that also converts most maternal T_4 to rT_3.[175, 185] In addition, the fetal sheep liver and kidney, in contrast to the adult liver and kidney, manifest little or no iodothyronine outer ring MDI activity, so that there is limited conversion of T_4 to active T_3.[175, 185] As a consequence, plasma T_3 levels in the fetus remain low until the last few weeks of gestation (see Fig. 20–5). Selected fetal tissues (brain, brown adipose tissue) have active iodothyronine outer ring MDI activities, which appear before birth in the rat and by midgestation in the sheep and contribute to local tissue T_3 concentrations; presumably this local T_3 is important in development.[185, 289, 290] Near term in the human fetus and in the neonatal period, the dramatic increase in plasma T_3 levels and presumably in T_3 production heralds the appearance of thyroid hormone actions on growth and development and on metabolism in the neonatal period.

Receptor or Postreceptor Immaturity

Human fetal tissues are largely unresponsive to thyroid hormones. This lack of response is true as well for other species. Fetal ovine liver and kidney thermogenesis (as evidenced by oxygen consumption, Na^+,K^+-ATPase activity, and mitochondrial α-glycerophosphate activity) is unresponsive to exogenous T_3 during the third trimester.[186, 187] Moreover, thyroid hormone responsiveness develops in a number of tissues (cardiac, hepatic, renal, and skin) only during the perinatal period; beta-adrenergic receptor binding in heart and lung of the ovine fetus is unresponsive to T_3 late in the third trimester but is responsive to T_3 in the neonatal period.[291] Rat pituitary GH concentrations become responsive to thyroid hormone only during the first weeks of extrauterine life.[292] Mouse submandibular gland EGF and NGF levels become responsive to thyroid hormone during the second week of life,[293, 294] as do urine and kidney EGF concentrations[294] and hepatic EGF receptor binding.[295] Mouse skin EGF levels and skin EGF receptors are responsive during the first neonatal week.[296, 297] Thus in spite of the presence of nuclear T_3 receptors in significant concentrations in developing rat and sheep,[187, 298] the appearance of many thyroid hormone actions in these species is delayed. The mechanism of this delayed thyroid hormone responsiveness is not clear, but delayed maturation of postnuclear receptor responsiveness seems likely.

The effect of the high circulating concentrations of GH in the fetus is also limited. Fetal somatic growth is not GH dependent; the GH-deficient fetus has little or no growth retardation.[113] The paucity of fetal GH effects is likely due to delayed maturation of GH receptors. In animals, such as sheep, hepatic GH receptor binding appears only during the neonatal period.[113, 135, 136] A deficiency of receptors may also be a factor in the limited PRL bioactivity in the fetus near term.[135, 136]

There is less information on fetal hormone responsiveness in other systems. Beta-adrenergic receptor binding in heart and lung of the sheep fetus is relatively low near term, and, as indicated earlier, increases in the neonatal period in response to thyroid hormones.[291] Moreover, premature lambs have an augmented plasma catecholamine surge at birth compared with term lambs, yet they have a relatively mild increase in plasma free fatty acid levels, which suggests reduced catecholamine responsiveness.[299] The high levels of progesterone and estrogens in fetal blood also seem to have limited effects in the fetus. Progesterone receptors are present in low concentration in fetal guinea pig kidney, lung, and uterus at midgestation and increase progressively to term.[300] Immunohistochemically, estrogen receptors appear in neonatal rat uterus, oviduct, cervix, and vagina during the first 10 d of extrauterine life.[301] The human neonate often manifests mild breast enlargement at birth, and vaginal estrogenation may be present in female infants at birth. Estrogen effects otherwise appear limited.

FETAL GROWTH

Somatomedins*

During the first two decades of postnatal life, growth and development are largely programmed by pituitary GH and thyroid hormones. Somatic growth is mediated by the somatomedins (IGF I and IGF II), molecules of approximately 7 kd and with 43 and 41% homologies, respectively, with insulin. Unlike most hormones, the somatomedins are synthesized in many tissues and act via ubiquitous (types I and II) receptors.[302] The somatomedins are active via autocrine and paracrine as well as endocrine routes. The liver is a major source of circulating IGF I, but other tissues contribute to circulating somatomedin levels as well.

The somatomedins circulate while bound to high-molecular-weight carrier proteins, which prolong the plasma half-life and provide a reservoir of circulating peptide available for target tissues.[302] The carrier proteins also may be essential for somatomedin actions by facilitating delivery to receptors. The type I receptor for IGF is a 300-kd heterotetramer composed of two 135-kd alpha and two 90-kd beta subunits. The beta subunit is a tyrosine kinase that is autophosphorylated subsequent to IGF I binding. The type II receptor is a single chain 250-kd protein without tyrosine kinase activity. The type I receptor binds IGF II and, with lower affinity, insulin, and it probably mediates the mitogenic responses to these molecules. Insulin-like actions of the somatomedins are mediated by insulin receptors. Amino acid uptake is stimulated by IGF I or insulin acting via both somatomedin type I and insulin receptors. The postnatal function of type II receptors is not clear.[302]

GH and nutritional status are the primary regulators of postnatal somatomedin production. GH receptors in liver and in most tissues can modulate IGF I mRNA levels. In adult rats GH has little effect on hepatic or pancreatic IGF

---

*Also see Chapter 21.

II mRNA levels but important effects on brain tissue. There is a negative feedback effect of IGF I on GH production mediated by a direct action on pituitary GH mRNA synthesis and by increased hypothalamic somatostatin release.[302] Food deprivation decreases tissue IGF I mRNA levels directly. Both dietary energy and protein appear to be involved. Thyroid hormones increase circulating somatomedin levels, predominantly via stimulation of pituitary GH production. Actions of estrogens and androgens on somatomedin levels also appear to be mediated via effects on GH production. Adrenal glucocorticoids inhibit the growth-promoting actions of somatomedins at the postreceptor tissue level.[302]

The somatomedins probably play an important role in the regulation of uterine and placental growth during pregnancy, as well as of early embryonic and fetal development. IGF I, EGF, and estrogens have all been shown to be in vitro mitogens for endometrial stromal cells, and the endometrial content of IGF I and IGF I mRNA is high at implantation and during early embryogenesis in the sow.[303] Uterine IGF I and IGF I mRNA levels decrease progressively with advancing gestation.[303] Placental tissue also contains IGF I and IGF II mRNAs and significant concentrations of the respective proteins, as well as IGF I receptors.[79, 80] Autocrine and paracrine roles for the IGFs in uterine and placental tissues are postulated. IGF I and insulin are produced by embryonic tissues during the prepancreatic stage of mouse development, and both factors have been shown to stimulate growth of embryonic mouse cells.[304]

Fetal growth is also importantly modulated by somatomedins. Immunoreactive IGF I is present in most fetal tissues.[305–307] IGF I and IGF II mRNAs can be demonstrated by in situ hybridization to be localized in mesenchymal and fibroblast-like cells in interstitial and perivascular connective tissues and surrounding capsular tissues.[307] In addition, immunoreactive IGF I is produced by in vitro explant cultures of fetal mouse tissues, and fibroblasts cultured from fetal rat lung and skin synthesize both IGFs.[308, 309] These data are consistent with a predominantly paracrine mode of action for these growth factors in the fetus.[305]

An endocrine role is also likely. Somatomedin-binding protein has been identified as early as 5 wk of gestation, and prenatally, as postnatally, circulating somatomedins are associated with binding proteins.[305] Thus during fetal and postnatal life, plasma concentrations of somatomedins are relatively high compared with tissue concentrations. In the fetus, in contrast to children and adults, IGF II levels are higher than those of IGF I (see Fig. 20–3). Fetal levels of both peptides at term are 30 to 50% of adult levels. In most studies cord blood IGF I concentrations correlate with birth size.[305, 310] In the rat, IGF II concentrations are elevated in fetal plasma relative to maternal serum, and levels fall to adult values during the early weeks of postnatal life; IGF I levels are low and increase postnatally.[311] Somatomedin receptors have been identified as early as 5 wk of gestation and are widespread in fetal tissues.[305, 312, 313] IGF I stimulates glycogenesis in cultured fetal rat hepatocytes and induces formation of myotubes in cultured myoblasts,[305, 314] and IGF II is active in cultured muscle and neonatal rat astroglial cells.[305, 313] Insulin receptors are relatively increased in fetal cells and are resistant to down-regulation;[287] there are no similar data available for the IGF I receptor.

As discussed earlier, GH receptors are relatively deficient, whereas receptors for hPL predominate in fetal tissues.[135, 136] Moreover, hPL stimulates IGF I production and augments amino acid transport and DNA synthesis in human fetal fibroblasts and muscle cells.[135, 136] In addition, nutrition influences somatomedins in developing mammals. IGF I levels fall in suckling rats deprived of milk,[305] and IGF I and IGF II levels are reduced in fetuses of protein-starved pregnant rats;[315] hPL reverses the low IGF II levels in these fetal animals.[315] There is no evidence that thyroid hormones modulate GH or somatomedin levels in the mammalian fetus, but, as mentioned earlier, glucocorticoids can inhibit fetal growth, presumably by inhibiting somatomedin action.[158]

These data support the view that the somatomedins are important in embryonic and fetal growth and that they are regulated, at least in part, in the fetus by hPL and nutritional substrate derived transplacentally. The hPL-somatomedin axis in the fetus thus resembles the postnatal GH-somatomedin system. The high levels of IGF II in fetal rat serum, the high levels of IGF II mRNA in fetal tissues, and the presence of a truncated form of IGF I in human fetal brain tissue suggest unique developmental actions of normal and variant forms of the peptides.[305, 311, 316]

Insulin

Insulin has been proposed to act as a fetal growth factor. Infants born to women with diabetes mellitus may have hyperinsulinemia associated with increased birth weight.[317] Most of this increased weight is accountable as body fat; there is little increase in body length, but some organomegaly may occur. Infants with hyperinsulinemia caused by nesidioblastosis or the Beckwith-Wiedemann syndrome may also have increased somatic growth in utero. Conversely, the human fetus with pancreatic agenesis is small and has decreased muscle bulk and little or no adipose tissue.[317] A 3-wk infusion of insulin into fetal monkeys near term increases fetal body weight and fetal heart, liver, and spleen weight but is without effect on lung, kidney, or brain weight.[318] A 2-wk infusion of insulin into fetal pigs does not alter body weight but does increase tissue glycogen stores and muscle RNA/DNA ratios.[319] These and other studies suggest that insulin may act as a fetal growth factor by promoting growth or hypertrophy of selected tissues. In clinical conditions associated with fetal hyperinsulinemia, insulin may act via insulin receptors (in adipose and liver tissues) or via type I IGF I receptors. Insulin may also have a role in regulating IGF I release.[317]

The Epidermal Growth Factor–Transforming Growth Factor α System

The EGF-TFG α system, like the somatomedin system, has been characterized in considerable detail.[320–324] EGF is a 6-kd peptide product of a large 1207-amino-acid precursor molecule and acts via a 170-kd membrane receptor glycoprotein.[322] This receptor, like the somatomedin receptor, has intrinsic tyrosine kinase activity, and tyrosine kinase–mediated autophosphorylation is a critical event in EGF signal transduction. TGF α, which has 35% amino acid homology with murine EGF and 44% homology with human EGF, also acts via the EGF receptor system.[321, 324]

EGF is a potent mitogen for ectodermal and mesodermal cells in tissue and organ culture.[243, 320, 321] These cells include keratinocytes derived from skin, conjunctival, and pharyngeal tissues; corneal endothelial cells; vascular smooth muscle cells; chondrocytes; fibroblasts; liver cells; thyroid follicular cells; granulosa cells; and mammary gland cells. EGF in adult humans is present in highest concentrations in sweat glands, salivary glands, Brunner (duodenal) glands, stomach, pancreas, bone marrow, prostate, kidney, and endocrine glands (pituitary, adrenal, and thyroid). High concentrations of EGF are also present in urine.[321]

The roles of EGF and TGF α in humans are incompletely understood. In rodents and sheep, EGF provokes precocious eyelid opening and tooth eruption in neonatal animals; stimulates lung maturation; promotes palatal development in organ culture; stimulates gastrointestinal maturation; evokes secretion of pituitary hormones including GH, PRL, and ACTH; and stimulates secretion of chorionic gonadotropin and placental lactogen by the placenta.[243, 320, 321] Both EGF and TGF α inhibit EGF receptor binding, and both factors accelerate eye opening and tooth eruption in the neonatal rodent, presumably via interaction with the same "EGF" receptor.[321, 325] Moreover, either TGF α or EGF in combination with TGF β stimulates colony proliferation of normal rat kidney cells in soft agar.[326]

In the postnatal rodent, EGF and pre-pro EGF mRNA are present in most tissues.[327] EGF and EGF mRNA are present in most adult mouse tissues, but mRNA levels are highest in salivary glands and kidneys.[327] EGF and pre-pro EGF mRNA levels are absent or low in the fetal rodent, and levels remain low in mouse tissues during the early neonatal period.[321] Tissue concentrations of both EGF and EGF mRNA increase in the mouse during the first 2 mo of postnatal life. Levels of EGF peptide in the salivary glands increase several thousand-fold between 3 wk and 2 to 3 mo of age. Mouse urine levels increase 200-fold and kidney concentrations increase 10-fold between 1 wk and 2 mo of age. EGF concentrations in mouse ocular tissues increase 100-fold during the first week of life.[321] Liver EGF concentrations increase more slowly, as do serum levels, and there is a high degree of correlation between serum and liver EGF levels in the developing mouse.[321, 328] Thus the production of EGF in the rodent is accelerated during the early neonatal period, and it is during this time that most hormone-stimulated growth and development occur.

There are few data on tissue TGF α concentrations in developing mammals.[321–329] Immunoreactive TGF α concentrations are measurable at relatively high levels in lung and brain tissues at 20 d of gestation in the rat and show minimal changes thereafter, through day 50 postnatal.[329] Liver, which also has high TGF α levels at 20 d of gestation, shows a progressive reduction in TGF α concentrations postnatally to nadir values in the young adult. Kidney tissue has low concentrations of TGF α in late gestation, and levels increase progressively during the first 2 mo of postnatal life. Thus the ontogenic pattern of TGF α is tissue specific, but most late fetal tissues studied contain TGF α, and levels persist or increase in most tissues through the period of growth and development.[329]

EGF has been proposed to play an important role in pregnancy and in fetal development. Maternal salivary gland and plasma EGF concentrations in the mouse increase four- to fivefold during pregnancy.[330] Removal of the salivary glands prevents the increase in plasma EGF; moreover, salivary gland removal reduces the number of mice completing term pregnancy (by 50%) and decreases the crown-rump length of fetuses delivered.[330] Administration of EGF antiserum to pregnant mice without salivary glands further increases the abortion rate, whereas administration of EGF improves pregnancy outcome.[330] These observations suggest an important role of EGF in pregnancy in the mouse. Maternal EGF is too large a molecule to traverse the placental barrier, so that an effect on maternal metabolism and an effect on the placenta are likely.[330] The placenta is richly endowed with EGF receptors, and placental tissue can readily bind and degrade EGF to constituent amino acids.[243, 321]

EGF receptors are present in embryonal and fetal tissues and in placenta, and EGF stimulates protein synthesis during the morula-blastocyst transition and in postimplantation mouse embryo tissue.[243, 331–334] However, EGF and EGF precursor mRNA levels are absent or present at low levels in selected fetal mouse tissues. In situ hybridization studies have revealed low levels of mRNA in embryonic mouse tooth, lung, dermis, and splenic tissues.[335] Low levels are also present in submandibular gland and kidney during the early neonatal period.[336, 337] Fetal mouse tissues have shown higher levels of a ligand that binds to the EGF receptor than of authentic EGF itself, and this ligand has chromatographic and immunological characteristics of TGF α.[338, 339] Thus the ligand for the fetal EGF receptor may be TGF α. TGF α is produced by the maternal decidua during the first half of gestation in rodents, and pro–TGF α mRNA is present in decidua.[338, 339] Decidual pro–TGF α mRNA levels peak at 8 d of gestation (term = 21 d) and decline through day 15, when the decidua is being absorbed. EGF receptors are present in decidua, and TGF α may stimulate proliferation of decidual tissue and may stimulate decidual hormone (PRL) production.[87]

A role for EGF in development of the palate has been demonstrated in the mouse.[335] Thorburn and co-workers[340] observed that the intravenous infusion of recombinant human EGF to the ovine fetus for 3 to 14 d produced skin hypertrophy and increased liver, kidney, adrenal, and thyroid weights; thymus gland weight was decreased. As indicated earlier, EGF receptors are present in a variety of fetal tissues. However, it is not clear whether EGF, TGF α, or both are produced by the ovine fetus. Freemark and Comer[88] reported the presence of TGF α–like transforming bioactivity in ovine fetal kidney and high-affinity EGF receptors in ovine fetal liver. These authors were unable to identify EGF in fetal kidney extracts and suggested that TGF α may play a role in ovine fetal development. Further evidence for a role of EGF in early mammalian development comes from studies of the effect of EGF antiserum administration to neonatal mice. EGF antiserum injected daily for the first 9 d after birth led to delayed eye and ear opening, delayed tooth eruption, accelerated hair growth, and reduced weight gain during the first 30 d of life.[341]

The control of EGF and TGF α production is poorly understood. The increases in EGF concentration in tissues, blood, and urine of the neonatal rodent correlate with and may be conditioned by the increases in thyroid and gonadal hormone levels.[321] EGF concentrations in the mouse submandibular gland are increased by thyroid hormones and testosterone. Thyroid hormones increase EGF concentrations in skin, ocular tissue, kidney, and urine in the developing mouse. Thyroid hormones also increase EGF receptor levels in developing mouse skin and liver.[295, 297, 321] GH increases urine EGF concentrations in the neonatal mouse, and estrogens increase EGF and EGF mRNA levels in mouse uterus.[342, 343] Testosterone stimulates EGF and EGF mRNA levels in submandibular gland and increases EGF receptor levels in prostatic tissue.[336, 344, 345] Thus EGF may mediate growth and developmental actions of a variety of hormones in selected tissues. There is little information about the regulation of TGF α production postnatally or prenatally. Other hormones, growth factors, or peptides may be involved in the control of fetal TGF α and/or EGF production and action.

Nerve Growth Factor

NGF is a 13-kd protein present at high concentrations in mouse salivary gland and at low concentrations in many adult tissues.[346, 347] It is also produced by human placental tissue.[81, 82] NGF binds to high-affinity plasma membrane receptors and is internalized and transported to subcellular organelles, including the nucleus, in responsive neurons of the peripheral nervous system.[346, 347] It promotes neurite outgrowth and induces tryosine hydroxylase and dopamine β-hydroxylase activities in developing sympathetic neurons. It acts on undifferentiated sympathetic cell precursors to evoke both hyperplastic and hypertrophic effects[243, 346] and plays a permissive role to stimulate development of immature autonomic neurons along either a sympathetic or a cholinergic pathway.[243]

Neonatal mice injected with NGF exhibit a marked increase in the volume of the superior cervical ganglia associated with significant increases in RNA polymerase, ornithine decarboxylase, and tyrosine hydroxylase activities. This growth factor also increases the nerve supply of body organs. Likewise, injection of NGF antiserum during early neonatal life results in a decrease in the size of the superior cervical ganglia, a reduction in tyrosine hydroxylase activity, and permanent sympathectomy.[243, 346] Studies of autoimmune immunosympathectomy models in rats and rabbits have shown that maternal NGF autoantibodies also impair autonomic nervous system development in utero.[348, 349] This impairment affects sympathetic and dorsal root ganglia and autonomic innervation of peripheral organs. NGF is produced by neonatal mouse astroglial cells in tissue culture, is present in developing mouse brain tissue, and may play a role in brain development.[350, 351] Thyroid hormones and testosterone modulate postnatal NGF levels in submandibular gland of the mouse.[344] There is no evidence that androgens or thyroid hormones modulate NGF production in the fetus.

Other Factors

A variety of incompletely characterized growth factors are also involved in fetal growth and development, including hematopoietic growth factors, fibroblast growth factors, PDGF, and others. Hematopoietic growth factors are known to be active in the fetus during development.[352] Erythropoietin (EP) in the fetal sheep is produced by the liver rather than the kidney, and a switch to kidney production occurs after parturition.[353] Postnatally, thyroid hormones, testosterone, and hypoxia modulate EP production. Although thyroid hormones have little effect on fetal hepatic EP production, their administration to the fetus accelerates the switching to kidney EP production.[353] Whether factors other than hypoxia modulate fetal EP production is not known.

Basic fibroblast growth factor may play a role in the growth and differentiation of endodermal and mesodermal tissues of mammalian embryos. Infusion of recombinant fibroblast growth factor into the renal artery of kidneys containing a subcapsular transplant of a 10-d-old rat embryo stimulated growth of the embryo.[354] Fibroblast growth factor antiserum retarded the growth of all tissues of endodermal origin and some of mesodermal origin.[354] Fibroblast growth factor, like EGF, stimulates the production of hCG from a choriocarcinoma cell line.[355] These observations and the fact that placental tissue contains fibroblast growth factor, NGF, TGF α, TGF β, IGF I, and IGF II suggest that the placenta may play a critical role in modulating fetal growth.[79–90]

THE TRANSITION TO EXTRAUTERINE LIFE

The transition to extrauterine life involves abrupt delivery from the protected intrauterine environment and succor by the placenta to the relatively cold extrauterine environment. The neonate must initiate air breathing and defend against hypothermia, hypoglycemia, and hypocalcemia as the placental supply of energy and nutritional substrate is removed. Both the adrenal cortex and the autonomic nervous system, including the para-aortic chromaffin system, are essential for extrauterine adaptation. Longer-term transition requires adaptation to an environment of intermittent nutrient supply and transient substrate deficiency and requires maturation of the hormone secretory control mechanisms for the PTH-CT system and the endocrine pancreas.

The Cortisol Surge

In most mammals a cortisol surge occurs near term and is mediated by increased cortisol production by the fetal adrenal and a decreased rate of conversion of cortisol to cortisone (see Fig. 20–4). The stimulus for the increased adrenal cortisol production is not clear; fetal plasma ACTH levels remain relatively unchanged. Whatever the mechanism, the cortisol surge augments surfactant synthesis in lung tissue; increases adrenomedullary phenylethanolamine N-methyltransferase activity, which in turn increases methylation of NE to epinephrine; increases hepatic iodothyronine outer ring MDI activity and hence increases conversion of T_4 to T_3; decreases sensitivity of the ductus arteriosus to prostaglandins, which facilitates ductus closure; induces maturation of several enzymes and transport processes of the small intestine; and stimulates maturation of hepatic enzymes.[138, 159, 161, 162] In some cases these events involve stimulation of synthesis of specific proteins or enzymes. In other instances, such as the action on the ductus arteriosus, the mechanism remains obscure. These effects are summarized in Figure 20–10. Secondary effects of the cortisol actions also promote extrauterine adaptations. The increased T_3 levels stimulate beta-adrenergic receptor binding and potentiate surfactant synthesis in lung tissue and increase the sensitivity of brown adipose tissue to NE.

The Catecholamine Surge

Parturition also evokes a dramatic catecholamine surge in the newborn, which produces extraordinarily high levels of NE, epinephrine, and dopamine in cord blood.[356] As indicated earlier, plasma NE concentrations exceed epinephrine levels because of peripheral as well as adrenomedullary and para-aortic catecholamine release. Cord blood NE levels of 15 nmol/L (2500 pg/mL) and epinephrine levels of 2 nmol/L (370 pg/mL) are common after spontaneous delivery of term infants.[357] Levels of 25 nmol/L (4200 pg/mL) of NE and 35 nmol/L (640 pg/mL) of epinephrine are common in cord blood of premature infants.[260] These changes evoke critical cardiovascular adaptations, including increased blood pressure and increased cardiac ventricular inotropic effects; increased glucagon secretion; decreased insulin secretion; increased brown adipose tissue thermogenesis with increased plasma free fatty acid levels; and pulmonary adaptation, including mobilization of pulmonary fluid and increased surfactant release.[249, 250, 356, 358, 359] These events are summarized in Figure 20–10.

Neonatal Brown Adipose Tissue Thermogenesis

Brown adipose tissue is the major site for thermogenesis in the newborn and is especially prominent in the mammalian fetus. The largest masses of brown adipose tissue envelop the kidneys and adrenal glands, and smaller masses surround the blood vessels of the mediastinum and neck.[360] The mass of brown adipose tissue peaks at the time of birth and gradually decreases in volume during the early weeks of life. Surgical removal of this tissue leads to neonatal hypothermia. NE, via beta-adrenergic receptors, stimulates brown adipose tissue thermogenesis, and optimal responsiveness of this

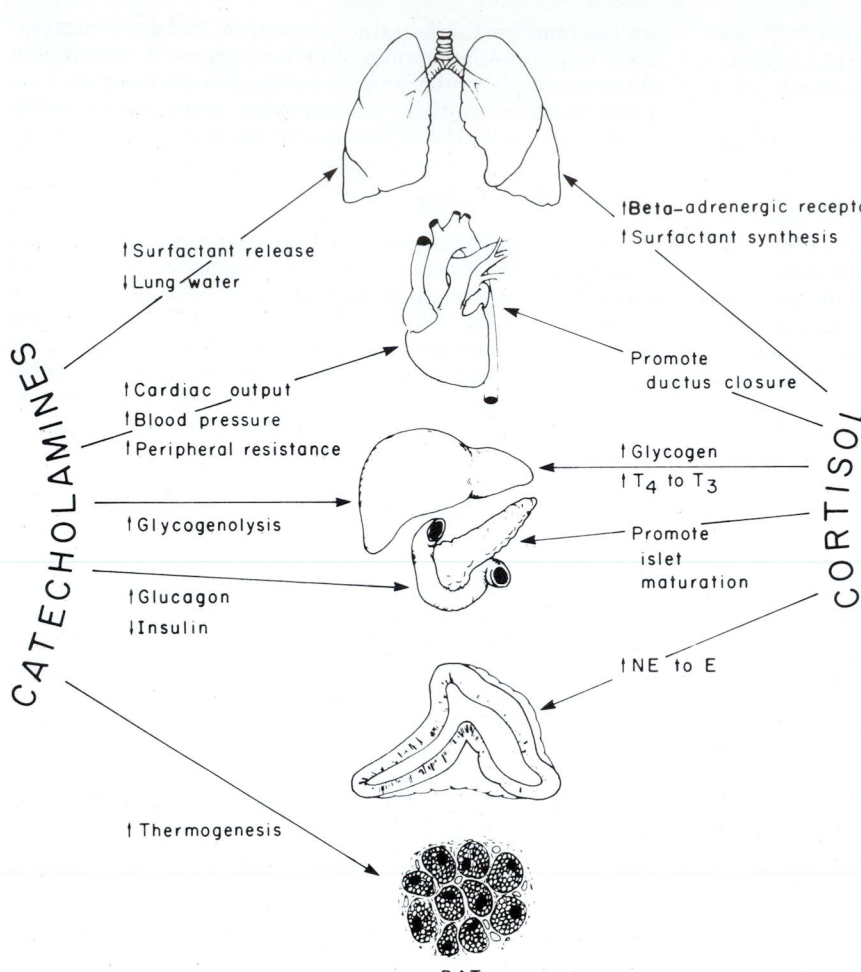

Figure 20–10. Actions of cortisol and catecholamines during fetal adaptation to the extrauterine environment. The prenatal cortisol surge acts to promote functional maturation of several organ systems as indicated. The neonatal catecholamine surge triggers or potentiates a number of the extrauterine cardiopulmonary and metabolic functional adaptations that are critical to extrauterine survival. See text for details.

tissue to NE is thyroid hormone dependent. Brown adipose tissue is rich in mitochondria containing a unique 32-kd uncoupling protein (thermogenin) that uncouples oxidation and phosphorylation of ADP to ATP and consequently enhances thermogenesis.[360] Thermogenin is T_3 dependent, and brown adipose tissue contains a 5'-monoiodothyronine deiodinase that synthesizes T_3 locally from T_4.[361] Full maturation of catecholamine-stimulated cellular respiration in brown adipose tissue occurs before delivery in the ovine fetus and requires thyroid hormone.[362, 363] Fetal thyroidectomy in this species leads to marked hypothermia, with low plasma free fatty acid levels and increased plasma epinephrine concentrations.[363] In vitro, basal brown adipose tissue thermogenesis and NE and dibutyryl cAMP–stimulated thermogenesis are decreased by fetal thyroidectomy.[363] Thus thyroid hormones and catecholamines are both essential for adequate brown adipose tissue thermogenesis and for the maintenance of body temperature in the extrauterine environment.

Calcium Homeostasis

The neonate must adjust rapidly from a high-calcium environment regulated by PTHRP and CT to an environment of low calcium requiring regulation by PTH and vitamin D. With removal of the placenta, plasma total calcium concentration falls and reaches a nadir of approximately 2.3 mmol/L (9 mg/dL) in term infants by 24 h of life.[262, 263, 364] The ionized calcium concentration reaches a low level of about 1.2 mmol/L (4.8 mg/dL).[364] Plasma PTH levels

in the neonate are relatively low in the neonatal period and are minimally responsive to hypocalcemia during the first 2 to 3 d of life.[365] CT concentrations are high in cord blood, about 2000 ng/L, increase further during the early neonatal period, and remain high for several days after birth.[262, 263, 366] The relatively obtunded PTH response and the high CT levels lead to a 2- to 3-d period of transient neonatal hypocalcemia.[336, 337] Progressive inhibition of CT secretion with progressive stimulation of PTH secretion gradually results in increased serum calcium levels in the neonate. The disappearance of PTHRP in the neonatal lamb is approximately coincident with the time of restoration of calcium levels to the adult range.[263] The mechanism for the transition from PTHRP to PTH secretion by the neonatal parathyroid glands is not clear.

Calcium homeostasis is also affected in the human newborn period by a low level of glomerular filtration, which persists for several days.[262] In addition, renal responsiveness to PTH is reduced for several days after birth.[262] These factors limit phosphate excretion and predispose the neonate to hyperphosphatemia, particularly if the diet includes high-phosphate milk such as unmodified cow's milk. Premature infants tend to have lower PTH and higher CT levels with more immature kidney function, and in these infants the neonatal hypocalcemia may be more marked and prolonged and the incidence of symptomatic hypocalcemia is much higher. Birth asphyxia also predisposes the neonate to hypocalcemia.[262, 366] Infants born to mothers with hypercalcemia caused by hyperparathyroidism have a high incidence of sympatomatic hypocalcemia. These infants have a more marked suppression of parathyroid function and a more prolonged period of transient hypoparathyroidism in the neonatal period. PTH secretion and calcium homeostasis usually normalize within 1 to 2 wk in full-term infants, but normalization may require 2 to 3 wk in the small premature infant.

Glucose Homeostasis

The abrupt withdrawal of the placental glucose supply leads to a prompt fall in plasma glucose in the term neonate.[277, 278, 367] The low glucose and high catecholamine levels stimulate glucagon secretion, and a transient peak in plasma glucagon level occurs within 2 h after birth.[277, 278, 356, 367] Plasma insulin levels are low at birth and tend to fall further secondary to the hypoglycemia. The early glucagon response is short-lived, but levels remain in the 100 ng/L range for the first 12 to 24 h and the glucagon/insulin ratio is high enough to stabilize glucose levels in the 2.8 to 4.0 mmol/L (50 to 70 mg/dL) range during this period. The early glucagon and catecholamine surges rapidly deplete hepatic glycogen stores, so that return of plasma glucose levels to normal after 12 to 18 h requires maturation of hepatic gluconeogenesis under the stimulus of a high plasma glucagon/insulin ratio.[278, 367] Glucagon secretion gradually increases during the early hours after birth, especially with protein feeding, which stimulates gut glucagon release and pancreatic glucagon secretion.[277, 278, 367] Premature infants have more severe and prolonged hypoglycemia because of relatively reduced glycogen stores and impaired hepatic gluconeogenesis.[277, 278, 367] Infants born to diabetic mothers have more severe neonatal hypoglycemia because of relative hyperinsulinism. In the healthy term infant, glucose homeostasis is achieved within 5 to 7 d of life; in premature infants 1 to 2 wk may be required.

Other Hormonal Adaptations

Changes in other hormone systems are summarized in Figures 20–3 to 20–6. Delivery of the placenta results in decreases in fetal blood levels of estrogens, progesterone, hCG, and hPL. The fall in estrogen levels (see Fig. 20–6) presumably removes the major stimulus to fetal PRL release, and PRL levels decrease within several weeks (see Fig. 20–3). The relatively delayed rate of fall may be due to lactotrope hyperplasia in the fetal pituitary or to delayed maturation of hypothalamic dopamine secretion. The gradual fall of GH levels during the early weeks of life is due to delayed maturation of hypothalamic-pituitary and feedback control of GH release.[113, 128, 134] In the neonatal primate there are concomitant decreases in plasma GH levels and GH responsiveness to exogenous GHRH.[368] The mechanisms remain unclear. Changes in secretion or in pituitary sensitivity to GHRH and/or somatostatin may be involved. Somatomedin levels fall to infantile values within a few days, presumably because of the removal of placental hPL and placental somatomedin production (see Fig. 20–3).

In male infants (see Fig. 20–6) after a transient fall in testosterone levels as the hCG stimulus abates, pituitary LH secretion rebounds, and there is a secondary surge of plasma testosterone that persists at significant levels for several weeks.[369] This surge is mediated by hypothalamic LHRH, and blockade of neonatal activation of the pituitary-testicular axis with an LHRH agonist in neonatal monkeys ablates the neonatal increments in LH and testosterone.[370] Such a blockade also results in subnormal increments in plasma LH and testosterone levels and subnormal testicular enlargement at puberty in these animals, which suggests that neonatal LHRH release with pituitary-testicular activation may be critical for normal sexual development of male primates.[370] In females a transient, secondary follicle-stimulating hormone surge may transiently elevate estrogen levels.

Delivery results in a reversal of the high fetal cortisone/cortisol ratio, and plasma cortisol concentrations remain relatively higher in the neonate in spite of relatively lower plasma ACTH concentrations (see Fig. 20–4). Presumably this increase relates to removal of estrogen inhibition of adrenal 3βHSD[138, 142] and perhaps to removal of a placental CRH action on fetal pituitary ACTH release. Plasma DHEAS and DHEA levels fall as the fetal adrenal atrophies (see Fig. 20–4).

The dramatic increase in serum TSH level during the early minutes after birth is due to cooling of the neonate in the extrauterine environment.[175, 176] The TSH surge peaks at 30 min, at TSH concentrations approximating 70 mU/L (see Fig. 20–5). This peak evokes increased thyroidal T_4 and T_3 secretion. In addition, increased peripheral conversion of T_4 to T_3 by liver and other tissues maintains the T_3 level in the extrauterine range of 1.6 to 3.4 nmol/L (105 to 220 ng/dL) (see Fig. 20–5).[175, 176] The re-equilibration of TSH levels to the normal extrauterine range probably relates to the readjustment of prevailing serum T_3 levels, as well as to continued maturation of feedback control of TSH by thyroid hormones during the early weeks of life. rT_3 production by fetal and neonatal tissues abates by 3 to 4 wk, at which time serum rT_3 concentrations fall to adult values.

THE IMPRINTING OF DEVELOPING ENDOCRINE SYSTEMS

There are now extensive data for several mammalian species supporting the concept of hormonal imprinting during a critical, usually perinatal, period of development. In the female rodent, transient neonatal androgen administration masculinizes the pattern of hypothalamic control of LHRH secretion and pituitary gonadotropin secretion, masculinizes adult behavior and adult sexual activity, permanently alters the pattern of GH secretion, increases longitudinal bone growth and body weight, and masculinizes the pattern of hepatic steroid metabolism.[371–374] Estrogen administration to pregnant rats during the last third of gestation produces cryptorchid male offspring and may permanently suppress spermatogenesis in adult males.[375] Perinatal estrogen administration to the developing female rodent produces long-term effects, including persistent vaginal cornification, hyperplastic vaginal lesions, and cervicovaginal cancer; synthetic nonsteroidal estrogen (diethylstilbestrol) has similar effects.[376] Chronic hyperprolactinemia also occurs, presumably secondary to the low-level continuous estrogen secretion in these anovulatory animals.[376] Female rats given a single neonatal dose of diethylstilbestrol manifest decreased uterine estradiol receptor binding as adults, and neonatal administration of dexamethasone causes decreased glucocorticoid binding in adult thymus tissue.[377] Transient levothyroxine administration to neonatal rodents leads to growth retardation, delayed puberty, decreased adult pituitary weight, decreased pituitary TRH concentrations, low serum TSH levels, and decreased TSH responsiveness to propylthiouracil challenge.[378–381] Adult adrenal function and EGF metabolism are also altered.[380, 382] Neonatal administration of insulin or alloxan to rats produces permanent alteration of glucose tolerance,[383, 384] and a single neonatal dose of vasopressin to the neonatal rat permanently enhances adult response to vasopressin.[385] Neonatal catecholamine administration alters the response of adult rat vascular tissue to NE.[377]

There is much less information about hormonal imprinting in primates and humans. Blockade of LHRH in neonatal monkeys with an LHRH agonist results in obtundation of plasma LH and testosterone levels and decreased testicular size at puberty.[370] Diethylstilbestrol administration to pregnant women increases the prevalence of vaginal adenocarcinoma in female offspring during the second and third decades of life.[386, 387] Congenital hypothyroidism in human infants may be associated with alteration of the set point for feedback control of TSH release such that serum TSH levels remain inappropriately elevated after return of serum T_4 levels to normal by treatment.[388, 389]

The mechanisms for these effects remain obscure. Permanent effects of neonatal administration of testosterone on brain structure have been demonstrated.[373] The effect in some instances may be transmitted to subsequent generations.[379, 383] A functional overlap of hormone-mediated imprinting has also been observed; both TSH and follicle-stimulating hormone given to the neonate alter the adult response to TSH, and neonatal oxytocin or vasopressin exposure can alter the adult response to vasopressin.[377, 385] Hormonal imprinting is also demonstrable in cell lines and in unicellular organisms in which a single exposure to a hormone produces a persistent alteration of the hormonal response characteristics.[377] These observations have suggested that hormone imprinting is due to a period of hormone receptor plasticity during a critical period of receptor maturation and that exposure to abnormal amounts of ligand during this period somehow alters the adult pattern of hormone receptor expression. Nuclear receptors as well as plasma membrane receptors may be involved. Plasticity of prohormone processing may also be involved, as in newborn rat intermediate pituitary lobe cells in vitro; dexamethasone exposure of such cells decreases production of α-MSH and increases production of ACTH-related peptides.[390] Whatever the mechanisms, the developing endocrine systems seem to have significant plasticity, and the maturation of endocrine control systems can be influenced by alterations in the prevailing hormone concentrations.

EPILOGUE

The foregoing review summarizes current understanding of the intrauterine endocrine milieu and highlights progress in this challenging frontier of medicine. This progress has set the stage for advances in the management of the infant of the diabetic mother, the infant with disordered sexual differentiation, and neonates with congenital thyroid, parathyroid, or pituitary disease. In addition, important advances in the management of premature labor and abnormalities of fetal growth have been seen. Most therapeutic approaches to intrauterine abnormalities to date have been indirect.

We are now entering a new era of direct access and management of the intrauterine environment, with all the potential advantages and risks that this entails.[391] With expansion of the application and scope of amniotic fluid and fetal cell sampling and the advent of fetal visualization and intrauterine fetal blood sampling, direct access to the fetus and diagnosis are now possible.[177, 392] Manipulation of the maternal menstrual cycle, artificial insemination, and in vitro fertilization are routine procedures. Selective embryocide has been utilized to control induced multiple embryo pregnancy.[393] Women are treated with glucocorticoids or glucocorticoids plus TRH to stimulate fetal lung maturation.[394] Tentative approaches have been made to intrauterine diagnosis and treatment of human fetal adrenal and thyroid disorders.[395-399] Intravenous nutritional supplementation of fetal sheep can prevent some forms of growth retardation,[400] and chronic fetal therapy via indwelling pumps is routinely used for treatment of fetal animals.[185] These approaches, coupled with increasing availability of synthetic hormones and growth factor agonists and antagonists, will facilitate direct fetal endocrine therapy.

In addition, transplantation of fetal neuroendocrine tissues in rodents can alter neuroendocrine, cognitive, and motor functions of the host. Transplantation of fetal preoptic area tissue restores mating and pregnancy in genetically hypogonadal mice;[401] transplantation of fetal hypothalamic vasopressin-containing neurons corrects diabetes insipidus in adult hosts;[402] and fetal brain grafts improve motor function in adults with nigrostriatal dopamine system lesions.[403] Fetal neuroendocrine tissue appears to survive after transplantation to adult rodent hosts, and preliminary studies demonstrate that cryopreserved human fetal brain tissue can be transplanted successfully to primate hosts.[404] The use of fetal tissues for transplantation involves difficult moral and ethical issues, but continuing progress in both technical and ethical areas is inevitable.[405] The next decades will witness continuing expansion of our understanding of the endocrinology and metabolism of the fetus and increasing effectiveness of efforts to diagnose and manage abnormal pregnancies, including direct fetal diagnosis and therapy and the utilization of fetal tissues in the treatment of adult disease.

REFERENCES

1. Chard T. Proteins of the human placenta: some general concepts. In: Grudzinskas JG, Teisner B, Seppala, eds. Pregnancy Proteins. New York: Academic, 1982: 3–21.
2. Osathanondh R, Tulchinsky D. Placental polypeptide hormones. In: Tulchinsky D, Ryan KJ, eds. Maternal-Fetal Endocrinology. Philadelphia: W. B. Saunders, 1980: 17–42.
3. Faber JJ. Diffusional exchange between foetus and mother as a function of the physical properties of the diffusing materials. In: Cross KW, Comline KS, Dawes GS, et al., eds. Foetal and Neonatal Physiology: Proceedings. New York: Cambridge University Press, 1973: 306–327.
4. Robinson NR, Atkinson DE, Jones CJP, et al. Permeability of the near-term rat placenta to hydrophilic solutes. Placenta 1988; 9:361–372.
5. Sodha RJ, Proegler M, Schneider H. Transfer and metabolism of norepinephrine studied from maternal to fetal and fetal to maternal sides in the in vitro perfused human placental life. Am J Obstet Gynecol 1984; 148:474–481.
6. Sandler M, Ruthven CRJ, Contractor SF. Transmission of noradrenaline across the human placenta. Nature 1963; 197:598.
7. Weaver DR, Namboodiri A, Reppert SM. Iodinated melatonin mimics melatonin action and reveals discrete binding sites in fetal brain. FEBS Lett 1988; 228:123–127.
8. Solomon S, Friesen HG. Endocrine relations between mother and fetus. Annu Rev Med 1968; 19:399–430.
9. Smith W, Adams W. Transplacental influence of androgens upon ovulatory mechanisms in the rat. J Endocrinol 1970; 48:477–478.
10. Pepe GJ, Albrecht ED. Transutero placental metabolism of cortisol and cortisone during mid and late gestation in the baboon. Endocrinology 1984; 115:1946–1951.
11. Murphy BEP. Cortisol and cortisone in human fetal development. J Steroid Biochem 1979; 11:509–513.
12. Boyard F, Ances IG, Tapper AJ, et al. Transplacental passage and fetal secretion of aldosterone. J Clin Invest 1970; 49:1389–1392.
13. Ron M, Levitz M, Chuba J, et al.Transfer of 25-hydroxyvitamin D_3 and 1,25-dihydroxyvitamin D_3 across the perfused human placenta. Am J Obstet Gynecol 1984; 148:370–374.
14. Roti E, Gnudi A, Braverman LE. The placental transport, synthesis and metabolism of hormone and drugs which affect thyroid function. Endocr Rev 1983; 4:131–149.
15. Glatz TH, Weitzman RE, Nathanielsz PW, et al. Metabolic clearance rate and transplacental passage of oxytocin in the pregnant ewe and fetus. Endocrinology 1980; 106:1006–1011.
16. Stegner H, Leake RD, Palmer SM, et al. Permeability of the sheep placenta to ^{125}I-arginine vasopressin. Dev Pharmacol Ther 1984; 7:140–144.
17. Sopelak VM, Hodgen GD. Infusion of gonadotropin releasing hormone agonist during pregnancy: maternal and fetal responses in primates. Am J Obstet Gynecol 1987; 156:755–760.

18. Garel JM, Milhaud G, Sizonenko PC. Inactivation de la calcitonine porcine par différents organes foetaux et maternels du rat. C R Acad Sci Paris 1970; 270:2469–2471.

19. Adam PAJ, King KC, Schwartz R, et al. Human placental barrier to ^{125}I-glucagon early in gestation. J Clin Endocrinol Metab 1972; 34:772–782.

20. Sperling MA, Erenberg A, Fiser RH, et al. Placental transfer of glucagon in sheep. Endocrinology 1973; 93:1435–1438.

21. Miyakawa I, Ikeda I, Maeyama M. Transport of ACTH across human placenta. J Clin Endocrinol Metab 1974; 39:440–442.

22. Campbell EA, Linton EA, Wolfe CDA, et al. Plasma corticotropin releasing hormone concentrations during pregnancy and parturition. J Clin Endocrinol Metab 1987; 64:1054–1059.

23. Wolf H, Sabata V, Frerichs H, et al. Evidence for impermeability of the human placenta for insulin. Horm Metab Res 1969; 1:224–227.

24. Balabanova S, Lang T, Wolf AS, et al. Placental transfer of parathyroid hormone. J Perinat Med 1986; 14:243–250.

25. King KC, Adam PAJ, Schwartz R, et al. Human placental transfer of human growth hormone. Pediatrics 1971; 48:534–539.

26. Foster DL, Karsch FJ, Nalbandov AV. Regulation of luteinizing hormone (LH) in the fetal and neonatal lamb. II Study of placental transfer of LH in the sheep. Endocrinology 1972; 90:589–592.

27. Symonds EM, Furler I. Plasma renin levels in the normal and anephric fetus at birth. Biol Neonate 1973; 23:133–138.

28. Blay J, Hollenberg MD. The nature and function of the polypeptide growth factor receptors in the human placenta. J Dev Physiol 1989; 12:237–248.

29. Luschinsky HL, Singher HO. Identification and assay of monoamine oxidase in the human placenta. Arch Biochem 1948; 19:95–107.

30. Iisalo E, Castren O. The enzymatic inactivation of noradrenaline in human placental tissue. Ann Med Exp Biol Fenn 1967; 45:253–257.

31. Siiteri PK, MacDonald PC. Placental estrogen biosynthesis during human pregnancy. J Clin Endocrinol Metab 1966; 26:751–761.

32. Ryan KJ. Placental synthesis of steroid hormones. In: Tulchinsky D, Ryan KJ, eds. Maternal-Fetal Endocrinology. Philadelphia: W. B. Saunders, 1980: 3–16.

33. Diczfalusy E. Endocrine functions of the human fetoplacental unit. Fed Proc 1964; 23:791–798.

34. Buster JE, Simon JA. Placental hormones, hormonal preparation for and control of parturition, and hormonal diagnosis of pregnancy. In: DeGroot LJ, Besser GM, Cahill GF Jr, et al., eds. Endocrinology. 2nd ed. Philadelphia: W. B. Saunders, 1989: 2043–2073.

35. Albrecht ED, Pepe GJ. Placental steroid hormone biosynthesis in primate pregnancy. Endocr Rev 1990; 11:124–150.

36. Khodr GS, Siler-Khodr TM. The effect of luteinizing hormone releasing factor on human chorionic gonadotropin secretion. Fertil Steril 1978; 30:301–304.

37. Siler-Khodr TM. Hypothalamic-like releasing hormones of the placenta. Clin Perinatol 1983; 10:553–566.

38. Radovick S, Wondisford FE, Nakayama Y, et al. Isolation and characterization of the human gonadotropin releasing hormone gene in the hypothalamus and placenta. Mol Endocrinol 1990; 4:476–480.

39. Ringler GE, Kallen CB, Strauss JF III. Regulation of human trophoblast function by glucocorticoids: dexamethasone promotes increased secretion of chorionic gonadotropin. Endocrinology 1989; 124:1625–1631.

40. Maruo T, Matsuo H, Ohtani T, et al. Differential modulation of chorionic gonadotropin (CG) subunit messenger ribonucleic acid levels and CG secretion by progesterone in normal placenta and choriocarcinoma cultured in vitro. Endocrinology 1986; 119:855–864.

41. Abu-Hakima M, Branchaud CL, Goodyear CG, et al. The effects of human chorionic gonadotropin on growth and steroidogenesis of the human fetal adrenal gland in vitro. Am J Obstet Gynecol 1987; 156:681–687.

42. Harada A, Hershman JM, Reed AW, et al. Comparison of thyroid stimulators and thyroid hormone concentrations in the sera of pregnant women. J Clin Endocrinol Metab 1979; 48:793–797.

43. Pekonen F, Alfthan H, Stenman UH, et al. Human chorionic gonadotropin (hCG) and thyroid function in early human pregnancy: circadian variation and evidence for intrinsic thyrotropic activity of hCG. J Clin Endocrinol Metab 1988; 66:853–856.

44. Miller WL, Eberhardt NL. Structure and evolution of the growth hormone gene family. Endocr Rev 1983; 4:97–130.

45. Barsh GS, Seeburg PH, Gelinas RE. The human growth hormone gene family: structure and evolution of the chromosomal locus. Nucleic Acids Res 1983; 11:3939–3985.

46. Chakravarti A, Phillips JA, Mellits KA, et al. Patterns of polymorphism and linkage disequilibrium suggest independent origins of the human growth hormone gene cluster. Proc Natl Acad Sci USA 1984; 81:6085–6089.

47. Hennen G, Frankenne F. Influence des hormones protéiques placentaires sur la physiologie maternelle. Ann Endocrinol (Paris) 1987; 48:278–288.

48. Golander A, Hurley T, Barrett J, et al. Prolactin synthesis by human chorion-decidual tissue. A possible source of prolactin in the amniotic fluid. Science 1978; 202:311–313.

49. Jara CS, Salud AT, Bryant-Greenwood GD, et al. Immunocytochemical localization of the human growth hormone variant in the human placenta. J Clin Endocrinol Metab 1989; 69:1069–1072.

50. Grino M, Chrousos GP, Margioris AN. The corticotropin releasing hormone gene is expressed in human placenta. Biochem Biophys Res Commun 1987; 148:1208–1214.

51. Chen CLC, Chang CC, Krieger DT, et al. Expression and regulation of proopiomelanocortin-like gene in the ovary and placenta: comparison with the testis. Endocrinology 1986; 118:2382–2389.

52. Laatikainen T, Saijonmaa O, Salminen K, et al. Localization and concentrations of β-endorphin and β-lipotrophin in human placenta. Placenta 1987; 8:381–387.

53. Margioris AN, Grino M, Protos P, et al. Corticotropin releasing hormone and oxytocin stimulate the release of placental proopiomelanocortin peptides. J Clin Endocrinol Metab 1988; 66:922–926.

54. Abboud TK. Maternal and fetal β endorphin: effects of pregnancy and labour. Arch Dis Child 1988; 63:707–709.

55. Egan DA, Grzegorczyk V, Tricarico KA, et al. Placental chorionic renin: production, purification and characterization. Biochim Biophys Acta 1988; 965:68–75.

56. Ihara Y, Taii S, Mori T. Expression of renin and angiotensinogen genes in the human placental tissues. Endocrinol Jpn 1987; 34:887–896.

57. Millan MA, Carvallo P, Izumi SI, et al. Novel sites of expression of functional angiotensin II receptors in the late gestation fetus. Science 1989; 244:1340–1342.

58. Rodda CP, Kubota M, Heath JA, et al. Evidence for a novel parathyroid hormone–related protein in fetal lamb, parathyroid glands and sheep placenta: comparisons with a similar protein implicated in humoral hypercalcemia of malignancy. J Endocrinol 1988; 117:261–271.

59. Jousset V, Legendre B, Besnard P, et al. Calcitonin-like immunoreactivity and calcitonin gene expression in the placenta and in the mammary gland of the rat. Acta Endocrinol 1988; 119:443–451.

60. Lee J, Seppala M, Chard T. Characterization of placental leuteinizing hormone releasing factor–like material. Acta Endocrinol 1981; 96:394–397.

61. Nowak RA, Bahr JM. Secretion of a gonadotropin-releasing hormone–(GnRH-)like factor by the rabbit fetal placenta in vitro. Placenta 1987; 8:299–304.

62. Seeburg PH, Adelman J. Characterization of cDNA for precursor of human luteinizing hormone releasing hormone. Nature 1984; 311:666–668.

63. Iwashita M, Evans MI, Catt KJ. Characterization of a gonadotropin releasing hormone receptor site in term placenta and chorionic villi. J Clin Endocrinol Metab 1986; 62:127–133.

64. Gibbons JM Jr, Mitnick M, Chieffo V. In vitro biosynthesis of TSH and LH releasing factors by the human placenta. Am J Obstet Gynecol 1975; 121:127–131.

65. Shambaugh GD, Kubek M, Wilber JF. Thyrotropin releasing hormone activity in the human placenta. J Clin Endocrinol Metab 1979; 48:483–486.

66. Youngblood WW, Humm J, Lipton MA, et al. Thyrotropin releasing hormone bioactivity in placenta: evidence for the existence of substances other than pyroglu-his-pro-NH$_2$ (TRH) capable of stimulating pituitary thyrotropin release. Endocrinology 1980; 106:541–546.

67. Polk DH, Reviczky AL, Lam RW, et al. Thyrotropin releasing hormone. Effect of thyroid status on tissue concentrations in fetal sheep. Clin Res 1988; 36:203A.

68. Kumasaka T, Nishi N, Yaoi Y, et al. Demonstration of immunoreactive somatostatin-like substance in villi and decidua in early pregnancy. Am J Obstet Gynecol 1979; 134:39–44.

69. Watkins WB, Yen SSC. Somatostatin in cytotrophoblast of the immature human placenta: localization by immunoperoxidase cytochemistry. J Clin Endocrinol Metab 1980; 50:969–971.

70. Shibasaki T, Dagiri E, Shizume K, et al. Corticotropin-releasing factor-like activity in human placental extracts. J Clin Endocrinol Metab 1982; 55:384–386.

71. Jones CT, Gu W, Parer JT. Production of corticotrophin releasing hormone by sheep placenta in vivo. J Dev Physiol 1989; 11:97–101.

72. Sasaki A, Liotta AS, Luckey MM, et al. Immunoreactive corticotropin releasing factor is present in human plasma during the third trimester of pregnancy. J Clin Endocrinol Metab 1984; 59:812–814.

73. Campbell EA, Linton EA, Wolfe CDA, et al. Plasma corticotropin-releasing hormone concentrations during pregnancy and parturition. J Clin Endocrinol Metab 1987; 64:1054–1059.

74. Jeske W, Soszyński P, Rogoziński W, et al. Plasma GHRH, CRH, ACTH, β-endorphin, human placental lactogen, GH, and cortisol concentrations at the third trimester of pregnancy. Acta Endocrinol 1989; 120:785–789.

75. Robinson BG, Emanuel RL, Frim DM, et al. Glucocorticoid stimulates expression of corticotropin-releasing hormone gene in human placenta. Proc Natl Acad Sci USA 1988; 85:5244–5248.

76. Frim DM, Emanuel RL, Robinson BG, et al. Characterization and gestational regulation of corticotropin releasing hormone messenger RNA in human placenta. J Clin Invest 1988; 82:287–292.

77. Goland RS, Stark RI, Wardlaw SL. Response to corticotropin-releasing hormone during pregnancy in the baboon. J Clin Endocrinol Metab 1990; 70:925–929.

78. Baird A, Wehrenberg WB, Bohlen P, et al. Immunoreactive and biologically active growth hormone releasing factor in rat placenta. Endocrinology 1985; 117:1598–1601.

79. Mills NC, D'Ercole AJ, Underwood LE, et al. Synthesis of somatomedin C/insulin-like growth factor I by human placenta. Mol Biol Rep 1986; 11:231–236.

80. Shen SJ, Daimon M, Wang CY, et al. Isolation of an insulin-like growth factor II cDNA with a unique 5′ untranslated region from human placenta. Proc Natl Acad Sci USA 1988; 85:1947–1951.

81. Goldstein LD, Reynolds CP, Perez Polo JR. Isolation of human nerve growth factor from placental tissue. Neurochem Res 1978; 3:185–193.

82. Walker P, Weichsel ME Jr, Fisher DA. Human nerve growth factor: lack of immunoreactivity with mouse nerve growth factor. Life Sci 1980; 26:195–200.

83. Frolick CA, Dart LL, Meyers CA, et al. Purification and initial characterization of a type B transforming growth factor from human placenta. Proc Natl Acad Sci USA 1983; 80:3676–3680.

84. Derynck R, Jarrett JA, Chen EY, et al. Human transforming growth factor α complimentary DNA sequence and expression in normal and transformed cells. Nature 1985; 316:701–705.

85. Hill DJ, Milner RDG. Mechanisms of fetal growth. In: Brook CDG, ed. Clinical Paediatric Endocrinology. Oxford: Blackwell Scientific, 1989: 3–31.

86. Hock RA, Hollenberg MD. Characterization of the receptor for epidermal growth factor–urogastrone in human placental membranes. J Biol Chem 19808 255:10731–10736.

87. Han VKM, Hunter ES III, Pratt RM, et al. Expression of rat transforming growth factor alpha mRNA during development occurs predominantly in the maternal decidua. Mol Cell Biol 1987; 7:2335–2343.

88. Freemark M, Comer M. Epidermal growth factor (EGF)–like transforming growth factor (TGF) activity and EGF receptors in ovine fetal tissues: possible role for TGF in ovine fetal development. Pediatr Res 1987; 22:609–615.

89. Morrish DW, Bhardwaj D, Dabbagh LK, et al. Epidermal growth factor induces differentiation and secretion of human chorionic gonadotropin and placental lactogen in normal human placenta. J Clin Endocrinol Metab 1987; 65:1282–1290.

90. Goustin AS, Betshultz C, Pfeifer-Ohlsson S, et al. Coexpression of the cis and myc proto-oncogenes in developing human placenta suggests autocrine control of trophoblast growth. Cell 1985; 41:301–312.

91. McGregor WG, Raymoure WJ, Kuhn RW, et al. Fetal tissue can synthesize a placental hormone. J Clin Invest 1981; 68:306–309.

92. Goldsmith PC, McGregor WG, Raymoure WJ, et al. Cellular localization of chorionic gonadotropin in human fetal liver and kidney. J Clin Endocrinol Metab 1983; 57:654–661.

93. Kapcala LP. Immunoassayable adrenocorticotropin in peripheral organs: concentrations during early development. Life Sci 1985; 37:2283–2290.

94. Martino E, Lernmark A, Seo H, et al. High concentration of thyrotropin releasing hormone in pancreatic islets. Proc Natl Acad Sci USA 1978; 75:4265–4267.

95. Pekary AE, Meyer NV, Vaillant C, et al. Thyrotropin releasing hormone and a homologous peptide in the male rat reproductive system. Biochem Biophys Res Commun 1980; 95:993–1000.

96. Suda T, Tomori N, Tozawa F, et al. Distribution and characterization of immunoreactive corticotropin-releasing factor in human tissues. J Clin Endocrinol Metab 1984; 59:861–866.

97. Petrusz P, Merchenthaler I, Maderdrut JL, et al. Corticotropin releasing factor (CRF)–like immunoreactivity in the vertebrate endocrine pancreas. Proc Natl Acad Sci USA 1983; 80:1721–1725.

98. Nieuwenhuyzen Kruseman AC, Linton EA, Ackland J, et al. Heterogeneous immunocytochemical reactivities of oCRF-41-like material in the human hypothalamus, pituitary and gastrointestinal tract. Neuroendocrinology 1984; 38:212–216.

99. Thompson RC, Seasholtz AF, Herbert E. Rat corticotropin releasing hormone gene: sequence and tissue specific expression. Mol Endocrinol 1987; 1:363–370.

100. Shibaski T, Kiyosawa Y, Masuda A, et al. Distribution of growth hormone releasing hormone–like immunoreactivity in human tissue extracts. J Clin Endocrinol Metab 1984; 59:263–268.

101. Koivusalo F, Leppaluoto J. High TRH immunoreactivity in purified pancreatic extracts of fetal and newborn rats. Life Sci 1979; 24:1655–1658.

102. Engler P, Scanlon MF, Jackson IMD. Thyrotropin releasing hormone in the systemic circulation of the neonatal rat is derived from the pancreas and other extraneural tissues. J Clin Invest 1981; 67:800–808.

103. McIntosh N, Pictet RL, Kaplan SL, et al. The developmental pattern of somatostatin in the embryonic and fetal rat pancreas. Endocrinology 1977; 101:825–829.

104. Koshimizu T. The development of pancreatic and gastrointestinal somatostatin-like immunoreactivity and its relationship to feeding in neonatal rats. Endocrinology 1983; 112:911–916.

105. Wu P, Jackson IMD. Identification, characterization and localization of thyrotropin releasing hormone precursor peptides in perinatal rat pancreas. Regul Pept 1988; 22:347–360.

106. Lamberton P, Wu P, Jackson IMD. Thyrotropin releasing hormone release from rat pancreas is stimulated by serotonin but inhibited by carbachol. Endocrinology 1985; 117:1834–1838.

107. Rahier J, Wallon J, Henquin JC. Abundance of somatostatin cells in the human neonatal pancreas. Diabetologia 1980; 18:251–254.

108. Leduque P, Aratan-Spire S, Czernichow P, et al. Ontogenesis of thyrotropin-releasing hormone in the human fetal pancreas. J Clin Invest 1986; 78:1028–1034.

109. Saito H, Saito S, Sano T, et al. Fetal and maternal plasma levels of immunoreactive somatostatin at delivery: evidence for its increase in the umbilical artery and its arterio-venous gradient in the feto-placental circulation. J Clin Endocrinol Metab 1983; 56:567–571.

110. Koshimizu T, Ohyama Y, Yokota Y, et al. Peripheral plasma concentrations of somatostatin-like immunoreactivity in newborns and infants. J Clin Endocrinol Metab 1985; 61:78–82.

111. Perelman AH, Klein AH, Fisher DA. Cord blood thyrotropin releasing hormone (TRH). Clin Res 1981; 29:111A.

112. Umans JG, Umans HR, Szeto HH. Effects of thyrotropin releasing hormone in the fetal lamb. Am J Obstet Gynecol 1986; 155:1266–1271.

113. Gluckman PD, Grumbach MM, Kaplan SL. The neuroendocrine regulation of growth hormone and prolactin in the mammalian fetus. Endocr Rev 1981; 2:363–395.

114. Stark RI, Frantz AG. ACTH–β-endorphin in pregnancy. Clin Perinatol 1983; 10:653–667.

115. Mulchahey JJ, DiBlasio AM, Martin MC, et al. Hormone production and peptide regulation of the human fetal pituitary gland. Endocr Rev 1987; 8:406–425.

116. Fisher DA. Maternal-fetal thyroid function in pregnancy. Clin Perinatol 1983; 10:615–626.

117. Falin LI. The development of human hypophysis and differentiation of cells of the anterior lobe during embryonic life. Acta Anat (Basel) 1961; 44:188–205.

118. Conklin JL. The development of the human fetal adenohypophysis. Anat Rec 1968; 160:79–91.

119. Thiveris JA, Currie RW. Observations in the hypothalamo-hypophyseal portal vasculature in the developing human fetus. Am J Anat 1980; 157:441–444.

120. Hyyppa M. Hypothalamic monoamines in human fetus. Neuroendocrinology 1972; 9:257–266.

121. Raiha N, Hjelt L. The correlation between the development of the hypophysial portal system and the onset of neurosecretory activity in the human fetus and infant. Acta Paediatr Scand 1957; 46:610–616.

122. Bresson JL, Clavequin MC, Fellman D, et al. Ontogeny of the neuroglandular system revealed with HPGRF-44 antibodies in human hypothalamus. Neuroendocrinology 1984; 39:68–73.

123. Bugnon C, Fellman D, Gouget A, et al. Corticolibrin neurons: cytophysiology, phylogeny and ontogeny. J Steroid Biochem 1984; 20:183–195.

124. Bresson JL, Clavequin MC, Fellman D, et al. Human corticolibrin hypothalamic neuroglandular system: comparative immunocytochemical study with anti-rat and anti-ovine corticotropin-releasing factor sera in the early stages of development. Dev Brain Res 1987; 32:241–246.

125. Bugnon C, Fellmann D, Block B. Immunocytochemical study of the ontogenesis of hypothalamic somatostatin-containing neurons in the human fetus. Cell Tissue Res 1977; 183:319–328.

126. Bugnon C, Block B, Lenys D, et al. Cytoimmunological study of the LH-RH neurons in humans during fetal life. In: Scott DE, Koslowski GP, Weindl A, eds. Brain Endocrine Interactions. III. Neural Hormones and Reproduction. Basel: S. Karger, 1978: 183–196.

127. Winters AJ, Eskay RL, Porter JC. Concentration and distribution of TRH and LRH in the human fetal brain. J Clin Endocrinol Metab 1974; 39:269–273.

128. Kaplan SL, Grumbach MM, Aubert ML. The ontogenesis of pituitary hormones and hypothalamic factors in the human fetus: maturation of central nervous system regulation of anterior pituitary function. Recent Prog Horm Res 1976; 32:161–243.

129. McNeilly S, Gilmore D, Dobbie G, et al. Prolactin releasing activity in the early foetal hypothalamus. J Endocrinol 1977; 73:533–534.

130. Baker BL, Jaffe RB. The genesis of cell types in the adenohypophysis of the human fetus as observed by immunohistochemistry. Am J Anat 1975; 143:137–161.

131. Begeot M, Dubois MP, Dubois PM. Immunologic localization of α- and β-endorphins and β-lipotropin in corticotrophic cells of the normal and anencephalic fetal pituitaries. Cell Tissue Res 1978; 193:413–422.

132. Suganuma N, Seo H, Yamamoto N, et al. The ontogeny of growth hormone in the human fetal pituitary. Am J Obstet Gynecol 1989; 160:729–733.

133. Goodyear CG, Sellen JM, Fuks M, et al. Regulation of growth hormone secretion from human fetal pituitaries, interactions between growth hormone releasing factor and somatostatin. Reprod Nutr Dev 1987; 27:461–470.

134. de Zegher F, Daaboul J, Grumbach MM, et al. Hormone ontogeny in the ovine fetus and neonate. XXII. The effect of somatostatin on the growth hormone (GH) response to GH-releasing factor. Endocrinology 1989; 124:1114–1117.

135. Freemark M, Comer M. Purification of a distinct placental lactogen receptor, a new member of the growth hormone/prolactin receptor family. J Clin Invest 1989; 83:883–889.

136. Hill DJ, Freemark M, Strain AH, et al. Placental lactogen and growth hormone receptors in human fetal tissues: relationship to fetal plasma hPL concentrations and fetal growth. J Clin Endocrinol Metab 1988; 66:1283–1290.

137. Carr BR, Casey ML. Growth of the adrenal gland of the normal human fetus during early gestation. Early Hum Dev 1982; 6:121–124.

138. Winter JSD. Fetal and neonatal adrenocortical physiology. In: Polin RA, Fox WW, eds. Neonatal and Fetal Medicine. Philadelphia: W. B. Saunders, 1992: 1829–1841.

139. Pepe GJ, Albrecht ED. Regulation of the primate fetal adrenal cortex. Endocr Rev 1990; 11:151–176.

140. Voutilainen R, Miller WL. Developmental expression of genes for the steroidogenic enzymes P450scc (20,20-desmolase), P450c17 (17 α-hydroxylase/17,20-lyase), and P450c21 (21-hydroxylase) in the human fetus. J Clin Endocrinol Metab 1986; 63:1145–1150.

141. John ME, Simpson ER, Carr BR, et al. Ontogeny of adrenal steroid hydroxylase: evidence for cAMP independent gene expression. Mol Cell Endocrinol 1987; 50:263–268.

142. Korte K, Hemsell PG, Mason JI. Sterol sulfate metabolism in the adrenals of the human fetus, anencephalic newborn and adult. J Clin Endocrinol Metab 1982; 55:671–675.

143. Nelson HP, Kuhn RW, Deyman ME, et al. Human fetal adrenal definitive and fetal zone metabolism of pregnenolone and corticosterone: alternative biosynthetic pathways and absence of detectable aldosterone synthesis. J Clin Endocrinol Metab 1990; 70:693–698.

144. Carr BR, Porter JC, MacDonald PC, et al. Metabolism of low density lipoprotein by human fetal adrenal tissue. Endocrinology 1980; 107:1034–1040.

145. Carr BR, Simpson ER. De novo synthesis of cholesterol by human fetal adrenal gland. Endocrinology 1981; 108:2154–2162.

146. Carr BR, Ohashi M, Simpson ER. Low density lipoprotein binding and de novo synthesis of cholesterol in the neocortex and fetal zones of the human fetal adrenal gland. Endocrinology 1982; 110:1994–1998.

147. Gray ES, Abramovitch DR. Morphologic features of the anencephalic adrenal gland in early pregnancy. Am J Obstet Gynecol 1980; 137:491–495.

148. Walsh SW, Norman RL, Novy MJ. In utero regulation of rhesus monkey fetal adrenals: effects of dexamethasone, adrenocorticotropin, thyrotropin-releasing hormone, prolactin, human chorionic gonadotropin, and α-melanocyte-stimulating hormone on fetal and maternal plasma steroids. Endocrinology 1979; 104:1805–1813.

149. Goland RS, Wardlow SL, Blum M, et al. Biologically active corticotropin-releasing hormone in maternal and fetal plasma during pregnancy. Am J Obstet Gynecol 1988; 159:884–890.

150. Winters AJ, Oliver C, Colston C, et al. Plasma ACTH levels in the human fetus and neonate as related to age and parturition. J Clin Endocrinol Metab 1974; 39:269–273.

151. Jones CT, Luther E, Ritchie JWK, et al. The clearance of ACTH from the adult and fetal sheep. Endocrinology 1975; 96:231–234.

152. Byrne GC, Perry YS, Winter JSD. Steroid inhibitory effects upon human adrenal 3β-hydroxysteroid dehydrogenase activity. J Clin Endocrinol Metab 1986; 62:413–418.

153. Beitins IZ, Bayard F, Ances FIG, et al. The metabolic clearance rate, blood production, interconversion and transplacental passage of cortisol and cortisone in pregnancy near term. Pediatr Res 1973; 7:509–519.

154. Dorr HG, Versmold HT, Sippell WG, et al. Antenatal betamethasone therapy: effects on maternal, fetal, and neonatal mineralocorticoids, glucocorticoids and progestins. J Pediatr 1986; 108:990–993.

155. Charnvises S, Fencl MD, Osathanondh R, et al. Adrenal steroids in maternal and cord blood after dexamethasone administration at midterm. J Clin Endocrinol Metab 1985; 61:1220–1222.

156. Rose JC, Turner CS, Ray DeW, et al. Evidence that cortisol inhibits basal adrenocorticotropin secretion in the sheep fetus by 0.70 gestation. Endocrinology 1988; 123:1307–1313.

157. Yang K, Jones SA, Challis JRG. Changes in glucocorticoid receptor number in the hypothalamus of the sheep fetus with gestational age and after adrenocorticotropin treatment. Endocrinology 1990; 126:11–17.

158. Johnson JW, Mitzner W, Beck JC, et al. Long term effects of betamethasone in fetal development. Am J Obstet Gynecol 1981; 141:1053–1064.

159. Ballard PL. Glucocorticoids and differentiation. In: Baxter JD, Rousseau GG, eds. Monographs on Endocrinology. Vol 12. Glucocorticoid Action. Berlin: Springer-Verlag, 1979: 493–575.

160. Pavlik A, Buresova M. The neonatal cerebellum: the highest level of glucocorticoid receptors in the brain. Dev Brain Res 1984; 12:13–20.

161. Liggins GC. Adrenocortical-related maturational events in the fetus. Am J Obstet Gynecol 1976; 126:931–941.

162. Fisher DA. The unique endocrine milieu of the fetus. J Clin Invest 1986; 78:603–611.

163. Beitins IZ, Bayard F, Levitsky L, et al. Plasma aldosterone concentrations at delivery and during the newborn period. J Clin Invest 1972; 51:386–394.

164. Beitins IZ, Graham GG, Kowarski A, et al. Adrenal function in normal infants and in marasmus and kwashiorkor: plasma aldosterone concentration and aldosterone secretion rate. J Pediatr 1974; 84:444–451.

165. Katz FH, Beck P, Makowski EL. The renin-aldosterone system in mother and fetus at term. Am J Obstet Gynecol 1974; 118:51–55.

166. Siegel SR, Fisher DA. Ontogeny of the renin-angiotensin-aldosterone system in the fetal and newborn lamb. Pediatr Res 1980; 14:99–102.

167. Ito Y, Matsumoto T, Ohbu K, et al. Concentrations of human atrial natriuretic peptide in the cord blood and the plasma of the newborn. Acta Paediatr Scand 1988; 77:76–78.

168. Cheung CY, Gibbs DM, Brace AA. Atrial natriuretic factor in maternal and fetal sheep. Am J Physiol 1987; 252:E279–E282.

169. Toran Allerand CD. Normal development of the hypothalamic-pituitary-thyroid axis. In: Ingbar SH, Braverman LE, eds. The Thyroid. Philadelphia: J. B. Lippincott, 1986: 7–23.

170. Fisher DA, Dussault JH. Development of the mammalian thyroid gland. In: Greer MA, Solomon DH, eds. Handbook of Physiology. Sect 7: Endocrinology. Vol III. The Thyroid. Washington DC: American Physiological Society, 1974: 21–38.

171. Fisher DA, Dussault JH, Sack J, et al. Ontogenesis of hypothalamic-pituitary-thyroid function and metabolism in man, sheep and rat. Recent Prog Horm Res 1977; 33:59–116.

172. Moseley JM, Matthews EW, Breed RH, et al. The ultimobranchial origin of calcitonin. Lancet 1968; 1:108–110.

173. Vulsma T, Gons MH, de Vijlder JJ. Maternal-fetal transfer of thyroxine in congenital hypothyroidism due to a total organification defect or thyroid agenesis. N Engl J Med 1989; 321:13–16.

174. Morreale De Escobar G, Calvo R, Obregon MJ, et al. Contribution of maternal thyroxine to fetal thyroxine pools in normal rats near term. Endocrinology 1990; 126:2765–2767.

175. Fisher DA, Klein AH. Thyroid development and disorders of thyroid function in the newborn. N Engl J Med 1981; 304:702–712.

176. Fisher DA, Polk DA. Development of the thyroid. Baillieres Clin Endocrinol Metab 1989; 3:627–657.

177. Ballabio M, Nicolini V, Jowett T, et al. Maturation of thyroid function in the normal human fetus. Clin Endocrinol 1989; 31:565–571.

178. Roti E. Regulation of thyroid stimulating hormone (TSH) secretion in the fetus and neonate. J Endocrinol Invest 1988; 11:145–158.

179. Jacobsen BB, Andersen H, Dige-Petersen H, et al. Pituitary-thyroid responsiveness to thyrotropin-releasing hormone in preterm and small-for-gestational age newborns. Acta Paediatr Scand 1977; 66:541–548.

180. Ingbar SH. Autoregulation of the thyroid: response to iodide excess and depletion. Mayo Clin Proc 1972; 47:814–823.

181. Sherwin JR. Development of regulatory mechanisms in the thyroid: failure of iodide to suppress iodide transport activity. Proc Soc Exp Biol Med 1982; 169:458–462.

182. Castaign H, Fournet JP, Leger FA, et al. Thyroid of the newborn and postnatal iodine overload. Arch Fr Pediatr 1979; 36:356–368.

183. Leonard JL, Visser TJ. Biochemistry of deiodination. In: Hennemann G, ed. Thyroid Hormone Metabolism. New York: Marcel Dekker, 1986: 189–229.

184. Fraser M, Liggins GC. Thyroid hormone kinetics during late pregnancy in the ovine fetus. J Dev Physiol 1988; 10:461–471.

185. Polk DH, Wu WY, Wright C, et al. Ontogeny of thyroid hormone effect on tissue 5′-monodeiodinase activity in fetal sheep. Am J Physiol 1988; 254:E337–E341.

186. Polk DH, Cheromcha D, Reviczky A, et al. Nuclear thyroid hormone receptors: ontogeny and thyroid hormone effects in sheep. Am J Physiol 1989; 256:E543–E549.

187. Fisher DA, Polk DH. Maturation of thyroid hormone actions. In: Delange F, Fisher DA, Glinoer D, eds. Research in Congenital Hypothyroidism. New York: Plenum, 1989: 61–77.

188. Bernal J, Pekonen F. Ontogenesis of nuclear 3,5,3′-triiodothyronine receptors in human fetal brain. Endocrinology 1984; 114:677–679.

189. Gonzales LW, Ballard PL. Identification and characterization of nuclear 3,5,3′-triiodothyronine–binding sites in fetal human lung. J Clin Endocrinol Metab 1981; 53:21–28.

190. Jost A. A new look at the mechanisms controlling sexual differentiation in mammals. Johns Hopkins Med J 1972; 130:38–53.

191. Wilson JD. Sexual differentiation. Annu Rev Physiol 1978; 40:279–306.

192. Pelliniemi LJ, Dym M. The fetal gonad and sexual differentiation. In: Tulchinsky D, Ryan KJ, eds. Maternal-Fetal Endocrinology. Philadelphia: W. B. Saunders, 1980: 252–280.

193. Page DC, Mosher R, Simpson EM, et al. The sex determining region of the human Y chromosome encodes a finger protein. Cell 1987; 51:1091–1104.

194. Schneider-Gädicke A, Beer-Romero P, Brown LG, et al. ZFX has a gene structure similar to ZFY, the putative human sex determinant, and escapes X inactivation. Cell 1989; 57:1247–1258.

195. Warren DW, Dufau ML, Catt KJ. Hormonal regulation of gonadotropin receptors and steroidogenesis in cultured fetal rat testes. Science 1982; 218:375–377.

196. Jost A, Vigier B, Prepin J, et al. Studies on sex differentiation in mammals. Recent Prog Horm Res 1973; 29:1–41.

197. Josso N. Antimullerian hormone: new perspectives for a sexist molecule. Endocr Rev 1986; 7:421–433.

198. Donahoe PK, Budzik GP, Trelstad M, et al. Mullerian inhibiting substance: an update. Recent Prog Horm Res 1982; 38:279–326.

199. Hutson JM, Fallat ME, Kamagata S, et al. Phosphorylation events during mullerian duct regression. Science 1984; 223:586–588.

200. Voutilainen R, Miller WL. Human mullerian inhibitory factor messenger

ribonucleic acid is hormonally regulated in the fetal testis and in adult granulosa cells. Mol Endocrinol 1987; 1:604–608.

201. Barraclough CA, Gorski RA. Evidence that the hypothalamus is responsible for androgen-induced sterility in the female rat. Endocrinology 1961; 68:68–79.

202. Naftolin F, Brawer JB. The effect of estrogens on hypothalamic structure and function. Am J Obstet Gynecol 1978; 132:758–765.

203. Ryan KJ, Naftolin F, Reddy V, et al. Estrogen formation in the brain. Am J Obstet Gynecol 1972; 114:454–460.

204. Sholl SA, Goy RW, Kim KL. 5α-Reductase, aromatase, and androgen receptor levels in the monkey brain during fetal development. Endocrinology 1989; 124:627–634.

205. Visser M, Swaab DF. Life span changes in the presence of melanocyte-stimulating-hormone-containing cells in the human pituitary. J Dev Physiol 1979; 1:161–178.

206. Perry RA, Mulvogue HM, McMillen IC, et al. Immunohistochemical localization of ACTH in the adult and fetal sheep pituitary. J Dev Physiol 1985; 7:397–404.

207. Silman RE, Chard T, Lowry PJ, et al. Human foetal pituitary peptides and parturition. Nature 1976; 260:716–718.

208. Silman RE, Holland T, Chard T, et al. The ACTH family tree of the rhesus monkey changes with development. Nature 1978; 276:526–528.

209. Osamura RY, Tsutsumi Y, Watanabe K. Light and electron microscopic localization of ACTH and proopiomelanocortin-derived peptides in human developmental and neoplastic cells. J Histochem Cytochem 1984; 32:885–893.

210. Glickman JA, Carson GD, Challis JRG. Differential effects of synthetic adrenocorticotropin and melanocyte stimulating hormone on adrenal formation in human and sheep fetus. Endocrinology 1979; 104:34–39.

211. Swaab DF, Martin JT. Functions of alpha melanotropin and other opiomelanocortin peptides in labour, intrauterine growth and brain development. Ciba Found Symp 1981; 81:196–217.

212. Facchinetti F, Storchi AR, Petraglia F, et al. Ontogeny of pituitary β-endorphin and related peptides in the human embryo and fetus. Am J Obstet Gynecol 1987; 156:735–739.

213. Fisher DA. Maternal-fetal neurohypophyseal system. Clin Perinatol 1983; 10:695–708.

214. Leake RD, Fisher DA. Ontogeny of vasopressin in man. In: Czernichow P, Robinson AG, eds. Diabetes Insipidus in Man. Frontiers in Hormone Research. Vol 13. Basel: S. Karger, 1985: 42–51.

215. Perks AM. Developmental and evolutionary aspects of the neurohypophysis. Am Zool 1977; 17:833–849.

216. Pavel S. Arginine vasotocin as a pineal hormone. J Neural Transm 1978; 13(Suppl):135–155.

217. Ervin MG, Leake RD, Ross MG, et al. Arginine vasotocin in ovine maternal and fetal blood, fetal urine, and amniotic fluid. J Clin Invest 1985; 75:1696–1701.

218. Bell RJ, Congiu M, Hardy KJ, et al. Gestation-dependent aspects of the response of the ovine fetus to osmotic stress induced by maternal water deprivation. Q J Exp Physiol 1984; 69:187–195.

219. Daniel SS, Stark RI, Husain MK, et al. Role of vasopressin in fetal homeostasis. Am J Physiol 1982; 242:F740–F744.

220. DeVane GW, Naden RP, Porter JC, et al. Mechanism of arginine vasopressin release in the sheep fetus. Pediatr Res 1982; 16:504–507.

221. Stark RI, Daniel SS, Hussain MK, et al. Vasopressin concentration in amniotic fluid as an index of fetal hypoxia: mechanisms of release in sheep. Pediatr Res 1984; 18:552–558.

222. Stegner H, Leake RD, Palmer SM, et al. The effect of hypoxia on neurohypophyseal hormone release in fetal and maternal sheep. Pediatr Res 1984; 18:188–191.

223. DeVane GW, Porter JC. An apparent stress-induced release of arginine vasopressin by human neonates. J Clin Endocrinol Metab 1980; 51:1412–1416.

224. Kelly RT, Rose JC, Meis PJ, et al. Vasopressin is important for restoring cardiovascular homeostasis in fetal lambs subjected to hemorrhage. Am J Obstet Gynecol 1983; 146:807–812.

225. Irion GL, Mack CE, Clark KE. Fetal hemodynamic and fetoplacental vascular response to exogenous arginine vasopressin. Am J Obstet Gynecol 1990; 162:1115–1120.

226. Jones CT, Ritchie JW. The effects of adrenergic blockade on fetal response to hypoxia. J Dev Physiol 1983; 5:211–222.

227. Norman LJ, Challis JRG. Dose dependent effects of arginine vasopressin on endocrine and blood gas responses of fetal sheep during the last third of pregnancy. Can J Physiol Pharmacol 1987; 65:2291–2296.

228. Norman LJ, Challis JRG. Synergism between systemic corticotropin-releasing factor and arginine vasopressin on adrenocorticotropin release in vivo varies as a function of gestational age in the ovine fetus. Endocrinology 1987; 120:1052–1058.

229. Brooks AN, White A. Activation of pituitary adrenal function in fetal sheep by corticotrophin-releasing factor and arginine vasopressin. J Endocrinol 1990; 124:27–35.

230. Benedetto MT, DeCicco F, Rossiello F, et al. Oxytocin receptor in human fetal membranes at term and during labor. J Steroid Biochem 1990; 35:205–208.

231. Tribollet E, Charpak S, Schmidt A, et al. Appearance and transient expression of oxytocin receptors in fetal, infant and peripubertal rat brain studied by autoradiography and electrophysiology. J Neurosci 1989; 9:1764–1773.

232. Ervin MG, Miller SJ, Ramseyer LJ, et al. Renal arginine vasopressin receptors in newborn and adult sheep. Clin Res 1990; 38:170A.

233. Robillard JE, Weitzman RE. Developmental aspects of the fetal renal response to exogenous arginine vasopressin. Am J Physiol 1980; 238:F407–F414.

234. Ervin MG, Ross MG, Leake RD, et al. Changes in steady state plasma arginine vasotocin levels affect ovine fetal renal and cardiovascular function. Endocrinology 1986; 118:759–765.

235. Ross MG, Ervin MG, Leake RD, et al. Fetal lung liquid regulation by neuropeptides. Am J Obstet Gynecol 1984; 150:421–425.

236. Cassin S, Perks AM. Studies of factors which stimulate lung fluid secretion in fetal goats. J Dev Physiol 1982; 4:311–325.

237. Perks AM, Cassin S. The effects of arginine vasopressin and epinephrine on lung liquid production in fetal goats. Can J Physiol Pharmacol 1989; 67:491–498.

238. Kullama LK, Balaraman V, Claybaugh JR, et al. Ontogeny of vasoconstrictor neurohypophysial hormone function in rats. Am J Physiol 1990; 258:R263–R268.

239. Manku MS, Mtabaji JB, Horrobin DF. Effect of cortisol, prolactin and ADH on the amniotic membrane. Nature 1975; 258:78–80.

240. Fisher DA, Pyle HR Jr, Porter JC, et al. Control of water balance in the newborn. Am J Dis Child 1963; 106:137–146.

241. Coupland RS. The prenatal development of the abdominal paraaortic bodies in man. J Anat 1952; 86:357–372.

242. Niemineva R, Pekkarinen A. The noradrenaline and adrenaline content of human fetal adrenal glands and aortic bodies. Ann Med Exp Biol Fenn 1952; 30:274–286.

243. Gospodarowicz D. Epidermal and nerve growth factors in mammalian development. Annu Rev Physiol 1981; 43:251–263.

244. Aloe L, Levi-Montalcini R. Nerve growth factor–induced transformation of immature chromaffin cells in vivo into sympathetic neurons: effect of antiserum to nerve growth factor. Proc Natl Acad Sci USA 1979; 76:1246–1250.

245. Wurtman RJ. Control of epinephrine synthesis in the adrenal medulla by the adrenal cortex: hormonal specificity and dose-response characteristics. Endocrinology 1966; 79:608–614.

246. Margolis EL, Rotti J, Jost A. Norepinephrine methylation in fetal rat adrenals. Science 1966; 154:275–276.

247. Comline RS, Silver M. Development of activity in the adrenal medulla of the foetus and newborn animal. Br Med Bull 1966; 22:16–20.

248. Shaul PW, Cha CJM, Oh W. Neonatal sympathoadrenal response to acute hypoxia: impairment after experimental intrauterine growth retardation. Pediatr Res 1989; 25:466–472.

249. Slotkin TA, Seidler FJ. Adrenomedullary catecholamine release in the fetus and newborn: secretory mechanisms and their role in stress and survival. J Dev Physiol 1988; 10:1–16.

250. Padbury JF, Agata Y, Polk DH, et al. Neonatal adaptation: naloxone increases the catecholamine surge at birth. Pediatr Res 1987; 21:590–593.

251. Stonestreet BS, Piasecki GJ, Susa JB, et al. Effects of insulin infusion on catecholamine concentration in fetal sheep. Am J Obstet Gynecol 1989; 160:740–745.

252. Cohen WR, Piasecki GJ, Cohn HE, et al. Plasma catecholamines in the hypoxaemic fetal rhesus monkey. J Dev Physiol 1987; 9:507–515.

253. Pryds O, Christensen NJ, Friis-Hansen B. Increased cerebral blood flow and plasma epinephrine in hypoglycemic, preterm neonates. Pediatrics 1990; 85:172–176.

254. Palmer SM, Oakes GK, Lam RW, et al. Catecholamine physiology in the ovine fetus. I. Gestational age variation in basal plasma concentrations. Am J Obstet Gynecol 1984; 149:420–425.

255. Palmer SM, Oakes GK, Lam RW, et al. Catecholamine physiology in the ovine fetus. II. Metabolic clearance rate of epinephrine. Am J Physiol 1984; 246:E350–E355.

256. Lewis AB, Evans WN, Sischo W. Plasma catecholamine responses to hypoxemia in fetal lambs. Biol Neonate 1982; 41:115–122.

257. Palmer SM, Oakes GK, Champion JA, et al. Catecholamine physiology in the ovine fetus. II. Maternal and fetal response to acute maternal exercise. Am J Obstet Gynecol 1984; 149:426–434.

258. Irestedt L, Lagercrantz H, Hjemdahl P, et al. Fetal and maternal plasma catecholamine levels at elective cesarean section under general or epidural anesthesia versus vaginal delivery. Am J Obstet Gynecol 1982; 142:1004–1010.

259. Padbury JF, Roberman B, Oddie TH, et al. Fetal catecholamine release in response to labor and delivery: the role of fetal acid-base status, sex, and heart rate patterns at term. Obstet Gynecol 1982; 60:607–611.

260. Newnham JP, Marshall JC, Padbury JF, et al. Fetal catecholamine release with preterm delivery. Am J Obstet Gynecol 1984; 149:888–893.

261. Seidler FJ, Brown KK, Smith PG, et al. Toxic effects of hypoxia on neonatal cardiac function in the rat: alpha-adrenergic mechanisms. Toxicol Lett 1987; 37:79–84.

262. Schedewie HK, Fisher DA. Perinatal mineral homeostasis. In: Tulchinsky D, Ryan KJ, eds. Maternal-Fetal Endocrinology. Philadelphia: W. B. Saunders, 1980: 355–386.

263. Care AD. Development of endocrine pathways in the regulation of calcium homeostasis. Baillieres Clin Endocrinol Metab 1989; 3:671–688.

264. Bouillon R, Van Assche FA. Perinatal vitamin D metabolism. Dev Pharmacol Ther 1982; 4(Suppl 1):38–44.

265. Stevenson JC. Mineral needs of the fetus. Curr Top Exp Endocrinol 1983; 5:177–196.

266. Moore ES, Langman CB, Favus MJ, et al. Role of fetal 1,25-dihydroxy-vitamin D production in intrauterine phosphorus and calcium homeostasis. Pediatr Res 1985; 19:566–569.

267. Abbas SK, Care AD, Van Baelen H, et al. Plasma vitamin D–binding protein and free 1,25-dihydroxyvitamin D_3 index in pregnant ewes and their fetuses in the last month of gestation. J Endocrinol 1987; 115:7–12.

268. Care AD, Caple IW, Abbas SK, et al. The effect of fetal thyroparathyroidectomy on the transport of calcium across the ovine placenta to the fetus. Placenta 1986; 7:417–424.

269. Brunette MG, Auger D, Lafond J. Effect of parathyroid hormone on PO_4 transport through the human placenta microvilli. Pediatr Res 1989; 25:15–18.

270. Lafond J, Auger D, Fortier J, et al. Parathyroid hormone receptor in human placental syncytiotrophoblast brush border and basal plasma membranes. Endocrinology 1988; 123:2834–2840.

271. Ross R, Halbert K, Tsang RC. Determination of the production and metabolic clearance rates of 1,25-dihydroxyvitamin D_3 in the pregnant sheep and its chronically catheterized fetus by primed infusion technique. Pediatr Res 1989; 26:633–638.

272. Austin LA, Heath N. Calcitonin, physiology and pathophysiology. N Engl J Med 1981; 304:269–278.

273. Takigawa M, Enomoto M, Shirai E, et al. Differential effects of 1α,25-dihydroxycholecalciferol and 24,25-dihydroxycholecalciferol on proliferation and the differentiated phenotype of rabbit costal chondrocytes in culture. Endocrinology 1988; 122:831–839.

274. Liu HM, Potter EL. Development of the human pancreas. Arch Pathol 1962; 74:439–452.

275. Steinke J, Driscoll S. The extractable insulin content of pancreas from fetuses and infants of diabetic and control mothers. Diabetes 1965; 14:573–578.

276. Assan R, Boillot J. Pancreatic glucagon and glucagon-like maternal in tissues and plasmas from human fetuses 6–26 weeks old. Pathol Biol 1973; 21:149–157.

277. Sperling MA. Carbohydrate metabolism: glucagon, insulin, and somatostatin. In: Tulchinsky D, Ryan KJ, eds. Maternal-Fetal Endocrinology. Philadelphia: W. B. Saunders, 1980: 333–354.

278. Girard J. Control of fetal and neonatal glucose metabolism by pancreatic hormones. Baillieres Clin Endocrinol Metab 1989; 3:817–836.

279. Ammon HP, Glocker C, Waldner RG, et al. Insulin release from pancreatic islets of fetal rats mediated by leucine, b-BCH, tolbutamide, glibenclamide, arginine, potassium chloride, and theophylline does not require stimulation of Ca^{2+} net uptake. Cell Calcium 1989; 10:441–450.

280. Formby B, Ullrich A, Coussens L, et al. Growth hormone stimulates insulin gene expression in cultured human fetal pancreatic islets. J Clin Endocrinol Metab 1988; 66:1075–1079.

281. Muntz DH, Levey GS, Schenk A. Adenosine 3′5′-cyclic monophosphate and phosphodiesterase activities in isolated fetal and neonatal rat pancreatic islets. Endocrinology 1973; 92:614–617.

282. Hole RL, Pian-Smith MCM, Sharp GWG. Development of the biphasic response to glucose in fetal and neonatal rat pancreas. Am J Physiol 1988; 254:E167–E174.

283. Hay WW Jr, Sparks JW, Wilkening RB, et al. Fetal glucose uptake and utilization as functions of maternal glucose concentration. Am J Physiol 1984; 246:E237–E242.

284. Duee PH, Pegorier JP, El Manoubi L, et al. Development of gluconeogenesis from different substrates in newborn rabbit hepatocytes. J Dev Physiol 1986; 8:387–394.

285. Herbin C, Duee PH, Pegorier JP, et al. Premature appearance of gluconeogenesis and fatty acid oxidation in the liver of the post term rabbit fetus. Pediatr Res 1988; 23:224–228.

286. Bloch CA, Menon RK, Sperling MA. Effects of somatostatin and glucose infusion on glucose kinetics in fetal sheep. Am J Physiol 1988; 255:E87–E93.

287. Kaplan SA. The insulin receptor. J Pediatr 1984; 104:327–336.

288. Devaskar SU, Ganguli S, Styer D, et al. Glucagon and glucose dynamics in sheep: evidence for glucagon resistance in the fetus. Am J Physiol 1984; 246:E256–E265.

289. Kaplan MM, Yakoski KA. Maturational patterns of iodothyronine phenolic and tyrosyl ring deiodinase activities in rat cerebrum, cerebellum and hypothalamus. J Clin Invest 1981; 67:1208–1214.

290. Ruiz de Ona C, Jesus Obregon M, Escobar del Rey F, et al. Developmental changes in rat brain 5′-deiodinase and thyroid hormones during the fetal period. The effects of fetal hypothyroidism and maternal thyroid hormones. Pediatr Res 1988; 24:588–594.

291. Padbury JF, Klein AH, Polk DH, et al. The effect of thyroid status in lung and heart beta adrenergic receptors in fetal and newborn sheep. Dev Pharmacol Ther 1986; 9:44–53.

292. Coulombe P, Ruel J, Dussault JH. Effects of neonatal hypo- and

293. Lakshmanan J, Beri U, Perheentupa J, et al. Acquisition of submandibular gland nerve growth factor (SMG-NGF) responsiveness to thyroxine in neonatal mice. J Neurosci Res 1984; 12:71–85.

294. Lakshmanan J, Perheentupa J, Macaso T, et al. Acquisition of urine, kidney and submandibular gland epidermal growth factor responsiveness to thyroxine administration in neonatal mice. Acta Endocrinol 1985; 109:511–516.

295. Alm J, Scott SM, Fisher DA. Epidermal growth factor receptor ontogeny in mice with congenital hypothyroidism. J Dev Physiol 1986; 8:377–385.

296. Hoath SB, Lakshmanan J, Fisher DA. Thyroid hormone effects on skin and hepatic epidermal growth factor concentrations in neonatal and adult mice. Biol Neonate 1984; 45:49–52.

297. Hoath SB, Lakshmanan J, Fisher DA. Epidermal growth factor binding to neonatal mouse skin explants and membrane preparations—effect of triiodothyronine. Pediatr Res 1985; 19:277–280.

298. Perez-Castillo A, Bernal J, Ferriero B, et al. The early ontogenesis of thyroid hormone receptor in the rat fetus. Endocrinology 1985; 117:2457–2461.

299. Padbury JF, Lam RW, Newnham JP, et al. Neonatal adaptation: greater neurosympathetic system activity in preterm than full term sheep at birth. Am J Physiol 1986; 248:E443–E449.

300. Pasqualini JR, Sumida C, Gelly C, et al. Progesterone receptors in the fetal uterus and ovary of the guinea pig: evolution during fetal development and induction and stimulation in estradiol-primed animals. J Steroid Biochem 1976; 7:1031–1038.

301. Yamashita S, Newbold RR, McLachlan JA, et al. Developmental pattern of estrogen receptor expression in female mouse genital tracts. Endocrinology 1989; 125:2888–2896.

302. D'Ercole AJ. Somatomedins/insulin-like growth factors. In: Brook CDG, ed. Clinical Paediatric Endocrinology. 2nd ed. Oxford: Blackwell Scientific, 1989: 74–95.

303. Simmen FA, Simmon RCM, Letcher LR, et al. IGF's in pregnancy: developmental expression in uterus and mammary gland and paracrine actions during embryonic and neonatal growth. In: LeRoith D, Raizada MK, eds. Molecular and Cellular Biology of Insulin-Like Growth Factors and Their Receptors. New York: Plenum, 1989: 195–208.

304. Spaventi R, Antica M, Pavelic K. Insulin and insulin-like growth factor I (IGF-I) in early mouse embryogenesis. Development 1990; 108:491–495.

305. D'Ercole AJ. Somatomedins/insulin-like growth factors and fetal growth. J Dev Physiol 1987; 9:481–495.

306. Han VKM, Hill DJ, Strain AJ, et al. Identification of somatomedin/insulin-like growth factor immunoreactive cells in the human fetus. Pediatr Res 1987; 22:245–249.

307. Han VKM, D'Ercole AJ, Lund PK. Cellular localization of synthesis of somatomedin (insulin-like growth factor) messenger RNA in the human fetus. Science 1987; 236:193–197.

308. D'Ercole AJ, Applewhite GT, Underwood LE. Evidence that somatomedins are synthesized by multiple tissues in the fetus. Dev Biol 1980; 75:315–328.

309. Adams SO, Nissley SP, Handwerger S, et al. Developmental patterns of insulin-like growth factor I and II synthesis and regulation in rat fibroblasts. Nature 1983; 302:150–153.

310. Bennett A, Wilson DM, Liu R, et al. Levels of insulin like growth factors I and II in human cord blood. J Clin Endocrinol Metab 1983; 57:609–612.

311. Moses AC, Nissley SP, Short PA, et al. Elevated levels of multiplication-stimulating activity, an insulin-like growth factor, in fetal rat serum. Proc Natl Acad Sci USA 1980; 77:3649–3653.

312. Sara VR, Hall K, Misaki M, et al. Ontogenesis of somatomedin and insulin receptors in the human fetus. J Clin Invest 1983; 71:1084–1094.

313. Han VKM, Lauder IM, D'Ercole AJ. Characterization of somatomedin–insulin like growth factor receptors and correlation with biological activity in cultured neonatal rat astroglial cells. J Neurosci 1987; 7:501–511.

314. Freemark M, D'Ercole AJ, Handwerger S. Somatomedin C stimulates glycogen synthesis in fetal rat hepatocytes. Endocrinology 1985; 116:2578–2582.

315. Pilistine SJ, Moses AC, Munro HN. Placental lactogen administration reverses the effect of low protein diet on maternal and fetal somatomedin levels in the pregnant rat. Proc Natl Acad Sci USA 1984; 81:5853–5857.

316. Sara VR, Carlsson-Skwirut C, Andersson C, et al. Characterization of somatomedins from human fetal brain: identification of a variant form of insulin-like growth factor I. Proc Natl Acad Sci USA 1986; 83:4904–4907.

317. Hill DJ, Milner RDG. Insulin as a growth factor. Pediatr Res 1985; 19:879–886.

318. Susa JB, McCormick KL, Widness JA, et al. Chronic hyperinsulinemia in the fetal rhesus monkey: effects on fetal growth and composition. Diabetes 1979; 28:1058–1063.

319. Spencer GSG, Hill D, Garsson G, et al. Somatomedin activity and growth

hormone levels in body fluids of the fetal pig: effect of chronic hyperinsulinemia. J Endocrinol 1983; 96:107–114.

320. Carpenter G, Cohen S. Epidermal growth factor. Annu Rev Biochem 1979; 48:193–216.

321. Fisher DA, Lakshmanan J. Metabolism and effects of EGF and related growth factors in mammals. Endocr Rev 1990; 11:418–442.

322. Schlessinger J, Schreiber AB, Levi A, et al. Regulation of cell proliferation by epidermal growth factor. CRC Crit Rev Biochem 1983; 14:93–111.

323. Schlessinger J. Allosteric regulation of the epidermal growth factor receptor kinase. J Cell Biol 1986; 103:2067–2072.

324. Marquardt H, Hunkapiller MW, Hood LE, et al. Transforming growth factors produced by retrovirus transformed rodent fibroblasts and human melanoma cells: amino acid sequence homology with epidermal growth factor. Proc Natl Acad Sci USA 1983; 80:4684–4688.

325. Smith JM, Sporn MB, Roberts AB, et al. Human transforming growth factor α causes precocious eyelid opening in newborn mice. Nature 1985; 315:515–516.

326. Anzano MA, Roberts AB, Meyers CA, et al. Synergistic interaction of two classes of transforming growth factors from murine sarcoma cells. Cancer Res 1982; 19:4776–4778.

327. Rall LB, Scott J, Bell GI, et al. Mouse prepro-epidermal growth factor synthesis by the kidney and other tissues. Nature 1985; 313:228–231.

328. Laborde NP, Grodin M, Buenaflor G, et al. Ontogenesis of epidermal growth factor in liver of BALB mice. Am J Physiol 1988; 255:E28–E32.

329. Brown PI, Lam R, Lakshmanan J, et al. Transforming growth factor alpha (TGF α) in the developing rat. Am J Physiol 1990; 259:E256–E260.

330. Tsutsumi O, Oka T. Epidermal growth factor deficiency during pregnancy causes abortion in mice. Am J Obstet Gynecol 1987; 156:241–244.

331. Adamson ED, Deller MJ, Warshaw JB. Functional EGF receptors are present on mouse embryo tissues. Nature 1981; 291:656–659.

332. Adamson ED, Meek J. Epidermal growth factor receptors during mouse development. Dev Biol 1984; 103:62–70.

333. Wood SA, Kaye PL. Effects of epidermal growth factor on preimplantation mouse embryos. J Reprod Fertil 1989; 85:575–582.

334. Nexo E, Hollenberg M, Figueroa A, et al. Detection of EGF-urogastrone and its receptor in fetal mouse development. Proc Natl Acad Sci USA 1980; 77:2782–2785.

335. Snead ML, Luo W, Oliver P, et al. Localization of epidermal growth factor precursor in tooth and lung during embryonic mouse development. Dev Biol 1989; 134:420–429.

336. Gubits RM, Shaw PA, Gresik EW, et al. Epidermal growth factor gene expression is regulated differently in mouse kidney and submandibular gland. Endocrinology 1986; 119:1382–1387.

337. Popliker M, Shatz A, Avivi A, et al. Onset of endogenous synthesis of epidermal growth factor in neonatal mice. Dev Biol 1987; 119:38–44.

338. Twardzik DH. Differential expression of transforming growth factor alpha during prenatal development of the mouse. Cancer Res 1985; 45:5413–5416.

339. Han VKM, Hunter ES III, Pratt RM, et al. Expression of rat transforming growth factor alpha mRNA during development occurs predominantly in the maternal decidua. Mol Cell Biol 1987; 7:2335–2343.

340. Thorburn GD, Waters MJ, Young IR, et al. Epidermal growth factor: a critical factor in fetal maturation? Ciba Found Symp 1981; 86:172–198.

341. Zschiesche W. Retardation of growth and epithelial differentiation in suckling mice by anti-EGF antisera. Biomed Biochim Acta 1989; 48:103–109.

342. Gonzales F, Lakshmanan J, Hoath S, et al. Effect of oestradiol-17β on uterine epidermal growth factor concentration in immature mice. Acta Endocrinol 1984; 105:425–428.

343. Korach KS, McLachlan JA, Teng CT. Influence of estrogens on mouse uterine epidermal growth factor precursor protein and messenger ribonucleic acid. Endocrinology 1988; 122:2355–2363.

344. Walker P, Weichsel ME Jr, Hoath SB, et al. Effect of T_4, testosterone and corticosterone on NGF and EGF concentrations in adult female mouse SMG: dissocation of EGF and NGF responses. Endocrinology 1981; 109:582–587.

345. Abdulmaged MT, Notiz HH. Prostatic epidermal growth factor receptors and their regulation by androgens. Endocrinology 1987; 121:1461–1467.

346. Levi-Montalcini R, Angeletti PU. Nerve growth factor. Physiol Rev 1968; 48:534–569.

347. Bradshaw RA. Nerve growth factor. Annu Rev Biochem 1978; 47:191–216.

348. Gorin PD, Johnson EM. Effects of exposure to nerve growth factor antibodies on the developing nervous system of the rat, an experimental autoimmune approach. Dev Biol 1980; 80:313–323.

349. Padbury JF, Lam RW, Polk DH, et al. Autoimmune sympathectomy in fetal rabbits. J Dev Physiol 1986; 8:369–376.

350. Tarris RH, Weichsel ME Jr, Fisher DA. Synthesis and secretion of a nerve growth stimulating factor by neonatal mouse astrocyte cells in vitro. Pediatr Res 1986; 20:367–372.

351. Lakshmanan J, Weichsel ME Jr, Tarris R, et al. β nerve growth factor in developing mouse cerebral cortical synaptosomes: measurement by competitive radioimmunoassay and bioassay. Pediatr Res 1986; 20:391–397.

352. Sieff CA. Hematopoietic growth factors. J Clin Invest 1987; 79:1549–1557.

353. Zanjani ED, Ascensau JL, McGlave PB. Studies on the liver to kidney switch of erythropoietin production. J Clin Invest 1981; 67:1183–1188.

354. Liu L, Nicoll CS. Evidence for a role of basic fibroblast growth factor in rat embryonic growth and differentiation. Endocrinology 1988; 123:2027–2031.

355. Oberbauer AM, Linkhart TA, Mohan S, et al. Fibroblast growth factor enhances human chorionic gonadotropin synthesis independent of mitogenic stimulation in Jar choriocarcinoma cells. Endocrinology 1988; 123:2696–2700.

356. Padbury JF. Functional maturation of the adrenal medulla and peripheral sympathetic nervous system. Baillieres Clin Endocrinol Metab 1989; 3:689–705.

357. Eliot RJ, Lam R, Leake RD, et al. Plasma catecholamine concentrations in infants at birth and during the first 48 hours of life. J Pediatr 1980; 96:311–315.

358. Padbury JF, Ludlow JK, Ervin MG, et al. Thresholds for physiological effects of plasma catecholamines in fetal sheep. Am J Physiol 1987; 252:E530–E537.

359. Padbury JF, Martinez AM. Sympathoadrenal system activity at birth: integration of postnatal adaptation. Semin Perinatol 1988; 12:163–172.

360. Polk DH. Thyroid hormone effects on neonatal thermogenesis. Semin Perinatol 1988; 12:151–156.

361. Obregon MJ, Pitamber R, Jacobsson A, et al. Euthyroid status is essential for the perinatal increase in thermogenin mRNA in brown adipose tissue of rat pups. Biochem Biophys Res Commun 1987; 148:9–14.

362. Klein AH, Reviczky A, Chou P, et al. Development of brown adipose tissue thermogenesis in the ovine fetus and newborn. Endocrinology 1983; 112:1662–1666.

363. Polk DH, Padbury JF, Callegari CC, et al. Effect of fetal thyroidectomy on newborn thermogenesis in lambs. Pediatr Res 1987; 21:453–457.

364. Longhead JL, Minouni F, Tsang RC. Serum ionized calcium concentrations in normal neonates. Am J Dis Child 1988; 142:516–518.

365. Dincsoy MY, Tsang RC, Laskarzewski P, et al. The role of postnatal age and magnesium on parathyroid hormone responses during exchange blood transfusion in the newborn period. J Pediatr 1982; 100:277–283.

366. Venkataraman PS, Tsang RC, Chen IW, et al. Pathogenesis of early neonatal hypocalcemia: studies of serum calcitonin, gastrin and plasma glucagon. J Pediatr 1987; 110:599–603.

367. Menon RK, Sperling MA. Carbohydrate metabolism. Semin Perinatol 1988; 12:157–162.

368. Wheeler MD, Styne DM. Longitudinal changes in growth hormone response to growth hormone–releasing hormone in neonatal rhesus monkeys. Pediatr Res 1990; 28:15–18.

369. Penny R, Parlow AF, Frasier O. Testosterone and estradiol concentrations in paired maternal and cord sera and their correlation with the concentration of chorionic gonadotropin. Pediatrics 1979; 64:604–608.

370. Mann DR, Gould KG, Collins DC, et al. Blockade of neonatal activation of the pituitary-testicular axis: effect on peripubertal luteinizing hormone and testosterone secretion and on testicular development in male monkeys. J Clin Endocrinol Metab 1989; 68:600–607.

371. Barraclough CA. Production of anovulatory sterile rats by single injection of testosterone propionate. Endocrinology 1961; 68:62–67.

372. Janson JD, Ekberg S, Isacksson D, et al. Imprinting of growth hormone secretion, body growth, and hepatic steroid metabolism by neonatal testosterone. Endocrinology 1985; 117:1881–1889.

373. Gorski RA. Sexual differentiation of brain structure in rodents. In: Serio M, Zanisi M, Martini L, eds. Sexual Differentiation: Basic and Clinical Concepts. New York: Raven, 1984: 65–77.

374. Dohler KD. The special case of hormonal imprinting. The neonatal influence on sex. Experientia 1985; 42:759–769.

375. Grocock CA, Charlton HM, Pike MC. Role of fetal pituitary in cryptorchidism induced by exogenous maternal oestrogen during pregnancy in mice. J Reprod Fertil 1988; 83:295–300.

376. Bern HA, Talamentes FJ Jr. Neonatal mouse models and their relation to disease in the human female. In: Herbst AL, Bern HA, eds. Developmental Effects of Diethylstilbestrol (DES) in Pregnancy. New York: Thieme-Stratton, 1981: 129–147.

377. Csaba G. Receptor ontogeny and hormonal imprinting. Experientia 1985; 42:750–759.

378. Bakke JL, Lawrence N. Persistent thyrotropin insufficiency following neonatal thyroxine administration. J Lab Clin Med 1966; 67:477–482.

379. Bakke JL, Lawrence NL, Bennet J, et al. Endocrine syndromes produced by neonatal hyperthyroidism, hypothyroidism, or altered nutrition and effects seen in untreated progeny. In: Fisher DA, Burrow GN, eds. Perinatal Thyroid Physiology and Disease. New York: Raven, 1975: 79–112.

380. Martin SM, Moberg GP. Effects of early neonatal thyroxine treatment on development of the thyroid and adrenal axes in rats. Life Sci 1981; 29:1683–1688.

381. Walker P, Courtin F. Transient neonatal hyperthyroidism results in hypothyroidism in the adult rat. Endocrinology 1985; 116:2246–2250.

382. Alm J, Lakshmanan J, Hoath S, et al. Neonatal hyperthyroidism alters

hepatic epidermal growth factor receptor ontogeny in mice. Pediatr Res 1988; 23:557–560.

383. Spiegel G, Levy LJ, Goldner MG. Glucose intolerance in the progeny of rats treated with single subdiabetogenic dose of alloxan. Metabolism 1971; 20:401–413.

384. Csaba G, Inczefi Gonda A, Dobozy O. Hereditary transmission in the F_1 generation of hormonal imprinting (receptor memory) induced in rats by neonatal exposure to insulin. Acta Physiol Hung 1984; 63:93–99.

385. Csaba G, Ronai A, Laszlo V, et al. Amplification of hormone receptors by neonatal oxytocin and vasopressin treatment. Horm Metab Res 1980; 12:28–31.

386. Herbst AL, Ulfelder H, Poskjanzer DC. Adenocarcinoma of the vagina: association of maternal stilbestrol therapy with tumor appearance in young women. N Engl J Med 1971; 284:878–881.

387. Herbst AL. The epidemiology of vaginal and cervical clear cell adenocarcinoma. In Herbst AL, Bern HA, eds. Developmental Effects of Diethylstilbestrol (DES) in Pregnancy. New York: Thieme-Stratton, 1981: 63–70.

388. Sato T, Suzuki Y, Taketani T, et al. Age related change in pituitary threshold for TSH release during thyroxine replacement therapy for cretinism. J Clin Endocrinol Metab 1977; 44:553–559.

389. McCrossin RB, Sheffield LJ, Robertson EF. Persisting abnormality in the pituitary-thyroid axis in congenital hypothyroidism. In: Stockigt JR, Nagataki S, eds. Thyroid Research VIII. Canberra: Australian Academy of Science, 1980: 37–40.

390. Sato SM, Mains RE. Plasticity in the adrenocorticotropin-related peptides produced by primary cultures of neonatal rat pituitary. Endocrinology 1988; 122:68–77.

391. Evans MI, Drugan I, Manning FA, et al. Fetal surgery in the 1990s. Am J Dis Child 1989; 143:1431–1436.

392. Thieriot-Prevost G, Daffos F, Forestier F, et al. Serum growth-promoting activity in normal and hypotrophic fetuses at midpregnancy. Pediatr Res 1987; 22:39–40.

393. O'Keane JA, Yuen BH, Farquharson DF, et al. Endocrine response to selective embryocide in a gonadotropin-induced quintuplet pregnancy. Am J Obstet Gynecol 1988; 158:364–367.

394. Morales WJ, O'Brien WF, Angel JL, et al. Fetal lung maturation: the combined use of corticosteroids and thyrotropin releasing hormone. Obstet Gynecol 1989; 73:111–116.

395. Forest MG, Betuel H, David M. Treatment anténatal de l'hyperplasie congénitale des surrénales par déficit en 21-hydroxylase: étude multicentrique. Ann Endocrinol (Paris) 1987; 48:31–34.

396. Kourides IA, Heath CV, Ginsberg-Fellner F. Measurement of thyroid stimulating hormone in human amniotic fluid. J Clin Endocrinol Metab 1982; 54:635–637.

397. Lightner ES, Fisher DA, Giles H, et al. Intraamniotic injection of thyroxine to a human fetus: evidence for conversion of T_4 to reverse T_3. Am J Obstet Gynecol 1977; 127:487–490.

398. Robinson PL, O'Mullane NM, Alderman B. Prenatal treatment of thyrotoxicosis. Br Med J 1979; 1:383–384.

399. Check JH, Rezvani I, Goodner D, et al. Prenatal treatment of thyrotoxicosis to prevent intrauterine growth retardation. Obstet Gynecol 1982; 60:122–124.

400. Charlton V, Johengen M. Fetal intravenous nutritional supplementation ameliorates the development of embolization-induced growth retardation in sheep. Pediatr Res 1987; 22:55–61.

401. Gibson MJ, Krieger DT, Charlton HM, et al. Mating and pregnancy can occur in genetically hypogonadal mice with preoptic area brain grafts. Science 1984; 225:949–951.

402. Gash D, Sladek JR Jr, Sladek CD. Functional development of grafted vasopressin neurons. Science 1980; 210:1367–1369.

403. Perlow MJ, Freed WJ, Hoffer BJ, et al. Brain grafts reduce motor abnormalities produced by destruction of nigrostriatal dopamine system. Science 1979; 204:643–647.

404. Redmond DE Jr, Naftolin F, Collier TJ, et al. Cryopreservation, culture and transplantation of human fetal mesencephalic tissue into monkeys. Science 1988; 242:768–771.

405. Annas GJ, Elias S. The politics of transplantation of human fetal tissue. N Engl J Med 1982; 320:1079–1082.

21

NORMAL AND ABERRANT GROWTH

Louis E. Underwood and Judson J. Van Wyk

Physical growth involves all the processes by which a fertilized egg attains the size, form, and function of an adult. In one sense, growth does not cease with the attainment of adulthood, because many cells replicate throughout life to replace those lost through normal attrition or those destroyed by injury or disease. The timing of various growth sequences and the capacity for growth are genetically encoded at the time of conception, and complex interactions among hormonal secretions, nutritional status, and specific disease states influence the expression of these genes.[1–6]

For many years, knowledge of how hormones affect growth and development was derived from the study of the effects of hormonal deficiency or hormonal excess on children and by observing the effect on experimental animals of organ ablation or hormone administration. Results from such studies have been amplified by the development of precise, specific methods for measuring the concentrations of hormones and hormone receptors and for assessing changes in the messenger RNAs (mRNAs) for these molecules. Attention is also being directed to the mechanisms by which hormones activate the intracellular events that lead either to mitosis or to the production of differentiated cell products. This chapter describes normal human growth and development, discusses the effects of hormones and peptide growth factors on these processes, and describes the role of hormones in various disorders of human growth and development.

PATTERNS OF NORMAL GROWTH

Physical Growth

PRENATAL GROWTH. By the end of gestation the fertilized human ovum has undergone about 42 successive cell divisions, and if all cells replicated in a uniform manner only five more duplications would be required to reach full adult size.[7] At the end of the first 10 wk of embryonic development, the fetus weights about 2.8 g and has a crown-rump length of 3.0 cm.[8] By this time, however, organogenesis is nearly complete. There then ensues profound acceleration in linear growth, with the peak velocity occurring about the 20th week. At this time, crown-heel length velocity may reach 2.5 cm/wk or 130 cm/y (Fig. 21–1). The maximal weight velocity occurs somewhat later, normally about 34 wk. This weight increment correlates with the acquisition of adipose tissue and results in a doubling of body weight in the last 8 wk of gestation. Toward the end of intrauterine life the rate of growth declines sharply, in part a consequence of uterine filling because growth decline occurs earlier in multiple pregnancies.

Knowledge of fetal age at birth makes it possible to distinguish prematurely born infants from those who are small as a consequence of intrauterine growth failure (small-for-gestational age [SGA] babies). In assessing gestational age, the convention of equating conception with the last

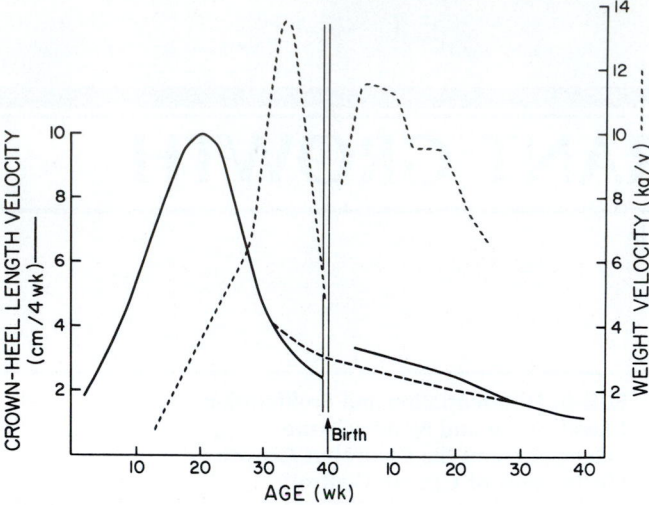

Figure 21–1. Rate of linear growth and weight gain in utero and during first 40 wk after birth. Note that length velocity is expressed as centimeters per week. The solid line depicts actual linear growth rate; the dashed line connecting the pre- and postnatal length velocity lines depicts the theoretical curve for no uterine restriction late in gestation. The lighter dashed line depicts weight velocity. (From data in Tanner JM. Fetus into Man. Cambridge, MA: Harvard University Press, 1978.)

missed menstrual period is misleading, because fertilization normally occurs 2 wk after menstruation; thus the actual duration of gestation is 38 rather than 40 wk. Errors in determining the age of the fetus at birth are compounded by variations in the interval between menstruation and fertilization and by mistaking early gestational bleeding for menstruation. It is often necessary, therefore, to determine gestational age on the basis of physical and neuromuscular maturity.[9]

The size of normal infants at birth is determined by poorly understood genetic and environmental factors. One factor is maternal size, because the slowing of fetal growth during the last few weeks of gestation is roughly proportional to maternal size and uterine space.[10–12] There are significant ethnic differences in growth during the prenatal period. For example, American Indians of the Cheyenne tribe have infants with mean birth weights of 3800 g, whereas infants of the Luni tribe of New Guinea have mean birth weights of 2400 g.[13] Environmental factors such as altitude also influence intrauterine growth. Infants born in the Andes Mountains of Peru average 1500 g lighter weight than infants born near sea level in Lima.[14] Many of the ethnic and environmental variations in birth weight are undoubtedly adaptational responses that improve the chances of the neonate for survival and of the mother for further reproductive function. For instance, a mother would rapidly become malnourished if she produced a succession of large infants in a nutritionally insufficient environment. Similarly, although a large size at birth may be advantageous under optimal environmental conditions, smaller size at birth improves fitness for survival when the nutrient supply is limited.

Less significant influences on birth weight in normal pregnancies include (1) the birth order of the infants: first-born infants are approximately 100 g lighter weight than later-born infants; (2) sex: male fetuses have higher average birth weights than females, and in mixed, multiple pregnancies the presence of a male fetus appears to enhance the growth of female fetuses;[15] and (3) maternal age: a reduction in birth weight occurs in first-born infants when maternal age is 38 or more.[16]

GROWTH FROM BIRTH TO PUBERTY. Growth during the first year of life is rapid, with more than doubling of birth weight and a 50% increase in body length. Linear growth velocities, which may reach 30 cm/y in the first 2 mo of life, decrease to one third of this rate by 10 mo of age and continue to decrease sharply until 2 to 3 y.[6, 17–19]

At birth the dominance of prenatal maternal influences is replaced by the influence of the genetic, nutritional, and hormonal status of the infant. Although the correlation coefficient between birth length and adult height is poor (r = .31), it is .8 by age 2 y. The latter correlation, which reflects the growth potential of the child, remains constant until the onset of puberty.

The linear growth of approximately two thirds of normal infants crosses percentile channels during the first 12 to 18 mo of life, the number shifting upward on the curve approximating the number shifting downward.[20] Prematurely born infants who are otherwise normal and some infants who are SGA undergo catch-up growth (Fig. 21–2). This accelerated rate of growth is most marked during the first 6 mo, but in the smallest infants it may continue for as long as 2 y before a stable growth rate is achieved. As a group, SGA infants catch up less well than prematurely born infants whose size is appropriate for their gestational age. In one group of SGA babies studied at age 4 y, 35% remained below the third percentile for both length and head circumference, and only 8% rose above the 50th percentile.[21] At the other end of the spectrum, infants who are exceptionally large at birth, such as those born of multiparous mothers, continue to grow rapidly for several months postnatally and do not begin deceleration to reach lower percentile standings until between the third and sev-

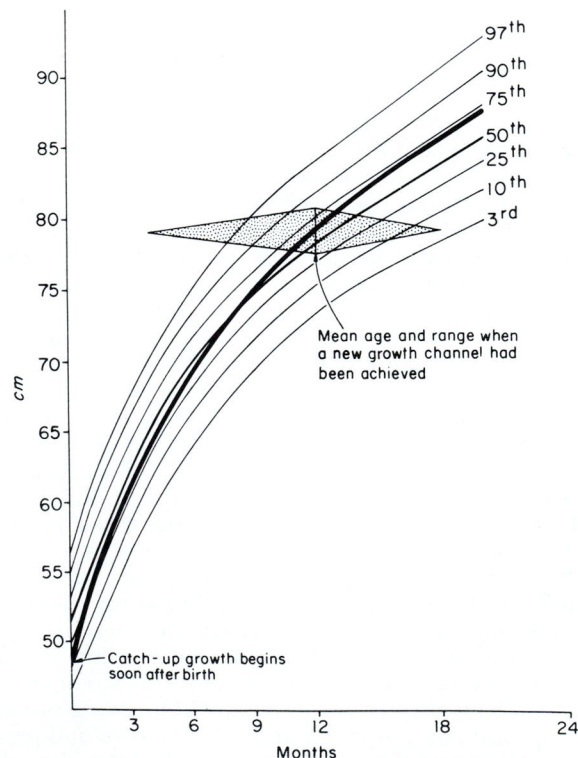

Figure 21–2. Mean growth curve of 10 normal male and 6 normal female infants whose lengths were close to the 10th percentile at birth and near the 70th percentile by 2 y. The curve shows that growth accelerates soon after birth, and that the phase of acceleration is complete at a mean age of 11.5 mo. (From Smith DW, Truog W, Rogers JE, et al. Shifting linear growth during infancy: illustration of genetic factors in growth from fetal life through infancy. J Pediatr 1976; 89:225–230.)

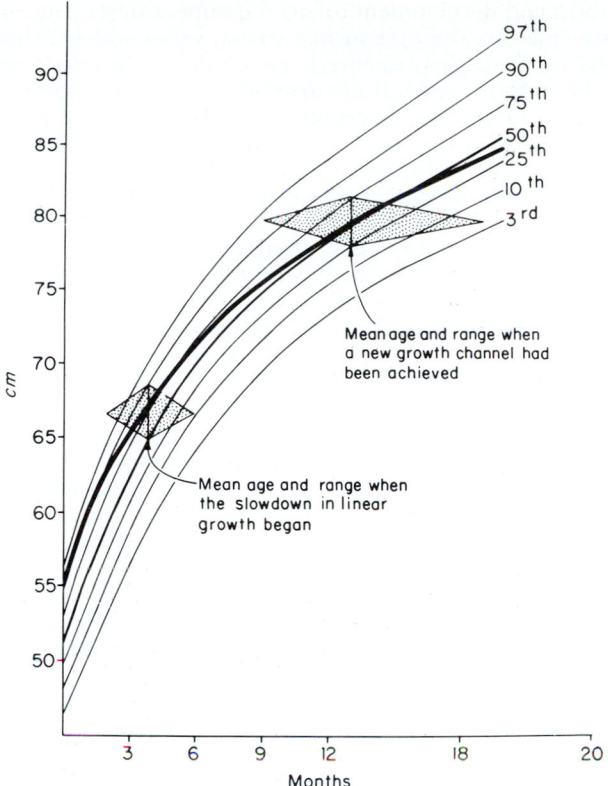

Figure 21–3. Mean growth curve of 11 normal male and 5 normal female infants who "lagged down" in growth during infancy. All were close to the 90th percentile for length at birth and near the 40th percentile by 2 y. The curve shows that this downward shift did not begin before 3 mo of age and was complete at a mean age of 13 mo. (From Smith DW, Truog W, Rogers JE, et al. Shifting linear growth during infancy: illustration of genetic factors in growth from fetal life through infancy. J Pediatr 1976; 89:225–230.)

enth months (Fig. 21–3). These children reach stable childhood growth channels early in the second year of life.[21]

After age 2 y the rates of gain in both height and weight show a slow downward trend and reach a nadir just before the beginning of the pubertal growth spurt. Before puberty the mean heights and weights of boys and girls are nearly equal. During the prepubertal period most children remain in a remarkably constant percentile channel for linear growth, and crossing of several percentile channels should be the occasion for investigation.

PUBERTAL GROWTH. The acceleration of somatic growth during puberty is one component of the dramatic changes that transform the child into an adult.[22, 23] The pubertal growth spurt occurs approximately 2 y later in boys than in girls, and this delay gives boys an average of two additional years of prepubertal growth than girls. Thus, at the onset of the pubertal growth spurt, boys are on the average 10 cm taller than girls at the corresponding developmental stage. The difference in average stature between men and women is due both to this longer period of prepubertal growth in boys and to a more intense pubertal growth spurt in boys. Furthermore, because the extremities grow faster than the trunk during the prepubertal period, the leg length of males is generally greater than of females, both in absolute terms and in relation to the trunk.

The pubertal growth spurt is relatively short, normally only about 2 y. The peak height velocity occurs in British boys at a mean age of 14.0 y and averages about 10.3 cm/y.[24] The peak height velocity in U.S. boys occurs between ages 13.5 and 14.[25] British girls have the maximal growth velocity

at a mean age of 12.1 y (U.S. girls ~12.5 y)[25] and at this time grow at an average rate of 9.0 cm/y.[26]

The appearance of secondary sexual characteristics and the hormonal changes of puberty are temporally related to the peak height velocity, regardless of when these events occur.[3, 22, 25] In normal girls, menarche predictably occurs on the descending limb of the height-velocity curve, but in girls with sexual precocity menarche may occur at the same time or slightly before the peak height velocity. Girls with delayed adolescence, on the other hand, have menarche later on the descending limb when growth has nearly ceased. The growth spurt of boys is late relative to that of girls, and male genital and pubic hair maturation is nearly complete by the time of the maximal pubertal growth rate. The relationship between the emergence of secondary sexual characteristics and pubertal growth is depicted in Figures 21–4 and 21–5.

Because linear growth curves represent a composite of early- and late-maturing children, those curves based on cross-sectional studies of large numbers of children give a misleading picture of individual growth patterns in later childhood. At the onset of the growth spurt, early-maturing children increase their percentile standing in an upward direction. Later, as growth rate decelerates, they cross percentile channels in a downward direction, as later-maturing children come into puberty. Similarly, children with delayed adolescence cross percentile channels downward for a time before they begin the growth spurt. The rapidity and duration of adolescent growth reflect hormonal and genetic

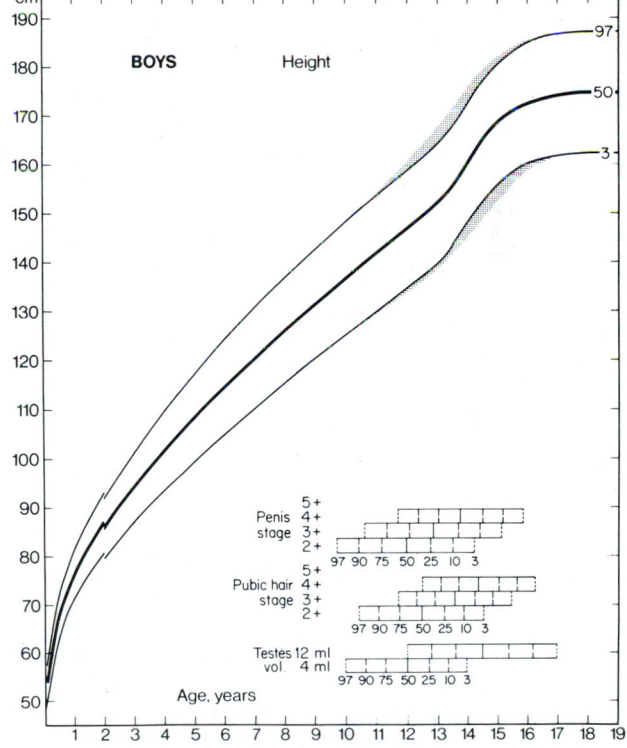

Figure 21–4. Cumulative (height-attained) growth chart for boys. The 97th, 50th, and 3rd percentile curves depict the normal growth pattern, from data collected by longitudinal as well as cross-sectional observations of British children. Outer (upper and lower) margins of shaded areas represent 97th and 3rd percentile standards collected by cross-sectional observations. The ages of attainment of stages of pubertal development (Tanner; see Table 21–8) are plotted by percentiles, the 97th percentile being the early limit of occurrence of a given pubertal stage and the 3rd being the late limit. (Modified from charts prepared by Tanner JM and Whitehouse RH from data published in refs. 17 and 18. [Original charts also contain 10th, 25th, 75th, and 90th percentile lines.] Reproduced with permission of Tanner JM and Castlemead Publications, Ward's Publishing Services, Herts, UK.)

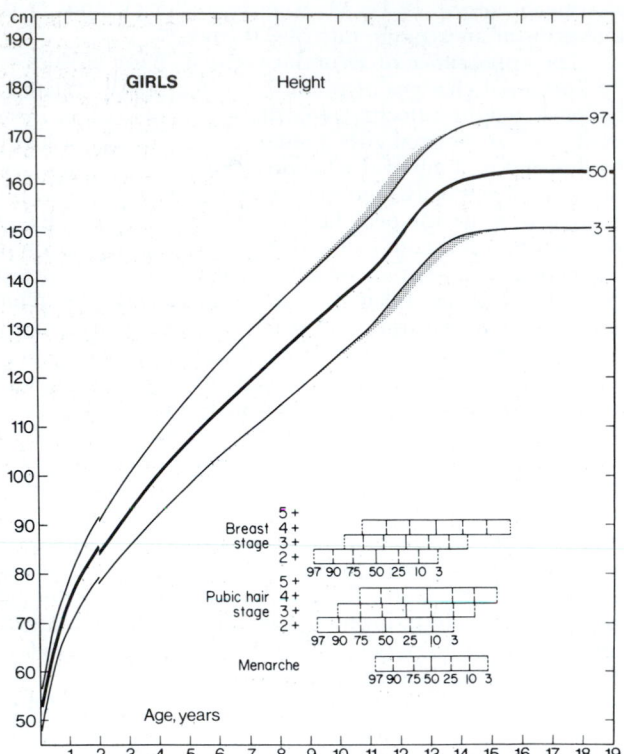

Figure 21–5. Cumulative growth chart for girls. See the legend to Figure 21–4. (Adapted and reproduced with permission of Tanner JM and Castlemead Publications, Ward's Publishing Services, Herts, UK.)

growth and development follow the same orderly pattern in most children, the pace of maturation varies widely. Thus a child's growth performance is better viewed in relationship to the stage of physical maturity than to chronological age. Because the ossification centers of the bony skeleton mature progressively from birth to adulthood, measurement of skeletal maturation provides an objective indication of maturity that is independent of chronological age, size, or growth rate.

Skeletal maturity, expressed as skeletal age, is best assessed after the neonatal period by radiography of the hand and the wrist. At minimal radiation dosage, this provides information on 30 bones, or about 10% of the total. Estimation of skeletal maturity traditionally has been made from the atlas of Greulich and Pyle,[37] in which radiographs of the left hand and wrist are matched with films obtained from "typical children" of various ages. Tanner and associates[38] devised a more objective method in which a numerical score is assigned to each stage of development of the individual bones of the hand and wrist. This method, although laborious, has less variance than the method of Greulich and Pyle.[39, 40]

In children with premature or delayed puberty, the skeletal age correlates better with the onset of the pubertal growth spurt and other events in pubertal development than do either chronological age or attained height. By using skeletal age, it is possible to predict the final adult stature with some degree of reliability[41–43] and to distinguish between children whose sexual maturity will occur early and those whose sexual development will be delayed. It should be emphasized, however, that height prediction data are derived from studies of normal children, and caution should be exercised in applying these techniques to children with diseases that influence the normal pattern of growth.

Organ Growth

DIFFERENTIAL GROWTH OF SPECIFIC ORGANS AND TISSUES. For the most part, growth of individual body parts parallels skeletal growth.[44] Tissues such as kidney, liver, spleen, and muscle grow rapidly early in life, grow slower during the prepubertal years, and accelerate in growth during puberty. Several tissues, however, differ from the general pattern. The brain and eyes are highly developed at birth and attain most of the adult size within the first few years of life. At the opposite end of the growth spectrum, the reproductive tissues, which grow little between the time of birth and the onset of puberty, reach adult size in the span of a few years. The lymphoid cell mass progressively increases throughout childhood, reaches a maximum before puberty, then slowly decreases in mass throughout adulthood.

CELL SIZE VERSUS CELL NUMBER. The rapid increase in external dimensions that characterizes childhood growth depends on increases both in the number of cells (hyperplasia) and in the size of individual cells (hypertrophy). In the early embryo, growth is almost exclusively due to increases in cell number; at succeeding stages of development the balance between hyperplasia and hypertrophy varies among tissues and at different stages of development. Patterns of growth can be assessed by determining the DNA and protein content of a tissue at different times. DNA content reflects cell number because the DNA content in each diploid nucleus is constant in each species. The ratio of protein to DNA is an index of cell size.

According to a classification proposed by Goss,[45–47] tissues increase or maintain their mass and function by renewal or expansion of the cell population or by maintenance of a static population. Renewing tissues (epidermis, gut mucosa,

mechanisms that differ from those that control growth during early childhood. Thus children entering puberty at exactly the same age and weight often show considerably greater scatter in adult heights than might have been anticipated from prepubertal growth patterns.

The rates of growth of different portions of the skeleton vary with the stage of puberty. In general, growth early in puberty is signaled by growth of the distal portion of the axial skeleton, the hands and the feet. Subsequently, arm and leg growth predominates, and still later trunk growth is relatively greater and is the more important determinant of growth during the latter stages of puberty.

The hormonal mechanisms involved in growth at puberty are not fully understood.[27, 28] In males both testosterone and growth hormone (GH) are essential for the pubertal growth spurt.[23, 29] GH secretion is increased, GH responses to provocative stimuli are greater,[30] and GH concentrations through the day are increased.[31] Testosterone augments the growth-promoting effect of GH and may stimulate growth in GH-deficient children, albeit at the cost of rapid advancement of skeletal maturation. We have observed[32] that testosterone does not affect basal serum concentrations of insulin-like growth factor I (IGF I, also called somatomedin-C) directly or increase the IGF I response to exogenous GH. The stimulation of growth by testosterone, therefore, appears to be mediated by increased IGF I, which is secondary to increased GH secretion, and perhaps by a direct androgen effect on growing tissues. Serum IGF I concentrations are high during puberty and reach maximal values at the time of the pubertal growth spurt.[33, 34]

In females, in whom elevations of plasma testosterone are less marked, pubertal growth is even less well understood. Estrogen may stimulate growth by increasing production of IGF I[35, 36] and by a direct anabolic effect.[23]

SKELETAL AGE AND PHYSICAL MATURITY. Although

male germ cells, and hematopoietic elements) grow by proliferating from undifferentiated cells that do not divide further once they reach the stage of differentiation. The rates of proliferation of hematopoietic cells, gut epithelium, and other renewing cell types are rapid, but they are balanced by corresponding rates of cellular destruction so that the rapid cell growth is not apparent unless disturbed by some pathological process or chemotherapeutic agent.

In expanding tissues all differentiated cells are capable of mitosis but exhibit little or no mitotic activity after appropriate organ size is achieved. During adult life growth may be reinitiated in response to tissue injury or loss of tissue mass. Examples of such tissues include endocrine and exocrine glands, liver, kidney, and lungs.

Neurons and skeletal muscle, which do not proliferate beyond certain developmental stages, are mitotically static tissues. They ordinarily survive for the life of the organism. If they sustain injury, however, they regrow only by cellular hypertrophy or axonal regeneration.

Some tissues such as the skeleton are more difficult to classify. Growth at the cartilaginous growth plate behaves like an expanding tissue because it ceases after epiphyseal fusion. Membranous and cancellous bone cells, however, proliferate throughout life to permit remodeling and replacement of cells lost by attrition and thus fulfill the requirements for renewing tissues.

THE ROLE OF TRADITIONAL HORMONES IN HUMAN GROWTH

Hormones that exert significant effects on skeletal and somatic growth include GH, thyroxine, cortisol, gonadal steroids, insulin, and a variety of peptide hormones that are loosely referred to as growth factors (Table 21–1).

Growth Hormone

GH, the most abundant hormone in the human pituitary, plays the primary role in controlling postnatal growth. Considerable progress has been made in elucidating the nature and actions of the hypothalamic factors that stimulate or inhibit GH release by the pituitary, but critical questions remain concerning the chemical nature of the active growth principle and the mechanisms by which GH produces its multiple effects.

The gene that encodes for human growth hormone (hGH) (GH1 or hGH N) is a member of the five-gene cluster of genes for GH and human placental lactogen (hPL, also called human chorionic somatomammotropin, hCS) located in a 50,000 base pair portion of the long arm of chromosome 17.[48, 49] The GH2 (hGH V or variant hGH) gene in this cluster encodes for a protein that differs from hGH by 13 amino acids and that is produced in abundance by the placenta.[50] The CSH1 (hPL) and CSH2 loci encode hPL proteins of identical sequence, and the CSH P1 locus encodes a protein that differs by 13 amino acids. Each of the five genes in the hGH-hPL cluster is organized similarly, having five exons interrupted by small introns at identical positions and of identical lengths. The five genes have 92 to 98% sequence homology.

A variety of abnormalities of the GH1 gene have been reported, and the consequences of these abnormalities attest to the importance of this gene for normal GH production and normal growth.[49] Deletions of the GH1 gene cause affected patients to be profoundly GH deficient and to have severe postnatal growth failure. No hGH is detectable in plasma. Treatment with hGH produces acceleration of growth, sometimes followed by the development of high-titer, growth-attenuating antibodies to GH.

Regardless of the modest variability in normal GH1 genes, hGH in pituitary extracts and in plasma is far from homogenous. These variant forms of hGH have diverse origins[51] and can be identified on the basis of charge or size. The major physiological component is a single chain peptide of 191 amino acids with a molecular mass of 22 kd. Several charge variants of hGH in pituitary gland extracts are generated by proteolytic digestion of 22-kd hGH. These isomers are more acidic and possess more biological activity than the parent molecule; they are not found in plasma, and their physiological significance is uncertain.[52] A 20-kd form of hGH is produced as a result of differential splicing of the mRNA for hGH. This form differs from 22-kd GH by the deletion of residues 32 to 46. The 20-kd GH makes up 5 to 10% of the total GH in pituitary and plasma and is equal in potency to 22-kd GH.

Whereas the growth-promoting actions of GH on muscle and skeletal tissue are like those of insulin, the long-term diabetogenic effects on carbohydrate metabolism and the lipolytic effects on fat are opposite to those of insulin. This apparent paradox is further illustrated by the interaction between GH and cortisol in different tissues: in muscle and cartilage, cortisol is catabolic and inhibits the action of GH; on the other hand, cortisol and GH are synergistic in producing the diabetogenic and lipolytic effects.

THE SOMATOMEDIN HYPOTHESIS OF GROWTH HORMONE ACTION. In 1957 Salmon and Daughaday[53] proposed that the growth-promoting effects of GH in vivo are not direct but are mediated by other GH-dependent factors in serum. It now appears that all or nearly all of the biological activities of human serum attributed to these factors are due

TABLE 21–1. Effect of Hormones on Growth and Development

Hormone	Linear Growth	Skeletal Maturation	Effect on Adult Stature (Untreated)
Growth hormone			
Excess	Increased	Normal	Increased
Deficiency	Decreased	Delayed	Decreased
Thyroxine			
Excess	Slightly increased	Slightly advanced	Minimal
Deficiency	Decreased	Delayed*	Decreased
Cortisol			
Excess	Decreased*	Delayed	Decreased
Androgen			
Excess	Increased	Advanced*	Decreased
Deficiency	Increased in extremities	Delayed (later childhood)	Eunuchoidal
Estrogen			
Excess	Increased	Advanced*	Decreased

*Denotes effect that usually predominates.

to two distinct peptides—IGF I and insulin-like growth factor II (IGF II)—collectively known as *somatomedins*. The somatomedin with the greater GH dependency was independently isolated and sequenced under the names of *insulin-like growth factor I*[54] and *somatomedin-C*.[55] The other somatomedin, IGF II, is similar in structure to IGF I but is less GH dependent and more potent in assays for insulin-like activity.[56, 57]

The somatomedins occupy a position of central importance in the growth of all tissues and are discussed in greater detail in a later section. Current concepts of the somatomedin hypothesis of GH action are illustrated in Figure 21–6. The major actions of GH in the living animal can be classified as direct or indirect. The direct actions are those on lipid and fat metabolism that are synergistic with cortisol and opposite to the actions of insulin and the somatomedins. The indirect anabolic and growth-promoting actions of GH are mediated by the somatomedins and include cell proliferation and protein synthesis in both skeletal and nonskeletal tissues. In contrast to the direct actions of GH, these growth-promoting actions are insulin-like and are opposed by cortisol. The somatomedin hypothesis does not presume that somatomedins are the only mediators of somatic growth, nor does it exclude the possibility that GH may stimulate growth directly by other mechanisms.

THE ROLE OF SOMATOMEDINS IN GROWTH HORMONE FEEDBACK. Strong support for the somatomedin hypothesis of GH action was provided by the demonstration that both IGF I and IGF II can mimic the growth-promoting action of GH in hypophysectomized rats.[58, 59] In addition, the somatomedins participate in a classic negative feedback loop in the regulation of GH secretion. At least two mechanisms appear to account for this effect: IGF I stimulates the production of somatostatin in hypothalamic remnants[60] and directly inhibits the action of growth hormone–releasing hormone (GHRH) on GH release from dispersed pituitary cell cultures.[61] IGF I also inhibits increase in GH mRNA in response to GHRH.[62] In adult normal rats, intraventricular

instillation of IGF I inhibits the episodic spikes of GH secretion that occur in control animals.[63]

DIRECT VERSUS INDIRECT ACTIONS OF GROWTH HORMONE ON SKELETAL GROWTH. Opposing views of the relative roles of GH and somatomedins on skeletal growth have become reconciled with recognition that growth factors are produced locally in many tissues in response to trophic hormone stimulation and that they act in these tissues by autocrine and paracrine modalities. For example, injection of GH into hypophysectomized rats leads to the appearance of both immunoreactive IGF I and mRNA for IGF I in the epiphyseal growth plate.[64, 65]

Green and colleagues[66] have attempted to reconcile the different roles of GH and somatomedins by proposing a "dual effector model of growth hormone action" in which GH and somatomedin act in tandem at the target site. In this model, GH stimulates local somatomedin production and stimulates chondrocyte precursor cells to undergo differentiation; the newly formed somatomedins then promote clonal growth of the differentiated cells (Fig. 21–7). This model was extrapolated from a preadipocyte cell line that requires the sequential actions of GH and somatomedin and may not be applicable to the interactions of GH and somatomedin in cartilage and other tissues. In certain other model systems the interactions between pituitary hormones and somatomedins are more complex in that IGFs and pituitary hormones act synergistically on both cytodifferentiation and cell proliferation.[67]

Thyroid Hormones

Thyroid hormones do not appear to play a significant role in the early growth and development of the human fetus because infants with congenital aplasia of the thyroid gland are of normal size at birth. In the primate fetus the major consequences of intrauterine thyroid deficiency are retardation of osseous and central nervous system development.[68, 69] Human infants with congenital hypothyroidism

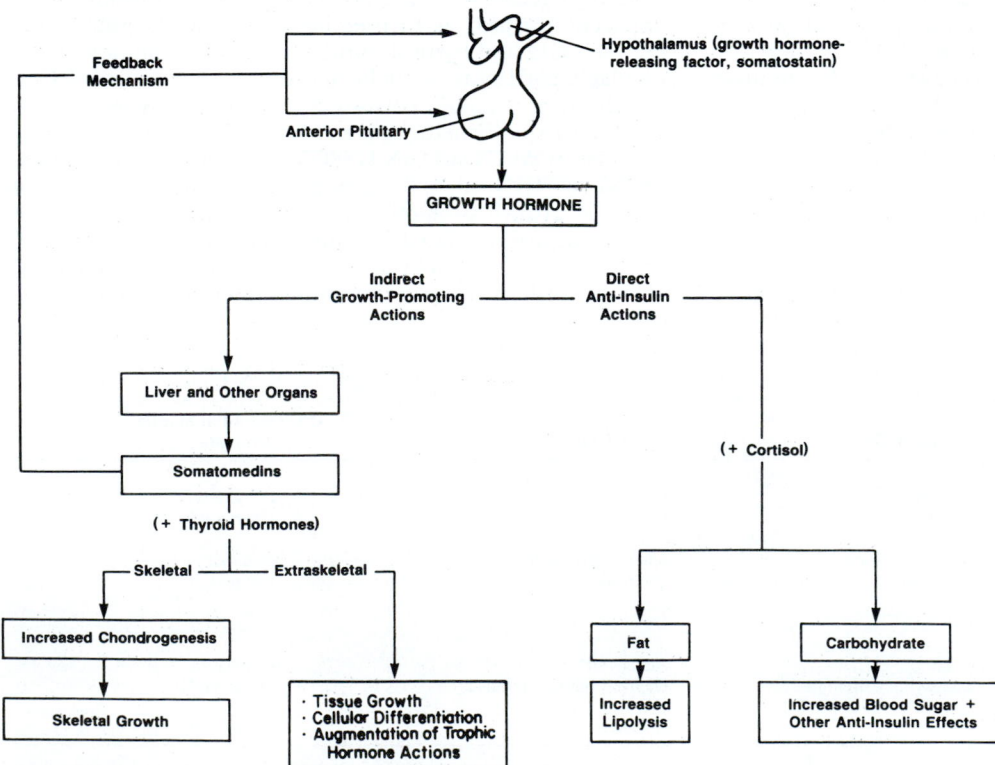

Figure 21–6. The somatomedin hypothesis of GH action. The direct actions of GH include diabetogenic and lipolytic actions and stimulatory action on several hepatic enzymes. These direct actions are antagonistic to insulin and are often synergistic with cortisol. The anabolic and growth-promoting actions of GH are mediated via the somatomedins. IGF I participates in the negative feedback on GH secretion at the hypothalamic level by stimulating somatostatin production and at the pituitary level by directly blocking the effect of GH-releasing hormone on the expression of the GH gene.

Effectors in Growth Hormone Action

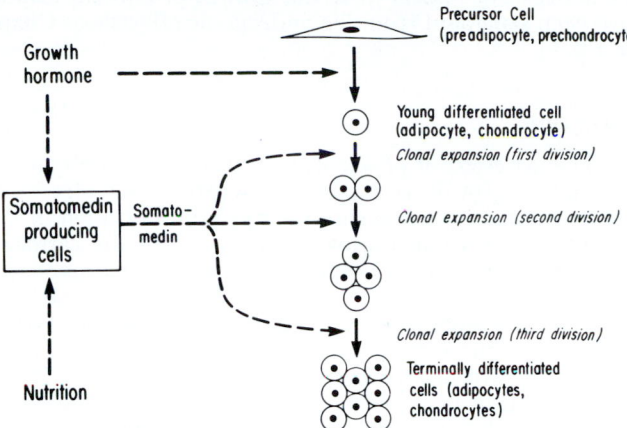

Figure 21–7. Green's dual effector hypothesis of GH action. According to this model, GH and IGFs act in tandem in target tissues. GH stimulates precursor cells (preadipocytes or prechondrocytes) to undergo differentiation and at the same time enhances the local production of somatomedins. Somatomedins then act on the differentiated precursor cells to stimulate their clonal expansion. (From Green H, Morikawa M, Nixon T. A dual effector theory of growth-hormone action. Differentiation 1985; 29:195–198.)

also exhibit immaturity of the skeleton and neurological immaturity. The critical period of thyroxine-dependent brain growth extends from the last portion of gestation to several months postnatally. Hypothyroidism during this period results in retarded growth of cell bodies, axons, and dendritic connections and delayed myelinization.[70] Although thyroid hormone may act directly on these processes, the administration of thyroxine to mature[71] and to neonatal[72] mice increases the concentration of nerve growth factor (NGF) in the brain. Thus the effects of thyroxine on neural maturation may be mediated through NGF.

Thyroid hormones play an important role in postnatal somatic growth, as exemplified by the severe growth failure that accompanies thyroid hormone deficiency. Whereas most disorders slow linear growth, hypothyroidism causes nearly absolute growth arrest. After correction of the thyroid hormone deficiency, growth is usually resumed at rapid rates, a period of so-called catch-up growth.

The role of thyroxine on skeletal growth appears to be permissive; GH does not stimulate growth in hypothyroid animals. The refractoriness of skeletal tissues to GH in such animals may be due to a defect in the response to IGFs at the cellular level. Thyroid hormone probably stimulates growth by two different mechanisms. Triiodothyronine (T_3) promotes cartilage growth in vitro by enhancing the effect of IGF I.[73, 74] More important, thyroid hormone accelerates cartilage maturation (see later Fig. 21–27).[75]

Thyroid hormone also influences the synthesis and secretion of GH by the pituitary gland. Hypothyroid patients frequently have severely blunted GH responses to provocative stimuli, and serum IGF I concentrations are sometimes low.[76] Administration of GH to such patients results in a prompt increase in serum IGF I level.[76] Growth retardation in hypothyroidism, therefore, is probably mediated both by deficient pituitary GH secretion and by deficient action of thyroid hormone on the cartilage growth plate.

Insulin

In addition to its primary role as the regulator of carbohydrate homeostasis, insulin may function as a stimulator of growth.[77, 78] The contrast between oversized, hyper-

insulinemic infants born to diabetic mothers and the poor growth of diabetic newborns with insulin deficiency suggests that insulin is a primary mediator of somatic growth in the fetus. Hyperinsulinism is present in overgrown infants with the Beckwith-Wiedemann syndrome, whereas insulinopenic newborns with pancreatic agenesis are small. Infants with insulin resistance also exhibit growth failure.[79, 80]

Insulin may augment fetal growth by stimulating somatomedin production. Administration of insulin to fetal rabbits increases plasma somatomedin activity and enhances endogenous cartilage growth.[81] Similarly, pig fetuses made chronically hyperinsulinemic between 90 and 104 d of gestation have elevated plasma somatomedin bioactivity.[82] It is not clear whether physiological amounts of insulin directly stimulate fetal growth; it is our bias that insulin exerts only a permissive action by stimulating uptake and utilization of substrates necessary for growth.

In postnatal life, insulin deficiency is associated with growth failure, and hyperinsulinism is accompanied by overgrowth in several conditions.[83] Examples of the former include malnutrition, inadequately treated diabetes mellitus, and untreated hypopituitarism. In otherwise normal children with exogenous obesity and in hyperphagic children who have had surgery for craniopharyngioma,[84] serum insulin concentrations may be increased and linear growth may be accelerated. In cultured cells high concentrations of insulin support cell growth, stimulate DNA synthesis,[85] and promote mitosis.[86] These actions of insulin may be mediated through the type I IGF receptor, which bears striking homology to the insulin receptor (see section on IGF I). A more important effect of high insulin levels in vivo may be to lower the levels of the low-molecular-weight, non–GH-dependent IGF-binding proteins. In many systems these binding proteins limit access of IGFs to their receptors, and lowering the concentrations of these binding proteins therefore may potentiate the action of IGFs.

Glucocorticoids

Glucocorticoids can inhibit the growth of immature animals. Indeed, only two to three times the normal daily secretion rate of cortisol is required to attenuate linear growth.[87, 88] The inhibitory effect on growth provides a useful means of differentiating children with states of cortisol excess from those with exogenous obesity (Fig. 21–8). In the former, growth failure is the rule, and the patient is nearly always short. In patients with exogenous obesity, however, linear growth is usually accelerated so that the heights of affected children are above the mean for age.

The growth-inhibitory effects of glucocorticoids are not limited to the skeleton. In weanling animals low doses of the hormone inhibit DNA synthesis in liver, heart, skeletal muscle, and kidney.[89] Tissues that renew and replenish themselves by cell proliferation are relatively resistant to the effects of glucocorticoids. These tissues include gut mucosa, testes, spleen, and the erythropoietic elements of bone marrow.

Glucocorticoids probably do not inhibit growth by suppression of GH secretion. Although large doses of cortisol inhibit GH secretion in adults, excess cortisol has only minimal effects on GH secretion in children.[90, 91] Furthermore, serum IGF I concentrations are not low in patients with glucocorticoid excess, and administration of GH in conjunction with glucocorticoid does not consistently reverse the growth attenuation.[92, 93] These and other lines of evidence suggest that glucocorticoids inhibit growth by direct action on the target tissue. For example, the addition of glucocorticoids to cartilage in vitro inhibits basal uptake of sulfate. Furthermore, high doses of glucocorticoids inhibit the syn-

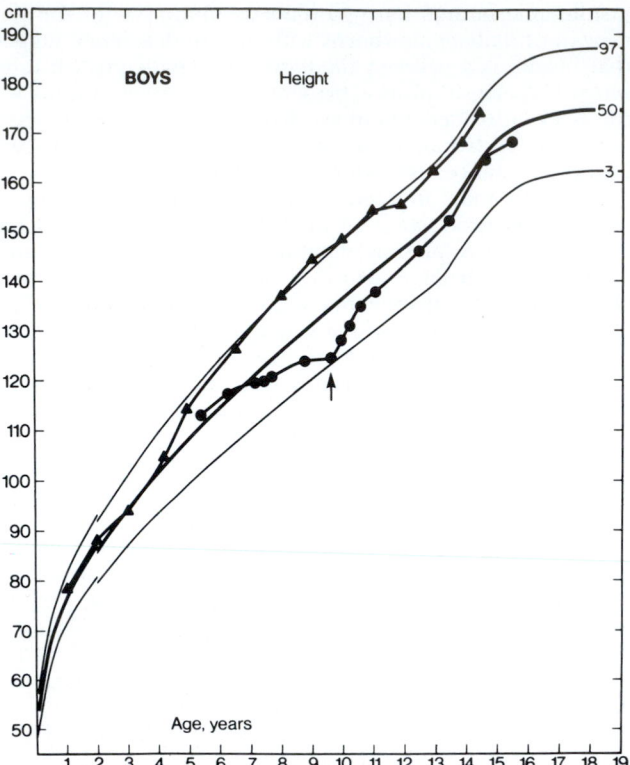

Figure 21–8. Growth curves of two boys with obesity. The boy depicted by circles (●—●) had cortisol excess related to Cushing disease. He experienced the onset of rapid weight gain associated with a decrease in linear growth at age 7 y. Diagnosis was made and adrenalectomy (arrow) was performed at age 9½ y; a period of catch-up growth followed. The boy whose growth is depicted by triangles ▲—▲) had exogenous obesity. At age 9½ y his weight was approximately the same as that of the patient with Cushing disease but his height was at the 97th percentile, which reflects stimulation of linear growth in patients with exogenous obesity.

thesis of glycosaminoglycans[94] and cause disruption in the ultrastructure of chondrocytes and extracellular matrix.[95] These changes are not completely reversible. Thus correction of cortisol excess may not be followed by the same degree of catch-up growth that characterizes other types of growth failure when the cause is removed.

Androgens

Testosterone and its metabolite dihydrotestosterone are potent anabolic agents that accelerate linear growth and weight gain and that increase lean muscle mass when administered to prepubertal children. States of androgen excess such as androgen-producing tumors, sexual precocity, and virilizing adrenal hyperplasia are uniformly associated with accelerated linear growth and weight gain.

The presence of GH is essential for the effective promotion of somatic growth by androgens.[29, 89] Administration of androgens to hypophysectomized rats has no effect on somatic growth;[96] the growth response to exogenous androgens is markedly diminished in humans with GH deficiency.[97] After GH replacement, however, androgens augment linear growth.[29, 98, 99] In addition androgens appear to enhance pituitary GH secretion.[23, 100]

Androgens cause disproportionate stimulation of epiphyseal maturation in prepubertal children and in children with growth arrest caused by either GH deficiency or glucocorticoid excess.[101] The ultimate effect of this discordance is loss of growth potential and diminution of eventual adult stature. Considerable effort has been expended in the search

for synthetic androgens that promote growth without producing virilization and stimulation of epiphyseal maturation, but it does not appear that the growth-promoting effects have been separated from the androgenic effects (see Chapter 13).

Estrogens

The net effect of pharmacological amounts of estrogens on somatic growth is inhibitory, whereas the effect on epiphyseal maturation is stimulatory. Administration of estrogen decreases linear growth and width of the cartilage growth plate in animals despite increased concentrations of GH in serum.[102, 103] In hypophysectomized animals the widening of the epiphyseal plate induced by exogenous GH is prevented by simultaneous estrogen treatment.[104] This inhibition of growth may be mediated by suppression of IGF I formation. Estrogens inhibit the GH-induced increase in IGF in hypophysectomized rats and in humans with hypopituitarism[89, 105, 106] and decrease the incorporation of sulfate by cartilage in animals. A direct inhibition by estrogens of IGF action is unlikely.[106, 107]

In humans, as in other species, estrogens increase basal plasma GH concentrations and enhance GH responses to provocative stimuli.[89] Administration of pharmacological doses of estrogens to tall girls leads to attenuation of growth rates and a decrease in predicted adult height.[108–112] Such treatment lowers the concentration of somatomedins in serum.[113, 114] Administration of estrogens to patients with acromegaly often produces clinical improvement such as reduction of soft tissue enlargement. This treatment is associated with increased GH and decreased IGF I concentrations.[115, 116]

Despite the fact that estrogens inhibit somatic growth, a paradoxical acceleration of growth is often observed in young children exposed to estrogens. This result is most likely related to a biphasic, dose-related effect of estrogens on growth:[114] at doses of 100 ng/kg/d ethinyl estradiol stimulates ulnar growth rate in girls with gonadal dysgenesis, but attenuation of growth occurs at higher doses. The low, growth-stimulating dose may not promote sexual maturation, which suggests that different tissues have variable sensitivities to the hormone.

Another factor that may contribute to the growth-promoting effect of estrogen is that estrogen treatment in children with intact pituitary, gonadal, and adrenal function causes a concomitant increase in androgens that secondarily cause acceleration of growth. Pubic hair develops and other androgen-related secondary sexual characteristics mature promptly after exposure to estrogens.

PEPTIDE GROWTH FACTORS OTHER THAN SOMATOMEDINS

The Relationship to Traditional Hormones: Paracrine and Autocrine Versus Endocrine Modes of Action

Although the hormones just discussed play pivotal roles in regulating overall body growth, their stimulatory effect on cell division in vitro is often less spectacular than the effects in vivo. A major reason for this discrepancy is that many traditional hormones influence growth in concert with peptide growth factors. In most respects peptide growth factors resemble the more traditional hormones in their behavior: they act through specific receptors, are subject to physiological regulation, and use similar mechanisms of signal transduction to produce biological effects in target tissues.

The most striking difference between peptide growth factors and classic hormones, however, is that growth factors are produced by many different tissues and exert many of their effects on neighboring tissues (paracrine effects) or even on their own cells of origin (autocrine effects) rather than on distant tissues that can be accessed only via the bloodstream (endocrine effects) (Fig. 21–9). These different modes of action are not mutually exclusive, however, because growth factors and other hormones can have different actions in different tissues. Somatostatin, for example, functions as a neurosecretory product in the hypothalamus, as a paracrine factor within the islets of Langerhans, and as a traditional hormone secreted by the pancreas and transported by portal blood to the liver.

The term *paracrine* was proposed half a century ago by Feyrter[117] to describe a network of epithelial clear cells distributed throughout the gut and other organs close to nerve endings and blood vessels (see Chapter 32). He postulated that these cells were "peripheral endocrine glands" and speculated that in addition to distant actions, these cells might have local "paracrine" effects in the regulation of gut function.

In 1980 Sporn and Todaro[118] added the concept of *autocrine* secretion to explain the endogenous production of autostimulatory growth factors by transformed cells. Although it was originally postulated that autocrine production of such "transforming growth factors" plays an etiological role in malignant transformation of cells, growth factors, including the so-called transforming growth factors, are produced by normal cells, and autocrine actions are central to normal cell biology rather than limited to malignant cells.

Direct evidence that locally produced growth factors are necessary for cell growth was provided by the observation that the growth of cultured cells can be inhibited by monoclonal antibodies directed at specific growth factors that are not present in the media in which the cells are grown.[119–121] An important consequence of autocrine and paracrine regulation is that the measurement of growth factor concentrations in blood or other fluids may poorly reflect physiological changes in the relevant tissues in which they are produced and in which they act. D'Ercole and colleagues,[122] for example, demonstrated that after injection of ovine GH to hypophysectomized rats, the tissue concentrations of IGF I rose several hours before a significant increase was detectable in serum.

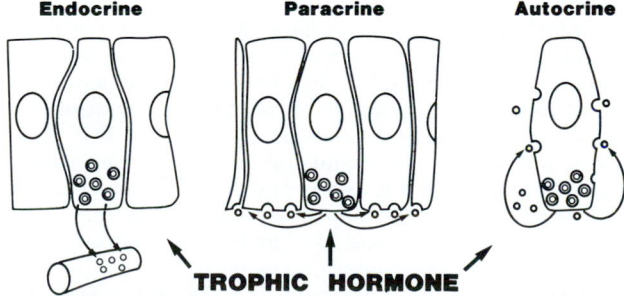

Figure 21–9. Schematic representation of modalities by which hormones and growth factors reach target tissues. Whereas traditional hormones are formed in glands of internal secretion and are transported to distant sites of action through the bloodstream (endocrine modality), peptide growth factors are more often produced locally by the target cells themselves (autocrine modality) or by neighboring cells (paracrine modality). Regardless of where they are formed, production is regulated in a similar fashion by trophic hormones and other regulatory influences.

Role in Differentiation and Proliferation

The effects of growth factors on cytodifferentiation are often overlooked. Most hormones and growth factors can stimulate either a mitogenic response or the development of differentiated cell functions depending on cell type, developmental stage, hormonal milieu, and other environmental circumstances. Some growth factors, such as transforming growth factor β (TGF β), are bifunctional and are able to either stimulate or inhibit growth. Thus the nature of the cellular response to hormones and growth factors is due less to the intrinsic properties of these chemical messengers than to the context in which they act. This was well stated by Sporn and Roberts,[123] who view growth factors as "part of a complex cellular signalling language, in which the individual peptides are the equivalent of characters of an alphabet code. . . . It is not surprising that meaning in this cellular language is contextual, because that is the case for all languages or codes."

Classification and Nomenclature

The naming of growth factors has followed no consistent pattern: some were named after some specialized property, others were assigned names corresponding to the tissue or cell type in which they were first encountered, and yet others were named according to the tissue on which they were presumed to act. Thus a mitogenic peptide isolated from bovine pituitary glands that stimulated cartilage growth was called *chondrocyte growth factor*,[124] and at the same time a mitogen for endothelial cells that had been isolated from cartilaginous tissues in young cows was called *cartilage-derived growth factor*.[125] Similarly, *endothelial cell growth factors* recovered from cultures of endothelial cells are confused with endothelial cell growth factors derived from fibroblasts or platelets but that stimulate endothelial cell growth. Qualification of the name *platelet-derived growth factor* (PDGF) led to even more confusion when it was recognized that platelets are a highly enriched source of at least four different growth factors including yet another endothelial growth factor.[126]

Confusion has also resulted from the fact that in several instances the same growth factors have been discovered independently by different investigators and therefore described under various different names. The best example of this is fibroblast growth factor (FGF), a substance that was originally isolated from bovine pituitary glands and brain as a highly basic mitogen for fibroblasts. Basic FGF was subsequently found to be widely distributed in many normal tissues derived from mesoderm and neuroectoderm. It is thus not surprising that FGF has been discovered and rediscovered under approximately 30 different names (Table 21–2). Such insights suggest that the number of growth factors may be finite and that many supposedly new growth factors may actually represent rediscoveries of previously recognized growth factors or homologous members of established superfamilies of growth factors. In this chapter we grouped currently recognized growth factors as members of such structurally related superfamilies or as members of categories that are based either on the organ systems that they regulate or on similarities in their effects (Table 21–3).

Major Growth Factor Families

The major superfamilies of growth factors are listed in Table 21–3. Because of their established importance the somatomedins (IGF-I and IGF-II) are discussed in detail in a separate section.

TABLE 21–2. Different Names for Fibroblast Growth Factor*

Basic FGF	Acidic FGF
Adipocyte growth factor	Astroglial growth factor I
Astroglial growth factor 2	Embryonic kidney–derived angiogenesis factor I
Cartilage-derived growth factor I	Endothelial cell growth factor
Cartilage growth factor (pituitary)	Endothelial growth factor
Chondrosarcoma growth factor	Eye-derived growth factor II
Embryonic kidney–derived angiogenesis factor 2	Heparin-binding growth factor class I
Embryonic carcinoma–derived growth factor	Retina-derived growth factor
Endothelial growth factor	
Eye-derived growth factor I	
Glial growth factor	
Heparin-binding growth factor	
Hepatoma growth factor	
Human pituitary growth factor	
Human placenta purified factor	
Leukemia growth factor (thymus)	
Mammary tumor–derived growth factor	
Macrophage growth factor	
Myogenic growth factor	
Prostatic osteoblastic factor	
Prostatic growth factor	
Prostatropin	
Tumor angiogenesis factor	
Uterine-derived growth factor	

*Heparin-binding growth factors have been extracted from many normal tissues as well as tumors and have been described by many different names. When their structures were determined, most of these proved to be identical with or closely related to basic FGF or acidic FGF.

Adapted from Gospadarowicz D. Fibroblast growth factor and its involvement in developmental processes. Curr Top Dev Biol 1990; 24:57–93.

THE EPIDERMAL GROWTH FACTOR/UROGASTRONE FAMILY

FAMILY MEMBERS. Mouse EGF. Epidermal growth factor (EGF) was discovered by Cohen in 1962 when he noted that extracts of salivary glands from adult male mice greatly accelerated eruption of the incisor teeth and opening of the eyelids of newborn mice.[127] He then proceeded to isolate and characterize EGF, delineate its interaction with receptors, and describe many of its biological effects.[128–130]

Mouse EGF is a single chain polypeptide of 53 amino acids with a molecular mass of 6045. It is extracted from mouse salivary gland as a heterotetramer composed of two EGF molecules and two identical 29-kd binding proteins with arginine esterase activity that reversibly bind to EGF at its COOH terminus.[131] The binding protein, which is encoded on a separate gene, liberates the active 53-amino-acid EGF from a 1217-amino-acid precursor.[132]

TABLE 21–3. Growth Factor Superfamilies

Somatomedins
  IGF I
  IGF II
Epidermal Growth Factor (EGF) Family
  EGF
  TGF α
  Amphiregulin
Fibroblast Growth Factors (Heparin-Binding Growth Factors)
  Acidic
  Basic
  Oncogenes (e.g., v-int-2, v-hst)
Platelet-Derived Growth Factors
  Beta,beta (v-sis oncogene)
  Alpha,beta
  Alpha,alpha
Transforming Growth Factor β Family
  TGF β types 1, 2, and 3
  Inhibins
  Activins
  Antimüllerian hormone
  Oncogenes (vg₁)
  Bone morphogenic proteins
  DPP-C (decapentaplegic transcript) (pattern formation in Drosophila)

Pre-proEGF is probably synthesized as a transmembrane protein because the amino acid structure has about 40% homology with residues from the extracellular domain of the cell-surface receptor for low-density lipoproteins.[133] Like the low-density lipoprotein receptor, the EGF precursor contains an internal region of hydrophobic residues that is believed to represent a transmembrane portion of the molecule. Pre-proEGF also contains certain repeated cysteine-rich sequences of amino acids similar to sequences in the EGF receptor.[134] In some tissues, such as the distal tubules of the kidney, pre-proEGF is synthesized but not processed to EGF.[135] Its function in these tissues is unclear, but the receptor-like structure suggests that it may participate in transmembrane signaling.

Human EGF/Urogastrone. The human homologue of mouse EGF was isolated from urine on the basis of its ability to inhibit acid release from gastric mucosa.[136] Although initially named urogastrone, this peptide has the biological properties of mouse EGF and is identical in 37 of the 53 amino acid residues. The mouse and human peptides cross-react with each other's receptors but differ considerably in the immunological cross-reactivities.[137, 138] The gene for human EGF maps to the same region of chromosome 4q as the gene for the T cell growth factor interleukin 2.[139]

Transforming Growth Factor α. Many tumors secrete an EGF-like peptide that is capable of interacting with EGF receptors in normal cells. This 50-amino-acid peptide was named *transforming growth factor α* (TGF α) because it was the first such peptide discovered. TGF α and EGF have a 35% sequence homology and apparently interact with the same receptor. TGF α is also produced by normal cells such as those in decidua, the central nervous system, and normal skin.[140] It is overexpressed in skin from patients with psoriasis.[141]

Amphiregulin. Amphiregulin is a 78-amino-acid glycoprotein that is 38% identical with EGF in the parts of the molecule that can be aligned. It was originally identified in cultures from human breast carcinoma cells because of its ability to inhibit the growth of several carcinoma cell lines while stimulating the proliferation of normal cells.[142] Unlike TGF α, amphiregulin reacts weakly with the EGF/TGF α receptor.

STRUCTURE AND FUNCTION. *EGF Regulation.* EGF concentrations in salivary glands are androgen dependent. Male submaxillary glands contain 15-fold more EGF than do female glands,[143] and salivary gland EGF content is increased after the administration of androgens to females and to castrated males.[144] Despite these pronounced sex-related differences, serum concentrations of EGF are comparable in male and female mice. In the skin (and in the submaxillary glands) EGF concentrations are also regulated by thyroid hormones, especially in the first 5 d of life.[145] Indeed, the acceleration by thyroid hormone administration of eyelid opening and tooth eruption in the neonatal mouse is probably mediated via EGF.

EGF Receptors and Postreceptor Events. The EGF receptor ranges in size in different tissues from 160 to 190 kd, depending on the degree of glycosylation.[146] The amino acid structure of the cytosolic portion is similar to that of the protein encoded by the v-*erb* B oncogene of avian erythroblastosis virus[147] and contains a tyrosine kinase that can both autophosphorylate itself and phosphorylate other cytosolic substrates.[148]

As for many other peptide hormones and growth factors, binding of EGF to its receptor is followed by internalization of the EGF-receptor complex and down-regulation of receptors on the cell surface.[149] A second EGF receptor-related gene may encode the amphiregulin receptor. A candidate for such a receptor is a protein with tyrosine kinase activity that was initially cloned from a tumor cell line on the basis of its homology with the EGF receptor gene.[150]

EGF Actions. Many of the biological effects of EGF stem from its ability to stimulate proliferation of the basal cell layers of ectodermally derived epithelia. EGF is present in amniotic fluid,[151, 152] and it, or its homologous family member TGF α, may be an important regulator of fetal development. When administered in utero to fetal lambs EGF induces maturation of airway epithelium and may protect against hyaline membrane disease.[153, 154] When administered to fetal lambs between 110 and 125 d of gestation, EGF also causes an increase in skin wrinkling and shedding of wool fibers.

EGF has potent effects on other developmental and proliferative processes. In the rat it appears to be essential for closure of the palate.[155, 156] Significant quantities of EGF are present in human breast milk, and its concentration in colostrum exceeds 300 μg/L. Colostral EGF may play a role in the maturation of the brush border and other gut functions in neonatal life.[157, 158]

FIBROBLAST GROWTH FACTORS*

PURIFICATION AND CHEMISTRY. Gospodarowicz and colleagues[160, 161] found that pituitary and brain extracts contain FGFs, which, together with small amounts of serum, are able to stimulate the proliferation of many cell lines of mesodermal and neuroectodermal origin.[160, 161] FGF was initially isolated from bovine brains as an acid labile, highly basic (pI 9.6) peptide of 13.4 kd that was indistinguishable from the FGF isolated from bovine pituitary glands.[162] An acidic form of FGF (pI 4.5) was subsequently isolated from bovine brain. The basic form is found in many tissues derived from mesoderm and neuroectoderm, whereas acidic FGF is confined mostly to nervous tissues and retina.

A unique property of the FGFs is a strong affinity for heparin, and heparin-binding growth factors have been isolated from a wide variety of cultured cells, organ extracts, and tumors.[162, 163] These FGF-like growth factors are the products of at least seven closely related genes, including the *int*-2 and *hst* proto-oncogenes.[164]

*See ref. 159.

BIOLOGICAL EFFECTS OF FGF. FGF stimulates cell proliferation in a manner similar to that of PDGF and can substitute for PDGF in defined media.[165] FGF induces mitosis in blastema cells in the stumps of frog limbs after amputation,[166] although a role in limb regeneration remains to be defined. FGF delays the senescence of cells maintained in culture, extending the life span of granulosa cells by 10 to 60 generations[167] and of corneal endothelial cells by up to 10-fold.[168]

Shing and co-workers[169] have drawn attention to the essential role of neovascularization in the growth of embryos, repair of wounds, and growth of tumors. FGF is a potent mitogen for vascular endothelial cells and now appears to account for most of the "angiogenesis factor" activities described by Folkman and other workers. The clinical utility of heparin-binding growth factors as a therapeutic agent in wound healing and in other clinical disorders is under active investigation[170] (Fig. 21–10).

FGF stimulates a host of biochemical processes within target tissues, including phosphorylation of intracytoplasmic proteins and induction of new protein synthesis. Although the FGFs are among the most potent growth factors described, their relevance to normal biological processes has not been delineated.[171] Unlike other hormones and growth factors, the gene for FGF lacks a signal peptide, and the mechanism of exiting its cells of origin is unknown. Nevertheless, FGF is found in the extracellular matrix of cultured

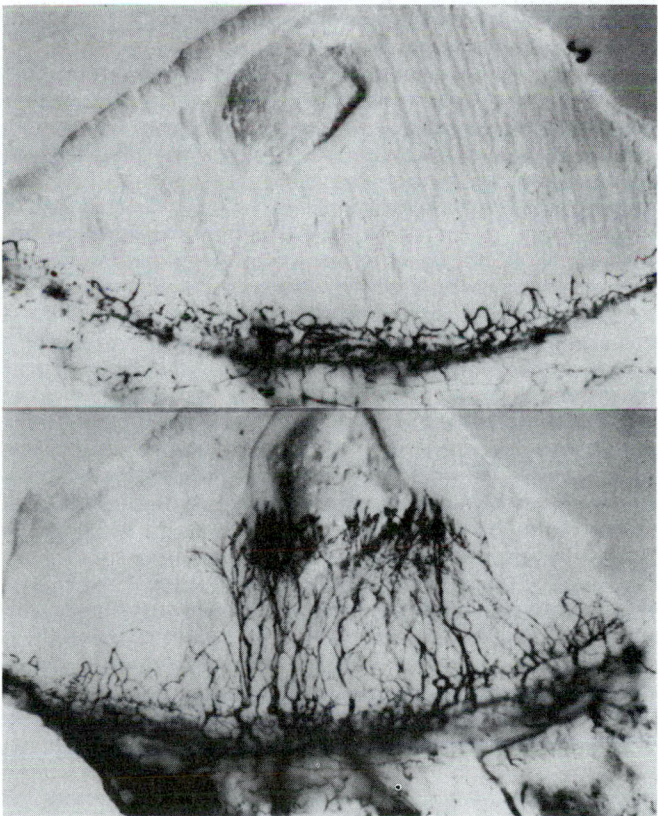

Figure 21–10. Stimulation of angiogenesis by basic FGF in rat cornea. Basic FGF (isolated from a rat chondrosarcoma) was incorporated into an ethylene vinyl acetate polymer and implanted by microsurgery into rat corneas. Control rats were implanted with polymer containing FGF that had been inactivated by boiling for 15 min. After 6 d the carotid arteries were injected with India ink, and the corneas were photographed. Note that the implant containing the active growth factor *(lower)* stimulated neovascularization by blood vessels originating from the limbus, whereas neovascularization did not occur in animals injected with polymer containing inactivated angiogenesis factor *(upper)*. (From Shing Y, Folkman J, Haudenschild C, et al. Angiogenesis is stimulated by a tumor-derived endothelial cell growth factor. J Cell Biochem 1985; 29:275–287. Copyright © 1985 John Wiley & Sons, Inc. Reprinted by permission of John Wiley & Sons, Inc.)

endothelial cells, where it is strongly bound to heparin-like substances. Furthermore, even in tissues that contain relatively high concentrations of FGF-like material by radioimmunoassay, it is frequently difficult or impossible to detect mRNAs for any of the known FGFs.

PLATELET-DERIVED GROWTH FACTOR*

DISCOVERY. It was long believed that the main function of platelets was to initiate blood coagulation by the release of clotting factors; an equally important platelet function is to release growth factors that initiate wound healing by reprogramming tissue cells to undergo division (see Fig. 21–10). Until the studies of Balk in 1971, it was not generally appreciated that plasma (the circulating fluid compartment of blood) is less effective than serum in supporting the proliferation of certain diploid cell lines.[174] He went on to postulate that serum contains a mitogen derived from the lysis of platelets during clotting that serves as a "wound hormone" for fibroblasts.[175] Rutherford and Ross[176] showed that, by supplementing platelet-poor plasma (made by separating the formed elements of blood before coagulation takes place) with a platelet extract, the enriched plasma is equipotent to whole serum in supporting the growth of dermal fibroblasts and aortic smooth muscle cells. PDGF is produced by a wide variety of cells in the embryo and in the adult and in many circumstances plays a pivotal role in growth regulation.

CHEMISTRY. In its unreduced state PDGF is a highly basic (pI 9.8 to 10.2) 30-kd dimeric peptide. The constituent A and B chains exhibit ~60% sequence identity but are encoded on separate genes on chromosome 22 that are similar in structural organization.[173, 177] The A chain occurs in two variants as a result of differential splicing. Each of the three possible isoforms of PDGF (AA, AB, and BB) have been isolated from natural sources.

The v-*sis* oncogene of simian sarcoma virus is a transduced PDGF B chain gene containing the entire region encoding proPDGF-B.[177–179] The presence of genes similar to v-*sis* together with the PDGF beta-receptor has been encountered in human sarcomas and glioma cell lines, which suggests that autocrine secretion of PDGF-like proteins may have a role in the genesis of certain human tumors.

PDGF ACTIONS. Two types of saturable high-affinity PDGF receptors of about 170 kd are present in a broad range of cells, largely of mesenchymal origin.[173, 180, 181] These receptors are designated alpha and beta. Because each of the two subunits in the dimeric PDGF molecule binds to one receptor molecule, two receptor molecules must also form a functional dimer for binding to take place (Fig. 21–11). The three isoforms of PDGF, AA, AB, and BB, bind with different affinities and specificities to these receptors so that the alpha-receptor binds all three isoforms with high affinity and the beta-receptor binds BB with high affinity, binds AB with a 10-fold lower affinity, and does not bind AA. These relationships provide diversity to the range of possibilities of PDGF regulation of cell proliferation. After PDGF binding, the receptor-ligand complex is rapidly internalized and degraded. As in the case of other growth factors, PDGF binding results in stimulation of tyrosine kinase activity.[182, 183]

THE ROLE OF PDGF IN CELL GROWTH. No large tissue stores of PDGF have been described. PDGF in blood is concentrated in the platelet alpha granules, where it is sequestered until cellular injury or some other stimulus leads to platelet degranulation.[184] Studies by Pledger and col-

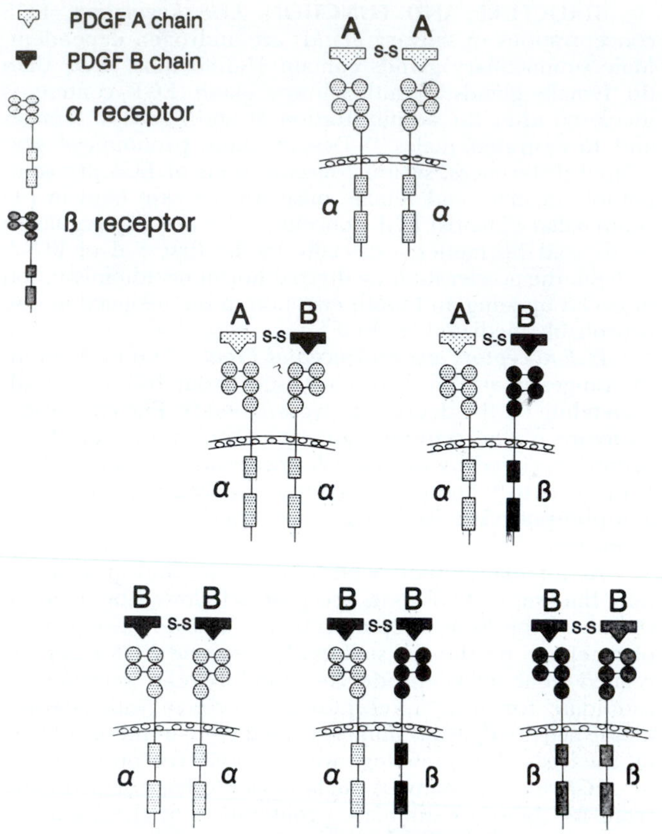

Figure 21–11. Schematic illustration of the abilities of the three isoforms of the PDGF dimer to bind to receptor composed of dimers of the alpha and beta receptor subunits. The model is based on the supposition that the PDGF A chain subunit binds only to alpha receptors, whereas the B chain subunit of PDGF binds to both alpha and beta receptors. The receptors are drawn to indicate that they are each composed of five extracellular immunoglobulin-like domains and a split cytoplasmic tyrosine kinase domain. (Adapted from Heldin CH, Westermark B. Platelet-derived growth factor: mechanism of action and possible in vivo function. Cell Regul 1990; 1:555–566.)

leagues indicated that transient exposure of BALB/c 3T3 cells to PDGF renders them "competent" to undergo DNA synthesis; however, IGFs and other substances in plasma (progression factors) are required for these competent cells to traverse the G_1 phase of the cell cycle and enter into DNA synthesis.[185] Other stimuli that can mimic the action of PDGF in cell replication include FGF, bombesin (gastrin-releasing factor), macrophage growth factor,[186] and exposure to precipitates of calcium phosphate or crystals of hydroxyapatite.[187]

In wound healing PDGF is a powerful chemotactic agent that recruits macrophages into wounds; furthermore, fibroblasts and endothelial cells are sensitive to the proliferative effects of PDGF, and replication of these cell types is essential to normal wound healing (Fig. 21–12).

Of equal importance from the standpoint of human pathophysiology is the possible role of PDGF in stimulating the proliferative changes associated with atherosclerotic plaques (see Fig. 21–12). A sequence of events beginning with intimal injury leads to platelet aggregation and degranulation, the release of PDGF, and the consequent migration of smooth muscle cells and their accumulation of lipids.[188] Agents that inhibit the degranulation of platelets diminish the atherosclerotic changes induced by homocystine administration in the rabbit.[189] FGF and other growth factors may also play important roles in the pathophysiology of the atherosclerotic plaque.[190]

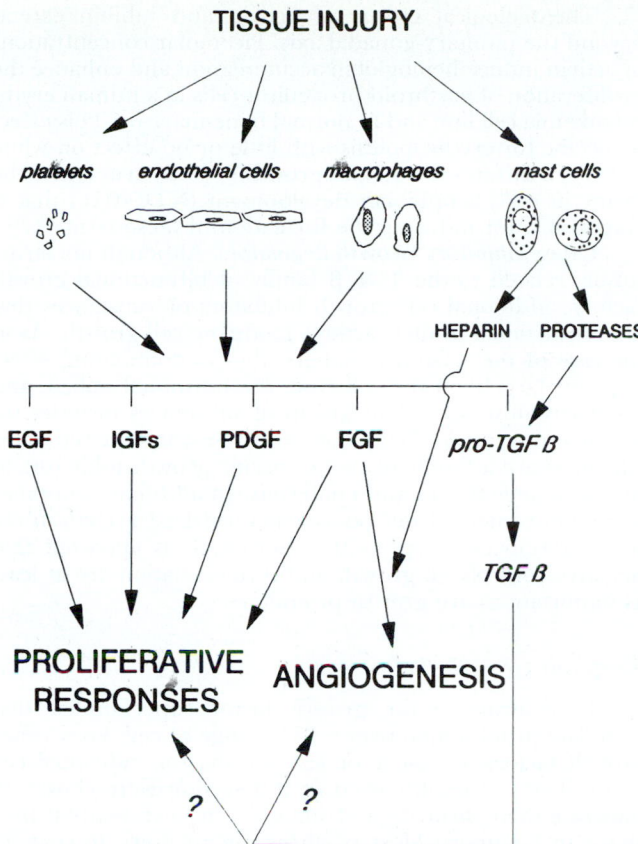

TISSUE INJURY

Figure 21-12. Some of the sources of the growth factors that are produced locally at sites of tissue injury and the important role of these factors in the healing process. Aggregation and lysis of platelets lead to the release of PDGF, TFG β, and other growth factors. Endothelial cells release FGF and other growth factors along with plasmin, which activates TGF β by releasing the active dimer from its latent precursor. TGF β is a powerful chemotactic agent that recruits macrophages into wounds, after which the macrophages become a further source of proteases and a variety of growth factors including interleukins, tumor necrosis factor, and other cytokines that are not shown. Heparin, released from mast cells, acts synergistically with FGF to stimulate neovascularization. Because TGF β can act as a mitogen under some circumstances and as a growth inhibitor under other circumstances, its most important role after injury may be to limit the proliferative response to tissue injury.

THE TRANSFORMING GROWTH FACTOR β FAMILY

The TGF β family of polypeptides includes three homologous members (TGF β_1, TGF β_2, and TGF β_3) localized in humans on chromosomes 19, 1, and 14, respectively, and a group of more distantly related polypeptides that nonetheless share sequence homology and biological activities.[191] The latter group includes antimüllerian hormone (AMH, also known as müllerian-inhibiting factor, MIF); inhibins and activins; several bone morphogenic proteins that may regulate cartilage and bone formation; vg$_1$, a *Xenopus* protein that may be involved in induction of mesoderm; and DPP-C, a *Drosophila* protein that regulates pattern formation.

THE TGF β MEMBERS

Chemistry. The three TGF β members are first synthesized as larger precursor polypeptides that are processed to yield 12.5-kd monomers.[191] The biologically active 25-kd polypeptide consists of two identical disulfide-linked monomers. Although the respective precursors differ, the three mature peptides are approximately 75% homologous, including all cysteine residues. The activins, inhibins, and AMH share 20 to 40% sequence identity with TGF β, and at least seven of the nine cysteine residues are conserved.

TGF β is secreted by cultured cells in an inactive or latent form that does not bind to TGF β cell-surface receptors. These latent forms of TGF β can be activated by transient acidification, treatment with chaotropic agents, or treatment with proteases such as plasmin. Indeed, plasmin inhibitors block some of the paracrine actions mediated by TGF β.[192] Inasmuch as latent forms of TGF β are secreted by nearly all types of cultured cells, the chemical mechanisms responsible for the latency and activation phenomena are central to understanding the regulation and biological roles of these peptides.

Receptors. Three distinct glycosylated binding proteins for TGF β have been identified in cell membranes by photoaffinity and cross-linking techniques. These proteins have M$_r$ values of 50,000 to 80,000 (type I), 115,000 to 140,000 (type II), and 280,000 to 330,000 (type III). The type III binding protein appears to differ from typical peptide hormone receptors because nearly half of the molecular mass is accounted for by heparan sulfate and chondroitin sulfate.[193] The biological effects of the TGF β in epithelial and perhaps other cell types are believed to be mediated by the type I receptor.

Biological Role of TGF β. Many growth factors are bifunctional, and the term *growth factor* rightly encompasses substances that inhibit as well as stimulate growth.[194] The TGF β members are particularly interesting because of bifunctionality. TGF β is a potent growth inhibitor, and production of TGF β2 by confluent monolayer cultures may be responsible for density-dependent inhibition of growth. Under appropriate circumstances TGF β inhibits the proliferation of most cell types, although its greatest effect is on epithelial cells. It is, for example, 10,000 times more potent than cyclosporine in suppressing T lymphocyte proliferation. TGF β does not kill cells, and its effects are reversible.

Under some circumstances TGF β stimulates the proliferation of mesenchymally derived cells such as fibroblasts and osteoblasts, but this effect is late and may be indirect. TGF β can transform normal cells so that they grow in soft agar only in the presence of EGF or TGF α. Indeed, its major role may be to prevent the proliferation of tumor cells rather than to stimulate their formation.

TGF β illustrates that the response of a cell to a hormonal signal may be determined more by the circumstances of the cell at that moment than by the nature of the signal. The growth of 3T3 fibroblasts, for example, is stimulated by TGF β in the presence of PDGF and is inhibited in the presence of EGF. Furthermore, in the presence of EGF or TGF α, TGF β stimulates the growth of rat kidney cells in soft agar and inhibits their growth in monolayer cultures.[195] It remains to be learned why these substances promote anchorage-dependent growth in some systems, act as transforming factors in other systems, and serve as growth inhibitors in yet other systems. The multifunctional capability of TGF β probably plays an extremely important role in embryonic development because in the early embryo it is primarily mitogenic, whereas in later stages it inhibits cell proliferation.

OTHER HOMOLOGOUS MEMBERS OF THE TGF β SUPERFAMILY

TGF β members are structurally related to AMH, inhibin, and activin and thus are members of one of the major growth factor superfamilies (Fig. 21-13).

Antimüllerian Hormone.[196, 197] AMH was first described by Jost as the testicular factor responsible for prenatal regression of the müllerian ducts in male embryos.[198] AMH was subsequently found to be homologous with TGF β and to be processed in a similar manner.[199, 200] AMH is present in the fetal ovary and postnatally in the mature graafian follicle. In boys the circulating blood levels are highest in the earliest months of life, but significant levels persist

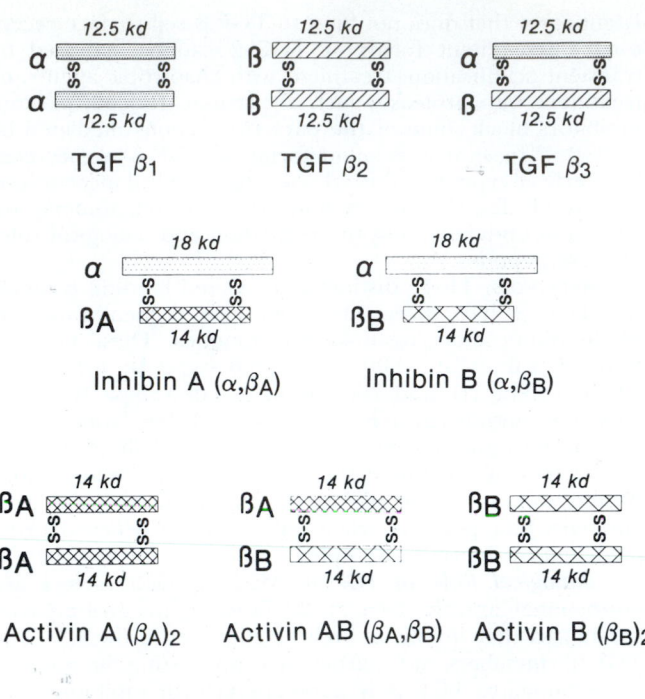

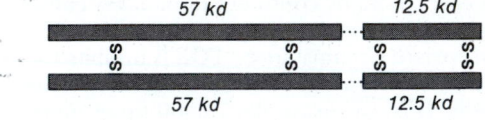

Antimüllerian hormone

Figure 21–13. Diagram of structural relationships among members of the TGF β family. TGF β$_1$ and TGF β$_2$ are homodimers (αα and ββ), whereas TGF β$_3$ is a heterodimer (αβ). The homology between the alpha and beta subunits is greater than 80%. The α subunits of inhibins A and B are unlike any other structures in the TGF β family. The β subunits of inhibin A and inhibin B (designated β$_A$ and β$_B$) are approximately 30% homologous to TGF β subunits. The activins consist of either homodimers or a heterodimer of the β$_A$ and/or β$_B$ subunits. Members of this family are isolated from intact cells and tissues as larger prohormones, which, in the case of the three patriarchal TGF β members, remain inactive until the mature dimers shown are liberated from their latent forms by exposure to acid conditions or proteases. An exception to this is AMH, which was isolated as a much larger active dimer, each element of which is 70 kd in size. The smaller homodimer consisting of identical 12.5-kd subunits cleaved from the precurser by plasmin digestion was found to retain the same biological activity as the larger form of AMH.

throughout childhood.[201] The functional significance of this peptide postnatally is unknown. In girls, AMH acts to inhibit meiosis of oocytes, possibly by inhibiting phosphorylation of the EGF receptor in response to EGF. The inhibitory effect of AMH on meiosis and on growth in a number of other systems can be counteracted by coincubation with EGF.[202]

Inhibin and Activin. It was postulated more than 50 y ago that the testis produces a nonsteroidal inhibitor of follicle-stimulating hormone (FSH) secretion.[203] Inhibins are now known to be present in both the testes and the ovaries. Inhibins are heterodimers with nonidentical alpha and beta subunits that are covalently linked by disulfide bridges. The beta subunits have sequence homology with TGF β and AMH. Activins are composed of two covalently linked beta subunits. Activins and inhibins are synthesized in the pituitary, the gonads, and probably other tissues as well.[204]

Activin and inhibin have opposite actions in the pituitary and gonads. In the pituitary, FSH secretion is inhibited by inhibin and stimulated by activin, whereas in the gonads, gonadotropin-dependent steroidogenesis and cell proliferation are potentiated by inhibin and inhibited by activin.[205, 206]

The biological effects of activin and inhibin extend beyond the pituitary-gonadal axis. Picomolar concentrations of activin induce hemoglobin accumulation and enhance the proliferation of erythroid progenitor cells in a human erythroleukemia cell line and in normal bone marrow. This effect is specific for erythropoiesis with little or no effect on white blood cell differentiation and growth.[207–209] Activin is also the factor in early amphibian development (XTC-MIF) that is responsible for inducing the formation of mesoderm.[210, 211]

Other Inhibitory Growth Regulators. Although not structurally related to the TGF β family of bifunctional growth factors, additional cell growth inhibitors or substances that are bifunctional in their actions modulate cell growth. As in the case of the TGF β members, the predominating effect depends largely on the cell type, the hormonal milieu, and other circumstances. This group of substances includes tumor necrosis factor (TNF), the interferons, and the retinoids. Chalones are a family of tissue-specific growth inhibitors in hematopoietic tissues and epidermis. In addition, a number of well-documented but poorly characterized growth-inhibiting substances are present in serum. It is apparent that negative controls on growth and differentiation are at least as important as are growth promoters.

Targeted Growth Factors

In contrast to the growth factor superfamilies that stimulate proliferation over a wide range of cell types, other growth factors are more or less specific for individual cell types. The factors discussed in this section were chosen to illustrate their diversity and some of the features that they share in common. Most of these agents were discovered because they regulate some highly specialized form of cytodifferentiation. As shown by further study, some are less specific than originally thought and have a wider range of action than implied by the names with which they were christened (Table 21–4).

NERVE GROWTH FACTOR

CHEMISTRY AND PURIFICATION. The existence of a diffusible neurotrophic substance was suggested by Levi-Montalcini and Hamburger in 1951 when they observed growth of dorsal root and sympathetic ganglia in chick embryos implanted with mouse sarcoma tissue.[212] Like EGF, NGF is found in large amounts in the male mouse submaxillary gland, a feature not shared with humans. It was while studying the biological effects of NGF in crude submaxillary gland extracts that Cohen[213] made the observations that led to the discovery of EGF.

TABLE 21–4. Examples of Targeted Growth Factors

Nerve growth factors
Hematopoietic growth factors
    Erythropoietin
    Colony-stimulating factors
        Granulocyte-macrophage CSF*
        Granulocyte CSF
        Macrophage CSF
        Multi-CSF (interleukin 3)
Other cytokines
    Interleukins 1–9
    Tumor necrosis factor
    Interferons
    Thymopoietins
Gastrointestinal hormones
    Bombesin (gastrin-releasing hormone)
    Enteroglucagon

*CSF, colony-stimulating factor.

NGF from submaxillary glands is a large 140-kd (7S) complex that can be dissociated into three types of subunits. The beta subunit is the biologically active component. This basically charged peptide has a molecular mass of 13 kd and about 25% homology with the A and B chains of human insulin.[214] It is associated with two alpha and two gamma subunits, and the entire complex is stabilized by two atoms of zinc. The gamma subunit is an arginine esterase that is analogous to the EGF-binding protein.[215]

NGF RECEPTORS. Two types of NGF receptor are present in neural cells: a high-affinity, low-capacity receptor with a relative molecular size between 75 and 80 kd and a low-affinity, high-capacity receptor. Lymphocytes and macrophages contain only the low-affinity receptor. Both the high- and low-affinity forms of the NGF receptor are believed to be derived from a single gene on human chromosome 17.[216]

BIOLOGICAL EFFECTS OF NGF. The predominant effect of NGF is to promote the survival, differentiation, and axonal outgrowth of sensory and sympathetic ganglia. Because neurons are terminally differentiated cells that do not replicate, NGF does not function as a mitogen for the mature nervous system. NGF is a weak mitogen for lymphoid tissue (vide infra), however, and it may be mitogenic for precursors of nervous tissue in the early embryo. Animals injected with neutralizing antibodies to NGF undergo degeneration of dorsal root and sympathetic ganglia,[217] and the injection of NGF into chick embryos prevents the preprogrammed cell death that characterizes the normal development of these neurons.[218] The effects of NGF on neuron survival appear to be developmentally regulated: the injection of blocking antibodies to NGF produces neuronal degeneration in fetal animals, but in adult animals the sensory neurons do not require NGF for survival.[219]

In addition to promoting the survival of this select population of developing neurons, NGF accelerates the biochemical and morphological differentiation of stem cells into sympathetic and sensory neurons.[220] A line of cells derived from a rat pheochromocytoma, PG-12, is induced morphologically and biochemically by NGF to become sympathetic neurons. The biochemical differentiation of these cells arises from the stimulatory effects of NGF on the synthesis of adrenergic and peptidergic neurotransmitters that are characteristic of sensory neurons.[221]

Selective NGF production during the development of peripheral tissues attracts the neurites of the appropriate sensory and sympathetic neurons along a chemotactic NGF gradient, which results in selective tissue innervation. NGF is then transported in a retrograde fashion to its target ganglia, where it is concentrated.[222] Relatively small amounts of NGF mRNA can be detected in the ganglia themselves.[223] This schema is believed to be the mechanism by which tissues determine both the specificity and the density of their axonal connections.[224]

NGF may also play a role in inflammatory and immune responses: NGF is a chemoattractant for neutrophilic leukocytes,[225] and the administration of the beta subunit of NGF to neonatal animals leads to an increased number of mast cells in a number of tissues.[226] NGF stimulates receptors for interleukin 2 on cultured human lymphocytes,[227] and low-affinity receptors for NGF are present on rat spleni mononuclear cells. NGF is a weak mitogen in mixed cultures of spleen mononuclear cells and potentiates the synthesis of DNA in response to several T cell and B cell mitogens.[228]

NGF IN HUMAN DISEASE. Several lines of evidence point to a role for NGF in disease. Fisher and colleagues have noted that the concentration of NGF in the brain of both adult and fetal mice is regulated by thyroxine and have suggested that the effects of thyroid hormones on brain development might result from alterations in NGF concentrations.[72, 229]

Increased amounts of serum NGF are present in patients with the peripheral form of neurofibromatosis[230] and in patients with multiple endocrine neoplasia type 2B (3).[231] The latter disorder is characterized by the growth of ganglioneuromas on the lips and throughout the alimentary tract and by a high incidence of medullary thyroid carcinoma and pheochromocytoma (also see Chapter 30).

ERYTHROPOIETIN

The importance of hematopoietic growth factors is made clear by the fact that approximately 9 billion red blood cells every hour turn over in normal adults.[232] All formed elements of the blood originate from a population of pleuripotential stem cells that differentiate during embryonic life into the various families of blood cells. Differentiation and maintenance of the different blood cell populations are governed to a large extent by a group of structurally unrelated sialoglycoproteins, each of which controls a specific population of cells.[233]

The possibility that hematopoiesis might be regulated by a humoral factor was initially suggested by the observation in 1906 that hypoxia in one rat of a parabiotic pair resulted in erythroid hyperplasia in the other.[234] It was found subsequently that extracts of blood and urine from hypoxic humans, sheep, and other species are enriched in a peptide growth factor called erythropoietin (EPO),[235] a 39-kd acidic sialoprotein that consists of a 166-amino-acid protein backbone (18.4 kd) plus carbohydrate.[236]

BIOLOGICAL CONTROL. The kidney is the major site of EPO production postnatally, and the liver is a major source in the fetus. The small amounts of hepatic EPO postnatally are insufficient to sustain red blood cell production in patients with end-stage renal disease. The major stimulus of EPO production is anoxia resulting from anemia, high altitude, or hypoventilation. Although renal arterial oxygenation is the major factor in its feedback regulation, EPO production is also under the control of both androgens and GH.[237, 238] The role of GH is to adjust red blood cell production to changes in body mass, and GH excess causes polycythemia only rarely. This effect of GH is mediated by IGF I, which potentiates both the production of EPO and the action of EPO at the cellular level.[239, 240] Under some circumstances IGF I may substitute for EPO; for example, IGF I was the major circulating erythropoietic factor in an anephric patient with low levels of EPO.[240a] The effect of androgens on erythropoiesis is reflected in the increased red blood cell mass in males after puberty and in females with elevated plasma testosterone concentrations. The use of androgens in patients with aplastic anemia is based on the ability of testosterone to stimulate EPO production. Because EPO originates in the kidney, androgen therapy is ineffective in the anephric state. It has been difficult to determine whether EPO is primarily a differentiation factor for existing cells or a true mitogen, because a single cell division may give rise to daughter cells with new functional properties. This confusion is due to the fact that EPO acts in concert with other growth factors including IGF I and activin. Most evidence suggests that EPO induces several cycles of proliferation in primitive stem cells before stimulating in proerythrocytes a terminal wave of mitosis that gives rise to cells that can synthesize hemoglobin.[241–243]

THERAPEUTIC USE. One of the most disabling features of end-stage renal disease is anemia resulting from hypoplasia of erythrocyte precursors. A spectacular triumph of recombinant DNA methodology is the provision of recombinant EPO to treat these patients (Fig. 21–14). In one study

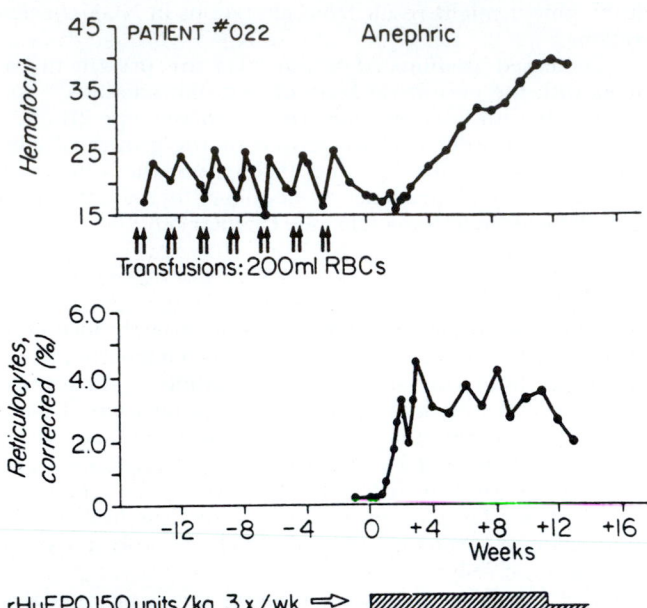

Figure 21–14. Effect of recombinant human EPO given three times a week on hematocrit *(upper)* and reticulocyte counts *(lower)* in an anephric patient who had previously remained anemic in spite of repetitive transfusions. Similar results have now been reported in several thousand patients. (From Eschbach JW, Egrie JC, Downing MR, et al. Correction of the anemia of end-stage renal disease with recombinant human erythropoietin. Results of a combined phase I and II clinical trial. Reprinted with permission from The New England Journal of Medicine 316, 73–78, 1987.)

of more than 2000 such patients, virtually all became independant of transfusions.[244]

GRANULOCYTE-MACROPHAGE COLONY-STIMULATING FACTORS*

The proliferation of white blood cells is controlled by peptide growth factors in a manner analogous to the control of red blood cell generation by EPO. The term *colony-stimulating factors* (CSFs) originated from the colony formation techniques designed to study the growth in soft agar of colonies of descendants of individual progenitor cells.[247] Cell division of these progenitor cells depends on specific mitogenic signals that may stimulate the growth of up to 10,000 progeny cells from the appropriate precursor. Like NGF and other tissue-specific growth factors, the CSFs also have important effects on cell survival, cell differentiation, and regulation of cell function.

The mouse granulocyte-macrophage CSFs are a family of at least four glycoproteins that cause bipotential precursor cells to differentiate into granulocytes, macrophages, or both.[248] These CSFs are *granulocyte-macrophage CSF* (GM-CSF), *granulocyte CSF* (G-CSF), *macrophage CSF* (M-CSF), and *multi-CSF*, which is identical with interleukin 3. The human CSFs are low-molecular-weight acidic glycoproteins that exhibit significant homology with mouse CSFs.

The main source of CSFs is the antigen-stimulated T lymphocyte, although some may also be produced by monocytes, fibroblasts, and endothelial cells after appropriate stimulation. Rich yields of CSFs have been obtained from lung, kidney, spleen, and salivary gland after treatment of animals with various lectins, antigens, or endotoxin.[249] Some CSFs can be easily detected in the circulation, whereas others are produced and act in a paracrine fashion on neighboring cells in the bone marrow.[250]

---

*See references 245, 246.

The CSFs exhibit considerable overlap in biological activity in different systems, and their interactions with each other and with other cytokines and growth factors are poorly understood. The production of large quantities of CSFs by recombinant DNA methodology should make it possible to determine the role of deficient CSF production in granulocytopenia of different etiologies and the clinical utility of these growth factors in treatment.[251] It has been suggested, for example, that the induction of differentiation by CSFs might be useful in the treatment of myeloid leukemias.[252] Perhaps their greatest promise is in ameliorating the myelosuppressive effect of cancer chemotherapy.[253]

OTHER CYTOKINES

INTERLEUKINS. The generic term *lymphokine* has been applied to all regulatory substances produced by lymphocytes other than antibodies. Because the term lymphokine (*monokine* in the case of substances produced by monocytes) connotes the cell of origin of these factors rather than their function, many substances of doubtful relevance to growth regulation are included under this designation along with those that clearly function in the same fashion as other peptide growth factors. The interleukins are lymphokines or monokines that regulate the growth and differentiation of lymphocytes. It is only out of historical convention that CSFs are usually not classified with interleukins or, for that matter, that substances that regulate the proliferation and maturation of lymphocytes are not called CSFs.

At least nine different interleukins are believed to have specific functions in the growth, differentiation, and regulation of the cells mediating immune responses. Although by every criterion the interleukins fit the category of growth factors, their role in the immune system is beyond the scope of this chapter and has been the subject of comprehensive reviews.[254–256]

As in the case of other growth factors, interleukins are also formed in cells that traditionally are not considered to be part of the immune system and have a wider range of biological actions than originally thought. For example, interleukin 1 (IL 1), which is produced by circulating monocytes and tissue macrophages from liver, functions as a hormone, whereas the IL 1 produced by more specialized cell types, such as keratinocytes and gingival epithelial cells, probably has a local paracrine function. IL 1 also releases corticotropin (ACTH, adrenocorticotropin), primarily by stimulating release of corticotropin-releasing hormone in the hypothalamus,[257] although IL 1 may also have direct actions at the pituitary level. This control of ACTH release by IL 1 thus serves the purpose of coordinating endocrine responses and other acute-phase responses to illness. In addition to its effects on lymphocyte and pituitary function, IL 1 together with interleukin 6 (IL 6) mediates other biological responses to acute inflammation, including fever, neutrophilia, and acute-phase protein production by the liver.[258, 259] Because of their multiple functions, most interleukins are known by several different names; for example, IL 6 is referred to as *hepatocyte-stimulating factor*.[260, 261]

TNF. Despite its name, TNF, or cachectin, is a typical pleiotropic cytokine, the activity of which is determined largely by the cell type to which it binds and the presence of other regulatory proteins.[262] Thus TNF can be a growth factor, a cytotoxin, a cytostatic agent, or an inducer of differentiation. TNF is also an inflammatory mediator regulating the activity of neutrophils, eosinophils, and T and B lymphocytes and modulating the properties of the vascular endothelium. Its discovery was due in large part to its ability to induce necrosis in malignant tumors.[263] TNF resembles lymphotoxin, another cytokine. Both are encoded on the short arm of chromosome 6 near the histocompatability locus[264] and share 30% amino acid homology. TNF is a mitogen for human diploid fibroblasts and acts synergistically with EGF, PDGF, and IGFs.[265] In low doses the administration of TNF causes hyperlipidemia, and TNF may play a role in the mobilization of fat depots in patients with cancer and other chronic diseases.[263] In higher dosages TNF can cause profound hypotension.[266]

INTERFERONS. *Interferon* is the term originally given to secreted glycoproteins capable of inducing an antiviral state in cells.[267] Interferon-α and interferon-β, originating in leukocytes and fibroblasts, respectively, differ in chemical and biological properties from interferon-γ, which is produced by stimulated T cells; indeed, the antiviral activity of interferon-γ appears to be in part secondary to its stimulation of interferon-α and interferon-β.[268] Studies with recombinant peptides and neutralizing antibodies have disclosed that the interferons are bifunctional regulators of normal cell growth; they stimulate cell replication under some circumstances and inhibit cell growth under others.[269] The predominant effect in most cell lines is to inhibit mitogenic signals (such as those from the proto-oncogenes c-*myc* and c-*fos*) in response to other growth factors.[270]

THYMOSINS AND THYMOPOIETINS. The long disputed role of the thymus as an endocrine organ was apparently resolved by the isolation of a family of peptides that control the proliferation and maturation of primitive lymphocytes into immunologically competent T cells.[271] Although lymphokines and thymic hormones stimulate apparently identical processes, there is a paucity of cross-reference to the thymic hormones in the lymphokine literature and to the interleukins (by any of their many aliases) in the thymic hormone literature.

Thymopoietin is a 49-amino-acid single chain peptide that induces the differentiation of prothymocytes into immunologically competent T cells with full expression of surface antigens.[272] A synthetic pentapeptide consisting of residues 32 to 36 is able to mimic the action of the native molecule[273] and has been tried for the treatment of rheumatoid arthritis.[274]

α$_1$-Thymosin is a 28-amino-acid peptide purified from bovine thymic extracts.[275] Injections of partially purified thymosin preparations into athymic dwarf nude mice lead to lymphocyte proliferation, increased somatic growth, and the capability of rejecting allografts.[275] Promising clinical results have been reported after injections of thymosin in children with genetic immunodeficiency disease and in patients with lymphocytopenia secondary to radiation or cancer chemotherapy.[276]

Oncogenes and the Control of Growth

A link between peptide growth factors and tumor-associated proteins was established with recognition that the gene products of tumor retroviruses are related to normal cell constituents and that analogues of tumor virus oncogenes also exist in normal cells.[277, 278] An oncogene is the portion of the viral genome that is responsible for imparting the neoplastic phenotype to its host. Retroviruses have the unique ability to incorporate DNA from the host cell into their own genome and to transfect a portion of their own RNA genome into the DNA genome of a host cell. Viral oncogenes are designated by a v- (for virus) followed by a cryptic three-letter code to designate the original source of the virus. The cellular proto-oncogenes, which are designated by a c- (for cellular), differ from viral oncogenes by the presence of noncoding sequences (introns) and by minor nucleotide differences.

The finding that oncogenes code for normal cell products led to an intensive effort to determine the mechanisms of malignant transformation. Although some proto-oncogenes encode peptide growth factors or growth factor receptors, most encode proteins involved in the postreceptor transduction of signals leading to cell differentiation or replication.[279] Studies of the mechanisms by which oncogenes cause malignant transformation provide insight into the mechanisms that regulate normal growth.[280, 281] Some of the various oncogenes and their products are shown in Table 21–5.

ONCOGENES ENCODING GROWTH FACTORS AND GROWTH FACTOR RECEPTORS. The first association of an oncogene with a peptide growth factor was established when the v-*sis* gene (simian sarcoma virus from the woolly monkey) was found to encode a protein that is almost identical with the NH$_2$-terminal 109 amino acids of the B chain of human PDGF.[282, 283] Soon thereafter, the v-*erb* B gene, obtained from an avian erythroblastosis virus, was shown to code a protein similar to a truncated portion of the EGF receptor and containing tyrosine kinase activity.[284] The *erb* A oncogene

---

TABLE 21–5. Some Oncogenes Related to Normal Growth Processes*

Oncogene	Homologues or Products
Growth factors	
sis	PDGF B chain
hst, int$_2$	FGF
vg$_1$	TGF β
Growth factor receptors	
erb B	Truncated EGF receptor
erb A	Steroid and thyroxine receptors
kit, fms	PDGF and CSF-1 receptors
Tyrosine-specific protein kinases	
src	Tyrosine-specific protein kinases
abl	
Ser/Thr-specific protein kinases	
mos	Substrates for growth factor–dependent tyrosine
raf	kinases (c-*mos* expressed primarily in gonads)
Signal transducers	
ras	GTP/GDP-binding protein (activates GTPase)
Nuclear oncogenes	
myc	Phosphoproteins that regulate gene transcription
myb	
fos	
jun	

*Examples of genes that were initially identified as the oncogenic moiety of tumor viruses and that were later shown to encode proteins that are homologous with proteins in normal cells that play important roles in growth regulation.

was then found to be homologous with the genes coding for receptors of the steroid/thyroid hormone family.[285]

ONCOGENES ENCODING PROTEIN KINASES. Several oncogenes such as *src* and *abl* code for cell membrane proteins that either are tyrosine kinases or stimulate tyrosine kinase activity.[286] Phosphorylation of tyrosine residues on specific proteins is a feature of the mitogenic actions of most growth factors. Some tyrosine kinases, such as *src* and *abl*, have no known functions apart from their kinase activity, whereas other tyrosine kinases such as the *erb* B gene product are embedded within the cytosolic portions of growth factor receptors. The tyrosine kinase function of growth factor receptors is essential for the mitogenic effects of the corresponding growth factor.[287] The gamma subunit of phospholipase C is a specific substrate for the tyrosine kinase of several growth factor receptors.[288]

Other oncogenes such as c-*mos* and c-*raf* encode kinases that preferentially phosphorylate serine and threonine residues. The expression of the c-*mos* oncogene is higher in the gonads than in any other tissue,[289] although the significance of this finding is unknown. The c-*raf* oncogene is one of the primary substrates for tyrosine phosphorylation in response to PDGF and certain other growth factors.[290]

ras **ONCOGENES.** Eucaryotic cells contain a highly conserved gene family encoding 21-kd proteins that are intimately involved in growth control. The family of *ras* oncogenes plays a crucial role in cell proliferation, and excessive expression or mutant forms of these genes occur in 10 to 40% of human tumors.[291] *ras* function is required for the mitogenic effects of many growth-promoting substances.[292] The *ras* proteins, together with the GTPase-activating protein, regulate the conversion of GTP to GDP in the cell membrane, a key step in the transduction of signals leading to the activation of protein kinase C.

ONCOGENES ENCODING NUCLEAR PROTEINS. The nuclear oncogenes c-*myc*, c-*fos*, and c-*jun* regulate gene transcription and are among the earliest genes transcribed after exposure of cells to growth factors. These nuclear oncogenes encode phosphoproteins that regulate gene transcription. Fos and Jun, the proteins encoded by the proto-oncogenes c-*fos* and c-*jun*, form a dimer through a leucine zipper motif. This dimer then mediates transcriptional regulation by binding to AP-1 DNA promoter elements.[293]

Interactions between growth factors and nuclear oncogenes were established with the discovery that PDGF stimulates in BALB/c 3T3 cells up to 40-fold increases in the c-*myc* mRNA, an oncogene that was originally found in avian myelocytomatosis virus.[294] Microinjection of this protein into BALB/c 3T3 cells bypasses the need for PDGF in traversing the G_1 phase of the cell cycle.[295] Expression of c-*myc* and other nuclear oncogenes is not sufficient or in some instances not even necessary for growth to occur.[296] In summary, nuclear oncogenes are among the few known genes that are expressed early in the passage through the cell cycle and that may hold a key to the cascade of cellular events that result in cell division.

Mechanisms of Growth Control

Although it is not possible to predict how all of this information will ultimately fit together, the large number of growth factors and products of oncogenes constitutes a major physiological growth-regulating system that may equal in importance the endocrine system as previously defined. These peptides operate by autocrine, paracrine, and even endocrine mechanisms to regulate processes as diverse as embryonic differentiation, aging, organ regeneration, and wound repair, as well as normal growth and development. Understanding of these factors is of potential importance in understanding the pathophysiology of many diseases that lie outside the traditional domain of endocrinology. Indeed, little information about these growth-regulating proteins and peptides has yet been incorporated into clinical endocrinology, and, except for the somatomedins, measurements of these substances have not been used diagnostically.

Now that recombinant DNA technology can provide much larger supplies of these growth-regulating substances to physiologists and clinical investigators, it may be possible to develop strategies to manipulate selectively the growth and differentiation of specific tissues and cell types. This, in turn, should facilitate the emergence of new therapies with specificity comparable to that of EPO in treating the anemia of end-stage renal disease. Furthermore, the explosion of knowledge concerning the mechanisms by which growth is regulated at the cellular level will extend the purview of endocrinology beyond the traditional boundaries.

THE SOMATOMEDINS

Introduction

Somatomedins were isolated on the basis of three properties: GH-like activities in cartilage (sulfation factor and thymidine factor),[297] insulin-like activity in adipose tissue and muscle (nonsuppressible insulin-like activities),[298, 299] and mitogenic properties in cell culture systems (multiplication-stimulating activity).[300, 301] *Insulin-like growth factor I*[54] and *somatomedin-C*[55] are different names for a 70-amino-acid, straight chain basic (pI 8.1 to 8.5) peptide that is homologous to human proinsulin. The other somatomedin, *insulin-like growth factor-II*, is a 67-amino-acid neutral peptide that is homologous to IGF I (Fig. 21–15). IGF I is more GH dependent and more potent in growth promotion than is IGF II, whereas IGF II has more insulin-like activity than does IGF I. The rat homologue of human IGF II was initially isolated and sequenced as multiplication-stimulating activity (MSA).[301, 302] There is now a consensus that the term *somatomedin* should be used only when referring to these peptides in a generic sense, and that *IGF I* and *IGF II* should be used when referring to the specific peptides. When necessary for clarity, species can be indicated by lower case prefixes and variant forms by suffixes.[303]

SOMATOMEDINS IN SPECIES OTHER THAN HUMANS. The structures of the somatomedins are highly conserved across species. Rats and probably other mammalian species have two forms of somatomedin that are homologous to human IGF I and IGF II. The amino acid sequence of bovine IGF I, for example, is identical with that of human IGF I. The basic GH-dependent rat somatomedin differs from human IGF I by only three amino acid residues,[304] and rat IGF II (multiplication-stimulating activity) is a 67-amino-acid peptide that differs in five residues from the structure of human IGF II.[302] IGFs and receptors for these factors have also been identified in birds, fish, and insects.

THE SOMATOMEDIN GENES. The somatomedins are encoded by single copy genes; the gene for pre-pro–IGF I is localized to the long arm of chromosome 12, and the gene for pre-pro–IGF II is localized to the short arm of chromosome 11.[305, 306] A variant form of IGF II exists in which the tetrapeptide Arg-Leu-Pro-Gly is substituted for the serine at position 29.[307]

The pre-pro–IGF II gene is close to the gene for preproinsulin, and the somatomedin loci on chromosomes 11 and 12 are also close to proto-oncogenes of the c-*ras* family. It has been suggested that chromosomes 11 and 12 have a common ancestry and that the close linkage of genes for

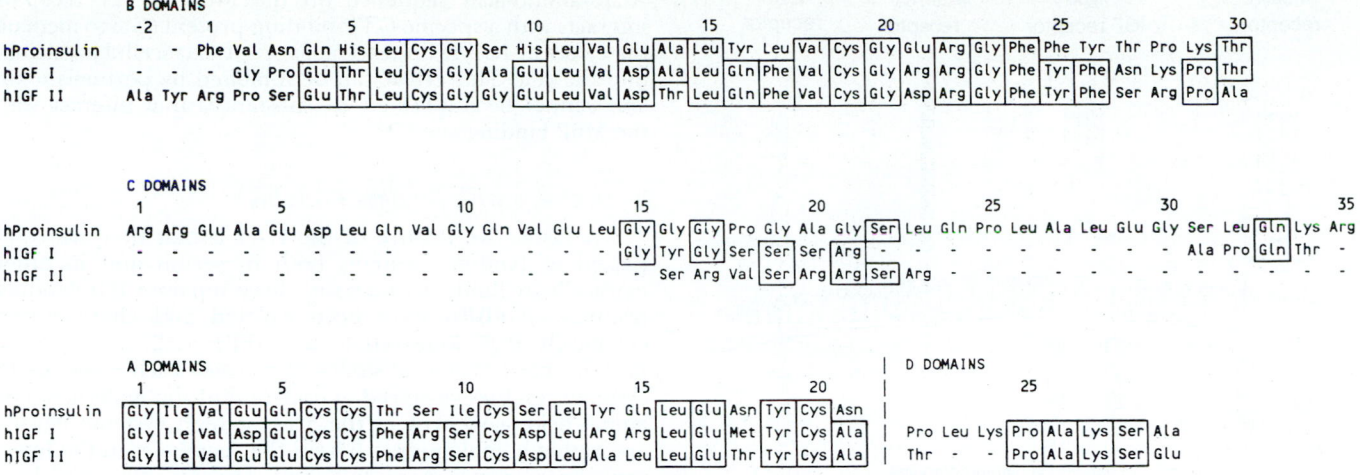

Figure 21–15. Homologies between human proinsulin and IGFs I (and IGF II). Although the three peptides exhibit striking homology in B and A domains, they diverge markedly in their connecting peptides (C domains). In addition, proinsulin lacks a D domain.

somatomedins with those for an important class of cellular oncogenes has both evolutionary and functional significance.[305]

Analysis of cDNAs encoding the somatomedins reveals that both IGF I and IGF II are synthesized like other secreted proteins with leader sequences of 25 and 24 amino acids, respectively, at the NH₂ termini. In addition, IGF I has an extension of 35 amino acids and IGF II has an extension of 89 residues at the respective COOH termini.[305, 308-310] Thus the pre-pro—forms of the hormones require post-translational processing to produce the mature forms. Variant cDNAs for IGFs arise from alternative splicing mechanisms and provide a mechanism by which gene expression can be modified in different tissues as a function of developmental status and environmental circumstance.[311]

Biological Actions of the Somatomedins

Interactions with Receptors

The overlapping biological effects of IGFs and insulin were initially attributed to the structural homologies between the peptides themselves,[297, 312] but this interpretation proved overly simplistic when it was shown that the receptors for insulin and IGF I are also structurally similar.[313, 314] Studies with radiolabeled IGFs have disclosed two types of receptors.

The type I receptor has a subunit structure similar to the heterotetrameric structure of the insulin receptor, with two disulfide-linked extracellular alpha subunits of about 130 kd and two 90-kd beta subunits that contain the transmembrane and cytosolic domains (Table 21–6 and Fig. 21–16). The type I receptor binds IGF I preferentially and has high-affinity binding sites for IGF II and, to a lesser extent, insulin. The fact that a monoclonal antibody to the type I receptor inhibits binding of IGF I more completely than the binding of IGF II suggests that IGF I and IGF II bind to different binding sites on the same receptor.[315] To complicate matters, chimeric receptors have been described in which an αβ subunit of the type I IGF receptor is covalently linked with an αβ subunit of the insulin receptor.[316]

The beta subunits of both the IGF type I and the insulin receptors contain a tyrosine kinase domain. Binding of ligand to receptor activates the tyrosine kinase, with resulting autophosphorylation of tyrosine residues on the receptor itself and tyrosine phosphorylation of other substrates. These phosphorylations are apparently essential for growth-promoting and other actions of the respective ligands.[317]

Type I IGF receptors are distributed throughout the body and are regulated by the hormones that act in concert with IGFs in eliciting biological responses. Thus PDGF stimulates an increase in IGF I binding in BALB/c 3T3 cells,[318] gonadotropins increase IGF I binding in the testis

TABLE 21–6. Comparison of Structure and Specificity of Receptors for Insulin, IGF I (Type I), and IGF II (Type II)

Receptor	Chemical Structure	Specificity for		
		Insulin	IGF I	IGF II
Insulin	Unreduced: heterotetramer > 300 kd			
	Reduced subunits			
	Alpha (binding): 130 kd	+ + + +*	+	+ +
	Beta (tyrosine kinase): 90 kd			
Type I IGF	Unreduced: heterotetramer > 300 kd			
	Reduced subunits			
	Alpha (binding): 130 kd	+	+ + + +	+ +
	Beta (tyrosine kinase): 90 kd			
Mannose 6-phosphate/IGF II (type II IGF)	Unreduced: 220 kd			
	Reduced: 260 kd	−†	+ +	+ + + +
	No known subunits			

*The relative affinity of each ligand for the respective receptors is indicated by the number of plus (+) marks.
†Although insulin does not itself bind to type II receptors, when insulin is incubated with intact cells containing type II receptors, the binding of IGF II is increased several-fold, because the number of type II receptors on the plasma membrane increases.

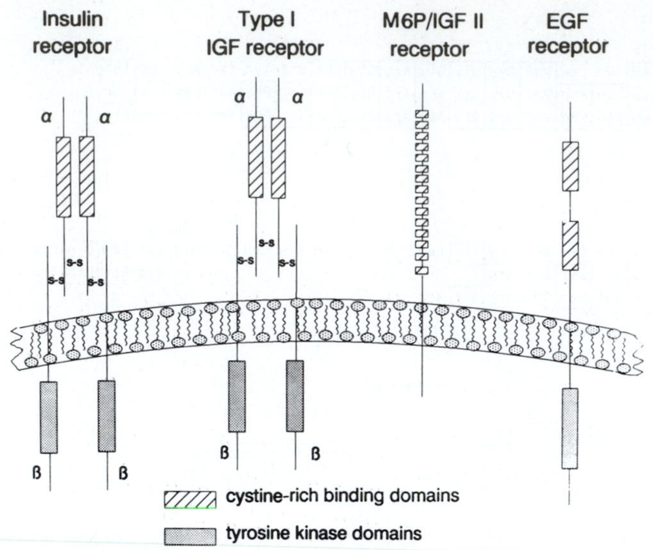

Insulin receptor | Type I IGF receptor | M6P/IGF II receptor | EGF receptor

[////] cystine-rich binding domains

[ ] tyrosine kinase domains

Figure 21–16. Diagram of structural organization of receptors for insulin, IGFs, and EGF. The insulin receptor and type I IGF receptor are heterotetramers with striking structural similarities and cross-reactivities, as summarized in Table 21–6. The alpha subunits, which constitute the extracellular binding domains, are rich in tertiary structure because of high cysteine content. The beta subunits contain an extracellular domain, a transmembrane domain, and a cytosolic domain with intrinsic tyrosine kinase activity. The mannose 6-phosphate (M6P)/IGF II receptor contains separate binding regions for IGF II and proteins that are complexed with M6P. The small boxes represent extracellular regions with repeating sequences. The M6P/IGF II receptor has 15 such cysteine-rich repeating units. Boxes with diagonal lines show tyrosine kinase domains. The M6P/IGF II receptor has no tyrosine kinase activity. The EGF receptor is a single chain protein with two cysteine-rich binding domains and a cytoplasmic tyrosine kinase domain.

and the ovary,[319, 320] and ACTH increases IGF I binding in the adrenal.[321] Type I receptors are subject to down-regulation in the same manner as are other peptide hormone receptors, and expression of the type I receptor gene varies inversely with serum levels of IGF I.[322, 323]

IGF II preferentially binds to the type II receptor, which has no dissociable subunits and no tyrosine kinase activity and which bears little resemblance to either the insulin or the type I IGF receptor (see Fig. 21–16). The type II receptor binds IGF I with lower affinity than does the type I receptor, and it does not bind insulin at all, although insulin causes a 3- to 10-fold increase in IGF II receptors on the plasma membrane.[324]

The amino acid composition of the type II receptor is essentially identical with that of the cation-independent mannose 6-phosphate (M6P) receptor.[325] The M6P/IGF II receptor is a single chain glycosylated transmembrane protein, the nonglycosylated form having a relative molecular size of 270 kd. This receptor has separate binding domains for IGF II and M6P.[326] At least one function of the M6P/IGF II receptor is to act as an intracellular shuttle by transporting acid hydrolases and other mannosylated proteins to the lysosomal compartment, with the unoccupied receptor then being recycled.[327] Approximately 80% of these receptors are localized to intracellular membranes, although they are in equilibrium with those on the plasma membrane. The M6P binding site mediates a variety of growth factor actions, such as processing the mannosylated precursor of TGF β into its active form[328] and serving as the receptor for proliferin, a prolactin-like molecule that is produced in mouse fibroblasts (BALB/c 3T3 cells) in response to mitogenic signals.[329]

Although most of the biological effects of IGF II are believed to be mediated through the type I or insulin receptors, several effects of IGF II have been ascribed to its interaction with the type II receptor.[330, 331] Nissley and colleagues[332] have provided a critical review of this subject.

A 13-amino-acid sequence on the M6P/IGF II receptor interacts with a specific GTP-binding protein (G_{i2}) to mediate the effect of IGF II on the transport of extracellular calcium into the cell. This effect can be inhibited by pertussis toxin and cannot be duplicated by substances that interact with the M6P binding site.[333, 334]

Interactions with Binding Proteins

A distinctive feature of the IGFs is that they are complexed to binding proteins both in serum and in other extracellular fluids. In humans, three separate IGF-binding proteins (IGFBPs) have been isolated and characterized chemically.[335, 336] Referred to as IGFBP 1, 2, and 3, these proteins have structural similarities in that each possesses 18 cysteine residues clustered at each end of the molecule. The amino acid sequences in the area of high cysteine density are highly homologous, whereas the sequences in the intervening regions are more divergent. The importance of these homologous cysteine clusters is not known, but site-directed mutagenesis in these regions results in loss of IGF-binding activity.[337]

IGFBP 1 was initially purified from amniotic fluid and was found to be a M_r 25,272 protein consisting of 259 amino acids.[338] It is also found in serum, lymph, CSF, and culture media from a variety of cell types. Liver, kidney, and brain appear to be major sites of production in vivo. IGFBP 1 is not GH dependent. Its serum concentrations are increased by conditions in which insulin secretion or insulin responsiveness is diminished, including fasting, when serum values rise during sleep; insulin resistance; pregnancy; and hypopituitarism. Values are reduced by hyperinsulinism whether caused by feeding, glucose infusion, GH, or glucocorticoids. In contrast to the levels of IGFBP 3, the concentrations of IGFBP 1 fluctuate markedly throughout a 24-h period (Fig. 21–17).

IGFBP 2 has been studied principally in rats; it was purified from Buffalo rat liver cell–conditioned media. It has a calculated M_r of 32,886 and is present in a variety of tissues. Its expression is particularly high in tissues of the rat fetus and decreases rapidly after birth.[339] Serum IGFBP 2 concentrations are increased by hypophysectomy and decreased by administration of GH and glucocorticoid. Like IGFBP 1, IGFBP 2 seems to be suppressed by insulin, because values in liver are increased in untreated diabetes mellitus and are suppressed by insulin administration.[340]

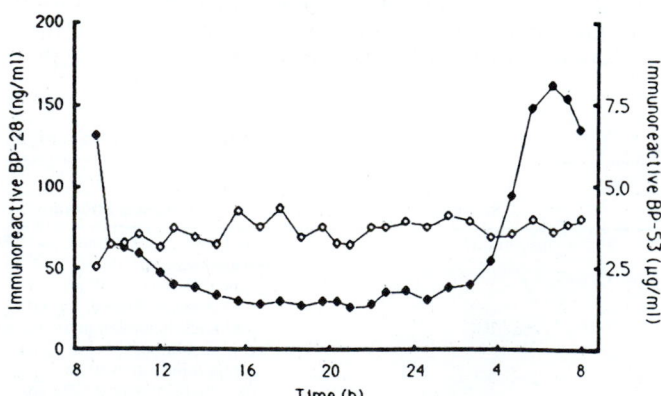

Figure 21–17. Fluctuations in serum concentration of (IGFBP 1) and IGFBP 3 in normal subjects. The filled symbols depict serum concentrations of IGFBP 1 (designated at left as BP-28). Note that values are increased between 4 and 9 AM, when serum insulin concentrations are low. The open symbols depict IGFBP 3 values (designated on the right as BP-53). (From RC Baxter, CT Cowell, Diurnal rhythm of growth hormone–independent binding protein for insulin-like growth factors in human plasma, J Clin Endocrinol Metab, 65, 432–440, 1987, © by The Endocrine Society.)

More than 70% of IGFs in serum circulate as part of a 150-kd binding protein complex known as IGFBP 3. This complex is composed of an acid-stable subunit of M_r 29,480 (or M_r ~54,000 when fully glycosylated), an acid-labile subunit of M_r 88,000, and IGF I or IGF II linked to the acid-stable subunit.[341, 342] IGFBP 3 levels in serum depend on GH and nutritional status. The levels are reduced in states of GH deficiency, restored by GH injections, and elevated in acromegaly and adolescence. The concentrations of IGFBP 3 are reduced when nutrients are restricted and are restored by feeding. IGFBP 3 concentrations are also IGF I dependent, being increased by IGF I infusion in animals that have been hypophysectomized or deprived of protein.[343]

In addition to different regulatory mechanisms, the IGFBPs are believed to have distinct functions. Because the concentration of IGFBP 3 is highest in serum, it may play the principal role as serum carrier protein for the IGFs. On the other hand, the concentrations of IGFBP 1 and IGFBP 2 are higher in lymph than in serum and may play a role in transporting IGFs out of the vascular space. Supporting this concept is the observation that IGFBP 1 can cross the intact vascular endothelium.[344]

Most studies have suggested that the predominant action of IGFBPs is to inhibit binding of IGFs to target cells and thereby attenuate IGF action.[345, 346] However, the addition of purified IGFBP 1 or 3 actually causes increased IGF binding and action. Also, preincubation of cultured human fibroblasts with IGFBP 3 followed by removal of the protein results in enhanced IGF I–induced thymidine incorporation.[347] IGFBP 1 also potentiates DNA synthesis in several cell types.[348]

Regulation of IGFs in Blood

IGF I concentrations in the serum of normal adults are about 200 µg/L, and IGF II concentrations are near 600 µg/L. The IGFBPs (particularly IGFBP 3) are the reason that serum IGF levels are higher and more stable than those of most peptide hormones. These relatively constant IGF serum concentrations make it possible to estimate the mean IGF value from a single specimen.

ASSAY METHODS AND ASSAY STANDARDS. IGF I and IGF II concentrations are measured by radioimmunoassay of extracted samples. In the past the IGF I concentration was also measured by using unextracted serum samples and pooled serum standards, so that 1 U/mL equaled the average of normal adult subjects.[349, 350] However, the binding proteins interfere with measurements in these direct assays.[351] Situations in which the interference by binding proteins causes aberrant results include chronic renal failure and pregnancy. As a result, serum should be extracted to remove IGFBPs before assays are done for IGFs.[352–354]

EFFECT OF AGE AND SEX. *Newborn and Early Childhood.* IGF levels are low at birth and during the first few years of life.[355, 356] In cord serum samples from full-term newborns, the IGF I level correlates with birth weight, birth length, and placental weight, and levels are lower in SGA infants (<2500 g) than in normal-sized infants.[357] The IGF II level is also low in newborns and correlates with birth weight.[358] Little postnatal change occurs in IGF I concentrations during the first 15 mo of life, and values do not correlate with either height percentile or growth rate.[359]

Values Through Childhood and Puberty. From about 1 y of age until puberty[356, 360] plasma concentrations of IGF I increase 2.5 times. There is an additional increase during puberty so that at midpuberty the mean value is 2.5 to 3 times higher than adult values (Fig. 21–18). This increment in IGF I concentrations in late childhood may be linked to the events of puberty, because girls achieve peak values between the ages of 11 and 13 y, whereas boys have their highest values between the ages of 13 and 15 y. When the pubertal rise in IGF I is plotted as a function of develop-

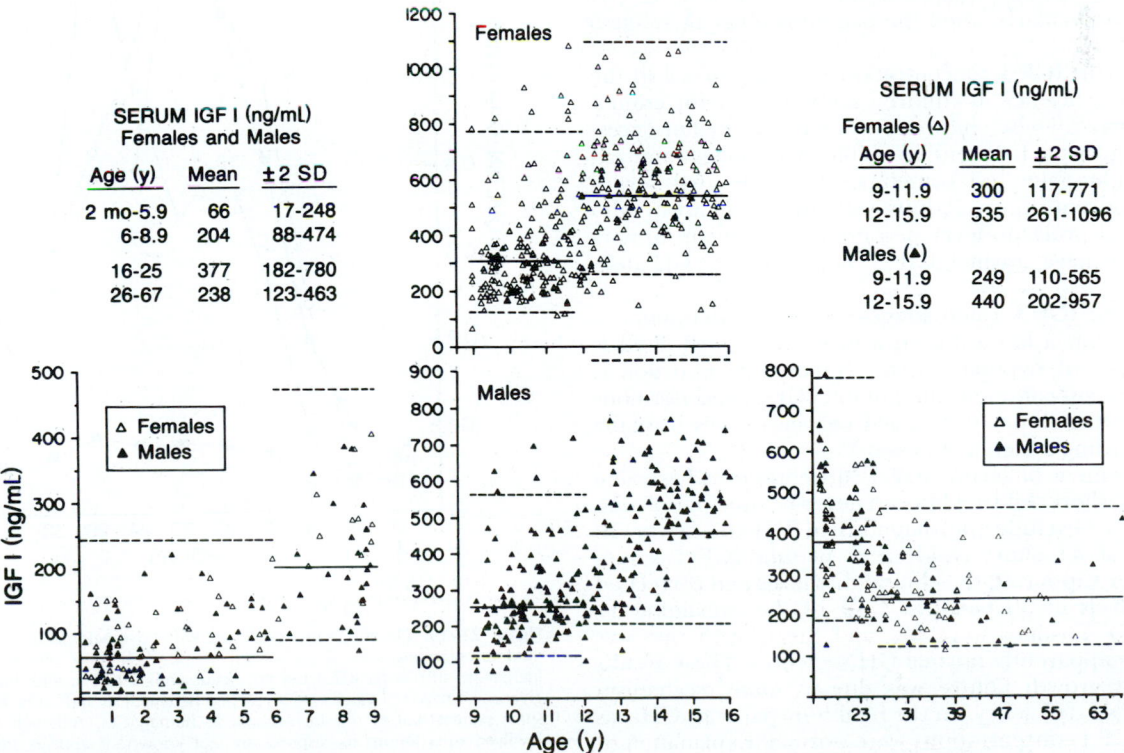

Figure 21–18. Serum concentrations of IGF I in 944 healthy volunteers, ages 2 mo to 68 y. Group means and 2 SD values are indicated in each panel, and numerical values are given above the left and right panels. IGF I levels were determined after serum samples were subjected to acid-ethanol extraction for removal of IGFBPs. (Data courtesy of Nichols Institute, San Juan Capistrano, CA.)

mental status rather than chronological age, maximal values occur in the midpubertal period (Tanner stage III for pubic hair, breasts, and genital development). Although more longitudinal studies are needed, the findings among cross-sectional studies[356, 361] and small-scale longitudinal studies of normal children[35] and of boys with constitutional growth delay[33] are in agreement. The causal role of GH in the pubertal IGF I rise is suggested by the observations that the responses of IGF I to GH injections correlate with bone age[362, 363] and that GH secretion is increased during puberty.[364–366]

The age dependence of IGF II is less clear. The values of IGF II are lower during the first year of life than in later childhood, and there is no rise during adolescence.[351]

The administration of low doses of ethinyl estradiol to girls with gonadal dysgenesis stimulates linear growth without increasing IGF I;[114] intermediate doses increase IGF I levels but do not stimulate growth,[114] and high-dose estrogen therapy arrests growth in tall girls and decreases IGF I concentrations, probably by direct inhibition of IGF I production.

Values in Adults. In adults there is an age-dependent downward trend so that IGF I values during the seventh decade are only half those in the second and third decades of life.[367] Adult females have slightly higher values than do males. Administration of GH to older adults causes a rise in IGF I levels, which suggests that the fall in IGF I with age is due to attenuated GH secretion.[368]

HORMONAL STATE. Hypopituitarism. In children with hypopituitarism, plasma IGF I concentrations are low and rise after injection of GH[369] (Fig. 21–19). In a group of GH-deficient subjects the mean concentration of IGF I was 12% of normal, whereas the mean IGF II level was 39% of normal.[351] Serum IGF I values should be interpreted with respect to normative data for developmental age (skeletal age or stage of puberty) rather than to chronological age. Nevertheless, a normal concentration of IGF I in a short child provides strong evidence against the diagnosis of GH deficiency, particularly when the patient is older than age 5 to 6 y.

The serum IGF I concentration may be normal in the face of GH deficiency in children after surgery for craniopharyngioma.[370] These children, who have normal or excessive linear growth, frequently exhibit hyperphagia and excessive weight gain and sometimes have elevated serum prolactin concentrations. Adults with hypopituitarism who have elevated prolactin levels secondary to pituitary tumors may likewise have normal IGF I values despite GH deficiency.[371]

A normal IGF I value suggests that GH deficiency is not present, but a low value in a growth-retarded child is not diagnostic of hypopituitarism. Suboptimal nutrition is perhaps the most common cause of low IGF I concentrations and may be the cause of reduced concentrations in many growth-retarding systemic illnesses.[369]

Measurement of serum IGF I concentrations has value for assessing short children but can never be used in isolation to make or to exclude the diagnosis of GH deficiency. In one study of 41 short children,[372] plasma IGF I values confirmed or supported the clinical diagnosis and correlated with GH levels in 30 patients. In 7 of the remaining 11 patients, IGF I values were low and the growth rate was slow despite apparently normal GH secretion. These results suggest that growth failure was due to some mechanism other than GH deficiency. In the final four patients, GH was low while IGF I concentrations were normal. Explanation of these discordant results must await clarification of the cause of growth failure in these children. In another study[373] the IGF I level was measured in 143 short children, and GH-

provocative tests were performed on 78 patients who had IGF I values below 0.5 U/mL. Half of these patients (values below 0.5 U/mL) were GH deficient, and IGF I screening for GH deficiency was as efficient and more convenient than measurement of exercise-induced GH. On the other hand, Dean and co-workers[374] concluded that IGF I measurements cannot be used to diagnose GH deficiency because approximately 15% of their patients with presumed hypopituitarism had serum values within the normal range. In summary, measurements of basal IGF I should be used in diagnosis of growth disorders in conjunction with clinical assessments and other tests.

Because concentrations of IGF I are GH dependent, one may assume that the short-term plasma IGF I responses to GH could be used to predict growth responses to long-term therapy. Unfortunately, our experience and that of others indicate that such measurements do not predict growth response. Chronic GH therapy raises the plasma IGF I level in most hypopituitary subjects, but some patients have low values even when growth is stimulated.[364]

Acromegaly. IGF I concentrations are uniformly elevated in the plasma of patients with acromegaly and in children with gigantism related to pituitary GH excess. In our initial study of 57 acromegalic adults, the mean value was 10 times higher than the value for control subjects.[375] The IGF I level correlated with indices of clinical severity such as heel pad thickness (r = .73), fasting glucose value (r = .74), and 1-h postprandial glucose value (r = .77). These

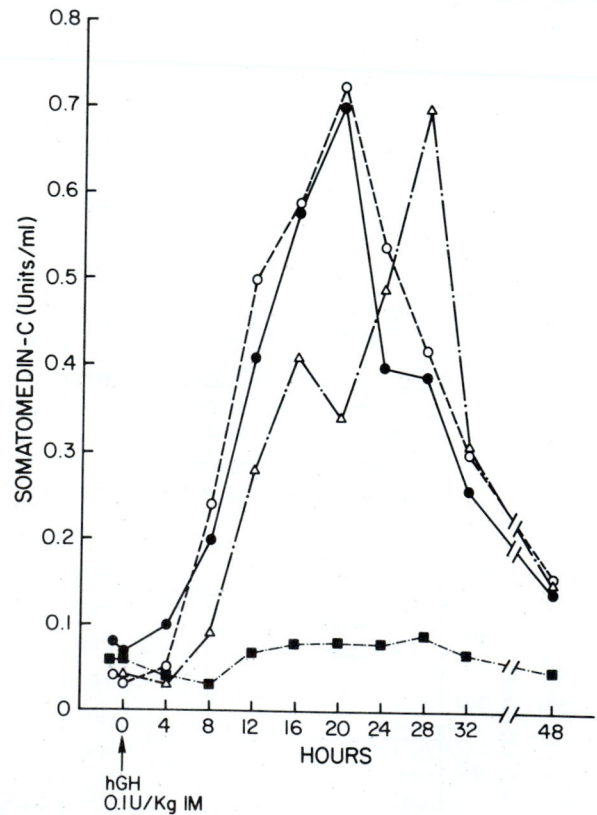

Figure 21–19. Plasma immunoreactive IGF I (somatomedin-C) responses to intramuscular injection of human GH in four children with hypopituitarism. Increments in plasma IGF I did not occur until 6 to 8 h after human GH was given, and maximal values were reached between 16 and 28 h. IGF I values of some patients fail to rise in response to human GH. Although all the factors involved in a failure to respond are not known, it appears that suboptimal nutritional status is one such factor. (From KC Copeland, LE Underwood, JJ Van Wyk, Induction of immunoreactive somatomedin-C in human serum by growth hormone: dose response relationships and effect on chromatographic profiles, J Clin Endocrinol Metab, 50, 690–697, 1980, © by The Endocrine Society.)

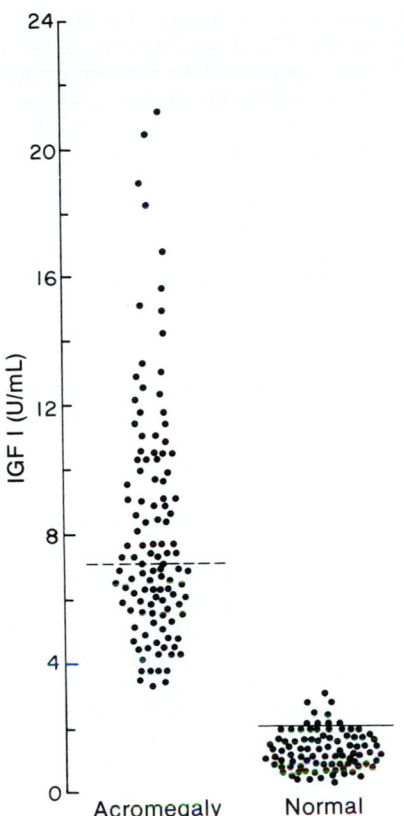

Figure 21–20. Scattergram comparing serum concentrations of IGF I for normal adults and for patients with active acromegaly. These measurements were made with a radioimmunoassay that uses a high-affinity polyclonal antibody to IGF I.

correlations are better than those between basal or glucose-suppressed GH levels and indices of clinical severity. Furthermore, in the more than 150 patients with active disease, we consistently found plasma IGF I to be elevated, even in those with low or marginal GH values (Fig. 21–20). Others have also documented the value of IGF I measurements in the diagnosis and management of acromegaly[376, 377] and in children with gigantism related to GH excess. During the pubertal growth spurt, however, caution must be observed in interpreting serum values, because normal pubertal children may have values four to five times higher than adult values. Pregnancy is likewise associated with high plasma levels of IGF I,[378] so that this test should be interpreted cautiously in diagnosing GH excess during pregnancy.

IGF I concentrations decrease dramatically in acromegalic patients who respond to treatment (also see Chapter 6). Although a single IGF I measurement provides the best available indicator of disease activity, it cannot be used as an index of how much treatment-related improvement has already occurred or as the sole means of determining whether additional therapy is needed. Serial measurements of IGF I, however, are useful for monitoring the course of acromegaly and the response to therapy.[375, 379]

Other Endocrinopathies. Plasma IGF I concentrations are nearly as low in thyroid hormone deficiency as in hypopituitarism and rise after thyroxine replacement.[76] Pharmacological administration of estrogens to normal subjects or acromegalic patients reduces IGF I levels.[380] Reduction of IGF I in response to high dosages of estrogen apparently provides the rationale for this form of treatment in girls in whom excessive height is predicted.

Prolactin has a weak stimulatory effect on IGF I and causes values to be normal in GH-deficient patients with prolactin-secreting tumors.[371] The relationship between hPL and IGF I is less well defined, although in hypophysectomized rats ovine placental lactogen is as effective as ovine GH in increasing IGF I levels.[381]

NUTRITIONAL STATE. Variations in nutritional status are as important as GH in modulating serum IGF I levels.[83, 382, 383] Whereas serum GH concentrations may be high in children with protein-calorie malnutrition, the IGF I level is low. In adult humans the IGF I level is reduced by fasting,[384] decreasing within 48 h of beginning the fast and reaching hypopituitary values within 10 d. With refeeding the serum IGF I level returns to normal within 4 to 6 d. The changes in IGF I concentration during fasting correlate with changes in nitrogen balance (r = .74). Furthermore, after a 3-d fast IGF I concentrations are not increased by administration of human GH.[385] Serum IGF I levels respond both to protein and energy[386] and to the quality of protein in the diet.[387] Indeed, IGF I could serve as a useful clinical indicator of nutritional sufficiency[388, 389] (Fig. 21–21). In rats GH receptors are reduced by fasting, but the principal cause of reduced IGF I in nutritional deprivation is at the postreceptor level of GH action. Decreased IGF I concentrations in nutritional restriction are accompanied by decreased levels of liver IGF I mRNA.[383]

HEPATIC FAILURE, CHRONIC ILLNESS, AND KIDNEY DISEASE. Hepatic failure is associated with low serum IGF I concentrations, but it is unclear whether this is due to destruction of tissue involved in IGF I generation or to malnutrition. In general, any cause of decreased protein synthesis results in decreased IGF I concentrations. The test therefore lacks specificity for many diseases in which IGF I levels are low. The effect of acute or chronic inflammation on IGF I is unknown. For these reasons, in patients with inflammatory bowel disease it may be unclear whether a low IGF I value is due to malnutrition or to a more specific effect of the inflammatory process.

In patients with renal failure, IGF I concentrations are

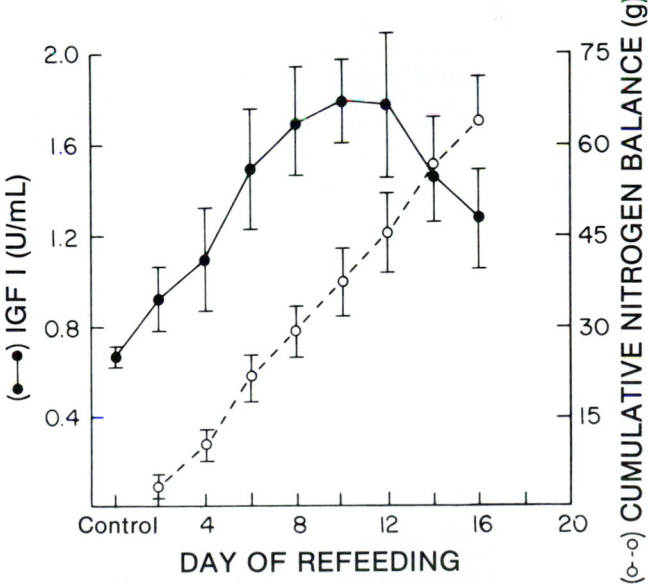

Figure 21–21. Effect on serum IGF I and nitrogen balance of refeeding malnourished adults. Six adults (22 to 65 y) with moderate malnutrition related to one of several bowel diseases were refed 32.7 to 42.6 kcal/kg body weight/d and 0.16 to 0.36 g/kg body weight/d of nitrogen. The mean serum IGF I level peaked at 10 d (individual peaks 9 to 12 d), and this apparent "overshot" in IGF I concentration decreased for several days thereafter to reach a more normal value for adults. The patients entered positive nitrogen balance promptly with refeeding. In this study, no changes in transferrin, retinol-binding protein, or prealbumin were observed during refeeding.

reduced, and the binding capacity for IGF I is increased.[390] The latter is due to a marked increase in IGFBP 3, probably related to decreased clearance.

The Role in Fetal Growth

The IGFs appear to play a central role in regulating embryonic and fetal growth and differentiation.[391] mRNAs have been identified in humans for IGF II from as early as 18 d[392] and for IGF I from at least 12 to 14 wk of gestation.[393] Both peptides are present in human fetal blood at least by as the second trimester.[391] Embryonal carcinoma cell lines have transcripts for both IGF I and IGF II and elaborate both peptides into culture media,[394] which suggests that synthesis of IGFs may commence at the time of blastocyst formation. In rodents IGF I is synthesized before organogenesis.[394, 395] IGF receptors and IGFBPs are also expressed during early development. Both type I and II IGF receptors are present at least from 9 wk of gestation in humans[396] and are found in undifferentiated embryonal carcinoma cells.[394] IGFBP 1 (the amniotic fluid–derived IGFBP) is ubiquitous in fetal fluids,[335, 336] and a similar or identical IGFBP is associated with mouse blastocysts.[395]

The fetal growth retardation in mice bearing a hemizygous disruption of the IGF II gene[397] establishes an essential role for IGF II during intrauterine growth. A crucial role for both IGF I and IGF II from early in development seems certain.

Actions at the Tissue Level

TISSUE DISTRIBUTION

IGFs are present in most tissues, although the concentrations are lower than those in blood. Most tissues from hypophysectomized rats contain less than 30% of normal IGF I levels[122] (Table 21–7). It is also possible to quantitate IGF mRNAs in tissues as a function of developmental status and other influences. In general, transcripts for IGF II are more abundant than are those for IGF I in the fetus, whereas IGF I mRNA predominates postnatally.[398] By Northern blot analysis mRNAs for IGF I are low in the liver of hypophysectomized rats and return to normal within 4 h after the administration of GH.[399] In contrast, messages for IGF II are barely detectable in most tissues of the postnatal rat, and there is no clear change after hypophysectomy or GH administration. A striking exception to this developmental pattern is present in brain, where IGF II mRNAs predominate over those for IGF I and appear to be regulated by GH.[400, 401] Similarly, as judged by radioimmunoassay, IGF II is the predominant somatomedin postnatally in certain other tissues, notably bone matrix[402, 403] and thyroid.

Although GH controls production of IGF I in liver and certain other tissues, estrogen controls IGF I production in the endometrium, a tissue in which GH has no effect on IGF I production.[404] Similarly, IGF I production is stimulated by ACTH, angiotensin II, and FGF in the adrenal[321] and by gonadotropic hormones in the gonads.[405, 406] Expression of IGF genes is also regulated by other growth factors, by nutritional status, and by injury. Regulation of growth factors (and in particular IGF) appears to be controlled by multiple signals that vary according to site in the body and physiological circumstance. It is perhaps not surprising, therefore, that the human gene for IGF II is under the control of at least four different response elements.[407]

The technique of in situ hybridization complements analysis of mRNAs in different tissues by localizing the cellular origin of IGF I and IGF II within a single tissue. In human fetal tissues hybridization is uniformly more intense in connective tissue of mesenchymal origin than in epithelial cells.[393] This distribution is different from the pattern of IGF distribution disclosed by immunocytochemistry, by which the peptides stain strongly in parenchymal cells.[408] This discrepancy suggests that IGFs are synthesized in cells lacking the capacity for storage in secretory granules and are then rapidly exported to the extracellular fluid and are taken up and utilized by neighboring cells in a paracrine manner.

ROLE IN CELL PROLIFERATION AND DIFFERENTIATION

Growth can occur either by cellular proliferation (hyperplasia) or by hypertrophy with concomitant synthesis of differentiated cell products. The number of differentiated cell functions regulated by the somatomedins is large, and the rate of expansion of this number suggests that these peptides play some yet undefined role that is essential for most cellular processes. The balance between proliferation and differentiation varies from tissue to tissue and may vary at different times in the same tissue depending on the developmental status and the rest of the hormonal milieu. The somatomedins act primarily as mitogens in some tissues, stimulate differentiation without obligatory proliferation in

TABLE 21–7. Extractable IGF I in Organs of Male Rats

| | U/g Wet Weight* | | |
| | | Hypophysectomized | |
Source	Normal Rats	Rats	% of Normal
Serum	28.7 ± 0.98	0.74 ± 0.12	2.6
Liver	1.91 ± 0.23	0.23 ± 0.08	12
Lung	2.04 ± 0.86	0.57 ± 0.13	27.9
Kidney	2.59 ± 0.80	0.77 ± 0.29	29.7
Heart	0.92 ± 0.33	0.48 ± 0.14	52.2
Muscle	0.42 ± 0.05	<0.08	<19.1
Testes	1.88 ± 0.42	0.52 ± 0.32	27.7
Prostate	1.06 (pooled)	0.40 (pooled)	37
Submaxillary gland	1.73 (pooled)	0.78 (pooled)	45
Brain	0.26 ± 0.09	0.28 ± 0.04	107.7

*Content of extractable IGF I in organs from normal and hypophysectomized rats. Male rats were hypophysectomized when they weighed ~100 g and were killed when they were 48–50 d old. Normal controls were the same age at the time of death and weighed ~250 g. There were six or seven rats per group, except for the pools as designated. Concentrations of IGF I, as determined by radioimmunoassay in tissue extracts, are corrected for contamination by residual blood. In this assay, 1 "unit" is equivalent to the IGF I content in 1 mL of a pool of plasma from normal human adults. Note that the content of IGF I in rat serum is much higher than that in human serum.

From D'Ercole AJ, Stiles AD, Underwood LE. Tissue concentrations of somatomedin C: further evidence for multiple sites of synthesis and paracrine or autocrine mechanisms of action. Proc Natl Acad Sci USA 1984; 81:935–939.

others, and in all responding tissues stimulate the production of cell products that are characteristic of that tissue.

EFFECT ON PROLIFERATION. Although somatomedins were first described as growth factors for skeletal tissue, IGF I or IGF II in fact stimulate DNA synthesis and cell proliferation in cells of diverse embryological origin and in organisms ranging from invertebrates to humans. Sato and colleagues found that few cells in culture proliferate under serum-free conditions unless micromolar concentrations of insulin are present in the medium.[409] At such high concentrations, insulin can function as a somatomedin surrogate by interacting with the type I IGF receptor. In most cells nanomolar concentrations of IGF promote cell replication as effectively as micromolar concentrations of insulin.

The interaction of IGFs with other growth factors has been studied extensively in the mouse BALB/c 3T3 fibroblast cell line. When cultures of these cells reach confluency they become arrested in the G_0 stage of the cell cycle, but if exposed to fresh serum they enter the G_1 phase of the cell cycle and undergo renewed DNA synthesis after a minimal lag of 12 h.[410] This stimulatory action of serum is caused by the sequential action of PDGF and of the growth factors contained in platelet-poor plasma.[411] IGFs are an essential component of the mitogenic activity of normal plasma because platelet-poor plasma loses the capacity to sustain progression through the cell cycle in the presence of a monoclonal antibody that neutralizes both IGF I and IGF II.[119] Although neither IGF I nor EGF alone can substitute for plasma in stimulating PDGF-treated cells to initiate DNA synthesis, the combination of IGF I plus EGF is as effective as plasma in this regard.[412, 413] Although both EGF and IGF I are required during the first 6 h of G_1, IGF I by itself can support the completion of the last half of G_1 and entry into DNA synthesis (Fig. 21–22).

Some cell types that do not appear to require added insulin or somatomedin produce their own somatomedins that function in an autocrine manner.[67, 414] Human fibroblasts, for example, produce IGF I, and the quantity of IGF I produced is increased by GH and by a variety of growth factors.[415, 416] Evidence that IGFs are made by many different cell types is supported by the fact that replication or specialized cell functions or both are attenuated by monoclonal

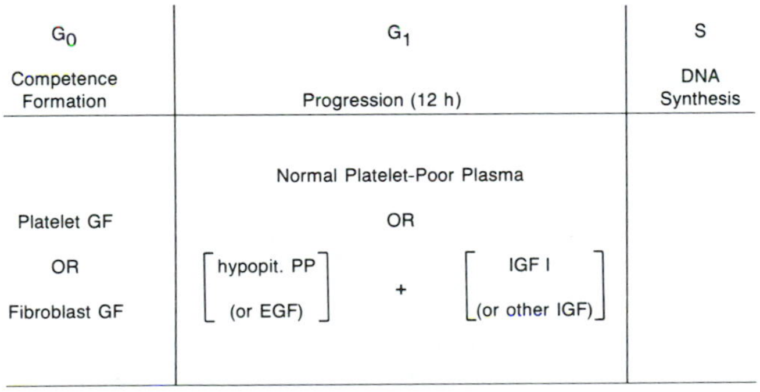

antibodies that neutralize endogenously produced IGFs. Immunoneutralization studies with monoclonal antibodies to IGFs or IGF receptors have further revealed that the mitogenic effect of several other hormones and growth factors is due in part to the ability to stimulate production of IGFs or IGF receptors in target tissues.[417]

Characteristically, in the absence of other hormones or growth factors the effects of IGF I or IGF II are weak, and many of these actions can be demonstrated only in the presence of other growth factors or hormones; thus amplification of the effect of other agonists is a common theme of IGF action.[418]

ROLE IN SPECIFIC TISSUES

The ubiquitous distribution of IGF receptors in virtually all tissues from early fetal life to old age suggests that IGFs play an important role in the growth, development, and function of most tissues, and they may also regulate responses to injury and disease.

EFFECT ON HEMATOPOIESIS IN BONE MARROW. Erythrocyte mass is closely coupled to the total body mass during the growth of mammals. Although EPO is the principal regulator of red blood cell mass, the coupling of red blood cell mass to growth is controlled by GH and, in turn, by IGF I.[239, 419] At the cellular level, the effect of EPO in stimulating colonies of erythroid stem cells requires IGFs (or high concentrations of insulin)[243] (Fig. 21–23). Similarly, IGF potentiates the action of CSF in bone marrow.

EFFECT IN ENDOCRINE TISSUES. IGFs are synthesized in the adrenals and the gonads in response to stimulation by their respective trophic hormones and then interact with the same trophic hormones in regulating cell proliferation and the specialized functions of the glands. Although inactive by themselves, IGFs potentiate the steroidogenic actions of ACTH and angiotensin II in the adrenals,[420] of follicle-stimulating hormone in ovarian granulosa cells,[421] and of LH on androgen production by theca-interstitial cells in the ovary[422] and Leydig cells in the testes[423] (Fig. 21–24).

Potentiation of trophic hormone action on steroidogenesis and other differentiated cell functions is accomplished by a variety of mechanisms, the most important of which appears to be amplification of the effect of trophic hormones on cyclic AMP generation. In addition, IGFs potentiate the action of ACTH in the adrenals and of gonadotropins in the gonads by inducing the cholesterol side-chain cleavage enzyme cytochrome P-450$_{scc}$.[424]

Effects in the Ovary. Compelling evidence that IGFs function as autocrine or paracrine regulators in the ovary has come from immunoneutralization studies in which the stimulation of progesterone production by porcine follicular fluid– or granulosa cell–conditioned media was attenuated by a monoclonal antibody to IGF I.[425] Although the local production of IGFs is regulated predominantly by gonadotropic hormones, the effect of IGFs in responsive cells is also regulated by IGFBPs.

The physiological importance of IGFBP in ovarian function was documented by Ling and colleagues during studies to identify naturally occurring inhibitors of FSH-stimulated functions in porcine follicular fluid. The first such inhibitor identified was the 53-kd subunit of the GH-dependent IGFBP[426] (Fig. 21–25). Additional IGFBPs have been identified in both human and animal ovaries. As discussed earlier, although such binding proteins act as agonists of IGF action under some conditions, under other circumstances they inhibit IGF action.[427]

These findings have been used to explain hirsutism and/or virilization of women with hyperinsulinism, as, for example, in women with the polycystic ovary syndrome. It

G_0	G_1		S
Competence Formation	Progression (12 h)		DNA Synthesis
	Normal Platelet-Poor Plasma		
Platelet GF	OR		
OR	[hypopit. PP	+	[IGF I
Fibroblast GF	(or EGF)]		(or other IGF)]

Figure 21–22. The BALB/c 3T3 mouse fibroblast cell line is frequently used as a model to determine the roles of various hormones and growth factors in cell proliferation. These cells become quiescent when grown to confluency, but if exposed to fresh serum they leave G_0, transit the G_1 phase of the cell cycle, and enter the S phase after a lag of 12 h. In this model the various components of serum act sequentially in stimulating this transit through the cell cycle. Lysis of platelets, such as occurs during blood coagulation, releases PDGF and perhaps other growth factors that confer a state of competence on cells stalled in G_0 so that they become capable of progressing through the G_1 phase of the cell cycle in response to the sequential actions of "progression factors" that circulate in platelet-poor plasma (PPP). Competent cells can progress to a point midway through G_1 in response to EGF plus IGF-deficient PPP from patients with hypopituitarism. Transit through the second half of G_1 requires only IGF I, IGF II, or unphysiologically high concentrations of insulin that act as a surrogate somatomedin by cross-reacting with the type I somatomedin receptor.

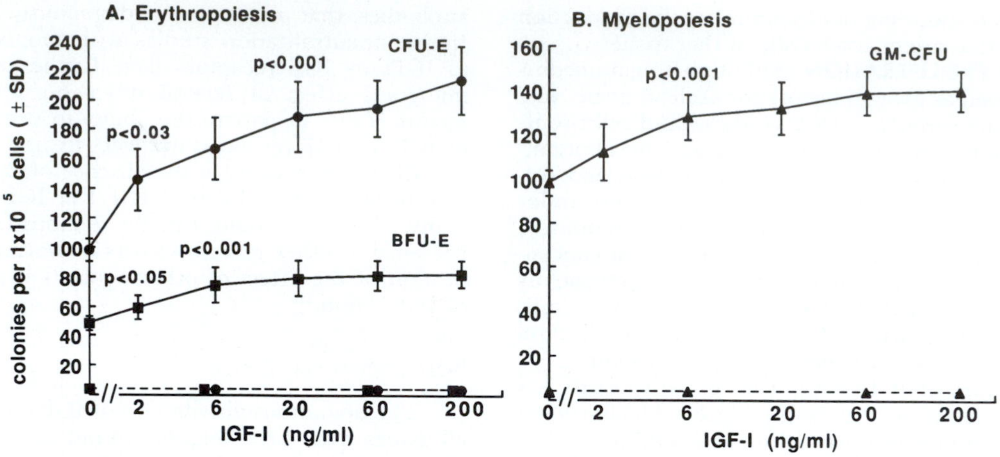

A. Erythropoiesis

B. Myelopoiesis

Figure 21–23. Effect of IGF I on the stimulation of hematopoiesis (erythropoiesis and myelopoiesis) by hemopoietic growth factors. Bone marrow cells from healthy human subjects were cultured in media containing increasing concentrations of recombinant human IGF I in the absence or the presence of saturating doses of hematopoietic growth factors. *Left*, Colonies originating either from primitive erythroid progenitors (BFU-E) or from relatively mature erythroid progenitors (CFU-E) were enumerated after 7 and 14 d of culture, respectively. CFU-E cultures contained 0.5 U/mL of partially purified sheep EPO (step III; Connaught Laboratories). BFU-E cultures contained 1 U/mL EPO plus 5% conditioned medium from a human T lymphoblast cell line (MoCM), the latter ingredient providing burst-promoting activity that is required for the initial stages of early erythroid progenitor cell growth. *Right*, Colonies originating from granulocyte-macrophage progenitors (GM-CFU) were enumerated on day 14. These cultures contained 5% MoCM as a source of GM-CSF. No erythroid or myeloid colony formation was observed in the presence of IGF I alone at concentrations up to 200 ng/mL. Concentrations of IGF I as low as 2 and 6 ng/mL, however, increased the number of erythroid and myeloid colonies above those stimulated by EPO or GM-CSF in the absence of IGF I. To convert IGF I values to nanomoles per liter, multiply by 0.13. (Adapted from Merchav S, Tatarsky I, Hochberg Z. Enhancement of erythropoiesis in vitro by human growth hormone is mediated by insulin-like growth factor-I. Br J Haematology 1988; 70:267–271; and from Merchav S, Tatarsky I, Hochberg Z. Enhancement of human granulopoiesis in vitro by biosynthetic insulin-like growth factor I/somatomedin C and human growth hormone. Reproduced from the Journal of Clinical Investigation, 1988, vol. 81, pp 791–797 by copyright permission of the American Society for Clinical Investigation.)

is possible that high concentrations of insulin can potentiate gonadotropin-dependent androgen production by cross-reacting with the type I IGF receptor. A more important effect of insulin on androgen secretion by polycystic ovaries, however, may be the suppression of IGFBP 1 by high insulin levels. Studies of surgical specimens from patients with polycystic ovarian disease have shown that the concentrations of this binding protein are lower than normal.[428] Thus insulin

at high levels mimics the action of somatomedins by interacting with the type I receptor and enhances the effects of somatomedins by lowering somatomedin-binding proteins.

Effects in the Thyroid. Investigation of the hormonal control of thyroid growth and function has been facilitated

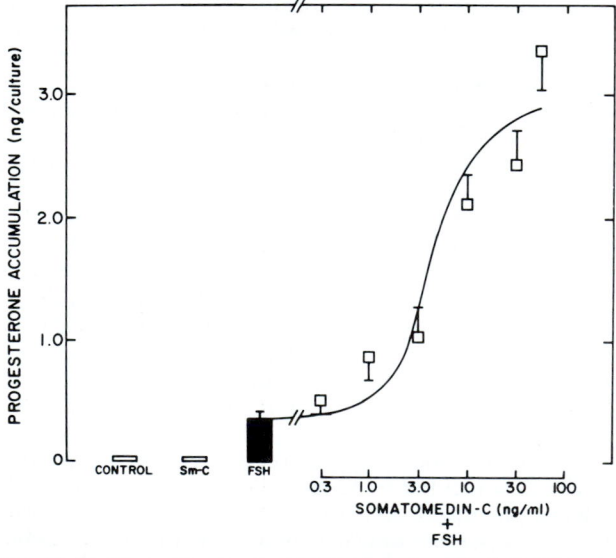

Figure 21–24. Effect of treatment with IGF I (somatomedin-C, Sm-C) on basal and FSH-stimulated progesterone accumulation by cultured rat granulosa cells. Cells were obtained from immature, hypophysectomized, diethylstilbestrol-treated female rats. Granulosa cells (1 × 10⁵/dish) were cultured for 72 h under serum-free conditions in the absence or the presence of FSH (20 ng/mL) with or without increasing concentrations (0.1 to 50 ng/mL) of IGF I. The concentration of progesterone in the medium was measured by radioimmunoassay. To convert IGF I values to nanomoles per liter, multiply by 0.13. (From EY Adashi, CE Resnick, ME Svoboda, et al., A novel role for somatomedin-C in the cytodifferentiation of the ovarian granulosa cell, Endocrinology, 115, 1227–1229, 1984, © by The Endocrine Society.)

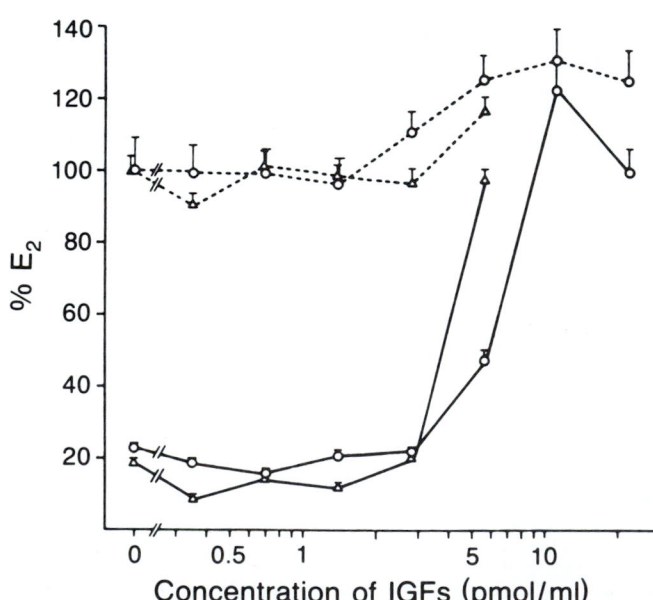

Figure 21–25. Inhibition of FSH dependent aromatase activity in rat granulosa cells by IGFBP and reversal by IGF I. Increasing concentrations of IGF I (○) or IGF II (△) were added to cultures of rat granulosa cells in the presence of 20 ng/mL ovine FSH and 0.5 μmol/L androstenedione (as a substrate for aromatase activity). Estradiol (E₂) was measured by radioimmunoassay after 72 h in the presence (solid lines) or absence (dashed lines) of an IGF inhibitor (4.6 pmol/mL) purified from porcine follicular fluid. The inhibitor was highly homologous with the 53-kd human GH-dependent IGFBP (IGFBP 3), and the inhibition of estradiol production could be reversed by increasing the concentration of either IGF I or IGF II. (From M Ui, M Shimonaka, S Shimasaki, et al, An insulin-like growth factor–binding protein in ovarian follicular fluid blocks follicle-stimulating hormone–stimulated steroid production by ovarian granulosa cells, Endocrinology, 125, 912–916, 1989, © by The Endocrine Society.)

by studies of a rat cell line (FRTL-5) that responds to TSH and to thyroid-stimulating immunoglobulins by cell division and appearance of some of the differentiated functions of thyroid follicular cells. The mitogenic response of these cells to either thyrotropin or IGF I alone is small, but thyrotropin causes more than a 30-fold increase in the response to IGF I[429] (Fig. 21–26). Thyrotropin accomplishes these effects by several mechanisms: it stimulates the production of an "amplification factor" for IGF I that possesses some of the characteristics of basic FGF, and it enhances tyrosine phosphorylation in response to IGF I.[430] IGF I has little or no effect on cyclic AMP production in these cells, either alone or in response to thyrotropin.

EFFECT IN MUSCLE. In muscle, the IGFs stimulate the proliferation of myoblasts and the differentiation into myotubes. The effect of IGF I on myoblasts is biphasic, so that at higher concentrations stimulation of differentiation ceases, and stimulation of [³H]thymidine incorporation into DNA becomes the dominant effect.[431] The effect of IGFs on differentiation does not depend on prior cell division, however, because myotube formation occurs even when DNA synthesis is blocked.[432] IGFs appear to induce terminal differentiation in myoblasts by stimulating expression of the gene encoding myogenin, a substance that mediates muscle differentiation.[433]

EFFECT ON DIFFERENTIATION OF LENS EPITHELIUM. The somatomedins also appear to be involved in proliferation and differentiation of lens epithelium. Cell proliferation in frog lens is GH dependent and can be stimulated in vivo by the administration of either GH or IGF I.[434] GH is not a mitogen for this cell type in vitro, however, whereas nanogram concentrations of IGFs stimulate DNA synthesis and mitosis in cultured rabbit lens epithelial cells.[435]

In the chick embryo, IGF I serves as a differentiation

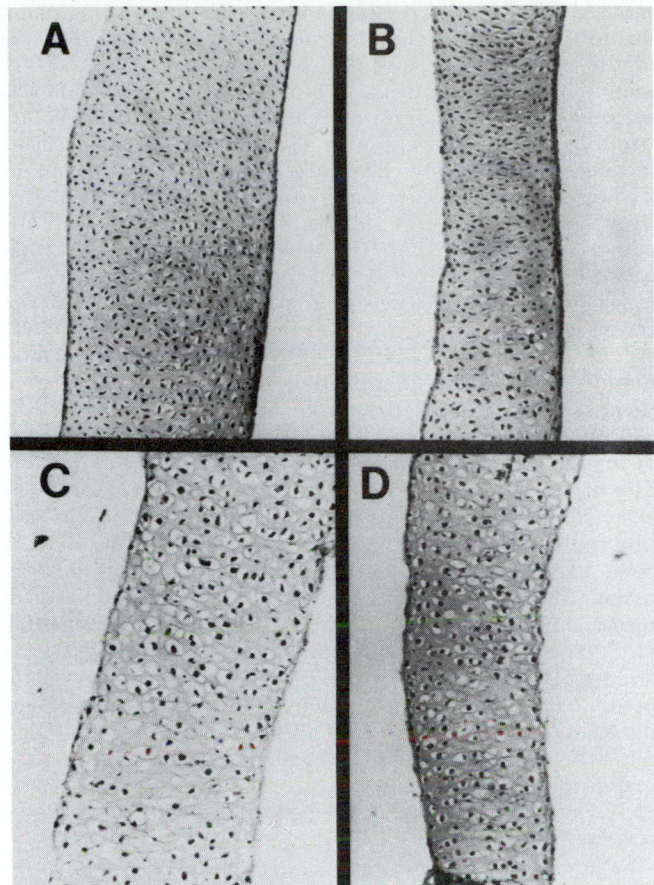

Figure 21–27. Effect of T_3 and IGF antibody on embryonic chick pelvis cartilage. Pelvic leaflets from 10-d chick embryos were placed in organ culture for 3 d in (A) serum-free medium containing no additions, (B) medium containing the monoclonal antibody to IGFs designated SM 1.20, (C) medium containing 1/nmol/L T_3, and (D) medium containing T_3 and SM 1.20. Cartilages were fixed, sectioned perpendicular to the long axes, and stained with hematoxylin and eosin. Original magnification × 100. The relative thinness of antibody-treated cartilage (B and D) is paralleled by lower cartilage weight, protein content, and cell number. T_3-treated cartilage has features of mature hypertrophic chondrocytes with lacunar formation. Although SM 1.20 treatment inhibited cartilage growth parameters, it did not affect the stimulatory effect of T_3 on cartilage maturation. (From Burch WM, Van Wyk JJ. Triiodothyronine stimulates cartilage growth and maturation by different mechanisms. Am J Physiol 1987; 252:E176–E182.)

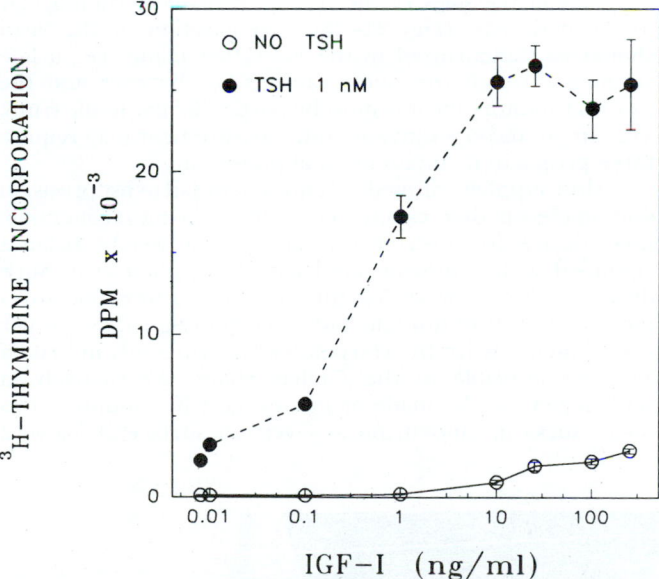

Figure 21–26. The effect of IGF I and thyrotropin on rat thyroid (FRTL-5) cells. FRTL-5 cells (5 × 10⁻⁴ cells/mL) were incubated for 48 h in increasing concentrations of IGF I in the presence or absence of bovine thyrotropin, 1 nM. [³H]thymidine (1 μCi) was added to each well 4 h before the experiment was terminated. Thyrotropin potentiated the mitogenic effects of IGF I both by increasing the amount of [³H]thymidine incorporated into the cells (an effect that may be explained by recruitment of additional quiescent cells into the cell cycle) and by sensitizing the cells to the mitogenic effects of IGF I, as evidenced by a significant reduction of the 50% effective concentration to IGF I. (From SI Takahashi, M Conti, JJ Van Wyk, Thyrotropin potentiation of insulin-like growth factor-I dependent deoxyribonucleic acid synthesis in FRTL-5 cells: mediation by an autocrine amplification factor(s), Endocrinology, 126, 736–745, 1990, © by The Endocrine Society.)

factor for lens epithelium, an effect characterized by elongation of the cells and synthesis of the specific lens protein δ-crystallin. Indeed, nanogram concentrations of IGF I stimulate full lens fiber differentiation within 18 h. The putative differentiation factor in the vitreous humor known as lentropin can be fully absorbed by a monoclonal antibody to IGF I.[436]

EFFECT ON CARTILAGE GROWTH. As discussed earlier, the growth-promoting actions of GH on skeletal growth are now believed to be mediated by the local production of IGF I by prechondrocytes or neighboring cells in the epiphyseal growth plate (Fig. 21–27). The relative roles of thyroid hormone and somatomedins in skeletal growth are less clear, however, because thyroid hormone deficiency causes as severe an arrest of skeletal growth and maturation as does GH deficiency.

In an in vitro model, cartilaginous pelvic leaflets from 10-d chick embryos were incubated with various combinations of IGF I or T_3 in the presence or absence of an antibody that neutralizes the effects of IGFs. Although the effects of T_3 and IGF I were similar in terms of increases in weight, protein, and cell number, T_3 uniquely stimulated marked cellular hypertrophy and cytoplasmic vacuoles similar to those seen in chondrocytes in the hypertrophic zone of the growth plate. The anti-IGF antibody, sm 1.2, completely blocked the normal growth that occurred in unsupplemented basal medium as well as that stimulated by exogenous IGF I. This antibody also attenuated the increases in weight, protein, and cell number stimulated by exogenous T_3 but had no effect on the hypertrophic changes induced by T_3 (see Fig. 21–27). These findings correlate with the clinical observation that GH (and by inference IGF I) has much less effect on epiphyseal maturation than it does on longitudinal growth, whereas thyroid hormones have a profound effect on both growth and epiphyseal maturation.

EFFECT IN CANCELLOUS BONE. Although the somatomedins were initially identified as mediators of GH-dependent skeletal growth, their role in growth of established cancellous bone is less well understood. Cancellous bone is in a state of continuous turnover throughout life, and the rate of cell loss is exactly balanced by replacement with new cells. Although numerous hormones and cytokines are implicated in bone homeostasis, a "skeletal growth factor" has been extracted from decalcified femora and other bony tissues. The amino acid sequence of purified skeletal growth factor is highly homologous, if not identical, to human IGF II.[437, 438] Similarly, certain cloned osteosarcoma cell lines secrete IGF II rather than IGF I as the principal somatomedin. These findings, together with studies with experimental bone models, have established that although IGF I plays the central role in epiphyseal growth, IGF II plays the major role in maintenance of cancellous bone. The effects of IGFs on skeletal tissue have been the subject of extensive reviews.[439, 440]

Effects of In Vivo Administration of IGF I

When given in vivo, IGF I produces anabolic effects and causes a lowering of blood glucose.[441] Whereas infusion of IGF I stimulates growth in GH-deficient mice and rats,[58, 442, 443] it has little growth-promoting effect in intact animals. In GH-deficient rats, 300 μg/d of IGF I is slightly less effective in stimulating longitudinal bone growth than approximately 80 μg/d of human GH,[444] but IGF I is more active than GH in increasing the weights of kidneys, spleen, and thymus. In humans the infusion of IGF I for several days produces nitrogen retention and decreases blood urea nitrogen.[445] Infusions of IGF I stimulate growth in rats made diabetic by treatment with streptozocin[446] and stimulate erythropoiesis in hypophysectomized rats.[239]

The predominant metabolic effect of IGF I is the reduction in blood glucose level, an effect that may be mediated via cross-reaction of IGF I with the insulin receptor. This result has suggested the possible therapeutic use of IGF I in the treatment of insulin-resistant diabetes mellitus, for which this peptide may be useful not only because it reduces the blood glucose level but also because it is not lipogenic. Notably, IGF I is less potent than insulin in adipose tissue but more potent than insulin in chondrocytes and osteoblasts.[441] IGF I also causes a prompt reduction in serum insulin and C peptide concentrations, perhaps by a direct effect on the pancreatic beta cells. In humans IGF I increases creatinine clearance (by 30%).

DISORDERS OF HUMAN GROWTH

Assessment of Growth and Development

Stature

The assessment of linear growth is one of the most sensitive means of evaluating the overall well-being of a child because it gives a net expression of genetic make-up, adequacy of nutrition and environment, and residual effects of previous disease. Well-kept growth records can provide the first clue to endocrine abnormalities, genetic or chromosomal disorders, malnutrition, and chronic systemic illness. In other instances, growth records may exclude suspected disorders and thereby eliminate the need for laboratory tests. Despite the simplicity of this method of evaluating child health, growth records frequently are incomplete or inaccurate.

TECHNIQUE OF MEASUREMENT. Errors in measurement, which may amount to several centimeters, may result from inadequacies of measuring instruments or improper positioning of the subject.[447] Supine length is generally taken from birth until 24 mo of age; thereafter, erect height is used. The best device for measuring the recumbent length of infants and young children is a box with an unyielding horizontal surface and a movable footboard of sufficient size to maintain the soles of the feet on a plane perpendicular to the body axis (Fig. 21–28). The position of the head should be standardized in the Frankfurt plane: i.e., a line running through the outer canthus of the eyes and the external auditory meatus must be perpendicular to the trunk axis. In an uncooperative infant, measurement may require three people to maintain optimal positioning.

Most suppliers of medical equipment fail to list precision stadiometers in their catalogues. Instead, the most commonly used device for measuring stature is a weight balance equipped with a moving (and usually flexible) arm. Such devices are nearly worthless for obtaining accurate measurements. A variety of durable stadiometers designed by Tanner and Whitehouse for the Harpenden Growth Study in Britain are now available in the United States. Alternatively, a stadiometer can be made at modest cost by mounting two meter sticks in tandem on any vertical surface at least 12

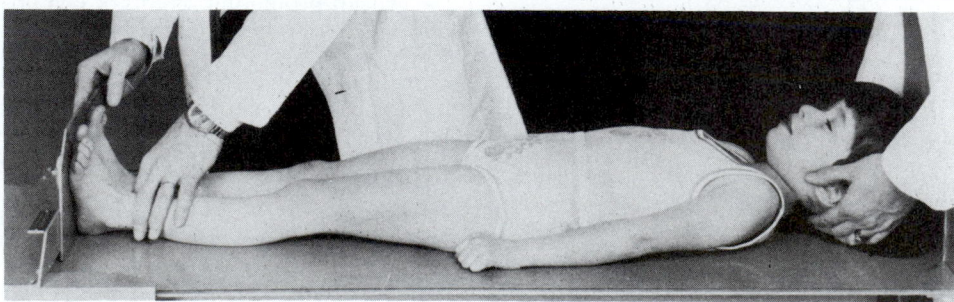

Figure 21–28. Technique for measuring recumbent length. (Photograph courtesy of Noel Cameron. A device suitable for measurement of length of infants can be purchased from Raven Equipment Limited, Unit 4, Ford Farm Industrial Complex, Braintree Rd, Dunmow Essex CMG 1HU, UK.)

inches wide and providing a sliding but rigid right-angle device of sufficient size to rest on the crown when the head is held in the Frankfurt plane. Wall-mounted stadiometers made of a heavy-grade plastic are also available from producers of GH and suppliers of infant foods.

Measurement of height should be done with the patient in bare feet with the heels, buttocks, and shoulders in contact with the stadiometer. Heels are placed together with medial malleoli touching, if possible, and lordosis is reduced by relaxing the shoulders and applying pressure to the abdomen (Fig. 21–29). Diurnal variations in height are minimized if modest upward pressure is applied to the mastoid processes or the mandibular angles.[448] When a young child is measured, it is often necessary for an assistant to ensure that the plantar surfaces of the heels remain in contact with the floor. The variation between observers of measurements obtained in such fashion should be no more than 0.3 cm. By using this technique, it is possible to determine a child's growth rate in only 3 to 4 mo. Because of seasonal variation in growth and other factors, however, it is inadvisable to make decisions about management until growth has been observed for an extended period.[449]

EVALUATION OF HEIGHT DATA. Accurate height meas-

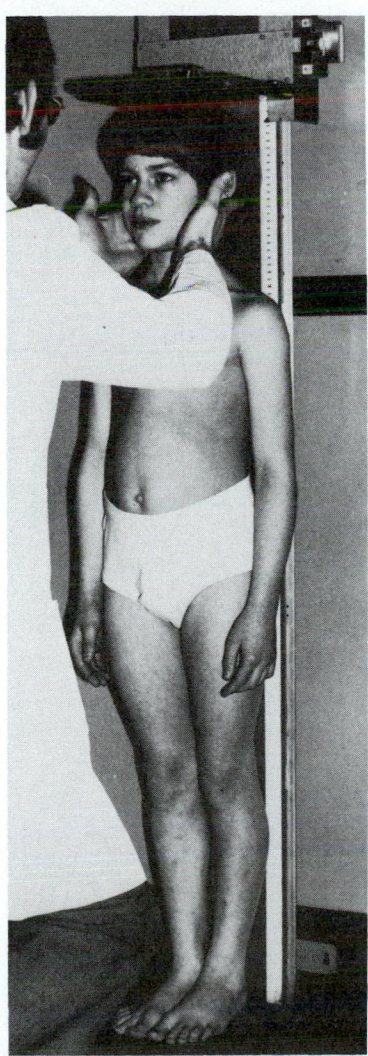

Figure 21–29. Technique for measuring erect height using the Harpenden stadiometer with a direct digital display of height. (Devices of this type are available from Holtain Ltd, Crosswell, Crymych, Dyfed SA41 3UF, Wales, UK. In the United States they may be obtained from Seritex Inc., 450 Barell Avenue, Carlstadt, NJ 07072.)

urements are of little value unless interpreted in the light of appropriate norms for children of the same age and sex and of comparable genetic and environmental background. Because growth is a dynamic process, sequential data from which the growth rate can be calculated are of more value than single measurements. Although many complex formulations have been proposed for the evaluation of linear growth, the most useful are simple cumulative growth and height-velocity charts. Many charts are based on data derived from cross-sectional studies in which large numbers of individual children, supposedly representative of a given population, are measured only once. Group means and population percentiles are calculated at each age for each sex. Alternatively, growth charts may be derived from longitudinal studies in which groups of subjects are measured periodically for a number of years.

The cross-sectional growth charts compiled by the National Center for Health Statistics provide the most accurate description of the size of children in the United States.[450] Growth charts from cross-sectional data tend to extend and flatten the growth spurt in a manner that does not reflect the rapid pubertal growth of individual children. The growth charts for British children prepared by Tanner contain longitudinal growth data and portray growth after the onset of the pubertal growth spurt more accurately.[17] Both cross-sectional and longitudinal data are needed to define growth completely. Cross-sectional data are useful for constructing prepubertal standards and for screening patients for growth disorders. Longitudinal data are better for assessment of pubertal growth and are most appropriate for repeated measurements in a given patient. In our own pediatric endocrine clinic we routinely use the British standard prepared by Tanner.

Height-velocity charts (Figs. 21–30 and 21–31) are useful in that they accentuate modest changes in growth rate and thereby make it easier to recognize growth-altering processes. They also make it possible to identify the onset of the pubertal growth spurt and the point of maximal height velocity and to anticipate the duration of statural growth. Such data are of prognostic value in the individual child and useful for evaluating the acute effects of any therapeutic intervention that may affect the growth process.

The height age of a child is obtained from the cumulative growth chart by determing the age at which the observed height intersects the 50th percentile. Calculation of the height age is useful for comparing the height with indices of development such as skeletal age, dental age, and mental age. Unlike skeletal age, however, the height age of a child is not a primary index of maturity because genetic factors are usually more important than maturational status in determining a child's height relative to peers.

A more precise method for relating a patient's height to that of age peers is the standard deviation score (SDS): $SDS = (X - Y)/SD$, where X is the actual measurement, Y is the mean height of children of the same age and sex, and SD is the standard deviation of the normal population at the same age and sex.

Weight

Measurements of weight should be interpreted in relation to stature rather than to age. In this context, body weight provides primarily an index of nutritional status and adipose tissue, although under special circumstances weight changes reflect alterations in extracellular fluid volume. Evaluation of birth weight in relation to the duration of gestation provides important information concerning the adequacy of the intrauterine environment and may supply clues to maternal drug or alcohol ingestion, intrauterine

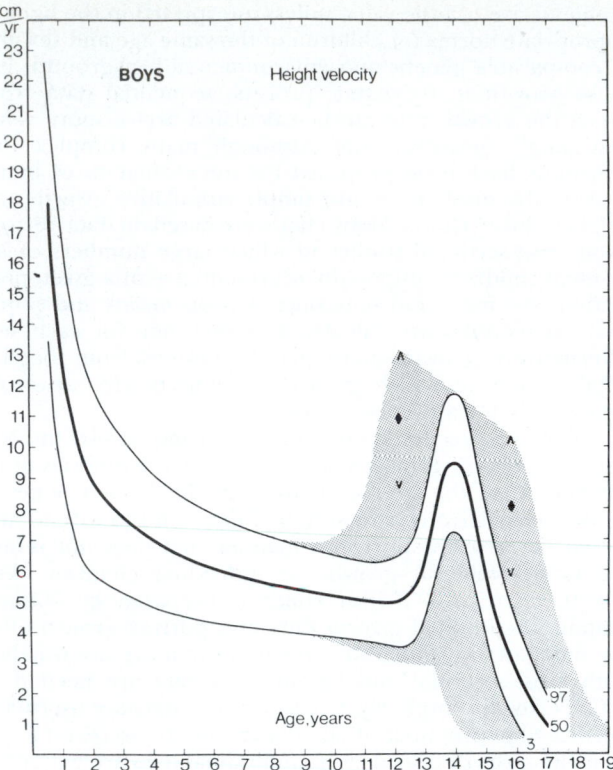

Figure 21–30. Height-velocity chart for boys constructed from longitudinal observations of British children. The 97th, 50th, and 3rd percentile curves define the general pattern of growth during puberty. Shaded areas define velocities of children who have peak velocities at ages up to 2 SD before or after the average age depicted by the percentile lines. Arrows and diamonds mark the 97th, 50th, and 3rd percentiles of peak velocity when the peak occurs at these early or late limits. (Modified from charts prepared by Tanner JM and Whitehouse RH from data published in refs. 17 and 18. Reproduced with permission of Tanner RH and Castlemead Publications, Ward's Publishing Services, Herts, UK.)

infection, various genetic disorders, or (in the case of large infants) diabetes mellitus in the mother.

In the older child, undernutrition is rarely a primary endocrine disturbance, except in long-standing hyperthyroidism. In underweight children, therefore, attention should be directed toward the detection of malabsorption syndromes, psychogenic feeding disorders, and systemic illnesses. Similarly, obesity is most commonly due to excessive ingestion of calories and sedentary habits, and a primary endocrine etiology such as primary hypothyroidism and Cushing syndrome is unusual. Both hypothyroidism and cortisol excess are associated with profound arrest of linear growth, whereas children with exogenous obesity are usually above the 50th percentile in stature and continue to grow at an accelerated rate (see Fig. 21–8). Thus serial stadiometer measurements in the obese child are usually sufficient to exclude the possibility of hypothyroidism or Cushing syndrome and may avert the need for expensive laboratory studies.

Segmental Proportions

Conclusions based on stature alone can be misleading in disorders that selectively affect the growth of the trunk or extremities. The first suspicion of chondrodystrophies, eunuchoidism, Marfan syndrome, and similar disorders often arises when it is observed that segmental measurements are disproportionate.

The ratio between the segments of the upper (trunk, neck, and head) and lower (leg) body diminishes from an

average value of 1.7 in term infants to slightly less than 1.0 at maturity. The upper segment can be measured accurately with a child sitting on a stool of fixed height. The back must be positioned against the stadiometer and the thighs must be horizontal to prevent pelvic tilt. The height of the stool is subtracted from the stadiometer reading to obtain the sitting height. The lower segment can be obtained directly by measuring with a steel tape the distance from the floor to the top of the pubic symphysis. Sitting height standards[451, 452] cannot be used for lower segment measurements, however. In children with deformities affecting only the trunk or legs, a fairly accurate estimate of nondeformed height can often be made after direct measurement of either the normal upper segment or lower segment and calculating the true height from the segmental proportions that are normal for an individual of that age and sex.

Pubertal Development

The rating scales advocated by Tanner[22] for grading stages of pubic hair and breast development in girls and pubic hair and genital development in boys are widely used as a type of shorthand for recording pubertal development (Table 21–8). These standards are of value in studies designed to relate such things as changes in growth velocity to specific pubertal changes in large populations of children. Tanner stagings by themselves are less satisfactory in following individual children, however, because they may be used differently by different examiners and because they fail to convey the gradations of development that are possible with precise descriptions and measurements of the breasts, pubic and axillary hair, and genital development.

In a majority of girls, breast budding precedes the appearance of pubic hair by a few months, and in some girls breast development may reach stage 3 before pubic hair

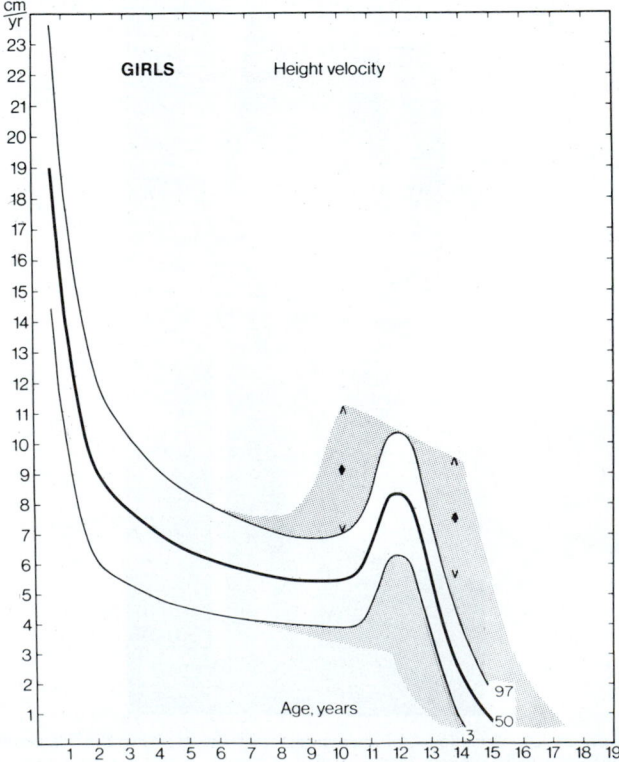

Figure 21–31. Height-velocity chart for girls. See the legend to Figure 21–30. (Modified and reproduced with permission of Tanner JM and Castlemead Publications, Ward's Publishing Services, Herts, UK.)

TABLE 21–8. Stages of Development of Secondary Sexual Characteristics

Boys: Genital (Penis) Development

Stage 1.   Prepubertal: testes, scrotum, and penis of about same size and proportion as in early childhood.

Stage 2.   Enlargement of scrotum and testes. Skin of scrotum reddens and changes in texture.

Stage 3.   Enlargement of penis, at first mainly in length. Further growth of testes and scrotum.

Stage 4.   Increased size of penis with growth in breadth and development of glans. Testes and scrotum larger; scrotal skin darkened.

Stage 5.   Genitalia adult in size and shape.

Girls: Breast Development

Stage 1.   Prepubertal: elevation of papilla only.

Stage 2.   Breast bud stage: elevation of breast and papilla as small mound. Enlargement of areola diameter.

Stage 3.   Further enlargement and elevation of breast and areola, with no separation of their contours.

Stage 4.   Projection of areola and papilla to form a secondary mound above level of breast.

Stage 5.   Mature stage: projection of papilla only, related to recession of areola to general contour of breast.

Both Sexes: Pubic Hair

Stage 1.   Prepubertal: vellus over pubes is not further developed than over abdominal wall.

Stage 2.   Sparse growth of long, slightly pigmented, downy hair, straight or slightly curled, chiefly at base of penis or along labia.

Stage 3.   Considerably darker, coarser, and more curled hair. Hair spreads sparsely over junction of pubes.

Stage 4.   Hair now adult in type, but area covered is still considerably smaller than in adult. No spread to medial surface of thighs.

Stage 5.   Adult in quantity and type with distribution of horizontal (or classically "feminine") pattern.

Stage 6.   Spread up linea alba (male-type pattern).

Modified from Tanner JM. Growth at Adolescence. 2nd ed. Oxford: Blackwell Scientific Publications, 1962.

appears. Conversely, pubic hair may reach stage 3 before breast development is apparent.[453, 454] As a rule, growth of axillary hair begins about the time that the breasts reach stage 3 or 4. The first menstrual period (menarche) is a relatively late pubertal event that must be preceded by secretion of sufficient estrogen to cause uterine growth and proliferation of endometrium. At menarche, the breasts and pubic hair usually have reached stage 4, the peak height velocity has been passed, and the linear growth rate is slowing.[455] The menarche of early-maturing girls occurs close to the point of peak height velocity, whereas late-maturing girls undergo menarche at a later point on the velocity curve. On the average, girls grow only 7.3 cm (range: 3 to 11 cm) after menarche.[456]

Although there are no standards for genital development in girls, considerable information about pubertal development can be obtained by inspecting the vulvar membranes for evidence of an estrogenic effect. During the prepubertal period the labial and vulvar membranes are bright red owing to the thinness of the epithelial layers. The labia minora have sharp edges and the vaginal secretions are watery. Early signs of estrogenic stimulation are thickening of the labia minora, development of a mucoid vaginal secretion, and a change in color from bright red to pastel pink. These changes are reflected in the transition in the estrogen-dependent tissues from predominantly sparse cuboidal cells with large nuclei to abundant squamous cells with pyknotic nuclei. Cytological examination of centrifuged urinary sediment (or of vaginal smear) is a sensitive method of ascertaining whether estrogen secretion has begun. Estrogen secretion can be confirmed by the finding on rectal examination of uterine enlargement.

In boys the testes change little in size between birth and the onset of puberty. As puberty begins, however, testicular

volume increases as the seminiferous tubules enlarge under gonadotropin stimulation. This testicular enlargement, which can usually be detected before other signs of puberty emerge, is followed by increased vascularity, wrinkling, and enlargement of the scrotum and the beginning of pubic hair growth.

The size of the testes may be estimated by direct measurement of length and width. During the prepubertal period the testes usually measure less than 2 cm along the long axis.[457] Length exceeding 2.5 cm is evidence of the onset of gonadotropin stimulation. Palpation of the testis and comparison with elliptical models of known volume[458] have shown that testicular volumes of 1 to 3 mL are typical for prepubertal boys, and a volume of 4 mL or greater signifies stimulation by gonadotropic hormones. The length of the stretched penis may also be measured.[459]

Growth of pubic hair in boys generally proceeds more slowly than genital development.[453, 454] Axillary and facial hair do not appear until genital development is well advanced, several years after the appearance of pubic hair. Deepening of the voice also occurs relatively late. Most pubertal males exhibit some enlargement of the areolae and underlying breast tissues, and many complain of breast tingling and tenderness during this period. In most instances, adolescent gynecomastia regresses after a few years.[460]

The timing of pubertal events relative to the growth spurt is different in boys and girls.[453] Whereas girls usually show acceleration of linear growth at the onset of puberty and reach peak height velocities relatively early in the pubertal process, boys typically reach peak height velocities when genital and pubic hair ratings are at stage 4 or 5.

Prediction of Adult Stature

There is a strong positive correlation between skeletal age and percentage of mature height achieved at any age, and this correlation becomes stronger as the child grows older. In a group of children of identical stature, therefore, those with the least advanced skeletal age tend to become taller adults than those whose skeletal development is more mature.

The most widely used tables for height prediction are those published originally by Bayley and Pinneau[41] and reproduced in the Greulich and Pyle Radiographic Atlas of Skeletal Development.[37] Two additional methods[461] are available: (1) the method of Tanner and associates[42] utilizes chronological age as well as skeletal age and height; and (2) that of Roche and colleagues[43] utilizes height, bone age, midparent height, chronological age, and weight. No matter which method is used, height prediction is often inaccurate in children with pathological growth patterns, probably because the standards are derived from data for normal children and the course of the disease of many short children cannot be predicted.

Tanner and associates have introduced another useful method for relating a child's height to expected growth based on parental stature. This technique permits a crude estimate of the range of target adult height for a given child, i.e., the range within which adult height may be expected to be, on the basis of genetic factors. For boys the father's height is plotted on the right ordinate of the growth chart at age 18 to 20, depending on the chart used. The mother's height is similarly plotted, but to adjust for sex, 13 cm (the difference in mean heights of adult men and women) is added to the mother's height. The mean of the paternal and maternal values (the midparent height) describes the center of the adult target height for the patient. The 3rd and 97th percentile range of midparent height is 20 cm (10 cm below and 10 cm above the mean) for boys. After the expected range for the adult height is determined, one can compare the child's height with the anticipated range. For girls the adjusted midparent height is similarly determined by using the mother's actual height and the father's height minus 13 cm. The 3rd and 97th percentiles for girls are from 9 cm below to 9 cm above the midparent adult target height.

Abnormalities of Fetal Growth

No hormone of maternal origin plays a direct, central role in fetal somatic growth.[462-465] Likewise, no classic hormone of fetal origin has been proved indispensable. Human anencephaly and intrauterine hypophysectomy in experimental animals do not curtail fetal growth. Athyreotic fetuses are of normal length at birth, as are agonadal infants and infants with virilizing conditions. For reasons stated earlier, the role of insulin in normal fetal growth is unclear, and the placenta may regulate fetal growth through the production of estrogens, peptide hormones, and growth factors. Indeed, placental hormones may play a more important role in fetal growth than hormones secreted by fetal endocrine glands.

Because fetal growth results largely from cell proliferation rather than hypertrophy, growth factors play a critical role as mitogenic and differentiating factors. Several findings suggest that somatomedins (IGFs) may play such a role (see previous section on IGFs in fetal growth). Cell membrane receptors for IGFs are abundant in fetal tissues, and multiple fetal tissues produce IGFs in vitro. The mRNAs for IGF II (less so for IGF I) are abundant and widespread in fetal tissues. IGFs stimulate growth of fetal cells in vitro. In humans the cord serum IGF levels correlate with birth weight, birth length, and placental weight.[466, 467] TGF β may participate in fetal growth because it stimulates the proliferation of fibroblasts from fetuses during the period of most rapid cell replication and inhibits the proliferation of fibroblasts from embryos near term. The possible importance of EGF and NGF in selected aspects of fetal and neonatal growth was discussed earlier.

Low-birth-weight newborns (<2500 g) may result from pregnancies terminating before the normal period of gestation is completed (premature infants) or from pregnancies in which intrauterine growth is retarded (SGA infants). Survival rates, perinatal complications, and postnatal growth patterns for the two groups often differ.[468, 469] Because dating the length of gestation by maternal history is unreliable, techniques based on physical, neurological, and laboratory findings are available to distinguish preterm from SGA infants.[9, 470] Charts for intrauterine growth similar to those for postnatal growth facilitate the identification of SGA infants.[468, 471, 472] Data are also available for the postnatal growth of low-birth-weight SGA infants.[473]

Causes of fetal growth retardation include intrinsic abnormalities of the fetus, abnormalities of the placenta, and maternal disorders (Table 21–9). Chromosomal, genetic, and infectious disorders intrinsic to the fetus account for perhaps 10% of all cases. Depending on the precise cause, the growth arrest of this category of infants may be due to decreased cell number, subnormal cell size, or both. In addition to retardation of somatic growth related to decreased cell number and cell size, these infants often exhibit disharmony in the growth of body parts resulting in congenital malformations, asymmetry, and unusual somatic features.

Maternal nutritional status is an important determinant of fetal growth.[474, 475] For example, there is a positive correlation between maternal weight gain during pregnancy and birth weight. Mild maternal malnutrition or malnutrition late in pregnancy affects only birth weight; however, more

TABLE 21–9. Classification of Causes of Fetal Growth Retardation

Intrinsic Abnormalities of the Fetus
Chromosomal and genetic abnormalities
  Autosomal aneuploidy–trisomy-21, -13, and -18; deletions of 4p, 5p−, and
    others
  Sex chromosome aneuploidy: 45,X, gonadal dysgenesis variants
  Primary growth failure syndromes: Russell-Silver syndrome, Seckel syndrome,
    leprechaunism, chondrodysplasias, and others
  Congenital infections
    Rubella, cytomegalovirus, toxoplasmosis
  Congenital anomalies
    Bilateral renal agenesis
Abnormalities of the Placenta
Abnormal implantation of placenta
Vascular malformations
Hemangiomas
Progressive vascular disease: infarction, premature aging
Maternal Disorders
Maternal malnutrition
Inherent uterine constraint to fetal growth
Vascular disorders: hypertension, toxemia, severe diabetes mellitus
Uterine malformations: fibroma, bifid uterus
Drug ingestion: alcohol, narcotics, tobacco

protracted, severe malnutrition causes a proportional reduction in length and head circumference.[476]

In general, the greater the mother's weight gain during pregnancy, the better the infant's growth during the first year of life. Although probably less important, the prepregnancy nutritional status of the mother is also a determinant of fetal growth. Maternal genetic factors also influence birth size, perhaps by the nature of uterine constraint to fetal growth.[477] For example, in mothers who have delivered one SGA infant, there is a 3.5% likelihood that the next infant will also be SGA; sisters of women delivering SGA infants are also more likely to have SGA newborns.

Consumption by a pregnant mother of as few as two alcoholic drinks per day may cause growth retardation in the fetus, and infants of alcoholic mothers exhibit profound growth retardation and morphogenic abnormalities.[478-481] The frequency of fetal loss and of abnormalities of fetal and postnatal growth and the severity of congenital anomalies relate to the amount of alcohol ingestion.[479, 482] Fetal growth retardation also correlates with the duration of alcohol consumption before pregnancy.[483, 484]

Maternal cigarette smoking attenuates fetal growth directly and produces deficits not only in birth weight but also in length, chest circumference, and head circumference.[485, 486] In addition to having a direct effect on fetal growth, maternal cigarette smoking produces low-birth-weight infants indirectly by increasing the likelihood of placental abruption and premature rupture of membranes. The reductions in birth weight range as high as 400 g, with a mean of 200 g, compared with infants of nonsmoking mothers. The more a woman smokes, the greater the reduction in the infant's birth weight. From several studies,[486] the mean decrease in birth weight of infants of women who smoked 20 cigarettes/d was 271 g (compared with infants of nonsmokers), and the percentage of low-birth-weight infants (<2500 g) was 13.4% compared with 4.8% for nonsmokers.

Maternal cocaine use also causes fetal growth retardation,[486, 487] presumably by causing uterine vasoconstriction and perhaps by decreasing maternal food intake. When used by mothers throughout pregnancy, cocaine produced a 600-g mean decrease in birth weight, a 3-cm decrease in length, and a 2-cm decrease in head circumference. When cocaine was used only in the first trimester, these adverse effects on growth did not occur.[488] Marihuana use during pregnancy also causes intrauterine growth retardation, although its effects are less severe than those of cocaine.[489]

Abnormalities of Postnatal Growth: Recognition and Diagnostic Assessment

The decision whether to embark on diagnostic studies in the short child is complicated by the lack of a bimodal distribution of height between normal individuals at the lower end of the normal distribution curve and those whose growth failure has pathological causes. Two to 3 million children in the United States have statures more than 2 SD below the mean for their age, but many of these children have no disease and do not need to be evaluated. On the other hand, a previously normal child who suddenly stops growing may be less than 2 SD below the mean for a number of years but requires investigation before the subnormal percentile standing calls attention to the problem. A current percentile standing, therefore, must be evaluated in light of the genetic background, gestational and medical history, physical findings, and (most important) the growth curve since birth and current growth rate.

In the absence of a universally accepted definition of a pathologically short individual, our clinic has adopted pragmatic guidelines for assessing children referred for retarded growth (Table 21–10). In any patient whose stature is more than 3 SD below the mean height for age, an immediate and thorough search is begun for an etiology. In children whose heights are between 2 and 3 SD below the mean, a limited number of screening tests for common causes of growth failure are obtained on the initial visit, and, if these results are unrevealing, no further studies are undertaken until the current rate of growth is documented for 6 mo or more. If this growth rate is subnormal, more extensive testing is undertaken. Children in whom a subnormal growth rate for age (less than 25th percentile on Tanner's incremental charts) is established by careful, serial measurements are evaluated without regard to whether the absolute height is subnormal. These decisions are tempered by the history and physical findings.

A complete family history is necessary to document the stature of family members and to determine whether there is any familial tendency toward delayed or early puberty. In the patient's history, note should be taken of nutritional adequacy, abnormal fecal elimination patterns, urinary frequency, symptoms of respiratory disease, recurrent or chronic infection, and headaches or other symptoms pointing to an intracranial lesion. The psychosocial environment should also be assessed.

The prenatal and early postnatal status of the patient is crucial. A history of intrauterine growth retardation may suggest some inherent deficiency in the capacity of cells to grow and divide. A history of slow growth in the first few postnatal months is a clue to abnormal mother-infant interaction, malabsorption, congenital heart disease, or other abnormalities of organ function. If growth failure occurred during a finite period in the distant past and normal growth has intervened since, the history taking should focus on the interval during which growth failure occurred, and the current evaluation may be restricted to periodic observations of the growth rate.

The physical examination is useful for separating nonendocrine organ or system malfunction from abnormalities of hormone secretion. In states of inadequate food intake, malabsorption, or other organic disease, the failure to gain weight is often more severe than the failure of linear growth. The nutritional status is evaluated by plotting the weight against height age rather than chronological age. Alternatively, measurement of skinfold thickness may provide a quantitative estimate of nutritional status. The physical examination may also provide clues to skeletal disorders, dysmorphic syndromes, diseases of specific organ systems, and endocrine disease, in particular hypothyroidism and Cushing syndrome.

When the history, physical examination, and growth data fail to provide a diagnostic clue, the patient should be screened for some of the relatively silent causes of growth failure. The screening should include assessment of renal function to rule out unrecognized renal failure and tubular disorders associated with acidosis or hypokalemia; measurement of serum calcium, phosphorus, and alkaline phosphatase levels to rule out rickets; thyroid function tests to exclude subclinical hypothyroidism; and measurement of serum IGF I concentration to screen for GH deficiency. The erythrocyte sedimentation rate should be checked in search of asymptomatic inflammatory bowel disease. All girls with growth retardation of unexplained cause should have an assessment of chromosomal karyotype even though no obvious stigmata of gonadal dysgenesis are present (see Table 21–10).

Radiological assessment of skeletal maturation has little value in differential diagnosis because most disorders that retard growth also retard bone age. Determination of skeletal age is useful, however, in assessing the growth potential of the short child. A normal bone age in a short child may suggest a previously unrecognized genetic abnormality such as chondrodysplasia. X-ray films of the sella turcica are frequently helpful for disclosing an unsuspected intrasellar tumor or, when the sella is abnormally small, for suggesting hypopituitarism. Cranial computed tomography is indicated when enlargement or erosion of the sella turcica is observed on plain x-ray examination, when suprasellar or intrasellar calcification is present, or when growth failure is accompanied by visual field abnormalities.

Hereditary Short Stature

The spectrum of postnatal growth patterns that fall within the range of normal reflects human genetic heterogeneity both between and within different ethnic groups.[455] The inheritance of growth potential is polygenic, with genes for stature located both on the sex chromosomes and the autosomes. Although stature does not follow strict mendelian laws of inheritance, Tanner and associates have provided charts that take mean parental height into consideration.[490]

TABLE 21–10. Guidelines for Assessment of Short Stature and Retarded Growth

Problem	Height is between mean and 2 SD below mean.	Height is between 2 and 3 SD below mean for age.	Height is more than 3 SD below mean for age.	Linear growth rate is less than the 25th percentile for age.
Action	No laboratory tests; observe growth rate as part of well-child care.	Screening studies; if normal results, observe growth rate at intervals of 3–4 mo.	Screening studies;* follow leads or undertake full assessment of pituitary function.	

*Screening studies, initial evaluation: (1) detailed history and physical examination; (2) analysis of growth trajectory from all available data; (3) urinalysis: assess ability to acidify and concentrate urine; (4) blood for urea nitrogen, creatinine, carbon dioxide, electrolytes, calcium, phosphorus, alkaline phosphatase, thyroid hormone, IGF I, and erythrocyte sedimentation rate; (5) x-ray films of hand and wrist for skeletal maturity; skull films for sella turcica size and abnormalities of sellar area; if the patient is female, karyotype for abnormalities of X chromosome.

With these charts one can determine whether a child whose height falls more than 2 SD below the population mean may still be normal, depending on parental size. Also, as indicated in the previous section on prediction of adult stature, relating the size of the child to the percentile of the midparent target height is useful for deciding whether a child is small for his or her family background.

Caution should be exercised in making the diagnosis of familial short stature, because applying this designation to the short child may preclude further efforts at diagnosis. For example, the diagnosis of familial short stature has been perpetuated in families in which impaired growth was the consequence of a single genetic defect such as hypophosphatemic rickets or renal tubular acidosis. Conversely, whereas the short stature of Japanese individuals was formerly thought to be solely genetic in origin, the improved growth of postwar Japanese children suggests that "ethnic" short stature may often be explained in part by nutritional and environmental effects. The terms *familial short stature* and *genetic short stature* should be reserved for situations in which all other causes of growth retardation have been excluded.

The term *constitutional short stature* is often used to describe short children whose height merely reflects their genetic constitution. Such a term has no real meaning and probably should not be used. For the patient who is short but otherwise healthy, has a delayed bone age, is growing at a normal rate, and is destined to have a significant delay in puberty, we prefer the descriptive phrase *constitutional growth delay*. Alternatively, the term *constitutional delay of growth and adolescence* is often used. These patients are discussed in a later section.

Differential Diagnosis of Growth Failure

The causes of short stature and growth failure may be grouped under three broad headings: (1) intrinsic defects of growing tissues, (2) abnormalities in the environment of growing tissues, and (3) hormonal abnormalities.

Intrinsic Defects of Growing Tissues

Generalized intrinsic defects, which include chromosomal abnormalities and some forms of intrauterine growth retardation, may result in slow or abnormal growth of most or all body tissues. On the other hand, the growth defect may be limited to certain tissues, as in the chondrodysplasias, where it may be expressed primarily in the growth of cartilage and bone.

SKELETAL DYSPLASIAS. The skeletal dysplasias are a heterogeneous group of disorders, more than 100 in number, characterized by short stature and abnormalities in shape and size of limbs, trunk, and skull. Most patients were previously classified according to physical findings as having either achondroplasia (short limbs) or Morquio disease (short trunk).[491, 492] The heterogenous clinical manifestations of these disorders led in turn to subclassifications based on Latin and Greek roots and eponyms derived from the observer who first reported the specific syndrome.

An international classification was proposed for grouping the skeletal dysplasias in 1970[493] and was subsequently revised.[494] The confusion about classification and the clinical features of these disorders can be expected to persist, however, until the pathophysiological mechanisms of each subgroup are clearly defined.[495]

Children with skeletal dysplasias almost always have abnormal skeletal proportions. Although mild skeletal disorders such as hypochondroplasia may not always be apparent on casual examination, their presence may be suggested

by measurements of sitting height and span and by calculations of the ratio of the upper segment of the body to the lower segment. If body proportions are abnormal, a detailed family history should be taken, other family members examined, and a radiological survey of the skeleton carried out. Particular note should be taken of which bones are affected (i.e., vertebral column, long bones, or both) and where within each bone the lesions are localized (i.e., epiphyses, metaphyses, or diaphyses). This information can provide important insight into anticipated adult height, possible complications later in life, and the genetic risks for siblings and offspring. In some instances the diagnosis can be confirmed by microscopic study of the enchondral growth plate.[495] Material for examination may be obtained from the iliac crest by biopsy or from other growth plates at the time of corrective surgery.

Clinically useful growth standards have been constructed for children with achondroplasia[496] and for those with other chondrodysplasias.[497] Early diagnosis of some of these disorders can be made by prenatal ultrasonography.[498] The short stature in some patients can be treated by surgical leg-lengthening procedures.[492]

CHROMOSOMAL ABNORMALITIES. *Abnormalities of Autosomes.* Abnormalities of autosome number or structure associated with short stature are usually accompanied by mental retardation and physical stigmata. In Down syndrome—the most common autosomal abnormality—growth failure is manifested early in life and is accompanied by delays in bone maturation and epiphyseal fusion.[499, 500] The mean height of girls younger than age 12 with Down syndrome is 1.5 to 2.0 SD below the population mean and more than 3 SD below the mean of girls aged 12 to 17 because Down syndrome patients have poor pubertal growth spurts. For boys, mean stature is 2 to 3 SD below the mean until age 13 and 2 to 4 SD below the mean thereafter. Women with Down syndrome are on average 20 cm shorter than population means, and men are approximately 25 cm shorter.[500] The reduction in adult stature is attributable primarily to shortness of the lower extremities. Growth of infants and children with Down syndrome may be delayed further by congenital or acquired hypothyroidism, both of which occur with increased frequency in patients with this syndrome.

Abnormalities of the X Chromosome. The most common chromosomal abnormalities causing short stature are those involving absence of or deletion from one of the sex chromosomes. The phenotypic and genotypic variants of gonadal dysgenesis are detailed in Chapter 14, and in reviews.[501] In the context of growth, the physician should be familiar with the phenotypic features of the syndrome and should be aware that girls with variants may have short stature and slow growth with few or no physical stigmata of the disease (Figs. 21–32 and 21–33).[502, 503] In our experience the most common variants presenting with few somatic abnormalities other than short stature are due to isochromosome abnormalities involving the long arm of the X chromosome, deletions of a portion of the X chromosome, or mosaic patterns of the 45,X/46,XX or 45,X/47,XXX variety.

Nuclear chromatin patterns in buccal mucosa are frequently misleading and should be abandoned in favor of a complete analysis of chromosomal karyotype, with one or more banding techniques. Chromosomal karyotypes of patients suspected of having gonadal dysgenesis are necessary no matter what the buccal smear shows. Girls with classic stigmata of the disorder and a negative buccal smear require karyotypic analysis to rule out the presence of a mosaic pattern involving all or part of a Y chromosome (see Chapter 14). Furthermore, buccal smears of girls with isochromosome or mosaic X chromosome abnormalities are likely to be

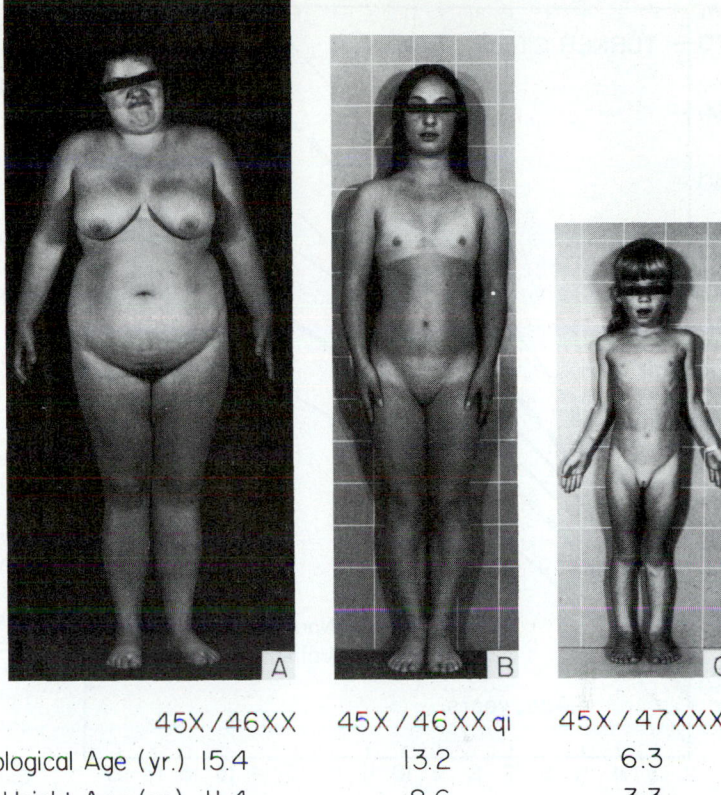

Figure 21–32. Three girls with variants of gonadal dysgenesis. The patient in *A* had no physical signs of the syndrome other than minimal shortening of the fourth metacarpal. Regular menses began at age 10. A cell line with 46,XX constitution predominated in peripheral lymphocytes. The patient in *B* had no physical stigmata of Turner syndrome other than short stature and sexual immaturity. She had markedly elevated serum gonadotropin concentrations and required cyclic estrogen-progesterone treatment. The patient in *C* had cubitus valgus and short stature, but no other stigmata. By age 15½ she showed partial feminization, had a serum FSH level within normal range, and had no menses.

	45X/46XX	45X/46XXqi	45X/47XXX
Chronological Age (yr.)	15.4	13.2	6.3
Height Age (yr.)	11.4	8.6	3.3

chromatin-positive, which causes the unwary physician to underdiagnose gonadal dysgenesis.

A small number of short girls who are later shown to have abnormalities of the X chromosome exhibit normal 46,XX karyotypes in peripheral lymphocytes. In such patients, analysis of skin fibroblasts may reveal a chromosomal abnormality. In several instances we have encountered short girls with normal lymphocyte and skin fibroblast karyotypes who had delayed sexual maturation accompanied by markedly elevated serum luteinizing hormone and FSH concentrations. In these girls cell lines with the abnormal karyotype may be localized to the ovaries and the tissues involved in skeletal growth.[504]

Girls with gonadal dysgenesis have slightly retarded intrauterine growth, followed by normal growth up to a bone age of about 3 y. Growth is quite slow in middle-childhood, and no pubertal growth spurt occurs[505, 506] (Fig. 21–34). Before the availability of recombinant GH to treat girls with gonadal dysgenesis, androgens were used widely. Low doses of androgens, usually in the form of a synthetic preparation (e.g., 0.1 mg of oxandrolone/kg body weight/d or 0.06 or 0.17 mg fluoxymesterone/kg body weight/d) sometimes cause two- to threefold increases in growth rate for a 1- to 2-y period.[507–509] However, recombinant GH therapy is effective in accelerating growth, either alone or in combination with androgens.[510] In a large multicenter study, treatment with GH (0.375 mg/kg body weight/wk) plus oxandrolone raised mean growth rates from 4.3 cm/y before therapy to 9.8, 7.4, and 6.1 cm/y in years 1, 2, and 3 of treatment, respectively.[511] Similar results have been reported by others.[510] Combination GH plus oxandrolone therapy seems to be more effective than GH alone. One study[511] shows evidence of an increase in predicted adult height (8.7 cm increase after 3 y of therapy). Regardless of whether this increase in predicted adult height is real, the attainment of milestones of growth and development at normal ages is almost certainly of psychological benefit to these girls.

Low doses of estrogens also stimulate growth.[114, 112] In a 6-mo study of the effect of 100 ng ethinyl estradiol/kg body

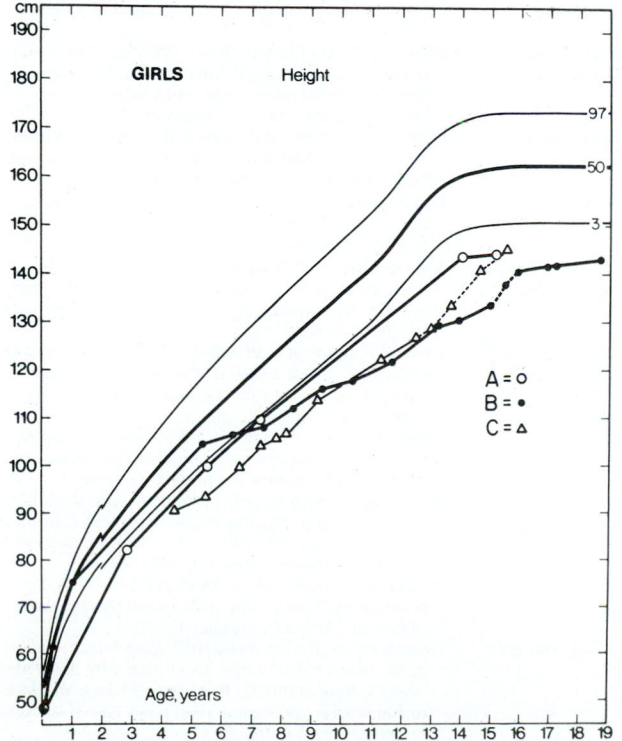

Figure 21–33. Growth curves for the three patients shown in Figure 21–32. Broken lines indicate growth during periods of treatment with oxandrolone.

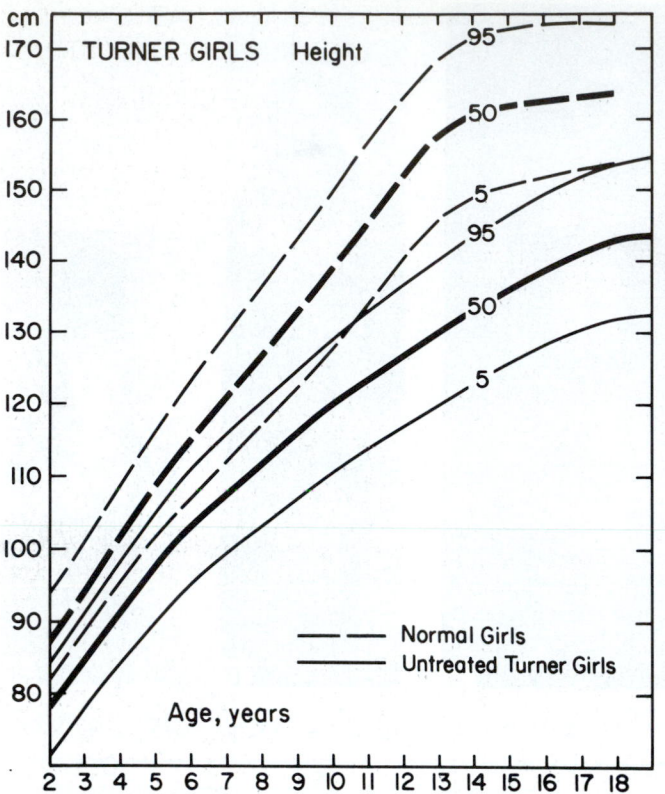

Figure 21–34. Comparison between growth curves of normal girls and girls with gonadal dysgenesis (Turner syndrome). The curves for girls with gonadal dysgenesis show the effects of intrauterine growth retardation and normal growth early in life, with later slowing and absence of the pubertal growth spurt. (From data in Ranke MB, Pfluger H, Rosendahl W, et al. Turner syndrome: spontaneous growth in 150 cases and review of the literature. Eur J Pediatr 1983; 141:81–88.)

bryogenesis. Typically, blood hormone concentrations are normal, and skeletal maturation is normal or only moderately delayed. The older term, primordial dwarfism, is rarely appropriate as the disorders are compartmentalized into specific syndromes. Some of the better-known entities are given in Table 21–11, and comprehensive descriptions are found in refs. 516 to 520.

Categorization of these conditions into specific syndromes serves a useful purpose in alerting the physician to associated abnormalities and in providing insight into the prognosis for physical and intellectual development and life expectancy.

Abnormalities in the Environment of Growing Tissues

This category of disorders encompasses the systemic diseases that impair growth by adversely affecting the general health and well-being of the growing child.[521] Such growth failure may occur by a variety of mechanisms including insufficient intake of calories and/or protein, insufficient oxygenation of tissues, and electrolyte imbalance. In many cases the exact mechanisms of growth retardation are not known. Patients with diseases of this type characteristically are poorly nourished and present with weights below the average for height. This situation contrasts with growth failure of endocrine origin in which body weight is often above the average for height.

NUTRITIONAL INSUFFICIENCY. Malnutrition is the most common cause of growth failure worldwide; it is

weight/d, the mean growth rate of girls with gonadal dysgenesis was 5.6 ± 0.5 cm/y (compared with 3.7 ± 0.2 cm/y in placebo-treated girls).[513, 514] In some studies the stimulatory effect of estrogens on growth is transient, and predicted adult height is not improved;[506, 515] also, girls treated with estradiol may have premature growth of breasts. Although it appears that estradiol therapy is not as beneficial for growth as GH combined with oxandrolone, studies of the combined use of GH and estradiol are in progress and could offer the advantage of avoidance of potential virilizing side effects of androgens and provide the psychologically satisfying benefits to the patient of receiving estrogen at an earlier, more appropriate age. Although administration of the larger dosages of estrogen required to promote maturation of secondary sexual characteristics should be postponed as long as possible to delay epiphyseal fusion, psychological considerations usually make some compromise mandatory. As one monitors the growth of girls with gonadal dysgenesis, it is important to keep in mind that such patients are susceptible to growth failure from causes other than chromosome abnormality. Specifically, autoimmune thyroiditis occurs with increased frequency in patients with gonadal dysgenesis, and sudden, unexpected deceleration of growth may herald the onset of hypothyroidism.

SHORT STATURE ASSOCIATED WITH DYSMORPHIC FEATURES (PRIMORDIAL DWARFISM). This term encompasses a variety of disorders characterized by intrauterine growth retardation, postnatal growth failure, and a spectrum of associated abnormalities. The disorders are of unknown etiology and can occur as a consequence of single- or multiple-gene defects or environmental insults during em-

TABLE 21–11. Dwarfism Associated with Dysmorphic Syndromes of Unknown Cause*

Syndrome	Principal Features
Prader-Willi syndrome	Intrauterine and postnatal hypotonia; obesity; mental deficiency; hypogonadism; small hands and feet; mild growth retardation possible
Russell-Silver syndrome	Asymmetry; small triangular face; short, incurred fifth finger; renal anomalies; prenatal onset of growth failure
Noonan syndrome (Turner-like)	Webbing of neck; low posterior hairline; shield chest; pectus excavatum; right-sided congenital heart disease; mental retardation; small penis and cryptorchidism; normal chromosomal karyotype
de Lange syndrome	Mental retardation; short nose and anteverted nostrils; abnormal lips and mouth; bushy eyebrows and long curly eyelashes; hypertonicity; abnormal cry
Bloom syndrome	Facial telangiectatic erythema; malar hypoplasia; microcephaly; prenatal onset of growth failure; predisposition to malignancy
Seckel syndrome (bird-headed dwarfism)	Microcephaly with premature synostosis; mental retardation; facial hypoplasia with prominent nose; low-set, malformed ears; crytorchidism; severe growth failure of prenatal onset
Progeria (Hutchinson-Gilford syndrome)	Premature aging with atherosclerosis; elevated plasma cholesterol level; alopecia; thinning of skin; nail hypoplasia; loss of subcutaneous fat; periarticular fibrosis; severe growth failure
Cockayne syndrome	Mental retardation; deafness; peripheral neuropathy; retinal pigmentation; optic atrophy; microcephaly; photosensitive dermatitis; premature aging
Leprechaunism	Intrauterine growth failure; prominent eyes; thick lips; large ears; large phallus; breast hyperplasia; hirsutism; islet cell hyperplasia with hyperinsulinism and insulin resistance; severe postnatal growth failure
Ellis–van Creveld syndrome	Intrauterine growth failure; short extremities; polydactyly; hypoplastic nails; small thorax; short upper lip; congenital cardiac defects
Aarskog syndrome	Growth failure during first year; hypertelorism; widow's peak; broad nasal bridge; short nose with anteverted nostrils; long philtrum; short, broad hands and feet; dorsal scrotal fold surrounding penis (shawl scrotum); cryptorchidism; probably X-linked recessive

*The reader is referred to refs. 516–520 for more complete coverage of these syndromes.

estimated that two thirds of the world's children are under-nourished. Severe growth retardation is associated with the clinical pictures of marasmus and kwashiorkor. In the former, in which the intake of both calories and protein is insufficient, disappearance of subcutaneous fat, muscle wasting, and shrinkage of internal organs are seen. Chronic diarrhea results from malnutrition-induced flattening of intestinal mucosa and from concomitant deficiencies of intestinal enzymes. These changes in turn aggravate the nutritional insufficiency. In kwashiorkor, caloric deprivation is usually less severe, but the quantity and quality of dietary protein are inadequate; in the pure form of kwashiorkor, some subcutaneous fat may persist despite severe protein deficiency.

In most affected children pictures of marasmus and kwashiorkor are merged. Affected patients may have elevated serum GH levels[522] but paradoxically depressed serum somatomedin concentrations.[83, 523] The high serum GH concentrations may serve a protein-sparing action via the effects of GH on carbohydrate and fat metabolism. The low somatomedin concentrations may prevent squandering of protein in growth. With refeeding and restoration of protein stores, the serum GH level falls to normal and is followed after some delay by an increase in somatomedin concentration and resumption of linear growth.

Although full-blown marasmus and kwashiorkor are relatively easy to diagnose, it is more difficult to recognize growth retardation secondary to modest nutritional deficiency. Not only are accurate dietary histories difficult to obtain, but it is often not clear whether the low caloric intake is a cause or a consequence of growth failure. This is because normal children expend a significant portion of caloric intake in growth; decreased caloric intake, therefore, may be anticipated when growth is arrested. In view of these practical problems, there is often no substitute for hospitalization to observe food intake and short-term weight gain when an adequate diet is provided.

Even in nations where food supplies are plentiful, growth retardation secondary to insufficient nutrition intake is still a problem. We have observed children, particularly girls in the second decade of life, with severe growth arrest secondary to anorexia nervosa. We also have cared for children with retarded linear growth and poor weight gain, whose mothers previously suffered from anorexia nervosa. These mothers, who express concern that their children may eat too much and become obese, purposefully limit the children's caloric intake. With refeeding, catch-up growth occurs. Even more commonly, growth failure can result from self-imposed restriction of caloric intake arising from a fear of becoming obese (Fig. 21–35).[524] Unlike children with anorexia, these children do not have a distorted body image; they do not vomit, abuse laxatives, hoard food, or exhibit compulsive exercise habits. Many have a preoccupation with achieving a slim figure and may recover without psychotherapy.

Growth retardation can also be associated with deficiencies of specific dietary components such as zinc and iron. Anemia is the primary manifestation of iron deficiency, but reduced appetite and growth failure, particularly failure to gain weight, may also occur.[525, 526] Zinc deficiency, which results in anorexia and failure to undergo pubertal development, is observed in children with malabsorption syndromes, chronic infection, sickle cell anemia, acrodermatitis enteropathica, and liver disease.[527, 528] It remains to be determined how often growth failure results from primary zinc deficiency in the absence of other disease.[529, 530]

MALABSORPTION AND CHRONIC INFLAMMATORY BOWEL DISEASE. In most children with malabsorption, growth failure is neither the initial presenting complaint nor

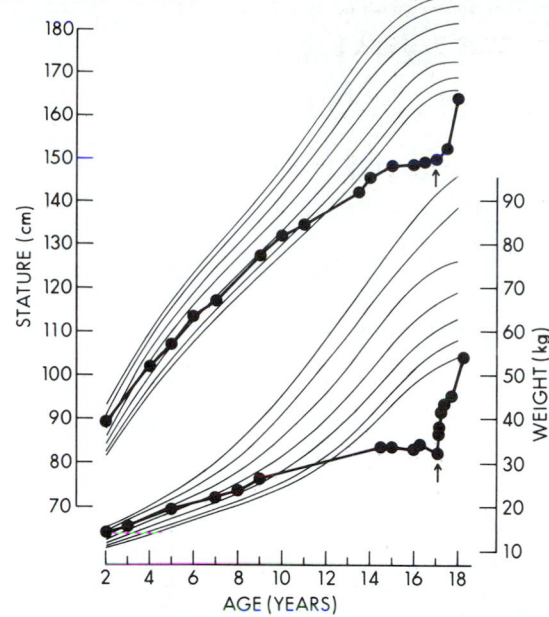

Figure 21–35. Curves of weight and height of a child who had growth failure resulting from prolonged self-imposed caloric restriction because of a fear of becoming obese. Note that crossing of percentiles on the weight curve preceded that for the height curve, and when caloric intake was normalized *(arrow)*, the gain in weight preceded the improvement in linear growth. Also note that at the end of the prolonged period of caloric restriction, weight age (10.2 y) was considerably less than height age (12 y). (From Pugilese MT, Lifshitz F, Grad F, et al. Fear of obesity: a cause of short stature and delayed puberty. Reprinted, by permission of The New England Journal of Medicine, 309; 513–518, 1983.)

the primary concern; nevertheless, severe growth failure can result from mild abnormalities of bowel function. This is particularly true for celiac disease (gluten-induced enteropathy)[531–533] and chronic inflammatory bowel disease. In celiac disease the time of onset of symptoms generally occurs in infancy when the patient begins to ingest wheat products containing gluten[534] (Fig. 21–36). In addition to having recurrent diarrhea, abdominal distention, and muscular inactivity, these children often exhibit apathy, irritability, and anorexia. The anorexia may contribute more to the growth failure than does fecal wastage of calories. It is therefore essential in children with growth failure of unknown cause and evidence of diminished body fat stores to take a careful history with regard to quantity and quality of stools and to measure stool fat. The diagnosis of celiac disease can be excluded only by a biopsy of the upper intestinal mucosa. Because asymptomatic celiac disease may cause growth failure,[531–533] jejunal biopsy may be indicated for patients with no explanation for growth failure even though there is no clinical evidence of celiac disease. Antigliadin immunoglobulin G antibodies are increased in virtually all affected patients but do not have high specificity for celiac disease.[534] On the other hand, antireticulum antibodies exhibit high specificity but low sensitivity, occurring in about half of affected patients.[534] Although useful, these antibody tests do not replace biopsy of the small bowel.

It is not appropriate to prescribe a gluten-free diet without first making a definite diagnosis of celiac disease. Further confusing the clinical picture is the observation that children with celiac disease may have low[533] or normal[535] GH secretion; in either case, IGF I concentrations are low.[535] The fact that IGF I level does not rise with GH administration but does increase with a gluten-free diet suggests that the GH resistance is caused by nutritional deficiency.

In Crohn disease (regional ileitis) and ulcerative colitis,

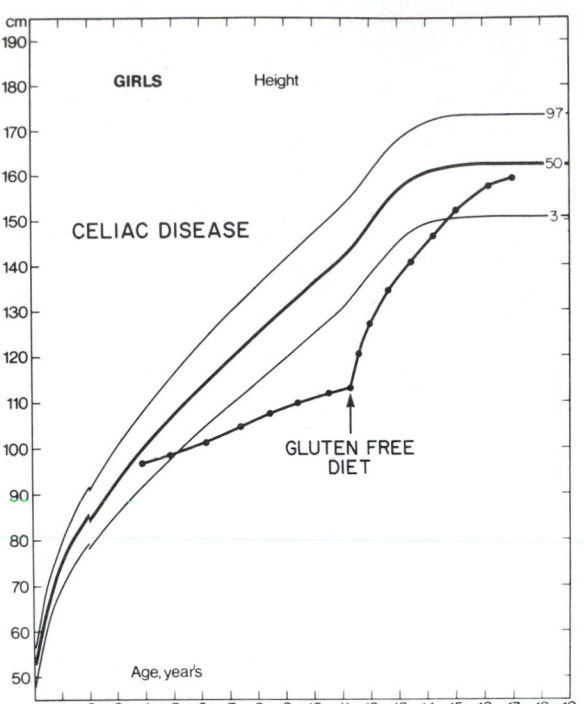

Figure 21–36. Catch-up growth in a girl with celiac disease. After 8 y of growth failure the patient was placed on a gluten-free diet and exhibited striking catch-up growth. Note the return to previous growth percentiles. (Courtesy of J. M. Tanner.)

growth failure may precede abdominal and bowel complaints by several years. Growth failure in inflammatory bowel disease is believed to be due to malnutrition.[521, 536–538] Energy intake is chronically inadequate in most growth-retarded children with inflammatory bowel disease. Likewise, exudation of proteins by the inflamed mucosa and interference with growth by drugs such as glucocorticoids may contribute to the pathogenesis. Losses of zinc because of diarrhea may also be a factor, as may an increased nutrient requirement secondary to chronic bowel inflammation. Basal serum GH levels and GH responses to provocative challenges are normal. Low IGF I values reflect the malnourished status. Finally, accelerated growth occurs when nutritional status is improved.[539–541] Because diagnosis of inflammatory bowel disease is sometimes difficult, the history should include a search for subtle bowel symptoms, abdominal pain, or recurrent fever. Measurement of the erythrocyte sedimentation rate is sometimes helpful, as is the finding of anemia or blood in the stools.

CHRONIC RENAL DISEASE. A variety of renal diseases, including chronic renal insufficiency, renal tubular acidosis, and Bartter syndrome, are associated with growth failure.[521, 542] Because clinical signs and symptoms may be minimal, all individuals with unexplained growth failure should have sufficient laboratory tests to exclude these disorders. In general, growth failure from renal disease is most profound in infancy and in the early years of life; it occurs when the glomerular filtration rate falls below 25 mL/min/1.73 m² surface area,[543] and the severity parallels the deficit in renal function. Multiple mechanisms contribute to the growth failure,[544, 545] including reduced intake of protein and calories, depletion of electrolytes such as potassium and calcium, bicarbonate wasting, diminished IGF concentrations, thyroid insufficiency, decreased androgen production, uremic inhibitors of growth, and long-term therapeutic use of glucocorticoids.

Hemodialysis often does not return growth to normal, and successful renal transplantation may not cause catch-up growth sufficient to erase the previous loss in height. Treatment of uremic rats with GH accelerates growth and improves food utilization,[546] and preliminary studies of children with chronic renal failure suggest that GH treatment produces significant acceleration of growth.[547]

Renal osteodystrophy also causes growth failure.[548] This syndrome is characterized by hypocalcemia, hyperphosphatemia, hyperphosphatasia, acidosis, and compensatory elevation of parathyroid hormone levels. Formation of 1,25-dihydroxycholecalciferol is attenuated because of loss of functional renal parenchyma. As a result of these alterations, formation and remodeling of bone are impaired. The therapeutic administration of calcitriol to these children causes acceleration of linear growth.[549–551]

CARDIAC DISEASE. The growth failure observed in infants and children with severe congenital heart disease reflects tissue hypoxia and the increased energy demands placed on the deformed heart. Growth failure frequently correlates with cyanosis, the size of the left-to-right shunt, the severity and chronicity of congestive heart failure, and the presence of obstructive pulmonary disease.[552, 553] Many patients, however, have low birth weight and a variety of extracardiac anomalies[554] and fail to undergo catch-up growth after successful correction of the cardiac defects.[555] The limited growth of these patients may in part be secondary to noncardiac, intrauterine factors.

CENTRAL NERVOUS SYSTEM DISEASE. Children with mental retardation or other central nervous system disorders may be short with no apparent cause. The mechanisms are largely undefined. In some cases caloric intake may be insufficient because of inability to recognize or respond to hunger or because of mechanical problems related to eating. Rarely, growth failure may be secondary to depressed GH secretion.[556]

HEMATOLOGICAL DISEASES. Children with sickle cell (SS) disease often have growth failure.[557–559] The failure to gain weight is usually more severe than the height deficit. Linear growth failure is apparent by age 2 y and continues through childhood. Puberty is delayed, which allows a longer period of growth and permits some affected individuals to reach normal adult height. Bone age is delayed in older children. Several mechanisms for growth retardation in sickle cell disease have been proposed, including chronic anemia, high energy cost of cardiovascular work, high cost of rapid erythropoietic turnover, suboptimal nutrition, and hormonal abnormalities. The precise mechanism is not known, but nutritional supplementation may ameliorate the growth retardation.[560]

Delays in growth and the onset of puberty are also common in patients with thalassemia major, but adult height is not significantly reduced from predicted height.[561] The severity of the growth retardation does not appear to correlate with the frequency of transfusions or of chelation therapy.[562] The mechanism for growth retardation is not certain, and more than one mechanism may be responsible in a given patient. Impaired ability to synthesize IGF I under the stimulus of GH is a common finding,[563, 564] but impaired serum GH responses to provocative stimuli and to GHRH have also been reported.[565]

DIABETES MELLITUS. In the preinsulin era and in the years immediately after insulin became available, growth failure was a prominent feature of diabetic children who survived for a prolonged period. Severe growth failure likewise was observed in the syndrome described by Mauriac, in which poorly controlled diabetic children developed hepatomegaly secondary to increased glycogen deposition and signs of cortisol excess.[566] The blood glucose level of such children oscillates between hypoglycemia and hyperglycemia, and diabetic ketoacidosis is common. Growth failure may be a manifestation of recurrent acidosis, chronic cortisol excess, inadequate intracellular nutrition, or other factors. Aside from these extreme cases of growth failure, which occur infrequently, diabetic children may have modest growth failure, even when diabetic control is good by other criteria.[567] In one study[568] a group of more than 100 diabetic children were of normal height at the onset of disease but showed a downward shift in percentile channels within 3 y. The primary effect on growth was a delayed and reduced pubertal growth spurt that was independent of diabetic control. It has been difficult to define specific factors that contribute to the growth failure observed in some diabetic children,[569] but intensive insulin therapy using continuous infusion techniques produces acceleration of linear growth in diabetics previously treated by conventional methods.[570]

The possibility that growth failure in diabetics may result from hypothyroidism secondary to Hashimoto thyroiditis or to celiac disease should be kept in mind. Each of these conditions occurs with increased frequency in patients with diabetes mellitus.[571]

VITAMIN D–RESISTANT RICKETS. This disorder, which is inherited as an X-linked trait, is characterized by short stature, hypophosphatemia, diminished renal tubular reabsorption of inorganic phosphate, decreased intestinal absorption of calcium, and rickets or osteomalacia unresponsive to physiological dosages of calciferol.[572] The growth of the upper segment in this disorder is normal, but the lower segment is shortened. The severity of the growth retardation correlates with the severity of the metabolic defect,[543] but short stature may occur in patients who exhibit no other signs of disease and have only hypophosphatemia. In patients with more severe disease, the serum alkaline phosphatase level is elevated. To achieve near-normal skeletal growth, it is essential to institute calciferol and phosphate treatment early and to monitor for adequacy of therapy. Calcitriol may be more effective than calciferol.[574]

OTHER METABOLIC DISORDERS. A variety of metabolic disorders may be associated with growth delay and short stature. In most instances the exact mechanism for the effects on growth are unknown. A detailed discussion of each of these disorders is beyond the scope of this chapter.[575]

Hormonal Abnormalities

DEFICIENCY. In a survey of 48,000 Scottish schoolchildren, severe GH deficiency was present in 1 in 4000.[576] The worldwide incidence, however, may be on the order of 1 in 10,000.[577, 578] Growth failure related to partial and more subtle GH deficiency may be more common.

Patients with GH disorders can be grouped into three broad categories: those with primary pituitary disease, those with hypothalamic dysfunction, and those who are unable to respond to GH (Table 21–12).

Primary Pituitary Failure. Genetic disorders that cause primary GH deficiency[579] include pituitary hypoplasia, pituitary aplasia, familial panhypopituitarism, and familial isolated GH deficiency. Six distinct genetic GH deficiency states have been reported, including two disorders in which there are multiple pituitary hormone deficiencies and four in which the GH deficiency is isolated. In the latter group, the nature of the defect varies from deletions of the gene for GH to defects in DNA that are not localized to the GH gene and sometimes cause structural abnormalities of the pituitary. Defective GH genes tend to produce severe GH defi-

TABLE 21–12. Classification of Pituitary Dwarfism

Primary Pituitary Disease
Genetic syndromes: aplasia, hypoplasia, familial panhypopituitarism, familial isolated GH deficiency, deletion of GH gene
Intrasellar tumors: adenomas, craniopharyngioma
Nontumorous destruction: trauma, infection, central nervous system radiation

Pituitary Deficiency Secondary to Hypothalamic Dysfunction
Idiopathic (many are the result of perinatal insult): multiple deficiencies (panhypopituitarism), primarily GH (isolated), constitutional growth delay (some cases)
Postinfectious deficiency
Postradiation deficiency
Histiocytosis
Hypothalamic tumor: craniopharyngioma, hamartoma, neurofibroma, germinoma
Psychosocial dwarfism

States of End-Organ Resistance to GH (High GH, Low IGF I)
Hereditary GH resistance (Laron-type dwarfism, ?Pygmies)
Biologically inactive GH ??
Protein-calorie malnutrition

ciency, sometimes with a tendency to form high titers of antibodies to exogenous GH. Primary hypopituitarism is associated with a variety of developmental defects. In anencephaly, the pituitary is small, deformed, and/or ectopic in location; in holoprosencephaly, absence or malformation of the pituitary gland is associated with impaired midline development of the embryonic forebrain and midline dysplasia of the face.[580, 581] The syndrome of septo-optic dysplasia[582] is characterized by optic nerve hypoplasia and abnormalities of the septum pellucidum and corpus callosum in association with GH deficiency. The clinical presentation of the latter syndrome varies in the severity of pituitary hormone deficiency, the loss of vision, and the severity of intracranial anomalies.[583, 584] Hypopituitarism also occurs with increased frequency in patients with cleft lip and palate,[585, 586] and children with cleft palate and short stature or slow growth should have studies done of pituitary function. Less common midline central nervous system and cranial defects associated with hypopituitarism are reviewed elsewhere.[581] In several of these disorders it is not known whether the primary lesion is in the pituitary or in the hypothalamus.

Pituitary destruction may also result from trauma, expanding intrasellar and suprasellar tumors, histiocytosis, granulomatous disease, therapeutic radiation of the central nervous system, and radiation of middle-ear tumors. GH deficiency secondary to cranial radiation for cancer is increasing in frequency.[587–590] Cranial radiation may also produce subnormal GH responses to provocative stimuli without impairing growth.[591] Some radiated children, on the other hand, have slowing of linear growth but normal GH responses to provocative testing.[592] In the latter group, GH secretion during sleep may be impaired, and growth is improved by GH therapy. Similarly, reduced pulsatile GH secretion may occur after cranial radiation for acute lymphoblastic leukemia.[593] Craniopharyngioma, the most common tumor to produce hypopituitarism in children, usually involves primarily the hypothalamus but may also destroy the pituitary.[594]

GH Deficiency Secondary to Hypothalamic Dysfunction. Pituitary hypofunction secondary to hypothalamic damage may be caused by a variety of insults: purulent meningitis, granulomas, hydrocephalus, histiocytosis, and hypothalamic tumors such as craniopharyngioma, germinoma, hamartoma, and neurofibroma. The largest number of patients in this group, however, are categorized under the term *idiopathic hypopituitarism.*[595]

Many cases of idiopathic hypopituitarism result from perinatal insult. A history of abnormal delivery and/or perinatal asphyxia is obtained in as many as 50 to 60% of children who are later shown to have hypopituitarism.[577, 596, 597] In a survey for perinatal abnormalities in our own patients (Table 21–13), 65% had at least one significant perinatal insult, and many had two or more insults.[598] Birth weights of these patients are generally normal; the sex ratio is 4:1 in favor of males. The inference that GH deficiency is secondary to hypothalamic dysfunction is based on the observation that most of these children have normal serum thyrotropin and prolactin responses after administration of thyrotropin-releasing hormone. Such children also secrete GH in response to injection of GHRH.[599–602]

Psychosocial Dwarfism (Emotional Deprivation Dwarfism). Failure to thrive in young children may occur as a result of an inadequate environment.[603–605] In 1967 Powell and associates[606, 607] described a group of emotionally disturbed children coming from hostile environments whose growth patterns resembled those caused by GH deficiency. Such children are withdrawn; have retarded speech development; and exhibit bizarre eating habits with polydipsia, tendencies to ingest spoiled food and drink, gorging, and vomiting. GH and ACTH secretion respond poorly to provocative testing. After a brief period of hospitalization or placement in a foster home, pituitary function, dietary habits, and mental status revert to normal, and linear growth is accelerated. These patients may have malabsorption, but the principal defect resides in the centers that regulate GH secretion. GH deficiency results from failure of the hypothalamus to stimulate the pituitary.

A clinical picture in infants, similar to the syndrome just described, is referred to as the *maternal deprivation syndrome.*[608–610] In these infants, failure to thrive is due to a combination of inadequate mothering, poor feeding practices, and insufficient caloric intake. GH secretion, rather than suppressed, is often normal or excessive, which supports the view that caloric deprivation is the major mechanism of growth failure.

We believe that the syndromes of psychosocial dwarfism and maternal deprivation represent the extremes of a spectrum. At one end, suppression of pituitary function is the primary mechanism for growth failure, and nutritional deficiency is a minor factor. At the other end, nutritional deprivation predominates, and pituitary function is appropriate.

Syndromes of Insensitivity to GH. The prototype of GH insensitivity was described as a familial form of short stature in Oriental Jewish persons and was characterized by normal or high serum GH and low somatomedin levels. This disorder, which is due to absent or defective GH receptors, is widely known as Laron-type dwarfism in recognition of the physician who described it.[611] Laron-type dwarfism, however, probably represents only one form of GH insensitivity, and we prefer the more general designation.

Most patients with GH insensitivity are from the Middle East and are the products of consanguineous marriages. The children have the physical appearance of severe GH deficiency but elevated basal serum GH concentrations and markedly exaggerated GH responses to provocative stimuli. The serum IGF I concentrations are low and do not increase in response to injection of human GH.[612] These children exhibit neither metabolic nor growth responses to administration of exogenous human GH.[613, 614] Hepatic cell membranes from children with GH insensitivity fail to bind radiolabeled GH, and the GH-binding protein in serum is absent.[615] Abnormalities of DNA restriction fragment length in some of these patients are consistent with defects in the gene encoding the GH receptor.[616]

Children with somewhat different clinical features have been noted in whom GH insensitivity was proposed as the mechanism for growth failure.[617, 618] These children have normal or high serum GH concentrations[617–619] and have been variously described as having syndromes of bioinactive GH, normal variant short stature, and GH-dependent growth failure. None have yet been shown to have abnormalities of the GH molecule, the GH receptor, or intracellular mechanisms involved in the response to GH.

Clinical Characteristics of Hypopituitarism in Children. Children with hypopituitarism are short and exhibit growth curves that deviate progressively from normal. Growth rates are commonly as low as 3 cm/y and almost always less than 4 to 5 cm/y (Fig. 21–37). In idiopathic hypopituitarism, growth failure may not be obvious until patients are 2 to 4 y old. In retrospect, however, it is often possible to establish that growth failure began in the first few months of life. Indeed, when growth failure does not occur until midchildhood, the possibility of a pituitary or a hypothalamic tumor or some other organic cause, should be considered. Children with hypopituitarism have normal skeletal proportions for age, tend to be somewhat overweight for height, and may have subcutaneous deposits of ripply abdominal fat (Fig. 21–38). Males who apparently have had prenatal onset of the disorder may have micropenis, small testes, and underdeveloped scrotum.[620] Congenital hypopituitarism may also be accompanied by prolonged neonatal hyperbilirubinemia[621] and hypoglycemia. Congenital hypopituitarism, therefore, should be considered when any one or more of the above-mentioned signs is present in a neonate. Although the head circumference of children with hypopituitarism is usually within the normal range for age, the growth of facial bones is retarded, thereby producing a disparity between the size of the face and that of the calvarium and an underdeveloped nasal bridge. In the first several years of life, approximately 10% of children with hypopituitarism have hypoglycemic convulsions. An additional 10% or more have asymptomatic fasting hypoglycemia.[622] Hypoglycemia is usually secondary to combined deficiencies of cortisol and GH and is corrected by replacement of both hormones.[623] Children with idiopathic hypopituitarism rarely have clinical hypothyroidism, but serum thyroid hormone levels are frequently low or in the low-normal range.

TABLE 21–13. Complication of Gestation, Labor and Delivery, and the Postnatal Period in Children with Idiopathic Hypopituitarism and in Sibling Controls

	No. of Complications in	
Complication	Patients with Hypopituitarism (n = 46)	Sibling Controls* (n = 54)
Gestation		
<37 wk long	7†	5
Bleeding	13	3‡
Toxemia	4	2
Labor and delivery		
3 h or less	8	3
24 h or more	5	3
Breech presentation	11	4
Difficult forceps	3	0
Cesarean section for fetal indications	2	0
Intrapartum distress and/or asphyxia	10	0
Postnatal complications		
Seizures	7§	0
Postnatal infection	2	0
Hyperpyrexia	1	0

*Control data were derived from siblings who immediately preceded or followed patients in birth order.
†Denominator is 42 patients; all others are 46 patients.
‡Hypopituitary vs. control; p < .005, by chi square method.
§Three were associated with hypoglycemia.
Data from Craft WH, Underwood LE, Van Wyk JJ. High incidence of perinatal insult in children with idiopathic hypopituitarism. J Pediatr 1980; 96:397–402.

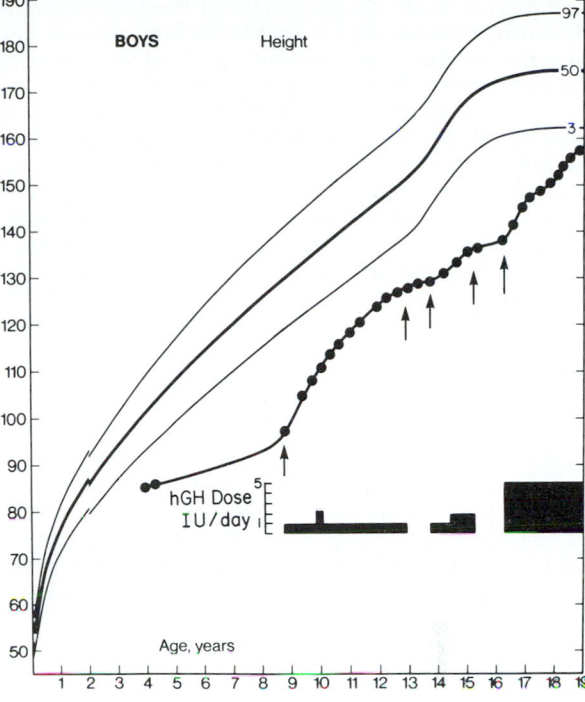

Figure 21–37. Growth curve of a male with idiopathic hypopituitarism who was treated for several years with pituitary human GH. Typical of such patients is the decrease in growth response as treatment is continued for long periods. Problems of this nature are less severe now that larger doses of GH can be given. At age 24 his height was 165 cm (65 inches).

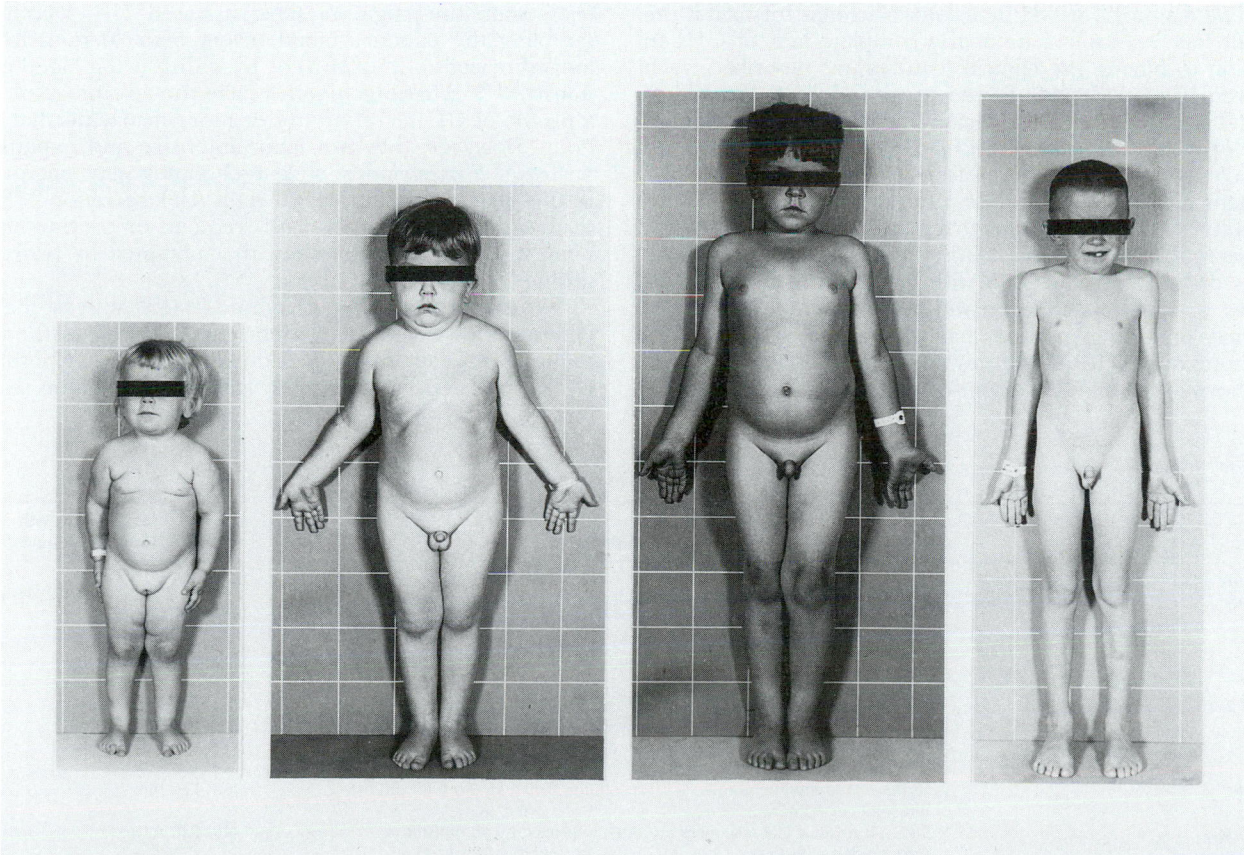

Figure 21–38. Four children with GH deficiency. All were more than 2 SD below the mean height for normal children when these photographs were taken. They exhibit normal body proportions, and with the exception of the boy at the right each has an excess of adipose tissue. The two boys at the right have small genitalia as well. (From Underwood LE, D'Ercole AJ. Anterior pituitary gland and hypothalamus: disorders affecting anterior pituitary function. In: Rudolph AM, Hoffman HIE, eds. Pediatrics. 19th ed. Norwalk, CT: Appleton & Lange, 1991:1572.)

Diagnosis of Hypopituitarism. The diagnosis of hypopituitarism is made by assessment of the history and physical features, documentation of the lifelong growth curve, assessment of the current growth rate, and analysis of pituitary function tests. This evaluation can be carried out in an ambulatory setting. The skeletal age is invariably delayed and usually is roughly equivalent to height age. This finding is of little specific diagnostic value. In patients with pituitary tumors or craniopharyngiomas, x-ray films may reveal enlargement or ballooning of the sella turcica, erosion of the sphenoid bone, or calcification of a suprasellar mass. On the other hand, the sella turcica is often small in idiopathic hypopituitarism. Sellar volume may be measured from standard skull radiographs and compared with normal standards for age and height.[624, 625] Approximately one third of our patients with idiopathic hypopituitarism had sellar volumes that were sufficiently small to be diagnostic of the disorder. When the possibility of a pituitary or a hypothalamic lesion is entertained seriously, a computed tomographic or magnetic resonance imaging scan is indicated.[626] Such a study is needed particularly for any child in whom an abnormality is suspected from the plain skull x-ray film, or for the older child who has late-onset growth failure and is therefore more likely to have an expanding lesion of the hypothalamus or the pituitary.

Measurement of serum IGF I concentrations by radioimmunoassay is also a useful screening method.[627, 628] Because caloric or protein malnutrition may depress IGF I concentrations, nutritional status must be taken into consideration in interpreting a low value. Furthermore, the IGF I value needs to be interpreted in light of developmental rather than chronological age.

The diagnosis of GH deficiency is straightforward if the patient has a complete or nearly complete lack of GH. In addition to having the clinical features just described, such children have evidence of little or no GH secretion, either spontaneously or after provocative testing. The diagnosis is more problematic, however, if the deficiency is partial rather than complete. Indeed, it is often difficult to separate GH-deficient children from those who are not deficient. This difficulty is due in large part to an inability to define normal GH secretion by available methods. Because GH measurements do not correlate well with GH-secretory capacity or predict which short children will benefit from GH therapy, a variety of testing methods have been devised (Table 21–14), none of which fully serves the purpose.

Normal serum GH responses to vigorous exercise sometimes exclude the diagnosis of GH deficiency. Because only 70% of normal children respond to this stimulus, however, low GH responses are not diagnostic. Measurement of GH during sleep may also be helpful. On a single sample taken 1 h after the onset of sleep, 60 to 70% of normal, non–GH-deficient children have serum GH concentrations greater than 7 µg/L. Fewer, however, reach a GH value that is now accepted as an unequivocal sign of normal GH secretion.

If provocative testing is to be used for diagnosis of GH deficiency, subnormal serum GH responses to two or more stimuli are required.[629–631] The definition of subnormal responses varies from one laboratory to another, in part because of the variability among GH assays. This variability is due to use of standards of different potency, antibodies that recognize different GH epitopes, and different assay systems. Most investigators consider responses of less than 7 to 10 µg/L (National Institutes of Health human GH standards) as suggesting impaired pituitary secretion. Because such cutoffs are arbitrary, the physician should always be cautious in the interpretation of tests of GH secretion.[632, 633] Of the provocative stimuli available, we use clonidine (4 µg/kg, orally) followed in 2 h by an intravenous infusion of L-arginine. Clonidine is a potent stimulator of GH secretion, although it produces sleepiness and a modest decrease in blood pressure. The latter is not troublesome if the patient is kept in bed for the 2-h test. We have abandoned the use of insulin-induced hypoglycemia. Although the risk of adverse consequences from the hypoglycemia is small, close monitoring by the physician is mandatory and the information obtained does not appear to be superior to that obtained with other tests.

Because of the limitation of pharmacological provocative tests, some investigators have assessed GH secretion by sampling the patient's blood (every 5 to 30 min) for prolonged periods (12 to 24 h) or by withdrawing blood continuously.[634, 635] These techniques have the advantage of giving a profile of GH secretion under more nearly normal conditions. However, they are labor intensive and expensive to perform. Furthermore, such techniques may not produce results that reflect the usual daily GH secretion,[635–637] and the accuracy of diagnosis with frequent or continuous sampling may not be better than that obtained by provocative testing.[638]

Studies with the hypothalamic GHRH suggest that most patients with isolated GH deficiency, as well as those with multiple pituitary hormone deficiencies, have hypothalamic GHRH deficiency; that is, they release some GH in response

---

TABLE 21–14. Clinical Tests of Growth Hormone Secretion

Test	Test Conditions*	Time of Growth Hormone Response
Screening Tests		
Exercise	Patient should be fasting; 15 min of moderate exercise, then 5 min of vigorous exercise.	20–40 min after exercise is begun
Sleep	GH rise occurs with deep sleep (stages 3, 4); awaken patient for sample; with EEG monitoring and frequent sampling, may be used as a more definitive test.	Initial peak within 1 h after onset of deep sleep
Formal Tests		
Insulin	Regular crystalline insulin 0.05–0.1 U/kg (IV); 50% fall in blood glucose is necessary for adequate test; nadir blood glucose level occurs 20–30 min after insulin is given.	45–75 min
Arginine	L-Arginine monohydrochloride, 5–10% solution, 0.5 g/kg (30 g for adults) infused over 30 min.	60–120 min
Levodopa	0.5 g/1.73 m² PO; GH responses are often improved by administering priming doses (0.25 g/1.73 m² for 1 d or more before test dose).	45–120 min
Glucagon	0.03 mg/kg IM or SC (maximum of 1 mg).	120–180 min
Clonidine	4 µg/kg PO.	60–120 min
Propranolol (used to augment responses to primary stimulus)	30–40 mg (children 0.75 mg/kg) PO 30–60 min before glucagon, insulin, arginine, or exercise tests.	As with primary stimuli

*EEG, electroencephalographic; IM, intramuscularly; IV, intravenously; PO, orally; SC, subcutaneously.

to the GHRH stimulus.[601, 602] The magnitude of the GH response to GHRH in individuals with hypopituitarism is usually lower in older patients and in patients with the most marked GH deficiency,[600] and the best responses are observed in those with partial GH deficiency. GHRH testing, therefore, is not a sensitive method for diagnosing GH deficiency. If GH deficiency is severe, the GH response will be absent or attenuated, but it may not be possible on a single test to distinguish pituitary disease from hypothalamic disease[639] because in patients with hypothalamic disease priming of the pituitary somatotrope with multiple doses of GHRH may be required. If the GH deficiency is milder, a GH-secretory response will be elicited.

Sensitive immunoassays that measure urinary GH have been developed, and they should reflect integrated GH secretion during the period of urine collection.[640–642] Although urinary GH excretion is low in GH-deficient patients, the ability of urinary GH to discriminate patients with milder GH deficiency from short children who do not have GH deficiency is not proved.

The diagnosis of hypopituitarism is on firmer footing if deficiencies of other hormones can be demonstrated. These may include low serum thyroxine level, low serum cortisol level, impaired cortisol response to hypoglycemia and ACTH, and impaired serum 11-desoxycortisol or urinary steroid responses to administration of metyrapone. Our protocol for evaluation of patients with suspected pituitary dwarfism is outlined in Table 21–15. Serum gonadotropin and thyrotropin levels are low in both normal children and those with hypopituitarism; this measurement, therefore, is usually not helpful. It needs to be determined whether the newer, more sensitive thyrotropin assays will be useful in this regard. Measurement of thyrotropin and gonadotropin levels is useful, however, if the patient has primary hypothyroidism or gonadal dysgenesis.

Treatment of Hypopituitarism. The focus of treatment of hypopituitarism is to promote normal growth rates by administration of GH. In the years before recombinant DNA–derived GH became available when only pituitary-derived GH was used, decisions about whom to treat and what dose to give were governed by the supply of hormone (see Fig. 21–37). With the usual dose of 0.05 mg (0.1U)/kg body weight three times weekly, the growth rates of GH-deficient children increased from a pretreatment rate of 3.5 to 4.0 cm/y before treatment to 8 to 10 cm/y during the first 12 mo of therapy.[643–645] The rate of growth in response to therapy decreases with time. Because the growth response is a function of the log-dose given,[646] treatment with recombinant GH at a dosage of 0.05 mg/kg/d produces slightly more rapid growth and no increase in the occurrence of side effects. The growth response is improved further by daily therapy. Intramuscular injection and subcutaneous injection are equally effective. Young children respond better than adolescents; the obese respond better than the thin; and severely GH-deficient children respond better than those with partial deficiencies. The price of GH at the time of this writing is approximately $40/mg, making the cost of treating a 30-kg child with 0.05 mg/kg/d more than $20,000/y. These costs may be mitigated in part by third-party payers and by grants of hormone from the suppliers to needy patients. Long-term treatment with recombinant GH is remarkably free from undesirable side effects. Nevertheless, concerns persist that GH treatment may precipitate the emergence of an occult tumor or other serious disease. An excess incidence of leukemia in GH-treated patients has been reported in Japan, but the experience worldwide has failed to confirm this association.[647]

When the growth response to GH is inadequate or decreases unexpectedly, several considerations are appropriate: (1) the original diagnosis should be reconsidered; (2) GH may be being administered improperly; (3) hypothyroidism may develop in patients receiving GH and attenuate growth; (4) intercurrent illness may tip the metabolic balance toward catabolism and attenuate the response to therapy; and (5) rarely, the formation of antibodies is associated with attenuation of responses. With the recombinant GH preparations currently in use, less than 20% of patients develop antibodies after prolonged use, and growth attenuation caused by antibodies is rare. A small number (probably <10%) of patients receiving GH develop clinical or chemical hypothyroidism during treatment.[648] The mechanism is unknown, but the hypothyroid state may attenuate the response to GH. Modest doses of levothyroxine (2 to 3 µg/kg) should be administered in conjunction with GH when the pretreatment serum thyroxine level is low or if thyroxine levels decrease during GH treatment.

Symptoms of adrenal insufficiency are uncommon in children with hypopituitarism, and we do not prescribe glucocorticoids in the absence of documented evidence of adrenal insufficiency (also see Chapter 9). When indicated, glucocorticoids should be given with caution (usually less than 10 mg/m² body surface area/d) because excessive doses may attenuate the growth response to GH. However, pharmacological doses of glucocorticoids may be necessary during periods of stress.

Diabetes insipidus is uncommon in patients with idiopathic hypopituitarism but does occur after pituitary surgery. It is most effectively treated by intranasal administration of desmopressin (DDAVP) (see Chapter 10).

Some boys with early-onset hypopituitarism have micropenis (<3 cm long when stretched), which should be treated early in life. We administer 50 mg of testosterone enanthate intramuscularly and evaluate the response 1 mo later. If penile growth is not satisfactory, the treatment can be repeated two or three times.

It is nearly impossible before puberty to predict which children with hypopituitarism will undergo sexual maturation. If needed, replacement therapy with androgens in boys produces a gratifying improvement in growth response to GH. We prefer testosterone enanthate, initially at 50 mg/mo intramuscularly. Over several years this dosage is gradually increased to doses as high as 300 mg every 2 to 3 wk. Despite this treatment, growth of sexual hair and beard is often suboptimal. Enlargment of the testes during therapy is taken

TABLE 21–15. A Scheme for Evaluation of Pituitary Function in Children Suspected of Having Hypopituitarism*

Test	Purpose
Skull x-ray films	Measurement of sella turcica volume; detection of intrasellar or suprasellar mass
Oral clonidine and L-arginine infusion	GH secretion (see Table 21–14)
Plasma IGF I by radioimmunoassay	GH-secretory status
Serum thyroxine	Detection of chemical hypothyroidism
Thyrotropin response to intravenous thyrotropin-releasing hormone	Localization of lesion (hypothalamic vs. pituitary)
Basal AM serum cortisol and cortisol level 45 min after administration of 0.25 mg synthetic 1,24-ACTH (cosyntropin)	Assessment of basal adrenal function Previous exposure of adrenal to endogenous ACTH (indicated by response to ACTH)
Serum 11-desoxycortisol response to metyrapone (300 mg/m² every 4 h for six doses)	Test of integrity of hypothalamic-pituitary-adrenal axis

*These tests can be completed in 24 h and can be performed on nonhospitalized patients. GH provocative tests may be performed in tandem after an overnight fast. The thyrotropin responses to thyrotropin-releasing hormone and the cortisol response to ACTH may be determined concurrently. Metyrapone testing is begun immediately on conclusion of GH testing, and a final blood sample for 11-desoxycortisol is drawn 24 h later.

as evidence of endogenous gonadotropin secretion, and testosterone therapy is discontinued. In girls, estrogen therapy may be required, and this can be accomplished with conjugated estrogens or ethinyl estradiol. After 9 to 12 mo of continuous estrogen therapy, cycling with estrogen and progestogen is advisable.

Delays in emotional development are common in GH-deficient children, particularly those who are short from an early age.[649] This delay results in part from low expectations on the part of those who come into contact with these children. As a result, affected children are immature and underachievers[650, 651] and have less than optimal adjustment in adulthood. Expectations of the patient and parents for growth when GH is given are almost always not reasonable. This frequently causes disappointment and depression after treatment has been in progress for several months to a few years. Counseling on a continuing basis is essential.

In one study of idiopathic GH deficiency,[652] only 50% of boys and 15% of girls treated for a long period with pituitary-derived GH achieved adult heights above the third percentile. Final height correlated best with midparent height and height at the start of treatment. The smaller the child at the beginning of therapy, the greater the ultimate height deficit and the poorer the prognosis. Patients with multiple pituitary hormone deficiencies achieve greater adult height than those with isolated GH deficiency. The best solution to insufficient growth with prolonged GH therapy is early diagnosis and treatment before significant growth delay occurs. Because recombinant GH is available and larger doses can be given, many patients reach percentile growth channels that are appropriate for midparent height (Figs. 21–39 and 21–40).

Constitutional Growth Delay. Many children are small for age because they mature slowly. The syndrome of growth

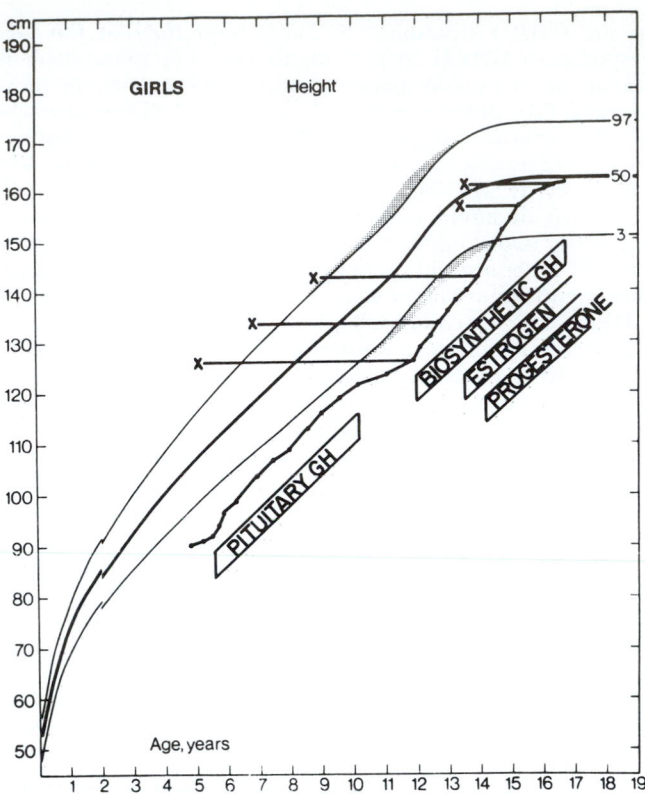

Figure 21–40. Growth curve of a GH-deficient girl who had prolonged treatment with GH. Note the impressive growth response at the time of the pubertal growth spurt. The Xs connected to horizontal lines indicate bone ages at corresponding chronological ages.

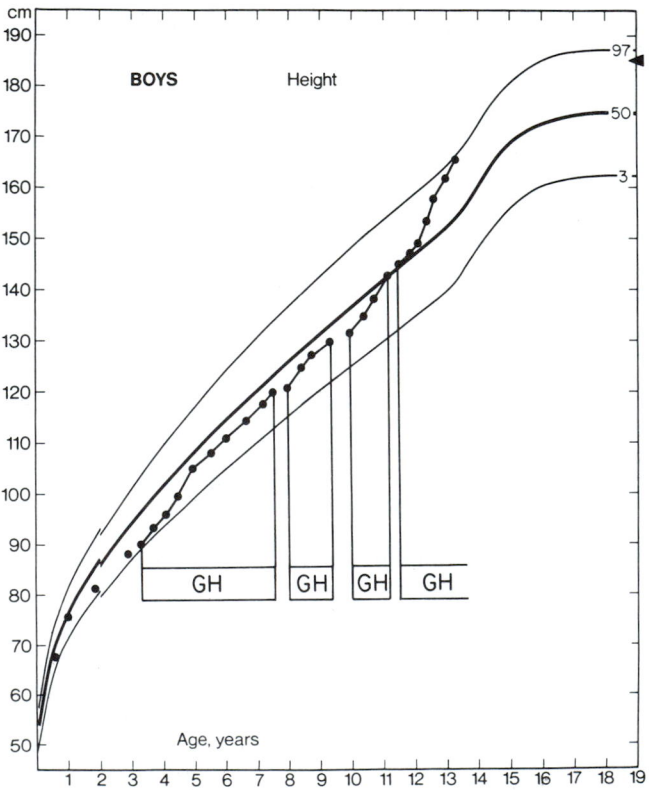

Figure 21–39. Growth curve of a GH-deficient boy treated with GH from an early age. The midparent target height, indicated by the arrowhead on the right, is above the 90th percentile. This curve illustrates the success achievable with early diagnosis and aggressive GH therapy.

retardation with delayed puberty, referred to as *constitutional growth delay,* accounts for a high proportion of referrals for growth evaluation, particularly in boys.[653, 654] These children commonly have slow growth in the first 4 to 5 y of life so that height falls below the third percentile. Subsequently, normal growth is resumed, and the curve parallels the third percentile (Fig. 21–41). Height and bone age are usually delayed by 2 to 4 y, and the onset of pubertal development is delayed by 2 y or more. Delay in growth and in pubertal development may have occurred in the father and other male relatives. Final adult stature, which may not be reached until age 20 or more, is often in the low-normal range, and sexual development and fertility are normal. There may also be a family history of relatively short stature, the combination producing enough impairment of growth to bring the patient to medical attention. The diagnosis of constitutional growth delay should be made only after the exclusion of other causes of delayed growth and puberty.

Most observers regard this syndrome as a normal growth variant. Although we agree, we believe that constitutional growth delay encompasses a spectrum of varying clinical severity ranging from the child with normal pituitary function and minimal delay in growth and pubertal development to the child whom many would identify with hypopituitarism. The gradation between these extremes, both in clinical severity and in GH responses, does not appear to have a bimodal distribution. Most of these boys experience acceleration of growth after administration of GH or androgens and continue to grow and develop sexually when therapy is withdrawn. Transient, functional hypopituitarism of this type (we use the term *lazy pituitary*) has been described by others.[100, 655] Gourmelen and associates[656] reported that as many as 20% of adolescent children with growth and pubertal delay had sluggish GH responses to provocative stimuli. When tested after the onset of puberty, however, almost all had normal GH secretion. Likewise, GH responses 48 h after exposure to exogenous androgens were also normal. Other authors have reported that patients with constitutional growth delay may secrete GH normally in response to pharmacological stimuli but have impaired spontaneous GH secretion.[657] For these various reasons, it is not surprising that patients with constitutional growth delay experience an accelerated growth rate with human GH therapy.[658, 659]

Slow-growing boys with delayed puberty often have feelings of physical and social inadequacy, and these psychological factors may affect decisions regarding therapy. For boys with modest growth failure and evidence of early testicular enlargement (>2.5 cm in length; >3 mL in volume), reassurance that they will mature normally is usually sufficient. For boys with more pronounced growth delay, a detailed search for causes of growth failure and a thorough assessment of pituitary function are warranted. If no abnormality is found, administration of androgens (50 to 100 mg of testosterone enanthate intramuscularly every month) may be indicated for psychological reasons. Treatment should be discontinued when the patient shows signs of testicular enlargement, which is an indication of endogenous gonadotropin secretion.

Therapy with GH in Short Children Who Are Presumed Not to Have GH Deficiency. The ability to produce unlimited amounts of GH by recombinant DNA methods has made it possible to pose the question as to whether short children who do not have GH deficiency should be treated. GH deficiency is not a prerequisite for response to GH therapy, and some children who are clearly not GH deficient grow when treated. Based on serum GH responses among short children, we believe a continuum exists between complete GH deficiency on the one hand and normal GH secretion on the other. When GH was scarce, children with serum GH values below 7 to 8 μg/L after provocative stimuli were considered to be candidates for treatment and those with values above this arbitrary cutoff were not. Such criteria fail to define who will benefit from GH therapy.

GH therapy of short normal children or those with constitutional growth delay does accelerate growth.[658–662] Indeed, a significant percentage (50% or more) of such children have acceleration of linear growth (>2 cm/y) over pretreatment growth rates with doses of exogenous GH that are no more than twice the average normal production rates. For the most part these studies have been carried out for only a year or so, and long-term benefits and effects on adult stature have not been determined.

Despite insufficient knowledge about the treatment of short stature with GH, parental and societal pressures to help short children are strong. Our society values tallness and places short individuals at a relative social and economic disadvantage. Body size correlates with self-concept, large size being associated with positive self-concept and small size being associated with negative self-image. The physician occupies the difficult position between societal pressures to relieve each child of the disadvantage of being short and the lack of insight into whether GH will accomplish this objective and whether there will be adverse side effects if GH is used.

We believe that the place of GH therapy for short stature cannot be defined until several questions are resolved. Until that time, GH should be prescribed in an ethical manner based on two considerations:[663] (1) comprehensive knowledge by the physician of all the issues related to treatment with GH and (2) extensive education and counseling about GH therapy for the patient and the family so that they can participate fully in decisions regarding treatment. The physician recommending and directing treatment should

1. Have in-depth knowledge of the processes of growth and development. We believe that it is inappropriate for physicians to prescribe GH for short stature unless they are thoroughly versed in the processes of growth and development.

2. Determine whether the patient is short compared with ancestors. Patients whose size is appropriate for their normal, relatively short ancestors may benefit more from counseling than from GH therapy.

3. Establish that the patient is growing slowly by collecting growth data for a sufficient length of time for a reliable baseline. Without such information, assessment of growth response is impossible, and decisions about continuing therapy are difficult.

4. Ensure that sufficient effort has been expended to exclude forms of growth failure that require specific treatments other than GH.

5. Define the needs of the patient by determining whether the child is under stress because of short stature.

6. Be certain that the family has realistic expectations about the possible responses to therapy and understands that years of therapy will be required.

7. Be certain that the family understands that treatment with GH may fail to accelerate growth and that a lack of response may have a negative psychological effect on the patient.

8. Ensure that the family knows that there is no good evidence that GH will make the patient a taller adult even when short-term acceleration of growth is achieved.

9. Set the goals of therapy by having the family define

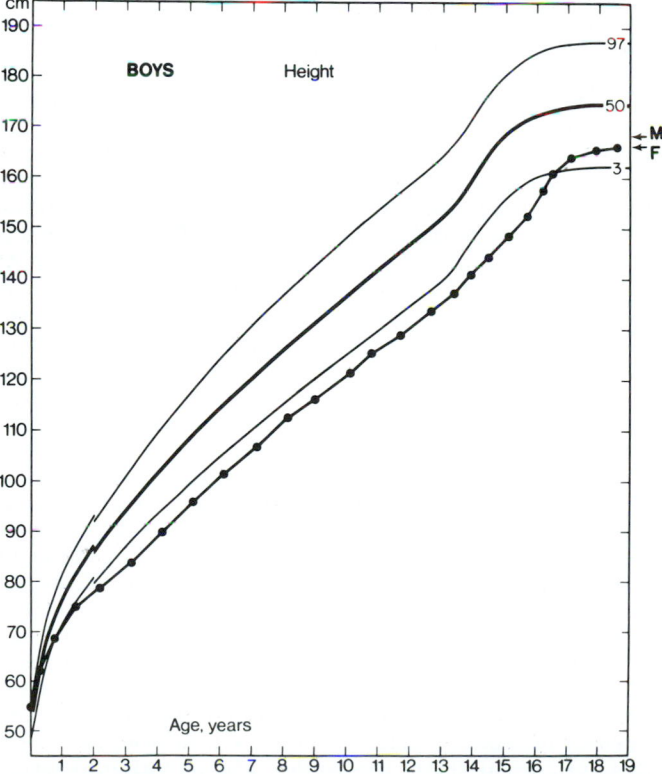

Figure 21–41. Growth curve of a typical boy with constitutional delay of growth and puberty. The curve illustrates the lag in growth in the first few years of life, maintenance of the position parallel to but below the 3rd percentile during most of childhood, and the late pubertal growth spurt allowing the patient to close the height gap between himself and his peers. M and F at the right indicate the mother's height (adjusted for sex) and the father's height, respectively.

how short-term acceleration of growth would benefit the patient socially and psychologically.

10. Ensure that the family is united in its commitment to therapy.

11. Develop an agreement with the family before therapy is begun as to the growth rate that will be acceptable during treatment and how decisions about continuing treatment will be made.

12. Ensure that the family is aware of the known physical and psychological risks of GH therapy and that there may be risks that are not known currently.

13. Ensure that psychological support and counseling are integral components of therapy, that the growth response and side effects are monitored regularly, and that post-treatment follow-up is accomplished.

THYROID HORMONE DEFICIENCY. Growth arrest is perhaps the most constant feature of primary hypothyroidism in infants and children. In newborns the disease should be suspected on the basis of poor feeding, unexplained attacks of choking and cyanosis, lethargy, hoarse cry, cutaneous vasomotor instability, and prolonged jaundice. In the past the diagnosis was frequently not made until full-blown signs emerged several weeks or months after birth. Fortunately, this delay has been largely eradicated by the measurement of blood thyroxine level in neonatal screening programs. Such programs are highly successful in preventing the mental retardation and other neurological sequelae that result from prolonged hypothyroidism during early infancy.[664–666]

In older children, acquired hypothyroidism is usually the result of Hashimoto thyroiditis or decompensation of an ectopic, dysgenetic thyroid gland. In these children the clinical signs and symptoms may be so subtle that hypothyroidism is not suspected (Fig. 21–42) for a prolonged period. In retrospective studies of growth records in our clinic, the average duration of acquired hypothyroidism before diagnosis was about 4 y. Inspection of serial photographs and previous growth records of these patients often reveals that growth failure preceded the appearance of other signs of myxedema (Fig. 21–43).

Diagnosis is made by showing that the serum thyroxine level is low and the thyrotropin level is elevated. Skeletal maturation is markedly delayed. In individuals with congenital hypothyroidism, the diagnosis of athyreosis or thyroid dysgenesis should be confirmed by technetium or radioiodide scanning. In older children in whom no thyroid can be palpated, scanning for an ectopic gland is indicated. When a gland is palpable, thyroid antibodies should be measured to determine whether Hashimoto thyroiditis is the cause. Also, genetic disorders of thyroid hormone biosynthesis should be considered.

Treatment of hypothyroidism is simple and inexpensive, and the results are gratifying. Levothyroxine dosages of 5 to 8 µg/kg body weight in the first year of life and 2 to 3 µg/kg body weight in late childhood[667] are usually sufficient. Adequacy of treatment can be judged from the growth curve, return of the serum thyrotropin level to normal, and the serum thyroxine concentration. Thyrotropin levels may not return to normal for several months in infants with congenital hypothyroidism, despite the fact that thyroid hormone replacement is adequate. In the first year or so of treatment, patients with prolonged growth arrest undergo catch-up growth, returning toward the growth channel they occupied before the onset of the disease (see Fig. 21–42). With treatment, all of the lost growth is not recovered,[668] the deficit in adulthood being related to the duration of the hypothyroidism before treatment. Excessive doses of levothyroxine should be avoided because they stimulate the disproportionate advancement of skeletal age and in infants premature closure of cranial sutures.

GLUCOCORTICOID EXCESS. Whether related to cortisol-secreting adrenal tumors, hypersecretion of ACTH, or therapy, glucocorticoid excess uniformly causes growth attenuation.[669] Cortisol-secreting adrenal tumors rarely may be associated with accelerated growth when androgens are the predominant secretory product of the tumor. Other signs of glucocorticoid excess include thinning of the skin, vascular fragility, osteoporosis, diminished muscle mass, weakness, obesity, glucose intolerance, and occasionally electrolyte disturbances. Truncal obesity in children may be less prominent than that in adults, and some children with Cushing disease show few signs of glucocorticoid excess other than growth failure.[92, 670] From data obtained in patients receiving exogenous glucocorticoids, it appears that two to three times (40 to 50 mg/m² of hydrocortisone) the normal daily production rate is sufficient to inhibit growth.[87, 88] Synthetic glucocorticoids are more likely to inhibit growth,[671] perhaps because the dosages tend to be excessive and because their metabolic clearance is slower than that of cortisol, thereby resulting in more prolonged exposure to the drug.

Glucocorticoid excess inhibits growth at the level of growing tissues because GH secretion is usually normal in affected children,[92] serum IGF I concentrations are normal, and treatment with GH or androgens does not reverse the effect of glucocorticoids.[672] Although most children with Cushing syndrome experience some degree of catch-up growth with treatment of their condition, the duration and intensity of growth acceleration may be insufficient to return them to normal height percentiles. The important determinants of catch-up growth appear to be the duration and intensity of the glucocorticoid exposure and the age of the patient at the time of exposure.[673] In this regard, glucocorticoid excess near puberty can have disastrous consequences.

The diagnosis of Cushing syndrome is often suspected

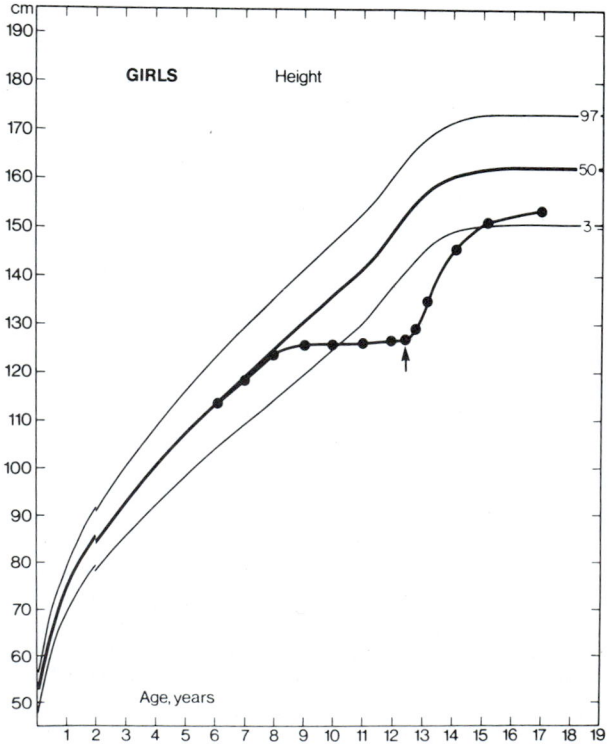

Figure 21–42. Growth chart of a girl with primary hypothyroidism diagnosed at age 12½ (arrow). Profound growth arrest began at age 8 to 9, and catch-up growth after levothyroxine replacement occurred over a 3- to 4-y period.

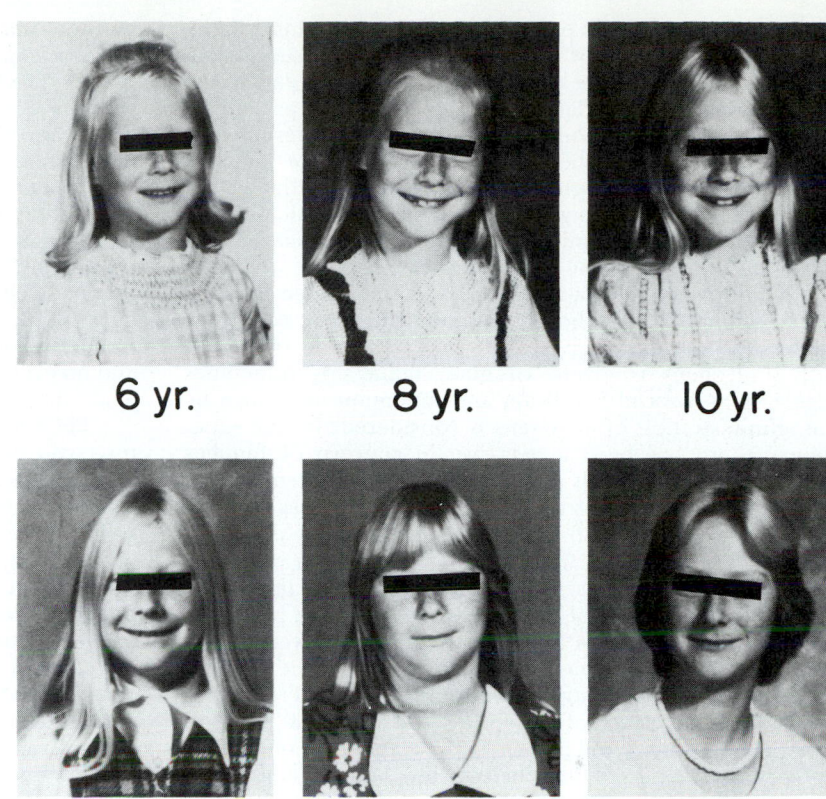

6 yr.   8 yr.   10 yr.

11 yr.   12 yr.   14 yr.

Figure 21–43. Serial photographs of a girl with primary hypothyroidism (growth curve shown in Fig. 21–42). Facial changes of hypothyroidism are apparent in photograph made at age 10. Goiter is present at age 12. Patient had been treated with replacement doses of levothyroxine for 1½ y at the time of the last photograph.

in children and adolescents with obesity, particularly if striae and glucose intolerance are present. Patients with exogenous obesity frequently exhibit accelerated linear growth, making costly laboratory tests unnecessary. In those cases in which the diagnosis remains uncertain, the diagnositic procedures described in Chapter 9 should be followed, with the dosages of dexamethasone and metyrapone reduced in proportion to the surface area of the child.[674]

Growth arrest secondary to administration of supraphysiological quantities of glucocorticoids can be reduced, along with other side effects, by giving single large doses of medication on alternate days;[675] this mode of administering glucocorticoids should be tried in all patients, provided the goals of therapy can be accomplished at the same time.

TALL STATURE

There are just as many children with stature greater than 2 SD above the mean as children with short stature. There are fewer pathological causes of excessive height, however, and concern over this problem is less frequent (Table 21–16). Because normal children now grow faster and reach greater adult stature than in the past, it is more difficult to segregate individuals with pathological tall stature from those whose tallness reflects optimal growth resulting from excellent health and nutrition. The most useful signs of overgrowth from pathological causes are the crossing of percentile channels upward on the growth chart and the association with abnormalities such as signs of virilization and abnormal body proportions.

FAMILIAL TALL STATURE. Most cases of suspected overgrowth represent variants of the normal growth pattern and reflect the more complete realization of genetic potential. These cases have been variously referred to as *constitutional*

or *familial tall stature*. In deciding whether tall stature is due to hereditary factors, it may be helpful to plot the height and, if possible, the entire growth record of the child's parents. Tall children whose parents are not tall should be

TABLE 21–16. Causes of Statural Overgrowth

Cause	Characteristics
Prenatal Onset	
Maternal diabetes mellitus	Cushingoid appearance with increased birth weight and length, neonatal hypoglycemia and hypocalcemia, respiratory distress, and jaundice
Beckwith-Wiedemann syndrome	See text
Cerebral gigantism	See text
Postnatal Onset	
Exogenous obesity	Accelerated linear growth accompanying rapid weight gain
Pituitary GH excess	See text
Marfan syndrome	See text
Sexual precocity and virilizing syndromes	See text
McCune-Albright syndrome	Associated GH excess related to pituitary tumor
Homocystinuria	Phenotypic characteristics of Marfan syndrome, mental retardation, excessive homocystine in urine, thromboembolic disease
Total lipodystrophy	Absence of adipose tissue, muscular hypertrophy, enlarged genitalia, diabetes mellitus, enlarged liver, hyperlipidemia; may be associated with acanthosis nigricans and increased GH secretion
Klinefelter syndrome (47,XXY)	Eunuchoid proportions both before and after puberty, small testes, gynecomastia
XYY karyotype	Elevated testosterone level in adult; sometimes impaired intellect and deviant behavior; hairy ears and varicose veins
Hyperthyroidism	Modest acceleration of growth

suspected of having a pathological disorder. Most of the gain in linear growth of normal tall children occurs in the first 4 y of life.[676] If the child is between ages 2 and 9, the child's height can be related to the height of the parents by using the charts of Tanner and associates.[490] Alternatively, the same insight can be gained by relating the patient's height to midparent height, as described earlier in the section on predicting adult height. In children with tall parents, diagnostic studies are unnecessary after it is established that the rate of growth is not accelerated.

Therapy for tall stature of boys in the United States is rarely requested or indicated, although in some countries, tallness in boys is not given the same value, and treatment with androgens is given. In girls, tallness is sometimes regarded as a social handicap, and limitation of growth by the administration of estrogens is considered. In our experience, there has been a decrease in concern of families about tall stature in girls and a reduction in the demand for treatment to attenuate growth. In the United States an adult height in women of 183 cm (72 inches) is widely accepted, and we have refrained from treating girls with a predicted adult height below this value. Before estrogen therapy is prescribed, it is essential that the adult height be predicted as accurately as possible and that the adverse psychological effects of excessive tallness be weighed against the possible harmful effects of estrogen administration. Treatment, which has the effect of hastening the onset of puberty, should be instituted well before the first signs of spontaneous puberty are expected and before the bone age is 12 y. Ethinyl estradiol in doses of 0.15 to 0.30 mg/d causes reductions from predicted adult heights of 4.9 to 5.8 cm in girls whose skeletal ages are 10.5 to 13.0 y at the beginning of therapy. Reductions of 1.8 to 3.6 cm can be anticipated in girls with skeletal ages of 14.0 to 15.5 y at the beginning of therapy.[109, 110, 677] The successful use of ethinyl estradiol at a dose of only 0.1 mg/d has also been reported.[111] Larger doses of estrogens (0.3 to 0.5 mg ethinyl estradiol/kg body weight; 7.5 to 10 mg of conjugated estrogen) are reasonably well tolerated and have been used in older girls to produce an abrupt attenuation (sometimes cessation) of growth. This effect of estrogens is likely to be mediated through the inhibition of IGF I synthesis.[678] When estrogen treatment is stopped, growth resumes unless the epiphyses are fused. Girls treated with estrogens may experience nausea, excessive weight gain, and, unless cyclic progestogens are added, breakthrough bleeding. In view of the long-term potential for adverse effects of estrogen administration, therapy should be undertaken only in extreme cases and after all known and potential side effects have been considered.[678]

PITUITARY GH EXCESS. Various aspects of excessive GH secretion are reviewed in Chapter 6. GH hypersecretion in children is usually associated with eosinophilic or chromophobe adenomas of the pituitary. This disease is characterized by rapid linear growth, overgrowth of soft tissues, and metabolic changes similar to those in acromegalic adults. The physical features of GH excess, such as enlargement of the lower jaw and thickening of the hands and feet, usually remain subtle until the disease is of long duration. If the tumor compresses normal pituitary tissues, thyrotropin, ACTH, and gonadotropin deficiency may be present. Diagnosis can be confirmed by showing that plasma IGF I and GH values are elevated and that GH is not suppressed after glucose loading (1.75 g glucose/kg body weight, up to a dose of 100 g). Abnormalities of the pituitary fossa are usually apparent on computed tomographic or magnetic resonance imaging scans. In children with pituitary gigantism, as in adults with acromegaly, the therapeutic challenge is to eradicate GH excess while preserving the remainder of pituitary function. In our experience, this goal is best accomplished by transsphenoidal pituitary adenectomy at the hands of a surgeon experienced with this technique.

CEREBRAL GIGANTISM (SOTOS SYNDROME). Children with this syndrome are usually above the 90th percentile for length and weight at birth and continue to grow rapidly for the first few years of life. After this, some decelerate in growth but remain parallel to the 97th percentile. Skeletal maturation is accelerated, and puberty occurs early.[679–681] Children with this syndrome have a large elongated head, prominent forehead, large ears and jaw, unusual slant to the eyes, elongated chin, and coarse facial features. Most have subnormal intelligence and impaired coordination. Endocrinologically, these children have normal GH secretion and no evidence of thyroid, adrenal, or gonadal dysfunction. The cause is not known.

BECKWITH-WIEDEMANN SYNDROME. Newborns with this syndrome exhibit marked macrosomia, macroglossia, omphalocele, and hypoglycemia. The hypoglycemia, which is often accompanied by islet cell hyperplasia and hyperinsulinism, usually disappears during infancy. Accelerated growth, however, continues. Skeletal maturation is also advanced, and individuals exhibit a tendency toward formation of tumors later in life.[682, 683] The mechanism of overgrowth in these patients in unclear, but hyperinsulinism may play a role. Serum concentrations of IGF I and IGF II are normal.

MARFAN SYNDROME. Patients with Marfan syndrome are usually above average in height but not outside the normal range. They exhibit long limbs with narrow hands and long, slender fingers (arachnodactyly). The arm span is greater than height, and the lower segment of the body is longer than the upper segment. Hyperextensible joints, kyphoscoliosis, rib cage deformities, and dislocation of the lens may be present. Death from dissecting aortic aneurysm can occur in early adult life.

SEXUAL PRECOCITY AND VIRILIZING DISORDERS. These conditions are the most common endocrine causes of statural overgrowth.[684] In affected children, acceleration of linear growth coincides with signs of premature sexual development or inappropriate virilization, regardless of whether the disorder is due to congenital adrenal hyperplasia, adrenal tumor, gonadal tumor, or the premature secretion of gonadotropic hormones. Rapid growth is accompanied by accelerated skeletal maturation so that the eventual adult stature is diminished rather than increased. If treatment of the primary disorder is successful, some patients exhibit "catch-down" growth (Fig. 21–44).

Administration of one of the luteinizing hormone–releasing hormone analogues is an effective means of suppressing pituitary gonadotropin secretion and is the treatment of choice for central precocious puberty.[685] The reader is referred to Chapter 22 for discussion of this therapy. In the context of growth, these agents reduce the accelerated growth rate and slow skeletal maturation, sometimes to below normal.

Two benign conditions that are not associated with accelerated linear growth but may be confused with sexual precocity are premature adrenarche and premature thelarche. In *premature adrenarche*, pubic hair emerges before age 7 in girls and before age 9 in boys, before there are other signs of pubertal development. Premature adrenarche is more common in girls than in boys and, in our experience, more common in black than in white girls. Sometimes it is associated with neurological defects or mental retardation. Plasma levels of adrenal androgens, such as dehydroepiandrosterone sulfate, are elevated, and urinary 17-ketosteroid levels may be high.[686–688] Height and bone age may be slightly advanced. It is important that this condition be differentiated from congenital adrenal hyperplasia and from adrenal tumors, in which there are multiple signs of androgen excess

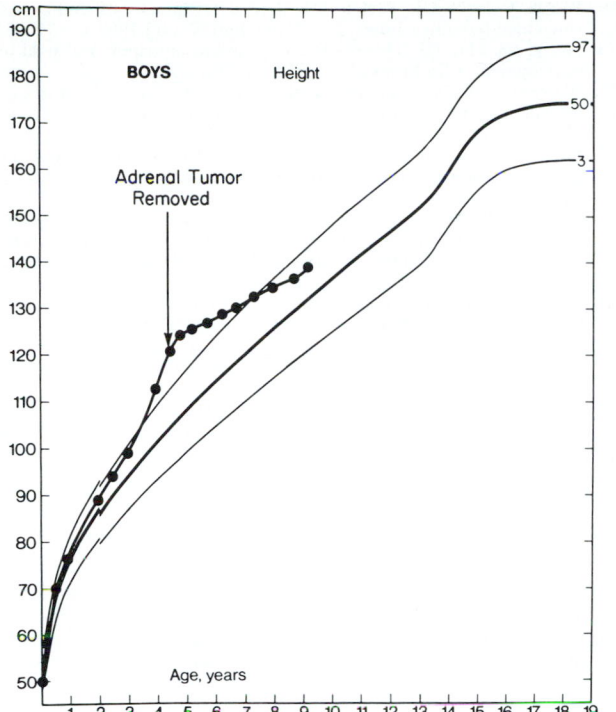

Figure 21–44. Growth curve of a boy with virilizing adrenal carcinoma. The patient had a 2-y history of progressive virilization accompanied by acceleration of linear growth. Soon after removal of the tumor, deceleration of growth occurred—so-called catch-down growth—until the height returned to the original percentile channel.

including accelerated linear growth, increased muscle mass, clitoral enlargement in girls, and deepening of the voice.

Premature thelarche, or benign infantile mammoplasia, is frequent in girls, particularly between the first and third years of life. It is characterized by enlargement of the breasts before age 8 without other signs of estrogenic effect. There is no associated pubic hair, and linear growth is not accelerated. Examination of the urinary sediment may reveal a slight degree of epithelial cornification; however, serum luteinizing hormone and estradiol levels are not consistently elevated, and the serum luteinizing hormone response to luteinizing hormone–releasing hormone is prepubertal in pattern.[689] This benign condition occurs predominantly in well-nourished girls. The only requirement for management is reassurance after the growth rate has been established to be normal and the presence of an ovarian tumor has been excluded by careful physical examination.

REFERENCES

General Reading

1. Falkner F, Tanner JM, eds. Human Growth: A Comprehensive Treatise. Vol 1. Developmental Biology, Prenatal Growth. 2nd ed. Vol 2. Postnatal Growth, Neurobiology. 2nd ed. New York: Plenum, 1986.
2. Falkner F, Tanner JM, eds. Human Growth: A Comprehensive Treatise. Vol 3. Methodology. Ecological, Genetic and Nutritional Effects on Growth. 2nd ed. New York: Plenum, 1986.
3. Tanner JM. Fetus into Man. Cambridge: Harvard University Press, 1978.
4. Marshall WA. Human Growth and Its Disorders. New York: Academic, 1977.
5. Smith DW. Growth and Its Disorders. Philadelphia: W. B. Saunders, 1977.
6. Tanner JM. Normal growth and techniques of growth assessment. Clin Endocrinol Metabl 1986; 15:411–451.

Normal Growth

7. Liggins GC. The drive to fetal growth. In: Beard RW, Nathanielsz PW, eds. Fetal Physiology and Medicine: The Basis of Perinatology. Philadelphia: W. B. Saunders, 1976: 254–270.
8. Hamilton WJ, Mossman HW. Human Embryology. Prenatal Developments of Form and Function. Baltimore: Williams & Wilkins, 1972.
9. Dubowitz LMS, Dubowitz V, Goldberg C. Clinical assessment of gestational age in the newborn infant. J Pediatr 1970; 77:1–10.
10. Thomson AM, Billewicz WZ, Hytten FE. The assessment of fetal growth. J Obstet Gynaecol Br Commonw 1968; 75:903–916.
11. Bulmer MG. The Biology of Twinning. Oxford: Clarendon, 1970.
12. Wilson RS. Growth and development of human twins. In: Falkner F, Tanner JM, eds. Human Growth: A Comprehensive Treatise. Vol III. Methodology. Ecological, Genetic and Nutritional Effects of Growth. New York: Plenum, 1986: 197–211.
13. Meredith HV. Body weight at birth of viable human infants: a worldwide comparative treatise. Hum Biol 1970; 42:217–264.
14. Kruger H, Arias-Stella J. The placenta and the newborn infant at high altitudes. Am J Obstet Gynecol 1970; 106:586–591.
15. Ounsted C, Ounsted M. Effect of Y chromosome on fetal growth-rate. Lancet 1970; 2:857–858.
16. Lobl M, Welcher DW, Mellits ED. Maternal age and intellectual functioning of offspring. Johns Hopkins Med J 1971; 128:347–361.
17. Tanner JM, Whitehouse RH, Takaishi M. Standards from birth to maturity for height, weight, height velocity and weight velocity, British children, 1965. Arch Dis Child 1966; 41:454–471, 613–635.
18. Tanner JM, Whitehouse RH. Clinical longitudinal standards for height, weight, height velocity, weight velocity and the stages of puberty. Arch Dis Child 1976; 51:170–179.
19. Tanner JM, Whitehouse RH. Height and weight charts from birth to 5 years allowing for length of gestation. Arch Dis Child 1973; 48:786–789.
20. Smith DW, Truog W, Rogers JE, et al. Shifting linear growth during infancy: illustration of genetic factors in growth from fetal life through infancy. J Pediatr 1976; 89:225–230.
21. Fitzhardinge PM, Steven EM. The small-for-date infant. 1. Later growth patterns. Pediatrics 1972; 49:671–681.
22. Tanner JM. Growth at Adolescence. 2nd ed. Oxford: Blackwell Scientific, 1962.
23. Prader A. Hormonal regulation of growth and the adolescent growth spurt. In: Grumbach MM, Sizonenko PC, Aubert ML, eds. Control of the Onset of Puberty. Baltimore: Williams & Wilkins, 1990: 534–546.
24. Marshall WA, Tanner JM. Variations in the pattern of pubertal changes in boys. Arch Dis Child 1970; 45:13–23.
25. Lee PA. Disorders of puberty. In: Lifshitz F, ed. Pediatric Endocrinology. New York: Marcel Dekker, 1985: 143.
26. Marshall WA, Tanner JM. Variations in the pattern of pubertal changes in girls. Arch Dis Child 1969; 44:291–303.
27. Sizonenko PC. Regulation of puberty and pubertal growth. In: Ritzen M, Aperia A, Hall K, et al., eds. The Biology of Normal Human Growth. New York: Raven, 1981: 297–308.
28. Goldstein S, Saenger P. The physiology of puberty. In: Moss AJ, ed. Pediatric Updates. New York: Elsevier Biomedical, 1984: 63–93.
29. Aynsley-Green A, Zachmann M, Prader A. Interrelation of the therapeutic effects of growth hormone and testosterone on growth in hypopituitarism. J Pediatr 1976; 89:992–999.
30. Frasier SD, Hilburn JM, Smith FG Jr. Effect of adolescence on the serum growth hormone response to hypoglycemia. J Pediatr 1970; 77:465–467.
31. Miller JD, Tannenbaum GS, Colle E, et al. Daytime pulsatile growth hormone secretion during childhood and adolescence. J Clin Endocrinol Metab 1982; 55:989–994.
32. Craft WH, Underwood LE. Effect of androgens on plasma somatomedin-C/IGF-I responses to growth hormone. Clin Endocrinol 1984; 20:549–554.
33. Hall K, Enberg G, Ritzen M, et al. Somatomedin A levels in serum from healthy children and from children with growth hormone deficiency or delayed puberty. Acta Endocrinol 1980; 94:155–165.
34. Underwood LE, Smith EP, Van Wyk JJ, et al. Somatomedin-C/IGF-I: regulation and clinical applications. In: Raiti S, Tolman RA, eds. Human Growth Hormone. New York: Plenum, 1986: 585–599.
35. Rosenfield RL, Furlanetto R, Bock D. Relationship of somatomedin-C concentration to pubertal changes. J Pediatr 1983; 103:723–728.
36. Rosenfield RL. Toward optimal estrogen-replacement therapy. N Engl J Med 1983; 309:1120–1121.
37. Greulich WW, Pyle SI. Radiographic Atlas of Skeletal Development of the Hand and Wrist. 2nd ed. Stanford, CA: Stanford University Press, 1959.
38. Tanner JM, Whitehouse RH, Marshall WA, et al. Assessment of Skeletal Maturity and Prediction of Adult Height. London: Academic, 1975.
39. Acheson RM, Fowler G, Fry EI, et al. Studies in the reliability of assessing skeletal maturity from x-rays. Hum Biol 1963; 35:317–349.
40. Roche AF, Davila GH, Eyman SL. A comparison between Greulich-Pyle and Tanner-Whitehouse assessments of skeletal maturity. Radiology 1971; 98:273–280.

41. Bayley N, Pinneau SR. Tables for predicting adult height from skeletal age: revised for use with the Greulich-Pyle hand standards. J Pediatr 1952; 40:423–441.
42. Tanner JM, Whitehouse RH, Marshall WA, et al. Prediction of adult height from height, bone age, and occurrence of menarche at ages 4–16 with allowance for midparent height. Arch Dis Child 1975; 50:14–26.
43. Roche AF, Wainer H, Thissen D. The RWT method for the prediction of adult stature. Pediatrics 1975; 56:1026–1033.
44. Brasel JA, Gruen RK. Cellular growth: brain, heart, kidney, lung, liver and skeletal muscle. In: Falkner F, Tanner JM, eds. Human Growth: A Comprehensive Treatise. Vol 2. Postnatal Growth, Neurobiology. 2nd ed. New York: Plenum, 1986: 53–65.
45. Goss RJ. Adaptive Growth. New York: Academic, 1964.
46. Goss RJ. Modes of growth and regeneration: mechanisms, regulations and distributions. In: Falkner F, Tanner JM, eds. Human Growth: A Comprehensive Treatise. Vol. 1. Developmental Biology, Prenatal Growth. 2nd ed. New York: Plenum, 1986: 3–26.
47. Goss RJ. The Physiology of Growth. New York: Academic, 1978.

Growth Hormone

48. Chawla RK, Parks JS, Rudman D. Structural variants of human growth hormone: biochemical, genetic and clinical aspects. Annu Rev Med 1983; 34:519–547.
49. Phillips JA. Genetic defects in processing growth hormone. In: Bercu B, ed. Basic and Clinical Aspects of Growth Hormone. New York: Plenum, 1988: 57–67.
50. Frankenne F, Closset J, Gomez F, et al. The physiology of growth hormones (GHs) in pregnant women and partial characterization of the placental GH variant. J Clin Endocrinol Metab 1988; 66:1171–1180.
51. Baumann G. Heterogenity of growth hormone. In: Bercu B, ed. Basic and Clinical Aspects of Growth Hormone. New York: Plenum, 1988: 13–31.
52. Lewis UJ, Singh RNP, Tutwiler GH, et al. Human growth hormone: a complex of proteins. Recent Prog Horm Res 1980; 36:477–508.
53. Salmon WD Jr, Daughaday WH. A hormonally controlled serum factor which stimulates sulfate incorporation by cartilage in vitro. J Lab Clin Med 1957; 49:825–836.
54. Rinderknecht E, Humbel RE. The amino acid sequence of human insulin-like growth factor I and its structural homology with proinsulin. J Biol Chem 1978; 253:2769–2776.
55. Klapper DG, Svoboda ME, Van Wyk JJ. Sequence analysis of somatomedin-C: confirmation of identity with insulin-like growth factor I. Endocrinology 1983; 112:2215–2217.
56. Zapf J, Froesch ER, Humbel RE. The insulin-like growth factors (IGF) of human serum: chemical and biological characterization and aspects of their possible physiological role. Curr Top Cell Regul 1981; 19:257–309.
57. Rinderknecht E, Humbel RE. Primary structure of human insulin-like growth factor II. FEBS Lett 1978; 89:283–286.
58. Schoenle E, Zapf J, Humbel RE, et al. Insulin-like growth factor I stimulates growth in hypophysectomized rats. Nature 1982; 296:252–253.
59. Schoenle E, Zapf J, Froesch ER. Insulin-like growth factors I and II stimulate growth of hypophysectomized rats. Diabetologia 1982; 23:199 (abstract).
60. Berelowitz M, Szabo M, Frohman LA, et al. Somatomedin-C mediates growth hormone negative feedback by effects on both the hypothalamus and the pituitary. Science 1981; 212:1279–1281.
61. Brazeau P, Guillemin R, Ling N, et al. Inhibition par les somatomédines de la sécrétion de l'hormone de croissance stimulée par le facteur hypothalamique somatocrinine (GRF) ou le peptide de synthèse hpGRF. C R Acad Sci [III] 1982; 295:651–654.
62. Yamashita S, Melmed S. Insulin-like growth factor I action on rat anterior pituitary cells: suppression of growth hormone secretion and messenger ribonucleic acid levels. Endocrinology 1986; 118:176–182.
63. Abe H, Molitch M, Van Wyk JJ, et al. Human growth hormone and somatomedin-C suppress the spontaneous release of growth hormone in unanesthetized rats. Endocrinology 1983; 113:1319–1324.
64. Nilsson A, Carlsson B, Isgaard J, et al. Regulation by GH of insulin-like growth factor I mRNA expression in rat epiphyseal growth plate as studied with in-situ hybridization. J Endocrinol 1990; 125:67–74.
65. Isaksson OG, Lindahl A, Nilsson A, et al. Mechanism of the stimulatory effect of growth hormone on longitudinal bone growth. Endocr Rev 1987; 8:426–438.
66. Green H, Morikawa M, Nixon T. A dual effector theory of growth hormone action. Differentiation 1985; 29:195–198.
67. Van Wyk JJ. The somatomedins: biological actions and physiologic control mechanisms. In: Li CH, ed. Hormonal Proteins and Peptides. Vol 12. New York: Academic, 1984: 81–125.

Thyroid Hormone

68. Alm J, Larsson A, Zetterstrom R. Congenital hypothyroidism in Sweden: psychomotor development in patients detected by clinical signs and symptoms. Acta Paediatr Scand 1981; 70:907–912.

69. Birrell J, Frost GJ, Parkin JM. The development of children with congenital hypothyroidism. Dev Med Child Neurol 1983; 25:512–519.
70. Hetzel BS, Hay ID. Thyroid function, iodine nutrition and fetal brain development. Clin Endocrinol 1979; 11:445–460.
71. Walker PA, Weichsel ME Jr, Fisher DA, et al. Thyroxine increases nerve growth factor concentration in adult mouse brain. Science 1979; 204:427–429.
72. Walker P, Weil ML, Weichsel ME Jr, et al. Effect of thyroxine on nerve growth factor concentration in neonatal mouse brain. Life Sci 1981; 28:1777–1787.
73. Froesch ER, Zapf J, Audhya TK, et al. Nonsuppressible insulin-like activity and thyroid hormones: major pituitary-dependent sulfation factors for chick embryo cartilage. Proc Natl Acad Sci USA 1976; 73:2904–2908.
74. Mosier HD Jr. Thyroid hormone. In: Daughaday WH, ed. Endocrine Control of Growth. New York: Elsevier, 1981: 25–66.
75. Burch WM, Van Wyk JJ. Triiodothyronine stimulates cartilage growth and maturation by different mechanisms. Am J Physiol 1987; 252:E176–E182.
76. Chernausek SD, Underwood LE, Utiger RD, et al. Growth hormone secretion and plasma somatomedin-C in hypothyroidism. Clin Endocrinol 1983; 19:337–344.

Insulin

77. Underwood LE, D'Ercole AJ. Insulin and insulin-like growth factors/somatomedins in fetal and neonatal development. Clin Endocrinol Metab 1984; 13:69–89.
78. Hill DJ, Milner RDG. Insulin as a growth factor. Pediatr Res 1985; 19:879–886.
79. D'Ercole AJ, Underwood LE, Groelke J, et al. Leprechaunism: studies of the relationship among hyperinsulinism, insulin resistance, and growth retardation. J Clin Endocrinol Metab 1979; 48:495–502.
80. Hill DE. The effect of insulin on fetal growth. Semin Perinatol 1978; 2:319–328.
81. Hill DJ, Milner RDG. Increased somatomedin and cartilage metabolic activity in rabbit fetuses injected with insulin in utero. Diabetologia 1980; 19:143–147.
82. Spencer GS, Hill DJ, Garssen GJ, et al. Somatomedin activity and growth hormone levels in body fluids of the fetal pig: effect of chronic hyperinsulinemia. J Endocrinol 1983; 96:107–114.
83. Phillips LS, Unterman TG. Somatomedin activity in disorders of nutrition and metabolism. Clin Endocrinol Metab 1984; 13:145–189.
84. Costin G, Kogut MD, Phillips LS, et al. Craniopharyngioma: the role of insulin in promoting postoperative growth. J Clin Endocrinol Metab 1976; 42:370–379.
85. Hollenberg MD, Cuatrecasas P. Insulin: interaction with membrane receptors and relationship to cyclic purine nucleotides and cell growth. Fed Proc 1975; 34:1556–1563.
86. Griffiths JB. Role of serum, insulin and amino acid concentration in contact inhibition of growth of human cells in culture. Exp Cell Res 1972; 75:47–56.

Glucocorticoids

87. Blodgett FM, Burgin L, Iezzoni D, et al. Effects of prolonged cortisone therapy on the statural growth, skeletal maturation and metabolic status of children. N Engl J Med 1956; 254:636–641.
88. Falliers CJ, Tan LS, Szentivanyi J, et al. Childhood asthma and steroid therapy as influences on growth. Am J Dis Child 1963; 105:127–137.
89. Widemann E. Adrenal and gonadal steroids. In: Daughaday WH, ed. Endocrine Control of Growth. New York: Elsevier, 1981: 67–119.
90. Morris HG, Jorgensen JR, Jenkins SA. Plasma growth hormone concentrations in corticosteroid-treated children. J Clin Invest 1968; 47:427–435.
91. Strickland AL, Underwood LE, Voina SJ, et al. Growth retardation in Cushing's syndrome. Am J Dis Child 1972; 123:207–213.
92. Solomon IL, Schoen EJ. Juvenile Cushing syndrome manifested primarily by growth failure. Am J Dis Child 1976; 130:200–202.
93. Matiasevic D, Gershberg H. Studies on hydroxyproline excretion and corticosteriod-induced dwarfism: treatment with human growth hormone. Metabolism 1966; 15:720–729.
94. Elders JM, Wingfield BS, McNatt ML, et al. Somatomedin and the regulation of skeletal growth. Ann Clin Lab Sci 1975; 5:440–451.
95. Mosier HD Jr, Jansons RA, Hill RR, et al. Cartilage sulfation and serum somatomedin in rats during and after cortisone-induced growth arrest. Endocrinology 1976; 99:580–589.

Androgens

96. Simpson ME, Marx W, Becks H, et al. Effect of testosterone propionate on the body weight and skeletal system of hypophysectomized rats. Synergism with pituitary growth hormone. Endocrinology 1944; 35:309–316.
97. Zachmann M, Prader A. Anabolic and androgenic effect of testosterone in sexually immature boys and its dependency on growth hormone. J Clin Endocrinol Metab 1970; 30:85–95.

98. MacGillivray M, Kolotkin M, Munschauer RW. Enhanced linear growth responses in hypopituitary dwarfs treated with growth hormone plus androgens versus growth hormone alone. Pediatr Res 1974; 8:103–108.

99. Howard CP, Takahashi H, Hayles AB. Children with growth hormone deficiency. Intermittent treatment with somatropin and oxandrolone. Am J Dis Child 1981; 135:326–328.

100. Illig R, Prader A. Effect of testosterone on growth hormone secretion in patients with anorchia and delayed puberty. J Clin Endocrinol Metab 1970; 30:615–618.

101. Kelley VC, Ruvalcaba RHA. Use of anabolic agents in treatment of short children. Clin Endocrinol Metab 1982; 11:25–39.

Estrogens

102. Lloyd HM, Meares JD, Jacobi J, et al. Effects of stilboestrol on growth hormone secretion and pituitary cell proliferation in the male rat. J Endocrinol 1971; 51:473–481.

103. Strickland AL, Sprinz H. Studies of the influence of estradiol and growth hormone on the hypophysectomized, immature rat epiphyseal cartilage growth plate. Am J Obstet Gynecol 1973; 115:471–477.

104. Josimovich JB, Mintz DH, Finster JL. Estrogenic inhibition of growth hormone-induced tibial epiphyseal growth in hypophysectomized rats. Endocrinology 1967; 81:1428–1430.

105. Phillips LS, Herington AC, Daughaday WH. Hormone effects on somatomedin action and somatomedin generation. In: Raiti S, ed. Advances in Human Growth Hormone Research. DHEW Publication No. (NIH) 74-612. Washington, DC; Government Printing Office, 1974: 50–67.

106. Weidemann E, Schartz E. Suppression of growth hormone–dependent human serum sulfation factor by estrogen. J Clin Endocrinol Metab 1972; 34:51–58.

107. Phillips LS, Herington AC, Daughaday WH. Steroid hormone effects on somatomedin. I. Somatomedin action in vitro. Endocrinology 1975; 97:780–786.

108. Whitelaw MJ. Experiences in treating excessive height in girls with cyclic oestradiol valerate. Acta Endocrinol 1967; 54:473–484.

109. Zachmann M, Ferrandez A, Murset G, et al. Estrogen treatment of excessively tall girls. Helv Paediatr Acta 1975; 30:11–30.

110. Wettenhall HNB, Cahill C, Roche AF. Tall girls: a survey of 15 years of management and treatment. J Pediatr 1975; 86:602–610.

111. Bartsch O, Weschke B, Weber B. Oestrogen treatment of constitutionally tall girls with 0.1 mg/day ethinyl estradiol. Eur J Pediatr 1988; 147:59–63.

112. Songo W, Scholler K, Heinze E, et al. Critical analysis of height reduction in oestrogen-treated tall girls. Eur J Pediatr 1988; 142:260–265.

113. Von Puttkamer K, Bierich JR, Brugger F, et al. Oestrogen treatment of girls with increased growth. Dtsch Med Wochenschr 1977; 102:983–988.

114. Ross JL, Cassorla FG, Skerda MC, et al. A preliminary study of the effect of estrogen dose on growth in Turner's syndrome. N Engl J Med 1983; 309:1104–1106.

115. Schwartz E, Echemendia E, Schiffer M, et al. Mechanism of estrogenic action in acromegaly. J Clin Invest 1969; 48:260–270.

116. Clemmons DR, Underwood LE, Ridgway EC, et al. Estradiol treatment of acromegaly. Reduction of immunoreactive somatomedin-C and improvement in metabolic status. Am J Med 1980; 69:571–575.

Peptide Growth Factors

117. Feyrter F. Ueber die These von den peripheren endokrinen Druesen. Wien Z Inn Med 1946; 27:9–38.

118. Sporn MB, Todaro GJ. Autocrine secretion and malignant transformation of cells. N Engl J Med 1980; 303:878–880.

119. Russell WE, Pledger WJ, Van Wyk JJ. Inhibition of the mitogenic effects of plasma by a monoclonal antibody to somatomedin-C. Proc Natl Acad Sci USA 1984; 81:935–939.

120. Clemmons DR, Van Wyk JJ. Evidence for a functional role of endogenously produced somatomedin-like peptides in the stimulation of human fibroblast and porcine smooth muscle cell DNA synthesis. J Clin Invest 1985; 75:1914–1918.

121. Van Wyk JJ, Casella SJ, Graves DR, et al. Evidence from monoclonal antibody studies that insulin stimulates deoxyribonucleic acid synthesis through the type I somatomedin receptor. J Clin Endocrinol Metab 1985; 61:639–643.

122. D'Ercole AJ, Stiles AD, Underwood LE. Tissue concentrations of somatomedin C: further evidence for multiple sites of synthesis and paracrine or autocrine mechanisms of action. Proc Natl Acad Sci USA 1984; 81:935–939.

123. Sporn MB, Roberts AB. Peptide growth factors are multifunctional. Nature 1988; 332:217–218.

124. Too CK, Murphy PR, Hamel AM, et al. Further purification of human pituitary-derived chondrocyte growth factor: heparin-binding and cross-reactivity with antiserum to basic FGF. Biochem Biophys Res Commun 1987; 144:1128–1134.

125. Davidson JM, Klagsbrun M, Hill KE, et al. Accelerated wound repair, cell proliferation, and collagen accumulation are produced by a cartilage-derived growth factor. J Cell Biol 1985; 100:1219–1227.

126. Miyazono K, Heldin CH. High-yield purification of platelet-derived endothelial cell growth factor: structural characterization and establishment of a specific antiserum. Biochemistry 1989; 28:1704–1710.

127. Cohen S. Isolation of a mouse submaxillary gland protein accelerating incisor eruption and eyelid opening in the newborn animal. J Biol Chem 1962; 237:1555–1562.

128. Cohen S, Taylor JM. Epidermal growth factor: chemical and biological characterization. Recent Prog Horm Res 1974; 30:533–550.

129. Cohen S, Savage CR Jr. Recent studies on the chemistry and biology of epidermal growth factor. Recent Prog Horm Res 1974; 30:551–574.

130. Carpenter G, Cohen S. Epidermal growth factor. Annu Rev Biochem 1979; 48:193–216.

131. Server AC, Shooter EM. Comparison of the arginine esteropeptidases associated with nerve and epidermal growth factors. J Biol Chem 1976; 251:165–173.

132. Gray A, Dull TJ, Ullrich A. Nucleotide sequence of epidermal growth factor cDNA predicts a 128,000-molecular weight protein precursor. Nature 1983; 303:722–725.

133. Russell DW, Schneider WJ, Yamamoto T, et al. Domain map of the LDL receptor-sequence homology with the epidermal growth factor precursor. Cell 1984; 37:577–585.

134. Yamamoto T, Davis CG, Brown MS, et al. The human LDL receptor: a cysteine-rich protein with multiple Alu sequences in its RNA. Cell 1984; 39:27–38.

135. Rall LB, Scott J, Bell GI, et al. Mouse prepro–epidermal growth factor synthesis by the kidney and other tissues. Nature 1985; 313:228–231.

136. Gregory H. Isolation and structure of urogastrone and its relationship to epidermal growth factor. Nature 1975; 257:325–327.

137. Gregory H, Holmes JE, Wilshire IR. Urogastrone levels in the urine of normal adult humans. J Clin Endocrinol Metab 1977; 45:668–672.

138. Hollenberg MD. Epidermal growth factor-urogastrone, a poly-peptide acquiring hormonal status. Vitam Horm 1979; 37:69–110.

139. Brissenden JE, Ullrich A, Francke U. Human chromosomal mapping of genes for insulin-like growth factors I and II and epidermal growth factor. Nature 1984; 310:781–784.

140. Han VK, D'Ercole AJ, Lee DC. Expression of transforming growth factor alpha during development. Can J Physiol Pharmacol 1988; 66:1113–1121.

141. Elder JT, Fisher GJ, Lindquist PB, et al. Overexpression of transforming growth factor alpha in psoriatic epidermis. Science 1989; 243:811–814.

142. Shoyab M, Plowman GD, McDonald VL, et al. Structure and function of human amphiregulin: a member of the epidermal growth factor family. Science 1989; 243:1074–1076.

143. Barthe PL, Bullock LP, Mowszowicz I, et al. Submaxillary gland epidermal growth factor: a sensitive index of biologic androgen activity. Endocrinology 1974; 95:1019–1025.

144. Byyny RL, Orth DN, Cohen S. Radioimmunoassay of epidermal growth factor. Endocrinology 1972; 90:1261–1266.

145. Hoath SB, Lakshmanan J, Scott SM, et al. Effect of thyroid hormones on epidermal growth factor concentration in neonatal mouse skin. Endocrinology 1983; 112:308–314.

146. Das M. Epidermal growth factor: mechanisms of action. Int Rev Cytol 1982; 78:233–256.

147. Downward J, Yarden Y, Mayes E, et al. Close similarity of epidermal growth factor receptor and v-erb-B oncogene protein sequences. Nature 1984; 307:521–527.

148. Carpenter G, King L Jr, Cohen S. Rapid enhancement of protein phosphorylation in A-431 cell membrane preparations by epidermal growth factor. J Biol Chem 1979; 254:4884–4891.

149. Carpenter G, Cohen S. ^{125}I-labeled human epidermal growth factor (hEGF): binding, internalization, and degradation in human fibroblasts. J Cell Biol 1976; 71:159–171.

150. Plowman GD, Whitney GS, Neubauer MG, et al. Molecular cloning and expression of an additional epidermal growth factor receptor–related gene. Proc Natl Acad Sci USA 1990; 87:4905–4909.

151. Barka T, van der Noen H, Greski EW, et al. Immunoreactive epidermal growth factor in human amniotic fluid. Mt Sinai J Med 1978; 45:679–684.

152. Nexo E, Lamberg SI, Hollenberg MD. Comparison of a receptor binding assay with a radioimmunoassay for measuring human epidermal growth factor-urogastrone in urine. Scand J Clin Lab Invest 1981; 41:577–582.

153. Sundell H, Serenius FS, Barthe P, et al. Effect of EGF on fetal lamb lung maturation. Pediatr Res 1975; 9:371–376.

154. Catterton WZ, Escobedo MB, Sexson WR, et al. Effect of epidermal growth factor on lung maturation in fetal rabbits. Pediatr Res 1979; 13:104–108.

155. Hassell JR, Pratt RM. Elevated levels of cAMP alters the effect of epidermal growth factor in vitro on programmed cell death in secondary palatal epithelium. Exp Cell Res 1977; 106:55–62.

156. Pratt RM, Yoneda T, Silver MH, et al. Involvement of glucocorticoids and EGF in secondary palate development. In: Pratt RM, Christiansen RL, eds. Current Research Trends in Prenatal Craniofacial Development. New York: Elsevier/North-Holland, 1980: 235–252.

157. St Hilaire RJ, Jones AL. Epidermal growth factor: its biologic and metabolic effects with emphasis on the hepatocyte. Hepatology 1982; 2:601–613.

158. Read LC, Upton FM, Francis GL, et al. Changes in the growth-promoting activity of human milk during lactation. Pediatr Res 1984; 18:133–139.
159. Baird A, Walicke PA. Fibroblast growth factors. Br Med Bull 1989; 45:438–452.
160. Gospodarowicz D. Purification of a fibroblast growth factor from bovine pituitary. J Biol Chem 1975; 250:2515–2520.
161. Gospodarowicz D, Bialecki H, Greenburg G. Purification of the fibroblast growth factor activity from bovine brain. J Biol Chem 1978; 253:3736–3743.
162. Bohlen P, Baird A, Esch F, et al. Isolation and partial molecular characterization of pituitary fibroblast growth factor. Proc Natl Acad Sci USA 1984; 81:5364–5368.
163. Burgess WH, Maciag T. The heparin-binding (fibroblast) growth factor family of proteins. Annu Rev Biochem 1989; 58:575–606.
164. Benharroch D, Birnbaum D. Biology of the fibroblast growth factor gene family. Isr J Med Sci 1990; 26:212–219.
165. Gospodarowicz D, Greene G, Moran J. Fibroblast growth factor can substitute for platelet factor to sustain the growth of BALB/c 3T3 cells in the presence of plasma. Biochem Biophys Res Commun 1975; 65:779–787.
166. Gospodarowicz D, Moran JS, Mescher AL. Cellular specificities of fibroblast growth factor and epidermal growth factor. In: Papaconstantinou J, Rutter WJ, eds. Molecular Control of Proliferation and Cyto-differentiation. 35th Symposium of the Society for Developmental Biology. New York: Academic, 1978: 33–61.
167. Gospodarowicz D, Bialecki H. Effects of epidermal and fibroblast growth factors on replicative life span of cultured bovine granulosa cells. Endocrinology 1978; 103:854–865.
168. Gospodarowicz D, Vlodavsky I, Savion N. The role of fibroblast growth factor and the extracellular matrix in the control of proliferation and differentiation of corneal endothelial cells. Vision Res 1981; 21:87–103.
169. Shing Y, Folkman J, Haudenschild C, et al. Angiogenesis is stimulated by a tumor-derived endothelial cell growth factor. J Cell Biochem 1985; 29:275–287.
170. Broadley KN, Aquino AM, Woodward SC, et al. Monospecific antibodies implicate basic fibroblast growth factor in normal wound repair. Lab Invest 1989; 61:571–575.
171. Rifkin DB, Moscatelli D. Recent developments in the cell biology of basic fibroblast growth factor. J Cell Biol 1989; 109:1–6.
172. Deuel TF, Huang JS. Platelet-derived growth factor. Structure, function, and roles in normal and transformed cells. J Clin Invest 1984; 74:669–676.
173. Heldin CH, Westermark B. Platelet-derived growth factor: mechanism of action and possible in vivo function. Cell Regul 1990; 1:555–566.
174. Balk SD. Calcium as a regulator of the proliferation of normal, but not of transformed, chicken fibroblasts in plasma-containing medium. Proc Natl Acad Sci USA 1971; 68:271–275.
175. Balk SD, Whitfield JF, Youdale T, et al. Roles of calcium, serum, plasma, and folic acid in the control of proliferation of normal and Rous sarcoma virus–infected chicken fibroblasts. Proc Natl Acad Sci USA 1973; 70:675–679.
176. Rutherford RB, Ross R. Platelet factors stimulate fibroblasts and smooth muscle cells quiescent in plasma serum to proliferate. J Cell Biol 1976; 69:196–203.
177. Johnsson A, Heldin CH, Wasteson A, et al. The c-sis gene encodes a precursor of the B chain of platelet-derived growth factor. EMBO J 1984; 3:921–928.
178. Josephs SF, Guo C, Ratner L, et al. Human protooncogene nucleotide sequences corresponding to the transforming region of simian sarcoma virus. Science 1984; 223:486–490.
179. Heldin CH, Betsholtz C, Claesson-Welsh L, et al. Subversion of growth regulatory pathways in malignant transformation. Biochim Biophys Acta 1987; 907:219–244.
180. Heldin CH, Westermark B, Wasteson A. Specific receptors for platelet-derived growth factor on cells derived from connective tissue and glia. Proc Natl Acad Sci USA 1981; 78:3664–3668.
181. Glenn K, Bowen-Pope DF, Ross R. Platelet-derived growth factor. 3. Identification of a platelet-derived growth factor receptor by affinity labeling. J Biol Chem 1982; 257:5172–5176.
182. Ek B, Westermark B, Wasteson A, et al. Stimulation of tyrosine-specific phosphorylation by platelet-derived growth factor. Nature 1982; 295:419–420.
183. Heldin CH, Wasteson A, Westermark B. Interaction of platelet-derived growth factor with its fibroblast receptor. Demonstration of ligand and receptor modulation. J Biol Chem 1983; 257:4216–4221.
184. Kaplan DR, Chao FC, Stiles CD, et al. Platelet alpha granules contain a growth factor for fibroblasts. Blood 1979; 53:1043–1052.
185. Pledger WJ, Leof EB, Chou BB, et al. Initiation of cell-cycle traverse by serum-derived growth factors. Cold Spring Harbor Conf Cell Prolif 1982; 9:259–273.
186. Leibovich SJ, Ross R. A macrophage-dependent factor that stimulates the proliferation of fibroblasts in vitro. Am J Pathol 1976; 84:501–513.
187. Cheung HS, Van Wyk JJ, Russell WE, et al. Mitogenic activity of hydroxyapatite: requirement for somatomedin C. J Cell Physiol 1986; 128:143–148.
188. Ross R, Glomset JA. The pathogenesis of atherosclerosis. N Engl J Med 1976; 295:369–377.
189. Harker LA, Ross R, Slichter SJ, et al. Homocystine-induced arteriosclerosis. The role of endothelial cell injury and platelet response in its genesis. J Clin Invest 1976; 58:731–741.
190. Klagsbrun M, Edelman ER. Biological and biochemical properties of fibroblast growth factors. Implications for the pathogenesis of atherosclerosis. Arteriosclerosis 1989; 9:269–278.
191. Barnard JA, Lyons RM, Moses HL. The cell biology of transforming growth factor β. Biochim Biophys Acta 1990; 1032:79–87.
192. Sata Y, Rifkin DB. Inhibition of endothelial cell movement by pericytes and smooth muscle cells: activation of a latent transforming growth factor-beta 1–like molecule by plasmin during co-culture. J Cell Biol 1989; 109:309–315.
193. Massague J, Cheifetz S, Boyd FT, et al. TGF-beta receptors and TGF-beta binding proteoglycans: recent progress in identifying their functional properties. Ann NY Acad Sci 1990; 593:59–72.
194. Roberts AB, Anzano MA, Wakefield LM, et al. Type beta transforming growth factor: a bifunctional regulator of cellular growth. Proc Natl Acad Sci USA 1985; 82:119–123.
195. Roberts AB, Thompson NL, Heine U, et al. Transforming growth factor-beta: possible roles in carcinogenesis. Br J Cancer 1988; 57:594–600.
196. Donahoe PK, Cate RL, MacLaughlin DT, et al. Mullerian inhibiting substance: gene structure and mechanism of action of a fetal regressor. Recent Prog Horm Res 1987; 43:431–467.
197. Josso N. Antimullerian hormone: new perspectives for a sexist molecule. Endocr Rev 1986; 7:421–433.
198. Jost A. Problems of fetal endocrinology: the gonadal and hypophyseal hormones. Recent Prog Horm Res 1953; 8:379–418.
199. Cate RL, Mattaliano RJ, Hession C, et al. Isolation of the bovine and human genes for mullerian inhibiting substance and expression of the human gene in animal cells. Cell 1986; 45:685–698.
200. Pepinsky RB, Sinclair LK, Chow EP, et al. Proteolytic processing of mullerian inhibiting substance transforming growth factor-beta–like fragment. J Biol Chem 1988; 263:18961–18964.
201. Baker ML, Metcalfe SA, Hutson JM. Serum levels of mullerian inhibiting substance in boys from birth to 18 years, as determined by enzyme immunoassay. J Clin Endocrinol Metab 1990; 70:11–15.
202. Coughlin JP, Donahoe PK, Budzik GP, et al. Mullerian inhibiting substance blocks autophosphorylation of the EGF receptor by inhibiting tyrosine kinase. Mol Cell Endocrinol 1987; 49:75–86.
203. McCullough, DR. Dual endocrine activity of the testes. Science 1932; 76:19–20.
204. Roberts V, Meunier H, Vaughan J, et al. Production and regulation of inhibin subunits in pituitary gonadotropes. Endocrinology 1989; 124:552–554.
205. Lin T, Calkins JH, Morris PL, et al. Regulation of Leydig cell function in primary culture by inhibin and activin. Endocrinology 1989; 125:2134–2140.
206. Gonzalez-Manchon C, Vale W. Activin-A, inhibin and transforming growth factor-beta modulate growth of two gonadal cell lines. Endocrinology 1989; 125:1666–1672.
207. Yu J, Shao L, Lemas V, et al. Importance of FSH-releasing protein and inhibin in erythrodifferentiation. Nature 1987; 330:765–767.
208. Yu J, Shao L, Vaughan J, et al. Characterization of the potentiation effect of activin on human erythroid colony formation in vitro. Blood 1989; 73:952–960.
209. Vale W, Rivier C, Hsueh A, et al. Chemical and biological characterization of the inhibin family of protein hormones. Recent Prog Horm Res 1988; 44:1–34.
210. Smith JC, Price BMJ, Van Nimmen K, et al. Identification of a potent *Xenopus* mesoderm-inducing factor as a homologue of activin A. Nature 1990; 345:729–731.
211. van den Eijnden-Van Raaij AJM, van Zoelent JJ, van Nimmen K, et al. Activin-like factor from a *Xenopus laevis* cell line responsible for mesoderm induction. Nature 1990; 345:732–734.
212. Levi-Montalcini R, Hamburger V. Selective growth stimulating effects of mouse sarcoma on the sensory and sympathetic nervous system of the chick embryo. J Exp Zool 1951; 116:321–362.
213. Cohen S. Purification of a nerve growth promoting protein from the mouse salivary gland and its neurocytotoxic antiserum. Proc Natl Acad Sci USA 1960; 46:302–311.
214. Frazier WA, Angletti RH, Bradshaw RA. Nerve growth factor and insulin: structural similarities indicate an evolutionary relationship reflected by physiological action. Science 1972; 175:482–488.
215. Thomas KA, Baglan NC, Bradshaw RA. The amino acid sequence of the gamma-subunit of mouse submaxillary gland 7S nerve growth factor. J Biol Chem 1981; 256:9156–9168.
216. Hempstead BL, Chao MV. The nerve growth factor receptor: biochemical and structural analysis. Recent Prog Horm Res 1989; 45:441–466.
217. Aloe L, Cozzari C, Calissano P, et al. Somatic and behavioural postnatal effects of fetal injections of nerve growth factor antibodies in the rat. Nature 1981; 291:412–415.
218. Hamburger V, Bruno-Bechtold JK, Yip JW. Neuronal death in the spinal ganglia of the chick embryo and its reduction by nerve growth factor. J Neurosci Res 1981; 1:60–71.

219. Gorin PD, Johnson EM Jr. Effects of long-term nerve growth factor deprivation on the nervous system of the adult rat: an experimental autoimmune approach. Brain Res 1980; 198:27–42.

220. Thoenen H, Barde YA. Physiology of nerve growth factor. Physiol Rev 1980; 60:1284–1335.

221. Acheson AL, Naujoks K, Thoenen H. Nerve growth factor–mediated enzyme induction in primary cultures of bovine adrenal chromaffin cells—specificity and level of regulation. J Neurosci 1984; 4:1771–1780.

222. Korsching S, Thoenen H. Quantitative demonstration of the retrograde axonal transport of endogenous nerve growth factor. Neurosci Lett 1983; 39:1–4.

223. Heumann R, Korsching S, Scott J, et al. Relationship between levels of nerve growth factor (NGF) and its messenger RNA in sympathetic ganglia and peripheral target tissues. EMBO J 1984; 3:3183–3189.

224. Thoenen H, Edgar D. Neurotropic factors. Science 1985; 229:238–242.

225. Gee AP, Boyle MDP, Munger KL, et al. Nerve growth factor: stimulation of polymorphonuclear leukocyte chemotaxis in vitro. Proc Natl Acad Sci USA 1983; 80:7215–7218.

226. Aloe L, Levi-Montalcini R. Mast cells increase in tissues of neonatal rats injected with the nerve growth factor. Brain Res 1977; 133:358–366.

227. Thorpe LW, Jerrells TR, Perez-Polo JR. Mechanisms of lymphocyte activation by nerve growth factor. Ann NY Acad Sci 1990; 594:78–84.

228. Thorpe LW, Perez-Polo JR. The influence of nerve growth factor on the in vitro proliferative response of rat spleen lymphocytes. J Neurosci Res 1987; 18:134–139.

229. Walker P, Weichsel ME Jr, Eveleth D, et al. Ontogenesis of nerve growth factor and epidermal growth factor in submaxillary glands and nerve growth factor in brains of immature male mice: correlation with ontogenesis of serum levels of thyroid hormones. Pediatr Res 1982; 16:520–524.

230. Fabricant RN, Todaro GJ. Increased serum levels of nerve growth factor in von Recklinghausen's disease. Arch Neurol 1981; 38:401–405.

231. Bigazzi M, Revoltella R, Casciano S, et al. High level of a nerve growth factor in the serum of a patient with medullary carcinoma of the thyroid gland. Clin Endocrinol 1977; 6:105–112.

232. Stewart WP, Scarffe JH. Clinical trials with hemopoietic growth factors. Prog Growth Factor Res 1989; 1:1–12.

233. Groopman JE, Molina JM, Scadden DT. Hematopoietic growth factors. Biology and clinical applications. N Engl J Med 1989; 321:1449–1459.

234. Carnot MP, Deflandre C. Sur l'activité hémopoietique du sérum au cours de la régénération du sang. C R Acad Sci 1906; 143:384–387.

235. Graber SE, Krantz SB. Erythropoietin and the control of red cell production. Annu Rev Med 1978; 29:51–66.

236. Jacobs K, Shoemaker C, Rudersdorf R, et al. Isolation and characterization of genomic and cDNA clones of human erythropoietin. Nature 1985; 313:806–810.

237. Alexanian R. Erythropoietin and erythropoiesis in anemic man following androgens. Blood 1969; 33:564–572.

238. Jepson JH, McGarry EE. Hemopoiesis in pituitary dwarfs treated with human growth hormone and testosterone. Blood 1972; 39:238–248.

239. Kurtz A, Zapf J, Eckardt KU, et al. Insulin-like growth factor I stimulates erythropoiesis in hypophysectomized rats. Proc Natl Acad Sci USA 1988; 85:7825–7829.

240. Claustres M, Chatelain P, Sultan C. Insulin-like growth factor I stimulates human erythroid colony formation in vitro. J Clin Endocrinol Metab 1987; 65:78–82.

240a. Congote LF, Brox A, Lin FK, et al. The N-terminal sequence of the major erythropoietic factor of an anephric patient is identical to insulin-like growth factor I. J Clin Endocrinol Metab 1991; 72:727–729.

241. Djaldetti M, Preisler H, Marks PA, et al. Erythropoietin effects on fetal mouse erythroid cells. II. Nucleic acid synthesis and the erythropoietin-sensitive cells. J Biol Chem 1972; 247:731–735.

242. Glass J, Lavidor LM, Robinson SH. Use of cell separation and short term culture techniques to study erythroid cell development. Blood 1975; 46:705–711.

243. Sawada K, Krantz SB, Dessypris EN, et al. Human colony-forming units-erythroid do not require accessory cells, but do require direct interaction with insulin-like growth factor I and/or insulin for erythroid development. J Clin Invest 1989; 83:1701–1709.

244. Adamson JW, Eschbach JW. Treatment of the anemia of chronic renal failure with recombinant human erythropoietin. Annu Rev Med 1990; 41:349–360.

245. Morstyn G, Burgess AW. Hemopoietic growth factors: a review. Cancer Res 1988; 48:5624–5637.

246. Platzer E. Human hemopoietic growth factors. Eur J Haematol 1989; 42:1–15.

247. Metcalf D. The Hemopoietic Colony-Stimulating Factors. Amsterdam: Elsevier/North-Holland, 1984.

248. Metcalf D. The granulocyte-macrophage colony-stimulating factors. Science 1985; 229:16–22.

249. Quesenberry P, Morley A, Stohlman F Jr, et al. Effect of endotoxin on granulopoiesis and colony-stimulating factor. N Engl J Med 1972; 286:227–232.

250. Sheriden JW, Metcalf D. Studies on the bone marrow colony stimulating factor (CSF): relation of tissue CSF to serum CSF. J Cell Physiol 1972; 80:129–139.

251. Klingemann HG. Clinical applications of recombinant human colony-stimulating factors. Can Med Assoc J 1989; 140:137–142.

252. Lotem J, Sachs L. Potential pre-screening for therapeutic agents that induce differentiation in human myeloid leukemia cells. Int J Cancer 1980; 25:561–564.

253. Gabrilove JL, Jakubowski A. Hematopoietic growth factors: biology and clinical application. Monogr J Natl Cancer Inst 1990; 10:73–77.

254. Bendtzen K. Biological properties of interleukins. Allergy 1983; 38:219–226.

255. Strober W, James SP. The interleukins. Pediatr Res 1988; 24:549–557.

256. Arai K, Lee F, Miyajima A, et al. Cytokines: coordinators of immune and inflammatory responses. Annu Rev Biochem 1990; 59:783–836.

257. Sapolsky R, Rivier C, Yamamoto G, et al. Interleukin-1 stimulated the secretion of hypothalamic corticotropin-releasing factor. Science 1987; 238:522–524.

258. Dinarello CA. Interleukin-1 and the pathogenesis of the acute-phase response. N Engl J Med 1985; 311:1413–1418.

259. Sehgal P. Interleukin-6: molecular pathophysiology. J Invest Dermatol 1990; 94:2S–6S.

260. Fuller GM, Grenett HE. The structure and function of the mouse hepatocyte stimulating factor. Ann NY Acad Sci 1989; 557:31–45.

261. Rokita H, Bereta J, Koj A, et al. Epidermal growth factor and transforming growth factor-beta differently modulate the acute phase response elicited by interleukin-6 in cultured liver cells from man, rat and mouse. Comp Biochem Physiol 1990; 95A:41–45.

262. Balkwill FR. Tumour necrosis factor. Br Med Bull 1989; 45:389–400.

263. Grunfeld C. Palladino MA Jr. Tumor necrosis factor: immunologic, antitumor, metabolic, and cardiovascular activities. Adv Intern Med 1990; 35:45–72.

264. Spies T, Morton CC, Nedospasov SA, et al. Genes for the tumor necrosis factors alpha and beta are linked to the human major histocompatibility complex. Proc Natl Acad Sci USA 1986; 83:8699–8702.

265. Vilcek J, Palombella VJ, Zhang Y, et al. Mechanisms and significance of the mitogenic and antiviral actions of TNF. Ann Inst Pasteur Immunol 1988; 139:307–311.

266. Perlmutter DH, Dinarello CA, Punsal PL, et al. Cachetin/tumor necrosis factor regulates hepatic acute-phase gene expression. J Clin Invest 1986; 78:1349–1354.

267. Isaacs A, Lindemann J. Virus interference: I. The interferon. Proc R Soc Lond [Biol] 1957; 147:258–267.

268. Hughes TK, Baron S. A possible role for IFNs α and β in the development of IFN-γ's antiviral state in mouse and human cells. In: Baron S, Dianzani F, Stanton GJ, et al., eds. The Interferon System. A Current Review to 1987. Austin: University of Texas Press, 1987: 187–196.

269. Opdenakker G, Cabeza-Arvelaiz Y, Van Damme J. Interaction of interferon with other cytokines. Experientia 1989; 45:497–598.

270. Romeo G, Fiorucci G, Rossi GB. Interferons in cell growth and development. Trends Genet 1989; 5:19–24.

271. Low TLK, Thurman GB, Chincarini C, et al. Current status of thymosin research: evidence for the existence of a family of thymic factors that control T-cell maturation. Ann NY Acad Sci 1979; 332:33–48.

272. Schlesinger DH, Goldstein G. The amino acid sequence of thymopoietin II. Cell 1975; 5:361–365.

273. Goldstein G, Scheid MP, Boyse EA, et al. A synthetic pentapeptide with biological activity characteristic of the thymic hormone thymopoietin. Science 1979; 204:1309–1310.

274. Veys EM, Huskisson EC, Rosenthal M, et al. Clinical response to therapy with thymopoietin pentapeptide (TP-5) in rheumatoid arthritis. Ann Rheum Dis 1982; 41:441–443.

275. Goldstein AL, Guha A, Zatz MM, et al. Purification and biological activity of thymosin, a hormone of the thymus gland. Proc Natl Acad Sci USA 1972; 69:1800–1803.

276. Wara DW, Goldstein AL, Doyle NE, et al. Thymosin activity in patients with cellular immunodeficiency. N Engl J Med 1975; 292:70–74.

277. Miller DM, Blume S, Borst M, et al. Oncogenes, malignant transformation, and modern medicine. Am J Med Sci 1990; 300:59–69.

278. Bishop JM. The molecular biology of RNA tumor viruses: a physician's guide. N Engl J Med 1980; 303:675–682.

279. Chiu IM. Growth factor genes as oncogenes. Mol Chem Neuropathol 1989; 10:37–48.

280. Druker BJ, Harvey J, Mamon BS, et al. Oncogenes, growth factors, and signal transduction. N Engl J Med 1989; 321:1383–1391.

281. Studzinski GP. Oncogenes, growth, and the cell cycle: an overview. Cell Tissue Kinet 1989; 22:405–424.

282. Doolittle RF, Hunkapiller MW, Hood LE, et al. Simian sarcoma virus onc gene, v-sis, is derived from the gene (or genes) encoding a platelet-derived growth factor. Science 1983; 221:275–277.

283. Waterfield MD, Scrace GT, Whittle N, et al. Platelet-derived growth factor is structurally related to the putative transforming protein p28sis of simian sarcoma virus. Nature 1983; 304:35–39.

284. Downward J, Yarden Y, Mayes E, et al. Close similarity of epidermal growth factor receptor and v-erb-B oncogene protein sequences. Nature 1984; 307:521–527.

285. Weinberger C, Thompson CC, Ong ES, et al. The c-erb-A gene encodes a thyroid hormone receptor. Nature 1986; 324:641–646.

286. Hunter T, Cooper JA. Protein-tyrosine kinase. Annu Rev Biochem 1985; 54:897–930.
287. Ullrich A, Schlessinger J. Signal transduction by receptors with tyrosine kinase activity. Cell 1990; 61:203–212.
288. Wahl MI, Olashaw NE, Nishibe S, et al. Platelet-derived growth factor induces rapid and sustained tyrosine phosphorylation of phospholipase C-gamma in quiescent BALB/c 3T3 cells. Mol Cell Biol 1989; 9:2934–2943.
289. Van de Woude GF, Blair DG, McGeady ML, et al. Properties of the mouse MOS proto-oncogene locus. Haematologica 1987; 72(Suppl 6):3–5.
290. Morrison DK, Kaplan DR, Rapp U, et al. Signal transduction from membrane to cytoplasm: growth factors and membrane-bound oncogene products increase Raf-1 phosphorylation and associated protein kinase activity. Proc Natl Acad Sci USA 1988; 85:8855–8859.
291. Konkel DA. What do *ras* oncogenes do? Mol Endocrinol 1988; 2:883–885.
292. Wigler MH. GAPs in understanding *ras*. Nature 1990; 346:696–697.
293. Sassone-Corsi P, Ransone LJ, Lamph WW, et al. Direct interaction between fos and jun nuclear oncoproteins: role of the "leucine zipper" domain. Nature 1988; 336:692–695.
294. Armelin HA, Armelin MC, Kelly K, et al. Functional role for *c-myc* in mitogenic response to platelet-derived growth factor. Nature 1984; 310:655–660.
295. Kaczmarek L, Hyland JK, Watt R, et al. Microinjected *c-myc* as a competence factor. Science 1985; 228:1313–1316.
296. Rollins BJ, Stiles CD. Regulation of *c-myc* and *c-fos* proto-oncogene expression by animal cell growth factors. In Vitro Cell Dev Biol 1988; 24:81–84.

The Somatomedins

297. Van Wyk JJ, Underwood LE, Hintz RL, et al. The somatomedins: a family of insulin-like peptides under growth hormone control. Recent Prog Horm Res 1974; 30:259–318.
298. Froesch ER, Burgi H, Ramseier EB, et al. Antibody-suppressible and non-suppressible insulin-like activities in human serum and their physiologic significance. J Clin Invest 1963; 42:1816–1834.
299. Rinderknecht E, Humbel RE. Polypeptides with nonsuppressible insulin-like and cell-growth promoting activities in human serum: isolation, chemical characterization, and some biological properties of forms I and II. Proc Natl Acad Sci USA 1976; 73:2365–2369.
300. Dulak NC, Temin HM. Multiplication-stimulating activity for chicken embryo fibroblasts from rat liver cell conditioned medium: a family of small polypeptides. J Cell Physiol 1973; 81:161–170.
301. Moses AC, Nissley SP, Short PA, et al. Purification and characterization of multiplication-stimulating activity: insulin-like growth factors purified from rat-liver-cell-conditioned medium. Eur J Biochem 1980; 103:387–400.
302. Marquardt H, Todaro GJ, Henderson LE, et al. Purification and primary structure of a polypeptide with multiplication-stimulating activity from rat liver cell cultures: homology with human insulin-like growth factor II. J Biol Chem 1981; 256:6859–6865.
303. Daughaday WH, Hall K, Salmon WD Jr, et al. On the nomenclature of the somatomedins and insulin-like growth factors. J Clin Endocrinol Metab 1987; 65:1075–1076 (letter).
304. Casella SJ, Smith EP, Van Wyk JJ, et al. Isolation of rat testis cDNAs encoding an insulin-like growth factor-I precursor. DNA 1987; 6:325–330.
305. Brissenden JE, Ullrich A, Francke U. Human chromosomal mapping of genes for insulin-like growth factors I and II and epidermal growth factor. Nature 1984; 310:781–784.
306. Tricoli JV, Rall LB, Scott J, et al. Localization of insulin-like growth factor genes to human chromosomes 11 and 12. Nature 1984; 310:784–786.
307. Jansen M, van Schaik FMA, van Tol H, et al. Nucleotide sequences of cDNAs encoding precursors of human insulin-like growth factor II (IGF-II) and an IGF-II variant. FEBS Lett 1985; 179:243–246.
308. Jansen M, van Schaik FMA, Ricker AT, et al. Sequence of cDNA encoding human insulin-like growth factor I precursor. Nature 1983; 306:609–611.
309. Bell GI, Merryweather JP, Sanchez-Pescador R, et al. Sequence of a cDNA clone encoding human preproinsulin-like growth factor II. Nature 1984; 310:775–777.
310. Dull TJ, Gray A, Hayflick JS, et al. Insulin-like growth factor II precursor gene organization in relation to insulin gene family. Nature 1984; 310:777–781.
311. Hoyt EC, Van Wyk JJ, Lund PK. Tissue and development specific regulation of a complex family of rat insulin-like growth factor I messenger ribonucleic acids. Mol Endocrinol 1988; 2:1077–1086.
312. Van Wyk JJ, Underwood LE, Hintz RL, et al. Exploration of the insulin-like effects and growth promoting properties of somatomedin by membrane receptor assays. In: Luft R, Hall K, eds. Advances in Metabolic Disorders. Vol 8. New York: Academic, 1975: 127–150.
313. Massague J, Czech MP. The subunit structures of two distinct receptors for insulin-like growth factors I and II and their relationship to the insulin receptor. J Biol Chem 1982; 257:5036–5045.
314. Chernausek SD, Jacobs S, Van Wyk JJ. Structural similarities between human receptors for somatomedin C and insulin: analysis by affinity labeling. Biochemistry 1981; 20:7345–7350.
315. Casella SJ, Han VK, D'Ercole AJ, et al. Insulin-like growth factor binding to the type I somatomedin receptor: evidence for two high affinity binding sites. J Biol Chem 1986; 261:9268–9273.
316. Moxham CP, Duronio V, Jacobs S. Insulin-like growth factor I receptor beta-subunit heterogeneity. Evidence for hybrid tetramers composed of insulin-like growth factor I and insulin receptor heterodimers. J Biol Chem 1989; 264:13238–13234.
317. Yardin Y, Ullrich A. Growth factor receptor tyrosine kinases. Annu Rev Biochem 1988; 57:443–478.
318. Clemmons DR, Van Wyk JJ, Pledger WJ. Sequential addition of platelet factor and plasma to BALB/c 3T3 fibroblast cultures stimulates somatomedin-C binding early in the cell cycle. Proc Natl Acad Sci USA 1980; 77:6644–6648.
319. Lin T, Blaisdell J, Haskell JF. Type I IGF receptors of Leydig cells are upregulated by human chorionic gonadotropin. Biochem Biophys Res Commun 1987; 149:852–858.
320. Adashi EY, Resnick CE, Svoboda ME, et al. Follicle-stimulating hormone enhances somatomedin C binding to cultured rat granulosa cells. J Biol Chem 1986; 261:3923–3926.
321. Penhoat A, Naville D, Jaillard C, et al. Hormonal regulation of insulin-like growth factor I secretion by bovine adrenal cells. J Biol Chem 1989; 264:6858–6862.
322. Lowe WJ Jr, Adamo M, Werner H, et al. Regulation by fasting of rat insulin-like growth factor I and its receptor. Effects on gene expression and binding. J Clin Invest 1989; 84:619–626.
323. Werner H, Woloschak M, Adamo M, et al. Developmental regulation of the rat insulin-like growth factor I receptor gene. Proc Natl Acad Sci USA 1989; 86:7451–7455.
324. Oppenheimer CL, Pessin JE, Massague J, et al. Insulin action rapidly modulates the apparent affinity of the insulin-like growth factor II receptor. J Biol Chem 1983; 258:4824–4830.
325. Oshima A, Nolan CM, Kyle JW, et al. The human cation-independent mannose 6-phosphate receptor. Cloning and sequence of the full-length cDNA and expression of functional receptor in COS cells. J Biol Chem 1988; 263:2553–2562.
326. Waheed A, Braulke T, Junghans U, et al. Mannose 6-phosphate/insulin like growth factor II receptor: the two types of ligands bind simultaneously to one receptor at different sites. Biochem Biophys Res Commun 1988; 152:1248–1254.
327. Kornfeld S. Trafficking of lysosomal enzymes. FASEB J 1987; 1:462–468.
328. Kovacina KS, Steele-Perkins G, Purchio AF, et al. Interactions of recombinant and platelet transforming growth factor-β_1 precursor with the insulin-like growth factor II/mannose 6-phosphate receptor. Biochem Biophys Res Commun 1989; 160:393–403.
329. Lee SJ, Nathans D. Proliferin secreted by cultured cells binds to mannose 6-phosphate receptors. J Biol Chem 1988; 263:3521–3527.
330. Blanchard MM, Barenton B, Sullivan A, et al. Characterization of the insulin-like growth factor (IGF) receptor in K562 erythroleukemia cells; evidence for a biological function for the type II IGF receptor. Mol Cell Endocrinol 1988; 56:235–244.
331. Mohan S, Linkhart T, Rosenfeld R, et al. Characterization of the receptor for insulin-like growth factor II in bone cells. J Cell Physiol 1989; 140:169–1976.
332. Nissley P, Kiess W, Sklar MM. The insulin-like growth factor II/mannose 6-phosphate receptor. In: LeRoith D, ed. Insulin-like Growth Factors: Cellular and Molecular Aspects. Boca Raton, FL: CRC Press, 1991: 111–150.
333. Okamoto T, Nishimoto I, Murayama Y, et al. Insulin-like growth factor II/mannose 6-phosphate receptor is incapable of activating GTP-binding proteins in response to mannose 6-phosphate, but capable in response to insulin-like growth factor II. Biochem Biophys Res Commun 1990; 168:1201–1210.
334. Okamoto T, Katada T, Murayama Y, et al. A simple structure encodes G protein–activating function of the IGF-II/mannose 6-phosphate receptor. Cell 1990; 62:709–717.
335. Ballard J, Baxter R, Binoux M, et al. On the nomenclature of IGF binding proteins. Acta Endocrinol 1989; 121:751–752.
336. Baxter RC, Martin JL. Binding proteins for insulin-like growth factors: structure, regulation and function. Prog Growth Factor Res 1989; 1:49–68.
337. Brinkman A, Groffen CAH, Kortleve DJ, et al. Identification of a domain in the low molecular weight IGF-I binding protein, IBP 1, which is essential for IGF-I binding. Endocr Soc Abstr 1989; 273.
338. Koistinen R, Huhtala ML, Stennian UH, et al. Purification of placental protein PP12 from human amniotic fluid and its comparison with PP12 from placenta by immunological, physiochemical and somatomedin-binding properties. Clin Chim Acta 1987; 164:293–303.
339. Brown AL, Chariotti L, Orlowski CC, et al. Nucleotide sequences and expression of a cDNA clone encoding a fetal rat binding protein for insulin-like growth factors. J Biol Chem 1989; 264:5148–5154.
340. Ooi GT, Orlowski CC, Brown AL, et al. Different tissue distribution and hormonal regulation of mRNAs encoding rat insulin-like growth factor binding proteins (IGFBP-1 and IGFBP-2). Mol Endocrinol 1990; 4:321–328.

341. Hintz RL. Plasma forms of somatomedin and the binding protein phenomenon. Clin Endocrinol Metab 1984; 13:31–42.

342. Furlanetto RW. The somatomedin-C binding protein: evidence for a heterologous subunit structure. J Clin Endocrinol Metab 1980; 51:12–19.

343. Clemmons DR, Thissen JP, Maes M, et al. Insulin-like growth factor I (IGF-I) infusion into hypophysectomized or protein-deprived rats induces specific IGF-binding proteins in serum. Endocrinology 1989; 125:2967–2972.

344. Bar RS, Clemmons Dr, Boes M, et al. Transcapillary permeability and subendothelial distribution of endothelial and amniotic fluid IGF binding proteins in rat heart. Endocrinology 1990; 127:1078–1086.

345. Zapf J, Schoenle E, Jagars G, et al. Inhibition of the action of nonsuppressible insulin-like activity on isolated rat fat cells by binding to its carrier protein. J Clin Invest 1979; 63:1077–1084.

346. Drop SLS, Valiquette G, Guyda HJ, et al. Partial purification and characterization of a binding protein for insulin-like activity (ILas) in human amniotic fluid: a possible inhibitor of insulin-like activity. Acta Endocrinol 1979; 90:505–518.

347. DeMellow JSM, Baxter RC. Growth hormone dependent insulin-like growth factor (IGF) binding protein both inhibits and potentiates IGF-I stimulated DNA synthesis in human skin fibroblasts. Biochem Biophys Res Commun 1988; 156:199–204.

348. Elgin RC, Busby WH, Clemmons DR. An insulin-like growth factor binding protein enhances the biological response to IGF-I. Proc Natl Acad Sci USA 1987; 84:3254–3258.

349. Furlanetto RW, Underwood LE, Van Wyk JJ, et al. Estimation of somatomedin-C levels in normals and patients with pituitary disease by radioimmunoassay. J Clin Invest 1977; 60:648–657.

350. Copeland KC, Underwood LE, Van Wyk JJ. Induction of immunoreactive somatomedin-C in human serum by growth hormone: dose response relationships and effect on chromatographic profiles. J Clin Endocrinol Metab 1980; 50:690–697.

351. Zapf J, Walter H, Froesch ER. Radioimmunological determination of insulin-like growth factors I and II in normal subjects and in patients with growth disorders and extrapancreatic tumor hypoglycemia. J Clin Invest 1981; 68:1321–1330.

352. Daughaday WH, Mariz IK, Blethen SL. Inhibition of access of bound somatomedin to membrane receptor and immunobinding sites: a comparison of radioreceptor and radioimmunoassay of somatomedin in native and acid-ethanol extracted serum. J Clin Endocrinol Metab 1980; 51:781–788.

353. Underwood LE, Murphy MG. Radioimmunoassay of the somatomedins/insulin-like growth factors. In: Patrono C, Peskar BA, eds. Handbook of Experimental Pharmacology. Vol 82. Berlin: Springer-Verlag, 1987: 501–574.

354. Davenport ML, Svoboda ME, Koerber KL, et al. Serum concentrations of insulin-like growth factor II (IGF-II) are not changed by short-term fasting and refeeding. J Clin Endocrinol Metab 1988; 67:1231–1235.

355. Foley TP, DePhilip R, Pericelli A, et al. Low somatomedin activity in cord serum from infants with intrauterine growth retardation. J Pediatr 1980; 96:605–610.

356. Bala RM, Lopatka J, Leung A, et al. Serum immunoreactive somatomedin levels in normal adults, pregnant women at term, children at various ages, and children with constitutionally delayed growth. J Clin Endocrinol Metab 1981; 52:508–512.

357. D'Ercole AJ, Underwood LE. Growth factors in fetal growth and development. In: Novy MJ, Resko JA, eds. Fetal Endocrinology. New York: Academic, 1981: 155–182.

358. Bennett A, Wilson DM, Liu F, et al. Levels of insulin-like growth factors I and II in human cord blood. J Clin Endocrinol Metab 1983; 57:609–612.

359. Kaplowitz PB, D'Ercole AJ, Van Wyk JJ, et al. Plasma somatomedin-C during the first year of life. J Pediatr 1982; 100:932–934.

360. Underwood LE, Smith EP, Van Wyk JJ, et al. Somatomedin-C/insulin-like growth factor I: regulation and clinical applications. In: Raiti S, Tolman RA, eds. Human Growth Hormone. New York: Plenum, 1986: 609–619.

361. Luna AM, Wilson DM, Wibbelsman CJ, et al. Somatomedins in adolescence: a cross-sectional study of the effect of puberty on plasma insulin-like growth factor I and II levels. J Clin Endocrinol Metab 1983; 57:268–271.

362. Blethen SL, Daughaday WH, Weldon VV. Kinetics of the somatomedin-C/insulin-like growth factor I: response to exogenous growth hormone in GH-dependent children. J Clin Endocrinol Metab 1982; 54:986–990.

363. Rosenfeld RG, Kemp SF, Hintz RL. Constancy of somatomedin response to growth hormone treatment of hypopituitary dwarfism, and lack of correlation with growth rate. J Clin Endocrinol Metab 1981; 53:611–617.

364. Illig R, Bucher H. Testosterone priming of growth hormone release, evaluation of growth hormone secretion. Pediatr Adolesc Endocrinol 1983; 12:75–85.

365. Maurus N, Blizzard RM, Link K, et al. Augmentation of growth hormone secretion during puberty. Evidence for a pulse amplitude–modulated phenomenon. J Clin Endocrinol Metab 1987; 64:596–601.

366. Martha PM, Rogol AD, Veldhuis JD, et al. Alterations in the pulsatile properties of circulating growth hormone concentrations during puberty in boys. J Clin Endocrinol Metab 1989; 69:563–570.

367. Rudman D, Kutner MH, Rogers CM, et al. Impaired growth hormone secretion in the adult population. J Clin Invest 1981; 67:1361–1369.

368. Johanson AJ, Blizzard RM. Low somatomedin-C levels in older men rise in response to growth hormone administration. Johns Hopkins Med J 1981; 149:115–117.

369. Underwood LE, D'Ercole AJ, Van Wyk JJ. Somatomedin-C and the assessment of growth. Pediatr Clin North Am 1980; 27:771–782.

370. Bucher H, Zapf J, Torresani T, et al. Insulin-like growth factors I and II, prolactin, and insulin in 19 growth hormone–deficient children with excessive, normal or decreased longitudinal growth after operation for craniopharyngioma. N Engl J Med 1983; 309:1142–1146.

371. Clemmons DR, Underwood LE, Ridgway EC, et al. Hyperprolactinemia is associated with increased immunoreactive somatomedin-C in hypopituitarism. J Clin Endocrinol Metab 1981; 52:731–735.

372. Reiter EO, Lovinger RD. The use of a commercially available somatomedin-C radioimmunoassay in patients with disorders of growth. J Pediatr 1981; 99:720–724.

373. Moore DC, Ruvalcaba RHA, Smith EK, et al. Plasma somatomedin-C as a screening test for growth hormone deficiency in children and adolescents. Horm Res 1982; 16:49–55.

374. Dean JH, Kellet JG, Bala RM, et al. The effect of growth hormone treatment on somatomedin levels in growth hormone–deficient children. J Clin Endocrinol Metab 1982; 55:1167–1173.

375. Clemmons DR, Van Wyk JJ, Ridgway EC, et al. Evaluation of acromegaly by radioimmunoassay of somatomedin-C. N Engl J Med 1979; 301:1138–1142.

376. Rieu M, Girard F, Bicaire H, et al. The importance of insulin-like growth factor (somatomedin) measurements in the diagnosis and surveillance of acromegaly. J Clin Endocrinol Metab 1982; 55:147–153.

377. Barken A, Beitins IZ, Kelch RP. Plasma insulin-like growth factor I/somatomedin C in acromegaly: correlation with the degree of growth hormone hypersecretion. J Clin Endocrinol Metab 1988; 67:69–73.

378. Furlanetto RW, Underwood LE, Van Wyk JJ, et al. Serum immunoreactive somatomedin-C is elevated late in pregnancy. J Clin Endocrinol Metab 1978; 47:695–698.

379. Wass JAH, Clemmons DR, Underwood LE, et al. Changes in circulating somatomedin-C levels in bromocriptine-treated acromegaly. Clin Endocrinol 1982; 17:369–377.

380. Clemmons DR, Underwood LE, Ridgway EC, et al. Estradiol treatment of acromegaly: reduction of immunoreactive somatomedin-C and improvement in metabolic status. Am J Med 1980; 69:571–575.

381. Hurley TW, D'Ercole AJ, Handwerger S, et al. Ovine placental lactogen induces somatomedin: a possible role in fetal growth. Endocrinology 1977; 101:1635–1638.

382. Phillips LS. Nutrition, metabolism and growth. In: Daughaday WH, ed. Endocrine Control of Growth. New York: Elsevier, 1981: 121–173.

383. Underwood LE, Smith EP, Clemmons DR, et al. The production and actions of insulin-like growth factors: their relationship to nutrition and growth. In: Tanner JM, ed. Auxology 88. London: Smith-Gordon, 1989: 235–249.

384. Clemmons DR, Klibanski A, Underwood LE, et al. Reduction of immunoreactive somatomedin-C during fasting in humans. J Clin Endocrinol Metab 1981; 53:1247–1250.

385. Merimee TJ, Zapf J, Froesch ER. Insulin-like growth factors in the fed and fasted states. J Clin Endocrinol Metab 1982; 55:999–1002.

386. Isley WL, Underwood LE, Clemmons DR. Dietary components that regulate serum somatomedin-C concentrations in humans. J Clin Invest 1983; 71:175–182.

387. Clemmons DR, Seek M, Underwood LE. Supplemental essential amino acids augment the somatomedin-C/insulin-like growth factor I response to refeeding after fasting. Metabolism 1985; 34:391–395.

388. Clemmons DR, Underwood LE, Dickerson RN, et al. Use of plasma somatomedin-C/insulin-like growth factor I measurements to monitor the response to nutritional repletion in malnourished patients. Am J Clin Nutr 1985; 41:191–198.

389. Unterman TG, Vazquez RM, Slas AJ, et al. Nutrition and somatomedin. XIII. Usefulness of somatomedin-C in nutritional assessment. Am J Med 1985; 78:228–234.

390. Goldberg AC, Trivedi B, Delmez JA, et al. Uremia reduces serum insulin-like growth factor I, increases insulin-like growth factor II and modifies their serum protein binding. J Clin Endocrinol Metab 1982; 55:1040–1045.

391. D'Ercole AJ. Somatomedins/insulin-like growth factors and fetal development. J Dev Physiol 1987; 9:481–495.

392. Brice AL, Cheetham JE, Bolton VN, et al. Temporal changes in the expression of the insulin-like growth factor II gene associated with tissue maturation in the human fetus. Development 1989; 106:543–554.

393. Han VK, D'Ercole AJ, Lund PK. Cellular localization of somatomedin (insulin-like growth factor) messenger RNA in the human fetus. Science 1987; 236:193–197.

394. Smith EP, Sadler TW, D'Ercole AJ. Somatomedins/insulin-like growth factors, their receptors and binding proteins are present during mouse embryogenesis. Development 1987; 101:73–82.

395. D'Ercole AJ. Somatomedins/insulin-like growth factors. In: Brook CGD, ed. Clinical Paediatric Endocrinology. 2nd ed. Oxford: Blackwell Scientific, 1989: 74–95.

396. Grizzard JD, D'Ercole AJ, Wilkins JR, et al. Affinity labeled somatomedin-C receptors and binding proteins from the human fetus. J Clin Endocrinol Metab 1984; 58:535–543.

397. DeChiara TM, Efstratiadis A, Robertson EJ. A growth-deficiency phenotype in heterozygous mice carrying an insulin-like growth factor II gene disrupted by targeting. Nature 1990; 345:78–80.

398. Lunk PK, Moats-Staats BM, Hynes MA, et al. Somatomedin-C/insulin-like growth factor-I and insulin-like growth factor-II mRNAs in rat fetal and adult tissues. J Biol Chem 1986; 261:14539–14544.

399. Hynes MA, Van Wyk JJ, Brooks PJ, et al. Growth hormone dependence of somatomedin-C/insulin-like growth factor-I and insulin-like growth factor-II messenger ribonucleic acids. Mol Endocrinol 1987; 1:233–242.

400. Hynes MA, Brooks PJ, Van Wyk JJ, et al. Insulin-like growth factor II messenger ribonucleic acids are synthesized in the choroid plexus of the rat brain. Mol Endocrinol 1988; 2:47–54.

401. Schoenle EJ, Haselbacher GK, Briner J, et al. Elevated concentration of IGF-II in brain tissue from an infant with macroencephaly. J Pediatr 1986; 108:737–740.

402. Mohan S, Jennings JC, Linkhart TA, et al. Primary structure of human skeletal growth factor: homology with human insulin-like growth factor-II. Biochim Biophys Acta 1988; 961:44–55.

403. Frolik CA, Ellis EF, Williams DC. Isolation and characterization of insulin-like growth factor-II from human bone. Biochem Biophys Res Commun 1988; 151:1011–1018.

404. Murphy LJ, Friesen HG. Differential effects of estrogen and growth hormone on uterine and hepatic insulin-like growth factor I gene expression in the ovariectomized hypophysectomized rat. Endocrinology 1988; 122:325–332.

405. Hammond JM, Hsu CJ, Klindt J, et al. Gonadotropins increase concentrations of immunoreactive insulin-like growth factor-I in porcine follicular fluid in vivo. Biol Reprod 1988; 38:304–308.

406. Naville D, Chatelain PG, Avallet O, et al. Control of production of insulin-like growth factor I by pig Leydig and Sertoli cells cultured alone or together. Cell-cell interactions. Mol Cell Endocrinol 1990; 70:217–224.

407. de Pagter Holthuizen P, Jansen M, van Schaik FM, et al. The human insulin-like growth factor-II gene contains two development-specific promoters. FEBS Lett 1987; 214:259–264.

408. Han VKM, Hill DJ, Strain AJ, et al. Identification of somatomedin/insulin like growth factor immunoreactive cells in the human fetus. Pediatr Res 1987; 22:245–249.

409. Bottenstein J, Hayashi L, Hutchings S, et al. The growth of cells in serum-free hormone-supplemented media. Methods Enzymol 1979; 58:94–109.

410. Pledger WJ, Stiles CD, Antoniades HN, et al. Induction of DNA synthesis in BALB/c 3T3 cells by serum components: a reevaluation of the commitment process. Proc Natl Acad Sci USA 1977; 74:4481–4485.

411. Stiles CD, Capone GT, Scher CD, et al. Dual control of cell growth by somatomedins and platelet derived growth factor. Proc Natl Acad Sci USA 1979; 76:1279–1283.

412. Leof EB, Van Wyk JJ, O'efe EJ, et al. Epidermal growth factor (EGF) is required only during the traverse of early G_1 in PDGF stimulated density-arrested BALB/c 3T3 cells. Exp Cell Res 1983; 147:202–208.

413. Leof EB, Wharton W, Van Wyk JJ, et al. Epidermal growth factor and somatomedin-C regulate G_1 progression in competent BALB/c 3T3 cells. Exp Cell Res 1982; 141:107–115.

414. Van Wyk JJ, Casella SJ, Graves DR, et al. Evidence from monoclonal antibody studies that insulin stimulates deoxyribonucleic acid synthesis through the type I somatomedin receptor. J Clin Endocrinol Metab 1985; 61:639–643.

415. Clemmons DR, Van Wyk JJ. Evidence for a functional role of endogenously produced somatomedin-like peptides in the stimulation of human fibroblast and porcine smooth muscle cell DNA synthesis. J Clin Invest 1985; 75:1914–1918.

416. Clemmons DR. Multiple hormones stimulate the production of somatomedin by cultured human fibroblasts. J Clin Endocrinol Metab 1984; 58:850–856.

417. Van Wyk JJ, Russell WE, Underwood LE, et al. Action of somatomedins on cell growth: effect of selective neutralization of somatomedin-C (insulin-like growth factor I) with a monoclonal antibody. In: Raiti S, Tolman RA, eds. Human Growth Hormone. New York: Plenum, 1986: 609–619.

418. Van Wyk JJ, Conti M, del Monte P, et al. The role of somatomedins in the growth and function of endocrine tissues. In: Sizonenko PC, Aubert ML, eds. The Endocrinology of Adolescence. New York: Raven, 1990: 127–140.

419. Merchav S, Tatarsky I, Hochberg Z. Enhancement of erythropoiesis in vitro by human growth hormone is mediated by insulin-like growth factor-I. Br J Haematol 1988; 70:267–271.

420. Penhoat A, Jaillard C, Saez JM. Synergistic effects of corticotropin and insulin-like growth factor-I on corticotropin receptors and corticotropin responsiveness in cultured bovine adrenocortical cells. Biochim Biophys Res Commun 1989; 165:355–359.

421. Adashi EY, Resnick CE, Hernandez JV, et al. Insulin-like growth factor I as an amplifier of follicle-stimulating hormone action: studies on mechanism(s) and site(s) of action in cultured rat granulosa cells. Endocrinology 1988; 122:1583–1591.

422. Magoffin DA, Kurtz KM, Erickson GF. Insulin-like growth factor-I selectively stimulates cholesterol side-chain cleavage expression in ovarian theca-interstitial cells. Mol Endocrinol 1990; 4:489–496.

423. Kasson BG, Hsueh AJ. Insulin-like growth factor-I augments gonadotropin-stimulated androgen biosynthesis by cultured rat testicular cells. Mol Cell Endocrinol 1987; 52:27–34.

424. Veldhuis JD, Rodgers RJ, Dee A, et al. The insulin-like growth factor, somatomedin-C, induces the synthesis of cholesterol side-chain cleavage cytochrome P-450 and adrenodoxin in ovarian cells. J Biol Chem 1986; 261:2499–2502.

425. Mondschein JS, Canning SF, Miller DQ, et al. Insulin-like growth factors (IGFs) as autocrine/paracrine regulators of granulosa cell differentiation and growth: studies with a neutralizing monoclonal antibody to IGF-I. Biol Reprod 1989; 41:79–85.

426. Shimasaki S, Shimonaka M, Ui M, et al. Structural characterization of a follicle-stimulating hormone action inhibitor in porcine ovarian follicular fluid. Its identification as the insulin-like growth factor–binding protein. J Biol Chem 1990; 265:2198–2202.

427. Ui M, Shimonaka M, Shimasaki S, et al. An insulin-like growth factor–binding protein in ovarian follicular fluid blocks follicle-stimulating hormone–stimulated steroid production by ovarian granulosa cells. Endocrinology 1989; 125:912–916.

428. Pekonen F, Laatikainen T, Buyalos R, et al. Decreased 34K insulin-like growth factor binding protein in polycystic ovarian disease. Fertil Steril 1989; 51:972–975.

429. Takahashi SI, Conti M, Van Wyk JJ. Thyrotropin potentiation of insulin-like growth factor-I dependent deoxyribonucleic acid synthesis in FRTL-5 cells: mediation by an autocrine amplification factor(s). Endocrinology 1990; 126:736–745.

430. Takahashi SI, Conti M, Prokop C, et al. Thyrotropin and insulin-like growth factor I regulation of tyrosine phosphorylation in FRTL-5 cells. J Biol Chem 1991; 266:7834–7841.

431. Florini JR, Ewton DZ, Falen SL, et al. Biphasic concentration dependency of the stimulation of myoblast differentiation by somatomedins. Am J Physiol 1986; 250:C771–C778.

432. Turo KA, Florini JR. Hormonal stimulation of myoblast differentiation in the absence of DNA synthesis. Am J Physiol 1982; 243:C278–C284.

433. Florini JR, Ewton DZ. Highly specific inhibition of IGF-I stimulated differentiation by an antisense oligodeoxyribonucleotide to myogenin mRNA. No effects on other actions of IGF-I. J Biol Chem 1990; 265:13435–13437.

434. Rothstein H, Van Wyk JJ, Hayden JH, et al. Somatomedin-C: restoration of in vivo cycle traverse in G_0/G_1 blocked cells of hypophysectomized animals. Science 1980; 208:410–412.

435. Reddan JR, Dziedzic DC. Insulin-like growth factors, IGF-I, IGF-2 and somatomedin C trigger cell proliferation in mammalian epithelial cells cultured in a serum-free medium. Exp Cell Res 1982; 142:293–300.

436. Beebe DC, Silver MH, Belcher KS, et al. Lentropin, a protein that controls lens fiber formation, is related functionally and immunologically to the insulin-like growth factors. Proc Natl Acad Sci USA 1987; 84:2327–2330.

437. Mohan S, Jennings JC, Linkhart TA, et al. Primary structure of human skeletal growth factor: homology with human insulin-like growth factor II. Biochim Biophys Acta 1988; 961:44–55.

438. Frolik CA, Ellis EF, Williams DC. Isolation and characterization of insulin-like growth factor II from human bone. Biochem Biophys Res Commun 1988; 151:1011–1018.

439. McCarthy TL, Centrella M, Canalis E. Insulin-like growth factor (IGF) and bone. Connect Tissue Res 1989; 20:277–282.

440. Canalis E, McCarthy T, Centrella M. Growth factors and the regulation of bone remodeling. J Clin Invest 1988; 81:277–281.

441. Froesch ER, Guler HP, Schmid C, et al. Therapeutic potential of insulin-like growth factor I. Trends Endocrinol Metab 1990; 1:254–260.

442. Van Buul-Offers S, Ueda I, Van den Brande JL. Biosynthetic somatomedin-C (Sm-C/IGF-I) increases the length and weight of Snell dwarf mice. Pediatr Res 1986; 20:825–827.

443. Hizuka N, Takano K, Asakawa K, et al. In vivo effects of insulin-like growth factor I in rats. Endocrinol Jpn 1987; 34(Suppl):115–121.

444. Guler HP, Zapf J, Schiewiller E, et al. Recombinant human insulin-like growth factor I stimulates growth and has distinct effects on organ size in hypophysectomized rats. Proc Natl Acad Sci USA 1988; 85:4889–4893.

445. Guler HP, Schmid C, Zapf J, et al. Effects of recombinant insulin-like growth factor I on insulin secretion and renal function in normal human subjects. Proc Natl Acad Sci USA 1989; 86:2868–2872.

446. Schiewiller E, Guler HP, Merryweather J, et al. Growth restoration in insulin-deficient diabetic rats by recombinant human insulin-like growth factor I. Nature 1986; 323:169–171.

Disorders of Human Growth

447. Cameron N. The methods of auxological anthropometry. In: Falkner F, Tanner JM, eds. Human Growth: A Comprehensive Treatise. Vol 2.

Postnatal Growth, Neurobiology. 2nd ed. New York: Plenum, 1986: 35–90.

448. Whitehouse RH, Tanner JM, Healy MJR. Diurnal variation in stature and sitting height in 12–14 year old boys. Ann Hum Biol 1974; 1:103–106.

449. Marshall WA. Evaluation of growth rate in height over periods of less than 1 year. Arch Dis Child 1971; 46:414–420.

450. Hamill PVV, Drizd TA, Johnson CL, et al. Physical growth: National Center for Health Statistics percentiles. Am J Clin Nutr 1979; 32:607–629.

451. Hamill PV, Johnson FE, Lemeshaw S. Body weight, stature and sitting height: white and Negro youths' 12–17 years. DHEW Publication No. (HRA) 74-1608. Series 11. No. 126. Washington, DC: Government Printing Office, 1973.

452. Tanner JM, Whitehouse RH. Sitting Height Charts. Herts, England: Castlemead Publications, Ward's Publishing Services.

453. Marshall WA. Puberty. In: Falkner F, Tanner JM, eds. Human Growth: A Comprehensive Treatise. Vol 2. Postnatal Growth, Neurobiology. 2nd ed. New York: Plenum, 1986: 141–181.

454. Lee PA. Normal ages of pubertal events among American males and females. J Adolesc Health Care 1980; 1:26–29.

455. Eveleth PB, Tanner JM. Worldwide Variation in Human Growth. London: Cambridge University Press, 1976.

456. Singleton A, Patois E, Pedron G, et al. Croissance de la taille, du segment supérieur et du diamètre biiliaque chez la fille après l'apparition des premières règles. Arch Fr Pediatr 1975; 32:859–870.

457. Laron Z, Zilka E. Compensatory hypertrophy of testicle in unilateral cryptorchidism. J Clin Endocrinol Metab 1969; 29:1409–1413.

458. Zachmann M, Prader A, Kind HP, et al. Testicular volume during adolescence: cross-sectional and longitudinal studies. Helv Paediatr Acta 1974; 29:61–72.

459. Schonfeld WA. Primary and secondary sexual characteristics: study of their development in males from birth through maturity, with biometric study of penis and testes. Am J Dis Child 1943; 65:535–549.

460. Roche AF, French NY, Davila GH. Areolar size during pubescence. Hum Biol 1971; 43:210–223.

461. Zachmann M, Sobradillo B, Frank M, et al. Bayley-Pinneau, Roche-Wainer-Thissen, and Tanner height predictions in normal children and in patients with various pathologic conditions. J Pediatr 1978; 93:749–755.

462. D'Ercole AJ, Underwood LE. Regulation of fetal growth by hormones and growth factors. In: Falkner F, Tanner JM, eds. Human Growth: A Comprehensive Treatise. Vol 1. Developmental Biology, Prenatal Growth. 2nd ed. New York: Plenum, 1986: 327–338.

463. Sizonenko PC, Aubert ML. Pre- and perinatal endocrinology. In: Falkner F, Tanner JM, eds. Human Growth: A Comprehensive Treatise. Vol 1. Developmental Biology, Prenatal Growth. 2nd ed. New York: Plenum, 1986: 339–376.

464. Milner RDG, Hill DJ. Fetal growth control: the role of insulin and related peptides. Clin Endocrinol 1984; 21:415–433.

465. Hill DJ. Peptide growth factors in fetal development. In: Tanner JM, Preece MA, eds. The Physiology of Human Growth. Cambridge: The Press Syndicate of the University of Cambridge, 1989: 141–166.

466. Gluckman PD, Brinsmead MW. Somatomedin in cord blood: relationship to gestational age and birth size. J Clin Endocrinol Metab 1976; 43:1378–1381.

467. Underwood LE, D'Ercole AJ, Furlanetto RW, et al. Somatomedin and growth: a possible role for somatomedin-C in fetal growth. In: Giordano G, Van Wyk JJ, Minuto F, eds. Somatomedin and Growth. New York: Academic, 1979: 215–223.

468. Gould JB. The low-birth-weight infant. In: Falkner F, Tanner JM, eds. Human Growth: A Comprehensive Treatise. Vol 1. Developmental Biology, Prenatal Growth. 2nd ed. New York: Plenum, 1986: 391–413.

469. Kitchen WH, Ryan MM, Rickards A, et al. Changing outcome over 13 years of very low birthweight infants. Semin Perinatol 1982; 6:373–389.

470. Lubchenco LO. Assessment of gestational age and development at birth. Pediatr Clin North Am 1970; 17:125–145.

471. Lubchenco LO, Hansman C, Boyd E. Intrauterine growth in length and head circumference as estimated from live births at gestational ages from 26–42 weeks. Pediatrics 1966; 37:403–408.

472. Tanner JM, Thomson AM. Standards for birthweight at gestation periods from 32–42 weeks, allowing for maternal height and weight. Arch Dis Child 1970; 45:566–569.

473. Brandt I. Growth dynamics of low-birth-weight infants with emphasis on the perinatal period. In: Falkner F, Tanner JM, eds. Human Growth: A Comprehensive Treatise. Vol. 1. Developmental Biology, Prenatal Growth. 2nd ed. New York: Plenum, 1986: 415–475.

474. Harding PGR. Fetal growth and nutrition. In: Goodwin JW, Gooden JO, Chance GW, eds. Perinatal Medicine. Baltimore: Williams & Wilkins, 1976: 255–269.

475. Edwards LE, Alton IR, Barrada MI, et al. Pregnancy in the underweight woman: course, outcome, and growth patterns of the infant. Am J Obstet Gynecol 1979; 135:297–302.

476. Winick M. Malnutrition and Brain Development. New York: Oxford University Press, 1976.

477. Jones OW. Genetic factors in the determination of fetal size. J Reprod Med 1978; 21:305–313.

478. Jones KL, Smith DW, Ulleland CN, et al. Pattern of malformation in offspring of chronic alcoholic mothers. Lancet 1973; 1:1267–1271.

479. Ouellette EM, Rosett HL, Rosman NP, et al. Adverse effects on offspring of maternal alcohol abuse during pregnancy. N Engl J Med 1977; 297:528–530.

480. Clarren SK, Smith DW. The fetal alcohol syndrome. N Engl J Med 1978; 298:1063–1067.

481. Fisher SE. The fetal alcohol syndrome. In: Lifshitz F, ed. Pediatric Endocrinology. New York: Marcel Dekker, 1985: 129–139.

482. Jones KL, Smith DW, Streissguth AP. Outcome in offspring of chronic alcoholic women. Lancet 1974; 1:1076–1078.

483. Russell M. Intrauterine growth in infants born to women with alcohol-related psychiatric diagnoses. Alcoholism 1977; 1:225–231.

484. Abel EL. Consumption of alcohol during pregnancy: A review of effects on growth and development of offspring. Hum Biol 1982; 54:421–453.

485. Jones KC, Chernoff GF. Drugs and chemicals associated with intrauterine growth deficiency. J Reprod Med 1978; 21:365–370.

486. Abel EL. Smoking during pregnancy: a review of effects on growth and development of offspring. Hum Biol 1980; 52:593–625.

487. MacGregor SN, Keith LG, Chasnoff IJ, et al. Cocaine use during pregnancy: adverse perinatal outcome. Am J Obstet Gynecol 1987; 157:686–690.

488. Chasnoff IJ, Griffith DR, MacGregor S, et al. Temporal patterns of cocaine use in pregnancy: perinatal outcome. JAMA 1989; 261:1741–1744.

489. Zuckerman B, Frank DA, Hingson R, et al. Effects of maternal marijuana and cocaine use on fetal growth. N Engl J Med 1989; 320:762–768.

490. Tanner JM, Goldstein H, Whitehouse RH. Standards for children's height at ages 2–9 years allowing for height of parents. Arch Dis Child 1970; 45:755–762.

491. Springer JW, Langer L Jr, Wiedemann HR. Bone Dysplasias: An Atlas of Constitutional Disorders of Skeletal Development. Philadelphia: W. B. Saunders, 1974.

492. Shapiro F. Epiphyseal disorders. N Engl J Med 1987; 317:1702–1710.

493. Maroteaux P. Nomenclature internationale des maladies osseuses constitutionnelles. Ann Radiol 1970; 13:455–464.

494. Rimoin DL. International nomenclature of constitutional diseases of bone: revision—May 1977. J Pediatr 1978; 93:614–616.

495. Stanescu V, Stanescu R, Maroteaux P. Pathogenic mechanisms in osteochondrodysplasias. J Bone Joint Surg 1984; 66A: 817–835.

496. Horton WA, Rotter JI, Rimoin DL, et al. Standard growth curves for achondroplasia. J Pediatr 1978; 93:435–438.

497. Horton WA, Hall JG, Scott CI, et al. Growth curves for height for diastrophic dysplasia, spondyloepiphyseal dysplasia congenita, and pseudoachondroplasia. Am J Dis Child 1982; 136:316–319.

498. Wladimiroff JW, Niermijer MF, Laar M, et al. Prenatal diagnosis of skeletal dysplasia by real-time ultrasound. Obstet Gynecol 1984; 63:360–364.

499. Cronk CE, Pueschel SM. Anthropometric studies. In: Pueschel SM, ed. The Young Child with Down Syndrome. New York: Human Science Press, 1984: 105–142.

500. Cronk C, Crocker AC, Pueschel SM, et al. Growth charts for children with Down syndrome: 1 month to 18 years of age. Pediatrics 1988; 81:102–110.

501. Rosenfeld RG, Grumbach MM. Turner Syndrome. New York: Marcel Dekker, 1988.

502. Hall JG, Sybert VP, Williamson RA, et al. Turner's syndrome. West J Med 1982; 137:32–44.

503. Kalousek D, Schiffrin A, Berguer AM, et al. Partial short arm deletions of the X chromosome and spontaneous pubertal development in girls with short stature. J Pediatr 1979; 94:891–894.

504. Goldstein DE, Kelly TE, Johanson AJ, et al. Gonadal dysgenesis with 45,XO/46,XX mosaicism demonstrated only in a streak gonad. J Pediatr 1977; 90:604–605.

505. Ranke MB, Pfluger H, Rosendahl W, et al. Turner syndrome: spontaneous growth in 150 cases and review of the literature. Eur J Pediatr 1983; 141:81–88.

506. Lyon AJ, Preece MA, Grant DB. Growth curve for girls with Turner syndrome. Arch Dis Child 1985; 60:932–935.

507. Urban MD, Lee PA, Dorst JP, et al. Oxandrolone therapy in patients with Turner syndrome. J Pediatr 1979; 94:823–827.

508. Moore DC, Tattoni DS, Ruvalcaba RH, et al. Studies of anabolic steroids. VI. Effect of prolonged administration of oxandrolone on growth in children and adolescents with gonadal dysgenesis. J Pediatr 1977; 90:462–466.

509. Lenko HL, Perheentupa J, Soderholm A. Growth in Turner's syndrome: spontaneous and fluoxymesterone stimulated. Acta Paediatr Scand Suppl 1979; 277:57–63.

510. Nilsson KO. What is the value of growth hormone treatment in short children with specified syndrome? Acta Paediatr Scand Suppl 1989; 362:61–68.

511. Rosenfeld RG, Hintz RL, Johanson AJ, et al. Three year results of a

randomized prospective trial of methionyl human growth hormone and oxandrolone in Turner syndrome. J Pediatr 1988; 113:393–400.

512. Lucky AW, Marynick SP, Rebar RW, et al. Replacement oral ethinyloestradiol therapy for gonadal dysgenesis: growth and adrenal androgen studies. Acta Endocrinol 1979; 91:519–528.

513. Ross JL, Long LM, Skerda M, et al. Effect of low doses of estradiol on 6-month growth rates and predicted height in patients with Turner syndrome. J Pediatr 1986; 109:950–958.

514. Ross JL, Cutler GB. Estrogen therapy in Turner syndrome. In: Rosenfeld R, Grumbach MM, eds. Turner Syndrome. New York: Marcel Dekker, 1990: 361–369.

515. Martinez A, Heinrich JJ, Domene H, et al. Growth in Turner's syndrome: long-term treatment with low dose ethinyl estradiol. J Clin Endocrinol Metab 1987; 65:253–257.

516. Smith DW. Recognizable Patterns of Human Malformation: Genetic, Embryologic and Clinical Aspects. 3rd ed. Philadelphia: W. B. Saunders, 1982.

517. Gorlin RJ, Pindborg JJ. Syndromes of the Head and Neck. 2nd ed. New York: McGraw-Hill, 1976.

518. Bergsma D. Birth Defects Compendium. 2nd ed. New York: Alan R. Liss, 1979.

519. Salmon MA, Lindenbaum RH. Developmental Defects and Syndromes. Aylesbury, England: HM & M Publishers, 1978.

520. McKusick VA. Mendelian Inheritance in Man. 4th ed. Baltimore: Johns Hopkins University Press, 1983.

521. Preece MA, Law CM, Davies PSW. The growth of children with chronic paediatric disease. Clin Endocrinol Metab 1986; 15:453–477.

522. Pimstone B, Barbezat G, Hansen JD, et al. Growth hormone and protein-calorie malnutrition. Impaired suppression during induced hyperglycaemia. Lancet 1967; 2:1333–1334.

523. Grant DB, Hambley J, Becker D, et al. Reduced sulphation factor in undernourished children. Arch Dis Child 1973; 48:596–600.

524. Pugliese MT, Lifhhitz F, Grad G, et al. Fear of obesity: a cause of short stature and delayed puberty. N Engl J Med 1983; 309:513–518.

525. Judisch JM, Naiman JL, Oski FA. The fallacy of the fat iron-deficient child. Pediatrics 1966; 37:987–990.

526. Woodruff CW. Iron deficiency in infancy and childhood. Pediatr Clin North Am 1977; 24:85–94.

527. Hambidge KM. The role of zinc and other trace metals in pediatric nutrition and health. Pediatr Clin North Am 1977; 24:95–106.

528. Gordon EF, Gordon RC, Passal DB. Zinc metabolism: basic, clinical and behavioral aspects. J Pediatr 1981; 99:341–349.

529. Lifshitz F, Zandsberg S. Disorders of growth. In: Lifshitz F, ed. Pediatric Endocrinology. New York: Marcel Dekker, 1985: 3–36.

530. Prasad AS. Clinical endocrinological and biochemical effects of zinc deficiency. Clin Endocrinol Metab 1985; 14:567–589.

531. Groll A, Candy D, Preece M, et al. Short stature as the primary manifestation of coeliac disease. Lancet 1980; 2:1097–1099.

532. Stenhammar L, Fallstrom SP, Jansson G, et al. Coeliac disease in children of short stature without gastrointestinal symptoms. Eur J Pediatr 1986; 145:185–186.

533. Verkasalo M, Kuitunen P, Leisti S, et al. Growth failure from symptomless celiac disease. A study of 14 patients. Hevl Paediatr Acta 1978; 33:489–495.

534. Auricchio S, Greco L, Troncone R. Gluten-sensitive enteropathy in childhood. Pediatr Clin North Am 1988; 35:157–187.

535. Lecornu M, David L, Francois R. Low serum somatomedin activity in celiac disease. Helv Paediatr Acta 1978; 33:509–516.

536. Kirschner BS. Nutritional consequences of inflammatory bowel disease on growth. J Am Coll Nutr 1988; 7:301–308.

537. Mock DM. Growth retardation in chronic inflammatory bowel disease. Gastroenterol 1986; 91:1019–1023.

538. Booth IW, Harries JT. Inflammatory bowel disease in childhood. Gut 1984; 25:188–202.

539. Layden T, Rosenberg J, Nemchausky B, et al. Reversal of growth arrest in adolescents with Crohn's disease after parenteral alimentation. Gastroenterology 1976; 70:1017–1021.

540. Kirschner BS, Klich JR, Kalmen SS, et al. Reversal of growth retardation in Crohn's disease with therapy emphasizing oral nutritional restitution. Gastroenterology 1981; 80:10–15.

541. Rosenthal SR, Snyder JD, Hendricks KM, et al. Growth failure and inflammatory bowel disease: approach to treatment of a complicated adolescent problem. Pediatrics 1983; 72:481–490.

542. Holliday MA, ed. Symposium on metabolism and growth in children with kidney disease. Kidney Int 1978; 14:299–382.

543. Betts PR, Magrath G. Growth pattern and dietary intake of children with chronic renal insufficiency. Br Med J 1974; 2:189–193.

544. Chesney RW. Growth retardation in childhood renal disease: a hormonal or nutritional problem? Am J Nephrol 1987; 7:253–256.

545. Rizzoni G, Broyer M, Guest G, et al. Growth retardation in childhood renal disease: scope of the problem. Am J Kidney Dis 1986; 7:256–261.

546. Mehls O, Ritz E, Hunziken EB, et al. Improvement of growth and food utilization by human recombinant growth hormone in uremia. Kidney Int 1988; 33:45–52.

547. Koch VH, Lippe BM, Nelson PA, et al. Accelerated growth after recombinant human growth hormone treatment of children with chronic renal failure. J Pediatr 1989; 115:365–371.

548. Avioli LV. Childhood renal osteodystrophy. Kidney Int 1978; 14:355–360.

549. Chesney RW, Moorthy AV, Eisman JA, et al. Increased growth after long-term oral 1,25-vitamin D_3 in childhood renal osteodystrophy. N Engl J Med 1978; 298:238–242.

550. Langman CB, Mazur AT, Baron R, et al. 25-Hydroxyvitamin D_3 (calcifediol) therapy of juvenile renal osteodystrophy: beneficial effect on linear growth velocity. J Pediatr 1982; 100:815–820.

551. Chan JCM, Kodroff MB, Landwehr DM. Effects of 1,25-dihydroxyvitamin-D_3 on renal failure. Pediatrics 1981; 68:559–571.

552. Feldt RH, Strickler GB, Weidman WH. Growth of children with congenital heart disease. Am J Dis Child 1969; 117:573–579.

553. Bayer LM, Robinson SJ. Growth history of children with congenital heart defects. Am J Dis Child 1969; 117:564–572.

554. Noonan JA. Association of congenital heart disease with syndromes or other defects. Pediatr Clin North Am 1978; 25:797–816.

555. Levy RJ, Rosenthal A, Miettinen OS, et al. Determinants of growth in patients with ventricular septal defect. Circulation 1978; 57:793–797.

556. Frasier SD, Hilburn JM, Smith FG Jr. Dwarfism and mental retardation: the serum growth hormone response to hypoglycemia. J Pediatr 1970; 77:136–138.

557. Stevens MCG, Maude GH, Cupidore L. Prepubertal growth and skeletal maturation in children with sickle cell disease. Pediatrics 1986; 78:124–132.

558. Platt OS, Rosenstock W, Espeland MA. Influence of sickle hemoglobinopathies on growth and development. N Engl J Med 1984; 311:7–12.

559. Phebus CK, Gloninger MF, Maciak BJ. Growth patterns by age and sex in children with sickle cell disease. J Pediatr 1984; 105:28–33.

560. Heyman MB, Vichinsky E, Katz R, et al. Growth retardation in sickle cell disease treated by nutritional support. Lancet 1985; 1:903–906.

561. DeLuca F, Simone E, Corona G, et al. Adult height in thalassaemia major without hormonal treatment. Eur J Pediatr 1987; 146:494–496.

562. Borgna-Pignatti C, De Stefano P, Zonta L, et al. Growth and sexual maturation in thalassemia major. J Pediatr 1985; 106:150–155.

563. Saenger P, Schwartz E, Markenson AL, et al. Depressed serum somatomedin activity in beta-thalassemia. J Pediatr 1980; 96:214–218.

564. Werther GA, Matthews RN, Burger HG, et al. Lack of response of non-suppressible insulin-like activity to short-term administration of human growth hormone in thalassemia major. J Clin Endocrinol Metab 1981; 53:806–809.

565. Pintor C, Cella SG, Manso P, et al. Impaired growth hormone (GH) response to GH-releasing hormone in thalassemia major. J Clin Endocrinol Metab 1986; 62:263–267.

566. Mandell F, Berenberg W. The Mauriac syndrome. Am J Dis Child 1974; 127:900–902.

567. Hjelt K, Braendholt V, Kamper J, et al. Growth in children with diabetes mellitus. Dan Med Bull 1983; 30:28–33.

568. Jivani SKM, Rayner PHW. Does control influence the growth of diabetic children? Arch Dis Child 1973; 48:109–115.

569. Herber SM, Dunsmore IR. Does control affect growth in diabetes mellitus? Acta Paediatr Scand 1988; 77:303–305.

570. Rudolf MCJ, Sherwin RS, Markowitz R, et al. Effect of intensive insulin treatment on linear growth in the young diabetic patient. J Pediatr 1982; 101:333–339.

571. Thain ME, Hamilton JR, Ehrlich RM. Coexistence of diabetes mellitus and celiac disease. J Pediatr 1974; 85:527–529.

572. Rasmussen H, Tenenhouse HS. Hypophosphatemias. In: Scriver CS, Beaudet AL, Sly WS, et al., eds. The Metabolic Basis of Inherited Disease. 6th ed. New York: McGraw-Hill, 1989: 2581–2604.

573. Herweijer TJ, Steendijk R. The relationship between attained adult height and the metaphyseal lesions in hypophosphataemic vitamin-D resistant rickets. Acta Paediatr Scand 1985; 74:196–200.

574. Chan JCM. Renal hypophosphatemic rickets—a review. Int J Pediatr Nephrol 1982; 3:305–310.

575. Scriver CS, Beaudet AL, Sly WS, et al., eds. The Metabolic Basis of Inherited Disease. New York: McGraw-Hill, 1989.

576. Vimpani GV, Vimpani AF, Lidgard GP, et al. Prevalence of severe growth hormone deficiency. Br Med J 1977; 2:427–430.

577. Rona RJ, Tanner JM. Aetiology of idiopathic growth hormone deficiency in England and Wales. Arch Dis Child 1977; 52:197–208.

578. Lacey KA, Parkin JM. Causes of short stature—a community study of children in Newcastle-upon-Tyne. Lancet 1974; 1:42–45.

579. Phillips JA. Genetic defects in processing growth hormone. In: Bercu B, ed. Basic and Clinical Aspects of Growth Hormone. New York: Plenum, 1988: 57–67.

580. Rimoin DL, Schimke RN. Genetic Disorders of the Endocrine Glands. St. Louis: C. V. Mosby, 1971.

581. Rimoin DL. Genetic disorders of the pituitary gland. In: Emery AEH, Rimoin DL, eds. Principles and Practices of Medical Genetics. Vol 2. Edinburgh: Churchill Livingstone, 1983: 1134–1151.

582. Hoyt WF, Kaplan SL, Grumbach MM, et al. Septo-optic dysplasia and pituitary dwarfism. Lancet 1970; 1:893–894.

583. Patel H, Tze WJ, Crichton JU, et al. Optic nerve hypoplasia with hypopituitarism. Am J Dis Child 1975; 129:175–180.

584. Izenberg N, Rosenblum M, Parks JS. The endocrine spectrum of septo-optic dysplasia. Clin Pediatr 1984; 23:632–636.

585. Roitman A, Laron Z. Hypothalamo-pituitary hormone insufficiency associated with cleft lip and palate. Arch Dis Child 1978; 53:952–955.

586. Rudman D, Davis GT, Priest JH, et al. Prevalence of growth hormone deficiency in children with cleft lip or palate. J Pediatr 1978; 93:378–382.

587. Shalet SM. Irradiation-induced growth failure. Ped Clin North Am 1986; 15:591–606.

588. Brauner R, Rappaport R. Pituitary hormone secretion and growth after cranial irradiation. In: Frisch H, Thorner MO, eds. Hormonal Regulation of Growth. New York: Raven, 1989: 245–253.

589. Albertsson-Wikland K, Lannering B, Márky I, et al. A longitudinal study on growth and spontaneous growth hormone (GH) secretion in children with irradiated brain tumors. Acta Paediatr Scand 1987; 76:966–973.

590. Lannering B, Albertsson-Wikland K. Growth hormone release in children after cranial irradiation. Horm Res 1987; 27:13–22.

591. Shalet SM, Price DA, Beardwell CG, et al. Normal growth despite abnormalities of growth hormone secretion in children treated for acute leukemia. J Pediatr 1979; 94:719–722.

592. Romshe CA, Zipf WB, Miser A, et al. Evaluation of growth hormone release and human growth hormone treatment in children with cranial irradiation–associated short stature. J Pediatr 1984; 104:177–181.

593. Blatt J, Bercu BB, Gillin JC, et al. Reduced pulsatile growth hormone secretion in children after therapy for acute lymphoblastic leukemia. J Pediatr 1984; 104:182–186.

594. Costin G. Endocrine disorders associated with tumors of the pituitary and hypothalamus. Pediatr Clin North Am 1979; 26:15–31.

595. Preece MA. Diagnosis and treatment of children with growth hormone deficiency. Clin Endocrinol Metab 1982; 11:1–24.

596. Steendijk R. Diagnostic and aetiologic features of idiopathic and symptomatic growth hormone deficiency in the Netherlands. A survey of 176 children. Helv Paediatr Acta 1980; 35:129–139.

597. Heinrich JJ, Martinez A, Bergada C. Etiology and association of growth hormone deficiency. Acta Endocrinol Suppl 279; 1986:113–117.

598. Craft WH, Underwood LE, Van Wyk JJ. High incidence of perinatal insult in children with idiopathic hypopituitarism. J Pediatr 1980; 96:397–402.

599. Borges JL, Blizzard RM, Gelato MC, et al. Effects of human pancreatic tumour growth hormone releasing factor on growth hormone and somatomedin-C levels in patients with idiopathic growth hormone deficiency. Lancet 1983; 2:119–124.

600. Schriock EA, Lustig RH, Rosenthal SM, et al. Effect of growth hormone–releasing factor on plasma growth hormone in relation to magnitude and duration of growth hormone deficiency in 26 children and adults with isolated growth hormone deficiency or multiple pituitary hormone deficiences: evidence for hypothalamic GRF deficiency. J Clin Endocrinol Metab 1984; 58:1043–1049.

601. Grossman A, Savage MO, Besser GM. Growth hormone releasing hormone. Clin Endocrinol Metab 1986; 15:607–627.

602. Thorner MO, Vance ML. Regulation of growth hormone secretion in man and the therapeutic implications of GHRH. In: Frisch H, Thorner MO, eds. Hormonal Regulation of Growth. New York: Raven, 1989: 19–29.

603. Widdowson EM. Mental contentment and physical growth. Lancet 1951; 1:1316–1318.

604. Patton RG, Gardner LI. Influence of family environment on growth: the syndrome of "maternal deprivation." Pediatrics 1962; 30:957–962.

605. Blizzard RM. Psychosocial short stature. In: Lifshitz F, ed. Pediatric Endocrinology. New York: Marcel Dekker, 1985: 87–107.

606. Powell GF, Brasel JA, Blizzard RM. Emotional deprivation and growth retardation simulating idiopathic hypopituitarism. I. Clinical evaluation of the syndrome. N Engl J Med 1967; 276:1271–1278.

607. Powell GF, Brasel JA, Raiti S, et al. Emotional deprivation and growth retardation simulating idiopathic hypopituitarism. II. Endocrinologic evaluation of the syndrome. N Engl J Med 1967; 276:1279–1283.

608. Krieger I, Mellinger RC. Pituitary function in the deprivation syndrome. J Pediatr 1971; 79:216–225.

609. Krieger I, Chen YC. Calorie requirements for weight gain in infants with growth failure due to maternal deprivation, undernutrition, and congenital heart disease. A correlation analysis. Pediatrics 1969; 44:647–654.

610. Whitten CF, Pettit MG, Fischoff J. Evidence that growth failure from maternal deprivation is secondary to undereating. JAMA 1969; 209:1675–1682.

611. Laron Z. Syndrome of familial dwarfism and high plasma immunoreactive growth hormone. Isr J Med Sci 1974; 10:1247–1253.

612. Daughaday WH, Laron Z, Pertzelan A, et al. Defective sulfation factor generation: a possible etiological link in dwarfism. Trans Assoc Am Physicians 1969; 82:129–138.

613. Laron Z, Pertzelan A, Karp M, et al. Administration of growth hormone to patients with familial dwarfism with high plasma immunoreactive growth hormone: measurement of sulfation factor, metabolic and linear growth responses. J Clin Endocrinol Metab 1971; 33:332–342.

614. Van den Brande JL, DuCaju MVL, Visser HKA, et al. Primary somatomedin deficiency. Arch Dis Child 1974; 49:297–304.

615. Baumann G, Shaw MA, Winter RJ. Absence of the plasma growth hormone binding protein in Laron-type dwarfism. J Clin Endocrinol Metab 1987; 65:814–816.

616. Godowski PJ, Leung DW, Meacham LR, et al. Characterization of the human growth hormone receptor gene and demonstration of a partial gene deletion in 2 parts with Laron-type dwarfism. Proc Natl Acad Sci USA 1989; 86:8083–8087.

617. Kowarski AA, Schneider J, Ben-Galim E, et al. Growth failure with normal serum RIA-GH and low somatomedin activity: somatomedin restoration and growth acceleration after exogenous GH. J Clin Endocrinol Metab 1978; 47:461–464.

618. Rudman D, Kutner MH, Blackston RD, et al. Children with normalvariant short stature: treatment with human growth hormone for 6 months. N Engl J Med 1981; 305:123–131.

619. Frazer T, Gavin JR, Daughaday WH, et al. Growth hormone dependent growth failure. J Pediatr 1982; 101:12–15.

620. Lovinger RD, Kaplan SL, Grumbach MM. Congenital hypopituitarism associated with neonatal hypoglycemia and microphallus: four cases secondary to hypothalamic hormone deficiencies. J Pediatr 1975; 87:1171–1181.

621. Copeland KC, Franks RC, Ramamurthy R. Neonatal hyperbilirubinemia and hypoglycemia in congenital hypopituitarism. Clin Pediatr 1981; 20:523–526.

622. Goodman HG, Grumbach MM, Kaplan SL. Growth and growth hormone. II. A comparison of isolated growth hormone deficiency and multiple pituitary hormone deficiencies in 35 patients with idiopathic hypopituitary dwarfism. N Engl J Med 1968; 278:57–68.

623. Underwood LE, Van den Brande JL, Antony GJ, et al. Islet cell function and glucose homeostasis in hypopituitary dwarfism: synergism between growth hormone and cortisone. J Pediatr 1973; 82:28–37.

624. Underwood LE, Radcliffe WB, Strickland AL, et al. Assessment of sella turcica volume in dwarfed children. J Clin Endocrinol Metab 1973; 36:734–741.

625. Underwood LE, Radcliffe WB, Guinto FC. New standards for the assessment of sella turcica volume in children. Radiology 1976; 119:651–654.

626. Smith SP, Wolpert SM, Sadeghi-Nejad A, et al. Value of computed tomographic scanning in patients with growth hormone deficiency. Pediatrics 1986; 78:601–605.

627. Rosenfeld RG, Wilson DM, Lee PDK, et al. Insulin-like growth factors I and II in evaluation of growth retardation. J Pediatr 1986; 109:428–433.

628. Rayner PHW, Rudd BT, Thomas PH, et al. Growth hormone deficiency and the measurement of somatomedin C/IGF-I: the influence of sexual maturation. Clin Endocrinol 1988; 28:361–371.

629. Frasier SD. A review of growth hormone stimulation tests in children. Pediatrics 1974; 53:929–937.

630. Joss EE. Growth hormone deficiency in childhood. Monogr Paediatr 1975; 5:1–83.

631. Hagenas L. Clinical tests as predictors of growth response in GH treatment of short normal children. Acta Paediatr Scand 1989; 362:36–43.

632. Bercu BB, Shulman D, Root AW, et al. Growth hormone (GH) provocative testing frequently does not reflect endogenous GH secretion. J Clin Endocrinol Metab 1986; 63:709–716.

633. Underwood LE, Sherman BM. Controversies in the treatment of short stature. In: Underwood LE, ed. Human Growth Hormone: Progress and Challenge. New York: Marcel Dekker, 1988: 145–191.

634. Albertsson-Wikland K, Rosberg S. Dynamics of GH secretion in children. In: Bercu B, ed. Basic and Clinical Aspects of Growth Hormone. New York: Plenum, 1988: 109–118.

635. Albertsson-Wikland K, Rosberg S. Analyses of 24-hour growth hormone profiles in children: relation to growth. J Clin Endocrinol Metab 1988; 67:493–500.

636. Donaldson DL, Hollowell JG, Pan FP, et al. Growth hormone secretory profiles: significant variation on consecutive nights. Pediatr Res 1988; 23:276A.

637. Lin TH, Kirkland RT, Sherman BM, et al. Growth hormone testing in short children and their response to growth hormone therapy. J Pediatr 1989; 115:57–63.

638. Rose SR, Ross JL, Uriarte M, et al. The advantage of measuring stimulated as compared with spontaneous growth hormone levels in the diagnosis of growth hormone deficiency. N Engl J Med 1988; 319:201–207.

639. Romer TE, Rymkiewicz-Kluczynska B, Olivier M, et al. Growth hormone–releasing hormone reverses secondary somatotroph unresponsiveness. J Clin Endocrinol Metab 1991; 72:503–506.

640. Albini CH, Quattrin T, Vandlen RL, et al. Quantitation of urinary growth hormone in children with normal and abnormal growth. Pediatr Res 1988; 23:89–92.

641. Sukegawa I, Hizuka N, Takano K, et al. Urinary growth hormone (GH) measurements are useful for evaluating endogenous GH secretion. J Clin Endocrinol Metab 1988; 66:1119–1123.

642. Hattori N, Shimatsu A, Yamanaka C, et al. Nocturnal urinary growth hormone excretion in children with short stature. Acta Endocrinol 1988; 119:113–117.
643. Milner RDG, Russell-Fraser T, Brook CGD, et al. Experience with human growth hormone in Great Britain: report of the MRC working party. Clin Endocrinol 1979; 11:15–38.
644. Tanner JM, Whitehouse RH, Hughes PCR, et al. Effect of human growth hormone treatment for 1 to 7 years on growth of 100 children, with growth hormone deficiency, low birthweight, inherited smallness, Turner's syndrome, and other complaints. Arch Dis Child 1971; 46:745–782.
645. Ranke MB, Bierich JR. Growth Hormone Deficiency. Baltimore: Urban & Schwarzenberg, 1983.
646. Frasier SD. Human pituitary growth hormone (hGH) therapy in growth hormone deficiency. Endocr Rev 1983; 4:155–170.
647. Fisher DA, Job JC, Preece M, et al. Growth hormone deficiency, human growth hormone and the occurrence of leukemia. Lancet 1988; 1:1159–1160.
648. Lippe BM, Van Herle AJ, LaFranchi SH, et al. Reversible hypothyroidism in growth-hormone deficient children treated with human growth hormone. J Clin Endocrinol Metab 1975; 40:612–618.
649. Stabler BS, Underwood LE, eds. Slow Grows the Child: Psychosocial Aspects of Growth Delay. Hillsdale, NJ: Lawrence Erlbaum, 1987.
650. Dean HJ, McTaggart TL, Fish DG, et al. Long-term social follow-up of growth hormone deficient adults treated with growth hormone during childhood. In: Stabler BS, Underwood LE, eds. Slow Grows the Child: Psychosocial Aspects of Growth Delay. Hillsdale, NJ: Lawrence Erlbaum, 1987: 73–82.
651. Mitchell CM, Libber S, Johanson AJ, et al. Psychosocial impact of long-term growth hormone therapy. In: Stabler BS, Underwood LE, eds. Slow Grows the Child: Psychosocial Aspects of Growth Delay. Hillsdale, NJ: Lawrence Erlbaum, 1987: 97–109.
652. Burns EC, Tanner JM, Preece MA, et al. Final height and pubertal development in 55 children with idiopathic growth hormone deficiency, treated for between 2 and 15 years with human growth hormone. Eur J Pediatr 1981; 137:155–164.
653. Clayton PE, Shalet SM, Price DA. Endocrine manipulation of constitutional delay in growth and puberty. J Endocrinol 1988; 116:321–323.
654. Shalet SM. Treatment of constitutional delay in growth and puberty (CDGP). Clin Endocrinol 1981; 31:81–86.
655. Eastman CJ, Lazarus L, Stuart MC, et al. The effect of puberty on growth hormone secretion in boys with short stature and delayed adolescence. Aust NZ J Med 1971; 1:154–159.
656. Gourmelen M, Pham-Huu-Trung MT, Girard F. Transient partial hGH deficiency in prepubertal children with delay of growth. Pediatr Res 1979; 13:221–224.
657. Bierich JR. Constitutional delay of growth and adolescent development. Eur J Pediatr 1982; 139:221–224.
658. Van Vliet G, Styne DM, Kaplan SL, et al. Growth hormone treatment for short stature. N Engl J Med 1983; 309:1016–1022.
659. Ivarsson SA. Can growth hormone increase final height in constitutional short stature? Acta Paediatr Scand 1989; 362(Suppl):56–60.
660. Gertner JM, Genel M, Gianfredi SP, et al. Prospective clinical trial of human growth hormone in short children without growth hormone deficiency. J Pediatr 1984; 104:172–176.
661. Underwood LE, Fisher DA, Frasier SD, et al. Growth hormone in the treatment of children with short stature. Pediatrics 1983; 72:891–894.
662. Grunt J, Howard C, Daughaday W. Comparison of growth and somatomedin C responses following growth hormone treatment in children with small-for-date short stature, significant idiopathic short stature and hypopituitarism. Acta Endocrinol 1984; 106:168–174.
663. Underwood LE, Rieser PA. Is it ethical to treat healthy short children with growth hormone? Acta Paediatr Scand 1989; 362(Suppl):18–23.
664. Burrow GN, Dussault JH. Neonatal Thyroid Screening. New York: Raven, 1980.
665. Fisher DA, Dussault JH, Foley TP, et al. Screening for congenital hypothyroidism: results of screening one million North American infants. J Pediatr 1979; 94:700–705.
666. Illig R, Largo RH, Weber M, et al. Sixty children with congenital hypothyroidism detected by neonatal thyroid: mental development at 1, 4 and 7 years: a longitudinal study. Acta Endocrinol Suppl 1986; 279:346–353.
667. Rezvani I, DiGeorge AM. Reassessment of the daily dose of oral thyroxine for replacement therapy in hypothyroid children. J Pediatr 1977; 90:291–297.
668. Rivkees SA, Bode HH, Crawford JD. Long-term growth in juvenile acquired hypothyroidism. N Engl J Med 1988; 318:599–602.
669. McArthur RG, Cloutier MD, Hayles AB, et al. Cushing's disease in children: findings in 13 cases. Mayo Clinic Proc 1972; 47:318–326.
670. Lee PA, Weldon VV, Migeon CJ. Short stature as the only clinical sign of Cushing's syndrome. J Pediatr 1975; 86:89–91.
671. Laron Z, Pertzelan A. The comparative effect of 6-fluoroprednisolone, 6-methylprednisolone, and hydrocortisone on linear growth of children with congenital adrenal virilism and Addison's disease. J Pediatr 1968; 73:774–782.
672. Morris HG, Jorgensen JR, Elrick H, et al. Metabolic effects of human growth hormone in corticosteroid-treated children. J Clin Invest 1968; 47:436–451.
673. Mosier HD, Smith FG, Schultz MA. Failure of catch-up growth after Cushing's syndrome in childhood. Am J Dis Child 1972; 124:251–253.
674. Streeten DHP, Faas FH, Elders MJ, et al. Hypercortisolism in childhood: shortcomings of conventional diagnostic criteria. Pediatrics 1975; 56:797–803.
675. Soyka LF. Treatment of the nephrotic syndrome in childhood: use of an alternate-day prednisone regimen. Am J Dis Child 1967; 113:693–701.
676. Dickerman Z, Loewinger J, Laron Z. The pattern of growth in children with constitutional tall stature from birth to age 9 years: a longitudinal study. Acta Paediatr Scand 1984; 73:530–536.
677. Sorgo W, Scholler K, Heinze F, et al. Critical analysis of height reduction in oestrogen-treated tall girls. Eur J Pediatr 1984; 142:260–265.
678. Report of the conference on estrogen treatment of the young. Pediatrics 1978; 62(Suppl):1087–1217.
679. Sotos JF, Dodge PR, Muirhead D, et al. Cerebral gigantism in childhood: a syndrome of excessively rapid growth with acromegalic features and a nonprogressive neurologic disorder. N Engl J Med 1964; 271:109–116.
680. Sotos JF, Cutler EA, Dodge P. Cerebral gigantism. Am J Dis Child 1977; 131:625–627.
681. Wit JM, Beemer FA, Barth PG, et al. Cerebral gigantism (Sotos syndrome). Compiled data of 22 cases. Eur J Pediatr 1985; 144:131–140.
682. Sotelo-Avila C, Gooch WM. Neoplasms associated with the Beckwith-Wiedemann syndrome. Perspect Pediatr Pathol 1976; 3:255–272.
683. Sotelo-Avila C, Gonzalez-Crussi F, Fowler JW. Complete and incomplete forms of Beckwith-Weidemann syndrome: their oncogenic potential. J Pediatr 1980; 96:47–50.
684. Kaplan SL, Grumbach MM. Pathogenesis of sexual precocity. In: Grumbach MM, Sizonenko PC, Aubert ML, eds. Control of the Onset of Puberty. Baltimore: Williams & Wilkins, 1990: 620–662.
685. Boepple PA, Mansfield MJ, Wierman ME, et al. Use of a potent, long acting agonist of gonadotropin-releasing hormone in the treatment of precocious puberty. Endocr Rev 1986; 7:24–33.
686. Korth-Schutz S, Levine LS, New MI. Evidence for the adrenal source of androgens in precocious adrenarche. Acta Endocrinol 1976; 82:342–352.
687. Sizonenko PC, Paunier L. Hormonal changes in puberty. III. Correlations of plasma dehydroepiandrosterone, testosterone, FSH and LH with stages of puberty and bone age in normal boys and girls and in patients with Addison's disease or hypogonadism or with premature or late adrenarche. J Clin Endocrinol Metab 1975; 41:894–904.
688. Cutler Jr GB, Schiebinger RJ, Albertson BD, et al. The adrenarche (human and animal). In: Grumbach MM, Sizonenko PC, Aubert ML, eds. Control of the Onset of Puberty. Baltimore: Williams & Wilkins, 1990: 506–524.
689. Caufriez A, Wolter R, Govaerts M, et al. Gonadotropins and prolactin pituitary reserve in premature thelarche. J Pediatr 1977; 91:751–753.

22

PUBERTY: ONTOGENY, NEUROENDOCRINOLOGY, PHYSIOLOGY, AND DISORDERS

Melvin M. Grumbach and Dennis M. Styne

INTRODUCTION

Puberty should not be considered as a de novo event but rather as a phase in the continuum of the development of gonadal function and the ontogeny of the hypothalamic-pituitary-gonadal system in the fetus, through puberty, to the attainment of full sexual maturation and fertility. During puberty secondary sexual characteristics appear, the adolescent growth spurt occurs, fertility is achieved, and profound psychological effects ensue.[1] These changes are a consequence of stimulation of the gonads by pituitary gonadotropins and increase in gonadal steroid output.

Historical evidence suggests that puberty occurs at an earlier age today than in the past.[2–6] The average age of menarche in industrialized European countries has decreased 2 to 3 mo per decade over the past 150 y, and in the United States the decrease has been approximately 2 to 3 mo per decade in the last century.[3–6] However, this secular trend has ceased in developed countries such as the United States since approximately 1940. Socioeconomic conditions, nutritional status, and states of health influence the age at onset and the progression of pubertal development.[7–9] The interaction of nutrition and puberty is of particular importance in areas of the world where nutrition is suboptimal.

If the age of puberty was later in past centuries compared with the present, the age of attaining adult height was also later. Surveys of army recruits, schoolchildren, and workers in Europe and America, as well as slave records, show that large portions of the population in the past two centuries grew considerably into their early 20s, whereas modern adolescents cease to grow and reach stable heights by 17 y of age.[4] The final heights attained during the 18th and 19th centuries were often at modern 25th percentiles or less.

The progressive decline in the age of puberty is probably a result of improvements in socioeconomic conditions, nutrition, and general health. In the nomadic Lapp culture, in which the standard of living changed little between 1870 and 1930, no trend toward earlier menarche was found.[9] The tendency for earlier menarche in Western Europe and the United States (Fig. 22–1) has slowed or ceased over the past 40 y,[3–6, 10–12] and the social class difference in menarcheal age has narrowed or disappeared in most countries. According to the most recent survey by the U.S. National Center for Health Statistics, the age of menarche in the United States is 12.8 y.[13, 14]

Nutrition even in those with generally good health also influences the age of puberty. Moderate obesity (up to 30%

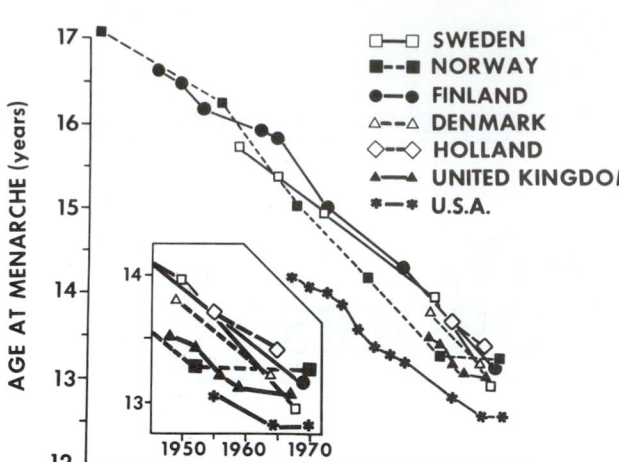

Figure 22–1. Changes in age at menarche, 1840 to 1978, illustrating the advance in the age of menarche in Western Europe and the United States since 1840 and the slowing of this trend over the last 30 y. (Modified from Tanner M, Eveleth PB. Variability between populations in growth and development at puberty. In: Berenberg SR, ed. Puberty, Biologic and Psychosocial Components. Leiden: H. E. Stenfert Kroese, 1975: 256–273. Reprinted by permission of Kluwer Academic Publishers.)

above normal weight for age) is associated with earlier menarche, although pathological obesity is associated with delayed menarche.[15] Delayed puberty is a feature of chronic disease and malnutrition; strenuous physical activity in girls, especially when associated with thinness, can delay or arrest puberty.[16] Inactive, bedridden children with mental retardation reach menarche at an earlier age and at a lower body fat value than do similarly retarded children who are more active.[17] The suggestion that blindness may advance the age of puberty[18] is not supported by more recent studies. Puberty starts at a later age and the period of pubertal development lasts longer at high altitudes than at low altitudes when nutritional status is similar.[19]

Genetic factors play an important role in the onset of puberty, as illustrated by the similar age of menarche in members of an ethnic population and in mother-daughter pairs. Secondary sexual development occurs earlier in black girls than in white girls in the United States, and there is no apparent effect of social or economic factors on this relationship. Thus when socioeconomic and environmental factors lead to good nutrition, general health, and infant care, the age of onset of puberty in normal children is determined largely by genetic factors.[20]

PHYSICAL CHANGES OF PUBERTY

Secondary Sexual Characteristics

Comparative description of the physical changes between individuals and populations requires an objective and reproducible method of describing the maturation of secondary sexual characteristics. Tanner[5] has developed standards of the most useful signs of sexual maturation that have been widely used throughout the world (see Figs. 22–2 to 22–4). A self-assessment scale of adolescent sexual maturation has been developed.[27]

Female

Two distinct phenomena occur in the female. The development of the breast and its modified apocrine glands

is primarily under the control of estrogens secreted by the ovaries (Fig. 22–2); the growth of pubic and axillary hair (Fig. 22–3) is mainly under the influence of androgens secreted by the adrenal and the ovary. The glandular and connective tissue of the mammary gland begins to develop at the onset of pubertal maturation. Thus lobules composed of small ductules and cellular connective tissue develop to a more pronounced degree in the female. Proliferation of fatty and connective tissue accounts for 80% of the volume of the adult, nonlactating female breast.[21] The classification of the stages of breast development[22] depends on specific characteristics common to the female breast but does not include size or inherent shape of the breasts, which are determined by genetic and nutritional factors (see Fig. 22–2). Four stages were described by Stratz,[23] a fifth was added by Reynolds and Wines,[24] and modifications were made to the schema by Tanner,[5, 22] who produced the most widely utilized staging. The initial breast development may be unilateral for several months and may be cause for un-

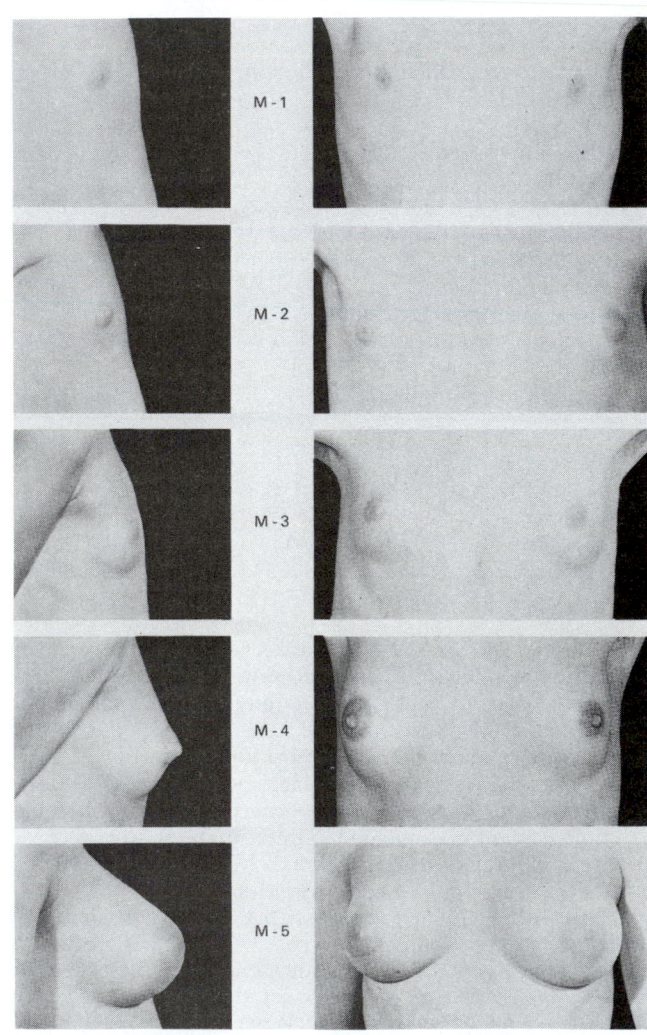

Figure 22–2. Stages of breast development according to Marshall and Tanner[22] and Reynolds and Wines.[24] Stage 1: preadolescent; elevation of papilla only. Stage 2: breast bud stage; elevation of breast and papilla as a small mound, enlargement of areolar diameter. Stage 3: further enlargement of breast and areola with no separation of their contours. Stage 4: projection of areola and papilla to form a secondary mound above the level of the breast. Stage 5: mature stage; projection of papilla only, resulting from recession of the areola to the general contour of the breast. (Photographs from Van Wieringen JD, Wafelbakker F, Verbrugge HP, et al. Growth Diagrams 1965 Netherlands: Second National Survey on 0–24 Year Olds. Netherlands Institute for Preventative Medicine TNO. Groningen: Wolters-Noordhoff, 1971. © Wolters-Noordhoff, Groningen.)

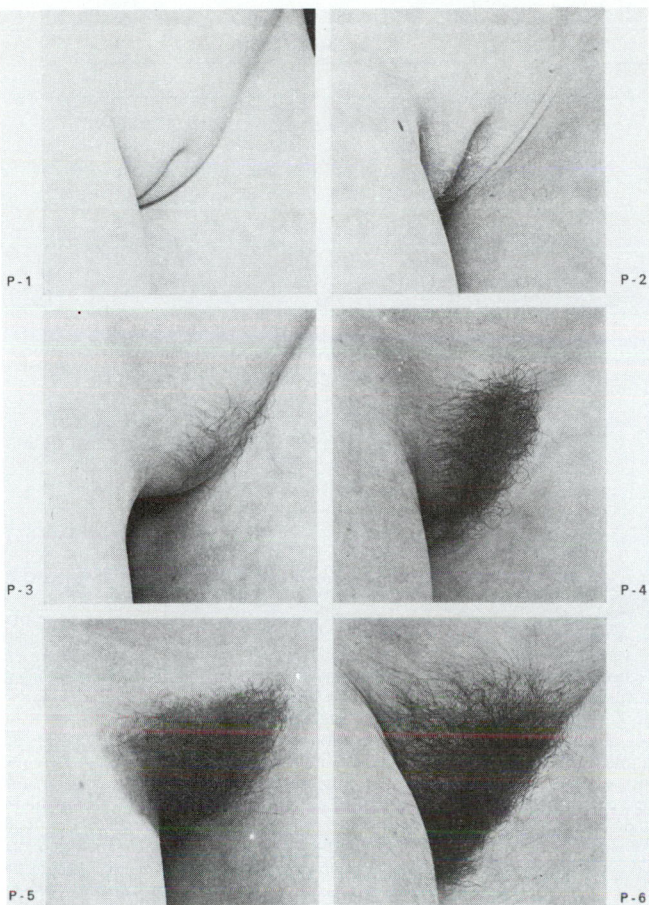

Figure 22–3. Stages of female pubic hair development, according to Marshall and Tanner,[22] Reynolds and Wines,[24] and Dupertuis et al.[717] Stage 1: preadolescent; the vellus over the pubes is not further developed than that over the anterior abdominal wall; i.e., there is no pubic hair. Stage 2: sparse growth of long, slightly pigmented, downy hair, straight or only slightly curled, appearing chiefly along the labia. This stage is difficult to see on photographs. Stage 3: hair is considerably darker, coarser, and curlier. The hair spreads sparsely over the junction of the pubes. Stage 4: hair is now adult in type, but the area covered by it is still considerably smaller than in most adults. There is no spread to the medial surface of the thighs. Stage 5: hair is adult in quantity and type, distributed as an inverse triangle of the classic feminine pattern. The spread is to the medial surface of the thighs but not up the linea alba or elsewhere above the base of the inverse triangle. (Photographs from Van Wieringen JD, Wafelbakker F, Verbrugge HP, et al. Growth Diagrams 1965 Netherlands: Second National Survey on 0–24 Year Olds. Netherlands Institute for Preventative Medicine TNO. Groningen: Wolters-Noordhoff, 1971. © Wolters-Noordhoff, Groningen.)

TABLE 22–1. Nipple Diameter Compared with Breast and Pubic Hair Stages: Comparison of Longitudinal and Cross-Sectional Data

| | Nipple Size (mm)* | |
Stage	Cross-Sectional Data	Longitudinal Data
Breast		
1	2.89 (0.81)	3.0 (0.77)
2	3.28 (0.89)	3.37 (0.96)
3	4.07 (1.32)	4.72 (1.40)†
4	7.74 (1.64)†	7.25 (1.46)†
5	9.94 (1.38)†	9.41 (1.45)†
Pubic hair		
1	2.95 (1.02)	3.14 (1.31)
2	3.32 (0.91)	3.69 (1.34)
3	4.11 (1.54)	4.44 (1.17)†
4	7.15 (1.81)†	6.54 (1.47)†
5	9.66 (1.59)†	8.98 (1.56)†

*Results are means ± standard deviation (SD; in parentheses).
†Significantly different from previous stage, $p < .05$.
Reprinted by permission of Elsevier Science Publishing Co., Inc. from Papilla (nipple) development during female puberty, by Rohn RD. Journal of Adolescent Health Care, Vol. 2, pp. 217–220. Copyright 1982 by The Society for Adolescent Medicine.

individual girls, increase in height velocity (rather than breast development) is actually the first sign of puberty in girls.

The pattern of development and growth of pubic hair in females is illustrated in Figure 22–3. Dulling and thickening of the vaginal mucosa from the prepubertal reddish glistening appearance occur, and secretion of clear or whitish discharge increases in the months before menarche as a result of estrogen action. The vaginal pH decreases as menarche approaches because of the increase of lactic acid produced by lactobacilli in the vaginal flora. The length of the vagina increases from about 8 cm at onset of puberty to 11 cm at menarche. Thickening, protrusion, and rugation of the labia majora and minora occur. Fat is deposited in the area of the mons pubis, and the labia majora becomes wrinkled in appearance. The clitoris enlarges slightly, and the urethral opening becomes more prominent. Photographic atlases of normal female prepubertal genitalia are now available and include standards for the variation in appearance of the hymenal opening.[26]

Male

The growth and maturation of the penis usually correlate closely with pubic hair development, because both features are under androgen control, but for the most accurate assessment the stages of pubic hair development and genital development should be determined independently and recorded separately (Fig. 22–4 and Table 22–3). Growth of the testes is usually the first sign of puberty in the male, and it begins approximately 6 mo after the initiation of breast development in girls. In general, when the longitudinal measurement of a testis is greater than 2.5 cm, pubertal testicular enlargement has begun. The testicular volume index ([length × width of right testis + length × width of left testis]/2) and testicular volume, measured by comparing the testes with ellipsoids of known volume, correlate with the stages of puberty[28] (Table 22–4). The right testis is usually larger than the left, and the left testis is located lower in the scrotum than the right testis. The phallus is best measured in the flaccid state stretched. The length of the erectile tissue (excluding the foreskin) increases from an average of 6.2 cm in the prepubertal state to 13.2 cm in the adult.

Limits of Normal Pubertal Development

Surveys of the attainment of various stages of puberty in the United States began with subjects at 12 y of age and,

founded concern by girls or parents. Indeed, surgical biopsies have been performed inappropriately in girls in whom it was not appreciated that asymmetrical development is normal. There are unusual cases of agenesis of the breast in which no glandular or fat enlargement occurs regardless of the level of estrogen stimulation. Changes in the diameter of the papilla of the nipple are sequential and linked to stages of pubertal development. Nipple papilla diameter does not increase much during pubic hair stage 1 to 3 or breast stage 1 to 3 (diameter is 3 to 4 mm) but does increase after breast stage 3, providing an objective method of differentiating stage 4 from 5 (final diameter is approximately 9 mm)[25] (Table 22–1). The stage of breast development is usually equal to the stage of pubic hair development in normal girls, but as different endocrine organs control these two processes, stages should be classified separately (Table 22–2). Areolar diameter also increases in boys at puberty, and most boys have palpable glandular enlargement of the breast (see Chapter 15). Although rarely evident clinically in

TABLE 22–2. Age at Stage of Puberty in Girls

| | British Girls* | | Swiss Girls† | |
Stage	Mean (y)	SD	Mean (y)	SD
Breast stage 2	11.50	1.10	10.9	1.2
Pubic hair stage 2	11.64	1.21	10.4	1.2
Peak height velocity	12.14	0.88	12.2	1.0
Breast stage 3	12.15	1.09	12.2	1.2
Pubic hair stage 3	12.36	1.10	12.2	1.2
Pubic hair stage 4	12.95	1.06	13.0	1.1
Breast stage 4	13.11	1.15	13.2	0.9
Menarche‡	13.47	1.12	13.4	1.1
Pubic hair stage 5	14.41	1.21	14.0	1.3
Breast stage 5	15.33	1.74	14.0	1.2

*Determined in a prospective study of sequential photographs by Marshall and Tanner.[22]
†Determined in a prospective longitudinal study of physical examinations as part of the First Zurich Longitudinal Study of Growth and Development. Reported by Largo and Prader.[32]
‡Mean age of menarche is 12.8 y ± 1.22 (SD) in American girls (from ref. 14).

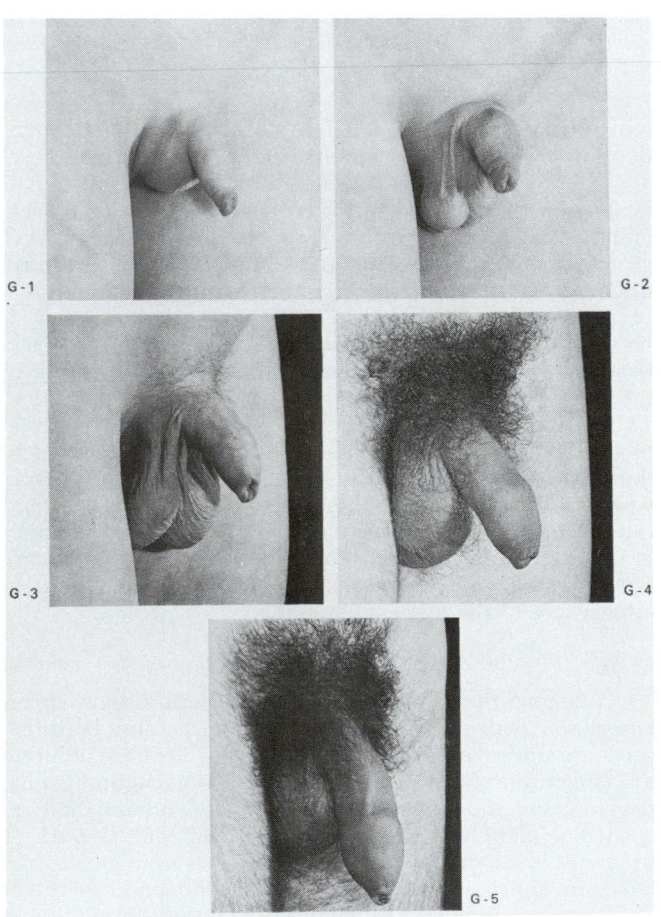

Figure 22–4. Stages of male genital development and pubic hair development, according to Marshall and Tanner,[31] Reynolds and Wines,[718] and Dupertuis et al.[717] *Genital development*: Stage 1: preadolescent. Testes, scrotum, and penis are about the same size and proportion as in early childhood. Stage 2: the scrotum and testes have enlarged; the scrotal skin shows a change in texture and also some reddening. Stage 3: growth of the penis has occurred, at first mainly in length but with some increase in breadth; there is further growth of the testes and scrotum. Stage 4: the penis is further enlarged in length and breadth with development of the glans. The testes and scrotum are further enlarged. The scrotal skin has further darkened. Stage 5: genitalia are adult in size and shape. No further enlargement takes place after stage 5 is reached. *Pubic hair development*: Stage 1: preadolescent. The vellus over the pubes is not further developed than that over the abdominal wall; i.e., there is no pubic hair. Stage 2: sparse growth of long, slightly pigmented, downy hair, straight or slightly curled, appearing chiefly at the base of the penis. Stage 3: hair is considerably darker, coarser, and curlier and spreads sparsely over the junction of the pubes. Stage 4: hair is now adult in type, but the area it covers is still considerably smaller than in most adults. There is no spread to the medial surface of the thighs. Stage 5: hair is adult in quantity and type, distributed as an inverse triangle. The spread is to the medial surface of the thighs but not up the linea alba or elsewhere above the base of the inverse triangle. Most men will have further spread of the pubic hair. (Photographs from Van Wieringen JD, Wafelbakker F, Verbrugge HP, et al. Growth Diagrams 1965 Netherlands: Second National Survey on 0–24 Year Olds. Netherlands Institute for Preventative Medicine TNO. Groningen: Wolters-Noordhoff, 1971. © Wolters-Noordhoff, Groningen.)

TABLE 22–3. Age at Stage of Puberty in Boys

| | British Boys* | | Swiss Boys† | |
Stage	Mean (y)	SD	Mean (y)	SD
Genitalia stage 2	11.64	1.07	11.2	1.5
Genitalia stage 3	12.85	1.04	12.9	1.2
Pubic hair stage 2	13.44	1.09	12.2	1.5
Genitalia stage 4	13.77	1.02	13.8	1.1
Pubic hair stage 3	13.90	1.04	13.5	1.2
Peak height velocity	14.06	0.92	13.9	0.8
Pubic hair stage 4	14.36	1.08	14.2	1.1
Genitalia stage 5	14.92	1.10	14.7	1.1
Pubic hair stage 5	15.18	1.07	14.9	1.0

*Determined in a prospective study of sequential photographs by Marshall and Tanner.[31]
†Determined in a prospective longitudinal study of physical examinations as part of the First Zurich Longitudinal Study of Growth and Development. Reported by Largo and Prader.[33]

TABLE 22–4. Correlation of Testicular Volume with Stage of Pubertal Development

Parameter	Pubertal Stage				
	1	*2*	*3*	*4*	*5*
TVI*	1.8	4.5	8.2	10.5	—
Volume (cm³)†	2.5	3.4	9.1	11.8	14
Volume (cm³)‡	1.8	4.2	10	11	15
Volume (cm³)§	1.8	5.0	9.5	12.5	17

*Testicular volume index calculated by (length × width of right testis and length × width of left testis) 2. Data from Burr et al.[120] and August et al.[121]
†Volume estimated by comparison with ellipsoid of known volume (orchidometer) that is equal to or smaller than the testes. Data from Zachmann et al.[28]
‡Volume by comparison with orchidometer. Data from Waaler et al.[705]
§Measurement with calipers and average volume of both testes calculated by 0.52 × longitudinal axis × transverse axis. Data from Waaler et al.[705]

although useful in defining the upper limits of normal pubertal development, are uninformative about the lower limits.[14, 29, 30] From the available data, American boys and girls are similar to British and Swiss children in age of attainment of most stages of pubertal development, except for menarche (see Tables 22–2 and 22–3).[22, 31–33] There is no difference between black and white boys in age of attainment of the stages of pubertal development. Black American girls are advanced in secondary sexual development compared with white American girls during the first three stages of puberty.[29] Some sign of puberty between ages 8 and 13 (mean 10.5) is shown by 95% of normal American girls, whereas 95% of boys enter puberty between ages 9 and 14 (mean 11.5).[11] English girls complete secondary sexual development in a mean of 4.2 y, but the range is 1.5 to 6 y; the mean for boys is 3.5 y, with a range of 2 to 4.5 y (Figs. 22–5 and 22–6).[22, 31]

Other Dimorphic Physical Changes

Although prepubertal children of both sexes have the same range of heights, other physical changes show sexual dimorphism. In boys, both the membranous and cartilaginous components of the vocal cords lengthen during puberty. In the peripubertal period the length of the vocal cords in both boys and girls is about 12 to 15 mm, of which the membranous portion is 7 to 8 mm. In adult men the vocal cords attain a length of 18 to 23 mm (membranous portion 12 to 16 mm), whereas in women the cords enlarge only slightly (13 to 18 mm). In the castrati whose vocal

brilliance had a great influence on the lyrical Italian operas, the membranous component of the vocal cords was the same length as in prepubertal boys and even shorter than in women.[34] During puberty the male larynx, cricothyroid cartilage, and laryngeal muscles enlarge; breaking of the voice occurs at approximately 13 y, and the adult voice is achieved by about 15 y.[35]

Facial hair in boys is first apparent on the corners of the upper lip and the upper cheeks; it then spreads to the midline of the lower lip and finally to the sides and the lower border of the chin. The first stage of facial hair development usually occurs during pubic hair stage 3 (average age of 14.9 in the United States), and the last stage occurs after pubic hair stage 5 and genital stage 5.

Axillary hair appears at approximately 13 y in American girls and 14 y in boys. Axillary sweat glands begin to function as the hair appears. The appearance of circumanal hair slightly precedes that of axillary hair in boys. Comedones, acne, and seborrhea of the scalp appear as a result of the increased secretion of gonadal steroids at about 13 y in girls; the most serious variety, acne fulminans, occurs mainly in pubertal males.[36]

Gonadal Development and Function

Female

OVARIAN DEVELOPMENT IN PUBERTY. (Also see Chapter 12.) Primordial follicles appear during the fourth to fifth month of fetal life and constitute the lifelong store of follicles

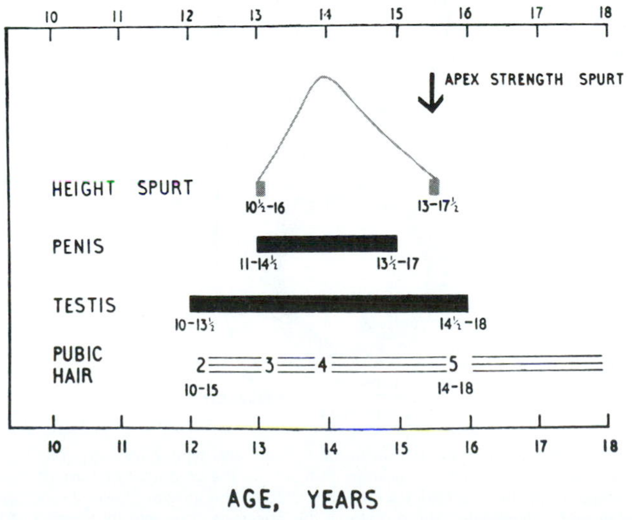

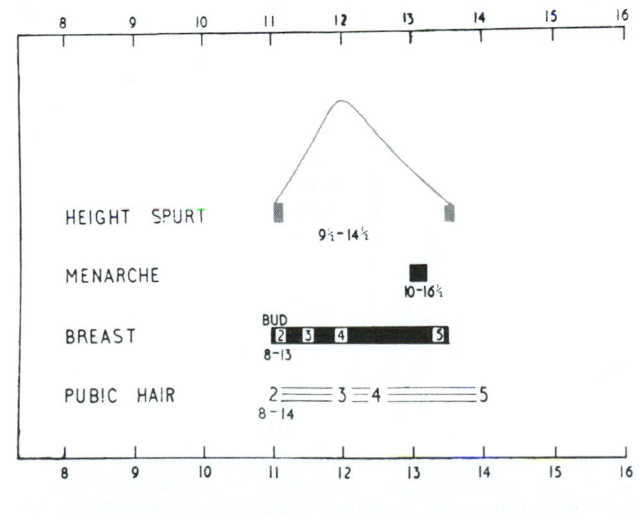

Figure 22–5. Diagram of the sequence of events at puberty in males. An average is represented in relation to the scale of ages; the range of ages within which some of the changes occur is indicated by the figures below. (From Marshall WA, Tanner JM. Variations in the pattern of pubertal changes in boys. Arch Dis Child 1970; 45:13–23.)

Figure 22–6. The sequence of events at puberty in females. The design of the figure is described in the legend of Figure 22–5. (From Marshall WA, Tanner JM. Variations in pattern of pubertal changes in girls. Arch Dis Child 1969; 44:291–303.)

for the individual. During fetal life and childhood, follicular growth to the large antral stage occurs, but before menarche all developing follicles are destined to undergo atresia (Fig. 22–7). Large preovulatory follicles are rarely present before puberty. During follicular growth, the oocyte enlarges and granulosa cells are transformed from spindle-shaped to cuboidal cells that, along with the ovum, secrete the zona pellucidum. The granulosa cells multiply with a substantial increase in volume of the follicle, and ultimately a plasma transudate, the follicular fluid, forms in response to follicle-stimulating hormone (FSH) and fills the antrum. The theca develops during the time of antrum formation. During reproductive life the follicle undergoes luteinization or terminal differentiation into a corpus luteum, which is the major source of gonadal steroids after ovulation. After 8 d of gonadal steroid secretion in the absence of fertilization, the follicle undergoes dedifferentiation, and cytolysis results in an avascular scar. If fertilization occurs, fetal tissue, through the secretion of human chorionic gonadotropin (hCG), supports the corpus luteum throughout pregnancy.[37, 38]

Ultrasonographic studies (Fig. 22–8) show that the corpus of the uterus increases during pubertal progression from an initial tubular shape to a bulbous structure and that the length of the uterus increases from 2 to 3 cm to 5 to 8 cm.[39] During prepuberty the ovaries measure 0.7 to 0.9 mL on ultrasound scans, and after the onset of puberty they increase in volume to 2 to 10 mL.[40]

MENARCHE. (See Chapter 12.) Anovulatory cycles are common in the first years after menarche. Apter and Vihko[41] reported a prevalence of 55% anovulation in the first 2 y after menarche that decreased to 20% anovulatory cycles by the fifth year; others have observed a lower number of ovulatory events shortly after menarche as well as 5 y after the event.[42, 43] The majority of pubertal females are infertile in terms of pregnancy risk, but a substantial number are fertile.

Male

TESTICULAR DEVELOPMENT IN PUBERTY. (Also see Chapter 13.) During pubertal development the testes increase in size, principally because of the growth of the seminiferous tubules associated with the onset of spermatogenetic activity, and testosterone production increases (reviewed in ref. 44) (Fig. 22–9 and Table 22–5). The Sertoli cells are the major cell type in the seminiferous cords in prepuberty, but in the adult, germ cells predominate. During progression through puberty, the Sertoli cells cease to undergo mitosis, differentiate into adult-type Sertoli cells, and form occlusive junctions with the development of the blood-testicular barrier. Although Leydig cells can be detected in early gestation and again during the neonatal period of testosterone secretion, during childhood the interstitial tissue is composed principally of undifferentiated mesenchyme-type cells. With pubertal development and rising serum luteinizing hormone (LH) levels, Leydig cells can be recognized again.

SPERMATOGENESIS. The first histological evidence of spermatogenesis appears between ages 11 and 15; sperm can be detected in the first morning urine specimen at a mean chronological age of 13.3, a phenomenon that probably reflects the maturation of spermatogenesis.[45, 46] Hence, spermarche is a relatively early pubertal event that occurs at

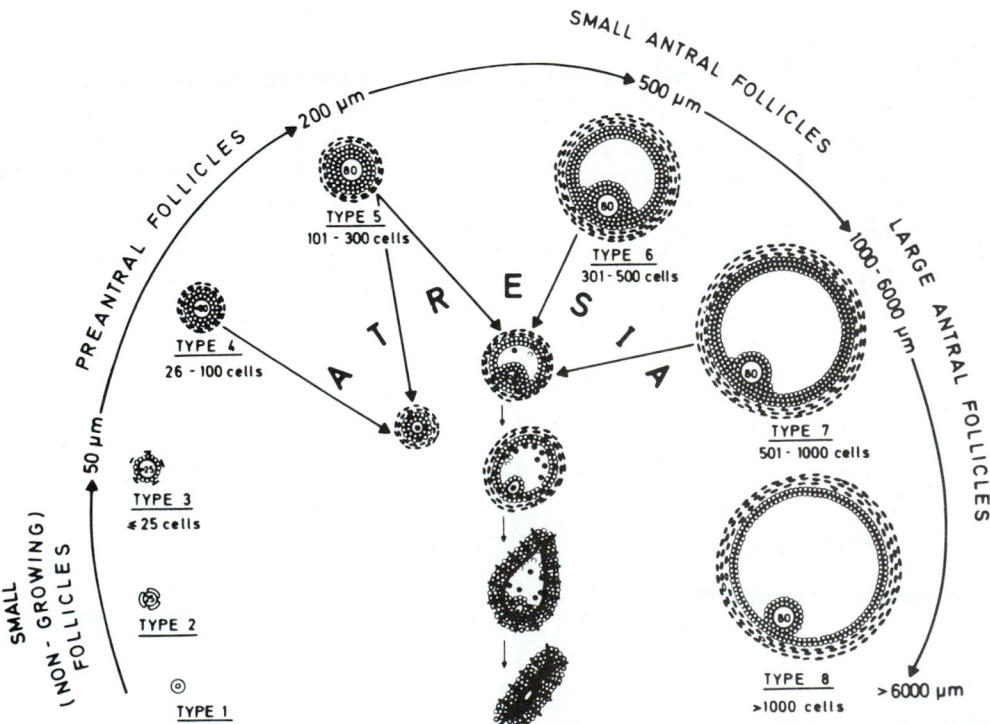

Figure 22–7. Schematic representation of the growth of ovarian follicles during infancy and childhood. Type 1 (primordial follicle) and type 2 (primary follicle) are composed of a small oocyte and a few to a ring of flat granulosa cells. In the diplotene (nesting) stage of prophase, primary follicles are the predominant form of oocyte and constitute the reservoir of cells from which follicular growth occurs. Types 3 to 5 (preantral follicles) are follicles that have entered the growth phase; the oocyte is enlarging and is surrounded by a zona pellucida, and granulosa cells increase in number and differentiate. The growth of the oocyte is complete by the end of the preantral stage, and the increased follicular size is due to follicular growth and fluid accumulation. Types 6 to 8 represent antral follicles (graafian follicles) and contain a fully grown oocyte, a large number of granulosa cells, a fluid-filled cavity, and a well developed theca external to the basement membrane. Large preovulatory follicles are absent (10,000 to 15,000 μm). Follicular growth and atresia take place throughout childhood; all follicles that enter the growth phase become atretic, and this can occur at any stage in their development but mainly involves large antral follicles. (From Peters H, Byskov AG, Grinsted J. Follicular growth in fetal and prepubertal ovaries of humans and other primates. Clin Endocrinol Metab 1978; 7:469–485.)

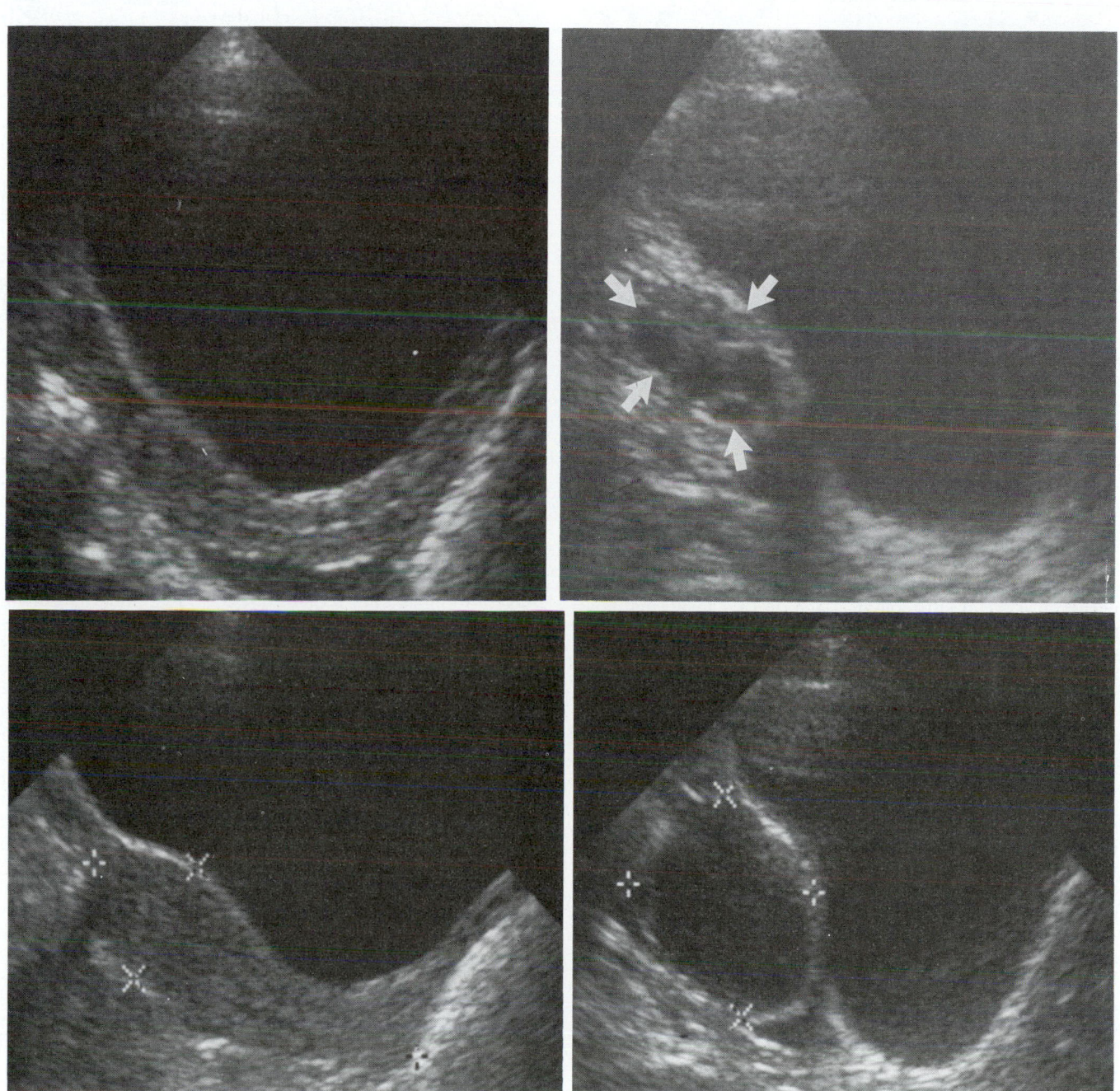

Figure 22–8. High-resolution pelvic ultrasonography. *Top left*, Prepubertal uterus. *Top right*, Prepubertal ovary demonstrating four small follicular cysts *(arrows)*. *Bottom left*, Pubertal postmenarchal uterus. *Bottom right*, Ovarian cyst in a girl with true precocious puberty.

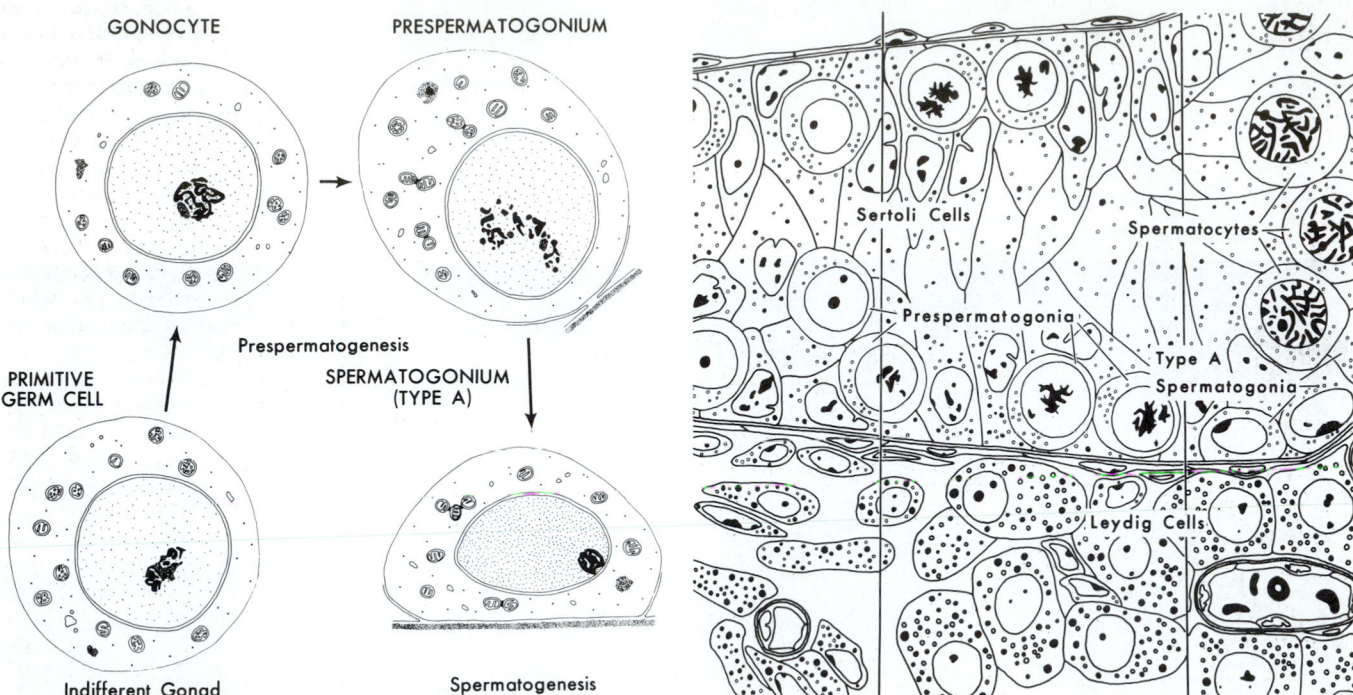

Figure 22–9. *Left,* Diagram illustrating developmental stages of testicular germ cells based on electron microscopic findings in the rabbit. Note differences between prespermatogonium and spermatogonium. *Right,* Diagram showing maturation of testicular cell types in the rabbit from prepubertal appearance at left to onset of spermatogenesis at right. Interstitial cells undergo changes in shape, size, and arrangement in the process of Leydig cell differentiation. (From Gondos B. Testicular development. In: Johnson AD, Gomes WR, eds. The Testis. Vol 4. New York: Academic, 1977: 1–37.)

a mean pubic hair stage of 2.5, before the attainment of adult plasma testosterone concentrations and before peak height velocity is reached.[46] The first conscious ejaculation occurs at a mean chronological age of 13½ in normal boys and at a mean bone age of 13½ in boys with delayed puberty.[47] The potential for fertility is reached before an adult phenotype is attained.

Adolescent Growth

Pubertal Growth Spurt

Prepubertal height and growth velocity are similar in boys and girls. The greatest growth occurs in infancy and decreases to the nadir known as the minimal prespurt velocity just before the pubertal growth spurt. During puberty boys and girls experience a growth velocity greater than at any time since infancy. The pubertal growth spurt may be divided for purposes of comparison into three stages: the time of minimal growth velocity in peripuberty just before the spurt (takeoff velocity); the time of most rapid growth, or peak height velocity; and the stage of decreased velocity and cessation of growth at epiphyseal fusion. Boys reach peak height velocity approximately 2 y later than girls

and are taller at takeoff (Fig. 22–10); peak height velocity occurs during stage 3 to 4 of puberty in most boys (see Tables 22–3 and 22–4 and Fig. 22–5) and is completed by stage 5 in more than 95% of boys.[31, 33] The pubertal growth spurt in girls occurs between stages 2 and 3 (see Table 22–2 and Fig. 22–6).[22, 32] Boys grew a mean of 28 cm and girls grew 25 cm between takeoff and cessation of growth in the United Kingdom study.[48] The mean height difference of 12.5 cm between adult men and women in the Zurich growth study resulted partly from the greater prespurt growth of boys (+1.5 cm); partly from the height difference at age of takeoff, with boys being taller at their later age of takeoff than girls (+6.5 cm); partly from the greater gain in height of boys during the pubertal growth spurt (+6 cm); and partly from the greater postspurt growth in girls (−1.5 cm).[48, 49]

A mathematical model of growth, based on longitudinal data, separates the infancy, childhood, and pubertal phases of growth and allows evaluation of growth in spite of the variation in the age of the onset of puberty. A slowly decelerating childhood component is the base, with a sigmoidal pubertal component added during secondary sexual development (Fig. 22–11). This model provides a new means of predicting adult height, the height adjusted for pubertal

TABLE 22–5. Cellular Activity in Human Testis at Different Stages of Development

Stage	Germ Cells	Sertoli Cells	Leydig Cells
Prepubertal	Prespermatogenic cells present	Predominant cells in seminiferous cords	Scattered, partially differentiated cells present
Pubertal	Initiation of spermatogenesis	Increased complexity, formation of occlusive junctions	Fully differentiated cells appear
Adult	Active spermatogenesis, predominant cells	Individual cells associated with groups of germ cells	Groups of fully differentiated cells present

From Gondos B, Kogan SJ: Testicular development during puberty. Grumbach MM, Sizonenko PC, Aubert ML, eds. Control of the Onset of Puberty. Baltimore: Williams & Wilkins, 1990: 387–398. © 1990, the Williams & Wilkins Co., Baltimore.

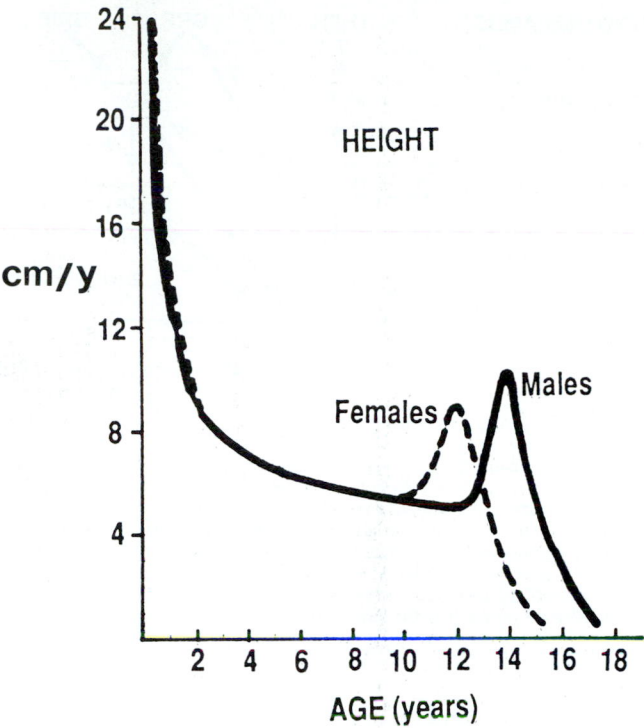

Figure 22–10. The adolescent growth spurt in boys and girls (growth velocity curves). Note the later onset and the greater peak height velocity in boys.

of peak height velocity and are purported to have greater validity for evaluation of growth of individual children during adolescence than the standard cross-sectional charts.

A host of other physiological and biochemical parameters change with the onset of puberty and must be interpreted in terms of the stage of pubertal development. The mean heart rate and maximal oxygen uptake do not change in boys with the passage of peak height velocity, but respiratory quotient increases at the time of peak height velocity.[52] Serum inorganic phosphate and alkaline phosphatase levels rise with growth rate during peak height velocity, and another measure of growth, the serum Gla-protein level, also reflects the increased growth rate at that time in both sexes.[53]

Because girls reach peak height velocity about 1.3 y before menarche, there is limited growth potential after menarche; most girls increase about 2.5 cm in height after menarche,[22] although there is a variation from 1 to as much as 7 cm. Boys have no comparable event to menarche during pubertal development to mark the amount of remaining growth; all that can be deduced by physical examination is that a boy in early puberty is likely to have significant growth left, whereas in late puberty limited growth is likely. The ages at menarche, takeoff, and peak height velocity are not good predictors of adult height; because the duration of pubertal growth is the more important determinant of final height, later onset of puberty and consequent increase in height at takeoff of the pubertal growth spurt can be balanced by a decrease in actual height achieved during peak height velocity and result in no net change in adult height. However, early onset of puberty can diminish ultimate adult stature,[54] and prolonged delay of puberty[51a] can increase stature. The age at peak height velocity and the age at initiation of puberty correlate well with the rate of passage through the stages of pubertal development in normal children.[48]

onset (HAPO) method.[50] Tanner and Davies[51] have constructed growth curves for American children using longitudinal data from the National Center for Health Statistics and calculated data from theoretical growth curves thereafter (see Chapter 21); these curves can be adjusted for time

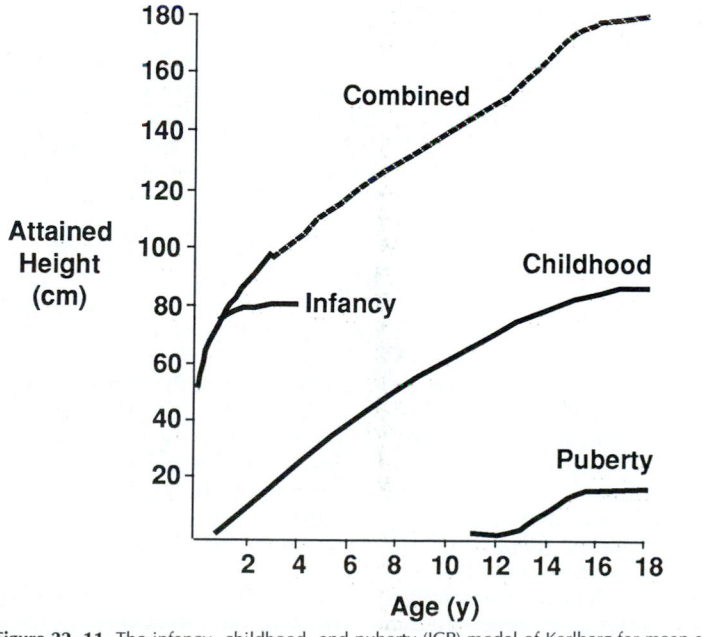

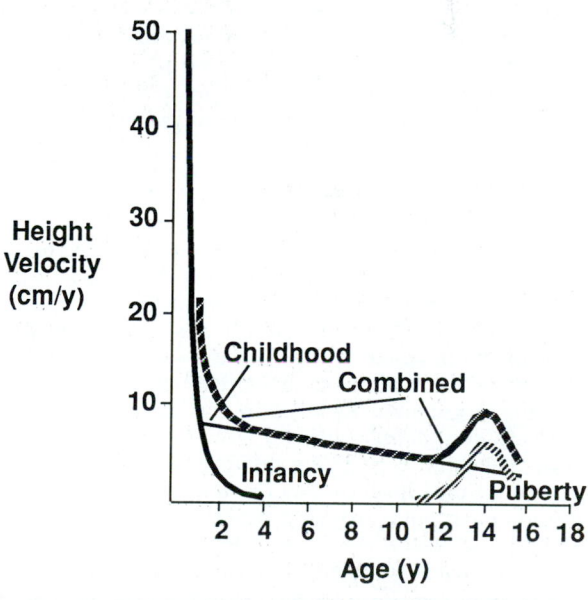

Figure 22–11. The infancy, childhood, and puberty (ICP) model of Karlberg for mean attained height *(left)* and height velocity *(right)* for boys. The mean value for each component (infancy, childhood, puberty) and their sums (combined growth, right; combined velocity, left) are plotted. The growth curve for an individual represents the additive effect of the three biological phases of the growth process (ICP). Karlberg has provided mathematical functions for each component of his model. *Infancy:* This component starts before birth and falls off by age 3–4 y. It can be described by the exponential function $y = a + b[1 - \exp(-ct)]$. Average total gain in height for Swedish boys is 79.0 cm (44.0% of final height) and for girls is 76.8 cm (46.2%). *Childhood:* This phase begins at the end of the first year of life and continues to mature height. A second-degree polynomial function describes this component: $y = a + bt + ct^2$. Average total gain in height for boys is 85.2 cm (47.4%) and for girls is 78.4 cm (47.3%). *Puberty:* The model for the pubertal growth spurt is a logistic function: $y = a/[1 + \exp(-b(t - t_v))]$. Average total gain in height for boys is 15.4 cm (8.6%) and for girls is 10.9 cm (6.5%); y designates attained height at time t in years from birth; a, b, and c are constants; t_v is the age at peak height velocity. (Adapted from Karlberg J. On the construction of the infancy-childhood-puberty growth standard. Acta Paediatr Scand [Suppl] 1989; 356:26–37.)

Both stature and the upper/lower segment ratio, defined as the length from the top of the pubic ramus to the top of the head divided by the distance from the top of the pubic ramus to the sole of the foot, change markedly during the peripubertal and early pubertal periods because of the elongation of the extremities.[55] The legs begin to grow before the trunk, although late in puberty, during the growth spurt, growth of the legs is similar to growth of the upper torso.[56] The mean upper/lower segment ratio of white adults is 0.92, and that of black adults is 0.85. There are no differences in upper/lower segment ratio between the sexes; however, the ratio of sitting height to standing height is higher in pubertal and adult females than in males.[3, 5] In general, hypogonadal patients have delayed epiphyseal fusion and lack a pubertal growth spurt; therefore, their extremities grow for a prolonged period, leading to a decreased upper/lower segment ratio and an increased span for height, a condition called eunuchoid proportions. The distal parts of the extremities, the hands and feet, grow before the proximal parts; a rapid increase in shoe size is a harbinger of the pubertal growth spurt.

The shoulders become wider in boys, whereas the hips enlarge more in girls; the ratio of biacromial (shoulder) breadth to bicrystal (hip) breadth remains constant in boys at about 1.37 but decreases in girls from 1.35 to 1.27.[5] The female pelvic inlet widens, mainly because of the growth of the os acetabuli.

Neural tissue reaches 95% of adult size by the onset of puberty.[5] The size of the head approaches the adult size by age 10, but changes in relationships of the parts of the face are apparent during puberty. Thus the mandible and nose enlarge more in boys, but they and the maxilla, brow, frontal sinuses, and middle and posterior fossae enlarge in both sexes, mainly during the pubertal growth spurt. Children with isosexual precocity have the facial appearance of older children, and individuals with delayed puberty have faces of younger children. The pituitary gland enlarges more in the female; in a magnetic resonance imaging (MRI) study the height of the pituitary glands was no greater than 6 mm before puberty, was 8 to 10 mm in teen-age females and had a spherical appearance in some, was no more than 7 mm in teen-age males, and decreased in young adults.[57]

Lymphoid tissue growth reaches a maximum at about age 12 and thereafter decreases with pubertal progression.

Hormonal Control of the Pubertal Growth Spurt

Hormonal control of the pubertal growth spurt is complex (Fig. 22–12). Growth hormone (GH) clearly is involved in increasing growth at puberty through the stimulation of insulin-like growth factor I (IGF I, also called somatomedin-C) production. Gonadal steroids have two effects on pubertal growth: (1) induction of an increase in GH secretion and thus the consequent increase in IGF I production, thereby indirectly stimulating pubertal growth, and (2) a direct effect on cartilage and bone by stimulating local production of IGF I, among other local factors (reviewed in ref. 58). Gonadal steroids have both growth-promoting and maturational actions on chondrocytes and osteoblasts; the latter action eventually leads to epiphyseal fusion and the cessation of longitudinal growth. Thyroid hormone also plays an important permissive role in pubertal growth.

The secretion of GH increases with pubertal development.[59–66] Increased GH pulse amplitude (not frequency) is mainly responsible for the augmented GH levels.[65] The increase in the concentration of serum gonadal steroids is the major factor in the higher GH secretion during puberty, as both estrogen and testosterone stimulate GH release.

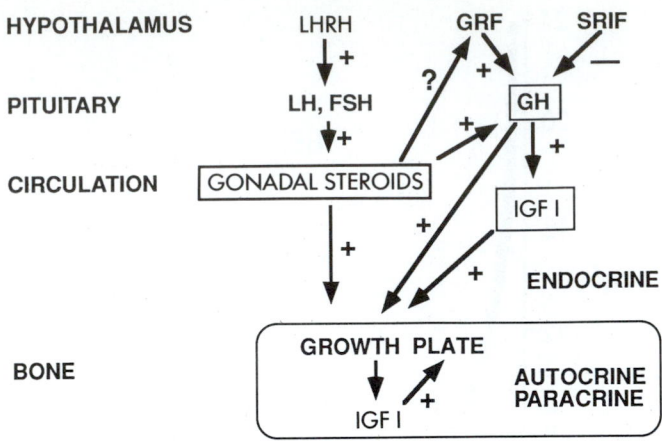

Figure 22–12. Interactions of the major growth-promoting hormones during puberty. Plus (+) indicates stimulatory action, minus (−) inhibitory action. Gonadal steroids in the circulation refer primarily to gonadal estrogens and androgens. Circulating IGF I arises mainly from liver, but other tissues also contribute (endocrine action). Growth hormone and gonadal steroids have a direct stimulatory effect on the generation of IGF I (paracrine action) locally in bone and cartilage cells. For simplification the feedback loops for IGF I and gonadal steroids on the hypothalamic-pituitary unit are omitted.

Increased GH secretion also occurs in sexual precocity. GH secretion decreases with the fall in gonadal steroid levels after treatment of children with true precocious puberty with potent luteinizing hormone–releasing hormone (LHRH) agonists.[60, 67]

Subjects with isolated GH deficiency[68] or GH resistance[69] have an impaired pubertal growth spurt, indicating the importance of GH in this time of rapid growth. Individuals with severe primary or secondary hypogonadism have a minimal or no pubertal growth spurt, demonstrating the primary role of gonadal steroids as well. Hypopituitary patients deficient in both GH and gonadotropins do not have an adolescent growth spurt when GH alone is replaced; gonadal steroids must also be given, substantiating the synergism between GH and gonadal steroids.[56, 70] Individuals with both true precocious puberty and GH deficiency (usually a consequence of cranial radiation) can exhibit a growth spurt indistinguishable from that of children with true precocious puberty and normal GH secretion; after treatment with an LHRH agonist for sexual precocity, subjects with GH deficiency and true precocious puberty have a significant decrease in growth velocity along with the suppression of their pubertal progression,[58] illustrating the direct effect of gonadal steroids on the pubertal growth spurt. The adolescent growth spurt in normal girls depends on both estradiol and GH. A pubertal growth spurt occurs in children with the complete form of androgen resistance (testicular feminization), a finding that supports a role for estrogen in the adolescent growth spurt in girls. Children with chronic adrenal insufficiency who are given appropriate replacement therapy have a normal pubertal growth spurt despite deficient adrenal androgen secretion, indicating a minimal impact of these adrenal androgens on normal growth at puberty.[71]

The concentration of plasma IGF I increases during puberty to reach an earlier peak in girls than in boys[72] and then decreases to adult levels (Fig. 22–13). Increased GH secretion at puberty induces the rise in IGF I level, and both increases are associated temporally with the pubertal growth spurt. The concentration of IGF I is high for chronological age in sexual precocity and low in delayed puberty. Although the precise role of gonadal steroids in the pubertal increase in IGF I concentration is uncertain, the major effect appears

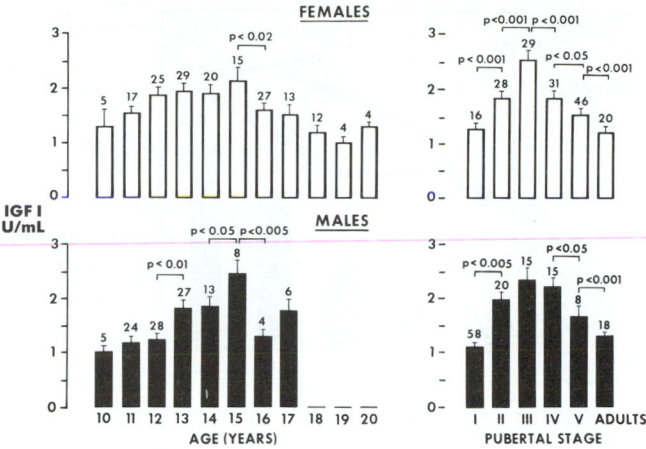

Figure 22–13. Serum IGF I (also called somatomedin C, SM-C) in females and males stratified by age *(left)* and by pubertal stage *(right)*. Males attain peak IGF I levels at 15 y (2.5 ± 0.2 U/mL) at pubertal (genital) stage 3 (2.3 ± 0.2 U/mL). IGF I concentrations reach a plateau between ages 12 and 15 (about 2 U/mL) and peak at pubertal (breast) stage 3 (2.5 ± 0.2 U/mL). The mean concentrations during puberty are higher than both adult and prepubertal values.

to be mediated through increased secretion of GH,[73] with an additional effect through the gonadal steroid–induced local generation of IGF I in cartilage and bone. Studies of patients with true precocious puberty before and after therapy with an LHRH agonist show elevated serum GH concentrations in the untreated state and suppressed GH concentrations for age and a decrease of serum IGF I concentration after therapy, further supporting the concept that GH is the major factor that raises circulating IGF I levels in puberty.[67]

Thyroid hormone is a requisite for normal growth. Patients with primary hypothyroidism may not have a growth spurt even when the disorder is accompanied by sexual precocity[74, 75] (see section on juvenile hypothyroidism).

Bone Age

Skeletal maturation is assessed by comparing radiographs of the hand, the knee, or the elbow with standards of maturation in a normal population.[74, 75] Ossification centers appear in early life, and finally the epiphyses or growth plates fuse with their shafts. Bone age, an index of physiological maturation, does not have a clear relationship in normal children to the onset of puberty; it is just as variable as chronological age. However, bone age is useful for predicting the age of menarche and in delayed puberty correlates better with the onset of secondary sexual development than does chronological age. In addition, bone age, height, and chronological age can be used for the prediction of final adult height from the Bayley-Pinneau tables[76] or the RWT,[77] Tanner-Whitehouse,[75] or Walker[78] technique. Separate standards are used for boys and girls; skeletal maturation is more advanced in girls than in boys of the same chronological age. For example, the bone ages of 11 in girls and 13 in boys (bone ages of early puberty in each sex) are equivalent stages of bone maturation. Although there are no separate standards of bone age, black children have slightly more advanced bone ages than do white children of the same chronological age.[79] A difference between bone age and chronological age must exceed 2 SD to be of biological significance. As commonly estimated, bone age is imprecise. The development of techniques for scanning radiographs coupled with computer analysis should increase the precision of the procedure. Bone density also increases during pubertal maturation.[80]

Body Composition

Striking changes in body composition occur during puberty along with the increase in gonadal hormone levels and maturation of secondary sexual characteristics. Lean body mass, skeletal mass, and body fat are equal in prepubertal boys and girls, but by maturity, men have 1.5 times the lean body mass and almost 1.5 times the skeletal mass of women, whereas women have twice as much body fat as men.[81–86] The increase in lean body mass starts at 6 y in girls and 9.5 y in boys and is the earliest change in body composition at puberty.

Abdominal fat accumulates[84] during pubertal development in girls, and the generalized distribution of fat in males (central fat or apple shaped) is different from that in females (lower body fat predominance or pear shaped).[85] Further, girls at breast stage 2 with predominant fat on the hips had higher gonadal steroid and gonadotropin concentrations, and girls with predominant fat in the abdomen had lower androgen/estrogen ratios, probably because of increased aromatization of androgens to estrogens in adipose tissue.[86] Some evidence suggests a relationship between fat distribution and testosterone-binding globulin (TeBG, also called sex hormone–binding globulin).

A "strength spurt" occurs during puberty after the pubertal growth spurt.[5] The discrepancy in adult strength between men and women is partly due to the fact that men have more muscle cells and partly a result of the greater size of individual muscle cells; the muscle mass is 54% of body weight in adolescent boys and 42% of body weight in adolescent girls. With the change in fat composition there is also a change in body water; body water increases 5% in men and decreases 5% in women. Whereas extracellular water is about 25% of body weight in boys and girls, intracellular water increases at puberty in boys from 36 to 39% and decreases in girls from 36 to 29%. Frisch and Revelle[87] point out that late-maturing girls gain fat more slowly; they relate menarche and the maintenance of menstrual function to the percentage and absolute amount of body fat.

Blood Pressure

Basal systolic and diastolic blood pressures increase with age, weight, height, surface area, and pubertal stage[88–93] at the time of puberty, as does the rise in systolic blood pressure induced by exercise. In sexual precocity, blood pressure rises above prepubertal levels to values commensurate with body size.[88]

Testosterone induces an increase in the concentration of hemoglobin and the red blood cell mass.

BEHAVIORAL CHANGES OF PUBERTY

The psychology and psychopathology of adolescence have not been studied carefully. A review of available publications is beyond the scope of this chapter, but certain aspects are of interest.[94–98d] In general, the more technologically advanced the society, the more protracted the adolescent psychological development.[94] At the beginning of the century, Hall[95] characterized the maturing child restrained by cultural influences as experiencing "Sturm und Drang" (storm and stress), and many depictions of adolescent turmoil followed. In an epidemiological study of 200 randomly selected 14- and 15-y-olds, although 50% reported themselves to be in misery, on evaluation only 12% of the boys and 15% of the girls were judged to be sad, and the prevalence of true psychiatric disorders was 16.3%.[96] In a longitudinal study of normal adolescents in the United States, of 320 first-year high school students followed for 4 y and 64 followed for 8 y, 21% were judged to be in turmoil (the tumultuous group) and the other 79% to have successful adaptive development.[97] A study of adolescent psychopathology demonstrated that many with adolescent turmoil "did not grow out of it" when studied 5 y later, in view of the eventual diagnosis of unipolar and bipolar depressive disorders.[98] The frequency of attempted suicide increases abruptly during puberty, and successful suicide now ranks fourth as a cause of death among 15- to 19-y-olds.[94, 96] The changes in behavior in adolescents are related to the changes in gonadal steroid levels.[94, 98b–d]

HORMONAL AND METABOLIC CHANGES IN PUBERTY

Puberty is a stage in a continuum extending from sexual differentiation and the ontogeny of the hypothalamic–pituitary gonadotropin–gonadal apparatus in the fetus to the completion of sexual maturation.[99, 100] This process involves changes in the central nervous system (CNS) and increased frequency and amplitude of LHRH secretion at puberty, which initiates and regulates the sequential increases in the secretion of pituitary gonadotropins and gonadal steroids that culminate in sexual maturity and fertility.

Gonadotropins

Because of the pulsatile secretion of LHRH, gonadotropin secretion is also episodic. Plasma levels of LH and FSH in the fetus rise after the establishment of the hypothalamic-pituitary portal system until midgestation and then fall toward term as higher inhibitory influences gain prominence; mean concentrations of fetal plasma FSH are higher in females than in males.[100–102] During the first 2 y after birth, plasma levels of LH and FSH rise intermittently to adult values and occasionally higher.[103] Then, from middle childhood, the plasma concentrations of FSH and LH remain low until puberty. Ultrasensitive assays for LH and FSH[104, 105] confirm earlier evidence of pulsatile secretion of the gonadotropins in prepuberty[106–108] and suggest that the immunoreactive levels of LH are lower than previously reported.[105] The serum FSH level is higher than the LH level in prepubertal boys and girls. There is a temporal concordance of LH pulses with FSH pulses of 43%. Primary testicular failure is associated with enhanced amplitude and frequency of FSH pulses.[107]

The peripubertal period is the time that immediately precedes the signs of sexual maturation. During this stage, enhanced release of LH can first be shown in response to intravenous LHRH, and augmented release of pulsatile LH occurs during sleep.[108–115] During puberty, the episodic secretion of FSH and LH becomes more clear-cut as the amplitude and frequency of the gonadotropin pulses increase.[113–115] Episodic LH secretion occurs mainly at night in late prepubertal boys; the amplitude and frequency of such peaks increase, and daytime secretion increases with the progression of pubertal development.[104, 105, 107, 112–118] Single daytime serum samples do not reliably indicate the stage of puberty because gonadotropin levels rise and fall in pulses and are elevated only during sleep in early puberty and during the day only later in puberty. Dynamic testing of gonadotropin release after LHRH administration offers more information than measurement of basal levels. Nonetheless, studies of a large number of individuals using single

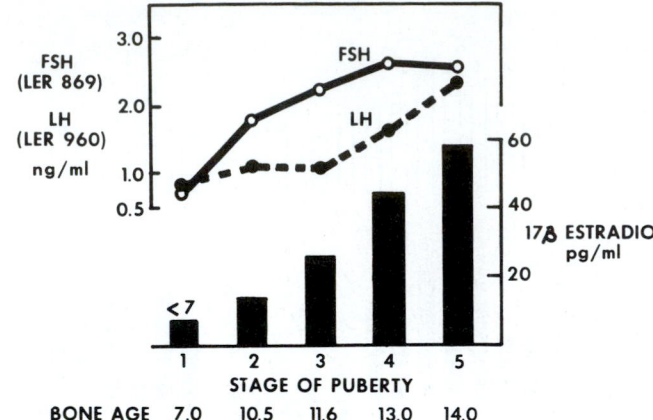

Figure 22–14. Mean plasma estradiol, FSH, and LH concentrations in prepubertal and pubertal females by pubertal stage of maturation (1 = prepubertal, 5 = menstruating adolescents) and the mean bone age for each stage. Single daytime values of gonadotropins have limited usefulness because of pulsatility of gonadotropin release and the increased amplitude of LH pulses during sleep through puberty. The gonadal steroid values, however, are useful in determining the stage of pubertal development. To convert FSH values (LER-869) to international units per liter, multiply by 8.4. To convert LH values (LER-960) to international units per liter, multiply by 3.8. To convert estradiol values to picomoles per liter, multiply by 3.671. (From Grumbach MM. Onset of puberty. In: Berenberg SR, ed. Puberty, Biologic and Social Components. Leiden: H. E. Stenfert Kroese, 1975: 1–21. Reprinted by permission of Kluwer Academic Publishers.)

daytime samples document a change in the mean serum gonadotropin levels between prepuberty and puberty.[119] In girls, FSH levels rise during the early stages of puberty, and LH levels tend to rise in the later stages; from beginning to late puberty, the LH concentration rises over 100-fold. In boys, FSH levels rise progressively through puberty, and LH levels rise and reach an early plateau (Figs. 22–14 and 22–15).[1, 120–123] Doses of exogenous LHRH that are ineffective in stimulating gonadotropin or gonadal steroid secretion before puberty become effective after the onset of pubertal development;[99] thus an amplification occurs in the hypothalamic-pituitary-gonadal axis with progression of puberty.[99, 109, 124]

Levels of biologically active LH as determined by rat or mouse interstitial cell assays and of biologically active FSH as assessed by rat Sertoli or granulosa cell assays have been compared with immunoreactive LH and FSH levels esti-

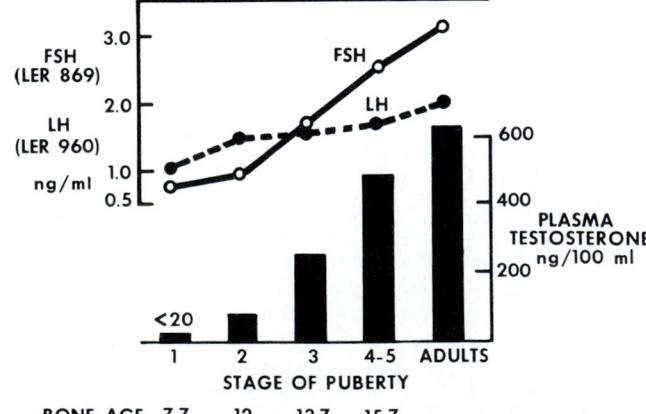

Figure 22–15. Mean plasma testosterone and gonadotropin levels in normal boys by stage of maturation (1 = prepubertal) and mean bone age for each stage. (See legend for Fig. 22–14.) To convert testosterone values to nanomoles per liter, multiply by 0.03467. (From Grumbach MM. Onset of puberty. In: Berenberg SR, ed. Puberty, Biologic and Social Components. Leiden: H. E. Stenfert Kroese, 1975: 1–21. Reprinted by permission of Kluwer Academic Publishers.)

mated by radioimmunoassay.[125–128] The increase in biologically active LH with the onset of puberty appears greater than that in immunoreactive LH. Measurement of biologically active LH may give a more accurate indication of the state of pubertal development than measurement of immunoreactive LH[125] (Fig. 22–16). This discordance may be related to changes in the glycosylation of the LH molecule or to technical factors such as the purity of LH standards, the quality of the radiolabeled LH, and the specificity of the antiserum.[126, 127] Bioactive LH peaks are not always concurrent with immunoactive LH pulses, further emphasizing the discrepancies between the two approaches.[128]

Although it has been difficult to characterize a diurnal variation of immunoreactive FSH secretion, secretion of bioactive FSH increases at night during sleep and is more resistant to testosterone-induced suppression than is immunoreactive LH.[125, 128]

Gonadal Steroids (Table 22–6)

Testosterone

The Leydig cells of the testes produce testosterone and, in lesser amounts, androstenedione, Δ^5-androstenediol, dihydrotestosterone, and estradiol. In addition to direct secretion, a small amount of testosterone is derived from extraglandular conversion of androstenedione secreted by the testes and the adrenal.[129] Although testosterone induces development of a male body habitus and voice change, dihydrotestosterone derived by 5α-reduction in the target cell is the major mediator of the development of the phallus and the prostate, temporal hair recession, and beard growth.[130] In the female, extraglandular conversion of ovarian androstenedione accounts for most circulating testosterone.

Prepubertal boys and girls have plasma testosterone concentrations of less than 0.3 nmol/L (0.1 ng/mL),[121, 132]

TABLE 22–6. Cardinal Hormonal Characteristics of Puberty

Increased amplitude and frequency of LH pulses (initially at night)
Increased LH response to intravenous LHRH
Increased estradiol secretion in girls and testosterone secretion in boys
Increased GH secretion
Increased serum IGF I concentration
Increased prolactin secretion in girls

except during the first 3 to 5 mo of infancy in the male, when pubertal levels are found.[103] Nighttime elevations of serum testosterone levels are detectable in the male during early puberty after the appearance of sleep-entrained secretion of LH[113, 131] and increased pituitary sensitivity to LHRH. In the daytime, increases in testosterone levels are detectable at approximately 11 y in boys, with a consistent increase throughout puberty.[121, 132] The steepest increment in testosterone occurs between pubertal stages 2 and 3 in males (see Fig. 22–14); testosterone concentrations can rise from 0.7 to 8 nmol/L (from 0.2 to 2.4 ng/mL) within 10 mo.[135]

Estrogens

In the female, the major estrogen, estradiol, is secreted principally (90%) by the ovary; a small fraction of circulating estradiol arises from the extraglandular conversion of testosterone and androstenedione. In the male, approximately 75% of estradiol is derived from extraglandular aromatization of testosterone and (indirectly) androstenedione and 25% is from testicular secretion.[129]

In the fetus and at term, levels of estrogen are high because of the conversion of fetal and maternal C_{19}-steroids to estrogen by the placenta. Plasma levels of estrogen drop precipitously in the first few days of life. Subsequently, the plasma estradiol level rises steadily through the stages of puberty until maturity (see Fig. 22–15), when concentrations of 180 pmol/L (50 pg/mL) are reached in the follicular stage and 550 pmol/L (150 pg/mL) or more in the luteal phase; estrone levels rise early and reach a plateau by mid-puberty.[1, 123] In all stages of puberty, boys have higher concentrations of estrone than estradiol, and levels of both estrogens are lower than those in girls at comparable stages.[133] Boys have higher levels of estrone and estradiol in pubertal stage 5 than in stage 1.

Adrenal Androgens

There is a progressive increase in plasma levels of Δ^5-steroids, dehydroepiandrosterone (DHEA) and dehydroepiandrosterone sulfate (DHEAS), in both boys and girls beginning by age 8 (skeletal age of 6 to 8) and continuing through ages 13 to 15 (Table 22–7); the increase in the secretion of adrenal androgen and its precursors is known as adrenarche. Plasma DHEA has a diurnal rhythm similar to that of cortisol, but plasma DHEAS shows less variation and is a useful biochemical marker of adrenarche. The role of adrenarche in puberty is discussed later (see under Adrenal Androgens and Adrenarche).

Testosterone-Binding Globulin

Between 97 and 99% of circulating testosterone and estradiol is reversibly bound to TeBG; only the free steroid is physiologically active.[134] TeBG is a glycoprotein of 90 to 100 kd, consists of heterogeneous monomers, and has one steroid binding site per dimeric molecule.[135] Prepubertal levels of TeBG are approximately equal in boys and girls, and a decrease in TeBG level occurs with advancing prepubertal age and the concomitant increase in the plasma

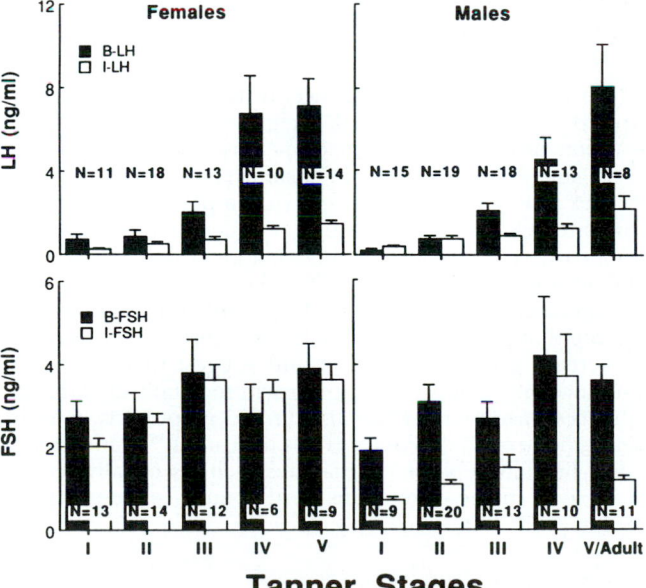

Figure 22–16. Bioactive and immunoreactive plasma LH and FSH levels in prepubertal and pubertal girls and boys. Filled bars designate bioactive LH and FSH and open bars immunoreactive LH and FSH. The concentration of LH is expressed as nanograms per milliliter (LER-960) and that of FSH as nanograms per liter (hFSH-I-3). For conversion to SI units, see the legend of Figure 22–14. (Data from Reiter EO, Beitins IZ, Ostrea TR, et al. Bioassayable luteinizing hormone during childhood and adolescence and in patients with delayed pubertal development. J Clin Endocrinol Metab 1982; 54:155–161; and from Beitins IZ, Padmanabhan V, Kasa-Vubu J, et al. Serum bioactive follicle-stimulating hormone concentrations from prepuberty to adulthood: a cross-sectional study. J Clin Endocrinol Metab 1990; 71:1022–1027. Figure courtesy of I.Z. Beitins.)

	Concentration, μmol/L (ng/mL), at Chronological Age					
	6–8 y	**8–10 y**	**10–12 y**	**12–14 y**	**14–16 y**	**16–20 y**
Boys	0.5 (188)	1.6 (586)	3.4 (1260)	3.6 (1330)	7.2 (2640)	7.2 (2640)
Girls	0.8 (306)	3.2 (1170)	3.1 (1130)	4.6 (1690)	6.9 (2540)	6.3 (2320)

	Concentration, μmol/L (ng/mL), at Bone Age				
	6–8 y	**8–10 y**	**10–12 y**	**12–14 y**	**14–16 y**
Boys	0.98 (360)	1.6 (574)	3.4 (1250)	5.8 (2150)	10.9 (4030)
Girls	0.73 (276)	3.1 (1130)	4.33 (1560)	7.1 (2610)	3.9 (1450)

Modified from Reiter EO, Fuldauer VG, Root AW. Secretion of the adrenal androgen, dehydroepiandrosterone sulfate, during normal infancy, childhood, and adolescence, in sick infants, and in children with endocrinologic abnormalities. J Pediatr 1977; 90:766–770.

gonadal steroid levels; at puberty there is a small decrease in TeBG levels in girls and a greater decrease in boys. The rise in adrenal androgen levels at adrenarche may explain the early drop in TeBG levels, which allows more free hormone at a given concentration of testosterone.[136] Although the plasma concentration of testosterone is 20 times greater in men than in women, the concentration of free testosterone is 40 times greater.[134, 137–139] Boys with hypogonadotropic hypogonadism and girls with androgen resistance show the same characteristic fall in TeBG levels at puberty, but values are intermediate between those of normal adult males and females.[140, 141] TeBG production is regulated by a number of factors. For example, it is down-regulated by GH administration in prepubertal children, perhaps by the action of IGF I.[142]

Prolactin

Prolactin levels rise in girls during puberty. Prepubertal mean (± standard error) plasma prolactin concentrations are 4.0 ± 0.5 μg/L in boys and 4.5 ± 0.6 μg/L in girls. Late pubertal girls and adult women have higher concentrations of prolactin (7.5 ± 0.7 and 8.3 ± 0.7 μg/L), whereas the mean concentration in adult men is 5.2 ± 0.4 μg/L.[143] This sex difference seems to be a consequence of the higher estradiol levels during puberty in girls and in women.

Inhibin

Inhibin, a heterodimeric glycoprotein product of the Sertoli cell of the testes and the ovarian granulosa cell (as well as the placenta), exerts a negative feedback action on the secretion of FSH from the pituitary. Inhibin is composed of an α subunit and one of two β subunits, β_A or β_B, which form inhibin A or inhibin B, dimers with apparently identical function. It is a member of a much larger family of glycoprotein hormones and growth factors that includes antimüllerian hormone (AMH, also called müllerian-inhibiting factor), transforming growth factor β, and the dimers of two inhibin subunits, activin A and activin B, which stimulate the release of FSH from pituitary cells. Production of inhibin is stimulated by FSH. Inhibin appears to play an important role in the feedback regulation of FSH secretion during puberty in males and the development of ovarian follicles in females, a period when Sertoli cells and granulosa cells, the target cells for FSH, divide.[144] Immunoreactive inhibin-like activity increases in both boys and girls during puberty, with mean plasma levels increasing in boys from 161 to 442 U/L and in girls from 97 to 231 U/L between stage 1 and stage 5.[145]

Antimüllerian Hormone

AMH, a 14-kd glycoprotein dimer structurally related to the subunit of inhibin and transforming growth factor β, is produced by the Sertoli cell of the fetal testis and later in gestation by granulosa cells of the fetal ovary.[146, 147] Immunoassayable concentrations are relatively high in newborn males, may rise further soon afterward, decrease by age 10, and decrease further during puberty. Newborn females have low or nondetectable levels, as do girls in early childhood, but after age 10 girls have levels varying from those in the male range[146] to nondetectable values.[147] Values were elevated in a man with a sex cord tumor and in a woman with a granulosa cell tumor; AMH may have potential as a tumor marker. Concentrations of AMH are slightly higher in individuals with delayed puberty than in pubertal age-matched controls and lower in those with testicular dysgenesis associated with impaired virilization than in normal boys. However, boys with isolated cryptorchidism have normal values of AMH.

Insulin-Like Growth Factor I

IGF I concentration rises during puberty to levels higher than those of prepubertal or adult subjects, remains elevated past the time of peak height velocity, and then falls to normal adult levels (see Fig. 22–13).[72, 73, 148, 149] The increase in testosterone level in boys and in estradiol level in girls correlates with the rise in IGF I concentration, but gonadal steroids are not the direct cause of the increase in circulating IGF I levels. Secretion of GH approximately doubles during puberty; the major effect of estrogen and testosterone on IGF I generation is mediated indirectly via augmented release of GH (see earlier). Children with true precocious puberty have plasma IGF I values characteristic of children in the same stage of normal puberty rather than children of the same chronological age.[73] After treatment of children with precocious puberty with LHRH agonists to lower plasma LH levels, IGF I values decrease along with the secretion of GH. In sexual precocity, as in normal puberty, gonadal steroid secretion appears to stimulate GH secretion, which in turn increases IGF I generation.

Insulin

Serum fasting insulin concentration likewise increases two- to threefold with peak height velocity, and insulin secretion after a glucose load increases over prepubertal levels, suggesting a degree of insulin resistance during puberty.[150–155] Puberty is associated with impairment of insulin-stimulated glucose metabolism as revealed by the euglycemic insulin clamp technique;[152] this change is more striking in adolescents with diabetes mellitus. However, it is limited to peripheral glucose metabolism. Hyperglycemic clamp studies indicate that pubertal individuals compensate for this defect by increasing insulin secretion and suggest that the insulin resistance does not involve amino acid metabolism. Thus the enhanced insulin response to glucose in puberty may increase the protein anabolic effects of insulin.[150] Patients with type I (insulin-dependent) diabetes mellitus usually require an increase in the dose of insulin for euglycemic control at puberty.[150, 154, 155]

Serum Lipids

Testosterone increases serum low-density lipoprotein (LDL) cholesterol and decreases high-density lipoprotein (HDL) cholesterol concentrations and thereby accounts for the adverse LDL/HDL ratio in adult males compared with adult females.[156] Postheparin hepatic lipase activity is increased by exogenous androgens (and decreased by estrogens), accounting for the decrease in HDL after androgen treatment or after a rise in endogenous androgen secretion.[157]

CENTRAL NERVOUS SYSTEM AND PUBERTY

The onset of puberty is a consequence of maturational changes that are incompletely understood.[99, 100, 158, 159] The development of secondary sexual characteristics, the adolescent growth spurt, the attainment of fertility, and the psychosocial changes entrain from the maturation of the gonads and the increase in gonadal steroid secretion. The events characterizing the development of gonadal function can be viewed as a continuum extending from sexual differentiation and the ontogenesis of the hypothalamic–pituitary gonadotropin–gonadal system through a juvenile pause (in which the system is largely quiescent) to the attainment of full sexual maturation and fertility during puberty. These developmental and maturational events have as their end point procreation. Two independent, but associated, processes (controlled by different mechanisms but closely linked temporally) are involved in the increased secretion of gonadal steroids in the peripubertal and pubertal period. The first, adrenarche, the increase in adrenal androgen secretion,[71] precedes by 2 y or so the second, gonadarche, or the pubertal reactivation of the hypothalamic–pituitary gonadotropin–gonadal apparatus.[100, 159] These two processes and their role in puberty will be considered separately.

Puberty is not an isolated de novo event but rather a critical stage, a developmental milestone that involves the reactivation of the hypothalamic LHRH pulse generator and gonadotropin secretion. This complex system, which operates actively during fetal life and infancy,[100, 101, 158-160] is suppressed to a low level of activity in childhood, as exemplified by the small amount of gonadotropin secretion.

Understanding the mechanisms involved in the restraint of gonadotropin secretion during childhood is essential for understanding the onset of puberty. Certain CNS lesions involving the hypothalamus and nearby structures can advance or delay the onset of human puberty.[99, 100, 161-164] For example, true precocious puberty (including cyclic ovulation in girls and spermatogenesis in boys) can occur secondary to a CNS tumor or an inflammatory lesion that involves the hypothalamus. Thus the hypothalamic-pituitary-gonadal complex can be activated prematurely (Table 22–8).

Several regulatory systems are involved in the control of human sexual maturation (Fig. 22–17):

1. In humans and nonhuman primates the neural component that controls gonadotropin secretion resides in the medial basal hypothalamus including the arcuate region[165]

TABLE 22–8. Hypothesis of the Control of the Onset of Human Puberty

1. *Central Dogma:* The CNS exercises the only major restraint on the onset of puberty. The neuroendocrine control of puberty is mediated by the hypothalamic LHRH-secreting neurosecretory neurons in the medial basal hypothalamus, which act as an endogenous pulse generator (oscillator).
2. The development of reproductive function is a continuum extending from sexual differentiation and the ontogeny of the hypothalamic-pituitary-gonadal system in the fetus to the attainment of full sexual maturation and fertility.
3. In the prepubertal child the LHRH pulse generator, operative in the fetus and infant, functions at a low level of activity (the juvenile pause) because of steroid-independent and steroid-dependent inhibitory mechanisms.
4. Puberty represents the *reactivation* (disinhibition) of the CNS suppressed LHRH pulse generator characteristic of late infancy and childhood, leading to increased amplitude and frequency of LHRH pulsatile discharges, to increased stimulation of the pituitary gonadotropes, and finally to gonadal maturation. Hormonally, puberty is initiated by the recrudescence of augmented pulsatile LHRH and gonadotropin secretion, mainly at night.

From Grumbach MM, Kaplan SL. The neuroendocrinology of human puberty: an ontogenetic perspective. In: Grumbach MM, Sizonenko PC, Aubert ML, eds. Control of the Onset of Puberty. Baltimore: Williams & Wilkins, 1990: 1–68. © 1990, the Williams & Wilkins Co., Baltimore.

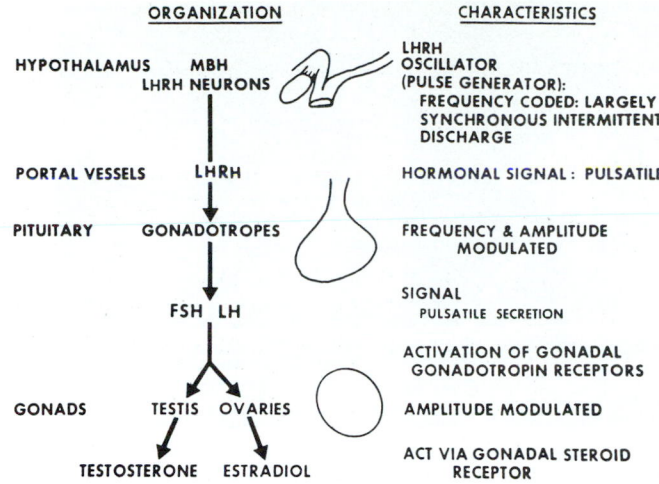

Figure 22–17. Organization and characteristics of the hypothalamic–pituitary gonadotrope–gonadal system. The medial basal hypothalamus (MBH) contains the transducer LHRH neurosecretory neurons. These neurons translate neural signals into a periodic, oscillatory chemical signal, LHRH. This MBH complex functions as an LHRH pulse generator (oscillator), which is frequency coded and releases LHRH from its axon terminals at the median eminence as a largely synchronous intermittent discharge into the primary capillary plexus of the hypothalamic-hypophyseal portal circulation. The LHRH pulse generator is influenced by biogenic amine neurotransmitters, peptidergic neuromodulators, neuroexcitatory amino acids, and neural pathways. During the follicular phase in the adult female and the adult male, an LHRH pulse (estimated indirectly by monitoring LH pulses in peripheral blood) occurs approximately every 90–120 min throughout the day. Changes in the frequency and probably in the amplitude of the LHRH-secretory episodes modulate the pattern of LH and FSH. The major site of action of testosterone and progesterone is on the LHRH pulse generator, as these two classes of steroids decrease LH pulse frequency, but a pituitary site of action has also been described. Estrogens have major direct inhibitory and stimulatory effects on the LHRH-primed pituitary gonadotrope; the inhibitory, or negative, feedback action is associated with a decrease in both the frequency and the amplitude of pituitary LH secretion. On the other hand, evidence also supports a negative and positive feedback action of estrogen on the LHRH pulse generator. Inhibin has a direct inhibitory effect on the pituitary gland and the secretion of FSH. The secretion of gonadal steroids by the gonads is controlled mainly by the amplitude of the gonadotropin signal. (Adapted from Grumbach MM, Kaplan SL. The neuroendocrinology of human puberty: an ontogenetic perspective. In: Grumbach MM, Sizonenko PC, Aubert ML, eds. Control of the Onset of Puberty. Baltimore: Williams & Wilkins, 1990: pp. 1–68. © 1990, the Williams & Wilkins Co., Baltimore.)

and its transducer LHRH neurosecretory neurons, which are dispersed and not segregated into a specific nucleus. These LHRH neurons act in a coordinated manner to translate neural signals into a periodic, oscillatory chemical signal, LHRH.[166] LHRH, a decapeptide, is synthesized as part of a larger precursor protein; the gene, which contains four exons and three introns,[167] is located on the short arm of chromosome 8. The LHRH neurosecretory neurons of the hypothalamic LHRH pulse generator exhibit spontaneous autorhythmicity[166, 168] and function intrinsically as a neuronal oscillator for the entrainment of the repetitive release of LHRH (Fig. 22–18). The mechanism for pulse generation, the coordinated synchronous discharge of LHRH, is unknown but may involve synaptic connections among LHRH neurons,[166, 169, 170] and LHRH itself may play a role. LHRH is synthesized in these neurons and released episodically from axon terminals at the median eminence into the primary plexus of the hypothalamic-hypophyseal portal circulation.[171] The hormone is then transported by the portal vessels to the anterior pituitary gland (see Chapter 5). LHRH is essential for the release of both FSH and LH. In some species, notably rodents, extrahypothalamic CNS structures, including the limbic system (hippocampus and amygdala),[172, 173] influence gonadotropin secretion. Further, the amplitude and frequency of the pulsatile LHRH signal are modified by catecholaminergic and serotoninergic neurons, through their effect on hypothalamic norepinephrine,

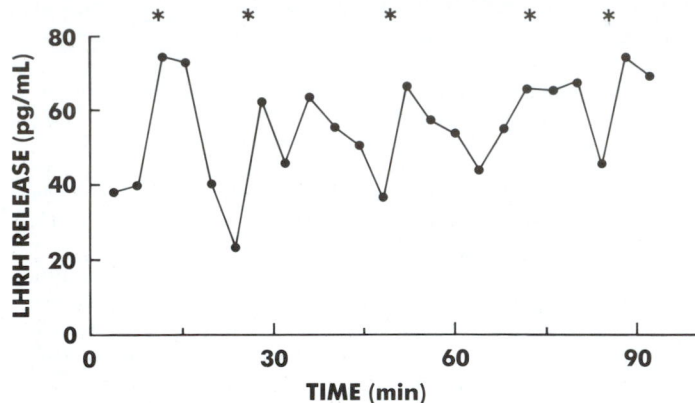

Figure 22–18. The immortalized hypothalamic LHRH neuronal cell line. *Left,* Phase contrast micrograph illustrating the neuronal phenotype (GT1–3 cell line) including the extension of multiple long neurites, cell-cell contacts, and growth cones. The neuroendocrine function of GT cells is limited to expression of LHRH and GAP. Magnification × 175. *Right,* Demonstration of autonomous LHRH (GnRH) pulses at about 20-min intervals by the LHRH neurons in culture. This is the same frequency as that for LH pulses in vivo, in castrated adult mice and rats. To convert LHRH values to picomoles per liter, multiply by 0.8460. (Micrograph from Mellon PL, Windle JJ, Goldsmith PC, et al. Immortalization of hypothalamic GnRH neurons by genetically targeted tumorigenesis. Neuron 1990; 5:1–10. Copyright by Cell Press. Graph courtesy of R. I. Weiner.)

dopamine, and serotonin, and by opioid peptide, corticotropin-releasing hormone, γ-aminobutyric acid, and excitatory amino acid neuronal networks.[171–174, 176] Whether the influence of extrahypothalamic factors on episodic LHRH release in humans is mediated by these pathways remains to be established; among these factors in humans, the inhibitory effects of opioid peptides and corticotropin-releasing hormone on the LHRH pulse generator are the most firmly established. Thus the hypothalamic–pituitary gonadotropin unit is influenced by gonadal steroids, inhibin, activin, and possibly follistatin[144, 145, 175] and by complex neural influences that integrate various intrinsic stimuli and environmental factors and cues. The LHRH pulse generator is a conceptual framework. In vitro studies suggest that the generation of the LHRH pulse is an intrinsic property of the LHRH neurosecretory neuronal network and that other factors modulate the fundamental autorhythmicity of the LHRH neuron.

2. The pituitary gonadotropes, in response to the LHRH rhythmic signal, release LH and FSH in a pulsatile manner. Each LH (and FSH) pulse is induced by a pulse of LHRH.

3. The gonads, which are modulated primarily by the amplitude of the gonadotropin pulse, transmit the episodic gonadotropin signal into pulsatile secretion of gonadal steroids.

This control mechanism, with its three principal components (medial basal hypothalamic LHRH neurosecretory neurons, pituitary gonadotropes, and gonadotropin-responsive elements of the gonad), is common to all mammalian species (see Fig. 22–17). At the last two levels—the pituitary gland and the gonad—the target cells contain receptors for the peptide hormones that mediate the cellular response to the signal.[177, 178]

Although the fundamental properties of the hypothalamic LHRH pulse generator–pituitary–gonadal complex are common to all mammalian species, diverse adaptive mechanisms and strategies have evolved among species and between the sexes that influence the biology and timing of puberty.[179, 180] Photoperiodicity and seasonal breeding, biological clocks, and pheromones are integral parts of the pubertal process in some species but not in the control of human puberty. Other environmental factors and cues that play a role in the human are less critical than in most mammals.

The hypothalamic LHRH pulse generator–pituitary system in the human functions during fetal life and early infancy. The system is suppressed to a low level of activity during childhood (the juvenile pause) and is derepressed or reactivated during puberty.[100, 101, 159, 181] In this light, puberty does not represent the initiation or first occurrence of pulsatile secretion of LHRH or pituitary gonadotropins but the reactivation or disinhibition of LHRH neurosecretory neurons in the medial basal hypothalamus and the endogenous, apparently self-sustaining oscillatory secretion of LHRH after the period of quiescent activity during childhood.

A large body of experimental and clinical studies supports the hypothesis that the CNS, and not the hypothalamic LHRH pulse generator, pituitary gland, gonads, or gonadal steroid target tissues, restrains activation of the hypothalamic-pituitary-gonadal system during the prepubertal years.[99, 100, 162, 163] This inhibitory effect of the CNS appears to be mediated through the hypothalamus and its neurosecretory neurons that synthesize and secrete LHRH in a pulsatile manner.

Pattern of Gonadotropin Secretion

There are two pulsatile secretory patterns of gonadotropins: tonic and cyclic. *Tonic,* or basal, secretion is regulated by a negative, or inhibitory, feedback mechanism in which changes in the concentration of circulating gonadal steroids and inhibin result in reciprocal changes in the secretion of pituitary gonadotropins. This is the pattern of secretion in the male and one of the control mechanisms in the female. *Cyclic* secretion involves a positive, or stimulatory, feedback mechanism in which an increase in circulating estrogens, to a critical level and of sufficient duration, initiates the synchronous release of LH and FSH (the preovulatory LH surge) that is characteristic of the normal adult woman before menopause. The secretion of FSH and LH is probably always *pulsatile* or *episodic,* whether the pattern is tonic or cyclic and regardless of age (i.e., in the fetus, infant, or child, during puberty, or in the adult). However, it is difficult to detect small pulses when the plasma gonadotropin concentration is low (as in prepubertal individuals) because of methodological limitations.

In men, the pulsatile release of LH has a variable periodicity of approximately 90 to 120 min and precedes testosterone secretion by about 40 min.[182] In women the overall pattern of LH pulse frequency and amplitude varies widely during the menstrual cycle from about one pulse per hour in the midfollicular phase to one pulse per 5 h in the late luteal phase.[183] Striking changes in the pattern of the pulsatile gonadotropin spikes and their circadian rhythm occur in the peripubertal period and during puberty. Even though LHRH stimulates the release of both FSH and LH, the pulsatile secretion of immunoreactive FSH in normal adults is less prominent; this discordance in FSH and LH pulses is attributed in part to the longer half-life of FSH than LH, to differences in the factors that modulate the action of LHRH on FSH and LH release by the gonadotropes (especially gonadal steroids, inhibin, and possibly activin), and to intrinsic differences in the secretory pattern of the two gonadotropins. For example, a change in the frequency of LHRH pulses can modify the ratio of FSH to LH released; midfollicular phase concentrations of estradiol and adult male concentrations of plasma testosterone have a greater inhibitory effect on the response of FSH than on that of LH to pulsatile injections of LHRH.[184–186]

The inherent oscillatory characteristic of gonadotropin secretion is a consequence of the pulsatile release of LHRH. However, the physiological significance of the episodic, rhythmic pattern of gonadotropic secretion was unclear until studies of the rhesus monkey by Knobil and associates[187, 279] revealed the essential nature of a periodic, oscillatory LHRH signal for the regulation of gonadotropin secretion. Inhibition of gonadotropin secretion results from the continuous infusion of LHRH because of desensitization of LHRH receptors on the gonadotrope.[177, 178, 188] Intermittent, or pulsatile, administration (e.g., LHRH 1 μg/min for 6 min every hour) restored pulsatile release of LH and FSH in adult monkeys in which hypothalamic lesions obliterated the arcuate nucleus region and thus eliminated endogenous LHRH secretion.[187, 279] Further, pulsatile LHRH administration re-established gonadotropin secretion in animals in which gonadotropin secretion had been suppressed by the continuous infusion of LHRH (Fig. 22–19). These studies provided evidence that the LHRH signal to the pituitary gonadotropes of the adult is frequency coded. Therapeutic pulsatile administration of natural LHRH has made possible the induction of ovarian or testicular maturation, including fertility, in patients with hypothalamic hypogonadism and the suppression of gonadotropin secretion by long-acting potent LHRH analogues in boys and girls with true precocious puberty (see later).

Ontogeny

Studies in the mouse,[189–191] rhesus monkey,[192] and human[193] indicate that LHRH neurons do not originate in the CNS. Instead they arise in the embryo from the epithelium of the olfactory placode and migrate along the pathway of the nervous terminalis-vermonasal complex to the forebrain; the latter also originates in the olfactory placode and forms a connection between the nasal septum and the forebrain (Fig. 22–20). In the mouse embryo (studied in detail by Schwanzel-Fukuda and Pfaff[189] and by Wray and associates[190, 191] by immunocytochemistry, [³H]thymidine autoradiography, and in situ hybridization histochemistry) the LHRH cells arise by embryonic day 9.5 (gestation days 18 and 19), exhibit a sharp peak of mitosis between days 10 and 11, and express LHRH messenger RNA and immunoreactive LHRH by day 10.5, and by day 12.5 all cells that make up the postnatal population of LHRH neurosecretory neurons are present. The cells migrate in a rostrocaudal direction through the nasal septum into the forebrain from day 12.5 to 15.5 along with the terminalis nerve. By day 16.5 the LHRH neurosecretory neurons have a postnatal distribution in the hypothalamus (see Fig. 22–20). LHRH cells were limited to the nasal region in the 36-d monkey embryo, were present in the basal hypothalamus by day 47, and after day 50 were in the same area of the medial basal hypothalamus as in the adult (Fig. 22–21).[192]

The Human Fetus

Schwanzel-Fukuda and co-workers[193] studied a 19-wk gestational male human fetus with Kallmann syndrome (see later). No LHRH neurosecretory neurons were detected in the brain, including the hypothalamus. However, dense clusters of LHRH cells and fibers were present in the nose, including the nasal septum and cribriform plate, and within the dural layers of the meninges under the forebrain. The olfactory bulbs were absent. In contrast, normal male fetuses at 19 wk of gestation had the expected distribution of LHRH neurons in the hypothalamus. These findings in the human

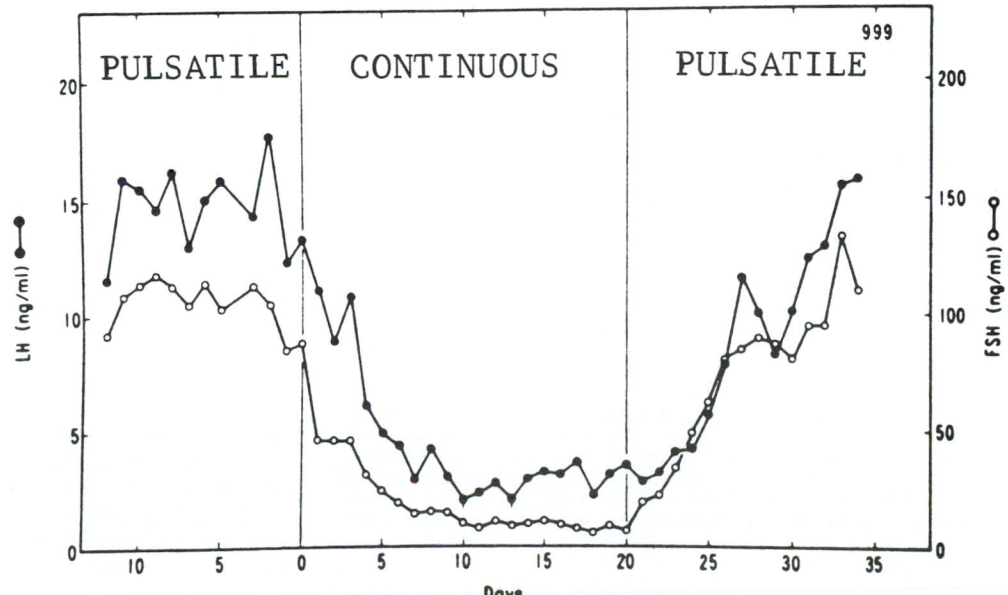

Figure 22–19. Effect of pulsatile administration of LHRH in contrast to continuous infusion of LHRH in adult oophorectomized rhesus monkeys in which gonadotropin secretion has been abolished by lesions that ablated the medial basal hypothalamic LHRH pulse generator. Note the high concentrations of plasma LH and FSH in monkeys given one LHRH pulse per hour, the suppression of gonadotropin secretion by continuous infusion of LHRH even though the total dose of LRF was the same, and the restoration of FSH and LH secretion when the pulsatile mode of LHRH administration was reinitiated. (From Belchetz PE, Plant TM, Nakai Y, et al. Hypophysial responses to continuous and intermittent delivery of hypothalamic gonadotropin releasing hormone. Science 1978; 202:631–633. Copyright 1978 by the AAAS.)

are consistent with the migration of LHRH neurosecretory neurons from the olfactory placode to the hypothalamus in other mammals. Adults have about 1500 hypothalamic LHRH neurons. In the mouse the number of LHRH neurons in the adult is similar to that in late fetal life.

LHRH has been detected in human embryonic brain extracts by 4.5 wk and in the fetal hypothalamus early in gestation (Table 22–9); further, the fetal pituitary gonadotropes are responsive to LHRH.[101, 102] The hypothalamic-hypophyseal portal system is functional by 11.5 wk of gestation.[194, 206] By 9 wk, LHRH neurons are detectable in the fetal hypothalamus, and by 16 wk axon fibers that contain LHRH are present in the median eminence and terminate in contact with capillaries of the portal system (reviewed in refs. 100 to 102). In fetal sheep the hypothalamus secretes LHRH in a pulsatile manner.[195, 196] Thus the available data are consistent with the development of a human fetal hypothalamic LHRH pulse generator by at least the end of the first trimester.

In the previous discussion of hormonal changes, the changing pattern of gonadotropin and gonadal steroid secretion was considered in relation to age. The human fetal gonad is affected by placental gonadotropins and by fetal pituitary FSH and LH. Early in gestation, the placental gonadotropin hCG may play an important role in the secretion of testosterone by the Leydig cells of the fetal testes during the virilization of the wolffian ducts and the external genitalia. However, it is uncertain whether functional hCG/LH and FSH receptors are present in the fetal testis by 12 wk of gestation[197–199] and whether the early fetal testis responds to hCG. In contrast to the adult testis, fetal Leydig cells do not demonstrate desensitization to chronic hCG/LH stimulation. FSH receptors have not been detected in the fetal ovary early in gestation.[199] It is only late in the second

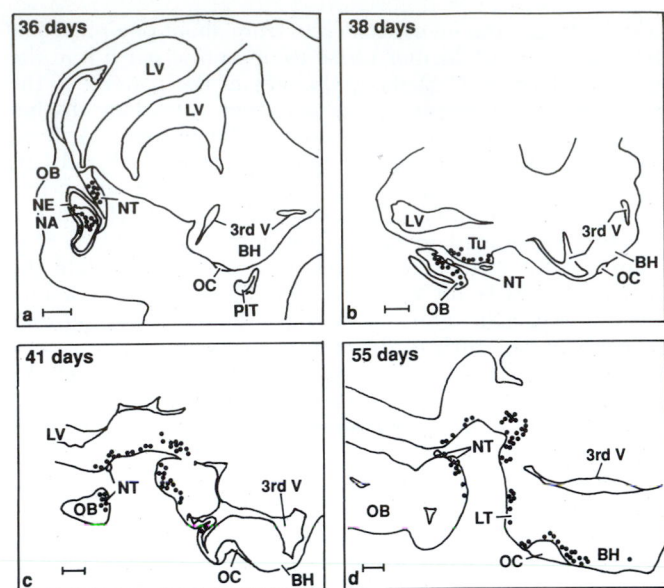

Figure 22–21. Ontogeny of the LHRH neurons in the rhesus monkey. In the 36-d embryo the LHRH cells (black dots) are located deep in the nasal septum along the path of the nervus terminalis but not within the brain. By day 38 LHRH cells are clustered along the dorsal region of the olfactory bulbs and nervus terminalis with a few cells arching back along the ventral surface of the forebrain. By 55 d the LHRH neurons are in the process of migration, but clusters of LHRH cells have entered the CNS and reached the basal hypothalamus. BH, basal hypothalamus; LT, lamina terminalis; LV, lateral ventricle; NA, nasal area; NE, nasal epithelium; NT, nervus terminalis; OB, olfactory bulb; OC, optic chiasm; Tu, olfactory tubercle. (Adapted from OK Ronnekiev, JA Resko, Ontogeny of gonadotropin-releasing hormone–containing neurons in early development of rhesus macaques, Endocrinology, 126, 498–511, 1990, © by The Endocrine Society.)

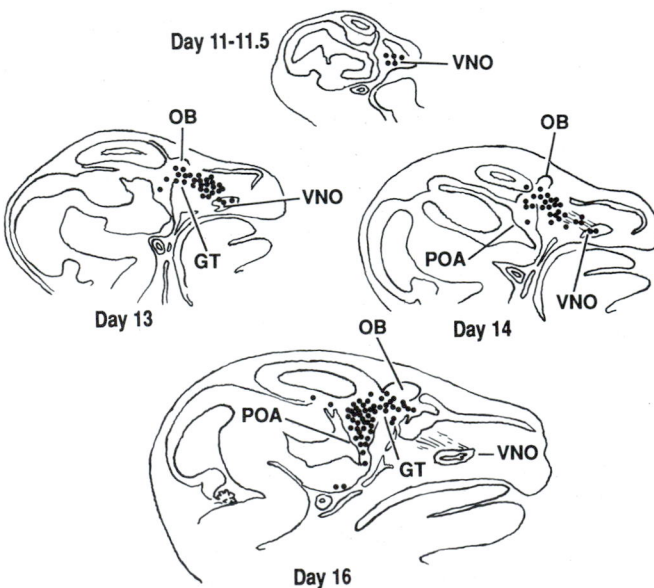

Figure 22–20. Ontogeny of LHRH neurons in the mouse. The route of migration of the LHRH neurosecretory neurons (black dots) in the mouse embryo is shown from their origin in the medial olfactory placode (a plate-like thickening of embryonic ectoderm) in the nasal region through the forebrain into the hypothalamus and preoptic areas. At embryonic (E) day 11 to 11.5 LHRH cells are in the anlage of the vomeronasal organ and medial wall of the olfactory placode. By E day 13 the number of LHRH neurons has increased, and most are in the nasal septum with the nervus terminalis and the vomeronasal nerves; only a few cells are in the brain. By E day 14 the majority of LHRH cells are in the ganglion terminale and the central root of the nervus terminalis and arch through the forebrain to the hypothalamus. By E day 16 most of the LHRH neurons are in the hypothalamus and preoptic areas, and the migration is almost complete. GT, ganglion terminale; OB, olfactory bulb; POA, preoptic area; VNO, vomeronasal organ. (Adapted from Schwanzel-Fukuda M, Pfaff DW. Origin of luteinizing hormone–releasing hormone neurons. Nature 1989; 338:161–164. Reprinted by permission from Nature, Vol. 338, pp. 161–164. Copyright © 1989 Macmillan Magazines Ltd.)

trimester, after completion of male phenotypic differentiation, that fetal FSH and LH have been documented to have an effect on the growth and maturation of the fetal testis and ovary. There is an apparent sex difference in the stage of gestation at which fetal pituitary gonadotropins have an important effect on the development of the fetal gonad. In the anencephalic fetus (which as a consequence of the severe CNS defect is deficient in hypothalamic LHRH and consequently deficient in pituitary gonadotropin) the testes appear hypoplastic by early in the third trimester; however, the ovaries in this disorder are normal until at least 32 wk of gestation.[102, 160, 200]

FSH and LH are detectable in the human fetal pituitary gland by 10 wk of gestation, and the content increases until approximately 25 to 29 wk of gestation[101, 158, 160, 201] (Figs. 22–22 and 22–23). The fetal pituitary gland not only can synthesize and store FSH and LH but also can secrete these hormones by 11 to 12 wk. The fetal serum LH and FSH concentrations rise to peak levels by midgestation and then decrease; the values in umbilical venous blood at term are low (see Figs. 22–22 and 22–23). In the ovine fetus, LH and FSH are secreted in a pulsatile manner in response to the episodic secretion of fetal hypothalamic LHRH (Fig. 22–24); human fetal pituitary gonadotropins are probably released in the same mode. The mean FSH and LH content of fetal pituitary glands and the concentration of fetal serum FSH are greater in female than in male fetuses at midgestation. This difference has been ascribed to the higher concentration of plasma testosterone between 11 and 24 wk in the male fetus (the only major difference in gonadal steroids between the male and female fetus), and the decrease in both serum FSH and LH concentrations toward term during late gestation has been attributed to the maturation of the negative feedback mechanism and the development of gonadal steroid receptors in the hypothalamic-pituitary unit.[101, 158, 201, 202]

TABLE 22–9. The Early Development of the Human Fetal Pituitary and Hypothalamus

Gestational Age (wk)	Hypothalamus	Pituitary	Portal Circulation
3	Forebrain appears		
4		Rathke pouch in contact with stomodeum	
5	Diencephalon differentiated	Rathke pouch separated from stomodeum and in contact with infundibulum; pituitary in culture can secrete ACTH, prolactin, GH, FSH	
6	Premamillary preoptic nucleus; LHRH detected	Intermediate-lobe primordia: cell cords penetrate mesenchyme around Rathke pouch	
7	Arcuate, supraoptic nucleus	Sphenoidal plate forms	
8	Median eminence differentiated: TRH detected*	Basophils appear	Capillaries in mesenchyme
9	Paraventricular nucleus; dorsal medial nucleus	Pars tuberalis formed: β-endorphin detected*	
10	Serotonin and norepinephrine detected*	Acidophils appear	
11	Mamillary nucleus; primary (hypothalamic) portal plexus present; β-endorphin and opoidergic neurons detected*	Secondary (pituitary) portal plexus present catecholamines (IF)†	Functional hypothalamic-hypophyseal portal system
12	Dopamine present		
13	Corticotropin-releasing hormone detected*	α-Melanocyte-stimulating hormone detected	
14	Fully differentiated hypothalamus	Adult form of hypophysis developed	

*Hormone detected at this gestational age but may be present earlier.
†IF, detected by immunofluorescence.
Modified from Gluckman P, Grumbach MM, Kaplan SL. The human fetal hypothalamus and pituitary gland. In: Tulchinsky D, Ryan KJ, eds. Maternal-Fetal Endocrinology. Philadelphia: W. B. Saunders, 1980: 196–232.

Consistent with this sequence of events, in vitro studies indicate that the human fetal pituitary gland is responsive to LHRH as early as 10 wk of gestation;[203] the LHRH-stimulated release of LH is greater in second-trimester fetal pituitary cells cultured from females than males and is augmented by estradiol in both sexes.[204] In vivo studies[205] during middle and late gestation demonstrate the stimulating action of exogenous LHRH on fetal FSH and LH release by 16 wk of gestation with a striking sex difference in the FSH response and a fall in responsivity to LHRH in late gestation (see Figs. 22–22 and 22–23). The anencephalic infant and some infants with neonatal hypothalamic hypopituitarism have an absent or diminished gonadotropin response to LHRH,[101, 102] in contrast to the brisk increase in gonadotropins elicited by LHRH in the normal infant.

The pattern of changes in FSH and LH concentration in the fetal pituitary glands and serum is consistent with a

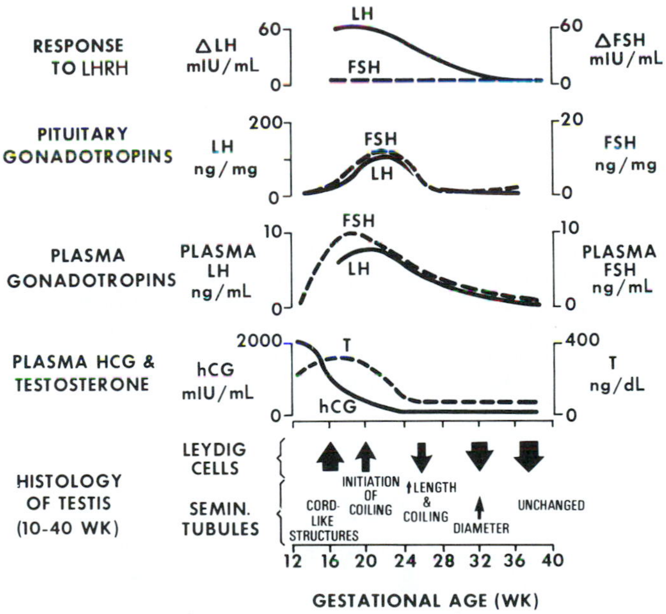

Figure 22–22. Comparison of the pattern of change of serum testosterone, hCG, and serum and pituitary LH (LER-960) and FSH (LER-869) levels in the human male fetus during gestation in relation to the morphological changes in fetal testis. The top graph illustrates the regression curve for the increment (Δ) between a baseline plasma LH and FSH level and the 15-min response to administration of LHRH to the male fetus plotted as a function of gestational age. The scale masks the slight increase in plasma FSH. Data were recalculated from Takagi et al.[205] The evidence supports the hypothesis that the hypothalamic LHRH pulse generator is functional early in gestation and mediates the rise in serum concentration of fetal pituitary gonadotropes. To convert plasma hCG values to international units per liter, multiply by 1.0. Other conversions are in the legends of Figures 22–14 and 22–15. (Modified from Kaplan SL, Grumbach MM. Pituitary and placental gonadotrophins and sex steroids in the human and sub-human primate fetus. Clin Endocrinol Metab 1978; 7:487–511; and Gluckman PD, Grumbach MM, Kaplan SL. The human fetal hypothalamus and pituitary gland. In: Tulchinsky D, Ryan KJ, eds. Maternal-Fetal Endocrinology. Philadelphia: W. B. Saunders, 1980: 196–232.

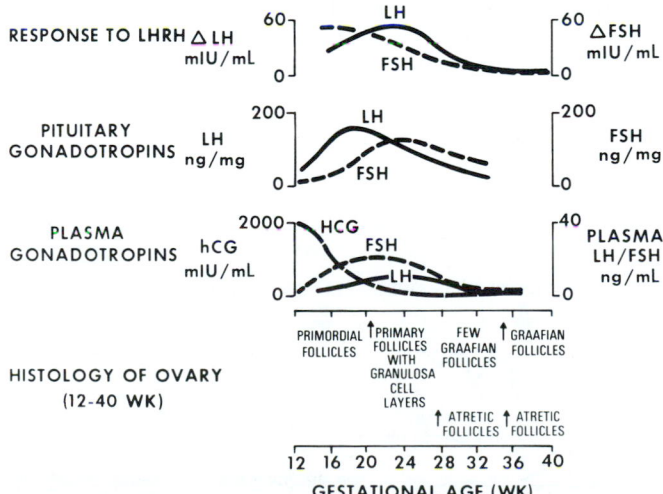

Figure 22–23. Pattern of change of serum FSH, LH, and hCG levels; concentration of pituitary FSH and LH; and increment (Δ) between baseline FSH and LH and the 15-min response to administration of LHRH in human female fetus during gestation with the development of the fetal ovary. See legends of Figures 22–14, 22–15, and 22–22 for conversions to SI units. (Modified from Kaplan SL, Grumbach MM. Pituitary and placental gonadotrophins and sex steroids in the human and sub-human primate fetus. Clin Endocrinol Metab 1978; 7:487–511.)

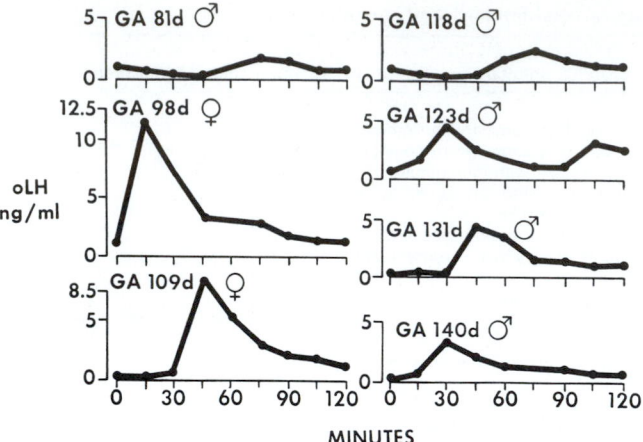

Figure 22–24. Pulsatile LH secretion in the ovine fetus. GA, gestational age. The length of gestation is 145 d in the sheep. (From SJ Clark, N Ellis, DM Styne, et al., Hormone ontogeny in the ovine fetus. XVII. Demonstration of pulsatile luteinizing hormone secretion by the fetal pituitary gland, Endocrinology, 115, 1774–1779, 1984, © by The Endocrine Society.)

sequence of increasing synthesis and secretion in which peak serum concentrations reach castrate levels, followed by a decline after midgestation that persists to term.[101] The high serum concentrations of FSH and LH in the female and LH in the male in early and midgestation are probably the result of relatively autonomous, unrestrained activity of the fetal hypothalamic LHRH pulse generator and subsequent stimulation of the fetal gonadotropes by LHRH.[101, 158] As a consequence of the pulsatile secretion of LHRH, the release of fetal LH and FSH is episodic (Figs. 22–24 and 22–25). As fetal development advances, the negative feedback mechanism matures and the hypothalamus secretes less LHRH, which in turn leads to decreased secretion of FSH and LH.[202] This inhibition of hypothalamic LHRH release and pituitary gonadotropin secretion appears to be a consequence of the increasing sensitivity of the hypothalamus and its LHRH pulse generator to the inhibitory effects of the high concentration of gonadal steroids (especially estrogens and progesterone) in the fetal circulation.[100, 101] The increasing CNS control of gonadotropin secretion seems to require the maturation of gonadal steroid receptors (intracellular or on the cell surface or both) in the fetal hypothalamus and in the pituitary gonadotropes.

The Sheep Fetus

Studies in the human fetus did not provide insight into the mechanisms of maturation or regulation of the hypothalamic LHRH–pituitary gonadotropin–gonadal apparatus. The fetal sheep model in which indwelling vascular catheters are placed in the fetus and pregnant ewe afford an opportunity for mechanistic studies.[194] The length of gestation in the sheep is about 145 d. The ontogeny of fetal gonadotropins, hypothalamic LHRH, and gonadal steroids is similar to that in the human fetus.[100–102] Fetal FSH and LH secretion in the ovine fetus is not autonomous.[100, 195, 196] By midgestation the secretion of fetal LH and FSH is pulsatile[196] and mediated by the hypothalamic LHRH pulse generator.[195] The ovine fetal hypothalamic–pituitary gonadotropin unit has the capacity to respond to gonadal steroid negative feedback by 0.6 gestation.[100, 202] A sex difference in gonadotropin secretion occurs in both the ovine and the human fetus,[100] as demonstrated by the fact that orchiectomy (but not oophorectomy) in the ovine fetus leads to an increase in pulsatile secretion of LH (and to a lesser degree FSH).[207] Opiodergic neurons have a tonic suppressive effect on the pulsatile release of LHRH in the fetus.[100] The excitatory amino acid analogue N-methyl-D-aspartate (NMDA) evokes an LH pulse mediated by LHRH, which provides additional evidence for the functional integrity of the fetal LHRH neurosecretory neurons and the capacity of glutamate and aspartate to stimulate, presumably directly, the LHRH pulse generator. Furthermore, FSH stimulates inhibin synthesis by the ovine testis and ovary, and administration of an inhibin-rich extract inhibits fetal FSH but not LH secretion, evidence of the functional capacity of the FSH–fetal gonadal inhibin feedback system.[208, 209] These observations in the human and ovine fetus, including the pattern of change of fetal FSH and LH, provide support for an operative hypothalamic LHRH–pituitary gonadotropin unit by at least 0.3 gestation in the human fetus and 0.4 gestation in the ovine fetus and for the central role of the CNS in this process.

The Human Neonate

The hypothalamic regulatory mechanisms for pituitary gonadotropins, as for other pituitary hormones, are not fully developed at birth.[100] Within a few minutes after birth in the male neonate, the concentration of LH increases abruptly in peripheral blood (about 10-fold) compared with that in cord blood. This short-lived surge in LH release is followed by

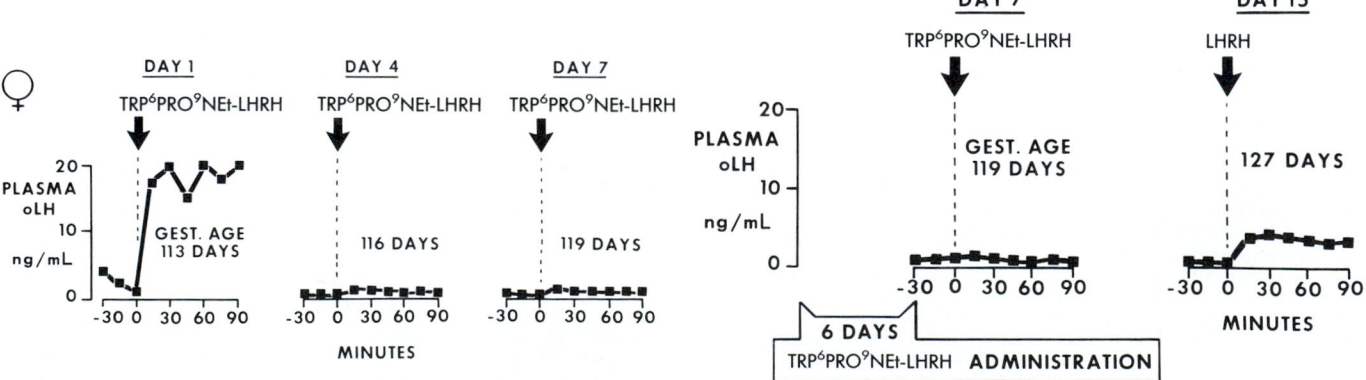

Figure 22–25. *Left*, The effect in the ovine fetus of administration for 7 d of LHRH agonist (10 μg intravenously daily) on the acute LH response to LHRH agonist. *Right*, Recovery of the LH response was impaired 8 d after discontinuing LHRH agonist administration to the ovine fetus. (From Grumbach MM, Kaplan SL. The neuroendocrinology of human puberty: an ontogenetic perspective. In: Grumbach MM, Sizonenko PC, Aubert ML, eds. Control of the Onset of Puberty. Baltimore: Williams & Wilkins, 1990:1–68. © 1990, the Williams & Wilkins Co., Baltimore.)

an increase in serum testosterone concentration during the first 3 h that persists for 12 h or more. In the female neonate this increase in LH release does not occur.[210] After the fall in circulating levels of steroids of placental origin (especially estrogens) after birth, the concentration of serum FSH and LH increases and exhibits a pulsatile pattern with wide perturbations during the first few months. FSH pulsatility is greater in the female infant and LH pulses are of greater magnitude in the male (Fig. 22–26). The high gonadotropin concentrations are associated with increased serum testosterone levels in male infants and increased estradiol levels in females.[211, 212] The mean FSH concentration is higher in females than in males during the first few years of life. By approximately 6 mo of age in the male and 1 to 2 y of age in the female, the concentration of plasma gonadotropins decreases to the low levels that are present until the onset of puberty. Thus the restraint of the hypothalamic LHRH pulse generator and the suppression of pulsatile LHRH secretion (and thus LH release) do not attain the prepubertal level of quiescence until late infancy or early childhood and earlier in boys than girls.[1, 100, 213]

Neural Control

The neural control of puberty involves two major factors: the timing of puberty and the mechanisms involved in control of the transition from the prepubertal or sexually infantile state through complete sexual maturation.

Timing and Onset of Puberty

The time of onset of puberty and its course are influenced by genetic factors and are modified by environmental factors operating through the CNS. The latter include socioeconomic factors, nutrition, general health, geography, and altitude.

The specific mechanisms involved in the timing of puberty are complex. Frisch and Revelle[87] have suggested

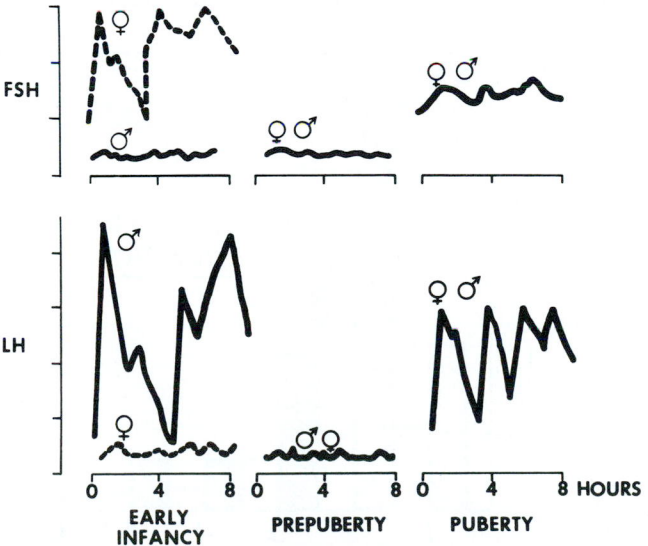

Figure 22–26. Change in the pattern of pulsatile FSH and LH secretion in early infancy, childhood, and puberty. The data for early infancy are derived from Waldhauser et al.[270] Note the pulsatile secretion in the infant and the striking difference in the amplitude of FSH and LH pulses between male and female infants. After infancy the amplitude and frequency of gonadotropin pulses decrease greatly for almost a decade (juvenile pause) until the onset of puberty. (From Grumbach MM, Kaplan SL. The neuroendocrinology of human puberty: an ontogenetic perspective. In: Grumbach MM, Sizonenko PC, Aubert ML, eds. Control of the Onset of Puberty. Baltimore: Williams & Wilkins, 1990: 1–68. © 1990, the Williams & Wilkins Co., Baltimore.)

that in healthy girls, despite different ages, there is an "invariant mean weight" (48 kg) for the initiation of the pubertal spurt in weight, the maximal rate of weight gain, and menarche.[214] The role of nutritional factors and body composition in the onset of menarche is supported by the earlier age of menarche in moderately obese girls;[15] delayed menarche in states of malnutrition and chronic disease, in twins, and after early athletic or ballet training; and the relationship of weight and diminished body fat to changes in gonadotropin secretion and amenorrhea in girls with anorexia nervosa, voluntary weight loss, and strenuous physical conditioning.[16, 215–217] Long-term studies of girls who had had malnutrition in infancy suggest that no permanent delay in puberty persists after early treatment.[218]

The proposed causal relationship of "critical body weight," "critical metabolic rate," and body fat to the time of *onset of puberty* has not been substantiated by direct measurements.[219–221] When increments in the excretion of urinary gonadotropins were correlated with changes in body composition at puberty, both developmental events occurred simultaneously rather than sequentially.[222] Moreover, menarche is a late event in the pubertal process and is remote from the factors that initiate the hormonal events and the first physical signs of sexual maturation. Nevertheless, some alteration of body metabolism may affect the CNS restraints on pubertal onset and progression.

The timing of puberty has been linked to the vague, but generally accepted, concept of "maturation" of the CNS; the maturation is the outcome or consequence of the totality of environmental and genetic factors that retard or accelerate the onset of puberty. It is a provocative but unproven hypothesis that a metabolic signal related to body composition is an important factor in the maturation or activation of the hypothalamic LHRH pulse generator and not a result of the early hormonal changes in puberty. In either event, clinical and experimental data support the contention that the factors influencing the timing of puberty are expressed finally through CNS regulation of the onset of puberty.[99, 100, 162, 165, 223–225] In the human, the pineal gland and melatonin do not appear to have a major effect on this control system.[100, 226, 227]

Mechanisms of Control

In some species, the neural control mechanism is exquisitely sensitive to the environment; for example, in the rat and the mouse, exteroceptive factors and cues, including light, olfaction, and pheromones, have an important influence, by way of the CNS, on gonadotropin secretion.[179, 180] In seasonal breeding species, such as sheep, the length of the light-dark cycle is critical and the pattern of gonadotropin secretion is different. In contrast, male and female primates exhibit an estrogen-provoked LH surge. Studies of the neural control of puberty in different species serve to emphasize the diversity of strategies and adaptive mechanisms that have evolved.[229–233]

In both the human and the subhuman primate, the increase in LH and FSH secretion in early infancy is followed by a long period in which the hypothalamic LHRH pulse generator is suppressed; as a consequence, the pituitary gonadotropin–gonadal axis is quiescent (see Table 22–9).[100, 159, 181] In humans, this prepubertal period or juvenile pause lasts approximately one decade. Two interacting mechanisms have been proposed to explain the prepubertal restraint of gonadotropin secretion.[100, 234] One is a gonadal steroid–dependent mechanism, a highly sensitive hypothalamic-pituitary-gonadal negative feedback system that is dominant in infancy and early childhood. The other is a steroid-independent mechanism that involves "intrinsic"

CNS inhibition of the LHRH pulse generator in the medial basal hypothalamus,[100, 181, 234] that is predominant throughout childhood (Fig. 22–27).

THE NEGATIVE FEEDBACK MECHANISM (GONADAL STEROID DEPENDENT). The principal evidence for an operative negative feedback mechanism in prepubertal children is as follows:[99, 100]

1. The pituitary of the prepubertal child secretes small amounts of FSH and LH, suggesting that the hypothalamic-pituitary-gonadal complex is operative in childhood but at a low level of activity.

2. In the absence of functional gonads in the prepubertal child, as in patients with the syndrome of gonadal dysgenesis or other congenital or postnatal gonadal deficiency, secretion of FSH and, to a lesser degree, LH is increased. The elevated gonadotropin levels in infancy and early childhood in patients with gonadal dysgenesis suggest that even low levels of hormones secreted by the normal prepubertal gonad inhibit gonadotropin secretion;[100, 234, 235] this inhibition supports the hypothesis that a sensitive, functional, tonic, negative feedback mechanism is active in infants and prepubertal children (Fig. 22–28).[99, 100]

3. The low level of gonadotropin secretion in childhood is shut off by administration of small amounts of gonadal steroids. The suppressive effect supports the idea that the hypothalamic–pituitary gonadotropin unit is highly sensitive to the feedback effect of gonadal steroids.[100, 236] However, as discussed later, this is not the dominant mechanism of LHRH and gonadotropin suppression during the juvenile pause.

Figure 22–29 shows the striking sensitivity of the

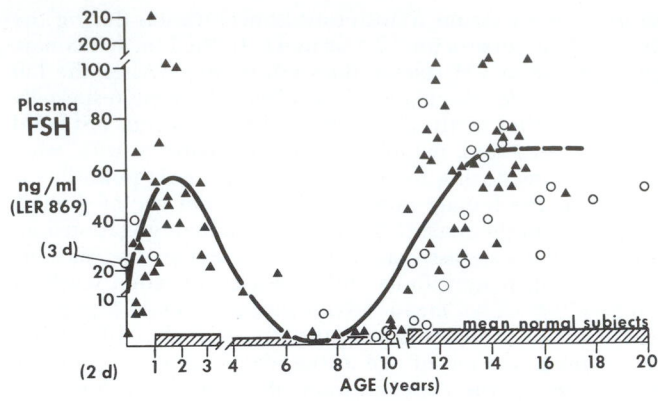

Figure 22–28. Change in pattern of the plasma concentration of FSH with age in 58 patients with the syndrome of gonadal dysgenesis. Mixed longitudinal (n = 23) and cross-sectional (n = 35) data. Triangles designated patients with 45,X karyotype. Circles indicate Turner syndrome patients with X chromosome mosaicism and/or structural abnormalities of the X chromosome. Note the values in the 2- and 3-d-old infants. The solid line represents a regression line of best fit. The hatched area indicates the mean plasma values in normal females. To convert FSH values to international units per liter, multiply by 8.4. (From FA Conte, MM Grumbach, SL Kaplan, A diphasic pattern of gonadotropin secretion in patients with the syndrome of gonadal dysgenesis, J Clin Endocrinol Metab, 40, 670–675, 1975, © by The Endocrine Society.)

hypothalamic–pituitary gonadotropin complex to the administration of small amounts of ethinyl estradiol. The prepubertal hypothalamic-pituitary unit appears to be approximately 6 to 15 times more sensitive than the adult system.[99]

The negative feedback mechanism becomes operative in the fetus during middle to late gestation[99, 100, 103, 202] (see Figs. 22–22 and 22–23). The lower pituitary content of FSH and LH and the lower serum concentration of FSH in the male fetus, as well as the decrease in serum FSH and LH in late gestation in both female and male fetuses, can be explained by the maturation of the gonadal steroid–dependent negative feedback mechanism. The sex differences in FSH and LH levels during midgestation appear to be a consequence of the high plasma testosterone concentration

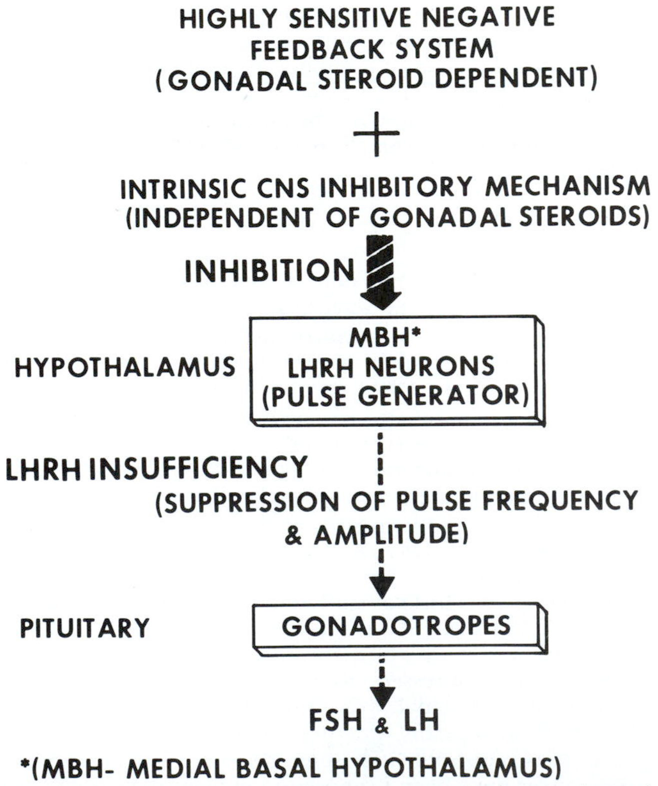

HIGHLY SENSITIVE NEGATIVE FEEDBACK SYSTEM (GONADAL STEROID DEPENDENT)

+

INTRINSIC CNS INHIBITORY MECHANISM (INDEPENDENT OF GONADAL STEROIDS)

INHIBITION

HYPOTHALAMUS | **MBH* LHRH NEURONS (PULSE GENERATOR)**

LHRH INSUFFICIENCY

(SUPPRESSION OF PULSE FREQUENCY & AMPLITUDE)

PITUITARY | **GONADOTROPES**

FSH & LH

*(MBH- MEDIAL BASAL HYPOTHALAMUS)

Figure 22–27. Postulated dual mechanism of restraint of puberty involves both gonadal steroid–dependent and gonadal steroid–independent (intrinsic CNS inhibitory mechanism) processes. (Modified from Grumbach MM, Kaplan SL. The neuroendocrinology of human puberty: an ontogenetic perspective. In: Grumbach MM, Sizonenko PC, Aubert ML, eds. Control of the Onset of Puberty. Baltimore: Williams & Wilkins, 1990: 1–68. © 1990, the Williams & Wilkins Co., Baltimore.)

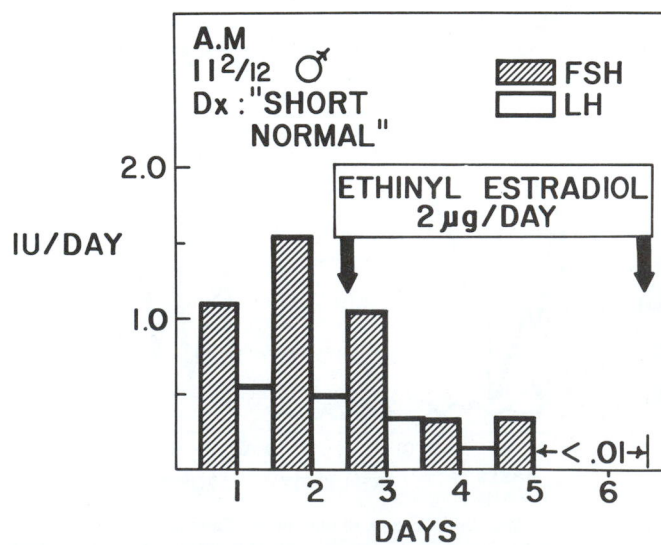

Figure 22–29. Effect of administration of ethinyl estradiol (2 μg/d) on the urinary excretion of LH and FSH in a prepubertal normal male aged 11 y, 2 mo. Note the rapid and significant decrease in LH and FSH levels by day 3 after treatment with estradiol; by day 4 the excretion of FSH and LH is less than 0.01 IU. (From Kelch RP, Kaplan SL, Grumbach MM. Suppression of urinary and plasma follicle-stimulating hormone by exogenous estrogens in prepubertal and pubertal children. Reproduced from the Journal of Clinical Investigation, 1973, vol. 52, pp. 1122–1128 by copyright permission of the American Society for Clinical Investigation.)

in the male fetus. Estrogen levels increase with advancing gestation in both sexes. However, in the newborn infant there is a sharp decrease in circulating levels of estrogen and other gonadal steroids during the first week of life. Consequently, the plasma levels of FSH and LH increase from the low levels at birth in response to the diminished feedback suppression of the hypothalamic–pituitary gonadotropin unit.[211, 212] The increased amplitude and frequency of pulsatile gonadotropin secretion in the second week of life evoke an increase in the plasma concentration of testosterone in male infants and of estradiol in female infants. The gonadal steroid values fall to prepubertal levels by approximately 6 mo of age, and by about 6 mo of age in the male and 1 to 2 y in the female, gonadotropin levels reach values characteristic of the prepubertal child.[211, 212]

"INTRINSIC" CNS INHIBITORY MECHANISM (GONADAL STEROID INDEPENDENT). The diphasic pattern of basal and LHRH-induced FSH and LH secretion from infancy to adulthood is similar in normal individuals and in agonadal patients, but in the latter gonadotropin concentrations are higher, except during the middle childhood nadir.[234, 235] The high concentration of plasma FSH and LH in agonadal children between infancy and age 4 y and the increased gonadotropin reserve reflect the absence of gonadal steroid inhibition (see Fig. 22–28) of the hypothalamic-pituitary unit by the low levels of plasma gonadal steroids.[100] However, the striking fall in gonadotropin secretion between ages 4 and 11 suggests the presence of a CNS inhibitory mechanism that, independent of gonadal steroid secretion, restrains the hypothalamic LHRH pulse generator during this pause. This mechanism suppresses LHRH and gonadotropin synthesis and pulsatile secretion and restrains the onset of puberty. The fall in gonadotropin secretion in agonadal children cannot be explained by gonadal steroid feedback (because functional gonads are lacking) or by increased secretion of adrenal steroids (because concentrations are low and glucocorticoid suppression of the adrenal does not augment the concentration of circulating gonadotropins).[100] Thus a steroid-independent inhibitory mechanism for suppression of the hypothalamic LRF pulse generator, located within the CNS, seems to be the dominant factor in restraint of puberty between ages 4 and 11.[100, 159] Gradual loss of this intrinsic CNS inhibitory mechanism would lead to disinhibition or reactivation of the LHRH pulse generator at puberty.

INTERACTION OF NEGATIVE FEEDBACK MECHANISM AND INTRINSIC CNS INHIBITORY MECHANISM. We believe that both of these mechanisms interact to restrain puberty (Fig. 22–30). During the first 2 to 3 y of life, the gonadal steroid negative feedback mechanism seems dominant, as evidenced by the striking difference in gonadotropin secretion between the agonadal and the intact infant and young child. Extrapolating from the changing pattern of plasma FSH and LH levels in agonadal infants and children, beginning at about 3 y of age the intrinsic CNS inhibitory mechanism becomes dominant and remains so during the rest of the juvenile pause, as evidenced by the fall in FSH and LH levels between ages 3 and 10 despite the lack of functional gonads. During this segment of the juvenile pause, the negative feedback mechanism is operative: agonadal patients in this age group have higher mean plasma FSH levels than normal prepubertal children and a greater FSH and LH response to the acute administration of LHRH.[234, 235] However, the negative feedback mechanism probably plays a secondary role. As puberty approaches, the CNS inhibitory mechanism gradually wanes, initially during nighttime sleep, and the hypothalamic LHRH pulse generator becomes less sensitive to gonadal steroid negative feedback (see Fig. 22–30).[100] After the onset of puberty gonadal

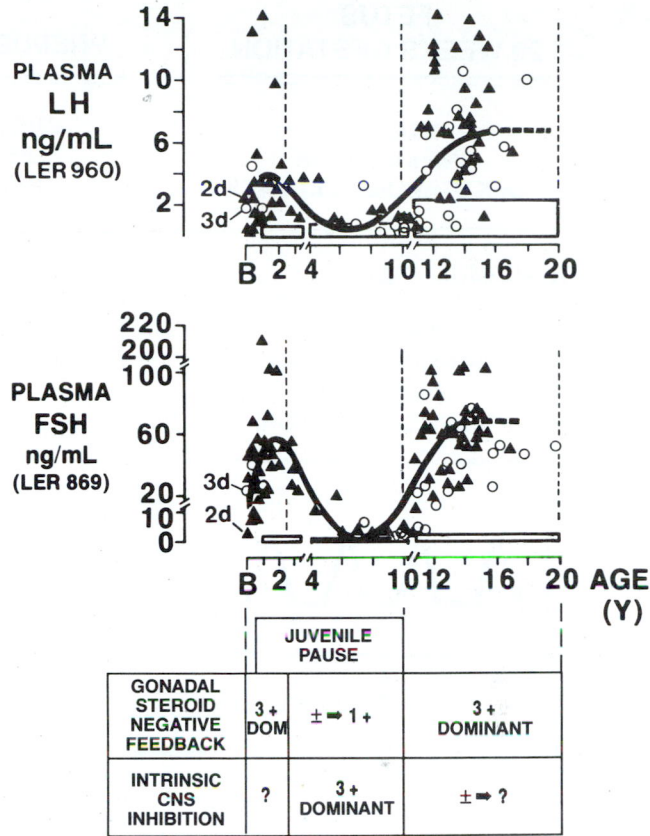

Figure 22–30. Interaction of the negative feedback mechanism and the putative intrinsic CNS inhibitory mechanism in restraining puberty as extrapolated from the pattern of change in the concentrations of FSH and LH in agonadal infants, children, and adolescents. (See Fig. 22–28 for key to symbols; the solid line is the regression curve of best fit; the solid bars connote the mean normal concentrations +1 SD of FSH and LH.) For about the first 3 y of life the sensitive gonadal steroid negative feedback mechanism has a dominant role in restraining gonadotropin secretion, as exemplified by the high gonadotropin concentrations in this age group in the absence of gonads (and gonadal steroid feedback). A major role of the intrinsic CNS inhibitory mechanism in this age group is unlikely in light of the rise in gonadotropins to castrate levels in the absence of functional gonads. From 4 to 6 y of age the postulated intrinsic CNS inhibitory mechanism is dominant, as indicated by the fall in FSH and LH concentrations in the absence of gonads. Even in this age group the augmented gonadotropin response evoked by LHRH and the slightly higher mean basal gonadotropin concentrations in agonadal individuals support a role, although a subsidiary one, for gonadal steroid negative feedback in the suppression of gonadotropin secretion during this period of the juvenile pause. We suggest that the intrinsic CNS inhibitory mechanism suppresses the functional LHRH pulse generator. Finally, after about 10 y of age the CNS inhibition gradually wanes, resulting in disinhibition of the LHRH pulse generator. The gonadal steroid negative feedback mechanism with an adult-type set point and inhibin play a dominant role in regulating the LHRH pulse generator–pituitary gonadotropin system. For conversion to SI units, see the legend of Figure 22–14. (Modified from Grumbach MM, Kaplan SL. The neuroendocrinology of human puberty: an ontogenetic perspective. In: Grumbach MM, Sizonenko PC, Aubert ML, eds. Control of the Onset of Puberty. Baltimore: Williams & Wilkins, 1990: 1–68. © 1990, the Williams & Wilkins Co., Baltimore.)

steroid negative feedback attains the set point characteristic of the adult and is again the dominant mechanism in restraining gonadotropin secretion (along with inhibin), as reflected in the increased gonadotropin concentrations characteristic of the adolescent with severe primary hypogonadism (see Fig. 22–30). A similar pattern has been described in the infant monkey.[237] The postulated ontogeny of this dual mechanism of restraint of puberty is illustrated in Figure 22–31.

Many neural, neurotransmitter/neuromodulator, hormonal, and metabolic factors as well as exteroceptive influences and cues[180] can influence the activity of the LHRH pulse generator, but the nature of the intrinsic inhibitory

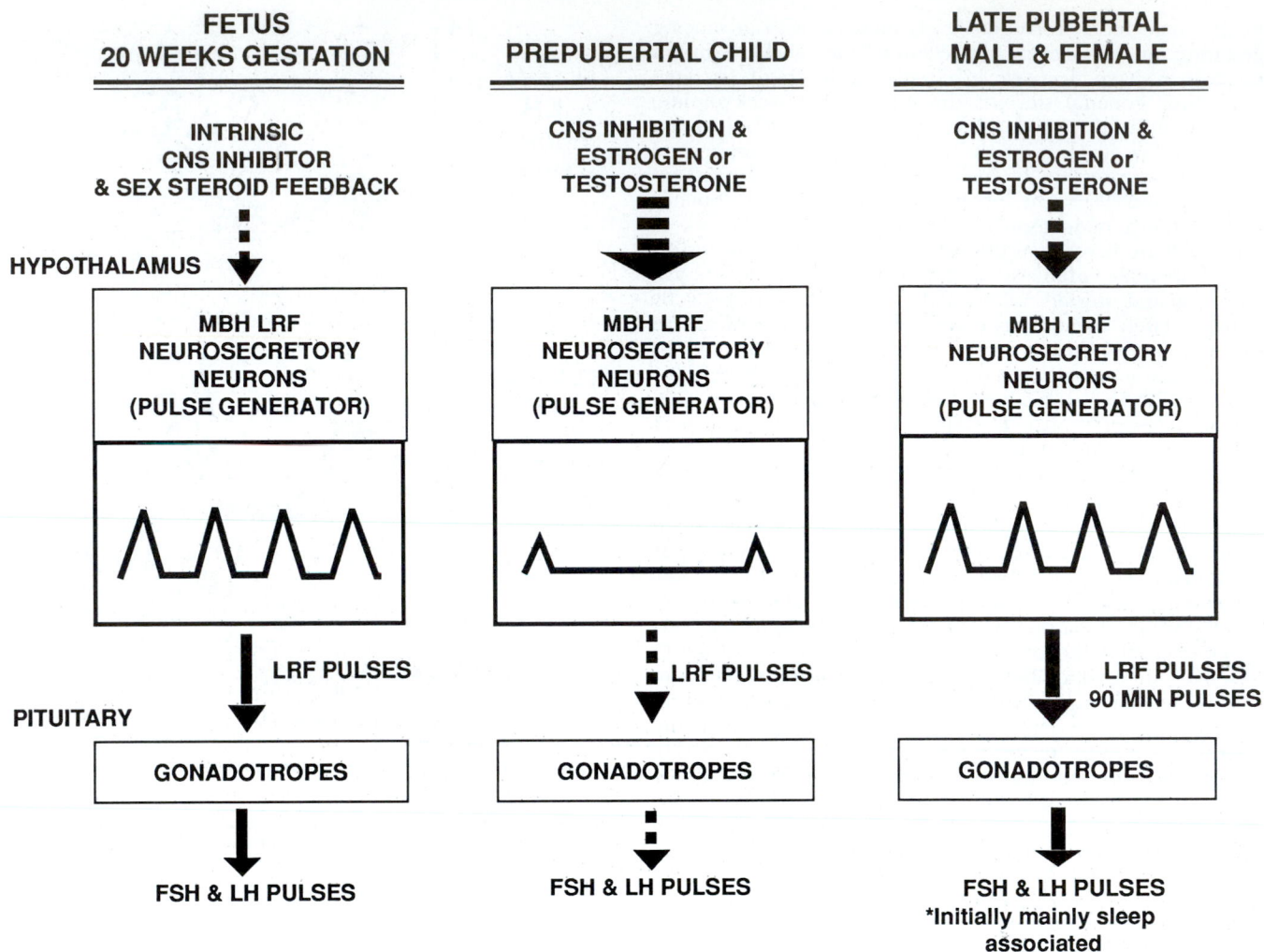

Figure 22–31. Postulated ontogeny of the dual mechanism for the inhibition of puberty. Interrupted arrows indicate inhibition. Note the action of both components during the juvenile pause (prepuberty). See Figure 22–30 for the relative role of these two mechanisms during development. LHRH is given as LRF in the figure; MBH, medial basal hypothalamus. (Modified from Grumbach MM, Kaplan SL. The neuroendocrinology of human puberty: an ontogenetic perspective. In: Grumbach MM, Sizonenko PC, Aubert ML, eds. Control of the Onset of Puberty. Baltimore: Williams & Wilkins, 1990: 1–68. © 1990, the Williams & Wilkins Co., Baltimore.)

mechanism remains speculative. In the rhesus monkey, despite the damping of the LHRH pulse generator during the juvenile pause,[238] the content of hypothalamic LHRH during this phase is similar to that in the infant and adult monkey,[239] nor does the amount of LHRH messenger RNA differ. It should be emphasized that quiescence of the LHRH pulse generator during the juvenile pause is not absolute. Infrequent LH and FSH pulses are detectable by sensitive and specific immunoradiometric assays.[104, 240] The end of the juvenile pause is marked by an increase in both LH pulse amplitude and frequency most evident during the early hours of sleep.[115, 118]

POTENTIAL COMPONENTS OF THE INTRINSIC CNS INHIBITORY MECHANISM. Indirect evidence for an inhibitory neural pathway that arises or projects through the posterior hypothalamus and suppresses the LHRH pulse generator has been derived from studies of children with organic forms of true (or central) precocious puberty (reviewed in ref. 100) and studies in the female monkey.[241, 242]

Children with true precocious puberty associated with posterior hypothalamic neoplasms (usually a pilocytic astrocytoma), radiation of the CNS, midline CNS developmental abnormalities such as septo-optic dysplasia with deficiency of one or more pituitary hormones, or other CNS lesions

Figure 22–32. *A,* True precocious puberty in a 2⁹⁄₁₂-y-old girl (SM) secondary to a large bilateral congenital suprasellar arachnoid cyst. Signs of sexual precocity were noted during the preceding year. The head circumference was +5 SD above the mean value for age, and frontal bossing was present. Breasts were Tanner stage 3. Serum estradiol, 26 pg/mL; estrone, 38 pg/mL; DHEAS, < 3 μg/dL. The serum LH concentration rose from 1.4 to 8.7 ng/mL (LER-960) after intravenous administration of LHRH, a pubertal response. Bone age, 3⁶⁄₁₂ y. Pelvic sonography showed pubertal-size uterus and ovaries. To convert estrone values to picomoles per liter, multiply by 3.699. To convert DHEAS values to micromoles per liter, multiply by 0.02714. For other conversions see legend of Figure 22–14. *B,* Cranial CT scans for SM showing low-density fluid collection in the middle cranial fossa, thinning of the cortex, and striking compression of the lateral and third ventricles. *C,* Cranial CT scans 8 mo later, after decompression of the arachnoid cyst and creation of a communication between the cyst and the basal cerebrospinal fluid cisterns and a cystoperitoneal shunt. Note the striking decrease in size of the fluid collections and expansion of the cerebral cortex. *D,* Basal and peak LH and FSH concentrations after LHRH administration in SM and serum estradiol values before and 2 wk and 9 mo after surgical decompression of the arachnoid cyst. Note prepubertal LH response to LHRH and fall in serum estradiol level by 9 mo after surgery. The bone age had increased by 3 y over an 11-mo period, but the velocity has now returned to normal. The patient remained prepubertal during follow-up. (From Grumbach MM, Kaplan SL. The neuroendocrinology of human puberty: an ontogenetic perspective. In: Grumbach MM, Sizonenko PC, Aubert ML, eds. Control of the Onset of Puberty. Baltimore: Williams & Wilkins, 1990: 1–68. © 1990, the Williams & Wilkins Co., Baltimore.)

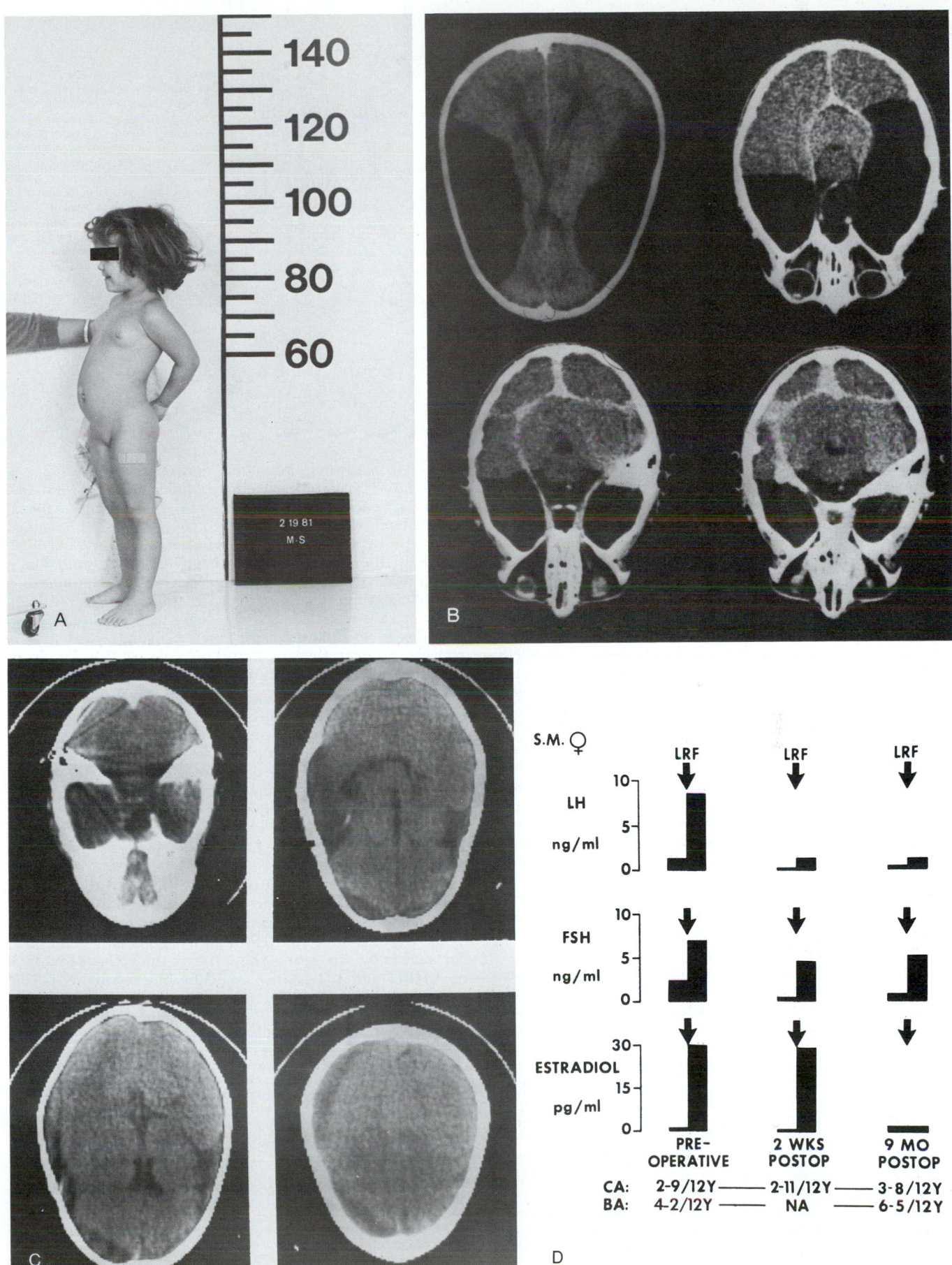

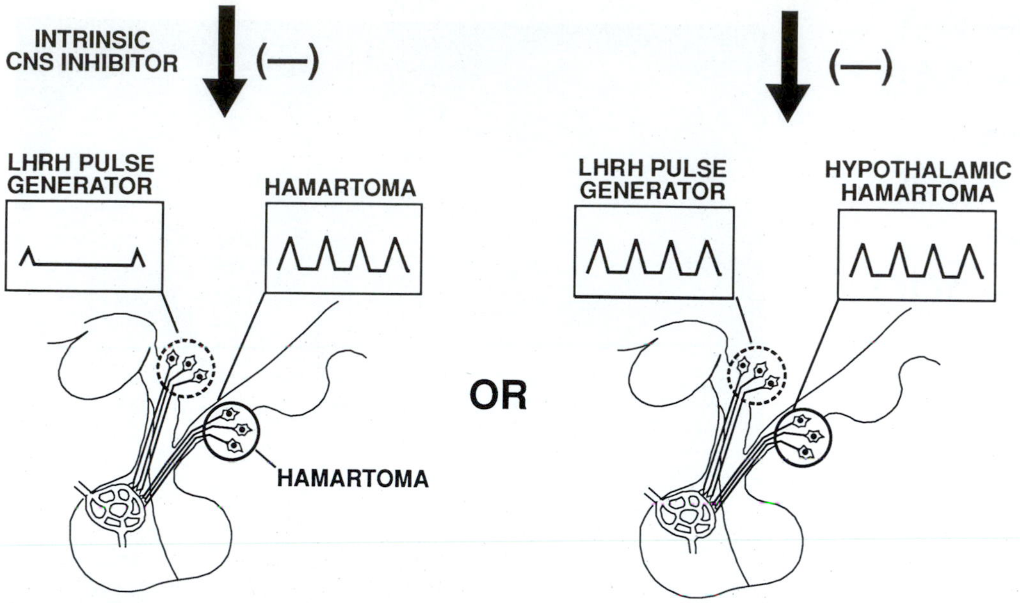

Figure 22–33. Hypothalamic hamartoma as an ectopic LHRH pulse generator that escapes the intrinsic CNS inhibitory mechanism and results in true precocious puberty. Two possible mechanisms are proposed. *Left,* The LHRH neurosecretory neurons in the hamartoma functioning as an LHRH pulse generator without activation of the suppressed normally located LHRH pulse generator. *Right,* The hamartoma acting as an ectopic LHRH pulse generator but communicating with and activating (possibly through axonic connections or by LHRH itself) the normally located hypothalamic LHRH pulse generator, which then functions synchronously with the hamartoma.

provide indirect evidence for an inhibitory neural component located in or projecting through the posterior hypothalamus. As a consequence of these lesions, the neural pathway inhibiting the hypothalamic LHRH pulse generator is compromised, resulting in its disinhibition and activation.[100] For example, a suprasellar arachnoid cyst can cause true precocious puberty by compressing and distorting the hypothalamus.[100] In some children with such cysts the puberty is reversed with regression of the hormonal and physical features of puberty after decompression of the cyst (Fig. 22–32). We suggest that the disinhibition of the CNS inhibitory mechanism was reversed by treatment of the cyst.

The LHRH-secreting hypothalamic hamartoma, a heterotypic mass of nervous tissue that contains LHRH neurosecretory neurons[243, 244] attached to the tuber cinereum or the floor of the third ventricle, can cause true precocious puberty. The LHRH neurons within the hamartoma with their axon fibers projecting to the median eminence secrete LHRH in pulsatile fashion. We consider the hypothalamic hamartoma an "ectopic LHRH pulse generator" that functions independently of the CNS inhibitory mechanism that normally restrains the hypothalamic LHRH pulse generator (Fig. 22–33).[100] An analogy can be drawn between the LHRH-secreting hypothalamic hamartoma and the rescue of fertility in the LHRH-deficient hypogonadal mouse (hyp/hyg) by transplantation of fetal or neonatal hypothalamic tissue into the third ventricle.[245, 246]

Moreover, the ontogeny of the fetal LHRH pulse generator suggests that its initial unrestrained function is followed by differentiation of inhibitory mechanisms in late gestation.[100] Similarly, the immortalized LHRH neurosecretory neuronal cell line exhibits spontaneous, synchronized autorhythmicity in the release of LHRH.[166, 168] Taken together, these observations suggest that a stimulatory input is not required for pulsatile LHRH secretion.

In addition, precocious sexual maturation can be induced in the juvenile female rhesus monkey by posterior hypothalamic lesions;[241] such lesions advance the age at onset of a pubertal increase in LH secretion and the time of the first positive feedback effects of estrogen.[242]

Table 22–10 lists some of the neural and neurotransmitter-neuromodulator factors that may play a role in the restraint of the LHRH pulse generator during the juvenile pause. Noradrenergic, dopaminergic, serotoninergic, and

opiotergic pathways; inhibitory neurotransmitters (e.g., γ-aminobutyric acid) and excitatory amino acids (e.g., glutamic and aspartic acids); and other brain peptides including pineal secretions (melatonin) and corticotropin-releasing hormone affect the hypothalamic LHRH pulse generator.[229, 230, 247–255] However, the precise mechanism of the CNS inhibition is not known. The studies of Plant[256] exclude melatonin as a critical restraining factor in primates (see review in ref. 100). Many studies have assessed the role of endogenous opioid peptides as possible mediators of the juvenile pause. None provide support for an important role of this family of neuropeptides in the juvenile pause.[257–261]

Studies of excitatory amino acid neurotransmitters using the analogue NMDA, which binds to the subtype of glutamate and aspartate receptors that mediates excitatory amino acid synaptic transmission, indicate that NMDA receptors are widely distributed throughout the CNS including the hypothalamus. NMDA stimulates LH release in neonatal[262] and adult[263] rats, fetal sheep,[248] and prepubertal[264] and adult[265] monkeys. NMDA evokes LHRH secretion from rat hypothalamic explants[266] but does not have a direct effect on pituitary gonadotropes.[248]

Studies by Plant and associates[253] indicate that in prepubertal monkeys, chronic intermittent administration of NMDA induces precocious puberty and complete activation of the hypothalamic LHRH–pituitary–gonadal system. Earlier studies by this group showed that the effect of NMDA on LHRH and LH release could be blocked by a specific

TABLE 22–10. Potential Components of the Intrinsic CNS Inhibitory Mechanism

A. Neural or neurohumoral
B. Neurotransmitter-neuromodulator pathways
  1. Neuroinhibitory (γ-aminobutyric acid) and neuroexcitatory (glutamic acid, aspartic acid) amino acids
  2. Endogenous opioid peptides
  3. Brain monoamines (and acetylcholine)
    a. Dopaminergic
    b. Noradrenergic
    c. Serotoninergic
  4. Pineal gland secretions
    a. Melatonin
    b. Vasotocin
    c. Others
  5. Other brain peptides

NMDA receptor antagonist, DL-2-amino-5-phosphonopentanoic acid. These observations suggest that the hypothalamic LHRH neurosecretory neuron is not a limiting factor in puberty. The pulse generator now joins the anterior pituitary gland, gonads, and gonadal steroid end organs as elements that are functionally intact prepubertally as well as in the fetus and can be fully activated before puberty as well as in the fetus by the appropriate stimulus. Hence, the CNS restraint of puberty lies above the level of the autorhythmic LHRH neurosecretory neurons in the hypothalamus.

SLEEP-ASSOCIATED LH RELEASE AND ONSET OF PUBERTY. Episodic, or pulsatile, secretion is the fundamental mode of release of pituitary LH and FSH and is evoked by the pulsatile LHRH signal originating from the hypothalamic LHRH oscillator. Discrete episodic bursts of LH release occur approximately once every 120 min (about 12 episodes over a 24-h period) in adult men[182, 267, 268] and about once every hour during the midfollicular phase in women.[183] In sensitive radioimmunoassays, secretory pulses of LH are detectable in prepubertal children;[104, 107, 118, 257, 272] the pulses are of lower amplitude and usually of lower frequency than those in pubertal children or adults. The low concentrations of plasma LH and FSH make it difficult to demonstrate pulsatile secretion for methodological and statistical reasons, but this problem has been overcome by the use of sensitive immunoassays. In adult men and in women during most phases of the menstrual cycle, little difference in the amplitude or frequency of these episodic pulses is apparent during a 24-h period. In pubertal children, however, Boyar and colleagues[112–114] described the mainly sleep-associated pulsatile release of LH in early and midpuberty; only in late puberty were prominent LH-secretory episodes detected during the day. Kulin and co-workers[271] noted significantly increased excretion of urinary LH in prepubertal children at night than during the day, although the absolute differences were small. In peripubertal, early and midpubertal, and even in prepubertal children, pulsatile LH secretion occurs largely during sleep (Fig. 22–34); in late puberty, the daytime LH pulses increase in amplitude but are still less than during sleep until the adult pattern is finally achieved.

The infant exhibits episodic gonadotropin secretion[270] (see Fig. 22–26); amplitude of the pulses is large and correlates with the increased plasma gonadotropin levels during the first 6 mo in boys and the first 1 to 2 y in girls.[211, 212] After this age, pulsatile secretion is more difficult to detect before the peripubertal period but it is demonstrable at low amplitude and frequency mainly at night[100, 104, 257, 269, 272] (see Fig. 22–26). In boys, augmented LH release during sleep leads to increased testosterone secretion and a rise in the plasma concentration of testosterone at night (see Fig. 22–34).[113] This pattern of sleep-associated LH secretion occurs in agonadal patients during the pubertal age period,[273] suggesting that it is not dependent on gonadal function. Furthermore, sleep-related gonadotropin release is demonstrable in children with idiopathic true precocious puberty[100, 274] and in glucocorticoid-treated children with congenital adrenal hyperplasia who have an advanced bone age and an early onset of true puberty.

Sleep-enhanced LH secretion can be viewed as a maturational phenomenon related to changes in the CNS and in the hypothalamic restraint of LHRH release. However, the neural factors involved in the initiation of this circadian rhythm are unclear. Episodic release of gonadotropins is suppressed by anti-LHRH antibodies and by the administration of gonadal steroids or of certain catecholaminergic agonists and antagonists and is augmented by the opioid antagonist naloxone.

We have suggested that an increase in endogenous LHRH secretion at puberty has a priming effect on the gonadotrope[99, 109] and leads to increased sensitivity of the

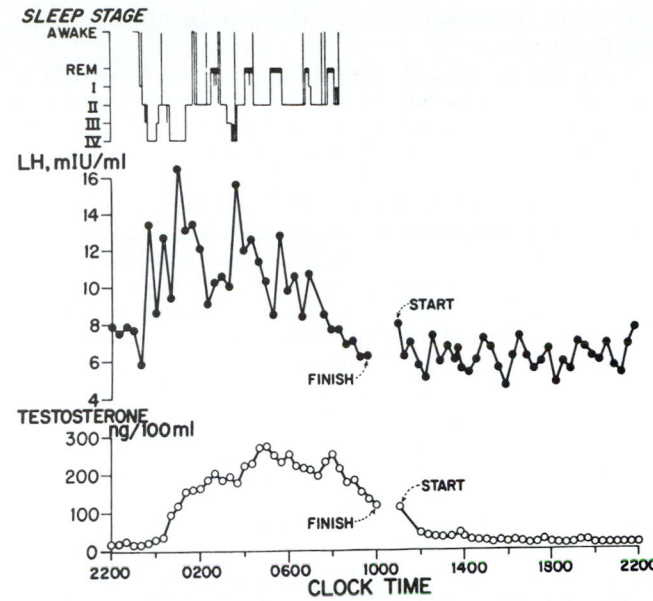

Figure 22–34. Plasma LH and testosterone sampled every 20 min in a 14-y-old boy in pubertal stage 2. The histogram displaying sleep stage sequence is depicted above the period of nocturnal sleep. Sleep stages are REM with stages I–IV shown by depth of line graph. Plasma LH is expressed as mIU/mL. Plasma testosterone is expressed as nanograms per 100 mL. To convert LH values to international units per liter, multiply by 1.0. To convert testosterone values to nanomoles per liter, multiply by 0.03467. (From Boyar RM, Rosenfeld RS, Kapen S, et al. Human puberty. Simultaneous augmented secretion of luteinizing hormone and testosterone during sleep. Reproduced from the Journal of Clinical Investigation, 1974, vol. 54, pp. 609–618 by copyright permission of the American Society for Clinical Investigation.)

pituitary to LHRH (either endogenous or exogenous). Sleep-associated LH release in the peripubertal period correlates with the increased sensitivity of the pituitary gonadotropes to administration of LHRH in the peripubertal period and puberty.

The augmented LH release at night in both sexes is evidence that the hypothalamic LHRH pulse generator initially is reactivated or disinhibited during sleep. Hence, the increased pulsatile secretion of gonadotropins that is entrained during sleep is the neuroendocrine hallmark of the onset of puberty.

PITUITARY AND GONADAL SENSITIVITY TO TROPIC STIMULI. Puberty encompasses orderly maturational changes that involve, sequentially, the extramedial basal hypothalamus, the hypothalamic LHRH pulse generator, the pituitary, the gonads, and the gonadal steroid target organs.[99, 100] At each level these structures may exhibit differences in responsiveness to neural or tropic stimuli, depending on their sensitivity and on the particular hormonal milieu. If the increased secretion of gonadotropins at the beginning of puberty is a consequence of changes in both neural and hormonal restraints on the synthesis and pulsatile secretion of LHRH, disinhibition of the LHRH pulse generator should lead to increased amplitude and frequency of pulses initially, followed by priming of the gonadotropes, increased pulsatile gonadotropin secretion from the pituitary, and finally augmented output of steroids by the gonad. LHRH release is not directly measurable in the human. However, endogenous LHRH secretion can be estimated indirectly and qualitatively by determining the pulsatile pattern of LH and by the gonadotropin response to exogenous LHRH. The pituitary sensitivity to synthetic LHRH and the dynamic reserve or readily releasable pool of pituitary gonadotropins have been studied at different stages of sexual maturation[99, 109–111] and in disorders of the hypothalamic-pituitary-gonadal system. The results support the concept that the prepubertal state is characterized by functional LHRH deficiency.[99, 100, 159, 181]

The release of LH after administration of LHRH is minimal in prepubertal children beyond infancy, increases during the peripubertal period and puberty[99, 100] (Fig. 22–35), and is still greater in adults (depending on the phase of the menstrual cycle in women).[277, 293] The change with maturation in the pattern of FSH release is different from that of LH and results in a striking reversal of the FSH/LH ratio after the administration of LHRH to both males and females between prepuberty and puberty.[99] FSH release after the administration of LHRH is comparable in prepubertal, pubertal, and adult males, indicating similar pituitary sensitivity to LHRH (see Fig. 22–35). Moreover, there is a sex difference in the FSH response: prepubertal and pubertal females release more FSH than males at all stages of sexual maturation.[99, 110] These observations suggest a striking change in pituitary sensitivity to LHRH in prepubertal and pubertal individuals as well as a sex difference in the "dynamic reserve" of pituitary FSH.[99] The sex difference in LH and FSH response to LHRH suggests that the pituitary gonadotropes of prepubertal females are more sensitive to

LHRH than those of prepubertal males, even though there is no apparent difference in the concentration of circulating gonadal steroids at this stage of maturation. Prepubertal girls have a larger readily releasable pool of pituitary FSH than prepubertal or pubertal males (see Fig. 22–35). The sex difference in sensitivity to LHRH and releasable FSH may be a factor in the higher frequency of idiopathic true precocious puberty in girls and in the occurrence of premature thelarche.[275] The available data are consistent with the hypothesis that less LHRH is required for FSH than for LH release. These findings also point out the difference between pituitary sensitivity and the actual secretory rate of FSH and LH.

The responses to LHRH in peripubertal children who do not yet exhibit physical signs of sexual maturation provide evidence that the self-priming effect[99] of endogenous LHRH augments pituitary responsiveness to exogenous LHRH and is an important factor in the increased gonadotropin secretion at puberty. This change in responsiveness of the gonadotropes is apparently mediated by increased pulsatile secretion of LHRH;[99, 100] the increased LH response to synthetic LHRH is one of the earliest hormonal markers of puberty onset.

The degree of previous exposure of gonadotropes to endogenous LHRH appears to affect both the magnitude and the quality of LH responses to a single intravenous dose of LHRH. Studies of the effects of acute and chronic administration of synthetic LHRH in hypergonadotropic hypogonadism, hypogonadotropic hypogonadism, constitutional delayed growth and adolescence, and idiopathic precocious puberty support this concept of "self-priming."[99, 109, 111, 124, 183, 282–286] The prepubertal pituitary gland has a smaller pool of releasable LH and decreased responsiveness to the acute administration of synthetic LHRH. With the approach of puberty, the derepression of the hypothalamic LHRH pulse generator and the increased pulsatile secretion of LHRH augment pituitary sensitivity to LHRH and enlarge the reserve of LH. The reason for the discordance in FSH and LH release prepubertally is not clear, but the frequency of LHRH pulses may be a factor.[184, 185, 187, 229, 278] In the adult rhesus monkey with ablative hypothalamic lesions that eliminate endogenous LHRH secretion, reduction in the frequency of exogenous LHRH pulses from one per hour to one every 3 h increased the FSH/LH ratio.[184] Furthermore, inhibin and endogenous gonadal steroids may also affect this ratio through action on the hypothalamus, the pituitary gland, or both.

These observations and the previously discussed role of the intermittence of the LHRH signal to the gonadotropes as an essential factor in the neural control of gonadotropin secretion have important implications for the induction of puberty. Pulsatile administration of LHRH to prepubertal monkeys promptly initiates puberty (and, in females, ovulatory menstrual cycles) and restores complete gonadal function in adult monkeys with hypothalamic lesions.[229, 256, 278, 280–281a] Similar studies in the human yielded comparable results in prepubertal children and in adults with hypothalamic hypogonadotropic hypogonadism.[185, 257, 272, 282–287] These results provide further support for reactivation of the hypothalamic LHRH pulse generator as the first hormonal change in the onset of puberty.

Responsiveness of the gonads to gonadotropins also increases during puberty. For example, the augmented testosterone secretion in response to administration of hCG at puberty in boys[288] is probably a consequence of the priming effect of the increase in endogenous secretion of LH (in the presence of FSH[289]) on the Leydig cell.

MATURATION OF POSITIVE FEEDBACK MECHANISM. In normal women, the midcycle surge in LH and FSH

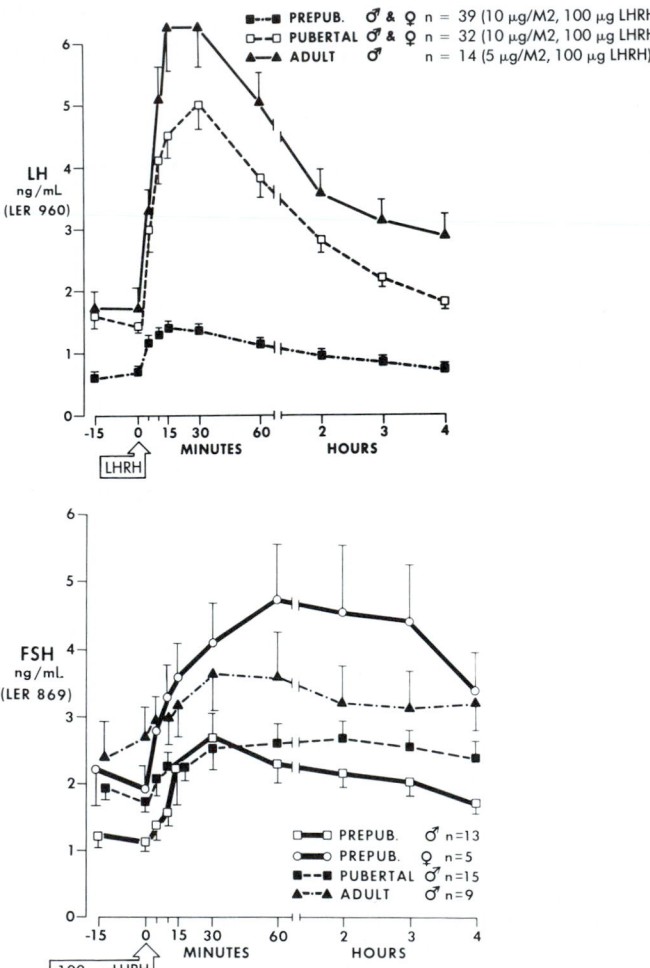

Figure 22–35. Changes in plasma LH (*top*) and FSH (*bottom*) levels in prepubertal, pubertal, and adult individuals. Note the limited LH response in prepubertal children compared with that of pubertal and adult subjects. The FSH response to LHRH is similar in prepubertal, pubertal, or adult males. In females, the FSH response is significantly greater than that of prepubertal, pubertal, or adult males. For conversion to SI units, see the legend of Figure 22–14. (Modified from Grumbach MM, Roth JC, Kaplan SL, et al. Hypothalamic-pituitary regulation of puberty in man: evidence and concepts derived from clinical research. In: Grumbach MM, Grave GD, Mayer FE, eds. Control of the Onset of Puberty. New York: John Wiley & Sons, 1974: 115–166.)

secretion is attributed to the positive feedback effect of an increased concentration of plasma estradiol for a sufficient length of time during the latter part of the follicular phase.[187, 276, 277] Estradiol has both negative and positive feedback effects on the hypothalamic-pituitary system. Although the suppressive effect is probably operative from late fetal life on, the positive action of estradiol on gonadotropin release has not been demonstrated in normal prepubertal and early pubertal children.[99, 100, 290] Hence, acquisition of positive feedback, a requisite for ovulation, is a late maturational event in puberty and, from the present evidence, probably does not occur before midpuberty in normal girls.[99, 100, 290, 291]

Among the requirements for a positive feedback action of estradiol on gonadotropin release at puberty[99] are (1) ovarian follicles primed by FSH to secrete sufficient estradiol to reach and maintain a critical level in the circulation, (2) a pituitary gland that is sensitized to LHRH and contains a large enough pool of releasable LH to support an LH surge, and (3) sufficient LHRH stores for the LHRH neurosecretory neurons to respond with an acute increase in LHRH release in addition to the usual adult pattern of pulsatile LHRH secretion.

Whether the main site of action of estradiol is at the level of the medial basal hypothalamus or the anterior pituitary is uncertain.[292] Knobil and Plant[280] have shown in the rhesus monkey that positive as well as negative feedback can occur in adult ovariectomized females in whom the medial basal hypothalamus is surgically disconnected from the remainder of the CNS. In monkeys with hypothalamic lesions, unvarying, intermittent LHRH administration leads to sufficient estradiol release from the ovary to induce an ovulatory LH surge in the absence of an increase in the dose of the LHRH pulses.[187, 281] Estradiol has a positive feedback effect directly on the pituitary gland in normal women, and prolonged administration of estradiol is accompanied by an augmented LH response to LHRH administration in women.[293] However, in women enhanced secretion of LHRH, as estimated by both bioassay and radioimmunoassay,[294] has been reported before and during the LH surge. These observations suggest that in women estradiol exerts its positive feedback action both at the pituitary gland and at the hypothalamic LHRH pulse generator but is demonstrable in the absence of an increase in pulsatile LHRH secretion. The failure to elicit a positive feedback action of estradiol could be related to the functional immaturity of either the CNS or the pituitary, manifested by inadequate LHRH pulses or insufficient LH reserve, respectively, or by both components.

The fact that gonadotropin cyclicity[295, 296] and estradiol-induced positive feedback can be demonstrated by midpuberty and before menarche does not imply that the positive feedback loop is complete.[1, 99, 213, 290, 291] Indeed, the modulating effect of the pubertal ovary and its output of estradiol on the hypothalamic–pituitary gonadotropin unit may be insufficient to induce an ovulatory LH surge even when there is an adequate pituitary store of readily releasable LH and FSH. The ovary, because of lack of sufficient gonadotropin stimulation, decreased responsivity, or other local factors, does not secrete estradiol at a high level or long enough to induce an ovulatory LH surge. We visualize the process leading to ovulation as a gradual one in which the ovary (the Zeitgeber for ovulation[187]) and the hypothalamic–pituitary gonadotropin complex become progressively more integrated and synchronous until, finally, an ovary primed for ovulation secretes sufficient estradiol to induce an ovulatory LH surge.[213]

Studies of basal body temperature[295] and of plasma progesterone concentrations[41, 297] suggest that as many as 55 to 90% of cycles are anovulatory during the first 2 y after menarche and that the proportion decreases to less than 20% of cycles by 5 y after menarche.[41] A cyclic surge of LH occurs during some anovulatory cycles in adolescence, but the mechanism of ovulation seems unstable and immature and does not appear to have attained the fine tuning and synchronization requisite for maintenance of regular ovulatory cycles.

Summary of Present Concept

Our present concept of the role of the hypothalamic-pituitary-gonadal system in the control of the onset of puberty is illustrated in Table 22–11. Clearly, the understanding of these complex maturational processes is incomplete.

Puberty is not an immutable process; it can be arrested or even reversed. Environmental factors and certain disorders that affect the onset or progression of puberty mediate their effects by direct or indirect suppression of the hypothalamic LHRH pulse generator and its periodic oscillatory signal, LHRH. For example, strenuous physical conditioning in girls (but not boys) and anorexia nervosa can delay or arrest puberty or lead to the reversion of the hypothalamic-

TABLE 22–11. Postulated Ontogeny of the Hypothalamic-Pituitary-Gonadal Circuit

Fetus
Medial basal hypothalamic LHRH neurosecretory neurons (pulse generator) operative by 80 d of gestation
Pulsatile secretion of FSH and LH by 80 d of gestation
Initially unrestrained secretion of LHRH (100 to 150 d)
Maturation of negative gonadal steroid feedback mechanisms by 150 d of gestation—sex difference
Low level of LHRH secretion at term

Early Infancy
Hypothalamic LHRH pulse generator functional after 12 d of age
Prominent FSH and LH episodic discharges until approximately 6 mo of age in males and 12 mo of age in females with transient increase in plasma levels of testosterone and estradiol in males and females, respectively

Late Infancy and Childhood
Intrinsic CNS inhibition of hypothalamic LHRH pulse generator operative; predominant mechanism in childhood; maximal sensitivity by approximately 4 y of age
Negative feedback control of FSH and LH secretion highly sensitive to gonadal steroids (low set point)
LHRH pulse generator inhibited; low amplitude and frequency of LHRH discharges
Low secretion of FSH, LH, and gonadal steroids

Late Prepubertal Period
Decreasing effectiveness of intrinsic CNS inhibitory influences and decreasing sensitivity of hypothalamic-pituitary unit to gonadal steroids (increased set point)
Increased amplitude and frequency of LHRH pulses, initially most prominent with sleep (nocturnal)
Increased sensitivity of gonadotropes to LHRH
Increased secretion of FSH and LH
Increased responsiveness of gonad to FSH and LH
Increased secretion of gonadal hormones

Puberty
Further decrease in CNS restraint of hypothalamic LHRH pulse generator and of the sensitivity of negative feedback mechanism to gonadal steroids
Prominent sleep-associated increase in episodic secretion of LHRH gradually changes to adult pattern of pulses about every 90 min
Pulsatile secretion of LH follows pattern of LHRH pulses
Progressive development of secondary sexual characteristics
Spermatogenesis in males
Middle to late puberty—operative positive feedback mechanism and capacity to exhibit an estrogen-induced LH surge
Ovulation in females

Modified from Grumbach MM, Roth JC, Kaplan SL, et al. Hypothalamic-pituitary regulation of puberty in man: evidence and concepts derived from clinical research. In: Grumbach MM, Grave GD, Mayer FE, eds. Control of the Onset of Puberty. New York: John Wiley & Sons, 1974: 115–166.

pituitary unit to a prepubertal state, depending on the magnitude of the functional LHRH insufficiency. With a decrease in physical activity in the former and with resumption of weight gain and attainment of sufficient body mass in the latter, the pubertal process is reactivated. In rare instances, true precocious puberty caused by an extrinsic mass lesion that impinges on the hypothalamus can be reversed by decompression or removal of the mass (a subarachnoid cyst, for example).[100, 161]

ADRENAL ANDROGENS AND ADRENARCHE

The adrenal component of pubertal maturation (the adrenarche) and the interactions between adrenal and gonadal hormones are poorly understood.[71, 299, 304, 305] Considerable speculation has focused on the mechanism of adrenarche, the fact that adrenarche occurs earlier than gonadarche (the maturation of the hypothalamic-pituitary-gonadal system), and the interaction between adrenal and gonadal hormones at puberty.

Nature and Regulation of Adrenal Androgens

The major androgens secreted by the adrenal cortex are DHEA, DHEAS, and androstenedione. By extraglandular metabolism, the adrenal androgens contribute to physiologically active testosterone and estradiol. In normal adult women, only androstenedione is an important precursor; DHEA and DHEAS contribute little to plasma testosterone and estradiol. However, scant information is available on the metabolism and kinetics of DHEA and DHEAS in prepubertal children. Androstenedione is the major androgen secreted by the ovary during and after puberty. It is more readily converted to potent androgens than DHEA or DHEAS. However, DHEA and DHEAS are useful biochemical markers of adrenal androgen secretion and the onset of adrenarche.

Cross-sectional and longitudinal studies have demonstrated a progressive increase in the plasma concentration of DHEA and DHEAS in boys and girls by the age of 7 or 8 (6 to 8 y skeletal age) that continues to age 13 to 15.[71, 300–302] During this 8-y period, a 20-fold increase in the concentration of DHEAS is accompanied by increased excretion of urinary 17-ketosteroids, especially 11-deoxy C_{19}-steroids. This increase serves as a mark of the onset of adrenarche and begins approximately 2 y before the increase in gonadotropin and gonadal steroid secretion. The increase is not associated with increased sensitivity of the pituitary gonadotropes to LHRH[275] or with sleep-associated LH secretion and occurs at an age when the hypothalamic-pituitary-gonadal complex is functioning at a low level.[71]

Changes in human adrenal microsomal enzyme activity during adrenarche are consistent with the alterations in adrenal androgen secretion. The increase in circulating adrenal androgen levels at adrenarche is associated with a rise in adrenal 17,20-desmolase and 17-hydroxylase activities (cytochrome P-450$_{c17}$), whereas 3β-hydroxysteroid dehydrogenase activity does not change significantly.[303, 304] These alterations in adrenal enzyme activity appear to be responsible for the increase in adrenal androgen secretion at adrenarche.

There are several hypotheses about the control of adrenal androgen secretion.[71, 299, 304] Evidence, although incomplete and indirect, suggests that the regulation of adrenal androgen secretion is based on a dual control mechanism: (1) corticotropin (ACTH, adrenocorticotropin) is obligatory

for (2) the action of an unidentified adrenal androgen–stimulating hormone, possibly pituitary in origin, or an intra-adrenal event.[71] This concept is illustrated in Figure 22–36. Rejected alternatives to a unique adrenal androgen–stimulating factor are the known pituitary hormones, such as ACTH, endorphin, prolactin, FSH or LH, and GH; estrogen; and a de novo maturational change in adrenal biogenesis with reactivation of 17,20-lyase and the C_{19}-steroid pathway. Despite much effort, a distinct hormone that stimulates adrenal androgen has not been isolated, and the mechanism of adrenarche remains unknown.

A distinct adrenal androgen–stimulating factor, whether of pituitary or other origin, could explain the following observations:[71]

1. The spurt in adrenal growth and the differentiation and growth of the zona reticularis at adrenarche occur independently of an increase in ACTH or cortisol secretion but correlate with the increase in plasma DHEAS (Fig. 22–37).

2. Cortisol and adrenal androgen secretions vary independently with age, during normal as well as premature adrenarche, and in Cushing disease, starvation, malnutrition, anorexia nervosa, and chronic disease.

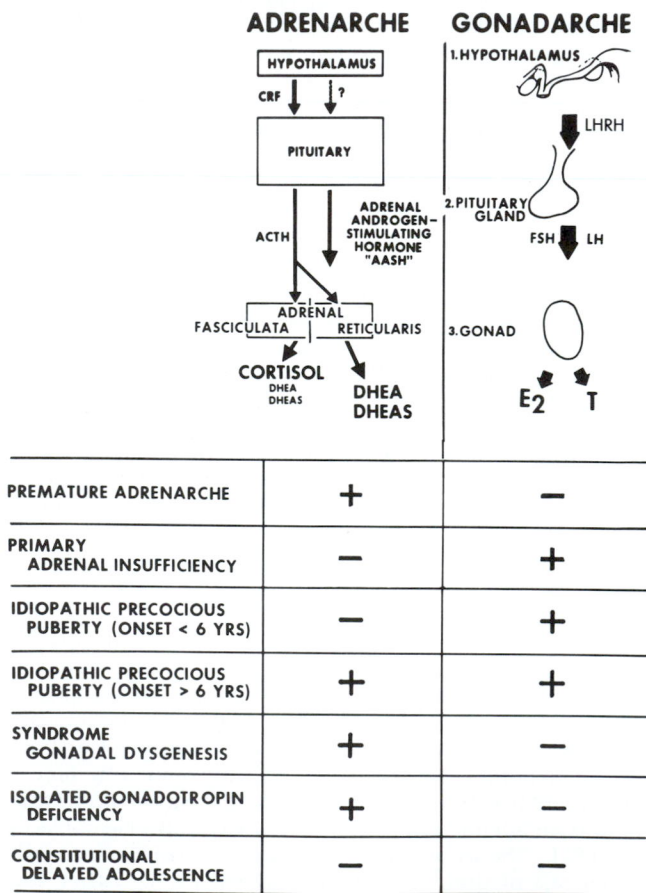

	ADRENARCHE	GONADARCHE
PREMATURE ADRENARCHE	+	−
PRIMARY ADRENAL INSUFFICIENCY	−	+
IDIOPATHIC PRECOCIOUS PUBERTY (ONSET < 6 YRS)	−	+
IDIOPATHIC PRECOCIOUS PUBERTY (ONSET > 6 YRS)	+	+
SYNDROME GONADAL DYSGENESIS	+	−
ISOLATED GONADOTROPIN DEFICIENCY	+	−
CONSTITUTIONAL DELAYED ADOLESCENCE	−	−

Figure 22–36. Hypothesis of the control of pituitary adrenal androgen secretion by a putative separate adrenal androgen–stimulating hormone acting on an ACTH-primed adrenal cortex. Although this diagram suggests that "AASH" arises from the pituitary gland, a distinct pituitary factor with "AASH" activity has not been isolated; an extrapituitary factor is not excluded. The lower part of the diagram shows the relationship of adrenarche to gonadarche, including dissociation in various clinical disorders of sexual development (+, present; −, absent). (Modified from CA Sklar, SL Kaplan, MM Grumbach, Evidence for dissociation between adrenarche and gonadarche: studies in patients with idiopathic precocious puberty, gonadal dysgenesis, isolated gonadotropin deficiency, and constitutionally delayed puberty, J Clin Endocrinol Metab, 51, 548–556, 1980, © by The Endocrine Society.)

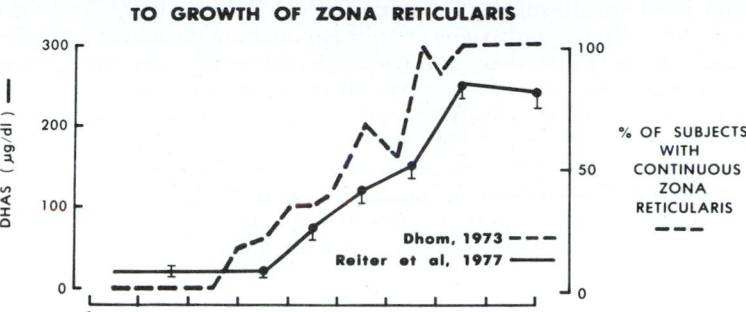

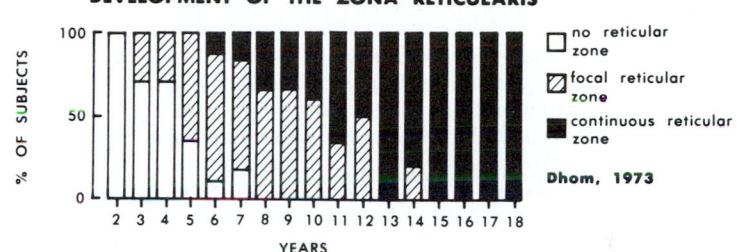

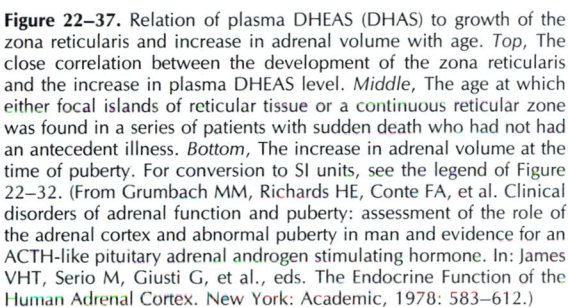

Figure 22–37. Relation of plasma DHEAS (DHAS) to growth of the zona reticularis and increase in adrenal volume with age. *Top,* The close correlation between the development of the zona reticularis and the increase in plasma DHEAS level. *Middle,* The age at which either focal islands of reticular tissue or a continuous reticular zone was found in a series of patients with sudden death who had not had an antecedent illness. *Bottom,* The increase in adrenal volume at the time of puberty. For conversion to SI units, see the legend of Figure 22–32. (From Grumbach MM, Richards HE, Conte FA, et al. Clinical disorders of adrenal function and puberty: assessment of the role of the adrenal cortex and abnormal puberty in man and evidence for an ACTH-like pituitary adrenal androgen stimulating hormone. In: James VHT, Serio M, Giusti G, et al., eds. The Endocrine Function of the Human Adrenal Cortex. New York: Academic, 1978: 583–612.)

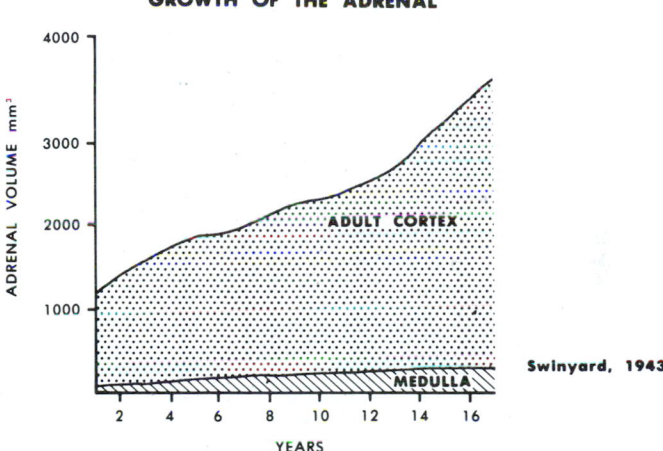

3. Unlike cortisol secretion, the secretion of DHEA and DHEAS in response to ACTH administration varies with age.

4. Dissociation of adrenarche and gonadarche occurs in a variety of disorders of sexual maturation (see Fig. 22–36), including premature adrenarche (onset of pubic or axillary hair before age 8), chronic adrenal insufficiency, true precocious puberty (when the onset is before age 6), primary hypogonadism, isolated gonadotropin deficiency, and anorexia nervosa.[305]

Adrenal Androgens and Puberty

The earlier onset of adrenarche than gonadarche and the contribution of adrenal androgens to the growth of pubic and axillary hair have led some to suggest that in normal children adrenal androgens are an important factor in the onset of puberty and the maturation of the hypothalamic-pituitary-gonadal complex. Although true precocious puberty may occur in circumstances in which the prepubertal child has previously been exposed to excessive levels of androgens from an endogenous or an exogenous source (e.g., after the initiation of glucocorticoid therapy in congenital virilizing adrenal hyperplasia),[71, 298] there is little evidence that adrenal androgens play an important qualitative or rate-limiting role in the onset of puberty in normal children.[71]

Most patients with premature adrenarche, who secrete excessive amounts of adrenal androgens for their age, enter puberty and experience menarche within the normal age range.[71] Moreover, prepubertal children who have congenital or acquired chronic adrenal insufficiency (Addison disease) and, consequently, have deficient or absent adrenal androgen secretion usually have a normal onset of and progression through puberty when given appropriate glucocorticoid and mineralocorticoid replacement therapy.[71] Thus early activation of adrenal androgen secretion does not commonly lead to sexual precocity, nor is deficient or absent adrenal androgen output usually associated with delayed puberty. Furthermore, growth studies in children with chronic adrenal insufficiency, isolated gonadotropin deficiency, hypergonadotropic hypogonadism, and androgen resistance (testicular feminization) suggest that in girls and boys adrenal androgens are not essential for the adolescent growth spurt, whereas gonadal steroids secreted by the testis and ovary are and act in concert with GH.[71] A transient increase in height velocity (about 1.5 cm/y in both sexes) that occurs in middle childhood (6 to 7 y) and lasts about 2 y has been attributed by some to adrenarche. However, the middle childhood spurt is related to the cyclic pattern of prepubertal growth and to genetic regulation of growth rather than an increase in either adrenal androgen or GH secretion.[304, 306]

DISORDERS OF PUBERTY

Delayed Puberty and Sexual Infantilism
(Table 22–12)

A useful definition of delayed puberty is lack of physical manifestations of sexual maturation in boys and girls at a chronological age that is 2 SD above the mean age at onset of puberty (or at which 95% of normal children have already entered puberty). Fewer than 2% of 14-y-old and 0.4% of 15-y-old white boys in the United States without evidence of organic disorders are prepubertal, and only 2.3% of white 12-y-old girls, 0.4% of white 13-y-old girls, and no 13-y-old black girls from the U.S. Health Examination Survey were prepubertal.[29, 30] Thus in the United States, the ages of 12 y in girls and 14 y in boys serve as practical guidelines to determine the need for evaluation. It is important to separate the patients destined to undergo spontaneous but delayed puberty from those with disorders associated with permanent sexual infantilism that require treatment. Diagnosis should determine whether a patient has constitutional (idiopathic) delay, hypogonadotropic hypogonadism, or primary gonadal failure with hypergonadotropic hypogonadism. Functionally, delayed puberty can be divided into disorders that affect the operation of the LHRH pulse generator, the pituitary gland, or the gonad.

Idiopathic (Constitutional) Delay in Growth and Puberty[164, 307]

Healthy individuals who spontaneously enter puberty after the age of 12 for girls and 14 for boys have constitutional delay in growth and adolescence. They usually are short (2 SD below the mean value for height for age) at evaluation and have been shorter than their classmates for years, although growth velocity and height are usually appropriate for bone age (Fig. 22–38). Family history often reveals that the mothers had delayed menarche and that the fathers and siblings did not enter puberty until late (age 14 to 18). Such individuals with a slow tempo of maturation have a constitutional delay at all stages of physical development and may be considered physiologically immature; as a result of the delay in the reactivation of the LHRH pulse generator, they have a functional deficiency of LHRH for chronological age but not for the stage of physiological development. Adrenarche and gonadarche occur later in subjects with constitutional (idiopathic) delay in growth and adolescence, whereas adrenarche usually occurs at a normal age in patients with isolated gonadotropin deficiency.[305, 308]

In patients with constitutional delay in growth and puberty, bone age correlates better with the onset of and progression through puberty than does chronological age. These patients have a retarded bone age at presentation but, on achieving a bone age of approximately 12 to 14 y for boys and 11 to 13 y for girls, they can be expected to

show the earliest stages of sexual maturation. The U.S. Health Examination Survey showed that 5.7% of boys with a bone age of 14 y lacked pubic hair (stage 1) and 4% were in genital stage 1, whereas at age 15 y only 0.2% were still in pubic hair stage 1 and 0.8% were still in genital stage 1. (Unfortunately the study started at an age at which the same descriptive information could not be determined for girls.[30]) In contrast to isolated gonadotropin deficiency, there is no impairment of olfaction and undescended testes are uncommon in constitutionally delayed patients. Plasma gonadal steroid levels may be low at the time of presentation (adrenarche as well as gonadarche is usually delayed), but as bone age advances, gonadotropin concentration and pulsatile LH

TABLE 22–12. Classification of Delayed Puberty and Sexual Infantilism

Idiopathic (Constitutional) Delay in Growth and Puberty (Delayed Activation of Hypothalamic LHRH Pulse Generator)

Hypogonadotropic Hypogonadism
CNS disorders
  Tumors
    Craniopharyngiomas
    Germinomas, astrocytomas, optic gliomas
  Congenital malformations, especially associated with craniofacial anomalies
  Radiation therapy
  Head trauma
  Other causes
    Hand-Schüller-Christian disease (histocytosis X, Langerhans cell histiocytosis)
    Postinfectious lesions of the CNS
    Vascular abnormalities of the CNS
    Granulomas
Isolated gonadotropin deficiency
  Kallmann syndrome with hyposmia or anosmia
  Without anosmia
  Congenital adrenal hypoplasia (X linked)
  Other disorders
Idiopathic and genetic forms of multiple pituitary hormone deficiencies
Miscellaneous disorders
  Prader-Willi syndrome
  Laurence-Moon-Biedl syndrome
  Functional gonadotropin deficiency
    Chronic systemic disease and malnutrition
    Hypothyroidism
    Diabetes mellitus
    Cushing disease
    Hyperprolactinemia
    Anorexia nervosa
    Bulimia
    Psychogenic amenorrhea
    Delayed puberty and/or menarche, especially in female athletes and ballet dancers (exercise amenorrhea)
  Marijuana use

Hypergonadotropic Hypogonadism
Males
  Syndrome of seminiferous tubular dysgenesis and its variants (Klinefelter syndrome)
  Other forms of primary testicular failure
    Chemotherapy
    Radiation therapy
    LH resistance
    Sertoli-only syndrome
    Testicular biosynthetic defects
  Anorchia and cryptorchidism
Females
  Syndrome of gonadal dysgenesis and its variants (Turner syndrome)
  46,XX and 46,XY gonadal dysgenesis
    Familial and sporadic 46,XX gonadal dysgenesis and its variants
    Familial and sporadic 46,XY gonadal dysgenesis and its variants
  Other forms of primary ovarian failure
    Premature menopause
    Radiation therapy
    Chemotherapy
    Autoimmune oophoritis
    Resistant ovary
    Polycystic ovary disease
    Pseudo-Turner syndrome
    Galactosemia

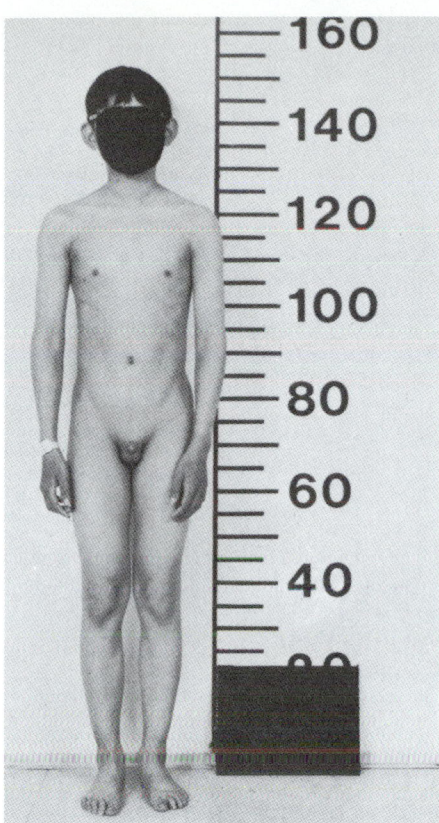

Figure 22–38. A boy 16 y, 2 mo of age, with constitutional delay in growth and puberty. Height, 149.5 cm (4 SD below the mean value for age); upper/lower body ratio, 1.1 (retarded for age); phallus, 6.0 × 1.6 cm; testes, 2.5 × 1.4 cm; the scrotum showed early thinning. At a chronological age of 15 y, 4 mo, the bone age was 11 y and the sella turcica was normal. The plasma concentration of LH was 0.7 ng/mL; FSH, 0.5 ng/mL. On LHRH testing the plasma concentration of LH increased to 2.2 ng/mL (an increment of 1.5 ng/mL), and the testosterone level rose from 52 to 77 ng/dL. The testes subsequently spontaneously enlarged, and the patient progressed through puberty. For conversion to SI units, see the legends of Figures 22–14 and 22–15. (From Styne DM, Grumbach MM. Puberty in the male and female: its physiology and disorders. In: Yen JCC, Jaffe RB, eds. Reproductive Endocrinology. 2nd ed. Philadelphia: W. B. Saunders, 1986: 313–384.)

secretion increase (initially at night), and the LH response to LHRH reflects maturation of the hypothalamic-pituitary system.

In most cases, the first signs of secondary sexual development occur within 1 y after LH rises more than 7.6 IU/L (2 ng/mL) (LER-960) after administration of 100 μg of synthetic LHRH intravenously or within 1 y after gonadotropin and testosterone or estradiol concentrations begin to increase spontaneously.[99, 100]

Constitutional delay in growth and adolescence in its pure form may be regarded as an extreme physiological variant of the normal velocity of development. It can be considered the counterpart of constitutional true precocious puberty. Thus a child usually reaches his or her full genetic potential in height and attains full sexual maturity, but it will take longer than usual. Patients with familial short stature alone do not have delayed pubertal development. Thus familial short stature is a physiological variant of growth distance in which the velocity of development and bone age are normal, whereas constitutional delay in growth and adolescence is a disorder of tempo that secondarily impairs growth distance. Of course, some children may have a combination of genetic short stature and constitutional delay, and these patients most often seek medical advice. The combination of delayed pubertal maturation and de-

creased stature during adolescence, superimposed on a strong familial tendency toward short stature, leads to conspicuous shortness, especially in the peripubertal period, more often than with either condition alone. Growth rate before the actual onset of puberty in these patients is often suboptimal, and for chronological age, GH secretion after provocative stimuli or after the administration of GH-releasing hormone may be decreased. Growth velocity and GH secretion in subjects with constitutional delay in growth and adolescence return to normal after the onset of puberty. The amplitude of GH secretion and the GH response to GH-releasing hormone increase after the administration of exogenous androgens or estrogens in subjects with constitutional delay in puberty.[64, 309–312] Thus constitutional delay in puberty may constitute a state of functional temporary GH insufficiency for chronological age but not for bone age. There is an interaction of IGF I and gonadotropins in the ovary and testis, and the relatively low secretion of GH (and presumably intragonadal IGF I) in constitutional delayed puberty may impair the gonadal response to gonadotropins.[313] Affected boys seem to be more distressed by short stature than by delay in sexual development.[314–314c]

Occasionally, individuals with constitutional delay in puberty are of normal stature. In such instances the genetic tendency for growth is greater than in cases characterized by short stature. In these patients, diagnostic and therapeutic decisions will focus on the pubertal status.

Hypogonadotropic Hypogonadism: Sexual Infantilism Related to Gonadotropin Deficiency

Insufficient pulsatile secretion of LHRH and the resulting FSH and LH deficiency lead to sexual infantilism. The magnitude of the LHRH deficiency and hence the phenotype can vary from severe sexual infantilism to instances in which the separation from constitutional delay of puberty is difficult. LHRH deficiency may be secondary to a genetic or developmental defect present at birth but undetected until the age of expected puberty, or it may be due to a tumor, inflammatory process, vascular lesion, or trauma. The deficiency of pulsatile LHRH may be quantitative—either absolute or relative—or qualitative, especially in females; it may involve abnormalities in the amplitude or frequency of LHRH pulses or in both components[182, 183, 315] (Fig. 22–39). Similarly, gonadotropin deficiency may arise from lesions or defects that involve the pituitary gland directly. When GH is affected as well as gonadotropins, impaired growth is manifested by decreased growth velocity and subsequent short stature. Patients with isolated deficiencies of FSH and LH usually are of normal height for age when seen in early or middle adolescent years, whereas patients with constitutional or idiopathic delay in growth and puberty usually have a normal growth rate for bone age but are short for chronological age. In contrast to subjects with constitutional delay in growth and puberty, gonadotropin-deficient patients usually do not exhibit a normal LH response to LHRH stimulation commensurate with bone age, and the concentrations of plasma FSH and LH and the excretion of urinary gonadotropins are frequently low.[101]

CNS DISORDERS: TUMORS. CNS tumors that lead to delayed puberty are usually extrasellar masses that interfere with LHRH synthesis, secretion, or stimulation of pituitary gonadotropes. Virtually all patients with hypothalamic-pituitary tumors and gonadotropin deficiency also have deficiency of one or more additional pituitary hormones (or, in the case of prolactin-secreting adenomas, an increased concentration of plasma prolactin). The patients with GH defi-

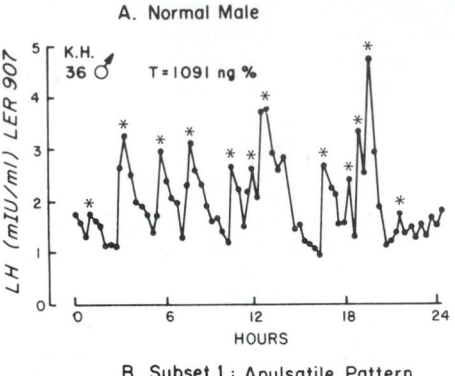

A. Normal Male

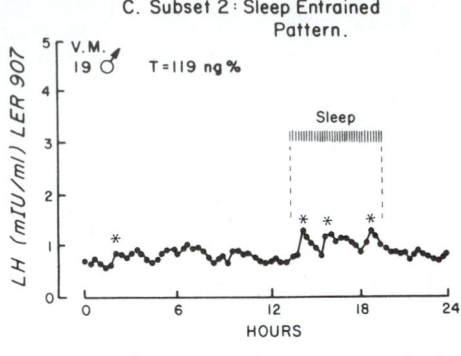

C. Subset 2: Sleep Entrained Pattern.

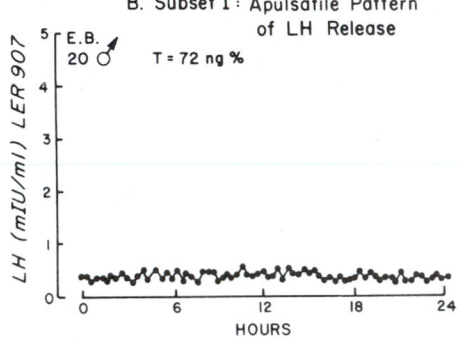

B. Subset 1: Apulsatile Pattern of LH Release

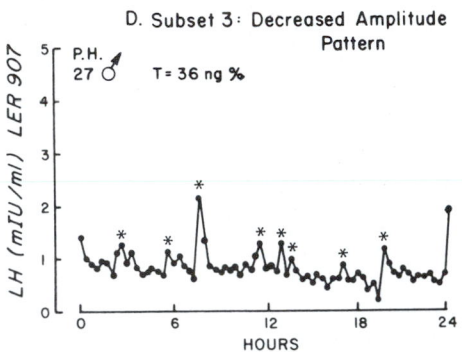

D. Subset 3: Decreased Amplitude Pattern

Figure 22–39. The various patterns of pulsatile LH secretion that can occur in isolated hypogonadotropic hypogonadism (*B–D*) compared with LH secretion in a normal man (*A*). *A,* The discrete LH pulses occurring about every 2 h in a normal 36-y-old man. *B,* Typical apulsatile LH pattern associated with a low testosterone concentration usually found in isolated hypogonadotropic hypogonadism. *C,* Pattern of developmental arrest with low-amplitude nocturnal LH pulses apparent only during sleep. *D,* Low-amplitude LH pulse pattern during sleep and wake periods. To convert LH values to international units per liter, multiply by 1.0. (From Spratt DI, Crowley WF. Hypogonadotropic hypogonadism: GnRH therapy. In: Krieger DT, Bardin CW, eds. Current Therapy in Endocrinology and Metabolism, 1985–1986. Toronto: B. C. Decker, 1985: 155–159.)

ciency caused by neoplasm often have a relatively late onset of growth failure compared with idiopathic and familial hypopituitary dwarfs, who usually exhibit growth failure early in life. Similarly, the presence of both anterior and posterior pituitary deficiencies suggests an expanding lesion or less commonly a midline developmental defect.

Craniopharyngioma. This is the most common neoplasm associated with hypothalamic-pituitary dysfunction and sexual infantilism (also see Chapters 5 and 6). This tumor of Rathke pouch originates from the pituitary stalk and is usually suprasellar, although it can be within the sella turcica; rarely, craniopharyngiomas are in the nasopharynx[316] or the third ventricle.[317] Craniopharyngiomas are usually symptomatic before age 20; the peak incidence is between ages 6 and 14.[318–320] CNS signs develop as the tumor encroaches on surrounding structures.

Clinical presentation and history include headache, visual disturbances, short stature, symptoms of diabetes insipidus, and weakness of one or more limbs.[319, 320] Signs on physical examination include visual defects (including bilateral temporal field deficits), optic atrophy or papilledema, and signs of GH deficiency, delayed puberty, and hypothyroidism.[319, 320] Although only a few patients seek evaluation because of short stature, most are below the mean in height and height velocity at the time of diagnosis.[320] Laboratory evaluation often indicates deficiencies in one or more pituitary hormones, including gonadotropin, GH, thyrotropin (TSH), ACTH, and vasopressin (AVP, also called antidiuretic hormone, ADH). The plasma concentration of prolactin may be normal or increased. Radiographic examination often shows retarded bone age.

Suprasellar or intrasellar calcification occurs in approximately 70% of patients but in less than 1% of normal individuals, and an abnormal sella is found in 70% of patients.[320] Some asymptomatic patients have been discovered by the coincidental finding of calcification or abnormalities of the sella on skull x-ray films taken for other indications.[318–321] Computed tomographic (CT) scans can reveal fine calcifications that are not apparent on routine roentgenograms, and CT or MRI scans can determine

whether the tumor is cystic or solid and indicate the presence of hydrocephalus (Fig. 22–40).[322] Smaller craniopharyngiomas, primarily intrasellar, can be resected or decompressed by transsphenoidal microsurgery, but larger or suprasellar masses usually require craniotomy. The combination of limited tumor removal and radiation therapy leads to as satisfactory a neurological prognosis as attempts at complete surgical extirpation and to a better endocrinological outcome.[320, 323, 324]

Other Extrasellar Tumors. Sexual infantilism may be caused by other extrasellar tumors that arise in or encroach on the hypothalamus. Germinomas (previously termed pinealomas, ectopic pinealomas, atypical teratomas, or dysgerminomas)[325] or other germ cell tumors of the CNS are the extrasellar tumors that most commonly cause sexual infantilism, although, when all primary CNS tumors are considered, germinomas are rare. The diagnosis is usually made during the second decade of life. Polydipsia and polyuria are among the most common symptoms, followed by visual difficulties and abnormalities of growth and puberty.[326] The most common endocrine abnormalities are deficiencies of vasopressin and GH, but other anterior pituitary hormone deficiencies (including gonadotropin deficiency) and elevated serum prolactin levels are frequent. Germinomas in boys may cause isosexual precocity by secretion of hCG. The tumor may be located in the suprasellar hypothalamic region, in the pineal region, or in another area of the CNS. Subependymal spread along the lining of the third ventricle is common, and seeding may lead to involvement of the lower spinal cord and corda equina. CT and MRI scans are useful in the diagnosis of tumors more than 0.5 cm in diameter.[327, 328] Germinomas are radiosensitive, and radiation is the preferred treatment; the clinical features and the response to radiation therapy are so characteristic that surgery is rarely indicated except for biopsy to establish a tissue diagnosis.[329] Hypothalamic and optic gliomas or astrocytomas, occurring either as part of neurofibromatosis (von Recklinghausen disease) or independently, can also cause sexual infantilism.[330–332]

Pituitary Tumors. Chromophobe adenomas are uncom-

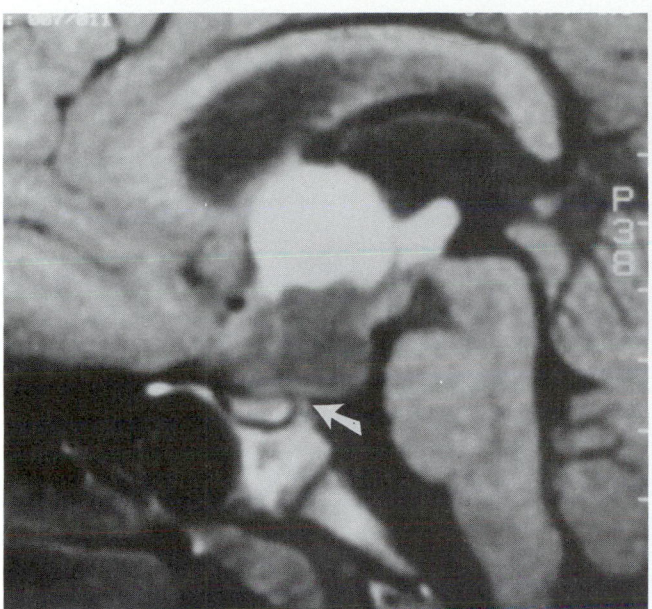 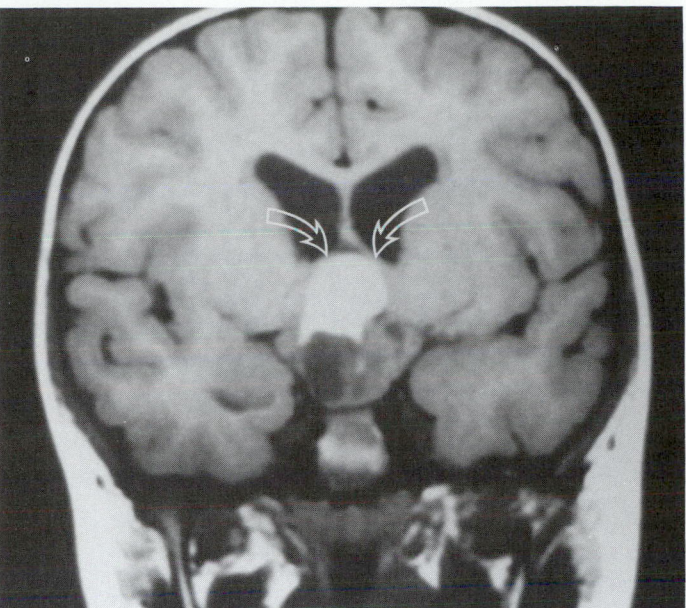

Figure 22–40. Craniopharyngioma in a short 5-y-old girl with a history of frontal headaches, impaired vision, and poor growth. *Left,* Midline sagittal T1-weighted image that shows a hyperintense region superiorly and an inferior hypointense region. The combination of hyper- and hypointense areas in a non–contrast enhanced examination is the most characteristic finding in craniopharyngioma. Note erosion of dorsum sellae (*solid white arrow*) and posterior pituitary bright spot. *Right,* Coronal-weighted T1 image shows tumor extending upward to the inferior frontal horns, narrowing the foramen of Monro and causing mild hydrocephalus. The open white arrows indicate the upper border of the hyperintense area of the tumor.

mon in children. Prolactin-secreting adenomas are also rare in childhood but occur more commonly in the later teenage years; delayed puberty or menarche or secondary amenorrhea may result. Hyperprolactinemia without demonstration of a pituitary tumor by imaging techniques has been associated with delayed puberty and galactorrhea without gynecomastia; bromocriptine suppresses the elevated prolactin secretion and the galactorrhea and allows progression of puberty.[333]

OTHER CNS DISORDERS LEADING TO DELAYED PUBERTY. *Hand-Schüller-Christian Disease, or Histiocytosis X (Langerhans Cell Histiocytosis).* This disorder is characterized by the infiltration of lipid-laden histiocytic cells or foam cells in the skin, viscera, and bone.[334, 335] Diabetes insipidus, usually resulting from infiltration of the hypothalamus, is the most common endocrine manifestation, and GH deficiency and delayed puberty may occur. There may be involvement of the lung, the liver, and the spleen. Other findings include cyst-like areas in flat bones of the skull, the ribs, the pelvis, and the scapula; in the long bones of the arms and legs; and in the dorsolumbar spine. Lesions of the mandible lead to the radiographic impression of "floating teeth" within rarefied bone and the clinical finding of absent or loose teeth. Infiltration of the orbit may lead to exophthalmos, and mastoid or temporal bone involvement may lead to chronic otitis media. Treatment with glucocorticoids, antineoplastic agents, and radiotherapy is of uncertain benefit. The natural waxing and waning course of this disease makes evaluation of therapy difficult.[335a]

Postinfectious Inflammatory Lesions of the CNS, Vascular Abnormalities, and Head Trauma. These are unusual causes of hypogonadotropic hypogonadism. Rarely, tuberculous or sarcoid granulomas of the CNS are associated with delayed puberty.[336] Hydrocephalus may cause delayed puberty that can be reversed with decompression.[337]

Radiation of the Head. Radiation of the head for treatment of CNS tumors, leukemia, or neoplasms of the head and the face may result in the gradual onset of hypothalamic-pituitary failure.[338] Although GH deficiency is the most common hormone disorder resulting from radiation, gonadotropin deficiency also occurs.

Developmental Defects. Midline malformations of the head and the CNS are associated with a variety of endocrine deficiencies. Septo-optic or optic dysplasia is caused by abnormal development of the prosencephalon. The optic nerve is usually affected, leading to small, dysplastic, pale optic discs and pendular nystagmus; severely affected patients may be blind. The midline hypothalamic defect can lead to GH deficiency and diabetes insipidus and may be associated with deficient ACTH, TSH, and gonadotropin secretion; as a consequence, short stature and delayed puberty result, although precocious puberty may occur (see later).[339] The septum pellucidum is often absent, and this is readily demonstrable by imaging techniques.[340] Other congenital midline defects from complete dysraphism and holoprosencephaly to cleft palate or lip can also be associated with hypothalamic-pituitary dysfunction.[337]

ISOLATED GONADOTROPIN DEFICIENCY (Table 22–13).[286, 287, 315, 341, 344] Isolated gonadotropin deficiency may occur in families or sporadically. In contrast to patients with CNS tumors, who usually have associated GH deficiency and growth failure, and to patients with constitutional delay in growth and adolescence, who are short for chronological age, patients with isolated gonadotropin deficiency are usually of appropriate height for their age (Fig. 22–41). Because concentrations of gonadal steroids are too low to fuse the

TABLE 22–13. Characteristics of Isolated Gonadotropin Deficiency

Males more commonly affected
Familial or sporadic
Height normal
Eunuchoid skeletal proportions
Delayed bone age
Small testes: diameter ≤ 2.5 cm
Normal adrenarche
Examine for anosmia or hyposmia (Kallmann syndrome)
Look for associated malformations (facial, skeletal, renal)

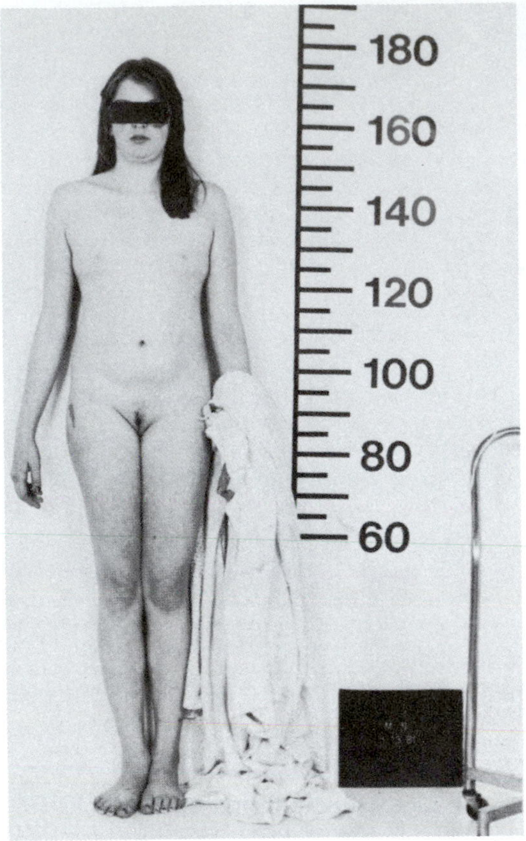

Figure 22–41. A girl 18 y, 8 mo of age, with isolated gonadotropin deficiency (sexual infantilism and primary amenorrhea). Height was 173 cm (+1 SD), weight was 66.5 kg (+1 SD), and skeletal age was 13 y. Adrenarche with pubic hair development occurred at age 13½ y. At the time of the photograph, pubic hair was in stage 3 and there was slight breast and nipple development resulting from a previous short course of estrogen therapy. Immature labia minora and majora were noted, and no estrogen effect was present on the vaginal mucosa. Olfactory testing was normal. The plasma LH (LER-960) level after LHRH administration rose from 0.5 to 1.8 ng/mL (a prepubertal response). Serum estradiol was undetectable. DHEAS level was 92 μg/dL (appropriate for pubic hair stage 2). Note the discrepancy between adrenarche and gonadarche. For conversion to SI units, see the legends of Figures 22–14 and 22–32. (From Styne DM, Grumbach MM. Puberty in the male and female: its physiology and disorders. In: Yen SCC, Jaffe RB, eds. Reproductive Endocrinology. 2nd ed. Philadelphia: W. B. Saunders, 1986: 313–384.)

TABLE 22–14. Features of Kallmann Syndrome

Clinical
  LHRH deficiency: absent or arrested puberty
  Anosmia or hyposmia
  In infancy: microphallus; cryptorchidism
  Normal stature and growth in childhood
  Normal adrenarche
  Eunuchoid proportions
  Associated midline defects (e.g., cleft lip, cleft palate, midline cranial anomalies)
  MRI: aplasia or hypoplasia of olfactory bulbs
Prevalence: approximately 1 in 7500 males, 1 in 50,000 females; one tenth prevalence of Klinefelter syndrome
Inheritance: sporadic and familial cases; genetic heterogeneity
  X linked
    X-linked recessive (Kallmann et al.[343])
    X chromosome deletion: Xp22.3 (Ballabio et al.[346])
  Autosomal
    Dominant (sex limitation) (Santen and Paulsen;[347] Merriam et al.[349])
    Recessive (White et al.[351])
Anatomy: developmental field defect
  Aplasia or hypoplasia of olfactory bulb
  Arrested migration of LHRH neurosecretory neurons from olfactory placode to medial basal hypothalamus

epiphyses at the normal age, these patients develop increased arm span for height and decreased upper/lower ratios and, if untreated, usually become tall adults. An autosomal recessive form has been described in the mouse (hyg/hyg) in which there is a deletion of a part of the LHRH gene. The mutant RNA is incapable of generating functional LHRH.[342]

Kallmann Syndrome (Table 22–14). This syndrome is the most common form of isolated hypogonadotropic hypogonadism in which anosmia or hyposmia resulting from agenesis or hypoplasia of the olfactory lobes is associated with LHRH deficiency.[343] The prevalence in boys is about six times that in girls (Fig. 22–42). Indeed, the extent of the defect in olfaction seems to correlate with the degree of LHRH deficiency; the extent of the LHRH deficiency correlates with the size of the testes[345] (Fig. 22–43). Affected individuals often do not notice impaired olfaction; testing with graded dilutions of pure scents is necessary. Undescended testes and gynecomastia are common in this and all types of hypogonadotropic hypogonadism in boys.[345] Associated defects are cleft lip, cleft palate, imperfect facial fusion, unilateral renal agenesis, epilepsy, and short meta-

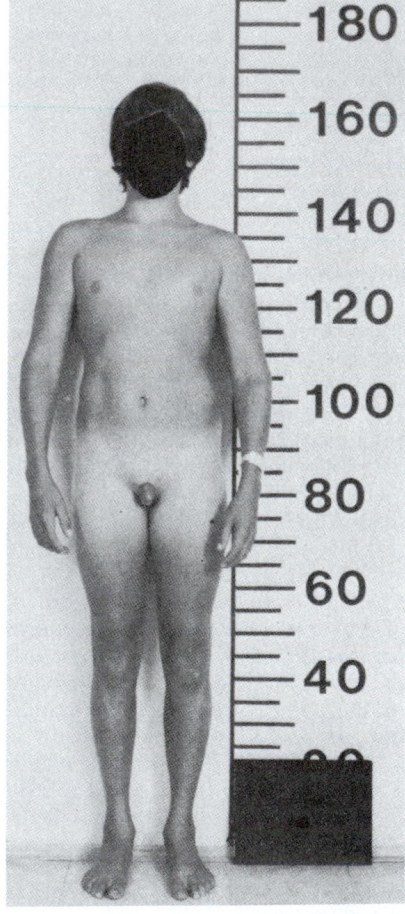

Figure 22–42. A boy of 15 y, 10 mo, with isolated gonadotropin deficiency and anosmia (Kallmann syndrome). He had undescended testes, but after administration of 10,000 U of hCG the testes descended and were palpable in the scrotum. Height, 163.9 cm (−1.5 SD); the upper/lower body ratio was 0.86, which is eunuchoid. The phallus measured 6.3 × 1.8 cm, and the testes were 1.2 × 0.8 cm. The concentration of plasma LH was less than 0.3 ng/mL; of FSH, 1.2 ng/mL; of testosterone, 16 ng/dL. After 100 μg of LHRH the plasma LH (LER-960) was 0.7 ng/mL and FSH (LER-869) 2.4 ng/mL. For conversion to SI units, see the legends of Figures 22–14 and 22–15. (From Styne DM, Grumbach MM. Puberty in the male and female: its physiology and disorders. In: Yen SCC, Jaffe RB, eds. Reproductive Endocrinology. 2nd ed. Philadelphia: W. B. Saunders, 1986: 313–384.)

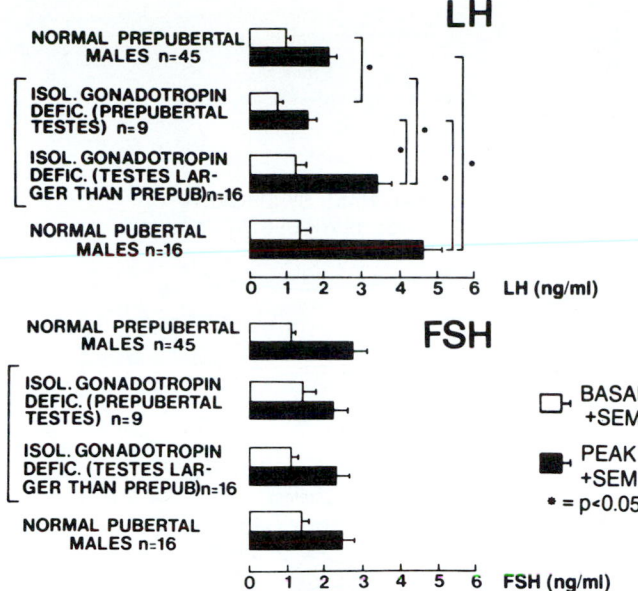

Figure 22–43. Serum LH and FSH responses to the administration of LHRH in 25 males with an isolated gonadotropin deficiency with or without anosmia, segregated according to whether the volume of the testes was prepubertal or >2.5 cm³; testicular volume in those with testes >2.5 cm³ were as large as 4 cm³. Basal and LHRH-stimulated gonadotropin levels after the intravenous injection of 100 μg LHRH (peak value) are shown. *p < .05. For conversion to SI units, see the legend of Figure 22–14. (From Van Dop C, Burstein S, Conte FA, et al. Isolated gonadotropin deficiency in boys: clinical characteristics and growth. J Pediatr 1987; 111:684–692.)

carpals (Table 22–15). This syndrome is genetically heterogeneous and can be transmitted as an X-linked, autosomal dominant or autosomal recessive trait. Reports of affected males who were infertile suggested an X-linked mode of inheritance,[343] and X linkage has been substantiated by gene mapping techniques, at Xp22.3. Contiguous gene deletions in this region of the X chromosome can lead to an association of Kallmann syndrome with X-linked ichthyosis caused by steroid sulfatase deficiency, mental retardation, and chondroplasia punctata.[346] (Also see Chapter 14.) Autosomal dominant inheritance of the phenotype is suggested by some studies,[347, 348] and this pattern of inheritance is supported by a report of an affected male who fathered an affected son after treatment with hCG.[349] Apparent autosomal recessive inheritance characterizes other kindreds.[351] Thus the various forms of Kallmann syndrome may be due to heterogeneous mutations.[347, 348, 351] A 20-y-old man with the complete picture of Kallmann syndrome had an identical twin brother (proved by genetic fingerprinting) with anosmia but a normal adult phenotype and normal plasma testosterone and gonadotropin concentrations.[350]

In Kallmann syndrome, fetal LHRH neurosecretory neurons fail to migrate from the olfactory placode, where they arise, to the medial basal hypothalamus, where they constitute the LHRH pulse generator. The defect may be absolute or relative. The fetal LHRH-containing cells and neurites are arrested in their migration to the brain and end in a tangle around the cribriform plate and in the dural layers adjacent to the meninges beneath the forebrain[193] (Fig. 22–44). Hence, Kallmann syndrome can be considered as a developmental malformation caused by a field defect.

Other Forms of Isolated Hypogonadotropic Hypogonadism. Hypogonadotropic hypogonadism may be transmitted by autosomal recessive inheritance with none of the other features of Kallmann syndrome. In the mouse, a genetic form of isolated gonadotropin deficiency secondary to absent or low levels of hypothalamic LHRH is transmitted as an autosomal trait (see earlier). Males with cerebellar ataxia and deficient gonadotropin production have been reported in kindreds with X-linked inheritance, and hypogonadotropic hypogonadism may be associated with the multiple lentigenes and basal cell nevus syndromes.

Congenital Adrenal Hypoplasia. Isolated gonadotropin deficiency has been reported in more than 16 males with the X-linked ("cytomegalic") form of congenital adrenal hypoplasia.[71, 352–355] These patients have deficient mineralocorticoid and glucocorticoid secretion and large vacuolated cells in the adrenal glands. Cryptorchidism is common. Congenital adrenal hypoplasia with gonadotropin deficiency is due to contiguous gene deletions in the Xp21 region involving a gene associated with congenital adrenal hypoplasia and a contiguous gene associated with hypogonadotropic hypogonadism.[356] Depending on the extent of the X chromosome deletion, glycerol kinase deficiency and Duchenne muscular dystrophy also may be features of the syndrome (see Chapter 14). As most of these patients die during childhood, it is not clear how many develop gonadotropin deficiency. In some patients, the defect may be at the level of the pituitary gonadotrope rather than the hypothalamus.[355]

Isolated LH Deficiency. Isolated LH deficiency (the fertile eunuch syndrome) is associated with deficient testosterone production in the presence of spermatogenesis and is probably an incomplete form of isolated gonadotropin deficiency;[357] the disorder may be idiopathic or secondary to a hypothalamic pituitary neoplasm. *Isolated FSH deficiency*, presumably caused by deficient production of the beta subunit of FSH, has also been described.[358]

IDIOPATHIC HYPOPITUITARY DWARFISM (Fig. 22–45). Idiopathic hypopituitarism is usually caused by a deficiency of hypothalamic releasing factors. In the untreated state, patients usually have delayed puberty. In contrast, patients with isolated GH deficiency ultimately undergo spontaneous pubertal development, without exogenous gonadal steroids, when the bone age reaches the pubertal stage of 11 to 13 y.[68, 359, 360] Those who have associated gonadotropin deficiency do not undergo spontaneous puberty, even when the bone age advances to the pubertal stage during GH therapy. Common to many patients with idiopathic hypopituitary dwarfism is early onset of growth failure; late onset of diminished growth suggests the presence of a CNS tumor.

TABLE 22–15. Isolated Gonadotropin Deficiency: Clinical Features in 20 Adolescent Boys

Classification	Age and Range* (y)	Testicular Enlargement	Undescended Testes	Gynecomastia	Ocular Anomalies	Other Anomalies
Euosmic	3⁵/₁₂–20⁶/₁₂	3/10	3/10	2/10	3/10	6/10†
Anosmic or hyposmic	7–18	2/10	8/10	6/10	7/10	7/10‡
Total		5/20	11/20	8/20	10/20	13/20

*First evaluated at University of California, San Francisco, Pediatric Endocrine Clinic. All of the patients had delayed puberty; mean height was normal for age.
†Cohen syndrome (1); congenital adrenal hypoplasia (1).
‡Absent kidney (1); talipes, camptodactyly (1).

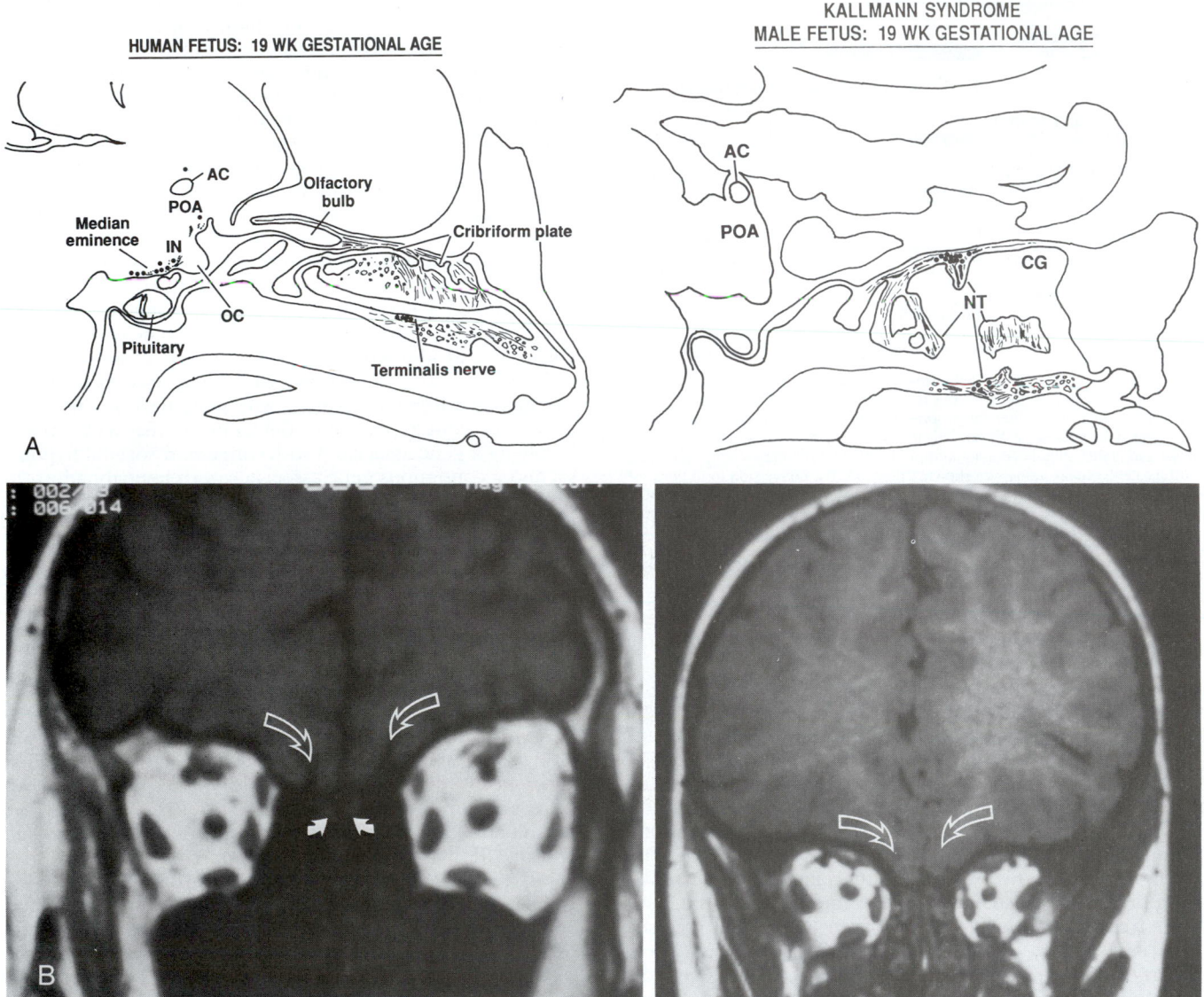

Figure 22–44. Comparison of the brain and nasal cavities of a normal 19-w-old male fetus *(upper left)* and those of a male fetus of similar age with Kallmann syndrome caused by an X chromosome deletion at Xp22.3 *(upper right)*. In the normal fetal brain the LHRH neurosecretory neurons (black dots) are located in the hypothalamic area including the medial basal hypothalamus; the anterior hypothalamic area; and, of interest regarding hypothalamic hamartoma as an ectopic LHRH pulse generator, in the premamillary and retromamillary areas. A small cluster of LHRH neurons is present among the fibers of the terminalis nerve on the floor of the nasal septum. In the male fetus with Kallmann syndrome, no LHRH neurons were detected in the hypothalamic region including the basal hypothalamus, median eminence, and preoptic area. The LHRH cells fail to migrate to and enter the brain from their origin in the nose; these cells end in a tangle beneath the forebrain on the dorsal surface of the cribriform plate and in the nasal cavity. AC, anterior commissure; CG, crista galli; IN, infundibular nucleus; NT, terminalis nerve; OC, optic chiasm; POA, preoptic area. Lower panels show MRI scans of brain (coronal section, T1-weighted image). *Lower left,* Normal olfactory sulci *(open white arrows)* and bulbs (small solid white arrow) in a 15-y-old boy. *Lower right,* Absent olfactory sulci *(open white arrows)* and bulbs in a 17-y-old anosmic, sexually infantile boy with Kallmann syndrome. (Adapted from Schwanzel-Fukuda M, Bick D, Pfaff DW. Luteinizing hormone–releasing hormone [LHRH]–expressing cells do not migrate normally in an inherited hypogonadal [Kallman] mouse. Mol Brain Res 1989; 6:311–326.)

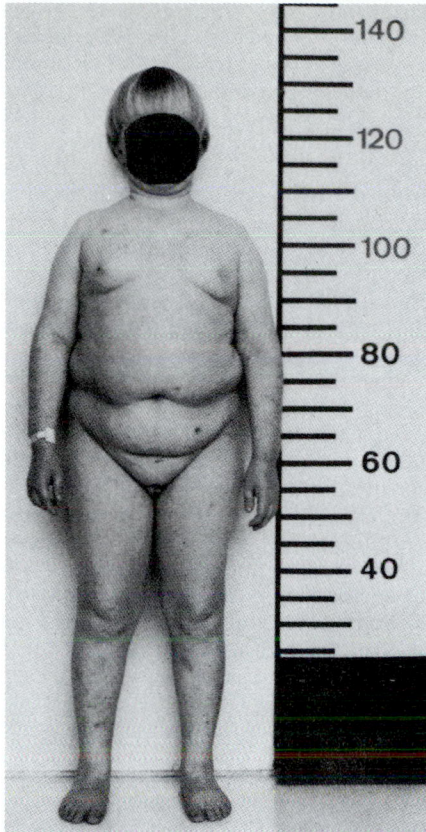

Figure 22–45. A 20-y-old male with idiopathic hypopituitary dwarfism and deficiencies of gonadotropins, thyrotropin, corticotropin, and GH, who had a history of arrested hydrocephalus. Height, 129 cm (−8 SD); the phallus was 2 cm in length, and the testes measured 1.5 × 1 cm. He had received thyroid and glucocorticoid replacement. Basal LH was less than 0.2 ng/mL, FSH was 0.5 ng/mL, and testosterone was less than 0.1 ng/mL. In response to 100 μg of LHRH, the plasma LH concentration increased slightly to 0.6 ng/mL and there was no increase in plasma testosterone. The excretion of urinary 17-ketosteroids was 1.1 mg/24 h. The bone age was 10 y, and the volume of the sella turcica was small on skull radiographs. For conversion to SI units, see the legends of Figures 22–14 and 22–15. (From Styne DM, Grumbach MM. Puberty in the male and female: its physiology and disorders. In: Yen SCC, Jaffe RB, eds. Reproductive Endocrinology. 2nd ed. Philadelphia: W. B. Saunders, 1986: 313–384.)

There is an association between breech delivery, especially in males, perinatal trauma, and idiopathic hypopituitarism,[359] and malformations of the pituitary stalk demonstrable by MRI are common in such patients. The familial forms of multiple pituitary hormone deficiencies with either autosomal recessive or X-linked inheritance are less common.[68, 69]

MISCELLANEOUS CONDITIONS. Prader-Willi Syndrome. This syndrome of massive obesity and carbohydrate intolerance, infantile hypotonia, poor fetal activity, short stature, small hands and feet, mental retardation, emotional instability, and characteristic facies with almond-shaped eyes is associated with delayed puberty caused by hypothalamic dysfunction.[362–366] Affected boys often have micropenis and cryptorchidism. Weight reduction has been associated with menarche in some females. Hence, severe obesity may play a role in the impaired puberty in some patients. This condition usually occurs sporadically. About half of affected individuals have a chromosomal deletion involving chromosome 15, usually an interstitial deletion of the long arm (del(15q11-12)),[361] although the location of the defect is variable among patients. In most and possibly all cases the deletion is on the paternally derived chromosome 15.[367] Several instances of the Prader-Willi syndrome have been

detected in which both members of the intact chromosome 15 pair were inherited from the mother, so-called uniparental disomy, which may occur with isodisomy or heterodisomy.[368] Thus lack of the paternal chromosome 15q11-13 region, caused by any of a variety of genetic mechanisms, can result in the syndrome.

Laurence-Moon-Biedl Syndrome. This autosomal recessive syndrome of polydactyly, obesity, mental retardation, and retinitis pigmentosa often includes delayed puberty and sexual infantilism. Hypogonadotropic hypogonadism and, less commonly, primary gonadal dysfunction have been reported.[369–371]

Functional Gonadotropin Deficiencies. Severe systemic and chronic disorders and malnutrition are associated with delayed puberty or failure to progress through the stages of puberty. It is necessary to distinguish the effects of malnutrition, which can lead to functional hypogonadotropic hypogonadism, from the primary effects of the disease. For example, a group of malnourished rural children from Kenya had chronological delay in pubertal development and excreted less urinary FSH and LH than well-nourished urban children of the same age. When the two groups were matched by pubertal stage rather than chronological age, there was no longer a difference in gonadotropin excretion.[372, 373] Another study of girls who had previously had kwashiorkor demonstrated no delay in breast development or peak height velocity but a delay in pubic hair development and menarche.[218] In general, weight loss of any cause to less than 80% of ideal weight for height can lead to gonadotropin deficiency;[374, 375] weight regain usually restores hypothalamic-pituitary gonadal function over a variable period.[376] If adequate nutrition and body weight are maintained in patients with regional enteritis or chronic pulmonary disease,[377, 378] gonadotropin secretion is usually adequate. Cystic fibrosis also delays puberty, in large part through malnutrition.[379, 380] However, even with normal pubertal progression, boys with cystic fibrosis may have oligospermia caused by obstruction of the spermatic ducts unrelated to their nutritional status.[381] Similarly, boys with sickle cell anemia often exhibit impaired Leydig cell function caused by ischemia of the testes, gonadotropin deficiency, or both factors.[382] Thalassemia major leads to abnormal sexual maturation in 80% of boys and complete absence of pubertal development in 40%[383] because of iron deposition in the pituitary. The gonads can be stimulated by exogenous gonadotropins, and satisfactory sexual development including fertility can be attained by the use of hCG and FSH.[384–387]

Chronic renal disease has been associated with delayed pubertal development[388, 389] and decreased pulsatile gonadotropin secretion; and successful renal transplantion usually restores gonadotropin secretion.[390] Patients with nephrotic syndrome have poor pubertal growth, poor secondary sexual development, and deficient gonadotropin secretion in a pattern resembling constitutional delay in puberty.[391] Children receiving renal or peritoneal dialysis often are delayed in reaching sequential pubertal stages and deficient in linear growth; gonadotropin concentrations may be elevated, presumably because of impaired renal clearance, but the response to LHRH is blunted in severe renal impairment.[389, 392] Improved growth and pubertal development usually ensue after renal transplantation, but the glucocorticoid treatment that follows transplantation presents its own problems. Survivors of renal transplantation who are having immune suppression and alternate-day steroid treatment often have delayed onset of puberty and decreased pulsatility of GH and gonadotropins at night.[393]

Advances in the treatment of *leukemia* have improved the prognosis. Children with early onset and long-term remission experience puberty at an appropriate age or with only slight delay, whereas patients with initial symptoms of leukemia in late childhood may have considerable delay of pubertal development.[394] The type of therapy also influences the age of puberty; radiation to the head may cause hypogonadotropic hypogonadism, and radiation to the abdomen or pelvis and certain types of chemotherapy, especially if administered during puberty, may impair gonadal function and cause primary hypogonadism.[395]

Hypothyroidism may delay the onset of puberty or menarche; treatment with levothyroxine will reverse this pattern.

Poorly controlled *diabetes mellitus* can lead to poor growth, fatty infiltration of the liver, and sexual infantilism (Mauriac syndrome),[396] probably related to poor nutritional status. The degree of control necessary to avoid these complications cannot be exactly quantified, but adolescents with even moderately poor control frequently manifest some degree of growth impairment and delayed puberty or irregular menses.[397]

Cushing disease can be associated with delayed onset or arrest of gonadarche, which usually is corrected by transsphenoidal removal of an ACTH-secreting pituitary adenoma.[398]

Anorexia nervosa is a functional disorder, apparently increasing in prevalence but rare in boys, characterized by a distorted body image, obsessive fear of obesity, and food avoidance that can cause severe weight loss, primary or secondary amenorrhea in affected females, and even death (also see Chapter 25). Other common features include onset in middle adolescence, hyperactivity, defective thermoregulation with hypothermia and sensitivity to cold, constipation, bradycardia and hypotension, decreased basal metabolic rate, dry skin, fine downy hypertrichosis, peripheral edema, and parotid enlargement.[399–401] The clinician should be aware of the subclinical form. Anorexia nervosa may rarely occur in association with a primary psychiatric disorder. It is important to rule out organic disease before the diagnosis of anorexia nervosa is made; one girl with a macroprolactinoma presented with signs consistent with anorexia nervosa.[402] The prevalence of anorexia nervosa is increased in gonadal dysgenesis. Hypogonadotropic hypogonadism has been documented in many patients with anorexia nervosa and, at least in part, is related to weight loss.[399, 400, 406] However, unidentified factors may contribute to the amenorrhea of anorexia nervosa, especially when the onset of amenorrhea precedes the onset of severe weight loss. Functional amenorrhea can also occur in women of normal weight and is characterized by normal levels of gonadotropin and normal gonadotropin response to LHRH stimulation but lack of or an inadequate midcycle LH surge and a decrease in normal pulsatile secretion (amplitude and/or frequency) of gonadotropins.[404] The consequences range in severity from severe estrogen deficiency to anovulation to a short luteal phase.

In anorexia nervosa the concentrations of plasma FSH, LH, and estradiol and the excretion of urinary gonadotropins are characteristically low. In adult women, there may be a reversion to a circadian rhythm of LH secretion and to the sleep-associated increase in episodic LH secretion characteristic of puberty; in severe cases, the amplitude of the pulsatile episodes is diminished and resembles the pattern in prepubertal children.[284] Similarly, the LH response to LHRH correlates with the severity of the weight loss.[402a, 403] In patients who weigh less than 75% of the appropriate weight, there is either a blunted or an absent LH response to the administration of synthetic LHRH and undetectable or small LH pulses. Administration of intravenous LHRH at 90- to 120-min intervals can stimulate the pituitary to produce LH pulses that are indistinguishable from the normal pubertal pattern.[284] This response further supports the important role of functional LHRH deficiency in the amenorrhea of anorexia nervosa. Other hormonal changes include an increased mean concentration of plasma GH and plasma cortisol; low levels of plasma IGF I, DHEAS, and plasma triiodothyronine with normal levels of thyroxine (unless associated with the "low thyroxine syndrome") and TSH; a decreased rise in serum prolactin after the administration of thyrotropin-releasing hormone (TRH) or insulin-induced hypoglycemia;[405] and a diminished capacity to concentrate urine.

The restoration of normal endocrine and metabolic function after weight gain suggests that many of these changes are secondary to starvation and severe weight loss; nevertheless, the amenorrhea may persist for months after weight gain, suggesting persistent hypothalamic dysfunction[406] (also see Chapter 25). Treatment of this disorder requires skillful management, understanding, patience, and psychiatric consultation. Various approaches have been used to increase the food intake. In view of the mortality, parenteral alimentation may be indicated in resistant patients with severe weight loss, especially in the presence of infection or an electrolyte imbalance (see Chapter 25).

Bulimia nervosa is thought to be a variant of anorexia nervosa[407] (also see Chapter 25). In this disorder the individual consumes large amounts of food, but food gorging is followed by induced vomiting.[406] Abuse of laxatives and diuretics is common. Although weight loss is not frequent, amenorrhea is common.[407] Bulimia is especially prevalent in high school and college students.

Cessation of growth can occur in infants and young children with *psychosocial dwarfism*. Stressful social situations can also inhibit growth and physical pubertal development at adolescence.[408]

Exercise, hypo-ovarianism, and amenorrhea: In healthy ballet dancers and female athletes, factors other than decreased body weight can impair pubertal progression and delay menarche through inhibition of the hypothalamic LHRH pulse generator.[215–217, 406, 409, 412] Teen-age ballet dancers are lighter, have less body fat than less physically active girls, and have a high incidence of delayed puberty and of primary and secondary amenorrhea. When the strenuous physical activity is interrupted (e.g., by injury), puberty advances, and menarche often occurs within a few months in those with amenorrhea, in some cases before significant change in body composition or weight.[406] Female athletes of normal weight who have less fat and more muscle than nonathletic girls (e.g., ice skaters or swimmers) are also at risk for delayed puberty and for primary and secondary amenorrhea.[16, 215] Thus both thinness and strenuous physical activity appear to act synergistically, but strenuous exercise training by itself may inhibit the LHRH pulse generator. The effect on pulsatile LHRH secretion may be mediated in part by endogenous opiodergic pathways involving β-endorphin. Even though gonadarche is retarded, adrenarche is not delayed.[16, 215] Athletes who began strenuous training before menarche had a delay in menarcheal age.[409] Osteopenia can result from the chronic hypoestrogenism.

Hyperprolactinemia related to micro- or macroprolactinomas of the pituitary is a rare cause of delayed puberty in both boys and girls.[341, 402, 410] Galactorrhea may be absent by history but it is often demonstrable by manual manipulation of the nipples. Pubertal progression in boys and girls and normal menstrual function in girls occur after treatment with bromocriptine and reduction in serum prolactin levels. Prolactin levels may be elevated in women athletes and may contribute to the delayed menarche.[411, 413]

Marijuana use has been associated with gynecomastia[414] and is a presumptive cause of pubertal delay.[415]

Hypergonadotropic Hypogonadism: Sexual Infantilism Caused by Primary Gonadal Disorders

Primary gonadal failure and the impaired secretion of gonadal steroids lead to decreased negative feedback and elevated LH and FSH levels. The most common forms of primary gonadal failure are associated with sex chromosome abnormalities and characteristic physical findings.[416] Testicular or ovarian dysfunction may rarely be an isolated finding.

KLINEFELTER SYNDROME (SYNDROME OF SEMINIFEROUS TUBULAR DYSGENESIS) AND ITS VARIANTS (see Chapter 14). Klinefelter syndrome, or seminiferous tubular dysgenesis, and its variants occur in approximately 1 in 1000 males and are the most common forms of male hypogonadism.[416, 417] The invariable clinical features include small, firm testes (less than 3.5 cm in length), impaired spermatogenesis, and a male phenotype, usually with gynecomastia and eunuchoid proportions[416] (Fig. 22–46). Elevated gonadotropin levels are found postpubertally; before the age of 12 gonadotropin concentrations are in the prepubertal range. Low gonadotropin concentrations occur rarely when hypogonadotropic hypogonadism is associated with 47,XXY Klinefelter syndrome.[418] Hyalinization and fibrosis of the seminiferous tubules and pseudoadenomatous changes of the Leydig cells develop after puberty; prepubertal testes show only subtle histological changes, although the testes are small and the germ cell content is reduced. Prepubertally, patients can be detected by the disproportion-

ate length of the extremities, decreased upper/lower body ratio, and increased arm span.[419] There is variation in Leydig cell function, but testosterone concentrations tend to be in the normal range until about age 14, after which they may fail to rise normally.[420, 421] The onset of puberty usually is not delayed, but impaired Leydig cell reserve and low testosterone levels may lead to slow progression or arrest of pubertal changes. Serum estradiol/testosterone ratios and TeBG levels are higher than those in normal males, which indicates an increased estrogen effect and decreased testosterone effect. These factors probably account, at least in part, for the gynecomastia characteristic of Klinefelter syndrome during adolescence.[421–423] Testosterone administration does not appear to reduce the gynecomastia, but dihydrotestosterone[424] may be effective. If the gynecomastia does not regress, a reduction mammoplasty is required. Tall stature for family size is common in this disorder.

Affected individuals detected by karyotype analysis at birth and in screening studies had minimal impairment (10 to 20 points) in verbal I.Q. compared with control subjects and normal full-scale I.Q. Severe retardation is uncommon, although there is an increased prevalence of speech and learning disorders and adjustment problems in adolescence. Psychopathology is rare in most studies, and a 20-y follow-up of 47,XXY individuals shows little or no variation from nonaffected controls in employment, social status, mental or physical health, or criminality.[425–427]

Conditions associated with Klinefelter syndrome include aortic valvular disease and ruptured berry aneurysms (six

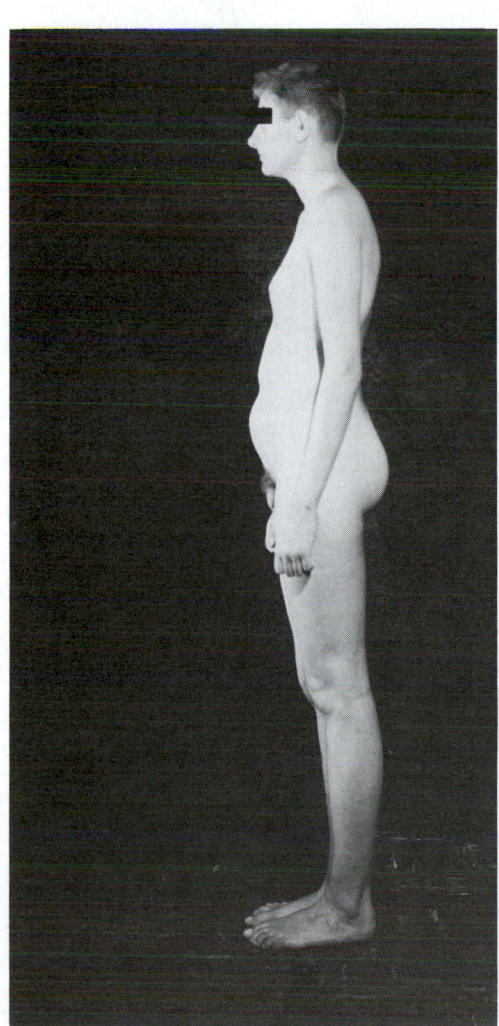 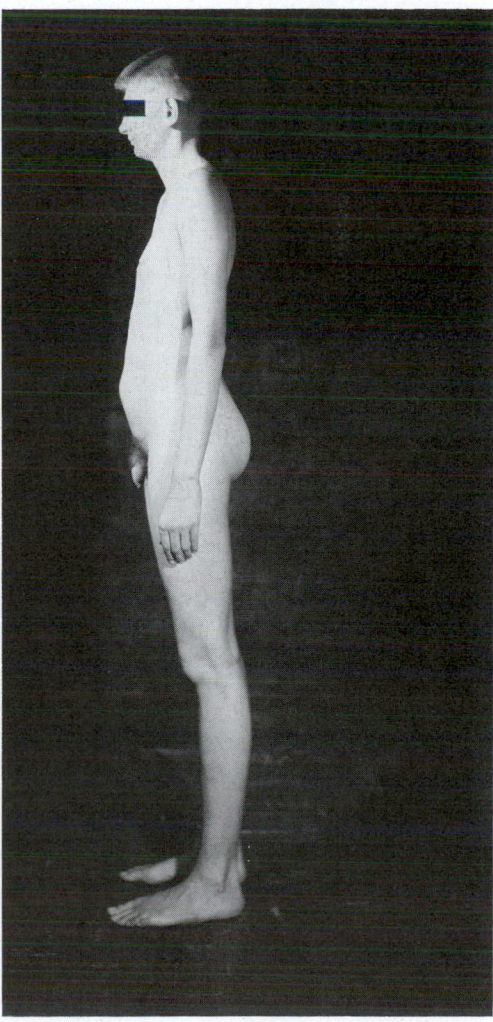

Figure 22–46. 47,XXY Klinefelter syndrome in 17-y-old identical twins. At age 15 gynecomastia was noted. The twins had a eunuchoid habitus and poorly developed male secondary sexual characteristics. Both were 187 cm in height; armspan 187 cm and 189.5 cm; the voices were high pitched; the testes measured 1.8 × 1.5 cm; penis length, 7.5 cm. Gynecomastia and signs of androgen deficiency were more evident in the twin on the left. Urinary gonadotropins, >50 mU/24 h. The testes exhibited extensive tubular fibrosis, small dysgenetic tubules, and clumping or pseudoadenomatous formation of Leydig cells; germ cells were rare. The microscopic appearance was typical of seminiferous tubule dysgenesis. Patients are described in Grumbach MM, Barr ML. Cytologic tests of chromosome sex in relation to sexual anomalies in man. Recent Prog Horm Res 1958; 14:255–324.

times the normal rate);[428] breast carcinoma (20 times the rate in normal men and one fifth that of women);[429] other malignancies such as acute leukemia, lymphoma, and germ cell tumor;[425] systemic lupus erythematosus;[430, 431] and osteoporosis.[432, 433] There is an increased incidence of fatigue, varicose veins, and essential tremor.

Most patients have a 47,XXY chromosomal karyotype. The next most common variant is 46,XY/47,XXY; 48,XXYY and 48,XXXY karyotypes are found with lower frequency and are associated with a higher incidence of mental retardation and somatic anomalies. The rare 46,XX male has some features of Klinefelter syndrome[416] (see Chapter 14). The 49,XXXXY karyotype is associated with a specific syndrome characterized by severe mental deficiency, skeletal abnormalities (such as radioulnar synostosis), and hypoplastic external genitalia with a small penis and undescended testes.[416]

OTHER FORMS OF PRIMARY TESTICULAR FAILURE.
Chemotherapeutic agents used in the treatment of nephrotic syndrome or leukemia, such as cyclophosphamide or chlorambucil, have led to Sertoli cell and germ cell damage in prepubertal patients; these effects are sometimes reversible.[434, 435] MOPP (Mustargen, Oncovin, procarbazine, prednisone) therapy for Hodgkin disease or, alternatively, adriamycin, bleomycin, vinblastine, and dacarbazine (ABVD) can also cause germ cell depletion. Although some degree of gonadal maturation such as that noted during puberty has been considered to be necessary before these drugs cause gonadal damage, gonadal damage can occur earlier as a result of therapy in the prepubertal period but may not be demonstrable until the age of puberty.[436] *Radiation* of the gonads can also cause primary testicular failure, usually resulting in azoospermia, although normal testosterone secretion may be associated with elevated LH and FSH values (compensated Leydig cell failure).[437]

Testicular biosynthetic defects (see Chapter 14): Male pseudohermaphroditism caused by 17α-hydroxylase (P-450$_{c17}$) deficiency is associated with sexual infantilism and a female phenotype; the testosterone biosynthetic defect blocks the synthesis of testosterone and adrenal androgens, impairing masculinization at all stages of development. Associated cortisol deficiency and increased mineralocorticoid secretion in this condition lead to hypertension, decreased serum potassium levels, and metabolic alkalosis. Glucocorticoid replacement suppresses ACTH and mineralocorticoid excess and corrects the electrolyte abnormalities, but no sexual development occurs unless exogenous gonadal steroids are administered. Partial deficiencies are compatible with ambiguous genitalia; one case of delayed puberty in a phenotypic male was attributed to partial deficiency of 17,20-desmolase and 17α-hydroxylase.[438]

A rarer autosomal recessive condition is cytochrome P-450$_{scc}$ deficiency (previously called 20,22-desmolase deficiency), in which the ability to produce C_{21}-, C_{19}-, and C_{18}-steroids is lost; severely affected patients have lipid-laden adrenal glands (the enzymatic block is just past the synthesis of cholesterol). The large adrenal glands may be visualized on sonographic, CT, or MRI scans. Death often occurs in infancy because of unrecognized glucocorticoid and mineralocorticoid deficiency. Affected individuals physically appear to be sexually infantile females, whether their karyotype is 46,XY or 46,XX; because of the absence of gonadal or adrenal estrogen or testosterone production, they do not develop secondary sexual characteristics.[416]

Luteinizing hormone resistance: Presumptive evidence of LH resistance caused by an LH receptor abnormality on the Leydig cell was reported in an 18-y-old boy with a male phenotype, no male secondary sexual development, gynecomastia, elevated plasma LH levels, and early pubertal

plasma testosterone concentrations that did not increase after hCG administration; there was no elevation of testosterone precursor levels.[439] The testes were prepubertal in size and had the microscopic appearance of normal prepubertal testes. Plasma membrane receptor preparations from the testes bound only one half as much radiolabeled hCG as control testes.

Anorchia and cryptorchidism: In the 46,XY male without palpable testes, it is important to determine whether any testicular tissue is present. The patient may have intra-abdominal testes, which carry an increased risk of malignant degeneration, or anorchia (the "vanishing testes syndrome"), in which no testes are found at laparotomy.[416, 440] The presence of a male phenotype and male internal ducts indicates that functioning fetal testes capable of secreting testosterone and AMH were present early during fetal life but degenerated thereafter. Administration of 2000 U of hCG intramuscularly usually evokes an increased concentration of plasma testosterone after 72 h when functional Leydig cells are present;[441] the lack of a rise in testosterone concentration, in conjunction with an increased plasma concentration of FSH and LH or an augmented gonadotropin response to LHRH,[443] is evidence for the diagnosis of bilateral anorchia. Cryptorchid testes may descend into the scrotum during more prolonged treatment with hCG (3000 U/m² surface area intramuscularly every other day for six doses), although some clinicians believe that such descent occurs only in retractile rather than true cryptorchid testes. Orchiopexy is necessary if hCG is ineffective. Because cryptorchidism may be due to a primary testicular defect, cryptorchid testes, even if replaced in the scrotum, may never have normal spermatogenic function; dysgenetic testes, even if located in the scrotum, carry a small, but definite, risk of malignant transformation.[416]

SYNDROME OF GONADAL DYSGENESIS AND ITS VARIANTS (see Chapter 14).[416, 442] The most common form of hypogonadism in the female is the syndrome of *gonadal dysgenesis* or *Turner syndrome* and its variants, with an incidence of 1 per 2500 to 10,000 liveborn girls.[442–445] The incidence of abnormalities of the X chromosome is even higher if pregnancies rather than newborns are considered because as many as 99% of 45,X conceptuses abort spontaneously and 1 in 15 spontaneous abortions has the 45,X karyotype.[446, 447] The 45,X karyotype is associated with female phenotype, short stature, sexual infantilism, and various somatic abnormalities. Sex chromosome mosaicism or structural abnormalities of an X or Y chromosome may modify the features of this syndrome. Thus we may view the syndrome of gonadal dysgenesis and its variants as a continuum ranging from the typical 45,X phenotype to a normal male or female phenotype.[416]

45,X Gonadal Dysgenesis (Fig. 22–47) (also see Chapter 14). Short stature and sexual infantilism are invariable features of sex chromatin–negative 45,X gonadal dysgenesis, or Turner syndrome. This karyotype is found in approximately half of cases of Turner syndrome.[448] Affected newborn infants may have lymphedema of the extremities and loose posterior cervical skin folds, which later develop into the webbed neck; the term Bonnevie-Ullrich syndrome has been applied to infants with these features of Turner syndrome. Other frequent features are distinct facies with micrognathia, fishmouth, high-arched palate with dental abnormalities, epicanthal folds, ptosis, and low-set or deformed ears; broad shield-like chest leading to the appearance of wide-spaced nipples, hypoplastic areolae, short neck with low hairline, and webbing (pterygium colli); recurrent otitis media, often leading to impaired hearing;[450] short fourth metacarpals and cubitus valgus that develop after birth; and extensive nevi, tendency to keloid formation, and

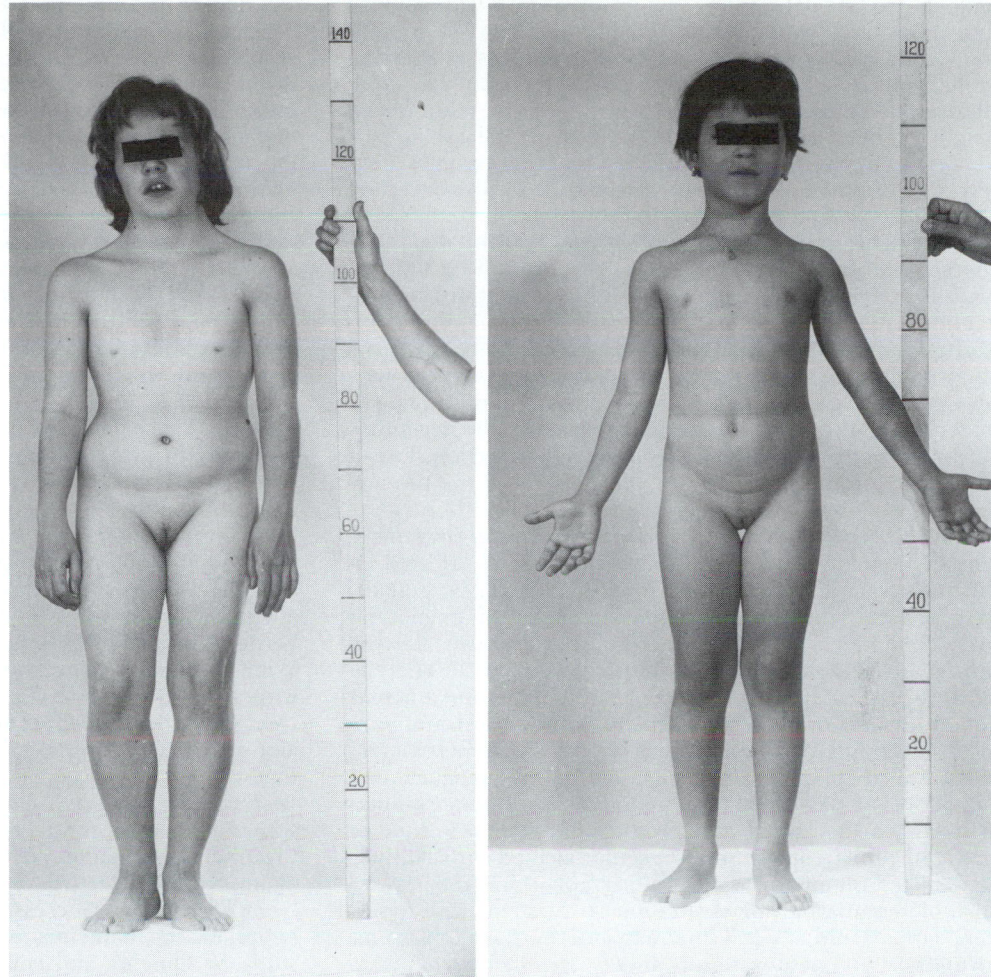

Figure 22–47. *Left,* A 14¹⁰/₁₂-y-old patient with the typical form of the syndrome of gonadal dysgenesis (Turner syndrome). The X chromatin pattern was negative and the karyotype was 45,X. She was short (height 134.5 cm; height age 9⁵/₁₂ y), sexually infantile except for the appearance of sparse pubic hair, and exhibited characteristic stigmata of the syndrome: a short webbed neck, shield-like chest with widely separated nipples, bilateral metacarpal signs, puffiness over the dorsum of the fingers, cubitus valgus, increased number of pigmented nevi, characteristic facies, and low-set ears. The bone age was 13⁶/₁₂ y; urinary 17-ketosteroids, 5.1 mg/d; urinary gonadotropin, >100 mU/d. Vaginal smears and the urocytogram showed an immature pattern in which cornified squamous cells were absent. With estrogen therapy, female secondary sexual characteristics were induced; the cyclic administration resulted in periodic estrogen-withdrawal bleeding. *Right,* A 45,X, 9¹¹/₁₂-y-old patient with Turner syndrome. Apart from short stature (height 118 cm; age 6¹⁰/₁₂ y), increased pigmented nevi, and subtle changes in the fingers and toes, she had few somatic anomalies. In contrast to the patient in the left panel, the main clinical feature was short stature.

hypoplastic nails.[416, 449] Lymphatic obstruction leads to the infantile puffiness of extremities and pterygium colli as well as a distinctive shape of the ears. Cardiovascular anomalies include coarctation of the aorta, aortic stenosis, and bicuspid aortic valves, and these subjects are at risk for dissecting aortic aneurysms.[452] Abnormal pelvocaliceal collecting systems, abnormal position or alignment of the kidneys, and abnormal vascular supply to the kidney are encountered.[451] Defects of the gastrointestinal system include intestinal telangiectasias and hemangiomatoses that can lead to massive gastrointestinal bleeding. Furthermore, the prevalence of inflammatory bowel disease is increased.[453–455] The uterus and fallopian tubes are infantile. Pelvic ultrasonography or MRI usually permits the detection of even a small uterus in these patients and commonly streak gonads. Autoimmune diseases, such as Hashimoto thyroiditis and Graves disease, are common. Glucose intolerance resulting from increased insulin resistance is also common after the age of puberty, although in some this may be due to associated obesity.[456, 457] Intelligence is normal,[459, 460] although specific tasks may be more difficult to complete. For example, spatiotemporal processing, visuomotor coordination,[458] and mathematical ability (particularly in geometry) may be impaired. Gender identity and sexual orientation are female.[459]

Patients are usually small at birth, grow slowly after the age of 3, fail to have a pubertal growth spurt,[461–463] and end up at a mean final height of approximately 142 to 143 cm.[462] Specific growth curves are available for plotting the growth of affected children.[462, 463]

As discussed earlier, the biphasic pattern of gonadotropin secretion in normal infancy and childhood (see Fig. 22–28) is exaggerated in gonadal dysgenesis. Thus baseline gonadotropin concentrations and peak LH and FSH values after LHRH administration are above normal between birth and 4 y of age and again after age 10. Baseline values of FSH are 3 to 10 times higher than LH values. However, between ages 4 and 10, mean gonadotropin concentrations in this syndrome are similar to the mean values in normal girls (see Figs. 22–28 and 22–30) and are lower than those before age 4 and after age 10.[234, 235]

The appearance of pubic hair is often delayed in the syndrome of gonadal dysgenesis, even though adrenarche, as assessed by the increase in concentration of plasma DHEAS, occurs at the normal age.[305] The pubic hair of affected individuals is sparse, but estrogen therapy increases the growth of pubic hair despite a lack of increase in adrenal androgen secretion.[464] The streak gonads result in sexual infantilism; rarely, probably in about 10% of cases, puberty, menarche, and, even more rarely, pregnancy may occur.[416]

Girls with gonadal dysgenesis have a tendency toward impaired glucose tolerance.[465] This finding may be of importance in view of the tendency to treat with GH, a diabetogenic agent. Furthermore, auxological studies demonstrate that patients with gonadal dysgenesis have intrauterine growth retardation, relatively normal growth until a bone age of 3 y, and then a decrease in growth with a profound reduction in growth rate at the time of expected puberty; this pattern of growth does not suggest that such patients are GH deficient.[463] In a group of girls with gonadal dysgenesis and spontaneous puberty, height velocity was transiently higher during puberty than in girls with amenorrhea, but final adult height was not different.[416] The adult stature of these patients correlates with midparental height.[448] The bone density is decreased, at least in part because of hypogonadism at puberty, and this becomes more severe with age in patients who discontinue or do not receive estrogen replacement therapy.

Sex Chromatin–Positive Variants of Gonadal Dysgenesis. Mosaicism of 45,X/46,XX, 45,X/47,XXX, or 45,X/46,XX/47,XXX chromosomes is associated with a chromatin-positive buccal smear and usually fewer manifestations of the syndrome of gonadal dysgenesis. Likewise, structural abnormalities of the X chromosome can be associated with fewer phenotypic features of the syndrome. Lack of genetic material on the long or the short arm of the second X chromosome can cause decreased gonadal function; loss of all or part of the short arm of the X leads to the physical findings of Turner syndrome (see Chapter 14).[416]

Sex Chromatin–Negative Variants of Gonadal Dysgenesis. These variants include 45,X/46,XY mosaicism. Affected individuals vary in phenotype from that of classic gonadal dysgenesis to that of ambiguous genitalia to phenotypic males.[416] Patients may present with short stature, delayed puberty, and a history of hypospadias repair.[466] There is variable testicular differentiation, ranging from a streak gonad to functioning testes. Patients with mosaicism involving a Y cell line or abnormalities of the Y chromosome are at risk for neoplastic transformation of the dysgenetic testes. Gonadoblastomas—benign nonmetastasizing tumors—may arise within the gonad and produce either testosterone or estrogens; the neoplasm may become calcified sufficiently to be detected on an abdominal radiograph. Thus the appearance of feminization or virilization in a patient with dysgenetic gonads and a Y cell line may indicate gonadoblastoma formation. Of greater significance is the increased prevalence of malignant germ cell tumors, arising within the dysgenetic gonad or gonadoblastoma.[467] Such tumors occur more often in postpubertal subjects and rarely in children.[468, 469] Because of this risk, we recommend the removal of all dysgenetic gonads in patients with a Y cell line.[416]

46,XX AND 46,XY GONADAL DYSGENESIS. Pure gonadal dysgenesis refers to phenotypic females with sexual infantilism and a 46,XX or 46,XY karyotype without chromosomal abnormalities.[416]

Familial and Sporadic 46,XX Gonadal Dysgenesis and Its Variants. The usual phenotype of 46,XX gonadal dysgenesis includes normal stature, sexual infantilism, bilateral streak gonad, normal female internal and external genitalia, and primary amenorrhea. The streak gonad occasionally produces estrogens or androgens, but malignant transformation is rare. Incomplete forms of this condition may result in hypoplastic ovaries that produce enough estrogen to cause some breast development and a few menstrual periods followed by secondary amenorrhea. The syndrome occurs sporadically or with autosomal recessive inheritance; some familial cases have been associated with sensorineural deafness.[416]

Familial and Sporadic 46,XY Gonadal Dysgenesis and Its Variants. A phenotype that includes female genitalia with or without clitoral enlargement, normal or tall stature, bilateral streak gonads, normal müllerian structures, sexual infantilism, and a eunuchoid habitus is typical of 46,XY gonadal dysgenesis. If the dysgenetic testes produce significant amounts of testosterone, slight clitoral enlargement may occur at birth and virilization may ensue at puberty. The incomplete form of 46,XY gonadal dysgenesis may involve

any degree of ambiguity of the external genitalia and internal ducts. The risk of neoplastic transformation of the streak gonads or dysgenetic testes is increased, and gonadectomy is indicated.[416] The disorder is usually transmitted as an X-linked or sex-limited autosomal dominant trait, less commonly as an autosomal recessive trait[416] (see Chapter 14).

OTHER CAUSES OF PRIMARY OVARIAN FAILURE. Premature menopause may occur at any age before the normal climacteric and has been reported in adolescent girls; cessation of ovarian function usually presents as secondary amenorrhea, but primary amenorrhea and delayed or arrested puberty may occur. Primary ovarian failure as a consequence of the long-term effects of cytotoxic chemotherapy and radiation is increasing in prevalence as these agents prolong life in children and adolescents with cancer.

Radiation therapy that includes the ovaries within the field can cause primary ovarian failure;[437] thus it is useful surgically to tack the ovaries out of the radiation field, if possible. Chemotherapy with nitroso compounds (carmustine and lomustine) or procarbazine for the treatment of brain tumors has been linked to primary gonadal failure manifested by elevated plasma gonadotropin levels in boys and girls; the boys had small testes but were able to secrete adequate testosterone for their pubertal stage.[436, 470] Prepubertal boys and girls treated with abdominal radiation for Wilms tumor plus chemotherapy (dactinomycin, vincristine with adriamycin, or cyclophosphamide in most) may experience gonadal damage, whereas those given chemotherapy alone usually do not.[471] Although it was previously thought that cancer therapy does not cause gonadal damage in prepubertal subjects, current evidence suggests otherwise.[472, 473] Attempts to protect the gonads by suppressing the pituitary-gonadal axis with gonadal steroids or LHRH agonists are ineffective.

Chemotherapy: Successful treatment of childhood acute lymphoblastic leukemia is now commonplace. In a large study by Quigley and colleagues,[474] after cytotoxic chemotherapy boys and girls had extensive germ cell damage as evidenced by increased FSH secretion and boys had decreased testicular size for the stage of puberty. The concentration of plasma inhibin was usually decreased. Many of the girls at puberty had evidence of a compensated decrease in ovarian follicular function. Quite likely as a result of cranial radiation, the mean age of menarche was advanced about 12 mo despite the ovarian damage; puberty was not advanced in the boys.

Autoimmune oophoritis can cause ovarian failure leading to primary amenorrhea, oligomenorrhea, arrest of puberty, and occasionally cystic enlargement of the ovaries.[475–477] Most often it is associated with other autoimmune endocrinopathies (see Chapter 31). Thirty-six percent of women with type I autoimmune polyglandular insufficiency (hypoparathyroidism, adrenal insufficiency, gonadal failure, diabetes mellitus, pernicious anemia, hypothyroidism, chronic hepatitis, mucocutaneous candidiasis, dystrophic nail hypoplasia, vitiligo, alopecia, keratinopathy, and intestinal malabsorption) exhibited ovarian failure before age 20, whereas only 4% of affected men had testicular failure by this age.[476] Autoimmune oophoritis is present in more than 20% of patients with autoimmune adrenal insufficiency. Various autoantibodies have been detected; some are organ specific, whereas others react with antigens in more than one tissue and more than one cell type.[475, 478] Glucocorticoid therapy may improve, at least temporarily, ovarian function.[479]

Resistant ovary is a rare form of primary hypogonadism, a syndrome associated with elevated concentrations of plasma FSH and LH and ovaries that contain primordial follicles.[480–482] Abnormality of FSH (and LH) receptors and signal transduction and antibodies to the FSH receptor are

TABLE 22–16. Differential Diagnostic Features of Delayed Puberty and Sexual Infantilism

Disorder	Stature	Plasma Gonadotropin Levels	LHRH Test: LH Response	Plasma Gonadal Steroid Levels	Plasma DHEAS Level	Karyotype	Olfaction
Constitutional delay in growth and adolescence	Short for chronological age, usually appropriate for bone age	Prepubertal, later pubertal	Prepubertal, later pubertal	Low, later normal	Low for chronological age, appropriate for bone age	Normal	Normal
Hypogonadotropic hypogonadism							
Isolated gonadotropin deficiency	Normal, absent pubertal growth spurt	Low	Prepubertal or no response	Low	Appropriate for chronological age	Normal	Normal
Kallmann syndrome	Normal, absent pubertal growth spurt	Low	Prepubertal or no response	Low	Appropriate for chronological age	Normal	Anosmia or hyposmia
Idiopathic multiple pituitary hormone deficiencies	Short stature and poor growth since early childhood	Low	Prepubertal or no response	Low	Usually low	Normal	Normal
Hypothalamic-pituitary tumors	Decrease in growth velocity of recent onset	Low	Prepubertal or no response	Low	Normal or low for chronological age	Normal	Normal
Primary gonadal failure							
Syndrome of gonadal dysgenesis and variants	Short stature since early childhood	High	Hyper-response for age	Low	Normal for chronological age	45,X or variant	Normal
Klinefelter syndrome and variants	Normal to tall	High	Hyper-response at puberty	Low or normal	Normal for chronological age	47,XXY or variant	Normal
Familial 46,XX or 46,XY gonadal dysgenesis	Normal	High	Hyper-response for age	Low	Normal for chronological age	46,XX or 46,XY	Normal

From Styne DM, Grumbach MM. Puberty in the male and female. In: Yen SCC, Jaffe RB, eds. Reproductive Endocrinology. 2nd ed. Philadelphia: W. B. Saunders, 1986: 313–384.

possible defects. In one report estrogen therapy for several months with suppression of the elevated gonadotropin levels was followed by spontaneous ovarian cycles.[482]

Galactosemia is commonly associated with primary ovarian failure. Most cases are detected by newborn screening programs.[483]

Polycystic ovary disease does not delay the onset of puberty but often delays menarche or causes menstrual abnormalities[484, 485] (see Chapter 12).

Noonan syndrome (pseudo-Turner syndrome, Ullrich syndrome): Subjects with Noonan syndrome have webbed neck, ptosis, short stature, cubitus valgus, and lymphedema, and hence this phenotype has been called pseudo-Turner syndrome.[416] Features that differentiate these individuals from those with Turner syndrome include triangular facies, pectus excavatum, right-sided heart disease (e.g., pulmonic stenosis or atrial septal defect), and an increased incidence of mental retardation. Females with Noonan syndrome have normal ovarian function. Males have normal differentiation of external genitalia but may have undescended testes; germinal aplasia or hypoplasia and impaired Leydig cell function may be present. Noonan syndrome is inherited as an autosomal dominant trait.[416] About 85% of patients are thought to be the result of new mutations.

Diagnosis of Delayed Puberty and Sexual Infantilism (Table 22–16)

Signs of puberty have not yet appeared in 0.4% of normal boys by age 15 and 0.4% of normal girls by age 13. Thus when prepubertal girls present at age 12 or prepubertal boys present at age 14, the physician must make a clinical judgment as to which are variants of the norm and which require extensive evaluation and treatment. Lack of pro-

gression through the stages of puberty, even if the age at onset is normal, may also require evaluation; a boy who has not completed secondary sexual maturation within 4.5 y after onset of puberty or a girl who does not menstruate within 5 y after onset may have a hypothalamic, pituitary, or gonadal disorder.

The diagnosis of hypergonadotropic hypogonadism is readily established by elevation of random plasma LH and FSH concentrations. However, the differential diagnosis of hypogonadotropic hypogonadism versus constitutional delay in growth and adolescence is more difficult because of the overlap in physical and laboratory findings in the two conditions, including inability to differentiate between normal and low concentrations of serum gonadotropins (Table 22–17).

A presumptive diagnosis can usually be formed during the initial evaluation on the basis of the history and physical examination. History taking must elicit all symptoms of chronic or intermittent illnesses and all details pertaining to growth and development as well as a history of olfaction. Disorders of pregnancy, abnormalities of labor and delivery, and birth trauma, if present in the patient's history, suggest that a congenital or neonatal event may be related to the delay in puberty. Poor linear growth and poor nutritional

TABLE 22–17. Endocrine Diagnosis of Constitutional Delayed Adolescence and Hypogonadotropic Hypogonadism

No single test reliably discriminates between the two diagnoses.
Onset of puberty in boys is indicated by
Testes > 2.5 cm in diameter
Serum testosterone concentration > 50 ng/dL
Pubertal LH response to LHRH bolus
Pubertal pattern of LH pulsatility

status during the neonatal period and childhood may reflect long-standing abnormalities of development. A growth chart is plotted to represent graphically the increase in stature and to assess growth velocity from birth (see Chapter 21). Family history may reveal disorders of puberty or infertility, anosmia, or hyposmia in relatives as well as delay in the age at onset of puberty in parents or siblings. A history of consanguinity is important in the detection of autosomal recessive disorders.

The physical examination starts with determining height and weight; the upper/lower segment ratio or sitting height is calculated and the arm span is measured and compared with the height. The height velocity should be documented over a period of at least 6 mo, preferably 12 mo. The signs of puberty are noted, and the stage of secondary sexual development is determined according to the standards presented earlier (see Figs. 22–2 to 22–4). The sizes of the testes and penis are measured in boys, and the diameter of glandular breast tissue and areolar size are noted in girls. The presence or absence of galactorrhea is defined. Obese boys often appear to have a small penis because of excessive adipose tissue surrounding the phallus; only when the fat is retracted can the full extent of phallic development be assessed. Cryptorchidism or retractile testes should be noted if no testes are palpated in the scrotum. Neurological examination, including examination of the optic discs and visual fields by frontal confrontation perimetry and evaluation of olfaction, may reveal findings suggesting the presence of a CNS neoplasm or a developmental defect (Kallmann syndrome). The stigmata of gonadal dysgenesis (Turner syndrome) or the small testes and gynecomastia of Klinefelter syndrome may suggest one of these diagnoses. Examination of the lungs, heart, kidney, and the gastrointestinal tract is also important.

Laboratory studies (Table 22–18) include determination of plasma LH and FSH concentrations, measurement of the rise in LH level after LHRH administration, determination of testosterone concentrations in boys and estradiol levels in girls, and measurements of thyroxine and prolactin concentrations in boys and girls if the clinical features warrant. Radiographic examination includes bone age determination and lateral skull x-ray films and, depending on the clinical findings, an MRI or CT scan of the brain. Ultrasound evaluation of the uterus and ovaries is not usually indicated initially in work-up of delayed puberty but provides useful information about the state of development of these structures.[39] One study demonstrated streak gonads in 50% of a group of 70 patients with Turner syndrome.[486] Assessment of chromosomal karyotype should be considered in all short girls, even in the absence of signs of the syndrome of gonadal dysgenesis, and in boys with Klinefelter stigmata.

A presumptive diagnosis of constitutional delay in growth and adolescence may be made if the history and growth chart reveal a history of short stature but consistent growth rate for skeletal age, if the family history includes parents or siblings with delayed puberty, if the physical examination (including assessment of the olfactory threshold) is normal, if optic discs and visual fields are normal, if the bone age is delayed, and if a lateral skull x-ray film is normal. The rate of growth in these patients is usually appropriate for bone age; a decrease in growth velocity occurs in some normal children just before the appearance of secondary sexual characteristics. Further, the onset at puberty correlates better with bone age than with chronological age. Elevated concentrations of gonadotropins and gonadal steroids precede pubertal development by several months; thus, measurements of LH, FSH, estradiol, or testosterone levels may help in predicting future development. In addition, an increase in concentration of LH of more than 7.6 IU/L (2 ng/ml LER-960) after intravenous administration of 100 μg of LHRH usually precedes the first sign of sexual maturation by about 1 y.

Clomiphene citrate, an antiestrogen with weak estrogenic effects, decreases secretion of gonadotropins in prepubertal patients but increases gonadotropin secretion in pubertal patients and in adults. However, we have not found administration of clomiphene citrate to be useful in the diagnosis of constitutional delay in growth and adolescence.

Various tests have been proposed for differentiating hypogonadotropic hypogonadism from constitutional delay in puberty. Trials assessing the prolactin response to TRH,[487] chlorpromazine,[488] metoclopramide,[489] or domperidone[490] for differential diagnosis either failed or gave inconsistent results.[489, 490] The combination of the prolactin response to metoclopramide and the gonadotropin response to LHRH has been suggested,[492] as has the use of priming doses of LHRH with subsequent evaluation of gonadotropin response to a subsequent dose of LHRH[491, 493] or to a superactive LHRH agonist.[494] A sensitive bioassay and immunofluorometric assay for LH may differentiate between constitutional delay in growth and adolescence and hypogonadotropic hypogonadism better than does radioimmunoassay.[495] Although the latter methods are promising, their efficacy remains to be confirmed. There is a tendency for hypogonadotropic patients to undergo adrenarche at a normal age and to have a higher DHEAS concentration than those with constitutional delay in growth.[305, 496, 497] At present there does not appear to be a practical and reliable endocrine test for differentiating between constitutional delay in growth and adolescence and hypogonadotropic hypogonadism.

A typical patient with isolated gonadotropin deficiency is of average height for age and has eunuchoid proportions; low plasma concentrations of gonadal steroids, LH, and FSH; and no increase or a blunted response of LH after LHRH administration. The amplitude and usually the frequency of LH pulses are decreased when serial blood samples are studied over a 24-h period. In Kallmann syndrome, the sense of smell is absent or impaired. However, differentiation of isolated gonadotropin deficiency in the absence of hyposmia or anosmia from constitutional delay in puberty may be difficult at initial study. Gonadotropin-deficient patients may be as short as those with constitutional delay in growth and adolescence, and concentrations of LH and FSH in hypogonadotropic hypogonadism may be indistinguishable from those of normal prepubertal children or children with constitutional delay. Sometimes, years of observation are necessary to detect the appearance of spontaneous and progressive signs of secondary sexual development or to document rising concentrations of gonadotropins or gonadal steroids before the diagnosis is clear. In general, but not in all cases, absence of the first signs of sexual maturation or

TABLE 22—18. Endocrine and Imaging Studies in Delayed Adolescence

Initial assessment
    Plasma testosterone or estradiol
    Plasma FSH and LH
    Plasma thyroxine (and prolactin)
    Bone age and lateral skull roentgenograph
    Test of olfaction

Follow-up studies
    Karyotype (short, phenotypic females)
    MRI and/or CT scan
    Pelvic sonography (females)
    LHRH test
    hCG test (males)
    Pattern of pulsatile LH secretion
    Visual acuity and visual fields

failure of a rise in gonadotropins or gonadal steroid levels by age 18 in the presence of a normal concentration of serum DHEAS for chronological age supports the diagnosis of isolated gonadotropin deficiency.

Patients with deficiency of gonadotropins combined with deficiency of other pituitary hormones require careful evaluation for a CNS neoplasm. Visual field or optic disc abnormalities support the diagnosis of CNS tumor; even if these tests are normal, radiographic examination of the skull should be done to evaluate the sella turcica and the suprasellar region for calcification or erosion. MRI and CT scans of the head are valuable in detecting mass lesions and developmental abnormalities of the hypothalamic-pituitary region.

Treatment of Delayed Puberty and Sexual Infantilism

Treatment of delayed puberty (Table 22–19) depends on the diagnosis and the nature of the disorder. Patients with constitutional delay in growth and adolescence ultimately have spontaneous onset and progression through puberty. Often, reassurance and continued observation to ensure that the expected sexual maturation occurs are sufficient. However, the stigma of appearing less mature than one's peers can cause psychological stress; such individuals may be unable to participate in the dating activities their friends are starting, smaller size may lead them to avoid participation in athletics, immature appearance may lead to ridicule especially in the locker room, and school work may suffer with their poor self-image.[498, 498a] Some children feel such intense peer pressure and low self-esteem that only the appearance of signs of puberty will reassure them and enable them to participate in sports and social activities with their peers. Poor self-image in late-maturing boys may carry into adulthood even after normal puberty ensues (reviewed in ref. 498 and 498a). For psychological reasons, in boys of age 14 or older who show no signs of puberty, a 6-mo course of testosterone enanthate (100 mg intramuscularly every 4 wk) may be helpful.[499–501] For girls of age 13 or older, a 3-mo course of ethinyl estradiol (5 to 10 μg/d orally) or conjugated estrogens (0.3 mg/d orally) may be used to initiate maturation of the secondary sexual characteristics without unduly advancing bone age or limiting final height.[502, 503] Psychological adjustment, self-image, and school performance of affected males can improve with such short-term androgen therapy.[504] If, during the 3 to 6 mo after discontinuing gonadal steroid therapy, spontaneous puberty does not ensue or the concentrations of plasma gonadotropins and plasma testosterone in boys or plasma estradiol in girls do not increase, the treatment may be repeated. Usually, only one or two courses of therapy are necessary. When treatment is discontinued after bone age has advanced, for example, to 13 or 14 y in boys, patients with constitutional delay continue pubertal development on their own, whereas those with gonadotropin deficiency do not progress and may, in fact, regress. The low dose of testosterone enanthate is generally considered to be safe but can raise LDL and lower HDL cholesterol values. A course of low-dose oxandrolone[505] (2.5 mg/d) is sometimes used as an oral alternative to testosterone enanthate.

Functional hypogonadotropic hypogonadism associated with chronic disease is treated by alleviating the underlying problem. Delayed puberty in this situation is usually a result of inadequate nutrition and low weight; when weight returns to normal values, puberty usually occurs spontaneously.

Treatment with thyroxine will allow normal pubertal development in hypothyroid patients with delayed puberty.

Congenital or acquired gonadotropin deficiency as a result of a lesion or surgery requires replacement therapy with gonadal steroids at an age approximating the normal age of onset of puberty (Tables 22–20 and 22–21). An exception may occur when GH deficiency coexists with gonadotropin deficiency; if bone age advancement and epiphyseal fusion are brought about by testosterone or estradiol replacement before therapy with GH causes adequate linear growth, adult height will be compromised. However, if puberty is not initiated early enough, the patient may well suffer psychological damage. It has been suggested that puberty should be initiated in such patients with low-dose gonadal steroids by age 14 in boys and age 13 in girls regardless of the definitive diagnosis of gonadotropin deficiency; thus these children with GH deficiency would be treated in a fashion similar to those with isolated delayed puberty. By contrast, clinical trials are in progress to determine the effects, if any, of artificially delaying puberty with

TABLE 22–19. Objectives in Management and Treatment and Therapy of Delayed Adolescence

Objectives
Determine site and etiology of abnormality
Induce and maintain secondary sexual characteristics
Induce pubertal growth spurt
Prevent the potential short-term and long-term psychological, personality, and social handicaps of delayed puberty
Ensure normal libido and potency
Attain fertility

Therapy
Concerned but not anxious or socially handicapped adolescent:
  Reassurance and follow-up (tincture of time)
  Repeat evaluation (including serum testosterone or estradiol) in 6 mo
Psychosocial handicaps, anxiety, highly concerned:
  Therapy for 4 mo with
    Boys: testosterone enanthate 100 mg intramuscularly every 4 wk at 14–14.5 y of age
    Girls: ethinyl estradiol 5–10 μg daily by mouth or conjugated estrogens 0.3 mg daily by mouth at 13 y of age
  No therapy for 4–6 mo; re-evaluate status including serum testosterone or estradiol; if indicated repeat treatment regimen

TABLE 22—20. Hormonal Substitution Therapy in Boys with Hypogonadism

Goal: to approximate normal adolescent development *when diagnosis is established*
Initial therapy: at 13 y of age, testosterone enanthate (or other long-acting testosterone ester) 50 mg intramuscularly every month for about 9 mo (6–12 mo)
Over the next 3 to 4 y: gradually increase dose to adult replacement dose of 200 mg every 2–3 wk
Begin *replacement therapy in boys with suspected hypogonadotropic hypogonadism* by bone age ≤14 y
To induce fertility at appropriate time: pulsatile LHRH or FSH and hCG therapy

TABLE 22–21. Hormonal Substitution Therapy in Girls with Hypogonadism

When diagnosis of hypogonadism is firmly established (e.g., girls with 45,X gonadal dysgenesis), begin hormonal substitution therapy at 12–13 y of age
Goal: to approximate normal adolescent development
Initial therapy: ethinyl estradiol 5 μg by mouth or conjugated estrogen 0.3 mg (or less) by mouth daily for 4–6 mo
After 6 mo of therapy (or sooner if "breakthrough" bleeding occurs) begin cyclic therapy:
  Estrogen: first 21 d of month
  Progestogen: (e.g., medroxyprogesterone acetate 5 mg by mouth) 12th to 21st day of month
  Gradually increase dose of estrogen *over next 2–3 y* to conjugated estrogen 0.6–1.25 mg or ethinyl estradiol 10–20 μg daily for first 21 d of month
In hypogonadotropic hypogonadism: to induce ovulation at appropriate time: pulsatile LHRH or FSH and hCG therapy

an LHRH analogue to attempt to achieve a greater final height in patients with isolated GH deficiency.[506]

Microphallus resulting from fetal androgen deficiency caused by a primary testicular defect or gonadotropin deficiency[508] can be successfully treated with small doses of testosterone enanthate (25 to 50 mg/mo intramuscularly), administered for short periods during infancy[507, 508] (also see Chapters 13 and 14).

As discussed earlier, episodic administration of LHRH can elicit pulsatile LH and FSH release and gonadal stimulation in prepubertal children or hypogonadotropic patients.[284–286] Portable pumps have been used to administer LHRH in episodic fashion over prolonged periods (see Chapters 12 and 13).[283, 509] Pulsatile LHRH therapy can induce puberty and promote the virilization of secondary sexual characteristics and spermatogenesis in men[509–511] and ovulation in women;[512, 513] pregnancy has been achieved with this regimen in women with hypogonadotropic hypogonadism. However, this approach is not practical for the routine induction of puberty in adolescent boys and girls with gonadotropin deficiency. hCG and human menopausal gonadotropin can be used as substitutes for LH and FSH, respectively, to produce full gonadal maturation, but these preparations are expensive and frequent injections are required. Thus, long-term gonadal steroid replacement therapy is the treatment of choice for hypothalamic or pituitary gonadotropin deficiency until fertility is desired.

Hypergonadotropic hypogonadism is treated by replacement of testosterone in boys and estradiol in girls. For treatment of gonadal dysgenesis, estrogen therapy should be initiated when the patient is age 12 to 13 to allow secondary sexual development at an appropriate chronological age. The Klinefelter syndrome is compatible with varying degrees of masculinization at puberty, but some patients require testosterone replacement.

Patients receiving gonadal steroid replacement follow the same treatment regimen whether the diagnosis is hypogonadotropic hypogonadism or hypergonadotropic hypogonadism (see Tables 22–20 and 22–21). Males receive testosterone enanthate, 100 mg/mo intramuscularly at the start; later the dosage is gradually increased to 200 to 300 mg every 2 to 3 wk. Low-dose replacement therapy is appropriate until well into the pubertal growth spurt[54] (also see Chapters 13 and 14). Initially, girls age 12 to 13 are given ethinyl estradiol, 5 μg/d orally, or conjugated estrogens, 0.3 mg/d by mouth, on the first 21 d of the month. The dose is gradually increased over the next 2 to 3 y to 10 μg of ethinyl estradiol or 0.6 to 1.25 mg of conjugated estrogen for the first 21 d of the month. The maintenance dose should be the minimal amount to maintain secondary sexual characteristics, sustain withdrawal bleeding, and prevent osteoporosis. After breakthrough bleeding occurs, or no later than 6 mo after the start of cyclic therapy, a progestogen (e.g., medroxyprogesterone acetate, 5 mg/d) is added on days 12 through 21 of the month. Undesirable effects are uncommon but may include weight gain, headache, nausea, peripheral edema, and mild hypertension (see Chapter 12).

The results of clinical trials of biosynthetic human hGH therapy in gonadal dysgenesis indicate an increase in growth rate and possibly final height[514] (also see Chapter 21).

Sexual Precocity

Sexual precocity (Table 22–22) is defined as the appearance of any sign of secondary sexual maturation at an age more than 2.0 SD below the mean. In fact, few modern data exist to establish the limits in North America, but extrapolating from studies in Switzerland, the ages of 8 in

TABLE 22–22. Classification of Sexual Precocity

True Precocious Puberty or Complete Isosexual Precocity (Premature Activation of the Hypothalamic LHRH Pulse Generator)
Idiopathic true precocious puberty
CNS tumors: hypothalamic hamartoma (ectopic LHRH pulse generator) and other tumors, especially optic glioma, hypothalamic astrocytoma
Other CNS disorders: developmental abnormalities, arachnoid cyst, hydrocephalus, infections, vascular, head trauma, cranial radiation
True precocious puberty after late treatment of congenital virilizing adrenal hyperplasia or previous chronic exposure to gonadal steroids

Incomplete Isosexual Precocity (Hypothalamic LHRH Independent)
Boys
  Gonadotropin-secreting tumors:
    hCG-secreting CNS tumors (e.g., chorioepithelioma, germinoma, teratoma)
    hCG-secreting tumors located outside the CNS (hepatoma, teratoma, choriocarcinoma)
  Increased androgen secretion by adrenal or testis
    Congenital adrenal hyperplasia (21-hydroxylase deficiency, 11β-hydroxylase deficiency)
    Virilizing adrenal neoplasm
    Leydig cell adenoma
    Familial testotoxicosis (sex-limited autosomal dominant pituitary gonadotropin–independent precocious Leydig cell and germ cell maturation)
Girls
  Estrogen-secreting ovarian or adrenal neoplasm
  Ovarian cyst
  Peutz-Jeghers syndrome
Both sexes
  McCune-Albright syndrome
  Hypothyroidism
  Iatrogenic or exogenous sexual precocity (including inadvertent exposure to estrogen in food, drugs, or cosmetics)

Variations of Pubertal Development
Premature thelarche
Premature adrenarche
Premature isolated menarche
Adolescent gynecomastia in boys

Contrasexual Precocity
Feminization in males
  Adrenal neoplasm
  Chorioepithelioma
  11α-Hydroxylase deficiency
  Late-onset adrenal hyperplasia
  Testicular neoplasm (Peutz-Jeghers syndrome)
  Increased extraglandular conversion of circulating adrenal androgens to estrogen
  Iatrogenic (exposure to estrogens)
Virilization in females
  Congenital adrenal hyperplasia
    21-Hydroxylase deficiency
    11-Hydroxylase deficiency
    3β-Hydroxydehydrogenase Δ[4,5]-isomerase deficiency
  Virilizing adrenal neoplasm
  Virilizing ovarian neoplasm (e.g., arrhenoblastoma)
  Iatrogenic (exposure to androgens)

Modified from Grumbach MM. True or central precocious puberty. In: Krieger DT, Bardin CW, eds. Current Therapy in Endocrinology and Metabolism, 1985–1986. Toronto: B. C. Decker, 1985: 5.

girls and 9 in boys can be set as the lower limits of the normal onset of puberty.[32, 33] If the sexual precocity results from premature reactivation of the hypothalamic LHRH pulse generator–pituitary gonadotropin–gonadal axis, the condition is called *complete isosexual precocity*, or *true* or *central precocious puberty*, and is LHRH dependent. Pulsatile LH release has a pubertal pattern and the rise in the concentration of LH after LHRH administration is indistinguishable from the normal pubertal pattern of serum LH. If extrapituitary secretion of gonadotropins or secretion of gonadal steroids independent of pulsatile LHRH stimulation leads to virilization in boys or feminization in girls, the condition is termed *incomplete isosexual precocity, pseudoprecocious puberty*, or *LHRH-independent sexual precocity*. The production of excessive estrogens in males leads to inappropriate feminization, and the production of increased androgen levels in females leads to inappropriate virilization; these conditions are termed *contrasexual precocity*. Hence, the disorders that cause sexual precocity can be separated into those in which the increased secretion of gonadal steroids depends on LHRH stimulation of pituitary gonadotropins and those in which it is unrelated to activation of the hypothalamic LHRH pulse generator.

In all forms of sexual precocity, the increased gonadal steroid secretion increases height velocity, somatic development, and the rate of skeletal maturation and, because of premature epiphyseal fusion, can lead to the paradox of tall stature in childhood but short adult height. Data on the final height in precocious puberty are scarce, but several studies of untreated females with idiopathic central precocious puberty demonstrated a mean final height of 151 to 155 cm.[161, 515–518, 522, 559, 560] There are few reports of final height in boys. In the four boys followed to adult stature by Thamdrup,[515] the mean height was 149.8 cm (range 145 to 155 cm), and all were well below midparent height and far below the fathers' height. Blood pressure matches that of height- and weight-related normal subjects rather than age-matched normal persons; thus elevated blood pressure for age may not indicate hypertension. Serum alkaline phosphatase and IGF I concentrations reflect the degree of sexual development rather than chronological age.[90]

True Precocious Puberty: Complete Isosexual Precocity (LHRH-Dependent Sexual Precocity)

In our series of over 200 patients with true precocious puberty,[161] girls had precocious puberty five times more commonly than boys, and the idiopathic form was eight times more common in girls than in boys (Table 22–23). Neurological abnormalities occurred at least as often as idiopathic true precocious puberty in boys, whereas in girls neurological lesions were a fifth as common as idiopathic disorders. Thus it is essential to search for a neurological etiology for true precocious puberty, especially in boys[161, 519] (Table 22–24).

LONG-TERM FOLLOW-UP OF TRUE PRECOCIOUS PUBERTY. Pregnancy has occurred in patients with true or central precocious puberty as early as 5 y of age.[521] Of course, such pregnancies are in fact the result of childhood sexual abuse. Fertility in later life is less well studied, but in our experience normal pregnancies have occurred in women who had idiopathic precocious puberty,[521, 523] a CNS abnormality triggering true precocious puberty,[522] or premature menarche. In the isosexual precocity of the McCune-Albright syndrome, there are also reports of adult fertility.[164, 524, 630]

IDIOPATHIC PRECOCIOUS PUBERTY. By definition, 2.5% of normal children develop signs of puberty before 9 y in boys and 8 y in girls. Although this definition is a useful guideline, a significant proportion of girls of age 6 to 8 with idiopathic precocious puberty represent one end of the bell-

TABLE 22–24. Etiology of True Precocious Puberty*

Etiology	Number and Sex
Idiopathic	121F, 13M
Other causes	
CNS-hypothalamic tumors	11F, 15M
Arachnoid cyst	2F, 1M
Hydrocephalus	6F, 1M
Head trauma (child abuse)	1F
Perinatal asphyxia, cerebral palsy	3F, 1M
Encephalitis or meningitis	3F, 1M
Sex chromosome abnormalities (47,XXY; 48,XXXY)	2M
Nonspecific seizure disorder or mental retardation	26F, 16M
Degenerative CNS disease	3M
Congenital virilizing adrenal hyperplasia with secondary true precocious puberty	3M

*Data from University of California, San Francisco, Pediatric Endocrine Clinic.

From Kaplan SL, Grumbach MM. Pathogenesis of sexual precocity. In: Grumbach MM, Sizonenko PC, Aubert ML, eds. Control of the Onset of Puberty. Baltimore: Williams & Wilkins, 1990: 620–660. © 1990, the Williams & Wilkins Co., Baltimore.

shaped curve for normal puberty onset and are examples of early normal puberty. Similarly, those with constitutional delay in growth and adolescence are healthy but late maturers in the older age segment of the normal distribution. There may be a history of early maturation in the family; rarely, true precocious puberty is transmitted as an autosomal recessive trait in boys and girls.[161, 525] A larger group of children, however, develop true precocious puberty with no familial tendency toward early maturation and no signs of organic disease; these children have idiopathic true precocious puberty. This condition, which may be manifest in infancy, is more common in girls than in boys and is commonly associated with electroencephalographic abnormalities.[526] The age at onset in girls in about 50% of cases is 6 to 7 y, in about 25% is 2 to 6 y, and in 18% in infancy[163] (Fig. 22–48).

In boys (Fig. 22–49) the testes usually enlarge under gonadotropin stimulation before any other signs of puberty are seen; in girls (Fig. 22–49) the appearance of breast development, enlargement of the labia minora, and maturational changes in the vaginal mucosa are the usual presenting signs, with variable manifestations of pubic hair depending on the age at onset. Progression of secondary

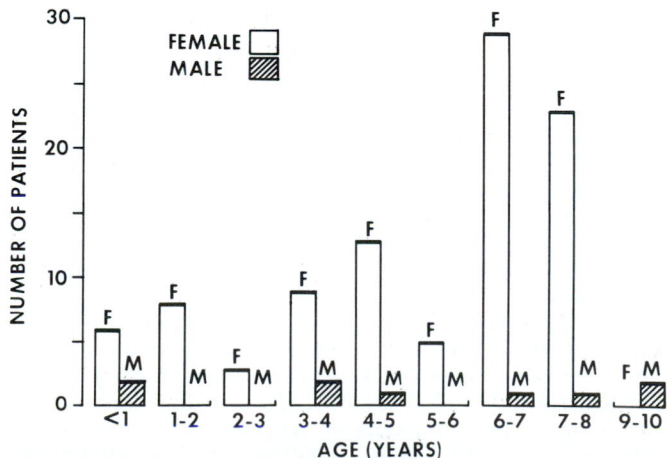

Figure 22–48. Age at onset of idiopathic true precocious puberty in 106 children. Open bars, female; hatched bars, male. At all ages, the frequency is greater in females than in males. The peak prevalence in girls is between ages 6 and 8 y. (From Kaplan SL, Grumbach MM. The neuroendocrinology of human puberty: an ontogenetic perspective. In: Grumbach MM, Sizonenko PC, Aubert ML, eds. Control of the Onset of Puberty. Baltimore: Williams & Wilkins, 1990: 1–68. © 1990, the Williams & Wilkins Co., Baltimore.)

TABLE 22–23. Distribution by Sex of Children with Idiopathic and Neurogenic Precocious Puberty

Series	Idiopathic		Neurogenic	
	Male	Female	Male	Female
Thamdrup (1961)[515]	4	34	7	11
Wilkins (1965)[164]	13	67	10	5
Sigurjonsdottir and Hayles (1968)[522]	8	54	16	16
University of California, San Francisco (1981)*	13	121	26	45

*Unpublished.

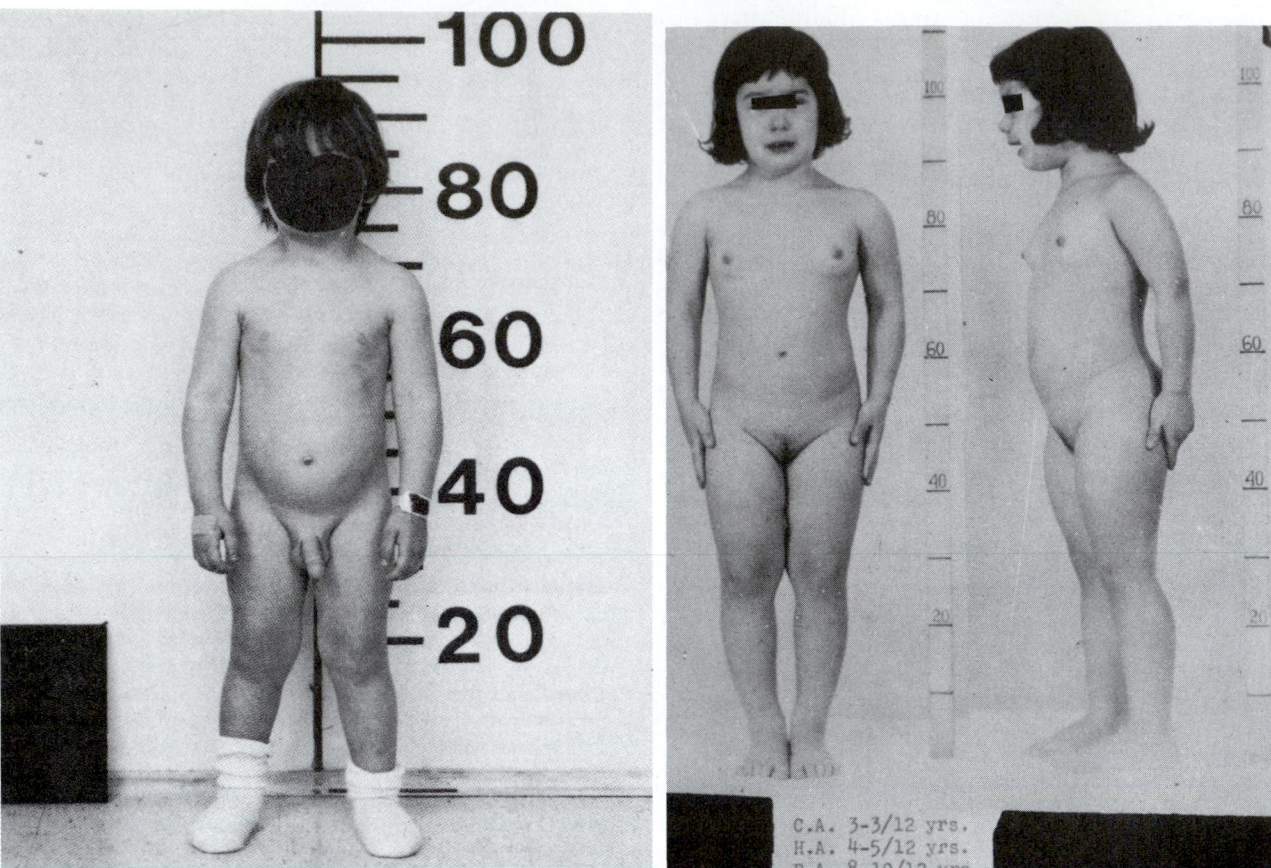

Figure 22–49. *Left*, A boy 2 y, 5 mo of age with idiopathic precocious puberty. He had pubic hair and phallic and testicular enlargement by 10 mo of age. At 1 y of age, his height was 86 cm (+4 SD); the phallus measured 10 × 3.5 cm, and the testes measured 2.5 × 1.5 cm. Plasma LH, 1.9 ng/mL; FSH, 1.2 ng/mL; and testosterone, 416 ng/dL. After 100 μg of LHRH, the plasma LH increased to 8.4 ng/mL and FSH to 1.8 ng/mL. When photographed, the patient had been treated with medroxyprogesterone acetate for 1.5 y. His height was 95.2 cm (+1 SD), the phallus was 6 × 3 cm, and the testes were 2.4 × 1.3 cm. Basal concentrations of LH (LER-960) were 0.9 ng/mL; FSH (LER-869), 0.8 ng/mL; and testosterone, 7 ng/dL. After 100 μg of LHRH, LH concentrations rose to 2.3 ng/mL, whereas FSH concentrations did not change when he was on treatment with medroxyprogesterone acetate. For conversion to SI units, see the legends of Figures 22–14 and 22–15. (Left panel from Styne DM, Grumbach MM. Puberty in the male and female: its physiology and disorders. In: Yen SCC, Jaffe RB, eds. Reproductive Endocrinology. 2nd ed. Philadelphia: W. B. Saunders, 1986: 313–384.) *Right*, A 3³/₁₂-y-old girl with idiopathic true precocious puberty who had recurrent vaginal bleeding since 9 mo of age. Height age, 4⁵/₁₂ years; bone age, 8¹⁰/₁₂ y.

sexual maturation is often more rapid than the normal pattern of pubertal maturation. A waxing and waning course of development may be encountered. The rapid growth is associated with increased GH secretion and elevation of serum IGF I levels because of stimulation by gonadal steroids.[60, 73] The ratio of bone age to chronological age and the rise of IGF I above normal values for age are predictive of outcome: more mildly affected children progress less rapidly and tend to maintain their target height.[527] However, slowly progressing cases occur, with little or no loss of predicted final height, and are characterized by the presence of normal or only slightly elevated estrogen and IGF I concentrations.[527] Spermatogenesis in males and ovulation in females often occur, and fertility is possible. True precocious puberty in females does not lead to premature menopause. However, in girls there is increased risk for the development of carcinoma of the breast in adulthood. Psychosexual development is not advanced in patients with sexual precocity.

The gonadotropin and gonadal steroid concentrations in plasma, the LH response to LHRH administration, and the amplitude and frequency of LH pulses are in the normal pubertal range[123, 274, 275] (Figs. 22–50 and 22–51). Adrenarche usually does not accompany gonadarche in girls with true precocious puberty younger than age 5 or 6: pubic hair is sparse or absent initially in girls of this age.[305] When the onset of true precocious puberty occurs after age 6, it may be associated with early adrenarche for chronological age but not for bone age.[305]

A small proportion of patients with central precocious puberty, including a pubertal response of LH to LHRH and increased pulsatile LH secretion at night, may either revert spontaneously to a more immature pubertal state, persist without further progression, or fluctuate between progression and regression.[161, 528] Thus in some patients the course need not be inexorably progressive.

CNS TUMORS CAUSING TRUE PRECOCIOUS PUBERTY. True precocious puberty resulting from CNS tumors (Tables 22–23, 22–24, and 22–25) has about the same prevalence in boys and girls; however, in boys, neurological abnormalities account for two thirds of those with true precocious puberty, and in our experience a CNS tumor was present in half of

TABLE 22–25. Classification of CNS Tumors Associated with Isosexual Sexual Precocity at University of California, San Francisco

10% of all true precocious puberty patients: CNS tumors, hypothalamic (n = 26)

Males—IPP*/organic precocious puberty = 13/15 = 0.9/1	
Females—IPP/organic precocious puberty = 121/11 = 12/1	
LHRH-dependent true precocious puberty	
Astrocytoma	3M, 5F
Hamartomas	3M, 3F
Neurofibromatosis	5M, 1F
Craniopharyngioma	2F
LHRH-independent incomplete sexual precocity	
hCG-secreting tumor†	4M

*IPP, idiopathic precocious puberty.
†CNS and extra-CNS neoplasms.

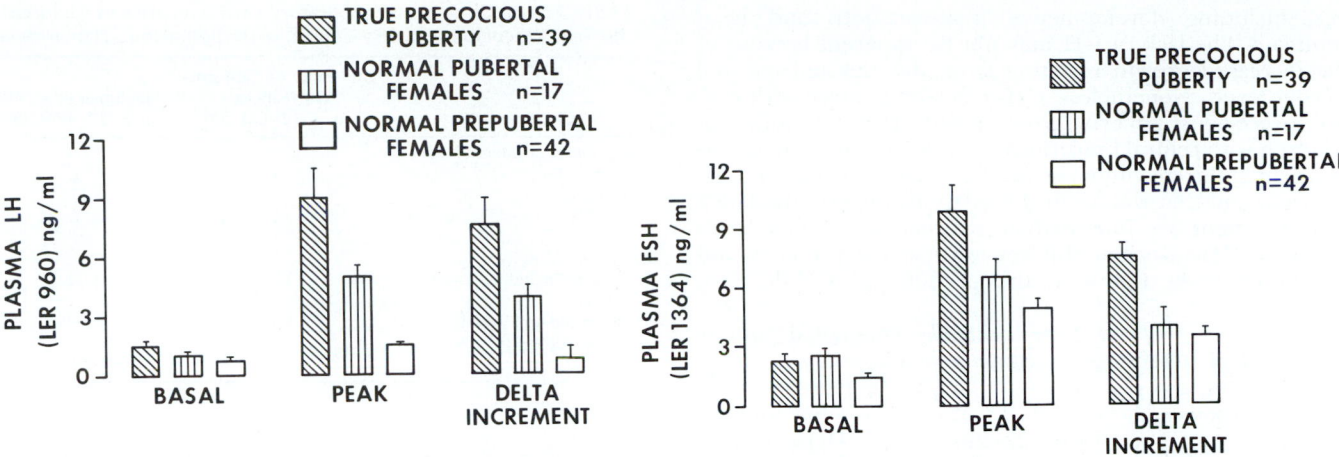

Figure 22–50. *Left,* Mean basal plasma LH level (LER-960) and mean peak and increment after intravenous LHRH (100 μg) in normal prepubertal and pubertal females and in females with idiopathic true precocious puberty. The mean peak and increments of plasma LH are higher in true precocious puberty than in normal puberty. *Right,* Basal FSH level (LER-1364) and mean peak and increment after intravenous LHRH (100 μg) in normal prepubertal and pubertal females with true precocious puberty. The concentration of FSH and the response to LHRH were greater in females with true precocious puberty and normal puberty than in prepubertal females. (From Kaplan SL, Grumbach MM. Pathogenesis of sexual precocity. In: Grumbach MM, Sizonenko PC, Aubert ML, eds. Control of the Onset of Puberty. Baltimore: Williams & Wilkins, 1990: 620–660. © 1990, the Williams & Wilkins Co., Baltimore.)

this group.[161] A CNS neoplasm must be considered in the differential diagnosis of any patient with true precocious puberty.[161, 164, 519, 522] Optic and hypothalamic gliomas (often associated with neurofibromatosis),[330, 331] astrocytomas, ependymomas, and, rarely, craniopharyngiomas may cause true precocious puberty, either by impinging on the neural pathways that inhibit the LHRH pulse generator in childhood

or as a consequence of cranial radiation for therapy. The prevalence of true precocious puberty is increased after cranial radiation for local tumors or leukemia.[58, 529, 530]

The unusual combination of GH deficiency and central precocious puberty can occur in children previously subjected to therapeutic radiation of the CNS in association with a CNS neoplasm or because of a variety of CNS abnormali-

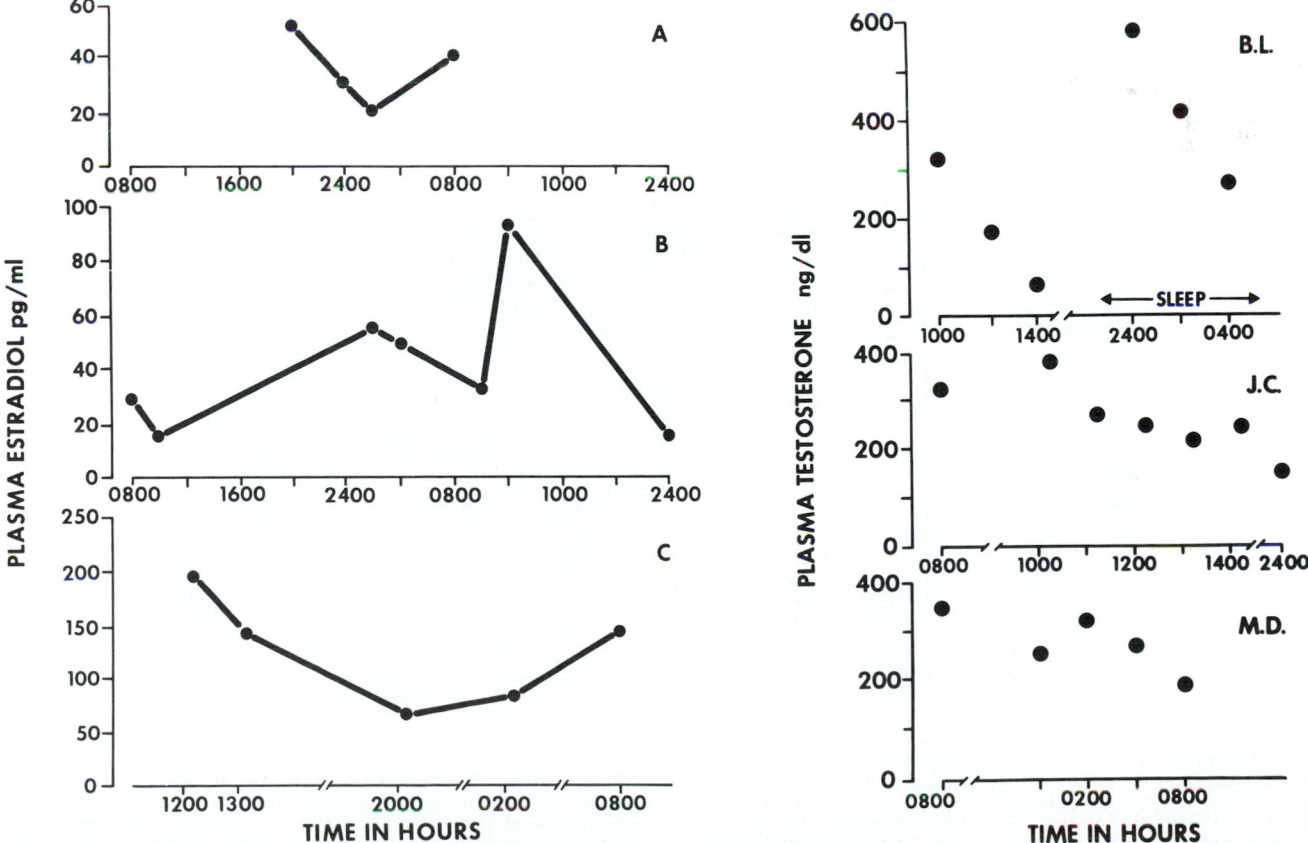

Figure 22–51. *Left,* Serial determinations of plasma estradiol in three girls with idiopathic true precocious puberty. Note the striking fluctuations in values. *Right,* Serial determinations of plasma testosterone in three boys with true precocious puberty (B.L. and J.C. have a hypothalamic hamartoma; M.D. has the idiopathic form). For conversion to SI units, see the legends of Figures 22–14 and 22–15. (From Kaplan SL, Grumbach MM. Pathogenesis of sexual precocity. In: Grumbach MM, Sizonenko PC, Aubert ML, eds. Control of the Onset of Puberty. Baltimore: Williams & Wilkins, 1990: 620–660. © 1990, the Williams & Wilkins Co., Baltimore.)

ties, including developmental malformations and head trauma.[58] The lack of GH may not be apparent because of the increased growth resulting from the elevated gonadal steroid levels. Nonetheless, GH-deficient children with central precocious puberty grow slower than GH-sufficient children with central precocious puberty but faster than GH-deficient children without sexual precocity. Further, in GH-deficient children with central precocious puberty the IGF I concentrations are intermediate between the higher levels found in GH-sufficient children with sexual precocity and the lower levels found in the prepubertal GH-deficient children.[58]

Hamartomas of the tuber cinereum—congenital tumors composed of heterotopic mass of neurosecretory neurons, fiber bundles, and glial cells—are frequently associated with true precocious puberty (Fig. 22–52), often before the patient is 3 y of age (Table 22–26).[161, 243, 532] Hypothalamic hamartomas that cause true precocious puberty can be associated with laughing (gelastic), petit mal, or generalized seizures; mental retardation; behavioral disturbances; and dysmorphic syndromes.[531, 532] With CT and MRI brain scans, hamartomas of the tuber cinereum are now being detected in young boys and girls previously thought to have idiopathic central precocious puberty (Fig. 22–53); before 1980 there were 37 patients in the literature with hamartomas of the tuber cinereum and since 1980 another 60 have been reported[532, 534, 536] (see Table 22–26). This increase is attributable to use of CT and MRI brain scans.[533] For example, Pescovitz and colleagues,[535] in reviewing the experience at the National Institutes of Health, reported that of 87 girls with true precocious puberty, 16% had a hypothalamic hamartoma, 40% had other CNS abnormalities, and 60% had idiopathic true precocious puberty. Among 20 boys with true precocious puberty, 2 had idiopathic true precocious puberty, 10 had a hypothalamic hamartoma, and 8 had other CNS abnormalities including hypothalamic neoplasms.

Hamartomas of the tuber cinereum are not true neoplasms but are midline spherical masses arising from the

TABLE 22–26. Clinical and Laboratory Characteristics of Children with True Precocious Puberty Caused by Hypothalamic Hamartoma

Characteristic	University of California, San Francisco (n = 12: 6M, 6F)	Hochman et al.,[243]* (n = 27: 18M, 9F)
Age at onset of pubertal signs		
Birth to 1 y	4	6
1 to 2 y	4	17
2 to 4 y	3	6
7 y	1	1
Neurological signs		
Seizures including gelastic type	3/12	11/24
Headache and visual symptoms	1/12	5/24
None	7/12	7/24

*Literature review.

third ventricle and composed of disordered but mature and differentiated neural elements.[243, 244, 534a, 536, 542] Usually the hamartomas are connected with the posterior portion of the tuber cinereum or mamillary body or the floor of the third ventricle by a distinct stalk. They appear on a CT scan as an isodense, abnormal fullness of the interpeduncular, prepontine, and posterior suprasellar cisterns, occasionally with distortion of the anterior third ventricle; they characteristically have a collar-button appearance.[537, 538] There is no enhancement with contrast material.[539] MRI gives the best visualization of the lesion[540, 541] (see Fig. 22–53). Analysis of hamartomas associated with true precocious puberty has revealed the presence of ectopic LHRH neurosecretory cells similar to the LHRH-containing neurons in the medial basal hypothalamus. This congenital tumor exerts its endocrine effects by the elaboration and pulsatile release of LHRH.[161, 519] Indeed, LHRH-containing fibers have been identified passing from the hamartoma toward the median eminence.[161, 534a] We have suggested that the LHRH-containing neurosecretory neurons in the tumor are unrestrained by the intrinsic

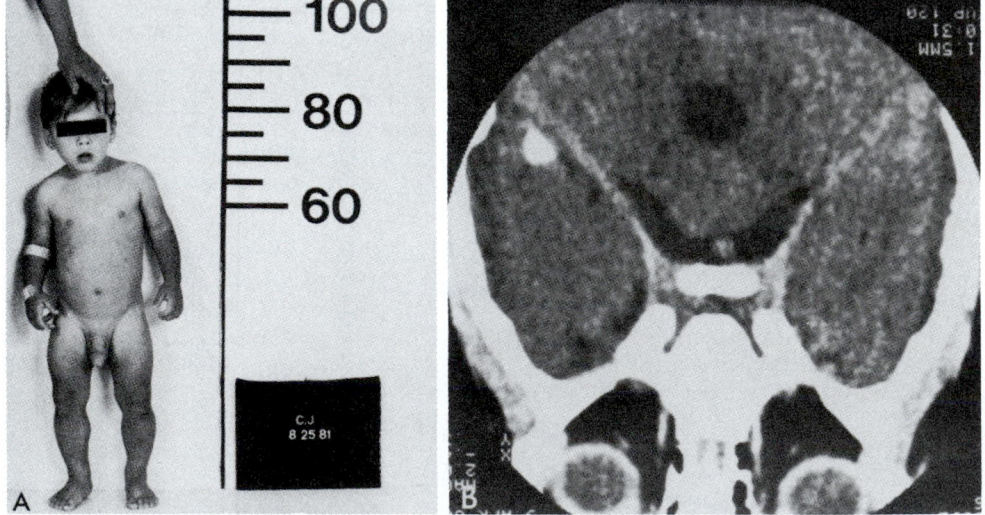

Figure 22–52. *A*, A 17-mo-old male infant with hamartoma of the tuber cinereum and true precocious puberty. At 8 mo of age, secondary sexual development was noted, and the patient was misdiagnosed as having congenital virilizing adrenal hyperplasia. He was treated with glucocorticoids, which slowed his growth but did not affect his sexual development and bone age advancement. When he was first seen at 17 mo, height was 84.2 cm; weight was 14.8 kg; the pubic hair stage was stage II; the penis was 10.4 × 2.2 cm; the testes were 1.5 × 2.8 cm; and the scrotum was thinned and rugated. The bone age was 4 9/12 y. After LHRH administration, the LH level rose from 0.5 to 3.1 ng/dL, the FSH level from 0.5 to 1.2 ng/mL, and the testosterone level from 409 to 450 ng/dL. DHEAS was 17 μg/dL (preadrenarchal value). The patient was treated with a potent long-acting LHRH-agonist deslorelin (D-Trp6Pro9NEt-LHRH), which resulted in arrest of his pubertal advancement and a striking decrease in the plasma concentration of testosterone, LH pulses, and the response to exogenous LHRH. *B*, CT scan of the patient, demonstrating a 1.5-cm mass posterior and rostral to the dorsum sella, which depresses the flow of the third ventricle. For conversion to SI units, see the legends of Figures 22–14, 22–15, and 22–32. (From Styne DM, Grumbach MM. Puberty in the male and female: its physiology and disorders. In: Yen SCC, Jaffe RB, eds. Reproductive Endocrinology. 2nd ed. Philadelphia: W. B. Saunders, 1986: 313–384.)

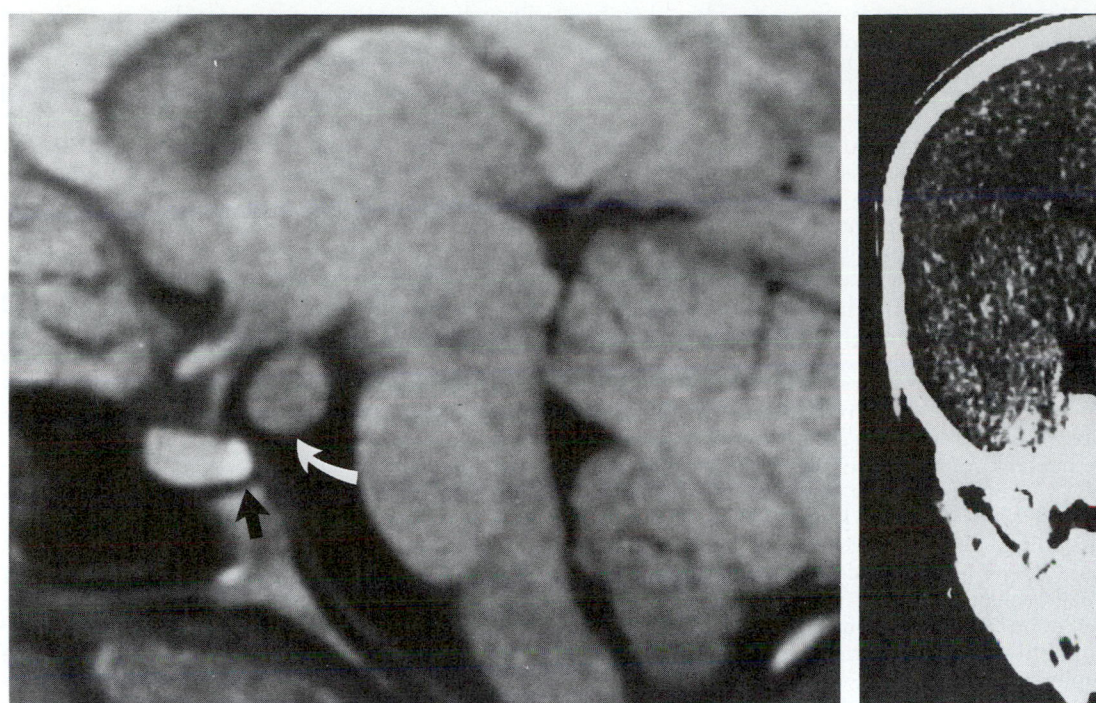
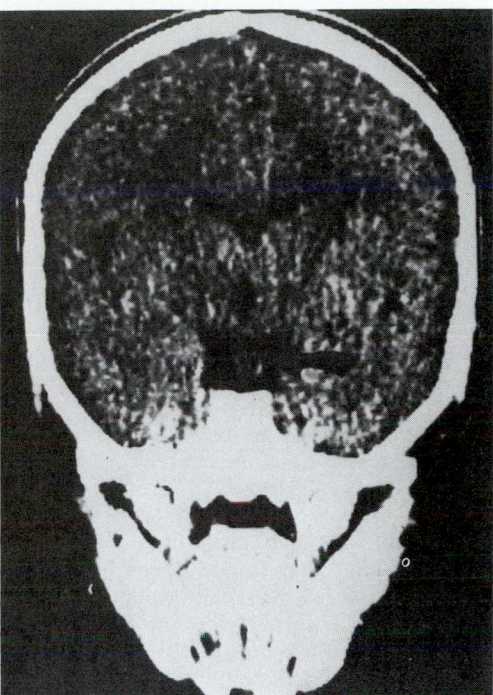

Figure 22–53. *Left,* MRI scan demonstrating a hypothalamic hamartoma *(solid white arrow)* in a 4-y-old boy with true precocious puberty; sagittal T1-weighted image. The posterior pituitary hot spot is designated by the solid black arrow. *Right,* CT brain scan (coronal section) showing an isodense, pedunculated, collar button–shaped hypothalamic hamartoma *(arrow)* in a 2-y-old girl with true precocious puberty.

CNS mechanism that inhibits the normal LHRH pulse generator and act as an ectopic LHRH pulse generator[100, 519] either independently or in synchrony with the LHRH neurosecretory neurons in the medial basal hypothalamus to produce intermittent secretory bursts of LHRH[100] (see Fig. 22–33); the LHRH is transported to the pituitary by way of the portal circulation and elicits pulsatile release of LH (Fig. 22–54). If the hamartoma were to secrete LHRH in a continuous fashion, true precocious puberty should not occur. (About 10% of hypothalamic hamartomas are not associated with true precocious puberty.)

Sexual precocity may be the first manifestation of a *hypothalamic tumor* of any cell type when it arises in or impinges on the posterior hypothalamus. However, neurological symptoms such as headaches and visual disturbances may develop, and children may have hydrocephalus or optic atrophy caused by an enlarging tumor.[161, 522]

The location of CNS tumors causing true precocious puberty makes surgical removal difficult. A conservative approach calls for biopsy of the neoplasm and radiation or chemotherapy or both depending on the pathological findings. An exception is the hypothalamic hamartoma. Although there are cases in which removal of a hypothalamic hamartoma has led to reversal of the pubertal process,[244, 534, 542] deaths have been reported after attempted operative removal.[243] Hamartomas grow slowly, if in fact they do enlarge, and any change in size can be detected readily on periodic CT or MRI scans. The precocious sexual development can be controlled by treatment with LHRH agonists.[543] Accordingly, we do not recommend neurosurgical extirpation in the absence of evidence of rapid growth of the tumor.[161, 519, 562]

OTHER CNS CONDITIONS. True precocious puberty may occur secondary to *hydrocephalus,*[544] *encephalitis, static cerebral encephalopathy, brain abscess,* or sarcoid *granulomas* or tuberculous granulomas of the hypothalamus, with or without tuberculous meningitis.[338] Central precocious puberty occurs after *head trauma*[58, 544] (usually in girls) and is associated with cerebral atrophy or focal encephalomalacia.[544]

Arachnoid cysts arising de novo, after infection, or after surgery can cause premature sexual development, possibly with associated GH deficiency.[100, 161, 546] Head nodding, ab-

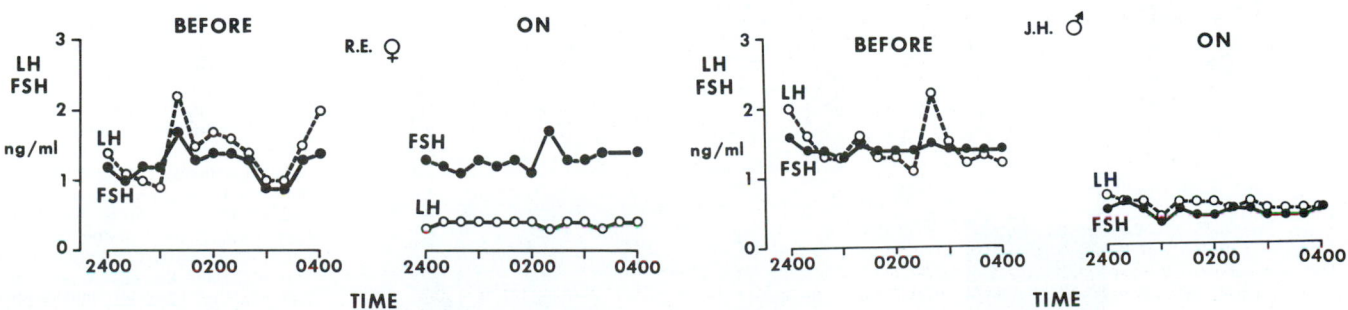

Figure 22–54. Pulsatile LH secretion before and during LHRH agonist therapy in a boy *(right)* and a girl *(left)* with true precocious puberty secondary to a hypothalamic hamartoma before. For conversion to SI units, see the legend of Figure 22–14.

normal gait, and abnormalities of visual fields are reported in 30 to 40% of cases. Erosion or enlargement of the sella turcica into a J shape may occur. Decompression and extirpation of suprasellar arachnoid cysts can reverse the sexual precocity[100, 547, 548] (see Fig. 22–32).

Neurofibromatosis type 1 (von Recklinghausen disease) may be associated with precocious puberty because of the propensity to develop CNS tumors. It is an autosomal disorder with dominant inheritance that has a prevalence of 1 in 3000 to 4000. It is characterized by multiple pigmented areas and overgrowth of nerve sheaths and fibrous tissue elements (Fig. 22–55).[330, 331, 549] Multiple café au lait spots are frequent and are smoother in outline than those of the McCune-Albright syndrome. The diagnosis is made if two or more of the following are observed: (1) six or more café au lait macules, the greatest diameter of which is more than 5 mm in prepubertal and more than 12.5 mm in postpubertal subjects; (2) two or more neurofibromas of any type or one plexiform neurofibroma; (3) freckling in the axilla or inguinal region; (4) optic glioma; (5) two or more Lisch nodules (ophthalmic hamartomas); (6) a distinctive osseous lesion such as sphenoid dysplasia or pseudoarthrosis; (7) a first-degree relative with neurofibromatosis type 1 according to the preceding criteria (reviewed in refs. 549 and 550).

Lesions of the skin in neurofibromatosis may be subcutaneous sessile or deep plexiform masses in children; pedunculated lesions develop in later childhood. Internal neurofibromas cause most of the complications. Bone abnormalities such as cysts and pseudoarthrosis, hemihypertrophy, bowing, scoliosis, and skull and facial defects are common (20%); dumbbell-shaped tumors of spinal nerve roots may cause pain, sensory and motor dysfunction, and bone erosions; gliomas or neurofibromas of any part of the CNS, including the optic nerves and hypothalamus, may calcify. Lisch nodules are frequent, particularly in adults.[550] Sarcomatous degeneration occurs in 5 to 15% of patients. Other neoplasms include CNS astrocytomas often involving the visual pathways, ependymomas, meningiomas, neurofibrosarcomas, rhabdomyosarcomas, and nonlymphocytic leukemias.[551] Pheochromocytoma may develop in affected adults.

The clinical manifestations include seizures, visual defects, and either delayed or true precocious puberty. Mental retardation occurs more often in this population but usually is not severe;[552] there is also an increased incidence of psychiatric disease.[553] Most affected children have some manifestations of the disease by 1 y of age.[330, 331, 549] The mutant gene is on the long arm of chromosome 17 (q11.2).[554–556]

Other CNS abnormalities associated with true precocious puberty but without demonstrable lesions on radiographic study include epilepsy,[526] laughing seizures,[557] mental retardation, and the post-traumatic state.[545] Septo-optic dysplasia (described earlier) may be associated not only with multiple pituitary hormone deficiencies and delayed puberty but also rarely with central precocious puberty.[58, 339, 530] Thus there may be coexisting deficiencies of some pituitary hormones and excessive secretion of others, including prolactin.[558]

TRUE PRECOCIOUS PUBERTY AFTER VIRILIZING DISORDERS. If a virilizing condition has been long-standing, correction of the virilization may be followed by development of true precocious puberty with activation of the hypothalamic–pituitary gonadotropin–gonadal system. This phenomenon occurs in boys and girls with congenital virilizing adrenal hyperplasia who were begun on glucocorticoid replacement therapy after age 4 to 8.[71, 164, 275] True precocious puberty has also been documented in children who received androgens for long periods during early childhood.

MANAGEMENT OF TRUE PRECOCIOUS PUBERTY. The objectives in the management and therapy of true precocious puberty are summarized in Table 22–27, which addresses the major psychosocial and clinical goals.[562] Psychosocial issues must be dealt with to provide optimal management of affected children.

Three principal agents have been used in the treatment of true precocious puberty whether idiopathic or neurological: medroxyprogesterone acetate, cyproterone acetate, and superactive LHRH agonists. Medroxyprogesterone and cy-

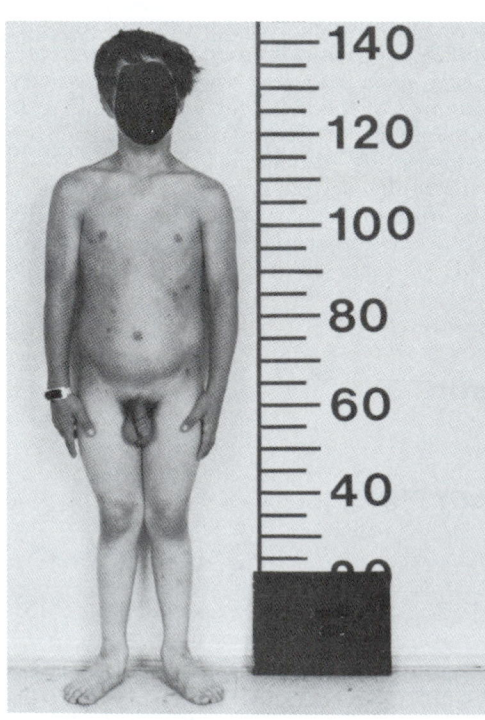
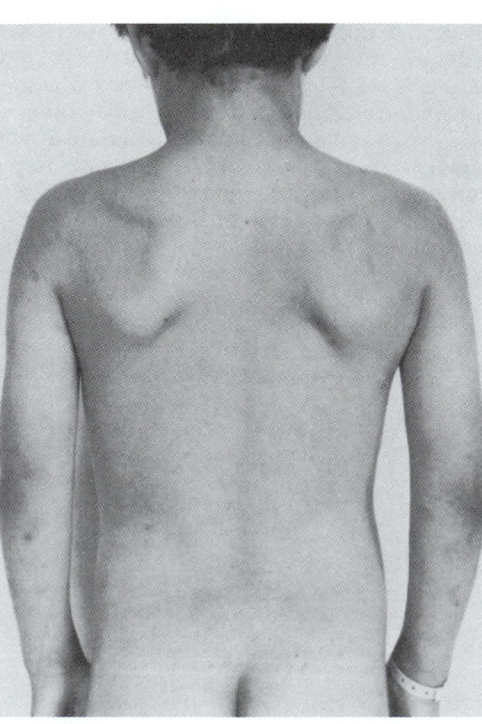

Figure 22–55. A boy of 8 y, 8 mo with neurofibromatosis and precocious puberty, secondary to a hypothalamic glioma. He had tonic-clonic seizures at 2½ y and rapid growth starting at 4 y; an enlarged penis and testes and the presence of pubic hair were first noted at 7½ y. At this time, his height was 139.9 cm (+1.4 SD); the phallus was 9 × 3 cm; the right testis measured 5.5 × 3.2 cm and the left measured 5.4 × 2.9 cm. He had stage 3 pubic hair and 24 large café au lait spots. CT scans and pneumoencephalography revealed a 1.5 × 2.5 cm hypothalamic mass, which was treated with radiation. The plasma concentration of LH was 0.5 ng/mL; FSH, 0.4 ng/mL; testosterone, 221 ng/dL. After 100 μg of intravenous LHRH the peak concentration of LH was 4.9 ng/mL and of FSH 1.4 ng/mL, a pubertal response. For conversion to SI units, see the legends of Figures 22–14 and 22–15. (From Styne DM, Grumbach MM. Puberty in the male and female: its physiology and disorders. In: Yen SCC, Jaffe RB, eds. Reproductive Endocrinology. 2nd ed. Philadelphia: W. B. Saunders, 1986: 313–384.)

TABLE 22–27. Objectives of the Management and Treatment of True Precocious Puberty

Detection and treatment of an expanding intracranial lesion
Arrest of premature sexual maturation until the normal age of onset of puberty
Regression of secondary sexual characteristics already present
Attainment of normal mature height; suppression of the rapid rate of skeletal maturation
Prevention of emotional disorders and handicaps and alleviation of parental anxiety; promotion of understanding by counseling, early sex education, and acceleration of social age
Reduction of risk of sexual abuse and of early sexual debut
Prevention of pregnancy in girls
Preservation of future fertility
Diminish the increased risk of breast cancer associated with early menarche

From Grumbach MM. True or central precocious puberty. In: Krieger DT, Bardin CW, eds. Current Therapy in Endocrinology and Metabolism, 1985–1986. Toronto: B. C. Decker, 1985: 5.

proterone reversed or arrested the progression of secondary sexual characteristics but had no apparent effect on final height, especially in affected girls.[161, 518, 559, 560] This failure may be due in part to the disproportionate action of the small amount of circulating estradiol on skeletal growth relative to its effect on secondary sexual characteristics. In any event, in none of the early studies with medroxyprogesterone or cyproterone was the concentration of plasma estradiol in girls and of testosterone in boys systematically monitored and the dosage of these agents adjusted accordingly. In addition, both medroxyprogesterone acetate and cyproterone acetate have undesirable effects in high doses.[561, 562]

Medroxyprogesterone Acetate and Cyproterone Acetate. The dosage of medroxyprogesterone acetate is 5 to 10 mg twice a day orally or 100 to 200 mg/m² surface area intramuscularly every 1 or 2 wk. We prefer the oral route.[163, 519] This agent inhibits gonadotropin secretion by its action on the hypothalamic LHRH pulse generator–pituitary gonadotropin unit and has a direct suppressive effect on gonadal steroidogenesis. Medroxyprogesterone acetate has glucocorticoid action and can suppress ACTH and cortisol secretion, increase appetite and lead to excessive weight gain, and induce hypertension and a cushingoid facies and appearance.[161, 519, 561]

Cyproterone acetate has antiandrogenic, antigonadotropic, and progestational properties. It has been used outside the United States for the treatment of true precocious puberty.[559, 560, 563] Its advantages and disadvantages are similar to those of medroxyprogesterone acetate.[519] The usual oral dose is 70 to 100 mg/m² surface area daily, given in two divided doses; the intramuscular dose is 100 to 200 mg/m² every 14 to 28 d. Cyproterone acetate suppresses the secretion of ACTH and the plasma concentration of cortisol. Fatigue and weakness are common side effects, probably as a consequence of secondary adrenal insufficiency. This agent lacks gluconeogenic activity and does not appear to produce cushingoid features. The long-term effects of either of these agents on fertility is not known.

For the treatment of true precocious puberty, medroxyprogesterone acetate has been replaced by the much more effective LHRH agonists; however, it is a back-up agent for the occasional patients who develop untoward effects from LHRH agonist therapy.

Superactive LHRH Agonists. The LHRH agonists, synthetic analogues of the amino acid sequence of the natural LHRH decapeptide, are the treatment of choice for true precocious puberty, whether idiopathic or organic (Table 22–28). Paradoxically, these pharmacological agents, when administered chronically, suppress pulsatile LH and FSH release, gonadal steroid output, and gametogenesis. In contrast to the effects of pulsatile administration at physiological doses and frequency,[564] continuous administration of natural LHRH also suppresses gonadotropin secretion[187, 279, 281] after an initial stimulation of gonadotropin release. Suppression results from binding of the agonist to the LHRH receptor on gonadotropes and subsequent desensitization of the gonadotrope to LHRH. Initially, down-regulation and loss of receptors occur. When receptor levels return to normal, desensitization persists as a result of uncoupling of the receptors from the intracellular signaling effector pathway.[565, 566] Administration of a potent LHRH agonist subcutaneously once a day, although initially stimulating gonadotropin release, induces desensitization of the gonadotropes to LHRH within a few days. In children with true precocious puberty this regimen blocks the effect of endogenous LHRH and functions as a selective, highly specific pharmacological clamp on the secretion of gonadotropins without interfering directly with release of the other pituitary hormones. In essence, the regimen produces a reversible medical gonadectomy (Table 22–29). The superactive agonist analogues of LHRH have about 15 to 200 times the potency of natural LHRH decapeptide, prolonged action, and low toxicity (see Table 22–28).

Replacing the glycine-amide terminus of LHRH with alkyl amines, as in [Pro⁹-ethylamide(NEt)]LHRH, substituting certain D-amino acids at position 6, as in [D-Trp⁶]LHRH, and making bulky hydrophobic alterations at position 6, as in [D-Nal(2)⁶]LHRH, increase the potency and duration of

TABLE 22–28. LHRH Agonists: Pharmacological Treatment of True Precocious Puberty

Structure of Natural LHRH and Substitutions in LHRH Agonist Analogues	Relative Potency	Formula	Dosage Form	Dose	References
<Glu-His-Pro-Ser-Trp-Gly-Leu-Arg-Pro-Gly-NH₂	1	LHRH			
1 2 3 4 5 6 7 8 9 10					
Deslorelin D-Trp⁶ -NEt	150	[D-Trp⁶Pro⁹NEt]LHRH	Subcutaneous Depot-intramuscular	4–8 µg/kg/d	519, 535, 543, 571–574, 577, 706
Nafarelin D-Nal(2)⁶	150	[D-Nal(2)⁶Pro⁹NEt]LHRH	Subcutaneous Intranasal	4 µg/kg/d 800–1600 µg/d	519, 577 519, 577, 707
Leuprolide D-Leu⁶ -NEt	20	[D-Leu⁶-Pro⁹NEt]LHRH	Subcutaneous Depot-intramuscular	20–50 µg/kg/d 140–300 µg/kg/mo	579, 708 580, Kaplan and Grumbach 1991*
Buserelin D-Ser(tBu)⁶ -NEt	20	[D-Ser(tBu)⁶Pro⁹NEt]LHRH	Subcutaneous Intranasal	20–40 µg/kg/d 1200–1800 µg/d	575, 581, 709, 710 575, 576, 581, 710–713
Tryptorelin D-Trp⁶	35	[D-Trp⁶]LHRH	Subcutaneous Depot-intramuscular	20–40 µg/kg/d 60 µg/kg/mo	714 582, 715
Histerelin D-His(Bzt)⁶ -NEt	150	[D-His(Bzt)⁶NEt]LHRH	Subcutaneous	8–10 µg/kg/d	Boepple and Crowley 1991*

*Not published.
Modified from Grumbach MM, Kaplan SL. Recent advances in the diagnosis and management of sexual precocity. Acta Paediatr Jpn 1988; 30(Suppl):155–175.

TABLE 22–29. Action of LHRH Agonists in True Precocious Puberty

A selective, highly specific pharmacological clamp on the secretion of
   gonadotropin that produces a "medical gonadectomy"
Chronic administration induces desensitization of the pituitary gonadotrope
   to the action of endogenous LHRH
As a consequence:
   Inhibition of pulsatile secretion of LH and FSH
   Inhibition of gonadotropin secretion results in a striking decrease in gonadal
      steroid output by testes or ovaries and reduction in gonadal size

action.[567] These changes make the molecule more resistant to enzymatic degradation, increase the binding affinity of the analogue for the receptor on the pituitary gonadotrope, increase hydrophobicity, and, with some analogues, increase binding to plasma proteins.[519, 565–567, 569, 570]

The suppressive effects of the agonists on gonadotropin secretion make them useful in the treatment of true precocious puberty.[519, 545, 571–577] Various agonists are available, some for subcutaneous administration, some for intranasal treatment, and some for injection intramuscularly in depot formulations (see Table 22–28). The bioavailability of agonists given intranasally is much reduced,[519, 568] as reflected in

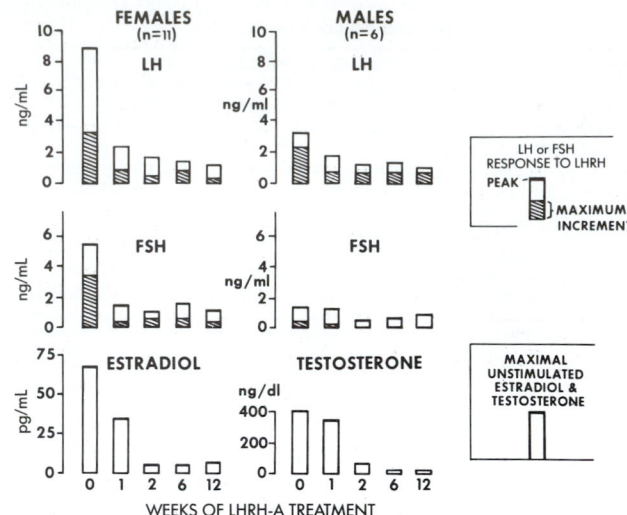

Figure 22–57. Deslorelin treatment (4 μg/kg/d subcutaneously) of girls and boys with true precocious puberty: effect during the first 12 wk of treatment on the LH and FSH response to a challenge with LHRH (mean peak response and maximum increment) and on the maximal unstimulated concentration of plasma estradiol in the girls and of plasma testosterone in the boys. Note the relatively rapid change from pubertal values to prepubertal values. For conversion to SI units, see the legends of Figures 22–14 and 22–15. (From DM Styne, DA Harris, CA Egli, et al., Treatment of true precocious puberty with a potent luteinizing-hormone releasing factor agonist: effect on growth, sexual maturation, pelvic sonography, and the hypothalamic-pituitary gonadal axis, J Clin Endocrinol Metab, 61, 142–151, 1985, © by The Endocrine Society.)

the need to use a high dose at more frequent intervals. The effectiveness of LHRH agonists in the treatment of true precocious puberty varies with the potency of the analogue, dose, route of administration, and compliance.[519, 577]

In both the idiopathic and organic forms of true precocious puberty, treatment with a potent LHRH agonist initially results in 1 to 3 d of increased FSH and LH release and a rise in circulating gonadal steroid levels; chronic therapy suppresses the pulsatile secretion of LH and FSH and blocks the pubertal LH response to the administration of native LHRH after 7 to 14 d of treatment (Figs. 22–56 and 22–57). Within 2 to 4 wk in girls and 6 wk in boys, gonadal steroid secretion is reduced to prepubertal levels and maintained in the prepubertal state by chronic treatment (Figs. 22–56 to 22–58). A plasma estradiol concentration of less than 36 pmol/L (10 pg/mL) in girls and a plasma testosterone level of less than 0.7 nmol/L (0.2 ng/mL) in boys indicate adequate gonadal suppression. LHRH agonist therapy does not affect the secretion of adrenal androgens.[519, 543, 573]

Changes in secondary sexual characteristics occur within the first 6 mo of therapy (see Fig. 22–58). In girls, these effects include reduction in breast size and pubic hair, cessation of menses if present before treatment, and decreased size of the uterus and ovaries as assessed by pelvic sonography. A small proportion of girls have recurrent episodes of hot flushes and moodiness. In boys, pubic hair thins, the testes decrease in size, acne and seborrhea regress, penile erections and masturbation become much less frequent, the high energy level and aggressive behavior diminish, and self-esteem improves.

Height velocity, expressed in centimeters per year or as standard deviations above the mean height velocity for chronological and bone age, decreases about 60% during the first year of therapy. Skeletal maturation slows dramatically during the first 3 y, to a rate often less than the progression in chronological age. From the second year on, height velocity for bone age is usually appropriate (Fig.

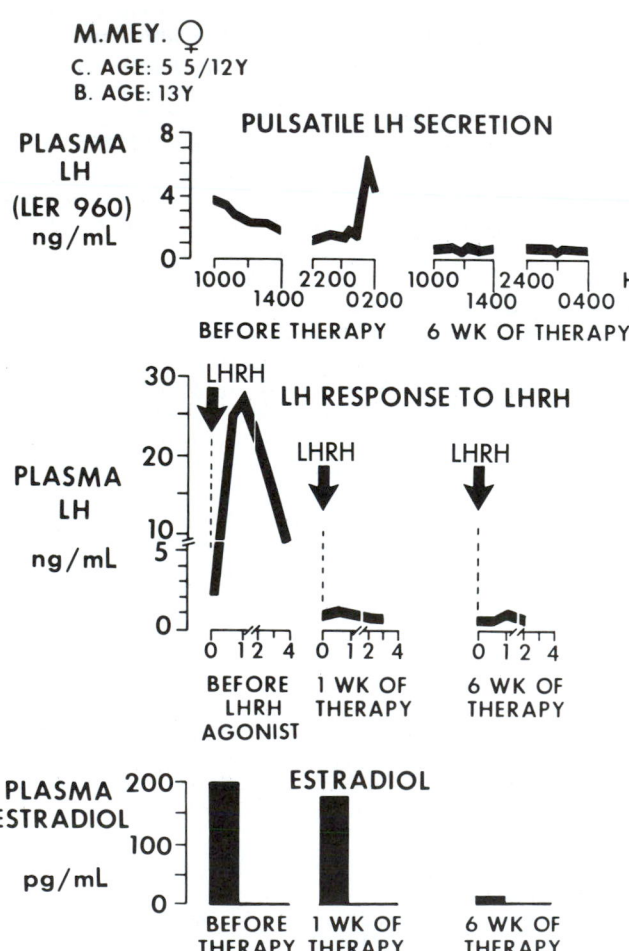

Figure 22–56. Effect of administration of the LHRH agonist deslorelin (4 μg/kg/d subcutaneously) on pulsatile secretion of LH (top), LH response to LHRH (middle), and plasma concentration of estradiol (bottom) in a 5½-y-old girl with idiopathic true precocious puberty. This patient, who had a bone age of 13 y when treatment was begun, has been administered deslorelin for 7 y. During this period, the estimated predicted final height increased by 15 cm. Surprisingly, the bone age advanced by only about 6 mo on serial examinations for several years. For conversion to SI units, see the legend of Figure 22–14. (Modified from Grumbach MM, Kaplan SL. Recent advances in the diagnosis and management of sexual precocity. Acta Paediatr Jpn 1988; 30[Suppl]:155–175.)

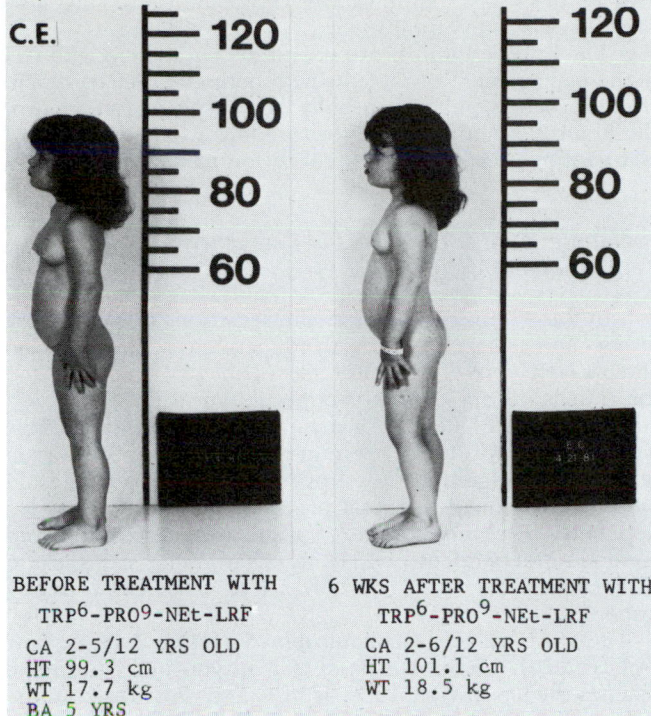

C.E.

BEFORE TREATMENT WITH
TRP^6-PRO^9-NEt-LRF

CA 2-5/12 YRS OLD
HT 99.3 cm
WT 17.7 kg
BA 5 YRS

6 WKS AFTER TREATMENT WITH
TRP^6-PRO^9-NEt-LRF

CA 2-6/12 YRS OLD
HT 101.1 cm
WT 18.5 kg

Figure 22–58. A 2$^{5/12}$-y-old girl with true precocious puberty after 6 wk of deslorelin therapy (4 µg/d subcutaneously). Note the regression in the size of the breasts; however, the rapid rate of growth had not decreased. At the end of 1 y of therapy, growth rate was suppressed to 4 cm/y, and bone age advanced only 1 y. CA, chronological age; HT, height; WT, weight; BA, bone age. (From Styne DM, Grumbach MM. Puberty in the male and female: its physiology and disorders. In: Yen SCC, Jaffe RB. Reproductive Endocrinology. 2nd ed. Philadelphia: W. B. Saunders, 1986: 313–384.)

final height in children treated with LHRH agonists support this contention.

Children with true precocious puberty have higher mean concentrations of circulating IGF I for chronological age, consistent with the increased secretion of gonadal steroids and comparable to the typical elevated IGF I levels of normal puberty. The IGF I concentration correlates best with the stage of puberty and the plasma concentration of testosterone or estradiol.[73] Treatment with LHRH agonists reduces the level of IGF I to the normal range for bone age but not for chronological age.[73] This indicates that gonadal steroids increase plasma IGF I concentrations in true precocious puberty as well as in normal puberty. Secretion of GH is increased in true precocious puberty to a level comparable to that in normal puberty.[60, 67] Treatment with LHRH agonists usually results in a decrease in GH secretion, most strikingly during sleep, and in a decrease in GH response to provocative stimuli. The reason for the fall in GH secretion is unclear, but it may involve both a decrease in plasma gonadal steroid levels and an increase in body mass index.[578]

When used chronically, LHRH agonists induce a pharmacological gonadectomy with reversion to a prepubertal level of gonadal steroid output. The use of depot formulations of LHRH agonists provides continuous exposure to the agonist with a single intramuscular injection every 4 wk and minimizes the problem of compliance.[378, 580, 582] However, irregular or inadequate treatment or poor compliance results in persistent or intermittent increase in the concentration of plasma gonadal steroids. Regular assessment is essential, initially at intervals of 1 to 3 mo. Such assessment involves periodic determinations of plasma testosterone levels in boys and estradiol levels in girls; the LH response to exogenous LHRH; measurement of growth, bone age, and secondary sexual characteristics; and in girls serial evaluations of ovarian morphology and uterine size by pelvic sonography. Regularly scheduled visits also provide the opportunity for continued counseling.

The criteria for treatment of patients with true precocious puberty are listed in Table 22–30. Therapy is not indicated if a pubertal pattern of pulsatile LH secretion is not present or if the LH response to exogenous LHRH is prepubertal. Before beginning treatment it is essential to establish the progressive nature of the sexual precocity. In a subset of girls, the tempo is relatively slow and the sexual precocity may not be sustained.[161, 577] The growth rate slows to normal for age, and skeletal maturation progresses in

22–59). At present, the growth data for compliant patients strongly suggest improved height potential as a result of therapy in young children with true precocious puberty, especially when treatment is begun soon after the onset of precocity and when the bone age is advanced only a few years. Even with the limitations of estimates of predicted height taken into account, effective therapy improves final height predictions or in young children maintains the normal target height for the individual. The accumulating data on

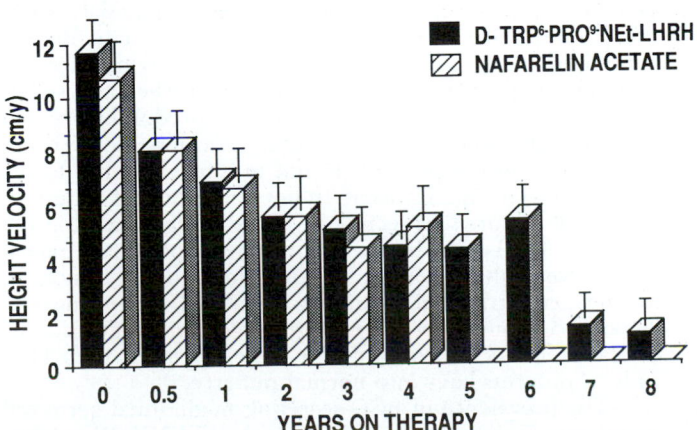

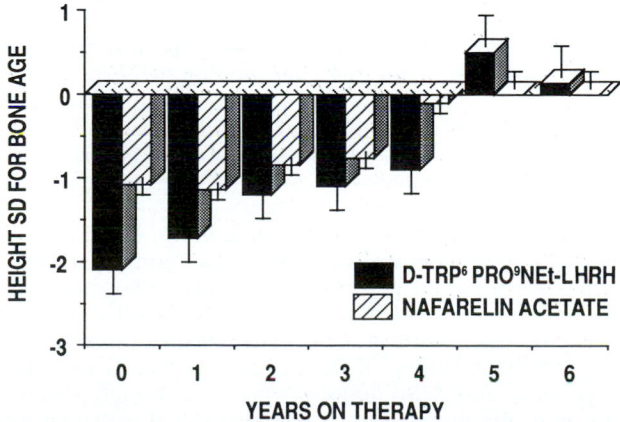

Figure 22–59. Effect of LHRH agonist therapy in true precocious puberty on growth. *Left,* Changes in mean height velocity (cm/y +1 SE) after the initiation of LHRH agonist therapy with D-Trp^{6}Pro^{9}NEt[LHRH] (deslorelin) (filled bars) or with nafarelin (hatched bars). A sharp decrease in height velocity occurred within 1 y. *Right,* Mean (±1 SE) height for bone age before and during LHRH agonist treatment. The discrepancy between height and the more advanced bone age decreases (reverts to normal) with chronic LHRH agonist treatment. (From Kaplan SL, Grumbach MM. True precocious puberty: treatment with GnRH-agonists. In: Delemarre-Van de Waal H, Plant TM, van Rees GP, et al., eds. Control of the Onset of Puberty III. Amsterdam: Elsevier, 1989: 357–373.)

TABLE 22–30. Indications for Therapy with LHRH Agonists in True Precocious Puberty

In children with clinical and unequivocal endocrine features of true precocious puberty:

Rapid advancement over a period of 6 mo to 1 y of secondary sexual characteristics, height, height velocity, and bone age in affected boys and girls

A serum testosterone concentration >3.5 nmol/L (>1 ng/mL) in boys less than 8 y of age

Onset of menarche (and recurrent menses) in girls less than 9 y of age

accordance with chronological age. In some girls we have observed within a 1- to 2-mo period the return of a pubertal pattern of LH pulsatility, of a pubertal LH response to LHRH, and of the concentration of plasma estradiol to a prepubertal state; in contrast to the typical patient, such girls do not exhibit the initial hyper-response of plasma estradiol and LH to the LHRH agonist. Many girls in this subset have clinical and hormonal features that fall between those of premature thelarche and true precocious puberty and are typical of neither condition.

Adverse Effects. Untoward reactions to LHRH agonists in the treatment of true precocious puberty have so far been minimal but include local and systemic allergic reactions in a few patients, including asthmatic episodes when the agent is given intranasally. When treatment is discontinued, even after 8 y, the gonadal suppression is reversed within a few weeks to months with a rise in the concentration of plasma gonadal steroids, progression of sexual maturation, and return of menses.[583] Despite these encouraging results, one must be alert to the possible emergence of unforeseen long-term side effects.

Psychosocial Aspects. Psychological management is a critical aspect of the care of children with true precocious puberty.[498a, 519, 562] With the advanced physical maturation for chronological age, they tend to seek friends closer to their size, strength, and physical development. Difficulties may arise because they lack the social skills of older children. Sex education of the child and the family is essential and must be given in a skillful, sensitive, and explicit manner; the risks of sexual abuse in both sexes and of pregnancy in girls need to be discussed. It is imperative to provide support in handling the increased height, the advanced sexual maturation, and the effects of gonadal steroids on behavior, activity, and emotional stability. The unrealistic demands and expectations that arise from the discrepancy between the physique and the chronological, mental, and psychosexual age require wise counseling, as do the reaction to ridicule by peers and the concern about being different from age mates. Some of these problems have been mitigated by school acceleration, advancing the child one or two grades, if this is consistent with the mental and emotional development. These comments are applicable to children with all forms of sexual precocity. The effectiveness of LHRH agonists has reduced but not eliminated many of these issues in true precocious puberty.[562]

LHRH agonists are effective in both boys and girls with idiopathic true precocious puberty, the androgen-induced form of secondary true precocious puberty following therapy of virilizing congenital adrenal hyperplasia with glucocorticoids, and organic forms of true precocious puberty associated with hamartomas of the tuber cinereum, hypothalamic neoplasms, and CNS lesions.[543, 573, 584] Although there are reports in the literature of surgical removal of hamartomas of the tuber cinereum,[244, 534, 542, 585, 586] the ease of medical treatment of this condition, the ability to follow the progress of this benign tumor with MRI or CT brain scans, and the risks of an adverse outcome of surgical intervention in this

area of the CNS[243] support the choice of LHRH agonists over surgical intervention.

The LHRH agonists are useful in conjunction with GH in the management of patients with both GH deficiency and true precocious puberty (usually as a result of radiation of the brain).[58] Such a regimen may allow a longer period of GH treatment before epiphyseal fusion in such subjects.[506]

Incomplete Form of Isosexual Precocity: LHRH-Independent Sexual Precocity

In this group of disorders the secretion of testosterone in boys and estrogen in girls is independent of the hypothalamic LHRH pulse generator (see Table 22–22). Affected individuals do not exhibit a pubertal-type LH response to administration of LHRH or a pubertal pattern of pulsatile LH secretion, nor do they respond to chronic administration of an LHRH agonist with suppression of gonadal steroid output. Incomplete isosexual precocity or precocious pseudopuberty is a consequence of gonadal or adrenal steroid secretion independent of LHRH, of iatrogenic exposure to gonadal steroids, or, in boys, of rare hCG- or LH-secreting tumors.

BOYS. *Chorionic Gonadotropin–Secreting Tumors.* Several types of tumors can secrete a glycoprotein hormone that has the bioactivity of LH or hCG and cross-reacts in the LH radioimmunoassay. Studies using highly specific antisera to the beta subunit of hCG confirm that the gonadotropin is hCG. Boys with these hCG-secreting neoplasms may have slightly enlarged testes and may be difficult to differentiate from boys with true precocious puberty on the basis of physical examination alone.[161, 228, 588] However, plasma hCG levels are elevated without an increase in the concentration of FSH or LH.[228] Hepatomas and hepatoblastomas are among the most serious of these tumors and cause firm, irregular nodular or smooth hepatic enlargement (Fig. 22–60). The hCG has been localized to the multinucleated tumor giant cells; in one case α-fetoprotein was found in the embryonal-type tumor cells spread throughout the hepatoblastoma.[587] The average survival is only 10.7 mo after diagnosis; the average age at onset is 2 y, 8 mo.[588–590]

Some teratomas or chorioepitheliomas in the hypothalamic region (or in the mediastinum, the gonads, or the retroperitoneum) and certain pineal tumors (usually a germinoma,[228, 520] less commonly a chorioepithelioma or its variants) cause sexual precocity in boys by secreting hCG rather than by activating the hypothalamic LHRH pulse generator and the pituitary gonadotropin–gonadal axis.[228] Such tumors are rare in girls and, if they occur, do not cause isosexual precocity because of the paucity of effects of hCG in females. However, germinomas in the suprasellar-hypothalamic region do not exhibit a sex predominance and are generally associated with pituitary hormone deficiencies. Calcification of the pineal is found in 8 to 11% of 8- to 11-y-old children and by itself is not indicative of a tumor. Germ cell tumors that secrete hCG are rarely located in the thalamus and basal ganglia. Germ cell tumors of the pineal region constitute less than 1% of primary CNS tumors in Western countries but account for 4.5% of such tumors in Japan.[591] Germinomas are radiosensitive, and regression of sexual precocity may occur if the bone age is less than 11 y, only to progress later into normal puberty.[228]

The prevalence of hCG-secreting mediastinal germ cell neoplasms is increased in boys with 47,XXY Klinefelter syndrome. Plasma α-fetoprotein is a useful additional marker for some of these germ cell tumors, although the cells in the tumor that secrete α-fetoprotein appear to differ from those that secrete hCG.

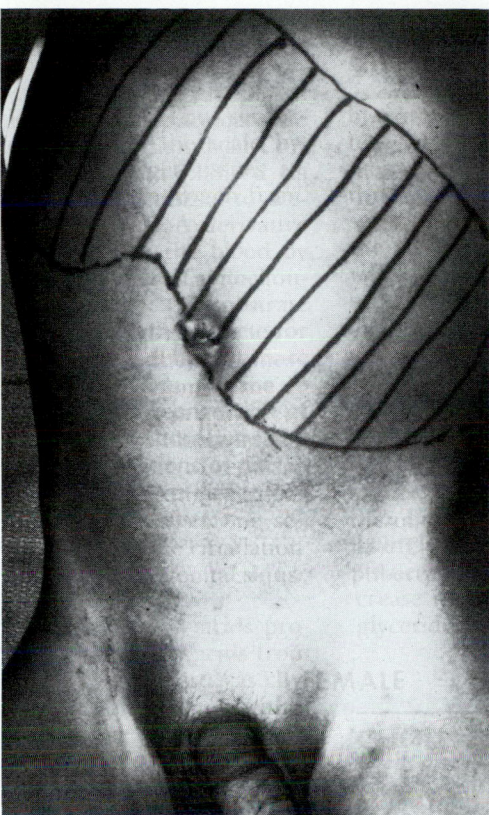 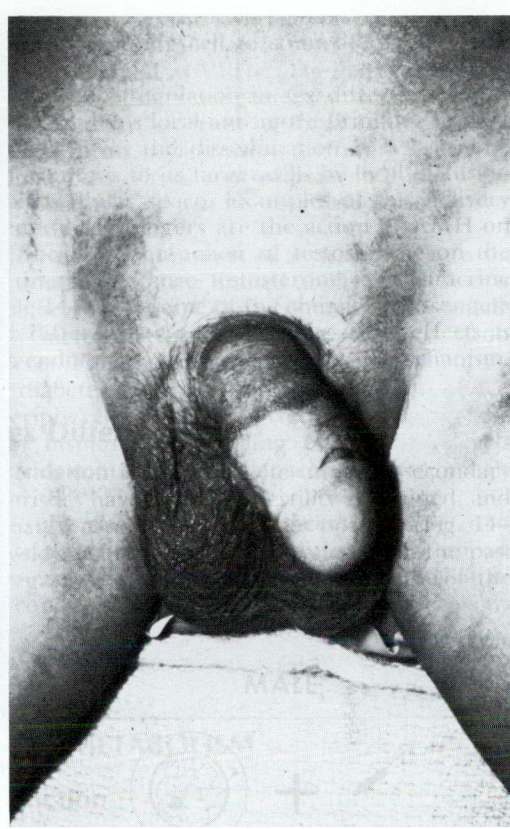

Figure 22–60. A 1⁹/₁₂-y-old boy with an hCG-secreting hepatoblastoma. Note the outline of the large liver (left) and the penile enlargement (right). The testes were 2 × 1 cm, and pubic hair was stage 2. The plasma hCG level was 50 mIU/mL; plasma testosterone, 168 ng/dL; and plasma α-fetoprotein, 160,000 ng/mL. Metastatic lesions in both lungs were seen on the roentgenogram of the chest. To convert testosterone values to SI units see the legend of Figure 22–14. To convert hCG values to international units per liter, multiply by 1.0. To convert α-fetoprotein values to micrograms per liter, multiply by 1.0. (From Kaplan SL, Grumbach MM. Pathogenesis of sexual precocity. In: Grumbach MM, Sizonenko PC, Aubert ML, eds. Control of the Onset of Puberty. Baltimore: Williams & Wilkins, 1990: 620–660. © 1990, the Williams & Wilkins Co., Baltimore.)

In one case, an LH- and prolactin-secreting pituitary tumor caused sexual precocity.[591] The concentration of serum LH was strikingly elevated (900 IU/L) and did not rise further after the administration of LHRH. The elevated serum testosterone 7 nmol/L (2 ng/mL) and prolactin (215 μg/L) levels and the high concentration of LH fell to prepubertal values after removal of a "chromophobe" adenoma with suprasellar extension.

Precocious Androgen Secretion Caused by Congenital Adrenal Hyperplasia, Virilizing Adrenal Tumor, or Leydig Cell Tumor. Virilizing congenital adrenal hyperplasia caused by a defect in 21-hydroxylation (cytochrome P-450$_{c21}$ deficiency) leads to elevated androgen concentrations and masculinization and is the most common cause of LHRH-independent sexual precocity in boys[416] (see Chapter 14). Approximately 75% of patients with P-450$_{c21}$ deficiency have salt loss resulting from impaired aldosterone secretion and have low serum sodium and high serum potassium concentrations. Increased plasma concentrations of 17-hydroxyprogesterone, increased levels of urinary 17-ketosteroids and pregnanetriol, and advanced bone age and rapid growth are characteristic. Treatment with glucocorticoids suppresses the abnormal androgen secretion and arrests virilization; treatment with mineralocorticoids, when necessary, corrects the electrolyte imbalance. A rarer form of virilizing adrenal hyperplasia is usually accompanied by hypertension and is caused by 11β-hydroxylase deficiency; the progressive virilization ceases and the blood pressure falls to normal with glucocorticoid therapy. All forms of congenital adrenal hyperplasia are inherited as autosomal recessive traits.[416] Virilizing congenital adrenal hyperplasia, if untreated, can cause anovulatory amenorrhea in females and oligospermia in males; with treatment, the infertility is usually corrected.

Virilizing adrenal carcinomas or adenomas secrete large amounts of DHEA and DHEAS and on occasion testosterone. Glucocorticoids do not suppress the increased secretion of adrenal androgens or the excretion of 17-ketosteroids to the normal range for age in carcinoma, but they readily decrease plasma 17-hydroxyprogesterone or 11-deoxycortisol levels and 17-ketosteroid excretion in congenital adrenal hyperplasia. Cushing syndrome resulting from adrenal carcinoma may cause isosexual precocity and growth failure in boys.

Adrenal rests, or heterotopic adrenal tissue in the testes, may enlarge with endogenous ACTH stimulation in boys with untreated or inadequately treated congenital adrenal hyperplasia and may mimic bilateral or unilateral interstitial cell tumors. Rarely, an *interstitial cell tumor* in boys is the cause of sexual precocity; unilateral enlargement (often nodular) of the testis occurs in this neoplasm, in contrast to the usually normal size of the testes for chronological age in boys with congenital adrenal hyperplasia or a virilizing adrenal tumor.[164]

Familial Testotoxicosis (Familial Gonadotropin-Independent Sexual Precocity with Premature Leydig Cell and Germ Cell Maturation). A unique form of sexual precocity in males is pituitary gonadotropin–independent familial premature Leydig cell and germ cell maturation, or testotoxicosis.[591–596] Although it has been recognized as an LHRH-independent form of male isosexual precocity only since 1981, this disorder was described more than 50 y ago. Affected boys have secondary sexual development with penile enlargement and bilateral enlargement of testes to the early or midpubertal range, although the testes may appear smaller than expected in relation to penile growth (Fig. 22–61). The testes show premature Leydig and Sertoli cell maturation and spermatogenesis; in some instances Leydig cell hyperplasia is present.[592, 593, 595] Serum hormone determinations reveal prepubertal basal and LHRH-stimulated gonadotropin concentrations and lack of a pubertal pattern of LH pulsatility, whether measured by immunological or bioassay techniques (Table 22–31). In affected boys, plasma testosterone values

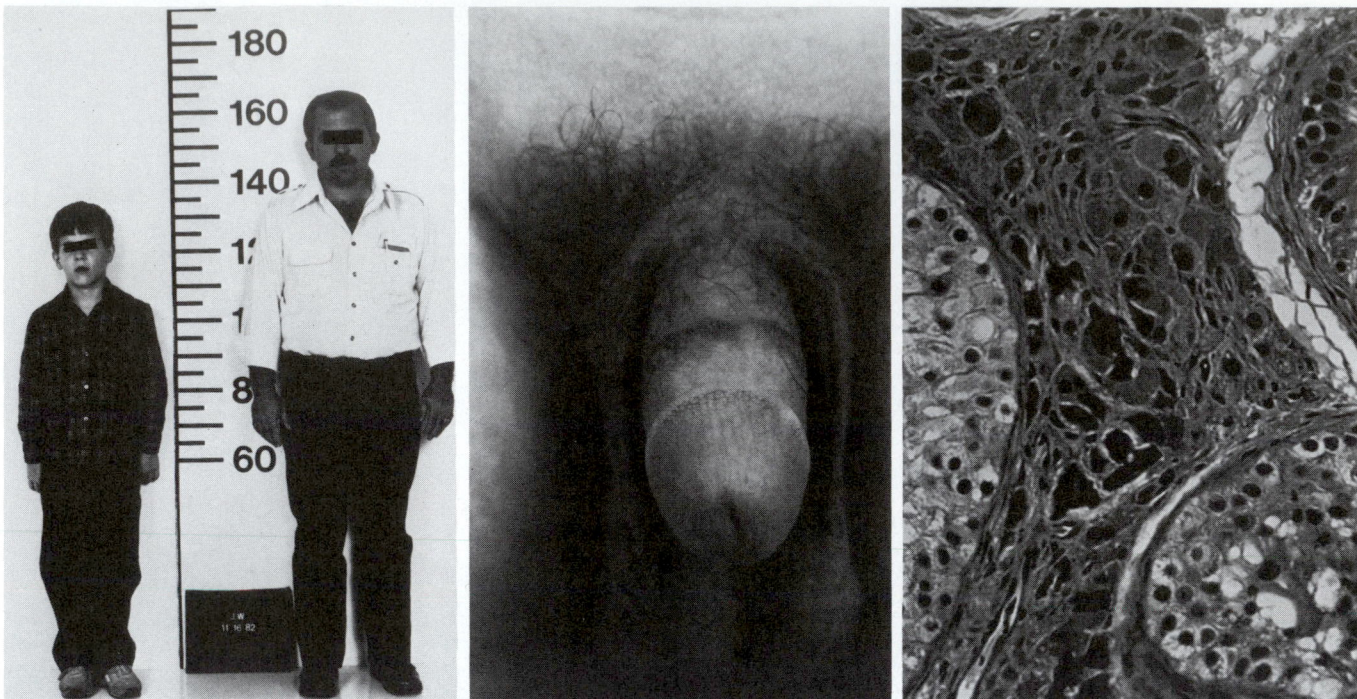

Figure 22–61. Familial testotoxicosis. *Left,* A 5½-y-old boy and his 28-y-old father with the disorder. The boy exhibited signs of sexual precocity by 3 y of age. Height, 130.6 cm (+4.8 SD); bone age, 12½ y. The plasma testosterone level was 267 ng/dL; dihydrotestosterone, 46 ng/dL; DHEAS, 23 μg/dL. The plasma LH and FSH levels were low and neither rose after treatment. Pulsatile LH secretion was not demonstratable. Treatment with deslorelin, an LHRH agonist, was without effect. The father had begun sexual maturation by 3 y of age and had reached a final height of 162.6 cm in his early teens. The plasma testosterone level was 294 ng/dL; LH, 0.5 ng/mL (LER-960); and FSH, 0.5 ng/mL (LER-869). The father had an adult-type LH and FSH response to LHRH; the LH level increased to 7.5 ng/mL and the FSH level to 2 ng/mL. At least 28 male family members over nine generations are affected. To convert dihydrotestosterone values to nanomoles per liter, multiply by 0.03467. For other conversions to SI units, see the legends of Figures 22–14 and 22–15. *Center,* External genitalia of the 5½-y-old boy. The penis measured 12 × 2.8 cm; the right testis was 4 × 2 cm and the left testis 3.5 × 2.5 cm. *Right,* Testis of the boy showed Leydig cell maturation without Reinke crystalloids and spermatogenesis. Mallory trichome.

are in the normal pubertal or adult range with normal clearance of testosterone. Treatment with an LHRH agonist does not suppress the testicular function or maturation.[593, 596] When most affected individuals reach adulthood, fertility is achieved and an adult pattern of LH secretion and response to LHRH is demonstrable.[594] In some adults, impaired spermatogenic function is associated with elevated concentrations of plasma FSH.[594] This disorder is inherited as a sex-limited autosomal dominant trait[594] and probably accounts for the earlier descriptions of "true" precocious puberty in families in which only males were affected. A kindred with nine generations of affected males has been reported.[594]

The pathogenesis of the LHRH-independent, pituitary gonadotropin–independent maturation of the testes is uncertain. No discordance in the ratio of bioactive to immunoactive endogenous LH was detected in affected boys in the rat Leydig cell bioassay for LH,[592, 593] nor have we found consistent discrepancies using the mouse Leydig cell assay for LH. These observations exclude the circulation of other

TABLE 22–31. Testotoxicosis: Salient Clinical and Laboratory Characteristics

Sex-limited autosomal dominant inheritance
Early onset of sexual precocity in boys with bilateral testicular enlargement
Prepubertal immunological and biological LH response to LHRH, prepubertal LH pulse secretory pattern
Concentration of plasma testosterone in pubertal range
Premature Leydig cell and seminiferous tubule maturation
No CNS, adrenal, or testicular abnormalities demonstrable by radiological or hormonal studies
Lack of suppression of plasma testosterone or physical signs of puberty by LHRH agonist

peptides with LH-like bioactivity but leave unanswered the question of an unidentified humoral factor that does not exhibit activity in the rat or mouse bioassay or that may act indirectly on the Leydig cell. Increased sensitivity of LH receptors on the Leydig cells is unlikely in view of the normal testosterone response to administration of a standard dose of hCG,[593] nor has a circulating immunoglobulin that binds to Leydig cells or other testicular components been detected.[593] Support for a circulating testis-stimulating factor in the plasma of affected boys has been obtained in a novel in vivo bioassay for LH activity using adult male monkeys pretreated with an LHRH antagonist.[597] Evidence has also been advanced for the existence of intratesticular paracrine regulatory mechanisms. Several locally generated factors including inhibin and activin, some uncharacterized, are believed to mediate interactions between the Sertoli and Leydig cells,[161, 593, 598–603] raising the possibility in familial testotoxicosis of an inherited abnormality in an intratesticular regulatory mechanism that leads to premature Leydig cell activation (and as a consequence premature onset of spermatogenesis).

Boys with this disorder do not respond to chronic administration of an LHRH agonist with suppression of testosterone secretion, in contrast to the characteristic response in patients with true precocious puberty.[593] However, testosterone secretion, height velocity and rate of bone maturation, and aggressive and hyperactive behavior have been decreased by treatment with oral medroxyprogesterone acetate.[519, 593]

Two other therapies have been used (Table 22–32). Ketoconazole, an orally active substituted imidazole derivative, suppresses gonadal and adrenal biosynthesis at several

TABLE 22–32. Pharmacological Therapy of Sexual Precocity

Disorder	Treatment	Action and Rationale
LHRH dependent		
True or central precocious puberty	LHRH agonists	Desensitization of gonadotropes; blocks action of endogenous LHRH
LHRH independent		
Incomplete sexual precocity		
Girls		
Autonomous ovarian cysts	Medroxyprogesterone acetate	Inhibition of ovarian steroidogenesis; regression of cyst (inhibition of FSH release)
McCune-Albright syndrome	Medroxyprogesterone acetate*	Inhibition of ovarian steroidogenesis; regression of cyst (inhibition of FSH release)
	Testolactone* or fadrozole	Inhibition of P-450 aromatase; blocks estrogen synthesis
Boys		
Familial testotoxicosis	Ketoconazole*	Inhibition of $P-450_{c17}$ (mainly 17,20-lyase activity)
	Spironolactone* or flutamide *and*	Antiandrogen
	testolactone or fadrozole	Inhibition of aromatase; blocks estrogen synthesis
	Medroxyprogesterone acetate*	Inhibition of testicular steroidogenesis

*If true precocious puberty develops, an LHRH agonist can be added.
Modified from Grumbach MM, Kaplan SL. Recent advances in the diagnosis and management of sexual precocity. Acta Paediatr Jpn 1988; 30(Suppl):155–175.

steps.[604] In the dosage used in testotoxicosis (200 mg every 8–12 h orally)[605, 606] ketoconazole mainly inhibits the enzyme cytochrome $P-450_{c17}$, which regulates both 17α-hydroxylation and the conversion of 17α-hydroxyprogesterone to androstenedione. However, even at the recommended dose, the agent produces a mild transient decrease in cortisol secretion and interferes with binding of testosterone to TeBG. Secondary true precocious puberty often occurs when the bone age advances to or has already reached the pubertal range (usually ≥11.5 y), at which time addition of an LHRH agonist is appropriate.[606] Ketoconazole can cause hepatic injury, which is usually mild and reversible, but rarely hepatotoxicity is severe.[604]

Another therapeutic approach has been the use of the antiandrogen (and antimineralocorticoid) spironolactone combined with testolactone, an inhibitor of cytochrome P-450 aromatase, a key enzyme in the conversion of androgens to estrogens.[607] More potent and specific nonsteroidal antiandrogens such as flutamide and nilutamide[608] and aromatase inhibitors such as fadrozole[609] are now available and potentially have greater therapeutic efficacy.

Table 22–32 lists the various agents used in the treatment of testotoxicosis; whether any of these agents or combination of agents will be effective and safe remains to be determined.

GIRLS. Incomplete isosexual precocity in girls (see Table 22–22) is caused by conditions in which estrogen is secreted autonomously by an ovarian cyst or tumor or by an adrenal neoplasm or by inadvertent exposure to estrogen. In a pure hCG-secreting tumor in girls, signs of isosexual precocity are absent. Girls harboring a teratoma or teratocarcinoma that secretes hCG have had sexual precocity caused by concurrent estrogen secretion by the tumor; these girls also may have galactorrhea, especially if human placental lactogen is also secreted.

Autonomous Ovarian Follicular Cysts. The most common childhood estrogen-secreting ovarian mass is the follicular cyst.[610] Antral follicles up to about 8 mm in diameter are common in the ovaries of normal prepubertal girls[38, 611–613] and may be seen in third-trimester fetuses and newborn infants.[614–616, 617a] They may appear and regress spontaneously. Large follicular cysts may be discovered because of the presence of an abdominal mass or abdominal pain, especially after torsion or as an unexpected finding on pelvic sonography performed for other reasons. Occasionally, the antral follicles secrete estrogen and may enlarge to form large masses, or the follicular cysts may recur and cause recurrent signs of sexual precocity and acyclic vaginal bleeding. Enlarged antral follicles or cysts occur in premature thelarche, true precocious puberty, and transient or incom-

plete sexual precocity.[161, 617, 617a–619] In some girls the transient or recurrent sexual precocity is LHRH independent (Fig. 22–62). The concentration of estradiol fluctuates, usually correlating with changes in the size of the cyst(s) when monitored by pelvic sonography,[620] and may increase to levels found in a granulosa cell tumor.[123, 161, 619] The concentration of gonadotropins is low, a pubertal pattern of pulsatile LH secretion is absent, and the LH rise induced by LHRH is prepubertal.[161, 617a, 618, 619]

An unusual syndrome of estradiol-secreting ovarian cysts in preterm infants born before 30 wk of gestation is associated with edema of the labia majora and, in some instances, of the lower abdominal wall.[616] In four preterm neonates the syndrome appeared weeks after birth and 1 to 4 wk before the putative date of a full term gestation. The follicular cysts, which may be unilateral or bilateral, were detected by abdominal and pelvic sonography. The LH and FSH response to LHRH suggested that the cysts were LHRH dependent. Treatment with medroxyprogesterone acetate was associated with regression of the cysts.

LHRH agonists are useful in the treatment of ovarian follicular cysts associated with true precocious puberty but not so-called autonomous cysts. However, girls with "autonomously" functioning ovarian follicular cysts, whether recurrent or an isolated episode, respond to treatment with oral medroxyprogesterone acetate. This agent also seems to prevent recurrence and accelerate involution of the follicular cysts.[161, 619] Surgical intervention is rarely indicated; a large or persistent cyst can be reduced by puncture at laparoscopy. The size of the cyst can be monitored readily by pelvic sonography.

Plasma estradiol concentrations in girls with recurrent cysts (≥7 cm) may increase to high levels indistinguishable from those in granulosa cell tumors of the ovary;[161, 619] alternatively, the levels of estrogen in blood and urine may be in the early pubertal range. A characteristic feature in girls with recurrent cysts is waxing and waning of estrogen levels that correlate with changes in the ovary on pelvic sonography. Pelvic ultrasonography is useful for visualization of ovarian cysts and estimation of functional activity.[620, 654] In some patients, exploratory laparotomy or laparoscopy may be necessary to differentiate these cysts from ovarian neoplasms or to rupture the cyst. The luteinization of follicular cysts may be related to subtle elevations and increased pulses of plasma FSH. A cyst that secretes estrogen autonomously differs from the follicular cysts that may occur in girls as a result of true precocious puberty. In the latter case, removal or reduction of the cyst does not correct the sexual precocity.[619, 623] Furthermore, the autonomously secreting cysts are not associated with augmented pulsatile LH

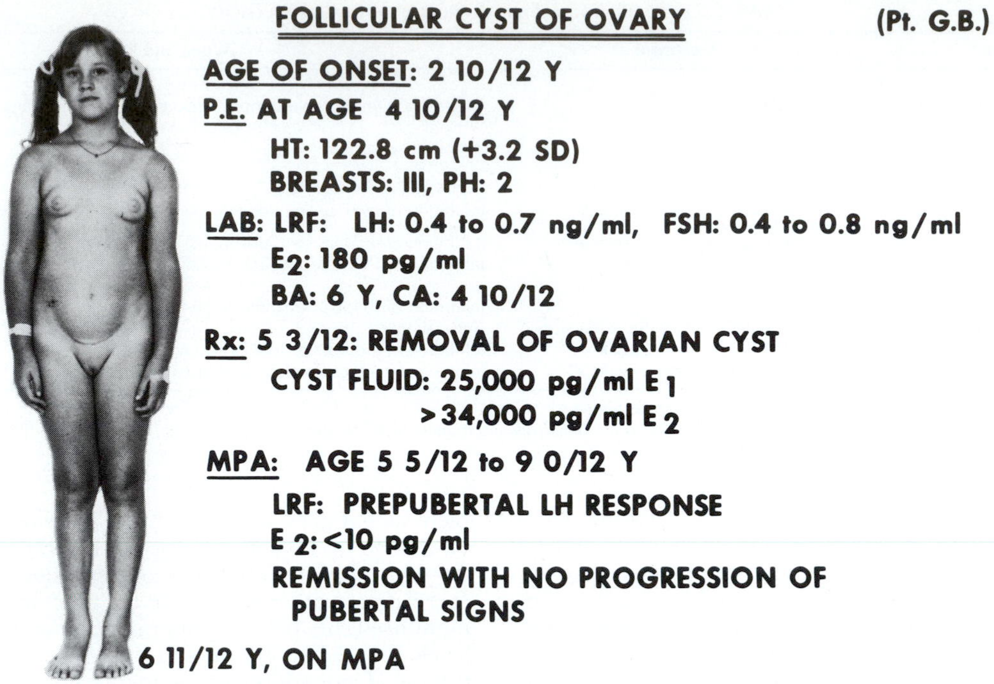

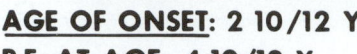

FOLLICULAR CYST OF OVARY   (Pt. G.B.)

AGE OF ONSET: 2 10/12 Y

P.E. AT AGE 4 10/12 Y

   HT: 122.8 cm (+3.2 SD)
   BREASTS: III, PH: 2

LAB: LRF: LH: 0.4 to 0.7 ng/ml,   FSH: 0.4 to 0.8 ng/ml
   E_2: 180 pg/ml
   BA: 6 Y, CA: 4 10/12

Rx: 5 3/12: REMOVAL OF OVARIAN CYST
   CYST FLUID: 25,000 pg/ml E_1
      >34,000 pg/ml E_2

MPA: AGE 5 5/12 to 9 0/12 Y

   LRF: PREPUBERTAL LH RESPONSE
   E_2: <10 pg/ml
   **REMISSION WITH NO PROGRESSION OF
   PUBERTAL SIGNS**

6 11/12 Y, ON MPA

Sequential Plasma Estradiol Levels in Patient with Recurrent Ovarian Cysts*

Age (y)	4 10/12	5 2/12	5 3/12	5 4/12	5 6/12	6 4/12	9 2/12	10 11/12	11 10/12
Estradiol (pg/mL)	180	10	796	10	500	55	12	22	193†
Treatment			Cyst removed		Start MPA Rx		Stop MPA Rx		

*Response of plasma gonadotropins to LHRH was prepubertal at ages 4½, 5 3/12, and 6 11/12 y. Six months after oral medroxyprogesterone acetate (MPA) was discontinued, normal cyclic menses began with evidence of ovulation. The subsequent course has been uneventful.
†Midcycle level.

Figure 22–62. A 4 10/12-y-old girl with recurrent "autonomous" follicular cysts of the ovary. MPA, medroxyprogesterone acetate (oral). For conversion to SI units, see the legend of Figure 22–14. (From Kaplan SL, Grumbach MM. Pathogenesis of sexual precocity. In: Grumbach MM, Sizonenko PC, Aubert ML, eds. Control of the Onset of Puberty. Baltimore: Williams & Wilkins, 1990: 620–660. © 1990, the Williams & Wilkins Co., Baltimore.)

secretion or with a pubertal LH response to LHRH administration. Ovarian cysts and sexual precocity have been associated with the fragile X syndrome in girls.[621]

Granulosa Cell Tumor of the Ovary. This tumor is rare in childhood, and theca cell tumors are even less common.[622, 623] Juvenile granulosa cell tumors have distinctive features that differentiate them from the tumors in adults. Characteristic histological features include nodular architecture, follicle formation, abundant interstitial and intrafollicular acid mucopolysaccharide–rich fluid, irregular microcysts, individual cell necrosis, and high mitotic activity (mean activity, 11 mitotic figures per 10 high-power fields). Size can vary from 2.5 to 25 cm with a mean diameter of 12 cm. The interstitial mucinous fluid consists predominantly of hyaluronic acid.[624] Prognosis is good, as only about 3% of patients die of the disease. Approximately 80% of granulosa cell tumors can be palpated on bimanual examination. Less than 5% are bilateral or clinically malignant. The concentration of plasma estradiol may increase to high levels;[123] FSH and LH concentrations are usually suppressed. Sonograms of the ovary facilitate diagnosis. After surgical removal, measurement of plasma estradiol levels is a useful screen for metastases; if the patient is younger than age 9, an elevated estradiol concentration suggests recurrence or metastasis.

Occasionally, *gonadoblastomas* in streak gonads, rare lipoid tumors, cystadenomas, and ovarian carcinomas secrete estrogens, androgens, or both hormones. Gonadal tumors composed of a mixture of germ cells and sex cord stromal cells that are distinct from gonadoblastoma are usually benign when discovered in female infants or children with 46,XX karyotypes,[625, 626] although neoplastic transformation is a risk.[627, 628] Two cases of metastasizing malignant mixed germ cell–sex cord–stromal tumors have been described in prepubertal girls with isosexual precocity.[628] Some of these neoplasms secrete α-fetoprotein and other tumor markers.

Peutz-Jeghers Syndrome. The syndrome of mucocutaneous pigmentation and gastrointestinal polyposis is associated with a rare sex cord tumor with annular tubules in both boys and girls.[629] Estrogen secretion by the tumor may lead to feminization and incomplete sexual precocity. Less frequently, an epithelial tumor of the ovary, dysgerminoma, or Sertoli-Leydig cell tumor has been found in patients with Peutz-Jeghers syndrome. Children with this disorder should be examined at regular intervals for the presence of gonadal tumors by pelvic sonography.

INCOMPLETE SEXUAL PRECOCITY: BOYS AND GIRLS. *McCune-Albright Syndrome.* This syndrome is characterized by the triad of irregularly edged hyperpigmented macules (café au lait spots); a slowly progressive bone disorder, polyostotic fibrous dysplasia, that can involve any bone and is frequently associated with facial asymmetry and hyperostosis of the base of the skull; and, most commonly in girls, LHRH-independent sexual precocity[630–632] (Fig. 22–63). Autonomous hyperfunction most commonly involves the ovary, but other endocrine involvement includes thyroid (nodular hyperplasia with thyrotoxicosis), adrenal (multiple hyperplastic nodules with Cushing syndrome), pituitary (adenoma or mammosomatotrope hyperplasia with gigantism and ac-

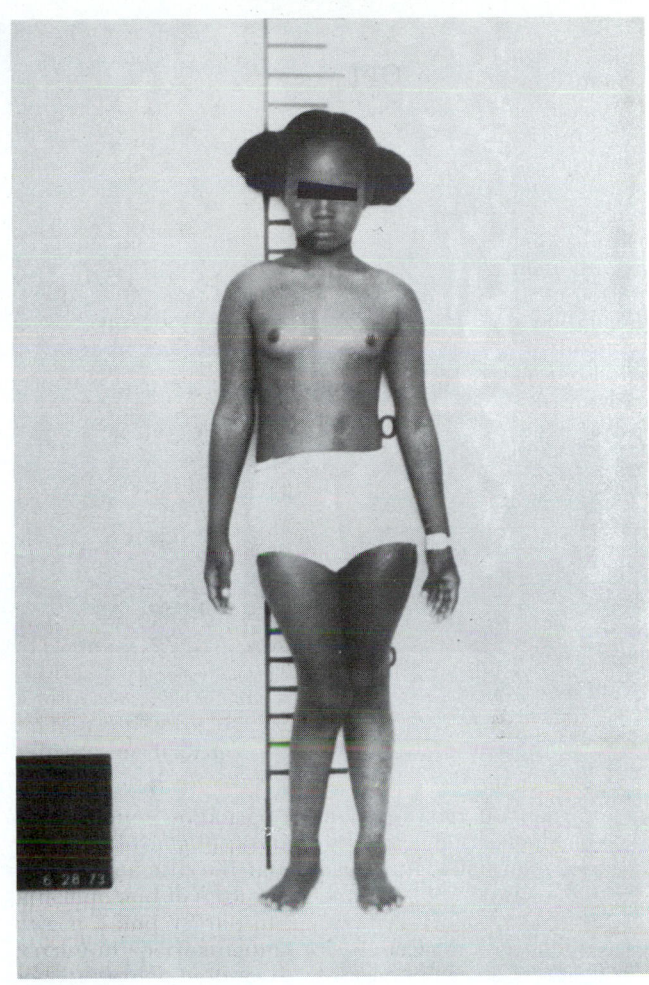

Figure 22–63. A 7⁴/₁₂-y-old girl with LHRH-independent sexual precocity associated with McCune-Albright syndrome. She had breast development since infancy and it increased noticeably at about 3 y of age; 6 mo later episodes of recurrent vaginal bleeding began. Growth of pubic hair was noted at about 4 to 5 y of age. At age 5³/₁₂ y the bone age was 6¹¹/₁₂ y; height was +1 SD above the mean value for age. By 6½ y of age, when she was seen at the University of California, San Francisco, the bone age had advanced to 9 y and height was at +1 SD. Breasts were at Tanner stage 4; pubic hair at stage 3. Extensive irregular café au lait macules cover the right side of the face, left lower abdomen and thigh, and both buttocks. A bone survey showed widespread involvement of the long bones with typical polyostotic fibrous dysplasia, and the floor of the anterior fossa of the skull was sclerotic and the diploic space widened. She has had two pathological fractures through bone cysts in the right upper femur. Note the osseous deformities. Plasma estradiol concentrations were consistently in the pubertal range; LH response to LHRH was prepubertal. Results of thyroid function studies were normal, including the TSH response to TRH administration, and antithyroid antibodies were not detected. Treatment with oral medroxyprogesterone acetate suppressed menses and arrested pubertal development but did not slow skeletal maturation. Her final height is 142 cm (−2.5 SD). Menstrual cycles are regular.

romegaly and hyperprolactinemia), and parathyroids (adenoma or hyperplasia with hyperparathyroidism).[630] The clinical and pathological findings have led to the suggestion that this disorder be considered a form of multiple endocrine adenomatosis.[630, 633, 634] In addition, hypophosphatemic vitamin D–resistant rickets or osteomalacia can occur in this syndrome, possibly because of a factor secreted by the bone lesions that inhibits 1α-hydroxylation of 25-hydroxycholecalciferol by the kidney.[630] At least two of the features must be present to consider the diagnosis.

The skin manifestations may not be conspicuous in infancy. The café au lait macules usually do not cross the midline and often are located on the same side as the main bone lesions and have a segmented distribution.[631]

The skeletal lesions in the cortex are dysplastic and are filled with spindle cells with poorly organized collagen support; they take the form of cystic areas of rarefaction on radiography and often result in pathological fractures and deformities[635] (Fig. 22–64). The bone lesions may be detected by a bone scan before they are visible radiographically. If the skull is involved, there may be compression of optic or auditory nerve foramina, which can lead to blindness, deafness (see Fig. 22–64), facial asymmetry, and ptosis.

The sexual precocity is due to an autonomously functioning luteinized follicular cyst of the ovary (see Table 22–23).[161, 630] The ovaries contain multiple follicular cysts and commonly exhibit asymmetrical enlargement as a result of a large solitary cyst (Fig. 22–65).[161, 596, 630, 633, 637, 638] The LH response to LHRH is prepubertal and the pubertal pattern of LH pulses is absent, at the onset and during the initial course.[161, 639, 640] Later in the course of the sexual precocity, when the bone age approaches 12 y, the LHRH pulse generator becomes operative and ovulatory cycles ensue. Thus, an affected girl may progress from LHRH-independent puberty to LHRH-dependent puberty[161, 639, 641] (Table 22–33). LHRH agonists are not effective for treatment, but testolactone, an aromatose inhibitor, has been useful in preliminary studies,[642] as has medroxyprogesterone acetate (see Table 22–32).

Sexual precocity is rare in boys with McCune-Albright syndrome.[630, 636] When affected, boys may have asymmetrical enlargement of the testes in addition to signs of sexual precocity. The seminiferous tubules are enlarged and exhibit spermatogenesis; Leydig cells may be hyperplastic.[636] The LH response to LHRH was prepubertal in two cases. The hormonal data (although scanty) and the testicular findings appear similar to those in boys with familial testotoxicosis (see ref. 630 for review).

The pathogenesis of the sporadic McCune-Albright syndrome is uncertain. Aside from occurrence in monozygotic twins, familial cases have not been described. Happle[643] has suggested that the disorder is caused by an autosomal "dominant" lethal gene that results in loss of the zygote in utero and that cells bearing this mutation survive only in embryos mosaic for the lethal gene. The mosaicism may arise by an early somatic mutation or by a gametic half-chromatid mutation. The severity of the disorder would depend on the proportion of mutant cells in the embryo. The description of somatic mutations in human endocrine tumors that convert the peptide chain of protein G_s into a

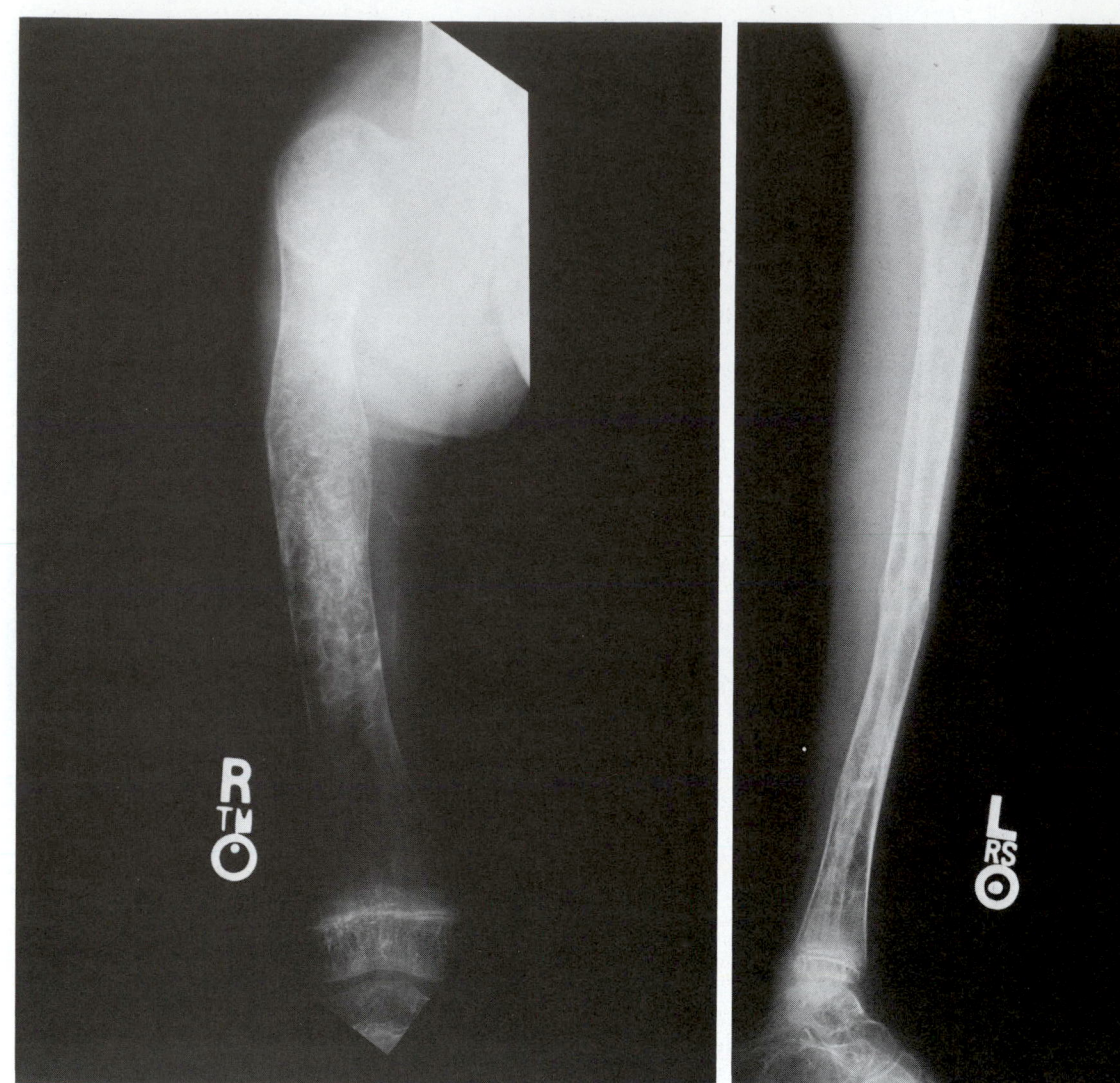

Figure 22–64. Bone lesions in McCune-Albright syndrome.

TABLE 22–33. A Patient with McCune-Albright Syndrome and Recurrent Ovarian Cysts

Chronological Age (y)	Bone Age (y)	Height (cm)	Physical Signs*	Basal and Post-LHRH‡	Plasma Estradiol, pmol/L (pg/mL)	X-Ray Films, Long Bones
1 4/12	1 3/12	81.1	Café au lait pigmentation, B2, PH1 Vaginal bleeding (× 2 mo)	LH 0.6–1.3† FSH 1.9–3.2† (DHEAS <0.14 μmol/L [<50 ng/mL])	40 (11)	Normal
1 8/12			B1, PH1			
2 6/12	2 6/12	92.4	B2, PH2 Vaginal bleeding	LH 0.6–1.1 FSH 1.9–3.2 (DHEAS <0.14 μmol/L [<50 ng/mL])	55–66 (15–18)	Normal
3 3/12		98.3	B1, PH1			
3 10/12	3 10/12		B2, PH1	LH 1.1–2.0 FSH 1–1.7	51–95 (14–26)	Normal
4 3/12			B1, PH1			
5 11/12	6	123.4	B3, PH2 Vaginal bleeding (× 2 mo)	LH 1.1–4.3 FSH 1.0–2.0	7.3–7.3 (20–20)	Polyostotic fibrous dysplasia of femurs
6 6/12	7 10/12	128.5	B3, PH2 Oral medroxyprogesterone acetate 10 mg bid started		<5	
7 10/12	8 10/12	136.8				
8 7/12		142.2				

*B2, breast stage 2; PH1, pubic hair stage 1.

†ng/mL. To convert ng/mL to IU/L, multiply LH value by 3.8 and FSH value by 8.4.

‡Note the prepubertal LH response to LHRH consistent with LHRH-independent sexual precocity until age 5 11/12 y, and the pubertal LH response at 5 11/12 y consistent with the development of secondary true precocious puberty (LHRH-dependent). Note discrepancy between gonadarche and adrenarche as evidenced by preadrenarchal concentration of DHEAS.

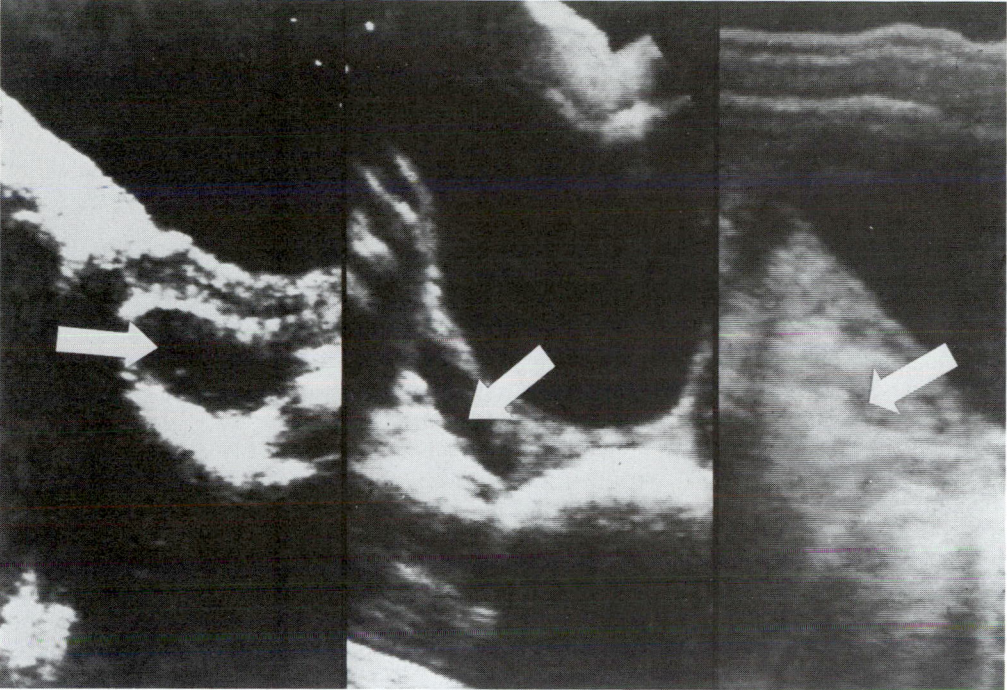

Figure 22–65. Serial pelvic sonograms at 2-wk intervals in a 6-y-old girl with McCune-Albright syndrome. Breast development and vaginal bleeding coincided with the enlargement of the ovarian cyst. With the spontaneous regression of the large ovarian cyst, the breasts regressed in size and vaginal bleeding ceased. (From Kaplan SL, Grumbach MM. Pathogenesis of sexual precocity. In: Grumbach MM, Sizonenko PC, Aubert ML, eds. Control of the Onset of Puberty. Baltimore: Williams & Wilkins, 1990:620–660. © 1990, the Williams & Wilkins Co., Baltimore.)

putative oncogene[644] raises the possibility of a similar defect in the McCune-Albright syndrome that both affects a differentiated function such as a signaling pathway and mediates the regulation of proliferation.

Juvenile Hypothyroidism. Long-standing untreated primary hypothyroidism, usually a consequence of Hashimoto thyroiditis, is an uncommon cause of incomplete isosexual precocity[645, 646] in both girls and boys and occurs in association with impaired growth and delayed skeletal maturation. If the concentration of plasma prolactin is elevated, galactorrhea may be demonstrable, more commonly in affected girls than boys (Fig. 22–66). The signs of sexual maturation are not accompanied by a pubertal growth spurt; rather growth is impaired (Fig. 22–67). Girls have breast development, enlarged labia minora, and estrogenic changes in the vaginal smear, usually without the appearance of pubic hair;[645, 648, 649, 652] some girls have irregular vaginal bleeding;[645] and solitary or multiple ovarian cysts may be demonstrable by pelvic sonography or by physical examination.[645] In boys the testes are enlarged because of an increase in the size of the seminiferous tubules, but signs of virilization and Leydig cell maturation are absent.[649] Enlargement of the sella turcica and the pituitary gland (see Fig. 22–67) has led to the misdiagnosis of a pituitary neoplasm. The hypothyroidism, incomplete sexual maturation, galactorrhea, and pituitary enlargement are reversed or corrected by levothyroxine therapy within a few months.[645]

In 1960 Van Wyk and Grumbach[645] suggested that the syndrome resulted from hormonal "overlap" in negative feedback regulation with increased secretion of gonadotropins, prolactin, and TSH as a consequence of the chronic hypothyroidism. With the advent of radioimmunoassays for pituitary hormones, increased prolactin secretion was documented in children[647] and adults with primary hypothyroidism and in affected girls with the syndrome.[648] Hyperprolactinemia correlated with the increased production of TSH.[647] GH release is usually decreased as in uncomplicated primary hypothyroidism.[650, 651] Hypothalamic TRH stimulates the release of both prolactin and TSH, and the increased TRH concentration in children with primary hypothyroidism

seems to account for the rise in serum prolactin and TSH levels.[647] However, the explanation for the sexual maturation remains uncertain. Pubertal development in primary hypothyroidism is usually delayed and is only rarely advanced for chronological age. By using radioimmunoassays for FSH and LH in which the cross-reaction with TSH is negligible, an increased concentration of plasma FSH but not LH has been detected.[650, 651] Bioactive LH activity is also low. In addition, increased FSH pulsatility, mainly at night, but not LH release was demonstrated in patients with the syndrome and in some children with primary hypothyroidism who did not exhibit premature sexual maturation.[650, 651] The increased FSH release and the high FSH/LH ratio (in contrast to that in normal puberty) seem to account for the increased estrogen secretion in girls and for the enlarged testes without signs of virilization in affected boys. The mechanism of increase in FSH but not LH release may be related to what occurs in premature thelarche, in which it is suspected that a low level of increased activity of the hypothalamic LHRH pulse generator increases FSH secretion but not LH secretion.[163] On the other hand, an LHRH-independent mechanism is also plausible. Pulsatile TSH release is increased at night and administration of TRH appears to increase FSH release in normal children (but not adults), and the FSH response to TRH is augmented in primary hypothyroidism.[651] If the latter observations are confirmed, it is likely that the incomplete sexual precocity and the increased prolactin secretion and galactorrhea are a consequence of the increased release of TRH, increased sensitivity of the mammotropes and gonadotropes to TRH, or both. This mechanism would explain the relatively rapid and complete reversal of the syndrome by levothyroxine treatment. The rare TSH-secreting pituitary tumors may also be associated with sexual precocity.[652]

Diagnosis of Sexual Precocity (Table 22–34)

The separation of patients with self-limited benign disorders, such as premature adrenarche or premature thelarche, from those with serious or even potentially fatal

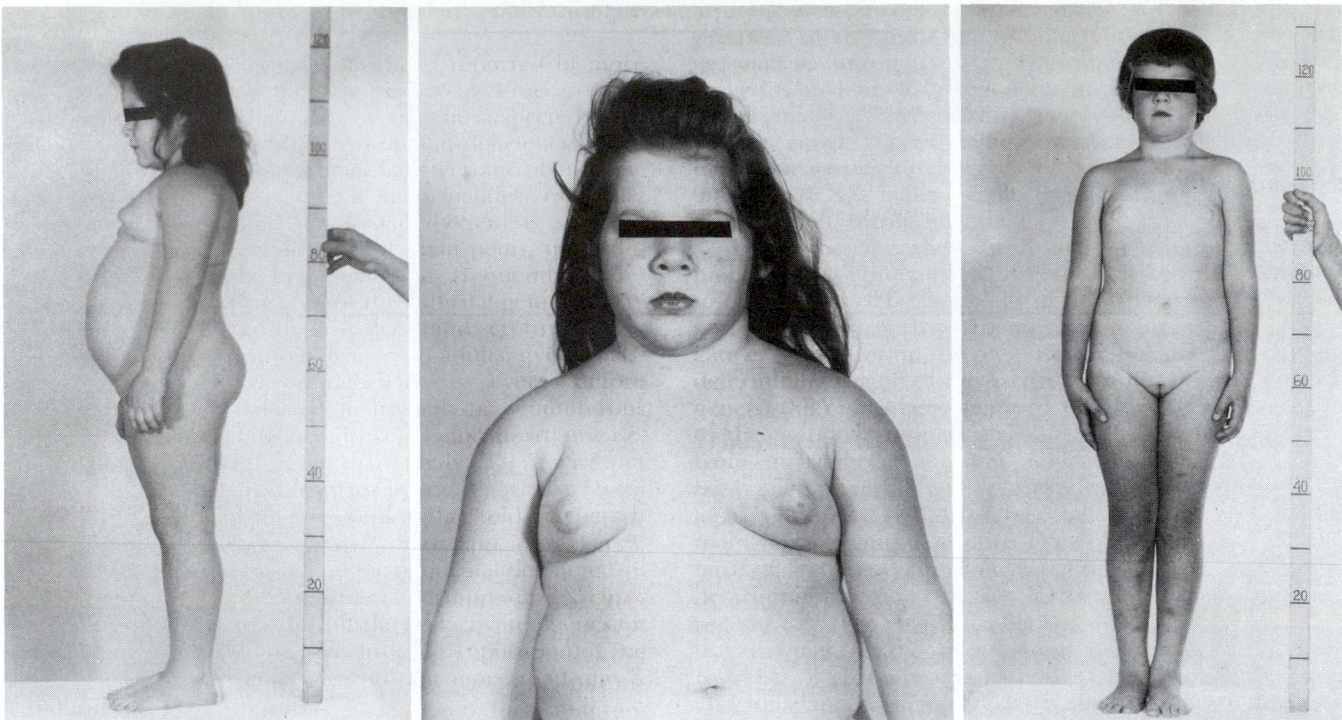

Figure 22–66. *Left and center,* Severe, chronic hypothyroidism of Hashimoto thyroiditis in a 7½-y-old girl with sexual precocity (without pubic or axillary hair), episodic vaginal bleeding, and galactorrhea. She had symptoms of hypothyroidism and a sharply decreased rate of growth over the previous 2 y (height, −1 SD; bone age, 5⁹⁄₁₂ y). Breast development was Tanner stage 3; the labia minora were enlarged, and the vaginal mucosa was dull pink, thickened, and rugated with evidence of an estrogenic effect. No acne, seborrhea, or hirsutism was present. The uterus was of adolescent size, and the endometrial mucosa was in a proliferative phase. Urinary gonadotropins were barely detectable by bioassay. *Right,* Striking change in appearance after 8 mo of thyroid hormone treatment. She had grown 7 cm in height and lost 8.1 kg in weight; the breasts had decreased in size, galactorrhea was no longer demonstrable, the labia minora had regressed, and the vaginal mucosa was pink and glistening (no estrogen effect). Ten weeks after the initiation of thyroid hormone replacement therapy, she developed a right slipped capital femoral epiphysis that was repaired surgically; recovery was uneventful.

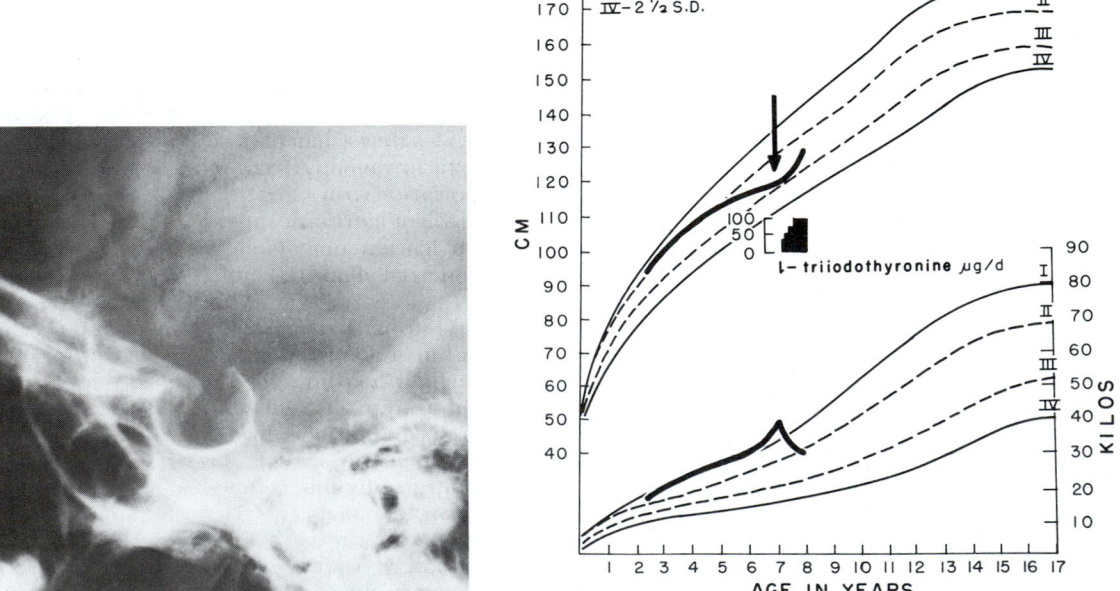

Figure 22–67. *Left,* Radiograph of the skull of a patient with hypothyroidism illustrating an enlarged pituitary fossa in the lateral view. The dorsum sellae was thin and demineralized, and the floor had a double contour line. The area of the sella turcica was 150 mm². Pneumoencephalography showed a suprasellar mass impinging on the cisterna chiasmatica. After thyroid hormone treatment for 8 mo, the area of the sella had decreased 30% in volume to 100 mm², the dorsum sellae had remineralized, and the double floor was no longer evident. *Right,* Growth curve illustrating the decrease in growth rate despite the sexual precocity and the catch-up growth induced by thyroid hormone therapy. (From Van Wyk JJ, Grumbach MM. Syndrome of precocious menstruation and galactorrhea in juvenile hypothyroidism: an example of hormonal overlap in pituitary feedback. J Pediatr 1960; 57:416–435.)

TABLE 22–34. Differential Diagnosis of Isosexual Precocity

Disorder	Serum Gonadotropin Concentration	LH Response to LHRH	Serum Sex Steroid Concentrations	Gonadal Size	Miscellaneous
True precocious puberty (premature reactivation of hypothalamic LRF pulse generator); LHRH dependent	Prominent LH pulses, initially during sleep	Pubertal LH response	Pubertal values of testosterone or estradiol	Normal pubertal testicular enlargement or ovarian and uterine enlargement (by sonography)	MRI or CT scan of brain to rule out a CNS tumor or other abnormality
Incomplete sexual precocity (LHRH independent)					
Males					
Chorionic gonadotropin-secreting tumor in males	High hCG	Prepubertal LH response	Pubertal value of testosterone	Slight to moderate uniform enlargement of testes	Hepatomegaly suggests hepatoblastoma; CT or MRI scan of brain if hCG-secreting CNS tumor suspected; α-fetoprotein determination
Leydig cell tumor in males	Prepubertal LH pulses	Prepubertal LH response	High testosterone levels	Irregular asymmetrical enlargement of testes	
Familial testoxicosis	Prepubertal LH pulses	Prepubertal LH response	Pubertal values of testosterone	Testes symmetrical and larger than 2.5 cm but smaller than expected for pubertal development; spermatogenesis occurs	Familial; sex-limited, autosomal dominant trait
Premature adrenarche	Prepubertal LH pulses	Prepubertal LH response	Prepubertal testosterone; ↑ DHEAS values appropriate for pubic hair stage 2	Testes prepubertal	Onset usually after 6 y of age; more frequent in brain-injured children
Females					
Granulosa cell tumor (follicular cysts may present similarly)	Low	Prepubertal LH response	Very high estradiol	Ovarian enlargement on physical, CT, or sonography	Tumor often palpable on abdominal examination
Follicular cyst	Low	Prepubertal LH response	Prepubertal to very high estradiol	Ovarian enlargement on physical, CT, or sonographic examination	Single or repetitive episodes; exclude McCune-Albright syndrome
Feminizing adrenal tumor	Low	Prepubertal LH response	High estradiol and DHEAS values	Ovaries prepubertal	Unilateral adrenal mass
Premature thelarche	Prepubertal LH pulses; nocturnal FSH pulses in some	Prepubertal LH response; often increased FSH response	Prepubertal or early pubertal estradiol	Ovaries prepubertal, usually with cysts; uterus prepubertal size	Onset usually before 3 y of age
Premature adrenarche	Prepubertal LH pulses	Prepubertal LH response	Prepubertal estradiol; ↑ DHEAS values appropriate for pubic hair stage 2	Ovaries prepubertal	Onset usually after 6 y of age; more frequent in brain-injured children

From Styne DM, Grumbach MM. Puberty in the male and female. In: Yen SCC, Jaffe RB, eds. Reproductive Endocrinology. 2nd ed. Philadelphia: W. B. Saunders, 1986: 313–384.

disorders is the first step in evaluation. The history may reveal symptoms suggesting perinatal abnormalities or injuries, previous infections, adventitious ingestion of or exposure to gonadal steroids, or the presence of similar conditions in family members. In addition, previous measurements should be plotted on a growth chart to determine height velocity and the age of onset of any increase in the rate of growth. Important aspects of the physical examination include description of the secondary sexual development according to Tanner stages; measurement of the penis and the testes in boys and breast tissue in girls; and examination for acne, oily skin, facial and body hair, pubic and axillary hair development, apocrine gland odor, muscular development, and galactorrhea. A careful examination of the external genitalia should be done with a nonrelated chaperone present, as the performance of such an examination has been interpreted by patients as sexual abuse in

several cases.[653] A thorough neurological examination is indicated, with emphasis on assessment of the visual fields and optic discs, and search for signs of increased intracranial pressure; evaluation for skin lesions of the McCune-Albright syndrome or neurofibromatosis; and examination for abdominal, gonadal, or adnexal masses and for coexisting endocrine disease. Radiographs should be obtained for determination of bone age and investigation of cranial or sellar abnormalities. Ultrasonography of the ovary and uterus is exceedingly useful in affected girls. Standards are available for the shape and volume of the uterus and the ovaries; the presence of microcysts and macrocysts of the ovary can be detected as well.[654] The upper limit of uterine length in the prepubertal state is 3.5 cm.[655] Measurements of plasma gonadotropin concentrations, testosterone levels in boys, estradiol levels in girls, and the LH response to administration of LHRH or the amplitude and frequency of LH pulses, especially at night, are of primary importance in diagnosis. Determination of thyroxine concentration is indicated when hypothyroidism is suspected.

True precocious puberty in males usually begins with enlargement of the testes, followed by other signs of secondary sexual maturation. A Leydig cell tumor or an adrenal rest usually causes asymmetrical enlargement of the testes, whereas an extragonadal hCG-secreting tumor is associated with less marked testicular enlargement than in true precocious puberty. An elevated hCG level with a prepubertal LHRH test indicates an ectopic, autonomous, gonadotropin-secreting tumor. If this tumor is in the CNS, abnormalities are present on MRI or CT brain scans; enlargement of the liver or a mediastinal mass in boys suggests an hCG-producing hepatic or germ cell tumor. Pubertal concentrations of LH and FSH, a pubertal mode of pulsatile LH secretion (initially during sleep), and/or pubertal LH response in the LHRH test confirms the diagnosis of true precocious puberty (and in boys differentiates true precocity from familial testotoxicosis); a CNS tumor must be considered as a potential cause of this premature activation of the hypothalamic LHRH pulse generator. The evaluation for a CNS tumor as a cause of true precocious puberty is similar to the investigation of an hCG-secreting tumor of the CNS. Although CT scanning is now a well-established procedure for determining the presence of a CNS abnormality,[656] MRI is more sensitive for the detection of small tumors in the hypothalamus, such as a hamartoma of the tuber cinereum[541, 657] (see Fig. 22–53).

The premature appearance of pubic hair, phallic enlargement, and other signs of virilization in a male without enlargement of the testes or the liver suggests the diagnosis of congenital virilizing adrenal hyperplasia, virilizing adrenal tumor, or, rarely, Cushing syndrome. Measurement of plasma 17-hydroxyprogesterone and DHEAS concentrations and the excretion of urinary 17-ketosteroids and their suppressibility with glucocorticoids will distinguish adrenal hyperplasia from a virilizing adrenal tumor. If growth rate is suppressed, the possibility of primary hypothyroidism or of Cushing syndrome is raised; elevated plasma concentrations of cortisol and urinary free cortisol and 17-hydroxycorticosteroid values confirm the latter diagnosis. The appearance in a girl of pubic hair and other signs of virilization, such as clitoral enlargement, acne, deepening voice, muscular development, or growth spurt, is caused by congenital virilizing adrenal hyperplasia, virilizing adrenal tumor, or virilizing ovarian tumor; Cushing syndrome caused by an adrenocortical carcinoma can cause virilization associated with growth failure. Virilizing ovarian tumors can often be palpated by bimanual examination or detected by pelvic ultrasound. The appearance of pubic hair without other signs of puberty in boys or girls is usually a result of premature adrenarche but may be the first sign of sexual precocity or adrenal virilism.

In a girl, breast development associated with dulling and thickening of the vaginal mucosa and enlargement of the labia minora indicates significant estrogen secretion or iatrogenic exposure to estrogen. In addition, the differential diagnosis includes true or central precocious puberty, an estrogen-secreting neoplasm, and a cyst of the ovary. If the plasma concentrations of gonadotropins are in the pubertal range, if LH pulses of pubertal amplitude are detected, or if a pubertal LH response to LHRH is elicited, true precocious puberty is present. Estrogen concentrations in girls early in normal or true precocious puberty are in the prepubertal range much of the day, and a single determination may be inadequate to reflect ovarian function[161] (see Fig. 22–51). A CNS tumor is less likely in girls than in boys to be the cause of this premature reactivation of the hypothalamic LHRH pulse generator–pituitary gonadal system.

However, studies using MRI or CT brain scans indicate that the hypothalamic hamartoma is more prevalent in both boys and girls with "idiopathic" true precocious puberty than was previously suspected. If the concentration of plasma estradiol is elevated but gonadotropin levels are low, an estrogen-secreting cyst or neoplasm is present. Ovarian tumors of moderate size can be palpated by bimanual examination. Advances in ultrasonographic techniques allow the delineation of ovarian cysts or tumors and the determination of uterine size, and this procedure has become an essential component of the diagnostic evaluation.[39] An estrogen-secreting neoplasm of the ovary is usually accompanied by high estradiol concentrations. However, some ovarian cysts are associated with concentrations of estradiol as high as those in granulosa cell tumors; the differential diagnosis between these cysts and ovarian neoplasms rarely requires exploratory laparotomy or laparoscopy and usually can be resolved by ultrasonography. Breast development in the absence of other estrogen effects is almost always a result of premature thelarche.

Iatrogenic Sexual Precocity

Prepubertal children are remarkably sensitive to exogenous gonadal steroids and may show signs of sexual maturation resulting from overlooked sources of androgens or estrogens, such as ingested or absorbed tonics, lotions, or creams that contain or are inadvertently contaminated with an estrogen.[658] Children who inhaled estrogen dust have developed sexual precocity. Likewise, estrogens can be absorbed from cosmetics. A short course of application of estrogen cream may be successful in treating labial adhesions, but long courses may lead to breast development or even withdrawal bleeding. In addition to breast development, pigmentation of the areolae and the linea alba and the appearance of pubic hair may be seen in children exposed to estrogen. Epidemics of gynecomastia in boys and thelarche in girls have occurred in schoolchildren in Italy and Puerto Rico;[659, 660] meat contaminated by estrogens was suspected in the Italian study and speculated about in the Puerto Rican cases. During a 10-y period more than 600 cases of gynecomastia in boys and premature thelarche or incomplete sexual precocity in girls were discovered in Puerto Rico. Ovarian cysts were demonstrated in two thirds of affected girls.[661, 661a] The wide publicity given these observations and the questions raised about contamination of the food supply by the clandestine use of estrogens as growth-promoting agents for meat production caused anxiety among parents, cattle raisers, and farmers. It was suggested that the use of estrogen preparations in animals to stimulate weight gain led to ingestion of estrogen-contaminated meat, but this idea has not been confirmed by extensive analyses of meat, poultry, and milk by the U.S. Department of Agriculture.[661a]

The administration of hCG to boys with undescended testes may induce secretion of testosterone sufficient to cause incomplete sexual precocity. From these examples it is clear that careful investigation of sources of possible exposure to exogenous hormones is mandatory in every case of sexual precocity.

Feminization in Boys and Virilization in Girls (Contrasexual Precocity)

BOYS. Feminization in a boy before the age of puberty is rare. Rarely, an *estrogen-secreting adrenal adenoma*[662] or a *chorionepithelioma* may cause gynecomastia. Gynecomastia has been reported in a 1-y-old boy with *11α-hydroxylase deficiency*[663] and in boys with *late-onset congenital adrenal hyper-*

plasia. Gynecomastia in prepubertal boys can also be caused by increased *extraglandular aromatization* of androstenedione and hence increased extraglandular estrogen production in sporadic or familial cases.[664, 665] Feminizing testicular tumors may cause gynecomastia in boys younger than age 6 with the *Peutz-Jeghers syndrome*. Both testes may be enlarged, and the histology indicates sex cord or Sertoli cell tumors that form annular tubules; increased estradiol secretion is noted in the basal state, and a further rise occurs after hCG administration. Ultrasonography or MRI scans of the testes may be useful in the diagnosis.[666]

GIRLS. Virilization in a girl indicates organic disease except for premature adrenarche. *Congenital adrenal hyperplasia* resulting from 21-hydroxylase or 11β-hydroxylase deficiency and *androgen-producing tumors* of the adrenal can cause virilization and were discussed earlier as occurring in males. 3β-Hydroxydehydrogenase/$\Delta^{4,5}$-isomerase deficiency is a rare type of congenital adrenal hyperplasia characterized by elevated Δ^5-17-hydroxypregnenolone, DHEA and DHEAS levels and, in the severe form, decreased secretion of aldosterone and cortisol. Severely affected patients have mineralocorticoid and glucocorticoid deficiency and may die in infancy. Excess adrenal androgens lead to virilization in utero and to ambiguous external genitalia, including clitoral enlargement in females with continued virilization after birth[416] (see Chapter 14). Milder forms of this disorder can cause hirsutism in women. 46,XY phenotypic women with incomplete forms of androgen resistance syndrome or with 17-oxidoreductase deficiency may have virilization as well as breast development at the time of expected puberty.

Cushing syndrome resulting from adrenal carcinoma usually manifests as growth failure with or without virilization, obesity, and moon facies; striae may not appear for months to years later.

Arrhenoblastoma, the most common virilizing ovarian tumor, is rare in children. Lipoid cell tumor of the ovary and gonadoblastoma are even more unusual sources of androgens.[667, 668]

Variations of Pubertal Development

PREMATURE THELARCHE. Unilateral or bilateral breast enlargement without other signs of sexual maturation (e.g., sexual hair and growth of the labia minora and the uterus) is not uncommon in infancy and childhood and has been referred to as premature thelarche. The disorder usually occurs by age 2 and rarely after age 4.[669–671a, 673–675] In a retrospective study in Minnesota, premature thelarche occurred with an incidence of 21.2 per 100,000 patient-years, 60% of cases were noted between 6 mo and 2 y of age, and most regressed in 6 mo to 6 y after diagnosis, although a few persisted until puberty. A 10- to 35-y follow-up was available in 25 cases, and no untoward effects on later health, growth, or fertility were evident.[670] The breast enlargement usually regresses after a few months[671, 671a] but occasionally persists for years or lasts until the onset of normal puberty; in about half of affected girls the breast development, which is characteristically cyclic, lasts 3 to 5 y. Usually, significant nipple development is absent and estrogen-induced thickening and dulling of the vaginal mucosa or enlargement of the uterus on ultrasonography is uncommon. Growth in stature is normal.[164, 669, 673, 673a, 679] This is a benign self-limited disorder compatible with normal pubertal development at an appropriate age; only reassurance and follow-up are necessary.[164, 673] Because the development may be unilateral, it is important to consider the condition in girls with unilateral breast development so that needless worry about breast cancer is not stimulated in the parents and no unnecessary surgical procedure is carried out. In selected instances,

sonography of the breast is useful in distinguishing unilateral premature thelarche from less benign conditions.

Plasma estrogen levels may be slightly elevated for age in premature thelarche,[123, 669, 677, 678] but some patients have nondetectable levels when studied, probably because samples are obtained after the transient episode of estrogen secretion. One report described a slight elevation of free estrogen.[678] However, there is no increase in plasma levels of TeBG or in TBG, indicators of estrogen action on circulating plasma proteins.[678a] The urocytogram often reveals an estrogen effect on squamous epithelial cells in the urine.[123, 674, 676] The concentration of serum FSH may be in the pubertal range, nocturnal FSH pulsatility has been detected, and the rise in FSH elicited by the administration of LHRH may be augmented for chronological age, with an FSH/LH ratio higher in precocious thelarche than in normal individuals or girls with central precocious puberty.[275, 669, 680, 681] However, these results overlap those in normal prepubertal girls. Sonograms of the ovary often show one or several cysts larger than 0.5 cm that disappear and reappear, usually correlating with changes in the size of the breasts.[654, 681] The uterus remains prepubertal in size. As noted, there is evidence for intermittent secretion of small amounts of estrogen from the ovary. Thus, as postulated for some recurrent ovarian cysts, premature thelarche appears to result from the ovarian response to transient increases in FSH levels and possible variations in ovarian sensitivity to FSH.[275, 676] The LH response to LHRH is prepubertal in all cases.[275, 672] Plasma inhibin and activin concentrations have not been reported. The use of contact thermography in girls with early breast development demonstrated findings in precocious thelarche closer to those of normal prepubertal controls than those of girls with true precocious puberty. Thermographic signs of increased vascularization were absent in precocious thelarche but present at least unilaterally in true precocious puberty.[682]

PREMATURE ISOLATED MENARCHE. Rarely, girls begin periodic vaginal bleeding at age 1 to 9 without any other signs of secondary sexual development.[683, 684] The bleeding can recur for 1 to 6 y and then cease. At the normal age of puberty (3 to 11 y later), secondary sexual development and menses ensue and follow a normal pattern, as does stature. Fertility was later demonstrated after a normal puberty in six patients with this variant of pubertal development. The etiology is uncertain, but it may be a counterpart of premature thelarche.

Isolated menarche may appear before other manifestations of sexual precocity in the McCune-Albright syndrome and in the precocious sexual maturation that can occur in juvenile hypothyroidism.

Before the diagnosis of premature menarche is accepted, all other causes of vaginal bleeding and precocious estrogen secretion and of exposure to exogenous estrogens should be excluded, including neoplasms, granulomas, infection of the vagina or cervix, or a foreign body. In a series of 50 girls who had vaginal bleeding before age 10, a local lesion was found in about 50%; half of the latter had a malignant neoplasm (usually a rhabdomyosarcoma) and other half had no discernible cause.[685] In another report, a foreign body was responsible for 25% of vaginal bleeding in prepubertal girls.[686] A careful examination for trauma such as that caused by sexual abuse is indicated. Urethral prolapse may be misdiagnosed as vaginal bleeding.

PREMATURE ADRENARCHE (PUBARCHE). Premature adrenarche[687–689]—the appearance of pubic hair, axillary hair, or both before age 8 in girls or age 9 in boys, without other signs of puberty or virilization—is caused by precocious secretion of adrenal androgens. The condition is more common in girls and usually occurs after age 6 y, although the onset may be as early as 6 mo.[687, 689] The prevalence is increased in children with CNS abnormalities. The electroencephalogram may be abnormal[71, 526] in the absence of other neurological findings. Familial transmission is rare.[690] Premature adrenarche is a nonprogressive disorder compatible with appropriate progression of further secondary sexual maturation at the normal age of puberty.

Plasma concentrations of DHEA, DHEAS, androstenedione, and testosterone and the excretion of urinary 17-ketosteroids are comparable to values normally found in pubic hair stage 2.[301, 679, 687, 691, 692] ACTH stimulation increases serum DHEA and DHEAS and urinary 17-ketosteroid levels, but the concentrations of plasma 17-hydroxyprogesterone and 17-hydroxypregnenolone do not increase to values found in individuals with congenital adrenal hyperplasia.[691, 693] As in congenital adrenal hyperplasia, dexamethasone suppresses adrenal androgen and androgen precursor secretion.[691, 692] Gonadotropin levels in the basal state and after LHRH are in the prepubertal range.[275, 694] Premature adrenarche occurs independently of gonadarche and is due to some factor other than increased secretion of LHRH or ACTH. Bone age and height are slightly advanced for chronological age. Minimal axillary hair growth and axillary odor may be noted in some patients.[688]

Variant forms of congenital virilizing adrenal hyperplasia caused by 21-hydroxylase (or more rarely 11β-hydroxylase or 3β-hydroxysteroid dehydrogenase) deficiency can be associated with precocious development of sexual hair without other signs of virilization. These patients exhibit an augmented plasma 17-hydroxyprogesterone response to an ACTH challenge. The frequency of patients with premature adrenarche who actually have late-onset congenital adrenal hyperplasia is not known. In one series the estimate was as high as 40%, but other studies suggest that there is at best a small increase in prevalence of late-onset congenital adrenal hyperplasia in patients with precocious pubarche. Bias in selection of patients and differences among ethnic groups may account for the discrepancy.[695] A family constellation is described with a dominant pattern of inheritance[690] of elevated adrenal androgens which presented as premature pubarche; later affected individuals developed hirsutism and amenorrhea.

ADOLESCENT GYNECOMASTIA. (Also see Chapter 15.) Normal pubertal boys in stages 2 and 3 may have either unilateral breast enlargement (approximately 25% of boys[696]) or bilateral breast enlargement (approximately 50 to 65%[697] of boys) of varying degrees, usually between chronological ages 14 to 14½ y or pubic hair stages 3 and 4. In these boys the plasma concentrations of testosterone and estrogen are normal for the stage of puberty. Pubertal gynecomastia is usually associated with an elevated ratio of serum estradiol level to testosterone level.[698–701] In a prospective study adolescent boys with gynecomastia had a lower mean free testosterone concentration, a lower weight, higher plasma TeBG levels, and a tendency toward earlier onset of puberty and more rapid progression through puberty.[696] However, in one study a significant decrease in the concentration ratio of plasma androstenedione to estrone and estradiol and a similarly low ratio of DHEAS to estrone and estradiol were described in boys with pubertal gynecomastia who had normal ratios of plasma testosterone to estrone and estradiol. It was postulated that either decreased adrenal production of androgens or increased peripheral conversion of adrenal androgens to estrogens was important in the development of pubertal gynecomastia.[702] Pubertal gynecomastia usually resolves spontaneously within 1 to 2 y of onset, and reassurance and continued observation are often adequate treatment. Nevertheless, some boys have conspicuous gynecomastia and sufficient psychological distress to warrant a reduction mammoplasty. Rarely, untreated gynecomastia persists into adulthood, as illustrated by a patient who had persistent unilateral gynecomastia that began during puberty and contralateral Poland syndrome of hypoplasia of the chest, breast tissue, and nipple.[703]

Gynecomastia is a component of the Klinefelter syndrome and of variants of the androgen resistance syndromes, including Rosewater syndrome (familial hypogonadism and gynecomastia) and Reifenstein syndrome (hypospadias, hypogonadism, and gynecomastia). These disorders usually have characteristic findings that allow ready differentiation from the normal gynecomastia of puberty[416] (see Chapter 14). Gynecomastia has been described in association with the administration of drugs such as cimetidine, spironolactone, digitalis, and phenothiazines (see Chapter 15).

Macro-Orchidism

The fragile X syndrome is associated with mental retardation, a long face and large prominent ears, and macro-orchidism in 80% of affected pubertal boys. Macro-orchidism may be evident only after careful measurements. The enlarged testes are due to increased interstitial volume and excessive connective tissue, including increased peritubular collagen fibers,[704] rather than to increase in the seminiferous tubules.

Macro-orchidism, without androgenization, is an occasional finding in prepubertal boys with long-standing primary hypothyroidism. This form of testicular enlargement appears to result from increased FSH secretion independent of a pubertal increase in LH secretion or a pubertal LH response to LHRH.

Disorders of Sexual Differentiation with Both Virilization and Feminization at Puberty

Virilization as well as feminization at puberty may occur in a phenotypic female who has a 46,XY karyotype in certain types of male pseudohermaphroditism (see Chapter 14). 17-Oxidoreductase deficiency (a testosterone biosynthetic defect) and incomplete forms of androgen resistance (resulting from defects in the androgen receptor) may present in this manner; however, ambiguous genitalia are usually noted early in life in these conditions. True hermaphrodites with ovarian and testicular tissue may undergo both virilization and feminization at puberty.[416]

REFERENCES

1. Grumbach, MM. Onset of puberty. In: Berenberg SR, ed. Puberty, Biologic and Social Components. Leiden: H. E. Stenfert Kroese, 1975: 1–21.
2. Aristotle. De generatione animalium. In: Tanner JM. A History of the Study of Human Growth. Cambridge: Cambridge University Press, 1981: 7.
3. Marshall WA, Tanner JM. Puberty. In: Falkner F, Tanner JM, eds. Human Growth. Vol 2. 2nd ed. New York: Plenum, 1986: 171–209.
4. Tanner JM. A History of the Study of Human Growth. Cambridge: Cambridge University Press, 1981: 286–298.
5. Tanner JM. Growth at Adolescence. Springfield, IL: Charles C Thomas, 1962.
6. Wyshak G, Frisch RE. Evidence for a secular trend in age of menarche. N Engl J Med 1982; 306:1033–1035.
7. Buffon H. Histoire naturelle. In: Tanner JM. A History of the Study of Human Growth. Cambridge: Cambridge University Press, 1981: 83.
8. Daw SF. Age of boys' puberty in Leipzig, 1727–49, as indicated by voice breaking in J. S. Bach's choir members. Hum Biol 1970; 42:87–89.
9. Kill V. Stature and growth of Norwegian men during past 200 years. Skr Nor Vidensk Akad 1939; 2(6):1–175.
10. Zacharias L, Wurtman RJ, Schatzoff M. Sexual maturation in contemporary American girls. Am J Obstet Gynecol 1970; 108:833–846.
11. Nicholson AB, Hanley C. Indices of physiological maturity: derivation and interrelationships. Child Dev 1953; 24:3–38.

12. Damon A. Larger body size and earlier menarche: the end may be in sight. Soc Biol 1974; 21:8–11.

13. Zacharias L, Rand M, Wurtman R. A prospective study of sexual development in American girls: the statistics of menarche. Obstet Gynecol Surv 1976; 31:325–337.

14. MacMahon B. Age at menarche. In: National Health Survey. DHEW Publication No. (HRA) 74-1615, Series 11, No. 133. Washington, DC: Government Printing Office, 1973: 1.

15. Hartz AJ, Barboriak PN, Wong A. The association of obesity with infertility and related menstrual abnormalities in women. Int J Obes 1979; 3:57–73.

16. Warren MP. The effects of exercise on pubertal progression and reproductive function in girls. J Clin Endocrinol Metab 1980; 51:1150–1157.

17. Osler DC, Crawford JD. Examination of the hypothesis of a critical weight at menarche in ambulatory and bedridden mentally retarded girls. Pediatrics 1973; 51:674–679.

18. Zacharias L, Wurtman RJ. Blindness: its relation to age of menarche. Science 1964; 144:1154–1155.

19. Freyre EA, Ortiz MV. The effect of altitude on adolescent growth and development. J Adolesc Health Care 1988; 9:144–149.

20. Zacharias L, Wurtman RJ. Age at menarche. N Engl J Med 1969; 280:868–875.

21. Drife JO. Breast development in puberty. Ann N Y Acad Sci 1986; 464:58–65.

22. Marshall WA, Tanner JM. Variations in pattern of pubertal changes in girls. Arch Dis Child 1969; 44:291–303.

23. Stratz CH. Der Korper des Kindes und Seine Pflege. Stuttgart: Ferdinand Enke, 1909: 245.

24. Reynolds EL, Wines JV. Individualized differences in physical changes associated with adolescence in girls. Am J Dis Child 1948; 75:329–350.

25. Rohn RD. Papilla (nipple) development during female puberty. J Adolesc Health Care 1982; 2:217–220.

26. McCann J. Color Atlas of Child Sexual Abuse. Chicago: Year Book Medical, 1989.

27. Duke PM, Litt IF, Gross RT. Adolescents self-assessment of sexual maturation. Pediatrics 1980; 66:918–920.

28. Zachmann M, Prader A, Kind HP, et al. Testicular volume during adolescence: cross-sectional and longitudinal studies. Helv Paediatr Acta 1974; 29:61–72.

29. Harlan WR, Harlan EA, Grillo GP. Secondary sex characteristics of girls 12 to 17 years of age: the U.S. Health Examination Survey. J Pediatr 1980; 96:1074–1078.

30. Harlan WR, Grillo GP, Coroni-Huntley J, et al. Secondary sex characteristics of boys 12 to 17 years of age: the U.S. Health Examination Survey. J Pediatr 1979; 95:293–297.

31. Marshall WA, Tanner JM. Variations in the pattern of pubertal changes in boys. Arch Dis Child 1970; 45:13–23.

32. Largo RH, Prader A. Pubertal development in Swiss girls. Helv Paediatr Acta 1983; 38:229–243.

33. Largo RH, Prader A. Pubertal development in Swiss boys. Helv Paediatr Acta 1983; 38:211–228.

34. Peschel ER, Peschel RE. Medical insights into the castrati in opera. Am Sci 1987; 75:578–583.

35. Karlberg P, Taranger J. The somatic development of children in a Swedish urban community. Acta Paediatr Scand [Suppl] 1976; 258:1–148.

36. Traupe H, von Mühlendahl KE, Brämswig J, et al. Acne of the fulminans type following testosterone therapy in three excessively tall boys. Arch Dermatol 1988; 124:414–417.

37. Ross GT. Follicular development: the life cycle of the follicle and puberty. In: Grumbach MM, Sizonenko PC, Aubert ML, eds. Control of the Onset of Puberty. Baltimore: Williams & Wilkins, 1990: 376–386.

38. Peters H, Byskov AG, Grinsted J. Follicular growth in fetal and prepubertal ovaries of humans and other primates. Clin Endocrinol Metab 1978; 7:469–485.

39. Fleischer AC, Shawker TH. The role of sonography in pediatric gynecology. Clin Obstet Gynecol 1987; 30:735–746.

40. Salardi S, Orsini LF, Cacciari E, et al. Pelvic ultrasonography in premenarcheal girls: relation to puberty and sex hormone concentrations. Arch Dis Child 1985; 60:120–125.

41. Apter D, Vihko R. Serum pregnenolone, progesterone, 17-hydroxyprogesterone, testosterone and 5α-dihydrotestosterone during female puberty. J Clin Endocrinol Metab 1977; 45:1039–1048.

42. Metcalf MG, MacKenzie JA. Incidence of ovulation in young women. J Biosoc Sci 1980; 12:345–352.

43. Lemarchand-Beraud T, Zufferey MM, Reymond M. Maturation of the hypothalamo-pituitary ovarian axis in adolescent girls. J Clin Endocrinol Metab 1982; 54:241–246.

44. Gondos B, Kogan SJ. Testicular development during puberty. In: Grumbach MM, Sizonenko PC, Aubert ML, eds. Control of the Onset of Puberty. Baltimore: Williams & Wilkins, 1990: 387–402.

45. Richardson DW, Short RV. Time of onset of sperm production in boys. J Biosoc Sci [Suppl] 1978; 5:15–24.

46. Nielsen CT, Skakkebaek NE, Darling JA, et al. Longitudinal study of testosterone and luteinizing hormone (LH) in relation to spermarche, pubic hair, height and sitting height in normal boys. Acta Endocrinol [Suppl] 1986; 279:98–106.

47. Laron Z, Arad J, Gurewitz R, et al. Age at first conscious ejaculation: a milestone in male puberty. Helv Paediatr Acta 1980; 35:13–20.

48. Tanner JM, Whitehouse RH, Marubini E, et al. The adolescent growth spurt of boys and girls of the Harpenden Growth Study. Ann Hum Biol 1976; 3:109–126.

49. Largo RH, Gasser TH, Prader A. Analysis of the adolescent growth spurt using smoothing spline functions. Ann Hum Biol 1978; 5:421–434.

50. Karlberg J, Fryer JG, Engstrom I, et al. Analysis of linear growth using a mathematical model. II. From 3 to 21 years of age. Acta Paediatr Scand [Suppl] 1987; 337:12–29.

51. Tanner JM, Davies PSW. Clinical longitudinal standards for height and height velocity for North American children. J Pediatr 1985; 107:317–329.

51a. Hägg U, Juranger J. Height and height velocity in early, average and late maturers followed to the age of 25: a prospective longitudinal study of Swedish urban children from birth to adulthood. Ann Hum Biol 1991; 18:47–56.

52. Vanden Eynde B, Vienne D, Vuylsteke-Wauters M, et al. Aerobic power and pubertal peak height velocity in Belgian boys. Eur J Appl Physiol 1988; 57:430–434.

53. Johansen JS, Giwercman A, Hartwell D, et al. Serum bone Gla-protein as a marker of bone growth in children and adolescents: correlation with age, height, serum insulin-like growth factor I, and serum testosterone. J Clin Endocrinol Metab 1988; 67:273–278.

54. Bourguignon JP. Linear growth as a function of age at onset of puberty and sex steroid dosage: therapeutic implications. Endocr Rev 1988; 9:467–488.

55. McKusick VA. Heritable Disorders of Connective Tissue. St. Louis: C. V. Mosby, 1972: 73–74.

56. Tanner JM, Whitehouse RH, Hughes PCR, et al. Relative importance of growth hormone and sex steroids for the growth at puberty of trunk length, limb length, and muscle width in growth hormone–deficient children. J Pediatr 1976; 89:1000–1008.

57. Elster AD, Chen MY, Key LL. Pituitary gland: MR imaging of physiologic hypertrophy in adolescence. Radiology 1990; 174:681–685.

58. Attie MK, Ramirez NR, Conte FA, et al. The pubertal growth spurt in eight patients with true precocious puberty and growth hormone deficiency: evidence for a direct role of sex steroids. J Clin Endocrinol Metab 1990; 71:975–983.

59. Miller JD, Tannenbaum GS, Colle E, et al. Daytime pulsatile growth hormone secretion during childhood and adolescence. J Clin Endocrinol Metab 1982; 55:989–994.

60. Ross JL, Pescovitz OH, Barnes K, et al. Growth hormone secretory dynamics in children with precocious puberty. J Pediatr 1987; 110:369–372.

61. Costin G, Kaufman FR. Growth hormone secretory patterns in children with short stature. J Pediatr 1987; 110:362–368.

62. Costin G, Kaufman FR, Brasel JA. Growth hormone secretory dynamics in subjects with normal stature. J Pediatr 1989; 115:537–544.

63. Garnier P, Raynaud F, Job JC. Growth hormone secretion during sleep. I. Comparison with GH responses to conventional pharmacologic stimuli in pubertal and early pubertal short subjects. Effects of treatment with human GH in patients with discrepant measurements of GH secretion. Horm Res 1988; 29:133–139.

64. Link K, Blizzard RM, Evans WS. The effect of androgens on the pulsatile release and twenty-four-hour mean concentration of growth hormone in peripubertal males. J Clin Endocrinol Metab 1986; 62:159–164.

65. Martha PM Jr, Rogol AD, Veldhuis JD. Alterations in the pulsatile properties of circulating growth hormone concentrations during puberty in boys. J Clin Endocrinol Metab 1989; 69:563–570.

66. Mauras N, Blizzard RM, Link K. Augmentation of growth hormone secretion during puberty: evidence for a pulse amplitude–modulated phenomenon. J Clin Endocrinol Metab 1987; 64:596–601.

67. Mansfield MJ, Rudlin CR, Crigler Jr, et al. Changes in growth and serum growth hormone and plasma somatomedin-C levels during suppression of gonadal sex steroid secretion in girls with central precocious puberty. J Clin Endocrinol Metab 1988; 66:3–9.

68. Rimoin DL, Merimee TJ, Rabinowitz D, et al. Genetic aspects of clinical endocrinology. Recent Prog Horm Res 1968; 24:365–437.

69. Phillips JA III. Inherited defects in growth hormone synthesis and action. In: Scriver CR, Beaudet AL, Sly WS, et al., eds. The Metabolic Basis of Inherited Disease. 6th ed. New York: McGraw-Hill, 1989; 1965–1983.

70. Aynsley-Green A, Zachmann M, Prader A. Interrelation of the therapeutic effects of growth hormone and testosterone on growth in hypopituitarism. J Pediatr 1976; 89:992–999.

71. Grumbach MM, Richards GE, Conte FA, et al. Clinical disorders of adrenal function and puberty: an assessment of the role of the adrenal cortex in normal and abnormal puberty in man and evidence for an ACTH-like pituitary adrenal androgen stimulating hormone. In: James VHT, Serio M, Giusti G, et al., eds. The Endocrine Function of the Human Adrenal Cortex, Serono Symposium. New York: Academic, 1977: 583–612.

72. Bala RM, Lopatka J, Leung A, et al. Serum immunoreactive somatomedin levels in normal adults, pregnant women at term, children at various ages, and children with constitutionally delayed growth. J Clin Endocrinol Metab 1981; 52:508–512.

73. Harris DA, Van Vliet G, Egli CA, et al. Somatomedin-C in normal puberty and in true precocious puberty before and after treatment with a potent luteinizing hormone–releasing hormone agonist. J Clin Endocrinol Metab 1985; 61:152–159.

74. Greulich WS, Pyle SI. Radiographic Atlas of Skeletal Development of the Hand and Wrist. Stanford, CA: Stanford University Press, 1959.

75. Tanner JM, Whitehouse RH, Marshall WA, et al. Assessment of Skeletal Maturity and Prediction of Adult Height: TW 2 Method. New York: Academic, 1975.

76. Bayley N, Pinneau SR. Tables for predicting adult height from skeletal age: revised for use with the Greulich-Pyle standards. J Pediatr 1952; 40:423–441.

77. Roche AF, Wainer H, Thissen D. The RWT method for the prediction of adult stature. Pediatrics 1975; 56:1026–1033.

78. Walker RN. Standards for somatotyping children. I. Prediction of young adult height from children's growth data. Ann Hum Biol 1974; 1:149–158.

79. Roche AF. Skeletal maturity of children 6–11 years: racial, geographic area of residence, socioeconomic differentials. In: National Health Survey. DHEW Vital and Health Statistics Series 11, No. 149. Washington, DC: Government Printing Office, 1975.

80. Gilsanz V, Gibbens DT, Roe TF, et al. Vertebral bone density in children: effect of puberty. Radiology 1988; 166:847–850.

81. Cheek DB. Body composition, hormones, nutrition and adolescent growth. In: Grumbach MM, Grave GD, Mayer FE, eds. Control of the Onset of Puberty. New York: John Wiley & Sons, 1974: 424–447.

81a. Malina RM. Growth of muscle tissue and muscle mass. In: Falkner F, Tanner JM, eds. Human Growth. Vol 2. 2nd ed. New York: Plenum, 1986: 77–99.

82. Forbes GB. Puberty: body composition. In: Berenberg SR, ed. Puberty, Biologic and Social Components. Leiden: H. E. Stenfert Kroese, 1975: 132–145.

83. Forbes GB. Body composition in adolescence. In: Falkner F, Tanner JM, eds. Human Growth. Vol 2. 2nd ed. New York: Plenum, 1986; 119–145.

84. Frisancho AR, Flegel PN. Advanced maturation with centripetal fat pattern. Hum Biol 1982: 54:717–727.

85. Garn SM. Fat weight and fat placement in the female. Science 1957; 125:1091–1092.

86. Ridder CM, Bruning PF, Zonderland ML, et al. Body fat mass, body fat distribution, and plasma hormones in early puberty in females. J Clin Endocrinol Metab 1990; 70:888–893.

87. Frisch RE, Revelle R. Height and weight at menarche and a hypothesis of critical body weights and adolescent events. Science 1970; 169:397–399.

88. Liker HR, Barnes KM, Comite F, et al. Blood pressure and body size in precocious puberty. Acta Paediatr Scand 1988; 77:294–298.

89. Voors AW, Webber LS, Frerichs RR, et al. Body height and body mass as determinants of basal blood pressure in children—the Bogalusa Heart Study. Am J Epidemiol 1977; 106:101–108.

90. Voors AW, Harsha DW, Webber LS, et al. Relation of blood pressure to stature in healthy young adults. Am J Epidemiol 1982; 115:833–840.

91. Hsu PH, Mathewson FAL, Rabkin SW. Blood pressure and body mass index patterns—a longitudinal study. J Chronic Dis 1977; 30:93–113.

92. Londe S, Johanson A, Kronemer NS, et al. Blood pressure and puberty. J Pediatr 1975; 87:896–900.

93. Report of the Second Task Force on Blood Pressure Control in Children—1987. Blood pressure nomograms. Pediatrics 1987; 79:1–25.

94. Michael RP, Zumpke D. Behavioral changes associated with puberty in higher primates and the human. In: Grumbach MM, Sizonenko PC, Aubert ML, eds. Control of the Onset of Puberty. Baltimore: Williams & Wilkins, 1990: 574–587.

95. Hall GS. Adolescence; Its Psychology and Its Relations to Physiology, Anthropology, Sociology, Sex, Crime, Religion and Education. New York: Appleton, 1904.

96. Weiner IB, del Gaudio AC. Psychopathology in adolescence. An epidemiological study. In: Chess S, Thomas A, eds. Annual Progress in Child Psychiatry and Child Development. New York: Brunner/Mazel, 1977: 471–488.

97. Offer D. The Psychological World of the Teenager: A Study of Normal Adolescent Boys. New York: Basic Books, 1969.

98. Masterson JF Jr. The psychiatric significance of adolescent turmoil. Am J Psychiatry 1968; 124:1549–1554.

98a. Rutter M, Graham P, Chadwick OFD, et al. Adolescent turmoil: fact or fiction? J Child Psychol Psychiatry 1976; 17:35–56.

98b. Udry RR, Billy JOG, Morris NM, et al. Serum androgenic hormones motivate sexual behavior in boys. Fertil Steril 1985; 43:90–94.

98c. Sussman EJ, Inoff-Germain G, Nottlemann ED, et al. Hormones, emotional dispositions and aggressive attitudes with early adolescents. Child Dev 1987; 58:1114–1134.

98d. Warren MP, Brooks-Gunn J. Mood and behavior at adolescence: evidence for hormonal factors. J Clin Endocrinol Metab 1989; 69:77–83.

99. Grumbach MM, Roth JC, Kaplan SL, et al. Hypothalamic-pituitary regulation of puberty in man: evidence and concepts derived from clinical research. In: Grumbach MM, Grave GD, Mayer FE, eds. Control of the Onset of Puberty. New York: John Wiley & Sons, 1974: 115–166.

100. Grumbach MM, Kaplan SL. The neuroendocrinology of human puberty: an ontogenetic perspective. In: Grumbach MM, Sizonenko PC, Aubert ML, eds. Control of the Onset of Puberty. Baltimore: Williams & Wilkins, 1990: 1–68.

101. Kaplan SL, Grumbach MM, Aubert ML. The ontogenesis of pituitary hormones and hypothalamic factors in the human fetus: maturation of central nervous system regulation of anterior pituitary function. Recent Prog Horm Res 1976; 32:161–243.

102. Gluckman PD, Grumbach MM, Kaplan SL. The human fetal hypothalamus and pituitary gland; the maturation of neuroendocrine mechanisms controlling the secretion of fetal pituitary growth hormone, prolactin, gonadotropin, and adrenocorticotropin-related peptides. In: Tulchinsky D, Ryan KJ, eds. Maternal-Fetal Endocrinology. Philadelphia: W. B. Saunders, 1980: 196–232.

103. Faiman C, Winter JSD. Gonadotropins and sex hormone patterns in puberty: clinical data. In: Grumbach MM, Grave GD, Mayer FE, eds. Control of the Onset of Puberty. New York: John Wiley & Sons, 1974: 32–61.

104. Dunkel L, Alfthan H, Stenman U, et al. Pulsatile secretion of LH and FSH in prepubertal and early pubertal boys revealed by ultrasensitive time-resolved immunofluorometric assays. Pediatr Res 1990; 27:215–219.

105. Dunkel L, Alfthan H, Stenman U, et al. Gonadal control of pulsatile secretion of luteinizing hormone and follicle-stimulating hormone in prepubertal boys evaluated by ultrasensitive time-resolved immunofluorometric assays. J Clin Endocrinol Metab 1990; 70:107–114.

106. Corley KP, Valk TW, Kelch RP, et al. Estimation of GnRH pulse amplitude during pubertal development. Pediatr Res 1981; 15:157–162.

107. Jakacki RI, Kelch RP, Sauder SE, et al. Pulsatile secretion of luteinizing hormone in children. J Clin Endocrinol Metab 1982; 55:453–458.

108. Kelch RP, Clemons LE, Markovs M, et al. Metabolism and effects of synthetic gonadotropin-releasing hormone (GnRH) in children and adults. J Clin Endocrinol Metab 1975; 40:53–61.

109. Roth JC, Kelch RP, Kaplan SL, et al. FSH and LH response to luteinizing hormone–releasing factor in prepubertal and pubertal children, adult males and patients with hypogonadotropic and hypergonadotropic hypogonadism. J Clin Endocrinol Metab 1972; 35:926–930.

110. Roth JC, Grumbach MM, Kaplan SL. Effect of synthetic luteinizing hormone–releasing factor on serum testosterone and gonadotropins in prepubertal, pubertal, and adult males. J Clin Endocrinol Metab 1973; 37:680–686.

111. Job JC, Garnier PE, Chaussain JL, et al. Elevation of serum gonadotropins (LH and FSH) after releasing hormone (LH-RH) injection in normal children and in patients with disorders of puberty. J Clin Endocrinol Metab 1972; 35:473–476.

112. Boyar R, Finkelstein J, Roffwarg H, et al. Synchronization of augmented luteinizing hormone secretion with sleep during puberty. N Engl J Med 1972; 287:582–586.

113. Boyar RM, Rosenfeld RS, Kapen S, et al. Simultaneous augmented secretion of luteinizing hormone and testosterone during sleep. J Clin Invest 1974; 54:609–618.

114. Kapen S, Boyar RM, Hellman L, et al. Twenty-four hour patterns of luteinizing hormone secretion in humans: ontogenic and sexual considerations. Prog Brain Res 1975; 42:103–113.

115. Hale PM, Khoury S, Foster CM, et al. Increased luteinizing hormone pulse frequency during sleep in early to midpubertal boys: effects of testosterone infusion. J Clin Endocrinol Metab 1988; 66:785–791.

116. Foster CM, Hassing JM, Padmanabhan V, et al. Testosterone infusion produces adult male luteinizing hormone secretory patterns in pubertal boys. J Clin Endocrinol Metab 1989; 69:1213–1220.

117. Hassing JM, Padmanabhan V, Kelch RP, et al. Differential regulation of serum immunoreactive luteinizing hormone and bioactive follicle-stimulating hormone by testosterone in early pubertal boys. J Clin Endocrinol Metab 1990; 70:1082–1089.

118. Wennink JM, Delemarre-Van deWaal HA, van Kessel H, et al. Luteinizing hormone secretion patterns in boys at the onset of puberty measured using a highly sensitive immunoradiometric assay. J Clin Endocrinol Metab 1988; 67:924–928.

119. Apter D, Cacciatore B, Alfthan H, et al. Serum luteinizing hormone concentrations increase 100-fold in females from 7 years to adulthood, as measured by time-resolved immunofluorometric assay. J Clin Endocrinol Metab 1989; 68:53–57.

120. Burr IM, Sizonenko PC, Kaplan SL, et al. Hormonal changes in puberty. I. Correlation of serum luteinizing hormone and follicle stimulating hormone with stages of puberty, testicular size, and bone age in normal boys. Pediatr Res 1970; 4:25–35.

121. August GP, Grumbach MM, Kaplan SL. Hormonal changes in puberty. III. Correlation of plasma testosterone, LH, FSH, testicular size and bone age with male pubertal development. J Clin Endocrinol Metab 1972; 34:319–326.

122. Sizonenko PC, Burr IM, Kaplan SL, et al. Hormonal changes in puberty. II. Correlation of serum luteinizing hormone and follicle stimulating hormone with stages of puberty and bone age in normal girls. Pediatr Res 1970; 4:36–45.

123. Jenner MR, Kelch RP, Kaplan SL, et al. Hormonal changes in puberty. IV. Plasma estradiol, LH, and FSH in prepubertal children, pubertal females, and in precocious puberty, premature thelarche, hypogonadism, and in a child with a feminizing ovarian tumor. J Clin Endocrinol Metab 1972; 34:521–530.

124. Spratt DI, Crowley WF Jr. Pituitary and gonadal responsiveness is enhanced during GnRH-induced puberty. Am J Physiol 1988; 254:E652–E657.

125. Beitins IZ, Padmanabhan V. Bioactivity of gonadotropins. Endocrinol Metab Clin North Am 1991; 20:85–120.

125a. Wang C, Zhong CQ, Leung A, et al. Serum bioactive follicle-stimulating hormone levels in girls with precocious sexual development. J Clin Endocrinol Metab 1990; 70:615–619.

126. Lucky AW, Rich BH, Rosenfield RL, et al. LH bioactivity increases more than immunoreactivity during puberty. J Pediatr 1980; 97:205–213.

127. Reiter EO, Beitins IZ, Ostrea T, et al. Bioassayable luteinizing hormone during childhood and adolescence and in patients with delayed pubertal development. J Clin Endocrinol Metab 1982; 54:155–161.

128. Reiter EO, Biggs DE, Veldhuis JD, et al. Pulsatile release of bioactive luteinizing hormone in prepubertal girls: discordance with immunoreactive luteinizing hormone pulses. Pediatr Res 1987; 21:409–413.

129. Weinstein RL, Kelch RP, Jenner MR, et al. Secretion of unconjugated androgens and estrogens by the normal and abnormal human testis before and after hCG. J Clin Invest 1974; 53:1.

130. Peterson RE, Imperato-McGinley J, Gautier T, et al. Male pseudohermaphroditism due to steroid 5α-reductase deficiency. Am J Med 1977; 62:170–191.

131. Judd HL, Parker DD, Yen SSC. Sleep-wake patterns of LH and testosterone release in prepubertal boys. J Clin Endocrinol Metab 1977; 44:865–869.

132. Knoor D, Bidlingmaier F, Butenandt O, et al. Plasma testosterone in male puberty. I. Physiology of plasma testosterone. Acta Endocrinol 1974; 75:181–194.

133. Angsusingha K, Kenny FM, Nankin HR, et al. Unconjugated estrone, estradiol and FSH and LH in prepubertal and pubertal males and females. J Clin Endocrinol Metab 1974; 39:63–68.

134. Anderson DC. Sex hormone–binding globulin. Clin Endocrinol 1974; 3:69–95.

135. Lindstedt G, Lundberg P, Hammond GL, et al. Sex hormone binding globulin—still many questions. Scand J Clin Lab Invest 1985; 45:1–6.

136. Maruyama Y, Aoki N, Suzuki S, et al. SHBG, testosterone, estradiol and DHA in prepuberty and puberty. Acta Endocrinol 1987; 114:60–67.

137. Horst HJ, Bartsch W, Dirksen-Thedens I. Plasma testosterone, sex hormone binding globulin capacity and per cent binding of testosterone and 5α-dihydrotestosterone in prepubertal and adult males. J Clin Endocrinol Metab 1977; 45:522–527.

138. Bartsch W, Horst HJ, Derwah KM. Interrelationships between sex hormone–binding globulin and 17β-estradiol, testosterone, 5α-dihydrotestosterone, thyroxine, and triiodothyronine in prepubertal and pubertal girls. J Clin Endocrinol Metab 1980; 50:1053–1056.

139. August GP, Tkachuk M, Grumbach MM. Plasma testosterone-binding affinity and testosterone in umbilical cord plasma, late pregnancy, prepubertal children and adults. J Clin Endocrinol Metab 1969; 29:891–899.

140. Cunningham SK, McKenna TJ. Evaluation of an immunoassay for plasma sex hormone–binding globulin: comparison with steroid-binding assay under physiological and pathological conditions. Ann Clin Biochem 1988; 25:360–366.

141. Cunningham SK, Loughlin T, Culliton M, et al. Plasma sex hormone–binding globulin levels decrease during the second decade of life irrespective of pubertal status. J Clin Endocrinol Metab 1984; 58:915–918.

142. Rudd BT, Rayner PH, Thomas PH. Observations on the role of GH/IGF-1 and sex hormone binding globulin (SHBG) in the pubertal development of growth hormone deficient (GHD) children. Acta Endocrinol Suppl 1986; 279:164–169.

143. Aubert ML, Sizonenko PC, Kaplan SL, et al. The ontogenesis of human prolactin from fetal life to puberty. In: Crosignani PG, Robyn C, eds. Prolactin and Human Reproduction. New York: Academic, 1977: 9–20.

144. De Jong FH. Inhibin. Physiol Rev 1988; 68:555–607.

145. Burger HG, McLachlan RI, Bangah M, et al. Serum inhibin concentrations rise throughout normal male and female puberty. J Clin Endocrinol Metab 1988; 67:689–694.

146. Hudson PL, Dougas I, Donahoe PK, et al. An immunoassay to detect human mullerian inhibiting substance in males and females during normal development. J Clin Endocrinol Metab 1990; 70:16–22.

147. Josso N, Legeai L, Forest MG, et al. An enzyme linked immunoassay for anti-mullerian hormone: a new tool for the evaluation of testicular function in infants and children. J Clin Endocrinol Metab 1990; 70:23–27.

148. Rosenfield RI, Furlanetto R, Bock D. Relationship of somatomedin-C concentrations to pubertal changes. J Pediatr 1983; 103:723–728.

149. Luna AM, Wilson DM, Wibbelsman CJ, et al. Somatomedins in adolescence: a cross-sectional study of the effect of puberty on plasma insulin-like growth factor I and II levels. J Clin Endocrinol Metab 1983; 57:268–271.

150. Amiel SA, Caprio S, Sherwin RS, et al. Insulin resistance of puberty: a defect restricted to peripheral glucose metabolism. J Clin Endocrinol Metab 1991; 72:277–282.

151. Bloch CA, Clemons P, Sperling M. Puberty decreases insulin sensitivity. J Pediatr 1987; 110:481–487.

152. Amiel SA, Sherwin RS, Simonson DC, et al. Impaired insulin action in puberty. A contributing factor to poor glycemic control in adolescents with diabetes. N Engl J Med 1986; 315:215–219.

153. Hindmarsh PC, Matthews DR, DiSilvio L, et al. Relation between height velocity and fasting insulin concentrations. Arch Dis Child 1988; 63:665–666.

154. Rosenbloom AL, Wheeler L, Bianchi R, et al. Age-adjusted analysis of insulin responses during normal and abnormal glucose tolerance tests in children and adolescents. Diabetes 1975; 24:820–828.

155. Hindmarsh P, Di Silvio L, Pringle PJ, et al. Changes in serum insulin concentration during puberty and their relationship to growth hormone. Clin Endocrinol 1988; 28:381–388.

156. Kirkland RT, Keenan BS, Probstfield JL, et al. Decrease in plasma high-density lipoprotein cholesterol levels at puberty in boys with delayed adolescence. Correlation with plasma testosterone levels. JAMA 1987; 257:502–507.

157. Sorva R, Kuusi T, Dunkel L, et al. Effects of endogenous sex steroids on serum lipoproteins and postheparin plasma lipolytic enzymes. J Clin Endocrinol Metab 1988; 66:408–413.

158. Grumbach MM, Kaplan SL. Fetal pituitary hormones and the maturation of central nervous system regulation of anterior pituitary function. In: Gluck L, ed. Modern Perinatal Medicine. Chicago: Year Book Medical, 1974: 247–271.

159. Grumbach MM. The neuroendocrinology of puberty. In: Krieger DT, Hughes JC, eds. Neuroendocrinology. Sunderland, MA: Sinauer Associates, 1980: 249–258.

160. Kaplan SL, Grumbach MM. Pituitary and placental gonadotropins and sex steroids in the human and sub-human primate fetus. Clin Endocrinol Metab 1978; 7:487–511.

161. Kaplan SL, Grumbach MM. Pathogenesis of sexual precocity. In: Grumbach MM, Sizonenko PC, Aubert ML, eds. Control of the Onset of Puberty. Baltimore: Williams & Wilkins, 1990: 620–660.

162. Donovan BT, van der Werff JJ. Physiology of Puberty. Baltimore: Williams & Wilkins, 1965.

163. Critchlow V, Bar-Sela ME. Control of the onset of puberty. In: Martini L, Ganong WF, eds. Neuroendocrinology. Vol II. New York: Academic, 1967: 101–162.

164. Wilkins L. The Diagnosis and Treatment of Endocrine Disorders in Childhood and Adolescence. Springfield, IL: Charles C Thomas, 1965.

165. King JC, Anthony ELP, Fitzgerald DM, et al. Luteinizing hormone–releasing hormone neurons in human preoptic/hypothalamus: differential intraneuronal localization of immunoreactive forms. J Clin Endocrinol Metab 1985; 60:88–97.

166. Mellon PL, Windle JJ, Goldsmith PC, et al. Immortalization of hypothalamic GnRH neurons by genetically targeted tumorigenesis. Neuron 1990; 5:1–10.

167. Adelman JP, Mason AJ, Hayflick JS, et al. Isolation of the gene and hypothalamic cDNA for the common precursor of gonadotropin-releasing hormone and prolactin release–inhibiting factor in human and rat. Proc Natl Acad Sci USA 1986; 83:179–183.

168. Martinez de la Escalera G, Choi ALH, Weiner RI. Dynamics of GnRH secretion from perfused GT1-1 cells. Soc Neurosci Abstr 1990; 16:284.

169. Marshall PE, Goldsmith PC. Neuroregulatory and neuroendocrine GnRH pathways in the hypothalamus and forebrain of the baboon. Brain Res 1980; 193:353–372.

170. Witkin JW, Silverman AJ. Synaptology of LHRH neurons in rat preoptic area. Peptides 1985; 6:263–271.

171. Reichlin S. Neuroendocrinology. In: Wilson JD, Foster DW, eds. Williams Textbook of Endocrinology. 8th ed. Philadelphia: W.B. Saunders, 1992; 135–219.

172. Gorski RA. Extrahypothalamic influences on gonadotropin secretion. In: Grumbach MM, Grave GD, Mayer FE, eds. Control of the Onset of Puberty. New York: John Wiley & Sons, 1974: 182.

173. Gorski RA. Maturation of neural mechanisms and the pubertal process. In: Grumbach MM, Sizonenko PC, Aubert ML, eds. Control of the Onset of Puberty. Baltimore: Williams & Wilkins, 1990: 259–281.

174. Gallo RV. Neuroendocrine regulation of pulsatile luteinizing hormone in the rat. Neuroendocrinology 1980; 20:122–131.

175. Ying S-Y. Inhibins, activins, and follistatins: gonadal proteins modulating the secretion of follicle-stimulating hormone. Endocr Rev 1988; 9:267–293.

176. Ojeda SR, Andrews WW, Advis JP. Recent advances in the endocrinology of puberty. Endocr Rev 1980; 1:228–257.

177. Huckle W, Conn PM. Molecular mechanisms of gonadotropin releasing hormone action. II. The effector system. Endocr Rev 1988; 9:387–395.

178. Hazum E, Conn PM. Molecular mechanism of gonadotropin releasing hormone (GnRH) action. I. The GnRH receptor. Endocr Rev 1988; 9:379–386. (Erratum in Endocr Rev 1989 10:229.)

179. Short RV. The evolution of human reproduction. Proc R Soc Med 1976; 195:3–24.

180. Bronson FH, Rissman EF. The biology of puberty. Biol Rev 1986; 61:157–195.

181. Reiter EO, Grumbach MM. Neuroendocrine control mechanisms and the onset of puberty. Annu Rev Physiol 1982; 44:595–613.

182. Spratt DI, O'Dea LSL, Schoenfeld D, et al. Neuroendocrine-gonadal axis in men: frequent sampling of LH, FSH, and testosterone. Am J Physiol 1988; 254:E658–E666.

183. Crowley WF, Filicori M, Spratt DI, et al. The physiology of gonadotropin releasing hormone (GnRH) secretion in men and women. Recent Prog Horm Res 1985; 41:473–526.

184. Wildt L, Hausler A, Marshall G, et al. Frequency and amplitude of gonadotropin-releasing hormone stimulation and gonadotropin secretion in the rhesus monkey. Endocrinology 1981; 109:376–385.

185. Gross KM, Matsumoto AM, Brenner WJ. Differential control of luteinizing hormone and follicle-stimulating hormone secretion by luteinizing hormone–releasing hormone pulse frequency in man. J Clin Endocrinol Metab 1987; 64:675–680.

186. Finkelstein JS, Budger TM, O'Dea SStL, et al. Effects of decreasing the frequency of gonadotropin-releasing hormone stimulation on gonadotropin secretion in gonadotropin-releasing hormone–deficient men and perifused rat pituitary cells. J Clin Invest 1988; 81:1725–1733.

187. Knobil E. The neuroendocrine control of the menstrual cycle. Recent Prog Horm Res 1980; 36:53–88.

188. Nett TM, Crowder ME, Moss GE, et al. GnRH-receptor interaction. v. Down-regulation of pituitary receptors for GnRH in ovariectomized ewes by infusion of homologous hormone. Biol Reprod 1981; 24:1145–1155.

189. Schwanzel-Fukuda M, Pfaff DW. Origin of luteinizing hormone–releasing hormone neurons. Nature 1989; 338:161–164.

190. Wray S, Grant P, Gainer H. Evidence that cells expressing luteinizing hormone-releasing hormone mRNA in the mouse are derived from progenitor cells in the olfactory placode. Proc Natl Acad Sci USA 1989; 86:8132–8136.

191. Wray S, Nieburgs A, Elkabes S. Spatiotemporal cell expression for luteinizing hormone–releasing hormone in the prenatal mouse: evidence for an embryonic origin in the olfactory placode. Dev Brain Res 1989; 46:309–318.

192. Ronnekleiv OK, Resko JA. Ontogeny of gonadotropin-releasing hormone–containing neurons in early fetal development of rhesus macaques. Endocrinology 1990; 126:498–511.

193. Schwanzel-Fukuda M, Bick D, Pfaff DW. Luteinizing hormone–releasing hormone (LHRH)–expressing cells do not migrate normally in an inherited hypogonadal (Kallmann) syndrome. Mol Brain Res 1989; 6:311–326.

194. Gluckman PD, Grumbach MM, Kaplan SL. The neuroendocrine regulation and function of growth hormone and prolactin in the mammalian fetus. Endocr Rev 1981; 2:363–395.

195. Clark SJ, Hauffa BP, Rodens KP, et al. Hormone ontogeny in the ovine fetus. XIX. The effect of a potent luteinizing hormone–releasing factor agonist on gonadotropin and testosterone release in the fetus and neonate. Pediatr Res 1989; 25:347–352.

196. Clark SJ, Ellis N, Styne DM, et al. Hormone ontogeny in the ovine fetus. XVII. Demonstration of pulsatile luteinizing hormone secretion by the fetal pituitary gland. Endocrinology 1984; 115:1774–1779.

197. Huhtaniemi I, Lautala P. Stimulation of steroidogenesis in human fetal testes by the placenta during perifusion. J Steroid Biochem 1979; 10:109–113.

198. Molsberry RL, Carr BR, Mendelson CR, et al. Human chorionic gonadotropin binding to human fetal testes as a function of gestational age. J Clin Endocrinol Metab 1982; 55:791–794.

199. Huhtaniemi IT, Yamamoto M, Ranta T, et al. Follicle-stimulating hormone receptors appear earlier in the primate fetal testis than in the ovary. J Clin Endocrinol Metab 1987; 65:1210–1214.

200. Baker RG, Scrimgeour JB. Development of the gonad in normal and anencephalic human fetuses. J Reprod Fertil 1980; 68:193–199.

201. Grumbach MM, Kaplan SL. Ontogenesis of growth hormone, insulin, prolactin, and gonadotropin in the human foetus. In: Foetal and Neonatal Physiology, Proceedings, Sir Joseph Barcroft Centenary Symposium. Cambridge: Cambridge University Press, 1973: 462–497.

202. Gluckman PD, Marti Henneberg C, Kaplan SL, et al. Hormone ontogeny in the ovine fetus. XIV. The effect of 17β-estradiol infusion on fetal plasma gonadotropins and prolactin and the maturation of sex steroid–dependent negative feedback. Endocrinology 1983; 112:1618–1623.

203. Groom GV, Boyns AR. Effect of hypothalamic releasing factor and steroids on release of gonadotrophins by organ culture of human fetal pituitary glands. J Endocrinol 1973; 59:511–522.

204. Jaffe AB, Mulcahey JJ, DiBabio AM, et al. Peptide regulation of pituitary and target tissue function and growth in the primate fetus. Recent Prog Horm Res 1988; 44:431–544.

205. Takagi ST, Yoshida T, Tsubata K, et al. Sex differences in fetal gonadotropins and androgens. J Steroid Biochem 1977; 8:609–620.

206. Thliveris JA, Currie RW. Observations on the hypothalamo-hypophyseal portal vasculature in the developing human fetus. Am J Anat 1980; 157:441–444.

207. Hart CS, Grumbach MM, Kaplan SL. The effect of fetal castration on hypothalamic pituitary gonadotropin unit in the ovine fetus. Endocr Soc Abstr 1990; 30.

208. Albers N, Bettendorf M, Hart CS, et al. Hormone ontogeny in the ovine fetus. XXIII. Pulsatile administration of follicle-stimulating hormone stimulates inhibin production and decreases testosterone synthesis in the ovine fetal gonad. Endocrinology 1989; 124:3089–3094.

209. Albers N, Hart CS, Kaplan SL, et al. Hormone ontogeny in the ovine fetus. XXIV. Porcine follicular fluid "inhibins" selectively suppress plasma follicle-stimulating hormone in the ovine fetus. Endocrinology 1989; 125:675–678.

210. Corbier P, Dehenin L, Castanier M, et al. Sex differences in serum luteinizing hormone and testosterone in the human neonate during the first few hours after birth. J Clin Endocrinol Metab 1990; 71:1347–1348.

211. Winter JSD, Faiman C, Hobson WC, et al. Pituitary-gonadal regulations in infancy. I. Patterns of serum gonadotropin concentrations from birth to four years of age in man and chimpanzee. J Clin Endocrinol Metab 1975; 40:545–551.

212. Forest MG. Pituitary gonadotropin and sex steroid secretion during the first two years of life. In: Grumbach MM, Sizonenko PC, Aubert ML, eds. Control of the Onset of Puberty. Baltimore: Williams & Wilkins, 1990: 451–478.

213. Grumbach MM. The central nervous system and the onset of puberty. In: Falkner F, Tanner JM, eds. Human Growth. Vol 2. New York: Plenum, 1978: 215–238.

214. Frisch RE. Fatness of girls from menarche to age 18 with a nomogram. Hum Biol 1976; 48:353–359.

215. Frisch RE, Wyshak G, Vincent L. Delayed menarche and amenorrhea in ballet dancers. Med Intell 1980; 303:17–18.

216. Frisch RE, Gotz-Welbergen AV, McArthur JW, et al. Delayed menarche and amenorrhea of college athletes in relation to age of onset of training. JAMA 1981; 246:1559–1564.

217. McArthur JW, Bullen BA, Beitins IZ, et al. Hypothalamic amenorrhea in runners of normal body composition. Endocr Res Commun 1980; 7:13–25.

218. Cameron N, Mitchell J, Meyer D, et al. Secondary sexual development of "Cape coloured" girls following kwashiorkor. Ann Hum Biol 1988; 15:65–75.

219. Johnston FE, Roche AF, Schell LM, et al. Critical weight at menarche. Am J Dis Child 1975; 129:19–23.

220. Cameron N. Weight and skinfold variation at menarche and the critical body weight hypothesis. Ann Hum Biol 1976; 3:279–282.

221. Billewicz WS, Fellowes HM, Hytten CA. Comments on the critical metabolic mass and the age of menarche. Ann Hum Biol 1976; 3:51–59.

222. Penny R, Goldstein IP, Frasier SD. Gonadotropin excretion and body composition. Pediatrics 1978; 61:294–300.

223. Odell WD, Swerdloff RS. Etiologies of sexual maturation: a model system based on the sexually maturing rat. Recent Prog Horm Res 1976; 32:245–288.

224. Davidson JM. Hypothalamic-pituitary regulation of puberty: evidence from animal experimentation. In: Grumbach MM, Grave GD, Mayer FE, eds. Control of the Onset of Puberty. New York: John Wiley & Sons, 1974: 79–103.

225. Ramirez VD. Endocrinology of puberty. In: Greep RO, Astwood EB, eds. Handbook of Physiology. Sect 7: Endocrinology. Vol II. Female Reproductive System. Part 1. Washington, DC: American Physiological Society, 1973: 1–28.

226. Lenko HL, Lang U, Aubert ML, et al. Hormonal changes in puberty. VII. Lack of variation of daytime plasma melatonin. J Clin Endocrinol Metab 1982; 54:1056–1058.

227. Cohen HN, Hay ID, Annesley TM, et al. Serum immunoreactive melatonin in boys with delayed puberty. Clin Endocrinol 1982; 17:517–521.

228. Sklar CA, Conte FA, Kaplan SL, et al. Human chorionic gonadotropin–secreting pineal tumor; relation to pathogenesis and sex limitation of sexual precocity. J Clin Endocrinol Metab 1981; 53:656–660.

229. Germak JA, Knobil E. Control of puberty in the rhesus monkey. In: Grumbach MM, Sizonenko PC, Aubert ML, eds. Control of the Onset of Puberty. Baltimore: Williams & Wilkins, 1990: 46–66.

230. Ojeda SR, Smith-White S, Advis JP, et al. First preovulatory gonadotropin surge in the rodent. In: Grumbach MM, Sizonenko PC, Aubert ML, eds. Control of the Onset of Puberty. Baltimore: Williams & Wilkins, 1990: 156–182.

231. Foster DL, Ryan KD. Puberty in the lamb: Sexual maturation of a seasonal breeder in a changing environment. In: Grumbach MM, Sizonenko PC, Aubert ML, eds. Control of the Onset of Puberty. Baltimore: Williams & Wilkins, 1990: 108–142.

232. Donovan BT. Puberty in the guinea pig and rabbit. In: Grumbach MM, Sizonenko PC, Aubert ML, eds. Control of the Onset of Puberty. Baltimore: Williams & Wilkins, 1990: 143–155.

233. Vandenbergh JG. Pheromones and mammalian reproduction. In: Kno-

bil E, Neill JD, eds. The Physiology of Reproduction. New York: Raven, 1988: 1679–1696.

234. Conte FA, Grumbach MM, Kaplan SL, et al. Correlation of LRF-induced LH and FSH release from infancy to 19 years with the changing pattern of gonadotropin secretion in agonadal patients: relation to the restraint of puberty. J Clin Endocrinol Metab 1980; 50:163–168.

235. Conte FA, Grumbach MM, Kaplan SL. A diphasic pattern of gonadotropin secretion in patients with the syndrome of gonadal dysgenesis. J Clin Endocrinol Metab 1975; 40:670–674.

236. Kelch RP, Kaplan SL, Grumbach MM. Suppression of urinary and plasma follicle-stimulating hormone by exogenous estrogens in prepubertal and pubertal children. J Clin Invest 1973; 52:1122–1128.

237. Plant TM. The effects of neonatal orchidectomy on the developmental pattern of gonadotropin secretion in the male rhesus monkey (Macaca mulatta). Endocrinology 1980; 106:1451–1454.

238. Watanabe G, Terasawa E. In vivo luteinizing hormone releasing hormone increases with puberty in the female rhesus monkey. Endocrinology 1989; 125:92–99.

239. Fraser MO, Pohl CR, Plant TM. The hypogonadotropic state of the prepubertal male rhesus monkey (Macaca mulatta) is not associated with a decrease in hypothalamic gonadotropin-releasing hormone content. Biol Reprod 1989; 40:972–980.

240. Wu FCW, Butler GE, Kelnar CJH, et al. Patterns of pulsatile luteinizing hormone secretion before and during the onset of puberty in boys: a study using an immunoradiometric assay. J Clin Endocrinol Metab 1990; 70:629–637.

241. Terasawa E, Noonan JJ, Nass TE, et al. Posterior hypothalamic lesions advance the onset of puberty in the female rhesus monkey. Endocrinology 1984; 115:2241–2250.

242. Schultz NJ, Terasawa E. Posterior hypothalamic lesions advance the time of the pubertal changes in luteinizing hormone release in ovariectomized female rhesus monkeys. Endocrinology 1988; 123:445.

243. Hochman HI, Judge DM, Reichlin S. Precocious puberty and hypothalamic hamartoma. Pediatrics 1981; 67:236–244.

244. Judge DM, Kulin HE, Santen R, et al. Hypothalamic hamartoma: a source of luteinizing-hormone–releasing factor in precocious puberty. N Engl J Med 1977; 296:7–10.

245. Krieger DT, Perlow MJ, Gibson MJ, et al. Brain grafts reverse hypogonadism of gonadotropin-releasing hormone deficiency. Nature 1982; 298:468–472.

246. Silverman AJ, Gibson M. Hypothalamic transplantation. Repair of defects in hypogonadal mice. Trends Endocrinol Metab 1990; 1:403–408.

247. Arslan M, Pohl CR, Plant TM. DL-2-Amino-5-phosphonopentanoic acid, a specific N-methyl-D-aspartic acid receptor antagonist, suppresses pulsatile LH release in the rat. Neuroendocrinology 1988; 47:465–468.

248. Bettendorf M, Albers N, de Zegher F, et al. A neuroexcitatory amino acid analogue, N-methyl-D,L-aspartate (NMDA), elicits LH and FSH release in the ovine fetus by a central mechanism. Endocr Soc Abstr 1988; p. 288.

249. Gambacciani M, Yen SS, Rasmussen D. GnRH release from the mediobasal hypothalamus: in vitro inhibition by corticotropin releasing factor. Neuroendocrinology 1986; 43:533–536.

250. Kuljis RO, Advis JP. Immunocytochemical and physiological evidence of a synapse between dopamine- and luteinizing hormone releasing hormone–containing neurons in the ewe median eminence. Endocrinology 1989; 124:1579–1581.

251. Leranth C, MacLusky NJ, Sakamoto H, et al. Glutamic acid decarboxylase–containing axons synapse on LHRH neurons in the rat medial preoptic area. Neuroendocrinology 1985; 40:536–539.

252. MacLusky NJ, Naftolin F, Leranth C. Immunocytochemical evidence for direct synaptic connections between corticotropin-releasing factor (CRF) and gonadotrophin-releasing hormone (GnRH)–containing neurons in the preoptic area of the rat. Brain Res 1988; 439:391–395.

253. Plant TM, Gay VL, Marshall GR, et al. Puberty in monkeys is triggered by chemical stimulation of the hypothalamus. Proc Natl Acad Sci USA 1989; 86:2506–2510.

254. Thind KK, Goldsmith PC. Infundibular gonadotropin-releasing hormone neurons are inhibited by direct opioid and autoregulatory synapses in juvenile monkeys. Neuroendocrinology 1988; 47:203–216.

255. Wilson RC, Kesner JS, Kaufman JM, et al. Central electrophysiologic correlates of pulsatile luteinizing hormone secretion in the rhesus monkey. Neuroendocrinology 1984; 39:256–260.

256. Plant TM. Puberty in primates. In: Knobil E, Neill JD, eds. The Physiology of Reproduction. New York: Raven, 1988: 1763–1788.

257. Kelch RP, Foster CM, Kletter GB, et al. Neuroendocrine regulation of puberty in boys. In: Sizonenko PC, Aubert ML, eds. Developmental Endocrinology. New York: Raven, 1990: 103–115.

258. Fraioli F, Cappa M, Fabbri A, et al. Lack of endogenous opioid inhibitory tone on LH secretion in early puberty. Clin Endocrinol 1984; 20:299–305.

259. Petraglia F, Bernasconi S, Iughetti L, et al. Naloxone-induced luteinizing hormone secretion in normal, precocious, and delayed puberty. J Clin Endocrinol Metab 1986; 63:1112–1116.

260. Mauras N, Veldhuis JD, Rogol AD. Role of endogenous opiates in pubertal maturation: opposing actions of naltrexone in prepubertal and late pubertal boys. J Clin Endocrinol Metab 1986; 62:1256–1263.

261. Saunder SE, Case GD, Hopwood NJ, et al. The effects of opiate antagonism on gonadotropin secretion in children and in women with hypothalamic amenorrhea. Pediatr Res 1984; 18:322–328.

262. Urbanski HF, Ojeda SR. Activation of luteinizing hormone–releasing hormone release advances the onset of female puberty. Neuroendocrinology 1987; 46:273–276.

263. Price MT, Olney JW, Cicero TJ. Acute elevations of serum luteinizing hormone induced by kainic acid, N-methyl aspartic acid or homocystic acid. Neuroendocrinology 1978; 26:352–358.

264. Gay VL, Plant TM. N-Methyl-D,L-aspartate elicits hypothalamic gonadotropin-releasing hormone release in prepubertal male rhesus monkeys (Macaca mulatta). Endocrinology 1987; 120:2289–2296.

265. Wilson RC, Knobil E. Acute effects of N-methyl-DL-aspartate on the release of pituitary gonadotropins and prolactin in the adult female rhesus monkey. Brain Res 1982; 248:177–179.

266. Bourguignon JP, Gerard A, Mathieu J, et al. Pulsatile release of gonadotropin-releasing hormone from hypothalamic explants is restrained by blockade of N-methyl-D,L-aspartate receptors. Endocrinology 1989; 125:1090–1096.

267. Judd HL. Biorhythms of gonadotropins and testicular hormone secretion. In: Krieger DT, ed. Endocrine Rhythms. New York: Raven, 1979: 299–324.

268. Rebar RW, Yen SSC. Endocrine rhythms in gonadotropins and ovarian steroids with reference to reproductive processes. In: Krieger DT, ed. Endocrine Rhythms. New York: Raven, 1979: 259–298

269. Penny R, Olambiwonnu NO, Frasier SD. Episodic fluctuations of serum gonadotropins in pre- and post-pubertal girls and boys. J Clin Endocrinol Metab 1977; 45:307–311.

270. Waldhauser F, Weissenbacher G, Frisch H, et al. Pulsatile secretion of gonadotropins in early infancy. Eur J Pediatr 1981; 137:71–74.

271. Kulin HE, Moore RC Jr, Santner SJ. Circadian rhythms in gonadotropin excretion in prepubertal and pubertal children. J Clin Endocrinol Metab 1976; 42:770–773.

272. Kelch RP, Marshall JC, Sauder SE. Pulsatile gonadotropin-releasing hormone and the induction of puberty in human beings. In: Grumbach MM, Sizonenko PC, Aubert ML, eds. Control of the Onset of Puberty. Baltimore: Williams & Wilkins, 1990: 82–107.

273. Boyar RM, Finkelstein JW, Roffwarg H, et al. Twenty-four patterns of luteinizing hormone and follicle-stimulating hormone secretory patterns in gonadal dysgenesis. J Clin Endocrinol Metab 1973; 37:521–525.

274. Boyar R, Finkelstein JW, David R, et al. Twenty-four hour patterns of plasma luteinizing hormone and follicle-stimulating hormone in sexual precocity. N Engl J Med 1973; 289:282–286.

275. Reiter EO, Kaplan SL, Conte FA, et al. Responsivity of pituitary gonadotropes to luteinizing hormone–releasing factor in idiopathic precocious puberty, precocious thelarche, precocious adrenarche and in patients treated with medroxyprogesterone acetate. Pediatr Res 1975; 9:111–116.

276. Ross GT, Cargille CM, Lipsett MB, et al. Pituitary and gonadal hormones in women during spontaneous and induced ovulatory cycles. Recent Prog Horm Res 1970; 26:1–62.

277. Yen SSC, Lasley BL, Wang FC, et al. The operating characteristics of the hypothalamic-pituitary system during the menstrual cycle and observations of biological action of somatostatin. Recent Prog Horm Res 1975; 31:321–363.

278. Pohl GR, Knobil E. The role of the central nervous system in the control of ovarian function in higher primates. Annu Rev Physiol 1982; 44:583–593.

279. Belchetz PE, Plant TM, Nakai Y, et al. Hypophyseal responses to continuous and intermittent delivery of hypothalamic gonadotropin-releasing hormone. Science 1978; 202:631–633.

280. Knobil E, Plant TM. The neuroendocrine control of gonadotropin secretion in the female rhesus monkey. Front Neuroendocrinol 1978; 4:249–264.

281. Knobil E, Plant TM, Wildt L, et al. Control of the rhesus monkey menstrual cycle: permissive role of the hypothalamic gonadotropin-releasing hormone. Science 1980; 207:1371–1373.

281a. Wildt L, Marshall G, Knobil E. Experimental induction of puberty in the infantile female rhesus monkey. Science 1980; 207:1373–1375.

282. Yoshimoto Y, Moridera K, Imura H. Restoration of normal pituitary gonadotropin reserve by administration of luteinizing hormone releasing hormone in patients with hypogonadotropic hypogonadism. N Engl J Med 1975; 292:242–245.

283. Jacobson RI, Seyler LE, Tamborlane WV, et al. Pulsatile subcutaneous nocturnal administration of Gn-RH by portable infusion pump in hypogonadotropic hypogonadism: initiation of gonadotropin responsiveness. J Clin Endocrinol Metab 1979; 49:652–654.

284. Marshall JC, Kelch RP. Low dose pulsatile gonadotropin-releasing hormone in anorexia nervosa: a model of human pubertal development. J Clin Endocrinol Metab 1979; 49:712–718.

285. Crowley WF Jr, McArthur JW. Stimulation of the normal menstrual cycle in Kallmann's syndrome by pulsatile administration of luteinizing hormone–releasing hormone (LHRH). J Clin Endocrinol Metab 1980; 51:173–175.

286. Valk TW, Corley KP, Kelch RP, et al. Hypogonadotropic hypogonadism: hormonal responses to low dose pulsatile administration of gonadotropin-releasing hormone. J Clin Endocrinol Metab 1980; 51:730–737.

287. Boyar RM, Finkelstein JW, Witkin M, et al. Studies of endocrine function in "isolated" gonadotropin deficiency. J Clin Endocrinol Metab 1973; 36:64–72.

288. Winter JSD, Tarasaka S, Faiman C. The hormonal response to hCG stimulation in male children and adolescents. J Clin Endocrinol Metab 1972; 34:348–353.

289. Sizonenko PD, Cuendet A, Paunier L. FSH. 1. Evidence for its mediating role on testosterone secretion in cryptorchidism. J Clin Endocrinol Metab 1973; 37:68–73.

290. Reiter EO, Kulin HE, Hamwood SM. The absence of positive feedback between estrogen and luteinizing hormone in sexually immature girls. Pediatr Res 1974; 8:740–745.

291. Presl J, Horejsi J, Stroufiova A, et al. Sexual maturation in girls and the development of estrogen-induced gonadotropic hormone release. Ann Biol Anim Biochim Biophys 1976; 16:377–383.

292. Gharib SD, Wierman ME, Shupnik MA, et al. Molecular biology of the pituitary gonadotropins. Endocr Rev 1990; 11:177–199.

293. Keye WR, Jaffe RB. Strength-duration characteristics of estrogen effects on gonadotropin response to gonadotropin-releasing hormone in women. I. Effects of varying duration of estradiol administration. J Clin Endocrinol Metab 1975; 41:1003–1008.

294. Elkind-Hirsch K, Ravnikar V, Schiff I, et al. Determinations of endogenous immunoreactive luteinizing hormone–releasing hormone in human plasma. J Clin Endocrinol Metab 1982; 54:602–607.

295. Doring GK. Uber die relativ Sterilitat in den Jahren nach der Menarche. Geburtsh Frauenheilkd 1963; 23:30–36.

296. Hansen JW, Hoffman HJ, Ross GT. Monthly gonadotropin cycles in premenarcheal girls. Science 1975; 190:161–163.

297. Winter JSD, Faiman C. Pituitary-gonadal relations in female children and adolescents. Pediatr Res 1973; 7:948–953.

298. Reiter EO, Grumbach MM, Kaplan SL, et al. The response of pituitary gonadotropes to synthetic LRF in children with glucocorticoid-treated congenital adrenal hyperplasia: lack of effect of intrauterine and neonatal androgen excess. J Clin Endocrinol Metab 1975; 40:318–325.

299. Cutler GB, Loriaux DL. Adrenarche and its relationship to the onset of puberty. Fed Proc 1980; 39:2384–2390.

300. Hopper BR, Yen SSC. Circulating concentrations of dehydroepiandrosterone and dehydroepiandrosterone sulfate during puberty. J Clin Endocrinol Metab 1975; 40:458–461.

301. Sizonenko PE, Paunier L. Correlation of plasma dehydroepiandrosterone, testosterone, FSH, and LH with stages of puberty and bone age in normal boys and girls and in patients with Addison's disease or hypogonadism or with premature or late adrenarche. J Clin Endocrinol Metab 1975; 41:894–904.

302. Reiter EO, Fuldauer VG, Root AW. Secretion of the adrenal androgen, dehydroepiandrosterone sulfate, during normal infancy, childhood, and adolescence, in sick infants, and in children with endocrinologic abnormalities. J Pediatr 1977; 90:766–770.

303. Schiebinger RJ, Albertson BD, Cassorla FG, et al. The developmental changes in plasma adrenal androgens during infancy and adrenarche are associated with changing activities of adrenal microsomal 17-hydroxylase and 17,20-desmolase. J Clin Invest 1981; 67:1177–1182.

304. Cutler GB Jr, Schiebinger RJ, Albertson BD, et al. The adrenarche (human and animal). In: Grumbach MM, Sizonenko PC, Aubert ML, eds. Control of the Onset of Puberty. Baltimore: Williams & Wilkins, 1990: 506–524.

305. Sklar CA, Kaplan SL, Grumbach MM. Evidence for dissociation between adrenarche and gonadarche: studies in patients with idiopathic precocious puberty, gonadal dysgenesis, isolated gonadotropin deficiency, and constitutionally delayed growth and adolescence. J Clin Endocrinol Metab 1980; 51:548–556.

306. Butler GE, McKie M, Ratcliffe SG. The cyclical nature of prepubertal growth. Ann Hum Biol 1990; 17:177–198.

307. Prader A. Delayed adolescence. Clin Endocrinol Metab 1975; 4:143–155.

308. Counts DR, Pescovitz OH, Barnes KM, et al. Dissociation of adrenarche and gonadarche in precocious puberty and in isolated hypogonadotropic hypogonadism. J Clin Endocrinol Metab 1987; 64:1174–1178.

309. Stanhope R, Hindmarsh P, Pringle PJ, et al. Oxandrolone induces a sustained rise in physiological growth hormone secretion in boys with constitutional delay of growth and puberty. Pediatrician 1987; 14:183–188.

310. Loche S, Corda R, Lampis A, et al. The effect of oxandrolone on the growth hormone response to growth hormone releasing hormone in children with constitutional growth delay. Clin Endocrinol 1986; 25:195–200.

311. Stolecke H, Gilessen G. Oxandrolone and spontaneous hGH secretion. Pediatr Res 1984; 18:1216 (abstract).

312. Clayton PE, Shalet SM, Price DA, et al. Growth and growth hormone responses to oxandrolone in boys with constitutional delay of growth and puberty (CDGP). Clin Endocrinol 1988; 29:123–130.

313. Cara JF, Rosenfield RL. Insulin-like growth factor I and insulin poten-

314. Apter D. Self-image in adolescents with delayed puberty and growth retardation. J Youth Adolesc 1981; 10:501–505.

314a. Mussen PH, Jones MC. Self conceptions, motivations and interpersonal attitudes of late and early maturing boys. Child Dev 1957; 28:243–256.

314b. Gordon M, Crouthamel C, Post EM, et al. Psychosocial aspects of constitutional short stature: social competence, behavior problems, self esteem and family functioning. J Pediatr 1982; 101:477–480.

314c. Crowne EC, Shalet SM, Wallace WHB, et al. Final height in boys with untreated constitutional delay in growth and puberty. Arch Dis Child 1990; 65:1109–1112.

315. Spratt DI, Carr DH, Merriam GR, et al. The spectrum of abnormal patterns of gonadotropin-releasing hormone secretion in men with idiopathic hypogonadotropic hypogonadism: clinical and laboratory correlations. J Clin Endocrinol Metab 1987; 64:283–291.

316. Byrne MN, Sessions DG. Nasopharyngeal craniopharyngioma. Case report and literature review. Ann Otol Rhinol Laryngol 1990; 99:633–639.

317. Fukushima T, Hirakawa K, Kimura M, et al. Intraventricular craniopharyngioma: its characteristics in magnetic resonance imaging and successful total removal. Surg Neurol 1990; 33:22–27.

318. Banna M. Craniopharyngioma: based on 160 cases. Br J Radiol 1976; 49:206–223.

319. Banna M, Hoare RD, Stanley P, et al. Craniopharyngioma in children. J Pediatr 1973; 83:781–785.

320. Thomsett JJ, Conte FA, Kaplan SL, et al. Endocrine and neurologic outcome in childhood craniopharyngioma: review of effect of treatment in 42 patients. J Pediatr 1980; 97:728–735.

321. Baumgartner JE, Wilson CB, Edwards MSB. Management of craniopharyngioma in children. Part 1. The effect of surgery and radiation therapy on outcome. J Neurosurg (in press).

322. Chakeres DW, Curtin A, Ford G. Magnetic resonance imaging of pituitary and parasellar abnormalities. Radiol Clin North Am 1989; 27:265–281.

323. Weiss M, Sutton L, Marcial V, et al. The role of radiation therapy in the management of childhood craniopharyngioma. Int J Radiat Oncol Biol Phys 1989; 17:1313–1321.

324. Fischer EG, Welch K, Shillito J Jr, et al. Craniopharyngioma in children. Long term effects of conservative surgical procedures combined with radiation therapy. J Neurosurg 1990; 73:534–540.

325. Dayan AD, Marshall AHE, Miller AA, et al. Atypical teratomas of the pineal and hypothalamus. J Pathol Bacteriol 1966; 92:1–28.

326. Sklar CA, Grumbach MM, Kaplan SL, et al. Hormonal and metabolic abnormalities associated with central nervous system germinoma in children and adolescents and the effect of therapy: Report of 10 patients. J Clin Endocrinol Metab 1981; 52:9–16.

327. Spiegel AM, Giovanni DC, Gordon P, et al. Diagnosis of radiosensitive hypothalamic tumors without craniotomy. Ann Intern Med 1976; 85:290–293.

328. Kilgore DP, Strother CM, Starshak RJ, et al. Pineal germinoma: MR imaging. Radiology 1986; 158:435–438.

329. Wara WM, Fellows FC, Sheline GE, et al. Radiation therapy for pineal tumors and suprasellar germinomas. Radiology 1977; 124:221–223.

330. Saxena KM. Endocrine manifestations of neurofibromatosis in children. Am J Dis Child 1970; 120:265–272.

331. Fienman NL, Yakovac WC. Neurofibromatosis in childhood. J Pediatr 1970; 76:339–346.

332. Kibirige MS, Birch JM, Campbell RH, et al. A review of astrocytoma in childhood. Pediatr Hematol Oncol 1989; 6:319–329.

333. Koenig MP, Zuppinger K, Leichti B. Hyperprolactinemia as a cause of delayed puberty: successful treatment with bromocriptine. J Clin Endocrinol Metab 1977; 45:825–828.

334. Vogel JM, Vogel P. Idiopathic histiocytosis: a discussion of eosinophilic granuloma, the Hand-Schüller-Christian syndrome, and the Letterer-Siwe syndrome. Semin Hematol 1972; 9:349–364.

334a. Komp DM. Langerhans cell histiocytosis. N Engl J Med 1987; 316:747–748.

334b. Writing Group of The Histiocyte Society. Histiocytosis syndromes in children. Lancet 1987; 1:208–209.

335. Sims DG. Histocytosis X: follow-up of 43 cases. Arch Dis Child 1977; 52:433–440.

335a. Lavin PT, Osband ME. Evaluating the role of therapy in histiocytosis X: clinical studies, staging, and scoring. Hematol Oncol Clin North Am 1987; 1:35–47.

336. Asherson RA, Jackson WPU, Lewis B. Abnormalities of development associated with hypothalamic calcification after tuberculous meningitis. Br Med J 1965; 2:839–843.

337. Fiedler R, Krieger DT. Endocrine disturbances in patients with congenital aqueductal stenosis. Acta Endocrinol 1975; 80:1–13.

338. Richards GE, Wara WM, Grumbach MM, et al. Delayed onset of hypopituitarism: sequelae of therapeutic irradiation of central nervous system, eye, and middle ear tumors. J Pediatr 1976; 89:553–559.

339. Hanna CE, Mandel SH, LaFranchi SH. Puberty in the syndrome of septo-optic dysplasia. Am J Dis Child 1989; 143:186–189.

tiate luteinizing hormone–induced androgen synthesis by rat ovarian theca-interstitial cells. Endocrinology 1988; 123:733–739.

340. Kaplan SL, Grumbach MM, Hoyt WF. A syndrome of hypopituitary dwarfism, hypoplasia of optic nerves, and malformation of prosencephalon: report of 6 patients. Pediatr Res 1970; 4:480–481 (abstract).

341. Job JC, Chaussain JL, Toublanc JE. Delayed puberty. In: Grumbach MM, Sizonenko PC, Aubert ML, eds. Control of the Onset of Puberty. Baltimore: Williams & Wilkins, 1990: 588–619.

342. Seeburg PH, Mason AJ, Steward TA, et al. The mammalian GnRH gene and its pivotal role in reproduction. Recent Prog Horm Res 1987; 43:69–107.

343. Kallmann F, Schonfeld WA, Barrera SW. Genetic aspects of primary eunuchoidism. Am J Ment Defic 1944; 48:203–236.

344. Weinstein RL, Reitz RE. Pituitary-testicular responsiveness in male hypogonadotropic hypogonadism. J Clin Invest 1974; 53:408–415.

345. Van Dop C, Burstein S, Conte FA, et al. Isolated gonadotropin deficiency in boys: clinical characteristics and growth. J Pediatr 1987; 111:684–692.

346. Ballabio A, Bardoni B, Carrozzo R, et al. Contiguous gene syndromes due to deletions in the distal short arm of the human X chromosome. Proc Natl Acad Sci USA 1989; 86:10001–10005.

347. Santen RJ, Paulsen CA. Hypogonadotropic eunuchoidism. I. Clinical study of the mode of inheritance. J Clin Endocrinol Metab 1973; 36:47–54.

348. Santen RJ, Paulsen CA. Hypogonadotropic eunuchoidism. II. Gonadal responsiveness to exogenous gonadotropins. J Clin Endocrinol Metab 1973; 36:55–63.

349. Merriam GR, Beitins IZ, Bode HH. Father to son transmission of hypogonadism with anosmia. Am J Dis Child 1977; 131:1216–1219.

350. Hipkin LJ, Casson IF, Davis JC. Identical twins discordant for Kallmann's syndrome. J Med Genet 1990; 27:198–199.

351. White BJ, Rogol AD, Brown KS, et al. The syndrome of anosmia with hypogonadotropic hypogonadism: a genetic study of 18 new families and a review. Am J Med Genet 1983; 15:417–435.

352. Prader A, Zachmann M, Illig KR. Luteinizing hormone deficiency in hereditary congenital adrenal hypoplasia. J Pediatr 1975; 86:421–422.

353. Kruse K, Sippell WG, Schnakenburg KV. Hypogonadism in congenital adrenal hypoplasia: evidence for a hypothalamic origin. J Clin Endocrinol Metab 1984; 58:12–17.

354. Hay ID, Smail PJ, Forsyth CC. Familial cytomegalic adrenocortical hypoplasia: an X-linked syndrome of pubertal failure. Arch Dis Child 1981; 56:715–721.

355. Kukishi K, Kaji M, Momoi T, et al. Failure to induce puberty in a man with X-linked congenital adrenal hypoplasia and hypogonadotropic hypogonadism by pulsatile administration of low dose gonadotropin-releasing hormone. Acta Endocrinol 1987; 114:153–160.

356. Goonewardena P, Dahl W, Ritzén M, et al. Molecular Xp deletion in a male: suggestion of a locus for hypogonadotropic hypogonadism distal to the glycerol kinase and adrenal hypoplasia loci. Clin Genet 1989; 35:5–12.

357. Smals AGH, Kloppenborg PWC, Van Haelst UJG, et al. Fertile eunuch syndrome versus classic hypogonadotrophic hypogonadism. Acta Endocrinol 1978; 87:389–399.

358. Rabin D, Spitz I, Bercovici B, et al. Isolated deficiency of follicle-stimulating hormone: clinical and laboratory features. N Engl J Med 1972; 287:1313–1317.

359. Goodman HG, Grumbach MM, Kaplan SL. Growth and growth hormone. II. A comparison of isolated growth-hormone deficiency and multiple pituitary-hormone deficiencies in 35 patients with idiopathic hypopituitary dwarfism. N Engl J Med 1968; 278:57–68.

360. Tanner JM, Whitehouse RH. A note on the bone age at which patients with true isolated growth hormone deficiency enter puberty. J Clin Endocrinol Metab 1975; 41:788–790.

361. Ledbetter DH, Mascarello JT, Riccardi VM. Chromosome 15 abnormalities and the Prader-Willi syndrome: a follow-up report of 40 cases. Am J Hum Genet 1982; 34:278–285.

362. Bray GA, Dahms WT, Swerdloff RS, et al. The Prader-Willi syndrome: a study of 40 patients and a review of the literature. Medicine 1983; 62:59–80.

363. Prader A, Labhart A, Willi H. Ein syndrom von Adipositas, Kleinwuchs, Kryptorchidismus und Oligophrenie nach Myatonieartigem Zustad im Neugeborenalter. Schweiz Med Wochenschr 1956; 86:1260–1261.

364. Tolis G, Lewis W, Verdy M, et al. Anterior pituitary function in the Prader-Labhart-Willi (PLW) syndrome. J Clin Endocrinol Metab 1974; 39:1061–1066.

365. Linde R, McNeil L, Rabin D. Induction of menarche by clomiphene citrate in a fifteen-year-old girl with the Prader-Labhart-Willi syndrome. Fertil Steril 1982; 37:118–120.

366. Cassidy SB, Ledbetter DH. Prader-Willi syndrome. Neurol Clin 1989; 7:37–54.

367. Knoll JHM, Nicholls RD, Magenis RE, et al. Angleman and Prader-Willi share a common chromosome 15 deletion but differ in parental origin of the deletion. Am J Med Genet 1989; 32:285–290.

368. Nicholls RD, Knoll JHM, Butler MG, et al. Genetic imprinting suggested by maternal hetero-disomy in non-deletion Prader-Willi syndrome. Nature 1989; 342:281–285.

369. Laurence JZ, Moon RC. Four cases of "retinitis pigmentosa," occurring in the same family, and accompanied by general imperfections of development. Ophthalmic Rev 1866; 2:32–41.

370. Bell J. The Laurence-Moon syndrome. In: The Treasury of Human Inheritance. Vol 5. Part 3. Cambridge: Cambridge University Press, 1958: 51–69.

371. Reinfrank RF, Nichols FL. Hypogonadotrophic hypogonadism in the Laurence-Moon syndrome. J Clin Endocrinol Metab 1964; 24:48–53.

372. Kulin HE, Bwibo N, Mutie D, et al. The effect of chronic childhood malnutrition on pubertal growth and development. Am J Clin Nutr 1982; 36:527–536.

373. Kulin HE, Bwibo N, Mutie D, et al. Gonadotropin excretion during puberty in malnourished children. J Pediatr 1984; 105:325–328.

374. Maki M, Kallonen K, Lahdeaho ML, et al. Changing pattern of childhood coeliac disease in Finland. Acta Paediatr Scand 1988; 77:408–412.

375. Frisch RE, McArthur JW. Menstrual cycles: fatness as a determinant of minimum weight for height necessary for their maintenance or onset. Science 1974; 185:949–951.

376. Vigersky R, Anderson AE, Thompson RH, et al. Hypothalamic dysfunction in secondary amenorrhea associated with simple weight loss. N Engl J Med 1977; 297:1141–1145.

377. Landon C, Rosenfeld RG. Short stature and pubertal delay in cystic fibrosis. Pediatrician 1987; 14:253–260.

378. Chaussain JL, Roger M, Couprie C, et al. Treatment of precocious puberty with a long-acting preparation of D-Trp^6-LHRH. Horm Res 1987; 28:155–163.

379. Reiter EO, Stern RC, Root AW. The reproductive endocrine system in cystic fibrosis. I. Basal gonadotropin and sex steroid levels. Am J Dis Child 1981; 135:422–426.

380. Stern RC, Boat TF, Doershuk CF, et al. Course of cystic fibrosis in 95 patients. J Pediatr 1976; 89:406–411.

381. Taussig LM, Lobeck CC, di Sant'Agnese PA, et al. Fertility in males with cystic fibrosis. N Engl J Med 1972; 287:586–589.

382. Olatunji Olambiwonnu N, Penny R, Frasier SD. Sexual maturation in subjects with sickle cell anemia: studies of serum gonadotropin concentration, height, weight, and skeletal age. J Pediatr 1975; 87:459–464.

383. Borgna Pignatti C, De Stefano P, Zonta L, et al. Growth and sexual maturation in thalassemia major. J Pediatr 1985; 106:150–155.

384. Celani MF, Rota C, Messori A, et al. Effect of increased haemoglobin levels on growth hormone (GH) secretion in beta-thalassaemia major: differences between prepubertal subjects and patients with delayed puberty. Exp Clin Endocrinol 1988; 92:225–230.

385. De Sanctis V, Vullo C, Katz M, et al. Gonadal function in patients with beta thalassaemia major. J Clin Pathol 1988; 41:133–137.

386. Sklar CA, Lew LQ, Yoon DJ, et al. Adrenal function in thalassemia major following long-term treatment with multiple transfusions and chelation therapy. Evidence for dissociation of cortisol and adrenal androgen secretion. Am J Dis Child 1987; 141:327–330.

387. Balducci R, Toscano V, Finocchi G, et al. Effect of hCG or hCG + treatments in young thalassemic patients with hypogonadotropic hypogonadism. J Endocrinol Invest 1990; 13:1–7.

388. Ferraris J, Saenger P, Levine L, et al. Delayed puberty in males with chronic renal failure. Kidney Int 1980; 18:344–350.

389. Ferraris JR, Domene HM, Escobar ME, et al. Hormonal problems in pubertal females with chronic renal failure: before and under hemodialysis and after renal transplantation. Acta Endocrinol 1987; 115:289–296.

390. Schaefer F, Stanhope R, Scheil H, et al. Pulsatile gonadotropin secretion in pubertal children with chronic renal failure. Acta Endocrinol 1989; 120:14–19.

391. Rees L, Greene SA, Adlard P, et al. Growth and endocrine function in steroid sensitive nephrotic syndrome. Arch Dis Child 1988; 63:484–490.

392. van Diemen-Steevoorde MD, Donckerwolcke RA, Brakel H, et al. Growth and sexual maturation in children after kidney transplantation. J Pediatr 1987; 110:351–356.

393. Rees L, Greene SA, Adlard P, et al. Growth and endocrine function after renal transplantation. Arch Dis Child 1988; 63:1326–1332.

394. Siris ES, Leventhal BG, Vaitukaitis JL. Effects of childhood leukemia and chemotherapy on puberty and reproductive function in girls. N Engl J Med 1976; 294:1143–1146.

395. Vilska S, Lahteenmaki P, Kaihola HL, et al. Endocrine status and growth after malignancy treated in childhood or adolescence. Int J Fertil 1988; 33:283–290.

396. Mauriac P. Hepatomégalie de l'enfance avec troubles de la croissance et du métabolisme des glucides. Paris Méd 1934; 2:525.

397. Bourgeois MJ, Travis LB. Diabetes Mellitus in Children and Adolescents. Philadelphia: W. B. Saunders, 1987: 206–208.

398. Styne DM, Grumbach MM, Kaplan SL, et al. Treatment of Cushing's disease in childhood and adolescence by transsphenoidal microadenomectomy. N Engl J Med 1984; 310:889–893.

399. Warren MP, Vande Wile RL. Clinical and metabolic features of anorexia nervosa. Am J Obstet Gynecol 1973; 117:435–449.

400. Schwabe AD, Lippe BM, Chang RJ, et al. Anorexia nervosa. Ann Intern Med 1981; 94:371–381.

401. Silverman JA. Anorexia nervosa: clinical and metabolic observations in a successful treatment plan. In: Vigersky RA, ed. Anorexia Nervosa. New York: Raven, 1977: 331–339.

402. Cheyne KL, Lightner ES, Comerci GD. Bromocriptine-unresponsive

prolactin macroadenoma in a prepubertal female. J Adolesc Health Care 1988; 9:331–334.

402a van Binsbergen CJM, Coelingh Bennink HJT, Odink J, et al. A comparative and longitudinal study on endocrine changes related to ovarian function in patients with anorexia nervosa. J Clin Endocrinol Metab 1990; 71:705–711.

403. Beaumont PJV, George GCW, Pimstone BL, et al. Body weight and the pituitary response to hypothalamic releasing hormones in patients with anorexia nervosa. J Clin Endocrinol Metab 1976; 43:487–496.

404. Yen SSC, Rebar R, VandenBerg G, et al. Hypothalamic amenorrhea and hypogonadotropinism: responses to synthetic LRF. J Clin Endocrinol Metab 1973; 36:811–816.

405. Waldhauser F, Toifl K, Spona J, et al. Diminished prolactin response to thyrotropin and insulin in anorexia nervosa. J Clin Endocrinol Metab 1984; 59:538–544.

406. Warren MP. Metabolic factors and the onset of puberty. In: Grumbach MM, Sizonenko PC, Aubert ML, eds. Control of the Onset of Puberty. Baltimore: Williams & Wilkins, 1990: 553–573.

407. Russell GFM. Bulimia nervosa: an ominous variant of anorexia nervosa. Psychol Med 1979; 9:429–448.

408. Eisenstein TD, Gerson MJ. Psychosocial growth retardation in adolescence. A reversible condition secondary to severe stress. J Adolesc Health Care 1988; 9:436–440.

409. Malina RM. Menarche in athletes: a synthesis and hypothesis. Ann Hum Biol 1983; 10:1–24.

410. Patton ML, Woolf PD. Hyperprolactinemia and delayed puberty: a report of three cases and their response to therapy. Pediatrics 1983; 71:572–575.

411. Noel GL, Suh HK, Stone JG, et al. Human prolactin and growth hormone release during surgery and other conditions of stress. J Clin Endocrinol Metab 1972; 35:840–851.

412. Loucks AV, Horvath SB. Athletic amenorrhea: a review. Med Sci Sports Exerc 1985; 17:56–72.

413. Brisson GR, Volle MA, Desharnais M, et al. Exercise induced dissociation of the blood prolactin response in young women according to their sports habits. Horm Metab Res 1980; 21:201–205.

414. Harmon J, Aliapoulios MA. Gynecomastia in marihuana user. N Engl J Med 1972; 287:936.

415. Copeland KC, Underwood LE, Van Wyk JJ. Marihuana smoking and pubertal arrest. J Pediatr 1980; 96:1079–1080.

416. Grumbach MM, Conte FA. Disorders of sex differentiation. In: Wilson JD, Foster DW, eds. Williams Textbook of Endocrinology. 8th ed. Philadelphia: W. B. Saunders, 1992: 853–951.

417. Klinefelter HF Jr, Reifenstein EC Jr, Albright F. Syndrome characterized by gynecomastia, aspermatogenesis without A-leydigism, and increased excretion of follicle-stimulating hormone. J Clin Endocrinol 1942; 2:615–627.

418. Wittenberg DF, Padayachi T, Norman RJ. Hypogonadotrophic variant of Klinefelter's syndrome. A case report. S Afr Med J 1988; 74:181–183.

419. Caldwell PD, Smith DW. The XXY (Klinefelter's) syndrome in childhood: detection and treatment. J Pediatr 1972; 80:250–258.

420. Sagawa I, Kazama T, Terada T, et al. Hormonal profiles in Klinefelters syndrome with and without testicular epidermoid cyst. Arch Androl 1988; 21:205–209.

421. Salbenblatt JA, Bender BG, Puck MH, et al. Pituitary-gonadal function in Klinefelter syndrome before and during puberty. Pediatr Res 1985; 19:82–86.

422. Plymate SR, Leonard JM, Paulsen CA. Sex hormone–binding globulin changes with androgen replacement. J Clin Endocrinol Metab 1983; 57:645–648.

423. Wieland RG, Zorn EM, Johnson MW. Elevated testosterone-binding globulin in Klinefelter's syndrome. J Clin Endocrinol Metab 1980; 51:1199–1200.

424. Eberle AJ, Sparrow JT, Keenan BS. Treatment of persistent pubertal gynecomastia with dihydrotestosterone heptanoate. J Pediatr 1986; 109:144–149.

425. Kleczkowska A, Fryns JP, Van den Berghe H. X-chromosome polysomy in the male: the Leuven experience 1966–1987. Hum Genet 1988; 80:16–22.

426. Nielsen J, Pelsen B. Follow-up 20 years later of 34 Klinefelter males with karyotype 47,XXY and 16 hypogonadal males with karyotype 46,XY. Hum Genet 1987; 77:188–192.

426a. Sorenson K. Klinefelter's Syndrome in Childhood, Adolescence and Youth: A Genetic, Clinical, Developmental, Psychiatric, and Psychologic Study. Lancaster, UK: Parthenon, 1988.

427. Porter ME, Gardner HA, DeFeudis P. Verbal deficits in Klinefelter (XXY) adults living in the community. Clin Genet 1988; 33:246–253.

428. Price WH, Clayton JF, Wilson J. Causes of death in X chromatin positive males (Klinefelter's syndrome). J Epidemiol Community Health 1985; 39:330–336.

429. Scheike O, Visfeldt J, Petersen B. Male breast cancer: III. Breast carcinoma in association with the Klinefelter syndrome. Acta Pathol Microbiol Scand Suppl 1973; 81:352–358.

430. Bizzaro A, Valentini G, DiMartino G. Influence of testosterone therapy on clinical and immunological features of autoimmune diseases associ-

ated with Klinefelter's syndrome. J Clin Endocrinol Metab 1987; 64:32–36.

431. Fialkow PJ. Genetic aspects of autoimmunity. Prog Med Genet 1969; 6:117–167.

432. Foresta C, Busnardo B, Zanatta G. Lower calcitonin levels in young hypogonadic men with osteoporosis. Horm Metab Res 1983; 15:206–207.

433. Foresta C, Zanatta GP, Busnardo B. Testosterone and calcitonin plasma levels in hypogonadal osteoporotic young men. J Endocrinol Invest 1985; 8:377–379.

434. Penso J, Lippe B, Ehrlich R, et al. Testicular function in prepubertal and pubertal male patients treated with cyclophosphamide for nephrotic syndrome. J Pediatr 1974; 84:831–836.

435. Callis L, Nieto J, Vila A, et al. Chlorambucil treatment in minimal lesion nephrotic syndrome: a reappraisal of its gonadal toxicity. J Pediatr 1980; 97:653–656.

436. Bramswig JH, Heimes U, Heiermann E, et al. The effects of different cumulative doses of chemotherapy on testicular function. Cancer 1990; 65:1298–1302.

437. Barrett A, Nicholls J, Gibson B. Late effects of total body irradiation. Radiother Oncol 1987; 9:131–135.

438. Bosson D, Wolter R, Toppet M, et al. Partial 17,20-desmolase and 17α-hydroxylase deficiencies in a 16-year-old boy. J Endocrinol Invest 1988; 11:527–533.

439. David R, Yoon DJ, Landin L, et al. A syndrome of gonadotropin resistance possibly due to a luteinizing hormone receptor defect. J Clin Endocrinol Metab 1984; 59:156–160.

440. Lustig RH, Conte FA, Kogan BA, et al. Ontogeny of gonadotropin secretion in congenital anorchism: sexual dimorphism versus syndrome of gonadal dysgenesis and diagnostic considerations. J Urol 1987; 138:587–591.

441. Saez J, Forest MG. Kinetics of human chorionic gonadotropin–induced steroidogenic reponse of the human testis. I. Plasma testosterone: implications for human chorionic gonadotropin stimulation test. J Clin Endocrinol Metab 1979; 49:278–283.

442. Rosenfeld RG, Grumbach MM, eds. Turner Syndrome. New York: Marcel Dekker, 1990: 1–512.

443. Hook EB, Hamerton JL. The frequency of chromosome abnormalities detected in consecutive newborn studies—differences studies. Results by sex and severity of phenotypic involvement. In: Hook EB, Porter IH, eds. Population Cytogenetics. New York: Academic, 1977: 63–79.

444. Hook EB, Warburton D. The distribution of chromosomal genotypes associated with Turner's syndrome: livebirth prevalence rates and evidence for diminished fetal mortality and severity in genotypes associated with structural X abnormalities or mosaicism. Hum Genet 1983; 64:24–27.

445. Turner HH. A syndrome of infantilism, congenital webbed neck and cubitus valgus. Endocrinology 1938; 23:566–574.

446. Carr DH, Gedeon M. Population cytogenetics in human abortuses. In: Hook EB, Porter IH, eds. Population Cytogenetics. New York: Academic, 1977: 1–9.

447. Warburton D, Kline J, Stein I. Monosomy X: a chromosomal anomaly associated with young maternal age. Lancet 1980; 1:167–169.

448. Massa G, Vanderschueren-Lodeweyckx M, Malvaux P. Linear growth in patients with Turner syndrome: influence of spontaneous puberty and parental height. Eur J Pediatr 1990; 149:246–250.

449. Palmer CG, Reichman A. Chromosomal and clinical findings in 110 females with Turner syndrome. Hum Genet 1976; 35:35–49.

450. Szpunar J. Middle ear disease in Turner's syndrome. Arch Otolaryngol Head Neck Surg 1968; 87:34–40.

451. Lippe BM, Geffner ME, Dietrich RB, et al. Renal malformations in patients with Turner syndrome: imaging with 141 patients. Pediatrics 1988; 82:852–856.

452. Lin AE, Lippe BM, Geffner ME, et al. Aortic dilation, dissection, and rupture in patients with Turner syndrome. J Pediatr 1986; 109:820–826.

453. Arulanantham K, Kramer MS, Gryboski JD. The association of inflammatory bowel disease and X-chromosomal abnormality. Pediatrics 1980; 66:63–67.

454. Knudtzon J, Svane S. Turner's syndrome associated with chronic inflammatory bowel disease: a case report and review of the literature. Acta Med Scand 1988; 223:375–378.

455. Price WH. A high incidence of chronic inflammatory bowel disease in patients with Turner's syndrome. J Med Genet 1979; 16:263–266.

456. Forbes AP, Engel E. The high incidence of diabetes mellitus in 41 patients with gonadal dysgenesis, and their close relatives. Metabolism 1963; 12:428–439.

457. Nielsen J, Johansen K, Yde H. The frequency of diabetes mellitus in patients with Turner's syndrome and pure gonadal dysgenesis. Acta Endocrinol 1969; 62:251–269.

458. Silbert A, Wolffe PH, Lilienthal J. Spatial and temporal processing in patients with Turner's syndrome. Behav Genet 1977; 7:11–21.

459. Nielsen J. Mental aspects of Turner syndrome and the importance of information and Turner contact groups. In: Rosenfeld RG, Grumbach MM, eds. Turner Syndrome. New York: Marcel Dekker, 1990: 451–467.

460. Garron DC. Intelligence among persons with Turner's syndrome. Behav Genet 1977; 7:105–127.
461. Brook CGD, Murset G, Zachmann M, et al. Growth in children with 45,XO Turner's syndrome. Arch Dis Child 1974; 73:789–795.
462. Lyon AJ, Preece MA, Grant DB. Growth curve for girls with Turner syndrome. Arch Dis Child 1985; 60:932–935.
463. Ranke MB, Stubbe P, Majewski F, et al. Spontaneous growth in Turner's syndrome. Acta Paediatr Scand Suppl 1988; 343:22–30.
464. Sklar CA, Kaplan SL, Grumbach MM. Lack of effect of oestrogens on adrenal androgen secretion in children and adolescents with a comment on oestrogens and pubic hair growth. Clin Endocrinol 1981; 14:311–320.
465. Cicognani A, Mazzanti L, Tassinari D, et al. Differences in carbohydrate tolerance in Turner syndrome depending on age and karyotype. Eur J Pediatr 1988; 148:64–68.
466. Aranoff GS, Morishima A. XO/XY mosaicism in delayed puberty. J Adolesc Health Care 1988; 9:501–504.
467. Scully RE. Gonadoblastoma: a review of 74 cases. Cancer 1970; 25:1340–1356.
468. Cuseen LJ, MacMahan RA. Germ cells and ova in dysgenetic gonads of a 46-XY female dizygotic twin. Am J Dis Child 1979; 133:373–375.
469. Khodr GS, Cadena GD, Ong TC. Y-autosome translocation, gonadal dysgenesis, and gonadoblastoma. Am J Dis Child 1979; 133:277–282.
470. Ahmed SR, Shalet SM, Campbell RH, et al. Primary gonadal damage following treatment of brain tumors in childhood. J Pediatr 1983; 103:562–565.
471. Perrone L, Sinisi AA, Sicuranza R, et al. Prepubertal endocrine follow-up in subjects with Wilms' tumor. Med Pediatr Oncol 1988; 16:255–258.
472. Nicosia SV, Matus Ridley M, Meadows AT. Gonadal effects of cancer therapy in girls. Cancer 1985; 55:2364–2372.
473. Matus Ridley M, Nicosia SV, Meadows AT. Gonadal effects of cancer therapy in boys. Cancer 1985; 55:2353–2363.
474. Quigley C, Cowell C, Jiminez M, et al. Normal or early development of puberty despite gonadal damage in children treated for acute lymphoblastic leukemia. N Engl J Med 1989; 321:143–151.
475. Irvine WJ. Autoimmunity in endocrine disease. Recent Prog Horm Res 1980; 36:509–556.
476. Ahonen P, Myllarniemi S, Sipila I, et al. Clinical variation of autoimmune polyendocrinopathy–candidiasis–ectodermal dystrophy (APECED) in a series of 68 patients. N Engl J Med 1990; 322:1829–1836.
477. Lucky AW, Rebar RW, Blizzard RM, et al. Pubertal progression in the presence of elevated serum gonadotropins in girls with multiple endocrine deficiencies. J Clin Endocrinol Metab 1977; 45:673–678.
478. Flora S, Bottazzo GF, Doniach D. Immunofluorescence studies on antibodies to steroid producing cells, and to germ line cells in endocrine disease and infertility. Clin Exp Immunol 1980; 39:97–111.
479. Eisenberg L. Normal child development. In: Kaplan HI, Freedman AM, Sadock BJ, eds. Comprehensive Textbook of Psychiatry. Baltimore: Williams & Wilkins, 1980: 2421–2442.
479a. Daniel WAJ. Adolescent growth and development. Semin Adolesc Med 1985; 1:1–96.
480. Starup J, Sele V, Henriksen B. Amenorrhea associated with increased production of gonadotropins and a morphologically normal ovarian follicular apparatus. Acta Endocrinol 1971; 66:248–256.
481. Dewhurst CJ, Dekoos EB, Ferreira HP. The resistant ovary syndrome. Br J Obstet Gynaecol 1975; 82:341–345.
482. Evers JLH, Rolland R. The gonadotropin resistant ovary syndrome: a curable disease? Clin Endocrinol 1981; 14:99–103.
483. Kaufman FR, Kogut MD, Donnell GN, et al. Hypergonadotropic hypogonadism in female patients with galactosemia. N Engl J Med 1981; 304:994–998.
484. Stanhope R, Adams J, Brook CG. Evolution of polycystic ovaries in a girl with delayed menarche: a case report. J Reprod Med 1988; 33:482–484.
485. Porcu E, Venturoli S, Magrini O, et al. Circadian variation of luteinizing hormone can have two different profiles in adolescent anovulation. J Clin Endocrinol Metab 1987; 65:488–493.
486. Massarano AA, Adams J, Preece MA, et al. Ovarian ultrasound appearances in the Turner syndrome. J Pediatr 1989; 114:568–573.
487. Spitz IM, Hirsch HJ, Trestian S. The prolactin response to thyrotropin-releasing hormone differentiates isolated gonadotropin deficiency from delayed puberty. N Engl J Med 1983; 308:575–579.
488. Winters SJ, Johnsonbaugh RE, Sherins RJ. The response of prolactin to chlorpromazine stimulation in men with hypogonadotrophic hypogonadism and early pubertal boys: relationship to sex steroid exposure. Clin Endocrinol 1982; 16:321–330.
489. Cristiano AM, Munabi A, el Sabbagh H, et al. Prolactin response to metoclopramide does not distinguish patients with hypogonadotrophic hypogonadism from delayed puberty. Clin Endocrinol 1988; 28:75–82.
490. Popovic V, Milosevic Z, Micic D. The prolactin response to TRH and domperidone does not differentiate male hypothalamic hypogonadism and constitutional delay of puberty. Exp Clin Endocrinol 1987; 89:211–215.
491. Gordon D, Cohen HN, Beastall GH, et al. Hormonal responses in pubertal males to pulsatile gonadotropin releasing hormone (GnRH) administration. J Endocrinol Invest 1988; 11:77–83.
492. Lanes R, Moncada G, Palacios A, et al. The metoclopramide test: a useful tool with the luteinizing hormone–releasing hormone test in distinguishing between constitutional delay of puberty and hypogonadotropic hypogonadism. Fertil Steril 1989; 52:55–59.
493. Partsch CJ, Hermanussen M, Sippell WG. Differentiation of male hypogonadotropic hypogonadism and constitutional delay of puberty by pulsatile administration of gonadotropin-releasing hormone. J Clin Endocrinol Metab 1985; 60:1196–1203.
494. Rosenfield RL, Burstein S, Cuttler L. Use of nafarelin for testing pituitary-ovarian function. J Reprod Med 1989; 34:1044–1050.
495. Haavisto A, Dunkel L, Pettersson K, et al. LH measurements by in vitro bioassay and a highly sensitive immunofluorometric assay improve the distinction between boys with constitutional delay of puberty and hypogonadotropic hypogonadism. Pediatr Res 1990; 27:211–214.
496. Cohen HN, Wallace AM, Beastall GH, et al. Clinical value of adrenal androgen measurement in the diagnosis of delayed puberty. Lancet 1981; 1:689–692.
497. Copeland KC, Paunier L, Sizonenko PC. The secretion of adrenal androgens and growth patterns of patients with hypogonadrotropic hypogonadism and idiopathic delayed puberty. Adolesc Med 1977; 91:985–990.
498. Lee PDK, Rosenfeld RG. Psychosocial correlates of short stature and delayed puberty. Pediatr Adolesc Endocrinol 1987; 4:851–863.
498a. Ehrhardt AA, Meyer-Bahlburg HFL. Psychologic correlates of abnormal pubertal development. Clin Endocrinol Metab 1975; 4:207–222.
499. Kaplowitz PB. Diagnostic value of testosterone therapy in boys with delayed puberty. Am J Dis Child 1989; 143:116–120.
500. Wilson DM, Kei J, Hintz RL, et al. Effects of testosterone therapy for pubertal delay. Am J Dis Child 1988; 142:96–99. (Erratum in Am J Dis Child 1988; 142:286.)
501. Richman RA, Kirsch LR. Testosterone treatment in adolescent boys with constitutional delay in growth and development. N Engl J Med 1988; 319:1563–1567.
502. Zachmann M, Studer S, Prader A. Short-term testosterone treatment at bone age of 12 to 13 years does not reduce adult height in boys with constitutional delay of growth and adolescence. Helv Paediatr Acta 1987; 42:21–28.
503. Rosenfield RL. Diagnosis and management of delayed puberty. J Clin Endocrinol Metab 1990; 70:559–562.
504. Rosenfeld RG, Northcraft GB, Hintz RL. A prospective, randomized study of testosterone treatment of constitutional delay of growth and development in male adolescents. Pediatrics 1982; 69:681–687.
505. Stanhope R, Buchanan CR, Fenn GC, et al. Double blind placebo controlled trial of low dose oxandrolone in the treatment of boys with constitutional delay of growth and puberty. Arch Dis Child 1988; 63:501–505.
506. Toublanc JE, Couprie C, Garnier P, et al. The effects of treatment combining an agonist of gonadotropin-releasing hormone with growth hormone in pubertal patients with isolated growth hormone deficiency. Acta Endocrinol 1989; 120:795–799.
507. Burstein S, Grumbach MM, Kaplan SL. Early determination of androgen-responsiveness is important in the management of microphallus. Lancet 1979; 2:983–986.
508. Reilly JM, Woodhouse CR. Small penis and the male sexual role. J Urol 1989; 142:569–571.
509. Santoro N, Filicori M, Crowley WF. Hypogonadotropic disorders in men and women: diagnosis and therapy with pulsatile gonadotropin-releasing hormone. Endocr Rev 1986; 7:11–23.
510. Aulitzky W, Frick J, Galvan G. Pulsatile luteinizing hormone–releasing hormone treatment of male hypogonadotropic hypogonadism. Fertil Steril 1988; 50:480–486.
511. Stanhope R, Brook CG, Pringle PJ, et al. Induction of puberty by pulsatile gonadotropin releasing hormone. Lancet 1987; 2:552–555.
512. Stanhope R, Adams J, Jacobs HS, et al. Ovarian ultrasound assessment in normal children, idiopathic precocious puberty, and during low dose pulsatile gonadotrophin releasing hormone treatment of hypogonadotrophic hypogonadism. Arch Dis Child 1985; 60:116–119.
513. Schoemaker J, van Kessel H, Simons AH, et al. Induction of first cycles in primary hypothalamic amenorrhea with pulsatile luteinizing hormone–releasing hormone: a mirror of female pubertal development. Fertil Steril 1987; 48:204–212.
514. Rosenfeld RG, Hintz RL, Johanson AJ, et al. Growth hormone therapy in Turner's syndrome. In: Rosenfeld RG, Grumbach MM, eds. Turner Syndrome. New York: Marcel Dekker, 1990: 393–405.
515. Thamdrup E. Precocious Sexual Development: A Clinical Study of 100 Patients. Springfield, IL: Charles C Thomas, 1961: 50.
516. Thamdrup E. Somatic development in puberty. A survey. Nord Med 1965; 74:1013–1018.
517. Kaplan SL, Grumbach MM. Clinical review 14: pathophysiology and treatment of sexual precocity. J Clin Endocrinol Metab 1990; 71:785–789.
518. Lee PA. Medroxyprogesterone therapy for sexual precocity in girls. Am J Dis Child 1981; 135:443–445.
519. Grumbach MM, Kaplan SL. Recent advances in the diagnosis and management of sexual precocity. Acta Paediatr Jpn (Overseas Ed) 1988; 30:155–175.

520. Reuben MS, Manning GR. Precocious puberty. Arch Pediatr 1923; 40:27–44.

521. Lenz J. Vorzeitige Mestruation, Geschlechtsreife und Entwicklung. Arch Gynaekol 1913; 99:67.

522. Sigurjonsdottir TJ, Hayles AB. Precocious puberty. A report of 96 cases. Am J Dis Child 1968; 115:309–321.

523. Muram D, Dewhurst J, Grant DB. Precocious puberty: a follow-up study. Arch Dis Child 1984; 59:77–78.

524. Benedict PH. Endocrine features in Albright's syndrome (fibrous dysplasia of bone). Metabolism 1962; 11:30–45.

525. Bierich JR. Sexual precocity. Clin Endocrinol Metab 1975; 4:107–142.

526. Liu N, Grumbach MM, De Napoli RA, et al. Prevalence of electroencephalographic abnormalities in idiopathic precocious puberty and premature pubarche: bearing on pathogenesis and neuroendocrine regulation of puberty. J Clin Endocrinol Metab 1965; 25:1296–1308.

527. Fontoura M, Brauner R, Prevot C, et al. Precocious puberty in girls: early diagnosis of a slowly progressing variant. Arch Dis Child 1989; 64:1170–1176.

528. Schwarz HP, Tschaeppeler H, Zuppinger K. Case report: unsustained central sexual precocity in four girls. Med Sci 1990; 299:260–264.

529. Leiper AD, Stanhope R, Kitching P, et al. Precocious and premature puberty associated with treatment of acute lymphoblastic leukaemia. Arch Dis Child 1987; 62:1107–1112.

530. Rappaport R, Brauner R. Growth and endocrine disorders secondary to cranial irradiation. Pediatr Res 1989; 25:561–567.

531. Genazzani AR, Facchinetti F, Pintor C, et al. Proopiocortin-related peptide plasma levels throughout prepuberty and puberty. J Clin Endocrinol Metab 1983; 57:56–61.

531a. Herman BH, Arthur-Smith A, Hammock MK, et al. Ontogeny of β-endorphin and cortisol in the plasma of children and adolescents. J Clin Endocrinol Metab 1988; 67:186–190.

532. Zuniga OF, Tanner SM, Wild WO, et al. Hamartoma of CNS associated with precocious puberty. Am J Dis Child 1983; 137:127–133.

533. Cacciari E, Frejaville E, Cicognani A. How many cases of true precocious puberty in girls are idiopathic? J Pediatr 1983; 102:357–360.

534. Starceski PJ, Lee PA, Albright L, et al. Hypothalamic hamartomas and sexual precocity. Am J Dis Child 1990; 144:225–228.

534a. Price RA, Lee PA, Albright AL, et al. Treatment of sexual precocity by removal of a luteinizing hormone–releasing hormone secreting hamartoma. JAMA 1984; 251:2247–2249.

535. Pescovitz DH, Comite F, Hench K, et al. The NIH experience with precocious puberty: diagnostic subgroups and response to short-term luteinizing hormone releasing hormone analogue therapy. J Pediatr 1986; 108:47–54.

536. Nishio S, Fujiwara S, Aiko Y, et al. Hypothalamic hamartoma. Report of two cases. J Neurosurg 1989; 70:640–645.

537. Diebler C, Ponsot G. Hamartomas of the tuber cinereum. Neuroradiology 1983; 25:93–101.

538. Lin SR, Bryson MM, Gobien R, et al. Neuroradiologic study of hamartomas of the tuber cinereum and hypothalamus. Neuroradiology 1978; 16:17–19.

539. Nakagawa N, Takahashi M, Kohrogi Y. Neuroradiologic findings of hypothalamic hamartoma with emphasis on computed tomography. J Comput Tomogr 1986; 10:77–83.

540. Peterman SB, Steiner RE, Bydder GM. Magnetic resonance imaging of intracranial tumors in children and adolescents. AJNR 1984; 5:703–709.

541. Hahn FJ, Leibrock LG, Huseman CA, et al. The MR appearance of hypothalamic hamartoma. Neuroradiology 1988; 30:65–68.

542. Sato M, Ushio Y, Arita N. Hypothalamic hamartoma: report of two cases. Neurosurgery 1985; 16:198–206.

543. Styne DM, Harris DA, Egli CA, et al. Treatment of true precocious puberty with a potent luteinizing hormone–releasing factor agonist: effect on growth, sexual maturation, pelvic sonography, and the hypothalamic-pituitary-gonadal axis. J Clin Endocrinol Metab 1985; 61:142–151.

544. Brauner R, Rappaport R, Nicod C, et al. True precocious puberty in non-tumor hydrocephalus. An analysis of 16 cases. Arch Fr Pediatr 1987; 44:433–436.

545. Sockalosky JJ, Kriel RL, Krach LE, et al. Precocious puberty after traumatic brain injury. J Pediatr 1987; 110:373–377.

546. Brauner R, Pierre-Kahn A, Nemedy-Sandor E. Precocious puberty caused by a suprasellar arachnoid cyst. Analysis of 6 cases. Arch Fr Pediatr 1987; 44:489–493.

547. Okamoto K, Nakasu Y, Sato M, et al. Isosexual precocious puberty associated with multilocular arachnoid cysts at the cranial base. Report of a case. Acta Neurochir (Wien) 1981; 57:87–93.

548. Clark SJ, Van Dop C, Conte FA, et al. Reversible true precocious puberty secondary to a congenital arachnoid cyst. Am J Dis Child 1988; 142:255–256.

549. Listernick R, Charrow J. Neurofibromatosis type 1 in childhood. J Pediatr 1990; 116:845–853.

550. Mulvihill JJ, Parry DM, Sherman JL, et al. NIH conference. Neurofibromatosis 1 (Recklinghausen disease) and neurofibromatosis 2 (bilateral acoustic neurofibromatosis). An update. Ann Intern Med 1990; 113:39–52.

551. Cohen BH, Rothner AD. Incidence, types, and management of cancer in patients with neurofibromatosis. Oncology 1989; 3:23–30.

552. Samuelsson B, Riccardi VM. Neurofibromatosis in Gothenburg, Sweden. II. Intellectual compromise. Neurofibromatosis 1989; 2:78–83.

553. Samuelsson B, Riccardi VM. Neurofibromatosis in Gothenburg, Sweden. III. Psychiatric and social aspects. Neurofibromatosis 1989; 2:84–106.

554. Xu GF, Lin B, Tanaka K, et al. The catalytic domain of the neurofibromatosis type 1 gene product stimulates ras GTPase and complements *ira* mutants of *S. cerevisiae*. Cell 1990; 63:835–841.

555. Ballester R, Marchuk D, Boguski M, et al. The NF1 locus encodes a protein functionally related to mammalian GAP and yeast IRA proteins. Cell 1990; 63:851–859.

556. Martin GA, Viskochil D, Bollag G, et al. The GAP-related domain of the neurofibromatosis type 1 gene product interacts with *ras* p21. Cell 1990; 63:843–849.

557. Money J, Hosta G. Laughing seizures with sexual precocity. Johns Hopkins Med J 1967; 120:326–336.

558. LaFranchi SH. Sexual precocity with hypothalamic hypopituitarism. Am J Dis Child 1979; 133:739–742.

559. Werder EA, Murset G, Zachmann M, et al. Treatment of precocious puberty with cyproterone acetate. Pediatr Res 1974; 8:248–256.

560. Sorgo W, Kiraly E, Homoki J, et al. The effects of cyproterone acetate on statural growth in children with precocious puberty. Acta Endocrinol 1987; 115:44–56.

561. Sadeghi-Nejad A, Kaplan SL, Grumbach MM. The effect of medroxyprogesterone acetate on adrenocortical function in children with precocious puberty. J Pediatr 1971; 78:616–624.

562. Grumbach MM. True or central precocious puberty. In: Kreiger DT, Bardin CW, eds. Current Therapy in Endocrinology and Metabolism, 1985–1986. Toronto: B. C. Decker, 1985: 4–8.

563. Stanhope R, Huen KF, Buzi F, et al. The effect of cyproterone acetate on the growth of children with central precocious puberty. Eur J Pediatr 1987; 146:500–503.

564. Marshall JC, Kelch RP. Gonadotropin releasing hormone: role of pulsatile secretion in the regulation of reproduction. N Engl J Med 1986; 315:1459–1468.

565. Hazum E, Conn PM. Molecular mechanism of gonadotropin releasing hormone (GnRH) action. I. The GnRH receptor. Endocr Rev 1988; 9:379–386.

566. Huckle W, Conn PM. Molecular mechanism of gonadotropin releasing hormone action. II. The effector system. Endocr Rev 1988; 9:387–395.

567. Karten MJ, Rivier JE. Gonadotropin-releasing hormone analog design. Structure-function studies toward the development of agonists and antagonists: rationale and perspective. Endocr Rev 1986; 7:44–66.

568. Holland FJ, Fishman L, Costigan DC, et al. Pharmacokinetic characteristics of the gonadotropin-releasing hormone analog D-Ser (tBU)-⁶Pro⁹NEt luteinizing hormone–releasing hormone (buserelin) after subcutaneous and intranasal administration in children with central precocious puberty. J Clin Endocrinol Metab 1986; 63:1065–1070.

569. Lemay A. Clinical appreciation of LHRH analogue formulation. Horm Res 1989; 32:93–101.

570. Handelsman DJ, Swerdloff RS. Pharmacokinetics of gonadotropin-releasing hormone and its analogs. Endocr Rev 1986; 7:95–105.

571. Comite F, Cutler GB Jr, Rivier J, et al. Short-term treatment of idiopathic precocious puberty with a long-acting analogue of luteinizing hormone–releasing hormone. A preliminary report. N Engl J Med 1981; 305:1546–1550.

572. Crowley WF Jr, Comite F, Vale W, and Cutler GB Jr. Therapeutic use of pituitary desensitization with a long-acting LHRH agonist: a potential new treatment for idiopathic precocious puberty. J Clin Endocrinol Metab 1981; 52:370–372.

573. Boepple PA, Mansfield MJ, Wierman ME, et al. Use of a potent, long acting agonist of gonadotropin-releasing hormone in the treatment of precocious puberty. Endocr Rev 1986; 7:24–33.

574. Comite F, Cassorla F, Barnes KM, et al. Luteinizing hormone releasing hormone analogue therapy for central precocious puberty. Long-term effect on somatic growth, bone maturation, and predicted height. JAMA 1986; 255:2613–2616.

575. Drop SL, Odink RJ, Rouwe C, et al. The effect of treatment with an LH-RH agonist (buserelin) on gonadal activity, growth and bone maturation in children with central precocious puberty. Eur J Pediatr 1987; 146:272–278.

576. Bourguignon JP, Van Vliet G, Vandeweghe M, et al. Treatment of central precocious puberty with an intranasal analogue of GnRH (buserelin). Eur J Pediatr 1987; 146:555–560.

577. Kaplan SL, Grumbach MM. True precocious puberty: treatment with GnRH-agonists. In: Delemarre-Van de Waal H, Plant TM, van Rees GP, et al., eds. Control of the Onset of Puberty. Amsterdam: Elsevier, 1989: 357–373.

578. Kamp GA, Manasco PK, Barnes KM, et al. Low growth hormone levels are related to body mass index and do not reflect impaired growth in luteinizing hormone–releasing hormone agonist–treated children with precocious puberty. J Clin Endocrinol Metab 1991; 72:301–307.

579. Kappy MS, Stuart T, Perelman A. Efficacy of leuprolide therapy in children with central precocious puberty. Am J Dis Child 1988; 142:1061–1064.

580. Kappy M, Stuart T, Perelman A, et al. Suppression of gonadotropin secretion by a long-acting gonadotropin-releasing hormone analog (leuprolide acetate, Lupron Depot) in children with precocious puberty. J Clin Endocrinol Metab 1989; 69:1087–1089.

581. Luder AS, Holland FJ, Costigan DC, et al. Intranasal and subcutaneous treatment of central precocious puberty in both sexes with a long-acting analog of luteinizing hormone–releasing hormone. J Clin Endocrinol Metab 1984; 58:966–972.

582. Roger M, Chaussain JL, Berlier P, et al. Long term treatment of male and female precocious puberty by periodic administration of a long-acting preparation of D-Trp⁶-luteinizing hormone–releasing hormone microcapsules. J Clin Endocrinol Metab 1986; 62:670–677.

583. Manasco PK, Pescovitz OH, Feuillan PP, et al. Resumption of puberty after long term luteinizing hormone–releasing hormone agonist treatment of central precocious puberty. J Clin Endocrinol Metab 1988; 67:368–372.

584. Pescovitz OH, Comite F, Cassorla F, et al. True precocious puberty complicating congenital adrenal hyperplasia: treatment with a luteinizing hormone–releasing hormone analog. J Clin Endocrinol Metab 1984; 58:857–861.

585. Roosen N, Cras P, Van Vyve M. Hamartoma of the tuber cinereum in a six-month-old boy, causing isosexual precocious puberty. Neurochirurgia (Stuttg) 1987; 30:56–60.

586. Markin RS, Leibrock LG, Huseman CA, et al. Hypothalamic hamartoma: a report of 2 cases. Pediatr Neurosci 1987; 13:19–26.

587. Morinaga S, Yamaguchi M, Watanabe I, et al. An immunohistochemical study of hepatoblastoma producing human chorionic gonadotropin. Cancer 1983; 51:1647–1652.

588. McArthur JW, Toll GD, Russfield AB, et al. Sexual precocity attributable to ectopic gonadotropin secretion by hepatoblastoma. Am J Med 1973; 54:390–403.

589. Braunstein GD, Bridson WE, Glass A, et al. In vivo and in vitro production of human chorionic gonadotropin and alpha-fetoprotein by a virilizing hepatoblastoma. J Clin Endocrinol Metab 1972; 35:857–862.

590. Heimann A, White PF, Riely CA, et al. Hepatoblastoma presenting as isosexual precocity. The clinical importance of histologic and serologic parameters. J Clin Gastroenterol 1987; 9:105–110.

591. Faggiano M, Criscuolo T, Perrone L, et al. Sexual precocity in a boy due to hypersecretion of LH and prolactin by a pituitary adenoma. Acta Endocrinol 1983; 102:167–172.

592. Schedewie HK, Reiter EO, Beitins IZ. Testicular Leydig cell hyperplasia as a cause of familial sexual precocity. J Clin Endocrinol Metab 1981; 52:271–278.

593. Rosenthal SM, Grumbach MM, Kaplan SL. Gonadotropin-independent familial sexual precocity with premature Leydig and germinal cell maturation (familial testotoxicosis): effects of a potent luteinizing hormone–releasing factor agonist and medroxyprogesterone acetate therapy in four cases. J Clin Endocrinol Metab 1983; 57:571–579.

594. Egli CA, Rosenthal SM, Grumbach MM, et al. Pituitary gonadotropin-independent male-limited autosomal dominant sexual precocity in nine generations: familial testotoxicosis. J Pediatr 1985; 106:33–40.

595. Gondos B, Egli CA, Rosenthal SM, et al. Testicular changes in gonadotropin-independent familial male sexual precocity. Familial testotoxicosis. Arch Pathol Lab Med 1985; 109:990–995.

596. Wierman ME, Beardsworth DE, Mansfield JM, et al. Puberty without gonadotropins: a unique mechanism of sexual development. N Engl J Med 1985; 312:65–72.

597. Manasco PK, Girton ME, Diggs RL, et al. Novel testis-stimulating factor in familial male precocious puberty. N Engl J Med 1991; 324:227–231.

598. de Kretser DM. Local regulation of testicular function. Int Rev Cytol 1987; 109:89–112.

599. Yee JB, Hutson JC. Effects of testicular macrophage–conditioned medium on Leydig cells in culture. Endocrinology 1985; 116:2682–2684.

600. Janecki A, Jakubowiak A, Lukaszyk A. Stimulatory effect of Sertoli cell in secretory products on testosterone secretion by purified Leydig cells in primary culture. Mol Cell Endocrinol 1985; 42:235–243.

601. Rommerts FFG, Hoogerbrugge JW, van der Molen HJ. Stimulation of steroid production in isolated rat Leydig cells by unknown factors in testicular fluid differs from the effects of LH or LH-releasing hormone. J Endocrinol 1986; 109:111–117.

602. Verhoeven G, Cailleau J. A Leydig cell stimulating factor produced by human testicular tubules. Mol Cell Endocrinol 1987; 49:137–147.

603. Schwall R, Schmelzer CH, Matsuyama E, et al. Multiple actions of recombinant activin-A in vivo. Endocrinology 1989; 125:1420–1423.

604. Feldman D. Ketoconazole and other imidazole derivatives as inhibitors of steroidogenesis. Endocr Rev 1986; 7:409–420.

605. Holland FJ, Fishman L, Bailey JD, et al. Ketoconazole in the management of precocious puberty not responsive to LHRH-analogue therapy. N Engl J Med 1985; 312:1023–1028.

606. Holland FJ, Kirsch SE, Selby R. Gonadotropin-independent precocious puberty ("testotoxicosis"): influence of maturational status on response to ketoconazole. J Clin Endocrinol Metab 1987; 64:328–333.

607. Laue L, Kenigsberg D, Pescovitz OH, et al. The treatment of familial male precocious puberty with spironolactone and testolactone. N Engl J Med 1989; 320:496–502.

608. Kuhn JM, Billebaud T, Navratil H. Prevention of the transient adverse effects of a gonadotropin-releasing hormone analogue (buserelin) in metastatic prostatic carcinoma by administration of an antiandrogen (nilutamide). N Engl J Med 1989; 321:413–418.

609. Kochak GM, Mangot S, Mulagha MT, et al. The pharmacodynamic inhibition of estrogen synthesis by fadrozole, an aromatase inhibitor and its pharmacokinetic disposition. J Clin Endocrinol Metab 1990; 71:1349–1355.

610. Towne BH, Mahour GH, Woolley MM, et al. Ovarian cysts and tumors in infancy and childhood. J Pediatr Surg 1975; 10:311–320.

611. Polhemus DW. Ovarian maturation and cyst formation in children. Pediatrics 1953; 11:588–594.

612. Peters H, Himelstein-Braw R, Faher M. The normal development of the ovary in childhood. Acta Endocrinol 1976; 82:617–630.

613. Peters H. The human ovary in childhood and early maturity. Eur J Obstet Gynecol Reprod Biol 1979; 3:137–144.

614. de Sa DJ. Follicular ovarian cysts in stillbirths and neonates. Arch Dis Child 1975; 50:45–50.

615. Zachariou Z, Roth H, Boos R, et al. Three years' experience with large ovarian cysts diagnosed in utero. J Pediatr Surg 1989; 24:478–482.

616. Sedin G, Bergquist C, Lindgren PG. Ovarian hyperstimulation syndrome in preterm infants. Pediatr Res 1985; 19:548–551.

617. Lyon AJ, De Bruyn R, Grant DB. Transient sexual precocity and ovarian cysts. Arch Dis Child 1985; 60:819–822.

617a. Liapi C, Evain-Brion D. Diagnosis of ovarian cysts from birth to puberty: a report of twenty cases. Acta Paediatr Scand 1987; 76:91–96.

618. Zipf WB, Kelch RP, Hopwood NJ, et al. Suppressed responsiveness to gonadotropin-releasing hormone in girls with unsustained isosexual precocity. J Pediatr 1979; 95:38–43.

619. Richards GE, Kaplan SL, Grumbach MM. Sexual precocity associated with functional follicular cysts, prepubertal gonadotropins and LRF response and fluctuating estrogen levels. Pediatr Res 1977; 11:431 (abstract).

619a. Tonetta SA, di Zerega GS. Intragonadal regulation of follicular maturation. Endocr Rev 1989; 10:205–229.

620. Fakhry J, Khoury A, Kotval PS, et al. Sonography of autonomous follicular ovarian cysts in precocious pseudopuberty. J Ultrasound Med 1988; 7:597–603.

621. Butler MG, Najjar JL. Do some patients with fragile X syndrome have precocious puberty. Am J Med Genet 1988; 31:779–781.

622. Young RH, Dickersin GR, Scully RE. Juvenile granulosa cell tumor of the ovary. A clinicopathologic analysis of 125 cases. Am J Surg Pathol 1984; 8:575–596.

623. Eberlein WR, Bongiovanni AM, Jones IT, et al. Ovarian tumors and cysts associated with sexual precocity. J Pediatr 1960; 57:484–497.

624. Biscotti CV, Hart WR. Juvenile granulosa cell tumors of the ovary. Arch Pathol Lab Med 1989; 113:40–46.

625. Masson P. Pflugerome. Bull Soc Anat (Paris) 1912; 14:403–404.

626. Talerman A. The pathology of gonadal neoplasm composed of germ cells and sex cord stroma derivatives. Pathol Res Pract 1980; 170:24–38.

627. Bhathena D, Haning RV, Shapiro S. Coexistence of a gonadoblastoma and mixed germ-cell cord stroma tumor. Pathol Res Pract 1985; 180:203–206.

628. Lacson AG, Gillis DA, Shawwa A. Malignant mixed germ-cell–sex cord–stromal tumors of the ovary associated with isosexual precocious puberty. Cancer 1988; 61:2122–2133.

629. Solh HM, Azoury RS, Najjar SS. Peutz-Jeghers syndrome associated with precocious puberty. J Pediatr 1983; 103:593–595.

630. Danon M, Crawford JD. The McCune-Albright syndrome. Ergeb Inn Med Kinderheilkd 1987; 55:81–115.

631. Albright F, Butler AM, Hampton AO, et al. Syndrome characterized by osteitis fibrosa disseminata, areas of pigmentation and endocrine dysfunction, with precocious puberty in females. N Engl J Med 1937; 216:727–746.

632. McCune DJ, Bruch H. Osteodystrophia fibrosa. Report of a case in which the condition was combined with precocious puberty, pathologic pigmentation of the skin, and hyperthyroidism, with a review of the literature. Am J Dis Child 1937; 54:806–848.

633. Danon MS, Robboy SH, Kin S, et al. Cushing syndrome, sexual precocity and polyostotic fibrous dysplasia. J Pediatr 1975; 87:917–921.

634. Lightner ES, Penny R, Frasier SD. Growth hormone excess and sexual precocity in polyostotic fibrous dysplasia. J Pediatr 1975; 87:922–927.

635. Nager GT, Kennedy DW, Kopstein E. Fibrous dysplasia: A review of the disease and its manifestations in the temporal bone. Ann Otol Rhinol Laryngol Suppl 1982; 92:1–52.

636. Giovanelli G, Bernasconi S, Banchini G. McCune-Albright syndrome in a male child: a clinical and endocrinologic enigma. J Pediatr 1978; 92:220–226.

637. Carani C, Pacchioni C, Baldini A, et al. Effects of cyproterone acetate, LHRH agonist and ovarian surgery in McCune-Albright syndrome with precocious puberty and galactorrhea. J Endocrinol Invest 1988; 11:419–423.

638. Reith KG, Comite F, Shawker T, et al. Pituitary and ovarian abnormalities demonstrated by CT and ultrasound in children with features of the McCune-Albright syndrome. Radiology 1984; 153:389–393.

639. Foster CM, Comite F, Pescovitz OH, et al. Variable response to a long-

acting agonist of luteinizing hormone–releasing hormone in girls with McCune-Albright syndrome. J Clin Endocrinol Metab 1984; 59:801–805.

640. Foster CM, Ross JL, Shawker T, et al. Absence of pubertal gonadotropin secretion in girls with McCune-Albright syndrome. J Clin Endocrinol Metab 1984; 58:1161–1165.

641. Pasquino AM, Tebaldi L, Cives C, et al. Precocious puberty in the McCune-Albright syndrome. Progression from gonadotrophin-independent to gonadotrophin-dependent puberty in a girl. Acta Paediatr Scand 1987; 76:841–843.

642. Feuillan PP, Foster CM, Pescovitz, OH, et al. Treatment of precocious puberty in the McCune-Albright syndrome with the aromatase inhibitor testolactone. N Engl J Med 1986; 315:1115–1119.

643. Happle R. The McCune-Albright syndrome: a lethal gene surviving by mosaicism. Clin Genet 1986; 29:321–324.

644. Lyons J, Landis CA, Harsh G, et al. Two G protein oncogenes in human endocrine tumors. Science 1990; 249:655–659.

645. Van Wyk JJ, Grumbach MM. Syndrome of precocious menstruation and galactorrhea in juvenile hypothyroidism: an example of hormonal overlap in pituitary feedback. J Pediatr 1960; 57:416–435.

646. Kendle FW. Case of precocious puberty in a female cretin. Br Med J 1905; 1:246.

647. Suter SN, Kaplan SL, Aubert ML. Plasma prolactin and thyrotropin and the response to thyrotropin-releasing factor in children with primary and tertiary hypothyroidism. J Clin Endocrinol Metab 1978; 47:1015–1020.

648. Hemady ZS, Siler-Khodr TM, Najjar S. Precocious puberty in juvenile hypothyroidism. J Pediatr 1978; 92:55–59.

648a. Piziak VK, Hahn HB. Isolated menarche in juvenile hypothyroidism. Clin Pediatr 1984; 23:177–179.

649. Laron Z, Karp M, Dolberg L. Juvenile hypothyroidism with testicular enlargement. Acta Paediatr Scand 1970; 59:317–322.

650. Pringle PJ, Stanhope R, Hindmarsh P, et al. Abnormal pubertal development in primary hypothyroidism. Clin Endocrinol 1988; 28:479–486.

651. Buchanan CR, Stanhope R, Adlard P, et al. Gonadotropin, growth hormone and prolactin secretion in children with primary hypothyroidism. Clin Endocrinol 1988; 29:427–436.

652. Wood LC, Olichney M, Locke H, et al. Syndrome of juvenile hypothyroidism associated with advanced sexual development: report of two new cases and comment on the management of an associated ovarian mass. J Clin Endocrinol Metab 1965; 25:1289–1295.

653. Money J, Lamacz M. Genital examination and exposure experienced as nosocomial sexual abuse in childhood. J Nerv Ment Dis 1987; 175:713–721.

654. Salardi S, Orsini LF, Cacciari E, et al. Pelvic ultrasonography in girls with precocious puberty, congenital adrenal hyperplasia, obesity, or hirsutism. J Pediatr 1988; 112:880–887.

655. Ivarsson SA, Nilsson KO, Persson PH. Ultrasonography of the pelvic organs in prepubertal and postpubertal girls. Arch Dis Child 1983; 58:352–354.

656. Rieth KG, Comite F, Dwyer AJ, et al. CT of cerebral abnormalities in precocious puberty. AJR 1987; 148:1231–1238.

657. Burton EM, Ball WS Jr, Crone K, et al. Hamartoma of the tuber cinereum: a comparison of MR and CT findings in four cases. AJNR 1989; 10:497–501.

658. Cook CD, McArthur JW, Berenberg W. Pseudoprecocious puberty in girls as a result of estrogen ingestion. N Engl J Med 1953; 248:671–674.

659. Precocious development in Puerto Rican children. Lancet 1986; 1:721–722 (editorial).

660. Fara GM, Del Corvo G, Bernuzzi S, et al. Epidemic of breast enlargement in an Italian school. Lancet 1979; 2:295–297.

661. Bongiovanni AM. An epidemic of premature thelarche in Puerto Rico. J Pediatr 1983; 103:245–246.

661a. Mills JL. Endocrinology of premature thelarche. In: McLachlan JA, ed. Estrogens in the Environment. II. Influences on Development. New York: Elsevier, 1985: 412–427.

662. Howard CP, Takahashi H, Hayles AB. Feminizing adrenal adenoma in a boy. Mayo Clin Proc 1977; 52:354–357.

663. MacLaren NL, Migeon CH, Raiti S. Gynecomastia with congenital virilizing adrenal hyperplasia (11-β-hydroxylase deficiency). J Pediatr 1975; 86:579–581.

664. Hemsell DL, Edman CD, Marks JF, et al. Massive extraglandular aromatization of plasma androstenedione resulting in feminization of a prepubertal boy. J Clin Invest 1977; 60:455–464.

665. Berkovitz GD, Guerami A, Brown TR, et al. Familial gynecomastia with increased extraglandular aromatization of plasma carbon19-steroids. J Clin Invest 1985; 75:1763–1769.

666. Wilson DM, Pitts WC, Hintz RL, et al. Testicular tumors with Peutz-Jeghers syndrome. Cancer 1986; 57:2238–2240.

667. Young RH, Scully RE. Ovarian Sertoli cell tumors: a report of 10 cases. Int J Gynecol Pathol 1984; 2:349–363.

668. Tavassoli FA, Norris HJ. Sertoli tumors of the ovary. A clinicopathologic study of 28 cases with ultrastructural observations. Cancer 1980; 46:2282–2297.

669. Ilicki A, Lewin P, Kauli LR, et al. Premature thelarche—natural history and sex hormone secretion in 68 girls. Acta Paediatr Scand 1984; 73:756–762.

670. Van Winter JT, Noller KL, Zimmerman D, et al. Natural history of premature thelarche in Olmsted County, Minnesota, 1940 to 1984. J Pediatr 1990; 116:278–280.

671. McKiernan J, Hull D. Breast development in the newborn. Arch Dis Child 1981; 56:525–529.

671a. McKiernan J, Coyne J, Cahalane S. Histology of breast development in early life. Arch Dis Child 1988; 63:136–139.

672. Caufriez H, Wolter R, Gouaerts M, et al. Gonadotropins and prolactin pituitary reserve in premature thelarche. J Pediatr 1977; 91:751–753.

673. Dresch PC, Arnal M, Prader A. A premature thelarche. Helv Paediat Acta 1960; 15:585–593.

673a. Caparo VJ, Bayonet-Rivera NP, Thomas A, et al. Premature thelarche. Obstet Gynecol Surg 1971; 26:2–7.

674. Silver HK, Sami D. Premature thelarche: precocious development of the breast. Pediatrics 1964; 34:107–111.

675. Mills JL, Stolley PD, Davies J, et al. Premature thelarche. Natural history and etiologic investigation. Am J Dis Child 1981; 135:743–745.

676. Collett-Solberg PR, Grumbach MM. A simplified procedure for evaluating estrogenic effects and the sex chromatin pattern in exfoliated cells in urine: studies in premature thelarche and gynecomastia of adolescence. J Pediatr 1965; 66:883–890.

677. Escobar ME, Rivarola MA, Bergada C. Plasma concentration of estradiol-17β in premature thelarche and in different types of sexual precocity. Acta Endocrinol 1976; 81:351–361.

678. Radfar N, Ansusinna K, Kenny FM. Circulating bound and free estradiol and estrone during normal growth and development and in premature thelarche and isosexual precocity. J Pediatr 1976; 89:719–723.

678a. Wenick GB, Chasalow FI, Blethen SL. Sex hormone–binding globulin and thyroxine-binding globulin levels in premature thelarche. Steroids 1988; 52:543–550.

678b. Rosner W. The functions of corticosteroid-binding globulin and sex hormone–binding globulin: recent advances. Endocr Rev 1990; 11:80–91.

679. Ferrier P, Shepard TH, Smith FK. Growth disturbances and values for hormone excretion in various forms of precocious sexual development. Pediatrics 1961; 28:258–275.

680. Pescovitz OH, Hench KD, Barnes KM, et al. Premature thelarche and central precocious puberty: the relationship between clinical presentation and the gonadotropin response to luteinizing hormone–releasing hormone. J Clin Endocrinol Metab 1988; 67:474–479.

680a. Stanhope R, Brook CC. Thelarche variant: a new syndrome of precocious sexual maturation? Acta Endocrinol 1990; 125:481–484.

681. Stanhope R, Abdulwahid NA, Adams J, et al. Studies of gonadotrophin pulsatility and pelvic ultrasound examinations distinguish between isolated premature thelarche and central precocious puberty. Eur J Pediatr 1986; 145:190–194.

682. Fréjaville E, Pagni G, Cacciari E, et al. Breast contact thermography for differentiation between premature thelarche and true precocious puberty. Eur J Pediatr 1988; 147:389–391.

683. Murram D, Dewhurst J, Grant DB. Premature menarche: a follow-up study. Arch Dis Child 1983; 58:142–143.

683a. Heller ME, Dewhurst J, Grant DB. Premature menarche without other evidence of precocious puberty. Arch Dis Child 1979; 54:472–475.

684. Blanco-Garcia M, Eva-Brion D, Roger M, et al. Isolated menses in prepubertal girls. Pediatrics 1985; 76:43–47.

685. Hill NCW, Oppenheimer LW, Morton KE. The aetiology of vaginal bleeding in children. A 20-year review. Br J Obstetr Gynaecol 1989; 96:467–470.

686. David L, Betand B, Berlier P, et al. Les hémorragie génitales de la fille avant la puberté. Ann Pediatr (Paris) 1984; 31:55–61.

687. Silverman SH, Migeon CJ, Rosenberg E, et al. Precocious growth of sexual hair without other secondary sexual development; "premature pubarche," a constitutional variation of adolescence. Pediatrics 1952; 10:426–431.

688. Thamdrup E. Premature pubarche, a hypothalamic disorder? Acta Endocrinol 1955; 18:564–567.

689. Rappaport R. Plasma androgens and LH in scoliotic patients with premature pubarche. J Clin Endocrinol Metab 1974; 38:401–406.

690. Lee PA, Migeon CJ, Bias WB, et al. Familial hypersecretion of adrenal androgens transmitted as a dominant, non–HLA linked trait. Obstet Gynecol 1987; 69:259–264.

691. Korth-Schutz S, Levine LS, New MI. Serum androgens in normal prepubertal and pubertal children and in children with precocious puberty. J Clin Endocrinol Metab 1976; 42:117–124.

692. Rosenfield RL. Plasma 17-ketosteroids and 17-beta-hydroxysteroid in girls with premature development of sexual hair. J Pediatr 1971; 79:260–266.

693. Doberne Y, Levine LS, New MI. Elevated urinary testosterone and androstanediol in precocious adrenarche. Pediatr Res 1975; 9:794–797.

694. Lee PA, Gareis FJ. Gonadotropin and sex steroid response to luteinizing hormone–releasing hormone in patients with premature adrenarche. J Clin Endocrinol Metab 1976; 43:195–197.

695. Oberfield SE, Mayes DM, Levine LS. Adrenal steroidogenic function in a black and Hispanic population with precocious pubarche. J Clin Endocrinol Metab 1990; 70:76–82.

696. Biro FM, Lucky AW, Huster GA, et al. Hormonal studies and physical maturation in adolescent gynecomastia. J Pediatr 1990; 116:450–455.

697. Nydick M, Bustos J, Dale JH, et al. Gynecomastia in adolescent boys. JAMA 1961; 178:449–454.

698. Large DM, Anderson DC. Twenty-four hour profiles of circulating androgens and estrogens in male puberty with and without gynecomastia. Clin Endocrinol 1979; 22:505–521.

699. Carlson SE. Gynecomastia. N Engl J Med 1980; 404:795–799.

700. LaFranchi SH, Parlow AF, Lippe BM, et al. Pubertal gynecomastia and transient elevation of serum estradiol level. Am J Dis Child 1975; 129:927–931.

701. Siiteri PK, MacDonald PC. The role of extraglandular estrogen in human endocrinology. In: Greep RO, Astwood EB, eds. Handbook of Physiology. Sect 7: Endocrinology. Vol II. Part 1. Female Reproductive System. Washington, DC: American Physiological Society, 1973: 615–629.

702. Moore DC, Schlaepfer LV, Paunier L, et al. Hormonal changes during puberty. V. Transient pubertal gynecomastia: abnormal androgen-estrogen ratios. J Clin Endocrinol Metab 1984; 58:492–499.

703. Mohoney J, Hynes B. Concurrent Poland's syndrome and gynecomastia: a case report. Can J Surg 1990; 33:58–60.

704. Chudley AE, Hagerman RJ. Fragile X syndrome. J Pediatr 1987; 110:821–830.

705. Waaler PE, Thorsen T, Stoa KF, et al. Studies in normal male puberty. Acta Paediatr Scand [Suppl] 1974; 1–36.

706. Manasco PK, Pescovitz OH, Hill SC, et al. Six-year results of luteinizing hormone releasing hormone (LHRH) agonist treatment in children with LHRH-dependent precocious puberty. J Pediatr 1989; 115:105–108.

707. Lin TH, LePage ME, Henzl M, et al. Intranasal nafarelin: an LH-RH analogue treatment of gonadotropin-dependent precocious puberty. J Pediatr 1986; 109:954–958.

708. Lee PA, Page JG. Effects of leuprolide in the treatment of central precocious puberty. J Pediatr 1989; 114:321–324.

709. Rappaport R, Fontoura M, Brauner R. Treatment of central precocious puberty with an LHRH agonist (buserelin): effect on growth and bone maturation after three years of treatment. Horm Res 1987; 28:149–154.

710. Suwa S, Hibi I, Kato K. LH-RH agonistic analog (buserelin) treatment of precocious puberty: collaborative study in Japan. Acta Paediatr Jpn Overseas Ed 1988; 30:176–184.

711. Donaldson MD, Stanhope R, Lee TJ, et al. Gonadotrophin responses to GnRH in precocious puberty treated with GnRH analogue. Clin Endocrinol 1984; 21:499–503.

712. Rime JL, Zumsteg U, Blumberg A, et al. Long-term treatment of central precocious puberty with an intranasal LHRH analogue: control of pituitary function by urinary gonadotropins. Eur J Pediatr 1988; 147:263–269.

713. Stanhope R, Pringle PJ, Brook CG. Growth, growth hormone and sex steroid secretion in girls with central precocious puberty treated with a gonadotrophin releasing hormone (GnRH) analogue. Acta Paediatr Scand 1988; 77:525–530.

714. Kauli R, Pertzelan A, Ben Zeev Z, et al. Treatment of precocious puberty with LHRH analogue in combination with cyproterone acetate—further experience. Clin Endocrinol 1984; 20:377–387.

715. Oostdijk W, Hummelink R, Odink RJ, et al. Treatment of children with central precocious puberty by a slow-release gonadotropin-releasing hormone agonist. Eur J Pediatr 1990; 149:308–313.

716. Van Wieringen JD, Wafelbakker F, Verbrugge HP. Growth Diagrams 1965 Netherlands: Second National Survey on 0–24 Year Olds. Netherlands Institute for Preventative Medicine TNO. Groningen: Wolters-Noordhoof Publishing, 1971.

717. Dupertuis CW, Atkinson WB, Elftman H. Sex differences in pubic hair distribution. Hum Biol 1945; 17:137–142.

718. Reynolds EL, Wines JV. Physical changes associated with adolescence in boys. Am J Dis Child 1951; 82:529–547.

719. Gondos B. Testicular development. In: Johnson AD, Gomes WR, eds. The Testes. Vol IV. New York: Academic, 1977: 1–37.

720. Styne DM, Grumbach MM. Puberty in the male and female: its physiology and disorders. In: Yen JCC, Jaffe RB, eds. Reproductive Endocrinology. Philadelphia: W. B. Saunders, 1986: 313–384.

721. Escomel E. La plus jeune mère du monde. Presse Med 1939; 47:875.

23

GLUCOSE HOMEOSTASIS AND HYPOGLYCEMIA

Philip E. Cryer

INTRODUCTION

Maintenance of the plasma glucose concentration is critical to survival, because plasma glucose is the predominant metabolic fuel utilized by the central nervous system under most conditions. The central nervous system cannot synthesize glucose, store more than a few minutes' supply, or concentrate glucose from the circulation. Thus brief hypoglycemia can cause profound brain dysfunction, and prolonged, severe hypoglycemia causes brain death. It is therefore not surprising that glucoregulatory systems have evolved to prevent or correct hypoglycemia.

The plasma glucose concentration is normally maintained within a relatively narrow range, roughly 3.9 to 8.3 mmol/L (70 to 150 mg/dL), despite wide variations in glucose influx and efflux such as those that follow meals and occur during exercise. Glucoregulatory failure caused by insulin deficiency and resulting in hyperglycemia (diabetes mellitus) is common (see Chapter 24). In contrast, hypoglycemia, except when produced as a side effect of treatment of diabetes, is not a common clinical disorder. This is because redundant glucose counterregulatory systems that raise the plasma glucose level are remarkably effective.

Elucidation of the physiology of glucoregulation in general and of glucose counterregulation in particular has provided major insights into the pathophysiology of hypoglycemia in humans. Nevertheless, there are major gaps in our understanding of the causes, mechanisms, and management of many hypoglycemic states. Hypoglycemia is the subject of two major books,[1, 2] and the physiology of glucose counterregulation and its pathophysiology in diabetes mellitus have been reviewed.[3, 4]

THE PHYSIOLOGY OF SYSTEMIC GLUCOREGULATION

Cellular and systemic glucoregulation is discussed in detail in Chapter 24. Therefore glucose metabolism and systemic glucose balance and their regulation are summarized here, with emphasis on those aspects relevant to glucose counterregulation. The physiology of human glucose counterregulation is then discussed in greater detail.

Glucose Metabolism

Glucose is derived from three sources: intestinal absorption that follows digestion of dietary carbohydrates; glycogenolysis, the breakdown of glycogen, the polymerized storage form of glucose; and gluconeogenesis, the formation of glucose from precursors, including lactate (and pyruvate), amino acids (especially alanine), and, to a lesser extent, glycerol (Fig. 23–1).

Although most tissues have the enzyme systems required to synthesize glycogen (glycogen synthase) and to hydrolyze glycogen (phosphorylase), only the liver and kidneys contain glucose–6-phosphatase, the enzyme necessary for the release of glucose into the circulation. The liver and kidneys also contain the enzymes necessary for gluconeogenesis (including the critical enzymes pyruvate carboxylase, phosphoenol-pyruvate carboxykinase, and fructose-1,6-bisphosphatase).

There are multiple potential metabolic fates of glucose transported into cells (external losses are normally negligible). It may be stored as glycogen. It may undergo glycolysis to pyruvate, which can be reduced to lactate, transaminated to form alanine, or converted to acetyl coenzyme A, which in turn can be oxidized to carbon dioxide and water via the tricarboxylic acid cycle, converted to fatty acids (and stored as triglycerides), or utilized for ketone body (acetoacetate, β-hydroxybutyrate) or cholesterol synthesis. Finally, glucose may be released into the circulation. As summarized in the following paragraphs, these fates differ in different organs.

The liver is remarkably flexible in its role in glucose homeostasis. It is, for practical purposes, the sole source of endogenous glucose production. Renal gluconeogenesis and glucose release contribute substantially to the systemic glucose pool only during prolonged starvation. Under conditions of high glucose output, the energy needs of the liver are largely provided by the beta-oxidation of fatty acids. On the other hand, the liver can also be an organ of net glucose uptake, with glucose stored as glycogen, oxidized for energy, or converted to fat, which can either remain in the liver or be transported to other tissues as very-low-density lipoproteins.

Muscle can either store or utilize glucose, the latter primarily through glycolysis to pyruvate, which is reduced to lactate or transaminated to form alanine. Lactate released from muscle is transported to the liver, where it serves as a

gluconeogenic precursor (Cori, or glucose-lactate, cycle); similarly, alanine may flow from muscle to the liver, where it, too, serves as a gluconeogenic precursor (glucose-alanine cycle). During a fast, muscle can reduce its glucose uptake to virtually zero, oxidize fatty acids for its energy needs, and, through proteolysis, mobilize amino acids for transport to the liver as gluconeogenic precursors.

Although quantitatively less important than muscle, adipose tissue can also utilize glucose for fatty acid synthesis or oxidation to glycerol-3-phosphate, which can then esterify fatty acids (derived largely from circulating very-low-density lipoproteins) to form triglycerides. During a fast, adipocytes can also decrease their glucose utilization and satisfy energy needs from the beta-oxidation of fatty acids. Other tissues, such as the formed elements of the blood and the renal medullae, do not have the capacity to decrease glucose utilization on fasting and therefore produce lactate at relatively fixed rates.

As mentioned earlier, glucose is the predominant metabolic fuel utilized by the brain under most conditions. Glucose undergoes terminal oxidation to carbon dioxide and water in the brain. When ketones are plentiful in the circulation, as during prolonged fasting, they can support the majority of the energy needs of the brain and reduce its glucose utilization.[5]

Systemic Glucose Balance

Maintenance of the normal plasma glucose concentration requires precise matching of glucose utilization and endogenous glucose production or dietary glucose delivery.

The postabsorptive state is the interdigestive period that begins approximately 5 to 6 h after a meal. However, the term is most commonly used to describe data obtained after a 10- to 14-h overnight fast. In the postabsorptive state, plasma glucose concentrations are relatively stable; thus glucose production and utilization rates are equal. They average 12 μmol/kg/min (2.2 mg/kg/min) and range from about 10 to 14 μmol/kg/min (1.8 to 2.6 mg/kg/min) in normal

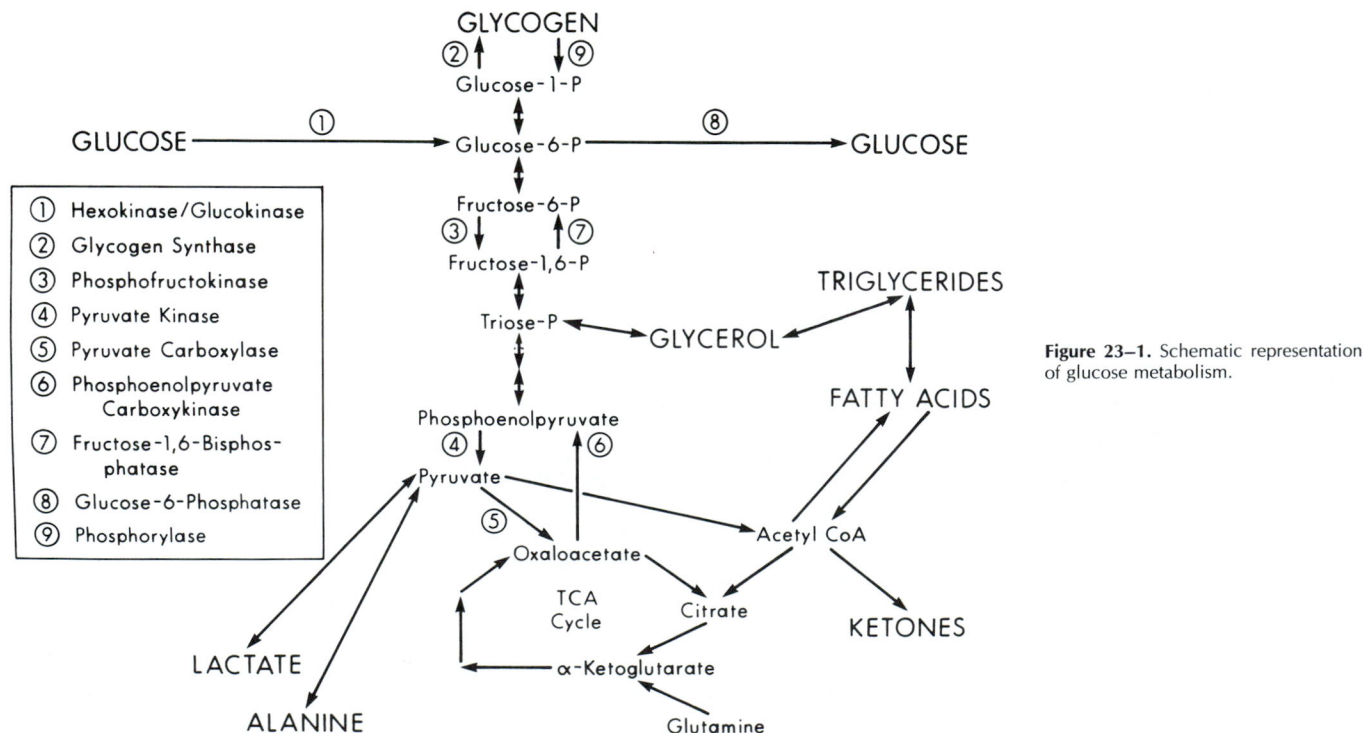

Figure 23–1. Schematic representation of glucose metabolism.

adults after an overnight fast.[6] Approximately 60% of basal glucose utilization is accounted for by the brain. The remainder is used by glycolyzing tissues such as the formed elements of the blood, the renal medullae, and, to some extent, muscle and fat. About three fourths of hepatic glucose production results from glycogenolysis and the remaining fourth from gluconeogenesis after an overnight fast. Gluconeogenesis from lactate, pyruvate, amino acids (especially alanine), and glycerol is estimated to represent 13, 1, 7 (4), and 4% of endogenous glucose production, respectively, and therefore 52, 4, 28 (16), and 16% of gluconeogenesis, respectively.[1]

The importance of gluconeogenesis in providing new glucose and supporting hepatic glycogen stores after an overnight fast becomes apparent when one considers the limited availability of preformed glucose. The glucose pool—free glucose in the extracellular fluid and that in the cells of certain tissues (primarily the liver but also small amounts in the kidneys, intestinal mucosa, pancreatic islets, brain, and blood cells)—is about 83 to 111 mmol (15 to 20 g) in the normal adult. Glycogen that can be mobilized to provide circulating glucose (i.e., hepatic glycogen) averages approximately 389 mmol (70 g), with a range of about 135 to 722 mmol (24 to 130 g).[7] Thus in an adult of average size, preformed glucose can provide as little as a 3-h supply and less than an 8-h supply of glucose on average, at the diminished rate of glucose utilization that occurs during the postabsorptive state. Clearly, therefore, gluconeogenesis is important for maintenance of the postabsorptive plasma glucose concentration.

If fasting is prolonged to 24 to 48 h, the plasma glucose level declines and then stabilizes, hepatic glycogen content falls to less than 56 mmol (10 g), and gluconeogenesis becomes the sole source of glucose production. Because amino acids are the gluconeogenic precursors that result in net glucose formation, muscle protein is degraded. Glucose utilization by muscle and fat virtually ceases. As lipolysis and ketogenesis accelerate and circulating ketone levels rise, ketones become a major source of fuel for the brain. Thus glucose utilization by the brain declines by about half, resulting in a decrease in the rate of glucose production required to maintain the plasma glucose concentration. This decrease in gluconeogenesis results in diminished protein wasting. After prolonged fasting (40 d), ketones provide an estimated 80 to 90% of the energy utilized by the brain, and renal gluconeogenesis provides up to half of the endogenous glucose production.[5, 8]

After a meal, glucose absorption results in rates of exogenous glucose delivery into the circulation that can be more than twice the rate of postabsorptive endogenous glucose production, depending on the carbohydrate content of the meal and the rate and degree of glucose absorption. As glucose is absorbed, endogenous glucose production is suppressed, and glucose utilization by liver, muscle, and fat accelerates.[9] Thus exogenous glucose is assimilated, and the plasma glucose concentration returns to approximately the postabsorptive level.

Exercise increases glucose utilization (by muscle) to rates that can be several-fold greater than those of the postabsorptive state. Endogenous glucose production normally accelerates to match utilization so that the plasma glucose concentration is maintained, but exhaustive exercise can result in rates of glucose utilization that exceed productive capacity and cause a decrease in the plasma glucose concentration.

From these examples it is clear that the plasma glucose concentration is normally maintained within a relatively narrow range despite wide variations in glucose flux, which is a remarkable homeostatic accomplishment.

Glucoregulatory Factors

The regulatory mechanisms that maintain systemic glucose balance involve hormonal, neural, and substrate factors. The cellular mechanisms of the actions of several of these[10] and details of their glycemic effects[11] have been reviewed.

Hormonal Factors

Glucoregulatory hormones include insulin, glucagon, epinephrine, cortisol, and growth hormone. Insulin is the dominant glucose-lowering hormone.[1-4] It suppresses endogenous glucose production and stimulates glucose utilization, thereby lowering the plasma glucose concentration. Insulin is secreted from the beta cells of the pancreatic islets into the hepatic portal circulation and has important actions on the liver as well as on peripheral tissues. It inhibits hepatic glycogenolysis and gluconeogenesis and, in concert with other factors (including hyperglycemia and hypoglucagonemia), converts the liver into an organ of net glucose uptake and fuel storage (glycogen and triglycerides). It also stimulates glucose uptake, storage, and utilization by other insulin-sensitive tissues such as muscle and fat. In the postabsorptive state, insulin regulates the plasma glucose concentration primarily by restraining hepatic glucose production.[12] Higher levels, such as those that occur after meals, are required to stimulate glucose utilization.[12] Insulin is a potent and critical hormone. Profound insulin deficiency and marked insulin excess can both be lethal. However, insulin is not the only physiologically important glucoregulatory hormone.

Glucose-raising, or counterregulatory, hormones include glucagon, epinephrine, growth hormone, and cortisol. Glucagon is secreted from the alpha cells of the pancreatic islets into the hepatic portal circulation and is commonly held to act exclusively on the liver under physiological conditions.[1-4] It is a potent activator of glycogenolysis and gluconeogenesis and increases hepatic glucose production within minutes. This increase is transient. Despite ongoing hyperglucagonemia, hepatic glucose production returns toward basal rates in about a 90-min period, although the hormone continues to support glucose production (i.e., withdrawal of glucagon results in a further decrease in glucose production thereafter).[13] Glucagon-induced hyperglycemia is also transient, because the glucagon-induced increase in glycogenolysis does not persist; during sustained hyperglucagonemia, gluconeogenesis increases progressively, at least for more than 4 h in dogs.[14] The transient glycogenolytic response to sustained hyperglucagonemia is not the result of glycogen depletion, as a further increase in glucagon causes additional glucose release. Instead, it is probably the result of glucose-induced insulin secretion coupled with the autoregulatory effect of hyperglycemia (see later), although other factors may be involved.

The hyperglycemic effect of the adrenomedullary hormone epinephrine is more complex. It both stimulates hepatic glucose production and limits glucose utilization. The actions of epinephrine are both direct and indirect and are mediated through both alpha- and beta-adrenergic mechanisms in humans.[15-17] Alpha-adrenergic limitation of insulin secretion is an important indirect hyperglycemic action of epinephrine. It allows the hyperglycemic response to occur, although an increase in insulin secretion as plasma glucose levels rise normally limits the magnitude of the glycemic response.[16, 17] Beta-adrenergic stimulation of glucagon secretion also occurs,[18, 19] but its contribution to the hyperglycemic effect of epinephrine under physiological conditions appears to be minor.[16, 17] Epinephrine also acts directly (i.e., independent of changes in other hormones) to increase hepatic glycogenolysis and gluconeogenesis. In humans the direct hepatic effect is mediated predominantly through beta-2–adrenergic mechanisms,[15, 17, 20] although direct alpha-adrenergic stimulation of hepatic glucose production has been reported.[21] Like glucagon, epinephrine acts within minutes and produces a transient increase in glucose production but continues to support glucose production at approximately basal rates thereafter. In contrast to glucagon, however, epinephrine also limits glucose utilization predominantly, if not exclusively, through direct beta-adrenergic mechanisms.[15–17] Because of this persistent effect on glucose utilization, sustained hyperepinephrinemia results in persistent hyperglycemia.

Long-term elevations of growth hormone and cortisol limit glucose utilization and stimulate glucose production. Initially, however, growth hormone has a plasma glucose–lowering (insulin-like) effect; its hyperglycemic effect does not appear for several hours.[22] Similarly, cortisol causes an increase in the plasma glucose level only after 2 to 3 h.[23]

The hyperglycemic effect of the combined infusion of glucagon, epinephrine, and cortisol is substantially greater than the sum of the effects of each hormone infused individually.[23] These synergistic interactions are potentially relevant to glucose counterregulation.

Neural Factors

The sympathetic neurotransmitter norepinephrine exerts hyperglycemic actions by mechanisms assumed to be similar to those of epinephrine discussed earlier, except that norepinephrine is released from axon terminals of sympathetic postganglionic neurons. These terminals are adjacent to adrenergic receptors on target cells within the innervated tissues. Electrical stimulation of hepatic sympathetic nerves decreases glycogen content, increases hepatic glucose release, and causes hyperglycemia in animals.[24] Direct periarterial hepatic nerve stimulation increases the plasma glucose level in humans.[25] Parasympathetic stimulation increases hepatic glycogen content and decreases hepatic glucose release in animals.[24] Direct muscarinic cholinergic inhibition of hepatic glucose production has been demonstrated in humans.[26] It is reasonable to anticipate that peptide neurotransmitters and neuromodulators will also be shown to affect glucose metabolism through indirect, or even direct, actions.

Substrate Factors

Glucose per se shifts hepatic metabolism in favor of glycogen storage.[27] The concept of hepatic glucose autoregulation (namely, that the rate of hepatic glucose production is an inverse function of the plasma glucose concentration, independent of hormonal and neural regulatory factors) has arisen as a result of findings in studies with dogs[28, 29] and humans.[30–32] Thus glucose autoregulation is potentially an important glucose counterregulatory factor. Effects of fatty acids and ketone bodies on glucose metabolism have also been described, but their physiological relevance remains to be established.

Control of Glucoregulatory Factors

Hypoglycemia suppresses the secretion of insulin and stimulates the release of glucagon, epinephrine, cortisol, and growth hormone, among other hormones.[3, 4] It also stimulates the release of norepinephrine and acetylcholine from sympathetic and parasympathetic postganglionic neurons, respectively. Regulation of the insulin and glucagon secretory responses to glucose deprivation does not appear to be critically dependent on the central nervous system. Recip-

rocal changes occur in insulin and glucagon release from pancreatic islets in vitro and from perfused pancreata in response to changes in medium glucose concentrations, and neither sympathetic nor parasympathetic neural connections are required for the glucagon-secretory response to hypoglycemia in vivo.[33–35] In contrast, the response of the adrenal medulla is mediated through the central nervous system. Although sympathetic reflexes mediated at the spinal cord level can be elicited by various stimuli in persons with cervical spinal cord transections,[36] sympathochromaffin responses to hypoglycemia[33] or to cellular glucopenia produced by 2-deoxyglucose[37] do not occur in such a situation. Thus brain centers are required to perceive hypoglycemia and to initiate the sympathochromaffin response. (Parenthetically, the plasma norepinephrine, as well as epinephrine, response to hypoglycemia is derived largely from the adrenal medullae.[38, 39]) The secretory responses of growth hormone and cortisol (via corticotropin [ACTH, adrenocorticotropin]) to hypoglycemia are also mediated through the brain.

Glucose Counterregulation

For purposes of discussion, the physiology of glucose counterregulation is divided into two categories: the correction of hypoglycemia and the prevention of hypoglycemia. This distinction is admittedly arbitrary, and the principles of both are fundamentally the same.

The Correction of Hypoglycemia

A series of studies have defined the physiological mechanisms that promote recovery from hypoglycemia produced by insulin administration in normal humans.[6, 38, 40, 41] These findings have been extended to identify the mechanisms of altered[42] and defective[43] glucose counterregulation in patients with insulin-dependent diabetes mellitus (IDDM) and are reviewed in refs. 3 and 4.

The simplest model of glucoregulation would be regulation of the plasma glucose concentration by insulin alone. As the plasma glucose level increases, insulin secretion increases, causing the glucose level to decrease; as the plasma glucose level decreases, insulin secretion decreases, causing the glucose level to increase. However, this model is too simple. First, it seems unlikely that maintenance of a variable as critical to survival as the plasma glucose concentration would depend solely on cessation of insulin secretion, clearance of secreted insulin, and dissipation of the cellular effects of insulin (which persist long after circulating insulin levels fall[44]). Second, the infusion of somatostatin (SRIF, somatotropin release–inhibiting factor) causes a decrease in insulin secretion and an initial decrease in plasma glucose level,[21] an observation incompatible with glucoregulation by insulin alone. Third, glucose counterregulation begins before insulin is dissipated[6, 40] and can be disrupted despite dissipation of insulin.[38, 41, 45–48] Partial counterregulation can occur in the presence of continuing hyperinsulinemia.[43] Thus glucose counterregulation involves a more complex model: the cessation of insulin secretion coupled with the activation of a glucose counterregulatory system or systems.

The temporal relationships between the kinetics of glucose counterregulation and the activation of glucose counterregulatory systems were first defined in humans by Garber and colleagues.[6] The former are illustrated in Figure 23–2. The rapid intravenous injection of regular insulin causes prompt suppression of hepatic glucose production and stimulation of glucose utilization. Thus the plasma glucose concentration falls. Subsequently, glucose utilization declines to the baseline level, and glucose production rises above baseline rates. Thus the plasma glucose concentration rises. The

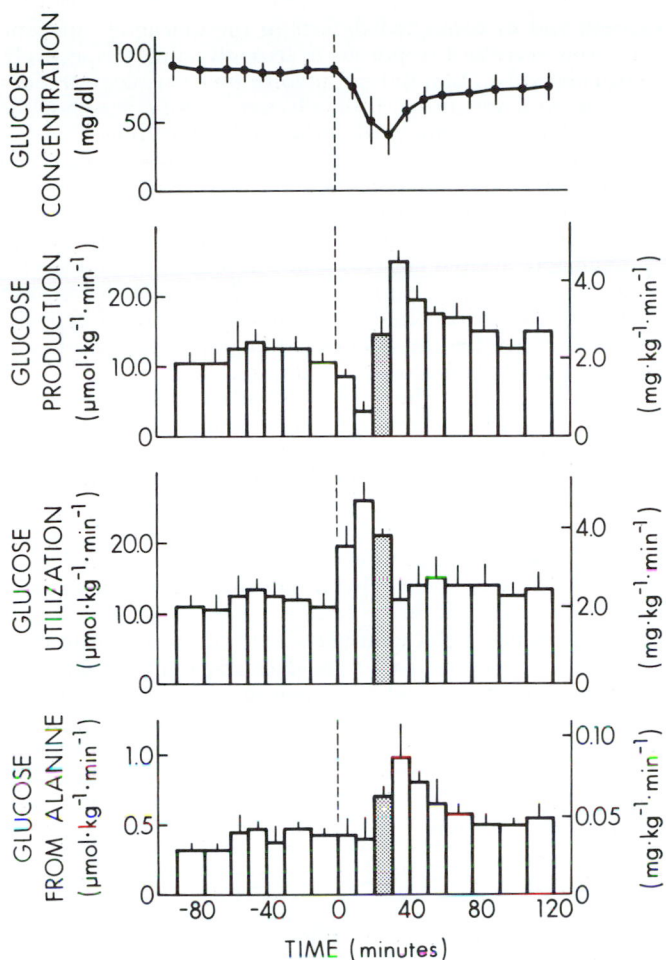

Figure 23–2. Mean (± SE) plasma glucose concentrations, glucose production and utilization rates, and rates of glucose formation from alanine (via gluconeogenesis) before and after rapid intravenous injection of insulin (0.05 U/kg) (*vertical dashed line*) in five normal humans. Shaded columns mark time frame of the onset of the glucose counterregulatory process. Data from ref. 40 are included. (From Cryer PE. The sympatho-adrenal system in human glucose counterregulation and diabetes mellitus. In: Ziegler MG, Lake CR, eds. Norepinephrine. Baltimore: Williams & Wilkins, 1984: 471. Copyright 1984, Alan R. Liss, New York.)

burst of glucose production that restores euglycemia after short-term hypoglycemia is largely the result of glycogenolysis, although gluconeogenesis accelerates as well.[6, 40] The onset of the glucose counterregulatory process is marked by a decline in glucose utilization and an increase in glucose production from its nadir (see shaded columns in Fig. 23–2). Clearly, any model of glucose counterregulation must include a component that acts within this time frame, generally less than 30 min after intravenous insulin injection.[6, 40] Plasma insulin concentrations continue to be increased 10- to 100-fold over baseline levels (depending on the amount injected) at the onset of the glucose counterregulatory process (Fig. 23–3).[6, 40] Thus dissipation of insulin cannot be the sole explanation for recovery from hypoglycemia. An additional counterregulatory factor or factors must be involved.

Insulin-induced hypoglycemia causes increases in plasma glucagon, epinephrine, and norepinephrine levels within the time frame of the onset of the glucose counterregulatory process (Fig. 23–4).[6, 40] Increases in plasma growth hormone and cortisol levels occur somewhat later but still in temporal relation to the counterregulatory process (Fig. 23–5).[6, 40] However, growth hormone and cortisol are not likely to be rapid glucose counterregulatory factors because of the delayed onset of their hyperglycemic actions, as discussed earlier.

The effects of selective deficiencies of the secretion or action of the potentially important glucose counterregulatory factors, alone and in combination, on the recovery from short-term hypoglycemia[38, 40, 41] are summarized in Figure 23–6. Recovery is impaired (by approximately 40%) by the infusion of somatostatin. Somatostatin inhibits the secretion of many hormones, including glucagon and growth hormone. The impaired glucose recovery is due to suppression of glucagon, rather than growth hormone, as evidenced by the fact that the defect is corrected by replacement of the former, but not the latter, during somatostatin infusion. Thus glucagon plays an important role in glucose counterregulation. However, substantial glucose recovery, to approximately 60% of normal, occurs in the absence of glucagon secretion (see Fig. 23–6). Thus an additional factor must be involved, at least when glucagon secretion is deficient. Epinephrine is the likely candidate because of its rapid and substantial secretion in response to hypoglycemia, its rapid hyperglycemic actions, and its enhanced secretion during the impaired glucose recovery produced by deficient glucagon secretion.[38]

Recovery from insulin-induced hypoglycemia is affected little by pharmacological adrenergic blockade[40, 42] or by the epinephrine-deficient state (e.g., in bilaterally adrenalectomized persons).[38] However, when adrenergic blockade is added to inhibition of glucagon secretion, recovery from

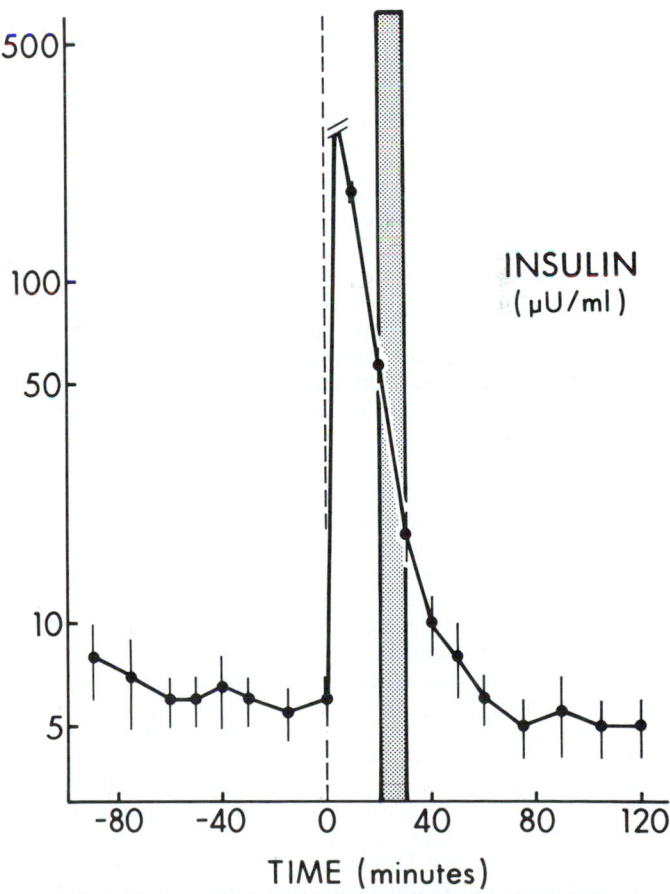

Figure 23–3. Mean (± SE) plasma insulin concentrations in the study shown in Figure 23–2. Regular insulin (0.05 U/kg) was injected intravenously (*vertical dashed line*) into five normal humans. The shaded column marks the time frame of the onset of the glucose counterregulatory process (see Fig. 23–2). Data from ref. 40 are included. To convert insulin values to picomoles per liter, multiply by 7.175. (From Cryer PE. The sympatho-adrenal system in human glucose counterregulation and diabetes mellitus. In: Ziegler MG, Lake CR, eds. Norepinephrine. Baltimore: Williams & Wilkins, 1984: 471. Copyright 1984, Alan R. Liss, New York.)

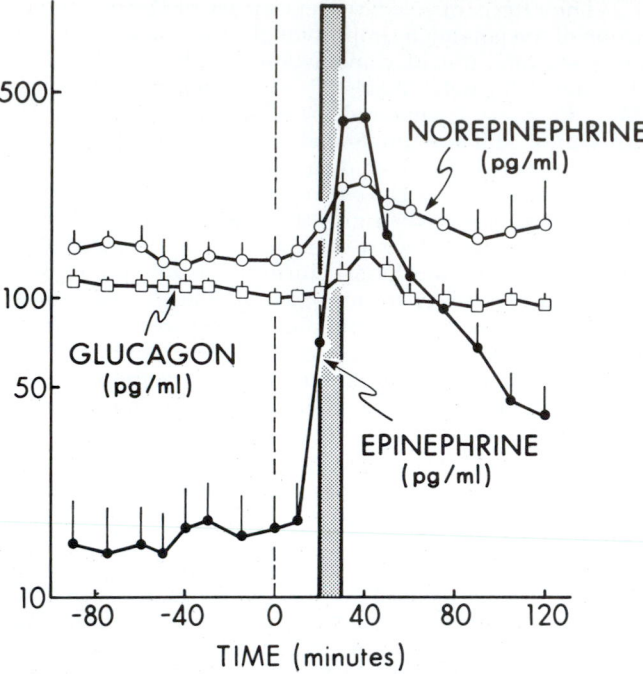

Figure 23–4. Mean (± SE) plasma glucagon, epinephrine, and norepinephrine concentrations in the study shown in Figure 23–2. Regular insulin (0.05 U/kg) was injected intravenously (*vertical dashed line*) into five normal humans. The shaded column marks the time frame of onset of the glucose counterregulatory process (see Fig. 23–2). Data from ref. 40 are included. To convert to SI units: epinephrine (pmol/L), multiply by 5.458; glucagon (pmol/L), multiply by 0.2871; norepinephrine (nmol/L), multiply by 0.005911. (From Cryer PE. The sympathoadrenal system in human glucose counterregulation and diabetes mellitus. In: Ziegler MG, Lake CR, eds. Norepinephrine. Baltimore: Williams & Wilkins, 1984: 471. Copyright 1984, Alan R. Liss, New York.)

hypoglycemia is markedly impaired (see Fig. 23–6). Furthermore, with combined deficiencies of glucagon and epinephrine secretion, glucose recovery fails to occur. This total disruption of hypoglycemic glucose counterregulation occurs despite the dissipation of insulin.

The foregoing data indicate that, in concert with decreasing insulin levels, glucagon plays a primary role in promoting glucose recovery from hypoglycemia; that epinephrine is not normally critical but compensates largely when glucagon secretion is deficient; and that recovery from insulin-induced hypoglycemia fails to occur only in the absence of both glucagon and epinephrine. Secretion of growth hormone and cortisol is not critical to recovery from short-term insulin-induced hypoglycemia.[38, 40, 41, 49] Neither norepinephrine release by the sympathetic nervous system nor glucose autoregulation is sufficiently potent to promote recovery from hypoglycemia in the absence of the key glucose counterregulatory hormones glucagon and epinephrine.

Absent or blunted glucagon-secretory responses to hypoglycemia and to physiological decrements in plasma glucose[50, 51] are common in patients with IDDM. To the extent that glucagon-secretory responses are deficient, such patients are dependent on epinephrine to promote recovery from hypoglycemia.[42] This finding provides further support for the role of glucagon in normal glucose counterregulation. The fact that patients with deficiencies of both glucagon and epinephrine are at substantial risk for severe hypoglycemia during intensive insulin therapy[43] provides additional support for the critical roles of these two hormones. Altered[42] glucose counterregulation and defective[43] glucose counterregulation in patients with IDDM are the results of disease-related deficiencies of the glucagon-secretory re-

sponse and of combined defects in the glucagon- and epinephrine-secretory responses to hypoglycemia, respectively. Their demonstration did not involve pharmacological intervention with somatostatin or adrenergic antagonists or the study of adrenalectomized individuals. The power of the counterregulatory systems is attested to by the fact that partial glucose counterregulation, sufficient to prevent symptomatic central nervous system glucose deprivation, occurs in nondiabetic subjects subjected to sustained, approximately fivefold elevations of the plasma insulin level.[43]

Pharmacological studies have disclosed roles for growth hormone and cortisol in defense against prolonged hypoglycemia.[4, 52, 53] Studies in patients with hypopituitarism support such a role (P. J. Boyle et al., unpublished data). There is also evidence that glucose autoregulation is operative in humans, albeit only during severe hypoglycemia.[4, 54, 55] Nonetheless, the fact that glucose counterregulation is disrupted, resulting in progressive hypoglycemia, when glucagon and epinephrine are deficient and insulin is present, despite normal growth hormone and cortisol secretion and intact autoregulatory mechanisms, indicates that these factors stand low in the hierarchy of glucose counterregulatory factors.

In summary, glucagon plays a primary role in promoting glucose recovery from hypoglycemia. Epinephrine compensates largely for deficient glucagon secretion. Glucose recovery from insulin-induced hypoglycemia fails to occur in the absence of both glucagon and epinephrine. Glucose counterregulation can be totally disrupted by combined deficiencies of glucagon and epinephrine despite substantial dissipation of insulin.

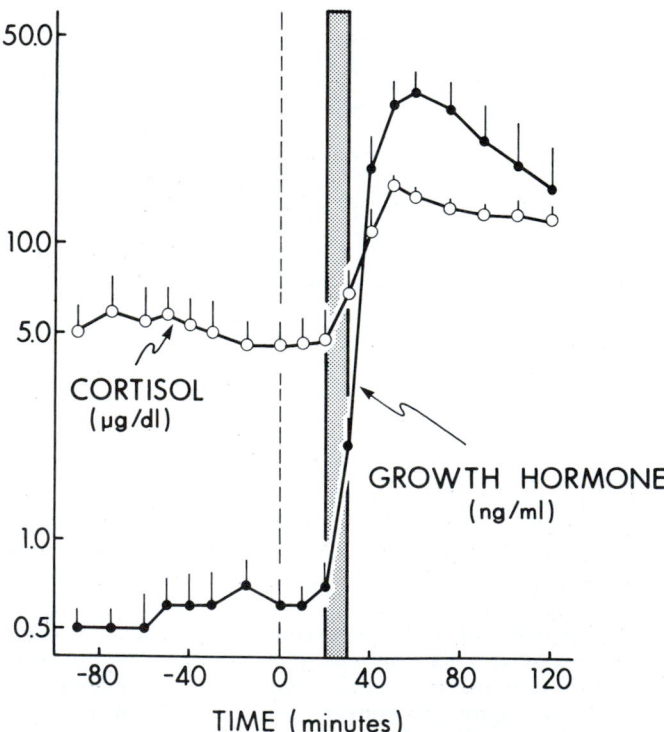

Figure 23–5. Mean (± SE) plasma cortisol and growth hormone concentrations in the study shown in Figure 23–2. Regular insulin (0.05 U/kg) was injected intravenously (*vertical dashed line*) into five normal humans. The shaded column marks the time frame of onset of the glucose counterregulatory process (see Fig. 23–2). Data from ref. 40 are included. To convert to SI units: cortisol (nmol/L); multiply by 27.59; growth hormone (nmol/L), multiply by 0.0465. (From Cryer PE. The sympatho-adrenal system in human glucose counterregulation and diabetes mellitus. In: Ziegler MG, Lake CR, eds. Norepinephrine. Baltimore: Williams & Wilkins, 1984: 471. Copyright 1984, Alan R. Liss, New York.)

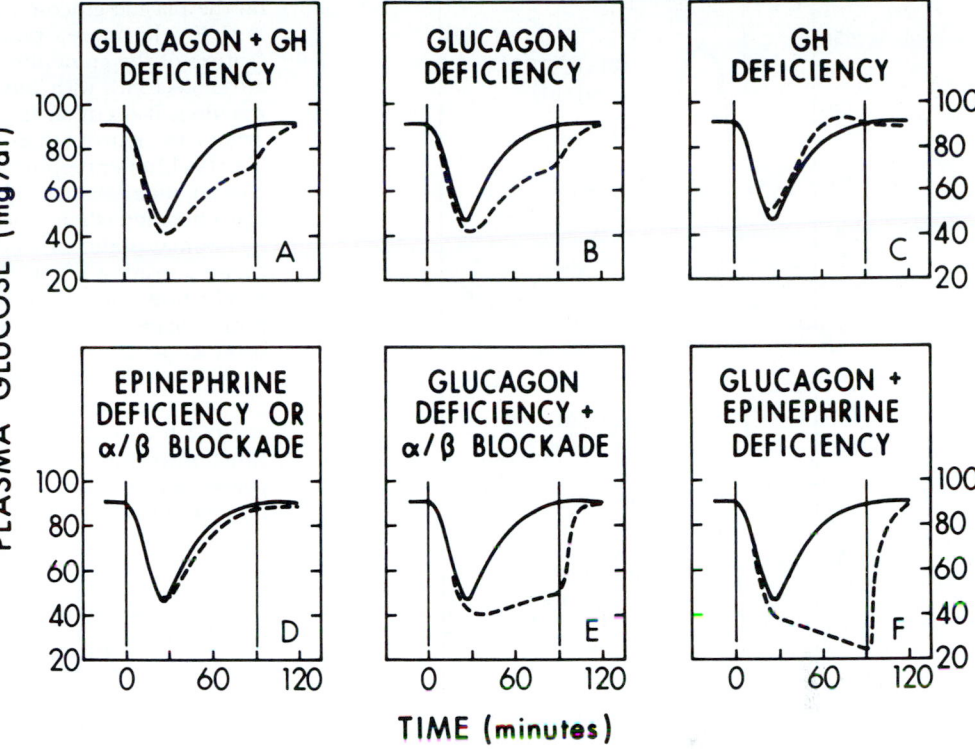

Figure 23–6. Plasma glucose curves during insulin-induced hypoglycemia in normal humans during control studies (*solid lines,* same in all panels) and as modified (*dashed lines*) by A, somatostatin infusion (glucagon + growth hormone [GH] deficiency); B, somatostatin + growth hormone replacement (glucagon deficiency); C, somatostatin + glucagon replacement (growth hormone deficiency); D, phentolamine and propranolol infusion (combined alpha- and beta-adrenergic blockade) or studies on bilaterally adrenalectomized individuals (epinephrine deficiency); E, somatostatin + phentolamine and propranolol infusion (glucagon deficiency + alpha- and beta-adrenergic blockade); and F, somatostatin infusion in bilaterally adrenalectomized individuals (glucagon + epinephrine deficiency). Insulin was injected intravenously at time zero. Infusions were performed from 0 to 90 min (between vertical lines in each panel). Curves are derived from data in refs. 38, 40, and 41. (From Cryer PE. Glucose counterregulation in man. Diabetes 1981; 30:261–264. Copyright 1981 by the American Diabetes Association. Reprinted with permission.)

The Prevention of Hypoglycemia

The mechanisms that blunt physiological decrements in the plasma glucose level, prevent hypoglycemia, and restore or maintain euglycemia have been studied in a model of the postprandial state—the transition from exogenous glucose delivery to endogenous glucose production late after glucose ingestion[45]—and in the postabsorptive state[46-48] in humans.

The possibility that classic counterregulatory hormones might be involved in the prevention, as well as in the correction, of hypoglycemia was suggested by the demonstration that physiological decrements in the plasma glucose level stimulate the secretion of these hormones.[51] The finding that the glycemic thresholds for activation of glucose counterregulatory systems lie within or just below the physiological plasma glucose concentration range and at glucose levels higher than those required to produce symptoms of hypoglycemia[56] (Fig. 23–7) is also consistent with that possibility.

POSTPRANDIAL STATE. The normal relationships between glucose absorption and endogenous glucose production immediately after glucose ingestion were demonstrated by isotopic studies with humans.[9] The normal plasma glucose curve is illustrated in Figure 23–8. After glucose ingestion, the plasma glucose concentration increases as the result of glucose absorption. Endogenous glucose production is markedly suppressed. Plasma glucose levels then decline rapidly as a result of accelerated glucose utilization coupled with diminishing glucose absorption. The venous plasma glucose level falls somewhat below the baseline concentration, but this is largely a reflection of glucose extraction across the forearm during this hyperinsulinemic condition. Although the cited study[9] was not carried through to completion of the counterregulatory process, the plasma glucose concentration is known to stabilize and then rise slightly (see Fig. 23–8). Because glucose absorption is complete by this time and glucose utilization continues, the rise in the plasma glucose concentration curve must be the result of resumption of endogenous glucose production. The text that follows

discusses the mechanisms that regulate this transition from exogenous glucose delivery to endogenous glucose production, blunt physiological decrements in plasma glucose, prevent hypoglycemia, and restore euglycemia late after glucose ingestion.

Transient increments in insulin secretion, transient decrements in glucagon release, and late rises in epinephrine (see Fig. 23–8) occur in response to glucose ingestion.[57] Such changes do not follow ingestion of water, xylose, or mannitol. Insulin concentrations do not fall below baseline levels late after glucose ingestion. Although the late increases in plasma epinephrine are significant,[57] plasma epinephrine concentrations do not commonly achieve the threshold level required

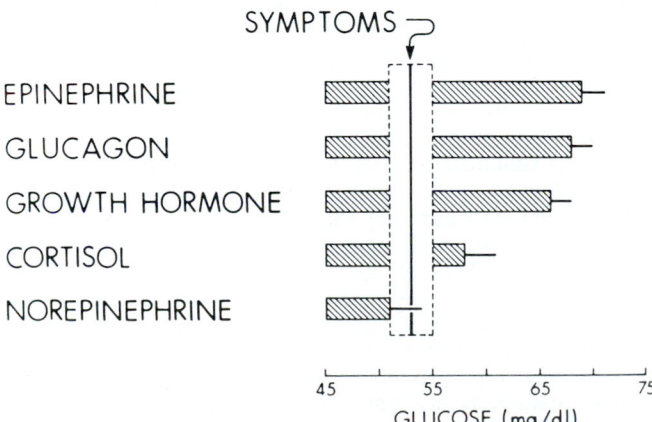

Figure 23–7. (Mean (± SE) arterialized venous glycemic thresholds for increments in plasma epinephrine, glucagon, growth hormone, cortisol, and norepinephrine and for symptoms of hypoglycemia during decrements in the plasma glucose concentration in normal humans. To convert glucose values to millimoles per liter, multiply by 0.05551. (From Schwartz NS, Clutter WE, Shah SD, et al. The glycemic thresholds for activation of glucose counterregulatory systems are at higher glucose levels than the threshold for symptoms. Reproduced from the Journal of Clinical Investigation, 1987, vol. 79, pp. 777–781 by copyright permission of the American Society for Clinical Investigation.)

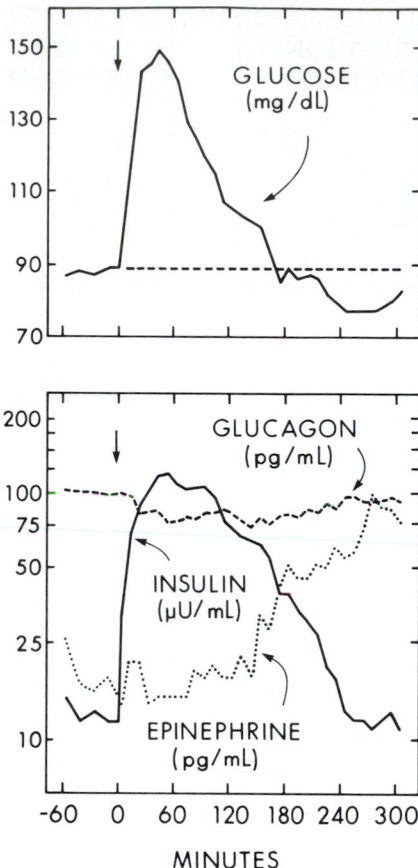

Figure 23–8. Mean plasma glucose concentrations (*top*) and glucose-specific variables (insulin, glucagon, and epinephrine) (*bottom*) after ingestion of 75 g of glucose (*arrows*) by normal humans. Curves are derived from data in ref. 57. Conversion factors for SI units are given in legends for Figures 23–3, 23–4, 23–5, and 23–7.

to affect basal glucose metabolism.[17, 58] Coupled with the physiology of glucose counterregulation discussed previously, these findings lead logically to the concept that the transition from exogenous glucose delivery to endogenous glucose production late after glucose ingestion is the result of coordinated diminution of insulin secretion and resumption of glucagon secretion, rather than dissipation of insulin alone, and that epinephrine does not normally play a critical role in this transition but compensates largely for deficient glucagon secretion. These hypotheses have been confirmed,[45] as summarized in Figure 23–9.

POSTABSORPTIVE STATE. Diminished insulin secretion is fundamental to maintenance of the postabsorptive plasma glucose concentration in that it permits hepatic glucose production to proceed, via hepatic glycogenolysis and gluconeogenesis, and limits glucose utilization by insulin-sensitive tissues (liver, muscle, and fat) so that obligate glucose utilization (central nervous system and glycolyzing tissues) does not result in hypoglycemia. As discussed later, hyperinsulinemia results in postabsorptive hypoglycemia. Nonetheless, insulin is not the sole determinant of the postabsorptive plasma glucose concentration.

The roles of selected glucoregulatory factors in maintenance of the postabsorptive plasma glucose concentration[21, 46] are summarized in Figure 23–10. After an overnight fast, pharmacological blockade of catecholamine actions with the nonselective beta-adrenergic antagonist propranolol and with the nonselective alpha-adrenergic antagonist phentolamine, individually or in combination, has little if any effect

on the plasma glucose concentration in normal humans.[21, 40, 46, 47] Furthermore, postabsorptive hypoglycemia is not a feature of the epinephrine-deficient state (e.g., as in bilateral adrenalectomy with adrenocortical hormone replacement), nor does it occur in the norepinephrine-deficient state that occurs in neuropathies of the autonomic nervous system. Thus neither epinephrine nor norepinephrine plays a critical role in maintenance of the postabsorptive plasma glucose concentration when other glucoregulatory systems are intact.

Somatostatin infusion suppresses both insulin and glucagon secretion but produces a biphasic change in glucose production and in the plasma glucose concentration in the postabsorptive state (see Fig. 23–10).[21, 59] Initially glucose production and the plasma glucose level decline, an effect attributable to suppression of glucagon secretion. Then glucose production increases, reaching baseline levels by about 2 h and then rising above baseline. This increase is a function of the suppression of insulin secretion in that it is prevented by insulin replacement. Glucose production and plasma glucose levels remain below baseline during isolated

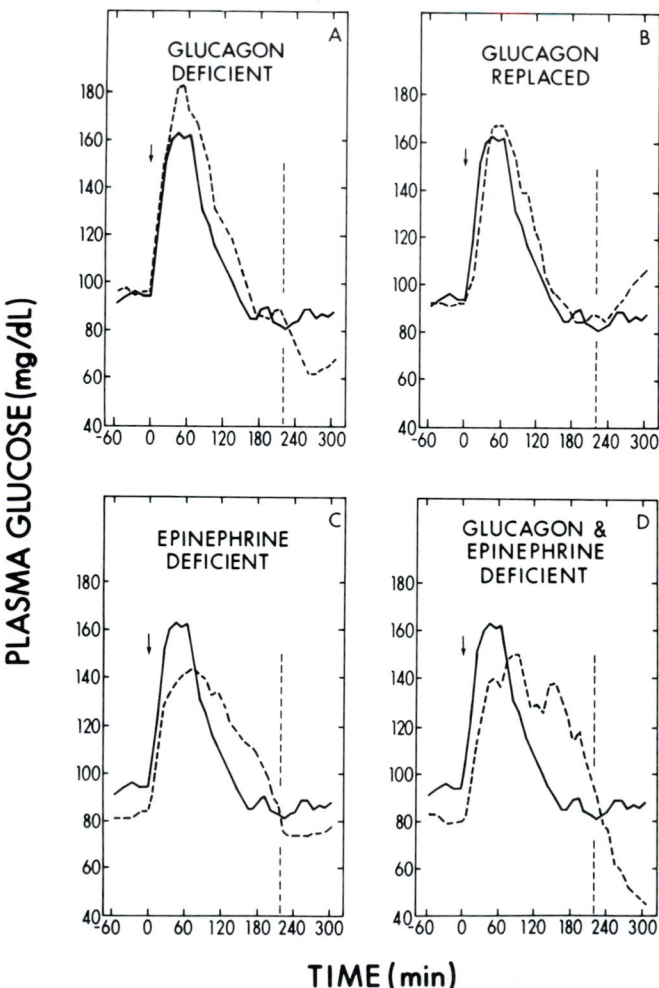

Figure 23–9. Mean plasma glucose curves before and after ingestion of 75 g of glucose (*arrows*) during control studies in normal humans (*solid lines,* same in all panels) and as modified (*dashed lines*) by somatostatin infusion with partial insulin replacement (glucagon deficient, *A*), somatostatin infusion with partial insulin replacement and glucagon replacement (glucagon replaced, *B*), studies in bilaterally adrenalectomized individuals (epinephrine deficient, *C*), and somatostatin infusion with partial insulin replacement in adrenalectomized individuals (glucagon and epinephrine deficient, *D*). Infusions were begun 225 min after the start of glucose ingestion (*vertical dashed line*) and continued through 305 min, the final sampling point. Curves are derived from data in ref. 45. To convert glucose values to millimoles per liter, multiply by 0.05551.

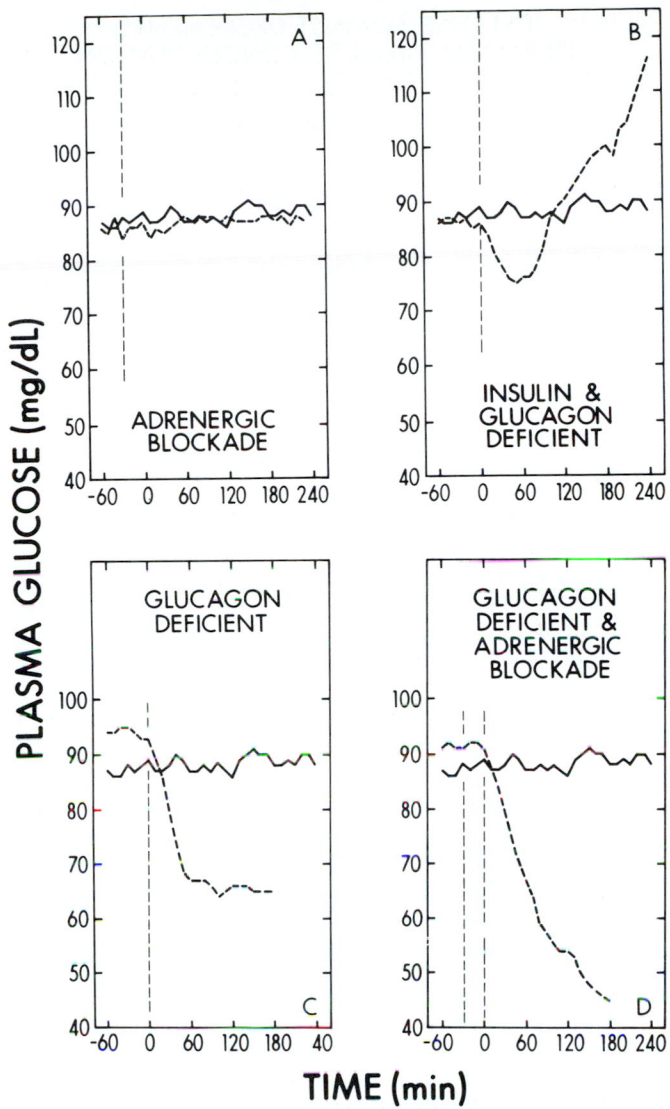

Figure 23–10. Mean plasma glucose concentrations in normal humans studied after an overnight fast during infusions of saline (*solid line,* same in all panels) and as modified (*dashed lines*) by the following interventions (begun at the *vertical dashed lines*): *A,* pharmacological combined alpha- and beta-adrenergic blockade; *B,* insulin and glucagon deficiency produced by infusion of somatostatin; *C,* glucagon deficiency produced by infusion of somatostatin with insulin replacement; and *D,* glucagon deficiency, again produced by infusion of somatostatin with insulin replacement, combined with pharmacological adrenergic blockade. Curves are derived from data in refs. 21 and 46. To convert glucose values to millimoles per liter, multiply by 0.05551.

glucagon deficiency (see Fig. 23–10). Adrenergic mechanisms are also involved, as adrenergic blockade reduces the late rises in glucose production and in plasma glucose level during somatostatin infusion.[21]

Thus glucagon supports postabsorptive glucose production and the postabsorptive plasma glucose concentration. Although the plasma glucose concentration decreases during isolated glucagon deficiency, it reaches a plateau at 3.3 to 3.9 mmol/L (60 to 70 mg/dL) and does not fall to hypoglycemic levels (see Fig. 23–10). Again, an additional counterregulatory factor must be operative under these conditions. Because adrenergic blockade during glucagon deficiency results in a progressive decline in the plasma glucose level to hypoglycemic levels (see Fig. 23–10), that factor is a catecholamine, almost certainly epinephrine.[46]

The mechanisms that prevent hypoglycemia during a more prolonged fast[47] are similar to those operative after an

overnight fast.[46] As shown in Figure 23–11, after a 3-d fast restoration of portal insulin levels to those present after an overnight fast results in a small decrement in plasma glucose concentration, but the glucose level plateaus, and hypoglycemia does not develop. Thus the prevention of hypoglycemia during a more prolonged fast is not due solely to decreased insulin secretion. Again, glucagon plays a primary counterregulatory role. Adrenergic mechanisms are not normally critical, but a catecholamine (presumably epinephrine) compensates and becomes important when glucagon is deficient. Progressive hypoglycemia develops when both glucagon and catecholamine actions are deficient.

Finally, as summarized in Figure 23–12, both decrements in insulin and increments in glucagon play major roles in the prevention of hypoglycemia during exercise.[48] Catecholamines are not normally critical, but progressive hypoglycemia develops when insulin and glucagon are held constant and catecholamine actions are blocked.

In short-term studies at least, other mechanisms (hormonal, neural, and substrate) are insufficient to prevent hypoglycemia when the key glucose counterregulatory hormones, glucagon and epinephrine, are deficient. However, chronic deficiencies of cortisol, growth hormone, or both, occasionally result in postabsorptive hypoglycemia, as discussed later in this chapter. The mechanisms producing this hypoglycemia have not been identified, but chronic deficiencies of cortisol and growth hormone would favor glucose

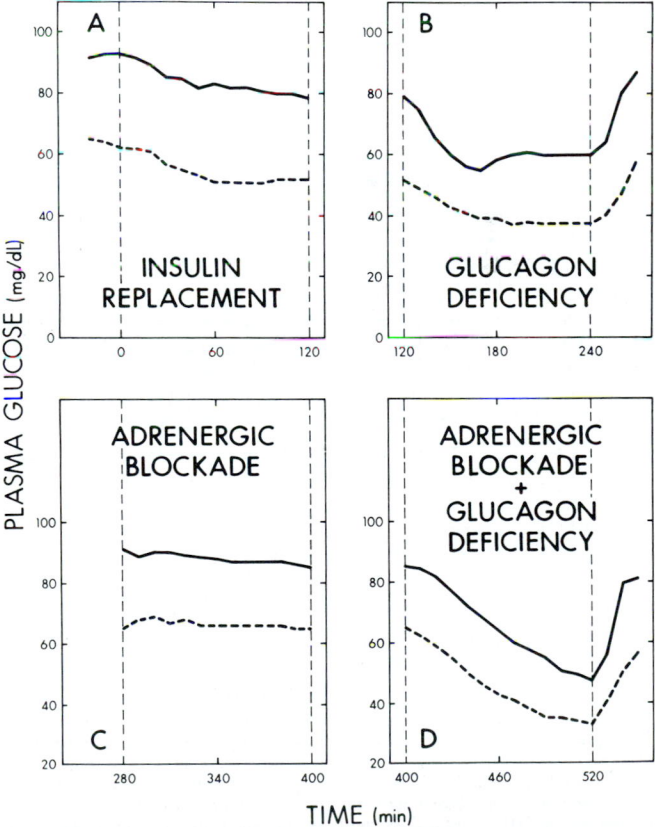

Figure 23–11. Mean plasma concentrations in normal humans studied after an overnight fast (*solid lines*) and after a 3-d fast (*dashed lines*) during the following interventions (begun at the *vertical dashed lines*): *A,* insulin replacement estimated to produce portal insulin concentrations after the 3-d fast that were comparable to those after the overnight fast; *B,* somatostatin infusion with insulin replacement (glucagon deficiency); *C,* phentolamine and propranolol infusions (combined alpha- and beta-adrenergic blockade); and *D,* phentolamine and propranolol infusions + somatostatin infusion with insulin replacement (adrenergic blockade + glucogon deficiency). Curves are derived from data in ref. 47. To convert glucose values to millimoles per liter, multiply by 0.05551.

utilization by insulin-sensitive tissues and limit, either directly or indirectly, hepatic glycogenolysis and gluconeogenesis.

Principles of Glucose Counterregulation

The principles of glucose counterregulation, outlined in Figure 23–13, can be summarized as follows:

1. Although decrements in insulin secretion normally play an important role, the prevention or correction of hypoglycemia is not due solely to the dissipation of insulin.

2. There are redundant glucose counterregulatory factors and a hierarchy among the glucoregulatory factors. Dissipation of insulin is likely the most important factor in defense against decrements in plasma glucose. Glucagon plays the primary counterregulatory role. Epinephrine, although not normally required, becomes critical when glucagon secretion is deficient. Epinephrine may also serve in concert with glucagon to prevent hypoglycemia under glucose-lowering conditions in which the action of glucagon alone may be insufficient. Glucose autoregulation may operate during severe hypoglycemia, and growth hormone and cortisol are involved in defense against prolonged hypoglycemia, but these stand low in the hierarchy of glucose counterregulatory factors. Other hormones, neurotransmit-

DEFENSE AGAINST DECREMENTS IN PLASMA GLUCOSE CONCENTRATION

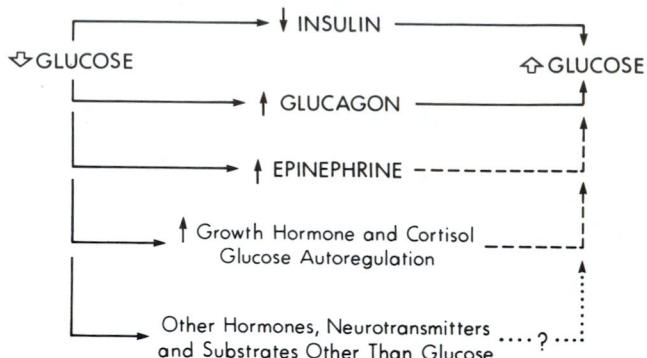

NORMAL GLUCOSE COUNTERREGULATION

Figure 23–13. Schematic representation of the normal hierarchy among the redundant glucose counterregulatory factors involved in the prevention or correction of hypoglycemia.

ters, and the effects of substrates other than glucose might be involved but, if so, play minor roles. Glucose counterregulation fails and hypoglycemia occurs when both glucagon and epinephrine are deficient and insulin is present or when insulin action is excessive.

The presence of redundant defenses against hypoglycemia accounts for the rarity of hypoglycemia in nondiabetics and the capacity of many intensively treated patients with IDDM to maintain the plasma glucose at levels sufficient for normal cerebral function despite hyperinsulinemia and deficient glucagon responses. The susceptibility to hypoglycemia of some patients with IDDM is a result of deficient glucagon and epinephrine secretion.[3, 4, 43]

These principles of human glucose counterregulation, developed from studies using somatostatin-induced glucagon deficiency, pharmacological adrenergic blockade, and surgical epinephrine deficiency, have been confirmed in that they predict the impact of disease-related deficiencies of glucagon, epinephrine, or both.[42, 43] Whether they can be applied to additional models of glucose counterregulation, and are thus general principles, remains to be established, but they provide a conceptual framework for understanding clinical hypoglycemia.

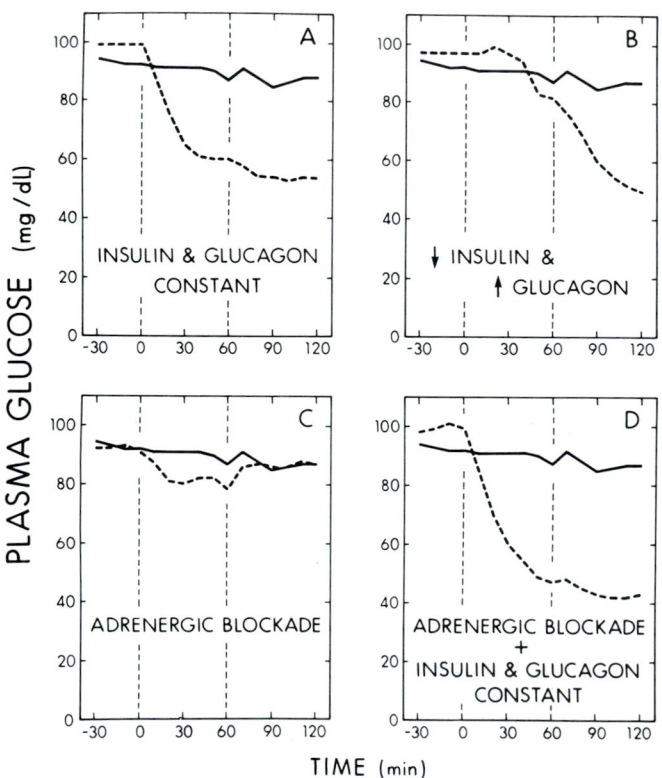

Figure 23–12. Mean plasma glucose concentrations in normal humans studied before, during (between the *vertical dashed lines*), and after moderate cycle exercise (~60% peak Vo₂max) in control studies (*solid lines*, same in all panels) and as modified (*dashed lines*) by *A*, somatostatin infusion with insulin, glucagon, and growth hormone replacement at fixed rates before, during, and after exercise to prevent normal exercise-associated decrements in insulin and increments in glucagon (insulin and glucagon constant); *B*, somatostatin infusion with growth hormone replaced at fixed rates, insulin replacement decreased during exercise, and glucagon replacement increased during exercise to reproduce the normal exercise-associated changes in these hormones (decreased insulin and increased glucagon); *C*, phentolamine and propranolol infusions before, during, and after exercise (adrenergic blockade); and *D*, phentolamine and propranolol infusions + somatostatin infusion with insulin, glucagon, and growth hormone replacement at fixed rates before, during, and after exercise (adrenergic blockade + insulin and glucagon constant). Curves are derived from data in ref. 48. To convert glucose values to millimoles per liter, mutliply by 0.05551.

THE PATHOPHYSIOLOGY OF HYPOGLYCEMIA

Clinical Manifestations of Hypoglycemia

The central nervous system manifestations that develop when the supply of glucose is inadequate are termed *neuroglycopenic symptoms and signs*, or *neuroglycopenia*.[60] These manifestations range from subtle impairment of mentation to coma and death. Between these extremes a variety of other expressions can occur, including visual symptoms, lethargy, confusion, behavioral changes, impaired performance of routine tasks, vertigo, paresthesias, incoordination, slurred speech, hunger, and focal neurological deficits (e.g., diplopia, hemiparesis). Seizures are common in children with hypoglycemia but are less frequent in adults. Hypothermia is often present, but hyperthermia sometimes follows hypoglycemia. Rarely, chronic hypoglycemia results in dementia or psychosis.

Some symptoms and signs of hypoglycemia are either directly or indirectly referable to central nervous system–mediated sympathochromaffin activity rather than to neuroglycopenia per se. These neurogenic manifestations include a nonspecific sense of arousal, anxiety, or impending doom coupled with palpitations (with a variable but often rather small increase in heart rate); tremulousness; cold feeling; and diaphoresis. All but the last can be reduced or prevented by adrenergic blockade. The diaphoretic response, which is not prevented but enhanced during adrenergic blockade, is prevented by cholinergic blockade. This response has been attributed to a sympathetic reflex involving cholinergic postganglionic neurons.[61]

The magnitude of the neuroendocrine response to hypoglycemia is clearly an inverse function of the glucose concentration at nadir.[51] As summarized in Figure 23–7, the arterialized venous glycemic thresholds for activation of several glucose counterregulatory systems during decrements in plasma glucose level normally lie within or just below the physiological plasma glucose concentration range and at glucose levels higher than those required to produce symptoms of hypoglycemia.[56] Thus glucose counterregulatory systems are activated at glucose levels of about 3.6 to 3.9 mmol/L (65 to 70 mg/dL), whereas symptoms develop at glucose concentrations of about 2.8 to 3.0 mmol/L (50 to 55 mg/dL) in normal humans.[56, 62] The rate of fall in plasma glucose level is not a determinant of the magnitude of the counterregulatory response.[51, 63]

Glucose metabolism, not transport, normally determines glucose utilization by the brain. The plasma glucose level at which the rate of glucose transport across the blood-brain barrier is half-maximal approximates normal plasma glucose concentrations.[64] Glucose transport becomes rate-limiting when the plasma glucose concentration falls to low levels, and brain function is impaired. The plasma glucose concentration at which this occurs differs among normal individuals and varies to a greater degree among patients with chronic disorders of glucoregulation. Patients with poorly controlled IDDM can suffer symptoms of hypoglycemia at higher plasma glucose concentrations than nondiabetic individuals.[3, 4, 65] In contrast, patients with well-controlled IDDM often tolerate subnormal plasma glucose levels without symptoms.[3, 4, 66] The mechanisms of these altered glycemic thresholds are not known. The possibility of central nervous system adaptation to antecedent glycemia by changes in the fraction of circulating glucose extracted by the brain has been hypothesized[67] but not proved.[3, 4] This is based on the findings of decreased fractional extraction of glucose by the brain in chronically hyperglycemic rats[68, 69] and increased fractional extraction of glucose by the brain in chronically hypoglycemic rats.[70] Similar tolerance of hypoglycemia occurs in other chronic hypoglycemic disorders, such as that resulting from an insulin-secreting tumor of the pancreatic islets.

Diagnosis of Hypoglycemia

The clinical manifestations of hypoglycemia are nonspecific. In addition, they vary among individuals and may vary from time to time in the same individual. They are also typically episodic. Thus although the history is of fundamental importance because it suggests the possibility of hypoglycemia, the diagnosis of hypoglycemia cannot be made on the basis of symptoms and signs alone.

The diagnosis of hypoglycemia should also not be made solely on the basis of plasma glucose measurements unless they are unequivocally subnormal. It is not possible to define a plasma glucose concentration below which neuroglycopenia invariably occurs and above which neuroglycopenia never occurs. Although neuroglycopenia commonly accompanies venous plasma glucose concentrations of less than 2.5 mmol/L (45 mg/dL),[1, 2] neuroglycopenia can occur at higher plasma glucose levels, especially in older persons[2] and in some patients with IDDM.[65] In addition, venous plasma glucose concentrations of substantially less than 2.5 mmol/L (45 mg/dL) may occur in overtly normal individuals late after glucose ingestion (arterial glucose levels are higher) and in some women and children during fasting without producing recognizable symptoms.[1, 2] This is not to say that distinctly low plasma glucose measurements should be ignored. Some patients with endogenous hyperinsulinism or intensively treated diabetes are asymptomatic at glucose levels that are unequivocally subnormal most of the time, as mentioned earlier. Because these patients can have neuroglycopenic symptoms at other times (presumably when glucose levels are even lower), it would be inappropriate to deny that they have hypoglycemia.

In general, venous plasma glucose concentrations obtained after an overnight fast are considered to be normal if greater than 3.3 mmol/L (60 mg/dL), those between 2.5 and 3.3 mmol/L (45 and 60 mg/dL) are suggestive of hypoglycemia, and those less than 2.5 mmol/L (45 mg/dL) are indicative of postabsorptive hypoglycemia. It should be recalled that substantial glucose extraction occurs across the forearm during hyperinsulinemic conditions. Thus arterial glucose concentrations (those relevant to brain function) are as much as 30% higher than venous glucose concentrations after an oral glucose load.[2] Low measured glucose levels can be the result of glycolysis in vitro (pseudohypoglycemia) if separation of plasma from the formed elements of the blood is delayed for several hours. This is particularly true if leukocytosis or polycythemia is present.

The diagnosis of hypoglycemia is most convincingly established when it is based on the Whipple triad:[71] symptoms consistent with hypoglycemia, low plasma glucose concentrations, and relief of those symptoms when plasma glucose concentrations are raised to normal levels.

Postabsorptive vs. Postprandial Hypoglycemia

Reproducible hypoglycemia in the postabsorptive state implies the presence of a serious disease and requires diagnostic explanation and therapy. This condition is commonly referred to as fasting hypoglycemia. However, it need not be apparent initially or exclusively during prolonged fasting or after an overnight fast. Postprandial hypoglycemia may become symptomatic during the latter portion of any interdigestive period, commonly associated with exercise. In contrast, postprandial (reactive, stimulative) hypoglycemia usually does not imply a serious underlying disorder. Thus the distinction between postabsorptive and postprandial hypoglycemia is fundamental.

Mechanisms of Hypoglycemia

A decrease in the plasma glucose concentration indicates that the rate of glucose efflux from the circulation exceeds that of glucose influx into the circulation. Theoretically hypoglycemia could result from excessive glucose efflux (excessive utilization or external losses), deficient glucose influx (deficient endogenous production), or both. There are conditions in which glucose utilization is increased markedly (e.g., exercise, pregnancy, large tumors) and in which renal losses occur at physiological plasma glucose concentrations (e.g., renal glycosuria, pregnancy). However, because of the normal capacity of the liver to increase glucose production several-fold, as discussed earlier, clinical hypoglycemia is rarely the result of excessive glucose efflux alone. Rather, it is commonly the result of hepatic glucose production that is either decreased absolutely or inappropriately low relative to the rate of glucose utilization.

In general, hypoglycemia can be the result of regulatory, enzymatic, or substrate defects. Glucoregulatory defects include those that result in excessive secretion, tissue levels, or sensitivity to insulin, or deficient secretion or action of counterregulatory hormones. Enzymatic defects may be primary or may result from generalized hepatic disease. Substrate defects include failure to mobilize or utilize gluconeogenic substrates.

Clinical Classification of Hypoglycemia

Hypoglycemia can be classified on the basis of glucose kinetic patterns, pathogenic mechanisms, or disease groups. The last approach is used in this chapter and is shown in Table 23–1. Hypoglycemia is divided into postabsorptive and postprandial varieties. Postabsorptive, or fasting, hypoglycemia can be the result of drugs, critical organ failure, hormonal deficiencies, non–beta cell tumors, endogenous hyperinsulinism (including that caused by pancreatic beta cell tumors), or disorders unique to infancy and childhood. Postprandial or reactive hypoglycemia is rarely due to congenital enzyme defects but can follow gastric surgery. It is uncommon as an idiopathic disorder.

The vast majority of episodes of hypoglycemia result from drugs, particularly insulin, sulfonylureas, or alcohol. In one series of patients treated for hypoglycemia in an emergency room, two thirds had diabetes mellitus and two thirds had been drinking alcohol.[72] Clearly, the combination of drug-treated diabetes and alcohol ingestion can be devastating. Nearly one fourth of the patients were septic, but diabetes or alcohol ingestion was common even in those patients. Drugs are also a common cause of hypoglycemia

TABLE 23–1. Clinical Classification of Hypoglycemia

I. Postabsorptive (fasting) hypoglycemia
  A. Drugs
    1. Especially insulin, sulfonylureas, alcohol
    2. Also pentamidine, quinine
    3. Rarely, salicylates, sulfonamides
    4. ? others
  B. Critical organ failure
    1. Hepatic disease
    2. Cardiac disease
    3. Renal disease
    4. Sepsis
    5. Inanition
  C. Hormonal deficiencies
    1. Cortisol, growth hormone, or both
    2. Glucagon and epinephrine
  D. Non–beta cell tumors
  E. Endogenous hyperinsulinism
    1. Pancreatic beta cell disorders
      a. Tumor (insulinoma)
      b. Nontumor
    2. Beta cell secretagogue (e.g., sulfonylureas)
    3. Autoimmune hypoglycemia
      a. Insulin antibodies
      b. Insulin receptor antibodies
      c. ? beta cell antibodies
    4. ? ectopic insulin secretion
  F. Hypoglycemias of infancy and childhood
    1. Neonatal hypoglycemias
    2. Congenital deficiencies of glucogenic enzymes
    3. Ketotic hypoglycemia of childhood
II. Postprandial (reactive) hypoglycemia
  A. Congenital deficiencies of enzymes of carbohydrate metabolism
    1. Galactosemia
    2. Hereditary fructose intolerance
  B. Alimentary hypoglycemia
  C. Idiopathic (functional) postprandial hypoglycemia

TABLE 23–2. Established and Putative Hypoglycemia-Causing Agents

	Agents Causing Hypoglycemia	
	Commonly	*Rarely*
Established		
Used commonly	Insulin	Salicylates
	Sulfonylureas	Sulfonamides
	Alcohol	
Used rarely	Pentamidine	
	Quinine	

Putative
Antihypertensives: beta-adrenergic antagonists (especially in IDDM, particularly those that block beta-2–adrenergic receptors); captopril
Analgesic/anti-inflammatory drugs: indomethacin, acetaminophen, propoxyphene, phenylbutazone, penicillamine
Antigout drugs: colchicine, sulfinpyrazone
Lipid-lowering drugs: clofibrate, bezafibrate
Antibiotics: chloramphenicol, ketoconazole, para-aminosalicylic acid
Antipsychotics: haloperidol
Antianginals: perhexilene
Others: monoamine oxidase inhibitors

in an inpatient setting.[73] Here, however, critical organ failure—particularly renal failure, but also hepatic failure, cardiac failure, and organ failure caused by sepsis or inanition—is a common factor. Hypoglycemia resulting from hormonal deficiencies is uncommon but worth finding, because it is often treatable by hormonal replacement. Hypoglycemia caused by non–beta cell tumors and that caused by endogenous hyperinsulinism are rare. Fewer than 1 in 1 million persons harbors an insulinoma. Diagnosis of insulinoma is challenging, but successful identification often leads to a gratifying outcome.

THE POSTABSORPTIVE (FASTING) HYPOGLYCEMIAS

Drugs

Drugs are the most common cause of hypoglycemia.[72, 73] The capacity of some drugs to cause hypoglycemia is well established. These drugs include insulin, sulfonylureas, alcohol, pentamidine, quinine, and, rarely, salicylates and sulfonamides. Many other drugs have been associated with hypoglycemia but often under complex clinical conditions in which a causative relationship cannot be considered established. Established and putative hypoglycemia-causing drugs are listed in Table 23–2.

Insulin

Hypoglycemia is a fact of life for persons with IDDM,[3, 4] who must take insulin to survive. The symptoms of hypoglycemic reactions and their prevalence in patients with IDDM are summarized in Table 23–3. Given the imperfections of insulin replacement therapy, distinctly low plasma glucose levels probably occur from time to time in virtually all such patients. Those using conventional therapy suffer an average of one episode of symptomatic hypoglycemia per week; patients practicing intensive therapy suffer an average of two such episodes per week. In a given year 10% of patients using conventional therapy and 25% of those on intensive regimens experience at least one episode of severe, temporarily disabling hypoglycemia requiring the assistance of another individual. Such events often include a seizure or loss of consciousness and require administration of intravenous glucose or of glucagon.[74] Four percent of deaths of patients with IDDM are attributed to hypoglycemia.[3, 4] Many patients are fearful of hypoglycemia and some feel guilty

TABLE 23–3. Prevalence of Hypoglycemic Symptoms in 172 Patients with Insulin-Dependent Diabetes Mellitus

Symptom	%
Sweating	49
Tremor	32
Blurred or double vision	29
Weakness	28
Hunger	25
Confusion	13
Vertigo	13
Odd behavior	11
Paresthesia of lips and tongue	10
Anxiety	10
Cold feeling	9
Incoordination	9
Fear of losing consciousness	8
Slurred speech	7
Palpitations	6
Nausea	5
Headache	4
Stupor	2
Vomiting	1

From Goldgewicht C, Slama G, Papoz L, et al. Hypoglycaemic reactions in 172 type 1 (insulin-dependent) diabetic patients. Diabetologia 1983; 24:95–99. Copyright Springer-Verlag, Heidelberg.

DEFENSE AGAINST DECREMENTS IN PLASMA GLUCOSE CONCENTRATION

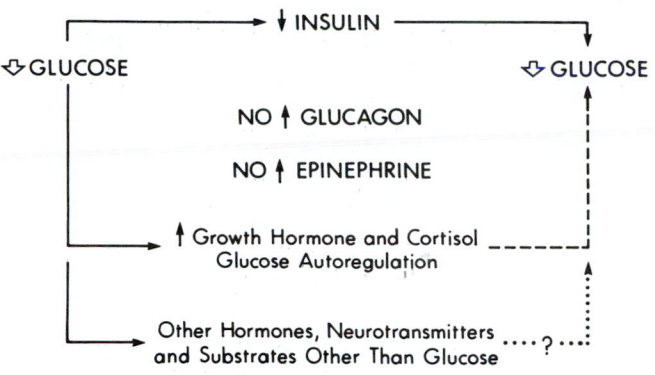

DEFECTIVE GLUCOSE COUNTERREGULATION

Figure 23–15. Defective glucose counterregulation, the result of combined deficiencies of the glucagon- and epinephrine-secretory responses to plasma glucose decrements, is present in many patients with IDDM.

about that fear. Hypoglycemia is the limiting factor in attempts to achieve near-normal plasma glucose levels. Clearly, iatrogenic hypoglycemia in IDDM is a problem that has not been solved.[4]

Deficient glucagon-secretory responses to decrements in plasma glucose are the rule in patients with IDDM.[3, 4, 50] This defect is an acquired one that commonly develops within the first few years of IDDM. It is selective, as the glucagon responses to other stimuli are intact. Although it is linked closely to immeasurably low C peptide levels,[75] which suggests that it might be the result of absolute insulin deficiency, its mechanism is unknown.[3, 4] To the extent that glucagon responses are deficient, patients with IDDM are largely dependent on epinephrine to prevent or correct hypoglycemia.[42] They have altered glucose counterregulation (Fig. 23–14), but it is often masked because epinephrine compensates.

Many patients with IDDM, typically but not invariably those with relatively long-standing disease, also have defi-

cient epinephrine-secretory responses to plasma glucose decrements.[3, 4] This defect, too, appears to be a selective one. Its mechanism is unknown. Although it is commonly viewed as one of the diabetic autonomic neuropathies,[76] the deficient epinephrine response is not closely linked to classic diabetic autonomic neuropathy, whether the latter is defined on clinical grounds, the results of reflex tests, or both.[77] It is, however, associated with the clinical syndrome of hypoglycemia unawareness discussed later.

Patients with combined deficiencies of glucagon- and epinephrine-secretory responses to decrements in plasma glucose have defective glucose counterregulation (Fig. 23–15).[3, 4, 43, 78] Prospective studies using insulin infusion tests to classify patients have demonstrated that those with defective glucose counterregulation (Fig. 23–16) have a 25-fold or greater increased risk for severe iatrogenic hypoglycemia during intensive therapy (Fig. 23–17).[43, 78]

Some patients with IDDM, typically those with relatively long-standing disease, lose the neurogenic symptoms of hypoglycemia. In the absence of these warning symptoms, they fail to recognize developing hypoglycemia and therefore do not act (e.g., eat) to prevent the development of severe hypoglycemia and its resultant neuroglycopenia. It is generally assumed that this syndrome of hypoglycemia unawareness contributes substantially to the frequency of severe hypoglycemia in affected patients. Although prospective studies have not been done, in cross-sectional studies 23% of 202 patients with IDDM had partial or complete hypoglycemia unawareness.[79] The frequency approached 50% in those with long-standing IDDM.[4]

The mechanism of hypoglycemia unawareness is not known,[4] although it is associated with a reduced plasma epinephrine response to experimental hypoglycemia.[80, 81] If reduced plasma epinephrine response is a marker for decreased sympathetic neural as well as adrenomedullary responses, the absence of warning symptoms normally attributable to the sympathochromaffin response to hypoglycemia could be explained.

Insulin excess is a well-recognized risk factor for iatrogenic hypoglycemia in patients with IDDM.[3, 4] It can occur, for example, when insulin doses are excessive or poorly timed, when the influx of exogenous glucose is decreased (as after missed meals or snacks, during an overnight fast, or with gastroparesis), or when endogenous glucose produc-

DEFENSE AGAINST DECREMENTS IN PLASMA GLUCOSE CONCENTRATION

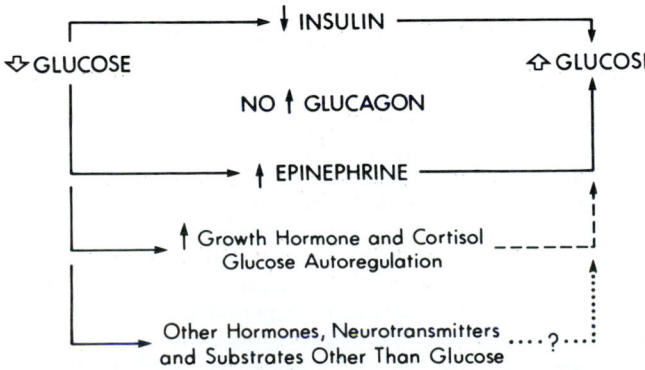

ALTERED GLUCOSE COUNTERREGULATION

Figure 23–14. Altered glucose counterregulation, the result of deficient glucagon-secretory responses to plasma glucose decrements, is the rule in patients with IDDM.

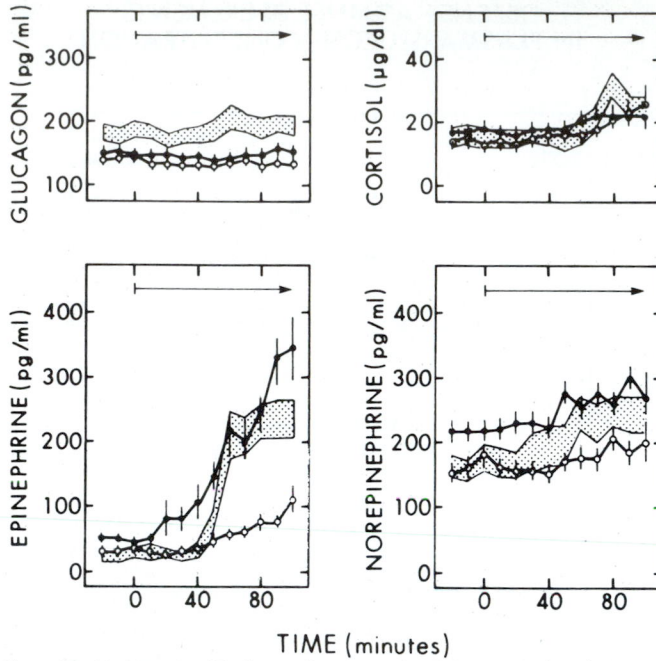

Figure 23–16. Mean (± SE) plasma glucagon, epinephrine, cortisol, and norepinephrine concentrations during intravenous infusion of regular insulin (40 mU/kg/h; *arrows*) in nondiabetic controls (*stipped areas*), patients with IDDM with adequate glucose counterregulation (*closed symbols*), and patients with IDDM with defective glucose counterregulation (*open symbols*). The last group was defined by development of neuroglycopenic symptoms, a plasma glucose concentration less then 1.9 mmol/L (35 mg/dL), or both during insulin infusion. For conversion factors to SI units, see Figures 23–3, 23–4, 23–5, and 23–7. (From White NH, Skor D, Cryer PE, et al. Identification of type I diabetic patients at increased risk for hypoglycemia during intensive therapy. Reprinted, by permission of the New England Journal of Medicine, 308; 485–491, 1983.)

tion is impaired (as after alcohol ingestion). It also can occur when insulin-independent glucose utilization is increased (as during exercise), when sensitivity to insulin is increased (as during intensive therapy or with chronic deficiencies of cortisol, growth hormone, or both), or when insulin clearance is delayed (as in the presence of high insulin antibody titers). However, analysis of clinical data has shown these risk factors to be weak predictors of high risk for severe hypoglycemia.[82] As just discussed, defective glucose counterregulation, likely in concert with hypoglycemia unawareness, is a much stronger indicator of risk for hypoglycemia.[43, 78] Thus the concept of risk factors for hypoglycemia in patients

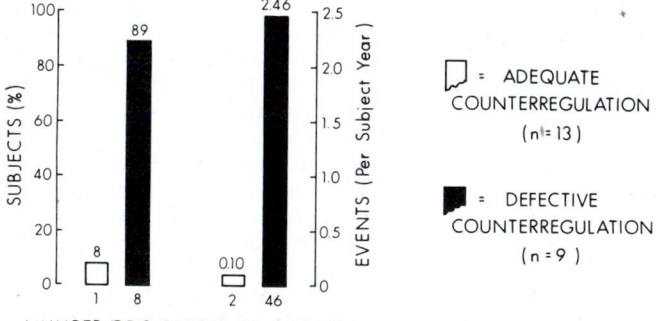

Figure 23–17. Percentage of patients affected and event rates for severe hypoglycemia during intensive therapy of IDDM in patients classified prospectively, by using an insulin infusion test, as having adequate (*open columns*) or defective (*shaded columns*) glucose counterregulation. The latter was defined by the development of neuroglycopenic symptoms, plasma glucose levels less than 2.8 mmol/L (50 mg/dL), or both during the insulin infusion test. Derived from data in ref. 43.

with IDDM has been broadened to include both insulin excess and compromised glucose counterregulation and, perhaps more reasonably, an interplay of both of these general mechanisms.[3, 4] Insulin excess of sufficient magnitude will cause hypoglycemia despite intact counterregulatory mechanisms. However, the integrity of the counterregulatory systems may well determine whether less marked hyperinsulinemia results in hypoglycemia.

The glucose counterregulatory hormones may also be involved in the pathogenesis of hyperglycemia in patients with IDDM.[76] For example, elevated levels occur in diabetic ketoacidosis and may well contribute to hyperglycemia and other metabolic derangements. It has been suggested plausibly that epinephrine, among other glucose-raising hormones, might be involved in hyperglycemia produced by physical or psychological stress. Nighttime to morning increments in plasma glucose—the dawn phenomenon—are best attributed to dissipation of previously injected insulin, nocturnal growth hormone secretion, or both.[83, 84] However, the magnitude of the dawn phenomenon is not great, averaging about 1.8 mmol/L (32 mg/dL). The clinical relevance of the Somogyi phenomenon—hyperglycemia resulting from the counterregulatory response to preceding hypoglycemia—has been questioned. Some investigators have concluded that nocturnal hypoglycemia does not appear to cause fasting or daytime postprandial hyperglycemia in patients with IDDM.[85, 86] Others, however, find postprandial glucose levels to be somewhat higher after nocturnal hypoglycemia in tightly controlled patients.[87]

Insulin therapy can, of course, also result in hypoglycemia in patients with non–insulin-dependent diabetes mellitus (NIDDM). Although defective glucose counterregulation has not been documented in NIDDM, it might occur in those with severe insulin deficiency. Finally, hypoglycemia can also be the result of surreptitious insulin injection, as discussed later.

Sulfonylureas

Sulfonylureas increase insulin secretion and also insulin action, thereby lowering the plasma glucose concentration. They are widely used to treat patients with NIDDM and can cause hypoglycemia.[88–90] In one survey of sulfonylurea-treated patients, 20% reported at least one episode of symptomatic hypoglycemia during a 6-mo period.[90] Tolbutamide (duration of action, 6 to 10 h), acetohexamide (12 to 18 h), and tolazamide (16 to 24 h) are metabolized in the liver; the metabolites of acetohexamide are potent, whereas those of tolazamide are weakly active. The hypoglycemic action of tolbutamide and tolazamide can be prolonged by hepatic disease or by the administration of other drugs that impair hepatic sulfonylurea metabolism (e.g., sulfonamides, chloramphenicol, coumarin, phenylbutazone, and clofibrate).[89] A striking feature of sulfonylurea-induced hypoglycemia is its long duration. Hypoglycemia can sometimes persist for days. Among the first-generation drugs, sulfonylurea-induced hypoglycemia is most commonly caused by chlorpropamide, probably because of its long duration of action (24 to 72 hours). Although the drug is in part metabolized, the activity of the metabolites is unknown; most of the chlorpropamide is excreted unchanged by the kidneys. It is therefore more likely to produce hypoglycemia in persons with renal insufficiency. Among the second-generation sulfonylureas, glyburide has been reported to cause hypoglycemia more commonly than glipizide.[88]

It is not difficult to recognize hypoglycemia resulting from insulin or sulfonylurea therapy in a patient with diabetes mellitus for which one of these drugs has been prescribed. However, insulin or a sulfonylurea is sometimes used surreptitiously, especially by persons knowledgeable about their use (e.g., patients with diabetes, their families, or medical personnel). These drugs have been used to commit suicide and to murder.[2] Hypoglycemia resulting from insulin injection is characterized by high plasma insulin but low plasma C peptide concentrations, as discussed later. Chronic insulin administration may lead to the formation of measurable insulin antibodies. Both plasma insulin and C peptide levels are inappropriately high in patients with sulfonylurea-induced hypoglycemia, a pattern similar to that of hyperinsulinism caused by pancreatic beta cell disorders, also discussed later. However, the sulfonylureas can be measured in plasma or urine.

Alcohol

Ethanol inhibits gluconeogenesis,[91, 92] presumably because its metabolism to acetaldehyde and then acetate by alcohol dehydrogenase and aldehyde dehydrogenase, respectively, depletes hepatic nicotinamide-adenine dinucleotide, a cofactor critical to the entry of most precursors into the gluconeogenic pathway (see Fig. 23–1). It does not inhibit glycogenolysis. Ethanol also inhibits cortisol[92, 93] and growth hormone[92–94] responses to hypoglycemia. Epinephrine responses are delayed.[92, 95] Glucagon release appears to be normal,[92] although a delayed response has been reported.[95]

In normal humans, ethanol administration does not produce postabsorptive hypoglycemia,[96] nor does it impair recovery from short-term hypoglycemia,[95] presumably because of intact glucagon secretion and responsive hepatic glycogenolysis, perhaps coupled with decreased sensitivity to insulin.[95–98] On the other hand, because gluconeogenesis becomes the dominant source of hepatic glucose production during prolonged hypoglycemia,[92] ethanol can contribute to the progression of hypoglycemia in insulin-treated patients with diabetes.

Clinical alcohol-induced hypoglycemia typically follows (by 6 to 24 h) a binge of moderate to heavy alcohol consumption during which the person eats little food (i.e., in the setting of glycogen depletion).[2, 93] Hypoglycemia can be profound. Mortality rates as high as 10% have been reported among hospitalized patients. Children appear to be particularly susceptible to hypoglycemia after the accidental ingestion of alcohol. Ethanol is usually still measurable in the blood at the time the patient presents with hypoglycemia. However, the levels may not be markedly elevated and correlate poorly with the plasma glucose concentration.[2, 93]

Other Drugs

Salicylates in relatively large doses (4 to 6 g/d) can lower the plasma glucose concentration[99] and can produce hypoglycemia in children and, rarely, in adults.[1, 2, 100] The mechanisms of salicylate-induced hypoglycemia are not known. Sulfonamides also rarely produce hypoglycemia through an unknown mechanism.[101]

Pentamidine[102, 103] produces hypoglycemia by causing insulin release. A beta cell toxin, pentamidine can also cause the late development of diabetes mellitus.[103] Hypoglycemia occurs frequently during pentamidine therapy (27%[102] and 14%[103] of patients treated in two series). Risk factors include pentamidine therapy of longer duration and increased dose, previous pentamidine therapy, and nephrotoxicity during therapy.[103]

Hypoglycemia occurs commonly in patients with severe malaria.[104–106] Although associated with relative hyperinsulinemia attributed to quinine-induced insulin release in one series,[104] hypoglycemia can occur in the absence of quinine therapy[105] and in the absence of hyperinsulinemia in quinine-treated patients.[106]

Hypoglycemia has been attributed rarely to many other drugs (see Table 23–2). In many of the reported cases, other potential causes of hypoglycemia have been present. The beta-adrenergic antagonists, such as propranolol, are prominent examples. Although hypoglycemia attributed to propranolol in otherwise healthy children has been reported,[107, 108] most of the reported patients have been diabetics using insulin. As discussed earlier, epinephrine-mediated beta-adrenergic mechanisms are not normally critical to glucose counterregulation, at least in adults, but become critical in glucagon-deficient patients with IDDM.[42, 43] Thus propranolol would be expected to increase the risk of hypoglycemia in such patients. In contrast, propranolol has little effect on glucoregulation when islet cell function is normal.

Critical Organ Failure

Among hospitalized patients, drugs, particularly insulin, are the most common cause of hypoglycemia,[73] and diseases that result in failure of one or more critical organ systems are the second most common.[73] These latter causes include hepatic, cardiac, and renal disease; sepsis; and inanition.

Hepatic Disease

In addition to appropriate regulatory signals and sufficient precursor supplies, maintenance of the postabsorptive plasma glucose concentration requires an enzymatically and structurally intact liver, the major source of endogenous glucose production via glycogenolysis and gluconeogenesis. Total hepatectomy results in profound hypoglycemia.[109] Specific enzyme deficiencies resulting in hypoglycemia are discussed later under Hypoglycemia in Infancy and Childhood. Hypoglycemia resulting from generalized hepatic damage is discussed here.

Because the normal liver has the capacity to increase its glucose production several-fold, extensive liver disease is required to produce hypoglycemia in the absence of markedly accelerated glucose utilization.[110] Hepatogenous hypoglycemia is most common when hepatic destruction is both rapid and massive[2] (e.g., in toxic hepatitis). Hypoglycemia has been reported in fulminant viral hepatitis,[111] in fatty liver attributed to starvation or alcohol ingestion, and in cholangitis and biliary obstruction.[2] It is unusual in the common forms of cirrhosis and hepatitis, although glucose metabolism is demonstrably altered—with lower postabsorptive plasma glucose concentrations, diminished glycemic responses to glucagon, and reduced hepatic glycogen—in patients with uncomplicated viral hepatitis.[112] Hypoglycemia occurs rather commonly in patients with primary malignant hepatic tumors but is probably the result of a glucoregulatory abnormality in such patients, as discussed later. It is unusual in metastatic liver disease, despite extensive displacement of normal tissue.[113]

Hypoglycemia in hepatic failure is plausibly viewed as the result of parenchymal dysfunction despite normal regulatory signals. In this construct, relative peripheral hyperinsulinemia would be attributed to shunting of blood from the portal to the peripheral circulation (i.e., decreased clearance of insulin by the diseased liver);[114] C peptide levels, an index of insulin secretion, might be expected to be appropriately suppressed. However, in a study of five patients with acute liver failure, Vilstrup and co-workers[115] found markedly elevated plasma C peptide and insulin levels under both euglycemic and hyperglycemic conditions. The patients were resistant to insulin and had elevated glucagon levels; they were not studied during hypoglycemia.

Cardiac Disease

Hypoglycemia occurs in occasional patients with severe cardiac failure of diverse etiologies. The pathogenesis is not known. Suggested possibilities include hepatic congestion, inanition, gluconeogenic substrate limitation, and hepatic hypoxia.[2] The finding of elevated blood lactate levels associated with hypoglycemia[116] raises the possibility of inhibited gluconeogenesis.

Renal Disease

Postabsorptive hypoglycemia occurs in some patients with renal failure.[117–121] The finding of a high frequency of renal insufficiency among hospitalized patients with low plasma glucose concentrations[73] suggests that compromised glucose counterregulation may be a common feature of renal failure. However, the pathogenesis of hypoglycemia in such patients is not known; multiple mechanisms may be involved.

Most, but not all, patients with hypoglycemia attributed to renal failure have been cachectic. One such patient had reduced glucose turnover, diminished gluconeogenesis from alanine, and reduced alanine turnover.[119] During fasting, plasma glucose declined, blood lactate did not increase, and blood alanine fell to very low levels. Hypoglycemia was attributed to substrate limitation of gluconeogenesis. However, at least one patient did not respond to substrate (glycerol, alanine) administration,[121] and patients have been reported with normal blood alanine concentrations and elevated blood lactate levels, which suggests inhibited gluconeogenesis.[121] Furthermore, decreased glycemic responses to exogenous glucagon have been reported,[121, 122] although this effect was not apparent in another study of uremic individuals.[123] It is notable that several of the patients with hypoglycemia attributed to renal failure have had diabetes mellitus.[117, 119] Presumably because of decreased renal metabolism of insulin, insulin requirements decrease with advancing renal failure in diabetes, thus enhancing the risk of insulin-induced hypoglycemia. Hypoglycemia can also occur during and after dialysis.[124]

Sepsis

Sepsis is not infrequently associated with hypoglycemia.[72, 73, 125] The pathogenesis in humans is not known but has been studied in animals. Increased glucose utilization characterizes experimental sepsis.[126, 127] Plasma glucose concentrations often rise initially because of increased glucose production. The development of hypoglycemia is associated with decreasing hepatic glucose production.[128] Increased glucose use by skeletal muscle accounts for only about 25% of the increase in glucose utilization;[129] increased glucose use by macrophage-rich tissues such as liver, spleen, and ileum appears to be responsible for most of the increment in glucose utilization.[130]

The factors responsible for increased glucose utilization and the failure of glucose production to match utilization are unclear, but there are interesting suggestive observations. For example, administration of the cytokine interleukin 1 causes hyperinsulinemia and decrements in plasma glucose in mice.[131] Under the appropriate conditions interleukin 1 enhances glucose-stimulated insulin secretion in vitro.[132]

Other cytokines, such as cachectin (tumor necrosis factor),[133] stimulate glucose transport into cells in vitro.

Inanition

Hypoglycemia can result from prolonged starvation,[134, 135] but nutritional hypoglycemia is unusual in developed countries.[2] Nonetheless, severe hypoglycemia associated with inanition and no other apparent cause has been reported in the United States.[136] Based on the observation of persistent hypoglycemia despite high rates of intravenous glucose infusion, these patients must have had high rates of glucose utilization. Beyond this, the pathogenesis of hypoglycemia is unknown. It is possible that glucose is the sole metabolic fuel in the setting of total body fat depletion.

Hormonal Deficiencies

Except in patients with IDDM, glucoregulatory abnormalities resulting in hypoglycemia are not common. The rarity of hypoglycemia caused by impaired glucose counterregulatory systems in nondiabetic subjects is testimony to the effectiveness of those systems under normal conditions and is best explained by the presence of redundant glucose counterregulatory mechanisms, as discussed earlier in this chapter. Thus the glucose-lowering actions of insulin are countered over the short term by glucagon or, if necessary, epinephrine. Over the longer term the modulating effects of other counterregulatory factors, notably growth hormone and cortisol, play a role. However, the rarity of clinical hypoglycemia in patients with deficient secretion of growth hormone, cortisol, or both provides further evidence that these are not major counterregulatory hormones.

Cortisol and Growth Hormone Deficiencies

The vast majority of adults with deficient secretion of cortisol, growth hormone, or both do not develop clinical hypoglycemia. Indeed, plasma glucose concentrations (and hepatic glucose production) after an overnight fast are indistinguishable from normal in glucocorticoid-withdrawn patients with primary adrenocortical failure[137] and in glucocorticoid-withdrawn patients with panhypopituitarism never treated with growth hormone (P. E. Cryer, unpublished results). However, postabsorptive hypoglycemia can occur in young children with chronic deficiencies of these hormones, particularly in the neonatal period and in children younger than 5 y.[138–140]

Clinically, hypoglycemia in such children is generally preceded by a period of caloric deprivation consistent with the observation that hypoglycemia can sometimes be provoked by 24 to 30 h of fasting in children with hypopituitarism who do not exhibit hypoglycemia after an overnight fast.[141, 142] This intolerance to fasting is largely corrected by glucocorticoid replacement, whereas growth hormone replacement has little effect.[141, 142] These findings suggest that a defect in gluconeogenesis causes hypoglycemia when hepatic glycogen stores are depleted. Cortisol tends to increase gluconeogenesis both by direct effects on hepatic gluconeogenic enzyme activities and by mobilizing gluconeogenic precursors to the liver.[11, 143, 144] Postabsorptive hypoglycemia is associated with low levels of circulating gluconeogenic precursors,[141, 145] suggesting a substrate limitation mechanism, but oral alanine administration does not reverse hypoglycemia completely.[145] Finally, in view of evidence that cortisol deficiency results in reduced epinephrine secretion,[146] presumably because of decreased induction of adrenomedullary phenylethanolamine *N*-methyltransferase by cortisol, one could postulate a contributing role for epinephrine deficiency in the pathogenesis of hypoglycemia. Glucagon secretion, however, has not been shown to be reduced in such patients. Thus it is not surprising that glucose recovery from short-term hypoglycemia is generally normal in patients with deficient secretion of cortisol, growth hormone, or both.[38, 49]

Adults with hypopituitarism can develop hypoglycemia when glucose utilization or losses are increased, as during exercise or pregnancy,[147] or when glucose production is impaired, as during alcohol ingestion.[148]

Glucagon and Epinephrine Deficiencies

Postabsorptive hypoglycemia occurs when both glucagon and epinephrine are deficient and insulin is present,[3, 4, 46, 47] as, for example, in some patients with IDDM,[3, 4, 43] discussed earlier. It has not been demonstrated convincingly in other conditions, perhaps because this constellation occurs only in patients with diabetes, because it is lethal when present from birth, or because it occurs but has not yet been well documented in postneonatal nondiabetic patients with postabsorptive hypoglycemia.

On the basis of current information concerning the physiology of glucose counterregulation, deficient epinephrine secretion alone should not result in postabsorptive hypoglycemia.[3, 4, 46, 47] As pointed out earlier, this conclusion is based on study of a limited number of adult human models; epinephrine may exert a primary counterregulatory role in other situations. However, hypoglycemia is not a feature of the epinephrine-deficient state that results from bilateral adrenalectomy when glucocorticoid and mineralocorticoid replacement is adequate,[39, 45] and hypoglycemia does not occur during pharmacological blockade of catecholamine action when other systems are intact.[40, 46, 47]

Diminished urinary[149, 150] and plasma[151] epinephrine responses to insulin-induced hypoglycemia occur in patients with ketotic hypoglycemia of childhood. Therapeutic responses to ephedrine, a catecholamine-releasing drug, have been reported in uncontrolled studies of such patients.[152, 153] Some patients have diminished glycemic responses to glucagon during fasting.[152–154] Thus patients with this disorder may have postabsorptive hypoglycemia as a result of deficient glucagon action coupled with deficient epinephrine secretion.

Hypoglycemia has been attributed to epinephrine deficiency in one member of each of three sets of twins.[155, 156] Compared with their unaffected twins, the hypoglycemic children had reduced, but not absent, urinary epinephrine responses to infused 2-deoxyglucose and to hypoglycemia induced by fasting. However, the glucagon-secretory status was not evaluated, and the affected children had inappropriately high insulin levels while hypoglycemic.[155] Thus it cannot be certain that the hypoglycemia was the result of epinephrine deficiency. Finally, reduced epinephrine excretion in infants of diabetic mothers is associated with neonatal hypoglycemia.[157]

In summary, coexistent hypoglycemia and deficient epinephrine secretion have been reported in several children. It is likely that the deficient epinephrine responses are pathogenically related to the hypoglycemia in some instances, although this relationship has not been established beyond doubt; epinephrine replacement has not been reported, and the beneficial effects of ephedrine were not observed under controlled conditions or accompanied by documented increments in epinephrine secretion. Even if one accepts a pathogenic role for epinephrine deficiency, however, it cannot be assumed that the hypoglycemia resulted solely from epinephrine deficiency. Thus coexistent abnormalities—particularly deficient glucagon or excessive insulin secretion or action—may have been present. Alternatively, epinephrine may play a primary glucose counterregulatory role in young children,[155] unlike its secondary role in adults.

Isolated glucagon deficiency would be expected to result in lowered postabsorptive plasma glucose concentrations but not hypoglycemia if epinephrine secretion were intact and insulin secretion were suppressed appropriately.[3, 4, 46, 47] Postabsorptive hypoglycemia attributed to isolated glucagon deficiency in an adult has been reported in an abstract.[158] A young man in whom insulinopenic hypoglycemia occurred after 18 h of fasting had plasma glucagon concentrations that were low during hypoglycemia and after arginine infusion. Glucagon infusion at a dose of 1.0 μg/min prevented hypoglycemia after 20 h of fasting. This dose of glucagon is supraphysiological.[38] The status of the patient's sympathochromaffin system is unknown. Postabsorptive hypoglycemia in another glucagon-deficient adult has been reported, but growth hormone secretion and cortisol secretion were also deficient, and the sympathochromaffin system was not assessed.[159] Neonatal hypoglycemia has also been attributed to glucagon deficiency.[160, 161] In one such patient hypoglycemia became refractory to conventional therapy but responded to glucagon (0.4 mg of zinc protamine glucagon twice daily) when the patient was 3 mo old.[160] The infant had low plasma glucagon levels during hypoglycemia; these did not rise in response to intravenous insulin, and glucose formation from [U-14C]alanine, an index of gluconeogenesis, was decreased. Urinary catecholamine excretion was judged to be normal. However, plasma insulin concentrations averaged 72 pmol/L (10 μU/mL) during hypoglycemia, and blood lactate, alanine, and ketone levels were low or in the low-normal range. Thus the hypoglycemia might have been the result of hyperinsulinism. Similar points apply to another patient with neonatal hypoglycemia attributed to glucagon deficiency.[161]

In summary, isolated deficiencies of epinephrine or glucagon rarely, if ever, cause postabsorptive hypoglycemia. On the other hand, combined deficiencies of both glucagon and epinephrine secretion increase the risk of hypoglycemia in patients with insulin-treated diabetes mellitus.[43] Whether such combined deficiencies result in postabsorptive hypoglycemia under other conditions remains to be established.

As a first step in the assessment of glucoregulatory hormone secretion, counterregulatory hormone concentrations in plasma can be measured during spontaneous or provoked hypoglycemia. Elevated values exclude deficient secretion (although deficient action remains a theoretical possibility). Random values not elevated during clinical hypoglycemic episodes do not convincingly document deficient secretion but provide a clue that requires specific testing. One can measure the plasma cortisol response to nonspecific stress or injected corticotropin or the plasma 11-deoxycortisol response to metyrapone and the plasma growth hormone response to oral doses of levodopa or clonidine or intravenous doses of arginine (see Chapter 6). On the other hand, if the clinical situation permits, the most relevant information is gained by systematic assessment of the counterregulatory response to rapid, insulin-induced decrements in the plasma glucose concentration. The insulin infusion test, designed to assess patients with IDDM before intensive therapy,[43] can be used for this purpose. This involves the infusion of regular insulin (40 mU/kg/h) with serial bedside measurements of the plasma glucose level and assessments of the mental status by a physician. Normally the plasma glucose concentration declines to a nadir (commonly between

2.2 and 2.8 mmol/L [40 to 50 mg/dL]) and then begins to rise. Symptoms, aside from sweating, palpitations, and anxiety (attributable to the sympathochromaffin response), do not occur. Neuroglycopenia sufficient to impair mentation is abnormal. A progressive decline in plasma glucose below 1.9 mmol/L (35 mg/dL) is also abnormal. The presence of either is an indication to stop the insulin infusion and to administer glucose intravenously. Such defective glucose counterregulation can be caused by defective secretion of counterregulatory hormones or by increased sensitivity to insulin. When this test is used to assess nondiabetic patients with postabsorptive hypoglycemia, serial measurements of plasma growth hormone and cortisol are in order. Measurements of plasma glucagon and epinephrine during the insulin infusion test are difficult to justify, as hypoglycemia resulting from combined glucagon and epinephrine deficiencies has been described only in patients with diabetes. Plasma C peptide can be measured if endogenous hyperinsulinism is a diagnostic consideration.

Deficiencies of Other Hormones

Hypoglycemia has been said to occur with hypothyroidism.[2, 162] Its mechanism is not known.

Non–Beta Cell Tumors

Postabsorptive hypoglycemia occurs in association with a variety of rare non–beta cell tumors. The majority are mesenchymal in origin: fibrosarcoma, mesothelioma, rhabdomyosarcoma, leiomyosarcoma, liposarcoma, hemangiopericytoma, neurofibroma, and lymphosarcoma. These are usually large tumors (0.3 to 20.0 kg).[2] More than one third are retroperitoneal, about one third are intra-abdominal, and the remainder are intrathoracic in location. In general, they are slow-growing, although many are malignant. Therefore even partial tumor resection can cause prolonged remission of hypoglycemia.

Epithelial non–beta cell tumors are occasionally associated with postabsorptive hypoglycemia. Hepatomas, adrenocortical tumors (usually malignant), and carcinoid tumors are the most common offenders. More than 25% of 142 patients with hepatomas reported from Hong Kong experienced hypoglycemia, and in 10%, hypoglycemia was a major recurrent problem during a period of several months.[163] Adrenocortical tumors associated with hypoglycemia are also generally large; they may or may not secrete excessive quantities of steroid hormones. Carcinoid tumors associated with hypoglycemia can be located in the ileum, bronchus, or pancreas.[2] They often produce clinical and biochemical manifestations of the carcinoid syndrome. Common carcinomas, including those of the stomach, colon, lung, breast, prostate, kidney, testis, and acinar pancreas, are only rarely associated with hypoglycemia. Hypoglycemia occurs occasionally in patients with leukemia, lymphoma, or multiple myeloma, as well as in patients with melanoma, teratoma, or pseudomyxoma. In patients with leukemias, pseudohypoglycemia (low glucose levels resulting from the metabolism of glucose in vitro by the large number of leukocytes present) is more likely than true hypoglycemia. Pseudohypoglycemia also occurs in patients with benign forms of leukocytosis.[164] It is suspected because of the absence of neuroglycopenia and is documented by the finding of normal concentrations of glucose in plasma promptly separated from the formed elements of the blood. Hypoglycemia has been reported in patients with neuroblastoma or paraganglioma, including pheochromocytoma.[2]

The pathogenesis of hypoglycemia associated with non–beta cell tumors is poorly understood. It likely differs among patients and may be multifactorial in a given patient. High rates of glucose turnover are common,[165, 166] consistent with the fact that large amounts of intravenous glucose may be required to prevent recurrent hypoglycemia in such patients.[167] Thus excessive glucose utilization may in itself explain hypoglycemia in some patients and play a role in the development of hypoglycemia in others. However, glucose utilization rates are not always increased.[168] Furthermore, as emphasized earlier, the liver normally has the capacity to increase glucose production several-fold, and increased glucose utilization per se may not cause hypoglycemia if hepatic glucoregulatory, enzymatic, and substrate supply mechanisms are intact. It is thus likely that reduced or inappropriately low hepatic glucose production plays a role in the development of non–beta cell tumor–associated hypoglycemia.[168]

Among the glucoregulatory factors, insulin and related peptides have been studied most extensively. Ectopic insulin secretion has not been demonstrated unequivocally, although relative hyperinsulinemia has been reported in hypoglycemic patients with fibrosarcomas,[169, 170] carcinoma of the cervix,[171] and carcinoid tumors.[172–174] However, insulin secretion is suppressed appropriately during hypoglycemia in the vast majority of patients. Thus insulin excess cannot explain most instances of non–beta cell tumor–associated hypoglycemia. Similarly, plasma levels of insulin-like growth factor I (IGF I, also called somatomedin-C), the peptide that mediates the growth-promoting effects of growth hormone and that is known to suppress plasma glucose levels, have not been found to be elevated in such patients.

Despite earlier controversy,[175–180] evidence indicates that excessive production of insulin-like growth factor II (IGF II) is involved in the pathogenesis of hypoglycemia in many patients with non–beta cell tumors. This evidence includes increased tumor content of IGF II and high levels of IGF II messenger RNA in mesenchymal tumors associated with hypoglycemia,[181–183] increased serum levels of IGF II in affected patients with mesenchymal tumors[182–184] and with hepatocellular carcinomas,[185] and the finding that IGF II circulates as 50- to 60-kd complexes with binding proteins rather than the predominant 150-kd complex of normal serum.[186] These smaller complexes cross the capillary membrane more readily and would be expected to exert a much stronger action on target tissues. This finding could explain how IGF II could cause hypoglycemia even though its circulating levels are not increased markedly.[186] In addition to the direct hypoglycemic actions of IGF II, IGF II–mediated suppression of growth hormone secretion (evidenced by low growth hormone and insulin-like growth factor I levels) might also contribute to hypoglycemia.[181, 182]

The glucose counterregulatory hormones have been little studied in patients with non–beta cell tumors and hypoglycemia. Diminished glucagon secretion[168] or action[187] has been noted in individual patients, but systematic studies have not been reported. The possibility that a tumor might elaborate an inhibitor of glucagon secretion has been suggested.[2, 168] However, there are no published data concerning sympathochromaffin function in patients with hypoglycemia associated with non–beta cell tumors. Metastatic destruction of the pituitary or the adrenal cortices could also contribute to the development of hypoglycemia. However, although metastases to the adrenal cortices are common, adrenocortical insufficiency is rare even in patients with advanced cancer.[188]

With respect to the enzymatic apparatus required to support glucose production, destruction of the liver by metastatic tumor could impair glucose production, but this is rare.[113]

The treatment of hypoglycemia associated with non–beta cell tumors involves short-term measures, such as parenteral doses of glucose, frequent feeding, and attention to specific identifiable glucoregulatory defects, as well as treatment of the primary tumor. Even partial reduction of tumor mass may result in remission of hypoglycemia. If the tumor cannot be treated and recurrent hypoglycemia is a problem, a trial of diazoxide, as discussed later, is reasonable. On theoretical grounds, a trial of growth hormone administration might be reasonable.[181, 182]

Endogenous Hyperinsulinism

Endogenous hyperinsulinism causing postabsorptive hypoglycemia can be the result of pancreatic beta cell disorders (including insulinoma), the presence of a beta cell secretagogue (e.g., a sulfonylurea), various autoimmune mechanisms, and perhaps the ectopic secretion of insulin.

Single, benign insulin-secreting tumors of the pancreatic islets (insulinomas) are present in 66%[189] to 85%[2] of patients with excessive secretion of insulin. In adults, solitary insulinomas are most common, although multiple adenomas or microadenomatosis also occurs. The majority of small children and some adults do not have discrete tumors. Hyperinsulinemia in these cases has been attributed to beta cell hyperplasia,[190] including a histological pattern termed *nesidioblastosis*—clusters of beta cells appearing to bud from pancreatic ducts. However, the specificity of the latter lesion is open to question, as it is found in the pancreata of individuals who did not have hypoglycemia.[191, 192] Thus there may be no specific histopathological findings in patients with endogenous hyperinsulinism who do not have insulinomas.

Insulinomas are rare; estimated occurrence is 1 in 1 million.[193] However, it is an often curable cause of potentially lethal hypoglycemia. Insulinomas occur in both sexes (approximately 60% in women) and at all ages in adults. In the Mayo Clinic series the median age at diagnosis was 50 in sporadic cases and 23 in patients with multiple endocrine neoplasia, type 1 (primary hyperparathyroidism, functioning pancreatic islet tumors, and functioning pituitary adenomas, inherited as an autosomal dominant trait; see Chapter 30).[1] Insulinomas occur within the substance of the pancreas in more than 99% of the cases; ectopic insulinomas have been found in areas of pancreatic heterotopia, including the wall of the duodenum, the porta hepatis, and the vicinity of the pancreas. Insulinomas are generally small, averaging 1 to 2 cm in diameter but ranging up to 15 cm.[1, 2] They almost always come to clinical attention because of the hypoglycemia that they produce, not because of local mass effects. Five to 10% of insulinomas are malignant, a diagnosis that can be made with confidence only when metastases are present. Islet cell carcinomas can secrete hormones in addition to insulin, including human chorionic gonadotropin, corticotropin, serotonin, gastrin, glucagon, somatostatin, and pancreatic polypeptide.[1, 2] Indeed, expression of the somatostatin, glucagon, and insulin genes was detected in all of four insulinomas tested in one report.[194] Correspondingly, apparent conversion of a malignant insulinoma to a glucagonoma syndrome has been reported,[195] and I have observed an aggressive gastrinoma syndrome (hypergastrinemia and perforated jejunal ulcers) in a patient treated surgically 15 y earlier for multiple insulinomas.

Normally insulin secretion declines during postabsorptive periods. This decrease in the plasma insulin level, coupled with glucagon secretion, results in maintenance of the plasma glucose concentration at levels sufficient to provide fuel for the brain between meals. Indeed, further suppression of insulin secretion permits maintenance of plasma glucose levels only 0.6 to 0.8 mmol/L (10 to 15 mg/dL) below postabsorptive values during a prolonged fast.[47]

The most consistent insulin secretory abnormality in patients with an insulinoma is failure of a normal decrease in insulin secretion as the plasma glucose level declines in the postabsorptive state. This failure results in relative hyperinsulinism (i.e., plasma insulin levels that are inappropriately high for the ambient plasma glucose concentration). Documentation of relative hyperinsulinism is fundamental to the diagnosis of endogenous hyperinsulinism. Hyperinsulinism in the portal and peripheral circulations results in low rates of glucose production with rates of glucose utilization that are not high in the absolute but are inappropriately high relative to the plasma glucose concentration.[196] Thus the plasma glucose concentration declines progressively in the postabsorptive state.

Less consistent abnormalities of insulin secretion include exaggerated insulin-secretory responses to the intravenous administration of tolbutamide, glucagon, calcium, and leucine; diminished insulin-secretory responses to the intravenous administration of glucose; and impaired suppression of insulin release in response to intravenous doses of somatostatin, epinephrine, or diazoxide.[2] All these have been utilized to diagnose insulinomas. However, they are not sufficiently precise (nor, for those that release insulin, sufficiently safe) for routine use. Nevertheless, the intravenous tolbutamide test has been used rather extensively to screen patients for hyperinsulinism.[197]

The common symptoms of hypoglycemia in patients with insulinomas are listed in Table 23–4. Although the fact that neuroglycopenic symptoms predominate is often emphasized, neurogenic symptoms also occur. Because the overnight fast is generally the longest interdigestive period, symptomatic episodes would be expected to occur commonly in the morning before breakfast. They do occur at that time but may also occur at other postabsorptive times, especially in the late afternoon, and are often associated with exercise.[1] As mentioned, symptoms referable to mass effects are unusual even when metastases are present.

The diagnosis of endogenous hyperinsulinism, which generally but not invariably implies the presence of an insulinoma, requires documentation of postabsorptive hypoglycemia with relative hyperinsulinism. Although this diagnosis occasionally can be made on the basis of biochemical findings alone, it most commonly includes the demonstration of the Whipple triad: biochemical hypoglycemia with symptoms that are relieved by elevation of the glucose level to normal.

The diagnosis of endogenous hyperinsulinism can be established with a single plasma sample (although multiple samples are desirable for confirmation) if that sample is obtained when the patient has symptomatic hypoglycemia in the postabsorptive state.[1, 2, 189, 198, 199] Under those conditions, a plasma glucose concentration less than 2.5 mmol/L (45 mg/dL) with a plasma insulin concentration greater than 72 pmol/L (10 μU/mL) and a plasma C peptide concentration

TABLE 23–4. Prevalence of Hypoglycemic Symptoms in Patients with Insulinomas

Symptom	%
Various combinations of diplopia, blurred vision, sweating, palpitations, or weakness	85
Confusion or abnormal behavior	80
Unconsciousness or amnesia	53
Grand mal seizures	12

From Service FJ, Dale AJD, Elveback LR, et al. Insulinoma. Clinical and diagnostic features of 60 consecutive cases. Mayo Clin Proc 1976; 51:417–429.

greater than 0.50 nmol/L (1.5 ng/mL) are diagnostic of endogenous hyperinsulinism in the broad sense and usually of primary beta cell disease (i.e., insulinoma or related disorders) if beta cell secretagogues such as sulfonylureas can be excluded. Indeed, plasma insulin levels greater than 36 pmol/L (5 μU/mL) and C peptide levels greater than 0.33 nmol/L (1.0 ng/mL) in such a hypoglycemic sample are suspicious and indicate that further study is required. It should be emphasized that these insulin and C peptide levels are not abnormal in the absence of hypoglycemia, and they are not necessarily abnormal in the postprandial state despite the presence of hypoglycemia. In theory, measurement of plasma C peptide should be more sensitive for diagnosis than that of insulin, because, in contrast to insulin, C peptide is degraded little, if at all, by the liver and its longer plasma halftime results in higher plasma concentrations despite equimolar secretion with insulin.[200] It is, of course, fundamental that the assays be reliable and designed to measure the relatively low plasma insulin and C peptide levels with precision.

Thus the critical samples are those obtained during postabsorptive hypoglycemia. This may be a random (but not postprandial) plasma sample. Often it is a sample obtained after a 12- to 14-h overnight fast. Indeed, Marks and Rose[2] found that endogenous hyperinsulinism could be diagnosed in more than 90% of the patients ultimately proven to have insulinomas using three or fewer plasma samples after overnight fasts. However, others have been able to demonstrate the Whipple triad and diagnose insulinomas in only 33% of the patients after a 12-h fast but in 71% at 24 h of fasting, 92% at 48 h, and 98% at 72 h.[1] Clearly, one should not interpret these percentages too literally, as patients who do not develop hypoglycemia during a diagnostic fast are less likely to undergo surgical explorations, and some may have undetected insulinomas. Although a plasma glucose level of less than 2.5 mmol/L (45 mg/dL) after an overnight fast is usually abnormal, it is not necessarily so during a prolonged fast, when lower values can occur in the absence of symptoms, especially in women and children.[1, 198, 199] Again, the critical issue is relative hyperinsulinemia.

When the plasma glucose concentration is not unequivocally low after an overnight fast in a patient in whom postabsorptive hypoglycemia is suspected, a diagnostic fast is in order. The patient must be hospitalized. Aside from noncaloric beverages, food is withheld until symptomatic hypoglycemia—preferably with a venous plasma glucose value of less than 2.5 mmol/L (45 mg/dL) develops or 72 h passes. Plasma glucose concentrations are measured serially; their frequency, based on the glucose level, is judgmental. Although bedside devices can be used to provide a quick estimate of the glucose level, plasma glucose concentrations must be measured in the laboratory. Critical decisions will be made on the basis of these glucose determinations; none of the bedside devices is sufficiently accurate for this purpose. It is not necessary to measure anything but glucose before hypoglycemia develops. However, when symptomatic hypoglycemia occurs, plasma insulin and C peptide (and proinsulin, if possible), as well as glucose, should be measured, and the serum or urine should be screened for sulfonylureas. Several samples for glucose, insulin, and C peptide should be obtained before the fast is terminated. If hypoglycemia does not develop during a diagnostic fast, many advocate a period of exercise before the fast is terminated; this exercise might provoke hypoglycemia in a patient with an insulinoma.

Another approach, which has not been found to be as effective as a diagnostic fast, is a C peptide suppression test. Hypoglycemia produced by the infusion or injection of

insulin normally suppresses insulin secretion and thus C peptide levels but generally does not do so in patients with endogenous hyperinsulinism. Thus a plasma C peptide value greater than 0.4 nmol/L (1.2 ng/mL) after intravenous infusion of regular insulin (0.1 U/kg over 60 min) to produce a plasma glucose level of 2.2 mmol/L (40 mg/dL) or less is abnormal and was found in 15 of 16 patients with insulinomas.[200] Counterregulatory hormone responses can also be assessed during insulin-induced hypoglycemia.

Rarely, an insulinoma is manifested by postprandial (reactive) hypoglycemia without postabsorptive hypoglycemia.[201] However, most patients with insulinomas and postprandial hypoglycemia also have postabsorptive hypoglycemia. When both forms of hypoglycemia are present, the differential diagnosis is that of postabsorptive hypoglycemia.

The differential diagnosis of postabsorptive hypoglycemia with inappropriately high immunoreactive insulin levels includes both endogenous and exogenous hyperinsulinism. Endogenous hyperinsulinism may be due to primary beta cell disease (e.g., insulinoma), the presence of a beta cell secretagogue (e.g., a sulfonylurea), autoimmune disorders with antibodies to insulin or to insulin receptors, or, rarely, ectopic insulin secretion. The presence of circulating antibodies to insulin was formerly thought to be diagnostic of exogenous insulin injection and indicative of factitious hypoglycemia caused by insulin injection,[202–205] a syndrome with poor prognosis most often seen in young women with medical knowledge or relatives with diabetes mellitus.[205] However, especially with the more purified insulins used currently, antibodies to insulin may not be present. Furthermore, insulin antibodies can develop in the absence of prior insulin administration and result in postabsorptive or postprandial hypoglycemia with high immunoreactive insulin levels.[206–210] Insulin antibodies invalidate standard insulin immunoassays; they result in artifactually high values when a double-antibody system is used. Indeed, reported insulin levels greater than 1400 pmol/L (200 μU/mL) during hypoglycemia should raise suspicion of this artifact.[211] Theoretically, plasma C peptide levels should be low in factitious or autoimmune hypoglycemia but, as discussed earlier, inappropriately high in patients with endogenous hyperinsulinism. Patients with insulin antibodies, whether as a result of insulin injections[211] or an autoimmune process,[209] do have suppressed plasma free C peptide levels. However, such patients may have elevated plasma total C peptide levels, because the insulin antibodies bind endogenous proinsulin, which contains the C peptide sequence and is recognized by human C peptide antisera.[209, 211] Thus an argument can be made for the routine measurement of insulin antibody levels in patients with postabsorptive hypoglycemia.

As determined with laborious gel filtration methods, plasma proinsulin levels are elevated in most patients with insulinomas.[212] By using sensitive radioimmunoassays, substantially elevated proinsulin concentrations were found after an overnight fast in all of 20 patients with insulinomas[213] and during hypoglycemia in all of 21 such patients.[214] With more widespread availability, the proinsulin radioimmunoassay may be a sensitive screening test for insulinomas. Interestingly, the insulin/proinsulin ratio was decreased from 6:1 in normal subjects to 1:1 in insulinoma patients, but was 10:1 in three patients with sulfonylurea-induced hypoglycemia. This suggests that proinsulin measurements might also be useful in distinguishing among the causes of endogenous hyperinsulinemia.

Hypoglycemia is rarely attributable to an antibody to the insulin receptor.[215–222] In such patients postabsorptive hypoglycemia is due to the insulin-like agonist action of the receptor antibodies. Insulin (and proinsulin) levels are elevated, perhaps because of decreased clearance.[222] Plasma C

TABLE 23–5. Differential Diagnosis of Hyperinsulinemic Postabsorptive Hypoglycemia*

Insulin†	C Peptide†	Proinsulin	Sulfonylureas†	Antibodies to			Diagnosis
				Insulin	Insulin Receptors	Beta Cells	
↑−↑↑↑‡	↓§	↓‖	−	+ or −	−	−	Exogenous hyperinsulinism
							Endogenous hyperinsulinism resulting from
↑	↑	↑	−	−	−	−	Insulinoma (? ectopic insulin secretion)
↑	↑	↑	+	−	−	−	Sulfonylurea ingestion
↑−↑↑↑‡	↓§	↓‖	−	+	−	−	Autoimmune, antibodies to insulin
↑	↓	↑	−	−	+	−	Autoimmune, antibodies to insulin receptors
↑‡	↑‖	↑‖	−	−	−	+	Autoimmune, antibodies to beta cells (?)

*−, negative; +, positive.

†Insulin, C peptide, and sulfonylureas must be measured in a sample obtained while the patient is hypoglycemic. Proinsulin has been reported to be elevated after an overnight fast in absence of hypoglycemia in patients with insulinomas, as well as during hypoglycemia in such patients.

‡Antibodies to insulin produce artificially elevated insulin values in a double-antibody radioimmunoassay. Even in the absence of antibodies to insulin, insulin concentrations are often elevated markedly after surreptitious insulin injection.

§Free C peptide levels are suppressed. Total C peptide levels may not be suppressed because of cross-reactivity with the C peptide sequence in antibody-bound proinsulin.

‖Theoretical.

peptide levels are suppressed appropriately.[219, 222] The presence of acanthosis nigricans and autoimmune phenomena may provide clues to the presence of antireceptor antibodies. Some patients have a history of glucose intolerance or diabetes mellitus. Finally, evidence for the presence of islet-stimulating antibodies in the sera of patients with hypoglycemia[223] suggests the possibility of still another form of autoimmune hypoglycemia.

The differential diagnosis of hyperinsulinemic postabsorptive hypoglycemia is summarized in Table 23–5. Briefly, a comprehensive biochemical assessment would include measurements, in samples obtained during symptomatic postabsorptive hypoglycemia, of plasma glucose, insulin, C peptide, proinsulin, and sulfonylureas, along with a test for antibodies to insulin. Clinical clues, such as acanthosis nigricans, evidence of an autoimmune disease, or both, should prompt a test for antibodies to the insulin receptor.

Once a diagnosis of postabsorptive hypoglycemia resulting from endogenous hyperinsulinism is established and sulfonylurea ingestion is excluded, a pancreatic beta cell lesion is often presumed to be present. This is reasonable, as ectopic insulin secretion, if it occurs, is rare,[169–174] as are (presumably) the autoimmune hypoglycemias.

The extent to which one should attempt to define the nature and anatomy of the beta cell lesion before surgery is a matter of judgment. A computed tomographic scan of the upper abdomen should be performed initially, although a study with negative results does not exclude insulinoma, as the tumors are often small. Detection rates of approximately 45 to 75% have been reported.[224, 225] Most malignant insulinomas are detected and staged with computed tomographic scans.[224] The value of magnetic resonance imaging remains to be determined. Preoperative ultrasonography is of relatively little value,[224, 225] but intraoperative ultrasonography is useful. The latter has high sensitivity and specificity, can detect tumors that are not palpable by the surgeon, and helps to define the relationship of the tumor to vital structures within the pancreas, such as the pancreatic duct and the great vessels.[225] Selective arteriography is also used to localize insulinomas.[1] Reported sensitivities range from 30 to 85%, but false-positive results occur.[2, 224] Because it is invasive, arteriography is not indicated if the tumor is localized with computed tomographic scans. In the presence of convincing clinical and biochemical evidence of an insulinoma, surgical exploration may be recommended without

arteriography in patients with negative computed tomographic scans, particularly in view of the utility of intraoperative ultrasonography. Pancreatic venous sampling for insulin, via the percutaneous transhepatic route, has successfully localized insulinomas.[224–226] However, false-positive localizations do occur and can sometimes be recognized if other pancreatic hormones (e.g., glucagon) are also measured.[226] This invasive technique should be reserved for difficult cases (e.g., patients in whom exploration has yielded inconclusive findings) and should be performed in a limited number of centers.

Because most patients with endogenous hyperinsulinism have solitary benign insulinomas, surgical therapy is generally effective. For solitary insulinomas, enucleation is sufficient. More extensive pancreatectomy is warranted for multiple adenomas or microadenomatosis. Even when total resection is not practical, reduction of the tumor mass often alleviates hypoglycemia, at least temporarily. When lesions are not apparent despite intraoperative ultrasonography, sequential resection starting with the tail of the pancreas is often performed. Total pancreatectomy is not advisable because of the associated morbidity and mortality, because partial pancreatectomy is often beneficial, and because of the availability of medical therapy for hypoglycemia. Some advocate a trial of diazoxide before exploration,[189] because conservative surgery is appropriate when hypoglycemia is shown to respond to this drug. Postoperative complications include pancreatitis, peritonitis, pancreatic fistulas, abscesses, and intestinal obstruction. In one large series surgical mortality was 10%,[227] although the figure is substantially lower in some reports.[1, 2] Hyperglycemia commonly follows effective surgery but is usually transient and disappears after a few days. Permanent diabetes mellitus occurs in about 10% of the cases.

Medical therapy is indicated in patients with malignant insulinomas and in those who will not, or cannot, undergo surgery. This therapy consists of measures designed to prevent hypoglycemia and, in patients with malignant tumors, to reduce the tumor burden. Diazoxide, which inhibits insulin secretion and may have additional hyperglycemic actions, is often effective in preventing hypoglycemia in patients with endogenous hyperinsulinism,[1, 2, 189, 228–231] as detailed later in this chapter. The somatostatin analogue octreotide is effective in some, but not all, patients.[232, 233–236] Available chemotherapeutic regimens are not effective in the treatment of malignant insulinomas. Streptozocin, alone or in combination with fluorouracil, has been used.[237, 238] Hepatic artery embolization has been used to palliate metastatic islet carcinomas.[239]

Hypoglycemia in Infancy and Childhood

Disorders unique to infancy and childhood include the neonatal hypoglycemias, specific enzyme deficiencies that result in hypoglycemia, and ketotic hypoglycemia of childhood. In many instances of hypoglycemia in infants and children the pathogenic mechanisms are fundamentally similar to those in adults (e.g., hypoglycemia can result from drugs, critical organ failure, hormonal deficiencies, non–beta cell tumors, and hyperinsulinism). Thus the differential diagnosis of hypoglycemia in infants and children is similar to that of hypoglycemia in adults but with additional unique disorders.[1, 240]

The fetus derives its glucose from the maternal circulation. Immediately after birth, the neonate must make a rapid transition from maternal glucose supply to endogenous glucose production. During the first 4 to 6 h of neonatal life, the plasma glucose concentration declines, stabilizes, and then begins to rise toward childhood-adult levels. Endogenous glucose production is initially the result of glycogenolysis and then of increasing gluconeogenesis.[1, 240] The glucoregulatory mechanisms that accomplish this transition to endogenous glucose production have not been defined precisely but probably include low insulin and high glucagon signals, perhaps in concert with increased catecholamine levels.[241] Whatever the mechanisms of this transition, the neonate is particularly vulnerable to hypoglycemia.

Infants and children have glucose turnover rates roughly three times higher than those in adults when expressed per unit of body weight.[242] Because of relatively high rates of glucose utilization, including that by the disproportionately large brain, and because of relatively limited stores of gluconeogenic precursors, children tolerate fasting less well than adults.[243] Hypoglycemia is the rule after 24 to 48 h of fasting in children.

Neonatal Hypoglycemia

Neonatal hypoglycemia—that developing in the first 72 h after birth—can be due to transient hyperinsulinism.[1, 240] This is best exemplified by hypoglycemic infants of diabetic mothers. If the mother's diabetes is not well controlled, the fetus is also hyperglycemic. This results in increased fetal insulin secretion and fetal hyperinsulinemia that persist into the neonatal period and cause transient hypoglycemia. Transient hyperinsulinism also underlies neonatal hypoglycemia in infants with Rh factor incompatibility or the Beckwith-Wiedemann syndrome (macroglossia, omphalocele, and visceromegaly), although the etiology of the hyperinsulinemia in these disorders is unknown. It can also follow exchange transfusion, resulting from hyperinsulinemia stimulated by the glucose administered during the procedure. It has also been caused by drugs given to the mother. These include agents that stimulate fetal insulin secretion (e.g., a sulfonylurea) or that produce maternal and fetal hyperglycemia and thus fetal hyperinsulinemia (e.g., administration of a beta-2–adrenergic agonist used to delay labor).

On the other hand, neonatal hypoglycemia can be due to factors other than hyperinsulinism. For example, as many as half the infants who are small for gestational age experience neonatal hypoglycemia.[244] This is not thought to be due to glucoregulatory defects or deficient mobilization of substrates, as the glucoregulatory hormones are normal and

blood lactate and alanine levels are elevated during hypoglycemia.[245] The latter data suggest impairment of gluconeogenesis, perhaps the result of delayed induction of one or more of the rate-limiting gluconeogenic enzymes. Neonatal hypoglycemia has also been attributed to hypoxia and to cold stress.[240]

Postabsorptive hypoglycemia caused by endogenous hyperinsulinism may persist from the neonatal period or may develop in the first year of life. Such patients rarely have discrete insulinomas. Many respond to therapy with diazoxide. Partial pancreatectomy should probably be limited to patients who do not respond adequately to diazoxide on the premise that this form of hyperinsulinism is usually transient. This premise remains to be proved.[1] On the other hand, hyperinsulinism that develops after the first year of life is more likely to be caused by an insulinoma.[2]

Congenital Deficiencies of Glucogenic Enzymes

A variety of specific congenital enzyme deficiencies, generally inherited as autosomal recessive traits, can cause recurrent hypoglycemia. If the disorder is compatible with survival, hypoglycemia persists into adult life but is usually first recognized in infancy or childhood. Although glucose metabolism is ultimately affected, the primary enzymatic defect may involve steps in the metabolism of carbohydrates, amino acids, or fatty acids.[1] Some of the relevant metabolic pathways are outlined in Figure 23–1.

Glucose-phosphatase deficiency (glycogen storage disease type I, or von Gierke disease) results in severe postabsorptive hypoglycemia and metabolic acidosis with elevated blood lactate, ketone, and alanine levels. The finding that ketonemia is less than that of normal children who have fasted for 24 to 30 h suggests a coexistent defect in ketogenesis.[246] Glycogen accumulation causes hepatomegaly. Hyperlipidemia, hyperuricemia, and growth retardation are common. With the exception of hepatomegaly, all these abnormalities can be reversed by the prevention of hypoglycemia with frequent feedings during waking hours and continuous intragastric glucose infusions during sleep.[247] Thus the abnormalities are the result of hypoglycemia and the activation of compensatory, but to some extent futile, glucoregulatory systems. Liver transplantation corrects hypoglycemia.[248] Interestingly, hepatic glucose-6-phosphatase enzyme activity is normal in some patients with otherwise clinically and chemically typical von Gierke disease. These patients appear to have a functional defect in glucose 6-phosphate hydrolysis.[249] Among the other glycogen storage diseases, glycogen synthase deficiency can cause severe postabsorptive hypoglycemia, whereas phosphorylase deficiency and debrancher enzyme deficiency cause asymptomatic hepatomegaly only.[1]

Deficiencies of gluconeogenic enzymes other than glucose-6-phosphatase (the final step in both gluconeogenic and glycogenolytic hepatic glucose release) include those of fructose-1,6-bisphosphatase, phosphoenolpyruvate carboxykinase, and pyruvate carboxylase.[1] Fructose-1,6-bisphosphatase deficiency causes severe postabsorptive hypoglycemia associated with metabolic acidosis and elevated blood lactate, ketone, and alanine levels.[250] Hyperlipidemia, hyperuricemia, and hepatomegaly occur as in von Gierke disease, although the hepatomegaly is the result of lipid, rather than glycogen, accumulation.

Postprandial, rather than postabsorptive, hypoglycemia is a feature of galactosemia and of hereditary fructose intolerance. The enzyme defect in the former, galactose-1-

phosphate uridyltransferase deficiency, results in hypoglycemia (often with vomiting and diarrhea) after galactose ingestion. The hypoglycemia has been attributed to acute inhibition of glycogenolysis.[251] Cataracts, hepatosplenomegaly, and mental retardation are the result of galactose 1-phosphate accumulation; their progression can be prevented by the elimination of galactose from the diet.[251] The enzyme deficiency is demonstrable in erythrocytes. Fructose 1-phosphate aldolase deficiency, the defect in hereditary fructose intolerance, causes hypoglycemia and vomiting after fructose ingestion and is associated with hepatomegaly. Fructose 1-phosphate accumulates and inhibits glycogenolysis.[252]

Deficient enzymes of amino acid metabolism can also cause hypoglycemia. For example, hypoglycemia occurs in patients with maple syrup urine disease,[253] which is caused by an enzyme deficiency that results in decreased decarboxylation of the α-ketoacids of leucine, isoleucine, and valine, the branched chain amino acids. The pathogenesis of the hypoglycemia is not clear, except that it results from defective gluconeogenesis.[253, 254] Hypoglycemia resulting from defective gluconeogenesis also occurs in methylmalonic aciduria.[255]

A variety of defects in long chain fatty acid oxidation can result in hypoglycemia along with hypoketonemia.[256–259] Normally, low-insulin, relatively high-glucagon states such as fasting (and these in addition to high catecholamine levels during stress) favor the mobilization of long chain fatty acids from fat (lipolysis) and their transport to the liver. These regulatory conditions also favor hepatic fatty acid oxidation and ketogenesis over triglyceride formation. Fatty acid oxidation requires that fatty acyl coenzyme A derivatives of the fatty acids be transported into mitochondria. Because the inner mitochondrial membranes are not permeable to fatty acyl coenzyme A esters, these are transesterified to fatty acyl carnitine at the outer surface of the membrane, transported across the membrane, and reconverted to fatty acyl coenzyme A esters at the inner surface of the membrane. The transesterifications are accomplished by carnitine palmitoyltransferases I and II, respectively. Within the mitochondrion, beta-oxidation of fatty acyl coenzyme A to acetyl coenzyme A occurs; among the fates of acetyl coenzyme A is conversion to hydroxymethylglutaryl coenzyme A, which can then be converted to ketones.

Recognized defects in long chain fatty acid metabolism resulting in hypoketonemia and postabsorptive hypoglycemia include systemic carnitine deficiency, carnitine palmitoyltransferase deficiency, and deficiencies of several enzymes involved in the initial step in beta-oxidation of fatty acids.[259] Systemic carnitine deficiency occurs as a primary disorder (of unknown mechanism) and can be secondary to a variety of genetic metabolic defects or to other conditions.[257–259] Liver and muscle carnitine levels are decreased; serum carnitine levels are variable. Hypotonia and hepatomegaly, the latter resulting from triglyceride accumulation, are common, and encephalopathy and cardiac failure may develop. Hypoglycemia can be the initial manifestation of systemic carnitine deficiency; early recognition may permit initiation of therapy before myopathy and encephalopathy develop.[260]

The pathogenesis of postabsorptive hypoglycemia in patients with defective long chain fatty acid oxidation has not been defined clearly, but glucose utilization may be inappropriately high.[256] Therapy includes avoidance of fasting and high-carbohydrate feedings.[1] Medium chain triglyceride feeding has been reported to be effective.[256] Responses to carnitine administration have been variable,[257, 258] perhaps because carnitine deficiency is not the primary abnormality in patients who do not respond. The key issue, however, is

avoidance of prolonged fasting as occurs, for example, with intercurrent illness.

Hypoglycemia occurs commonly in young children with Reye syndrome (vomiting, liver disease, and encephalopathy, typically after a viral illness). Hypoglycemia is the result of defective gluconeogenesis, perhaps an acquired form of pyruvate carboxylase deficiency.[1]

Ketotic Hypoglycemia of Childhood

Ketotic hypoglycemia of childhood has its onset between the ages of 2 and 5 and typically remits spontaneously before the age of 10. Postabsorptive hypoglycemia, with appropriate hypoinsulinemia and hyperketonemia, develops after 8 to 16 h of fasting, often associated with or as the result of an intercurrent illness. Because similar biochemical changes follow a longer period of fasting in normal children, so-called ketotic hypoglycemia may represent only one end of the normal distribution of glycemic tolerance to fasting.[261] Alternatively, this category may include several different specific disorders. This diagnosis is now made less frequently.

The pathogenesis of ketotic hypoglycemia appears to involve diminished provision of a major hepatic gluconeogenic substrate, alanine, from muscle.[262, 263] Blood alanine levels are low during postabsorptive hypoglycemia, and alanine infusion results in an increase in plasma glucose. Glycogenolytic and gluconeogenic systems remain intact, and aside from low epinephrine levels,[149–154] glucoregulatory signals are appropriate.[1] Deficient epinephrine secretion could cause decreased alanine mobilization, as epinephrine accelerates alanine turnover in humans.[264] Nonetheless, at least in adults, epinephrine deficiency per se does not cause postabsorptive hypoglycemia, as discussed earlier.

Treatment includes the avoidance of prolonged fasting and the provision of glucose during intercurrent illnesses that ordinarily result in prolonged fasting, with the expectation that the disorder will remit spontaneously.

THE POSTPRANDIAL (REACTIVE) HYPOGLYCEMIAS

Postprandial (reactive, stimulative) hypoglycemia occurs exclusively after meals, typically within 4 h after food ingestion. Any of the disorders that cause postabsorptive hypoglycemia can result in hypoglycemia detected after a meal. The diagnostic and therapeutic approach is identical with that of postabsorptive hypoglycemia in such a patient.

Congenital deficiencies of enzymes of carbohydrate metabolism, such as galactosemia[251] and hereditary fructose intolerance,[252] are rare causes of postprandial hypoglycemia early in life. Postprandial hypoglycemia is common in patients who have undergone gastric surgery that results in rapid movement of swallowed food into the small intestine (e.g., gastrectomy, gastroenterostomy, pyloroplasty, gastric bypass).[265, 266] This type of postprandial hypoglycemia, termed *alimentary hypoglycemia*, is thought to be the result of marked early hyperinsulinemia caused by rapid absorption of ingested nutrients, the enhanced secretion of insulinotropic gut factors, or both. Hypoglycemia, which is sometimes severe enough to cause neuroglycopenic symptoms including loss of consciousness,[2] occurs early after food ingestion, typically within 1½ to 3 h. Symptoms of hypoglycemia must be distinguished from those of the dumping syndrome—abdominal fullness, nausea, and weakness—which occur less than 1 h after meals. A pattern of postprandial hypoglycemia similar to that of alimentary hypoglycemia has also been described in rare patients who have not undergone gastric surgery.[267]

There is no question that clinical postprandial hypoglycemia occurs in some patients with the specific disorders of glucose metabolism mentioned in the preceding paragraph. However, the frequency, and even the existence, of clinically relevant idiopathic (or functional) postprandial hypoglycemia is a matter of intense debate.[1,2] Some have suggested that hypoglycemia is a common problem, responsible for much illness in society. Others deny the existence of idiopathic postprandial hypoglycemia. The truth likely lies between these extremes and is probably closer to the latter view.[268–272]

Idiopathic postprandial hypoglycemia is all too often erroneously diagnosed by patients and by physicians. For example, only 16 of 118 patients evaluated for suspected postprandial hypoglycemia in one series had both a plasma glucose concentration lower than the 10th percentile of asymptomatic individuals and typical symptoms after an oral glucose load; only 5 of those 16 had similar symptoms after their regular meals.[268] Other investigators have also found that most patients thought to have hypoglycemic symptoms as well as low glucose levels after glucose ingestion have normal glucose levels after a mixed meal.[269, 271] In one series employing glucose measurements during symptomatic episodes, only 5% of 132 episodes were associated with blood glucose levels of 2.8 mmol/L (50 mg/dL) or less.[271] Some authorities[273] have endorsed the view that the term *idiopathic postprandial hypoglycemia* should be abandoned and that the designation *idiopathic postprandial syndrome*[268] should be substituted.

A diagnosis of postprandial hypoglycemia should not be made on the basis of plasma glucose concentration alone. The lower limits of normal for plasma glucose concentrations late after glucose ingestion can be defined in statistical terms. For example, in 650 individuals who remained asymptomatic after ingestion of 100 g of glucose, glucose concentrations at nadir were: lower 2.5th percentile, 2.2 mmol/L (30 mg/dL); 5th percentile, 2.4 mmol/L (43 mg/dL); 10th percentile, 2.6 mmol/L (47 mg/dL); and 25th percentile, 3.0 mmol/L (54 mg/dL).[269] However, because the lowest glucose levels in these subjects cause no recognizable symptoms, have no known long-term ill effects, are self-limited, and do not imply the presence of a disease that requires treatment, there is no reason to arbitrarily classify 2.5 or 5.0% of the population as having a disease. Thus the diagnosis of reactive hypoglycemia requires appropriate symptoms temporally related to a low plasma glucose concentration after a mixed meal and relief of symptoms as the plasma glucose concentration rises (Whipple triad). The diagnosis should not be made on the basis of an oral glucose tolerance test.[2, 268–270, 272]

The pathogenesis of true postprandial hypoglycemia (Whipple triad fulfilled) in general is poorly defined. That of idiopathic postprandial hypoglycemia (or syndrome) is unknown. There is no evidence that insulin secretion is excessive. Increased sensitivity to insulin[274, 275] and normal monocyte insulin receptors[274] have been reported. These data are consistent with either increased cellular responsiveness to insulin at a site or sites of insulin action distal to the insulin receptors, or decreased counterregulatory hormone secretion or action. As discussed earlier, glucagon, in concert with dissipation of insulin, normally regulates the transition from exogenous glucose delivery to endogenous glucose production late after glucose ingestion. Epinephrine is not normally critical but compensates partially and becomes critical when glucagon secretion is deficient.[45] Thus deficient glucagon secretion would plausibly explain the pathogenesis of the postprandial syndrome, including compensatory enhancement of epinephrine secretion, the production of symptoms attributable to the sympathochromaffin response, and the prevention of severe hypoglycemia and restoration of euglycemia. In accord with this possibility, lower pancreatic glucagon concentrations have been reported to occur in persons with glucose nadirs less than 2.8 mmol/L (50 mg/dL), when compared with those with higher glucose nadirs after glucose ingestion.[276] However, glucagon levels were lower at baseline as well and were not discernibly lower in two patients with "severe" hypoglycemia (nadirs of 1.5 and 1.3 mmol/L).[276] Whether those with lower glucose nadirs had symptoms was not stated. Moreover, similarly selected patients (glucose nadir less than 2.8 mmol/L) in another study had elevated glucagon-like immunoreactivity and normal pancreatic glucagon levels after glucose ingestion.[277] The occurrence of a markedly enhanced, and presumably compensatory, epinephrine response in patients with symptoms or signs such as sweating, tremor, and increased heart rate temporally related to the low glucose nadir late after glucose ingestion has been documented.[278]

Diets low in carbohydrate and high in protein are commonly recommended to patients designated as having reactive hypoglycemia. Their efficacy has not been established by controlled studies. Frequent feedings and avoidance of simple sugars are also advised. Anticholinergic drugs have been reported to be beneficial in patients with idiopathic reactive hypoglycemia but commonly produce undesirable side effects.[279] Propranolol has been reported to reduce symptoms (except diaphoresis) in patients with postgastrectomy hypoglycemia. Pectin has been stated to decrease postprandial hypoglycemia after gastric surgery.[280] Such patients have also been treated surgically with reversal of a segment of proximal jejunum.[281]

THE TREATMENT OF POSTABSORPTIVE HYPOGLYCEMIA

Emergency Treatment

Because of the vulnerability of the brain to prolonged hypoglycemia, the plasma glucose concentration must be raised at least to normal levels as rapidly as possible, and recurrence of hypoglycemia must be prevented thereafter. Postprandial hypoglycemia, because it is self-limited, rarely requires emergency treatment. In contrast, postabsorptive hypoglycemias are typically persistent or progressive and require short-term as well as long-term therapy.

Oral administration of glucose is preferred if the hypoglycemic patient is alert enough to swallow. A reasonable dose is 10 to 20 g of carbohydrate.[282, 283] If the patient is not able (or willing) to take oral feedings, glucose should be given intravenously. A commonly used dose is 25 g (50 mL of a 50% glucose solution). Glucagon (1.0 mg) is an effective alternative[284] and can be given intramuscularly or even subcutaneously. Thus family members of patients prone to recurrent hypoglycemia without glycogen depletion (e.g., those with diabetes mellitus) can be trained to administer glucagon when the patient is unable to take carbohydrate orally and is known or presumed to be hypoglycemic. After the initial response to glucagon, patients should be urged to eat to prevent recurrent hypoglycemia in view of the transient effect of glucagon on glucose production.

Clinical improvement should occur less than 10 min after the plasma glucose level is raised and maintained, provided brain damage has not occurred. Whenever possible, the presence of hypoglycemia should be documented before therapy, and the plasma glucose response to therapy should be followed by measurements of the plasma glucose level. If these are not available and there is no clinical response within 15 min, the initial therapy should be repeated, and access to plasma glucose monitoring and intravenous glucose infusion should be attained as soon as possible. These are available in hospitals and from many emergency medical services. To aid communication with medical personnel in such emergencies, persons prone to hypoglycemia should wear tags identifying their disorder.

Even if there is a response to initial therapy, glucose monitoring to ensure maintenance of the plasma glucose concentration is desirable. Recurrence of hypoglycemia is a function of the hypoglycemic mechanism, its magnitude, and its duration, and of the adequacy of therapy. For example, recurrent hypoglycemia is the rule after chlorpropamide overdosage, whereas it is unusual after recovery from hypoglycemia produced by regular insulin. Inadequate rates of glucose infusion or too small an oral feeding may contribute to recurrence.

Although prompt recovery of central nervous system function commonly follows restoration of the plasma glucose concentration, recovery is sometimes delayed, perhaps because of cerebral edema. Unconsciousness lasting more than 30 min after the plasma glucose concentration has been raised to normal and maintained is referred to as *posthypoglycemic coma*.[285] It has been treated with mannitol given intravenously (40 g as a 20% solution over 20 min), glucocorticoids (e.g., dexamethasone, 10 mg), or both,[2, 285–287] along with maintenance of the plasma glucose concentration.

In some instances hypoglycemia persists despite the intravenous infusion of seemingly large doses of glucose, implying massive glucose overutilization. Although the primary short-term therapeutic approach is to infuse large enough amounts of glucose to bring the plasma concentration to normal, measures designed to reduce glucose utilization can be added. For example, when the hypoglycemia is caused by endogenous hyperinsulinism, including that resulting from sulfonylurea overdosage, the addition of diazoxide (see the following section) is effective.[288–290]

Long-Term Treatment

Definitive treatment of the postabsorptive hypoglycemias requires correction of the underlying hypoglycemic mechanism whenever possible. When that is not possible, attempts to increase exogenous or endogenous glucose delivery and to limit glucose utilization should be made. Long-term therapy may involve dietary modifications, medications, surgery, radiation, or a combination of these.

Although the judicious use of snacks is a useful component of therapeutic regimens for patients with IDDM, frequent feedings are a less than ideal approach to the long-term treatment of chronic hypoglycemic disorders. One problem is unwanted weight gain. However, frequent feedings, even overnight gastric infusions, are sometimes necessary when other measures are inadequate.

Hypoglycemia caused by drugs is limited to the duration of action of the offending drug. If the causative agent is known, the management is straightforward: discontinuation of the drug (at least temporarily), maintenance of the plasma glucose level while drug action continues, and adjustment of subsequent drug regimens to avoid recurrent hypoglycemia. Therapy is more difficult if the drug is used surreptitiously.

As discussed earlier, postabsorptive hypoglycemia resulting from endogenous hyperinsulinism is often curable by surgical removal of an insulinoma. If this is not possible because of multiple or metastatic tumors or the absence of a definable lesion, diazoxide is often effective.[228–231, 291] Diaz-

oxide has also been used in the short-term treatment of sulfonylurea-induced hypoglycemia[288–290] and has been tried, with variable success, in other forms of postabsorptive hypoglycemia.

Diazoxide (100 to 800 mg/d in adults and 5 to 30 mg/ kg body weight/d in infants and children) raises the plasma glucose concentration in large part by suppressing insulin secretion. The finding of an exaggerated insulin-secretory response to tolbutamide during diazoxide administration[292] suggests inhibition of insulin release with ongoing insulin biosynthesis. Beta-adrenergic mechanisms also participate in the hyperglycemic action of diazoxide;[293, 294] beta-adrenergic antagonists are said to reduce the action of the drug.[2]

Diazoxide is bound tightly to albumin and has a plasma half-time of 20 to 30 h.[295] When given by rapid intravenous injection it is a potent hypotensive drug, but when given orally or by slow intravenous infusion it has little hypotensive action; indeed, hypertensive responses have occurred. Although chemically related to the thiazide diuretics, diazoxide causes sodium retention. Coadministration of a thiazide diuretic both limits sodium retention and potentiates the hyperglycemic action of diazoxide.[230, 231, 291] Both edema formation and gastrointestinal side effects (anorexia, nausea, and sometimes vomiting) are dose related. A bothersome problem is that of generalized growth of lanugo hair (hypertrichosis lanuginosa) during prolonged therapy. Allergic reactions, including rashes and agranulocytosis, are rare.

The treatment of hypoglycemia associated with non–beta cell tumors involves short-term measures pending effective medical, surgical, or radiotherapeutic treatment of the tumor. Hypoglycemia resulting from glucocorticoid deficiency is corrected by replacement therapy. Hypoglycemia is rarely an indication for growth hormone replacement. Remissions of autoimmune hypoglycemias have been associated with immunosuppressive, particularly glucocorticoid, therapy.[216, 217, 219–221] The treatment of hypoglycemia caused by inanition, hepatic or renal disease, cardiac failure, or sepsis includes short-term measures and, when possible, treatment or management of the underlying disease process. The treatment of the hypoglycemias of infancy and childhood and of postprandial hypoglycemia was already discussed.

THE APPROACH TO THE PATIENT WITH HYPOGLYCEMIA

The first step in the care of a patient suspected of having hypoglycemia is clear documentation that the patient does in fact have this abnormality. Establishment of the relationship between documented hypoglycemia and symptoms and signs attributable to hypoglycemia is fundamental, as is the distinction between postprandial and postabsorptive hypoglycemic states. As emphasized throughout this chapter, the presence of postabsorptive hypoglycemia raises the distinct possibility of a progressive, potentially fatal disorder and demands conclusive diagnostic assessment, treatment, and follow-up. The presence of postprandial hypoglycemia is diagnostically irrelevant in a patient with postabsorptive hypoglycemia. In contrast, isolated postprandial hypoglycemia is self-limited, rarely produces ominous symptoms, and is not progressive.

Hypoglycemia is often suspected on the basis of symptoms that are nonspecific. It is much more often suspected than diagnosed. In some patients plasma drawn for reasons other than suspected hypoglycemia is reported to have a low glucose concentration. Although artifact (e.g., glycolysis in vitro) is reasonably suspected under these conditions, true hypoglycemia must be considered. Occasionally patients are found to be hypoglycemic at the time of presentation to a hospital. This represents a frequently missed diagnostic opportunity; plasma should be saved for subsequent measurements of insulin, C peptide, and drugs if the hypoglycemia should be persistent or recurrent and its cause not apparent.

If hypoglycemia is documented in the absence of an obvious cause, three questions need to be addressed: Is hypoglycemia a recurrent phenomenon? Are there associated symptoms that are relieved when the plasma glucose concentration is raised to normal levels (Whipple triad)? Is this postabsorptive hypoglycemia? These questions are approached initially by measurement of the plasma glucose concentration after an overnight fast, repeated if necessary. The same procedure is the proper approach in suspected hypoglycemia. If this measurement answers all three questions in the affirmative, then determination of the hypoglycemic mechanism must proceed. If the plasma glucose concentration is normal after an overnight fast, a judgment must be made regarding the need for a prolonged diagnostic fast. Once postabsorptive hypoglycemia is excluded, the physician must decide whether postprandial hypoglycemia is likely enough to warrant further testing by frequent plasma glucose measurements after meals.

A conservative approach in patients demonstrating affirmative answers to the foregoing questions is as follows: if a plausible hypoglycemic mechanism (e.g., drugs, adrenocortical insufficiency) is apparent and is treatable or self-limited, further diagnostic evaluation should not be undertaken with the expectation that hypoglycemia will not be a continuing problem. This approach requires documentation that hypoglycemia resolves. Rarely, two different causes for hypoglycemia coexist. Obviously it would be a serious error to assume an untreatable hypoglycemic mechanism and miss a treatable one.

If a plausible hypoglycemic mechanism is not apparent after the initial history, physical examination, and routine laboratory determinations in a patient with documented postabsorptive hypoglycemia, the initial diagnostic considerations should include hyperinsulinism caused by an insulinoma or related beta cell disorder or the surreptitious use of sulfonylureas or insulin. Clinically occult hormonal deficiencies or a non–beta cell tumor, the surreptitious use of alcohol, autoimmune hypoglycemias, and occult defects in glucogenic enzyme systems are less likely possibilities. Thus at the time of postabsorptive hypoglycemia, plasma insulin and C peptide levels (and proinsulin if possible) should be measured, the blood or urine should be screened for sulfonylureas, and the blood alcohol level should be determined. Insulin antibody determinations, measurement of serum tumor markers such as β-human chorionic gonadotropin, radiographic tumor search, and provocative tests for hormonal deficiencies are logically deferred until the results of the initial studies are known. However, it may be cost effective to proceed with these studies if the short-term management of hypoglycemia requires continuous hospitalization.

With respect to the assessment for possible hormone deficiencies, insulin-induced hypoglycemia offers several advantages. It permits assessment of cortisol and growth hormone secretion, as well as of glucagon and epinephrine, if indicated; it provides insight into the adequacy of glucose recovery from acute hypoglycemia; and it permits assessment of the suppressibility of C peptide levels.

In children, the various enzymatic defects discussed earlier and the syndrome of ketotic hypoglycemia need to be included in the differential diagnosis of postabsorptive hypoglycemia. Otherwise the differential diagnosis is similar, except in neonates, to that detailed earlier in this chapter.

It has been emphasized in this chapter that except when produced as a side effect of the treatment of diabetes, hypoglycemia is not common. Because of its danger, however, it is a tragedy to miss the diagnosis or to treat the condition improperly.

REFERENCES

1. Service FJ, ed. Hypoglycemic Disorders. Boston: G. K. Hall, 1983.
2. Marks V, Rose FC. Hypoglycemia. 2nd ed. Oxford: Blackwell, 1981.
3. Cryer PE. Hypoglycemia and insulin dependent diabetes mellitus. In: Alberti KGMM, Krall LP, eds. The Diabetes Annual/4. New York: Elsevier, 1988: 272–310.
4. Cryer PE, Binder C, Bolli GB, et al. Hypoglycemia in insulin dependent diabetes mellitus. Diabetes 1989; 38:1193–1199.
5. Owen OE, Morgan AP, Kemp HG, et al. Brain metabolism during fasting. J Clin Invest 1967; 46:1589–1595.
6. Garber AJ, Cryer PE, Santiago JV, et al. The role of adrenergic mechanisms in the substrate and hormonal response to insulin induced hypoglycemia in man. J Clin Invest 1976; 58:7–15.
7. Nilsson LH. Liver glycogen content in man in the postabsorptive state. Scand J Clin Lab Invest 1973; 32:317–323.
8. Owen OE, Felig P, Morgan AP, et al. Liver and kidney metabolism during prolonged starvation. J Clin Invest 1969; 48:574–583.
9. Radziuk J, McDonald TJ, Rubenstein D, et al. Initial splanchnic extraction of ingested glucose in normal man. Metabolism 1978; 27:657–669.
10. Exton JH. Mechanisms of hormonal regulation of hepatic glucose metabolism. Diabetes Metab Rev 1987; 3:163–183.
11. Frizell RT, Campbell PJ, Cherrington AD. Gluconeogenesis and hypoglycemia. Diabetes Metab Rev 1988; 4:51–70.
12. Rizza RA, Mandarino L, Gerich JE. Dose-response characteristics for the effects of insulin on production and utilization of glucose in man. Am J Physiol 1981; 240:630–639.
13. Rizza RA, Gerich JE. Persistent effect of hyperglucagonemia on glucose production in man. J Clin Endocrinol Metab 1979; 48:352–353.
14. Cherrington AD, Williams PE, Shulman GI, et al. Differential time course of glucagon's effect on glycogenolysis and gluconeogenesis in the conscious dog. Diabetes 1981; 30:180–187.
15. Rizza RA, Cryer PE, Haymond MW, et al. Adrenergic mechanisms for the effect of epinephrine on glucose production and clearance in man. J Clin Invest 1980; 65:682–689.
16. Berk MA, Clutter WE, Skor DA, et al. Enhanced glycemic responsiveness to epinephrine in insulin dependent diabetes mellitus is the result of the inability to secrete insulin. J Clin Invest 1985; 75:1842–1851.
17. Clutter WE, Rizza RA, Gerich JE, et al. Regulation of glucose metabolism by sympathochromaffin catecholamines. Diabetes Metab Rev 1988; 4:1–15.
18. Gerich JE, Lorenzi M, Tsalikian E, et al. Studies on the mechanisms of epinephrine induced hyperglycemia in man. Diabetes 1976; 25:65–71.
19. Gray DE, Lickley HLA, Vranic M. Physiologic effects of epinephrine on glucose turnover and plasma free fatty acid concentrations mediated independently of glucagon. Diabetes 1980; 29:600–608.
20. Deibert DC, DeFronzo RA. Epinephrine induced insulin resistance in man. J Clin Invest 1980; 65:717–721.
21. Rosen SG, Clutter WE, Shah SD, et al. Direct, α-adrenergic stimulation of hepatic glucose production in postabsorptive man. Am J Physiol 1983; 245:E616–E626.
22. MacGorman LR, Rizza RA, Gerich JE. Physiological concentrations of growth hormone exert insulin-like and insulin antagonist effects on both hepatic and extrahepatic tissues in man. J Clin Endocrinol Metab 1981; 53:556–559.
23. Shamoon H, Hendler R, Sherwin RS. Synergistic interactions among anti-insulin hormones in the pathogenesis of stress hyperglycemia in humans. J Clin Endocrinol Metab 1981; 52:1235–1241.
24. Lautt WW. Hepatic nerves: a review of their functions and effects. Can J Physiol Pharmacol 1980; 58:105–123.
25. Nobin A, Falck B, Ingemansson S, et al. Organization and function of the sympathetic innervation of the human liver. Acta Physiol Scand 1977; Suppl 452:103–106.
26. Boyle PJ, Liggett SB, Shah SD, et al. Direct muscarinic cholinergic inhibition of hepatic glucose production in humans. J Clin Invest 1988; 82:445–449.
27. Hers HG. The control of glycogen metabolism in the liver. Annu Rev Biochem 1976; 45:167–189.
28. Shulman GI, Liljenquist JE, Williams PE, et al. Glucose disposal during insulinopenia in somatostatin treated dogs. The roles of glucose and glucagon. J Clin Invest 1978; 62:487–491.
29. Sacca L, Cryer PE, Sherwin RS. Blood glucose regulates the effects of insulin and counterregulatory hormones on glucose production in vivo. Diabetes 1979; 28:533–536.

30. Sacca L, Hendler R, Sherwin RS. Hyperglycemia inhibits glucose production in man independent of changes in glucoregulatory hormones. J Clin Endocrinol Metab 1979; 47:1160–1963.

31. Liljenquist JE, Mueller GL, Cherrington AD, et al. Hyperglycemia per se (insulin and glucagon withdrawn) can inhibit hepatic glucose production in man. J Clin Endocrinol Metab 1979; 48:171–174.

32. Sacca L, Sherwin R, Hendler R, et al. Influence of continuous physiologic hyperinsulinemia on glucose kinetics and counterregulatory hormones in normal and diabetic humans. J Clin Invest 1979; 63:849–857.

33. Palmer JP, Henry DP, Benson JW, et al. Glucagon response to hypoglycemia in sympathectomized man. J Clin Invest 1976; 57:522–525.

34. Palmer JP, Werner PL, Hollander P, et al. Evaluation of the control of glucagon secretion by the parasympathetic nervous system in man. Metabolism 1979; 28:549–552.

35. Werner PL, Benson JW, Brodsky JB, et al. Comparison of glucagon response to 2-deoxy-D-glucose and hypoglycemia in man. Am J Physiol 1980; 239:E227–E231.

36. Mathias CJ, Christensen NJ, Corbett JL, et al. Plasma catecholamines during paroxysmal neurogenic hypertension in quadriplegic man. Circ Res 1976; 39:204–208.

37. Brodows RG, Pi-Sunyer FX, Campbell RG. Neural control of counterregulatory events during glucopenia in man. J Clin Invest 1973; 52:1841–1844.

38. Gerich JE, Davis J. Lorenzi M, et al. Hormonal mechanisms of recovery from insulin induced hypoglycemia in man. Am J Physiol 1979; 236:E380–E385.

39. Shah SD, Tse TF, Clutter WE, et al. The human sympathochromaffin system. Am J Physiol 1984; 247:E380–E384.

40. Clarke WL, Santiago JV, Thomas L, et al. Adrenergic mechanisms in recovery from hypoglycemia in man: adrenergic blockade. Am J Physiol 1979; 236:E147–E152.

41. Rizza RA, Cryer PE, Gerich JE. Role of glucagon, epinephrine and growth hormone in human glucose counterregulation: effects of somatostatin and adrenergic blockade on plasma glucose recovery and glucose flux rates following insulin induced hypoglycemia. J Clin Invest 1979; 64:62–71.

42. Popp DA, Shah SD, Cryer PE. The role of epinephrine mediated β-adrenergic mechanisms in hypoglycemic glucose counterregulation and posthypoglycemic hyperglycemia in insulin-dependent diabetes mellitus. J Clin Invest 1982; 69:315–326.

43. White NH, Skor D, Cryer PE, et al. Identification of type 1 diabetic patients at increased risk for hypoglycemia during intensive therapy. N Engl J Med 1983; 308:485–491.

44. Gray RS, Scarlett JA, Griffin J, et al. In vivo deactivation of peripheral, hepatic and pancreatic insulin action in man. Diabetes 1982; 31:929–936.

45. Tse TF, Clutter WE, Shah SD, et al. The mechanisms of postprandial glucose counterregulation in man: physiologic roles of glucagon and epinephrine vis-à-vis insulin in the prevention of hypoglycemia late after glucose ingestion. J Clin Invest 1983; 72:278–286.

46. Rosen SG, Clutter WE, Berk MA, et al. Epinephrine supports the postabsorptive plasma glucose concentration, and prevents hypoglycemia, when glucagon secretion is deficient in man. J Clin Invest 1984; 73:405–411.

47. Boyle PJ, Shah SD, Cryer PE. Insulin, glucagon and catecholamines in the prevention of hypoglycemia during fasting in humans. Am J Physiol 1989; 256:E651–E661.

48. Hirsch I, Marker J, Smith L, et al. Glucoregulation during exercise: a reassessment. Diabetes 1989; 38:21A (abstract).

49. Voorhees ML, Jakubowski AF, MacGillivray MH. The adrenomedullary and glucagon responses of hypopituitary children to insulin induced hypoglycemia. Pediatr Res 1981; 15:912–915.

50. Gerich JE, Langlois M, Noacco C, et al. Lack of glucagon response to hypoglycemia in diabetes: evidence for an intrinsic pancreatic alpha cell defect. Science 1973; 182:171–173.

51. Santiago JV, Clarke WL, Shah SD, et al. Epinephrine, norepinephrine, glucagon and growth hormone release in association with physiologic decrements in the plasma glucose concentration in normal and diabetic man. J Clin Endocrinol Metab 1980; 51:877–883.

52. DeFeo P, Periello G, Torlone E, et al. Demonstration of a role for growth hormone in glucose counterregulation. Am J Physiol 1989; 256:E835–E843.

53. DeFeo P, Periello G, Torlone E, et al. Contribution of cortisol to glucose counterregulation. Am J Physiol 1989; 257:E35–E42.

54. Bolli G, DeFeo P, Periello G, et al. Role of hepatic autoregulation in defense against hypoglycemia in humans. J Clin Invest 1985; 75:1623–1631.

55. Hansen I, Firth R, Haymond M, et al. The role of autoregulation of hepatic glucose production in man. Diabetes 1986; 35:186–191.

56. Schwartz NS, Clutter WE, Shah SD, et al. The glycemic thresholds for activation of glucose counterregulatory systems are higher than the threshold for symptoms. J Clin Invest 1987; 79:777–781.

57. Tse TF, Clutter WE, Shah SD, et al. Neuroendocrine responses to glucose ingestion in man: specificity, temporal relationships and quantitative aspects. J Clin Invest 1983; 72:270–277.

58. Clutter WE, Bier DM, Shah SD, et al. Epinephrine plasma metabolic

59. Lins PE, Efendic S. Hyperglycemia induced by somatostatin. Horm Metab Res 1976; 8:497–498.

60. Marks V, Marrack D, Rose FC. Hyperinsulinism in the pathogenesis of neuroglycopenic syndromes. Proc R Soc Med 1961; 54:747–749.

61. Robertshaw D. Hyperhidrosis and the sympatho-adrenal system. Med Hypotheses 1979; 5:317–322.

62. Mitrakou A, Ryan C, Veneman T, et al. Hierarchy of glycemic thresholds for activation of counterregulatory hormone secretion, initiation of symptoms, and onset of cerebral dysfunction in normal humans. Am J Physiol 260:E67–E74, 1991.

63. Amiel SA, Simonson DC, Tamborlane WV, et al. Rate of glucose fall does not affect counterregulatory hormone responses to hypoglycemia in normal and diabetic humans. Diabetes 1987; 36:518–522.

64. Lund-Andersen H. Transport of glucose from blood to brain. Physiol Rev 1979; 59:305–352.

65. Boyle PJ, Schwartz NS, Shah SD, et al. Plasma glucose concentrations at the onset of hypoglycemic symptoms in patients with poorly controlled diabetes and nondiabetics. N Engl J Med 1988; 318:1487–1492.

66. Amiel SA, Tamborlane WV, Simonson DC, et al. Defective glucose counterregulation after strict glycemic control of insulin-dependent diabetes mellitus. N Engl J Med 1987; 316:1376–1383.

67. Cryer PE. Does central nervous system adaptation to antecedent glycemia occur in patients with insulin dependent diabetes mellitus? Ann Intern Med 1985; 103:284–286.

68. Gjedde A, Crone A. Blood-brain glucose transfer: repression in chronic hyperglycemia. Science 1981; 214:456–457.

69. McCall AL, Millington WR, Wurtman RJ. Metabolic fuel and amino acid transport into the brain in experimental diabetes mellitus. Proc Natl Acad Sci USA 1982; 79:5406–5410.

70. McCall AL, Fixman LB, Fleming N, et al. Chronic hypoglycemia increases brain glucose transport. Am J Physiol 1986; 251:E442–F447.

71. Whipple AO. The surgical therapy of hyperinsulism. J Int Chir 1938; 3:237–276.

72. Malouf R, Brust JCM. Hypoglycemia: causes, neurological manifestations, and outcome. Ann Neurol 1985; 17:421–430.

73. Fischer KF, Lees JA, Newman JH. Hypoglycemia in hospitalized patients. Causes and outcomes. N Engl J Med 1986; 315:1245–1250.

74. The DCCT Research Group. Diabetes control and complications trial (DCCT): results of feasibility study. Diabetes Care 1987; 10:1–19.

75. Fukuda M, Tanaka A, Tahara Y, et al. Correlation between minimal secretory capacity of pancreatic β-cells and stability of diabetic control. Diabetes 1988; 37:81–88.

76. Cryer PE. Decreased sympathochromaffin activity in IDDM. Diabetes 1989; 38:405–409.

77. Ryder REJ, Vora JP, Atica JA, et al. Hypoglycemic unawareness and inadequate hypoglycaemic counterregulation are not due to autonomic neuropathy. Diabetologia 1987; 30:576A (abstract).

78. Bolli GB, DeFeo P, DeCosmo S, et al. A reliable and reproducible test for adequate glucose counterregulation in type I diabetes mellitus. Diabetes 1984; 33:732–737.

79. Frier BM, Hepburn DA, Eadington DW, et al. How common is hypoglycaemic unawareness in insulin-dependent diabetes and what is its relationship to autonomic neuropathy? Diabetes Res Clin Pract 1988; 5:5622 (abstract).

80. Hoeldtke RD, Boden G, Shuman CR, et al. Reduced epinephrine secretion and hypoglycemia unawareness in diabetic autonomic neuropathy. Ann Intern Med 1981; 96:459–462.

81. Heller SR, Herbert M, Macdonald IA, et al. Influence of sympathetic nervous system on hypoglycaemic warning symptoms. Lancet 1987; 2:359–363.

82. Lorenz R, Siebert C, Cleary P, et al. Epidemiology of severe hypoglycemia in the DCCT. Diabetes 1988; 37:3A (abstract).

83. Campbell PJ, Bolli GB, Cryer PE, et al. Pathogenesis of the dawn phenomenon in patients with insulin-dependent diabetes mellitus. N Engl J Med 1985; 312:1473–1479.

84. Periello G, DeFeo P, Bolli GB. The dawn phenomenon: nocturnal blood glucose homeostasis in insulin-dependent diabetes mellitus. Diabetic Med 1988; 5:13–21.

85. Tordjman KM, Havlin CE, Levandoski LA, et al. Failure of nocturnal hypoglycemia to cause fasting hyperglycemia in patients with insulin-dependent diabetes mellitus. N Engl J Med 1987; 317:1552–1559.

86. Hirsch IB, Smith LJ, Havlin CE, et al. Failure of nocturnal hypoglycemia to cause daytime hyperglycemia in patients with insulin dependent diabetes mellitus. Diabetes Care 1990; 13:133–142.

87. Periello G, DeFeo P, Torlone E, et al. The effect of asymptomatic nocturnal hypoglycemia on glycemic control in diabetes mellitus. N Engl J Med 1988; 319:1233–1239.

88. Gerich JE. Oral hypoglycemia agents. N Engl J Med 1989; 321:1231–1245.

89. Ferner RE, Neil HAW: Sulphonylureas and hypoglycaemia. Br Med J 1988; 296:949–950.

90. Jennings AM, Wilson RM, Ward JD. Symptomatic hypoglycemia in NIDDM patients treated with oral hypoglycemic agents. Diabetes Care 1989; 12:203–208.

91. Kriesberg RA, Owen W, Siegal AM. Ethanol-induced hyperlacticacidemia: inhibition of lactate utilization. J Clin Invest 1971; 50:166–174.

92. Lecavalier L, Bolli G, Cryer P, et al. Contributions of gluconeogenesis and glycogenolysis during glucose counterregulation in normal humans. Am J Physiol 1989; 256:E844–E851.

93. Marks V. Alcohol and carbohydrate metabolism. Clin Endocrinol Metab 1978; 7:33–41.

94. Wilson N, Brown P, Juil S, et al. Glucose turnover and metabolic and hormonal changes in ethanol induced hypoglycemia. Br Med J 1982; 282:849–853.

95. Kolaczynski JW, Ylikahri R, Härkonen M, et al. The acute effect of ethanol on counterregulatory response and recovery from insulin induced hypoglycemia. J Clin Endocrinol Metab 1988; 67:384–388.

96. Yki-Järvinen H, Koivisto VA, Ylikahri R, et al. Acute effects of ethanol and acetate on glucose kinetics in normal subjects. Am J Physiol 1988; 254:E175–E180.

97. Shelmet JJ, Reichard GA, Skutches CL, et al. Ethanol causes acute inhibition of carbohydrate, fat and protein oxidation and insulin resistance. J Clin Invest 1988; 81:1137–1145.

98. Shah JH. Alcohol decreases insulin sensitivity in healthy subjects. Alcohol Alcohol 1988; 23:103–109.

99. Fang V, Foyle WO, Robinson SM, et al. Hypoglycemic activity and chemical structure of salicylates. J Pharm Sci 1968; 57:2111–2116.

100. Arena FP, Dugowson C, Saudek CD: Salicylate-induced hypoglycemia and ketoacidosis in a nondiabetic adult. Arch Intern Med 1978; 138:1153–1156.

101. Poretsky L, Moses AC. Hypoglycemia associated with trimethoprim/sulfamethoxazole therapy. Diabetes Care 1984; 7:508–509.

102. Stahl-Bayliss CM, Kalman CM, Laskin OL. Pentamidine-induced hypoglycemia in patients with the acquired immunodeficiency syndrome. Clin Pharmacol Ther 1986; 39:271–275.

103. Waskin H, Stehr-Green JK, Helmick CG, et al. Risk factors for hypoglycemia associated with pentamidine therapy for pneumocystis pneumonia. JAMA 1988; 260:345–347.

104. White NJ, Warrell DA, Chanthavanich P, et al. Severe hypoglycemia and hyperinsulinemia in falciparum malaria. N Engl J Med 1983; 309:61–66.

105. White NJ, Miller KD, Marsh K, et al. Hypoglycaemia in African children with severe malaria. Lancet 1987; 1:708–711.

106. Taylor TE, Molyneux ME, Wirima JJ, et al. Blood glucose levels in Malawian children before and during the administration of intravenous quinine for severe falciparum malaria. N Engl J Med 1988; 319:1040–1047.

107. Hesse B, Pedersen JT. Hypoglycemia after propranolol in children. Acta Med Scand 1973; 193:551–552.

108. McBride JT, McBride MC, Vites PH. Hypoglycemia associated with propranolol. Pediatrics 1973; 51:1085–1087.

109. Mann FC, Magath TB. Studies on the physiology of the liver. II. The effect of the removal of the liver on the blood sugar level. Arch Intern Med 1922; 30:73–84.

110. Zimmerman HJ, Thomas LJ, Scherrr EH. Fasting blood sugar in hepatic disease with reference to infrequency of hypoglycemia. Arch Intern Med 1953; 91:577–584.

111. Samson RL, Trey C, Timme AH, et al. Fulminant hepatitis with recurrent hypoglycemia and hemorrhage. Gastroenterology 1967; 53:291–300.

112. Felig P, Brown WV, Levine RA, et al. Glucose homeostasis in viral hepatitis. N Engl J Med 1970; 283:1436–1440.

113. Younus S, Soterakis J, Sossi AJ, et al. Hypoglycemia secondary to metastases to the liver. Gastroenterology 1977; 72:334–337.

114. Johnston DG, Alberti KGMM. Hyperinsulinism of hepatic cirrhosis: diminished degradation or hypersecretion. Lancet 1977; 1:10–13.

115. Vilstrup H, Iversen J, Tygstrup N. Glucoregulation in acute liver failure. Eur J Clin Invest 1986; 16:193–197.

116. Medalle R, Webb R, Waterhouse C. Lactic acidosis and hypoglycemia. Arch Intern Med 1971; 128:273–278.

117. Block MB, Rubenstein AH. Spontaneous hypoglycemia in diabetic patients with renal insufficiency. JAMA 1970; 213:1863–1866.

118. Frizell M, Larsen PR, Field JB. Spontaneous hypoglycemia associated with chronic renal failure. Diabetes 1973; 22:493–498.

119. Garber AJ, Bier DM, Cryer PE, et al. Hypoglycemia in compensated chronic renal insufficiency. Diabetes 1974; 23:982–986.

120. Peitzman SJ, Agarwal BN. Spontaneous hypoglycemia in end-stage renal disease. Nephron 1977; 19:131–139.

121. Rutsky EA, McDaniel HG, Tarpe DL, et al. Spontaneous hypoglycemia in chronic renal failure. Arch Intern Med 1978; 138:1364–1368.

122. Schmitz O. Peripheral and hepatic resistance to insulin and hepatic resistance to glucagon in uraemic patients. Acta Endocrinol 1988; 118:125–134.

123. Baylor P, Shilo S, Zonszein J, et al. β-Adrenergic contribution to glucagon-induced glucose production and insulin secretion in uremia. Am J Physiol 1986; 251:E322–E327.

124. Greenblatt DJ. Fatal hypoglycaemia occurring after peritoneal dialysis. Br Med J 1972; 2:270–271.

125. Miller SI, Wallace RJ Jr, Musher DM, et al. Hypoglycemia as a manifestation of sepsis. Am J Med 1980; 68:649–653.

126. Hargrove DM, Bagby GJ, Lang CH, et al. Adrenergic blockade does not abolish elevated glucose turnover during bacterial infection. Am J Physiol 1988; 254:E16–E22.

127. Hargrove DM, Bagby GJ, Lang CH, et al. Adrenergic blockade prevents endotoxin-induced increases in glucose metabolism. Am J Physiol 1988; 255:E629–E635.

128. Naylor JM, Kronfeld DS. In vivo studies of hypoglycemia and lactic acidosis in endotoxic shock. Am J Physiol 1985; 248:E309–E316.

129. Meszaros K, Bagby GJ, Lang CH, et al. Increased uptake and phosphorylation of 2-deoxyglucose by skeletal muscles in endotoxin-treated rats. Am J Physiol 1987; 253:E33–E39.

130. Meszaros K, Lang CH, Bagby GJ, et al. In vivo glucose utilization by individual tissues during nonlethal hypermetabolic sepsis. FASEB J 1988; 2:3083–3086.

131. del Ray A, Besedovsky H. Interleukin 1 affects glucose homeostasis. Am J Physiol 1987; 253:R794–R798.

132. Commens PJ, Wolf BA, Enanue ER, et al. Interleukin 1 is a potent modulator of insulin secretion from isolated rat islets of Langerhans. Diabetes 1987; 36:963–970.

133. Lee MD, Zentella A, Pekala PH, et al. Effect of endotoxin-induced monokines on glucose metabolism in the muscle cell line L6. Proc Natl Acad Sci USA 1987; 84:2590–2594.

134. Gounelle H, Marche J. Spontaneous coma due to hypoglycemia in undernourished persons. Occup Med 1946; 1:48–59.

135. Wharton B. Hypoglycaemia in children with kwashiorkor. Lancet 1970; 1:171–173.

136. Elias AN, Gwinup G. Glucose-resistant hypoglycemia in inanition. Arch Intern Med 1982; 142:743–746.

137. Maleribi D, Liberman B, Giurno-Filho A, et al. Glucocorticoids and glucose metabolism: hepatic glucose production in untreated Addisonian patients and on two different levels of glucocorticoid administration. Clin Endocrinol 1988; 28:415–422.

138. Artavia-Loria E, Chaussain JL, Bougnères PF, et al. Frequency of hypoglycemia in children with adrenal insufficiency. Acta Endocrinol [Suppl] 1986; 279:275–278.

139. Brasel JA, Wright JC, Wilkins L, et al. Evaluation of seventy-five patients with hypopituitarism beginning in childhood. Am J Med 1965; 38:484–498.

140. Goodman HG, Grumbach MM, Kaplan SL. Growth and growth hormone. II. A comparison of isolated growth hormone deficiency and multiple pituitary hormone deficiencies in 35 patients with idiopathic hypopituitary dwarfism. N Engl J Med 1968; 278:57–68.

141. Haymond MW, Karl I, Weldon VV, et al. The role of growth hormone and cortisone in glucose and gluconeogenic substrate regulation in fasted hypopituitary children. J Clin Endocrinol Metab 1976; 42:846–856.

142. Wolfsdorf JI, Sadeghi-Nejad A, Senior B. Hypoketonemia and age-related fasting hypoglycemia in growth hormone deficiency. Metabolism 1983; 32:457–462.

143. Ashmore J, Morgan D. Metabolic effects of adrenal glucocorticoid hormones. In: Eisenstein AB, ed. The Adrenal Cortex. Boston: Little, Brown, 1967: 249–267.

144. Rizza RA, Mandarino L, Gerich JE. Cortisol induced insulin resistance in man: impaired suppression of glucose production and stimulation of glucose utilization due to a postreceptor defect of insulin action. J Clin Endocrinol Metab 1981; 54:131–138.

145. Aynsley-Green A, Moncrieff MW, Ratter S, et al. Isolated ACTH deficiency. Arch Dis Child 1978; 53:499–502.

146. Rudman D, Moffitt SD, Fernhoff PM, et al. Epinephrine deficiency in hypocorticotropic hypopituitary children. J Clin Endocrinol Metab 1981; 53:722–729.

147. Smallridge RC, Corrigan DF, Thomason AM, et al. Hypoglycemia in pregnancy. Occurrence due to adrenocorticotropic hormone and growth hormone deficiency. Arch Intern Med 1980; 140:564–565.

148. Steer P, Marnell R, Werk EE Jr. Clinical alcohol hypoglycemia and isolated adrenocorticotropic hormone deficiency. Ann Intern Med 1969; 71:343–348.

149. Broberger O, Jungner I, Zetterstrom R. Studies in spontaneous hypoglycemia in childhood. Failure to increase epinephrine secretion in insulin-induced hypoglycemia. J Pediatr 1959; 55:713–719.

150. Tietze HU, Zurbrug RP, Zuppinger KA, et al. Occurrence of impaired cortisol regulation in children with hypoglycemia associated with adrenal medullary hyporesponsiveness. J Clin Endocrinol Metab 1972; 34:948–958.

151. Christensen NJ. Hypoadrenalinemia during insulin hypoglycemia in children with ketotic hypoglycemia. J Clin Endocrinol Metab 1974; 38:107–112.

152. Rosenbloom AL, Tiwary CM. Ketotic (idiopathic glucagon unresponsive) hypoglycemia. Catecholamine excretion and effects of ephedrine therapy. Arch Dis Child 1972; 47:924–926.

153. Court JM, Dunlop ME, Boulton TJC. Effect of ephedrine in ketotic hypoglycemia. Arch Dis Child 1974; 49:63–65.

154. Sizonenko PC, Paunier L, Vallotton MB, et al. Response to 2-deoxyglucose and to glucagon in "ketotic hypoglycemia" of childhood: evidence for epinephrine deficiency and altered alanine availability. Pediatr Res 1973; 7:983–993.

155. Kerr DS, Brooke OG, Robinson HM. Fasting energy utilization in the smaller of twins with epinephrine-deficient hypoglycemia. Metabolism 1981; 30:6–17.

156. Kerr DS, Picou DIM. Fasting glucose production in the smaller of twins with epinephrine-deficient hypoglycemia. Metabolism 1981; 30:18–26.

157. Light IJ, Sutherland JM, Loggie JM, et al. Impaired epinephrine release in hypoglycemic infants of diabetic mothers. N Engl J Med 1967; 277:394–398.

158. Bleicher SJ, Levy LJ, Zarowitz H, et al. Glucagon deficiency hypoglycemia: a new syndrome? Clin Res 1970; 19:355 (abstract).

159. Starke AAR, Valverde I, Botazzo GF, et al. Glucagon deficiency associated with hypoglycemia and the absence of islet cell antibodies in the polyglandular failure syndrome before the onset of insulin-dependent diabetes mellitus: a case report. Diabetologia 1983; 25:336–339.

160. Vidnes J, Oyasaeter S. Glucagon deficiency causing severe neonatal hypoglycemia in a patient with normal insulin secretion. Pediatr Res 1977; 11:943–949.

161. Kollee LA, Monnens LA, Cejka V, et al. Persistent neonatal hypoglycemia due to glucagon deficiency. Arch Dis Child 1978; 53:422–424.

162. McDaniel HG, Pittman CS, Oh SJ, et al. Carbohydrate metabolism in hypothyroid myopathy. Metabolism 1977; 26:867–873.

163. McFadzean AJS, Yeung RTT. Further observations of hypoglycaemia in hepato-cellular carcinoma. Am J Med 1969; 47:220–235.

164. Arem R, Jeang MK, Blevens TC, et al. Polycythemia rubra vera and artifactual hypoglycemia. Arch Intern Med 1982; 142:2199–2201.

165. Kreisberg RA, Hershman JM, Spenney JC, et al. Biochemistry of extrapancreatic tumor hypoglycemia. Diabetes 1970; 19:248–258.

166. Chandalia HB, Boshell BR. Hypoglycemia associated with extrapancreatic tumors. Arch Intern Med 1972; 129:447–456.

167. Crawford WH. Hypoglycemia with coma in a case of primary carcinoma of the liver. Am J Med Sci 1931; 181:496–502.

168. Silbert C, Rossini AA, Ghazvinian S, et al. Tumor hypoglycemia: deficient splanchnic glucose output and deficient glucagon secretion. Diabetes 1976; 25:202–206.

169. Oleesky S, Bailey I, Samols E, et al. A fibrosarcoma with hypoglycaemia and a high serum insulin level. Lancet 1962; 2:378–380.

170. Lyall SS, Marieb MJ, Wise JK, et al. Hyperinsulinemic hypoglycemia associated with a neurofibrosarcoma. Arch Intern Med 1975; 135:865–867.

171. Kiang DT, Bauer GE, Kennedy BJ. Immunoassayable insulin in carcinoma of the cervix associated with hypoglycemia. Cancer 1973; 31:801–805.

172. Shames JM, Dhurandhar NE, Blackard WG. Insulin-secreting bronchial carcinoid tumor with widespread metastases. Am J Med 1968; 44:632–636.

173. Appleyard TN, Losowsky MD. A pancreatic tumor with carcinoid syndrome and hypoglycemia. Postgrad Med J 1970; 46:159–171.

174. Marks V, Samols E. Hypoglycemia of nonendocrine origin. Proc R Soc Med 1966; 59:338–340.

175. Megyesi K, Kahn CR, Roth J, et al. Hypoglycemia in association with extrapancreatic tumors: demonstration of elevated plasma NSILA-s by a new radioreceptor assay. J Clin Endocrinol Metab 1974; 38:931–934.

176. Hyodo T, Megyesi K, Kahn CR, et al. Adrenocortical carcinoma and hypoglycemia: evidence for production of nonsuppressible insulin-like activity by the tumor. J Clin Endocrinol Metab 1977; 44:1175–1184.

177. Gorden P, Hendricks CM, Kahn CR, et al. Hypoglycemia associated with non-islet-cell tumor and insulin-like growth factors. N Engl J Med 1981; 305:1452–1455.

178. Daughaday WH, Trivedi B, Kapadia M. Measurement of insulin-like growth factor II by a specific radioreceptor assay in serum of normal individuals, patients with abnormal growth hormone secretion, and patients with tumor-associated hypoglycemia. J Clin Endocrinol Metab 1981; 53:289–294.

179. Zapf J, Walter H, Froesch ER. Radioimmunological determination of insulin-like growth factors I and II in normal subjects, in patients with growth disorders and extrapancreatic tumor hypoglycemia. J Clin Invest 1981; 68:1321–1330.

180. Widmer Zu, Zapf J, Froesch ER. Is extrapancreatic tumor hypoglycemia associated with elevated levels of insulin-like growth factor II? J Clin Endocrinol Metab 1982; 55:833–840.

181. Daughaday WH, Emanuelle MA, Brooks MH, et al. Synthesis and secretion of insulin-like growth factor II by a leiomyosarcoma with associated hypoglycemia. N Engl J Med 1988; 319:1434–1440.

182. Ron D, Powers AC, Pandian MR, et al. Increased insulin-like growth factor II production and consequent suppression of growth hormone secretion: a dual mechanism of tumor-induced hypoglycemia. J Clin Endocrinol Metab 1989; 68:701–706.

183. Lowe WL, Roberts CT, LeRoith D, et al. Insulin-like growth factor-II in nonislet cell tumors associated with hypoglycemia: increased levels of messenger ribonucleic acid. J Clin Endocrinol Metab 1989; 69:1153–1159.

184. Merimee TJ. Insulin-like growth factors in patients with nonislet cell tumors and hypoglycemia. Metabolism 1986; 35:360–363.

185. Wu J-C, Daughaday WH, Lee S-D, et al. Radioimmunoassay of serum IGF-I and IGF-II in patients with chronic liver disease and hepatocellular carcinoma with or without hypoglycemia. J Lab Clin Med 1988; 112:589–594.

186. Daughaday WH, Kapadia M. Significance of abnormal serum binding of insulin-like growth factor II in the development of hypoglycemia in patients with non–islet-cell tumors. Proc Natl Acad Sci USA 1989; 86:6778–6782.

187. Li TCM, Reed CE, Stubenbord WT JR, et al. Surgical cure of hypoglycemia associated with cystosarcoma phyllodes and elevated nonsuppressible insulin-like protein. Am J Med 1983; 74:1080–1084.

188. Cedermark BJ, Sjoberg HE. Clinical significance of metastases to the adrenal glands. Surg Gynecol Obstet 1981; 152:607–610.

189. Fajans SS, Floyd JC Jr. Diagnosis and medical management of insulinomas. Annu Rev Med 1979; 30:313–329.

190. Brennan MD, Service FJ, Carpenter A-M, et al. Diagnosis of pancreatic islet hyperplasia causing hypoglycemia in a patient with portocaval anastomosis. Am J Med 1980; 68:941–948.

191. Witte DP, Greider MH, DeSchryver-Kecskemeti K, et al. The juvenile human endocrine pancreas: normal v. idiopathic hyperinsulinemic hypoglycemia. Semin Diagn Pathol 1984; 1:30–42.

192. Rahier J. Relevance of endocrine pancreas nesidioblastosis to hyperinsulinemic hypoglycemia. Diabetes Care 1989; 12:164–166.

193. Kalvie H, White TT. Pancreatic islet β-cell tumors and hyperplasia. Ann Surg 1972; 175:326–335.

194. Philippe J, Powers AC, Mojsov S, et al. Expression of peptide hormone genes in human islet cell tumors. Diabetes 1988; 37:647–651.

195. D'Arcangues CM, Awoke S, Lawrence GD. Metastatic insulinoma with long survival and glucagonoma syndrome. Ann Intern Med 1984; 100:233–235.

196. Rizza RA, Haymond MW, Verdonk CA, et al. Pathogenesis of hypoglycemia in insulinoma patients. Suppression of hepatic glucose production by insulin. Diabetes 1981; 30:377–381.

197. McMahon MM, O'Brien PC, Service FJ. Diagnostic interpretation of the intravenous tolbutamide test for insulinoma. Mayo Clin Proc 1989; 64:1481–1488.

198. Fajans SS, Floyd JC Jr. Fasting hypoglycemia in adults. N Engl J Med 1976; 294:766–771.

199. Merimee TJ, Fineberg SF. Homeostasis during fasting II. Substrate differences between men and women. J Clin Endocrinol Metab 1973; 37:698–702.

200. Service FJ, Horwitz DL, Rubenstein AH, et al. C-peptide suppression test for insulinoma. J Lab Clin Med 1977; 90:180–186.

201. Rayfield EJ, Pulini M, Golub A, et al. Nonautonomous function of a pancreatic insulinoma. J Clin Endocrinol Metab 1976; 43:1307–1310.

202. Palumbo PJ, Molnar GD, Taylor WF, et al. Insulin antibody binding in diabetes mellitus and factitious hypoglycemia. Mayo Clin Proc 1969; 44:725–737.

203. Berkowitz S, Parish JE, Field JB. Factitious hypoglycemia: why not diagnose before laparotomy? Am J Med 1971; 51:669–674.

204. Service FJ, Palumbo PJ. Factitial hypoglycemia: three cases diagnosed on the basis of antibodies. Arch Intern Med 1974; 134:336–340.

205. Grunberger G, Weiner JL, Silverman R, et al. Factitious hypoglycemia due to surreptitious administration of insulin. Ann Intern Med 1988; 108:252–257.

206. Hirata Y, Ishizu H. Elevated insulin binding capacity of serum proteins in a case with spontaneous hypoglycemia and mild diabetes not treated with insulin. Tohoku J Exp Med 1972; 107:277–286.

207. Hirata Y, Tominaga M, Ito J-I, et al. Spontaneous hypoglycemia with insulin autoimmunity in Graves' disease. Ann Intern Med 1974; 81:214–218.

208. Ichihara K, Shima K, Saito Y, et al. Mechanism of hypoglycemia observed in a patient with autoimmune syndrome. Diabetes 1977; 26:500–506.

209. Anderson JH Jr, Blackard WG, Goldman J, et al. Diabetes and hypoglycemia due to insulin antibodies. Am J Med 1978; 64:868–872.

210. Goldman J, Baldwin D, Rubenstein AH, et al. Characterization of circulating insulin and proinsulin binding antibodies in autoimmune hypoglycemia. J Clin Invest 1979; 63:1050–1059.

211. Scarlett JA, Mako ME, Rubenstein AH, et al. Factitious hypoglycemia. diagnosis by measurement of serum C-peptide immunoreactivity and insulin binding antibodies. N Engl J Med 1977; 297:1029–1032.

212. Gutman RA, Lazarus NR, Penhos JC, et al. Circulating proinsulin-like material in patients with functioning insulinomas. N Engl J Med 1971; 284:1003–1008.

213. Cohen RM, Given BD, Licinio-Paixao J, et al. Proinsulin radioimmunoassay in the evaluation of insulinomas and familial hyperproinsulinemia. Metabolism 1986; 35:1137–1146.

214. Hampton SM, Beyzavi K, Teale D, et al. A direct assay for proinsulin in plasma and its application in hypoglycaemia. Clin Endocrinol 1988; 29:9–16.

215. Taylor SI, Barbetti F, Accili D, et al. Syndromes of autoimmunity and hypoglycemia. Endocrinol Metab Clin North Am 1989; 18:123–143.

216. Elias D, Cohen IR, Shecter Y, et al. Antibodies to insulin receptor followed by anti-idiotype. Diabetes 1987; 36:348–354.

217. Braund WJ, Naylor BA, Williamson DH, et al. Autoimmunity to insulin receptor and hypoglycaemia in patient with Hodgkin's disease. Lancet 1987; 1:237–240.

218. Walters EG, Tavaré JM, Denton RM, et al. Hypoglycaemia due to an insulin-receptor antibody in Hodgkin's disease. Lancet 1987; 1:241–243.

219. Selinger S, Tsai J, Pulini M, et al. Autoimmune thrombocytopenia and primary biliary cirrhosis with hypoglycemia and insulin receptor autoantibodies. Ann Intern Med 1987; 107:686–688.

220. Moller DE, Ratner RE, Borenstein DG, et al. Autoantibodies to the insulin receptor as a cause of autoimmune hypoglycemia in systemic lupus erythematosus. Am J Med 1988; 84:334–338.

221. Rochet N, Blanche S, Carel JC, et al. Hypoglycaemia induced by antibodies to insulin receptor following a bone marrow transplantation in an immunodeficient child. Diabetologia 1989; 32:167–172.

222. Kiyokawa H, Kono N, Hamaguchi T, et al. Hyperinsulinemia due to impaired insulin clearance associated with fasting hypoglycemia and postprandial hyperglycemia: an analysis of a patient with antiinsulin antibodies. J Clin Endocrinol Metab 1989; 69:616–621.

223. Wilkin TJ, Hammonds P, Mirza JH, et al. Graves' disease of the β-cell: glucose dysregulation due to islet-cell stimulating antibodies. Lancet 1988; 2:1155–1158.

224. Clark LR, Jaffe MH, Choyke PL, et al. Pancreatic imaging. Radiol Clin North Am 1985; 23:489–501.

225. Fraker DL, Norton JA. Localization and resection of insulinomas and gastrinomas. JAMA 1988; 259:3601–3605.

226. Kinoshita Y, Nonaka H, Suzuki S, et al. Accurate localization of insulinomas using percutaneous transhepatic portal venous sampling—usefulness of simultaneous measurement of plasma insulin and glucagon levels. Clin Endocrinol 1985; 23:587–593.

227. Stefanini P, Carboni M, Patrassi N, et al. Beta-islet tumors of the pancreas: results of a study on 1,067 cases. Surgery 1974; 75:597–609.

228. Marks V, Rose FC, Samols E. Hyperinsulinism due to metastasizing insulinoma: treatment with diazoxide. Proc R Soc Med 1965; 58:577–578.

229. Graber AL, Porte D Jr, Williams RH. Clinical use of diazoxide and mechanism for its hyperglycemic effects. Diabetes 1966; 15:143–148.

230. Fajans SS, Flogel JC Jr, Thiffault CA, et al. Further studies on diazoxide suppression of insulin release from abnormal and normal islet tissue in man. Ann NY Acad Sci 1968; 150:261–280.

231. Marks V, Samols E. Diazoxide therapy of intractable hypoglycemia. Ann NY Acad Sci 1968; 150:442–454.

232. Osei K, O'Dorisio TM. Malignant insulinoma: effects of a somatostatin analog (compound 201–995) on serum glucose, growth and gastroentero-pancreatic hormones. Ann Intern Med 1985; 103:223–225.

233. Kvols LK, Buck M, Moertel CG, et al. Treatment of metastatic islet cell carcinoma with a somatostatin analogue (SMS 201–995). Ann Intern Med 1987; 107:162–168.

234. Alberts AS, Falkson G. Rapid reversal of life-threatening hypoglycaemia with a somatostatin analogue (octreotide). S Afr Med J 1988; 74:75–76.

235. Hearn PR, Ahmed M, Woodhouse NJY. The use of SMS 201–995 (somatostatin analogue) in insulinomas. Horm Res 1988; 29:211–213.

236. Boden G, Ryan IG, Shuman CR. Ineffectiveness of SMS 201–995 in severe hyperinsulinemia. Diabetes Care 1988; 11:664–668.

237. Broder LE, Carter SK. Pancreatic islet cell carcinoma. II. Results of therapy with streptozotocin in 52 patients. Ann Intern Med 1973; 79:108–118.

238. Moertel CG, Hanley JA, Johnson LA. Streptozotocin alone compared with streptozotocin plus fluorouracil in the treatment of advanced islet cell carcinoma. N Engl J Med 1980; 303:1189–1195.

239. Ajani JA, Carrasco H, Charnsangavej C, et al. Islet cell tumors metastatic to the liver: effective palliation by sequential hepatic artery embolization. Ann Intern Med 1988; 108:340–344.

240. Cowett RM. Pathophysiology, diagnosis and management of glucose homeostasis in the neonate. In: Lockhart JD, ed. Current Problems in Pediatrics. Vol. 15. Chicago: Year Book Medical, 1985: 1–47.

241. Sperling MA, Garguli S, Leslie N, et al. Fetal-perinatal catecholamine secretion: role in perinatal glucose homeostasis. Am J Physiol 1984; 247:E69–E74.

242. Bier DM, Leake RD, Haymond MW, et al. Measurement of "true" glucose production rates with 6,6-dideutero-glucose. Diabetes 1977; 26:1016–1023.

243. Haymond MW, Karl IE, Clarke WL, et al. Differences in circulating gluconeogenic substrates during short term fasting in men, women and children. Metabolism 1982; 31:33–42.

244. Jones MD Jr, Battaglia FC. Intrauterine growth retardation. Am J Obstet Gynecol 1977; 127:540–549.

245. Haymond MW, Karl IE, Pagliara AS. Increased gluconeogenic substrates in small for gestational age infants. N Engl J Med 1974; 291:322–328.

246. Binkiewicz A, Senior B. Decreased ketogenesis in von Gierke's disease (type I glycogenosis). J Pediatr 1973; 83:973–978.

247. Greene HL, Slonim AE, Burr IM, et al. Type 1 glycogen storage disease. Five years of management with nocturnal intragastric feeding. J Pediatr 1989; 96:590–595.

248. Malatack JJ, Iwatsuki S, Gartner JC, et al. Liver transplantation for type I glycogen storage disease. Lancet 1983; 1:1073–1075.

249. Lange AJ, Arion WJ, Beaudet AL. Type 1b glycogen storage disease is caused by a defect in the glucose-6-phosphate translocase of the microsomal glucose-6-phosphatase system. J Biol Chem 1980; 255:8381–8384.

250. Pagliara AS, Karl IE, Keating JP, et al. Hepatic fructose-1,6-diphosphatase deficiency: a cause of lactic acidosis and hypoglycemia in infancy. J Clin Invest 1972; 51:2115–2123.

251. Segal S. Disorders of galactose metabolism. In: Stanbury JB, Wyngaarden JB, Fredrickson DS, eds. The Metabolic Basis of Inherited Disease. 4th ed. New York: McGraw-Hill, 1978: 160–181.

252. Kaufman U, Froesch ER. Inhibition of phosphorylase-a by fructose-1-phosphate, alpha-glycerophosphate and fructose-1,6-diphosphate: explanation for fructose-induced hypoglycemia in hereditary fructose intolerance and fructose-1,6-diphosphatase deficiency. Eur J Clin Invest 1973; 3:407–413.

253. Haymond MW, Karl IE, Feigin RD, et al. Hypoglycemia and maple syrup urine disease: defective gluconeogenesis. Pediatr Res 1973; 7:500–508.

254. Haymond MW, Ben-Galim E, Strobel KE. Glucose and alanine metabolism in children with maple syrup urine disease. J Clin Invest 1978; 62:398–405.

255. Cheema-Dhadli S, Lernoff CC, Halperin ML. Effect of 2-methylcitrate on citrate metabolism: implications for the management of patients with propionic acidemia and methylmalonic aciduria. Pediatr Res 1975; 9:905–908.

256. Glasgow AM, Engel AG, Bier DM, et al. Hypoglycemia, hepatic dysfunction, muscle weakness, cardiomyopathy, free carnitine deficiency, and long chain acylcarnitine excess responsive to medium chain triglyceride diet. Pediatr Res 1983; 17:319–326.

257. Robouche CJ, Engel AG. Carnitine metabolism and deficiency. Mayo Clin Proc 1983; 58:533–540.

258. Angelini C, Trevisan C, Isaya G, et al. Clinical varieties of carnitine and carnitine palmitoyltransferase deficiency. Clin Biochem 1987; 20:1–7.

259. Nyhan WL. Abnormalities of fatty acid oxidation. N Engl J Med 1988; 319:1344–1346.

260. Slonim AE, Borum PR, Mark RE, et al. Nonketotic hypoglycemia: an early indicator of systemic carnitine deficiency. Neurology 1983; 33:29–33.

261. Senior B. Ketotic hypoglycemia. J Pediatr 1973; 82:555–556.

262. Pagliara AS, Karl IE, DeVivo DC, et al. Hypoalaninemia: a concomitant of ketotic hypoglycemia. J Clin Invest 1972; 51:1440–1449.

263. Haymond MW, Karl IE, Pagliara AS. Ketotic hypoglycemia: an amino acid substrate limited disorder. J Clin Endocrinol Metab 1974; 38:521–530.

264. Miles JM, Nissen S, Gerich J, et al. Effects of epinephrine infusion on leucine and alanine kinetics in humans. Am J Physiol 1984; 247:E166–E172.

265. Leichter SB, Permutt MA. Effect of adrenergic agents on postgastrectomy hypoglycemia. Diabetes 1975; 24:1005–1010.

266. Shultz KT, Neelon FA, Nilsen LB, et al. Mechanism of postgastrectomy hypoglycemia. Arch Intern Med 1971; 128:240–246.

267. Permutt MA, Kelly J, Bernstein R, et al. Alimentary hypoglycemia in the absence of gastrointestinal surgery. N Engl J Med 1973; 288:1206–1210.

268. Charles MA, Hofeldt F, Shackelford A, et al. Comparison of oral glucose tolerance tests and mixed meals in patients with apparent idiopathic postabsorptive hypoglycemia. Diabetes 1981; 30:465–470.

269. Lev-Ran A, Anderson RW. The diagnosis of postprandial hypoglycemia. Diabetes 1981; 30:996–999.

270. Betteridge DJ. Reactive hypoglycemia. Br Med J 1987; 295:286–287.

271. Palardy J, Havrankova J, Lepage R, et al. Blood glucose measurements during symptomatic episodes in patients with suspected postprandial hypoglycemia. N Engl J Med 1989; 321:1421–1425.

272. Service FJ. Hypoglycemia and the postprandial syndrome. N Engl J Med 1989; 321:1472–1473.

273. Foster DW, Rubenstein AH. Hypoglycemia, insulinoma, and other hormone-secreting tumors of the pancreas. In: Petersdorf RG, Adams RD, Braunwald E, et al., eds. Harrison's Principles of Internal Medicine. 10th ed. New York: McGraw-Hill, 1983: 682–689.

274. Goldman J. Pathogenesis of functional or idiopathic reactive hypoglycemia: hyperresponsiveness to insulin and increased receptor effector coupling. In: Andreani D, DePirro R, Lauro R, et al., eds. Current Views on Insulin Receptors. New York: Academic, 1981: 499–505.

275. Tamburrano G, Leonetti F, Sbraccia P, et al. Increased insulin sensitivity in patients with idiopathic reactive hypoglycemia. J Clin Endocrinol Metab 1989; 69:885–890.

276. Foa PP, Dunbar JC, Klein SP, et al. Reactive hypoglycemia and A-cell ("pancreatic") glucagon deficiency in the adult. JAMA 1980; 244:2281–2285.

277. Shima K, Tabata M, Tanaka A, et al. Exaggerated response of plasma glucagon-like immunoreactivity to oral glucose in patients with reactive hypoglycemia. Endocrinol Jpn 1981; 28:249–256.

278. Chalew SA, McLaughlin JV, Mersey J, et al. The use of the plasma epinephrine response in the diagnosis of idiopathic postprandial syndrome. JAMA 1984; 251:612–615.

279. Permutt MA, Keller D, Santiago JV. Cholinergic blockade in reactive hypoglycemia. Diabetes 1977; 26:121–127.

280. Jenkins DJA, Bloom SR, Albuquerque RH, et al. Pectin and complications after gastric surgery: normalization of postprandial glucose and endocrine responses. Gut 1980; 21:574–579.

281. Fink WJ, Hucke ST, Gray TW, et al. Treatment of postoperative reactive hypoglycemia by a reversed intestinal segment. Am J Surg 1976; 131:19–22.

282. Brodows RG, Amatruda JM. A modification of the glucose clamp technique for studying treatment of hypoglycemic reactions. Diabetes 1983; 32(Suppl 1):64A (abstract).

283. Havlin CE, Cryer PE. Hypoglycemia: the limiting factor in the management of insulin dependent diabetes mellitus. Diabetes Educator 1988; 14:407–411.

284. Collier A, Steedman DI, Patrick AW, et al. Comparison of intravenous glucagon and dextrose in treatment of severe hypoglycemia in an accident and emergency department. Diabetes Care 1987; 10:712–715.

285. Kay WW. The treatment of prolonged insulin coma. J Ment Sci 1961; 107:194–238.

286. MacCuish AC, Munro JF, Duncan LJP. Treatment of hypoglycaemic coma with glucagon, intravenous dextrose, and mannitol infusion in a hundred diabetics. Lancet 1970; 2:946–949.

287. Hoffbrand BI, Sevitt LH. Use of mannitol in prolonged coma due to insulin overdosage. Lancet 1966; 1:402.

288. Johnson SF, Schade DS, Peake GT. Chlorpropamide-induced hypoglycemia. Successful treatment with diazoxide. Am J Med 1977; 63:799–804.

289. Pfieffer MA, Wolter CF, Samols E. Management of chlorpropamide-induced hypoglycemia with diazoxide. South Med J 1978; 71:606–608.

290. Jacobs RF, Nix RA, Paulus TE, et al. Intravenous infusion of diazoxide in the treatment of chlorpropamide-induced hypoglycemia. J Pediatr 1978; 93:801–803.

291. Seltzer HS, Allen EW. Hyperglycemia and inhibition of insulin secretion during administration of diazoxide and tri-chloromethiazide in man. Diabetes 1969; 18:19–28.

292. Anderson JH, Byrd GW, Blackard WG. Hyperresponsiveness to tolbutamide of dogs pretreated with diazoxide. Metabolism 1971; 20:1023–1030.

293. Staquet M, Yabo R, Viktora J, et al. An adrenergic mechanism for hyperglycemia induced by diazoxide. Metabolism 1965; 14:1000–1009.

294. Walfish PG, Natale R, Chang C. Beta adrenergic receptor mechanisms in the metabolic effects of diazoxide in fasted rats. Diabetes 1970; 19:228–233.

295. Koch-Weser J. Diazoxide. N Engl J Med 1976; 294:1271–1273.

24

DIABETES MELLITUS

Roger H. Unger and Daniel W. Foster

INTRODUCTION

Diabetes mellitus comprises an etiologically and clinically heterogeneous group of hyperglycemic disorders. The hyperglycemia is the consequence of a relative or absolute deficiency of insulin in the presence of a relative or absolute excess of glucagon. When the insulin deficiency is extreme, these hormonal abnormalities are responsible for the tendency to develop ketoacidosis. Diabetes is associated with a set of late complications involving the eyes, kidneys, nerves, and blood vessels. It is now a leading cause of adult blindness in the United States and a major cause of renal failure, gangrene, myocardial infarction, and stroke.[1]

DIAGNOSIS OF DIABETES

The diagnosis of symptomatic diabetes is not difficult. The symptoms of increased thirst, polyuria, polyphagia, and

1255

TABLE 24–1. Glucose Levels Recommended as Diagnostic for Diabetes by Oral Glucose Tolerance Testing

	Mosenthal-Barry	Fajans-Conn	National Diabetes Data Group
1-h value*	9.2 mmol/L (165 mg/dL)	10.3 mmol/L (185 mg/dL)	11.1 mmol/L (200 mg/dL)
2-h value	6.4 mmol/L (115 mg/dL)	7.8 mmol/L (140 mg/dL)	11.1 mmol/L (200 mg/dL)

*"True glucose" measurements in plasma (measurements in whole blood are 15% lower). The Hoffman ferricyanide method generally used in autoanalyzers is approximately 0.3 mmol/L (5 mg/dL) above the true glucose value.

weight loss coupled with an elevation of the plasma glucose level are pathognomonic. When diabetes is suspected in an asymptomatic patient, the primary diagnostic test is measurement of the fasting plasma glucose concentration. If the value is not elevated, an oral glucose tolerance test can be done. Other procedures are of less value.

Fasting Plasma Glucose

The "gold standard" for the diagnosis of diabetes is an elevated glucose concentration in the plasma after an overnight fast. The diagnostic value usually cited is 7.8 mmol/L (140 mg/dL) or above on at least two occasions.[2] Some investigators have argued that 8.3 mmol/L (150 mg/dL) more accurately divides diabetic from nondiabetic subjects.[3]

The Oral Glucose Tolerance Test

Because the distribution curve of oral glucose tolerance tests (OGTTs) in the general population is unimodal, no single set of glucose values will separate all nondiabetics from all diabetics. Various diagnostic standards for diabetes have been recommended (Table 24–1). The most sensitive, those of Mosenthal and Barry,[4] gave positive results in 40% of a random population,[5] making them too nonspecific for general diagnostic purposes. However, the fact that less than 1% of individuals who were classified as normal by these criteria developed overt diabetes within the subsequent 10 y indicates that when postglucose values are below 8.3 mmol/L (150 mg/dL) future development of diabetes is unlikely. The least sensitive but most specific diagnostic criteria are those of the National Diabetes Data Group (Table 24–2), which selected 11.1 mmol/L (200 mg/dL) as the separation point between nondiagnostic and diagnostic OGTT values. This choice was consistent with the actual separation point between nondiabetic and diabetic OGTT modes in the Pima Indians, a population that does have a bimodal distribution of OGTT values.[6] The diagnostic validity of the 11.1 mmol/L (200 mg/dL) line in Pimas is buttressed by the demonstration that microaneurysms almost never developed in subjects whose glucose levels were below this value after a glucose load.[7]

TABLE 24–2. Criteria for the Diagnosis of Diabetes, National Diabetes Data Group

1. Fasting plasma glucose: ≥7.8 mmol/L (140 mg/dL) on at least two occasions
2. Oral glucose tolerance test (1.75 g glucose/kg body weight; 75 g maximum):
   a. Diabetes mellitus: plasma glucose ≥ 11.1 mmol/L (200 mg/dL) at 2 h and one other point in the test
   b. Impaired glucose tolerance: plasma glucose between 7.8 and 11.1 mmol/L (140 and 200 mg/dL) at 2 h and ≥ 11.1 mmol/L (200 mg/dL) between zero time and 2 h
   c. Gestational diabetes: two or more values greater than
      fasting—5.8 mmol/L (105 mg/dL)
      1 h—10.6 mmol/L (190 mg/dL)
      2 h—9.2 mmol/L (165 mg/dL)

Adapted with permission from National Diabetes Data Group, Classification and diagnosis of diabetes mellitus and other categories of glucose intolerance, Diabetes vol. 28, pp. 1038–1057, 1979. Copyright 1979 by the American Diabetes Association.

The problem with the OGTT is that it is influenced by many factors other than diabetes. Age, diet, state of health, gastrointestinal function, medications, and emotional state are among these variables. After age 50 glucose tolerance declines progressively as a consequence of changes in insulin sensitivity of target tissues.[8, 9] This may be a nonpathological aspect of aging. Thus in a middle-aged or elderly individual a diagnosis of diabetes based on the Mosenthal-Barry or Fajans-Conn standards for oral glucose tolerance (see Table 24–1) would probably serve no useful clinical purpose and might needlessly jeopardize employability or insurability. By contrast, the same abnormality in a child would usually indicate an early phase of autoimmune diabetes.

Standards for the OGTT were derived from tests performed in normal, healthy, well-nourished populations; their application to patients who are acutely or chronically ill, carbohydrate restricted, physically inactive, or taking certain medications results in a high percentage of false-positive results. Therefore, an OGTT should be performed only in well persons who have been consuming a normal diet with adequate carbohydrate for 3 d before the test. Because an abnormal glucose tolerance test result in an acutely or chronically ill person may reflect stress hyperglycemia rather than diabetes, the test should be deferred until after the individual has fully recovered. The procedure is not necessary if a diagnostic elevation of the fasting plasma glucose level is consistently present.

The Intravenous Glucose Tolerance Test (K Value)

The intravenous glucose tolerance test is not useful as a routine diagnostic test for diabetes because of its insensitivity, but it constitutes a clinical research tool for reproducible assessment of glucose disposal. Results are reported as K values, a reflection of the time required for glucose to clear the circulation. ($K = 0.69/T_{1/2} \times 100$, where $T_{1/2}$ is the time required for glucose to reach one half of the calculated zero-time concentration.) The normal value for K is 1.2 or greater. The insulin response to intravenously injected glucose provides a useful index of residual beta cell function during the development of autoimmune diabetes.

Glycosylated Hemoglobin (Hemoglobin A₁c)

In persons without hemoglobinopathy, an increased level of hemoglobin A_{1c} constitutes presumptive evidence of diabetes, although verification by standard procedures is required. A normal hemoglobin A_{1c} level does not exclude impaired glucose tolerance or mild diabetes. Hemoglobin A_{1c} determinations for diagnostic purposes correlate well with the fasting serum glucose level.[10, 11] Absolute values for hemoglobin A_{1c} vary from laboratory to laboratory, but the distributions of glycosylated hemoglobin concentrations in normal persons and diabetic patients do not overlap.[11] The hemoglobin A_{1c} levels of patients with impaired glucose tolerance are intermediate between those of normal individuals and diabetic patients. A value greater than 3 standard deviations above the normal mean is more than 99% specific for diabetes, although it is rather insensitive. A hemoglobin A_{1c} determination is a convenient way to obtain an integrated assessment of antecedent glycemia over an extended period under real life conditions. A single blood sample is sufficient and no preparation of the patient is required.

Muscle Capillary Basement Membrane Thickening

A characteristic lesion of diabetes is thickening of the capillary basement membranes in tissues throughout the body. Quantitatively reliable measurement of capillary basement membrane thickness is most conveniently performed in specimens of quadriceps muscle. The pathogenetic implications of this lesion are uncertain, but it is generally accepted that a muscle capillary basement membrane width greater than 180 nm (1800 Å) is diagnostic of diabetes provided vascular disease such as lupus erythematosus is not present. Although originally proposed as a genetic marker of diabetes independent of hyperglycemia,[12] basement membrane thickening is now regarded as a consequence of the metabolic disorder. This follows from studies of monozygotic twins discordant for hyperglycemia in whom the muscle capillary basement membranes were normal or less thick in the normoglycemic twin[13-15] and from the observation that muscle capillary basement membrane thickness appears to recede after 2 y of near-normalization of the plasma glucose level throughout the day by aggressive insulin therapy.[16, 17] Whatever the eventual interpretation of muscle capillary basement membrane thickening in diabetes, it is a research, not a clinical, tool and is not routinely used for diagnosis.

NOMENCLATURE AND DEFINITIONS

Diabetes mellitus can be divided into two major categories depending on whether endogenous insulin secretion is sufficient to prevent diabetic ketoacidosis. In most previous classifications, including that of the National Diabetes Data Group[2] (Table 24–3), the terms insulin-dependent diabetes mellitus (IDDM) and type 1 diabetes are used synonymously,[18] a practice that has been criticized.[19] In this chapter minor modifications have been introduced. The term *insulin-dependent diabetes mellitus* will be applied to all forms of diabetes in which exogenous insulin is required to prevent diabetic ketoacidosis, regardless of etiology. The term *type 1* will be applied only to diabetes resulting from autoimmune destruction of beta cells regardless of whether the destruction is sufficiently complete to result in ketoacidosis-prone IDDM.

Similarly, non–insulin-dependent diabetes mellitus (NIDDM) and type 2 diabetes are generally used synony-

TABLE 24–3. Classification of Diabetes Recommended by the National Diabetes Data Group

I. Idiopathic diabetes mellitus
  1. Insulin-dependent or type 1
  2. Non–insulin-dependent or type 2
    a. Nonobese
    b. Obese*
II. Gestational diabetes
III. Impaired glucose tolerance
IV. Previous abnormality of glucose tolerance
V. Potential abnormality of glucose tolerance
VI. Secondary diabetes

*Obesity is defined as 120% or more of ideal body weight (Metropolitan Life Tables) or body mass index greater than 25 in women or 27 in men (body mass index = weight [kg] ÷ height [m]²). Revised tables of acceptable weights were published in the Metropolitan Life Foundation Statistical Bulletin 1983 (January–June); 64:2–9.

mously. In this chapter, the term *non–insulin-dependent diabetes mellitus* will be applied to any form of diabetes, regardless of etiology, in which endogenous insulin production is sufficient to prevent diabetic ketoacidosis. The term *type 2 diabetes* will be restricted to patients with NIDDM who do not have autoimmune destruction of beta cells (type 1 disease), diabetes secondary to pancreatic disease, or other rare causes of hyperglycemia. Thus in this formulation IDDM and NIDDM indicate only the absence or presence of beta cell function, whereas type 1 and type 2 distinguish between autoimmune and nonautoimmune forms of diabetes. For example, if a patient with autoimmune diabetes were to pass through a transient non–insulin-dependent period during which beta cell destruction is incomplete, he or she would be classified as having type 1 NIDDM until such time as insulin dependence appeared, whereupon the classification would change to type 1 IDDM.

GENETICS AND ETIOLOGY OF TYPE 1 INSULIN-DEPENDENT DIABETES MELLITUS

Demography

Prevalence

Type 1 IDDM is predominantly a disease of whites or populations with a substantial white genetic admixture, such as American blacks. It is rare in Japanese, Chinese, Filipinos, Asiatic Indians, American Indians, African blacks, Polynesians, Eskimos, Micronesians, and Melanesians (Table 24–4).[20–23] In Israeli children of European parentage the prevalence of IDDM is almost three times that in Israeli children of Asiatic or African parentage.[24]

These differences may not be entirely racial, because there are said to be striking regional differences in preva-

TABLE 24–4. Prevalence of Insulin-Dependent Diabetes in General Populations (1970–1980)*

Country	Age Group (y)	Method of Ascertainment	Prevalence/1000
Australia	20-y-old men	Interview and screening for national service	3.7
Cuba	0–14	National registry	0.13
France	0–19	Central registry	0.3
Japan	6–15	Urine tests on 25,000 persons	0.12
Sweden	0–15	Known cases	2.2
United States	0–15	Household interviews	0.38
United States	0–16	Known cases	1.3
United States	6–18	School records	1.9

*As evidenced by the three studies in the United States, estimates of prevalence vary depending on method of ascertainment. If the criteria of Table 24–2 were applied, different prevalence values would be found.

Adapted from West KM. Epidemiology of Diabetes and Its Vascular Lesions. New York: Elsevier, 1978: 292–293.

lence in the same country.[25] An environmental impact is also suggested by seasonal variations in rate of appearance[26, 27] and by the fact that 50% or fewer of identical twins are concordant for IDDM.[28]

The prevalence of type 1 insulin-dependent diabetes in the United States is about 260 per 100,000 (0.26%) by age 20.[29] Although some patients develop typical type 1 IDDM at a later age, the number of such late-onset patients is probably low. In England the prevalence of type 1 IDDM is 220 per 100,000 (0.22%) by age 20.[30] The equivalent figure in Denmark at age 19 is 240 per 100,000 (0.24%).[31] Although in Great Britain the prevalence of autoimmune diabetes appears to have been constant between 1946 and 1958, the disease seems to be manifesting itself at an earlier age.[32] In midwestern Poland the incidence almost doubled from 3.5 per 100,000 in the period 1970 to 1981 to 6.6 per 100,000 in 1982 to 1984.[33] The increase was largely in younger children.

Incidence

In countries in which the population is predominantly white the reported yearly appearance rate of IDDM ranges from 3.7 to 20.0 per 100,000.[29, 34] The Pittsburgh registry in the United States showed an incidence ranging from 10 per 100,000 per year for nonwhite males to 16 per 100,000 per year for white males. Rates in women were intermediate between those in nonwhite and white males.[29] The overall incidence in Rochester, Minnesota, was 8.4 per 100,000 per year.[34] In Denmark the incidence has been estimated to be 13.2 per 100,000 per year between 0 and 29 y of age.[27, 35] In both the United States and Denmark the peak age of onset is between 10 and 14 y.[29, 31] Some workers think that the incidence of type 1 diabetes has increased over the last several decades,[33, 35] but this view is not universally shared.[22, 29]

Family Studies

Familial aggregation of type 1 IDDM is uncommon. In the first large family study of diabetes, less than 4% of the parents and 6% of the siblings of a proband with IDDM had diabetes.[36] In another study diabetes was present in 11% of the parents and 11% of siblings.[37] The concordance rate of 50% or less for IDDM in monozygotic twins has already been mentioned and contrasts sharply with the familial aggregation and the almost 100% concordance in monozygotic twins observed in type 2 NIDDM.[38] In a cohort of 493 families studied after identification of a proband with IDDM,[39] the risk of insulin-dependent diabetes in siblings was significantly higher (8.5%) when the diabetic proband was diagnosed before age 10 than when it was diagnosed after age 10 (4.6%). Only 79 (16%) of the families had one or more siblings or parents with IDDM. Family histories of 1280 subjects admitted to the Children's Hospital of Pittsburgh showed 2.6% of the parents to have IDDM and 2.4% to have NIDDM.[40] The risk to siblings was 3.3% overall but increased to 10.5% if one parent also had diabetes. No differences were found between blacks and whites. An evaluation of seven studies involving 9000 families revealed a mean risk for diabetes of 1.3% in parents, 4.2% in siblings, and 1.9% in offspring.[40] Thus familial transmission of IDDM is not common.

Offspring of type 1 diabetic fathers are at much higher risk for autoimmune diabetes than offspring of type 1 diabetic mothers.[41] This remarkable difference is apparently confined to fathers with a DR4 allele[42] and is not the result of a selective loss of diabetes-susceptible fetuses in the perinatal period.[41]

Genetics

The Major Histocompatibility Complex

The major histocompatibility complex (MHC) is important in diabetes both because susceptibility to type 1 IDDM appears to be linked to certain human leukocyte antigen (HLA) alleles and because the region controls immune response. A brief review is therefore provided.

The MHC in humans is located on the short arm of the sixth chromosome. The gene products of this region include the HLAs, glycoprotein molecules that are located in the plasma membranes of cells (Fig. 24–1).[43–45] Other known products include the C2 and C4 components of the classic complement pathway and the properdin factor Bf of the alternative complement pathway. Because the major histocompatibility region is large in genetic terms, it is probable that additional undiscovered proteins are encoded there. A number of loci have been firmly established and are designated by the letters A, B, C, and D (Fig. 24–2). A series of alleles are present at each site, identified by arabic numerals (e.g., HLA-B8). The addition of a lowercase w indicates that identification of the antigen is provisional (e.g., Dw2). Additional loci such as DQ (formerly DC) have been described.[46, 47] A nomenclature has been developed that classifies gene products of the MHC according to their function. Class I molecules include gene products of the HLA-A, -B, and -C loci; class II molecules are encoded at D (and D-related sites); and class III molecules represent the complement-related proteins.

CLASS I SURFACE ANTIGENS. Class I surface antigens are expressed on all nucleated cells. The human antigens are equivalent to gene products coded for in mice by the K and D sites of the H-2 locus (MHC) on the 17th chromosome. The antigens consist of two chains (see Fig. 24–1). The larger chain, a glycosylated polypeptide with an apparent molecular mass of about 43 kd, is encoded on chromosome 6; the smaller chain, β_2-microglobulin (apparent molecular mass of 12 kd), is encoded on chromosome 15. The two chains are associated noncovalently. Genetic variability is accounted for by the larger chain. Class I molecules are involved in cell-mediated immunity. They are required for recognition and rejection of foreign (nonself) cells and

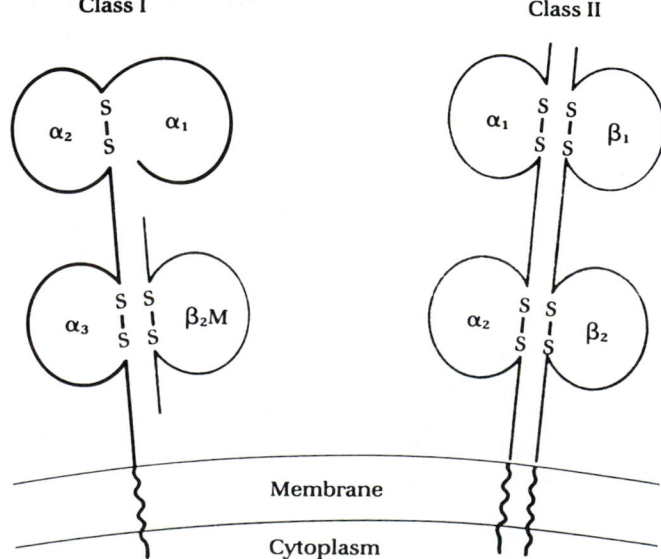

Figure 24–1. Structure of class I and class II MHC molecules. In class I the alpha chain is variable but β_2-microglobulin (β_2M) is invariant. In class II both alpha and beta chains are variable. (From Golub ES. Immunology: A Synthesis. Sunderland, MA: Sinauer Associates, 1987: 222–233.)

Human Chromosome 6

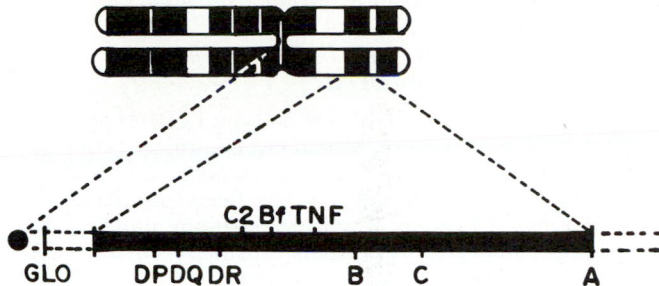

Figure 24–2. Schematic representation of the major histocompatibility complex in humans. Loci are approximate. C2 and Bf are complement-related sites, and TNF is the tumor necrosis factor gene. See text for details. (Adapted from Irvine WJ. Immunological aspects of diabetes mellitus: a review [including the salient points of the NDDG report on the classification of diabetes]. In: Irvine WJ, ed. Immunology of Diabetes. Edinburgh: Teviot Scientific Publications, 1980: 1–53.)

intrinsic (self) cells that have been altered by viral infection or malignant disease.[43] The mechanism is through activation of quiescent T lymphocytes, which become capable of inducing cell lysis. These T cells, called cytotoxic or killer (K) T cells, are activated by exposure to antigen-presenting cells, macrophages that process antigens such as viral proteins and present selected peptide fragments of such antigens in association with the class I molecule expressed on the cell surface. Only the subset of T lymphocytes with receptors for both the viral antigen and the class I molecule (i.e., the "neoantigen" formed by a viral protein complexed to the class I antigen) become activated.[48] This obligate requirement for class I molecules in the recognition of and response to foreign antigens, so-called MHC restriction, ensures that only cells bearing the processed foreign antigen–class I molecule complex will by lysed by the activated cytotoxic T cell.

CLASS II MOLECULES. Class II molecules are equivalent to Ia antigens in the murine system and are often so designated. Figure 24–2 shows the orientation of the human HLA-D region on the short arm of chromosome 6, and Figure 24–3 provides a map of the class II loci of this region. DR specificities can be determined by mixed lymphocyte culture and serological testing or DNA sequencing. DQ can

be assayed either immunologically or by DNA sequencing. However, the polymerase chain reaction is now routinely employed to obtain the most complete and pertinent analysis for genetic screening. Class II molecules normally are expressed only on B lymphocytes, tissue and circulating macrophages, endothelial cells, and some activated T lymphocytes. They are not normally present on connective tissue cells or epithelial cells. This limited expression protects against inappropriate T cell activation and autoimmunity.[49] Class II antigens consist of a heavy alpha chain, apparent molecular mass of 33 kd (range of 29 to 34 kd), and a lighter beta chain, apparent molecular mass of 28 kd (range of 25 to 28 kd) (see Fig. 24–1). The alpha chain is probably invariant, whereas the beta chain is highly polymorphic. In a manner analogous to that described for activation of cytotoxic T cells, helper T cells are triggered into activity by exposure to cells presenting a foreign antigen or an autoantigen in association with the class II molecule; i.e., helper T lymphocyte activation is also MHC restricted. The activation of helper-inducer T lymphocytes involves a receptor complex composed of a monomeric antigen designated T3 and a heterodimer called Ti to which antigen-presenting cells bind[50] (Fig. 24–4). Activated helper T cells then interact with B lymphocytes and plasma cells expressing the same antigen–class II complex expressed by the activating macrophage to enhance antibody formation.

How helper T cells interact with the cytotoxic T cell population involved in rejection of transplanted allografts is not completely understood, although it is clear that survival

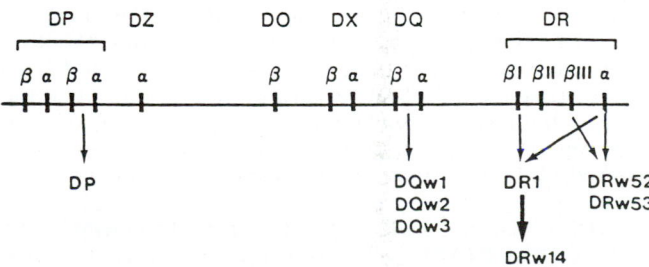

Figure 24–3. Map of the class II loci of the human HLA-D region on the short arm of chromosome 6. The DRβ₁ and DRα gene products associate to form a cell-surface heterodimeric glycoprotein. The resulting molecule reacts with the alloantisera that define the major DR allotypes. The relatively nonpolymorphic DRβ₃ gene products are utilized in several DR allotypes. DRβ₂ is a pseudogene. The DQα and DQβ genes encode the DQ serological specificities (DQw1, DQw2, and DQw3). Only one DPα and DPβ gene is expressed. The second DPα and DPβ and DXα and DXβ genes are not expressed. DOβ and DZα are expressed only in very small amounts. (From Todd JA, Bell JI, McDevitt HO. HLA-DQβ gene contributes to susceptibility and resistance to insulin-dependent diabetes mellitus. Reprinted by permission from Nature, Vol. 329, pp. 599–604. Copyright © 1987 Macmillan Magazines Limited.)

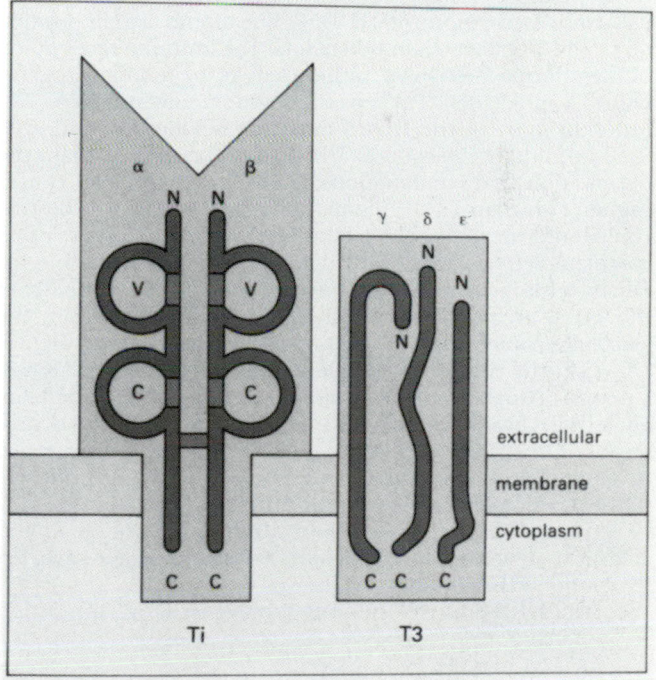

Figure 24–4. Structure of the human T cell receptor. The T cell receptor is a complex of the Ti molecule, which binds antigen/MHC, and the T3 molecular complex. Ti consists of a disulfide-linked heterodimer formed of alpha and beta chains. Each of these chains consists of variable (V) and constant (C) domains stabilized by intrachain disulfide bonds, a short "hinge-like" segment, and transmembrane and intracytoplasmic portions. The Ti portion of the molecule is polymorphic and carries the T cell idiotype. The T3 complex consists of three noncovalently associated peptides, each of which probably traverses the cell membrane. They are monomorphic and appear to transduce the activation signal from Ti to the cell itself. The monoclonal antibody CD3 recognizes primarily the delta chain of T3. (From Male D, Champion B, Cooke A. The T cell antigen receptor. In: Advanced Immunology. London: Gower Medical Publishing, 1987: 7.1–7.7. Courtesy of Male D, Champion B, and Cooke A and Gower Medical Publishing.)

is prolonged by antibodies directed against class II (Ia) molecules on the antigen-presenting cell.[51, 52]

Both class I and class II molecules could be important in the immune reactions that characterize development of type 1 IDDM, although the mechanism is unknown. It might be speculated, for example, that high-risk class I and/or class II molecules confer susceptibility for insulin-dependent diabetes through more effective presentation of antigen.

It has also been noted that cells that do not usually express DR antigens (e.g., the beta cells of the pancreas) might do so in predisposed individuals, leading to activation of inducer and cytotoxic T cells that would then cause diabetes.[49]

Associations Between HLA Antigens and Type 1 IDDM

Approximately 95% of white type 1 IDDM patients have either DR3 or DR4 antigens[53–56] and 55 to 60% have both DR3 and DR4. (In other ethnic groups HLA-linked susceptibility to diabetes may involve different alleles.[57])

It was previously thought that a susceptibility gene was linked to the DR3 and DR4 loci. Today it is thought that the alleles of HLA-DQ beta chain primarily determine susceptibility and resistance to autoimmune destruction of beta cells. If an aspartic acid residue occupies position 57 in both alleles of that chain, autoimmune diabetes will not occur. Full susceptibility requires that both alleles be Asp-57–negative[58] (Table 24–5). However, Asp-57 does not appear to be protective in DR4/DR4 individuals,[59] suggesting that other amino acids may be involved in susceptibility. Seventy percent of DR4 IDDM patients are DQw3.2-positive, a serotype that is closely associated with DR4 and accounts for its strong association with IDDM. The amino acid in position 45 of the DQ beta chain determines the immune recognition of the epitope as DQw3.2 rather than as the nondiabetogenic DQw3.1 molecule.[59] Perhaps the segment encompassing residues 45 to 57 of the DQw3 molecule is somehow critical to the autoimmune response. These findings may explain the observation that combinations of DR and DQ alleles confer higher risk than either alone.[60] The DQ alleles can best be considered as analogous to the "extended haplotypes" that correlate better with risk for diabetes than simple testing for DR in serological tests.[61] Terminology changes frequently in the HLA area. What we call DQw3.1 in this chapter, the aspartate-containing allele, is now designated DQw7. DQw3.2, the nonaspartate allele, has been renamed DQw8. Current evidence suggests that the primary susceptibility allele is DQw3.2 (DQw8) and that DQw3.1 (DQw7) is protective. Other aspartate-containing alleles are nonprotective or neutral.[61a] The fact that some subjects with HLA-DR3 or -DR4 develop diabetes whereas others do not likewise may be explained by the presence or absence of a single amino acid at a structurally critical site, a difference not revealed by routine HLA typing.

DR2/DR2-positive subjects enjoy striking protection

from type 1 IDDM. When type 1 IDDM develops in DR2-positive individuals, it is the consequence of an unusual clustering of a DQβ susceptibility gene with DR2, a combination not ordinarily found.[62] The DR2 allele also occurs in patients with the IDDM of Wolfram syndrome.[63]

Subclassification of Type 1 IDDM: Is There Heterogeneity Within IDDM?

It would be useful to subclassify type 1 IDDM according to HLA haplotype if there were in fact clinical and etiological distinctions between DR3/DR3-associated diabetes and DR4/DR4-associated disease. It has been postulated that homozygous DR3 results in a primary autoimmune disorder and homozygous DR4 represents a primary environmental insult with a secondary autoimmune response.[62, 64–67] Subjects in the DR3 subgroup were reported to have an increased prevalence of other autoimmune disease (e.g., adrenal insufficiency, Hashimoto thyroiditis), a female preponderance, an older age at onset, and a low capacity for forming antibodies to insulin. By contrast, subjects with the DR4 alleles supposedly had little, if any, association with immune endocrine disease but exhibited a male predominance, a tendency to younger onset, and a high capacity to form insulin antibodies. A subsequent analysis of 745 patients with type 1 diabetes that began between 1 and 19 y of age revealed that those with HLA-DR3 but not HLA-DR4 had milder disease with less ketonuria at diagnosis and a greater tendency for partial remissions.[68] In that series DR4 diabetes was more severe and more common in females. Although heterogeneity of autoimmune diabetes seems inherently plausible, it has not yet been convincingly established that serologically detected differences in DR alleles or even extended haplotypes reflect clinical differences in the disease.

Inheritance

The mode of inheritance of type 1 IDDM is unknown. Dominant, recessive, intermediate, and polygenic mechanisms have all been proposed.

THE EVIDENCE FOR AND AGAINST AN AUTOSOMAL DOMINANT INHERITANCE. Support for a dominant mode of inheritance in humans initially came from an evaluation of IDDM in black Americans.[69] Because about 20% of genes in the black population are derived from whites and the prevalence of IDDM is roughly equivalent in blacks and whites, it was argued that autosomal recessive inheritance could be ruled out and that dominant inheritance was possible. However, the greater prevalence of diabetes in American blacks than in their West African counterparts could be consequent to environmental factors. Another family study of the frequency of transmission of DR4 from diabetic parents to diabetic offspring was also interpreted as favoring the possibility of dominant inheritance.[70] However, the rarity of IDDM in parents, siblings, and offspring of affected subjects virtually excludes simple dominant inheritance.[37, 39, 71]

THE EVIDENCE FOR AND AGAINST AUTOSOMAL RECESSIVE INHERITANCE. Recessive inheritance is suggested by the high frequency of HLA identity (two shared haplotypes) in concordant siblings with type 1 IDDM.[72] The fact that concordance rates for diabetes are only about 50% in HLA-identical siblings does not eliminate the recessive interpretation, because only half or less of monozygotic twins are concordant for IDDM.[28, 38, 73] The apparent decrease in expressivity may simply reflect an environmental requirement, to be discussed.

Against the recessive theory is the observation that homozygosity for the DR3 or DR4 allele does not greatly

---

TABLE 24–5. Predicted Susceptibility for Autoimmune Diabetes of DR3 and/or DR4 Subjects in General Population Based on DNA Sequence of DQ Beta Chain Gene*

Susceptibility	Asp-57
Full	Neg/neg
10%	Neg/pos
0	Pos/pos

*See text for details.

From Todd JA, Bell JI, McDevitt HO. HLA-DQβ gene contributes to susceptibility and resistance to insulin-dependent diabetes mellitus. Reprinted by permission from Nature, Vol. 329, pp. 599–604. Copyright © 1987 Macmillan Magazines Limited.

increase the risk for diabetes, whereas a specific heterozygosity, DR3/DR4, does.[74] This argument has been used to conclude that the recessive hypothesis can be rejected,[75] although such a view has been challenged.[76]

OTHER MODELS OF INHERITANCE. The observation that heterozygosity for DR3/DR4 significantly increases the risk for diabetes relative to homozygosity for other high-risk alleles has suggested that at least two susceptibility genes exist and that they act synergistically.[64] According to the two-gene hypothesis, one gene would be sufficient to put the subject at risk for diabetes and the presence of the second gene would enhance that risk. A three-gene model has also been proposed.[77, 78] It is interesting that in nonobese diabetic (NOD) mice, which develop a syndrome of autoimmune diabetes that resembles the human disorder, at least three recessive loci are required for expression of the disease.[79] These include the major histocompatibility locus and a Thy-1/Alp-1–linked locus. If human susceptibilities also are polygenic, a locus proximal to Thy-1 and Alp-1 on the long arm of chromosome 11 should be looked for.

Another area of interest is the T cell receptor gene.[80] The autoimmune process requires recognition of the class II molecule–antigen complex by this receptor. If it is assumed that only two loci are required for maximal susceptibility to diabetes in humans, the risk of a homozygous Asp-57–negative person with diabetogenic T cell receptor alleles should theoretically approach that of an unaffected identical twin of a type 1 diabetic (see Table 24–5). Whether this will prove to be the case is not yet known.

At the time of this writing we conclude that the mode of inheritance in type 1 IDDM remains masked. Relative risk and prevalence of autoimmune diabetes in siblings of diabetic probands[81] are shown in Table 24–6.

Type 1 Insulin-Dependent Diabetes Mellitus: Environmental-Genetic Interactions

The relative contributions of genetics and environment in the pathogenesis of individual cases of type 1 diabetes may vary (Fig. 24–5) (see ref. 82 for a review). Anecdotal reports, such as the development of diabetes in two haplo-nonidentical siblings within 1 wk after mumps infection, raise the possibility of primary environmental input. A case of massive beta cell necrosis also seems to bypass genetic requirements and fit this category.[83] This would be comparable to the nonautoimmune destruction of beta cells by a high dose of streptozocin or alloxan in animals or by the poison Vacor in humans.[84] Other environmental factors of uncertain importance include N-nitroso compounds used in curing mutton; an increase in autoimmune diabetes in Icelandic boys has been attributed to maternal ingestion of such chemicals at the time of conception.[85] At the other end of the spectrum of environmental-genetic interaction is the spontaneous diabetes that develops in the Bio-Breeding/Worcester (BB/W) rat[86] and the NOD mouse.[87] In neither of these forms of autoimmune diabetes is any environmental factor apparent, and the syndrome is therefore listed in Figure 24–5 as primary (1°) autoimmunity. Except for the rare instances of fulminating virally or chemically induced destruction of beta cells cited earlier, human type 1 diabetes requires a genetic background of susceptibility. The concept that an environmental agent is involved in precipitating autoimmunity to beta cells in genetically susceptible individuals is based entirely on inheritance and concordance patterns in identical twins and family studies, as already discussed. From such studies it has been postulated that type 1 IDDM results whenever an environmental

TABLE 24–6. Prevalence of and Relative Risk for Autoimmune Diabetes in 16-Year-Old Siblings of Diabetic Probands

	Prevalence (%)	Relative Risk
Identical twin	50	
HLA-identical sibs	14	118
Haplo-identical sibs	4	31
Nonidentical sibs	1	NS
All sibs	5	36

Adapted with permission from Gorsuch AN, Spencer KM, Lister J, et al., Can future type I diabetes be predicted? Diabetes vol. 31, pp. 862–866, 1982. Copyright 1982 by the American Diabetes Association.

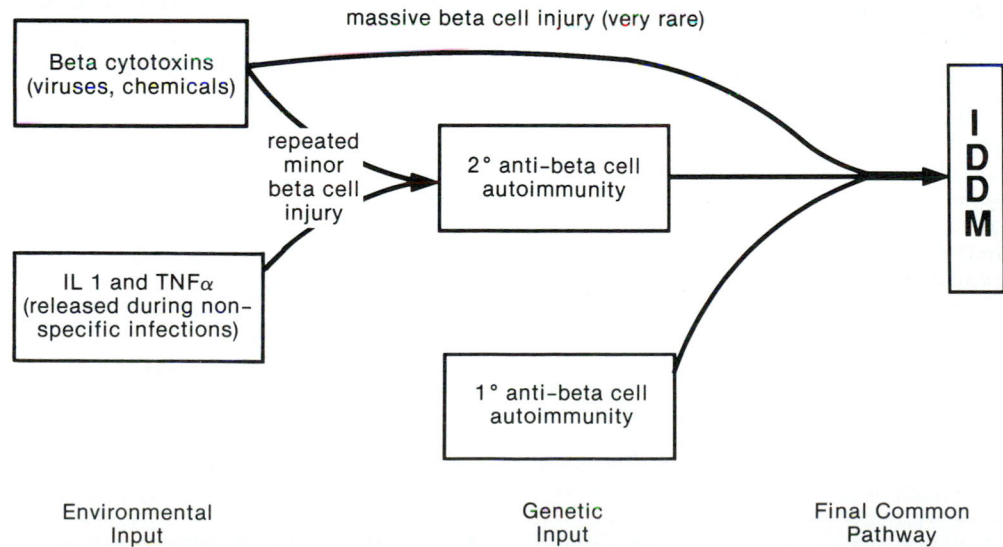

massive beta cell injury (very rare)

Beta cytotoxins (viruses, chemicals)

repeated minor beta cell injury

IL 1 and TNFα (released during non-specific infections)

2° anti–beta cell autoimmunity

1° anti–beta cell autoimmunity

IDDM

Environmental Input

Genetic Input

Final Common Pathway

Figure 24–5. Putative pathogenic pathways to IDDM. Injury may be entirely environmental, a combination of environmental and genetic factors (most common), or a purely genetic event (theoretical). Potential environmental factors include viruses and chemicals. They may act specifically or injure beta cells nonspecifically through generation of cytokines such as interleukin 1 or tumor necrosis factor α. Genetic factors are presumed to be permissive and determine susceptibility to autoimmunity after the initial injury to beta cells. Rarely an autoimmune requirement may be bypassed if massive beta cell injury results from specific betatoxic substances. A more common scenario is repeated minor beta cell injuries that produce secondary anti–beta cell autoimmunity in genetically susceptible individuals. In theory, such autoimmunity might occur on a primary basis without any external environmental input. The final common pathway of beta cell death refers to the theory that destruction is mediated by toxic oxygen radicals.

TABLE 24–7. Possible Environmental Triggers for Diabetes Mellitus

Viruses
Mumps virus
Rubella virus
Cytomegalovirus
Coxsackieviruses B4 and B5
Retroviruses with type C particles
Retrovirus with type A particles and p73 antigen production
Reoviruses
Encephalomyocarditis virus

Betacytotoxins
Nitroso compounds
Vacor
Others?

insult to the beta cells exceeds the genetically determined tolerance of that individual to beta cell injury. Stated differently, the genetic contribution is necessary but ordinarily insufficient to cause the disease; usually an environmental factor is required as the trigger for its initiation. This concept permits one to attribute discordance for diabetes in monozygotic twins to differences in environmental experience. Possible environmental triggers are listed in Table 24–7.

Is the Environmental Factor in Type 1 Insulin-Dependent Diabetes Mellitus a Virus?

The onset of type 1 IDDM sometimes coincides with or follows infection with mumps, rubella, cytomegalic, measles, influenza, encephalitis, polio, and Epstein-Barr viruses.[88] Congenital rubella appears to impose a very real risk, inducing diabetes in about 20% of affected individuals in the United States and Australia (but not England).[88] If the affected child is DR3 or DR4 the prevalence may increase to 40%, an astonishingly high risk.[89] Congenital infection with rubella probably is a bona fide instance of autoimmune diabetes resulting from a prior viral infection. Despite these rare associations and the demonstration that viruses cause diabetes in experimental animals, it has not been proved that viruses are an important environmental agent in human type 1 diabetes. Two thirds of children with new-onset diabetes in Sweden had immunoglobulin M antibodies against coxsackievirus B, compared with 12% of control children.[90] However, this finding appears to be offset by failure to demonstrate differences in antiviral antibody titers in identical twins discordant for diabetes.[91] IDDM is not consistently associated with viral epidemics or with increased virus antibody titers, and an epidemic of IDDM has never been reported.

Although coxsackievirus B4 has been isolated from a patient who died in ketoacidosis with apparent postinfectious diabetes,[92] this case may fit into the category of fulminating beta cell destruction rather than a virally triggered autoimmune disorder. The virus was obtained from the pancreas and caused hyperglycemia when injected into mice, proving its betacytotropism. Beta cell destruction with acute and chronic inflammation of the islets was observed in 4 of 7 cases of fatal coxsackievirus B infection, 20 of 45 cases of cytomegalovirus infection, 2 of 14 cases of varicella-zoster infection, and 2 of 45 cases of congenital rubella.[93] However, in this study viruses were not isolated from tissues, and again there is no evidence that autoimmune diabetes would have supervened if the patients had lived. Of greater potential interest is the report that cytomegalovirus is incorporated in the genome of 22% of type 1 diabetics.[94] However, no cause-and-effect relationship has thus far been established.

The etiological implications of clinical findings such as rising viral titers are called into question by the observation that marked differences in susceptibility to the same inoculum of virus occur in different strains of mice.[95] Resistance or susceptibility appears to be genetically determined.[96] Thus, two persons (e.g., siblings) exposed to the same viral infection might express the same rise in viral titers, yet diabetes would develop in only one because of intrinsic genetic susceptibility factors. Susceptibility could mean sensitivity of beta cells to a particular dose of virus or the propensity to develop an autoimmune response to a viral antigen expressed in beta cells or to autoantigens released in the course of the subtle beta cell damage. Similarly, antiviral titers might be taken as evidence against a causal role of viruses when in fact the virus was the requisite environmental factor. It is also known that viruses that attack the pancreas vary in virulence and that virulence can be increased by serial passage through islet tissue.[97] Thus the same strain of virus could be dangerous or innocuous depending on its history. Concomitant exposure to other nonviral islet toxins enhances host susceptibility to viral damage and may represent another variable.[98] Interestingly, retrovirus-like particles have been identified in NOD mice and are presumed to be vertically transmitted.[99] One could envision, therefore, that viral inhabitants of normal beta cells are triggered to produce viral proteins by some seemingly innocuous event. For example, type A particles are linked to the insulin promoter of db/db mice and mild hyperglycemia may therefore increase their expression together with that of insulin.[100]

In summary, although incontrovertible evidence of their role in type 1 IDDM is lacking, viruses remain the environmental agents most likely to induce diabetes in susceptible persons. However, their modus operandi may be more subtle and more complex than the simple concepts heretofore conceived. In this regard we note that exposure to certain viruses may actually protect susceptible individuals from autoimmune diabetes; thus discordance might be environmentally associated with viral protection rather than viral damage. (See under Strategies for Preventing Autoimmune Diabetes.)

Is Type 1 Insulin-Dependent Diabetes Mellitus an Immune-Mediated Disease?

The evidence that type 1 IDDM is an immune-mediated disease can be summarized as follows (Table 24–8). First, it

TABLE 24–8. Evidence for a Role of Autoimmunity* in Type 1 IDDM

1. Linkage of type 1 IDDM to specific class II antigens associated with autoimmune disease
2. Coexistence of type 1 IDDM with autoimmune endocrinopathy (e.g., thyrotoxicosis, Hashimoto thyroiditis, Addison disease)
3. Familial aggregation of type 1 diabetes and other autoimmune conditions, such as pernicious anemia, vitiligo, myasthenia gravis, rheumatoid arthritis, and collagen diseases
4. Lymphocytic insulitis in the islets of Langerhans of type 1 diabetic subjects dying soon after diagnosis
5. Presence of islet cell antibodies in a high proportion of type 1 diabetic subjects at the time of diagnosis
6. Presence of islet cell surface antibodies in human survivors of poisoning by the beta-cytotoxic rodenticide Vacor
7. Islet cell antibodies precede overt diabetes in discordant monozygotic twins and triplets destined to become concordant
8. Increased numbers of killer T lymphocytes in 50 to 60% of newly diagnosed diabetic children
9. Pancreas transplanted from nondiabetic to diabetic monozygotic twin develops insulitis without graft rejection accompanied by return of diabetes after initial reversal of hyperglycemia
10. Remissions of new-onset type 1 IDDM can be induced by immunosuppression therapy

*Autoimmunity is used to indicate immune mechanisms directed against self. It is recognized that the immune response may be initiated by environmental factors.

is linked with class II (D region) antigens known to be associated with autoimmune disease.[52–62] Second, type 1 IDDM may occur with other forms of immune endocrinopathy, such as Hashimoto thyroiditis, adrenal insufficiency, pernicious anemia, myasthenia gravis, and vitiligo.[101] Third, the diabetes–immune endocrinopathy coupling may cluster in families.[101] Fourth, a very early (initial?) lesion in diabetes in both animals[102] and humans[103, 104] is an infiltration of lymphocytes in the islets of Langerhans ("insulitis") that is characteristic of lymphocytic infiltrations in other autoimmune diseases. Fifth, islet cell antibodies directed against both cytoplasmic and cell-surface determinants are present in a high percentage of type 1 diabetic subjects at the time of diagnosis.[64, 65, 82] Such antibodies are also found after other types of beta cell injury, e.g., in survivors of Vacor poisoning who develop diabetes[105] and in rats made diabetic with low doses of streptozocin[106] or infected with small quantities of diabetogenic viruses.[107] It is not clear whether the anti-islet antibodies found in experimental diabetes and in human disease are causally linked to the pathophysiological process or are the consequence of it—a nonpathogenic epiphenomenon resulting from islet cell injury.

The fact that overt diabetes can be prevented by immunotherapy in the low-dose streptozocin model of diabetes[102] and in the spontaneously diabetic BB/W rat[108] suggests that autoimmunity plays a role in these forms of diabetes. Further evidence in support of this thesis is the observation that diabetes can be induced in prediabetic BB rats by splenic lymphocytes from diabetic BB animals activated with concanavalin A.[109] Diabetes can also be induced in diabetes-resistant BB/W rats by pretreatment with cyclophosphamide, by partial thymectomy, or by injections of anti-RT6 antibody.[110, 111] These maneuvers apparently eliminate RT6$^+$ T lymphocytes, a population that presumably restrains the effector T lymphocytes responsible for beta cell destruction. Conversely, treatment with whole blood from a diabetes-resistant BB strain prevents diabetes in a susceptible strain,[112] the blood presumably containing functional or potentially functional suppressor T lymphocytes. The observation that Ia antigen–bearing lymphocytes are increased in type 1 diabetes, as in other autoimmune diseases, is in accord with the immune hypothesis.[113] (Ia antigen in rodents is equivalent to human class II HLA, and the terms are commonly used interchangeably in the jargon of immunologists.) Activated T lymphocytes from type 1 diabetic patients include both helper and cytotoxic cells, consistent with a role for both humoral and cell-mediated immunity in the induction of type 1 diabetes. Additional support for the autoimmune theory comes from the observation that remissions in type 1 diabetes in humans can be induced for as long as 1 y by altering the immune response with cyclosporine.[114] Perhaps the most compelling evidence is the report of rapid development of insulitis and destruction of beta cells in pancreata transplanted from unaffected monozygotic twins into the twins with diabetes.[115]

Whether abnormalities in ratios of helper (CD4) to suppressor (CD8) T lymphocytes might predispose to autoimmune pathogenesis is unknown. It is conceivable that an increased helper/suppressor ratio might augment the immune response on exposure to self-antigens. Early reports suggested disproportionate deficiencies of suppressor T cells,[116] but other studies have emphasized modest lymphopenia with greater depression of cells expressing CD4 than those expressing CD8.[117, 118] Failure to find an elevated helper/suppressor ratio may reflect the time of testing, because the ratio tends to be elevated early after diagnosis, returning toward normal with time.[119] Although conceptionally attractive, an increased helper/suppressor T lymphocyte ratio cannot be considered established.

To summarize, we believe the evidence persuasive that type 1 IDDM is an autoimmune disease.[120, 121] In the sections that follow we discuss certain aspects of the immune response that appear to be important.

Islet Cell Cytoplasmic Antibodies

In sections of fresh human pancreas, cytoplasmic antibodies reacting with islets are detected in the serum of 60 to 90% of newly diagnosed patients with type 1 diabetes compared with 0.5% of nondiabetic controls.[122] These antibodies generally react with all four islet cell types: alpha cells (glucagon), beta cells (insulin), delta cells (somatostatin), and pancreatic polypeptide–secreting cells. Occasionally antibodies specific for a single cell type are seen.[123] Only the insulin-secreting cells are destroyed in diabetes. The other cell types are normal or increased in number.[124, 125] The lymphocytes in insulitis are confined to islets containing beta cells, further implying a killing specificity for the insulin-producing sites.[104, 126] Alpha, delta, and pancreatic polypeptide cells are also spared in diabetes produced by chemical beta-cytotoxins, such as streptozocin,[127] and by viruses.[128]

Islet cell cytoplasmic antibodies (ICA-cyt) disappear in 85 to 90% of type 1 patients within 2 y after onset of the IDDM.[129] It has been claimed that the 10 to 15% of the patients in whom these antibodies persist for more than 2 to 3 y exhibit (1) a high prevalence of thyroid and gastric autoantibodies compared with that in patients with IDDM of a similar duration who do not possess islet antibodies; (2) frequent coexistence of autoimmune endocrinopathy; (3) a strong family history of other autoimmune disorders; (4) a female preponderance; (5) a strong association with HLA-DR3/B8, the HLA axis associated with other organ-specific antibodies; and (6) reduced levels of immunoglobulin G antibodies to exogenous insulin compared with those in patients with DR4 IDDM.[64, 130–132] The possibility of heterogeneity within the type 1 IDDM category has been reviewed.[133] It should be noted, however, that a later survey of 375 children indicated that 62% were still islet cell antibody positive after 3 y.[134] In this study no correlation with sex, age, or DR type was noted. Although this might be explained by differences in populations or assay techniques,[120] the idea that persistent antibody titers identify a special form of autoimmune diabetes cannot be considered proved.

Why patients with type 1 diabetes sometimes exhibit disease in several endocrine glands is not known (see Chapter 31), but one possibility is that islet cell antibodies cross-react with a common antigenic determinant in different tissues.[135] Such interaction might be taken as support for a pathogenetic role for these antibodies, but the weight of evidence suggests that they are simply markers of beta cell damage. Indeed the growing list of antibodies observed at the onset of this disease now includes, in addition to islet cell antibodies (cytoplasmic and surface),[136] autoantibodies directed against insulin,[137] islet 64- and 38-kd proteins,[138] proinsulin,[139] immunoglobulins,[140] and insulin receptors.[141] The 64-kd antigen appears to be glutamic acid decarboxylase, but could also be a heat shock protein.[138, 138a]

Islet Cell Surface Antibodies

With human insulinoma cells as the detection system, islet cell surface antibodies were originally reported to be present in 90% of new-onset IDDM patients.[142] The yield is lower when a rat islet system is used for detection.[143] With human fetal islets almost all newly diagnosed type 1 diabetics are positive.[144] The surface antibodies lyse islets in the presence of complement and impair islet function.[145–148] They bind to, specifically damage, and preferentially lyse beta cells.[149, 150] Thus if any of the islet cell antibodies are responsible for beta cell destruction, it is more likely that surface rather than cytoplasmic antibodies play the critical role. Islet cell cytoplasmic and surface antibodies may be present simultaneously in the same patient, but either can occur alone.[149, 151] Surface antibodies are seldom used for clinical testing because of the difficulties in obtaining viable islet or insulinoma cell preparations on a routine basis and because of the simplicity of tests for cytoplasmic antibodies, which have recently been improved[152] and standardized.[153]

Islet Cell Antibodies and the Natural History of Type 1 Diabetes Mellitus

Table 24–9 shows the approximate prevalence of ICA-cyt in different types of diabetes. The highest percentage is in newly diagnosed type 1 patients, with decreasing prevalence in non–insulin-dependent and gestational diabetes.[122, 154–157] The prevalence of ICA-cyt in first-degree relatives of subjects with type 1 diabetes is six times that in the control population of nondiabetic persons. Islet cell surface antibodies are also present in highest percentage in newly diagnosed young patients with type 1 disease but are likewise found in a significant number of subjects with non–insulin-dependent diabetes.[158]

It was initially claimed that diabetes ultimately develops in nondiabetic subjects who are positive for ICA-cyt[159] and that about 80 to 85% of positive patients with non–insulin-dependent diabetes eventually require insulin therapy, as opposed to only 15% of negative subjects.[122] It is now recognized that type 1 diabetes usually proceeds through the following sequence: prediabetes → impaired glucose tolerance → non–insulin-dependent diabetes → insulin-de-

TABLE 24–9. Prevalence of Islet Cell Cytoplasmic Antibodies*

Population	% Positive
Normal	0.5
New-onset type 1 IDDM	60–90
New-onset nonobese NIDDM	20
Gestational diabetes	10
First-degree relatives of patients with type 1 IDDM	3

*Approximate percentage from a variety of studies in the literature.

pendent diabetes (Fig. 24–6).[160] The appearance of diabetes in discordant monozygotic twins or triplets after long latent periods is in accord with this construct.[161, 162] We now know, however, that progression from ICA-cyt positivity to overt diabetes is not inevitable, especially in adults.[163] ICA-cyt positivity has a greater predictive value in children. Patients with apparent NIDDM who are ICA-cyt–positive usually have type 1 diabetes in slow evolution (subtotal beta cell damage). Antibodies to the 64-kd islet antigen also appear to be highly predictive of diabetes in both children and adults, but the assay is not routinely available.[163]

Cell-Mediated Immunity

The early evidence favoring cell-mediated immune mechanisms in the pathogenesis of type 1 diabetes includes the following: (1) Lymphocytes from children with IDDM adhere to insulinoma cells in coculture, forming rosettes and causing more killing than control lymphocytes.[164] (2) Killer T lymphocyte levels and antibody-dependent cytotoxicity are increased in newly diagnosed type 1 diabetic subjects and in islet cell antibody–positive unaffected children with one or more haplotypes in common with a diabetic sibling.[165] (3) Insulitis is present in islets of acute diabetes of recent

Stages in the Development of Diabetes Mellitus

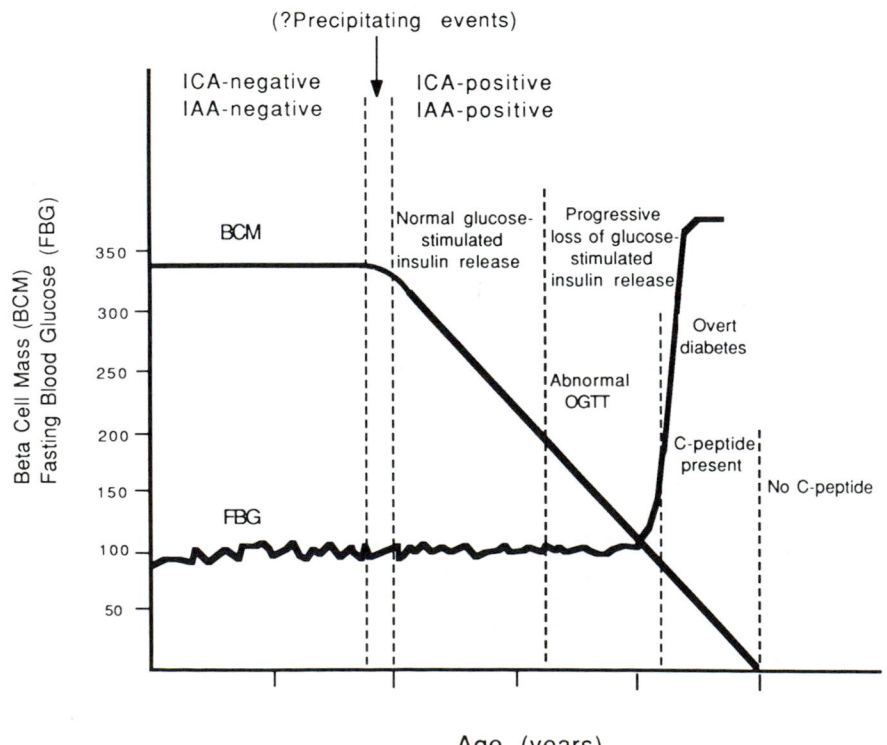

Figure 24–6. Hypothetical depiction of the natural history of autoimmune diabetes. Genetically susceptible people begin their lives without any detectable abnormality. A precipitating event (e.g., viral infection) causing minimal destruction of beta cells is followed by autoimmunity. This is reflected by positive tests for islet cell antibodies (ICA) and insulin autoantibodies (IAA). Although beta cell mass decreases, the functional reserve of beta cells is more than enough to maintain normal glucose levels. Continual injury results in sufficient loss of beta cell mass to cause diminution in glucose-stimulated insulin release and ultimately an abnormal OGTT. As the destruction of beta cells continues, fasting glucose levels will rise above normal but the patient may remain asymptomatic. In the strict sense this is NIDDM, a state that may be relatively short-lived. Then the classic manifestations of IDDM may appear with marked hyperglycemia, glycosuria, and ketonemia, which will culminate in ketoacidosis unless treated. At the onset of this overt phase of the diabetes, C peptide is still present, indicating that some beta cells have survived. Ultimately these will disappear and C peptide levels will become unmeasurable. (Modified from Eisenbarth GS. Type 1 diabetes mellitus. A chronic autoimmune disease. Modified with permission from the New England Journal of Medicine, 314, 1360–1368, 1986.)

onset.[104, 126] Although defective suppressor T lymphocyte function has been reported, the importance of this defect in cell-mediated immunity is not clear.[166]

Subsequent evidence provides further support for the importance of cell-mediated immunity in the pathogenesis of autoimmune destruction of beta cells. In the BB rat the regulatory role of RT6+ cells in preventing spontaneous and adoptively transferred insulitis and diabetes has been demonstrated.[112] Insulitis and diabetes have been adoptively transferred to radiated diabetes-resistant nonobese normal (NON) mice via cells from bone marrow,[167] spleen,[168, 169] and lymph nodes.[170] The transfused spleen cells migrate to the spleen and to immature lymph nodes within 24 h.[171] There they undergo proliferation and maturation before beginning the autoimmune process in the islets on about the fifth day after the transfusion. Adoptive transfer of L3T4+ cells (the murine equivalent of CD4+ helper T cells in humans) will cause insulitis without T cell–induced destruction or diabetes. Both L3T4+ and Lyt2+ T cells (the equivalent of CD8+ cytotoxic T cells in humans) are required for adoptive transfer of the full syndrome.[170, 172, 173]

The identity of the putative K cells is still a matter of controversy. In BB rats cytotoxic T cells are virtually absent; this suggests that natural killer (NK) cells are the predominant cytotoxic cell type in this model.[174] NK cell number and activity are increased in diabetes-prone BB rats.[174, 175] These cells are responsive to activation by interleukin 2 (IL 2) and are thought to be centrally involved in the beta cell destruction.[176] It is not certain that these findings apply to other forms of autoimmune diabetes, however. IL 2, the activator of NK cells secreted by the L3T4+ helper T cells, is reportedly deficient in human type 1 diabetes.[177] Because IL 2

deficiency may be an acquired epiphenomenon related somehow to beta cell destruction (IL 2 deficiency is not present in nondiabetic monozygotic twins of type 1 patients), it remains possible that this lymphokine is important in the autoimmune attack.

Mechanisms of Cellular Killing

Direct killing of beta cells by various cytotoxic lymphocytes can be separated into three phases:[178] (1) effector cell–target cell interaction involving recognition and cell-cell contact between immunocytes and beta cells; (2) effector cell preparation for delivery of the lethal blow; and (3) K cell–independent destruction of target cells.

Two major populations of lymphocytes are involved in killing: cytotoxic T cells and enlarged granular lymphocytes that do not bear the classic T and B cell markers. The latter can be separated into NK cells and K cells.

Most of the T cells utilize alpha and beta chains of their T cell receptor to recognize antigens associated with class I molecules on the target cell (Fig. 24–7); a few recognize target cells through another receptor mechanism that has not yet been identified. K cells recognize targets via binding of their high-affinity Fc receptor to immunoglobulin G antibodies coating the target cells.

After the lymphocytes conjugate with target cells they undergo a series of changes culminating in the secretion of cytolysins present in their granules (Fig. 24–8). The granules congregate at the pole of the cytotoxic cell that is in contact with the target cell and are released by exocytosis. These granules contain pore-forming proteins called *perforins*, which in the presence of Ca^{2+} bind to target cell membranes

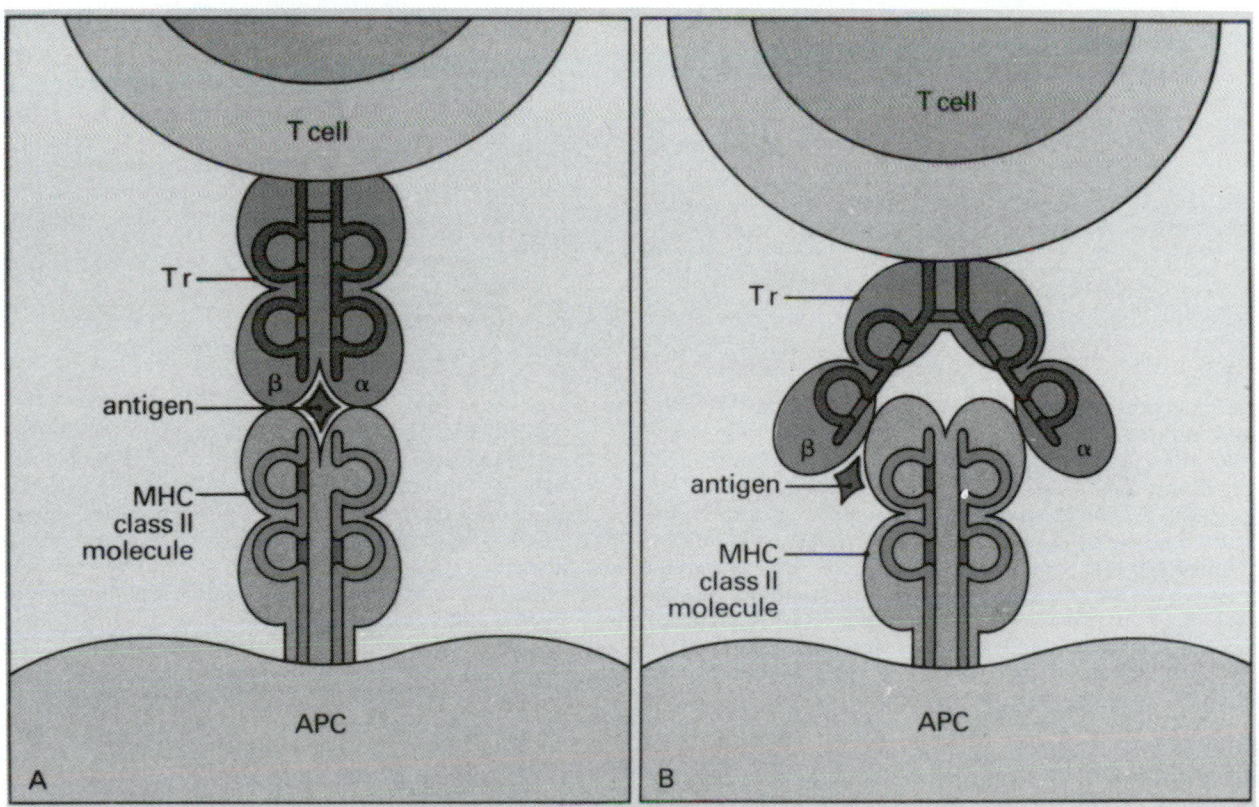

Figure 24–7. Two models depicting the roles of the alpha and beta chains of the T cell receptor in interacting with antigen/MHC. In model *A*, the alpha and beta chains associate to form a single combining site that interacts with antigen and both chains of the class II HLA molecule. In model *B*, a single antigen-binding site is formed by interaction between one chain of the T cell receptor (beta in this case) and one chain of the class II molecule. The other T cell receptor chain (alpha) might interact with the class II molecule to further stabilize the T cell–APC interaction. MHC, major histocompatibility complex; APC, antigen-presenting cell. (From Male D, Champion B, Cooke A. Antigen processing and presentation. In: Advanced Immunology. London: Gower Medical Publishing 1987: 7.1–7.7. Courtesy of Male D, Champion B, and Cooke A and Gower Medical Publishing.)

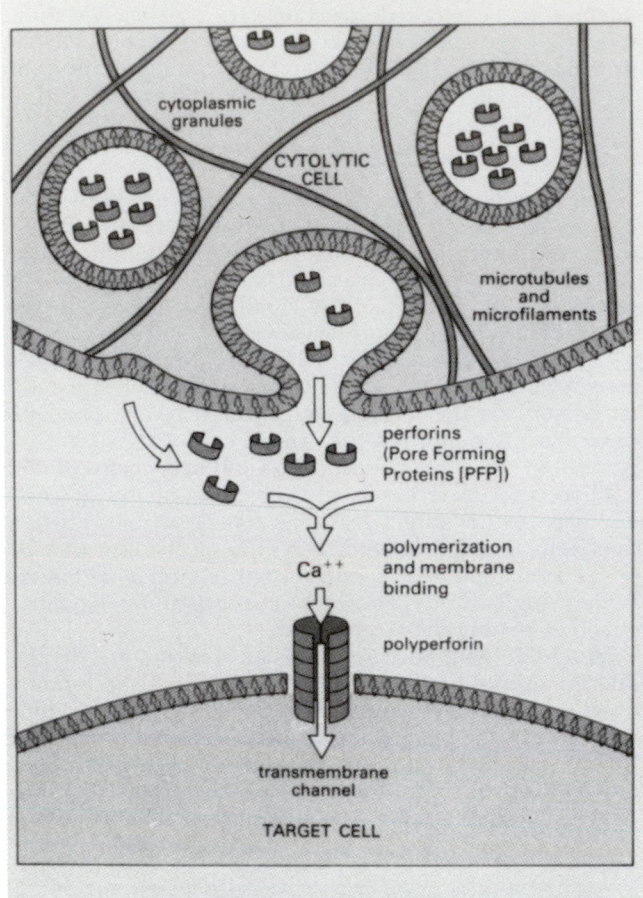

Figure 24–8. Exocytosis of perforins leads to transmembrane channel formation in target cells. Killing of target cells by cytolytic lymphocytes involves the secretion of granule contents into the intercellular environment between the closely apposed effector and target cells. Perforins, monomeric pore-forming proteins, are one of the major constituents of granules; in the presence of Ca^{2+} they bind to the target cell membrane and polymerize to form polyperforins, which are inserted into the membrane to create transmembrane channels. This appears to be essential, although not sufficient, for target cell killing by cytotoxic effector cells. The nature of other mediators is not yet known. (From Male D, Champion B, Cooke A. Cytotoxic cells. In: Advanced Immunology. London: Gower Medical Publishing, 1987: 7.1–7.7. Courtesy of Male D, Champion B, and Cooke A and Gower Medical Publishing.)

and polymerize to form *polyperforins*. Polyperforins are then inserted into the membrane, creating transmembrane channels. At this point other mediators, as yet incompletely identified, proceed with the process of killing. The killing process that occurs through this mechanism differs from that caused by complement. The attack complex of complement initially induces reversible swelling of the cell, which progresses to irreversibility through disruption of the plasma membrane. Cellular cytotoxicity appears to occur via a mechanism called *apoptosis*. The mitochondrial structure is preserved but the cell forms blebs and ultimately becomes fragmented, forming so-called apoptotic bodies that have intact plasma membranes. These bodies undergo secondary necrosis.[178, 179]

In addition to direct killing by cell-cell contact, indirect killing can be caused by cytotoxic substances released from lymphocytes and macrophages. Resident macrophages are normally present in the tissues surrounding the islets, but these are ED2$^+$ cells considered to be only weakly responsive to immunogenic stimuli. A few weeks before the onset of

diabetes there is recruitment of ED1$^+$ macrophages, which aggregate at periductal and perivascular locations adjacent to noninfiltrated islets.[180] Infiltration of islets by ED1$^+$ macrophages is a very early event. It has been demonstrated that at least two macrophage-produced peptide hormones, interleukin 1 (IL 1) and tumor necrosis factor α (TNF-α), have destructive effects on beta cells. IL 1 is a selective beta cell cytotoxin that is effective in picomolar concentrations.[181, 182] Its effects on beta cells are potentiated by TNF-α.[183, 184] How IL 1 kills beta cells and how its action is potentiated by TNF-α are not known. Interestingly, the effects of IL 1 on isolated islets in vitro are bimodal. At very low concentrations pre-proinsulin messenger RNA (mRNA) production and proinsulin biosynthesis are stimulated and glucose-induced insulin secretion is potentiated,[185] whereas at higher concentrations these functions are inhibited and cytotoxicity occurs.[186]

It has been postulated that all of the IL 1 effects on beta cells are mediated by oxygen-derived free radicals.[187] Beta cells are exquisitely sensitive to free radicals and have the lowest free radical scavenger potential of any cell in the body.[188–191] Superoxide anions, hydrogen peroxide, and hydroxyl radicals are produced intracellularly during electron transfer in the respiratory chain but may also arise from other mechanisms. Normally they are scavenged by antioxidant mechanisms. When production of free radicals exceeds the capacity of the antioxidant defenses, disorganization of intracellular enzymes and membranes will result. The defense consists of a team of enzymes: superoxide dismutase, catalase, and glutathione peroxidase. High levels of superoxide, whether they result from increased production or decreased enzymatic scavenging, will result in cessation of growth, mutagenesis, and cell death (see ref. 192 for review). The damage to the DNA caused by the oxidants activates poly(ADP ribose) synthetase, which depletes NAD by converting it to nicotinamide in the course of ADP-ribosylation.[191] Nicotinamide treatment presumably prevents autoimmune diabetes in rodents by repleting NAD.[189] The hydroxyl radical may be important because hydroxyl scavengers can prevent diabetes induced by alloxan injection.[193] It must be emphasized, however, that there is no evidence that oxygen toxicity is operative in spontaneous human autoimmune diabetes.

Aberrant Expression of Class II Molecules as a Cause of Type 1 Diabetes: Status of the Controversy

In 1983 it was reported that normal human thyroid cells in tissue culture can express HLA class II molecules after stimulation with mitogens.[194] Normally class II molecules are present only on certain cells of the immune system. This quickly led Bottazzo and co-workers to propose the concept of aberrant HLA-DR expression and antigen presentation by endocrine cells as a factor in endocrine autoimmunity.[47, 183, 195] Soon thereafter, the death of a child in ketoacidotic coma made it possible to study in a relatively fresh condition the pancreas of a patient with new-onset autoimmune diabetes.[196] Class II molecule expression was found on insulin-containing cells but not on other endocrine or exocrine cells. In addition, levels of class I molecules, which are normally expressed in virtually all nucleated cells, including beta cells, were markedly increased in this specimen. Subsequent examination of other pancreata appears to have confirmed the original report.[197] The intriguing hypothesis that emerged from these observations was that the antigen-presenting function, which normally belongs to the macrophage lineage of cells, could be usurped by beta cells, which could then process antigens, whether exogenously or endogenously derived, and present them to helper T lymphocytes. Even more provocative was the reported presence on beta cells of type 1 diabetic patients of immunoreactive interferon-α (IFN-α).[198] If confirmed, this might provide an explanation for the hyperexpression of class I molecules, which IFN-α could induce. The in vitro induction of class II molecule expression in cultured beta cells from human pancreas occurs in the presence of interferon-γ (IFN-γ) plus tumor necrosis factor β (TNF-β; lymphotoxin).[199] IFN-γ alone is not sufficient.[200]

A number of more recent developments have tended to challenge this provocative hypothesis. First, it has been suggested that the DR-expressing insulin-containing cells observed in vivo are not beta cells but are macrophages that have engulfed insulin granules.[201] In the islets of NOD mice class II expression by endocrine cells was not observed at any age, whereas about 30% of mononuclear cells infiltrating the islets were class II-positive. Similar conclusions have been reached by others.[202] Second, transgenic technology has been employed to produce mice that express class II molecules on beta cells. This was done by constructing a transgene containing the gene for class II molecules linked to the insulin promoter.[203, 204] All of these mice developed diabetes but none exhibited any evidence of insulitis or autoimmune destruction of beta cells. When a class I MHC gene was linked to the insulin promoter, causing overexpression of class I molecules in beta cells, mice also developed a nonautoimmune form of diabetes.[205] Perhaps beta cell dysfunction and even death may result from aberrant overexpression of a foreign protein, which in contrast to insulin is not secreted and therefore accumulates in large quantities within the beta cell, impairing cellular function. The failure of these transgenic mice to develop autoimmune diabetes strongly suggests that aberrant expression of DR molecules cannot in and of itself cause autoimmune destruction of beta cells, at least in mice. It has also been demonstrated in transgenic mice that expression of class II molecules on beta cells does not endow them with an antigen-presenting function that could be responsible for autoimmunity.[206] In fact, expression of class II molecules on beta cells induced by cytokines released during nonspecific infections might actually prevent initiation of a "bystander" autoimmune reaction.[206]

On the other hand, transgenic mice that express IFN-γ on beta cells do develop an inflammatory disease of the islets that culminates in diabetes.[203] The capillaries in such islets were *addressin*-positive. Addressins constitute a unique endothelial cell recognition system that controls lymphocyte traffic into inflamed tissues.[207] This finding raises the possibility that IFN-γ is a primary or at least early trigger of a cascade that involves the stimulation of IL 1 and TNF-α secretion by macrophages. As was mentioned previously and will be discussed further later, these lymphokines may be responsible for beta cell death.

Despite the difficulties just discussed, the Bottazzo theory remains attractive. Conceptually the sequence would involve viral infection (or some other stimulus) followed by cytokine-induced appearance of class II molecules on the beta cell surface. The mere appearance of D region products would not be sufficient to impart risk; only the appearance of certain alleles (e.g., DQw3.2/DQw8) would be able to activate the immune response. A further necessary element would be a T cell receptor of the proper configuration to recognize the neoantigen. At the time of this writing we believe that the aberrant expression theory is viable but unproved.

A Summary of Current Immunological Information

1. Autoimmune diabetes develops almost exclusively in individuals expressing DR3 and/or DR4 molecules. Susceptibility is most closely linked with two Asp-57–negative DQ beta chain alleles, except in DR4/DR4 homozygotes, in whom the amino acid at position 45 may be critical.

2. Susceptibility phenotypes are necessary but not sufficient to cause the disease.

3. Any sublethal injury to beta cells, whether caused by viruses or by beta-cytotoxic substances, can result in an autoimmune insulitis that results in progressive destruction of beta cells.

4. Although viruses and beta-cytotoxins have been implicated as triggers in autoimmune diabetes of humans, no clear-cut associations have been established to explain the vast majority of cases.

5. Autoimmune diabetes in humans is a slowly progressive disorder that becomes clinically overt only after more than 90% of beta cells have been destroyed; evidence of autoimmunity is present in the form of antibodies to various proteins both in the cytoplasm and on the cell surface of beta cells long before this stage has been reached.

6. Antibodies are generally regarded as markers of the destructive process rather than its cause.

7. Macrophages, T helper lymphocytes, and T cytotoxic/suppressor lymphocytes are present in insulitis, and both helper and cytotoxic/suppressor subsets are required for adoptive transfer of the disease. The evidence is persuasive that the destructive process is cell mediated rather than antibody mediated and that NK cells may play an important role.

8. IL 1 in picomolar concentrations can damage and destroy beta cells in isolated islets without destroying alpha and delta cells. Its effects are greatly potentiated by TNF-α and by stimulation of beta cell secretory activity.

9. Beta cells are exquisitely sensitive to free radicals—perhaps the most sensitive cells in the body. Antioxidant depletion enhances and antioxidant supplementation decreases beta cell destruction in both experimental and spontaneous diabetes of animals.

Working Hypothesis for the Pathogenesis of Autoimmune Diabetes (Fig. 24–9)

A hypothesis that seems plausible is based largely on the work and concepts of Nerup and associates[182] and on the Like-Rossini model of insulitis induced by multiple low-dose streptozocin injections.[106] The autoimmune basis of the latter model, which is sex and strain specific, is suggested by the fact that the insulitis can be passively transferred[208] and prevented by immunosuppression. It probably follows that any beta cell injury, regardless of cause, could theoretically induce in susceptible individuals an autoimmune process that may or may not progress to complete destruction of the beta cell mass. The failure thus far to incriminate definitively any viral or chemical beta-cytotoxic agent as a common factor in autoimmune diabetes could mean that the common injurious factor is not externally derived but rather an internal agent. The internal environment does contain an extremely potent and selective beta cell toxin, IL 1, the toxicity of which is greatly potentiated by TNF-α. These substances are secreted by macrophages, some of which are in permanent residence in normal islets of Langerhans, as in other tissues. It is notable that HLA-DR2–positive individuals who are resistant to autoimmune

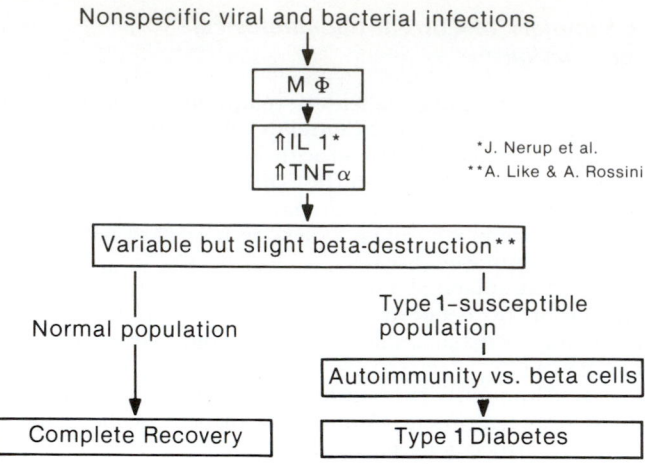

Nonspecific viral and bacterial infections

M Φ

⇑ IL 1*
⇑ TNF α

*J. Nerup et al.
**A. Like & A. Rossini

Variable but slight beta-destruction**

Normal population

Type 1–susceptible population

Autoimmunity vs. beta cells

Complete Recovery

Type 1 Diabetes

Figure 24–9. The lymphokine hypothesis for the pathogenesis of type 1 diabetes. In response to nonspecific infections macrophages release IL 1 and TNF α, which exert a streptozocin-like action on beta cells. The resulting destruction of beta cells is slight and is followed in the normal population by complete recovery without any evidence of impaired beta cell function. In genetically susceptible individuals, an autoimmune process is initiated. The final common pathway involved in beta cell death is thought by some to be the generation of toxic oxygen radicals. Beta cell death can presumably be prevented through the activity of superoxide dismutase, chemical antioxidants, scavenging molecules, or stimulation of DNA repair with nicotinamide.

diabetes are low secretors of TNF-α,[209] the gene for which is located in the HLA region of chromosome 6.[210]

Secretion of IL 1 and TNF by macrophages is currently thought to require MHC-restricted activation of T helper lymphocytes via IFN-γ. Their production may be limited to a specific tissue. However, during stressful events such as viral infections, endotoxin-producing bacterial infections, and trauma there may be an increase in IL 1 and TNF-α in the systemic circulation.[211] In normal persons beta cells may be intermittently damaged or destroyed by repeated transient elevations of these circulating beta-cytotoxins but an autoimmune response is not elicited and the lost beta cells are quickly replaced via the remarkable compensatory capability of the islets of Langerhans. In susceptible individuals, however, these multiple episodes of relatively minor beta cell injury incite an autoimmune response that results in progressive loss of beta cells at a rate exceeding the replacement capacity (see Fig. 24–9). By bypassing the requirement for an injurious factor in the external environment, this as-yet unproven hypothesis would accommodate all known features of type 1 diabetes.

Prevention of Autoimmune Diabetes

The criteria for preventability of a disease are listed in Table 24–10. Type 1 diabetes qualifies with respect to the first four criteria. First, it has been unequivocally identified as an autoimmune process, even though the specific envi-

TABLE 24–10. Criteria of Disease Preventability

The type of disease process, if not the actual cause, must be known.

High-risk groups must be identifiable.

The preovert phase (the time between the onset of the process and the onset of overt disease) must be sufficiently long to provide time for diagnosis and treatment.

There must be clinical tests to diagnose and track the preovert destructive process.

There must be an effective intervention with a low risk/reward ratio.

TABLE 24–11. Strategies for Preventing Type 1 Diabetes

Blocking antigen presentation	Blocking effector cells
Anti–class II monoclonal antibodies	Monoclonal antibody
Macrophage depletion with silica	Cyclosporine-like agents
Blocking antigen recognition	Inducing tolerance
Lymphocytic choriomeningitis virus	
Anti-CD4 monoclonal antibodies	Selective clonal deletion

ronmental factors, if any, have yet to be identified. Second, the maximal-risk groups are identifiable. (However, maximal risk is probably still extremely low, even among the homozygous DQ beta, Asp-57–negative, DR3/DR4 population. A random prediabetes screening effort among schoolchildren intended to prevent overt diabetes would require testing for islet cell antibodies as well as for susceptibility.) Third, the time between the onset of beta cell destruction and the onset of clinically overt diabetes is now thought to average 3 y or more, which is ample for diagnosis and intervention. Fourth, there are immunological and functional tests that permit meaningful tracking of the immunological process and its effects on beta cell function. Tests for ICA-cyt and insulin autoantibodies are suitable procedures for most clinical laboratories, as are functional tests of glucose-stimulated insulin secretion.

Unfortunately, however, there is as yet no known effective risk-free intervention that can be justified for use in otherwise normal healthy children. Cyclosporine might be effective if administered before most of the beta cells were destroyed, inasmuch as it prevents autoimmune diabetes in rodents[212, 213] and may reverse clinical diabetes in humans if given within 1 mo of the onset of symptoms.[114] However, because of cyclosporine-related nephropathy and the fact that at present there are no clear-cut criteria for establishing the inevitability of overt diabetes, one cannot at this point justify an intervention that would entail a significant risk.

Strategies for Preventing Autoimmune Diabetes (Table 24–11)

The advances summarized in the preceding pages provide reason for hope that a safe and effective means of intervention may not be far away. If one accepts the working hypothesis that has been outlined for the pathogenesis of diabetes, the disease could be prevented by intervention at one or more of the three loci (environment, autoimmunity, final common pathway) portrayed in Figure 24–5.

PREVENTING THE INITIAL INJURY. Intervention at the level of the external environment to prevent beta cell injury is not realistic because of the uncertainty that any single viral or chemical agent is an important factor in most human diabetes. If the lymphokine hypothesis is correct, prevention of injury by macrophage-derived IL 1 (and/or other cytokines) is theoretically possible but probably impractical in humans. This approach has been used effectively in BB rats[214] and NOD mice.[215] Intraperitoneal injections of silica, which is selectively toxic to macrophages that infiltrate the islets at the early stage of insulitis, completely prevent development of diabetes. The salutary effect of antimacrophage treatment could, of course, have been due to interference with antigen presentation by the macrophages rather than prevention of cytokine-mediated damage. Even if possible, macrophage depletion might result in an unacceptable immunological deficit.

PREVENTING ANTIGEN PRESENTATION. Intervention at the level of antigen presentation can be accomplished either by eliminating the macrophages as just described or by using monoclonal antibodies to react with the class II molecules that present antigens.[216] A more selective potential strategy would involve administration of a nonimmunogenic peptide that is homologous with a portion of the beta cell antigen and would therefore compete with the natural antigen for binding in the cleft of the class II molecule.[217] The problem with this approach is that the antigen (or antigens) of type 1 diabetes has not been identified, although a leading candidate is the 64-kd islet glutamic acid decarboxylase previously mentioned.[138]

PREVENTING ANTIGEN RECOGNITION OR AUTOIMMUNE EFFECTOR FUNCTION. At a level of antigen recognition by helper T cells, administration of monoclonal antibodies against the L3T4 determinant (equivalent to CD4-bearing helper cells in humans) effectively prevents autoimmune diabetes in NOD mice.[218, 219] After a course of treatment, antibody therapy can be discontinued without the subsequent appearance of diabetes. Interestingly, infection of NOD mice with lymphocytic choriomeningitis virus reduces the incidence of diabetes by attacking the T helper subset of L3T4+ cells.[220] Inhibition of macrophage function

with silica, as previously mentioned, may prevent antigen presentation and initiation of the autoimmune process.[221] Antibodies against cytotoxic T cells or NK cells are effective in preventing diabetes in rodents.[221, 223] An antibody against asialo-GM$_1$ ganglioside that depletes NK cell activity in the peripheral blood also protects.[224] Blockade of IL 2 and/or interferon-induced activation of NK cells might also serve to block effector function.[225]

BLOCKADE OF FINAL COMMON PATHWAY (Fig. 24–10). Finally, blockade of the so-called final common pathway by administration of antioxidants to prevent free radical–induced damage is an area of potential interest. Such measures have proved effective in preventing both autoimmune islet damage in mice and destruction of islet allografts.[189, 226]

OTHER INTERVENTIONS. A streptococcal preparation (OK-432) suppresses anti-islet autoimmunity and prevents diabetes in NOD mice[227] and BB rats,[228] apparently without immunosuppression. It is unlikely that this preparation will be used in humans. Theoretically, the induction of immune tolerance to the principal antigens of the beta cells might

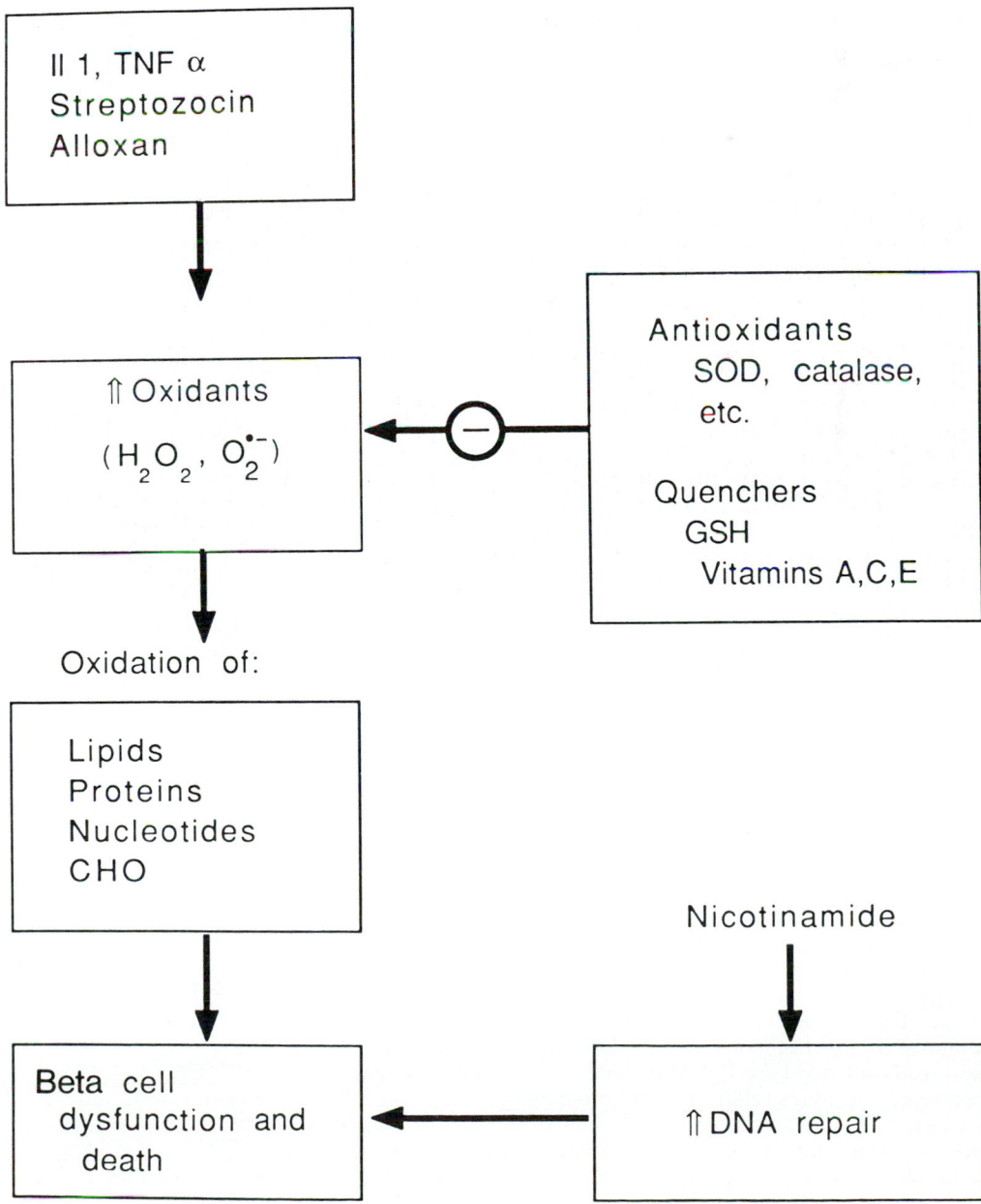

Figure 24–10. The "final common pathway" of beta cell destruction refers to the hypothesis that beta-cytotoxic events involve the same mechanism, i.e., macromolecular damage resulting from an increase in the level of oxidants (H_2O_2, $O_2^{\bullet-}$) relative to antioxidants (superoxide dismutase [SOD], catalase, glutathione peroxidase) and quenchers such as glutathione (GSH) and vitamins A, C, and E. The basis for this idea is the fact that antioxidants are capable of preventing beta cell damage resulting from the administration of streptozocin or alloxan to animals. Oxidants are also thought to mediate damage to cells resulting from autoimmunity and rejection. See also Figure 24–5. Nicotinamide is thought to protect beta cells by repleting NAD, which is reduced by the increased poly(ADP ribose) synthetase activity required for repair of DNA breakage caused by the free radicals.

TABLE 24–12. Comparison of Pancreatic Weight and Mass of Endocrine Cells at Autopsy

	Total Pancreatic Weight (Mean and Range) (g)	Weight of Pancreatic Endocrine Component (mg)	Total Mass of Endocrine Cells (mg)				Alpha/Beta Ratio
			Beta	Alpha	Delta	Pancreatic Polypeptide	
Normals	82 (67–110)	1395	850	225	125	190	0.26
Type 1 IDDM	40 (26–51)	413	0	150	90	185	∞
Type 2 NIDDM	73 (55–100)	1449	825	375	100	180	0.45

Data from Rahier J, et al. Cellular composition of the human diabetic pancreas. Diabetologia 1983; 24:366–371. Mass of endocrine cells was estimated from Figure 3 of the cited reference and should be considered approximate.

prevent the disease in susceptible persons. Alternatively, destroying specific helper T cell clones by presenting the key beta cell antigen(s) coupled to a toxic substance such as ricin might arrest the autoimmune attack once it had begun. Both of the interventions must await the identification of the important antigen(s) involved in this disease.

Pathology of the Islets of Langerhans in Type 1 Insulin-Dependent Diabetes Mellitus

Early Pathology

Acute insulitis, the infiltration of the pancreatic islets of type 1 IDDM patients by lymphocytes and macrophages, was first described in 1910.[229] It was subsequently reported that two thirds of diabetics studied at autopsy within 6 mo after the initial symptoms of IDDM exhibited the lesion.[104] Lymphocytes were largely confined to the 10% of islets with surviving beta cells and were absent in islets of long-standing IDDM. Lymphocytic infiltration of the pancreas in type 1 IDDM has been demonstrated noninvasively using radiolabeled lymphocytes and scanning techniques.[230] It has been suggested that insulitis is secondary to subtotal islet injury rather than its cause.[231] This conclusion is based on the observations that beta cell volume decreases before the development of insulitis[231] and that islet damage can occur after treatment with low-dose streptozocin in thymectomized, T lymphocyte–depleted mice without lymphocytic infiltration of the beta cell areas.[232] Whether these findings apply to human diabetes is not known.

Focal regeneration of beta cells is observed soon after the onset of diabetes[126] but occurs less frequently as the disease progresses. The hydropic changes in beta cells described in the preinsulin era are seen today only in the rare untreated patient.

Late Pathology

The reduction in pancreatic weight in type 1 diabetic subjects studied at autopsy 1.5 to 34 y after diagnosis (Table 24–12)[233] is the consequence of atrophy of exocrine tissue, which constitutes about 98% of the normal pancreas. The atrophy may result from loss of the high levels of insulin that normally perfuse the acinar tissue via the pancreatic vasculature.[234, 235] These high intrapancreatic concentrations of insulin may exert a tropic effect on acini that is not attained by subcutaneous insulin therapy. Thus, no matter how well controlled the IDDM patient, the exocrine pancreas remains at all times relatively insulin deficient.

The islets in IDDM are fewer and often smaller than normal, weighing in total less than one third of those of nondiabetic controls or patients with type 2 NIDDM.[233] Beta cells are virtually absent. The islets consist almost entirely of cells that secrete glucagon (alpha) and somatostatin (delta) and, in the dorsal part of the head of the pancreas, pancreatic polypeptide (PP or F cells) (Fig. 24–11). The normal islet architecture with its nonrandom arrangement of the islet cell types is lost.[125] Because insulin, glucagon, and somatostatin each exerts major effects on various islet cells (Table 24–13), the architectural disruption may have profound functional consequences. The number of alpha and delta cells per islet is normal or increased,[125] and the total alpha and delta cell mass per pancreas is within the normal range.[236]

GENETICS AND ETIOLOGY OF TYPE 2 NON–INSULIN-DEPENDENT DIABETES MELLITUS

Demography

Prevalence

NIDDM is the most common of the hyperglycemic states. The disease exists in all populations, but prevalence varies greatly, e.g., 1% in Japan,[237] 34% in the Micronesians of Nauru,[21, 238] and greater than 40% in the Pima Indians of Arizona.[6] In whites the figure is probably between 1 and 2%, using modern criteria for the definition of diabetes.[239] The high prevalence of NIDDM among Nauruans and Pimas appears to be a relatively recent development that followed a change in the pattern of food intake from one of chronic caloric deprivation, in which both obesity and diabetes were rare, to one of caloric abundance, in which both abnormalities are common. A similar phenomenon (usually called urbanization) has been described in other American Indian tribes,[20] Pacific Islanders,[21] Australian aboriginals,[240] and Asiatic Indian groups.[241] Presumably the changes in lifestyle that accompany urbanization result in obesity, which facilitates expression of a predisposition for NIDDM.[21] The urbanization phenomenon has been most carefully studied in nonwhite groups, but it is probably ethnically and racially nonspecific.

TABLE 24–13. Effects of Islet Hormones on Secretion by Islet Cells*

Hormone	Alpha Cells	Beta Cells	Delta Cells	Pancreatic Polypeptide Cells
Glucagon	—	↑	↑	?
Insulin	↓	↓	↓ ?	↓ ?
Somatostatin	↓	↓	↓	↓

*Key: increase ↑ ; decrease ↓ ; no effect — .

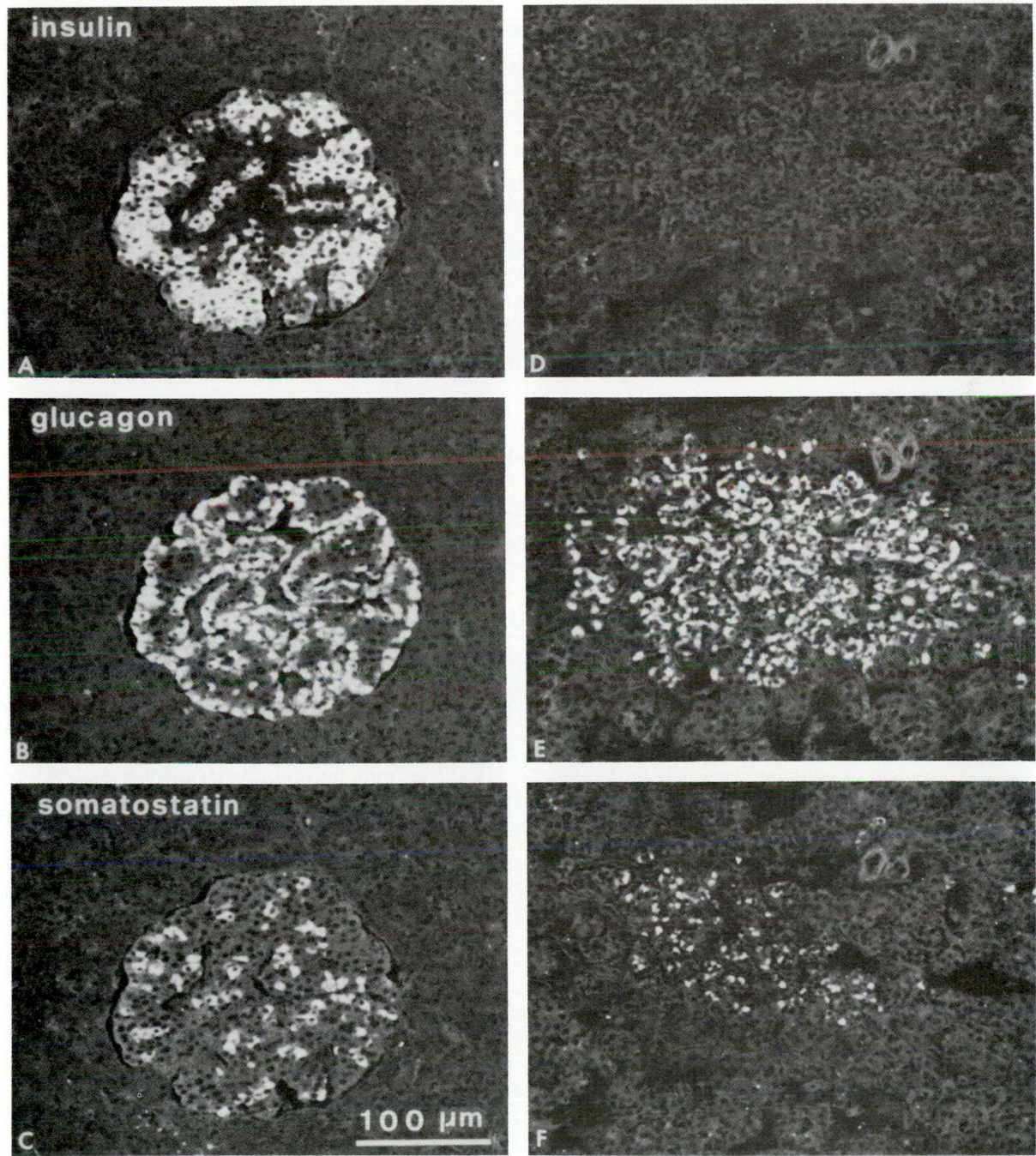

Figure 24–11. Consecutive serial sections of an islet from the tail of the normal human pancreas *(A–C)* and an islet from the tail of the pancreas of a patient with type 1 diabetes mellitus of 5 y duration *(D–F)* treated for immunofluorescence with anti-insulin, antiglucagon, and antisomatostatin antisera. In the diabetic islet there are no insulin-containing cells but there are numerous glucagon- and somatostatin-containing cells, which have lost their normal distribution pattern and appear scattered throughout the islets. (Courtesy of L. Orci.)

Incidence

Few reliable studies of the incidence of NIDDM are available. The Pima Indians have an appearance rate of 2650 cases per 100,000 population per year, the highest in the world.[242] This value is approximately 20 times that in whites (134 per 100,000 per year).[242] In Rochester, Minnesota, the incidence in whites was 158 per 100,000 per year in men and 113 per 100,000 per year in women.

Family Studies

Familial aggregation of type 2 NIDDM is very common, in contrast to type 1 IDDM. Thirty-eight percent of siblings and one third of the offspring of individuals with NIDDM exhibit diabetes or abnormal glucose tolerance.[243, 244] The percentage of affected siblings varies inversely with the obesity of the proband.[243] Concordance for identical twins for type 2 NIDDM has been reported to be 90 to 100%,[38, 245] compared with 50% or less in type 1 IDDM. The National Heart, Lung and Blood Institute study of 250 monozygotic twins[246] reported that 58% of co-twins of type 2 diabetic patients were diabetic but only 1 of 15 originally discordant co-twins remained nondiabetic during a 10-y interval.

Genetics

HLA and Type 2 NIDDM

There is no association between HLA and NIDDM in whites, although HLA-A2 levels are significantly higher in diabetic Pima Indians[247] and in South African Xhosas[248] than in nondiabetic controls from the same population. Because the frequency of the A2 allele in the general population is high, a relationship to NIDDM is doubtful.

Linkage with Other Genes

The structural gene for insulin, located on the short arm of chromosome 11 in humans, contains a 5'-flanking region that is polymorphic with respect to the number and arrangement of a family of tandemly repeated nucleotides beginning 363 base pairs upstream from the transcription site.[249] Homozygosity for a long (>1500 base pairs) fragment was initially reported to be associated with susceptibility to type 2 NIDDM.[250–252] However, subsequent studies have failed to confirm the relationship.[253, 254]

Restriction fragment length polymorphism in the insulin receptor gene has been reported in 12 of 51 NIDDM subjects but in only 4 of 52 nondiabetic control subjects.[255] The nondiabetic subjects with the polymorphism were found to have hyperinsulinemia and/or a nondiagnostic glucose tolerance, implying an association between an insulin receptor gene polymorphism and insulin resistance.[255] If confirmed, this observation might be relevant to the report of defective insulin receptor tyrosine kinase activity in human skeletal muscle from obese and type 2 diabetic subjects[256] and to the apparent familial aggregation of in vivo insulin resistance in Pima Indian families.[257]

Finally, an association has been reported among NIDDM, Rh blood group, and haptoglobin phenotype. A single dose of the haptoglobin 1 allele was associated with an approximately 50% increase in the prevalence of NIDDM and a double dose of this allele with a 100% increase. This raises the possibility of a linkage disequilibrium between the haptoglobin gene and a putative susceptibility gene for NIDDM.[258]

Chlorpropamide-Alcohol Flush

Chlorpropamide-primed alcohol-induced flushing has been proposed as a genetic marker for certain types of NIDDM.[259] This phenomenon has been reported to be present in 38% of patients with NIDDM and 87% of patients with maturity-onset diabetes in the young (MODY) compared with 10% of controls.[260] The flush consists of redness of the face and neck, a sense of warmth or burning, and a more intense and prolonged rise in facial skin temperature than occurs in controls. It is blocked by naloxone[260] and by indomethacin and aspirin,[261, 262] implying a mediating role for endogenous opioids and prostaglandins in the phenomenon. Acetaldehyde levels rise during flushing,[263, 264] suggesting a chlorpropamide-induced block of acetaldehyde dehydrogenase activity.[265] The significance of the chlorpropamide-alcohol flush is not established, some laboratories confirming[266] and others failing to confirm[267, 268] the original findings. Evidence against the flush as a marker for a specific genetic subset of type 2 NIDDM comes from the observation that administration of chlorpropamide for 1 wk converted negative responders to positive responders regardless of whether the type of diabetes was IDDM or NIDDM.[268]

Inheritance

The mode of inheritance in the common form of type 2 NIDDM is unknown. If the mechanism were autosomal recessive, 100% of offspring of conjugal diabetics would become diabetic. This is not the case,[269] although in one study all such offspring over age 50 were reported to have a diabetic oral glucose tolerance test.[270] Recessive inheritance with low penetrance is unlikely because concordance in monozygotic twins is close to 100%. Inheritance must, therefore, be multifactorial.[270]

Inheritance in one form of NIDDM, MODY, is known to be autosomal dominant.[271, 272] It is the only form of diabetes in which the mechanism of transmission is clear. The clinical syndrome is usually mild, and many affected individuals are asymptomatic.[272] Most are not obese. Late degenerative complications are perhaps less common than in other forms of diabetes but do occur.[273] There are no associations with HLA[274] or with polymorphic sequences in DNA near the insulin gene.[275] Heterogeneity may exist in MODY because the insulin response to glucose is low in some patients and high in others.[273]

Is There Heterogeneity Within Ordinary Type 2 NIDDM?

The premise that all obese and nonobese patients with type 2 NIDDM have variants of the same disorder is now being questioned. As discussed, some lean NIDDM patients seem pathophysiologically and perhaps etiologically closer to those with type 1 IDDM than to those with obese type 2 NIDDM (Table 24–14). They tend to be hypoinsulinemic rather than hyperinsulinemic, and, as in type 1 IDDM patients, their exaggerated glucagon response to an arginine infusion[276] or to a protein meal[277] is reduced by appropriate insulin administration.[278] In contrast, obese type 2 IDDM subjects appear to be less sensitive to insulin-mediated improvement in glucagon response to these signals.[276, 277] The 20% of NIDDM patients who are positive for islet cell antibodies at the time of diagnosis (see Table 24–9) could represent a form of type 1 autoimmune insulopathy in which beta cell destruction is incomplete,[279] as mentioned earlier. Despite initial responsiveness to oral hypoglycemic drugs, these patients ultimately require insulin treatment.[154] It

TABLE 24–14. Possible Heterogeneity in Non–Insulin-Dependent Diabetes: Functional Characteristics

Characteristic	Type 1 IDDM	Nonobese NIDDM (Type 1 Subset)*	Obese NIDDM (Type 2 Subset)*
Cytoplasmic islet cell antibodies	Positive	Positive	Negative
Insulin and C peptide in plasma	Absent or very low	Low	High
Glucagon in plasma	Relative or absolute elevation	Relative or absolute elevation	Relative elevation
Effect of insulin on abnormal alpha cell response to arginine	Corrected	Corrected	Not corrected

*Non–insulin dependent diabetes is considered to have two subsets, one (largely nonobese) progressing to type 1 IDDM and the other (largely obese) remaining non–insulin dependent. See text for additional details.

seems likely that NIDDM, as currently classified, is heterogeneous, with some of the nonobese patients probably representing type 1 diabetes in slow evolution without complete beta cell destruction.

Environmental-Genetic Interactions

Despite the powerful genetic influence indicated by the nearly 100% concordance rate in monozygotic twins with NIDDM, environment also plays a role in pathogenesis (for reviews, see refs. 280 and 281). This is best illustrated by the effects of urbanization on the prevalence of diabetes in populations who previously inhabited rural or underdeveloped areas.[280] Presumably the major factor is greater food availability, which in turn permits obesity to develop.[20, 21] As discussed subsequently, obesity induces insulin resistance,[282, 283] which, unless adequately compensated for, can convert previously normoglycemic subjects into hyperglycemic patients.[284]

It has been postulated that ready availability of food is necessary but is not the sole requirement for development of obesity in NIDDM. The term "thrifty gene" was introduced to describe a condition of efficient metabolism that evolved in certain populations exposed to alternating availability of food.[285, 286] According to this idea, evolution selected for individuals who preferentially utilized food for useful work or energy storage and wasted fewer calories as heat, a distinct advantage in "feast or famine" cycles. Presumably evolutionary pressure for such an adaptation was greatest in hunting-fishing tribes, but it also could have occurred in agrarian peoples under conditions in which the water supply was marginal, as is the case in many parts of the world. The appearance of the putative thrifty gene would induce vulnerability to obesity directly and to diabetes indirectly if food were freely available and freely eaten. Despite the attractiveness of this concept, there is no convincing evidence that thrifty genes exist in humans. The existence of metabolic defects in obesity has been difficult to confirm, as discussed in Chapter 25.

Pathology of the Islets of Langerhans in Non–Insulin-Dependent Diabetes Mellitus

Endocrine Cell Composition

The islet cell mass is not reduced in patients with NIDDM (see Table 24–12),[233] although earlier studies had suggested otherwise.[287] The content of glucagon-producing alpha cells is increased while the beta cell mass is normal in size.[236] The ratio of alpha to beta cells in type 2 patients is twice that in controls (see Table 24–12). In the forms of NIDDM that were designated type 1 NIDDM in our classification, the changes in the islets might resemble those found in early type 1 IDDM.

Amyloid and Amylin

Pancreatic islet deposits of amyloid are found frequently in type 2 diabetic patients but only rarely in matched controls.[288] The amyloid is deposited between the endocrine cells and the capillaries, often penetrating into plasma membrane invaginations of beta cells. Analysis of insular amyloid led to the discovery of a 37-amino-acid peptide, known variously as diabetes-associated peptide, islet-amyloid polypeptide or amylin. Amylin, which is derived from an 89-amino-acid precursor,[289] has major homology with calcitonin gene–related peptide.[290, 291] In normal islets amylin is copackaged with insulin in beta cell granules.[292] However, in type 2 diabetic patients amyloid is deposited outside beta cells. The fact that amylin is expressed in normal human and rat islets (Fig. 24–12)[289, 291] and copackaged with insulin suggests that it must be cosecreted with insulin and may therefore have a hormonal role (Fig. 24–13). Cosecretion has now been demonstrated in perfused rat pancreas. Impairment of amylin secretion accompanies beta cell damage or depletion.[292a] It has been reported that amylin inhibits insulin-stimulated glycogen synthesis in isolated skeletal muscle,[293] which raises the possibility that it may influence the disposition of insulin-mediated glucose metabolism by increasing flux through the Cori cycle. If amylin is oversecreted in type 2 diabetes and accumulates and crowds out beta cells, it would provide a link between the defects in insulin secretion and those in insulin action that coexist in most patients with this form of diabetes.

NORMAL ISLET CELL FUNCTION

Insulin, glucagon, and somatostatin have profound effects on secretion of other islet hormones (see Table 24–13). Because the metabolic abnormalities that characterize diabetes mellitus are hormonally induced, normal islet cell function will be discussed before the changes that induce the diabetic state are outlined.

Interactions of Islet Cell Hormones

Normally, glucagon secretion is suppressed by insulin,[294] even by relatively small increases in its concentration. Conversely, insulin secretion is directly stimulated by small changes in the concentration of glucagon.[295] Minute increments of somatostatin suppress both insulin and glucagon in vitro[296, 297] and in vivo,[298] whereas modest increases of glucagon stimulate somatostatin.[296] These facts and the nonrandom arrangement of the three major types of cells[299] within the normal islets have inspired the concept of a paracrine system by which the three peptides influence neighboring cells via the intervening interstitium.[300] There is, however, evidence against free communication between islet cells via the interstitial spaces. The interstitium sur-

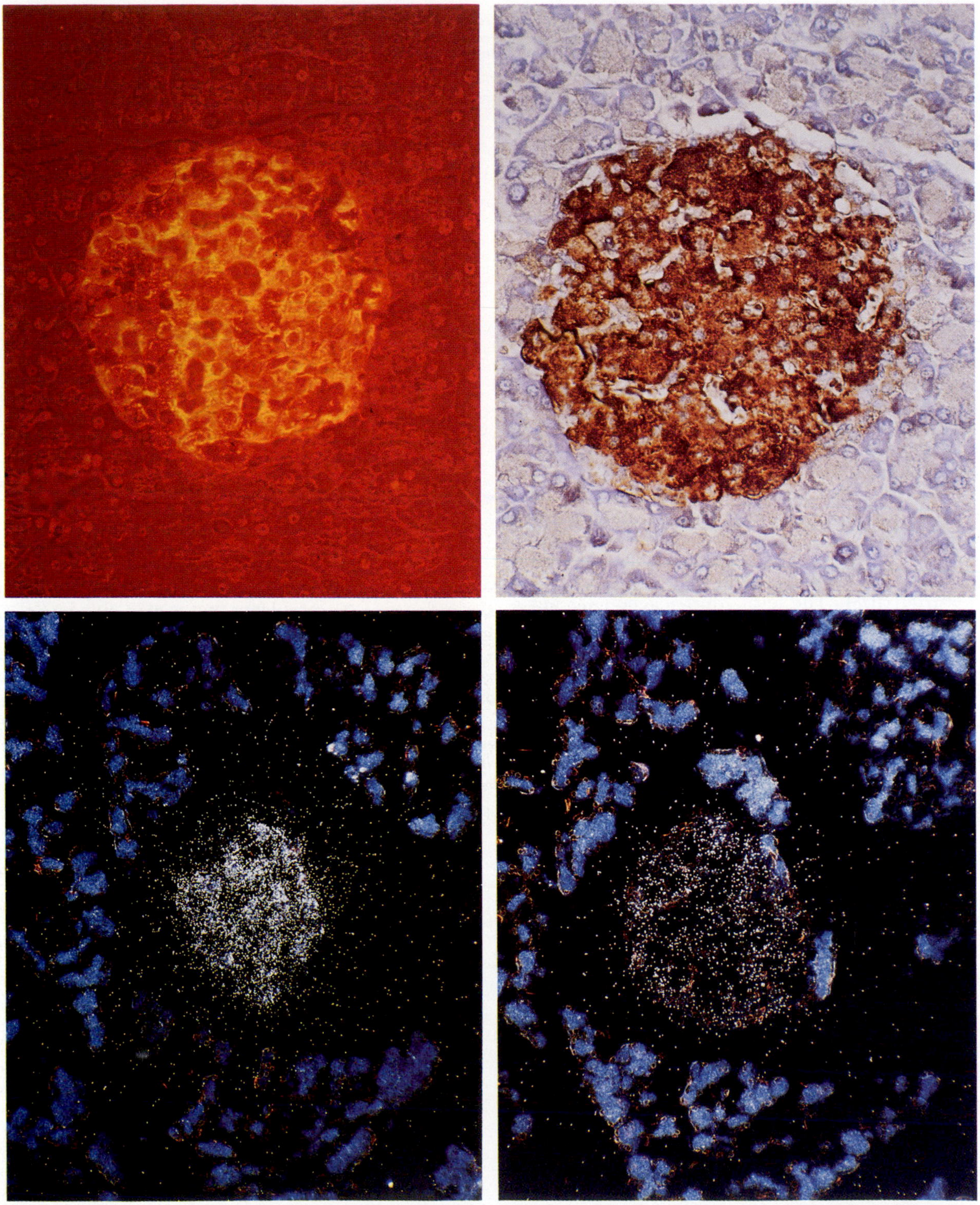

Figure 24–12. Immunofluorescence and rhodamine immunostaining of a normal rat islet for insulin *(upper left)* and amylin *(upper right)* and in situ hybridization of two different islets for proinsulin *(left)* and proamylin *(right)* mRNA. (Courtesy of Drs. Juan Lechago, Ling Chen, and Tausif Alam.)

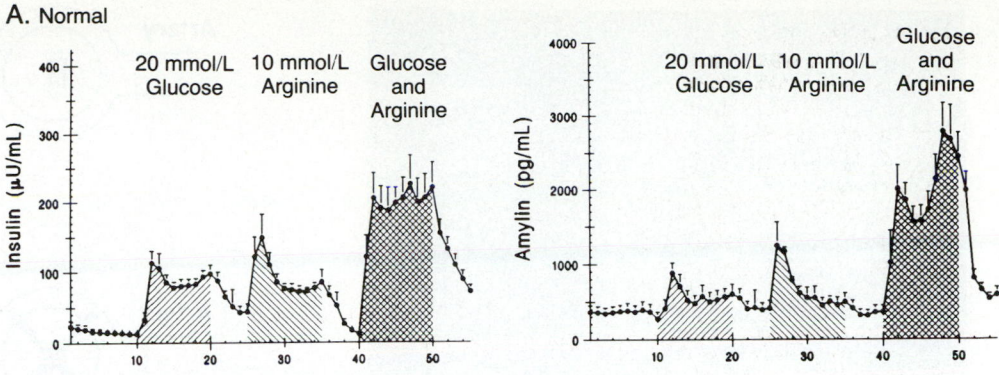

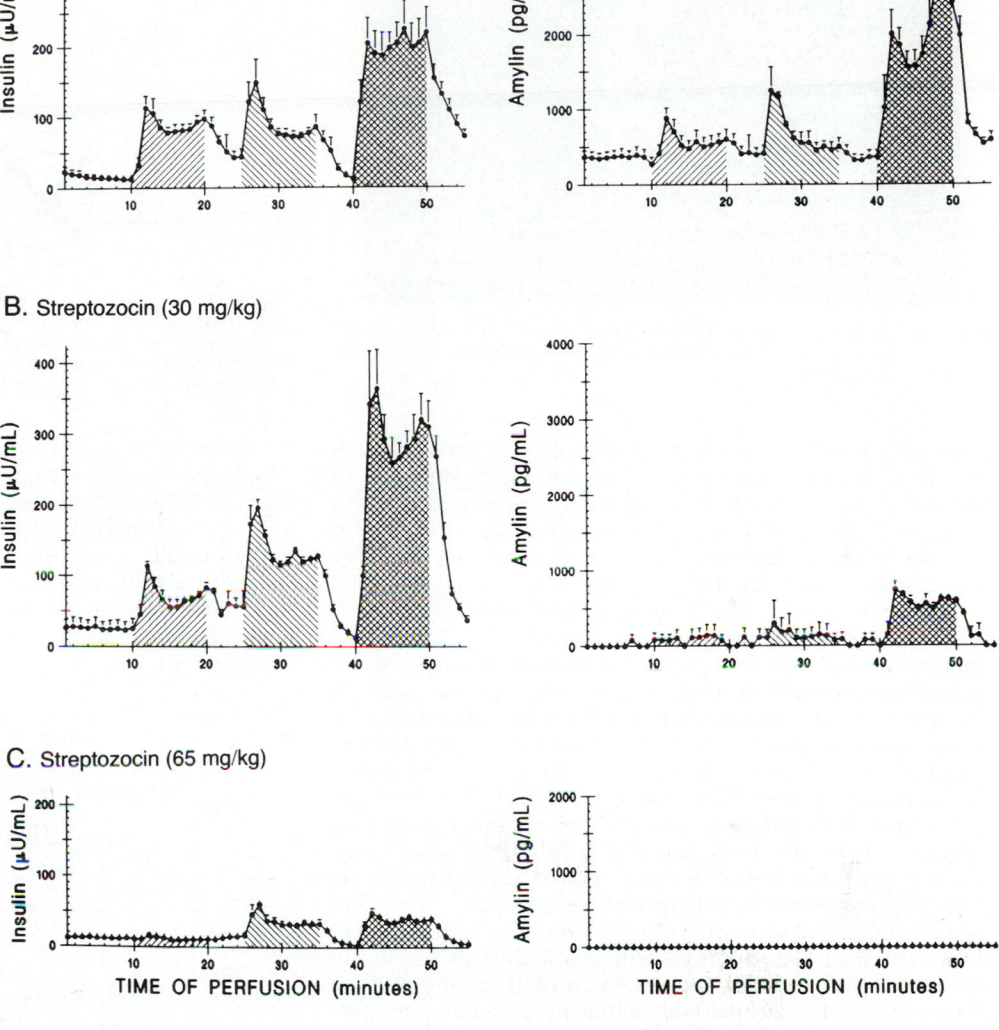

Figure 24–13. Insulin and amylin secretion from isolated, perfused pancreata of normal and streptozocin-treated rats. *A,* Male Wistar rats (n = 6) were anesthetized and the isolated pancreas was perfused with 20 mmol/L glucose, 10 mmol/L arginine, and the combination. Samples were assayed for insulin *(left)* and amylin *(right)*. Male Wistar rats (n = 3) received a single injection of *(B)* 30 mg/kg streptozocin or *(C)* 65 mg/kg streptozocin and after 6 to 10 d the pancreata were perfused to quantitate insulin and amylin secretion. All perfusate samples were analyzed in duplicate and the data represent the mean ± SEM.

rounding the afferent capillaries to the islet cells must be a hormone-poor space to explain the fact that the cells respond to doses of arterially perfused somatostatin that are but a minute fraction of the somatostatin concentration at the secretory pole of the delta cells.[296] Very small increments in arterial insulin[294] concentrations also exert profound effects, so it seems likely that the hormone receptors of islet cells receive communication via the circulation rather than via the interstitium.

Gap junctions are patches of closely arrayed globular proteins called *connexons* (Fig. 24–14), through which intercellular channels connect the cytosol of contiguous cells to one another to form syncytial domains (Fig. 24–15). These channels may provide another mechanism for cell-cell communication by small molecules such as nucleotides or ions.[301, 302] But the major route of within-islet communication between cells may be the local circulation, which appears (in the rat at least) to flow from the beta cell–rich medulla of the islet to the alpha cell–rich cortex (Fig. 24–16).[303] This circulatory arrangement exposes alpha cells (and delta cells) to the highest circulating insulin concentrations in the body and facilitates action of insulin as a release-inhibiting factor for glucagon (Fig. 24–17).[304, 305] The beta cell, on the other

hand, receives systemic blood and is thus exposed to much lower concentrations of glucagon than would be the case if there were direct flow from alpha cell to beta cell.

Islet Cell Hormone Responses in Fuel Regulation

The responses of alpha and beta cells to various stimuli depend on the ambient and antecedent plasma glucose concentrations. The alterations that occur in response to glucose need and glucose abundance will be considered separately.

Glucose Need

Whatever the mechanisms, coordinated secretion of insulin and glucagon vigorously defends against glycemic fluctuations below or above the normal range (for a review, see ref. 306). Maintenance of glucose constancy can be considered a vital function of the islets, with defense against hypoglycemia its most critical mission. This follows from the fact that in the nonketotic state the energy needs of the brain can be met only by glucose; the absence of glucose

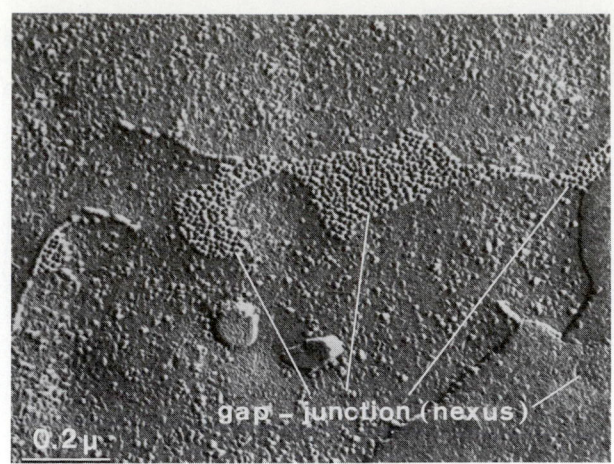

Figure 24–14. A freeze-fracture electron photomicrograph showing a gap junction, an aggregation of intramembranous particles or connexons (see also Fig. 24–15). (Courtesy of L. Orci.)

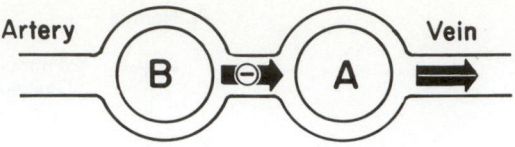

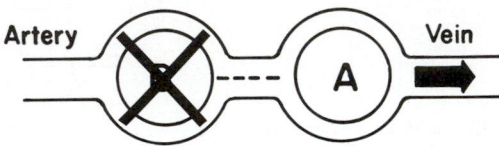

Figure 24–16. Schematic representation of blood flow from beta cell to alpha cell. Locally secreted insulin would restrain glucagon release as indicated by the minus sign *(top)*. Glucagon is presumed to reach the beta cell only through the systemic (not local) circulation. In diabetes, absent or dysfunctional beta cells *(bottom)* would remove this restraint, accounting for hyperglucagonemia.

ultimately results in death of central nervous system tissues. A fall in glucose concentration toward the lower level of normal elicits a prompt fall in insulin concentration and a reciprocal rise in glucagon secretion (Fig. 24–18). Thus if glucose utilization increases from the resting state (Fig. 24–19*a*), as in exercise, the following events occur: (1) glucagon (and catecholamine) levels increase and stimulate hepatic glucose production, primarily via glycogen breakdown; (2) there is a concomitant decrease in insulin secretion, which contributes to the rise in glucagon concentration; and (3) decreased insulin concentration reduces peripheral glucose utilization, potentiates hepatic actions of glucagon, and enhances free fatty acid release from adipocytes.[307] Hypoglycemia is thereby prevented, and glucose delivery to both the brain and the exercising muscles is maintained. A similar decrease in insulin level and rise in glucagon level occur during starvation (Fig. 24–19*c*),[308] with a resulting increase in both glycogenolysis and gluconeogenesis; again the fall in insulin reduces nonessential glucose utilization and enhances free fatty acid release from adipocytes, thus providing an alternative source of fuel. Conversion of free fatty acids to the ketone bodies (acetoacetate and β-hydroxybutyrate) provides a back-up substrate that can substitute for glucose in the brain.[309] In prolonged starvation the shift of the body to a lipid-based energy supply (free fatty acids and ketones)

minimizes protein wastage by reducing the need for protein-derived gluconeogenesis.[310]

To summarize, in circumstances of glucose need, the fall in insulin concentration and rise in glucagon concentration increase glycogen breakdown, enhance gluconeogenesis, and ultimately favor a shift to the use of fat for energy by providing increased levels of free fatty acids and ketone bodies.

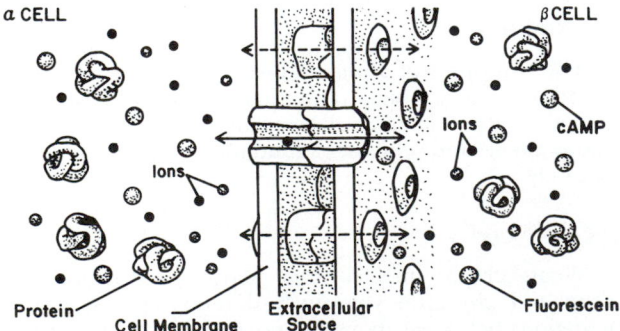

Figure 24–15. Schematic representation of gap junctions. Conduits through which small molecules such as ions, nucleotides, or fluorescein pass from the cytosol of one cell to that of a contiguous cell without entering the intercellular space are called connexons. The gap junction is an aggregation of connexons in a differentiated portion of the cell membranes. (Courtesy of L. Orci.)

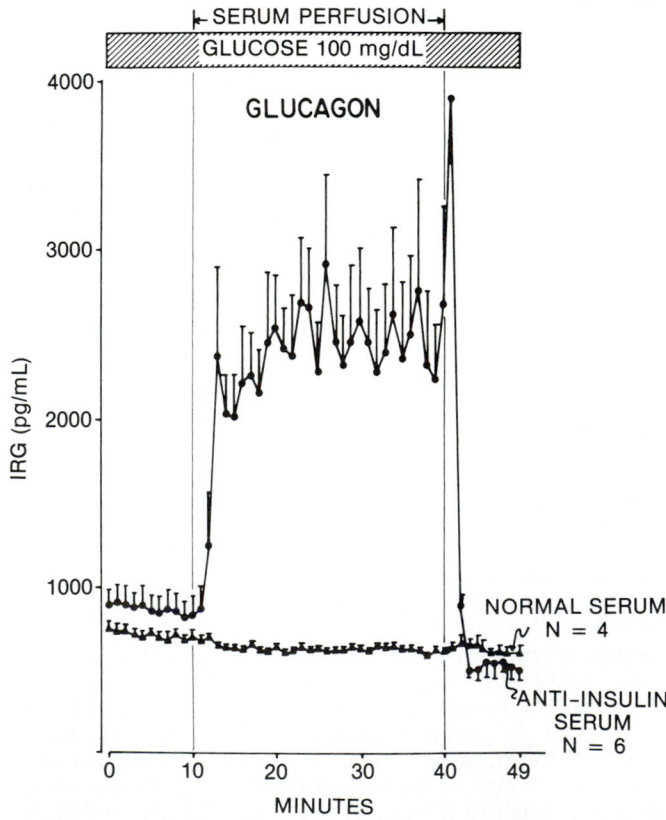

Figure 24–17. The effect of anti-insulin serum (●) on glucagon secretion (mean ± SEM) in the isolated perfused rat pancreas. Normal guinea pig serum (▲) was used as a control. The rapid rise in glucagon during perfusion of the antiserum is consistent with intravascular neutralization of newly secreted insulin as it passes through the islet from beta cells to alpha cells.

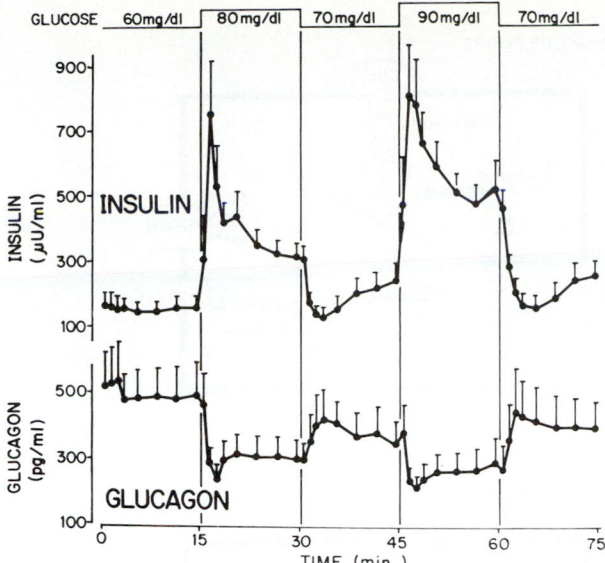

Figure 24–18. Response of insulin and glucagon to modest changes in glucose concentration in the isolated perfused dog pancreas. Note the reciprocal changes in glucagon and insulin release. (Unpublished work of K. Kawai and R. H. Unger.)

Glucose Abundance

Infusion of glucose (see Fig. 24–18) or ingestion of carbohydrate elicits a prompt rise in insulin level and a decrease in glucagon level (Figs. 24–19e and 24–20, left).[311] The increase in insulin level, which occurs before ("anticipates") the rise in arterial glucose levels,[312] is thought to be mediated largely via hormonal[313] and parasympathetic[314] signals arising in the gastrointestinal tract, which form the so-called enteroinsular axis.[315] The early insulin release allows increased glucose disposal during absorption and prevents hyperglycemia. If the rise in insulin level occurred only after glucose entered the circulation, much higher concentrations of the hormone would be required to correct the large change in glucose concentration that would result if absorption were unaccompanied by an early increase in utilization. When a carbohydrate-free protein meal is ingested (Fig. 24–20, right), insulin concentrations rise slightly to promote incorporation of amino acids into protein; a parallel rise in glucagon concentration[311] prevents hypoglycemia from the protein-induced insulin secretion.[316]

ISLET CELL FUNCTION IN DIABETES

Islet Cell Function in Insulin-Dependent Diabetes Mellitus

IDDM can be defined pathophysiologically as a state in which insulin secretion is at all times insufficient to suppress glucagon or to counter glucagon-mediated enhancement of hepatic glucose and ketone production. Insulin lack in IDDM is always associated with relative or absolute hyperglucagonemia,[311, 317] resulting from loss of the restraining influence of insulin[295] on the secretion of glucagon by the alpha cell (see Fig. 24–19f).[304] The enhanced basal secretion of glucagon in the insulin-deficient state is accompanied by disturbed glucoregulatory function. A rise in glucose concentration appears not to suppress glucagon release[306, 318] as it does in normal individuals. It may, paradoxically, cause glucagon release to increase.[319] The normal increase in glucagon

elicited by insulin-induced hypoglycemia is also impaired in type 1 IDDM[320] but not until the disease has been present for about 2 y.[321]

Whatever the mechanism, diabetic alpha cells seem to be functionally "blind" to changes in the glucose concentration (see Fig. 24–19f). Glucagon response to a protein meal[311] (Fig. 24–21) and to arginine infusion[317] is excessive in IDDM and is not blunted by hyperglycemia, although it is readily corrected by insulin.[277] Control of the plasma glucose to nearly normal levels with long-term insulin treatment corrects the basal hyperglucagonemia[322] as well as the exaggerated glucagon response to an arginine infusion[277] or a protein meal.[278] The suppressive effect of insulin on glucagon is the result of an immediate somatostatin-like block of glucagon release[323] together with a slower inhibitory effect (within an hour) on glucagon gene expression by alpha cells[324] (Fig. 24–22).

The Importance of Disordered Insulin-Glucagon Relationships in Insulin-Dependent Diabetes Mellitus

The bihormonal defect just described implies that major overproduction of glucose and ketones by the liver cannot occur unless glucagon is present.[325] The basis for this conclusion is shown in Figure 24–19a to d. In normal fasting individuals at rest, hepatic glucose production and steady-state glucose utilization by peripheral tissues are equal—about 10 g/h (see Fig. 24–19a).[326, 327] The brain at all times requires about 6 g of glucose per hour if significant ketosis is not present.[309] Glucose metabolism in the brain does not require the mediation of insulin. In humans about 75% of hepatic glucose production is mediated by glucagon,[328] whereas only about 40% of total glucose utilization occurs in insulin-sensitive tissues. Therefore, if both insulin and glucagon were completely lacking (Fig. 24–23), glucose production would decrease by 75% to approximately 2.5 to 4 g/h, but utilization would decrease by only 40% to approximately 6 g/h.[329] Thus, instead of the hyperglycemia that occurs with insulin deficiency in the *presence* of glucagon (see Fig. 24–19f), glucose levels would remain constant or even fall. This has been shown both experimentally[330, 331] and in the syndrome of congenital glucagon deficiency, which is associated with intractable hypoglycemia.[332] In the absence of glucagon, ketone production is limited despite insulin deficiency.[333, 334]

Five forms of bihormonal deficiency of insulin and glucagon have provided insight into this problem: (1) somatostatin-induced glucagon suppression in insulin-deprived type 1 diabetes;[335] (2) somatostatin-secreting tumors;[336] (3) hypophysectomized, depancreatized (Houssay) dogs;[337] (4) surgically induced bihormonal deficiency in a human[338] (Figs. 24–23 and 24–24) and in dogs;[325] and (5) diabetes in rats treated with a glucagon receptor antagonist that blocks glucagon action.[339]

Glucagon suppression by somatostatin prevents both the severe endogenous hyperglycemia and the hyperketonemia that otherwise occur in insulin-deprived IDDM patients, in a sense transforming IDDM into a mild NIDDM (ketoacidosis resistant) for the duration of the glucagon suppression.[333] This effect has been maintained experimentally for up to 48 h.[335] When glucagon is infused, hyperglycemia and ketonemia rapidly appear (Fig. 24–25). In somatostatinoma, suppression of both insulin and glucagon by endogenous somatostatin causes a mild diabetes without overproduction of glucose or ketones.[336] Similarly, in dogs after hypophysectomy, which causes a profound deficiency of pancreatic and extrapancreatic glucagon,[337] total pancreatectomy results in

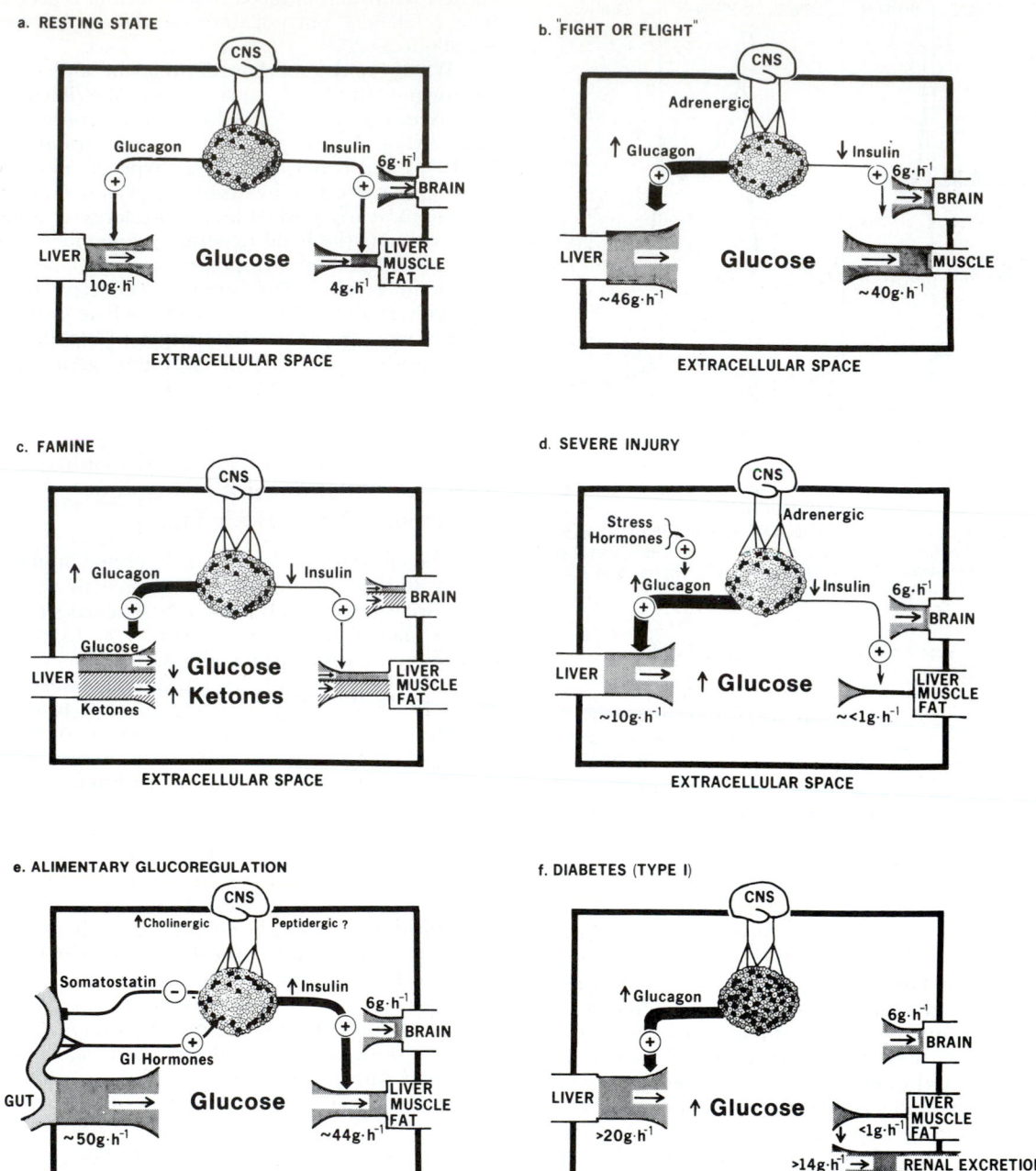

Figure 24–19. Regulation of glucose by insulin and glucagon under various conditions of fuel need and availability. The islet of Langerhans is depicted with neural connections to the central nervous system (CNS). The extracellular space is indicated by a box (heavy border) into which glucose flows from the liver or gut and from which it flows, independent of insulin action, to the brain and, under insulin mediation, into other tissues. Values given for rates of glucose utilization and production are estimates.

In the resting state *(a)*, insulin and glucagon maintain equality between the rate of glucose utilization and that of hepatic glucose production. Approximately 75% of basal glucose production is estimated to be glucagon mediated.

In "fight or flight" *(b)*, the huge increase in glucose utilization by muscle would cause hypoglycemia if the liver did not replace this glucose precisely—in large part through an adrenergically mediated increase in glucagon level and a decrease in insulin level. The latter minimizes the uptake of endogenously produced glucose by tissues other than exercising muscles and brain.

In famine (starvation) *(c)*, the rise in glucagon level, coupled with a decrease in insulin level, promotes glycogenolysis and gluconeogenesis; within 1 wk, a shift to ketone production occurs (hatched area). This shift is required for continued survival.

In severe injury *(d)*, an adrenergically mediated increase in glucagon level and a decrease in insulin secretion stimulate hepatic glucose production and minimize glucose utilization by insulin-responsive tissues. The stress hormones—growth hormone, β-endorphin, epinephrine, and cortisol—all increase glucagon secretion.

In alimentary glucoregulation *(e)*, signals arising in the gastrointestinal tract immediately after a meal (gastrointestinal hormones, cholinergic and perhaps peptidergic neurotransmitters) reach the islets of Langerhans and elicit an anticipatory response of insulin secretion, thereby avoiding major perturbations in the concentration of glucose and other ingested nutrients. Ambient glucose concentration is the major determinant of the magnitude of insulin response to these signals.

In type 1 diabetes *(f)*, islets consist primarily of cells secreting glucagon and somatostatin but little or no insulin. In insulin deprivation there is marked hyperglucagonemia and overproduction of glucose and ketones (not shown) by the liver. Unrestrained secretion and unopposed actions of glucagon are unbuffered by an insulin-mediated increase in glucose uptake into insulin-sensitive tissues. Consequently, the rise in plasma glucose is limited only by glucose excretion and glucose utilization by insulin-independent tissues such as brain. If glucagon is absent, the lack of insulin does not generate massive hepatic overproduction of ketones and glucose. (From Unger RH, Orci L. Glucagon and the A cell. Physiology and pathophysiology. Reprinted, by permission of The New England Journal of Medicine, 304; 1518–1524, 1981.)

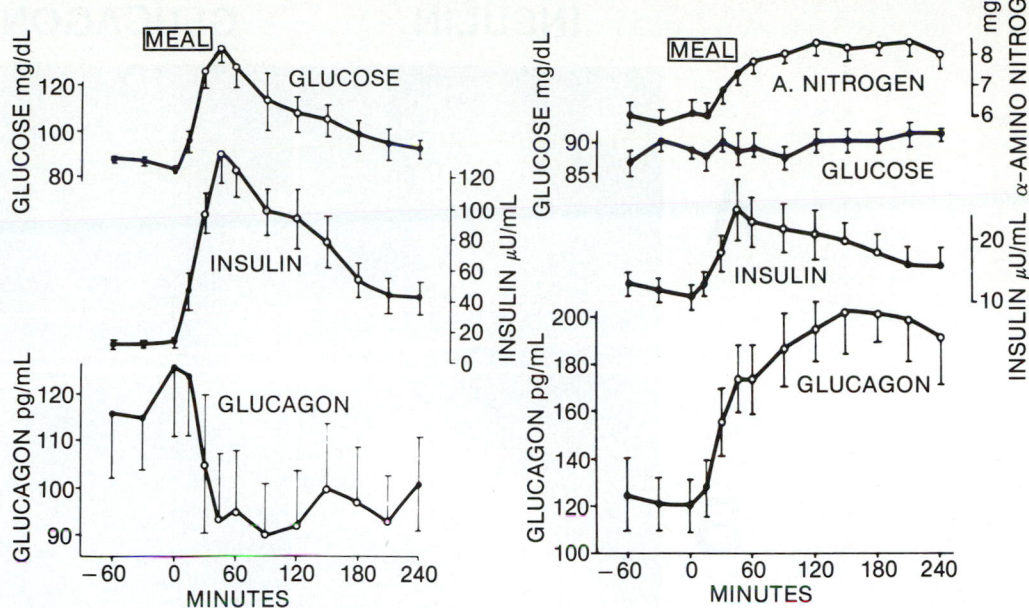

Figure 24–20. *Left,* Response of plasma glucagon of normal subjects to a large carbohydrate meal (mean ± SEM). *Right,* Response of plasma glucagon of normal subjects to a large protein meal (mean ± SEM).

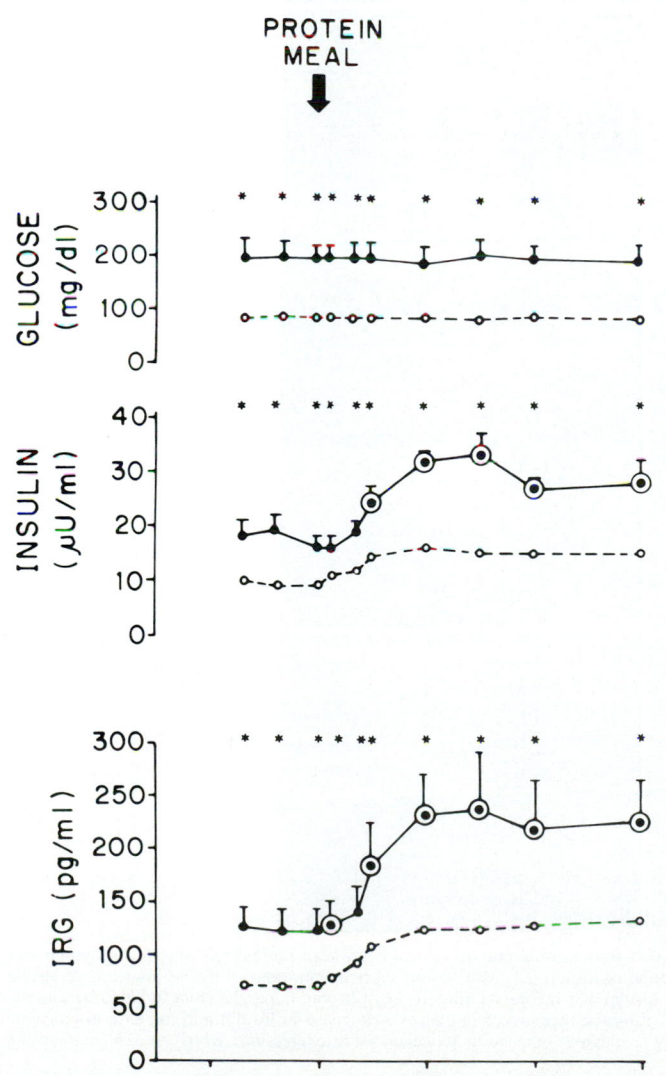

Figure 24–21. The plasma glucose, insulin, and immunoreactive glucagon (IRG) responses to a protein meal in 10 subjects with adult-onset diabetes and 12 subjects who received constant infusion of insulin at 1 U/h. (●) diabetic subjects; (○) nondiabetic subjects; (*) p < 0.05 diabetic versus nondiabetic subjects; (◉) p < 0.05 versus baseline. (From Raskin P, Aydin I, Yamamoto T, et al. Abnormal alpha cell function in human diabetes. The response to oral protein. Am J Med 1978; 64:988–997.)

INSULIN   GLUCAGON

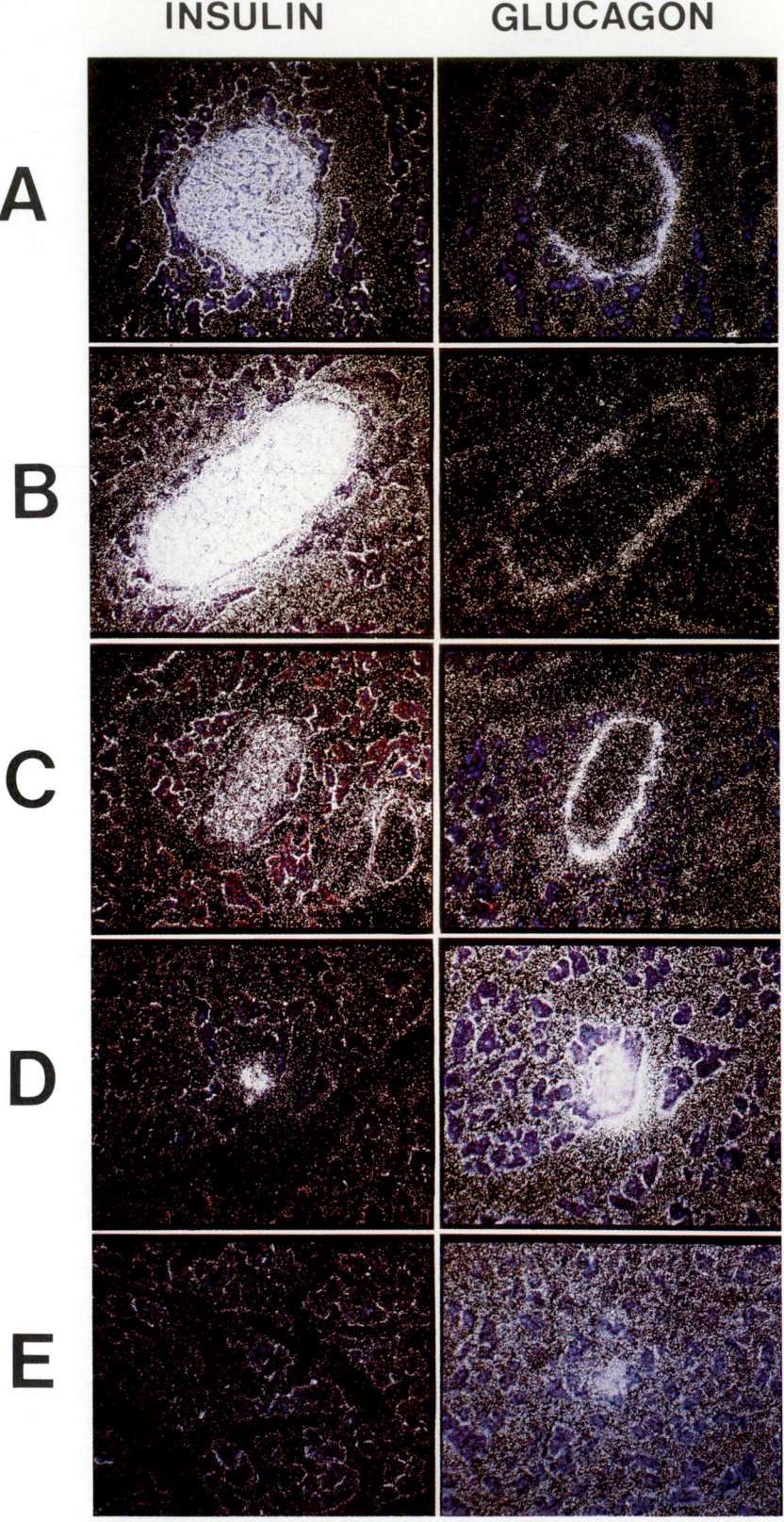

Figure 24–22. In situ hybridization for proinsulin mRNA and proglucagon mRNA of islets from normal rats *(A)* and of islets from normal rats after 5 d of continuous intravenous infusion of 50% glucose *(B)*, after chronic hypoglycemia induced by infusion of insulin *(C)*, with severe streptozocin-induced IDDM after 2 d of insulin deprivation *(D)*, and after 2 d of insulin deprivation followed by injection of regular insulin 1 h before sacrifice *(E)*. *B*, Chronic hyperglycemia induced by glucose infusion causes an increase in insulin and a decrease in glucagon gene expression. *C*, Chronic hypoglycemia causes a decrease in insulin and increase in glucagon gene expression. *D*, Insulin deprivation in severe streptozocin-induced IDDM causes a marked increase in glucagon gene expression, which at 1 h after insulin administration is profoundly rreduced *(E)*.

BIHORMONAL DEFICIENCY

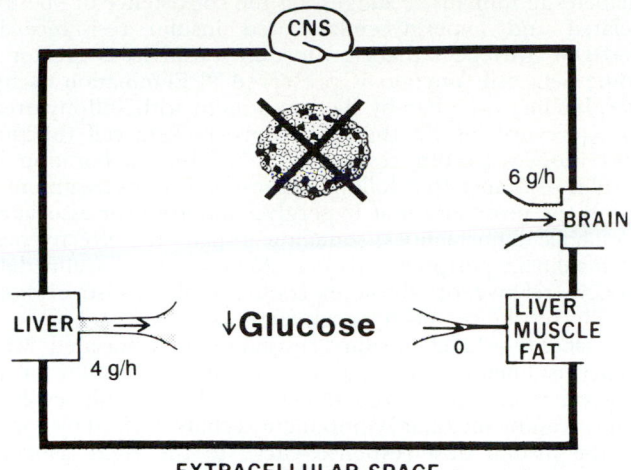

Figure 24–23. Schematic representation of combined insulin and glucagon deficiency. In the absence of both hormones, hepatic glucose production is low (~4 g/h) after an overnight fast. Plasma glucose concentration is normal or below normal because, despite low insulin-mediated glucose utilization, non–insulin-mediated uptake in the brain continues (~6 g/h). Replacement of glucagon would cause hyperglycemia (see Fig. 24–24).

an NIDDM-like syndrome with fasting normoglycemia or mild hyperglycemia and postprandial hyperglycemia. If glucagon is replaced, severe insulin-dependent diabetes supervenes.

Pancreatectomized humans have variable plasma glucagon concentrations depending on the level of therapeutic insulin and the state of metabolic control at the moment of sampling.[338, 340–342] When they receive insulin, glucagon may be unmeasurable in plasma. When such patients are deprived of exogenous insulin and become totally insulin deficient, levels of glucagon will rise to a concentration sufficient to increase hepatic glucose and ketone production, but the process occurs more slowly than in type 1 IDDM patients.[341] The extraordinary biological potency of glucagon, demonstrable in hepatocytes in vitro at concentrations as low as 10^{-13} mol/L,[343] is greatly enhanced by the absence of insulin. Only rarely is glucagon deficiency truly complete, but in one such totally depancreatectomized patient immu-

noreactive pancreatic glucagon, gut glucagon-like immunoreactivity, and insulin were unmeasurable by radioimmunoassay (see Fig. 24–24). When deprived of insulin, this patient maintained normoglycemia throughout a 12-h study.[338] Other depancreatectomized persons appear to have virtually normal levels of plasma glucagon,[342] which probably arises from extrapancreatic sites.

The explanation for the minimal metabolic consequences of insulin deficiency in the absence of glucagon lies in the fact that the major direct effect of insulin on the liver is to oppose the effects of glucagon;[344] i.e., insulin can have only a minimal influence on hepatic glucose and ketone metabolism when glucagon is not present. The biochemical mechanisms of these interactions are discussed subsequently.

Islet Cell Function in Non–Insulin-Dependent Diabetes Mellitus

Although NIDDM is not generally considered a primary islet cell disorder, there is substantial evidence for abnormal islet cell function, whether on a primary or secondary basis.[281] In obese NIDDM subjects the insulin response to a glucose load decreases and glucose tolerance progressively deteriorates, even though in absolute terms insulin levels may exceed those of nonobese controls.[345] Whatever the insulin level, if hyperglycemia exists, the insulin concentration can be viewed as low in the relative sense, because the functional mission of the beta cells is to secrete enough insulin to maintain normoglycemia. Support for this interpretation comes from the observation that induction of a comparable level of hyperglycemia in weight-matched nondiabetic subjects elicits hyperinsulinemia well above that of the NIDDM patient. The insulin response to glucose is delayed in mild cases,[346] but in severe NIDDM it may be virtually absent.[347, 348] The magnitude of loss of the acute insulin response to intravenously administered glucose is related to the degree of fasting hyperglycemia.[347] The loss of the first-phase insulin response to intravenous glucose but not to nonglucose stimuli[348] indicates that the initial functional lesion of the beta cell in NIDDM, as in IDDM, is selective in nature. The selective loss of glucose-stimulated insulin secretion at the time that fasting hyperglycemia appears is a feature of both NIDDM and IDDM. This abnormality is now believed to be, at least in part, the consequence of decreased activity of the normal glucose transporter of beta cells.[348a] It is thus prob-

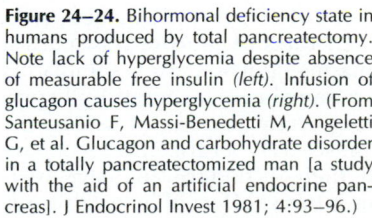

Figure 24–24. Bihormonal deficiency state in humans produced by total pancreatectomy. Note lack of hyperglycemia despite absence of measurable free insulin *(left)*. Infusion of glucagon causes hyperglycemia *(right)*. (From Santeusanio F, Massi-Benedetti M, Angeletti G, et al. Glucagon and carbohydrate disorder in a totally pancreatectomized man [a study with the aid of an artificial endocrine pancreas]. J Endocrinol Invest 1981; 4:93–96.)

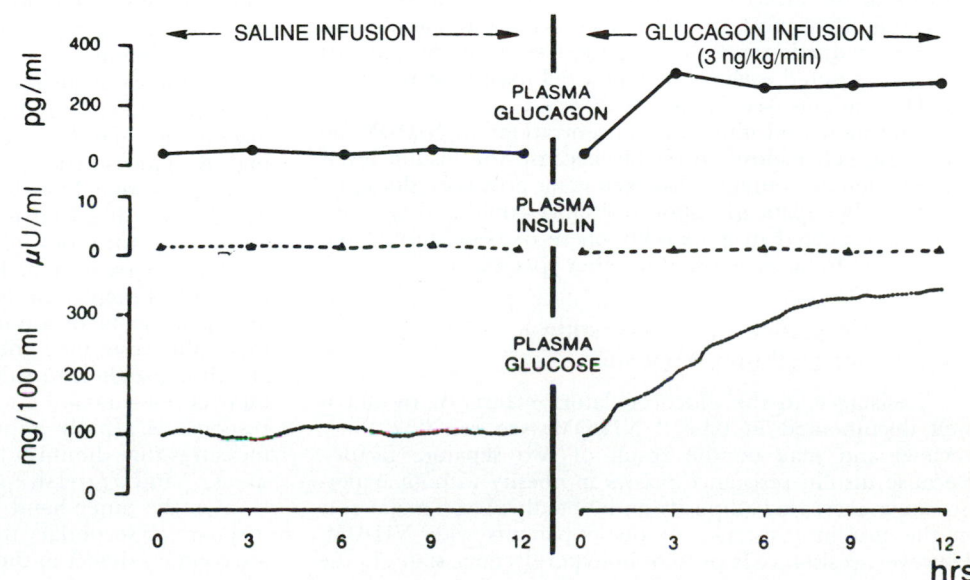

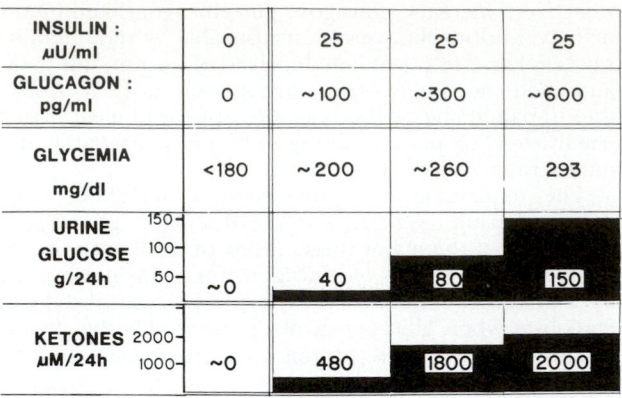

INSULIN : µU/ml	0	25	25	25
GLUCAGON : pg/ml	0	~100	~300	~600
GLYCEMIA mg/dl	<180	~200	~260	293
URINE GLUCOSE g/24h	~0	40	80	150
KETONES µM/24h	~0	480	1800	2000

Figure 24–25. Roles of insulin and glucagon in hepatic fuel overproduction in IDDM. When both insulin and glucagon are absent, the massive hyperglycemia and hyperketonemia observed in the presence of glucagon do not occur. In patients in whom insulin was clamped at approximately 25 µU/mL for 3 d, hyperglycemia, glycosuria, and ketonuria increased progressively as glucagon levels rose consequent to glucagon infusion. Thus, deficiency of insulin does not result in massive overproduction of fuels by the liver unless glucagon is present. (From Unger RH. The milieu interieur and the islets of Langerhans. Diabetologia 1981; 20:1–11.)

able that in all common forms of diabetes loss of glucose-stimulated insulin secretion is a prerequisite, i.e., that fasting hyperglycemia could not occur if the insulin response to hyperglycemia were still present. A more subtle abnormality in patients with NIDDM is lack of the normal secretion of insulin in 12- to 15-min bursts.[349] Glucose-intolerant first-degree relatives of NIDDM patients also exhibit this defect.[350]

Steady-state glucagon levels in NIDDM, although normal or above normal in absolute terms, are always high in the relative sense, because comparable hyperglycemia in nondiabetics suppresses plasma glucagon to subfasting values.[317, 351] Glucagon suppression after an oral glucose load is impaired in NIDDM in proportion to loss of the insulin response.[352] As in type 1 IDDM, this loss of glucose-induced glucagon suppression can be improved or corrected by appropriate infusion of exogenous insulin.[353] However, in obese patients with type 2 NIDDM the hyperglucagonemia is hyporesponsive to insulin. The high glucagon levels are probably responsible for the high hepatic glucose output demonstrated in such patients.[354] In dogs 70% of the insulin-induced fall in glucose output is due to concomitant insulin-mediated suppression of glucagon; if exogenous glucagon is coinfused, the effect of insulin on the liver is abolished,[355] indicating that most of the effect of insulin on hepatic glucose production is exerted at the level of alpha cells. At autopsy, as noted earlier, the alpha cell mass is increased in NIDDM patients (see Table 24–12).[233]

The increased glucagon concentrations in NIDDM do not cause ketoacidosis, probably because the insulin levels are sufficient to counteract the ketogenic effects of glucagon. Conceivably hepatic glucagon resistance could also be operative, as reported in genetically obese diabetic mice,[356] but this has yet to be established in other species.

Insulin Resistance in Non–Insulin-Dependent Diabetes Mellitus

Resistance to the glucoregulatory effects of insulin is well documented in type 2 NIDDM (see ref. 357 for a review) and may be the result of two separate factors. Because insulin resistance occurs in obesity without hyperglycemia, increased adiposity undoubtedly plays a major role in the insulin resistance of obese patients with NIDDM. However, resistance is present in hyperglycemic states in the

absence of obesity, as in alloxan-diabetic dogs[358] and type 1 diabetes in humans,[359] suggesting the coexistence of obesity-related and hyperglycemia-related insulin resistance in NIDDM. In type 1 diabetes, insulin sensitivity is greater if some beta cell function is preserved.[360] Elimination of hyperglycemia, whether by diet, treatment with sulfonylurea, or aggressive insulin therapy, improves beta cell function and reduces insulin resistance.[361, 362] The amelioration in insulin resistance that follows aggressive insulin treatment[362] raises the possibility that hyperglycemia itself (or associated metabolic abnormalities) somehow impairs the effectiveness of insulin in peripheral tissues. Alternatively, insulin deficiency (relative or absolute) could be the cause of both insulin resistance and hyperglycemia.

Obesity-related insulin resistance is associated with hyperinsulinemia[282] and reduced numbers of insulin receptors on monocytes,[363] red blood cells,[364] and adipocytes.[365] The receptor-mediated component is characterized by a shift in the insulin dose-response curve to the right. Normal maximal rates of glucose transport are achieved but at the price of increased insulin concentrations. The capacity of the increased insulin to overcome receptor-mediated resistance reflects the fact that in the normal state, maximal effects of insulin are achieved when only a small percentage of receptors are occupied; i.e., many unoccupied ("spare") receptors can be brought into action by extra insulin.[366]

If the defect in glucose transport cannot be overcome at any insulin concentration, insulin unresponsiveness is said to be present, a condition described as "postreceptor resistance."[366] It appears to be caused by failure of activation of tyrosine kinase in the beta subunit of the insulin receptor despite insulin occupancy of the alpha subunit.[367] Tyrosine kinase appears to be necessary for all metabolic actions of insulin (see later).[367]

The Relationship Between Beta Cell Dysfunction and Peripheral Insulin Resistance in Non–Insulin-Dependent Diabetes Mellitus

Islet dysfunction and peripheral insulin resistance are both present in type 2 NIDDM as noted. Does one defect cause the other or at least precede the other? The answer is uncertain. An increased beta cell content of islets has been found in nonobese infants who died of various causes within 7 mo of birth to nondiabetic Pima Indian mothers (personal communication, L. Orci and Y. Stefan). Conceivably this could signify a primary islet abnormality manifested by hyperinsulinemia.

In theory hyperinsulinemia could induce insulin resistance by down-regulation of insulin receptors. Hyperinsulinemia may be caused by replacement of the normal high-K_m glucose transporter of the beta cell with a low-K_m transporter that has also been demonstrated in beta cells. The latter could lead to high rates of glucose transport at lower concentrations of plasma glucose, thus stimulating insulin hypersecretion. Hyperamylinemia caused by hyperactive islets might also be important because of its capacity to impair insulin action in muscle. Hyperglycemia secondary to insulin resistance could then secondarily damage islets and decrease their function. A direct effect of hyperglycemia on beta cell function is suggested by the fact that the insulin response is rapidly improved in patients with NIDDM by measures that diminish hyperglycemia, i.e., diet,[368] sulfonylureas,[369] and aggressive insulin therapy.[370, 371]

On the other hand, it is possible that insulin resistance (primary or secondary to obesity) is the initial lesion causing a secondary defect in the beta cell via "exhaustion" or direct

TABLE 24–15. Effects of Stress-Related Hormones on Secretion of Islet Hormones and on Metabolism of Liver and Other Tissues*

	Islets		Extrapancreatic Tissues		
Hormone	Insulin Secretion	Glucagon Secretion	Adipocytes: Lipolysis	Muscle: Glucose Utilization	Liver: Glucose Production
Catecholamines	↓	↑	↑	↓	↑
Corticotropin	—	—	↑	—	—
Cortisol	±	↑	↑	↓	↑
Growth hormone	↑	↑	↑	↓	↑
β-Endorphin	—	↑	—	—	—
Vasopressin	—	↑	—	—	↑

*Key: increase ↑; decrease ↓; no effect or not known —.

damage from hyperglycemia. A possible model exists in rats given a 90% pancreatectomy.[372] Such animals demonstrate the characteristic loss of first-phase insulin response to glucose that is seen in human disease, suggesting dysfunction of normal beta cells secondary to a driven demand for insulin. Damage to islet function by amyloid deposition in the islet interstitium secondary to oversecretion of amylin could also play a role.

At present it is not possible to assign primacy to either process; one must state that both an islet cell defect and peripheral insulin resistance are present in overt type 2 NIDDM and that both are probably required for the appearance of clinical diabetes.[373] However, in the preovert phase of NIDDM in Pima Indians with impaired glucose tolerance, the major defect is insulin insensitivity without impairment of insulin secretion.[374] The latter appears only after the disease becomes overt.

PATHOPHYSIOLOGY OF THE DIABETIC STATES

Hormonal Physiology

A decrease in insulin production and release and/or diminished insulin activity in target tissues is critical to the development of symptomatic diabetes. Consequent to insulin deficiency, as noted earlier, glucagon concentrations rise. A fall in the insulin/glucagon ratio causes increased production of glucose by the liver while the absolute decrease in plasma insulin concentration (or insulin action) reduces glucose utilization in peripheral tissues. In consequence, basal hyperglycemia and postprandial hyperglycemia supervene. A further decrease in the insulin/glucagon ratio leads to more serious syndromes of decompensation: diabetic ketoacidosis and hyperosmolar nonketotic coma. A rapid fall in the insulin/glucagon ratio may result from omission of insulin in the insulin-treated subject or from the development of some other condition leading to release of catecholamines and other stress hormones.[375] These hormones act in multiple ways: they block secretion of residual endogenous insulin (if any), they stimulate further glucagon secretion, and they enhance the consequences of insulin deficiency in fat and muscle and glucagon excess in liver (Table 24–15).

Insulin deficiency blocks glucose utilization by insulin-requiring tissues, activates lipolysis in adipose tissue, enhances proteolysis in muscle, causes hyperglucagonemia, and intensifies glucagon effects on liver. Glucagon, when unopposed by a normal insulin response, is primarily responsible for the hepatic components of diabetic decompensation: increased glycogenolysis, gluconeogenesis, and ketogenesis (Table 24–16).[344] At the risk of oversimplifying, insulin deficiency is the cause of augmented delivery to the liver of the substrates for glucose and ketone production (amino acids and free fatty acids, respectively) and glucagon is the switch that activates the hepatic production machinery for glucose and ketones.

Stress-induced secretions of epinephrine, norepinephrine, cortisol, growth hormone, β-endorphin, angiotensin, and vasopressin may play auxiliary roles in development of diabetic ketoacidosis (see Table 24–16).[376] Their hyperglycemic impact is exaggerated because of insulin deficiency.[377] Extreme hyperglucagonemia may develop as a consequence of infection,[378] myocardial infarction,[379] trauma,[380] or burns,[381] in addition to diabetic ketoacidosis itself.[382] All these conditions may be associated with hyperglycemia. Epinephrine at concentrations observed in surgical stress and diabetic ketoacidosis causes a marked decrease in peripheral tissue sensitivity to physiological elevation of insulin. In addition, it inhibits insulin-mediated reduction in hepatic glucose production by direct action or by blocking insulin-mediated suppression of glucagon.[383] The levels of stress hormones are occasionally so high that they can convert a mild type 2 diabetic state into a catabolic facsimile of insulin-deprived type 1 IDDM, even to the point of causing ketoacidosis. If renal excretion of glucose is impaired during the foregoing events, extreme hyperglycemia with hyperosmolality will result.

Molecular Physiology

Peptide hormones such as insulin and glucagon initiate their metabolic effects by binding to receptors on the cell surface (see Chapter 4). The interaction of insulin with its receptor has been studied extensively (for review, see refs. 367, 384, and 385). The receptor is a symmetrical peptide oligomer consisting of two alpha and two beta subunits (Fig. 24–26). The alpha subunit has an apparent molecular mass of 125 to 135 kd and is the site of insulin binding. Linked to one another and the pair of beta subunits by disulfide bridges, the pair of alpha subunits lie entirely outside the plasma membrane. The beta subunits, which have an apparent molecular mass of 95 kd, are tyrosine kinases. They are the effector units of the insulin receptor.

TABLE 24–16. Contribution of Hormonal Abnormalities to Metabolic Derangements of Severe Diabetes*

Derangement	Insulin Deficiency	Glucagon Excess
Underutilization of glucose	+ + + +	0
Overproduction of glucose	+	+ + + +
Increased glycogenolysis	+	+ + + +
Increased gluconeogenesis	+	+ + + +
Increased release of amino acids	+ + + +	0
Increased lipolysis	+ + + +	+ (?)
Increased hepatic ketogenesis	+ (?)	+ + + +

*The pluses are semiquantitative indices of the magnitude of effect, from minor (+) to major (+ + + +); 0 is no effect; ? is uncertain.

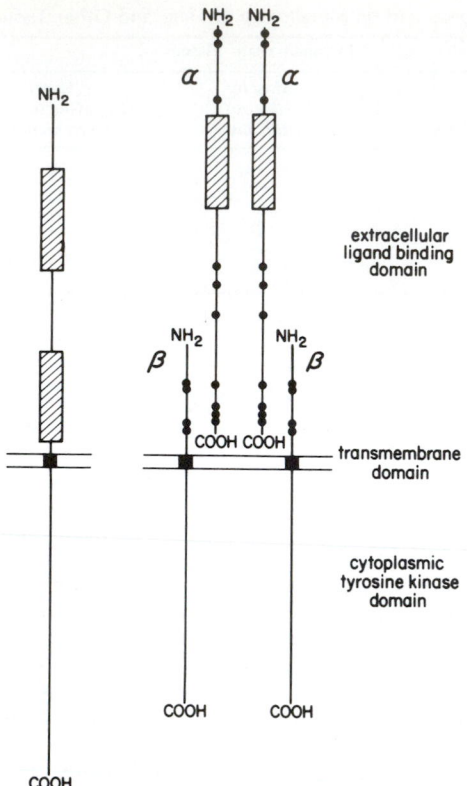

Figure 24–26. Schematic comparison of the epidermal growth factor *(left)* and insulin *(right)* receptors. Regions of high cysteine residue concentration are shown as hatched boxes; transmembrane domains as filled boxes; and single cysteine residues, possibly involved in formation of the α_2-β_2 insulin receptor complex, as filled circles. (From Ulrich A, Bell JR, Chen EY, et al. Human insulin receptor and its relationship to the tyrosine kinase family of oncogenes. Reprinted by permission from Nature, Vol. 313, pp. 756–761. Copyright © 1985 Macmillan Magazines Limited.)

Understanding of how the interactions between insulin and the insulin receptor mediate biological effects is still incomplete. These effects include inhibition of lipolysis; stimulation of protein biosynthesis and lipogenesis; activation of glucose, amino acid, and ion transport; dephosphorylation of the enzymes glycogen synthase, hormone-sensitive lipase, and pyruvate dehydrogenase; phosphorylation of seryl residues of ribosomal S6, of ATP citrate-lyase, and of acetyl-CoA carboxylase; promotion of cell growth; redistribution of certain proteins such as the insulin-sensitive glucose transporter of fat and muscle (GLUT 4),[385a] and insulin-like growth factor II; stimulation of gene expression for certain enzymes; and suppression of glucagon gene expression.[324, 385] The chronology of some of these effects is shown in Table 24–17. The binding of insulin activates a tyrosine-specific protein kinase that is the beta subunit of the receptor (see Fig. 24–26).[384–386] This autophosphorylation of the beta subunit activates its kinase activity toward other external substrates.[385] In the liver, insulin has the capacity to decrease cyclic AMP levels, possibly by enhancing phosphodiesterase activity, but its major effect on hepatic glucose production may be via inhibition of the cyclic AMP–dependent protein kinase.[387] This would oppose glucagon effects in the liver (see later).

In the case of glucagon, metabolic events are initiated by the binding of hormone to the regulatory subunit of the glucagon receptor, which is somehow coupled to the catalytic subunit of adenylate cyclase by a guanine nucleotide–binding regulatory protein (G_s). The latter activates the cyclase.[388] There is also an inhibitory guanine nucleotide–binding pro-

TABLE 24–17. Chronology of Insulin Action

Seconds
Binding to receptor
Activation of receptor protein tyrosine kinase
Receptor autophosphorylation

Seconds to Minutes
Changes in gene transcription
Stimulation of hexose and ion transport
Ligand-mediated receptor internalization
Alterations in intracellular enzyme activities
Seryl and threonyl phosphorylation of the receptor

Hours
Synthesis of protein, lipid, and nucleic acid
Maximal down-regulation of the receptor
Cell growth

From Rosen O. After insulin binds. Science 1987; 237:1452–1458. Copyright 1987 by the AAAS.

tein (G_i) identified by its capacity to bind islet-activating protein, a product of *Bordetella pertussis*.[389, 390] Cyclic AMP concentrations in liver rise within seconds after the administration of glucagon, the final levels depending on the balance between activities of the synthesizing enzyme adenylate cyclase and the degrading enzyme phosphodiesterase. Glucagon is now thought to have a second receptor through which cyclic AMP–independent action leads to rapid breakdown of phosphatidylinositol 4,5-bisphosphate, elevation of Ca^{2+} levels, and activation of protein kinase C (see ref. 391 for review).

Cytosolic cyclic AMP binds to the inactive dimeric form of the cyclic AMP–dependent protein kinase; activation of this kinase initiates all the known actions of glucagon (Fig. 24–27). The activated enzyme promotes phosphorylation of a series of intracellular enzymes with ATP serving as the phosphoryl donor. Phosphorylation of these enzymes alters their functional activity, in some cases activating and in others inactivating. For example, phosphorylation of phosphorylase *b* kinase enables it to phosphorylate phosphorylase *b* to the active form, phosphorylase *a*, the rate-limiting enzyme for glycogenolysis in liver (see Fig. 24–27). On the other hand, phosphorylation of the active *a* form of glycogen synthase inactivates it to the inactive *b* form, thus reducing glycogen formation. The end result is simultaneous enhancement of glycogenolysis and inhibition of glycogen synthesis.[392]

Glucagon also enhances hepatic gluconeogenesis and inhibits glycolysis. These actions likewise are exerted via the cyclic AMP–mediated increase in protein kinase activity (see Fig. 24–27, top). The key step in glycolysis involves the conversion of fructose 6-phosphate to fructose 1,6-bisphosphate by the enzyme 6-phosphofructo-1-kinase; the equivalent regulatory step in gluconeogenesis involves conversion of fructose 1,6-bisphosphate to fructose 6-phosphate by fructose-1,6-bisphosphatase. The activity of 6-phosphofructo-1-kinase is allosterically increased by fructose 2,6-bisphosphate while that of fructose-1,6-bisphosphatase is reciprocally inhibited.[393–396] Thus fructose 2,6-bisphosphate promotes glycolysis and inhibits gluconeogenesis by controlling the two key enzymes in the opposing pathways. Fructose 2,6-bisphosphate is formed from fructose 6-phosphate by the enzyme 6-phosphofructose-2-kinase/fructose-2,6-bisphosphatase. This interesting enzyme is bifunctional, the activity expressed being determined by the phosphorylation state.[395, 397] When dephosphorylated it is a kinase, when phosphorylated a phosphatase. Glucagon thus works by the sequence: ↑ cyclic AMP → ↑ cyclic AMP–dependent protein kinase → ↑ phosphorylation of 6-phosphofructose-2-kinase/fructose-2,6-bisphosphatase → ↓ fructose 2,6-bisphosphate → ↓ glycolysis and ↑ gluconeogenesis (Fig. 24–

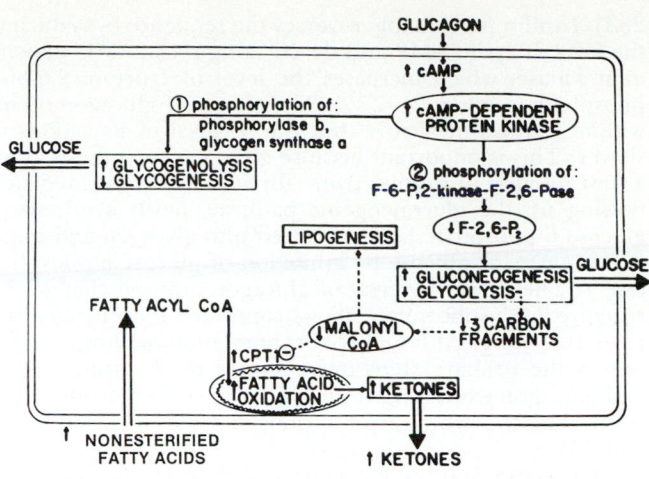

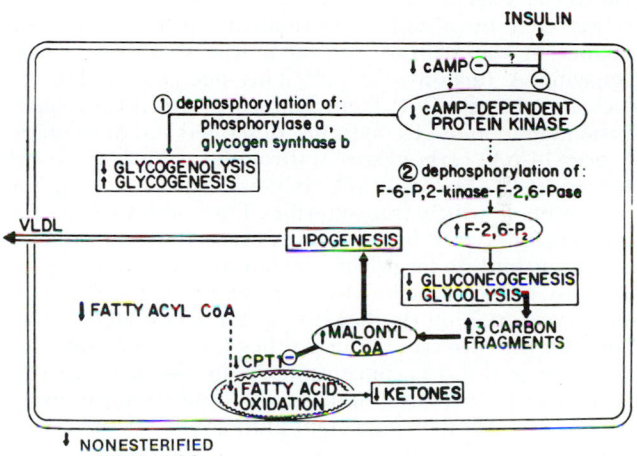

Figure 24–27. *Top,* Glucagon-induced catabolic cascade in hepatocytes. Binding of glucagon to the regulatory subunit of its receptor activates adenylate cyclase to increase cyclic AMP levels. This activates cyclic AMP–dependent protein kinase, which initiates all the known actions of glucagon by phosphorylating certain key enzymes, thereby redirecting their activities toward catabolism. Phosphorylation of inactive phosphorylase b ① converts it to the active a form, thereby promoting glycogenolysis and enhanced glucose production. Phosphorylation of glycogen synthase a inactivates it to the b form and reduces glycogen formation. Phosphorylation of the bifunctional enzyme ② that regulates fructose 2,6-bisphosphate (F-2,6-P_2) synthesis and degradation, 6-phosphofructose-2-kinase/fructose-2,6-bisphosphatase (F-6,P,2-kinase-F-2,6-Pase), lowers its kinase activity and increases its phosphatase action. This depletes F-2,6-P_2, a stimulator of glycolysis and inhibitor of gluconeogenesis. The result of F-2,6-P_2 depletion is enhanced glucose production from nonglucose precursors and diminished formation of pyruvate, the substrate for lipogenesis. Consequently, levels of malonyl-CoA, the product of the first committed step in lipogenesis, are reduced. This abolishes the inhibitory action of malonyl-CoA on carnitine palmitoyltransferase I (CPT I), the enzyme responsible for transesterification of fatty acyl–CoA to fatty acyl carnitine, allowing fatty acids to enter into the mitochondria, the site of beta-oxidation to ketones. The level of fatty acyl–CoA derived from free fatty acids delivered to liver from adipocytes is increased as the consequence of deficiency of insulin, an antilipolytic hormone. Thus, the high glucagon–low insulin mixture induces the full catabolic syndrome of increased glucose production and accelerated ketogenesis.

Bottom, Insulin-induced anabolic cascade. Insulin, when present in sufficient concentration, lowers glucagon release and reverses the glucagon-mediated catabolic cascade. The cyclic AMP concentration is lowered, probably by an insulin-mediated increase in phosphodiesterase activity. The major effect of insulin may be to inactivate the cyclic AMP–dependent protein kinase (see text). Dephosphorylation of enzymes at ① and ② promotes glycogen formation and increases F-2,6-P_2 levels, thereby stimulating glycolysis and inhibiting gluconeogenesis. Pyruvate becomes available for lipogenesis, increasing malonyl-CoA levels and inhibiting CPT I. Ketone formation slows and fatty acid synthesis increases. Fatty acids are esterified to triglycerides, which are then packaged and released as VLDL. Plasma free fatty acid levels are much lower but continue to contribute to triglyceride and VLDL formation.

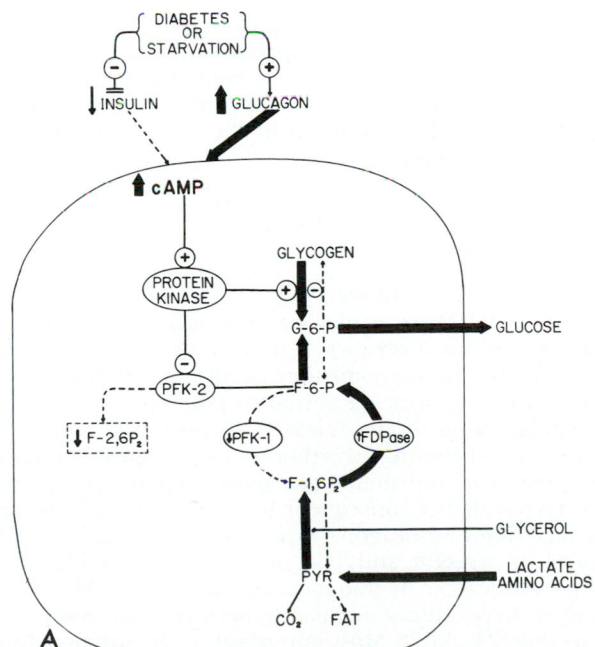

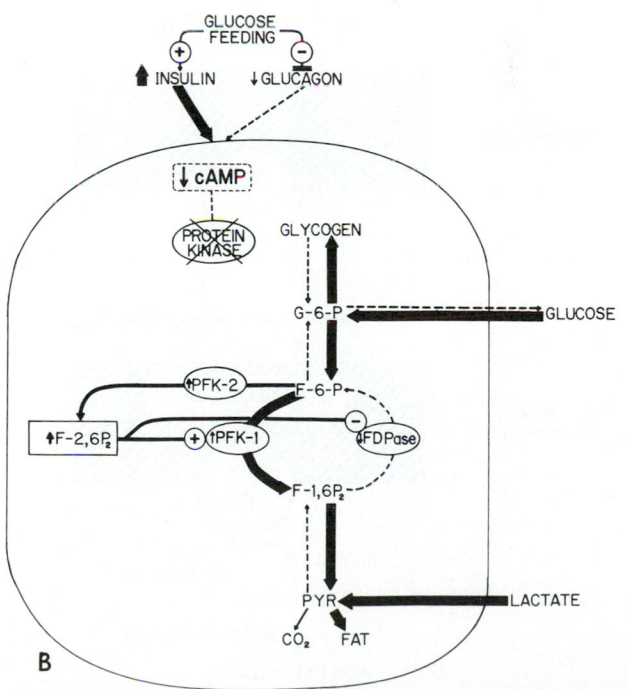

Figure 24–28. *A,* Enhancement of gluconeogenesis and glycogenolysis by glucagon in diabetes and starvation. Both processes are activated by an increase in cyclic AMP concentration in the hepatocyte. Phosphofructokinase 1 (PFK-1) catalyzes the formation of fructose 1,6-bisphosphate (F-1,6P_2) in the glycolytic pathway, and PFK-2 synthesizes fructose 2,6-bisphosphate (F-2,6P_2), a regulator of PFK-1 activity. PFK-2 and fructose-2,6-bisphosphatase activities are contained in the same protein (see text). Cyclic AMP–induced phosphorylation of the enzyme decreases the former and increases the latter. Decreased levels of F-2,6P_2 result in decreased glycolysis and increased gluconeogenesis.

B, Inhibition of gluconeogenesis and activation of glycogen synthesis, glycolysis, and lipogenesis by insulin. Insulin decreases the cyclic AMP level, deactivates protein kinase, and reverses changes in F-2,6P_2 and substrate flux over the glycolytic-gluconeogenic pathway produced by glucagon. Glycogen synthesis and lipogenesis are also increased.

28A). Insulin presumably reverses the sequence by reducing the level of cyclic AMP and deactivating cyclic AMP–dependent kinase, which increases the level of fructose 2,6-bisphosphate (see Fig. 24–28B). The effects of glucagon occur within minutes in vitro,[398] but the reversal of its actions is slower. This is important because glycogen resynthesis after a fast occurs primarily from three-carbon intermediates flowing up the gluconeogenic pathway, newly synthesized glucose 6-phosphate being diverted into glycogen and away from release as glucose by inhibition of glucose-6-phosphatase.[399] The slower reversal of glucagon-induced changes in fructose 2,6-bisphosphate allows continued gluconeogenesis after refeeding. Although phosphorylation-dephosphorylation is the primary short-term control mechanism, insulin and glucagon exert long-term control via other means, as by controlling the synthesis of various enzymes (e.g., refs. 400 and 401).

Glucagon induces ketogenesis and blocks hepatic lipogenesis (see Figs. 24–27 and 24–28).[402] These two events are orchestrated by a fall in intrahepatic levels of the first product in the pathway of fatty acid synthesis, malonyl coenzyme A (malonyl-CoA).[403] This decrease is due to a block in substrate flow from glucose to acetyl-CoA caused by the inhibition of glycolysis just described and by inhibition of acetyl-CoA carboxylase[404] through a phosphorylation mechanism.[405] Malonyl-CoA inhibits carnitine palmitoyltransferase I, which transesterifies fatty acyl–CoA to fatty acyl carnitine, enabling it to traverse the mitochondrial membrane and undergo beta-oxidation to ketones (Fig. 24–29).[406] By reducing malonyl-CoA levels, glucagon disinhibits the enzyme, poising the hepatocyte for accelerated acetoacetate and β-hydroxybutyrate synthesis as soon as fatty acid and fatty acyl–CoA concentrations in the liver increase consequent to increased lipolysis resulting from the insulin deficiency.[407] Another important glucagon-mediated event is an increase in hepatic carnitine levels, although the mechanism is unknown.[408] The combination of increased fatty acyl–CoA and carnitine levels and activated carnitine palmitoyltransferase I ensures brisk rates of ketogenesis.

The molecular physiology of uncontrolled diabetes has of necessity been elucidated in experimental animals. Although some aspects, such as malonyl-CoA control of carnitine palmitoyltransferase I, have been confirmed in humans,[409] others remain to be tested.

CLINICAL PICTURE

Type 1 Insulin-Dependent Diabetes Mellitus

Uncomplicated Onset

Symptomatic diabetes is due to the foregoing hormonal and biochemical changes, which initiate a pattern of progressive pathophysiological deterioration. The insulin lack reduces glucose utilization and increases glucagon secretion. Neither ingested glucose nor glucose produced at an enhanced rate by the glucagon-stimulated liver can be disposed of normally via insulin-mediated pathways. This leads to hyperglycemia and glycosuria. Progressive osmotic diuresis causes dehydration, thirst, and, if glucose losses are extensive, weight loss despite polyphagia. When the rate of glucose excretion approximates the rate of hepatic glucose overproduction, hyperglycemia reaches a plateau. This generally occurs when glucose is in the range of 17 to 28 mmol/L (300 to 500 mg/dL).

In children the onset of symptoms often occurs over a short period; families can sometimes give the precise time the illness appears even if the onset is not heralded by ketoacidosis. Because the symptoms are not subtle, there is usually no difficulty in diagnosis. This does not mean that the pathological process leading to overt diabetes is brief or that the symptoms always appear suddenly.[160–162] As discussed previously, destruction of beta cells usually requires more than a year. The diagnosis of diabetes in children is being increasingly recognized in the non–insulin-requiring phase of the disease.

Acute Decompensation: Diabetic Ketoacidosis

Diabetic ketoacidosis may be the initial event in the course of IDDM, or it may occur at any time subsequently (see ref. 392 for a review). It may be precipitated by stress, other illness, or the omission of insulin. It may develop slowly after a protracted period of poor control. The counterregulatory hormones released during stress oppose insulin action and stimulate further glucagon release. They may also potentiate and mimic glucagon's action (see Table 24–15). Hypovolemia consequent to diuresis directly increases the secretion of glucagon,[382] catecholamines, and other hormones of stress[376] and, via decreasing renal blood flow, reduces glucagon degradation by the kidney. The result is marked hyperglucagonemia, hyperglycemia, and ketoacidosis (Fig. 24–30).[392] Most important, if the osmotic diuresis is prolonged, a decrease in glomerular filtration rate occurs, closing off the "safety valve" for hyperglycemia (i.e., renal excretion of glucose). This results in a rapid rise of the plasma glucose level from its previous plateau because hepatic production continues unabated (see Fig. 24–30). Hyperosmolality thus becomes a factor and water moves out of cells. Substantial urinary losses of sodium, potassium, mag-

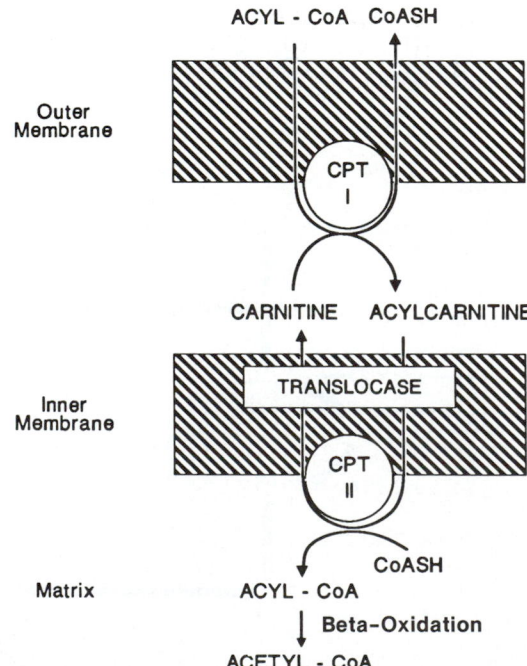

Figure 24–29. Fatty acid oxidation system in liver. The inner mitochondrial membrane is impermeable to long chain fatty acyl–CoA but permeable to fatty acylcarnitine. Formation of the carnitine ester is catalyzed by CPT I, the rate-limiting step in the sequence. This enzyme is inhibited by malonyl-CoA. The transesterification reaction is reversed inside mitochondria by CPT II. Most of the fatty acid molecules entering the mitochondria are converted to ketones, only a small amount of the acetyl-CoA generated being oxidized in the tricarboxylic acid cycle.

DIABETIC KETOACIDOSIS

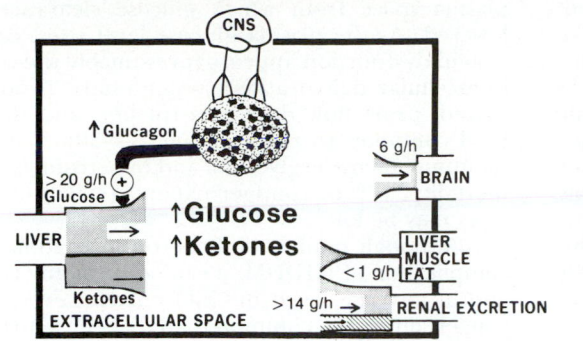

NONKETOTIC HYPEROSMOLAR COMA

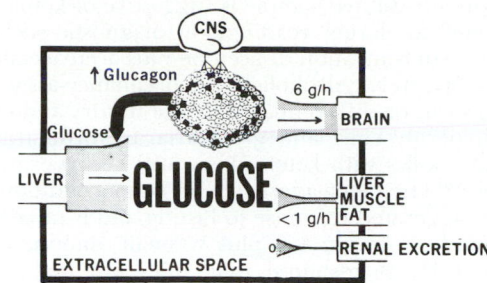

Figure 24–30. Acute decompensation in diabetes mellitus. Diabetic ketoacidosis is usually associated with unmeasurable insulin levels and extremely high glucagon levels. The resulting overproduction of glucose, coupled with negligible glucose utilization by tissues other than brain, causes hyperglycemia, which reaches a plateau when glucose excretion plus cerebral glucose uptake equals hepatic glucose production. Ketone production rises sharply to produce a metabolic acidosis.

In nonketotic hyperosmolar coma, insulin levels may also be quite low, although the islets may contain functioning beta cells in patients with NIDDM. A stressful precipitating illness with a prolonged osmotic diuresis reduces the effective extracellular space, thereby increasing discharge of insulin-inhibiting and glucagon-stimulating hormones (see also Table 24–13). Glucose utilization is reduced, and glucose production is increased. In contrast to the situation early in the development of diabetic ketoacidosis, renal excretion of glucose is reduced because of more severe volume depletion, thereby permitting a rapid increase in plasma concentration to extreme levels. Why ketone production does not increase to ketoacidosis levels is not known (see text).

nesium, bicarbonate, and chloride take place, and hyperketonemia increases the hydrogen ion concentration of the body fluids. Loss of the extracellular constancy of fuels, fluids, solutes, and pH places the function of all cells at jeopardy. Central nervous system dysfunction, for example, is common, being primarily due to intracellular dehydration.[410] Death is inevitable without appropriate intervention.

ADMISSION FINDINGS. The history usually reveals polyuria, polydipsia, polyphagia, and weight loss for a variable period of time, although in some children the onset can be abrupt. Abdominal pain, nausea, and vomiting are common and may be due to the ketoacidosis or to an associated disorder. The mental status may vary from slight drowsiness to profound lethargy, but deep coma is rare. The rapid, deep respirations of Kussmaul partially compensate for the metabolic acidosis by blowing off carbon dioxide; rarely respiration is depressed if central nervous system impairment is severe and the pH is very low.[411] A high plasma acetone level imparts a fruity odor to the breath. Skin turgor is decreased, and mucous membranes are dry. Tachycardia is usual and hypotension may be present. Fever strongly suggests infection, but leukocytosis may be present without infection. The initial examination usually suggests the diagnosis, but documentation of hyperglycemia and ketosis is required.

Typical admission laboratory findings in diabetic ketoacidosis are shown in Table 24–18. The metabolic acidosis is due primarily to increased concentrations of acetoacetic and β-hydroxybutyric acids, with free fatty acids, lactate, and organic acids usually playing only a minor role. Serum osmolality is almost always high when consciousness is impaired. Although sodium losses in the urine and vomitus may be substantial, the relative or absolute hyponatremia in large part reflects a shift of intracellular water into the extracellular space in response to hyperglycemia. Hypertriglyceridemia can cause spurious hyponatremia; a sodium value below 120 mmol/L generally is due to hyperlipemia, although occasionally it is due to acute dilution caused by vomiting combined with water intake. Hypertriglyceridemia may be manifested by milkiness of serum or lipemia retinalis. Despite urinary potassium losses, hyperkalemia is usual on admission, a consequence of the metabolic acidosis. A normal or low potassium level before treatment suggests a severe total body deficit of potassium. Increased serum levels of myoglobin and creatine kinase consistent with nontraumatic

rhabdomyolysis may be present in the more seriously ill patients.[412]

DIFFERENTIAL DIAGNOSIS. Altered consciousness related to ketoacidosis is usually easily differentiated from hypoglycemia in diabetic subjects on clinical grounds, so the routine administration of 50% glucose pending laboratory confirmation is not indicated. Measurement of urinary ketones and plasma glucose in capillary blood by a reflectance meter or chemical strip should provide adequate guidelines pending formal laboratory confirmation. Rarely cerebrovascular accidents lead to glycosuria and ketonuria, but the initial diagnostic confusion in such cases usually is rapidly resolved by the clinical course.

Diabetic ketoacidosis is an anion gap acidosis, meaning that the unmeasured anion fraction is greater than 16 mmol/L (calculated by subtracting the plasma concentration of chloride plus bicarbonate from that of sodium plus potassium). There are five major causes of anion gap acidosis: diabetic ketoacidosis, alcoholic ketoacidosis, lactic acidosis, renal failure, and certain poisonings (e.g., ethylene glycol, methyl alcohol).[392] Starvation in late pregnancy or during lactation[413] may rarely cause an anion gap acidosis of the ketoacidosis type. Ketoacidosis can be differentiated from other forms of metabolic acidosis accompanied by fasting ketosis (positive urinary ketones) by measuring ke-

TABLE 24–18. Initial Laboratory Findings in Severe Diabetic Decompensation

	Diabetic Ketoacidosis*	Hyperosmolar Coma†
Glucose (mmol/L [mg/dL])	216 (475)	65 (1166)
Sodium (mmol/L)	132	144
Potassium (mmol/L)	4.8	5
Bicarbonate (mmol/L)	<10.0	17
Blood urea nitrogen (mmol/L [mg/dL])	9 (25)	31 (87)
Acetoacetate (mmol/L)	4.8	ND‡
β-Hydroxybutyrate (mmol/L)	13.7	ND
Free fatty acids (mmol/L)	2.1	0.73
Lactate (mmol/L)	4.6	ND
Osmolarity (mmol/kg)	310	384

*Based on 88 consecutive episodes of diabetic ketoacidosis at Parkland Memorial Hospital (D.W. Foster, unpublished study).

†From Al Arieff, HJ Carroll, Nonketotic hyperosmolar coma with hyperglycemia, Medicine 51, 73–74, © by Williams & Wilkins, 1972.

‡ND, not done.

tones semiquantitatively in serial dilutions of plasma with reagent sticks that detect acetone and acetoacetate. Because even prolonged starvation rarely causes total ketone concentrations greater than 4 to 6 mmol/L,[309, 310] a moderate to large response in any diluted sample is suggestive of ketoacidosis ("moderate" to "large" readings on diagnostic sticks usually indicate a concentration of acetone plus acetoacetate of 4 mmol/L or greater). Alcoholic- and pregnancy-associated ketoacidosis can be differentiated by the history and by the fact that hyperglycemia and glycosuria are ordinarily absent. Some alcoholics with ketoacidosis may be hyperglycemic, however.[414] The ketoacidosis in the latter conditions represents an exaggerated response to fasting and is rapidly reversible by glucose or glucose plus a small amount of insulin (5 to 10 U), a response that rules out diabetic ketoacidosis. The diagnosis of lactic acidosis requires the measurement of lactate in the plasma, but the initial clue is severe metabolic acidosis with absent urinary ketones or a plasma ketone result that is positive only in the undiluted state despite a large urinary acetone content. (Tests for urinary ketones may be positive in lactic acidosis because nausea and vomiting induce a fasted state.)

Type 2 Non–Insulin-Dependent Diabetes Mellitus

Uncomplicated Onset

Type 2 NIDDM varies widely in severity. Most patients are asymptomatic, and the diagnosis is made by the detection of hyperglycemia or glycosuria on routine examination. In such patients the mean concentration of glucose in the plasma throughout the day is below the renal threshold, and glycosuria either does not occur or occurs intermittently such that symptomatic osmotic diuresis does not supervene. Other patients with NIDDM develop frank hyperglycemia, but because the onset is gradual the diagnosis is delayed for weeks or months. Only rarely is the onset of symptoms as acute as in IDDM; when this occurs it is usually the result of the stress of an acute intercurrent illness. Occasionally the presenting symptom of type 2 NIDDM is a diabetic complication such as peripheral neuropathy, gangrene, or a vascular event that leads the physician to test for hyperglycemia or perform a glucose tolerance test.

Acute Decompensation: Nonketotic Hyperosmolar Coma

The characteristic acute catabolic complication of type 2 NIDDM, analogous to diabetic ketoacidosis in type 1 IDDM, is nonketotic hyperosmolar coma, a syndrome of extreme hyperglycemia and dehydration. The pathophysiology involves an imbalance between glucose production and its excretion in the urine. As noted earlier, maximal hepatic production of glucose results in a plateau of plasma glucose level no higher than 17 to 28 mmol/L (300 to 500 mg/dL) provided urine output is maintained. Hyperosmolar coma results when the sum of glucose excretion plus metabolism is less than the rate at which glucose enters the extracellular space. The blood glucose level then rises above the aforementioned plateau. Many clinical scenarios can produce this syndrome, but whatever the initiating event, the common denominator is the inability to excrete glucose as rapidly as it enters the extracellular space (see Fig. 24–30). Hyperosmolar coma most frequently occurs in older patients in whom an intercurrent illness increases glucose production secondary to stress hormones and impairs the capacity to ingest fluids. As the extracellular fluid and plasma volumes shrink, two consequences ensue: the capacity to excrete

glucose decreases or disappears as urine volume falls, while hepatic glucose production pours glucose into a shrinking plasma space from which glucose clearance is markedly lowered. As the plasma glucose level rises, central nervous system dysfunction appears (presumably the consequence of intracellular dehydration), water intake is additionally impaired, urine flow decreases further, and the blood sugar level continues to rise (see Fig. 24–30). The end result is monumental hyperglycemia and hyperosmolality with a high mortality.[415, 416] In younger patients (<50 y of age) mortality rates may be lower.[417]

Although nonketotic hyperosmolar coma is generally a complication of NIDDM, it can occur in any type of diabetes and at any age, even in children. However, hyperosmolar coma is much less common than diabetic ketoacidosis in type 1 IDDM. If enough insulin is present to prevent ketoacidosis but is insufficient to control the blood sugar level (a not uncommon occurrence), osmotic diuresis coupled with inadequate water intake leads to falling urine output and nonketotic hyperosmolar coma.

The mechanism by which ketoacidosis is suppressed when extreme hyperglycemia occurs is not known. Hyperosmolality inhibits lipolysis in vitro,[418] and free fatty acid levels in hyperosmolar coma average 0.7 mmol/L,[415, 416] compared with 2.0 mmol/L in diabetic ketoacidosis,[419] presumably providing less substrate for ketogenesis in the liver. However, the syndrome can occur in patients with free fatty acid concentrations of 1.4 to 4.0 mmol/L.[420] The absence of serious ketosis is not due to lower concentrations of glucagon in hyperosmolar coma, because the concentrations equal or surpass those seen in ketoacidosis.[421] This suggests that extreme hyperglycemia somehow breaks through the glucagon-mediated lipogenic block, permitting synthesis of sufficient malonyl-CoA (perhaps from glucose-derived lactate) to restrain the production of acetoacetate and β-hydroxybutyrate.

ADMISSION FINDINGS. The events that culminate in hyperosmolar coma are usually a consequence of another serious disorder affecting a patient who happens to have type 2 NIDDM. The precipitating disease may color or dominate the clinical presentation; conversely, the underlying disorder may be camouflaged by the dramatic metabolic crisis. Stroke, myocardial infarction, pneumonia and other infections, burns, and heat stroke are common precipitating events. Acute pancreatitis is frequent, although it is not always clear whether it initiates the syndrome or is a consequence of it. Pancreatitis has dual detrimental consequences: a drop in residual insulin release coupled with sequestration of large amounts of extracellular fluid in the "third space"— the inflammatory bed surrounding the pancreas. This provides both of the prerequisites for hyperosmolar coma: reduced insulin level coupled with reduced capacity to excrete glucose. Abdominal pain may be a transient accompaniment of the metabolic disturbance, or it may reflect important precipitating intra-abdominal disease.[422]

On examination, patients with hyperosmolar coma exhibit extreme dehydration and may have supine or orthostatic hypotension. Hypothermia may be present. Kussmaul respiration is usually absent, an important clinical clue in differentiating the disorder from diabetic ketoacidosis. Hyperpnea may be present, however, if lactic acidosis supervenes. Gastric distention, ileus, and hematemesis are common and may recede with treatment.[422] Functional impairment of the central nervous system ranges from confusion to coma. Seizures are common and may be either focal or generalized.[423] Other neurological findings, such as rapidly reversible hemiplegia, may be noted. Neurological signs may be metabolic in etiology, in which case they recede with treatment, or they may result from underlying disease worsened by the metabolic insult, in which case reversibility may not occur. Pleural or pericardial friction rubs together with electrocardiographic changes may be due to metabolic alterations and disappear with rehydration, or may indicate infection or pulmonary infarction.[422]

Lactic acidosis is common because of the marked fluid deficits that lead to hypotension and decreased tissue perfusion. Because the patients frequently have not eaten for hours to days before admission, the urine may be positive for ketones, causing confusion with ketoacidosis. Differentiation can usually be made by semiquantitative analysis of ketones in dilute plasma as already described, but plasma should be drawn for the quantitative measurement of lactate (and ketones, if available) to confirm the clinical impression.

Typical laboratory findings are shown in Table 24–18. Plasma osmolality is markedly elevated. Although the glucose concentration in plasma is, on average, about 67 mmol/L (1200 mg/dL), values as high as 267 mmol/L (4800 mg/dL) have been reported.[424] If plasma osmolality cannot be measured directly, a close estimate may be obtained from routine analyses:

$$\text{Plasma osmolality (mmol/L)} =$$
$$2[Na^+ + K^+] \text{ (mmol/L)} + \text{glucose (mmol/L)}$$
$$+ \text{ BUN (mmol/L)}$$

Virtually all patients have elevated blood urea nitrogen (BUN) (average, 31 mmol/L [87 mg/dL]) and creatinine (average, 486 μmol/L [5.5 mg/dL]) levels.[416]

DIFFERENTIAL DIAGNOSIS. The differential diagnosis of nonketotic hyperosmolar coma is not a problem once laboratory values showing extreme hyperglycemia are returned. The diagnostic challenge consists in the detection of underlying disease and elucidation of the precipitating mechanism. The range of possibilities is large because of the broad spectrum of complicating illnesses. Occasionally the disorder occurs solely because of insufficient insulin or sulfonylureas, particularly if the patient replaces the fluid loss with sugar-containing soft drinks.[422] The syndrome may be caused iatrogenically by the administration of drugs[425–427] (phenytoin, glucocorticoids, thiazide diuretics, cimetidine, or furosemide) or by maneuvers such as high-calorie tube feedings, intravenous hyperalimentation, intravenous infusion of hypertonic glucose, or peritoneal dialysis with glucose-containing solutions.

In hyperosmolar coma without apparent precipitating illness the differential diagnosis is that of altered central nervous system function, usually stroke, head injury, or brain tumor. For this reason a computed tomographic scan of the head is frequently needed, especially if the patient's neurological deficit fails to respond as the metabolic disorder recedes.

Management of the acute metabolic syndromes is discussed in the section on treatment.

THE COMPLICATIONS OF DIABETES

Since the availability of insulin, the number of deaths from acute metabolic complications has markedly decreased. Increasingly, therefore, disability and death in both IDDM and NIDDM result from the degenerative complications of the disease. We note, however, that overall mortality may be decreasing. A study in Denmark of 2930 patients showed a 30 to 40% decrease in mortality for subjects diagnosed after 1956 compared to those diagnosed between 1933 and 1946.[428] If confirmed, this suggests a decrease in death rates from both acute and chronic complications. Traditionally,

retinopathy, neuropathy, and nephropathy have been designated *microvascular* complications, whereas atherosclerosis and its sequelae (stroke, myocardial infarction, gangrene) have been called *macrovascular* complications. In this section the pathogenesis of these complications and their clinical manifestations will be discussed.

The Role of Metabolic Control

The relationship of diabetic complications to the metabolic derangements of diabetes has been the subject of controversy for more than four decades.[429] The possibility that the microvascular, nonatherosclerotic diabetic complications may be independent of the metabolic abnormalities is suggested by the fact that many diabetics endure decades of poor control without developing complications. Rarely, diabetic glomerulosclerosis[430] and retinopathy[431, 432] occur in patients without known hyperglycemia or are found at the first diagnosis of diabetes. Thickening of the quadriceps muscle capillary basement membranes has been reported in 50% of normoglycemic, glucose-tolerant offspring of two diabetic patients[12] and in nondiabetic HLA-DR4–positive parents of type 1 diabetic children.[433] However, the relationship of such changes to clinically overt microangiopathy has not been established. For example, there appears to be a lack of correlation between muscle capillary basement membrane thickness and parameters of renal dysfunction such as creatine clearance, albuminuria, and fractional volume of the glomerular mesangium.[434] Muscle capillary basement membrane width may reflect glycemic control and may even be correlated with the thickness of the glomerular basement membrane, but changes in its thickness are not reflected in functional and structural changes of progressive diabetic nephropathy. Although it has been shown that meticulous glycemic control can reduce muscle capillary basement membrane thickness,[17] such treatment does not reverse long-standing microalbuminuria.[435] However, aggressive treatment early in the course slows progression of microalbuminuria and may even reverse it.

Extensive evidence favors a relationship between metabolic abnormalities of diabetes and its microangiopathic complications. The cited reports of diabetic complications in the absence of hyperglycemia are extremely rare and not compelling when compared to the fact that the 98% of the human race that is normoglycemic is untouched by the microvascular complications characteristic of diabetes. Nodular glomerulosclerosis, which is present in 55% of hyperglycemic Pima Indians, has never been demonstrated in a normoglycemic Pima.[436] The 6-y incidence of diabetic retinopathy was negligible in Pima Indians with a 2-h OGTT glucose level below 11 mmol/L (200 mg/dL) but increased to 20% when 2-h glucose levels were above that value.[7] A similar relationship between retinopathy and 2-h blood glucose levels has been observed in London,[437] Athens,[438] and Oxford, Massachusetts.[439]

The facts that glomerular basement membranes are normal at the onset of both primary type 1 IDDM and secondary acquired diabetes but are thickened 3.5 to 5 y later[440, 441] and that diabetic nephropathy develops in normal kidneys transplanted from nondiabetic donors into diabetic recipients[442] strongly support a pathogenic influence of the metabolic milieu. Consistent with this view is the observation that a kidney transplanted into a diabetic "cured" by successful pancreatic transplantation remained normal for 4 y thereafter,[443] at which time the patient died of a myocardial infarction. In other studies light microscopic and electron microscopic examination showed that biopsy specimens of glomerular basement membranes in transplanted kidneys appeared normal and without thickening 2 to 3 y after combined kidney and pancreas transplantation.[444] A remarkable report has appeared that diabetic kidneys transplanted into nondiabetic recipients revert to normal within 7 mo.[445] On the other hand, successful pancreatic transplantation did not prevent progression of established diabetic retinopathy, again suggesting that hyperglycemia per se is not the sole issue in the development of complications.[446] It is possible that genetic factors play a determining role.[429]

Will Meticulous Control Prevent the Complications of Diabetes?

Evidence that diabetic complications occur only in the presence of diabetic metabolic derangements does not necessarily prove that such complications can be prevented by meticulous control of glycemia. None of the studies designed to test this critical question has provided a conclusive answer. The study from Malmö, Sweden,[447] is perhaps the most noteworthy of the retrospective evaluations. Before 1935, diabetic subjects were treated with multiple injections of regular insulin. In 1935 long-acting insulins were introduced and were routinely used thereafter. The pre-1935 treatment group had less retinopathy and nephropathy than the post-1935 group, suggesting that better control of postprandial hyperglycemia provided by multiple injections of regular insulin played a role.

Of the prospective studies, the most ambitious involved 4400 patients followed continuously for 25 y.[448] After 12 y of type 1 diabetes, retinopathy was correlated with the duration and severity of hyperglycemia. In another study patients receiving multiple injections of regular insulin developed fewer microaneurysms than those receiving a single injection of long-acting insulin.[449] This study was criticized because of problems in the experimental design, but a reassessment and further follow-up resulted in similar conclusions.[450] A 2-y randomized prospective study of patients with advanced background retinopathy at first suggested that intensive glucoregulation prevented deterioration of renal and sensory nerve function but not retinopathy.[451] More recently it was reported that background retinopathy progressed to proliferative retinopathy in both aggressively controlled patients receiving continuous subcutaneous insulin infusion and control patients receiving conventional insulin treatment. However, improvement in retinal morphology was much more common in the former group.[452] As noted earlier, pancreatic transplantation in one series did not prevent progression of retinopathy.[446] The Diabetes Control and Complications Trial, a large multicenter prospective trial designed to test the effect of control on development of diabetic retinopathy, is under way in the United States, sponsored by the National Institutes of Health. Results are not available at the time of this writing. On balance, the answer to the question of prevention by meticulous control is "maybe."

Can Meticulous Control Reverse Established Complications?

Although good control may cause a reduction in the width of thickened muscle capillary basement membranes,[17] it does not appear to reverse established, clinically manifest diabetic microvascular disease.[453] It may help preserve renal and sensory nerve function over a 2-y period.[454] Occasionally, initial worsening of diabetic retinopathy is observed after a period of intensive therapy.[453, 455] The cause of deterioration in retinopathy is unknown. Perhaps retinal glycopenia resulting from reduced glucose delivery to ischemic areas of the glucose-dependent retina may play a role in this therapeutic paradox. As mentioned earlier, clinically manifest diabetic nephropathy may progress despite a reduction in muscle capillary basement membrane width induced by meticulous control (unpublished observations, P. Raskin, A. O. Pietri, R. H. Unger, et al.). This dichotomy suggests that in muscle, a tissue in which new capillary formation can occur, basement membrane thickening in new capillaries is being prevented by metabolic normalization. By contrast, no such turnover of retinal and glomerular capillaries occurs; damaged capillaries are thus the permanent legacy of the past metabolic trauma. Motor nerve conduction velocity may improve,[456] but improvement in symptoms is minimal. Vibration sense is unimproved.[452]

To summarize: (1) Diabetic microangiopathy rarely, if ever, occurs in the absence of the metabolic abnormalities of diabetes. (2) Many patients tolerate the metabolic abnormalities of diabetes for decades without developing diabetic vasculopathy,[429, 457, 458] suggesting the presence of some pathogenetic factor in addition to the metabolic abnormalities. This factor could be genetic. Thus some persons with only mildly elevated blood sugar levels may have complications while others with constant, major hyperglycemia are exempt.[429, 457] (3) Correction of the metabolic and hormonal abnormalities of diabetes may prevent or retard the development of complications, but this is unproved. (4) There is no evidence that meticulous control of a diabetic patient reverses clinically established microangiopathic complications; progression of diabetic retinopathy may be accelerated, at least in the initial period after meticulous control is instituted.

Potential Mechanisms in the Pathogenesis of Complications

Pathogenesis of the various diabetic complications may not be uniform. Distinct abnormalities might operate in nerve and kidney, for example, or several abnormalities might act in concert. Three possible mechanisms have received considerable attention: (1) the glycosylation of proteins, (2) the polyol pathway, and (3) the hemodynamic hypothesis.

Glycation Modifies Proteins

Enzymatic glycosylation is a normal post-translational process that greatly expands the structural and functional repertoire of proteins that can be synthesized from only 20 amino acids.[459] Basement membrane protein, α_2-macroglobulin, collagen, some cell-surface receptors, HLA antigens, immunoglobulins, and certain hormones are but a few of the important glycoproteins synthesized enzymatically. When a protein is exposed to a high glucose concentration, nonenzymatic incorporation of glucose can occur, resulting in unregulated glycosylation. The term favored for nonenzymatic glycosylation is glycation, but in this chapter glycosylation will be used interchangeably. The reaction involves the rapid formation of a Schiff base (aldimine), followed by a much slower internal shift (Amadori rearrangement; Fig. 24–31).[460] Lysine and valine residues are the primary sites of glucose addition. Such unregulated glycation changes protein structure and may alter function. In nondiabetics this is prevented by appropriate insulin secretion whenever the extracellular glucose concentration approaches the range in which nonenzymatic glycosylation becomes a potential problem. Some glycation occurs at normal plasma glucose concentrations, but detrimental glycation requires hyperglycemia.

In the case of hemoglobin, the most extensively studied of the glycated proteins, epsilon-amino groups of interchain lysines are glycosylated, but it is glycosylation of the terminal

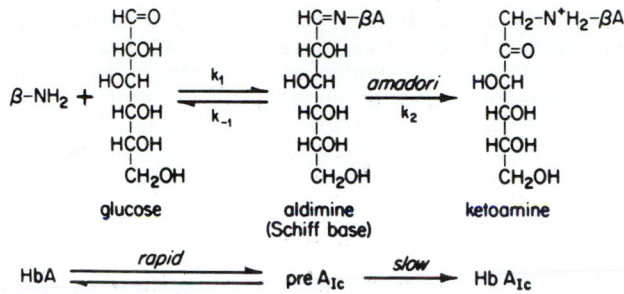

Figure 24–31. Nonenzymatic glycosylation of hemoglobin to form hemoglobin A$_{1c}$. This reaction is prototypical for glycosylation of proteins in general. Amino acids primarily glycosylated are lysine and valine. (From Higgins PJ, Bunn HF. Kinetic analysis of the nonenzymatic glycosylation of hemoglobin. J Biol Chem 1981; 256:5204–5208.)

valine of the beta chain that alters its surface charge and fortuitously converts it to fast-moving hemoglobin A$_{1c}$ on electrophoresis.[461] The level of hemoglobin A$_{1c}$ provides an index of integrated glucose concentration over the life span of the red blood cell, which normally is about 100 to 120 d. The measurement of glycated albumin, which turns over more rapidly than hemoglobin, provides a short-term clinical index of diabetic control.[462] After a week of intensive glucose control, levels of glycated serum proteins decrease by approximately 40% while the hemoglobin A$_{1c}$ level drops only 10%.[463] Although hemoglobin was the first protein to receive attention, it is likely that every protein in the body can undergo glycosylation provided intracellular glucose or glucose 6-phosphate concentrations reflect plasma glucose levels. Intracellular proteins in insulin-requiring tissues of the diabetic subject may be partially protected from glycation despite extracellular hyperglycemia, because glucose is excluded from entering the cell by the deficiency of insulin.[464] Nevertheless, at autopsy, tissues from diabetic subjects reflect a generalized increase in glycosylation.[465]

Nonenzymatically glycosylated proteins slowly form fluorescent cross-linked protein adducts (usually called advanced glycosylation end products), a process known as browning. Formation increases with the ambient glucose concentration. Assay for browning products by measuring collagen-linked fluorescence in skin biopsy specimens from patients with long-standing diabetes reveals levels twice that of normal subjects.[466] Fluorescence is increased in patients with severe retinopathy and nephropathy, suggesting a relationship between cumulative hyperglycemia and the severity of diabetic complications. The specific chemical product bestowing fluorescence was identified as 2-(2-furoyl)-4(5)-(2-furanyl)-1*H*-imidazole, but there is now a question about its role.[467]

Can Overglycosylation of Proteins in Diabetes Produce Disease?

The level of glycosylation of a protein in vivo is determined in part by its time of contact with a given level of hyperglycemia. In addition, the turnover rate of the protein influences the extent of glycosylation. Proteins in plasma that turn over slowly, such as red blood cell membranes,[468] hemoglobin,[460] albumin,[462] low-density lipoproteins (LDLs),[469] high-density lipoproteins (HDLs),[470] and immunoglobulin G,[471] become significantly glycosylated in diabetes. Outside the circulation, increased glycation has been found in lens,[472] glomerular basement membrane,[473] aorta, coronary arteries, and femoral nerve.[465] It should be pointed out that false estimates of the extent of nonenzymatic glycation may be obtained if the thiobarbituric acid (colorimetric) method is

used because it measures glycosylation regardless of mechanism; in glomeruli of diabetic humans the glycosylation of lysine and hydroxylysine residues by enzymatic mechanisms turned out to be far greater than the glycosylation by nonenzymatic reactions when the two processes were differentiated.[474]

Interference with function of a protein by glycation requires either that the affected intrachain lysines be close to the active site(s) of the molecule or that stereochemical configuration of the protein be distorted. The function of some proteins is known to be altered by glycosylation, and in other cases the possibility is suspected but unproved. In the former category are hemoglobin, albumin, lens protein, fibrin, collagen, lipoproteins, the glycoprotein recognition system of hepatic endothelial cells,[475] and antithrombin III.[476] In the latter category are immunoglobulin G, red blood cell membranes, circulating white blood cells, myelin, and von Willebrand factor.

Glycosylation of hemoglobin blocks the reaction of 2,3-diphosphoglycerate with positively charged residues on the beta chain, causing a slight but clinically insignificant increase in oxygen affinity.[477, 478] Glycosylated albumin inhibits the hepatic uptake of glycoproteins[477] and is taken up into small blood vessels more rapidly than native albumin, but a report that it binds to glomerular basement membranes[479] has not been confirmed.[480] Glycated fibrin is less susceptible to digestion by plasmin,[481] which might account for its extensive accumulation in diabetic tissues.[482] Nonenzymatic glycosylation of the crystalline proteins of the lens may promote the formation of disulfide links between protein molecules;[472] aggregates of crystalline protein with molecular weights in excess of 5×10^6 scatter light, i.e., constitute a cataract.

It is not known whether glycosylation of collagen in glomerular basement membranes is related to their thickening in diabetes. There appears to be a generalized increase in basement membrane synthesis.[483] Glycosylated collagen is more insoluble and resistant to digestion because of increased intramolecular cross-linking,[484] which may decrease its degradation. It has also been postulated that decreased proteoglycan synthesis causes increased permeability of basement membranes and that thickening is a compensatory response.[485]

It has been reported that glycosylated collagen is antigenic in rats and that rats with streptozocin-induced diabetes form antibodies to glycosylated but not native collagen.[486] If this is true, antibodies to glycosylated collagen could damage the glomerular basement membranes either directly or via immune complexes. Conceivably, the absence of severe microangiopathy in some poorly controlled diabetics could represent a reduced immunological response to glycosylated collagen.

Glycated skin collagen is resistant to digestion by collagenase.[487] It is not clear whether glycation is responsible for connective tissue changes, such as tight waxy skin and limited joint mobility, that are said to indicate an increased risk of late complications.[488, 489]

Glycosylation of the red cell membrane could play a role in the 15% reduction in erythrocyte survival time[490] and perhaps in the loss of the normal red blood cell deformability that occurs in poorly controlled diabetes.[491, 492] Normal red blood cells pass easily through capillaries with luminal diameters smaller than their own because they are deformable; loss of flexibility could cause sludging of blood and contribute to retinal and renal ischemia.[492, 493] Glycosylation of myelin protein[494] may account in part for the functional changes in nerve conduction.

Theoretically, overglycosylation of insulin receptors could contribute to the reduced sensitivity to insulin that occurs in chronic hyperglycemia[359, 495] and is reversed by meticulous control.[361, 362] Membrane glycosylation in leukocytes conceivably might account for the reduced chemotaxis,[496] diapedesis,[497] phagocytosis,[498] bactericidal activity,[498] and cell-mediated immunity[499] reported in diabetes, although this has not yet been explored. The defective response of T cells and B cells to mitogens can be restored by the normalization of glucose.[499, 500] Overglycosylation of von Willebrand factor could contribute to the increased platelet aggregation reported in poorly controlled diabetes.[501] The previously mentioned advanced glycosylation end products have been proposed as a major factor in diabetic macrovascular disease.[502] By cross-linking matrix and plasma proteins, they may accelerate development of atherosclerosis.

The Polyol Pathway

A second general mechanism possibly underlying diabetic complications is activation of the polyol pathway.[503] In this pathway glucose is reduced to sorbitol under the influence of the enzyme aldose reductase (D-aldose:NADP⁺ 1-oxidoreductase) with NADPH as cofactor. Sorbitol can then be oxidized to fructose with the production of NADH by the enzyme sorbitol dehydrogenase (L-iditol dehydrogenase). Aldose reductase is present in the retina, kidney papillae, lens, Schwann cells, and aorta, tissues that are frequently damaged in diabetes. Polyols have been implicated in the pathogenesis of cataracts,[504] retinopathy,[505] neuropathy,[506] and aortic disease.[507] In the lens, sorbitol may cause osmotic swelling, which is initially reversible, but subsequently Na⁺,K⁺-ATPase activity falls.[504] How the latter interacts with the postulated role of glycosylated lens proteins in the genesis of cataracts[472, 508] is not known. In nerves polyols also inhibit Na⁺,K⁺-ATPase,[509, 510] a lesion that accompanies the characteristic *myo*-inositol deficiency found in experimental diabetic neuropathy.[506, 509–511] Although *myo*-inositol deficiency is routinely observed in nerves from diabetic rats and repaired by *myo*-inositol feeding,[509, 511] biopsy specimens of sural nerve from humans with diabetic neuropathy failed to show diminished levels of *myo*-inositol.[512] Further studies will be required to understand the discrepancy. Experimentally, retinopathy,[505] cataracts,[504] nephropathy,[503] and the metabolic abnormalities of peripheral nerve[506, 510] can be prevented by inhibition of the polyol pathway. Sorbinil, an aldose reductase inhibitor tested in human trials, may relieve symptoms in painful diabetic neuropathy[513] and in long-term treatment appears to enhance nerve regeneration in diabetic humans.[514] The use of these inhibitors as prophylaxis for complications has not been reported.

Nonenzymatic glycation of proteins and the polyol pathway may not be unrelated mechanisms. It is now known that fructose generated in the polyol sequence can nonenzymatically bind to protein (called fructation) and that fluorescence of collagen from diabetic animals is decreased by inhibitors of aldol reductase.[515] It is thus possible that an active polyol pathway may contribute significantly to nonenzymatic glycation of proteins.

Hemodynamic Hypothesis

A third postulated general mechanism of tissue injury is based on the observation that blood flow is increased in patients studied shortly after the onset of IDDM (for a review see ref. 516). Because the blood pressure is usually normal in such patients, it is likely that arteriolar resistance is decreased. The increased hydrostatic pressure in the capillary beds is thought to increase filtration of potentially damaging proteins and other macromolecules (including immune complexes) into the walls of blood vessels and mesangium, secondarily stimulating synthesis of mesangial

and basement membrane components. The latter step is presumed to enhance capillary "leakiness," setting up a vicious cycle. The hemodynamic hypothesis has received most attention in connection with diabetic renal disease.[517] In view of the wide spectrum of dysfunctions that characterize the diabetic state, the probability that a single abnormality like hyperperfusion, by itself, could cause microangiopathy is low.

Atherosclerosis

Diabetes is a risk factor for atherosclerosis, particularly in women.[517] Age, hypertension, and smoking further increase its frequency. The atherosclerotic risk is greatest in poorly controlled individuals, possibly because of associated hypercholesterolemia and hypertriglyceridemia. Coronary, cerebral, and peripheral vessels are involved, leading to an increased incidence of myocardial infarction, stroke, and gangrene. The atherosclerotic syndromes in diabetes are not distinguishable from those occurring in persons without diabetes except that the incidence of silent myocardial infarction is said to be higher.[518]

How Poor Diabetic Control May Cause Hypertriglyceridemia and Hypercholesterolemia

Marked hypertriglyceridemia is common in diabetes both as a transient accompaniment of poor metabolic control and as a persistent finding in some relatively well-controlled patients. In the latter situation a genetic form of hyperlipidemia may coexist with diabetes, a fact that usually can be established by study of nondiabetic family members.[519] Patients with type 1 IDDM frequently have normal triglyceride levels if they are in good glycemic control. However, if significant insulin deficiency develops they may become severely hypertriglyceridemic with increases in both chylomicrons and very-low-density lipoprotein (VLDL) triglycerides (Fig. 24–32A). Two mechanisms may be operative. First, the synthesis of lipoprotein lipase may be greatly curtailed because of insulin deficiency;[520, 521] this produces a defect in lipolysis of triglyceride-rich lipoproteins. Second, high levels of free fatty acids present because of poor control provide substrate to the liver for overproduction of VLDL triglycerides. Insulin therapy will reverse both of these defects and restore triglyceride levels to normal.[521]

Moderate hypertriglyceridemia also may occur in type 2 NIDDM patients even in the presence of normal or elevated insulin levels. The elevation of VLDL triglycerides in some patients may be due in part to obesity and a high caloric intake. Overloading the liver with substrate (carbohydrate from the diet and free fatty acids from adipocytes) will stimulate the production of VLDL triglycerides.[522, 523] Free fatty acid elevation is probably due to peripheral insulin resistance.[524] NIDDM patients also do not clear triglycerides well because they have a moderate reduction in lipoprotein lipase levels.[525] The defect in triglyceride metabolism (overproduction of VLDL triglycerides and defective lipolysis of triglyceride-rich lipoproteins) (see Fig. 24–32A) is not as marked in patients with NIDDM as in patients with severe insulin deficiency. However, when insulin levels fall in advanced NIDDM, severe hypertriglyceridemia similar to that of IDDM can develop, and insulin therapy is then required for reduction of triglyceride levels.

Both IDDM and NIDDM patients can have elevated LDL cholesterol, but in the absence of concomitant genetic defects, increases are minimal. Several factors can contribute to an increase in LDL cholesterol concentrations (see Fig. 24–32A). First, overproduction of VLDL particles in obese

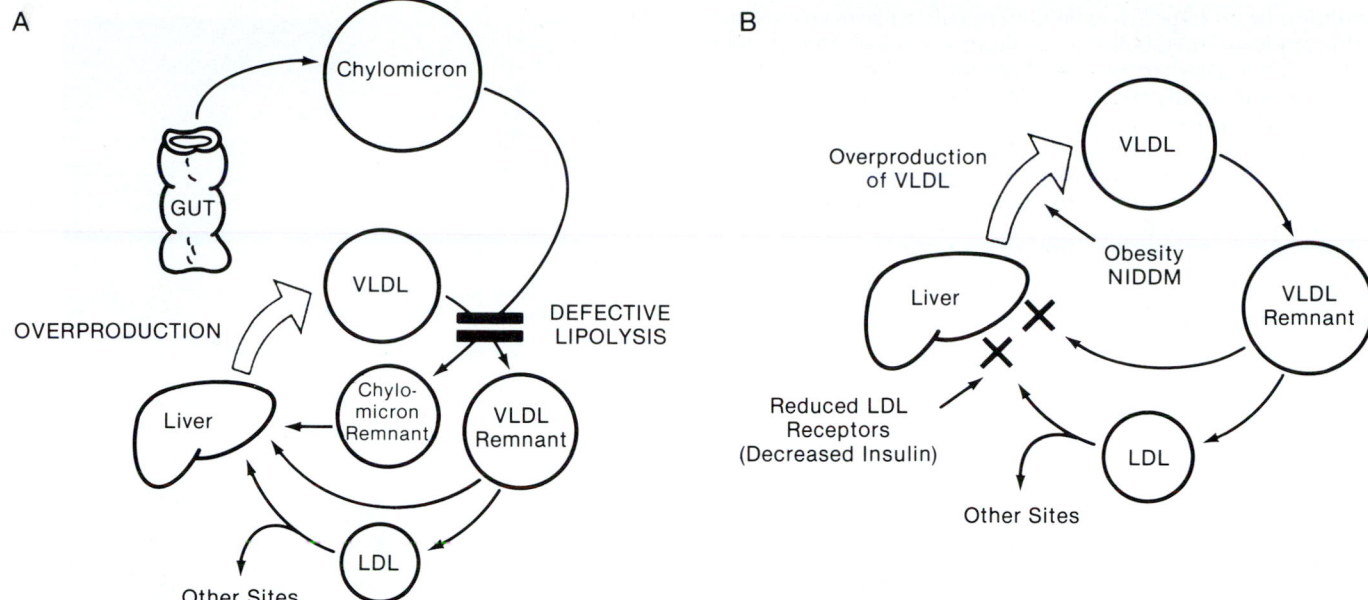

Figure 24–32. *A,* Defects in metabolism of triglyceride-rich lipoproteins in diabetes. The triglyceride-rich lipoproteins are derived from two sources, the gut and the liver. The gut secretes chylomicrons after ingestion of dietary fat. In the circulation, triglycerides of chylomicrons are hydrolyzed by lipoprotein lipase, which degrades these lipoproteins to chylomicron remnants. The latter are removed by the liver. The liver secretes VLDL, which likewise undergoes lipolysis by lipoprotein lipase. The resulting VLDL remnants can have two fates; they can be taken up by the liver or converted to LDL. LDL is removed mainly by the liver and to a lesser extent by other tissues. Most LDL and VLDL remnants are cleared from the circulation by LDL (*apo* B/E) receptors. Chylomicron remnants are removed by a separate receptor, usually designated the chylomicron remnant or *apo* E receptor. In diabetes, two abnormalities may exist in triglyceride metabolism: overproduction of VLDL and defective lipolysis of triglyceride-rich lipoproteins by lipoprotein lipase. Both contribute to the hypertriglyceridemia of diabetes.

B, Mechanisms of hypercholesterolemia in diabetes mellitus. Two factors can elevate LDL levels in diabetic patients. These are overproduction of VLDL, which can lead to increased production of both intermediate-density lipoprotein and LDL, and reduced activity of LDL receptors. The overproduction of VLDL can be due to both obesity and NIDDM. Reduced levels of LDL receptors are the consequence of relative and absolute decreases in insulin action secondary to insulin deficiency or insulin resistance or both. This leads to decreased clearance of both LDL and VLDL remnants, both of which contribute to a rise in LDL concentrations. (Courtesy of Dr. S. Grundy.)

patients with NIDDM can lead to increased conversion of VLDL to LDL; i.e., LDL synthesis is increased.[526] Second, insulin deficiency may reduce the activity of LDL receptors, impairing LDL clearance. Third, if obese diabetics consume an excess of saturated fatty acids and cholesterol, this too can suppress the activity of LDL receptors and accentuate the rise in LDL levels. Overall, the frequency of elevated LDL cholesterol levels in diabetic patients is increased, but to a much lesser degree than is hypertriglyceridemia.

The mechanism by which VLDL and LDL induce or enhance the atherosclerotic process is not known, although they probably act through formation of foam cells (cholesterol ester–laden macrophages and smooth muscle cells) within the arterial wall. The formation of these cells represents a crucial first step in the development of the atherosclerotic plaque. It is likely that oxidative modification of LDL enhances uptake in macrophages destined to become foam cells. The receptor involved here is not the normal LDL receptor but the alternate acetyl LDL (scavenger) receptor.[527] It is not known whether diabetes alters oxidative rates for LDL.

High-Density-Lipoprotein Cholesterol

HDL cholesterol levels often are low in poorly controlled diabetic patients, especially in those with NIDDM.[528] HDL cholesterol may protect against the development of atherosclerosis,[529] and this could be one factor contributing to coronary heart disease in diabetics, particularly in women.[530] Low levels of HDL may be due to glycation, which accelerates its turnover.[470] The composition of HDL is also abnormal in non–insulin-dependent diabetes.[531] HDL levels become normal after rigorous metabolic control.[532, 533]

Platelets, Prostaglandins, and Vascular Disease

Increased platelet aggregation has been postulated as a factor in diabetic atherogenesis and in the disseminated intravascular coagulation that has been reported in diabetic ketoacidosis.[534, 535] Enhanced adhesiveness is observed in both IDDM and NIDDM before the development of clinically apparent atherosclerosis and may be related in part to the elevated levels of von Willebrand factor characteristic of diabetes.[536] The accelerated second phase of platelet aggregation in diabetes may be due to increased thromboxane A_2 synthesis by diabetic platelets,[537] because it is reversed by inhibitors of prostaglandin synthase. Finally, synthesis of prostacyclin, a vasodilator and inhibitor of platelet aggregation, is diminished in the blood vessels of type 1 diabetic patients.[538] Such abnormalities could play a role in the large vessel disease or the microangiopathy of diabetes. However, in careful studies of plasma and urinary metabolites of thromboxane, presumed to be of platelet origin, and of prostacyclin, derived from endothelial cells, no differences between diabetic patients with or without retinopathy and nondiabetic controls were noted.[539] There were likewise no differences between diabetics and controls in platelet granule constituents, in the aggregation response to adenosine diphosphate and arachidonic acid, or in the serum levels of thromboxane B_2. Although these studies suggest that platelet activation does not precede microvascular complications, other authors disagree.[540]

It has been observed that high concentrations of insulin, such as might occur in insulin-treated patients, inhibit prostacyclin production in rat aorta in vitro, presumably by lowering cyclic AMP concentrations.[541] However, acute insulin-induced hypoglycemia does not alter plasma or urinary thromboxane metabolites,[539] making it unlikely that platelet activation related to overinsulinization causes the acceleration in retinopathy sometimes observed in meticulously controlled patients.

To summarize, the cause of the accelerated atherosclerosis of diabetes has yet to be fully explained. It is almost certainly multifactorial with contributions from abnormalities in lipid metabolism, hemostatic factors, and the endothelium/smooth muscle unit of the vessel wall itself.

Cardiomyopathy

The possibility of a specific diabetes-related cardiomyopathy was suggested by the description in 1972 of four middle-aged patients with diabetes who died of congestive heart failure without evidence of valvular, hypertensive, atherosclerotic, congenital, or alcoholic heart disease.[542] Postmortem examination revealed only cardiomegaly and myocardial fibrosis. In one of the patients subendothelial thickening and acid mucopolysaccharide deposits in capillaries suggested diabetic microangiopathy.[542] The possibility that this cardiomyopathy was related to diabetes is supported by the finding of an increased prevalence of unexplained congestive heart failure in diabetes[543] and by autopsy reports of cardiac hypertrophy in the absence of specific cardiac disease. Interstitial and perivascular fibrosis has been observed, associated with periodic acid–Schiff (PAS)–positive deposits,[544] myocardial capillary basement membrane thickening,[545] and capillary microaneurysms.[546] Functional alterations in the heart have been demonstrated in diabetic animals[547] and humans[548] in the absence of coronary atherosclerosis, and changes in cardiac myosin have been observed in diabetic rats.[549] Echocardiographic abnormalities resembling those of cardiomyopathy induced by alcohol, doxorubicin hydrochloride (Adriamyacin), or viral infection were found in one sixth of young IDDM patients, independent of the duration of diabetes or the level of hyperglycemia.[548] Another echocardiographic study of 80 type 1 diabetic patients without signs of ischemic heart disease revealed cardiac hyperfunction, particularly in patients who were developing nephropathy.[550] This was attributed to hyperperfusion. Impaired peak diastolic filling rate has been demonstrated by radionuclide left ventricular angiography in type 1 diabetic patients without diabetic complications or demonstrable coronary artery disease.[551] This defect may be the earliest functional manifestation of diabetic cardiomyopathy. In a larger study of 63 asymptomatic type 1 patients aged 30 to 50 y radionuclide ventriculography revealed a smaller than normal rise in left ventricular ejection fraction during dynamic exercise in 29% of patients. Some of these individuals had arteriolar thickening and interstitial fibrosis on endocardial biopsy but conspicuous basement membrane thickening was not common.[552] A role of an intracellular Ca^{2+} overload in diabetic cardiomyopathy is supported by the fact that cardiac function and ultrastructural status in streptozocin-diabetic rats are improved by the Ca^{2+} antagonist verapamil.[553] Increasingly diabetic cardiomyopathy is being accepted as a clinical reality, although the pathogenesis of this putative entity is varied and multifactorial.

Dermopathy

Skin changes in diabetes mellitus include shin spots (Fig. 24–33), diabetic bullae, and necrobiosis lipoidica diabeticorum (Fig. 24–34).[554] It is doubtful that microangiopathy is solely responsible for diabetic dermopathy, because capillary basement membranes are thickened both in the shin spots and in nearby normal skin. Such spots are present in more

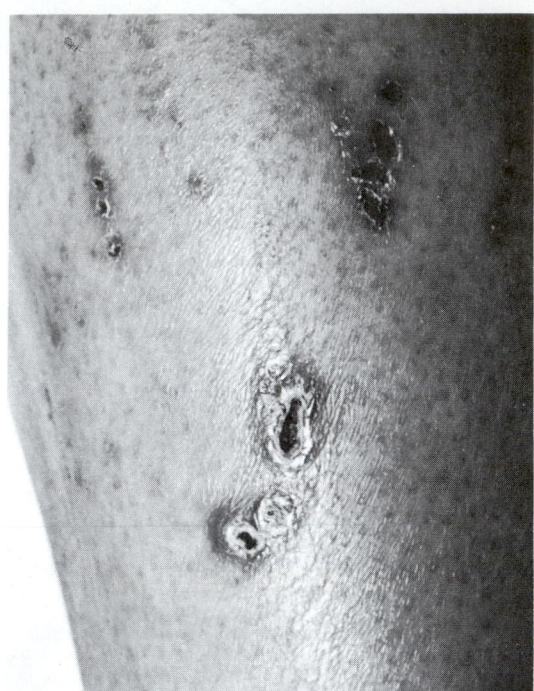

Figure 24–33. Early lesions of dermopathy showing central crusting; in this patient the lesions appear in a somewhat linear arrangement. (From Binkley GW. Dermopathy in the diabetic syndrome. Arch Dermatol 1965; 92:625. Copyright 1965, American Medical Association.)

than half the men and approximately one third of the women with diabetes who are over the age of 30. They are not specific for diabetes and may be seen after trauma in nondiabetic subjects.

Necrobiosis lipoidica diabeticorum consists of round, firm, reddish brown to yellow plaques that most commonly involve the legs. The hands, arms, abdomen, and head are occasionally affected. The lesions may appear within the first year of the diabetes.

Diabetic Foot Syndrome

The diabetic foot syndrome is the consequence of coexisting vascular insufficiency and neuropathy.[555, 556] The latter is probably more important, as evidenced by the fact that ulcers indistinguishable from those of diabetes occur in other neuropathic diseases such as leprosy. The vascular insufficiency may involve large vessels, arterioles, and capillaries. There is extensive arteriovenous shunting at the precapillary level, and tissue oxygenation is impaired in areas at risk.[557, 558] The neuropathy is predominantly sensory and is characterized by a diminution of pain, vibratory perception, and position sense. Normally the integrity of the skin of the feet is protected by the ability to sense pain, which prompts an unconscious shift in gait or position whenever minimal trauma occurs. In diabetes, by contrast, such pain-mediated adjustments may not occur, permitting continuing trauma and leading to the breakdown of skin. This defect may be present even though routine sensory examination is normal. If the capacity to sweat is lost because of autonomic neuropathy, the resulting dryness of the skin leads to cracking, superficial inflammation, or chronic dermatitis.[556] The normal increase in blood flow required for healing after trivial trauma or infection may not occur because of vascular disease. Callus formation secondary to abnormal distribution of pressure because of the proprioceptive defect predisposes to pressure ischemia, and microthrombi contribute to ulcer development or gangrene.

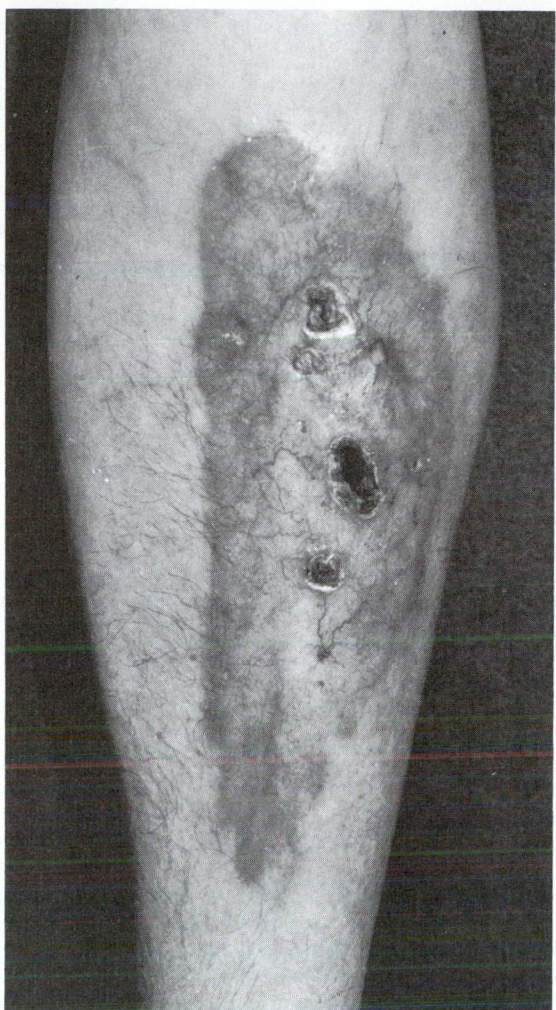

Figure 24–34. Extensive dry ulcerative plaque of necrobiosis lipoidica diabeticorum. (Courtesy of Dr. George Odland.)

The most important aspect of management for the diabetic foot syndrome is prophylaxis. Diabetic patients should inspect their feet daily, searching for redness and other signs of trauma, which may not be symptomatic. Soaking the feet for 20 min in warm water followed by an application of oil-based lotions may help keep the skin soft. Well-fitting shoes are imperative, and, if possible, a different pair of shoes should be worn each half-day to minimize pressure in the same areas. Jogging shoes are ideal. Calluses should be treated by sanding with paper or an emery board. Trimming of calluses should be done only by a podiatrist, physician, or specially trained nurse. Once an ulcer develops, the most important treatment is bed rest to remove pressure, coupled with débridement, soaks, and antibiotics if infection is present. Some physicians treat ulcers by placing a well-fitting orthopedic walking cast to remove pressure. The advantage is that the patient can continue to work. X-ray examination of the foot is indicated in every patient with an ulcer, because foreign bodies (pins, tacks, glass, nails) are commonly present, often unrecognized because of impaired pain sensation. A corollary is that diabetic subjects should never go barefoot.

The diabetic foot is perhaps the most preventable of all diabetic complications, utilizing the relatively simple measures just mentioned. It is tragic that such measures do not always receive adequate attention.

Nephropathy

Diabetic nephropathy now accounts for close to half of the patients receiving long-term renal dialysis in the United States. Estimates of the prevalence of end-stage nephropathy in IDDM vary widely. It has been reported in 50% of the cases of childhood-onset IDDM and 30% of those of IDDM beginning before age 31.[559] Yet a 40-y follow-up of IDDM patients indicates that the majority did not develop proteinuria[458] and only 8% developed end-stage nephropathy.[560] Death from renal disease is less frequent in type 2 diabetes, perhaps because of the shorter duration of disease and the higher cardiovascular mortality. In Japan renal disease was the cause of death in 11.9% of the 201 subjects who died in a 20-y follow-up of 1221 diabetic patients.[561] On the other hand, nephropathy appears to be rare in Japanese-American men with diabetes.[562] Although end-stage renal disease is uncommon in type 2 diabetes, 65% of diabetic Pima Indians, all with NIDDM, had histological evidence of diabetic glomerulosclerosis at autopsy.[563] Widely differing prevalence rates are probably the consequence of genetic factors. This follows from the observation that some families with multiple members who have diabetes rarely exhibit nephropathy, whereas in other multiplex families more than 80% of affected siblings have renal disease.[564]

Pathology

Diabetic glomerulosclerosis is ordinarily divided into two classes, a common diffuse form and a nodular form that represents accelerated disease (Fig. 24–35).[565] The two patterns may coexist. In the diffuse form the entire mesangium is thickened. The nodular form consists of capsular drops, fibrin caps and adhesions in the glomeruli, microaneurysms, and large spherical accumulations of PAS-positive material in the mesangium at the periphery of the glomerular tufts.[565] The latter are the glomerular nodules of Kimmelstiel and Wilson.

Diabetic nephropathy begins with thickening of the glomerular basement membrane, an increase in the mesangial matrix (a forerunner of diffuse glomerulosclerosis), and subintimal hyaline thickening of both afferent and efferent arterioles. These changes are not present at the onset of diabetes but begin to appear 1.5 to 2.5 y after the metabolic abnormality has been recognized.[440, 441] The mesangial matrix between the glomerular capillaries, which together with the afferent and efferent glomerular vessels form the glomerular hilum, contains nerve endings, smooth muscle, and cells with angiotensin II receptors. Normally the mesangium takes up and processes macromolecules from the circulation.[566] In rodents such molecules move from the periphery of the mesangium to the hilum of the glomerulus and leave the area via the distal tubular cells.[567] The capacity to clear macromolecules is impaired in diabetes.[566] Accumulation of albumin and larger proteins within the glomerular wall and in the mesangium may stimulate mesangial matrix production and lead to the diffuse and nodular changes of diabetic nephropathy.[566] In humans, plasma proteins, particularly albumin, are deposited along the tubular basement membrane and Bowman capsule in the kidney (see Fig. 24–35D)[568] as well as in basement membranes of muscle and skin.[569] Five years after the onset of diabetes, hyalinosis of the efferent glomerular arterioles and early Kimmelstiel-Wilson nodules, the two most specific changes of diabetic nephropathy, may be present.[570] Normal kidneys transplanted into diabetic recipients develop these changes within 4 y,[571] suggesting that the abnormal metabolic environment is required. Conversely, as noted earlier, transplantation of

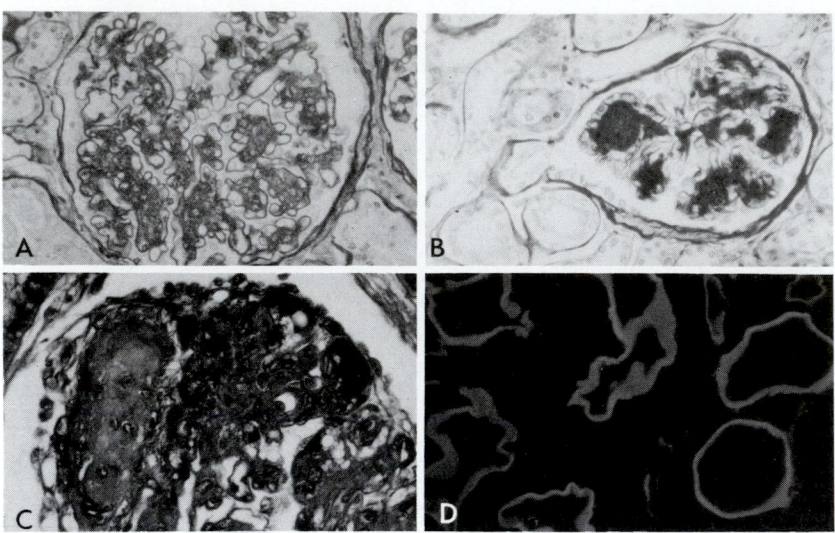

Figure 24–35. Representative lesions of diabetic nephropathy. *A,* Glomerulus showing diffuse diabetic glomerulosclerosis. There is diffuse thickening of all mesangial areas by a moderate increase in mesangial matrix. PAS, light microscopy. Magnification × 400.

B, Glomerulus showing nodular diabetic glomerulosclerosis. There is focal accentuation of the mesangial matrix into rounded nodules (Kimmelstiel-Wilson nodules). PAS, light microscopy. Magnification × 400.

C, Portion of glomerulus showing mesangial nodule of Kimmelstiel-Wilson at the left and regions of fuchsinophilic "fibrin caps." Trichrome stain. Magnification × 600.

D, Small segment of renal cortex from a diabetic patient showing diffuse intense linear staining along all tubular basement membranes with antisera to human albumin. Immunofluorescence microscopy. Magnification × 600.

(Photomicrographs courtesy of Drs. Fred G. Silva, Conrad L. Pirani, and Edwin H. Elgenbrodt.)

kidneys with established diabetic nephropathy into nondiabetic recipients resulted in normalization of the thickened mesangial matrix and glomerular capillary basement membranes and disappearance of arteriolar subintimal deposits,[445] although this unique report will be difficult to confirm.

Natural History

The natural history of diabetic nephropathy is summarized in Table 24–19 and Figure 24–36. At the onset of diabetes the kidneys are usually enlarged[572] owing to increased glomerular and tubular size.[440, 441] When metabolic control is poor, the glomerular filtration rate is high.[572, 573] Microproteinuria (<550 mg protein/24 h), mainly albumin of glomerular rather than tubular origin, is present in suboptimally controlled, conventionally treated patients and recedes after 72 h of intensive insulin treatment,[574] although the glomerular size remains above normal. Microproteinuria is not detected by reagent strips for urinary protein and requires immunoassay. The reversible component of microproteinuria is attributed to the combination of hemodynamic abnormalities and loss of charge selectivity of the glomerular membranes.[575, 576]

In the absence of macroproteinuria (>550 mg/24 h, reagent strip–positive) end-stage diabetic nephropathy rarely, if ever, develops, because renal hyperfunction continues until significant proteinuria appears.[577] However, if microproteinuria exceeds 50 mg/24 h, there is a high risk of future macroproteinuria.[578] At first microalbuminuria is present only after a provocative exercise test.[577] Persistent macroproteinuria in excess of 550 mg/24 h indicates glomerular basement membrane disease and is said to predict future renal failure.[579] In one large study macroproteinuria appeared an average of 17 y after the onset of the IDDM.[580] From this point on, glomerular filtration wanes inexorably by about 11 mL/min/y[579] and renal failure is inevitable. The presence of hypertension accelerates the process.[581] The nephrotic syndrome is common, and diabetic retinopathy is almost always present. In one study of 134 patients in whom diabetes was not classified as to type but in most cases began after age 40, only 28% survived 10 y after the onset of continuous proteinuria.[582] This is a little over half the expected survival rate for diabetic patients without proteinuria. At the end stage of diabetic nephropathy the kidney is reduced in size but not to the degree seen in end-stage glomerulonephritis or pyelonephritis. The clinical course of diabetic nephropathy is summarized in Table 24–19.

Pathophysiological Hypotheses

The pathogenic mechanism of diabetic nephropathy is unknown, but it probably results from several causes. The initial abnormality may be chronic renal hyperperfusion. Vasodilation of afferent and efferent glomerular arterioles increases renal plasma flow, and the transcapillary hydraulic pressure gradient across the glomerular basement membrane rises, accounting for the early proteinuria.[583, 584] One important factor in the induction of hyperperfusion may be renal hypoxia, presumably the consequence of interactions among increased levels of glycosylated hemoglobin, decreased levels of red blood cell 2,3-diphosphoglycerate,[585] increased plasma viscosity,[586] and diminished red blood cell deformability.[491] In addition, glucagon[587] and growth hormone,[588] both of which are elevated in poorly controlled diabetes,[589, 590] and hyperglycemia itself[591] increase renal blood flow. Hyperglucagonemia correlates with increased glomerular RNA in diabetic rats.[592] Various other factors have been postulated to play a role: atrial natriuretic peptide, vasodilator prostaglandins, ketone bodies, excess protein intake, renin deficiency, hyporesponsiveness to catecholamines or angiotensin, and altered calcium metabolism.[517] However, their importance remains unknown.

The hyperperfusion model is supported by the fact that reduction in renal perfusion seems to protect the kidney from diabetic nephropathy.[593] In diabetic rats unilateral renal

TABLE 24–19. Typical Clinical Course of Diabetic Nephropathy

Years After Onset of Diabetes (Approximate)	Clinical Course
0	Enlarged kidneys, supernormal function, microalbuminuria reversed by meticulous insulin treatment
2	Thickening of glomerular basement membrane and increase in mesangial matrix
10–15	Silent period: no overt proteinuria; microalbuminuria may be present, especially after exercise (>30 μg/min indicative of future proteinuria)
10–20	Proteinuric period intermittent at first, then persistent (>0.5 g/24 h); this means that a relentless decline in glomerular function has begun
>15	Azotemic period begins on average 17 y after onset
20	Uremic period: diabetic retinopathy, hypertension, and nephrotic syndrome may be present

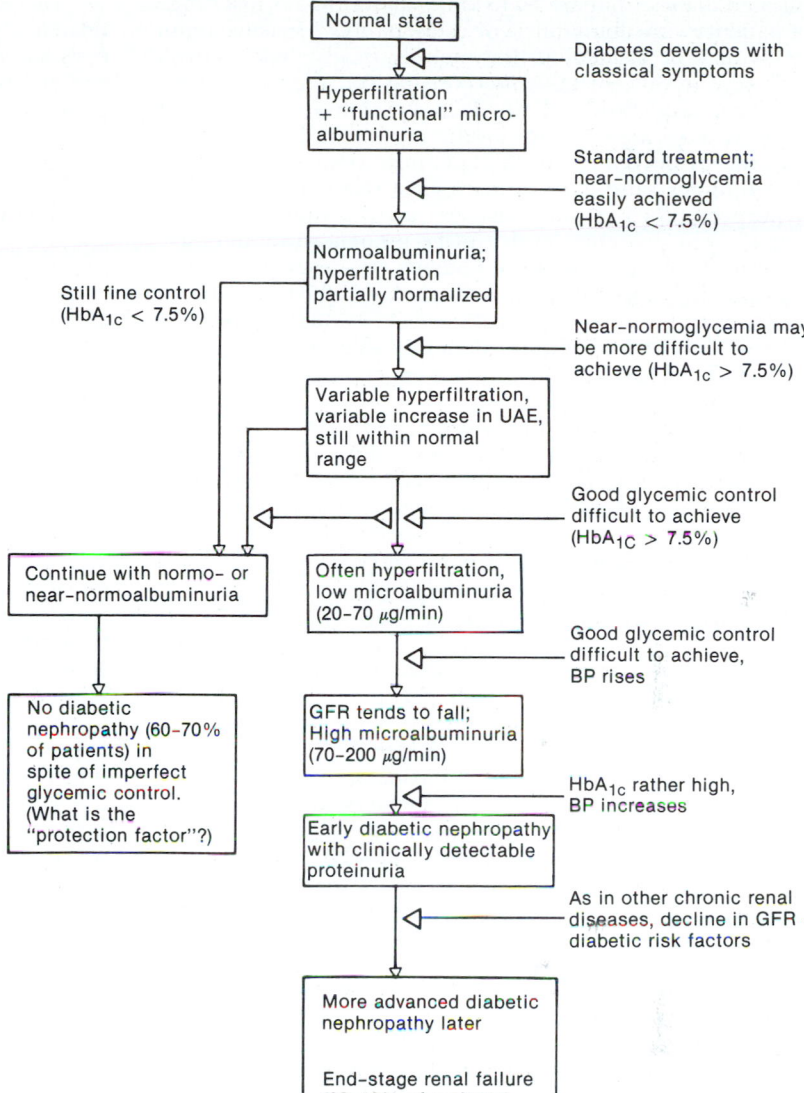

Figure 24–36. Natural history of nephropathy in untreated diabetes mellitus. UAE, urinary albumin excretion; BP, blood pressure; GFR, glomerular filtration rate; HbA$_{1c}$, hemoglobin A$_{1c}$. (From Mogensen CE. Therapeutic interventions in nephropathy of IDDM. Diabetes Care 1988; 11[Suppl 1]:10–15. Reproduced with permission of the American Diabetes Association, Inc.)

artery stenosis reduces both the mesangial thickening and the deposition of immunoglobulin and complement in the stenotic kidney while accelerating the diabetic glomerulopathy in the normally perfused kidney.[593] Interestingly, a diabetic patient with unilateral renal artery stenosis developed severe unilateral diabetic nephropathy in the normal kidney.[594]

Glomerular basement membrane thickening has been ascribed to a rapid increase in membrane production, there being no definitive evidence of decreased removal of membrane components. The sialic acid content of the membrane is reduced, and the content of collagen-related components (glycine, hydroxylysine, hydroxyproline, and disaccharide) is increased.[483] Decreased levels of heparan sulfate proteoglycan may increase porosity of the basement membranes, especially to anionic molecules, and elicit a compensatory increase in the synthesis of type IV collagen to account for basement membrane thickening.[485, 595] However, increased porosity has not been demonstrated in early human diabetes.[596] Altered permeability, if it occurs, could be due to a loss of negative charge secondary to increased glycosylation of the membrane or decreased levels of heparan sulfate. Laminin levels are increased in diabetic mice[485] but are decreased in glomerular basement membranes from diabetic

subjects.[595] Whatever the mechanisms, mesangial expansion ultimately encroaches on the subendothelial space and the glomerular capillary lumen, causing a decline in glomerular blood flow and filtration.[597]

Hyporeninemic Hypoaldosteronism

Hyporeninemic hypoaldosteronism is common in diabetic nephropathy. The appropriate renin response to postural change or sodium restriction is lost, blunting aldosterone release.[598] Basal aldosterone levels are normal, and the aldosterone response to angiotensin II is intact.[599] Hyperkalemia and hyperchloremic metabolic acidosis are the clinical clues to diagnosis.

Hyporeninemic hypoaldosteronism is probably a heterogeneous group of disorders. It may result from direct damage to the juxtaglomerular apparatus, to macula densa cells, to efferent autonomic nerves, or to receptors that respond to changes in pressure and ions. In some patients a defect in renin biosynthesis is suggested by the presence of a "big renin" in plasma; indeed, the level of inactive renin may be abnormally high in uncomplicated diabetes without proteinuria.[600] However, a study of 293 diabetic patients indicated that inactive prorenin levels are normal in uncomplicated diabetes but are 50 to 200% above the normal range in patients with albuminuria or retinopathy.[601] Inactive renin levels may be related to the intensity of glycemic control: they rose in 30% of patients receiving conventional insulin treatment and followed for 1 to 3 y but in only 7% of patients receiving intensive insulin treatment. Prorenin concentrations decreased in 43% of those treated intensively. The findings raise the possibility of a relationship between hyperproreninemia and microvascular complications and suggest that prorenin levels can be influenced by intensive control of glycemia. In some patients renin may be physiologically suppressed by an increased extracellular volume, in which case it is corrected by diuresis.[602] In fact, despite the relative hypoaldosteronism demonstrable by provocative tests, sodium wasting and volume depletion are uncommon in the syndrome.

The hyperkalemia of hyporeninemic hypoaldosteronism is accentuated by coexisting renal failure. An additional major contributing factor is the inability of diabetic patients to mount a normal insulin response to a rising serum potassium level. Ordinarily insulin buffers the serum potassium level by stimulating potassium entry into cells.[603]

Other Renal Diseases in Diabetes

Urinary tract infection is a common problem in patients with diabetes. It is probable that cystitis and pyelonephritis are no more frequent than in the general population, but symptoms may be more severe.[604] A rare but potentially fatal illness is emphysematous pyelonephritis characterized by gas in the renal parenchyma or perirenal space.[605] Mortality rates as high as 80% have been reported. Antibiotic therapy is often ineffective and nephrectomy may be required. Such a therapeutic decision is difficult, especially if underlying nephropathy is present or gas is present in both kidneys. A trial of antibiotics is always indicated together with early urological consultation.

A second serious complication of diabetes is papillary necrosis.[606] Manifestations include fever, flank pain, and ultimately septicemia and shock. Red and white blood cells, bacteria, and fragments of the papilla may be present in the urinary sediment. Intravenous urography or angiographic procedures must be avoided in patients suspected of having papillary necrosis because of the high risk of acute renal failure when the serum creatinine level is above 220 μmol/L (2.5 mg/dL). Similarly, nephrotoxic antibiotics should be given with care and in reduced doses in the presence of azotemia.

Diabetic patients have also been reported to have unrelated primary renal diseases such as arteriolar nephrosclerosis, interstitial nephritis, membranous glomerulonephritis, and lupus nephritis. The clinician must be alert to these possibilities, although statistically they are rare.

Treatment of Diabetic Nephropathy

There is no specific treatment of diabetic nephropathy apart from the hope that meticulous control may slow its progression. Therapeutic interventions used to prevent progression of early nephropathy include aggressive treatment of glycemia (as can be achieved with insulin pumps), antihypertensive therapy (particularly with angiotensin-converting enzyme inhibitors), and a low-protein diet (Table 24–20). Reversibility of the early signs of diabetic nephropathy has been reported when tight control is initiated early in the course, but treatment is less successful after changes have been present for some time. Early aggressive treatment may cause microalbuminuria and increased glomerular filtration to disappear,[607, 608] but this is relatively rare. Strict control also can prevent progression to macroproteinemia.[609] Progressive renal disease characterized by gross proteinuria, blood pressure elevation, and diminished glomerular filtration rate has not been helped by insulin pump therapy. Kidney size has been reported to decrease in some studies[610] but not others.[608] Thus the pump option should be restricted to patients with early nephropathy. Once renal failure has appeared, the risks of tight control are particularly high and the expected benefits negligible.[611]

Hypertension appears to be the single most important deleterious factor in the progression of diabetic nephropathy, even more important than glycemic control. Control of blood pressure is therefore an obligatory goal. This is true both in incipient nephropathy and in more advanced renal disease.[576, 612, 613] In a 6-mo study, treatment of normotensive patients who had fixed albuminuria with angiotensin-converting enzyme inhibitors was shown to slow the decrease in filtration fraction and reduce microalbuminuria,[614] but long-term results are not yet available to determine the effects on progression of established nephropathy. However, the demonstrated benefits of conventional antihypertensive treatment with cardioselective beta-blockers, diuretics, and vasodilators in patients with overt diabetic nephropathy[576, 612–615] suggest that results will be favorable.

Unless renal insufficiency is present, the goal of antihypertensive therapy should be 120/80 mm Hg (standing). Side effects of antihypertensive drugs may be a greater

TABLE 24–20. Effects of Intervention Modalities*

Test Parameter	Insulin (Insulin Pumps)	Antihypertensive: ACE Inhibition	Antihypertensive: Non–ACE Inhibition	Low-Protein Diet
Hyperfiltration (and elevated filtration fraction)	Long-term GFR ↓ ~5% (Aarhus)	Filtration fraction ↓ by ACE	No studies	↓ Hyperfiltration (Aarhus)
Borderline elevated UAE	Total normalization in a 4-y follow-up study (Oslo)	No studies	No studies	No studies
Persistent microalbuminuria (30–300 mg/24 h)	Stabilization (Gentofte)	Microalbuminuria somewhat ↓ (Paris)	Long-term regression of microalbuminuria (Aarhus)	Reduced in a small series on a short-term basis (London)
Proteinuria without ↑ BP, possibly with ↓ GFR	No studies	Studies ongoing	No studies	Reduction of fall rate in GFR and reduced proteinuria according to preliminary studies (London, Dallas)
Proteinuria, ↑ BP, ↓ GFR	No effect seen in a small series (does not rule out an effect) (London)	In patients conventionally treated, additional ACE inhibitor may reduce progression (Göteborg)	Long-term treatment with cardioselective beta-blockers, diuretics, and vasodilators considerably reduces decline in GFR (Aarhus, Copenhagen)	

*ACE, angiotensin-converting enzyme; UAE, urinary albumin excretion; BP, blood pressure; GFR, glomerular filtration rate; ↑, increased; ↓, decreased.
From Mogensen CE. Therapeutic interventions in nephropathy of IDDM. Diabetes Care 1988; 11(Suppl 1):10–15. Reproduced with permission of the American Diabetes Association, Inc.

problem in diabetic than in nondiabetic subjects. Hyperglycemia and impotence may be aggravated by thiazides and other antihypertensives, and the counterregulatory response to hypoglycemia may be reduced by beta-adrenergic blockade, predisposing to serious episodes of hypoglycemia. Potassium must be administered with caution because tolerance to exogenous potassium is greatly impaired when the increase in insulin secretion normally stimulated by potassium is inadequate or absent.[603] Coexisting hyporeninemic hypoaldosteronism, which may precede serious renal failure, accentuates this problem.

There is preliminary evidence that a low-protein diet may reduce diabetic hyperfiltration,[616] diminish proteinuria,[617] and slow the rate of disease progression.[618] However, further evaluation is required. These findings are summarized in Table 24–20.

When creatinine clearance falls below 20 mL/min, planning for the treatment of uremia, whether by dialysis or kidney transplantation, must begin. Hemodialysis, originally thought to be contraindicated in diabetes, is now an accepted form of treatment. Survival rates are about 50% at 3 y, 30% at 5 y, and 10% at 9 y.[619, 620] Some diabetic subjects tolerate dialysis well, but for most the quality of life is seriously compromised by cardiac, peripheral vascular, and opthalmological complications.[620, 621] Continuous ambulatory peritoneal dialysis is another option,[622] but in most centers only a small percentage of patients utilize this method.

Renal transplantation is very successful, with 5-y survival rates in some centers as high as 65% and 10-y survivals reaching 45%.[620] Related-donor transplants and transplants between HLA-matched donors give even higher values.[620, 623] It has been claimed that retinopathy is arrested or improved after successful renal transplantation in 80% of the recipients.[624] Meticulous control of diabetes is indicated postoperatively in the hope that this will prevent the development of nephropathy in the transplanted kidney.

Hyporeninemic hypoaldosteronism with hyperchloremic acidosis should be treated with Shohl solution (sodium citrate–citric acid) titrated to bring the bicarbonate concentration of plasma to about 22 mmol/L. In some cases fludrocortisone is required to control hyperkalemia.[599]

Pyelonephritis is an absolute indication for hospitalization in diabetic subjects. Treatment requires the systemic administration of antibiotics.

Diabetic Retinopathy

Although diabetes is a leading cause of adult blindness in the United States, the risk of blindness in an individual patient is low, probably less than 10%.[625, 626] Nevertheless, it is a serious problem and a constant fear for those afflicted with the disease. The retinopathic syndromes are usually categorized as background (simple) and proliferative (Table 24–21). Presumably they represent different stages of the same pathophysiological process, but this has never been proved.

Background Retinopathy

Background retinopathy was found in 3% of diabetic Pima Indians at the time of diagnosis.[7] The prevalence of background retinopathy increases with age, and after 25 to 30 y of disease about 90% of the patients have demonstrable retinal lesions.[627] In a 5-y longitudinal study of 231 type 1 patients with an average age of 17.6 ± 4.0 y and a mean duration of diabetes of 8.5 ± 4.9 y by the end of the study, 47% developed some kind of retinal change.[628] These changes were minimal in half of the subjects. Definite background retinopathy appeared in 17%, and 4% developed

TABLE 24–21. Lesions of Diabetic Retinopathy

Background	Proliferative
Increased capillary permeability	New vessels
Capillary closure and dilation	Scar (retinitis proliferans)
Microaneurysms	Vitreal hemorrhage
Arteriovenous shunts	Retinal detachment
Dilated veins	
Hemorrhages (dot and blot)	
Cotton-wool spots	
Hard exudates	

proliferative disease. After 18 y of diabetes every patient had at least incipient structural abnormalities in the retina.[628]

Background or simple retinopathy includes dilation, constriction, and tortuosity of vessels; microaneurysms; dot-shaped inner retinal hemorrhages; dot-blot, linear, or flame-shaped preretinal hemorrhages; and hard or soft exudates.[629] Hard exudates are due to leakage of proteins and lipids from hyperpermeable capillaries and tend to form rings, often in the macular area. Cotton-wool exudates represent microinfarctions. A sudden increase in cotton-wool spots usually heralds a rapid progression of retinopathy. Hard exudates may coalesce into yellow patches and impair vision if they extend into the macular region. Microaneurysms, which are thought to develop consequent to loss of supporting pericytes, are transient, lasting from months to years (Fig. 24–37); they frequently become hyalinized and appear as whitish spots. Macular edema is common and can lead to serious loss of vision.

Proliferative Retinopathy

Proliferative retinopathy, the most serious complication of diabetic ophthalmopathy, carries a high risk of vitreous hemorrhage, scarring, retinal detachment, and blindness (see Table 24–21).[627, 630] Although estimates vary widely, up to 10% of the patients with IDDM are said to develop proliferative retinopathy within 15 y and more than 25% are afflicted after 20 to 50 y.[631] Blindness is reported to occur in 43% of IDDM patients and 61% of NIDDM patients within 5 y after the onset of proliferative retinopathy.[627] Because of associated nephropathy and coronary artery disease, proliferative retinopathy indicates poor prognosis for life as well as for vision. The initiating event in proliferative disease is new vessel formation.[625–627, 630] The new vessels, radiating out from the optic disc or peripheral vessels, initially lie on the retinal surface unsupported by

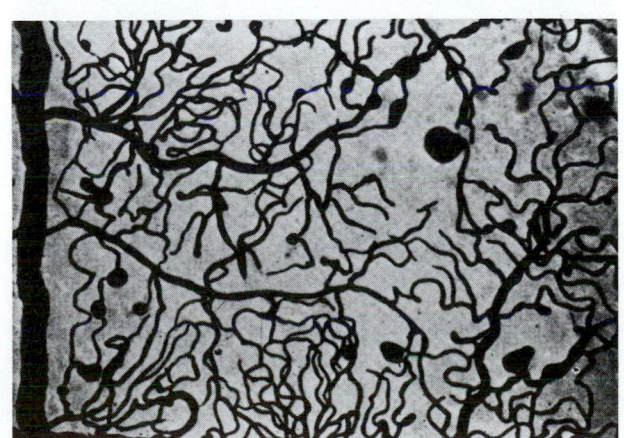

Figure 24–37. Capillary microaneurysms in diabetic retinopathy. India ink perfusion of retinal vessels. (From Ashton N. Arteriolar involvement in diabetic retinopathy. Br J Ophthalmol 1953; 37:282–292.)

connective tissue and may rupture and bleed into the vitreo-retinal space. Ultimately they become encased in connective tissue, forming adhesions between the vitreal gel and the retina. Traction from the vitreous humor caused by glial proliferation may result in either hemorrhage or retinal detachment. Vitreal hemorrhage itself may stimulate contraction, leading to a lifting off of the retina attached to it by scar tissue. Glial proliferation from the disc may also occur independently of vascularization and, if it covers the macula, will cause blindness.

Pathogenesis of Diabetic Retinopathy

Capillary vasodilation and hyperpermeability, basement membrane thickening, loss of endothelial cells and pericytes, focal occlusion of capillaries, and formation of arteriovenous shunts are thought to combine with abnormalities in the blood to cause retinal ischemia, the presumed first step in the pathogenesis of retinopathy (Fig. 24–38).[632] Factors leading to decreased blood flow in the retina are identical to those previously postulated to play a role in renal disease. These include increased blood viscosity,[633, 634] red blood cell sludging and aggregation,[491, 492] increased levels of fibrinogen, and diminished fibrinolysis related to inhibition of plasmin by increased concentrations of alpha-2–globulin.[490, 635, 636] High levels of von Willebrand factor,[476, 536] increased production of thromboxane A_2 by platelets,[534] and reduced prostacyclin production by endothelial cells[538] are thought to favor platelet aggregation. Other evidence,[539] discussed previously, argues against this provocative formulation. Impaired release of oxygen from hemoglobin,[477, 585] resulting from the combined effect of increased hemoglobin A_{1c} and reduced 2,3-diphosphoglycerate levels, may contribute to local hypoxia.

Increased vascular permeability is a very early lesion in the pathogenetic sequence.[626] It may represent endothelial dysfunction resulting from an opening of tight junctions consequent to osmotic stress or increased vesicular transport.[637, 638]

Ischemia probably stimulates compensatory new vessel formation, because similar neovascularization occurs in other conditions in which retinal oxygen content is diminished such as sickle cell–hemoglobin C disease, polycythemia vera, and central retinal vein occlusion.[639] Capillary closure is regarded as the first step in neovascularization.[640, 641] There

is fragmentation of the vascular basement membrane followed by migration of endothelial cells from the wall of the vessel into the interstitium to form capillary sprouts.[642] A local capillary growth factor may be involved, because fluid samples from eyes of patients with ocular neovascularization stimulate vascular endothelial cell migration and proliferation.[642] Insulin-like growth factor I (IGF I, also called somatomedin-C) appears to be elevated in type 1 diabetic patients with rapidly deteriorating vision from proliferative and exudative retinopathy.[643]

The proximate cause of diabetic retinopathy is not known. However, it is considered a consequence of the altered metabolic state accompanying insulin deficiency because background retinopathy appears in secondary diabetes caused by cystic fibrosis,[644] chronic pancreatitis, or total pancreatectomy.[645] The possibility that polyol pathway activity is involved is suggested by results of experiments with galactose-fed animals. Galactose causes basement membrane thickening[505] and capillary microaneurysms[646] indistinguishable from the lesions seen in experimental and naturally occurring diabetes. The lesions can be prevented by treatment with an aldose reductase inhibitor.[505] The enzymatic machinery for sorbitol formation is present in the retina.[647] Direct support for a causal role of the polyol pathway in the genesis of diabetic retinopathy comes from studies indicating that experimental retinopathy in animals[506] and alteration of the blood-retinal barrier in humans[648] can be prevented or reversed by inhibitors of aldose reductase.

Although metabolic factors are considered primary, it is possible that genetic determinants are also operative.[649] In type 1 diabetes, predisposition to retinopathy had been reported to be linked to HLA-DR4 and not to HLA-DR3,[649] but other workers have failed to confirm this.[650] In identical twins, retinopathic concordance was observed in all but 1 of 15 pairs of NIDDM patients with the same duration of diabetes but in only 5 of 10 comparable IDDM pairs, suggesting the importance of nongenetic factors in the latter group.[651]

Evaluation and Treatment of Diabetic Retinopathy

Intravenous fluorescein angiography with retinal photography is the most sensitive diagnostic procedure for diabetic retinopathy, although plain color photographs are also helpful. Early breakdown of the blood-retinal barrier can be evaluated by quantitative vitreous fluorophotometry.[652]

Photocoagulation with the xenon arc or an argon laser is the most effective treatment for proliferative retinopathy. Originally laser therapy was prescribed only if new vessels were present on or within one disc diameter of the optic nerve or elsewhere if associated with a recent hemorrhage. Therapy is now offered much earlier in many cases.[626] The laser destroys new capillaries, leaky vessels, and microaneurysms and can diminish retinal edema. The incidence of hemorrhage and gliosis is clearly reduced by photocoagulation. Destruction of hypoxic retinal regions may result in diminished release of the putative growth factor for new vessel formation. Panretinal photocoagulation has been extensively used to diminish retinal oxygen demands and preserve blood flow (oxygenation) in unaffected areas. A total of 2000 to 3000 lesions is produced over a 10- to 14-d period.[630, 653] Pars plana vitrectomy may be required when blindness is the result of vitreous hemorrhage or opacification, provided serious proliferative retinopathy is not present.[626, 654] The risks of the procedure include iatrogenic retinal tears, recurrent hemorrhage, precipitation of cataracts, neovascular glaucoma, infection, and loss of the eye,

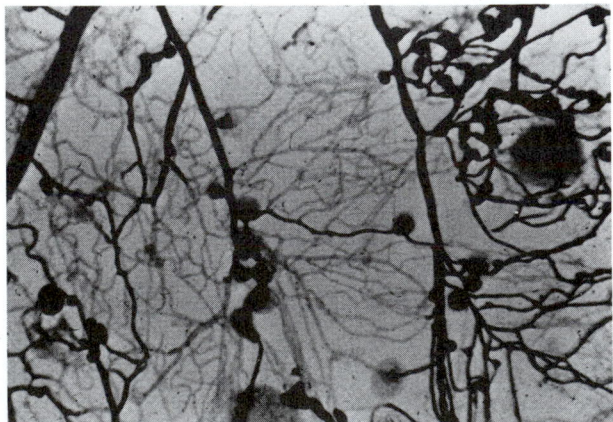

Figure 24–38. Retinal nonperfusion in diabetic retinopathy. Combined India ink, trypsin digestion. Note central area of nonperfusion with remaining acellular capillaries. (Photograph by N. Ashton. From Bresnick GH, Segal P, Mattson D. Fluorescein angiographic and clinicopathologic findings. In: Little HL, Jack RL, Patz A, et al., eds. Diabetic Retinopathy. New York: Thieme-Stratton, 1983: 37–71.)

but they appear to be at an acceptable level when the procedure is performed by a highly qualified surgeon. Hypophysectomy is no longer considered a therapeutic option.

Cataracts

So-called snowflake cataracts, fine flecks within the lens cortex, are identical to senile cataracts of nondiabetic subjects but seem to occur earlier and more often in diabetes, their reported frequency in type 1 disease ranging from 4 to 10%.[655, 656] Current hypotheses concerning their pathogenesis have been reviewed earlier in this chapter. The treatment is surgical and the risks and results are similar to those in nondiabetics.[657]

Diabetic Neuropathy

There are three recognized forms of diabetic neuropathy: mononeuropathy involving a peripheral or cranial nerve, symmetrical peripheral polyneuropathy (the most common), and autonomic neuropathy.[658] The last two are considered to be metabolic in etiology, whereas mononeuropathy is usually attributed to disease of the vasa nervorum.[659, 660]

Mononeuropathy

Diabetic mononeuropathy may involve the femoral, obturator, sciatic, median, or ulnar nerve or may affect a cranial nerve in isolation. The usual picture is the sudden appearance of wristdrop, footdrop, or paralysis of the third, fourth, or sixth cranial nerve. Several nerves may be involved at the same time (mononeuritis multiplex), but this is unusual.[658] Radiculopathy is a rare syndrome causing chest or abdominal wall pain that can mimic herpes or a "surgical abdomen." Under ordinary circumstances the mononeuropathic syndromes subside spontaneously after a few days to a few weeks.

Diabetic amyotrophy is a syndrome characterized by atrophy, pain, and fasciculations in muscles of the limb girdle distribution.[660, 661] Interosseous, thenar, and hypothenar muscles of the hands may also be involved. The disorder is considered to be a severe manifestation of vasculopathic peripheral neuropathy, although anterior spinal artery thrombosis can produce a similar picture. Patients with this form of neuropathy usually have had IDDM or NIDDM for at least 20 y.

Symmetrical Peripheral Polyneuropathy

The most common manifestation of the peripheral neuropathy of diabetes is symmetrical sensory loss in the distal lower extremities.[658] Motor deficits and upper extremity involvement are less common, although the Achilles reflex is frequently absent, sometimes even at the time of diagnosis of diabetes. The most common symptoms are numbness, tingling, and burning that is worse at night. Lancinating or lightning pain (tabes-like) may become extremely severe, and suicides are known to have occurred because of it. Such patients should be advised that their pain is not permanent and will subside spontaneously within months to years as the involved neurons become destroyed. Many diabetic patients are symptomless despite impairment of conduction velocity, loss of stretch reflexes, and absence of pain and vibratory perception in the feet on physical examination. The diminished sensory perception of diabetic neuropathy, even when asymptomatic, may lead to unperceived injuries to the skin and joints, causing calluses, ulceration, and neuropathic

arthropathy (Charcot joints). Painless tarsal and leg fractures may occur, especially in those who walk or jog for exercise.

The rare syndrome of neuropathic cachexia may simulate the neuromyopathic syndrome that sometimes accompanies malignant disease. There may be a loss of up to 60% of the body weight, anorexia, severe depression, impotence, and symmetrical peripheral neuropathy associated with long-standing mild diabetes. It occurs predominantly in men in the sixth decade of life, and other diabetic complications are absent. The prognosis is excellent, with uniform recovery within 1 y.[661]

Autonomic Neuropathy

The manifestations of autonomic neuropathy include anhidrosis of the lower extremities (sometimes associated with hyperhidrosis of the upper half of the body), orthostatic hypotension, sexual dysfunction, and motility disturbances of the bladder, esophagus, stomach, gallbladder, small intestine, and colon.[662, 663] The syndrome of counterregulatory failure leading to hypoglycemia may also be related to autonomic neuropathy. (This is discussed in the section on insulin treatment.) The normal fluctuations in pupil size, known as pupillary unrest, are reduced by about 35% in diabetic patients of age 25 to 43 y.[664] The ability to maintain miosis in a continuous light is also impaired.

The most serious consequence of autonomic neuropathy is an alteration in cardiac sympathetic innervation with Q-T interval prolongation, which can be associated with sudden arrhythmia and death.[665] Nonuniform loss of adrenergic neurons in the heart has been demonstrated by *meta*-iodo-benzylguanidine scintigraphy in a patient who subsequently died unexpectedly.

GENITOURINARY DISTURBANCES. Rarely bladder dysfunction may be the presenting sign of diabetes.[666] Paralysis of the bladder may progress without symptoms other than gradually increasing intervals between voidings. This may escape detection until an infection or urinary retention occurs. Examination reveals suprapubic dullness to percussion or, less commonly, a palpable mass. Suprapubic percussion should therefore be a routine part of the physical examination in diabetes. An asymptomatic neurogenic bladder is present in over 80% of patients with diabetic neuropathy. The diagnosis is made by cystometric or x-ray examination; the picture is that of a thin, distended, atonic bladder.[667] Treatment is unsatisfactory. In patients with hypourination, scheduled voidings every 3 h and the administration of bethanechol supplemented with phenoxybenzamine may reduce residual urine to 100 mL or less and decrease the risk of infection. Complicating obstructive disease such as prostatic hypertrophy should be relieved. Chronic prophylactic treatment with trimethoprim-sulfamethoxazole may be helpful in preventing infections. With complete paralysis, in-and-out self-catheterization or an indwelling catheter may be required. Occasionally bladder neck resection may be useful.[667]

Impotence ultimately occurs in up to 75% of men with prolonged diabetes.[658] It may be due to either neuropathy or vascular disease. Destruction of the nervi erigentes, the parasympathetic nerves that dilate the penile arteries and allow the engorgement of the corpora cavernosa and the corpus spongiosum of the penis, results in complete and irreversible impotence. Endothelium-derived relaxation factors are probably also important.[668] The syndrome is particularly disturbing because the libido is intact. Obviously, non-neuropathic causes of sexual dysfunction can also occur in diabetic subjects and should be considered in the differential diagnosis. A common precipitating factor is antihypertensive drugs. Autonomic neuropathy is suggested if on physical examination the bulbocavernosus reflex is missing and perianal stroking fails to elicit anal contraction. Treatment is implantation of a penile prosthesis or, rarely, intermittent papaverine injection (see Chapter 19).

DIABETIC GASTROENTEROPATHY. Gastrointestinal symptoms may occur in up to three quarters of diabetic patients.[669] Any portion of the system, from esophagus to anus, may be involved. Esophageal symptoms are usually mild, varying from heartburn to dysphagia.[658] In one study[670] one fifth of asymptomatic patients had radiological evidence of gastric retention. Vagal neuropathy delays gastric emptying and impairs the gastric acid response to sham feeding,[671] but episodes of intractable nausea and vomiting may be due to other unidentified factors. Variability of gastric emptying may be a factor in instability of the blood sugar level in some patients. Loss of the normal migrating interdigestive motor complexes that sweep the stomach and upper gut free of debris and bacteria[672] may permit bacterial growth in the stomach and upper intestine.[672, 673] These complexes are stimulated by motilin[674] and suppressed by somatostatin.[675] Perhaps the high levels of somatostatin reported in insulin deficiency[676] play an auxiliary role in this syndrome. Metoclopramide is the treatment of choice if decompression by gastric suction fails to relieve the problem. It increases gastric emptying and has a central antiemetic effect.[677-679]

Constipation, the most common gastrointestinal symptom of diabetic subjects, occurs in about two thirds of the patients.[669] It is present in almost 90% of the patients with evidence of extensive neuropathy but also in almost one third of individuals without neuropathic symptoms. Constipation is usually intermittent and may alternate with diarrhea.

Diabetic diarrhea, defined as a stool volume greater than 200 g/d, occurs in patients with poorly controlled, longstanding, insulin-requiring diabetes and is usually chronic and intermittent. However, frequent passage of small semiformed stools due to anal sphincter dysfunction and fecal incontinence are often confused with diabetic diarrhea.[680, 681] Careful measurement of the 24-h stool volume should precede an extensive work-up for diarrhea.

True diarrhea in diabetics may be neuropathic, or it may have a nondiabetic etiology, such as bacterial overgrowth in the small bowel,[672, 673] gluten-induced enteropathy,[682] or pancreatic insufficiency,[683] all of which are more common in diabetics than in the general population. Bacterial overgrowth can lead to bile acid deconjugation[684] and cause mild steatorrhea, as in the blind-loop syndrome.[685] Not all patients with diabetic diarrhea exhibit bacterial overgrowth in the small intestine,[686] although the occasional success of treatment with tetracycline favors a bacterial role in some patients.[687] If steatorrhea is severe, a nondiabetic etiology should be sought.

Strict glycemic control may reduce symptoms of diabetic gastroenteropathy,[688] perhaps by improving nerve function[689] or lowering somatostatin levels.[676] Metoclopramide may be useful in some cases of diarrhea. Ordinarily there is a good response to loperamide or diphenoxylate and atropine. A trial of tetracycline may be undertaken if symptomatic treatment does not work, particularly if steatorrhea is present. Cholestyramine is not usually helpful.[690] The treatment of diabetic diarrhea is usually carried out empirically on a trial-and-error basis without an extensive diagnostic work-up.

CARDIOVASCULAR NEUROPATHY AND POSTURAL HYPOTENSION. Baroreceptors of the aortic arch and the carotid sinus, together with catecholamines and the renin-angiotensin-aldosterone system, maintain blood pressure and cerebral blood flow during a change in position. Impairment of this system may cause light-headedness, syncope, and rarely sudden death. When baroreceptor impairment is superimposed on underlying cerebrovascular disease, transient focal manifestations may occur. About one fourth of insulin-dependent diabetic men were found to have cardiovascular manifestations of autonomic neuropathy in one study, the prevalence increasing with age.[691] Detailed investigations in large populations or other forms of the disease are not available. Parasympathetic functions, which are usually lost before sympathetic functions in diabetic autonomic neuropathy, are evaluated by determining beat-to-beat variation of the heart and the effect of the Valsalva maneuver and carotid massage on the heart rate.[692] The heart rate is often high at rest in affected individuals and may be virtually fixed.[693] Cardiorespiratory arrest may occur in young diabetics with severe autonomic neuropathy involving the heart.[694] The risk is greatest during surgery. Impaired ability to maintain miosis in a continuous light[664] and an abnormal pupillary response to darkness are useful markers of generalized autonomic neuropathy.[695]

Sympathetic nerve function can be assessed by determining the blood pressure response during standing or static exercise[663] and by measuring catecholamine responses to positional change and to exercise.[696, 697] Baroreceptor insufficiency,[663] reduction in catecholamine secretion,[697, 698] and inability to increase the pulse rate[693] combine to cause orthostatic hypotension. A subset of patients with postural hypotension have elevated levels of plasma norepinephrine; this has been attributed to vascular insensitivity to catecholamines induced by sodium depletion in association with hyporeninemic hypoaldosteronism.[699] Insulin may accentuate postural hypotension over a 1- to 3-h period after injection.[700]

Treatment involves elevation of the head of the bed with blocks, wearing elastic stockings, supplementary salt intake, and, in resistant cases, fludrocortisone.[599]

TESTS OF AUTONOMIC FUNCTION. Because tests of autonomic function are simple to perform but perhaps not widely known in the general medical community, a brief summary will be given.[658, 701] Measurement of variations in the electrocardiographic R-R interval in one of several tests has been advocated as the simplest and most reliable means of testing for autonomic dysfunction.[702] Heart rate response to the Valsalva maneuver is tested by having the subject blow against an aneroid or mercury manometer to 40 mm Hg for 15 s. The test is performed three times with a rest of 1 min between. An electrocardiogram is taken continuously during the test. The Valsalva ratio has the longest R-R interval after release as the numerator and the shortest R-R interval during the maneuver as the denominator. Heart rate variation during deep breathing is evaluated using six deep breaths per minute with the electrocardiogram running and marked at inspiratory and expiratory points. Maximal and minimal R-R intervals are measured and converted to heart rate. Immediate heart rate response to standing is tested by measuring the R-R interval at the 15th and 30th beats after the patient rises from a supine to an upright posture. The result is reported as the 30:15 ratio.

Blood pressure response to standing is determined by using the fall in systolic blood pressure on standing as the test marker. Blood pressure response to static exercise is tested with a hand grip dynamometer. Maximal effort is determined first, and the blood pressure is assessed after 5 min of exertion at 30% of maximum. The blood pressure normally rises during isometric exercise. Three basal diastolic pressures are coupled with the highest diastolic pressure developed during hand grip.

Although normal values for these tests have to be established for each laboratory,[691] standard interpretations are given in Table 24–22.

TABLE 24–22. Normal and Abnormal Values in Tests of Autonomic Function

Test*	Normal	Borderline	Abnormal
Parasympathetic (heart rate response)			
Valsalva (Valsalva ratio)	≥1.21	1.11–1.20	≤1.10
Deep breathing (max:min HR)	≥15 beats/min	11–14 beats/min	≤10 beats/min
Standing (30:15 ratio R-R)	≥1.04	1.01–1.03	≤1.00
Sympathetic (blood pressure response)			
Standing (↓ systolic)	≤10 mm Hg	11–29 mm Hg	≥30 mm Hg
Exercise (↑ diastolic)	≥16 mm Hg	11–15 mm Hg	≤10 mm Hg

*See text for description of tests.

Adapted from Dyrberg T, Benn J, Christiansen JS, et al. Prevalence of diabetic autonomic neuropathy measured by simple bedside tests. Diabetologia 1981; 20:190–194.

The Cause of Neuropathy

The cause of diabetic neuropathy is unknown. Three hypotheses have received most attention: the vascular hypothesis, the axonal hypothesis, and the metabolic hypothesis.[659, 703, 704] Ischemic disease of arterioles is generally acknowledged as a primary cause of mononeuropathy, but microvascular disease is also considered as a primary contributor to other forms of neuropathy.[704] The axonal hypothesis supposes early functional changes, such as slow axonal transport, followed by structural degeneration.[705]

Understanding of the metabolic abnormalities of the diabetic nerve comes from studies in rats. In experimental diabetes the *myo*-inositol content of nerves and motor conduction velocity decrease in parallel.[511] However, because the *myo*-inositol content measured in sural nerves was not decreased in diabetic patients either with or without neuropathy,[512] the role of *myo*-inositol deficiency in the pathogenesis of human diabetic neuropathy is uncertain. Mean endoneural glucose, fructose, and sorbitol values are higher in diabetic patients than in controls and the sorbitol content of nerves is inversely related to the number of myelinated fibers. In animals both defects can be repaired by meticulous control of diabetes or feeding *myo*-inositol. Hyperglycemia lowers the *myo*-inositol content of Schwann cells and axons, probably by increasing the sorbitol-fructose content of the nerve via the polyol pathway.[503, 506, 659, 703] The sequence appears to be as follows: hyperglycemia → increased sorbitol-fructose → decreased *myo*-inositol in Schwann cells and axons → decreased phosphoinositol turnover → decreased Na$^+$,K$^+$-ATPase activity → abnormal energy metabolism → nerve dysfunction → structural damage. Treatment of affected animals with a polyol pathway inhibitor prevents both the fall in *myo*-inositol content and the decreased ATPase activity, thereby reversing the functional abnormalities. Inhibition of aldose reductase has likewise been reported to partially restore structural defects in sural nerves of patients with diabetic neuropathy.[514]

As noted later, however, therapy with polyol pathway inhibitors in humans produces only small changes in measurable nerve function. Part of the problem may be that in established neuropathy secondary structural changes are so advanced that it is too late to expect improvement from correction of metabolic abnormalities. The role of glycosylated myelin, if any, is not known.[494]

Treatment of Diabetic Neuropathy

There is no specific therapy for diabetic neuropathy. Aggressive glucoregulation with insulin may improve nerve conduction but vibration sense does not change[452] and clinical benefit is usually limited. In fact, in 13 diabetic patients who had been "cured" by combined pancreatic and renal transplants, 2 y of normoglycemia failed to reverse the neuropathy and autonomic dysfunction to a clinically important degree even though nerve conduction improved.[706] Because there was very little difference in the degree of clinical improvement between this group and the diabetic patients who received only a kidney graft, it appears that it was the cure of uremia rather than "cure" of hyperglycemia that played the more important ameliorating role. Painful neuropathy should be treated first with mild analgesics, followed by nonsteroidal anti-inflammatory drugs.[707] Although phenytoin[708] and carbamazepine[709] have been recommended, the authors do not find them helpful. In severe cases a trial of amitriptyline, 75 mg at bedtime, with or without fluphenazine, 1 mg three times daily, is indicated.[710]

Aldose reductase inhibitors are experimental drugs intended to inhibit polyol accumulation in tissues in the hope of preventing certain diabetic complications despite hyperglycemia. Diabetic neuropathy is one of several complications that might theoretically benefit from this approach. The reduced nerve conduction velocity associated with experimental diabetes in rats can be reversed by correction of hyperglycemia with insulin,[511] by supplementation of the diet with *myo*-inositol,[511, 710, 711] or by administration of an aldose reductase inhibitor.[712] Both sorbinil[713] and ONO-2235[714] improve nerve conduction velocity in animals. As noted earlier, sorbinil prevents fluorescence of collagen in streptozocin-diabetic rats,[515] which suggests a link between the polyol pathway and nonenzymatic glycosylation.

The results in humans have been less clear-cut. Sorbinil therapy in patients has been associated with a high incidence of skin rash that disappears when the drug is discontinued.[715] Because the benefits of the drug in the treatment of diabetic neuropathy have been marginal,[716, 717] its status is in doubt. However, in uncontrolled human trials the inhibitors ONO-2235 and tolrestat reportedly improved motor nerve conduction, pain, and numbness.[718, 719] Because sorbinil has been reported to reduce sural nerve sorbitol content by 42%, to increase numbers of regenerating myelinated nerve fibers by almost fourfold, and to produce electrophysiological and clinical evidence of improved nerve function,[514] aldose reductase inhibitors still hold promise for the prevention of neuropathy in patients who are not well controlled by antihyperglycemic treatment. On the other hand, a placebo-controlled double-blind crossover trial of sorbinil in which each treatment period lasted 6 mo demonstrated no improvement in either peripheral or autonomic nerve function despite highly significant inhibition of aldose reductase activity.[720] Like the rashes, side effects such as leukopenia and lymphadenopathy associated with the use of sorbinil also disappear when administration of the drug is stopped.

Peripheral Vascular Disease

Peripheral macrovascular disease in diabetic patients is similar to that found in nondiabetic subjects, but it begins at an earlier age, advances more rapidly, and is more common.[721, 722] Leg and foot amputations are five times more frequent in diabetic than in nondiabetic persons.[723] Diabetic women are not spared. Bilateral lesions and distal arterial occlusions of small and medium-sized arteries below the knee are common in diabetes,[721, 724] and, together with microvascular involvement and neuropathic lesions, are responsible for the increase in gangrene. Coexisting renal, cardiac, cerebrovascular, and metabolic problems increase the mortality associated with amputation. Lipid abnormalities, smoking, and hypertension are added risk factors for this complication.[725]

The history may reveal intermittent claudication in the calf, thigh, or buttocks. Pain at rest can be due to either diabetic neuropathy or ischemia; it tends to be relieved by dependency of the lower extremities. The need to sleep in a chair may lead to the development of dependent edema. The skin of the leg may be atrophic, hairless, and cold with thickened toenails related to fungal infection. There is pallor and a delayed refilling after elevation and subsequent lowering of the leg. Despite evidence of advanced vascular insufficiency, the dorsalis pedis or posterior tibial pulse may be palpable.

Noninvasive evaluation of peripheral vascular disease has traditionally utilized Doppler-assisted blood pressure measurements, but these may not be accurate in diabetic subjects.[558] Measurement of the transcutaneous oxygen tension appears to be a more promising technique.[726, 727] Definitive study requires arteriography, but there is a significant risk as noted later.

The treatment of peripheral vascular disease is unsatisfactory. Vasodilators are of little value and may be harmful by reducing collateral blood flow to an ischemic area.[728] Sympathectomy is also ineffective, perhaps because autonomic neuropathy has already produced an "autosympathectomy."[729] Vascular surgery is the only option, but the risks of injecting radiographic dye are extremely high. After intravenous pyelography, for example, exacerbation of renal disease occurred in about three fourths of patients whose creatinine levels exceeded 180 μmol/L (2 mg/dL).[730] Indications for arteriography include nocturnal or rest pain, ulcerations that fail to respond to optimal medical treatment, and gangrene. Obstructions of the aorta and iliac arteries can be treated by endarterectomy. For obstructions below the inguinal ligament a saphenous vein bypass graft is performed. Most such grafts lose function within a decade and reoperation is generally unsuccessful.[731] The value of catheter angioplasty to fracture obstructing plaques is under study.[732, 733]

Although conservative surgery for gangrene should be attempted, failure rates for distal amputations are high (50% for digits and >30% for transmetatarsal amputation), requiring more proximal amputations. Arteriography and segmental pressure and pulse measurements have been disappointing in predicting stump healing, but measurements of blood flow have been helpful. In one study amputations at sites with a blood flow of more than 2.6 mL/100 g of tissue/min invariably healed, but healing never occurred if the flow was less than 2.0 mL/100 g of tissue/min.[731]

PREGNANCY IN DIABETES

Maternal Fuel-Hormone Physiology in Normal Pregnancy

In the first trimester of a nondiabetic pregnancy, insulin's action is enhanced by estrogens and progesterone and glucose levels tend to decrease.[734] (See also Chapter 17.) By contrast, in late pregnancy glucose tolerance is slightly reduced and insulin levels increase,[735] suggesting insulin resistance.[736] This resistance is in part related to human placental lactogen, an insulin antagonist without circadian rhythm or feedback control by plasma glucose, which increases in concentration in proportion to the placental mass.[735, 737] The insulin resistance of pregnancy appears to be a postreceptor phenomenon.[738] Because delivery to the fetus of the fuels required for its growth and oxidative needs is a function of the maternal fuel concentration times the placental blood flow, resistance to insulin action in the maternal circulation raises the mother's postprandial levels of glucose and other nutrients, thereby shunting a larger share of glucose and amino acids from the mother to the fetus in the last half of pregnancy, the time of maximal fetal growth.[739] Increased maternal free fatty acid and VLDL levels during pregnancy provide alternative substrates for her use.

The maternal adjustment to fetal needs has been characterized as "accelerated starvation." Experiments in animals have revealed that a fast during pregnancy elicits higher rates of lipolysis,[740] ketogenesis,[741] and gluconeogenesis[742] than occur in the nonpregnant state. It is presumed that similar changes occur in women. Thus the omission of a single meal, which is a routine procedure before laboratory tests, may have a significant metabolic impact on the pregnant woman and could be dangerous if ketone bodies are teratogenic as has been claimed.[735, 743]

In a mother with borderline beta cell function the foregoing metabolic changes of pregnancy result in gestational diabetes. With pre-existing diabetes the same changes will require an increased insulin dosage.

The Infant of the Diabetic Mother

In the United States there are over 400,000 diabetic women of reproductive age, and approximately 1 in 100 pregnant nondiabetic women has carbohydrate intolerance.[744] Despite attempts to treat diabetes aggressively during pregnancy, the fetal and neonatal death rates of infants of diabetic mothers remain in excess of those in normal population.[745] Table 24–23 lists some of the disorders encountered in such infants. Infants of mothers with gestational diabetes experience fewer perinatal problems than those of overtly diabetic mothers.

Macrosomia (oversized fetus) is the most common neonatal abnormality in diabetic pregnancy. Because insulin does not cross the placenta, the metabolism of maternal substrates received by the fetus depends entirely on fetal insulin. In a normal pregnancy the slight increase in postprandial levels of the maternal nutrients that cross to the fetus, paticularly the amino acids, constitutes an important stimulus for the secretion of fetal insulin and other growth factors. The fetal glucose concentration also parallels the very narrow range of blood glucose levels of the nondiabetic mother. In a diabetic pregnancy, likewise, fetal nutrient levels reflect the maternal levels, which will exceed the normal range. If the mother is poorly controlled, the fetus

TABLE 24–23. Abnormalities Encountered in Neonates of a Diabetic Mother

Macrosomia	Renal vein thrombosis
Hypoglycemia	Persistence of fetal circulation
Hypocalcemia	Cardiomyopathy
Respiratory distress syndrome	Congenital heart disease
Polycythemia	Caudal regression syndrome
Hyperbilirubinemia	Miscellaneous congenital anomalies

Adapted by permission of Elsevier Science Publishing Co., Inc. from The infant of the diabetic mother and diabetes in infancy, by Fleischman AR, Finberg L. In: Eilenberg M, Rifkin H, eds. Diabetes Mellitus. Theory and Practice. 3rd ed. New Hyde Park, NY: Medical Examination Publishing, 1983: 715–725. Copyright 1983 by Medical Examination Publishing Company, Inc.

will therefore be hyperglycemic and hyperaminoacidemic. This causes fetal hyperinsulinemia and hyperplasia of beta cells in the fetal pancreas. Whereas in a nondiabetic pregnancy the fetal beta cells are stimulated predominately by amino acids rather than by glucose,[746] in a poorly controlled diabetic pregnancy the fetal beta cells respond to glucose as vigorously as in the adult.[747, 748] The resulting hyperinsulinemia stimulates fetal growth, which from the 30th week of gestation onward correlates well with amniotic fluid insulin levels[749] and the maternal hemoglobin A_{1c} concentration.[750] The birth weight and length of infants of poorly controlled diabetic mothers average 550 g and 1.5 cm above normal, respectively.[751] Subcutaneous adipose tissue is increased, and hypertrophy and hyperplasia of most organs, including the liver, are evident.[749] The brain size is not increased. Because of hyperinsulinism, all infants of diabetic mothers should be carefully monitored for hypoglycemia during the first hours and days of life.

Fetal hyperglycemia is associated with delayed lung maturation. The incidence of respiratory distress syndrome is increased sixfold in neonates of diabetic mothers until the 38th week of gestation.[752] In animal studies depletion of lung glycogen is delayed by maternal diabetes.[753] This may be important because lung glycogen is thought to be a precursor of surface-active phospholipids (surfactants). Glucose infusion into fetal lambs reduces the amount of surface-active material in tracheal fluid, suggesting that the defect is due to hyperglycemia.[754] Newborns of diabetic mothers must be monitored carefully for signs of respiratory distress regardless of birth weight.

The normal polycythemia of the newborn is exaggerated in neonates of diabetics.[755] The resulting hyperviscosity can result in thrombus formation in the brain and other organs and contribute to persistence of the fetal circulation (cyanosis related to right-to-left shunts through a patent foramen ovale or ductus arteriosus).[756] Renal vein thrombosis, a consequence of hyperviscosity;[757] hyperbilirubinemia;[758] and hypocalcemia[745] are also observed.

The incidence of malformations involving many organ systems is increased approximately two- to threefold in infants of diabetic mothers, and such malformations account for 30 to 50% of the neonatal mortality.[759] A malformation seen almost exclusively in infants of diabetic mothers is the caudal regression syndrome, in which there is hypoplasia of the lower segment of the body.[760] This syndrome ranges from minor defects of the lower extremities and spine to agenesis of these structures. Congenital heart disease, including transposition of the great vessels, coarctation of the aorta, and atrial and ventricular septal defects, is five times more common in offspring of diabetic mothers.[761] Generalized myocardial hypertrophy involving, in particular, the intraventricular septum is the most common cardiac abnormality and may cause poor contractility and death.[761] Short left colon syndrome can also occur.[759]

Management of the Diabetic Pregnancy

Obstetrical Management

Multidisciplinary teams for the management of diabetic pregnancy have reduced perinatal mortality from trauma secondary to macrosomia and from the respiratory distress syndrome.[759] In the past, fetoplacental function was monitored by determining urinary estriol levels[762] but this is no longer considered reliable.[763] The primary means of detecting fetal distress is measurement of fetal heart rate.[763–765] The normal fetus should accelerate the heart rate spontaneously twice during 20 min of observation with the rate increasing by 15 beats/min for at least 15 s.[765] Maternal reports of fetal movement and ultrasonic determination of

fetal activity and size are also important. Sonography provides an index of gestational age, shows malformations of the heart and other organs, and allows estimation of fetal weight. It is not always possible to predict lung maturity, but a lecithin/sphingomyelin ratio greater than 2, coupled with measurable levels of phosphatidylglycerol in amniotic fluid, is accompanied by a low instance of respiratory distress syndrome.[765] By utilizing these signs, the optimal time of delivery usually can be calculated.

Management of the Blood Glucose in Pregnancy

Perinatal mortality in diabetic pregnancies has fallen to 2 to 6% in specialized centers in the United States.[735, 765] In offspring of diabetics with severe vascular complications, the mortality is much higher. The persistence of congenital malformations is thought to reflect the fact that fetal vulnerability to malformations is maximal in the first few days to weeks after fertilization.[766, 767] Delayed early growth of the fetus in diabetic mothers may prolong the period of risk of skeletal malformation.[768, 769] If this is correct, it follows that normalization of the plasma glucose level even relatively late in pregnancy may prevent macrosomia and respiratory distress, but prevention of congenital malformations requires normoglycemia before impregnation.[770] According to this thesis, diabetic women must be started on aggressive insulin therapy at the time of planning for a new infant if the risk of congenital defects is to be minimized. However, a multicenter study was unable to demonstrate a relationship between increased malformation rates in infants of diabetic mothers and the level of glycemic control during organogenesis; blood glucose and glycosylated hemoglobin levels during early pregnancy were not significantly higher in women whose infants were malformed.[771] Neither was hypoglycemia more common.[771] Nevertheless, among infants of diabetic women in whom good metabolic control was instituted less than 21 d after conception, major malformations occurred in 4.9%, compared with 9% of infants of diabetic women in whom good control was instituted later. The incidence of major malformation was 2.1% in infants of nondiabetic control patients. The fact that infants of early-entry women have a more favorable outcome justifies efforts to achieve reasonably good control from the time of conception through the period of organogenesis.[771] Because of the possible neurological consequences of fetal hypoglycemia, the position that preprandial blood glucose levels should be below 5 mmol/L (90 mg/dL) and postprandial levels below 9 mmol/L (160 mg/dL) requires serious reexamination. Even though perinatal mortality in infants of mothers with mean blood glucose levels of less than 5.5 mmol/L (100 mg/dL) during the third trimester is far below that in infants of mothers with mean levels above 8 mmol/L (150 mg/dL),[772] the fact that brain development continues throughout the entire pregnancy[773] demands careful avoidance of recurrent hypoglycemic episodes. Self-monitoring of blood glucose during pregnancy will allow the properly trained diabetic patient to avoid poor control without experiencing frequent or severe hypoglycemic episodes. Dietary recommendations during pregnancy include energy intake of 30 to 35 kcal/kg ideal body weight and a carbohydrate intake at or above 200 g/d. The recommended distribution of calories is 20 to 25% protein, 40 to 50% carbohydrate, and 30 to 35% fat.[759]

Maternal Complications

Maternal risk during pregnancy is largely confined to patients with serious complications such as proliferative retinopathy and coronary artery disease. The impact of these factors on maternal outcome should be a consideration in counseling a potential mother with severe diabetic complications. The pregnant diabetic patient should be hospitalized for any acute illness, deterioration in diabetic control, or evidence of poor adherence to therapy. She is carried to near term (usually 36 wk) unless a threat to fetal well-being requires that the pregnancy be interrupted. During labor, glucose and insulin are administered intravenously at a rate that maintains the plasma glucose level in the normal fasting range.

Gestational Diabetes

There are 30,000 to 90,000 cases of gestational diabetes per year in the United States.[735] In untreated subjects the infant mortality is 7%.[774] Screening for diabetes both during the initial visit and again after the 24th week of pregnancy, when gestational diabetes is most prevalent, is, therefore, mandatory. Gestational diabetes is diagnosed when, after a 100-g oral glucose load, plasma glucose values of 10.6 mmol/L (190 mg/dL) at 1 h, 9.2 mmol/L (165 mg/dL) at 2 h, and 8 mmol/L (145 mg/dL) at 3 h are exceeded at two or more points (see Table 24–2).[2] Some workers recommend insulin therapy in gestational diabetes.[775] This is said to reduce the incidence of macrosomia, but controlled studies of fetal-neonatal outcome have not appeared.

Approximately half the mothers who develop gestational diabetes revert to normal after delivery. Gestational diabetes may reappear in subsequent pregnancies.

SURGERY IN THE DIABETIC PATIENT

Surgery, like other forms of trauma, elicits a sympathetic discharge, which enhances hepatic fuel production and reduces insulin-mediated fuel utilization. This combination of metabolic changes causes so-called stress hyperglycemia, which maintains the flow of fuels to the brain in anticipation of a possible decrease in cerebral blood flow. Table 24–15 summarizes current understanding of the hormonal basis for stress hyperglycemia.

Patients with type 1 IDDM ideally should be admitted to the hospital at least 2 d before an elective operation to establish optimal metabolic regulation.[776] Diabetes per se is not a consideration in the choice of anesthesia. The glucose level should be maintained between 8 and 11 mmol/L (150 and 200 mg/dL) during surgery to provide protection against hypoglycemia. Monitoring can be accomplished using capillary blood and glucose-sensitive testing sticks if a glucose analyzer is not available in the operating suite. Intermediate insulin is omitted on the day of surgery. Patients with type 2 diabetes who do not normally need insulin may require it during surgery. Again, modest hyperglycemia is desirable during the operative procedure.

Control of the plasma glucose level during surgery usually can be achieved by the infusion of 5% dextrose containing regular insulin in a concentration of 10 to 20 U/L at a rate of 100 to 150 mL/h. Alternatively, short-acting insulin can be given subcutaneously. With the subcutaneous method about one third of the daily dose is administered before surgery and hypoglycemia is prevented by the intravenous administration of dextrose. No single protocol will meet the needs of all patients. The important requirement is careful glucose monitoring during the operative and postoperative periods to guide insulin therapy. Adjustments are made as needed from estimates of the plasma glucose level. Postoperatively the plasma glucose level is monitored

every 4 to 6 h. During procedures such as renal transplantation, an effort to achieve more meticulous control of the plasma glucose is indicated. Here, glucose testing is done hourly with adjustment of the intravenous insulin drip as needed.

TREATMENT

Treatment of Insulin-Dependent Diabetes Mellitus

Metabolic Goals

By definition, all patients with IDDM require daily injections of insulin to avoid the catabolic cascade that leads to ketoacidosis, coma, and death. The possible therapeutic objectives with insulin therapy in IDDM are listed in order of increasing difficulty: (1) elimination of the catabolic state and its symptoms, (2) elimination of glycosuria, and (3) achievement of pre- and postprandial euglycemia with normalization of the hemoglobin A_{1c} level. Reversal of a catabolic state is, of course, obligatory and together with control of glycosuria can be achieved by conventional insulin treatment. Conventional insulin treatment is defined as a regimen in which the patient receives one or two daily injections of an intermediate-acting insulin (NPH or Lente) with or without added regular insulin. Traditionally dosage was based primarily on semiquantitative analysis of the urinary glucose level monitored by the patient together with periodic measurement of the fasting plasma glucose level determined in a laboratory. Today even conventional therapy is now usually based on home glucose monitoring by the patient unless financial restraints preclude purchase of the expensive dextrose-measuring sticks or a home glucose monitor.

Achievement of a normal plasma glucose level, by contrast, requires a more complex insulin delivery program based on frequent determinations of the plasma glucose concentration by the patient, who must, in effect, assume the roles of physician's assistant, laboratory technician, and dietitian. Home monitoring of plasma glucose is required because semiquantitative urine methods are insensitive in estimating hyperglycemia and incapable of detecting hypoglycemia.

Available Insulin Preparations

Insulins currently available in the United States include rapidly acting preparations suitable for intravenous, intramuscular, and subcutaneous use with a peak activity at 2 to 4 h, intermediate-acting preparations such as NPH (isophane) and Lente with a 6- to 12-h span of peak activity, and long-acting preparations such as Ultralente and protamine zinc insulin (PZI) with a 14- to 24-h span of maximal action. The duration and peak of insulin activity may vary substantially among patients and from day to day in the same patient. Differences may also be seen between diabetic and nondiabetic subjects, especially with regular insulin.[777] If a mixture of rapidly acting and intermediate-acting insulins is used, it should be injected promptly after mixing to prevent delayed absorption of regular insulin caused by interactions with protamine of the NPH or the excess zinc of the Lente insulins.[778] Commercially mixed insulin, 70% NPH and 30% regular, is available but has the disadvantage of a fixed ratio. It can be helpful for patients who have difficulty mixing accurately.

Most insulins are packaged at a concentration of 100 U/mL (U-100). Standard animal insulin is now much purer (as judged by contamination with proinsulin) than the conventional or partially purified insulin of the past.[779, 780] Most preparations have proinsulin contents of less than 50 parts per million (ppm). Beef or pork insulin labeled "purified" has a proinsulin content of less than 10 ppm, usually in the range of 1 to 5 ppm. Human insulin, i.e., synthetic insulin with a structure identical to that of the human hormone, has to a large extent replaced animal insulin in the United States and Europe. It is produced either by chemical synthesis, exchanging the terminal alanine at position B30 of pork insulin for the threonine found in that position in human insulin, or by recombinant DNA techniques. The biological effects of pork insulin and synthetic human insulin are essentially identical,[781, 782] although the human hormone is less antigenic.[783] However, this difference has not proved to be of clinical importance.[784, 785] One study reported that 36% of 176 patients with insulin-dependent diabetes who were switched from beef-pork insulin to human insulin experienced symptoms related to neuroglycopenia rather than those attributable to sympathoadrenal activation during hypoglycemia.[786] This observation has not been confirmed by carefully controlled blinded studies and should be considered unproved. The great achievement of manufacturing insulin ensures adequate supplies of the hormone for all times.

The use of human proinsulin and insulin analogues has also been studied. Although proinsulin has only a fraction (~10%) of the biological activity of insulin, it is purported to have a disproportionate effect on hepatic glucose production. Proinsulin development has been put on hold, however, because of a report of increased myocardial infarctions in one study.[780] Analogue development is focusing on point mutations in the molecule that might accentuate hepatic or peripheral effects of the hormone.

Conventional Insulin Therapy: Titrating the Insulin Dose

Patients with type 1 IDDM are best regulated as outpatients because insulin requirements during hospitalization may differ from those during customary daily activities. In either case a week of close supervision throughout the day coupled with intensive training and education is highly desirable. Insulin therapy is usually begun with a single prebreakfast dose of 25 U of NPH or Lente insulin. This is increased in 5- to 10-U increments at 2- to 4-d intervals until daytime glycosuria becomes minimal. In many patients a single dose of intermediate-acting insulin does not provide adequate control of glycosuria. The amount of NPH required to abolish glycosuria between breakfast and lunch, when insulin requirements are usually highest, may cause hypoglycemic symptoms in the afternoon; if so, regular insulin should be substituted for intermediate-acting insulin in 5-U increments at 2- to 4-d intervals until morning glycosuria and afternoon hypoglycemia have both been eliminated. If hyperglycemia or glycosuria is excessive before breakfast, a second dose of intermediate-acting insulin should be given either before the evening meal or at bedtime. A small amount of regular insulin may be required before the evening meal. In such a split-dose regimen, two thirds of the total daily dose is generally given before breakfast. Whenever the dose of insulin is increased, its effects should be observed for at least 2 or 3 d before making another increase. However, if unexplained hypoglycemia occurs (not accounted for by a skipped meal or unusual exercise), an immediate reduction in insulin dose is required.

In most patients with IDDM, control of symptoms is achieved with relative ease with conventional regimens. Although the catabolic state is eliminated and glycosuria is minimized, postprandial hyperglycemia and levels of glycosylated hemoglobin are not normalized. For other patients life is a series of dose readjustments that never succeed in eliminating either hyperglycemic or hypoglycemic fluctuations.[787] The reasons for this brittleness are not understood. Dietary inconsistency doubtless plays a role. Stress or tension, acting via counterregulatory hormone release, probably is important in many. Variations in the absorption of insulin and fluctuating insulin antibody levels may contribute in others.[787, 788] The maintenance of even minimal secretory capacity of residual beta cells is an important factor in the glycemic stability of insulin-dependent diabetic patients.[789] The C peptide response to glucose (a measure of endogenous insulin secretion) is correlated with stability; that is, patients with little or no response tend to be unstable. Intravenous glucagon testing may stimulate a rise in C peptide levels in diabetics previously considered to have no residual beta cells.[789] C peptide nonresponders are more apt to develop neuroglucopenia during insulin clamping tests and are less able to mount a response of endogenous glucagon to hypoglycemia than are C peptide responders. Alterations in gastric emptying may also contribute to instability. Deficiency of amylin (see Fig. 24–13) may also play a role. Usually the precise problem is never identified. The presence of brittle diabetes is usually an indication for attempts at meticulous control. In some patients a chronic catabolic state may leave the liver depleted of glycogen, thereby removing the primary substrate for defense against hypoglycemia; if so, a period of a high-carbohydrate feeding and increased insulin may be useful to replenish glycogen stores.

Patients who monitor their metabolic control solely by urine testing should obtain the prebreakfast specimen 30 min after voiding the overnight contents of the bladder. They should be taught that 4+ glycosuria in a small volume of urine does not signify as much glucose loss as 4+ glycosuria in a large volume of urine. If home glucose monitoring is not possible, measurement of the glycosylated hemoglobin level gives a more accurate picture of control than do random glucose determinations in the physician's office.[789–791] In fact, glycosylated hemoglobin values are useful in all patients because the test provides a check on the accuracy of patients who monitor capillary blood values at home.

Meticulous Control

Multicenter studies now under way should determine whether meticulous control of diabetes (maintenance of the plasma glucose level in the normal range throughout the day) will prevent complications that develop over a period of 10 y or more in patients who have conventional regimens. To achieve such control the patient must be willing and able to make a formidable commitment of time, effort, and money. Before advising such a course, the physician must first determine whether the clinical situation justifies the effort. First, the patient's competence and willingness to assume the role of physician's assistant must be determined. Second, the potential clinical benefit must justify the venture. For example, pregnancy and renal transplantation in diabetic patients *demand* meticulous control. In all other patients with complication-free IDDM the hope of a prophylactic advantage from meticulous control makes it a reasonable, but not obligatory, therapeutic option. For persons whose life expectancy is limited by advanced age, by the presence of established diabetic complications, by cardiovascular or cerebrovascular disease, or by any life-shortening condition, a rigorous program is difficult to justify on the basis of potential benefits.[611] Indeed, successful pancreatic transplantation resulting in permanent normoglycemia failed to reverse or even to stem the progression of either early or advanced proliferative retinopathy.[446] Put simply, the use of aggressive insulin therapy with a goal of achieving normoglycemia should be considered mandatory only in pregnancy and renal transplantation. If ongoing studies prove that meticulous control prevents or slows development of complications, then it would be offered to all IDDM patients at the onset of their disease.

Regimens of Meticulous Control

Regimens intended to achieve meticulous control must attempt to mimic the normal diurnal profile of endogenous insulin release. In nondiabetic subjects insulin levels rise spontaneously in response to an increase in glucose concentrations in plasma. In the patient with IDDM the normal glucose-sensing system and the endogenous insulin source are missing, so the patient must be trained to substitute for both. Plasma glucose levels must be measured several times each day and appropriate doses of insulin supplied. This can be accomplished in two ways: intensified multiple subcutaneous injections or the use of a continuous subcutaneous insulin infusion (CSII) device.

INTENSIFIED MULTIPLE SUBCUTANEOUS INSULIN INJECTIONS. Several doses of insulin are administered throughout the day, the amounts based on self-monitoring of glucose by a reflectance meter or chemical strip. Various programs are available, and the physician "custom designs" a system with which she or he feels comfortable (Table 24–24). In general, regular insulin is given before each meal.[792–794] Basal coverage is provided by either intermediate-acting insulin (NPH or Lente) given before bedtime or long-acting insulin (PZI or Ultralente) injected together with regular insulin before the evening meal. In the former schedule four injections a day are required: evening intermediate insulin plus regular insulin before each meal. With long-acting insulin only three injections are needed: regular before breakfast and lunch, long-acting plus regular insulin before supper. For patients who object to multiple injections, devices such as a button infuser, which permits injections through a needle port that is inserted once daily, may be tried. Alternatively, a 23- or 25-gauge butterfly needle may be inserted into the abdomen and replaced every 5 d.[795, 796]

For the initiation of therapy in a person not previously treated with insulin, 0.6 to 0.7 U/kg/d is a reasonable starting dose.[792] For persons already taking insulin, a slight reduction of 20 to 30% is suggested if the daily dose is greater than 1.0 U/kg. In the four-dose schedule, about 25% of the daily insulin is given as NPH before bedtime (9 to 10 PM), with the remaining 75% administered as regular insulin distributed such that a slightly larger amount is given before breakfast—e.g., 30% breakfast, 22.5% lunch, 22.5% supper. Adjustment of intermediate insulin is based on the fasting plasma glucose level, changes being made at 2-d intervals. Similarly, the regular insulin dosage is altered depending on the postprandial values during the previous day (see Table 24–24). Once a reasonable pattern is obtained, a sliding scale is prescribed to guide daily dosage adjustments. Capillary glucose measurement can be decreased to fasting and premeal measurements during stable periods, with periodic resumption of a full seven- or eight-point schedule to confirm that the shorter profile is accurate.

Three-dose insulin schedules using Ultralente can be handled according to the same general scheme, although a higher percentage of the total daily dose is given as Ultralente, usually 40 to 60%.

Intensive conventional therapy can be extremely effective. Results equivalent to those obtained with insulin infusion pumps have been demonstrated using a crossover design.[792, 797] However, such therapy requires never-ending surveillance, which only the patient can provide. Consequently, intensive practical training in blood glucose measurement, insulin therapy, and meal composition is essential. Simple lectures and films are not sufficient. After a training program the patient's competence should be tested to certify qualifications for assuming the responsibility for self-care.

CONTINUOUS SUBCUTANEOUS INSULIN INFUSION. Meticulous glucoregulation together with greater flexibility of lifestyle can be achieved by CSII provided by a portable insulin infusion device.[798–801] The available instruments vary in cost and sophistication. Insulin is delivered through a 25-gauge scalp vein indwelling needle positioned under the abdominal skin and connected to the pump by a catheter. The needle site is changed at least every other day to avoid cutaneous infections and needle blockage.

Insulin is infused at a constant basal rate (usually 0.5 to 2.0 U/h) with a bolus given before meals. The basal state can be programmed for automatic delivery of up to four different basal rates in a 24-h period.[802] Most patients require only one or two basal rates per day, the lower rate because of reduced nocturnal requirements and the higher rate to

---

TABLE 24–24. Intensified Multiple Subcutaneous Insulin Injections: Typical Schedule*

	Plasma Glucose, mmol/L (mg/dL)		Appropriate Change in Insulin Dosage	
	Fasting	*Pre- or Postprandial*	*Intermediate Units*	*Regular Units*
Initiation or readjustment of therapy	>5 (>90)	>7.8 (>140)	+2	+2
	<3.3 (<60)	<3.3 (<60)	−2	−2
Daily therapy		<3.3 (<60)		−2
		3.3–5 (60–90)		No change
		5–6.7 (90–120)		+1
		6.7–8.3 (120–150)		+2
		8.3–11.1 (150–200)		+3
		11.1–13.9 (200–250)		+4
		>13.9 (250)		+6

*For initial therapy 0.6–0.7 U/kg/d is given, 25% NPH or Lente, 75% regular. Intermediate insulin is given at 2100 h and is changed every 48 h solely on the basis of the fasting plasma glucose level. In the initiation phase the regular insulin dose for each meal is based on the postprandial glucose value from the previous day. Once the therapeutic plan is developed, alterations in the daily insulin dose are based on immediate preprandial glucose values. If seven- or eight-point glucose testing shows the overall pattern of glycemia to have changed, readjustment can be carried out in a fashion similar to initiation. This plan should be considered only a guide. Responses vary, so that treatment in each patient must be custom designed.

Data from Schiffrin A, Belmonte MM. Comparison between continuous subcutaneous insulin infusion and multiple injections of insulin. Diabetes 1982; 31:255–264. Copyright 1982 by the American Diabetes Association.

TABLE 24–25. Typical Variable Insulin Schedule for a Patient Receiving CSII*

Capillary Blood Glucose (mmol/L [mg/dL])		Units of Insulin Before					
		Breakfast	Snack	Lunch	Snack	Dinner	Snack
<2.8	(<50)	5	0	3	0	3	0
2.8–5.6	(51–100)	6	0.5	4	0.5	5	0
5.6–8.3	(101–150)	7	1	5	1	6	1
8.3–11.1	(151–200)	8	1.5	6	1.5	7	1.5
11.1–13.9	(201–250)	9	2	7	2	8	2
13.9–16.7	(251–300)	10	2.5	8	2.5	9	2.5
>16.7	(>300)				Call health care team		

*About 50% of the daily insulin dose is given at a constant basal rate, the remainder being administered as a bolus 15 to 30 min before meals, depending on preprandial glucose value; e.g., if blood glucose is 230 before dinner, 7 U of insulin is given. Basal rate adjustments are usually made from the 3 AM glucose level, being decreased for any value below 80 mg/dL (see text).

Adapted from Raskin P. Treatment of insulin-dependent diabetes mellitus with portable insulin infusion device. Med Clin North Am 1982; 66:1269–1283.

cope with early morning hyperglycemia, the so-called dawn phenomenon. The pump is programmed for delivery of premeal boluses 30 min before eating. Conversion to pump therapy requires 3 to 5 d of inpatient training to obtain best results. One may begin with the same total daily dose of insulin that the patient had been receiving with conventional treatment or decrease it by 20 to 30% if large amounts (>1 U/kg/d) are being used. For first-time therapy, 0.6 to 0.7 U/kg/d is reasonable. From 40 to 50% of the dose is administered basally at a constant rate, the remainder being given before the three meals in burst fashion over a 30-min period. For example, a 60-kg patient who had been receiving 24 U of intermediate insulin per day with conventional therapy would begin with a basal rate of 12 U/d (0.5 U/h), which would be adjusted downward if the 3 AM glucose level were below 4.4 mmol/L (80 mg/dL) or upward if the 7 AM value were over 7.8 mmol/L (140 mg/dL). The remaining 50% of the previous dose would be used to mimic normal meal-induced insulin release. A typical preprandial variable insulin dose schedule appears in Table 24–25. Despite its lower caloric content, breakfast requires a larger bolus than the evening meal. The technique can result in near-normalization of diurnal glucose concentrations, at least in an ideal setting. Such results may not be achievable when large groups of patients are followed in a busy clinical practice. For example, in a group of 100 patients cared for in a private clinic, the mean fasting glucose value decreased from 11 mmol/L (200 mg/dL) during conventional therapy to 8.8 mmol/L (158 mg/dL) during pump therapy. Equivalent figures for nonfasting values were 11.8 mmol/L (213 mg/dL) and 8 mmol/L (145 mg/dL), respectively.[802] Children have more difficulty in attaining good control than adults.[802] The requirements for education and training of patients are even more stringent than those recommended earlier for intensive conventional therapy.

Specific complications of pump therapy include cutaneous abscesses that have on occasion been serious (in one case fatal sepsis resulted), subcutaneous lumps, severe diabetic decompensation (including ketoacidosis) caused by undetected interruption of insulin delivery, hypoglycemia, and death.[803]

Benefits of Meticulous Control

Whether diabetic complications can be prevented or delayed by meticulous control is under study. At present the known benefits include improvement or a return to normal of blood glucose profiles and concentrations of amino acids, plasma glycoproteins, free fatty acids, triglyceride, LDL and HDL cholesterol, lactate, and pyruvate.[804, 805] The plasma glucagon level becomes normal, as do the responses of growth hormone and catecholamine to exercise. An im-

proved sense of well-being and greater flexibility of lifestyle may justify this therapy for some patients. Rapid healing of recalcitrant foot ulcers has been reported after 6 to 8 wk of continuous subcutaneous insulin infusion, and, if confirmed, this would become an indication for its use.[806] Neuropathic components of the diabetic syndrome such as gastroparesis may improve with enhanced diabetic control.[688] Deterioration of parasympathetic and somatosensory nerve function was reported to be less in type 1 patients after 2 y of CSII treatment than after conventional insulin treatment.[807]

As stated earlier, good control without hypoglycemia is obligatory in every diabetic pregnancy and should be started before conception to protect the fetus from congenital disease. The same applies to the recipient of a renal transplant, the goal of meticulous control being protection of the transplanted kidney from the microvascular disease that afflicts the host.

Risks of Meticulous Control

The hoped-for and the known benefits of meticulous control must be carefully weighed against the risks, the most important of which is hypoglycemic encephalopathy. Acceleration of retinopathy is a less common complication,[453–455, 803] but all patients must understand that amelioration of retinopathy cannot be expected. Although deterioration is always a matter of concern when patients with this complication are subjected to CSII,[808, 809] one study of 30 type 1 patients who received CSII for over 31 mo reported a slowing in the progression of early retinopathy.[809] Established proliferative retinopathy does not appear to improve or even to stabilize after "cure" of diabetes by pancreas transplantation as noted earlier.[446] In alloxan-diabetic dogs microaneurysms and other lesions that develop during 60 mo of hyperglycemia can be inhibited by good control beginning at the onset of the diabetes. But if 30 mo of poor control precedes 30 mo of good control, retinopathy will develop during the period of good control.[810] If these findings can be extrapolated to humans, they suggest that good control at the onset of diabetes may prevent retinopathy but that once the process has begun, good glycemic control cannot be expected to be beneficial. Although there may be rare exceptions, pump therapy and intensive conventional therapy are relatively contraindicated in patients with coronary artery disease, cerebrovascular disease, renal failure, proliferative retinopathy, or advanced autonomic neuropathy.[611] Background retinopathy is not a contraindication, but frequent ophthalmological surveillance is required to detect accelerated neovascularization.[453, 455] Although frank renal failure is a strong contraindication, proteinuria with or without mild azotemia does not preclude aggressive insulin therapy. Such therapy may reverse microproteinuria[574] but has not been shown to reduce renal failure.[811]

During the initial period after its introduction 35 mostly unexpected deaths in patients given CSII therapy were reported in North America.[812] Many occurred at night during sleep, strongly suggesting hypoglycemia. There was little evidence of deliberate or inadvertent overdosing of insulin. Pump malfunction was not found to be a problem. However the death rate in subjects given CSII was not excessive for IDDM.[812] Moreover, some of the deaths occurred in patients with the relative contraindications for meticulous control just outlined. In others, incompetence, psychiatric problems, or motivational defects made them unsuitable for a self-care regimen.[611] Had stringent criteria for selection of patients been applied, most of these mishaps might have been avoided. Recommended criteria for selection of patients for meticulous control by multiple subcutaneous injections or by CSII are listed in Table 24–26. Despite these difficulties, CSII is now a commonly used means of obtaining superior glycemic control in insulin-dependent diabetic patients.[813]

Why the Vulnerability for Hypoglycemia in Insulin-Dependent Diabetes Mellitus?

During exercise or extended fasting, nondiabetic persons are protected from hypoglycemia by a decrease in insulin level and a rise in glucagon and catecholamine levels, which themselves modulate changes in islet hormone secretion (see Fig. 24–19b). The decrease in insulin level reduces glucose utilization by nonexercising insulin-requiring tissues, enhances the release of free fatty acids from adipocytes, and disinhibits glucagon secretion, thereby increasing hepatic glucose production to a rate sufficient to maintain normoglycemia and ensure the normal flow of fuel to the brain. In the patient with insulin-treated IDDM, insulin levels obviously cannot decrease with exercise or fasting. Thus glucose utilization does not decrease, and inhibition of free fatty acid release continues. Moreover, continuing suppression of glucagon secretion by insulin and its opposition to the hepatic effects of the low levels of glucagon limit hepatic glucose and ketone production. These combined effects, and perhaps the deficiency of amylin, render the diabetic patient extremely vulnerable to hypoglycemia under conditions that do not impose risks for normal persons.

An impaired ability to prevent hypoglycemia is probably characteristic of insulin-dependent diabetes, but correction is usually possible through adequate secretion of counterregulatory hormones (see Table 24–15).[321, 814–818] However, in some patients with long-standing IDDM this ability wanes.[816–818] In normal subjects insulin-induced hypoglycemia elicits an increase in glucagon, catecholamine, cortisol, and growth hormone levels, the first two being of major

importance in the acute defense response, which depends on glycogen breakdown.[814] If the glucagon response is blocked experimentally during insulin-induced hypoglycemia, the catecholamine response restores normoglycemia; if catecholamine action in response to hypoglycemia is blocked experimentally, the glucagon response restores glucose levels to normal. However, if both are blocked, hypoglycemia persists.[814, 815] In IDDM of more than 2 y duration, the glucagon response to insulin-induced hypoglycemia is generally reduced[816, 817] but a normal catecholamine response provides adequate protection. However, after about 15 y of diabetes, the catecholamine response may wane, leaving the patient relatively defenseless against hypoglycemia.[818, 819] The defect appears to be specific for insulin-induced hypoglycemia because catecholamine release in response to other stimuli is intact.[818] Counterregulatory failure in diabetes carries a high risk of prolonged hypoglycemia, permanent brain damage, and death. Because it may not be associated with other evidence of autonomic neuropathy, its etiology is uncertain.

Nocturnal hypoglycemia is a danger for any patient being treated by intensive conventional or pump therapy, and that danger is enhanced if counterregulatory defenses are impaired. In many patients given meticulous treatment regimens, glucose levels reach a nadir at 3 AM and rise by 1 to 6 mmol/L (20 to 100 mg/dL) at 7 AM. This early morning rise is known as the dawn phenomenon. Nocturnal surges in growth hormone are thought to be primarily responsible for this phenomenon, which is a result of a major increase in hepatic glucose production coupled with the substantial reduction in glucose clearance.[820] When a constant overnight insulin infusion was administered to six insulin-dependent diabetic patients, plasma glucose levels rose from 5.4 mmol/L (98 mg/dL) at midnight to 12.5 mmol/L (225 mg/dL) at 8 AM; this suggests that a normal 7 AM glucose level may signify that the glucose concentration was dangerously low at 3 AM. Only a glucose determination in the early morning hours provides an adequate answer. In pumps with programming capabilities it is possible to reduce the basal rate after midnight and increase it before 7 AM. Alternatively, one can accept a slightly elevated 7 AM glucose level and, by drastically reducing the breakfast and raising the prebreakfast insulin bolus, achieve near-normalization of the glucose profile by midmorning.

Exercise-induced hypoglycemia tends to be less dangerous than nocturnal hypoglycemia because the patient is awake and can usually take appropriate measures or obtain help. Counterregulatory hormone release does not appear to be significantly impaired in type 2 NIDDM, although the number of patients examined is small.[821]

Avoidance of hypoglycemia should have an even higher priority than avoidance of hyperglycemia. It seems probable that if the criteria for selection of patients listed in Table 24–26 were stringently applied, together with a strategy for avoidance of hypoglycemia, meticulous control would be as safe as conventional therapy. Some investigators have suggested that all patients considered for intensive insulin therapy be tested for counterregulatory response beforehand.[822]

TABLE 24–26. Criteria for Selection of Patients for Meticulous Control in Diabetes

Indications	Contraindications
Absolute	Absolute
Pregnancy	Counterregulatory failure
Postrenal transplantation	Unwillingness or inability for any reason to assume full responsibility for acceptable implementation of a diabetes self-care program
Relative	Relative
Otherwise healthy patient unable to normalize hemoglobin A_{1c} or achieve other therapeutic objectives*	Life expectancy < 10 y Diabetic retinopathy or nephropathy Cerebrovascular disease Cardiovascular disease

*Other objectives could include greater well-being, greater resistance to infection, improved healing of foot ulcers, normalization of lipid profile, improvement in gastroparesis.

Complications of Insulin Therapy

HYPOGLYCEMIA. Hypoglycemia of a mild degree occurs occasionally in most patients receiving insulin (see Chapter 23). It is particularly common in subjects with counterregulatory defects and those with renal failure. Clinical manifestations of hypoglycemia are due to hyperepinephrinemia or neuroglycopenia. The hyperepinephrinemic symptoms (perspiration, tachycardia, tremor, pallor, and a subjective feeling of uneasiness) occur early, before the hypoglycemia becomes profound. The neuroglycopenic manifestations include changes in personality or behavior, confusion, obtundation, convulsions, and coma. They develop after the arterial glucose level has fallen too low to meet cerebral needs. Nocturnal hypoglycemia may be manifested by nightmares, night sweats, and morning headache. Occasionally patients with cerebrovascular disease experience focal neurological manifestations as a result of reduction in the delivery of glucose to hypoperfused areas of the brain. This may occur in the absence of profound systemic hypoglycemia. In such patients meticulous control imposes a high risk of further neurological damage.

If the patient is conscious, ingestion of a sweet drink, sugar, or candy is the treatment of choice. All insulin-treated patients should carry carbohydrate and identification that indicates that they have diabetes. In unconscious subjects, the intravenous administration of glucose is required. Intramuscular injection of 1 mg of glucagon can also be utilized. Glucagon availability is particularly important for insulin-treated diabetic subjects who live in rural areas without quick access to medical facilities, but any hypoglycemia-prone, insulin-requiring diabetic patient should have a vial of glucagon on hand.

The term *Somogyi phenomenon* is employed to designate rebound hyperglycemia after an episode of undetected hypoglycemia.[823] Rebound hyperglycemia is reduced by decreasing the dose of insulin.[824] Although this phenomenon does exist, glucose profiling throughout the day indicates that it is less common than was previously thought. In fact, deliberate induction of nocturnal hypoglycemia by infusing insulin in insulin-dependent diabetic patients failed to cause fasting hyperglycemia.[825] It may be more frequent in children. In one study 6 of 34 children were found to have evidence of asymptomatic nocturnal hypoglycemia with hyperglycemic rebound.[826] If glycosuria and hyperglycemia persist throughout the day, the possibility of rebound hyperglycemia and overinsulinization is unlikely.

INSULIN LIPODYSTROPHY AND LIPOATROPHY. Atrophy or hypertrophy of subcutaneous tissue may occur at insulin injection sites. The problem is usually seen with nonpurified animal insulins and has almost disappeared when synthetic insulins are used. Hypoesthetic masses may develop, and these become tempting sites for insulin injections. The absorption of insulin from such areas is unpredictable and may lead to erratic or poor control. The patient should be taught to rotate the injection sites and avoid such areas. Lipoatrophy tends to develop during the first year of insulin therapy and regress thereafter. It is prevalent in children and women and may involve an immune reaction to some contaminant of the older insulins, because it improves when purified or synthetic insulin is injected into the affected region. Occasionally lipoatrophy develops at sites never used for insulin injection.

INSULIN ALLERGY. Significant cutaneous reactions to insulin occur in up to 5% of patients treated with the hormone.[827] The reactions are mediated primarily by immunoglobulin E antibodies, although immunoglobulin G may participate. Allergy may develop with initiation of insulin therapy, usually appearing within the first month, but severe reactions ordinarily occur in patients resuming therapy after an insulin-free period. Many patients with insulin allergy have histories of sensitivity to other drugs as well. Local insulin allergy is characterized by erythema, pruritus, and induration at the injection site, whereas systemic allergy is manifested by generalized urticaria, angioneurotic edema, or frank anaphylaxis. In a study of 117 patients with insulin allergy, 87 were found to have cuta-

neous reactions only, 18 had both cutaneous and systemic manifestations, and 12 had only systemic reactions.[828]

Local insulin reactions should be treated with an antihistamine. In patients using animal insulins a switch to biosynthetic human insulin should be made. If the patient does not respond to these measures, desensitization is required. Desensitization is mandatory if systemic reactions occur.[829] Once this is accomplished, insulin therapy should not be stopped for any reason.

INSULIN RESISTANCE. As noted earlier, insulin resistance plays a prominent role in non–insulin-dependent diabetes, in this country mediated largely by obesity. Modest insulin resistance is also present in the absence of obesity in type 1 IDDM[359] and recedes with good control.[360] The rare syndromes of insulin resistance have been reviewed.[830] The pathophysiological defect may be at the prereceptor level (e.g., antibodies to the insulin molecule), at the level of binding to the receptor (e.g., type A binding defects or type B insulin resistance with anti–insulin receptor antibodies), or at a postbinding site (e.g., obesity, leprechaunism). Many insulin-resistant states are associated with acanthosis nigricans. We will comment here only on immunological insulin resistance due to anti-insulin antibodies and the poorly understood insulin resistance associated with impaired insulin absorption. Diabetes caused by a primary state of insulin resistance is considered at the end of the chapter.

IMMUNOLOGICAL RESISTANCE. Clinically significant immunological resistance in which antibodies are directed against insulin occurs in only about 0.01% of insulin-treated subjects, even though essentially all patients have low levels of insulin antibodies after 3 mo of therapy. True resistance, arbitrarily defined as an insulin requirement of at least 200 U/d,[831] can be attributed to insulin antibodies only when their titer is high enough to bind large amounts of insulin.[832] Anti-insulin antibodies are usually the consequence of insulin therapy but may rarely develop spontaneously in patients without diabetes who have unrelated monoclonal gammopathy[833] or autoimmune endocrinopathy, particularly thyroid disease.[834] Autoantibodies against insulin can cause either insulin-resistant hyperglycemia or, if they release bound insulin inappropriately, hypoglycemia.[834]

Insulin requirements may be extremely high in patients with antibodies against insulin.[827, 831] The use of human insulin usually is of no benefit in preventing or reversing the syndrome. Concentrated insulin (U-500) has been effective in some cases,[835] as has sulfated insulin, presumably because it has a higher affinity for the insulin receptor than for the insulin antibody.[836] If none of the foregoing maneuvers are successful, high-dose steroids (80 to 100 mg prednisone/d) should be given, with rapid tapering after the response is obtained. This may occur in as little as 48 h. About three fourths of patients so treated will respond.[827, 831]

SUBCUTANEOUS DEGRADATION OR MALABSORPTION OF INSULIN. Insulin resistance may also result from abnormal absorption or enhanced degradation of injected hormone.[837–839] The clinical diagnosis of increased subcutaneous destruction is usually based on the observation that large amounts of insulin given subcutaneously are ineffective but intravenous insulin works normally.[840] In one patient 5000 U given subcutaneously was required for adequate control.[837] Increased degradation of insulin may also occur in the plasma.[841] Addition of aprotinin, a protease inhibitor, to the insulin solution may provide improvement,[840] although its effects might be due to local enhancement of blood flow rather than to inhibition of the peptide-degrading activity of tissue.[842] Alterations in local blood flow have been considered important in the brittle diabetic syndrome even in persons not characterized as resistant.[843] Anaphylactic reactions to aprotinin have been reported, and only about one third of patients presumed to have the subcutaneous insulin resistance syndrome respond to the drug.[787, 788] A peculiar characteristic of this syndrome is that it appears to come and go spontaneously. Although emphasis has been placed on enhanced insulin degradation, there is some doubt that this is the sole operative factor. Studies reporting enhanced insulin degradation in biopsy specimens have been handicapped by insufficient tissue to perform assays. Interestingly, a candidate enzyme for this degradation has homologies with a protease found in *Escherichia coli*.[844]

Treatment is difficult. Basically one can give large amounts of insulin subcutaneously with or without aprotinin, utilizing intravenously administered insulin for acute complications such as ketoacidosis, or administer insulin into the peritoneal cavity.[845] The latter approach has been recommended, but the authors of this chapter are aware of one patient who failed to respond to the intraperitoneal administration of insulin. Thus the syndrome of non–antibody-mediated insulin resistance has to be considered an unsolved problem.

Insulin Delivery Systems Under Development

CLOSED-LOOP GLYCEMIC SYSTEMS. A closed-loop system is one in which insulin is automatically delivered in accordance with need as dictated by the ambient glucose concentration. To our knowledge no practical closed-loop device suitable for implantation has yet been developed. However, a closed-loop glycemic sensor with a wearable artificial endocrine pancreas has undergone testing.[846] Glucose is continuously monitored by a glucose sensor inserted into the subcutaneous tissue of the arm. The feedback control system apparently gives better glycemic profiles than either multiple-dose insulin therapy or CSII regimens.

CONTROLLED RELEASE OF INSULIN FROM IMPLANTABLE MATRICES. Implantable ethylene–vinyl acetate copolymer matrices[847] and cholesterol-matrix implants[848] have been shown to provide therapeutically effective controlled release of insulin in streptozocin-diabetic rats. If such a system could be perfected to provide a reliable basal rate of insulin delivery in human diabetic patients, perhaps premeal boluses could be delivered via the nasal route (see following section), thus completely circumventing the need for injections.

INTRANASAL INSULIN DELIVERY. Intranasal aerosolized insulin with the surfactant laureth 9 was found to give glycemic control comparable to that of CSII over a 3-mo period in a group of eight insulin-dependent diabetic patients.[849] The most striking finding was the ability of intranasally administered insulin to limit 2-h postprandial glucose increments to only 2.1 mmol/L (38 mg/dL) above premeal glucose levels. A major problem has been the irritating effect of detergents used to facilitate absorption. A new adjuvant, sodium taurodihydrofusidate, appears to represent a significant advance.[780] The efficacy of Ultralente insulin administered to provide a basal rate of insulin delivery and intranasal insulin in lieu of regular insulin has been studied in nine patients.[852] Levels of glycosylated hemoglobin rose significantly after substitution of intranasal therapy and three patients were considered to be treatment failures. The remaining six subjects expressed preference for the intranasal regime and the level of glycemic control was considered to be acceptable. However, achievement of glycemic control equivalent to that obtained with subcutaneously administered insulin required an intranasal dose 21 times as high as the subcutaneous dose. The resulting expense, coupled with uncertainty about the long-term local effects of intranasal treatment, is the major concern at the moment. In general the intranasal route of administration appears to be effective

in about 50% of patients and may therefore be a useful addition to current therapeutic options.[850]

IMPLANTED BIOLOGICAL INSULIN DELIVERY SYSTEMS. Permselective tubular membranes containing fragments of human insulinomas and implanted in the peritoneal cavity of streptozocin-diabetic rats have reduced fasting glucose levels and brought insulin levels to within the normal range.[851] Their removal results in prompt reappearance of hyperglycemia. The insulinoma cells remain morphologically intact despite long-term implantation. It appears from this study that immunoseparation of insulin-secreting cells by synthetic membranes may provide a means of implanting pancreatic xenografts derived from animal islets. This may yet become the most practical and effective means of beta cell replacement.

Diet Therapy

In normal persons the postprandial influx of nutrients is greeted by a rise in insulin levels timed to prevent or minimize change in nutrient concentration, particularly that of glucose. The early phase of insulin response seems to be triggered largely by hormones released from the gut[315] and/or by parasympathetic signals, inasmuch as it precedes the rise in glucose concentration.[312] Regimens designed to provide meticulous control with pump therapy or multiple insulin injections attempt to duplicate this by providing an anticipatory premeal dose of insulin given early enough to minimize any postprandial change in glycemia. The timing of meals must be carefully matched with insulin injections if normoglycemia is to be achieved.

All patients of normal weight with IDDM should be given a diet that contains approximately 35 kcal/kg body weight. The American Diabetes Association favors a carbohydrate content of 50 to 60%,[852] whereas others advocate that carbohydrate contribute 40 to 45% of the energy.[853] Although it is likely that the diet with the more restricted carbohydrate intake facilitates glucoregulation, the atherogenic risk of its increased fat content outweighs the hoped-for benefits of better glycemic control. This problem appears to have been minimized by substituting monounsaturated and polyunsaturated for saturated fats.[854] A diet containing 35% carbohydrate and 50% fat, 33% of which was monounsaturated, resulted in lower mean plasma glucose levels, reduced insulin requirements, and lowered plasma levels of triglycerides and VLDL while increasing HDL cholesterol levels. LDL levels were not affected. If LDL cholesterol is elevated and cannot be significantly reduced without pharmacological intervention, agents such as lovastatin appear to be as effective in diabetics as in nondiabetics and are devoid of any apparent side effects during short-term treatment.[855]

Many clinicians prefer to divide food intake into three meals and three snacks, with 20% of the calories at breakfast, 20% at lunch, and 30% at dinner time. Midmorning, mid-afternoon, and bedtime snacks make up the remaining 30%. In patients who object to a midmorning snack, this 10% can be added to the bedtime snack, thus providing additional protection against nocturnal hypoglycemia. Because blood glucose levels and insulin requirements are highest between breakfast and lunch, it seems reasonable to shift much of the carbohydrate from breakfast to the evening meal and bedtime snack. The caloric intake should be appropriately adjusted if the weight increases or decreases. Ordinarily sweets and refined sugar are not permitted, although this proscription need not be absolute.[856, 857]

Despite the importance of diet, few physicians or patients are truly knowledgeable in this area. The distribution of pamphlets and food exchange lists does little to promote dietary adherence. The most effective way to manage the diabetic diet is to provide the patient with practical training in meal preparation under the supervision of a skilled nutritionist. In communities where this approach is not available, the physician and patient must follow written guidelines to diet therapy.[858]

Exercise in Insulin-Dependent Diabetes Mellitus

The role of exercise in the therapy of IDDM has not been systematically addressed; it has been noted that exercise can be either helpful or harmful.[859] Presumably, as in normal persons, regular exercise is of benefit for the cardiovascular system. It may also help in lowering plasma glucose levels. On the other hand, exercise may cause hypoglycemia. In normal persons the plasma glucose level rises slightly with vigorous exercise and decreases if exercise is prolonged (>90 min). Moderate exercise for short periods does not change glucose concentrations because enhanced glucose utilization in skeletal muscle is matched by increased hepatic production.[860] If a poorly controlled diabetic subject exercises, plasma glucose concentrations may rise because insulin is inadequate to allow a maximal increase in its utilization in muscle in the presence of elevated production of glucose.[860] Conversely, in the well-controlled patient, hypoglycemia may supervene because hepatic glucose production remains restrained by the undiminished circulating insulin levels while glucose utilization in muscle is increased consequent to exercise.[861, 862] This problem is in part the result of the injection of insulin subcutaneously in an area where exercise may increase the absorption rate of the hormone.[862] However, hypoglycemia may occur independently of increased insulin absorption because additional capillaries open up in the exercising muscle, enhancing glucose utilization in previously inactive fibers.[859–863] To prevent exercise-induced hypoglycemia in patients treated with insulin infusion pumps, a reduction or omission of the premeal bolus may be required.[864, 865] All diabetic patients requiring insulin must be warned of the danger of exercise-induced hypoglycemia. Self-testing of the plasma glucose response to exercise may be valuable for those who exercise regularly so as to formulate a program for appropriate modification of the insulin dose on exercise days. This is even more important if meticulous control is being attempted.

Treatment of Non–Insulin-Dependent Diabetes Mellitus

Metabolic Goals

The therapeutic objectives in NIDDM do not differ from those in IDDM: return of metabolic abnormalities to normal in the hope of maintaining health and extending life. However, there is within the NIDDM category a broad clinical spectrum of islet cell function and body weight that permits a greater choice of therapeutic options. At the same time, the older age of the patients and the greater frequency of other clinical problems require individualization of therapeutic regimens.

The Therapeutic Options

By definition, insulin is not an obligatory form of therapy in patients with NIDDM. These patients can be divided into three therapeutic categories according to beta cell function relative to insulin sensitivity: those with sufficient islet cell reserve and insulin sensitivity to maintain relatively normal glucose levels provided the intake of calories and carbohydrate is restricted, those who require in addition to dietary restriction the oral administration of antihyperglycemic drugs, and those in whom control of hyperglycemia is not possible without the administration of exogenous insulin.

Patients must also be separated for therapeutic purposes into obese and nonobese groups, inasmuch as beta cell function and sensitivity can be improved in the former by weight reduction.[368] Pima Indians with obese type 2 NIDDM experienced remarkable improvement in beta cell function and amelioration of glucose intolerance after 3 wk of caloric restriction and evidenced improved sensitivity of target tissues after 18 wk.[361] Such remissions occurred only in patients with fasting glucose levels below 14 mmol/L (250 mg/dL) and diabetes of less than 5 y duration.

Unfortunately, dietary adherence and weight reduction are seldom achieved.

Orally Administered Antihyperglycemic Drugs

In principle, these drugs should be used only for the treatment of hyperglycemia that persists despite full adherence to the prescribed diet. In practice, obesity is rarely corrected, and dietary prescriptions are usually ignored. The antihyperglycemic drugs are therefore frequently employed inappropriately as the initial therapy rather than as adjuvant to a dietary regimen.

Sulfonylureas are the only orally administered antihyperglycemic drugs approved for use in the United States. Their pharmacological characteristics are summarized in Table 24–27. The mechanism of action is debated. Acute administration of a sulfonylurea stimulates insulin release. Their important action may be to lower the glycemic threshold required for a given insulin secretory response.[866] During long-term administration of the drugs, insulin levels tend to decrease as hyperglycemia recedes, suggesting increased beta cell sensitivity to hyperglycemia or improvement of insulin resistance in target tissues. Sulfonylureas have been reported to cause an increase in insulin binding to fibroblasts[867] and

TABLE 24–27. The Sulfonylureas

Agent	Daily Dose (mg)	Doses/Day	Duration of Hyperglycemic Action (h)	Metabolism/Excretion
Acetohexamide	250–1500	1 or 2	12–18	Liver/kidney
Chlorpropamide	100–500	1	60	Kidney
Tolazamide	100–1000	1 or 2	12–14	Liver
Tolbutamide	500–3000	2 or 3	6–12	Liver
Glyburide* (glybenclamide)	1.25–20	1 or 2	Up to 24	Liver/kidney
Glipizide	2.5–40	1 or 2	Up to 24	Liver/kidney
Glibornuride	12.5–100	1 or 2	Up to 24	Liver/kidney

*Glyburide is the generic name in the United States; glybenclamide is the international nonproprietary name.

Adapted by permission of Elsevier Science Publishing Co., Inc. from The oral hypoglycemic agents, by Lebovitz HE, Feinglos MN. In: Ellenberg M, Rifkin H, eds. Diabetes Mellitus. Theory and Practice. 3rd ed. New Hyde Park, NY: Medical Examination Publishing, 1983: 591–610. Copyright 1983 by Medical Examination Publishing Company, Inc.

hepatocytes[868] secondary to an increase in receptor number, but this has been disputed.[869] The importance of this effect in regard to sulfonylureas is not clear, because the drugs potentiate insulin action in the absence of increased binding.[868, 870] Sulfonylureas appear to act synergistically with insulin in vivo by enhancing glucose disposal.[871] Some of the second-generation drugs also appear to decrease hepatic glucose production.[872] However, there is little indication for use of sulfonylureas together with insulin in NIDDM because, in practice, control is only rarely improved with combined therapy. Because sulfonylureas are ineffective in type 1 IDDM or pancreatectomized animals, it is safe to conclude that their major mechanism of action is to enhance beta cell function.

Therapeutic Efficacy of Sulfonylureas

Although there are exceptions, patients with fasting glucose levels in excess of 16.7 mmol/L (300 mg/dL) generally do not respond to sulfonylureas, whereas most patients with levels below 14 mmol/L (250 mg/dL) exhibit at least a partial response. Overall, about 85% of unselected patients with NIDDM respond initially to the drugs but secondary failure occurs in about 25%.[873] Transient failures may be due to intercurrent infection, surgery, or other stress, with a return of responsiveness after the removal of that stress. Failure to adhere to diet and continued weight gain play a role in many patients. In other secondary failures, unresponsiveness to sulfonylureas may reflect the progression of what in reality was type 1 autoimmune insulinopathy rather than type 2 NIDDM.[66] Finally, bona fide type 2 NIDDM may well be a slowly progressive disorder despite conventional assumptions to the contrary.

Most studies have failed to show a salutary effect of sulfonylureas on glucose intolerance, progression to overt diabetes, or development of cardiovascular disease. However, a long-term Swedish study revealed remarkable improvement in all three categories in glucose-intolerant men given tolbutamide at 1.5 g/d over a 10-y follow-up period.[874] This remains to be confirmed.

Toxicity of Sulfonylureas

Toxic side effects of sulfonylureas occur in about 3% of the patients.[873] They include bone marrow depression, hemolytic anemia, rash (including the Stevens-Johnson syndrome), nausea and vomiting, abnormal liver function (especially increased levels of alkaline phosphatase), vasomotor flushing with alcohol, and antidiuresis, which may cause hyponatremia. The antidiuretic effect, most commonly seen with chlorpropamide, is due to increased vasopressin release and sensitization of the renal tubule to its action. Concern that sulfonylureas predispose to coronary artery disease has dissipated.[873]

Serious hypoglycemia associated with sulfonylureas may occur with fasting in patients with renal disease given chlorpropamide or acetohexamide and as a consequence of drug interaction.[873] Because sulfonylurea-induced hypoglycemia tends to be prolonged, hospitalization is mandatory.

The Biguanides

The biguanides, phenformin and metformin, are not used in the United States because of the enhanced risk of lactic acidosis.[875] The mechanisms by which these drugs cause or worsen lactic acidosis are not known, although many biochemical effects have been described.[876] In pathophysiological terms both overproduction of lactate in nonhepatic tissues and decreased uptake by the liver are important.

Metformin appears to be safer than phenformin.[876] The drug is mildly effective in treatment of certain cases of NIDDM, particularly when combined with sulfonylureas.[877] Biguanides should not be used in patients with renal insufficiency and should be withdrawn during intercurrent illnesses other than mild viral infections of the upper respiratory tract.

Experimental Drugs

ACARBOSE. This drug, which is not available for general use in the United States, is an α-glucosidase inhibitor that interferes with the intestinal absorption of carbohydrates[878] and thereby reduces postprandial hyperglycemia.[879] It is not yet clear whether its therapeutic effects in diabetes outweigh its side effects, which include flatulence.

MIDAGLIZOLE. Midaglizole, (±)-2-[α-(2-imadazolin-2-ylmethyl)benzyl]pyridine, is a new type of antihyperglycemic agent that has alpha-2–adrenoreceptor–antagonizing activity and is thought to lower plasma glucose levels largely via stimulation of endogenous insulin secretion. It also inhibits epinephrine-induced platelet aggregation. In 20 patients with mild non–insulin-dependent diabetes baseline glucose levels fell from a pretreatment mean of 10.4 mmol/L (187 mg/dL) on diet alone to 6.7 mmol/L (120 mg/dL) after 4 wk of treatment with the drug.[880] Postprandial glucose levels were also reduced. The only side effect was diarrhea or soft stools, which occurred in 8.5% of patients.

CIGLITAZONE. The most interesting of the experimental pharmacological drugs is ciglitazone, 5-[[4-[(1-methylcyclohexyl)methoxy]phenyl]methyl]-2,4-thiazolidinedione. In ob/ob and db/db mice a dramatic fall in the blood glucose level occurs after 2 d of treatment at a dose of 100 mg/kg. Its effectiveness is limited to animals with insulin-resistant diabetes. It increases the basal rate of glucose metabolism, lipogenesis, insulin receptor number, and the postreceptor response to insulin.[881, 882] Trials in humans have not yet been reported.

MODIFIERS OF FATTY ACID METABOLISM. Because inhibition of fatty acid oxidation increases glucose utilization, the hypoglycemic effects of agents that modify fatty acid metabolism are being explored. Etomoxir, (±)-ethyl 2-[6-(p-chlorophenoxy)hexyl]glycidate, is such a compound. Etomoxir lowers the glucose level in streptozocin-diabetic rats by about 8.3 mmol/L (150 mg/dL) in 4 h in association with a striking increase in plasma free fatty acid and triglyceride concentrations.[883] Concomitant nicotinic acid administration prevents the lipid abnormalities and doubles the hypoglycemic effects of therapy. It remains to be seen whether this treatment will be applicable to humans.

Immunomodulatory Intervention in Autoimmune Diabetes

Unlike the other experimental agents mentioned in this section, immunosuppressive drugs are currently available to physicians. It must therefore be stressed that *at the present time no immunosuppressant drug currently on the market should be used for treating any form of diabetes or prediabetes.*

Cyclosporine has little or no effect in patients with diabetes of more than 2 mo duration.[884] However, in carefully selected patients with diabetes of 2 mo or less cyclosporine may induce a remission such that insulin treatment may no longer be required. For example, in a group of patients with a mean age of 15.4 ± 8.2 y and a duration of diabetes of 39 ± 62 d, orally administered cyclosporine in a dose of 10 mg/kg/d induced a 12-mo non–insulin-requiring remission in 45% of patients. Such favorable results were strongly related to age at onset of diabetes; patients over 16 y of age benefited six times more frequently than younger patients. Duration of the diabetes was a critical variable; patients who began the drug within 3 wk of initiation of insulin treatment benefited five times more often than those who started later. In the successfully treated patients, levels of glycosylated hemoglobin decreased to normal and levels of glucagon-stimulated C peptide rose toward normal. When cyclosporine was discontinued, a relapse invariably followed within a few weeks, indicating that continuous treatment for an indefinite time is required for lasting benefit. Initial remissions in up to two thirds of patients and year-long remissions in nearly half have been reported in other studies.[114] In two subsequent randomized controlled trials, non–insulin-requiring remissions of 12 mo duration were induced in 24%[885] and 32%[886] of cyclosporine-treated patients compared with 10%[885] and 3%[886] remission rates in placebo-treated controls.

The cyclosporine studies provide powerful support for the autoimmune nature of type 1 diabetes and provide unequivocal evidence that a substantial complement of beta cells is still intact or at least viable at the onset of metabolic decompensation. This is consistent with findings in BB rats, in which 20% of the normal complement of insulin-containing cells was still present on the first day of overt diabetes.[887] Patients in a non–insulin-requiring remission induced by cyclosporine exhibit a markedly diminished response to glucose but a relatively normal response to nonglucose nutrients.[888]

The reluctance to sanction the use of cyclosporine for the treatment of diabetes is based on its known side effects, of which nephrotoxicity is the most common.[889] The effects of the drug on renal function are reversible upon its discontinuation even after several years of treatment. However, because the diabetes invariably reappears when cyclosporine treatment is discontinued, there seems to be little gain for diabetic patients treated with this drug. Moreover, renal biopsy specimens from some cyclosporine-treated patients have exhibited histopathological changes,[890] which in the presence of diabetes could increase the risk of permanent renal disease. Lymphoma has been reported in patients treated with cyclosporine for other disorders but has not thus far been encountered in cyclosporine-treated diabetic patients.

The therapeutic benefits of immunosuppression would almost certainly be far greater if intervention were instituted during the preovert phase of the disease when a far greater complement of beta cells is still present. However, at present this would seem even less justifiable than cyclosporine therapy at the onset of the diabetes, inasmuch as the criteria for predicting inevitability of progression from a preovert to an overt phase of the disease have not yet been established.

Conceivably, further carefully controlled studies may modify the current view concerning the use of cyclosporine in autoimmune diabetes and prediabetes. Until then, or until the development of a less toxic immunosuppressive agent, the clinician has no option but to continue to manage the disease in a conventional manner.

Treatment of Ketoacidosis

The treatment of diabetic ketoacidosis has been extensively reviewed.[392, 891, 892]

Replacement of Fluid and Electrolytes

Hypovolemia and vascular collapse are the cause of death in uncomplicated ketoacidosis, and correction is the most urgent therapeutic priority. Volume repletion alone without insulin administration can lower plasma glucose levels and decrease counterregulatory hormone concentrations but may not reverse the acidosis.[376] For this reason insulin is always required.

The average fluid deficit in adults is 3 to 5 L, and the rate of volume replacement is determined by clinical assessment. Generally 1 or 2 L of isotonic saline is administered rapidly during the first 2 h, but if hypotension, extreme hyperglycemia, and oliguria are present, more should be given. If hypernatremia develops, 0.45% sodium chloride can be substituted for isotonic saline, but this is usually not necessary. Free water is ordinarily provided by the infusion of 5% dextrose begun as the plasma glucose level falls below 16.7 mmol/L (300 mg/dL). Correction of the extracellular fluid volume deficit takes precedence over correction of the free water deficit. Ringer's lactate can be used in lieu of saline to minimize the chloride load. Large amounts of sodium chloride contribute to the hyperchloremic acidosis that commonly occurs during and after therapy. Long-standing disagreement concerning the best repair solution probably reflects the fact that sodium chloride and balanced electrolyte solutions are equally effective, particularly if underlying renal function is normal.

The hyperkalemia usually present on admission recedes when insulin action begins and potassium moves back into cells. Potassium replacement is required at this point to prevent hypokalemia. *Potassium given before insulin has begun to act is potentially lethal.* During the first 4 h of therapy, potassium should be administered only if the initial level is normal or low on direct measurement. Even then, it should be given only after insulin action has begun; without insulin potassium cannot enter cells effectively, and hyperkalemia may quickly reach cardiotoxic levels.[496] An appropriate initial rate is 20 to 40 mEq/h, but the serum potassium level should be monitored every 2 to 4 h. If laboratory results are delayed, serial electrocardiograms can be obtained to provide clues to the presence of hypokalemia. The total amount of potassium required ordinarily does not exceed 160 mEq in the first 24 h. Potassium should be given with extreme care, if at all, in the anuric patient.

Phosphate deficits usually range from 0.5 to 1.5 mmol/kg of body weight but may be larger,[893, 894] becoming apparent only when insulin action shifts phosphate back into cells with restoration of glucose metabolism. Rhabdomyolysis, impaired cardiac function, hemolysis, and respiratory failure are potential consequences of phosphate deficiency, but they are rare. Reduced levels of red blood cell 2,3-diphosphoglycerate lower tissue oxygenation by no more than 20%, but even this may be significant if associated microvascular disease, autonomic neuropathy, or hypovolemia prevents a compensatory increase in capillary blood flow. Phosphate depletion is usually silent clinically, and phosphate replacement has little effect on the course of diabetic ketoacidosis.[893, 894] If initial phosphate values are low, the potassium can be administered in the form of potassium phosphate to provide 40 to 60 mmol of the anion.

The matter of bicarbonate administration is unsettled.[895] Severe acidosis impairs myocardial contractility and, when coupled with volume depletion, may cause shock.[392] If the pH is below 7.0 or the bicarbonate level is less than 5 mmol/L, it is prudent to infuse sodium bicarbonate (100 mmol NaHCO$_3$ per liter of 0.45% saline) as initial therapy,[896] although in one retrospective study this failed to produce clinical benefit.[897] Opposition to bicarbonate therapy is based on the fact that when the red blood cell 2,3-diphosphoglycerate level is low, a sudden rise in pH may reduce oxygen release to tissues by shifting the oxygen dissociation curve to the left, thereby predisposing to lactic acidosis. It is also thought that bicarbonate induces paradoxical intracellular acidification, especially in the heart, thereby decreasing left ventricular function. Bicarbonate administration should be halted when the pH reaches 7.2.

Insulin Therapy

All patients in diabetic ketoacidosis require regular insulin administered by vein or, in the absence of venous access, by intramuscular injection. Traditionally insulin was recommended in doses of 50 to 100 U/h,[392] but low-dose treatment using 6 to 10 U/h is equally effective.[896] The advantage of the low-dose regimen is its simplicity. Its disadvantage is delayed recovery from acidosis in the rare patient with significant insulin resistance because of a high titer of insulin antibodies or other factors. The authors believe that an initial bolus of 50 U followed by a constant infusion of 10 to 20 U/h is a reasonable approach. Larger doses of insulin will be required if acidosis does not begin to respond over a 3- to 4-h period as indicated by a rise in pH or a reduction in the anion gap. Insulin must be given until the urine is free of ketones because continued ketosis, even in the absence of acidosis, indicates that the enzymes mediating hepatic fatty acid oxidation and acetoacetate and β-hydroxybutyrate synthesis have not been deactivated. Under these circumstances any rise in free fatty acid concentration (e.g., because of medical complications or hypoglycemia) results in recurrent ketoacidosis. It is likely that high concentrations of insulin overcome insulin resistance through binding to the IGF I receptor, which exerts insulin-like effects.

Glucose Administration

Once insulin has restored glucose uptake by the insulin-requiring tissues and suppressed the hyperglucagonemia,[392] hypoglycemia will supervene unless exogenous glucose is provided. Because glucose levels always fall before ketone levels decrease, exogenous glucose must be provided to cover the insulin needed to reverse the ketosis. Infusions are ordinarily begun when the plasma glucose level reaches 14 to 17 mmol/L (250 to 300 mg/dL) to minimize the risk of cerebral edema. Hypoglycemia is never a problem when glucose is started early.

The Mechanisms by Which Appropriate Therapy Reverses Diabetic Ketoacidosis

Replacement of fluid and electrolyte deficits restores perfusion of tissues to normal, corrects or prevents hypoxia, and lowers the high levels of counterregulatory hormones. Insulin-mediated suppression of glucagon lowers the hepatic cyclic AMP level and the activity of cyclic AMP–dependent protein kinases; this re-establishes hepatic glycogenesis, stops glycogenolysis, and raises fructose 2,6-bisphosphate levels (see Fig. 24–27, lower). The increase in fructose 2,6-bisphosphate concentration blocks gluconeogenesis and activates hepatic glycolysis, thereby providing substrate for lipogenesis. The consequent rise in malonyl-CoA concentration inhibits carnitine palmitoyltransferase I activity and blocks ketogenesis. The levels of ketones fall as a consequence of continued catabolism in the face of inhibited synthesis. In adipocytes, insulin inhibits lipolysis and reduces free fatty acid delivery to the liver. Simultaneously, insulin action in the periphery increases glucose uptake by muscle and lowers blood glucose levels. Anabolic processes are thus re-established and catabolism is inhibited.

Complications of Diabetic Ketoacidosis

Death is rare in properly treated diabetic ketoacidosis. Precipitating or complicating illness, such as myocardial infarction, sepsis, or acute pancreatitis, accounts for most of the mortality.[892] Death can result from shock (caused by volume depletion, reduced myocardial contractility, and diminished responsiveness of the arteries to catecholamines) or from therapeutic errors.

INFECTION. Although leukocytosis may occur in diabetic ketoacidosis in the absence of infection, fever generally indicates infection and demands a careful hunt for pneumonia, pyelonephritis, and septicemia. Infections that are ordinarily trivial—e.g., apical tooth abscesses or furunculosis—can sometimes precipitate diabetic ketoacidosis. Mucormycosis of the paranasal sinuses is a rare but uniquely ketoacidosis-associated infection manifested by facial pain, bloody nasal discharge, orbital swelling, proptosis, blurred vision, and impairment of consciousness. The pathogenicity of this ubiquitous fungus in diabetic ketoacidosis is said to result from an acidosis-induced block in the binding of iron to transferrin, which provides the pathogen with free iron, an obligatory growth factor.[898]

VASCULAR THROMBOSIS. A thrombotic event may occur during or after apparently successful management of hyperosmolar coma or ketoacidosis. Both disorders predispose to thrombosis, the result of a combination of volume contraction, low cardiac output, increased viscosity of the blood, underlying atherosclerosis, direct damage to endothelium by the hyperosmolar milieu, and changes in clotting factors and platelet function.[899] Factor VIII activity is increased while partial thromboplastin time is shortened and the level of antithrombin III is reduced. Platelets from patients with ketoacidosis exhibit increased in vivo aggregation,[535] perhaps because of increased synthesis of prostaglandin E_2 and thromboxanes coupled with reduced synthesis of prostacyclin by endothelium. Spontaneous aggregation of platelets and disseminated intravascular coagulation thus can occur in uncontrolled diabetes and can be reversed by improvement in the metabolic state.

CEREBRAL EDEMA. In children and adolescents, cerebral edema may develop during the course of treatment of ketoacidosis.[900] The syndrome is rare in adults. The complication should be suspected when a patient with ketoacidosis who had no underlying neurological illness begins to deteriorate 3 to 10 h into treatment with increasing stupor or coma coupled with signs of increased intracranial pressure. Papilledema, pupillary dysfunction, hyperpyrexia, and a variety of other neurological manifestations may be present. The treatment involves the administration of hypertonic mannitol and dexamethasone.[901] The cause of the cerebral edema is not known, although osmotic disequilibrium between intracellular and extracellular fluids probably plays a role. A fall in the plasma oncotic pressure during treatment may be contributory.[902]

RESPIRATORY DISTRESS SYNDROME. Another complication of an uncontrolled diabetes, occurring in both ketoacidosis and hyperosmolar coma, is the adult respiratory distress syndrome.[903] The picture is heralded by unexplained hypoxemia and dyspnea in the absence of pneumonia or underlying pulmonary or cardiac disease. Physical findings may be absent early although subsequently rales are heard. The x-ray findings resemble those in pulmonary edema, but the capillary wedge pressure is normal or low as determined by Swan-Ganz catheter. Mortality is high despite treatment with positive end-expiratory pressure and careful fluid management.

Clinical Errors

Clinical errors contribute importantly to the mortality in diabetic ketoacidosis (Table 24–28). The erroneous administration of hypertonic glucose at the outset increases intracellular dehydration. In patients with major volume depletion, the administration of insulin without sufficient fluids may shift extracellular water into cells, further shrinking the extracellular fluid volume and impairing blood flow to critical vascular beds or, conceivably, precipitating vascular collapse. The premature administration of potassium before insulin has begun to act may cause fatal hyperkalemia early, whereas later, when insulin is acting, failure to administer potassium may lead to fatal hypokalemia in potassium-depleted patients.

Common nonlethal conditions resulting from therapeutic errors include recurrent ketoacidosis caused by failure to maintain glucose and insulin treatment until ketones have been cleared and depleted glycogen stores restocked and hypoglycemia caused by insufficient glucose administration.

Treatment of Nonketotic Hyperosmolar Coma

Fluid repletion is the most important aspect of treatment. The deficit, which may reach 10 L or more, far exceeds that of diabetic ketoacidosis.[415, 416] The first 2 or 3 L should be given rapidly, even in elderly individuals with uncertain cardiac function. Careful monitoring of the central venous pressure permits rapid repletion of volume without a risk of overexpansion. The initial serum sodium level may be high, normal, or low, depending on the relative losses of sodium and water in the urine in the face of a shift of water out of cells secondary to hyperglycemia. Treatment should begin with normal saline at a rate that will replete at least half of the estimated fluid deficit within 6 h, after which 0.45% saline can be given to complete volume replacement. Re-expansion of the extracellular fluid volume reduces the levels of glucagon, catecholamines, and the other hormones of stress and re-establishes glucose excretion if renal function is intact.[392] This reduces hyperglycemia independently of insulin action.

Insulin should be given. A low-dose schedule consisting of a 10-U bolus and 5 to 10 U/h thereafter is appropriate. Because of the high rate of infection, particularly with gram-negative organisms,[416] antibiotics should be given empirically to any patient with fever pending the outcome of blood, urine, or sputum (transtracheal aspirate) cultures. Although mortality rates are generally high in hyperosmolar coma (>50%), some authors report a much lower percentage of deaths (<14%).[417] The mortality is highest in older patients.

Prevention and Treatment of Macrovascular and Microvascular Complications

Macrovascular Disease

Macrovascular disease accounts for much of the morbidity and mortality seen in diabetic patients. Elimination of risk factors such as hypertension and cigarette smoking seems mandatory in diabetic patients. It seems almost futile to attempt to correct hyperglycemia without also eliminating the other risk factors.

Management of hypercholesterolemia by dietary means in diabetic patients represents a special problem as noted earlier. The most appropriate diet is said to be one in which monounsaturated or polyunsaturated fats are substituted for unsaturated fats and carbohydrate intake is limited.[854] If dietary management fails to control hypercholesterolemia or hypertriglyceridemia, medications such as lovastatin, bile salt–binding resins, nicotinic acid, probucol, and gemfibrozil can be employed as in nondiabetic patients.[855, 904] Early

TABLE 24–28. Errors in the Therapy of Diabetic Ketoacidosis

Time	Therapeutic Error	Consequences
Initial 4 h	Hypertonic glucose administered because of erroneous diagnosis of hypoglycemia	Further increase in hyperosmolality and intracellular dehydration
	Inappropriate potassium administration	Hyperkalemic cardiotoxicity
	Overly rapid correction of hyperglycemia	Cerebral edema
	Insufficient saline solution	Hypotension
	Too much insulin without enough fluid	Decreased blood pressure due to shift of volume from extracellular to intracellular space
After 6–12 h	Insufficient potassium	Hypokalemic cardiotoxicity
	Insufficient glucose	Hypoglycemia; reappearance of ketosis

attention to atherogenic risk factors will be of far greater value than interventions after these complications have become clinically apparent.

More specific treatment for atherosclerosis in diabetes is not available. Aminoguanidine, an agent that prevents cross-linking between arterial wall proteins in experimental diabetes, might be useful in human disease, but no data are yet available.[905]

Microvascular Disease

The serious problem of diabetic microvascular disease and the possible role of hyperglycemia were discussed earlier, together with the possible importance of the polyol pathway as mediator of the pathological process. We noted that although aldose reductase inhibitors prevent microvascular complications in experimental diabetes, their effects in established complications in humans are minimal.

A means of inhibiting new vessel formation would be helpful in diabetic retinopathy approaching the proliferative stage. A promising lead is the observation that a heparin analogue, β-cyclodextrin tetradecasulfate, is a powerful inhibitor of neovascularization in the rabbit cornea.[906] Other factors regulating angiogenesis are known and could also be exploited.[907] For the present, however, it must be concluded that microvascular disease is untreatable.

Pancreatic Transplantation

The cure of diabetes by transplantation of a normal pancreas or isolated islets remains an unfulfilled hope in routine clinical practice. Studies in rodents suggested that isolated islets might be transplantable across genetic barriers without immunosuppression.[908] However, transplantation of fetal islets[909] or human fetal pancreatic allografts[910] has little effect, probably because the amount of transplanted tissue is too small to provide meaningful insulin production. Whole or segmental pancreatic transplants are more successful but require ongoing immunosuppression. In general, pancreatic transplants are done at the time of kidney replacement in patients with renal failure.[911] As new techniques are developed, such as bladder drainage of exocrine secretions (which allows monitoring of graft rejection by following amylase values in the urine), pancreatic grafting may become more common in patients with early renal disease.[912] The risks of the procedure, graft failure rates near 50% at 1 y, and the dangers of prolonged immunosuppression have persuaded diabetologists that pancreatic transplantation in patients without complications is not indicated.[911]

RARE CAUSES OF DIABETES

In this chapter we have concentrated on the common forms of diabetes. Hyperglycemia or glucose intolerance occurs in a wide variety of other genetic and acquired diseases.[913] Because most of these diseases are rare, little detail is available regarding the metabolic abnormality, and in some cases glucose intolerance may simply be the consequence of accompanying stress. A list of these disorders is available.[913]

Three of the rare diabetic syndromes are of particular interest because of insight provided into the physiological actions of insulin. The first is due to an abnormal insulin.[914, 915] The usual clinical picture is mild hyperglycemia with hyperinsulinemia and decreased binding of the mutant insulin to target tissues. The response to normal insulin is intact. The defect in one of these insulins (insulin Chicago) is a point mutation (cytidylate-to-guanylate transversion) in the insulin gene that causes a leucine → phenylalanine substitution at position 25 of the beta chain.[916] The treatment is straightforward because the response to exogenous insulin is normal.

The second condition is due to antibodies arising not against the insulin molecule but against the insulin receptor. Originally described in middle-aged women with clinical and laboratory features suggesting collagen-vascular disease, this disorder is also recognized to be a feature of androgen excess in women, particularly those with polycystic ovary disease.[917] Insulin resistance can be extreme and hyperglycemia severe, although some patients exhibit normal glucose values at the expense of extremely high insulin levels.[918] Other affected individuals may experience hypoglycemia or alternating phases of hypoglycemia and hyperglycemia.[919] Experiments in animals suggest that in relatively low doses the antireceptor antibody acts as an agonist, binding to the insulin receptor and producing hypoglycemia.[920] At high concentrations the antibody causes hyperglycemia by desensitizing the receptor to endogenous (or exogenous) insulin. Treatment requires immunosuppression.[921] In severe cases plasmapheresis may be tried.[922]

A third syndrome is insulin resistance caused by mutations in the insulin receptor itself.[923–925] These genetic defects provide strong evidence that tyrosine kinase activity is necessary for insulin action in humans, confirming the findings with immunological blockade and experimentally induced mutations.[367]

REFERENCES

1. National Diabetes Advisory Board. Diabetes in the 1980's. Challenges for the future. U.S. Department of Health and Human Services, Public Health Service. NIH Publication No. 82-2143. Washington, DC: Government Printing Office, 1982.
2. National Diabetes Data Group. Classification and diagnosis of diabetes mellitus and other categories of glucose intolerance. Diabetes 1979; 28:1039–1057.
3. Ito C, Mito K, Hara H. Review of criteria for diagnosis of diabetes mellitus based on results of follow-up study. Diabetes 1983; 32:343–351.
4. Mosenthal HO, Barry E. Criteria for and interpretation of normal glucose tolerance tests. Ann Intern Med 1950; 33:1175–1194.
5. Unger RH. The standard two-hour oral glucose tolerance test in the diagnosis of diabetes mellitus in subjects without fasting hyperglycemia. Ann Intern Med 1957; 47:1138–1153.
6. Bennett PH, Rushforth NB, Miller M, et al. Epidemiologic studies of diabetes in the Pima Indians. Recent Prog Horm Res 1976; 32:333–376.
7. Pettitt DG, Knowler WC, Lisse JR, et al. Development of retinopathy and proteinuria in relation to plasma-glucose concentrations in Pima Indians. Lancet 1980; 2:1050–1052.
8. Fink RI, Kolterman OG, Griffin J, et al. Mechanisms of insulin resistance in aging. J Clin Invest 1983; 71:1523–1535.
9. Rowe JW, Minaker KL, Pallotta JA, et al. Characterization of the insulin resistance of aging. J Clin Invest 1983; 71:1581–1587.
10. Dunn PJ, Cole RA, Soeldner JS, et al. Temporal relationship of glycosylated haemoglobin concentrations to glucose control in diabetics. Diabetologia 1979; 17:213–220.
11. Singer DE, Coley CM, Sarnat JH, et al. Tests of glycemia in diabetes mellitus. Their use in establishing a diagnosis and in treatment. Ann Intern Med 1989; 110:125–137.
12. Siperstein MD, Unger RH, Madison LL. Studies of muscle capillary basement membranes in normal subjects, diabetic, and prediabetic patients. J Clin Invest 1968; 47:1973–1999.
13. Karam JH, Rosenthal M, O'Donnell JJ, et al. Discordance of diabetic microangiopathy in identical twins. Diabetes 1976; 25:24–28.
14. Ganda OP, Williamson JR, Soeldner JS, et al. Muscle capillary basement membrane width and its relationship to diabetes mellitus in monozygotic twins. Diabetes 1983; 32:549–556.
15. Barnett AH, Spiliopoulos AJ, Pyke DA, et al. Muscle capillary basement membrane in identical twins discordant for insulin-dependent diabetes. Diabetes 1983; 32:557–560.
16. Peterson CM, Jones RL, Esterly JA, et al. Changes in basement membrane thickening and pulse volume concomitant with improved glucose control and exercise in patients with insulin-dependent diabetes mellitus. Diabetes Care 1980; 3:586–589.
17. Raskin P, Pietri A, Unger RH, et al. The effect of diabetic control on skeletal muscle capillary basement membrane width in patients with type I diabetes mellitus. N Engl J Med 1983; 309:1546–1550.
18. Bennett PH. Classification of diabetes. In: Ellenberg M, Rifkin H, eds. Diabetes Mellitus. Theory and Practice. 3rd ed. New Hyde Park, NY: Medical Examination Publishing, 1983:409–414.
19. Keen H. Problems in the definition of diabetes mellitus and its subtypes. In: Köbberling J, Tattersall R, eds. The Genetics of Diabetes Mellitus. Proceedings of the Serono Symposia. Vol 47. London: Academic, 1982: 1–11.
20. West KM. Epidemiology of Diabetes and Its Vascular Lesions. New York: Elsevier, 1978: 292–293.
21. Zimmet P. Epidemiology of diabetes and its macrovascular manifestations in Pacific populations: the medical effects of social progress. Diabetes Care 1979; 2:144–153.
22. Gamble DR. The epidemiology of insulin dependent diabetes, with particular reference to the relationship of virus infection to its etiology. Epidemiol Rev 1980; 2:49–70.
23. Holmgren G, Samuelson G, Hermansson B. The prevalence of diabetes mellitus: a study of children and their relatives in a northern Swedish county. Clin Genet 1974; 5:465–468.
24. Cohen T. Juvenile diabetes in Israel. Isr J Med Sci 1971; 7:1558–1561.
25. Teuscher A, Zuppinger K, Lüschner R, et al. Häufigkeit des jugendlichen Diabetes mellitus in Kanton Bern (Schweiz). Schweiz Med Wochenschr 1975; 105:1218–1223.
26. Bloom A, Hayes TM, Gamble DR. Register of newly diagnosed diabetic children. Br. Med J 1975; 3:580–583.
27. Christau B, Kromann H, Andersen OO, et al. Incidence, seasonal and geographical patterns of juvenile-onset insulin-dependent diabetes mellitus in Denmark. Diabetologia 1977; 13:281–284.
28. Tattersall RB, Pyke DA. Diabetes in identical twins. Lancet 1972; 2:1120–1125.
29. LaPorte RE, Fishbein HA, Drash AL, et al. The Pittsburgh insulin-dependent diabetes mellitus (IDDM) registry. The incidence of insulin-dependent diabetes mellitus in Allegheny County, Pennsylvania (1965–1976). Diabetes 1981; 30:279–284.
30. Wadsworth MEJ, Jarrett RJ. Incidence of diabetes in the first 26 years of life. Lancet 1974; 2:1172–1174.
31. Green A, Andersen PK. Epidemiological studies of diabetes mellitus in Denmark. 3. Clinical characteristics and incidence of diabetes among males aged 0 to 19 years. Diabetologia 1983; 25:226–230.
32. Kurtz Z, Peckham CS, Ades AE. Changing prevalence of juvenile-onset diabetes mellitus. Lancet 1988; 2:88–90.
33. Rewers M, LaPorte RE, Walczak M, et al. Apparent epidemic of insulin-dependent diabetes mellitus in midwestern Poland. Diabetes 1987; 36:106–113.
34. Melton LJ III, Palumbo PJ, Chu C-P. Incidence of diabetes mellitus by clinical type. Diabetes Care 1983; 6:75–86.
35. Christau B, Kromann H, Christy M, et al. Incidence of insulin-dependent diabetes mellitus (0–29 years at onset) in Denmark. Acta Med Scand (Suppl) 1979; 624:54–60.
36. Simpson NE. The genetics of diabetes: a study of 233 families of juvenile diabetics. Ann Hum Genet 1962; 26:1–21.
37. Tattersall RB, Fajans SS. A difference between the inheritance of classical juvenile-onset and maturity-onset type diabetes of young people. Diabetes 1975; 24:44–53.
38. Barnett AH, Eff C, Leslie RDG, et al. Diabetes in identical twins. A study of 200 pairs. Diabetologia 1981; 20:87–93.
39. Chern MM, Anderson VE, Barbosa J. Empirical risk for insulin-dependent diabetes (IDD) in sibs. Further definition of genetic heterogeneity. Diabetes 1982; 31:1115–1118.
40. Wagener DK, Sacks JM, LaPorte RE, et al. The Pittsburgh study of

of IDDM. Diabetes 1982; 31:136–144.
41. Warram JH, Krowlewski AS, Gottlieb MS, et al. Differences in risk of insulin-dependent diabetes in offspring of diabetic mothers and diabetic fathers. N Engl J Med 1984; 311:149–152.
42. Vadheim CM, Rotter JI, Maclaren NK, et al. Preferential transmission of diabetic alleles within the HLA gene complex. N Engl J Med 1986; 315:1314–1318.
43. Benacerraf B. Role of MHC gene products in immune regulation. Science 1981; 212:1229–1238.
44. Steinmetz M, Hood L. Genes of the major histocompatibility complex in mouse and man. Science 1983; 222:727–733.
45. Shackelford DA, Kaufman JF, Korman AJ, et al. HLA-DR antigens: structure, separation of subpopulations, gene cloning and function. Immunol Rev 1982; 66:133–187.
46. Corte G, Calabi F, Damiani G, et al. Human Ia molecules carrying DC1 determinants differ in both α- and β-subunits from Ia molecules carrying DR determinants. Nature 1981; 292:357–360.
47. Strominger JL. Biology of the human histocompatibility leukocyte antigen system and a hypothesis regarding the generation of autoimmune diseases. J Clin Invest 1986; 77:1411–1415.
48. Kämpe O, Bellgrau D, Hammerling U, et al. Complex formation of class I transplantation antigens and a viral glycoprotein. J Biol Chem 1983; 258:10594–10598.
49. Bottazzo GF, Pujol-Borrell R, Hanafusa T, et al. Role of aberrant HLA-DR expression and antigen presentation in induction of endocrine autoimmunity. Lancet 1983; 2:1115–1119.
50. Acuto O, Reinherz EL. The human T-cell receptor. Structure and function. N Engl J Med 1985; 312:1100–1111.
51. Faustman D, Hauptfeld V, Lacy P, et al. Prolongation of murine islet allograft survival by pretreatment of islets with antibody directed to Ia determinants. Proc Natl Acad Sci USA 1981; 78:5156–5159.
52. Bach FH, Sachs DH. Current concepts. Immunology. Transplantation immunology. N Engl J Med 1987; 317:489–492.
53. Barbosa J, King R, Noreen H, et al. The histocompatibility system in juvenile, insulin-dependent diabetic multiplex kindreds. J Clin Invest 1977; 60:989–998.
54. Spielman RS, Baker L, Zmijewski CM. Gene dosage and susceptibility to insulin-dependent diabetes. Ann Hum Genet 1980; 44:135–150.
55. Walker A, Cudworth AG. Type I (insulin-dependent) diabetic multiplex families. Mode of genetic transmission. Diabetes 1980; 29:1036–1039.
56. Nerup J, Mandrup-Poulsen T, Mølvig J. The HLA-IDDM association: implications for etiology and pathogenesis of IDDM. Diabetes Metab Rev 1987; 3:779–802.
57. Sakurami T, Ueno Y, Nagaoka K, et al. HLA-DR specifications in Japanese with juvenile-onset insulin-dependent diabetes mellitus. Diabetes 1982; 31:105–116.
58. Todd JA, Bell JI, McDevitt HO. HLA-DQβ gene contributes to susceptibility and resistance to insulin-dependent diabetes mellitus. Nature 1987; 329:599–603.
59. Kwok WW, Lotshaw C, Milner ECB, et al. Mutational analysis of the HLA-DQ3.2 insulin-dependent diabetes mellitus susceptibility gene. Proc Natl Acad Sci USA 1989; 86:1027–1030.
60. Sheehy MJ, Scharf SJ, Roe JR, et al. Diabetes-susceptible HLA haplotype is best defined by a combination of HLA-DR and -DQ alleles. J Clin Invest 1989; 83:830–835.
61. Segall M. Perspectives in diabetes. HLA and genetics of IDDM. Holism vs. reductionism. Diabetes 1988; 37:1005–1008.
61a. Baisch JM, Weeks T, Giles R, et al. Analysis of HLA-DQ genotypes and susceptibility in insulin-dependent diabetes mellitus. N Engl J Med 1990; 322:1836–1841.
62. Cohen N, Brantbar C, Font MP, et al. HLA-DR2–associated DW-subtypes correlate with RFLP clusters: most DR2 IDDM patients belong to one of these clusters. Immunogenetics 1986; 23:47–51.
63. Monson JP, Boucher BJ. HLA type and islet cell antibody status in family with (diabetes insipidus and mellitus, optic atrophy, and deafness) DIDMOAD syndrome. Lancet 1983; 1:1286–1287.
64. Bottazzo GF, Mirakian R, Dean BM, et al. How immunology helps to define heterogeneity in diabetes mellitus. In: Köbberling J, Tattersall R, eds. The Genetics of Diabetes Mellitus. Proceedings of the Serono Symposia. Vol 47. London: Academic, 1982: 79–90.
65. Bottazzo GF, Doniach D. Pancreatic autoimmunity and HLA antigens. Lancet 1976; 2:800.
66. Irvine WJ. Classification of idiopathic diabetes. Lancet 1977; 1:638–642.
67. Rotter JI, Rimoin DL. Heterogeneity in diabetes mellitus—update, 1978. Evidence for further genetic heterogeneity within juvenile-onset insulin-dependent diabetes mellitus. Diabetes 1978; 27:599–608.
68. Ludvigsson J, Samuelsson U, Beuforts C, et al. HLA-DR3 is associated with a more slowly progressive form of type 1 (insulin-dependent) diabetes. Diabetologia 1986; 29:207–210.
69. MacDonald MJ. Hypothesis: the frequencies of juvenile diabetes in American blacks and Caucasians are consistent with dominant inheritance. Diabetes 1980; 29:110–114.
70. MacDonald MJ, Gottschall J, Hunter JB, et al. HLA-DR4 in insulin-dependent diabetic parents and their diabetic offspring: a clue to dominant inheritance. Proc Natl Acad Sci USA 1986; 83:7049–7053.

71. Barbosa J, Chern MM, Anderson VE, et al. Linkage analysis between the major histocompatibility system and insulin-dependent diabetes in families with patients in two consecutive generations. J Clin Invest 1980; 65:592–601.
72. Rubinstein P, Suciu-Foca N, Nicholson JF. Genetics of juvenile diabetes mellitus. A recessive gene closely linked to HLA D and with 50 per cent penetrance. N Engl J Med 1977; 297:1036–1040.
73. Pyke DA. Diabetes: the genetic connections. Diabetologia 1979; 17:333–343.
74. Nerup J. HLA studies in diabetes mellitus: a review. Adv Metab Disord 1978; 9:263–277.
75. Rotter JI, Anderson CE, Rubin R, et al. HLA genotypic study of insulin-dependent diabetes. The excess of DR3/DR4 heterozygotes allows rejection of the recessive hypothesis. Diabetes 1983; 32:169–174.
76. Williams RC. Has the recessive hypothesis for susceptibility to insulin-dependent diabetes mellitus been firmly and unequivocally rejected? Diabetes 1983; 32:774–776.
77. Hodge SE, Rotter JI, Lange KL. A three-allele model for heterogeneity of juvenile onset insulin-dependent diabetes. Ann Hum Genet 1980; 43:399–412.
78. Louis EJ, Thomson G. Three-allele synergistic mixed model for insulin-dependent diabetes mellitus. Diabetes 1986; 35:958–963.
79. Prochazka M, Leiter EH, Serreze DV, et al. Three recessive loci required for insulin-dependent diabetes in nonobese-diabetic mice. Science 1987; 237:286–289.
80. Millward BA, Walsh KI, Leslie RDG, et al. T-cell receptor beta dependent diabetes. Clin Exp Immunol 1987; 70:152–157.
81. Gorsuch AN, Spencer KM, Lister J, et al. Can future type I diabetes be predicted? A study in families of affected children. Diabetes 1982; 31:862–866.
82. Cahill GF Jr, McDevitt HO. Insulin-dependent diabetes mellitus: the initial lesion. N Engl J Med 1981; 304:1454–1465.
83. Foulis AK, Francis ND, Farquharson MA, et al. Massive synchronous B-cell necrosis causing type 1 (insulin-dependent) diabetes—a unique histopathological case report. Diabetologia 1988; 31:46–50.
84. Karam JH, Lewitt PA, Young CW, et al. Insulinopenic diabetes after rodenticide (Vacor) ingestion. A unique model of acquired diabetes in man. Diabetes 1980; 29:971–978.
85. Helgason T, Jonasson MR. Evidence for food additive as a cause of ketosis prone diabetes. Lancet 1981; 2:716–720.
86. Mordes JP, Desemone J, Rossini AA. The BB rat. Diabetes Metab Rev 1987; 3:725–750.
87. Kataoka S, Satoh J, Fujiya H, et al. Immunologic aspects of the nonobese diabetic (NOD) mouse: abnormalities of cellular immunity. Diabetes 1983; 32:247–253.
88. Yoon J-W, Ray UR. Perspectives on the role of viruses in insulin-dependent diabetes. Diabetes Care 1985; 8(Suppl 1):39–44.
89. Menser MA, Forrest JM, Bransby RD. Rubella infection and diabetes mellitus. Lancet 1978; 1:57–60.
90. Frisk G, Fohlman J, Kobbah M, et al. High frequency of coxsackie-B-virus–specific IgM in children developing type 1 diabetes during a period of high-diabetes morbidity. J Med Virol 1985; 17:219–227.
91. Nelson PG, Pyke DA, Gamble DR. Viruses and the aetiology of diabetes: a study in identical twins. Br Med J 1975; 4:249–251.
92. Yoon J-W, Austin M, Onodera T, et al. Virus-induced diabetes mellitus. Isolation of a virus from the pancreas of a child with diabetic ketoacidosis. N Engl J Med 1979; 300:1173–1179.
93. Jenson AB, Rosenberg HS, Notkins AL. Pancreatic islet-cell damage in children with fatal viral infections. Lancet 1980; 2:354–358.
94. Pak CY, Eun H-M, McArthur RG, et al. Association of cytomegalovirus infection with autoimmune type 1 diabetes. Lancet 1988; 2:1–4.
95. Yoon J-W, Onodera T, Notkins AL. Virus-induced diabetes mellitus. XV. Beta cell damage and insulin-dependent hyperglycemia in mice infected with coxsackie virus B4. J Exp Med 1978; 148:1068–1080.
96. Yoon J-W, Notkins AL. Virus-induced diabetes mellitus. VI. Genetically determined host differences in the replication of encephalomyocarditis virus in pancreatic beta cells. J Exp Med 1976; 143:1170–1185.
97. Yoon J-W, Onodera T, Notkins AL. Virus-induced diabetes mellitus. VIII. Passage of encephalomyocarditis virus and severity of diabetes in susceptible and resistant strains of mice. J Gen Virol 1977; 37:225–232.
98. Toniolo A, Takashi O, Yoon J-W, et al. Induction of diabetes by cumulative environmental insults from viruses and chemicals. Nature 1980; 288:383–385.
99. Fujita H. Retrovirus-like particles in pancreatic β-cells of NOD mice. Biomed Res 1984; 5:67–70.
100. Leiter EL, Fewell JW, Kuff EL. Glucose induces type A retroviral gene transcription and translation in pancreatic beta cells. J Exp Med 1986; 163:87–100.
101. Nerup J, Cathelineau C, Seignalet J, et al. HLA and endocrine disease. In: Dausset J, Svejgaard A, eds. HLA and Disease. Copenhagen: Munksgaard, 1977: 149–167.
102. Rossini AA, Like AA, Chick WL, et al. Studies of streptozotocin-induced insulitis and diabetes. Proc Natl Acad Sci USA 1977; 74:2485–2489.
103. Bottazo GF. β-cell damage in diabetic insulitis: are we approaching a solution? Diabetologia 1984; 26:241–249.
104. Gepts W, In't Veld P. Islet morphologic changes. Diabetes Metab Rev 1987; 3:859–872.

105. Karam JH, Prosser PR, LeWitt PA. Islet-cell surface antibodies in a patient with diabetes mellitus after a rodenticide ingestion. N Engl J Med 1978; 299:1191.

106. Like AA, Rossini AA. Streptozotocin-induced pancreatic insulitis: new model of diabetes mellitus. Science 1976; 193:415–417.

107. Craighead JE. The role of viruses in the pathogenesis of pancreatic disease and diabetes mellitus. Prog Med Virol 1975; 19:161–214.

108. Like AA, Rossini AA, Guberski DL, et al. Spontaneous diabetes mellitus: reversal and prevention in the BB/W rat with antiserum to rat lymphocytes. Science 1979; 206:1421–1423.

109. Koevary S, Rossini A, Stoller W, et al. Passive transfer of diabetes in the BB/W rat. Science 1983; 220:727–728.

110. Like AA, Weringer EJ, Holdash A, et al. Nature of resistance to autoimmune diabetes in BioBreeding/Worcester control rats. Diabetologia 1983; 25:175.

111. Greiner DL, Mordes JP, Handler ES, et al. Depletion of RT6.1$^+$ T-lymphocytes induces diabetes in resistant BioBreeding/Worcester (BB/W) rats. J Exp Med 1987; 166:461–475.

112. Rossini AA, Mordes JP, Pelletier AM, et al. Transfusions of whole blood prevent spontaneous diabetes mellitus in the BB/W rat. Science 1983; 219:975–977.

113. Jackson RA, Morris MA, Haynes BF, et al. Increased circulating Ia-antigen–bearing T cells in type I diabetes mellitus. N Engl J Med 1982; 306:785–788.

114. Bougneres PF, Carel JC, Castino L, et al. Factors associated with early remission of type 1 diabetes in children treated with cyclosporine. N Engl J Med 1988; 318:663–670.

115. Sibley RK, Sutherland DER, Groetz F, et al. Recurrent diabetes mellitus in the pancreas iso- and allograft: a light and electron microscopic and immunohistochemical analysis of four cases. Lab Invest 1985; 53:132–144.

116. Pozzilli P, Zuccarini O, Iavicoli M, et al. Monoclonal antibodies defined abnormalities of T-lymphocytes in type 1 (insulin-dependent) diabetes. Diabetes 1983; 32:91–94.

117. Quinion-Debrie MC, Debray-Sachs M, Dardenne M, et al. Anti-islet cellular and humoral immunity. T-cell subsets and thymic function in type 1 diabetes. Diabetes 1985; 34:373–379.

118. Hitchcock CL, Riley WJ, Alamo A, et al. Lymphocyte subsets and activation in prediabetes. Diabetes 1986; 35:1416–1422.

119. Buschard K, Röpke C, Madsbad S, et al. T lymphocyte subsets in patients with newly diagnosed type 1 (insulin-dependent) diabetes: a prospective study. Diabetologia 1983; 25:247–251.

120. Lernmark Å, Li S, Baekkeskov S, et al. Islet-specific immune mechanisms. Diabetes Metab Rev 1987; 3:959–980.

121. Barbosa J, Bach FH. Cell-mediated autoimmunity in type 1 diabetes. Diabetes Metab Rev 1987; 3:981–1004.

122. Irvine WJ, Gray RS, Steel JM. Islet cell antibody as a marker for early stage type 1 diabetes mellitus. In: Irvine WJ, ed. Immunology of Diabetes. Edinburgh: Teviot Scientific Publications, 1980: 117–154.

123. Bottazzo GF, Landrum R. Separate autoantibodies to human pancreatic glucagon and somatostatin cells. Lancet 1976; 2:873–876.

124. Volk BW, Wellmann KF. The pathology of the diabetic pancreas. In: Ellenberg M, Rifkin H, eds. Diabetes Mellitus. Theory and Practice. 3rd ed. New Hyde Park, NY: Medical Examination Publishing, 1983: 309–321.

125. Orci L, Baetens D, Rufener C, et al. Hypertrophy and hyperplasia of somatostatin-containing D-cells in diabetes. Proc Natl Acad Sci USA 1976; 73:1338–1342.

126. Gepts W, LeCompte PM. The pancreatic islets in diabetes. Am J Med 1981; 70:105–115.

127. Orci L. The microanatomy of the islets of Langerhans. Metabolism 1976; 25(Suppl 1):1303–1313.

128. Stefan Y, Malaisse-Lagae F, Yoon J-W, et al. Virus-induced diabetes in mice: a quantitative evaluation of islet cell population by immunofluorescence technique. Diabetologia 1978; 15:395–401.

129. Irvine WJ, McCallum CJ, Gray RS, et al. Pancreatic islet-cell antibodies in diabetes mellitus correlated with the duration and type of diabetes, coexistent autoimmune disease, and HLA type. Diabetes 1977; 26:138–147.

130. Bottazzo GF, Cudworth AG, Moul DJ, et al. Evidence for a primary autoimmune type of diabetes mellitus. Br Med J 1978; 2:1253–1255.

131. Cudworth AG, Spencer KM, Gorsuch AN, et al. Immunogenetic heterogeneity in insulin-dependent diabetes. In: Köbberling FJ, Tattersall R, eds. The Genetics of Diabetes Mellitus. Proceedings of the Serono Symposia. Vol 47. London: Academic, 1982: 63–78.

132. Schernthaner G, Ludwig H, Mayr WR. Immunoglobulin G–insulin antibodies and immune region–associated alloantigens in insulin-dependent diabetes mellitus. J Clin Endocrinol Metab 1979; 48:403–407.

133. Rotter JI, Rimoin DL. Genetics of insulin-dependent diabetes. In: Martin JM, Ehrlich RM, Holland FJ, eds. Etiology and Pathogenesis of Insulin-Dependent Diabetes Mellitus. New York: Raven, 1981: 37–59.

134. Kolb H, Dannehl K, Grüneklee D, et al. Prospective analysis of islet cell antibodies in children with type 1 (insulin-dependent) diabetes. Diabetologia 1988; 31:189–194.

135. Satoh J, Prabhakar BS, Haspel MV, et al. Human monoclonal autoantibodies that react with multiple endocrine organs. N Engl J Med 1983; 309:217–220.

136. Lernmark A. Islet cell antibodies. Diabetic Med 1982; 4:285–292.

137. Srikanta S, Ricker AT, McCulloch DK, et al. Autoimmunity to insulin, beta cell dysfunction, and development of insulin-dependent diabetes mellitus. Diabetes 1986; 35:139–142.

138. Baekkeskov S, Aanstoot H-J, Christgan S, et al. Identification of the 64K autoantigen in insulin-dependent diabetes as the GABA-synthesizing enzyme glutamic acid decarboxylase. Nature 1990; 347:151–156.

138a. Jones DB, Hunter NR, Duff GW. Heat-shock protein 65 as a β-cell antigen of insulin-dependent diabetes. Lancet 1990; 336:583–585.

139. Kuglin B, Gries FA, Kolb H. Evidence of IgG autoantibodies against human proinsulin in patients with IDDM before insulin treatment. Diabetes 1988; 37:130–132.

140. Di Mario U, Dotta F, Crisa L, et al. Circulating anti-immunoglobulin antibodies in recent-onset type I diabetic patients. Diabetes 1988; 37:462–466.

141. Ludwig SM, Faiman C, Dean HJ. Insulin and insulin-receptor autoantibodies in children with newly diagnosed IDDM before insulin therapy. Diabetes 1987; 36:420–425.

142. Maclaren NK, Huang S-W, Fogh J. Antibody to cultured human insulinoma cells in insulin-dependent diabetes. Lancet 1975; 1:997–1000.

143. Lernmark Å, Freedman ZR, Hofmann C, et al. Islet-cell surface antibodies in juvenile diabetes mellitus. N Engl J Med 1978; 299:375–380.

144. Pujol-Borrell R, Khoury EL, Bottazzo GF. Islet cell surface antibodies in type 1 (insulin-dependent) diabetes mellitus: use of human fetal pancreas cultures as substrate. Diabetologia 1982; 22:89–95.

145. Lernmark Å, Sehlin J, Täljedal I-B, et al. Possible toxic effects of normal and diabetic patient serum on pancreatic B cells. Diabetologia 1978; 14:25–31.

146. Rittenhouse HG, Oxender DL, Pek S, et al. Complement-mediated cytotoxic effects on pancreatic islets with sera from diabetic patients. Diabetes 1980; 29:317–322.

147. Eisenbarth GS, Morris MA, Scearce RM. Cytotoxic antibodies to cloned rat islet cells in serum of patients with diabetes mellitus. J Clin Invest 1981; 67:403–408.

148. Kanatsuna T, Baekkeskov S, Lernmark Å, et al. Immunoglobulin from insulin-dependent diabetic children inhibits glucose-induced insulin release. Diabetes 1983; 32:520–524.

149. Dobersen MJ, Scharff JE, Ginsberg-Fellner F, et al. Cytotoxic autoantibodies to beta cells in the serum of patients with insulin-dependent diabetes mellitus. N Engl J Med 1980; 303:1493–1498.

150. Dobersen MJ, Scharff JE. Preferential lysis of pancreatic B-cells by islet cell surface antibodies. Diabetes 1982; 31:459–462.

151. Lernmark Å, Baekkeskov S. Islet cell antibodies—theoretical and practical implications. Diabetologia 1981; 21:431–435.

152. Bright GM. Quantitative assay for human cytoplasmic islet cell antibodies. Diabetes 1987; 36:1183–1186.

153. Gleichmann H, Bottazzo GF. Progress towards standardization of cytoplasmic islet cell–antibody assay. Diabetes 1987; 36:578–584.

154. Irvine WJ. Immunological aspects of diabetes mellitus: a review (including the salient points of the NDDG report on the classification of diabetes). In: Irvine WJ, ed. Immunology of Diabetes. Edinburgh: Teviot Scientific Publications, 1980: 1–53.

155. Rodger B, Whittingham S, Martin FIR, et al. A population survey of pancreatic islet cell antibodies. Clin Exp Immunol 1980; 39:125–129.

156. Steel JM, Irvine WJ, Clarke BF. The significance of pancreatic islet cell antibody and abnormal glucose tolerance during pregnancy. J Clin Lab Immunol 1980; 4:83–85.

157. Irvine WJ, McCallum CJ, Gray RS, et al. Clinical and pathogenic significance of pancreatic-islet-cell antibodies in diabetics treated with oral hypoglycemic agents. Lancet 1977; 1:1025–1027.

158. Van De Winkel M, Smets G, Gepts W, et al. Islet cell surface antibodies from insulin-dependent diabetics bind specifically to pancreatic B cells. J Clin Invest 1982; 70:41–49.

159. Irvine WJ, Gray RS, McCallum CJ. Pancreatic islet-cell antibody as a marker for asymptomatic and latent diabetes and prediabetes. Lancet 1976; 2:1097–1102.

160. Eisenbarth GS, Connelly J, Soeldner JS. The "natural" history of type 1 diabetes. Diabetes Metab Rev 1987; 3:873–891.

161. Srikanta S, Ganda OP, Jackson RA, et al. Type I diabetes mellitus in monozygotic twins: chronic progressive beta cell dysfunction. Ann Intern Med 1983; 99:320–326.

162. Srikanta S, Ganda OP, Eisenbarth GS, et al. Islet-cell antibodies and beta-cell function in monozygotic triplets and twins initially discordant for type I diabetes mellitus. N Engl J Med 1983; 308:322–325.

163. Maclaren NK. Perspectives in diabetes. How, when and why to predict IDDM. Diabetes 1988; 37:1591–1594.

164. Huang S-W, Maclaren NK. Insulin-dependent diabetes: a disease of autoaggression. Science 1976; 192:64–66.

165. Pozzilli P, Sensi M, Gorsuch A, et al. Evidence for raised K-cell levels in type-1 diabetes. Lancet 1979; 2:173–175.

166. Rossini AA. Immunotherapy for insulin-dependent diabetics? N Engl J Med 1983; 308:333–335.

167. Serreze DV, Leiter EH, Worthen SM, et al. NOD marrow stem cells adoptively transfer diabetes to resistant (NOD × NON) F1 mice. Diabetes 1988; 37:252–255.

168. Bendelac A, Carnand C, Bortard C, et al. Syngeneic transfer of autoimmune diabetes from diabetic NOD mice to healthy neonates. Requirement for both L3T4+ and Lyt-2+ T cells. J Exp Med 1987; 166:823–832.

169. Wicker LS, Miller BJ, Mullen Y. Transfer of autoimmune diabetes mellitus with splenocytes from nonobese diabetic (NOD) mice. Diabetes 1986; 35:855–860.

170. Hanafusa T, Sugihara S, Fujina-Kurihara H, et al. Induction of insulitis by adoptive transfer with L3T4+ Lyt2− lymphocytes in T-lymphocyte–depleted NOD mice. Diabetes 1988; 37:204–208.

171. Logothetopoulos J, Valiquette N, MacGregor I, et al. Adoptive transfer of insulitis and diabetes in neonates of diabetes-prone and -resistant rats. Tissue localization of injected blasts. Diabetes 1987; 36:1116–1123.

172. Miller BJ, Appel MC, O'Neill JJ, et al. Both Lyt-2+ and L3T4+ T cell subsets are required for the transfer of diabetes in nonobese diabetic mice. J Immunol 1988; 440:52–58.

173. Charlton B, Mandel TE. Progression from insulitis to beta-cell destruction requires L3T4+ T-lymphocytes. Diabetes 1988; 37:1108–1112.

174. Woda BA, Biron CA. Natural killer cell number and function in the spontaneously diabetic BB/W rat. J Immunol 1986; 137:1860–1866.

175. Woda BA, Padden C. BioBreeding/Worcester (BB/Wor) rats are deficient in the generation of functional cytotoxic T cells. J Immunol 1987; 139:1514–1517.

176. Pukel C, Baquerizo H, Rabinovitch A. Interleukin 2 activates BB/W diabetic rat lymphoid cells cytotoxic to islet cells. Diabetes 1987; 36:1217–1222.

177. Kaye WA, Adri MNS, Soeldner JS, et al. Acquired defect in interleukin-2 production in patients with type I diabetes mellitus. N Engl J Med 1986; 315:920–924.

178. Male D, Champion B, Cooke S. Cytotoxic lymphocytes. In: Advanced Immunology. London: Gower Medical, 1987: 7.1–7.7.

179. Podack ER. The molecular mechanism of lymphocyte-mediated tumour cell lysis. Immunol Today 1985; 6:21–27.

180. Walker R, Bone AJ, Cooke A, et al. Distinct macrophage subpopulations in pancreas of BB/E rats. Possible role for macrophages in the pathogenesis of IDDM. Diabetes 1988; 37:1301–1304.

181. Bendtzen K, Mandrup-Poulsen T, Nerup J, et al. Cytotoxicity of human pI 7 interleukin-1 for pancreatic islets of Langerhans. Science 1986; 232:1545–1547.

182. Nerup J, Mandrup-Poulsen T, Mølvig J, et al. Mechanisms of pancreatic β-cell destruction in type I diabetes. Diabetes Care 1988; 11(Suppl 1):16–23.

183. Bottazzo GF, Pujol-Borrel R, Hanafusa T, et al. Role of aberrant HLA-DR expression and antigen presentation in the induction of endocrine autoimmunity. Lancet 1983; 2:1115–1119.

184. Mandrup-Pouslen T, Bendtzen K, Dinarello CA, et al. Human tumor necrosis factor potentiates human interleukin-1 mediated rat pancreatic β-cell toxicity. J Immunol 1987; 139:4077–4082.

185. McDaniel ML, Hughes JH, Wolf BA, et al. Descriptive and mechanistic considerations of interleukin 1 and insulin secretion. Diabetes 1988; 37:1311–1315.

186. Sandler S, Andersson H, Hellerström C. Inhibitory effects of interleukin 1 on insulin secretion, insulin biosynthesis, and oxidative metabolism of isolated rat pancreatic islets. Endocrinology 1987; 121:1424–1431.

187. Nerup J, Mandrup-Poulsen J, Mølvig J, et al. Immune interactions with islet cells—implications for the pathogenesis of IDDM. In: Pipeleers D, ed. Pathology of the Endocrine Pancreas in Diabetes. Berlin: Springer-Verlag, 1988.

188. Dulin WE, Wyse BM. Reversal of streptozotocin diabetes with nicotinamide. Proc Soc Exp Biol Med 1969; 130:992–994.

189. Yamada K, Nonaka K, Hanafusa T, et al. Preventive and therapeutic effects of large dose nicotinamide injections on diabetes associated with insulitis. An observation in nonobese diabetic (NOD) mice. Diabetes 1982; 31:749–753.

190. Okamoto H. The role of poly(ADP-ribose) synthetase in the development of insulin-dependent diabetes and islet β-cell regeneration. Biomed Biochim Acta 1985; 44:15–20.

191. Asayama K, Kooy NW, Burn IM. Effect of vitamin E deficiency and selenium deficiency on insulin secretory reserve and free radical scavenging systems in islets: decrease of islet manganosuperoxide dismutase. J Lab Clin Med 1986; 107:459–464.

192. Halliwell B, ed. Oxygen Radicals and Tissue Injury. Proceedings of a Brook Lodge Symposium, Apr 27–29, 1987. Bethesda: FASEB (for Upjohn), 1988.

193. Heikkila RE, Winston B, Cohen G, et al. Alloxan-induced diabetes: evidence for the hydroxyl radical as a cytotoxic intermediate. Biochem Pharmacol 1976; 25:1085–1092.

194. Pujol-Borrell R, Hanafusa T, Chiovato L, et al. Lectin-induced expression of DR antigen on human cultured follicular thyroid cells. Nature 1983; 304:71–73.

195. Bottazzo GF. Death of a beta cell: homicide or suicide? Diabetic Med 1986; 3:119–130.

196. Bottazzo GF, Dean BM, McNally JM, et al. In situ characterization of autoimmune phenomena and expression of HLA molecules in the pancreas in diabetic insulitis. N Engl J Med 1985; 313:353–360.

197. Foulis AK, Farquharson MA. Aberrant expression of HLA-DR antigens

198. Foulis AK, Farquharson MA, Meager A. Immunoreactive α-interferon in insulin-secreting β cells in type 1 diabetes mellitus. Lancet 1987; 2:1423–1427.

199. Pujol-Borrell R, Todd I, Doshi M, et al. HLA class II induction in human islet cells by interferon-gamma plus tumour necrosis factor or lymphotoxin. Nature 1987; 326:304–306.

200. Campbell IL, Bizilj K, Coleman PG, et al. Interferon-gamma induces the expression of HLA-A, B, C but not HLA-DR on human pancreatic beta-cells. J Clin Endocrinol Metab 1986; 62:1101–1109.

201. Signore A, Cooke A, Pozzilli P, et al. Class-II and IL2 receptor positive cells in the pancreas of NOD mice. Diabetologia 1987; 30:902–905.

202. In't Veld PA, Pipellers DG. In situ analysis of pancreatic islets in rats developing diabetes. Appearance of nonendocrine cells with surface MHC class II antigens and cytoplasmic insulin immunoreactivity. J Clin Invest 1988; 82:1123–1128.

203. Sarvetnick N, Liggitt D, Pitts SL, et al. Insulin-dependent diabetes mellitus induced in transgenic mice by ectopic expression of class II MHC and interferon-gamma. Cell 1988; 52:773–782.

204. Lo D, Burkely LC, Widora G, et al. Diabetes and tolerance in transgenic mice expressing class II MHC molecules in pancreatic beta cells. Cell 1988; 53:159–168.

205. Allison J, Campbell IL, Morahan G, et al. Diabetes in transgenic mice resulting from over-expression of class I histocompatibility molecules in pancreatic β cells. Nature 1988; 333:529–533.

206. Markmann J, Lo D, Naji A, et al. Antigen presenting function of class II MHC expressing pancreatic β-cells. Nature 1988; 336:475–479.

207. Jalkenen S, Steere AC, Fox RI, et al. A distinct endothelial cell recognition system that controls lymphocyte traffic into inflamed synovium. Science 1986; 233:556–558.

208. Buschard K, Rygaard J. Passive transfer of streptozotocin induced diabetes with spleen cells. Acta Pathol Microbiol Scand 1977; 85:469.

209. Mølvig J, Baek L, Christensen P, et al. Endotoxin stimulated human monocyte secretion of interleukin 1, tumor necrosis factor alpha and protoglandin E$_2$ shows stable interindividual differences. Scand J Immunol 1988; 27:705–716.

210. Spies T, Morton CC, Nedospasov SA, et al. Genes for the tumor necrosis factors α and β are linked to the human histocompatibility complex. Proc Natl Acad Sci USA 1986; 83:8699–8702.

211. Dinarello CA, Mier JW. Lymphokines. N Engl J Med 1987; 317:940–945.

212. Mori Y, Suko M, Oyudaira H, et al. Preventive effects of cyclosporin on diabetes in NOD mice. Diabetologia 1986; 29:244–247.

213. Like AA, Dirodi V, Thomas S, et al. Prevention of diabetes mellitus in the BB/W rat with cyclosporin-A. Am J Pathol 1984; 117:92–97.

214. Lee K-U, Pak CY, Yoon J-W. Prevention of lymphocytic thyroiditis and insulitis in diabetes-prone BB rats by depletion of macrophages. Diabetologia 1988; 31:400–402.

215. Lee KU, Amano K, Yoon J-W. Evidence for initial involvement of macrophage in development of insulitis in NOD mice. Diabetes 1988; 37:989–991.

216. Baitard C, Michie S, Serrurier P, et al. In vivo prevention of thyroid and pancreatic autoimmunity in the BB rat by antibody to class II major histocompatibility complex gene products. Proc Natl Acad Sci USA 1985; 82:6627–6631.

217. Adorini L, Muller S, Cardinaux F, et al. In vivo competition between self peptides and foreign antigens in T-cell activation. Nature 1988; 334:623–625.

218. Koike T, Itoh Y, Ishii T, et al. Preventive effect of monoclonal anti L3T4 antibody on development of diabetes in NOD mice. Diabetes 1987; 36:534–541.

219. Shizuru JA, Taylor-Edwards C, Banks BA, et al. Immunotherapy of the nonobese diabetic mouse: treatment with an antibody to T-helper cells. Science 1988; 240:659–662.

220. Oldstone MB. Prevention of type I diabetes in nonobese diabetic mice by virus infection. Science 1988; 239:500–502.

221. Charlton B, Bacelj A, Mandel TE. Administration of silica particles or anti-Lyt2 antibody prevents beta-cell destruction in NOD mice given cyclophosphamide. Diabetes 1988; 37:930–935.

222. Herold KC, Montac AG, Fitch FW. Treatment with anti-T-lymphocyte antibodies prevents induction of insulitis in mice given multiple doses of streptozotocin. Diabetes 1987; 36:796–801.

223. Like AA, Biron CA, Weringer EJ, et al. Prevention of diabetes with monoclonal antibodies that recognize T lymphocytes or natural killer cells. J Exp Med 1986; 164:1145–1159.

224. Jacobson JD, Markmann JF, Brayman KL, et al. Prevention of recurrent autoimmune diabetes in BB rats by anti-asialo-GM$_2$ antibody. Diabetes 1988; 37:838–841.

225. Nair MP, Lewis EW, Schwartz SA. Immunoregulatory dysfunctions in type I diabetes: natural and antibody-dependent cellular cytotoxic activities. J Clin Immunol 1986; 6:363–372.

226. Nomikos IN, Prowse SJ, Carotenuto P, et al. Combined treatment with nicotinamide and desferrioxamine prevents islet allograft destruction in NOD mice. Diabetes 1986; 35:1302–1304.

227. Toyota T, Satoh J, Oya K, et al. Streptococcal preparation (OK-432)

inhibits development of diabetes in NOD mice. Diabetes 1986; 35:476–499.

228. Satoh J, Shinutani S, Oya K, et al. Treatment with streptococcal preparation (OK-432) suppresses anti-islet autoimmunity and prevents diabetes in BB rats. Diabetes 1988; 37:1188–1194.

229. Weichselbaum A. Uber dei Veränderungen des Pankreas bei Diabetes Mellitus. Sitzungsber Kais Akad Wiss Wien Math Naturwiss Kl Abt 1 1910; 119:73–281.

230. Kaldany A, Hill T, Wentworth S, et al. Trapping of peripheral blood lymphocytes in the pancreas of patients with acute-onset insulin-dependent diabetes mellitus. Diabetes 1982; 31:463–466.

231. Bonnevie-Nielsen V, Steffes MW, Lernmark Å. A major loss in islet mass and B-cell function precedes hyperglycemia in mice given multiple low doses of streptozotocin. Diabetes 1981; 30:424–429.

232. Leiter EH, Beamer WG, Shultz LD. The effect of immunosuppression on streptozotocin-induced diabetes in C57BL/KsJ mice. Diabetes 1983; 32:148–155.

233. Rahier J, Goebbels RM, Henquin JC. Cellular composition of the human diabetic pancreas. Diabetologia 1983; 24:366–371.

234. Korc M, Owerback D, Quinto C, et al. Pancreatic islet–acinar cell interaction: amylase messenger RNA levels are determined by insulin. Science 1981; 213:351–353.

235. Kawai K, Orci L, Unger RH. High somatostatin uptake by the isolated perfused dog pancreas consistent with an "insuloacinar" axis. Endocrinology 1982; 110:660–662.

236. Stefan Y, Orci L, Malaisse-Lagae F, et al. Quantitation of endocrine cell content in the pancreas of nondiabetic and diabetic humans. Diabetes 1982; 31:694–700.

237. Kawate R, Yamakido M, Nishimoto Y, et al. Diabetes mellitus and its vascular complications in Japanese migrants on the island of Hawaii. Diabetes Care 1979; 2:161–170.

238. Zimmet P, Taft P, Guinea A, et al. The high prevalence of diabetes mellitus on a Central Pacific island. Diabetologia 1977; 13:111–115.

239. Genuth SM, Houser HB, Carter JR Jr, et al. Community screening for diabetes by blood glucose measurement. Results of a five year experience. Diabetes 1976; 25:1110–1117.

240. Wise PH, Edwards FM, Craig RJ, et al. Diabetes and associated variables in the south Australian aboriginal. Aust NZ J Med 1976; 6:191–196.

241. Zimmet P, Kirk R, Serjeantson S, et al. Diabetes in Pacific populations—genetic and environmental interactions. In: Melish JS, Hanna J, Baba S, eds. Genetic-Environmental Interaction in Diabetes Mellitus. Amsterdam: Excerpta Medica, 1982: 9–17.

242. Knowler WC, Bennett PH, Hamman RF, et al. Diabetes incidence and prevalence in Pima Indians: a 19-fold greater incidence than in Rochester, Minnesota. Am J Epidemiol 1978; 108:497–505.

243. Köbberling J. Studies on the genetic heterogeneity of diabetes mellitus. Diabetologia 1971; 7:46–49.

244. Köbberling J, Tillil H. Empirical risk figures for first degree relatives of non–insulin dependent diabetics. In: Köbberling J, Tattersall R, eds. The Genetics of Diabetes Mellitus. Proceedings of the Serono Symposia. Vol 47. London: Academic, 1982: 201–209.

245. Barnett AH, Spiliopoulos AJ, Pyke DA, et al. Metabolic studies in unaffected co-twins of non–insulin-dependent diabetics. Br Med J 1981; 282:1656–1658.

246. Newman B, Selby JV, King MC, et al. Concordance for type 2 (non–insulin-dependent) diabetes mellitus in male twins. Diabetologia 1987; 30:763–768.

247. Knowler WC, Savage PJ, Nagulesparan M, et al. Obesity, insulin resistance and diabetes mellitus in the Pima Indians. In: Köbberling J, Tattersall R, eds. The Genetics of Diabetes Mellitus. Proceedings of the Serono Symposia. Vol 47. London: Academic, 1982: 243–250.

248. Briggs BR, Jackson WPU, DuToit ED, et al. The histocompatibility (HLA) antigen distribution in diabetes in southern African blacks (Xhosa). Diabetes 1980; 29:68–71.

249. Owerbach D, Bell GI, Rutter WJ, et al. The insulin gene is located on the short arm of chromosome 11 in humans. Diabetes 1981; 30:267–270.

250. Owerback D, Nerup J. Restriction fragment length polymorphism of the insulin gene in diabetic individuals. Diabetologia 1981; 21:311.

251. Rotwein P, Chyn R, Chirgwin J, et al. Polymorphism in the 5'-flanking region of the human insulin gene and its possible relation to type 2 diabetes. Science 1981; 213:1117–1120.

252. Owerbach D, Nerup J. Restriction fragment length polymorphism of the insulin gene in diabetics. In: Köbberling J, Tattersall R, eds. The Genetics of Diabetes Mellitus. Proceedings of the Serono Symposia. Vol 47. London: Academic, 1982: 281–282.

253. Bell GI, Horita S, Karam JH. A polymorphic locus near the human insulin gene is associated with insulin-dependent diabetes mellitus. Diabetes 1984; 33:176–183.

254. Elbein SC, Corsetti L, Goldgar D, et al. Insulin gene in familial NIDDM. Lack of linkage in Utah Mormon pedigrees. Diabetes 1988; 37:569–576.

255. McClain DA, Henry RR, Ullrich A, et al. Restriction-fragment-length polymorphism in insulin-receptor gene and insulin resistance in NIDDM. Diabetes 1988; 37:1071–1075.

256. Arner P, Pollare T, Lithall H, et al. Defective insulin receptor tyrosine kinase in human skeletal muscle in obesity and type 2 (non–insulin-dependent) diabetes mellitus. Diabetologia 1987; 30:437–440.

257. Lillioja S, Mott DM, Zawadzki JK, et al. In vivo insulin action is familial characteristic in nondiabetic Pima Indians. Diabetes 1987; 36:1329–1335.

258. Stern MP, Ferrell RE, Rosenthal M, et al. Association between NIDDM, Rh blood group, and haptoglobin phenotype. Results from the San Antonio Heart Study. Diabetes 1986; 35:387–391.

259. Leslie RDG, Pyke DA. Chlorpropamide-alcohol flushing: a dominantly inherited trait associated with diabetes. Br Med J 1978; 2:1519–1521.

260. Pyke DA, Leslie RDG, Barnett AH, et al. Chlorpropamide alcohol flushing. In: Köbberling J, Tattersall R, eds. The Genetics of Diabetes Mellitus. Proceedings of the Serono Symposia. Vol 47. London: Academic, 1982: 271–279.

261. Barnett AH, Spiliopoulos AJ, Pyke DA. Blockade of chlorpropamide-alcohol flushing by indomethacin suggests an association between prostaglandins and diabetic vascular complications. Lancet 1980; 2:164–166.

262. Strakosch CR, Jeffreys DB, Keen H. Blockade of chlorpropamide alcohol flush by aspirin. Lancet 1980; 1:394–396.

263. Jerntorp P, Öhlin H, Bergström B, et al. Elevation of plasma acetaldehyde—the first metabolic step in CPAF? Diabetologia 1980; 19:286.

264. Barnett AH, Gonzalez-Auvert C, Pyke DA, et al. Blood concentrations of acetaldehyde during chlorpropamide-alcohol flush. Br Med J 1981; 293:939–941.

265. Podgainy H, Bressler R. Biochemical basis of the sulfonylurea-induced Antabuse syndrome. Diabetes 1968; 17:679–682.

266. Köbberling J, Weber M. Facial flush after chlorpropamide-alcohol and enkephalin. Lancet 1980; 1:538–539.

267. Köbberling J, Bengsch N, Brüggeboes B, et al. The chlorpropamide alcohol flush. Lack of specificity for familial non–insulin dependent diabetes. Diabetologia 1980; 29:359–363.

268. Fui SNT, Keen H, Jarrett J, et al. Test for chlorpropamide-alcohol flush becomes positive after prolonged chlorpropamide treatment in insulin-dependent and non–insulin-dependent diabetics. N Engl J Med 1983; 309:93–96.

269. Tattersall R. Diabetes in the offspring of conjugal diabetic parents. In: Creutzfeldt W, Köbberling J, Neel JV, eds. The Genetics of Diabetes Mellitus. New York: Springer-Verlag, 1976: 188–193.

270. Goto Y, Kakizaki M, Toyota T. Heredity of diabetes mellitus. In: Melish JS, Hanna J, Baba S, eds. Genetic-Environmental Interaction in Diabetes Mellitus. Amsterdam: Excerpta Medica, 1982: 18–29.

271. Tattersall RB, Fajans SS. A difference between the inheritance of classical juvenile-onset and maturity-onset type diabetes of young people. Diabetes 1975; 24:44–53.

272. Tattersall RB. Mild familial diabetes with dominant inheritance. Q J Med 1974; 43:339–357.

273. Fajans SS. Heterogeneity between various families with non–insulin-dependent-diabetes of the MODY type. In: Köbberling J, Tattersall R, eds. The Genetics of Diabetes Mellitus. Proceedings of the Serono Symposia. Vol 47. London: Academic, 1982: 47:251–260.

274. Barbosa J, King R, Goetz FC, et al. HLA in maturity-onset type of hyperglycemia in the young. Arch Intern Med 1978; 138:90–93.

275. Owerbach D, Thomsen B, Johansen K, et al. DNA insertion sequences near the insulin gene are not associated with maturity-onset diabetes of young people. Diabetologia 1983; 25:18–20.

276. Raskin P, Aydin I, Unger RH. Effect of insulin on the exaggerated glucagon response to arginine stimulation in diabetes mellitus. Diabetes 1976; 25:227–229.

277. Raskin P, Aydin I, Yamamoto T, et al. Abnormal alpha cell function in human diabetes. The response to oral protein. Am J Med 1978; 64:988–997.

278. Kawamori R, Shichiri M, Kikuchi M, et al. Perfect normalization of excessive glucagon responses to intravenous arginine in human diabetes mellitus with the artificial beta-cell. Diabetes 1980; 29:762–765.

279. Groop L, Miettinen A, Groop PH, et al. Organ-specific autoimmunity and HLA-DR antigens as markers for beta-cell destruction in patients with type II diabetes. Diabetes 1988; 37:99–103.

280. Zimmet P. Type 2 (non–insulin-dependent) diabetes—an epidemiological overview. Diabetologia 1982; 22:399–411.

281. DeFronzo RA, Ferrannini E. The pathogenesis of non–insulin-dependent diabetes. An update. Medicine 1982; 61:125–140.

282. Bagdade JD, Bierman EL, Porte D Jr. The significance of basal insulin levels in the evaluation of the insulin response to glucose in diabetic and nondiabetic subjects. J Clin Invest 1967; 46:1549–1557.

283. Beard JC, Ward WK, Halter JB, et al. Relationship of islet function to insulin action in human obesity. J Clin Endocrinol Metab 1987; 65:59–64.

284. Knowler WC, Pettitt DJ, Savage PJ, et al. Diabetes incidence in Pima Indians: contributions of obesity and parental diabetes. Am J Epidemiol 1981; 113:144–156.

285. Neel JV. Diabetes mellitus: a "thrifty" genotype rendered detrimental by "progress"? Am J Hum Genet 1962; 14:353–362.

286. Neel JV. The thrifty genotype revisited. In: Köbberling J, Tattersall R, eds. The Genetics of Diabetes Mellitus. Proceedings of the Serono Symposia. Vol 47. London: Academic, 1982: 283–293.

287. Maclean N, Ogilvie RF. Observation on the pancreatic islet tissue of young diabetic subjects. Diabetes 1959; 8:83–91.

288. Clark A, Cooper CJ, Lewis CE, et al. Islet amyloid formed from diabetes-associated peptide may be pathogenic in type-2 diabetes. Lancet 1987; 2:231–234.

289. Sanke T, Bell GI, Sample C, et al. An islet amyloid peptide is derived from an 89-amino acid precursor by proteolytic processing. J Biol Chem 1988; 263:17243–17246.

290. Westermark P, Wilander E, Westermark GT, et al. Islet amyloid poly-peptide-like immunoreactivity in the islet B cells of type 2 (non–insulin-dependent) diabetic and non-diabetic individuals. Diabetologia 1987; 30:887–892.

291. Leffert JD, Newgard CB, Okamoto H, et al. Rat amylin: cloning and tissue-specific expression in pancreatic islets. Proc Natl Acad Sci USA 1989; 86:3127–3130.

292. Johnson KH, O'Brien TD, Hayden DW, et al. Immunolocalization of islet amyloid polypeptide (IAPP) in pancreatic beta cells by means of peroxidase-antiperoxidase (PAP) and protein A–gold techniques. Am J Pathol 1988; 130:1–8.

292a. Ogawa A, Harris V, McCorkle SK, et al. Amylin secretion from the rat pancreas and its selective loss after streptozotocin treatment. J Clin Invest 1990; 85:973–976.

293. Leighton B, Cooper GJS. Pancreatic amylin and calcitonin gene–related peptide cause resistance to insulin in skeletal muscle in vitro. Nature 1988; 335:632–635.

294. Raskin P, Fujita Y, Unger RH. Effect of insulin-glucose infusions on plasma glucagon levels in fasting diabetics and nondiabetics. J Clin Invest 1975; 56:1132–1138.

295. Samols E, Marri G, Marks V. Promotion of insulin secretion by glucagon. Lancet 1965; 2:415–416.

296. Kawai K, Ipp E, Orci L, et al. Circulating somatostatin acts on the islets of Langerhans by way of a somatostatin-poor compartment. Science 1982; 218:477–478.

297. Samols E, Harrison J. Remarkable potency of somatostatin as a glucagon suppressant. Metabolism 1976; 25(Suppl 1):1495–1497.

298. Zyznar ES, Pietri AO, Harris V, et al. Evidence for the hormonal status of somatostatin in man. Diabetes 1981; 30:883–886.

299. Orci L, Unger RH. Functional subdivision of islet of Langerhans and possible role of D cells. Lancet 1975; 2:1243–1244.

300. Unger RH, Orci L. Hypothesis: possible roles of the pancreatic D-cell in the normal and diabetic states. Diabetes 1977; 26:241–244.

301. Orci L, Malaisse-Lagae F, Ravazzola M, et al. A morphological basis for intercellular communication between α- and β-cells in the endocrine pancreas. J Clin Invest 1975; 56:1066–1070.

302. Meda P, Kohen E, Kohen C, et al. Direct communication of homologous and heterologous endocrine islet cells in culture. J Cell Biol 1982; 92:221–226.

303. Bonner-Weir S, Orci L. New perspectives on the microvasculature of the islets of Langerhans in the rat. Diabetes 1982; 31:883–889.

304. Samols E, Weir GC, Bonner-Weir S. Intraislet insulin-glucagon-soma-tostatin relationships. In: Lefebvre PJ, ed. Glucagon II. Berlin: Springer-Verlag, 1983: 133–173.

305. Maruyama H, Hisatomi A, Orci L, et al. Insulin within islets is a physiologic glucagon release inhibitor. J Clin Invest 1984; 74:2296–2299.

306. Unger RH. The milieu intérieur and the islets of Langerhans. Diabetologia 1981; 20:1–11.

307. Kemmer FW, Vranic M. The role of glucagon and its relationship to other glucoregulatory hormones in exercise. In: Unger RH, Orci L, eds. Glucagon. Physiology, Pathophysiology, and Morphology of the Pancreatic A-Cells. New York: Elsevier, 1981: 297–331.

308. Aguilar-Parada E, Eisenтraut AM, Unger RH. Effects of starvation on plasma pancreatic glucagon in normal man. Diabetes 1969; 18:717–723.

309. Owen OE, Morgan AP, Kemp HG, et al. Brain metabolism during fasting. J Clin Invest 1967; 46:1589–1595.

310. Cahill GF, Herrera MG, Morgan AP, et al. Hormone-fuel interrelationships during fasting. J Clin Invest 1966; 45:1751–1769.

311. Müller WA, Faloona GR, Aguilar-Parada E, et al. Abnormal alpha-cell function in diabetes. Response to carbohydrate and protein ingestion. N Engl J Med 1970; 283:109–115.

312. Fischer U, Hommel H, Ziegler M, et al. The mechanism of insulin secretion after oral glucose administration. I. Multiphasic course of insulin mobilization after oral administration of glucose in conscious dogs. Differences to the behavior after intravenous administration. Diabetologia 1972; 8:104–110.

313. Unger RH, Ketterer H, Dupré J, et al. The effects of secretin, pancreozymin, and gastrin on insulin and glucagon secretion in anesthetized dogs. J Clin Invest 1967; 46:630–645.

314. Bloom SR, Vaughan NJA, Russell RCG. Vagal control of glucagon release in man. Lancet 1974; 2:546–549.

315. Unger RH, Eisenтraut AM. Entero-insular axis. Arch Intern Med 1969; 48:810–822.

316. Unger RH, Ohneda A, Aguilar-Parada E, et al. The role of aminogenic glucagon secretion in blood glucose homeostasis. J Clin Invest 1969; 48:810–822.

317. Unger RH, Aguilar-Parada E, Müller WA, et al. Studies of pancreatic alpha cell function in normal and diabetic subjects. J Clin Invest 1970; 49:837–848.

318. Unger RH, Madison LL, Müller WA. Abnormal alpha cell function in diabetics. Response to insulin. Diabetes 1972; 21:301–307.

319. Buchanan KD, McCarroll AM. Abnormalities of glucagon metabolism in untreated diabetes mellitus. Lancet 1972; 2:1394–1395.

320. Gerich JE, Langlois M, Noacco C, et al. Lack of glucagon response to hypoglycemia in diabetes: evidence for an intrinsic pancreatic alpha cell defect. Science 1973; 182:171–173.

321. Bolli G, DeFeo P, Compagnucci P, et al. Abnormal glucose counter-regulation in insulin-dependent diabetes mellitus. Interaction of anti-insulin antibodies and impaired glucagon and epinephrine secretion. Diabetes 1983; 32:134–141.

322. Raskin P, Pietri A, Unger RH. Changes in glucagon levels after four to five weeks of glucoregulation by portable insulin infusion pumps. Diabetes 1979; 28:1033–1035.

323. Starke A, Imamura T, Unger RH: Relationship of glucagon suppression by insulin and somatostatin to the ambient glucose concentration. Implications for the etiology of diabetic hyperglucagonemia. J Clin Invest 1987; 79:20–24.

324. Chen L, Komiya I, Inman L, et al. Molecular and cellular responses of islets during perturbations of glucose homeostasis determined by in situ hybridization histochemistry. Proc Natl Acad Sci USA 1989; 86:1367–1371.

325. Dobbs R, Sakurai H, Sasaki H, et al. Glucagon: role in the hyperglycemia of diabetes mellitus. Science 1975; 187:544–547.

326. Wahren J, Felig P, Cerasi E, et al. Splanchnic and peripheral glucose and amino acid metabolism in diabetes mellitus. J Clin Invest 1972; 51:1870–1878.

327. Owen OE, Reichle FA, Mozzoli MA, et al. Hepatic, gut, and renal substrate flux rates in patients with hepatic cirrhosis. J Clin Invest 1981; 68:240–252.

328. Liljenquist JE, Mueller GL, Cherrington AD, et al. Evidence for an important role of glucagon in the regulation of hepatic glucose production in normal man. J Clin Invest 1977; 59:369–374.

329. Unger RH, Orci L. Glucagon and the A cell. Physiology and pathophysiology. N Engl J Med 1981; 304:1518–1524, 1575–1580.

330. Koerker DJ, Ruch W, Chideckel E, et al. Somatostatin: hypothalamic inhibitor of the endocrine pancreas. Science 1974; 184:482–484.

331. Sakurai H, Dobbs R, Unger RH. Somatostatin-induced changes in insulin and glucagon secretion in normal and diabetic dogs. J Clin Invest 1974; 54:1395–1402.

332. Vidnes J, Oyasaeter S. Glucagon deficiency causing severe neonatal hypoglycemia in a patient with normal insulin secretion. Pediatr Res 1977; 11:943–949.

333. Gerich JE, Lorenzi M, Bier DM, et al. Prevention of human diabetic ketoacidosis by somatostatin: evidence for an essential role of glucagon. N Engl J Med 1975; 292:985–989.

334. Scheen AJ, Krzentowski G, Castillo M, et al. A 6-hour nocturnal interruption of a continuous subcutaneous insulin infusion. 2. Marked attenuation of the metabolic deterioration by somatostatin. Diabetologia 1983; 24:319–325.

335. Raskin P, Unger RH. Hyperglucagonemia and its suppression: importance in the metabolic control of diabetes. N Engl J Med 1978; 299:433–436.

336. Unger RH. Somatostatinoma. N Engl J Med 1977; 296:998–1000.

337. Nakabayashi H, Dobbs RE, Unger RH. The role of glucagon deficiency in the Houssay phenomenon of dogs. J Clin Invest 1978; 61:1355–1362.

338. Santeusanio F, Massi-Benedetti M, Angeletti G, et al. Glucagon and carbohydrate disorder in a totally pancreatectomized man (a study with the aid of an artificial endocrine pancreas). J Endocrinol Invest 1981; 4:93–96.

339. Johnson DG, Goebel CU, Hruby VJ, et al. Hyperglycemia of diabetic rat decreased by a glucagon receptor antagonist. Science 1982; 215:1115–1116.

340. Boden G, Master RW, Rezvani I, et al. Glucagon deficiency and hyper-aminoacidemia after total pancreatectomy. J Clin Invest 1980; 65:706–716.

341. Barnes AJ, Bloom SR. Pancreatectomised man: a model for diabetes without glucagon. Lancet 1976; 1:219–221.

342. Holst JJ, Pedersen JH, Baldissera F, et al. Circulating glucagon after total pancreatectomy in man. Diabetologia 1983; 25:396–399.

343. Richards CS, Furuya E, Uyeda K. Regulation of fructose-2,6-P_2 concentration in isolated hepatocytes. Biochem Biophys Res Commun 1981; 100:1673–1679.

344. Boyd ME, Albright EB, Foster DW, et al. In vitro reversal of the fasting state of liver metabolism in the rat. J Clin Invest 1981; 68:142–152.

345. Perley J, Kipnis DM. Plasma insulin responses to oral and intravenous glucose: studies in normal and diabetic subjects. J Clin Invest 1967; 46:1954–1962.

346. Seltzer HS, Allen EW, Herron AL Jr, et al. Insulin secretion in response to glycemic stimulus: relation of delayed initial release to carbohydrate intolerance in mild diabetes mellitus. J Clin Invest 1967; 46:323–335.

347. Brunzell JD, Robertson RP, Lerner RL, et al. Relationships between

fasting plasma glucose levels and insulin secretion during intravenous glucose tolerance tests. J Clin Endocrinol Metab 1976; 42:222–229.

348. Pfeifer MA, Halter JB, Porte D Jr. Insulin secretion in diabetes mellitus. Am J Med 1981; 70:579–588.

348a. Johnson JH, Ogawa A, Chen L, et al. Underexpression of β cell high Km glucose transporters in noninsulin-dependent diabetes. Science 1990; 250:546–549.

349. Polonsky KS, Given BD, Hirsch LJ, et al. Abnormal patterns of insulin secretion in non–insulin-dependent diabetes mellitus. N Engl J Med 1988; 318:1231–1239.

350. O'Rahilly S, Turner RC, Matthews DR. Impaired pulsatile secretion of insulin in relatives of patients with non–insulin-dependent diabetes. N Engl J Med 1988; 318:1225–1230.

351. Reaven GM, Chen YD, Golay A, et al. Documentation of hyperglucagonemia throughout the day in nonobese and obese patients with noninsulin-dependent diabetes mellitus. J Clin Endocrinol Metab 1987; 64:106–110.

352. Hatfield HH, Banasiak MF, Driscoll T, et al. Glucose suppression of glucagon: relationship to pancreatic beta cell function. J Clin Endocrinol Metab 1977; 44:1080–1087.

353. Aydin I, Raskin P, Unger RH. The effect of short-term intravenous insulin administration on the glucagon response to a carbohydrate meal in adult onset and juvenile type diabetes. Diabetologia 1977; 13:629–636.

354. Barron AD, Schaeffer LD, Shragg P, et al. Role of hyperglucagonemia in maintenance of increased rates of hepatic glucose output in type II diabetes. Diabetes 1987; 36:274–283.

355. Stevenson RW, Williams PE, Cherrington AD. Role of glucagon suppression on gluconeogenesis during insulin treatment of the conscious dog. Diabetologia 1987; 30:782–790.

356. Yen TT, Stamm NB, Fuller RW, et al. Hepatic insensitivity to glucagon in ob/ob mice. Res Commun Chem Pathol Pharmacol 1980; 30:29–40.

357. Olefsky JM, Kolterman OG. Mechanisms of insulin resistance in obesity and noninsulin dependent (type II) diabetes. Am J Med 1981; 70:151–168.

358. Reaven GM, Sageman WS, Swenson RS. Development of insulin resistance in normal dogs following alloxan-induced insulin deficiency. Diabetologia 1977; 13:459–462.

359. DeFronzo RA, Hendler R, Simonson D. Insulin resistance is a prominent feature of insulin-dependent diabetes. Diabetes 1982; 31:795–801.

360. Bonora E, Coscelli C, Butturini U. Residual B cell function and insulin sensitivity in type I (insulin-dependent) diabetes mellitus. Diabetologia 1983; 25:298.

361. Andrews WJ, Vasquez B, Nagulesparan M, et al. Insulin therapy in obese noninsulin-dependent diabetes induces improvements in insulin action and secretion which are maintained for two weeks after insulin withdrawal. Diabetes 1984; 33:634–642.

362. Scarlett JA, Gray RS, Griffin J, et al. Insulin treatment reverses the insulin resistance of type II diabetes mellitus. Diabetes Care 1982; 5:353–363.

363. Bar RS, Gordon P, Roth J, et al. Fluctuations in the affinity and concentration of insulin receptors on circulating monocytes of obese patients: effects of starvation, refeeding and dieting. J Clin Invest 1976; 58:1123–1135.

364. Gambhir KK, Archer JA, Bradley CJ. Characteristics of human erythrocyte insulin receptors. Diabetes 1978; 27:701–708.

365. Olefsky JM. Decreased insulin binding to adipocytes and circulating monocytes from obese subjects. J Clin Invest 1976; 57:1165–1172.

366. Olefsky JM. Insulin resistance and insulin action. An in vitro and in vivo perspective. Diabetes 1981; 30:148–162.

367. Kahn CR, White MF. The insulin receptor and molecular mechanism of insulin action. J Clin Invest 1988; 82:1151–1156.

368. Savage PJ, Bennion LJ, Flock EV, et al. Diet-induced improvement of abnormalities in insulin and glucagon secretion and in insulin receptor binding in diabetes mellitus. J Clin Endocrinol Metab 1979; 48:999–1007.

369. Kosaka K, Kuzuya T, Akanuma Y, et al. Increase in insulin response after treatment of overt maturity-onset diabetes is independent of the mode of treatment. Diabetologia 1980; 18:23–28.

370. Hidaka H, Nagulesparan M, Klimes I, et al. Improvement of insulin secretion but not insulin resistance after short term control of plasma glucose in obese type II diabetics. J Clin Endocrinol Metab 1982; 54:217–222.

371. Vague P, Moulin J-P. The defective glucose sensitivity of the B cell in non insulin dependent diabetes. Improvement after twenty hours of normoglycaemia. Metabolism 1982; 31:139–142.

372. Bonner-Weir S, Trent DF, Weir GC. Partial pancreatectomy in the rat and subsequent defect in glucose-induced insulin release. J Clin Invest 1983; 71:1544–1553.

373. Weir GC. Non–insulin-dependent diabetes mellitus: interplay between B-cell inadequacy and insulin resistance. Am J Med 1982; 73:461–464.

374. Lillioja S, Mott DM, Howard BV, et al. Impaired glucose tolerance as a disorder of insulin action. N Engl J Med 1988; 318:1217–1225.

375. Unger RH. Glucagon and the insulin:glucagon ratio in diabetes and other catabolic illnesses. Diabetes 1971; 20:834–838.

376. Waldhausl W, Kleinberger G, Korn A, et al. Severe hyperglycemia: effects of rehydration on endocrine derangements and blood glucose concentrations. Diabetes 1979; 28:577–584.

377. Shamoon H, Hendler R, Sherwin RS. Altered responsiveness to cortisol, epinephrine, and glucagon in insulin-infused juvenile-onset diabetics. Diabetes 1980; 29:284–291.

378. Rocha DM, Santeusanio F, Faloona GR, et al. Abnormal pancreatic alpha-cell function in bacterial infections. N Engl J Med 1973; 288:700–703.

379. Willerson JT, Hutcheson DR, Leshin SJ, et al. Serum glucagon and insulin levels and their relationship to blood glucose values in patients with acute myocardial infarction and acute coronary insufficiency. Am J Med 1974; 57:747–753.

380. Lindsey CA, Faloona GR, Unger RH. Glucagon and the insulin:glucagon ratio in severe trauma. Trans Assoc Am Physicians 1973; 86:264–271.

381. Wilmore DW, Moylan JA, Pruitt BA, et al. Hyperglucagonaemia after burns. Lancet 1974; 1:73–75.

382. Müller WA, Faloona GR, Unger RH. Hyperglucagonemia in diabetic ketoacidosis: its prevalence and significance. Am J Med 1973; 54:52–57.

383. Diebert DC, DeFronzo RA. Epinephrine-induced insulin resistance in man. J Clin Invest 1980; 65:717–721.

384. Kahn CR. The insulin receptor and insulin: the lock and key to diabetes. Clin Res 1983; 31:326–335.

385. Rosen O. After insulin binds. Science 1987; 237:1452–1458.

385a. Bell GI, Kayano T, Buse JB, et al. Molecular biology of mammalian glucose transporters. Diabetes Care 1990; 13:198–208.

386. Kasuga M, Zick Y, Blithe DL, et al. Insulin stimulates tyrosine phosphorylation of the insulin receptor in a cell-free system. Nature 1982; 298:667–669.

387. Gabbay RA, Lardy HA. Site of insulin inhibition of cAMP-stimulated glycogenolysis. cAMP-dependent protein kinase is affected independent of cAMP changes. J Biol Chem 1984; 259:6052–6055.

388. Rodbell M. The actions of glucagon at its receptor: regulation of adenylate cyclase. In: Lefebvre PJ, ed. Glucagon I. Berlin: Springer-Verlag, 1983: 263–290.

389. Northrup JK, Sternweis PC, Gilman AG. The subunits of the stimulatory regulatory component of adenylate cyclase. Resolution, activity, and properties of the 35,000-dalton (β) subunit. J Biol Chem 1983; 258:11361–11368.

390. Gilman AG. Guanine nucleotide–binding regulatory proteins and dual control of adenylate cyclase. J Clin Invest 1984; 73:1–4.

391. Exton JH. Mechanisms of hormonal regulation of hepatic glucose metabolism. Diabetes Metab Rev 1987; 3:163–183.

392. Foster DW, McGarry JD. The metabolic derangements and treatment of diabetic ketoacidosis. N Engl J Med 1983; 309:159–169.

393. Furuya E, Uyeda K. A novel enzyme catalyzes the synthesis of activation factor from ATP and D-fructose-6-P. J Biol Chem 1981; 256:7109–7112.

394. Van Schaftingen E, Davies DR, Hers HG. Inactivation of phosphofructokinase 2 by cyclic AMP–dependent protein kinase. Biochem Biophys Res Commun 1981; 103:362–368.

395. El-Maghrabi MR, Claus TH, Pilkis J, et al. Regulation of rat liver fructose 2,6-bisphosphatase. J Biol Chem 1982; 257:7603–7607.

396. Hers H-G, Van Schaftingen E. Fructose-2,6-bisphosphate two years after its discovery. Biochem J 1982; 206:1–12.

397. El-Maghrabi MR, Fox E, Pilkis J, et al. Cyclic AMP dependent phosphorylation of rat liver 6-phosphofructo 2-kinase/fructose 2,6-bisphosphatase. Biochem Biophys Res Commun 1982; 106:794–802.

398. Richards CS, Uyeda K. The effect of insulin and glucose on fructose-2,6-P_2 in hepatocytes. Biochem Biophys Res Commun 1982; 109:394–401.

399. Newgard CB, Moore SV, Foster DW, et al. Efficient hepatic glycogen synthesis in refeeding rats requires continued carbon flow through the gluconeogenic pathway. J Biol Chem 1984; 259:6958–6963.

400. Spence JT. Levels of translatable mRNA coding for rat liver glucokinase. J Biol Chem 1983; 258:9143–9146.

401. Veneziale CM, Donofrio JC, Nishimura H. The concentration of P-enolpyruvate carboxykinase protein in murine tissues in diabetes of chemical and genetic origin. J Biol Chem 1983; 258:14257–14262.

402. McGarry JD, Foster DW. Hormonal control of ketogenesis. Adv Exp Med Biol 1979; 111:79–96.

403. McGarry JD, Takabayashi Y, Foster DW. The role of malonyl-CoA in the coordination of fatty acid synthesis and oxidation in isolated rat hepatocytes. J Biol Chem 1978; 253:8294–8300.

404. Cook GA, Nielsen RC, Hawkins RA, et al. Effect of glucagon on hepatic malonyl coenzyme A concentration and on lipid synthesis. J Biol Chem 1977; 252:4421–4424.

405. Lent BA, Lee K-H, Kim K-H. Regulation of rat liver acetyl-CoA carboxylase. Stimulation of phosphorylation and subsequent inactivation of liver acetyl-CoA carboxylase by cyclic 3':5'-monophosphate and effect on the structure of the enzyme. J Biol Chem 1978; 253:8149–8156.

406. McGarry JD, Leatherman GF, Foster DW. Carnitine palmitoyltransferase I: The site of inhibition of hepatic fatty acid oxidation by malonyl-CoA. J Biol Chem 1978; 253:4128–4136.

407. McGarry JD, Foster DW. Regulation of hepatic fatty acid oxidation and ketone body production. Annu Rev Biochem 1980; 49:385–420.

408. McGarry JD, Robles-Valdes C, Foster DW. Role of carnitine in hepatic ketogenesis. Proc Natl Acad Sci USA 1975; 72:4385–4388.

409. McGarry JD, Mills SE, Long CS, et al. Observations on the affinity for carnitine, and malonyl-CoA sensitivity of carnitine palmitoyltransferase I in animal and human tissues. Demonstration of the presence of malonyl-CoA in non-hepatic tissues of the rat. Biochem J 1983; 214:21–28.

410. Fulop M, Rosenblatt A, Kreitzer SM, et al. Hyperosmolar nature of diabetic coma. Diabetes 1975; 24:549–599.

411. Verdon F, van Mele G, Perret C. Respiratory response to acute metabolic acidosis. Bull Eur Physiopathol Respir 1981; 17:223–235.

412. Møller-Petersen J, Andersen PT, Hjørne N, et al. Nontraumatic rhabdomyolysis during diabetic ketoacidosis. Diabetologia 1986; 29:228–234.

413. Chernow B, Finton C, Rainey TG, et al. "Bovine ketosis" in a nondiabetic postpartum woman. Diabetes Care 1982; 5:47–49.

414. Levy LJ, Duga J, Girgis M, et al. Ketoacidosis associated with alcoholism in nondiabetic subjects. Ann Intern Med 1973; 78:213–219.

415. Gerich JE, Martin MM, Recant L. Clinical and metabolic characteristics of hyperosmolar nonketotic coma. Diabetes 1971; 20:228–238.

416. Arieff AI, Carroll HJ. Nonketotic hyperosmolar coma with hyperglycemia: clinical features, pathophysiology, renal function, acid-base balance, plasma–cerebrospinal fluid equilibria and the effects of therapy in 37 cases. Medicine 1972; 51:73–94.

417. Carroll P, Matz R. Uncontrolled diabetes mellitus in adults: experience in treating diabetic ketoacidosis and hyperosmolar nonketotic coma with low-dose insulin and uniform treatment regimen. Diabetes Care 1983; 6:579–585.

418. Gerich J, Penhos JC, Gutman RA, et al. Effect of dehydration and hyperosmolarity on glucose, free fatty acid and ketone body metabolism in the rat. Diabetes 1973; 22:264–271.

419. Beigelman PM. Severe diabetic ketoacidosis (diabetic "coma"). 482 episodes in 257 patients; experience of three years. Diabetes 1971; 20:490–500.

420. Vinik AI, Joffe BI, Joubert SM. Metabolic findings in a patient with hyperosmolar non-ketoacidotic diabetic stupor. Br Med J 1970; 4:155–156.

421. Lindsey CA, Faloona GR, Unger RH. Plasma glucagon in nonketotic hyperosmolar coma. JAMA 1974; 229:1771–1773.

422. Matz R. Coma in the nonketotic diabetic [hyperosmolar nonketotic coma (HNKC) in the diabetic]. In: Ellenberg M, Rifkin H, eds. Diabetes Mellitus. Theory and Practice. New York: Medical Examination Publishing, 1983: 655–666.

423. Guisado R, Arieff AI. Neurologic manifestations of diabetic comas: correlation with biochemical alterations in the brain. Metabolism 1975; 24:665–679.

424. Knowles HC Jr. Syrupy blood. Diabetes 1966; 15:760–761.

425. Curtis J, Horrigan F, Ahearn D, et al. Chlorthalidone-induced hyperosmolar hyperglycemic nonketotic coma. JAMA 1972; 220:1592–1593.

426. Pomare EW. Hyperosmolar non-ketotic diabetes and cimetidine. Lancet 1978; 1:1202.

427. Lavender S, McGill RJ. Nonketotic hyperosmolar coma and furosemide therapy. Diabetes 1974; 23:247–248.

428. Borch-Johnsen K, Kreiner S, Deckert T. Mortality of type I (insulin-dependent) diabetes mellitus in Denmark: a study of relative mortality in 2930 Danish type I diabetic patients diagnosed from 1933 to 1972. Diabetologia 1986; 29:767–772.

429. Siperstein MD. Diabetic microangiopathy, genetics, environment and treatment. Am J Med 1988; 85(Suppl 5A):119–130.

430. Strauss FG, Argy WP Jr, Schreiner GE. Diabetic glomerulosclerosis in the absence of glucose intolerance. Ann Intern Med 1971; 75:239–242.

431. Soler NG, FitzGerald MG, Malins JM, et al. Retinopathy at diagnosis of diabetes, with special reference to patients under 40 years of age. Br Med J 1969; 3:567–569.

432. Hutton WL, Snyder WB, Vaiser A, et al. Retinal microangiopathy without associated glucose intolerance. Trans Am Acad Ophthalmol Otolaryngol 1972; 76:968–978.

433. Marks JF, Raskin P, Stastny P. Increase in capillary basement membrane width in parents of children with type I diabetes mellitus. Association with HLA-DR4. Diabetes 1981; 30:475–480.

434. Ellis EN, Mauer SM, Goetz FC, et al. Relationship of muscle capillary basement membrane to renal structure and function in diabetes mellitus. Diabetes 1986; 35:421–425.

435. Feldt-Rasmussen B, Mathiesen ER, Hegedüs L, et al. Kidney function during 12 months of strict control in insulin-dependent diabetic patients with incipient nephropathy. N Engl J Med 1986; 314:665–670.

436. Kamenetzky SA, Bennett PH, Dippe SE, et al. A clinical and histologic study of diabetic nephropathy in the Pima Indians. Diabetes 1974; 23:61–68.

437. Jarrett RJ, Keen H. Hyperglycaemia and diabetes mellitus. Lancet 1976; 2:1009–1012.

438. Katsilambros N. Diabetic retinopathy and blood sugar. Lancet 1976; 2:1253.

439. O'Sullivan JB, Cosgrove J, McCaughan D. Blood sugars, vascular abnormalities and survival. The Oxford study after 17 years. Postgrad Med J 1968; 44(Suppl):955–959.

440. Osterby R. Early phases in the development of diabetic glomerulopathy. Acta Med Scand 1974; Suppl 574:3–82.

441. Osterby R, Gundersen HJG. Glomerular size and structure in diabetes mellitus. I. Early abnormalities. Diabetologia 1975; 11:225–229.

442. Mauer SM, Miller K, Goetz FC, et al. Immunopathology of renal extracellular membranes in kidneys transplanted into patients with diabetes mellitus. Diabetes 1976; 25:709–712.

443. Gliedman ML, Tellis VA, Soberman R, et al. Long-term effects of pancreatic transplant function in patients with advanced juvenile-onset diabetes. Diabetes Care 1978; 1:1–9.

444. Bohmann SO, Tydén G, Wilcek H, et al. Prevention of kidney graft diabetic nephropathy by pancreas transplantation in man. Diabetes 1985; 34:306–308.

445. Abouna GM, Kremer GD, Daddah SK, et al. Reversal of diabetic nephropathy in human cadaveric kidneys after transplantation into nondiabetic recipients. Lancet 1983; 2:1274–1276.

446. Ramsay RC, Goetz FC, Sutherland DER, et al. Progression of diabetic retinopathy after pancreas transplantation for insulin-dependent diabetes mellitus. N Engl J Med 1988; 318:208–214.

447. Johnsson S. Retinopathy and nephropathy in diabetes mellitus: comparison of the effects of two forms of treatment. Diabetes 1960; 9:1–8.

448. Pirart J. Diabetes mellitus and its degenerative complications: a prospective study of 4400 patients observed between 1947 and 1973. Diabetes Care 1978; 1:168–188, 252–263.

449. Job D, Eschwege E, Guyot-Argenton C, et al. Effect of multiple daily insulin injections on the course of diabetic retinopathy. Diabetes 1976; 25:463–469.

450. Eschwege E, Job D, Guyot-Argenton C, et al. Delayed progression of diabetic retinopathy by divided insulin administration: a further follow-up. Diabetologia 1979; 16:131–135.

451. Lauritzen T, Frost-Larsen K, Larsen H-W, et al. The effect of near-normal blood glucose levels upon retinopathy: two-year follow-up. Diabetologia 1983; 25:174 (abstract).

452. Lauritzen T, Frost-Larsen K, Larsen HW, et al. Two-year experience with continuous subcutaneous insulin infusion in relation to retinopathy and neuropathy. Diabetes 1985; 34(Suppl 3):74–79.

453. Tamborlane WV, Pulkin JE, Bergman M, et al. Long-term improvement of metabolic control with the insulin pump does not reverse diabetic microangiopathy. Diabetes Care 1982; 5(Suppl 1):58–64.

454. Holman RR, Mayon-White V, Orde-Peackar C, et al. Prevention of deterioration of renal and sensory-nerve function by more intensive management of insulin-dependent diabetic patients. A two-year randomised prospective study. Lancet 1983; 1:204–208.

455. Drash AL, Daneman D, Travis L. Progressive retinopathy with improved metabolic control in diabetic dwarfism (Mauriac's syndrome). Diabetes 1980; 29(Suppl 2):1A.

456. Pietri A, Ehle AL, Raskin P. Changes in nerve conduction velocity after six weeks of glucoregulation with portable insulin infusion pumps. Diabetes 1980; 29:668–671.

457. Rosenstock J, Raskin P. Diabetes and its complications: blood glucose control vs. genetic susceptibility. Diabetes Metab Rev 1988; 4:417–435.

458. Kofoed-Enevoldsen A, Borch-Johnsen K, Kreiner S, et al. Declining incidence of persistent proteinuria in type I (insulin-dependent) diabetic patients in Denmark. Diabetes 1987; 36:205–209.

459. Uy R, Wold EF. Posttranslational covalent modification of proteins. Only 20 amino acids are used in protein synthesis, yet some 140 "amino acids" are found in various proteins. Science 1977; 198:890–896.

460. Bunn HF. Evaluation of glycosylated hemoglobin in diabetic patients. Diabetes 1981; 30:613–617.

461. Higgins PJ, Bunn HF. Kinetic analysis of the nonenzymatic glycosylation of hemoglobin. J Biol Chem 1981; 256:5204–5208.

462. Dolhofer R, Wieland OH. Glycosylation of serum albumin: elevated glycosyl albumin in diabetic patients. FEBS Lett 1979; 103:282–286.

463. Dolhofer R, Renner R, Wieland OH. Different behaviour of haemoglobin A_{1a-c} and glycosyl-albumin levels during recovery from diabetic ketoacidosis and non-acidotic coma. Diabetologia 1981; 21:211–215.

464. Higgins PJ, Garlick RL, Bunn HF. Glycosylated hemoglobin in human and animal red cells. Role of glucose permeability. Diabetes 1982; 31:743–748.

465. Vogt BW, Schleicher ED, Wieland OH. ε-Amino-lysine–bound glucose in human tissues obtained at autopsy. Increase in diabetes mellitus. Diabetes 1982; 31:1123–1127.

466. Monnier VM, Vishwanath V, Frank KE, et al. Relation between complications of type I diabetes mellitus and collagen-linked fluorescence. N Engl J Med 1986; 314:403–408.

467. Horinchi S, Shiga M, Arakie N, et al. Evidence against in vivo presence of (2-furoyl)-4(5)-(2-furanyl)-1H-imidazole, a major fluorescent advanced end product generated by nonenzymatic glycosylation. J Biol Chem 1988; 263:18821–18826.

468. Miller JA, Gravallese E, Bunn HF. Nonenzymatic glycosylation of erythrocyte membrane proteins. Relevance to diabetes. J Clin Invest 1980; 65:896–901.

469. Witzum JL, Mahoney EM, Branks MJ, et al. Nonenzymatic glucosylation of low-density lipoprotein alters its biologic activity. Diabetes 1982; 31:283–291.

470. Witzum JL, Fisher M, Pietro T, et al. Nonenzymatic glucosylation of high-density lipoprotein accelerates its catabolism in guinea pigs. Diabetes 1982; 31:1029–1032.
471. Kaneshiga H. Nonenzymatic glycosylation of serum IgG and its effect on antibody activity in patients with diabetes mellitus. Diabetes 1987; 36:822–828.
472. Cerami A, Stevens VJ, Monnier VM. Role of nonenzymatic glycosylation in the development of the sequelae of diabetes mellitus. Metabolism 1979; 28(Suppl 1):431–437.
473. Cohen MP, Urdanivia E, Surma M, et al. Increased glycosylation of glomerular basement membrane collagen in diabetes. Biochem Biophys Res Commun 1980; 95:765–769.
474. Garlick RL, Bunn HF, Spiro RG. Nonenzymatic glycation of basement membranes from human glomeruli and bovine sources. Diabetes 1988; 37:1144–1150.
475. Summerfield JA, Vergall J, Jones EA. Modulation of a glycoprotein recognition system on rat hepatic endothelial cells by glucose and diabetes mellitus. J Clin Invest 1982; 69:1337–1347.
476. Villanueva GB, Allen N. Demonstration of altered antithrombin III activity due to nonenzymatic glycosylation at glucose concentration expected to be encountered in severely diabetic patients. Diabetes 1988; 37:1103–1107.
477. Arturson G, Garby L, Robert M, et al. Oxygen affinity of whole blood in vivo and under standard conditions in subjects with diabetes mellitus. Scand J Clin Lab Invest 1974; 34:19–22.
478. Flückiger R, Winterhalter KH. Glycosylated hemoglobins. In: Caughey WS, ed. Biochemical and Clinical Aspects of Hemoglobin Abnormalities. New York: Academic, 1978: 205–214.
479. McVerry BA, Fisher C, Hopp A, et al. Production of pseudodiabetic renal glomerular changes in mice after repeated injections of glucosylated proteins. Lancet 1980; 1:738–740.
480. Jeraj KP, Michael AF, Mauer SM, et al. Glucosylated and normal human or rat albumin do not bind to renal basement membranes of diabetic and control rats. Diabetes 1983; 32:380–382.
481. Brownlee M, Vlassara H, Cerami A. Nonenzymatic glycosylation reduces the susceptibility of fibrin to degradation by plasmin. Diabetes 1983; 32:680–684.
482. Davies MJ, Woolf N, Carstairs KC. Immunohistochemical studies in diabetic glomerulosclerosis. J Pathol Bacteriol 1966; 92:441–445.
483. Beisswenger PJ, Spiro RG. Human glomerular basement membrane: chemical alteration in diabetes mellitus. Science 1970; 168:596–598.
484. Kohn RR, Schnider SL. Glucosylation of human collagen. Diabetes 1982; 31(Suppl 3):47–51.
485. Rohrbach DH, Hassell JR, Kleinman HK, et al. Alterations in the basement membrane (heparan sulfate) proteoglycan in diabetic mice. Diabetes 1982; 31:185–188.
486. Bassiouny AR, Rosenberg H, McDonald TL. Glucosylated collagen is antigenic. Diabetes 1983; 32:1182–1184.
487. Schnider SL, Kohn RR. Effects of age and diabetes mellitus on the solubility and nonenzymatic glucosylation of human skin collagen. J Clin Invest 1981; 67:1630–1635.
488. Rosenbloom AL, Silverstein JH, Lezotte DC, et al. Limited joint mobility in childhood diabetes mellitus indicates increased risk for microvascular disease. N Engl J Med 1981; 305:191–194.
489. Rosenbloom AL, Silverstein JH, Riley WJ, et al. Limited joint mobility in childhood diabetes: family studies. Diabetes Care 1983; 6:370–373.
490. Petersen CM, Jones RL, Koenig RJ, et al. Reversible hematologic sequelae of diabetes mellitus. Ann Intern Med 1977; 86:425–429.
491. Schmid-Schönbein H, Volger E. Red-cell aggregation and red-cell deformability in diabetes. Diabetes 1976; 25(Suppl 2):897–902.
492. McMillan DE, Utterback NG, La Puma J. Reduced erythrocyte deformability in diabetes. Diabetes 1978; 27:895–901.
493. Kohner EM, McLeod D, Marshall J. Diabetic eye disease. In: Keen H, Jarret J, eds. Complications of Diabetes. London: Edward Arnold, 1982: 19–108.
494. Vlassara H, Brownlee M, Cerami A. Excessive nonenzymatic glycosylation of peripheral and central nervous system myelin components in diabetic rats. Diabetes 1983; 32:670–674.
495. Yki-Järvinen H, Helve E, Koivista VA. Hyperglycemia decreases glucose uptake in type I diabetes. Diabetes 1987; 36:892–896.
496. Mowat AG, Baum J. Chemotaxis of polymorphonuclear leukocytes from patients with diabetes mellitus. N Engl J Med 1971; 284:621–627.
497. Tan JS, Anderson JL, Watanakunakorn C, et al. Neutrophil dysfunction in diabetes mellitus. J Lab Clin Med 1975; 85:26–33.
498. Bagdade JD. Phagocytic and microbicidal function in diabetes mellitus. Acta Endocrinol 1976; 83(Suppl 201):27–34.
499. Casey JI, Heeter BJ, Klyshevich KA. Impaired response of lymphocytes of diabetic subjects to antigen of Staphylococcus aureus. J Infect Dis 1977; 136:495–501.
500. Selam J-L, Clot J, Andary M, et al. Circulating lymphocyte subpopulations in juvenile insulin-dependent diabetes. Correction of abnormalities by adequate blood glucose control. Diabetologia 1979; 16:35–40.
501. Jones RL, Peterson CM. Hematologic alterations in diabetes mellitus. Am J Med 1981; 70:339–352.
502. Brownlee M, Cerami A, Vlassara H. Advanced products of nonenzymatic glycosylation and the pathogenesis of diabetic vascular disease. Diabetes Metab Rev 1988; 5:437–451.
503. Winegrad AI. Banting lecture 1986. Does a common mechanism induce the diverse complications of diabetes? Diabetes 1986; 36:396–406.
504. Kinoshita JH. Mechanisms initiating cataract formation. Invest Ophthalmol 1974; 13:713–724.
505. Robison WG Jr, Kador PF, Kinoshita JH. Retinal capillaries: basement membrane thickening by galactosemia prevented with aldose reductase inhibition. Science 1983; 221:1177–1179.
506. Greene DA, Lattimer SA, Sima AAF. Are disturbances of sorbitol, phosphoinositide, and Na⁺-K⁺-ATPase regulation involved in pathogenesis of diabetic neuropathy? Diabetes 1988; 37:688–693.
507. Morrison AD, Clements RS Jr, Winegrad AI. Effects of elevated glucose concentrations on the metabolism of the aortic wall. J Clin Invest 1972; 51:3114–3123.
508. Chiou S-H, Chylack LT Jr, Bunn HF, et al. Role of nonenzymatic glycosylation in experimental cataract formation. Biochem Biophys Res Commun 1980; 95:894–901.
509. Greene DA, Lattimer SA. Impaired rat sciatic nerve sodium-potassium adenosine triphosphatase in acute streptozotocin diabetes and its correction by dietary myo-inositol supplementation. J Clin Invest 1983; 72:1058–1063.
510. Greene DA, Lattimer SA. Action of sorbinil in diabetic peripheral nerve: relationship of polyol (sorbitol) pathway inhibition to a myo-inositol-mediated defect in sodium-potassium ATPase activity. Diabetes 1984; 33:712–716.
511. Greene DA, de Jesus PV Jr, Winegrad AI. Effects of insulin and dietary myoinositol on impaired peripheral motor nerve conduction velocity in acute streptozotocin diabetes. J Clin Invest 1975; 55:1326–1336.
512. Dyck PJ, Zimmerman BR, Viles TH, et al. Nerve glucose, fructose, sorbitol, myo-inositol and fiber degeneration and regeneration in diabetic neuropathy. N Engl J Med 1988; 319:542–548.
513. Young RJ, Ewing DJ, Clarke BF. A controlled trial of sorbinil, an aldose reductase inhibitor, in chronic painful diabetic neuropathy. Diabetes 1983; 32:938–942.
514. Sima AAF, Bril V, Nathaniel V, et al. Regeneration and repair of myelinated fibers in sural-nerve biopsy specimens from patients with diabetic neuropathy treated with sorbinil. N Engl J Med 1988; 319:548–555.
515. Suárez G, Rajaram R, Oronsky AL, et al. Nonenzymatic glycation of bovine serum albumin by fructose (fructation). Comparison with the Maillard reaction initiated by glucose. J Biol Chem 1989; 264:3674–3679.
516. Parving H-H, Viberti GC, Keen H, et al. Hemodynamic factors in the genesis of diabetic microangiopathy. Metabolism 1983; 32:943–949.
517. Anderson S, Brenner B. Pathogenesis of diabetic glomerulopathy: hemodynamic considerations. Diabetes Metab Rev 1988; 4:163–177.
518. Soler NG, Bennett MA, Pentecost BL, et al. Myocardial infarction in diabetics. Q J Med 1975; 44:125–132.
519. Brunzell JD, Hazzard WR, Motulsky AG, et al. Evidence for diabetes mellitus and genetic forms of hypertriglyceridemia as independent entities. Metabolism 1975; 24:1115–1121.
520. Eckel RH. Lipoprotein lipase. A multifunctional enzyme relevant to common metabolic diseases. N Engl J Med 1989; 320:1060–1068.
521. Taskinen M-R, Nikkila EA. Lipoprotein lipase activity of adipose tissue and skeletal muscle in insulin-deficient human diabetes. Relation to high density and very-low-density lipoproteins and response to treatment. Diabetologia 1979; 17:351–356.
522. Greenfield M, Kolterman O, Olefsky J, et al. Mechanism of hypertriglyceridemia in diabetic patients with fasting hyperglycemia. Diabetologia 1980; 18:441–446.
523. Abrams JJ, Ginsberg H, Grundy SM. Metabolism of cholesterol and plasma triglycerides in nonketotic diabetes mellitus. Diabetes 1982; 31:903–910.
524. Yki-Järvinen H, Taskinen M-R. Interrelationships among insulin's antilipolytic and glucoregulatory effects and plasma triglycerides in nondiabetic and diabetic patients with endogenous hypertriglyceridemia. Diabetes 1988; 37:1271–1278.
525. Brunzell JD, Porte D Jr, Bierman EL. Abnormal lipoprotein lipase–mediated triglyceride removal in untreated diabetes mellitus associated with hypertriglyceridemia. Metabolism 1979; 28:901–907.
526. Howard BV, Abbott WGH, Beltz WF, et al. Integrated study of low density lipoprotein metabolism and very low density lipoprotein metabolism in non–insulin-dependent diabetes. Metabolism 1987; 36:870–877.
527. Steinberg D, Parthasarathy S, Carew TE, et al. Beyond cholesterol. Modifications of low-density lipoprotein that increase its atherogenicity. N Engl J Med 1989; 320:915–924.
528. Hollenbeck CB, Chen Y-DI, Greenfield MS, et al. Reduced plasma high density lipoprotein–cholesterol concentrations need not increase when hyperglycemia is controlled with insulin in non–insulin-dependent diabetes mellitus. J Clin Endocrinol Metab 1985; 62:605–608.
529. Miller GJ. High density lipoproteins and atherosclerosis. Annu Rev Med 1980; 31:97–108.
530. Gordon T, Castelli WP, Hjortland MC, et al. Diabetes, blood lipids, and

the role of obesity in coronary heart disease risk for women. The Framingham study. Ann Intern Med 1977; 87:393–397.

531. Biesbroeck RC, Albers JJ, Wahl PW, et al. Abnormal composition of high density lipoproteins in non–insulin-dependent diabetics. Diabetes 1982; 31:126–131.

532. Nikkila EA. High density lipoproteins in diabetes. Diabetes 1981; 30(Suppl 2):82–87.

533. Dunn FL, Raskin P, Bilheimer DW, et al. The effect of diabetic control on very low density lipoprotein–triglyceride metabolism in patients with noninsulin-dependent diabetes mellitus and hypertriglyceridemia. Metabolism 1984; 33:117–123.

534. Butkus A, Skrinska VA, Schumacher OP. Thromboxane production and platelet aggregation in diabetic subjects with clinical complications. Thromb Res 1980; 19:211–223.

535. Kwaan HC, Colwell JA, Suwanwela N. Disseminated intravascular coagulation in diabetes mellitus, with reference to the role of increased platelet aggregation. Diabetes 1972; 21:108–113.

536. Lufkin EG, Fass DN, O'Fallon WM, et al. Increased von Willebrand factor in diabetes mellitus. Metabolism 1979; 28:63–66.

537. Sagel J, Colwell JA, Crook L, et al. Increased platelet aggregation in early diabetes mellitus. Ann Intern Med 1975; 82:733–738.

538. Johnson M, Harrison HE, Raftery AT, et al. Vascular prostacyclin may be reduced in diabetes in man. Lancet 1979; 1:325–326.

539. Alessandrini P, McRae J, Feman S, et al. Thromboxane biosynthesis and platelet function in diabetes mellitus. N Engl J Med 1988; 319:208–212.

540. Colwell JA, Lopez-Virella MF. A review of the development of large-vessel disease in diabetes mellitus. Am J Med 1988; 85(Suppl 5A):113–118.

541. Lasche EM, Larson RE. Interaction of insulin and prostacyclin production in the rat. Diabetes 1982; 31:454–458.

542. Rubler S, Dlugash J, Yuceoglu YZ, et al. New type of cardiomyopathy associated with diabetic glomerulosclerosis. Am J Cardiol 1972; 30:595–602.

543. Kannel WB, Hjortland M, Castelli WP. Role of diabetes in congestive heart failure: the Framingham Study. Am J Cardiol 1974; 34:29–34.

544. Regan TJ, Lyons MM, Ahmed SS, et al. Evidence for cardiomyopathy in familial diabetes mellitus. J Clin Invest 1977; 60:885–899.

545. Fischer VW, Barner HB, Leskiw ML. Capillary basal laminar thickness in diabetic human myocardium. Diabetes 1979; 28:713–719.

546. Factor SM, Okun EM, Minase T. Capillary microaneurysms in the human diabetic heart. N Engl J Med 1980; 302:384–388.

547. Regan TJ, Ettinger PO, Khan MI, et al. Altered myocardial function and metabolism in chronic diabetes mellitus without ischemia in dogs. Circ Res 1974; 35:222–237.

548. Sanderson JE, Brown DJ, Rivellese A, et al. Diabetic cardiomyopathy. An echocardiographic study of young diabetics. Br Med J 1978; 1:404–407.

549. Dillman WH. Diabetes mellitus induces changes in cardiac myosin of the rat. Diabetes 1980; 29:579–582.

550. Thuesen L, Christiansen JS, Mogensen CE, et al. Cardiac hyperfunction in insulin-dependent diabetic patients developing microvascular complications. Diabetes 1988; 37:851–856.

551. Ruddy TD, Schumak SL, Liu PP, et al. The relationship of cardiac diastolic function to concurrent hormonal and metabolic status in type I diabetes mellitus. J Clin Endocrinol Metab 1988; 66:113–118.

552. Fisher BM, Gillen G, Lindop GB, et al. Cardiac function and coronary arteriography in asymptomatic type I (insulin-dependent) diabetic patients: evidence for a specific diabetic heart disease. Diabetologia 1986; 29:706–712.

553. Afzal N, Ganguly PK, Dhalla KS, et al. Beneficial effects of verapamil in diabetic cardiomyopathy. Diabetes 1988; 37:936–942.

554. Gilgor RS, Lazarus GS. Skin manifestations of diabetes mellitus. In: Ellenberg M, Rifkin H, eds. Diabetes Mellitus. Theory and Practice. New Hyde Park, NY: Medical Examination Publishing, 1983: 879–893.

555. Ward JD. The diabetic leg. Diabetologia 1982; 22:141–147.

556. Brand PW. The diabetic foot. In: Ellenberg M, Rifkin H, eds. Diabetes Mellitus. Theory and Practice. New Hyde Park, NY: Medical Examination Publishing, 1983: 829–849.

557. Edmonds ME, Roberts VC, Watkins PJ. Blood flow in the diabetic neuropathic foot. Diabetologia 1982; 22:9–15.

558. Boulton AJM. The diabetic foot. Med Clin North Am 1988; 72:1513–1530.

559. Marks HH. Longevity and mortality of diabetics. Am J Public Health 1965; 55:416–423.

560. Lestradet H, Papoz L, Hellouis de Menibus C, et al. Long-term study of mortality and vascular complications in juvenile-onset (type I) diabetes. Diabetes 1981; 30:175–179.

561. Sasaki A, Uehara M, Horiuchi N, et al. A long-term follow-up study of Japanese diabetic patients: mortality and causes of death. Diabetologia 1983; 25:309–312.

562. Fujimoto WY, Leonetti DL, Kinyanu JL, et al. Prevalence of complications among second-generation Japanese-American men with diabetes, impaired glucose tolerance, or normal glucose tolerance. Diabetes 1987; 36:730–739.

563. Kamenetzky SA, Bennett PH, Dippe SE, et al. A clinical and histologic study of diabetic nephropathy in the Pima Indians. Diabetes 1974; 23:61–68.

564. Seaquist ER, Goetz FC, Rich S, et al. Familial clustering of diabetic renal disease. Evidence for genetic susceptibility and diabetic nephropathy. N Engl J Med 1989; 320:1161–1165.

565. Salinas-Madrigal L, Pirani CL, Pollak VE. Glomerular and vascular "insudative" lesions of diabetic nephropathy: electron microscopic observations. Am J Pathol 1970; 59:369–397.

566. Mauer SM, Steffes MW, Chern M, et al. Mesangial uptake and processing of macromolecules in rats with diabetes mellitus. Lab Invest 1979; 41:401–406.

567. Leiper JM, Thomson D, MacDonald MK. Uptake and transport of Imposil by the glomerular mesangium in the mouse. Lab Invest 1977; 37:526–533.

568. Miller K, Michael AF. Immunopathology of renal extracellular membranes in diabetes mellitus. Specificity of tubular basement-membrane immunofluorescence. Diabetes 1976; 25:701–708.

569. Barbosa J, Cohen RA, Chavers B, et al. Muscle extracellular membrane immunofluorescence and HLA as possible markers of prediabetes. Lancet 1980; 2:330–333.

570. Takazakura E, Nakamoto Y, Hayakawa H, et al. Onset and progression of diabetic glomerulosclerosis. A prospective study based on serial renal biopsies. Diabetes 1975; 24:1–9.

571. Mauer SM, Barbosa J, Vernier RL, et al. Development of diabetic vascular lesions in normal kidneys transplanted into patients with diabetes mellitus. N Engl J Med 1976; 295:916–920.

572. Christiansen JS, Gammelgaard J, Frandsen M, et al. Increased kidney size, glomerular filtration rate and renal plasma flow in short-term insulin-dependent diabetics. Diabetologia 1981; 20:451–456.

573. Mogensen CE, Andersen MJF. Increased kidney size and glomerular filtration rate in untreated juvenile diabetes: normalization by insulin treatment. Diabetologia 1975; 11:221–224.

574. Viberti GC, Pickup JC, Jarrett RJ, et al. Effect of control of blood glucose on urinary excretion of albumin and β_2 microglobulin in insulin-dependent diabetes. N Engl J Med 1979; 300:638–641.

575. Hostetter TH, Rennke HG, Brenner BM. The case for intrarenal hypertension in the initiation and progression of diabetic and other glomerulopathies. Am J Med 1982; 72:375–380.

576. Viberti GC, Walker JD. Diabetic nephropathy: etiology and prevention. Diabetes Metab Rev 1988; 4:147–162.

577. Mogensen CE, Østerby R, Gundersen HJG. Early functional and morphologic vascular renal consequences of the diabetic state. Diabetologia 1979; 17:71–76.

578. Viberti GC, Hill RD, Jarrett RJ, et al. Microalbuminuria as a predictor of clinical nephropathy in insulin-dependent diabetes mellitus. Lancet 1982; 1:1430–1432.

579. Mogensen CE. Renal function changes in diabetes. Diabetes 1976; 25:872–879.

580. Goldstein HH. Discussion: the problem of end-stage diabetic nephropathy. Kidney Int 1974; 6(Suppl 1):S21–S26.

581. Mogensen CE. Progression of nephropathy in long-term diabetics with proteinuria and effect of initial antihypertensive treatment. Scand J Clin Lab Invest 1976; 36:383–388.

582. Caird FI. Survival of diabetics with proteinuria. Diabetes 1961; 10:178–181.

583. Hostetter TH, Troy JL, Brenner BM. Glomerular hemodynamics in experimental diabetes mellitus. Kidney Int 1981; 19:410–415.

584. Deen WM, Bohrer MP, Brenner BM. Macromolecule transport across glomerular capillaries: application of pore theory. Kidney Int 1979; 16:353–365.

585. Ditzel J. Oxygen transport impairment in diabetes. Diabetes 1976; 25(Suppl 2):832–838.

586. McMillan DE. Disturbance of serum viscosity in diabetes mellitus. J Clin Invest 1974; 53:1071–1079.

587. Parving H-H, Christiansen JS, Noer I, et al. The effect of glucagon infusion on kidney function in short-term insulin-dependent juvenile diabetics. Diabetologia 1980; 19:350–354.

588. Corvilain J, Abramow J. Some effects of human growth hormone on renal hemodynamics and on tubular phosphate transport in man. J Clin Invest 1962; 41:1230–1235.

589. Unger RH. Glucagon physiology and pathophysiology. N Engl J Med 1971; 285:443–449.

590. Unger RH. High growth hormone levels in diabetic ketoacidosis. A possible cause of insulin resistance. JAMA 1965; 191:945–947.

591. Christiansen JS, Frandsen M, Parving H-H. Effect of intravenous glucose infusion on renal function in normal man and in insulin-dependent diabetics. Diabetologia 1981; 21:368–373.

592. Cortes P, Dumler F, Venkatachalam KK, et al. Alterations in glomerular RNA in diabetic rats: roles of glucagon and insulin. Kidney Int 1981; 20:491–499.

593. Mauer SM, Steffes MW, Azar S, et al. The effects of Goldblatt hypertension on development of the glomerular lesions of diabetes mellitus in the rat. Diabetes 1978; 27:738–744.

594. Berkman J, Rifkin H. Unilateral nodular diabetic glomerulosclerosis (Kimmelstiel-Wilson): report of a case. Metabolism 1973; 22:715–722.

595. Shimomura H, Spiro RG. Studies on macromolecular components of

human glomerular basement membrane and alterations in diabetes: decreased levels of heparan sulfate proteoglycan and laminin. Diabetes 1987; 36:374–381.

596. Mogensen CE. Kidney function and glomerular permeability to macromolecules in early juvenile diabetes. Scand J Clin Lab Invest 1971; 28:79–90.

597. Steffes MW, Brown DM, Basgen JM, et al. Amelioration of mesangial volume and surface alterations following islet transplantation in diabetic rats. Diabetes 1980; 29:509–515.

598. Christlieb AR, Kaldany A, D'Elia JA, et al. Aldosterone responsiveness in patients with diabetes mellitus. Diabetes 1978; 27:732–737.

599. DeFronzo RA. Hyperkalemia and hyporeninemic hypoaldosteronism. Kidney Int 1980; 17:118–134.

600. DeLeiva A, Christlieb AR, Belby JC, et al. Big renin and biosynthetic defect of aldosterone in diabetes mellitus. N Engl J Med 1976; 295:639–643.

601. Luetscher JA, Kraemer FB, Wilson DM, et al. Increased plasma inactive renin in diabetes mellitus. A marker of microvascular complications. N Engl J Med 1985; 312:1412–1417.

602. Oh MS, Carroll HJ, Clemmons JE, et al. A mechanism for hyporeninemic hypoaldosteronism in chronic renal disease. Metabolism 1974; 23:1157–1166.

603. Santeusanio F, Faloona GR, Knochel JP, et al. Evidence for a role of endogenous insulin and glucagon in the regulation of potassium homeostasis. J Lab Clin Med 1973; 81:809–817.

604. Axelrod L. Infections in the diabetic patient. Clin Diabetes 1985; 3:97–105.

605. Cook DJ, Achong MR, Dobranowski J. Emphysematous pyelonephritis. Complicated urinary tract infection in diabetes. Diabetes Care 1989; 12:229–232.

606. Groop L, Laasonen L, Edgren J. Renal papillary necrosis in patients with IDDM. Diabetes Care 1989; 12:198–202.

607. Dahl-Jørgensen K, Hanssen KF, Kierulf P, et al. Reduction of urinary albumin excretion after 4 years of continuous subcutaneous insulin infusion in insulin-dependent diabetes mellitus: the Oslo study. Acta Endocrinol 1988; 117:19–25.

608. Wiseman MJ, Saunders AJ, Keen H, et al. Effect of blood glucose control on increased glomerular filtration rate and kidney size in insulin-dependent diabetes. N Engl J Med 1985; 312:617–621.

609. Feldt-Rasmussen B, Mathiesen E, Deckert T. Effect of two years of strict metabolic control in the progression of incipient nephropathy in insulin-dependent diabetes. Lancet 1986; 2:1300–1304.

610. Kleinman KS, Fine LG. Prognostic implications of renal hypertrophy in diabetes mellitus. Diabetes Metab Rev 1988; 4:179–189.

611. Unger RH. Meticulous control of diabetes: benefits, risks, and precautions. Diabetes 1982; 31:479–483.

612. Mogensen CE. Antihypertensive treatment inhibiting the progression of diabetic nephropathy. Acta Endocrinol (Suppl 238) 1980; 94:103–111.

613. Mogensen CE, Schmitz A, Christensen CK. Comparative renal pathophysiology relevant to IDDM and NIDDM patients. Diabetes Metab Rev 1988; 4:453–483.

614. Marre M, Leblanc H, Suárez L, et al. Converting enzyme inhibition and kidney function in normotensive diabetic patients with persistent microalbuminuria. Br Med J 1987; 294:1448–1452.

615. Parving H-H, Andersen AR, Smidt UM, et al. Effect of antihypertensive treatment on kidney function in diabetic nephropathy. Br Med J 1987; 294:1443–1447.

616. Pedersen O, Jørgensen FS, Pedersen MM, et al. The effect of moderate protein restriction in normoalbuminuric type I (insulin-dependent) diabetic patients. Diabetologia 1988; 31:530A (abstract).

617. Cohen D, Dodds R, Viberti GC. Effect of protein restriction in insulin-dependent diabetics at risk of nephropathy. Br Med J 1987; 247:795–798.

618. Evanoff GV, Thompson CS, Brown J, et al. Effect of dietary protein restriction on the progression of diabetic nephropathy. Arch Intern Med 1987; 147:492–495.

619. Comty CM, Kjellsen D, Shapiro FL. A reassessment of the prognosis of diabetic patients treated by chronic hemodialysis (CHD). Trans Am Soc Artif Intern Organs 1976; 22:404–410.

620. Jacobson SH, Fryd D, Sutherland DER, et al. Treatment of the diabetic patient with end-stage renal failure. Diabetes Metab Rev 1988; 4:191–200.

621. Friedman EA. Diabetic renal disease. In: Ellenberg M, Rifkin H, eds. Diabetes Mellitus. Theory and Practice. 3rd ed. New Hyde Park, NY: Medical Examination Publishing, 1983: 759–776.

622. Amair P, Khanna R, Leibel B, et al. Continuous ambulatory peritoneal dialysis in diabetics with end-stage renal disease. N Engl J Med 1982; 306:625–630.

623. Kjellstrand CM, Goetz FC, Najarian JS. Transplantation and dialysis in diabetic patients. An update. In: Friedman EA, L'Esperance FA Jr, eds. Diabetic Renal-Retinal Syndrome. New York: Grune & Stratton, 1980: 342–352.

624. Ramsay RC, Knobloch WH, Barbosa JJ, et al. The visual status of diabetic patients after renal transplantation. Am J Ophthalmol 1979; 87:305–310.

625. Palmberg PF. Diabetic retinopathy. Diabetes 1977; 26:703–709.

626. Davis MD. Diabetic retinopathy: a clinical overview. Diabetes Metab Rev 1988; 4:291–322.

627. Burditt AF, Caird FI, Draper GJ. The natural history of diabetic retinopathy. Q J Med 1968; 37:303–317.

628. Burger W, Hövener G, Düsterhus R, et al. Prevalence and development of retinopathy in children and adolescents with type I (insulin-dependent) diabetes mellitus. A longitudinal study. Diabetologia 1986; 29:17–22.

629. Murphy RP, Patz A. The natural history and management of nonproliferative diabetic retinopathy. In: Little HL, Jack RL, Patz A, et al., eds. Diabetic Retinopathy. New York: Thieme-Stratton, 1983: 225–241.

630. Little HL. Proliferative diabetic retinopathy: pathogenesis and treatment. In: Little HL, Jack RL, Patz A, et al., eds. Diabetic Retinopathy. New York: Thieme-Stratton, 1983: 257–273.

631. Caird FI, Pirie A, Ramsell TG. Diabetes and the Eye. Oxford: Blackwell Scientific, 1968.

632. Ashton N. Pathogenesis of diabetic retinopathy. In: Little HL, Patz A, Jack RL, et al., eds. Diabetic Retinopathy. New York: Thieme-Stratton, 1983: 85–106.

633. McMillan DE. Plasma protein changes, blood viscosity and diabetic microangiopathy. Diabetes 1976; 25(Suppl 2):858–864.

634. Little HL. Role of blood elements in the pathogenesis of diabetic retinopathy. In: Little HL, Patz A, Jack RL, et al., eds. Diabetic Retinopathy. New York: Thieme-Stratton, 1983: 136–147.

635. Little HL. The role of abnormal hemorheodynamics in the pathogenesis of diabetic retinopathy. Trans Am Ophthalmol Soc 1976; 74:573–636.

636. Almér L-O, Pandolfi M. Fibrinolysis and diabetic retinopathy. Diabetes 1976; 25(Suppl 2):807–810.

637. Ishibashi T, Tanaka K, Taniguchi Y. Disruption of blood-retinal barrier in experimental diabetic rats: an electron microscopic study. Exp Eye Res 1980; 30:401–410.

638. Wallow IHL, Engerman RL. Permeability and patency of retinal blood vessels in experimental diabetes. Invest Ophthalmol Vis Sci 1977; 16:447–461.

639. Henkind P. Ocular neovascularization. Am J Ophthalmol 1978; 85:287–301.

640. Kohner EM. Dynamic changes in the microcirculation of diabetics as related to diabetic microangiopathy. Acta Med Scand 1975; Suppl 578:41–47.

641. Patz AI. Studies on retinal neovascularization. Invest Ophthalmol Vis Sci 1980; 19:1133–1149.

642. Glaser BM, Patz A. Neovascularization: current concepts. In: Little HL, Patz A, Jack RL, et al., eds. Diabetic Retinopathy. New York: Thieme-Stratton, 1983: 377–390.

643. Merimee TJ, Zapf J, Froesch ER. Insulin-like growth factors. Studies in diabetics with and without retinopathy. N Engl J Med 1983; 309:527–530.

644. Rodman HM, Waltman SR, Krupin T, et al. Quantitative vitreous fluorophotometry in insulin-treated cystic fibrosis patients. Diabetes 1983; 32:505–508.

645. Tiengo A, Segato T, Briani G, et al. The presence of retinopathy in patients with secondary diabetes following pancreatectomy or chronic pancreatitis. Diabetes Care 1983; 6:570–574.

646. Engerman RL, Kern TS. Experimental galactosemia produces diabetic-like retinopathy. Diabetes 1984; 33:97–100.

647. MacGregor LC, Rosecan LR, Laties AM, et al. Altered retinal metabolism in diabetes. I. Microanalysis of lipid, glucose, sorbitol, and *myo*-inositol in the choroid and in the individual layers of the rabbit retina. J Biol Chem 1986; 261:4046–4051.

648. Cunha-Vaz JG, Mota CC, Leite EC, et al. Effect of sorbinil on blood-retinal barrier in early diabetic retinopathy. Diabetes 1986; 35:574–578.

649. Dornan TL, Ting A, McPherson CK, et al. Genetic susceptibility to the development of retinopathy in insulin-dependent diabetics. Diabetes 1982; 31:226–231.

650. Bodansky HJ, Wolf E, Cudworth AG, et al. Genetic and immunologic factors in microvascular disease in type I insulin-dependent diabetes. Diabetes 1982; 31:70–74.

651. Leslie RDG, Pyke DA. Diabetic retinopathy in identical twins. Diabetes 1982; 31:19–21.

652. Waltman SR, Oestrich C, Krupin T, et al. Quantitative vitreous fluorophotometry. A sensitive technique for measuring early breakdown of the blood-retinal barrier in young diabetic patients. Diabetes 1978; 27:85–87.

653. Frank RN. Visual fields and electroretinography following extensive photocoagulation. Arch Ophthalmol 1975; 93:591–598.

654. Mandelcorn MS, Blankenship G, Machemer R. Pars plana vitrectomy for the management of severe diabetic retinopathy. Am J Ophthalmol 1976; 81:561–570.

655. Waite JH, Beetham WP. The visual mechanism in diabetes mellitus. (A comparative study of 2002 diabetics, and 457 non-diabetics for control.) N Engl J Med 1935; 212:367–379, 429–443.

656. O'Brien CS, Molsberry JM, Allen JH. Diabetic cataract. Incidence and morphology in 126 young diabetic patients. JAMA 1934; 103:892–897.

657. Caird FI, Hutchinson M, Pirie A. Cataract extraction and diabetes. Br J Ophthalmol 1965; 49:466–471.

658. Vinik A, Mitchell B. Clinical aspects of diabetic neuropathies. Diabetes Metab Rev 1988; 4:223–253.

659. Greene DA, Lattimer SA, Sima AAF. Pathogenesis and prevention of diabetic neuropathy. Diabetes Metab Rev 1988; 4:201–221.

660. Raff MS, Sangalang V, Asbury AK. Ischemic mononeuropathy multiplex associated with diabetes mellitus. Arch Neurol 1968; 18:487–499.

661. Ellenberg M. Diabetic neuropathic cachexia. Diabetes 1974; 23:418–423.

662. Hosking DJ, Bennett T, Hampton JR. Diabetic autonomic neuropathy. Diabetes 1978; 27:1043–1054.

663. Hilsted J. Pathophysiology in diabetic autonomic neuropathy: cardiovascular, hormonal, and metabolic studies. Diabetes 1982; 31:730–737.

664. Hreidarsson AB, Gundersen HJ. Reduced pupillary unrest. Autonomic nervous system abnormality in diabetes mellitus. Diabetes 1988; 37:446–451.

665. Kahn JK, Sisson JC, Vinik AI. QT interval prolongation and sudden cardiac death in diabetic autonomic neuropathy. J Clin Endocrinol Metab 1987; 64:751–754.

666. Ellenberg M. Diabetic complications without manifest diabetes. Complications as presenting clinical symptoms. JAMA 1963; 183:926–930.

667. Balfour J, Ankenman GJ. Atonic neurogenic bladder as a manifestation of diabetic neuropathy. J Urol 1956; 76:746–752.

668. Saenz de Tejada I, Goldstein I, Azadzoi K, et al. Impaired neurogenic and endothelium-mediated relaxation of penile smooth muscle from diabetic men with impotence. N Engl J Med 1989; 320:1025–1030.

669. Feldman M, Schiller LR. Disorders of gastrointestinal motility associated with diabetes mellitus. Ann Intern Med 1983; 98:376–384.

670. Kassander P. Asymptomatic gastric retention in diabetics (gastroparesis diabeticorum). Ann Intern Med 1958; 48:797–812.

671. Feldman M, Corbett DB, Ramsey EJ, et al. Abnormal gastric function in longstanding, insulin-dependent diabetic patients. Gastroenterology 1979; 77:12–17.

672. Vantrappen G, Janssens J, Hellemans J, et al. The interdigestive motor complex of normal subjects and patients with bacterial overgrowth of the small intestine. J Clin Invest 1977; 59:1158–1166.

673. Goldstein F, Wirts CW, Kowlessar OD. Diabetic diarrhea and steatorrhea. Microbiologic and clinical observations. Ann Intern Med 1970; 72:215–218.

674. Weisbrodt NW. Motility of the small intestine. In: Johnson LR, ed. Physiology of the Gastrointestinal Tract. New York: Raven, 1981: 411–443.

675. Aizawa I, Itoh Z, Harris V, et al. Plasma somatostatin-like immunoreactivity during the interdigestive period in the dog. J Clin Invest 1981; 68:206–213.

676. Schusdziarra V, Rouiller D, Harris V, et al. The response of plasma somatostatin-like immunoreactivity to nutrients in normal and alloxan diabetic dogs. Endocrinology 1978; 103:2264–2273.

677. Snape WJ, Battle WM, Schwartz SS, et al. Metoclopramide to treat gastroparesis due to diabetes mellitus. A double-blind controlled trial. Ann Intern Med 1982; 96:444–446.

678. McCallum RW, Ricci DA, Rakatansky H, et al. A multicenter placebo-controlled clinical trial of oral metoclopramide in diabetic gastroparesis. Diabetes Care 1983; 6:463–467.

679. Pinder RM, Brogden RN, Sawyer PR, et al. Metoclopramide: a review of its pharmacological properties and clinical use. Drugs 1976; 12:81–131.

680. Read NW, Harford WV, Schmulen AC, et al. A clinical study of patients with fecal incontinence and diarrhea. Gastroenterology 1979; 76:747–756.

681. Schiller LR, Santa Ana CA, Schmulen AC, et al. Pathogenesis of fecal incontinence in diabetes mellitus. Evidence for internal-anal-sphincter dysfunction. N Engl J Med 1982; 307:1666–1671.

682. Thompson MW. Heredity, maternal age, and birth order in the etiology of celiac disease. Am J Hum Genet 1951; 3:159–166.

683. Frier BM, Saunders JHB, Wormsley KG, et al. Exocrine pancreatic function in juvenile-onset diabetes mellitus. Gut 1976; 17:685–691.

684. Scarpello JHB, Hague RV, Cullen DR, et al. The ^{14}C-glycocholate test in diabetic diarrhoea. Br Med J 1976; 2:673–675.

685. Sumi SM, Finlay JM. On the pathogenesis of diabetic steatorrhea. Ann Intern Med 1961; 55:994–997.

686. Whalen GE, Soergel HK, Geenen JE. Diabetic diarrhea. A clinical and pathophysiological study. Gastroenterology 1969; 56:1021–1032.

687. Malins JM, French JM. Diabetic diarrhoea. Q J Med 1957; 26:467–480.

688. Aylett P. Gastric emptying and secretion in patients with diabetes mellitus. Gut 1965; 6:262–265.

689. Graf RJ, Halter JB, Pfeifer MA, et al. Glycemic control and nerve conduction abnormalities in non–insulin-dependent diabetic subjects. Ann Intern Med 1981; 94:307–311.

690. Molloy AM, Tomkin GH. Altered bile in diabetic diarrhoea. Br Med J 1978; 2:1462–1463.

691. Dyrberg T, Benn J, Christiansen JS, et al. Prevalence of diabetic autonomic neuropathy measured by simple bedside tests. Diabetologia 1981; 20:190–194.

692. Ewing DJ. Cardiovascular reflexes and autonomic neuropathy. Clin Sci 1978; 55:321–327.

693. Wheeler T, Watkins PJ. Cardiac denervation in diabetes. Br Med J 1973; 4:584–589.

694. Page MM, Watkins PJ. Cardiorespiratory arrest and diabetic autonomic neuropathy. Lancet 1978; 1:14–16.

695. Hreidarsson AB. Pupil size in insulin-dependent diabetes. Relationship to duration, metabolic control, and long-term manifestations. Diabetes 1982; 31:442–448.

696. Smith AA, Dancis J. Catecholamine release in familial dysautonomia. N Engl J Med 1967; 277:61–64.

697. Leveston SA, Shah SD, Cryer PE. Cholinergic stimulation of norepinephrine release in man. Evidence of a sympathetic postganglionic axonal lesion in diabetic adrenergic neuropathy. J Clin Invest 1979; 64:374–380.

698. Christensen NJ. Plasma catecholamines in long-term diabetics with and without neuropathy and in hypophysectomized subjects. J Clin Invest 1972; 51:779–787.

699. Cryer PE, Silverberg AB, Santiago JV, et al. Plasma catecholamines in diabetes. The syndromes of hypoadrenergic and hyperadrenergic postural hypotension. Am J Med 1978; 64:407–416.

700. Page MM, Watkins PJ. Provocation of postural hypotension by insulin in diabetic autonomic neuropathy. Diabetes 1976; 25:90–95.

701. Ewing DJ, Clark BF. Diagnosis and management of diabetic autonomic neuropathy. Br Med J 1982; 285:916–918.

702. Genovely H, Pfeifer MA. RR-variation. The autonomic test of choice in diabetes. Diabetes Metab Rev 1988; 3:255–271.

703. Finegold D, Lattimer SA, Nolle S, et al. Polyol pathway activity and myo-inositol metabolism. A suggested relationship in the pathogenesis of diabetic neuropathy. Diabetes 1983; 32:988–992.

704. Asbury AK. Understanding diabetic neuropathy. N Engl J Med 1988; 319:577–578.

705. Sidenius P. The axonopathy of diabetic neuropathy. Diabetes 1982; 31:356–363.

706. Solders G, Wilczek H, Gunnarsson R, et al. Effects of combined pancreatic and renal transplantation on diabetic neuropathy: a two-year follow-up study. Lancet 1987; 2:1232–1235.

707. Thomas PK, Ward JD, Watkins PJ. Diabetic neuropathy. In: Keen H, Jarrett J, eds. Complications of Diabetes. London: Edward Arnold, 1982: 109–136.

708. Saudek CD, Werns S, Reidenberg MM. Phenytoin in the treatment of diabetic symmetrical polyneuropathy. Clin Pharmacol Ther 1977; 22:196–199.

709. Rull JA, Quibrera R, González-Millán H, et al. Symptomatic treatment of peripheral diabetic neuropathy with carbamazepine (Tegretol): double blind crossover trial. Diabetologia 1969; 5:215–218.

710. Davis JL, Lewis SB, Gerich JE, et al. Peripheral diabetic neuropathy treated with amitriptyline and fluphenazine. JAMA 1977; 238:2291–2292.

711. Greene DA, Lewis RA, Lattimer SA, et al. Selective effects of myo-inositol administration on sciatic and tibial motor nerve conduction parameters in the streptozotocin-diabetic rat. Diabetes 1982; 31:573–578.

712. Yue DK, Hanwell MA, Satchell PM, et al. The effect of aldose reductase inhibition on motor nerve conduction velocity in diabetic rats. Diabetes 1982; 31:789–794.

713. Greene DA, Lattimer SA, Sima AAF. Sorbitol, phosphoinositides, and sodium-potassium ATPase in the pathogenesis of diabetic complications. N Engl J Med 1987; 316:599–606.

714. Kikkawa R, Hatanaka J, Yasada H, et al. Effect of a new aldose reductase inhibitor, (E)-3-carboxymethyl-5-[(2E)-methyl-3-phenylpropenylidene] rhodamine (ONO-2235) on peripheral nerve disorders in streptozotocin-diabetic rats. Diabetologia 1983; 24:290–292.

715. Young RJ, Ewing DJ, Clarke BF. A controlled trial of sorbinil, an aldose reductase inhibitor, in chronic painful diabetic neuropathy. Diabetes 1983; 32:938–942.

716. Lewin IG, O'Brian IAD, Morgan MH, et al. Clinical and neurophysiological studies with the aldose reductase inhibitor, sorbinil, in symptomatic diabetic neuropathy. Diabetologia 1984; 26:445–448.

717. Fagins J, Brattberg A, Jameson S, et al. Limited benefit of treatment of diabetic polyneuropathy with an aldose reductase inhibitor: a 24 week controlled trial. Diabetologia 1985; 28:323–329.

718. Hotta N, Kakuta H, Kimura M, et al. Experimental and clinical trial of aldose reductase inhibitor in diabetic neuropathy. Diabetes 1985; 34(Suppl 1):98A (abstract).

719. Koglan L, Clark C, Ryder S, et al. The results of long-term open-label administration of ALREDASE in the treatment of diabetic neuropathy. Diabetes 1985; 34(Suppl 1):202A (abstract).

720. Martyn CN, Reid W, Young RJ, et al. Six-month treatment with sorbinil in asymptomatic diabetic neuropathy. Failure to improve abnormal nerve function. Diabetes 1987; 36:987–990.

721. Warren S, LeCompte PM, Legg MA. Pathology of Diabetes Mellitus. Philadelphia: Lea & Febiger, 1966.

722. Brownlee M, Cahill GF Jr. Diabetic control and vascular complications. In: Paoletti R, Gotto AM Jr, eds. Atherosclerosis Reviews. Vol 4. New York: Raven, 1979: 29–70.

723. Report of the National Commission on Diabetes to the Congress of the

United States. DHEW Publication No. (NIH) 76-1022, Vol 3, Part 2. Washington, DC: Government Printing Office, 1976: 64.

724. Strandness DE Jr, Priest RE, Gibbons GE. Combined clinical and pathologic study of diabetic and nondiabetic peripheral arterial disease. Diabetes 1964; 13:1366–1372.

725. Beach KW, Strandness DE Jr. Arteriosclerosis obliterans and associated risk factors in insulin-dependent and non–insulin-dependent diabetes. Diabetes 1980; 29:882–888.

726. White RA, Nolan L, Harley D, et al. Noninvasive evaluation of peripheral vascular disease using transcutaneous oxygen tension. Am J Surg 1982; 144:68–75.

727. Railton R, Newman P, Hislop J, et al. Reduced transcutaneous oxygen tension and impaired vascular response in type 1 (insulin-dependent) diabetes. Diabetologia 1983; 25:340–342.

728. Coffman JD. Vasodilator drugs in peripheral vascular disease. N Engl J Med 1979; 300:713–717.

729. Smith RB III, Dratz AF, Coberly JC, et al. Effect of lumbar sympathectomy on muscle blood flow in advanced occlusive vascular disease. Am Surg 1971; 37:247–251.

730. Harkonen S, Kjellstrand CM. Exacerbation of diabetic renal failure following intravenous pyelography. Am J Med 1977; 63:939–946.

731. Levin ME, O'Neal LW. Peripheral vascular disease. In: Ellenberg M, Rifkin H, eds. Diabetes Mellitus. Theory and Practice. 3rd ed. New Hyde Park, NY: Medical Examination Publishing, 1983: 803–828.

732. Abbott WM. Percutaneous transluminal angioplasty: surgeon's view. Am J Roentgenol 1980; 135:917–920.

733. Greenfield AJ. Femoral, popliteal, and tibial arteries: percutaneous transluminal angioplasty. Am J Roentgenol 1980; 135:927–935.

734. Kalkhoff RK, Kissebah AH, Kim H-J. Carbohydrate and lipid metabolism during normal pregnancy: relationship to gestational hormone action. Semin Perinatol 1978; 2:291–307.

735. Freinkel N. Of pregnancy and progeny. Diabetes 1980; 29:1023–1035.

736. Tsibris JCM, Raynor LO, Buhi WC, et al. Insulin receptors in circulating erythrocytes and monocytes from women on oral contraceptives or pregnant women near term. J Clin Endocrinol Metab 1980; 51:711–717.

737. Gewolb IH, Warshaw JB. Influences on fetal growth. In: Warshaw JB, ed. The Biological Basis of Reproductive and Developmental Medicine. New York: Elsevier Biomedical, 1983: 365–389.

738. Moore P, Kolterman O, Weyant J, et al. Insulin binding in human pregnancy: comparisons with the postpartum, luteal, and follicular states. J Clin Endocrinol Metab 1981; 52:937–941.

739. Kimura RE, Warshaw JB. Metabolism during development. In: Warshaw JB, ed. The Biological Basis of Reproductive and Developmental Medicine. New York: Elsevier Biomedical, 1983: 337–364.

740. Knopp RH, Herrera E, Freinkel N. Metabolism of adipose tissue isolated from fed and fasted pregnant rats during late gestation. J Clin Invest 1970; 49:1438–1446.

741. Herrera E, Knopp RH, Freinkel N. Plasma fuels, insulin, liver composition, gluconeogenesis, and nitrogen metabolism during late gestation in the fed and fasted rat. J Clin Invest 1969; 48:2260–2272.

742. Freinkel N, Metzger BE. Some considerations of fuel economy in the fed state during late human pregnancy. In: Camerini-Davalos RA, Cole HS, eds. Early Diabetes in Early Life. New York: Academic, 1975: 289–301.

743. Horton WE Jr, Sadler TW. Effects of maternal diabetes on early embryogenesis. Alterations in morphogenesis produced by the ketone body, β-hydroxybutyrate. Diabetes 1983; 32:610–616.

744. Health Interview Survey. Washington, DC: National Center for Health Statistics, 1973.

745. Fleischman AR, Finberg L. The infant of the diabetic mother and diabetes in infancy. In: Ellenberg M, Rifkin H, eds. Diabetes Mellitus. Theory and Practice. 3rd ed. New Hyde Park, NY: Medical Examination Publishing, 1983: 715–725.

746. Chez RA, Mintz DH, Horger EO III, et al. Factors affecting the response to insulin in the normal subhuman pregnant primate. J Clin Invest 1970; 49:1517–1527.

747. Mintz DH, Chez RA, Hutchinson DL. Subhuman primate pregnancy complicated by streptozotocin-induced diabetes mellitus. J Clin Invest 1972; 51:837–847.

748. Obenshain SS, Adam PAJ, King KC, et al. Human fetal insulin response to sustained maternal hyperglycemia. N Engl J Med 1970; 283:566–570.

749. Ogata ES, Sabbagha R, Metzger BE, et al. Serial ultrasonography to assess evolving fetal macrosomia. Studies in 23 pregnant diabetic women. JAMA 1980; 243:2405–2408.

750. Widness JA, Schwartz HC, Thompson D, et al. Glycohemoglobin (HbA$_{1c}$): a predictor of birth weight in infants of diabetic mothers. J Pediatr 1978; 92:8–12.

751. Osler M, Pedersen J. The body composition of newborn infants of diabetic mothers. Pediatrics 1960; 26:985–992.

752. Robert MF, Neff RK, Hubbell JP, et al. Association between maternal diabetes and the respiratory-distress syndrome in the newborn. N Engl J Med 1976; 294:357–360.

753. Gewolb IH, Barrett C, Wilson CM, et al. Delay in pulmonary glycogen degradation in fetuses of streptozotocin diabetic rats. Pediatr Res 1982; 16:869–873.

754. Warburton D. Chronic hyperglycemia reduces surface active material flux in tracheal fluid of fetal lambs. J Clin Invest 1983; 71:550–555.

755. Oski FA, Naiman JL. Polycythemia and hyperviscosity in the neonatal period. In: Hematologic Problems in the Newborn. 3rd ed. Philadelphia: W. B. Saunders, 1982: 87–96.

756. Gersony WM. Persistence of the fetal circulation: a commentary. J Pediatr 1973; 82:1103–1106.

757. Avery ME, Oppenheimer EH, Gordon HH. Renal-vein thrombosis in newborn infants of diabetic mothers. Report of two cases. N Engl J Med 1957; 256:1134–1138.

758. Taylor PM, Wofson JH, Bright NH, et al. Hyperbilirubinemia in infants of diabetic mothers. Biol Neonate 1963; 5:289–298.

759. Gabbe SG. Diabetes mellitus in pregnancy: have all the problems been solved? Am J Med 1981; 70:613–618.

760. Rusnak SL, Driscoll SG. Congenital spinal anomalies in infants of diabetic mothers. Pediatrics 1965; 35:989–995.

761. Rowland TW, Hubbell JP Jr, Nadas AS. Congenital heart disease in infants of diabetic mothers. J Pediatr 1973; 83:815–820.

762. Gabbe SG, Mestman JH, Freeman RK, et al. Management and outcome of pregnancy in diabetes mellitus, classes B to R. Am J Obstet Gynecol 1977; 129:723–732.

763. Whittle MJ, Anderson D, Lowensohn RI, et al. Estriol in pregnancy. VI. Experience with unconjugated plasma estriol assays and antepartum fetal heart rate testing in diabetic pregnancies. Am J Obstet Gynecol 1979; 135:764–772.

764. Visser GH, Huisjes HJ. Diagnostic value of the unstressed antepartum cardiotocogram. Br J Obstet Gynaecol 1977; 84:321–326.

765. Landon MB, Gabbe SG. Diabetes and pregnancy. Med Clin North Am 1988; 72:1493–1511.

766. Eriksson UJ, Dahlstrom E, Hellerstrom C. Diabetes in pregnancy. Skeletal malformations in the offspring of diabetic rats after intermittent withdrawal of insulin in early gestation. Diabetes 1983; 32:1141–1145.

767. Mills JL, Baker L, Goldman AS. Malformations in infants of diabetic mothers occur before the seventh gestational week. Implications for treatment. Diabetes 1979; 28:292–293.

768. Pedersen JF, Molsted-Pederson L. Early fetal growth delay detected by ultrasound marks increased risk of congenital malformation in diabetic pregnancy. Br Med J 1981; 283:269–271.

769. Pedersen JF, Molsted-Pederson L. Early growth delay predisposes the fetus in diabetic pregnancy to congenital malformation. Lancet 1982; 1:737.

770. Pedersen J, Molsted-Pedersen L. Congenital malformations: the possible role of diabetes care outside pregnancy. Ciba Found Symp 1979; 63:265–271.

771. Mills JF, Knaff RH, Simpson JL, et al. Lack of relation of increased malformation rates in infants of mothers to glycemic control during organogenesis. N Engl J Med 1988; 318:671–676.

772. Karlsson K, Kjellmer I. The outcome of diabetic pregnancies in relation to the mother's blood sugar level. Am J Obstet Gynecol 1972; 112:213–220.

773. Dobbing J. Prenatal nutrition and neurological development. In: Craviots J, Hambraeus L, Vahlquist B, eds. Symposia of the Swedish Nutrition Foundation XII—Early Malnutrition and Mental Development. Uppsala: Almquist and Wiksell, 1974: 96–110.

774. O'Sullivan JB, Charles D, Mahan CM, et al. Gestational diabetes and perinatal mortality rate. Am J Obstet Gynecol 1973; 116:901–904.

775. Roversi GD, Gargiulo M, Nicolini U, et al. Maximal tolerated insulin therapy in gestational diabetes. Diabetes Care 1980; 3:489–494.

776. Schade DS. Surgery and diabetes. Med Clin North Am 1988; 72:1531–1543.

777. Roy B, Chou MCY, Field JB. Time-action characteristics of regular and NPH insulin in insulin-treated diabetics. J Clin Endocrinol Metab 1980; 50:475–479.

778. Nolte MS, Poon V, Grodsky GM, et al. Reduced solubility of short-acting soluble insulins when mixed with longer-acting insulin. Diabetes 1983; 32:1177–1181.

779. Skyler JS. Insulin pharmacology. Med Clin North Am 1988; 72:1337–1354.

780. Zinman B. The physiologic replacement of insulin. An elusive goal. N Engl J Med 1989; 321:363–370.

781. Sonnenberg GE, Chantelau E, Sundermann S, et al. Human and porcine regular insulins are equally effective in subcutaneous replacement therapy. Results of a double-blind crossover study in type I diabetic patients with continuous subcutaneous insulin infusion. Diabetes 1982; 31:600–602.

782. Home PD, Massi-Benedetti M, Shepherd GAA, et al. A comparison of the activity and disposal of semi-synthetic human insulin and porcine insulin in normal man by the glucose clamp technique. Diabetologia 1982; 22:41–45.

783. Heding LG, Marshall MO, Persson B, et al. Immunogenicity of monocomponent human and porcine insulin in newly diagnosed type I (insulin-dependent) diabetic children. Diabetologia 1984; 27(Suppl):96–98.

784. Skyler JS, Pfeiffer EF, Raptis S, et al. Biosynthetic human insulin: progress and prospects. Diabetes Care 1981; 4:140–143.

785. Zuppinger K, Aebi C, Fankhauser S, et al. Comparison of human and porcine insulin therapies in children with newly diagnosed diabetes mellitus. Diabetologia 1987; 30:912–915.

786. Teuscher A, Berger WG. Hypoglycemia unawareness in diabetics transferred from beef/pork insulin to human insulin. Lancet 1987; 2:382–385.

787. Schade DS. Brittle diabetes: strategies, diagnosis, and treatment. Diabetes Metab Rev 1988; 4:371–390.

788. Schade DS, Santiago JV, Skyler JS, et al. Unstable diabetes and insulin resistance. In: Schade DS, Santiago JV, Skyler JS, et al., eds. Intensive Insulin Therapy. Princeton: Excerpta Medica, 1983: 264–283.

789. Fukuda M, Tanaka A, Tahara Y, et al. Correlation between minimal secretory capacity of pancreatic beta-cells and stability of diabetic control. Diabetes 1988; 37:81–88.

790. Nathan DM, Singer DE, Hurxthal K, et al. The clinical information value of the glycosylated hemoglobin assay. N Engl J Med 1984; 310:341–346.

791. Goldstein DE. Is glycosylated hemoglobin clinically useful? N Engl J Med 1984; 310:384–385.

792. Schiffrin A, Belmonte MM. Comparison between continuous subcutaneous insulin infusion and multiple injections of insulin. A one-year prospective study. Diabetes 1982; 31:255–264.

793. Skyler JS, Skyler DL, Seigler DE, et al. Algorithms for adjustment of insulin dosage by patients who monitor blood glucose. Diabetes Care 1981; 4:311–318.

794. Rizza RA, Gerich JE, Haymond MW, et al. Control of blood sugar in insulin-dependent diabetes: comparison of an artificial endocrine pancreas, continuous subcutaneous insulin infusion, and intensified conventional insulin therapy. N Engl J Med 1980; 303:1313–1318.

795. Raskin P. Open and closed insulin infusion systems: newer methods of insulin delivery. In: Ellenberg M, Rifkin H, eds. Diabetes Mellitus. Theory and Practice. 3rd ed. New Hyde Park, NY: Medical Examination Publishing, 1983: 941–957.

796. Slama G, Garrel D, Tchobroutsky G. Multiple daily insulin injections through subcutaneously implanted needle. Lancet 1980; 1:1078.

797. Reeves ML, Seigler DE, Ryan EA, et al. Glycemic control in insulin-dependent diabetes mellitus. Comparison of outpatient intensified conventional therapy with continuous subcutaneous insulin infusion. Am J Med 1982; 72:673–680.

798. Pickup JC, Keen H, Parsons JA, et al. Continuous subcutaneous insulin infusion: improved blood-glucose and intermediary-metabolite control in diabetics. Lancet 1979; 1:1255–1258.

799. Tamborlane WV, Sherwin RS, Genel M, et al. Reduction to normal of plasma glucose in juvenile diabetes by subcutaneous administration of insulin with a portable infusion pump. N Engl J Med 1979; 300:573–578.

800. Felig P, Bergman M. Intensive ambulatory treatment of insulin-dependent diabetes. Ann Intern Med 1982; 97:225–230.

801. Kitabchi AE, Fisher JN, Matteri R, et al. The use of continuous insulin delivery systems in treatment of diabetes mellitus. Adv Intern Med 1983; 28:449–490.

802. Mecklenburg RS, Benson JW Jr, Becker NM, et al. Clinical use of the insulin infusion pump in 100 patients with type I diabetes. N Engl J Med 1982; 307:513–518.

803. Schade DS, Santiago JV, Skyler JS, et al. Hazards of intensive insulin therapy. In: Schade DS, Santiago JV, Skyler JS, et al., eds. Intensive Insulin Therapy. Princeton: Excerpta Medica, 1983: 287–301.

804. Schade DS, Santiago JV, Skyler JS, et al. Effects of intensive treatment on substrate and hormonal abnormalities. In: Schade DS, Santiago JV, Skyler JS, et al., eds. Intensive Insulin Therapy. Princeton: Excerpta Medica, 1983: 71–87.

805. Rosenstock J, Vega GL, Raskin P. Effect of intensive diabetes treatment on low-density lipoprotein apolipoprotein β kinetics in type I diabetics. Diabetes 1988; 37:393–397.

806. Rubinstein A, Pierce CE Jr II, Bloomgarden Z. Rapid healing of diabetic foot ulcers with continuous subcutaneous insulin infusion. Am J Med 1983; 75:161–165.

807. Jakobsen J, Christiansen JS, Kristoffersen I, et al. Autonomic and somatosensory nerve function after 2 years of continuous subcutaneous insulin infusion in type I diabetes. Diabetes 1988; 37:452–455.

808. Canny CL, Kohner EM, Trautman J, et al. Comparison of stereofundus photographs in patients with insulin-dependent diabetes during conventional insulin treatment or continuous subcutaneous insulin infusion. Diabetes 1985; 34(Suppl 3):50–55.

809. Kohner EM, Lawson PM, Ghosh G, et al. Conference on insulin pump therapy in diabetes. Multicenter study of effect on microvascular disease. Assessment of fluorescein angiograms. Diabetes 1985; 34(Suppl 3):56–60.

810. Engerman RL, Kern TS. Progression of incipient diabetic retinopathy during good glycemic control. Diabetes 1987; 36:808–812.

811. Rosenstock J, Friberg T, Raskin P. Effect of glycemic control on microvascular complications in patients with type I diabetes mellitus. Am J Med 1986; 81:1012–1018.

812. Teutsch SM, Herman WH, Dwyer DM, et al. Mortality among diabetic patients using continuous subcutaneous insulin-infusion pumps. N Engl J Med 1984; 310:361–368.

813. Mecklenburg RS, Benson JW Jr, Blumenstein BA, et al. Long-term metabolic control with insulin pump therapy. Report of experience with 127 patients. N Engl J Med 1985; 313:464–468.

814. Cryer PE. Glucose counterregulation in man. Diabetes 1981; 30:261–264.

815. Gerich J, Davis J, Lorenzi M, et al. Hormonal mechanisms of recovery from insulin-induced hypoglycemia in man. Am J Physiol 1979; 236:E380–E385.

816. Bolli G, De Feo P, Compagnucci P, et al. Important role of adrenergic mechanisms in acute glucose counterregulation following insulin-induced hypoglycemia in type I diabetes. Evidence for an effect mediated by beta-adrenoreceptors. Diabetes 1982; 31:641–647.

817. De Feo P, Bolli G, Perriello G, et al. The adrenergic contribution to glucose counterregulation in type I diabetes mellitus. Dependency on A-cell function and mediation through beta$_2$-adrenergic receptors. Diabetes 1983; 32:887–893.

818. Boden G, Reichard GA Jr, Hoeldtke RD, et al. Severe insulin-induced hypoglycemia associated with deficiencies in the release of counterregulatory hormones. N Engl J Med 1981; 305:1200–1205.

819. Cryer PE. Decreased sympathochromaffin activity in IDDM. Diabetes 1989; 38:405–409.

820. Campbell PJ, Bolli GB, Cryer PE, et al. Pathogenesis of the dawn phenomenon in patients with insulin-dependent diabetes mellitus. Accelerated glucose production and impaired glucose utilization due to nocturnal surges in growth hormone secretion. N Engl J Med 1985; 312:1472–1479.

821. Boden G, Soriano M, Hoeldtke RD, et al. Counterregulatory hormone release and glucose recovery after hypoglycemia in noninsulin-dependent diabetic patients. Diabetes 1983; 32:1055–1059.

822. White NH, Skor DA, Cryer PE, et al. Identification of type I diabetic patients at increased risk for hypoglycemia during intensive therapy. N Engl J Med 1983; 308:485–491.

823. Somogyi M. Exacerbation of diabetes by excess insulin action. Am J Med 1959; 26:169–191.

824. Wilson DE. Excessive insulin therapy: biochemical effects and clinical repercussions. Current concepts of counterregulation in type I diabetes. Ann Intern Med 1983; 98:219–227.

825. Tordjman KM, Havlin CE, Levandoski LA, et al. Failure of nocturnal hypoglycemia to cause fasting hyperglycemia in patients with insulin-dependent diabetes mellitus. N Engl J Med 1987; 317:1552–1559.

826. Winter RJ. Profiles of metabolic control in diabetic children—frequency of asymptomatic nocturnal hypoglycemia. Metabolism 1981; 30:666–672.

827. Kahn CR, Rosenthal AS. Immunologic reactions to insulin: insulin allergy, insulin resistance, and the autoimmune insulin syndrome. Diabetes Care 1979; 2:283–295.

828. Kahn CR, Mann D, Rosenthal AS, et al. The immune response to insulin in man. Interaction of HLA alloantigens and the development of the immune response. Diabetes 1982; 31:716–723.

829. Galloway JA, Bressler R. Insulin treatment in diabetes. Med Clin North Am 1978; 62:663–680.

830. Kahn CR. Role of insulin receptors in insulin-resistant states. Metabolism 1980; 29:455–466.

831. Shipp JC, Cunninham RW, Russell RO, et al. Insulin resistance: clinical features, natural course and effects of adrenal steroid treatment. Medicine 1965; 44:165–186.

832. Kurtz AB, Nabarro JDN. Circulating insulin-binding antibodies. Diabetologia 1980; 19:329–334.

833. Rhie FH, Ganda OP, Bern MM, et al. Insulin resistance and monoclonal gammopathy. Metabolism 1971; 30:41–45.

834. Goldman J, Baldwin D, Rubenstein AH, et al. Characterization of circulating insulin and proinsulin-binding antibodies in autoimmune hypoglycemia. J Clin Invest 1979; 63:1050–1059.

835. Nathan DM, Axelrod L, Flier JS, et al. U-500 insulin in the treatment of antibody-mediated insulin resistance. Ann Intern Med 1971; 94:653–656.

836. Davidson JK, DeBra DW. Immunologic insulin resistance. Diabetes 1978; 27:307–318.

837. Paulsen EP, Courtney JW III, Duckworth WC. Insulin resistance caused by massive degradation of subcutaneous insulin. Diabetes 1979; 28:640–645.

838. Kitabchi AE, Stentz FB, Cole C, et al. Accelerated insulin degradation: an alternate mechanism for insulin resistance. Diabetes Care 1979; 2:414–417.

839. Pickup JC, Home PD, Bilous RW, et al. Management of severely brittle diabetes by continuous subcutaneous and intramuscular insulin infusions: evidence for a defect in subcutaneous insulin absorption. Br Med J 1981; 282:347–350.

840. Freidenberg GR, White N, Cataland S, et al. Diabetes responsive to intravenous but not subcutaneous insulin: effectiveness of aprotinin. N Engl J Med 1981; 305:363–368.

841. McElduff A, Eastman CJ, Haynes SP, et al. Apparent insulin resistance

due to abnormal enzymatic insulin degradation: a new mechanism for insulin resistance. Aust NZ J Med 1980; 10:56–61.

842. Williams G, Pickup JC, Bowcock S, et al. Subcutaneous aprotinin causes local hyperaemia. A possible mechanism by which aprotinin improves control in some diabetic patients. Diabetologia 1983; 24:91–94.

843. Williams G, Pickup J, Clark A, et al. Changes in blood flow close to subcutaneous insulin injection sites in stable and brittle diabetics. Diabetes 1983; 32:466–473.

844. Affholter JA, Fried VA, Roth RA. Human insulin-degrading enzyme shares structural and functional homologies with *E. coli* protease III. Science 1988; 242:1415–1418.

845. Schade DS, Eaton RP, Warhol RM, et al. Subcutaneous peritoneal access device for type I diabetic patients nonresponsive to subcutaneous insulin. Diabetes 1982; 31:470–473.

846. Shichiri M, Kawamori R, Hakui N, et al. Closed-loop glycemic control with a wearable artificial endocrine pancreas. Variations in daily insulin requirements to glycemic response. Diabetes 1984; 33:1200–1202.

847. Brown L, Muhoz C, Siemer L, et al. Controlled release of insulin from polymer matrices. Control of diabetes in rats. Diabetes 1986; 35:692–697.

848. Wang PY. Prolonged release of insulin by cholesterol-matrix implant. Diabetes 1987; 36:1068–1072.

849. Salzman R, Manson JE, Griffin GT, et al. Intranasal aerosolized insulin. Mixed-meal studies and long term use in type I diabetes. N Engl J Med 1985; 312:1078–1084.

850. Frauman AG, Cooper ME, Parsono BJ, et al. Long-term use of intranasal insulin in insulin-dependent diabetic patients. Diabetes Care 1987; 10:573–578.

851. Altman JJ, Houlbert D, Callerd P, et al. Long-term plasma glucose normalization in experimental diabetic rats with microencapsulated implants of benign human insulinomas. Diabetes 1986; 35:625–633.

852. American Diabetes Association. Principles of nutrition and dietary recommendations for individuals with diabetes mellitus: 1979. Diabetes 1979; 28:1027–1030.

853. Hollenbeck CB, Coulston AM, Reaven GM, et al. Opinion leaders forum. The diabetic dietary prescription: an ongoing controversy. Diab Nutr Metab 1988; 3:239–254.

854. Garg A, Bonanome A, Grundy SM, et al. Comparison of a high-carbohydrate diet in patients with non–insulin-dependent diabetes mellitus. N Engl J Med 1988; 319:829–834.

855. Garg A, Grundy SM. Lovastatin for lowering cholesterol levels in non–insulin-dependent diabetes mellitus. N Engl J Med 1988; 318:81–86.

856. Bantle JP, Laine DC, Castle GW, et al. Postprandial glucose and insulin responses to meals containing different carbohydrates in normal and diabetic subjects. N Engl J Med 1983; 309:7–12.

857. Crapo PA, Olefsky JM. Food fallacies and blood sugar. N Engl J Med 1983; 309:44–45.

858. Arky RA. Nutritional management of the diabetic. In: Ellenberg M, Rifkin H, eds. Diabetes Mellitus. Theory and Practice. 3rd ed. New Hyde Park, NY: Medical Examination Publishing, 1983: 539–566.

859. Kemmer FW, Berger M. Therapy and better quality of life: the dichotomous role of exercise in diabetes mellitus. Diabetes Metab Rev 1986; 2:53–68.

860. Wahren J, Felig P, Hagenfeldt L. Physical exercise and fuel homeostasis in diabetes mellitus. Diabetologia 1978; 14:213–222.

861. DeFronzo RA, Ferrannini E, Sato Y, et al. Synergistic interaction between exercise and insulin on peripheral glucose uptake. J Clin Invest 1981; 68:1468–1474.

862. Zinman B, Murray FT, Vranic M, et al. Glucoregulation during moderate exercise in insulin-treated diabetics. J Clin Endocrinol Metab 1977; 45:641–652.

863. Kemmer FW, Berchtold P, Berger M, et al. Exercise-induced fall of blood glucose in insulin-treated diabetics unrelated to alteration of insulin mobilization. Diabetes 1979; 28:1131–1137.

864. Martin MJ, Robbins DC, Bergenstal R, et al. Absence of exercise-induced hypoglycaemia in type I (insulin-dependent) diabetic patients during maintenance of normoglycaemia by short-term, open-loop insulin infusion. Diabetologia 1982; 23:337–342.

865. Poussier P, Zinman B, Marliss EB, et al. Open-loop intravenous insulin waveforms for postprandial exercise in type I diabetes. Diabetes Care 1983; 6:129–134.

866. Pfeifer MA, Halter JB, Porte D Jr. Insulin secretion in diabetes mellitus. Am J Med 1981; 70:579–588.

867. Prince MJ, Olefsky JM. Direct in vitro effect of a sulfonylurea to increase human fibroblast insulin receptors. J Clin Invest 1980; 66:608–611.

868. Salhanick AI, Konowitz P, Amatruda JM. Potentiation of insulin action by a sulfonylurea in primary cultures of hepatocytes from normal and diabetic rats. Diabetes 1983; 32:206–212.

869. Vigneri R, Pezzino V, Wong KY, et al. Comparison of the in vitro effect of biguanides and sulfonylureas on insulin binding to its receptors in target cells. J Clin Endocrinol Metab 1982; 54:95–100.

870. Maloff BL, Lockwood DH. In vitro effects of a sulfonylurea on insulin action in adipocytes. Potentiation of insulin-stimulated hexose transport. J Clin Invest 1981; 68:85–90.

871. Putnam WS, Andersen DK, Jones RS, et al. Selective potentiation of insulin-mediated glucose disposal in normal dogs by the sulfonylurea glipizide. J Clin Invest 1981; 67:1016–1023.

872. Groop L, Luzi L, Melander A, et al. Different effects of glyburide and glipizide on insulin secretion and hepatic glucose production in normal and NIDDM subjects. Diabetes 1987; 36:1320–1328.

873. Lebovitz HE, Feinglos MN. The oral hypoglycemic agents. In: Ellenberg M, Rifkin H, eds. Diabetes Mellitus. Theory and Practice. 3rd ed. New Hyde Park, NY: Medical Examination Publishing, 1983: 591–610.

874. Sartor G, Scherstén B, Carlstöm S, et al. Ten-year follow-up of subjects with impaired glucose tolerance. Prevention of diabetes by tolbutamide and diet regulation. Diabetes 1980; 29:41–49.

875. Misbin RI. Phenformin-associated lactic acidosis: pathogenesis and treatment. Ann Intern Med 1977; 87:591–595.

876. Cohen RD, Woods HF. Lactic acidosis revisited. Diabetes 1983; 32:181–191.

877. Unger RH, Madison LL, Carter NW. Tolbutamide-phenformin in ketoacidosis-resistant patients. JAMA 1960; 174:2132–2136.

878. Caspary WF. Sucrose malabsorption in man after ingestion of α-glucosidehydrolase inhibitor. Lancet 1978; 1:1231–1233.

879. Taylor RH, Jenkins DJA, Barker HM, et al. Effect of acarbose on the 24-hour blood glucose profile and pattern of carbohydrate absorption. Diabetes Care 1982; 5:92–96.

880. Kawazu S, Suzuki M, Negishi K, et al. Initial phase II clinical studies on midaglizole (DG-5128). A new hypoglycemic agent. Diabetes 1987; 36:221–226.

881. Chang AY, Wyse BM, Gilchrist BJ, et al. Ciglitazone, a new hypoglycemic agent. I. Studies in ob/ob and db/db mice, diabetic Chinese hamsters, and normal and streptozotocin-diabetic rats. Diabetes 1983; 32:830–838.

882. Chang AY, Wyse BM, Gilchrist BJ. Ciglitazone, a new hypoglycemic agent. II. Effect on glucose and lipid metabolisms and insulin binding in the adipose tissue of C57BL/6J-ob/ob and −+/? mice. Diabetes 1983; 32:839–845.

883. Reaven GM, Chang H, Hoffman BB. Additive hypoglycemic effects of drugs that modify free-fatty acid metabolism by different mechanisms in rats with streptozotocin-induced diabetes. Diabetes 1988; 37:28–32.

884. Stiller CR, Dupré J, Gent M, et al. Effects of cyclosporine immunosuppression in insulin-dependent diabetes mellitus of recent onset. Science 1984; 223:1362–1367.

885. Assan R, Bach JF, DuRostu H, et al. Metabolic and immunological effect of cyclosporine in recently diagnosed type I diabetes mellitus. Lancet 1985; 1:67–71.

886. Canadian-European Randomized Control Trial: cyclosporin in insulin-dependent diabetes mellitus (IDDM). Clin Invest Med 1987; 10:1365 (abstract).

887. Tominaga M, Komiya I, Johnson JH, et al. Loss of insulin response to glucose but not arginine during development of autoimmune diabetes in BB/W rats: relationship to islet volume and glucose transport rate. Proc Natl Acad Sci USA 1986; 83:9749–9753.

888. Dupré J, Stiller CR, Jenner M, et al. Responses to nutrients in non–insulin-requiring (NIR) remission of type I diabetes during administration of cyclosporine. Diabetes 1987; 36(Suppl 1):74A (abstract).

889. Myers BD, Ross J, Newton L, et al. Cyclosporin-associated nephropathy. N Engl J Med 1984; 311:699–705.

890. Mihatsch MJ, Thiel G, Ryffel B. Ciclosporin-associated nephropathy. In: Schindler R, ed. Ciclosporin in Autoimmune Diseases. Berlin: Springer-Verlag, 1985: 50–58.

891. Alberti KGMM, Hockaday TDR. Diabetic coma: a reappraisal after five years. Clin Endocrinol Metab 1977; 6:421–455.

892. Clements RS Jr, Vourganti B. Fatal diabetic ketoacidosis: major causes and approaches to their prevention. Diabetes Care 1978; 1:314–325.

893. Wilson HK, Keuer SP, Lea AS, et al. Phosphate therapy in diabetic ketoacidosis. Arch Intern Med 1982; 142:517–520.

894. Keller U, Berger W. Prevention of hypophosphatemia by phosphate infusion during treatment of diabetic ketoacidosis and hyperosmolar coma. Diabetes 1980; 29:87–95.

895. Matz R. Diabetic acidosis. Rationale for not using bicarbonate. NY State J Med 1976; 76:1299–1303.

896. Kitabchi AE. Low-dose insulin therapy in diabetic ketoacidosis: fact or fiction? Diabetes Metab Rev 1989; 5:337–363.

897. Lever E, Jaspan JB. Sodium bicarbonate therapy in severe diabetic ketoacidosis. Am J Med 1983; 75:263–268.

898. Artis WM, Fountain JA, Delcher KH, et al. A mechanism of susceptibility to mucormycosis in diabetic ketoacidosis: transferrin and iron availability. Diabetes 1982; 31:1109–1114.

899. Paton RC. Haemostatic changes in diabetic coma. Diabetologia 1981; 21:172–177.

900. Rosenbloom AL, Riley WJ, Weber FT, et al. Cerebral edema complicating diabetic ketoacidosis in childhood. J Pediatr 1980; 96:357–361.

901. Franklin B, Liu J, Ginsberg-Fellner F. Cerebral edema and ophthalmoplegia reversed by mannitol in a new case of insulin-dependent diabetes mellitus. Pediatrics 1982; 69:87–90.

902. Fein IA, Rackow EC, Sprung CL, et al. Relation of colloid osmotic pressure to arterial hypoxemia and cerebral edema during crystalloid volume loading of patients with diabetic ketoacidosis. Ann Intern Med 1982; 96:570–575.

903. Carroll P, Matz R. Adult respiratory distress syndrome complicating severely uncontrolled diabetes mellitus: report of nine cases and a review of the literature. Diabetes Care 1982; 5:574–580.

904. Grundy SM. Drug therapy: HMG-CoA reductase inhibitors for treatment of hypercholesterolemia. N Engl J Med 1988; 319:24–32.

905. Brownlee M, Vlassara H, Kooney A, et al. Aminoguanidine prevents diabetes-induced arterial wall cross-linking. Science 1986; 232:1629–1632.

906. Folkman J, Weisz PB, Joullié MM, et al. Control of angiogenesis with synthetic heparin substitutes. Science 1989; 243:1490–1493.

907. Folkman J. Successful treatment of an angiogenic disease. N Engl J Med 1989; 320:1211–1212.

908. Faustman D, Hauptfeld V, Lacy P, et al. Demonstration of active tolerance in maintenance of established islet of Langerhans allografts. Proc Natl Acad Sci USA 1982; 79:4153–4155.

909. Voss F, Brewin A, Dawidson I, et al. Transplantation of proliferated preislet cells into diabetic patient with renal transplants. Transplant Proc 1989; 21:2751–2756.

910. Jovanovic-Peterson L, Williams K, Brennan M, et al. Studies of human fetal pancreatic allografts in diabetic recipients without immunosuppression. J Diabetic Complications 1989; 3:107–112.

911. Sutherland DER. Who should get a pancreas transplant? Diabetes Care 1988; 11:681–685.

912. The University of Michigan Pancreas Transplant Committee. Pancreatic transplantation as treatment for IDDM. Proposed candidate criteria before end-stage diabetic nephropathy. Diabetes Care 1988; 11:669–675.

913. Rotter JI, Anderson CE, Rimoin DL. Genetics of diabetes mellitus. In: Ellenberg M, Rifkin H, eds. Diabetes Mellitus. Theory and Practice. 3rd ed. New Hyde Park, NY: Medical Examination Publishing, 1983: 481–503.

914. Given BD, Mako ME, Tager HS, et al. Diabetes due to secretion of an abnormal insulin. N Engl J Med 1980; 302:129–135.

915. Shoelson S, Haneda M, Blix P, et al. Three mutant insulins in man. Nature 1983; 302:540–543.

916. Kwok SCM, Steiner DF, Rubenstein AH, et al. Identification of a point mutation in the human insulin gene giving rise to a structurally abnormal insulin (insulin Chicago). Diabetes 1983; 32:872–875.

917. Taylor SI, Dons RF, Hernandez E, et al. Insulin resistance associated with androgen excess in women with autoantibodies to the insulin receptor. Ann Intern Med 1982; 97:851–855.

918. Flier JS, Bar RS, Muggeo M, et al. The evolving clinical course of patients with insulin receptor autoantibodies: spontaneous remission or receptor proliferation with hypoglycemia. J Clin Endocrinol Metab 1978; 47:985–995.

919. Taylor SI, Grunberger G, Marcus-Samuels B, et al. Hypoglycemia associated with antibodies to the insulin receptor. N Engl J Med 1982; 307:1422–1426.

920. Dons RF, Havlik R, Taylor SI, et al. Clinical disorders associated with autoantibodies to the insulin receptor. Simulation by passive transfer of immunoglobulins to rats. J Clin Invest 1983; 72:1072–1080.

921. Kawanishi K, Kawamura K, Nishina Y, et al. Successful immunosuppressive therapy in insulin resistant diabetes caused by anti–insulin receptor autoantibodies. J Clin Endocrinol Metab 1977; 44:15–21.

922. Muggeo M, Flier JS, Abrams RA, et al. Treatment by plasma exchange of a patient with autoantibodies to the insulin receptor. N Engl J Med 1979; 300:477–480.

923. Kahn CR, Goldstein BJ. Molecular defects in insulin action. Science 1989; 245:13.

924. Taira M, Taira M, Hashimoto N, et al. Human diabetes associated with a deletion of the tyrosine kinase domain of the insulin receptor. Science 1989; 245:63–66.

925. Odawara M, Kodowaki T, Yamamoto R, et al. Human diabetes associated with a mutation in the tyrosine kinase domain of the insulin receptor. Science 1989; 245:66–68.

25

EATING DISORDERS: OBESITY, ANOREXIA NERVOSA, AND BULIMIA NERVOSA

Daniel W. Foster

Although obesity and anorexia nervosa are not primary endocrine disorders, patients with either condition are often referred for evaluation to ensure that hormonal dysfunction is not primary. Moreover, both conditions are accompanied by changes in the endocrine system. For these reasons, it seems appropriate to review the illnesses in a textbook devoted to endocrinology.

OBESITY

Obesity refers to an excess of body fat. In most cases it develops in the absence of any underlying disease process; rarely it is due to another primary disorder (e.g., Cushing syndrome). At one level the cause of obesity is understood. It is always due to greater energy intake than is expended. The mystery lies in the cause of the energy imbalance. In an organism in which precisely regulated feedback systems normally function to maintain steady-state conditions of health, the fundamental question is why caloric intake becomes disproportionate to body needs. This is especially so in the case of the extreme obesity categorized as massive or morbid, a condition that makes life dysfunctional for both cosmetic and physiological reasons before it extracts a higher cost: premature death.[1, 2] Although numerous investigations have been carried out since the last edition of this book, definitive answers remain elusive. What is known is reviewed in this chapter.

Definitions of Obesity

All definitions of obesity are arbitrary because the distribution of weight in the general population describes a curve rather than segregating into distinct populations of obese and nonobese.[3] Unfortunately, the various methods for evaluating fatness do not give the same answers when compared directly.[4, 5] It is therefore not easy to derive precise criteria for diagnosis.

Several approaches have been taken. The first utilizes techniques designed to measure the amount of fat in the body directly. Values are established for persons presumed to be normal, and obesity is defined by a percentage of body fat outside the normal range in statistical terms. A second approach depends on indirect estimates of body fat by using methods that have been correlated with the direct measurements. A third technique is to define obesity in terms of risk to life, i.e., significant obesity is the level of overweight that causes excess mortality relative to an idealized normal weight. This approach depends on life insurance data and utilizes tables of desirable weights for height and age. Finally, fatness can be defined visually: a person who looks fat probably is fat.[6] This technique is the only one that is not statistically based; only two groups are identified, fat and nonfat.

DIRECT TECHNIQUES FOR ESTIMATING BODY FAT. A number of procedures are available for measurement of body fat, some clinically applicable and others research tools. They include densitometry, estimates of total body water, measurement of total body potassium, neutron activation techniques, computed tomographic (CT) and magnetic resonance imaging (MRI) scans, and electrical methods measuring impedance and conductivity.[5] All have limitations because fixed assumptions are made that may not hold for the individual under study.

Densitometry. Densitometry is generally considered to be the "gold standard" for estimating body fat. Underwater weighing is the usual approach for assessment of body volume. It is assumed that fat-free tissue and fat have different densities, which are fixed. Standard formulas also assume that hydration of tissues is constant and that bone mineral content is fixed. The data supporting these assumptions are minuscule. One widely used "reference body" was based on measurements from only three cadavers. Formulas in the literature vary considerably in their constants.[4, 5] Four examples illustrate:

$$\% \text{ fat} = 100 \left(\frac{5.053}{\text{density}} - 4.164 \right) \quad (1)$$

$$\% \text{ fat} = 100 \left(\frac{4.201}{\text{density}} - 3.813 \right) \quad (2)$$

$$\% \text{ fat} = 100 \left(\frac{4.570}{\text{density}} - 4.142 \right) \quad (3)$$

$$\% \text{ fat} = 100 \left(\frac{4.950}{\text{density}} - 4.50 \right) \quad (4)$$

All give roughly the same answers, however, the usual error probably not exceeding 4%.[7] In the four formulas listed, a measured body density of 1.060 would give percent fat values of 15, 15, 17, and 17%, respectively.

Total Body Water Estimates. Measurements of total body water are usually carried out with tritiated or deuterated water, although ^{18}O can also be used as a label for water. Isotope dilution is measured at steady state, usually 2 to 3 hours after administration. It is assumed that water in the body is limited to fat-free mass. The lean body mass is calculated from the assumption of a fixed percentage of water in lean tissue, usually 70 to 72%. Body fat is then taken as the difference between weight and calculated lean body mass, with a correction for the skeleton. Even if total water content is accurately measured, the percentage of water in the tissues varies in individuals. In lean tissue taken at autopsy, water content ranges from 69.3 to 77.5%.[4] The effects of such differences can be dramatic; a change of constant from 70 to 77% can result in a 10-kg difference in estimated body fat content.

Total Body Potassium Measurements. Estimates of lean body weight can also be made via measurement of total potassium in the body, if it is assumed that potassium is essentially limited to the fat-free compartment.[8] This measurement can be done either by isotope dilution using ^{42}K or by determining ^{40}K in a whole body counter. Various constants have been suggested.[5] Once again the assumption of a fixed constant renders estimated values suspect because the potassium content per kilogram of intracellular water in lean tissue varies from individual to individual.

Other Methods.[5, 9] Other methods for estimation of fat content have been reported, but experience with them is limited. Neutron activation appears to be accurate, although constants are based on data from a few dogs. It is claimed that the technique can give values for body water, ash, lean tissue, and fat mass. Expense precludes wide use. Regional fat content can be assessed by CT or MRI, but values applied to the whole body are problematic. Measurement of electrical impedance is inexpensive and appears to be fairly accurate. Dual photon beam absorptiometry also has promise.

In summary, methods for directly estimating body fat utilize constants often based on minimal data. They are probably adequate for broad comparisons of groups of patients and for longitudinal study of individual subjects, but absolute values may not be accurate. Validation by chemical measurement of total fat in the body is obviously not possible in humans. The upper limit of normality for percent fat has been listed as 19% for men and 22% for women,[10] but other studies have shown higher values in nonobese subjects.[8]

INDIRECT TECHNIQUES FOR ESTIMATING BODY FAT.
Skinfold Measurements. The percentage of body fat can be estimated by measuring the width of subcutaneous skinfolds with calibrated calipers.[4, 11] The best correlations appear to require four skinfold measurements (biceps, triceps, subscapular, and suprailiac), but acceptable values can be obtained with two measurements.[11–13] Equations and nomograms are available for conversion of skinfold thickness to body fat.[12, 13] Although there are some technical problems, such as the amount of pressure that should be applied to the calipers, the primary difficulty is that fat distribution may differ in individuals who have the same amount of total adipose tissue. Thus in some forms of obesity the fat distribution is generalized, whereas in others the fat is largely abdominal.[14] Estimates of percent fat will be inaccurate insofar as distribution is skewed. In addition to these anatomical variations, the ratio of subcutaneous fat to deep fat also varies, values being reported to range from 0.1 to 0.7.[11] This variation is important because in some patients the bulk of new fat may be deposited in the abdomen and not be accurately reflected by skinfold measurement. For example, body fat increases with aging, whereas skinfold thickness does not.[9] Despite these potential difficulties, skinfold measurements are adequate for longitudinal study of body composition in individuals and appear to provide useful information in cross-sectional studies of the population.[15, 16]

Obesity is usually delineated by comparison of skinfold measurements in the test subject with values obtained in young men and nonpregnant women. Data from the Health and Nutrition Examination Survey 1971–1974 (HANES) in the United States were used to define severe obesity as a combined skinfold measurement (triceps and subscapular) above the 95th percentile for ages 20 to 29.[16] The absolute value for the upper limits of normal was 51 mm in men and 70 mm in women. A different definition of obesity was utilized in the Ten State Nutritional Survey; any value above the 85th percentile (triceps measurement alone) was considered to be abnormal.[3] Thus attention to definitions of obesity is imperative when comparing the results of surveys.

Weight/Height Ratios. The most widely used clinical tool for the assessment of obesity is the body mass index (BMI), defined as weight divided by the square of the height (W/H²), in kilograms per meter. Correlation with body fat measured directly by densitometry is quite good.[17] Although the denominator in the BMI is generally taken as H² in adults, a variable formula is preferable in children.[17] A BMI of 25 is ordinarily taken as the upper limit of normal, with the span 25 to 29.9 considered to be overweight, and 30 or greater, obesity.[17] Some investigators set the figures for women slightly lower (the upper limit of normal is 23.8),[17] but in practice this does not appear to be necessary. Formulas have been derived for calculating percent fat in the body from the BMI: (1) for men: % fat = 1.218(W/H²) − 10.13; (2) for women, % fat = 1.48(W/H²) − 7.[17]

Morbidity and mortality can be predicted from BMI values.[18] Excess mortality begins to appear in the range 25 to 30, but significant increases in mortality occur only at BMI values higher than 30. Bray[9, 18] has categorized risks as follows: BMI value of 20 to 25, very low; 25 to 30, low; 30

to 35, moderate; 35 to 40, high; and above 40, very high. Risk can be further assessed by measurement of waist/hip ratios (see next section). Thus a person with a BMI value between 30 and 35, who is normally considered to be at moderate risk, would be reclassified as high risk if the waist/hip ratio were elevated.[9]

Waist/Hip Ratios. All fat is not equal. A large number of studies indicate that complications of obesity correlate with abdominal fat and less well with lower body fat (buttocks and legs).[14, 19] The term *android* is sometimes used for central ("beer belly") obesity; *gynoid* is the adjective chosen for obesity of the lower body that is often seen in women. The distal localization of fat in some women may be so extreme as to suggest a forme fruste of partial lipodystrophy—the ribs easily visible, the waist not enlarged, but the buttocks and legs significantly, even massively, obese. Distribution is assessed clinically by measuring the circumference of the waist and hips and expressing the values as a ratio. The waist is measured at the narrowest point between the rib cage and iliac crests; the hips are measured at the maximal point for the buttocks. Although values higher than 0.72 are considered abnormal,[9] complication rates increase substantially at ratios higher than 1.0 for men and 0.9 for women,[18] which suggests that these values are threshold levels for assignment of clinical risk. The impact of fat distribution is not minor. For example, although obesity imparted a relative risk for diabetes of 3.7 in a group of white women, central obesity increased the risk to 10.3.[19] (It is not that obesity of the lower body has no risk, only that the risks are much lower.) The relation is even more complicated in that deep abdominal fat appears to be more detrimental than subcutaneous fat.[20] Deep and superficial fat can be differentiated by CT, but clinically this is unnecessary. The larger the abdominal girth, the greater the amount of deep fat.

STANDARD TABLES. The most widely used standards for acceptable weight of adults in the United States have been those provided by the Metropolitan Life Insurance Company. These tables base the definition of acceptable weights on mortality experience in age- and sex-ranked weights per height at the time of entry into the life insurance system; i.e., the acceptable ranges were those encompassing the lowest mortality of the insured in each height/weight category. Separate ranges were established for small, medium, and large frames, although no definitions for these categories were ever provided. For this reason the Fogarty Conference on obesity in America suggested a modification in which "average weight" was considered to be the median value for medium frame at each height, and the acceptable range was bracketed by the lowest weight for a small frame and highest weight for a large frame.[21] One little-recognized alteration was that the original heights and weights from the Metropolitan tables were obtained with subjects clothed and wearing shoes, whereas the Fogarty tables list acceptable weights and heights that were obtained without clothes or shoes. It has been recommended that 2.54 cm (1 inch) be added to the heights and 2.3 and 1.4 kg (5 and 3 lb) to the weights of men and women, respectively, in the Fogarty tables when making comparisons with the data from the 1979 Build Study.[10] The convention of using an acceptable range of weights without referral to frame size has been widely accepted.[17]

New tables of desirable weight were published in 1983 based on the 1979 Build Study of the Society of Actuaries and Association of Life Insurance Medical Directors of America.[10] The new standards, modified to conform to the Fogarty Conference style, are shown in Table 25–1.

The interpretation of these data is complicated by several factors. First, the data are based on a preselected sample of the population defined by willingness or ability to purchase life insurance; presumably, those of lower socioeconomic status are under-represented. Second, the data are not broken down by age or race. Third, persons accepted for insurance probably had no obvious major illness, which suggests that the sample was likely healthier at the start than the population as a whole. Fourth, 10% of the weights and heights were taken from history rather than by measurements, and a bias toward rounding off weights in 2.3-kg (5-lb) increments and heights in even inches was acknowledged.[10] Despite these difficulties, the data are valuable because they are based on large numbers (nearly 4 million

TABLE 25–1. Acceptable Weights from the 1983 Metropolitan Height and Weight Tables*

| Height | | Women | | | | Men | | | |
| Height | | Average Weight | | Acceptable Range | | Average Weight | | Acceptable Range | |
cm	in	KG	LB	KG	LB	KG	LB	KG	LB
147	58	52	115	46–60	102–131	—	—	—	—
150	59	53	117	46–61	103–134	—	—	—	—
152	60	54	120	47–62	104–137	—	—	—	—
155	61	55	122	48–64	106–140	—	—	—	—
157	62	57	125	49–65	108–143	62	136	58–68	128–150
160	63	58	128	50–67	111–147	63	138	59–70	130–153
163	64	60	131	52–69	114–151	64	140	60–71	132–156
165	65	61	134	53–70	117–155	65	143	61–73	134–160
168	66	62	137	54–72	120–159	66	145	62–75	136–164
170	67	64	140	56–74	123–163	67	148	63–76	138–168
173	68	65	143	57–76	126–167	69	151	64–78	140–172
175	69	66	146	59–77	129–170	70	154	65–80	142–176
178	70	68	149	60–79	132–173	71	157	65–82	144–180
180	71	69	152	61–80	135–176	73	160	66–84	146–184
183	72	70	155	63–81	138–179	75	164	68–85	149–188
185	73	—	—	—	—	76	167	69–87	152–192
188	74	—	—	—	—	78	171	70–90	155–197
190	75	—	—	—	—	80	175	72–92	158–202
193	76	—	—	—	—	81	179	74–94	162–207

*Average weight is midpoint for acceptable range of weights listed for medium frame in Metropolitan tables. The acceptable range is bracketed by the lowest acceptable weight for a small frame and the highest acceptable weight for a large frame. Heights are measured with the person wearing shoes and weights, indoor clothing. To convert to height without shoes, the recommendation is subtraction of 2.5 cm or 1 inch. For weight without clothes, subtract 2.3 kg (5 lb) for men and 1.4 kg (3 lb) for women.

Adapted with permission from Metropolitan Life Insurance Company from tables published in Metropolitan Life Foundation Statistical Bulletin 1983 (Jan.-June); 64:2–9. Raw data from Build Study, 1979. Society of Actuaries and Association of Life Insurance Medical Directors of America, 1980.

policies in men and almost 600,000 policies in women) and because they are related to actual experience insofar as mortality is concerned.

How the tables should be used to estimate obesity in the population is uncertain. Some authors consider 20% above average weight as defined in Table 25–1 to be equivalent to obesity,[15] whereas the working party of the Royal College of Physicians[17] chose the defining line as 20% above the upper limit of acceptable range of the Fogarty table (i.e., 20% above the highest acceptable weight for a large frame at each height). The latter appears to be preferable because this value correlates best with data showing risk per excess weight.

Tables of standard weights are also available for children,[17, 22] and the same problems apply. Again, 20% above average weight for height, age, and sex is often chosen as the dividing point between obese and nonobese.[23]

Life insurance data indicate that average weights of men increase up to age 50 and then fall off, whereas those of women continue to increase to age 60. Similar results were obtained by using measurements of skinfold thickness to assess body fat.[3] Some authors believe that the age-related increase in mean weight is not necessarily normal or healthy and therefore define desirable weight as that found in men and nonpregnant women in young adulthood, usually ages 20 to 29.[16, 21] The prevalence of obesity will obviously be judged higher with such a standard than in the 1979 Build Study, which accepts increasing weight with age as normal.[10] Because there are no firm data on the relationship between body weight and morbidity, relative mortality rates probably give the best indication of the level of obesity that places a person at risk to health, the difficulties already mentioned notwithstanding. The 1979 Build Study indicates that the lowest mortality for men was bracketed by the span −15 to +5% of average weight. Average weight was defined as the mean weight per height for all patients in a given age interval. Although absolute mean weights increase each decade, mortality experience was related to percent over- or underweight for the given age interval, so that age factors out and data can be related to the entire male and female population in the study. The lowest mortality in women was found in the span −15 to −5% of average weight. Table 25–2 shows the ratios of actual to expected mortality relative to percent deviations of weight. Significant excess mortality begins to appear in men in the +15 to +25% bracket (117%) but does not clearly manifest itself in women until the +45 to +55% range. This difference suggests that use of a single criterion for obesity in men and women[17] may be

in error. From the data of Table 25–2 it appears that 20% above average weight might be proper for diagnosis of obesity in men, whereas the appropriate figure for women might be as high as 50% above average weight. The findings seem to indicate that women tolerate obesity better than men from the standpoint of accelerated mortality. Other data suggest that even mild obesity in women confers increased risk of death from cardiovascular disease.[1]

SUMMARY. For research purposes densitometry is probably the method of choice for estimating body fat content. However, even densitometry has to be supplemented by assessment of fat distribution for meaningful interpretations to be drawn. Risk may be assessed clinically by calculating the BMI and a waist/hip ratio. More sophisticated techniques are usually not necessary.

Prevalence of Obesity

The prevalence of obesity varies depending on the definition used. With the data of the 1979 Build Study and a figure of 20% or more above average weight as representing obesity, only 4% of men and 10% of women would be judged obese.[10] This method obviously understates the problem because a rise in weight with age was considered normal. If one compares values with ideal weights at ages 20 to 29, higher figures are obtained: 14% of men and 24% of women are more than 20% above acceptable levels. In the United Kingdom, 39% of men and 32% of women were considered *overweight* on the basis of a BMI of 25 or higher, but only 6% of men and 8% of women were defined as *obese* (BMI 30 or higher).[17] If obesity is defined as skinfold thickness greater than the 95th percentile of adults between the ages of 20 and 29, 5% of men and 7% of women were judged obese in the first HANES survey.[16] If the cutoff point was decreased to the 85th percentile, 13% of men and 22.7% of women were ranked as fat. There was a lower prevalence in black men than in white men (11.6 vs. 13.3%), whereas black women were more likely to be fat than their white counterparts (31.2 vs. 21.8%).[24] Highest percentages (49%) were seen in black women aged 45 to 64 whose incomes were below the poverty level. The National Institutes of Health Consensus Development Conference on Health Implications of Obesity, utilizing the data of HANES 2 (1976 to 1980), accepted an estimate that 26% of Americans are overweight, although not all of these individuals would be considered obese.[25] On balance, utilizing the least stringent definitions, it appears that serious adult obesity has an upper limit of prevalence in both the United States and the United Kingdom (uncorrected for age, sex, or race) of no more than 15% for men and 25% for women. These values seem surprising given the general impression that major obesity is a common affliction, at least in the United States. However, when 5291 persons were observed making food choices in public eating places and classified by appearance against profiles of body type into normal, overweight, or obese, only 10% were placed in the obese category.[6] It seems likely that gross obesity would have been readily recognized and so classified. Despite statements to the contrary, there is likewise no firm evidence that the prevalence of obesity is increasing. With the criterion of 20% above desirable weight, the figures in the United States for 1960 to 1962 were 14.5% in men and 25% in women; equivalent figures in 1971 to 1974 were 14% in men and 23.8% in women.[21] Caution regarding acceptance of the conclusions that prevalence of obesity is no greater than 25% at a maximum and that the prevalence of obesity is not increasing would seem warranted because no large population survey is available from the 1980s. It is conceivable that significant change could have occurred in the last decade. The 1979 Build Study indicates that the

TABLE 25–2. Ratio of Actual to Expected Mortality as a Function of Relative Weight*

| | Actual/Expected Mortality × 100 | |
% Deviation	Men	Women
−25 to −35	117	128
−15 to −25	102	111
− 5 to −15	95	93
±5	95	97
+ 5 to +15	106	100
+15 to +25	117	109
+25 to +35	130	103
+35 to +45	139	109
+45 to +55	168	131
+55 to +65	186	140

*Percent deviation refers to excess or deficit above mean weight per height, stratified according to age. Data shown are cumulative values for all ages. Mortality ratio represents actual deaths in deviating range relative to overall mortality in sample.

Data from Build Study, 1979. Society of Actuaries and Association of Life Insurance Medical Directors of America, 1980.

general population became heavier in the interval 1955 to 1979. Shift of the weight-per-height curves to the heavier side would mean that the "fatness" of the truly fat would be more prominent. This could account for the fact that the population looks fatter, although the statistical definition of obesity based on percentages above a population-derived acceptable weight range has not changed.

Natural History of Obesity

It is not possible to describe a single natural history of obesity because the abnormality is not a single disease and because long-term, large-scale follow-up in individuals is not available. Thus one is limited to cross-sectional surveys in the population and some clinical judgments. A typical cross-sectional picture of fatness in a sample of the general population, assessed by measurement of the triceps skinfold, is shown in Figure 25–1. The results affirm that fat content is greater in women than in men and that there is a gradual overall increase in fat from prepuberty until the sixth or seventh decade of life, when adiposity decreases. The illustration shown is for white persons, but the pattern is qualitatively similar in black individuals. In the Ten State Nutritional Survey, from which these data are taken, black girls had less fat than their white counterparts until ages 17 to 18, after which the curves crossed; i.e., in adulthood, black women were fatter than white women.[3] Black men persistently had thinner skinfolds than white men. The pattern shown in Figure 25–1 is thought to reflect the usual sequence of modest obesity that characterizes middle age. Maturity-onset obesity presumably simply represents an exaggerated weight gain occurring against the background curve that characterizes the population as a whole.

The more critical issue has to do with prolonged obesity, i.e., obesity that is present throughout life or that begins at a very early age. The clinical impression is that such obesity tends to be more severe and that distribution of fat is generalized, involving extremities as well as the trunk, in contrast to adult-onset obesity, which frequently is central in type and spares the arms and legs. The question then becomes, does obesity as a child predispose to obesity as an adult? Arguments have been advanced on both sides.[17, 26–31]

Part of the problem is that prospective longitudinal studies have never been done. Moreover, when cohorts of children have been analyzed retrospectively, heights and weights at early ages tend to be taken from measurements in physicians' records and thus are reasonably accurate, whereas adult data often reflect patient recall.[27, 30] Subject-reported weights tend to be underestimated and heights overestimated when checked by actual measurement.[27] On balance it can be stated that fat infants have a higher chance of being obese in adulthood than nonfat infants, but that obesity is not inevitable for those in the high percentiles of weight for height, age, and sex in the early years.[17] In a typical study, 36% of infants in the 90th percentile for weight remained obese in adulthood, compared with 14% of infants below the 75th percentile.[27] Other data are similar and suggest that 40% of children with weights 20% higher than the standard remain overweight as adults.[30]

How excess weight in infancy might influence adult development is not yet known. One theory is that overnutrition might increase the total number of adipocytes or preadipocytes in the body, thus predetermining ultimate weight (or at least potential capacity for weight gain) in those whose obesity begins early in life.[31] Although focus has been placed on postnatal feeding patterns in the predisposition to adult obesity,[16] it is conceivable that intrauterine nutrition is also important. This idea follows from two observations. First, children born to mothers exposed to the Dutch famine of 1944 to 1945 during the last trimester of pregnancy and first few months of life showed a lower prevalence of adult obesity than counterparts delivered from mothers not in the famine belt.[32] Offspring of mothers experiencing famine in only the first two trimesters, by contrast, had increased rates of subsequent obesity. The differences, although statistically significant, were small. The authors suggested that undernutrition in the first two trimesters might predispose to obesity by increasing the hypothalamic drive to eat, whereas caloric deprivation in the third trimester and early infancy might limit the ultimate size of the adult adipose tissue mass. Neither interpretation could be tested.

The second observation was that the offspring of Pima Indian women with diabetes mellitus had a higher prevalence of obesity than did children of nondiabetic mothers (47.7 vs. 22.9%, respectively),[33] despite similar levels of maternal obesity estimated from the BMI. The implication is that maternal hyperglycemia, inducing fetal hyperinsulinism, caused "excessive nutrition," which would not only result in increased birth weights but also predispose to subsequent obesity.[33] Although intrauterine events may influence subsequent degrees of fatness, environmental factors (e.g., family eating patterns) are probably more important in most cases.[3, 21]

To summarize, obesity can begin at any age, but two overall patterns can be discerned. One begins in childhood or adolescence and tends to be lifelong; the other appears in middle age and represents an exaggeration of the normal pattern of adiposity shown in Figure 25–1.

What Causes Obesity?

Weight gain requires an intake of energy that is greater than its expenditure. It therefore follows that obesity occurs only in response to sustained caloric excess. Food intake need not be abnormally high during development provided physical activity is limited, although the ontogeny of obesity is ordinarily accompanied by high caloric intake. Once attained, the obese state is commonly maintained at a level of caloric intake insufficient to produce obesity because accompanying morbidity precludes active exercise. The factors predisposing to serious obesity are not completely under-

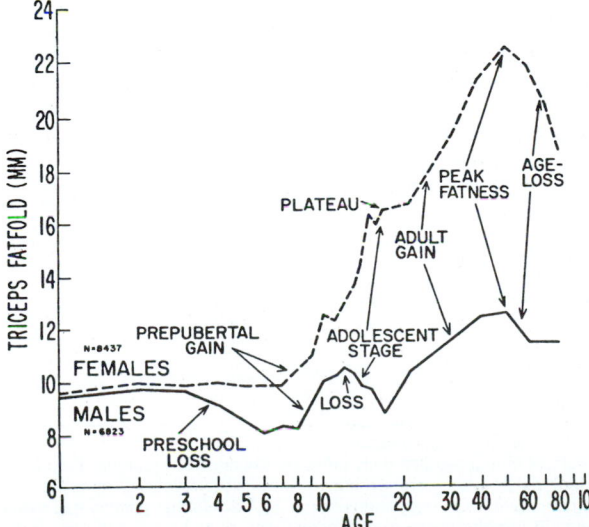

Figure 25–1. Trends in fatness related to age as assessed by triceps skinfold in a sample of the general population (n = 15,000). (From Garn SM, Clark DC. Trends in fatness and the origins of obesity. Pediatrics 1976; 57:443–456. Copyright American Academy of Pediatrics 1976.)

stood despite numerous investigations. In this section, potentially important issues are briefly reviewed.

A METABOLIC DEFECT? Obese patients frequently claim that they gain weight on amounts of food that do not cause obesity in other persons. This would imply a more efficient use of ingested calories than would be the case in lean individuals. There seems to be little doubt that some persons can maintain weight near normal despite wide swings in the amount of food eaten.[17] The example of an individual who normally ate 3000 kcal/d, but who gained only a few kilograms after ingesting 5750 kcal daily for months, is widely cited.[34] In the overfeeding experiment at the University of Vermont, volunteers of normal weight were made obese and compared with spontaneously obese subjects. It was found that 2700 kcal/m² body surface was required to maintain body weight in the volunteers at steady state, compared with an estimated 1100 to 1400 kcal/m² in the spontaneously obese.[35] The excess calories necessary to gain 1 kg of weight varied considerably even among normal subjects; for example, on a high-fat diet one subject required only 4703 kcal/kg, whereas another needed 8471 kcal/kg.[36] These findings strongly suggested a difference in metabolic efficiency between lean and obese, the former presumably having a capacity to waste calories as heat not shared by the latter. The attractiveness of this postulate was enhanced by observations in genetically obese rodents indicating a thermoregulatory defect on exposure to cold.[37] Similarly, the Kalahari Bushmen and aborigines of Australia have been shown to have a defect in defending body temperature on exposure to cold.[38] The latter are known to be highly susceptible to obesity in an urban setting where food is plentiful. Thus the idea that major obesity might be caused by or associated with a metabolic defect has received much attention.

In simple terms, heat generation in the body falls into four categories: (1) that induced by physical activity (also called the thermic effect of exercise, TEE); (2) that produced in sustaining basal metabolism (maintenance of resting structure and function in the body); (3) that released after the absorption of food (also called the thermic effect of food, TEF, or diet-induced thermogenesis, DIT); and (4) that developed to sustain body temperature (thermoregulatory or facultative thermogenesis).[39] Each is potentially a site of metabolic regulation wherein lean persons may have the capacity to modulate weight gain or loss in response to a given food intake by increasing or decreasing the fraction of calories wasted as heat. Because ingested energy can be utilized for work, heat generation, or energy storage, it follows that the greater the conversion of excess calories to heat, the lesser will be their availability for storage as fat, given a fixed requirement for work. On the basis of animal studies, it has been proposed that the propensity to develop obesity is genetically influenced through alterations in thermogenic capacity.[38–40] The idea would be that in the past, when food supply was intermittent, genetic pressure would be toward efficient metabolism so that a high percentage of food eaten would be stored to sustain the individual during periods when food was not available. This genetic defect would be manifested as obesity in societies in which food was constantly available.

Attractive as the theory is, evidence in support is inconclusive at best. Metabolic rates are usually estimated by indirect calorimetry in which oxygen uptake and carbon dioxide production are measured over short intervals. Although a number of assumptions are required and technical problems are real, results from both indirect and direct calorimetry (in which heat production is not calculated but measured) are generally comparable.[41, 42] If resting metabolic rates are reported in absolute terms, it is clear that obese subjects generate *more* heat than their lean counter-

parts.[39, 41–45] Because absolute energy expenditure relative to energy intake determines weight gain or loss, this figure would appear critical even though oxygen uptake is lower in obese than in lean controls when related to surface area, current weight, or metabolic mass (weight^0.75).[43–45] Because the resting metabolic rate increases as body mass increases, it is not possible from these data to know what the resting metabolic rate (and metabolic efficiency) was in obese persons before weight gain; i.e., it is conceivable that metabolic efficiency may be high in potentially obese persons at the beginning of weight gain (and through the dynamic phase of the development of obesity) but eventually return to normal in response to massive obesity by some sort of compensatory mechanism. It is not surprising that absolute metabolic rates are higher in obese than in normal subjects, even though adipose tissue is considered to be metabolically less active than nonfat tissues, because lean body mass always increases in the obese state.[8]

To address the question of metabolic efficiency before development of obesity, assessment of energy balances has been carried out in children who had a parent currently or previously overweight and compared with values for children whose parents had never been obese.[46] The experiment was based on the observation that obese children tend to have obese parents (see later). The heights and weights of the two groups were essentially identical, but energy expenditure in the offspring of the obese was only about 80% of that found in the children of nonobese parents (Table 25–3). Oxygen demands both at rest and during activity were less, suggesting the possibility of more efficient metabolism in the children presumably at risk for subsequent obesity because of parental involvement. The children of the obese appeared to maintain their weights at normal levels by restricting food intake.[46] The implication would be that at young age the children were eating physiologically (to meet needs) but that any subsequent increase in caloric intake might result in obesity. Energy intake was measured by bomb calorimetry in this study, but expenditures were estimated from integrated pulse rates during 4 to 7 d. Although each child had oxygen uptake calibrated with pulse rate at rest and during exercise at the beginning of the experiment, the possibility of error is greater than with direct calorimetry. It likewise is uncertain that the children characterized as potentially obese on the basis of parental weight would, in fact, become obese. Overall these data are soft and of questionable reliability.

The issue of possible differences in postprandial thermogenesis between obese and normal subjects is unsettled. Normal persons given excess calories increase heat produc-

TABLE 25–3. Daily Energy Balance in Children of Normal-Weight and Obese Parents*

	Normal Parents (n = 12)	Obese Parents (n = 8)
Height (cm)	111.3	110.7
Weight (kg)	19.1	19.5
Body fat (%)	14.3	16.8
Lean body mass (kg)	16.2	17.0
Energy intake (kcal)	1433	1115
Energy expenditure (kcal)	1508	1174
Rest	1183	999
Activity	371	190

*Energy intake was measured by bomb calorimetry. Energy expenditure was calculated from integrated daily pulse rates obtained by monitor. Before the study period, pulse rates were calibrated with oxygen uptakes at rest and during exercise. Each child was studied for 4 to 7 d. Normal parents had never been obese; in the obese group, one parent was or had been 20% above desirable weight.

Adapted from Griffiths M, Payne PR. Energy expenditure in small children of obese and non-obese parents. Reprinted by permission from Nature, Vol. 260, pp. 698–700. Copyright © 1976 Macmillan Magazines Ltd.

tion; conversely, when calories are restricted, they decrease heat production, as demonstrated by direct calorimetry.[42] In one study five currently obese and five previously obese women had about 50% less heat production after a meal than did five lean controls when assessed by indirect calorimetry.[47] Glucose-induced thermogenesis may also be impaired by obesity, presumably as a consequence of insulin resistance, although the changes are small.[48] On the other hand, other investigators have failed to show diminished dietary thermogenesis in obesity.[41, 45] An analysis of five studies of postprandial thermogenesis in which measurements were carried out by indirect calorimetry has been published.[41] The data are summarized in Table 25–4. On average, obese persons expend 7.8% of ingested calories as heat compared with 10% in normal persons, a difference that is not significant. By direct calorimetry the percentage of meal energy disposable as heat was 7% in obese and 5.9% in lean subjects.[41] In another experiment in which food intake was increased by 50%, only about 12.5% of the extra calories was recovered as heat.[42] Although most of these experiments were short term, similar results have been reported in more prolonged studies.[42] In 11 of 18 studies, dietary thermogenesis was lower in the obese than in the lean subjects, whereas in 7 there was no difference.[48] Studies with direct calorimetry show that total energy expenditure by the obese is always higher than that by the lean, including the energy utilized in postprandial thermogenesis.[49] The key factor was fat-free mass, determined by densitometry, which accounted for 81% of the variance between individuals. In most of the cited studies, meals of identical caloric content were given to lean and obese subjects. When the energy content of the test meal is made proportional to the resting metabolic rate, which in turn is determined by the lean body mass, the thermic response to a meal is not influenced by obesity.[50] Essentially all authors, even those reporting an obesity-associated defect in postprandial thermogenesis, agree that alterations in this mechanism cannot be of major importance in causing the disorder.[41, 47]

Exercise-induced thermogenesis is also not impaired in established obesity,[41, 48, 49, 51] doubtless because more energy is required to move an increased body mass. One study showed a defect in thermogenesis in obese women when exercise was combined with food, but the effect was subtle and physiologically unimportant (a 10-kcal difference for 40 min of exercise).[51]

Finally, lowering ambient temperature results in normal heat generation in obese white subjects, at least over a narrow range of temperatures.[41] It is not certain that this would be the case with more extreme changes. In one small study in which environmental temperature was dropped from 32 to 8°C, the fall in core body temperature in four women varied almost fourfold.[52] The leanest subject had the greatest increase in oxygen uptake and least fall in core temperature, and the subject with the most body fat had the least increase in oxygen uptake and the greatest fall in core temperature, but none of the subjects was truly obese. Studies with four men were also inconclusive because of the narrow range of body fat. More extensive examination of response to large temperature changes in lean and obese groups is needed.

The thermogenic response to food appears to be mediated by the sympathetic nervous system, with carbohydrate playing the major role.[48, 53, 54] When norepinephrine is infused into humans there is a small but definite rise in resting metabolic rate.[55] Some studies, reflecting results with obese rodents, have reported diminished thermogenic responses to norepinephrine in currently obese and previously obese subjects.[56, 57] This result led to speculation that heat production from brown fat, which is a key thermogenic tissue activated by norepinephrine, might be deficient or dysfunctional in obese humans (see later).[58] However, other careful studies failed to confirm a blunted response to norepinephrine in obesity.[55] Differences that have been reported might be genetically determined because obesity in Pima Indians reduced the thermogenic response to norepinephrine with overfeeding but did not do so in non–Pima Indians.[55, 57]

An intriguing observation is that heat production in individual white adipocytes taken from obese subjects by biopsy is less than it is in cells from lean controls.[59] With weight reduction, heat production per cell increased about 40%. The findings could be due to diminished futile cycle (heat-wasting) activity in the adipocytes of obese persons independent of sympathetic nervous system activity. In animals the behavior of fat cells is determined by their environment; e.g., hypertrophied fat cells from obese animals rapidly revert to normal when transplanted into lean recipients.[60, 61] It cannot be assumed, therefore, that the defect shown by microcalorimetry in the fat cells is genetically determined.

To sum up, no definitive statement can be made regarding the possibility that a metabolic defect renders heat generation from ingested food, exercise, or exposure to cold deficient in major obesity. Clinical experience and some in vivo experiments with humans suggest that differences in metabolic efficiency exist between the obese and their lean counterparts, which enables the former to gain or maintain weight more easily than the latter. On the other hand, studies of thermogenesis in patients with established obesity fail, for the most part, to show significant differences from

TABLE 25–4. Dietary Thermogenesis in Lean and Obese Subjects*

Study	Nutrient	Energy Content (kcal)	Lean Basal Expenditure (kcal/min)	Lean Thermic Effect (% of Test Meal)	Obese Basal Expenditure (kcal/min)	Obese Thermic Effect (% of Test Meal)
1	Glucose	200	1.24	4.8	1.15	11.2
2	Protein	200	1.82	8.6	1.24	31.8
3	Protein					
	a.	1000	1.13	5.4	1.04	7.2
	b.	500	1.12	4.4	0.93	9.7
4	Mixed	560	1.07	1.5	0.88	3.0
5	Glucose	300	1.26	6.9	1.09	5.7
	Protein	300	1.24	17.7	1.10	12.1
	Fat	300	1.25	8.3	1.09	4.5
Weighted mean			1.26	7.8	1.07	10.0

*Energy content of diets is rounded off to nearest 10. Conversion to kilocalories from watts reported in original table utilized conversion factors listed by authors. Weighted means were based on number of subjects in each study.

Adapted from Blaza S, Garrow JS. Thermogenic response to temperature, exercise and food stimuli in lean and obese women, studied by 24 h direct calorimetry. Br J Nutr 1983; 49:171–180, by permission of Cambridge University Press.

lean controls. It is conceivable that short-term experiments in thermogenesis fail to uncover the putative defects. Alternatively, small changes in several types of thermogenesis may function additively to account for accelerated weight gain over long periods. Perhaps more attractive is the view that metabolic efficiency is supranormal before the onset of obesity or in its dynamic phase of development, but that subsequently the defect in heat generation is overcome as obesity becomes marked.[46, 49] According to this formulation a tight coupling would exist between caloric intake and fat formation before obesity becomes major, but progressive uncoupling would occur (toward the level seen in lean persons) as a compensatory mechanism under the pressure of increasing degrees of fatness. However, the cumulative evidence is not impressive in establishing metabolic efficiency as a major contributing cause of obesity.

Although the issue of a metabolic defect in obesity is not settled, a consideration of the general principles and the possible sites of such defects may be helpful. The energy released in the oxidation of substrates is, for the most part, captured in high-energy nucleotides, especially ATP, which are then utilized to drive thermodynamically unfavorable reactions in the body. These reactions include such disparate activities as contraction of muscles and synthesis of fat. Even in the most efficient systems, energy is lost as heat; e.g., in contracting skeletal muscle, heat wastage is 30 to 50%. For regulatory purposes such as minimizing weight gain from excess calories or generating heat in the cold, focus has been placed on ATP-utilizing, heat-releasing reactions that are not coupled to useful ends.[62] Several potential sites will be discussed.

Futile Cycles in the Glycolytic-Gluconeogenic Pathway.
An example of a heat-wasting system would be the coupled reactions catalyzed by phosphofructokinase and fructose-bisphosphatase, which are key enzymes regulating reciprocal flow over glycolytic and gluconeogenic pathways in liver (Fig. 25–2). Under normal circumstances these reactions do not operate simultaneously.[63] Should they do so, fructose 6-phosphate would be converted to fructose 1,6-bisphosphate, which in turn would be hydrolyzed back to fructose 6-phosphate, with the net result that ATP would be broken down and would release heat in the absence of change in substrate concentrations, thus fulfilling the criterion of a futile cycle. Substrate cycling with ATP breakdown has been directly demonstrated at the phosphofructokinase/fructose-bisphosphatase step in humans, as has futile cycling between glucose and glucose 6-phosphate.[64] Hypothyroidism decreases cycling, but hyperthyroidism does not increase activity at these sites. A defect in catecholamine activation of

phosphofructokinase in hearts from the genetically obese Zucker rat has been reported, which raises the possibility that heat production at the phosphofructokinase/fructose-bisphosphatase site might be defective in this animal.[65]

Na+,K+-ATPase. A second potential site is the Na+,K+-ATPase of the plasma membrane. This enzyme is primarily responsible for the extrusion of sodium from intracellular water, a reaction that is catalyzed by the breakdown of ATP. Two observations focused attention on this ATPase. First, it was suggested that the metabolic effects of thyroid hormone were mediated by the enzyme, a ouabain-inhibitable protein.[66] The presumption was that the heat generation and weight loss that are characteristic of thyrotoxicosis could be accounted for in major part by increased synthesis and activity of the Na+,K+-ATPase. Second, activity of the Na+,K+-ATPase was found to be decreased in livers of mice with genetic obesity.[67] These animals could not maintain body temperature against a cold challenge, which suggests that the defect in Na+,K+-ATPase was functionally important and that it accounted for the defective capacity to expend energy as heat. The animals were thus at risk for hypothermia from cold and obesity from food.

Subsequently it was reported by some[68–70] but not all[71, 72] authors that the Na+,K+-ATPase in erythrocytes of obese humans was reduced. Interpretation of the findings is complicated by the fact that some obese patients have *increased* numbers of erythrocyte Na+,K+-ATPase units,[68] even though functional characteristics of the enzyme were abnormal in one such patient.[73]

A major question is whether Na+,K+-ATPase activity of red blood cells reflects equivalent activity in other tissues. Hepatic Na+,K+-ATPase activity was reported to be higher in six obese subjects than in three normal control subjects.[74] Unfortunately, simultaneous values for the erythrocytes were not obtained, and interpretation was further clouded by the fact that weight loss had occurred secondary to either diet or surgery. Concern about adequacy of the erythrocyte as a marker for Na+,K+-ATPase activity in heat-generating sites is also raised by the observation that pump units in erythrocytes from hyperthyroid patients are decreased rather than increased,[75] which is the expected response from animal studies.[66] Likewise, Na+,K+-ATPase activity in lymphocytes obtained from hyperthyroid patients was not increased.[76] For these reasons the role of this enzyme in the etiology of human obesity remains uncertain.

Brown Fat. A third potential site of heat generation is brown fat. This tissue is responsible for up to 60% of the heat generated during nonshivering thermogenesis in newborn, cold-acclimated, and hibernating animals.[58, 77, 78] Brown fat is present in adult humans, but the amount is highest in infancy and decreases with age.[79] It is located around the kidneys, adrenal glands, pericardium, and large vessels of the mediastinum and neck. It rarely makes up over 2% of body weight in humans.[80] Heat generation by brown fat in animals can be increased by exposure to cold or by food ingestion.[58, 77, 81] A good deal is now known about the mechanism through which respiration and heat production are controlled in this tissue. A unique uncoupling protein called *thermogenin* (32 kd) makes up 10 to 15% of the inner mitochondrial membrane in brown fat.[82] Thermogenin is a proton channel that has the capacity to dissipate proton gradients across the inner mitochondrial membrane. In normal coupled electron transport in which oxidation of NADH is linked to ATP synthesis, protons are pumped from the mitochondrial matrix across the inner mitochondrial membrane to the inner membrane space, which is in equilibrium with the cytoplasm by the action of electron-transporting respiratory enzymes. The protons then re-enter

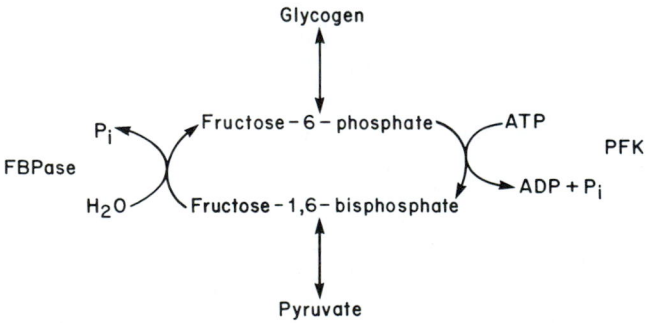

Figure 25–2. A potential futile cycle in the glycolytic-gluconeogenic pathway. Simultaneous activity of phosphofructokinase (PFK) and fructose-bisphosphatase (FBPase) results in ATP breakdown and heat release, with no net change in fructose 6-phosphate or fructose 1,6-bisphosphate.

the matrix through a complex ATP synthase consisting of a transmembrane proton channel (F_0) and a larger matrix subunit of multiple chains (F_1) that functions as an ATPase when detached from the membrane.[83] The energy of re-entrant protons provides the energy for ATP synthesis. Thermogenin effectively bypasses the proton-translocating ATP synthase by allowing proton entry through its own channel. This allows fatty acid oxidation to proceed in unimpeded (uncoupled) fashion with concomitant release of heat. Proton transport by thermogenin is inhibited by the binding of ATP, GTP, ADP, and GDP.

Regulation of heat generation in brown fat occurs by both acute and adaptive mechanisms. The former is mediated by norepinephrine released via sympathetic nerves. Norepinephrine acts through the generation of cyclic AMP after binding to a beta-adrenergic receptor.[82] The probable mechanism of action is stimulation of a lipase that generates rapid increases in long chain fatty acid concentration.[84] The fatty acids are thought to alter the capacity of ATP to inhibit thermogenin, although activation of an ATPase may contribute to the loss of inhibition.[85, 86] Adaptive, or long-term, regulation of thermogenic capacity appears to involve increased synthesis of thermogenin because the content of messenger RNA (mRNA) coding for the protein is increased by cold exposure, overeating, or action of a beta-receptor agonist.[87]

The beta-receptor of brown adipose tissue is distinct from the classic beta-1 and beta-2 subtypes and has been called the beta-3–receptor.[88] A gene for the human beta-3–receptor has been identified.[89] It has been postulated that this beta-receptor may be uniquely coupled to accelerated metabolism in humans, but direct experimental evidence is not available.

Activity of brown fat appears to be diminished in the Zucker obese rat,[81] in obesity induced in animals by ventromedial hypothalamic lesions,[90] and in ob/ob mice.[91] No information is available on the functional response of brown adipose tissue in humans, although an increased temperature response in skin thought to overlie brown fat sites has been observed after ephedrine administration.[58] This finding is compatible with the possibility of hormone-responsive brown adipocytes in humans but clearly is not definitive.

To conclude, no direct evidence exists to indicate that brown fat plays a significant role in human metabolism.[80] As noted earlier, it is difficult to show defects in dietary, exercise-induced, or facultative thermogenesis in human obesity. A defect in brown fat function or a diminished brown fat mass thus seems unlikely as a primary defect in obesity.

Glycerol-3-Phosphate Dehydrogenase. Another possible site for caloric wastage is the α-glycerophosphate shuttle, which functions as one of the transport systems for transfer of reducing equivalents from cytosol into the mitochondria.[92] In this shuttle, dihydroxyacetone phosphate is reduced to *sn*-glycerol-3-phosphate (α-glycerophosphate), by use of NADH as the hydride ion donor under the influence of the enzyme glycerol-3-phosphate dehydrogenase. Inside the mitochondria the reaction is reversed, except that the hydride ion receptor is flavin adenine dinucleotide rather than NAD. The importance of this difference is that oxidation of reduced flavin adenine dinucleotide in the electron transport chain bypasses the first ATP generation site, potentially allowing loss of about one third more energy as heat than would be the case if NADH were regenerated intramitochondrially; i.e., a mole of NADH potentially can generate 3 mol of ATP but a mole of reduced flavin adenine dinucleotide can generate only 2. Activities of both cytosolic and intramitochondrial glycerol-3-phosphate dehydrogenases appear to be decreased in adipose tissue from obese persons,[93] theoretically favoring utilization of the more efficient NADH-linked shuttles.

ABNORMAL EATING PATTERNS. Body weight seems somehow to be regulated in that lean persons tend to remain lean, whereas obese persons almost always remain obese for prolonged periods, if not for life. Even if weight loss is achieved by obese subjects, maintenance of the loss appears to be almost impossible.[94] Because the absolute metabolic rate goes up with increasing size,[39, 41, 43, 49] it follows that obese persons by and large eat more than their normal-sized counterparts (if weight is being maintained), even though energy expenditure by exercise may be lower than normal. It has been estimated that patients weighing more than 114 kg require up to 3500 kcal/d just to maintain weight; higher levels would be needed if weight gain were progressing.[95] Obesity in childhood likewise appears to be triggered by overeating.[96]

Why do fat people continue to eat in the face of obesity? The answer to this question is not known. It has been traditional to say that food intake is regulated by both external and internal signals. The former refers to such things as availability and attractiveness of food; the latter reflects unknown physiological indicators of hunger and satiety. The two types of signals should not be considered independent, because metabolic events may alter emotional responses and emotional factors may trigger or modulate physiological control of food intake.[97]

A popular theory regarding eating patterns in obesity suggests that the sequence begins with overfeeding in infancy so that the infant learns to eat nonphysiologically; i.e., because the mother supplies breast or bottle in response to crying or irritation, even if it is not the normal feeding time, a learning disorder is induced in which emotions such as anger or tension are interpreted as hunger.[98] A second consequence of this induced behavior would be a tendency to eat primarily in response to external signals, especially the availability of food. Both of these interpretations have been questioned. For example, obese mothers, who historically tend to have obese children,[3] actually underfeed their infants relative to nonobese controls.[99] Similarly, although considerable literature suggests that obese subjects respond preferentially to external cues for eating, significant overlap exists between obese and lean subjects, which renders the externality theory nondecisive for development of obesity.[100–102] In other words, almost everyone responds to external eating cues, and in both lean and obese subsets of the population there are those who are highly responsive to extrinsic signals. This is in accord with experiments showing that excess weight gain to the point of obesity can be induced in normal rats by making the diet attractive ("cafeteria diet").[103] Because variety in meals increases food intake in humans, easy access to an appealing, nonuniform diet may contribute to the problem of obesity in Western nations.[104] Although both lean and obese persons can be high responders to external signals, a greater percentage of the latter may exhibit this phenomenon.[100]

Cultural changes may also contribute to the trend toward fatness in the United States and other developed countries. With many families having both parents working, there is increasing dependence on fast-food meals obtained outside the home and on microwave preparations with short cooking times.[105] Such foods tend to be high in fat. Adiposity in humans correlates positively with fat content of the diet and negatively with content of carbohydrate and plant protein.[106] The same is true for animals. Whether this effect is due solely to the higher caloric value of fat relative to protein and carbohydrate on a per weight basis or is due to regulatory effects caused by the carbohydrate/fat ratio[107] is not clear.

How food intake is controlled physiologically is not known. Both short- and long-term control mechanisms probably exist. The former likely relate to intrameal and intermeal satiety signals; the latter may be coupled in some way to steady-state body weight.[108] Short-term signals for hunger and satiety are probably multifactorial and involve both the gastrointestinal tract and the central nervous system.[109] In the gastrointestinal tract, stretch receptors, chemoreceptors, or osmotic receptors may initiate signals to the central nervous system via either neural or humoral mechanisms. Substrates such as glucose, ketones, or amino acids may be involved.[108, 110, 111] Much effort has been spent in the search for circulating satiety signals that might be absent in obesity. Studies with parabiotic mice and rats strongly suggest the existence of such an appetite-suppressing factor.[112–114] Implantation of pancreatic islets from normal animals has been reported to reverse genetically determined obesity in mice,[115] presumably by means of release of pancreatic polypeptide.[116] Pancreatic polypeptide secretion in response to a protein meal is reduced in obese humans,[117] but its role as a satiety factor is uncertain because the polypeptide is also released in response to hypoglycemia or administration of 2-deoxy-D-glucose, which impairs glucose metabolism in tissues.[117, 118]

A variety of other neuropeptides and hormones have been proposed as modulators of food intake (for review see ref. 109). Perhaps most attention has been paid to cholecystokinin. Endogenous cholecystokinin decreases food intake in animals,[119] and blockade of cholecystokinin receptors in the brain prevents satiety and increases food intake.[120] Acute administration of cholecystokinin in humans produces small but measurable decreases in food intake.[109] Other candidate regulatory molecules include bombesin, motilin, somatostatin, satietins, insulin, glucocorticoids, dynorphin, endorphins, neuropeptide Y, galanin, growth hormone–releasing hormone, corticotropin-releasing hormone (CRH), catecholamines, and γ-aminobutyric acid.[109] The conclusion from reviewing multiple studies is that many factors affect hunger and satiety under experimental conditions. Their role in normal humans is problematic, and no single major signal for either feeding or satiety has been identified.

Long-term regulation of eating has been postulated to be related to adipose tissue mass. The idea is that a set point for body weight in each individual somehow signals the need to eat more or less (gain or lose weight) because of deviations between current weight and the preferred value.[121] Presumably the putative "ponderostat" or "lipostat" could be reset after weight had been maintained at a new level for some fixed period. How the adipose tissue mass or stored triglyceride might signal hunger or satiety (if indeed it does) is not known. An intriguing candidate molecule is adipsin, which is a serine protease with the same enzymatic activity as complement factor D.[122] Adipsin is deficient in adipocytes of genetically obese rodents and rats with monosodium glutamate–induced hypothalamic obesity but not in rats with dietary obesity. The expression of the adipsin gene is regulated by glucocorticoids, which decrease adipsin mRNA.[123] The potential importance is that glucocorticoid excess is associated with increased appetite and eventual obesity in both rodents and humans. It is not established that adipsin plays a role in human obesity. Even in animals there is no evidence that it is a satiety signal maintaining fat mass. At least one form of a fat-losing syndrome, however, partial lipodystrophy, is associated with increased levels of an autoantibody (C3 nephritic factor) that increases levels of C3b, an intermediate necessary for the action of both adipsin and factor D in the alternative complement pathway.[122]

Despite the near-certainty that short- and long-term controls of satiety and weight exist in humans, the set point theory has been increasingly questioned.[124] The basic set point theory is that the body has the capacity to autoregulate weight over a narrow range and defends that weight by alterations in food intake and metabolic energy expenditure.[121] Thus the body's response to overeating would be an increased metabolic rate (and presumably decreased food intake), whereas weight loss would result in a decreased metabolic rate (efficiency of caloric use would increase). However, weight in normal persons may vary considerably. For example, in a study of nearly 3000 men and women followed in Framingham, Massachusetts, for 18 years, the average deviation in weight for 10 examinations was 9.6 kg (highest to lowest).[125] There was no difference in findings between men and women. Other studies have not found predicted changes in metabolic rates required for defense of a set point.[124] On the basis of experiments utilizing altered caloric density (same volume of food but varying caloric content), it is clear that adjustments of intake to maintain weight are imperfect.[17] This situation almost certainly is due to the fact that physiological controlling signals, whether derived from the gut, peripheral tissues, or central nervous system, can be overridden by conditioning factors that may be psychological, cultural, or economic.[17, 19] There is no evidence that the physiological controls for eating or the response to internal signals of hunger or satiety are qualitatively different in the lean and the obese.

To summarize, obese persons eat too much in absolute terms and particularly in relation to body weight. As a group, they may be more dependent on external cues and less dependent on internal signals than their lean counterparts, but considerable overlap exists.

FAT CELL SIZE, NUMBER, AND DISTRIBUTION. The observation that fat cell number and size could be altered by feeding patterns in the neonatal rat[126] led to the concept of hyperplastic and hypertrophic obesity; in the former the total number of adipose tissue cells in the body is increased and the cells are larger, whereas in the latter only size is altered. The general concept has been that early-onset obesity is hyperplastic and that the distribution of body fat is generalized, whereas adult-onset obesity is hypertrophic and the distribution of fat more restricted. In analogy to the rodent model it might be supposed, as mentioned earlier, that overfeeding in infancy could increase the number of preadipocytes and adipocytes so that a foundation for the subsequent development of massive obesity was laid. In other words, an increase in adipocyte or preadipocyte number spread throughout the body would increase the potential capacity for storage of fat in the face of caloric excess. This concept is not universally accepted.[17, 31] It does seem likely, on the basis of cross-sectional and longitudinal studies, that major childhood obesity is hyperplastic (Fig. 25–3).[31, 127] Furthermore, sequential biopsies in the same child indicate that weight loss does not decrease cell number, at least over periods up to 3 mo.[127] It has been suggested that fat cell number in children normally increases significantly when body fat reaches 25% of total weight.[31, 127] Children destined to be obese can usually be identified by age 2 because the fat cell size is much larger than that of lean controls, who actually appear to show a decrease in size between ages 1 and 2.[31] Massively obese adults tend to have increased numbers of fat cells, but it is uncertain when the increase occurs.[128] Preadipocytes from obese subjects may replicate more rapidly in culture than similar cells from lean controls.[129] As noted earlier, fat cells in animals are intrinsically normal in the obese state.[60, 61] Overall, the concepts of hyperplastic and hypertrophic obesity are of little clinical consequence.

Of perhaps more import is the observation that not all fat cells behave alike. The problem of insulin resistance in adipocytes, an essentially constant feature of obesity, illus-

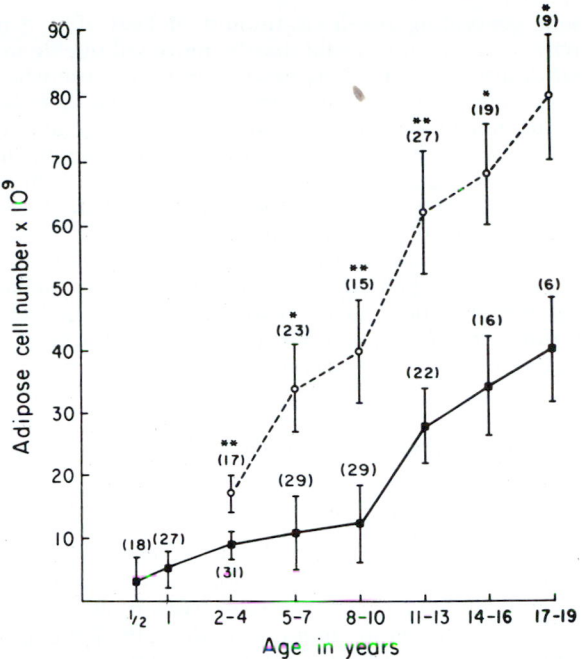

Figure 25–3. Cross-sectional study of adipose cell number as a function of age in humans. Open circles represent obese subjects, solid squares nonobese. The number of subjects at each age is listed in parentheses. Asterisks represent statistically significant differences between obese and nonobese groups for the appropriate age range (*P < .05; **P < .01). (From Knittle JL, Timmers K, Ginsberg-Fellner F, et al. The growth of adipose tissue in children and adolescents. Cross-sectional and longitudinal studies of adipose cell number and size. Reproduced from The Journal of Clinical Investigation, 1979, vol. 63, pp. 239–246 by copyright permission of The American Society for Clinical Investigation.)

which is an indicator of lipolysis, is increased in central obesity despite the fact that responsiveness to both epinephrine and insulin is impaired.[140] In addition to the question of whether hormone-sensitive lipase and LPL are rate-limiting in adipocyte triglyceride metabolism, there is also the question of cause and effect. Most changes in adipocyte function in obesity are probably secondary to changes in cell volume.[135] Whether changes in LPL and hormone-sensitive lipase in regional fat have anything to do with the greater risk of hyperinsulinemia, glucose intolerance, hypertriglyceridemia, and elevated blood pressure that accompanies increases in upper body fat is not known.[141]

BODY IMAGE. Massively obese persons exhibit detrimental psychological responses on losing weight.[142] The concept has developed that they are somehow "imprinted" with an image of themselves as fat that exerts a powerful influence on eating patterns. Presumably this image of fatness could contribute to development of obesity and, more important, override the need or desire to lose weight after obesity was established. As attractive as the hypothesis is, the evidence for a distortion in perception of self as a major determinant of obesity is not persuasive. Adult-onset obesity is uncommonly associated with a perceptual disorder of body size.[143] Moreover, changes in self-assessment of body image in response to weight loss appear to go in opposite directions in adults and adolescents, the former overestimating body size[144] and the latter underestimating.[145] It may be that with examination of large numbers of obese subjects and properly matched controls, the concept of a major abnormality in image perception will disappear, as seems to be the case in anorexia nervosa.[146]

DIMINISHED EXERCISE. The role of diminished physical activity as a causal agent in development of obesity is unsettled. The literature on the subject is large, but the problem is that most studies have compared lean and already obese subjects, so that diminished physical activity could be consequence rather than cause. As cited earlier, nonobese children of obese parents appear to expend less energy per day than nonobese children of nonobese parents,[46] which suggests a causal role. This subject has been reviewed by the working party of the Royal College of Physicians with the conclusion that "there is little evidence to show that physical inactivity is the specific cause of weight gain in most overweight individuals."[17] This conclusion seems entirely reasonable, although it would be expected that diminished activity consequent to development of massive obesity plays a role in maintaining weight and rendering weight loss more difficult in the face of caloric restriction. The working party did note that a societal decrease in physical activity (sports and work), as appears to have occurred in the United Kingdom, would tend to single out individuals predisposed to obesity for other reasons. This view is supported by a study of a large group of subjects in which it was found by direct calorimetry that a significant part of variance in 24-h energy expenditure is due to physical activity ("fidgeting").[49] However, obese subjects were not less active than lean subjects and because of increased weight and lean body mass the obese expended more energy in activity. The authors concluded only that diminished activity might identify persons at risk for obesity.[49]

SOCIOECONOMIC FACTORS. Although serious obesity can occur in any stratum of society, statistically a higher prevalence is found in lower socioeconomic groups.[19, 147] The presumption is made that in high social classes slimness is considered both fashionable and important to success in the world of commerce. Presumably the desire for slimness is capable of counteracting the drive to eat in this population.

GENETICS. Although genetic forms of obesity occur in humans (see later section on secondary obesity), ordinary

trates the point. Adipocytes isolated from patients with childhood obesity do not exhibit as severe a defect in insulin binding as fat cells taken from older obese subjects.[130] Subcutaneous fat cells from the thigh are smaller than adipocytes obtained simultaneously from subcutaneous tissue in the abdomen and are less responsive to epinephrine-induced lipolysis.[131] Even fat cells taken from the same region of the body differ in metabolic responses. Thus adipocytes obtained from the subcutaneous tissue of the abdominal wall were more resistant to epinephrine-induced lipolysis and more sensitive to insulin-mediated antilipolysis than fat cells obtained simultaneously from the omentum.[131–133] These differences appear to be due to variations in beta-receptor concentrations.[134] The question then becomes: do differences in catecholamine-induced lipolysis and insulin-induced antilipolysis play a role in the development and maintenance of obesity? On balance, the regulatory actions of catecholamines and insulin on adipocyte lipolysis appear to be normal in common obesity.[135]

The role of lipoprotein lipase (LPL) has also received considerable attention, the thesis being that increased activity of the enzyme might predispose to fat deposition even if lipolytic rates were unchanged.[136] Enzyme activity is higher in the obese in response to heparin and meals.[137] It also appears that LPL activity does not diminish normally or actually increases after weight reduction in obese subjects.[138, 139] It is presumed that these changes would predispose to weight gain by enhancing fat filling of adipocytes or preadipocytes. A common problem with these types of studies is that conclusions about regulation in the adipocyte in vivo are risky. In other words, it is not known if the increased LPL activity causes increased fatty acid transport and triglyceride synthesis for a given triglyceride load. Illustrative of the general problem is that free fatty acid turnover,

fatness is not inherited by simple mendelian patterns. There is no question that obese children tend to have obese parents. In four series covering 2002 children, one or both parents were obese an average 72% of the time.[148] Fat mothers appeared to be more frequent than fat fathers. The clustering of obesity in families could be an example of pseudoheredity, based on the fact that such families have common attitudes toward food, eating, and exercise; i.e., they like to eat and do not like to exercise.[3] Thus fat parents may have fat children not because of genetic predisposition but because of behavioral factors. The importance of environment is emphasized by the fact that monozygotic twins, raised apart, may differ in weight by 4.5 kg or more.[17, 148] Other studies suggest a genetic influence in obesity. Adopted children in Denmark have weights more closely related to biological than to adoptive parents.[149] Monozygotic twins resemble each other more than dizygotic twins, a finding that holds whether they are raised together or apart.[148, 150] When monozygotic twin pairs are overfed, weight gain is much closer within pairs than between pairs.[151]

The genetic influences in obesity are almost certainly multifactorial. Genetic contribution to subcutaneous fat is low but may approach 25 to 30% for visceral fat.[151, 152] The response to overfeeding may also be influenced by genetic factors, which could contribute up to 40% of observed differences in energy expenditure among individuals.[152]

The clustering of obesity in families does mean that prophylactic measures to prevent lifelong obesity should focus on children of fat parents, especially those with fat mothers. The pediatrician should initiate dietary restriction and exercise prescriptions early, because adult fate in terms of weight may be set in children as young as age 2.[127]

OVERVIEW. The pathophysiology of obesity is, in one sense, clear: energy intake is greater than energy expenditure. What causes this is less clear. The simplest explanation is that fat people overeat because food is good and readily available. The higher fat content of Western diets is also important. No study has failed to show less energy expenditure in the obese than in the lean; thus food intake is always greater in obese than in lean subjects. Animal studies clearly show that obesity can be produced simply by exposure to unlimited amounts of a tasty diet. Other factors probably play a role (Fig. 25–4). Genetic influences are manifested primarily in the arena of energy expenditure. If metabolic efficiency in the population represents a bell-shaped curve,

persons generating the least amount of heat after eating, exercise, or exposure to cold may be more vulnerable to the threat of attractive or inexpensive food than those who are less efficiently coupled. It is likely, however, that there is not a specific genetic defect (certainly not a single gene defect) leading to metabolic efficiency but simply movement down a normal distribution curve. Although disturbances in body image, an altered set point (ponderostat), differences in perinatally determined fat cell number, and diminished exercise may play a role, these effects are difficult to prove. Absence of or a failure to respond to a satiety signal or signals would appear to be reasonable but so far remain undocumented. A major problem is separating primary and secondary events. For example, physical activity always decreases with massive obesity, but this does not imply its presence during the genesis of obesity. What can be said with certainty is that fat people are fat because they overeat.

Clinical Picture

Because weight distribution in the general population is not bimodal, the diagnosis of obesity, as noted earlier, is not clear-cut or definitive. For the same reason, attribution of symptoms to the obese condition is difficult. Persons who are mildly overweight by statistical standards have no symptoms, whereas those massively obese both suffer and are at risk for life. Young persons with obesity have less difficulty than adults because many of the complications influenced by the obese state (such as heart disease) are age related. Obesity in childhood has been reported to predispose to infection and hypertension, but critical evaluation of the studies suggests methodological flaws that render the conclusions suspect.[153]

Obesity has psychological, behavioral, and medical consequences. Psychological responses are derived from the subject's and society's reaction to fatness. Because obesity is considered to be cosmetically unattractive in Western cultures, obese persons (especially women) tend to have negative self-images that may progress to the point of self-hate.[154, 155] Obesity may be considered as disease, sin, or simple ugliness,[154] with the result that the seriously obese person may express anxiety, depression, hostility, guilt, or somatic complaints.[156]

In terms of behavior, obesity may result in diminished activity because of shortness of breath, joint pain, stasis edema, and muscle fatigue even before overt medical complications supervene. It is not uncommon to see a withdrawal syndrome in which the person avoids social contact in the hope of escaping embarrassment. Although there are increasing efforts to counter negative self-images in the obese by advocating "fat pride,"[154] it remains common for the obese person to experience underemployment or frank rejection by schools and businesses.

The medical problems can be serious.[18] With massive obesity there is clearly an increased prevalence of cardiovascular disease, hypertension, diabetes, pulmonary disorders, and gallstones.[2, 10, 17] Mortality in morbidly obese men is 12-fold higher than that in the general population in the 25- to 34-y-old age range (Fig. 25–5). The degree of excessive deaths decreases with age, but the probability of dying remains twice as high as normal even in the 65- to 74-y-old range.[2] Excess mortality in women is qualitatively similar.[10, 157] The causes of death in a cohort of 200 morbidly obese men followed prospectively for an average of 7.5 y are shown in Figure 25–6. Cardiovascular disease represents the greatest risk, as expected.[2, 10, 17, 157] Some studies also show excessive mortality from cirrhosis of the liver.[157] For men, death from malignancy appears to be less than that in the general population,[2] although statistically there is increased

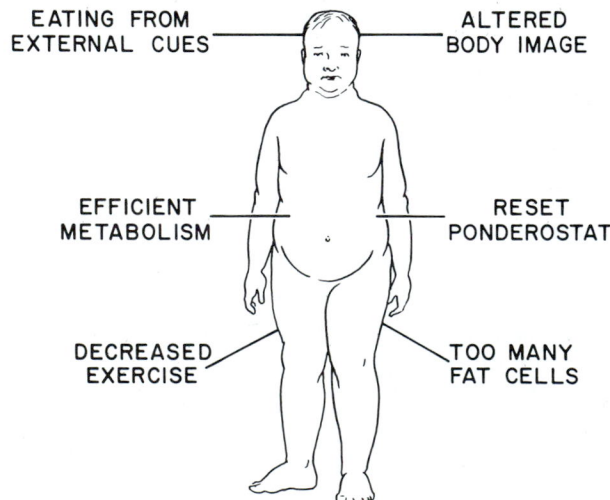

EATING FROM
EXTERNAL CUES

ALTERED
BODY IMAGE

EFFICIENT
METABOLISM

RESET
PONDEROSTAT

DECREASED
EXERCISE

TOO MANY
FAT CELLS

Figure 25–4. Potential factors in development of morbid obesity. See text for details.

mortality from cancer of the colon, rectum, and prostate.[17] Women show increased risk of malignancy in breast, uterus, and cervix. The fact that the death rate from appendicitis is twice as high in obese men and women as in nonobese subjects highlights the risk of surgery in fat persons.[157]

Massive obesity no doubt imposes a risk to life, but it is uncertain whether this is the case for mild or moderate obesity (see Table 25–2). The role of moderate fatness has been examined in a longitudinal study of nearly 1000 men in Sweden.[158] Degrees of fatness were evaluated by several indices, and the study group was divided into quintiles for subsequent evaluation. Even small increases in body fat were associated with an increased risk of developing hypertension, diabetes, gallstones, kidney stones, and cerebrovascular disease. Surprisingly, ischemic heart disease did not appear to correlate with moderate degrees of fatness, in contrast to women in the United States in whom even slight obesity imposes a cardiovascular risk.[1] Overall, it seems likely that even moderate obesity is a health risk. The degree of that risk is doubtless modified by environmental factors (type of diet, smoking, stress) and genetic background. This genetic influence is illustrated by the report that obese black women in South Africa are resistant to hypertension, glucose intolerance, and lipid abnormalities, whereas obese white women in the same society exhibit these complications.[159] Apart from the more serious complications, obese persons have a high prevalence of gout, osteoarthritis, and varicose veins.[17]

CARDIOVASCULAR DISEASE. There has been considerable discussion about the reality of risk of cardiovascular disease from obesity per se. Some authors have argued that for modest obesity the risk is low.[158] However, most investigations indicate an increased threat, even when confounding variables such as smoking are factored out.[17] In the Framingham study, obesity was associated with enhanced appearance of coronary artery disease (angina and death from myocardial infarction), congestive heart failure, and, in women, stroke.[15] It is not clear whether the effects of obesity are direct (obesity is an independent risk factor) or indirect

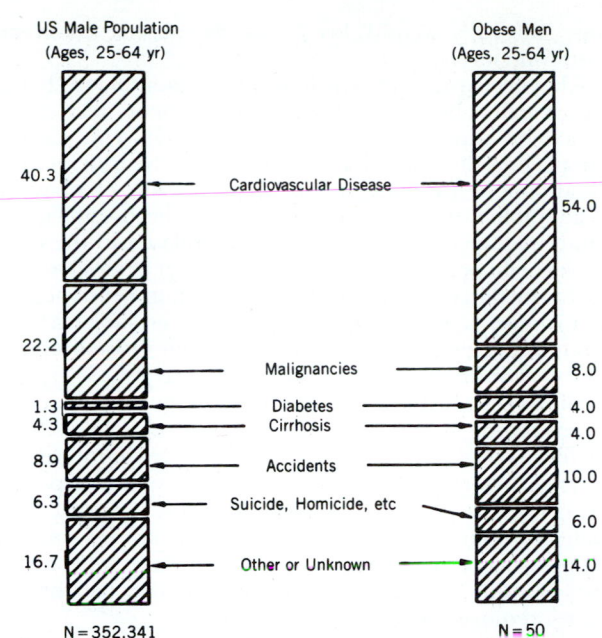

Figure 25–6. Frequency of common causes of death in morbidly obese men and in the general male population in the United States. (From Drenick EJ, Bale GS, Seltzer F, et al. Excessive mortality and causes of death in morbidly obese men. JAMA 1980; 243:443–445. Copyright 1980, American Medical Association.)

(obesity acts by predisposing to diabetes, hypertension, and hyperlipidemia, which are then the direct risk factors). The indirect thesis is perhaps more likely. The lipid abnormalities of obesity are those expected to be atherogenic: increased low-density lipoprotein and cholesterol, increased very-low-density lipoprotein and triglyceride, and decreased high-density lipoprotein cholesterol.[15, 160] Space precludes a detailed discussion of mechanisms, but overproduction of very-low-density lipoprotein is probably key, with low-density lipoprotein increasing via the sequence very-low-density lipoprotein → intermediate-density lipoprotein → low-density lipoprotein.[161] As in the other metabolic defects of obesity, atherogenic lipid abnormalities appear to correlate with abdominal obesity.[162, 163] Factors other than lipids doubtless play a role in the atherosclerosis/myocardial infarction syndrome of obesity. For example, the inhibitor of tissue plasminogen activator appears to be increased in obesity, a response that presumably favors dysregulated thrombosis.[164]

Obesity imposes circulatory changes because of the necessity to perfuse the increased mass of tissue (lean and fat). Pulmonary and systemic blood volumes are increased, and stroke volume and cardiac output are high.[165] The increased workload on the heart leads to dilatation and hypertrophy, particularly if systemic resistance is elevated by hypertension. Simultaneously, myocardial oxygen demand is increased. These circulatory adjustments predispose to congestive heart failure and, if coronary atherosclerosis is present, may lead to infarction and death as oxygen demand exceeds supply. Weight reduction decreases ventricular mass.[166]

HYPERTENSION. Obesity is associated with hypertension,[15, 17, 158, 160] which improves or reverses with weight reduction.[160, 167] Obesity appears to influence blood pressure adversely, even in students of high school age.[168] The cause of the hypertension is uncertain. Peripheral resistance appears to be increased, coupled with a high cardiac output.[169] Obese subjects also have increased basal and stimulated levels of norepinephrine relative to age-, sex-, and race-matched controls,[170] and this increase could conceivably play an important role in raising peripheral resistance. Norepinephrine

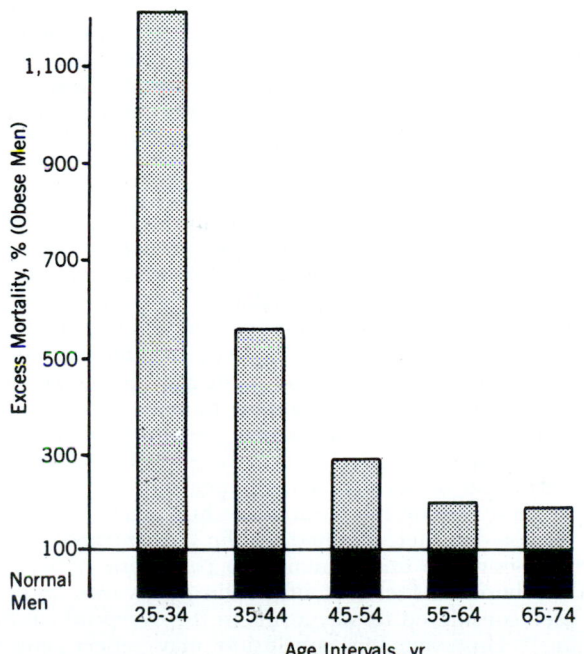

Figure 25–5. Probability of death in morbidly obese men (average weight 144 kg) relative to U.S. men as a whole. (From Drenick EJ, Bale GS, Seltzer F, et al. Excessive mortality and causes of death in morbidly obese men. JAMA 1980; 243:443–445. Copyright 1980, American Medical Association.)

values fall with weight loss,[170] as do plasma renin and aldosterone levels.[167, 170]

The mechanisms by which the above-mentioned changes occur remain obscure. Enhanced sympathetic nervous system activity appears to be mediated by diet, with carbohydrate playing the major stimulatory role.[171] Sensitivity to salt may also be a problem in the hypertension of obesity.[172] Considerable attention has been paid to the possibility that insulin resistance in obesity is causally related to the development of hypertension, either alone or in association with diabetes mellitus and dyslipidemia.[173] Insulin resistance may also produce a similar effect in nonobese subjects.[174] Although interesting, a causal role for insulin resistance in the hypertension of obesity is unproved.

DIABETES MELLITUS. A high percentage of patients with non–insulin-dependent diabetes mellitus are obese.[175] Presumably, excessive caloric intake and obesity induce insulin resistance, which leads to hyperglycemia in those patients bearing diabetic gene(s).[176] According to this construct, obese patients without diabetes can synthesize and secrete sufficient insulin to overcome the insulin-resistant state, whereas impaired insulin synthesis and release in the patient with diabetes remove the capacity to do so.

The cause of non–insulin-dependent diabetes mellitus remains unknown (see Chapter 24), but insulin resistance plays a primary role.[176, 177] The threshold for development of insulin resistance is 120% of ideal body weight.[178] Maximal impairment of glucose disposal in nondiabetic subjects is reached when percent body fat reaches about 30%; i.e., increasing fatness beyond this level does not cause a further fall in insulin sensitivity.[177] The insulin resistance is multifactorial. It is partly due to distribution defects of insulin in muscle. Insulin does not increase blood flow to muscle in obese humans,[179] and the ratio of capillaries to muscle fibers is decreased, resulting in lower levels of tissue insulin relative to plasma insulin in obese compared with normal subjects.[177] Insulin receptor number and function are clearly decreased.[176, 180] Postreceptor defects also exist, likely caused by uncoupling of hormone-occupied receptor from activation of the tyrosine kinase that is critical to insulin action.[181] Physiologically, a defect in glucose transport is likely due to a deficiency of intracellular glucose transporters that normally move to the plasma membrane in response to insulin.[182, 183] After glucose enters the cell, resistance is manifested by a block in glucose storage, with little effect on glucose oxidation.[177] Impaired glycogen synthesis may be due to deactivation of glycogen synthase by the insulin-resistant state. Insulin resistance in the liver is manifested by increased glucose production,[176, 184] a defect that is seen even in children with developing obesity.[185] Elevated insulin levels in plasma are due primarily to pancreatic hypersecretion.[186, 187] Decreased hepatic extraction of insulin accentuates the problem in severe insulin resistance and correlates with an increased waist/hip ratio. Pulsatile patterns of insulin secretion are normal in obesity.[188]

PULMONARY DYSFUNCTION. Pulmonary dysfunction is common in severe obesity, especially in the supine position.[165, 169, 189] Obese patients tend to take rapid and shallow breaths. Functional residual capacity and expiratory reserve volume of the lung are low. Maximal expiratory flow rates are low in obese men (not women), even if they have never smoked.[190] Ventilation takes place predominantly in the upper lobes, whereas perfusion occurs primarily in the lower segments, resulting in a ventilation-perfusion mismatch and hypoxemia.[189] Seriously overweight patients are also at risk for hypoventilation, the presence of which is defined by elevated P_{CO_2}. Hypoxemia alone may occur in simple obesity, but hypoxemia and carbon dioxide retention together justify the diagnosis of obesity-hypoventilation syndrome. The cause of the hypoventilation appears to be a diminished ventilatory response to both hypoxia and hypercapnia, although mechanical factors and respiratory muscle weakness doubtless also play a role. It is uncertain whether diminished sensitivity of respiratory centers is a complication of obesity or an antecedent lesion; an acquired defect appears intuitively more likely. Sleep apnea is not unusual in obese patients manifesting alveolar hyperventilation. What is not clear is whether the prevalence is more common in obesity than in a normal-weight population.[191] Sleep apnea in obesity has more severe consequences because of the coexisting pulmonary disorder. Apnea in this syndrome may be central (no respiratory movements), obstructive (no airflow despite respiratory movements), or mixed (initial absence of respiratory muscle activity followed by ineffective activity). The obstructive form is probably more common in obesity and may require tracheostomy.[192] Sleep studies are required to differentiate central from obstructive apnea. Central apnea may respond to medroxyprogesterone therapy.[193] Even if obstructive apnea is present, a trial of the drug may be indicated because an element of primary hypoventilation may coexist with predominant obstruction.

Pulmonary hypertension, polycythemia, and frank cor pulmonale may result from combined respiratory dysfunction. Morbidly obese subjects with compromised pulmonary function are at particular risk during anesthesia and may die suddenly (presumably from arrhythmias) during surgery or in the immediate postoperative period.[165]

GALLSTONES. Gallstones are present in a higher percentage of obese than of normal subjects.[17] The reason is that the bile of the former is supersaturated because of enhanced biliary secretion of cholesterol.[194] Saturability markedly increases in the fasting state because the concentration of solubilizing phospholipids falls while cholesterol output remains high. Hypocaloric diets, on the other hand, do not produce this change. From the standpoint of cholelithiasis, fasting, especially prolonged fasting, is not an optimal therapeutic regimen.

Endocrine Abnormalities

A number of endocrine changes accompany the obese state, but most, if not all, are secondary, because they can be induced by overfeeding previously normal persons and can be reversed by weight loss.[195] The obesity-associated changes in endocrine function are summarized in Table 25–5.[196]

ENDOCRINE PANCREAS. The fact that obesity is associated with insulin resistance and hyperinsulinism was described earlier. The only syndrome of obesity in which insulin excess may be causally related to weight gain is that related to ventromedial hypothalamic lesions in animals.[197] Removal of the pancreatic islets from neural (vagal) control by autotransplantation reverses hyperinsulinemia, diminishes food intake, and restores weight gain to control levels. Hyperinsulinism is also present in humans with hypothalamic obesity,[198] but it is not known whether the increased levels are primary, as in rodents with ventromedial hypothalamic damage, or secondary, as appears to be the case in simple obesity occurring naturally in humans.[195, 199]

As noted earlier, elevated insulin concentrations in ordinary obesity are due primarily to pancreatic hypersecretion.[187] Abnormal feedback of insulin on its own secretion has been considered to play a role in the overproduction of insulin.[200] However, this conclusion may reflect only the higher starting levels of insulin in the obese because per cent decreases in C peptide (a marker of endogenous insulin secretion) are similar in lean and obese subjects.

In summary, hyperinsulinism is common in obesity, and

TABLE 25–5. Endocrine Changes in Obesity*

Endocrine Pancreas	**Adrenal Gland**
↑ insulin (insulin resistance)	→ cortisol
→ or ↑ glucagon	↑ cortisol production
↓ pancreatic polypeptide	→ urinary free cortisol
→ somatostatin	→ dexamethasone suppression
	→ norepinephrine, epinephrine
	↑ androgen in women
Hypothalamus and Pituitary Gland	**Testis**
↓ growth hormone (→ somatomedin)	↓ total testosterone
→ gonadotropins	→ free testosterone
→ thyrotropin	↑ estradiol
→ prolactin	↑ estrone
abnormal regulation of vasopressin	→ androstenedione, dihydrotestosterone
Thyroid Gland	**Ovary**
→ thyroxine	→ or ↑ total and free estradiol
→ or ↑ triiodothyronine	→ or ↑ total and free estrone
↓ triiodothyronine receptors	
Adipose Tissue	
↑ conversion of androgen to estrogen	

*Symbols: ↓, decreased; ↑, increased; →, normal. Hormone values refer to concentrations in plasma.

insulin resistance is characteristic when major weight gain occurs. Insulin resistance is probably due to obesity, but several factors may contribute.

Less information is available for the other pancreatic hormones. The glucagon level has been reported to be normal, elevated, or decreased in obesity, but pancreatic glucagon (as opposed to total glucagon) is elevated in at least some subjects.[201] Whether this elevation is a manifestation of relative insulin resistance or of some other mechanism is not known. Glucagon resistance has been demonstrated in obese animals[202–204] and could conceivably play a role, although it has not yet been reported in humans. Basal pancreatic polypeptide concentrations are low in human obesity, and the response to a protein meal is blunted.[117, 205] These low concentrations are of potential importance because pancreatic polypeptide, as noted earlier, has been reported to function as a satiety factor in rodents.[116, 206] Release of somatostatin from the pancreas of obese Zucker rats is increased after stimulation by amino acids,[207] although elevation of somatostatin content of gastrointestinal tissue consequent to starvation appears no different in lean and obese animals.[208] Metabolism of somatostatin has not been fully evaluated in human obesity, but plasma levels appear to be normal in the basal state and after glucose stimulation in obese Pima Indians.[209]

THYROID GLAND. Because of the possibility that obesity is related to a metabolic defect, there has been extensive study of thyroid function in overweight humans.[196, 210] Basically, thyroid hormone concentrations are normal in obesity, although a few subjects have an elevated triiodothyronine (T_3) level, probably consequent to carbohydrate overfeeding.[211] With caloric restriction the T_3 level falls, and the reverse T_3 concentration rises in obese subjects, as in normal persons.[196, 212, 213] The thyrotropin (TSH) response to thyrotropin-releasing hormone (TRH) is normal in obesity.[212–214] A small percentage of patients have low radioactive iodine uptake that is unresponsive to TSH.[196] This change is probably due to subclinical thyroiditis rather than to obesity. Receptors for T_3 in nuclear extracts of monocytes are reported to be low in human obesity.[215] Nuclear T_3 receptors are low in the liver and lung of ob/ob mice, which may be the cause of decreased activity of Na^+,K^+-ATPase in these tissues.[216]

ADRENAL GLAND. A common problem in differential diagnosis is that of Cushing syndrome versus simple obesity because glucose intolerance and hypertension are common

in both. Simple obesity may be accompanied by a central distribution of fat and striae. The latter are ordinarily white but occasionally purplish, so as to be indistinguishable from those seen in adrenocortical hyperfunction. Although cortisol production rates and 24-h urinary 17-hydroxysteroid values may be elevated in obesity, basal plasma cortisol and urinary free cortisol values tend to be normal.[196, 217] Overnight dexamethasone suppression is normal in about 90% of obese controls but in only 2% of subjects with Cushing syndrome.[217] Thus about 10% of obese patients in whom Cushing syndrome is in question will need the standard (long) dexamethasone suppression test. Obese subjects almost invariably show suppression in the standard test.[217, 218] Other tests for Cushing syndrome, such as continuous 7-h dexamethasone infusion,[219] have not been applied to large numbers of obese subjects but have given normal results in small series.[220]

Norepinephrine turnover appears to be decreased in several forms of animal obesity.[221] In humans basal norepinephrine concentrations are normal, decreasing appropriately with diminished caloric intake and increasing with upright posture.[222, 223] Epinephrine response to isometric exercise is deficient in obese women but normal in obese men.[223] Thermogenic response to infused norepinephrine is blunted in the obese,[222] possibly accounting for the fact that in some studies the rise in oxygen uptake after a meal is less in obese than in normal subjects.[224] Insulin produces equivalent rises in plasma norepinephrine values in lean and obese subjects.[224]

TESTIS. The concentration of testosterone in plasma of massively obese men is low.[196, 225] Levels of testosterone-binding globulin are decreased while the percentage of free testosterone is elevated, resulting in normal absolute concentrations of free testosterone in most subjects. A few massively obese men have low free concentrations of testosterone.[225] Plasma levels of androstenedione and dihydrotestosterone are normal.[196] The hypothalamic-pituitary-testicular axis is intact.[196, 225, 226] Thus the administration of clomiphene citrate results in appropriate rises in follicle-stimulating hormone (FSH), luteinizing hormone (LH), and testosterone concentrations.[226]

Concentrations of estradiol and estrone are both increased in obese men, and estrogen production rates are high.[226, 227] Most of the increase comes from conversion of androgen precursors, but there may be some increase in estradiol secretion from the testis.[226] The increased estrogenization of obese men is usually clinically silent; gynecomastia, impotence, and feminization are rare.[227]

The abnormal sex hormone concentrations are reversible by weight loss.[227]

OVARY. Obese women, like obese men, have a decreased concentration of testosterone-binding globulin.[228] Total estradiol and estrone levels have been reported to be normal or increased, with the percentage of free hormone elevated.[196, 229, 230] Conflicting results may be due to failure to discriminate between upper and lower body obesity. Free and total estradiol levels are elevated in persons with upper but not lower body obesity phenotypes.[231] Serum estrone levels are not different in the two types of obesity, although estrone production rates are high in lower body obesity. Estrone production derives from aromatization in peripheral fat, whereas estradiol (in premenopausal women) arises primarily from the ovary.[196, 232] The conversion rate of androstenedione to estrone is increased disproportionately in lower body obesity.[231] It has been reported that cultured omental preadipocytes from obese women are stimulated to release mitogenic factors by the presence of estradiol, but it cannot be assumed that the hormone is causally related to development of the obese state.[233] Continued overproduction of estrogens peripherally may be important in menopausal obese women, in whom it could play a role in both dysfunctional bleeding and development of uterine cancer. A factor that may be important in development of estrogen-linked abnormalities during reproductive life is an obesity-associated decrease in hydroxylation at the 2α and 17α positions of estradiol.[234] This decrease would be expected to enhance biological activity of secreted estrogens because conversion to the metabolites results in a loss of estrogenic function. Basal gonadotropin concentrations are usually normal in obese women, and the response to luteinizing hormone–releasing hormone (LHRH, also called gonadotropin-releasing hormone, GnRH) is intact.[196, 228, 229, 235] Some studies have indicated increased LH/FSH ratios, and low levels of gonadotropins have been reported.[196] Secondary amenorrhea and hirsutism are not uncommon. However, the major cause appears to be increased androgen production with concomitant elevations of plasma testosterone, 5α-dihydrotestosterone, and dehydroepiandrosterone.[196, 225, 229, 236] Unbound levels of androgens are high because of decreased testosterone-binding globulin and correlate with oligomenorrhea and hirsutism.[236] Androgen levels are higher in upper body obesity.[231] A significant proportion of the androgen excess appears to derive from the adrenal gland because it is dexamethasone suppressible.[235] Androgen excess and amenorrhea are reversible with weight loss.[235, 237]

HYPOTHALAMUS AND PITUITARY GLAND. The only consistent abnormality of the hypothalamic-anterior pituitary system involves growth hormone. Plasma levels and response to a variety of stimuli are impaired,[196] and 24-h integrated values are lower in young obese subjects than in lean controls, although the difference tends to disappear with age.[238, 239] Despite the low growth hormone levels, concentrations of insulin-like growth factor I (IGF I, also called somatomedin-C) are normal.[196, 240] The decrease in growth hormone may be mediated by negative feedback action of IGF I.[196] Enhanced sensitivity of pituitary somatotrophes to IGF I may be due to chronically depressed hypothalamic cholinergic tone because pyridostigmine tends to restore the response to growth hormone–releasing hormone.[241, 242] Gonadotropin and TSH concentrations and their regulation are intact.[196] The mean prolactin concentration is also normal, although some patients fail to demonstrate a rise in prolactin after hypoglycemia or other stimulating maneuvers.[196, 243] After insulin hypoglycemia, some formerly obese women exhibit an exaggerated rise in plasma cortisol and a failure to increase plasma norepinephrine.[243] The former was interpreted as residual hypothalamic dysfunction; the latter was taken to represent an abnormal sympathetic nervous system. However, as noted earlier, there is little evidence for significant abnormality in the hypothalamic-pituitary-adrenal axis.

Concentrations of vasopressin (AVP, also called antidiuretic hormone, ADH) are normal in the basal state but do not suppress properly after a water load.[244]

MISCELLANEOUS. Other hormonal abnormalities have been reported, but none are thought to be of major importance.[196] Parathyroid hormone levels are often elevated for unknown reasons. Vitamin D deficiency and hypercalciuria have been postulated but are unproved. β-Endorphin levels are increased and do not return to normal after weight loss. Plasma renin and aldosterone concentrations are normal, although the aldosterone response to furosemide is said to be enhanced.

Treatment

In principle the treatment of obesity is simple, but in practice long-term weight loss is nearly impossible to achieve.[245] Almost everything works for a short time, but over a period of several years the results are dismal.[93, 94, 245, 246] Therapeutic reports that fail to consider dropouts must be regarded with skepticism, because those that cannot be located are likely to represent failures.[245, 247] Because the long-term results with all techniques are dismal, only a brief review of therapy will be provided here.

DIET. If energy intake is less than energy expenditure, weight loss will occur.[248, 249] No adult patient studied by direct calorimetry in a metabolic chamber has ever needed less than 1200 kcal/d to maintain body weight.[248] It follows that anyone truly eating 1000 kcal/d or less will lose weight. For fixed energy intake the absolute loss of weight per given calorie restriction is greater in the more obese than in the less obese because total energy requirements increase with increasing weight. The rate of weight loss varies, depending on fluid shifts and a variety of other factors such as change in exercise patterns and alterations in metabolic rate,[93, 95, 250, 251] but in general a negative balance of around 7500 kcal is required to lose 1 kg of weight if evaluation is carried out beyond the first few days of intervention (to avoid confusion from fluid loss).[252] This means that a 100-kcal deficit per day should approximate a 5-kg weight loss in a year—a trivial change in intake and yet one that cannot usually be accomplished. For this reason, more radical regimens have been tried, including total fasts,[94] very-low-calorie (240 to 330 kcal) diets,[253] and low-calorie (about 800 kcal) diets.[251, 254] There has been extensive discussion about the safety of very-low-calorie diets.[253] There is no question that excessive deaths occurred with liquid protein diets derived from gelatin and collagen that were deficient in essential amino acids.[255, 256] The danger appears to be due to cardiac arrhythmias.[257] If a protein source such as egg albumin or milk/soya is used, the very-low-calorie diets do not appear to cause excessive mortality rates.[253, 258] Some regimens are supplemented with 25 to 50 g of carbohydrate for the express purpose of diminishing protein requirements, minimizing fluid and electrolyte abnormalities, and maintaining serum T_3 concentrations.[248] Vitamins, minerals, and unsaturated fatty acids have to be added to the basic protein-carbohydrate mixture to avoid deficiency states. Weight loss occurs rapidly, and in many obese diabetic patients plasma glucose levels return to normal.[248, 259] Side effects are usually minimal, but hair loss, a sense of coldness, and thinning of the skin have been observed.

The problem is that weight loss can rarely be maintained after the very-low-calorie diet is stopped.[259] Thus, as with all forms of diet, the incidence of long-term improvement is low. Fasting or "supplemental fasting," as the very-low-calorie diets are sometimes called, is probably acceptable as a short-term tool to initiate a weight loss program, but radical diets cannot be counted on for the long term because weight gain tends to occur with reintroduction of food.

Much discussion has focused on the possibility that obese subjects "turn down" their metabolic rates when placed on dietary restriction, the fall in resting metabolic rate exceeding the fall in weight.[48, 260] Metabolic rates do fall with caloric restriction, but with reinstitution of energy intake to provide weight maintenance they return to previous levels;[261] i.e., the percent changes in body weight and resting metabolic rates are equivalent. This suggests that failure to maintain weight loss after severe caloric restriction is due to resumption of overeating rather than to a metabolic defect.

BEHAVIORIAL THERAPY. Behavioral therapy is designed to change eating patterns by guided training.[17, 102, 262] The method requires extensive self-monitoring of dietary practice—not only how much is eaten or drunk, but where and when. Attempts are also made to identify stimuli for eating. Behavioral therapy tries to change habits in a beneficial way by slowing food intake (e.g., putting utensils down between bites, increasing chewing time); separating eating from triggering events (e.g., eating in a room devoid of television or radio); eliminating energy-rich foods; controlling impulses to eat between meals when tired, bored, or under stress; and increasing exercise. Behavioral programs, too, have limited long-term success.[263, 264] Results may be marginally better if behavioral training is applied to the family unit rather than to the obese subject alone.[17]

EXERCISE. Exercise is almost invariably included in therapy for fat people. In theory the utilization of calories should be as valuable as the restriction of caloric intake. In practice this turns out not to be true because extensive exercise is needed to increase caloric expenditure significantly. For example, if one spent 5 kcal/min on a brisk walk[265] it would require a full hour to achieve a deficit of 300 kcal/d. Repetitive exercise regimens require tremendous dedication, a drive that may be absent from massively or even moderately obese people. Thus the dropout rates from exercise programs, like those for diet, are high.[17] Increased adherence may occur if training is carried out in groups under supervision.[266, 267] Ideally, protocols should be individually prescribed with the aim of achieving a specific level of training. Progress can be monitored by heart rate if oxygen uptakes cannot be measured.[267] Although long-term gains from exercise are minimal,[17] training can be accomplished in the obese[268] with beneficial side effects such as diminution of hypertension.[269] There has been speculation that some patients, identified as having increased adipose cellularity in contrast to a primary increase in cell size, may respond to exercise by gaining weight rather than losing because of increased food intake.[269]

Overall, exercise is of marginal benefit in the treatment of obesity.[248, 270] However, despite the cited reservations, an exercise component is appropriate to therapy for the obese, especially if support is available to enhance adherence.

DRUGS. Because of the extreme difficulty in achieving weight loss in major obesity, there has been a recurrent hope that drugs might help.[9] Thus far, that hope has not been fulfilled. T_3 has been added to very-low-calorie diets in an attempt to counteract the fall in plasma concentrations of T_3 that occur with semistarvation. Modest increases in the rate of weight loss are produced in the short term.[271, 272] However, nitrogen loss is accelerated by T_3 therapy so that three fourths of the extra loss comes from the lean body mass, not adipose tissue stores.[272]

Appetite-suppressant drugs are usually analogues of amphetamine. The most extensively evaluated have been diethylpropion, mazindol, phentermine, and fenfluramine.[17] All are central nervous system stimulants except fenfluramine, which has depressant qualities.[273] Fluoxetine, a serotonin reuptake inhibitor, has been reported to be effective in assisting weight loss.[248] Most patients with major obesity have received these drugs at some time during the course of their treatment. Although double-blind studies show short-term efficacy, weight gain essentially always recurs after withdrawal, which indicates that these agents should be used sparingly if at all.[9, 273, 274]

A variety of other drugs have been tested in weight loss programs, including human chorionic gonadotropin, levodopa, bromocriptine, opioid antagonists, and γ-linolenic acid.[248, 274] There is no evidence that any are of benefit. Sucrose polyester, a nonabsorbable mixture of six- to eight-carbon fatty acids in ester linkage with sucrose, has been used as a caloric diluent with modest decreases in total caloric intake (about 25%).[275] A beneficial side effect is a slight lowering of low-density lipoprotein cholesterol and triglyceride levels in plasma. Sucrose polyester appears to be safe, although prolonged use may produce deficiencies of fat-soluble vitamins.[275] Thus far, only short-term studies have been carried out, leaving the question of clinical usefulness unresolved.[276]

Some reports suggest that growth hormone injections may enhance the loss of body fat.[277, 278] It is interesting that such fat loss was accompanied by an increase in lean body mass in elderly men.[278] The effects of growth hormone in treatment of ordinary obesity are unknown, and potential side effects have not been evaluated.

Overall, there is considerable skepticism that drugs are useful, although this opinion is not universal.[279]

SURGERY. Because of the lack of success in medical therapy for massive obesity, attempts to reverse the condition by surgery were clearly justified. The most widely used procedure has been the jejunoileal bypass.[246] The first two forms of jejunoileal bypass were the Payne procedure (35 cm of jejunum anastomosed end to side to 10 cm of ileum) and the Scott operation (30 cm of jejunum anastomosed end to end with 15 cm of ileum, the proximal cut portion of the latter being inserted into the transverse colon).[280] Operative mortality is ordinarily around 4% but can be higher.[246] Large weight loss follows surgery and is sustained; it is due to both decreased food intake and malabsorption. The loss of appetite may be related to bacterial overgrowth in the bypassed segment.[281] On the other hand, significant complications follow both procedures,[282] including diarrhea (essentially universal); vitamin D deficiency with osteomalacia; diminished plasma levels of vitamins B_{12} and A and folic acid; arthritis; renal calculi (oxalate); hyperuricemia; deficiencies of magnesium, calcium, and potassium; and liver disease, which in some cases progresses to cirrhosis and hepatic coma. Because of these problems, jejunoileal bypass is no longer performed in most centers.[9, 246, 282, 283] Variants have been tried, including biliopancreatic and biliointestinal bypass operations.[9, 248, 284] In the former, drainage from the stomach is divided so that the fundus is isolated from the antrum, which is drained along with pancreatic and biliary ducts. In the latter, the bypassed loop is attached to the gallbladder, which allows bile salt reabsorption in the ileum. The patient must have a functioning gallbladder for this procedure.

A second procedure is the gastric bypass, which appears to be effective in producing weight loss without the serious late complications seen with the jejunoileal procedure.[285–287] Gastric plication (gastroplasty), involving a stapling procedure, is also widely used. The staples are applied either transversely across the stomach two fingers below the esophagogastric junction (leaving a 30- to 45-cm³ pouch and a channel along the greater curvature) or vertically along the lesser curvature. In controlled studies gastric bypass appears slightly more effective than gastroplasty. Although successful initially in almost all patients, the failure rate for both procedures is high when evaluated rigorously (up to 50% according to some assessments).[247] For this reason, it is not clear that gastric stapling or bypass surgery should be recommended as routine therapy for patients with morbid obesity.[288] Operative mortality is usually under 1%, but iron, vitamin B_{12}, and thiamine deficiencies may be late complications.[9]

Other procedures include jaw wiring and placement of gastric balloons.[9, 248, 284] The former causes weight loss, but the latter in controlled trials is no more effective than a sham operation.[248] Liposuction is useful for only cosmetic purposes.

OVERVIEW. Treatment of mild obesity is probably not necessary, but if desired for cosmetic reasons it can usually be accomplished by dietary restriction and an increase in exercise. On the other hand, results of therapy for seriously overweight persons, particularly the morbidly obese who are

50 kg or more overweight, are poor. The initial approach should be moderate dietary restriction with emphasis on long-term weight loss. Fasting or very-low-calorie, high-protein diets ordinarily should be used only for initiation of therapy or for circumstances in which rapid weight loss is required because of a medical complication: diabetes mellitus, cardiac disease, pulmonary distress, or the need for elective surgery. Drugs are not recommended. Exercise should be added both for an improved sense of well-being and for its effect on caloric balance, with the recognition that the limitation of caloric intake is more important. Gastric bypass surgery or plication should probably be reserved for patients with major medical complications of obesity, although these complications may themselves increase the operative risk. Conceivably, surgery is justified in patients with uncomplicated obesity whose illness has precluded employment or otherwise ruined the personal life, especially for individuals whose professions require extensive contact with the public. Physicians who deal with obese subjects have extensive experience with ministers, teachers, and police officers who have been discriminated against because of a weight problem. It should be remembered that surgery is expensive and not always reimbursable by insurance.

The patient with serious obesity should be seen regularly (probably weekly) by the professionals directing care: the nutritionist in every case, the behavioral therapist if such services are available, and the physician. Occasionally it may be worthwhile for those who can afford it to enter a special resident program as a form of shock treatment to reinforce the seriousness of the problem.[160]

The conclusion is inescapable that morbid obesity is an unsolved therapeutic problem.

Secondary Obesity

Almost every person who has morbid obesity believes that there is an underlying "glandular" reason. In consequence, endocrinologists are often consulted. In fact, secondary obesities are rare. The term *secondary* means that obesity accompanies another illness that is considered to be the primary disease state. In adults, one has to consider Cushing syndrome and hypothyroidism. In children, hypothalamic lesions may be the most common form. Craniopharyngioma heads the list, but other solid tumors, infections, and trauma can also occur.[198]

Acquired obesity (not present from infancy) coupled with headache, growth disorder, or endocrine dysfunction merits a CT or MRI examination of the head. The genetic diseases associated with obesity include the Prader-Willi syndrome, the Alström syndrome, the Laurence-Moon-Biedl syndrome, the Carpenter syndrome, the Cohen syndrome, and Blount disease.[289-291] The pathophysiology of the obesity in these syndromes is not known. One possibility is that sedentary behavior may play a significant role in the skeletal disorders and the syndromes with blindness.[292] The *Prader-Willi syndrome* consists of short stature, mental retardation, cryptorchidism, small hands and feet, neonatal hypotonia, and obesity. The face is also characteristic, with almond-shaped eyes and a fish-like mouth. Insulin resistance and glucose intolerance or diabetes mellitus are thought to be consequent to obesity. The disorder is associated with a deletion in the 15th chromosome.[293] The *Alström syndrome* is manifested by childhood blindness related to retinal degeneration, infantile obesity (which may disappear in adulthood), nerve deafness, diabetes mellitus with insulin resistance, acanthosis nigricans, chronic nephropathy, and hypogonadism in males but not females.[292] There appears to be primary testicular failure because testes are small, testosterone concentrations in plasma are low, and gonado-

tropin levels are high. Patients with the *Laurence-Moon-Biedl syndrome* exhibit retinitis pigmentosa, mental retardation, obesity, polydactyly, and hypogonadism. The last is associated with low gonadotropin levels, in contrast to the Alström syndrome.[289, 292] Glucose intolerance, deafness, and renal disease are rare. The *Carpenter syndrome* is characterized by obesity, mental retardation, male hypogonadism, acrocephaly, polydactyly, and syndactyly.[289] *Cohen syndrome* patients have microcephaly, severe mental retardation, short stature, facial abnormalities, and modest obesity.[290] *Blount disease* consists of bowed legs, tibial torsion, and obesity.[291] Although obesity is common, it is uncertain whether it really is intrinsic to the disorder.

In summary, secondary forms of obesity are uncommon. In adults, thyroid function and dexamethasone suppression tests may be required in some patients to rule out hypothyroidism and Cushing syndrome. The genetic disorders in children are usually clinically evident. Hypothalamic disease may manifest itself solely by obesity, but it usually presents with other clinical clues.

ANOREXIA NERVOSA–BULIMIA NERVOSA

Anorexia nervosa and bulimia nervosa are common syndromes characterized by bizarre eating patterns that become the central focus of the patient's life. Occurring primarily in young women, they represent life-disrupting illnesses for the afflicted and their families, and they lead to death in a significant number of cases. In this chapter, anorexia and bulimia will be considered variant expressions of the same underlying disorder. Although the clinical manifestations and outcome of the two syndromes are distinctive, overlapping features suggest that the root disorder is the same: an obsessive fear of being fat. In anorexic patients the primary reactive mechanism is the rigid restriction of food intake; with bulimia a loss of control in the drive to eat is compensated for by induced vomiting and laxative use.

History and Prevalence

Anorexia nervosa was described by Richard Morton in 1689, who reported the case of a girl aged 17 who was "like a skeleton only clad with skin."[294] He concluded that she had "a nervous consumption." The name *anorexia nervosa* appears to have been coined by Sir William Gull. Gull and Charles Lasègue, a French contemporary, both published accurate descriptions of the clinical manifestations. Anorexia nervosa became confused with pituitary apoplexy for a number of decades because of Simmonds' report of death by "emaciation" in a woman with pituitary destruction, but the issue was reclarified in 1930 when Berkman published his experience with 117 patients and emphasized that the physiological abnormalities were due to a psychic disturbance.[294, 295]

The true prevalence of anorexia and bulimia is unknown. Anorexia has been estimated to be present in 1% of upper-class adolescent girls in the United Kingdom[296] and in 2.9% of South African schoolgirls.[297] In the epidemiological archives of disease in Rochester, Minnesota, the incidence was 7.3 per 100,000 patient-years, with an overall prevalence of 0.1% (0.2% in women, 0.02% in men).[298] Discrepancies in prevalence doubtless derive from different criteria for diagnosis and different methods of ascertainment. Although subclinical disease may be present in up to 5% of the population,[299] most authorities accept a value of around 1% in whites. Similar figures have been found for bulimia,[300] although estimates of 1 to 4% have been cited.[301]

Diagnosis

The diagnosis of anorexia nervosa or bulimia nervosa is usually not difficult from a clinical standpoint when the full syndromes are present. Since 1972, the criteria of Feighner and colleagues[302] have been most widely used in research studies (Table 25–6). These include (1) onset before age 25; (2) weight loss of at least 25% of original body weight accompanied by anorexia; (3) fixed and distorted attitude toward eating and weight (denial of illness, enjoyment of weight loss, body image of thinness, unusual hoarding or handling of food); (4) absence of medical illness to account for weight loss; (5) absence of primary psychiatric disorder; and (6) presence of at least two of the following: amenorrhea, lanugo, bradycardia, periods of overactivity, episodes of bulimia, and emesis. The criteria given by the Diagnostic and Statistical Manual of Mental Disorders, third edition (DSM-III) of the American Psychiatric Association are less specific.[303] Both sets of criteria have been attacked as being too rigid, especially the 25% requirement for weight loss.[304, 305] Children in particular may be severely ill without having lost one fourth of their original body weight. For this reason the revised 1987 edition of DSM-III (DSM-III-R) lowers the diagnostic level for weight loss from 25 to 15% (see Table 25–6).[306] Also added are requirements for fear of fatness, a feeling that one is fat, and amenorrhea, either primary or secondary. The Feighner criteria, if one substitutes 15% for the 25% weight loss, appear to be the more useful for research studies. In practice the spectrum of eating disorders includes mild forms that do not meet either set of criteria. Such variants may progress to the full-blown syndrome but do not necessarily do so.

From a clinical standpoint the major features are an intense fear of becoming fat; a history of significant weight loss either currently (classic anorexia nervosa) or in the past (bulimia nervosa); absence of organic illness sufficient to cause weight loss; absence of primary psychiatric illness leading to loss of interest in eating; and the presence of unusual eating habits, either extreme dieting or gorging/regurgitation. Absence of one or more of the other features mentioned by Feighner and colleagues[302] should not exclude the diagnosis—including amenorrhea, which is perhaps the most constant biological expression of classic anorexia nervosa.[305] Although a disturbance of body image is common, this finding is not a specific, as discussed later.

The DSM-III-R has now provided diagnostic criteria for bulimia nervosa as well as anorexia nervosa[306] (see Table 25–6). Patients are required to have at least two recurrent episodes of binge eating per week for a minimum of 3 mo; a sense of lost control over eating binges; chronic self-induced vomiting, laxative or diuretic use, strict dieting, or extensive exercise; and, finally, a persistent overconcern with body shape or weight.

In either form of eating disorder care must be taken not to overlook other illnesses that may cause weight loss, vomiting, or increased food intake. Occult malignancy, diabetes mellitus, renal failure, and inflammatory bowel disease are common illnesses that must be considered. At times a classic eating disorder may coexist with organic illness, e.g., anorexia nervosa with diabetes mellitus.

Clinical Picture

ANOREXIA NERVOSA. The clinical features of anorexia nervosa are well delineated in reviews that provide access to the literature on this subject.[307–311]

Demographic Features. Anorexia nervosa is primarily a disease of women, only 4 to 6% of affected subjects being males. The age at onset ranges from prepuberty to the early

TABLE 25–6. Diagnostic Criteria for Anorexia Nervosa and Bulimia Nervosa

Anorexia Nervosa

Feighner et al.	DSM-III-R

1. Onset prior to age 25
2. Anorexia with weight loss of at least 25% of original body weight
3. Distorted attitude toward eating, food, or weight that overrides hunger, admonitions, reassurances, and threats
4. No known medical illness that could account for the weight loss
5. No other known psychiatric disorder
6. At least two of the following manifestations:
  a. Amenorrhea
  b. Lanugo hair
  c. Bradycardia (persistent resting pulse of 60 beats per minute or less)
  d. Periods of overactivity
  e. Episodes of bulimia
  f. Vomiting (may be self-induced)
	1. Refusal to maintain body weight over a minimal normal weight for age and height, e.g., weight loss leading to maintenance of body weight 15% below that expected; or failure to make expected weight gain during period of growth, leading to body weight 15% below that expected
	2. Intense fear of gaining weight or becoming fat, even though underweight
	3. Disturbance in the way in which one's body weight, size, or shape is experienced, e.g., the person claims to "feel fat" even when emaciated, believes that one area of the body is "too fat" even when obviously underweight
	4. In females, absence of at least three consecutive menstrual cycles when otherwise expected to occur (primary or secondary amenorrhea) (a woman is considered to have amenorrhea if her periods occur only following hormone, e.g., estrogen, administration)

Bulimia Nervosa

DSM-III-R
1. Recurrent episodes of binge eating (rapid consumption of a large amount of food in a discrete period of time) 2. A feeling of lack of control over eating behavior during the eating binges 3. The person regularly engages in either self-induced vomiting, use of laxatives or diuretics, strict dieting or fasting, or vigorous exercise in order to prevent weight gain 4. A minimum average of two binge-eating episodes a week for at least 3 mo 5. Persistent overconcern with body shape and weight

Adapted from Feighner JP, Robins E, Guze SB, et al. Diagnostic criteria for use in psychiatric research. Arch Gen Psychiatry 1972; 26:57–63, copyright 1972, American Medical Association; and with permission from the Diagnostic and Statistical Manual of Mental Disorders, Third Edition, Revised. Copyright 1987 American Psychiatric Association.

30s. The most common time of appearance is 4 to 5 y after menarche.[309] The disease appears to occur primarily in whites, usually in families from the middle or upper class. A disproportionate number are Jewish. There is an increased prevalence of anorexia in parents and siblings of index cases.[312] In one study, 29 of 102 patients had a primary family member who was at least 20% below the mean weight of a matched population.[309] Only 10 family members were as much as 20% overweight. Because the prevalence of obesity in the general population is greater than 10%, it can be concluded that fatness in families of subjects with anorexia is not excessive. This conclusion is important because in the past it was considered that the disorder might have something to do with a reaction to obesity in a parent. Onset of disease frequently follows a stressful event in the subject's life.

Behavioral Characteristics. The term anorexia is really inappropriate because true loss of appetite does not occur until late in the course of disease, if at all. Patients are not free of hunger; rather, they are obsessed with the fear of being fat so that hunger sensations are ignored or denied. An intense preoccupation with food is usually discernible. Although anorexic patients drastically restrict their own food intake, it is not unusual for them to enjoy preparing elaborate meals for others and to collect recipes and hoard food in the home. Most subjects appear knowledgeable about nutritional matters, particularly the caloric content of food, although some show lesser insight than matched controls.[313] It is usually stated that carbohydrates are avoided, but this is not always the case. Fat intake tends to be low and protein intake is high. Sporadic dieting usually begins about a year before the start of the disease proper, often at the point at which maximal weight was reached.[309]

To assist weight loss, it is common for patients to exercise excessively, often in ritualistic fashion. A significant percentage induce vomiting and use laxatives or diuretics. Periodic gorging of the type seen in the bulimic variant of the disease may also occur in classic anorexia nervosa.

Perceptual Abnormalities. Patients with anorexia nervosa characteristically deny illness, at least until the disease is far advanced. Resistance to treatment is profound. They deny hunger, fatigue, and change in physical appearance. Affected subjects may have a disturbance of body image that makes them see themselves as continually fat.[314] Several types of objective evaluation show the propensity of anorexic patients to overestimate true body size while the capacity to assess other objects accurately is maintained. However, there are doubts about the specificity of distorted body image in anorexia nervosa.[146, 314–317] Similar distortions can be seen in control populations. The tendency to overestimate body size is usual in adolescence and tends to ameliorate or disappear with age or maturation. For this reason it has been suggested that disturbance of body image be deleted from the diagnostic criteria for anorexia nervosa.[146]

Symptoms. The denials that characterize anorexia nervosa tend to minimize spontaneous revelation of symptoms, although almost all patients will discuss amenorrhea when asked. Sleep disturbances are fairly common.[309, 312, 318] Constipation is not unusual, although diarrhea may occur with laxative use.[310] Complaints of early satiety and abdominal pain are frequent. The cause of these gastrointestinal symptoms is not known, although abnormally slow gastric emptying has been reported.[319] Gastric rupture can occur, usually in bulimic patients, but it may be seen with classic anorexia nervosa during refeeding.[320] Cold intolerance is often acknowledged, and true hypothermia has been reported.[307] Traditionally cold intolerance has been attributed to "functional hypothyroidism," but abnormality of the hypothalamic temperature-regulating centers may be a more likely expla-

nation.[321] Patients with anorexia nervosa do not defend well against either heat or cold challenge. Heat production in muscle, measured directly by microcalorimetry, is diminished about 50% per unit muscle mass in anorexia nervosa compared with normal controls.[322] Heat generation in platelets is not impaired, nor is the defect in muscle seen in bulimic subjects. Whether this defect is regulated locally or by the central nervous system is not known. Anorexic patients may also develop excessive vasoconstriction, cyanosis, and numbness of the extremities on exposure to cold, which reflects an abnormal sensitivity of the vessels to low temperatures.[323] Raynaud phenomenon has been noted. Finally, CT studies show that subcutaneous fat loss is greater than deep fat loss in anorexia.[324] Subcutaneous fat provides thermal insulation, and its absence allows greater heat loss.

Physical Findings. The physical examination in classic anorexia nervosa is characterized pre-eminently by cachexia so severe as to be reminiscent of concentration camp victims in World War II. In the fully dressed state the degree of weight loss may not be appreciated because the victims tend to wear masking clothes (long sleeves, long skirts, slacks). Parotid enlargement related to malnutrition may soften the angularity of the face expected with this degree of weight loss. As in other forms of semistarvation, the pulse rate is slow, and blood pressure is on the low side. The basal metabolic rate is decreased, consequent to diminished body mass. Peripheral edema is common. It is usually due not to hypoalbuminemia but to a failure to mobilize the normal extracellular fluid volume with starvation. An increase in body hair, usually quite fine, may be present. A yellow cast to the skin related to carotenemia is a helpful clue because carotene levels are characteristically low in other forms of malnutrition. A summary of the physical findings in 65 anorexic patients is shown in Table 25–7.[325]

BULIMIA NERVOSA. The term *bulimia* means literally "ox hunger" or a voracious appetite. It has come to stand for a syndrome of astonishing food intake during short periods in young women who usually have a previous or present picture of anorexia nervosa. The gorging is then followed by induced vomiting and often by the use of laxatives in large amounts. If one selects patients for anorexia nervosa by the Feighner criteria, about 40 to 50% of subjects admit bulimia-vomiting,[326, 327] but some patients may exhibit binge eating without ever going through an anorexic phase.[328] Two fundamental features characterize the syndrome: (1) an irresistible urge to overeat and (2) a marked fear of becoming fat. The former predominates in this form of the illness, but other features distinguish it from anorexia nervosa. In simple terms, patients with nonbulimic anorexia nervosa deal with the fear of being fat by restricting food intake (restrictors). Their phobia of being fat appears to be so powerful that control over eating is not lost. Bulimic patients, on the other hand, lose such control and thus become gorgers. They control weight gain only by vomiting

TABLE 25–7. Physical Findings in 65 Patients with Anorexia Nervosa

Abnormality	% Affected
Skin (e.g., hairiness, dryness)	88
Hypothermia (<96.6°F, rectal)	85
Bradycardia (<60 beats/min)	80
Cachexia	72
Bradypnea (<15 breaths/min)	66
Hypotension (<70 mm Hg systolic)	52
Heart murmur	38
Edema	23

Adapted from Silverman JA. Anorexia nervosa: clinical and metabolic observations in a successful treatment plan. In: Vigersky RA, ed. Anorexia Nervosa. New York: Raven, 1977: 331–339.

and using laxatives. A careful study of 30 patients illustrates the ontogeny of the bulimic syndrome.[328] Eleven of 30 patients began bulimic behavior after a period of weight gain, whereas 19 started during a period of weight loss. Eventually all patients began to gain weight. At the time treatment was sought, 24 subjects were still underweight, two were of normal weight, and four were above healthy weight. In every case, however, bulimia was interpreted to be a signal of actual or anticipated failure in control of food intake.

Demographic Features. As with typical anorexia nervosa, most patients are women. Major demographic features are similar in the two groups, although the premorbid weight and weight at time of assessment appear to be higher in bulimic subjects.[327] Maximal weight loss during the course of illness is also less. Mothers of bulimic patients have a higher prevalence of obesity than mothers of restrictors, but the percentage is still not excessive relative to the general population.

Behavioral Characteristics. The drive to eat in bulimic patients is overwhelming. Thoughts are constantly on food, and even dreams may focus on eating. The drive is not from hunger. One patient described it as follows: "It is not hunger. Hunger is a feeling of a gap inside you. You eat something small to stop that feeling. I go on eating after I've satisfied that hunger. I want to keep on eating until I feel full—it's the final limit—you can then eat no more."[328] The amount of food ingested can be enormous, up to 50,000 cal/d. In a series of 40 patients, the mean duration of binge-eating episodes was 1.2 h, but an episode could last as long as 8 h.[329] On average gorging occurred 12 times a week, but the range was from as few as 1 to as many as 46 times. The mean number of calories ingested per episode was 3415, but the number could reach 11,500 at one sitting. In these 40 patients the major foods eaten, in descending order of frequency, were ice cream, bread or toast, candy, doughnuts, soft drinks, and other foods. Usually more than one food was used in an episode. Overeating is ordinarily carried out secretly and alone, generally in the afternoon and evening.[328, 329] Often the episodes appear to be precipitated by ingestion of a "forbidden" high-carbohydrate food, which sets up an unstoppable chain reaction. If the urge to eat the first morsel can be controlled, binges do not occur. (Some have likened this situation to the "first drink" phenomenon in alcoholics.) There may thus be an all-or-none pattern to the eating. The term *dietary chaos* has been coined to describe the eating behavior in bulimic subjects,[330] and it is an accurate description.

After gorging, essentially all patients with bulimia induce vomiting,[328, 329] most often by activating the gag reflex with the fingers or a toothbrush, although some subjects learn to regurgitate spontaneously. Ipecac may be used by as many as 20% of patients and may cause myopathy and, possibly, cardiomyopathy.[331] Vomiting may become ritualistic, with a fixed number of retchings required to allow satisfaction that all food has been removed. A high percentage of patients also use laxatives,[331] although cathartic abuse is not as common as vomiting. Other forms of weight control, such as excessive exercise and use of diuretics, probably occur to a similar extent in both anorexic and bulimic syndromes.

A striking feature of bulimia is the propensity to carry out antisocial behavior.[326–328, 332, 333] Twelve to 14% of patients with bulimia admit stealing (most often food); the actual percentage may be higher. Stealing is not a feature of anorexia nervosa with major weight loss.[332] Patients in the bulimic phase use both street drugs and alcohol to a greater extent than do anorexic subjects.[311] Self-mutilation and suicide attempts are three to four times more common in

TABLE 25–8. Behavioral Patterns in Anorexia Nervosa and Bulimia Nervosa

	% of Patients	
Behavior	Anorexia Nervosa	Bulimia Nervosa
Use of alcohol	4.8	20.4
Use of illicit drugs	11.6	28.6
Stealing	0	12.1
Self-mutilation	1.5	9.2
Suicide attempts	7.1	23.1

Adapted from Garfinkel PE, Moldofsky H, Garner DM. The heterogeneity of anorexia nervosa. Bulimia as a distinct subgroup. Arch Gen Psychiatry 1980; 37:1036–1040. Copyright 1980, American Medical Association.

bulimia than in anorexia (Table 25–8). Although most patients with eating disorders are uninterested in sex, sexual promiscuity can occur.[328]

Perceptual Abnormalities. Formal testing of body image perception in the bulimic subset has not been reported, although it has been stated that overestimation of body size was greater in bulimics than in a control group.[326] There is probably no major difference from classic anorexia.

Symptoms. In contrast to classic anorexia nervosa, amenorrhea was present in only 11 of 28 subjects when cessation of menses was not used as part of the selection criteria.[328] This difference is probably because weight loss was less severe in the bulimic group. Although amenorrhea is not frequently seen, irregular menses and oligomenorrhea are common.[334] The other major complaint, often spontaneously voiced, is of depression. So ubiquitous is recognizable depression that some authors considered bulimia a variant of the affective disorder. However, it is now thought that bulimia and depression are distinct syndromes that share some endocrine and affective features.[335] In view of the recurrent vomiting with hypokalemia, one would expect complaints of weakness to be frequent, but this was not obvious in the cited series. Convulsions and tetany occur but are rare.[328] The cause of the former is not known; hypokalemia presumably accounted for the latter. Constipation, abdominal pain, and cold intolerance do not appear to be major complaints.

Physical Findings. Bulimic patients are usually not emaciated and as a consequence do not exhibit bradycardia, relative hypotension, or hypothermia. Parotid enlargement may follow binges. They may have scars from self-mutilation or suicide attempts.

Laboratory Abnormalities

Although many systems of the body are affected in severe anorexia nervosa, most of the laboratory changes are of little consequence and not unique because they occur in other forms of semistarvation. Laboratory abnormalities in bulimia are less common. Unless specified otherwise, the changes described in this section are for anorexia. Hematological findings include anemia, leukopenia (relative neutropenia, lymphocytosis), thrombocytopenia, low erythrocyte sedimentation rate, and decreased fibrinogen levels in plasma.[307, 308, 310, 311, 336] The anemia and occasional pancytopenia appear to be due to hypoplasia of the bone marrow, which is filled with a gelatinous mucopolysaccharide. Peripheral blood smears may show acanthosis. Hypokalemia may occur in both anorexia and bulimia secondary to vomiting or laxative use.

Plasma protein levels tend to be normal, although hypoalbuminemia may be seen.[308, 310] Essential amino acid values are not low, in contrast to those in kwashiorkor, probably because of the relatively high protein intake of anorexic subjects.

β-Carotene levels in plasma are high, together with vitamin A and its derivatives.[310] The mechanism of this elevation is not clear. However, the fact that anorexic subjects who vomit have serum carotene levels only one half those of nonvomiters suggests that dietary intake plays a major role.[337]

Mild hypercholesterolemia is frequent in anorexia nervosa. The cholesterol elevation is in the low-density lipoprotein fraction; both high-density and very-low-density lipoprotein levels are normal.[338] Plasma triglyceride concentrations are normal despite low values for hepatic and LPL activities. The cause of the hypercholesterolemia is not known, although neutral sterol and bile acid secretion appears to be low.[339] The failure of ovulation and amenorrhea that is almost universal in anorexia doubtless plays a major role. The ritualized exercise of anorexia would be expected to lower low-density and increase high-density lipoprotein levels, but this beneficial effect is neutralized in amenorrheic women.[340] It is presumed that estrogen deficiency is the primary cause, probably acting through a diminution in hepatic low-density lipoprotein receptor number.

In view of the known relationship between malnutrition and depressed immune function (variable effect on humoral immune function; profound effect on cellular immunity), there has been considerable interest in the immune response in anorexia nervosa. In a series of five patients,[341] mean levels of immunoglobulin G, immunoglobulin M, and transferrin were low before hyperalimentation. The deficiencies were reversed by feeding. A number of alternative complement pathway proteins were also low. The mechanism was thought to be decreased synthesis. When 22 consecutively admitted patients were studied by an anergy panel to test delayed hypersensitivity, only 6 showed defective responses.[342] This number is in accord with the view that most patients with anorexia nervosa are surprisingly free of infection.[342-344] Occasionally infection does occur, as indicated by a death from herpes simplex encephalitis.[343]

Other abnormalities have been reported, but none is of major clinical significance. The glomerular filtration rate is generally slightly low, and prerenal azotemia with blood urea nitrogen levels as high as 21 to 25 mM (60 to 70 mg/dL) may be seen.[325] Renal concentrating ability is impaired and polyuria may occur.[345] Arginine vasopressin is not released normally in response to an osmotic stimulus, and its action in the kidney may be impaired.[308, 345, 346] Levels of vasopressin in the cerebrospinal fluid are elevated relative to those in plasma.[345] Nonspecific ST-T changes may be seen on electrocardiographic examination. Serum amylase levels may be elevated in the absence of clinical signs of pancreatitis. High levels of amylase are more common in bulimia than in anorexia.[331, 347] In 30 hospitalized patients with anorexia nervosa, plasma zinc and copper values were low, although the content of these metals in hair was normal.[348] Iron-binding capacity was decreased, but plasma iron and ceruloplasmin levels were normal. Hypogeusia (taste impairment) was noted, most marked for bitter and sour stimuli.

Endocrine Findings

Considerable interest has focused on the endocrine system in anorexia nervosa for two reasons. First, the earlier period of confusion between pituitary insufficiency and anorexia nervosa needed to be clarified. Second, amenorrhea is an almost constant feature in the typical form of the disease. It now seems clear that the endocrine changes are all secondary; i.e., there is no evidence for primary dysfunction in the pituitary gland, gonads, thyroid, or adrenal

glands. A summary of endocrine changes in anorexia and bulimia is shown in Table 25–9. For reviews, see refs. 334 and 349.

AMENORRHEA. About one half of patients with anorexia nervosa develop secondary amenorrhea concomitant with the onset of dieting, whereas one fifth cease menses before the onset of overt disease. The remaining patients undergo secondary failure of menses only after weight loss is significant.[310, 350] Presumably, early amenorrhea is due to psychological stress antedating clinical illness.[351] It is now generally accepted that the primary defect is localized in the hypothalamus and operates via impaired release of LHRH. Baseline LH and FSH values are low, and the 24-h LH profile regresses to either a prepubertal pattern (all values low) or a pubertal pattern (sleep-dependent LH release only).[352] The prepubertal pattern is most common.[353] With weight gain, reversal of the abnormalities occurs, the pubertal pattern appearing at about 70% ideal body weight and the adult pattern near 80% ideal body weight. The pituitary response to LHRH is abnormal with severe weight loss, but reverses to normal with weight gain.[354] Pituitary responsiveness to LHRH can be restored either by low-dose LHRH treatment (given by infusion) or by pulsatile injection.[354, 355] Characteristically FSH responds first and then LH, the pattern mirroring the events that take place during normal puberty. Presumably, the lack of pituitary responsiveness to acute stimulation by LHRH represents removal of a trophic effect of LHRH with prolonged semistarvation. Why the hypothalamus is unable to release LHRH in anorexia nervosa is not known, although abnormalities in norepinephrine and dopamine metabolism in the central nervous system have been postulated.[310, 334] Bromocriptine, a dopaminergic agonist, has no effect on the abnormalities, however.[354] The hypothalamic-pituitary axis is likewise unresponsive to clomiphene.[356]

Low estrogen levels and failure to ovulate in anorexia appear to be solely due to gonadotropin deficiency, because ovulation can be induced by either exogenous gonadotropins or LHRH administration for prolonged periods.[357, 358] Although menses usually return with weight gain, this is not invariably so as psychological factors can continue to override the reversal of cachexia. It has been claimed that after secondary amenorrhea a body weight about 10% greater than that needed for menarche is required.[359]

Men with anorexia nervosa appear to have the same abnormalities in gonadotropins seen in females, and in consequence testosterone levels are low.[360]

As noted earlier, amenorrhea is not as common in bulimia as in anorexia. Studies of gonadotropic function in bulimia are not in agreement. Part of the problem may be that menstruating and anovulatory patients were pooled. It is likely that basal LH levels are low in bulimic women with menstrual irregularities and that as a consequence estradiol and progesterone concentrations are also low.[349] It has been reported that in bulimic women the LH response to LHRH was enhanced, in contrast to the diminished response characteristic of anorexia nervosa with weight loss.[349, 361]

OTHER PITUITARY HORMONES. Basal growth hormone values are elevated in some patients with both anorexia nervosa and bulimia.[321, 334, 349] Overall about one third to one half of patients have elevated basal levels, although the response to provocative stimuli may be impaired in others.[250, 334, 349, 362] IGF I levels are low in both anorexia nervosa and bulimia nervosa.[334, 349, 363] It is possible that elevated growth hormone levels are the consequence of diminished feedback activity by IGF I. IGF I levels are probably low because of both decreased synthesis and the presence of inhibitors of somatomedins in plasma, which are features characteristic of malnutrition and weight loss of any cause. Plasma prolac-

TABLE 25–9. Endocrine Changes in Anorexia Nervosa and Bulimia Nervosa*

Anorexia Nervosa	Bulimia Nervosa
Hypothalamus and Pituitary Gland	
↓ LH (↓ response to LHRH)	→ or ↓ LH (↑ response to LHRH)
↓ FSH	→ or ↓ FSH
↑ or → growth hormone (↓ IGF I)	↑ or → growth hormone (↓ IGF I)
→ TSH (delayed response to TRH)	→ TSH (delayed response to TRH)
→ corticotropin (↓ response to CRH)	→ corticotropin (↓ or → response to CRH)
→ or ↓ prolactin (↓ response to TRH)	→ or ↓ prolactin (↑ response to TRH)
Abnormal regulation vasopressin	? vasopressin regulation
Thyroid Gland	
↓ thyroxine	→ thyroxine
↓ T$_3$	→ or ↓ T$_3$
↑ reverse T$_3$	? reverse T$_3$
Adrenal Gland	
→ or ↑ cortisol	→ or ↑ cortisol
↑ urinary free cortisol	→ urinary free cortisol
Abnormal dexamethasone suppression	Abnormal dexamethasone suppression
↓ dehydroepiandrosterone and its sulfate	
Ovary	
↓ estradiol	→ or ↓ estradiol
↓ estrone	→ or ↓ estrone
↓ progesterone	→ or ↓ progesterone
Testis	
↓ testosterone	

*Symbols: ↓, decreased; ↑, increased; →, normal.

tin levels are usually normal in anorexia.[321, 364, 365] Prolactin levels have been reported as both normal and low in bulimia.[349] Prolactin response to TRH is said to be blunted[366] in anorexia, whereas some subjects have a paradoxical rise after LHRH.[367] Bulimic patients are said to have an increased release of prolactin after TRH. Abnormal control of vasopressin was cited earlier.[345] TSH and corticotropin (ACTH, adrenocorticotropin) will be discussed later.

THYROID. Despite the slow pulse and low basal metabolic rate that characterize anorexia nervosa and other forms of weight loss, there is no evidence of hypothyroidism.[368, 369] The usual picture is low-normal thyroxine (T$_4$), low T$_3$, and increased reverse T$_3$ levels. There are two forms of the euthyroid sick syndrome: one in which the T$_3$ value is low and both T$_4$ and reverse T$_3$ levels are elevated,[370] and the other in which both T$_4$ and T$_3$ levels are low.[371] The former mimics hyperthyroidism, the latter hypothyroidism. The low-normal T$_4$ is thought to be due to an inhibitor that blocks binding of T$_4$ to thyroid-binding globulin.[371] The TSH response to TRH may be abnormal in the low T$_4$, T$_3$ syndrome.[371] A common pattern is delay in the peak response to TRH, although absolutely blunted responses are also seen.[334] Reversal of the thyroid abnormalities occurs with weight gain. Some patients have an overshoot of T$_3$ accompanied by symptoms of mild hyperthyroidism in the recovery phase.[372] Some investigators have found low levels of T$_3$ in bulimia, but large numbers of patients have not been studied.[349] TSH levels are normal, but a delayed time to peak release after TRH is seen, as in anorexia.

ADRENAL GLAND. Adrenal function has been extensively studied in the eating disorders but is still not completely understood.[334] Chemical findings suggest hypercortisolism, but no clinical features of cortisol excess are noted.[373] Plasma cortisol levels are high-normal or elevated. Urinary free cortisol is also elevated. The half-life of plasma cortisol is prolonged, and urinary metabolites are decreased.[374] Cortisol production rates are normal or slightly elevated, particularly if body mass is considered.[334, 375] Many explanations for elevated cortisol levels have been offered, including peripheral resistance to the hormone.[373] Cortisol binding in plasma is normal. The present consensus is that the primary defect is localized in the hypothalamus, but the mechanism is unknown. Dexamethasone suppression is abnormal in anorexia, and the ACTH response to CRH is blunted.[373, 376] CRH levels in the cerebrospinal fluid are elevated,[376, 377] whereas ACTH levels are low.[378] The presumption is that the initial lesion is hypersecretion of CRH, hypersecretion of ACTH, overproduction of cortisol, and hyperplasia of the adrenals, with subsequent feedback of cortisol on the pituitary so that ACTH levels fall into the normal range.[373] It is assumed that feedback on the hypothalamus is impaired, which would account for the elevated CRH levels. Although the ACTH response to synthetic CRH is blunted, the cortisol response expected from a given rise in ACTH is increased.[373]

Bulimic subjects without weight loss have normal urinary free cortisol levels, with high-normal concentrations in plasma. Failure of dexamethasone suppression is common.[349] The ACTH response to CRH has been reported to be both normal[373] and impaired.[379]

Levels of dehydroepiandrosterone and its sulfate are low in anorexia.[380] A number of enzyme defects have been reported (e.g., 5α-reductase deficiency), but their significance is unknown.[307, 310, 381]

The abnormalities in hypothalamic-pituitary-adrenal function are restored by weight gain.

MISCELLANEOUS. Melatonin levels have generally been found to be increased with higher than normal day/night ratios,[382, 383] although night concentrations were not increased in one study.[384] The response of glucagon to hypoglycemia is impaired, whereas release after administration of arginine is normal.[385]

Complications of Anorexia Nervosa and Bulimia Nervosa

Serious complications may develop when the eating disorders are severe or prolonged. Osteoporosis in anorexia nervosa can involve both the spine and peripheral bones.[386–388] Osteopenia progresses most rapidly if dieting begins before the peak bone mass has been attained and if amenorrhea is primary or begins early.[389] The primary mechanism appears to be estrogen deficiency, but dietary calcium or vitamin D deficiency and hypercortisolism may play ancillary roles. Teeth are not affected except for enamel wear in patients who vomit.[390]

Atrophy of the brain with dilated ventricles was found by CT in both anorexia[391] and bulimia.[392] Because the bulimic patients studied were not underweight, the explanation for the atrophy is not forthcoming. It is claimed that an inverse relationship exists between plasma concentrations of T_3 and ventricular size in both types of eating disorders,[392] but the meaning of this negative correlation is not clear. Electroencephalographic abnormalities have also been seen, predominantly in binge eaters.[331] Some consider the changes to be nonspecific.

Heart disease is a potentially fatal complication of anorexia nervosa and may cause sudden death.[393] Ventricular tachyarrhythmias are the major mechanism, similar to the deaths occurring with liquid protein diets. All patients should be followed with electrocardiograms, a prolonged Q-T interval being a distinct sign of danger. In addition, severe weight loss leads to both systolic and diastolic dysfunction of the ventricles, with the possibility of congestive heart failure, especially on refeeding.[394] Heart rate and blood pressure responses to exercise are routinely blunted. Mitral valve prolapse is common in women with anorexia nervosa and resolves with weight gain.[395] The mechanism is thought to be a valvuloventricular mismatch; i.e., decreased left ventricular volume caused by starvation leaves the normal leaflets too long. Heart disease is relatively rare in normal-weight bulimic subjects, although hypokalemia related to vomiting may cause arrhythmias.[331] As mentioned earlier, heavy use of ipecac can potentially cause cardiomyopathy.

The serious complications of bulimia nervosa are the consequence of binge eating and vomiting. Tears or ruptures of the esophagus may result in pneumomediastinum or pneumoperitoneum.[331] Spontaneous rupture of the stomach may follow gorging or may occur with refeeding in anorexic patients.[320, 331] If vomiting is severe, hypotension related to volume depletion and metabolic acidosis may ensue. Finally, fatal pulmonary aspiration with asphyxiation may follow giant gorges.

Psychological Accompaniments

Although the diagnosis of anorexia nervosa is designed to exclude primary psychiatric illnesses such as schizophrenia or severe depression, a significant percentage of patients have psychoneurotic symptoms,[396] depression,[397] and transient psychoses.[398] Considerable emphasis has been placed on impaired psychosexual maturation in girls with anorexia, but this problem has not been confirmed in all series.[399]

Etiology

The cause of anorexia nervosa is not known. It has been argued[400] that hypothalamic dysfunction is primary, but the evidence appears persuasive that the disorder is a psychiatric one. The psychodynamics are not clear and in fact may not be fixed. Whatever other factors operate in the genesis of the disease, the families tend to be "enmeshed": there are blurred generational boundaries so that parents and children are constantly involved in each other's problems.[310, 401] Some workers suggest that both major eating disorders—the anorexia nervosa and bulimia nervosa syndromes and obesity—have as a fundamental characteristic a paralyzing sense of ineffectiveness induced by early events in family life.[98] Subjects experience themselves as acting only in response to demands coming from others and as not doing anything because they want to. This has been colorfully stated as

follows: "The development of anorexia may be conceived as a shouting and unrelenting 'No' which extends to every area of living, though most conspicuous in the food refusal. Uncontrolled obesity, on the other hand, is the manifest expression of despair, of having given up all efforts to establish a sense of inner control and independent identity."[98] The family members of bulimic subjects have a higher prevalence of affective disorders, alcoholism, and drug use than is the case with classic anorexia nervosa.[402] Some have thought that traditional explanations of enmeshed families are oversimplified,[403] but others continue to favor the classic view.[404]

Although family structure appears to play a primary role in the genesis of anorexia nervosa, culture is also important.[311, 405] In contemporary Western society the ideal female figure is that of a slender prepubertal girl bearing the secondary sexual characteristics of a mature woman. Preoccupation with diets and weight loss is common in normal teen-age girls in these societies: up to 70% in the 12th grade.[406] The prevalence of anorexia nervosa in dancers is 10 times that in the general population, which suggests that even occupation may play a role. Anorexia-like syndromes have been seen with increasing frequency in athletes who want to reduce their fat to 5 to 7% of body weight.[407, 408] Thus, if there is a rising prevalence of anorexia nervosa, it may be due to relentless cultural pressures to diet, stay slim, and exercise, this pressure selecting those predisposed to develop the illness.

How the psychodynamic dysfunction is translated into biological disease remains a mystery. Numerous neurotransmitter systems are altered in anorexia and bulimia[409] and may play a mediating role. For example, cholecystokinin secretion is impaired in bulimia[410] and could represent a failed satiety signal. But what caused it? These are the questions of future research.

Treatment

There is no specific treatment for anorexia or bulimia, although multiple approaches have been tried.[411] A partial list includes insulin, thyroid hormone, gonadotropins, antidepressants, antipsychotics, tranquilizers, electroconvulsive therapy, appetite stimulants, and leukotomy. From a psychological and psychiatric standpoint, behavior modification and individual and group psychotherapy have been tried, singly and in combination. Most experts in the field agree that there is no one way to approach what is an incredibly difficult problem. However, certain general principles can be developed.[311, 411, 412, 413]

First, some attempt must be made to provide insight to the patient about the problem. Second, behavior has to be modified. Third, families must be involved. In general, both individual and group psychotherapy will be required. Antidepressant drugs are often prescribed,[311, 414] but results are marginal. The possibility of inducing cardiac arrhythmias with tricyclic antidepressants in wasted subjects has to be considered. Cyproheptadine has been tried but probably is of little use. In short, no specific pharmacotherapy is available.

Most therapy is done on an outpatient basis. It may be preferable to initiate treatment in the hospital when weight loss is extreme.[411, 412] Hospitalization is always indicated with complications such as arrhythmias, aspiration, or rupture of the gastrointestinal tract. The immediate aim of hospitalization is weight gain. Every attempt should be made to do this by having the patient eat. Tube feeding or intravenous hyperalimentation should be undertaken only as a last resort. Care must be taken to keep electrolyte values within normal limits. Phosphate depletion is especially dangerous and may lead to cardiac or respiratory failure.[394, 415] The patient must be encouraged to eat and must be repeatedly assured of the "safety" of eating. It may be useful for the physician to state specifically: "I will not let you get fat" and set up a contractual relationship as a guarantee; e.g., "If you gain x pounds, which is necessary for your safety, we will stop there for several months before proceeding." During the initial phases of therapy, whether as an inpatient or an outpatient, every effort should be made to keep the patient from eating alone. As in anorexia, no specific therapy is available for bulimia.

To summarize, there is no definitive therapy for the eating disorders. Patience is an absolute requirement for the health care team, who must be thought trustworthy by the patient. Many patients are followed in special clinics for eating disorders, but many are managed by nonpsychiatrists.[416, 417] The long-term outlook in anorexia and bulimia is difficult to ascertain and impossible to relate to treatment programs.

Attempts have been made to evaluate the results of follow-up studies.[418-422] The problem is that the range of responses is so broad for each parameter as to make firm conclusions impossible. Best estimates for patients followed 2 y or longer suggest that about 50% achieve normal weight, 20% are improved but underweight, 20% are unchanged from the anorexic state, 5% are obese, and 4 to 6% are dead. Eighty-eight deaths from anorexia were recorded in the latest tabulation of follow-up studies but none in patients with bulimia.[422] Of the deaths, 44 (50%) were due to complications of anorexia, 21 (24%) were suicides, 5 (6%) were due to pulmonary disease, 5 (6%) were secondary to accidents or another illness, and 13 (15%) were of unknown cause. Perhaps 50 to 75% start menses again, although irregularity is common. Despite the fact that most patients gain weight, eating disorders (restriction, bulimia, vomiting, laxative use) continue to be common (up to 70%). As many as 50% of patients have recognizable psychiatric difficulties not directly related to the eating disturbance. Thus although many patients with anorexia nervosa get better and are able to function in society, the prognosis for normal physical and mental health is poor. Earlier evidence suggested that nonbulimic patients fare better than bulimic subjects,[328, 421] but subsequent studies have not confirmed this prediction.[422]

REFERENCES

Obesity

1. Manson JE, Colditz GA, Stampfer MJ, et al. A prospective study of obesity and risk of coronary heart disease in women. N Engl J Med 1990; 322:882–889.
2. Drenick EJ, Bale GS, Seltzer F, et al. Excessive mortality and causes of death in morbidly obese men. JAMA 1980; 243:443–445.
3. Garn SM, Clark DC. Trends in fatness and the origins of obesity. Pediatrics 1976; 57:443–456.
4. Grande F. Assessment of body fat in man. In: Bray GA, ed. Obesity in Perspective. DHEW Publication No. (NIH) 75–708. Washington, DC: Government Printing Office, 1975:189–203.
5. Lukaski HC. Methods for the assessment of human body composition: traditional and new. Am J Clin Nutr 1987; 46:537–556.
6. Coll M, Meyer A, Stunkard AJ. Obesity and food choices in public places. Arch Gen Psychiatry 1979; 36:795–797.
7. Pearson AM, Purchas RW, Reineke EP. Theory and potential usefulness of body density as a predictor of body composition. In: Body Composition in Animals and Man. Publication 1598. Washington, DC: National Academy of Sciences, 1968:153–169.
8. Forbes GB, Welle SL. Lean body mass in obesity. Int J Obes 1983; 7:99–107.
9. Bray GA. Obesity: basic considerations and clinical approaches. Dis Mon 1989; 35:449–537.
10. Build Study, 1979. Society of Actuaries and Association of Life Insurance Medical Directors of America, 1980.
11. Durnin JVGA, Womersley J. Body fat assessed from total body density and its estimation from skinfold thickness: measurements on 481 men and women aged 16 to 72 years. Br J Nutr 1974; 32:77–97.
12. Lohman TG. Skinfolds and body density and their relation to body fatness: a review. Hum Biol 1981; 53:181–225.
13. Sloan AW, Weir JB. Nomograms for prediction of body density and total body fat from skinfold measurements. J Appl Physiol 1970; 28:221–222.
14. Kissebah AH, Vydelingum N, Murray R, et al. Relation of body fat distribution to metabolic complications of obesity. J Clin Endocrinol Metab 1982; 54:254–260.
15. Hubert HB, Feinleib M, McNamara PM, et al. Obesity as an independent risk factor for cardiovascular disease: a 26-year follow-up of participants in the Framingham Heart Study. Circulation 1983; 67:968–977.
16. Abraham S, Johnson CL. Prevalence of severe obesity in adults in the United States. Am J Clin Nutr 1980; 33:364–369.
17. Black D, James WPT, Besser GM, et al. Obesity. A report of the Royal College of Physicians. J R Coll Physicians Lond 1983; 17:5–65.
18. Bray GA. Overweight is risking fate. Definition, classification, prevalence, and risks. Ann NY Acad Sci 1987; 499:14–28.
19. Kissebah AH, Peiris AN. Biology of regional body fat distribution: relationship to non–insulin-dependent diabetes mellitus. Diabetes Metab Rev 1989; 5:83–109.
20. Després, Nadeau A, Tremblay A, et al. Role of deep abdominal fat in the association between regional adipose tissue distribution and glucose tolerance in obese women. Diabetes 1989; 38:304–309.
21. Bray GA. Obesity in America: an overview. In: Bray GA, ed. Obesity in America. DHEW Publication No. (NIH) 79-359. Washington, DC: Government Printing Office, 1979:1–19.
22. Merrit RJ. Obesity. Curr Probl Pediatr 1982; 12:1–58.
23. Ginsberg-Fellner F, Jagendorf LA, Carmel H, et al. Overweight and obesity in preschool children in New York City. Am J Clin Nutr 1981; 34:2236–2241.
24. Health, United States, 1978. DHEW Publication No. (PHS) 78-1232. Washington, DC: Government Printing Office, 1978:215.
25. Van Itallie TB. Health implications of overweight and obesity in the United States. Ann Intern Med 1985; 103:983–988.
26. Eid EE. Follow-up study of physical growth of children who had excessive weight gain in first six months of life. Br Med J 1970; 2:74–76.
27. Charney E, Goodman HC, McBride M, et al. Childhood antecedents of adult obesity. Do chubby infants become obese adults? N Engl J Med 1976; 295:6–9.
28. Will a fat baby become a fat child? Nutr Rev 1977; 35:138–140.
29. Poskitt EME, Cole TJ. Do fat babies stay fat? Br Med J 1977; 1:7–9.
30. Stark O, Atkins E, Wolff OH, et al. Longitudinal study of obesity in the National Survey of Health and Development. Br Med J 1981; 283:13–17.
31. Knittle JL, Timmers K, Ginsberg-Fellner F, et al. The growth of adipose tissue in children and adolescents. Cross-sectional and longitudinal studies of adipose cell number and size. J Clin Invest 1979; 63:239–246.
32. Ravelli G-P, Stein ZA, Susser MW. Obesity in young men after famine exposure in utero and early infancy. N Engl J Med 1976; 295:349–353.
33. Pettitt DJ, Baird HR, Aleck KA, et al. Excessive obesity in offspring of Pima Indian women with diabetes during pregnancy. N Engl J Med 1983; 308:242–245.
34. Sims EAH. Experimental obesity, dietary-induced thermogenesis, and their clinical implications. Clin Endocrinol Metab 1976; 5:377–395.
35. Sims EAH, Danforth E Jr, Horton ES, et al. Endocrine and metabolic effects of experimental obesity in man. Recent Prog Horm Res 1973; 29:457–496.
36. Goldman RF, Haisman MF, Bynum G, et al. Experimental obesity in man: metabolic rate in relation to dietary intake. In: Bray GA, ed. Obesity in Perspective. DHEW Publication No. (NIH) 75-708. Washington, DC: Government Printing Office, 1975: 165–186.
37. Trayhurn P, Thurlby PL, Woodward CJH, et al. Thermoregulation in genetically obese rodents: the relationship to metabolic efficiency. In: Festing MFW, ed. Animal Models of Obesity. New York: Oxford University Press, 1979: 191–203.
38. James WPT, Trayhurn P. An integrated view of the metabolic and genetic basis for obesity. Lancet 1976; 2:770–773.
39. James WPT, Trayhurn P. Thermogenesis and obesity. Br Med Bull 1981; 37:43–48.
40. Coleman DL. Diabetes and obesity: thrifty mutants? Nutr Rev 1978; 36:129–132.
41. Blaza S, Garrow JS. Thermogenic response to temperature, exercise and food stimuli in lean and obese women, studied by 24 h direct calorimetry. Br J Nutr 1983; 49:171–180.
42. Dauncey MJ. Metabolic effects of altering the 24 h energy intake in man, using direct and indirect calorimetry. Br J Nutr 1980; 43:257–269.
43. James WPT, Davies HL, Bailes J, et al. Elevated metabolic rates in obesity. Lancet 1978; 1:1122–1125.
44. Feurer ID, Crosby LO, Buzby GP, et al. Resting energy expenditure in morbid obesity. Ann Surg 1983; 197:17–21.
45. Felig P, Cunningham J, Levitt M, et al. Energy expenditure in obesity in fasting and postprandial state. Am J Physiol 1983; 244:E45–E51.
46. Griffiths M, Payne PR. Energy expenditure in small children of obese and non-obese parents. Nature 1976; 260:698–700.

47. Shetty PS, Jung RT, James WPT, et al. Postprandial thermogenesis in obesity. Clin Sci 1981; 60:519–525.
48. Jéquier E, Schutz Y. Energy expenditure in obesity and diabetes. Diabetes Metab Rev 1988; 4:583–593.
49. Ravussin E, Lillioja S, Anderson TE, et al. Determinants of 24-hour energy expenditure in man. Methods and results using a respiratory chamber. J Clin Invest 1986; 78:1568–1578.
50. D'Alessio DA, Kavle EC, Mozzoli MA, et al. Thermic effect of food in lean and obese men. J Clin Invest 1988; 81:1781–1789.
51. Segal KR, Gutin B. Thermic effects of food and exercise in lean and obese women. Metabolism 1983; 32:581–589.
52. Andrews F, Jackson F. Increasing fatness inversely related to increase in metabolic rate but directly related to decrease in deep body temperature in young men and women during cold exposure. Ir J Med Sci 1978; 147:329–330.
53. Thorin D, Golay A, Simonson DC, et al. The effect of selective beta adrenergic blockade on glucose-induced thermogenesis in man. Metabolism 1986; 35:524–528.
54. Berne C, Fagius J, Niklasson F. Sympathetic response to oral carbohydrate administration. Evidence from microelectrode nerve recordings. J Clin Invest 1989; 84:1403–1409.
55. Katzeff HL, O'Conell M, Horton ES, et al. Metabolic studies in human obesity during overnutrition and undernutrition: thermogenic and hormonal responses to norepinephrine. Metabolism 1986; 35:166–175.
56. Jung RT, Shetty PS, James WPT, et al. Reduced thermogenesis in obesity. Nature 1979; 279:322–323.
57. Kush RD, Young JB, Katzeff HL, et al. Effect of diet on energy expenditure and plasma norepinephrine in lean and obese Pima Indians. Metabolism 1986; 35:1110–1120.
58. Rothwell NJ, Stock MJ. A role for brown adipose tissue in diet-induced thermogenesis. Nature 1979; 281:31–35.
59. Sörbris R, Monti M, Nilsson-Ehle P, et al. Heat production by adipocytes from obese subjects before and after weight reduction. Metabolism 1982; 31:973–978.
60. Ashwell M, Meade CJ. Obesity: do fat cells from genetically obese mice (C57BL/6J ob/ob) have an innate capacity for increased fat storage? Diabetologia 1978; 15:465–470.
61. Ashwell M, Meade CJ. Adipose tissue in genetically obese rodents. In: Festing MFW, ed. Animal Models of Obesity. New York: Oxford University Press, 1979: 107–130.
62. Newsholme Ea. A possible metabolic basis for the control of body weight. N Engl J Med 1980; 302:400–405.
63. Hers HG, Hue L. Gluconeogenesis and related aspects of glycolysis. Annu Rev Biochem 1983; 52:617–653.
64. Shulman GI, Landenson PW, Wolfe MH, et al. Substrate cycling between gluconeogenesis and glycolysis in euthyroid, hypothyroid and hyperthyroid man. J Clin Invest 1985; 76:757–764.
65. Patten GS, Filsell OH, Clark MG. Obesity and the regulation of phosphofructokinase in heart: an apparent insensitivity to adrenergic activation in mature-age genetically obese rats. Metabolism 1982; 31:1137–1141.
66. Edelman IS. Thyroid thermogenesis. N Engl J Med 1974; 290:1303–1308.
67. Bray GA, York DA, Yukimura Y. Activity of (Na$^+$ + K$^+$)-ATPase in the liver of animals with experimental obesity. Life Sci 1978; 22:1637–1642.
68. DeLuise M, Blackburn GL, Flier JS. Reduced activity of the red-cell sodium-potassium pump in human obesity. N Engl J Med 1980; 303:1017–1022.
69. DeLuise M, Rappaport E, Flier JS. Altered erythrocyte Na$^+$ + K$^+$ pump in adolescent obesity. Metabolism 1982; 31:1153–1158.
70. Klimes I, Nagulesparan M, Unger RH, et al. Reduced Na$^+$,K$^+$-ATPase activity in intact red cells and isolated membranes from obese man. J Clin Endocrinol Metab 1982; 54:721–724.
71. Mir MA, Charalambous BM, Morgan K, et al. Erythrocyte sodium-potassium-ATPase and sodium transport in obesity. N Engl J Med 1981; 305:1264–1268.
72. Simat BM, Mayrand RR, From AHL, et al. Is the erythrocyte sodium pump altered in human obesity? J Clin Endocrinol Metab 1983; 56:925–929.
73. DeLuise M, Flier JS. Functionally abnormal Na$^+$–K$^+$ pump in erythrocytes of a morbidly obese patient. J Clin Invest 1982; 69:38–44.
74. Bray GA, Kral JG, Björntorp P. Hepatic sodium-potassium–dependent ATPase in obesity. N Engl J Med 1981; 304:1580–1582.
75. Cole CH, Waddell RW. Alteration in intracellular sodium concentration and ouabain-sensitive ATPase in erythrocytes from hyperthyroid patients. J Clin Endocrinol Metab 1976; 42:1056–1063.
76. Arnott RD, White R, Jerums G. Effect of thyroid status on ouabain binding to the human lymphocyte. J Clin Endocrinol Metab 1982; 54:1150–1156.
77. Alexander G. Body temperature control in mammalian young. Br Med Bull 1975; 31:61–68.
78. Foster DO, Frydman ML. Nonshivering thermogenesis in the rat. II. Measurements of blood flow with microspheres point to brown adipose tissue as the dominant site of calorigenes is induced by noradrenaline. Can J Physiol Pharmacol 1978; 56:110–122.
79. Heaton JM. The distribution of brown adipose tissue in the human. J Anat 1972; 112:35–39.
80. Rothwell NJ, Stock MJ. Brown adipose tissue: does it play a role in the development of obesity? Diabetes Metab Rev 1988; 4:595–601.
81. Rothwell NJ, Stock MJ. Acute effects of fat and carbohydrate on metabolic rate in normal, cold-acclimated and lean and obese (fa/fa) Zucker rats. Metabolism 1983; 32:371–376.
82. Bouillaud F, Weissenbach J, Ricquier D. Complete cDNA-derived amino acid sequence of rat brown fat uncoupling protein. J Biol Chem 1986; 261:1487–1490.
83. Boyer PD. A perspective of the binding change mechanism for ATP synthesis. FASEB J 1989; 3:2164–2178.
84. Bukowiecki LJ, Folléa N, Lupien J, et al. Metabolic relationships between lipolysis and respiration in rat brown adipocytes. The role of long chain fatty acids as regulators of mitochondrial respiration and feedback inhibitors of lipolysis. J Biol Chem 1981; 256:12840–12848.
85. LaNoue KF, Strzelecki T, Strzelecka D, et al. Regulation of the uncoupling protein in brown adipose tissue. J Biol Chem 1986; 261:298–305.
86. Rothwell NJ, Stock MJ, Wyllie MG. Na$^+$,K$^+$-ATPase activity and noradrenaline turnover in brown adipose tissue of rats exhibiting diet-induced thermogenesis. Biochem Pharmacol 1981; 30:1709–1712.
87. Ricquier D, Bouillaud F, Toumelin P, et al. Expression of uncoupling protein mRNA in thermogenic or weakly thermogenic brown adipose tissue. Evidence for a rapid β-adrenoreceptor-mediated and transcriptionally regulated step during activation of thermogenesis. J Biol Chem 1986; 261:13905–13910.
88. Arch JRS, Ainsworth AT, Cawthorne MA, et al. Atypical β-adrenoceptor on brown adipocytes as target for anti-obesity drugs. Nature 1984; 309:163–165.
89. Emorine LJ, Marullo S, Briend-Sutren MM, et al. Molecular characterization of the human β$_3$-adrenergic receptor. Science 1989; 245:1118–1121.
90. Seydoux J, Ricquier D, Rohner-Jeanrenaud F, et al. Decreased guanine nucleotide binding and reduced equivalent production by brown adipose tissue in hypothalamic obesity. Recovery after cold acclimation. FEBS Lett 1982; 146:161–164.
91. Hogan S, Himms-Hagen J. Abnormal brown adipose tissue in obese (ob/ob) mice: response to acclimation to cold. Am J Physiol 1980; 239:E301–E309.
92. Bray GA. Is corpulence catching? In: Björntorp P, Cairella M, Howard AN, eds. Recent Advances in Obesity Research: III. London: John Libbey, 1981:374–387.
93. Bray GA. Effect of caloric restriction on energy expenditure in obese patients. Lancet 1969; 2:397–398.
94. Drenick EJ, Johnson D. Weight reduction by fasting and semistarvation in morbid obesity: long-term follow-up. Int J Obes 1978; 2:123–132.
95. Bray GA. The myth of diet in the management of obesity. Am J Clin Nutr 1970; 23:1141–1148.
96. Waxman M, Stunkard AJ. Caloric intake and expenditure of obese boys. J Pediatr 1980; 96:187–193.
97. Sahakian BJ. The interaction of psychological and metabolic factors in the control of eating and obesity. Hum Nutr Appl Nutr 1982; 36A:262–271.
98. Bruch H. Developmental considerations of anorexia nervosa and obesity. Can J Psychiatry 1981; 26:212–217.
99. Rodin J. Psychological factors in obesity. In: Björntorp P, Cairella M, Howard AN, eds. Recent Advances in Obesity Research: III. London: John Libbey, 1981:106–123.
100. Rodin J. The externality theory today. In: Stunkard AJ, ed. Obesity. Philadelphia: W. B. Saunders, 1980:226–239.
101. Rodin J, Schank D, Striegel-Moore R. Psychological features of obesity. Med Clin North Am 1989; 73:47–66.
102. Rodin J, Wing RR. Behavioral factors in obesity. Diabetes Metab Rev 1988; 4:701–725.
103. Sclafani A, Springer D. Dietary obesity in adult rats: similarities to hypothalamic and human obesity syndromes. Physiol Behav 1976; 17:461–471.
104. Rolls BJ, Rowe EA, Rolls ET, et al. Variety in a meal enhances food intake in man. Physiol Behav 1981; 26:215–221.
105. Cassell JA. Commentary: American food habits in the 1980's. Top Clin Nutr 1989; 4:47–58.
106. Dreon DM, Frey-Hewitt B, Ellsworth N, et al. Dietary fat: carbohydrate ratio and obesity in middle-aged men. Am J Clin Nutr 1988; 47:995–1000.
107. Flatt JP. Importance of nutrient balance in body weight regulation. Diabetes Metab Rev 1988; 4:571–581.
108. Van Itallie TB, Vanderweele DA. The phenomenon of satiety. In: Björntorp P, Cairella M, Howard AN, eds. Recent Advances in Obesity Research: III. London: John Libbey, 1981:289.
109. Morley JE. Neuropeptide regulation of appetite and weight. Endocr Rev 1987; 8:256–287.
110. Bray GA. The Obese Patient. Philadelphia: W. B. Saunders, 1976:44–93.
111. Bray GA, Teague RJ, Lee CK. Brain uptake of ketones in rats with differing susceptibility to dietary obesity. Metabolism 1987; 36:27–30.

112. Coleman DL. Effects of parabiosis of obese with diabetes and normal mice. Diabetologia 1973; 9:294–298.

113. Parameswaran SV, Steffens AB, Hervey GR, et al. Involvement of a humoral factor in regulation of body weight in parabiotic rats. Am J Physiol 1977; 232:R150–R157.

114. Nishizawa Y, Bray GA. Evidence for a circulating ergostatic factor: studies on parabiotic rats. Am J Physiol 1980; 239:R344–R351.

115. Gates RJ, Hunt MI, Lazarus NR. Further studies on the amelioration of the characteristics of New Zealand obese (NZO) mice following implantation of islets of Langerhans. Diabetologia 1974; 10:401–406.

116. Gates RJ, Lazarus NR. The ability of pancreatic polypeptides (APP and BPP) to return to normal the hyperglycemia, hyperinsulinemia and weight gain of New Zealand obese mice. Horm Res 1977; 8:189–202.

117. Marco J, Zulueta MA, Correas I, et al. Reduced pancreatic polypeptide secretion in obese subjects. J Clin Endocrinol Metab 1980; 50:744–747.

118. Hedo JA, Villanueva ML, Marco J. Stimulation of pancreatic polypeptide and glucagon secretion by 2-deoxy-D-glucose in man: evidence for cholinergic mediation. J Clin Endocrinol Metab 1978; 47:366–371.

119. Weller A, Smith GP, Gibbs J. Endogenous cholecystokinin reduces feeding in young rats. Science 1990; 247:1589–1591.

120. Dourish CT, Rycroft W, Iversen SD. Postponement of satiety by blockade of brain cholecystokinin (CCK-B) receptors. Science 1989; 245:1509–1511.

121. Keesey RE. Physiological regulation of body weight and the issue of obesity. Med Clin North Am 1989; 73:15–27.

122. Rosen BS, Cook KS, Yaglom J, et al. Adipsin and complement factor D activity: an immune-related defect in obesity. Science 1989; 244:1483–1487.

123. Spiegelman BM, Lowell B, Napolitano A, et al. Adrenal glucocorticoids regulate adipsin gene expression in genetically obese mice. J Biol Chem 1989; 264:1811–1815.

124. Garrow JS. Energy balance in man—an overview. Am J Clin Nutr 1987; 45:1114–1119.

125. Gordon T, Kannel WB. The effects of overweight on cardiovascular diseases. Geriatrics 1973; 28:80–88.

126. Hirsch J, Han PW. Cellularity of rat adipose tissue: effects of growth, starvation, and obesity. J Lipid Res 1969; 10:77–82.

127. Ginsberg-Fellner F, Knittle JL. Weight reduction in young obese children. I. Effects on adipose tissue cellularity and metabolism. Pediatr Res 1981; 15:1381–1389.

128. Hirsch J, Batchelor B. Adipose tissue cellularity in human obesity. Clin Endocrinol Metab 1976; 5:299–311.

129. Roncari DAK, Lau DCW, Kindler S. Exaggerated replication in culture of adipocyte precursors from massively obese persons. Metabolism 1981; 30:425–427.

130. Olefsky JM. Decreased insulin binding to adipocytes and circulating monocytes from obese subjects. J Clin Invest 1976; 57:1165–1172.

131. Lafontan M, Dang-Tran L, Berlan M. Alpha-adrenergic antilipolytic effect of adrenaline in human fat cells of the thigh: comparison with adrenaline responsiveness of different fat deposits. Eur J Clin Invest 1979; 9:261–266.

132. Östman J, Arner P, Engfeldt P, et al. Regional differences in the control of lipolysis in human adipose tissue. Metabolism 1979; 28:1198–1205.

133. Bolinder J, Kager L, Östman J, et al. Differences at the receptor and postreceptor levels between human omental and subcutaneous adipose tissue in the action of insulin on lipolysis. Diabetes 1983; 32:117–123.

134. Wahrenberg H, Lönnqvist F, Arner P. Mechanisms underlying regional differences in lipolysis in human adipose tissue. J Clin Invest 1989; 84:458–467.

135. Arner P. Control of lipolysis and its relevance to development of obesity in man. Diabetes Metab Rev 1988; 4:507–515.

136. Eckel RH. Lipoprotein lipase. A multifunctional enzyme relevant to common metabolic diseases. N Engl J Med 1989; 320:1060–1068.

137. Ong JM, Kern PA. Effect of feeding and obesity on lipoprotein lipase activity, immunoreactive protein, and messenger RNA levels in human adipose tissue. J Clin Invest 1989; 84:305–311.

138. Eckel RH, Yost TJ. Weight reduction increases adipose tissue lipoprotein lipase responsiveness in obese women. J Clin Invest 1987; 80:992–997.

139. Kern PA, Ong JM, Saffari B, et al. The effects of weight loss on the activity and expression of adipose-tissue lipoprotein lipase in very obese humans. N Engl J Med 1990; 322:1053–1059.

140. Jensen MD, Haymond MW, Rizza RA, et al. Influence of body fat distribution on free fatty acid metabolism in obesity. J Clin Invest 1989; 83:1168–1173.

141. Krotkiewski M, Björntorp P, Sjöström L, et al. Impact of obesity on metabolism in men and women. Importance of regional adipose tissue distribution. J Clin Invest 1983; 72:1150–1162.

142. Hirsch J. The psychological consequences of obesity. In: Bray GA, ed. Obesity in Perspective. DHEW Publication No. (NIH) 75-708. Washington, DC: Government Printing Office, 1975:81–94.

143. Stunkard A, Burt V. Obesity and the body image: II. Age at onset of disturbances in the body image. Am J Psychiatry 1967; 123:1443–1447.

144. Glucksman ML, Hirsch J. The response of obese patients to weight reduction: III. The perception of body size. Psychosom Med 1969; 31:1–7.

145. Speaker JG, Schultz C, Grinker JA, et al. Body size estimation and locus of control in obese adolescent boys undergoing weight reduction. Int J Obes 1983; 7:73–83.

146. Hsu LKG. Is there a disturbance in body image in anorexia nervosa? J Nerv Ment Dis 1982; 170:305–307.

147. Whitelaw AGL. The association of social class and sibling number with skinfold thickness in London schoolboys. Hum Biol 1971; 43:414–420.

148. Bray GA. The inheritance of corpulence. In: Cioffi LA, James WPT, Van Itallie TB, eds. The Body Weight Regulatory System: Normal and Disturbed Mechanisms. New York: Raven, 1981:185–195.

149. Stunkard AJ, Søorensen TIA, Hanis C, et al. An adoption study of human obesity. N Engl J Med 1986; 314:193–198.

150. Stunkard AJ, Harris JR, Pedersen NL, et al. The body-mass index of twins who have been reared apart. N Engl J Med 1990; 322:1483–1487.

151. Bouchard C, Tremblay A, Després J-P, et al. The response to long-term overfeeding in identical twins. N Engl J Med 1990; 322:1477–1482.

152. Bouchard C. Genetic factors in obesity. Med Clin North Am 1989; 73:67–81.

153. Mallick MJ. Health hazards of obesity and weight control in children: a review of the literature. Am J Public Health 1983; 73:78–82.

154. Allon N. The stigma of overweight in everyday life. In: Bray GA, ed. Obesity in Perspective. DHEW Publication No. (NIH) 75-708. Washington, DC: Government Printing Office, 1975:83–102.

155. Dwyer J, Mayer J. The dismal condition: problems faced by obese adolescent girls in American society. In: Bray GA, ed. Obesity in Perspective. DHEW Publication No. (NIH) 75-708. Washington, DC: Government Printing Office, 1975: 103–110.

156. Charles SC, Blumberg P. Assessment of psychiatric status among the morbidly obese. Obesity/Bariatric Med 1982; 11:71–78.

157. Heald FP. The natural history of obesity. Adv Psychosom Med 1972; 7:102–115.

158. Larsson B, Björntorp P, Tibblin G. The health consequences of moderate obesity. Int J Obes 1981; 5:97–116.

159. Walker ARP, Segal I. The puzzle of obesity in the African black female. Lancet 1980; 1:263 (letter).

160. Nelius SJ, Heyden S, Hansen JP, et al. Lipoprotein and blood pressure changes during weight reduction at Duke's Dietary Rehabilitation Clinic. Ann Nutr Metab 1982; 26:384–392.

161. Wolf RN, Grundy SM. Influence of weight reduction on plasma lipoproteins in obese patients. Arteriosclerosis 1983; 3:160–169.

162. Peeples LH, Carpenter JW, Israel RG, et al. Alterations in low-density lipoproteins in subjects with abdominal adiposity. Metabolism 1989; 38:1029–1036.

163. Ostlund RE Jr, Staten M, Kohrt WM, et al. The ratio of waist-to-hip circumference, plasma insulin level, and glucose intolerance as independent predictors of the HDL_2 cholesterol level in older adults. N Engl J Med 1990; 322:229–234.

164. Vague P, Juhan-Vague I, Chabert V, et al. Fat distribution and plasminogen activator inhibitor activity in nondiabetic obese women. Metabolism 1989; 38:913–915.

165. Vaughan RW, Conahan TJ. Cardiopulmonary consequences of morbid obesity. Life Sci 1980; 26:2119–2127.

166. MacMahon SW, Wilcken DEL, MacDonald GJ. The effect of weight reduction on left ventricular mass. A randomized controlled trial in young, overweight hypertensive patients. N Engl J Med 1986; 314:334–339.

167. Tuck ML, Sowers J, Dornfeld L, et al. The effect of weight reduction on blood pressure, plasma renin activity, and plasma aldosterone levels in obese patients. N Engl J Med 1981; 304:930–933.

168. Goldring D, Hernandez A, Choi S, et al. Blood pressure in a high school population. II. Clinical profile of the juvenile hypertensive. J Pediatr 1979; 95:298–304.

169. Messerli FH, Ventura HO, Reisin E, et al. Borderline hypertension and obesity: two prehypertensive states with elevated cardiac output. Circulation 1982; 66:55–60.

170. Sowers JR, Whitfield LA, Beck FWJ, et al. Role of enhanced sympathetic nervous system activity and reduced Na^+,K^+-dependent adenosine triphosphatase activity in maintenance of elevated blood pressure in obesity: effects of weight loss. Clin Sci 1982; 63:121s–124s.

171. Landsberg L, Krieger DR. Obesity, metabolism, and the sympathetic nervous system. Am J Hypertens 1989; 2:125S–132S.

172. Rocchini AP, Key J, Bondie D, et al. The effect of weight loss on the sensitivity of blood pressure to sodium in obese adolescents. N Engl J Med 1989; 321:580–585.

173. Kaplan NM. The deadly quartet. Upper-body obesity, glucose intolerance, hypertriglyceridemia, and hypertension. Arch Intern Med 1989; 149:1514–1520.

174. Zavaroni I, Bonora E, Pagliara M, et al. Risk factors for coronary artery disease in healthy persons with hyperinsulinemia and normal glucose tolerance. N Engl J Med 1989; 320:702–706.

175. National Diabetes Data Group. Classification and diagnosis of diabetes mellitus and other categories of glucose intolerance. Diabetes 1979; 28:1039–1057.

176. Olefsky JM. Insulin resistance and insulin action. An in vitro and in vivo perspective. Diabetes 1981; 30:148–162.

177. Lillioja S, Bogardus C. Obesity and insulin resistance: lessons learned from the Pima Indians. Diabetes Metab Rev 1988; 4:517–540.
178. Campbell PJ, Gerich JE. Impact of obesity on insulin action in volunteers with normal glucose tolerance: demonstration of a threshold for the adverse effect of obesity. J Clin Endocrinol Metab 1990; 70:1114–1118.
179. Laakso M, Edelman SV, Brechtel G, et al. Decreased effect of insulin to stimulate skeletal muscle blood flow in obese man. A novel mechanism for insulin resistance. J Clin Invest 1990; 85:1844–1852.
180. Kolterman OG, Insel J, Saekow M, et al. Mechanisms of insulin resistance in human obesity. Evidence for receptor and postreceptor defects. J Clin Invest 1980; 65:1272–1284.
181. Kahn CR, White MF. The insulin receptor and the molecular mechanism of insulin action. J Clin Invest 1988; 82:1151–1156.
182. Ciaraldi TP, Kolterman OG, Olefsky JM. Mechanism of the postreceptor defect in insulin action in human obesity. Decrease in glucose transport system activity. J Clin Invest 1981; 68:875–880.
183. Hissin PJ, Karnieli E, Simpson IA, et al. A possible mechanism of insulin resistance in the rat adipose cell with high-fat/low-carbohydrate feeding. Depletion of intracellular glucose transport systems. Diabetes 1982; 31:589–592.
184. Prager R, Wallace P, Olefsky JM. In vivo kinetics of insulin action on peripheral glucose disposal and hepatic glucose output in normal and obese subjects. J Clin Invest 1986; 78:472–481.
185. Bougnères P-F, Artavia-Loria E, Henry S, et al. Increased basal glucose production and utilization in children with recent obesity versus adults with long-term obesity. Diabetes 1989; 38:477–483.
186. Peiris AN, Mueller RA, Smith GA, et al. Splanchnic insulin metabolism in obesity. Influence of body fat distribution. J Clin Invest 1986; 78:1648–1657.
187. Polonsky KS, Given BD, Hirsch L, et al. Quantitative study of insulin secretion and clearance in normal and obese subjects. J Clin Invest 1988; 81:435–441.
188. Polonsky KS, Given BD, Van Cauter E. Twenty-four-hour profiles and pulsatile patterns of insulin secretion in normal and obese subjects. J Clin Invest 1988; 81:442–448.
189. Luce JM. Respiratory complications of obesity. Chest 1980; 78:626–631.
190. Rubinstein I, Zamel N, DuBarry L, et al. Airflow limitation in morbidly obese, nonsmoking men. Ann Intern Med 1990; 112:828–832.
191. Block AJ, Boysen PG, Wynne JW, et al. Sleep apnea, hypopnea and oxygen desaturation in normal subjects. A strong male predominance. N Engl J Med 1979; 300:513–517.
192. Kryger M, Quesney LF, Holder D, et al. The sleep deprivation syndrome of the obese patient. A problem of periodic nocturnal upper airway obstruction. Am J Med 1974; 56:531–539.
193. Sutton FD Jr, Swillich CW, Creagh CE, et al. Progesterone for outpatient treatment of pickwickian syndrome. Ann Intern Med 1975; 83:476–479.
194. Grundy SM. Mechanism of cholesterol gallstones formation. Semin Liver Dis 1983; 3:97–111.
195. Horton ES, Danforth E Jr, Sims EAH, et al. Endocrine and metabolic alterations in spontaneous and experimental obesity. In: Bray GA, ed. Obesity in Perspective. DHEW Publication No. (NIH) 75-708. Washington, DC: Government Printing Office, 1975:323–334.
196. Glass AR. Endocrine aspects of obesity. Med Clin North Am 1989; 73:139–160.
197. Inoue S, Bray GA, Mullen YS. Transplantation of pancreatic β-cells prevents development of hypothalamic obesity in rats. Am J Physiol 1978; 235:E266–E271.
198. Bray GA, Gallagher TF Jr. Manifestations of hypothalamic obesity in man: a comprehensive investigation of eight patients and a review of the literature. Medicine 1975; 54:301–330.
199. Maruhama Y, Abe R. A familial form of obesity without hyperinsulinism at the outset. Diabetes 1981; 30:14–18.
200. Elahi D, Nagulesparan M, Hershcopf RJ, et al. Feedback inhibition of insulin secretion by insulin: relation to the hyperinsulinemia of obesity. N Engl J Med 1982; 306:1196–1202.
201. Starke AAR, Erhardt G, Berger M, et al. Elevated pancreatic glucagon in obesity. Diabetes 1984; 33:277–280.
202. Ma GY, Gove CD, Hems DA. Effects of glucagon and insulin on fatty acid synthesis and glycogen degradation in the perfused liver of normal and genetically obese (ob/ob) mice. Biochem J 1978; 174:761–768.
203. McCune SA, Durant PJ, Jenkins PA, et al. Comparative studies on fatty acid synthesis, glycogen metabolism, and gluconeogenesis by hepatocytes isolated from lean and obese Zucker rats. Metabolism 1981; 30:1170–1178.
204. Malewiak MI, Griglio S, Kalopissis AD, et al. Oleate metabolism in isolated hepatocytes from lean and obese Zucker rats. Influence of a high fat diet and in vitro response to glucagon. Metabolism 1983; 32:661–668.
205. Lassmann V, Vague P, Vialettes B, et al. Low plasma levels of pancreatic polypeptide in obesity. Diabetes 1980; 29:428–430.
206. Malaisse-Lagae F, Carpentier J-L, Patel YC, et al. Pancreatic polypeptide: a possible role in the regulation of food intake in the mouse. Hypothesis. Experientia 1977; 33:915–917.
207. Boden G, Baile CA, McLaughlin CL, et al. Effects of starvation and obesity on somatostatin, insulin, and glucagon release from an isolated perfused organ system. Am J Physiol 1981; 241:E215–E220.
208. Voyles NR, Awoke S, Wade A, et al. Starvation increases gastrointestinal somatostatin in normal and obese Zucker rats: a possible regulatory mechanism. Horm Metab Res 1982; 14:392–395.
209. Sasaki H, Nagulesparan M, Dubois A, et al. Hyperinsulinemia in obesity: lack of relation to gastric emptying of glucose solution or to plasma somatostatin levels. Metabolism 1983; 32:701–705.
210. Jung RT, Shetty PS, James WPT. Nutritional effects on thyroid and catecholamine metabolism. Clin Sci 1980; 58:183–191.
211. Danforth E Jr, Horton ES, O'Connell M, et al. Dietary-induced alterations in thyroid hormone metabolism during overnutrition. J Clin Invest 1979; 64:1336–1347.
212. Azizi F. Effect of dietary composition on fasting-induced changes in serum thyroid hormones and thyrotropin. Metabolism 1978; 27:935–942.
213. Carlson HE, Drenick EJ, Chopra IJ, et al. Alterations in basal and TRH-stimulated serum levels of thyrotropin, prolactin, and thyroid hormones in starved obese men. J Clin Endocrinol Metab 1977; 45:707–713.
214. Wilcox RG. Triiodothyronine, TSH, and prolactin in obese women. Lancet 1977; 1:1027–1029.
215. Burman KD, Latham KR, Djuh YY, et al. Solubilized nuclear thyroid hormone receptors in circulating human mononuclear cells. J Clin Endocrinol Metab 1980; 51:106–116.
216. Guernsey DL, Morishige WK. Na^+ pump activity and nuclear T_3 receptors in tissues of genetically obese (ob/ob) mice. Metabolism 1979; 28:629–632.
217. Crapo L. Cushing's syndrome: a review of diagnostic tests. Metabolism 1979; 28:955–977.
218. Eddy RL, Jones AL, Gilliland PF, et al. Cushing's syndrome: a prospective study of diagnostic methods. Am J Med 1973; 55:621–630.
219. Biemond P, de Jong FH, Lamberts SWJ. Continuous dexamethasone infusion for seven hours in patients with the Cushing syndrome. A superior differential diagnostic test. Ann Intern Med 1990; 112:738–742.
220. Abou Samra AB, Dechaud H, Estour B, et al. β-Lipotropin and cortisol response to an intravenous infusion dexamethasone suppression test in Cushing's syndrome and obesity. J Clin Endocrinol Metab 1985; 61:116–119.
221. Yoshida T, Kemnitz JW, Bray GA. Lateral hypothalamic lesions and norepinephrine turnover in rats. J Clin Invest 1983; 72:919–927.
222. Jung RT, Shetty PS, James WPT, et al. Plasma catecholamines and autonomic responsiveness in obesity. Int J Obes 1982; 6:131–141.
223. Gustafson AB, Kalkhoff RK. Influence of sex and obesity on plasma catecholamine response to isometric exercise. J Clin Endocrinol Metab 1982; 55:703–708.
224. O'Hare JA, Minaker KL, Meneilly GS, et al. Effect of insulin on plasma norepinephrine and 3,4-dihydroxyphenylalanine in obese men. Metabolism 1989; 38:322–329.
225. Glass AR, Swerdloff RS, Bray GA, et al. Low serum testosterone and sex-hormone-binding-globulin in massively obese men. J Clin Endocrinol Metab 1977; 45:1211–1219.
226. Schneider G, Kirschner MA, Berkowitz R, et al. Increased estrogen production in obese men. J Clin Endocrinol Metab 1979; 48:633–638.
227. Stanik S, Dornfeld LP, Maxwell MH, et al. The effect of weight loss on reproductive hormones in obese men. J Clin Endocrinol Metab 1981; 53:828–832.
228. Kopelman PG, Pilkington TRE, White N, et al. Abnormal sex steroid secretion and binding in massively obese women. Clin Endocrinol 1980; 12:363–369.
229. O'Dea JPK, Wieland RG, Hallberg MC, et al. Effect of dietary weight loss on sex steroid binding, sex steroids, and gonadotropins in obese postmenopausal women. J Lab Clin Med 1979; 93:1004–1008.
230. Zumoff B, Strain GW, Kream J, et al. Obese young men have elevated plasma estrogen levels but obese premenopausal women do not. Metabolism 1981; 30:1011–1014.
231. Kirschner MA, Samojlik E, Drejka M, et al. Androgen-estrogen metabolism in women with upper body versus lower body obesity. J Clin Endocrinol Metab 1990; 70:473–479.
232. Edman CD, MacDonald PC. Effect of obesity on conversion of plasma androstenedione to estrone in ovulatory and anovulatory young women. Am J Obstet Gynecol 1978; 130:456–461.
233. Cooper SC, Roncari DA. 17-Beta-estradiol increases mitogenic activity of medium from cultured preadipocytes of massively obese persons. J Clin Invest 1989; 83:1925–1929.
234. Schneider J, Bradlow HL, Strain G, et al. Effects of obesity on estradiol metabolism: decreased formation of nonuterotropic metabolites. J Clin Endocrinol Metab 1983; 56:973–978.
235. Glass AR, Dahms WT, Abraham G, et al. Secondary amenorrhea in obesity: etiologic role of weight-related androgen excess. Fertil Steril 1978; 30:243–244.
236. Hosseinian AH, Kim MH, Rosenfield RL. Obesity and oligomenorrhea are associated with hyperandrogenism independent of hirsutism. J Clin Endocrinol Metab 1976; 42:765–769.
237. Newmark SR, Rossini AA, Naftolin FI, et al. Gonadotropin profiles in fed and fasted obese women. Am J Obstet Gynecol 1979; 133:75–80.

238. Pasquali R, Antenucci D, Casimirri F, et al. Clinical and hormonal characteristics of obese amenorrheic hyperandrogenic women before and after weight loss. J Clin Endocrinol Metab 1989; 68:173–179.

239. Meistas MT, Foster GV, Margolis S, et al. Integrated concentrations of growth hormone, insulin, C-peptide and prolactin in human obesity. Metabolism 1982; 31:1224–1228.

240. Phillips LS, Vassilopoulou-Sellin R. Somatomedins. N Engl J Med 1980; 302:371–380, 438–446.

241. Cordido F, Casanueva FF, Dieguez C. Cholinergic receptor activation by pyridostigmine restores growth hormone (GH) responsiveness to GH-releasing hormone administration in obese subjects: evidence for hypothalamic somatostatinergic participation in the blunted GH release of obesity. J Clin Endocrinol Metab 1989; 68:290–293.

242. Ghigo E, Mazza E, Corrias A, et al. Effect of cholinergic enhancement by pyridostigmine on growth hormone secretion in obese adults and children. Metabolism 1989; 38:631–633.

243. Jung RT, Campbell RG, James WPT, et al. Altered hypothalamic and sympathetic responses to hypoglycemia in familial obesity. Lancet 1982; 1:1043–1046.

244. Drenick EJ, Carlson HE, Robertson GL, et al. The role of vasopressin and prolactin in abnormal salt and water metabolism of obese patients before and after fasting and during refeeding. Metabolism 1977; 26:309–317.

245. Drenick EJ. The prognosis of conventional treatment in severe obesity. In: Björntorp P, Cairella M, Howard AN, eds. Recent Advances in Obesity Research: III. London: John Libbey, 1981:80–84.

246. Joffe SN. Surgical management of morbid obesity. Gut 1981; 22:242–254.

247. Freeman JB, Burchett H. Failure rate with gastric partitioning for morbid obesity. Am J Surg 1983; 145:113–119.

248. Bray GA, Gray DS. Treatment of obesity: an overview. Diabetes Metab Rev 1988; 4:653–679.

249. Atkinson RL. Low and very low calorie diets. Med Clin North Am 1989; 73:203–215.

250. Runcie J, Hilditch TE. Energy provision, tissue utilization, and weight loss in prolonged starvation. Br Med J 1974; 2:352–356.

251. Yang M-U, Van Itallie TB. Composition of weight lost during short-term weight reduction. Metabolic responses of obese subjects to starvation and low-calorie ketogenic and nonketogenic diets. J Clin Invest 1976; 58:722–730.

252. Passmore R, Strong JA, Ritchie FJ. The chemical composition of the tissue lost by obese patients on a reducing regimen. Br J Nutr 1958; 12:113–122.

253. Howard AN. The historical development, efficacy and safety of very-low-calorie diets. Int J Obes 1981; 5:195–208.

254. Bogardus C, LaGrange BM, Horton ES, et al. Comparison of carbohydrate-containing and carbohydrate-restricted hypocaloric diets in the treatment of obesity. Endurance and metabolic fuel homeostasis during strenuous exercise. J Clin Invest 1981; 68:399–404.

255. Isner JM, Sours HE, Paris AL, et al. Sudden, unexpected death in avid dieters using the liquid-protein-modified-fast diet. Observations in 17 patients and the role of the prolonged QT interval. Circulation 1979; 60:1401–1412.

256. Sours HE, Frattali VP, Brand CD, et al. Sudden death associated with very low calorie weight reduction regimens. Am J Clin Nutr 1981; 34:453–461.

257. Lantigua RA, Amatruda JM, Biddle TL, et al. Cardiac arrhythmias associated with a liquid protein diet for the treatment of obesity. N Engl J Med 1980; 303:735–738.

258. Vertes V, Genuth SM, Hazelton IM. Supplemented fasting as a large-scale outpatient program. JAMA 1977; 238:2151–2153.

259. Genuth SM, Vertes V, Hazelton I. Supplemented fasting in the treatment of obesity. In: Bray GA, ed. Recent Advances in Obesity Research: II. Westport, CT: Food and Nutrition Press, 1978: 370–378.

260. Miller DS, Parsonage S. Resistance to slimming. Adaptation or illusion? Lancet 1975; 1:773–775.

261. Wadden TA, Foster GD, Letizia KA, et al. Long-term effects of dieting on resting metabolic rate in obese outpatients. JAMA 1990; 264:707–711.

262. Brownell KD, Kramer FM. Behavioral management of obesity. Med Clin North Am 1989; 73:185–201.

263. Stunkard AJ, Penick SB. Behavior modification in the treatment of obesity: the problem of maintaining weight loss. Arch Gen Psychiatry 1979; 36:801–806.

264. Stunkard AJ, Craighead LW, O'Brien R. Controlled trial of behaviour therapy, pharmacotherapy, and their combination in the treatment of obesity. Lancet 1980; 2:1045–1047.

265. Passmore R, Durnin JVGA. Human energy expenditure. Physiol Rev 1955; 35:801–840.

266. Hanefeld M, Zschornack M, Weck M, et al. Physical training in obese subjects: selection, motivation, organization and follow-up problems. In: Björntorp P, Cairella M, Howard AN, eds. Recent Advances in Obesity Research: III. London: John Libbey, 1981:290–294.

267. Foss ML. Exercise prescription and training programs for obese subjects. In: Björntorp P, Cairella M, Howard AN, eds. Recent Advances in Obesity Research: III. London: John Libbey, 1981:307–314.

268. Kukkonen K, Rauramaa R, Siitonen O, et al. Physical training of obese middle-aged persons. Ann Clin Res 1982; 14(Suppl 34):80–85.

269. Krotkiewski M, Mandroukas K, Sjöström L, et al. Effects of long-term physical training on body fat, metabolism, and blood pressure in obesity. Metabolism 1979; 28:650–658.

270. Segal KR, Pi-Sunyer FX. Exercise and obesity. Med Clin North Am 1989; 73:217–236.

271. Moore R, Grant AM, Howard AN, et al. Treatment of obesity with triiodothyronine and a very-low-calorie liquid formula diet. Lancet 1980; 1:223–226.

272. Koppeschaar HPF, Meinders AE, Schwarz F. Metabolic responses in grossly obese subjects treated with a very-low-calorie diet with and without triiodothyronine treatment. Int J Obes 1983; 7:133–141.

273. Munro JF. General principles of drug therapy in obesity. In: Björntorp P, Cairella M, Howard AN, eds. Recent Advances in Obesity Research: III. London: John Libbey, 1981: 180–183.

274. Munro JF, Ford MJ. Drug treatment of obesity. In: Silverstone T, ed. Drugs and Appetite. London: Academic, 1982:125–157.

275. Glueck CJ, Hastings MM, Allen C, et al. Sucrose polyester and covert caloric dilution. Am J Clin Nutr 1982; 35:1352–1359.

276. Mellies MJ, Vitale C, Jandacek RJ, et al. The substitution of sucrose polyester for dietary fat in obese, hypercholesterolemic outpatients. Am J Clin Nutr 1985; 41:1–12.

277. Snyder DK, Clemmons DR, Underwood LE. Dietary carbohydrate content determines responsiveness to growth in energy-restricted humans. J Clin Endocrinol Metab 1989; 69:745–752.

278. Rudman D, Feller AG, Nagraj HS, et al. Effects of human growth hormone in men over 60 years old. N Engl J Med 1990; 323:1–6.

279. Weintraub M, Bray GA. Drug treatment of obesity. Med Clin North Am 1989; 73:237–249.

280. Gaspar MR, Movius HJ II, Rosental JJ, et al. Comparison of Payne and Scott operations for morbid obesity. Ann Surg 1976; 184:507–515.

281. Maxwell JD, McGouran RC. Jejuno-ileal bypass: clinical and experimental aspects. Scand J Gastroenterol 1982; 17(Suppl 74):129–147.

282. Halverson JD, Wise L, Wazna MF, et al. Jejunoileal bypass for morbid obesity. A critical appraisal. Am J Med 1978; 64:461–475.

283. Hocking MP, Duerson MC, O'Leary JP, et al. Jejunoileal bypass for morbid obesity. Late follow-up in 100 cases. N Engl J Med 1983; 308:995–999.

284. Kral JG. Surgical treatment of obesity. Med Clin North Am 1989; 73:251–264.

285. Mason EE, Printen KJ, Hartford CE, et al. Optimizing results of gastric bypass. Ann Surg 1975; 182:405–414.

286. Griffen WO Jr, Young VL, Stevenson CC. A prospective comparison of gastric and jejunoileal bypass procedures for morbid obesity. Ann Surg 1977; 186:500–509.

287. Alden JF. Gastric and jejunoileal bypass. A comparison in the treatment of morbid obesity. Arch Surg 1977; 112:799–806.

288. Alpers DH. Surgical therapy for obesity. N Engl J Med 1983; 308:1026–1027.

289. Rimoin DL, Schimke RN. Genetic Disorders of the Endocrine Glands. St. Louis: C. V. Mosby, 1971.

290. Goecke T, Majewski F, Kauther KD, et al. Mental retardation, hypotonia, obesity, ocular, facial, dental, and limb abnormalities (Cohen syndrome). Eur J Pediatr 1982; 138:338–340.

291. Dietz WH Jr, Gross WL, Kirkpatrick JA Jr. Blount disease (tibia vara): another skeletal disorder associated with childhood obesity. J Pediatr 1982; 101:735–737.

292. Goldstein JL, Fialkow PJ. The Alström syndrome. Report of three cases with further delineation of the clinical, pathophysiological, and genetic aspects of the disorder. Medicine 1973; 52:53–71.

293. Ledbetter DH, Riccardi VM, Airhart SD, et al. Deletions of chromosome 15 as a cause of the Prader-Willi syndrome. N Engl J Med 1981; 304:325–329.

Anorexia Nervosa–Bulimia Nervosa

294. Lucas AR. Toward the understanding of anorexia nervosa as a disease entity. Mayo Clin Proc 1981; 56:254–264.

295. Berkman JM. Anorexia nervosa, anorexia, inanition, and low basal metabolic rate. Am J Med Sci 1930; 180:411–424.

296. Crisp AH, Palmer RL, Kalucy RS. How common is anorexia nervosa? A prevalence study. Br J Psychiatry 1976; 128:549–554.

297. Ballot NS, Delaney NE, Erskine PJ, et al. Anorexia nervosa—a prevalence study. S Afr Med J 1981; 59:992–993.

298. Lucas AR, Beard CM, O'Fallon WM, et al. Anorexia nervosa in Rochester, Minnesota: a 45-year study. Mayo Clin Proc 1988; 63:433–442.

299. Button EJ, Whitehouse A. Subclinical anorexia nervosa. Psychol Med 1981; 11:509–516.

300. Ben-Tovim DI, Subbiah N, Scheutz B, et al. Bulimia: symptoms and syndromes in an urban population. Aust NZ J Psychiatry 1989; 23:73–80.

301. Herzog DB, Copeland PM. Bulimia nervosa—psyche and satiety. N Engl J Med 1988; 319:716–718.

302. Feighner JP, Robins E, Guze SB, et al. Diagnostic criteria for use in psychiatric research. Arch Gen Psychiatry 1972; 26:57–63.

303. American Psychiatric Association. Diagnostic and Statistical Manual of Mental Disorders. 3rd ed. Washington, DC: American Psychiatric Association, 1980.

304. Irwin M. Diagnosis of anorexia nervosa in children and the validity of DSM-III. Am J Psychiatry 1981; 138:1382–1383.

305. Kirstein L. Diagnostic issues in primary anorexia nervosa. Int J Psychiatry Med 1981–82; 11:235–244.

306. American Psychiatric Association. Diagnostic and Statistical Manual of Mental Disorders. 3rd ed., revised. Washington, DC: American Psychiatric Association, 1987.

307. Halmi KA. Anorexia nervosa: recent investigations. Annu Rev Med 1978; 29:137–148.

308. Drossman DA, Ontjes DA, Heizer WD. Anorexia nervosa. Gastroenterology 1979; 77:1115–1131.

309. Crisp AH, Hsu LKG, Harding B, et al. Clinical features of anorexia nervosa. A study of a consecutive series of 102 female patients. J Psychosom Res 1980; 24:179–191.

310. Schwabe AD, Lippe BM, Chang RJ, et al. Anorexia nervosa. Ann Intern Med 1981; 94:371–381.

311. Herzog DB, Copeland PM. Eating disorders. N Engl J Med 1985; 313:295–303.

312. Halmi KA. Anorexia nervosa: demographic and clinical features in 94 cases. Psychosom Med 1974; 36:18–26.

313. Beumont PJV, Chambers TL, Rouse L, et al. The diet composition and nutritional knowledge of patients with anorexia nervosa. J Hum Nutr 1981; 35:265–273.

314. Strober M, Goldenberg I, Green J, et al. Body image disturbance in anorexia nervosa during the acute and recuperative phase. Psychol Med 1979; 9:695–701.

315. Ben-Tovim DI, Whitehead J, Crisp AH. A controlled study of the perception of body width in anorexia nervosa. J Psychosom Res 1979; 23:267–272.

316. Garfinkel PE, Moldofsky H, Garner DM. The stability of perceptual disturbances in anorexia nervosa. Psychol Med 1979; 9:703–708.

317. Garner DM. Body image in anorexia nervosa. Can J Psychiatry 1981; 26:224–227.

318. Halmi KA, Goldberg SC, Eckert E, et al. Pretreatment evaluation in anorexia nervosa. In: Vigersky RA, ed. Anorexia Nervosa. New York: Raven, 1977:43–54.

319. Holt S, Ford MJ, Grant S, et al. Abnormal gastric emptying in primary anorexia nervosa. Br J Psychiatry 1981; 139:550–552.

320. Saul SH, Dekker A, Watson CG. Acute gastric dilatation with infarction and perforation. Report of fatal outcome in patient with anorexia nervosa. Gut 1981; 22:978–983.

321. Vigersky RA, Loriaux DL. Anorexia nervosa as a model of hypothalamic dysfunction. In: Vigersky RA, ed. Anorexia Nervosa. New York: Raven, 1977:109–121.

322. Fagher B, Monti M, Theander S. Microcalorimetric study of muscle and platelet thermogenesis in anorexia nervosa and bulimia. Am J Clin Nutr 1989; 49:476–481.

323. Luck P, Wakeling A. Increased cutaneous vasoreactivity to cold in anorexia nervosa. Clin Sci 1981; 61:559–567.

324. Mayo-Smith W, Hayes CW, Biller BM, et al. Body fat distribution measured with CT: correlations in healthy subjects, patients with anorexia nervosa, and patients with Cushing syndrome. Radiology 1989; 170:515–518.

325. Silverman JA. Anorexia nervosa: clinical and metabolic observations in a successful treatment plan. In: Vigersky RA, ed. Anorexia Nervosa. New York: Raven, 1977:331–339.

326. Casper RC, Eckert ED, Halmi KA, et al. Bulimia. Its incidence and clinical importance in patients with anorexia nervosa. Arch Gen Psychiatry 1980; 37:1030–1035.

327. Garfinkel PE, Moldofsky H, Garner DM. The heterogeneity of anorexia nervosa. Bulimia as a distinct subgroup. Arch Gen Psychiatry 1980; 37:1036–1040.

328. Russell G. Bulimia nervosa: an ominous variant of anorexia nervosa. Psychol Med 1979; 9:429–448.

329. Mitchell JE, Pyle RL, Eckert ED. Frequency and duration of binge-eating episodes in patients with bulimia. Am J Psychiatry 1981; 138:835–836.

330. Palmer RL. The dietary chaos syndrome: a useful new term? Br J Med Psychol 1979; 52:187–190.

331. Mitchell JE, Seim HC, Colon E, et al. Medical complications and medical management of bulimia. Ann Intern Med 1987; 107:71–77.

332. Crisp AH, Hsu LKG, Harding B. The starving hoarder and voracious spender: stealing in anorexia nervosa. J Psychosom Res 1980; 24:225–231.

333. Herzog DB. Bulimia: the secretive syndrome. Psychosomatics 1982; 23:481–487.

334. Newman MM, Halmi KA. The endocrinology of anorexia nervosa and bulimia nervosa. Endocrinol Metab Clin North Am 1988; 17:195–212.

335. Levy AB, Dixon KN, Stern SL. How are depression and bulimia related? Am J Psychiatry 1989; 146:162–169.

336. Myers TJ, Perkerson MD, Witter BA, et al. Hematologic findings in anorexia nervosa. Conn Med 1981; 45:14–17.

337. Bhanji S, Mattingly D. Anorexia nervosa: some observations on "dieters"

338. Mordasini R, Klose G, Greten H. Secondary type II hyperlipoproteinemia in patients with anorexia nervosa. Metabolism 1978; 27:71–79.

339. Nestel PJ. Cholesterol metabolism in anorexia nervosa and hypercholesterolemia. J Clin Endocrinol Metab 1974; 38:325–328.

340. Lamon-Fava S, Fisher EC, Nelson ME, et al. Effect of exercise and menstrual cycle status on plasma lipids, low density lipoprotein particle size, and apolipoproteins. J Clin Endocrinol Metab 1989; 68:17–21.

341. Wyatt RJ, Farrell M, Berry PL, et al. Reduced alternative complement pathway control protein levels in anorexia nervosa: response to parenteral alimentation. Am J Clin Nutr 1982; 35:973–980.

342. Pertschuk MJ, Crosby LO, Barot L, et al. Immunocompetency in anorexia nervosa. Am J Clin Nutr 1982; 35:968–972.

343. George GCW. Anorexia nervosa with herpes simplex encephalitis. Postgrad Med J 1981; 57:366–367.

344. Bowers TK, Eckert E. Leukopenia in anorexia nervosa. Lack of increased risk of infection. Arch Intern Med 1978; 138:1520–1523.

345. Gold PW, Kaye W, Robertson GL, et al. Abnormalities in plasma and cerebrospinal-fluid arginine vasopressin in patients with anorexia nervosa. N Engl J Med 1983; 308:1117–1123.

346. Nishita JK, Ellinwood EH Jr, Rockwell WJ, et al. Abnormalities in the response of plasma arginine vasopressin during hypertonic saline infusion in patients with eating disorders. Biol Psychiatry 1989; 26:73–86.

347. Gwirtsman HE, Kaye WH, George DT, et al. Hyperamylasemia and its relationship to binge-purge episodes: development of a clinically relevant laboratory test. J Clin Psychiatry 1989; 50:196–204.

348. Casper RC, Kirschner B, Sandstead HH, et al. An evaluation of trace metals, vitamins, and taste function in anorexia nervosa. Am J Clin Nutr 1980; 33:1801–1808.

349. Levy AB. Neuroendocrine profile in bulimia nervosa. Biol Psychiatry 1989; 25:98–109.

350. Fries H. Studies on secondary amenorrhea, anorectic behavior, and body-image perception: importance for the early recognition of anorexia nervosa. In: Vigersky RA, ed. Anorexia Nervosa. New York: Raven, 1977:163–176.

351. Lachelin GCL, Yen SSC. Hypothalamic chronic anovulation. Am J Obstet Gynecol 1978; 130:825–831.

352. Boyar RM, Katz J. Twenty-four hour gonadotropin secretory patterns in anorexia nervosa. In: Vigersky RA, ed. Anorexia Nervosa. New York: Raven, 1977:177–187.

353. Pirke KM, Fichter MM, Lund R, et al. Twenty-four hour sleep-wake pattern of plasma LH in patients with anorexia nervosa. Acta Endocrinol 1979; 92:193–204.

354. Beumont PJV, Abraham SF. Continuous infusion of luteinizing hormone releasing hormone (LHRH) in patients with anorexia nervosa. Psychol Med 1981; 11:477–484.

355. Marshall JC, Kelch RP. Low dose pulsatile gonadotropin-releasing hormone in anorexia nervosa: a model of human pubertal development. J Clin Endocrinol Metab 1979; 49:712–718.

356. Wakeling A, Marshall JC, Beardwood CJ, et al. The effects of clomiphene citrate on the hypothalamic-pituitary-gonadal axis in anorexia nervosa. Psychol Med 1976; 6:371–380.

357. Espinosa-Campos J, Robles C, Gual C, et al. Hypothalamic, pituitary, and ovarian function assessment in a patient with anorexia nervosa. Fertil Steril 1974; 25:453–458.

358. Nillius SJ, Fries H, Wide L. Successful induction of follicular maturation and ovulation by prolonged treatment with LH-releasing hormone in women with anorexia nervosa. Am J Obstet Gynecol 1975; 122:921–928.

359. Frisch RE. Food intake, fatness, and reproductive ability. In: Vigersky RA, ed. Anorexia Nervosa. New York: Raven, 1977:149–161.

360. McNab D, Hawton K. Disturbances of sex hormones in anorexia nervosa in the male. Postgrad Med J 1981; 57:254–256.

361. Devlin MJ, Walsh BT, Katz JL, et al. Hypothalamic-pituitary-gonadal function in anorexia nervosa and bulimia. Psychiatry Res 1989; 28:11–24.

362. Brambilla F, Ferrari E, Cavagnini F, et al. Alpha 2–adrenoceptor sensitivity in anorexia nervosa: GH response to clonidine or GHRH stimulation. Biol Psychiatry 1989; 25:256–264.

363. Rappaport R, Prevot C, Czernichow P. Somatomedin activity and growth hormone secretion. I. Changes related to body weight in anorexia nervosa. Acta Paediatr Scand 1980; 69:37–41.

364. Issacs AJ, Leslie RDG, Gomez J, et al. The effect of weight gain on gonadotrophins and prolactin in anorexia nervosa. Acta Endocrinol 1980; 94:145–150.

365. Skrabanek P, Devlin J, McDonald D, et al. Plasma prolactin and gonadotrophins in anorexia nervosa and amenorrhoea due to weight loss. Acta Endocrinol 1981; 97:433–435.

366. Waldhauser F, Toifel K, Spona J, et al. Diminished prolactin response to thyrotropin and insulin in anorexia nervosa. J Clin Endocrinol Metab 1984; 59:538–541.

367. Beumont PJV, Abraham SF, Turtle J. Paradoxical prolactin response to gonadotropin-releasing hormone during weight gain in patients with anorexia nervosa. J Clin Endocrinol Metab 1980; 51:1283–1285.

368. Burman KD, Vigersky RA, Loriaux DL, et al. Investigations concerning

thyroxine deiodinative pathways in patients with anorexia nervosa. In: Vigersky RA, ed. Anorexia Nervosa. New York: Raven 1977: 255–261.

369. Moshang T Jr, Utiger RD. Low triiodothyronine euthyroidism in anorexia nervosa. In: Vigersky RA, ed. Anorexia Nervosa. New York: Raven, 1977: 263–270.

370. Schimmel M, Utiger RD. Thyroidal and peripheral production of thyroid hormones. Review of recent findings and their clinical implications. Ann Intern Med 1977; 87:760–768.

371. Kaptein EM, Grieb DA, Spencer CA, et al. Thyroxine metabolism in the low thyroxine state of critical nonthyroidal illnesses. J Clin Endocrinol Metab 1981; 53:764–771.

372. Moore R, Mills IH. Serum T_3 and T_4 levels in patients with anorexia nervosa showing transient hyperthyroidism during weight gain. Clin Endocrinol 1979; 10:443–449.

373. Gold PW, Gwirtsman H, Avgerinos PC, et al. Abnormal hypothalamic-pituitary-adrenal function in anorexia nervosa. Pathophysiologic mechanisms in underweight and weight-corrected patients. N Engl J Med 1986; 314:1335–1342.

374. Boyar RM, Hellman LD, Roffwarg H, et al. Cortisol secretion and metabolism in anorexia nervosa. N Engl J Med 1977; 296:190–193.

375. Walsh BT, Katz JL, Levin J, et al. The production rate of cortisol declines during recovery from anorexia nervosa. J Clin Endocrinol Metab 1981; 53:203–205.

376. Hotta M, Shibasaki T, Masuda A, et al. The responses of plasma adrenocorticotropin and cortisol to corticotropin-releasing hormone (CRH) and cerebrospinal fluid immunoreactive CRH in anorexia nervosa patients. J Clin Endocrinol Metab 1986; 62:319–324.

377. Kaye WH, Gwirtsman HE, George DT, et al. Elevated cerebrospinal fluid levels of immunoreactive corticotropin-releasing hormone in anorexia nervosa: relation to state of nutrition, adrenal function, and intensity of depression. J Clin Endocrinol Metab 1987; 64:203–208.

378. Gwirtsman HE, Kaye WH, George DT, et al. Central and peripheral ACTH and cortisol levels in anorexia nervosa and bulimia. Arch Gen Psychiatry 1989; 46:61–69.

379. Mortola JF, Rasmussen DD, Yen SSC. Alterations of the adrenocorticotropin-cortisol axis in normal weight bulimic women: evidence for a central mechanism. J Clin Endocrinol Metab 1989; 68:517–522.

380. Zumoff B, Walsh BT, Katz JL, et al. Subnormal plasma dehydroisoandrosterone to cortisol ratio in anorexia nervosa: a second hormonal parameter of ontogenic regression. J Clin Endocrinol Metab 1983; 56:668–672.

381. Doerr P, Fichter M, Pirke KM, et al. Relationship between weight gain and hypothalamic pituitary adrenal function in patients with anorexia nervosa. J Steroid Biochem 1980; 13:529–537.

382. Ferrari E, Foppa S, Bossolo PA, et al. Melatonin and pituitary-gonadal function in disorders of eating behavior. J Pineal Res 1989; 7:115–124.

383. Tortosa F, Puig-Domingo M, Peinado MA, et al. Enhanced circadian rhythm of melatonin in anorexia nervosa. Acta Endocrinol 1989; 120:574–578.

384. Kennedy SH, Garfinkel PE, Parienti V, et al. Changes in melatonin levels but not cortisol levels are associated with depression in patients with eating disorders. Arch Gen Psychiatry 1989; 46:73–78.

385. Fujii S, Tamai H, Kumai M, et al. Impaired glucagon secretion to insulin-induced hypoglycemia in anorexia nervosa. Acta Endocrinol 1989; 120:610–615.

386. Newman MM, Halmi KA. Relationship of bone density to estradiol and cortisol in anorexia nervosa and bulimia. Psychiatry Res 1989; 29:105–112.

387. Hay PJ, Hall A, Delahunt JW, et al. Investigation of osteopaenia in anorexia nervosa. Aust NZ J Psychiatry 1989; 23:261–268.

388. Biller BM, Saxe V, Herzog DB, et al. Mechanisms of osteoporosis in adult and adolescent women with anorexia nervosa. J Clin Endocrinol Metab 1989; 68:548–554.

389. Klibanski A, Biller BMK, Rosenthal DI, et al. Effects of prolactin and estrogen deficiency in amenorrheic bone loss. J Clin Endocrinol Metab 1988; 67:124–130.

390. Milosevic A, Slade PD. The orodental status of anorexics and bulimics. Br Dent J 1989; 167:66–70.

391. Krieg JC, Lauer C, Leinsinger G, et al. Brain morphology and regional cerebral blood flow in anorexia nervosa. Biol Psychiatry 1989; 25:1041–1048.

392. Krieg JC, Lauer C, Pirke KM. Structural brain abnormalities in patients with bulimia nervosa. Psychiatry Res 1989; 27:39–48.

393. Isner JM, Roberts WC, Heymsfield SB, et al. Anorexia nervosa and sudden death. Ann Intern Med 1985; 102:49–52.

394. Schocken DD, Holloway JD, Powers PS. Weight loss and the heart. Effects of anorexia nervosa and starvation. Arch Intern Med 1989; 149:877–881.

395. Meyers DG, Starke H, Pearson PH, et al. Leaflet to left ventricular size disproportion and prolapse of a structurally normal mitral valve in anorexia nervosa. Am J Cardiol 1987; 60:911–914.

396. Hsu LKG, Crisp AH. The Crown-Crisp experiential index (CCEI) profile in anorexia nervosa. Br J Psychiatry 1980; 136:567–573.

397. Eckert ED, Goldberg SC, Halmi KA, et al. Depression in anorexia nervosa. Psychol Med 1982; 12:115–122.

398. Grounds A. Transient psychoses in anorexia nervosa: a report of 7 cases. Psychol Med 1982; 12:107–113.

399. Beumont PJV, Abraham SF, Simson KG. The psychosexual histories of adolescent girls and young women with anorexia nervosa. Psychol Med 1981; 11:131–140.

400. Vande Wiele RL. Anorexia nervosa and the hypothalamus. Hosp Pract 1977; 12:45–51.

401. Norris DL. Clinical diagnostic criteria for primary anorexia nervosa. An analysis of 54 consecutive admissions. S Afr Med J 1979; 56:987–993.

402. Strober M, Salkin B, Burroughs J, et al. Validity of the bulimia-restricter distinction in anorexia nervosa. Parental personality characteristics and family psychiatric morbidity. J Nerv Ment Dis 1982; 170:345–351.

403. Marcus D, Wiener M. Anorexia nervosa reconceptualized from a psychosocial transactional perspective. Am J Orthopsychiatry 1989; 59:346–354.

404. Humphrey LL. Observed family interactions among subtypes of eating disorders using structural analysis of social behavior. J Consult Clin Psychol 1989; 57:206–214.

405. Garfinkel PE. Some recent observations on the pathogenesis of anorexia nervosa. Can J Psychiatry 1981; 26:218–223.

406. Huenemann RL, Shapiro LR, Hampton MC, et al. A longitudinal study of gross body composition and body conformation and their association with food and activity in a teen-age population. Views of teen-age subjects on body conformation, food and activity. Am J Clin Nutr 1966; 18:325–338.

407. Smith NJ. Excessive weight loss and food aversion in athletes simulating anorexia nervosa. Pediatrics 1980; 66:139–142.

408. Yates A, Leehey K, Shisslak CM. Running—an analogue of anorexia? N Engl J Med 1983; 308:251–255.

409. Fava M, Copeland PM, Schweiger U, et al. Neurochemical abnormalities of anorexia nervosa and bulimia nervosa. Am J Psychiatry 1989; 146:963–971.

410. Geracioti TD Jr, Liddle RA. Impaired cholecystokinin secretion in bulimia nervosa. N Engl J Med 1988; 319:683–688.

411. Piazza E, Piazza N, Rollins N. Anorexia nervosa: controversial aspects of therapy. Compr Psychiatry 1980; 21:177–189.

412. Russell G. The current treatment of anorexia nervosa. Br J Psychiatry 1981; 138:164–166.

413. Balaa MA, Drossman DA. Anorexia nervosa and bulimia: the eating disorders. Dis Mon 1985; 31:1–52.

414. Goldbloom DS, Kennedy SH, Kaplan AS, et al. Anorexia nervosa and bulimia nervosa. Can Med Assoc J 1989; 140:1149–1154.

415. Gustavsson CG, Eriksson L. Acute respiratory failure in anorexia nervosa with hypophosphataemia. J Intern Med 1989; 225:63–64.

416. Bhanji S. Anorexia nervosa: physicians' and psychiatrists' opinions and practice. J Psychosom Res 1979; 23:7–11.

417. Health and Public Policy Committee, American College of Physicians. Position paper. Eating disorders: anorexia nervosa and bulimia. Ann Intern Med 1986; 105:790–794.

418. Crisp AH. Therapeutic outcome in anorexia nervosa. Can J Psychiatry 1981; 26:232–235.

419. Hsu LKG. Outcome of anorexia nervosa. A review of the literature (1954 to 1978). Arch Gen Psychiatry 1980; 37:1041–1046.

420. Schwartz DM, Thompson MG. Do anorectics get well? Current research and future needs. Am J Psychiatry 1981; 138:319–323.

421. Crisp AH, Kalucy RS, Lacey JH, et al. The long-term prognosis in anorexia nervosa: some factors predictive of outcome. In: Vigersky RA, ed. Anorexia Nervosa. New York: Raven, 1977:55–65.

422. Herzog DB, Keller MB, Lavori PW. Outcome in anorexia nervosa and bulimia nervosa. A review of the literature. J Nerv Ment Dis 1988; 176:131–143.

26

DISORDERS OF LIPID METABOLISM

Edwin L. Bierman and John A. Glomset

INTRODUCTION

Knowledge of the metabolism of lipids and lipoproteins has increased rapidly during the past few years. In particular, there has been an explosion of information regarding the role of receptors and apolipoproteins in lipoprotein physiology, which has led to a re-evaluation of our understanding of hyperlipidemic disorders in humans. A framework of pathophysiological concepts can now be formulated as a guide to diagnosis and therapy and as an aid to following developments in this field.

The aim of this chapter is to describe lipid metabolism and transport with specific attention to hormone-lipid interrelationships and then to discuss current knowledge about hyperlipidemia in relation both to specific primary disorders and to diabetes, atherosclerosis, and other endocrine disorders closely associated with it.

TRIGLYCERIDE METABOLISM

A major function of triglyceride is to provide an efficient storage form for energy. The importance of triglyceride as a fuel can be appreciated from the fact that enough is usually stored to support many weeks of fasting, whereas carbohydrate is stored in amounts sufficient to last only a few hours.[1] An advantage of triglyceride is that it yields more than twice as many calories per gram as either carbo-

hydrate or protein and requires less than half the amount of intracellular water for storage. Both properties depend on its long chain fatty acid constituents. Fatty acids contain a high proportion of carbon and hydrogen relative to oxygen and thus yield a large amount of energy when oxidized. In addition, they tend to promote self-association of triglycerides and to prevent mixing with water. This allows efficient fuel storage but imposes special requirements for transport and metabolism. These requirements are discussed here in relation to pathways that lead to the formation and utilization of triglyceride stores.

Digestion and Absorption

Human diets contain variable amounts of triglyceride (fat) provided by both plant and animal foods. Typical Western diets provide as much as 40% of the total calories in the form of triglyceride, but, on a worldwide scale, this type of diet is geographically as well as historically unusual. Less affluent people often consume a lower proportion of triglyceride than carbohydrate.

Most dietary triglyceride is absorbed in the duodenum and proximal jejunum after undergoing partial hydrolysis in the gut lumen. The events that precede absorption of the dietary triglyceride are schematically illustrated in Figure 26–1. First, the triglyceride is mechanically mixed with the aqueous secretions of the gastrointestinal tract to form large fat droplets. Then a stable emulsion of smaller fat droplets is formed as bile acids, and phospholipids from the diet and

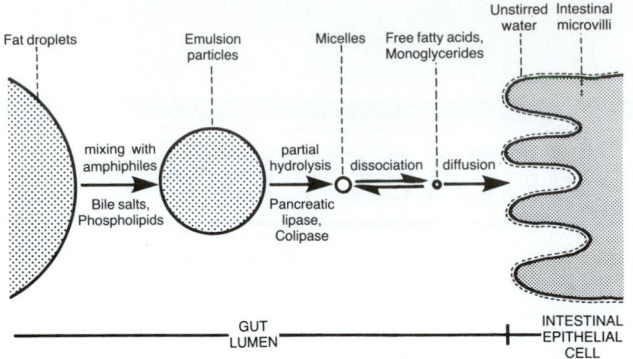

Figure 26–1. Schematic representation of events during hydrolysis and absorption of dietary triglyceride.

bile become associated with the droplet surface. These substances are amphophilic, i.e., partly hydrophilic and partly hydrophobic, and thus promote the formation of a stable oil-water interface.[2] The conversion of large fat droplets to many small droplets greatly increases the total surface area of fat exposed to the action of water-soluble gut lipases. These lipases include a lingual lipase that begins to act in the stomach and a lipase in pancreatic juice that acts within the lumen of the intestine. Both lipases preferentially hydrolyze triglycerides that are present as insoluble aggregates.

Action of pancreatic lipase on the small droplets of dietary triglyceride leads to the formation of monoglycerides and free fatty acids (FFAs). At the same time, action of a pancreatic phospholipase on the phospholipid associated with the droplet surface leads to the formation of lysophospholipids and FFAs. As more and more triglyceride and phospholipid are hydrolyzed, the hydrolytic products leave the droplet surface and, in association with the bile acids, form aggregates termed *micelles*.

The micelles are small enough (about 5 nm in diameter) to enter the spaces between the microvilli of intestinal epithelial cells and there can approach the unstirred aqueous layer that is immediately adjacent to the cell surface. When micelles at the boundary of this layer dissociate, they provide monomeric FFAs and monoglycerides that can diffuse through the unstirred layer and penetrate the cell membranes. Within the cells the FFAs, the monoglycerides, and the small amounts of free glycerol that are formed during digestion are reconverted into triglyceride, packaged into lipoproteins, and secreted into lymph (Fig. 26–2). These processes occur rapidly, as can be demonstrated by sequential electron microscopy. Within 20 to 30 min after the introduction of fat into the intestinal lumen, the Golgi region of the intestinal epithelial cells is crowded with lipid, and

within 1 h the lipid can be observed in the extracellular space at the base of the cell, ready for entrance into the lymphatic system.

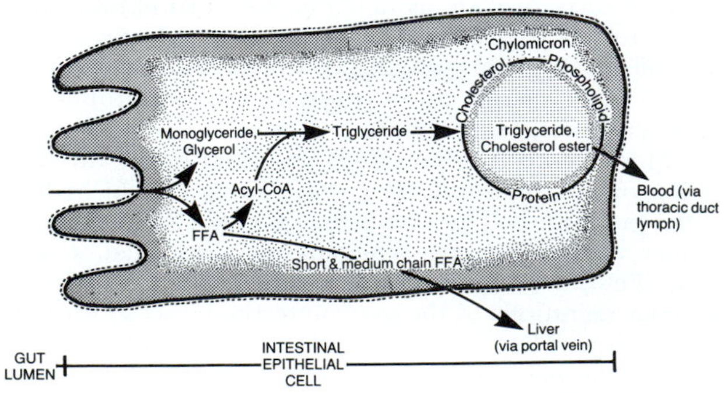

The FFAs and monoglycerides that are converted to triglycerides within intestinal epithelial cells are those that have chains at least 14 carbon atoms long. Shorter chain fatty acids largely pass through the epithelial cells and are transported via the portal vein to the liver. Before long chain FFAs can be converted to triglycerides, they must first be activated by reaction with ATP and coenzyme A (CoA) to form fatty–acyl CoA derivatives that in turn react with monoglycerides or with glycerol 3-phosphate (Fig. 26–3). Other fatty acyl–CoA derivatives can react with absorbed lysophosphatidylcholine to form phosphatidylcholine or with cholesterol to form cholesteryl esters. All of these lipids then associate with proteins to form large particles termed *chylomicrons*.

Chylomicrons normally vary from about 75 to about 600 nm in diameter, depending on the fat load ingested.[3] They typically contain about 90% triglyceride, 1% each of cholesterol and cholesteryl ester, 6 to 8% phospholipid, and 1 to 2% protein. The protein includes four separate apolipoproteins that are synthesized by the intestinal epithelial cell: apolipoprotein (apo) AI, apo AII, apo AIV, and apo B48.[3,4] Although the functional role of these apolipoproteins in chylomicron metabolism is not completely understood, all contribute to an amphophilic surface layer of phospholipid, cholesterol, and protein that stabilizes a large core of triglyceride and cholesteryl ester within the chylomicron particle. Furthermore, apo B48 is known to play a special role in chylomicron formation and secretion. Patients afflicted with abetalipoproteinemia[5] are unable to synthesize this apolipoprotein and, apparently because of this, do not form and secrete chylomicrons. They absorb and re-esterify dietary lipids, but these lipids accumulate within mucosal cells.

Transport and Metabolism of Chylomicron Triglyceride

After being secreted by intestinal epithelial cells, chylomicrons pass through the mesenteric and thoracic duct lymph and enter the bloodstream. Then the triglyceride of

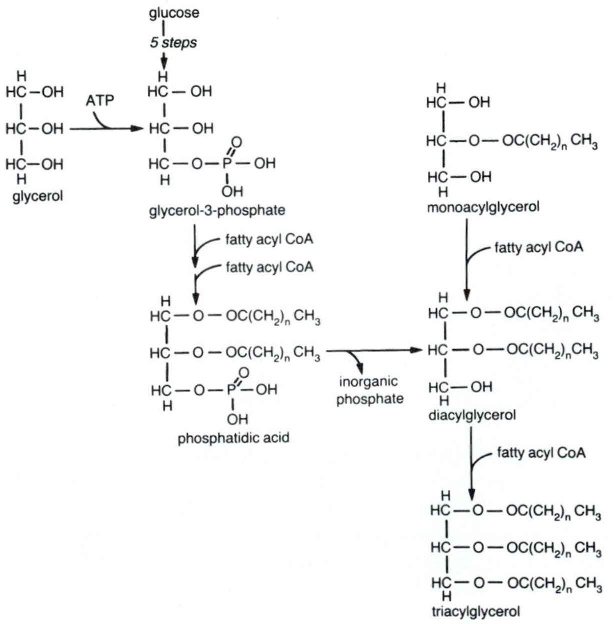

Figure 26–2. Schematic representation of conversion of absorbed monoglycerol and FFAs into chylomicron triglyceride.

Figure 26–3. Synthesis of triglyceride within the mucosal cell. Note that the major pathway utilizes monoglyceride formed during digestion.

chylomicrons is rapidly hydrolyzed by lipoprotein lipase (LPL) adsorbed to the luminal surface of capillaries (Fig. 26–4). Most of the FFAs released in this way are taken up by adipose cells, re-esterified, and stored as adipose tissue triglyceride. Several metabolic events contribute to this aspect of chylomicron metabolism. First, chylomicrons change in composition as they mix with other lipoproteins (Table 26–1) in the lymph and plasma. They lose phospholipid and apolipoproteins AI, AII, and AIV and take up cholesterol and apolipoproteins CI, CII, CIII, and E. Although the significance of these changes is not fully understood, apo CII, primarily acquired through transfer from high-density lipoprotein (HDL), is known to affect profoundly the clearance of chylomicron triglyceride from the plasma. apo CII activates LPL in vitro, whereas patients afflicted with familial apo CII deficiency[6, 7] develop hypertriglyceridemia and hyperlipemia when they ingest fat because chylomicrons accumulate in the plasma. Patients who have familial LPL deficiency[7] develop similar abnormalities, providing additional evidence for the importance of this enzyme in the normal clearance of chylomicrons.

Studies both in humans and in experimental animals have produced considerable information about the normal biochemistry and physiology of LPL.[8] The cells of several different tissues, including adipose tissue, muscle, and mammary tissue, seem able to synthesize and secrete LPL activity, although enzymes from different tissues may vary.[9] After secretion into the extracellular fluid, LPL becomes associated with the luminal surface of nearby capillary endothelial cells. Once adsorbed onto this surface, LPL effectively hydrolyzes the triglycerides of chylomicrons that transiently adsorb to the same surface (Fig. 26–5). It attacks the ester bonds 1 and 3 of chylomicron triglycerides, producing 2-monoglycerides and FFAs. The 2-monoglycerides may be further hydrolyzed by intracellular enzymes, whereupon an additional molecule of FFA and a molecule of glycerol are released. The FFA becomes available for uptake by tissue cells and—in the case of adipose tissue—is largely reconverted into triglyceride. The liberated glycerol, on the other hand, re-enters the bloodstream and is metabolized mainly by the liver and the kidney.

Different mechanisms normally affect the concentration of LPL in different tissues.[10] The activity of LPL in adipose tissue decreases during fasting and in diabetes, is increased by carbohydrate feeding, and is highest in animals that have been fasted and then refed. In contrast, the activity of heart muscle LPL increases during prolonged fasting, whereas mammary tissue LPL activity is relatively low until parturition, when it increases as much as 10-fold. The fact that the content of LPL in different tissues differs under varying

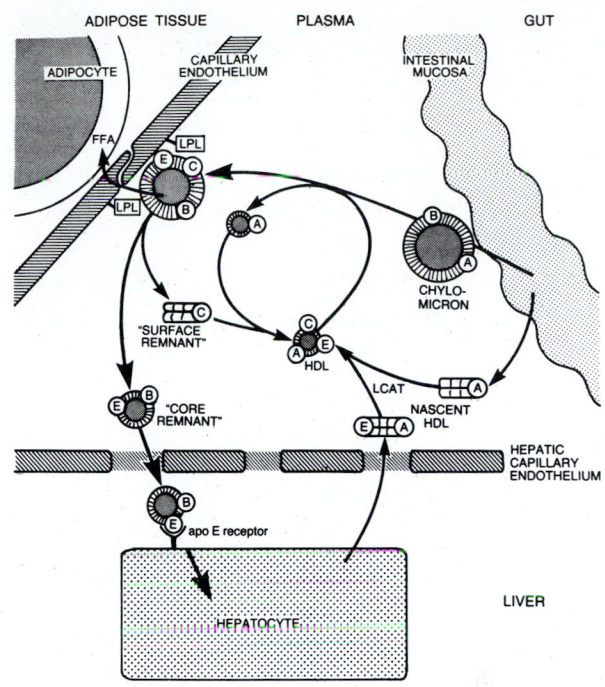

Figure 26–4. Schematic representation of the metabolism of chylomicrons and chylomicron remnants. A, B, C, and E designate apolipoproteins A, B, C, and E. -IIII- designates lipoprotein surface film composed of phospholipid and unesterified cholesterol. Stippled areas within lipoprotein particles and in the single adipocyte designate core triglyceride and cholesteryl ester. Note that the hepatic endothelium is fenestrated.

physiological circumstances suggests that LPL not only plays a general role in chylomicron clearance but also specifically directs chylomicron-derived FFAs into different tissues. It should be noted in this regard that high concentrations of glucose and insulin in the plasma direct chylomicron-derived FFAs to adipose tissue not only by stimulating adipose tissue LPL activity but also by stimulating the intracellular re-esterification of FFA in adipocytes (Fig. 26–6).

After the bulk of the triglyceride in a given chylomicron has been hydrolyzed by LPL, the remainder of the chylomicron desorbs from the endothelial surface and enters the circulation. Part of the phospholipid and cholesterol of the original circulating chylomicron, 10 to 15% of the original triglyceride, and most if not all of the cholesteryl ester, apo B48, and apo E together form a lipoprotein particle referred to as a *chylomicron remnant*. As will be discussed later, both this particle and additional phospholipid and cholesterol

TABLE 26–1. Composition and Properties of Major Plasma Lipoproteins

Designation; Electrophoretic Mobility	Size; Density	Major "Core" Lipid*	Major Apolipoproteins†	Source of Nascent Particles	Direct Enzymatic Attack by‡
Chylomicrons	70–600 nm; <0.940 g/mL	TG	apo C, E, B48	Gut	LPL
VLDL; prebeta	30–70 nm; <1.006 g/mL	TG	apo C, E, B100	Liver	LPL
IDL; slow prebeta	10–30 nm; 1.006–1.019 g/mL	CE	apo E, B100	VLDL	LPL?
LDL; beta	20–25 nm; 1.019–1.063 g/mL	CE	apo B100	VLDL, IDL	HL?
HDL; alpha	7–10 nm; 1.063–1.21 g/mL	CE	apo AI, AII, AIV, C, E	Liver, gut	LCAT, HL
Lp(a); sinking prebeta	30–40 nm; 1.047–1.12 g/mL	CE	apo(a), B100	Liver	—

*TG, triglyceride; CE, cholesteryl ester.
†Major apolipoproteins of circulating particles.
‡LPL, lipoprotein lipase; HL, hepatic lipase; LCAT, lecithin-cholesterol acyltransferase.

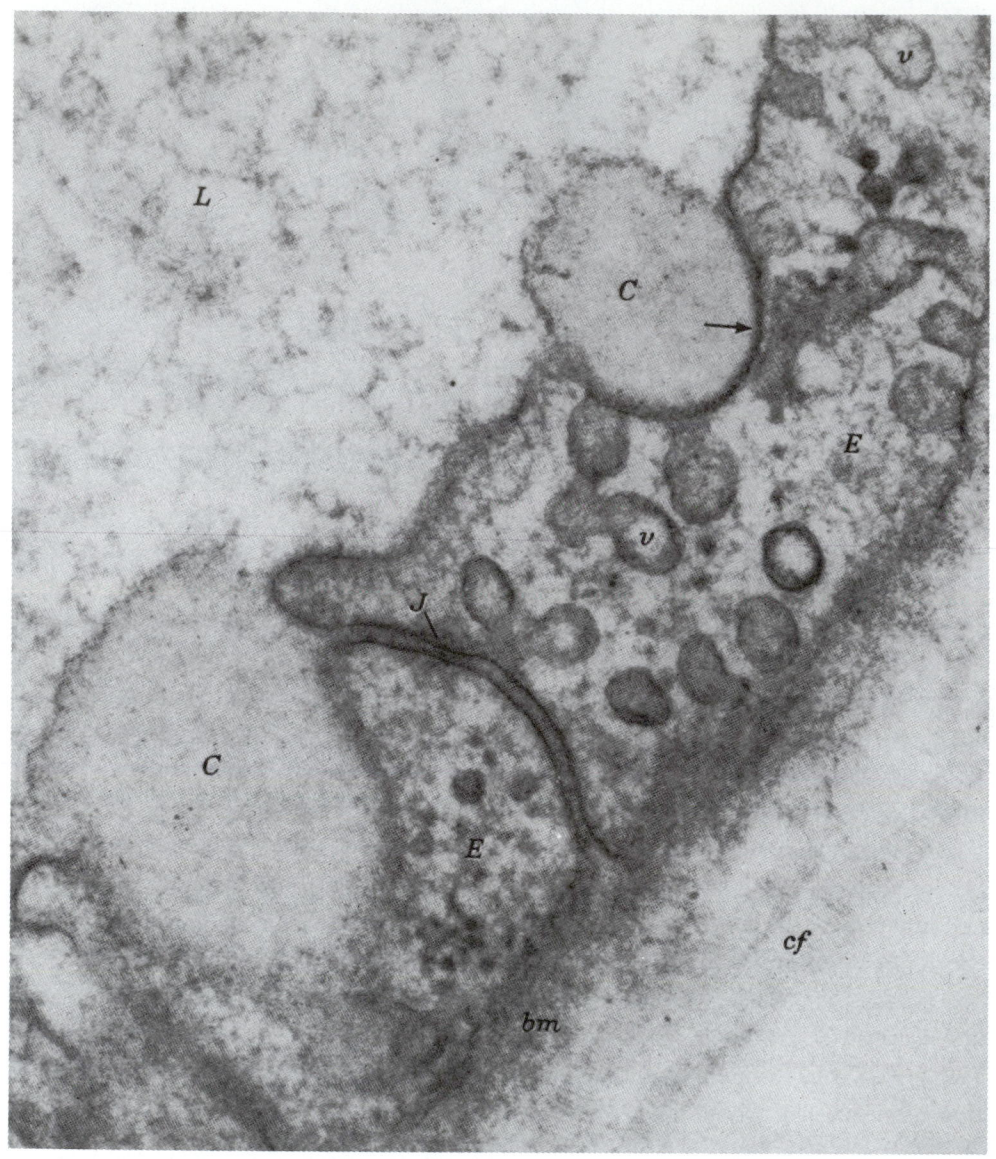

Figure 26–5. Detail of the capillary endothelium of a rat mammary gland 10 min after intravenous injection of chyle. L, capillary lumen; C, chylomicron; E, endothelium; J, cell junction; v, vesicle; bm, basement membrane; cf, collagen fiber. Lead citrate stain; magnification × 140,000. (From Schoefl GI, French JE. Vascular permeability to particulate fat: morphological observations on vessels of lactating mammary gland and of lung. Proc R Soc Lond [Biol] 1968; 169:53.)

derived from the original chylomicron are normally cleared from the plasma by mechanisms that involve the liver.

Production of Triglyceride from Carbohydrate

When dietary fat is replaced by carbohydrate in humans, endogenous synthesis of fatty acid increases in the liver and, to a lesser extent, in adipose tissue. This biosynthesis depends on glucose and insulin. Fatty acids synthesized in the liver are converted mainly to triglyceride, packaged into very-low-density lipoprotein (VLDL), secreted into the plasma, and then cleared from the plasma within minutes to hours by mechanisms similar to those involved in removal of chylomicron triglyceride.

The pathways of fatty acid biosynthesis and the mechanisms that control them appear to be similar in adipose tissue and liver. Fatty acids are synthesized from two-carbon units and hydrogen, both of which are mainly derived from glucose. Activated two-carbon units (acetyl-CoA) are formed from pyruvate within the mitochondria by the pyruvate dehydrogenase reaction (see Chapters 23 and 24). Because fatty acid biosynthesis occurs outside the mitochondria, the two-carbon units must be transferred across the relatively impermeable mitochondrial membrane. The principal pathway of transfer appears to involve condensation of acetyl-CoA with oxalacetate to form citrate. Citrate is transferred across the membrane by a membrane carrier protein, or permease, and reconverted to acetyl-CoA and oxalacetate outside the mitochondria by a cleavage reaction that requires ATP and CoA. Eight acetyl-CoA molecules are required for

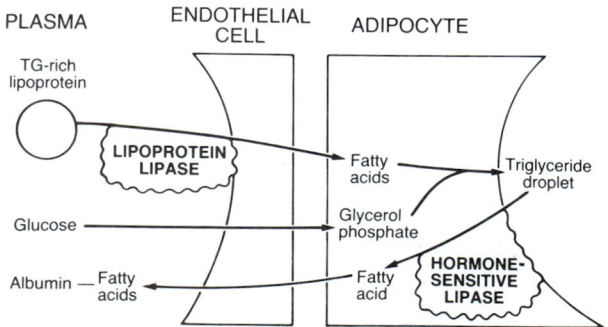

Figure 26–6. Regulatory role of LPL and hormone-sensitive lipase in deposition and mobilization of adipose tissue triglyceride. Insulin promotes triglyceride storage by enhancing LPL activity and fatty acid esterification via glycerol phosphate formation from glucose and simultaneously limits fatty acid mobilization by inhibiting hormone-sensitive lipase activity.

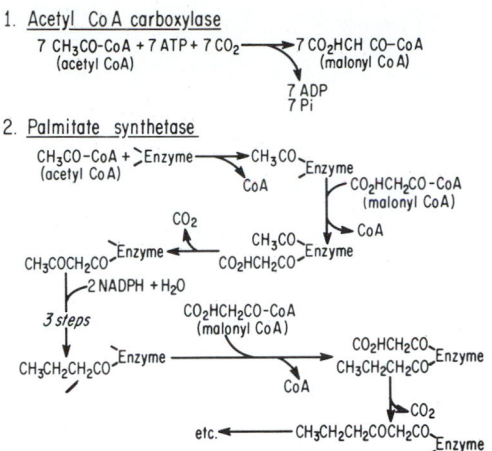

1. Acetyl Co A carboxylase

$$7 \; CH_3CO\text{-}CoA + 7 \; ATP + 7 \; CO_2 \longrightarrow 7 \; CO_2HCH \; CO\text{-}CoA$$
(acetyl CoA) → (malonyl CoA)
7 ADP
7 Pi

2. Palmitate synthetase

Figure 26–7. Schematic representation of formation of palmitic acid in the extramitochondrial fluid. Pi, inorganic phosphate.

synthesis of one molecule of palmitic acid (16 carbon atoms). One acetyl group appears to be transferred directly to a carrier protein–enzyme complex (fatty-acid synthase). The remaining seven are first carboxylated by a key enzyme, acetyl-CoA carboxylase, to form malonyl-CoA (Fig. 26–7). Subsequently, the malonyl groups are successively transferred to fatty-acid synthase and condensed to form a long hydrocarbon chain. With each transfer of a malonyl group, one molecule of CoA and one of CO_2 are released. At each step, four atoms of hydrogen, transferred from two molecules of NADPH, are required to convert the elongated chain into a saturated hydrocarbon.

The NADPH appears to be derived from two separate pathways, the pentose shunt, which produces two molecules of NADPH during the oxidation of glucose 6-phosphate and 6-phosphogluconate, and the malic enzyme pathway. In the latter, the oxalacetate produced by the citrate cleavage reaction is first reduced by NADH to form malate. Then the malate is reoxidized by NADP in the presence of malic enzyme (malate dehydrogenase) to form NADPH, pyruvate, and CO_2. Palmitic acid synthesized by this sequence of condensation and reduction steps can be activated to form palmitoyl-CoA and directly esterified to form triglycerides and other lipids, or it can be elongated or dehydrogenated or both to form other fatty acids. Elongation occurs within the mitochondria or in association with the endoplasmic reticulum (microsomes). Dehydrogenation occurs in the endoplasmic reticulum and is coupled to chain elongation.

The major fatty acids synthesized from palmitic acid in this way are stearic acid, a saturated fatty acid containing 18 carbon atoms, and oleic acid, a fatty acid containing 18 carbon atoms and one double bond. Major fatty acids that cannot be synthesized by animal tissues are linoleic acid (18 carbon atoms, two double bonds) and γ-linolenic acid (18 carbon atoms, three double bonds). These fatty acids and their metabolic products, e.g., arachidonic acid and docosahexaenoic acid, are essential for normal health and development[11–13] and must be provided directly or indirectly by plant foods.

The rate of biosynthesis of palmitic acid and its fatty acid products by mammalian liver is highest for hypercaloric, high-carbohydrate diets; low for fat-rich diets; and lowest during prolonged starvation or diabetes. The factors that cause these differences are only partially understood, but some potential mechanisms of fine and coarse control have been identified. For example, both pyruvate dehydrogenase and acetyl-CoA carboxylase are regulated by allosteric effectors and by phosphorylation-dephosphorylation mechanisms. Both enzymes can be phosphorylated by protein

kinases and thereby inactivated, and both are dephosphorylated to their active forms by protein phosphatases[14–16] that seem to be affected by insulin. These phosphorylation-dephosphorylation reactions in conjunction with allosteric control mechanisms involving key substrates and products[17] appear at least partly to explain the rapid changes in fatty acid biosynthesis noted in various physiological conditions, but slower changes in the concentrations of other enzymes appear to explain more long-term physiological effects. Thus the rates of biosynthesis of glucokinase, the citrate cleavage enzyme, acetyl-CoA carboxylase, fatty-acid synthase, glucose-6-phosphate dehydrogenase, 6-phosphogluconate dehydrogenase, and malic enzyme are all coordinately affected by diet, producing long-term control of fatty acid biosynthesis.

Whether fatty acids are synthesized slowly or rapidly by liver cells, VLDLs are still formed and secreted into the plasma because the liver also forms VLDL triglyceride from circulating FFA.[18] VLDLs can be recognized in the Golgi region of the cell before secretion. Like chylomicrons, they contain a large core of triglyceride surrounded by a layer of protein, phospholipid, and unesterified cholesterol. Although the apolipoproteins of freshly secreted human or primate VLDL have not yet been studied, human VLDLs isolated from plasma contain mainly apolipoproteins B100, C, and E.[19] As in the case of the apo B48 of chylomicrons, the apo B100 of VLDL seems to be required for lipoprotein formation and secretion. Patients afflicted with abetalipoproteinemia[4] form neither apo B48 nor apo B100 and synthesize neither chylomicrons nor VLDLs. The fact that a single genetic defect affects both apo B48 and apo B100 in this disease suggests that the two apolipoproteins are closely related. The apolipoproteins differ in molecular weight, however, and patients have been described[20] who seem able to form apo B48 but not apo B100.

After VLDLs appear in plasma, they circulate for several hours and apparently interact repeatedly with LPL on the luminal surface of tissue capillaries (Fig. 26–8). As a result,

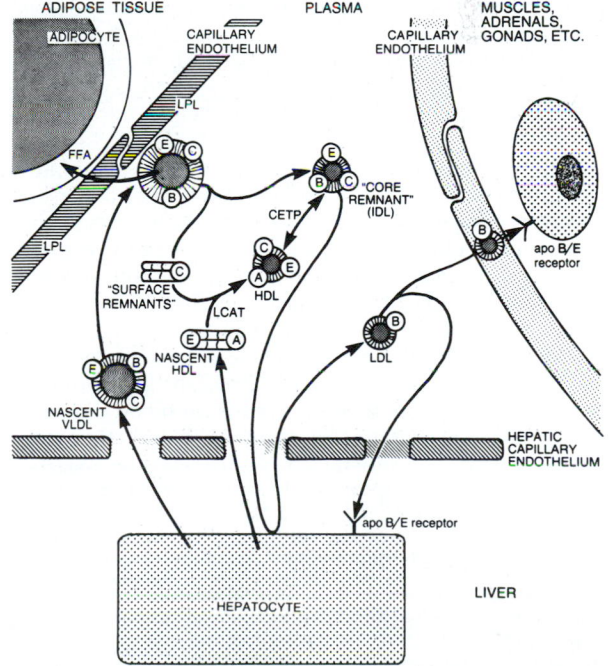

Figure 26–8. Schematic representation of metabolism of VLDLs and their lipoprotein remnants. A, B, C, and E designate apolipoproteins A, B, C, and E. -IIII- designates lipoprotein surface film composed of phospholipid and unesterified cholesterol. Stippled areas within lipoprotein particles and in the single adipocyte designate core triglyceride and cholesteryl ester. Note that the hepatic capillary endothelium is fenestrated.

they progressively lose triglyceride and become smaller. As in the case of chylomicrons, the LPL reaction is promoted by apo CII associated with the lipoprotein surface. In the presence of glucose and insulin the reaction largely occurs in adipose tissue, and the FFAs released are taken up by fat cells and stored in the form of triglyceride.

The fate of the lipoprotein products formed by the action of LPL on VLDL differs from that of chylomicron remnants, as will be discussed later in detail. Instead of being rapidly removed from plasma, VLDL "remnants" interact with other proteins and enzymes and are thereby successively converted into smaller, denser lipoproteins that play an important role in cholesterol metabolism.

Release of Fatty Acids from Adipose Tissue Stores

Net release of FFA and glycerol from adipose tissue triglyceride occurs during several physiological conditions, including exercise, stress, and fasting, as well as in uncontrolled diabetes. Hormones play an important part in this release. Some hormones and autonomic nervous stimulation (Table 26–2) increase lipolysis within minutes by promoting formation of cyclic AMP (cAMP), which stimulates a protein kinase that activates a rate-limiting triglyceride hydrolase, "hormone-sensitive lipase"[21] (Fig. 26–9). Thyroid hormone appears to increase the sensitivity of adipose tissue to these hormones, whereas insulin and prostaglandin E_1 inhibit their action. Studies with rats suggest that growth hormone may stimulate lipolysis in a different way. In vitro, in the presence of dexamethasone, it increases release of FFA from adipose tissue but only after a time lag of about 2 h. This effect can be inhibited by agents that block protein synthesis, which suggests that the biosynthesis of new protein is involved. Once the effect has developed, however, it is insensitive to agents that block protein synthesis but is sensitive to inhibition by insulin. This suggests that the new protein synthesized is the hormone-sensitive triglyceride hydrolase. The synergism between growth hormone and glucocorticoids and the relatively long time lag are of interest because both features characterize the action of growth hormone in vivo.

Fate of Plasma Free Fatty Acids

When glycerol and FFAs are released from adipose tissue, they circulate briefly in the plasma. If lipolysis is brisk, the plasma concentrations of these metabolites rise. The rise only partially reflects the rate of lipolysis, however, because uptake by the tissues is proportional to the concentration in the plasma. The glycerol is mainly metabolized in the kidney and the liver, where it is phosphorylated by glycerol kinase and either reutilized for triglyceride formation or used for gluconeogenesis. The fatty acids circulate as albumin complexes. Their disposal depends greatly on blood flow. During intense exercise, when the flow of blood through the splanchnic bed is reduced, they are largely oxidized in muscle. Those taken up by the liver are activated by reaction

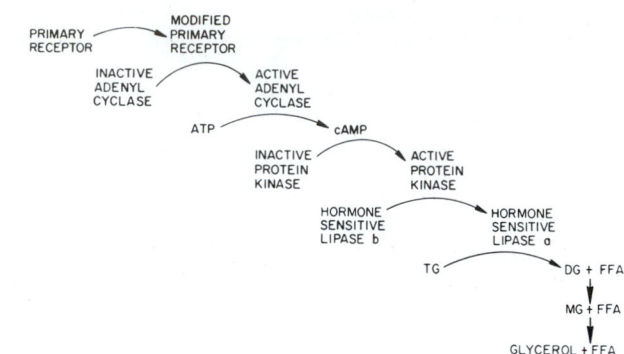

Figure 26–9. Cascade of reactions involved in activation of hormone-sensitive lipase. (From Steinberg D, Huttunen JK. The role of cyclic AMP in activation of hormone-sensitive lipase of adipose tissue. Adv Cyclic Nucleotide Res 1972; 1:47–62.)

with ATP and CoA to form acyl-CoA. The activated acyl groups are then converted to triglyceride or other lipids and secreted as VLDL, oxidized to CO_2 or converted into ketone bodies, depending on nutritional and hormonal conditions. In the presence of glucose and insulin, conversion to VLDL triglyceride predominates. During fasting or in diabetes, when glucose or insulin or both are diminished, most of the acyl groups are oxidized or converted into ketone bodies.

Fatty Acid Oxidation and Ketogenesis

For oxidation and ketogenesis to occur, activated fatty acids must be transported into the mitochondria by a specific mechanism. Neither FFAs nor their CoA derivatives formed outside the mitochondria readily penetrate the inner mitochondrial membrane, but an enzyme present in this membrane, carnitine palmitoyltransferase I, reversibly transfers fatty acyl groups from acyl-CoA to carnitine, and acylcarnitine derivatives can enter the mitochondria (see Chapter 24). Once they are inside, a second enzyme, carnitine palmitoyltransferase II, causes essentially irreversible transfer of the acyl groups from acylcarnitine to mitochondrial CoA, thus effectively preventing the fatty acids from returning to the cytosol. The fatty acyl–CoA derivatives then enter the beta-oxidation pathway and contribute to the formation of reduced coenzymes (NADH and FADH) and acetyl-CoA.

When small amounts of fatty acids are oxidized, the reduced coenzymes largely enter the electron transport pathway within the mitochondria and yield ATP and H_2O. The acetyl-CoA condenses with oxalacetate to form citrate and is either transported across the mitochondrial membrane by the permease system and reconverted to fatty acid or oxidized to CO_2 by the enzymes of the citric acid cycle. During fasting and in uncontrolled diabetes, however, the flow of FFAs into the liver is greatly increased. Under these conditions, production of VLDL triglyceride from these fatty acids is limited, and reduced coenzymes and acetyl-CoA within the mitochondria accumulate. The acetyl-CoA molecules then condense successively to form acetoacetyl-CoA and hydroxymethylglutaryl CoA (HMG CoA), whereupon the latter is cleaved to yield acetoacetate and acetyl-CoA. This causes the release of CoA, which can then be used in the metabolism of additional fatty acids by the beta-oxidation pathway. In addition, the free acetoacetate formed can be reduced by the excess mitochondrial NADH to form β-hydroxybutyrate, thus liberating NAD for use in beta-oxidation. Alternatively, it can decompose spontaneously to yield acetone, which accounts for the increased concentrations of all three metabolites in the plasma during ketogenesis.

TABLE 26–2. Hormones That Affect Lipolysis In Vitro

Rapid Stimulation	Slow Stimulation
Catecholamines (beta-1–agonists)	Growth hormone
Corticotropin	Glucocorticoids
Glucagon	**Suppression**
Secretin	Insulin
Thyrotropin	Oxytocin
Prolactin	Prostaglandin (PGE₁)
Placental lactogen	Somatomedins
Vasopressin	Gastric inhibitory polypeptide
Vasoactive intestinal peptide	

The fate of the plasma ketones, like that of the plasma fatty acids, depends on nutritional and hormonal conditions. After a short period of fasting, acetoacetate and β-hydroxybutyrate increase in concentration in plasma and are metabolized in muscle, heart, and brain. In muscle, the acetoacetate is activated to acetoacetyl-CoA utilizing mitochondrial CoA stores before being cleaved to acetyl-CoA and oxidized via the citric acid cycle. (β-Hydroxybutyrate is oxidized to acetoacetate for activation; it does not form a CoA derivative directly.) Because fatty acids taken up from the blood by muscle also must be converted into derivatives of mitochondrial CoA before they can be metabolized, the two substrate types compete with each other. Moreover, both compete for the CoA ordinarily utilized by the pyruvate dehydrogenase reaction in converting pyruvate derived from glucose to acetyl-CoA. This competition, along with the conversion of pyruvate dehydrogenase to its less active phosphorylated form in the presence of increased concentrations of acetyl-CoA, may partially account for the decreased utilization of glucose by muscle noted during fasting and diabetes.

Summary: Hormonal Effects

Adipocyte triglyceride is formed from fatty acids provided by either dietary fat or biosynthesis. Fatty acids from dietary fat are largely transported to adipose tissue as chylomicrons. Those formed by biosynthesis arise mainly within the liver and are transported to adipose tissue as VLDL triglycerides. Formation of triglyceride within adipocytes and liver depends on the availability of glucose and insulin. Both are required for fatty acid biosynthesis and for formation of triglyceride glycerol, and both promote transport of triglyceride to adipose tissue by increasing the activity of adipose tissue LPL.

Glucose and insulin also diminish release of FFAs from adipocytes. Insulin blocks activation of a cAMP-dependent, intracelluar, hormone-sensitive triglyceride hydrolase by epinephrine, corticotropin (ACTH, adrenocorticotropin), and other hormones; glucose and insulin promote re-esterification of hydrolyzed fatty acid.

The availability of glucose and insulin also appears to determine the fate of FFA taken up by the liver. In the absence of one or both, and in conjunction with an excess of glucagon, only a small proportion of the FFA is converted to triglyceride and secreted as VLDL. The bulk of the FFA is converted to acylcarnitine, transported into the mitochondria, and either oxidized or used to form ketone bodies. The reaction that forms acylcarnitine (carnitine palmitoyltransferase I) may be a critical control point in this process. It is blocked by malonyl-CoA, an intermediate in the biosynthesis of fatty acids.

The transfer of large amounts of acylcarnitine into the mitochondria, coupled with the limited ability of the liver to oxidize the fatty acyl groups to CO_2, accounts at least partially for the greatly increased formation of ketone bodies observed in diabetes. Finally, lack of insulin may contribute to the ketosis of diabetes by decreasing the utilization of acetoacetate by peripheral tissues. This effect probably depends on the role of insulin in controlling plasma FFA levels, because fatty acids compete with acetoacetate for mitochondrial CoA.

Lack of insulin also affects the concentration of circulating plasma triglyceride. In insulin deficiency, the adipose tissue LPL concentration is diminished, leading to an increase in the concentration of VLDL and chylomicron triglyceride.

CHOLESTEROL METABOLISM

Form and Function

Cholesterol is both a key constituent of cell membranes and lipoproteins and a precursor of bile acids and steroid hormones. Its function in membranes apparently depends on its amphophilic character and its unique, wedge-like shape (Fig. 26–10), which allows it to intercalate in a special way between molecules of membrane phospholipid. This intercalation markedly decreases the permeability of membranes to water-soluble compounds and also decreases membrane fluidity.[22] The water insolubility of cholesterol and the inability of most tissues to degrade it even partially presumably contribute to its value as a cell membrane constituent, but, as in the case of triglyceride, its hydrophobic properties complicate the processes of transport and metabolism. These processes are discussed in relation to two general pathways of cholesterol circulation and transport: (1) the circulation of cholesterol and its products between the liver and the intestine and (2) the circulation of cholesterol between the liver and other peripheral tissues.

Enterohepatic Circulation of Cholesterol and Bile Acids

Although a dietary requirement for cholesterol does not exist, cholesterol in food normally contributes significantly to a pool of cholesterol and its bile acid products that circulate several times each day between the intestine and the liver. Western diets, rich in eggs, dairy products, and meat (see under Therapy of Hyperlipidemia), can provide up to 0.5 to 1.0 g of exogenous cholesterol per day. A considerable proportion of this cholesterol is in the form of cholesteryl ester and probably is not directly absorbed. But pancreatic juice contains a cholesteryl ester hydrolase that in the presence of certain bile acids catalyzes the hydrolysis of cholesteryl esters in the intestinal lumen to release FFAs and unesterified cholesterol. The latter mixes with the unesterified cholesterol of food, bile, and possibly desquamated mucosal cells, and considerable amounts can be absorbed. The process of absorption is not well understood, but it

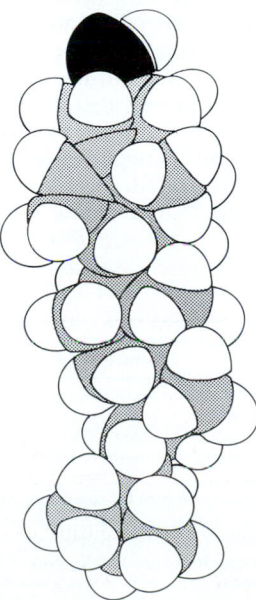

Figure 26–10. Space-filling model of the molecular size and shape of unesterified cholesterol. Hydrogen atoms are white; carbon atoms are gray; oxygen atom is black.

seems to be passive rather than active. Unesterified cholesterol in the intestinal lumen is taken up by mixed micelles of bile acid and FFA, monoglyceride, or phospholipid. As a component of these micelles, cholesterol then enters the spaces between the microvilli of the mucosal cells and becomes available for net transfer into the cell. When net transfer occurs, it is probably to replace mucosal unesterified cholesterol that has been incorporated on the surfaces of newly formed chylomicrons or intestinal HDL or that has been esterified within the cell and incorporated into the interior "cores" of these lipoproteins. If net transfer of cholesterol into mucosal cells does not occur but FFAs, monoglycerides, or lysophospholipids are taken up, the micelles are disrupted and cholesterol precipitates, no longer capable of being absorbed. Overall, cholesterol absorption is incomplete; only about 30 to 60% of cholesterol in the intestinal lumen appears to enter body pools.[23]

How cholesterol transfers from the microvillus membrane to the intracellular site of lipoprotein synthesis has not yet been determined, but the intestinal mucosa contains a soluble, lipid-carrier protein that might function in this regard. A considerable proportion of the cholesterol involved in lipoprotein synthesis becomes associated with the lipoprotein surface, particularly when a large amount of fat is being absorbed. When a relatively small amount of fat is being absorbed, more cholesterol becomes esterified and is incorporated into the lipoprotein interior. Cholesteryl esters are formed from fatty acyl–CoA and cholesterol by a reaction catalyzed by acyl CoA:cholesterol acyltransferase (ACAT).[24]

The amount of chylomicron cholesterol that is secreted each day into the intestinal lymph can be estimated by assuming that approximately 100 g of triglyceride is packaged in chylomicrons each day and that about 2% of the mass of chylomicrons is cholesterol. After chylomicrons enter the plasma and are attacked by LPL, much of this cholesterol, particularly the cholesteryl ester, becomes associated with chylomicron remnants. The remainder of the cholesterol and also the remaining phospholipid apparently become associated with HDL.

Chylomicron remnants are rapidly removed from the plasma by a process that involves the liver (see Fig. 26–4). The remnant particles are about 75 nm in diameter and thus are small enough to pass through pores in the capillary endothelium of the liver into the space of Disse. Because the particles contain apo E, they bind to receptors for this lipoprotein located on the surface of hepatocytes[25] (Table 26–3). The receptors mediate uptake of the remnant particles into hepatocytes and thus effect clearance of the particles from the plasma.

The importance of apo E in remnant clearance is dramatically illustrated by familial dysbetalipoproteinemia, a disease that will be discussed later in more detail. Patients with this condition show different amino acid sequence abnormalities, for example, a cysteine-arginine interchange in a critical segment of apo E that normally interacts with the apo E receptor. These abnormalities lead to defective binding of chylomicron remnants to the hepatocyte surface and to an increase in the concentration of remnant particles in the plasma.

Under normal circumstances, however, remnant particles that bind to the apo E receptors of hepatocytes are rapidly taken up into the cell by adsorptive endocytosis. The ingested particles are then hydrolyzed within secondary lysosomes to yield amino acids, FFAs, and unesterified cholesterol. Lysosomal cholesteryl ester hydrolase evidently plays a critical role in the hydrolytic process, because patients who are unable to synthesize this enzyme accumulate intracellular cholesteryl esters.[26]

One effect of the influx of chylomicron remnant cholesterol into the liver is the decreased synthesis of endogenous cholesterol. Thus hepatocytes, like most cells, can synthesize cholesterol from acetyl-CoA by a multistage series of condensation reactions (Fig. 26–11). Studies with perfused rat livers[27, 28] have suggested that uptake of chylomicron remnants leads to a decrease in the activity of hydroxymethylglutaryl-CoA reductase (HMG-CoA reductase), the rate-limiting enzyme of cholesterol biosynthesis. This enzyme catalyzes the conversion of HMG CoA to mevalonic acid, the first committed metabolite in the biosynthesis of cholesterol. It is subject to multivalent feedback suppression by sterols and by nonsterol products of mevalonic acid,[29] as well as to phosphorylation and dephosphorylation.[30, 31] Down-regulation and inactivation of HMG-CoA reductase by these mechanisms leads to diminished formation of hepatic cholesterol, which limits the tendency of dietary cholesterol to increase hepatic cholesterol levels.

Much of the cholesterol taken up or synthesized by the liver is either converted into bile acids[32] or secreted directly into bile. Conversion into bile acids occurs by a series of reactions located in the endoplasmic reticulum, cytosol, and mitochondria (Fig. 26–12). In dogs and rats this conversion increases several-fold when the animals are fed cholesterol. In humans, however, the response appears to be much more limited, and increased amounts of unesterified cholesterol are secreted into the bile instead. This important species difference may predispose humans to the formation of cholesterol gallstones.[33] Why humans are unable to increase bile acid formation in response to dietary cholesterol is not understood, but it may depend on the 7α-hydroxylase that catalyzes the first step in bile acid formation. It is generally agreed that this step is an important control point in bile acid biosynthesis,[34] and its negative feedback control by bile acids has been demonstrated.

The mechanisms that promote the direct secretion of

TABLE 26–3. Lipoprotein Receptors

Organ/Cell	Major Lipoprotein Bound	Apolipoprotein Specificity	Postulated Function
Liver	Chylomicron remnant	apo E	Exogenous cholesterol removal
	VLDL remnant	apo B100, E	Endogenous cholesterol removal
	LDL	apo B100, E	Endogenous cholesterol removal
	HDL	apo AI, AII, AIV	Endogenous cholesterol removal
Adrenals, gonads	Chylomicron remnant	apo E	Provide cholesterol for steroid hormone synthesis
	LDL	apo B100, E	Provide cholesterol for steroid hormone synthesis
	HDL	apo AI	Provide cholesterol for steroid hormone synthesis
Macrophage	B VLDL	apo E, B100	Scavenger for excess cholesterol
	Modified LDL	Modified apo B + ?	Scavenger for excess cholesterol
	LDL	apo B100, E	Unknown
Other tissues	LDL	apo B100, E	Provide cholesterol for cell growth and replication
	VLDL remnant	apo B100, E	Provide cholesterol for cell growth and replication
	HDL	apo AI, AII, AIV	Reverse cholesterol transport

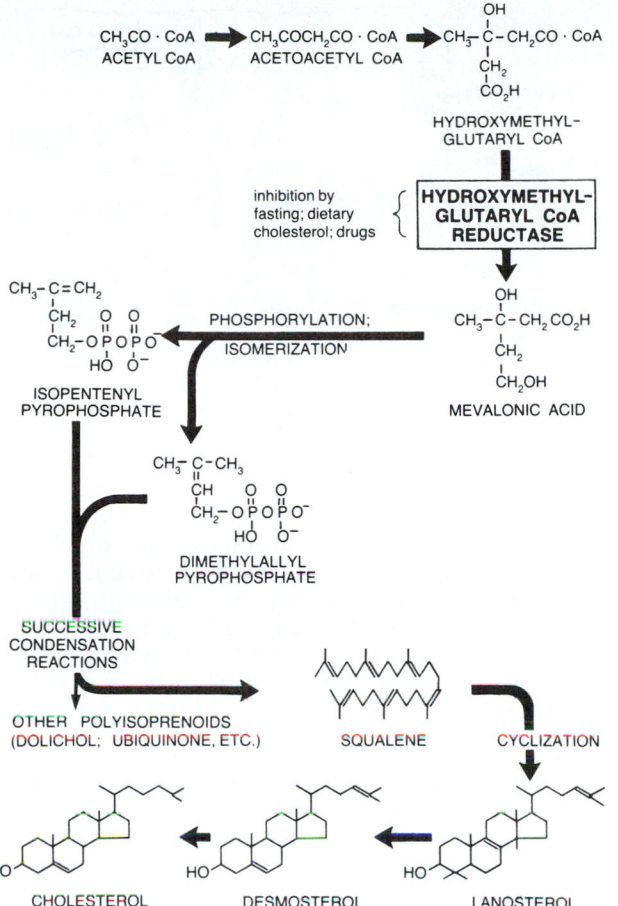

Figure 26–11. Partial representation of reactions involved in cholesterol biosynthesis. Note that the enzyme HMG-CoA reductase catalyzes the principal rate-limiting reaction.

Circulation of Cholesterol Between Liver and Peripheral Tissues

Because most peripheral cells can synthesize cholesterol but few cells can even partially degrade it, special mechanisms are required to maintain cholesterol balance in peripheral tissues. The liver contributes to these mechanisms by secreting at least two types of plasma lipoprotein and at least one plasma enzyme that together promote the transport of cholesterol to and from peripheral cells. One type of lipoprotein secreted by the liver has already been discussed in connection with the transport of hepatic triglyceride. Thus VLDL of hepatic origin consists of a core of triglyceride that is stabilized by a thin film of phospholipid, unesterified cholesterol, and apolipoproteins B100, C, and E. In addition, in some species at least, VLDL can contain ACAT-derived cholesteryl esters of hepatic origin. On being secreted into plasma, VLDLs transport triglyceride to tissues that contain LPL, whereupon LPL catalyzes the partial hydrolysis of the triglyceride, producing remnant lipoproteins that are analogous to chylomicron remnants (see Fig. 26–8). These cholesterol-rich remnants may be taken up directly by the liver[35] or may continue to circulate in the plasma and be gradually converted into small lipoproteins known as low-density lipoproteins (LDLs) that deliver cholesterol to peripheral cells. The mechanisms of conversion and the role of the liver in this process remain to be clarified.

In addition to secreting VLDL, the liver secretes lipoproteins referred to as nascent HDL. These lipoproteins mainly include disc-shaped particles that contain phosphatidylcholine, unesterified cholesterol, and apo AI or E. After being secreted into plasma, nascent HDLs interact with a plasma enzyme that also is synthesized and secreted by the liver. This enzyme, lecithin-cholesterol acyltransferase (LCAT),

cholesterol in bile are not understood, but it has been established that bile acids stimulate the secretion of biliary phosphatidylcholine and that bile acids and phosphatidylcholine together form micelles that can solubilize cholesterol. Bile containing these micelles is stored in the gallbladder and released into the intestine in response to fatty meals. Within the intestinal lumen, the micelles are presumably disrupted as the bile salts participate in the hydrolysis and transport of dietary fat. The phosphatidylcholine is partially hydrolyzed by pancreatic phospholipase, and the cholesterol mixes with that of the diet. Substantial recirculation (enterohepatic circulation) of each of these bile components occurs, however, because the bile salts are efficiently absorbed by an active mechanism in the distal ileum and return to the liver complexed to the albumin of the portal blood; the phosphatidylcholine (resynthesized in the mucosa) and cholesterol return to the liver as components of chylomicrons, as mentioned earlier. Nevertheless, a small proportion of the bile acids and a considerably larger proportion of the bile cholesterol escape reabsorption during each recirculation of the bile, and because the number of recirculations per day has been estimated to be as great as 10, a substantial amount of cholesterol and bile acid is lost in the feces. This loss of bile acids and cholesterol, up to 1.0 to 1.5 g/d, coupled with loss of cholesterol by desquamation of skin and intestinal mucosa cells, approximately balances the amount of cholesterol that is absorbed by the intestine and the amount of endogenous cholesterol that is synthesized.

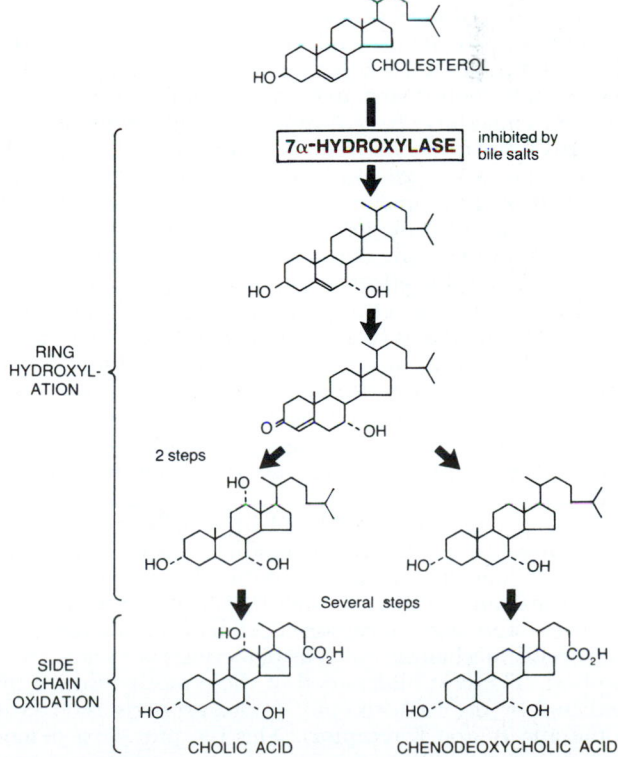

Figure 26–12. Partial representation of the reactions that convert cholesterol to primary bile acids. Note that the enzyme 7α-hydroxylase catalyzes the principal rate-limiting reaction.

forms cholesteryl esters in plasma by transferring fatty acids from HDL phosphatidylcholine to HDL unesterified cholesterol. The LCAT reaction is activated by apolipoproteins, particularly apo AI, the principal apolipoprotein component of mature, circulating HDL. The cholesteryl esters formed by the reaction spontaneously form a core within the HDL particle, thus converting disc-shaped HDL to spherical HDL. The cholesteryl esters can also be transferred to other plasma lipoproteins by a plasma cholesteryl ester exchange protein.[36] By supplying LCAT-derived cholesteryl esters to VLDL and VLDL remnants, the plasma cholesteryl ester exchange protein appears to play a major role in converting these remnants to LDL. The following sequence of events is thought to be involved. LPL hydrolyzes the triglyceride of VLDL, effectively diminishing the core volume and thereby decreasing the requirement for surface phosphatidylcholine, unesterified cholesterol, and protein. Superfluous phosphatidylcholine, unesterified cholesterol, and C apolipoproteins dissociate from the VLDL remnant particle and interact with HDL. LCAT converts the phosphatidylcholine and unesterified cholesterol to HDL cholesteryl ester. Finally, the cholesteryl ester transfer protein transfers cholesteryl esters from the HDL to VLDL and VLDL remnants.

The importance of these reactions in providing cholesteryl esters to VLDL and LDL is illustrated by experiments with the plasma of patients with familial LCAT deficiency.[37] This plasma contains abnormally high concentrations of phosphatidylcholine and unesterified cholesterol and exceedingly low concentrations of cholesteryl ester. It also contains both disc-shaped HDL and unusual particles that appear to be surface remnants of chylomicrons and VLDL. However, when the plasma is incubated with LCAT from normal individuals, the phosphatidylcholine and unesterified cholesterol are converted to cholesteryl esters, and as an indirect consequence the disc-shaped HDLs become spherical, the putative surface remnants decrease in concentration, and the content of cholesteryl ester in VLDL and LDL increases toward normal.

Other processes evidently also contribute to the formation of normal LDL because more than conversion of VLDL phosphatidylcholine and unesterified cholesterol to VLDL remnant cholesteryl ester is required. Both additional lipid and apo E must be removed to produce LDL because LDL particles are about 20 nm in diameter, i.e., one fourth to one third of the diameter of the parent VLDL, and chiefly contain a core of cholesteryl ester surrounded by phospholipid, unesterified cholesterol, and apo B. It is not yet clear how this removal is effected, although a hepatic lipase may be involved.[38] The net effect is the formation of a cholesterol-rich lipoprotein that is small enough to be transported across the endothelial cells of peripheral capillaries. Thus the fate of exogenous cholesterol transported via chylomicron remnants and that of endogenous cholesterol transported via VLDL remnants differ (see Figs. 26–4 and 26–8), because none of the chylomicron remnants appears to be converted to LDL.[39]

The conversion of VLDL to LDL usually requires about 12 h, after which LDLs are gradually cleared from the plasma during the course of several days. Clearance from the plasma can be effected either by peripheral tissues or by the liver, and both receptor-dependent mechanisms and nonspecific mechanisms such as pinocytosis are known to be involved. The best understood of these mechanisms is that mediated by the LDL receptor (more properly referred to as the apo B–apo E receptor). This receptor, first demonstrated in experiments with human skin fibroblasts,[40] binds lipoproteins that contain apo B and/or apo E with high affinity (see Table 26–3; Fig. 26–13). On binding these lipoproteins, the receptor-lipoprotein complex is transferred

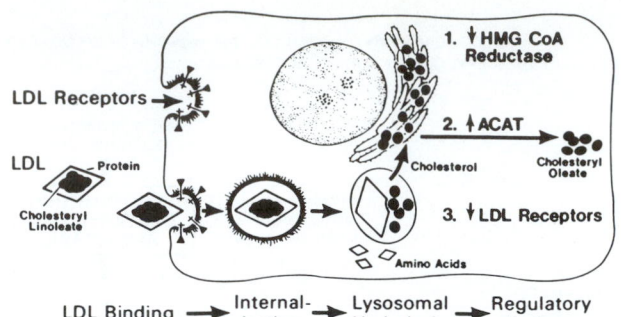

Figure 26–13. Schematic representation of metabolism of LDL by peripheral cells. (From Goldstein JL, Brown MS. The LDL receptor defect in familial hypercholesterolemia. Implications for pathogenesis and therapy. Med Clin North Am 1982; 66:335–362.)

to a special region of the cell surface referred to as a coated pit, where the lipoproteins are internalized by adsorptive endocytosis. Lipoprotein-containing intracellular vesicles formed by this process subsequently fuse with lysosomes, whereupon the lipoproteins are degraded by lysosomal hydrolases and unesterified cholesterol is released into the cytosol. As cytosolic cholesterol accumulates, it is esterified by an intracellular ACAT or used to form membranes. At the same time, it activates feedback mechanisms that reduce intracellular HMG-CoA reductase activity and down-regulate the LDL receptor. These feedback mechanisms clearly limit both the intracellular synthesis of cholesterol from acetyl CoA and the uptake of excessive amounts of LDL cholesterol.

The importance of the apo B–apo E receptor in mediating the normal clearance of LDL from the plasma is emphasized by the strikingly high concentrations of LDL that are typically found in the plasma of homozygous patients with familial hypercholesterolemia.[41] These high concentrations of LDL develop primarily because cells that normally have receptors for LDL either lack the ability to form functioning apo B–apo E receptors or are unable to internalize lipoproteins that have been bound. Clearance of LDL from the plasma must therefore be mediated by other, less effective mechanisms.

Cells that normally have LDL receptors include fibroblasts, smooth muscle cells, adrenocortical cells, and luteal cells from the ovary. Indeed, LDL receptors seem to mediate cholesterol uptake into most cells (see Table 26–3) and account for about two thirds of the removal of LDL particles from plasma.[41] The number of LDL receptors associated with a given cell seems to be regulated by intracellular requirements for cholesterol. For example, the number of LDL receptors associated with skin fibroblasts in culture increases after mitogenic stimulation,[42] presumably reflecting the increased requirement for cell membrane cholesterol that develops during cell replication. Moreover, LDL seems to play a key role in delivering cholesterol to endocrine cells that synthesize steroid hormones because the number of LDL receptors associated with adrenocortical cells is high and increases in response to corticotropin.[43] Similarly, the number of LDL receptors associated with ovarian luteal cells increases in response to chorionic gonadotropin.[44]

LDL is not the only lipoprotein that can deliver cholesterol to cells, however (see Table 26–3). HDL can deliver cholesterol to the rat adrenal, ovary, and testis.[45] Moreover, macrophages have receptors that bind abnormal lipoproteins including chemically modified LDL and the cholesteryl ester–rich VLDL of patients with familial dysbetalipoproteinemia.[46]

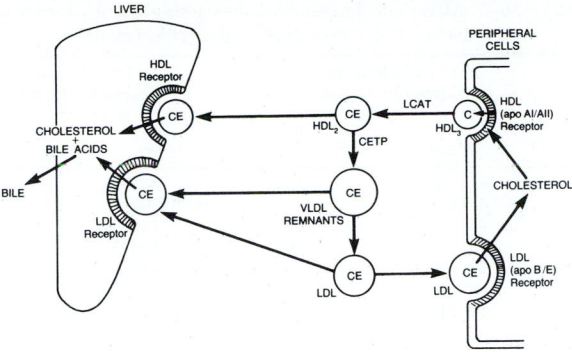

Figure 26–14. Schematic representation of current concepts concerning the role of HDL, LCAT, and cholesteryl ester transfer protein (CETP) in reverse cholesterol transport. C, cholesterol; CE, cholesteryl ester.

Lipoproteins not only deliver cholesterol to cells but apparently also contribute to reverse cholesterol transport. Thus the removal of cholesterol from peripheral cells is currently thought to involve the following intracellular and extracellular events (Fig. 26–14). First, cholesterol in peripheral cells in the form of cholesteryl esters is hydrolyzed by an intracellular cholesteryl ester hydrolase.[46] Then, on interaction of cells with HDL that is transiently bound to HDL receptors on the cell surface,[47] the liberated unesterified cholesterol transfers to the plasma membrane and becomes associated with the HDL. The HDL cholesterol is subsequently esterified by the LCAT reaction and either transferred to other lipoproteins by lipid transfer protein, also called cholesteryl ester transfer protein,[48] or removed directly by the liver. Macrophages may facilitate the removal of cholesterol by the liver by synthesizing and secreting apo E.[46] According to this concept, apo E binds to HDL and thereby promotes binding and internalization of HDL by the liver.

Evidence that HDL contributes importantly to reverse cholesterol transport is provided by the abnormalties that accompany Tangier disease.[49] This inborn error of metabolism is characterized by abnormally low concentrations of HDL in the plasma and by the presence of cholesteryl ester–rich foam cells in peripheral lymph nodes. The concentrations of HDL are thought to be low in the patient's plasma because of a defect in the processing of apo AI that leads to defective binding of lipid.[50]

Reverse cholesterol transport has attracted considerable interest because of the possibility that cholesterol derived from peripheral cells and then internalized by the liver might be excreted from the body via the enterohepatic circulation. That this is a possibility is suggested by the observation[51] that ingestion of the bile acid–binding resin cholestyramine leads to an increase in the number of apo B–apo E receptors in the hepatocytes of experimental animals. Ingestion of this resin increases both the conversion of cholesterol to bile acids and the net excretion of bile acids in the stool, and this presumably increases the uptake of cholesteryl ester–rich lipoproteins into the cell.

Pharmacological doses of estrogens also increase the number of apo B–apo E receptors associated with hepatocytes[52] and decrease the concentration of cholesterol-rich VLDL in dysbetalipoproteinemia (see later). Because high doses of estrogen are known to increase the flow of bile, these effects may be connected. Neither cholestyramine nor estrogens appear to affect the hepatic receptor for chylomicron remnants. Because of this and because the chylomicron remnant receptor appears to recognize apo E but not apo B, at least two different receptors for lipoproteins are clearly present on the hepatocytes.

Summary

Cholesterol can be synthesized by essentially all animal cells. Animal cells cannot, however, degrade it, although adrenals, ovaries, and testes convert it to steroid hormones and the liver can convert it to bile acids. Thus there is no dietary requirement for cholesterol, but there is a requirement for mechanisms that effect cholesterol balance.

The liver plays an important role in this regard because it secretes bile containing both bile acids and unesterified cholesterol. Although these components circulate several times each day between the liver and the intestine, a portion is swept into the distal gastrointestinal tract and ultimately degraded by intestinal bacteria and excreted in the stool. This causes a daily loss of bile acids and cholesterol that approximately balances the cholesterol that is formed by biosynthesis and absorbed from the diet.

The liver also contributes to cholesterol balance by secreting plasma lipoproteins and at least one enzyme that promote the transport of cholesterol to and from peripheral cells. The transport of cholesterol to peripheral cells is closely linked to the transport of triglyceride. Thus a relatively large amount of cholesterol enters the plasma each day in association with triglyceride-rich lipoproteins. After the triglyceride in these lipoproteins is hydrolyzed by LPL, remnant lipoproteins that are relatively rich in cholesterol can be taken up by cells that have receptors for apo B and/or apo E. The cholesterol that enters the cells in this way affects feedback mechanisms that reduce both the synthesis of cholesterol and the synthesis of the apo B–apo E receptor. Meanwhile, cholesterol that accumulates intracellularly is converted to cholesteryl ester.

The transport of cholesterol from peripheral cells appears to depend on HDL. These lipoproteins can bind to cells without being internalized and remove unesterified intracellular cholesterol. Subsequently, the cholesterol can be esterified by LCAT and transferred to lipoproteins that contain apo B or E. Either these lipoproteins or HDL can then return cholesterol to the liver.

Thus the liver plays a central role in the regulation of plasma cholesterol traffic. It not only secretes cholesterol into both bile and plasma (as a component of VLDL) but also controls removal of cholesterol via receptors for chylomicron remnants, VLDL remnants, LDL, and HDL. Each of these steps appears to be regulated by and subject to dietary, hormonal, and genetic influences.

DISORDERS OF LIPID METABOLISM

Hyperlipidemia: Definition and Overview

Hyperlipidemia consists of an excessive accumulation of one or more of the major lipids transported in plasma and is a manifestation of one or more abnormalities of lipid metabolism or transport (Table 26–4). For clinical purposes,

TABLE 26–4. Pathogenesis of Hyperlipidemic Disorders

Locus of Abnormality	Example
Intracellular enzymes of lipid synthesis or catabolism	Familial hypertriglyceridemia?
Extracellular enzymes of lipoprotein transport	LPL deficiency
	LCAT deficiency
	HL deficiency*
	LTP deficiency*
Apoprotein structure	Dysbetalipoproteinemia (type III)
	Familial defective apo B100
Cell-surface lipoprotein receptors	Familial hypercholesterolemia

*HL, hepatic lipase; LTP, lipid transfer protein.

hyperlipidemia may be manifested as hypercholesterolemia or hypertriglyceridemia or both. Thus levels of the triglyceride- and cholesterol-rich lipoproteins (see Table 26–1) are elevated (hyperlipoproteinemia). The older terms lipemia and hyperlipemia refer to the turbid or lactescent plasma visible when the large, triglyceride-rich particles accumulate.

Aside from producing overt signs and symtoms such as xanthoma, lipemia retinalis, and acute abdominal crises (pancreatitis), elevated plasma concentrations of certain lipids and lipoproteins are associated with an increased risk of atherosclerotic disease. It is this risk that is generally used as the guideline for deciding which lipid or lipoprotein levels are abnormally high. Although there is an exponential gradient of risk associated with increasing cholesterol levels throughout the population,[53] which has become the focus of national screening and prevention programs,[54] particular attention has been focused on individuals whose triglyceride or cholesterol levels are in the upper 5% for their age and sex. Consequently, such persons have been arbitrarily defined as hyperlipidemic (Table 26–5). Genetic abnormalities of lipoprotein transport associated with increased risk for atherosclerosis commonly raise lipid levels above the 95th percentile and, often, the 99th percentile. Thus unless an inherited biochemical marker is present (e.g., LPL deficiency, LDL receptor defect), the definition of "disease" is somewhat arbitrary, because there are continuous distributions of both plasma levels and morbidity risk in the population. Also, because populations vary widely, it is meaningless to select arbitrary limits for normality and apply them to all populations. Ultimately, the level at which preventive management can be successfully achieved will influence our definition of abnormality.

Excessive lipid accumulation in plasma in one or more lipoprotein classes can result from defective removal from plasma or excessive endogenous production or both. These abnormalities may be primary or may occur as a secondary result of other diseases, such as endocrine disorders (diabetes or hypothyroidism, for example), or consequent to therapy with certain hormones or drugs (Table 26–6).

TABLE 26–5. Mean and Upper 95th Percentile Values for Fasting Plasma Cholesterol and Triglyceride Levels*

Age (y)	Cholesterol (mmol/L [mg/dL]) Mean	95th Percentile	Triglyceride (mmol/L [mg/dL]) Mean	95th Percentile
MALES	4.1 (160)	5.2 (200)	0.6 (55)	1.1 (100)
0–10	4.0 (155)	5.2 (200)	0.8 (70)	1.6 (140)
10–20	4.5 (175)	5.9 (230)	1.2 (110)	2.5 (225)
20–30	5.0 (195)	6.7 (260)	1.5 (135)	3.3 (290)
30–39	5.4 (210)	7.0 (270)	1.7 (150)	3.6 (320)
40–49	5.6 (215)	7.1 (275)	1.6 (145)	3.4 (305)
50–59	5.6 (215)	7.1 (275)	1.6 (140)	3.2 (280)
60–69	5.3 (205)	7.0 (270)	1.5 (130)	2.9 (260)
70 +				
FEMALES				
0–10	4.1 (160)	5.2 (200)	0.7 (60)	1.2 (110)
10–20	4.1 (160)	5.2 (200)	0.8 (75)	1.5 (130)
20–30	4.3 (165)	5.7 (220)	0.8 (75)	1.6 (140)
30–39	4.7 (180)	6.1 (235)	1.0 (85)	1.8 (160)
40–49	5.2 (200)	6.7 (260)	1.1 (100)	2.3 (200)
50–59	5.8 (225)	7.6 (295)	1.4 (120)	2.8 (250)
60–69	5.9 (230)	7.8 (300)	1.5 (130)	2.7 (240)
70 +	5.9 (230)	7.5 (290)	1.5 (130)	2.7 (235)

*Adapted from data derived from cross-sectional plasma lipid distributions among 48,431 white participants in Visit 1 of the Lipid Research Clinics Prevalence Study of 11 North American populations (The Lipid Research Clinics Program Data Book: Selective Variables in 11 North American Populations. Vol 1. Physiologic and Sociodemographic Characteristics, 1979). Ninety-fifth percentile values approximately +2 SD above the mean for cholesterol. Because triglyceride levels are not normally distributed, mean values will be higher than median values. Data for females are restricted to those not taking estrogen-containing drugs, because women taking sex hormones have altered plasma lipid levels.

From Wallace RB, Hoover J, Sandler D, et al. Altered plasma-lipids associated with oral contraceptive or oestrogen consumption. The Lipid Research Clinic Program. Lancet 1977; 2:11–14.

The primary forms of hyperlipidemia are generally divided into familial, in which there is clear evidence of a genetic predisposition (monogenic or polygenic) based on the presence of the disorder in closely related family members, and sporadic, in which neither known genetic nor

TABLE 26–6. Secondary Hyperlipidemia

Cause of Hyperlipidemia	Chylomicrons (I)	Chylomicrons + VLDL (V)	VLDL (IV)	Remnants (III)	LDL (IIA)	LDL + VLDL (IIB)
ENDOCRINE						
Diabetes mellitus						
Severe, untreated	+	+				
Moderate		+	+	+		+
Corticosteroid therapy						
High dose	+	+				
Low dose or Cushing syndrome			+		+	+
Hypothyroidism		+	+	+	+	+
Hypopituitarism (ateliotic dwarfism)		+	+			
Acromegaly			+			
Anorexia nervosa					+	
Estrogen or oral contraceptive therapy		+	+			
Lipodystrophy (congenital or acquired)		+	+			
NONENDOCRINE						
Renal disease						
Nephrotic syndrome		+	+		+	+
Uremia		+	+	+		
Alcohol		+	+			
Dysglobulinemia	+	+		+	+	
Glycogen storage disease	+	+				
Werner syndrome					+	+
Acute intermittent porphyria					+	
Liver disease					LP-X*	
Isotretinoin therapy		+	+			
Antihypertensive therapy (thiazides; beta-blockers)			+	+		

*LP-X, lipoprotein-X.

TABLE 26–7. Pathophysiological Classification of the Hyperlipidemias

| Mechanism | Disorders | | Lipoprotein Abnormalities | Common Xanthomas | Early Atherosclerosis |
	Primary	Secondary			
Increased triglyceride production: Increased endogenous VLDL synthesis	Familial hypertriglyceridemia	Hyperinsulinemic states Obesity Estrogen therapy Glucocorticoid therapy Type II diabetes mellitus (treated) Growth hormone excess Alcohol Pregnancy	↑ VLDL ↑ VLDL, chylomicrons	None Eruptive	None (?)
Decreased triglyceride removal: Abnormal LPL function	LPL deficiency LPL activator (apo CII) deficiency LPL inhibition	Low insulin (untreated diabetes mellitus) Hypothyroidism Uremia Dysglobulinemia (systemic lupus erythematosus, myeloma, lymphoma, macroglobulinemia)	↑ VLDL, chylomicrons	Eruptive	None
Decreased remnant removal: Core lipid accumulation	Dysbetalipoproteinemia (broad-beta disease)	Hypothyroidism	↑ remnants, VLDL, chylomicrons Abnormal apo E	Planar (palmar); tuberous, tuberoeruptive disease	Coronary; peripheral vascular
Surface lipid accumulation	LCAT deficiency	Liver disease	Disc-shaped HDL LP-X		
Decreased LDL removal	Familial hypercholesterolemia Familial defective apo B100	Hypothyroidism Anorexia nervosa	↑ LDL	Tendon	Coronary
Mechanisms unknown: Combined hyperlipidemias (multiple lipoprotein phenotypes)	Familial combined hyperlipidemia	Hypothyroidism Nephrotic syndrome Glucocorticoid therapy	↑ LDL and/or VLDL ↑ Apo B		Coronary

known secondary factors appear to play a role. The primary and secondary hyperlipidemias are generally characterized by similar laboratory abnormalities. Thus differentiation between primary and secondary hyperlipidemia is sometimes difficult but is the cornerstone of successful therapy, because the secondary hyperlipidemias may be corrected simply by treatment of the causative disease, when possible, or by withdrawal of the offending drug.

Hyperlipidemia has been classified into six types, based on the specific electrophoretic patterns of the various lipoproteins in plasma[55] (see Table 26–1). Excess chylomicrons have been designated as type I hyperlipoproteinemia, excess LDL as type IIA, excess remnant lipoproteins in VLDL and intermediate-density lipoproteins as type III, excess VLDL as type IV, and an excess of both chylomicrons and VLDL as type V. Increases of both LDL and VLDL levels characterize type IIB.

However, these types of patterns are not specific, and the plasma lipoprotein pattern may change with time in any individual, a phenomenon to be expected because of the precursor-product relationships in the metabolism of VLDL and LDL (see under Circulation of Cholesterol Between Liver and Peripheral Tissues) and the profound effects of diet on VLDL transport. Classification solely by this method, furthermore, does not reflect the pathophysiological or genetic mechanisms responsible for the disorders. A single mechanism may lead to several different lipoprotein patterns, and, conversely, a single pattern may result from a variety of diseases or mechanisms. Table 26–7 presents a classification of hyperlipoproteinemias based on pathophysiological characteristics. Removal defects occur at three general sites along the lipoprotein transport pathway, and more has been learned about mechanisms responsible for these

abnormalities than about alterations in lipoprotein production. The common secondary causes of lipid disorders and the types of associated hyperlipoproteinemias are depicted in Table 26–6. Discrete familial hyperlipidemic disorders that have been defined are summarized in Table 26–8. These more comprehensive classifications are useful for diagnostic purposes; they also provide a more complete understanding of the rationale for different approaches to therapy. As pathophysiological and molecular mechanisms continue to be defined, diagnostic and therapeutic approaches will be sharpened further.

Increased Triglyceride Production

Increased triglyceride-rich lipoprotein production (see under Production of Triglyceride from Carbohydrate) is a normal response to caloric excess and alcohol ingestion and frequently occurs during the third trimester of pregnancy. However, in some individuals increased triglyceride production is abnormal; it appears to be characteristic of common primary forms of hyperlipidemia, such as familial hypertriglyceridemia, and of hyperinsulinemic states secondary to endocrine abnormalities. In its mildest form, this abnormality is manifest by a modest elevation of triglyceride levels in VLDL (type IV lipoprotein pattern). However, when hypertriglyceridemia is more marked, LPL-dependent removal mechanisms for triglyceride-rich lipoproteins become saturated, leading to varying degrees of chylomicronemia and a type V lipoprotein pattern.[56] This commonly occurs when two causes of increased triglyceride production are present simultaneously, e.g., estrogen treatment in a patient with familial hypertriglyceridemia. It also occurs when triglyceride removal defects are associated with factors promoting

TABLE 26–8. Genetic Hyperlipidemias

Disorder	Plasma Lipoprotein Pattern	Genetic Mechanism	Primary Defect	Estimated Population Frequency
Familial hypercholesterolemia	IIA, IIB	Autosomal dominant	LDL receptor	1–2/1,000
Polygenic hypercholesterolemia	IIA, IIB	Polygenic	Unknown	—
Familial hypertriglyceridemia	IV, V	Autosomal dominant	Unknown	2/1,000
Familial combined hyperlipidemia	IIA, IIB, IV, V	Autosomal dominant	Unknown	3–5/1,000
Familial dysbetalipoproteinemia	III	Autosomal recessive*	apo E	1/10,000
LPL deficiency	I, V	Autosomal recessive	Lipoprotein lipase	Rare
Hepatic lipase deficiency	—	Unknown	Hepatic lipase	Rare
apo CII deficiency	I, V	Autosomal recessive	apo CII	Rare
LCAT deficiency	—	Autosomal recessive	Lecithin-cholesterol acyltransferase	Rare
Lipid transfer protein deficiency	—	Unknown	Lipid transfer protein	Rare

*The genetic mechanism for the common abnormal apoprotein E phenotype; a superimposed cause of hyperlipidemia is necessary for expression of the disease.

triglyceride synthesis, such as excess alcohol intake.[57] These multiple abnormalities can occur in some diabetics.

Increased production of triglyceride-rich VLDL often occurs during therapy with corticosteroids[58] or estrogenic agents[59] and in Cushing syndrome.[60] Estrogen-containing oral contraceptive steroids have been shown to mildly increase plasma triglyceride levels;[61] in some individuals, gross hypertriglyceridemia has been unmasked (see under Hyperlipidemia and Estrogens). Hypertriglyceridemia of this kind also has been observed as a consequence of non-nephrotic chronic renal disease (untreated patients and those undergoing chronic peritoneal dialysis, hemodialysis, or renal transplantation).

FAMILIAL HYPERTRIGLYCERIDEMIA. In monogenic familial hypertriglyceridemia, all affected family members have elevated basal plasma triglyceride levels but not hypercholesterolemia. The pathophysiological abnormality appears to be related to overproduction of VLDL triglycerides.[62] Because the synthesis of VLDL apo B is normal, VLDL particles in this disorder are large and triglyceride rich. A specific defect in hepatic lipogenesis has not been demonstrated; however, the synthetic regulatory mechanism appears to be unusually sensitive to insulin, resulting in a higher plasma triglyceride level for a given insulin concentration.[63] Thus triglyceride levels in patients with familial hypertriglyceridemia may be particularly responsive to weight gain, estrogens, alcohol, or high carbohydrate ingestion. HDL cholesterol levels are very low with a reciprocal increase in HDL triglyceride.

Hypertriglyceridemia usually does not emerge until adulthood. The disorder is not associated with xanthomas or other symptoms unless hyperchylomicronemia supervenes. This particular familial form of hypertriglyceridemia occurs frequently (see Table 26–8) but may not be associated with a high incidence of premature atherosclerosis,[64] in contrast to the situation in which high triglyceride and VLDL levels are present in individuals who are members of families with familial combined hyperlipidemia.

Because of the elevated fasting triglyceride levels in these patients after consumption of high-carbohydrate, fat-free diets, it was once thought that their metabolic defect was related specifically to carbohydrate, and the disorder was termed *carbohydrate-induced lipemia*. It is now clear, however, that "carbohydrate induction" is a normal phenomenon because the basal triglyceride levels of healthy subjects not accustomed to eating high-carbohydrate, low-fat diets transiently increase in response to fat-free diets.[65] The distinguishing feature in patients with endogenous lipemia is abnormal triglyceride regulation in the basal state after ingestion of normal amounts of carbohydrate and fat. Increasing the proportion of carbohydrate in the diet accentuates the hypertriglceridemia but does not cause it.

Triglyceride Removal Defects

The catabolism of triglyceride-rich lipoproteins, particularly chylomicrons, is critically dependent on LPL activity (see under Transport and Metabolism of Chylomicron Triglyceride). Thus factors affecting LPL influence chylomicron clearance. Impaired LPL activity leads to defective removal of all triglyceride-rich lipoproteins, but it usually produces a predominance of chylomicrons (type I lipoprotein pattern), which are large and normally are not taken up as such by cells.[66] An accumulation of chylomicrons together with VLDL (type V) occurs frequently, because VLDL is normally catabolized by a similar mechanism involving LPL and this mechanism is readily saturated.[56] This accumulation may vary with age (children have less VLDL) and diet (fat ingestion increases the concentration of chylomicrons).

LIPOPROTEIN LIPASE DEFICIENCY. Although LPL deficiency may occasionally be seen in its inherited autosomal recessive form (see Table 26–8), it is more frequently acquired, as in severe insulin-deficient diabetes mellitus, hypothyroidism, and uremia (see Table 26–7). The type I pattern is more likely to occur in the rare familial disorder, manifesting itself in childhood with typical episodes of eruptive xanthoma and with the acute abdominal pain of pancreatitis. On the other hand, the type V pattern is more frequent in adults, largely because they accumulate more endogenous VLDL than do children.

Regardless of underlying cause or age of onset, hyperchylomicronemia can be associated with a syndrome (chylomicronemia syndrome)[7, 67] that includes milky plasma, lipemia retinalis, acute pancreatitis, and eruptive xanthoma caused by deposits of chylomicrons in the skin.[68] The xanthomas (Fig. 26–15) are usually located over extensor surfaces of the arms, lower extremities, buttocks, or back and often wax and wane with dietary fat content and the degree or duration of the disorder. Dyspnea, dementia, and pseudohyponatremia may also be associated with hyperchylomicronemia. Hepatomegaly resulting from foam cell accumulation may be prominent in children. The vast majority of patients with chylomicronemia and marked hypertriglyceridemia (plasma triglyceride levels greater than 23 mmol/L [2000 mg/dL]) do not have one of the rare genetic disorders associated with abnormal LPL function. Rather, chylomicronemia is usually associated with an acquired disorder secondary to another disease or drug (e.g., untreated diabetes mellitus or estrogen or antihypertensive therapy), causing decreased LPL activity superimposed on an underlying familial form of hypertriglyceridemia.

Chylomicronemia may be recognized easily by the characteristic milky appearance of fresh plasma after centrifugation of blood or brief refrigeration. Diagnosis of LPL deficiency is suggested by findings of a markedly elevated

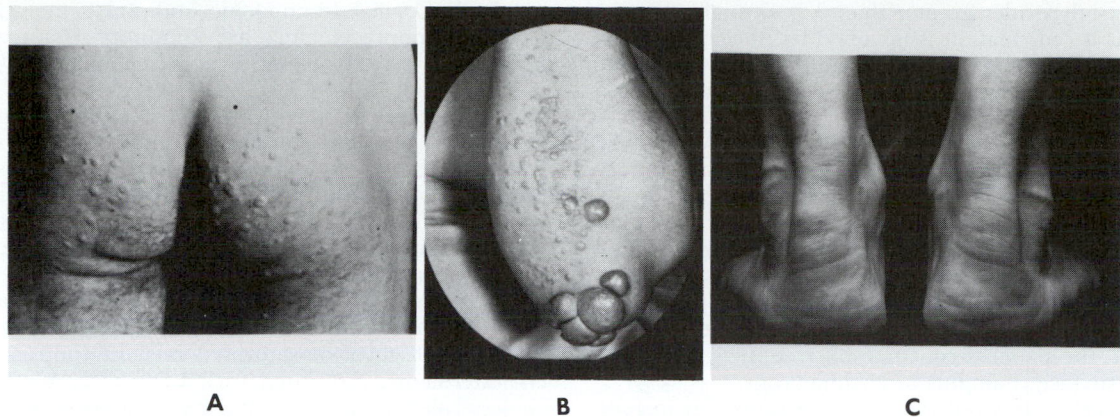

Figure 26–15. Various types of xanthomas seen in different hyperlipidemic disorders. *A,* Eruptive xanthomas distributed over the skin of the buttocks. *B,* Tuberous xanthomas on the elbow. Eruptive xanthomas are also present. *C,* Tendinous xanthomas of the Achilles tendons.

plasma triglyceride level accompanied by normal or only slightly increased cholesterol concentrations, and it is confirmed by subnormal LPL activity in postheparin plasma or in biopsy samples of adipose tissue.

The underlying molecular defects are heterogeneous; some patients fail to make any enzyme protein, and others synthesize abnormal enzyme—either catalytically defective or unable to bind to capillary endothelium.[7]

IMPAIRED LIPOPROTEIN LIPASE FUNCTION. Defective function of LPL may occur and may produce milder degrees of hypertriglyceridemia, with or without chylomicronemia. Enzyme assay in plasma may be normal. However, mild decreases in adipose tissue or muscle LPL can be demonstrated.[69] Many hypertriglyceridemic patients with impaired LPL function are also moderately severe diabetics, and the degree of the lipoprotein abnormality seems to be directly related to the magnitude of the fasting hyperglycemia in the untreated state, suggesting that insulin deficiency is responsible for the impaired LPL activity. (This is described further under Hyperlipidemia and Diabetes Mellitus.) The defect appears to be related to low LPL activity in adipose tissue and, possibly, muscle. Another common cause of decreased LPL function is chronic renal failure.[70] Rare causes of impaired LPL function include an inherited deficiency of the activator apo CII or the familial presence of circulating LPL inhibitors.[71]

Defective Remnant Removal

Action of LPL on triglyceride-rich lipoproteins produces small spherical particles (chylomicron and VLDL core remnants) relatively poor in triglyceride and rich in cholesteryl ester. During this process, redundant surface lipids and apoproteins (surface remnants) are lost from the particles. Remnant removal disorders can affect either core remnants or surface remnants.

FAMILIAL DYSBETALIPOPROTEINEMIA. In this disorder LPL activity is normal, but core remnants appear to accumulate. These remnants contain apo E and either apo B48 (chylomicron remnants) or B100 (VLDL remnants).[72] Remnant lipoproteins separate by density with VLDL and intermediate-density lipoprotein but have the electrophoretic mobility of β- rather than pre–β-lipoproteins ("β-VLDL," type III lipoprotein pattern), hence the origin of the descriptive terms for the disorder, dysbetalipoproteinemia and broad-beta disease. Remnant accumulation in this disorder appears to be due to defective remnant removal,[73] presumably the result of inherited homozygous defects in apo E

structure[74] (see Table 26–3). These defects can result from one of a number of mutations of the apo E gene, leading to failure of recognition of the defective apo E lipoproteins by hepatic receptors.[74] The structural defects in apo E usually lead to functionally defective apo E associated with complete absence of one of the apo E isoforms, apo E3, that is normally detectable by isoelectric focusing. An additional abnormality is necessary for the emergence of hyperlipidemia and complete expression of the disease, because the heterozygous trait is extremely common (about 15% of the general population).[74, 75] About 1% of unselected asymptomatic normolipidemic individuals are homozygous for the E3 deficiency (phenotype E2/E2), yet only about 1 in 50 of the individuals with this phenotype has the disease. The remainder actually tend to have low plasma cholesterol and LDL levels, presumably as a result of impaired conversion of VLDL to LDL. The associated abnormality necessary to produce hyperlipidemia in the presence of functionally defective apo E is usually a familial form of hypertriglyceridemia leading to overproduction of VLDL (e.g., familial combined hyperlipidemia). This thesis is consistent with the frequent occurrence of hyperlipidemia without apo E abnormalities among relatives of patients with dysbetalipoproteinemia.[72] The disorder may also occasionally emerge in the presence of acquired disorders such as hypothyroidism.[76] As with several other inherited lipoprotein disorders, patients with this form of hyperlipidemia are prone to develop coronary atherosclerosis at an early age; peripheral vascular disease is particularly prominent.[77] The disorder is rare in premenopausal women and is usually not expressed in men before adulthood. The sex difference may be related to the effect of exogenous estrogens in lowering β-VLDL levels by increasing remnant catabolism,[73] possibly by an effect on hepatic apo B–apo E receptors.[52] Obesity and hyperuricemia frequently coexist with this disorder.

Diagnosis of the disease is strongly suggested by the finding of palmar xanthomas (orange-yellow discoloration of the palmar creases) and/or tuberous and tuberoeruptive xanthomas, which are almost pathognomonic when present (see Fig. 26–15). Levels of both plasma triglycerides and cholesterol are elevated in approximately a 1:1 ratio, and a type III lipoprotein pattern on paper or agarose electrophoresis is common. For a definitive diagnosis, however, preparative ultracentrifugation of plasma and electrophoretic and compositional analysis of VLDL are required, particularly in asymptomatic patients. The presence of beta-migrating VLDL, low levels of LDL, and an abnormally cholesterol-rich VLDL fraction (ratio of VLDL cholesterol to total serum triglycerides greater than 0.3) strongly suggests the diagnosis. Confirmation is obtained by isoelectric focusing of VLDL apoproteins. Atypical rare forms of the disease are associated with complete absence of all apo E or with a structural abnormality of apo E3.[74, 77]

FAMILIAL LECITHIN-CHOLESTEROL ACYLTRANSFERASE DEFICIENCY. This disorder, characterized by absence or near absence of LCAT from the plasma,[37] is associated with many plasma lipoprotein abnormalities including an accumulation of disc-shaped HDL. The content of cholesteryl ester in all of the lipoproteins is low; abnormal particles, rich in unesterified cholesterol and phospholipid, are found in the LDL fraction. Because the concentration of these particles decreases when the patients consume fat-free diets, the particles may be surface remnants of chylomicrons.[78]

The clinical features of the rare disease usually include moderate anemia and proteinuria as well as corneal opacities. In middle age, renal dysfunction can progress to the nephrotic syndrome and, ultimately, renal failure. Laboratory features include β-VLDL that contain low amounts of cholesteryl ester and absent or barely detectable β-lipoproteins. Liver function tests are normal, in contrast to those of patients with biliary obstruction or hepatitis, which yield similar, although less pronounced, plasma lipoprotein abnormalities.[79]

FAMILIAL HEPATIC LIPASE DEFICIENCY. This rare autosomal recessive disorder[80] is associated with the accumulation of large, buoyant, triglyceride-rich LDL[38] and HDL,[80] suggesting a role for hepatic lipase in the formation of normal LDL and HDL.

Defective Low-Density Lipoprotein Removal

LDL is normally formed as a result of catabolism of VLDL and VLDL remnants and is removed and catabolized by cellular mechanisms largely dependent on the LDL (apo B100–apo E) receptor. Most disorders that cause marked hypercholesterolemia in the absence of hypertriglyceridemia affect LDL removal.

FAMILIAL HYPERCHOLESTEROLEMIA. This disorder, whose primary monogenic form was originally called essential hypercholesterolemia, is characterized by an accumulation of the cholesterol-rich low-density (beta) lipoproteins (type II lipoprotein pattern) as a result of defective catabolism. Most affected individuals are heterozygotes for the mutant gene. Skin fibroblasts and mononuclear cells from the rare homozygous individuals with familial hypercholesterolemia have absent or defective LDL receptors and therefore cannot normally bind, internalize, or catabolize LDL.[41] Various molecular abnormalities affecting in common the function of the LDL receptor, have been described.[41, 81] The more common heterozygotes[41, 81] are affected to a lesser degree. Familial hypercholesterolemia is expressed early in life and has been documented in cord blood samples.[41] Elevated LDL and plasma cholesterol levels (in heterozygotes, ranging from about 9 to 15 mmol/L [350 to 600 mg/dL] or above the 99th percentile for age and sex) are present throughout life; most symptoms and signs become apparent as early as the third or fourth decade. Hypercholesterolemia is markedly aggravated by coexistent hypothyroidism.[82]

Polygenic hypercholesterolemia describes patients in whom the LDL cholesterol level is above the 95th percentile for age and sex but simple monogenic inheritance cannot be demonstrated. This form is poorly understood, is undoubtedly heterogeneous, may be influenced by the apo E isoform pattern, and may underlie plasma cholesterol sensitivity to dietary cholesterol in some individuals.

Both familial (monogenic and polygenic) varieties of hyperbetalipoproteinemia are common. Heterozygous familial hypercholesterolemia occurs in about 1 in 500 individuals (see Table 26–8). LDL elevation also occurs secondary to hypothyroidism, in which the removal rate appears to be decreased,[84] and in the nephrotic syndrome, in which VLDL and LDL production may be increased.[85] Occasionally, it occurs in patients with acute intermittent porphyria[86] or with myeloma,[87] in which an abnormal paraprotein is thought to bind to β-lipoprotein and diminish its clearance rate. Hypercholesterolemia associated with increased LDL levels may also be seen in patients with anorexia nervosa,[88] and it may occur in those who have ingested excessive amounts of dietary cholesterol or saturated fats. In contrast to hypercholesterolemia associated with LDL accumulation, hypercholesterolemia in obstructive liver disease is associated with accumulation of an abnormal cholesterol-rich lipoprotein (LP-X).[79]

Regardless of the cause of accumulation of these cholesterol-rich lipoproteins, the risk of coronary atherosclerosis is high and cardiovascular complications are frequent. Severe hypercholesterolemia is associated with a specific kind of xanthoma, the tendinous xanthoma, which may be nodular or diffuse but usually appears bilaterally on the extensor forearm tendons, Achilles tendons (see Fig. 26–15), or tendons of the hand. Its presence strongly suggests familial hypercholesterolemia; it typically appears during early adulthood in heterozygotes and during the first decade of life in individuals with the rare homozygous form of the disorder. Xanthelasma and corneal arcus also may appear at an early age.

FAMILIAL DEFECTIVE APO B100. Study of moderately hypercholesterolemic individuals with decreased removal of their own LDL, in contrast to normal removal of normal LDL, revealed a family whose affected members had LDL that bound poorly to normal LDL receptors on fibroblasts.[89] The defective LDL was due to a mutation in the gene for apo B100. Other similar individuals have been found.

Combined Hyperlipidemias

Combined hyperlipidemia refers to the presence of multiple lipoprotein phenotypes either in the same individual over time or among family members. Usually levels of LDL, VLDL, or both are increased in plasma. Combined hyperlipidemia frequently occurs in association with a primary familial disorder[90] or with hypothyroidism or nephrotic syndrome. It can also be seen in patients with chronic renal disease who have undergone renal transplantation and are subsequently maintained on glucocorticoid therapy.[91] Mechanisms for combined hyperlipidemia are poorly understood but may involve both overproduction of VLDL and impaired removal of both triglyceride-rich and cholesterol-rich lipoproteins.[92] In the case of hypothyroidism, impaired lipoprotein removal predominates. In nephrotic syndrome, both increased VLDL production, apparently linked to hypoalbuminemia, and diminished lipoprotein catabolism, possibly related to urinary loss of apoproteins, can occur.

FAMILIAL COMBINED HYPERLIPIDEMIA. Frequently associated with coronary atherosclerosis, this disorder (multiple lipoprotein-type hyperlipidemia) was described as a distinct entity in 1973.[93–95] The precise pathophysiological and molecular mechanisms have not yet been established but may be related to increased production of apo B, which can appear in excess in VLDL, LDL, or both.[96] Thus this disease may be seen with a variety of lipoprotein types (IIB, IIA, or IV) in affected individuals in the same family. Patients may have hypertriglyceridemia, hypercholesterolemia, or both; phenotypic expression in any individual may be related to the degree of obesity, diet, drugs, and other factors and can change with time. VLDL particles are small, LDL may be heterogeneous, and HDL may be abnormal.[90, 96] One hypothesis for overproduction of apo B in this disorder involves impaired feedback regulation of synthesis.

Hyperlipidemia usually does not emerge until the third decade and is accentuated by common disorders (see Table 26–6). There are no specific xanthomas. Premature coronary artery atherosclerosis usually becomes clinically evident in men by about age 40.[64] At present, diagnosis can be established only by family studies; both plasma cholesterol and triglyceride levels are elevated, and lipoprotein analysis shows a pattern of elevated LDL, VLDL, or both in affected family members. In patients with hypertriglyceridemia in whom secondary causes have been excluded, a strongly positive family history of early atherosclerosis (before age 55 in men) favors the diagnosis of familial combined hyperlipidemia.

The characteristic feature of this disorder is increased plasma levels of apo B, regardless of the type of hyperlipidemia or whether lipid levels actually exceed the 95th percentile. The condition in which total cholesterol and LDL cholesterol levels are in the normal range in the presence of high apo B levels has been termed *hyperapobetalipoproteinemia*.[97] It is likely that many of these patients are part of the spectrum of this familial disorder.[90] Some individuals with similar clinical, laboratory, and family findings appear to be heterozygous for LPL deficiency.[98] The extent of heterogeneity of familial combined hyperlipidemia remains to be determined.

Hyperlipidemia and Diabetes Mellitus

Alterations in fat transport often resulting in hypertriglyceridemia are well-recognized concomitants of diabetes mellitus. In large groups of diabetic subjects, elevated plasma triglyceride levels are present in about one third and appear to be related to the critical role of insulin in both the production and removal from plasma of triglyceride-rich lipoproteins.[99] Abnormalities in insulin availability are associated with two distinct pathophysiological disturbances that affect the production and removal of triglyceride. These abnormalities appear to be extremes of a spectrum influenced by varying effects of obesity and insulin resistance (high insulin levels) and untreated diabetes (low insulin levels).

Insulin availability appears to be necessary for normal function of LPL (see under Triglyceride Metabolism); thus the extreme insulin deficiency associated with severe, uncontrolled diabetes mellitus leads to hypertriglyceridemia secondary to an acquired LPL deficiency.[100] "Diabetic lipemia" with milky plasma and eruptive xanthoma (a form of the chylomicronemia syndrome) may occur as a result of the frequent coexistence of untreated insulin-deficient diabetes with a familial form of hypertriglyceridemia.[101]

LPL activity, assessed either indirectly in postheparin plasma or directly in adipose tissue, is low in patients with the diabetic lipemia syndrome. Although this disorder was recognized in about 5% of diabetic subjects before the insulin era, it is now relatively rare. When it occurs, the underlying enzyme deficiency is promptly reversed with appropriate insulin repletion, which improves triglyceride removal and reduces plasma triglyceride levels. Hypertriglyceridemia can be produced by brief withdrawal of insulin from insulin-dependent juvenile diabetics; LPL activity decreases, and triglyceride levels rise within 48 h.[102] The diabetic lipemia syndrome has also been observed in association with alcohol ingestion and during prolonged treatment with high doses of corticosteroids.[103]

Marked hypertriglyceridemia (plasma triglyceride levels above 23 mmol/L [2000 mg/dL]) with chylomicronemia appears to result from the interaction of two different diseases in the same patient—in the case of diabetes mellitus, insulin deficiency superimposed on a separately inherited familial form of hypertriglyceridemia.[104] Insulin treatment restores triglyceride levels to those seen in nondiabetic hypertriglyceridemic relatives.

More subtle effects of insulin deficiency occur in patients with less severe diabetes, i.e., those with moderate, fasting hyperglycemia in the range of 2.3 mmol/L (200 mg/dL). Patients with moderate diabetes may have mild abnormalities of adipose and muscle LPL[69, 105] that appear to be related to the degree of insulin deficiency as judged by fasting glucose or glycohemoglobin levels. Most untreated diabetics with hypertriglyceridemia fall into this category. As with severe insulin-deficient diabetics, these persons respond to replacement therapy. When chylomicronemia, and presumably LPL deficiency, occurs in a patient who is being treated for diabetes, it indicates either that therapy is suboptimal or that an additional cause of hypertriglyceridemia is involved.

By a completely different mechanism, excess insulin associated with the obese, insulin-resistant patient with impaired glucose tolerance or non–insulin-dependent diabetes leads to an acquired form of overproduction hypertriglyceridemia. This abnormality also may be seen in insulin-dependent diabetic patients who have been well treated. Aside from its effect on LPL activity, insulin (among other factors) appears to act on the liver to promote VLDL production,[106] presumably by enhancing lipogenesis and lipoprotein packaging and by preventing hepatic triglyceride breakdown. Elevated serum insulin levels, both in the basal state and after glucose stimulation, are directly related to basal plasma triglyceride levels and lipoprotein abnormalities in normal subjects as well as in those with hypertriglyceridemia.[106, 107]

Obesity is the most prevalent of several secondary factors (see Table 26–6) that induce hypertriglyceridemia by impairing the action of insulin on glucose metabolism in peripheral tissue. This reduced responsiveness (insulin resistance) is "sensed" by some unknown process by the pancreas, which attempts to compensate and secrete additional insulin. The hyperinsulinemia associated with adiposity is well documented. The basal hyperinsulinemia often observed in persons with a mild degree of hypertriglyceridemia is usually accounted for by the degree of coexisting adiposity. In one disorder, familial hypertriglyceridemia, the triglyceride-regulatory mechanism appears to be more sensitive to insulin, however, resulting in higher plasma triglyceride levels for a given insulin level.[63] Correlations between adiposity and plasma triglyceride (or VLDL) levels have been observed with indices of adiposity distributed around the abdomen, such as the waist/hip ratio.[108] Furthermore, studies have shown that obese individuals, with or without diabetes, have higher VLDL triglyceride production rates than control subjects of normal weight.[109, 110]

Most patients with hypertriglyceridemia and mild hyperglycemia have abdominal (upper body) obesity. As might be expected, obesity-related hypertriglyceridemia responds dramatically to weight reduction, which reverses basal hyperinsulinemia, hypertriglyceridemia, and impaired glucose tolerance. The other forms of hypertriglyceridemia associated with hyperinsulinemia respond to reduction or removal of the offending hormone or drug or to correction of a causative disorder.

Hypercholesterolemia associated with increased LDL levels may also occur in diabetes mellitus. The carbohydrate-restricted, high-fat (and high-cholesterol) diet formerly used by some to manage insulin-dependent diabetes was associated with increased cholesterol levels, which were restored to normal by use of low-fat diets.[111] Because insulin enhances receptor-mediated LDL degradation,[112] insulin deficiency may impair LDL catabolism, leading to hypercholesterolemia. In harmony with this interpretation, intensive insulin therapy lowers LDL as well as VLDL levels in insulin-dependent diabetes[113] and in non–insulin-dependent diabetes.[114] In non–insulin-dependent diabetes, increased LDL and cholesterol levels may occur as a result of increased rates of synthesis of LDL and cholesterol whether associated with obesity or not.[115, 116] The potential role of glycosylation of LDL in decreasing LDL catabolism[117] remains speculative (see Chapter 24).

Hyperlipidemia and Hypothyroidism

In addition to the hypercholesterolemia and elevated LDL levels frequently observed in hypothyroidism, deficiency of thyroid hormone exerts profound effects on triglyceride transport, often leading to hypertriglyceridemia.[118] The severity of the effect is in large part related to the degree of hormone deficiency and is independent of whether the condition is primary or secondary to pituitary disorders. Thus the presence or absence of hypertriglyceridemia or hypercholesterolemia offers no diagnostic aid in the differentiation between primary and secondary hypothyroidism. Furthermore, no fundamental differences in alterations of lipoprotein metabolism between primary and secondary hypothyroidism have been observed.[119]

Availability of adequate thyroid hormone is essential for normal activity of LPL. In hypothyroidism, low LPL activity appears to be reciprocally related to hypertriglyceridemia, and the abnormalities are reversible with thyroid replacement.[119, 120] As with insulin deficiency, the triglyceride-rich lipoprotein accumulation may vary in degree and type with diet and age and results from impaired VLDL catabolism.[118] Reversible hypertriglyceridemia associated with low LPL activity has been reported in a 14-mo-old hypothyroid infant.[121]

Although fatty acid mobilization from adipose tissue may be decreased in hypothyroidism, thereby reducing fatty acid flux to the liver, diminished hepatic production of triglyceride-rich lipoproteins is presumably insufficient to counterbalance impairment of their removal.

The normal removal of chylomicron and VLDL remnants also appears to be affected by hypothyroidism, because a type III lipoprotein pattern and all the features of dysbetalipoproteinemia can become clinically manifest with thyroid insufficiency and can be reversed with treatment.[76] LDL clearance and catabolism are impaired in hypothyroidism, resulting in the hypercholesterolemia characteristic of the hypothyroid state. This impaired LDL removal from plasma presumably is associated with decreased receptor-mediated LDL degradation, which is reversible with thyroid replacement.[84, 122]

Thus a wide variety of patterns of hyperlipoproteinemia can be produced by hypothyroidism (see Table 26–6). In a large series of patients with primary myxedema,[123] the majority (53%) were hyperlipidemic, with increased VLDL or LDL levels or both. In addition, intermediate-density lipoprotein and fasting chylomicronemia were not unusual. Individuals with untreated hypothyroidism may be predisposed to atherosclerosis, but the role of these varieties of secondary hyperlipidemia in that regard is unknown.

Hyperlipidemia and Estrogens

Estrogens, like insulin, influence both the production and the removal of plasma lipoproteins. In most women receiving estrogen-containing oral contraceptive steroids, some increase in plasma triglyceride and VLDL levels occurs.[124] This increase appears to be proportional to the estrogen (but not the progestogen) content of the medication and to the pretreatment triglyceride levels. In population surveys, women below age 25 taking oral contraceptives have plasma triglyceride levels averaging 48% higher than those of women not taking drugs.[61] These levels remain in the normal range in most instances, however, and the long-term effect of this increase remains unknown. In a few instances, massive hypertriglyceridemia, chylomicronemia, and life-threatening pancreatitis ensue,[125] usually when estrogen therapy is given to a woman with a previously unrecognized familial form of hypertriglyceridemia (such as familial hypertriglyceridemia or familial combined hyperlipidemia). Thus plasma triglyceride levels should be measured before starting estrogen or estrogen-containing oral contraceptive therapy, and these drugs should be avoided in patients with pre-existing hypertriglyceridemia. The mechanism of the estrogen-induced increase in plasma triglyceride levels appears to be related to an enhanced hepatic VLDL triglyceride production rate,[59] perhaps modulated by increased insulin levels. Efficiency of triglyceride removal may also be enhanced by estrogen but not enough to keep pace with accelerated triglyceride input. Adipose tissue LPL activity is not altered.

In contrast to these effects on triglyceride-rich lipoproteins, estrogens appear to enhance the clearance of cholesterol-rich lipoproteins and thus may be therapeutic in certain familial hyperlipidemias. In women with dysbetalipoproteinemia, exogenous estrogens dramatically lower cholesterol and triglyceride levels, return the altered VLDL lipid composition and apoprotein concentration to normal, and correct the impaired removal of remnants.[73, 126] The inherited apo E3 deficiency persists, however. Enhanced remnant removal produced by estrogens may be related to the increased activity of hepatic apo B–apo E receptors seen in rats given high estrogen doses.[52] Estrogen may also lower LDL cholesterol levels in postmenopausal women with heterozygous familia hypercholesterolemia,[127] perhaps by enhancing receptor-mediated catabolism.

Estrogens exert profound effects on HDL metabolism. Women characteristically have higher levels of HDL cholesterol (mainly the lighter HDL_2 density subclass) than men at all ages after puberty. Although this difference can be explained by androgenization of males at puberty (male HDL levels decrease, whereas female HDL levels remain at prepubertal values),[128] exogenous estrogens raise HDL_2 concentrations in both sexes. Thus estrogens may play a role in regulating HDL metabolism, but the metabolic mechanisms are as yet unknown. Estrogen-containing oral contraceptives have variable effects on HDL cholesterol, depending on their estrogen and progestogen content.[129] More potent progestogens lower HDL and raise LDL levels.[130] Whether the intrinsically higher HDL_2 levels of women are related to their lower risk of premature atherosclerosis (see later) is speculative. Atherosclerotic complications related to oral contraceptive use may be mediated only in part by effects on lipid transport and appear to be related to the dose of estrogen and progestogen in the product.[131] In contrast, postmenopausal estrogen therapy in most,[132, 133] but not all,[134] studies appears to reduce risk of death from atherosclerotic heart disease among older women.

Hyperlipidemia and Atherosclerosis

Premature atherosclerosis is often associated with lipoprotein abnormalities. In both cross-sectional and longitudinal population studies, lipoprotein abnormalities may be highly predictive of the development of coronary atherosclerosis and as such are considered among the major risk factors. The prominent alterations that are consistently related to atherogenesis, whether directly or indirectly, include hypercholesterolemia (reflecting increased concentration of LDL),[53] hypertriglyceridemia (reflecting increased concentration of VLDL and/or remnants and triglyceride enrichment of LDL and HDL),[135] increased apo B levels,[136] and reduced levels of HDL (particularly the HDL_2 particle subfraction)[137] and its major apolipoprotein, apo AI.[138]

Hypercholesterolemia resulting from increased LDL levels is frequently associated with premature atherosclerosis, whether genetically determined, as in familial hypercholesterolemia, familial combined hyperlipidemia, or polygenic hypercholesterolemia, or as a secondary manifestation of untreated hypothyroidism, nephrotic syndrome, or high cholesterol and saturated fat intake. Hypertriglyceridemia may be associated with premature atherosclerosis in some specific disorders; this association may not be apparent in studies of whole populations. Patients with elevated VLDL levels who come from families with familial combined hyperlipidemia appear to be at increased risk.[64] Patients with comparably elevated VLDL levels from families with familial hypertriglyceridemia may not have an increased risk. Hypertriglyceridemia in association with impaired remnant removal (dysbetalipoproteinemia) puts patients at increased risk.[77] In addition, increased VLDL levels may increase the risk for premature atherosclerosis when associated with other risk factors such as diabetes mellitus[139, 140] and in patients who smoke and are hypertensive while having chronic hemodialysis.[141]

In a study of 500 consecutive 3-mo survivors of myocardial infarction in Seattle, in which more than 2600 relatives were tested, Goldstein and colleagues[93, 142] found that familial combined hyperlipidemia was associated with 30% of the cases of myocardial infarction in patients who had hyperlipidemia (one third of all cases), whereas familial hypertriglyceridemia occurred in 14% and familial hypercholesterolemia occurred in only 10% (Fig. 26–16). Among families of patients with hypertriglyceridemia in another study,[64] myocardial infarction was four times more prevalent and occurred at younger ages in affected individuals with familial combined hyperlipidemia compared with controls or with those with familial hypertriglyceridemia.

Population studies in which apo B has been measured have shown a close correlation between high apo B levels and coronary atherosclerosis with or without coexisting hypercholesterolemia.[136] Because increased apo B levels appear to be characteristic of familial hypercholesterolemia and familial combined hyperlipidemia,[90] the relation of high apo B levels to atherosclerosis may in large part reflect the presence of these common genetic disorders.

An unusual variant of LDL called Lp(a) (see Table 26–1) is highly correlated with coronary atherosclerosis.[5] It contains a protein, apo(a) that is somewhat homologous to plasminogen and is linked to apo B100 or the lipoprotein. Lp(a) levels vary widely in plasma from undetectable to 100 mg/dL. High levels appear to be genetically determined[143] and are not influenced by diet and only minimally influenced by drugs such as niacin (nicotinic acid).

Individuals in whom remnants of triglyceride-rich lipoprotein metabolism accumulate with resultant hypertriglyceridemia and/or hypercholesterolemia (e.g., familial dysbetalipoproteinemia) are also at risk for development of early atherosclerosis (peripheral as well as coronary).[77] These remnants are relatively rich in cholesteryl ester and apo E and may be particularly atherogenic.

According to current concepts of atherogenesis,[144, 145] cholesterol-rich and triglyceride-rich lipoproteins may play a direct role in lesion formation. Both arterial endothelial cells and smooth muscle cells take up LDL cholesterol and remnant cholesterol via both the cellular LDL receptor–mediated and LDL receptor–independent pathways.[146] Chylomicron and VLDL remnants, cholesterol-rich β-VLDL produced by high cholesterol intake, and altered LDL also can be taken up by monocyte-derived macrophages,[46] which enter the arterial wall during atherogenesis. LDL can be altered by oxidative modification, chemical modification (with endogenous compounds such as malondialdehyde, produced during platelet aggregation), and glycosylation. The role of these modifications of LDL in vivo remains to be determined. However, modified forms of LDL are present in atheroma.[147, 148] Excessive cellular accumulation of cholesterol (as cholesteryl ester) leads to foam cell formation and fatty plaques. Elevated LDL levels may also damage endothelial cells[149] and stimulate the proliferation of arterial smooth muscle cells, processes that occur during atherogenesis.

A variety of hormones and other circulating or cell-derived growth factors may also play a role in atherogenesis.[150] Insulin (in concentrations commonly found in type II and treated type I diabetes mellitus), insulin-like growth factor I (IGF I, also called somatomedin-C), and platelet-derived growth factor can stimulate arterial smooth muscle cell proliferation. These mitogens also increase flux of LDL into cells by increasing their LDL receptor level and promoting cholesterol biosynthesis in the cell. On the other hand, insulin deficiency (and thyroid hormone deficiency) may influence atherogenesis via impaired LDL receptor–mediated catabolism, resulting in high circulating LDL and VLDL remnant levels. Glucocorticoids, estrogens, and progestogens may play a role by influencing lipoprotein concentration and composition and by direct effects on arterial cell function.

HDL may confer protection against the development of premature atherosclerosis and therefore might be considered an antirisk factor.[137] That is, individuals with high HDL cholesterol levels have less atherosclerosis, whereas those with low HDL levels have more. This relationship has been established for coronary, peripheral, and cerebrovascular atherosclerosis. Women characteristically have HDL levels about 25% higher than those of men; HDL can be increased by estrogen and reduced by androgen. In women, low HDL cholesterol levels, particularly when associated with diabetes mellitus and obesity, markedly raise the risk for premature

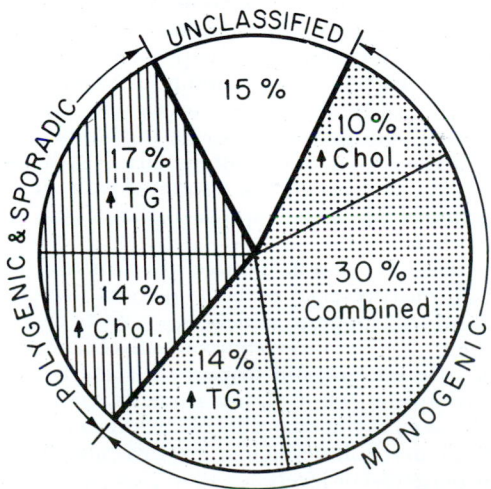

Figure 26–16. Genetic analysis of hyperlipidemia in 164 myocardial infarction survivors.

TABLE 26–9. Factors Affecting HDL Cholesterol Levels

Increase	Decrease
Estrogens	Puberty in males
Exercise	Androgens; progestogens
Leanness	Obesity
Hypotriglyceridemic drugs	Hypertriglyceridemia
Alcohol	Type II diabetes mellitus
Phenytoin	Cigarette smoking
Familial hyperalphalipoproteinemia syndromes	Familial HDL deficiency syndromes

atherosclerosis.[151] Rare genetic hyperalphalipoproteinemia syndromes (high HDL levels) are associated with increased longevity.[152] Conversely, hypoalphalipoproteinemia syndromes are usually associated with increased risk for atherosclerosis.[153] Obesity and cigarette smoking are also associated with low HDL levels (Table 26–9). These associations are specific for the less dense HDL_2 subfraction of HDL particles and also correlate closely with reduced apo AI concentrations. Very high HDL cholesterol levels have also been reported in families with lipid transfer protein deficiency.[154]

One hypothesis for the inverse correlation between HDL cholesterol (or apo AI) levels and the risk of development of coronary atherosclerosis is that HDL can remove cholesterol from arterial wall cells as the first step in reverse cholesterol transport (see Fig. 26–14). A specific receptor for HDL in extrahepatic cells, distinct from the LDL receptor,[47] appears to promote cholesterol efflux from cells and prevent intracellular cholesterol accumulation. HDL and apo AI levels also are directly linked to LPL-related triglyceride removal,[155] and therefore HDL and VLDL levels vary inversely. Patients with one of several rare deficiencies or abnormalities of HDL and/or apoAI (low-HDL syndromes such as Tangier disease) usually have premature atherosclerosis, even if LDL cholesterol levels are low.[153] The role of the inverse relationship between HDL and VLDL triglyceride (perhaps mediated by LPL) and the association of HDL with other atherosclerosis-modifying factors such as diabetes, exercise, and alcohol remain speculative.

Hypolipidemia

Although rare and usually genetically determined, hypolipidemia may be secondary to other disorders. It is usually defined by cholesterol or triglyceride levels below the fifth percentile of age- and sex-matched population norms. In patients with hyperthyroidism, advanced liver disease, intestinal malabsorption, or severe malnutrition, serum cholesterol and triglyceride levels may be very low. Familial LDL deficiency occurs in abetalipoproteinemia, a rare autosomal recessive syndrome in which patients cannot produce chylomicrons or VLDL as a result of absence of apo B48 and apo B100 (see under Production of Triglyceride from Carbohydrate). Manifestations include malnutrition, steatorrhea, ataxia, acanthocytosis, and pigmentary retinal degeneration.[156] Vitamin E has been used successfully for symptomatic therapy. In accordance with the role of LDL in providing cholesterol for synthesis of steroid hormones in the gonads and adrenal gland,[157] these patients have subnormal luteal-phase progesterone levels[158] and an impaired glucocorticoid response to corticotropin.[159] In hypobetalipoproteinemia, a distinct familial disorder, serum LDL levels are low but not zero and there are fewer clinical manifestations. Individuals homozygous for dysfunctional apo E (phenotype E2/E2) (see under Defective Remnant Removal) are also hypocholesterolemic with low LDL levels, unless an additional hyperlipidemic disorder supervenes. Individuals have been described who cannot produce apo

B100 in the liver and hence have low VLDL and LDL levels but can produce apo B48 in the intestine and consequently can absorb fat normally and make chylomicrons.[20, 160] The presence of an abnormal apo B species (apo B37) also has been associated with familial hypobetalipoproteinemia.[161]

Tangier disease, one type of familial HDL deficiency, is a rare syndrome characterized by storage of cholesteryl esters throughout the body, particularly in reticuloendothelial cells and Schwann cells, leading to orange tonsils, corneal opacities, and peripheral neuropathy.[50] There appears to be a defect in the regulation of HDL transport, and hypertriglyceridemia may be present. Less severe defects are seen in several varieties of hypoalphalipoproteinemia (low-HDL syndromes) that appear to predispose to atherosclerosis.[153] HDL levels are also low in familial LCAT deficiency, the rare disorder in which patients are unable to form cholesteryl esters in serum and accumulate free cholesterol in tissues.

Diagnosis of Hyperlipidemia

The first step in the diagnostic approach to the patient with hyperlipidemia is routine quantitative measurement of both cholesterol and triglyceride levels in plasma obtained after an overnight (10- to 15-h) fast. When values are above normal (exceed the 95th percentile matched for age and sex; see Table 26–4) and are verified at least once more, a combination of personal, dietary, drug, and family histories; a thorough examination; and laboratory tests are necessary to define the specific disorder accurately. Usually these are sufficient to implicate other diseases or drugs that cause hyperlipidemia (see Table 26–6). At a minimum, tests for thyroid and liver function, plasma glucose and protein, and urinary protein should be performed. When cholesterol or triglyceride values or both are above the 99th percentile, in the absence of another cause, the likelihood of a monogenic familial disorder is increased.

A family history of premature coronary atherosclerosis (with or without known hyperlipidemia) is important in establishing a genetic diagnosis and deciding on a therapeutic approach. Physical examination should focus on the presence of characteristic xanthomas (see Fig. 26–15), which, when present, are virtually pathognomonic of several of the genetic disorders and reflect elevated levels of a particular class of lipoproteins. Thus, tendon xanthomas are characteristic of familial hypercholesterolemia (increased LDL levels); tuberous, tuberoeruptive, and palmar crease xanthomas are typical of dysbetalipoproteinemia (increased levels of chylomicron and VLDL remnants); and eruptive xanthomas are features of LPL deficiency (increased chylomicron levels). Rarely, individuals may have tendon xanthomas without hyperlipidemia associated with compositional abnormalities in lipoproteins (e.g., in cerebrotendinous xanthomatosis or hyperbetasitosterolemia). Corneal arcus and xanthelasmas may be seen in younger patients with increased LDL levels but are less specific in older individuals. Xanthelasmas in normolipidemic subjects may be associated with the presence of a structurally abnormal apo E or increased levels of apo B.[162]

Inspection of a plasma sample after an overnight fast can indicate the presence of chylomicrons (lactescent appearance), which suggests a deficiency in triglyceride removal. When a high concentration of triglyceride-rich VLDL is present, the plasma also appears turbid. For practical purposes, completely clear plasma suggests a normal triglyceride level and rules out disorders of chylomicron and VLDL transport. Hypercholesterolemia in this situation usually reflects increased LDL levels.

Because lipoproteins carry varying amounts of triglyceride and cholesterol, the relative degree of elevation of these two lipids in whole plasma is sometimes helpful. In hyperchylomicronemia, the triglyceride/cholesterol ratio is high, 10:1 or higher. With increased VLDL levels, the ratio is somewhat lower but still high. Because cholesterol is a component of these triglyceride-rich lipoproteins, hypercholesterolemia may ensue if VLDL or chylomicron levels are high enough. With accumulation of LDL alone, the triglyceride/cholesterol ratio may be as low as 1:2 or less, and in dysbetalipoproteinemia the ratio is about 1:1. On the other hand, in combined hyperlipidemias, in which both LDL and VLDL levels may be increased in varying proportions, ratios of lipids in plasma can be misleading.

Plasma lipoprotein electrophoresis, which can be used to define a qualitatively abnormal lipoprotein pattern, is usually not necessary[163] and ordinarily is not helpful for diagnostic or therapeutic decisions. When serum measurements show only an elevated cholesterol level, there is a close correlation between serum cholesterol and LDL cholesterol levels. Occasionally, in certain individuals (usually young women or those involved in strenuous exercise), a mildly increased serum cholesterol level may be due to elevated HDL levels. These can be distinguished by precipitation methods that measure HDL cholesterol. With marked degrees of hypertriglyceridemia, electrophoretic studies are inadequate for diagnosis, because high levels of triglycerides produce a smearing effect and lipoprotein patterns merge. Furthermore, electrophoretic analysis fails to define disease or distinguish discrete genetic disorders, such as familial hypercholesterolemia, from familial combined hyperlipidemia. In some situations, ultracentrifugation of plasma (and/or isoelectric focusing of apoproteins) will lead to an answer (as in the definition of dysbetalipoproteinemia); in others, more detailed family studies, including measurement of fasting cholesterol and triglyceride levels among first-degree relatives, are most helpful. Familial hypercholesterolemia in affected children can be detected in cord blood samples. Aside from that disorder, familial LPL deficiency, and familial LCAT deficiency, other familial forms of hyperlipidemia are not detectable before puberty.

Much interest has been generated in the measurement of HDL cholesterol levels, because low HDL levels have been associated with increased risk of myocardial infarction in population studies. The value of HDL cholesterol measurements for predicting the occurrence of myocardial infarction in an individual patient has not been established, however. The analytical error of HDL measurements in some laboratories exceeds the differences in HDL levels associated with risk. Measurements of HDL are most helpful for estimation of LDL cholesterol.[164] Because of the inverse relationship between plasma triglyceride (or VLDL) and HDL levels, measurement of HDL cholesterol in most hypertriglyceridemic patients, with or without hypercholesterolemia, gives little additional useful information because HDL cholesterol levels are predictably low. HDL cholesterol levels are difficult to interpret in the presence of even modest increases of plasma triglyceride levels. Drugs that raise plasma triglyceride levels (e.g., thiazides, beta-adrenergic blocking agents) lower HDL cholesterol levels, and those that reduce triglyceride levels (e.g., clofibrate, gemfibrozil, niacin) usually raise HDL cholesterol levels (see Table 26–9).

An estimate of LDL concentration can be simply obtained from measurements of serum cholesterol and triglycerides coupled with an independent measurement of HDL cholesterol. This estimate (serum cholesterol minus serum triglycerides/5 minus HDL cholesterol, all in milligrams per deciliter) correlates closely with LDL cholesterol measured directly by ultracentrifugation.[164] It is a reliable approximation for patients with triglyceride levels below about 4.5

mmol/L (400 mg/dL) but cannot be used for those with dysbetalipoproteinemia whose VLDL triglyceride/cholesterol ratio is much less than the normal value of about 5:1.

Thus from inspection of a fasting plasma sample, measurement of cholesterol and triglyceride levels, and measurement of HDL cholesterol, an approximate assessment of lipoprotein levels can be made. A specific lipoprotein disorder can often be diagnosed from a consideration of the history, laboratory tests that differentiate primary and secondary hyperlipidemias, and examination of any xanthomas present. When special tests are indicated (e.g., quantification of lipoproteins after ultracentrifugation of plasma or measurements of postheparin plasma LPL; apolipoproteins CII, B, or AI; isoforms of apo E; LP(a); lipid transfer protein; or LCAT), referral to a lipid clinic is in order.

Therapy of Hyperlipidemia

Before a therapeutic program for hyperlipidemia is undertaken, the possible underlying secondary causes should be thoroughly investigated because some occur frequently (see Table 26–6). Treatment is usually a matter of withdrawal of inciting pharmacological agents or therapy of the underlying illness. When underlying causes cannot be elucidated, it must be assumed that the disorder is primary, either familial or sporadic. Although diet and drugs are the mainstays of treatment for hyperlipidemia, therapy must be aimed at the pathophysiology associated with the disorder rather than at a particular lipoprotein pattern, which often is nonspecific.

Goals of therapy are directed either at prevention of life-threatening episodes of acute pancreatitis (chylomicronemia syndrome) or reduction of risk for atherosclerosis (see later). In deciding whom to treat, how vigorously, and by what modalities, consideration should be given to the patient's past dietary history, prior bouts of acute abdominal pain, family history of hyperlipidemia, presence of xanthomas or early atherosclerosis, age, and presence of other diseases. Treatment is usually lifelong, and a decision to intervene with drugs (or surgery) must be considered carefully and reserved for those at high risk for development of accelerated atherosclerosis. In addition to chylomicronemia syndrome, which must be treated vigorously, individuals who are younger, have a positive family history, or have associated risk factors for atherosclerosis, such as diabetes or hypertension, generally are candidates for treatment of hyperlipidemia.

With hypertriglyceridemia, regardless of cause, fasting plasma triglyceride levels above about 11 mmol/L (1000 mg/dL) are associated with a high risk for the development of pancreatitis and the chylomicronemia syndrome. Because these untoward consequences are potentially fatal and repeated triglyceride measurements vary widely when levels above 5.8 mmol/L (500 mg/dL) are reached, such levels usually indicate a need for lipid-lowering management, at least by dietary means.

Individuals with fasting plasma triglyceride levels between 2.9 and 5.8 mmol/L (250 and 500 mg/dL) present a different problem, because in the aggregate such levels are associated with a twofold excessive risk of cardiovascular disease.[165] About 5% of U.S. men above age 30 have levels exceeding 2.9 mmol/L (250 mg/dL) (see Table 26–5). In an individual patient these levels may be normal, may reflect lifestyle influences (obesity, cigarette smoking), or may be a marker for an underlying genetic form of hyperlipidemia that might be associated with an increased risk of accelerated atherosclerosis and require some form of therapy. Therefore, if such a patient has a positive family history of hyperlipidemia or premature cardiovascular disease (e.g., myocardial infarction in a first-degree male relative before age 50 or female relative before age 60) or coexistent hypercholesterolemia, further investigation is indicated to define the nature of the disorder before institution of appropriate therapy. Other than the promotion of lifestyle changes, the majority of patients with triglyceride levels within this range do not require a specific form of therapy.

Plasma cholesterol levels above about 6.2 mmol/L (240 mg/dL) (corresponding to an LDL cholesterol level of 4.1 mmol/L [160 mg/dL]) are also associated with a high risk of cardiovascular disease. When coupled with other risk factors (Table 26–10) or when cardiovascular disease is already present, total cholesterol levels above 5.2 mmol/L (200 mg/dL) (LDL cholesterol > 3.4 mmol/L [>130 mg/dL]) also confer high risk. These observations form the basis for the recommendations of the National Cholesterol Education Program (Table 26–11).[54] Most of these individuals in the high-risk range have polygenic hypercholesterolemia, and dietary modification is generally sufficient to lower cholesterol levels. More intensive therapy, beginning with a dietary approach, is usually advised for patients found to have hypercholesterolemia on the basis of one of the familial disorders.

DIET. Dietary intervention alone can be effective in lowering blood lipid levels in many individuals with hyperlipidemia and should be the first approach to therapy. Some genetic disorders, such as familial hypercholesterolemia, respond minimally; optimal diet alone rarely achieves more than a 20% reduction in cholesterol levels. Nevertheless, in all primary familial or sporadic disorders, dietary therapy should always be attempted initially. Only when the hyperlipidemia proves refractory and the patient remains at high risk for the development of atherosclerosis should pharmacological agents be considered.

LPL deficiency, in which hypertriglyceridemia is aggravated by dietary fat, is best handled by stringent restriction of fat intake to reduce chylomicron input and optional substitution of medium chain triglycerides. The rationale for this substitution is that medium chain triglycerides, in contrast to long chain triglycerides, are absorbed directly via the portal vein, bypassing chylomicron formation and transport through intestinal lymphatics. Dietary adherence is critical because none of the available drugs is effective in this disorder, although clofibrate, gemfibrozil, or niacin, by lowering VLDL levels, can help prevent frequent episodes of life-threatening severe chylomicronemia and acute pancreatitis.[67] Fish oils rich in omega-3 fatty acids can also be used because they effectively lower VLDL levels (see later).[166] When severe insulin deficiency is the cause of LPL deficiency, the patient should be vigorously treated with insulin. In hypertriglyceridemia associated with impaired LPL activity in conjunction with hyperglycemia, insulin is effective in correcting the disorder.[167]

TABLE 26–10. Risk Factors for Atherosclerosis

Male sex
Family history of premature coronary artery disease (before age 55 in a parent or sibling)
Cigarette smoking (currently smoking more than 10 cigarettes per day)
Hypertension
Low HDL cholesterol (below 0.9 mmol/L [35 mg/dL])
Diabetes mellitus
Personal history of cerebrovascular disease or occlusive peripheral vascular disease
Severe obesity (>30% overweight)

Most other types of hyperlipidemia respond to a basic diet that is low in cholesterol and saturated fat. Because obesity aggravates many hyperlipidemias by promoting production of VLDL, the diet should be hypocaloric until the patient achieves ideal body weight. Such a diet most likely will contain a high proportion of carbohydrate (more than 50% of total calories), but in most instances this is of little concern, even in patients with hypertriglyceridemia. Although basal triglyceride levels are highest with high-carbohydrate diets, this occurs only transiently during periods of a few weeks of adaptation. The 24-h patterns of triglyceride levels in patients with hypertriglyceridemia after a period of adaptation[168] are actually lower with higher-carbohydrate diets than with diets higher in fat. If control of hypertriglyceridemia is meant to reduce levels throughout the day, as in diabetic therapy, a calorie-restricted, relatively low-fat, high-carbohydrate diet would be desirable for the control of the hypertriglyceridemias. Even for lowering overnight fasting triglyceride levels, a low-fat diet may be more effective than a low-carbohydrate diet for long-term management.[169]

Thus a disproportionate restriction of carbohydrates in the diet of these patients is not usually justified. Alcohol, which may increase triglyceride production by altering the caloric balance and directly stimulating hepatic syntheses, should be discouraged in patients with any disorder in the transport of VLDL. Dietary management will be ineffective unless drugs such as estrogens, glucocorticoids, thiazide diuretics, or beta-adrenergic blockers, which aggravate many forms of hypertriglyceridemia, can be withdrawn or the dosage lowered.

In patients with hypercholesterolemia, particular emphasis must be placed on lowering the intake of cholesterol-containing foods[170] (Table 26–12). Decreasing the cholesterol intake of the average American from 400 to 700 mg/d to less than 300 mg/d is an essential step in therapy, because dietary cholesterol will accumulate beyond the body's ability to compensate by reducing the amount synthesized and increasing the amount secreted, thus leading to an increase in plasma cholesterol level (Fig. 26–17). Furthermore, cho-

TABLE 26–11. Guideline for Treatment of High Blood Cholesterol (C) Levels in Adults

Decision	Basis	Cholesterol, mmol/L (mg/dL)		
		Desirable	*Borderline High*	*High*
Screening	All patients			
LDL estimation	High total C	<5.2 (<200)	5.2–6.2 (200–239)*	≥6.2 (≥240)
Treatment				
Diet	High LDL C	<3.4 (<130)	3.4–4.1 (130–159)*	≥4.1 (≥160)
Drug†	High LDL C	—	—	≥4.9 (≥190) or ≥4.1 (≥160)*

*Becomes high risk if definite coronary heart disease or two or more risk factors (Table 26–10) are present.
†After a trial of diet alone.
Data from Report of the National Cholesterol Education Program; Expert Panel on Detection, Evaluation, and Treatment of High Blood Cholesterol in Adults. Arch Intern Med 1988; 148:36–69.

TABLE 26–12. Cholesterol and Saturated Fat Content in Some Common Foods

Food	Cholesterol (mg/100 g)	Saturated Fat (g/100 g)
Eggs	500	3
Organ meats (liver, kidney)	>300	2
Butter	230	50
Shrimp, crab, lobster	110	1
Cheese	110	21
Meat (beef, pork, lamb)	90–100	5–13
Poultry (no skin)	90	1
Fish	70	1
Ice cream (10% fat)	40	7
Sherbet; frozen yogurt	4	<1
Milk, whole (3.5% fat)	14	2
Milk, skim	2	0
Cottage cheese	6	<1
Margarine, soft	0	16
Vegetable oil	0	13
Coconut oil, cocoa butter	0	75

Adapted from Connor WE, Connor SL. The dietary treatment of hyperlipidemia. Med Clin North Am 1982; 66:485–518.

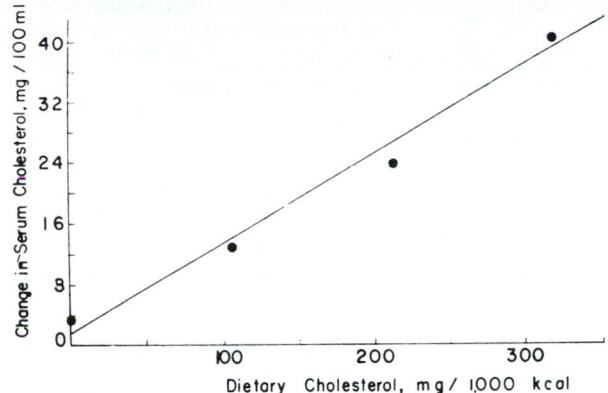

Figure 26–17. Relation between cholesterol intake and change in serum cholesterol after 21 d on a cholesterol-free formula diet of constant fatty acid composition. (Adapted from Mattson FH, Erickson BA, Kligman AM. Effect of dietary cholesterol on serum cholesterol in man. Am J Clin Nutr 1972; 25:589–594. © Am J Clin Nutr. American Society for Clinical Nutrition.)

lesterol feeding has been reported to increase LDL synthesis and reduce receptor-mediated LDL catabolism.[171] Saturated fat intake should also be curtailed to less than 10% of total calories,[54] because saturated fatty acids appear to raise serum cholesterol levels, primarily by decreasing receptor-mediated LDL clearance.[172, 173] Cholesterol and saturated fat usually occur in many of the same foods, however, so they are restricted by similar dietary regimens. Because they have such a high risk of developing premature atherosclerosis, children of patients with familial hypercholesterolemia should be screened in infancy and childhood, and appropriate management should be instituted as early in life as possible, although improvement in outcome has not yet been proved. Dietary management can reduce cholesterol levels during the first year of life in infants with familial hypercholesterolemia.[174]

The value of substituting polyunsaturated fat for saturated fat in diets for patients with hypercholesterolemia is debatable. A diet high in polyunsaturated fats appears to be less efficient in lowering cholesterol levels than restriction of cholesterol and saturated fats without the substitution. Furthermore, the long-term effects of diets containing highly unsaturated fats are unknown.[175] A highly polyunsaturated fat containing long chain fatty acids of the omega-3 series, such as eicosapentaenoic acid (found in large amounts in certain fish oils such as salmon or mackerel), in contrast to the fatty acids of the omega-6 series, such as linoleic acid (found in vegetable oil), markedly lowers VLDL levels in normal subjects and has been associated with the very low lipid levels and diminished incidence of atherosclerosis in populations that subsist on high-fish diets.[166] The role of these highly polyunsaturated marine fats in the management of various hyperlipidemic states is controversial. Although VLDL levels are consistently lowered, many patients with hypertriglyceridemia respond to fish oil with increased LDL levels.[176] LDL cholesterol and apo B levels are not lowered in individuals with familial combined hyperlipidemia;[177] conversely, LDL and apo B levels decrease in patients with

familial hypercholesterolemia.[178] Fish oil supplementation worsens glucose control in patients with type II diabetes mellitus.[179] High dietary intake of omega-3 fatty acids can also prolong bleeding time in conjunction with altered prostaglandin synthesis.[165] Current recommendations of the American Heart Association for the population at large[180] limit intake of polyunsaturated fats to no more than 10% of total calories. Increase of the ratio of polyunsaturated to saturated fat to about 1.0 from the usual value of about 0.3 is achieved mainly by reduction of saturated fat intake. Reduction of the proportion of fat calories to 30 to 35% of the total calories requires a reciprocal increase in the proportion of carbohydrate calories to 50% or more. This diet is also the recommended first phase in the management of all hyperlipidemic states. Additional steps are a progressive reduction in total fat, saturated fat, and cholesterol and, when obesity is present, caloric restriction (Table 26–13).

Thus there is a *single basic diet* for all the common forms of hyperlipidemia. This low-calorie, low-saturated-fat, low-cholesterol diet is appropriate for patients with hyperlipidemia and is prudent for the population at large. In practice, it translates into limitation of animal fats and emphasis on vegetable oils, fish, and carbohydrates. It carries little known risk in adults and is effective in lowering the levels of both cholesterol- and triglyceride-rich lipoproteins. It should be individualized to fit the particular lipid disorder of the patient; for example, special attention should be paid to dietary fat and cholesterol restriction for patients with familial hypercholesterolemia (to as little as 20 to 25% fat calories and 200 to 150 mg cholesterol) and to alcohol and calorie restriction for those with hypertriglyceridemia and elevated VLDL levels. The role of various dietary fibers is being evaluated. Addition of soluble fibers such as psyllium and oat bran to the diet can lower LDL cholesterol levels by about 10%.[181] Increasing physical activity is a useful adjunct to the dietary management of many hyperlipidemic states.[182]

DRUGS. When dietary management is ineffective, phar-

TABLE 26–13. Basic Diet for Treatment of the Hyperlipidemias

Step	Total Fat (% calories)	Saturated Fatty Acids (% calories)	Polyunsaturated Fatty Acids (% calories)	Monounsaturated Fatty Acids (% calories)	Cholesterol (mg/d)
1	<30	<10	<10	10–15	<300
2	<30	<7	<10	10–15	<200

Data from AHA Recommendations for Treatment of Hyperlipidemia in Adults. Circulation 1985; 69:1065–1090a; and from Report of the National Cholesterol Education Program. Expert Panel on Detection, Evaluation, and Treatment of High Blood Cholesterol in Adults. Arch Intern Med 1988; 148:36–69.

A. Elevated triglyceride-rich lipoproteins
   1. Fibric acid derivatives (clofibrate, gemfibrozil)
   2. Niacin
B. Elevated cholesterol-rich lipoproteins
   1. Bile acid–binding resins (cholestyramine, colestipol)
   2. Niacin
   3. HMG-CoA reductase inhibitors (lovastatin)
C. Both types of lipoproteins increased
   1. Niacin
   2. Drug combinations (A plus B)

macological agents may be added to the therapeutic regimen. Drugs often must be added for the management of patients with monogenic forms of hyperlipoproteinemia (Table 26–14), particularly those with familial hypercholesterolemia, familial combined hyperlipidemia, and/or a positive family history of early atherosclerosis or prior episodes of acute pancreatitis. There is no evidence to support the use of lipid-lowering drugs for the prevention of atherosclerosis in the general population.[183] Drug therapy is recommended for patients whose LDL cholesterol level remains above 4.9 mmol/L (190 mg/dL) (or above 4.1 mmol/L [>160 mg/dL] in the presence of other risk factors) after a trial of diet therapy (see Table 26–11) or whose triglyceride levels remain above 5.8 mmol/L (500 mg/dL).[184]

Drugs that act by reducing hepatic VLDL triglyceride production (e.g., clofibrate, gemfibrozil, niacin) are effective in treating several forms of hypertriglyceridemia (Table 26–15). Clofibrate appears to act both by enhancing LPL-mediated clearance of triglyceride-rich lipoproteins and by reducing hepatic lipid and VLDL synthesis.[185] Clofibrate is effective in preventing recurrent bouts of abdominal pain in many patients with chylomicronemia syndrome.[67] It is also useful in the therapy of dysbetalipoproteinemia,[77, 186] in which it markedly lowers triglyceride and cholesterol levels in conjunction with reducing β-VLDL levels. Such therapy induces regression of xanthomas, improves peripheral blood flow, and reduces symptoms (intermittent claudication and angina pectoris). Gemfibrozil, another fibric acid derivative, has similar effects on lipid transport. These drugs raise HDL cholesterol and apo AI levels. Niacin probably acts primarily by inhibiting VLDL production, secondarily by lowering LDL levels.[187] It is of interest that the amide of niacin (niacinamide) can substitute for the vitamin but does not possess the lipid-lowering properties of niacin. As a result of decreased HDL catabolism, niacin also raises HDL cholesterol and apo AI levels.[188] Its role as a potent inhibitor of adipose tissue hormone-sensitive lipase in reducing fatty acid mobilization and consequently lowering VLDL triglyceride levels remains speculative.

By directly diverting cholesterol and bile acids from the intestine to the feces, bile acid–binding resins, such as cholestyramine and colestipol, enhance cholesterol excretion, reduce body cholesterol pools, reduce enterohepatic recycling, and increase hepatic LDL (apo B100–apo E) receptor activity and thus receptor-mediated catabolism[189] (see under Circulation of Cholesterol Between Liver and Peripheral Tissues). Consequently, these agents are useful in lowering plasma cholesterol levels in patients with hypercholesterolemia associated with increased LDL levels. Although dextrothyroxine reduces both plasma cholesterol and triglyceride levels by 10 to 15%, presumably by stimulating removal processes more than synthesis, it was withdrawn from a large, secondary drug prevention trial because of higher incidences of mortality and morbidity among male patients with coronary heart disease treated with the drug.[190] It is likely that the lipid-lowering action of thyroid hormone and its analogues is not separable from the stimulating effect on tissue oxygen consumption. Estrogens in high doses were also withdrawn from this trial because of adverse effects on mortality. However, in lower doses, estrogens appear to be effective in lowering LDL levels of postmenopausal women with hypercholesterolemia[127] and are uniquely effective in lowering chylomicron and VLDL remnant levels in familial dysbetalipoproteinemia. However, in that disorder, use of estrogen remains experimental because of its tendency to provoke atherosclerotic and thrombotic complications; its use should be restricted to selected women who fail to respond to diet and a fibric acid derivative. Probucol, an antioxidant that also lowers LDL levels modestly, is used in the treatment of hypercholesterolemia; however, in contrast to bile acid binders, it lowers HDL cholesterol as well. Its role in therapy is uncertain. It prevents LDL oxidation in vitro and atherosclerosis in hypercholesterolemic, LDL receptor–deficient rabbits.[191, 192] However, no long-term trials in humans have been reported.

Thus a bile acid–binding resin (colestipol or cholestyramine) is the treatment of choice for patients with familial hypercholesterolemia, and a fibric acid derivative (clofibrate or gemfibrozil) or niacin is appropriate for patients with hypertriglyceridemia at high risk (see Table 26–14). Combined therapy with a resin and niacin has resulted in return of LDL cholesterol levels to normal in patients with heterozygous familial hypercholesterolemia, even when plasma cholesterol levels initially exceeded 10.4 mmol/L (400 mg/dL).[193, 194] The effect of this and other combined drug approaches on regression (or interruption of progression) of atherosclerotic lesions and its use in the treatment of familial combined hyperlipidemia are being evaluated.

One therapeutic approach to reduction of LDL levels aims at increasing LDL receptor activity and thereby enhancing LDL receptor–mediated catabolism. Drugs, such as

TABLE 26–15. Drugs Available for Treatment of the Hyperlipidemias

Class of Drug	Drugs Available	Major Lipoprotein Decreased	Mechanism	Usual Daily Dose	Common Side Effects
Fibric acid derivatives	Clofibrate Gemfibrozil	VLDL (LDL)	Decreases VLDL synthesis; enhances LPL action	2 g 1–2 g	Gallstones; myopathy
Niacin (nicotinic acid)	Niacin	VLDL (LDL)	Decreases VLDL synthesis	3–7 g	Pruritus; flushing; hyperglycemia; hepatic dysfunction
Bile acid–binding resins	Cholestyramine Colestipol	LDL	Promotes sterol excretion; increases LDL receptor-mediated removal	16–24 g 15–20 g	Gastrointestinal symptoms
Nonabsorbable sterol binders	Neomycin Sitosterol	LDL	Promotes sterol excretion	1–2 g 3–6 g	Gastrointestinal symptoms
Probucol	Probucol	LDL	Unknown	1 g	Diarrhea; lower HDL
Steroids	Norethindrone Oxandrolone	Chylomicrons (VLDL)	Enhances LPL action	5 mg 5 mg	Fluid retention; hypertension; hirsutism
HMG-CoA reductase inhibitors	Lovastatin	LDL	Blocks cholesterol synthesis; increases LDL receptor-mediated removal	20–40 mg	Gastrointestinal symptoms; myopathy

lovastatin, that block cholesterol synthesis by inhibiting the rate-limiting enzyme in cholesterol biosynthesis, HMG-CoA reductase, decrease LDL cholesterol and apo B levels in patients with heterozygous familial hypercholesterolemia[195] and with polygenic hypercholesterolemia.[196] Cellular LDL receptor activity increases as a counterregulatory response, resulting in accelerated hepatic LDL clearance and lower plasma LDL cholesterol levels.[197] Combined therapy with a bile acid–binding resin is particularly effective.[198]

Side effects of these lipid-lowering agents need to be considered, particularly because they are needed for long-term use in the primary hyperlipidemias. Clofibrate and gemfibrozil in usual adult doses are associated with an increased incidence of gallstones. In patients with impaired ability to metabolize the drugs, such as those with uremia or hepatic disease, these drugs may cause an acute myopathy associated with increased serum creatine levels; in such instances, doses should be drastically reduced to 1.0 to 1.5 g/wk.[199] Clofibrate potentiates the action of warfarin, necessitating a reduction of the anticoagulant dosage. In some patients reduction of VLDL levels is associated with an increase in LDL levels. Niacin is associated with severe flushing; this can be minimized by the use of small doses of aspirin and by a gradual increase in dose (no more than 2 g/d/mo) from an initial dose of 100 mg three times daily with meals to a total daily dose of 3 to 7 g in four divided doses. Because of its potential to promote hyperglycemia, to impair hepatic function, and to activate peptic ulcers, the drug should not be given to patients with diabetes mellitus or with liver or peptic ulcer disease. Bile acid–binding agents are constipating, and while lowering serum cholesterol levels they may actually increase VLDL synthesis and aggravate hypertriglyceridemia in some patients; this effect may be transient, however, and can be ameliorated by the addition of one of the drugs that interfere with VLDL triglyceride synthesis.

SURGERY AND OTHER PROCEDURES. Partial ileal bypass operations have been performed on patients with hypercholesterolemia after myocardial infarction.[200] This experimental procedure results in increased excretion of cholesterol degradation products in the stool, lowering of LDL cholesterol levels, and reduction of morbidity from coronary heart disease. A lowering of LDL and cholesterol levels has been obtained in some, but not all, young patients with the rare and severe homozygous form of familial hypercholesterolemia after portacaval shunt procedures.[201] Its mechanism remains unknown, but it appears to result in a net efflux of accumulated tissue cholesterol and a striking reduction of xanthoma size.[202] A remarkable lowering of LDL levels in a patient with homozygous hypercholesterolemia has been achieved after successful liver transplantation.[41]

Plasmapheresis can be used as an alternative therapeutic approach to severe familial hypercholesterolemia.[203] Repeated plasmapheresis about three times monthly will maintain LDL cholesterol levels within or near the normal range. Because this procedure also drains HDL as well as other phasma constituents, specific LDL-pheresis has been explored in which LDL is immunoabsorbed by exposure of plasma to solid-phase LDL antibody;[204] marked reduction of LDL levels and xanthoma size has been reported.[205]

Rationale for Therapy

The association between hypercholesterolemia, hypertriglyceridemia, and atherosclerotic disease in persons with and without hyperglycemia has been amply confirmed in a variety of population studies. Although various factors have

thus far been implicated, the mechanisms that account for this relationship are yet to be completely elucidated.

The rationale for treating symptomatic hyperlipidemia is obvious. Prevention of the potentially fatal complication of acute pancreatitis is an absolute indication for treatment of marked hypertriglyceridemia with chylomicronemia. Treatment of asymptomatic disorders is based on the "lipid hypothesis"—that lowering lipid levels will decrease morbidity and mortality from associated atherosclerosis. Results of the large clofibrate trial under the auspices of the World Health Organization in a normal population[206] provided evidence favoring the lipid hypothesis. Cholesterol lowering (and presumably triglyceride lowering) was associated with a reduced incidence of nonfatal myocardial infarctions. The increase in total mortality in that study remains unsettling, however, and its relevance to the management of specific hyperlipidemic states is unknown. Niacin given to patients without regard to the presence of hyperlipidemia reduced the incidence of myocardial infarctions in the coronary drug trial. Several reports[207, 208] suggest that lipid-lowering therapy that causes a decrease in LDL and an increase in HDL levels inhibits progression of pre-existing coronary or femoral atherosclerosis studied angiographically. The most convincing evidence to date favoring lipid-lowering therapy for high-risk patients to prevent morbidity and mortality from atherosclerotic disease has emerged from the multicenter Lipid Research Clinics trial.[209] By using both diet and drug (cholestyramine) to reduce plasma cholesterol levels for at least 5 y in asymptomatic hypercholesterolemic middle-aged men, it has been shown that sustained reduction of LDL levels decreases morbidity and mortality from atherosclerosis, the degree of decrease being proportional to the degree of LDL reduction. Bile acid–binding resins (with niacin and diet therapy) also decrease progression and even induce regression of existing coronary lesions (determined by angiography) in conjunction with lipid lowering in patients who have had coronary artery bypass graft surgery.[210] A fibric acid drug, gemfibrozil, has been shown in Helsinki to reduce mortality from coronary heart disease in association with lowered triglyceride and cholesterol and raised HDL cholesterol levels in a hypertriglyceridemic subgroup of hyperlipidemic patients.[211] Use of calestipol together with lovastatin or niacin decreased progression and induced regression of coronary artery lesions in men with high levels of apo B and a familial history of premature atherosclerosis.[212] Further definition of candidates for lipid-lowering drugs must await the results of additional studies that are needed to define the long-term efficacy and safety of lipid-lowering agents and develop procedures for identifying additional subsets of individuals at risk (e.g., women, younger men, the elderly, those with specific familial disorders) who should be treated by lipid-lowering management for the prevention of atherosclerosis and its sequelae.

REFERENCES

1. Cahill GF Jr. Starvation in man. N Engl J Med 1970; 282:668–675.
2. Carey MC, Small DM, Bliss CM. Lipid digestion and absorption. Annu Rev Physiol 1983; 45:651–677.
3. Bisgaier CL, Glickman RM. Intestinal synthesis, secretion, and transport of lipoproteins. Annu Rev Physiol 1983; 45:625–636.
4. Kane JP. Apolipoprotein B: structural and metabolic heterogeneity. Annu Rev Physiol 1983; 45:637–650.
5. Kane JP, Havel RJ. Disorders of the biogenesis and secretion of lipoproteins containing the B-apolipoproteins. In: Scriver CR, Beaudet AL, Sly WS, et al., eds. The Metabolic Basis of Inherited Disease. 6th ed. New York: McGraw-Hill, 1989: 1139–1164.
6. Breckenridge WC, Little JA, Steiner G, et al. Hypertriglyceridemia associated with deficiency of apolipoprotein C-II. N Engl J Med 1978; 298:1265–1273.
7. Brunzell JD. Familial lipoprotein lipase deficiency and other causes of the chylomicronemia syndrome. In: Scriver CR, Beaudet AL, Sly WS,

et al., eds. The Metabolic Basis of Inherited Disease. 6th ed. New York: McGraw-Hill, 1989; 1165–1180.

8. Nilsson-Ehle P, Garfinkel AS, Schotz MC. Lipolytic enzymes and plasma lipoprotein metabolism. Annu Rev Biochem 1980; 49:667–693.

9. Fielding PE, Shore VG, Fielding CJ. Lipoprotein lipase. Isolation and characterization of a second enzyme species from postheparin plasma. Biochemistry 1977; 16:1896–1900.

10. Kuwajima M, Foster DW, McGarry JD. Regulation of lipoprotein lipase in different rat tissues. Metabolism 1988; 37:597–601.

11. Needleman P, Turk J, Jakschik BA, et al. Arachidonic acid metabolism. Annu Rev Biochem 1986; 55:69–102.

12. Neuringer M, Anderson GJ, Connor WE. The essentiality of N-3 fatty acids for the development and function of the retina and brain. Annu Rev Nutr 1988; 8:517–541.

13. Crawford MA, Hassam AG, Stevens PA. Essential fatty acid requirements in pregnancy and lactation with special reference to brain development. Prog Lipid Res 1982; 20:31–40.

14. Reed LJ, Yeaman SJ. Pyruvate dehydrogenase. In: Boyer PD, Krebs EG, eds. The Enzymes. Vol XVIII. Control by Phosphorylation. 3rd ed. San Diego: Academic, 1987: 77–95.

15. Brownsey RW, Denton RM. Acetyl–coenzyme A carboxylase. In: Boyer PD, Krebs EG, eds. The Enzymes. Vol XVIII. Control by Phosphorylation. 3rd ed. San Diego: Academic, 1987: 123–146.

16. Witters LA, Watts TD, Daniels DL, et al.: Insulin stimulates the dephosphorylation and activation of acetyl-CoA carboxylase. Proc Natl Acad Sci USA 1988; 85:5473–5477.

17. Wakil SJ, Stoops JK, Joshi VC. Fatty acid synthesis and its regulation. Annu Rev Biochem 1983; 42:537–579.

18. Duerden JM, Gibbons GF. Secretion and storage of newly synthesized hepatic triacylglycerol fatty acids in vivo in different nutritional states and in diabetes. Biochem J 1988; 255:929–935.

19. Kane JP, Sata T, Hamilton RL, et al. Apolipoprotein composition of very low density lipoproteins of human serum. J Clin Invest 1975; 56:1622–1634.

20. Malloy MJ, Kane JP, Hardman DA, et al. Normotriglyceridemic abetalipoproteinemia. Absence of the B-100 apolipoprotein. J Clin Invest 1981; 67:1441–1450.

21. Strålfors P, Olsson H, Belfrage P. Hormone-sensitive lipase. In: Boyer PD, Krebs EG, eds., The Enzymes. Vol XVIII. Control by Phosphorylation. 3rd ed. San Diego: Academic, 1987: 147–177.

22. Demel RA, de Kruyff B. The function of sterols in membranes. Biochim Biophys Acta 1976; 457:109–132.

23. Grundy SM. Cholesterol metabolism in man. West J Med 1978; 128:13–25.

24. Helgerud P, Saarem K, Norum KR. Acyl-CoA:cholesterol acyltransferase in human small intestine: its activity and some properties of the enzymic reaction. J Lipid Res 1981; 22:271–277.

25. Mahley RW, Innerarity TL. Lipoprotein receptors and cholesterol homeostasis. Biochim Biophys Acta 1983; 737:197–222.

26. Assman G, Fredrickson DS. Acid lipase deficiency: Wolman's disease and cholesteryl ester storage disease. In: Scriver CR, Beaudet AL, Sly WS, et al., eds. The Metabolic Basis of Inherited Disease. 6th ed. New York: McGraw-Hill, 1989: 1626–1644.

27. Nervi FO, Dietschy JM. Ability of six different lipoprotein fractions to regulate the rate of hepatic cholesterogenesis in vivo. J Biol Chem 1975; 250:8704–8711.

28. Sherrill BC, Dietschy JM. Characterization of the sinusoidal transport process responsible for uptake of chylomicrons by the liver. J Biol Chem 1978; 253:1859–1867.

29. Nakanishi M, Goldstein JL, Brown MS. Multivalent control of 3-hydroxy-3-methylglutaryl coenzyme A reductase. J Biol Chem 1988; 263:8929–8937.

30. Beg ZH, Stonik JA, Brewer HB. Modulation of the enzymic activity of 3-hydroxy-3-methylglutaryl coenzyme A reductase by multiple kinase systems involving reversible phosphorylation: a review. Metabolism 1987; 36:900–917.

31. Easom RA, Zammit VA. Acute effects of starvation and treatment of rats with anti-insulin serum, glucagon and catecholamines on the state of phosphorylation of hepatic 3-hydroxy-3-methyglutaryl-CoA reductase in vivo. Biochem J 1987; 241:183–188.

32. Björkhem I. Mechanism of bile acid biosynthesis in mammalian liver (review). In: Danielsson H, Sjovall J, eds. Comprehensive Biochemistry. Amsterdam: Elsevier, 1985: 231–278.

33. Bennion LJ, Grundy SM. Risk factors for the development of cholelithiasis in man. N Engl J Med 1978; 299:1161–1167, 1221–1227.

34. Myant NB, Mitropoulos KA. Cholesterol 7 alpha-hydroxylase. J Lipid Res 1977; 18:135–153.

35. Brown MS, Goldstein JL. Lipoprotein receptors in the liver. Control signals for plasma cholesterol traffic. J Clin Invest 1983; 72:743–747.

36. Zilversmit DB, Morton RE, Hughes LB, et al. Exchange of retinyl and cholesteryl esters between lipoproteins of rabbit plasma. Biochim Biophys Acta 1982; 712:88–93.

37. Norum KR, Gjone E, Glomset JA. Familial lecithin:cholesterol acyltransferase deficiency and related disorders. In: Scriver CR, Beaudet AL, Sly WS, et al., eds. The Metabolic Basis of Inherited Disease. 6th ed. New York: McGraw-Hill, 1989: 1181–1194.

38. Auwerx JH, Marzetta CA, Hokanson JE, et al. Large buoyant LDL-like particles in hepatic lipase deficiency. Arteriosclerosis 1989; 9:1–7.

39. Goldstein JL, Kita T, Brown MS. Defective lipoprotein receptors and atherosclerosis. N Engl J Med 1983; 309:288–296.

40. Goldstein JL, Brown MS. The low-density lipoprotein pathway and its relation to atherosclerosis. Annu Rev Biochem 1977; 46:897–930.

41. Goldstein JL, Brown MS. Familial hypercholesterolemia. In: Scriver CR, Beaudet AL, Sly WS, et al., eds. The Metabolic Basis of Inherited Disease. 6th ed. New York: McGraw-Hil, 1989: 1215–1250.

42. Chait A, Ross R, Albers JJ, et al. Platelet-derived growth factor stimulates activity of low density lipoprotein receptors. Proc Natl Acad Sci USA 1980; 77:4084–4088.

43. Kovanen PT, Goldstein JL, Chappell DA, et al. Regulation of low density lipoprotein receptors by adrenocorticotropin in the adrenal gland of mice and rats in vivo. J Biol Chem 1980; 255:5591–5598.

44. Hwang J, Jairam Menon KM. Characterization of low density and high density lipoprotein receptors in the rat corpus luteum and regulation by gonadotropin. J Biol Chem 1983; 258:8020–8027.

45. Andersen JM, Dietschy JM. Regulation of sterol synthesis in 15 tissues of rat. II. Role of rat and human high and low density lipoproteins and of rat chylomicron remnants. J Biol Chem 1977; 252:3652–3659.

46. Brown MS, Goldstein JL. Lipoprotein metabolism in the macrophage: implications for cholesterol deposition in atherosclerosis. Annu Rev Biochem 1983; 52:223–261.

47. Oram JF, Brinton EA, Bierman EL. Regulation of high density lipoprotein receptor activity in cultured human skin fibroblasts and human arterial smooth muscle cells. J Clin Invest 1983; 72:1611–1621.

48. Albers JJ, Tollefson JH, Chen CH, et al. Isolation and characterization of human plasma lipid transfer proteins. Arteriosclerosis 1984; 4:49–58.

49. Assman G, Schmitz G, Brewer HB Jr. Familial high density lipoprotein deficiency: Tangier disease. In: Scriver CR, Beaudet AL, Sly WS, et al., eds. The Metabolic Basis of Inherited Disease. 6th ed. New York: McGraw-Hill, 1989: 1267–1282.

50. Schaefer EJ, Kay LL, Zech LA, et al. Tangier disease: High density lipoprotein deficiency due to defective metabolism of an abnormal apolipoprotein A-I (APOA-I Tangier). J Clin Invest 1982; 70:934–945.

51. Kovanen PT, Bilheimer DW, Goldstein JL, et al. Regulatory role for hepatic low density lipoprotein receptors in vivo in the dog. Proc Natl Acad Sci USA 1981; 78:1194–1198.

52. Windler EE, Kovanen PT, Chao Y-S, et al. The estradiol-stimulated lipoprotein receptor of rat liver. A binding site that mediates the uptake of rat lipoproteins containing apoproteins B and E. J Biol Chem 1980; 255:10464–10471.

53. Martin MJ, Hulley SB, Browner WS, et al. Serum cholesterol, blood pressure, and mortality: implications from a cohort of 361,662 men. Lancet 1986; 2:933–936.

54. Report of the National Cholesterol Education Program; Expert Panel on Detection, Evaluation, and Treatment of High Blood Cholesterol in Adults. Arch Intern Med 1988; 148:36–69.

55. Beaumont JL, Carlson LA, Cooper GR, et al. Classification of hyperlipidaemias and hyperlipoproteinaemias. Bull WHO 1970; 43:891–915.

56. Brunzell JD, Hazzard WR, Porte D Jr, et al. Evidence for a common, saturable, triglyceride removal mechanism for chylomicrons and very low density lipoproteins in man. J Clin Invest 1973; 52:1578–1585.

57. Janus ED, Lewis B. Alcohol and abnormalities of lipid metabolism. Clin Endocrinol Metab 1978; 7:321–332.

58. Ettinger WH Jr, Hazzard WR. Prednisone increases very low density lipoprotein and high density lipoprotein in healthy men. Metabolism 1988; 37:1055–1058.

59. Glueck CJ, Fallat RW, Scheel D. Effects of estrogenic compounds on triglyceride kinetics. Metabolism 1975; 24:537–545.

60. Taskinen MR, Nikkilä EA, Pelkonen R, et al. Plasma lipoproteins, lipolytic enzymes, and very low density lipoprotein triglyceride turnover in Cushing's syndrome. J Clin Endocrinol Metab 1983; 57:619–626.

61. Wallace RB, Hoover J, Sandler D, et al. Altered plasma-lipids associated with oral contraceptive or oestrogen consumption. The Lipid Research Clinic Program. Lancet 1977; 2:11–14.

62. Chait A, Albers JJ, Brunzell JD. Very low density lipoprotein overproduction in genetic forms of hypertriglyceridemia. Eur J Clin Invest 1980; 10:17–22.

63. Brunzell JD, Bierman EL. Plasma triglyceride and insulin levels in familial hypertriglyceridemia. Ann Intern Med 1977; 87:198–199.

64. Brunzell JD, Schrott HG, Motulsky AG, et al. Myocardial infarction in the familial forms of hypertriglyceridemia. Metabolism 1976; 25:313–320.

65. Little JA, McGuire V, Derksen A. Available carbohydrates. In: Levy R, Rifkind B, Dennis B, et al., eds. Nutrition, Lipids, and Coronary Disease. New York: Raven, 1979: 119–148.

66. Floren CH, Albers JJ, Kudchodkar BJ, et al. Receptor-dependent uptake of human chylomicron remnants by cultured skin fibroblasts. J Biol Chem 1982; 256:425–433.

67. Brunzell JD, Bierman EL. Chylomicronemia syndrome. Med Clin North Am 1982; 66:455–468.

68. Parker F, Bagdade JD, Odland GF, et al. Evidence for the plasma chylomicron origin of lipids accumulating in diabetic eruptive xantho-

mas: a correlative lipid biochemical, histochemical and electron microscopic study. J Clin Invest 1970; 49:2172–2187.

69. Taskinen M-R, Nikkilä EA. Lipoprotein lipase activity of adipose tissue and skeletal muscle in insulin-deficient human diabetes. Diabetologia 1979; 17:351–356.

70. Goldberg A, Sherrard D, Brunzell JD. Adipose tissue lipoprotein lipase in chronic hemodialysis: role in plasma triglyceride metabolism. J Clin Endocrinol Metab 1978; 47:1173–1182.

71. Brunzell JD, Miller NE, Alaupovic P, et al. Familial chylomicronemia due to a circulating inhibitor of lipoprotein lipase activity. J Lipid Res 1983; 24:147–155.

72. Havel RJ. Familial dysbetalipoproteinemia. Med Clin North Am 1982; 66:441–454.

73. Chait A, Brunzell JD, Albers JJ, et al. Type III hyperlipoproteinaemia ("remnant removal disease"): insight into the pathogenetic mechanism. Lancet 1977; 1:1176–1178.

74. Mahley RW, Rall SC Jr. Type III hyperlipoproteinemia (dysbetalipoproteinemia): the role of apolipoprotein E in normal and abnormal lipoprotein metabolism. In: Scriver CR, Beaudet AL, Sly WS, et al., eds. The Metabolic Basis of Inherited Disease. 6th ed. New York: McGraw-Hill, 1989: 1195–1214.

75. Utermann G, Pruin N, Steinmetz A. Polymorphism of apolipoprotein E. III. Effect of a single polymorphic gene locus on plasma lipid levels in man. Clin Genet 1979; 15:63–72.

76. Hazzard WR, Bierman EL. Aggravation of broad-beta disease (type III hyperlipoproteinemia) by hypothyroidism. Arch Intern Med 1972; 130:822–828.

77. Brewer HB Jr. Type III hyperlipoproteinemia: diagnosis, molecular defects, pathology and treatment. Ann Intern Med 1983; 98(Part I):623–640.

78. Glomset JA, Norum KR, Nichols AV, et al. Plasma lipoproteins in familial lecithin: cholesterol acyltransferase deficiency: effects of dietary manipulation. Scand J Clin Lab Invest 1975; 35(Suppl 142):3–29.

79. Sabesin SM, Hawkins HL, Kuiken L, et al. Abnormal plasma lipoproteins and lecithin-cholesterol acyltransferase deficiency in alcoholic liver disease. Gastroenterology 1977; 72:510–518.

80. Breckenridge WC, Little JA, Alaupovic P, et al. Lipoprotein abnormalities associated with a familial deficiency of hepatic lipase. Atherosclerosis 1982; 45:161–179.

81. Tollenhanz H, Hobgood KK, Brown MS, et al. The LDL receptor locus in familial hypercholesterolemia: multiple mutations disrupt transport and processing of a membrane receptor. Cell 1983; 32:941–951.

82. Illingworth DR, McClung MR, Connor WE, et al. Familial hypercholesterolaemia and primary hypothyroidism: coexistence of both disorders in a young woman with severe hypercholesterolaemia. Clin Endocrinol 1981; 14:145–152.

83. Davignon J, Gregg RE, Sing CF. Apolipoprotein E polymorphism and atherosclerosis. Arteriosclerosis 1988; 8:1–21.

84. Thompson GR, Soutar AK, Spengel FA, et al. Defects of receptor mediated low density lipoprotein catabolism in homozygous familial hypercholesterolemia and hypothyroidism in vivo. Proc Natl Acad Sci USA 1981; 78:2591–2595.

85. Kekki M, Nikkilä EA. Plasma triglyceride metabolism in the nephrotic syndrome. Eur J Clin Invest 1971; 1:345–351.

86. Lees RS, Song CS, Levere RD, et al. Hyperbetalipoproteinemia in acute intermittent porphyria. N Engl J Med 1970; 282:432–433.

87. Taylor JS, Lewis LA, Battle JD, et al. Plane xanthoma and multiple myeloma with lipoprotein-paraprotein complexing. Arch Dermatol 1978; 114:425–431.

88. Mordasini R, Klose G, Greten H. Secondary type II hyperlipoproteinemia in patients with anorexia nervosa. Metabolism 1978; 27:71–79.

89. Innerarity TL, Weisgraber KH, Arnold KS, et al. Familial defective apolipoprotein B-100: low density lipoproteins with abnormal receptor binding. Proc Natl Acad Sci USA 1987; 84:6919–6923.

90. Grundy SM, Chait A, Brunzell JD. Familial combined hyperlipidemia workshop. Arteriosclerosis 1987; 7:203–207.

91. Ibels LS, Alfrey AC, Weil R III. Hyperlipidemia in adult, pediatric, and diabetic renal transplant patients. Am J Med 1978; 64:634–642.

92. Beil U, Grundy SM, Crouse JR, et al. Triglyceride and cholesterol metabolism in primary hypertriglyceridemia. Arteriosclerosis 1982; 2:44–57.

93. Goldstein JL, Schrott HG, Hazzard WR, et al. Hyperlipidemia in coronary heart disease. II. Genetic analysis of lipid levels in 176 families and delineation of a new inherited disorder: combined hyperlipidemia. J Clin Invest 1973; 52:1544–1568.

94. Rose HG, Kranz P, Weinstock M, et al. Inheritance of combined hyperlipoproteinemia: evidence for a new lipoprotein phenotype. Am J Med 1973; 54:148–160.

95. Nikkilä EA, Aro A. Family study of serum lipids and lipoproteins in coronary heart-disease. Lancet 1973; 1:954–959.

96. Brunzell JD, Albers JJ, Chait A, et al. Plasma lipoproteins in familial combined hyperlipidemia and monogenic familial hypertriglyceridemia. J Lipid Res 1983; 24:147–155.

97. Sniderman A, Shapiro S, Marpole D, et al. Association of coronary atherosclerosis with hyperapobetalipoproteinemia [increased protein but normal cholesterol levels in human plasma low density (B) lipoproteins] Proc Natl Acad Sci USA 1980; 77:604–608.

98. Babirak SP, Iverius PH, Fujimoto WY, et al. The detection and characterization of the heterozygote state for lipoprotein lipase deficiency. Arteriosclerosis, 1989; 9:326–334.

99. Bierman EL. Insulin and hypertriglyceridemia. Isr J Med Sci 1972; 8:303–308.

100. Bagdade JD, Bierman EL, Porte D Jr. Diabetic lipemia—a form of acquired fat-induced lipemia. N Engl J Med 1967; 276:427–433.

101. Chait A, Brunzell JD. Severe hypertriglyceridemia: role of familial and acquired disorders. Metabolism 1983; 32:209–214.

102. Bagdade JD, Porte D Jr, Bierman EL. Acute insulin withdrawal and the regulation of plasma triglyceride removal in diabetic subjects. Diabetes 1968; 17:127–132.

103. Bagdade JD, Porte D Jr, Bierman EL. Steroid-induced lipemia. Arch Intern Med 1970; 125:125–129.

104. Brunzell JD, Hazzard WR, Motulsky AG, et al. Evidence for diabetes mellitus and genetic forms of hypertriglyceridemia as independent entities. Metabolism 1975; 24:1115–1121.

105. Taskinen M-R, Nikkilä EA, Kuusi T, et al. lipoprotein lipase activity and serum lipoproteins in untreated type 2 (insulin-independent) diabetes associated with obesity. Diabetologia 1982; 22:46–50.

106. Tobey TA, Greenfield M, Kraemer F, et al. Relationship between insulin resistance, insulin secretion, very low density lipoprotein kinetics, and plasma triglyceride levels in normotriglyceridemic man. Metabolism 1981; 30:165–171.

107. Modan M, Halkin H, Lusky A, et al. Hyperinsulinemia is characterized by jointly disturbed plasma VLDL, LDL, and HDL levels. Arteriosclerosis 1988; 8:227–236.

108. Anderson AJ, Sobocinski KA, Freedman DS, et al. Body fat distribution, plasma lipids, and lipoproteins. Arteriosclerosis 1988; 8:88–94.

109. Grundy SM, Mok HYI, Zech L, et al. Transport of very low density lipoprotein triglycerides in varying degrees of obesity and hypertriglyceridemia. J Clin Invest 1979; 63:1274–1283.

110. Kissebah AH, Alfarsi S, Evans DJ, et al. Integrated regulation of very low density lipoprotein triglyceride and apolipoprotein B kinetics in noninsulin dependent diabetes mellitus. Diabetes 1982; 31:217–225.

111. Blanc MH, Ganda OP, Gleason RE, et al. Improvement of lipid status in diabetic boys: the 1971 and 1979 Joslin Camp lipid levels. Diabetes Care 1983; 6:64–66.

112. Chait A, Bierman EL, Albers JJ. Low density lipoprotein receptor activity in cultured human skin fibroblasts. Mechanism of insulin-induced stimulation. J Clin Invest 1979; 64:1309–1319.

113. Rosenstock J, Vega GL, Raskin P. Effect of intensive diabetes treatment on low-density lipoprotein apolipoprotein B kinetics in type I diabetes. Diabetes 1988; 37:393–397.

114. Taskinen MR, Kuusi T, Helve E, et al. Insulin therapy induces antiatherogenic changes of serum lipoproteins in noninsulin-dependent diabetes. Arteriosclerosis 1988; 2:168–177.

115. Kesaniemi YA, Grundy SM. Increased low density lipoprotein production associated with obesity. Arteriosclerosis 1983; 3:170–177.

116. Kissebah A, Alfarsi S, Evans DJ, et al. Plasma low density lipoprotein transport kinetics in noninsulin-dependent diabetes mellitus. J Clin Invest 1983; 71:655–667.

117. Witztum JL, Mahoney EM, Branks MJ, et al. Nonenzymatic glucosylation of low-density lipoprotein alters its biologic activity. Diabetes 1982; 31:283–291.

118. Abrams JJ, Grundy SM, Ginsberg H. Metabolism of plasma triglycerides in hypothyroidism and hyperthyroidism in man. J Lipid Res 1981; 22:307–322.

119. Valdermarsson S, Hedner P, Nilsson-Ehle P. Dyslipoproteinemia in hypothyroidism of pituitary origins: effects of L-thyroxine substitution on lipoprotein lipase, hepatic lipase, and on plasma lipoproteins. Acta Endocrinol 1983; 103:192–197.

120. Pykälistö O, Goldberg AP, Brunzell JD. Reversal of decreased human adipose tissue lipoprotein lipase and hypertriglyceridemia after treatment of hypothyroidism. J Clin Endocrinol Metab 1976; 43:591–600.

121. Baum D, Guthrie R, Brunzell JD, et al. An abnormality of triglyceride metabolism in infantile hypothyroidism. Am J Dis Child 1973; 125:612–613.

122. Chait A, Bierman EL, Albers JJ. Regulatory role of triiodothyronine in the degradation of low density lipoprotein by cultured human skin fibroblasts. J Clin Endocrinol Metab 1979; 48:887–889.

123. Koppers LE, Palumbo PJ. Lipid disturbances in endocrine disorders. Med Clin North Am 1972; 56:1013–1020.

124. Knopp RH, Walden CE, Wahl PW, et al. Oral contraceptive and postmenopausal estrogen effects on lipoprotein triglyceride and cholesterol in an adult female population: relationships to estrogen and progestin potency. J Clin Endocrinol Metab 1981; 53:1123–1132.

125. Davidoff F, Tischler S, Rosoff C. Marked hyperlipidemia and pancreatitis associated with oral contraceptive therapy. N Engl J Med 1973; 289:552–555.

126. Kushwaha RS, Hazzard WR, Gagne C, et al. Type III hyperlipoproteinemia: paradoxical hypolipidemic response to estrogen. Ann Intern Med 1977; 87:517–525.

127. Tikkanen MJ, Nikkilä EA, Vartiainen E. Natural estrogen as an effective treatment for type-II hyperlipoproteinemia in postmenopausal women. Lancet 1978; 2:490–491.

128. Heiss G, Tamir I, Davis CE, et al. Lipoprotein-cholesterol distribution in selected North American populations: the Lipid Research Clinics Program Prevalence Study. Circulation 1980; 61:302–315.

129. Bradley DD, Wingerd J, Pettiti DB, et al. Serum high density lipoprotein cholesterol in women using oral contraceptives, estrogens, and progestins. N Engl J Med 1978; 299:17–20.

130. Wahl P, Walden C, Knopp R, et al. Effect of estrogen/progestin potency on lipid/lipoprotein cholesterol. N Engl J Med 1983; 308:862–867.

131. Stadel BV. Oral contraceptives and cardiovascular disease. N Engl J Med 1981; 305:672–677.

132. Bush TL, Barrett-Connor E, Cowan LD, et al. Cardiovascular mortality and noncontraceptive use of estrogen in women: results from the Lipid Research Clinics Program Follow-up Study. Circulation 1987; 75:1102.

133. Stampfer MJ, Willett WC, Colditz GA, et al. A prospective study of postmenopausal estrogen therapy and coronary heart disease. N Engl J Med 1985; 313:1044–1049.

134. Wilson PWF, Garrison RJ, Castelli WP. Postmenopausal estrogen use, cigarette smoking, and cardiovascular morbidity in women over 50: the Framingham study. N Engl J Med 1985; 313:1038–1043.

135. Austin MA. Plasma triglyceride as a risk factor for coronary heart disease: the epidemiologic evidence and beyond. Am J Epidemiol 1989; 129:249–259.

136. Brunzell JD, Sniderman AD, Albers JJ, et al. Apoprotein B and AI and coronary artery disease in man. Arteriosclerosis 1984; 4:79–83.

137. Miller GJ. High density lipoproteins and atherosclerosis. Annu Rev Med 1980; 31:97–108.

138. Maciejko JJ, Holmes DR, Kottke BA, et al. Apolipoprotein A-I as a marker of angiographically assessed coronary-artery disease. N Engl J Med 1983; 309:385–389.

139. Laakso M, Pyorala K, Sarlund H, et al. Lipid and lipoprotein abnormalities associated with coronary heart disease in patients with insulin-dependent diabetes mellitus. Arteriosclerosis 1986; 6:679–684.

140. West KM, Ahuja MMS, Bennett PH, et al. The role of circulating glucose and triglyceride concentrations and their interactions with other "risk factors" as determinants of arterial disease in nine diabetic population samples from the WHO multinational study. Diabetes Care 1983; 6:361–369.

141. Haire HM, Sherrard DJ, Scardapane DM, et al. Smoking, hypertension and mortality in maintenance dialysis population. Cardiovasc Med 1978; 3:1163–1168.

142. Goldstein JL, Hazzard WR, Schrott HG, et al. Hyperlipidemia in coronary heart disease. I. Lipid levels in 500 survivors of myocardial infarction. J Clin Invest 1973; 52:1533–1543.

143. Utermann G, Kraft HG, Menzel HJ, et al. Genetics of the quantitative Lp(a) lipoprotein trait. I. Relation of Lp(a) glycoprotein phenotypes to Lp(a) lipoprotein concentrations in plasma. Hum Genet 1988; 78:41–46.

144. Ross R. Medical progress: the pathogenesis of atherosclerosis—an update. N Engl J Med 1986; 413:488–500.

145. Steinberg D. Lipoproteins and atherosclerosis. Arteriosclerosis 1983; 3:283–301.

146. Chait A, Ross R, Bierman EL. Stimulation of receptor-dependent and receptor-independent pathways of low-density lipoprotein degradation in arterial smooth muscle cells by platelet-derived growth factor. Biochim Biophys Acta 1988; 960:183–189.

147. Steinberg D, Parthasarathy S, Carew TE, et al. Beyond cholesterol: modifications of low density lipoprotein that increase its atherogenicity. N Engl J Med 1989; 320:915–924.

148. Haberland ME, Fong D, Cheng L. Malondialdehyde-altered protein occurs in atheroma of Watanabe heritable hyperlipidemic rabbits. Science 1988; 241:215–218.

149. Hessler JR, Robertson AL Jr, Chisolm GM. LDL-induced cytotoxicity and its inhibition by HDL in human vascular smooth muscle and endothelial cells in culture. Atherosclerosis 1979; 32:213–229.

150. Stout RW. Hormones and Atherosclerosis. Boston: MTP Press, 1982.

151. Gordon T, Castelli WP, Hjortland MC, et al. Diabetes, blood lipids, and the role of obesity in coronary heart disease risk for women. The Framingham study. Ann Intern Med 1977; 87:393–397.

152. Glueck CJ, Gartside PS, Steiner PM, et al. Hyperalpha- and hypobeta-lipoproteinemia in octogenarian kindreds. Atherosclerosis 1977; 27:387–406.

153. Schaefer EJ. Clinical, biochemical and genetic features in familial disorders of high density lipoprotein deficiency. Arteriosclerosis 1984; 4:303–322.

154. Yamashita S, Matsuzawa Y, Okazaki M, et al. Small polydisperse low density lipoproteins in familial hyperalphalipoproteinemia with complete deficiency of cholesteryl ester transfer activity. Atherosclerosis 1988; 70:7–12.

155. Magill P, Rao SN, Miller NE, et al. Relationships between the metabolism of high-density and very-low-density lipoproteins in man: studies of apolipoprotein kinetics and adipose tissue lipoprotein lipase activity. Eur J Clin Invest 1982; 12:113–120.

156. Malloy MJ, Kane JP. Hypolipidemia. Med Clin North Am 1982; 66:469–484.

157. Carr BR, Simpson ER. Lipoprotein utilization and cholesterol synthesis by the human fetal adrenal gland. Endocr Rev 1981; 2:306–326.

158. Illingworth DR, Corbin DK, Kemp ED, et al. Hormone changes during the menstrual cycle in abetalipoproteinemia: reduced luteal phase progesterone in a patient with homozygous hypobetalipoproteinemia. Proc Natl Acad Sci USA 1982; 79:6685–6689.

159. Illingworth DR, Orwoll ES, Connor WE. Impaired cortisol secretion in abetalipoproteinemia. J Clin Endocrinol Metab 1980; 50:977–979.

160. Herbert PN, Hyams JS, Bernier DN, et al. Apolipoprotein B-100 deficiency: intestinal steatosis despite apolipoprotein B-48 synthesis. J Clin Invest 1985; 76:403–412.

161. Young SG, Bertics SJ, Curtiss LK, et al. Characterization of an abnormal species of apolipoprotein B, apolipoprotein B-37, associated with familial hypobetalipoproteinemia. J Clin Invest 1987; 79:1831–1841.

162. Douste-Blazy P, Marcel YL, Cohen L, et al. Increased frequency of APO E-ND phenotype and hyperapobetalipoproteinemia in normolipidemic subjects with xanthelasmas of the eyelids. Ann Intern Med 1982; 96:164–169.

163. Fredrickson DS. It's time to be practical. Circulation 1975; 51:209–211 (editorial).

164. Friedewald WT, Levy RI, Fredrickson DS. Estimation of the concentration of low-density lipoprotein cholesterol in plasma, without use of the preparative ultracentrifuge. Clin Chem 1972; 18:499–502.

165. Hulley SB, Rosenman RH, Bawol RD, et al. Epidemiology as a guide to clinical decisions. The association between triglyceride and coronary heart disease. N Engl J Med 1980; 302:1383–1389.

166. Goodnight SH Jr, Harris WS, Connor WC, et al. Polyunsaturated fatty acids, hyperlipidemia, and thrombosis. Arteriosclerosis 1982; 2:87–113.

167. Brunzell JD, Porte D Jr, Bierman EL. Reversible abnormalities in postheparin lipolytic activity during the late phase of release in diabetes mellitus. Metabolism 1975; 24:1123–1137.

168. Schlierf G, Reinhemer W, Stosberg V. Diurnal patterns of plasma triglycerides and free fatty acids in normal subjects and in patients with endogenous (type IV) hyperlipemia. Nutr Metab 1971; 13:80–91.

169. Cominacini L, Zocce I, Gorbin U, et al. Long-term effect of a low-fat, high-carbohydrate diet on plasma lipids of patients affected by familial endogenous hypertriglyceridemia. Am J Clin Nutr 1988; 48:57–65.

170. Connor WE, Connor SL. The dietary treatment of hyperlipidemia. Med Clin North Am 1982; 66:485–518.

171. Packard CJ, McKinney L, Carr K, et al. Cholesterol feeding increases low density lipoprotein synthesis. J Clin Invest 1983; 72:45–51.

172. Shepherd J, Packard CJ, Grundy SM, et al. Effects of saturated and polyunsaturated fat diets on the chemical composition and metabolism of low density lipoproteins in man. J Lipid Res 1980; 21:91–99.

173. Glueck CJ, Tsang RC. Pediatric familial type II hyperlipoproteinemia: effects of diet on plasma cholesterol in the first year of life. Am J Clin Nutr 1972; 25:224–230.

174. Spady DK, Dietschy JM. Dietary saturated triacylglycerols suppress hepatic low density lipoprotein receptor activity in the hamster. Proc Natl Acad Sci USA 1985; 82:4526–4530.

175. Ahrens EH Jr. Dietary fats and coronary heart disease: unfinished business. Lancet 1979; 2:1345–1348.

176. Sullivan DR, Sanders TAB, Trayner IM, et al. Paradoxical elevation of LDL apoprotein B levels in hypertriglyceridaemic patients and normal subjects ingesting fish oil. Atherosclerosis 1986; 61:129–134.

177. Failor RA, Childs MT, Bierman EL: The effects of ω3 and ω6 fatty acid–enriched diets on plasma lipoproteins and apoproteins in familial combined hyperlipidemia. Metabolism 1988; 37:1021–1028.

178. Friday KE, Failor RA, Childs MT, et al. Omega 3 (ω3) fatty acid enriched diets lower plasma LDL cholesterol and apolipoprotein B (apoB) in subjects with familial hypercholesterolemia (FH) but not familial combined hyperlipidemia (FCHL). Clin Res 1988; 36:759a.

179. Friday KE, Childs MT, Tsunehara CH, et al. Omega-3 fatty acid supplementation raises plasma glucose while lowering triglyceride levels in type II diabetes. Diabetes Care 1989; 12:276–281.

180. Dietary guidelines for healthy American adults. Circulation 1988; 77:721a–724a.

181. Anderson JW, Story L, Sieling B, et al. Hypocholesterolemic effects of oat-bran or bean intake for hypercholesterolemic men. Am J Clin Nutr 1984; 40:1146–1155.

182. Gordon DJ, Witztum JL, Hunninghake D, et al. Habitual physical activity and high-density lipoprotein cholesterol in men with primary hypercholesterolemia. Circulation 1983; 67:512–520.

183. Oliver MF. Risks of correcting the risks of coronary disease and stroke with drugs. N Engl J Med 1983; 306:297–298.

184. Treatment of hypertriglyceridemia. NIH consensus development conference summary. Arteriosclerosis 1984; 4:296–301.

185. Kissebah AH, Adams PW, Harrigan P, et al. The mechanism of action of clofibrate and tetranicotinoyl fructose (Bradilan) on the kinetics of plasma free fatty acid and triglyceride transport in type IV and type V hypertriglyceridemia. Eur J Clin Invest 1974; 4:163–174.

186. Stuyt PMJ, Demacker PNM, Van 'T Laar A. Long-term treatment of type III hyperlipoproteinemia with clofibrate. Atherosclerosis 1981; 40:329–336.

187. Grundy SM, Mok HYI, Zech L, et al. Influence of nicotinic acid on metabolism of cholesterol and triglycerides in man. J Lipid Res 1981; 22:24–36.
188. Packard CJ, Stewart JM, Third JLHC, et al. Effects of nicotinic acid therapy on high density lipoprotein metabolism in type IV and type V hyperlipoproteinemia. Biochim Biophys Acta 1980; 618:53–62.
189. Shepard J, Packard CJ, Bicker S, et al. Cholestyramine promotes receptor mediated low density lipoprotein catabolism. N Engl J Med 1980; 302:1219–1222.
190. Stamler J. The Coronary Drug Projects: findings leading to further modifications of its protocol with respect to dextrothyroxine. JAMA 1972; 220:996–1008.
191. Kita T, Nagano Y, Yokode M, et al. Probucol prevents the progression of atherosclerosis in Watanabe heritable hyperlipidemic rabbit, an animal model for familial hypercholesterolemia. Proc Natl Acad Sci USA 1987; 84:5928–5931.
192. Carew TE, Schwenke DC, Steinberg D. Antiatherogenic effect of probucol unrelated to its hypocholesterolemic effect: evidence that antioxidants in vivo can selectively inhibit low density lipoprotein degradation in macrophage-rich fatty streaks and slow the progression of atherosclerosis in the Watanabe heritable hyperlipidemic rabbit. Proc Natl Acad Sci USA 1987; 84:7725–7729.
193. Kane JP, Malloy MJ, Tun P, et al. Normalization of LDL levels in heterozygous familial hypercholesterolemia with a combined drug regimen. N Engl J Med 1981; 304:251–258.
194. Illingworth DR, Phillipson BE, Rapp JH, et al. Cholestipol plus nicotinic acid in treatment of heterozygous familial hypercholesterolemia. Lancet 1981; 1:296–298.
195. Havel RJ. Lowering cholesterol, 1988: rationale, mechanisms, and means. J Clin Invest 1988; 81:1653–1660.
196. Lovastatin Study Group II. Therapeutic response to lovastatin (mevinolin) in nonfamilial hypercholesterolemia. JAMA 1986; 256:2829–2834.
197. Bilheimer DW, Grundy SM, Brown MS, et al. Mevinolin and colestipol stimulate receptor-mediated clearance of low density lipoprotein from plasma in familial hypercholesterolemia heterozygotes. Proc Natl Acad Sci USA 1983; 80:4124–4128.
198. Mabuchi H, Sakai T, Sakai Y, et al. Reduction of serum cholesterol in heterozygous patients with familial hypercholesterolemia. N Engl J Med 1983; 308:609–613.
199. Sherrard DJ, Goldberg AP, Haas LB, et al. Chronic clofibrate therapy in maintenance hemodialysis patients. Nephron 1980; 25:219–221.
200. Buchwald H, Varco RL, Motts JP, et al. Effect of partial ileal bypass surgery on mortality and morbidity from coronary heart disease in patients with hypercholesterolemia. N Engl J Med 1990; 323:946–955.
201. Forman MB, Baker SG, Mieny CJ, et al. Treatment of homozygous familial hypercholesterolemia with portacaval shunt. Atherosclerosis 1982; 41:349–361.
202. McNamara DJ, Ahrens EH Jr, Kolb R, et al. Treatment of familial hypercholesterolemia by portacaval anastomosis: effect on cholesterol metabolism and pool sizes. Proc Natl Acad Sci USA 1983; 80:564–568.
203. Thompson GR. Plasma exchange for hypercholesterolemia. Lancet 1981; 1:1246–1248.
204. Stoffel W, Borberg H, Greve V. Application of specific extracorporeal removal of low density lipoprotein in familial hypercholesterolemia. Lancet 1981; 2:1005–1007.
205. Thompson GR. Plasma exchange for hypercholesterolaemia. Lancet 1981; 2:1246–1248.
206. World Health Organization (WHO). Cooperative trial on primary prevention of ischemic heart disease using clofibrate to lower serum cholesterol. Lancet 1980; 2:379–384.
207. Duffield RGM, Miller NE, Brunt JNH, et al. Treatment of hyperlipidemia retards progression of symptomatic femoral atherosclerosis. Lancet 1983; 2:639–641.
208. Brensike JF, Levy RI, Kelsey SF, et al. Effect of therapy with cholestyramine on progression of coronary arteriosclerosis: results of the NHLBI type II coronary intervention study. Circulation 1984; 69:313–324.
209. Lipid Research Clinics Program. The lipid research clinics coronary primary prevention trial results. I. Reduction in incidence of coronary heart disease. JAMA 1984; 251:351–364.
210. Blankenhorn DH, Nesim SA, Johnson RL, et al. Beneficial effects of combined colestipol-niacin therapy on coronary atherosclerosis and coronary venous bypass grafts. JAMA 1987; 257:3233–3240.
211. Frick MH, Elo O, Happa K, et al. Helsinki heart study: primary-prevention trial with gemfibrozil in middle-aged men with dyslipidemia. N Engl J Med 1987; 317:1237–1245.
212. Brown G, Albers JJ, Fisher LD, et al. Regression of coronary artery disease as a result of intensive lipid-lowering therapy in men with high levels of apolipoprotein B. N Engl J Med 1990; 323:1289–1298.

27

PARATHYROID HORMONE, CALCITONIN, AND THE CALCIFEROLS

Gerald D. Aurbach, Stephen J. Marx, and Allen M. Spiegel

INTRODUCTION

In this chapter we present a broad survey of endocrine control of mineral (calcium, magnesium, and phosphate) metabolism and the disturbances of these systems in medical practice. Parathyroid hormone (PTH), calcitonin (CT), and the calciferols are the principal calcitropic hormones. Together with extracellular calcium, they synergize with and feed back on each other to determine their own secretion rates and actions. They regulate processes as diverse as skeletal turnover and availability of cytoplasmic calcium for intracellular signaling.

The chapter begins with a review of mineral metabolism, its endocrine regulation, and the hormones involved. Utilization of the laboratory and the manifestations and treatment of clinical disorders of calcium metabolism are described. In the final section we discuss disturbances in phosphate and magnesium metabolism and disorders of calcitonin.

CALCIUM, MAGNESIUM, AND PHOSPHATE METABOLISM

Evolution of Roles for Calcium, Magnesium, and Phosphate

Complex organic molecules evolved in the primordial atmosphere and oceans, and the development of membranes permitted the compartmentalization of biochemical reactions in a medium of regulated composition.[1] The cytoplasm of animal cells has a composition different from that of present-day oceans and lakes (Table 27–1). To maintain a consistent cytoplasmic ionic composition, cells recognize and respond to changes in plasma membrane permeability. Such changes influence transmembrane fluxes of ions in the presence of concentration gradients. Fluxes of ions with large transmembrane concentration gradients (sodium, potassium, and calcium) have a central role in transmission of information into and between cells.

The evolutionary pressures that led to selection of magnesium and phosphorus as major cytoplasmic components are poorly understood. Many cellular reactions depend on the availability of organic and inorganic phosphate. Phosphate* functions as a major cytoplasmic buffer, participates in energy exchange, and is an essential component of membranes and nucleic acids. Phosphorus is scarce in the earth's crust and must be concentrated by all plant and animal species; its availability in the sea and soil is one limiting factor for population growth of all organisms. Calcium salts are limited in solubility at physiological pH and could precipitate if in millimolar concentrations in cytosol. The solubility of magnesium salts and the greater abundance of magnesium than of calcium in ocean water (see Table 27–1) may help explain why magnesium evolved as the principal cytoplasmic divalent cation.

With the evolution of multicellular life forms, extracellular fluids replaced ocean water as the immediate cellular environment. Adaptation to fresh water and then to a terrestrial habitat was accompanied by increasing capacity to regulate the extracellular concentrations of important minerals such as calcium, magnesium, and phosphate.

In mammals the bulk of body calcium, magnesium, and phosphate is in the skeleton (Table 27–2). An endoskeleton composed of crystalline molecules such as hydroxyapatite, $Ca_{10}(PO_4)_6(OH)_2$, provides mechanical support and serves as a reservoir of these important but sparingly soluble minerals.

Extracellular Compartments

EXTERNAL SOURCES AND NUTRITION. Large amounts of calcium, magnesium, and phosphate must be regularly supplied to the body.[2] The recommended daily allowances for children and adults in the United States are 800 to 1200 mg of calcium, 300 to 400 mg of magnesium, and 800 to 1200 mg of phosphate. True requirements for minerals in the diet have not been established and remain an issue of controversy.[3, 4] Phosphate and magnesium are present in most dietary components, and any but a grossly unbalanced diet will meet the minimal requirements. Symptomatic nutritional deficiency of phosphate develops in normal subjects only with dietary restriction of phosphate combined with ingestion of phosphate binders (such as aluminum hydroxide antacid preparations). Selective and symptomatic nutritional deficiency of magnesium has been observed only with synthetic diets designed for the purpose of inducing this state. Calcium content is high in dairy products (Table 27–3).

TABLE 27–1. Mineral Composition of Solutions

Solution	Calcium (mmol/L)	Magnesium (mmol/L)	Inorganic Phosphate (mmol/L)
Ocean (Pacific)	10	48	0.001
Lake (Huron)	0.90	0.25	0.003
Cytoplasma—squid axon			
Total	0.3	6.7	3.0
Ionized	0.0001	3.5	1.5
Plasma			
Hagfish*	5.4	10.4	1.0
Salmon (ocean phase male)	2.3	1.0	4.7
Salmon (fresh-water phase male)	2.9	1.8	4.5
Human	2.4	0.9	1.2

*The hagfish is a primitive ocean dweller with a skeleton.

---

*Because organic phosphorus is in the form of phosphate, the latter term is employed in this chapter. Quantitation of phosphate, by convention, is in units of phosphorus content.

TABLE 27–2. Distribution of Calcium, Magnesium, and Phosphate in the Body of a 70-kg Human Adult*

Compartment	Calcium (g)	Magnesium (g)	Phosphate (g)
Bones and teeth	1300 (99)	14 (54)	600 (86)
Extracellular fluid	1 (0.1)	0.3 (1)	0.2 (0.03)
Cells	7 (1.0)	12 (46)	100 (14)

*Numbers in parentheses indicate percentage of total for each element.

Dietary calcium intake as nondairy components is relatively constant (200 to 300 mg/d) among most human populations, but there are major population differences in average intake of dairy products throughout the world, ranging from 100 to more than 1000 mg of calcium per day. In the United States, dairy products contribute approximately 500 mg of calcium to the average daily diet of an adult.[5] The consequences for humans of a diet critically low in calcium or calcium/phosphate ratio are not established. In rats a low-calcium diet retards skeletal growth. The usual calcium/phosphate ratio (weight/weight) in the diet of most species is approximately 1.0, and large decreases in this ratio by administration of a diet high in phosphate promote increased parathyroid secretion and increased skeletal resorption rates.[6] In the United States the recommended dietary calcium/phosphate ratio is 1.0, but average dietary ratios range from 0.3 to 0.9. The higher values reflect greater consumption of cow's milk with a calcium/phosphate ratio of 1.3 (see Table 27–3).

PLASMA AND EXTRACELLULAR FLUID. Less than 2% of body calcium, magnesium, and phosphate is in the plasma and extracellular fluid (ECF) (see Table 27–2), yet the concentrations of these minerals in ECF are controlled within narrow limits. Plasma calcium participates in multiple processes, including proteolysis (e.g., the clotting and kinin generation cascades), regulation of plasma membrane potential, and exocytosis. Its normal concentration in plasma is

2.2 to 2.6 mmol/L (8.8 to 10.3 mg/dL), with minor variation dependent on laboratory methods. Normal plasma concentrations of magnesium (0.8 to 1.2 mmol/L [1.8 to 3.0 mg/dL]) and phosphate (0.8 to 1.6 mmol/L [2.5 to 5 mg/dL]) encompass larger fractional variations from their means. Calcium introduced into the ECF rapidly equilibrates with a calcium pool of much greater calcium content.[7] The anatomical locations of this portion of the miscible or central pool are not well defined but undoubtedly include mitochondria and surfaces of bone mineral.

Plasma is a complex solution, and only the ionized fraction of calcium participates directly in most biological reactions (Table 27–4). The focal point of the regulation of mineral metabolism is the concentration of ionized calcium in plasma, but owing to major technical problems this remains difficult to measure accurately.[8] The minute-to-minute and interindividual variations are small, however. Change in circulating ionized calcium concentration is a major signal for modification of secretion rates of PTH and CT. The concentration of ionized calcium differs among the compartments of the ECF. For example, in the cochlear endolymph of rats the total calcium concentration is 30 µmol/L, of which most is ionized. It may change in one compartment without changing in others. Ionized calcium concentrations are reduced 20% in the cerebrospinal fluid adjacent to cerebellar cells undergoing repetitive stimulation and are reduced 90% with severe depression of central nervous system function.

Albumin accounts for 70% of the protein binding of calcium in serum, and some myeloma globulins can bind enough calcium to increase total serum calcium concentration without affecting the ionized fraction. Albumin contains approximately 12 calcium-binding regions per molecule. In vivo, only 20% of these sites are occupied at any time. Proportional binding increases with rise in pH such that, within the physiological range, ionized calcium concentration changes approximately -0.05 mmol/L for each $+0.1$ unit change in pH. The concentration of albumin in the circulation varies independently of that of ionized calcium and is a major source of intra- and interindividual variations in total concentration of calcium in serum. A simple correction for this effect is to increase total serum calcium concentration $+0.25$ mmol/L for each 10 g/L reduction of albumin concentration below the normal mean and to apply an opposite correction for high serum albumin concentrations. Serum concentrations of albumin are higher in males than in females by 2 g/L, increase with the hemoconcentration of upright posture or use of tourniquets, and decrease in certain chronic illnesses (such as chronic hepatic disease and nephrotic syndrome).

A small portion of circulating calcium is in the form of complexes, half with bicarbonate and the remainder with phosphate, citrate, and other anions.[9] The ionized plus complexed forms of calcium constitute the free or filterable calcium. The small radii of these complexes allow free diffusion through small pores and inclusion in the renal glomerular filtrate. The concentration of complexed calcium

TABLE 27–3. Calcium, Magnesium, and Phosphate Content of Foods*

Food	Calcium	Magnesium	Phosphate
Vegetables			
Carrots	37	23	36
Peas	26	35	116
Lima beans	52	67	142
Spinach	93	88	51
Tomato	13	14	27
Lettuce	35	11	26
Potato (peeled)	7	22	53
Corn	3	48	111
Fruit			
Apple	7	5	10
Orange	41	11	20
Banana	8	33	26
Meat			
Fish steak (flounder)	54	30	885
Beef steak	10	20	150
Liver (beef)	8	13	352
Chicken	12	20	200
Miscellaneous			
Bread (rye)	75	42	147
Almond (shelled)	234	270	504
Chicken egg (white and yolk)	54	11	205
Salt	253	120	0
Dairy			
Bovine milk	119	13	93
Bovine skim milk	123	11	101
Human milk	33	4	14
Butter	24	2	23
Brick cheese	674	24	451
Cottage cheese	60	5	132

*All entries expressed as mg/100 g edible portion.
From U.S. Department of Agriculture Handbooks 8 (1975) and 8–1 (1976).

TABLE 27–4. States of Calcium, Magnesium, and Phosphate in Human Plasma*

State	Calcium (mmol/L)	Magnesium (mmol/L)	Phosphate (mmol/L)
Protein-bound	1.15 (47)	0.27 (29)	0.15 (13)
Filtrable or free†			
Complexed	0.25 (10)	0.07 (8)	0.40 (35)
Ionized	1.07 (43)	0.58 (63)	0.60 (52)

*Numbers in parentheses indicate percentage of total for each mineral.
†Free = complexed + ionized.

in serum increases during renal failure because of accumulation of phosphate, sulfate, and other small anions. Rapid infusion of calcium chelators such as edetate (EDTA) or citrate (often a preservative in banked blood) can complex enough calcium to cause hypocalcemia.

The proportional distribution of magnesium as ionized, protein bound, and complexed is similar to that of calcium in serum (see Table 27–4). Magnesium binds to the same sites on albumin as does calcium; lower binding affinity of these sites for magnesium than for calcium results in a larger proportion of magnesium in free or diffusible forms. The homeostatic mechanisms regulating magnesium in the ECF are poorly understood.[10] Ionized magnesium elicits responses similar to those induced by calcium ion with regard to secretion of PTH and CT, although the parathyroid gland is more sensitive to calcium than to magnesium.

Seventy percent of the phosphate in the circulation is covalently bound in phospholipids and phosphoproteins. The remaining 30% is inorganic phosphate in serum. Serum phosphate concentrations are higher in infants than in adults, and there is a diurnal pattern with peak levels during sleep.[11] Small amounts of serum phosphate (5 to 15%) are noncovalently bound to protein. The majority circulates as ions or complexes of HPO_4^{2-} and $H_2PO_4^-$, with the usual molar ratio of these anions being 4:1. Changes in total body phosphate stores modulate the activity of the renal 25-hydroxycholecalciferol (25-OHD) 1α-hydroxylase enzyme and thereby participate in the regulation of circulating concentrations of 1,25-dihydroxycholecalciferol ($1,25(OH)_2D$). Phosphate depletion leads to increased activity of this enzyme even in the total absence of the parathyroid glands. Phosphate ion does not have direct effects on the rates of secretion of PTH or CT; however, each of the major calcitropic hormones—PTH, CT, and the calciferols—affects phosphate fluxes into and out of the plasma compartments.

Calcium, Magnesium, and Phosphate Transport Across Organs

Large amounts of calcium, magnesium, and phosphate continuously enter and leave plasma via intestine, kidney, and bone. Each of the organs contributes to regulation of plasma concentrations of these minerals. Each employs independent mechanisms to regulate ion influx to plasma and other mechanisms to regulate efflux; each contains ion-transporting cells that are polarized with a redundant plasma membrane on the side not exposed to plasma—renal tubular and intestinal mucosal cells possess a brush border, whereas the analogous structure in bone is the ruffled border on the bone face of actively resorbing osteoclasts; and each is responsive to one or more of the three major calcitropic hormones.

INTESTINE. Calcium absorption in vivo and in vitro is a composite of saturable and nonsaturable processes (Fig. 27–1).[12] The saturable components provide short-term compensation for variation in dietary calcium availability and ensure that net calcium absorption varies less than exogenous supply. Within the physiological range, net absorption of phosphate (and magnesium) varies linearly with dietary supply. Thus the intestine plays a greater role in the adaptation to changes in exogenous availability of calcium than in that of phosphate or magnesium.

Net absorption is the difference between lumen-to-plasma flux and plasma-to-lumen flux (the latter includes the contents of all the digestive juices). The interrelations of absorption of calcium, magnesium, and phosphate are complex. In rats the net absorption rate for calcium is greatest in the duodenum in vitro, although considerable absorption occurs in the jejunum in vivo because of the rapid transit of

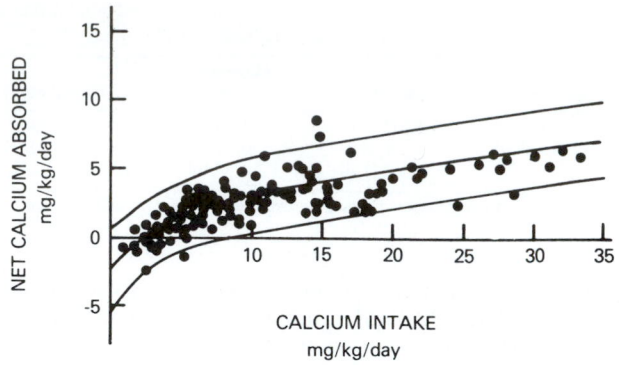

Figure 27–1. Relationship between net absorbed calcium and dietary calcium intake in normal subjects. Data from 212 balance studies on healthy individuals aged 19 to 83. Note the suggestion of a multicomponent process, saturable (decreasing slope) at low dietary calcium intake and nonsaturable (constant slope) at intakes above 10 mg/kg/d. (From Wilkinson R. Absorption of calcium, phosphorus, and magnesium. In: Nordin BEC, ed. Calcium, Phosphate and Magnesium Metabolism. Edinburgh: Churchill Livingstone, 1976.)

food through the duodenum. Net lumen-to-plasma flux for phosphate is greater in the jejunum than in the duodenum; in this segment, net movement of phosphate to plasma is far greater than that of calcium. The intestinal absorption of calcium, magnesium, and phosphate is depressed in vitamin D deficiency and increased with vitamin D excess; although net calcium absorption varies over a wide range—from 15 to 70% of intake, depending on calciferol status—magnesium and phosphate absorptions show much smaller deviations from their norms.

Calcium absorption is increased by dietary sugars; lactose stimulates calcium absorption even in vitamin D–deficient animals. The lactose effect occurs whether lactose is administered before or together with calcium, suggesting that it is an effect on mucosal energy metabolism.

Net intestinal absorption of calcium is subject to metabolic regulation. Long-term adaptations are determined by alterations in calciferol metabolism and alterations in intestinal responsiveness to the calciferol metabolites. Deficiency of either calcium or phosphorus leads to increased production of $1,25(OH)_2D$. PTH probably has no direct action on the intestinal translocation of minerals but affects control indirectly by regulating $1,25(OH)_2D$ synthesis. CT does not significantly influence intestinal calcium fluxes.

KIDNEYS. Ions and complexes not bound to proteins cross the renal glomerulus.[13, 14] In a 70-kg adult with a glomerular filtration rate (GFR) of 120 mL/min and an ECF volume of 12 L, a volume equivalent to the ECF traverses the glomerulus each 100 min. Approximately 65% of the glomerular filtrate (GF) is reabsorbed in the proximal tubule. Phosphate is avidly reabsorbed by the early portion of the proximal convoluted tubule. This sodium-dependent process is under inhibitory regulation by PTH and other factors that decrease fractional sodium reabsorption by the proximal tubule (sodium loading, volume expansion, and carbonic anhydrase inhibition). Large differences in phosphate delivery from the proximal tubule are not compensated for in the distal segments, although there is uncertainty concerning the contributions of phosphate secretion and reabsorption in distal segments. Phosphate secretion does occur in the nephrons of nonmammalian species. Phosphate reabsorption by the mammalian kidney can be modeled simply as a high-affinity system operating near saturation. When filtered phosphate rises beyond a threshold concentration, the overflow is excreted into the urine. When filtered phosphate load drops below the threshold, phosphate is efficiently reabsorbed (Fig. 27–2). The urine content is equivalent to 5

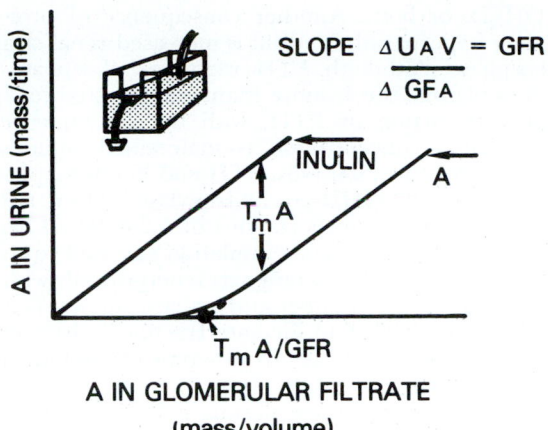

Figure 27–2. Relationship between urinary excretion and filtered load of solutes (A) for which the kidney has a threshold of excretion. For inulin (or creatinine) there is no threshold and excretion is a fixed fraction of load, the fraction being identical to that for renal clearance. For A (calcium, phosphate, or magnesium), clearance is a function of filtered load. Beyond the load at maximal resorption, the slope is identical to GFR. Maximal tubular resorption of A is the vertical distance between the lines or its equivalent, the y (abscissa) intercept. The x (ordinate) intercept of the extrapolated line is T_mA/GFR or the "theoretical renal threshold" of A. Inset shows how level of tank outlet (threshold) influences content of tank (serum concentration) when there is equilibrium of influx and outflux.

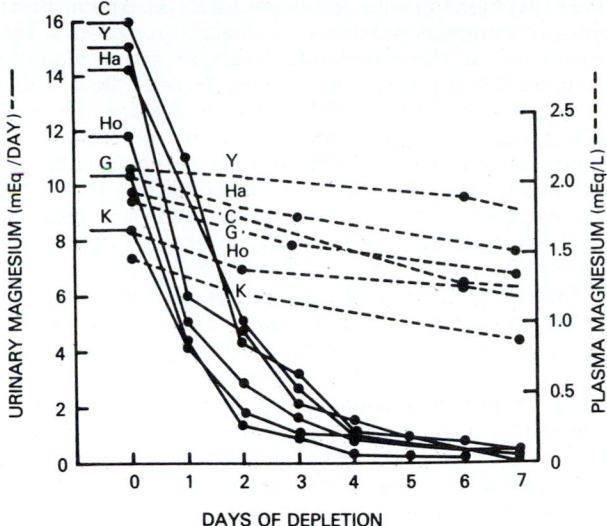

Figure 27–3. Effect of a synthetic magnesium-deficient diet on plasma magnesium concentration and urinary magnesium excretion in six patients. (Modified from ME Shils, Experimental human magnesium depletion, Medicine, 48, 61–85, © by Williams & Wilkins, 1969.)

to 20% of the filtered load for phosphate but only 0.5 to 5% for calcium and 2 to 10% for magnesium.

Calcium and magnesium concentrations of late proximal fluid are similar to those in GF. These divalent cations are translocated in the proximal tubules with sodium-driven bulk flow. The major regulation of divalent cation exchange between plasma and renal filtrate occurs in the distal tubules. Calcium is actively reabsorbed in the thick ascending limb of the distal tubule. Distal calcium transport sites are also capable of translocating magnesium, but there are mechanisms for transporting one or the other divalent cation preferentially. Thiazide diuretics and lithium preferentially decrease the renal clearance of calcium with little effect on renal magnesium clearance. In contrast, restriction of dietary magnesium leads, by unknown mechanisms, to rapid and selective renal conservation of magnesium without large decreases in serum concentration of magnesium (Fig. 27–3). PTH increases distal tubular reabsorption of calcium and probably magnesium. For this reason, the maintenance of normocalcemia in hypoparathyroidism may be possible only with a high rate of calcium flow into the urine (i.e., hypercalciuria). CT increases the renal clearance of sodium, calcium, magnesium, and phosphate; in human adults these actions may be significant only at high concentrations of CT. Calciferol metabolites have minor effects on the renal handling of calcium, magnesium, and phosphate.

URINARY EXCRETION OF CALCIUM. Calcium concentration in the urine is determined by filtered load of calcium and multiple factors that modulate the renal handling of filtered calcium, other solutes, and free water.[13, 14] With a 400-mg calcium diet the 24-h urinary calcium excretion should be less than 6.2 mmol (250 mg) in adult men and less than 5.0 mmol (200 mg) in women; these upper limits rise only by 1.2 mmol/d (50 mg/d) with a 1000-mg calcium diet. Hypercalciuria is associated with an increased incidence of calcium-containing stones (see Chapter 29). The term hypercalciuria is applied in a statistical sense that need not imply any underlying disorder, however. The only recognized disturbance directly attributable to hypercalciuria is a reversible decrease in the capacity of the kidneys to concentrate urine.

Many agents and disorders are associated with increases in total urinary excretion of calcium. The filtered load of calcium is increased in states with elevated concentrations of ultrafiltrable calcium in plasma; in general, this is equivalent to hypercalcemia. With subnormal PTH secretion caused by hypercalcemia, the renal tubular reabsorption of calcium decreases, producing particularly severe hypercalciuria. Similarly, with partial parathyroid suppression (serum calcium level at the upper normal range), the renal clearance of calcium is high. This occurs with increased influx of calcium to plasma from the intestine (absorptive hypercalciuria: vitamin D excess) or from bone (resorptive hypercalciuria: Paget disease of bone, thyrotoxicosis, skeletal metastases, immobilization). In temperate regions there is a seasonal variation in average urinary calcium excretion, with a peak in August and a nadir in December (Fig. 27–4). This may

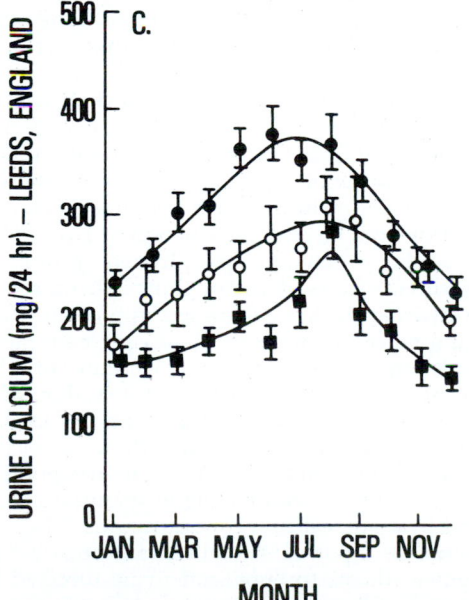

Figure 27–4. Seasonal variation in urinary calcium excretion in population of Leeds, England (low annual ultraviolet exposure): (●) stone formers, (○) normal males, and (■) normal women. (From Robertson WG, Gallagher JC, Marshall DH, et al. Seasonal variations in urinary excretion of calcium. Br Med J 1974; 4:436–437.)

reflect variations in solar exposure with consequent fluctuations in cutaneous synthesis of cholecalciferol and hence fluctuations in the circulating levels of active vitamin D metabolites. Many natriuretic agents decrease distal tubular reabsorption of calcium. These include dietary salt, certain diuretics (furosemide and ethacrynic acid), mineralocorticoid escape, and CT. With systemic acidosis, renal calcium clearance also increases by unknown mechanisms. Urinary calcium excretion rate doubles after a moderate protein or carbohydrate load, and this may be exaggerated in stone formers.[15]

BONES. The extracellular pools of calcium, magnesium, and phosphate are in equilibrium with much larger intracellular pools. A large portion of these pools is in bone,[15] the blood supply of which accounts for 5 to 25% of the cardiac output. This equilibrium damps the amplitude of changes in plasma concentration that result from variation in exchange across the intestines. In normal adults, ECF calcium efflux to bone (bone apposition) and influx from bone (bone resorption) are each approximately 0.2 mmol (8 mg)/kg body weight/d, a composite of passive exchange with crystal faces and active transport by bone cells. Bone cells can participate in regulation of ECF mineral concentration by two mechanisms, one a balance between osteoblastic apposition and osteoclastic resorption and the other involving osteocytic exchange of minerals between ECF and bone. The relative importance of these two mechanisms is not known. Bidirectional and net fluxes of calcium and phosphate between plasma and bone are determined, in large part, by circulating PTH and vitamin D metabolites.

Endocrine Regulation of Calcium, Phosphate, and Magnesium Concentrations in Extracellular Fluid

Maintenance of plasma ionized calcium concentration within a narrow range is the central theme in mineral homeostasis. The parathyroid gland serves as principal regulator of this process. Although secretion of CT by the thyroid is also regulated by ionized calcium, CT does not function as a major regulator of the plasma calcium concentration. PTH regulates serum calcium concentration through its direct actions on mineral transport in bone and kidney and its secondary actions on mineral transport in intestine (mediated directly by $1,25(OH)_2D$).

In the absence of PTH, plasma calcium can be maintained in the range of 1.2 to 1.5 mmol/L (5 to 6 mg/dL) by the combination of near-complete renal tubular reabsorption plus small net influx of calcium to the central (miscible with ECF) pool from bone or intestine. Without PTH, hypophosphatemia alone can increase production of $1,25(OH)_2D$ modestly; however, when the parathyroid gland functions normally, direct effects of serum phosphate on the renal 25-OHD 1α-hydroxylase system are less important. Under normal circumstances a decrease in serum concentration of ionized calcium results in increased secretion of PTH. With elevation of plasma PTH renal conservation of calcium becomes even more effective than can be explained by decreased filtered load alone, and influx of calcium from bone to plasma also increases. Acute interruption of intestinal calcium input, as with fasting, does not lead to perceptible drops in serum calcium concentrations. The decrement of net intestinal input of 4 mmol/d (150 mg/d) is balanced by changes in fluxes to bone and urine directed by PTH. The response of bone reflects increased activation of osteocytes and osteoclasts. If hypocalcemia persists for longer than 1 to 2 d, the skeletal response becomes progressively larger as osteoclast activity and numbers increase. The increases are a consequence of prolonged stimulation by PTH,

$1,25(OH)_2D$, or both. Another consequence of prolonged secondary hyperparathyroidism is increased renal clearance of phosphate. Although PTH mobilizes phosphate from bone into plasma, this is more than compensated for by the phosphaturic action of PTH, with the consequence that serum calcium concentration is maintained while serum phosphate concentration falls. PTH and hypophosphatemia each stimulate 25-OHD 1α-hydroxylase. After approximately 24 h, serum concentrations of $1,25(OH)_2D$ begin to rise (Fig. 27–5). Continued stimulation can lead to fivefold elevations. $1,25(OH)_2D$ not only acts synergistically with PTH to increase osteoclast number and activity but also functions independently of PTH to increase fractional absorption of calcium across the intestines from a typical baseline of 25% to a maximum of 75%.

The response to hypercalcemia is largely the opposite of the response to hypocalcemia. Whereas changes in skeletal balance buffer large hypocalcemic challenges, changes in urinary excretion buffer the major portion of hypercalcemic challenge. Secretion of PTH decreases within seconds of a rise in serum calcium level. Because the normal parathyroid gland secretes hormone at about 20% of the maximal value, the absolute decrease in response to hypercalcemia is less than the absolute increase in response to hypocalcemia. Plasma calcium level reaches a peak 3 h after an oral dose of calcium. Even with a large dose (on the order of 25 mmol

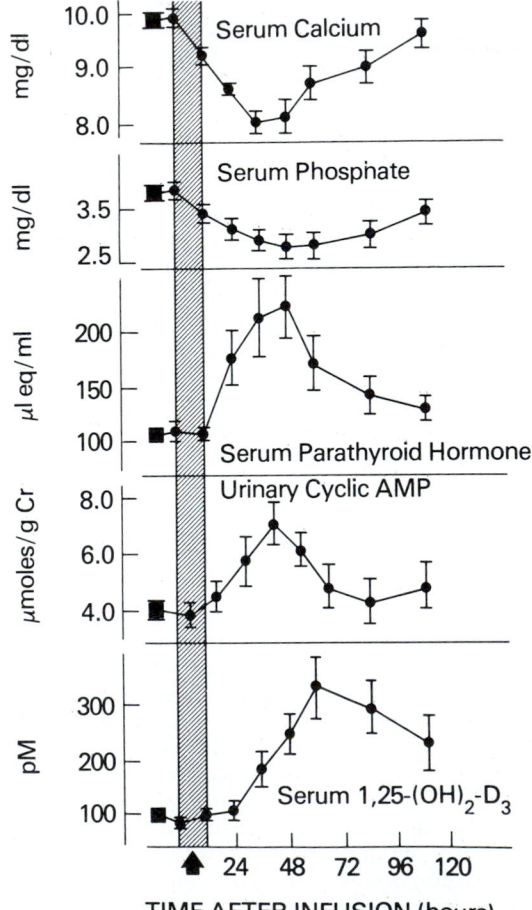

Figure 27–5. Response of PTH-calciferol axis to hypocalcemia. Eight patients with Paget disease received plicamycin (25 μg/kg) by infusion (*hatched band*). Note that response of serum $1,25(OH)_2D$ lags 12 to 24 h behind changes in serum PTH and urinary cAMP. (Modified from Bilezikian JP, Canfield RE, Jacobs TP, et al. Response of 1 alpha, 25-dihydroxyvitamin D_3 to hypocalcemia in human subjects. Reprinted with permission from The New England Journal of Medicine, 299, 437–441, 1978.)

[1000 mg] elemental calcium), the peak plasma calcium rises only 0.25 mmol/L (1 mg/dL) above the baseline. A small rise in ionized calcium concentration leads to suppression of PTH secretion with a consequent increased renal clearance of calcium. With suppression of PTH, renal clearance of phosphate decreases, raising the serum phosphate level. Lower PTH and higher serum phosphate levels each inhibit $1,25(OH)_2D$ production and, therefore, decrease intestinal absorption of calcium. Hypercalcemia raises CT concentrations, but CT does not make an important contribution in the response to hypercalcemia (unless the hypercalcemia is associated with intense osteoclastic activity).

Phosphate concentration in ECF is less stringently controlled than calcium concentration; it usually is maintained within 30% of the mean (0.8 to 1.5 mmol/L [2.5 to 4.5 mg/dL]). No known endocrine factor serves to regulate this function primarily. The main determinants of plasma phosphate modulation are the threshold for renal excretion and the filtrable load (see Fig. 27–2). Phosphate withdrawal does not evoke an immediate response, but over several days serum phosphate concentrations fall, leading to a rise in production of $1,25(OH)_2D$. This increases intestinal absorption of calcium, which raises the serum calcium level minimally and suppresses PTH secretion. This derivative suppression of PTH decreases the renal clearance of phosphate and increases renal clearance of calcium. Renal clearance of phosphate also decreases independently of changes in PTH secretion. Within 3 to 4 d of phosphate withdrawal, urinary excretion of phosphate can decrease from a baseline of 25 mmol/d (1000 mg/d) to immeasurable levels. The phosphaturic response to exogenous PTH becomes blunted, although the response of nephrogenous cyclic AMP (cAMP) to PTH is conserved. Thus, although serum concentrations of phosphate are not regulated as rapidly and narrowly as those of calcium, the body pool of phosphate is conserved with avidity.

Plasma phosphate concentration reaches a peak 1.5 h after an oral load. An oral dose of 1.5 g can raise the serum concentration by 0.5 mmol/L (1.5 mg/dL). There is no acute hormonal response to a single phosphate load; the excess is cleared principally by virtue of its surpassing the maximal transport capacity of the kidney. The normal diet does not contain large amounts of phosphate, so the problem of disposal of acute loads is rare.

Serum magnesium concentration is maintained largely independently of known calcitropic hormones. Magnesium exerts effects on PTH secretion similar in direction to those of calcium; however, the magnesium-related control is small in comparison to that of calcium under physiological conditions. The steady-state concentration of serum magnesium is determined principally by the threshold for renal excretion of magnesium (see Fig. 27–2). Intestinal absorption is a fixed fraction of dietary intake, and dramatic changes in intake are not normally encountered.

Steady State and Normal Variation

At zero net external mineral exchange (zero mineral balance), skeletal mineral apposition must equal skeletal mineral resorption.[2, 15] Calcium, magnesium, and phosphate content in urine approximates that of net intestinal absorption; losses by perspiration are negligible. Typical daily exchanges of calcium, magnesium, and phosphate in the body are illustrated in Figure 27–6. Many short-term and long-term deviations from the steady state occur. Some of the common ones are considered here.

After ingestion of calcium, total calcium concentration in plasma reaches a peak 2.5 to 3 h later; the maximal increase in total serum calcium concentration is approximately 0.25 mmol/L (1 mg/dL) after a large oral calcium load (25 mmol or 1000 mg). Because magnesium and phosphate are absorbed less efficiently than calcium in the duodenum, their net intestinal absorption varies less with sudden inputs (meals). Other nutrients interact with mineral home-

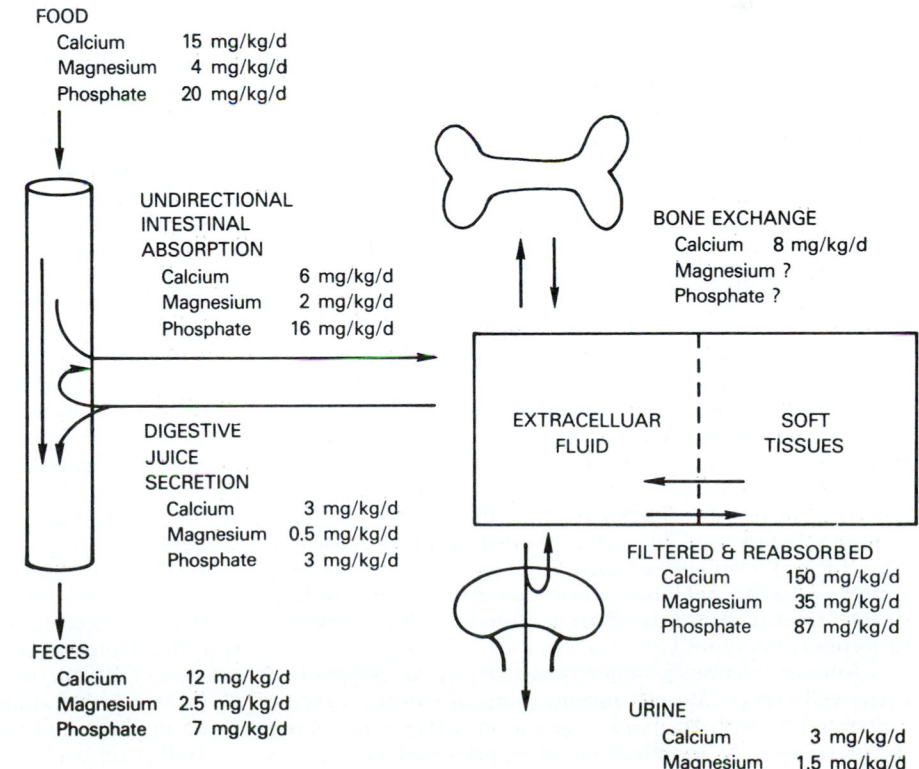

Figure 27–6. Typical daily exchanges of calcium, magnesium, and phosphate among anatomical compartments in adults.

ostasis. For example, carbohydrate loads influence changes in phosphate concentration because phosphate enters cells during glucose uptake.[16] Furthermore, the renal clearances of calcium and magnesium increase after an oral glucose load. The mediators of these changes are not known. CT secretion blunts the rise in serum calcium concentration after the administration of oral calcium loads to the rat. The increase in CT secretion may be controlled through hormones released by the intestines, because it occurs with minimal or no change in serum calcium concentration.[17]

Bone mineral mass is responsive to alterations in physical activity. Weightlessness or immobilization leads to net loss of mineral from skeletal stores. Prolonged immobilization, particularly during periods of high bone turnover, leads to loss of skeletal mineral with negative calcium balances of 5 mmol/d (200 mg/d) in adults. It causes hypercalciuria and sometimes nephrocalcinosis or hypercalcemia. The skeletal loss reflects increased mineral resorption rate and variable changes in mineral apposition.

Pregnancy and lactation influence maternal mineral homeostasis. The calcium demands of shell formation in fowl represent the extreme case.[18] In domestic chickens the calcium content of the eggshell is 50 mmol (2 g) or approximately 10% of the calcium mass of the maternal skeleton, yet the process of shell mineralization requires less than 24 h. In anticipation of shell formation, the chicken develops a specialized form of medullary bone with high mineral turnover rates. In comparison, the human neonate contains 500 to 750 mmol (20 to 30 g) of calcium; most mineralization occurs in the last trimester, requiring an average of 6 mmol (250 mg) of calcium daily during this period. A similar quantity is secreted each day in milk during normal lactation. Maternal skeletal turnover increases by approximately 50% in the second trimester, even before fetal mineral accumulation reaches high daily rates. Current recommendations are for an increase of maternal calcium intake by 400 mg/d during pregnancy and lactation; however, this practice may not be necessary because of high $1,25(OH)_2D$ levels and absorptive hypercalciuria in the first and second trimesters of pregnancy.[19]

Changes in bone mineral mass occur during growth and senescence. During the pubertal growth spurt, net daily positive calcium balance approximates 10 mmol/d (400 mg/d). Skeletal bone mass reaches a plateau in the third decade and then gradually falls. After the menopause, annual losses of skeletal mass average 1 to 2%/y in women, equivalent to 0.7 to 1.5 mmol (30 to 60 mg) calcium per day.

Calcium, Magnesium, and Phosphate in Cytosol

Each of these three ions is important in the metabolism of all cells, but little is known about regulation of their concentrations within the cells. The concentrations of magnesium and phosphate in cytoplasm are within an order of magnitude of those in plasma. Of the magnesium in cytosol, 50 to 90% is complexed to phosphate, citrate, and other anions such as the adenosine phosphates. In particular, enzymes utilizing ATP interact with it in the form of $MgATP^{2-}$. Phosphate is covalently incorporated in many proteins, lipids, and nucleic acids. Many enzymes undergo dramatic shifts in activity when modified by phosphorylation or dephosphorylation.

Ionized calcium has been measured in the cytoplasm of many cell types.[20] Basal concentrations are in the range of 100 nmol/L, with dramatic rises after plasma membrane depolarization or mobilization of sequestered intracellular calcium, as during muscle contraction. With small localized fluxes of calcium into the cytosol, the change in concentration is restricted to a portion of the cytosolic volume because of the limited mobility of calcium ions in cytoplasm and the effectiveness of calcium-sequestering systems that restore the cytosolic ionized calcium concentration to the baseline.

Ionized calcium in cytoplasm is under complex control, and calcium in turn modulates many functions, making it one of the cell's important second messengers. The processes that can increase the ionized calcium concentration in cytoplasm include electrical impulses, hormones, drugs, and intracellular signals. A small number of agents, such as somatostatin, decrease the ionized calcium concentration in cytosol. Cytosolic calcium carries information by interacting with proteins such as the calcium-binding proteins (see later), protein kinase C, and ion channels. A rise of cytosolic calcium concentration is central in activating secretion by most exocrine and endocrine cells; for example, in chromaffin cells synexin is a calcium-binding protein that promotes the secretory process. The parathyroid cell, showing decreased secretion with rise of extra- or intracellular calcium level, is an important exception to this rule.

Sudden rises of cytosolic calcium level result from rapid calcium influx to cytoplasm down its concentration gradient from one or more of several compartments (including extracellular fluid, sarcoplasmic reticulum, calciosome, and mitochondrion). Calcium may move down these gradients by ion channel opening or by less defined processes. Calcium can enter through ion-selective pores known as calcium channels; these can be opened or closed by electrical potential (voltage-gated channels) or by ligands such as hormones and drugs, many of which have widespread use in pharmacotherapy (calcium channel blockers).[21] The calcium channels have been subclassified with regard to their electrical properties and interactions with drugs; most or all calcium channel subtypes are multimeric structures with a principal transmembrane protein component that is homologous to a component of sodium channels and potassium channels.[22] Structurally related calcium channels have been identified in plasma membranes and in sarcoplasmic reticulum. Inositol 1,4,5-trisphosphate (IP_3) discharges calcium from a subset of cytoplasmic organelles (called calciosomes) that may or may not have distinct morphology; one IP_3 receptor protein shows striking homology to a principal calcium channel protein.[23] This calcium release process is the subject of intense study. Calcium may also be discharged into cytoplasm from mitochondria (see later).

Under certain circumstances the calcitropic hormones themselves use rises of cytoplasmic calcium level as a portion of their signaling mechanism. PTH can elevate the cytoplasmic calcium level in renal tubule cells and osteoblasts, CT can elevate the calcium level in bone cells, and $1,25(OH)_2D$ may cause either rapid (over minutes) or slow (over hours) increases of cytoplasmic calcium level in certain cells. The rapid PTH-induced changes in target cell calcium concentration may account for the early (first 60 min) drop in serum calcium level after PTH administration before mobilization of calcium from extracellular pools into plasma (Fig. 27–7).

Sudden drops of cytoplasmic calcium concentration reflect active or passive transport against the calcium gradient. Ca-ATPase enzymes in several membrane compartments (plasma membrane, sarcoplasmic reticulum) serve this function.[24] Their high affinity for calcium increases calcium efflux from cytosol whenever cytosolic calcium concentration rises. Calcium is also transported from cytoplasm by exchange with sodium; this low-calcium-affinity exchange may be important in the plasma membranes of excitable tissues and in mitochondrial membranes. In non-nucleated erythrocytes the plasma membrane calcium pump ejects calcium

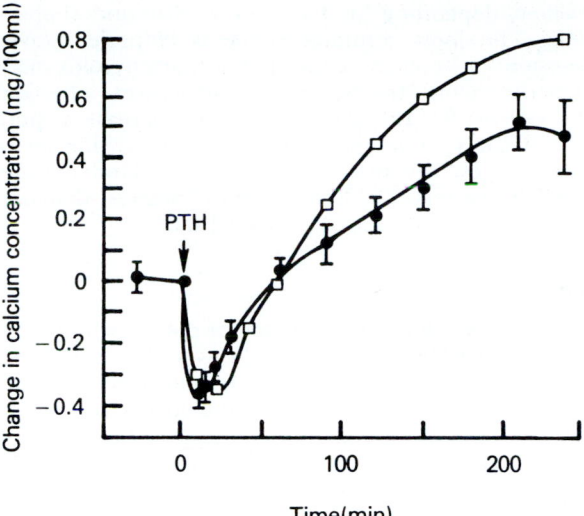

Figure 27–7. Comparison of extracellular calcium concentrations in response to PTH in vitro and in vivo. Serum calcium concentration change after administration of PTH to dogs (□); medium calcium concentration change after exposure of mouse calvaria bones to PTH (●). (Modified from JA Parsons, RM Neer, JT Potts Jr, Initial fall of plasma calcium after intravenous injection of parathyroid hormone, Endocrinology, 89, 735–740, 1971, © by The Endocrine Society, and from Robertson WG, Peacock M, Atkins D, et al. The effect of parathyroid hormone on the uptake and release of calcium by bone in tissue culture. Clin Sci 1972; 43:715–718.)

from the cytosol. In cardiac muscle cells the plasma membrane represents only 0.1% of the total membrane surface exposed to cytosol; in these cells the mitochondria and other organelles have a major role in mediating calcium efflux from cytosol. Contracted striated muscle relaxes with rapid removal of cytoplasmic calcium into sarcoplasmic reticulum. In many cells small changes in ionized calcium concentration can be buffered by the plasma membrane calcium pump or even by passive binding to calcium-binding proteins in the cytoplasm. At physiological concentrations of magnesium, calcium pumps in mitochondria and sarcoplasmic reticulum show reduced affinity for calcium. Because these organelles have a weak affinity but a high capacity for calcium, they are well suited for removal of calcium after ionized calcium concentration rises abruptly, as during striated muscle contraction.

Plasma membranes undergo complex interactions with cytosolic calcium. Not only do changes in membrane permeability and pump activity regulate calcium fluxes into and out of cytosol, but cytosolic calcium in turn affects several membrane properties. In the erythrocyte and in many other cells, an increased ionized calcium level in cytosol increases potassium permeability. In contrast, a large local rise in cytosolic calcium level to 5×10^{-5} mol/L in blowfly salivary gland cells leads to closure of intercellular plasma membrane pores, thereby isolating the cell from direct cytoplasmic contact with neighboring cells.

Generally, mitochondria contain most of the intracellular calcium. Large amounts of amorphous calcium phosphate can be sequestered in mitochondria without forming organized crystals. Mitochondrial calcium accumulation is particularly prominent in dystrophic cells or cells exposed to prolonged hypercalcemia; accumulation is also high in calcifying cartilage and in healing bone fractures. Mitochondria have a mechanism for active accumulation of calcium that is effective when cytoplasmic ionized calcium concentration is above normal (10^{-7} mol/L in squid axon). Factors that cause calcium discharge from mitochondria include sodium, phosphate, prostaglandins, and an oxidized state of the pyridine nucleotide equilibrium in the matrix or its coupled adenylate nucleotide equilibrium in the cytosol. Slow release of calcium by relatively oxidized mitochondria could activate a series of enzymes (phosphorylase kinase, pyruvate dehydrogenase phosphatase, lipases, and enzymes involved in mitochondrial oxidation of β-hydroxybutyrate) to restore reducing potential in the cell and its mitochondria.

Intracellular Calcium-Binding Proteins

Many cytoplasmic enzyme activites are sensitive to changes in ionized calcium concentration within the physiological range. These include adenylate cyclase, guanylate cyclase, cAMP phosphodiesterase, actomyosin ATPase, and protein kinase C. The types of modulation and the relative concentrations of these enzymes determine, in part, the message that changes in cytoplasmic calcium concentration will convey to the remainder of the cell. The calcium sensitivity of many enzymes is conveyed by interactions with regulatory proteins that have critical calcium binding sites (Fig. 27–8).[25] Changes in cytoplasmic ionized calcium concentration also regulate contractile proteins and thus affect processes such as striated muscle contraction, secretory gran-

Figure 27–8. Calcium as a cytoplasmic messenger. Extra- or intracellular signals change the ionized calcium concentration in cytosol until active pumps restore the basal concentration. This change in ionic calcium activity causes rapid conformational shifts in calcium-binding proteins (troponin C, vitamin D–dependent calcium-binding protein, and calmodulin) that modulate cytosol enzyme activities. The enzyme active site is schematized as a solid bar on the enzyme protein.

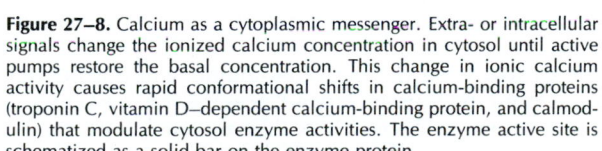

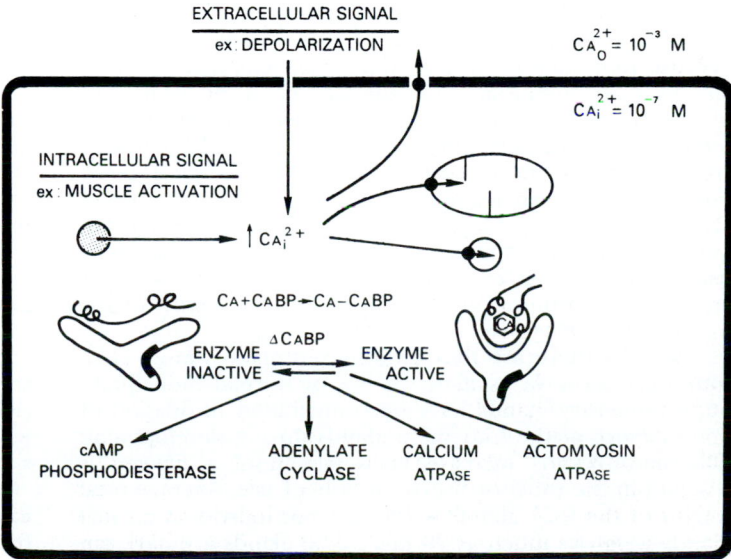

ule exocytosis, mitotic spindle function, and ciliary beating. Muscle contraction is effected by the sliding of actin and myosin filaments along their long axes, energized by ATP hydrolysis. This activity, actomyosin ATPase, is inhibited by a mixture of several cytosolic proteins (tropomyosin, troponin C, troponin I, and troponin T) in the absence of calcium. Increases in ionized calcium concentration to more than 10^{-7} mol/L abolish this inhibition. The actomyosin ATPase inhibitory activity is a property of the tropomyosin-troponin complex, whereas the calcium-dependent release from inhibition is a property of troponin C. Rabbit striated muscle troponin C contains four homologous regions (presumably the result of successive gene duplications) that bind divalent cations. Calcium binding to troponin C leads to conformational changes that modulate the interaction of tropomyosin with actomyosin ATPase. The amino acid sequences of C troponins from several species show homologies to the sequences of other major calcium-binding proteins (parvalbumins, myosin light chains, calmodulins, and vitamin D–dependent calcium-binding proteins). The vitamin D–dependent calcium-binding proteins are considered in more detail in the section on intestinal action of calciferol.

PARATHYROID GLANDS

Embryology

The parathyroid glands are derived from the endodermal germ layer of the third and fourth pairs of branchial pouches. The lower pair of glands develop (in association with the thymus) from the third branchial pouch. They migrate caudally with the thymus until, at the 18-mm embryo stage, they separate from the thymus and assume their final position at the lower pole of the thyroid gland. The upper parathyroids derive from the fourth (more caudal) branchial pouch but remain almost stationary during embryological development, accounting for their final location at the upper pole of the thyroid.

Anatomy

The upper parathyroids are usually located near the junction of the middle thyroid artery and the recurrent laryngeal nerve. They may be flattened against the posterior thyroid capsule or, rarely, embedded within the thyroid. Aberrant locations include the tracheoesophageal groove and retroesophageal space. The blood supply is from the inferior thyroid artery.

The lower parathyroids are more variable in position because they migrate farther during development. Generally, they are found lateral to the trachea at the lower pole of the thyroid, but they may be present in the anterior mediastinum in association with thymic tissue if separation from the thymus fails to occur during embryological development. Other aberrant locations[26] include the carotid sheath and, rarely, the pharyngeal submucosa (possibly related to failure to migrate caudally). The blood supply is usually from the inferior thyroid artery, but glands in the anterior mediastinum may be supplied by a branch of the internal mammary artery.

Usually there are four parathyroid glands. More than four may occur in as many as 6% of normal individuals. Supernumerary glands have been attributed to division of one or more of the four main glands during development. The parathyroids increase in weight until a plateau is reached in the third or fourth decade of life. Average total weight of the four glands is 120 mg, but individual normal glands weigh as much as 70 mg.[27] The glands are dark tan

to yellow, depending on fat content. Size and shape vary widely. The most common shape is ellipsoidal (average dimension: $6 \times 5 \times 2$ mm), but parathyroids may be flattened or elongated by adjacent structures. The content of fat cells within the glands begins to increase at puberty and continues to increase with age. According to early autopsy series, the normal parathyroid gland consists of about 50% stromal fat. Later studies[27] suggest that normal glands contain less than 20% stromal fat.

Histology

The chief cell is the major cell of the parathyroid gland and is responsible for PTH synthesis and secretion. Chief cells are usually arranged in cords and sheets within the gland, but follicular and acinar arrangements are sometimes observed.[28] The chief cell is 4 to 8 μm in diameter, with a small central nucleus containing dense chromatin. Chief cells have been segregated into two types on the basis of ultrastructural appearance. The "active" chief cell contains parallel arrays of endoplasmic reticulum in which the precursor protein of PTH is synthesized. A prominent Golgi region (the probable site of hormone packaging) and membrane-bound granules (presumed to contain PTH) are present. There are generally few secretory granules, and little hormone is stored in the cell. Secretion occurs as granule membranes fuse with the plasma membrane. Microtubules in the cell may be important in movement of secretory granules toward the cell periphery. Secretory mechanisms are discussed subsequently.

The "inactive" chief cell contains a dispersed endoplasmic reticulum, a smaller Golgi region, abundant glycogen-containing vacuoles, and lipofuscin granules. In the normal gland the ratio of inactive to active chief cells is about 3:1, but in suppressed glands the ratio may approach 10:1. There is a continuous cycle from active to inactive forms of chief cell (including transitional forms).

Oxyphil cells appear after puberty. They are 6 to 10 μm in diameter and contain a small central pyknotic nucleus, bright eosinophilic cytoplasm, and abundant mitochondria. Oxyphil cells usually show a sparse endoplasmic reticulum and a poorly developed Golgi region and normally may not secrete PTH. Oxyphil cells, which increase in number with age, may represent a degenerative form of chief cell.

PARATHYROID HORMONE

Chemistry

PTH was purified in 1959, about 35 years after the first active extract of PTH was prepared by Collip. The principal form of PTH stored in and released from the parathyroid glands is an 84-amino-acid, single chain polypeptide that is synthesized within the parathyroid gland through precursor forms. After secretion into the circulation, the hormone is metabolized to smaller polypeptide fragments that are inactive.

The structures of the native 84-amino-acid polypeptide hormones from the human, bovine, porcine, rat, and chicken species are shown in Table 27–5. The molecules are similar in charge and length and are highly homologous. Also shown is the NH_2-terminal portion of the PTH-related peptide (PTHRP) responsible for certain hypercalcemias associated with malignancies.[29] It activates PTH receptors but does not share immunoreactivity with the PTHs.

Certain other chemical properties[30, 31] are also of significance. The NH_2-terminal third of the molecule is critical for binding of the hormone to specific receptors on cells,

TABLE 27–5. Structure of Parathyroid Hormones*

					10															20					
hPTHRP	A	—	—	—	H	—	—	L	—	D	K	—	—	S	I	Q	D	L	R	—	R	F	F	—	H
hPTH	S	V	S	E	I	Q	L	M	H	N	L	G	K	H	L	N	S	M	E	R	V	E	W	L	R
bPTH	A	—	—	—	—	—	—	—	—	—	—	—	—	—	—	—	—	—	—	—	—	—	—	—	—
pPTH	—	—	—	—	—	—	—	—	—	—	—	—	—	—	L	—	—	—	—	—	—	—	—	—	—
rPTH	A	—	—	—	—	—	—	—	—	—	—	—	—	A	—	V	—	—	M	Q	—	—	—	—	—
cPTH	—	—	—	—	M	—	—	—	—	E	—	R	H	T	V	—	—	G	D	—	—	Q			

				30										40								50		
hPTHRP	H	L	I	A	E	I	—	T	A	E	I	R	A	T	S	E	V	S	P	N	S	K	P	S
hPTH	K	K	L	Q	D	V	H	N	F	V	A	L	G	A	P	L	A	P	R	D	A	G	S	Q	R
bPTH	—	—	—	—	—	—	—	—	—	—	—	—	S	I	—	Y	R	—	G	S	—	—	—	—
pPTH	—	—	—	—	—	—	—	—	—	—	—	—	S	I	V	H	—	G	—	—	—	—
rPTH	—	—	—	—	—	—	—	S	—	—	V	Q	M	—	A	—	E	G	S	Y
cPTH	M	—	—	—	—	S	A	L	E	.	.	.	.	D	—	R	T

					60									70						
hPTHRP	—	N	T	—	N	H	P	—	R	F	G	S	D	D	E	G	R	Y	L	T	.	.	.	.	.
hPTH	P	R	K	K	E	D	N	V	L	V	E	S	H	E	K	S	L	G	E	A	.	.	.	.	.
bPTH	—	—	—	—	—	—	—	—	—	—	Q	—	—	—	—	—	—	—	—	.	.	.	.
pPTH	—	—	—	—	—	—	—	—	—	—	Q	—	—	—	—	—	—	—	—	.	.	.	.
rPTH	—	T	—	—	E	—	—	—	—	D	G	N	S	—	—	—	—	G	.	.	.	.
cPTH	—	—	N	—	—	I	—	—	G	—	I	R	N	R	R	—	L	P	E	H	L	R	A	A

									80											90			
hPTHRP	.	.	.	.	.	.	.	.	E	T	N	K	—	E	T	Y	K	E	Q	P	L	K	T	P	G	K	K	K	K
hPTH	.	.	.	.	.	.	.	.	D	K	A	D	V	N	V	L	T	K	A	K	S	Q
bPTH	.	.	.	.	.	.	.	—	—	—	—	—	D	—	—	I	—	—	—	P	—
pPTH	.	.	.	.	.	.	.	—	—	—	—	—	D	—	—	I	—	—	—	P	—
rPTH	.	.	.	.	.	.	.	—	—	—	—	—	D	—	—	V	—	—	—	P	—
cPTH	V	Q	K	K	S	I	D	L	—	—	—	Y	M	—	—	—	P	—	T	—	P	.

*Complete amino acid sequences of human parathyroid hormone–related peptide (hPTHRP), human PTH (hPTH), bovine PTH (bPTH), porcine PTH (pPTH), rat PTH (rPTH), and chicken PTH (cPTH). Single-letter codes for amino acids are shown. The numbering system refers to the mammalian peptides. Chicken PTH is longer (lengthened in segment 61–71 and shortened in segment 32–45) than the mammalian PTHs. Only the first 91 amino acids of the total of 141 amino acids are shown for human PTHRP. The latter shares 50% homology with the parathyroid hormones in the first 16 amino acids.

See refs. 25–27 and 34 and Heinrich GK, Kronenberg HM, Potts JT Jr, et al. Gene encoding parathyroid hormone. Nucleotide sequence of the rat gene and deduced amino acid sequence of rat preproparathyroid hormone. J Biol Chem 1984; 259:3320–3223; and Khosla S, Demay M, Pines M, et al. Nucleotide sequence of cloned cDNAS encoding chicken preproparathyroid hormone. J Bone Miner Res 1988; 3:689–698.

for activation of adenylate cyclase, and for biological activity. Removal of the two NH_2-terminal amino acids destroys biological activity but not receptor-binding activity. Binding to the receptor depends on two regions within the molecule (residues 10 to 27 and 25 to 34). The latter regions are highly conserved among the species of PTH. The sequence 1 to 27 is the minimum required for detectable biological activity. Synthetic polypeptides encompassing the first 34 amino acids generally are fully as active (and some analogues more active) on a molar basis as the entire sequence 1 to 84. The bovine hormone can be iodinated to the extent of 1 mol/mol of polypeptide on the single tyrosine (position 43) residue with retention of biological activity. Oxidation of the methionines in the NH_2 terminus destroys biological activity; substitution of norleucine for methionine yields synthetic peptides resistant to oxidative inactivation. Many antisera developed against intact human, porcine, or bovine PTH recognize predominantly the COOH-terminal antigenic sites of the hormone. Removal of even a single NH_2-terminal amino acid causes more than 90% loss of biological potency but little or no loss of reactivity with such antisera. These features account for marked discrepancies found in the past between biological and immunological reactivity of peptide fragments of the hormone identified in gland extracts and in plasma. A synthetic peptide lacking two amino acids (Ala-Ser) at the NH_2 terminus is a competitive inhibitor of PTH action in vitro, and an analogue with residues 7 to 34 is a low-affinity blocker of PTH action in vivo.[30]

Bioassay of Parathyroid Hormone

The original bioassay devised by Collip and Clark was based on the hormone-induced rise in serum calcium concentration of dogs. This method allowed development of the first active extract of parathyroid glands. The in vivo assays now used commonly are based on serum calcium measurements in parathyroidectomized rats or in calcium-injected chicks or quail (Table 27–6). The most commonly used in vitro assay depends on activation of renal adenylate cyclase in response to PTH. In this assay the conversion of ^{32}P-labeled ATP to radioactive cAMP is determined in vitro. These various bioassays have been utilized in evaluating the biological activity of synthetic parathyroid-related polypeptides. Results obtained with these methods generally agree. Certain synthetic hormone analogues, however, may show discrepant results (e.g., peptides shortened at the NH_2 terminus are more active in the chick than in the rat hypercalcemia assay). These discrepancies, as well as those between in vitro and in vivo assays, represent in part differences in distribution and metabolism of the several peptides in the different systems.

Bioassay of Hormone in Plasma

The highly sensitive technique of quantitative cytochemistry allows detection of hormone at dilutions 100 to 1000 times greater than those used in other bioassays. This method is the only one that has been applicable to date for bioassays of PTH in plasma. This assay for PTH is based on determination of the activity of glucose-6-phosphate dehydrogenase, an enzyme specifically activated by PTH, in the distal convoluted tubules of the guinea pig kidney. Active PTH can be detected at the femtogram level, corresponding to 1:1000 dilutions of normal human plasma. Unfortunately, the technique is cumbersome and time-consuming and is not likely to find clinical utility. Other methods that can be applied in concentrated plasma are the modified adenylate cyclase assay[32] and the modified cAMP assay using rat osteosarcoma cells in vitro.[33]

TABLE 27–6. Bioassays for Parathyroid Hormone

Preparation	Parameter	Dose Range (USP U/Animal or U/mL)
Parathyroidectomized rat	Serum calcium	5–40
Calcium-injected chick or quail	Serum calcium	1–12
Mouse calvaria	Calcium release in vitro	0.01–1.0
Rat long bone	^{45}Ca release in vitro	0.01–1.0
Mouse calvaria	$^{14}CO_2$ produced in vitro from ^{14}C-citrate	0.0025–0.15
Renal adenylate cyclase	^{32}P-cyclic 3′,5′-AMP produced from ^{32}P-ATP	1.4–12
Renal adenylate amplified with GppNHp	^{32}P-cyclic 3′,5′-AMP produced from ^{32}P-AMP	10^{-4}–10^{-2}*
Isolated bone cells	Cyclic 3′,5′-AMP	0.1–2.0
Rat osteosarcoma cells†	Cyclic 3′,5′-AMP	10^{-4}
Guinea pig kidney segments‡	Glucose-6-phosphate dehydrogenase cytochemical determination	10^{-10}–10^{-6}

*Nissenson RA, Abbott SR, Teitelbaum AP, et al. Endogenous biologically active human parathyroid hormone: measurement by a guanyl nucleotide-amplified renal adenylate cyclase assay. J Clin Endocrinol Metab 1981; 52:840–846.

†Pines M, Santora A, Spiegel A. Effects of phorbol esters and pertussis toxin on agonist-stimulated cyclic AMP production in rat osteosarcoma cells. Biochem Pharmacol 1986; 35:3639–3641.

‡Fenton S, Somers S, Heath DA. Preliminary studies with the sensitive cytochemical assay for parathyroid hormone. Clin Endocrinol 1978; 9:381–384; and Chambers DJ, Dunham J, Zanelli M, et al. A sensitive bioassay of parathyroid hormone in plasma. Clin Endocrinol 1978; 9:375–379.

References for other methods may be found in Aurbach GD, Chase LR. In: Greep RO, Astwood EB, eds. Handbook of Physiology. Sect 7: Endocrinology. Vol VII. Parathyroid Gland. Bethesda: American Physiological Society, 1977: 353–381.

IMMUNOREACTIVITY AND IMMUNOASSAY OF PARATHYROID HORMONE. Domains that are immunogenic within polypeptides do not necessarily correspond to the segments specifically required for biological activity. Thus radioimmunoassay for any polypeptide hormone activity does not necessarily reflect the bioactivity. PTH is one polypeptide showing striking divergences between biological and immunological reactivities. Multiple types of immunoreactive fragments of PTH are present in the circulation. The first observation suggesting heterogeneity of PTH-immunoreactive material in the circulation was reported by Berson and Yalow (reviewed in refs. 30, 31). They developed two different antisera to bovine PTH. With one antiserum the apparent half-life of the hormone in the circulation was long. The other antiserum detected a peptide that rapidly disappears from the plasma after parathyroidectomy. They concluded that more than one form of PTH is present in the circulation. Furthermore they found that the half-life of both forms of the hormone was prolonged in uremic subjects and that the hormone extracted from human parathyroids differed in immunological reactivity from that in the circulation. These observations were followed by others in several laboratories, with the following general conclusions: (1) Immunological reactivity in bovine and human glands differs from that in the general circulation. (2) The discrepancies vary in degree depending on the antiserum used. (3) In some instances, the immunological reactivity secreted into medium by parathyroid explants differs from that extracted directly from the explant; these discrepancies are common in long-term (greater than 24 h) incubations in vitro. (4) Gel filtration (a means of separation of molecules by size) of peripheral plasma indicates that immunoreactive PTHRPs of different sizes are present in the circulation. (5) Selective antisera directed specifically at the NH₂ terminus, at the midregion of the molecule, or at the COOH-terminal region

provide discrepant estimates of PTH concentration in the peripheral circulation.

RADIOIMMUNOASSAYS FOR CLINICAL USE. COOH-terminal–, midregion–, and NH₂-terminal–"specific" radioimmunoassays have been developed by immunization with synthetic parathyroid peptides or with intact PTH. The most clinically useful assays are the NH₂-terminal assays and the midregion assays.[34–36] The midregion assays are preferable to COOH-terminal assays in providing higher sensitivity (up to 100% of normal subjects show detectable activity), more facile assay characteristics, and closer correlation with clinical state.

Highly sensitive and specific two-site immunoassays have been developed that allow detection of "intact" PTH (form secreted from the gland) and circumvent many of the problems of earlier radioimmunoassays. These methods utilize two independent antibodies, one developed against NH₂-terminal PTH peptides and the other against mid- or COOH-terminal sequences, plus highly sensitive immunoradiometric or chemiluminescence detection systems. This technology provides analyses tantamount to those obtained by bioassay and permits determination of even the minute concentrations of hormone in hypoparathyroid plasma. Correlation with clinical state is excellent (see section on hyperparathyroidism).

Biosynthesis

The base sequences for the entire coding regions of the genes for human, bovine, rodent and avian PTH have been determined by using complementary DNA (cDNA) copies of messenger RNA (mRNA). These analyses[31, 37] (also see Table 27–5) confirm by an independent method the sequences obtained by peptide analytical techniques. PTH is synthesized on the ribosome first as a 110-amino-acid chain polypeptide called pre-proPTH.[30, 38] This form of the hormone was first identified in in vitro experiments utilizing purified bovine PTH mRNA in a cell-free wheat germ extract capable of carrying out mRNA-directed peptide synthesis. The pre-pro form of the hormone is illustrated in Figure 27–9. In the intact parathyroid cell, proPTH and PTH are synthesized. The amino acids constituting the

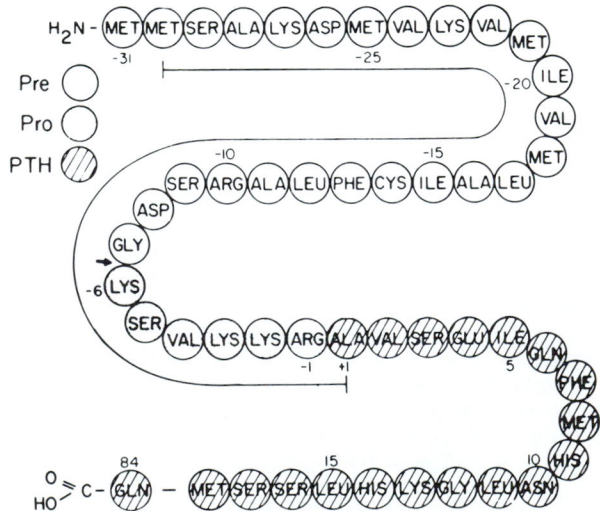

Figure 27–9. Structures of biosynthetic intermediates of PTH. Pre-proPTH is the form in which the molecule is biosynthesized on the ribosomes and includes residues −31 to 84. This form is rapidly converted to proPTH (residues −6 to 84), which is then converted to PTH, the form stored in and elaborated from secretory granules in the gland. See also Figure 27–10. (From Habener JF, Kemper BW, Rich A, et al. Biosynthesis of parathyroid hormone. Recent Prog Horm Res 1977; 33:249–308.)

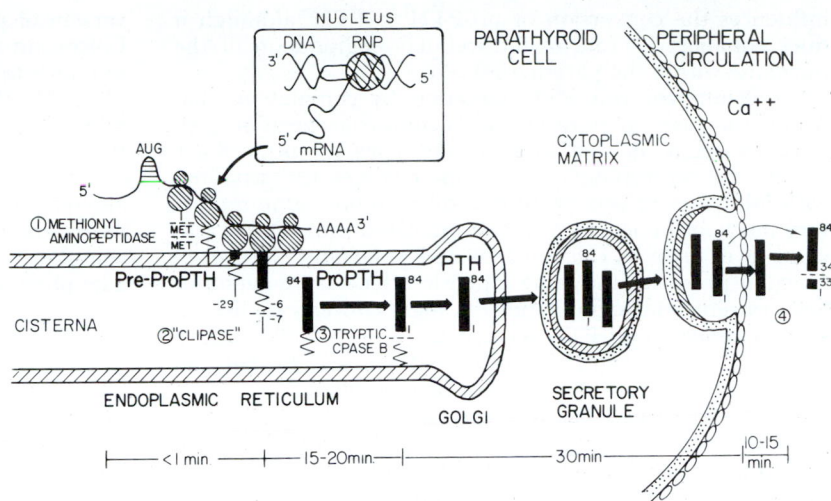

Figure 27–10. Scheme depicting biosynthesis of precursor and secretory forms of PTH. The pre-proPTH form is biosynthesized on the ribosome and then transported across the membranes of the endoplasmic reticulum with concomitant cleavage to the pro form of the hormone. The pre-pro segment may serve a transport function in translocating the biosynthetic precursor across the endoplasmic reticulum membrane. Within the cisterna of the endoplasmic reticulum, the prohormone is converted to the 84-amino-acid PTH for packaging in secretory granules. This PTH molecule is elaborated from secretory granules into the circulation for subsequent interaction with specific PTH receptors in target tissues. The hormone also undergoes degradation to inert forms after secretion from the gland. In addition, some fragments of the molecule may be elaborated directly into the circulation from the parathyroid gland. (From Habener JF, Kemper BW, Rich A, et al. Biosynthesis of parathyroid hormone. Recent Prog Horm Res 1977; 33:249–308.)

additional 25-amino-acid leader peptide representing the pre-prohormone are probably removed as the synthesized polypeptide is released from the cytoplasmic matrix of the rough endoplasmic reticulum. A synthetic analogue of the leader sequence blocks processing of pre-proPTH to proPTH. The pre sequence is hydrophobic and probably facilitates movement of the nascent peptides onto or across membranes. The structure of the COOH-terminal portion of this segment is critical for proper processing of pre-proPTH to PTH.[39] Figure 27–10 depicts the possible intracellular pathway for biosynthesis of PTH. After biosynthesis, proPTH is converted by another proteolytic process to PTH in the Golgi region of the cell. Transport from the Golgi region may involve microtubular function in that vinblastine and colchicine inhibit the conversion of the proPTH to PTH and cause accumulation of the prohormone. PTH synthesized in parathyroid glands is processed by this sequence (Fig. 27–11).[38, 40] The prohormone contains six additional amino acids at the NH_2 terminus (see Fig. 27–9). ProPTH possesses little biological activity (less than 0.2% of that of native hormone). Thus conversion of prohormone within the gland to native hormone generates a potent polypeptide from one that is inactive.

Secretion of Parathyroid Hormone

The concentration of calcium in the circulation is an important factor for PTH secretion. This concept is based on analyses by bioassay or radioimmunoassay of secreted hormone as well as on determination of peptides secreted by glands in vitro. In addition to calcium, biological amines, peptides, steroids, and several classes of drugs influence PTH secretion.[41, 42]

cAMP AND PARATHYROID HORMONE SECRETION. Although calcium is the major factor controlling secretion, cAMP is an important cellular regulator of PTH secretion. Dopamine and epinephrine stimulate PTH secretion in cattle. Beta-adrenergic catecholamines, dopamine, secretin, and prostaglandin E_2 each activate adenylate cyclase and cause increased concentrations of cAMP in parathyroid cells or tissue slices in vitro. In addition, some adenomatous or hyperplastic human parathyroid cells respond to glucagon, vasoactive intestinal peptide, and histamine.[41, 43] Inhibitors of cyclic-nucleotide phosphodiesterase also stimulate release of PTH. Conversely, agents that inhibit PTH release or secretion (e.g., calcium, alpha-adrenergic catecholamines, and prostaglandin $F_{2\alpha}$) inhibit cAMP accumulation in parathyroid cells. Thus PTH secretion appears to be intimately related to cAMP content of parathyroid tissue. The major

effects of ions and related agents in controlling secretion, however, are by mechanisms outside the cAMP pathway (see later). cAMP seems to influence secretion from a preformed hormone pool, presumably that stored in mature secretory granules. Calcium, on the other hand, controls secretion of newly synthesized as well as preformed pools of hormone.[44] The parathyroid cell contains cAMP-regulated protein kinase,[8] and at least two parathyroid cell membrane proteins become phosphorylated in response to kinase activation by cAMP generation.[45]

EFFECTS OF IONS ON SECRETION. Calcium is the major regulator of PTH secretion. The precise mechanism whereby calcium exerts this effect has not been established. Part of the effect may be mediated by a decrease in cAMP content through calcium stimulation of calmodulin-activated phosphodiesterase. This mechanism, however, cannot account for the major effect of calcium in inhibiting parathyroid secretion. The effect of calcium on cAMP accumulation is less marked than its capacity to inhibit PTH release.[41] Calcium does not affect acutely the rate of synthesis of PTH, but over a period of days changes in calcium concentration regulate (hypocalcemia stimulates) steady-state concentrations of PTH mRNA.[46] There is no evidence that calcium

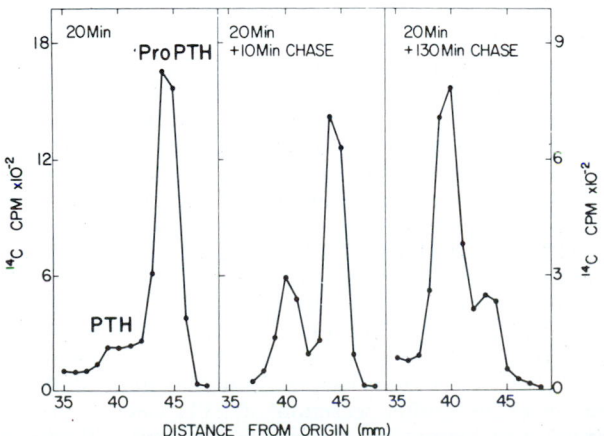

Figure 27–11. Biosynthesis of proPTH and conversion to PTH. Analyses by gel electrophoresis were carried out at the intervals shown after adding radioactive amino acids to parathyroid gland slices. This illustrates early production of radioactive proPTH and later appearance of radioactivity on PTH molecules. (From Habener JF, Kemper BW, Rich et al. Biosynthesis of parathyroid hormone. Recent Prog Horm Res 1977; 33:249–308, as adapted from Kemper B, Habener J, Potts JT Jr, et al. Proparathyroid hormone: identification of a biosynthetic precursor to parathyroid hormone. Proc Natl Acad Sci USA 69:643–649, 1972.)

influences the conversion of proPTH to PTH, although it does enhance the rate of intracellular degradation of the hormone within the parathyroid cell.

Calcium controls PTH secretion by complex mechanisms. Increases in extracellular calcium concentration produce transient as well as sustained rises in intracellular calcium concentration,[42, 47] and these changes are associated with inhibitory effects of calcium on secretion. One regulatory mechanism activated by the increased intracellular calcium level involves calcium-activated potassium channels.[48] Calcium produces the same biphasic effects (stimulation at low concentrations, inhibition at high concentrations) on such channels as on PTH secretion.[48] The calcium-sensitive potassium channel in the parathyroid cell may explain the depolarizing response[49] of these cells to calcium.

Changes in ECF calcium level also induce a rise in the intracellular level of IP$_3$, a mediator that causes mobilization of intracellular stores of calcium.[50]* Activators of protein kinase C activity (phorbol esters and diacylglycerol) also increase IP$_3$ and intracellular calcium levels. Specifically, calcium promotes mobilization of this kinase to the cell membrane,[51] and a consequence in the parathyroid cell is phosphorylation of two proteins of molecular mass 20 and 100 kd, respectively.[52] Whether these phosphoproteins are involved in regulating secretion is unknown.

Effects of extracellular calcium on both IP$_3$ and intracellular calcium appear to be mediated through a cell membrane signaling system. These observations have led to the concept that a cell-surface "receptor" for calcium is required for transmitting the signal.[42, 47] Interaction with voltage-regulated calcium channels is also involved,[53, 54] and such channels might be the receptors of concern. Further, transmission of the calcium signal across the membrane may require a GTP-binding protein (G protein) because incubation with pertussis toxin blocks the calcium signal at some point beyond interaction with the calcium channel.[53] Moreover, GTP and analogues can stimulate hormone release in permeabilized cells,[42] implying further that G proteins are involved in PTH secretion.

EFFECTS OF OTHER FACTORS ON PTH SECRETION. A number of divalent and trivalent ions affect secretion in a manner similar to calcium, albeit at varying apparent affinities. Magnesium, strontium, manganese, barium, and lanthanum may act through the same receptor as calcium, although there are differences between their effects and those of calcium. Lithium increases secretion and decreases sensitivity of the parathyroid cell to inhibition by calcium.[42] Potassium stimulates secretion; increases in cellular sodium concentration in response to ouabain suppress secretion.[55, 56]

In summary, considerable progress has been made in understanding calcium regulation of PTH secretion. This phenomenon, however, is complex and involves more than one intracellular signaling processes. There is still too little information to formulate an overall integrated scheme to explain calcium regulation of PTH secretion.

EFFECTS OF OTHER AGENTS ACTING AT THE SUBCELLULAR LEVEL. Microtubules and microfilaments are important for several types of cellular function, including intracellular transport and release of secretory products. Certain classes of drugs, colchicine, and vinblastine cause disruption of microtubular and microfilamentous function. Vinblastine and colchicine inhibit secretion of PTH (see ref. 41 for a review). Colchicine and vinblastine interfere with the con-

version of proPTH to PTH in the bovine parathyroid cell. Colchicine also is known to cause hypocalcemia in vivo and to interfere with the peripheral action of PTH.

EFFECTS OF OTHER DRUGS, HORMONES, AND VITAMINS. 1,25(OH)$_2$D inhibits release of PTH and suppresses the cellular content of PTH mRNA.[57] Several amines, including tromethamine (TRIS), diethylamine, and lysine amide, interfere with conversion of proPTH to PTH in vitro. These amines may interfere at the level of the Golgi complex. Vitamin A and cortisol stimulate PTH secretion. The physiological significance of these effects is not known.

Nature of Products Released from Parathyroid Glands

The major biologically active product secreted from the parathyroid gland is the 84-amino-acid hormone.[31] In addition, other immunoactive peptides are released, including NH$_2$-terminal and COOH-terminal fragments. The proportion of COOH-terminal fragments is increased in hypercalcemia.[58] PTH is a substrate for protein kinases in the parathyroid cell, and some of the secreted peptides may be phosphorylated. Perhaps some of the heterogeneity of PTH is engendered by these phosphorylated derivatives of the hormone.

Another product, parathyroid secretory protein (molecular mass 70 kd),[59, 60] is secreted in response to calcium or magnesium in a manner similar to PTH. Parathyroid secretory protein, a glycosylated protein, is similar or identical to chromogranin-A in secretory granules of the adrenal medulla.[61] Carbohydrate is added just before secretion, suggesting that glycosylation is involved in processing of secretory granules or in secretion itself. Parathyroid secretory protein can also undergo phosphorylation within the cell, and part of this protein is elaborated from the cell in the phospho form.[62]

Metabolism of Parathyroid Hormone

Multiple immunoreactive forms of PTH circulate in plasma and include fragments of approximately 5.5 to 7 kd. The liver, kidney, and parathyroid gland generate similar fragments, at least in vitro.[63–65] Cathepsin-like enzymes catalyze cleavage of the native hormone to such forms in the parathyroid gland[66] and in Kupffer cells.[65] Indeed the latter can generate biologically active NH$_2$-terminal peptides from PTH(1–84).[65] The parathyroid gland itself does not release NH$_2$-terminal fragments of the hormone. Although bioactive NH$_2$-terminal products of PTH(1–84) can be generated in vitro, normally there are no circulating bioactive fragments of the hormone.[67, 68]* Virtually all bioactive hormone in plasma represents PTH(1–84), the form of the hormone secreted from the gland. Moreover, with the two-site immunoassays (see section on hyperparathyroidism) that do not detect immunologically reactive fragments, the problems with early radioimmunoassays created by metabolism of the secreted hormone have been circumvented.

Physiology

The primary function of PTH is to control calcium concentration in the ECF. The concentration of calcium is a function of the rate of transfer of calcium into and out of bone, the GF, and the gastrointestinal tract (see Fig. 27–6). PTH stimulates the reabsorption of calcium from the GF, enhances calcium resorption from bone, and influences

---

*On the other hand, under certain conditions changes in intracellular calcium and IP$_3$ levels are dissociated from effects on secretion. Moreover, pertussis toxin does not inhibit calcium effects on IP$_3$ and intracellular calcium. However, some G proteins are not substrates for pertussis toxin–catalyzed ADP-ribosylation.

*A smaller circulating bioactive component is present only in severe renal failure.[68]

absorption of calcium from the gastrointestinal tract secondarily through its influence on the renal formation of active vitamin D metabolites. Although the overall influence of PTH on these three tissues—kidney, bone, and gut—is to increase the calcium level in the ECF, the effects of the hormone on the different tissues do not occur simultaneously. The effect on the kidney is the most rapid, and clearance of calcium increases promptly after removal of the parathyroid glands.[69] Changes in resorption of calcium from bone in vitro occur in two phases.[70] The earlier phase is manifested by release of calcium within 2 to 3 h after addition of PTH and does not depend on protein synthesis. The later phase presumably involves biosynthesis of new proteins, particularly lysosomal enzymes, including collagenase and other hydrolytic enzymes, and is blocked by inhibitors of protein synthesis. In vivo the hypercalcemic effect of enhanced absorption of calcium from the gut is relatively slow to develop. This phenomenon depends on formation of active vitamin D metabolites, which reach intestinal cells through the circulation. In the intestinal cells the metabolites induce synthesis of new proteins, in particular proteins involved in calcium and phosphate transport across the intestinal wall. This indirect effect of the hormone on calcium absorption from the gut develops over a period of 24 h or longer.

PTH influences phosphate concentration in the ECF through two mechanisms. A reduction in plasma phosphate is produced by the direct phosphaturic action of PTH on the kidney, the predominant effect of the hormone under usual conditions.[69] A rise in plasma phosphate level may follow massive hormone-induced bone resorption with increased release of phosphate and other minerals from bone. If renal function is impaired, this effect may predominate. PTH also causes an increase in urinary hydroxyproline excretion, secondary to effects on collagen metabolism.

EFFECTS OF PARATHYROID HORMONE ON KIDNEY

Calcium Reabsorption. Excessive secretion of PTH causes a rise in urinary calcium excretion. This effect is secondary to the hypercalcemia (and thus a high filtered load of calcium) produced by the hormone. The direct action of the hormone on the kidney is to enhance fractional reabsorption of calcium from the GF. This renal effect is readily apparent in experiments in which calcium clearance is measured at various plasma calcium concentrations with or without the influence of PTH. At any given calcium load, calcium clearance is decreased under the influence of PTH and is increased in the absence of parathyroid secretion. Thus in the first few hours after parathyroidectomy the urinary excretion of calcium increases. It is not until hypocalcemia has developed that urinary calcium excretion decreases. The renal effect of PTH is especially apparent in the golden hamster, which is extremely sensitive to this function of PTH. Parathyroidectomy in this animal causes a marked loss of calcium into the urine, and the hypocalcemia attendant on parathyroidectomy is due to the increased renal loss. In humans, PTH also regulates the reabsorption of calcium from the GF. Measurement of renal clearance of calcium as a function of serum calcium level can provide a useful clinical parameter (Fig. 27–12).

Calcium clearance is closely linked to sodium clearance in the kidney,[71] and calcium and sodium transports may be coupled, particularly in the proximal tubule. Replacement of sodium by choline or lithium inhibits calcium reabsorption in the proximal tubule, and ouabain, which inhibits Na^+,K^+-ATPase, abolishes active calcium reabsorption in the kidney of the golden hamster. The bulk of calcium is reabsorbed in the proximal tubule, and in that segment PTH actually decreases calcium absorption. The major physiological effect of PTH (i.e., enhancement of calcium reabsorption) occurs

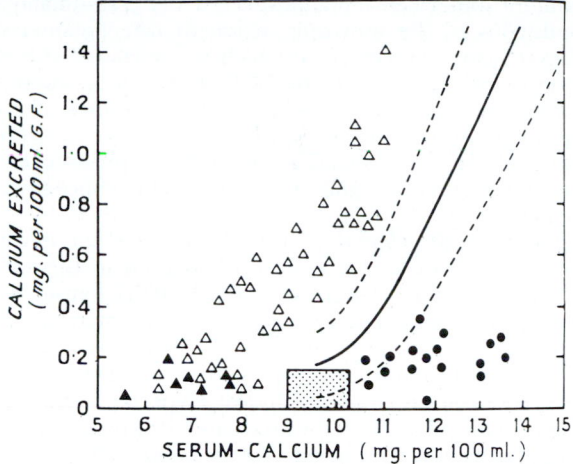

Figure 27–12. Urinary excretion of calcium as a function of serum calcium concentration in normal subjects (solid line; dashed lines show ±2 SD) and in patients with hypoparathyroidism (△, ▲) and hyperparathyroidism (●). Shaded area represents the normal physiological situation. (From Nordin BEC, Peacock M. Role of the kidney in regulation of plasma-calcium. Lancet 1969; 2:1280–1283.)

beyond the proximal tubule in the thick ascending and the granular portions of the distal tubule.[72, 73] cAMP is the intracellular mediator of this effect.[73–76]

Phosphaturic Effect. The enhancement of phosphate excretion was among the first physiological effects of PTH discovered. The mechanism of this effect appears to involve actions at distinct loci within the nephron in the proximal and distal convoluted tubules. The phosphaturic effect is thought to result from a direct inhibition of phosphate transport (sodium-dependent phosphate transport).[77] An additional action may be secondary to changes in reabsorption of sodium or bicarbonate (or both). In the dog, PTH causes a 30 to 40% reduction in proximal tubular reabsorption of sodium and phosphate, although this results in minimal or undetectable natriuresis. Infusion of dibutyryl cAMP has a similar effect on proximal reabsorption of sodium and phosphate. Thus PTH causes a net decrease in proximal reabsorption of phosphate, and this effect is mediated through cAMP generation.[77, 78] In addition, there is a distal tubular effect of PTH that similarly produces decreased reabsorption of phosphate.[72]

Sodium reabsorption is inhibited by PTH in the proximal tubule,[72] and inhibition of phosphate reabsorption appears to be dependent on sodium. Dibutyryl cAMP has a similar influence on sodium and phosphate in the proximal tubule, and cAMP regulates sodium transport in a number of tissues. Phosphaturia may also be affected by changes in intraluminal pH or proximal transport of bicarbonate. Increases in pH and bicarbonate content of the urine were also among the earliest physiological effects observed for PTH. PTH enhances bicarbonate clearance (see later) and also decreases intracellular pH through a cAMP mechanism that regulates an Na^+/H^+ antiporter in kidney cells.[79] A rise in pH would change the ratio of HPO_4^{2-} to $H_2PO_4^-$ and consequently decrease the likelihood of reabsorption of phosphate; monovalently charged phosphate is more readily translocated across cell membranes than is the divalently charged ion. Phosphate permeability is less in the distal than in the proximal nephron; thus phosphate rejected by any mechanism in the proximal tubule causes increased elaboration of phosphate into the urine. Micropuncture studies have identified a direct action of the hormone on inhibition of phosphate reabsorption in the distal tubule.[72] Another factor in the phosphaturic effect is a general increase in proximal tubular cell metabolism by PTH. Presumably this is analogous to the inotropic action of catecholamines on perfused heart preparations, which is associated with elaboration of phosphate into the ECF. This is a manifestation of increased utilization of ATP, because the rate of elaboration of phosphate into the ECF corresponds to a decrease in intracellular concentration of creatine phosphate (the intracellular reservoir that maintains ATP concentrations constant).

Effects on Bicarbonate. Alkalinization and increased bicarbonate content in urine were discovered in the earliest tests of biological responses to PTH. PTH causes a net inhibition of bicarbonate reabsorption in the proximal renal tubule; this leads to a type of proximal renal tubular acidosis. Proximal renal tubular acidosis has been observed in hyperparathyroidism (see under Primary Hyperparathyroidism), and marked increases in bicarbonate clearance have been observed after infusion of parathyroid extract.[80]

Other Effects on the Kidney. PTH inhibits isotonic fluid reabsorption in the proximal tubule.[72] The sodium excluded from proximal reabsorption passes to the distal nephron, where part of it is reabsorbed. The water associated with the sodium is incompletely reabsorbed, giving rise to a net increase in free water clearance[81] and an increase in urine flow. This effect is similar to that of catecholamines, another class of hormones influencing ion transport through a cAMP-controlled mechanism. Catecholamines also inhibit proximal sodium reabsorption and give rise to increased free water clearance. PTH and dibutyryl cAMP also enhance magnesium absorption in the cortical ascending limb.[76a]

PTH also affects vitamin D metabolism through cAMP-mediated actions on renal vitamin D hydroxylases. PTH increases activity of the 1α-hydroxylase and inhibits the 24-hydroxylase.[82]

ACTIONS OF PARATHYROID HORMONE ON BONE. In addition to a direct action on the kidney in maintaining serum calcium, PTH acts on bone, the chief reservoir of calcium within the body. As noted earlier, the effect of PTH in mobilizing calcium from bone occurs in two or more phases:[70] an early phase characterized by mobilization of calcium from areas of bone in rapid equilibrium with the ECF and a later phase associated with increased synthesis of bone enzymes, particularly lysosomal enzymes that promote bone resorption and influence bone remodeling. Bone remodeling, the resorption of older osteons and subsequent replacement with new bone formation, is due to degradation of bone by osteoclasts and subsequent infiltration of osteoblasts that synthesize new collagen and allow remineralization of replacement osteons.

PTH stimulates both bone formation and bone resorption. The major initial effect of PTH on bone is increased resorption. This is associated with inhibited osteoblast function and enhanced osteoclast activity and later with enhancement of bone formation. Parathyroid grafts to bone cause resorption at the surface immediately adjacent to the transplant. At the opposite surface there is increased bone deposition. PTH, moreover, causes an increase in bone apposition in rats,[83, 84] and areas of increased bone formation (osteosclerosis) are present in the bones of some subjects with primary hyperparathyroidism.[85] PTH effects on bone formation may be mediated through the action of other substances such as bone growth factors (coupling factors) linking bone formation to bone resorption rate.[86]

Cell Types Involved. There is an increase in the ratio of osteoclasts to osteoblasts in bone on administration of PTH to animals and in hyperparathyroidism. Originally it was thought that PTH caused an actual conversion of osteoblasts to osteoclasts or that it induced an increased rate of conversion of osteoprogenitor cells to osteoclasts. However, osteo-clasts do not originate in skeletal tissue per se but migrate from marrow, thymus, and other extraskeletal reticuloendothelial sources. PTH influences all three bone cell types—osteoclasts, osteoblasts, and osteocytes. Administration of hormone in vivo causes an increase in the extracellular space of bone lacunae, presumptive evidence for resorption of bone immediately surrounding the osteocyte (osteocytic osteolysis). Scanning electron microscopy studies provide further evidence for direct effects of PTH on osteocytes and osteoblasts. PTH brings about a rapid elongation and extension of cellular processes and changes in shape to a stellate form.

Effects on Bone and Bone Cells in Vitro. PTH causes direct resorption of bone fragments in vitro. This enhanced osteolysis is accompanied by increased activity of osteoclasts and, initially, by inhibition of osteoblast activity. PTH stimulates RNA synthesis in osteoclasts, increases the number of nuclei per osteoclast, and increases the number of osteoclasts. Moreover, there are increases in content and release of lysosomal enzymes,[87, 88] increases in carbonic anhydrase activity, and an increase in uptake and incorporation of uridine. The increases in enzyme activity depend on the new RNA and protein synthesis. Lysosomal enzymes are released rapidly from bone by PTH. β-Glucuronidase is released as early as or earlier than detectable release of calcium. Other effects of PTH on bone include enhanced synthesis of hyaluronate, inhibition of citrate decarboxylation, inhibition of collagen synthesis, and changes in alkaline phosphatase activity. Alkaline phosphatase activity detected in cytochemical assays increases rapidly (3 min) in bone in vitro after exposure to PTH. At later times alkaline phosphatase activity may be reduced and acid phosphatase content of osteoclasts increased.[90] Only some of the mechanisms bringing about these changes are known; some may be mediated by increases in cellular cAMP content. Changes in calcium fluxes represent another intracellular signal modulating some of these events. PTH stimulates calcium uptake in isolated bone cells.[91–93]

Isolation of Cell Types Sensitive to Parathyroid Hormone. The varied effects, some inhibitory, some stimulatory, of PTH on bone in vitro have been clarified somewhat by studies of separated bone cells. A technique for liberating cells from fetal calvaria was developed by Peck and associates.[94] Cells released early in the course of digestion are sensitive to both PTH and CT for several days, whereas those released later in digestion are sensitive only to PTH (Fig. 27–13). The first cell type released is osteoclast-like; the later cells show osteoblast-like features. These two cell types are distinct in their responses to PTH, 1,25(OH)$_2$D, and CT.[95] Most of the stimulatory influences of PTH are on the osteoclast-like cells and include increases in the levels of lysosomal enzymes. Conversely, the inhibitory influences of PTH, on citrate decarboxylation, collagen synthesis, and alkaline phosphatase activity, are manifestations of PTH action on osteoblast-like cells. 1,25(OH)$_2$D or high concentrations of calcium affect enzyme activities in a manner similar to PTH or dibutyryl cAMP, suggesting that a change in cellular calcium level might be a mediator of the effects of increased cellular cAMP content.

The effects of the hormone on the different cell types suggest that more than one type of bone cell contains receptors for PTH. The response of a particular cell to the hormone depends on the nature of the cell; PTH can produce anabolic as well as catabolic effects on bone.

Osteoclasts actually may be devoid of receptors for PTH. Osteoblasts (and the related cells, osteocytes) are probably the primary bone cells that interact directly with PTH. Changes in cell shape have been observed only in osteoblasts after exposure to PTH, and responses (increased cAMP

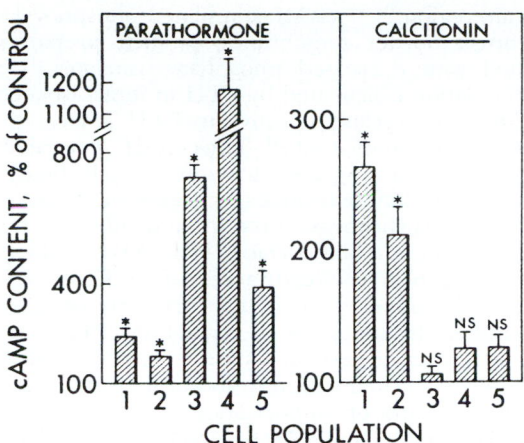

Figure 27–13. Distinct bone cell populations sensitive to PTH and CT, respectively. Cells are released at different rates from bone treated with collagenase in vitro. Cells bearing receptors for CT (osteoclast-like cells) are released early in the course of digestion. Another group of cells (osteoblast-like), released later in the course of digestion, is sensitive to PTH but not to CT. (From R Luben, G Wong, D Cohn, Biochemical characterization with parathormone and calcitonin of isolated bone cells, Endocrinology, 99, 526–534, 1976, © by The Endocrine Society.)

content) are normal in the bone of osteopetrotic rats (which lacks normal osteoclasts).[96] The postulate that osteoblasts respond primarily and directly to PTH implies that activation of osteoclasts on exposure to PTH is secondary to the interaction of the hormone with osteoblasts. Indeed, osteoblast-like cells release a factor that stimulates osteoclastic resorption,[97, 98] and osteoblasts are required for PTH control of osteoclastic resorption.[99]

EFFECTS ON THE INTESTINE. Although the intestine is one of the major organs supplying calcium to the ECF, PTH does not directly affect gastrointestinal absorption of calcium. Nevertheless, intestinal absorption of calcium reflects parathyroid status; absorption is low in hypoparathyroidism and high in hyperparathyroidism and increases after treatment with PTH (Fig. 27–14). The effect of PTH on absorption of calcium is mediated indirectly through regulation of synthesis of $1,25(OH)_2D$ in the kidney. The latter metabolite of vitamin D ($1,25(OH)_2D$) causes enhanced absorption of calcium from the gastrointestinal tract. This is discussed further in the section on vitamin D metabolism.

OTHER EFFECTS OF PARATHYROID HORMONE. Intravenous injections of PTH cause transient hypocalcemia that may reflect entry of calcium into cells (see Fig. 27–7). Parathyroid-mediated calcium flux into and out of cells may represent part of the mechanism of action of PTH and has been observed in vitro. Other effects of PTH include actions on rates of mitosis of lymphocytes in vitro, changes in blood flow through the celiac axis, increased concentrations of calcium in the mammary gland, enhanced lipolysis in isolated fat cells, and increased gluconeogenesis in liver and kidney.

Mechanism of Action of Parathyroid Hormone

RECEPTORS, INTRACELLULAR MESSENGERS, AND CELL ACTIVATION. PTH interacts with specific receptors on cells in bone and kidney. Receptors for PTH have been identified by determining binding of ^{125}I-labeled PTH to cells or cell membranes. Many physiological effects of PTH on the kidney and bone are mediated by PTH receptor activation of adenylate cyclase and generation of the intracellular messenger cAMP.[100–102] PTH also can directly activate cellular

calcium transport[103–105] and the phosphatidylinositol[106] pathway independently of the adenylate cyclase pathway. This raises the question of whether, as with the catecholamines, arginine vasopressin (AVP, also called antidiuretic hormone, ADH), and certain other hormones, there may be more than one kind of PTH receptor. cAMP can itself, however, produce some of the calcium transport effects. Progress is being made in identification and purification of PTH receptors.[107–111] The chemistry of PTH and studies of its receptors have allowed development of peptide inhibitors of PTH action.[112] Further work in this area may provide inhibitors for treatment of certain types of hypercalcemia.

MECHANISMS OF ACTION IN THE KIDNEY. PTH activates adenylate cyclase predominantly in the renal cortex, whereas AVP stimulates the enzyme in the medulla.[100–102] These findings fit the physiological concept that AVP acts predominantly on collecting ducts and that calcium and phosphate transport, presumably under the regulation of PTH, occurs in the cortical portions of the nephron. Earlier studies also indicated that areas responsive to CT could be distinguished from the principal loci for either PTH or AVP action. Later studies[113, 114] provided precise localization of hormone-sensitive loci in the nephron. PTH receptors are distributed in the cortical regions of both the proximal and the distal tubules. Two areas of the proximal cortical tubule, the early convoluted and the straight portion, respond to PTH. In the distal cortical tubule, parathyroid-sensitive enzyme is found in the granular portion and the cortical ascending limb. Distinct sites are found for CT (primarily cortical ascending limb), AVP (collecting tubule), and catecholamines. Catecholamines also act in the distal convoluted tubule but at a site proximal to the distal site for PTH (Fig. 27–15). The distribution of PTH-sensitive adenylate cyclase agrees with the physiological findings that PTH influences phosphate transport at proximal and at distal tubular sites. In the proximal convoluted tubule, PTH also causes activation of alkaline phosphatase and carbonic anhydrase. In the distal convoluted tubule, PTH at low concentrations causes activation of glucose-6-phosphate dehydrogenase.[114]

MECHANISM OF ACTIVATION OF ADENYLATE CYCLASE. Activation of adenylate cyclase by polypeptide or amine hormones does not depend solely on hormone-receptor interaction. (Also see Chapter 4.) Hormonal activation

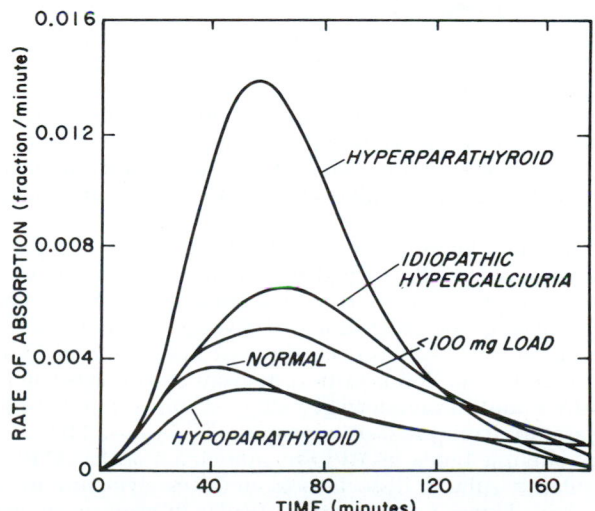

Figure 27–14. Rates of gastrointestinal absorption of calcium as a function of parathyroid status in humans. (Modified from Birge SJ, Peck WA, Berman M, et al. Study of calcium absorption in man: a kinetic analysis and physiologic model. Reproduced from the Journal of Clinical Investigation, 1969, vol. 48, pp. 1705–1713 by copyright permission of the American Society for Clinical Investigation.)

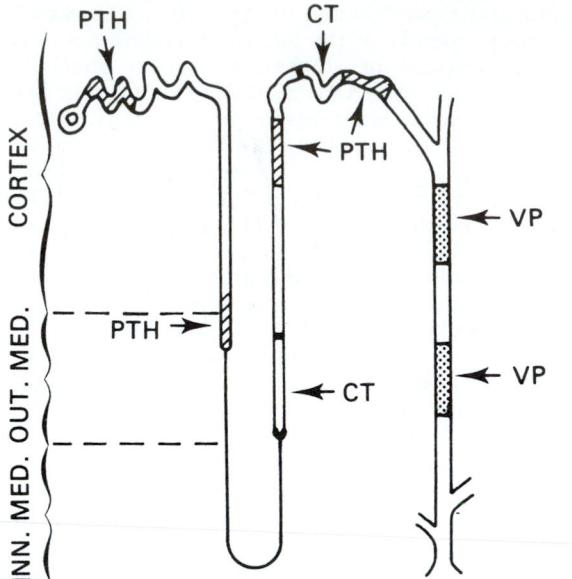

Figure 27–15. Schematic depicting regions of nephron of rabbit sensitive to PTH and CT. Discontinuities in hormone response from one region to another are not as abrupt as shown here for illustrative purposes. (Modified from Chabardes D, Imbert-Teboul M, Gagnan-Brunette M, et al. Distribution of adenylate-cyclase–linked hormone receptors in the nephron. In: Copp DH, Talmage RV, eds. Endocrinology of Calcium Metabolism. Amsterdam: Excerpta Medica, 1978: 209–214.)

of adenylate cyclase depends on at least three or four interacting proteins or enzymes: (1) hormone receptor, (2) guanine nucleotide–binding (coupling) protein, (3) the adenylate cyclase catalytic unit, and (4) GTPase. The coupling component of the complex is itself composed of alpha and beta subunits. On interaction with GTP, the protein dissociates and the GTP-bound alpha subunit then activates the adenylate cyclase complex. Some forms of pseudohypoparathyroidism, a disorder of PTH responsiveness, are due to deficient guanine nucleotide–regulatory components (see section on pseudohypoparathyroidism). A guanosine triphosphatase (GTPase) activity deactivates adenylate cyclase. GTP and nonhydrolyzable (stable to GTPases) GTP analogues (e.g., guanylylimidodiphosphate) facilitate activation of PTH-stimulatable adenylate cyclase.[32]

cAMP ACCUMULATION IN THE KIDNEY AND EFFECTS ON PROTEIN KINASE. PTH causes a rapid increase in cAMP concentration[102] in kidney slices and renal tubules incubated in vitro. This reflects activation of adenylate cyclase in the plasma membranes of the cells. cAMP accumulation in turn causes activation of enzymes and ion transport systems. These systems are activated through another class of enzymes, protein kinases, which respond to cAMP accumulation and catalyze phosphorylation of enzyme and transport systems.

Protein kinases catalyze the transfer of the gamma phosphate of ATP to a hydroxy amino acid (usually serine) in the acceptor protein. Kinase activation by cAMP has been implicated in the inactivation of glycogen synthase and the activation of phosphorylase, adipocyte lipase, steroidogenesis in the testis, and ion transport in avian erythrocytes, in toad bladder, and in mammalian kidney. cAMP-sensitive protein kinases are composed of two types of subunits. The regulatory subunit binds cAMP. On interaction with cAMP, the regulatory subunit dissociates from the catalytic unit to yield an active kinase enzyme. Of particular interest in the nephron is the polarity of distribution of cAMP-dependent protein kinase. After injection of PTH there is aggregation of cAMP at the luminal surface of tubular cells.[115] Moreover, cAMP–protein kinase is located in the luminal (brush border

microvilli) region.[116, 117] cAMP-stimulated phosphorylation of renal brush border membranes in such preparations is associated with decreased phosphate transport.[118] Similar phosphorylation is activated by PTH in intact isolated renal cells. Adenylate cyclase sensitive to PTH is located in the basolateral portion of the cell. Thus cAMP generated at the plasma membrane migrates through the cell, binds to the cAMP–receptor kinase complex, activates the kinase,[119] phosphorylates a brush border protein, and inhibits phosphate transport at the luminal surface. The cAMP at the luminal surface may explain the ready access of cAMP to the luminal fluid and the appearance in the urine of nephrogenous cAMP under the influence of circulating PTH. PTH also causes activation of protein kinase C in renal cells.[120] This activation is associated with translocation of the kinase to the cell membrane and phosphorylation of membrane protein.

ACTIVATION OF ENZYME AND TRANSPORT PROCESSES IN THE RENAL TUBULE. The activation by PTH of alkaline phosphatase, glucose-6-phosphate dehydrogenase, gluconeogenesis, and transport of sodium, bicarbonate, and calcium depends on the mediation of cAMP, based on the observation that exogenous dibutyryl cAMP can stimulate each of these processes. The facts that cAMP is found in the tubular fluid and that cAMP-dependent kinases are located in the luminal border of cells raise the question of whether cAMP is a mediator of cell-cell communication along the course of the nephron. This would allow activation of enzymes within the nephron at sites distant from the cell immediately activated by PTH interaction.

MICROTUBULAR FUNCTION OF cAMP. Certain functions mediated by cAMP involve microtubules of cells. Microtubular systems bind colchicine, vinblastine, and cytochalasin, and these agents disrupt microtubular function. Colchicine causes hypocalcemia and interferes with the action of PTH in maintaining calcium concentrations in the ECF. Colchicine and vinblastine also interfere with cell transport processes in the kidney[121] and the action of PTH on bone. Thus microtubules may be involved in the cAMP–protein kinase–mediated actions of PTH on both bone and kidney.

PARATHYROID HORMONE ACTION IN BONE. Bone cells have receptors for PTH and, like kidney cells, respond to hormone-receptor interaction with activation of adenylate cyclase and generation of cAMP. The rise in cAMP can account for the bone-resorbing action of the hormone.[101] Prostaglandins of the E series produce bone resorption and also cause an increase in cAMP content of bone.[101] Further evidence that cAMP is a mediator of bone resorption includes induction by dibutyryl cAMP of lysosomal enzymes in bone and of resorption in vitro.[87] Indeed, the majority of responses of bone to PTH appear to be mediated by cAMP.[86, 87, 89, 91, 100, 101, 122–125] The response to cAMP in bone cells is specific. cAMP mediates the stimulatory effect of PTH on osteoblasts and the inhibitory effect of CT on osteoclasts. The effects of PTH on osteoclasts are dependent and secondary to actions of the latter hormone on osteoblasts.[97–99] CT (see section on CT) stimulates cAMP formation in osteoclasts and thereby inhibits their function. Whether all effects of PTH on bone are mediated by cAMP is not known. As noted earlier, the hormone may also activate transcellular calcium fluxes (perhaps by directly activating calcium channels) and the phosphatidylinositol–C kinase pathway independently of cAMP.[92, 93]

The biological effects of PTH on bone, like those on the kidney, probably involve activation of protein kinases. cAMP kinases have been identified in osteoblasts and in osteosarcoma cells.[126] Microtubules and microfilaments may be substrates for cAMP-dependent kinases in these cells. PTH induces changes in cell shape of osteoblasts through disruption of microfilaments. Colchicine in vitro disrupts microtubule assemblies in osteoclasts, decreases ruffled borders on osteoclasts, and prevents hormone-induced resorption of bone.[127]

Cyclic Nucleotides in Extracellular Fluids

The observations of Sutherland and collaborators[128] indicated that cyclic nucleotides appear in the ECF and that changes in hormonal status can influence the concentration of cyclic nucleotides therein. They showed that hypophysectomy reduces the urinary excretion of cGMP and that this was restored toward normal by administering thyroxine or pituitary hormones. In the same studies, however, hypophysectomy was without effect on urinary excretion of cAMP. Part of the cAMP generated intracellularly in response to specific hormones is extruded into the surrounding medium or body fluid. For example, the cAMP content of the hepatic vein plasma reflects stimulation by glucagon of hepatic cells; in the adrenal vein it reflects stimulation by corticotropin (ACTH, adrenocorticotropin). Thus plasma cAMP is derived from diverse tissues, and ablation of a single organ does not cause a major change in its plasma concentration.[129]

CLEARANCE OF CYCLIC NUCLEOTIDES FROM THE PLASMA. Half-lives for disappearance of cAMP and cGMP from plasma are similar and approximate 30 min.[129] Both cyclic nucleotides distribute in a space exceeding the extracellular volume. Renal clearance accounts for 20 to 30% of the clearance of cyclic nucleotides from the miscible pool. About two thirds of this renal clearance is accounted for by excretion. The remainder is the result of enzymatic destruction within the kidney.

The major sources of plasma cAMP are unknown. Although PTH, catecholamines, corticotropin, and glucagon can each cause a rise in the plasma cAMP level, none of the corresponding receptor tissues—liver, kidney, or adrenal—seems to be the major source of plasma cAMP under resting conditions.

URINARY EXCRETION OF cAMP. Fifty to sixty percent of cAMP in the urine is cleared from plasma by glomerular filtration, and the remaining 40 to 50% is contributed by the kidney (nephrogenous cAMP).

The fact that PTH is a major influence on urinary cAMP made it possible to use this parameter for clinical diagnosis. Injection of PTH causes an increase in urinary cAMP level; parathyroidectomy causes a rapid reduction in urinary cAMP level.[129–132] Similarly, infusion of calcium inhibits parathyroid secretion and leads to decreased urinary cAMP excretion.[131, 132] This effect of PTH is due to the direct activation of adenylate cyclase in the renal tubule and release of cAMP into the luminal fluid. Extensive analyses have been carried out on cAMP clearance.[132] Determinations of creatinine and cAMP in plasma and urine allow calculations of urinary cAMP excretion in nanomoles per minute, in nanomoles per milligram of creatinine, and in nanomoles per deciliter of GF; cAMP clearance; cAMP/creatinine clearance ratio; and nephrogenous cAMP in nanomoles per deciliter of GF. Presentation of the data as nephrogenous cAMP in nanomoles per deciliter of GF gives the sharpest differentiation among hypoparathyroid, normal, and hyperparathyroid groups (see Fig. 27–36). The discrimination between these groups was almost as good when the data were expressed as nanomoles of cAMP per deciliter of GF. The latter parameter corrects the urinary cAMP/creatinine ratio for plasma creatinine ($[U_{cAMP}/U_{Cr}] \times P_{Cr}$) without determining the plasma cAMP level. The parameters expressing cAMP as a function of GF circumvent the disadvantages of expressing urinary cAMP as a rate (per unit time or per milligram of creatinine). Rate per se can vary with several

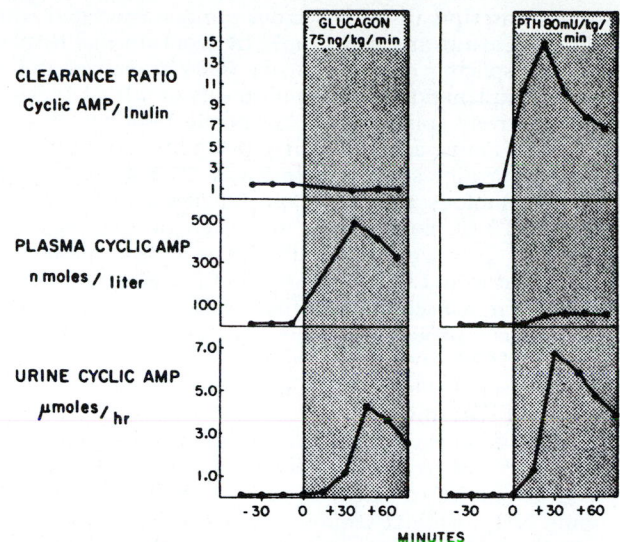

Figure 27–16. cAMP response patterns to glucagon and PTH in humans. Both glucagon and PTH cause an increase in urinary excretion of cAMP. PTH causes an increase in nephrogenous cAMP level and a marked increase in the clearance ratio of cAMP to creatinine. The increase caused by glucagon reflects cAMP cleared from the plasma by glomerular filtration. (From Kaminsky NI, Broadus AE, Hardman JG, et al. Effects of parathyroid hormone on plasma and urinary adenosine 3′,5′ monophosphate in men. Reproduced from the Journal of Clinical Investigation, 1970, vol. 49, pp. 2387–2395 by copyright permission of the American Society for Clinical Investigation.)

other functions, including sex (women excrete less creatinine and thus show a higher basal cAMP/creatinine ratio than men), illness (e.g., hyperthyroidism), or any disturbance that decreases creatinine production.

OTHER PHYSIOLOGICAL INFLUENCES ON URINARY cAMP EXCRETION. Administration of glucagon, AVP, and catecholamines also influences urinary cAMP. AVP, like PTH, activates adenylate cyclase in specific regions of the nephron. Nevertheless, AVP causes only minor changes in excretion of cAMP. Glucagon causes an increase in urinary cAMP excretion, but the effect reflects the action of this hormone on the liver. As a consequence, the concentration of cAMP in plasma (Fig. 27–16) increases and is cleared by glomerular filtration. The effects of glucagon and PTH on urinary cAMP can be differentiated by the simultaneous measurement of plasma and urinary cAMP levels. Volume expansion also increases urinary cAMP excretion, and this effect is mediated in part by increased secretion of PTH. Under basal conditions none of these latter factors significantly influences the parameter cAMP excreted per deciliter of GF.

PARATHYROID HORMONE–RELATED PROTEIN

Chemistry and Molecular Biology

In the humoral hypercalcemia of malignancy (see under Hypercalcemia), tumors secrete a factor that mimics most of the actions of PTH (including increased urinary cAMP excretion) but is immunochemically distinct from PTH.[133] Recognition of this syndrome led three groups to the purification of a PTHRP from tumors associated with humoral hypercalcemia.[133–135] The cDNA encoding PTHRP was then cloned, and the sequence of the primary gene product was defined.[29, 136] The gene is localized on the short arm of chromosome 12. RNA blot hybridization analysis reveals multiple transcripts in mRNA from tumors associated with the humoral syndrome and in mRNA from normal tissues. Alternative splicing of the primary RNA transcript is the most likely explanation for the multiplicity of mRNA species.

Alternatively spliced mRNAs encode peptides of 175, 177, and 209 amino acids. The first 36 amino acids represent a presumed leader sequence, functionally comparable but with low homology to the pre-pro segment of PTH (see section on PTH biosynthesis). Cleavage of the relatively hydrophobic pre segment would leave a short basic pro sequence that would be cleaved to yield the mature protein. The NH$_2$-terminal sequence of the resulting 139-, 141-, and 177-amino-acid proteins matches that determined for the purified PTHRP and shows homology to PTH through residue 13 (see Table 27–5). Thereafter, the sequences of PTH and PTHRP diverge.

PTHRP has been purified from tumor cell–conditioned medium[134, 135] and from tumor tissue.[133] Purified peptides of 3.4, 6 to 9, and 16 to 18 kd all show PTH-like activity and the same NH$_2$-terminal sequence; the smaller peptides are presumably NH$_2$-terminal fragments. It is unclear whether cells secrete the intact protein (which may subsequently undergo physiological and/or artifactual proteolysis) or whether the protein is cleaved intracellularly and NH$_2$-terminal fragments are secreted.

Assay

PTHRP was identified and purified as a factor that activates adenylate cyclase in bone- and kidney-derived cells. PTHRP is also active in the guinea pig kidney cytochemical bioassay for PTH[136] and in bone resorption assays. Availability of synthetic peptides and expressed forms of PTHRP[137] permits development of radioimmunoassays. An antiserum against a synthetic peptide representing residues 1 to 10 of PTHRP reacts with purified PTHRP but shows less than 1% cross-reactivity with PTH NH$_2$-terminal peptides.[134] Most PTH antisera, including those directed against NH$_2$-terminal epitopes, show little, if any, cross-reactivity with PTHRP.[133]

Physiology and Mechanism of PTHRP Action

The biological activity of PTH resides in the NH$_2$-terminal residues 1 to 34. The homology between PTHRP and PTH in the NH$_2$-terminal 13 residues presumably accounts for the actions of PTHRP in mimicking most, if not all, of the effects of PTH. Intact PTHRP and NH$_2$-terminal fragments of PTHRP purified from hypercalcemia-producing tumors,[135] recombinant PTHRP (1 to 141) expressed in bacteria,[137] and synthetic peptides corresponding to residues 1 to 34 or 1 to 36 of PTHRP[138–140] activate adenylate cyclase in kidney membranes and in osteoblast cell lines, inhibit phosphate uptake in a kidney cell line, and stimulate calcium release in in vitro bone resorption assays. Data on the relative potency of PTHRP versus PTH in in vitro assays are inconsistent, perhaps reflecting differences in assay conditions and hormone preparations. In intact animals, infusion of PTHRP leads to hypercalcemia, decreases renal phosphate reabsorption, increases urinary cAMP excretion, increases renal calcium reabsorption, stimulates 1,25(OH)$_2$D formation, and increases osteoclastic bone resorption. In nude mice bearing human PTHRP-secreting tumors, infusion of neutralizing antisera to PTHRP lowers serum calcium and urinary cAMP excretion.[141]

These results led to the conclusion that PTHRP and PTH bind to closely related or identical receptors in kidney and bone cells. Evidence supporting this conclusion comes from finding that the PTH antagonist synthetic PTH(3–34) antagonizes activation of adenylate cyclase in bone and kidney cells by PTHRP. Direct binding studies also suggest that PTH and PTHRP bind to a common, approximately 80-kd receptor in osteoblasts and kidney cells.[142, 143] Receptor activation by either PTH or PTHRP would then lead to stimulation of cAMP formation (see section on mechanism of PTH action) and to stimulation of other intracellular signaling pathways.

The physiological role of PTHRP, if any, remains conjectural. Definition of such a role awaits development of sensitive and specific assays to characterize any secreted hormone. Although attention has been focused on humoral actions of PTHRP that mimic those of PTH, PTHRP may normally function as a paracrine rather than an endocrine factor and may possess biological activities in addition to PTH-like actions. Such activities could reside in portions of the molecule that diverge in sequence from PTH.

mRNA blot hybridization analysis has identified specific PTHRP mRNA transcripts in a range of endocrine and nonendocrine tissues.[144] Notably, the mRNA is overexpressed in some human parathyroid adenomas. Expression of mRNA in human keratinocytes correlates with the isolation of PTHRP from cultured keratinocyte-conditioned medium.[145] These findings and the demonstration[146, 147] that dermal fibroblasts respond to PTHRP with increased cAMP formation suggest that PTHRP may regulate some aspect of skin physiology. mRNA encoding PTHRP is present in lactating mammary glands of rats.[148] The mRNA appears and disappears within hours as a function of the suckling stimulus. These data suggest a role for PTHRP in transfer of calcium to milk.

CALCITONIN

Parafollicular Cells

Calcitonin is produced by the parafollicular or C cells of the thyroid gland.

EMBRYOLOGY. In submammalian vertebrates, the most caudal (fifth) branchial pouch gives rise to a distinct structure, the ultimobranchial body, that contains CT-secreting cells. In mammals, the ultimobranchial body and the medial portion of the fourth branchial pouch become incorporated into the lateral lobes of the thyroid, accounting for the intrathyroidal location of the parafollicular cells. The primordial cells that give rise to the parafollicular cells are derived from ectodermal neural crest precursors that migrate ventrally into the branchial pouch rather than from branchial endoderm.

DISTRIBUTION, HISTOLOGY, AND ULTRASTRUCTURE. Parafollicular cells compose about 0.1% of the mass of the normal thyroid and are localized in the central region of the middle third of each lateral lobe. They may occur singly or in clusters; C cells are present *within* follicles and are separated from the colloid by the follicular cell cytoplasm and from the interstitium by the follicular basement membrane.

The parafollicular cells are larger than follicular cells and have a large clear nucleus. These morphological criteria permit tentative identification, but definitive confirmation requires histochemical and immunochemical techniques. Thus parafollicular cells stain with silver nitrate (argyrophilia) and display masked metachromasia (staining by toluidine blue after mineral acid hydrolysis). Like several other polypeptide-secreting cells (e.g., pancreatic islet cells), parafollicular cells take up and decarboxylate amine precursors such as 5-hydroxytryptophan. The relationship of this property (amine precursor uptake and decarboxylation) to polypeptide synthesis and secretion has not been clarified.

Immunochemical studies provide direct evidence for the role of parafollicular cells in the synthesis and secretion of CT. Immunofluorescence and immunoperoxidase techniques (Fig. 27–17) are the most sensitive and specific methods for identifying parafollicular cells.

Electron microscopy of parafollicular cells shows membrane-bound granules, abundant mitochondria, microtubules, a well-developed Golgi region, free ribosomes, and relatively poorly developed rough endoplasmic reticulum. The presence of adrenergic nerve terminals abutting on parafollicular cells has provoked speculation regarding sympathetic modulation of CT secretion.

Acute hypercalcemia causes degranulation of parafollicular cells. Chronic hypercalcemia can lead to hypertrophic changes, including an increase in cell content of free ribosomes, rough endoplasmic reticulum, and Golgi elements.

Chemistry of Calcitonins

CT polypeptides from different species uniformly consist of a 32-amino-acid polypeptide with an NH_2-terminal seven-member disulfide ring and a COOH terminus of prolineamide.[149] As many as 19 of the 32 amino acids differ in the most diverse (human versus ovine) forms of the polypeptide (Table 27–7). A number of features are common to the molecules in addition to the NH_2-terminal disulfide bridge and constant chain length that terminates in prolineamide. Six of the seven NH_2-terminal residues are identical, and the variability of the middle region of the molecule (residues 10 to 27) is more apparent than real. An acidic residue (aspartic acid or glutamic acid) is generally found at position 15, and the only other acidic residues are at position 26 or 30. Basic residues are also limited to a few positions, and wherever there are substitutions for basic residues, asparagine and glutamine are the most common replacements. Aromatic residues may exist at positions 12, 13, 16, 19, 22, and 27 but have never been found within the 11 NH_2-terminal residues. All variants contain at least one aromatic amino acid, but some contain neither tryptophan nor tyrosine. The ovine molecule contains three tyrosines.

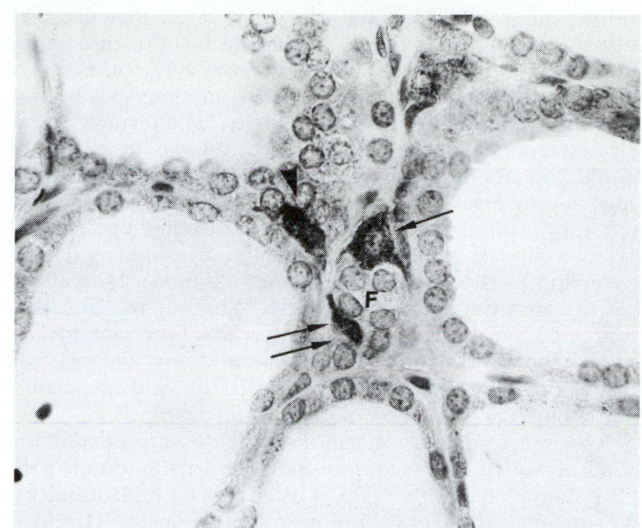

Figure 27–17. Normal adult thyroid gland stained according to the Steinberger peroxidase-antiperoxidase technique, employing a primary antiserum to human CT and with a methyl green counterstain. The C cell lying in the center (*single arrow*) has a triangular shape with elongated cytoplasmic processes. Portions of two other C cells (*arrowhead and double arrows*) are also present in this section. Magnification × 640. (Courtesy of Dr. Ronald A. DeLellis.)

The fish and chicken CTs are immunologically similar and represent the most potent of the CT molecules. The human and rat hormones are related in amino acid sequence and show a high degree of immunological cross-reactivity.

Structure-Function Relationships

The availability of natural and synthetic CT congeners has led to development of considerable information concerning structure and activity.[149] Virtually the complete structure of the 32-amino-acid peptide is required for significant biological activity. It is possible to delete serine[2] from the

---

TABLE 27–7. Amino Acid Sequence of the Calcitonins*

Species		2		4		6		8		10		12		14		16
Eel	—	Ser	—	—	—	—	—	Val	—	—	Lys	Leu	Ser	—	Glu	Leu
Salmon I	—	Ser	—	—	—	—	—	Val	—	—	Lys	Leu	Ser	—	Glu	Leu
Salmon II	—	Ser	—	—	—	—	—	Val	—	—	Lys	Leu	Ser	—	—	Leu
Salmon III	—	Ser	—	—	—	—	—	Met	—	—	Lys	Leu	Ser	—	—	Leu
Human	Cys	Gly	Asn	Leu	Ser	Thr	Cys	Met	Leu	Gly	Thr	Tyr	Thr	Gln	Asp	Ph
Rat	—	—	—	—	—	—	—	—	—	—	—	—	—	—	—	Leu
Porcine	—	Ser	—	—	—	—	—	Val	—	Ser	Ala	—	Trp	Arg	Asn	Leu
Bovine	—	Ser	—	—	—	—	—	Val	—	Ser	Ala	—	Trp	Lys	—	Leu
Ovine	—	Ser	—	—	—	—	—	Val	—	Ser	Ala	—	Trp	Lys	—	Leu
Chick	—	Ala	Ser	—	—	—	—	Val	—	—	Lys	Leu	Ser	—	Gln	Leu

Species		18		20		22		24		26		28		30		32
Eel	His	—	Leu	Gln	—	Tyr	—	Arg	—	Asp	Val	—	Ala	—	Thr	—
Salmon I	His	—	Leu	Gln	—	Tyr	—	Arg	—	Asn	Thr	—	Ser	—	Thr	—
Salmon II	His	—	Leu	Gln	—	—	—	Arg	—	Asn	Thr	—	Ala	—	Val	—
Salmon III	His	—	Leu	Gln	—	—	—	Arg	—	Asn	Thr	—	Ala	—	Val	—
Human	Asn	Lys	Phe	His	Thr	Phe	Pro	Gln	Thr	Ala	Ile	Gly	Val	Gly	Ala	Pro-NH$_2$
Rat	—	—	—	—	—	—	—	—	—	Ser	—	—	—	—	—	—
Porcine	—	Asn	—	—	Arg	—	Ser	Gly	Met	Gly	Phe	—	Pro	Glu	Thr	—
Bovine	—	Asn	Tyr	—	Arg	—	Ser	Gly	Met	Gly	Phe	—	Pro	Glu	Thr	—
Ovine	—	Asn	Tyr	—	Arg	Tyr	Ser	Gly	Met	Gly	Phe	—	Pro	Glu	Thr	—
Chick	His	—	Leu	Gln	—	Tyr	—	Arg	—	Asp	Val	—	Ala	—	Thr	—

*The entire sequence is shown for human CT. Dashes indicate residues identical to those in the human molecule. Residues are shown for other CTs only where they differ from those of human CT.

Table modified from Potts JT Jr, Aurbach GD. Chemistry of the calcitonins. In: Greep RO, Astwood EB, eds. Handbook of Physiology. Sect 7: Endocrinology. Vol VII. Parathyroid Gland. Bethesda: American Physiological Society, 1977: 423. Results for rat CT are those of Raulais D, Hagaman J, Ontjes DA, et al. The complete amino acid sequence of rat thyrocalcitonin. Eur J Biochem 1976; 64:607–611. For chick CT results are those of Minvielle S, Cressent M, Delehaye MC, et al. Sequence and expression of the chicken calcitonin gene. FEBS Lett 1987; 223:63–68.

seven-member NH₂-terminal dicysteine ring structure with no loss of biological activity.[150] Removal of even one amino acid at position 16,[151] however, destroys 80% or more of activity, and shortening the chain in any way other than noted causes almost total loss of activity. The tertiary alpha-helical structure in the region of residues 8 to 22 of the peptide appears most important for activity.[152] The disulfide bridge is not essential for activity.[153] Methionine, when located at position 8 immediately adjacent to the heptapeptide ring, is a site of potential inactivation through oxidation. Conversion of the methionine to methionine sulfone at this locus destroys the biological activity. When methionine is at position 25, oxidation does not alter biological activity. An acidic carboxyl function is not essential for activity, and substitution of asparagine for the aspartic acid at position 15 in bovine CT enhances biological potency.

The fish and avian hormones have enhanced potency compared with other CTs. One possible explanation for the high potency of salmon CT I is its enhanced hydrophilicity; this property, however, is not seen in salmon CT II and in eel CT, which are similarly potent. Salmon CT also has the highest net positive charge of the CTs known to date. Deamidation of the COOH-terminal proline (with consequent increase in negative charge in the molecule) leads to reduced biological activity. Areas of increased positive charge may be of importance in binding to receptors. The loss of activity with deletion of Leu-16 (salmon) or Phe-16 (human) has been attributed to loss of alpha-helical structure required for correct orientation of hydrophobic and charged groups.[152]

Biological Assay of Calcitonin

Biological assays for CT generally are based on the hypocalcemic effect. The simplest bioassays depend on injection of test material in rats. Generally the minimal amount of hormone detected by in vivo bioassay is 0.1 to 1 mU. An in vitro bioassay may be performed with renal membrane adenylate cyclase or with tumor cells and measurement of cAMP response.[151] The latter are sensitive to the nanogram range of salmon CT and may be adaptable for general use.

Biosynthesis of Calcitonin

Calcitonin is the product of a gene that directs synthesis of two different peptides, calcitonin in the thyroid (or ultimobranchial gland) and calcitonin gene–related peptide (CGRP) in the central nervous system. The gene contains six exons that are initially transcribed to a precursor of two different mRNAs. The pre-mRNA is processed differently in the C cells than in the central nervous system, and this processing is controlled by differential splicing.[154, 155] This is depicted diagrammatically in Figure 27–18. The mRNA for CT codes for a large (approximately 17 kd) precursor peptide that is processed to the 32-amino-acid CT.[156] The first 25 amino acids of the precursor represent the leader or signal sequence. The secretory product, CT itself, represents a segment beginning 84 amino acids from the first residue in the leader sequence and ending 20 amino acids proximal to the COOH terminus of the 17-kd precursor. Although CGRP production and CT production are normally discrete, C cell tumors may cosecrete the two peptides.[157] CGRP has a number of pharmacological actions on the cardiovascular and central nervous systems,[155] but its physiological significance is still to be defined. The peptide immediately NH₂-terminal to CT itself (NH₂-terminal proCT) is mitogenic for bone cells.[158]

Radioimmunoassays

Radioimmunoassays for human CT are based on antibodies to synthetic or isolated human CT. In either event, the antigen corresponds to the amino acid sequence of CT in medullary carcinoma of the thyroid. The structures of porcine, salmon, and human CT differ (see Table 27–7), and there is poor immunological cross-reactivity between them. The rat and human hormones are similar, however, and a radioimmunoassay for rat CT was developed by immunizing rats with human CT. The immunoassay for human CT is useful in the diagnosis and management of medullary carcinoma of the thyroid. A high-sensitivity, specific two-site radioimmunoassay has been developed.[159]

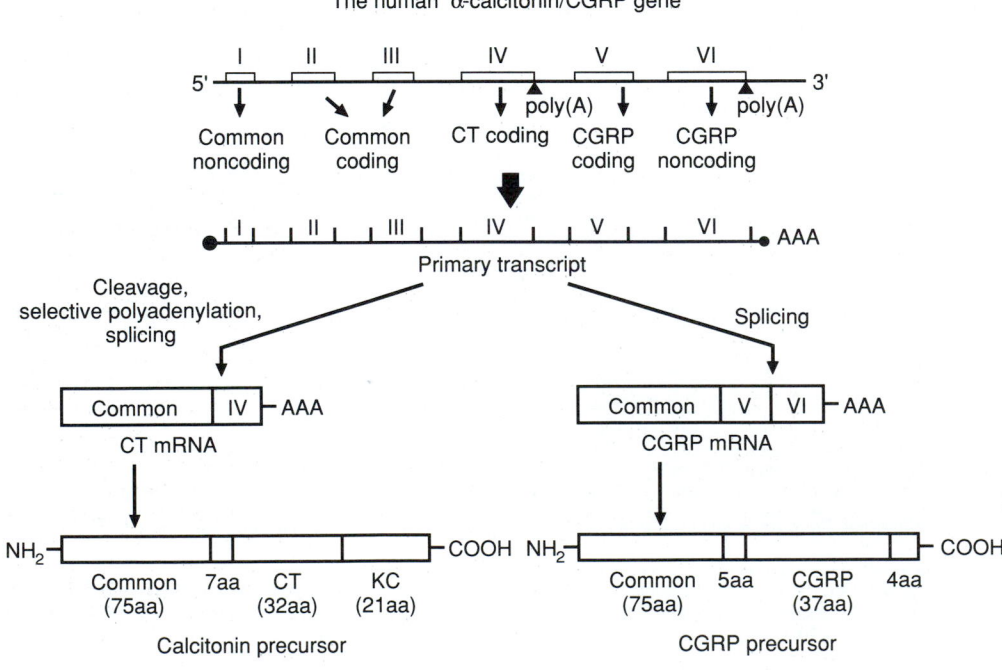

The human α-calcitonin/CGRP gene

Figure 27–18. Transcription and translation of the human α-calcitonin/CGRP gene. The gene contains six exons. The initial transcript is processed differently in the thyroid (C cell) and the central nervous system. In the C cell the primary transcript is cleaved to produce mRNA representing exons I to IV. From this the CT precursor molecule (exon I is not translated) is synthesized. This precursor peptide is processed to CT. The final transcript in the central nervous system represents exons I to III plus V and VI. Again, exon I is not translated. The peptide precursor in the central nervous system is then processed to CGRP. (Data from Breimer LH, MacIntyre I, Zaidi M. Peptides from the calcitonin genes: molecular genetics, structure and function. Biochem J 1988; 255:377–390.)

Secretion of Calcitonin

Calcium stimulates secretion of CT. In addition, beta-adrenergic catecholamines and several peptides, including glucagon (in dogs), cholecystokinin, gastrin, and ceruletide (cerulein), cause release of CT. Ceruletide and cholecystokinin share the tetrapeptide COOH terminus of pentagastrin. (Pentagastrin and calcium are the principal secretagogues in testing for medullary carcinoma.) Beta-adrenergic catecholamines and glucagon act in receptor tissues by increasing the cAMP level, and theophylline and dibutyryl cAMP also stimulate CT release. Thus cAMP in the C cell is an intracellular mediator for secretion of CT and for secretion of PTH.[160]

The concentration of calcium in the circulation influences the content of CT in the thyroid gland. Hypocalcemia in parathyroidectomized rats is associated with increased CT content of the thyroid gland, whereas hypercalcemia causes depletion of secretory granules from the C cells of the thyroid and reduced CT content of the thyroid gland. In some species, CT secretion is important for control of blood calcium.[17] Instillation of calcium into the stomach of normal rats causes little or no change in plasma calcium but in thyroidectomized animals causes hypercalcemia. These observations suggest that a gastrointestinal hormone (most likely cholecystokinin[161]) is released in response to calcium or a calcium-containing meal in the rat and that this hormone is a secretagogue for CT. In the pig, instillation of calcium into the stomach causes release of gastrin and of CT. Thus gastrin may be a significant secretagogue for CT in response to alimentary intake of calcium in this species. Of further interest is the fact that, in the pig, PTH is capable of stimulating gastrin release. Interrelationships between gastrointestinal and calcitropic hormones appear to be important in regulation of calcium metabolism in the pig, rat, and other subprimates. Although there is no proven significance for human physiology, such hormone-secretagogue interactions may be relevant in the understanding of multiple endocrine neoplasia (see Chapter 30).

Immunoreactive CT exists in human plasma in multiple forms including CT monomer, oxidized monomer, a dimer, and possibly a precursor of CT approximately 12 kd in size.[162] These peptides vary with clinical status, renal function, and nature of tissue elaborating CT. High-molecular-weight species seem to accumulate in chronic renal disease. Multiple forms are secreted by medullary thyroid carcinoma as well as by tumors that produce CT ectopically. The dimer of CT in plasma can be formed from the native hormone. The dimer is inactive but can be converted to the monomer with restoration of biological activity through reduction with sulfhydryl reagents. Of the various forms of immunoreactive CT in the circulation, some may represent peptides elaborated from the secretory source and others represent peripheral forms. Too little is known about the metabolism of CT to determine the origin of the several high-molecular-weight forms of immunoreactive CT.

Physiology

GENERAL. The lowering of serum calcium concentration is the principal physiological action of the hormone. Hypophosphatemia accompanies the hypocalcemia, suggesting that the effects are brought about through reduction of bone resorption.[160, 163] Studies of radioactive calcium kinetics in vivo as well as in vitro show changes in specific activity of plasma calcium interpretable as inhibition of release of calcium from a major calcium pool, presumably bone (Fig. 27–19). In vitro, CT inhibits the PTH effect on release of radioactive calcium from bone. Actions of CT on bone are

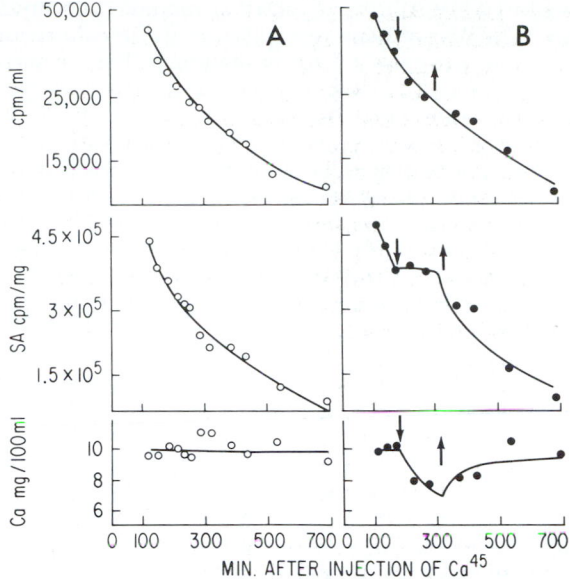

Figure 27–19. Changes in calcium metabolism in the rat in response to CT. Groups of rats were given radioactive calcium intravenously, and serial determinations were made of radioactivity and calcium levels in blood. Serum calcium level remains constant and specific activity changes continuously in plasma of control rats. Rats injected with CT *(first arrow)* develop acute hypocalcemia and abrupt retardation of the decrease in specific activity of plasma calcium. Results are interpreted as reflecting inhibition of bone resorption (interruption of supply of stable calcium to the plasma compartment) by CT in vivo. (From JL O'Riordan, GD Aurbach, Mode of action of thyrocalcitonin, Endocrinology, 82, 377–383, 1968, © by The Endocrine Society.)

also evident in the decrease of alkaline phosphatase and pyrophosphatase activity and hydroxyproline production, each accompanying the inhibition of bone resorption. The hypophosphatemic action reflects inhibition of bone resorption[130] plus promotion of phosphate entry into bone. In addition, CT causes a modest degree of phosphaturia that can contribute to hypophosphatemia.

ACTIONS ON BONE. The hypocalcemic activity of CT in vivo is effected predominantly by inhibiting calcium resorption from bone and is not dependent on a functioning kidney, gastrointestinal tract, or parathyroid gland. A direct action on bone was also implied by radioactive calcium kinetic studies in the intact animal. CT inhibits bone functions mediated by osteoclasts, including direct inhibition of bone resorption.[164–169] CT inhibits osteoclasts via a cAMP-mediated mechanism.[100, 170] Other functions of resorbing bone, particularly enzymatic activities stimulated by PTH, are inhibited by CT.

Bone resorption in vitro, whether spontaneous or induced by any of several agents including PTH, vitamin A, vitamin D, dibutyryl cAMP, and prostaglandins, is inhibited by CT. Virtually all resorptive effects, including lysosomal enzyme changes, mineral release, and degradation of collagen, are inhibited.[100] The magnitude of the inhibitory effect on bone is a function of the rate of bone resorption. At low rates of bone resorption, effects of CT are minimal. At high rates of bone resorption, the effects are greater. After prolonged incubation of skeletal tissue with CT in vitro, the inhibition of resorption is lost. This effect has been termed an escape phenomenon. Refractoriness to the in vitro effects of CT might be directly related to loss of CT receptors (down-regulation of receptors) from the target tissue and consequently decreased production of cAMP in response to the hormone.

MECHANISM OF ACTION OF CALCITONIN. The effects of CT, particularly those on osteoclasts, appear to be mediated by cAMP. Dibutyryl cAMP at modest concentrations causes induction of bone resorption in tissue culture and at higher concentrations causes inhibition of bone resorption and of the effects of PTH. Thus the effects of high concentrations of dibutyryl cAMP mimic the effects of CT, which itself causes increased accumulation of cAMP in bone through specific activation of adenylate cyclase. CT also causes activation of renal adenylate cyclase and increased formation of cAMP in the renal tubule. Effects of diverse CT congeners on cAMP production show orders of potency in vitro that parallel closely biological effects in vivo.[149] This parallelism in dose response for physiology and biochemistry (cyclic nucleotide production) supports the concept that cAMP is the mediator of action of CT.

RECEPTORS FOR CALCITONIN AND DISTRIBUTION AMONG CELL TYPES. The discussion of the mechanism of action of PTH indicated that adenylate cyclase responses to CT and PTH appear in different regions along the course of the nephron. CT activates adenylate cyclase in the medullary ascending thick limb of the nephron as well as in the "bright" segment of the distal cortical tubule (see Fig. 27–16). These CT-sensitive areas respond relatively little to PTH, which activates adenylate cyclase in the proximal convoluted tubule as well as in a more distal region of the distal convoluted tubule of the rabbit. There are significant differences in response of bone cells as well. Osteoclast activity is stimulated by PTH and is inhibited by CT. Osteoclast-like cells respond primarily to CT, whereas osteoblast-like cells respond only to PTH.

IDENTIFICATION OF CALCITONIN RECEPTORS. Specific receptors are present in renal plasma membranes, membranes from fetal rat calvaria (Fig. 27–20), and osteoclasts.[168] $1,25(OH)_2D$ regulates osteoclast formation (see Chapter 28) and increases the apparent number of CT receptors on osteoclasts.[168] Radioiodinated salmon CT binds with high affinity to membranes in these tissues.[171] CT analogues inhibit binding of iodinated CT to the receptor, and the apparent affinities of binding of these analogues parallel the biological activity (see Fig. 27–20). The CT analogues have the same order of effectiveness in stimulating adenylate cyclase in kidney and bone. Specific receptors for CT are also present in human lymphocyte tumor cell lines[172] and brain cells.[173] The receptors on human cells are similar to those in rat kidney or bone. The human hormone shows similar potency when tested in human tissues and with receptors from other species.

CALCIFEROLS

Vitamin Terminology

The D vitamins (calciferols) are steroid molecules in which one of the four rings has been opened (secosteroids).[174] The bond between C-9 and C-10 of the B ring has been cleaved, giving a conjugated triene structure. The metabolism and mechanism of action of the calciferols are in many ways analogous to those of other steroid hormones.[175–178]

Metabolic Pathways

SOURCES OF INACTIVE PRECURSORS—ROLE OF SUNLIGHT. The precursors of vitamin D_2* and vitamin D_3 are produced in plants (ergosterol) and animals (7-dehydrocholesterol), respectively. Vitamins D_2 and D_3 differ only with respect to the side-chain structure (Fig. 27–21) and are generated nonenzymatically by radiation of the precursors. Lanosterol is a precursor of both ergosterol and 7-dehydrocholesterol. 7-Dehydrocholesterol is an intermediate in cholesterol biosynthesis in some tissues, and its conversion to cholesterol is irreversible. 7-Dehydrocholesterol is present in the human dermis and epidermis. Radiation with near-ultraviolet light (230 to 313 nm wavelength) penetrates as far as the upper portion of the dermis, causing generation of several sterols, including some with antirachitic (vitamin D–like) bioactivity (see Fig. 27–21). Skin pigments influence the efficiency of light penetration.[179] At a wavelength of 295 nm there is little generation of products other than previtamin D_3. Previtamin D_3 and vitamin D_3 are isomers that attain a physicochemical equilibrium that favors vitamin D_3. Exposure of ergosterol to heat and light produces a series of reactions analogous to those seen with 7-dehydrocholesterol (see Fig. 27–21). Vitamin D_2 (ergocalciferol) or vitamin D_3 (cholecalciferol) can be used as dietary supplements. Ergocalciferol and cholecalciferol appear to have identical biological properties in humans, and requirements for the vitamin can be fully satisfied by dietary or endogenous sources. The vitamin D content of an unfortified diet can be highly variable but is generally low.

In the temperate zones there is usually adequate sunlight to allow synthesis and release of sufficient cholecalciferol by the epidermis to obviate dependence on dietary sources of these sterols. Mean serum concentrations of vitamin D and most of its metabolites reflect season, global latitude, and average hours of solar exposure.

Ergocalciferol and cholecalciferol are inert when incubated in vitro with vitamin D target tissues and, after administration to vitamin D–deficient animals, cause physiological responses only after a time lag of 6 to 12 h. This time lag reflects the requirement that the calciferols undergo activation by a sequence of hydroxylations (Fig. 27–22), then gain access to the interior of target tissues, from which they direct changes in cell composition and function. This mechanism of action was uncovered by the use of radiolabeled calciferol as a probe. For example, after administration of labeled calciferol to vitamin D–deficient animals, a series of mono- and dihydroxylated (polar) metabolites were detected (Fig. 27–23); intestinal target tissue accumulated a metabolite subsequently identified as $1,25(OH)_2D$.

CALCIFEROL 25-HYDROXYLATION. The initial step in vitamin D activation is introduction of a hydroxyl group at C-25. 25-OHD acts more rapidly in vivo than does the precursor and shows intrinsic activity on intestine and bone in vitro. The liver is the principal site of vitamin D 25-hydroxylation, although it can also occur in the intestines and kidneys of certain species. Vitamin D 25-hydroxylase activity is present in microsomal and mitochondrial fractions of the liver.[180] The enzyme is not stimulated by rachitogenic diets.

CALCIFEROL 1α-HYDROXYLATION. $1,25(OH)_2D$ is the most potent known natural metabolite of vitamin D. The rate of synthesis in normal adults is 0.8 to 2.4 nmol/d (0.3 to 1.0 μg/d). In humans the normal circulating concentration of $1,25(OH)_2D$ is approximately one thousandth that of 25-OHD. The 1α-hydroxylation of 25-OHD and other vitamin D analogues is the major recognized control point in calciferol metabolism. Nephrectomy, but not ureteral ligation, leads to an abrupt cessation of this activity in vivo. The normal renal 25-OHD 1α-hydroxylase activity is present in proximal convoluted tubules.[181] Potentially important extrarenal sites of 1α-hydroxylation are the placenta and granuloma tissue.

Most studies of the enzyme system have used 25-OHD

---

*The subscripts for vitamin D denote the order in which the compounds were isolated. In the absence of a subscript, the term vitamin D refers to either or both compounds.

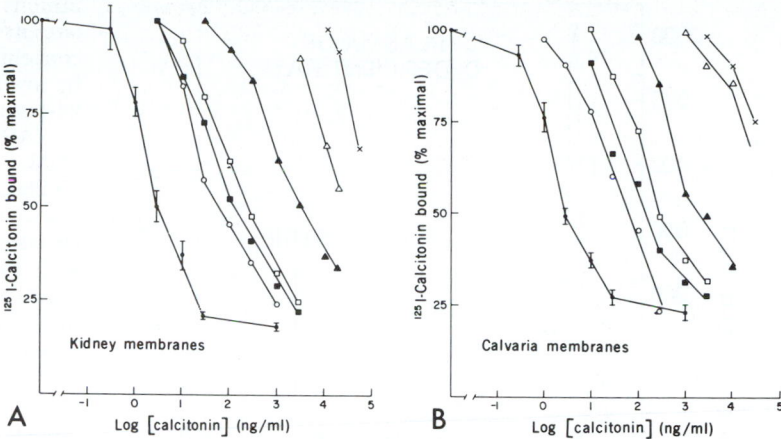

Figure 27–20. Receptor-ligand interactions with CT polypeptides. Renal *(A)* or skeletal *(B)* cell membranes were incubated in vitro with ^{125}I-labeled salmon CT and indicated amounts of unlabeled congeners. The CT peptides specifically inhibited binding of labeled CT to receptor sites on the membranes. The apparent affinities (taken as concentrations required for half-maximal inhibition) paralleled the biological effectiveness of the polypeptides. ●, salmon CT; ○, porcine CT; ■, ovine CT; □, bovine CT; ▲, human CT; △, human CT fragment amide; X, human CT sulfoxide. (From Marx SJ, Woodward CJ, Aurbach GD, et al. Calcitonin receptors of kidney and bone. Science 1972; 178:999–1001. Copyright 1972 by the American Association for the Advancement of Science.)

as a substrate, and it is generally assumed that the same enzyme system can also use as substrates $24,25(OH)_2D$, $25,26(OH)_2D$, and probably other 25-hydroxylated metabolites. The enzyme system shares many properties with other steroidogenic mixed-function oxidase systems. Each requires molecular oxygen, magnesium, NADPH, an iron-sulfur protein (the chicken kidney protein cross-reacts immunologically with adrenal ferredoxin), and a ferredoxin reductase (thought to be flavoprotein). Cytochrome P-450 serves as the terminal electron donor and oxygenase in the adrenal mitochondrial steroid monooxygenase; a similar hemoprotein is involved in the renal system. The renal 25-OHD 1α-hydroxylase–associated cytochrome binds aminoglutethimide, metyrapone, and carbon monoxide with kinetics similar to those of the adrenal cytochrome P-450.

The renal enzyme may be regulated by modifications of enzyme synthesis, enzyme degradation, or enzyme action (for example, modifications of cofactors). In renal tubules, the activity decays with a half-time of 3.5 to 4 h when either protein or RNA synthesis is inhibited, indicating a rapid turnover of both mRNA and protein. Even when protein synthesis is inhibited, however, total activity can be increased in vitro by incubation with dibutyryl cAMP. Dietary vitamin D deprivation leads to a 5- to 20-fold increase in this activity, and this reverts to normal within several days after acute vitamin D repletion. Administration of excess vitamin D to chickens and humans results in accumulation of large amounts of 25-OHD in serum, whereas the serum concentration of $1,25(OH)_2D$ does not rise outside the normal range. The mechanism whereby the renal tubules respond to excess or deficiency of calcium involves an intermediary action of PTH. The renal 25-OHD 1α-hydroxylase activity decreases to unstimulated levels within 24 h of parathyroidectomy in vitamin D–depleted chickens. It increases with systemic infusion of PTH, cAMP, or dibutyryl cAMP into thyroparathyroidectomized, vitamin D–deficient rats.

Phosphate depletion regulates the renal 25-OHD 1α-hydroxylase activity by mechanisms independent of PTH (Fig. 27–24); the phosphate-associated changes are of a lower magnitude than those caused by changes in parathyroid status. Phosphate depletion leads to increased serum concentrations of $1,25(OH)_2D$ and increased intestinal absorption of calcium and phosphate. PTH causes major changes in renal phosphate transport, so some of the actions of PTH on this hydroxylase system may be mediated by changes in the intracellular or extracellular phosphate compartment.

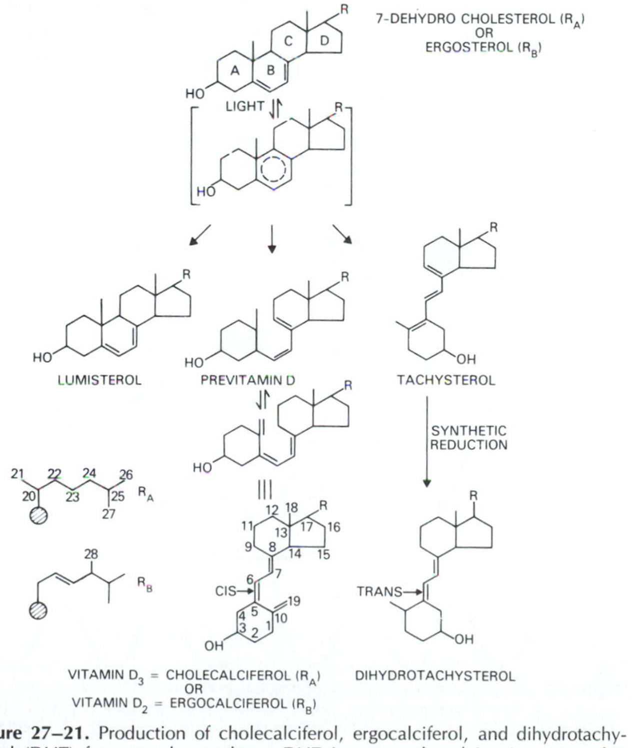

Figure 27–21. Production of cholecalciferol, ergocalciferol, and dihydrotachysterol (DHT) from sterol preculsors. DHT is not produced in vivo. Note that modification of C-5–C-6 configuration places 3-hydroxyl group of DHT in a pseudo–1-hydroxyl configuration.

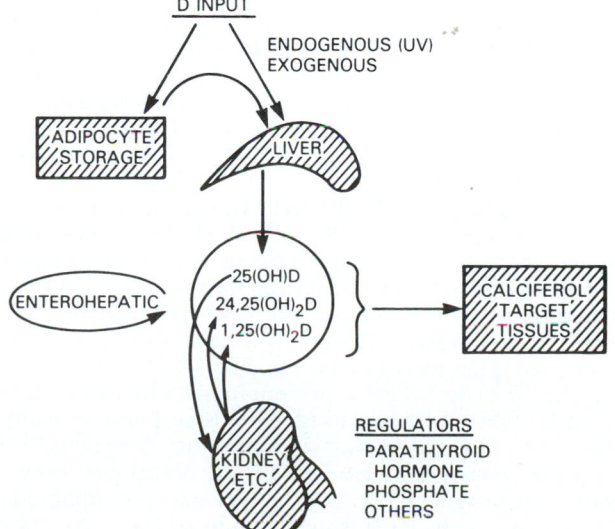

Figure 27–22. Metabolic pathways for production of major biologically active vitamin D metabolites.

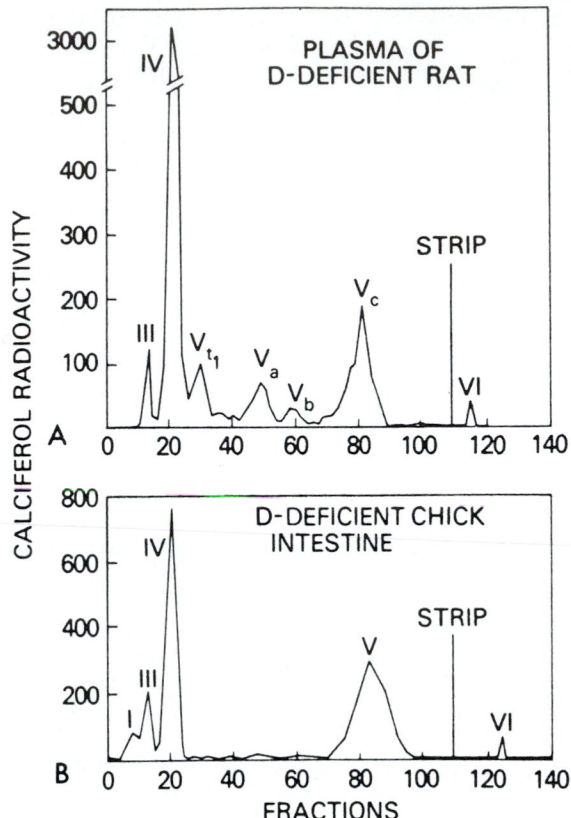

Figure 27–23. *Top,* 2.5 µg tritiated cholecalciferol was injected into a calciferol-deficient rat, and plasma was obtained 24 h later. Lipids were extracted with an organic solvent and chromatographed on a column of Sephadex LH-20. The probable major components of the peaks are as follows: III, D_3; IV, 25-OHD$_3$; V_a, 24,25(OH)$_2$D$_3$; V_c, 25,26(OH)$_2$D$_3$. 1,25(OH)$_2$D$_3$ (V, *bottom*) cochromatographed with peak V_c in top panel. *Bottom,* Calciferol-deficient chicks were injected with 0.25 µg tritiated cholecalciferol. Lipids were extracted from the small intestine and chromatographed on a similar column. (Modified from Holick MF, DeLuca HF. A new chromatographic system for vitamin D_3 and its metabolites; resolution of a new vitamin D_3 metabolite. J Lipid Res 1971; 12:460–465.)

Several additional factors influence renal 25-OHD 1α-hydroxylase activity. For example, 1,25(OH)$_2$D in vitro acts via its receptor to inhibit renal 25-OHD 1α-hydroxylase activity. In fowl the needs of egg production require sex-dependent controls of mineral metabolism. The male Japanese quail produces far less 1,25(OH)$_2$D than does the female. Acute administration of estrogen to the male increases the renal 25-OHD 1α-hydroxylase activity strikingly within 24 h.[182] Lactation may also place major stresses on mineral regulation. The serum 1,25(OH)$_2$D level is increased during lactation in rats. Stimulation of 1α-hydroxylase has also been observed with prolactin, growth hormone, insulin, and CT.[181]

CALCIFEROL 24-HYDROXYLATION. Another major metabolite of vitamin D is 24,25(OH)$_2$D. Under normal circumstances in humans, its serum concentration is approximately one tenth that of 25-OHD and 100 times that of 1,25(OH)$_2$D. The kidney is the principal site of 24-hydroxylation of 25-OHD, and anephric humans produce this metabolite in decreased quantities. The rat renal 25-OHD 24-hydroxylase, like the 1α-hydroxylase, is present in mitochondria. The two renal 25-OHD hydroxylating systems respond to many of the same modulators but in opposing directions.[183] For example, variation of either PTH or phosphate levels can cause contrasting changes in the two activities; inhibition of 24-hydroxylase by PTH is mediated by cAMP,[183] and administration of 1,25(OH)$_2$D to vitamin D–deficient chicks or rats

inhibits metabolism of 25-OHD to 1,25(OH)$_2$D and stimulates its metabolism to 24,25(OH)$_2$D$_3$. In humans, circulating concentrations of 24,25(OH)$_2$D are in large part determined by availability in plasma of the 25-OHD substrate for the 24-hydroxylase system.[184]

ADDITIONAL PATHWAYS OF CALCIFEROL METABOLISM. Calciferol metabolites of uncertain role include 25,26(OH)$_2$D, 25-OHD-26,23-lactone, 1,24,25(OH)$_3$D, 24 keto metabolites, 5,6-*trans*-25-OHD, and C-17 side-chain cleavage metabolites. In tissues, vitamin D may be esterified with palmitate, stearate, oleate, and linoleate. These esters retain antirachitic potency and may be major storage forms of the vitamin. Many unidentified metabolites are excreted in bile. One of the major components is a glucuronide. A water-soluble glycoside of 1,25(OH)$_2$D has been identified in certain plants and can cause hypercalcemia in grazing animals.

Calciferol Absorption, Transport, Storage, and Excretion

Normally, 60 to 90% of dietary calciferol is absorbed by the small intestine by mechanisms similar to those that allow the absorption of cholesterol and other fat-soluble sterols. Impairment of fat absorption causes proportional reduction in absorption of vitamin D. Absorbed calciferols are initially incorporated into chylomicra. In chylomicron-free blood, vitamin D circulates principally bound to alpha-globulin, which shows preferential affinity for the 25-hydroxylated forms of the calciferols.

Thirty percent of radiolabeled vitamin D, administered intravenously to vitamin D–deficient rats, is rapidly sequestered within the liver to be hydroxylated and released within several hours as 25-OHD. In the vitamin D–replete state the percentage of conversion to 25-OHD is low, and a large portion, probably over half, of circulating vitamin D is partitioned into body fat pools. Adipose tissue provides a limitless reservoir for vitamin D storage.[185] Consequently, when vitamin D is ingested in excessive amounts, much is retained in lipid stores. Several months may be required before the content of these pools returns to normal levels. The mechanism for entry of epidermal vitamin D into the

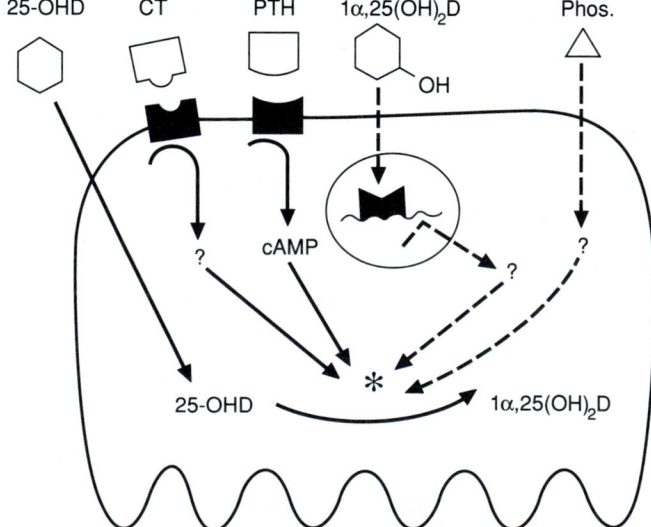

Figure 27–24. Multiple mechanisms for regulation of the 25-OHD 1α-hydroxylase system. Positively acting factors (*solid arrows*) and negatively acting factors (*dashed arrows*) converge by widely different mechanisms onto the 25-OHD 1α-hydroxylase system (*). All these processes occur in the renal proximal tubule; however, not all these regulatory pathways need occur within the same cell.

circulation is probably diffusion down a concentration gradient facilitated by binding to carrier proteins in ECF.

Unlike the parent compounds, 25-OHD shows intrinsic activity in vitro. Although more polar than the parent compound, 25-OHD is also sparingly soluble in aqueous solutions and circulates bound to the same alpha-globulin (transcalciferin) that transports most of vitamin D in chylomicron-free plasma.[186] This alpha-globulin is 55 kd in size and is identical with a protein previously referred to in studies of population genetics as group-specific component (Gc). It shows amino acid sequence homology with albumin and α-fetoprotein (fetuin). Two major forms of the protein are the expressions of codominant alleles. Multiple other allelic forms occur rarely, but no variation in their effectiveness for vitamin D transport in humans has been detected. The 25-OHD transport globulin is synthesized in the liver, and its concentration rises moderately with estrogenic stimulation, as during pregnancy or treatment with estrogenic contraceptives. Under usual conditions men and women have similar levels, however. The protein contains a single high-affinity vitamin D binding site per molecule, with preferential affinity for the 25-hydroxylated forms. This feature favors partition of the nonhydroxylated forms into adipose tissue while the active 25-hydroxylated metabolites are retained within the circulation. Normally, less than 5% of its vitamin D binding sites are occupied. The concentration of the protein in plasma is similar in states of calciferol excess or deficiency. The 25-OHD–binding globulin of the chicken shows preferential affinity for the vitamin D_3 series over the vitamin D_2 series of analogues, and this accounts for the relative ineffectiveness of ergocalciferol analogues in chickens. The stability and high affinity of binding for 25-OHD make it possible to use the protein in competitive binding assays for vitamin D metabolites. Transcalciferin also binds actin with high affinity and may serve to inactivate any actin in the circulation, where actin has highly toxic properties.

Approximately half of the body pool of 25-OHD is bound in the circulation to transcalciferin. This bound form turns over with a half-time of 15 d in normal humans and approximately 45 d in anephric humans (Table 27–8). Most of the remainder of the 25-OHD pool is inside cells. 25-OHD–binding proteins are present in the cytosol, and like the plasma 25-OHD transport globulin, cytosolic proteins are useful as reagents for competitive binding assays of vitamin D metabolites. The 25-OHD binder in cytosol is either a translocated form of the plasma 25-OHD transport globulin that has associated with actin or a contaminating artifact from serum.

25-OHD, like other calciferol metabolites, goes through an enterohepatic circulation. Estimates of the fraction of the circulating pool cycling through this pathway each day vary from less than 5% to over 30%.[187] 25-OHD can be hydroxylated in the 1α, 24, and 26 positions; these reactions occur primarily in the kidney and are subject to varying degrees of metabolic regulation. $1,25(OH)_2D$ can decrease serum 25-OHD levels by increasing hydroxylation at residues other than 1.

The hydroxy metabolites of 25-OHD, like their precursors, are sparingly soluble in water and also circulate bound

to the 25-OHD transport globulin. The half-life of intravenously injected $1,25(OH)_2D$ in the circulation is approximately 5 h in humans. During a 6-d period, approximately 15% is excreted as urinary metabolites and 50% is excreted as fecal metabolites. The total turnover of $1,25(OH)_2D$ in adults is 0.3 to 1.0 μg/d. Like 25-OHD, $1,25(OH)_2D$ undergoes enterohepatic circulation.

Actions of Calciferols

INTESTINAL ACTIONS. In the vitamin D–deficient animal, the intestine shows the most dramatic response to vitamin D administration which induces large increases in fractional absorption of calcium and lesser increases in absorption of phosphate and magnesium.[12, 177] Calcium transport along the small and large intestine is regulated by vitamin D. In the rat, the rates of basal and stimulated transport show a hierarchy with duodenum > jejunum > ileum > colon; phosphate absorption by the small intestine in the rat shows a different hierarchy of rates with jejunum > duodenum > ileum. Active metabolites of vitamin D control intestinal calcium and phosphate transport even in the total absence of PTH.

In the vitamin D deficiency state, administration of calciferol analogues in vivo or in vitro produces important alterations in the composition of the intestinal mucosa. These changes develop at approximately the same time as the increase in mucosal-to-serosal translocation of calcium. The mediator of $1,25(OH)_2D$–dependent calcium transport has not been identified with certainty. However, intestinal mucosal epithelia contain a water-soluble calcium-binding protein (calbindin), and its concentration in tissue mirrors, to a limited degree, calcium transport rates. Its concentration increases as early as 2 h after administration in vivo or in vitro of $1,25(OH)_2D$. The size of the major mammalian intestinal calbindin is 9 kd; this calbindin contains two domains that bind calcium with high affinity. A second and larger (28 kd) calbindin, containing four calcium binding domains, is found in brain and kidney. It is encoded by a different gene remotely related to the 9-kd calbindin. The 28-kd calbindin gene is regulated by $1,25(OH)_2D$ in kidney but not in brain. The amino acid sequences show major homologies to those of myosin light chain, troponin C, parvalbumin, and calmodulin. These proteins bind calcium with high affinity at a highly conserved domain with structural features described as an "EF hand." Calmodulin shows high affinity for and critical interactions with cytoplasmic calcium. The function of the intestinal calbindin is not known, but its high content in the intestinal mucosa suggests that it may function as a calcium buffer rather than as a calcium sensor.[188]

SKELETAL ACTIONS. The antirachitic action of vitamin D has traditionally been measured by the increase in osteoid calcification produced by vitamin D administration to vitamin D–depleted animals. There are two schools of thought regarding the mechanisms of its skeletal effects. According to one view, the antirachitic effect results from provision of suitable concentrations of calcium and phosphate in ECF (because of increased intestinal absorption) for mineralization of osteoid.[189]

The alternative view is that, in addition to the just-cited actions, calciferols produce direct anabolic effects on bone. Many in vitro evaluations of the direct skeletal actions have utilized calvaria or long bones of young animals. In these systems the active metabolites can mobilize skeletal mineral and matrix.[190, 191] Similar effects occur at high doses in vivo in normal or in parathyroidectomized animals.[192] $1,25(OH)_2D$ is the most potent analogue in eliciting these actions. There is also evidence for direct anabolic effects of

TABLE 27–8. Distribution Space and Clearance of Calciferols

Metabolite	Body Pool (μg)	Circulation Half-Time (d)	Turnover (μg/d)
Vitamin D*	1000	30	15
25-OHD	200	15	7
$1,25(OH)_2D$	0.5	0.2	1

*D refers to D_2 plus D_3.

1,25(OH)₂D on bone. Under certain conditions, 1,25(OH)₂D at modest doses can increase bone mass in vitamin D–replete animals. Furthermore, in cultures of osteoblast-like cells 1,25(OH)₂D can increase proliferation, alkaline phosphatase activity, and synthesis and secretion of osteocalcin (see Chapter 28).[193, 194]

DIRECT ACTIONS OUTSIDE INTESTINE AND SKELETON. 1,25(OH)₂D influences directly several steps in the calciferol metabolic pathway.[175–177] In the skin, 1,25(OH)₂D increases the accumulation of 7-dehydrocholesterol; in the proximal renal tubule, it inhibits activity of 25-OHD 1α-hydroxylase; in kidney and in cells cultured from several organs, 1,25(OH)₂D increases activity of 25-OHD 24-hydroxylase. Each of these three actions on calciferol metabolism is probably mediated through the cytoplasmic receptor for 1,25(OH)₂D.

1,25(OH)₂D influences secretion of several peptides including PTH, prolactin, and osteocalcin (by osteoblast-like cells).[194] Direct inhibitory effects on PTH secretion, PTH biosynthesis, and proliferation in the parathyroid gland are a potentially important step in the feedback control of this gland,[195] perhaps even contributing to parathyroid hyperplasia independent of hypocalcemia when renal failure results in a defect in 1,25(OH)₂D synthesis.

1,25(OH)₂D induces differentiation of the HL-60 and other human leukemia cell lines toward monocyte function.[196] This raises the possibility that 1,25(OH)₂D is important in formation of the osteoclast, a multinucleate cell thought to derive from fusion of monocyte-like precursors. The occurrence of total alopecia in patients with resistance to 1,25(OH)₂D suggests that the hormone also influences maturation or function of the hair follicle. Many tissues contain receptors for 1,25(OH)₂D and proteins that cross-react in immunoassays for vitamin D–dependent calcium-binding protein.

BIOCHEMICAL MECHANISM OF ACTION. The secosteroid hormones are analogous to other steroid hormones in their biochemical mechanisms of action (Fig. 27–25) (also see Chapter 3). The most detailed studies have employed intestinal tissues, but there is evidence for analogous mechanisms in other tissues.

The chicken intestinal mucosa contains two proteins with high affinity for 1,25(OH)₂D. One is presumably the translocated or contaminating serum 25-OHD transport globulin; the other shows the high affinity and specificity for 1,25(OH)₂D characteristic of a receptor molecule.[197] Its specificity for interaction with vitamin D analogues correlates

well with the biological activities in vitro and in vivo. This receptor molecule determines the localization of 1,25(OH)₂D in nuclear chromatin. The number of receptors for 1,25(OH)₂D in a tissue can vary over time. Receptors are not found in fetal rat intestine, and their appearance postnatally correlates with acquisition of 1,25(OH)₂D–responsive active transport of calcium.[198] Glucocorticoids modulate receptor numbers in vivo and in vitro. In the rat, glucocorticoids increase receptor numbers, whereas in the mouse they decrease receptor numbers.[199] A major molecular action of 1,25(OH)₂D is to increase concentrations of mRNA for 9- or 28-kd vitamin D–dependent calcium-binding protein in selected tissues; other actions include increase in level of mRNA for osteocalcin (in osteoblasts) and decrease in level of mRNA for PTH (in parathyroid cells). These changes in mRNA concentration can result from transcriptional and/or post-transcriptional actions.

Calciferol Assays

BIOASSAYS. Antirachitic potency has traditionally been assessed by the line test. Nutritional rickets is induced in test rats. Animals then receive a single dose of standard or test compound, and 7 d later the degree of linear (therefore the name line test) calcification in the radial epiphysis is quantitated. A dose of 1 IU (25 ng) of vitamin D per rat will produce a detectable response. In this assay, vitamin D is almost equipotent to 1,25(OH)₂D because of the efficient conversion of vitamin D to 1,25(OH)₂D by the vitamin D–deficient animal. In contrast, calciferol analogues, such as the 5,6-trans series, that are low in intrinsic activity even after 25-hydroxylation are weak in this system.

In a different type of assay, metabolites are tested for potency in raising the serum calcium concentration in normal or hypoparathyroid animals. Because the renal 25-OHD 1α-hydroxylation operates at low efficiency in these animals, the assay is biased toward analogues possessing a 1α-hydroxy or pseudo–1α-hydroxy configuration. In these "calcemic" assays, the analogues of the 5,6-trans series are approximately equipotent on a molar basis to vitamins D₂ and D₃, which have a 5,6-cis configuration.

Some of the most sensitive detection systems take advantage of the high affinities and specificities of target tissues and transport proteins. With fetal rat bones in organ culture, as little as 2 pg of 1,25(OH)₂D/mL in the medium will cause detectable bone resorption after a 72-h incubation.[200] Alternatively, analogues can be quantitated by competition with radiolabeled 1,25(OH)₂D for binding to receptor proteins from thymus or from intestinal mucosa (Fig. 27–26).[201, 202] The serum or cytosolic 25-OHD–binding proteins are utilized for competitive radioligand assays to quantitate 25-hydroxy metabolites of the calciferols (Fig. 27–27). The specificities of the serum transport globulin and 1,25(OH)₂D receptor protein are quite different (compare the curves for 1,25(OH)₂D and 25-OHD in Figs. 27–26 and 27–27). With either system a specific metabolite can be assayed only after separation from other cross-reacting metabolites.

Antisera developed by immunization with conjugates of calciferol analogues may make it possible to develop radioimmunoassay techniques already useful in the assessment of other steroid hormones.

PHYSICOCHEMICAL ASSAYS. High concentrations of vitamin D can be quantitated colorimetrically after reaction with antimony trichloride. The calciferol triene structure has a peak absorbance at 264 nm. Because of high concentrations in normal plasma, 25-OHD can be isolated and quantitated by ultraviolet absorbance. The same method is applicable to the quantitation of vitamins D₂ and D₃ and 24,25(OH)₂D in serum.

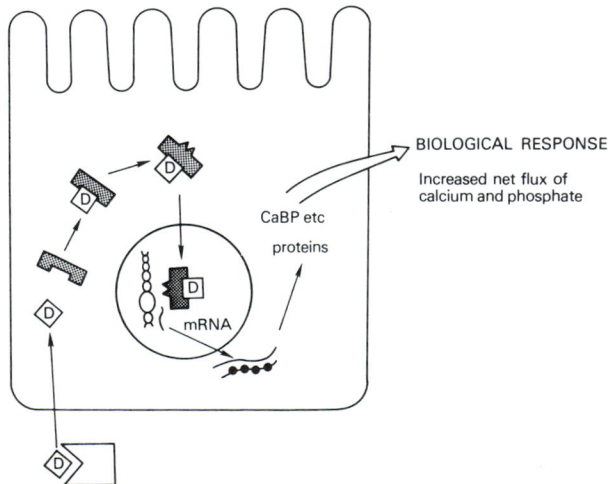

Figure 27–25. Major steps in target cell response to bioactive vitamin D metabolites.

BIOLOGICAL RESPONSE

Increased net flux of calcium and phosphate

CaBP etc proteins

mRNA

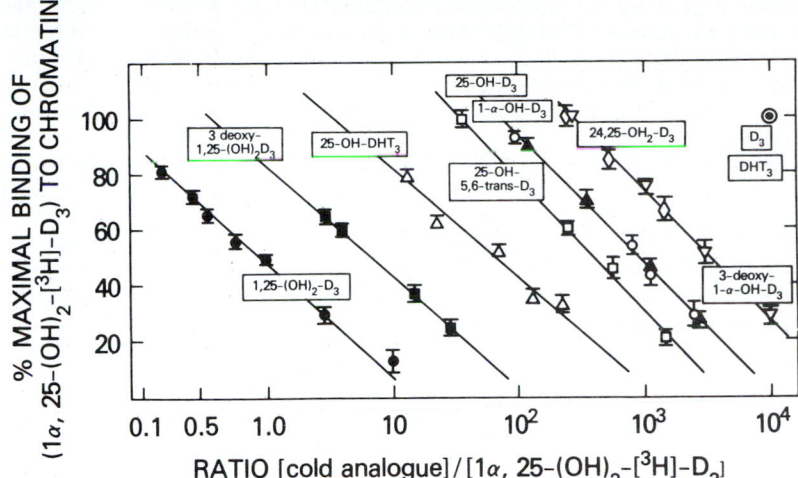

Figure 27–26. Competition of structural analogues of 1,25(OH)$_2$D$_3$ for its chick intestinal mucosal receptor system. (From Procsal DA, Okamura WH, Norman AW. Structural requirements for the interaction of 1α,25-(OH)$_2$-vitamin D$_3$ with its chick intestinal system. J Biol Chem 1975; 250:8382–8388.)

All biochemical and physicochemical assays in present use must contend with two problems. The first is the need to separate calciferol metabolites from interfering lipids. This is particularly difficult in assays based on ultraviolet absorbance. The second is the need to separate multiple cross-reacting vitamin D metabolites. The most sensitive and specific assays generally require a multistep purification (organic extraction together with radioactive markers for recovery and identification plus a chromatographic procedure before measurement by absorbance or by one of the sensitive bioassays).

STRUCTURE-FUNCTION RELATIONS. The most potent natural metabolite is 1,25(OH)$_2$D. Its biological potency is attributable to high-affinity interactions with a receptor protein in target tissues. The mammalian serum vitamin D transport globulins interact preferentially with 25-hydroxy analogues of vitamin D. Lack of the 25-hydroxyl group favors partition of analogues into adipose stores when these are administered in vivo. The affinity of 24,25(OH)$_2$D for the binding globulin is similar to that of 25-OHD. Side-chain lengthening or shortening by one carbon decreases binding affinity to transcalciferin by 10-fold. The transport globulin of the chicken (unlike that of the human) interacts only weakly with the C-17 side chain of the vitamin D$_2$ series, so that in chickens the vitamin D$_2$ analogues are more rapidly cleared and thus less potent than are analogues of the vitamin D$_3$ series. A-ring modifications of 25-OHD such as insertion of the 1α-hydroxyl or deletion of the 3β-hydroxyl cause a 10-fold loss of affinity for the serum transport globulin.

The requirements for direct binding to the intestinal "receptor" have also been analyzed in detail. Substitution with a different side-chain hydroxyl (i.e., 1,24(OH)$_2$D) causes no substantial loss of receptor affinity. Several other features of the C-17 side chain are critical. Removal of the 25-hydroxyl group (i.e., 1α-OHD) leads to a 900-fold drop in receptor affinity, and insertion of an extra hydroxyl group (i.e., 1,24R,25(OH)$_3$D) decreases the affinity two- to fivefold. The calciferol A ring is flexible in natural solutions with a rapid equilibrium between chair-chair configurations. The consequences of the associated shifts of the 1α-hydroxyl group from axial to equatorial positions may be important in receptor interaction. Deletion of the 1α-hydroxyl group causes a 900-fold loss in affinity for the intestinal receptor. Synthetic 1β-OHD, in which the 1-hydroxyl is below the plane of the A ring, has undetectable activity in vivo (less than 1% the antirachitic activity of vitamin D). The 5,6-cis configuration is not essential, but conversion to a trans configuration results in an approximately 100-fold decrease in intrinsic affinity of the 25-hydroxylated forms for the receptor. This rotates the 3-hydroxyl group to a pseudo-1α configuration (Fig. 27–28), producing analogues that are active (albeit showing low receptor affinity) without a need for 1α-hydroxylation. From this it can be inferred that neither the 3β-hydroxyl group nor the C-19 methylene

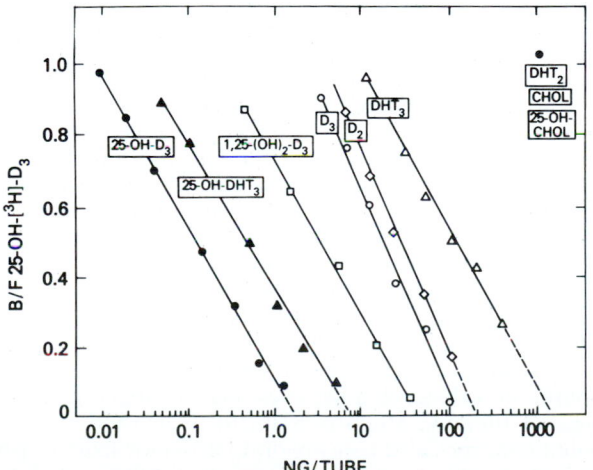

Figure 27–27. Competition of structural analogues of 25-OHD$_3$ for its transport globulin (transcalciferin) from rat serum. (From Belsey R, Clark MB, Bernat M, et al. The physiologic significance of plasma transport of vitamin D and metabolites. Am J Med 1974; 57:50–56.)

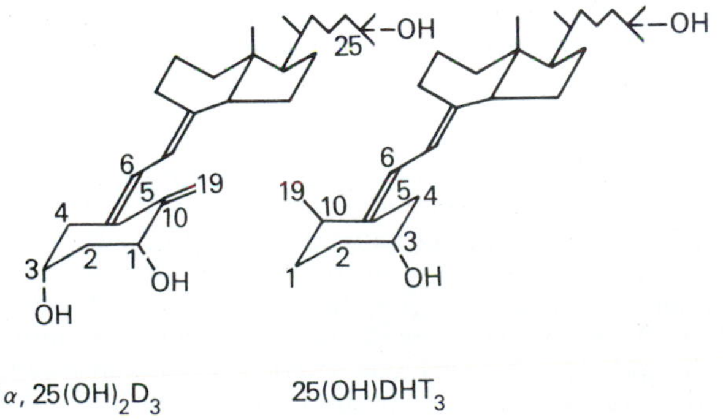

1α, 25(OH)$_2$D$_3$ 25(OH)DHT$_3$

Figure 27–28. Possible conformations of 1α,25(OH)$_2$D$_3$, and 25-OH-dihydro-tachysterol.

group is essential. In most bioassays 24,25(OH)$_2$D has actions similar to those of 25-OHD. Occasional reports of unique effects of 24,25(OH)$_2$D in other systems (neonatal or fetal rat chondrocyte;[203] bone mass in the vitamin D–replete state[204]) have raised the possibility of effector systems with specificities different from those of the receptor in intestinal mucosa.[205]

Pharmacology

Conditions responsive to calciferol analogues include hypoparathyroidism, neonatal hypocalcemia, many forms of rickets and osteomalacia, and secondary hyperparathyroidism of uremia. Low circulating concentration of 1,25(OH)$_2$D is a common feature in most of these states, making treatment with calciferol analogues logical. Details of therapy are discussed in sections dealing with the pathological states; the general pharmacology of calciferol is outlined here.

In most organic solvents these sterols are quite soluble. They can be crystallized from alcohol solutions in the form of long prisms that undergo decomposition at room temperature over 2 d. Stability is increased by protection from light, oxygen, and heat. Ergocalciferol and cholecalciferol are stable for prolonged periods in fats, oils, or propylene glycol. An active water-soluble form of 1,25(OH)$_2$D has been discovered in plants (*Solanum malacoxylon, Cestrum diurnum,* and *Tricetium flavescens*) known to cause calcinosis in grazing animals. In these extracts 1,25(OH)$_2$D is linked to one or more glycoside groups. This indicates the feasibility of development of synthetic water-soluble analogues of the calciferols. Features that determine the utility of an analogue are rate of onset and offset of action. The calciferols have half-times to onset or offset of action of approximately 2 wk in treatment of hypoparathyroidism. Most of the administered drug accumulates in body fat, and that in the circulation must be activated by both 25- and 1α-hydroxylation. These features make these drugs useful in patients retaining intact parathyroid-renal axes responsive to variations in mineral availability. Prolonged storage in body fat is the basis for "stoss therapy," wherein a large dose of vitamin D is given orally once every 2 to 6 mo for prevention or treatment of vitamin D deficiency.[206] Vitamins D, by generating the 25-hydroxylated metabolites, may be effective even in the anephric patient. Their storage characteristics also make them useful when daily drug administration is not practical or when parenteral therapy is required. Nutritional vitamin D deficiency in adults responds to 5 to 100 μg/d (200 to 4000 IU/d) of cholecalciferol or ergocalciferol; typical requirements are 10-fold higher in most states with abnormal calciferol metabolism. Calcifediol differs from vitamin D$_3$ insofar as a smaller proportion is stored in body fat and it bypasses hepatic 25-hydroxylation. Thus the onset and offset of action are faster, and it is effective when there is impairment of hepatic 25-hydroxylation, as in primary biliary cirrhosis or some cases of neonatal hypocalcemia. Because calcifediol has intrinsic agonist activity, it retains some effectiveness even without the renal 25-OHD 1α-hydroxylase system.

The half-time of calcitriol for onset or offset of action is 1 to 3 d. Thus it is extremely useful when rapid responses are important, as in symptomatic neonatal hypocalcemia or rapidly changing clinical status (bone remineralization after parathyroidectomy). One microgram per day increases intestinal calcium absorption in normal or vitamin D–deficient adults. This drug bypasses the principal regulatory influence of the parathyroid-renal axis. If PTH or the renal 25-OHD 1α-hydroxylase response is absent, treatment with any calciferol metabolite will provide unregulated circulating metabolite levels and a constant degree of activation of

1,25(OH)$_2$D receptors. 1α-OHD$_3$ and dihydrotachysterol are synthetic analogues that do not require renal activation to produce a metabolite with an active A ring; each requires 25-hydroxylation by the liver, and 1α-OHD$_3$, perhaps because it is more polar, is more rapid in onset and offset (3- to 5-d half-time) than is dihydrotachysterol (7- to 25-d half-time).

All the active calciferol analogues cited are similar in effects on mineral metabolism in humans. Their initial and major site of action is the intestine, where mucosal-to-serosal movement of calcium is promoted. Secondary hyperparathyroidism is gradually suppressed by elimination of hypocalcemia and perhaps also by direct action of calciferol metabolites on the parathyroid glands. High concentrations of calciferol metabolites also cause mobilization of calcium and phosphate from skeletal store.[207] As the serum calcium concentration rises, calcium excretion into the urine increases. In the absence of PTH secretion, high renal calcium excretion may occur even before a normal serum calcium concentration is attained. Hypercalciuria is a potential problem whenever calciferol analogues are used for treatment of hypoparathyroidism. It may cause deterioration in renal-function even in the absence of hypercalcemia. If uncorrected, this imposes a risk of nephrocalcinosis, nephrolithiasis, and/or irreversible decrease in glomerular filtration. Decreasing glomerular filtration with continued calcium mobilization from the intestine or skeleton or both leads to progressive hypercalcemia and worsening renal damage. The potentially nephrotoxic effects of the calciferols are thus indirect, resulting from excesses of calcium in urine and plasma. Vitamin D intoxication can occur independently of the renal 25-OHD 1α-hydroxylase system. In normal persons, the 1α-hydroxylase is suppressed effectively when high concentrations of calciferol substrate are present. Thus excessive intakes of vitamin D can be associated with normal or even low serum concentrations of 1,25(OH)$_2$D but toxic concentrations of 25-OHD.

A variety of considerations influence dosage requirement. Dietary calcium determines the quantity of calcium available to be absorbed from the intestinal lumen. Fluctuations in dietary calcium make therapy difficult in states with compromised parathyroid and renal regulatory function. This problem can be minimized by giving supplemental calcium by mouth, so that dietary variations contribute in only a minor way to the high baseline intake. Calcium equivalent to an elemental calcium level of 15 mg/kg (for example, 3 g/d of calcium carbonate for adults) blunts diet-associated fluctuations and can be abruptly withdrawn if calciferol overdose should occur. Daily flux of calcium out of the central or circulating pool also determines calciferol requirements. At early points in treatment of osteomalacia, large amounts of calcium may be deposited each day in the skeleton. As skeletal pools are repleted, whole body calcium needs, and thus whole body calciferol needs, diminish. Renal excretion of calcium may change abruptly if the patient is given thiazide diuretics (which decrease renal calcium clearance) or loop diuretics (such as ethacrynic acid, furosemide, and related compounds) (which increase renal calcium clearance). A number of other drugs interact with mineral or calciferol metabolism by mechanisms that are often poorly understood. Interactions with glucocorticoids, estrogens, and anticonvulsants are considered subsequently. Last, the metabolism of calciferol analogues may change during the course of therapy. Much remains to be learned about metabolite clearance and conversion to active or inactive products during periods of changing mineral status.

Because calciferol therapy is often a long-term commitment, cost and facility of monitoring serum metabolite concentrations should also be considered. Serum 25-OHD (because of its slow turnover and ease of measurement) is simple to monitor during therapy with vitamin D or calcifediol; serum $1,25(OH)_2D$ (because of its rapid turnover and difficulty of measurement) is more difficult to monitor during therapy with calcitriol; however, its concentrations fluctuate much less during therapy with $1\alpha\text{-OHD}_3$, which is not currently available in the United States.

The following principles should serve as general guidelines. (1) Underlying disorders such as malabsorption should receive appropriate treatment. (2) With low serum concentrations of 25-OHD, one should utilize analogues that restore normal serum concentrations and allow normal regulation of mineral metabolism by the parathyroid-renal axis. (3) With impaired 25-OHD 1α-hydroxylation in parathyroid or renal disease, any metabolites that generate active forms will have similar effects. Selection should then be based on considerations of rapidity of action, cost, and facility of monitoring. (4) All analogues have a potential to cause hypercalciuria and irreversible renal damage. (5) Dosage requirements may vary during treatment, particularly if there are changes in calcium needs or interacting drugs. (6) Treatment with calcium minimizes effects of variations in dietary calcium.

MISCELLANEOUS HUMORAL CALCITROPIC FACTORS

GONADAL STEROIDS. Lifelong or premature deficiency of the principal estrogens in women or of androgens in men is associated with an increased incidence of osteoporosis. The endocrine changes at menopause cause increased rate of loss of bone mass. In addition, among perimenopausal women, the incidence of primary hyperparathyroidism is increased. The skeletal actions of PTH seem accentuated in estrogen lack, but the mechanism for this has not been established. A direct action of estrogen on the osteoblast[208] or chondrocyte[209] may be important.

Administration of estrogens to menopausal women in physiological replacement amounts leads to the following: slight fall of serum calcium concentration, rise in serum concentration of PTH and $1,25(OH)_2D$, decreased urinary excretion of calcium, and retention of total body calcium for at least 6 to 12 mo. All these changes could reflect estrogenic interference with net skeletal resorption. Estrogen administration to patients receiving calciferol analogues may increase the requirement. Occasionally pharmacological doses of estrogen cause decreases in serum calcium level in patients with refractory hypercalcemia (bone metastases or parathyroid cancer).

GLUCOCORTICOIDS. States of glucocorticoid excess are associated with accelerated loss of skeletal mass, particularly from regions of trabecular bone such as vertebrae.[190] Glucocorticoids antagonize the action of calciferol analogues in states of hypoparathyroidism or calciferol excess. Glucocorticoids may have additional therapeutic effects in certain hypercalcemic states; they can inhibit some tumors that release calcemic factors (myeloma, lymphoma, and some prostaglandin-producing neoplasms) and may inhibit the direct skeletal action of certain osteoclast-activating factors (OAFs).

The histological effect of glucocorticoids on the skeleton suggests decreased bone formation and increased bone resorption. The decrease in bone formation has been attributed principally to direct inhibition of osteoblast differentiation. The increase in bone resorption may be multifactorial in cause. Glucocorticoid administration may cause increased circulating PTH levels. Furthermore, incubation of rat calvaria with physiological concentrations of glucocorticoids leads to an increase in tissue cAMP response to PTH; glucocorticoid suppression of skeletal cAMP phosphodiesterase activity accounts in part for this. Glucocorticoids interfere directly with intestinal calcium absorption and also may interfere with the maintenance of normal plasma concentrations of both 25-OHD and $1,25(OH)_2D$. Glucocorticoids do not compete with the calciferols for binding to their high-affinity serum transport proteins or target issue cytoplasmic receptors. However, they can modulate the number of receptors for $1,25(OH)_2D$ in ways that are species specific (increase in rat, decrease in mouse).

THYROID HORMONES. Thyrotoxicosis, like immobilization, is associated with hypercalciuria, decrease in bone mass, and mild hypercalcemia.[210] Thyroid hormone in vitro leads to a direct stimulation of bone resorption. The histological features of bone in thyrotoxicosis suggest increased skeletal resorptive and formative activities. An increased quantity of osteoid is the result of an increase in the numbers, not the width, of osteoid borders, reflecting intense osteoblastic activity without any defect in osteoid mineralization. The parathyroid glands are suppressed; the combination of normal to elevated concentrations of calcium with secondary decrease of circulating PTH level accounts for a high incidence of hypercalciuria in thyrotoxicosis. Hypothyroidism in children causes growth retardation (with stippled epiphyses). In vitro, thyroid hormones directly stimulate maturation of cartilage in the region of the growth plate.[211]

OSTEOCLAST-ACTIVATING FACTORS. Factors that activate osteoclasts and stimulate bone resorption in vitro are present in culture media of activated human leukocytes and of cells from patients with multiple myeloma or lymphoma.[192] OAFs are a series of small proteins structurally distinct from PTH (for example, interleukin 1[212] and tumor necrosis factor β or lymphotoxin[213]). The resorptive activity of some OAF preparations, unlike that of PTH, is blocked by glucocorticoid concentrations achievable in vivo. The term OAF has been applied to several factors, some of which stimulate cAMP in bone and others of which do not. Mediators such as these or the prostaglandins may account for the bone resorption associated with some skeletal metastases or inflammatory disorders of the skeleton (periodontal disease, arthritis, osteomyelitis). Most act by being released within bone and not via the systemic circulation.

UTILIZATION OF THE LABORATORY IN ASSESSING CALCITROPIC HORMONES

Standard evaluations of clinical history, radiographs, and mineral concentrations in serum or urine are usually inadequate to allow definitive diagnosis and therapy. This section outlines the utility and limitations of specialized tests in disorders of mineral metabolism.

Assessment of the State of Calcium in Blood

Total calcium concentration in serum can be determined by atomic absorption, colorimetry, or compleximetry (EDTA titration). Ionically active calcium, however, determines membrane excitability and chemical reactivity and regulates the secretion of PTH and CT. Total serum calcium does not accurately reflect ionically active calcium when the fraction complexed to proteins and other anions is abnormal.

Calcium ionic activity can be measured directly with

electrodes analogous to those used for measuring pH.[8] Serum or plasma is difficult to work with, however, because of change in specimen pH and because of protein interference. In most laboratories, total calcium is determined with greater precision than is calcium ion activity. Ion-specific electrodes are useful when major distortions exist in the calcium-binding activity of serum proteins and when high circulating concentrations of calcium chelators such as citrate, oxalate, edetate, or unidentified factors are present.

The filtered load of calcium is of great relevance to urinary excretion of calcium.[9] Filtrable calcium can be assessed in vitro with artificial membranes under conditions that simulate glomerular filtration. This fraction correlates better with serum ionized calcium concentration than does total calcium level. Unfortunately, the precision of determinations of ultrafiltrable calcium is generally lower than that for ionized calcium.

Direct Assays of the Calcitropic Hormones in Blood

PARATHYROID HORMONE. Most of the immunoreactive PTH in peripheral blood represents inactive metabolites of the hormone. The concentrations are determined by distribution volume, secretion rate, and metabolic clearance. The mixture of PTH fragments in serum depends on serum calcium concentration and on variations in function of parathyroid gland, kidney, and liver. However, useful assays have been developed with four major types of specificity (intact, NH_2-terminal, midregion, or COOH-terminal). Clinical validation is more important than region specificity. With the best-validated PTH radioimmunoassays, directed at either NH_2- or COOH-terminal antigens, the range of values in primary hyperparathyroidism overlaps with the normal range.[35] PTH assays that require an epitope at the NH_2 terminus and another at the COOH terminus (for example, two-site immunoradiometric assays) give information that correlates well with the level of intact, biologically active PTH. Such assays have achieved great clinical utility, particularly as they are little affected by differences in renal clearance of inactive PTH fragments. Measurement of the concentration of immunoreactive PTH is important in assessing patients with hypocalcemia or hypercalcemia. The PTH immunoassay is also useful for the localization of PTH-secreting tissues by assessment of samples directly aspirated from a suspicious lesion or taken from venous beds of the parathyroids. Protocols for stimulating or inhibiting secretion of PTH have not been helpful.

CALCITONIN. The methodological difficulties of this radioimmunoassay are similar in type to but less in degree than those of the radioimmunoassay for PTH. A two-site immunoradiometric assay is also available for measurement of CT. Unlike the heterogeneous forms attributable to small fragments of PTH, CT heterogeneity represents multiple high-molecular-weight forms. Normal basal concentrations are below the lower detection limits of many assays, and results with different antisera may not agree as the antisera react with different components of the multiple circulating forms. The difficulty in detecting basal concentrations can, to some extent, be overcome by assessing the concentration after stimulating hormone secretion. Useful stimuli include calcium or pentagastrin or combinations of the two (ethanol and glucagon have also been used). Tests with both secretagogues give similar information when performed in a standardized manner. The CT immunoassay is useful for the diagnosis of medullary carcinoma of the thyroid, which virtually always secretes CT. The CT immunoassay of serum after secretagogue administration sometimes allows diagno-

sis of the premalignant phase of this tumor (see Chapter 30). CT is sometimes a useful marker for tumors outside the C cells.

CALCIFEROL METABOLITES. Radioligand assays for the calciferol metabolites have the same limitations as those for all compounds at low concentrations. Often serum must be purified by extraction with organic solvents and by one or more chromatography procedures to eliminate interfering lipids. 25-OHD can be measured in serum extracts by ultraviolet absorption or by competitive radioligand assay. The binding proteins used include serum 25-OHD transport globulin, cytosol 25-OHD-binding globulin, or antibodies against calciferol conjugates. Purification methods can resolve 25-OHD$_2$ from 25-OHD$_3$, but this is not necessary in clinical application. These assays are sufficiently sensitive to detect concentrations below the normal range and are useful in assessing calciferol excess, calciferol deficiency, or certain abnormalities in calciferol metabolism (malabsorption, decreased hepatic 25-hydroxylation, or increased 25-OHD clearance). Normal serum concentrations of $1,25(OH)_2D$ are about 0.1% of those of 25-OHD. Most assays of $1,25(OH)_2D$ in serum, therefore, require extensive sample purification. The binding phase has included dispersed osteosarcoma cells, bovine thymus nuclear extract, and antibodies against a calciferol conjugate. Although the assays are technically demanding, they may provide clinically useful information. Features limiting the utility of assays for $1,25(OH)_2D$ are technical difficulty, expense, rapid fluctuations in serum concentrations, and the general utility of assay for 25-OHD in evaluating the calciferol metabolic pathway.

Renal Clearance of Solutes as Indices of Circulating PTH Activity

cAMP. Normally approximately 50% of urinary cAMP excretion is accounted for by glomerular filtration of cAMP from plasma. The remainder is synthesized and excreted by the kidney under direct control by circulating PTH. Correction can be made for variations in serum concentrations of cAMP and in GFR (nephrogenous urinary cAMP excretion rate corrected by GFR).

$$\frac{cAMP}{GFR} = \frac{U_{cAMP} \times V}{C_{Cr}}$$

which simplifies to

$$\frac{cAMP}{GFR} = U_{cAMP} \times \frac{P_{Cr}}{U_{Cr}}$$

where U = urine; P = plasma; V = volume; C = clearance; and Cr = creatinine. This assay is compromised by the fact that many cancers are associated with increased urinary cAMP excretion. Determination of renal cAMP excretion after PTH administration is also useful in defining states of PTH resistance.

PHOSPHATE. Another prominent action of PTH is regulation of renal clearance of phosphate. Indices that reflect this action include serum phosphate concentration, renal tubular reabsorption of phosphate (TRP), and theoretical renal phosphate threshold. TRP is derived from the following simple relationship:

$$TRP = \frac{C_{Cr} - C_P}{C_{Cr}} = 1 - \frac{U_P \times S_{Cr}}{U_{Cr} \times S_P}$$

where C = clearance; S = serum; P = phosphate; U = urine; and Cr = creatinine. The clearance study is performed in the morning over 2 to 4 h with the patient fasting. Because renal excretion of phosphate is determined by multiple factors in addition to PTH activity, these tests have been largely replaced by the radioimmunoassay of PTH in serum or of cAMP in urine.

CALCIUM. PTH decreases the renal clearance of calcium. Analysis of the relation between serum calcium concentration and urinary calcium excretion thus provides indirect information about status of the PTH-calciferol axis (see Fig. 27–13). At any serum concentration of calcium, PTH suppression or deficiency is characterized by relative hypercalciuria, whereas PTH excess is characterized by relative hypocalciuria. Because factors other than PTH also modulate renal clearance of calcium, these tests complement but do not replace the radioimmunoassay for PTH in serum. Assessment of urinary calcium excretion and solubility is also important for the evaluation of patients with nephrolithiasis (see Chapter 29).

Intestinal Interaction with Calcitropic Hormones

CELLULAR RESPONSE TO CALCIFEROLS. Assessment of vitamin D receptors and vitamin D–dependent calcium-binding proteins in intestinal mucosa may eventually become useful for assessing cellular responsiveness to calciferols. Receptors for $1,25(OH)_2D$ can be assessed in circulating mononuclear cells or in cultured skin fibroblasts. Several markers of bioresponse to $1,25(OH)_2D$ are undergoing exploration, including skeletal release of osteocalcin and hormonal induction of 25-OHD 24-hydroxylase in cells.

MINERAL BALANCE. The net balance for any metabolic component is the difference between input and output. Thus the net balance is the difference between the dietary input and the output in urine and feces. In practice, mineral input and output are difficult to quantitate. Slow intestinal transit and intestinal mixing prevent segregation of the fecal output remaining from one meal; thus balance studies require evaluation periods of several days. Quantitation of input over such a long period requires rigid control of diet and is possible only with a metabolic kitchen and a cooperative subject. Optimal equilibration of mineral homeostasis to a constant diet requires several weeks. Balance differences of as little as 50 mg/d could be important; thus meticulous analysis of total intake and output is demanding but essential. Balance studies are now rarely done even in a research setting.[2]

ISOTOPIC EVALUATION OF CALCIUM ABSORPTION. Unidirectional and net (the difference between lumen-to-plasma and plasma-to-lumen flux) intestinal absorption can be assessed with calcium isotopes.[7] An isotope (usually ^{47}Ca) is administered orally with a standard meal containing a fixed amount of ^{40}Ca, usually 100 mg. Use of stable isotopes (^{44}Ca or ^{42}Ca), which are not widely available, can make it possible to perform these tests in children and pregnant women. Unidirectional absorption can be estimated from kinetic analysis of the isotope in blood samples obtained during the following ½ to 6 h. The accuracy of the calculations can be enhanced by solving and correcting for clearance of circulating calcium. This is accomplished by simultaneously administering a different calcium isotope intravenously or by giving the same isotope at a different time and assuming that the patient is in the same metabolic state. Net absorption can also be quantitated by determining the difference between the administered isotope dose and the quantity excreted in feces over the following 7 to 10 d

or by measuring the whole body isotope retention more than 7 d later, when the nonabsorbed tracer (plus that secreted by the intestines) has been eliminated from the intestines. Increased calcium absorption rates occur with calciferol excess, hyperparathyroidism, calcium nephrolithiasis, and sarcoidosis. Decreased rates occur with renal failure, hypoparathyroidism, malabsorption, and other calciferol deficiency states.

Response to Oral or Intravenous Calcium

Challenge with oral or intravenous calcium has been advocated in the evaluation of urolithiasis (oral calcium), parathyroid autonomy (oral or intravenous calcium), and C cell function. The greatest utility is in subclassification of idiopathic hypercalciuria (see Chapter 29).

PRIMARY HYPERPARATHYROIDISM

Primary hyperparathyroidism is a state of hypersecretion of PTH by the parathyroid gland. The etiology has not been clearly defined, but mutations may be involved. There is a history of prior radiation to the neck[214, 215] in a fraction of the cases. Moreover, genetic rearrangements and deletions involving the q13 region of chromosome 11 have been detected in adenomas as well as hyperplastic tissue (the latter from subjects with familial multiple endocrine neoplasia type 1 [MEN 1]) removed from patients with hyperparathyroidism.[216-218] Further of interest is that MEN 1, a hereditary syndrome associated with parathyroid hyperplasia, is linked to the same region of chromosome 11.[219, 220] Parathyroid tumors in the hyperplastic glands of patients with MEN 1, as well as adenomas, are frequently monoclonal.[216-218]

Primary hyperparathyroidism may also arise from the long-term consequences of secondary hyperparathyroidism, as in chronic renal disease (therein dubbed tertiary hyperparathyroidism) or long-standing osteomalacia. Chronic loss of calcium through the kidney might likewise represent a stimulus to hyperplasia and ultimate adenomatous growth of the glands and uncontrolled hypersecretion of hormone.

Prevalence

The prevalence of primary hyperparathyroidism appears to have increased with the advent of more widespread recognition of the disorder and with routine analysis of serum calcium. In one consecutive series of 26,000 serum calcium measurements, the prevalence of primary hyperparathyroidism was approximately 1:1000.[221] This is a prevalence approximately 10-fold that ascertained in early studies of hyperparathyroidism. The high prevalences in surveys based on serum calcium measurements do not provide an estimate of cases requiring treatment. Ascertainment on the basis of hypercalcemia alone includes asymptomatic hyperparathyroidism as well as familial hypocalciuric hypercalcemia (FHH) (the exact prevalence of the latter disorder is unknown). Because parathyroidectomy is usually contraindicated in FHH, it is important that such cases be separated from primary hyperparathyroidism.

Pathology

Hypersecretion of PTH with primary hyperparathyroidism may be caused by a single adenoma, primary chief cell or clear cell hyperplasia of all parathyroid glands, or carcinoma.

Histopathology

ADENOMA. Parathyroid adenomas may be composed of chief cells, transitional forms between chief and oxyphil cells, and, rarely, only oxyphil cells (Figs. 27–29 and 27–30). Unlike normal oxyphil cells, those in adenomas contain abundant endoplasmic reticulum and Golgi vesicles. Immunoperoxidase staining for PTH indicates that these oxyphil cells do in fact synthesize PTH.[222] An even rarer form of parathyroid adenoma is the so-called lipoadenoma or hamartoma. These lesions tend to be large and soft and consist of a fatty fibrillar stroma with nests of parathyroid glandular tissue interspersed.[223] The weight of parathyroid adenomas varies from 100 mg to more than 20 g. Larger lesions are often cystic and show areas of hemorrhage. There may be considerable cellular pleomorphism and atypia and even visible mitoses in adenomas.

CHIEF CELL HYPERPLASIA. Chief cell hyperplasia is diagnosed on finding more than one parathyroid grossly or microscopically abnormal. Several forms of chief cell hyperplasia have been described. The classic variety is the simplest form to diagnose because there is obvious enlargement of several parathyroids. In pseudoadenomatous hyperplasia, a single gland may be grossly enlarged with subtle, if any, enlargement of remaining glands. The minimally enlarged glands, however, have an abnormal histological appearance

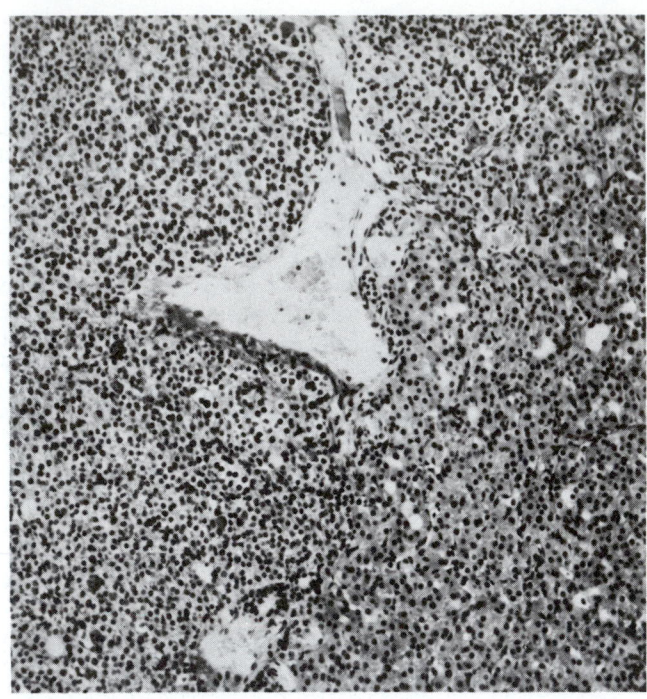

Figure 27–30. Sheets of minimally pleomorphic chief cells with a few intermixed transitional oxyphil cells *(lower right)* but no stromal fat cells in a patient with primary chief cell hyperplasia. Magnification × 120. (Courtesy of Dr. Benjamin Castleman.)

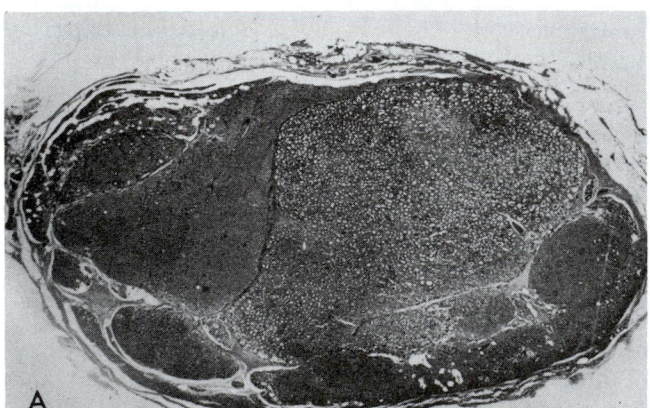

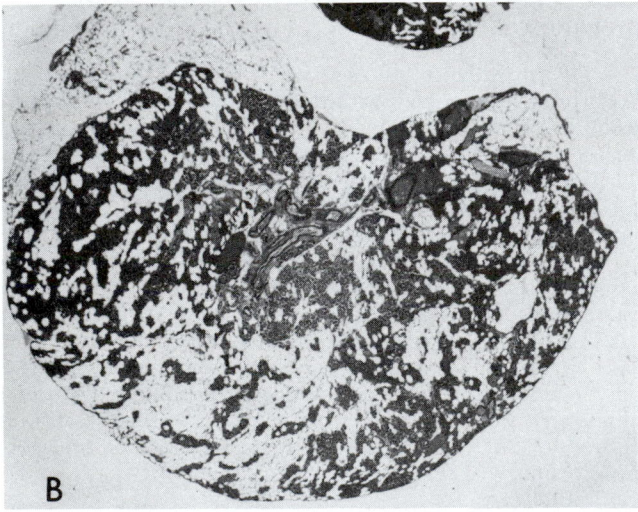

Figure 27–29. *A,* Cross-section of an entire hyperplastic parathyroid gland, showing islands of parathyroid cells in varying patterns. The small solid islands are made up predominantly of oxyphil cells, with the largest island of chief cells in an acinar pattern. Magnification × 11. *B,* Cross-section of an entire normal parathyroid gland, demonstrating usual amount and distribution of stromal fat in a middle-aged person. Magnification × 15. (Courtesy of Dr. Benjamin Castleman.)

with nodularity and an increased chief cell/fat cell ratio. In occult hyperplasia, there is subtle enlargement of all four glands and a reduction in fat cell content.

DIFFERENTIAL DIAGNOSIS OF ADENOMA, MULTIPLE ADENOMAS, AND CHIEF CELL HYPERPLASIA. Adenoma can be diagnosed only when there is a single abnormal parathyroid gland and the remaining glands are normal. Hyperplasia implies abnormality of all parathyroid glands. Accurate pathological diagnosis requires that there be clear-cut criteria for differentiating adenoma from hyperplastic glands and from normal glands. Unfortunately, no conclusive criteria exist. Although the existence of a compressed rim of normal tissue outside the capsule of an enlarged gland is evidence for the diagnosis of adenoma, a similar appearance may occur in nodular (pseudoadenomatous) chief cell hyperplasia.[224] Thus the distinction between adenoma and hyperplasia cannot be made by examining a single gland. Two studies provide conflicting evidence on the distinction between adenoma and hyperplasia. In one,[225] the ratio of glucose-6-phosphate dehydrogenase isoenzymes was studied in parathyroid tumor cells from women heterozygous at the X chromosome–linked locus for this enzyme. In each case both isoenzymes were present, suggesting that parathyroid "adenomas" have a multicellular rather than clonal origin and are therefore similar to hyperplastic glands. In the other study,[226] significant differences were found in ABO(H) cell-surface antigens in adenomatous versus hyperplastic glands. Most adenomatous cells lose these surface antigens, whereas they are retained in hyperplastic cells. Although there was some overlap, the findings suggest a qualitative difference between adenomatous and hyperplastic cells. This question requires further study.

The distinction between normal and abnormal parathyroid glands is usually based on size, weight, and percentage of stromal cells (or, conversely, parenchymal cellularity). In extreme cases the distinction is simple, but the fact that normal glands contain less fat than was hitherto appreciated[27] makes this a poor criterion. Thus it may not be possible to distinguish normal from abnormal tissue solely on the basis of light microscopic evaluation of the proportion of glandular fat versus parenchyma. Therefore, other methods, including intracellular fat staining, measurement of glandular density, and flow cytometric analysis of intranuclear DNA content, have been employed in an effort to distinguish normal from abnormal tissue. Some reports suggest that these techniques are useful,[227] but no method provides unequivocal differentiation between normal and abnormal glands.

This lack of conclusive criteria causes variability in the reported incidence of adenoma versus hyperplasia. Certain authors suggest that virtually all cases of primary hyperparathyroidism are due to hyperplasia,[228] but the general experience is that the majority (>80%) are due to single adenomas and that a minority are due to hyperplasia. In virtually all cases of familial hyperparathyroidism (including FHH and the MEN syndromes), hyperplasia is the underlying lesion. A further point of controversy concerns the existence of multiple or double adenomas. Some contend that enlargement of more than one gland implies hyperplasia, but in several series about 2% of all cases of primary hyperparathyroidism are attributed to enlargement of two glands.[229] Support for this contention comes from biopsy proof of normal remaining parathyroid glands, absence of affected family members, and long-term follow-up showing no evidence for recurrent disease. Accurate pathological diagnosis has important implications for surgical therapy. Correlation of pathological diagnoses and long-term responses to therapy will be necessary to validate methods for assessment of parathyroid pathology.

WATER-CLEAR CELL HYPERPLASIA. This lesion occurs in about 1% of all cases of primary hyperparathyroidism. Grossly, the superior glands are usually disproportionately enlarged. The empty appearance of water-clear cells is attributable to large membrane-lined vacuoles filling the cytoplasm.

CARCINOMA. Parathyroid carcinoma accounts for 3 to 4% of cases of primary hyperparathyroidism in most series, but some evidence[230] suggests a lower figure. The malignant lesion may be palpable in the neck in as many as half of the cases and at surgery is often firm and densely adherent to local structures. Characteristic histological features include capsular and vascular invasion; cells are usually organized into trabeculae separated by thick fibrous bands (Fig. 27–31). Mitotic figures are almost always present. Local invasion, spread to regional lymph nodes, and distant metastases (lung, liver, and bone in order of decreasing frequency) have been described. Hypercalcemia greater than 3.6 mmol/L (14.5 mg/dL) and marked elevations in levels of circulating PTH are characteristic of parathyroid cancer.[230]

Clinical Manifestations

GENERAL. Primary hyperparathyroidism is a disease with protean manifestations varying from asymptomatic to systemic symptoms and signs such as weakness, fatigability, headache, weight loss, and depression. The disease tends to segregate into three categories in terms of clinical presentation. In the mildest form there may be no symptoms or signs, and discovery is made only through routine determination of serum calcium. The second form develops insidiously over a period of years and presents predominantly as renal colic. In the third group, the interval between development of symptoms and diagnosis may be much shorter, with hypercalcemia, debility, bone pain, and sometimes pathological fracture. Weight loss, anemia, and elevated erythrocyte sedimentation rate may suggest systemic malignancy. Polydipsia, polyuria, pruritus, anorexia, and nausea and vomiting may develop secondary to hypercalcemia.

RENAL MANIFESTATIONS. Renal colic is one of the most common symptoms of hyperparathyroidism. Nephrocalcinosis and metabolic acidosis may also occur. Most stones in hyperparathyroidism are calcium oxalate, but calcium phosphate stones also occur. Development of either should alert the physician to the possible diagnosis. Correlation has been reported between $1,25(OH)_2D$ concentrations in plasma and nephrolithiasis in primary hyperparathyroidism.[231]

SKELETAL MANIFESTATIONS. Bone disease in hyperparathyroidism may present as bone pain, pathological fracture, bone cysts, or localized swellings of bone encountered as "epulis" of the jaw or "brown tumors" (areas of accumulated osteoclasts, osteoblasts, and fibrous tissue) of bones.[224] The skeletal lesion observed in hyperparathyroidism, osteitis fibrosa cystica, is discussed in Chapter 28.

Several symptoms and signs are referable to the joints. Gout and pseudogout may be complications of the disease.[232] Chondrocalcinosis and predisposition to attacks of pseudogout occur with greater frequency than in the general population. Nonspecific arthralgias involving all of the joints of the hands or sometimes centered in the proximal interphalangeal joints are also reported. The etiology of these nonspecific arthralgias is unknown, but they usually disappear after correction of the underlying disorder.

GASTROINTESTINAL MANIFESTATIONS. Peptic ulcer occurs with increased frequency in primary hyperparathyroidism. Hypercalcemia per se can cause an increase in serum gastrin level and an increase in gastric acid secretion. Moreover, hyperparathyroidism as part of the MEN 1 syndrome may be the first manifestation of endocrine disease in the syndrome and in these families may precede the Zollinger-Ellison syndrome[233, 234] (see Chapter 30). In the latter instance, pancreatic islet tumors secrete massive amounts of gastrin, causing huge increases in acid production by the stomach. The concentrations of gastrin in serum in the Zollinger-Ellison syndrome usually exceed 600 ng/L. Chronic pancreatitis also may be associated with primary hyperparathyroidism. The pathophysiology leading to this association is unknown. Pancreatitis may be exacerbated in subjects with worsening hyperparathyroidism and in the postoperative phase of parathyroidectomy.

NEUROLOGICAL MANIFESTATIONS. Neurological abnormalities in hyperparathyroidism include emotional labil-

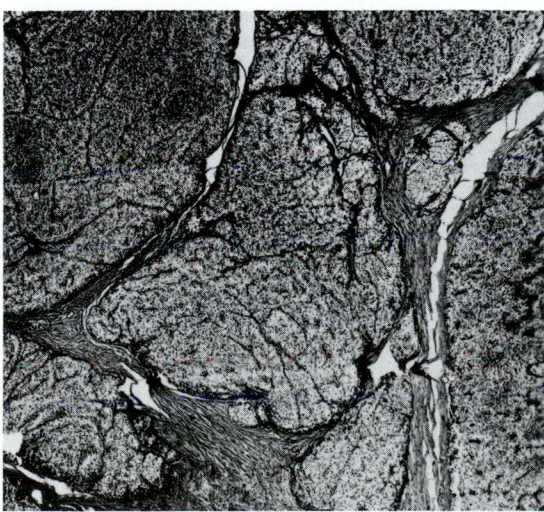

Figure 27–31. Parathyroid carcinoma. Prominent acellular dense fibrous bands separating islands of tumor cells. Magnification × 28. (Courtesy of Dr. Benjamin Castleman.)

ity, slow mentation, poor memory, depression, and neuromuscular abnormalities.[235] Easy fatigability is one of the most prominent symptoms. Muscle weakness, particularly involving the proximal groups of the extremities, can be demonstrated by objective muscle examination in many cases. Occasional patients complain of decreased hearing, dysphasia, anosmia, and dysesthesias. Abnormal tongue movements resembling fasciculations may be present. Frequently, reflexes are hyperactive. Less common neurological abnormalities include atrophy of the tongue, decreased vibratory sense in the feet, and glove-and-stocking sensory loss.

NEUROMUSCULAR ABNORMALITY. Proximal muscle weakness may range from barely detectable to weakness that limits activity. The patient may complain of muscle aches and pains and heaviness in the lower extremities with difficulty climbing stairs, getting out of a chair, or getting out of a bathtub. Symptoms in the lower extremities precede those in the upper extremities. Loss of muscle strength correlates with changes evident on muscle biopsy. The characteristic finding is muscle atrophy that is most prominent in type II fibers (Fig. 27–32). Type II fiber atrophy is characteristic of a neuropathic lesion, and these fibers are the first to undergo atrophy on denervation. Thus the muscle lesion in hyperparathyroidism represents a neuropathy[226] and not a myopathy. The electromyogram shows a polyphasic potential pattern compatible with denervation. Small-amplitude potentials of short duration on myograms also are observed and again represent neuropathic changes. Muscle weakness improves on correction of hyperparathyroidism.[236]

OTHER ASSOCIATED ABNORMALITIES. Some of the signs and symptoms in hyperparathyroidism are secondary to hypercalcemia itself. Polyuria (related to associated hypercalciuria), polydipsia, and constipation are probably due to hypercalcemia. In severe hypercalcemia the electrocardiogram may reveal a shortened Q-T interval. Other infrequent abnormalities include "band keratopathy," pruritus, subconjunctival deposits of calcium, and ectopic calcifications in lungs, kidneys, arteries, and skin. Ectopic calcification is more likely in association with renal impairment and phosphate retention. Band keratopathy is recognized as opaque material in parallel lines within the limbus of the eye. Pruritus may be secondary to microscopic deposits of calcium within the skin. Loosening of the teeth and hypermobility of the joints also have been described.

Anemia and elevated erythrocyte sedimentation rate are common.[232] Indeed, anemia was reported in half of the original series from the Massachusetts General Hospital.[237]

The cause of the anemia is unknown. Monoclonal gammopathy has been reported as an unrelated coexistent disorder in hyperparathyroidism. These hematological abnormalities and weight loss in some cases may suggest that hypercalcemia may be due to malignancy. Clearly, these abnormalities should not deter evaluation for hyperparathyroidism.

Hypertension is observed in 20 to 60% of patients. The mechanism is unknown. Some have implicated hypercalcemia, hyper-reninemia, or renal impairment; others have not found these factors to correlate with hypertension.[238, 239] Saralasin, an angiotensin inhibitor, does not lower blood pressure in the disease, and few cases show significant improvement in hypertension after correction of hyperparathyroidism.[240]

ASSOCIATED ENDOCRINE DISORDERS. Sporadic occurrence of Hashimoto thyroiditis and Cushing syndrome has been reported in hyperparathyroidism, unrelated to the various types of MEN. Endocrinopathies in familial hyperparathyroidism are discussed separately.

RADIOLOGICAL ABNORMALITIES IN PRIMARY HYPERPARATHYROIDISM. Radiographic evidence of hyperparathyroidism is expressed as subperiosteal resorption (best recognized in the phalanges and distal portions of the clavicles), generalized osteopenia or osteoporosis, demineralization ("salt and pepper pattern") of the skull, bone cysts or brown tumors (evidenced as areas of radiolucency, particularly in the long bones), and occasionally patchy or diffuse areas of increased bone density (osteosclerosis). The symphysis pubis and sacroiliac joints may appear widened. Nephrocalcinosis as well as nephrolithiasis may be evident on x-ray films of the kidney. Tomograms of the kidney may show nephrocalcinosis not detected by routine roentgenograms. Demineralization around the teeth is evidenced as loss of the lamina dura. Chondrocalcinosis is apparent in up to 10% of patients (Fig. 27–33). In severe cases resorption of the distal phalangeal tufts and clubbing of the fingers may be present (Fig. 27–34).

Occasional roentgenographic features include deviation of the esophagus on esophagogram as a result of impingement by a parathyroid adenoma. Rarely, a mediastinal adenoma is of sufficient size and location to be recognized as an abnormal mass on lateral chest x-ray. Computed tomographic scans, magnetic resonance imaging, and arteriography allow more precise characterization of mediastinal lesions[241] (and see under Preoperative Localization of Abnormal Parathyroid Glands).

There may be signs of ectopic calcification. Several cases

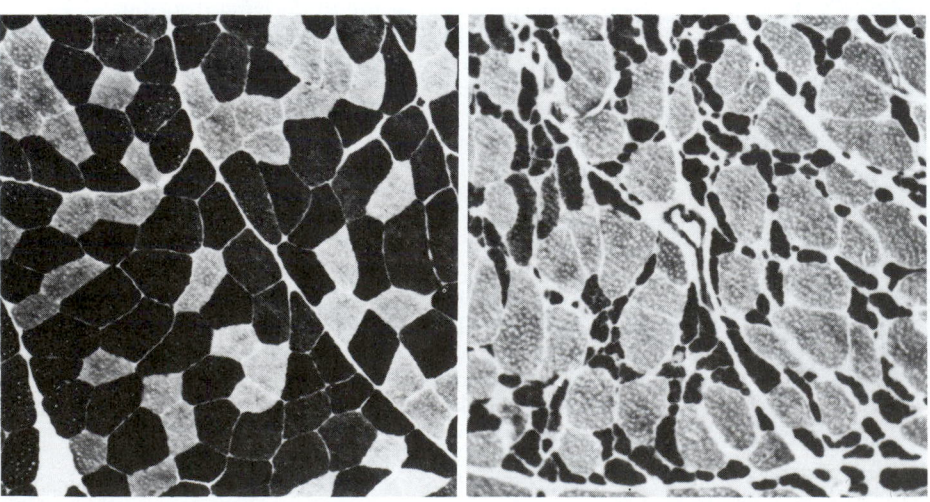

A **B**

Figure 27–32. Biopsy specimens of muscle. *A,* Section showing normal quadriceps muscle specimen with slightly larger type II (dark-stained) than type I (light) fibers. *B,* Specimen from patient with primary hyperparathyroidism and marked muscle weakness. Note marked atrophy, particularly of type II fibers. (ATPase stain). (Reproduced, with permission, from Patten BM, Bilezikian JP, Mallette LE, et al. Neuromuscular disease in primary hyperparathyroidism. Ann Intern Med 1974; 80:182–193.)

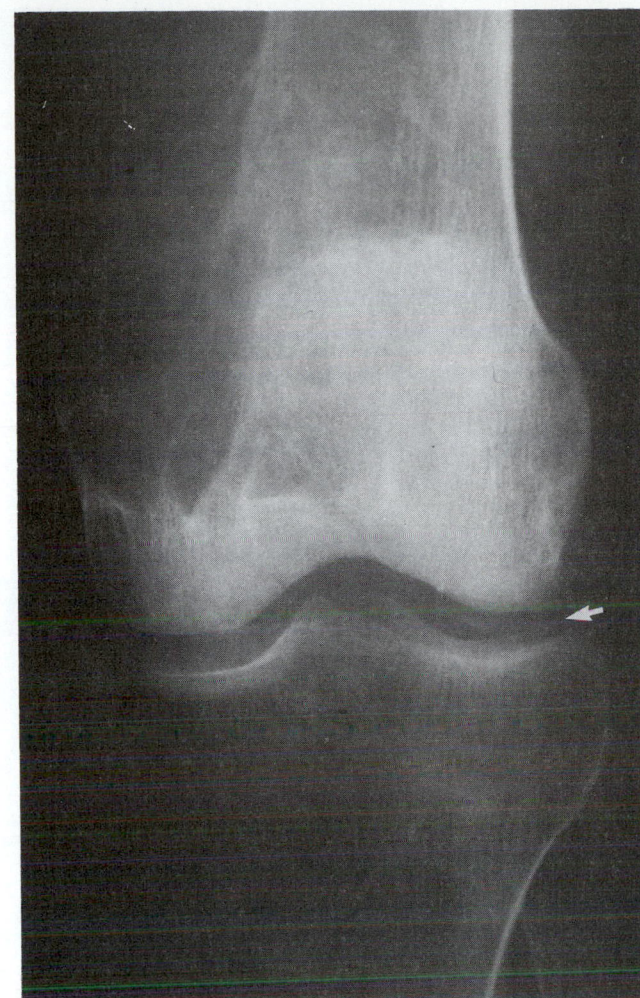

Figure 27–33. Chondrocalcinosis in a patient with osteitis fibrosa cystica. Note intraarticular calcification *(arrow)*.

of pulmonary calcification have been described. This may develop consequent to intercurrent viral pulmonary infection in subjects with hypercalcemia. Cholelithiasis has been reported in hyperparathyroidism, but the incidence does not seem to be greater than that in the general population. Abnormalities on gastrointestinal x-ray films can reflect associated diseases or evidence of MEN. For example, chronic pancreatitis may be evident with calcifications in the pancreas. Coexisting peptic ulcer and hypertrophic rugae in the stomach in association with Zollinger-Ellison syndrome may be recognized on upper gastrointestinal series. Patients who have received intravenous phosphate therapy may show evidence of calcification of small arteries, including the digital arteries.

Laboratory Studies

Hypercalcemia and hypophosphatemia are the laboratory hallmarks of primary hyperparathyroidism. Hypercalcemia is almost always present. This reflects the action of PTH on the kidney and the skeleton to increase resorption of calcium from bone and reabsorption from the GF and to stimulate $1,25(OH)_2D$ production with consequent increased calcium absorption from the gut. Hypophosphatemia is a consequence of the direct action of PTH on the kidney and can be aggravated by hypercalcemia. Serum calcium determination and PTH immunoassay are the two most important tests. Other laboratory parameters for evaluating parathyroid function include urinary cAMP clearance and deter-

mination of vitamin D metabolites in plasma. An outline of laboratory tests for hyperparathyroidism is provided in Table 27–9.

HYPERCALCEMIA. High blood calcium concentration is almost always present. In any one patient, however, particularly in early or mild cases, serial analyses may reveal fluctuations of serum calcium concentration into and out of the normal range. Some cases of "normocalcemic hyperparathyroidism" represent sampling bias—serum calcium being analyzed near the nadir of such fluctuations. Other causes of apparent normocalcemic hyperparathyroidism or masked hypercalcemia include coexistent vitamin D deficiency, hypoalbuminemia, and acidosis. In the latter instances the ionized calcium level is high even though total serum calcium concentration is normal. Hypercalcemia that is masked by vitamin D deficiency becomes evident on administration of vitamin D. Hypercalcemia detected in the general clinic population is due to primary hyperparathyroidism in about half the cases, and hypercalcemia detected in surveys of healthy populations is usually caused by primary hyperparathyroidism.[221] The differential diagnosis of hypercalcemia is discussed later.

PLASMA PHOSPHATE IN HYPERPARATHYROIDISM. Blood phosphate level tends to be low as a consequence of the renal effects of PTH in increasing the clearance of phosphate into urine. Hypophosphatemia, however, is a less reliable parameter for diagnosis than hypercalcemia. Plasma phosphate level varies with phosphate intake, time of sampling, and renal function. True hypophosphatemia is found

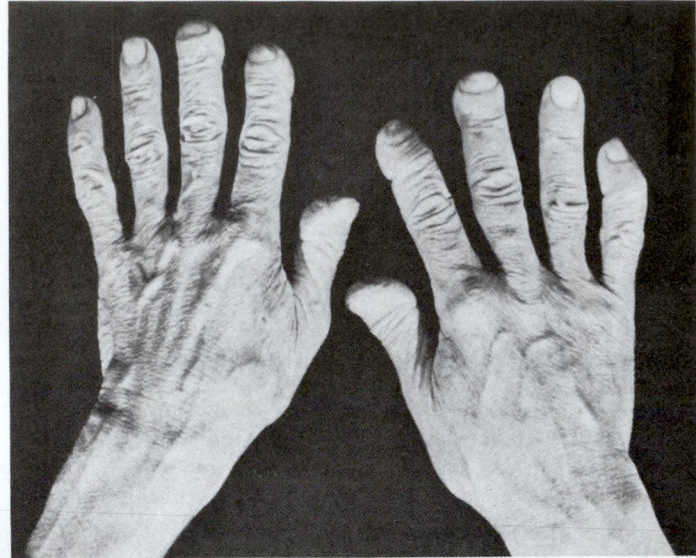

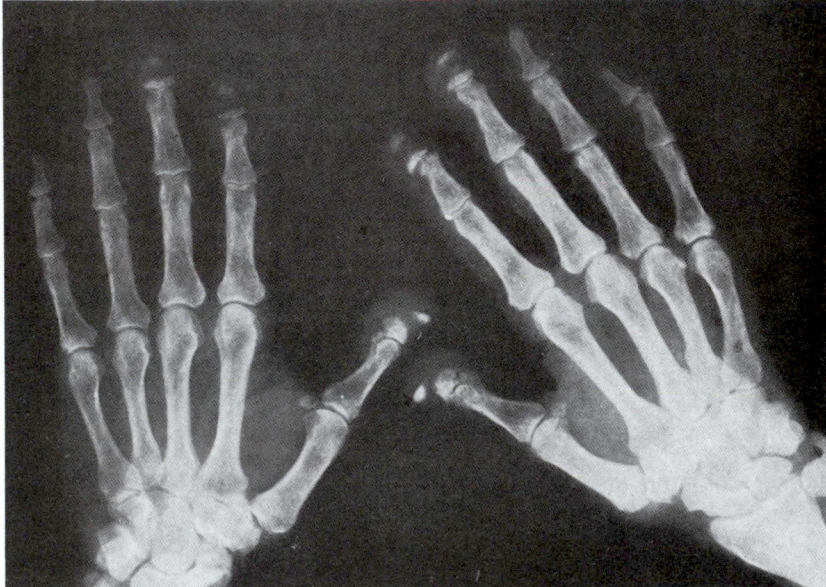

Figure 27–34. Marked periosteal bone erosion in the terminal phalanges of a patient with primary hyperparathyrodism. Erosion has been so extensive that clubbing has resulted.

in only about half of cases. Several suggestions have been made in attempts to improve the diagnostic efficacy of serum phosphate concentration as a discriminant in diagnosis. Phosphate clearance, TRP, a phosphate excretion index expressing phosphate excretion per deciliter of GF, and T_m phosphate (tubular maximum for phosphate reabsorption) have all been proposed as better diagnostic indices. None, however, is adequate for diagnosis. In one series of surgically documented hyperparathyroidism, determinations of phosphate clearance or of TRP were abnormal in only 50 to 60% of cases.

IMMUNOASSAY FOR PARATHYROID HORMONE. Immunoassay for PTH is a primary diagnostic parameter in hyperparathyroidism. Diagnostic utility was previously hampered by detection of circulating biologically inert COOH-terminal metabolic products of the hormone (see sections on radioimmunoassay and peripheral metabolism), and this problem was amplified in patients with renal impairment. The development of two-site assays[34-36] has improved the sensitivity and specificity of PTH immunoassay. The assay measures intact PTH almost exclusively, and sensitivity allows detection of even the suppressed concentrations found in some patients with hypoparathyroidism (Fig. 27–35). With

the new assays, coexistence of high concentrations of calcium and inappropriately high levels of PTH in plasma virtually makes the diagnosis of primary hyperparathyroidism. Conversely, high blood calcium levels with low concentrations of PTH suggest non–parathyroid-related hypercalcemia. PTH immunoassay can also be used to monitor the course of parathyroid surgery.[241a]

URINARY cAMP. The role of cAMP in the mechanism of action of PTH has been discussed. Because certain cells in the renal tubule bear specific receptors for PTH, respond to the hormone with an increased concentration of cAMP, and elaborate cAMP directly into the luminal fluid, the rate of excretion of cAMP in the urine reflects the circulating concentration of biologically active PTH. The total amount of cAMP excreted represents cAMP cleared from the plasma by glomerular filtration plus the nephrogenous contribution itself. In primary hyperparathyroidism the total excretion of cAMP in the urine is increased,[126, 232] and assessments of parathyroid secretory activity have been based on this observation (Fig. 27–36). Urinary cAMP determinations, like PTH immunoassay,[241a] can also be used to monitor the course of parathyroid surgery (see discussion under Postoperative Course).

TABLE 27–9. Laboratory Tests in Hyperparathyroidism

Major Significance

Total serum calcium	Almost always increased; may be intermittent; masked in coexistent vitamin D deficiency; hypoalbuminemia
PTH (two-site immunoassay)	Normal compatible with hyperparathyroidism (HPT); ↑ diagnostic with significant hypercalcemia. ↓ indicates non–parathyroid-related hypercalcemia
Urinary cAMP	
UcAMP/dL GF*	↑ diagnostic of HPT if malignancy excluded
NcAMP/dL GF†	↓ excludes HPT if renal function normal
Urinary calcium excretion‡	Usually ↑ ; ↓ in FHH; highest in non–parathyroid-related hypercalcemia
Alkaline phosphatase	Increased bone fraction indicates significant bone disease (osteitis fibrosis cystica)

Lesser Significance

Prednisone challenge (30 mg/d × 10)	Little or no effect in HPT; calcium falls to normal—suspect vitamin D toxicity; sarcoidosis; myeloma (sometimes); milk-alkaline syndrome
Protein electrophoresis; bone marrow; Bence Jones protein	Helps rule out hypercalcemia of malignancy
Bone x-ray films	May show signs of HPT—subperiosteal resorption; "salt-and-pepper skull"; bone cysts
	Helps rule out malignancy
Arteriography (selective)	Localize parathyroid tissue before reoperation in failed surgery
Venous (selective) catheterization	Localize parathyroid tissue before reoperation in failed surgery
Computed tomographic scan; radiothallium scan; ultrasonography; magnetic resonance imaging	Adjuncts in localization, even new cases

Ancillary

Thyroid scan	Indicated before arteriography or venography and as part of radiothallium scan procedure
Serum gastrin	↑ in coexistent Zollinger-Ellison syndrome
TRP/phosphate clearance	Abnormal in 50–60% of cases
Hematology	↑ erythrocyte sedimentation rate, anemia in 25% of HPT
Serum chemistry	↑ chloride ↓ CO_2 in some cases
Kidney x-ray films	If suspected nephrolithiasis, nephrocalcinosis
Serum phosphate	Usually decreased; normal or ↑ in coexistent renal disease; if high or normal suspect nonparathyroid hypercalcemia
1,25(OH)$_2$D assay	Elevated in HPT, particularly those with nephrolithiasis
Ionized calcium	Elevated in HPT, may be test of choice in future but generally not equal to total calcium determination as diagnostic parameter
Serum magnesium	Usually normal or ↓ ; may be ↑ in FHH

*Total urinary cAMP expressed as nmol/dL GF; normal range 1.83–4.55 nmol/dL GF.
†Nephrogenous cAMP (NcAMP) = (cAMP/dL GF) − plasma cAMP; normal range 0.29–2.81 nmol/dL GF.
‡May be expressed as mass per 24 h or per dL GF, or as calcium/creatinine clearance ratio.

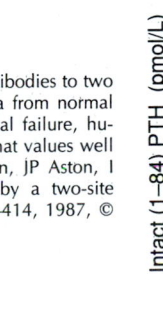
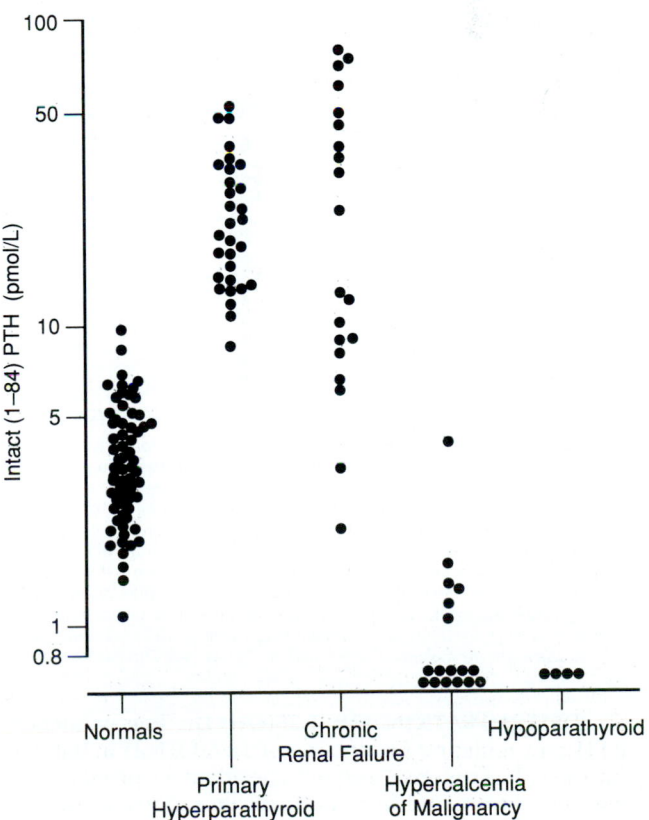

Figure 27–35. Chemiluminescence immunoassay for PTH utilizing antibodies to two different epitopes of PTH. Results shown were obtained with plasma from normal persons and subjects with primary hyperparathyroidism, chronic renal failure, humoral hypercalcemia of malignancy, and hypoparathyroidism. Note that values well below the normal range can be detected. (Adapted from RC Brown, JP Aston, I Weeks, et al., Circulating intact parathyroid hormone measured by a two-site immunochemiluminometric assay, J Clin Endocrinol Metab, 65, 407–414, 1987, © by The Endocrine Society.)

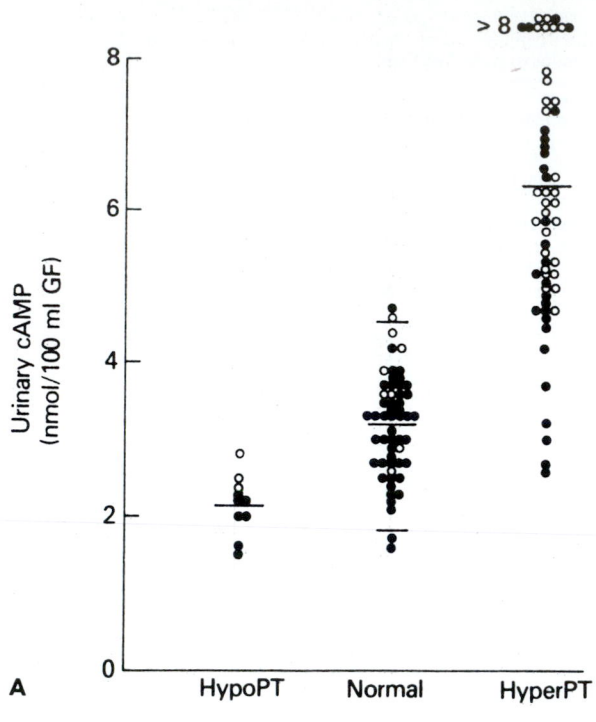

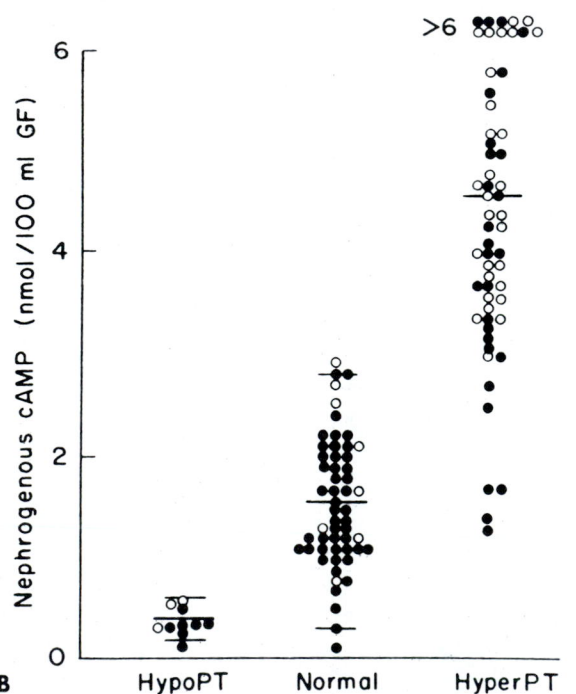

Figure 27–36. Urinary cAMP excretion as a function of parathyroid status. *A*, Total urinary cAMP excretion expressed as nmol cAMP excreted per 100 mL of GF. *B*, Nephrogenous cAMP expressed as nmol nephrogenous cAMP per 100 mL of GF. Parameter shown in *A* is satisfactory for routine clinical testing. Nephrogenous cAMP *(B)* gives slightly greater discrimination between parathyroid secretory states. Note that each of the parameters affords differentiation of parathyroid hypofunction as well as hyperfunction. Open symbols represent subjects with renal impairment. (From Broadus AE, Mahaffey JE, Bartter FC, et al. Nephrogenous cyclic adenosine monophosphate as a parathyroid function. Reproduced from the Journal of Clinical Investigation, 1977, vol. 60, pp. 771–783 by copyright permission of the American Society for Clinical Investigation.)

DETERMINATION OF 1,25(OH)₂D. The influence of PTH on regulating production of $1,25(OH)_2D$ in the kidney via the 1-hydroxylase enzyme is evident in primary hyperparathyroidism, and increased concentrations of the metabolite are present in plasma. There is considerable overlap between normal and hyperparathyroid subjects, however. Patients with high concentrations of $1,25(OH)_2D$ appear more prone to develop hyperabsorption of calcium, hypercalciuria, and renal lithiasis.[231]

GASTROINTESTINAL ABSORPTION OF CALCIUM IN PRIMARY HYPERPARATHYROIDISM. Gastrointestinal absorption of calcium is increased. Calcium absorption tends to return toward normal with surgical correction of the disease.[242] The increase in gastrointestinal absorption of calcium in hyperparathyroidism is presumably secondary to the enhanced rates of generation of $1,25(OH)_2D$ by the kidney in response to PTH.

URINARY CALCIUM AND PHOSPHATE DETERMINATIONS. Urinary phosphate clearance is increased in primary hyperparathyroidism. Parametric expression of urinary phosphate excretion was discussed earlier. In general, these parameters are not valuable discriminatory indices. Determination of urinary calcium excretion is important, however, in differentiating among types of hypercalcemia. Urinary calcium excretion is best expressed as a function of GFR (calcium clearance/creatinine clearance). Such parameters help in segregating subjects with FHH and in differentiating parathyroid-related hypercalcemia from that with nonparathyroid causes. Because PTH causes reabsorption of calcium from the GF, urinary calcium excretion is generally reduced relative to serum calcium level in primary hyperparathyroidism. Conversely, in non–parathyroid-related hypercalcemia, parathyroid secretion is inhibited and urinary calcium level is high for any given serum calcium level (see Fig. 27–13).

METABOLIC ACIDOSIS. Hyperchloremia with reduction of plasma bicarbonate level is common, whereas metabolic alkalosis (cause not defined) with low plasma chloride level occurs in non–parathyroid-related hypercalcemias. PTH causes decreased proximal reabsorption of bicarbonate.[243] Patients with hereditary fructose intolerance and Fanconi syndrome develop proximal renal tubular acidosis with bicarbonate loss that resolves with parathyroidectomy. Moreover, part of the metabolic acidosis in early renal impairment is attributable to secondary hyperparathyroidism, inducing proximal tubular rejection of bicarbonate and aggravating the acidosis of renal disease. There is also a defect in proximal reabsorption of bicarbonate in primary hyperparathyroidism (Fig. 27–37). This is evidenced by estimation of the tubular maximum T_m for bicarbonate reabsorption, which is carried out by infusing sodium bicarbonate intravenously, attempting to achieve a constant increment in plasma bicarbonate concentration without increasing ECF volume (see Fig. 27–37). The abnormality in bicarbonate reabsorption is corrected after parathyroidectomy.[244]

Impaired T_m for bicarbonate under the influence of PTH probably explains the metabolic acidosis in primary hyperparathyroidism. Occasionally the acidosis becomes even more severe in the first few days after removal of the parathyroid adenoma. The worsening of acidosis may be related to several causes: deterioration in renal function after surgery, phosphate depletion, release of hydrogen ions from recalcifying bone, and return of function of residual parathyroid tissue. Phosphate depletion per se causes a similar type of proximal tubular bicarbonate wasting.[245]

PARATHYROID SECRETORY CONTROL IN PRIMARY HYPERPARATHYROIDISM. PTH secretion in primary hyperparathyroidism has been generally assumed to be "autonomous" and not suppressible by increasing concentrations of calcium perfusing the glands. Conversely, the glands of secondary hyperparathyroidism are considered normally suppressible by elevated concentrations of calcium. The concept of strict autonomy is now in doubt. Certain parathyroid adenomas respond to increments in calcium concen-

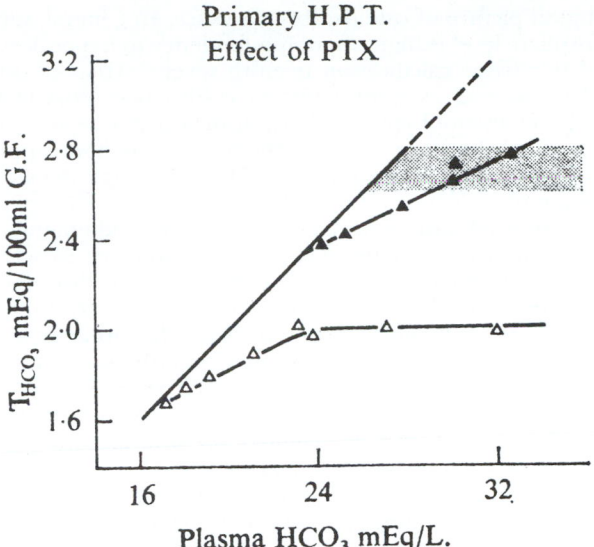

Figure 27–37. Renal capacity for bicarbonate reabsorption in hyperparathyroidism and effect of parathyroidectomy. Bicarbonate reabsorption, expressed as T_m bicarbonate, is reduced under the influence of PTH. This phenomenon can lead to proximal tubular acidosis in hyperparathyroidism and is corrected after removal of a parathyroid adenoma. (From Muldowney FP, Carroll DV, Donohoe JF, et al. Correction of renal bicarbonate wastage by parathyroidectomy. Q J Med 1971; 40:487–498, by permission of Oxford University Press.)

tration with reduction in rates of secretion. Other studies indicate that patterns of response in primary hyperparathyroidism are not absolute. Some glands show no suppressibility in vivo; others show suppressed secretion in response to high concentrations of calcium, but the concentrations of calcium required for inhibition (K_i) are greater than normal. Development of isolated parathyroid cell preparations allows study of secretion in vitro from normal or abnormal glands removed surgically.[246] One group of adenomatous glands is sensitive to inhibition by calcium with apparently normal K_i both in vivo and in vitro (Fig. 27–38). Others are resistant to suppression by calcium. Again, results in vitro compare favorably to those in vivo. Cells from hyperplastic glands generally show suppression normally (see Fig. 27–38). Even this may be abnormal in that normal glands from patients undergoing resection of parathyroid adenomas show apparent K_i values for calcium that are below normal. Occasionally, cases of sporadic parathyroid hyperplasia show nonsuppressibility.

Beta-adrenergic responses vary in abnormal parathyroid cells. Whereas normal bovine parathyroid cells uniformly show beta-2–type adrenergic receptors, parathyroid cells from patients show varying beta-1– to beta-2–type receptors and responses. Moreover, the response in vitro of parathyroid tissue from hyperparathyroid patients to beta-adrenergic agonists ranges from no increment in cAMP concentration to normal amounts. PTH release in response to beta-adrenergic agonists and to dibutyryl cAMP varies in pathological parathyroid tissue. Response to unusual secretagogues has also been characterized in adenomatous tissue. Parathyroid cells have shown substantial increases in cAMP concentration in response to glucagon, vasoactive intestinal peptide, and histamine.[41, 42] These agonists have small effects with normal bovine tissue. Because tumors may contain "ectopic receptors," it is possible that some of the human parathyroid responses may be due to receptors not normally on parathyroid cells.

OTHER LABORATORY ABNORMALITIES. Hypokalemia is infrequent in hyperparathyroidism. In some cases it re-

flects coincidental hyperaldosteronism. It also may develop in patients treated with phosphate by mouth. There is a tendency toward hypomagnesemia, and this may be aggravated after surgical correction. Hypomagnesemia may be due to impaired renal reabsorption of magnesium or long-term bone demineralization (bone is an important repository for magnesium) in response to hypersecretion of PTH. Low or normal plasma levels of magnesium help differentiate this disorder from FHH, which is frequently characterized by high normal or elevated concentrations of magnesium in plasma. There is also an increased incidence of hyperuricemia.

Anemia and elevation of the erythrocyte sedimentation rate occur in severe disease. There are no specific changes in marrow aspirates or peripheral blood smears, although this form of anemia may represent a type of myelofibrosis.

SUMMARY. Increased total calcium concentration on repeated analysis of plasma remains the hallmark of the disorder. The two-site immunoassays for PTH permit differentiation between non–parathyroid-related hypercalcemia (functionally suppressed parathyroid glands) and primary hyperparathyroidism. Determination of total urinary cAMP (expressed as cAMP excretion per deciliter of GF) or nephrogenous cAMP may also be helpful in difficult situations. Tests of interest in the diagnosis are summarized in Table 27–9.

Differential Diagnosis

The differential diagnosis of primary hyperparathyroidism includes the nonparathyroid causes of hypercalcemia, demineralization of bone, nephrolithiasis, and hypophosphatemia. The differential diagnosis of hypercalcemia is discussed separately. It is convenient to group those disorders associated with high rates of secretion of PTH, such as primary hyperparathyroidism, ectopic hyperparathyroidism, secondary hyperparathyroidism, or FHH. This group is characterized by laboratory results compatible with the increased rates of parathyroid secretion—high concentrations of PTH in plasma, increased excretion of urinary cAMP, and low urinary calcium levels. Virtually all other causes of

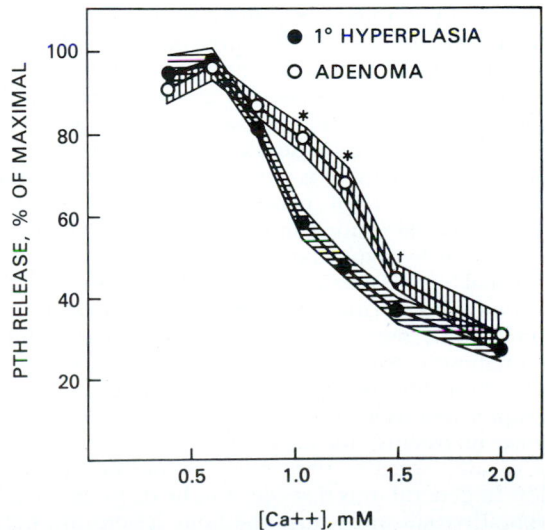

Figure 27–38. Relationship of PTH release to calcium concentration with isolated parathyroid cells in vitro. Most hyperplastic cells show calcium inhibition curves that are indistinguishable from normal ones. Adenoma cells show significantly higher K_i values for calcium. (From EM Brown, MF Brennan, S Hurwitz, et al., Dispersed cells prepared from human parathyroid glands: distinct calcium sensitivity of adenomas vs. primary hyperplasia, J Clin Endocrinol Metab, 46, 267–276, 1978, © by The Endocrine Society.)

hypercalcemia are associated with reduced PTH secretion. Significant renal impairment with hypercalcemia complicates interpretation of PTH radioimmunoassay as well as cAMP excretion. The last parameter, however, is severely affected only as GFR drops below 30% of normal.

Other effects of PTH secretion in hyperparathyroidism include hyperchloremic acidosis (reflecting the action of PTH on the rejection of bicarbonate in the proximal tubule of the kidney) and hypophosphatemia, a manifestation of the phosphaturic action of PTH. In nonparathyroid causes of hypercalcemia there is a tendency to metabolic alkalosis and hyperphosphatemia. The two latter parameters, however, are not specific enough to be precise diagnostic parameters. Certain non–parathyroid-related causes of hypercalcemia respond to glucocorticoid therapy.

"Ectopic hyperparathyroidism" in which a nonparathyroid tumor produces PTH may be difficult to diagnose because the laboratory findings do not differ from those of hyperparathyroidism caused by parathyroid adenoma or hyperplasia. Diagnosis of this rare disorder depends on localizing the associated malignancy and proving that it is the source of ectopic production of PTH. Too often this diagnosis has been made without adequate justification. Venous catheterization studies with sampling for PTH can be the sole means, other than surgical exploration, of distinguishing between ectopic hyperparathyroidism and cancer with coexistent primary hyperparathyroidism.

DIFFERENTIAL DIAGNOSIS OF OSTEITIS FIBROSA CYSTICA. Several metabolic diseases of bone may be associated with generalized demineralization of the skeleton, radiolucent areas of bone, or areas of osteosclerosis or increased bone density similar to that found in primary hyperparathyroidism. They may be differentiated on the basis of radiological appearance as well as of laboratory parameters (see also Chapter 28). Disorders include Paget disease of bone, osteoporosis, osteomalacia, multiple myeloma, malignancy metastatic to bone, polyostotic fibrous dysplasia, secondary hyperparathyroidism, pseudohypoparathyroidism, and solitary bone cysts. Hypercalcemia may be associated with Paget disease in patients with extensive involvement who are at bed rest. Generally, Paget disease can be differentiated by roentgenography. The laboratory features are distinct from those in primary hyperparathyroidism, and plasma calcium level is usually normal. In osteoporosis, serum levels of calcium, phosphate, and alkaline phosphatase and all parameters of parathyroid function are normal. Clinical characteristics of malignant disease as well as roentgenographic appearance should alert the physician to the possibility of malignant metastases in bone. Bone marrow examination is indicated whenever there is suspicion of underlying skeletal malignancy. Analysis of plasma and urine for myeloma proteins should be routine in suspected cases. Osteomalacia may be caused by hypovitaminosis D, resistance to vitamin D, intestinal malabsorption, or renal tubular acidosis. In these conditions serum calcium level is normal or low, sometimes with tetany. Bone biopsy may be helpful in differentiating osteomalacia from osteitis fibrosa cystica.

Polyostotic fibrous dysplasia is a challenge in that roentgenographic lesions in bone and bone biopsy samples resemble those in osteitis fibrosa cystica. In some cases sexual precocity and somatic precocity are present in affected females. In general, this disorder can be differentiated from hyperparathyroidism because the bone lesions are not generalized as in primary hyperparathyroidism, and laboratory parameters of parathyroid function are normal. Polyostotic fibrosa dysplasia may also be associated with pigmented skin. Primary hyperparathyroidism and polyostotic fibrous dysplasia of bone may rarely coexist.

Secondary hyperparathyroidism may produce the histological picture of osteitis fibrosa cystica. In general, serum phosphate level is high, there is a tendency to hypocalcemia, and soft tissue calcification is more severe. Areas of osteomalacia as well as osteitis fibrosa cystica may exist in this condition. Pseudohypoparathyroidism also may be associated with osteitis fibrosa cystica. In these cases the bone appears to be sensitive to the actions of PTH even though the kidney is resistant.

Nephrolithiasis may be associated with idiopathic hypercalciuria, gout, hyperoxaluria, or cystinuria, as well as primary hyperparathyroidism. None of these disorders is associated with hypercalcemia, and parathyroid function tests are generally normal (one form of idiopathic hypercalciuria is associated with increased parathyroid secretory activity). Five to 20% of cases of nephrolithiasis, however, are due to primary hyperparathyroidism. Thus serum calcium level should be determined on several occasions in cases of nephrolithiasis or renal colic.

NEPHROCALCINOSIS. Nephrocalcinosis occurs in several disorders including renal tubular acidosis, pyelonephritis, and primary hyperparathyroidism. The general laboratory features of primary hyperparathyroidism, however, should establish the correct diagnosis.

Preoperative Localization of Abnormal Parathyroid Glands

Surgical correction of primary hyperparathyroidism is effective in most cases. Indeed, the limiting factor is the availability of an experienced parathyroid surgeon. In new cases the use of preoperative localization procedures probably cannot be economically justified. Cases of recurrent or persistent hyperparathyroidism, failed surgery, or prior neck surgery, however, warrant use of all available means to localize abnormal parathyroid glands before further surgery is undertaken. The approaches include computed tomography,[241] ultrasonography, radiothallium-technetium subtractive scintigraphy* (hereafter referred to as radiothallium scanning), arteriography, and selective venous sampling with immunoassay for PTH. There are claims of 60 to 90% success rates for computed tomography, ultrasonography,[247, 248] or radiothallium[249] scanning in previously unoperated cases. When surgery is required again, however, the authors have found lower rates of success.

Arteriography and selective venous catheterization should be reserved for recurrent hyperparathyroidism or persistent hyperparathyroidism after initial cervical exploration. Arteriography should be carried out first to search for lesions and to delineate venous anatomy. Arteriography in experienced hands reveals an abnormal mass in approximately 60% of adenomas missed at prior surgery.[250] Selective venous sampling of the small veins of the neck provides lateralizing information in a similar percentage of cases. Fine-needle aspiration of masses identified by computed tomography or ultrasonography can obviate the need for venous sampling.[251] Arteriographic identification of a hormone concentration gradient in a vein draining the lesion proves the nature of the lesion. No single procedure is successful in every case requiring reoperation. For this reason, arteriography, venous sampling, ultrasonography, computed tomography and magnetic resonance imaging, and radiothallium scanning should all be considered in the approach to any case before undertaking a second surgical exploration (Fig. 27–39).

---

*Obtained by scanning with radiothallium and radiotechnetium separately, then substracting the image of the latter from that of the former.

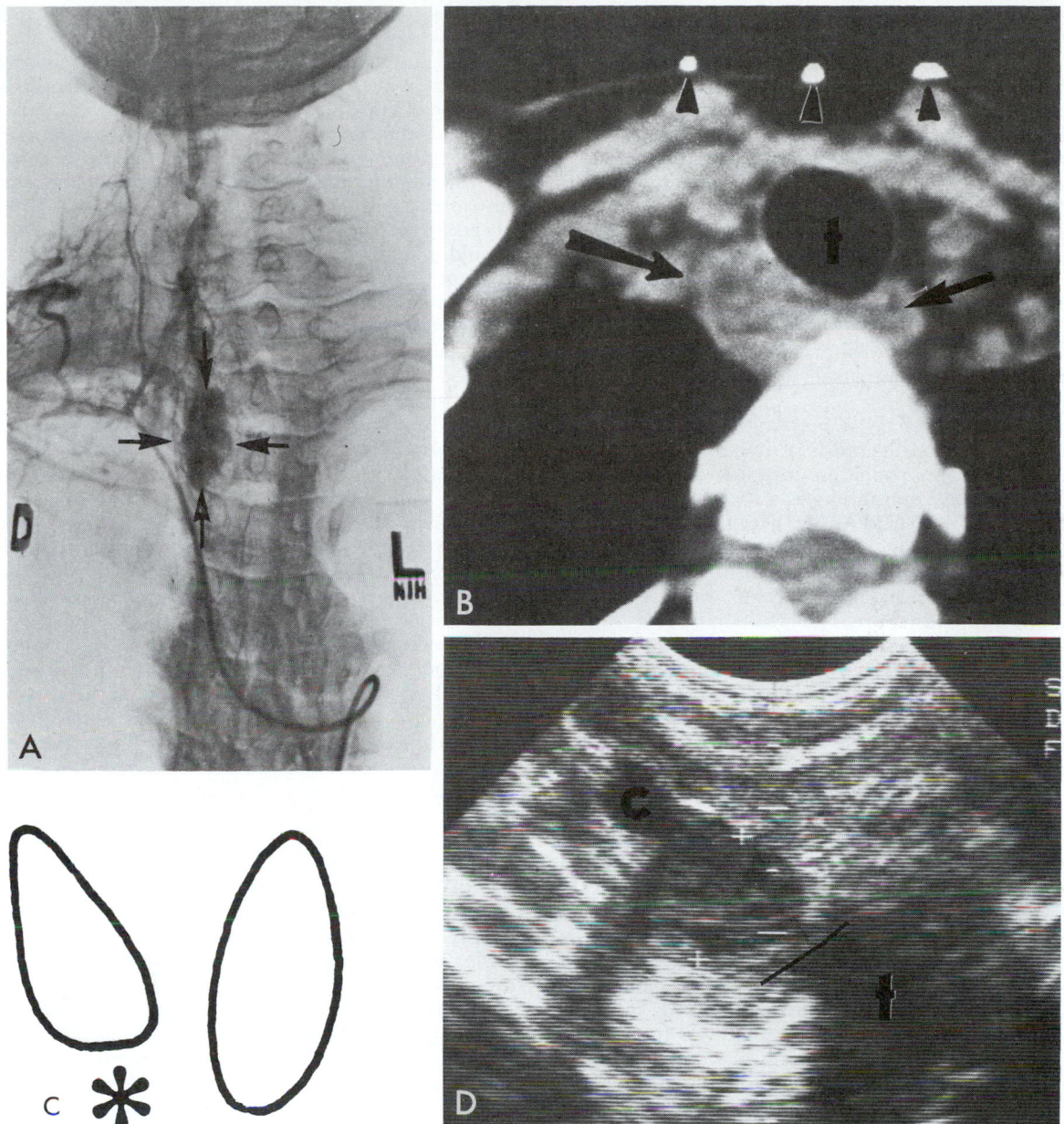

Figure 27–39. Localization studies for parathyroid lesions. *A*, Arteriographic localization of parathyroid adenoma *(arrows)*. *B*, Computed tomographic scan localizing parathyroid adenoma (same case as in *A*); t, trachea; thin arrow points to esophagus *(small dark area)*; arrowheads indicate barium markers on skin over manubrium. *C*, Diagram of radiothallium localization of parathyroid adenoma. Asterisk represents remaining density after subtracting (by computer) radiotechnetium image from radiothallium image. Thyroid outline, representing perimeter of radiotechnetium image, is superimposed. *D*, Ultrasonogram of parathyroid adenoma. t, trachea; C, right carotid; parathyroid adenoma between two white crosses. Right lobe of thyroid lies just anterior *(toward top)* and medial to adenoma. (Courtesy of Drs. Adrian Krudy and Eric Jones.)

Treatment of Primary Hyperparathyroidism

ASYMPTOMATIC HYPERPARATHYROIDISM. In early series, hyperthyroidism was diagnosed via symptoms and signs of the disease. Now the diagnosis is commonly made in asymptomatic subjects who are initially ascertained by discovery of hypercalcemia. Experience with the asymptomatic disorder makes it likely that some patients with mild hyperparathyroidism have normal life expectancy without developing symptomatic disease. Some patients previously diagnosed as having asymptomatic hyperparathyroidism may have hypocalciuric hypercalcemia.

Management of asymptomatic hyperparathyroidism is a problem because we do not know the risk for development of renal and osseous complications in any given patient. A study at the Mayo Clinic[252] of 134 patients with mild or asymptomatic hyperparathyroidism over a 5-y period showed the following results: 20% eventually required surgery, 58% showed no change in clinical status, 4% died of unrelated causes, and 18% were lost to follow-up. In 12 cases the original diagnosis was probably incorrect.

The risk of progression of the disease, the cost of long-term follow-up, and psychological factors must be weighed against the morbidity, cost, and risk of surgical failure in subjects who might otherwise live normal lives without surgical intervention. An approach that we find useful is as follows: (1) Obtain detailed family history in attempt to exclude FHH, familial hyperparathyroidism, or MEN type 1 or type 2A. These disorders are frequently associated with multiple gland hyperplasia, which in asymptomatic cases may militate against surgical intervention. (2) Evaluate renal function, urinary calcium excretion, and skeletal integrity by x-ray and bone densitometry. If all these results are normal, surgery may be postponed, but the patient must be re-evaluated for renal, gastrointestinal, and skeletal status at regular periods, e.g., every 6 to 12 mo. Progression of the disease at subsequent examination is indication for surgical intervention. (3) Subjects with definite abnormalities in skeletal or renal function, even though clinically asymptomatic, are candidates for surgery. (4) The need for therapeutic decisions on these subjects is not urgent. Patients in the asymptomatic hyperparathyroidism group followed at the Mayo Clinic and at the National Institutes of Health have not developed rapid progressive disease or hypercalcemic crisis requiring emergency surgery. Nevertheless, careful monitoring is required.

Normocalcemic primary hyperparathyroidism was discussed in the section on diagnosis of hyperparathyroidism. Subjects in this category should be managed as outlined for primary hyperparathyroidism in general.

SYMPTOMATIC HYPERPARATHYROIDISM: MEDICAL MANAGEMENT. There is no wholly satisfactory medical treatment for primary hyperparathyroidism. Mild disease in postmenopausal women has been treated with estrogen;[253] hypercalcemia improves, there is no effect on PTH secretion, and the long-term effectiveness of such therapy is not known. Other procedures can be useful until surgery is possible or when surgery is not feasible or is refused. Such patients have been treated for up to 12 mo or longer by use of oral phosphate.[254] Phosphate equivalent to 2 g of phosphorus per day in divided doses should be given for the first 2 or 3 d. The dose should be reduced to 1 to 1.5 g daily thereafter (see under Treatment of Hypercalcemia). This treatment can reduce plasma calcium level, urinary calcium excretion, and plasma $1,25(OH)_2D$ concentration, but it stimulates parathyroid secretion and increases urinary cAMP excretion. This accentuation of the hyperparathyroid state may cause further demineralization of bone. Certain of the newer diphosphonates might also be helpful in managing these cases.[255] If treatment with phosphate is contraindicated or not effective, plicamycin may be used but only in emergency and then with caution. Repeated use of the drug is associated with bone marrow toxicity. CT is not efficacious in controlling hypercalcemia in primary hyperparathyroidism. Glucocorticoids are ineffective, and use of these drugs complicates management before, during, and after surgery.

EMERGENCY TREATMENT. Occasionally hypercalcemia may become progressive and severe (hypercalcemic crisis), leading to weakness, dehydration, mental deterioration, coma, uremia, and death. Aggressive intervention with intravenous fluids and furosemide is indicated (see under Hypercalcemia). Plicamycin may be required. Intensive use of these measures usually allows stabilization of the clinical state pending definitive surgery. Occasionally, hemodialysis may be required. Some have advocated emergency surgery as soon as the clinical situation is stabilized.

Surgery

The surgical approach may be influenced by the particular experience with parathyroid pathology at each medical center. Some reports suggest a high incidence of four-gland parathyroid hyperplasia. The majority of clinics, however, continue to find that primary hyperparathyroidism is accounted for in more than 80% of cases by a single parathyroid adenoma. Exceptions are subjects with a family history of hypercalcemia, hyperparathyroidism, or other manifestations of MEN. The latter groups almost always show multiple gland hyperplasia as the pathological basis for primary hyperparathyroidism.

For cases with single parathyroid adenomas, some surgeons favor the following approach. One side of the neck is searched meticulously first. If an adenoma and a normal gland on that side are each proved by biopsy (frozen sections), the adenoma is removed and the wound closed. This leaves the contralateral side undisturbed and suitable for future exploration in the unlikely event that this becomes necessary. If the lesion is not found initially, the surgeon should extend the procedure to the contralateral side and attempt to identify all four parathyroid glands. Biopsy identification of all glands (results of frozen section at surgery should be confirmed by analysis of permanent sections) is essential to aid in deciding whether to undertake subsequent surgical exploration or to support the diagnosis of hyperplasia.[256] In multiple gland hyperplasia all parathyroid tissue should be removed save for approximately 50 mg of the most normal-appearing gland. Total parathyroidectomy with autotransplantation of 50 to 100 mg of tissue to the arm is used in some centers.[257–259] If neither hyperplastic nor adenomatous glands are found, dissection should be extended to the retroesophageal and retropharyngeal space and to retrieve, if possible, the thymic fat pad through the cervical incision. If two normal glands (biopsy identification) have been found on one side of the neck, the surgeon may consider excising the thyroid lobe on the opposite side. Occasional parathyroid adenomas are entirely within the bed of the thyroid and are undetectable by visual inspection. If, after extensive exploration, no abnormal parathyroid tissue is found, a mediastinal exploration should be considered, but only at a later date. Before further surgery is carried out, detailed localization studies should be performed in an attempt to localize the abnormal tissue. The patient's interest is best served by a surgeon with extensive experience in parathyroid surgery.

REOPERATION FOR PERSISTENT OR RECURRENT HYPERPARATHYROIDISM. Failure of initial surgery to cure hyperparathyroidism is an indication for temporizing, re-evaluating the diagnosis, and performing localizing procedures before further surgical intervention. It is best not to proceed with mediastinal exploration at the time of original neck surgery because most adenomas missed at the time of initial surgical exploration are within the neck. Moreover, after a prolonged dissection of the neck, neither the surgeon nor the patient is ideally suited to proceed with a further major procedure. It is best to allow a period of several weeks of recovery, if the clinical condition permits, before undertaking localization procedures and considering further surgery. The full gamut of localizing procedures (see Preoperative Localization of Abnormal Parathyroid Glands) should be utilized. Prior parathyroid or thyroid surgery may distort the vascular tree as well as produce sufficient scar tissue to lend additional morbidity to further surgery without localization. Preoperative localization allows the surgeon to plan the type of operation needed and to concentrate on dissecting areas where the pathology is to be found.[250] High mediastinal tumors may be reached through a cervical incision or through a relatively simple "hockey stick" sternum-splitting maneuver. The latter is associated with less morbidity than is a complete sternum-splitting exploration. The locations found for parathyroid lesions in 25 successful reoperative procedures are shown in Figure 27–40. Note that only five of the lesions represented mediastinal adenomas, and of these only three required sternotomy, the remaining two being retrieved from the neck. This experience is borne out by reports from several centers and is one reason for cautioning against extending the procedure to sternotomy at the initial operation. Repeat surgery in the

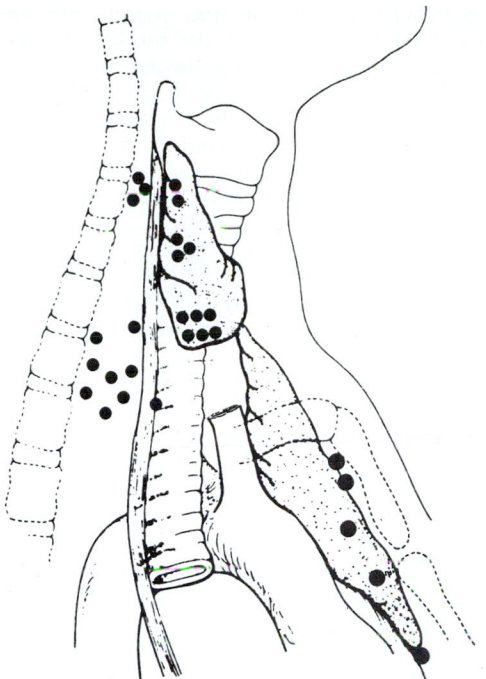

Figure 27–40. Location of parathyroid adenomas missed at initial surgery but found upon subsequent successful surgical exploration. (From Brennan MF, Doppman JL, Marx SJ, et al. Reoperative parathyroid surgery for persistent hyperparathyroidism. Surgery 1978; 83:669–676.)

hands of those experienced in the procedure is successful in approximately 90% of cases of true hyperparathyroidism not caused by parathyroid cancer.

PARATHYROID CARCINOMA. Parathyroid carcinoma is a rare cause of primary hyperparathyroidism[228] and probably accounts for less than 3 to 4% of cases. A palpable gland, hypercalcemia greater than 3.5 mmol/L (14 mg/dL), and high circulating concentrations of free subunits of human chorionic gonadotropin are more common in parathyroid cancer than in primary hyperparathyroidism not due to malignancy.[230, 260] Carcinomas tend to be slow-growing and are curable in the early stages by adequate local excision. Local spread or dissemination may develop through rupture of the tumor capsule at the initial operation. Parathyroid carcinoma is one cause of persistent or recurrent primary hyperparathyroidism. Local recurrences and isolated metastases also may be amenable to excision and thereby afford improvement in the hyperparathyroid state.

POSTOPERATIVE COURSE. After successful removal of the parathyroid adenoma there is rapid correction of most of the biochemical abnormalities of hyperparathyroidism. The concentration of PTH in the circulation falls rapidly (half-time $\cong$ 10 min),[29] and urinary cAMP excretion usually drops 50% within 30 to 90 min. Indeed, rapid assays for cAMP[261, 262] and PTH can be utilized as intraoperative indices of successful parathyroidectomy. Serum calcium level begins to fall within hours, may drop through the normal range within 4 to 12 h after surgery, and usually reaches a nadir 4 to 7 d later. Immediately after parathyroidectomy there is a transient increase in urinary calcium level; subsequently it falls to the undetectable range as hypocalcemia develops.

Marked and prolonged hypocalcemia may develop after parathyroidectomy as a result of several metabolic perturbations. (1) The most common cause is accelerated skeletal uptake of calcium ("hungry bones")[263] attendant on abrupt cessation and correction of the excessive bone resorption induced by long-term hyperparathyroidism. The severity

and duration of this phenomenon are functions of the degree of bone demineralization present. This form of bone disease is associated with marked osteoblastic activity in the bone and large amounts of unmineralized osteoid tissue. (2) Prolonged hyperparathyroidism with marked bone demineralization may lead to total body depletion of magnesium. After parathyroidectomy and restoration of bone formation, hypomagnesemia may interfere with secretion or action of PTH from residual normal glands. (3) Permanent or temporary hypoparathyroidism may develop, particularly in subjects who have undergone prior parathyroidectomy (the adenoma ultimately excised may represent the sole remaining parathyroid tissue) or in patients who have undergone aggressive resection of multiglandular parathyroid hyperplasia. Determination of urinary cAMP level in the postoperative period (Fig. 27–41) allows differentiation of hypocalcemia related to hypoparathyroidism, permanent or temporary, from that related to accelerated skeletal remineralization (hungry bones).[263] Permanent hypoparathyroidism is also associated with hyperphosphatemia. In one series[232] the achievement of serum phosphate levels greater than 2 mmol/L (6 mg/dL) heralded permanent hypoparathyroidism. Hungry bones is a form of osteomalacia, and hypocalcemia may be preventable by administration of vitamin D metabolites preoperatively. Modest hypocalcemia in the postoperative period need not be treated beyond ensuring an adequate calcium intake. Significant and symptomatic hypocalcemia may require administration of calcium by vein (5 to 15 mg/kg body weight of calcium in 500 to 1500 mL of saline) given slowly over the course of 6 to 24 h with or without administration of vitamin D analogues. Calcitriol is the most useful because it is rapid in onset and offset of action, allowing ready adjustment of treatment. Therapy should be withdrawn as rapidly as clinical progress allows. Definite signs of recovery are usual within 7 to 10 d postoperatively. It is probably best to allow some degree of hypocalcemia as long as symptoms are controlled because hypercalcemia tends to inhibit recovery of remaining parathyroid tissue. Excessive use of calcium or vitamin D analogues should be avoided. Magnesium deficiency should be

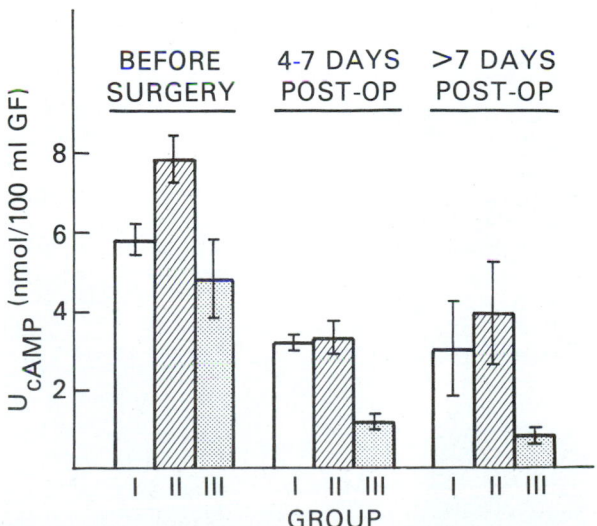

Figure 27–41. Urinary cAMP excretion before parathyroidectomy (set on left), in early postoperative period (middle set), and 7 to 10 d after parathyroidectomy (set on right). Three types of results were obtained. Group I was normocalcemic postoperatively. Group II required vitamin D transiently for hypocalcemia (because of "hungry bones"). Group III became permanently hypoparathyroid upon removal of sole remaining parathyroid tissue. (From Spiegel AM, Marx SJ, Brennan MF, et al. Parathyroid function after parathyroidectomy: evaluation by measurement of urinary cAMP. Clin Endocrinol 1981; 15:65–73.)

corrected by intravenous administration (if renal function is satisfactory) of 80 to 120 mEq of magnesium. Serum magnesium concentration alone may not reflect the severity of total body depletion. In magnesium depletion, urinary magnesium excretion will be low so long as significant total depletion of magnesium exists (see Fig. 27–6).

Permanent hypoparathyroidism is usually treated with vitamin D analogues. An experimental program has been developed to correct permanent hypoparathyroidism attendant on removal of multiple hyperplasic glands or sole remaining adenomatous glands with autotransplantation of part of the tissue to the forearm. One approach is to freeze some of the parathyroid tissue removed at surgery. If hypoparathyroidism develops later, the cryopreserved tissue can then be implanted in the forearm.

Unexplained complications in the postoperative period include gout, pseudogout, and pancreatitis. Arthralgia or arthritis in the postoperative period should alert the physician to the possibility of gout or pseudogout; the latter in particular should be suspected in patients with intra-articular calcification. In some cases, particularly those with compromised renal function, metabolic acidosis may develop or become worse in the postoperative period. The cause has not been defined. Rarely, bone cysts may be so extensive as to lead to fracture of long bones in patients who return too quickly to vigorous activity. Bone cysts can be differentiated from brown tumors on the basis of remineralization evident on roentgenograms. Brown tumors show dense remineralization within 6 to 12 mo after surgery (Fig. 27–42). Cysts do not remineralize and, if major in extent, may require orthopedic intervention and packing with bone chips. In general, restoration of bone mineral content ensues once hyperparathyroidism is corrected. Within 6 mo much of the loss in bone density, as determined by bone densitometry, is recovered, and by 12 mo recovery is almost complete.[264]

Hyperparathyroidism in Pregnancy

Hyperparathyroidism in pregnancy can pose difficult clinical management problems. In addition to the usual clinical expression of the disease—renal, gastrointestinal, and musculoskeletal—for which the mother is at risk, there is the potential risk to the fetus if surgery is required during the first trimester and the danger of neonatal hypocalcemia in the postnatal period. Although hyperparathyroidism is not rare—representing approximately 0.1% of the general clinic population—its prevalence appears to be less in pregnancy. Fewer than 100 cases have been reported.[265, 266] The apparent low incidence might reflect differences in diagnostic screening in prenatal versus medical clinics, a difference in the age of populations surveyed, differences in laboratory methods, masking of the diagnosis by hypoproteinemia, or protection against hyperparathyroidism by the pregnant state.

In pregnancy several mechanisms allow the rapid assimilation of calcium by the fetus.[267, 268] Calcium absorption in the mother increases from approximately 150 to 400 mg/d at 20 wk. The placenta develops an efficient calcium transport mechanism that allows the fetal serum calcium level to exceed that of the mother. PTHRP peptide is thought to regulate this process.[269] This mechanism in the fetus may aggravate the hypercalcemia of hyperparathyroidism in the mother. The major detrimental influences of maternal hyperparathyroidism on the fetus are death (as high as 30% stillbirth, abortion, or neonatal death), failure to thrive in the postnatal period, and delayed neonatal hypocalcemia. Even in the normal fetus PTH secretion apparently is suppressed and is not initiated until approximately 48 h after birth. The accentuated fetal hypercalcemia attendant upon maternal hyperparathyroidism causes prolonged suppression of PTH secretion until very late in the postnatal period. This late neonatal hypocalcemia may be the first clue to the existence of maternal hyperparathyroidism. Of 11 cases of postnatal hypocalcemia in progeny of 25 mothers with primary hyperparathyroidism, 9 of the babies developed hypocalcemia in the first few weeks of life. One developed hypocalcemia only during weaning at the age of 5 mo. In larger series, however, the incidence of neonatal hypocalcemia in progeny of hyperparathyroid mothers is only 12 to 15%.[265, 266]

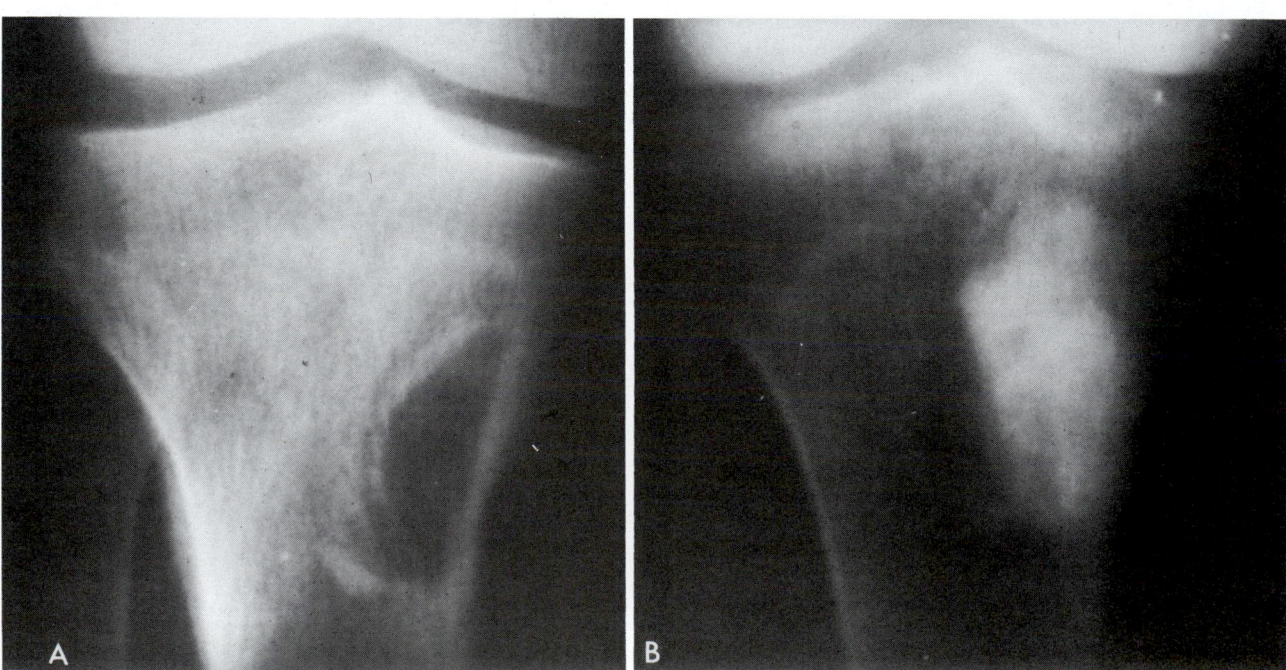

Figure 27–42. Brown tumor of bone before (A) and 1 y after (B) correction of primary hyperparathyroidism.

TREATMENT OF HYPERPARATHYROIDISM IN PREGNANCY. Symptomatic hyperparathyroidism should be corrected surgically. The optimal period for surgical intervention is the second trimester. The possible teratogenic risk of anesthetic agents during the first trimester is a relative contraindication to surgery. This risk must be weighed against the risk to the mother should severe hyperparathyroidism develop. There are no available data to evaluate the prognosis of mild primary hyperparathyroidism during pregnancy, but it probably has minimal morbidity for mother and fetus.

Neonatal Primary Hyperparathyroidism

Primary hyperparathyroidism in the neonatal period is rare. Approximately one quarter of reported cases with severe neonatal primary hyperparathyroidism occurred in kindreds with FHH (see later).[270, 271] In its most severe form, the disease is characterized by hypotonia, poor feeding, constipation, and respiratory distress. Generalized bone undermineralization, multiple fractures, and a deformed, narrow chest may be present. Histologically, the parathyroids have shown hyperplasia but never adenoma. Recognition and treatment of the severe form are crucial because the 1-y survival rate in untreated cases is below 50%. The high prevalence of multiple gland hyperplasia and of postoperative recurrence may require total parathyroidectomy as the surgical approach.

The asymptomatic form of neonatal primary hyperparathyroidism is common in kindreds with FHH, occurring in half the offspring of any affected parent. Transient neonatal hyperparathyroidism can also occur in the offspring of a mother who was hypocalcemic during pregnancy. Because the principal determinant of serum calcium level in the fetus is the maternal serum calcium concentration, maternal hypocalcemia causes secondary parathyroid stimulation in the fetus. Typically the infant exhibits parathyroid bone disease.

Familial Hypercalcemia

Several distinct syndromes of familial hypercalcemia have been delineated. In most, primary hyperparathyroidism is the cause. A survey in Sweden indicated a 0.013% prevalence of familial hypercalcemia in a population with a 0.6% prevalence of hypercalcemia.[272] Among patients with primary parathyroid hyperplasia, familial hypercalcemia occurs in about half, depending on the definition of hyperplasia and on referral bias.

MULTIPLE ENDOCRINE NEOPLASIA, TYPE 1 (MEN 1). (Also see Chapter 30.) This disorder of multiple tissues is usually benign and is associated with hypersecretion of hormones[273] (Table 27–10). It has also been called multiple endocrine adenomatosis and Wermer syndrome. It is inherited as an autosomal dominant trait. Primary hyperparathyroidism is the most common clinical manifestation in the syndrome, being present in 97% of cases with clinical manifestations. Less common features include excessive secretion

of gastrin (20 to 40% of cases), insulin (2 to 10% of cases), other pancreatic islet peptides (rarely glucagon or vasoactive intestinal peptide), and anterior pituitary peptides (prolactin 15 to 25% or, less frequently, corticotropin or growth hormone). Pancreatic tumors are rare causes of hypercalcemia independent of PTH excess. Nonsecreting tumors occur as well but rarely metastasize. These include lipomas (20%), pituitary chromophobe adenomas, carcinoid tumors, and adrenal and thyroid adenomas. Expression of the trait tends to follow consistent patterns within each kindred. In some kindreds there is a high incidence of hypergastrinemia, whereas in others prolactinomas are common. Affected persons usually manifest endocrine hyperfunction between ages 18 and 35.

Many small kindreds seem to express primary hyperparathyroidism alone. These may represent distinct hereditary syndrome(s) of familial hyperparathyroidism such as familial cystic parathyroid adenomatosis or may simply be due to the possibility that in small kindreds MEN 1 is manifested as isolated primary hyperparathyroidism.

The biochemical features of MEN 1 are those related to excessive secretion by the affected endocrine cells. Because hyperparathyroidism occurs in almost 95% of affected members, the most useful test for family screening is serum calcium level. Excessive basal secretion of gastrin or prolactin may occur in asymptomatic family members, but hypercalcemia is evident in most and in 85% of those with Zollinger-Ellison syndrome.

The cause of the abnormal activation (proliferation and secretion) of endocrine cells in MEN 1 is not known. Plasma from MEN 1 patients contains high concentrations of a substance that stimulates proliferation of parathyroid cells.[275] The MEN 1 growth factor, which is closely related to basic fibroblast growth factor, is a mitogen for cloned endothelial cells from the parathyroid but not for cloned epithelial (chief) cells from the parathyroid. The MEN 1 gene, which is on the long arm of chromosome 11, is thought to be a recessive oncogene analogous to the gene for retinoblastoma.[276] The normal alleles are hypothesized to encode a growth-suppressive function; inactivation of both alleles (thus "recessive") is necessary to transform a cell of specified type into the precursor of a benign or malignant tumor clone. One inactivated allele is inherited as the germ line mutation; the second allele is inherited in normal form from the unaffected parent but becomes inactivated by a somatic mutation in the tumor precursor cell. Clonal loss of an MEN 1 allele has been documented in malignant insulinomas and in benign parathyroid tumors in MEN 1;[217, 276] this criterion for clonality established that many parathyroid tumors in MEN 1 are monoclonal adenomas rather than multiclonal hyperplasia. The relation between this somatic mutation in the tumor precursor cell and the production or action of the MEN 1 growth factor is not known.

Treatment of MEN 1 depends on the manifestations. Recurrence of primary parathyroid hyperplasia in MEN 1, sometimes many years after apparently successful subtotal parathyroidectomy, is more common than in sporadic parathyroid hyperplasia. On the other hand, hypercalcemia may

TABLE 27–10. Major Features in Syndromes of Familial Hypercalcemia

Feature	Multiple Endocrine Neoplasia Type 1	Multiple Endocrine Neoplasia Type 2A*	Hypocalciuric Hypercalcemia
Inheritance	Autosomal dominant	Autosomal dominant	Autosomal dominant
Incidence of hypercalcemia during first decade	Low	Low	High
Associated endocrinopathy	Islet cell; anterior pituitary	Medullary thyroid cancer; pheochromocytoma	None
Unique biochemical features	Hypergastrinemia	Hypercalcitoninemia	Relative hypocalciuria
Subtotal parathyroidectomy	Useful	Useful	Rarely useful

*MEN type 2B (3) rarely has hypercalcemia or hyperparathyroidism.

exacerbate the degree of hypergastrinemia and the amount of gastric acid secreted at any serum concentration of gastrin. Thus active primary hyperparathyroidism makes management of the gastrin-gastric axis difficult.

OTHER MULTIPLE ENDOCRINE NEOPLASIAS. Primary hyperparathyroidism occurs in 20 to 30% of patients with MEN type 2A (see Table 27–10). More commonly, in patients without known parathyroid disturbance, diffusely hyperplastic parathyroid glands may be discovered at thyroid surgery for C cell hyperplasia or medullary carcinoma. MEN 2B (formerly 3) is a similar but distinct syndrome of more aggressive hyperfunction of thyroid C cells and adrenal chromaffin cells in which there is a low incidence of primary hyperparathyroidism. Distinguishing features include mucosal neuromas, ganglioneuromas, and a marfanoid habitus (see Chapter 30). The genes for MEN 2A and MEN 2B are on the long arm of chromosome 10.

FAMILIAL HYPOCALCIURIC HYPERCALCEMIA. FHH, also called familial benign hypercalcemia, is an autosomal dominant trait (see Table 27–10) with a high incidence of expression of hypercalcemia at all ages. Its prevalence is similar to that of MEN 1.[270, 271] Most affected persons show no severe symptoms clearly attributable to the underlying process. Easy fatigability and muscle weakness are common but generally mild. Nephrolithiasis and peptic ulcer disease have similar incidences to those in the general population. Subtotal parathyroidectomy almost inevitably is followed by persistence or rapid recurrence of hypercalcemia. The parathyroid glands are only minimally enlarged.

Hypercalcemia and hypophosphatemia are similar in magnitude to those of typical primary hyperparathyroidism. The main biochemical feature that differentiates these patients from those with typical primary hyperparathyroidism is lower renal clearance of filtered calcium (Fig. 27–43). Indices of parathyroid function (immunoreactive PTH, urinary cAMP excretion, and calculated renal threshold for phosphate excretion) suggest inappropriately normal circulating PTH activity in FHH.

The etiology of this disorder is not known. It appears to affect divalent cation interactions in both the parathyroid gland and the kidneys. The clinical and biochemical features are distinct from those of MEN syndromes. The most useful diagnostic features are the typical familial pattern with onset of hypercalcemia early in the first decade, absence of features of MEN 1 or MEN 2A serum magnesium concentrations that are high or in the upper normal range, and low renal clearance of calcium (calcium clearance/creatinine clearance usually below 0.01). Differentiation of this disorder from typical primary hyperparathyroidism may be impossible without the characteristic family history. The homozygous state of the FHH mutation results in severe neonatal primary hyperparathyroidism (see earlier).

The hypercalcemia is not responsive to glucocorticoids, natriuretic agents, or subtotal parathyroidectomy. In general these patients have an excellent prognosis and long life expectancy without parathyroidectomy. The only measure that consistently causes the serum calcium concentration to return to normal is total parathyroidectomy and subsequent treatment with calcium or vitamin D analogues or both. This should be undertaken only if severe complications exist (such as severe neonatal primary hyperparathyroidism or recurrent pancreatitis).

SECONDARY HYPERPARATHYROIDISM

Secondary hyperparathyroidism is a state of compensatory hypersecretion of PTH and may occur in any condition in which there is a tendency toward hypocalcemia. Secondary hyperparathyroidism has been described in chronic renal disease, rickets and osteomalacia, intestinal malabsorption syndromes, Fanconi syndrome, and renal tubular acidosis. Persistent hypersecretion of PTH in these disorders can produce all of the characteristics of hyperparathyroid bone disease, including osteitis fibrosa and osteosclerosis. A subclass of nephrolithiasis associated with a renal leak for calcium may also be due to secondary hyperparathyroidism. The latter form of nephrolithiasis is associated with modest hypophosphatemia and increased excretion of urinary cAMP.

CHRONIC RENAL FAILURE AND SECONDARY HYPERPARATHYROIDISM. The finding of parathyroid hyperplasia and hyperparathyroid bone disease in patients with chronic renal failure and documentation that animals made uremic are resistant to the effects of PTH led to the recognition that secondary hyperparathyroidism can result from chronic renal disease. The tacit assumption of excessive secretion of PTH in this state was confirmed when radioimmunoassays for PTH became available. High concentrations of immunoassayable PTH are usually found in renal failure. Much of the immunoactive hormone that accumulates is biologically inert COOH-terminal fragments of the hormone molecule. Intact PTH, however, also circulates in high concentration (see Fig. 27–35) in renal impairment. Stimuli that enhance the release of PTH in normal subjects produce a rise in urinary cAMP, and biologically active hormone in plasma has been detected in cases of chronic renal failure.[32] Multiple factors are involved in the pathogenesis of the hyperparathyroidism. These include hyopocalcemia, hyperphosphatemia, decreased production of 1,25(OH)$_2$D, reduced gastrointestinal absorption of calcium, peripheral resistance to the action of PTH, and probably others yet to be recognized. (Aluminum toxicity[167] in some cases produces an osteomalacic-type abnormality with suppressed PTH secretion.) The initial stimulus appears to be a chronic reduction of ionized calcium in the ECF because of renal retention of phosphate; indeed, there is a tendency toward frank hypocalcemia as a result of the hyperphosphatemia. Hyperphosphatemia, moreover, decreases renal production of 1,25(OH)$_2$D. Hypocalcemia is exaggerated further by de-

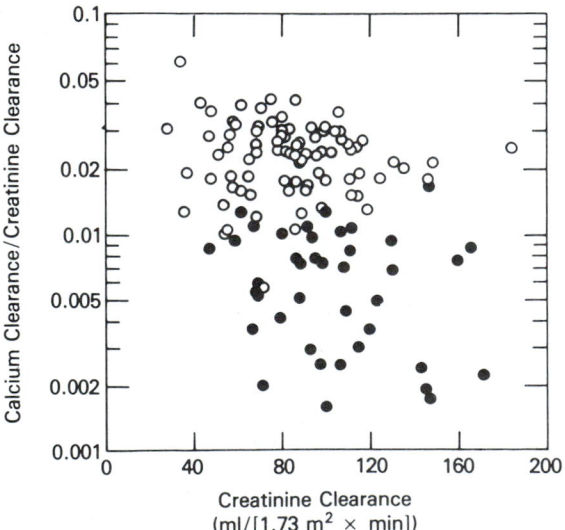

Figure 27–43. Ratio of calcium clearance to creatinine clearance ([Ca$_U$ × Cr$_P$]/[Cr$_U$ × Ca$_P$]) in 90 patients with typical primary hyperparathyroidism (O) and 40 patients with familial hypocalciuric hypercalcemia (●). These data are based on average 24-h urinary excretion values and average fasting serum samples (total nonfiltrable calcium).

creased intestinal absorption of calcium caused by reduced production of the active vitamin D metabolite. A further contributing factor to hypocalcemia is relative skeletal resistance to PTH.[277] The concerted actions of these factors foster development of hypocalcemia, which is a recognized stimulus to secretion of PTH. Renal impairment, moreover, causes accumulation (decreased renal clearance) of biologically active, intact PTH in the circulation. Other hormones including catecholamines also are cleared at reduced rates in chronic renal disease. Catecholamines are secretagogues for PTH, but their contribution to excessive PTH secretion in secondary hyperparathyroidism is unknown.

RENAL OSTEODYSTROPHY. The skeletal abnormalities in chronic renal failure include osteitis fibrosa cystica, osteomalacia, osteosclerosis, and generalized osteopenia. The degree of involvement of each form of bone disease varies, presumably as a function of the competing effects of resistance to PTH,[277] defective production of vitamin D metabolites, and effects of PTH on bone. Any of the classic lesions of primary hyperparathyroidism can occur, although bone cysts are less common. Early in the course of renal impairment the major skeletal pathology may reflect osteitis caused by the excessive production of PTH.[278] In later stages osteomalacia may be more significant as the effects of impaired formation of $1,25(OH)_2D$ become evident. Osteosclerosis can also be seen. Generalized osteopenia may lead to development of multiple pathological fractures, particularly in subjects undergoing chronic hemodialysis.

Clinically, osteodystrophy causes bone pain. In addition, proximal muscle weakness may be similar to that in primary hyperparathyroidism.

MANAGEMENT OF RENAL OSTEODYSTROPHY. The general approach is to control plasma phosphate and calcium levels and to correct osteomalacia.[279] Control of serum phosphate concentration is important to prevent the adverse effects of hyperphosphatemia. Generally this can be effected with calcium carbonate. Aluminum hydroxide–containing antacids, it is now recognized, should not be used because they predispose to aluminum toxicity of bone. Serum calcium concentration can be controlled by giving calcium supplements by mouth and by use of calcitriol to increase calcium absorption from the gut.[280] In resistant cases successful control has been effected through use of intravenous calcitriol.[281] Patients undergoing dialysis can be regulated partially by raising the calcium concentration in the dialysate. This may cause hypercalcemia in the immediate postdialysis period.

Renal transplantation may correct, to a major degree, secondary hyperparathyroidism of chronic renal disease. In some cases, however, hyperparathyroidism may persist after transplantation.[282, 283] Parathyroidectomy in this instance may be warranted but should be reserved for those in whom disabling bone disease shows no promise of improvement for prolonged periods beyond transplantation.

The vitamin D metabolites, calcitriol and 1α-hydroxycholecalciferol (not available in the United States), make possible effective correction of poor gastrointestinal absorption of calcium and osteomalacia. These short-acting metabolites, as well as dihydrotachysterol, previously used for this purpose, are advantageous if hypercalcemia develops and the dosage must be reduced. Use of these agents requires careful monitoring of blood phosphate because vitamin D therapy causes an increase not only in calcium absorption but also in phosphate absorption from the gut. Aluminum toxicity,[284] a complication of hemodialysis and treatment with phosphate-binding gels, can cause a form of osteomalacia resistant to treatment with vitamin D analogues. This aggravates further skeletal resistance to the actions of PTH.

VITAMIN D DEFICIENCY/DEPENDENCY AND SECONDARY HYPERPARATHYROIDISM. Osteomalacia or rickets due to vitamin D deficiency or "vitamin D dependency" can be associated with hypocalcemia and consequent secondary hyperparathyroidism. In each instance the hypocalcemia is secondary to decreased intestinal transport of calcium, a function dependent on normal action of vitamin D metabolites. The secondary hyperparathyroidism in these disorders is readily correctible by appropriate treatment with vitamin D analogues.

Vitamin D–resistant rickets or phosphate diabetes usually is an X-linked disorder characterized by a renal reabsorptive defect for phosphate. Chronic phosphate wasting leads to development of an osteomalacia-like skeletal disorder with pseudofractures and stunting of growth. Usually these subjects do not show hypocalcemia and do not express severe secondary hyperparathyroidism unless hypocalcemia develops in the course of treatment with phosphate. The Fanconi syndrome encompasses another type of renal reabsorptive defect involving amino acids, glucose, and phosphate. The renal loss of phosphate (phosphate diabetes) leads to demineralization, rickets, or osteomalacia. Usually serum calcium is normal, and severe secondary hyperparathyroidism does not develop unless there is progressive glomerular insufficiency.

HYPERCALCEMIA

Introduction

Hypercalcemia is a metabolic disturbance with formidable diagnostic and therapeutic problems. The clinical spectrum ranges from a life-threatening disorder to an asymptomatic biochemical abnormality. Malignancy is probably the leading cause of hypercalcemia in hospitalized patients, but primary hyperparathyroidism is the most common diagnosis in hypercalcemia discovered on routine biochemical screening.

Pathogenesis

Hypercalcemia represents an imbalance in calcium flux into and out of the blood compartment (Fig. 27–44). Normally, movements of calcium into and out of bone are equal because of close coupling between bone resorption and bone formation. In various pathological states, resorption may exceed formation and cause increased net flow of calcium from bone to blood. The ability of the body to compensate (e.g., increase renal calcium excretion) for increased calcium flux from the large (~1000 g) skeletal calcium reservoir is limited. From the foregoing it is clear that osteolytic factors are of primary pathogenetic importance in most hypercalcemic states. Numerous osteolytic factors have been identified (PTH, prostaglandins, PTHRP, lymphokines such as interleukin 1, transforming growth factors, thyroid hormone, and $1,25(OH)_2D$), and others undoubtedly exist.

Decreased renal calcium excretion and increased intestinal calcium absorption often contribute to increased serum calcium concentration but are rarely the sole cause of hypercalcemia. Reduced renal calcium excretion may be a consequence of renal failure, volume depletion, or humoral factors. A slight reduction in renal calcium excretion may be sufficient to cause hypercalcemia if increased bone turnover or increased intestinal calcium absorption (or both) is present. PTH, PTHRP, and thiazide diuretics reduce renal calcium excretion even when renal function is normal. Increased circulating levels of vitamin D and increased sensi-

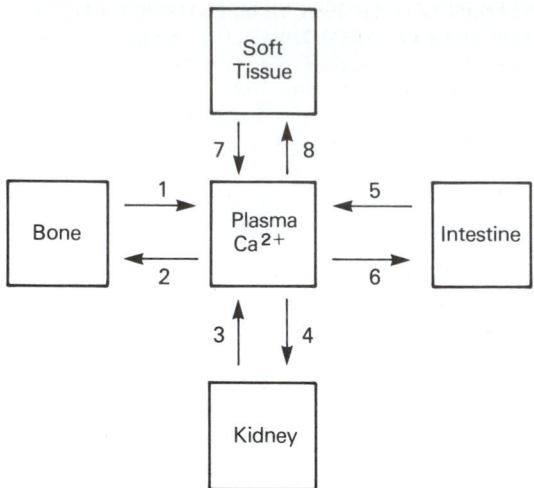

Figure 27–44. Schematic diagram of compartments involved in calcium homeostasis. *Hypercalcemia* is caused by (1) increased calcium flux from bone to blood produced by osteolytic factors and osteolytic metastases, (4) decreased renal calcium excretion, either functional (e.g., PTH or thiazides) or resulting from impaired renal function, (5) increased intestinal calcium absorption, and (7) increased flux of calcium from soft tissues to blood. *Hypocalcemia* is caused by (1) decreased calcium flux from bone to blood produced by PTH deficiency, (2) increased flux of calcium from blood to bone (e.g., healing osteitis fibrosa, osteoblastic metastases), (3) decreased renal calcium reabsorption associated with PTH deficiency, (5) decreased intestinal calcium reabsorption associated with 1,25(OH)$_2$D deficiency, and (8) increased calcium deposition in soft tissues (e.g., hyperphosphatemia).

tivity to vitamin D are the major factors leading to increased intestinal calcium absorption. Increased flux of calcium into blood from soft tissue calcium deposits is a theoretical but unproven cause of hypercalcemia.

Clinical Manifestations

Hypercalcemia of any etiology can seriously disrupt normal neurological, gastrointestinal, and renal functions. The severity of symptoms in a given patient is a function of the degree and rapidity of onset of hypercalcemia. Routine determination of serum calcium is important in evaluating patients with a wide variety of complaints, because the symptoms of hypercalcemia are varied and nonspecific.

NEUROLOGICAL. Central nervous system manifestations range from lethargy to confusion and coma. The electroencephalogram shows slowing and nonspecific abnormalities that revert to normal (with a variable lag period) after correction of hypercalcemia. In some patients, headache is prominent. Depression, paranoia, and other neuropsychiatric syndromes have been described and may resolve after correction of hypercalcemia. Generalized muscle weakness and hyporeflexia are characteristic findings in severe hypercalcemia. Neuromuscular function can improve dramatically with lowering of serum calcium concentration. Cerebrospinal fluid protein level, in the absence of primary neurological disease, is normal.

GASTROINTESTINAL. Constipation, anorexia, nausea, and vomiting are frequent. Poor fluid intake and fluid loss because of emesis contribute to acute hypercalcemic crisis. Hypercalcemia probably increases gastric acid secretion, but the relationship between hypercalcemia, increased gastric acid secretion, and peptic ulcer disease is complex. Hyperparathyroidism, particularly the hereditary form, is associated with an increased incidence of peptic ulcer disease, but there is no clear-cut association between other causes of hypercalcemia and peptic ulcer. Acute pancreatitis, although frequently associated with hyperparathyroidism, may occur with other hypercalcemic disorders as well. Indeed, pancreatitis has been reported in patients with hypercalcemia

related to metastatic breast carcinoma and to calcium infusion.

CARDIOVASCULAR. Hypercalcemia decreases the plateau phase of the cardiac action potential. This is reflected in a shortened S-T segment and consequently a reduced Q-T interval (corrected for heart rate) on the electrocardiogram (Fig. 27–45). With hypercalcemia in excess of 4 mmol/L (16 mg/dL) the T wave widens, tending to *increase* the Q-T interval. For this reason, the Q_o-T_c segment (distance from onset of QRS complex to onset of T wave corrected for heart rate) is a more reliable indication of hypercalcemia. Arrhythmias are uncommon, but with acute elevation of serum calcium concentration, bradycardia and first-degree heart block may occur. Theoretically, hypercalcemia sensitizes the heart to digitalis, but the clinical evidence for this is scant. One should, nonetheless, exercise caution in administering digitalis to hypercalcemic patients.

Acute elevation of serum calcium concentration may cause a rise in blood pressure, possibly through direct vasoconstriction, but the hypertension of chronic hypercalcemia may be due to renal damage. Although some reports suggest that hypertension is corrected with cure of hypercalcemia, this is not the general experience.

RENAL. Hypercalcemia impairs renal function in several ways. It causes polyuria and polydipsia by interfering with the action of AVP on the collecting ducts. Renal blood flow and GFR are reduced. Proximal tubular function may be impaired, causing excessive urinary sodium loss. With persistent hypercalcemia (especially in patients with elevated serum phosphorus concentration), calcium phosphate salts are deposited in the tubules. Focal scarring and inflammation (interstitial nephritis) may develop. In severe cases, nephrocalcinosis is visible on x-ray films, but histological evidence of renal parenchymal calcification is often present in the absence of detectable nephrocalcinosis. Hypercalciuria and urolithiasis may also occur. Superimposed urinary tract infection may aggravate hypercalcemic nephropathy. In the absence of primary glomerular disease, proteinuria is slight.

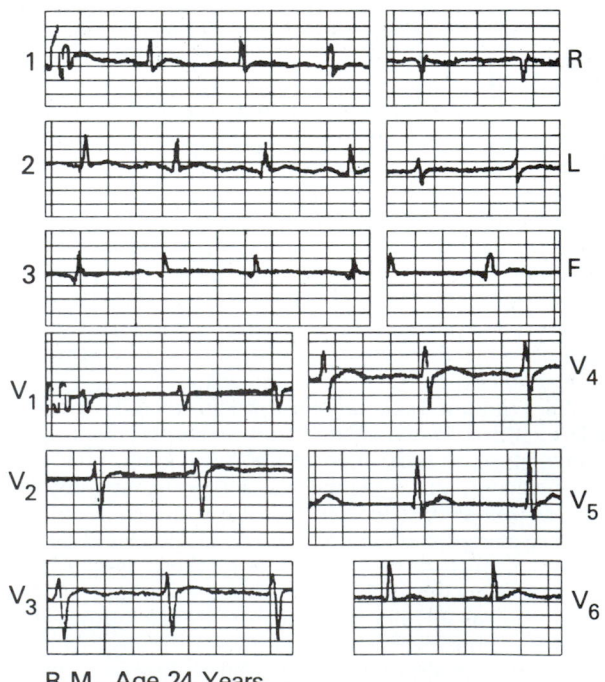

R.M. Age 24 Years

Figure 27–45. Absent S-T segments and short Q-T intervals in hypercalcemia. (From VanderArk CR, Ballantyne F III, Reynolds EW Jr. Electrolytes and the electrocardiogram. Complex electrocardiography. Cardiovasc Clin 1973; 5:285–294.)

Hypercalcemia-induced renal impairment is reversible if the hypercalcemia is of short duration and promptly corrected. Significant improvement in renal function after correction of hypercalcemia cannot be expected in patients with irreversible anatomical damage such as nephrocalcinosis.

OTHER. Soft tissue calcification may occur. Pruritus may be due to deposits of calcium phosphate in the skin and may improve after correction of hypercalcemia. Calcium activates several of the factors in the clotting system. This may in part account for occasional reports of widespread thrombosis in hypercalcemic patients.

Treatment of Hypercalcemia

Hypercalcemia can be corrected (see Fig. 27–44) by (1) inhibiting bone resorption, (2) increasing calcium excretion, and (3) decreasing intestinal calcium absorption. (Soft tissue calcium deposition may be associated with significant reduction in hypercalcemia but is obviously hazardous and should be avoided if at all possible.) Because increased bone resorption is the most important cause of hypercalcemia, agents capable of inhibiting bone resorption are generally the most effective therapy.

Therapy of hypercalcemia often must be instituted without a specific diagnosis. Many forms of therapy are nonspecific. Thus, hydration and increasing calcium excretion by forced sodium diuresis lowers serum calcium level regardless of the underlying cause. Plicamycin lowers serum calcium concentration by antagonizing the bone resorptive effects of a wide variety of agents. On the other hand, identification of factors that cause hypercalcemia allows institution of specific therapy. Destruction of a malignancy (by surgery, radiation, or chemotherapy), correction of thyrotoxicosis, and removal of a parathyroid adenoma are examples of specific treatments. In addition, several agents often used nonspecifically are considerably more effective when used selectively. For example, glucocorticoids are particularly effective in treatment of vitamin D intoxication and sarcoidosis.

Rigid guidelines cannot be set, but degree of hypercalcemia, severity of symptoms, and overall status of the patient are factors in deciding whether and how to treat. The mildly hypercalcemic, asymptomatic patient may not require therapy, but a specific diagnosis should be made. Severely symptomatic patients (hypercalcemia crisis) require emergency measures to correct hypercalcemia. Sampling blood for PTH and urine for cAMP determinations may be feasible even in acutely ill patients and may assist in subsequent attempts to diagnose the underlying disease. If severe hypercalcemia is corrected, chronic therapy may be necessary to avoid recurrence. Unfortunately, chronic therapy of hypercalcemia is generally unsatisfactory, so that, whenever feasible, one should treat the underlying disease.

FORMS OF THERAPY

Mobilization. Every effort should be made to avoid immobilization, which accelerates bone resorption and aggravates hypercalcemia. In some patients mobilization may be impossible, but activity should be encouraged as soon as other therapeutic measures have reduced the serum calcium concentration and relieved acute symptoms.

Hydration. Decreased fluid intake (nausea and vomiting) and inability to excrete a concentrated urine cause the dehydration that invariably accompanies severe hypercalcemia. Dehydration lowers GFR and reduces renal calcium excretion; hypercalcemia is in turn aggravated. Rehydration (generally with intravenous saline solution) is an important initial step in treating severely hypercalcemic patients. A rapid fall of 0.5 to 0.75 mmol/L (2 to 3 mg/dL) in total serum calcium concentration is typical after rehydration

alone. Maintaining adequate hydration is vital in chronic management. If adequate oral intake is not feasible, intermittent parenteral hydration may be required.

Sodium Diuresis. Because increased sodium excretion leads to increased calcium excretion, sodium diuresis is effective short-term therapy for hypercalcemia of all etiologies. Effective therapy requires infusion of large amounts (5 to 10 L/d) of isotonic saline together with potent diuretics (e.g., furosemide in doses of 100 mg every 2 h) to ensure maximal urinary sodium excretion. With appropriate therapy, urinary calcium excretion of 25 to 50 mmol/d (1 to 2 g/d) can be achieved, and serum calcium concentration may decrease by 0.5 to 1 mmol/L (2 to 4 mg/dL) in 24 h. Infusion of sodium sulfate has been reported to be even more effective, but in practice sodium sulfate offers little advantage over saline plus diuretics.

Hypokalemia, hypomagnesemia, and congestive heart failure are potential complications of forced sodium diuresis. They can be avoided by monitoring the central venous pressure (or pulmonary capillary wedge pressure) and by adequately replacing urinary losses of potassium (which may reach 200 mmol/d) and magnesium. A urinary catheter may be required, especially in obtunded patients. Forced sodium diuresis has been effective even in patients with impaired renal function (creatine clearance ~20 mL/min). Indeed, renal function often improves after correction of hypercalcemia. Severe renal failure, however, precludes use of this form of therapy.

Dialysis. This technique has been used effectively in patients with severe renal failure. Calcium (>25 mmol/d[>1 g/d]) can be removed from the blood either by peritoneal dialysis or by hemodialysis using calcium-free dialysates. Significant quantities of phosphate may also be dialyzed from the blood; because phosphate depletion aggravates hypercalcemia, serum phosphorus concentration should be monitored and phosphate supplements must be given as required.

Edetate. Edetate (EDTA) forms complexes with ionized calcium; the complexes are rapidly excreted by the kidney. Reports of severe renal injury attributed to such infusion have caused this form of therapy for hypercalcemia to be abandoned.[285]

Plicamycin. This cytotoxic agent was initially evaluated as a cancer chemotherapeutic agent, but its use was associated with serious toxicity. The observation that plicamycin (previously termed mithramycin) caused significant reduction in serum calcium concentration (93% of patients in a large series) prompted evaluation of its efficacy in the treatment of hypercalcemia.[286] The agent is a potent inhibitor of bone resorption and probably acts directly on the osteoclast. Reduction in serum calcium concentration is accompanied by reduced urinary calcium and hydroxyproline levels; PTH secretion is not inhibited and may indeed be stimulated by plicamycin-induced hypocalcemia (Fig. 27–46).

The agent can be given in a bolus injection or in an intravenous infusion over several hours. The usual dose is 25 μg/kg body weight. A single dose corrected hypercalcemia within 48 h in 30 of 41 cases of malignancy.[286] Normocalcemia may persist for days after a single dose, and recurrence depends on the underlying illness. Repeat administration is usually effective, but cumulative toxicity limits the frequency with which this agent can be given.

Anorexia and nausea frequently follow administration. Hemorrhage and liver and renal damage are the most serious toxic effects. Bleeding is due to thrombocytopenia and inhibition of hepatic clotting factor synthesis. A rise in prothrombin time and release of hepatic enzymes (aspartate aminotransferase, lactate dehydrogenase, alkaline phospha-

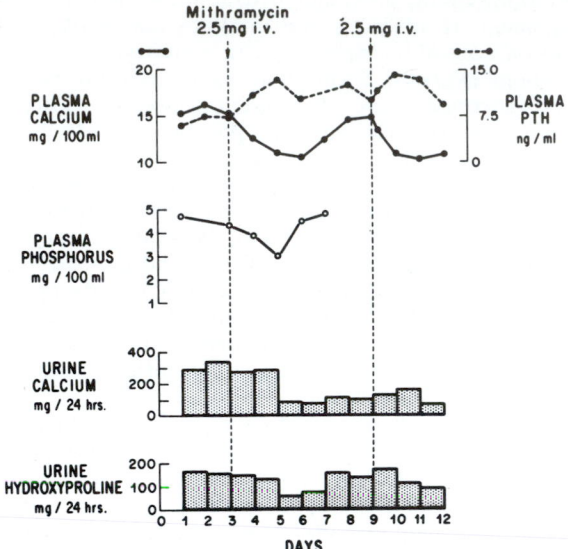

Figure 27–46. Effects of plicamycin (mithramycin) on plasma calcium, phosphorus, and PTH and urinary calcium and hydroxyproline levels in a patient with hypercalcemia caused by parathyroid carcinoma. Note that urinary calcium and hydroxyproline levels decrease, as does plasma calcium level, indicating decreased bone resorption. In contrast to these parameters, plasma PTH level is *not* reduced. (From Singer FR, Neer RM, Murray TM, et al. Mithramycin treatment of intractable hypercalcemia due to parathyroid carcinoma. Reprinted with permission from The New England Journal of Medicine, 283, 634–636, 1970.)

tase) indicate liver damage. Proteinuria and azotemia may develop. Toxic effects are most likely after repeated administration and in patients with pre-existing compromise of bone marrow, liver, and renal function.

Calcitonin. CT, which is effective in inhibiting bone resorption and is relatively free of toxicity, is not uniformly effective in lowering serum calcium concentration. Patients with hyperparathyroidism, malignancies, vitamin D intoxication, and other diseases have had good responses, but many "escape" from the effects during continued administration. It has been suggested without good evidence that combining phosphate therapy with CT may prevent escape.[287] The possibility that combining CT with low doses of other more toxic agents such as plicamycin might reduce toxicity without reducing efficacy has not been adequately evaluated. One study suggested that combined CT and glucocorticoid therapy is more effective in treating hypercalcemia of malignancy than either agent alone,[288] but another study showed that the combination of glucocorticoids and CT was less effective than either plicamycin or a diphosphonate in treating hypercalcemia of malignancy.[289]

Salmon CT is the most effective congener. The amount given should probably not exceed 8 MRC units/kg body weight intramuscularly or intravenously every 6 h, because higher doses are not likely to be more effective. For infusions, dilute gelatin or albumin solution may be used as vehicle. Nausea and vomiting may occur with high doses.

Phosphate. Administration of phosphate intravenously is an effective method for lowering serum calcium concentration. Phosphate has a direct inhibitory effect on bone resorption in vitro, and this may in part explain its in vivo hypocalcemic action. Unfortunately, acutely raising the serum phosphorus concentration in hypercalcemic subjects also leads to the precipitation of calcium phosphate salts.[290] Extensive metastatic calcification (sometimes associated with hypocalcemia, hypotension, renal failure, and death) has been reported in hypercalcemic patients after intravenous phosphate therapy. The true incidence of soft tissue calcification with either phosphate therapy may be low, and metastatic calcification can be a feature of hypercalcemia itself.[290] The likelihood of developing metastatic calcification after intravenous phosphate therapy may depend on the dose administered, the pretreatment serum phosphorus concentration, and the renal function. A situation analogous to intravenous phosphate infusion occurs in patients undergoing chemotherapy of certain malignancies (Burkitt lymphoma, lymphoblastic leukemia).[291] Rapid lysis of tumor cells releases a large amount of inorganic phosphate. Hyperphosphatemia, hypocalcemia, renal failure, and metastatic calcification have been reported in both hypercalcemic and normocalcemic patients.

Phosphate has been generally given intravenously in doses up to 50 mmol (1.5 g of elemental phosphorus) over 6 to 8 h. The decrease in serum calcium concentration is directly related to the dose of phosphate and to the maximal rise in serum phosphorus concentration achieved. Extreme hyperphosphatemia (>2.6 mmol/L [>8 mg/dL]) may occur with doses in excess of 50 mmol.

The anorexia of hypercalcemia may preclude oral administration of phosphates in the acute treatment of hypercalcemia. Once acute symptoms have been relieved by other measures, chronic therapy with oral phosphates may prevent recurrence of hypercalcemic crisis. Phosphate by mouth is probably less hazardous because the serum phosphorus level is increased more gradually. Nonetheless, chronic therapy even orally may cause metastatic calcification, particularly if hyperphosphatemia is produced. Serum phosphorus concentration must be closely monitored (peak concentration may be checked about 2 h after a dose), particularly in patients with impaired renal function. Therapy is usually initiated with four divided doses to give the equivalent of 2 to 3 g of elemental phosphorus per day. (Elemental phosphorus constitutes one fifth to one fourth of the weight of most phosphate salt preparations.) The dose may be reduced subsequently, depending on the serum phosphorus concentration. Diarrhea and gastrointestinal symptoms force reduction in dose in some patients.

Diphosphonates. Diphosphonates (bisphosphonates), analogues of pyrophosphate with a carbon atom rather than an oxygen bridging the two phosphates, are stable to cleavage by pyrophosphatases and inhibit hydroxyapatite crystal formation and dissolution. Many derivatives of the basic diphosphonate structure have been synthesized. Of these, ethane-1-hydroxy-1,1-diphosphonate (etidronate disodium), amino-hydroxypropane diphosphonate (APD), and dichloromethylene diphosphonate (Cl_2 MDP) have been tested clinically. All three compounds inhibit bone resorption, but the last two are more potent than etidronate and produce less inhibition of bone mineralization than etidronate at comparable doses. Several studies[289, 292, 293] have demonstrated the efficacy of APD and Cl_2 MDP in reducing serum calcium level in patients with hypercalcemia of malignancy. Both are effective parenterally as well as orally, although onset of action is slower with the oral route of administration. Etidronate is ineffective orally but shows some activity in correcting hypercalcemia when given parenterally. Doses of 7.5 mg/kg body weight/d infused over 2 h for 2 to 4 consecutive days returned serum calcium concentration to normal in 19 of 26 patients with hypercalcemia of malignancy.[294] At present, only etidronate is licensed for clinical use in the United States.

Glucocorticoids. Glucocorticoids are not uniformly effective in lowering serum calcium concentration. In pharmacological doses they increase urinary calcium excretion, but this effect is minor. Glucocorticoids antagonize the effects of vitamin D by undefined mechanisms. They reduce intestinal calcium absorption and bone resorption and lower serum calcium concentration and urinary calcium excretion in hypervitaminosis D. Glucocorticoids also lower serum 1,25(OH)$_2$D concentration in granulomatous disorders such as sarcoidosis and may be effective in some forms of hypercalcemia of malignancy. Multiple myeloma, leukemias, lymphomas, and some breast carcinomas are the most responsive tumors. Part or all of the effect may be due to destruction of tumor. Some glucocorticoid-responsive tumors (e.g., multiple myeloma, certain lymphomas) produce cytokines (such as interleukin 1 and tumor necrosis factor β) that act as osteoclast-activating factors (OAFs). The ability of glucocorticoids to block the bone resorptive effect of OAFs in vitro may explain the efficacy of this form of therapy in hypercalcemia due to OAF-producing malignancies. Glucocorticoids are ineffective against PTH-mediated bone resorption.

Doses of 40 to 100 mg/d of prednisone or the equivalent have been used to treat hypercalcemia. The side effects of excess corticosteroids are well known. In patients who do not appear to respond (a fall in serum calcium level usually occurs within 1 wk), treatment should be discontinued.

Indomethacin. Indomethacin (25 mg orally every 6 h) and aspirin (in doses sufficient to cause serum salicylate concentrations of 1.4 to 2.2 mmol/L [20 to 30 mg/dL]) are prostaglandin synthetase inhibitors and may correct hypercalcemia caused by production of prostaglandins by tumors. Although prostaglandins may be critical intermediates in osteoclast-mediated bone resorption, prostaglandin synthesis inhibitors are generally ineffective in treating most forms of hypercalcemia.[295]

Other Agents. Gallium nitrate has shown promise in treatment of hypercalcemia. It was more effective than salmon CT in a randomized double-blind study of subjects with hypercalcemia of malignancy.[296] The drug acts by inhibiting bone resorption. Although the incidence of adverse reactions has been low, further studies are needed to establish the safety and efficacy. Ethiofos (WR-2721) is another experimental drug with hypocalcemic activity. The drug acts in part by inhibiting PTH secretion but may also inhibit bone resorption. Ethiofos reduced serum calcium and serum PTH levels in a subject with parathyroid carcinoma.[297] The utility of this agent will require further investigation.

SUMMARY. Acute treatment of hypercalcemia must be designed on an individual basis. Rehydration and early mobilization are generally applicable. In severely symptomatic patients, additional measures are often required. Forced saline diuresis can be used safely in most patients if cardiovascular status and serum electrolyte concentrations are monitored. Plicamycin is probably the agent of first choice provided major contraindications (bone marrow, liver, or renal failure) are not present. Intravenous etidronate may prove equally effective and is less toxic than plicamycin. CT shows low toxicity but is not consistently effective. Intravenous phosphate, because of its potential acute toxicity, should be used only in life-threatening hypercalcemia and if etidronate disodium is ineffective and plicamycin is contraindicated.

There is no entirely satisfactory form of therapy for chronic hypercalcemia. Glucocorticoid therapy is useful in vitamin D intoxication and sarcoidosis. Chronic therapy with phosphate by mouth, if tolerated, can be used in all forms of hypercalcemia. The serum phosphorus concentration and renal function should be monitored closely, and the patient should be examined at frequent intervals for signs of soft tissue calcification.

Differential Diagnosis of Hypercalcemia

The initial step in evaluating a patient with confirmed hypercalcemia should be assignment to one of two broad categories: PTH-mediated or non–PTH-mediated hypercalcemia. This division is of clinical importance because subsequent diagnostic and therapeutic maneuvers in the two categories are different (Fig. 27–47). Assessment of circulating PTH activity using the two-site assay usually separates hypercalcemic patients into one of these two groups because hypercalcemia unrelated to parathyroid gland activity causes suppression of endogenous PTH secretion. Indeed, two-site PTH immunoassays (see section on PTH immunoassays) generally provide excellent discrimination between subjects with primary hyperparathyroidism and those with non–PTH-mediated hypercalcemia (including those related to PTHRP secretion).

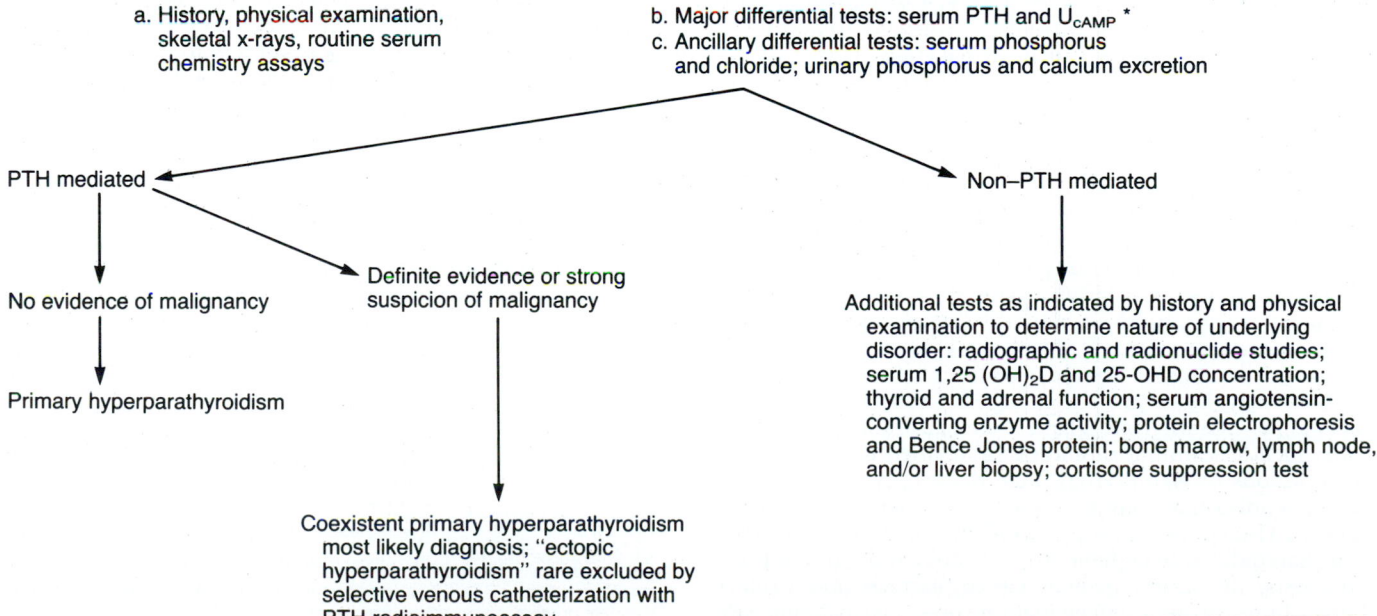

Figure 27–47. Flow diagram for evaluation of hypercalcemia. Hypercalcemia confirmed by multiple determinations; thiazides discontinued; emergency therapy given to severely hypercalcemic patients. *Elevation of both PTH and urinary cAMP (U$_{cAMP}$) levels diagnostic of PTH mediated; low PTH and U$_{cAMP}$ levels diagnostic of non–PTH mediated; combination of low PTH and high U$_{cAMP}$ levels highly suggestive of tumor secretion of PTHRP. See text for discussion of pitfalls in interpretation.

The renal effects of PTH have been discussed. Measurement of serum phosphorus, chloride, and bicarbonate levels and of urinary calcium and phosphorus excretion (normalized for filtered load) sometimes provides suggestive indices for PTH-dependent or -independent mechanisms. Results, however, show considerable overlap among these parameters, and complicating factors may negate the differential value of these measurements.[298] Thus nausea and vomiting or diuretic therapy renders serum chloride and bicarbonate measurement difficult to interpret. A further diagnostic complication is that PTHRP, which is secreted by certain tumors, mimics many of the actions of PTH, e.g., phosphaturia. Renal failure may limit the value of urine calcium and phosphorus estimation, even when corrections for reduced creatinine clearance are applied. Several groups have attempted to combine these parameters (e.g., serum chloride/phosphate ratio) in an effort to increase diagnostic utility, but the limitations of the individual measurements apply to the combined indices. Radiographic evidence of subperiosteal resorption is specific for PTH-mediated hypercalcemia but is rarely present.

Measurements of serum immunoreactive PTH concentration and urinary cAMP excretion are the most useful tests for differentiating PTH-mediated from non–PTH-mediated hypercalcemia, but both must be interpreted cautiously, particularly with compromised renal function. Unequivocal elevations in both urinary cAMP and serum PTH levels strongly favor PTH-mediated hypercalcemia, but nomograms suggesting that values for serum PTH in the normal range are "inappropriately elevated" in the presence of hypercalcemia must be interpreted with caution. Urinary cAMP excretion may be elevated in some patients with hypercalcemia of malignancy without concomitant elevation in serum PTH levels by radioimmunoassay. This is generally due to tumor secretion of PTHRP (see earlier under Physiology and Mechanism of PTHRP Action). Elevation in urinary cAMP level alone, then, cannot be taken as evidence for primary hyperparathyroidism.

Most patients with PTH-mediated hypercalcemia have primary hyperparathyroidism. Ectopic secretion of PTH itself is extremely rare. Selective venous catheterization to detect a gradient for PTH in neck veins draining the parathyroids is the only way to exclude a malignancy ectopically secreting PTH; this procedure is usually unnecessary, particularly in the absence of evidence suggestive of malignant disease. Patients with non–PTH-mediated hypercalcemia require further diagnostic investigation.

The history may be helpful: (1) chronicity of symptoms argues against malignancy; (2) family history of hypercalcemia or other endocrinopathy suggests MEN 1 or 2A or FHH; and (3) clues to other specific disorders, e.g., vitamin D ingestion, should be sought. On physical examination, there may be evidence for specific pathology, e.g., malignancy or sarcoid skin lesions. The presence of soft tissue calcification (e.g., band keratopathy) argues against uncomplicated hyperparathyroidism. A neck mass generally represents an incidental thyroid nodule but in hyperparathyroidism may be a grossly enlarged (and not necessarily malignant) parathyroid gland. Skeletal radiography and radionuclide scanning should be performed to detect metastatic lesions or parathyroid bone disease. Additional laboratory studies that may be appropriate, particularly in the non–PTH-mediated group, include (1) liver function tests (e.g., sarcoidosis, malignancy), (2) thyroid and adrenal function tests, (3) serum protein electrophoresis and urinary Bence Jones protein determination (note that patients with primary hyperparathyroidism may show coincidental benign monoclonal gammopathy), (4) bone marrow aspiration, (5) serum 25-OHD and 1,25(OH)$_2$D determination, (6) addi-

tional radiographic or biopsy studies to localize malignancy or provide evidence of sarcoidosis, and (7) serum angiotensin-converting enzyme activity, which is generally elevated in patients with sarcoidosis and is lowered by glucocorticoid therapy. However, elevated enzyme activity has also been reported[299] in patients with primary hyperparathyroidism and malignancy.

In difficult cases, the steroid suppression test may be useful; 60 mg of prednisone or equivalent glucocorticoid is administered daily for 7 to 10 d with daily measurements of serum calcium. A prompt (within 2 to 3 d) decrease in serum calcium level is characteristic of vitamin D intoxication and sarcoidosis. A positive response may also be seen in certain malignancies, thyrotoxicosis, and, of course, in hypercalcemia associated with adrenal insufficiency. Hypercalcemia refractory to corticosteroids is characteristic of primary hyperparathyroidism. Hypercalcemia associated with most types of malignancy is also unresponsive to glucocorticoid. In summary, careful clinical and laboratory evaluations permit specific diagnosis in most cases. Neck exploration and parathyroidectomy should not be performed as diagnostic maneuvers but rather as therapeutic procedures in patients in whom there is a high likelihood of finding abnormal parathyroid tissue.

Specific Hypercalcemic Disorders

MALIGNANCY. Malignancy is a common cause of hypercalcemia. In patients with disseminated and untreatable malignant disease, the development of hypercalcemia may have little clinical importance, but with the advent of newer and more aggressive forms of cancer treatment, the diagnosis and correction of hypercalcemia may be lifesaving. Occasionally, hypercalcemia may be the first manifestation of otherwise occult malignancy; evaluation of hypercalcemia in such cases may permit cure of the underlying disease.

Increased bone resorption is the final common pathway for tumor-induced hypercalcemia. The role of metastatic bone lesions in this regard has long been appreciated. The observation that some patients with malignancy and hypercalcemia lacked bone metastases raised the possibility of tumor production of a humoral osteolytic factor (humoral hypercalcemia of malignancy [HHM] syndrome). Early speculation centered on ectopic production of PTH, and the term *pseudohyperparathyroidism* was applied to this syndrome. It is now clear that ectopic secretion of authentic PTH is rare. HHM instead is caused by secretion of other osteolytic factors, in particular PTHRP.[133] The known mechanisms of hypercalcemia associated with malignancy are outlined in Table 27–11. Classification of tumors with and without bone metastases into separate categories (Table 27–11) is somewhat arbitrary because humoral factors may also play a role in hypercalcemia associated with bone metastases. Indeed, a poor correlation exists between extent of metastatic bone

TABLE 27–11. Mechanisms of Hypercalcemia Associated with Malignancy

Hypercalcemia Caused by	Tumor Type(s)	Mediator(s)
Hematogenous malignancy	Myeloma, Burkitt lymphoma	OAFs, e.g., lymphotoxin
	Hodgkin lymphoma	1,25(OH)$_2$D
Solid malignancy with bone metastases*	Breast, lung carcinoma	Prostaglandin E (?); other
Solid malignancy without bone metastases	Hypernephroma, various squamous carcinomas	PTHRP; others (?) (e.g., growth factors)
Coexistent primary hyperparathyroidism	All types	PTH

*Humoral secretion of factors such as PTHRP can contribute to hypercalcemia in such cases.

disease, assessed radiographically, and serum calcium level.[300] The anticalciuretic action of tumor-secreted humoral factors such as PTHRP may synergize with increased calcium release from skeletal metastases to account for hypercalcemia in selected cases.[301] Nonetheless, certain malignancies almost invariably cause hypercalcemia in association with bone metastases, whereas others commonly cause hypercalcemia without evidence of direct bone invasion by tumor.

MALIGNANCY WITH BONE METASTASES

Breast Cancer. Hypercalcemia in patients with breast cancer is almost always associated with bone metastases. The high incidence of breast cancer in the general population and the frequent occurrence (about 65%) of metastatic bone disease make this malignancy the leading cause of tumor-associated hypercalcemia, which may occur spontaneously or after administration of estrogens, androgens, or antiestrogens such as tamoxifen. The latter phenomenon is restricted to patients with pre-existing metastatic bone disease and may be due to transient stimulation of the tumor by the hormone or hormone analogue. Estrogens and antiestrogens may also lead to release of bone-resorbing activity from breast cancer cells.[302] In severe cases it may be necessary to discontinue steroid or tamoxifen administration to control hypercalcemia with other measures.[303]

The pathogenesis of hypercalcemia associated with breast cancer is unclear. Breast cancer cells are capable of resorbing bone directly, without activating osteoclasts.[304] Various substances (osteolytic sterols, prostaglandins) have also been suggested as bone-resorbing factors in breast cancer–related hypercalcemia, but conclusive evidence for any is lacking. Hypercalcemia in cases of breast cancer without evidence of bone metastases is most likely due to another disease. If serum PTH and urinary cAMP levels are elevated, the most likely diagnosis is coexistent primary hyperparathyroidism. In rare instances hypercalcemia has been attributed to breast cancer without bone involvement,[305] and this may be due to secretion of PTHRP.[133] Prostaglandin synthetase inhibitors (see later) are *not* effective in treating hypercalcemia in patients with breast cancer. A good response to glucocorticoids often but not invariably occurs.

Multiple Myeloma, Lymphoma, Leukemia. Skeletal or bone marrow involvement (or both) is characteristic of these malignancies. In myeloma, skeletal involvement may take the form of focal lytic lesions or diffuse osteoporosis. Some evidence implicates a cytokine, OAF, in the mechanism of hypercalcemia associated with multiple myeloma and some lymphomas (e.g., Burkitt lymphoma). OAF activity is present in culture fluid of myeloma cells (but not from peripheral plasma) and has potent bone-resorbing activity.[306] OAF production has been correlated with the extent of bone disease in myeloma but not with hypercalcemia (Fig. 27–48). OAF activity may be due to any of several leukocyte monokines such as interleukin 1, lymphotoxin, and tumor necrosis factor, each of which possesses potent bone-resorbing activity. Indeed, OAF secreted by myeloma cell lines was identified as lymphotoxin.[307] In some lymphomas, hypercalcemia is associated with an increased serum level of $1,25(OH)_2D$.[308] The mechanism is presumably identical to that in hypercalcemia of sarcoidosis (see later), i.e., unregulated production of $1,25(OH)_2D$ by tumor cells. Lymphomas with a granulomatous component such as Hodgkin disease[309] are likely to cause hypercalcemia by this mechanism. Hypercalcemia is common in patients with cutaneous T cell lymphomas and T cell leukemias from whom a type C retrovirus (human T cell lymphotrophic virus I, HTLV-I) has been isolated.[310] This disease is endemic in parts of Japan and the Caribbean, but cases have been reported in other countries including the United States. Lytic bone lesions have been described, but the role of direct tumor invasion versus indirect osteoclast activation is not yet clear. Although an elevated serum $1,25(OH)_2D$ level was found in one reported case,[308] normal or low values for serum $1,25(OH)_2D$ were found in five other hypercalcemic subjects with this malignancy.[311] Glucocorticocoids are often effective in correcting hypercalcemia associated with myeloma, lymphoma, and leukemia. This may in part reflect tumoricidal activity; the facts that glucocorticoids block OAF-mediated bone resorption in vitro and inhibit excessive $1,25(OH)_2D$ formation suggest additional therapeutic mechanisms.

Miscellaneous. Many other tumors metastasize to bone and may be associated with hypercalcemia. Because the correlation between extent of bone lesions and hypercalcemia is poor, other factors, including production of osteolytic and anticalciuretic substances, are probably operative in many of these cases.[301]

MALIGNANCY WITHOUT BONE METASTASES.

Tumors may cause hypercalcemia without metastasizing to bone by producing humoral osteolytic factors. However, it should be recognized that skeletal radiographs do not detect all bone metastases; radionuclide bone scans are more sensitive, but in some cases clinically inapparent lesions are observed at autopsy. Correction of hypercalcemia by treatment of the primary tumor (e.g., surgical removal) provides stronger evidence that tumor production of osteolytic substances is

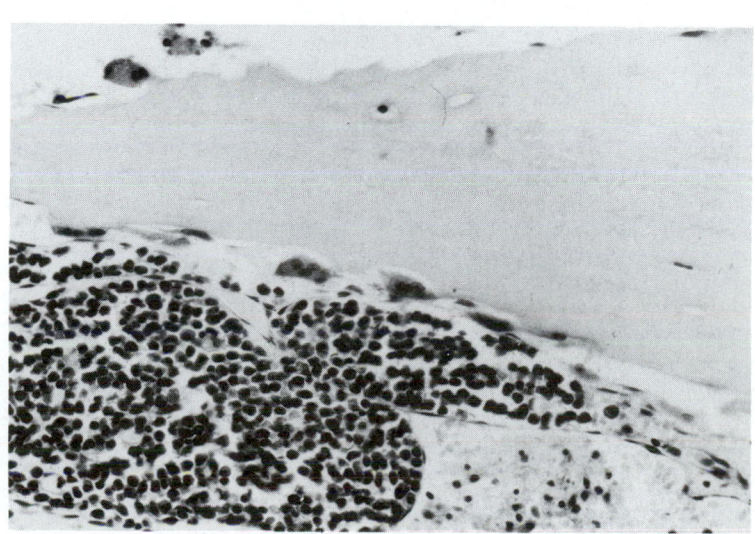

Figure 27–48. Histological section of an osteolytic lesion in the clavicle of patient with multiple myeloma, showing increased numbers of osteoclasts in resorption lacunae lying adjacent to myeloma cells. (From Mundy GR, Raisz LG, Cooper RA, et al. Evidence for the secretion of an osteoclast-stimulating factor in myeloma. Reprinted with permission from The New England Journal of Medicine, 291, 1041–1046, 1974.)

involved. Still more direct is demonstration of bone-resorbing activity by bioassay in extracts of the tumor. These criteria have been fulfilled in few cases reported as hypercalcemia caused by tumor production of osteolytic factors. Nonetheless, there is strong evidence that many tumor types, in particular hypernephroma; pancreatic carcinoma; squamous carcinoma of lung, cervix, and esophagus; and other head and neck tumors, cause hypercalcemia by producing osteolytic factors. The identity of such a factor (or factors) has important implications for understanding pathogenesis and designing therapy. Many, if not most, cases of HHM are due to tumor secretion of PTHRP,[133] but additional osteolytic factors, alone or in combination with PTHRP, may be involved.

Ectopic Hyperparathyroidism. With the initial recognition of the syndrome of malignancy-associated hypercalcemia without bone metastases, it was widely assumed that ectopic production of PTH by the tumor (by analogy with other ectopic hormone secretion syndromes) was responsible. However, the vast majority of patients with HHM have low or normal serum PTH levels.[133] In patients with HHM related to secretion of PTHRP, increased immunoreactive serum PTH is not found because homology of PTH and PTHRP (see Table 27–5) is limited to the extreme NH2 terminus and NH2-terminal–specific PTH antisera usually do not cross-react with PTHRP. In summary, most cases of HHM are not due to ectopic PTH secretion, but in rare cases tumors secrete PTH.[312]

Prostaglandins. Prostaglandins, particularly of the E series, are potent bone-resorbing agents and may be involved in some cases of tumor-associated hypercalcemia. Data supporting this mechanism include the finding of elevated urinary excretion of prostaglandin metabolites in some hypercalcemic patients with solid tumors and concomitant lowering of urinary prostaglandin and serum calcium levels after administration of prostaglandin synthase inhibitors such as indomethacin (Fig. 27–49). The source of prostaglandin, i.e., tumor production versus local production in bone secondary to some other tumor factor (see later), has not been identified. The frequency of prostaglandin-mediated hypercalcemia in cancer patients is unknown. The initial success reported in treating malignancy-associated hypercalcemia with prostaglandin synthesis inhibitors has not been confirmed.[295] Indiscriminate use of indomethacin to treat tumor-associated hypercalcemia is, therefore, not advisable. Even in patients with elevated urinary prostaglandin E metabolite levels, indomethacin may not lower serum calcium concentration, especially if bone metastases are present.

PTHRP. Urinary cAMP measurements in patients with cancer-associated hypercalcemia revealed a subgroup with elevated nephrogenous cAMP (Fig. 27–50). Most such patients show few or no bone metastases, suggesting that a humoral factor is responsible for the hypercalcemia. A PTH-like factor had been suggested as responsible for this syndrome because, as with PTH hypersecretion, renal phosphate threshold is depressed and urinary cAMP level is elevated. Radioimmunoassay of serum PTH, however, discloses suppressed or low-normal values. The PTH-like factor is not recognized by antisera that readily detect PTH in patients with primary hyperparathyroidism. PTH-like activity, however, is present in serum of patients with HHM tested by a sensitive radioimmunoassay (see under Assays for PTH) as well as in tumor extracts tested by a canine renal cortical adenylate cyclase assay. Production of cAMP in bone and kidney cells was used as an assay in purifying the PTH-like factor (here termed PTHRP) from tumor extracts. PTHRP was then sequenced, and the cDNA was cloned (see earlier section on PTHRP). The limited NH2-terminal sequence homology to PTH (see Table 27–5) explains the fact that PTHRP mimics many actions of PTH. The potent bone-resorbing activity of this peptide suggests that it alone could cause hypercalcemia in HHM. Other factors (see later) may synergize with PTHRP to give rise to the full syndrome of HHM.

Patients with malignancy-associated hypercalcemia and high nephrogenous cAMP levels may have elevated fasting calcium excretion, low serum 1,25(OH)2D levels, and, on bone biopsy, an uncoupling characterized by increased bone resorption without compensatory formation.[133] These characteristics are different from those in patients with hypersecretion of PTH.

It is not clear whether these differences between HHM associated with PTHRP secretion and primary hyperparathyroidism are due to differences in the biological activities of PTHRP and PTH or whether factors released by malignant cells (e.g., transforming growth factors) inhibit bone formation, renal calcium reabsorption, and 1,25(OH)2D formation, thereby altering the clinical expression of HHM. Immobilization of cancer patients may contribute to reduced osteoblastic activity. Low serum 1,25(OH)2D levels are not invariable in HHM; indeed, in patients with renal cell carcinoma, serum 1,25(OH)2D levels may be normal or elevated.[313] Many, if not most, cases of HHM are associated

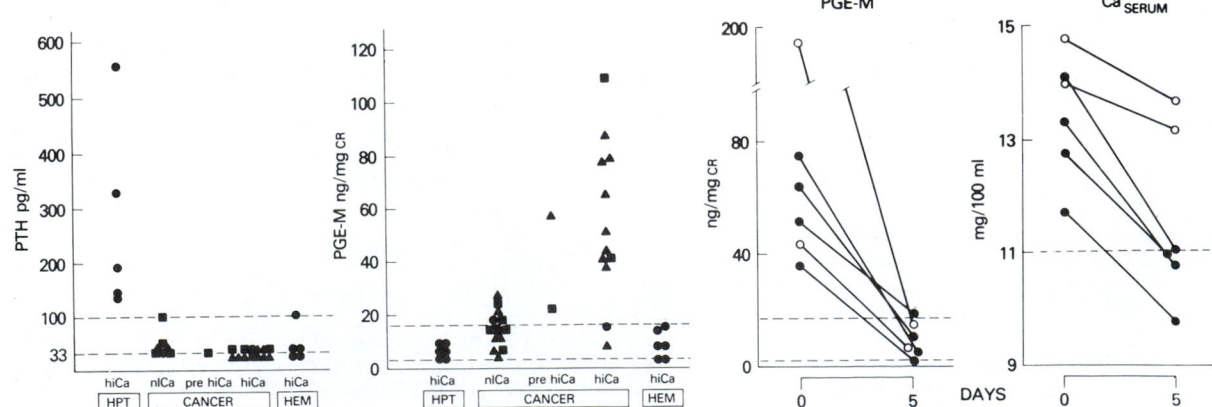

Figure 27–49. Plasma PTH *(left)* and urinary prostaglandin E metabolites (PGETM) *(left center)* in patients with hyperparathyroidism (HPT), solid tumors (cancer) with varying serum calcium concentrations, and hematogenous malignancies (HEM) with hypercalcemia. Response of urinary PGE-M *(right center)* and serum calcium *(right)* to indomethacin therapy is shown in hypercalcemic patients with (○) or without (●) bone metastases. (From Seyberth HW, Segre GV, Morgan JL, et al. Prostaglandins as mediators of hypercalcemia associated with certain types of cancer. Reprinted with permission from The New England Journal of Medicine, 293, 1278–1283, 1975.)

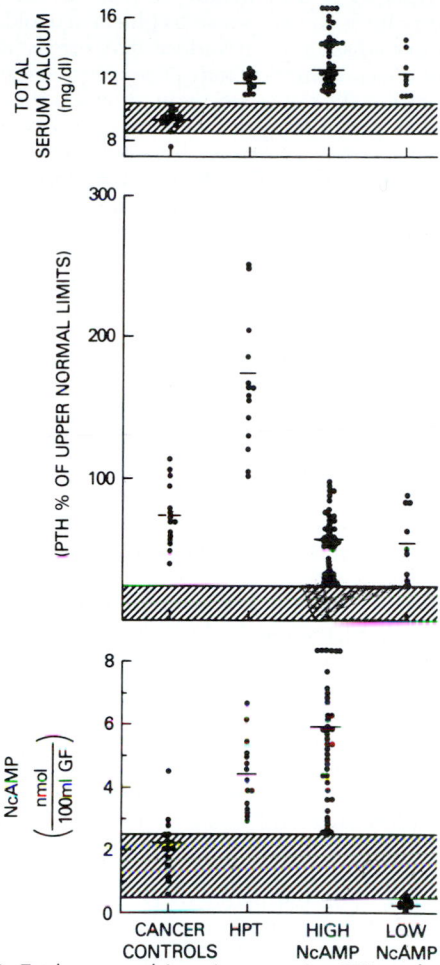

Figure 27–50. Total serum calcium, immunoactive PTH, and nephrogenous urinary cAMP levels in normocalcemic patients with cancer (cancer controls), patients with hyperparathyroidism (HPT), and hypercalcemic patients with cancer with high (HIGH NcAMP) and low (LOW NcAMP) nephrogenous urinary cAMP levels. Shaded areas for serum calcium *(top)* and NcAMP *(bottom)* indicate normal ranges. Serum immunoactive PTH level *(middle)* was measured with a multivalent antiserum (GP101). Data are expressed as a percentage of upper limit of normal range. Shaded area indicates detection limit. (From Stewart AF, Horst R, Deftos LJ, et al. Biochemical evaluation of patients with cancer-associated hypercalcemia. Reprinted with permission from The New England Journal of Medicine, 303, 1377–1383, 1980.)

with PTHRP secretion. Further studies should clarify the role of additional osteolytic factors in this syndrome.

Transforming Growth Factors. Tumor cells may release transforming growth factors of both the α and β types. Both types of transforming growth factors and cytokines such as interleukin 1 stimulate bone resorption. Colony-stimulating factors that act to stimulate formation and recruitment of osteoclast precursors could also increase bone resorption. Tumors associated with hypercalcemia and production of one or more of such factors have been reported (for example, see ref. 314). A tumor factor that stimulates prostaglandin formation and bone resorption has also been reported.[315] Further studies are required to determine the importance of these and other factors in malignancy-associated hypercalcemia.

THYROTOXICOSIS. Thyrotoxicosis is associated with reduced intestinal calcium absorption, hypercalciuria, and occasional hypercalcemia; the incidence of hypercalcemia in patients with thyroid hormone excess varies widely (2 to 20%).[316] Part of this variability may be attributed to failure to exclude coexistent primary hyperparathyroidism. More

than 40 patients with coexistent hyperthyroidism and hyperparathyroidism have been reported. Serum albumin is often depressed in thyrotoxicosis, so the ionized calcium level may be higher than expected based on measurement of total serum calcium concentration.[205] Hypercalcemia should not be attributed to hyperthyroidism unless the serum calcium concentration returns to normal and remains normal after antithyroid therapy. Serum PTH concentration should be low or normal and nephrogenous cAMP concentration should be reduced if hypercalcemia is due to thyrotoxicosis. Hypercalcemia in thyrotoxicosis is generally mild, but, rarely, severe hypercalcemia causes symptoms (constipation, anorexia, mental slowing) that obscure the diagnosis. Increased bone resorption in thyrotoxicosis is due to a direct effect of thyroid hormone. Propranolol (given orally or intravenously) rapidly corrects hypercalcemia associated with thyrotoxicosis.[317]

VITAMIN D INTOXICATION. Hypercalcemia associated with vitamin D intoxication usually occurs in patients treated for hypoparathyroidism and presents no diagnostic difficulties provided serum calcium concentration is monitored. Rarely, hypercalcemia is due to surreptitious or inadvertent ingestion of excess vitamin D; correct diagnosis may be difficult unless one has a high index of suspicion and takes a careful history (including a check of all medications and vitamins). If surreptitious calciferol intake is suspected, the serum 25-OHD level should be determined. Hypercalcemia in hypervitaminosis D causes suppression of PTH, but occurrence of renal failure may complicate interpretation of measurements of PTH and nephrogenous cAMP levels. Soft tissue calcification (nephrocalcinosis and band keratopathy) may be due to increased serum calcium *and* phosphate concentrations. The half-life of vitamin D is long, and vitamin D intoxication may persist for months. Vitamin D excess leads to hypercalcemia by increasing both intestinal calcium absorption and bone resorption. The initial hypercalciuria may dissipate as renal failure progresses. 25-OHD is the principal metabolite responsible for vitamin D intoxication, although calcitriol, given in excess, is a potent inducer of hypercalcemia.[201] Discontinuation of vitamin D and treatment with glucocorticoids effectively lower serum calcium concentration in most patients (often within 3 to 4 d). Prolonged therapy as just mentioned may be necessary. CT is of secondary importance in treatment of vitamin D intoxication. In cases of massive vitamin D overdose, treatment with inducers of hepatic microsomal enzyme synthesis (e.g., glutethimide) may be useful[318] because such agents enhance the rate of catabolism of vitamin D by the liver.

HYPERVITAMINOSIS A. At least six cases of hypercalcemia attributed to hypervitaminosis A have been reported.[319] Affected patients consumed in excess of 75,000 IU/d, an amount capable of causing increased bone resorption. Because most of the patients also consumed small doses of vitamin D, the hypercalcemia may not be due solely to vitamin A excess but rather to a synergistic action of vitamins A and D. Periosteal calcifications, if present, should suggest vitamin A intoxication because they are not seen with other causes of hypercalcemia. Serum vitamin A concentrations are raised in chronic renal failure. Hypervitaminosis A may contribute to hypercalcemia in patients with renal failure, particularly if they are taking vitamin A supplements. Discontinuation of vitamin A ingestion corrects the hypercalcemia. There is suggestive evidence that glucocorticoids hasten return of serum calcium concentration to normal in this condition. Hypercalcemia has also been reported in patients with acne given the vitamin A derivative isotretinoin (13-*cis*-retinoic acid).[320] The incidence of this complication is unclear, but patients given this agent should have the serum calcium level checked periodically.

SARCOIDOSIS AND OTHER GRANULOMATOUS DISEASES. The incidence of hypercalcemia in sarcoidosis is approximately 17%. Hypercalcemia is more likely in chronic and disseminated sarcoidosis than in transient or localized disease. Direct bone involvement occurs but is *not* a prerequisite for development of hypercalcemia. Spontaneous fluctuations in serum calcium concentration are common, and mild hypercalcemia may remit without therapy. Occasional patients show severe hypercalcemia and develop nephrocalcinosis and uremia. There is increased intestinal absorption of calcium, increased urinary calcium excretion, and hypercalcemia, in decreasing order of frequency. These abnormalities in calcium homeostasis and their correction by glucocorticoids, as well as the observation that many patients with sarcoidosis given small amounts of vitamin D ($\sim$10,000 IU/d) become hypercalcemic, have led to the hypothesis of disordered vitamin D metabolism in this condition. Serum concentrations of bioactive vitamin D and of 25-OHD are normal, but serum $1,25(OH)_2D$ concentration is elevated. Normocalcemic subjects with sarcoidosis, moreover, may show an abnormal rise in serum $1,25(OH)_2D$ level when challenged with modest doses (e.g., 10,000 IU/d) of vitamin D. These data suggest that the abnormal calcium metabolism is due to enhanced formation or decreased degradation of serum $1,25(OH)_2D$.[321, 322] Hypercalcemia with elevated serum $1,25(OH)_2D$ in a bilaterally nephrectomized subject with sarcoidosis (Fig. 27–51) suggests extrarenal formation of the metabolite, perhaps in the granuloma itself. Indeed, $1,25(OH)_2D$ is produced by pulmonary alveolar macrophages from subjects with active sarcoidosis.[323] Interferon-γ, a lymphokine secreted in high concentrations by pulmonary inflammatory cells from subjects with sarcoidosis, induces formation of $1,25(OH)_2D$ by pulmonary alveolar macrophages from normal subjects. Glucocorticoids decrease serum calcium concentration in sarcoidosis, apparently by reducing formation of $1,25(OH)_2D$. Chloroquine is also effective in lowering serum calcium concentration in sarcoidosis. Like glucocorticoids, it acts by decreasing formation of $1,25(OH)_2D$ and can be used for patients who cannot tolerate glucocorticoids.[324]

Hypercalcemia in sarcoidosis is associated with suppressed serum PTH and urinary cAMP levels. A further differential point is the response to glucocorticoids. Primary hyperparathyroidism and sarcoidosis may coexist in the same patient, and the combination may pose diagnostic difficulties. Neck exploration should be performed only if there is strong biochemical evidence for primary hyperparathyroidism and if glucocorticoids fail to correct hypercalcemia in a patient with sarcoidosis. Conversely, persistent hypercalcemia after removal of abnormal parathyroid tissue and correction of PTH hypersecretion may be due to a coexistent hypercalcemic disorder such as sarcoidosis. Indeed, hypercalcemia related to sarcoidosis can occur in patients with long-standing hypoparathyroidism.[325]

Hypercalcemia has been reported in other granulomatous disorders as well. Although definitive evidence is lacking, the increased sensitivity of serum calcium to vitamin D supplements and correction of hypercalcemia by glucocorticoids make it plausible that the pathophysiology in some of these cases is similar to that of sarcoidosis. It is likely that sarcoidosis, tuberculosis, fungal infections, berylliosis, and certain lymphomas cause hypercalcemia through unregulated production of $1,25(OH)_2D$ by the granulomatous tissue.[326]

IDIOPATHIC HYPERCALCEMIA IN INFANCY. This rare syndrome is characterized by hypercalcemia and abnormal growth and development. The hypercalcemia may be associated with the features of Williams syndrome including hypoplastic mandible and low-set ears, giving rise to the characteristic elfin facies; cardiac anomalies, most typically supravalvular aortic stenosis; mental retardation; growth retardation; scoliosis; accessory nipples; and abnormal teeth (peg-like, widely spaced).[327] The hypercalcemia causes constipation and hypotonia and may lead to nephrocalcinosis and uremia. Affected infants who survive may become normocalcemic. The pathogenesis is unknown. Evidence in favor of a role for vitamin D in the syndrome includes the observation that offspring of rabbits given excessive amounts of vitamin D during pregnancy have facial and aortic anomalies similar to those seen in humans with the disease. Autopsy studies have disclosed normal parathyroids. There is suggestive evidence for increased sensitivity to vitamin D in affected patients. In one study,[327] an abnormal but mild rise in serum 25-OHD was seen after a pharmacological challenge with vitamin D. Another study, however, reported increased concentrations of $1,25(OH)_2D$ in infants with hypercalcemia and elfin facies syndrome.[328] The defect in vitamin D metabolism presumptively responsible for hypercalcemia remains to be defined. Therapy consists of reduction in calcium intake and discontinuation of vitamin D ingestion. Glucocorticoids and CT have also been used.

ADRENAL INSUFFICIENCY. Hypercalcemia is as frequent in adrenal insufficiency as are hyponatremia and hyperkalemia. Diagnostic confusion may result from the similarity in symptoms of adrenal insufficiency and severe hypercalcemia. The correct diagnosis has been made in some cases only after a "steroid suppression" test for hypercalcemia. The mechanism responsible for hypercalcemia in adrenal insufficiency is not entirely clear.[329] Both decreased renal clearance of calcium and increased influx of calcium from bone to ECF have been observed. The former is due to the decreased ECF volume and decreased sodium excretion characteristic of adrenal insufficiency; the latter may involve loss of glucocorticoid antagonism of vitamin D metabolite action on bone. The hypercalcemia of adrenal insufficiency is readily corrected by appropriate therapy with glucocorticoids.

MILK-ALKALI SYNDROME. In 1949 Burnett and co-workers (reviewed in ref. 330) described six patients with hypercalcemia, normal to elevated serum phosphorus con-

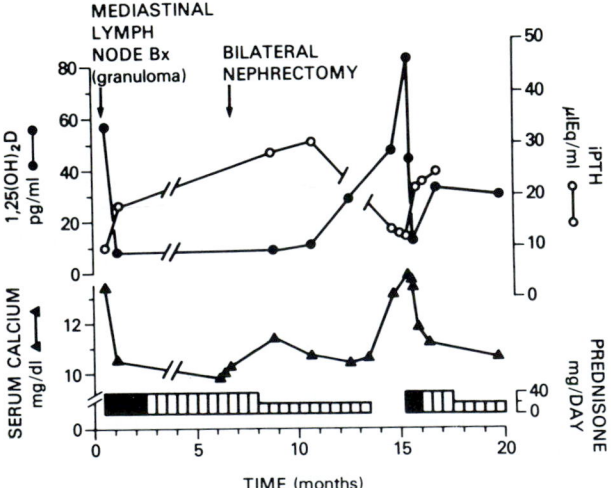

Figure 27–51. Serum concentrations of $1,25(OH)_2D$, immunoactive PTH (iPTH), and calcium in relation to prednisone treatment in a patient with sarcoidosis in whom bilateral nephrectomy was performed. Solid portion of bar representing prednisone administration indicates daily therapy, and open portion indicates alternate-day therapy. Bx, biopsy. (From Barbour GL, Coburn JW, Slatopolsky E, et al. Hypercalcemia in an anephric patient with sarcoidosis: evidence for extrarenal generation of 1,25-dihydroxyvitamin D. Reprinted with permission from The New England Journal of Medicine, 305, 440–443, 1981.)

centration, renal insufficiency, and soft tissue calcification (including band keratopathy and nephrocalcinosis). All had consumed large amounts of milk and absorbable alkali (generally sodium bicarbonate) as treatment for peptic ulcer. Reduction of calcium and alkali intake ameliorated the condition. Normal parathyroids were observed at surgery in only one patient, but the authors concluded that hyperparathyroidism was not responsible for the hypercalcemia. Excessive calcium and alkali intake was postulated to cause soft tissue calcification, reduction in renal function and urinary calcium excretion, and ultimately hypercalcemia. According to this formulation, PTH secretion should be suppressed, but this has not been adequately documented with modern methods for assessment of PTH secretion.[330] At present, the milk-alkali syndrome is rarely encountered, probably because absorbable alkali is no longer used in the treatment of ulcer disease. Several over-the-counter antacids, however, contain absorbable calcium and alkali and thus have the potential for causing the syndrome. Additional factors, in particular thiazide diuretic therapy, an established cause of hypocalciuria and alkalosis, may act synergistically with ingestion of absorbable calcium and alkali to cause hypercalcemia.

Diagnosis of the milk-alkali syndrome is based on obtaining a history of calcium and alkali ingestion and observing the response to withdrawal of these agents. "Inappropriately detectable" serum PTH should not be accepted as evidence for primary hyperparathyroidism in this setting, because renal impairment is commonly present. Conversely, the coexistence of hypercalcemia and peptic ulcer disease should prompt thorough evaluation for evidence of MEN 1 with primary hyperparathyroidism and Zollinger-Ellison syndrome. Generally, cessation of calcium and alkali ingestion is sufficient to correct hypercalcemia. Severe hypercalcemia may require other measures (see section on therapy), including dialysis if renal function is severely compromised.

THIAZIDES. Therapy with thiazide diuretics may lead to hypercalcemia. Unlike other natriuretic agents, thiazides *increase* renal calcium reabsorption. In subjects with normal mineral homeostasis, a transient elevation in *total* serum calcium concentration (secondary to hemoconcentration) may occur during the first days of thiazide treatment. Thiazides rarely if ever cause a sustained elevation in serum ionized calcium concentration in normal subjects. In patients with high rates of bone resorption and a tendency to hypercalciuria, however, thiazide diuretics, because of their hypocalciuric effect, may precipitate or aggravate hypercalcemia.

Thiazides may also raise serum calcium concentration by extrarenal mechanisms. Thiazide-induced hypercalcemia has been observed in uremic patients given chronic hemodialysis and in vitamin D–treated hypoparathyroid patients. Thiazides do not decrease urinary calcium excretion significantly in either group. Potentiation of PTH action on bone and a direct effect of thiazides on bone appear to be the most likely mechanisms. Thiazide therapy should be promptly discontinued in patients discovered to be hypercalcemic. Persistent hypercalcemia (>1 mo after discontinuation of thiazide) should alert one to seek another cause for the hypercalcemia. In one study,[331] 20 of 95 patients discovered to be hypercalcemic on routine screening were receiving thiazides. Hypercalcemia persisted in 14 of 20 after discontinuation of thiazide therapy, and primary hyperparathyroidism was proved surgically in each. If hypercalcemia remits after thiazides are stopped, continued follow-up is appropriate. Such patients may have mild primary hyperparathyroidism or other abnormalities and may again develop hypercalcemia.

IMMOBILIZATION. Immobilization is an infrequent cause of hypercalcemia (fewer than 50 cases have been reported). Because serum calcium determinations are not routinely performed in immobilized patients, the true incidence of immobilization hypercalcemia may be higher. A prospective study showed that 6 of 12 patients (ages 4 to 15 y) immobilized after single limb fractures developed hypercalcemia.

Hypercalcemia has been reported after immobilization in patients with single or multiple fractures, in quadriplegics, and in patients with extensive burns. Although usually mild, severe hypercalcemia and hypercalcemic crisis may occur. Hypercalcemia generally develops only several weeks after the onset of immobilization. The nonspecific nature of hypercalcemic symptoms makes it advisable to measure serum calcium level routinely in such patients.

Immobilization causes an increase in the bone resorption/formation ratio. Patients with high rates of bone turnover (adolescents, Paget disease) are at greatest risk for hypercalcemia. Excess calcium released from bone is largely excreted by the kidney. Resulting hypercalciuria may lead to renal and bladder stones, urinary obstruction, and impaired renal function. Reduction in renal function leads to reduced calcium excretion and may be sufficient to cause hypercalcemia.

Increased bone resorption is central to the pathogenesis of immobilization hypercalcemia, but increased PTH secretion is not responsible for increased bone resorption.[332] Fasting and 24-h urinary calcium excretion are elevated, but serum phosphorus and renal phosphorus thresholds are also increased; $1,25(OH)_2D$ and PTH levels in serum are decreased, and urinary cAMP level is reduced. It appears then that PTH secretion is suppressed by increased calcium flux from bone caused by an as-yet unidentified factor(s).

Serum PTH level should be interpreted cautiously in immobilized hypercalcemic patients (particularly if renal impairment has also developed). Neck exploration should not be performed solely because of mild PTH elevation in this circumstance.

Mild hypercalcemia in an immobilized patient may not require any therapy. Symptomatic patients, who require therapy, should be mobilized as soon as feasible, because this is the most effective and safest form of therapy. Exercises while in bed do not appear to be effective. Glucocorticoids have been used to treat immobilized hypercalcemic patients but without convincing effectiveness. Phosphate given by mouth may be useful and may reduce urinary calcium excretion if serum phosphate level is not elevated; it must be given carefully, if at all, if serum phosphorus is already high. High fluid intake, furosemide, and CT may also be effective.

ACUTE RENAL FAILURE. More than 20 patients with hypercalcemia and acute renal failure have been reported. In virtually every case, renal failure was caused by myoglobinuria secondary to skeletal muscle injury. Hypercalcemia developed most commonly during the diuretic phase and was often severe but transient (the longest duration recorded being 5 mo). In several cases, soft tissue calcification (often involving the injured muscles) was seen on x-ray examination. The cause of hypercalcemia has not been elucidated. Release of calcium from soft tissue deposits during the diuretic phase has been invoked, but this theory is unproved. In acute renal failure associated with muscle necrosis, hyperphosphatemia is more severe and often leads to calcification of necrotic muscle. The role of PTH is controversial; difficulties in measuring bioactive PTH in patients with renal failure probably account for the discrepant results in various reports with PTH immunoassay. One study[333] of six patients with rhabdomyolysis-induced acute renal failure showed hypocalcemia, marked hyperphosphatemia, and reduced serum 1,25(OH)₂D level in the acute phase. During recovery there was moderate hypercalcemia, increased serum $1,25(OH)_2D$ level, and persistent elevation in serum PTH level. The authors suggested that hypercalcemia was due to increased serum $1,25(OH)_2D$ concentration, which in turn was caused by excessive PTH secretion. According to this hypothesis, there is a disequilibrium between recovery of renal function and regression of the secondary hyperparathyroidism provoked by the initial hypocalcemia. Another study of four subjects with hypercalcemia in the diuretic phase of acute renal failure caused by rhabdomyolysis found elevation in $1,25(OH)_2D$ level with undetectable PTH and suggested that extrarenal or unregulated renal production of $1,25(OH)_2D$ may be responsible.[334] Further studies with the more specific two-site PTH immunoassay are needed. Parathyroidectomy is probably never indicated because the hypercalcemia is transient. If severe, it may be treated by conservative measures.

HYPOPARATHYROIDISM

Introduction

Hypoparathyroidism is a state of decreased secretion or peripheral action of PTH and can be due to inadequate secretion, biologically ineffective hormone, or organ insensitivity to PTH (Fig. 27–52). Diminution of PTH action on kidney and bone leads to hypocalcemia and hyperphosphatemia.

Clinical Manifestations

Hypocalcemia and hyperphosphatemia lead to signs and symptoms that are independent of the specific cause of hypoparathyroidism (Table 27–12). Decreased serum ionized calcium concentration increases neuromuscular excitability and may permit the examiner to elicit Chvostek or Trousseau sign. (Many normal subjects also show Chvostek sign, so it should always be sought *before* contemplated neck surgery.) Symptoms may range in severity from mild paresthesias (circumoral tingling and numbness, "needles and pins" feeling in hands and feet) to tetany with muscle cramps, carpopedal spasms, laryngeal stridor, and convulsions. Hypocalcemic seizures are usually not associated with loss of consciousness or incontinence and are rarely preceded by an aura. There may be nonspecific electroencephalographic abnormalities, particularly an increase in high-voltage slow waves; the electroencephalogram reverts to normal with correction of hypocalcemia. Mental changes include irritability, paranoia, depression, and frank psychosis. Papille-

TABLE 27–12. Signs and Symptoms in Types of Hypoparathyroidism

Sign or Symptom	"Classic"* Pseudo	Idiopathic	Postsurgical
Increased neuromuscular excitability	+	+	+
Cataracts	+	+	+†
Basal ganglia calcification	+	+	+†
Prolonged Q-T interval on electrocardiogram	+	+	+
Papilledema	+	+	+
Dental defects	+	+	+‡
Alopecia	−	+	−
Vitiligo	−	+	−
Moniliasis	−	+	−
Hypothyroidism§	+	+	+
Hypoadrenalism	−	+	−
Primary hypogonadism	+‖	+	−
Albright hereditary osteodystrophy (brachydactyly, short, obese, round face)	+	−	−
Subcutaneous calcification (and bone formation)	+	−	−

*Classic refers to patients with features of Albright osteodystrophy.
†Uncommon unless long-standing disease present.
‡Uncommon because postsurgical hypoparathyroidism is rarely seen in children.
§The mechanism of hypothyroidism differs in each of the three forms of hypoparathyroidism. Hypothyroidism is a rarer accompaniment of hypoparathyroidism than of hypoadrenalism.
‖Primary and/or secondary amenorrhea is common in classic PHP. The mechanism may involve resistance to gonadotropins.

dema, elevated cerebrospinal fluid pressure, and neurological signs mimicking a cerebral tumor may occur in chronic hypocalcemia.

Intracranial calcifications, particularly in the basal ganglia, are visible on skull x-ray films in approximately 20% of patients. With the more sensitive computed tomographic scan, intracranial calcifications have been demonstrated in patients with normal standard skull x-ray films. A parkinsonian-like syndrome may occur in patients with basal ganglia calcification. Increased sensitivity to the dystonic effects of phenothiazines may also be present, even in the absence of radiographic evidence of basal ganglia calcification. Calcified basal ganglia may also occur on a familial basis without abnormal parathyroid function.

Calcification of the lens can lead to cataract formation. Correction of hypocalcemia does not lead to regression of cataracts once formed. Development of calcified basal ganglia and cataracts is probably a function of the duration of the hypoparathyroid state and is more common in pseudohypoparathyroidism and idiopathic hypoparathyroidism than in postsurgical hypoparathyroidism.

Electrocardiographic manifestations of hypocalcemia include prolongation of the Q-T interval (particularly the Q-T corrected for rate) and T wave changes such as peaking and inversion. The Q-T interval returns to normal rapidly

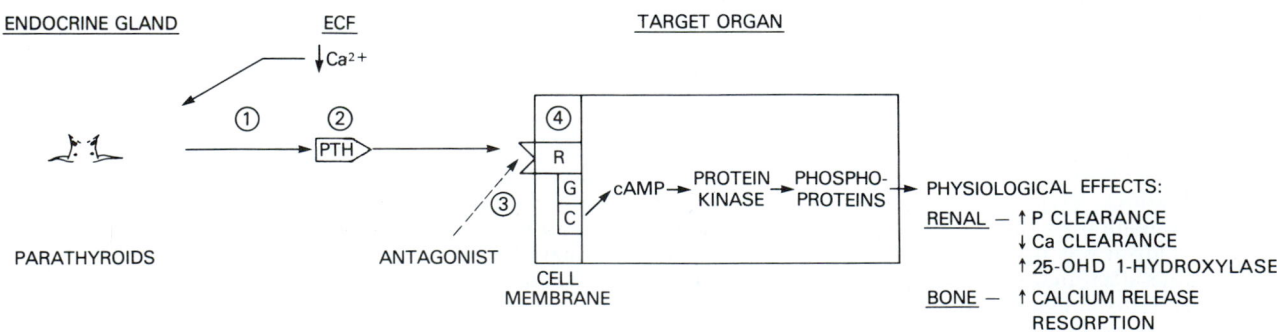

Figure 27–52. Sites of defect potentially leading to deficient PTH action: (1) deficient PTH secretion; (2) biologically inactive PTH; (3) PTH antagonist; (4) target cell defects—these could involve the PTH receptor (R), the guanine nucleotide–coupling protein (G), the catalytic unit (C) of adenylate cyclase, cAMP-dependent protein kinase, or the protein substrate(s) of the kinase.

after correction of hypocalcemia, but T wave abnormality may be slower to regress. A prolonged Q-T interval should theoretically predispose to ventricular tachycardia, but this arrhythmia is rare in association with hypoparathyroidism. Similarly, hypocalcemia might be expected to cause resistance to the effect of cardiac glycosides, and one case of atrial fibrillation apparently refractory to digitalis has been reported. Reversion to normal sinus rhythm occurred only after normocalcemia was restored. Congestive heart failure associated with severe hypocalcemia has been reported in neonates and rarely in children and adults. Return of serum calcium concentration to normal improves cardiac function in hypocalcemic patients with congestive heart failure.[335]

Dental abnormalities occur frequently.[336] Depending on the age at onset of the disorder, one may find enamel hypoplasia (manifest clinically as circumferential bands or pits traversing the crowns of the affected teeth), dental hypoplasia, defective root formation, and failure of adult teeth to erupt. The dental abnormalities help to date the onset of hypocalcemia.

Poorly controlled hypoparathyroidism in pregnancy may lead to a form of secondary hyperparathyroidism in the fetus and severe skeletal demineralization in the neonate. Although neonatal hyperparathyroidism is transient in such cases, death can result from complications of skeletal fractures.[337] Thus it is important to control serum calcium level in pregnant subjects with hypoparathyroidism.

DIFFERENTIAL DIAGNOSIS. Hypocalcemia, hyperphosphatemia, and normal renal function strongly suggest hypoparathyroidism. The type may be indicated by the history and physical examination. The patient should be asked about previous neck surgery and about other affected family members. On physical examination there may be a neck scar suggesting postsurgical hypoparathyroidism; features of Albright hereditary osteodystrophy, suggesting pseudohypoparathyroidism; or vitiligo, alopecia, and moniliasis, suggesting "idiopathic" hypoparathyroidism. Definitive characterization of the form of hypoparathyroidism (see Fig. 27–52) requires determination of plasma PTH and urinary cAMP levels and measurement of the response of urinary cAMP and urinary phosphate to exogenous PTH (Table 27–13). Bovine parathyroid extract, previously used in the standard PTH infusion test, is no longer available commercially. A comparable test based on infusion of the synthetic NH_2-terminal (1–34) fragment of human PTH (teriparatide acetate) gives equivalent results. True hypoparathyroid patients show low or undetectable PTH levels and respond normally to exogenous PTH, indicating PTH deficiency. These patients may be grouped as to the cause of PTH deficiency, e.g., hypomagnesemia, postsurgical, idiopathic. Elevated concentration of serum PTH coupled with a normal response to exogenous PTH suggests secretion of a biologically inactive form of PTH. Elevated serum PTH and an abnormal response to exogenous PTH signify resistance to PTH and may be further subdivided according to the site of defect (see Fig. 27–52).

There is a spectrum of parathyroid disfunction in these disorders. Measurement of serum calcium and PTH levels after a standard edetate infusion may reveal "decreased parathyroid reserve" or "latent hypoparathyroidism" manifest by prolonged hypocalcemia and inadequate rise in serum PTH level. Such individuals may be at risk for symptomatic hypocalcemia under conditions that demand compensatory PTH secretion, such as pregnancy and lactation.

Specific Forms of Hypoparathyroidism

DEFICIENT PARATHYROID HORMONE SECRETION

Postsurgical. The incidence of permanent hypoparathyroidism after thyroidectomy varies widely in surgical series (a range of 0.2 to 33% has been reported).[339] The extent of thyroid resection, the experience of the surgeon, and the diligence in diagnosing hypocalcemia all contribute to the variation in incidence. In some patients, postoperative hypocalcemia is transient, suggesting that sufficient viable parathyroid tissue remains to restore normal mineral homeostasis. Such patients, however, may show "decreased parathyroid reserve." There may be a long latent period before symptoms develop and hypocalcemia is diagnosed. Increased CT secretion and bone hunger may contribute to transient hypocalcemia after thyroidectomy, but injury to parathyroid tissue is the likeliest cause in these cases, as in permanent hypocalcemia.

Hypoparathyroidism is an extremely rare complication of radioactive iodine therapy. Both permanent and reversible forms have been reported.[340] Onset is generally delayed (between 5 and 18 mo after therapy). Surprisingly, most cases are associated with therapy of Graves disease rather than thyroid carcinoma. Patients with intrathyroidal parathyroids may be at greatest risk for this complication, because beta particles emitted by ^{131}I destroy tissue only to a depth of about 2 mm.

Permanent hypoparathyroidism develops in 1% of patients after initial surgery for primary hyperparathyroidism. The risk of permanent hypoparathyroidism increases in subtotal parathyroidectomy for parathyroid hyperplasia and after repeated neck surgery for recurrent or persistent disease. In some cases autotransplantation of parathyroid tissue to the forearm is indicated to prevent hypoparathyroidism in these high-risk patients. Deliberate parathyroidectomy and autotransplantation have also been advocated by some surgeons for patients undergoing thyroid cancer resection. Precise indications for autotransplantation of parathyroids, however, have not been established. Because grafts may either fail or hyperfunction, it is unwise to perform parathyroid transplants indiscriminately.

Idiopathic Hypoparathyroidism. Deficient PTH secretion without a defined cause (e.g., surgical injury) is termed *idiopathic hypoparathyroidism.* This disease is rare and may occur on a sporadic or familial basis. The mode of inheritance of the familial variety is uncertain, possibly because several forms of the disease exist. Symptoms often begin in

---

TABLE 27–13. Biochemical Characteristics in Types of Hypoparathyroidism

Characteristic	Serum PTH	U_{cAMP}	Exogenous PTH*	
			U_{cAMP} Response	U_P Response
Deficient PTH secretion	Low	Low	Normal	Normal
Secretion of ineffective PTH	High†	Low	Normal	Normal
Resistance to PTH—defective receptor–adenylate cyclase complex	High	Low	Low	Low
Resistance to PTH—defect distal to receptor–adenylate cyclase complex	High	High	Normal	Low

*5 U/kg body weight, 200 U maximum, of synthetic (1–34) NH_2-terminal fragment of PTH administered intravenously over 10 min. Urine collected before and after infusion for measurement of cAMP, phosphorus, and creatinine.[338] U_{cAMP}, urinary cAMP; U_P, urinary phosphate.

†High if species secreted cross-reacts with antiserum used in radioimmunoassay.

childhood but may appear later, particularly in sporadic cases. The few histological studies available show parathyroid atrophy with fatty replacement. An autoimmune etiology has been suggested by the finding of antibodies directed against parathyroid tissue in many affected individuals. In one study[341] antibodies to antigenic determinants on the surface of human parathyroid cells were detected in the sera of 8 of 23 adult patients with idiopathic hypoparathyroidism. In three of these subjects, binding of antibodies to dispersed human parathyroid cells inhibited PTH release. Another study found anti–endothelial cell antibodies in the sera of all six subjects (ages 12 to 24) with idiopathic hypoparathyroidism and suggested a role for such antibodies in the endocrine dysfunction.[342] Patients with this disorder may also develop primary adrenal insufficiency and, more rarely, primary hypothyroidism, primary hypogonadism, diabetes mellitus, and pernicious anemia[343] (see Chapter 31). Affected individuals should be monitored for these additional endocrine deficiencies. Chronic mucocutaneous moniliasis (resulting from a defect in cellular immunity), alopecia areata, and vitiligo (with antibodies directed against melanocytes) all occur in patients with idiopathic hypoparathyroidism and bolster the hypothesis that a disordered immune system is responsible for deficient PTH secretion. Monilial lesions may be seen on physical examination and are generally not affected by serum calcium status. Idiopathic hypoparathyroidism is also rarely associated with other syndromes of uncertain etiology, e.g., Kearns-Sayre syndrome (ophthalmoplegia, retinal degeneration, myopathy, and ataxia), Kenny syndrome (growth retardation and other anomalies),[344] and the syndrome of hereditary nephrosis with nerve deafness.

Hypomagnesemia. Hypomagnesemia may be caused by chronic alcoholism, malabsorption, increased renal clearance in therapy with aminoglycoside antibiotics, prolonged parenteral nutrition, cisplatin administration, or an isolated defect in intestinal absorption of magnesium. Hypocalcemia is frequently associated with hypomagnesemia and can be corrected by magnesium replacement, suggesting a role for magnesium depletion in the genesis of the hypocalcemia. Hypomagnesemia-induced peripheral resistance to the effects of PTH has been invoked to explain hypocalcemia, but the results of studies testing the effect of hypomagnesemia on the renal response to PTH (increase in urinary cAMP level and phosphaturia) are contradictory. Serum PTH concentrations in patients with hypocalcemia associated with hypomagnesemia have been undetectable, normal, or elevated.[345] There is an acute rise in serum PTH level in patients with hypocalcemia and hypomagnesemia given magnesium intravenously (Fig. 27–53). (In normal subjects, magnesium infusion either suppresses or does not affect PTH secretion.) The increase in serum PTH level was not accompanied by acute changes in serum calcium level and occurred even in patients with elevated basal serum PTH. The major effect of hypomagnesemia probably is to impair PTH release (as opposed to synthesis); peripheral resistance to PTH may also contribute to hypocalcemia because, as mentioned, some patients have elevated basal serum PTH. Effects of hypomagnesemia on peripheral metabolism and clearance of PTH have not been carefully studied.

Suppressed PTH Secretion. Elevation of serum calcium concentration by nonparathyroid mechanisms suppresses normal PTH secretion. Acute reduction in serum calcium in this setting (e.g., after administration of plicamycin to a patient with hypercalcemia caused by malignancy) may be followed by a brief period of parathyroid suppression leading to hypocalcemia. An analogous situation may occur after removal of a parathyroid adenoma, except that in this case normal parathyroid tissue is suppressed by hypercalcemia.

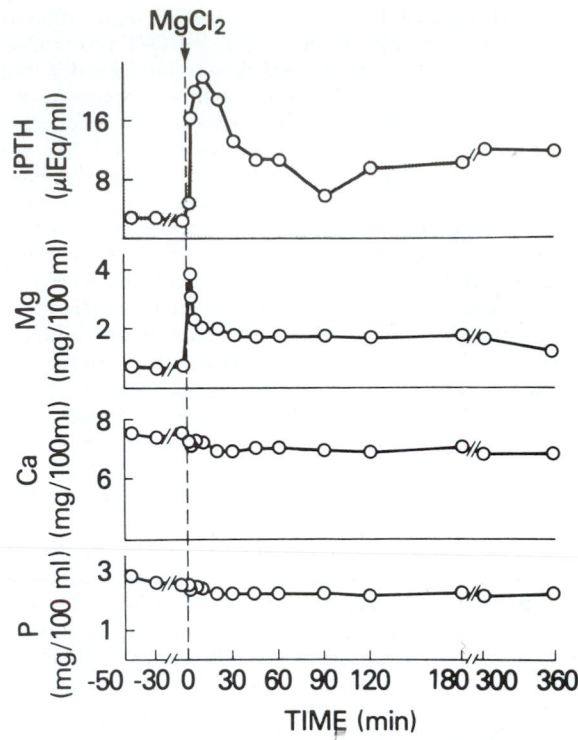

Figure 27–53. Serum immunoactive PTH (iPTH), magnesium, calcium, and phosphorus concentrations before and after intravenous infusion of magnesium chloride (3 mg/kg body weight infused over 30 s) in a hypomagnesemic, hypocalcemic patient. (From S Anast, JL Winnacker, LR Forte, TW Burns, Impaired release of parathyroid hormone in magnesium deficiency, J Clin Endocrinol Metab, 42, 707–717, 1976, © by The Endocrine Society.)

Hypocalcemia in the first 2 to 3 d of life and hypocalcemia in infants of hypercalcemic mothers are other examples of this mechanism. Normal parathyroids recover function quickly (generally within 1 wk), even after prolonged suppression by hypercalcemia. Hypocalcemia and hypermagnesemia have been reported in women receiving magnesium intravenously for toxemia of pregnancy. Hypermagnesemia most likely causes hypocalcemia by suppressing PTH secretion.[346]

Miscellaneous Causes of Deficient PTH Secretion. Any process that replaces or destroys sufficient normal parathyroid tissue may cause hypoparathyroidism. Metastases to the parathyroids are seen at autopsy in 12% of patients dying of malignant disease; breast cancer is the most common primary tumor.[347] Despite the relatively frequent finding of metastases to the parathyroids, hypoparathyroidism is rarely caused by invasion with tumor. Cancer chemotherapy, particularly with doxorubicin and cytarabine (cytosine arabinoside), can cause hypocalcemia and deficient PTH secretion,[348] and similar findings were reported in a patient who developed a toxic reaction (agranulocytosis and rash) during propylthiouracil therapy for thyrotoxicosis.

Iron storage disease (secondary to idiopathic hemochromatosis or transfusional overload) causes gonadal and islet beta cell dysfunction and has been considered a rare cause of hypoparathyroidism. Studies of larger numbers of patients with transfusion-dependent thalassemia suggest that parathyroid dysfunction is common.[349] The disorders range from mild dysfunction (manifest as isolated hyperphosphatemia) to frank hypoparathyroidism. The incidence of parathyroid dysfunction is positively correlated with age and number of transfusions. Hypoparathyroidism has also been reported in Wilson disease and may, by analogy with thalassemia, be due to copper deposition in the parathyroids.[350]

The syndrome may occur on a familial basis. The anomalies include thymic aplasia (with resulting T cell abnormalities) and cardiac malformations. Latent hypoparathyroidism in subjects with the partial syndrome may be unmasked by edetate infusion.[351] Defects in embryogenesis involving the branchial pouches may cause agenesis of the parathyroids in DiGeorge syndrome.

Secretion of Biologically Inactive Parathyroid Hormone.
Theoretically, hypoparathyroidism could be caused by a defect in PTH biosynthesis (see Fig. 27–52) with either failure to secrete PTH or secretion of an abnormal, biologically inactive form of the hormone.[352] With normal feedback regulation of the parathyroid gland, hypocalcemia should cause increased secretion of the defective PTH in the latter situation. Because an altered form of the hormone may retain immunoreactivity, serum PTH level determined by radioimmunoassay might be elevated in this syndrome. Patients with such a disorder should respond normally to exogenous PTH and thus be distinguished from patients with resistance to PTH (see Table 27–13). Hypothetical secretion of an aberrant form of the hormone that is capable of antagonizing the effect of exogenous PTH is discussed later.

Two cases of hypoparathyroidism putatively caused by secretion of ineffective PTH have been reported.[352] In neither case were the data for such a mechanism definitive. The structure of the human gene for PTH has been elucidated,[37] and it is now feasible to identify specific defects in PTH synthesis caused by mutations in the gene. Linkage analysis, using restriction fragment length polymorphisms of the PTH gene, has excluded a primary defect within the PTH gene itself in the majority of families with familial hypoparathyroidism, but in one family preliminary evidence suggests a genetic defect in the pre portion of the molecule (see section on PTH biosynthesis) that may impair processing of the hormone.[353]

RESISTANCE TO PARATHYROID HORMONE (PSEUDOHYPOPARATHYROIDISM).
In 1942 Albright and co-workers described three patients with hypocalcemia, hyperphosphatemia, a blunted phosphaturic and calcemic response to exogenous PTH, and a characteristic physical appearance subsequently termed *Albright hereditary osteodystrophy* (AHO).[354] They suggested that hypoparathyroidism in these patients is due to target organ unresponsiveness to PTH rather than to PTH deficiency. Subsequent studies have confirmed this hypothesis, so that *pseudohypoparathyroidism* (PHP), as Albright termed the disorder, is the first true hormone resistance syndrome. Many cases of hypoparathyroidism associated with PTH resistance, including many without AHO, have been reported subsequently. PHP is a heterogeneous syndrome with multiple underlying causes.

Pathogenesis.
Resistance to PTH might reflect defects at any of multiple sites (see Fig. 27–52): circulating antagonist of PTH action, abnormal PTH receptor, abnormal adenylate cyclase component (not limited to PTH receptor tissue, e.g., the guanine nucleotide–binding protein [G_s] that couples hormone receptors to stimulation of adenylate cyclase), abnormal cAMP-dependent protein kinase, or defective kinase substrate.

After the discovery that many of the actions of PTH are mediated by cAMP, it was shown[130] that subjects with PHP, with few exceptions (see under PHP Type II), lacked the normal brisk rise in urinary cAMP excretion after intravenous infusion of PTH (Fig. 27–54). This observation implies that hormone resistance in PHP type I is due to a proximal defect in hormone action, presumably in the receptor–adenylate cyclase complex.

Other studies[355, 356] indicate that tissues (including erythrocytes, fibroblasts, platelets, lymphoblasts, and in one case

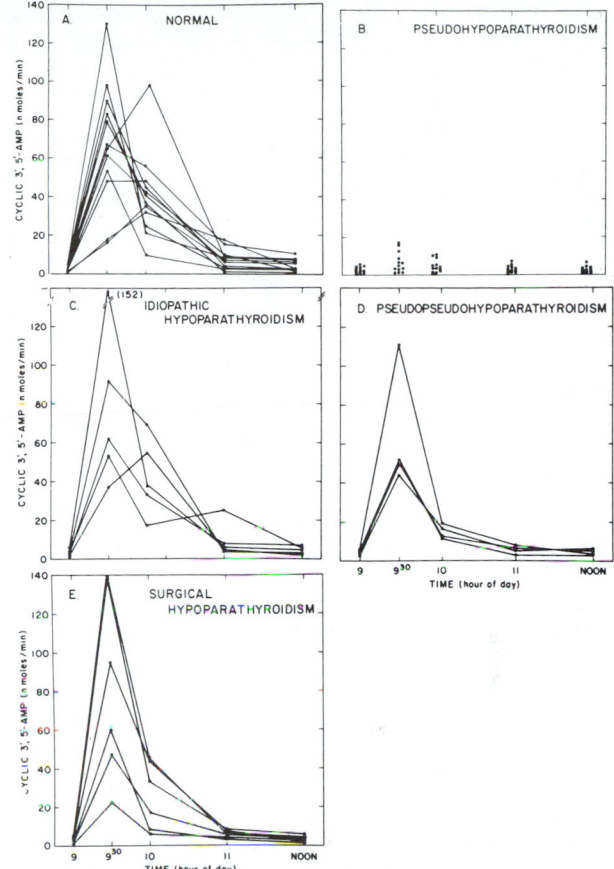

Figure 27–54. Response of urinary cAMP concentration to PTH infusion (300 U given between 9 AM and 9:15 AM) in normal subjects and in patients with various forms of hypoparathyroidism. (From Chase LR, Melson GL, Aurbach GD. Pseudohypoparathyroidism: defective excretion of 3′,5′-AMP in response to parathyroid hormone. Reproduced from the Journal of Clinical Investigation, 1969, vol. 48, pp. 1832–1844 by copyright permission of the American Society for Clinical Investigation.)

kidney) from some patients with PHP show about a 50% reduction in activity of G_s (Fig. 27–55). Most patients with reduced G_s activity show reduction in steady-state mRNA level for the alpha subunit of the G_s protein.[357] Deficient G_s activity apparently limits intracellular cAMP production and thereby impairs hormone responsiveness. Virtually all patients with G_s deficiency show the characteristic features of AHO (see later), whereas those with normal G_s activity and PHP generally do not display features of AHO (see Fig. 27–55). Subjects with PHP and deficient G_s activity show a high incidence of resistance to additional hormones.[358] This finding is consistent with a defect in a component of the hormone response mechanism not limited to PTH target organs. Patients with PHP and normal G_s activity, by contrast, usually have no evidence for resistance to hormones other than PTH. The defect in the latter group presumably involves a PTH-specific component such as the PTH receptor itself. Still other cases with normal G_s activity and multiple hormone resistance may represent defects in another general component of the hormone response mechanism (or a G_s defect not evident with available assays).

Studies utilizing the sensitive cytochemical bioassay for PTH suggest that biologically inactive PTH or an inhibitor of PTH may be secreted in some cases of PHP. An aberrant form of PTH (or another agent such as an antibody) capable of binding to the PTH receptor but incapable of activating adenylate cyclase could explain resistance to exogenous PTH in some forms of PHP.

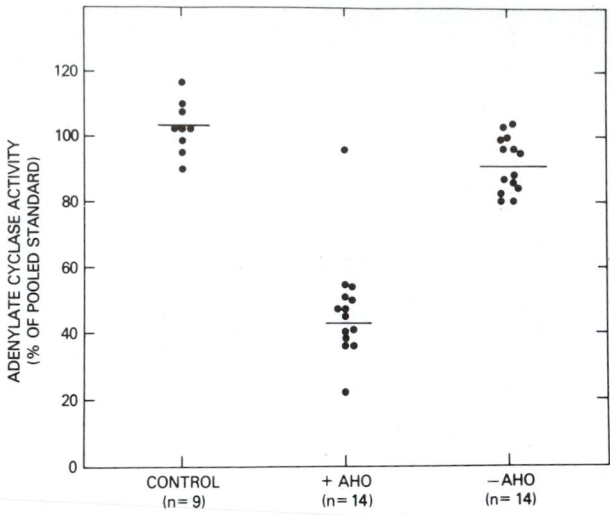

Figure 27–55. Erythrocyte G_s activity in PHP. Erythrocyte G_s activity was measured by adding detergent extracts of erythrocyte membranes (containing G) to membranes of a G_s-deficient mutant mouse cell line and assaying resultant adenylate cyclase activity. Results are expressed as a percentage of the value of a standard pool of normal erythrocyte membranes. Controls (normal subjects and others with PTH-deficient hypoparathyroidism) show values close to 100%, as do subjects with PHP without the features of AHO. Patients with PHP and AHO (with few exceptions) show reduced activity (about 50% of normal). (From Spiegel AM, Levine MA, Aurbach GD, et al. Deficiency of hormone receptor–adenylate cyclase coupling protein: basis for hormone resistance in pseudohypoparathyroidism. Am J Physiol 1982; 243:E37–E42.)

Clinical Features

PHP with Deficient G_s Activity (PHP Ia). Essentially all patients with this form of the disorder show the physical features of AHO, including short stature, round face, short thick neck, obesity, reduced intelligence, subcutaneous calcifications or ossification, and a variety of bone anomalies, the most characteristic being shortening of the metacarpals and metatarsals (Figs. 27–56 and 27–57). Associated endocrine abnormalities are common.[358] Some, such as primary hypothyroidism and hypogonadism, may be clinically mani-

fest. Other defects are more subtle and evident only upon provocative testing. Almost all patients show an elevated basal thyroid-stimulating hormone level and a hyper-response to thyrotropin-releasing hormone. Antithyroid antibody titers are low or absent, and a goiter is generally not found. PHP Ia may on occasion present as infantile hypothyroidism.[359] Primary thyroid resistance to thyroid-stimulating hormone is a likely explanation for these findings.

PHP Ia is often familial, suggesting a genetic basis for the disease. An X-linked inheritance was originally suggested based on lack of well-documented cases of male-to-male transmission. Other data, compatible with either autosomal dominant or recessive inheritance, have been obtained in studies utilizing erythrocyte G_s activity as a marker (clinically unaffected relatives showed normal G_s activity).[360]

The term *pseudopseudohypoparathyroidism* (PPHP) was originally applied by Albright to a patient with the phenotypic features of AHO but with no demonstrable metabolic abnormality. This led to indiscriminate use of this term. Because the features of AHO are not absolutely specific and because other entities, such as gonadal dysgenesis and familial brachydactyly, share certain of the clinical features, some have questioned whether PPHP is a true entity. In our opinion, this term should be reserved for patients meeting the following criteria: (1) clear-cut phenotypic features of AHO, (2) first-degree relative with PHP, and (3) relatively normal urinary cAMP response to PTH. The mothers of several patients with PHP fulfill these criteria. Subjects with PPHP show reduction in G_s activity comparable to that in subjects with PHP and may show subtle signs of hormone resistance such as elevated basal serum PTH and/or basal serum TSH levels despite apparently normal urinary cAMP response to PTH.[361] Such a phenomenon raises important questions about the genetic basis for PHP and about the relationship between the features of AHO and the fundamental defect responsible for hormone resistance. The phenotypic expression of G_s deficiency may depend on the product of another gene that differs in subjects with PHP and PPHP.[360, 361] Further work is needed to evaluate this hypothesis.

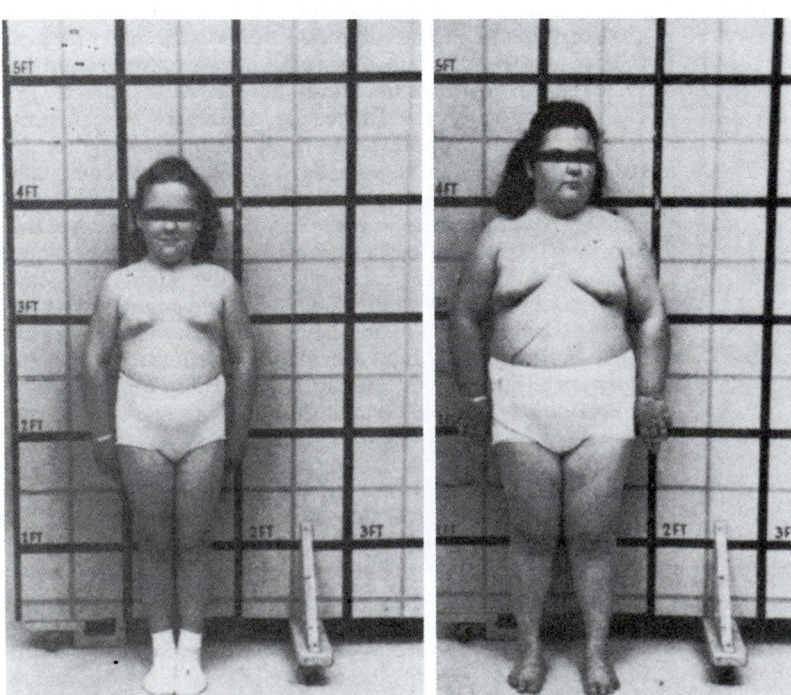

Figure 27–56. Daughter *(left)* and mother *(right)* with pseudohypoparathyroidism.

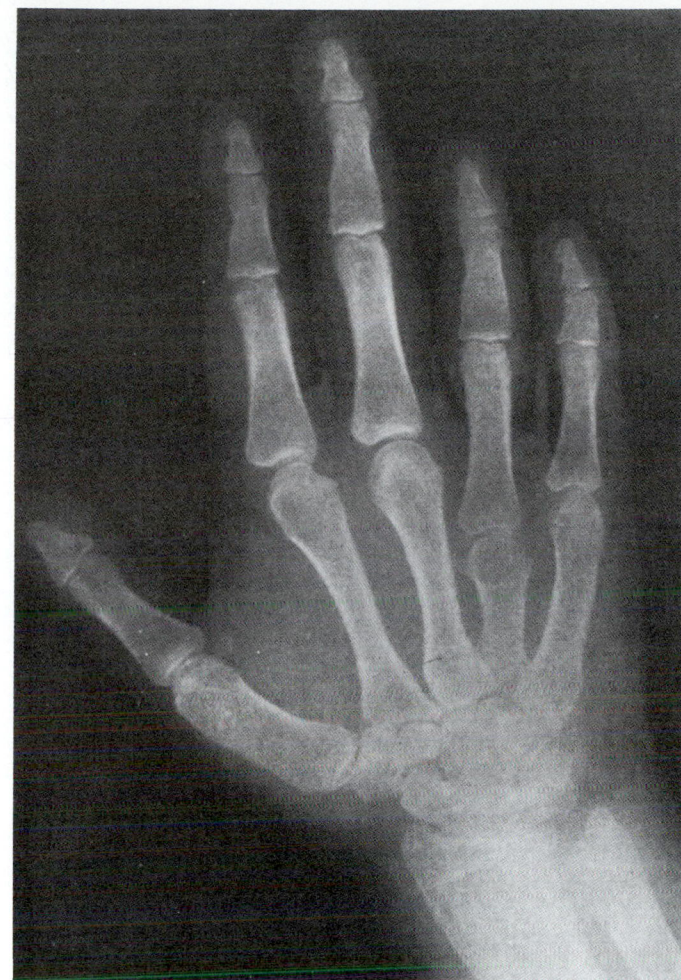

Figure 27–57. Radiograph of hand of patient with PHP. Note shortened fourth metacarpal.

PHP with Normal G_s Activity (PHP Ib). Most of these patients are normal in appearance. A few show the typical features of AHO. Detailed endocrine testing has generally disclosed no abnormality other than PTH resistance, but there have been some exceptions. Another abnormality in these subjects and in those with PHP and G_s deficiency is reduced serum prolactin concentration, both basally and on stimulation.[362] The significance and mechanism for this abnormality are as yet unclear. There are several well-documented examples of inheritance of PHP with normal G_s activity. Skin fibroblasts from 7 of 10 subjects with PHP Ib showed selective resistance to PTH in terms of cAMP response.[363] These results are compatible with the possibility of an intrinsic abnormality in the PTH receptor in subjects with PHP Ib.

PHP Type II. A small number of cases have been reported with biochemical features of hypoparathyroidism, elevated serum PTH level, normal urinary cAMP level, but subnormal phosphaturic response to PTH. In such cases, the defect in the kidney appears to be distal to cAMP formation. In the original report[364] it was suggested that a defective cAMP-dependent protein kinase could be responsible, but there are no direct data on this point. Because hypocalcemia may blunt the phosphaturic response to PTH, it is important to test the phosphaturic response after restoration of normocalcemia before diagnosing PHP type II. Patients with hypocalcemia associated with vitamin D depletion, for example, may have findings resembling those of PHP type II, but their deficient phosphaturic response to PTH returns to normal on restoration of normocalcemia.[365]

PHP with Osteitis Fibrosa Cystica. There is no direct evidence for skeletal resistance to PTH in PHP. A deficient calcemic response to PTH may reflect renal rather than skeletal resistance, because normal serum concentration of $1,25(OH)_2D$ may be required for a normal calcemic response. Reduced renal production of $1,25(OH)_2D$ in response to PTH has been reported in PHP.[366] (The response to dibutyryl cAMP is normal, suggesting that the response mechanism distal to cAMP is intact.)

Some patients with biochemical findings of hypoparathyroidism and elevated serum PTH level also have radiographic evidence of excessive parathyroid action on bone, i.e., osteitis fibrosa cystica. Some have defective urinary cAMP response to PTH. Presumably, hypocalcemia is due to reduced urinary excretion of phosphate with resulting hyperphosphatemia and to reduced absorption of calcium from the intestine secondary to low serum $1,25(OH)_2D$ level. Hypocalcemia is not overcome by increased mobilization of calcium from bone. Most have not shown the features of AHO. The basis for this form of PHP is unclear. This may be a unique entity involving a selective renal defect. Alternatively, there may be a spectrum of skeletal responsiveness in PHP, and these patients may represent one end of this spectrum.[367] Further study of this problem is required, particularly because such patients may represent a clue to differences in the mechanism of PTH action on bone versus kidney. Treatment of such patients with vitamin D in amounts sufficient to bring serum calcium into the normal range and suppress serum PTH leads to healing of bone lesions.

Therapy

Vitamin D and calcium supplements are the mainstay of therapy of all forms of hypoparathyroidism (with the exception of deficient PTH secretion associated with hypomagnesemia, which should be treated by replacing magnesium). Vitamin D, 50,000 to 100,000 U/d (1 to 2 mg/d), together with calcium salts (1 to 2 g elemental calcium/d), corrects hypocalcemia in most patients, but the precise dose varies from patient to patient and in a given patient over time. More potent vitamin D metabolites, such as calcitriol or 1α-hydroxycholecalciferol (not available in the United States), provide more rapid onset and offset of action but require close monitoring of serum calcium level to avoid toxicity. In the absence of PTH, urinary calcium concentration is higher than normal at any given serum calcium concentration (see Fig. 27–13). To avoid hypercalciuria and nephrolithiasis, serum calcium concentration should generally be maintained in the range of 2 to 2.2 mmol/L (8 to 9 mg/dL), which should prevent neuromuscular symptoms. Patients taking glucocorticoids, e.g., those with the autoimmune form of hypoparathyroidism associated with adrenal insufficiency, require close monitoring of therapy because of antagonistic effects on vitamin D action.

Therapy directed at reduction in serum phosphorus, e.g., antacids or acetazolamide, is generally not required because restoration of serum calcium concentration decreases renal threshold of phosphorus excretion and lowers serum phosphorus concentration. One report[368] suggests that combined therapy with thiazide diuretics and sodium restriction allows maintenance of a normal serum calcium level in patients with hypoparathyroidism. Vitamin D was not given to these patients. A potential advantage of this approach is the prevention of hypercalciuria, but reduced urinary calcium content alone could not account for the elevation in serum calcium concentration. Long-term studies are needed to assess the role of this approach. Patients with hypoparathyroidism may be uniquely sensitive to the calciuretic effects of diuretics such as furosemide. Development of symptomatic hypocalcemia during furosemide therapy emphasizes the need for careful monitoring of serum calcium level in patients who require diuretics.[369]

HYPOCALCEMIC DISORDERS

Introduction

Hypocalcemia occurs in a variety of acquired and hereditary diseases. It may be the principal manifestation, as in hypoparathyroidism, or merely one of a constellation of abnormalities, as in chronic renal failure. Regardless of cause, patients with a low ionized serum calcium concentration often develop symptoms of neuromuscular irritability, including paresthesias, muscle cramps, and seizures. Development of symptoms is not well correlated with the absolute degree of hypocalcemia. The clinical impression that the rate of fall in serum calcium level is the critical determinant of tetany has not been substantiated by studies of edetate-induced hypocalcemia in dogs. Decreased total serum calcium concentration, with a normal ionized fraction, can exist with hypoproteinemia or acidosis. These possibilities should be excluded by measuring serum protein concentration and calculating the corrected serum calcium level or by directly measuring ionized calcium concentration. Alkalosis decreases ionized (but not total) serum calcium concentration (a change from pH 7.4 to 7.6 may decrease ionized calcium by 0.25 mmol/L) and may precipitate tetany.

Pathophysiology

Hypocalcemia can represent a defect of any of several control points in the homeostatic regulation of calcium concentration (see Fig. 27–44). In most cases the cause is diminished secretion or action of PTH or $1,25(OH)_2D$ or both. As a consequence of deficient PTH, calcium fluxes from bone to ECF and from renal tubular lumen to ECF are reduced; renal clearance of phosphate is decreased, leading to hyperphosphatemia. Deficient PTH action also leads to reduced renal formation of $1,25(OH)_2D$ (either directly or secondary to hyperphosphatemia). Low $1,25(OH)_2D$ concentration leads to reduced calcium flux from intestinal lumen to blood. Thus diminished calcium entry into the ECF from three anatomical pools (see Fig. 27–44, 1, 3, and 5) accounts for hypocalcemia in states of PTH deficiency.

In states of reduced vitamin D effect, calcium flux from intestine to blood is decreased; in addition, PTH mobilization of calcium from bone to blood is impaired. Both of these factors (see Fig. 27–44, 1 and 5) may produce hypocalcemia. Although reduced intestinal calcium absorption and decreased calcium release from bone are the most frequent causes of hypocalcemia, reduction in serum calcium level may also result from increased loss of calcium into soft tissue (see Fig. 27–44, 8), bone (see Fig. 27–44, 2), or other pools (hemodialysis, transplacental). Frank hypocalcemia may develop if compensatory actions of PTH or $1,25(OH)_2D$ are inadequate.

Differential Diagnosis

The clinical and biochemical features depend on the underlying cause of hypocalcemia. Renal function (serum creatinine, creatinine clearance) and gastrointestinal function (D-xylose tolerance test, serum carotene concentration, quantitation of stool fat) should be evaluated because renal failure and malabsorption are common causes of hypocalcemia. Skeletal x-ray films should be examined for abnormalities, including features suggestive of secondary hyperparathyroidism, osteomalacia, osteoblastic tumor metastases, or bone anomalies suggesting PHP.

History and physical examination may provide diagnostic clues, e.g., cataracts or evidence of neck surgery in the past. Measurements of serum PTH, phosphate, 25-OHD, $1,25(OH)_2D$, and urinary cAMP levels are essential in defining the category of hypocalcemia (Table 27–14).

Specific Causes of Hypocalcemia

HYPOPARATHYROIDISM. Disorders involving deficient PTH action on kidney and bone are discussed in detail in the preceding section.

ABNORMALITIES IN VITAMIN D METABOLISM. Hypocalcemia may develop in deficiency of vitamin D or its active metabolites 25-OHD and $1,25(OH)_2D$. Both acquired (principally chronic renal failure) and hereditary forms exist and are described fully in Chapter 28.

DISPROPORTIONATE NET CALCIUM INFLUX INTO BONE. Albright described severe hypocalcemia after removal of a parathyroid adenoma from a patient with osteitis fibrosa cystica. Bone biopsy in the early postoperative period showed increased osteoid formation and osteoblast numbers, with reduction in osteoclasts. Approximately 4 mo after surgery, serum calcium concentration became normal, with radiographic and bone biopsy evidence of healing of bone. The hypocalcemia is due to the hungry bone syndrome discussed earlier.

TABLE 27–14. Biochemical Categorization of Hypocalcemic Disorders

Disorder	Serum PTH and U_{cAMP}	Serum P	Alkaline P	25-OHD	$1,25(OH)_2D$
Hypoparathyroidism	Low*	High	Normal	Normal	Low
Vitamin D deficiency (e.g., nutritional, malabsorption, liver disease)	High	Low	High	Low	Low-normal
Deficient $1,25(OH)_2D$ formation or action (e.g., renal failure, hereditary vitamin D dependency)	High	Low	High	Normal	Low†
Increased bone formation (e.g., healing osteitis fibrosa, osteoblastic metastases)	Normal to high	Low-normal	High	Normal	(? high)
Increased soft tissue calcification (e.g., tumor lysis or phosphate infusion)	Normal to high	High	Normal	Normal	(? low)

*PTH-resistant forms have high serum PTH and low (PHP, type I) or high (PHP, type II) urinary cAMP (U_{cAMP}).
†Elevated in $1,25(OH)_2D$ insensitivity.

Hypocalcemia can also occur after either total or subtotal thyroidectomy. Surgical injury to the parathyroids appears to be the major cause of hypocalcemia after thyroidectomy; bone hunger secondary to long-standing Graves disease may play a minor role.

OSTEOBLAST METASTASES. Hypocalcemia is common in patients with cancer but usually represents a reduction in the total rather than ionized fraction because of associated hypoalbuminemia. Ionized hypocalcemia may occur in association with skeletal metastases, particularly in patients with cancer of prostate and of breast. Twenty-three of 143 patients with bone metastases in one series showed hypocalcemia.[370] When hypoproteinemia and renal failure have been excluded, hypocalcemia is attributed to increased calcium flux into osteoblastic lesions. Evidence against hypoparathyroidism in such patients includes normal or low concentration of phosphate in serum, but few reported cases include measurements of PTH concentration. Careful measurement of calcium kinetics is also lacking.

ACUTE HYPERPHOSPHATEMIA. An increase in serum phosphate concentration may decrease serum calcium concentration by inhibiting bone resorption, by promoting extraskeletal calcification, or by a combination of the two. Exogenous phosphate can be a cause, e.g., intravenous phosphate infusion given to treat hypercalcemia or administration of phosphate enemas to infants. Hypocalcemia associated with endogenous phosphate loads also occurs, e.g., secondary to rhabdomyolysis[334] or during chemotherapy of highly responsive tumors such as Burkitt lymphoma or acute lymphoblastic leukemia. Extensive soft tissue calcification, renal failure, and death have occurred in several cases. Hypocalcemia may persist beyond the hyperphosphatemic phase. In one case of tumor lysis syndrome, prolonged hypocalcemia was associated with depressed serum $1,25(OH)_2D$ concentration.[371]

PANCREATITIS. The etiology of hypocalcemia in acute pancreatitis is uncertain. Calcium soap deposits in areas of fat necrosis have been described in autopsied cases; the amount of elemental calcium deposited in this manner may exceed 2 g and could account for hypocalcemia in some cases.[372] Humoral mechanisms involving glucagon release from the injured pancreas and secondary increase in CT secretion also have been invoked. Elevated serum glucagon and CT concentrations have not been observed in all studies; the relatively weak hypocalcemic effect of these hormones, moreover, makes it unlikely that they account for hypocalcemia. Inadequate PTH response to hypocalcemia may be related to the frequently associated hypomagnesemia.

CRITICAL ILLNESS. Low serum ionized calcium concentration is relatively frequent in critically ill adults[373] and children,[374] particularly those with sepsis. A combination of factors, including renal failure, hypomagnesemia, and transfusion with citrate-anticoagulated blood (see later), may be responsible in individual cases. Absolute or relative hypoparathyroidism also occurs in many hypocalcemic subjects with critical illness. In subjects whose clinical status improves, resumption of normal parathyroid function also occurs.

TOXIC SHOCK SYNDROME. The toxic shock syndrome is characterized by extreme fever, hypotension, erythroderma, headache, and liver and occasional renal abnormalities. It has been reported most frequently in young women with onset during the menses and is thought to be related to a toxic product of certain strains of staphylococci. Hypocalcemia is a frequent finding,[375] occurring within a few hours of onset of the disease and lasting several days. Multiple mechanisms are probably responsible for the hypocalcemia, including the often profound hypoalbuminemia and acute renal failure. Hypomagnesemia and hyperphosphatemia are generally not involved. The possibility of relative PTH deficiency is unclear. Extreme elevations in serum CT level have been reported in several patients and were in a higher range than expected with renal impairment alone. The significance of this observation and its relation to the pathogenesis of the hypocalcemia are obscure, because other diseases with elevations in CT level are not associated with hypocalcemia (see later).

MALABSORPTION. In certain cases of malabsorption, hypocalcemia may occur even though absorption of vitamin D and magnesium is normal. Fecal fat in excess of 10 g/d may be associated with sufficient calcium malabsorption to cause hypocalcemia.

CALCIUM CHELATORS. Substances such as citrate or edetate reduce ionized (but not total) serum calcium concentration by forming complexes. Clinically this may be encountered during transfusion of blood anticoagulated with citrate, e.g., in infants undergoing exchange transfusion or in adults receiving massive amounts of blood (especially with reduced liver function, which delays citrate metabolism). Such patients should be monitored closely, and ionized calcium concentration should be measured if possible to guide treatment with calcium. Certain radiographic contrast media also contain calcium-complexing substances such as edetate and citrate. These agents, together with intrinsic properties (hypertonicity, calcium binding) of the contrast media, may lead to acute lowering of ionized calcium concentration after injections, e.g., during arteriographic studies. The clinical significance of this phenomenon is not established, but regional hypocalcemia (e.g., after coronary artery injections) may have deleterious effects on cardiac function.

HYPERCALCITONINEMIA. Hypercalcitoninemia is generally *not* associated with hypocalcemia because CT is a relatively weak hypocalcemic agent in adult humans. Thus in patients with medullary carcinoma of the thyroid secreting excess CT, hypocalcemia is rare. In states of increased bone resorption, e.g., Paget disease, administration of CT (or other inhibitors of bone resorption such as plicamycin) may lower serum calcium concentration.

NEONATAL HYPOCALCEMIA. Hypocalcemia in the first 2 to 3 d of life occurs with increased frequency in infants who are premature, are born to diabetic mothers, or suffer respiratory distress syndrome. High calcium concentration in normal cord blood at term reflects active placental transfer of calcium from mother to fetus and may account for the low serum PTH and high serum CT concentration measured during the first 2 to 3 d of life. Hypocalcemia occurring later (about 1 wk post partum) is often associated with feeding of cow's milk or other high-phosphate formula. Inability to excrete sufficient phosphate in the urine at this stage may be involved. Immaturity of the hepatic 25-hydroxylase system may contribute to rapid depletion of 25-OHD stores. In cases of maternal hyperparathyroidism, neonatal hypocalcemia may occur after the first week of life, reflecting prolonged (but temporary) suppression of parathyroid function in the infant.

Therapy

Whenever possible, any underlying disorder should be treated; resolution of hypocalcemia will generally ensue. When this is not possible, chronic therapy with vitamin D and calcium may be required. Acute symptomatic hypocalcemia of any cause can be treated by intravenous calcium infusion. Adults requiring urgent treatment can be given 10 to 20 mL of 10% calcium gluconate (which contains about 10 mg elemental calcium/mL) intravenously over 10 min. (In patients taking digitalis, rapid intravenous administration of calcium may be hazardous.) In less urgent situations, calcium gluconate may be administered by slow intravenous infusion (the equivalent of 20 mg elemental calcium/kg body weight) over 4 to 8 h as needed to alleviate symptoms.

DISTURBANCES OF PHOSPHATE AND MAGNESIUM IN SERUM

Hypophosphatemia

CLINICAL FEATURES. Hypophosphatemia usually occurs in the setting of a multisystem disturbance;[376] symptoms depend in part on the duration and degree of hypophosphatemia. The major finding in acute hypophosphatemia is nonspecific neuroencephalopathy developing with serum phosphate concentrations below 0.8 mg/dL. It may include features such as muscle weakness, paresthesias, depressed reflexes, cranial nerve palsies, tremor, and confusion. The main symptoms of chronic hypophosphatemia are attributed to depletion of cellular energy stores (e.g., ATP and creatine phosphate) and to impaired oxygen delivery to tissues (consequent to low concentrations of 2,3-diphosphoglycerate in erythrocytes). Milder chronic hypophosphatemia may cause vague musculoskeletal complaints, but the incidence and etiology of this phenomenon have not been established. Symptoms of chronic hypophosphatemia typically occur with phosphate concentrations below 0.5 mmol/L (1.5 mg/dL). The principal symptoms of chronic hypophosphatemia are debility, weakness, and anorexia. A neuropathy typically presents with distal paresthesias, but in severe form it may include cranial nerve dysfunction, paralysis, or seizures. Manifestations of muscle dysfunction include impaired function of respiratory and cardiac muscles and rhabdomyolysis. Chronic hypophosphatemia leads to dysfunction in all tissues tested (polymorphonuclear leukocytes, platelets, erythrocytes). Depletion of erythrocyte phosphate stores can cause hemolytic anemia. There is also mild resistance to insulin. Hypercalciuria is primarily caused by increased renal production of $1,25(OH)_2D$ but may also reflect independent effects of hypophosphatemia to increase resorption of skeletal mineral and to increase renal clearance of calcium. Hypophosphatemia over many years leads to osteomalacia and, in children, to rickets and retardation of growth. This topic is covered in Chapter 28.

ETIOLOGIES OF HYPOPHOSPHATEMIA. Circulating phosphate is in equilibrium with four pools: the cell interior, intestinal lumen, renal lumen, and bone mineral. Most causes of hypophosphatemia involve an imbalance between the plasma and one of these four pools.

Increased Efflux into Cells. Hypophosphatemia may develop acutely over minutes or hours without prior chronic phosphate depletion. Extracellular phosphate is in rapid equilibrium with a much larger pool of intracellular phosphate (see Table 27–2); acute hypophosphatemia reflects rapid transfer of phosphate into cells. Because symptoms are attributed to depletion of intracellular phosphate pools, there is an apparent paradox that phosphate flux into cells could cause symptoms. However, shifts are not uniform among organs, and even within a given cell phosphate may be compartmentalized. Phosphate can be sequestered in cells during glucose uptake (increased formation of 1,3-diphosphoglycerate during glycolysis), glycogenolysis (formation of glucose 1-phosphate and then glucose 6-phosphate), or conversion of ADP to ATP. Some manipulations that can cause hypophosphatemia by these mechanisms include hyperventilation with respiratory alkalosis or high plasma levels of glucose, fructose, insulin, or epinephrine. Carbohydrate transport into cells accounts for most of the drop of serum phosphate (a decrease of 0.05 to 0.15 mmol/L [0.15 to 0.45 mg/dL]) after meals. In comparison, that caused by hyperventilation is larger in magnitude (decrease of 0.6 to 1 mmol/L [2 to 3 mg/dL]) and more rapid in onset (beginning within 3 to 5 min). Combinations of glucose and insulin can cause acute hypophosphatemia with refeeding after starvation, treatment of diabetic ketoacidosis, and use of intravenous alimentation. Hypophosphatemia with total parenteral nutrition is prevented by inclusion of sufficient phosphate in the nutrition solutions. Total body phosphate depletion always occurs with diabetic ketoacidosis, and hypophosphatemia is common in the 4th through 24th hours of therapy, but several controlled studies have not shown significant benefit from administration of phosphate. It is appropriate to monitor serum phosphate concentration early during treatment. Hemodialysis lowers serum phosphate concentration in a similar manner by combination of efflux into cells and loss to dialysis fluid.

Impaired Intestinal Flux. Hypophosphatemia does not develop from deficiencies in natural diets because phosphate is common to the cytoplasm of plants and animals. Phosphate absorption is not severely compromised by malabsorption of fat; the associated secondary hyperparathyroidism and phosphaturia are more important. Hypophosphatemia can present as one component of the metabolic imbalances with profuse diarrhea. Selective deficiency of phosphate can be induced by consumption of agents that render phosphate unavailable for absorption. Aluminum-containing antacids (including sucralfate) are the only class of agents that has been implicated.[377] They may depress serum phosphate level below 0.3 mmol/L (1 mg/dL) within 2 wk. Chronic ingestion has been implicated as a cause of osteomalacia; but the fact that aluminum per se may induce a low-turnover osteomalacia (see Chapter 28) indicates that this phenomenon must be re-examined.

Impaired Skeletal Flux. High flux rates of phosphate from plasma to bone occur during remineralization of demineralized bone. This is a component of the hungry bone syndrome, and it may cause hypophosphatemia after parathyroidectomy even in anephric patients.

Impaired Renal Flux. Serum phosphate concentration is determined by relatively constant inflow to plasma and the theoretical threshold for phosphate excretion (see Fig. 27–2). Most causes of chronic hypophosphatemia reflect decreases in renal threshold for phosphate excretion by the kidney. For this reason, analysis of urine phosphate content to derive an index of renal phosphate transport is central in distinguishing renal from other etiologies of hypophosphatemia. PTH is the principal known humoral determinant of this threshold and accounts for the hypophosphatemia in primary and secondary (nonazotemic) hyperparathyroidism. In some cancers with hypercalcemia, unidentified factors may exert PTH-like actions on the renal transport of phosphate. Many disorders of the proximal tubule (most but not all with associated impairment of renal 25-OHD 1α-hydroxylase) decrease this threshold. The threshold is also decreased by most diuretics. Glucocorticoids and estrogens decrease the renal threshold for phosphate excretion; this may be an indirect effect on the kidney (secondary hyperparathyroidism or other processes may be responsible). The threshold is depressed in idiopathic hypercalciuria; this may result from intrinsic or extrinsic influences on the kidney.

Hypophosphatemia can be prominent in several complex disturbances of uncertain or multifactorial etiology. In ketoacidosis, for example, vomiting, osmotic diuresis, and imbalance between intra- and extracellular pools may all contribute. Other states associated with hypophosphatemia of multifactoral cause include alcoholism, septicemia, hypokalemia, and burns.

MANAGEMENT OF HYPOPHOSPHATEMIA. Phosphate may be poorly tolerated by mouth, and parenteral therapy may be necessary. Begin therapy with 0.16 mmol (5 mg)/kg body weight of phosphate as the neutral sodium or potassium salt over 6 h intravenously. This dose is below that for repletion of depleted phosphate stores, and subsequent therapy must be determined by monitoring serum phosphate concentrations.

With chronic phosphate depletion, treatment of the underlying cause (antacid abuse, primary hyperparathyroidism, or secondary hyperparathyroidism) is usually sufficient. Chronic phosphate depletion as opposed to acute hypophosphatemia requires high doses of oral phosphorus dietary supplement; normal maintenance requires 0.5 mmol (15 mg)/kg/d orally. Therapy of severe depletion or of renal wasting requires doses three times this. Primary disturbances of the renal tubule may require therapy for many years, particularly in children, in whom phosphate is essential for normal growth. Phosphate preparations are distasteful and may cause gastric irritation or diarrhea. Side effects can be minimized by administration every 4 h while awake and by increasing dosage gradually over 1 to 2 wk.

Hyperphosphatemia

CLINICAL FEATURES. No specific symptoms are directly attributable to hyperphosphatemia. Rather, symptoms evolve from secondary changes in calcium flux. Acute hyperphosphatemia can lead to hypocalcemic tetany or precipitation of calcium phosphates in vascular structures with consequent vascular collapse. Hypocalcemia results from these primary effects on calcium fluxes and from the inhibitory effect of hyperphosphatemia on renal synthesis of $1,25(OH)_2D$. The principal consequence of chronic hyperphosphatemia is calcification of soft tissues. Interstitial calcification of the kidney may contribute to renal compromise.[378] Masses of mineralized tissue can accumulate about large joints in chronic renal failure and in nonazotemic tumoral calcinosis (Fig. 27–58). The masses do not cause pain, but they are subject to breakdown and chronic inflammation. Associated changes in bone vary from acute decrease in resorption to chronic increases in resorption and in new bone formation (the latter two reflect, in part, secondary hyperparathyroidism).

ETIOLOGIES OF HYPERPHOSPHATEMIA. Hyperphosphatemia can be renal or extrarenal in etiology, and analysis of renal handling of phosphate establishes the appropriate category. The most common cause of pathological hyperphosphatemia is uremia. Although a renal problem, it can also be thought of as a pure abnormality in filtered load per nephron. This is one rationalization for therapy with phosphate-binding drugs. Phosphate restriction in uremia slows secondary hyperparathyroidism, but there is controversy over whether it actually slows progression of azotemia. Four states cause elevations of the theoretical renal threshold for phosphate excretion: deficiency of PTH, high concentrations of growth hormone, tumoral calcinosis, and drugs. Serum phosphorus concentration is higher in children than in adults, for reasons that are not known. Hyperphosphatemia is a central chemical feature of hypoparathyroidism and presumably accounts for the soft tissue calcifications that can

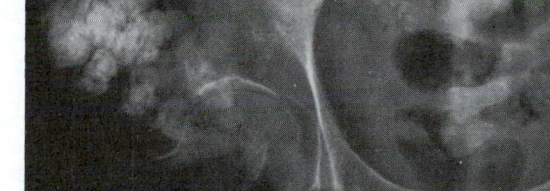

Figure 27–58. Periarticular masses in a patient with nonazotemic hyperphosphatemic tumoral calcinosis.

be associated (cornea and basal ganglia). Growth hormone excess causes lesser degrees of hyperphosphatemia.

Nonazotemic tumoral calcinosis is frequently an autosomal dominant disorder associated with hyperphosphatemia but may occur sporadically. Chronic low-grade infection in huge calcified masses can cause fevers of "unknown" origin and amyloidosis. Serum concentrations of $1,25(OH)_2D$ are higher than appropriate for the degree of hyperphosphatemia, suggesting that a single renal defect affects phosphate transport and 1-hydroxylation of 25-OHD.[379] Drugs capable of raising the renal threshold for phosphate excretion would be of potential value in therapy of disorders with renal wasting of phosphate; however, the only drug in this category is etidronate. Because it causes hyperphosphatemia only at high doses and moreover causes osteomalacia at such doses, this drug is not useful in therapy of phosphate wasting states.

The filtered load of phosphate can rise pathologically from either exogenous or endogenous sources. Certain laxatives contain phosphate as the active ingredient, and this ingredient can be absorbed by either the oral or rectal route. Phosphate can also be absorbed across the skin; this route contributes to the hyperphosphatemia associated with skin burns produced by "white phosphate" in incendiary bombs. Endogenous sources of phosphate may overwhelm renal excretory mechanisms. Endogenous phosphate comes from inside cells, and cell death is the usual cause. Phosphate is released with rhabdomyolysis, heat stroke, malignant hyperpyrexia, cardiac surgery, and lactic acidosis. Chemotherapy, particularly in lymphoproliferative disorders of children, can cause severe hyperphosphatemia;[380] diuresis is often required to prevent renal failure caused by the combination of hyperphosphatemia and hyperuricemia. Episodic acute hyperphosphatemia with seizures and polyuria has been reported in a sibship.[381]

MANAGEMENT OF HYPERPHOSPHATEMIA. Acute hyperphosphatemia is rarely severe enough (3.2 mmol/L [10 mg/dL]) to require therapy. When the hyperphosphatemia is of endogenous origin, the basic therapy is life support. Useful measures include forced natriuresis and administration of glucose plus insulin. If these measures are not effective, hemodialysis should be used.

Therapy for chronic hyperphosphatemia can be tailored to etiology. The hyperphosphatemia of hypoparathyroidism is improved (although not completely) by return of serum calcium concentration to normal even in the complete absence of PTH; this is presumed to result from a direct action of calcium on the renal transport of phosphate. Therapy of growth hormone excess (another poorly understood cause of hyperphosphatemia) is evident. There is no specific cure for tumoral calcinosis, but calcium administration is contraindicated. Phosphate binders given orally can decrease phosphate load sufficiently to cause regression of calcific masses. The only alternative is surgical excision of masses that produce symptoms.

Hypomagnesemia

Regulation of magnesium in ECF is similar to that of phosphate. For both, the plasma concentration is determined by filtrable load and a theoretical renal threshold for excretion. Unlike serum phosphate concentration, serum magnesium concentration does not commonly show rapid change in fluxes to and from cells and does not show major age or sex dependence. Whereas specific symptoms of cellular phosphate depletion are identifiable and require prolonged therapy, the features of magnesium depletion are those of low magnesium concentration in plasma, and the symptoms caused by chronic depletion can evolve over hours when transcellular fluxes lower plasma levels acutely.[382]

CLINICAL FEATURES. Symptoms can be classified as directly attributable to hypomagnesemia, secondary to hypocalcemia, or secondary to potassium wasting. Symptoms attributable to hypomagnesemia occur at concentrations below 0.5 mmol/L (1.2 mg/dL) and include anorexia, nausea, tremor, and mood alterations (apathy, depression, anxiety, agitation, or confusion). Similar symptoms have been attributed to magnesium depletion without hypomagnesemia under the term *latent tetany*, but there is not adequate documentation that this is a valid clinical entity. Claims that low magnesium content in water (soft water) leads to increased death rate from cardiac disease are based on insufficient evidence. There are no universally accepted criteria for establishing a diagnosis of magnesium depletion without hypomagnesemia. Erythrocyte magnesium level is an index of magnesium concentration at time of erythropoiesis; muscle magnesium level can be expressed in relation to intracellular protein content; or magnesium retention can be quantitated by evaluating urinary excretion (usually 75 to 80%) over 24 h after administration of an intravenous load. The magnesium load test can be misleading if there is excessive loss through the intestine or kidney.

Hypocalcemia begins after 10 to 20 d of magnesium depletion and can present as symptomatic hypocalcemic tetany.[383] The principal etiology is reversible impairment of secretory function of the parathyroid gland. Acute administration of magnesium immediately corrects the hormone secretory function of the parathyroid gland (see Fig. 27–53). Diminished calcemic response to PTH and a decreased urinary cAMP response to PTH may be found at the same time, suggesting that hypocalcemia may be multifactorial in origin.

Chronic hypomagnesemia causes depletion of cellular potassium, impairment of renal potassium conservation with hypokalemia, and ventricular irritability (with increased susceptibility to intoxication by cardiac glycosides). These three effects may reflect dysfunction of Na^+,K^+-ATPase, a magnesium-dependent enzyme.

ETIOLOGIES OF HYPOMAGNESEMIA. As with hypophosphatemia, hypomagnesemia can evolve from a disordered flux between plasma and any one of several pools. Redistribution of magnesium from plasma into soft tissues or bone can occur acutely in pancreatitis or in therapeutic hyperthermia, after parathyroidectomy, or during recovery from ketoacidosis, starvation, or azotemic acidosis. In all except the first two, the underlying disorder may be associated with loss of cell mass with disproportional loss of magnesium.

Chronic hypomagnesemia resulting from impaired intestinal absorption of magnesium is found in generalized malabsorption or in selective deficiency of magnesium transport. Hypomagnesemia occurs in 20 to 40% of cases of steatorrhea. Restriction of dietary magnesium sufficient to cause hypomagnesemia is effected only with artificial diets.

Impaired renal conservation is the second major cause of chronic hypomagnesemia, and this can develop in treatment with most diuretics (except acetazolamide), uncontrolled diabetes mellitus, volume expansion, Bartter syndrome, hypercalcemia, or hypoparathyroidism. Although PTH causes a mild increase in renal resorption of magnesium, the hypercalcemia in primary hyperparathyroidism often overrides this. Intrinsic renal causes include aminoglycoside nephropathy,[384] chronic tubulointestitial disease, and, rarely, hereditary defects in tubular transport of magnesium. Additional causes of negative magnesium balance include extensive burns, profuse sweating, excessive lactation, nasogastric suction, and biliary fistula.

In the United States the disorder most commonly associated with hypomagnesemia is alcoholism. The cause of hypomagnesemia in alcoholism is probably multifactorial, including starvation, diarrhea, and impaired renal conservation (the latter caused by alcohol, aldosterone, and ketoacidosis).

TREATMENT OF HYPOMAGNESEMIA. Most cases of hypomagnesemia can be managed by measures directed at the underlying etiology without administration of magnesium. Prophylaxis in patients with restricted oral intake requires approximately 4 mmol of magnesium per day in the form of magnesium gluconate. Acute symptoms (convulsions) can be managed with 8 mmol of magnesium sulfate diluted to 100 mL. Deficits causing symptoms can be replaced intravenously over 4 to 5 d; renal losses may be between 10 and 50% of infused amounts. Intramuscular dosage (as 50% magnesium sulfate) is quite painful. Adult patients with intestinal malabsorption or renal wasting of magnesium may require 30 to 50 mmol/d indefinitely. This is usually below the dosage that induces diarrhea.

Hypermagnesemia

CLINICAL FEATURES OF HYPERMAGNESEMIA. Mild elevations in serum magnesium concentration cause no symptoms or signs.[385] Symptoms begin with concentrations of 3.6 to 6 mmol/L (9 to 15 mg/dL); these are comparable to concentrations attained during treatment of eclampsia (3 to 4 mmol/L [7 to 10 mg/dL]). Symptoms are attributable to impairment of neuromuscular transmission. These include depression of the sinoatrial and atrioventricular conduction in the heart, depression of sympathetic ganglia (vasodilation, pupillary dilation), and loss of deep tendon reflexes. Other associated symptoms include nausea, lethargy, confusion, and respiratory depression. Rare complications include refractory hypotension, smooth muscle paralysis, and hypocalcemia caused by suppression of PTH secretion.

CAUSES OF HYPERMAGNESEMIA. Hypermagnesemia resulting from a high renal threshold for magnesium is always mild and without clinical symptoms. The causes include familial hypocalciuric hypercalcemia, occasionally primary hyperparathyroidism, hypothyroidism, and deficiency of mineralocorticoids.

With normal GFR, the filtered load of magnesium would have to rise fivefold to cause even modest hypermagnesemia. Symptomatic hypermagnesemia is usually due to a combination of increased load of magnesium and decreased GFR. Endogenous sources of increased load include all causes of cell catabolism, such as tumor lysis or ketoacidosis. Exogenous sources include Epsom salts (magnesium sulfate), antacids or laxatives, errors in preparation of dialysis fluids, and overly vigorous treatment of eclampsia.

TREATMENT OF HYPERMAGNESEMIA. Symptomatic hypermagnesemia usually reflects life-threatening illness requiring multisystem support. Calcium antagonizes the effects of hypermagnesemia; associated hypocalcemia should be corrected, and acute administration of 100 to 200 mg calcium may be effective even with normocalcemia. Although diuresis is effective, it often is not feasible because of uremia. In this setting, hemodialysis is the most effective treatment.

HYPERCALCITONINISM

Medullary Carcinoma of the Thyroid*

Medullary thyroid cancer, which arises in the parafollicular or C cells, accounts for less than 10% of thyroid cancers.

---

*Also see Chapters 8 and 30.

Its epidemiological, histological, and biochemical features differ from those of neoplasms arising from thyroid follicular cells.[386] The male/female ratio is 1:1. The tumor is also important because of frequent hereditary occurrence, association with other endocrine abnormalities, and use as a model for cancerous processes that may be diagnosed on the basis of secretory product markers and, therefore, treated at early stages.

CLINICAL FEATURES. The tumor typically presents in patients aged about 50 as one or more palpable thyroid nodules. It grows slowly, spreading via contiguous lymphatics; rapid growth and hematogenous metastases occur infrequently. The sporadic disease may be unicentric in origin, but hereditary tumors are multicentric, beginning most commonly at the junctions of the middle and upper thirds of the thyroid lobes, where normal C cells are present in largest numbers.[386] The tumor may contain or secrete hormones other than CT. These include serotonin, prostaglandins, somatostatin, and corticotropin. It also secretes other peptide products of the CT gene. Approximately 20% of affected patients develop diarrhea, variably attributed to intestinal actions of secreted CT, prostaglandins, or serotonin. Diarrhea as a manifestation of the humoral tumor product usually indicates the presence of a large tumor bulk and metastases. In MEN 2B, diarrhea may reflect intestinal ganglioneuromatosis (see later). Other than diarrhea, there are no humorally mediated signs clearly linked to C cell cancer except for the rare occurrence of hypocalcemia.

LABORATORY ANALYSES. Radioactive thyroid scans are often unremarkable at early stages of the tumor. The tumor may contain large calcifications, unlike the fine, stippled calcifications seen with papillary thyroid carcinoma (Fig. 27–59); large, calcified, nodular metastases are also characteristic. Another characteristic radiographic feature is a fibrotic reaction about metastases in the lungs. Skeletal metastases may assume a lytic or, less commonly, sclerotic appearance. There are distinctive histological features; the cells are polyhedral or spindle shaped with variable amounts of stroma and stromal calcification. Almost all contain amyloid resulting from agglomeration of peptides encoded by the CT gene. The tumor cells contain CT and often contain enzymes related to the biogenic amine pathways character-

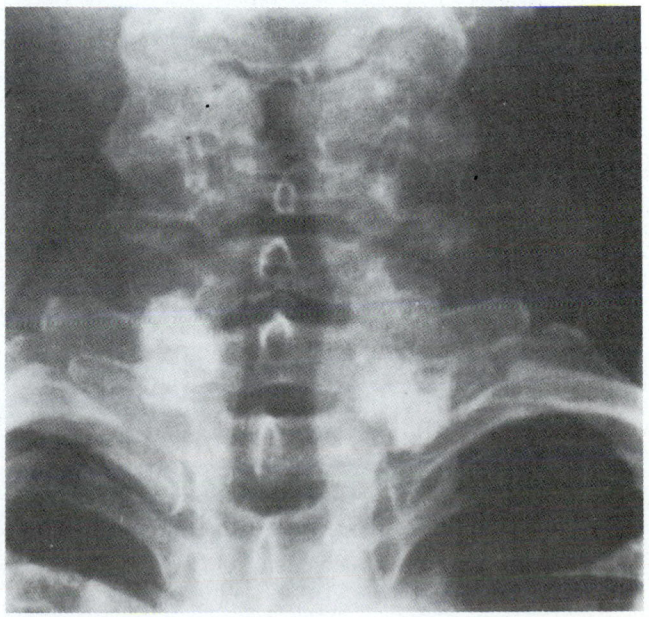

Figure 27–59. Large, calcified, intrathyroidal masses characteristic of medullary thyroid carcinoma. (Courtesy of Dr. H. Keiser.)

istic of neuroectodermal cells. These include dopa decarboxylase and histaminase. Serum calcium and phosphate concentrations are generally normal. In small numbers of patients evaluated by bone biopsy, no uniform abnormalities attributable to CT have been found. The radioimmunoassay of CT in serum is applicable for diagnosis (see later) and follow-up; it has also been used with selective venous sampling to localize metastases.

Serum immunoreactive CT may also be increased in neonates, in azotemia, and in hypercalcemia or hypergastrinemia (both of which may act as C cell secretagogues). Circulating concentrations of other tumor products, such as histaminase and carcinoembryonic antigen, are increased in many of patients with metastatic medullary thyroid carcinoma.

THERAPY. Surgery is the treatment of choice, although no studies have yet documented its efficacy in increasing survival. The usual approach is total thyroidectomy with a degree of node removal dependent on evidence of tumor stage. No thyroid tissue should be left because of the malignant potential of residual C cells. Residual thyroid tissue inaccessible to surgery can be ablated with radioactive iodine. Because of aggressive thyroidectomy and simultaneous therapy for parathyroid hyperplasia, these patients are at high risk for postoperative hypoparathyroidism. The disease presenting as a thyroid mass is associated with a 10-y postoperative survival of approximately 67%.[387] Family testing allows early diagnosis. Local radiotherapy, radioactive iodine as primary therapy, and chemotherapy have been used with little success.

Familial Medullary Carcinoma of the Thyroid

Familial medullary carcinoma of the thyroid occurs as an expression of two distinct traits, each with autosomal dominant transmission.[386] The eponym Sipple syndrome has been applied to both of these hereditary forms, although Sipple's description did not include the multiple neuroma variant. Unlike the sporadic tumor that is often unicentric in origin, familial disease is usually multifocal in the thyroid gland. An early phase of diffuse C cell hyperplasia can be diagnosed by serial testing (see later).

MULTIPLE ENDOCRINE NEOPLASIA, TYPE 2A. (See also Chapters 8 and 30.) For this autosomal dominant trait, there is approximately a 100% incidence of medullary thyroid carcinoma in adults. Approximately one third of affected family members also have abnormalities of other endocrine tissues (primary parathyroid hyperplasia or pheochromocytoma or both) (see Table 27–10). The initial hyperplasia[388] of these tissues progresses to a nodular phase. Malignant change is rare in the adrenal medulla and has not been reported for the parathyroids of these patients. Approximately 10% of affected adults develop hypercalcemia or nephrolithiasis or both. More commonly, the surgeon recognizes diffusely hyperplastic parathyroid glands at the time of surgery directed at the thyroid gland of a normocalcemic patient. It is not known if the parathyroid hyperplasia is a secondary response to a C cell product; CT, for example, might cause PTH resistance or a direct agonist effect on the parathyroid cell. However, parathyroid hyperplasia is not common in patients with sporadic medullary carcinoma of the thyroid or with the multiple neuroma variant of familial medullary carcinoma of the thyroid (see later). Pheochromocytoma may occur, sometimes subtly expressed in members of families with MEN 2A or 2B. This diagnosis should always be considered before administration of general anesthesia. The usual provocative tests for pheochromocytoma are often not helpful for diagnosis in asymptomatic cases of MEN 2A, but a biochemically silent adrenomedullary mass may be recognized with computed tomography of the adrenal. In several families, affected persons have manifested a disproportionate increase in urinary excretion of epinephrine.

MULTIPLE ENDOCRINE NEOPLASIA, TYPE 2B. The C cell and adrenomedullary abnormalities in these patients are indistinguishable from those of patients with MEN 2A. However, these tumors are expressed at an earlier age and metastasize more readily in patients with MEN 2B.[389] Another major distinguishing feature of this disorder is overgrowth of elements of nerve tissue with the result that the patients develop multiple mucosal neuromas, thickened cor-

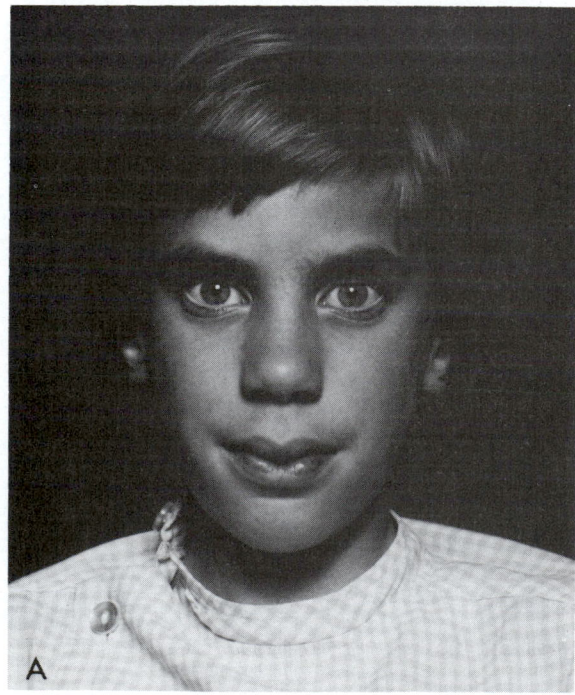

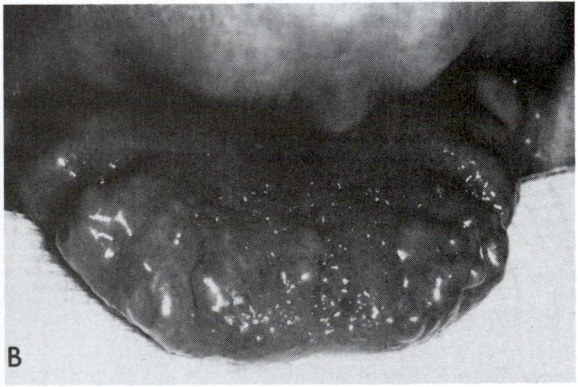

Figure 27–60. *A,* Characteristic facies of patient with MEN 2B. Note bumpy lips and thickened tarsal plates of eyelids. *B,* Surface of tongue is studded with nodular mucosal neuromas. (*A* from Carney JA, Hayles AB. Alimentary tract manifestations of multiple endocrine neoplasia, type 2b, Mayo Clin Proc 1977; 52:543–548. *B* from Carney JA, Sizemore GW, Lovestedt SA. Mucosal ganglioneuromatosis, medullary thyroid carcinoma, and pheochromocytoma: multiple endocrine neoplasia, type 2b. Oral Surg 1976; 41:739–752.)

neal nerves, and ganglioneuromatosis of the intestine.[386] The mucosal neuromas result in a characteristic facial appearance of buccal and lingual nodules, thick bumpy lips, and thickened tarsal plates (Fig. 27–60). This phenotype can often be diagnosed in the first decade of life. The thickened corneal nerves are best appreciated by slit lamp examination, and an ophthalmologist may be the first to suspect the presence of the underlying disorder. Intestinal ganglioneuromatosis leads to frequent abnormalities of intestinal transit, including diarrhea, constipation, diverticulosis, and megacolon. General muscle development is often poor. Lax joints and the tall, slender body habitus with pectus excavatum or carinatum result in an external appearance resembling that in Marfan syndrome. No lenticular or vascular abnormalities occur, however.

PATHOGENESIS OF MULTIPLE ENDOCRINE NEOPLASIA, TYPES 2A AND 2B. The clinical phenotypes of MEN 2A and MEN 2B are close, and the genes for each of these and for familial isolated medullary thyroid carcinoma have been localized to the pericentromeric region of chromosome 10. Evidently each of these hereditary syndromes reflects a similar type of mutation. Unlike the gene for MEN 1, that for MEN 2A and 2B does not seem to behave as a recessive oncogene in a tumor precursor cell. Rather, the tumors in MEN 2A and 2B may show somatic deletion of a gene on chromosome 1.[390] Stepwise deletion of genes other than that causing the germ line transmission of the tumor susceptibility has also been found in other hereditary tumors such as colon cancer/familial adenomatous polyposis of the colon.

EARLY DIAGNOSIS. Recognition of the familial pattern and progression through a premalignant phase makes possible diagnosis of hereditary cases long before development of a palpable neck mass. Early diagnosis and treatment may improve the life expectancy of these patients.[391] Direct testing for the MEN 2A gene(s) or its encoded product(s) may soon be possible. CT radioimmunoassay allows diagnosis of premalignant phases of the disorder in the majority. High basal concentration of CT in plasma without other conditions known to cause this (pregnancy, uremia, hypergastrinemia, other cancers) is virtually diagnostic of the cancerous phase of the trait. Increased diagnostic sensitivity during the early phases of C cell hyperfunction is obtained by measuring serum CT concentration after administration of a standardized CT secretagogue. The most potent stimulus is an infusion of calcium gluconate (equivalent to 2 mg of elemental calcium/kg body weight) over 1 min followed by pentagastrin (0.5 µg/kg body weight) over 5 s. This also evokes an unpleasant sensation of retrosternal distress. Serial testing of persons at risk for inheritance of the trait allows diagnosis of the malignant and premalignant phases of C cell dysfunction in many cases before the age of 10 (Fig. 27–61).[392] However, rigorous standardization of the CT radioimmunoassay is critical. Some unaffected persons have undergone inappropriate thyroid surgery because of misuse of CT radioimmunoassay results.

Other Calcitonin-Producing Tumors

High circulating concentrations of CT may be found in patients with diverse neoplasms and might be caused by CT production by the tumor or increased thyroidal secretion of CT under the influence of subtle hypercalcemia or other tumor-mediated processes. Some tumors that produce and release CT derive from cells of neuroectodermal origin (small cell cancer of the lung, carcinoid tumors, pancreatic islet cell cancer, pheochromocytoma), so CT secretion by them may not be "ectopic" but an exaggeration of normal secretion. Certain other tumors such as breast cancer, not

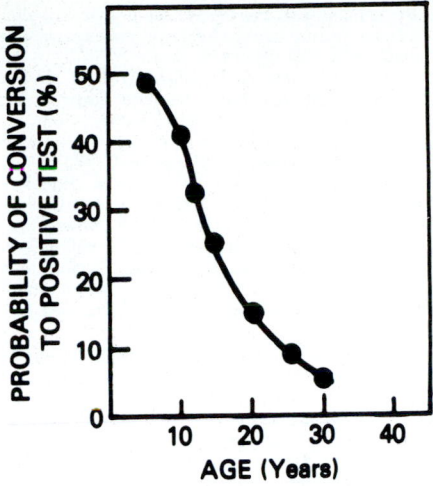

Figure 27–61. Likelihood of conversion to a positive C cell challenge test among persons at 50% risk for the gene. Data are derived from analysis of subjects followed serially in 11 kindreds with MEN 2A. (From Gagel RF, Jackson CE, Block MA, et al. Age-related probability of development of hereditary medullary thyroid carcinoma. J Pediatr 1982; 101:941–946.)

recognized as neuroectodermal in origin, also may secrete CT.

REFERENCES

1. Urist MR. Biogenesis of bone: calcium and phosphorus in the skeleton and blood in vertebrate evolution. In: Greep RO, Astwood EB, eds. Handbook of Physiology. Sect 7: Endocrinology. Vol VII. Parathyroid Gland. Washington, DC: American Physiological Society, 1976: 183–214.
2. Nordin BEC, ed. Calcium, Phosphate, and Magnesium Metabolism. New York: Churchill-Livingstone, 1976.
3. Heaney RP, Gallagher JC, Johnston CC, et al. Calcium nutrition and bone health in the elderly. Am J Clin Nutr 1982; 36:986–1013.
4. Harper AE. Evolution of recommended dietary allowances—new directions? Annu Rev Nutr 1987; 7:509–537.
5. Pennington JA, Young BE, Wilson DB, et al. Mineral content of foods and total diets: the selected minerals in foods survey, 1982 to 1984. J Am Diet Assoc 1986; 86:876–891.
6. Bell RR, Draper HH, Tzeng DYM, et al. Physiological responses of human adults to foods containing phosphate additives. J Nutr 1977; 107:42–50.
7. Heaney RP. Calcium kinetics in plasma: as they apply to the measurements of bone formation and resorption rates. In: Bourne GH, ed. Biochemistry and Physiology of Bone Calcification and Physiology. Vol 4. New York: Academic, 1976: 105–133.
8. Engel K, Pederson KO, Nielsen SP, et al., eds. Ionized Calcium Workshop No 1. Scand J Clin Lab Invest 1983; 43:1–126.
9. Tofaletti J. Physiological importance of calcium complexes. In: Anghileri LJ, Tuffet-Anghileri AM, eds. Role of Calcium in Biological Systems. Vol 2. Boca Raton, FL: CRC Press, 1982: 69–78.
10. Livingston DM, Wacker WEC. Magnesium metabolism. In: Greep RO, Astwood EB, eds. Handbook of Physiology. Sect 7: Endocrinology. Vol VII. Parathyroid Gland. Washington, DC: American Physiological Society, 1976: 215–224.
11. Markowitz ME, Rosen JF, Laxaminarayan S, Mizruchi M. Circadian rhythms of blood minerals during adolescence. Pediatr Res 1984; 18:456–462.
12. Bronner F. Intestinal calcium absorption and transport. In: Carafoli E, ed. Membrane Transport of Calcium. New York: Academic, 1982: 237–262.
13. Walser M. Divalent cations: physicochemical state in glomerular filtrate and urine and renal excretion. In: Orloff J, Berliner RW, eds. Handbook of Physiology. Sect 8: Renal Physiology. Washington, DC: American Physiological Society, 1973: 555–586.
14. Sullivan RAL, Dirks JH. Renal handling of calcium, phosphorus, and magnesium. In: Brenner BM, Rector FC, eds. The Kidney. Vol 1. 2nd ed. Philadelphia: W. B. Saunders, 1981: 551–618.
15. Parfitt AM, Kleerekoper M. The divalent ion homeostatic system—physiology and metabolism of calcium, phosphorus, magnesium, and bone. In: Maxwell MH, Kleeman CR, eds. Clinical Disorders of Fluid and Electrolyte Metabolism. 3rd ed. New York: McGraw-Hill, 1980: 269–398.

16. Lennon EJ, Lemann J Jr, Piering WF, et al. Effect of glucose on urinary cation excretion during extracellular volume expansion in normal man. J Clin Invest 1974; 53:1424–1433.
17. Cooper CN, Bolman RM III, Linehan WM, et al. Interrelationships between calcium, calcemic hormones and gastrointestinal hormones. Recent Prog Hormone Res 1978; 34:259–283.
18. Hurwitz S. Calcium metabolism in birds. In: Florkin M, Scheer BI, eds. Zoology. Vol 10. New York: Academic, 1978: 273–306.
19. Gertner JM, Coustan DR, Kliger AS, et al. Pregnancy as state of physiologic absorptive hypercalciuria. Am J Med 1986; 81:451–456.
20. Cobbold H, Rink TJ. Fluorescence and bioluminescence measurements of cytoplasmic free calcium. Biochem J 1987; 248:313–328.
21. Vanhoutte PM, Paoletti R, Govoni S, eds. Calcium antagonists: pharmacology and clinical research. Ann NY Acad Sci 1988; 522:1–798.
22. Catterall WA. Structure and function of voltage-sensitive ion channels. Science 1988; 242:50–61.
23. Furuichi T, Yoshikawa S, Miyawaki A, et al. Protein predicted by inositol 1,4,5-triphosphate receptor cDNA is homologous to a calcium channel protein. Nature 1989; 342:32–38.
24. Carafoli E. The plasma membrane calcium transporting systems in the regulation of cell calcium. In: Adelstein R, Klee C, Rodbell M, eds. Advances in Second Messenger and Phosphoprotein Research. Vol 21. New York: Raven, 1988: 147–155.
25. Cohen P, Klee CB, eds. Calmodulin. New York: Elsevier, 1988.
26. Thompson NW, Eckhauser FE, Harness JK. The anatomy of primary hyperparathyroidism. Surgery 1982; 92:814–821.
27. Dufour DR, Wilkerson SY. The normal parathyroid revisited: percentage of stromal fat. Hum Pathol 1982; 13:717–721.
28. Capen CC, Roth SI. Ultrastructural and function relationships of normal and pathologic parathyroid cells. Pathobiol Annu 1973; 3:129–175.
29. Suva LJ, Winslow GA, Wettenall REH, et al. A parathyroid hormone–related protein implicated in malignant hypercalcemia: cloning and expression. Science 1987; 237:893–896.
30. Potts JT Jr, Kronenberg HM, Rosenblatt M. Parathyroid hormone: chemistry, biosynthesis, and mode of action. Adv Protein Chem 1982; 35:323–396.
31. Habener JF, Rosenblatt M, Potts JT Jr. Parathyroid hormone: biochemical aspects of biosynthesis, secretion, action, and metabolism. Physiol Rev 1984; 64:985–1053.
32. Nissenson RA, Abbott SR, Teitelbaum AP, et al. Endogenous biologically active human parathyroid hormone: measurement by a guanyl nucleotide–amplified renal adenylate cyclase assay. J Clin Endocrinol Metab 1981; 52:840–846.
33. Pines M, Santora A, Spiegel A. Effects of phorbol esters and pertussis toxin on agonist-stimulated cyclic AMP production in rat osteosarcoma cells. Biochem Pharmacol 1986; 35:3639–3641.
34. Nussbaum SR, Zahradnik RJ, Lavigne JR, et al. A highly sensitive two-site immunoradiometric assay of parathyrin (PTH) and its clinical utility in evaluating patients with hypercalcemia. Clin Chem 1987; 33:1364–1367.
35. Aston JP, Wheeler MH, Brown RC, et al. Studies on in vivo and in vitro release of intact parathyroid hormone using a new two-site immunochemiluminometric assay. World J Surg 1988; 12:454–462.
36. Brown RC, Aston JP, Weeks I, et al. Circulating intact parathyroid hormone measured by a two-site immunochemiluminometric assay. J Clin Endocrinol Metab 1987; 65:407–414.
37. Kronenberg HM, McDevitt BE, Hendy GM, et al. Studies of parathyroid hormone biosynthesis using recombinant DNA technology. In: Cohn DV, Talmage RV, Matthews JL, eds. Hormonal Control of Calcium Metabolism. Princeton: Excerpta Medica, 1981: 5–18.
38. Rosenblatt M. Pre-proparathyroid hormone, proparathyroid hormone, and parathyroid hormone: the biologic role of hormone structure. Clin Orthop 1982; 170:260–276.
39. Wiren KM, Ivashkiv L, Ma P, et al. Mutations in signal sequence cleavage domain of preproparathyroid hormone alter protein translocation, signal sequence cleavage, and membrane-binding properties. Mol Endocrinol 1989; 3:240–250.
40. Cohn DV, MacGregor RR, Chu LLH, et al. Calcemic fraction A: biosynthetic peptide precursor of parathyroid hormone. Proc Natl Acad Sci USA 1972; 69:1521–1525.
41. Brown EM. Parathyroid secretion in vivo and in vitro. Regulation by calcium and other secretagogues. Miner Electrolyte Metab 1982; 8:130–150.
42. Brown EM, Chen CJ. Calcium, magnesium and the control of PTH secretion. Bone Miner 1989; 5:249–257.
43. Brown EM. Histamine receptors on dispersed parathyroid cells from pathological human parathyroid tissue. J Clin Endocrinol Metab 1980; 51:1325–1329.
44. Cohn DV, Kumarasamy R, Ramp WW. Internal processing and secretion of parathyroid gland proteins. Vitam Horm 1986; 43:283–316.
45. Lasker RD, Spiegel AM. Endogenous substrates for cAMP-dependent phosphorylation in dispersed bovine parathyroid cells. Endocrinology 1982; 111:1412–1414.
46. Yamamoto M, Igarashi T, Muramatsu M, et al. Hypocalcemia increases and hypercalcemia decreases the steady-state level of parathyroid hormone messenger RNA in the rat. J Clin Invest 1989; 83:1053–1056.
47. Nemeth EF, Scarpa A. Are changes in intracellular free calcium neces-

sary for regulating secretion in parathyroid cells? Ann NY Acad Sci 1987; 493:542–551.
48. Jia M, Ehrenstein G, Iwasa K. Unusual calcium-activated potassium channels of bovine parathyroid cells. Proc Natl Acad Sci USA 1988; 85:7236–7239.
49. Lopez-Barneo J, Armstrong CM. Depolarizing response of rat parathyroid cells to divalent cations. J Gen Physiol 1983; 82:269–294.
50. Membreño L, Chen TH, Woodley S, et al. The effects of protein kinase-C agonists on parathyroid hormone release and intracellular free Ca^{2+} in bovine parathyroid cells. Endocrinology 1989; 124:789–797.
51. Abou-Samra AB, Jueppner H, Westerberg D, et al. Parathyroid hormone causes translocation of protein kinase-C from cytosol to membranes in rat osteosarcoma cells. Endocrinology 1989; 124:1107–1113.
52. Morrissey JJ. Effect of phorbol myristate acetate on secretion of parathyroid hormone. Am J Physiol 1988; 254:E63–E70.
53. Fitzpatrick LA, Brandi ML, Aurbach GD. Control of PTH secretion is mediated through calcium channels and is blocked by pertussis toxin treatment of parathyroid cells. Biochem Biophys Res Commun 1986; 138:960–965.
54. Fitzpatrick LA, Chin H, Nirenberg M, et al. Antibodies to an alpha subunit of skeletal muscle calcium channels regulate parathyroid cell secretion. Proc Natl Acad Sci USA 1988; 85:2115–2119.
55. Brown EM, Adragna N, Gardner DG. Effect of potassium on PTH secretion from dispersed bovine parathyroid cells. J Clin Endocrinol Metab 1981; 53:1304–1306.
56. Dempster DW, Tobler PH, Olles P, et al. Potassium stimulates parathyroid hormone release from perifused parathyroid cells. Endocrinology 1982; 111:191–195.
57. Naveh-Many T, Friedlaender MM, Mayer H, et al. Calcium regulates parathyroid hormone messenger ribonucleic acid (mRNA), but not calcitonin mRNA in vivo in the rat. Dominant role of 1,25-dihydroxyvitamin D. Endocrinology 1989; 125:275–280.
58. Mayer GP, Keaton JA, Hurst JG, et al. Effects of plasma calcium concentration on the relative proportion of hormone and carboxyl fragments in parathyroid venous blood. Endocrinology 1979; 104:1778–1784.
59. Kemper B, Habener JF, Rich A, et al. Parathyroid secretion: discovery of a major calcium-dependent protein. Science 1974; 184:167–169.
60. Cohn DV, Morrissey MM, Hamilton JW, et al. Isolation and partial characterization of secretory protein I from bovine parathyroid glands. Biochemistry 1981; 7:4135–4140.
61. Cohn DV, Zangerle R, Fischer-Colbrie R, et al. Similarity of secretory protein I from parathyroid gland to chromogranin A from adrenal medulla. Proc Natl Acad Sci USA 1982; 79:6056–6059.
62. Bhargava G, Russell J, Sherwood LM. Phosphorylation of parathyroid secretory protein. Proc Natl Acad Sci USA 1983; 80:878–881.
63. MacGregor RR, Cohn DV, Hamilton JW. The content of carboxyl-terminal fragments of parathormone in extracts of fresh bovine parathyroid. Endocrinology 1983; 112:1019–1025.
64. Bringhurst FR, Segre GV, Lampman GW, et al. Metabolism of parathyroid hormone by Kupffer cells: analysis by reverse-phase high-performance liquid chromatography. Biochemistry 1982; 21:4252–4258.
65. Pillai S, Zull JE. Production of biologically active fragments of parathyroid hormone by isolated Kupffer cells. J Biol Chem 1986; 261:14919–14923.
66. MacGregor RR, Jilka RL, Hamilton JW. Formation and secretion of fragments of parathormone. Identification of cleavage sites. J Biol Chem 1986; 261:1929–1934.
67. Bringhurst FR, Stern AM, Yotts M, et al. Peripheral metabolism of PTH: fate of biologically active amino terminus in vivo. Am J Physiol 1988; 255:E886–E893.
68. Goltzman D, Bennett HP, Koutsilieris M, et al. Studies of the multiple molecular forms of bioactive parathyroid hormone and parathyroid hormone–like substances. Recent Prog Horm Res 1986; 42:665–703.
69. Talmage RV, Meyer RA Jr. Physiological role of parathyroid hormone. In: Greep RO, Astwood RF, eds. Handbook of Physiology. Sect 7: Endocrinology. Vol VII. Parathyroid Gland. Washington, DC: American Physiological Society, 1976: 343–351.
70. Raisz LG. Mechanisms of bone resorption. In: Greep RO, Astwood RF, eds. Handbook of Physiology. Sect 7: Endocrinology. Vol VII. Parathyroid Gland. Washington, DC: American Physiological Society, 1976: 117–136.
71. Agus ZS, Goldfarb S, Wasserstein A. Calcium transport in the kidney. Rev Physiol Biochem Pharmacol 1981; 90:155–169.
72. Dennis VW, Brazy PC. Divalent anion transport in isolated renal tubules. Kidney Int 1982; 22:498–506.
73. Bourdeau JE, Burg MB. Effect of PTH on calcium transport across the cortical thick ascending limb of Henle's loop. Am J Physiol 1980; 239:F121–F126.
74. Biddulph DM, Wrenn RW. Effects of parathyroid hormone on cyclic AMP, cyclic GMP, and efflux of calcium in isolated renal tubules. J Cyclic Nucleotide Res 1977; 3:129–138.
75. Agus ZS, Wasserstein A, Goldfarb S. PTH, calcitonin, cyclic nucleotides, and the kidney. Annu Rev Physiol 1981; 41:583–595.
76. Friedman PA. Basal and hormone-activated calcium absorption in mouse renal thick ascending limbs. Am J Physiol 1988; 254:F62–F70.
76a. Shareghi GR, Agus ZS. Magnesium transport in the cortical thick

ascending limb of Henle's loop of the rabbit. J Clin Invest 1982; 69:759–769.

77. Quamme G, Pfeilschifter J, Murer H. Parathyroid hormone inhibition of Na$^+$/phosphate cotransport in OK cells: generation of second messengers in the regulatory cascade. Biochem Biophys Res Commun 1989; 158:951–957.

78. Caverzasio J, Rizzoli R, Bonjour JP. Sodium-dependent phosphate transport inhibited by parathyroid hormone and cyclic AMP stimulation in an opossum kidney cell line. J Biol Chem 1986; 261:3233–3237.

79. Pollock AS, Warnock DG, Strewler GJ. Parathyroid hormone inhibition of Na$^+$-H$^+$ antiporter activity in a cultured renal cell line. Am J Physiol 1986; 250:F217–F225.

80. Jaeger P, Jones W, Kashgarian M, et al. Parathyroid hormone directly inhibits tubular reabsorption of bicarbonate in normocalcaemic rats with chronic hyperparathyroidism. Eur J Clin Invest 1987; 7:415–420.

81. Winaver J, Chen TC, Fragola J, et al. Alterations in renal tubular water transport induced by parathyroid hormone: evidence for both antidiuretic hormone-mediated and independent effects. J Lab Clin Med 1982; 99:457–473.

82. Shigematsu T, Horiuchi N, Ogura Y, et al. Human parathyroid hormone inhibits renal 24-hydroxylase activity of 25-hydroxyvitamin D3 by a mechanism involving adenosine 3',5'-monophosphate in rats. Endocrinology 1986; 118:1583–1589.

83. Tam CS, Heersche JNM, Murray TM, et al. Parathyroid hormone stimulates the bone apposition rate independently of its resorptive action: differential effects of intermittent and continuous administration. Endocrinology 1982; 110:506–512.

84. Hock JM, Gera I, Fonseca J, et al. Human parathyroid hormone-(1–34) increases bone mass in ovariectomized and orchidectomized rats. Endocrinology 1988; 122:2899–2904.

85. Genant HK, Baron JM, Paloyan E, et al. Osteosclerosis in primary hyperparathyroidism. Am J Med 1975; 59:104–113.

86. Canalis E, Centrella M, Burch W, et al. Insulin-like growth factor I mediates selective anabolic effects of parathyroid hormone in bone cultures. J Clin Invest 1989; 83:60–65.

87. Vaes G. Parathyroid hormone–like action of N^6-2'-O-dibutyryladenosine-3',5'-(cyclic) monophosphate on bone explants in tissue culture. Nature 1968; 219:939–940.

88. Eilon G, Raisz LG. Comparison of the effects of stimulators and inhibitors of resorption on the release of lysozomal enzymes and radioactive calcium from fetal bone in organ culture. Endocrinology 1978; 103:1969–1975.

89. Hall GE, Kenny AD. Bone resorption induced by parathyroid hormone and dibutyryl cyclic AMP: role of carbonic anhydrase. J Pharmacol Exp Ther 1986; 238:778–782.

90. Braidman IP, St John JG, Anderson DC, et al. Effects of physiological concentrations of parathyroid hormone on acid phosphatase activity in cultured rat bone cells. J Endocrinol 1986; 111:17–26.

91. Dziak R, Stern PH. Calcium transport in isolated bone cells. III. Effects of parathyroid hormone and cyclic 3',5'-AMP. Endocrinology 1975; 97:1281–1287.

92. van Leeuwen JP, Bos MP, Lowik CW, et al. Effect of parathyroid hormone and parathyroid hormone fragments on the intracellular ionized calcium concentration in an osteoblast cell line. Bone Miner 1988; 4:177–188.

93. Donahue HJ, Fryer MJ, Eriksen EF, et al. Differential effects of parathyroid hormone and its analogues on cytosolic calcium ion and cAMP levels in cultured rat osteoblast-like cells. J Biol Chem 1988; 263:13522–13527.

94. Peck WA, Birge SJ, Fedak SA. Bone cells: biochemical and biological studies after enzymatic isolation. Science 1964; 146:1476–1477.

95. Cohn DV, Wong GL. The actions of parathormone calcitonin and 1,25-dihydroxycholecalciferol on osteoclast- and osteoblast-like cells in culture. In: Copp DH, Talmage RV, eds. Endocrinology of Calcium Metabolism. Amsterdam: Excerpta Medica, 1978: 241.

96. Rodan GA, Rodan SB, Marks SC. Parathyroid hormone stimulation of adenylate cyclase activity and lactic acid accumulation in calvaria of osteopetrotic (ia) rats. Endocrinology 1978; 102:1501–1505.

97. Perry HM, Skogen W, Chappel JC, et al. Conditioned medium from osteoblast-like cells mediate parathyroid hormone induced bone resorption. Calcif Tissue Int 1987; 40:298–300.

98. McSheehy PM, Chambers TJ. Osteoblast-like cells in the presence of parathyroid hormone release soluble factor that stimulates osteoclastic bone resorption. Endocrinology 1986; 119:1654–1659.

99. Jilka RL. Are osteoblastic cells required for the control of osteoclast activity by parathyroid hormone? Bone Miner 1986; 1:261–264.

100. Aurbach GD, Chase LR. Cyclic nucleotides and biochemical actions of parathyroid hormone and calcitonin. In: Greep RO, Astwood EB, eds. Handbook of Physiology. Sect 7: Endocrinology. Vol VII. Parathyroid Gland. Washington, DC: American Physiological Society, 1976: 353–381.

101. Peck WA, Klahr S. Cyclic nucleotides in bone and mineral metabolism. Adv Cyclic Nucleotide Res 1979; 11:89–130.

102. Klahr S, Peck WA. Cyclic nucleotides in bone and mineral metabolism. II. Cyclic nucleotides and the renal regulation of mineral metabolism. Adv Cyclic Nucleotide Res 1980; 13:133–180.

103. Bourdeau JE, Lau K. Effects of parathyroid hormone on cytosolic free calcium concentration in individual rabbit connecting tubules. J Clin Invest 1989; 83:373–379.

104. Fujii Y, Fukase M, Tsutsumi M, et al. Parathyroid hormone control of free cytosolic Ca^{2+} in the kidney. J Bone Miner Res 1988; 3:525–532.

105. Yamada H, Tsutsumi M, Fukase M, et al. Effects of human PTH-related peptide and human PTH on cyclic AMP production and cytosolic free calcium in an osteoblastic cell clone. Bone Miner 1989; 6:45–54.

106. Civitelli R, Reid IR, Westbrook S, et al. PTH elevates inositol polyphosphates and diacylglycerol in a rat osteoblast-like cell line. Am J Physiol 1988; 255:E660–E667.

107. Nissenson RA, Karpf D, Bambino T, et al. Covalent labeling of a high-affinity, guanyl nucleotide sensitive parathyroid hormone receptor in canine renal cortex. Biochemistry 1987; 26:1874–1878.

108. Karpf DB, Arnaud CD, King K, et al. The canine renal parathyroid hormone receptor is a glycoprotein: characterization and partial purification. Biochemistry 1987; 26:7825–7833.

109. Coltrera MD, Potts JT Jr, Rosenblatt M. Identification of a renal receptor for parathyroid hormone by photoaffinity radiolabeling using a synthetic analogue. J Biol Chem 1981; 256:10555–10559.

110. Forte LR, Langeluttig SG, Poelling RE, et al. Renal parathyroid hormone receptors in the chick: down-regulation in secondary hyperparathyroid animal models. Am J Physiol 1982; 242:E154–E163.

111. Brennan DP, Levine MA. Characterization of soluble and particulate parathyroid hormone receptors using a biotinylated bioactive hormone analog. J Biol Chem 1987; 262:14795–14800.

112. Goldman ME, McKee RL, Caulfield MP, et al. A new highly potent parathyroid hormone antagonist: [D-Trp$_{12}$,Tyr34]bPTH-(7–34)NH$_2$. Endocrinology 1988; 123:2597–2599.

113. Morel F, Chabardes D, Imbert-Teboul M, et al. Multiple hormonal control of adenylate cyclase in distal segments of the rat kidney. Kidney Int [Suppl] 1982; 11:555–567.

114. Chambers DJ, Schafer DH, Laughran JA Jr, et al. Dose-related activation by PTH of specific enzymes in various regions of the kidney. In: Copp DH, Talmage RV, eds. Endocrinology of Calcium Metabolism. Amsterdam: Excerpta Medica, 1978: 216.

115. Dousa TP, Steiner AL. Immunofluorescent localization of cyclic nucleotides in the nephron. In: Copp DH, Talmage RV, eds. Endocrinology of Calcium Metabolism. Amsterdam: Excerpta Medica, 1978: 221.

116. Insel P, Balakir R, Sacktor B. Binding of cyclic AMP to renal brush-border membranes. J Cyclic Nucleotide Res 1975; 1:107–122.

117. Shlatz LJ, Schwartz IL, Kinne-Saffran E, et al. Distribution of parathyroid hormone–stimulated adenylate cyclase in plasma membranes of cells of the kidney cortex. J Membr Biol 1975; 24:131–144.

118. Hammerman MR, Hansen VA, Morrissey JJ. Cyclic AMP–dependent protein phosphorylation and dephosphorylation alter phosphate transport in canine renal brush border vesicles. Biochim Biophys Acta 1983; 755:10–16.

119. Noland TA Jr, Henry HL. Protein phosphorylation in chick kidney. Response to parathyroid hormone, cyclic AMP, calcium, and phosphatidylserine. J Biol Chem 1983; 258:538–546.

120. Tamura T, Sakamoto H, Filburn CR. Parathyroid hormone 1-34, but not 3-34 or 7-34, transiently translocates protein kinase C in cultured renal (OK) cells. Biochem Biophys Res Commun 1989; 159:1352–1358.

121. Bacon RA, Wu KI, Ying AL, et al. Colchicine blocks the action of parathyroid hormone but not nicotinamide on renal phosphate transport. Biochim Biophys Acta 1987; 905:268–272.

122. Centrella M, McCarthy TL, Canalis E. Parathyroid hormone modulates transforming growth factor beta activity and binding in osteoblast-enriched cell cultures from fetal rat parietal bone. Proc Natl Acad Sci USA 1988; 85:5889–5893.

123. Yee JA, Sutton JK. Parathyroid hormone regulation of proline uptake by cultured neonatal mouse osteoblastlike cells. J Bone Miner Res 1989; 4:23–27.

124. Yee JA. Effect of parathyroid hormone on amino acid transport by cultured neonatal mouse calvarial bone cells. J Bone Miner Res 1988; 3:211–218.

125. Fritsch J, Edelman A, Balsan S. Early effects of parathyroid hormone on membrane potential of rat osteoblasts in culture: role of cAMP and Ca^{2+}. J Bone Miner Res 1988; 3:547–554.

126. Livesey SA, Kemp BE, Re CA, et al. Selective hormonal activation of cyclic AMP–dependent protein kinase isoenzymes in normal and malignant osteoblasts. J Biol Chem 1982; 257:14983–14987.

127. Holtrop ME, Raisz LG, Simmons HA. The effects of parathyroid hormone, colchicine, and calcitonin on the ultrastructure and the activity of osteoclasts in organ culture. J Cell Biol 1974; 60:346–355.

128. Sutherland EW. On the biological role of cyclic AMP. JAMA 1970; 214:1281–1288.

129. Broadus AE. Clinical cyclic nucleotide research. Adv Cyclic Nucleotide Res 1977; 8:509–548.

130. Chase LR, Melson GL, Aurbach GD. Pseudohypoparathyroidism: Defective excretion of 3',5'-AMP in response to parathyroid hormone. J Clin Invest 1969; 48:1832–1844.

131. Chase LR, Aurbach GD. Parathyroid function and the renal excretion of 3',5'-adenylic acid. Proc Natl Acad Sci USA 1967; 58:518–525.

132. Broadus AE. Nephrogenous cyclic AMP. Recent Prog Horm Res 1981; 37:667–701.

133. Broadus AE, Mangin M, Ikeda K, et al. Humoral hypercalcemia of cancer: identification of a novel parathyroid hormone–like peptide. N Engl J Med 1988; 319:556–563.
134. Moseley JM, Kubota M, Diefenbach-Jagger H, et al. Parathyroid hormone–related protein purified from a human lung cancer cell line. Proc Natl Acad Sci USA 1987; 84:5048–5052.
135. Strewler GJ, Stern PH, Jacobs JW, et al. Parathyroid hormonelike protein from human renal carcinoma cells. J Clin Invest 1987; 80:1803–1807.
136. Mangin M, Webb AC, Dreyer BE, et al. Identification of a cDNA encoding a parathyroid hormone–like peptide from a human tumor associated with humoral hypercalcemia of malignancy. Proc Natl Acad Sci USA 1988; 85:597–601.
137. Thorikay M, Kramer S, Reynolds FH, et al. Synthesis of a gene encoding parathyroid hormone–like protein (1–141): purification and biological characterization of the expressed protein. Endocrinology 1989; 124:111–118.
138. Horiuchi N, Caulfield MP, Fisher JE, et al. Similarity of synthetic peptide from human tumor to parathyroid hormone in vivo and in vitro. Science 1987; 238:1566–1568.
139. Kemp BE, Moseley JM, Rodda CP, et al. Parathyroid hormone–related protein of malignancy: active synthetic fragments. Science 1987; 238:1568–1570.
140. Stewart AF, Mangin M, Wu T, et al. Synthetic human parathyroid hormone–like protein stimulates bone resorption and causes hypercalcemia in rats. J Clin Invest 1988; 81:596–600.
141. Kukreja SC, Shevrin DH, Wimbiscus SA, et al. Antibodies to parathyroid hormone–related protein lower serum calcium in athymic mouse models of malignancy-associated hypercalcemia due to human tumors. J Clin Invest 1988; 82:1798–1802.
142. Nissenson RA, Diep D, Strewler GJ. Synthetic peptides comprising the amino-terminal sequence of a parathyroid hormone–like protein from human malignancies. J Biol Chem 1988; 263:12866–12871.
143. Juppner H, Abou-Samra AB, Uneno S, et al. The parathyroid hormone–like peptide associated with humoral hypercalcemia of malignancy and parathyroid hormone bind to the same receptor on the plasma membrane of ROS 17/2.8 cells. J Biol Chem 1988; 263:8557–8560.
144. Ikeda K, Weir EC, Mangin M, et al. Expression of messenger ribonucleic acids encoding a parathyroid hormone–like peptide in normal human and animal tissues with abnormal expression in human parathyroid adenomas. Mol Endocrinol 1988; 2:1230–1236.
145. Merendino JJ, Insogna KL, Milstone LM, et al. A parathyroid hormone–like protein from cultured human keratinocytes. Science 1986; 231:388–390.
146. Silve C, Santora A, Spiegel A. A factor produced by cultured rat Leydig tumor cells associated with humoral hypercalcemia stimulates adenosine 3′,5′-monophosphate production via the parathyroid hormone receptor in human skin fibroblasts. J Clin Endocrinol Metab 1985; 60:1144–1147.
147. Wu TL, Insogna KL, Hough LM, et al. Skin-derived fibroblasts respond to human parathyroid hormone–like adenylate cyclase–stimulating proteins. J Clin Endocrinol Metab 1987; 65:105–109.
148. Thiede MA, Rodan GA. Expression of a calcium-mobilizing parathyroid hormone–like peptide in lactating mammary tissue. Science 1988; 242:278–280.
149. Potts JT Jr, Aurbach GD. Chemistry of the calcitonins. In: Greep RO, Astwood EB, eds. Handbook of Physiology. Sect 7: Endocrinology. Vol VII. Parathyroid Gland. Washington, DC: American Physiological Society, 1976: 423–430.
150. Schwartz KE, Orlowski RC, Marcus R. des-Ser^2 salmon calcitonin, a biologically potent synthetic analog. Endocrinology 1981; 108:831–835.
151. Findlay DM, Michelangeli VP, Orlowski RC, et al. Biological activities and receptor interactions of des-Leu^{16} salmon and des-Phe^{16} human calcitonin. Endocrinology 1983; 112:1288–1291.
152. Findlay DM, Michelangeli VP, Martin TJ, et al. Conformational requirements for activity of salmon calcitonin. Endocrinology 1985; 117:801–805.
153. Orlowski RC, Epand RM, Stafford AR. Biologically potent analogues of salmon calcitonin which do not contain an N-terminal disulfide-bridged ring structure. Eur J Biochem 1987; 162:399–402.
154. Rosenfeld MG, Amara SG, Evans RM. Alternative RNA processing: determining neuronal phenotype. Science 1984; 225:1315–1320.
155. Zaidi M, Chambers TJ, Bevis PJ, et al. Effects of peptides from the calcitonin genes on bone and bone cells. Q J Exp Physiol 1988; 73:471–485.
156. Jacobs JW, Goodman RH, Chin WW, et al. Calcitonin messenger RNA encodes multiple polypeptides in a single precursor. Science 1981; 213:457–459.
157. Seitz PK, Cooper CW. Cosecretion of calcitonin and calcitonin gene–related peptide from cultured rat medullary thyroid C cells. J Bone Miner Res 1989; 4:129–134.
158. Burns DM, Forstrom JM, Friday KE, et al. Procalcitonin: amino-terminal cleavage peptide (N-procalcitonin) is a bone-cell mitogen. Proc Natl Acad Sci USA 1989; 86:9519–9523.
159. Seth R, Motte P, Kehely A, et al. A sensitive and specific two-site enzyme-immunoassay for human calcitonin using monoclonal antibodies. J Endocrinol 1988; 119:351–357.
160. Talmage RV, Cooper CW, Toverud SU. The physiological significance of calcitonin. Bone Miner Res 1983; 1:74–143.
161. Persson P, Gunditz T, Axelson J, et al. Cholecystokinins but not gastrin-17 release calcitonin from thyroid C-cells in the rat. Regul Pept 1988; 21:45–56.
162. Tobler PH, Tschopp FA, Dambacher MA, et al. Identification and characterization of calcitonin forms in plasma and urine of normal subjects and medullary carcinoma patients. J Clin Endocrinol Metab 1983; 57:749–754.
163. Munson PL. Physiology and pharmacology of thyrocalcitonin. In: Greep RO, Astwood EB, eds. Handbook of Physiology. Sect 7: Endocrinology. Vol VII. Parathyroid Gland. Washington, DC: American Physiological Society, 1976: 443–464.
164. Chambers TJ, Magnus CJ. Calcitonin alters behaviour of isolated osteoclasts. J Pathol 1982; 136:27–39.
165. Jones SJ, Boyde A. Scanning electron microscopy of bone cells in culture. In: Copp DH, Talmage RV, eds. Endocrinology of Calcium Metabolism. Amsterdam: Excerpta Medica, 1978: 97.
166. Holtrop ME, King GJ, Raisz LG. Factors influencing osteoclast activity as measured by ultrastructural morphometry. In: Copp DH, Talmage RV, eds. Endocrinology of Calcium Metabolism. Amsterdam: Excerpta Medica, 1978: 91.
167. Holtrop ME, King GJ. The ultrastructure of the osteoclast and its functional implications. Clin Orthop 1977; 123:177–196.
168. Takahashi N, Akatsu T, Sasaki T, et al. Induction of calcitonin receptors by 1 alpha, 25-dihydroxyvitamin D3 in osteoclast-like multinucleated cells formed from mouse bone marrow cells. Endocrinology 1988; 123:1504–1510.
169. Murrills RJ, Shane E, Lindsay R, et al. Bone resorption by isolated human osteoclasts in vitro: effects of calcitonin. J Bone Miner Res 1989; 4:259–268.
170. Nicholson GC, Moseley JM, Sexton PM, et al. Abundant calcitonin receptors in isolated rat osteoclasts. Biochemical and autoradiographic characterization. J Clin Invest 1986; 78:355–360.
171. Marx SJ, Woodard C, Aurbach GD, et al. Renal receptors for calcitonin: binding and degradation of hormone. J Biol Chem 1973; 248:4797–4802.
172. Moseley JM, Findlay DM, Martin TJ, et al. Covalent cross-linking of a photoactive derivative of calcitonin to human breast cancer cell receptors. J Biol Chem 1982; 257:5846–5851.
173. van Houten M, Rizzo AJ, Goltzman D, et al. Brain receptors for blood-borne calcitonin in rats: circumventricular localization and vasopressin-resistant deficiency in hereditary diabetes insipidus. Endocrinology 1982; 111:1704–1710.
174. Bell PA. The chemistry of the vitamins D. In: Lawson DEM, ed. Vitamin D. New York: Academic, 1978: 1–50.
175. De Luca HF. Metabolism and mechanism of action of vitamin D—1982. In: Peck WA, ed. Bone and Mineral Research Annual 1. Princeton: Excerpta Medica, 1983: 7–73.
176. Marx SJ, Liberman UA, Eil C. Calciferols: actions and deficiencies in action. Vitam Horm 1983; 40:235–308.
177. Norman AW, Roth J, Orci L. The vitamin D endocrine system: steroid metabolism, hormone, receptors, and biological response (calcium binding proteins). Endocr Rev 1982; 3:331–366.
178. Clemens TL, Adams JA, Henderson SL, et al. Increased skin pigment reduces the capacity of skin to synthesize vitamin D$_3$. Lancet 1983; 1:74–76.
179. Webb AR, Holick MF. The role of sunlight in the cutaneous production of vitamin D$_3$. Annu Rev Nutr 1988; 8:375–399.
180. Masumoto O, Ohyama Y, Okuda K. Purification and characterization of vitamin D 25-hydroxylase from rat liver mitochondria. J Biol Chem 1988; 263:14256–14260.
181. Kawashima H, Kraut JA, Kurokawa K. Metabolic acidosis suppresses 25-hydroxyvitamin D$_3$-1alpha-hydroxylase in the rat kidney. J Clin Invest 1982; 70:135–140.
182. Tanaka Y, Castillo L, Wineland MJ, et al. Synergistic effect of progesterone, testosterone, and estradiol in the stimulation of chick renal 25-hydroxyvitamin D$_3$-1-hydroxylase. Endocrinology 1978; 103:2035–2039.
183. Shigematsu T, Horiuchi N, Ogura Y, et al. Human parathyroid hormone inhibits renal 24-hydroxylase activity of 25-hydroxyvitamin D$_3$ by a mechanism involving adenosine 3′,5′-monophosphate in rats. Endocrinology 1986; 118:1583–1589.
184. Markestad T. Plasma concentrations of 1,25-dihydroxyvitamin D, 24,25-dihydroxyvitamin D, and 25,26-dihydroxyvitamin D in the first year of life. J Clin Endocrinol Metab 1983; 57:755–759.
185. Mawer EB, Blackhouse J, Holman CA, et al. The distribution and storage of vitamin D and its metabolites in human tissue. Clin Sci 1972; 43:413–431.
186. Cooke NE, Haddad JG. Vitamin D binding protein (Gc-globulin). Endocr Rev 1989; 10:294–307.
187. Clements MR, Chalmers TM, Fraser DR. Enterohepatic circulation of vitamin D: a reappraisal of the hypothesis. Lancet 1984; 1:1376–1379.
188. Christakos S, Gabrielides C, Rhoten WB. Vitamin D–dependent calcium binding proteins: chemistry, distribution, functional considerations, and molecular biology. Endocr Rev 1989; 10:3–26.

189. Underwood JL, DeLuca HF. Vitamin D is not directly necessary for bone growth and mineralization. Am J Physiol 1984; 246:E493–E498.

190. Raisz LG, Kream BE. Regulation of bone formation. (Parts I and II). N Engl J Med 1983; 309:29–35, 83–89.

191. Raisz LG. Local and systemic factors in the pathogenesis of osteoporosis. N Engl J Med 1987; 318:818–828.

192. Holtrop ME, Cox KA, Clark MB, et al. 1,25-Dihydroxycholecalciferol stimulates osteoclasts in rat bones in the absence of parathyroid hormone. Endocrinology 1981; 108:2293–2301.

193. Beresford JN, Gallagher JA, Russell RGG. 1,25-Dihydroxyvitamin D_3 and human bone-derived cells in vitro: effects on alkaline phosphatase, type I collagen, and proliferation. Endocrinology 1986; 119:1776–1785.

194. Price PA, Baukol SA. 1,25-Dihydroxyvitamin D_3 increases synthesis of the vitamin K–dependent bone protein by osteosarcoma cells. J Biol Chem 1980; 255:11660–11663.

195. Okazaki T, Igarashi T, Kronenberg HM. 5'-Flanking region of the parathyroid hormone gene mediates negative regulation by 1,25-$(OH)_2$ vitamin D_3. J Biol Chem 1988; 263:2203–2208.

196. Suda T, Miyaura C, Abe E, et al. Modulation of cell differentiation, immune responses and tumor promotion by vitamin D compounds. In Peck WA, ed. Bone and Mineral Research/4. New York: Elsevier, 1986: 1–48.

197. Haussler MR, Mangelsdorf DJ, Komm BS, et al. Molecular biology of the vitamin D hormone. Recent Prog Horm Res 1988; 44:263–296.

198. Halloran BP, De Luca HF. Appearance of the intestinal cytosolic receptor for 1,25-dihydroxyvitamin D_3 during neonatal development in the rat. J Biol Chem 1982; 256:7338–7342.

199. Hirst MA, Feldman D. Glucocorticoids downregulate the number of 1,25-dihydroxyvitamin D_3 receptors in mouse intestine. Biochem Biophys Res Commun 1981; 105:1590–1596.

200. Stern PH, Hamstra AJ, DeLuca HF, et al. A bioassay capable of measuring 1 picogram of 1,25-dihydroxy vitamin D_3. J Clin Endocrinol Metab 1978; 46:891–896.

201. Hughes MR, Baylink DJ, Jones PG, et al. Radioligand receptor assay for 25-hydroxyvitamin D_2/D_3 and 1-alpha,25-dihydroxyvitamin D_2/D_3: application to hypervitaminosis D. J Clin Invest 1976; 58:61–70.

202. Porteous CE, Coldwell RD, Trafford DJ, et al. Recent developments in the measurement of vitamin D and its metabolites in human body fluids. J Steroid Biochem 1987; 28:785–801.

203. Binderman I, Somjen D. 24,25-Dihydroxycholecalciferol induces the growth of chick cartilage in vitro. Endocrinology 1984; 115:430–432.

204. Nakamura T, Kurokawa T, Orimo H. Increase of bone volume in vitamin D–repleted rats by massive administration of 24R,25-$(OH)_2D_3$. Calcif Tissue Int 1988; 43:235–243.

205. Brommage R, DeLuca HF. Evidence that 1,25-dihydroxyvitamin D_3 is the physiologically active metabolite of vitamin D_3. Endocr Rev 1985; 6:491–507.

206. Markestad T, Hesse V, Siebenhuner M, et al. Intermittent high-dose vitamin D prophylaxis during infancy: effect on vitamin D metabolites, calcium, and phosphorus. Am J Clin Nutr 1987; 46:652–658.

207. Maierhofer WJ, Lemann J Jr, Graw RW, et al. Dietary calcium and serum 1,25-$(OH)_2$–vitamin D concentrations as determinants of calcium balance in healthy men. Kidney Int 1984; 26:752–759.

208. Ernst M, Schmid C, Froesch ER. Enhanced osteoblast proliferation and collagen gene expression by estradiol. Proc Natl Acad Sci USA 1988; 85:2307–2310.

209. Corvol MT, Carrascosa A, Tsagris L, et al. Evidence for a direct in vitro action of sex steroids on rabbit cartilage cells during skeletal growth: influence of age and sex. Endocrinology 1987; 120:1422–1429.

210. Burman KD, Monchik JM, Earll JM, et al. Ionized and total serum calcium and parathyroid hormone in hyperthyroidism. Ann Intern Med 1976; 84:668–671.

211. Burch WM, Lebovitz HE. Triiodothyronine stimulates maturation of porcine growth-plate cartilage in vitro. J Clin Invest 1982; 70:496–504.

212. Dewhirst FE, Stashenko PP, Mole JE, et al. Purification and partial sequence of human osteoclast-activating factor: identity with interleukin 1B. J Immunol 1985; 135:2562–2568.

213. Garrett IR, Durie BGM, Nedwin GE, et al. Production of lymphotoxin, a bone-resorbing cytokine by cultured human myeloma cells. N Engl J Med 1987; 317:526–532.

214. Katz A, Braunstein GD. Clinical, biochemical, and pathologic features of radiation-associated hyperparathyroidism. Arch Intern Med 1983; 143:79–82.

215. Beard CM, Heath H 3d, O'Fallon WM, et al. Therapeutic radiation and hyperparathyroidism. A case-control study in Rochester, Minn. Arch Intern Med 1989; 149:1887–1890.

216. Arnold A, Kim HG, Gaz RD, et al. Molecular cloning and chromosomal mapping of DNA rearranged with the parathyroid hormone gene in a parathyroid adenoma. J Clin Invest 1989; 83:3024–3040.

217. Friedman E, Sakaguchi K, Bale AE, et al. Clonality of parathyroid tumors in familial multiple endocrine neoplasia type I. N Engl J Med 1989; 321:213–218.

218. Thakker RV, Bouloux P, Wooding C, et al. Association of parathyroid tumors in multiple endocrine neoplasia type I with loss of alleles on chromosome 11. N Engl J Med 1989; 321:218–224.

219. Larsson C, Skogseid B, Oberg K, et al. Multiple endocrine neoplasia type I gene maps to chromosome 11 and is lost in insulinoma. Nature 1988; 332:85–87.

220. Bale SJ, Bale AE, Stewart K, et al. Linkage analysis of multiple endocrine neoplasia type I with Int2 and other markers on chromosome 11. Genomics 1989; 4:320–322.

221. Boonstra CE, Jackson CE. Serum calcium survey for hyperparathyroidism: results in 50,000 clinic patients. Am J Clin Pathol 1971; 55:523–526.

222. Poole GV Jr, Albertson DA, Marshall RB, et al. Oxyphil cell adenoma and hyperparathyroidism. Surgery 1982; 92:799–805.

223. Geelhoed GW. Parathyroid adenolipoma: clinical and morphologic features. Surgery 1982; 92:806–810.

224. Black WC III, Utley Jr. The differential diagnosis of parathyroid hyperplasia and chief cell adenoma. Am J Clin Pathol 1968; 49:761–774.

225. Fialkow PJ, Jackson CJ, Block MA, et al. Multicellular origin of parathyroid "adenomas." N Engl J Med 1977; 297:696–698.

226. Woltering EA, Emmot RC, Javadpour N, et al. ABO (H) cell surface antigens in parathyroid adenoma and hyperplasia. Surgery 1981; 90:1–9.

227. Dekker A, Watson CG, Barnes EL Jr. The pathologic assessment of primary hyperparathyroidism and its impact on therapy. Ann Surg 1979; 190:671–675.

228. Paloyan E, Lawrence AM. Primary hyperparathyroidism: pathology and therapy. JAMA 1981; 246:1344.

229. Verdonk CA, Edis AJ. Parathyroid "double adenomas": fact or fiction? Surgery 1981; 90:523–526.

230. Shane E, Bilezikian JP. Parathyroid carcinoma: a review of 62 patients. Endocr Rev 1982; 3:218–226.

231. Broadus AE, Horst RL, Llang R, et al. The importance of circulating 1,25-dihydroxyvitamin D in the pathogenesis of hypercalciuria and renal stone formation in primary hyperparathyroidism. N Engl J Med 1980; 302:421–426.

232. Mallette LE, Bilezikian JP, Heath DA, et al. Primary hyperparathyroidism: clinical and biochemical features. Medicine 1974; 53:127–146.

233. Norton JA, Cornelius MJ, Doppman JL, et al. Effect of parathyroidectomy in patients with hyperparathyroidism, Zollinger-Ellison syndrome, and multiple endocrine neoplasia type I: a prospective study. Surgery 1987; 102:958–966.

234. Betts JB, O'Malley BP, Rosenthal FD. Hyperparathyroidism: a prerequisite for Zollinger-Ellison syndrome in multiple endocrine adenomatosis type I—report of further family and a review of the literature. Q J Med 1980; 49:69–76.

235. Patten BM, Bilezikian JP, Mallette LE, et al. Neuromuscular disease in hyperparathyroidism. Ann Intern Med 1974; 80:182–193.

236. Wersall-Robertson E, Hamberger B, Ehren H, et al. Increase in muscular strength following surgery for primary hyperparathyroidism. Acta Med Scand 1986; 220:233–235.

237. Albright F, Aub JC, Bauer W. Hyperparathyroidism. JAMA 1934; 102:1276–1287.

238. Sangal AK, Beevers DG. Parathyroid hypertension. Br Med J 1983; 286:498–499.

239. Resnick LM, Laragh JH, Sealey JE, et al. Divalent cations in essential hypertension. N Engl J Med 1983; 309:888–891.

240. Salahudeen AK, Thomas TH, Sellars L, et al. Hypertension and renal dysfunction in primary hyperparathyroidism: effect of parathyroidectomy. Clin Sci 1989; 76:289–296.

241. Doppman JL, Krudy AG, Brennan MF, et al. CT appearance of enlarged parathyroid glands in the posterior superior mediastinum. J Comput Assist Tomogr 1982; 6:1099–1102.

241a. Flentje D, Schmidt-Gayk H, Fischer S, et al. Intact parathyroid hormone in primary hyperparathyroidism. Br J Surg 1990; 77:168–172.

242. Mallette LE, Sode JE, Marx SJ, et al. Total body retention of orally administered calcium in primary hyperparathyroidism. J Clin Endocrinol Metab 1975; 40:582–588.

243. Jaeger P, Jones W, Kashgarian M, et al. Parathyroid hormone directly inhibits tubular reabsorption of bicarbonate in normocalcaemic rats with chronic hyperparathyroidism. Eur J Clin Invest 1987; 17:415–420.

244. Muldowney FP, Carroll DV, Donohoe JF, et al. Correction of renal bicarbonate wastage by parathyroidectomy. Q J Med 1971; 40:487–498.

245. Gold LW, Massry SG, Arieff AI, et al. Renal bicarbonate wasting during phosphate depletion: a possible cause of altered acid-base homeostasis in hyperparathyroidism. J Clin Invest 1973; 52:2556–2562.

246. Brown EM, LeBoff MS, Oetting M, et al. Secretory control in normal and abnormal parathyroid tissue. Recent Prog Horm Res 1987; 43:337–382.

247. Simeone JF, Mueller PR, Gerrucci JT, et al. High-resolution real-time sonography of the parathyroid. Radiology 1981; 141:745–751.

248. Reading CC, Cargoneau JW, James EM, et al. High-resolution parathyroid sonography. AJR 1982; 139:539–546.

249. Young AE, Gaunt JI, Croft DN, et al. Location of parathyroid adenomas by thallium-201 and technetium-99m subtraction scanning. Br Med J 1983; 286:1384–1386.

250. Brennan MF, Doppman JL, Krudy AG, et al. Assessment of techniques for preoperative parathyroid gland localization in patients undergoing reoperation for hyperparathyroidism. Surgery 1982; 91:6–11.

251. Doppman JL, Krudy AG, Marx SJ, et al. Aspiration of enlarged parathyroid glands for parathyroid hormone assay. Radiology 1983; 148:31–35.

252. Scholz DA, Purnell DC. Asymptomatic primary hyperparathyroidism. 10-year prospective study. Mayo Clin Proc 1981; 56:473–478.

253. Selby PL, Peacock M. Ethinyl estradiol and norethindrone in the treatment of primary hyperparathyroidism in postmenopausal women. N Engl J Med 1986; 314:1481–1485.

254. Broadus AE, Magee JS, Mallette LE, et al. A detailed evaluation of oral phosphate therapy in selected patients with primary hyperparathyroidism. J Clin Endocrinol 1983; 56:953–961.

255. Shane E, Baquiran DC, Bilezikian JP. Effects of dichloromethylene diphosphonate on serum and urinary calcium in primary hyperparathyroidism. Ann Intern Med 1981; 95:23.

256. Castleman B, Schwartz A, Roth SI. Parathyroid hyperplasia in primary hyperparathyroidism. Cancer 1976; 38:1668–1675.

257. Wells SA Jr, Farndon JR, Dale JK, et al. Long-term evaluation of patients with primary parathyroid hyperplasia managed by total parathyroidectomy and heterotopic autotransplantation. Ann Surg 1980; 192:451–458.

258. Wells SA Jr, Ellis GJ, Gunnells JC, et al. Parathyroid autotransplantation in primary parathyroid hyperplasia. N Engl J Med 1976; 295:57–62.

259. Brennan MF, Marx SJ, Doppman JL, et al. Results of reoperation for persistent and recurrent hyperparathyroidism. Ann Surg 1981; 194:671–676.

260. Stock JL, Weintraub BD, Rosen SW, et al. Human chorionic gonadotropin subunit measurement in primary hyperparathyroidism. J Clin Endocrinol Metab 1982; 54:57–63.

261. Spiegel AM, Eastman ST, Attie MF, et al. Intraoperative measurements of urinary cyclic AMP to guide surgery for primary hyperparathyroidism. N Engl J Med 1980; 303:1457–1460.

262. Norton JA, Brennan MF, Saxe AW, et al. Intraoperative urinary cyclic adenosine monophosphate as a guide to successful reoperative parathyroidectomy. Ann Surg 1984; 200:389–395.

263. Albright F, Reifenstein EC Jr. The Parathyroid Glands and Metabolic Bone Disease. Baltimore: Williams & Wilkins, 1948: 113.

264. Leppla DC, Snyder W, Pak CYC. Sequential changes in bone density before and after parathyroidectomy in primary hyperparathyroidism. Invest Radiol 1982; 17:604–606.

265. Shangold MM, Dor N, Welt SI, et al. Hyperparathyroidism and pregnancy: a review. Obstet Gynecol Surv 1982; 37:217–228.

266. Kristoffersson A, Dahlgren S, Lithner F, et al. Primary hyperparathyroidism in pregnancy. Surgery 1985; 97:326–330.

267. Cushard WG, Creditor MA, Canterbury JM, et al. Physiologic hyperparathyroidism in pregnancy. J Clin Endocrinol Metab 1976; 34:767–771.

268. Delmonico FL, Neer RM, Cosimi AB, et al. Hyperparathyroidism during pregnancy. Am J Surg 1976; 131:329–337.

269. Abbas SK, Pickard DW, Rodda CP, et al. Stimulation of ovine placental calcium transport by purified natural and recombinant parathyroid hormone–related protein (PTHrP) preparations. Q J Exp Phys 1989; 74:549–552.

270. Marx SJ, Attie MR, Spiegel AM, et al. An association between neonatal severe primary hyperparathyroidism and familial hypocalciuric hypercalcemia in three kindreds. N Engl J Med 1982; 306:257–264.

271. Marx SJ, Spiegel AM, Levine AM, et al. Familial hypocalciuric hypercalcemia: the relation to primary parathyroid hyperplasia. N Engl J Med 1982; 307:416–426.

272. Christensson T. Familial hyperparathyroidism. Ann Intern Med 1976; 85:614–615.

273. Brandi ML, Marx SJ, Aurbach GD, et al. Familial multiple endocrine neoplasia type 1: a new look at pathophysiology. Endocr Rev 1987; 8:391–405.

274. Mallette LE, Malini S, Rappoport MP, et al. Familial cystic parathyroid adenomatosis. Ann Intern Med 1987; 107:54–60.

275. Brandi ML, Aurbach GD, Fitzpatrick LA, et al. Parathyroid mitogenic activity in plasma from patients with familial multiple endocrine neoplasia type 1. N Engl J Med 1986; 314:1287–1293.

276. Larsson C, Skogseid B, Oberg K, et al. Multiple endocrine neoplasia type 1 gene maps to chromosome 11 and is lost in insulinoma. Nature 1988; 332:85–87.

277. Massry SG, Coburn JW, Lee DBN, et al. Skeletal resistance to parathyroid hormone in renal failure. Ann Intern Med 1973; 78:357–364.

278. Llach F, Massry SG, Singer FR, et al. Skeletal resistance to endogenous parathyroid hormone in patients with early renal failure: a possible cause for secondary hyperparathyroidism. J Clin Endocrinol Metab 1975; 41:339–345.

279. Hanley DA, Sherwood LM. Secondary hyperparathyroidism in chronic renal failure: pathophysiology and treatment. Med Clin North Am 1978; 62:1319–1339.

280. Quarles LD, Davidai GA, Schwab SJ, et al. Oral calcitriol and calcium: efficient therapy for uremic hyperparathyroidism. Kidney Int 1988; 34:840–844.

281. Andress DL, Norris KC, Coburn JW, et al. Intravenous calcitriol in the treatment of refractory osteitis fibrosa of chronic renal failure. N Engl J Med 1989; 321:274–279.

282. Conceicao SC, Wilkinson R, Feest TG, et al. Hypercalcemia following renal transplantation: causes and consequences. Clin Nephrol 1981; 16:235–244.

283. Parfitt AM. Hypercalcemic hyperparathyroidism following renal transplantation: differential diagnosis, management, and implications for cell population control in the parathyroid gland. Miner Electrolyte Metab 1982; 8:92–112.

284. Cannata JF, Briggs JD, Junor BJ, et al. Effect of acute aluminum overload on calcium and parathyroid-hormone metabolism. Clin Nephrol 1981; 16:235–244.

285. Dudley HR, Ritchie AC, Schilling A, et al. Pathologic changes associated with the use of sodium ethylene diamine tetra-acetate in the treatment of hypercalcemia. N Engl J Med 1955; 252:331–337.

286. Perlia CP, Gubisch NJ, Wolter J, et al. Mithramycin treatment of hypercalcemia. Cancer 1970; 25:389–394.

287. Brautbar N, Luboshitzky R. Combined calcitonin and oral phosphate treatment for hypercalcemia in multiple myeloma. Arch Intern Med 1977; 137:914–916.

288. Binstock ML, Mundy GR. Effect of calcitonin and glucocorticoids in combination on the hypercalcemia of malignancy. Ann Intern Med 1980; 93:269–272.

289. Ralston S, Gardner MD, Dryburgh FJ, et al. Comparison of aminohydroxypropylidene diphosphonate, mithramycin, and corticosteroids/calcitonin in treatment of cancer-associated hypercalcemia. Lancet 1985; 2:907–910.

290. Heath DA. The use of inorganic phosphate in the management of hypercalcemia. Metab Bone Dis Relat Res 1980; 2:213–215.

291. Spiegel AM, Greene M, Magrath I, et al. Hypercalcemia with suppressed parathyroid hormone in Burkitt's lymphoma. Am J Med 1978; 64:691–695.

292. Jacobs TP, Siris ES, Bilezikian JP, et al. Hypercalcemia of malignancy: treatment with intravenous dichloromethylene diphosphonate. Ann Intern Med 1981; 94:312–316.

293. van Breukelen FJM, Bijvoet OLM, Frijlink WB, et al. Efficacy of aminohydroxypropylidene biphosphonate in hypercalcemia: observations on regulation of serum calcium. Calcif Tissue Int 1982; 34:321–327.

294. Ryzen E, Martodam RR, Troxell M, et al. Intravenous etidronate in the management of malignant hypercalcemia. Arch Intern Med 1985; 145:449–452.

295. Mundy GR, Wilkinson R, Heath DA. Comparative study of available medical therapy for hypercalcemia of malignancy. Am J Med 1983; 94:421–432.

296. Warrell RP Jr, Israel R, Frisone M, et al. Gallium nitrate for acute treatment of cancer-related hypercalcemia. Ann Intern Med 1988; 108:669–674.

297. Glover DJ, Shaw L, Glick JH, et al. Treatment of hypercalcemia in parathyroid cancer with WR-2721, S-2-(3-aminopropylamino)ethylphosphorothioic acid. Ann Intern Med 1985; 103:55–57.

298. Fisken RA, Heath DA, Somers S. Hypercalcemia in hospital patients: clinical and diagnostic aspects. Lancet 1981; 1:202–207.

299. Lufkin EG, DeRemee RA, Rohrbach MS. The predictive value of serum angiotensin-converting enzyme activity in the differential diagnosis of hypercalcemia. Mayo Clin Proc 1983; 58:447–451.

300. Ralston S, Fogelman I, Gardner MD, et al. Hypercalcemia and metastatic bone disease: is there a causal link? Lancet 1982; 2:903–905.

301. Ralston SH, Gardner MD, Jenkins AS, et al. Malignancy-associated hypercalcemia: relationship between mechanisms of hypercalcemia and response to antihypercalcemic therapy. Bone Miner 1987; 2:227–242.

302. Valentin-Opran A, Eilon G, Saez S, et al. Estrogens and antiestrogens stimulate release of bone resorbing activity by cultured human breast cancer cells. J Clin Invest 1985; 75:726–731.

303. Legha SS, Powell K, Buzdar AU, et al. Tamoxifen-induced hypercalcemia in breast cancer. Cancer 1981; 47:2803–2806.

304. Eilon G, Mundy GR. Direct resorption of bone by human breast cancer cells in vitro. Nature 1978; 276:726–728.

305. Hickey RC, Samaan NA, Jackson GL. Hypercalcemia in patients with breast cancer. Arch Surg 1981; 116:545–552.

306. Mundy GR, Raisz LG, Cooper RA, et al. Evidence for the secretion of an osteoclast stimulating factor in myeloma. N Engl J Med 1974; 291:1041–1046.

307. Garrett IR, Durie BGM, Nedwin GE, et al. Production of lymphotoxin, a bone-resorbing cytokine, by cultured human myeloma cells. N Engl J Med 1987; 317:526–532.

308. Breslau NA, McGuire JL, Zerwekh JE, et al. Hypercalcemia associated with increased serum calcitriol levels in three patients with lymphoma. Ann Intern Med 1984; 100:1–7.

309. Jacobson JO, Bringhurst FR, Harris NL, et al. Humoral hypercalcemia in Hodgkin's disease. Cancer 1989; 63:917–923.

310. Blayney DW, Jaffe ES, Fisher RI, et al. The human T-cell leukemia/lymphoma virus, lymphoma, lytic bone lesions, and hypercalcemia. Ann Intern Med 1983; 98:144–151.

311. Dodd RC, Winkler CF, Williams ME, et al. Calcitriol levels in hypercal-

cemic patients with adult T-cell lymphoma. Arch Intern Med 1986; 146:1971–1972.

312. Yoshimoto K, Yamasaki R, Sakai H, et al. Ectopic production of parathyroid hormone by small cell lung cancer in a patient with hypercalcemia. J Clin Endocrinol Metab 1989; 68:976–981.

313. Yamamoto I, Kitamura N, Aoki J, et al. Circulating 1,25-dihydroxyvitamin D concentrations in patients with renal cell carcinoma–associated hypercalcemia are rarely suppressed. J Clin Endocrinol Metab 1987; 64:175–179.

314. Linkhart TA, Mohan S, Jennings JC, et al. Copurification of osteolytic and transforming growth factor β activities produced by human lung tumor cells associated with humoral hypercalcemia of malignancy. Cancer Res 1989; 49:271–278.

315. Bringhurst FR, Bierer BE, Godeau F, et al. Humoral hypercalcemia of malignancy: release of a prostaglandin-stimulating bone-resorbing factor in vitro by human transitional carcinoma cells. J Clin Invest 1986; 77:456–464.

316. Daly JG, Greenwood RM, Himsworth RL. Serum calcium concentration in hyperthyroidism at diagnosis and after treatment. Clin Endocrinol 1983; 19:397–404.

317. Mallette LE, Rubenfeld S, Silverman V. A controlled study of the effects of thyrotoxicosis and propranolol treatment on mineral metabolism and parathyroid hormone immunoreactivity. Metabolism 1985; 34:999–1006.

318. Iqbal SJ, Taylor WH. Treatment of vitamin D_2 poisoning by induction of hepatic enzymes. Br Med J 1982; 285:541–542.

319. Frame B, Jackson CE, Reynolds WA, et al. Hypercalcemia and skeletal effects in chronic hypervitaminosis A. Ann Intern Med 1974; 80:44–48.

320. Valentic JP, Elias AN, Weinstein GD. Hypercalcemia associated with oral isotretinoin in the treatment of severe acne. JAMA 1983; 250:1899–1900.

321. Bell NH, Stern PH, Pantzer E, et al. Evidence that increased circulating 1,25-dihydroxyvitamin D is the probable cause for abnormal calcium metabolism in sarcoidosis. J Clin Invest 1979; 64:218–225.

322. Papapoulos SE, Clemens TL, Fraher LJ, et al. 1,25-Dihydroxycholecalciferol in the pathogenesis of the hypercalcemia of sarcoidosis. Lancet 1979; 1:627–630.

323. Singer FR, Adams JS. Abnormal calcium homeostasis in sarcoidosis. N Engl J Med 1986; 315:755–757.

324. O'Leary TJ, Jones G, Yip A, et al. The effects of choloroquine on serum 1,25-dihydroxyvitamin D and calcium metabolism in sarcoidosis. N Engl J Med 1986; 315:727–730.

325. Zimmerman J, Holick MF, Silver J. Normocalcemia in a hypoparathyroid patient with sarcoidosis: evidence for parathyroid hormone–independent synthesis of 1,25 dihydroxyvitamin D. Ann Intern Med 1983; 98:338–339.

326. Lemann J Jr, Gray RW. Calcitriol, calcium, and granulomatous disease. N Engl J Med 1984; 311:1115–1117.

327. Taylor AB, Stern PH, Bell NH. Abnormal regulation of circulating 25-hydroxyvitamin D in the Williams syndrome. N Engl J Med 1982; 306:972–975.

328. Garabedian M, Jacqz E, Guillozo H, et al. Elevated plasma 1,25-dihydroxyvitamin D concentrations in infants with hypercalcemia and elfin facies. N Engl J Med 1985; 312:948–952.

329. Mills E, Bouillon JE, Boelaert J, et al. Etiology of hypercalcemia in a patient with Addison's disease. Calcif Tissue Int 1982; 34:523–526.

330. Orwoll ES. The milk-alkali syndrome: current concepts. Ann Intern Med 1982; 97:242–248.

331. Christensson T, Hellstrom K, Wengle B. Hypercalcemia and primary hyperparathyroidism: prevalence in patients receiving thiazides as detected in a health screen. Arch Intern Med 1977; 137:1138–1142.

332. Stewart AF, Adler M, Byers CM, et al. Calcium homeostasis in immobilization: an example of resorptive hypercalciuria. N Engl J Med 1982; 306:1136–1140.

333. Llach F, Felsenfeld AJ, Haussler MR. The pathophysiology of altered calcium metabolism in rhabdomyolysis-induced acute renal failure. N Engl J Med 1981; 305:117–123.

334. Akmal M, Bishop JE, Telfer N, et al. Hypocalcemia and hypercalcemia in patients with rhabdomyolysis with and without acute renal failure. J Clin Endocrinol Metab 1986; 63:137–142.

335. Connor TB, Rosen BL, Blaustein MB, et al. Hypocalcemia precipitating congestive heart failure. N Engl J Med 1982; 307:869–872.

336. Jensen SB, Illum F, Dupont E. Nature and frequency of dental changes in idiopathic hypoparathyroidism and pseudohypoparathyroidism. Scand J Dent Res 1981; 89:26–37.

337. Stuart C, Aceto T Jr, Kuhn JP, et al. Intrauterine hyperparathyroidism. Am J Dis Child 1979; 133:67–70.

338. Mallette LE. Synthetic human parathyroid hormone 1–34 fragment for diagnostic testing. Ann Intern Med 1988; 109:800–804.

339. Gann DS, Paone JF. Delayed hypocalcemia after thyroidectomy for Graves' disease is prevented by parathyroid autotransplantation. Ann Surg 1979; 190:508–513.

340. Burch WM, Posillico JT. Hypoparathyroidism after I-131 therapy with subsequent return of parathyroid function. J Clin Endocrinol Metab 1983; 57:398–401.

341. Posillico JT, Wortsman J, Srikanta S, et al. Parathyroid cell surface autoantibodies that inhibit parathyroid hormone secretion from dispersed human parathyroid cells. J Bone Miner Res 1986; 1:475–483.

342. Fattorossi A, Aurbach GD, Sakaguchi K, et al. Anti–endothelial cell antibodies: detection and characterization in sera from patients with autoimmune hypoparathyroidism. Proc Natl Acad Sci USA 1988; 85:4015–4019.

343. Neufeld M, Maclaren NK, Blizzard RM. Two types of autoimmune Addison's disease associated with different polyglandular autoimmune (PGA) syndromes. Medicine 1981; 60:355–362.

344. Bergada I, Schiffrin A, Abu Srair H, et al. Kenny syndrome: description of additional abnormalities and molecular studies. Hum Genet 1988; 80:39–42.

345. Rude RK, Oldham SB, Sharp CF Jr, et al. Parathyroid hormone secretion in magnesium deficiency. J Clin Endocrinol Metab 1978; 47:800–806.

346. Cholst IN, Steinberg SF, Tropper PJ, et al. The influence of hypermagnesemia on serum calcium and parathyroid hormone levels in human subjects. N Engl J Med 1984; 310:1221–1225.

347. Horwitz CA, Myers WPL, Foote FW Jr. Secondary malignant tumors of the parathyroid glands. Am J Med 1972; 52:797–808.

348. Freedman DB, Shannon M, Dandona P, et al. Hypoparathyroidism and hypocalcemia during treatment for acute leukemia. Br Med J 1982; 284:700–702.

349. Brezis M, Shaley O, Leibel B, et al. The spectrum of parathyroid function in thalassemia subjects with transfusional iron overload. Miner Electrolyte Metab 1982; 8:307–313.

350. Carpenter TO, Carnes DL Jr, Anast CS. Hypoparathyroidism in Wilson's disease. N Engl J Med 1983; 309:873–877.

351. Gidding SS, Minciotti AL, Langman CB. Unmasking of hypoparathyroidism in familial partial DiGeorge syndrome by challenge with disodium edetate. N Engl J Med 1988; 319:1589–1591.

352. Breslau NA, Pak CYC. Hypoparathyroidism. Metabolism 1979; 28:1261–1276.

353. Ahn TG, Antonarakis SE, Kronenberg HM, et al. Familial isolated hypoparathyroidism: a molecular genetic analysis of 8 families with 23 affected persons. Medicine 1986; 65:73–81.

354. Albright F, Burnett C, Smith PH, et al. Pseudo-hypoparathyroidism—an example of "Seabright-Bantam" syndrome. Endocrinology 1942; 30:922–932.

355. Levine MA, Downs RW Jr, Singer M, et al. Deficient activity of guanine nucleotide regulatory protein in erythrocytes from patients with pseudohypoparathyroidism. Biochem Biophys Res Commun 1980; 94:1319–1324.

356. Farfel Z, Brickman AS, Kaslow HR, et al. Defect of receptor-cyclase coupling protein in pseudohypoparathyroidism. N Engl J Med 1980; 303:237–242.

357. Carter A, Bardin C, Collins R, et al. Reduced expression of multiple forms of the alpha subunit of the stimulatory GTP-binding protein in pseudohypoparathyroidism type Ia. Proc Natl Acad Sci USA 1987; 84:7266–7269.

358. Levine MA, Downs RW Jr, Moses AM, et al. Resistance to multiple hormones in patients with pseudohypoparathyroidism: association with deficient activity of guanine nucleotide regulatory protein. Am J Med 1983; 74:545–556.

359. Levine MA, Jap TS, Hung W. Infantile hypothyroidism in two sibs: an unusual presentation of pseudohypoparathyroidism type Ia. J Pediatr 1985; 107:919–922.

360. Van Dop C, Bourne HR. Pseudohypoparathyroidism. Annu Rev Med 1983; 34:259–266.

361. Levine MA, Jap TS, Mauseth RS, et al. Activity of the stimulatory guanine nucleotide binding protein is reduced in erythrocytes from patients with pseudohypoparathyroidism and pseudopseudohypoparathyroidism: biochemical, endocrine, and genetic analysis of Albright's hereditary osteodystrophy in 6 kindreds. J Clin Endocrinol Metab 1986; 62:497–502.

362. Brickman AS, Carlson HE, Deftos LJ. Prolactin and calcitonin responses to parathyroid hormone infusion in hypoparathyroid, pseudohypoparathyroid, and normal subjects. J Clin Endocrinol Metab 1981; 53:661–664.

363. Silve C, Santora A, Breslau N, et al. Selective resistance to parathyroid hormone in cultured skin fibroblasts from patients with pseudohypoparathyroidism type Ib. J Clin Endocrinol Metab 1986; 62:640–644.

364. Drezner M, Neelon FA, Lebovitz HE. Pseudohypoparathyroidism type II: a possible defect in the reception of the cyclic AMP signal. N Engl J Med 1973; 289:1056–1060.

365. Rao DS, Parfitt AM, Kleerekoper M, et al. Dissociation between the effects of endogenous parathyroid hormone on adenosine 3′,5′-monophosphate generation and phosphate reabsorption in hypocalcemia due to vitamin D depletion: an acquired disorder resembling pseudohypoparathyroidism type II. J Clin Endocrinol Metab 1985; 61:285–290.

366. Breslau NA, Weinstock RS. Regulation of 1,25(OH)$_2$D synthesis in hypoparathyroidism and pseudohypoparathyroidism. Am J Physiol 1988; 255:E730–E736.

367. Breslau NA, Moses AM, Pak CYC. Evidence for bone remodeling but

lack of calcium mobilization response to parathyroid hormone in pseu-dohypoparathyroidism. J Clin Endocrinol Metab 1983; 57:638–644.

368. Porter RH, Cox BG, Heaney D, et al. Treatment of hypoparathyroid patients with chlorthalidone. N Engl J Med 1978; 298:577–581.

369. Gabow PA, Hanson TJ, Popovtzer MM, et al. Furosemide-induced reduction in ionized calcium in hypoparathyroid patients. Ann Intern Med 1977; 86:579–581.

370. Raskin P, McClain CJ, Medsger TA Jr. Hypocalcemia associated with metastatic bone disease. Arch Intern Med 1973; 132:539–543.

371. Dunlay RW, Camp MA, Allon M, et al. Calcitriol in prolonged hypocal-cemia due to the tumor lysis syndrome. Ann Intern Med 1989; 110:162–164.

372. Stewart AF, Longo W, Kreutter D, et al. Hypocalcemia associated with calcium-soap formation in a patient with a pancreatic fistula. N Engl J Med 1986; 315:496–498.

373. Zaloga GP, Chernow B. The multifactorial basis for hypocalcemia during sepsis. Ann Intern Med 1987; 107:36–41.

374. Cardenas-Rivero N, Chernow B, Stoiko MA, et al. Hypocalcemia in critically ill children. J Pediatr 1989; 114:946–951.

375. Chesney RW, McCarron DM, Haddad JG, et al. Pathogenic mechanisms of the hypocalcemia of the staphylococcal toxic-shock syndrome. J Lab Clin Med 1983; 101:576–585.

376. Berner YN, Shike M. Consequences of phosphate imbalance. Annu Rev Nutr 1988; 8:121–148.

377. Lotz M, Zisman E, Bartter FC. Evidence for a phosphorus-depletion syndrome in man. N Engl J Med 1968; 278:409–415.

378. Haut LL, Alfrey AC, Guggenheim S, et al. Renal toxicity of phosphate in rats. Kidney Int 1980; 17:722–731.

379. Prince MJ, Schaeffer PC, Goldsmith RS, et al. Hyperphosphatemic tumoral calcinosis: association with elevation of serum 1,25-dihydroxy-cholecalciferol concentrations. Ann Intern Med 1982; 96:586–591.

380. Cohen LF, Balow JE, Macgrath IT, et al. Acute tumor lysis syndrome: a review of 37 patients with Burkitt's lymphoma. Am J Med 1980; 68:486–491.

381. Miller WL, Meyer WJ, Bartter FC. Intermittent hyperphosphatemia, polyuria, and seizures—a new familial disorder. J Pediatr 1975; 86:233–235.

382. Elin RJ. Magnesium in health and disease. Dis Mon 1988; 34:161–219.

383. Shils ME. Experimental human magnesium depletion. Medicine 1969; 48:61–85.

384. Bar RS, Wilson HE, Mazzaferri EL. Hypomagnesemic hypocalcemia secondary to renal magnesium wasting: a possible consequence of high-dose gentamycin therapy. Ann Intern Med 1975; 82:646–649.

385. Somjen GN, Hilmy M, Stephen CR. Failure to anesthetize human subjects by intravenous administration of magnesium sulfate. J Pharmacol Exp Ther 1966; 154:652–659.

386. Khairi MRA, Dexter RN, Burzynski NJ, et al. Pheochromocytoma and medullary thyroid carcinoma: multiple endocrine neoplasia type III. Medicine 1975; 54:89–112.

387. Chong GC, Beahrs OH, Sizemore GW, et al. Medullary carcinoma of the thyroid gland. Cancer 1975; 35:695–704.

388. DeLellis RA, Nunnemacher G, Wolfe HJ. C-cell hyperplasia: an ultra-structural analysis. Lab Invest 1977; 36:237–248.

389. Norton JA, Froome LC, Farrell RE, et al. Multiple endocrine neoplasia type IIb: the most aggressive form of medullary thyroid carcinoma. Surg Clin North Am 1979; 59:109–118.

390. Mathew CGP, Smith BA, Thorp K, et al. Deletion of genes on chromosome 10 in endocrine neoplasia. Nature 1987; 328:524–526.

391. Graze K, Spiler IJ, Tashjian AH Jr, et al. Natural history of familial medullary thyroid carcinoma. Effect of a program for early diagnosis. N Engl J Med 1978; 299:980–985.

392. Gagel RF, Jackson CE, Block MA, et al. Age-related probability of development of hereditary medullary thyroid carcinoma. J Pediatr 1982; 101:941–946.

28

METABOLIC BONE DISEASE

Gerald D. Aurbach, Stephen J. Marx, and Allen M. Spiegel

INTRODUCTION

This chapter addresses generalized disorders of bone formation and resorption. The first section is a discussion of the biology of bone, bone cells, and mineralization. Skeletal formation and resorption are coupled by concerted actions of osteoblasts and osteoclasts, which, in turn, are regulated by hormones and a series of systemic as well as local factors, some of which are involved in disorders of bone. Next is presented an outline of laboratory tests of bone function, followed by a discussion of rickets and osteomalacia, parathyroid bone disease, Paget disease, osteoporosis, osteogenesis imperfecta, and osteopetrosis. Ectopic calcification, a related but not truly metabolic bone disease, and extraskeletal ossification are presented in the closing section.

BONE STRUCTURE

Skeletal tissue consists of extracellular matrix containing organic (35%) and inorganic (65%) components and cells. The cells account for a minor fraction of bone volume but carry out the dual functions of the skeletal system: (1) regulation of the distribution and content of the inorganic component, thereby helping maintain the serum calcium concentration within a narrow range (mineral homeostasis) and (2) continuous resorption and formation of the matrix (remodeling), allowing the skeletal system to respond to the mechanical forces generated by weight bearing and physical activity (skeletal homeostasis).

Bone Histology

The three main types of bone cells are osteoblasts, osteocytes, and osteoclasts. Osteoblasts are located at the bone-forming surface and are responsible for elaborating the organic components of the extracellular matrix. The unmineralized matrix forms the osteoid seam or zone; approximately 10 d after the osteoid is formed, mineralization begins. During this interval modification of collagen (maturation) facilitates calcification. The junction between mineralized bone and unmineralized osteoid is known as the *calcification front*. This region selectively incorporates tetracyclines, and this property can be exploited to calculate the linear rate of mineral deposition (Fig. 28–1).

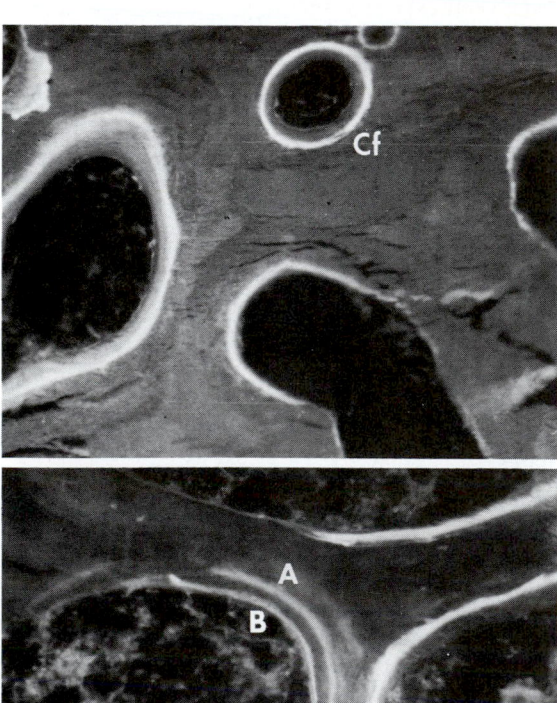

Figure 28–1. Tetracycline labels sites of active mineralization and is deposited at the calcification front (Cf) *(top)*. A double-label technique can be used to measure the rate of mineralization; label A was administered about 10 d before label B *(bottom)*. Undecalcified iliac crest, ultraviolet light, magnification × 113. (From Aaron J. Histology and microanatomy of bone. In: Nordin BEC, ed. Calcium, Phosphate and Magnesium Metabolism. Edinburgh: Churchill Livingstone, 1976: 298–356.)

Osteoblasts, after forming the organic matrix, become surrounded by it and are then termed *osteocytes*. This arbitrary distinction does not imply an abrupt alteration in functional properties, and young osteocytes show many osteoblastic features. Osteoclasts, like osteoblasts, are found at the bone surface and are localized to regions of active bone resorption.

Bone Cell Origin

Labeling studies with tritiated thymidine have been used to identify proliferating osteoprogenitor cells at the bone surface. These cells are indistinguishable from fibroblasts by light microscopy. The preosteoblast is believed to be derived from primitive mesenchymal cells. The transformation of preosteoblasts to osteoblasts and finally to osteocytes takes about 5 d in rats.

Osteoclasts are not derived from an endogenous bone cell but rather from a circulating or resident monocytic precursor, ultimately derived from hematopoietic stem cells. Some forms of osteopetrosis, a disorder caused by abnormal osteoclast function, can be cured in mice and humans by the transplantation of normal marrow or spleen cells.[1] The monocytes and osteoclasts of beige mice contain giant lysosomes. Bone marrow preparations from beige mice injected intravenously into irradiated osteopetrotic mice cure the disorder, and osteoclasts containing giant lysosomes are then found in the bones of the recipient.[2]

OSTEOBLASTS. Active osteoblasts are cuboidal and approximately 20 μm in diameter. The cytoplasm is basophilic, reflecting the extensive rough endoplasmic reticulum characteristic of cells actively engaged in protein synthesis. The Golgi apparatus, which may be important in collagen processing and extrusion, is prominent, and alkaline phosphatase activity is abundant. Osteoblast cell processes may extend within the osteoid zone and communicate with osteocytes. The inactive osteoblast assumes a more flattened fibroblastic appearance; a layer of flattened osteoblasts covering the bone surface may act like a barrier controlling the flow of ions across the bone surface.

OSTEOCYTES. As noted, osteoblasts, once surrounded by matrix, are termed osteocytes. Each cell is surrounded by its own lacuna, but an extensive canlicular system connects osteocytes and surface osteoblasts and probably serves as a channel for the flow of ions and nutrients. The ultrastructure of osteocytes is variable; intracellular organelles may be poorly developed, suggesting a metabolically inactive cell, or a well-developed Golgi apparatus and endoplasmic reticulum may be seen, reflecting active synthetic function. The presence of numerous mitochondria and cytoplasmic vacuoles in certain osteocytes implies a function in bone resorption. In states of excessive parathyroid hormone (PTH) secretion, enlargement of the osteocytic perilacunar space is often observed. This has been interpreted to signify PTH stimulation of osteocytic osteolysis. The importance of this process in mineral homeostasis is not clear, but osteocytic osteolysis may be responsible for the rapid movement of calcium from bone into the extracellular fluid. As bone ages, the number of viable osteocytes decreases with hypermineralization of the osteocytic canaliculi.

OSTEOCLASTS. These multinucleated cells may reach 100 μm in diameter. The osteoclast is highly mobile, moving along the bone surface, actively resorbing bone, and leaving resorption lacunae in its wake. The cytoplasm contains abundant mitochondria, vacuoles, vesicles, and lysosomes containing acid hydrolases important for the bone resorption process. Tartrate-resistant acid phosphatase is a lysosomal enzyme present in the osteoclast. At one surface, the plasma membrane of the osteoclast displays a redundant membrane

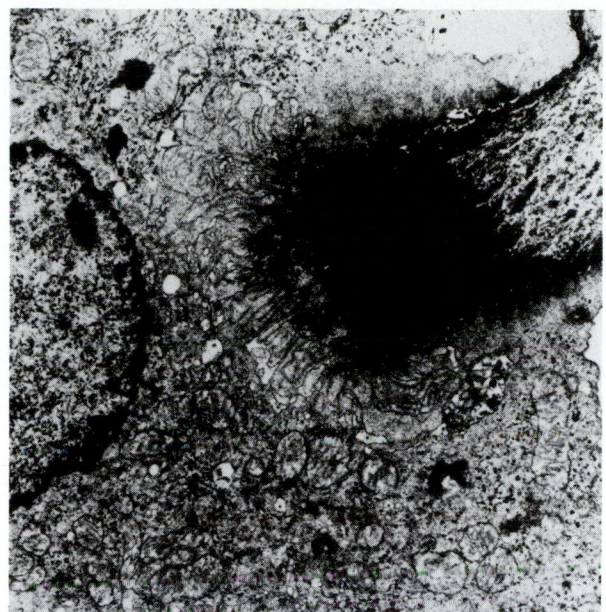

Figure 28–2. Electron micrograph of an osteoclast from a fetal rat bone cultured with PTH. The clear zone of the osteoclast surrounds a bone spicule. Invaginations of the cell membrane adjacent to the one spicule constitute the ruffled border responsible for resorbing mineral and matrix. Magnification × 9100. (From Holtrop ME, Raisz LG, Simmons HA. The effects of parathyroid hormone, colchicine, and calcitonin on the ultrastructure and the activity of osteoclasts in organ culture. Reproduced from the Journal of Cell Biology, 1974, vol. 60, pp. 346–355 by copyright permission of the Rockefeller University Press.)

structure, the ruffled border (Fig. 28–2), under which the clear zone is found, separating bone from osteoclast and representing the area where bone resorption takes place. Acid is released along with acid hydrolases and acid phosphatase into the clear zone region. The ruffled border contains a proton pump that promotes release of acid into the clear zone.[3] Carbonic anhydrase in the osteoclast is also required for acid release. Indeed, one form of osteopetrosis is attributed to carbonic anhydrase deficiency.[4] Osteoclasts normally do not resorb unmineralized osteoid, and the complete sequence of steps in bone resorption is still unknown. For example, it is not known whether organic matrix removal precedes mineral removal. Crystals of hydroxyapatite and collagen fibrils have both been identified between the resorbing surface and the ruffled border.

OTHER CELLS. Other cells found in bone include endothelial cells, fibroblasts, preosteoclasts (of hemopoietic stem cell origin), and preosteoblasts (mesenchymal stem cells).

Cortical and Trabecular Bone

Eighty percent of the skeletal mass is made up of cortical (compact) bone, and 20% is composed of trabecular (cancellous, spongy) bone. The former is found principally in the shafts of long bones, and the latter is present in vertebrae, most flat bones, and the ends of long bones. Microscopic analysis of cortical bone reveals closely packed osteons (haversian systems) consisting of concentric lamellae of bone surrounding a central (haversian) canal; interstitial lamellae, which represent the remains of remodeled osteons; and circumferential lamellae at the periosteal and endosteal surfaces of the bone. The dense structure of cortical bone is pierced by the osteonal central canals as well as the so-called Volkmann canals, which radiate from the central canals to connect neighboring osteons and to form an anastomotic network through which blood and lymph vessels course from the cortex to the periosteum. In trabecular bone,

lamellae are arranged in longitudinal bundles. The individual trabeculae anastomose within the marrow cavity, and their arrangement is dictated by the mechanical stresses on the bone. Although cortical bone makes up the majority of the skeletal mass, its surface area (about 3.2 m²) is smaller than that of trabecular bone (about 16 m²).

Woven and Lamellar Bone

The organic extracellular bone matrix may be arranged in woven or lamellar fashion. This distinction is readily apparent in decalcified bone examined with the polarizing microscope. In woven bone, coarse collagen bundles are irregularly distributed, and osteocytes are randomly positioned. In lamellar bone, collagen bundles are highly ordered; under polarized light one observes alternating isotropic and anisotropic bands (2 to 3 μm thick). Osteocytes are evenly distributed, and their long axes run parallel to those of the lamellae. Woven bone (also termed *immature* or *fibrous*) is seen in embryonic bone and is not normally found after age 2. It appears to be associated with states of rapid bone formation and remodeling and is thus found in fracture callus as well as in Paget disease and osteitis fibrosa (Fig. 28–3).

Control of Bone Formation and Resorption

The skeleton is a dynamic organ that undergoes growth and remodeling until adult height is attained; remodeling

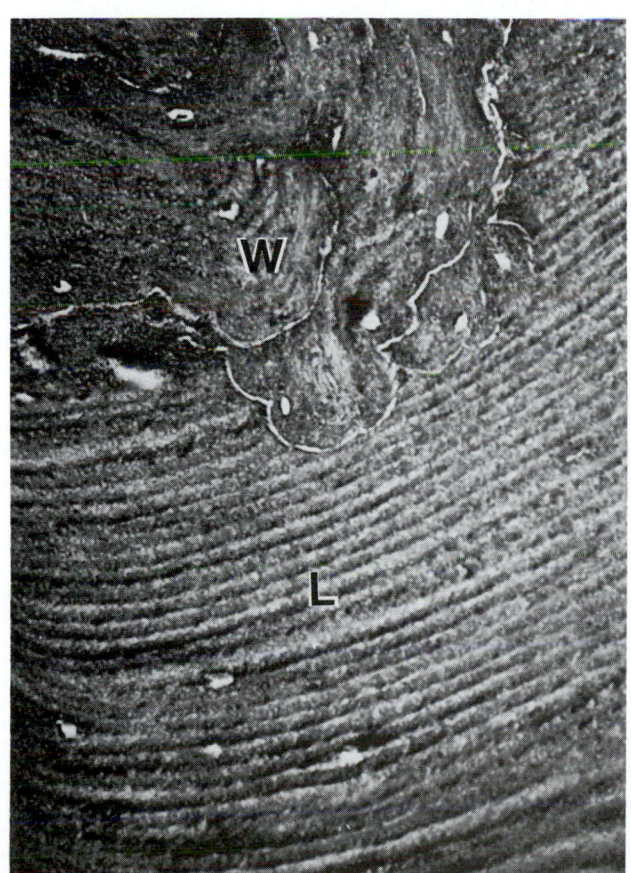

Figure 28–3. Lamellar (L) and woven (W) bone from a patient with Paget disease. Decalcified, hematoxylin and eosin stain, differential contrast optics, magnification × 280. (From Aaron J. Histology and microanatomy of bone. In: Nordin BEC, ed. Calcium, Phosphate and Magnesium Metabolism. Edinburgh: Churchill Livingstone, 1976: 298–356.)

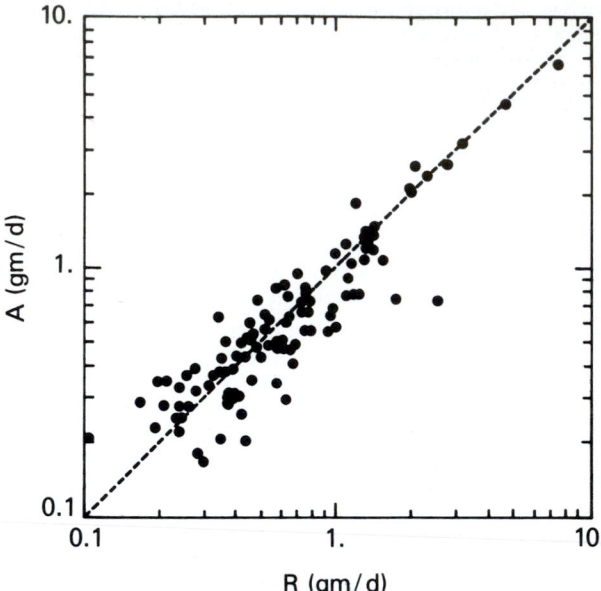

Figure 28–4. Calcium removal (R) from bone plotted as a function of calcium accretion (A) in 108 patients with various disorders of calcium metabolism. (From Harris WH, Heaney RP. Skeletal renewal and metabolic bone disease. Reprinted with permission from The New England Journal of Medicine, 280, 253–259, 1969.)

continues throughout life in response to mechanical and other regulatory factors. Skeletal homeostasis is achieved through the interplay of bone resorption and formation. There is close coupling of formation and resorption (Fig. 28–4). The mechanisms by which this tight regulation is achieved have not yet been elucidated.

In addition to its structural function, the skeleton constitutes the predominant reservoir of calcium in the body and is important in mineral homeostasis. Regulation of serum calcium may involve the transfer of calcium from bone to the extracellular fluid by osteocytes without matrix degradation.[5] Conversely, there may be major changes in the rates of bone formation and resorption (e.g., in Paget disease) without significant changes in the serum calcium. In part, this may be due to the coupling mechanism mentioned earlier. The serum calcium level may change as a consequence of uncoupling of bone formation and resorption (e.g., the hypercalcemia of malignant disease). Stimulation of bone formation and inhibition of bone resorption are critical to the successful therapy of many metabolic bone diseases.

Bone Formation

Bone formation is a complex process that involves migration and proliferation of primitive mesenchymal cells, differentiation into osteoblast precursor cells, maturation of osteoblasts, formation of matrix, and, finally, mineralization.[6] Differentiation and growth of chondrocytes, formation and mineralization of cartilage, vascular invasion, and resorption of cartilage are additional intermediate steps in the process of endochondral bone formation. Bone formation is controlled at multiple loci, including osteoblast differentiation, proliferation, and matrix formation.

Bone contains several growth factors and lymphokines that affect bone cell function in vitro, and probably in vivo as well (Table 28–1).[7–23] Transforming growth factor β (TGF β) is produced by osteoblasts and can stimulate mitogenesis and collagen synthesis. TGF β also is released from cells in response to bone-resorbing agents.[14] Depending on concentration it can either stimulate or inhibit bone cell growth. Both insulin-like growth factors, IGF I (also called somatomedin-C) and IGF II, are also mitogenic for bone cells and also stimulate collagen formation. A substance earlier described as skeletal growth factor has now been identified as IGF II.[9] The structure of another regulatory factor in bone, so-called bone morphogenetic protein, has been deduced by analyzing the cDNA for the proteins.[16] The biologically active material consists of three related proteins, two of which share homology with TGF β. When injected subcutaneously this class of proteins causes infiltration of bone cells into the injection site, cartilage formation, and calcification. Other mitogenic proteins for bone cells include platelet-derived growth factor, basic and acidic fibroblast growth factors, and α_2-microglobulin. Two or more growth factors may serve as the coupling factor (coupling bone formation to resorption), as some of them (such as TGF β and IGF II) are released from bone cells on exposure to bone-resorbing agents such as PTH or 1,25-dihydroxycholecalciferol (1,25(OH)$_2$D). A partial list of growth factors and related substances that act on or are produced in bone is given in Table 28–1. In addition to these factors a number of systemic hormones, including PTH, 1,25(OH)$_2$D, calcitonin, glucocorticoids, insulin, thyroxine, growth hormone, and gonadal steroids, influence bone formation (see Tables 28–1 and 28–3). In vivo, physiological concentrations of 1,25(OH)$_2$D and thyroid hormone promote net bone formation. 1,25(OH)$_2$D acts on osteoblasts (see earlier), but the mechanism (or mechanisms) of thyroid hormone action on bone cells has not been defined. Presumably, one of the thyroid hormone receptors in the retinoic acid receptor protein family is involved. PTH causes bone resorption and also stimulates bone formation, perhaps secondary to production of coupling factors such

TABLE 28–1. Growth Factors and Bone

Factor	Cell Source	Effects/Comments	Reference
IGF I*	Osteoblast	↑ mitogenesis;† ↑ collagen ↑ osteocalcin	7, 8
IGF II	Osteoblast	↑ mitogenesis; also called skeletal growth factor	8, 9
TGF β*	Osteoblast	↑ mitogenesis; ↑ collagen	10–14
Platelet-derived growth factor	Osteoblast	↑ mitogenesis	15, 15a
Bone morphogenetic proteins	Osteoblast	Promotes cartilage and bone formation	16, 16a
Interleukin 1	Osteoblast	↑ resorption; ↑ mitogenesis, ↑ collagen (decreases at high doses)	17
Fibroblast growth factor, basic	Osteoblast	↑ collagen; ↑ mitogenesis	18
Fibroblast growth factor, acidic	—‡	↑ mitogenesis	19, 20
Interferon	—	↑ resorption	21
Tumor necrosis factor α	Osteoblast	↑ resorption	22, 22a
Lymphotoxin (tumor necrosis factor β)	—	↑ resorption	23

*Estrogen stimulates production of insulin-like growth factors (IGFs)[22] and transforming growth factor β (TGF β).[23]
†Mitogenesis: mitogenic effect shown on bone cells or cloned bone tumor cells.
‡Undetermined.

as TGF β and IGF II. Calcitonin does not affect osteoblasts primarily but may enhance bone formation by inhibiting action of osteoclasts. Glucocorticoids initially increase collagen synthesis and later inhibit collagen synthesis. In vivo, reduced bone formation is the predominant effect. Insulin at low concentrations stimulates osteoblast collagen synthesis; at higher concentrations it is mitogenic for osteoblasts. The effects of growth hormone on the skeleton are presumably mediated by local production of IGF I. It was long believed that gonadal steroids such as estrogens also act indirectly on bone, as estrogen receptors had not been identified in bone cells. However, osteoblasts and osteoblast-like tumor cells contain estrogen receptors,[24] and these cells respond to estrogen with production of growth factors and other proteins (see Tables 28–1 and 28–3).

Bone Matrix Mineralization

The mechanism of mineralization of bone matrix is not fully understood. Several factors are believed to be important.[26] Calcium and phosphate ions in the extracellular fluid are in metastable equilibrium (i.e., their concentrations exceed the solubility product [Ca × P]), and they may be kept from forming a solid phase by inhibitors of calcification such as inorganic pyrophosphate. Synthetic analogues of pyrophosphate, the diphosphonates, bind to bone matrix and may prevent mineralization. Osteoblasts contain abundant alkaline phosphatase activity, and the serum concentration of this enzyme is increased in states of increased bone formation. Alkaline phosphatase activity may facilitate mineralization by cleaving phosphate groups, either decreasing the effectiveness of inhibitors of calcification or increasing the local phosphate concentration in sites of mineralization. Evidence to prove either hypothesis is lacking, but mineralization is defective in patients with hypophosphatasia, a hereditary deficiency of alkaline phosphatase activity.

Calcium and phosphate concentrations at the site of mineralization may be regulated by the membrane-like action of the osteoblast layer on the bone-forming surface. Calcium is taken up by intracellular organelles, in particular mitochondria. Calcium- and phosphate-rich, membrane-lined vesicles are also extruded into the extracellular matrix; these calcium- and phosphate-filled matrix vesicles may initiate mineralization, but evidence for such a role has been obtained only in states of rapid matrix formation and mineralization.

Organic matrix components may play a role in calcification. The concentration of minor glycoprotein components decreases abruptly in sites where bone matrix is being mineralized. Glycoproteins may act as inhibitors of calcification that must be degraded before the process can begin. Specific noncollagenous matrix proteins such as osteocalcin and osteonectin may also be important in initiating mineralization.

Several hormonal factors influence mineralization, but they likely act through the regulation of serum calcium and phosphate concentrations.[26] Thus 1,25(OH)$_2$D is necessary for normal bone mineralization, probably because it enhances intestinal calcium absorption, not because it exerts direct effects on bone.

The major organic component of bone matrix, collagen, is vital in normal mineralization. The unique structure of collagen encompasses gap regions (hole zones) sufficiently large to accommodate the mineral phase of bone without disruption of the fibrils themselves (Fig. 28–5). The majority of the solid-phase calcium and phosphate is located within the collagen fibrils and is highly ordered (i.e., the long axes of the crystals run parallel to the collagen fibrils, and the mineral has the same periodicity [64 to 70 nm] as the collagen

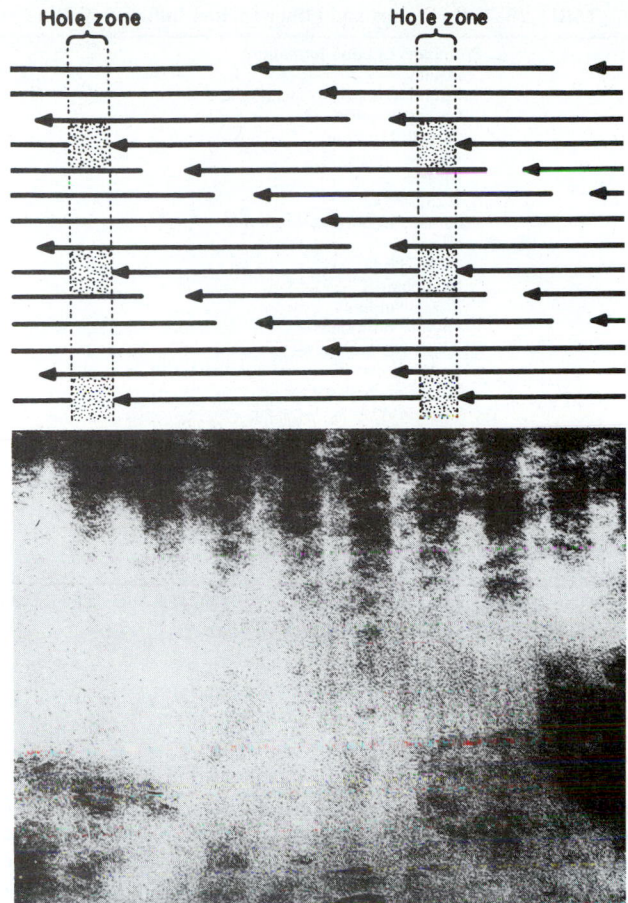

Figure 28–5. The staggered arrangement of individual molecules in collagen fibers results in hole zones between the head of one molecule and the tail of the next. Mineral deposition *(bottom)* begins within the hole zones. (From Glimcher MJ, Krane SM. Treatise on Collagen 2. Part B. New York: Academic, 1968: 67–251.)

fibril). In addition, the collagen fibril itself may serve as a heterogeneous nucleation catalyst in the mineralization process. The binding of calcium, phosphate, or both to side-chain groups on collagen amino acid residues could be the initiating factor in further calcium and phosphate precipitation and ultimate calcification.

Once mineralization is initiated, it proceeds rapidly, so that within 6 to 12 h, 60 to 70% of the final amount of mineral is deposited (primary mineralization phase). Subsequently mineralization occurs more slowly and may not be complete until 1 to 2 mo later (secondary mineralization phase).

Bone Resorption

Bone resorption is accomplished by osteoclasts, the multinucleated giant cells derived from circulating or marrow monocyte precursor cells. Early osteoclasts, or osteoclast precursors, are recruited to the bone surface by substances released from bone matrix or from osteoblasts. After reaching the bone surface, the osteoclast precursors attach, fuse, and become multinucleated. These processes are regulated by 1,25(OH)$_2$D, PTH, and other factors. Bone-resorbing substances (Table 28–2) stimulate production of increased numbers of multinucleated osteoclasts and increased osteoclast activity. Osteoclast resorption in response to PTH, prostaglandins, interleukin 1 (IL 1), and 1,25(OH)$_2$D (and

TABLE 28–2. Hormones and Other Factors Influencing Bone

Promoters of bone formation
  Insulin
  Insulin-like growth factors I and II
  Estrogens, androgens
  Growth hormone
  Thyroid hormone
  PTH*
  1,25(OH)$_2$D
Promoters of bone resorption
  PTH
  1,25(OH)$_2$D
  Interleukin 1
  Prostaglandins
  Thyroid hormone
  Epidermal growth factor
  Lymphotoxin (tumor necrosis factor β)
  Tumor necrosis factor α
  Vitamin A
Inhibitors of bone resorption
  Calcitonin
  Phosphate
  Plicamycin
  Diphosphonates
  Glucocorticoids
  Aspirin, indomethacin

*Promotes bone formation indirectly, possibly through stimulation of bone resorption and hence coupling to bone formation.

perhaps other factors as well) requires the presence of osteoblasts.[27] Indeed, osteoblasts, not osteoclasts, contain receptors for PTH and 1,25(OH)$_2$D. In response to PTH or 1,25(OH)$_2$D, osteoblasts release factors, including prostaglandins, TGF β, and IL 1, that stimulate osteoclast activity. PTH induces changes in the shape of osteoblasts, and these changes may be important in exposing the bone matrix surface to osteoclastic dissolution. PTH and 1,25(OH)$_2$D induce differentiation of immature osteoclast precursors, known as *tartrate-resistant acid phosphatase–negative* (TRAC-negative) cells, to TRAC-positive cells, which eventually fuse into multinucleated mature osteoclasts.[28] Osteoclasts bear receptors for calcitonin, which inhibits maturation and fusion of osteoclast precursors. Calcitonin also inhibits function of osteoclasts and may accelerate destruction of multinucleated osteoclasts.

Osteoclasts are replete with lysosomal acid hydrolases, including cysteine proteinases as well as tartrate-resistant acid phosphatase. These enzymes are released in response to bone-resorbing agents such as PTH, 1,25(OH)$_2$D, IL 1, and prostaglandins.[28]

Thyroid hormones directly increase bone resorption in long-term bone cultures. Several of the growth factors, such as epidermal growth factor and platelet-derived growth factor, cause bone resorption, most likely by stimulating prostaglandin release. Other substances such as vitamin A and lipopolysaccharides can also increase bone resorption.[5]

Calcitonin, both in vitro and at pharmacological doses in vivo, is an effective inhibitor of bone resorption. Phosphate inhibits bone resorption, but its use in vivo may cause ectopic calcification. Plicamycin is a cytotoxic antibiotic that inhibits osteoclast function at doses below those leading to nonspecific cell death. The diphosphonates are pyrophosphate analogues that resist cleavage by pyrophosphatases. Substitutions on the diphosphonate backbone confer different potency and properties.[29] Certain diphosphonates inhibit both mineralization and resorption, some are more potent in inhibiting resorption than in blocking mineralization, and still others selectively inhibit resorption. The mechanism by which diphosphonates inhibit bone resorption is not clear but appears to involve a direct action on osteoclasts rather than merely rendering the mineral phase less susceptible to

dissolution.[30] The treatment of newborn rats with one diphosphonate produces osteopetrotic bone and abnormal thymic function,[31] suggesting that the agent may act by impairing T lymphocyte function (e.g., by inhibiting release of osteoclast-activating factor). Glucocorticoids, which may indirectly lead to increased bone resorption, inhibit bone resorption in certain disorders such as multiple myeloma. This effect appears to be due to inhibition by glucocorticoids of osteoclast-activating factor–mediated bone resorption.[5] Inhibitors of prostaglandin synthesis such as aspirin and indomethacin also reduce bone resorption under certain conditions.

Skeletal Homeostasis

Skeletal Growth and Modeling

With the exception of flat bones such as the skull, bones grow by a process termed *endochondral ossification*. Early in embryonic development, primitive mesenchymal cells form a cartilage rudiment similar in shape to the bone ultimately formed. Along the shaft (diaphysis) osteoblasts lay down a collar of bone. Continued periosteal formation of new lamellae enlarges this collar, and late in fetal life haversian remodeling begins, leading to development of the definitive cortex. Resorption proceeds at the endosteal surface but does not keep pace with periosteal apposition; thus the cortex thickens as the marrow cavity is enlarged. At the metaphyseal ends of the bone, trabeculae of calcified cartilage form the primary spongiosa. These are resorbed and replaced by bony trabeculae in the secondary spongiosa. An epiphyseal ossification center develops at each end; this region is responsible for the linear growth of bone. Successive layers of cartilage—resting, proliferating, maturing, and calcifying zones—make up the epiphyseal growth plate. With maturity the epiphyseal plates ossify, and further linear growth ceases. Cartilage remains only on the articular surface.

The shape of individual bones is controlled by a process termed *modeling*, which is operative during growth.[32] So-called osteoblastic and osteoclastic drifts model the bone's architecture, moving the periosteal and cortical endosteal surfaces through space.[32] In response to specific mechanical forces, modeling leads to characteristic details of bone structure such as inwaisting of vertebral bodies and long bone metaphyses (reviewed in ref. 32).

Skeletal Remodeling

Bone modeling and remodeling require continuous cycles of bone formation and resorption under regulation of systemic hormones and local bone cell paracrine and autocrine factors. There is constant skeletal remodeling in response to changing mineral concentrations and the structural requirements of the body.[33] Under normal conditions the mechanical competence of the skeleton is maintained during remodeling. Remodeling involves the concerted action of osteoclasts and osteoblasts in bone resorption and formation at the periosteal surface, at the trabecular and cortical endosteal surfaces, and within the cortex. Intracortical (haversian) remodeling requires resorption of previously deposited bone to make room for new bone formation. This is accomplished by a "cutting cone" of osteoclasts that removes everything in its path parallel to the long axis of the bone and is followed by capillaries and osteoblasts that line the newly formed cavity with concentric bone lamellae. The newly formed osteons (haversian systems) may be 200 μm in diameter and several millimeters long. The remains of old, partially resorbed osteons form the interstitial lamellae

TABLE 28–3. Characteristic Proteins and Enzymes of Bone

Protein	Source*	Properties/Comments	Reference
Osteonectin	OB	Extracellular support matrix	35, 36
Osteocalcin (bone gla protein)	OB	Contains γ-carboxyglutamic acid; ↑ by 1,25(OH)$_2$D, dependent on vitamins K and C chemotactic for OCs	37, 38
Matrix gla protein (MGP)	OB	Contains γ-carboxyglutamic acid; ↑ by 1,25(OH)$_2$D, dependent on vitamin K	38
Osteopontin	OB	↑ by 1,25(OH)$_2$D	35
Bone sialoprotein	—†	May be unique to bone; partial sequence homology with osteopontin	39
Alkaline phosphatase	OB	Marker for OBs; regulated by PTH, 1,25(OH)$_2$D, and estrogen	40, 41
Procollagenase	OB	After conversion to collagenase, degrades unmineralized collagen	42
Collagen type I	OB	Characteristic abundant bone protein; ↑ by estrogen	43
Proteoglycans	—	Bone matrix component	44
Tartrate-resistant acid phosphatase	OC	Marker for OCs, released on activation of OCs	45
Lysosomal hydrolases, cysteine peptidases	OC	Degrade bone matrix; degrade bone collagen; released on activation of OCs	28

*OB, osteoblast; OC, osteoclast.
†Undetermined.

without a central canal. A cement line demarcates the border between resorbed bone and newly formed bone.

The basic structural units of bone are visible under polarized light. In cortical bone they look like ellipses or circles, depending on the plane of section, and correspond to haversian systems. In trabecular bone they are arch-like.[34] The basic structural unit represents the end product of continuous bone remodeling by functional bone units, termed *basic multicellular units* (BMUs). Each BMU cycle is characterized by the activation of osteoclasts, resorption, activation of osteoblasts, and formation. Because osteoblastic bone formation is coupled to osteoclast resorption, the overall rate of bone turnover is determined by the rate of osteoclast activation. The total bone mass reflects cumulative bone balance at the BMU level. The magnitude and direction of changes in bone mass depend on the ratio of bone formation to bone resorption at the BMU level and on the "birth rate" of BMUs per unit volume of bone tissue. Because the ratio of endosteal surface to bone volume is greater for trabecular than for cortical bone, any excess bone resorption at endosteal surfaces produces larger decreases in trabecular than in cortical bone volume. This relationship presumably explains the greater involvement of trabecular bone (e.g., vertebrae) in osteoporosis.

Chemistry of Bone and Bone Proteins

A number of proteins and enzymes (Table 28–3)[28, 35–45] are produced by bone cells. Collagen, osteonectin, osteocalcin, osteopontin, and proteoglycans are important for physical structure as well as biochemical function of bone. The content of these proteins in bone is controlled by local autocrine and paracrine regulators as well as by systemic hormones.

Collagen

Thirteen forms of collagen[43, 46] have been identified, more than eight in connective tissue alone. Collagen is broadly classified according to groups and more specifically as types. Group 1 includes types I to III, V, and K; displays an apparent molecular size of 95 kd; and is fibrillar and continuously helical in structure. Group 2 (types IV and VI to VIII) is similar in size but is nonfibrillar, with nonhelical peptide segments. Group 3 (types IX and X) is smaller (apparent molecular size of 95 kd).[43]

Collagen is the major protein component of bone. The collagen molecule is a rigid, rod-like structure (1.5 × 300 nm) composed of three polypeptide (alpha) chains held together in a helical fashion by covalent and noncovalent forces (see refs. 43, 46, and 47 for reviews on collagen structure, synthesis, and regulatory control). Multiple colla-

gen molecules are assembled together end to end to form fibrils that are approximately five to seven molecules thick; the fibrils in turn are arranged in bundles or fibers that are visible by light microscopy in the extracellular bone matrix. Electron microscopy of collagen fibrils reveals cross-striations with a characteristic periodicity (64 to 70 nm). The striations result from the staggered arrangement of individual molecules within the fibril (see Fig. 28–5). In regions where adjacent molecules overlap (overlap zone), an increase in charge density accounts for the striations noted by electron microscopy. Gaps (40 nm) between the end of one molecule and the head of the next represent the hole zones visualized on electron microscopy by negative staining; these are the initial sites of mineral deposition.

The primary amino acid sequences of several collagen chains have been elucidated. Bone collagen molecules are composed of two identical alpha-1 chains and a homologous but distinct alpha-2 chain. This so-called type I collagen is also found in skin but differs from collagens in cartilage (type II), elastic tissue (type III), and basement membranes (type IV). Collagen contains glycine at every third amino acid position and high contents of proline and lysine.

COLLAGEN BIOSYNTHESIS. With more than 50 exons and numerous intervening sequences, the collagen gene is one of the most complex genes yet studied. Transcription to messenger RNA (mRNA) involves numerous splices, and errors in this process are a potential cause of genetic abnormalities in collagen structure.

Biosynthesis of collagen is depicted in Figure 28–6. Individual alpha chains are synthesized in a precursor form (pre-pro alpha chain) that contains a signal (leader) segment as well as additional NH$_2$- and COOH-terminal prosequences. The signal sequence of about 100 residues (longer than for most secreted proteins) is cleaved as the peptide chain enters the rough endoplasmic reticulum. Within this compartment, separate enzymes catalyze the hydroxylation of lysine and proline residues; ascorbic acid is a necessary cofactor for these hydroxylations. Triple helix formation may be initiated by noncovalent forces, but interchain disulfide bridges between cysteines in the COOH-terminal prosequence portions of the alpha chains help to stabilize the conformation. Enzymatic glycosylation begins shortly after the NH$_2$-terminal ends of the newly synthesized collagen polypeptides move into the cisternae of the rough endoplasmic reticulum and hydroxylysine is synthesized. Glycosylation of hydroxylysines may facilitate extrusion of the procollagen molecule from the cell. Several enzymes, collectively termed *procollagen peptidases*, act extracellularly to cleave the NH$_2$- and COOH-terminal propeptide extensions, leaving a largely triple helical molecule. The copper-requiring enzyme, lysyl oxidase, converts certain of the lysine and hydroxylysine residues to α-aminoadipic acid semialdehyde

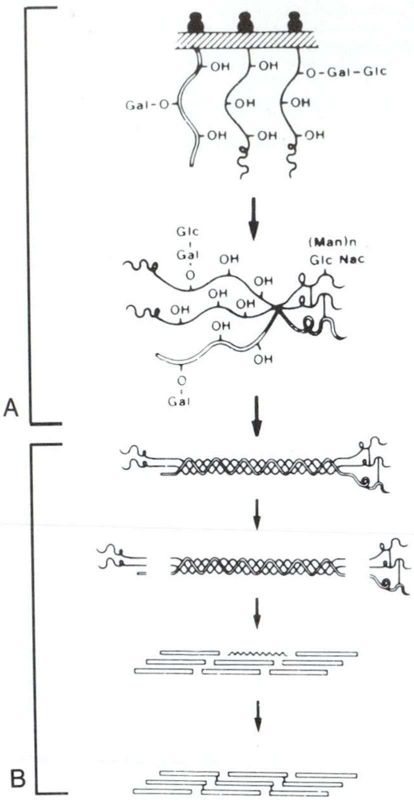

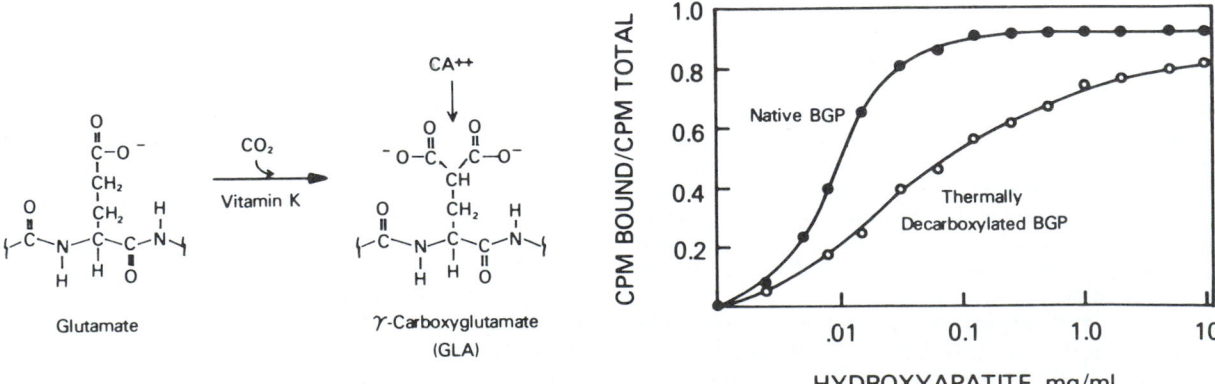

Figure 28–6. Synthesis and assembly of collagen fibrils. *A*, Intracellular post-translational modifications of pro alpha chains, association of propeptide domains, and folding into triple-helical conformation. Gal, galactose; Glc, glucose; Glc Nac, *N*-acetylglucosamine; (Man)n, mannose. *B*, Enzymatic cleavage of procollagen to collagen, self-assembly of collagen monomers into fibrils, and cross-linking of fibrils. (Modified from Prockop DJ, Kivirikko K. Heritable diseases of collagen. Reprinted with permission from The New England Journal of Medicine, 311, 376–386, 1984.)

and 5-hydroxy-α-aminoadipic acid semialdehyde, respectively. These modified residues interact with each other and with other amino groups to form intra- and intermolecular cross-links that help to bind collagen molecules into fibrils. Several inherited disorders of collagen synthesis involve defective lysyl oxidase activity.

Noncollagen Organic Matrix Components

A fraction (about 10%) of the organic matrix consists of noncollagen components, including proteins (see Table 28–3), acid mucopolysaccharides, and lipids. Some of these components may be important in bone cell biology and mineralization.

OSTEOCALCIN (BONE GLA PROTEIN). Osteocalcin composes 1 to 2% of the total bone protein and is also found in dentin, sites of ectopic calcification, and plasma.[37] The structure of the protein from several species, including humans, is highly conserved, suggesting some important function. The molecular mass is about 6 kd, and the isoelectric point is acidic (pH 4.0). The protein contains three γ-carboxyglutamic acid (gla) residues (hence, bone gla protein). The gla residues are formed through post-translational modifications of glutamic acid residues in the protein catalyzed by a vitamin K–requiring enzyme. (Osteocalcin differs in structure from other vitamin K–dependent proteins, such as clotting factors, that contain gla.) The gla residues bind calcium relatively weakly but show much higher affinity for hydroxyapatite (1 mg of osteocalcin may bind 17 mg of hydroxyapatite). The binding of hydroxyapatite to osteocalcin is dependent on the gla content of the protein and is reduced when osteocalcin is decarboxylated or in vitamin K–deficient animals (Fig. 28–7). Osteocalcin may also be important in recruiting osteoclasts or precursors to the bone surface.[38]

Osteocalcin is synthesized by the osteoblast, and the mRNA is detected exclusively in bone. Production of osteocalcin depends on three vitamins: vitamin D, actually $1,25(OH)_2D$; vitamin K, for carboxylation to produce gla residues; and vitamin C, for conversion of proline at residue 9 to hydroxyproline.[38] The osteocalcin gene contains three introns. Transcription of the gene is regulated by $1,25(OH)_2D$ and factors operative during mineralization of bone tissue. mRNA for osteocalcin increases at least 10-fold with $1,25(OH)_2D$ and 200-fold in mineralizing matrix.[48] $1,25(OH)_2D$ response elements responsible for regulation of synthesis of the protein have been identified on the osteocalcin gene. $1,25(OH)_2D$ stimulates secretion of osteocalcin by osteosarcoma cells. PTH, calcitonin, and changes in the calcium concentration of the medium are without effect.

Osteocalcin circulates in the plasma of humans and other animals. The mean plasma concentration in adults is about 5 μg/L. Plasma osteocalcin is derived from newly synthesized bone osteocalcin and not from resorption of old bone. The implication is that plasma osteocalcin could serve as a sensitive and specific marker of osteoblast activity. In patients with Paget disease, primary hyperparathyroidism, and other metabolic bone disorders, increases in plasma osteocalcin usually correlate with bone-derived serum alkaline phosphatase activity. The half-life for osteocalcin (cleared by the kidney) in plasma is about 5 min. Plasma

Figure 28–7. *Left*, Vitamin K–dependent gamma-carboxylation of glutamate and site of calcium binding. *Right*, Role of γ-carboxyglutamic acid residues in binding of synthetic hydroxyapatite to BGP (bone gla protein). The extent of binding was assayed by measuring ^{125}I-labeled BGP in the supernatant after sedimentation of hydroxyapatite. (From Price P. Osteocalcin. In: Peck WA, ed. Bone and Mineral Research Annual 1. Amsterdam: Excerpta Medica, 1983: 157–190.)

Bone Scanning with Isotopes

Bone-seeking isotopic tracers, particularly diphosphonates labeled with radioactive technetium (^{99m}Tc), adsorb to bone crystal surfaces, allowing the imaging of zones of increased turnover or increased vascularity. This technique is particularly valuable in identifying local nonhomogeneities such as tumor, fracture, Paget disease, and abscess. This procedure can also be calibrated to identify diffusely increased rates of skeletal turnover, as in hyperparathyroidism and thyrotoxicosis.

Quantitation of Skeletal Mass

Because skeletal strength bears a rough relation to mineral content, mineral content is a useful indicator of the skeletal status. Current definitions of osteoporosis are based on the total or regional content of bone.

QUANTITATIVE RADIOGRAMETRY. The status of cortical bone can be evaluated by quantitating the metacarpal cortical thickness or metacarpal cortical area from standard radiographs. This technique has poor reproducibility and does not allow for variations in cortical porosity.

NEUTRON ACTIVATION ANALYSIS. Exposure to a neutron flux activates a portion of the stable isotope ^{48}Ca to the unstable isotope ^{49}Ca. Gamma emissions from the decay of ^{49}Ca are an index of the body calcium content. This can be used to measure calcium in the total body or in segments. Although the technique is the standard against which other techniques are compared, errors of as much as 10% in elderly subjects can result from extraosseous calcium (e.g., osteophyte or arterial plaque).

PHOTON ABSORPTIOMETRY. In photon absorptiometry a collimated beam of ^{125}I is passed through bone, and the attenuation of radiation is measured to indicate density. Reproducibility is better than that of quantitative radiogrametry. Cortical porosity influences the readings. This method has been applied principally to analysis of the radius. The midradius contains 95% cortical bone, and results from this segment correlate well with estimates of the total body calcium. The distal radius has been used to assess spongy bone; however, arm positioning is more variable at this site, and 75% of the bone at this site is cortical.

COMPUTED TOMOGRAPHY, DUAL-PHOTON ABSORPTIOMETRY, AND DUAL-ENERGY RADIOGRAPHY. Computed tomography, dual-photon absorptiometry, and dual-energy radiography for selectively measuring spongy or cortical bone are undergoing development and testing.[56] They can be applied to vertebrae, which consist of 75% spongy and 25% compact elements. Single-energy computed tomography is used to quantitate spongy bone within one or multiple vertebrae, but the measurement is limited by the variable contribution from marrow elements. With dual-photon absorptiometry, two energy channels are used to resolve contributions from soft tissue and bone. This method requires a radiation source of ^{153}Gd, with associated problems of source stability. Dual-energy radiography is a new technique under development that combines the advantages of the reproducibility of x-ray sources with the selectivity from computed tomography using two energies.[57]

These techniques are widely available, depending on cost and local preferences. Although clearly important in research, their roles in the screening and monitoring of patients are not established.[58]

RICKETS AND OSTEOMALACIA

Nutritional Deficiency of Vitamin D

Before 1920 nutritional rickets and osteomalacia were major problems, particularly in cities in temperate zones.

TABLE 28–4. Vitamin D Content of Unfortified Foods*

Food	Content (IU/100 g or IU/dL)*
Egg yolk	50
Halibut	40
Herring (fresh or canned)	320
Sardines (canned)	1100–1500
Shrimp	150
Liver (chicken, beef, calf)	0–70
Butter	35
Cheese	12–15
Milk (bovine)	0.3–4
Milk (human)	0–10

*1 IU is equivalent to 25 ng of ergocalciferol or cholecalciferol.
Modified with permission from Yendt ER. Vitamin D: part II. In: Rasmussen H, ed. Pharmacology of the Endocrine System and Related Drugs, Copyright 1970, Pergamon Press PLC.

Understanding the antirachitic properties of light and of cod liver oil was one of the great accomplishments in medical investigation. In the United States, needs for the vitamin generally are satisfied through conversion, in the skin, of 7-dehydrocholesterol to cholecalciferol (vitamin D_3) under the influence of ultraviolet radiation. Endogenous production of vitamin D_3 is normally 10 to 100 μg/d. The minimal requirement for vitamin D (ergocalciferol or cholecalciferol) is approximately 1.25 to 1.75 μg/d (50 to 70 IU/d) in children and adults. The recommended dietary allowance of vitamin D for adults is 5 μg/d (200 IU/d). In the United States, ergocalciferol (or in some regions cholecalciferol) is added routinely to cow's milk, at 10 μg/qt, and many other foods are similarly fortified.

Factors predisposing to nutritional vitamin D deficiency include prematurity, rapid growth with a consequent need for adequate skeletal calcium and phosphorus, inadequate light exposure, and avoidance of vitamin D–supplemented foods. In a person deficient in solar exposure, a diet unfortified with vitamin D is not adequate to avoid deficiency (Table 28–4). In particular, human milk and cow's milk are inadequate sources. Thus mild rickets can occur during the winter months in otherwise healthy breast-fed infants who are not given vitamin D supplements or fed fortified foods.

Severe nutritional deficiency of vitamin D is rare in the United States, but vitamin D supplements deficiency remains a public health problem in many other nations. For example, among children of Asian immigrants in Bradford, England, the prevalence of biochemical features of vitamin D deficiency was 45% in 1973. The clinical and biochemical features of nutritional vitamin D deficiency are relevant to an understanding of many disorders with hereditary or acquired abnormalities of vitamin D metabolism.[59]

Clinical Features

The characteristic skeletal disturbance in vitamin D deficiency and in some other metabolic disorders is osteomalacia, which means literally soft bones. The malacic bone is subject to distortion in shape and to fracture; deformity is particularly likely to develop with vitamin D deficiency in infancy or childhood. The deformities of bone represent the characteristic skeletal appearance seen in rickets. Congenital nutritional rickets occurs only in the offspring of mothers with severe vitamin D deficiency. However, nutritional rickets may be manifest between the ages of 6 and 24 mo, and somewhat earlier in premature infants, who often have small adipose depots and delayed maturation of the hepatic enzymes catalyzing 25-hydroxylation of calciferols. Deficiencies in bone mineralization are particularly evident in regions of rapid bone growth and turnover. In the first year of life the most rapidly growing bones are in the cranium, wrists, and ribs. Rickets at this time leads to widened cranial sutures, frontal bossing, posterior flattening of the skull (craniotabes), bulging of the costochondral junctions (rachitic rosary), indentation of the ribs at the diaphragmatic insertions (Harrison groove), and enlargement of the wrists. The rib cage may be so deformed as to compromise respiratory function. Dental eruption is often delayed, and the teeth show irregular pits, grooves, and enamel hypoplasia. There is severe muscular hypotonia and weakness, resulting in a lax, protuberant abdomen. Although growth and weight are adequate, the infant may be unable to stand without support until age 3. In older children, proximal muscle weakness may be prominent. Compromised respiratory musculature contributes to the high incidence of pneumonia. Signs of other vitamin deficiencies may also be present. Tetany and laryngeal stridor are uncommon, as hypocalcemia is usually mild. After the first year of life, the deformities are most severe about the legs because of their rapid growth and weight-bearing function. Most deformities are the result of pressure on weakened growth plates, but in severe rickets the bony shafts of the long bones also are deformed and subject to fracture. The ends of the long bones become visibly enlarged. Bowleg (genu varum) or knock-knee (genu valgum) worsens progressively. In long-standing disease there may be coxa vara and rachitic saber shins. Moderate deformities before age 4 may resolve after adequate vitamin D treatment, but later defects result in lasting deformity, compromise in adult height, or both. When rickets begins later in childhood (about age 10), the shafts of the long bones may remain straight while the knee metaphyses become angulated. There is an increased susceptibility to pathological fracture.

Osteomalacia in the adult causes less severe clinical features. In the mature skeleton, only 5% or less of calcium is newly laid down each year. Thus a mineralization defect in adults must be present for several years to produce clinical manifestations. The characteristic symptom is pain when weight or pressure is applied to the affected bones. Low backache relieved by recumbency is an early complaint, but the pain may involve other portions of the spine, ribs, and feet. A narrowing of the pelvic outlet from inward pressure of the hips may cause difficulties during childbirth and was once a cause of widespread morbidity. Loss of vertebral height can lead to kyphosis. The skeletal deformities may be associated with other features of malnutrition. Associated proximal muscle weakness contributes to a waddling gait or severe crippling. Patients with osteomalacia may be thought initially to have neurological disorders because of weakness. There is often a series of relapses and remissions. The first manifestation may be an acute fracture, the most common sites being the femoral neck, pubic ramus, spine, or ribs. This description is applicable to severe osteomalacia. The incidence and morbidity of mild osteomalacia are less well understood, but with increasing use of bone biopsy and assays for circulating vitamin D metabolites in blood, this process is becoming better defined. Although osteomalacia can cause fractures, vitamin D deficiency is probably not an important contributor to osteoporosis in most industrialized nations.[60]

Radiographic Features

In children the failure of cartilage calcification is manifested by delayed opacification of the epiphyses and widening of growth plates. In vitamin D deficiency the ends of the growing metaphyses are frayed or irregular, and the usually straight transverse appearance becomes concave or cupped. They widen owing to the pressure borne by a large mass of poorly calcified cartilage (Fig. 28–9). In the diaphyses, the cortex is thin, the periosteum may be fuzzy, and bone trabeculae are sparse and coarse. In childhood the characteristic shaft deformities (i.e., genu varum, genu valgum, and coxa vara) are present, but pseudofractures are uncommon. Variable manifestations of secondary hyperparathyroidism include irregular lacy subperiosteal erosions, especially about the metaphyses of long bones; the bone cysts and phalangeal lesions present in adults are rare in children. Fluctuations in disease severity result in the appearance of thin, radiodense growth arrest lines (Harris lines) in the metaphyses parallel to the growth plates. The earliest radiographic feature in healing rickets appears at days 8 to 30 of treatment as a dense line of calcified cartilage

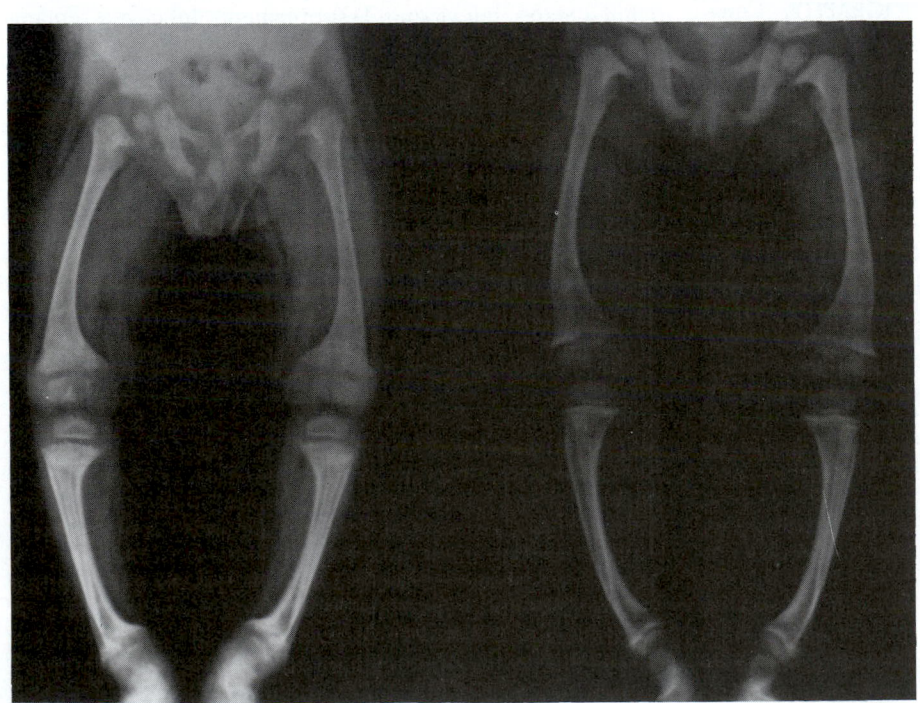

Figure 28–9. *Left,* Active rickets in a patient with tissue resistance to 1,25(OH)$_2$D at age 21 mo with genu varum, irregular metaphyses, and widened growth plates. *Right,* Inactive rickets in the same patient at age 27 mo after treatment with massive doses of ergocalciferol. (From SJ Marx, AM Spiegel, EM Brown, et al., Familial syndrome of decrease in sensitivity to 1,25-hydroxyvitamin D, J Clin Endocrinol Metab, 47, 1303–1310, 1978, © by The Endocrine Society.)

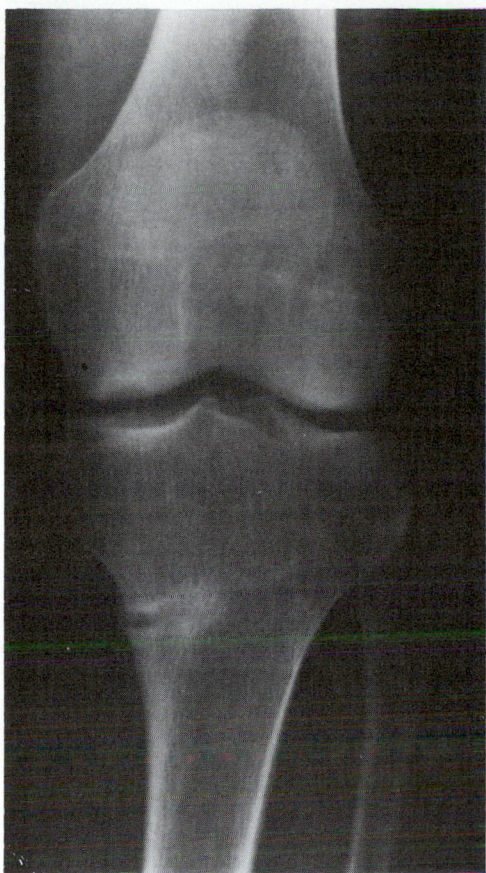

Figure 28–10. Active osteomalacia in a patient (a sibling of the patient in Fig. 28 9) with hereditary tissue resistance to 1,25(OH)₂D at age 18 with pseudofracture of the left tibia. (From SJ Marx, AM Spiegel, EM Brown, et al., Familial syndrome of decrease in sensitivity to 1,25-hydroxyvitamin D, J Clin Endocrinol Metab, 47, 1303–1310, 1978, © by The Endocrine Society.)

separated from the metaphysis by a small zone of uncalcified cartilage.

Significant osteomalacia may exist without radiographic manifestations, but a generalized decrease in bone density and in total skeletal mineral content is common. However, in certain forms of osteomalacia (e.g., in half of adults with familial X-linked hypophosphatemia), the total bone mineral content is increased, albeit with excessive quantities of unmineralized osteoid. The characteristic radiographic feature of adult osteomalacia is the pseudofracture, a straight transverse ribbon-like band. Pseudofractures (Looser zones or Milkman syndrome) localize, often symmetrically, at the concave sides of the shafts of long bones, as well as the ribs, scapulae, and pubic rami (Fig. 28–10). They probably originate from repeated microfractures with a build-up of uncalcified callus. In some locations they may result from the pressure of pulsating arteries. The medullary cavities are narrowed, with trabeculae that are coarse and reduced in number. The bone cortex is thinned and, on fine-grain radiographs, exhibits small intracortical striations of decreased density. Long-standing disease leads to deformities that include bowing of long bones, biconcave vertebrae, and a distorted pelvic outlet that has a triangular appearance on standard anteroposterior views. Fractures (sometimes superimposed on pseudofractures) heal slowly.

The selective malabsorption of calcium leads to secondary hyperparathyroidism with subperiosteal resorption, especially on the medial border of the middle phalanges, and erosion of the digital tufts. In severe cases the associated soft tissue changes have an outward appearance that resembles clubbing. The long bones may contain sharp-margined cysts, and the symphysis pubis and the sacroiliac joints become widened.

Bone Histology and Biochemistry

The defect common to rickets and osteomalacia is lack or deficiency of mineralization of bone. The bone mineral density is decreased, and osteoid borders are increased in length, width, and volume. In growing bones regions of endochondral ossification show the most striking abnormality. Systematic histological studies have been done with rats rendered rachitic by diets deficient in vitamin D and phosphorus. The histological appearance of the zones of resting and proliferating cartilage is normal. In the zone of maturing cartilage, however, the usually regular columns of chondrocytes are disorganized and greatly increased in length (Fig. 28–11). The zone of hypertrophic cartilage at the diaphyseal end of the columns is sparse. At the diaphyseal end, the calcification front and zone of vascular invasion are distorted or unrecognizable.

Mechanical stress on the unsupported cellular growth plate leads to the epiphyseal bulging characteristic of rickets. After epiphyseal fusion, these changes can no longer occur. Whenever remodeling occurs, mineralization is deficient. The result is osteomalacia, or softening of bones.

The definition of osteomalacia that is most broadly used is a deficient rate of mineral accumulation at the mineralization front. This is best estimated through quantitative histomorphometry after labeling bone in vivo with tetracycline given in two doses separated by a 14-d interval. Unfortunately the term osteomalacia has been given several definitions dependent principally on the method of analysis: (1) a decrease in mineralization of osteoid, (2) an increase in osteoid width, and (3) an increase in the proportion of bone surface covered by osteoid independent of width. With vitamin D deficiency, all three definitions are acceptable. Prominent osteoid seams reflect an imbalance of osteoid synthesis and osteoid mineralization. For example, in vitamin D–deficient rats, osteoid deposition rate is slowed, but the maturation and mineralization of osteoid are inhibited to an even greater extent, with the result that osteoid seams are increased in length and width. Unmineralized osteoid is also prominent in hyperparathyroidism, thyrotoxicosis, Paget disease, and fluorosis and after diphosphonate administration, but should not obfuscate proper interpretation of the skeletal abnormalities of these other disorders (see later discussion).

In vitamin D deficiency the mineralization front is lost or decreased in prominence. This is also evident in the periosteocytic lacunae. The latter location is disproportionally affected by X-linked hypophosphatemia. The normal lamellar structure of osteoid is preserved, but with polarized light the number of lamellae is increased in proportion to the increase in osteoid thickness. Extensive coating of bone surfaces with unmineralized osteoid probably helps account for the resistance to mobilization of mineral from bones by PTH. Small zones of unmineralized osteoid may persist deep within mineralized bone even after therapy, and these may contribute to a porotic skeletal appearance. If secondary hyperparathyroidism develops, osteoclast numbers are increased. Regions of reactive tissue with trabeculae of woven (immature) bone correspond to radiographic regions of pseudofracture.

There is disagreement about whether the osteoid in vitamin D deficiency is normal in mineralization potential. Clearly the composition of bone and cartilage is abnormal. In addition to the gross deficiency of mineral, there is an

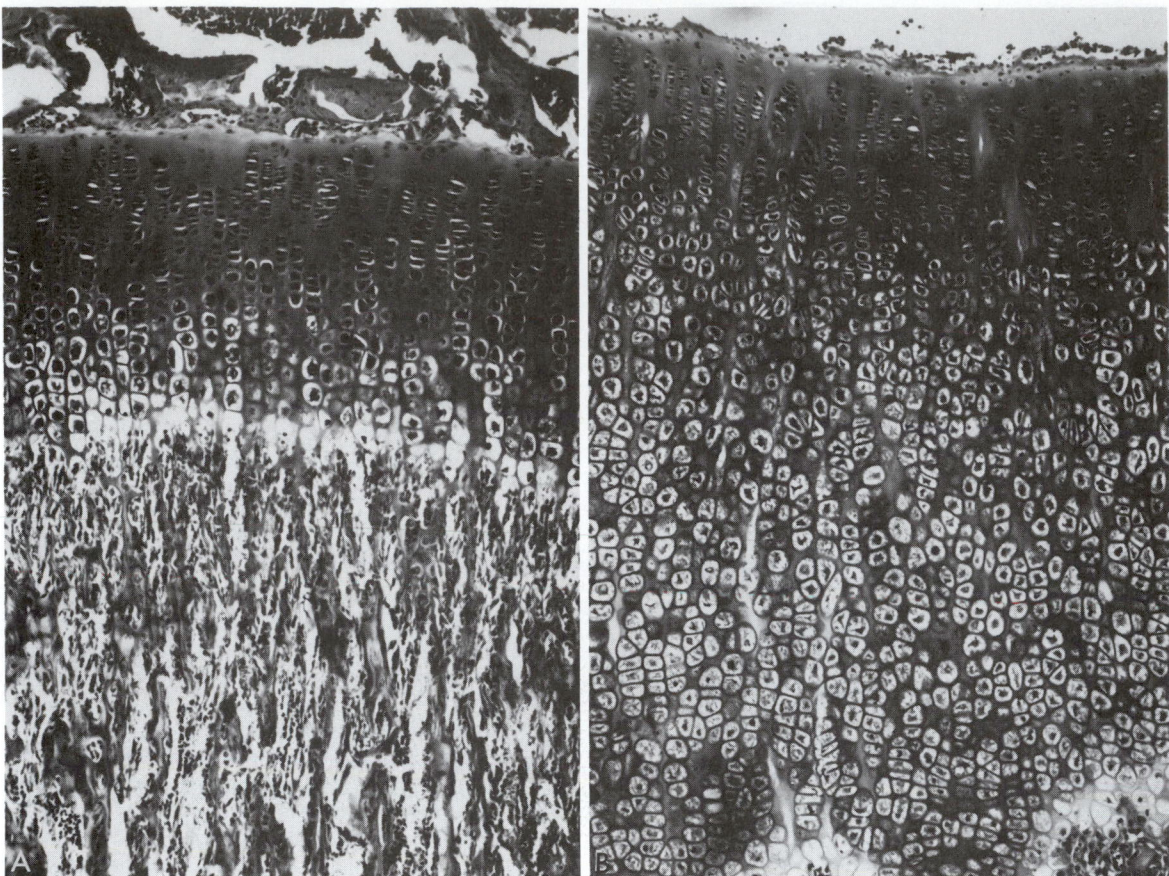

Figure 28–11. *A*, Normal epiphyseal plate of an immature rat, with the articular aspect at top. *B*, Epiphyseal plate from a rat after 6 wk on a diet deficient in phosphorus and vitamin D. Note the increase in axial height of cartilage mass. Normal orderly columns are replaced by increased numbers of cells in irregular rows. Magnification × 400. (Courtesy of Dr. H. J. Mankin.)

increase of lipid within chondrocytes and a decrease in the synthetic rates of RNA, protein, and polysaccharide in the epiphyseal maturation zone. Increased hydroxylation of lysine in vitamin D–deficient bone collagen is similar to that in fetal bone collagen. All these changes, however, may be secondary to the structural distortions in the malacic bone. In the proliferative zone of the growth plate, DNA synthesis is not abnormal, rachitic cartilage contains a normal quantity and distribution of matrix vesicles, and these retain a normal capacity to accumulate apatite when provided with sufficient mineral substrate in vitro. In contrast, in the rickets and osteomalacia induced in chickens by the administration of diphosphonates, the matrix vesicles do not accumulate mineral normally in vitro.

Laboratory Tests

The principal laboratory features of vitamin D deficiency can be understood by considering the intestinal actions of vitamin D. Deficient calcium absorption leads to mild hypocalcemia. This promotes secondary hyperparathyroidism. The manifestations of secondary hyperparathyroidism include an increased plasma PTH concentration, a decreased renal threshold for phosphate excretion and hypophosphatemia, and increased circulating concentrations of skeletal alkaline phosphatase. Often, as a result of secondary hyperparathyroidism, the serum calcium concentration is maintained within the lower portion of the normal range. Urinary calcium is low owing to the reduced filtered load and the action of elevated serum concentrations of PTH on the renal transport of calcium. In time, skeletal

changes become evident first on histological and later on radiographic evaluations. The circulating concentrations of vitamin D and 25-hydroxycholecalciferol (25-OHD) are low. The serum $1,25(OH)_2D$ values may be in the normal range, however, although inappropriately low for the degree of secondary hyperparathyroidism. Assessment of the total serum 25-OHD concentration, which may include the D_2 and D_3 forms of 25-OHD, 24,25-dihydroxycholecalciferol ($24,25(OH)_2D$), 25,26-dihydroxycholecalciferol ($25,26(OH)_2D$), $1,25(OH)_2D$, and perhaps other metabolites, is a useful indicator of the state of vitamin D nutrition. A low 25-OHD concentration alone is not diagnostic of dietary deficiency, as it may also reflect malabsorption, defective hepatic 25-hydroxylation of vitamin D, or increased clearance of circulating 25-OHD.

During the early phases of treatment, when skeletal mineralization may be rapid, the serum calcium concentration may actually decrease, and the serum alkaline phosphatase level may rise. The serum concentration of alkaline phosphatase, after peaking, generally returns to normal over several months. The time course of resolution of the secondary hyperparathyroidism is not well delineated, but there may be a disproportionate incidence of primary hyperparathyroidism among people with remote histories of treated vitamin D deficiency.

Treatment of Nutritional Vitamin D Deficiency

The treatment and prevention of nutritional vitamin D deficiency are straightforward. Low doses of ergocalciferol

(2 to 5 μg/d) or even ultraviolet radiation of the skin will effect a satisfactory cure (see also Chapter 27).[61, 62] In practice, ergocalciferol is given orally in doses of 125 μg/d (5000 IU/d) for the treatment of nutritional deficiency in infants and adults. Because the vitamin can be stored in body fat, regimens of intermittent high-dose parenteral treatment (stosstherapy) have been employed when day-to-day cooperation is not optimal.[63] These regimens incur a mild risk of hypercalcemia because of differences in individual responses. The response to ergocalciferol begins within days, but if an active metabolite such as calcitriol is given, a change in intestinal calcium absorption is measurable within hours. The early biochemical changes may include decreases in serum and urinary calcium values during early active skeletal mineralization. This can be avoided by supplying extra calcium by mouth (2 to 3 g of elemental calcium in four divided doses). Calcitriol may be useful for acute symptoms of tetany but is not recommended for maintenance therapy, as it does not replete body calciferol stores or allow regulation of the endogenous production of 1α-hydroxylated calciferol metabolites. Severe symptomatic hypocalcemia, which is rarely a feature of nutritional vitamin D deficiency, should be considered a medical emergency and can be treated with intravenous calcium infusion (15 mg of calcium/kg body weight infused over 6 to 24 h). Bone deformities may require orthopedic intervention after the metabolic deficit is corrected, because deficient bone may never be completely repaired.[64]

Defects in Vitamin D Metabolism and Action

General Considerations in Differential Diagnosis

A large number of conditions can cause the histological and radiological features of rickets and osteomalacia. Several states associated with active osteoblast function should be differentiated from the more typical osteomalacic disorders. Active osteoblast function is associated with a mild dispro-

portion between osteoid production and calcification, so-called high-turnover osteomalacia. During periods of rapid growth, severe limitation of dietary calcium can be manifest as rickets, although the more typical lesion in calcium deficiency is osteoporosis. Bone in the region of a healing fracture develops increased osteoid within 5 d. Disproportionate osteoid may also be found in active Paget disease, thyrotoxicosis, and primary hyperparathyroidism. In the last condition, true vitamin D deficiency may be present simultaneously, even resulting in normocalcemic or masked primary hyperparathyroidism.

Some generalized skeletal disorders may mimic rickets or osteomalacia. The metaphyseal chondrodystrophies are a group of disorders generally manifested as short-limbed dwarfism. These individuals may be given large doses of a calciferol in the belief that they have vitamin D–resistant rickets; the consequence is repeated episodes of vitamin D intoxication. In the metaphyseal chondrodystrophies, metaphyseal growth plates are distorted but not osteomalacic. The radiographic features mimic rickets, but the frayed metaphyses have a characteristic sclerotic appearance unlike that of the undermineralized zone in rickets. Most of the metaphyseal chondrodystrophies are associated with normal serum calcium, phosphorus, and alkaline phosphatase concentrations, except a severe juvenile form (Jansen type) that may cause hypercalcemia and its complications. In adults, generalized bone demineralization can occur in several disorders, osteoporosis often being a major concern. The diagnosis of osteomalacia is best made by recognizing the underlying cause and characteristic biochemical abnormalities. An adequate history and several simple laboratory analyses (for example, serum calcium, phosphorus, alkaline phosphatase, creatinine, and 25-OHD; Fig. 28–12) will exclude most diagnoses. A bone biopsy may be useful when serum and radiographic features are inconclusive, although experience with the technique is limited in most hospitals.

Deficiency of 25-OHD

Malabsorption of fat may cause vitamin D deficiency through a combination of malabsorption and increased loss

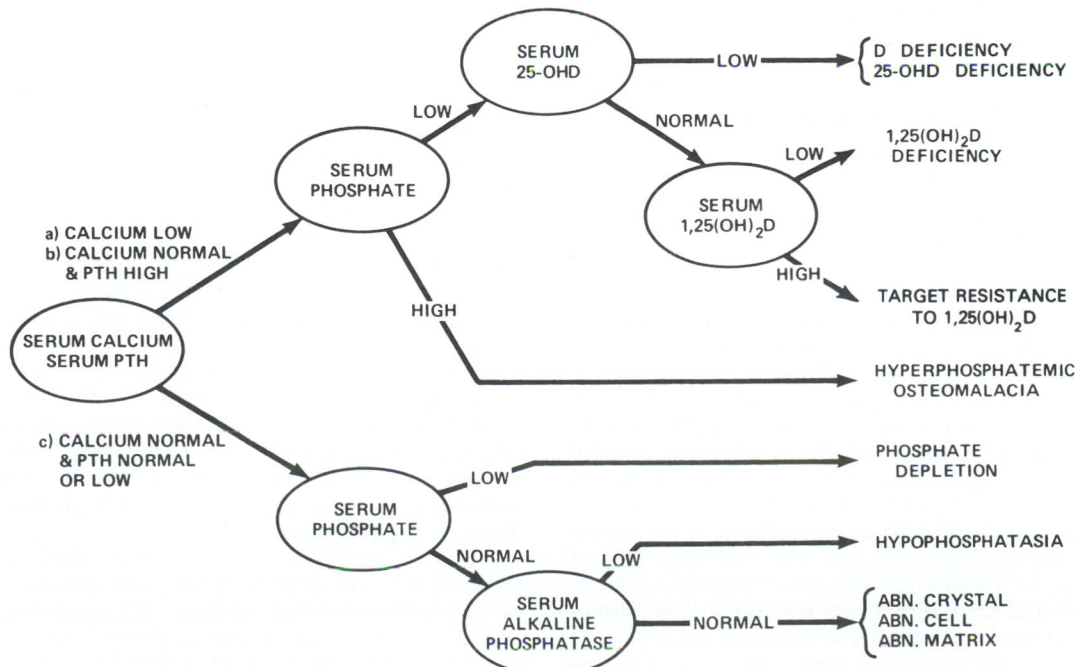

Figure 28–12. Algorithm for evaluation of patients with rickets or osteomalacia. Refer to descriptions of diagnostic categories for further details.

of 25-OHD and endogenous vitamin D owing to disruption of the enterohepatic circulation. Often there is also an element of light deprivation or body fat depletion that contributes to compromise of vitamin D stores. Rickets and osteomalacia may be early complications of gluten-sensitive enteropathy, pancreatic insufficiency, or intestinal bypass surgery. Children with malabsorption and vitamin D deficiency may be dwarfed. Vitamin D deficiency caused by malabsorption is associated with reduced concentrations of vitamin D and 25-OHD in serum.

The serum concentration of 25-OHD may also be depressed in patients with liver disease. Malabsorption and impairment of the enterohepatic circulation of vitamin D metabolites contribute to this picture, as does a decreased capacity to 25-hydroxylate the vitamin in the liver. A similar defect in hepatic production as well as increased metabolism of 25-OHD can contribute to neonatal hypocalcemia and neonatal rickets.[65] The serum concentration of 25-OHD drops progressively after birth in premature but not full-term infants. This can be prevented or treated by giving ergocalciferol in doses 4- to 10-fold greater than those recommended for normal neonates.

The goal of treatment is the restoration of normal serum concentrations of 25-OHD. The underlying disorder should be corrected if possible. Otherwise the vitamin D deficiency can be managed with oral or parenteral preparations of ergocalciferol or calcifediol.

Anticonvulsant-Induced Osteomalacia

Certain drugs interfere with vitamin D metabolism and action by mechanisms that are incompletely understood. Chronic use of anticonvulsants (phenytoin and barbiturates, particularly when taken in combination) may cause rickets or osteomalacia, with an attendant increase in the risk of fracture during seizures. Secondary hyperparathyroidism develops, and serum concentrations of 25-OHD tend to be mildly diminished but sometimes not sufficiently to explain the severity of the skeletal disorder. A reduced plasma 25-OHD level may be due to proliferation of hepatocyte smooth endoplasmic reticulum and shunting of vitamin D metabolism to other unidentified polar metabolites. Concentrations of $1,25(OH)_2D$ in the plasma are inappropriately low for the degree of secondary hyperparathyroidism.[66] Anticonvulsants partially inhibit the responses to active calciferol metabolites by both intestine and bone in vitro. Whatever the cause, anticonvulsant osteomalacia can be prevented or treated with calciferol analogues.

Decreased Renal 25-OHD 1α-Hydroxylase Activity

CHRONIC RENAL DISEASE. Low serum concentrations of $1,25(OH)_2D$ are common to many forms of rickets or osteomalacia. 25-OHD 1α-hydroxylase, the enzyme that catalyzes the most critical and most highly regulated step in calciferol metabolism, is found primarily in the kidney. A number of disease processes impinge on this system. Chronic renal failure leads to widespread disturbances in mineral regulation,[67] including several distinctive skeletal disturbances.

The normal intake and absorption of phosphate in the diet require that the kidneys excrete approximately 10% of the filtered load of phosphate. Phosphate retention, developing early in renal compromise, contributes to renal osteodystrophy. In animal models and in humans, restriction of gastrointestinal absorption of phosphate prevents or delays the early manifestations of renal osteodystrophy. A likely

sequence is as follows: renal compromise leads to decreased function of the 25-OHD 1α-hydroxylase system and to phosphate retention; phosphate retention inhibits the renal 25-OHD 1α-hydroxylase system further; and azotemia per se inhibits the intestinal absorption of calcium. Thus several factors lower the serum calcium concentration, and secondary hyperparathyroidism develops early. Advanced renal failure is associated with low serum concentrations of $1,25(OH)_2D$, even in the presence of severe secondary hyperparathyroidism. Acidosis develops both because of damage to the acid excretory mechanisms and because of the bicarbonate wasting of secondary hyperparathyroidism.

In other disorders such as primary renal tubular acidosis, some of the Fanconi syndromes, and the syndrome of tumor osteomalacia, decreased production of $1,25(OH)_2D$ undoubtedly also contributes significantly to the pathophysiology (discussed later).

HEREDITARY DEFICIENCY OF 25-OHD 1α-HYDROXYLASE. Hereditary vitamin D pseudodeficiency (vitamin D–dependent rickets) type I is a rare autosomal recessive disorder.[68] Affected persons develop early-onset vitamin D deficiency with hypocalcemia, secondary hyperparathyroidism, and hypophosphatemia. Typically rickets is diagnosed between the ages of 4 and 12 mo and is unresponsive to amounts of ergocalciferol or calcifediol that are effective in nutritional rickets. Complete cure is attainable but dependent on continuous treatment with high doses of either of these drugs. Before treatment, circulating concentrations of $1,25(OH)_2D$ are low. The disorder is responsive to physiological doses of calcitriol, making it highly likely that an abnormality of the 25-OHD 1α-hydroxylase system causes vitamin D pseudodeficiency type I. In some of these cases serum concentrations of $1,25(OH)_2D$ remain low even during effective treatment with ergocalciferol, suggesting profound deficiency of the enzyme and a clinical response that is dependent on pharmacological serum concentrations of 25-OHD or other weak vitamin D agonists. These patients must be differentiated from those with the more common X-linked familial hypophosphatemia. In the latter condition, patients may remain stable without therapy after adolescence; in vitamin D pseudodeficiency, however, manifestations eventually recur whenever therapy is withdrawn.

Hereditary Generalized Resistance to $1,25(OH)_2D$

Some patients with vitamin D pseudodeficiency have high serum concentrations of $1,25(OH)_2D$ before and during treatment (vitamin D pseudodeficiency type II). This disorder is presumably due to defects in the response of target tissues to $1,25(OH)_2D$. The affected patients in half the kindreds show partial or total alopecia, which reflects the most severe underlying defect. Treatment is of three types, depending on severity. (1) Moderate defects can be managed with extremely high doses of ergocalciferol or cholecalciferol, which allow patients to maintain high serum $1,25(OH)_2D$ levels from endogenous production. (2) More severe defects require still higher serum $1,25(OH)_2D$ concentrations that can be achieved only with high doses of calciferol analogues such as calcitriol that do not require 1α-hydroxylation. (3) Patients with no calcemic response to any form or amount of calciferol require high doses of calcium orally or intravenously.

Studies with cells cultured from these patients have shown a series of defects in function of $1,25(OH)_2D$ receptors: hormone-binding defects, DNA-binding defects, or cytosol-to-nucleus translocation defects.[69] Analyses on several such patients have characterized the specific mutations in the gene for the vitamin D receptor (Fig. 28–13).[70]

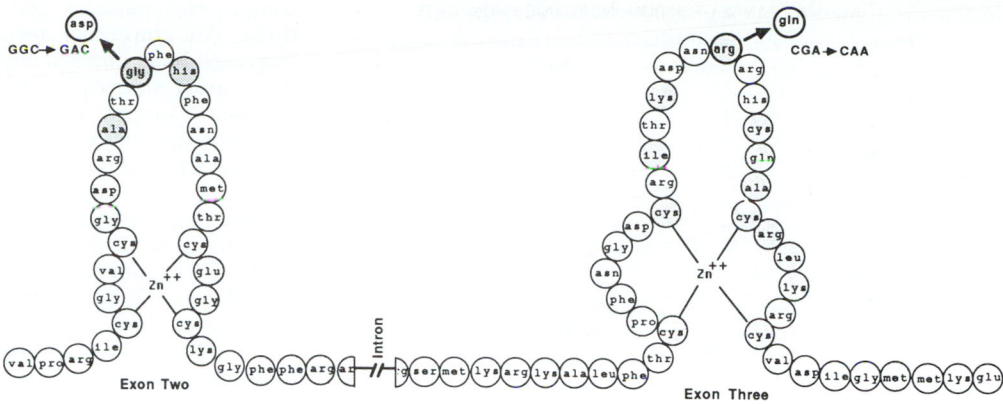

Figure 28–13. Amino acid sequence and hypothetical structure of the vitamin D receptor DNA binding domain. The amino acids are shown as two potential zinc finger arrays. The conserved residues from receptors for steroids, thyroid hormone, and retinoic acid are shaded. The single nucleotide change causing an amino acid change in one of two kindreds with hereditary resistance to 1,25(OH)₂D (and vitamin D receptors showing abnormal binding to DNA) is shown at the tip of the zinc fingers. (Modified from Hughes MR, Malloy PJ, Kieback DG, et al. Point mutations in the human vitamin D receptor gene associated with hypocalcemic rickets. Science 1988; 242: 1702–1705. Copyright 1988 by the American Association for the Advancement of Science.)

Defects in Mineral Metabolism

Calcium Deficiency Syndromes

Calcium-deficient rickets with high concentrations of serum 1,25(OH)₂D has been documented in three circumstances; in each the skeletal requirement for calcium exceeds the capacity of the intestines to supply this mineral:

1. Rickets can develop during rapid adolescent growth in children who consume a diet low in calcium (such as African Bantu children). In this group the serum calcium concentration is maintained at a normal level by compensatory increases in serum PTH and 1,25(OH)₂D.[71]

2. Rickets caused by deficiency of vitamin D or 25-OHD is associated with high serum concentrations of 1,25(OH)₂D during the remineralization phase of therapy. If treatment provides 25-OHD, the mineral flux to bone sustains hypocalcemia and secondary hyperparathyroidism so that serum concentrations of 1,25(OH)₂D may become three times the upper normal concentration for 1 to 2 mo.

3. Among survivors of extreme prematurity, the growing skeleton does not get sufficient calcium and phosphate from intestinal absorption;[72] this could reflect combinations of undeveloped intestinal capacity to respond to 1,25(OH)₂D and an imbalance between skeletal needs and dietary supply.

Phosphate Deficiency Syndromes

The importance of phosphate metabolism in the osteomalacias is underscored by the fact that in rats the serum phosphate concentration is normally 3 mmol/L (9.0 mg/dL) (double that in mature humans), and only combined restriction of vitamin D and phosphate will foster development of nutritional rickets or osteomalacia. Food faddism in humans generally cannot cause a nutritional deficiency of phosphate, because phosphate is uniformly distributed in all foodstuffs (see Table 27–3). Severe phosphate deficiency can develop with consumption of effective phosphate chelators such as aluminum hydroxide. Phosphate depletion states may also arise during unbalanced alimentation, intravenous feeding, or dietary restriction in combination with hemodialysis against a low-phosphate solution.

Within 5 d after phosphate restriction, renal clearance of phosphate becomes nearly undetectable. Continued phosphate depletion leads to hypophosphatemia with increased intestinal absorption of calcium and increased renal excretion of calcium. Both these effects on calcium flux are the result of phosphate-associated changes in vitamin D metabolism.[73] Phosphate restriction causes an increase in renal 25-OHD 1α-hydroxylase that is independent of parathyroid

function and an increased accumulation of 1,25(OH)₂D in intestinal target tissues. Even with high serum concentrations of 1,25(OH)₂D, osteomalacia develops if insufficient phosphate is available in serum to support mineralization of osteoid. If this process continues for several months, patients manifest muscle weakness, anorexia, bone pain, and occasionally elevation of serum alkaline phosphatase activity. Depletion of phosphate also may compromise cellular energy metabolism, leading to defective function of muscle cells, leukocytes, monocytes, and erythrocytes.

Rickets and osteomalacia may also develop in conditions causing a reduced renal threshold for phosphate excretion. This, of course, is an integral feature of secondary hyperparathyroidism and contributes an element of phosphate depletion to all vitamin D deficiency states except those associated with hyperphosphatemia. Decreases in the renal threshold for phosphate excretion can also produce severe osteomalacia in the absence of secondary hyperparathyroidism.

X-Linked Familial Hypophosphatemia

X-linked familial hypophosphatemia was the first rachitic process recognized to be refractory to vitamin D and is the most common form of hereditary rickets.[68] As with most X-linked processes, the disturbance is most severe in males, who may manifest florid rickets during childhood. Females often exhibit only hypophosphatemia. Bone age is retarded, and stature is decreased, with the shortening most severe in the legs. Dental caries are increased in frequency. Muscle weakness is less common than in hypocalcemic rickets. In adults the disease may stabilize without treatment.

The radiographic features are basically those of rickets and osteomalacia. Another radiographic feature in adults is a paradoxically radiopaque skeleton with an increase in the total mineral mass. This is a manifestation of mineralization, albeit deficient, of a very large mass of osteoid and may cause confusion with osteopetrosis. In addition, osteophytes may limit motion at the elbows, shoulders, and hips or cause spinal ankylosis. The histological features resemble those of typical rickets or osteomalacia. Although adults may not exhibit symptoms, histological evidence of osteomalacia persists. The major biochemical features in the serum are a normal calcium concentration and a significantly depressed phosphate concentration. A normal serum calcium concentration and an absence of severe secondary hyperparathyroidism are major diagnostic features. Hypophosphatemia during fasting and postprandially is a manifestation of a low threshold for renal phosphate excretion and is detectable from age 6 mo until old age (Fig. 28–14). The alkaline

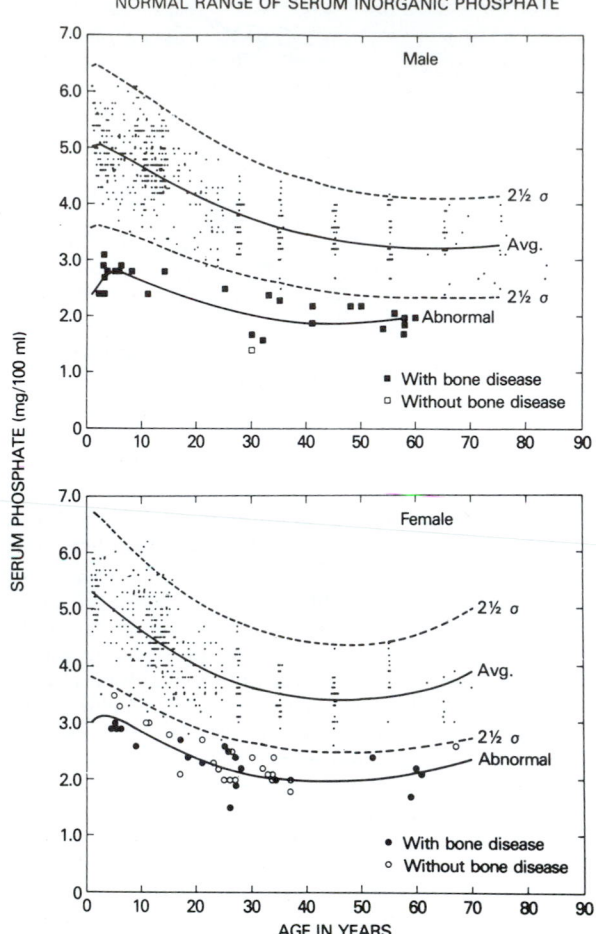

NORMAL RANGE OF SERUM INORGANIC PHOSPHATE

Figure 28–14. Normal serum phosphate concentrations in males and females (dotted curves are computerized fits ±2.5 SD to the estimate range for 99% of normal) compared with concentrations in affected members from five families with X-linked hypophosphatemia. Note that at all ages, serum phosphate concentrations are outside 99% confidence limits for normal. (Modified from BG Greenberg, RW Winters, JB Graham, The normal range of serum inorganic phosphorus and its utility as a discriminant in the diagnosis of congenital hypophosphatemia, J Clin Endocrinol Metab, 20, 364–379, 1960, © by The Endocrine Society.)

phosphatase activity in the plasma may be high when rickets is the most active but is otherwise normal. Intestinal absorption of calcium is mildly decreased, and the serum calcium level is maintained at normal by mild secondary hyperparathyroidism. These features differ from those of pure phosphate depletion with activation of production of $1,25(OH)_2D$. In fact, defective response of the renal 25-OHD 1α-hydroxylase (to either PTH or phosphorus depletion) is an integral part of this disorder. The cause of hypophosphatemia is unclear. A parallel defect in intestinal phosphate transport may be present. Whether a humoral factor or an intrinsic target tissue defect is the cause has not been settled. In mice with X-linked hypophosphatemic rickets, renal transport and intestinal transport of phosphate are abnormal; the skeletal manifestations can be prevented by adding phosphate to the diet but are not improved by treatment with cholecalciferol or calcitriol. A defect in sodium-dependent phosphate transport is found in brush border membrane vesicles from kidneys of affected animals.[74]

Although X-linked familial hypophosphatemia varies in severity, phenotypic expression is generally uniform. However, genetic heterogeneity does exist. Kindreds have been described with autosomal dominant or autosomal recessive

transmission patterns and with differences in clinical features. An autosomal recessive variant is associated with increased bone mineral content at early ages, early fusion of the cranial sutures, and nerve deafness. One autosomal dominant variant is associated with glucose intolerance. Mutation in either of two separate loci on the X chromosome (hyp or gyr) of the mouse produces a hypophosphatemic phenotype, and one of these mutations also causes cochlear defects (gyr, for gyration). Sensorineural hearing defects are also common in X-linked hypophosphatemia in humans, perhaps for similar reasons.

Many of these patients have been treated with pharmacological doses of the calciferols. Although skeletal healing may occur, hypophosphatemia persists, suggesting the primacy of the phosphate transport abnormality. Moreover, such therapy incurs a high risk of episodic vitamin D intoxication and irreversible renal damage. Treatment with calcifediol or calcitriol alone is similarly unsatisfactory. Satisfactory results have been attained by the administration of inorganic phosphate at doses equivalent to 1 to 4 g of elemental phosphorus per day. This must be given by mouth at inconvenient 4-h intervals to maintain a nearly normal serum concentration of phosphate. Simultaneous treatment with calcitriol improves bone mineralization and allows use of lower doses of phosphates (1 to 2 g/d).[75] Because the renal defect causes both phosphate wasting and defective 25-OHD 1α-hydroxylase, combination therapy with phosphate and a calciferol is logical. However, this therapy introduces a risk of renal damage from hyperphosphaturia and hypercalciuria and requires careful monitoring of urine and blood chemistry.

Renal Tubular Damage

Several renal tubular disorders may be associated with rickets or osteomalacia disproportionate to the degree of renal failure. Some of the disorders affect the proximal tubule, with a stereotyped pattern of renal wastage of phosphate, glucose, bicarbonate, and amino acids (Fanconi syndrome). The causes include inborn errors of metabolism (cystinosis, galactosemia, glycogen storage disease, the hepatorenal form of hereditary tyrosinemia, hereditary fructose intolerance, hepatolenticular degeneration, and the oculocerebrorenal syndrome), intoxications (lead, mercury, cadmium, outdated tetracycline, streptozocin, and Lysol), immunopathies (amyloidosis, Bence Jones proteinuria, and Sjögren syndrome), and idiopathic factors. It is not known to what extent phosphate depletion or deficient production of $1,25(OH)_2D$ contributes to these syndromes. Models for rickets caused by proximal tubular disorders have been developed by administering either maleic acid or strontium to rats. Such proximal tubular dysfunction causes decreased production of $1,25(OH)_2D$, and the skeletal manifestations can be prevented by the administration of calcitriol. A rachitic state also occurs in proximal renal tubular acidosis;[76] in this disorder, however, the skeletal manifestations can be prevented simply by treatment with sufficient bicarbonate (5 to 15 mmol/kg body weight/d) to return the serum pH to normal. Osteomalacia may also develop with acidosis after ureterosigmoidostomy. Low serum concentrations of $1,25(OH)_2D$ have been implicated.

Renal Wasting of Phosphate with High Serum $1,25(OH)_2D$ Levels

There are two rare hereditary disorders with activation of 25-OHD 1α-hydroxylase by chronic hypophosphatemia. The first is a combination of hypophosphatemia with absorptive hypercalciuria, resulting from the high serum

1,25(OH)$_2$D level. In its mildest expression in some members of a large kindred, it showed many features similar to those of idiopathic hypercalciuria.[77] The second disorder is a combination of hereditary Fanconi syndrome with high serum levels of 1,25(OH)$_2$D.[78]

These unusual syndromes highlight the fact that the defects in X-linked hypophosphatemia or most Fanconi syndromes have a broader impact on the kidney, compromising not only solute transport but also the renal 25-OHD 1α-hydroxylase activity.

Tumor Osteomalacia

Another syndrome of renal phosphate wastage occurs with several neoplastic processes. Typically a previously healthy adult develops progressive hypophosphatemic osteomalacia with a normal serum calcium concentration. Removal of a small, usually benign, tumor leads to dramatic reversal of the metabolic disturbance. The tumors include sclerosing or cavernous hemangiomas and ossifying and nonossifying mesenchymal tumors of bone. Analogous disturbances have occurred in prostatic cancer, fibrous dysplasia of bone, the basal cell nevus syndrome, and neurofibromatosis. The cell of origin and the presumed humoral mediators are not known. A low serum level of 1,25(OH)$_2$D has been documented in some,[79] and the tumor may release factors that inhibit the renal 25-OHD 1α-hydroxylase system. This etiology should be considered in any normocalcemic adult with a phosphate-wasting disorder of unknown origin. The offending tumor may be difficult to locate.

Hyperphosphatemic Osteomalacia

Osteomalacia or rickets can also be associated with hyperphosphatemia. Cases have been described in Asian immigrants to Britain who had nutritional vitamin D deficiency and parathyroid failure of unknown origin, in a patient with idiopathic hypoparathyroidism and normal 25-OHD stores, and in three siblings in a single family. In the presence of hypocalcemia and secondary hyperparathyroidism, the deficient phosphaturic response to PTH had led to diagnoses such as pseudohypoparathyroidism type II or hypohyperparathyroidism. The serum concentration of 1,25(OH)$_2$D is low or inferred to be low. In some cases, the hyperphosphatemia is a result of hypocalcemia-induced impairment of renal phosphate excretion.[80] The association with osteomalacia, which is usually associated with phosphate depletion, is particularly puzzling.

Disturbances of Bone Cells and Bone Matrix

Familial Hypophosphatasia

Hypophosphatasia is an autosomal recessive disorder of variable severity.[81] In Toronto the incidence is approximately 1 in 100,000 live births. Its most severe manifestation is infantile rickets with craniostenosis and death at 1 to 2 y of age from complications of hypercalcemia (vomiting, nephrocalcinosis, and renal failure). A less severe manifestation in childhood causes premature loss of primary teeth, pseudofractures, and radiolucent zones in long bones with characteristic notching at the borders of the frayed metaphyses. The bone cortices are often thickened, with subperiosteal new bone formation and calcification of the paraspinal ligaments. The least severe grade presents in adulthood with premature loss of teeth, fractures, and nephrolithiasis. These persons may give a history of rickets in childhood. The mild adult form may also occur as an autosomal dominant trait.

The characteristic biochemical features are low serum concentrations of alkaline phosphatase reflecting deficient isoenzyme from bone, a marked increase in serum and urinary phosphorylethanolamine, and lesser increases in pyrophosphate. Some affected individuals intermittently show normal levels of alkaline phosphatase. The urinary hydroxyproline excretion rate is low. Analysis of bone from affected persons reveals an absence or severe deficiency of alkaline phosphatase activity in osteoblasts, and point mutation in the alkaline phosphatase gene has been documented in the lethal form of the disorder.[82] Increased urinary excretion of phosphorylethanolamine and pyrophosphate is the result of elevation in the plasma levels of these compounds, which are substrates for osteoblast alkaline phosphatase. It is not known whether the accumulation of these phosphoesters relates to the mineralization defect. Some substrates for the alkaline phosphatase enzyme may be mineralization inhibitors that must be cleaved to allow normal mineralization. This possibility is supported by the production of an osteomalacic state by the administration of diphosphonates (see later discussion) that are phosphatase-resistant analogues of pyrophosphate. No satisfactory treatment for hypophosphatasia is available.

Low-Turnover Osteomalacia

Low-turnover osteomalacia is a state with decreased activity of bone cells (osteoblasts and osteoclasts). The disorder occurs in patients undergoing hemodialysis and in those treated with total parenteral nutrition. Proposed causative factors include relative deficiency of PTH (such as after parathyroidectomy) and aluminum accumulation in bone. The hemodialysis group exhibits bone pain, fractures, and suppression of parathyroid function; there is a propensity to develop hypercalcemia, particularly during therapy with calciferols. Aluminum accumulates at the bone mineralization front in these patients, but the role of aluminum in the disorder has not been established.[83] In the group undergoing total parenteral nutrition, the clinical features are similar except that hypercalciuria is common. Speculation about the etiology has focused on aluminum in casein hydrolysates and on the use of ergocalciferol supplements.[84]

Fibrogenesis Imperfecta Ossium and Axial Osteomalacia

Fibrogenesis imperfecta ossium is a rare disorder in patients older than age 50.[85] It leads to severe skeletal pain, tenderness, and progressive immobilization. Radiographs show a symmetrical distribution of coarse dense trabeculae with a periosteal reaction and soft tissue calcifications. This may resemble Paget disease, and the serum alkaline phosphatase level is similarly elevated. Demonstration of the loss of the usual birefringence of bone collagen fibrils under polarized light is diagnostic. Electron microscopy shows disorganized bone collagen fibrils. This disorder may be an acquired disturbance in matrix structure that will not support normal mineralization.

Axial osteomalacia is another rare disorder developing after age 60. Symptoms are mild and are limited to the spine, pelvis, and ribs. Matrix qualities have not been described, but the disorder resembles fibrogenesis imperfecta ossium.

Mineralization Inhibitors: Fluorides and Diphosphonates

Diphosphonates are analogues of pyrophosphate in which a P–C–P bond replaces the P–O–P bond, rendering the bond less susceptible to hydrolysis. They adsorb to bone mineral and are useful as bone-scanning agents. In vitro and in vivo they inhibit apatite crystal deposition and resorption. Certain analogues may block bone resorption but not bone deposition. In animals they also block the renal 25-OHD 1α-hydroxylase.

Inorganic fluoride also accumulates in bone mineral. Chronic ingestion of fluoride (more than 20 mg of fluoride ion/d) leads to skeletal fluorosis, a potentially crippling disorder associated with arthralgias, periosteal new bone formation, osteophyte formation, osteosclerosis, and kyphosis. Osteoid surface area and width increase. There are also degenerative changes in osteocytes and the accumulation of periosteal new bone with a disordered lamellar structure. The fluoride content of bone is increased, and the size of bone crystals is increased. Whether fluorides cause osteomalacia by a direct interaction with bone crystals is not known. Fluorides at lower and briefer dosages are used to treat osteoporosis.

OSTEITIS FIBROSA CYSTICA

Osteitis fibrosa cystica is the characteristic bone abnormality of primary or secondary hyperparathyroidism (see Fig. 28-8D). (Also see Chapter 27.) It is manifested as generalized osteopenia, increased bone resorption (particularly at the subperiosteal surfaces), and the formation of cysts or cyst-like areas (brown tumors). The usual bones involved (as observed on roentgenograms) are the phalanges, distal clavicles, and skull. In severe cases the long bones, patella, and ribs may become involved, and resorption may take place in the distal tufts of the phalanges. Brown tumors may present as swellings of the long bones or phalanges with distortion and distention of cortical bone and, in severe cases, fractures. Bone pain can occur.

Histologically, the bones show increased numbers of multinucleated osteoclasts and osteoblasts as well as areas of increased resorption, increased numbers of trabecular surfaces showing resorption, and fibroblastic proliferation.[86] The lacunae around osteocytes increase in size as a result of osteocytic osteolysis. Proliferation of osteoclasts and fibroblasts is also evident in marrow spaces.[87] Areas of unmineralized osteoid may also be found. Brown tumors are collections of multinucleated osteoclasts in a spindle cell stroma. Bone formation as well as resorption is increased. Increased bone formation is evidenced by increased osteoblast numbers and islands of newly formed bone and is reflected by areas of osteosclerosis on radiographs and by an increase in the plasma alkaline phosphatase level.[87] Because osteoclast activity exceeds osteoblast activity, the net result is bone resorption. Nevertheless, overall bone structure is virtually normal, unlike the disorganized mosaic appearance of bone in Paget disease. Bone demineralization of osteitis fibrosa cystica differs from that in osteoporosis, in which no increase in either osteoblast or osteoclast activity occurs (see Fig. 28-8).

RENAL OSTEODYSTROPHY

Bone disease is a major complication of chronic renal failure. The longer life is preserved, as by hemodialysis, the greater the osteodystrophy. More than 90% of the patients maintained for 2 y with hemodialysis have radiological evidence of bone disease.[88] Renal osteodystrophy is a complex disturbance of bone comprising varying degrees of osteomalacia, osteitis fibrosa cystica, and osteosclerosis. The etiology is not completely understood, but impaired vitamin

D metabolism, secondary hyperparathyroidism, diminished gastrointestinal absorption of calcium, and sometimes aluminum toxicity are involved. The use of heparin during dialysis may also contribute. Reduction of the renal mass impairs normal physiological production of $1,25(OH)_2D$ in response to PTH. This in turn leads to malabsorption of calcium from the gut. Hypocalcemia is due to both hyperphosphatemia and diminished calcium absorption and causes secondary hyperparathyroidism (see Chapter 27). The basic defect is caused by $1,25(OH)_2D$ deficiency, and hypersecretion of PTH causes osteitis fibrosa cystica and osteosclerosis.

Manifestations of osteodystrophy include bone pain and fractures. Accompanying abnormalities include muscle weakness (a consequence of uremic neuropathy), soft tissue and vascular calcification, and pruritus.

Treatment of renal osteodystrophy is generally directed toward reduction of serum phosphate level and use of calciferol analogues to enhance calcium absorption and suppress PTH secretion.[89–91] Aluminum toxicity is due to the incorporation into bone of aluminum from two sources: gastrointestinal absorption from aluminum hydroxide gels given to diminish phosphate absorption, and aluminum in the water used in hemodialysis. Aluminum is toxic to bone and produces an osteomalacia-like disturbance that sharply reduces calcification of matrix.[92] The clinical manifestations are severe bone pain, spontaneous fractures, and sometimes hypercalcemia. This syndrome can be difficult to differentiate from the usual osteomalacia of renal osteodystrophy or hyperparathyroidism. The intact PTH (two-site) immunoassay is useful in this regard. In aluminum bone disease the PTH level in blood is low or normal. The deferoxamine challenge test[92] may also be useful for this purpose. Aluminum bone disease can be prevented by eliminating aluminum-containing gels and using aluminum-free water in hemodialysis. Some success has been achieved in treating aluminum bone disease with infusions of deferoxamine.[93] Treatment of renal osteodystrophy by using calcium carbonate by mouth plus calcifediol[94] or calcitriol[90] appears to be a useful alternative to administration of aluminum-containing phosphate binders and in some cases corrects renal osteodystrophy.

Severe secondary hyperparathyroidism may be an indication for parathyroidectomy. This is definitely indicated if tertiary hyperparathyroidism develops, which is defined by absolute and persistent hypercalcemia after a long period of secondary hyperparathyroidism. In other forms of secondary hyperparathyroidism, parathyroidectomy may also be indicated, usually in those with severe osteitis fibrosa cystica. Indiscriminate parathyroidectomy causes worsening of bone disease, severe osteomalacia,[92] and tetany that is difficult to control. Renal transplantation, in many cases, leads to resolution of renal osteodystrophy.[89]

PAGET DISEASE (OSTEITIS DEFORMANS)

Paget disease affects about 3% of people older than age 40, and the incidence rises with age. Men are affected more commonly than women.

Pathophysiology

The hallmark of Paget disease is disordered bone remodeling. The lesions may occur singly or at multiple sites. Initially, excessive bone resorption results in a lytic appearance on x-ray views (osteoporosis circumscripta in the skull). Histologically, abundant osteoclasts are seen that have ac-

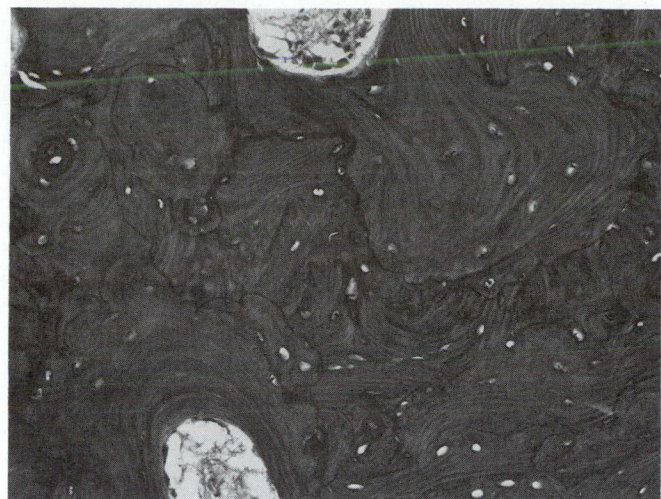

Figure 28–15. Bone biopsy specimen from a patient with Paget disease showing the typical mosaic pattern (i.e., disorganized lamellar bone and cement lines). Decalcified bone magnified × 80. (From Singer FR. Paget's Disease of Bone. New York: Plenum, 1977.)

tively resorbed bone. Later the marrow spaces are occupied by a fibrovascular stroma, and an increase in osteoblast activity (presumably because of normal coupling of bone formation and resorption) leads to excessive bone formation. The combination of disorganized resorption and formation leads to the characteristic mosaic pattern—areas of lamellar bone randomly connected by cement lines at the borders of prior resorption (Fig. 28–15). In the final stage, increased cellular activity is not found. Bone in Paget disease may show increased density on x-ray views, but the abnormal structure makes bone weaker than normal (see Fig. 28–15).

Etiology

Numerous theories (e.g., abnormalities in collagen structure and calcitonin deficiency) have been proposed as to the pathogenesis. A genetic basis is suggested by its familial occurrence (more than 87 families with multiple involved members have been reported). An autosomal dominant pattern of inheritance has been postulated.

The finding of intranuclear inclusions in osteoclasts from pagetic bone has suggested a possible viral origin.[95] Essentially all patients have these inclusions, and they are not found in hyperparathyroidism, osteomalacia, multiple myeloma, or fibrous dysplasia. Similar inclusions are present in giant cell tumors of bone; this is of interest because of the possible relationship of such tumors to Paget disease. Therapy with calcitonin can correct metabolic abnormalities but does not lead to disappearance of the intranuclear inclusions. In contrast, therapy with diphosphonate may lead to disappearance of intranuclear inclusions.[96] The inclusions are present in 20 to 40% of the osteoclasts in Paget disease and consist of microfilaments in a paracrystalline array (occasional single microfilaments may also be seen) (Fig. 28–16). The similarity to the paramyxovirus inclusions in brain cells of patients with subacute sclerosing panencephalitis suggests that a slow virus may be involved. Features compatible with such a possibility include the late onset and long subclinical course, the absence of acute inflammation, the presence of multinucleated giant cells, and the geographic and familial clustering of the disease. Geographic clustering, which is rare in Asia and Africa but common in Western Europe and the United States, could be due to an infectious agent. Familial clustering could result from genetic susceptibility to infection by a viral agent. However, no genetic marker for susceptibility to Paget disease has been found.

Immunofluorescent staining of the intranuclear inclusions with antimeasles virus serum has been reported.[95] Despite this finding and despite the similarity of the intranuclear inclusions to the subacute sclerosing panencephalitis agent, patients with Paget disease do not show high titers of antimeasles antibodies. Thus the measles-like agent of subacute sclerosing panencephalitis is probably not responsible for Paget disease. One group has reported that osteoclasts from pagetic lesions in a long-term culture show specific

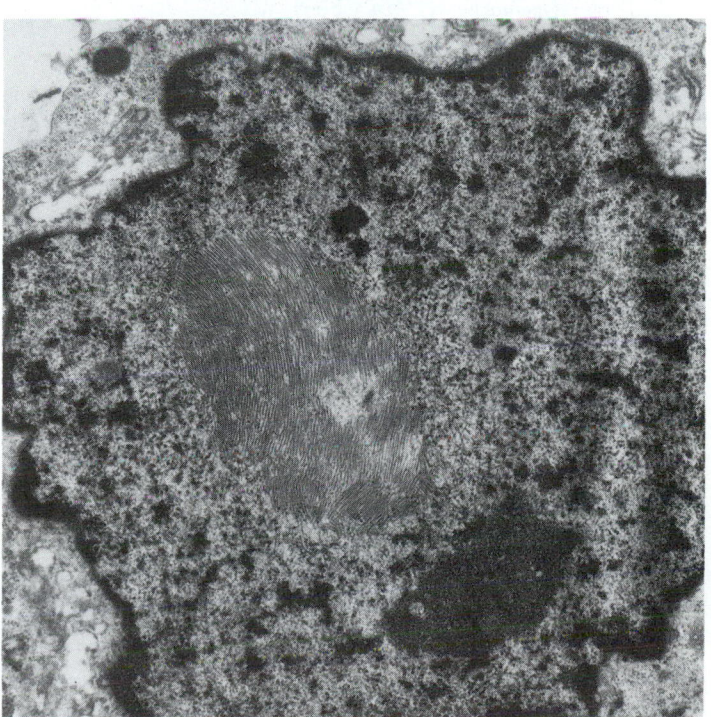

Figure 28–16. Electron micrograph of an osteoclast nucleus from a patient with Paget disease showing characteristic intranuclear inclusion (consisting of 125 Å diameter microfilaments). Decalcified bone magnified × 32,400. (Courtesy of Dr. Barbara G. Mills and Dr. Frederick R. Singer.)

immunofluorescent staining with antisera against both measles virus and respiratory syncytial virus,[97] and genomic RNA of the measles virus has been detected in pagetic bone cells by in situ hybridization.[98] Ultimate proof of a viral pathogenesis and identification of the responsible agent will require isolation of the virus from bone cells and documentation that it can cause the disease.

Clinical Features

The clinical spectrum of Paget disease ranges from asymptomatic patients with involvement of a single bone detected incidentally on x-ray examination to crippling deformities and serious neurological complications (Fig. 28–17). The axial skeleton is more commonly affected than the appendicular skeleton. In several series (including autopsy and retrospective radiological surveys), the sites affected (in decreasing order) are pelvis, lumbar spine, sacrum, femur, skull, shoulders, thoracic spine, cervical spine, and ribs.[99]

The manifestations are due to abnormal bone structure, increased skeletal blood flow, or a combination.[100] Pain may be caused by direct involvement of bone or by secondary osteoarthritis in joints (commonly hip or knee) adjacent to pagetic bone. Inadequate tensile strength of involved bone may lead to deformities, typically bowing of the femur or tibia, which may impair walking. Fissuring or partial fractures in the long bones at sites of active resorption may progress to complete transverse fractures; pathological fractures (again most commonly in the femur and tibia) may also occur in weakened bones. The incidence of fracture in patients with multiple bone involvement is about 18%. Several types of bone tumor may complicate Paget disease. Malignant lesions, usually osteogenic sarcoma or fibrosarcoma, occur in less than 1% and carry a poor patient prognosis. The femur and humerus are the most common sites of malignant transformation, which is heralded by increased pain, rapid soft tissue swelling, or a marked increase in the alkaline phosphatase level. Benign tumors such as giant cell tumors also occur. These lesions, more properly termed *giant cell reparative granulomas of bone*,[101] are polyostotic in distribution, are limited to pagetic bone, and may show familial or geographic clustering. Local radiation is effective for benign tumors, but no treatment is effective for sarcomas.

Increased skeletal blood flow may lead to high-output cardiac failure. Increased bone vascularity also makes surgery on pagetic bone more difficult. Neurological complications are relatively rare (with the exception of deafness) but potentially serious[102] and may be caused by the direct neural encroachment of pagetic bone or by "steal" syndromes produced by increased skeletal vascularity. Deafness occurs in 12 to 50% of the patients with extensive Paget disease and may be conductive (middle-ear ossicle involvement) or sensorineural (cochlear invasion or eighth nerve compression in the auditory canal). Platybasia (invagination of the base of the skull by cervical vertebrae) may lead to vertebral-basilar insufficiency with vertigo, hydrocephalus, cerebellar herniation, ataxia, and lower cranial nerve lesions. Spinal cord compression is rare despite the frequency of lumbar vertebral involvement[103] but can be produced by narrowing of the spinal canal by pagetic bone (demonstrable by myelography) or by vascular mechanisms. Extramedullary hematopoiesis is a rare cause of spinal cord compression.

It has been suggested that Paget disease can lead to the development of primary hyperparathyroidism.[104] However, the coincidence is more likely because both diseases are relatively common. Secondary hyperparathyroidism has been documented in untreated patients, particularly those with severe Paget disease.[105] Increased demand for calcium during periods of accelerated bone formation is the postulated mechanism. Secondary hyperparathyroidism can also occur with medical therapy of Paget disease,[96] because therapy blocks bone resorption before bone formation.

Diagnostic Evaluation

On physical examination the long bones may be deformed and the skull may be enlarged. The skin over involved bone may be warm because of increased cutaneous blood flow. Funduscopic examination reveals angioid streaks in about 15% of the patients with polyostotic involvement. These lesions are due to cracks in the Bruch membrane.

The bone lesions of Paget disease show a characteristic radiographic appearance reflecting the disordered bone remodeling (Fig. 28–18). Osteoblast tumor metastases, especially pelvic metastases from prostatic carcinoma, may present a similar appearance. Thickening of the pelvic brim and iliopectineal line and widening of the pubic and ischial bones serve to distinguish Paget disease from osteoblast metastases. Biopsy may rarely be necessary to make the diagnosis.

Radiographic evidence of bone involvement does not necessarily reflect continued metabolic activity in Paget disease. Scanning with bone-seeking radioactive agents such as technetium Tc 99m diphosphonate allows a distinction to be made between active lesions with a high uptake and burned-out lesions with a minimal uptake. Scanning also can be used to follow the effects of therapy, but this is ordinarily unnecessary because more sensitive and easier biochemical tests are available. Increased uptake of tracer, however, may be

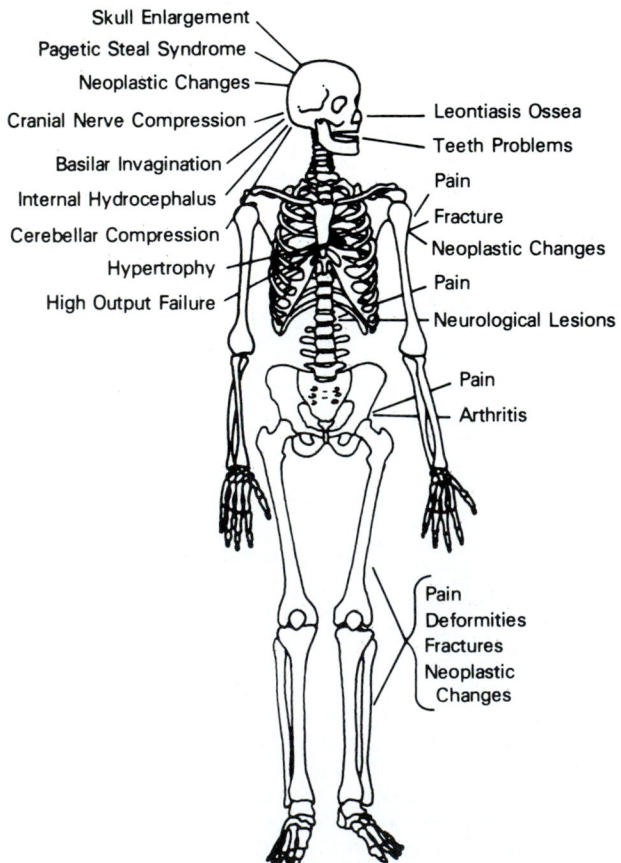

Figure 28–17. Features and complications of Paget disease. (Reprinted by permission of Greenwood Publishing Group, Inc., Westport, CT, from Paget's Disease of Bone: Assessment and Management by R. C. Hamdy. Copyright © 1981 by Praeger Publishers.)

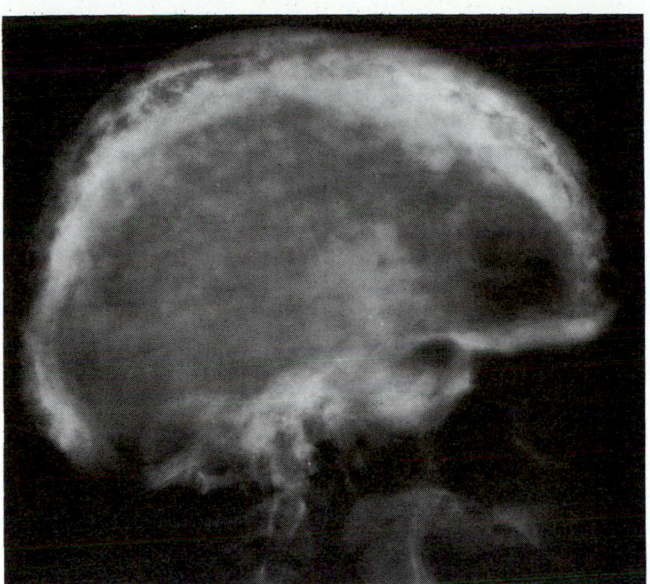

Figure 28–18. Radiograph of the skull in a patient with advanced Paget disease showing thickening, disordered new bone formation (cotton-wool patches), and basilar impression. (From Singer FR. Paget's Disease of Bone. New York: Plenum, 1977.)

the earliest indication of recurrence of disease after stopping treatment.[106] Conventional radiography may show serial changes in a given bone but requires meticulous attention to positioning and radiographic technique.

Biochemical indices of bone resorption and formation are increased and are useful parameters for diagnosis and evaluation of therapy.[100] Increased resorption is reflected in the elevated urinary excretion of hydroxyproline. (In about one fifth of patients, however, hydroxyproline excretion is normal.) This parameter returns to normal with therapy. Increased bone formation is reflected by elevated serum alkaline phosphatase activity, but about one tenth of patients have normal values for total activity. Even these normal values may decline with therapy. The serum alkaline phosphatase level declines more slowly than the urinary hydroxyproline excretion during treatment. This feature supports the hypothesis that increased bone formation is a secondary phenomenon resulting from coupling. Elevations in serum osteocalcin levels in patients with active Paget disease correlate with the serum alkaline phosphatase level,[107] but this parameter is less sensitive at lower levels of disease activity than serum alkaline phosphatase.[105]

Serum calcium and phosphate concentrations are normal despite the increased bone turnover. Hypercalcemia may occur in patients who are immobilized, but concomitant hyperparathyroidism (and other causes of hypercalcemia) should be excluded. An increased incidence of hyperuricemia may be due to increased bone cell turnover.

Treatment

Indications for treatment include pain, neurological complications, hypercalcemia caused by immobilization, multiple fractures, and, rarely, high-output cardiac failure.[100] Treatment may also be indicated before orthopedic surgery to decrease blood loss. Pain, the most common indication for treatment, can be relieved when caused by direct bone involvement but not when caused by secondary osteoarthritis. A brief trial of therapy may be indicated to help make the distinction. Improvement in neurological symptoms with effective medical therapy has been reported.[102, 103] The ra-

pidity of response in some cases suggests a vascular basis for neurological dysfunction rather than encroachment of bone on neural tissue. Deafness rarely improves. There is no evidence that prophylactic therapy is beneficial in the asymptomatic patient, although it may be tried in younger subjects with severe progressive but asymptomatic disease.

Treatment is primarily based on drugs that inhibit bone resorption. Decreased bone formation is due to removal of the osteoclast induction of osteoblast activity. A transient imbalance between bone formation and resorption with therapy commonly leads to an initial decrease in the serum calcium level. Secondary hyperparathyroidism may develop. Treatment suppresses but does not cure the underlying lesion. Effective drugs include calcitonin, the diphosphonates, and plicamycin.

Surgery is indicated on an individual basis. In rare cases diagnostic biopsy or surgical correction of a deformed limb may be appropriate; surgical treatment is also appropriate for fractures, tumors, and osteoarthritis complicating Paget disease. Neurological syndromes unresponsive to medical therapy may require surgery.

Calcitonin

Salmon calcitonin, the most potent form of the hormone, has been used in the United States for several years; the porcine and human forms of the hormone have been used mainly in Europe. For salmon calcitonin the usual starting dose is 20 to 50 MRC units/d. The drug may be given parenterally (intramuscularly or subcutaneously) or by intranasal or rectal routes of administration. It is free of major toxicity. Nausea is the major side effect (in perhaps 10% of patients); flushing may also occur. Serum alkaline phosphatase and urinary hydroxyproline levels usually fall about 50% with treatment. In patients with severe disease these parameters frequently remain abnormal.[108] Nonetheless, x-ray studies may demonstrate restoration of a normal appearance to bone. Most patients experience rapid relief of pain and decreased skeletal blood flow. In some, a reversal of neurological complications occurs. After stopping treatment, beneficial effects may persist but usually not as long as with diphosphonates. Most authors[108, 109] favor intermittent rather than prolonged maintenance therapy. Resistance to calcitonin may develop. This may be caused by antibodies, particularly after treatment with salmon or porcine calcitonin,[109] but there is a poor correlation between antibody titer and resistance. Although transient hypocalcemia may occur, overt secondary hyperparathyroidism after calcitonin administration is uncommon.

Diphosphonates

The diphosphonates produce effects on bone resorption and formation. Etidronate sodium is available in the United States for the treatment of Paget disease. In high doses (20 mg/kg body weight) it inhibits both resorption and formation of bone. At lower doses (5 mg/kg body weight) it selectively inhibits bone resorption. Dichloromethylene diphosphonate selectively inhibits bone resorption but was withdrawn from clinical testing in the United States because of potential toxicity. Aminopropylidene diphosphonate inhibits bone formation at doses 500 times greater than those that suppress bone resorption but is not available in the United States. The diphosphonates are effective orally, but low and variable intestinal absorption causes difficulty in establishing the appropriate dose. Etidronate, unlike the other drugs, causes increased tubular absorption of phosphate and thus may elevate the serum phosphate level. Response of serum phosphate level can be used as an index of patient compliance and absorption of the drug.

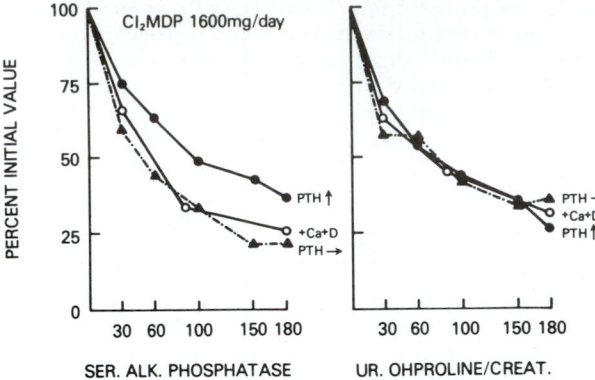

Figure 28–19. Reduction in mean percentages of pretreatment serum alkaline phosphatase *(left)* and urinary hydroxyproline *(right)* values in 21 patients with Paget disease treated with dichloromethylene diphosphonate (1600 mg/d) with (9 patients) or without (12 patients) calcium and vitamin D. Values of patients treated with dichloromethylene diphosphonate alone are plotted on two separate curves according to their respective plasma PTH values (normal or increased). The abscissa indicates days of diphosphonate treatment. (From PD Delmas, MC Chapuy, E Vignon, et al., Long term effects of dichloromethylene diphosphonate in Paget's disease of bone, J Clin Endocrinol Metab, 54, 837–844, 1982, © by The Endocrine Society.)

Etidronate causes alkaline phosphatase and urinary hydroxyproline levels to return to the normal range in many patients. Although more effective than placebo in relieving bone pain in controlled studies, it may cause increased pain at high doses (20 mg/kg/d). Although some studies have reported x-ray evidence of healing of bone lesions, progression of lytic lesions has also been observed with low doses (7 mg/kg) of etidronate.[110] This may be due to inhibition of bone mineralization, resulting in osteomalacia. Such patients may well be at risk for fracture. For this reason treatment should be restricted to 5 to 10 mg/kg body weight for no longer than 6 mo. Not all patients respond to lower doses, and the time required for the return of biochemical parameters to normal is longer. For this reason some authors recommend the use of higher doses for shorter intervals.[110] Patients with predominantly lytic disease should probably not be treated with higher doses because of the increased risk of fracture. Remission may persist for long periods after discontinuation of the agent.

Because of the incomplete response to calcitonin in some patients and because of the potential hazards of etidronate in higher doses, combined treatment with calcitonin may be advantageous.[108] Thus one might achieve an increased and persistent benefit while preventing the adverse effects on bone formation. Etidronate (7.5 mg/kg) combined with calcitonin gave better responses than calcitonin alone in one study, but it is uncertain that the combination was better than etidronate alone.[108]

Dichloromethylene diphosphate is effective in the treatment of Paget disease[96] but, as noted, is not available in the United States. Bone biopsy specimens from treated patients showed decreased resorption without evidence of a mineralization defect. The reduction in alkaline phosphatase and urinary hydroxyproline levels may persist for 1 y after discontinuing therapy. The lowest effective dose is 800 mg/d. The addition of oral calcium (1 g of elemental calcium per day) and vitamin D (8000 IU/d) prevents development of secondary hyperparathyroidism, which is otherwise common after treatment. Higher alkaline phosphatase activity persists in patients who are not suppressed (Fig. 28–19).

Aminopropylidene diphosphonate has similar efficacy in Paget disease and does not inhibit bone mineralization.[111] Transient fever occurs in half the patients treated with the drug.

Plicamycin

Plicamycin is administered intravenously, and regimens for Paget's disease utilize either daily infusions for limited periods or weekly infusions of longer duration.[98a, 100] Although this therapy may return biochemical parameters to normal and relieve bone pain, side effects, including nausea and vomiting and hepatic and renal toxicity, are relatively common. Consequently, plicamyin should be reserved for patients who fail to respond to other therapies.

Summary

Several therapies are available for Paget disease. Each has advantages and drawbacks. Calcitonin is relatively free of serious toxicity but is not completely effective and must be given parenterally. Etidronate works well but at higher doses may impair bone mineralization and cause increased pain and risk of fracture. If low-dose etidronate is not effective, a combination of calcitonin and etidronate may be advantageous. Plicamycin, because of toxicity, should be reserved for patients who are resistant to other therapies.

PRIMARY OSTEOPOROSIS

Osteoporosis is a state of reduced bone mass per unit volume with a normal ratio of mineral to matrix. The risk of fracture with minimal trauma is increased in osteoporotic bone, and this risk correlates with the degree of reduced bone mass (Fig. 28–20). Age, race, and sex are important influences on skeletal mass. Bone mass is lost in almost all persons older than age 50, and a high percentage of the population older than age 70 is at risk for fracture.

Bone remodeling is normally regulated by systemic and locally produced agents and metabolic, nutritional, and mechanical factors; it is not surprising that osteoporosis can be

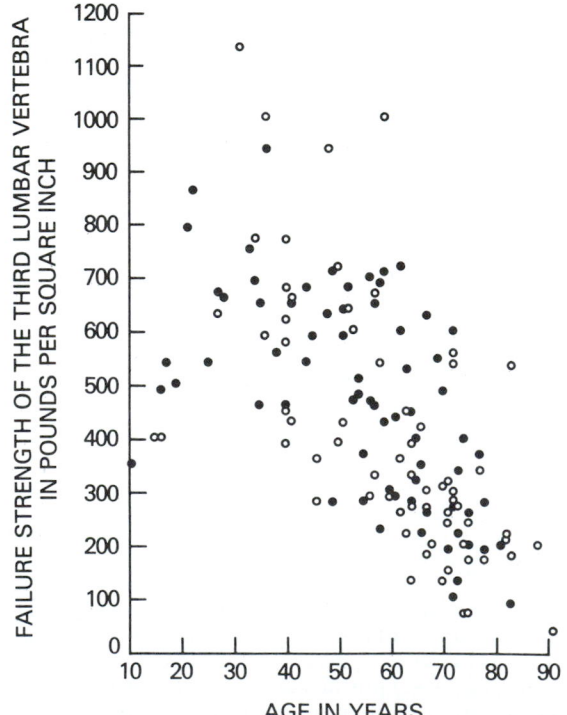

Figure 28–20. Change in vertebral compressive strength with advancing age in 137 cadavers (o = female; ● = male). (From Weaver JV, Chalmers J. Cancellous bone: its strength and changes with aging and an evaluation of some methods for measuring its mineral content. J Bone Joint Surg 1966; 48A:289–298.)

TABLE 28–5. Causes of Osteoporosis

Cause unknown
  Primary osteoporosis (senile, postmenopausal)
  Juvenile osteoporosis
Endocrine abnormalities
  Glucocorticoid excess
  Thyrotoxicosis
  Hypogonadism
  Hyperprolactinemia
  Diabetes mellitus
  Hyperparathyroidism
Malignant disease
  Multiple myeloma
  Leukemia
  Lymphoma
  Mastocytosis
Drugs
  Heparin
  Ethanol
Immobilization
Genetic abnormalities in bone collagen synthesis
  Homocystinuria
  Ehlers-Danlos syndrome
  Osteogenesis imperfecta
Hepatic disease
  Primary biliary cirrhosis

due to diverse disease processes (Table 28–5). Osteoporosis caused by obvious pathogenetic factors, such as excess cortisol in Cushing disease, is termed *secondary*. The most common forms of osteoporosis, variously referred to as *senile, postmenopausal, involutional,* or *primary,* are of uncertain pathogenesis. The distinction between primary and secondary forms of osteoporosis is somewhat arbitrary, because secondary factors such as overtreatment with thyroid hormones may contribute to bone loss in patients with primary disease.

Epidemiology and Clinical Significance

Primary osteoporosis is a major public health problem.[112] An estimated 4 to 6 million persons are affected in the United States. In one fourth of white women older than age 60, osteoporosis is radiographically detectable in the spine. Loss of bone mass in critical weight-bearing areas (e.g., proximal femur and vertebrae) may have disastrous consequences. In the United States there are about 1 million fractures per year in women older than age 45, and approximately 70% of these are attributable to osteoporosis. The incidence of hip fractures resulting from minor trauma increases from 2 per 1000 per year in women age 50 to 64 to more than 10 per 1000 per year in women older than age 75, paralleling the rising incidence of osteoporosis. The morbidity and mortality from hip fractures are considerable. The short-term medical costs have been estimated at $1 billion a year, and the total costs related to osteoporosis are estimated at $6 billion annually in the United States. Prevention of bone loss would reduce dramatically the incidence of fractures in the elderly.

Pathogenesis

The pathogenesis of primary osteoporosis has been difficult to elucidate for the following reasons:

1. Bone loss leading to clinically significant disease is usually gradual. A negative balance as small as 30 mg/d of calcium can lead to loss of one third of the bone mass over a 30-y period. Most clinical studies are performed over short intervals (6 mo to 2 y), and precise techniques are required to document bone loss over such intervals.

2. Bone loss is not uniform throughout the skeleton. Trabecular bone is affected disproportionately, and this phenomenon is reflected in the most common fracture sites: vertebrae, proximal femur, and distal radius. In the past, sensitive noninvasive methods for assessing trabecular bone volume were not available. More than 30% of the skeletal mass must be lost before becoming radiographically detectable by conventional skeletal x-ray examination. The development of reliable noninvasive methods (dual-photon absorptiometry, dual-energy x-ray scanning, and quantitative computed tomography) for measuring trabecular bone in the lumbar vertebrae and proximal femur represents a breakthrough.

3. Clinical diagnosis ordinarily requires detection of one or more vertebral crush fractures. Patients so affected may not be appropriate for the study of dynamic or early pathogenetic factors leading to bone loss. Unfortunately, definite criteria for diagnosing early disease do not exist.

4. Osteoporosis is heterogeneous. Multiple factors, acting alone or in combination, may give rise to primary osteoporosis. This heterogeneity may require histomorphometric analysis of bone for detection.

Theories of Pathogenesis

Progressive loss of bone mass is part of the normal aging process. It begins between the third and fifth decades of life (earlier in women than in men), develops more rapidly in trabecular than in cortical bone, and is accelerated in women after the menopause (Fig. 28–21). Although qualitative abnormalities in the mineral or organic matrix have been reported in primary osteoporosis,[113] susceptibility to fracture is usually due to deficient bone mass rather than defective bone.

One view of the disease is that the group destined to suffer fractures is not distinct but represents the end of the spectrum of age-dependent bone loss. If this is correct, attention should be focused on the mechanisms underlying the age-dependent process. An alternative view is that bone loss may be due solely to the aging process, but individual

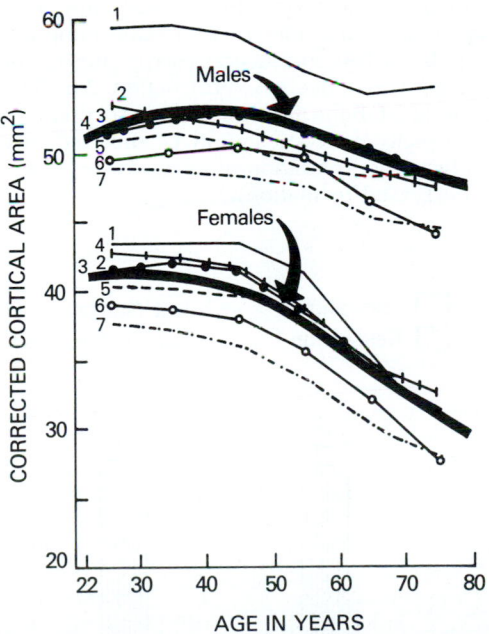

Figure 28–21. Age-related decrease in metacarpal cortical area of males and females from seven different countries. Heavy black lines represent pooled weighted means from all subjects (a total of 5834). (From Garn SM, Rohmann CG, Wagner B, et al. Population similarities in the onset and rate of adult endosteal bone loss. Clin Orthop 1969; 65:51–60.)

fracture susceptibility is determined by the initial skeletal mass at maturity (peak bone mass). Thus those individuals with smaller amounts of bone (corrected for body size) at maturity are more likely to fall below a critical fracture threshold with aging. A third view is that the group destined to suffer fractures is distinct and subject to accelerated bone loss for reasons other than age.

Each of the foregoing views of primary osteoporosis may be valid.[112, 114] With dual-photon absorptiometry in normal volunteers and in patients with nontraumatic hip and vertebral fractures, one finds a linear decrease in bone density with age in the spine and femur of men and women. The rate of loss is greater in women than in men, and this difference is more marked for the vertebrae than for the femur. The bone mineral density of the proximal femur in patients with hip fractures is not different from age-adjusted values in control subjects; in contrast, the bone mineral density of the lumbar spine in patients with vertebral fractures is below the age-adjusted normal mean, especially in women aged 51 to 65. Thus primary osteoporosis may consist of two syndromes.[112] Postmenopausal osteoporosis affects a subset of women in the early postmenopausal period and is characterized by excessive trabecular bone loss, leading to vertebral fractures. Senile osteoporosis involves essentially all elderly women (and to a lesser extent elderly men) and is characterized by proportionate loss of cortical and trabecular bone, leading to hip or vertebral fractures. This formulation is consistent with epidemiological data showing an 8:1 ratio of women to men for vertebral fractures compared with a 2:1 ratio for hip fractures and with the younger age of patients with nontraumatic vertebral fractures compared with those with hip fractures.

A reduction in the bone mass ultimately must evolve from an increase in the ratio of bone resorption to bone formation. An increased rate of resorption may be responsible (Fig. 28–22),[115] but the overall rates of bone turnover vary in affected individuals. Subgroups show high, normal, or low rates of turnover, but the importance of these differences is unclear. Age-dependent increases in markers of bone turnover (serum osteocalcin and alkaline phosphatase and urinary hydroxyproline levels) and an inverse correlation of these parameters with bone mineral density suggest that bone loss in osteoporosis is due to increased resorption rather than decreased formation. An abnormality in the coupling of bone formation to resorption could be involved.[112] Ideally, therapy should be directed to the underlying defect (e.g., inhibition of excess resorption or stimulation of decreased formation).

Specific Pathogenetic Factors

GENETIC AND RACIAL FACTORS. Bone mineral density in the lumbar spine and proximal femur is more highly correlated in monozygotic than dizygotic twins.[116] This relation implies that genetic factors influence bone mass at these sites. Premenopausal daughters of women with postmenopausal osteoporosis show lower lumbar vertebral bone mass than normal controls of similar age.[117] The relative deficits in lumbar spine bone mass in daughters of women with osteoporosis are approximately half of the relative deficits of their mothers. These findings support the idea that genetic factors are a determinant of peak bone mass and imply that relatively low peak bone mass rather than excessive bone loss may be the primary determinant of postmenopausal osteoporosis in a fraction of women.

Racial differences in bone mass (black men > white men > black women > white women) are reflected in racial differences in fracture incidence (Fig. 28–23). Premenopausal black women have higher mean bone mineral density of the radius, hip, and spine than premenopausal white women of comparable age and weight.[118] The basis for these racial differences is unclear, but a reduction in bone formation rate has been reported in black adults.[119] This paradoxical finding (given the greater bone mass in black persons than in white persons) leads to speculation that an overall reduction in rates of bone remodeling in black persons may lead to increased bone mass.[119]

ESTROGEN DEFICIENCY. Estrogen deficiency after natural or surgical menopause is an important factor leading to bone loss.[120] Bone mass declines more rapidly after menopause. One cross-sectional study of normal women, by dual-photon absorptiometry of the lumbar spine, showed a linear relationship between bone mineral density and age.[114] A 2-y longitudinal study, however, using quantitative computed tomography of the lumbar vertebrae, showed an accelerated loss of bone in women after surgical menopause. It is likely that bone loss is more rapid after surgical than after natural menopause, given the more gradual diminution in estrogen secretion after the latter. Studies in perimenopausal women indicate that bone loss from the spine, femoral neck, and, to a lesser extent, the radius occurs before menopause. The extent of bone loss correlates with various measures of circulating estrogens, which also begin to decline even before menopause.[121, 122]

Estrogen deficiency also correlates with the incidence of fracture.[123, 124] In retrospective studies employing case-control methods, estrogen treatment caused a 50% reduction in the risk of hip and Colles fractures in postmenopausal

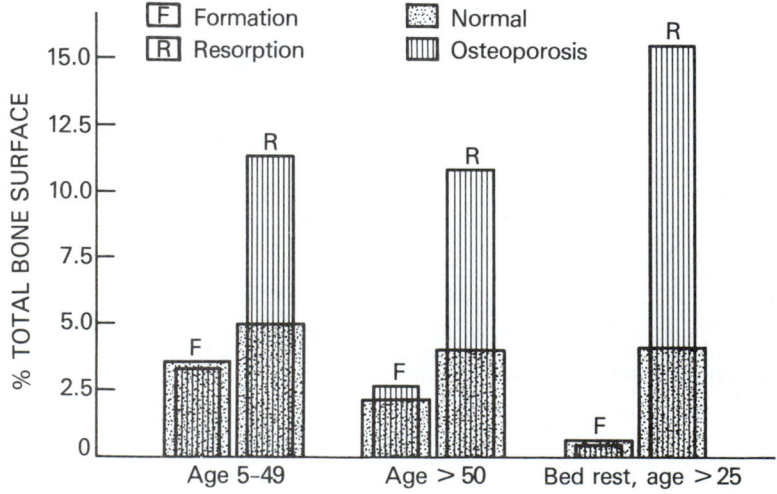

Figure 28–22. Values for bone resorption and formation in patients with juvenile and idiopathic osteoporosis *(left)* and postmenopausal osteoporosis *(center)*, and in osteoporotic patients who have been confined to bed rest *(right)*; each group has age-matched controls. Resorption is greater than normal in all three groups, whereas formation is not different from normal and is depressed in the normal and osteoporotic bed rest groups *(right)*. (From Jowsey JOM, Offord KD. Osteoporosis: juvenile, idiopathic, and post-menopausal. In: Horton JE, Tarpley TM, Davis WF, eds. Mechanisms of Localized Bone Loss. [A Special Supplement to Calcified Tissue Abstracts.] London: IRL, 1978: 345–364, by permission of Oxford University Press.)

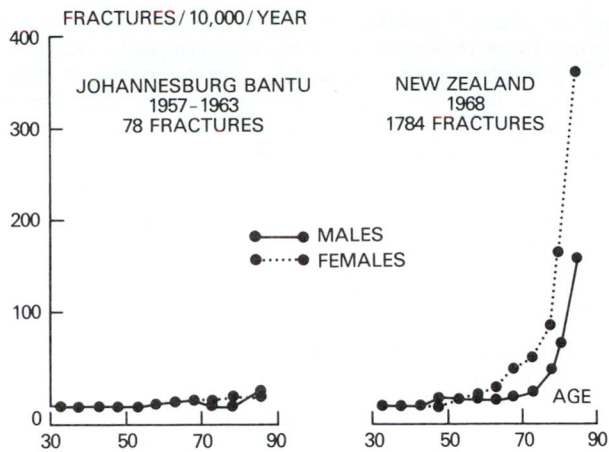

FRACTURES / 10,000 / YEAR

JOHANNESBURG BANTU
1957–1963
78 FRACTURES

NEW ZEALAND
1968
1784 FRACTURES

●——● MALES
●·····● FEMALES

AGE

Figure 28–23. Incidence of femoral neck fractures as a function of age in the Johannesburg Bantu population *(left)* and in New Zealanders *(right)*. (From Cave W, Nordin BEC. International fracture survey; first year report to the International Health Foundation. Privately printed, 1972. Reproduced in Horsman A. Bone mass. In: Nordin BEC, ed. Calcium, Phosphate and Magnesium Metabolism. Edinburgh: Churchill Livingstone, 1976: 357–404.)

women. Moreover, osteoporosis of the spine was less frequent in women taking estrogens compared with postmenopausal women not taking estrogens. No dosage effect was found, but the duration of estrogen therapy and the proximity of initiation of therapy to the time of menopause correlated with reduced fracture risk. In a large retrospective cohort study (the Framingham study) the relative risk of hip fracture in subjects taking any estrogen was 0.65 after adjustment for age and weight.[125]

Positive correlations have been found in perimenopausal women not only between serum estrogen level and bone density[121, 122] but also between serum free testosterone level and bone density.[122] Trabecular bone density is higher in young women with excess androgens (both otherwise normal, including serum estrogens) than in normal young women.[126] Thus in both men (see section on secondary forms of osteoporosis) and women, androgens contribute to maintenance of normal bone mass. Obese women have higher estrogen levels as a result of conversion of adrenal and ovarian androgens to estrogens in adipose tissue. Slender women show a greater prevalence of osteoporosis[122] and are at greater risk for fracture.[125] Additional factors, such as increased weight-bearing stress on the skeleton in obese women, may be involved in this difference.

The mechanism whereby estrogen deficiency predisposes to bone loss is unknown but may involve increased sensitivity of bone to PTH, resulting in increased net bone resorption.[112] Previous speculations centered on indirect effects of gonadal steroids, but identification of estrogen and androgen receptors in osteoblasts[24, 25] makes direct modulation of bone remodeling by gonadal steroids plausible. Another hypothesis suggests that ovarian steroids may act by blocking a postmenopausal increase in IL 1 release.[127] Because IL 1 is a potent bone-resorbing agent, local release of this factor in bone by monocytes or other skeletal cells could be relevant to the pathogenesis of osteoporosis. Because estrogen deficiency is a universal concomitant of menopause, the specific factors responsible for clinically evident disease in affected postmenopausal women also require identification. Differences in peak bone mass achieved may be a critical variable in this regard.

VITAMIN D METABOLITES. Intestinal calcium absorption decreases with age. Greater reductions in calcium absorption have been reported in patients with osteoporosis compared with age-matched controls.[128] Because vitamin D,

in particular $1,25(OH)_2D$, is the major determinant of calcium absorption, a role for vitamin D in the pathogenesis of osteoporosis has been sought. Most, but not all, studies have found reduced levels of serum $1,25(OH)_2D$ in osteoporotic patients compared with age- and sex-matched controls.[112] The differences are small, and the mean values for osteoporotic patients are generally within the normal range. Nonetheless these slight reductions in serum $1,25(OH)_2D$ level may be related to the reduction in calcium absorption referred to earlier.

The reduction in the serum $1,25(OH)_2D$ level is presumably not due to reduced substrate availability because serum 25-OHD concentrations are usually normal. Increased catabolism is unlikely but has not been excluded. 1α-Hydroxylase activity decreases with age in rats, and a similar phenomenon could operate in humans. Renal function also deteriorates with age, and this or other unknown factors could lead to reduced formation of $1,25(OH)_2D$. In one study osteoporotic patients showed a substantially reduced serum $1,25(OH)_2D$ response to infusion of PTH.[129] Controls were younger, however, so that the findings may primarily reflect the effects of age. Other studies have shown no difference in the response of the serum $1,25(OH)_2D$ level to pharmacologic doses of PTH.[130, 131] The endogenous PTH response to oral phosphate challenge was lower in a group of postmenopausal osteoporotic women than in age-matched controls.[132] Serum $1,25(OH)_2D$ actually fell in response to oral phosphate in the osteoporotic group but did not change in the controls. In a group of younger subjects, the serum $1,25(OH)_2D$ was unaffected by phosphate, but the PTH response was also less. On balance it is likely that the reduction in serum $1,25(OH)_2D$ levels in osteoporotic patients is due both to decreased stimulation of the 1α-hydroxylase by PTH and to an age-related decrease in the capacity of the enzyme to respond. It is not known whether the decreased PTH level is due to estrogen deficiency, but short-term estrogen administration to osteoporotic patients can increase both the serum $1,25(OH)_2D$ level and intestinal calcium absorption.[128] In one study[133] estrogen administration increased the serum $1,25(OH)_2D$ level in healthy postmenopausal women but failed to augment the rise in $1,25(OH)_2D$ after edetate-induced hypocalcemia. Against the hypothesis that early postmenopausal bone loss is related to vitamin D deficiency are data from a longitudinal study of 19 normal perimenopausal women in whom serum estrogen level and appendicular bone mass decreased without a concomitant reduction in either 25-OHD or $1,25(OH)_2D$ levels.[134]

PARATHYROID HORMONE. Measurements of serum PTH levels in patients with osteoporosis have yielded inconsistent results.[112] Because nonbiologically active fragments of the hormone are usually measured in such experiments, the results must be interpreted cautiously. The possibility of an increase in the serum PTH level with age must be taken into account when evaluating PTH in osteoporosis. A slight reduction in the serum PTH level in a small subgroup of patients with osteoporosis may be related to estrogen deficiency, as discussed earlier. Elevation of the serum PTH level is uncommon in patients with a decreased bone mass. Another theory suggests that primary reduction in renal 1α-hydroxylase activity leads to secondary hyperparathyroidism, which then causes or contributes to osteoporosis in these patients.

CALCITONIN DEFICIENCY. The role of calcitonin deficiency in the pathogenesis of osteoporosis is uncertain. Studies of basal and calcium-stimulated serum calcitonin levels in humans show lower levels of basal and calcium-stimulated serum calcitonin in women compared with men. Older women have lower values than younger women.[135] Estrogen treatment of postmenopausal women was reported to increase basal serum calcitonin values,[136] but no such increase was found in another study.[137] In one study[138] the calcitonin production rate was reduced in postmenopausal osteoporotic women. In contrast, no difference was found in the calcitonin-secretory reserve in a group of 25 post-menopausal women with untreated osteoporosis when compared with normal age-matched controls.[139] The basal calcitonin value was actually higher in the osteoporotic subjects. Therefore, if calcitonin deficiency occurs in osteoporosis, it is unlikely to be of significance in pathogenesis.

DEFICIENT DIETARY CALCIUM. The recommended dietary allowance for calcium for nonpregnant adults in the United States is 800 mg/d. The median calcium intake in postmenopausal women is below this value, leading to the suggestion that a deficiency of dietary calcium is a significant factor in the development of postmenopausal osteoporosis[140] and to the recommendation that calcium intake be increased (1000 mg/d for premenopausal and 1500 mg/d for post-menopausal women). The evidence linking reduced calcium intake to development of osteoporosis is tenuous. A comparison of two regions of Yugoslavia in which dietary calcium intake varied did show a reduction in cortical bone density and an increase in incidence of femoral neck fractures in the group with reduced calcium intake, but racial and nutritional differences other than dietary calcium may have confounded these results.[141] More impressive results were obtained in a 14-y prospective study of a relatively homogeneous population in southern California.[142] An inverse association was found between dietary calcium and subsequent risk of hip fracture, even after adjustment for confounding factors such as smoking, alcohol intake, exercise, and obesity. Nonetheless, the majority of studies (see, for example, ref. 143) have failed to reveal a relation between dietary calcium and either bone mineral density or rates of bone loss. Furthermore, most controlled studies have failed to show an effect of calcium supplementation (up to 2000 mg/d) on bone loss in postmenopausal women.[144] Given these conflicting results, it is difficult to justify routine high-dose (>1000 mg/d) calcium supplementation. It is still possible that variation in calcium intake during skeletal growth and maturation may influence peak bone mass, and it is reasonable to emphasize the importance of adequate calcium intake during this period.

PHYSICAL ACTIVITY. Immobilization with decreased weight bearing is an important stimulus to bone resorption. A rapid initial rate of bone loss after immobilization is followed by a lower rate of loss or a plateau.[145] Normal volunteers subjected to bed rest show similar changes. Weightlessness in space travel also leads to a negative calcium balance, with a 33% reduction in trabecular bone volume occurring over 25 wk. Cortical bone is lost at a lower rate. At the opposite extreme, athletes tend to have increased bone mass. Studies of normal men and women (i.e., nonathletes) indicate that measures of physical fitness and muscle strength correlate positively with bone mineral density in the femoral neck and spine.[146, 147] Various measures of body mass also correlated with bone mineral density of the radius, hip, and spine.[118, 146, 147] Part of this effect may be due to increased estrogen production in obese women (see earlier discussion), but an independent effect of weight per se may also contribute. Thus integrated physical load (a function of physical activity, muscle strength, and weight) may be a determinant of peak bone mass and may thereby help to determine the population at risk for osteoporosis. If this concept is correct, prophylactic exercise programs (initiated well before menopause) should reduce the incidence of fractures.

OTHER PATHOGENETIC FACTORS. Alcohol and smoking have been implicated as risk factors in some epidemiological studies.[148] Smoking may predispose persons to osteoporosis by increasing the hepatic metabolism of estrogens.[149] The protective effect of obesity has been noted. Factors other than bone mass per se may contribute to fracture risk. For example, psychotropic drug use by the elderly increases the risk of falling and thereby the risk of hip fracture.[150]

Clinical Features

Many subjects with osteoporosis are asymptomatic (despite having vertebral crush fractures) and are identified incidentally by radiographs taken for other purposes. When symptoms occur, they may be of two general types. Immediately after a vertebral crush fracture (occurring by definition after minimal trauma or exertion), there may be sharp pain over the involved region. This generally subsides within 1 mo regardless of therapy. Analgesics, temporary splinting, and rest are appropriate. Some patients have chronic, dull, diffuse back pain. Neurological signs resulting from nerve root compression are uncommon and if present should prompt a search for other lesions. Vertebral collapse causes a loss in height and may lead to dorsal kyphosis (dowager's hump). Fractures of the proximal femur and distal radius are also common.

Laboratory and Radiological Evaluation

Vertebral changes on radiographs, in order of increasing severity, include loss of horizontal trabeculations (Fig. 28–24), biconcavity caused by ballooning of the intervertebral discs (codfish vertebrae), anterior wedge fractures, and compression fractures. The lowest thoracic and upper lumbar vertebrae are most commonly affected. Fractures of vertebrae above T-6 are almost never due to primary osteoporosis and should prompt a search for malignant disease. Changes in the appendicular skeleton include cortical thinning and loss of trabecular bone in areas such as the femoral neck.

Relatively precise, noninvasive methods for measuring forearm, spine, and hip bone density are now available (see section on laboratory assessments of bone metabolism). These include single- and dual-photon absorptiometry, dual-wavelength x-ray absorptiometry, and quantitative computed tomography. These tests are useful in research on the pathogenesis of osteoporosis and in assessment of the response to therapy. However, the utility and cost-effectiveness of these tests in screening the general population to identify individuals at risk for osteoporosis are not clearly established. Screening for osteoporosis has been evaluated[150] on the basis of several criteria: Does the condition cause sufficient morbidity to warrant screening? Is effective prophylactic treatment available? Is screening safe and inexpensive? Does the screening test have adequate predictive value? On the basis of these criteria, the use of forearm bone densitometry is questionable because wrist fractures cause relatively little morbidity and results for the forearm cannot be used to predict the risk of vertebral or hip fracture in the individual patient.[112] Hip fractures cause considerable morbidity and, indirectly, mortality, but because there is overlap of hip bone mass between women with and those without hip fractures, measurement of bone density of the hip lacks predictive value.[112, 151]

Measurement of vertebral bone density may be helpful in predicting individuals at risk for vertebral fractures,[112, 151] and estrogen therapy may protect such individuals from development of osteoporosis. Even in this instance, screening would be relevant only when a decision regarding estrogen replacement therapy would be influenced by the test results. In general, then, widespread screening of the population does not appear to be justified.[151]

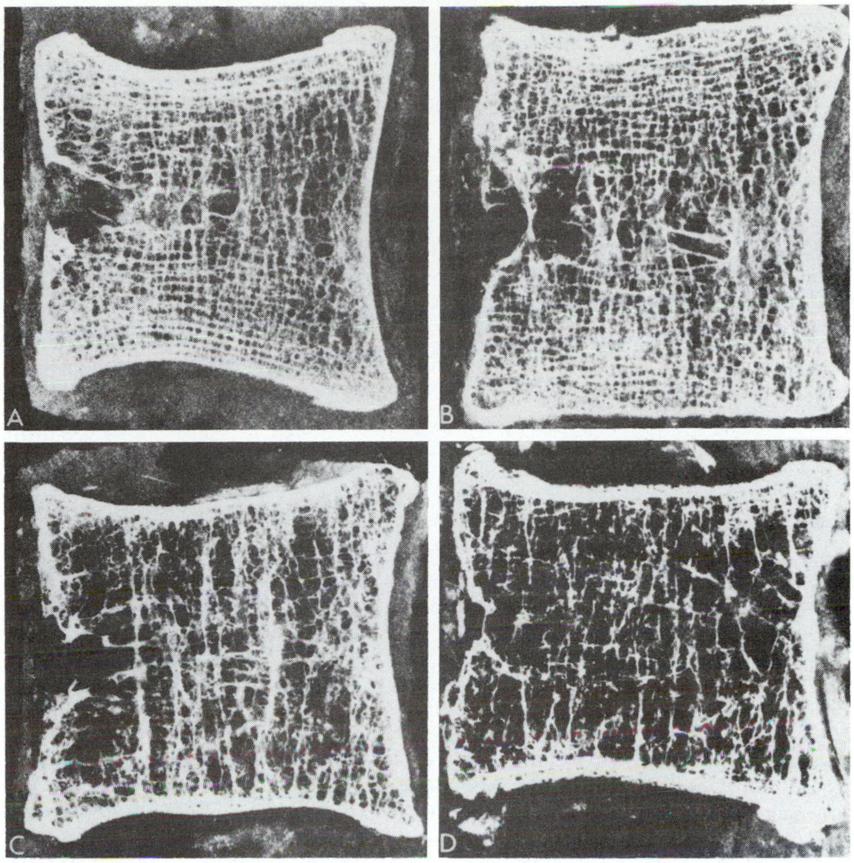

Figure 28–24. Radiographs of sagittal sections taken from second lumbar vertebral body of female subjects of different ages. *A,* Age 29, regular trabecular pattern. *B,* Age 40, some thinning of transverse trabeculae. *C,* Age 84, loss of horizontal trabeculae, thickening of vertical trabeculae. *D,* Age 92, further loss of normal trabecular pattern. (From Atkinson PJ. Variation in trabecular structure of vertebrae with age. Calcif Tissue Res 1967; 1:24–37.)

Because primary osteoporosis is a diagnosis of exclusion, secondary forms of bone loss should be excluded (see Table 28–5). Secondary forms of osteoporosis should be suspected in groups with a low prevalence of the primary form of the disease (i.e., white men, young white women, and black persons of both sexes and all ages).

A complete history (including all drugs) and physical examination are important in delineating secondary causes of bone loss. Laboratory evaluation should include thyroid function tests, serum protein electrophoresis, and a 24-h urinary free cortisol determination to screen for subtle thyrotoxicosis, myeloma, and cortisol excess, respectively. Serum calcium and phosphate concentrations and alkaline phosphatase activity are generally normal, although the serum alkaline phosphatase level may increase transiently after a fracture. Serum vitamin D metabolite and PTH levels are also usually normal, although subtle abnormalities (slightly decreased serum $1,25(OH)_2D$ or slightly increased serum PTH level) may be present. Osteomalacia may be difficult to distinguish from osteoporosis on skeletal x-ray films but should be accompanied by increased serum alkaline phosphatase and depressed serum 25-OHD or $1,25(OH)_2D$ levels. Primary hyperparathyroidism may present initially as osteoporosis but should be manifested by increased serum calcium and PTH levels.

In certain cases, bone biopsy and histomorphometric analysis may help to distinguish osteomalacia from osteoporosis and provide information about the rate of bone turnover. High rates may be a clue to secondary causes of bone loss such as clinically inapparent thyrotoxicosis.

Therapy

In patients with established disease, definitive therapy requires a restoration of lost bone mass. This objective may not be achievable in advanced disease. A more realistic objective is stabilization of bone mass or a decrease in the rate of bone loss. Obviously prevention is preferable to treatment and should be considered in high-risk subjects (i.e., individuals with low peak bone mass or accelerated rates of bone loss). With current noninvasive methods for measurement of bone mass, it may be possible to identify subjects at high risk for vertebral but not hip fractures (see earlier discussion).

Drugs Useful in Treatment

ESTROGEN. Treatment of postmenopausal women with estrogen delays or halts bone loss and reduces the incidence of fractures.[125, 152] In some studies estrogen therapy caused a slight increase in bone mass. The minimal effective dose appears to be between 0.15 and 0.6 mg/d of conjugated estrogens. Progestogens may also be effective but have no clear-cut advantage over estrogens. An important unresolved question is the duration of therapy required to provide significant protection. In one study bone loss rapidly ensued after cessation of hormone administration (Fig. 28–25). The fracture incidence is lowest when estrogen therapy is begun promptly after menopause and maintained continuously. In another study no acceleration of bone loss occurred after stopping treatment.[153] The basis for the discrepant results is not clear. Because long-term estrogen therapy may be associated with slightly increased risk of endometrial and breast carcinoma,[154] the shortest course of treatment offering protection from fractures is desirable. Because this period is not known, the decision to initiate estrogen therapy in a given woman must be based on an individual assessment of risk for osteoporosis (e.g., a slender white woman is more likely to be chosen for therapy than an obese black woman). Women with premature menopause are obvious candidates

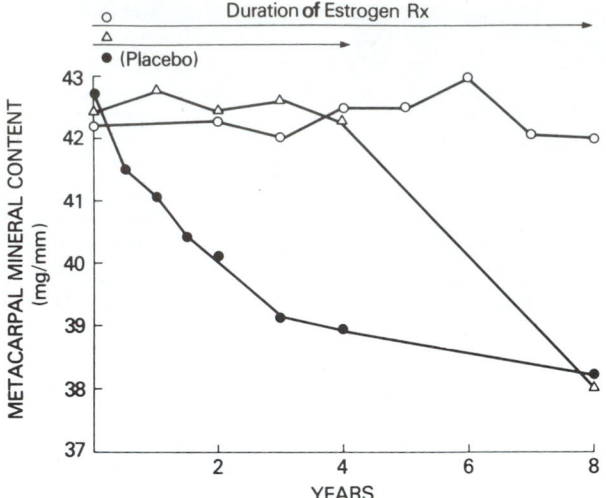

Figure 28–25. Effect of estrogen therapy on postmenopausal bone loss. Metacarpal mineral content (third metacarpal, right hand) was measured by photon absorptiometry over an 8-y period in ovariectomized women maintained with placebo (●), with estrogen (25 μg mestranol/d) for all 8 y (○), or with estrogen for the first 4 y only (△). (From Lindsay R, Hart DM, MacLean A, et al. Bone response to termination of oestrogen treatment. Lancet 1978; 1:1325–1327.)

for estrogen therapy. In the risk-benefit assessment of prospective treatment with estrogens, protection from cardiovascular disease may prove to be an overriding consideration.

CALCIUM, CALCIFEROL, AND CALCITRIOL. Because intestinal calcium absorption decreases with age and because calcium intake is reduced in many older individuals, administration of calcium by mouth with or without calciferol has been advocated to help prevent bone loss. The efficacy of this approach has not been established.[140] In fact, in several reports significant bone loss occurred when only calcium supplements were given to control groups.[144] Studies of calcitriol treatment of osteoporosis have provided conflicting results. Two similarly designed (2-y, double-blind, randomized, placebo-controlled) studies of calcitriol treatment have been reported. In one,[155] no benefit from calcitriol in terms of bone density or fracture rate was observed. In the other,[156] vertebral bone density stabilized and radial bone density increased in the calcitriol group, but no significant reduction in fracture incidence occurred. The dose in the latter study (mean = 0.8 mg/d) was twice that in the former, and some nephrotoxicity occurred. Thus it is not clear that calcitriol is useful therapy in most subjects with osteoporosis.

THIAZIDES. Thiazides have a significant hypocalciuric effect. This action could result in a positive calcium balance and prevent bone loss. Japanese men taking thiazides over a long term showed increased bone mineral density in the radius.[157] In contrast, in a 2-y study of postmenopausal women, treatment with thiazides reduced urinary calcium excretion but failed to retard bone loss from the radius.[158] Genetic differences or variations in dose or duration of therapy might account for the discrepant results. In a case-control study of elderly subjects, long-term thiazide use (>6 y) was associated with a 50% reduction in incidence of hip fractures.[159]

FLUORIDE. Fluoride increases osteoblast number and stimulates trabecular bone formation in the axial skeleton but by itself may lead to osteomalacia, reduced tensile strength of bone, and an increase in fractures. Calcium and calciferol given with fluoride may prevent the osteomalacia. A regimen of 40 to 100 mg/d of sodium fluoride (yielding concentrations in serum between 5 and 10 μmol/L), 1 to 2 g/d of elemental calcium (as the carbonate), and 50,000 U of calciferol once or twice a week has been tested. Prelimi-

nary results suggest that fluoride given in this way can reduce vertebral fractures, the effect being observed even in patients taking estrogens.[160] Although these results suggest that fluoride-induced bone is fracture resistant, several points are noteworthy. The beneficial effect is less marked in the first year, suggesting a delay in response. Fluoride-treated patients, moreover, appear to segregate into responsive and unresponsive subgroups. In the former, radiographic evidence of fluoride effect includes coarsening of vertebral trabeculations and thickening of end plates. Fracture protection is limited to this group. The reason for unresponsiveness in the other group is not clear, but it may reflect a primary osteoblast defect or poor absorption of fluoride.

Fluoride also produces side effects, including development of osteophytes and calcification of ligaments, nausea and vomiting, synovitis, and pain and tenderness over the feet (plantar fascial syndrome). In one study 40% of patients showed significant side effects, and one tenth had to discontinue the drug.[160] To overcome these side effects, a slow-release form of sodium fluoride has been tested. Although favorable results (reduced frequency of vertebral fractures and fewer side effects) were obtained, a larger number of subjects need to be studied.[161] The most serious concern is an increase in incidence of hip fractures with fluoride therapy. To date, conflicting results have been obtained, with some studies showing no increase in hip fracture incidence[162] and others showing a large (10-fold) increased incidence.[163]

Fluoride is an experimental drug not yet approved for general use. It is specifically contraindicated in patients with renal failure.

CALCITONIN. Calcitonin treatment causes short-term decrease in bone loss. In subjects defined as showing high-turnover osteoporosis (based on biochemical indices and total body retention of bone-seeking radioisotope), calcitonin treatment for 1 y increased vertebral bone mineral density, but subjects with normal-turnover osteoporosis showed no increase.[164] The long-term efficacy of the hormone, particularly its capacity to reduce the incidence of fractures, is not established.

DIPHOSPHONATES. Diphosphonates, like calcitonin, can inhibit bone resorption, and the newer drugs do so without inhibiting bone formation. Diphosphonates may be useful in selected situations characterized by high rates of bone resorption (e.g., immobilization, as in paraplegics). Diphosphonates have also been incorporated into a form of therapy known as *ADFR* (activate, depress, free, repeat; also termed cyclic or coherence therapy). In one regimen tested in an uncontrolled short-term trial, oral phosphate was given for 7 d to activate bone resorption; next a high dose of diphosphonate (etidronate) was given for 5 d to depress bone resorption; and then oral calcium supplements were given for 48 d (free); the cycle was then repeated. The rationale is to increase bone mass by sequential activation of resorption (e.g., oral phosphate provokes an increase in endogenous PTH) and formation. Preliminary results from this trial were encouraging, but controlled, long-term studies demonstrating a reduction in fracture incidence are required.[165]

HUMAN PTH(1–34). Low doses of PTH may induce an anabolic effect on bone. Preliminary results in a multicenter trial of synthetic PTH(1–34) showed no significant changes in calcium balance or cortical bone density, but there was an increased rate of bone turnover and an increase in trabecular bone volume as measured in a limited number of iliac crest biopsy specimens.[166] In a subsequent trial[167] of daily subcutaneous injection of PTH(1–34) combined with 0.25 μg/d of calcitriol, trabecular bone density (as measured by computed tomography of lumbar vertebrae) and total body calcium retention both increased. The study subjects were men, and it is not known whether similar results can be achieved in women.

EXERCISE. Although immobilization causes loss of bone mass, it is not clear whether exercise is effective in preventing bone loss. It is difficult to show an effect of physical activity in retrospective studies because of the problem of assessing previous levels of exercise. Several short-term studies show reductions in the rate of bone loss in postmenopausal women participating in exercise programs.[168] Exercise may also be beneficial in increasing flexibility and agility, thereby decreasing the likelihood of falls. Long-term studies are needed to evaluate the utility of exercise programs in preventing fracture. In women with exercise-induced amenorrhea, any positive effects of exercise on bone mass are outweighed by estrogen deficiency (see under Secondary Forms of Osteoporosis).

Summary

In patients with far advanced disease, symptomatic treatment is probably all that is indicated. Additional measures to prevent further bone loss can be taken but may not affect the clinical course. In patients with significant bone loss and in those at risk for fracture (assessed with dual-wavelength absorptiometry or quantitative computed tomography of the vertebrae), therapy should be directed at increasing bone mass and preventing further loss. At present, fluoride in combination with calcium and calciferol is the only regimen that appears to effect an increase in bone mass. There are many side effects, and the long-term safety and efficacy of the treatment remain to be established. For prevention, estrogen therapy, an adequate calcium and vitamin D intake, and perhaps a mild exercise program are probably most useful. The benefits of estrogen treatment should be weighed against the risks. Certainly, all women who undergo premature menopause (surgical or spontaneous) should seriously be considered for estrogen therapy. Given the strong evidence that estrogen prevents bone loss, most other postmenopausal women are candidates for estrogen replacement as well.

SECONDARY FORMS OF OSTEOPOROSIS

Endocrine Causes

Generalized osteoporosis may be caused by a number of endocrine abnormalities, including primary hyperparathyroidism, hypercortisolism, and hyperthyroidism.[51] Patients with acromegaly show an increased bone mass; osteoporosis in acromegaly is probably due to concomitant secondary hypogonadism.

GLUCOCORTICOID EXCESS. Osteoporosis is a consequence of cortisol excess from endogenous or exogenous sources. Children and the elderly, particularly women, are at greatest risk for developing significant bone loss. There is a positive correlation between the duration (but not dose) of steroid therapy and the degree of bone loss. Alternate-day administration causes less bone loss in animals than does daily therapy, but data for humans suggest that significant bone loss occurs even with alternate-day steroid treatment.[169]

Osteoporosis may be the principal manifestation of endogenous cortisol excess in young adults with adrenal hyperplasia, in patients with relatively indolent malignancies that secrete corticotropin (ACTH, adrenocorticotropin) ec-

topically (such as medullary carcinoma of the thyroid, carcinoid, or thymoma), and, rarely, in patients with the usual form of bilateral adrenal hyperplasia.[170] Osteoporosis is also an important complication of glucocorticoid therapy. Asthmatic patients taking glucocorticoids over a prolonged period have an increased incidence of rib and vertebral fractures and diminished bone mineral density.[171]

Glucocorticoids inhibit bone formation, apparently through a direct action on the osteoblast, and increase bone resorption through an indirect mechanism.[172] The latter effect is due to antagonism of $1,25(OH)_2D$-mediated intestinal calcium absorption, which leads to secondary hyperparathyroidism. The precise mechanism of glucocorticoid interference with vitamin D action has not been clarified. No abnormality in $1,25(OH)_2D$ metabolism has been found in subjects receiving glucocorticoid treatment[173] or in patients with Cushing syndrome.[174] Glucocorticoids also increase urinary calcium excretion, further diminishing calcium balance. Areas of trabecular bone are disproportionately affected.

Correction of endogenous cortisol excess allows restoration of bone mass; whether discontinuation (or substantial reduction) of exogenous glucocorticoid therapy leads to restoration of bone mass is not clear.[175] Prophylactic therapy may be appropriate in high-risk subjects. One approach is to monitor patients taking glucocorticoids with serial measurements of trabecular bone density (e.g., distal radius or vertebrae) at 3- to 6-mo intervals and to institute therapy if substantial bone loss occurs.[172] Appropriate measures include thiazide treatment (in patients showing excessive urinary calcium excretion) and calcium and calciferol supplements to enhance intestinal calcium absorption, thereby suppressing secondary hyperparathyroidism. Careful monitoring to avoid vitamin D intoxication is essential. In a controlled study, 2 µg/d of 1α-hydroxycholecalciferol reduced serum PTH and urinary hydroxyproline excretion and increased calcium absorption and bone mass in patients taking glucocorticoids.[176] Fluoride therapy may also counteract the inhibitory effect of glucocorticoids on bone formation.[172]

THYROTOXICOSIS. Thyroxtoxicosis may lead to the development of osteoporosis, but significant bone loss is rare, possibly because of relatively early diagnosis and treatment. Bone loss is presumably a direct result of thyroid hormone excess because thyroid hormone causes resorption of bone in vitro. The bone loss is characterized by accelerated bone turnover and a marked increase in osteoclast activity.[177] Bone formation is also increased but presumably is insufficient to match the accelerated turnover. Elevated serum alkaline phosphatase activity derives from either bone or liver. (Correction of thyrotoxicosis leads to restoration of bone mass.[178]) Significant bone loss has also been observed with exogenously administered thyroid hormone.

HYPOGONADISM. Hypogonadism, whether caused by primary gonadal failure or secondary to gonadotropin deficiency, is associated with osteoporosis, particularly of trabecular bone. Given the critical role of estrogens in preventing bone loss in normal premenopausal women (see earlier discussion), it is not surprising that estrogen deficiency of sufficient duration can lead to osteoporosis. Iatrogenic gonadotropin deficiency (e.g., treatment of women with analogues of luteinizing hormone–releasing hormone [LHRH, also called gonadotropin-releasing hormone, GnRH] for endometriosis) causes reversible reductions in serum estradiol level and in trabecular bone density.[179] Similar findings occur in women with hypothalamic amenorrhea.[180] Female runners with exercise-related amenorrhea also have reduced lumbar spinal bone mineral content.[181] Estrogen deficiency apparently outweighs any possible benefit of physical activity on bone formation. Young women with anorexia nervosa, particularly with onset during adolescence and of long duration, may show severe osteopenia and spinal crush fractures. Reduced bone density in this disease may reflect failure to attain normal peak bone mass because of estrogen deficiency during adolescence. An elevated serum cortisol concentration may also contribute to osteoporosis in anorexia nervosa.[182] Estrogen deficiency is likely the major factor responsible for the osteoporosis associated with syndromes of gonadal dysgenesis.[183] Estrogen treatment in subjects with gonadal dysgenesis causes increased bone density, but prospective studies are needed to verify the beneficial effects of estrogen treatment in this and other estrogen-deficient states.

Hypogonadal men are also at increased risk for osteoporosis and vertebral fractures.[184] Testosterone deficiency appears to be the major factor responsible for deficient bone mass in men with hypogonadism associated with Klinefelter syndrome and gonadotropin deficiency, whether primary or associated with disorders such as hemochromatosis.[185]

HYPERPROLACTINEMIA. Hyperprolactinemia can be associated with osteoporosis, as evidenced by a reduced bone mineral content in both the distal radius and the lumbar vertebrae. In women with hyperprolactinemia, reduced estrogen secretion appears to be the key factor in reduced bone mineral content. Amenorrheic hyperprolactinemic women have lower bone density than eumenorrheic women with comparable elevation in serum prolactin.[180] Women with hyperprolactinemia in whom regular menses are restored by treatment have higher bone density than untreated or unsuccessfully treated women.[186] In hyperprolactinemic men, radial and vertebral bone density may likewise be reduced because of associated hypogonadism, as bone mineral content increases only in treated subjects in whom normal gonadal function (reflected in increased serum testosterone level) is restored.[186, 187] These results suggest that prevention of osteoporosis may be an indication for treatment of hyperprolactinemia. Such recommendations must be tempered by the fact that the clinical importance of reduced bone density (i.e., increased fracture rate) in hyperprolactinemia has not been established.

DIABETES MELLITUS. There is a reduction in bone mass in patients with insulin-dependent (type I) diabetes mellitus.[188] The mechanism is unclear. In diabetic rats there is a reduced serum $1,25(OH)_2D$ level, reduced intestinal calcium absorption, secondary hyperparathyroidism, and accelerated bone loss. Hypercalciuria is common in human diabetics.[189, 190] Plasma levels of PTH and vitamin D metabolites are generally normal,[188, 189] although decreased plasma PTH and elevated serum $24,25(OH)_2D$ levels have been reported.[190] In insulin-dependent diabetic subjects, elevated urinary calcium levels and reduced tubular reabsorption of phosphate are improved by restoration of normoglycemia.[189] Excessive calcium (and possibly phosphate) loss in the urine may contribute to bone loss in patients with diabetes. A primary decrease in bone formation caused by reduced insulin action has also been postulated. Whether these abnormalities or the decreases in bone mass are clinically significant is uncertain. In a study of 28 women with non–insulin-dependent (type II) diabetes, bone mineral density was not reduced.[191] A study of approximately 1000 diabetic patients and an equal number of age-, sex-, and race-matched controls showed no difference in incidence of fractures at any site (vertebrae, proximal femur, or distal radius).[192]

Malignant Disease

Several malignant tumors, primarily of myeloid or lymphocytic cell types, may cause diffuse osteopenia. Multiple myeloma is perhaps the most common. The neoplastic plasma cell secretes osteoclast-activating factor, which may be involved in mediating bone loss. Certain leukemias and lymphomas may also cause diffuse bone loss. For example, T cell lymphoma can induce hypercalcemia and diffuse osteopenia.[193] A specific mediator equivalent to osteoclast-activating factor has not been identified in this disease. Systemic mastocytosis can also cause diffuse osteopenia;[194] bone marrow biopsy and metachromatic staining may be necessary to detect granuloma-like aggregates of mast cells in such cases. Heparin or possibly other agents released by mast cells may be the effector molecule.

Immobilization

Increased bone resorption resulting from decreased weight bearing is a well-recognized cause of bone loss.[145] This phenomenon is discussed in the section on physical activity in the pathogenesis of primary osteoporosis.

Drugs

Long-term heparin administration is associated with bone loss and an increased incidence of fractures.[194] Heparin-induced potentiation of PTH-mediated bone resorption and activation of collagenase may underlie the bone loss. Patients given warfarin sodium for prolonged periods show no reduction in bone mass.[195] Ethanol ingestion may also cause or contribute to bone loss.

Hepatic Disease

Liver disease can cause osteomalacia secondary to malabsorption or defective metabolism of vitamin D. Some patients with liver disease, particularly primary biliary cirrhosis, develop osteopenia even with calciferol treatment.[196] They may malabsorb calcium and phosphate as well as vitamin D.

Juvenile Osteoporosis

This rare disease of heterogeneous etiology occurs in children between the ages of 8 and 15. Manifestations include bone pain, fractures with minimal trauma (most commonly metaphyseal fractures of the distal tibia and vertebral crush fractures), reduced bone density at areas of new bone growth, and loss of height. Calcium, phosphate, and alkaline phosphatase levels in serum are generally normal for the age. Spontaneous recovery occurs within 4 or 5 y, but deformities may persist. It is important to exclude other causes of osteoporosis such as Cushing disease and osteogenesis imperfecta. Most forms of treatment (e.g., calcitonin, vitamin D, and gonadal steroids) are ineffective, but one patient treated with diphosphonates showed marked improvement.[197]

Lysinuric Protein Intolerance

This autosomal recessive defect impairs dibasic amino acid transport. Growth retardation and episodic hyperammonemia are generally the earliest manifestations, but osteopenia is a nearly constant complication and may be the presenting feature.[198] Citrulline therapy corrected the skeletal and other clinical abnormalities in one patient.[198]

OSTEOGENESIS IMPERFECTA

Osteogenesis imperfecta, the brittle bone syndrome, is a heterogeneous group of diseases with increased bone fragility leading to fracture and deformity as major manifestations.[199] Substantial progress has been made in elucidating the biochemical and genetic bases for the various subtypes of this syndrome (reviewed in refs. 47, 200, and 201). An additional challenge will be to understand how specific abnormalities in collagen synthesis and structure lead to increased bone fragility and extraskeletal manifestations.

Classification, Genetics, and Clinical Manifestations

Osteogenesis imperfecta has an estimated incidence of 1 in 20,000 to 50,000.[198] Heterogeneity is evident in the mode of inheritance and in the clinical features.[199] The most common form is inherited as an autosomal dominant trait and is relatively mild in terms of fracture and deformity (type I). Type II is a rare severe form (generally lethal in the perinatal period). Initially thought to be inherited in an autosomal recessive fashion, it is now clear that infants with type II disease have dominant mutations rather than an autosomal recessive disorder.[200] Type III osteogenesis imperfecta is characterized by severe bone fragility, progressive deformity, and probable autosomal recessive inheritance.[200, 201] Type IV is differentiated from type I disease only by the lack of blue sclerae.

The skeletal manifestations are fractures, commonly of the long bones, and deformities, which may include scoliosis. Extraskeletal manifestations are blue sclerae, deafness, thin skin, and cardiac abnormalities such as aortic insufficiency and floppy mitral valves. These features are likely related to abnormal collagen synthesis. Opalescent teeth resulting from abnormal dentin synthesis (dentinogenesis imperfecta) occur in subgroups within both type I and type II categories.[200] Because type I collagen is present in both dentin and bone, it is not clear why all patients with osteogenesis imperfecta do not have abnormal teeth. Lax ligaments and joints and, in severe cases, hyperplastic callus formation are additional features. Short stature is probably secondary to repeated fracture and deformity.

Osteoporosis in osteogenesis imperfecta may be secondary to the treatment of fractures by immobilization. An abnormal organic matrix of bone rather than a reduction in the bone mass may be the primary cause of bone fragility. Histomorphometric studies of bone in patients with osteogenesis imperfecta have yielded conflicting results. In some there was an increased bone turnover, but again this may represent a secondary change. Reduced bone formation resulting from decreased osteoblast activity is likely to be more important.

In the less severe types I and IV, the fracture rate peaks in childhood, decreases to relatively low values during adolescence, and, in men, remains low in adulthood. In women, however, the fracture rate rises again after the menopause.[202] The fracture rate in postmenopausal women is about seven times that in the general population and encompasses fractures of both long bones and vertebrae. This increased risk likely reflects the combination of age-related bone loss and the primary abnormality in collagen synthesis. Estrogen treatment may be particularly relevant for this subgroup of postmenopausal women.

Pathogenesis

A number of biochemical abnormalities have been characterized in bone and skin collagen, and in skin fibroblasts cultured from patients with osteogenesis imperfecta. These include decreased synthesis of type I collagen, anomalous presence of type III or V collagen in bone, increased hydroxylation of lysine residues, and abnormalities in cross-linking of collagen fibrils.[199] Given the complexity of the collagen genes (each contains more than 50 exons) and the number of post-translational modifications involved in collagen formation (see Fig. 28–6), the possibilities for errors in synthesis are great.

The molecular basis for many of the biochemical abnormalities of collagen in osteogenesis imperfecta has been defined. Restriction fragment length polymorphism analysis of kindreds has made it possible to link specific disease subtypes to either the COL1A1 or COL1A2 genes encoding the alpha-1 (I) and alpha-2 (I) chains of collagen, respectively.[200] The phenotypic heterogeneity of osteogenesis imperfecta is reflected in genetic heterogeneity, but it is not possible to segregate precisely the clinical variants (types I to IV) into discrete groups based on the genetic defect. Some general patterns, however, have emerged. Reduced synthesis of type I collagen and reduced pro-alpha-1 (I) mRNA are characteristic of type I osteogenesis imperfecta.[203] A single mutant allele may eliminate collagen production. This limits overall type I collagen synthesis to about 50% of normal.[201] In contrast, the lethal type II variant of the disease is most commonly associated with qualitative defects in type I collagen. Deletions (see, for example, ref. 204) and insertions in the COL1A1 gene that alter alpha-1 (I) chain length have been reported, but point mutations, particularly involving key glycine residues, appear to be more common.[201] For example, substitution of cysteine for Gly-904 of the alpha-1 (I) chain was found in a subject with type II disease.[205] A single abnormal allele can profoundly reduce (>75%) overall synthesis of normal collagen molecules; apparently the mutant gene product combines with normal chains to form an unstable triple helix. Type III disease has been associated with homozygosity for a deletion in the COL1A2 gene. In contrast, in type IV disease dominant structural mutations in the COL1A2 gene have been reported.[200] In general, mutations in the alpha-1 (I) chain produce a more severe phenotype than those in the alpha-2 (I) chain. The position of the mutation also appears to be critical in determining phenotype. For example, mutations substituting cysteine for glycine in the alpha-1 (I) chain can give rise to type I, II, or III disease, depending on whether Gly-94, -718, or -526, respectively, is substituted.[206] Mutations in the NH_2-terminal propeptide region of the alpha chain give rise to a form (type VII) of Ehlers-Danlos syndrome (see later).[47]

Expression of naturally occurring and engineered mutant COL1A1 genes in cells and transgenic mice has permitted detailed analysis of the phenotypic consequences of specific mutations. Expression of a Gly-859-to-cysteine substitution mutant of the COL1A1 gene in transgenic mice, for example, results in death in the perinatal period of all progeny carrying the mutant gene. The overall phenotype closely resembles that of human type II osteogenesis imperfecta.[201]

Diagnosis

The diagnosis of the most common form of the disease usually poses no problem. Fragile bones, blue sclerae, early deafness, and multiple affected family members are reasonably specific clues. In less common forms without blue sclerae, the disease may be confused with other causes of bone fragility. Thus in adolescents it may be difficult to differentiate the disease from juvenile osteoporosis. Intrauterine diagnosis is theoretically feasible if linkage between a DNA polymorphism and the abnormal phenotype has been established or if a mutation has previously been sequenced in other affected family members.[201]

Therapy

No form of treatment is effective. The use of calcitonin is of dubious value, as increased bone resorption is unlikely to be the primary problem. Therapy with fluoride and calciferol has also been unsuccessful.[199, 200] Surgery, primarily internal fixation to prevent deformity, is appropriate in selected cases.

Other Genetic Disorders of Collagen Synthesis

Other inherited disorders of collagen synthesis may cause increased fragility of bone.[47] These include certain forms of the Ehlers-Danlos syndrome, Menkes syndrome, and homocystinuria. The defect in most of these disorders appears to involve abnormal collagen synthesis. In certain forms of the Ehlers-Danlos syndrome there is a deficiency of lysyl oxidase, the enzyme required for normal cross-link formation. In Menkes syndrome, abnormal intestinal copper transport leads to copper deficiency, which in turn impairs lysyl oxidase (a copper-requiring enzyme) activity. In homocystinuria, a high circulating homocysteine level (caused by a deficiency of cystathionine synthetase) apparently interferes with the normal cross-linking of collagen.

ACRO-OSTEOLYSIS SYNDROMES

Several rare genetic and acquired diseases cause lysis of the bones of the distal extremities and may also be associated with generalized osteoporosis.[207] The basis for either local or generalized bone loss has not been determined for any of these. An example is the Hajdu-Cheney syndrome, characterized by dissolution of the terminal phalanges of the hands and feet, malformations of the skull, generalized skeletal demineralization (affecting in particular the vertebrae), fractures, premature loss of teeth, scoliosis, and coarse hair. Autosomal dominant inheritance has been found in some families. Disappearance of the distal tufts of the phalanges or transverse lucent bands in the distal phalanges may be noted on x-ray films. The fingers may show changes that mimic clubbing. Bone biopsy and biochemical studies have not revealed specific abnormalities, and the cause remains unknown. A study of vitamin D metabolites in one case did not reveal significant abnormalities.[208]

OSTEOECTASIA WITH HYPERPHOSPHATASIA (JUVENILE PAGET DISEASE)

Osteoectasia with hyperphosphatasia is a rare hereditary disorder of bone remodeling.[209] Among the approximately 30 reported cases, there is a clustering of Puerto Rican and American Indian families. Inheritance appears to be autosomal recessive. The disease begins in infancy and is generally fatal in adulthood; death occurs from arterial complications. There is an accelerated turnover of membranous bone and chronic elevation of both alkaline phosphatase activity in the serum and the urinary hydroxyproline level. The cause is unknown. Skeletal lesions on x-ray examination resemble those in adult Paget disease, but there is symmetrical involvement of the long bones. Abnormal remodeling leads to widened diaphyses and lack of a distinct corticomedullary separation. There may be bowing of the femur and tibia and an increased head size. Histopathological studies demonstrate thickened osteoid seams and a predominance of woven bone. Calcitonin may be capable of reversing the metabolic, histological, and radiographic abnormalities.

FIBROUS DYSPLASIA

Patients with this rare disease show fibrous replacement of bone at one (monostotic form) or more (polyostotic form) sites. The femur, proximal tibia, and craniofacial bones are the most commonly affected. Lesions appear cystic on radiographs, may show sclerotic margins, and can be difficult to distinguish from those of osteitis fibrosa cystica or other cystic bone lesions. The histological appearance, characterized by a cellular fibroblastic stroma between rare bone spicules, generally permits a specific diagnosis. Serum calcium and phosphate concentrations are normal, but serum alkaline phosphatase activity and the urinary hydroxproline level may be elevated. Fractures and skeletal deformity may occur. The disease generally appears during childhood but may develop after age 20. There is no specific treatment.

Pigmented skin lesions (café au lait spots) with irregular borders (coast of Maine) are common. Several endocrine abnormalities have been reported in the polyostotic form. These include isosexual precocity in girls,[210] hyperthyroidism, acromegaly,[211] gigantism,[212] glucose intolerance with hyperinsulinism (perhaps secondary to growth hormone excess), and adrenal hyperplasia. The triad of polyostotic fibrous dysplasia, pigmented skin lesions, and sexual precocity in girls is called the *McCune-Albright syndrome*. The cause of the bone lesions and their relationship to the reported endocrine abnormalities remain unexplained.

Acquired hypophosphatemia and osteomalacia have been observed in several patients with fibrous dysplasia. The coexistence of primary hyperparathyroidism and fibrous dysplasia has also been reported.[213] It is not clear whether the coexistence of the two represents anything more than coincidence.

OSTEOPENIA IN ERYTHROPOIETIC DISORDERS

Hematological disorders causing marrow hyperplasia (e.g., thalassemia) are frequently accompanied by osteoporosis.[214] Reduced bone formation and either normal or increased[215] bone resorption have been found on bone biopsy. The mechanism by which marrow influences bone has not been elucidated, but factors such as osteoclast-activating factor or prostaglandins could be involved.[216]

OTHER SKELETAL DYSPLASIAS

A host of congenital bone dysplasias have been described, each different with respect to pattern of skeletal involvement, genetics, and associated nonskeletal abnormalities. Few metabolic defects have been identified. The mucopolysaccharide storage diseases are a notable exception. These disorders are due to a deficiency of specific lysosomal enzymes.[217]

The chondrodysplasias are disorders of defective endochondral ossification that cause abnormal skeletal growth. Some may be due to defects in the structure of type II collagen. In a family with spondyloepiphyseal dysplasia, for example, a deletion of exon 48 of the type II collagen gene was found.[218] This presumably leads to abnormal and unstable procollagen trimers in cartilage consisting of normal and shortened chains.

OSTEOPETROSIS

Osteopetrosis (the Albers-Schonberg syndrome or marble bone disease) constitutes a heterogeneous group of disorders characterized by increased bone mineral content. There are at least three distinct forms. Other hereditary and acquired diseases also show increased bone mass (osteosclerosis) as a prominent feature. Acquired causes include heavy metal poisoning, fluorosis, metastatic cancer, myelofibrosis, mastocytosis, Paget disease, sarcoidosis, tuberous sclerosis, and uremia.

Osteopetrosis is the result of failure of the normal coupling of bone resorption and formation. Loss of normal osteoclast function leads to defective modeling and remodeling of bone and increased skeletal radiopacity. Animal models of the disease (e.g., gray-lethal mice) can be cured by transfer of hematopoietic stem cells from normal to affected mice.[2] Conversely, transfer of stem cells from affected animals to normal animals irradiated to destroy endogenous hematopoietic stem cells produces osteopetrosis. These experiments have established that osteoclasts originate from circulating hematopoietic stem cells rather than from mesenchymal cells and have localized the cause of the disease in mice to osteoclast dysfunction. The molecular abnormality within the osteoclast has not been defined at the molecular level. One form is attributable to genetic deficiency of carbonic anhydrase.[4]

Infantile (Lethal) Osteopetrosis

This rare autosomal recessive disorder develops shortly after birth. Generalized skeletal sclerosis leads to obliteration of the marrow spaces. Calcified metaphyseal cartilaginous bars are characteristic. Extramedullary hematopoiesis leads to hepatosplenomegaly. The face shows frontal bossing, hypertelorism, and exophthalmos. Thickening of the skull encroaches on cranial nerve foramina and produces cranial nerve palsies, including optic atrophy. Pathological fractures occur because the apparently dense bone is, nonetheless, fragile. Death generally occurs within the first decade of life from hemorrhage or infection. A defect in phagocytosis by peripheral blood monocytes may predispose to infection and is of interest because of the relation between circulating monocytes and osteoclasts. Skeletal x-ray films show increased density, deficient modeling, sclerotic foci within bone (endobones), and thickened vertebral end plates. Bone biopsy studies may show an increased number of osteoclasts but no evidence of active resorption (lack of Howship lacunae).

As a result of studies in animal models of the disease, allogeneic bone marrow transplantation has been attempted.[1, 219] By using either busulfan or total body radiation, along with cyclophosphamide to prevent rejection, successful results have been obtained in at least five cases in which HLA-identical donors were available. Additional therapy to avert graft-versus-host disease has been given in some cases. With HLA-nonidentical donors the results have been less clear-cut. Successful grafting results in a reduction in bone density (Fig. 28–26), the appearance of normal bone modeling, and an improvement in hematological and neurological parameters. Definitive proof of engraftment was obtained in a case in which an affected female received marrow

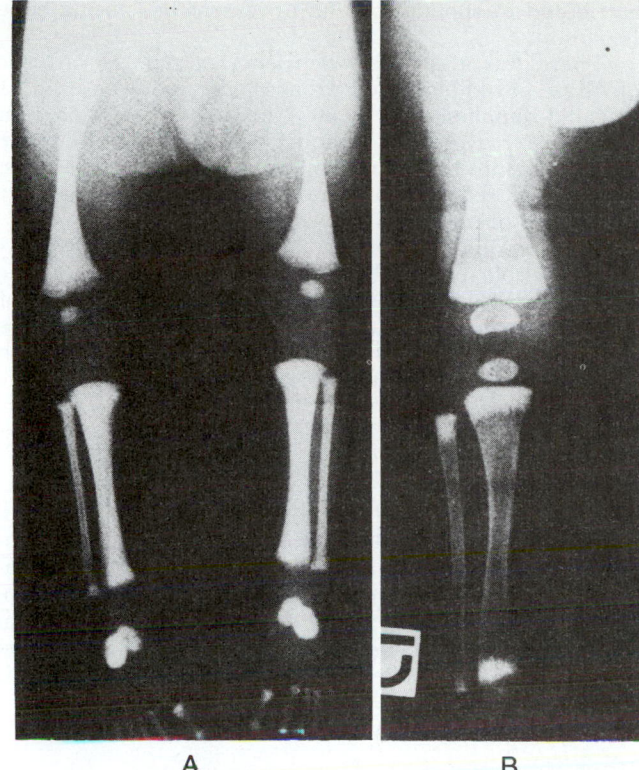

Figure 28–26. Radiographs of the lower limb in a patient with osteopetrosis (A) at age 2 mo before a bone marrow transplant and (B) at age 9 mo after the transplant, showing formation of normal medullary bone. (From Ballet JJ, Griscelli C. Lymphoid cell transplantation in human osteopetrosis. In: Horton JE, Tarpley TM, Davis WF, eds. Mechanisms of Localized Bone Loss. [A Special Supplement of Calcified Tissue Abstracts.] London: IRL, 1978: 399–414, by permission of Oxford University Press.)

from her HLA-identical brother.[1] Osteoclasts contained a Y chromosome, proving their donor origin, whereas osteoblasts lacked a Y chromosome. In addition, peripheral mononuclear phagocytes showed improved bacterial killing after engraftment. Thus in humans, as in animals, lethal osteopetrosis is due to an osteoclast defect that can be cured by engraftment with normal hematopoietic stem cells. The long-term efficacy and safety of this form of therapy have not been established. An 11-mo-old female for whom a suitable marrow transplant donor could not be found was treated with high-dose (up to 32 μg/d) calcitriol.[220] Morphological and biochemical evidence showed increased bone resorption in vivo during treatment, and in vitro evidence of increased bone resorption by the patient's monocytes was also obtained. Nonetheless, after 3 mo of treatment there was minimal clinical improvement in the neurological and hematological manifestations in this individual.[220] These results, however, support the possibility that impaired osteoblast or osteoclast precursors' response to calcitriol may form part of the pathogenesis of some forms of osteopetrosis.

Early-Onset Nonlethal Osteopetrosis

An autosomal recessive form of osteopetrosis that presents in early childhood differs from other childhood forms in that it is not lethal. There may be multiple fractures, increased bone density, reduced bone modeling, and mild anemia. Additional features include basal ganglion calcification and type I (distal) renal tubular acidosis. Three siblings with this disorder showed spontaneous improvement in skeletal abnormalities with time.[221] Acidosis may have contributed to spontaneous improvement by causing bone dissolution.

There was a complete deficiency of type II carbonic anhydrase in red blood cells from 18 affected subjects in 11 unrelated families, and a 50% deficiency was noted in obligate heterozygotes.[221] Although direct studies of enzyme activity have not been performed for kidney or bone cells, the red blood cell defect may reflect a widespread deficiency of this form of the enzyme.

The implications are that carbonic anhydrase type II plays a key role in osteoclast-mediated bone resorption. The type II isozyme may also be important for secretion of hydrogen ion in the distal tubule in the kidney. The basis for the cerebral ganglion calcification is unclear, although the type II isozyme is the only soluble form of the enzyme in brain homogenates.[222]

Late-Onset Osteopetrosis

This disorder, which is more common and milder in expression than the childhood form, shows autosomal dominant inheritance.[223] The disease may be discovered incidentally on skeletal radiographs. Mild anemia, cranial nerve palsies, and pathological fractures may occur. The variation in clinical severity among families may reflect the heterogeneity of the disease. The basis for osteoclast dysfunction is unknown.

Other Inherited Bone Dysplasias with Increased Bone Density

Congenital skeletal dysplasias with increased bone density include pycnodysostosis, osteopoikilosis, diaphyseal dysplasia, and osteopathia striata.[224] Each shows unique phenotypic features, and the mode of inheritance has been defined in some. Specific metabolic defects have not been identified.[209]

EXTRASKELETAL CALCIFICATION AND OSSIFICATION

Calcium may be deposited in soft tissues despite normal serum calcium and phosphate concentrations in response to injury (dystrophic calcification). It may also occur secondary to abnormal serum calcium and phosphate concentrations in the absence of injury. Calcium deposits in the skin may cause pruritus and draining ulcers; deposits in muscle and in joint capsules may impair mobility. Calcification of spinal and extraspinal ligaments and tendons has been reported in patients treated for long periods with synthetic derivatives of vitamin A.[225] Parenchymal calcifications can cause serious disturbance in renal, cardiac, and pulmonary function, and arterial calcification can cause ischemia. Extraskeletal calcification may be detected on x-ray examination. Some forms of soft tissue calcification (e.g., tumoral calcinosis and pulmonary parenchymal calcification[226]) can be detected by technetium Tc 99m diphosphonate scanning before they are radiographically apparent. The calcification of bone matrix in extraskeletal sites is termed ectopic ossification. This too may be dystrophic, or it may be a feature of a genetic disease.

Dystrophic Calcification

Soft tissue calcification is a nonspecific response to tissue damage. Examples include calcified granulomas with tuberculous infection, pleural calcification in asbestosis, and periarticular calcification after joint trauma.

Amorphous calcium phosphate or hydroxyapatite deposits in skin and subcutaneous tissue often occur in scleroderma and may be seen in dermatomyositis and systemic lupus erythematosus as well. Similar deposits without associated disease have been termed calcinosis universalis.

Ectopic Ossification

Fibrodysplasia Ossificans Progressiva

Fibrodysplasia ossificans progressiva (also termed myositis ossificans progressiva) is a rare disorder of unknown etiology in which bone is formed in the connective tissues of skeletal muscles, ligaments, and tendons. The disease is inherited as an autosomal dominant trait, with an equal incidence in men and women.[227] There are many associated skeletal abnormalities, but most appear to be secondary to ectopic ossification.[228] About 80% of the patients show valgus deformity of the great toe; other abnormalities of the metatarsals and metacarpals may also be seen.[229]

It develops shortly after birth or in childhood. The back and neck are often affected first; the hands, diaphragm, and viscera are spared. Biopsy of early lesions may show degenerating muscle fibers, fibroblast proliferation, and mononuclear cell infiltration. Ectopic cartilage and bone matrix form within the fibrosing muscle, and the lesion is successively mineralized and converted into ectopic bone. Progression leads to impaired mobility; thoracic involvement complicated by pneumonia is the usual cause of death. The disease may be fatal before adulthood.[227] Spontaneous fluctuations make evaluation of therapy difficult.

Dystrophic Ossification

Ectopic ossification may be secondary to trauma or neurological injury (e.g., spinal cord lesions). The sites most commonly affected are adjacent to the hip joint and along the medial side of the thigh. Ankylosis and severely impaired mobility may result.

Therapy of Dystrophic Calcification and Ossification

Many forms of therapy have been tried in calcinosis and in fibrodysplasia ossificans progressiva. There have been reports of success with etidronate disodium, but controlled studies have not been performed. In ectopic ossification complicating total hip replacement or spinal cord injury, one study has shown a decreased incidence and severity of ossification with diphosphonate therapy.[230]

Calcification in Hypercalcemic or Hyperphosphatemic States

Hypercalcemic Disorders

Soft tissue calcification may complicate any hypercalcemic disorder but occurs most frequently when the serum phosphate concentration is also elevated (e.g., with renal impairment secondary to vitamin D intoxication) rather than depressed (e.g., in uncomplicated primary hyperparathyroidism). Therapeutic administration of phosphate salts, particularly intravenously, may also cause soft tissue calcification in hypercalcemic patients. Calcium phosphate precipitates preferentially in sites of localized alkalosis—kidney tubules, lungs, gastric mucosa, and eyes. Other local factors may allow calcification in the skin and arterial walls.

Hyperphosphatemic Disorders

Extraskeletal calcification may develop in eucalcemic or even hypocalcemic states if the serum phosphate concentration is high. Thus soft tissue calcification is observed in uremia, in idiopathic hypoparathyroidism, and in pseudo-hypoparathyroidism (ectopic ossification may also occur in the last condition). In uremia, hypermagnesemia may contribute to soft tissue mineral deposition. A potentially lethal calcinosis syndrome, with soft tissue ulceration and diffuse vascular calcification, has been reported in some uremic patients with severe secondary hyperparathyroidism. The syndrome has been reported before or after renal transplantation.[231] Extreme hyperphosphatemia with consequent ectopic calcification and renal failure (caused by nephrocalcinosis) has also been observed as a complication of chemotherapy of tumors such as lymphomas.[232] Alkalinization of the urine (to avoid urate deposition) may be inappropriate in such patients in view of the reduced solubility of calcium phosphate in alkaline urine. Tumoral calcinosis is a rare, often familial disease characterized by massive deposition of calcium phosphate periarticularly. The serum phosphate level is often elevated (see also Chapter 27).

Therapy for Ectopic Calcification in Hypercalcemia or Hypophosphatemia

Treatment of the underlying disorder, when feasible, and correction of hypercalcemia constitute the appropriate therapy for soft tissue calcification complicating hypercalcemic states. Hyperphosphatemic disorders are best treated by a reduction in the serum phosphate concentration. A diet low in phosphate plus administration of phosphate-binding antacids may be effective. Regression of lesions has been documented in tumoral calcinosis after phosphate deprivation.

REFERENCES

1. Coccia PF, Krivit W, Cervenka J, et al. Successful bone-marrow transplantation for infantile malignant osteopetrosis. N Engl J Med 1980; 302:701–708.
2. Ash P, Loutit JF, Townsend KMS. Osteoclasts derived from hematopoietic stem cells. Nature 1980; 283:669–670.
3. Blair HC, Teitelbaum SL, Ghiselli R, et al. Osteoclastic bone resorption by a polarized vacuolar proton pump. Science 1989; 245:855–857.
4. Ohlsson A, Cumming WA, Paul A, et al. Carbonic anhydrase II deficiency syndrome: recessive osteopetrosis with renal tubular acidosis and cerebral calcification. Pediatrics 1986; 77:371–381.
5. Ibbotson KJ, D'Souza SM, Kanis JA, et al. Physiological and pharmacological regulation of bone resorption. Metab Bone Dis Rel Res 1980; 2:177–189.
6. Reddi AH. Local and systemic mechanisms regulating bone formation and remodeling: an overview. In: Silberman M, Slavkin HC, eds. Current Advances in Skeletogenesis. Amsterdam: Excerpta Medica, 1982: 77–86.
7. Canalis E, McCarthy T, Centrella M. Isolation and characterization of insulin-like growth factor I (somatomedin-C) from cultures of fetal rat calvariae. Endocrinology 1988; 122:22–27.
8. McCarthy TL, Centrella M, Canalis E. Regulatory effects of insulin-like growth factors I and II on bone collagen synthesis in rat calvarial cultures. Endocrinology 1989; 124:301–309.
9. Mohan S, Jennings JC, Linkhart TA, et al. Primary structure of human skeletal growth factor: homology with human insulin-like growth factor-II. Biochim Biophys Acta 1988; 966:44–55.
10. Robey PG, Young MF, Flanders KC, et al. Osteoblasts synthesize and respond to transforming growth factor-type beta (TGF-beta) in vitro. J Cell Biol 1987; 105:457–463.
11. Centrella M, McCarthy TL, Canalis E. Transforming growth factor beta is a bifunctional regulator of replication and collagen synthesis in osteoblast-enriched cell cultures from fetal rat bone. J Biol Chem 1987; 262:2869–2874.
12. Centrella M, McCarthy TL, Canalis E. Parathyroid hormone modulates transforming growth factor beta activity and binding in osteoblast-enriched cell cultures from fetal rat parietal bone. Proc Natl Acad Sci USA 1988; 85:5889–5893.
13. Tashjian AH Jr, Voelkel EF, Lazzaro M, et al. Alpha and beta human transforming growth factors stimulate prostaglandin production and bone resorption in cultured mouse calvaria. Proc Natl Acad Sci USA 1985; 82:4535–4538.
14. Pfeilschifter J, Mundy GR. Modulation of type beta transforming growth factor activity in bone cultures by osteotropic hormones. Proc Natl Acad Sci USA 1987; 84:2024–2028.
15. Hauschka PV, Mavrakos AE, Iafrati MD, et al. Growth factors in bone matrix. Isolation of multiple types by affinity chromatography on heparin-Sepharose. J Biol Chem 1986; 261:12665–12674.
15a. Graves DT, Valentin-Opran A, Delgado R, et al. The potential role of platelet-derived growth factor as an autocrine or paracrine factor for human bone cells. Connect Tissue Res 1989; 23:209–218.
16. Wozney JM, Rosen V, Celeste AJ, et al. Novel regulators of bone formation: molecular clones and activities. Science 1988; 242:1528–1534.
16a. Celeste AJ, Iannazzi JA, Taylor RC, et al. Identification of transforming growth factor beta family members present in bone-inductive protein purified from bovine bone. Proc Natl Acad Sci USA 1990; 87:9843–9847.
17. Hanazawa S, Amano S, Nakada K, et al. Biological characterization of interleukin-1–like cytokine produced by cultured bone cells from newborn mouse calvaria. Calcif Tissue Int 1987; 41:31–37.
18. Canalis E, Centrella M, McCarthy T. Effects of basic fibroblast growth factor on bone formation in vitro. J Clin Invest 1988; 81:1572–1577.
19. Globus RK, Patterson-Buckendahl P, Gospodarowicz D. Regulation of bovine bone cell proliferation by fibroblast growth factor and transforming growth factor beta. Endocrinology 1988; 123:98–105.
20. Rodan SB, Wesolowski G, Thomas K, et al. Growth stimulation of rat calvaria osteoblastic cells by acidic fibroblast growth factor. Endocrinology 1987; 121:1917–1923.
21. Gowen M, MacDonald BR, Russell RG. Actions of recombinant human gamma-interferon and tumor necrosis factor alpha on the proliferation and osteoblastic characteristics of human trabecular bone cells in vitro. Arthritis Rheum 1988; 31:1500–1507.
22. Bertolini DR, Nedwin GE, Bringman TS, et al. Stimulation of bone resorption and inhibition of bone formation in vitro by human tumour necrosis factors. Nature 1986; 319:516–518.
22a. Gowen M, Chapman K, Littlewood A, et al. Production of tumor necrosis factor by human osteoblasts is modulated by other cytokines, but not by osteotropic hormones. Endocrinology 1990; 126:1250–1255.
23. Garrett IR, Durie BG, Nedwin GE, et al. Production of lymphotoxin, a bone-resorbing cytokine, by cultured human myeloma cells. N Engl J Med 1987; 317:526–532.
24. Komm BS, Terpening CM, Benz DJ, et al. Estrogen binding, receptor mRNA, and biologic response in osteoblast-like osteosarcoma cells. Science 1988; 241:81–84.
25. Gray TK, Mohan S, Linkhart TA, et al. Estradiol stimulates in vitro the secretion of insulin-like growth factors by the clonal osteoblastic cell line, UMR106. Biochem Biophys Res Commun 1989; 158:407–412.
26. Raisz, LG, Kream BE. Regulation of bone formation. N Engl J Med 1983; 309:29–35, 83–89.
27. McSheehy PM, Chambers TJ. Osteoblast-like cells in the presence of parathyroid hormone release soluble factor that stimulates osteoclastic bone resorption. Endocrinology 1986; 119:1654–1659.
28. Vaes G. Cellular biology and biochemical mechanism of bone resorption. Clin Orthop 1988; 231:239–271.
29. Fleisch H. Bisphosphonates: mechanisms of action and clinical applications. In: Peck WA, ed. Bone and Mineral Research Annual 1. Amsterdam: Excerpta Medica, 1983: 319–357.
30. Reitsma PH, Teitelbaum SL, Bijvoet OLM, et al. Differential action of the bisphosphonates (3-amino-1-hydroxypropylidene)-1,1-bisphosphonate (APD) and disodium dichloromethylidene bisphosphonate (C12MDP) on rat macrophage-mediated bone resorption in vitro. J Clin Invest 1982; 70:927–933.
31. Milhaud G, Labat ML, Moricard Y. (Dichloromethylene)diphosphonate-induced impairment of T-lymphocyte function. Proc Natl Acad Sci USA 1983; 80:4469–4473.
32. Frost HM. Mechanical determinants of bone modeling. Metab Bone Dis Rel Res 1982; 4:217–229.
33. Jaworski ZFG. Physiology and pathology of bone remodeling. Orthop Clin North Am 1981; 12:485–512.
34. Courpron P. Bone tissue mechanisms underlying osteoporoses. Orthop Clin North Am 1981; 12:513–545.
35. Heinegard D, Oldberg A. Structure and biology of cartilage and bone matrix noncollagenous macromolecules. FASEB J 1989; 3:2042–2051.
36. Bolander ME, Young MF, Fisher LW, et al. Osteonectin cDNA sequence reveals potential binding regions for calcium and hydroxyapatite and shows homologies with both a basement membrane protein (SPARC) and a serine proteinase inhibitor (ovomucoid). Proc Natl Acad Sci USA 1988; 85:2919–2923.
37. Price P. Osteocalcin. In: Peck WA, ed. Bone and Mineral Research Annual 1. Amsterdam: Excerpta Medica, 1983: 157–190.
38. Hauschka PV, Lian JB, Cole DEC, et al. Osteocalcin and matrix gla protein: vitamin K–dependent proteins in bone. Physiol Rev 1989; 69:990–1047.

39. Oldberg A, Franzen A, Heinegard D. The primary structure of a cell-binding bone sialoprotein. J Biol Chem 1988; 263:19430–19432.

40. Noda M, Yoon K, Thiede M, et al. cDNA cloning of alkaline phosphatase from rat osteosarcoma (ROS 17/2.8) cells. J Bone Miner Res 1987; 2:161–164.

41. Boyan BD, Schwartz Z, Bonewald, LF, et al. Localization of 1,25-(OH)$_2$D$_3$-responsive alkaline phosphatase in osteoblast-like cells (ROS 17/2.8, MG63, and MC 3T3) and growth cartilage cells in culture. J Biol Chem 1989; 264:11879–11886.

42. Delaisse JM, Eeckhout Y, Vaes G. Bone-resorbing agents affect the production and distrubution of procollagenase as well as the activity of collagenase in bone tissue. Endocrinology 1988; 123:264–276.

43. Miller EJ. The structure of fibril-forming collagens. Ann NY Acad Sci 1985; 460:1–12.

44. Beresford JN, Fedarko NS, Fisher LW, et al. Analysis of the proteoglycans synthesized by human bone cells in vitro. J Biol Chem 1987; 262:17164–17172.

45. Andersson GN, Marks SC Jr. Tartrate-resistant acid ATPase as a cytochemical marker for osteoclasts. J Histochem Cytochem 1989; 37:115–117.

46. Tikka L, Pihlajaniemi T, Henttu P, et al. Gene structure for the alpha 1 chain of a human short-chain collagen (type XIII) with alternatively spliced transcripts and translation termination codon at the 5′ end of the last exon. Proc Natl Acad Sci USA 1988; 85:7491–7495.

47. Prockop DJ, Kivirikko K. Heritable diseases of collagen. N Engl J Med 1984; 311:376–386.

48. Lian J, Stewart C, Puchacz E, et al. Structure of the rat osteocalcin gene and regulation of vitamin D–dependent expression. Proc Natl Acad Sci USA 1989; 86:1143–1147.

49. Hauschka PV, Frenkel J, DeMuth R, et al. Presence of osteocalcin and related higher molecular weight 4-carboxyglutamic acid–containing proteins in developing bone. J Biol Chem 1983; 258:176–182.

50. Riggs BL, Wahner HW, Dunn WL, et al. Differential changes in bone mineral density of the appendicular and axial skeleton with aging: relationship to spinal osteoporosis. J Clin Invest 1981; 67:328–335.

51. Seeman E, Wahner HW, Offord KP, et al. Differential effects of endocrine dysfunction on the axial and appendicular skeleton. J Clin Invest 1982; 69:1302–1309.

52. Meunier PJ. Histomorphometry of the skeleton. In: Peck WA, ed. Bone and Mineral Research Annual 1. Amsterdam: Excerpta Medica, 1983: 191–222.

53. Epstein S. Serum and urinary markers of bone remodeling: assessment of bone turnover. Endocr Rev 1988; 9:437–449.

54. Krane SM, Kantrowitz FG, Byrne M, et al. Urinary excretion of hydroxylysine and its glycosides as an index of collagen degradation. J Clin Invest 1977; 59:819–827.

55. Jung A. Methods for analyzing calcium kinetics. In: Anghileri LJ, Tuffet-Anghileri AM, eds. The Role of Calcium in Biological Systems. Boca Raton, FL: CRC Press, 1982: 107–118.

56. Dequeker J, ed. Proceedings of the Second International Workshop on Non-Invasive Bone Measurement. Leuven, Belgium: Leuven University Press, 1988.

57. Kelly TL, Slovik DM, Schoenfeld DA, et al. Quantitative digital radiography versus dual photon absorptiometry of the lumbar spine. J Clin Endocrinol Metab 1988; 67:839–844.

58. Cummings SR. Health and Public Policy Committee, American College of Physicians position paper: bone mineral densitometry. Ann Intern Med 1987; 107:932–936.

59. David L. Common carential rickets. In: Glorieux FH, ed. Rickets. New York: Raven, 1991: 107–122.

60. Lips P, Netelenbos JC, Jongen MJM, et al. Histomorphometric profile and vitamin D status in patients with femoral neck fractures. Metab Bone Dis Rel Res 1982; 4:85–93.

61. Marx SJ. Rickets and osteomalacia. In: Conn HF, ed. Current Therapy 1983. Philadelphia: W. B. Saunders, 1983: 451–454.

62. Paunier L. Prevention of rickets. In: Glorieux FH, ed. Rickets. New York: Raven, 1991: 263–272.

63. Markestad T, Hesse V, Siebenhuner M, et al. Intermittent high-dose vitamin D prophylaxis during infancy: effect on vitamin D metabolites, calcium, and phosphorus. Am J Clin Nutr 1987; 46:652–658.

64. Parfitt AM, Rao DS, Stanciu J, et al. Irreversible bone loss in osteomalacia: comparison of radial photon absorptiometry with iliac bone histomorphometry during treatment. J Clin Invest 1985; 76:2403–2412.

65. Hillman LS, Haddad JG. Hypocalcemia and other abnormalities of mineral homeostasis during the neonatal period. In: Heath DA, Marx SJ, eds. Calcium Disorders. Boston: Butterworth Scientific, 1982: 248–276.

66. Christensen CK, Lund B, Lund BJ, et al. Reduced 1,25-dihydroxyvitamin D and 24,25-dihydroxyvitamin D in epileptic patients receiving chronic combined anticonvulsant therapy. Metab Bone Dis Rel Res 1981; 3:17–22.

67. Liebross BA, Coburn JW. Renal osteodystrophy. In: Heath DA, Marx SJ, eds. Calcium Disorders. Boston: Butterworth Scientific, 1982: 151–188.

68. Scriver CR, Fraser D, Kooh SW. Hereditary rickets. In: Heath DA, Marx SJ, eds. Calcium Disorders. Boston: Butterworth Scientific, 1982: 1–46.

69. Marx SJ. 1,25-Dihydroxyvitamin D$_3$ receptors and resistance: implications in rickets, osteomalacia, and other conditions. In: Glorieux FH, ed. Rickets. New York: Raven, 1991: 167–184.

70. Hughes MR, Malloy PJ, Kieback DG, et al. Point mutations in the human vitamin D receptor gene associated with hypocalcemic rickets. Science 1988; 242:1702–1705.

71. Pettifor JM. Dietary calcium deficiency. In: Glorieux F, Guesry PR, eds. Rickets and Osteomalacia. New York: Raven (in press).

72. Steichen JJ, Tsang RC, Greer FR, et al. Elevated serum 1,25-dihydroxyvitamin D concentration in rickets of very low-birth-weight infants. J Pediatr 1981; 99:293–297.

73. Dominguez JH, Gray RW, Lemann J Jr. Dietary phosphate deprivation in women and men: effects on mineral acid balances, parathyroid hormone, and the metabolism of 25-OH-vitamin D. J Clin Endocrinol Metab 1976; 43:1056–1068.

74. Tenenhouse HS, Scriver CR, McInnes RR, et al. Renal handling of phosphate in vivo and in vitro by the X-linked hypophosphatemic male mouse: evidence for a defect in the brush border membrane. Kidney Int 1978; 14:236–244.

75. Glorieux FH, Chabot G, Tau C. Familial hypophosphatemic rickets. In: Glorieux FH, ed. Rickets. New York: Raven, 1991: 185–202.

76. Brenner RJ, Spring DB, Sebastian A, et al. Incidence of radiographically evident bone disease, nephrocalcinosis, and nephrolithiasis in various types of renal tubular acidosis. N Engl J Med 1982; 307:217–221.

77. Tieder M, Modai D, Shaked U, et al. "Idiopathic hypercalciuria" and hereditary hypophosphatemic rickets: two phenotypical expressions of a common genetic defect. N Engl J Med 1987; 316:125–129.

78. Tieder M, Arie R, Modai D, et al. Elevated serum 1,25-dihydroxyvitamin D concentrations in siblings with primary Fanconi's syndrome. N Engl J Med 1988; 319:845–849.

79. Ryan EQ, Reiss E. Oncogenous osteomalacia: a review of the world literature of 42 cases and report of two new cases. Am J Med 1984; 77:501–512.

80. Rao DS, Parfitt AM, Kleerekoper M, et al. Dissociation between the effects of endogenous parathyroid hormone on adenosine 3′,5′-monophosphate generation and phosphate reabsorption in hypocalcemia due to vitamin D depletion: an acquired disorder resembling pseudohypoparathyroidism type II. J Clin Endocrinol Metab 1985; 61:285–290.

81. Rasmussen H. Hypophosphatasia. In: Stanbury JB, Wyngaarden JB, Fredrickson DS, et al., eds. The Metabolic Basis of Inherited Disease. 5th ed. New York: McGraw-Hill, 1983: 1497–1507.

82. Weiss MJ, Cole DE, Ray K, et al. A missense mutation in the human liver/bone/kidney alkaline phosphatase gene causing a lethal form of hypophosphatasia. Proc Natl Acad Sci USA 1988; 85:7666–7669.

83. Kanis JA, Cundy TF, Hamdy NAT. Renal osteodystrophy. Ballieres Clin Endocrinol Metab 1988; 2:193–241.

84. Shike M, Sturtridge WC, Tam CS, et al. A possible role of vitamin D in the genesis of parenteral-nutrition–induced metabolic bone disease. Ann Intern Med 1981; 95:560–568.

85. Swan CHJ, Shah K, Brewer DB, et al. Fibrogenesis imperfecta ossium. Q J Med 1976; 178:233–253.

86. Hunter D, Turnbull HM. Hyperparathyroidism: generalized osteitis fibrosa. Br J Surg 1931–1932; 19:203–239.

87. Jowsey J. Bone histology and hyperparathyroidism. Clin Endocrinol Metab 1974; 3:267–284.

88. Avioli LV. Renal osteodystrophy. In: Avioli LV, Krane SM, eds. Metabolic Bone Disease. Vol II. New York: Academic, 1978: 149–215.

89. Muirhead N, Adami S, Sandler LM, et al. Long-term effects of 1,25-dihydroxy vitamin D$_3$ and 24,25-dihydroxy vitamin D$_3$ in renal osteodystrophy. Q J Med 1982; 51:427–444.

90. Quarles LD, Davidai GA, Schwab SJ, et al. Oral calcitriol and calcium: efficient therapy for uremic hyperparathyroidism. Kidney Int 1988; 34:840–844.

91. Andress DL, Norris KC, Coburn JW, et al. Intravenous calcitriol in the treatment of refractory osteitis fibrosa of chronic renal failure. N Engl J Med 1989; 321:274–279.

92. Teitelbaum SL. Histological manifestations of abnormal parathyroid hormone metabolism in renal osteodystrophy. Contrib Nephrol 1988; 64:1–4.

93. Boyce BF, Mocan MZ, Byars J, et al. Treatment and histological healing of aluminum-related osteomalacia. Contrib Nephrol 1988; 64:151–159.

94. Hercz G, Andress DL, Nebeker HG, et al. Reversal of aluminum-related bone disease after substituting calcium carbonate for aluminum hydroxide. Am J Kidney Dis 1988; 11:70–75.

95. Rebel A. Paget's disease. Clin Orthop 1987; 217:2–170.

96. Delmas PD, Chapuy MC, Vignon E, et al. Long term effects of dichloromethylene diphosphonate in Paget's disease of bone. J Clin Endocrinol Metab 1982; 54:837–844.

97. Mills BG, Singer FR, Weiner LP, et al. Evidence for both respiratory syncytial virus and measles virus antigens in the osteoclasts of patients with Paget's disease of bone. Clin Orthop 1984; 183:303–311.

98. Basle MF, Fournier JG, Rozenblatt S, et al. Measles virus RNA detected in Paget's disease of bone by in situ hybridization. J Gen Virol 1986; 67:907–913.

99. Guyer PB. Paget's disease of bone: the anatomical distribution. Metab Bone Dis Rel Res 1981; 4,5:239–242.

99a. Lebbin D, Ryan WG, Schwartz TB. Outpatient treatment of Paget's disease of bone with mithramycin. Ann Intern Med 1974; 81:635–637.

100. Kanis JA, Evanson JM, Russell RGG. Paget's disease of bone: diagnosis and management. Metab Bone Dis Rel Res 1981; 4,5:219–230.

101. Upchurch KS, Simon LS, Schiller AL, et al. Giant cell reparative granuloma of Paget's disease of bone: a unique clinical entity. Ann Intern Med 1983; 98:35–40.

102. Chen JR, Rhee RSC, Wallach S, et al. Neurologic disturbances in Paget disease of bone: response to calcitonin. Neurology 1979; 29:448–457.

103. Douglas DL, Kanis JA, Duckworth T, et al. Paget's disease: improvement of spinal cord dysfunction with diphosphonates and calcitonin. Metab Bone Dis Rel Res 1981; 4,5:327–336.

104. Chapuy MC, Zucchelli P, Meunier PJ. Parathyroid function in Paget's disease of bone. Miner Electrolyte Metab 1981; 6:112–118.

105. Siris ES, Clemens TP, McMahon D, et al. Parathyroid function in Paget's disease of bone. J Bone Miner Res 1989; 4:75–79.

106. Vellenga CJLR, Pauwels EKJ, Bijvoet OLM, et al. Bone scintigraphy in Paget's disease treated with combined calcitonin and diphosphonate (EHDP). Metab Bone Dis Rel Res 1981; 4,5:103–111.

107. Deftos LJ, Parthemore JG, Price PA. Changes in plasma bone GLA protein during treatment of bone disease. Calcif Tissue Int 1982; 34:121–124.

108. Hosking DJ. Calcitonin and diphosphonate in the treatment of Paget's disease of bone. Metab Bone Dis Rel Res 1981; 4,5:317–326.

109. Levy F, Muff R, Dotti-Sigrist S, Formation of neutralizing antibodies during intranasal synthetic salmon calcitonin treatment of Paget's disease. J Clin Endocrinol Metab 1988; 67:541–545.

110. Krane SM. Etidronate disodium in the treatment of Paget's disease of bone. Ann Intern Med 1982; 96:619–625.

111. Frijlink WB, Bijvoet OLM, Velde JT, et al. Treatment of Paget's disease with (3-amino-1-hydroxypropylidene)-1,1-bisphosphonate (A.P.D.). Lancet 1979; 1:799–803.

112. Riggs BL, Melton LJ III. Involutional osteoporosis. N Engl J Med 1986; 314:1676–1686.

113. Burnell JM, Baylink DJ, Chestnut CH, et al. Bone matrix and mineral abnormalities in postmenopausal osteoporosis. Metabolism 1982; 31:1113–1120.

114. Riggs BL, Wahner HW, Seeman E, et al. Changes in bone mineral density of the proximal femur and spine with aging. J Clin Invest 1982; 70:716–723.

115. Nordin BEC, Aaron J, Speed R, et al. Bone formation and resorption as the determinants of trabecular bone volume in postmenopausal osteoporosis. Lancet 1981; 2:277–279.

116. Pocock NA, Eisman JA, Hopper JL, et al. Genetic determinants of bone mass in adults: a twin study. J Clin Invest 1987; 80:706–710.

117. Seeman E, Hopper JL, Bach LA, et al. Reduced bone mass in daughters of women with osteoporosis. N Engl J Med 1989; 320:554–558.

118. Liel Y, Edwards J, Shary J, et al. The effects of race and body habitus on bone mineral density of the radius, hip, and spine in premenopausal women. J Clin Endocrinol Metab 1988; 66:1247–1250.

119. Weinstein RS, Bell NH. Diminished rates of bone formation in normal black adults. N Engl J Med 1988; 319:1698–1701.

120. Richelson LS, Wahner HW, Melton LJ III, et al. Relative contributions of aging and estrogen deficiency to postmenopausal bone loss. N Engl J Med 1984; 311:1273–1275.

121. Johnston CC Jr, Hui SL, Witt RM, et al. Early menopausal changes in bone mass and sex steroids. J Clin Endocrinol Metab 1985; 61:905–911.

122. Steinberg KK, Freni-Titulaer LW, DePuey EG, et al. Sex steroids and bone density in premenopausal and perimenopausal women. J Clin Endocrinol Metab 1989; 69:533–539.

123. Hutchinson TA, Polansky SM, Feinstein AR. Postmenopausal estrogens protect against fractures of distal hip and radius. Lancet 1979; 2:705–709.

124. Weiss NS, Ure CL, Ballard JH, et al. Decreased risk of fractures of the hip and lower forearm with postmenopausal use of estrogen. N Engl J Med 1980; 303:1195–1198.

125. Kiel DP, Felson DT, Anderson JJ, et al. Hip fracture and the use of estrogens in postmenopausal women. N Engl J Med 1987; 317:1169–1174.

126. Buchanan JR, Hospodar P, Myers C, et al. Effect of excess endogenous androgens on bone density in young women. J Clin Endocrinol Metab 1988; 67:937–942.

127. Pacifici R, Rifas L, McCracken R, et al. Ovarian steroid treatment blocks a postmenopausal increase in blood monocyte interleukin 1 release. Proc Natl Acad Sci USA 1989; 86:2398–2402.

128. Gallagher JC, Riggs BL, DeLuca HF. Effect of estrogen on calcium absorption and serum vitamin D metabolites in postmenopausal osteoporosis. J Clin Endocrinol Metab 1980; 51:1359–1364.

129. Slovik DM, Adams JS, Neer RM, et al. Deficient production of 1,25-dihydroxyvitamin D in elderly osteoporotic patients. N Engl J Med 1981; 305:372–374.

130. Riggs BL, Hamstra A, DeLuca HF. Assessment of 25-hydroxyvitamin D 1 alpha-hydroxylase reserve in postmenopausal osteoporosis by administration of parathyroid extract. J Clin Endocrinol Metab 1981; 53:833–835.

131. Sorensen OH, Lumholtz B, Lund B, et al. Acute effects of parathyroid hormone on vitamin D metabolism in patients with bone loss of aging. J Clin Endocrinol Metab 1982; 54:1258–1261.

132. Silverberg SJ, Shane E, Cruz LDL, et al. Abnormalities in parathyroid hormone secretion and 1,25-dihydroxyvitamin D_3 formation in women with osteoporosis. N Engl J Med 1989; 320:277–281.

133. Cheema C, Grant BF, Marcus R. Effects of estrogen on circulating "free" and total 1,25-dihydroxyvitamin D and on the parathyroid–vitamin D axis in postmenopausal women. J Clin Invest 1989; 83:537–542.

134. Falch JA, Oftebro H, Haug E. Early postmenopausal bone loss is not associated with a decrease in circulating levels of 25-hydroxyvitamin D, 1,25-dihydroxyvitamin D, or vitamin D–binding protein. J Clin Endocrinol Metab 1987; 64:836–841.

135. Deftos LJ, Weisman MH, Williams GW, et al. Influence of age and sex on plasma calcitonin in human beings. N Engl J Med 1980; 302:1351–1353.

136. Stevenson JC, Abeyasekera G, Hillyard CJ, et al. Calcitonin and the calcium-regulating hormones in postmenopausal women: effect of estrogens. Lancet 1981; 1:693–695.

137. Body JJ, Struelens M, Borkowski A, et al. Effects of estrogens and calcium on calcitonin secretion in postmenopausal women. J Clin Endocrinol Metab 1989; 68:223–226.

138. Reginster JY, Deroisy R, Albert A, et al. Relationship between whole plasma calcitonin levels, calcitonin secretory capacity, and plasma levels of estrone in healthy women and postmenopausal osteoporotics. J Clin Invest 1989; 83:1073–1077.

139. Tiegs RD, Body JJ, Wahner HW, et al. Calcitonin secretion in postmenopausal osteoporosis. N Engl J Med 1985; 312:1097–1100.

140. Heaney RP. Calcium intake requirement and bone mass in the elderly. J Lab Clin Med 1982; 100:309–312.

141. Matkovic V, Kostial K, Simonovic I, et al. Bone status and fracture rates in two regions of Yugoslavia. Am J Clin Nutr 1979; 32:540–549.

142. Holbrook TL, Barrett-Connor E, Wingard DL. Dietary calcium and risk of hip fracture: 14-year prospective population study. Lancet 1988; 2:1046–1048.

143. Riggs BL, Wahner HW, Melton LJ III, et al. Dietary calcium intake and rates of bone loss in women. J Clin Invest 1987; 80:979–982.

144. Riis B, Thomsen K, Christiansen C. Does calcium supplementation prevent postmenopausal bone loss? N Engl J Med 1987; 316:173–177.

145. Mazess RB, Whedon GD. Immobilization and bone. Calcif Tissue Int 1983; 35:265–267.

146. Pocock N, Eisman J, Gwinn T, et al. Muscle strength, physical fitness, and weight but not age predict femoral neck bone mass. J Bone Miner Res 1989; 4:441–448.

147. Bevier WC, Wiswell RA, Pyka G, et al. Relationship of body composition, muscle strength, and aerobic capacity to bone mineral density in older men and women. J Bone Miner Res 1989; 4:421–432.

148. Stevenson JC, Lees B, Devenport M, et al. Determinants of bone density in normal women: risk factors for future osteoporosis? Br Med J 1989; 298:924–928.

149. Jensen J, Christiansen C, Rodbro P. Cigarette smoking, serum estrogens, and bone loss during hormone-replacement therapy early after menopause. N Engl J Med 1985; 313:973–975.

150. Ray WA, Griffin MR, Schaffner W, et al. Psychotropic drug use and the risk of hip fracture. N Engl J Med 1987; 316:363–369.

151. Cummings SR, Black D. Should perimenopausal women be screened for osteoporosis? Ann Intern Med 1986; 104:817–823.

152. Ettinger B, Genant HK, Cann CE. Postmenopausal bone loss is prevented by treatment with low-dosage estrogen with calcium. Ann Intern Med 1987; 106:40–45.

153. Christiansen C, Christensen MS, Transbol I. Bone mass in postmenopausal women after withdrawal of estrogen/gestagen replacement therapy. Lancet 1981; 1:459–461.

154. Barrett-Connor E. Postmenopausal estrogen replacement and breast cancer. N Engl J Med 1989; 321:319–320.

155. Ott SM, Chestnut CH III. Calcitriol treatment is not effective in postmenopausal osteoporosis. Ann Intern Med 1989; 110:267–274.

156. Aloia JF, Vaswani A, Yeh JK, et al. Calcitriol in the treatment of postmenopausal osteoporosis. Am J Med 1988; 84:401–408.

157. Wasnich RD, Benfante RJ, Yano K, et al. Thiazide effect on the mineral content of bone. N Engl J Med 1983; 309:344–347.

158. Transbol I, Christensen MS, Jensen FG, et al. Thiazide for the postponement of postmenopausal bone loss. Metabolism 1982; 31:383–386.

159. Ray WA, Griffin MR, Downey W, et al. Long term use of thiazide diuretics reduces risk of hip fracture. Lancet 1989; 2:687–690.

160. Riggs BL, Seeman E, Hodgson SF, et al. Effect of the fluoride/calcium regimen on vertebral fracture occurrence in postmenopausal osteoporosis. N Engl J Med 1982; 306:446–450.

161. Pak CYC, Sakhaee K, Zerwekh JE, et al. Safe and effective treatment of osteoporosis with intermittent slow release sodium fluoride: augmentation of vertebral bone mass and inhibition of fractures. J Clin Endocrinol Metab 1989; 68:150–159.

162. Mamelle N, Meunier PJ, Dusan R, et al. Risk-benefit ratio of sodium fluoride treatment in primary vertebral osteoporosis. Lancet 1988; 2:361–365.

163. Hedlund LR, Gallagher JC. Increased incidence of hip fracture in

osteoporotic women treated with sodium fluoride. J Bone Miner Res 1989; 4:223–225.

164. Civitelli R, Gonnelli S, Zacchei F, et al. Bone turnover in postmenopausal osteoporosis: effect of calcitonin treatment. J Clin Invest 1988; 82:1268–1274.

165. Mallette LE, LeBlanc AD, Pool JL, et al. Cyclic therapy of osteoporosis with neutral phosphate and brief, high-dose pulses of etidronate. J Bone Miner Res 1989; 4:143–148.

166. Reeve J, Meunier PJ, Parsons JA, et al. Anabolic effect of human parathyroid hormone fragment on trabecular bone in involutional osteoporosis: a multicentre trial. Br Med J 1980; 280:1340–1344.

167. Slovik DM, Rosenthal DI, Doppelt SH, et al. Restoration of spinal bone in osteoporotic men by treatment with human parathyroid hormone (1–34) and 1,25-dihydroxyvitamin D. J Bone Miner Res 1986; 1:377–381.

168. Krolner B, Toft B, Nielsen SP, et al. Physical exercise as prophylaxis against involutional vertebral bone loss: a controlled trial. Clin Sci 1983; 64:541–546.

169. Reid IR. Pathogenesis and treatment of steroid osteoporosis. Clin Endocrinol 1989; 30:83–103.

170. Hough S, Teitelbaum SL, Bergfeld MA, et al. Isolated skeletal involvement in Cushing's syndrome: response to therapy. J Clin Endocrinol Metab 1981; 52:1033–1038.

171. Adinoff AD, Hollister JR. Steroid-induced fractures and bone loss in patients with asthma. N Engl J Med 1983; 309:265–268.

172. Baylink DJ. Glucocorticoid-induced osteoporosis. N Engl J Med 1983; 309:306–308.

173. Hahn TJ, Halstead LR, Baran DT. Effects of short term glucocorticoid administration on intestinal calcium absorption and circulating vitamin D metabolite concentrations in man. J Clin Endocrinol Metab 1981; 52:111–115.

174. Seeman E, Kumar R, Hunder GG, et al. Production, degradation, and circulating levels of 1,25-dihydroxyvitamin D in health and in chronic glucocorticoid excess. J Clin Invest 1980; 66:664–669.

175. Dempster DW. Bone histomorphometry in glucocorticoid-induced osteoporosis. J Bone Miner Res 1989; 4:137–141.

176. Braun JJ, Birkenhager-Frenkel DH, Rietveld AH, et al. Influence of 1-alpha-hydroxyvitamin D administration on bone and bone mineral metabolism in patients on chronic glucocorticoid treatment. Clin Endocrinol 1983; 18:265–273.

177. Fallon MD, Perry HM, Bergfeld M, et al. Exogenous hyperthyroidism with osteoporosis. Arch Intern Med 1983; 143:442–444.

178. Bayley TA, Harrison JE, McNeill KG, et al. Effect of thyrotoxicosis and its treatment on bone mineral and muscle mass. J Clin Endocrinol Metab 1980; 50:916–922.

179. Johansen JS, Riis BJ, Hassager C, et al. The effect of a gonadotropin-releasing hormone agonist analog (nafarelin) on bone metabolism. J Clin Endocrinol Metab 1988; 67:701–706.

180. Klibanski A, Biller BMK, Rosenthal DI, et al. Effects of prolactin and estrogen deficiency in amenorrheic bone loss. J Clin Endocrinol Metab 1988; 67:124–130.

181. Fisher EC, Nelson ME, Frontera WR, et al. Bone mineral content and levels of gonadotropins and estrogens in amenorrheic running women. J Clin Endocrinol Metab 1986; 62:1232–1236.

182. Biller BMK, Saxe V, Herzog DB, et al. Mechanisms of osteoporosis in adult and adolescent women with anorexia nervosa. J Clin Endocrinol Metab 1989; 68:548–554.

183. Stepan JJ, Musiolva J, Pacovsky V. Bone demineralization, biochemical indices of bone remodeling, and estrogen replacement therapy in adults with Turner's syndrome. J Bone Miner Res 1989; 4:193–198.

184. Francis RM, Peacock M, Aaron JE, et al. Osteoporosis in hypogonadal men: role of decreased plasma 1,25-dihydroxyvitamin D, calcium malabsorption, and low bone formation. Bone 1986; 7:261–268.

185. Diamond T, Stiel D, Posen S. Osteoporosis in hemochromatosis: iron excess, gonadal deficiency, or other factors? Ann Intern Med 1989; 110:430–436.

186. Schlechte J, El-Khoury G, Kathol M, Walkner L. Forearm and vertebral bone mineral in treated and untreated hyperprolactinemic amenorrhea. J Clin Endocrinol Metab 1987; 64:1021–1026.

187. Greenspan SL, Oppenheim DS, Klibanski A. Importance of gonadal steroids to bone mass in men with hyperprolactinemic hypogonadism. Ann Intern Med 1989; 110:526–531.

188. Heath H III, Lambert PW, Service FJ, et al. Calcium homeostasis in diabetes mellitus. J Clin Endocrinol Metab 1979; 49:462–466.

189. Gertner JM, Tamborlane WV, Horst RL, et al. Mineral metabolism in diabetes mellitus: changes accompanying treatment with a portable subcutaneous insulin infusion system. J Clin Endocrinol Metab 1980; 50:862–866.

190. Witt MF, White NH, Santiago JV, et al. Use of oral calcium loading to characterize the hypercalciuria of young insulin-dependent diabetics. J Clin Endocrinol Metab 1983; 57:94–100.

191. Weinstock RS, Goland RS, Shane E, et al. Bone mineral density in women with type II diabetes mellitus. J Bone Miner Res 1989; 4:97–101.

192. Heath H III, Melton LJ, Chu CP. Diabetes mellitus and risk of skeletal fracture. N Engl J Med 1980; 303:567–570.

193. Blayney DW, Jaffe ES, Fisher RI, et al. The human T-cell leukemia/lymphoma virus, lymphoma, lytic bone lesions, and hypercalcemia. Ann Intern Med 1983; 98:144–151.

194. Fallon MD, Whyte MP, Teitelbaum SL. Systemic mastocytosis associated with generalized osteopenia. Hum Pathol 1981; 12:813–820.

195. Piro LD, Whyte MP, Murphy WA, et al. Normal cortical bone mass in patients after long term coumadin therapy. J Clin Endocrinol Metab 1982; 54:470–473.

196. Epstein O, Kato Y, Dick R, et al. Vitamin D, hydroxyapatite, and calcium gluconate in treatment of cortical bone thinning in postmenopausal women with primary biliary cirrhosis. Am J Clin Nutr 1982; 36:426–430.

197. Hoekman K, Papalous SE, Peters ACB, et al. Characteristics and bisphosphonate treatment of a patient with juvenile osteoporosis. J Clin Endocrinol Metab 1985; 61:952–956.

198. Carpenter TO, Levy HL, Holtrop ME, et al. Lysinuric protein intolerance presenting as childhood osteoporosis. N Engl J Med 1985; 312:290–294.

199. Smith R, Francis MJO, Houghton GR. The Brittle Bone Syndrome. London: Butterworths, 1983.

200. Cole WG. Osteogenesis imperfecta. Clin Endocrinol Metab 1988; 2:243–266.

201. Cole WG, Jaensich R, Bateman JF. New insights into the molecular pathology of osteogenesis imperfecta. Q J Med 1989; 70:1–4.

202. Paterson CR, McAllion S, Stellman JL. Osteogenesis imperfecta after the menopause. N Engl J Med 1984; 310:1694–1696.

203. Rowe DW, Shapiro JR, Poirier M, et al. Diminished type I collagen synthesis and reduced alpha 1 (I) collagen messenger RNA in cultured fibroblasts from patients with dominantly inherited (type I) osteogenesis imperfecta. J Clin Invest 1985; 76:604–611.

204. Chu ML, Williams CJ, Pepe G, et al. Internal deletion in a collagen gene in a perinatal lethal form of osteogenesis imperfecta. Nature 1983; 304:78–80.

205. Constantinou CD, Nielsen KB, Prockop DJ. A lethal variant of osteogenesis imperfecta has a single base mutation that substitutes cysteine for glycine 904 of the $alpha_1$ (I) chain of type I procollagen. J Clin Invest 1989; 83:574–584.

206. Starman BJ, Eyre D, Charbonneau H, et al. Osteogenesis imperfecta: the position of substitution for glycine by cysteine in the triple helical domain of the pro-$alpha_1$ (I) chains of type I collagen determines the clinical phenotype. J Clin Invest 1989; 84:1206–1214.

207. Elias AN, Pinals RS, Anderson HC, et al. Hereditary osteodysplasia with acro-osteolysis (the Hajdu-Cheney syndrome). Am J Med 1978; 65:627–636.

208. Sakano T, Hyodo S, Nishi Y, et al. Levels of vitamin D metabolites in a case of acro-osteolysis syndrome. Acta Paediatr Scand 1983; 72:617–620.

209. Beighton P. Sclerosing bone dysplasias. In: Papadatos CJ, Bartsocas CS, eds. Skeletal Dysplasias. New York: Alan R. Liss, 1982: 173–194.

210. D'Armiento M, Reda G, Camagna A, et al. McCune-Albright syndrome: evidence for autonomous multiendocrine hyperfunction. J Pediatr 1983; 102:584–586.

211. Lipson A, Hsu TH. The Albright syndrome associated with acromegaly: report of a case and review of the literature. Johns Hopkins Med J 1981; 149:10–14.

212. Albin J, Wu R. Abnormal hypothalamic-pituitary function in polyostotic fibrous dysplasia. Clin Endocrinol 1981; 14:435–443.

213. Rosen IB, Palmer JA. Fibrosseous tumors of the facial skeleton in association with primary hyperparathyroidism: an endocrine syndrome or coincidence. Am J Surg 1981; 142:494–498.

214. Vernejoul MC, Girot R, Gueris J, et al. Calcium phosphate metabolism and bone disease in patients with homozygous thalassemia. J Clin Endocrinol Metab 1982; 54:276–281.

215. Pootrakul P, Hungsprenges S, Fucharoen S, et al. Relation between erythropoiesis and bone metabolism in thalassemia. N Engl J Med 1981; 304:1470–1473.

216. Raisz LG. What marrow does to bone. N Engl J Med 1981; 304:1485–1486.

217. McKusick VA, Neufeld EF. The mucopolysaccharide storage diseases. In: Stanbury JB, Wyngaarden JB, Frederickson DS, et al., eds. The Metabolic Basis of Inherited Disease. 5th ed. New York: McGraw-Hill, 1983: 751–777.

218. Lee B, Vissing H, Ramirez F, et al. Identification of the molecular defect in a family with spondyloepiphyseal dysplasia. Science 1989; 244:978–980.

219. Sieff CA, Chessells JM, Levinsky RJ, et al. Allogeneic bone-marrow transplantation in infantile malignant osteopetrosis. Lancet 1983; 1:437–441.

220. Key L, Carnes D, Cole S, et al. Treatment of congenital osteopetrosis with high-dose calcitriol. N Engl J Med 1984; 310:409–415.

221. Whyte MP, Murphy WA, Fallon MD, et al. Osteopetrosis, renal tubular acidosis, and basal ganglion calcification in three sisters. Am J Med 1980; 69:64–74.

222. Sly WS, Whyte MP, Sundaram V, et al. Carbonic anhydrase II deficiency in 12 families with the autosomal recessive syndrome of osteopetrosis with renal tubular acidosis and cerebral calcification. N Engl J Med 1985; 313:139–145.

223. Bollerslev J. Autosomal dominant osteopetrosis: bone metabolism and epidemiological, clinical, and hormonal aspects. Endocr Rev 1989; 10:45–67.

224. Papadatos CJ, Bartsocas CS. Skeletal Dysplasias. New York: Alan R. Liss, 1982.

225. DiGiovanna JJ, Helfgott RK, Gerber LH, et al. Extraspinal tendon and ligament calcification associated with long-term therapy with etretinate. N Engl J Med 1986; 315:1177–1182.

226. Herry JY, Chevet D, Moisan A, et al. Pulmonary uptake of Tc-99m-labelled methylene diphosphonate in a patient with a parathyroid adenoma. J Nucl Med 1981; 22:888–890.

227. Connor JM, Evans DAP. Genetic aspects of fibrodysplasia ossificans progressiva. J Med Genet 1982; 19:35–39.

228. Cremin B, Connor JM, Beighton P. The radiological spectrum of fibrodysplasia ossificans progressiva. Clin Radiol 1982; 33:499–508.

229. Schroeder HW Jr, Zasloff M. The hand and foot malformations in fibrodysplasia ossificans progressiva. Johns Hopkins Med J 1980; 147:73–78.

230. Finerman GAM, Stover SL. Heterotopic ossification following hip replacement and spinal cord injury. Metab Bone Dis Rel Res 1981; 4,5:337–342.

231. Perloff LJ, Spence RK, Grossman RA, et al. Lethal post-transplantation calcinosis. Transplantation 1979; 27:21–25.

232. Kanfer A, Richet G, Roland J, et al. Extreme hyperphosphataemia causing acute anuric nephrocalcinosis in lymphosarcoma. Br Med J 1979; 2:1320–1321.

KIDNEY STONES

Charles Y. C. Pak

Kidney stones (nephrolithiasis, renal calculi) are concretions composed of crystalline components and organic matrix. The morbidity is caused by obstruction, bleeding, or infection.

Although the symptomatic presentations may be similar, the disorder is heterogeneous as to composition and etiology. Some stones are made of calcium salts (calcareous renal stones); others are not. Likewise, stones of the same chemical composition can result from different metabolic or environmental disturbances. Some stones are due to generalized metabolic derangements, involving alterations of calcium and phosphorus metabolism, parathyroid function, or vitamin D status, as in the hypercalciurias associated with calcium stones.

Recognition of the complex nature of nephrolithiasis has led to classification of the disorders in a more physiological manner on the basis of underlying metabolic or environmental derangements.[1] As a consequence, therapies can be specifically selected for the ability to "reverse" the particular disturbances.[2]

This chapter will consider the pathogenesis, diagnosis, and management of nephrolithiasis with a special emphasis on underlying metabolic derangements.

BACKGROUND

Epidemiology

Nephrolithiasis is common. As many as 0.2% of the population of the United States may have renal stones each year. The prevalence of stones within the urinary tract at necropsy is around 5%. The lifetime prevalence rate of nephrolithiasis may be as high as 10%; i.e., 10% of the population may form renal stones in their lifetime.[3] In the United States, stones originating in the kidneys (kidney stones) predominate over those originating in the bladder (bladder stones). Bladder stones are rare in industrialized countries except in association with a foreign body (e.g., indwelling catheter), although they were common in antiquity and are still frequent in Southeast Asia.[4]

A high prevalence of kidney stones has been reported in regions of hot climate, where they are probably due to dehydration and low urine output. The southeastern United States has often been referred to as the "stone belt." However, the prevalence and presentation of stone-forming patients residing in this region do not differ from those of patients living elsewhere.

Nephrolithiasis is a disease of high probability of recurrence and requires adequate long-term therapy directed at correcting the underlying defect.

Chemical Composition of Stones

Stones can be categorized according to whether they are composed predominantly of calcium salts.[5] Calcareous renal stones, which constitute approximately 75% of all stones, are composed mainly of calcium oxalate alone (35%) or in combination with hydroxyapatite (35%). The remaining calcareous stones (5%) are principally hydroxyapatite or brushite ($CaHPO_4 \cdot 2H_2O$).

The most common noncalcareous stones, 15 to 20% of the total, are composed of struvite ($MgNH_4PO_4 \cdot 6H_2O$). Often called "infection" stones, they typically occur as mixtures with carbonate apatite, tricalcium diphosphate, or calcium oxalate. Pure struvite stones are rare. Stones of uric acid (approximately 5%) or cystine (1 to 3%) usually occur alone but may be found as mixtures with calcium oxalate or calcium phosphate. Rarely, stones are composed of sodium urate, xanthine, 2,8-dihydroxyadenine,[6] or triamterene.

Calcium oxalate stones are more common in men than in women, and middle-aged white men are particularly susceptible. Struvite and calcium phosphate stones are more common in women. Chemical composition of the stone may sometimes provide the diagnosis (e.g., cystine stones for cystinuria, struvite stones for urinary tract infection with urea-splitting organisms, and uric acid stones for gout). The finding of calcium phosphate as the predominant component suggests the diagnosis of distal renal tubular acidosis or primary hyperparathyroidism. However, the identification of the most common, calcium oxalate stones, has limited diagnostic value because they can result from a wide variety of metabolic and environmental disturbances.

Physical Chemistry of Stone Formation

Three major theories have been invoked to explain stone formation. The precipitation-crystallization theory considers stone formation to be a physicochemical process of precipitation of salts from a supersaturated urinary environment.[7] In the matrix theory the stone is thought to form in an organic matrix, analogous to the formation of bone.[8] The inhibitor theory assumes that deficiency of inhibitors in urine leads to stone formation.[9]

A current scheme for stone formation, based on physicochemical principles, considers the process to begin by nucleation of a crystal nidus, followed by transformation of the nidus into a stone through crystal growth, epitaxial growth, and crystal aggregations.[10] This scheme is consistent with all three of the major theories, because stones could form without or within an organic matrix, and lack of inhibitors could facilitate the process.

Nucleation, the mechanism by which a crystal nidus is formed, can be defined by the degree of saturation of the urine with respect to the crystal nidus and by the limit of metastability.

STATE OF SATURATION. The concentration products or the concentrations of individual ions such as calcium or oxalate generally provide a poor measure of urinary saturation. Urinary activity products of the ions making up stones provide the best estimates of the state of saturation. Activity of an ion is the product of ionic concentration and activity coefficient, where activity coefficient is an inverse function of ionic strength. Although several techniques have been described for estimating the state of saturation from activity products, the different methods have yielded varying results.

Two general approaches have been used for this purpose. In one, the activity product is calculated from an estimate of ionic activities and compared with the thermodynamic solubility product.[11, 12] The ratio of the activity product to the thermodynamic solubility product yields the relative saturation ratio. This technique is not precise because the relative saturation ratio of calcium oxalate may overestimate the true state of saturation by as much as a factor of 3.[13]

In another approach (activity product ratio method),[14] the activity product is calculated for a urine sample before and after incubation of that urine to "equilibrium" with a synthetic solid phase, against which the state of saturation is being measured. The ratio of activity products before and after incubation represents the state of saturation; the ratio of 1 indicates saturation, greater than 1 supersaturation, and less than 1 undersaturation. The activity product ratio has physicochemical validity because it indicates the extent to which the synthetic solid phase undergoes growth or dissolution in urine. When the urine sample is supersaturated, there is growth of the solid phase, as indicated by a decrease in concentration of constituent ions in the ambient fluid. When the urine sample is undersaturated, there is dissolution of the solid phase, with an increase in concentration of constituent ions in the ambient fluid.

The urinary environment of patients with stones is typically supersaturated with respect to stone constituents. The urine of subjects without stones may also be supersaturated, but it is generally less supersaturated than the urine of stone-forming patients.[14]

METASTABILITY. Metastability is the condition in which spontaneous nucleation or precipitation of stone-forming salts does not occur during the period of observation, even though urine may be supersaturated with respect to those salts.[10] Urine supports varying degrees of metastable supersaturation with respect to stone-forming salts because of the presence of inhibitors that increase and promoters that reduce metastability. The limit of metastability indicates the point at which nucleation (or formation of a crystal nidus) occurs; it may be defined by the formation product ratio.

The formation product ratio[14] represents the lowest supersaturated state at which nucleation is initiated. Above this value, nucleation proceeds. It is measured in urine samples free of crystalline constituents, as follows. For brushite, the urine sample is rendered increasingly supersaturated with respect to calcium phosphate by adding a solution of calcium chloride. The lowest calcium concentration that elicits spontaneous precipitation of calcium phosphate at the prescribed time is then noted. The corresponding activity product of Ca^{2+} and HPO_4^{2-} represents the formation product. The ratio of the formation product and the activity product at saturation is the formation product ratio. Thus the formation product ratio is a direct measure of the degree to which urine must be supersaturated for spontaneous precipitation to occur. The formation product ratio of calcium oxalate is obtained similarly by adding increasing amounts of oxalate (as oxalic acid or sodium oxalate) to urine. Because of the particle "impurities" in urine, the nucleation that proceeds in urine may be nonhomogeneous. The formation product ratio of brushite and calcium oxalate is sensitive to both low- and high-molecular-weight inhibitors. Thus it is augmented by pyrophosphate, citrate, and glycopeptide.

The urine of patients with calcium stones not only is supersaturated with calcium oxalate and calcium phosphate but also has a reduced formation product ratio.[14] Thus the nucleation process is facilitated in the "stone-forming" urinary environment. This increased propensity for nucleation is reflected by the reduced amount of soluble oxalate or calcium required to elicit spontaneous precipitation of calcium oxalate and calcium phosphate in urine of stone-forming patients.[15]

CRYSTAL GROWTH. The growth of crystals of the same chemical composition may be measured by adding to solution a small amount of a synthetic solid phase (representing stone) and determining its rate of growth.[10] Because the rate of growth is a function of the amount of solid phase added, the duration of growth, and the extent of metastable supersaturation, these variables must be controlled. This technique is difficult to apply to whole urine because large amounts of inhibitors are normally present. Therefore, crystal growth is typically measured in a standard synthetic metastable solution to which a small amount of urine (1 to 5%) has been added.[16] Unfortunately, such assessments with diluted urine samples may have limited biological significance.

The inhibition of crystal growth of calcium phosphate in urine is largely due to low-molecular-weight substances (e.g., citrate and pyrophosphate),[17] whereas the inhibition of crystal growth of calcium oxalate is largely due to high-molecular-weight substances (glycopeptides and glycosaminoglycans).[16, 18-20] The rate of crystal growth of calcium oxalate and calcium phosphate may be increased in the urine of patients with calcium stones.[14]

CRYSTAL AGGREGATION. Crystal aggregation is the process by which preformed crystals (25 to 50 μm in diameter individually) aggregate into large clusters.[21] Crystal aggregates of calcium oxalate 100 to 200 μm in diameter have been found in stone-forming urine. Normal urine may contain substances that inhibit the aggregation of calcium oxalate crystals, thereby allowing passage of the crystals through the urinary tract. These inhibitors may be deficient or absent in stone-forming urine. For example, rapid aggregation of calcium oxalate crystals has been reported in urine of patients with hypocitraturic nephrolithiasis.[22]

HETEROGENEOUS NUCLEATION. Nucleation from a metastably supersaturated solution can be induced by a heterologous "seed." This process of heterogeneous nucleation may be the basis for the formation of stones of mixed crystalline composition. Because the solution is metastable, spontaneous precipitation would not occur without seeding. To be biologically meaningful, the heterogeneous nucleation should have some degree of specificity.

Several forms of heterogeneous nucleation have been described. An example is nucleation of calcium oxalate by seeds of calcium phosphate or monosodium urate.[23, 24] For some systems, epitaxial fit or crystalline spatial conformity has been demonstrated between the seed crystal and the induced phase.[25]

CLASSIFICATION OF NEPHROLITHIASIS

One method of diagnostic differentiation of nephrolithiasis is based on the categorization of underlying metabolic or environmental abnormalities, assuming that these disturbances are important in stone formation (Table 29–1). Although complete validation is lacking, excessive renal excretion of calcium, uric acid, oxalate, or cystine or defective excretion of citrate (hypocitraturia) or magnesium may contribute to stone formation. This classification is based on the presumed principal abnormality. Several disturbances may, in fact, coexist in a given disorder. Pathogenetic significance of the metabolic disturbances in stone formation is described in Table 29–2.

Role of Hypercalciuria

Hypercalciuria plays a major role in calcium stone formation. First, it increases the saturation of urine with respect to stone-forming calcium salts. There is a direct correlation between urinary saturation of calcium oxalate or brushite and urinary calcium concentration.[14] Although a rise in urinary calcium concentration may reduce the ionic oxalate concentration through increased complexation of oxalate, this effect is generally less prominent than the increase in ionic calcium concentration. Second, hypercalciuria induced by a high calcium intake raises the urinary saturation of calcium salts.[26] Despite suggestions to the contrary, the opposing effect of the reduction in urinary oxalate concentration binding by calcium in the intestinal tract is

TABLE 29–1. Classification of Nephrolithiasis

Type of Nephrolithiasis	Sole Occurrence* (%)	Combined Occurrence* (%)
Calcium nephrolithiasis		
Hypercalciuric nephrolithiasis		
Absorptive	20	40
Renal	5	8
Resorptive	3	5
Other	15	25
Renal phosphate leak		
Primary 1,25(OH)$_2$D excess		
Combined renal tubular disturbances		
Hyperuricosuric calcium nephrolithiasis	10	40
Hyperoxaluric calcium nephrolithiasis	2	15
Enteric hyperoxaluria		
Primary hyperoxaluria		
Dietary hyperoxaluria		
Hypocitraturic calcium nephrolithiasis	10	50
Distal renal tubular acidosis		
Chronic diarrheal syndrome		
Hypomagnesiuric calcium nephrolithiasis	5	10
Gouty diathesis	15	30
Cystinuria	1	1
Infection stones	1	5
Low urine volume	10	50
No disturbance and miscellaneous causes	3	3

*The range in percentage for each diagnosis is an approximate estimate based on experience in Dallas. Some patients present with more than one abnormality. Thus, unlike sole occurrence percentages, the combined occurrence percentages add up to more than 100%.

modest. Third, hypercalciuria reduces the urinary inhibitor activity against the crystallization of calcium salts through binding and inactivation of negatively charged inhibitors.[27] In synthetic solutions, the inhibitor activity of citrate and chondroitin sulfate against the spontaneous precipitation of calcium oxalate is attenuated by a rise in calcium concentration, although the inhibitor activity of glycopeptide is accentuated. Fourth, persistent hypercalciuria is one of the most important determinants of continued stone formation during therapy.[28] Finally, correction of hypercalciuria by administration of thiazide or sodium cellulose phosphate restores the normal urinary physicochemical environment[29] and retards the formation of new stones.[30]

An important role for hypercalciuria in stone formation does not exclude the operation of other factors that may coexist in individual patients, such as relative hyperoxaluria, hyperuricosuria, and hypocitraturia.

Role of Hyperuricosuria

Recurrent calcium nephrolithiasis (stones of calcium oxalate and/or calcium phosphate) can occur in subjects with hyperuricosuria and no other discernible cause for nephrolithiasis, provided that the urinary pH is greater than the dissociation constant (pK_a) of 5.47 for the first proton of uric acid.[31] The association of hyperuricosuria with calcium nephrolithiasis has led to the suggestion that hyperuricosuria is pathogenetically important in calcium stone formation.[32] The following scheme has been proposed: the urine may be supersaturated with respect to monosodium urate because it has a high content of uric acid and a pH (>5.5) in which monosodium urate is stable.[33] Either a colloidal or crystalline monosodium urate can form in such a supersaturated environment[34, 35] and initiate the formation of calcium stones by (1) direct induction of heterogeneous nucleation of cal-

TABLE 29–2. Pathogenetic Significance of Various Derangements in Stone Formation

Derangement	Physicochemical Effect in Urine
Hypercalciuria	Increased saturation of calcium oxalate and calcium phosphate
	Attenuation of inhibitor activity of citrate and chondroitin sulfate
Hyperuricosuria	Increased saturation of monosodium urate
	Facilitated urate-induced crystallization of calcium oxalate
Hyperoxaluria	Increased saturation of calcium oxalate
Hypocitraturia	Increased saturation of calcium salts via reduced calcium complexation by citrate
	Reduced inhibitor activity against crystallization of calcium salts resulting from loss of inhibitor activity of citrate
Hypomagnesiuria	Increased saturation of calcium oxalate because of reduced binding of oxalate
Low urinary pH	Low uric acid solubility
Cystinuria	Increased saturation of cystine
High urinary pH	Increased phosphate dissociation
	Increased saturation of calcium phosphate and struvite (if ammonium ion concentration is high)
Low urine volume	Increased saturation of stone-forming salts (because of the rise in concentration of stone-forming constituents)

cium oxalate[23] or (2) adsorption of glycosaminoglycans (which are inhibitors of crystal aggregation or spontaneous nucleation of calcium oxalate).[34, 36]

This scheme is supported by the demonstration of supersaturation of urine with monosodium urate,[23] by the ability of monosodium urate to induce heterogeneous nucleation of calcium oxalate,[23] and by the capacity of monosodium urate to attenuate the inhibitory activity of heparin (model mucopolysaccharide)[36] or naturally occurring urinary macromolecules.[37] Moreover, the induction of hyperuricosuria by oral purine loading facilitates spontaneous precipitation of calcium oxalate in urine, commensurate with a rise in urinary saturation of monosodium urate.[35] Unfortunately, the presence of crystalline monosodium urate in urine has not yet been documented.

Role of Hyperoxaluria

A role for hyperoxaluria in stone formation is suggested by its identification as a risk factor for stone formation and by its frequent association with calcium nephrolithiasis. Hyperoxaluria probably facilitates stone formation by increasing urinary saturation of calcium oxalate.

Role of Hypocitraturia

Hypocitraturia may be a risk factor for the formation of calcium stones because citrate is known to inhibit stone formation. Citrate reduces urinary saturation of calcium oxalate or calcium phosphate by forming a soluble complex with calcium and thereby reducing calcium ion activity.[38] Although citrate is an effective inhibitor of calcium phosphate crystal growth,[17] it has only modest inhibitory activity against calcium oxalate crystal growth.[16] However, citrate directly inhibits spontaneous nucleation of calcium oxalate.[39] Citrate may also be a potent inhibitor of the agglomeration of preformed calcium oxalate crystals.[22]

Other simple (low-molecular-weight) and complex (macromolecular) inhibitors of the crystallization of calcium salts in urine include pyrophosphate, glycopeptides,[40] glycosaminoglycans,[20] ribonucleic acids, and glycoproteins. Renal excretion of these substances may be disturbed in certain patients with nephrolithiasis, but this has never been fully substantiated. However, the finding that a specific urinary glycoprotein in patients with calcium nephrolithiasis may be abnormal structurally and functionally is intriguing and could be important pathogenetically.[19] Measurement of these inhibitors may have diagnostic or predictive utility if simple and reliable assays could be developed. Furthermore, therapeutic approaches to augmenting the activity of these inhibitors in urine may be developed.

Role of Hypomagnesiuria

Magnesium is a weak direct inhibitor of the crystallization of stone-forming calcium salts. It attenuates the crystallization of calcium oxalate indirectly by complexing oxalate,[16] thereby reducing the ionic oxalate concentration and the urinary saturation of calcium oxalate. Thus calcium oxalate crystallization could be enhanced in the setting of hypomagnesiuria.

Role of Altered Urinary pH

Persistent passage of unusually acidic urine (pH < 5.5) may cause both uric acid and calcium stones. When urinary pH is close to or less than the dissociation constant of uric acid,[31] the concentration of undissociated uric acid is high, promoting uric acid crystallization. The uric acid crystals in turn may promote the crystallization of calcium oxalate by the mechanism described for monosodium urate. Although uric acid is less efficient than monosodium urate in inducing heterogeneous nucleation of calcium oxalate (on a weight basis), its crystalline dimensions are more compatible with crystalline overgrowth.[25] Moreover, uric acid can remove naturally occurring urinary macromolecular inhibitors of stone formation, thereby attenuating their activity.[27]

In contrast, a high urinary pH (neutral or alkaline) favors formation of calcium phosphate stones. It increases urinary saturation of calcium phosphate by enhancing the dissociation of phosphate and raising the concentration of trivalent phosphate ion. If a high concentration of ammonium ion is also present (e.g., as a result of infection with urea-splitting organisms), struvite (magnesium ammonium phosphate) saturation could increase, promoting formation of infection stones.[41]

Role of Urinary Cystine

Cystine is sparingly soluble in urine. Its solubility is greater at higher pH and is enhanced by electrolytes and macromolecules;[42] however, it rarely exceeds 1.7 mmol/L (400 mg/L). Cystine stones may form when urinary cystine concentration exceeds the solubility of cystine.

Role of Low Urine Volume

Low urine volume contributes to stone formation by increasing the concentration of stone-forming constituents and raising the saturation of stone-forming salts.[43] Volume changes affect both cationic and anionic components of the stone-forming salt (e.g., calcium and oxalate in calcium oxalate). For instance, a reduction in urine output by one half generally increases urinary saturation by more than twofold. Therefore, marked urinary supersaturation may result from reduced urine output even when the total renal excretion of stone-forming constituents is normal.

PATHOPHYSIOLOGICAL DERANGEMENTS

Hypercalciuria

The association of hypercalciuria with calcium nephrolithiasis has long been recognized. The term idiopathic hypercalciuria has been used to denote this entity.[44] Progress in pathophysiological elucidation mandates that this term be discarded because hypercalciuria of nephrolithiasis is composed of several entities of different origin (Fig. 29–1).[45]

ABSORPTIVE HYPERCALCIURIA. The primary abnormality in absorptive hypercalciuria is intestinal hyperabsorption of calcium, presumed to occur independently of 1,25-dihydroxycholecalciferol $(1,25(OH)_2D)$.[46] (This category excludes patients with high serum $1,25(OH)_2D$ levels.) The consequent increase in the circulating concentration of calcium increases the renal filtered load and suppresses parathyroid function. Hypercalciuria ensues from the increased filtered load and the reduced tubular reabsorption of calcium associated with parathyroid hormone (PTH) suppression. The excessive renal loss of calcium compensates for the high calcium absorption from the intestinal tract and helps to maintain serum calcium concentration in the normal range.

The exact cause of the enhancement of intestinal calcium absorption is not known. It may be a primary jejunal abnormality,[47, 48] because the high calcium absorption has been observed only in the jejunum and the absorption of magnesium and phosphate is normal. The primary nature of this disturbance is indicated by persistence of intestinal hyperabsorption of calcium during treatment with glucocorticoids (which lower intestinal calcium absorption in sarcoidosis),[49] thiazide (which lowers the urinary calcium level),[50] and orthophosphate (which reduces the serum concentration of $1,25(OH)_2D$).[51] Thiazide treatment of absorptive hypercalciuria may provoke positive calcium balance and skeletal calcium retention.[38] Moreover, absorptive hypercalciuria appears to be inherited as an autosomal dominant trait.[52, 53] The concept that the syndrome is due to a hereditary defect

is supported by similar biochemical findings in inbred hypercalciuric rats.[54]

There is no evidence that the skeleton is adversely affected in this condition, consistent with the lack of parathyroid stimulation, hypophosphatemia, or $1,25(OH)_2D$ excess. Normal values have been reported for serum osteocalcin and serum alkaline phosphatase concentrations, urinary hydroxyproline concentration, and bone density in the radius (shaft) and lumbar vertebrae.[45] Calcium balance is close to zero to begin with; it does not turn more negative when calcium absorption is partially blocked by sodium cellulose phosphate.

In the usual case of absorptive hypercalciuria, there is no evidence for a "primary" renal calcium leak. Fasting urinary calcium concentration may be increased secondary to the primary enhancement of intestinal calcium absorption. That is, if the duration of fast is inadequate and the absorbed calcium is incompletely cleared by the kidneys, the high calcium absorption may cause fasting hypercalciuria by increasing the renal filtered load of calcium and by suppressing parathyroid function, thus impairing renal tubular reabsorption of calcium.[55] However, fasting hypercalciuria can be eliminated by prolongation of the fast or by prior administration of sodium cellulose phosphate (which binds calcium in the intestinal tract and reduces calcium absorption), without provoking hyperparathyroidism. Lack of a primary disturbance in renal proximal tubular function is substantiated by the normal calciuric response to carbohydrate load[56] and by the normal natriuretic response to thiazide.[57]

RENAL HYPERCALCIURIA. The primary abnormality in renal hypercalciuria is thought to be impairment of renal tubular reabsorption of calcium.[58] The consequent reduction in the circulating concentration of calcium stimulates parathyroid function. There may be excessive mobilization of calcium from bone and enhanced intestinal absorption of calcium because of excess of PTH and ensuing stimulation of the renal synthesis of $1,25(OH)_2D$. These compensatory mechanisms restore the serum calcium level toward normal. Unlike the situation in primary hyperparathyroidism, the serum calcium concentration is normal and the state of hyperparathyroidism is secondary.

Some patients with hypercalciuric nephrolithiasis, albeit a minority in most series, have a biochemical presentation in keeping with the forgoing scheme. The combination of high serum PTH or urinary cyclic AMP concentration, elevated serum $1,25(OH)_2D$ concentration, and enhanced intestinal calcium absorption has been shown in such patients in the setting of normal serum calcium level and fasting hypercalciuria (indicative of renal calcium leak).[46] Correction of the renal calcium leak by thiazide restores the normal serum $1,25(OH)_2D$ level and fractional calcium absorption commensurate with the correction of hyperparathyroidism.[50] These findings support the contention that $1,25(OH)_2D$ synthesis is enhanced by secondary parathyroid stimulation and that intestinal calcium absorption is high because of $1,25(OH)_2D$ excess.

The occurrence of a primary renal calcium leak is supported by three lines of evidence. First, fasting hypercalciuria is associated with parathyroid stimulation and is poorly corrected by inhibition of intestinal calcium absorption (and removal of any effect of absorbed calcium) with sodium cellulose phosphate.[55] Second, there is a unique natriuretic response to thiazide. When thiazide is given to block reabsorption of calcium and sodium in the distal (renal) tubule, impaired proximal tubular function causes an exaggerated renal excretion of these cations. The enhanced natriuretic and calciuric responses to thiazides are encountered only in patients with renal hypercalciuria with secondary hyperparathyroidism.[57] Third, an exaggerated calciuric

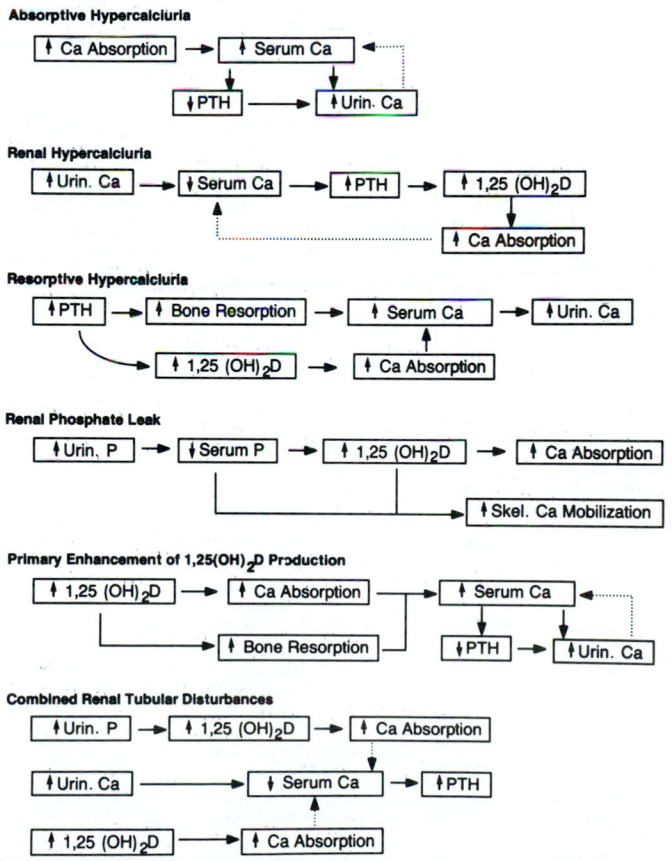

Figure 29–1. Pathophysiological schemes for the various forms of hypercalciuria associated with nephrolithiasis.

response to a glucose load occurs in patients with renal hypercalciuria but not in those with absorptive hypercalciuria.[56] Ingestion of readily metabolizable carbohydrate (without calcium) normally augments renal calcium excretion, probably through an alteration in renal proximal tubular function.[59]

It has been suggested that renal calcium leak might be secondary to an excessive dietary intake of sodium.[60] However, institution of a low sodium intake (9 mmol/d) does not eliminate fasting hypercalciuria in patients with renal hypercalciuria.

That renal calcium leak (and secondary hyperparathyroidism) can be long-standing is shown by changes in bone density. Although clinical bone disease is rare, mean bone density as measured by photon absorptiometry in the distal third of the radius is reduced in subjects with renal hypercalciuria (compared with age- and sex-matched controls).[61] These results indicate that secondary hyperparathyroidism has deleterious effects on the skeleton. The lack of more serious involvement is probably due to the compensatory intestinal hyperabsorption of calcium that results from the PTH-induced renal synthesis of $1,25(OH)_2D$. This compensation is often inadequate, and negative calcium balance can occur when the urinary calcium level exceeds calcium absorption.

To summarize, specific features distinguish absorptive hypercalciuria and renal hypercalciuria[62] (Table 29–3). Renal hypercalciuria is characterized by fasting hypercalciuria and secondary hyperparathyroidism. Intestinal calcium absorption is increased primarily in absorptive hypercalciuria, as shown by independence of $1,25(OH)_2D$ action, lack of correction by thiazide diuretics, and involvement of the gastrointestinal tract localized to the jejunum only. In contrast, in renal hypercalciuria, the intestinal calcium absorption is secondarily stimulated by $1,25(OH)_2D$ action and is corrected by thiazide. The disturbance in renal tubular function in renal hypercalciuria may be generalized, as shown by an exaggerated natriuretic response to thiazide and enhanced calciuric response to carbohydrate load.

RESORPTIVE HYPERCALCIURIA. Resorptive hypercalciuria resulting in kidney stones is generally due to primary hyperparathyroidism (also see Chapter 27). Other causes of excessive bone resorption, such as oncogenic hypercalcemia, thyrotoxicosis, and sarcoidosis, occasionally result in stone formation. In primary hyperparathyroidism, the initial event is excessive resorption of bone resulting from hypersecretion of PTH. Intestinal absorption of calcium is frequently elevated because of PTH-mediated stimulation of the renal synthesis of $1,25(OH)_2D$.[63] These effects increase the circu-

lating concentration and the filtered load of calcium in urine. Development of hypercalciuria in primary hyperparathyroidism seems paradoxical because the primary effect of PTH in the kidney is to stimulate tubular reabsorption of calcium. However, hypercalciuria occurs in primary hyperparathyroidism when the PTH-dependent augmentation of renal tubular reabsorption of calcium is "overcome" by an increase in the renal filtered load and by a suppressive effect of hypercalcemia on the renal reabsorption of calcium.

Stone formation has become less common in primary hyperparathyroidism, probably because of earlier diagnosis. The biochemical and clinical features of patients with primary hyperparathyroidism who develop nephrolithiasis may be different from those of patients without stones. Patients with stones are thought to have a longer duration of the disease process, less severe hypercalcemia, and a smaller amount of abnormal parathyroid tissue than patients who present with bone disease.[64] Hypercalciuria is characteristic of stone-forming patients with primary hyperparathyroidism and may be one of the causes of renal stone formation, because it is also a frequent finding in normocalcemic patients with calcium nephrolithiasis. The hypercalciuria may result from excessive PTH-dependent bone resorption and/or enhanced intestinal absorption of calcium resulting from PTH-dependent synthesis of $1,25(OH)_2D$. The component of the hypercalciuria that is due to enhanced intestinal absorption may be of particular importance for the formation of kidney stones.[65] Thus a predilection for nephrolithiasis has been reported in patients with primary hyperparathyroidism who have a high circulating concentration of $1,25(OH)_2D$ and increased intestinal absorption of calcium. Conversely, patients presenting with bone disease are reported to have lower glomerular filtration, lower levels of 25-hydroxycholecalciferol (25-OHD), and higher values of serum PTH than those without bone disease. Impairment of renal function and/or decreased levels of vitamin D prohormones might lead to impaired synthesis of $1,25(OH)_2D$, further increasing PTH secretion and worsening bone disease.[66]

However, many patients with primary hyperparathyroidism who present with renal stones cannot be distinguished from those without stones on the basis of biochemical or physicochemical features.[67] First, there is no unique histological pattern in the parathyroid glands characteristic of stone formation. The prevalence of nephrolithiasis is similar in patients with parathyroid hyperplasia and those with parathyroid adenoma. Second, mean bone density as assayed by photon absorptiometry is reduced in both the stone-forming and the non–stone-forming groups.[67] The

TABLE 29–3. Evidence That Absorptive and Renal Hypercalciurias Are Physiologically Distinct

Physiological Parameter	Absorptive Hypercalciuria Type I or Type II	Renal Hypercalciuria
Parathyroid function	Normal or suppressed	Stimulated
Renal calcium leak	Secondary	Primary
Effect of sodium cellulose phosphate	Correctable	Noncorrectable
Natriuretic response to thiazide	Normal	Exaggerated
Intestinal calcium absorption	Primarily increased	Secondarily increased
Jejunal absorption	Increased	Increased
Ileal absorption	Normal	Increased
Intestinal magnesium absorption	Normal	Increased
Serum $1,25(OH)_2D$ vs. calcium absorption	No correlation	Correlated
Effect of treatment with		
Thiazide on serum $1,25(OH)_2D$ and calcium absorption	No change	Decreased
Sodium cellulose phosphate on		
Urinary calcium	Markedly decreased	Less marked
Calcium conservation	Intact	Impaired
Skeletal status		
Bone density (radial shaft)	Normal	Decreased
Calcium balance	Normal	Normal or negative

mean value for the fractional change in bone density is actually lower in patients with stones than in those without stones, although the difference is not significant. It thus seems clear that skeletal involvement is a characteristic feature of PTH excess. Third, biochemical findings for patients with stones cannot be distinguished from those for patients without stones, at least in a group with surgically proven primary hyperparathyroidism.[67] Patients with stones and those without stones have similar degrees of elevation of serum calcium, serum PTH, and serum $1,25(OH)_2D$ levels; fractional calcium absorption; and urinary calcium levels.[67] Most patients without stones have high fractional calcium absorption, and some patients with stones have normal absorption.

Finally, the urine of patients with stones cannot be distinguished from that of non–stone-forming patients by measurements of urinary composition or saturation with stone-forming salts.[67] Reduced inhibitor activity in urine might contribute to the predilection for stone formation; for example, it has been reported[68] that the urinary citrate concentration is lower in patients with primary hyperparathyroidism who present with stones than in those without stones, although it is not different from that in normal subjects without stones. A similar reduction in urinary pyrophosphate level has also been reported in stone-forming patients.

Although the overall scheme for resorptive hypercalciuria in primary hyperparathyroidism is generally accepted, the mechanisms by which intestinal calcium absorption is controlled are not entirely clear. The high intestinal calcium absorption is customarily ascribed to the enhanced PTH-mediated synthesis of $1,25(OH)_2D$. Thus the fractional calcium absorption is directly related to serum $1,25(OH)_2D$ levels.[69] However, in some patients with primary hyperparathyroidism, the intestinal hyperabsorption of calcium persists after parathyroidectomy and after restoration of normal serum $1,25(OH)_2D$ levels.[70] Therefore, factors other than $1,25(OH)_2D$ may contribute to the maintenance of high intestinal calcium absorption in hyperparathyroid patients in the postoperative state.

RENAL PHOSPHATE LEAK. Hypophosphatemia ensuing from renal phosphate leak is thought to cause intestinal hyperabsorption of calcium by stimulating the renal synthesis of $1,25(OH)_2D$.[71] This concept is supported by the findings of (1) low tubular threshold concentration of phosphate and hypophosphatemia in some patients with hypercalciuric nephrolithiasis in the absence of hyperparathyroidism, (2) stimulation of the renal synthesis of $1,25(OH)_2D$ by inhibition of intestinal phosphate absorption, and (3) significant inverse correlation between serum $1,25(OH)_2D$ concentration and serum phosphorus concentration.[72] Moreover, the presence of hypophosphatemia and/or high serum $1,25(OH)_2D$ concentration provides an explanation (other than PTH excess) for the occurrence of fasting hypercalciuria, poor calcium conservation, reduced bone density, and abnormal histomorphometric picture of bone[73] in some hypercalciuric patients with normal parathyroid function.

PRIMARY ENHANCEMENT OF $1,25(OH)_2D$ SYNTHESIS. Many of the biochemical characteristics of absorptive hypercalciuria can be explained by overproduction of $1,25(OH)_2D$, whether it occurs independently or is secondary to the renal phosphate leak. These characteristics include intestinal hyperabsorption of calcium and parathyroid suppression. The high fasting urinary calcium level sometimes encountered can be produced secondarily by parathyroid suppression through the loss of PTH-dependent stimulation of renal tubular reabsorption of calcium.[74] This interpretation is supported by the fact that absorptive hypercalciuria resembles the state induced in normal subjects by calcitriol therapy.[74] Thus the combination of fasting hypercalciuria and suppressed parathyroid function could cause an acquired renal calcium leak through a primary increase in $1,25(OH)_2D$ synthesis.

Fasting hypercalciuria could also result from the $1,25(OH)_2D$-dependent stimulation of bone resorption.[75] Calcitriol augments urinary calcium excretion even when patients are placed on a low-calcium diet and increases levels of urinary hydroxyproline (a marker of bone resorption) and serum osteocalcin (a marker of bone formation and turnover).[76]

A role for excessive $1,25(OH)_2D$ production is supported by the finding of high serum $1,25(OH)_2D$ levels in some patients with absorptive hypercalciuria and the finding of accelerated $1,25(OH)_2D$ synthesis in vivo in the subset of patients with absorptive hypercalciuria and high serum $1,25(OH)_2D$ levels.[77] This type of absorptive hypercalciuria probably occurs in only a fraction of the patients and is distinguished from the usual absorptive hypercalciuria (previously described), in which a pathogenetic role of $1,25(OH)_2D$ is not implicated.

COMBINED RENAL TUBULAR DISTURBANCES. Fasting hypercalciuria with normal parathyroid function could result from a variety of disturbances in renal proximal tubular function, including calcium leak, abnormal phosphate transport, and accelerated $1,25(OH)_2D$ synthesis.[78] Stated otherwise, a defect in the kidney could lead to both renal and absorptive hypercalciurias. Renal calcium leak would lead to renal hypercalciuria with secondary hyperparathyroidism. Enhancement of $1,25(OH)_2D$ synthesis, either independently or secondarily as a result of renal phosphate leak, would cause absorptive hypercalciuria by enhancing intestinal calcium absorption and masking parathyroid stimulation. The occurrence of both renal calcium leak and renal phosphate leak or increased $1,25(OH)_2D$ synthesis could also cause fasting hypercalciuria without parathyroid stimulation. Thus renal hypercalciuria need not be accompanied by hyperparathyroidism, and absorptive hypercalciuria could result secondarily from $1,25(OH)_2D$-mediated stimulation of intestinal calcium absorption.

GENERAL COMMENTS. Additional factors may be involved in the pathogenesis of hypercalciuria. For example, enhanced renal excretion of prostaglandin E_2 has been reported in patients with hypercalciuric nephrolithiasis. Treatment with inhibitors of prostaglandin synthesis corrected the hypercalciuria in such patients and reduced urinary calcium in normocalcemic patients with nephrolithiasis but not in normal subjects.[79]

The preceding discussion emphasizes the variable role of $1,25(OH)_2D$ in the pathogenesis of hypercalciuria. Synthesis of $1,25(OH)_2D$ is enhanced in renal hypercalciuria, resorptive hypercalciuria of primary hyperparathyroidism, renal phosphate leak, primary enhancement of $1,25(OH)_2D$ synthesis, and combined renal tubular disturbances. Enhanced $1,25(OH)_2D$ production could cause hypercalciuria by stimulating intestinal calcium absorption and skeletal calcium mobilization. On the other hand, normal or suppressed $1,25(OH)_2D$ synthesis occurs in classic absorptive hypercalciuria. Increased intestinal calcium absorption in the presence of normal or low levels of the vitamin could be due to up-regulation of $1,25(OH)_2D$ receptor levels or exaggerated expression of the receptor.[80] However, the unique intestinal absorptive profile encountered in absorptive hypercalciuria suggests that calcium absorption is independent of vitamin D, at least in some patients with this syndrome.

In the usual case of absorptive hypercalciuria, fasting urinary calcium concentration and parathyroid function are normal, whereas fasting hypercalciuria and secondary hyperparathyroidism accompany renal hypercalciuria. In contrast, fasting hypercalciuria with normal parathyroid function may be encountered in renal phosphate leak, primary $1,25(OH)_2D$ excess, or combined renal tubular disturbances. The fasting urinary calcium level may be high because of excessive skeletal mobilization of calcium resulting from hypophosphatemia or $1,25(OH)_2D$ excess. These conditions are infrequent causes of hypercalciuria; the absorptive and renal forms account for most cases.

Fasting hypercalciuria with normal parathyroid function can also be an artifact produced by incomplete exclusion of the effects of absorbed calcium.[55] When calcium and sodium restriction is not adequate and the duration of fast is insufficient, there may be incomplete clearance of absorbed calcium, leading to fasting hypercalciuria.

Hyperuricosuria

Uric acid is an end product of purine metabolism and cannot be degraded in humans because they lack uricase, which is present in other mammalian species. A major site of disposal of uric acid is the kidney, where filtration, reabsorption, and secretion all occur.

Hyperuricosuria may ensue when the serum concentration and the renal filtered load of uric acid are increased as a result of (1) the availability of an excessive amount of substrate, e.g., from a diet high in purine-rich foods[81] or from accelerated degradation and turnover of nucleic acids, or (2) a disturbance in purine biosynthesis that causes overproduction of purine substrates for uric acid synthesis (Table 29–4). A high urinary uric acid level can occur transiently when renal tubular reabsorption of uric acid is impaired, as during early stages of extracellular volume expansion or after administration of uricosuric agents such as probenecid. In the steady state, however, normal urinary uric acid concentration is restored in the latter conditions because of the secondary decline in the serum concentration and renal filtered load of uric acid, even though renal tubular reabsorption of uric acid remains impaired.[82]

Hyperuricosuria may be the only observed physiological abnormality in patients with calcium nephrolithiasis. Such a defect (hyperuricosuric calcium oxalate nephrolithiasis or hyperuricosuric calcium urolithiasis) exists alone in approximately 10% of patients with renal calculi.[62] Although hy-peruricosuria may coexist with the various forms of hypercalciuria, only the pure disorder is considered in this section.

The most common cause of hyperuricosuria in patients with hyperuricosuric calcium oxalate nephrolithiasis is probably dietary overindulgence in purine-rich foods.[81] Such individuals have a history of a liberal intake of meat, poultry, and fish, and their estimated purine intake is higher than that of control groups. Hyperuricosuria in such patients can be ameliorated by dietary purine deprivation.[35, 81, 83]

However, about 30% of patients with hyperuricosuric calcium oxalate nephrolithiasis have hyperuricosuria as the result of uric acid overproduction. Hyperuricosuria persists despite long-term purine deprivation. No further studies have been performed to elucidate the nature of this apparent urate overproduction.

Hyperoxaluria

Oxalate is derived from both in vivo synthesis and intestinal absorption. Once synthesized or absorbed, it is not further degraded, and the principal route of excretion is the kidney. Data on renal handling of oxalate are limited and conflicting. Of the 30 mg of oxalate excreted normally, 80% is derived from in vivo synthesis and the remainder is derived from the diet.

No primary derangement in renal handling of oxalate has been recognized. Rather, hyperoxaluria is due to increased serum concentrations and increased renal filtered loads resulting from (1) high substrate availability, as caused by administration of methoxyflurane or ascorbic acid; (2) enzymatic disturbances in the oxalate biosynthetic pathway that cause overproduction, as in primary hyperoxaluria (rare); or (3) increased intestinal absorption of oxalate (see Table 29–4), as in the hyperoxaluria of ileal disease.[84, 85]

Two factors probably act in concert to cause intestinal hyperabsorption of oxalate: (1) intestinal transport of oxalate may be primarily increased because of the action of bile salts and fatty acids on the permeability of intestinal mucosa to oxalate, and (2) the total amount of oxalate absorbed may be increased because of an enlarged intraluminal pool of oxalate available for absorption. For example, the intestinal fat malabsorption characteristic of ileal disease may exaggerate soap formation with divalent cations, limit the amount of "free" divalent cations available to complex oxalate, and thereby enlarge the available oxalate pool.

The formation of calcium oxalate stones has multifactorial causes. In addition to the disturbance in oxalate metabolism, the intestinal absorption and renal excretion of calcium are often decreased in enteric hyperoxaluria, probably because of loss of the intestinal site of calcium absorption as a result of disease or resection, intraluminal binding of calcium by nonabsorbed fatty acids, and vitamin D deficiency associated with fat malabsorption. Urine volume may be reduced because of fluid loss from the intestinal tract. Urinary citrate concentration may be depressed because of hypokalemia and metabolic acidosis,[86, 87] and urinary magnesium concentration may be low because of impaired intestinal magnesium absorption. Saturation of urine with calcium oxalate may be increased because of the high oxalate concentration, even though the urinary calcium level may be low, and low urine volume exaggerates urinary supersaturation. Moreover, inhibitor activity against crystallization of calcium salts is reduced because of low renal excretion of citrate and magnesium.

Hypocitraturia

Urinary citrate excretion is a function of filtration, reabsorption, peritubular transport, and synthesis by the

TABLE 29–4. Derangements Other Than Hypercalciuria That Can Cause Nephrolithiasis

Derangement	Causes
Hyperuricosuria	Primary overproduction Dietary purine overindulgence or increased cellular degradation
Hyperoxaluria	High substrate availability (e.g., vitamin C or oxalate intake) Primary overproduction intestinal hyperabsorption of oxalate (enteric hyperoxaluria)
Hypocitraturia	Renal tubular acidosis Enteric hyperoxaluria Hypokalemia (e.g., thiazide therapy) Diet high in animal protein Urinary tract infection Other
Hypomagnesiuria	Insufficient dietary intake of magnesium
Low urinary pH (uric acid stones)	Gout and chronic diarrheal syndrome Diet high in animal protein
Cystinuria	Impaired renal tubular reabsorption of cystine
High urinary pH and ammonium (struvite stones)	Infection with urea-splitting organisms

renal tubular cell. Approximately 80 to 90% of filtered citrate is normally reabsorbed, and citrate secretion is usually negligible. Peritubular transport (citrate flux between peritubular blood and tubular cell) and tubular synthesis do not directly influence citrate excretion in urine; they do so indirectly by affecting the renal tissue content and ultimately the filtered load of citrate.

Although the exact physiology of renal handling of citrate has not been elucidated, several factors influence citrate excretion. Citrate excretion is enhanced by alkalosis,[87] PTH, vitamin D, growth hormone, and estrogen and decreased by acidosis,[88] hypokalemia,[89] androgen, and urinary tract infection (probably because of bacterial degradation of citrate). Acid-base status probably plays the most important role in citrate excretion. For example, acidosis reduces the urinary citrate concentration by both enhancing renal tubular reabsorption and impairing peritubular uptake and synthesis of citrate. This mechanism accounts for the occurrence of hypocitraturia in distal renal tubular acidosis (complete or incomplete),[90] chronic diarrheal states (resulting from intestinal alkali loss),[91] hypokalemia (from intracellular acidosis), thiazide therapy (from hypokalemia),[89] and a diet high in animal protein (from elevated acid-ash content) (see Table 29–4).[92] Urinary citrate concentration may also be low after strenuous physical exercise (because of lactic acidosis)[93] and after high-sodium intake (probably because of sodium-induced potassium loss).

Distal acidification defect (type I) is the only form of renal tubular acidosis associated with nephrolithiasis. The stone formation is the result of high urinary pH and calcium levels and low urinary citrate levels. Calcium phosphate crystallization is promoted by increased urine saturation (resulting from increased dissociation of phosphate and hypercalciuria) and reduced inhibitor activity (from hypocitraturia). Crystallization of calcium oxalate may also be enhanced because of increased saturation (resulting from hypercalciuria and reduced citrate complexation of calcium) and impaired inhibitor activity (from hypocitraturia). The predominant stone constituent is calcium phosphate (hydroxyapatite), but calcium oxalate is also typically present as a minor constituent. Nephrocalcinosis commonly coexists with nephrolithiasis.

Nephrolithiasis is not associated with proximal renal tubular acidosis (type II) or hyporeninemic hypoaldosteronism (type IV). In these disorders, the urinary citrate level may be low because of acidosis but the urinary calcium level is also low because of bicarbonaturia in type II and renal insufficiency in type IV. Moreover, urinary pH is normal in type IV.

Distal renal tubular acidosis should not be confused with calcium oxalate nephrolithiasis of the chronic diarrheal syndrome. In the latter disorder, metabolic acidosis is secondary to intestinal alkali loss in the stool. Stone (calcium) formation is due to low urinary citrate concentration and low urine volume. Gastrointestinal disorders that cause this syndrome include the postgastrectomy state, inflammatory disease of the small bowel, bowel resection or bypass, and colitis. States of malabsorption of fat, hyperoxaluria, and low urinary magnesium level may contribute to calcium oxalate stone formation. Uric acid lithiasis may develop as a result of low urinary pH.

In many patients with hypocitraturic calcium nephrolithiasis, the cause of low urinary citrate concentration is unknown.

Hypomagnesiuria

Urinary magnesium concentration may be low in chronic diarrheal states, especially in the setting of fat malabsorption, because of impaired intestinal absorption of magnesium.[94] Hypomagnesiuria may also occur in the absence of gastrointestinal disease in a minority of patients with calcium nephrolithiasis.[95] It is probably due to a diet insufficient in magnesium content.

Gouty Diathesis

This entity is exemplified by primary gout, which is usually associated with low urinary pH, hyperuricosuria, and stones. More commonly, hyperuricosuria represents a forme fruste or early phase of primary gout before the onset of arthritic manifestations.[96] It is noteworthy that stone disease often precedes the onset of articular symptoms in patients with primary gout.[97]

Gouty diathesis[96] is characterized by a low urinary pH, less than 5.5, of unknown etiology, occurring independently of excessive alkali loss or consumption of a diet rich in acid-ash content. Stones may be composed of uric acid alone, calcium alone, or both calcium and uric acid. Finally, some patients present with hyperuricemia, hypertriglyceridemia, frank gouty arthritis, and a family history of gout.

The stone formation in gouty diathesis is probably due to the increased amount of undissociated uric acid in the acidic urinary environment, which leads to the development of uric acid stones.[62] Calcium stones could form by heterogeneous nucleation or binding of inhibitors by uric acid itself or its salt (monosodium urate).

Noncalcareous Stones

URIC ACID LITHIASIS. Critical determinants for uric acid lithiasis are a urinary pH lower than the dissociation constant for uric acid (5.47) and/or hyperuricosuria.[33] Besides primary gout, other causes of uric acid nephrolithiasis include certain inborn errors of uric acid metabolism, secondary causes of urate overproduction, chronic diarrheal states, and use of uricosuric agents. Three well-studied enzymatic disorders of uric acid metabolism are hypoxanthine-guanine phosphoribosyltransferase deficiency (Lesch-Nyhan syndrome), phosphoribosyl pyrophosphate synthetase overactivity, and glucose-6-phosphatase deficiency (type I glycogen storage disease). Affected patients have marked overproduction of uric acid. In myeloproliferative disorders, leukemia, neoplasia, and hemolytic anemia, hyperuricemia and hyperuricosuria occur because of an increased rate of nucleic acid turnover. As many as half of patients with myeloproliferative disorders may form uric acid stones, which may be the initial clinical manifestation.

Certain drugs such as probenecid, high-dose salicylates, and x-ray contrast agents may produce an acute uricosuria by inhibiting net uric acid reabsorption and increasing the fractional excretion of uric acid. Chronic administration of these agents, however, results in a new steady state in which the rate of uric acid excretion should be no greater than the pretreatment rate. Thus the risk of stone formation occurs early, except in the setting of urate overproduction. A high incidence of uric acid lithiasis is associated with gastrointestinal disorders, including ulcerative colitis and regional enteritis, and with the presence of ileostomy.[98] Uric acid stones in these cases are related to variable degrees of dehydration and bicarbonate loss resulting in an unusually acidic and concentrated urine. The excretion rate of uric acid is usually normal.

CYSTINURIA. Normally, cystine is filtered and almost completely reabsorbed in the proximal nephron, so that less than 20 mg is excreted in urine each day. In cystinuria, the serum concentration and hence the renal filtered load of cystine are reduced. Exaggerated cystine excretion under this circumstance suggests a disturbance in renal handling of cystine. More than one defect can impair tubular reabsorption and back diffusion of cystine.[99]

Similar defects in transport of other dibasic amino acids are present. However, exaggerated renal excretion of these amino acids and cystine may not be due to a single transport defect.[100] Increasing the filtered load of one of these amino acids does not necessarily augment the excretion of others.[101]

The intestinal transport of dibasic amino acids may also be defective in cystinuria. The disorder has been classified into three types based on varying intestinal transport disturbances for these amino acids.[102] The intestinal transport has been assessed by the in vitro uptake of radiolabeled amino acid by specimens of jejunal mucosa obtained by peroral biopsy and by studies of plasma cystine levels after oral cystine administration. In type I cystinuria, there is no uptake of cystine, lysine, or arginine by jejunal mucosa, and plasma cystine concentration is not elevated after an oral cystine load. Thus there is defective intestinal transport of all three dibasic amino acids. In types II and III, the intestinal transport of dibasic amino acids is disturbed but less severely than in the type I presentation. In type II, some cystine is taken up by jejunal mucosa but at a reduced rate, and oral cystine loading does not increase the plasma cystine level. In type III cystinuria, cystine and lysine uptake by jejunal mucosa is variably reduced and the increment in plasma cystine after oral cystine loading is blunted but present. In the homozygous state, all three types of cystinuria involve excessive renal excretion of all four dibasic amino acids.[102] In the heterozygous state, type I cystinuria is characterized by normal cystine excretion, whereas types II and III have elevated cystine and lysine excretion (although not quite up to the level encountered in the homozygous state), probably because of a prevailing (although reduced) intestinal uptake of these amino acids.

INFECTION STONES. Infection of the urinary tract with urea-splitting organisms may be associated with renal stones of struvite and calcium carbonate apatite.[41] The critical determinant is the formation of ammonia in urine because of enzymatic degradation of urea by bacterial urease. The ammonia is hydrated to form ammonium and hydroxyl ions. The resulting alkalinity of the urine augments dissociation of phosphate to form triphosphate ions and reduces the solubility of struvite. Thus the urinary environment becomes supersaturated with struvite. Although struvite stones may form de novo from infection alone, they also occur as a complication of other causes of renal calculi, such as hypercalciuria.

DIAGNOSTIC CONSIDERATIONS

Most diagnostic protocols are based on underlying metabolic-environmental derangements or on stone composition. Such protocols differ in the exactness of diagnostic separation, especially of the hypercalciurias. Most protocols include analysis of urine for certain stone-forming risk factors (calcium, uric acid, oxalate, citrate, sodium, magnesium, pH, and volume) and screening of blood for calcium, phosphorus, electrolytes, and uric acid.[1, 103] Urinary risk factors are typically assessed in urine collected from patients with a random diet and fluid intake. Some measurements are repeated after imposition of a restricted diet (e.g., with limited calcium and sodium content) to assess the contribution of dietary factors.[1] Differentiation of the different hypercalciurias requires determination of the fasting urinary calcium level (to obtain a measure of renal calcium leak),[104] the calciuric response to oral calcium load (for an indirect

measure of intestinal calcium absorption),[104] and the serum PTH level and may necessitate assessment of response to sodium cellulose phosphate therapy (to remove the effect of absorbed calcium on fasting urinary calcium).[55] A qualitative cystine determination, stone analysis, urine culture, and appropriate radiological examination of stones are necessary for a full examination. Diagnostic criteria for the major forms of nephrolithiasis are summarized in Table 29–5.

Absorptive hypercalciuria type I[1] is characterized by normal serum calcium and phosphorus levels; normal fasting urinary calcium level (<0.03 mmol/L [<0.11 mg/100 mL] glomerular filtrate), increased urinary calcium level after an oral calcium load (>5 mmol/mg [>0.2 mg/mg] creatinine), normal or suppressed parathyroid function (normal serum immunoreactive PTH level), and urinary calcium level for a restricted diet (10 mmol [400 mg] calcium and 100 mmol sodium/d) of more than 5 mmol/d (200 mg/d). These values reflect increased intestinal calcium absorption, resulting parathyroid suppression, and hypercalciuria.

Absorptive hypercalciuria type II[1] is characterized by the same biochemical features as type I except for normal urine calcium level (<5 mmol/d [<200 mg/d]) for a restricted diet of 10 mmol (400 mg) calcium and 100 mmol sodium/d. If these patients are placed on a diet of 25 mmol/d (1000 mg/d) calcium and 100 mmol/d sodium, urinary calcium level exceeds 0.1 mmol/kg body weight/d (4 mg/kg/d) or 6 mmol/d (250 mg/d).

Renal hypercalciuria[1] has the following features: normal serum calcium level, fasting urinary calcium level greater than 0.03 mmol/L glomerular filtrate (>0.11 mg/100 mL glomerular filtrate), and enhanced parathyroid activity (high serum immunoreactive PTH level). These results indicate a renal leak of calcium with compensatory parathyroid stimulation. Evidence of parathyroid stimulation (high serum PTH level) is critical for the diagnosis of renal hypercalciuria. Bone density may be low in patients with renal hypercalciuria, and osteopenia may occur in some.

Primary hyperparathyroidism is characterized by hypercalcemia, hypophosphatemia, hypercalciuria, and increased or inappropriately high serum PTH level. Bone density in the radial diaphysis is often low. Hypercalcemic symptoms, peptic ulcer, or bone disease (osteitis, pathological fractures, osteoporosis) may be present.

Fasting hypercalciuria with a normal serum PTH concentration characterizes renal phosphate leak, primary enhancement of 1,25(OH)$_2$D synthesis, and combined renal tubular disturbances. In renal phosphate leak, the serum phosphorus level and renal threshold concentration of phosphorus are less than 0.8 mmol/L (2.5 mg/dL) and remain low even when dietary phosphate is restricted.

Hyperuricosuric calcium oxalate nephrolithiasis[105] is characterized by hyperuricosuria (urinary uric acid > 3.6 mmol/d [>600 mg/d] in at least two of three urine samples), normal serum calcium level, normal fasting and calcium load response, normal urinary calcium level, normal urinary oxalate level (<500 μmol/d [<45 mg/d]), and calcium nephrolithiasis. Hyperuricosuria, defined functionally here by the upper normal limit of 3.6 mmol/d (600 mg/d), correlates with the urinary supersaturation with monosodium urate and with the propensity for calcium stone formation.[33] (Other laboratories employ a higher upper limit for urinary uric acid, e.g., 4.5 mmol/d [750 mg/d] for women and 4.8 mmol/d [800 mg/d] for men.) Urinary pH is typically greater than 5.5. Hyperuricosuria may be the only abnormality in patients with calcium stones, or it may coexist with various forms of hypercalciuria.

Hypocitraturic calcium nephrolithiasis in the pure presentation is the condition in which hypocitraturia (urinary citrate < 1.7 mmol/d [<320 mg/d]) is present alone without

TABLE 29–5. Diagnostic Criteria for Major Forms of Nephrolithiasis*

Form	Serum				Urine								
	Ca	P	PTH	1,25-(OH)$_2$D	Ca (Fasting)	Ca (Ca Load)	Ca (24 h)	Uric Acid	Ox	Cit	pH	α	BD
AH-I	N	N	N	N	N	↑	↑	N	N	N	N	↑	N
AH-II	N	N	N	N	N	↑	N	N	N	N	N	↑/N	N
RH	N	N	↑	↑	↑	N/↑	↑	N	N	N	N	↑	↓
P leak	N	↓	N	↑	↑	↑	↑	N	N	N	N	↑	↓
1,25(OH)$_2$D excess	N	N	N	↑	↑	↑	↑	N	N	N	N	↑	N
Combined	N	N/↓	N	↑	↑	↑	↑	N	N	N	N	↑	N/↓
HUCU	N	N	N	N	N	N	N	↑	N	N	N	N	N
EH	N/↓	N/↓	N/↑	N	↓	↓	↓	↓	↑	↓	N	↓	↓
Hypocit	N	N	N	N	N	N	N	N	N	↓	N	N	N
RTA	N	N	N/↑	N	↑	N	N/↑	N	N	↓	N	↓	↓
Gouty diathesis	N	N	N	N	N	N	N	N/↑	N	N	↓	N	N

*Fasting samples represent 2-h collections obtained in the morning after an overnight fast. Ca load samples were obtained over a 4-h period after oral ingestion of 1 g Ca; they provide an indirect measure of intestinal Ca absorption. Fractional Ca absorption (α) was estimated from fecal recovery of radioactivity after oral administration of radiocalcium with 100 mg Ca. BD represents bone density measured in distal third of radius by photon absorptiometry. PTH is immunoreactive parathyroid hormone. ↑, high; ↓, low; N, normal; Ox, oxalate; Cit, citrate; AH-I, absorptive hypercalciuria type I; AH-II, absorptive hypercalciuria type II; RH, renal hypercalciuria; P leak, renal phosphate leak; 1,25(OH)$_2$D excess, primary 1,25(OH)$_2$D excess; Combined, combined renal tubular disturbances; HUCU, hyperuricosuric calcium nephrolithiasis; EH, enteric hyperoxaluria; Hypocit, idiopathic hypocitraturic calcium nephrolithiasis; RTA, incomplete renal tubular acidosis. Data reflect criteria for sole presentations.

other physiological derangements (such as hypercalciuria or hyperuricosuria).[91] Hypocitraturia may be caused by distal renal tubular acidosis, metabolic acidosis of chronic diarrheal states, or thiazide-induced hypokalemia. Complete distal renal tubular acidosis is characterized by hyperchloremic metabolic acidosis (high serum chloride and low serum potassium and carbon dioxide levels) and high urinary pH (>6.8) in the absence of infection of the urinary tract. Incomplete renal tubular acidosis is characterized by normal serum electrolyte levels but an impaired ability to acidify the urine after ammonium chloride load. Both complete and incomplete forms may be associated with hypercalciuria, hypocitraturia, calcium nephrolithiasis, and nephrocalcinosis. Stone analysis typically shows a preponderance of hydroxyapatite with calcium oxalate as a minor constituent.

Chronic diarrheal states[91] capable of producing hypocitraturia and calcium nephrolithiasis include ileal disease or ileal resection, gastrectomy, ulcerative colitis, and colectomy. The degree of hypocitraturia is generally proportional to the severity of intestinal fluid loss. In severe diarrheal states, urinary citrate concentration may be very low (<0.3 mmol/d [<50 mg/d]); serum electrolyte abnormalities of acquired metabolic acidosis (caused by intestinal fluid loss) and low urinary pH may also be present. Some patients show full features of enteric hyperoxaluria.

In thiazide-induced hypocitraturia,[88] serum potassium level is low or low normal and urinary citrate level is low (<1.7 mmol/d [<320 mg/d]). Thiazide action may also cause a high serum bicarbonate and a low serum chloride concentration.

The invariant feature in gouty diathesis is the persistent passage of an acidic urine (pH < 5.5).[96] The cause of low urinary pH is not always evident. Some patients may give a personal or family history of gouty arthritis. Others may present with hyperuricemia or hypertriglyceridemia. The stones may be composed of uric acid alone, calcium oxalate-phosphate alone, or a mixture of the two. Some patients may form pure uric acid stones on one occasion and calcium stones on another occasion. Uric acid stones are radiolucent.

In cystinuria, the cyanide-nitroprusside test provides a qualitative measure of the cystine content of urine. If positive, a quantitative test should be performed. In patients with cystine stones, urinary cystine concentration is greater than 1 mmol/g creatinine (>250 mg/g creatinine).

Lithiasis resulting from infection is diagnosed by showing that the stones are composed of magnesium ammonium phosphate. Such struvite stones are often associated with pyuria, positive urine culture for urea-splitting organisms (*Proteus*, certain species of *Staphylococcus*, *Pseudomonas*, or *Klebsiella*), and high urinary pH (>7.5). Struvite stones are radiopaque and sometimes may attain a large (staghorn) size; they usually occur as mixtures with calcium carbonate apatite or less commonly with calcium oxalate.

RATIONAL THERAPY FOR NEPHROLITHIASIS

Elucidation of the pathophysiology and formulation of diagnostic criteria for different causes of nephrolithiasis make it possible to devise individual and specific treatment programs.[2, 106] Such regimens ideally should (1) reverse the underlying physicochemical and physiological derangements, (2) inhibit new stone formation, (3) prevent nonrenal complications of the disease process, and (4) be free of serious side effects.[106] The underlying assumption is that the physicochemical and physiological aberrations identified are etiologically important in the formation of renal stones (as previously discussed) and that the correction of such disturbances will prevent new stone formation. Moreover, such a selected treatment program is assumed to be more effective and safer than a "random" treatment. Despite a lack of conclusive verification, these hypotheses appear reasonable and logical. For some treatment programs for nephrolithiasis, considerable information is available about the physicochemical and physiological effects (Table 29–6).

Primary Hyperparathyroidism

Parathyroidectomy is the optimal treatment for nephrolithiasis of primary hyperparathyroidism (also see Chapter 27). After successful surgery, urinary calcium excretion, serum concentration of calcium, and intestinal calcium absorption are restored to normal.[107] The urine becomes less saturated with calcium oxalate and brushite, and the limit of metastability (formation product ratio) for these calcium salts increases.[108] The rate of new stone formation is reduced unless urinary tract infection is present. Parathyroidectomy is contraindicated in secondary hyperparathyroidism of renal hypercalciuria and in absorptive hypercalciuria.

There is no established medical treatment for the nephrolithiasis of primary hyperparathyroidism. Although orthophosphates have been recommended for disease of mild to

TABLE 29–6. Optimal Treatment Programs for Nephrolithiasis

Indication	Treatment	Physiological Action*	Physicochemical Action*
Absorptive hypercalciuria type I (also 1,25(OH)$_2$D excess)	Sodium cellulose phosphate	↓ intestinal calcium (Ca) absorption ↓ urinary Ca	↓ urinary saturation of Ca oxalate ↓ Ca phosphate saturation
	Thiazide	= intestinal Ca absorption ↓ urinary Ca (transient) ↓ urinary citrate	↓ urinary saturation of Ca salts
Absorptive hypercalciuria type II	Low-Ca diet	↓ intestinal Ca absorption ↓ urinary Ca	↓ urinary saturation of Ca oxalate and Ca phosphate
Renal hypercalciuria (also combined renal tubular disturbances)	Thiazide	↓ urinary Ca (sustained) ↓ intestinal Ca absorption	↓ urinary saturation of Ca salts
Renal phosphate leak	Orthophosphate	↓ 1,25(OH)$_2$D ↓ intestinal Ca absorption ↓ urinary Ca ↑ urinary citrate and pyrophosphate	↓ urinary saturation of Ca oxalate ↑ inhibitor activity
Hyperuricosuric Ca nephrolithiasis	Allopurinol	↓ urinary uric acid	↓ urate-induced crystallization of Ca salts
	Potassium citrate	↑ urinary citrate	↓ urinary saturation of Ca oxalate ↓ urate-induced crystallization of Ca salts
Enteric hyperoxaluria	↓ oxalate intake	↓ urinary oxalate	↓ urinary saturation of Ca oxalate
	Potassium citrate	↑ urinary citrate ↑ urinary pH	↓ urinary saturation of Ca oxalate ↑ inhibitor activity
	Magnesium gluconate Calcium citrate	↑ urinary Mg ↑ urinary citrate ↑ urinary pH	↓ urinary saturation of Ca oxalate ↑ inhibitor activity
Hypocitraturic Ca nephrolithiasis	Potassium citrate	↑ urinary citrate ↑ urinary pH ↓/= urinary Ca	↓ urinary saturation of Ca oxalate ↑ inhibitor activity
Gouty diathesis	Potassium citrate	↑ urinary pH ↓ undissociated uric acid ↑ urinary citrate	↓ urinary saturation of uric acid ↓ Ca oxalate crystallization
Cystinuria	Penicillamine or tiopronin †	Mixed disulfide with cysteine ↓ urinary cystine	↓ urinary saturation of cystine
Infection stones	Acetohydroxamic acid	↓ urease activity ↓ NH$_4$$^+$ ↓ pH	↓ urinary saturation of struvite

*↓, decrease; ↑, increase; =, no change.
† α-Mercaptopropionylglycine.

moderate severity, their safety and efficacy have not yet been proved.[109] The use of estrogen in postmenopausal women with this condition has shown some promise.[110] A medical approach should be applied only when parathyroid surgery cannot be undertaken.

Absorptive Hypercalciuria Type I

No treatment program is capable of correcting the basic abnormality of absorptive hypercalciuria, although several drugs restore normal calcium excretion. Sodium cellulose phosphate administration is probably the optimal therapy.[106] When given orally, this nonabsorbable ion-exchange resin binds calcium and inhibits calcium absorption.[45, 111] However, decreased calcium absorption is due to limitation of the amount of intraluminal calcium available for absorption and not to correction of the disturbance in calcium transport.

There are two potential complications of sodium cellulose phosphate therapy.[106, 112] First, the agent may cause magnesium depletion by binding dietary magnesium. Second, sodium cellulose phosphate may produce secondary hyperoxaluria[113] by binding divalent cations in the intestinal tract, reducing formation of divalent cation–oxalate complexes, and making more oxalate available for absorption. These complications may be prevented by oral magnesium supplementation (magnesium citrate, 10 mEq given twice a day separately from sodium cellulose phosphate) and moderate dietary restriction of oxalate. Under such circumstances, sodium cellulose phosphate (10 to 15 g/d, given with meals) lowers urinary calcium level, reduces urinary saturation of calcium salts, and retards new stone formation

without significantly altering urinary oxalate or magnesium levels.[2] This drug is contraindicated in other forms of hypercalciuria because it may further stimulate parathyroid function and worsen negative calcium balance. Because of this potential complication, sodium cellulose phosphate should be given only in severe cases of absorptive hypercalciuria type I and in thiazide-resistant hypercalciuria.

Thiazide does not decrease intestinal calcium absorption,[46] but it is widely used to treat this disorder because of its hypocalciuric action. However, thiazide may have limited long-term effectiveness in absorptive hypercalciuria type I.[114] It is usually effective in reducing the urinary calcium level during the first 2 y of treatment, but thereafter urinary calcium generally returns to the pretreatment range (Fig. 29–2). Intestinal calcium absorption persistently remains elevated throughout thiazide treatment. Thiazide may cause accretion of calcium in bone during the early years of therapy; eventually a low turnover state of bone interferes with continued calcium accretion in the skeleton.[38] The "rejected" calcium would then be excreted in urine. In contrast, calcium retention does not occur in renal hypercalciuria because thiazide causes a decrease in intestinal calcium absorption commensurate with the reduction in urinary calcium level.[114]

The following guidelines for the use of these two agents are recommended until more selective therapies are found: Sodium cellulose phosphate is appropriate for patients with severe absorptive hypercalciuria type I (urinary calcium > 8.75 mmol/d [>350 mg/d]) and for patients resistant to or intolerant of thiazide therapy. In patients at risk for bone disease (growing children, postmenopausal women, or el-

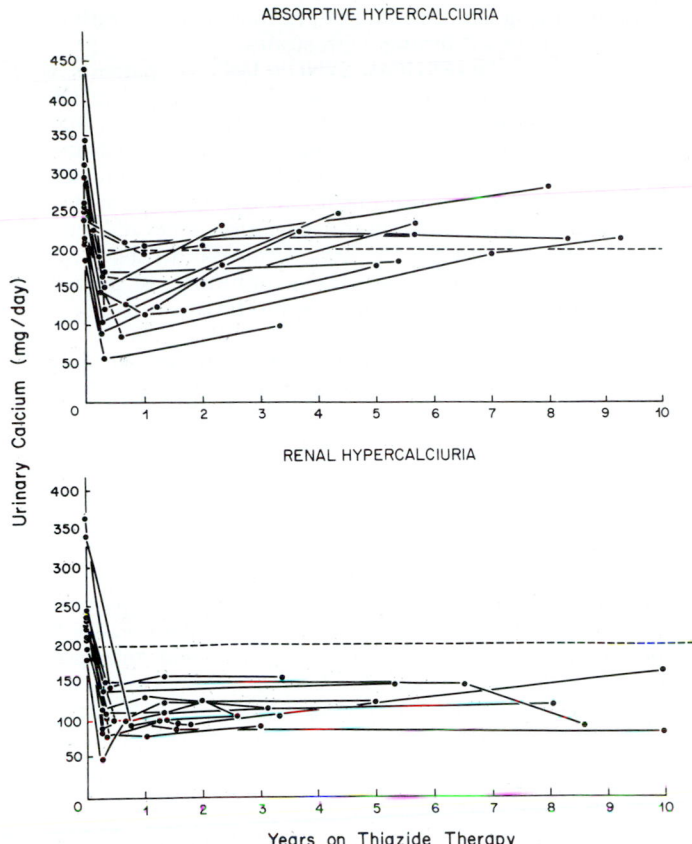

ABSORPTIVE HYPERCALCIURIA

RENAL HYPERCALCIURIA

Years on Thiazide Therapy

Figure 29–2. Contrasting effect of thiazide on urinary calcium in absorptive hypercalciuria versus renal hypercalciuria. (From CYC Pak, Medical management of nephrolithiasis in Dallas: update 1987, J Urol, 140, 461–467, © by Williams & Wilkins, 1988.)

derly men), thiazide is the first choice. When thiazide becomes ineffective in lowering the urinary calcium level, this treatment may be temporarily replaced by sodium cellulose phosphate or orthophosphate treatment (for approximately 6 mo). Restoration of hypocalciuric response to thiazide may then ensue, permitting resumption of thiazide therapy. Potassium citrate (e.g., 15 to 20 mEq twice a day) should be given along with thiazide (e.g., trichlormethiazide 4 mg/d) to prevent hypokalemia and to augment citrate excretion.[115]

In absorptive hypercalciuria type II, a low-calcium diet (10 to 15 mmol/d [400 to 600 mg/d]) and a high fluid intake (sufficient to maintain urine output greater than 2 L/d) are appropriate[2] because normocalciuria can be restored by dietary calcium restriction alone and because increased urine volume reduces urinary saturation of calcium oxalate, brushite, and monosodium urate and inhibits spontaneous nucleation of calcium oxalate.

Renal Hypercalciuria

Thiazide is the treatment of choice for renal hypercalciuria.[46, 50] This agent corrects the renal leak of calcium directly by augmenting calcium reabsorption in the distal tubule and by causing extracellular volume depletion, which stimulates proximal tubular reabsorption of calcium. The ensuing correction of secondary hyperparathyroidism restores normal serum 1,25(OH)$_2$D levels and intestinal calcium absorption. Physicochemically, the urine becomes less saturated with calcium oxalate and brushite, largely because of the reduced calcium excretion.[116] Moreover, urinary in-

hibitor activity, as reflected by an increase in the limit of metastability, occurs by an unknown mechanism. These effects are shared by hydrochlorothiazide (50 mg twice a day), chlorthalidone (50 mg/d), and trichlormethiazide (4 mg/d). Potassium supplementation (15 to 20 mEq twice a day) may be required to prevent hypokalemia and attendant hypocitraturia. Concurrent use of triamterene, a potassium-sparing agent, should be undertaken with caution because of the possibility of triamterene stone formation.[117] Amiloride may be used with thiazide, because it may also exert a hypocalciuric action, to exaggerate the hypocalciuric action of thiazide and to prevent hypokalemia.[118] However, amiloride does not augment citrate excretion. Thus in patients with hypercalciuric nephrolithiasis and hypocitraturia, in whom the use of potassium citrate is contemplated, it is probably wise to use thiazide alone without a potassium-sparing diuretic. Thiazide is contraindicated in primary hyperparathyroidism because of potential aggravation of hypercalcemia.

Renal Phosphate Leak

Administration of orthophosphate (neutral or alkaline salt of sodium and/or potassium, 0.5 g phosphorus three to four times a day) appears to be a logical treatment because of its potential for inhibiting 1,25(OH)$_2$D synthesis.[119] However, there is no convincing evidence that this treatment restores intestinal calcium absorption in this condition. Orthophosphate reduces urinary calcium concentration probably by directly enhancing the renal tubular reabsorption of calcium. Urinary phosphorus concentration is markedly increased during therapy. Physicochemically, orthophosphate reduces urinary saturation of calcium oxalate but increases that of brushite.[29] Moreover, the urinary inhibitor activity is increased, probably because of the increased concentration of pyrophosphate and citrate. Although contrary reports have appeared, this treatment program has been reported to cause soft tissue calcification and parathyroid stimulation.[120] It is contraindicated in nephrolithiasis complicated by urinary tract infection.

Hyperuricosuric Calcium Oxalate Nephrolithiasis

Allopurinol (300 mg/d) is the drug of choice in hyperuricosuric calcium oxalate nephrolithiasis resulting from uric acid overproduction, because of its ability to reduce uric acid synthesis and to lower urinary uric acid concentration.[32] Its use in hyperuricosuria associated with dietary purine overindulgence is also reasonable, because dietary purine restriction may be impractical. Physicochemical changes ensuing from restoration of a normal urinary uric acid level include an increase in the urinary limit of metastability of calcium oxalate.[35] Thus the spontaneous nucleation of calcium oxalate is retarded by treatment, probably by inhibition of monosodium urate–induced stimulation of calcium oxalate crystallization.[36] Because of the potential exaggeration involved in the latter process, a moderate sodium restriction (<150 mmol/d) may be advisable.

Potassium citrate is an effective alternative to allopurinol for treatment of this condition.[121] Citrate can inhibit the heterogeneous nucleation of calcium oxalate by monosodium urate.[121] When potassium citrate is given to patients with hyperuricosuric calcium oxalate nephrolithiasis, the urinary citrate concentration rises. Not only does the induced hypercitraturia reduce urinary saturation of calcium oxalate (by complexing calcium), it also inhibits urate-induced crystallization of calcium oxalate.

Enteric Hyperoxaluria

Stone formation in enteric hyperoxaluria is multifactorial. The treatment should therefore be directed at correcting the various disturbances, including hyperoxaluria, hypocitraturia and low urinary pH, hypomagnesiuria, and low urine volume.

Oral administration of large amounts of calcium (0.25 to 1.0 g four times a day) or magnesium has been recommended for the control of calcium nephrolithiasis of ileal disease. Although urinary oxalate concentration may decrease (probably because of binding of oxalate by divalent cations), the concurrent rise in urinary calcium concentration may obviate the beneficial effect of this therapy, at least in some patients.[122] Cholestyramine does not cause a sustained reduction in oxalate excretion, but limitation of dietary oxalate intake and partial replacement of dietary fat with medium chain fatty acids may be helpful in patients with malabsorption.

The treatment of low urinary citrate and pH levels with potassium citrate will be considered under Chronic Diarrheal Syndrome. Hypomagnesiuria is due to impaired intestinal absorption of magnesium. It contributes to calcium oxalate stone formation because of reduced complexation of oxalate by magnesium and consequent rise in the urinary saturation of calcium oxalate. Oral magnesium supplementation can partially correct hypomagnesiuria, although it may worsen diarrhea. In our experience, magnesium citrate (10 mEq two to four times a day) is better tolerated and absorbed than magnesium oxide or hydroxide. Magnesium chloride is contraindicated because it exaggerates metabolic acidosis.

A high fluid intake is recommended to ensure adequate urine volume. Control of excessive intestinal fluid loss with an antidiarrheal agent may be necessary before a sufficient urine output can be achieved.

Calcium citrate may theoretically have a role in the management of enteric hyperoxaluria. This treatment may lower urinary oxalate level by binding oxalate in the intestinal tract and increase urinary citrate and pH levels by providing an alkali load.[123] Finally, it may correct the malabsorption of calcium and reverse demineralization of the skeleton by enhancing calcium absorption. If hypercalciuria develops, thiazide may be added.

Hypocitraturic Calcium Nephrolithiasis

RENAL TUBULAR ACIDOSIS (DISTAL). Potassium citrate therapy is capable of correcting both metabolic acidosis and hypokalemia.[90] Moreover, it may restore normal urinary citrate concentration, although large doses (up to 120 mEq/d) may be required in severe acidotic states. Urinary calcium concentration typically decreases with the correction of acidosis. The overall rise in urinary pH is small because the urinary pH is high to begin with; urinary pH is generally below 7.5 during treatment unless a urinary tract infection is present.

Thus potassium citrate treatment produces a sustained decline in the urinary saturation of calcium oxalate (through a reduction in urinary calcium level and rise in citrate complexation of calcium). The urinary saturation of calcium phosphate does not increase because the rise in phosphate dissociation is relatively small (as a result of the modest rise in pH) and is adequately compensated by a decrease in ionic calcium concentration. Moreover, inhibitor activity against the crystallization of calcium oxalate and calcium phosphate is augmented by the direct action of citrate.

If renal sodium leak is significant, alkali might be provided as a mixed sodium-potassium salt. However, renal sodium wasting is not prominent in most patients with renal tubular acidosis presenting with stones.

CHRONIC DIARRHEAL SYNDROME. In patients with mild to moderate severity of intestinal fluid loss in whom hypocitraturia is not severe (urinary citrate in the range of 0.5 to 1.5 mmol/d [100 to 300 mg/d]), potassium citrate (40 to 60 mEq in three or four divided doses in a liquid form) is generally effective in restoring normal urinary citrate and pH levels.[91] Urinary calcium concentration generally remains low. In those with severe hypocitraturia (urinary citrate < 0.5 mmol/d [<100 mg/d]), even high doses of potassium citrate (up to 120 mEq/d) may be ineffective in restoring a normal urinary citrate level.

A liquid preparation of potassium citrate is preferable to a slow-release tablet preparation in these states because some of the patients may have abnormal intestinal motility and may be more prone to obstruction caused by a tablet preparation. Furthermore, a slow-release medication may be poorly absorbed because of rapid intestinal transit.

A frequent dose schedule (three or four times a day) is recommended for the liquid preparation because of the relatively short duration of biological action. In other hypocitraturic conditions, the solid slow-release preparation is preferable or is better tolerated. A less frequent dose schedule (twice a day) is acceptable for the solid preparation because of its slow-release characteristic.

THIAZIDE-INDUCED HYPOKALEMIA. Hypokalemia resulting from thiazide may cause hypocitraturia, probably by causing intracellular acidosis, and may thereby attenuate the beneficial hypocalciuric effect of therapy on renal stone formation.[115]

It has been suggested that potassium citrate may be less effective than potassium chloride in correcting the thiazide-induced hypokalemia because of the poor reabsorbability of citrate from the renal tubules.[124] However, severe chloride depletion is uncommon in patients with thiazide-induced hypocitraturia. Potassium citrate (15 to 20 mEq twice a day) is usually effective in preventing hypokalemia and maintaining normal urinary citrate levels.

IDIOPATHIC HYPOCITRATURIC CALCIUM NEPHROLITHIASIS. Idiopathic hypocitraturic calcium oxalate nephrolithiasis can be the result of isolated hypocitraturia with calcium stones or of hypocitraturia occurring in conjunction with absorptive and renal hypercalciurias or with hyperuricosuric calcium oxalate nephrolithiasis.[125] Stones formed are composed predominantly of calcium oxalate.

Potassium citrate treatment (15 to 30 mEq twice a day) produces a sustained increase in urinary citrate excretion.[125] Urinary pH can be maintained at 6.5 to 7.0. Along with these changes, the urinary saturation of calcium oxalate declines to normal limits.

Gouty Diathesis

Potassium citrate is the treatment of choice for this condition. A dosage of 30 to 60 mEq/d in divided doses increases the low urinary pH (<5.5) to the desired range (<6).[96] Because of the resulting enhanced dissociation of uric acid, the amount of undissociated uric acid decreases to levels found in normal controls (<0.9 mmol/d [<150 mg/d]). Thus potassium citrate therapy increases the solubility of uric acid, preventing uric acid stone formation. Moreover, this treatment inhibits formation of calcium stones by reducing urinary saturation of calcium oxalate and retarding the crystallization of calcium oxalate.

Sodium alkali is as effective as potassium citrate in preventing uric acid nephrolithiasis because it has a similar capacity for raising urinary pH. However, calcium stones

Cystine Stones

A low-methionine diet has often been recommended for the control of cystine nephrolithiasis because methionine is a precursor of cystine. Although such a dietary maneuver may reduce cystine excretion, rigid methionine restriction is impractical. Dietary sodium restriction may also reduce cystine excretion, but this beneficial effect may be neutralized by reduced solubility of cystine resulting from loss of the "solubilizing" action of sodium.

In patients with cystine calculi and moderate cystinuria (1 to 2 mmol/d [250 to 500 mg/d]), conservative measures of high fluid intake and alkali administration should be attempted. The aim of fluid therapy is to increase urine volume sufficiently to reduce the cystine concentration below the solubility limit. At least 3 L of fluid should be provided, including two 8-oz glassfuls with each meal and at bedtime. Patients should be directed to wake up at night to urinate and drink water. Additional fluids should be consumed when excessive sweating or intestinal fluid loss is present. A minimum urine output of 2 L/d on a consistent basis is attainable by most patients with proper and persistent instruction.

In theory, alkali therapy would enhance cystine solubility by raising urinary pH. However, excessive alkali therapy is not indicated,[100] and substantial increases in cystine solubility do not occur until the urinary pH exceeds 7.5. The provision of alkali, no matter how much, rarely raises urinary pH above 7.5. When urinary pH increases above 7.0 with alkali therapy, calcium phosphate nephrolithiasis may be enhanced because of the enhanced urinary supersaturation of hydroxyapatite in an alkaline environment.

Thus a modest amount of alkali is recommended to maintain urinary pH in a high normal range (6.5 to 7.0). Potassium citrate has the advantages over sodium citrate that it does not cause hypercalciuria, is less likely to promote development of calcium stones,[96, 126] and does not induce increased cystine excretion.[127]

The object of penicillamine treatment is to reduce total cystine excretion by complexing cysteine, the monomeric form of cystine. Penicillamine may be added to the conservative treatment program in patients with moderate cystinuria when the conservative treatment is ineffective in controlling stone formation. In patients with severe cystinuria (>2 mmol/d [>500 mg/d]), in whom conservative management alone is not likely to be effective, penicillamine therapy (together with conservative measures) may be begun.

Penicillamine shares with cysteine a free sulfhydryl group.[128] Thus it undergoes thiol-disulfide exchange with cystine to form penicillamine-cysteine disulfide, which is much more soluble than cystine. After oral administration, a sufficient amount of penicillamine can be excreted in urine to complex cysteine and thereby lower cystine excretion. Unfortunately, penicillamine therapy is associated with frequent and sometimes severe side effects, including nephrotic syndrome, dermatitis, and pancytopenia.[129]

Tiopronin (α-mercaptopropionylglycine) has biochemical and clinical actions similar to those of penicillamine.[130] However, it has a lower toxicity profile than penicillamine.

Infection Stones

If long-standing control of infection with urea-splitting organisms can be achieved, new stone formation may be averted and some existing stones may be dissolved. Unfortunately, such control is difficult to obtain with antibiotic therapy. If a struvite stone is present, it is difficult to eradicate infection completely because the stone may harbor the organisms within its interstices. Even if "sterilization" of urine can be achieved by antibiotic therapy, reinfection by organisms harbored by the stones can occur. For this reason, surgical removal of the struvite stones is usually recommended.

Acetohydroxamic acid, a urease inhibitor, reduces urinary saturation of struvite by preventing the formation of ammonium and hydroxyl ions.[131] It may prevent stone growth and sometimes cause dissolution of existing stones. However, it may cause hemolytic anemia, thrombophlebitis, and nonspecific neurological symptoms (disorientation, tremulousness, and headache).[132]

Conservative Management

The conservative measures of high fluid intake and avoidance of dietary excesses should be applied in all patients with nephrolithiasis.[133] They may be applied alone in patients with a single stone episode and inactive stone disease but should be instituted together with a specific medical treatment program in patients with recurrent stone disease, particularly if extrarenal manifestations are present. Some conservative programs are applicable to all forms of stone disease, whereas others are useful for particular causes.

High fluid intake is the only nutritional modification that is useful in all forms of nephrolithiasis. By increasing urine output, urinary concentration of constituent ions and saturation of stone-forming salts are lowered. Although dietary restriction of oxalate may be beneficial in all types of nephrolithiasis, it is particularly indicated when intestinal absorption of oxalate is increased, as in ileal disease and when calcium absorption is increased. Rigid calcium restriction (<10 mmol/d [<400 mg/d]) is ill advised, even in patients who have high intestinal calcium absorption, because it is difficult to adhere to, may adversely affect general nutrition, and may cause negative calcium balance. However, moderate calcium restriction (10 to 15 mmol/d [400 to 600 mg/d]) may be useful in absorptive hypercalciuria because it alone may control the hypercalciuria in the less severe (type II) presentation and permit reduction of the dosage of medication necessary to restore normal urinary calcium concentration in the more severe (type I) presentation. Calcium restriction is neither necessary nor indicated in patients with nephrolithiasis with normal intestinal absorption of calcium.

Moderate sodium restriction (100 mmol/d) may be helpful in all forms of nephrolithiasis.

REFERENCES

1. Pak CYC, Britton F, Peterson R, et al. Ambulatory evaluation of nephrolithiasis: classification, clinical presentation and diagnostic criteria. Am J Med 1980; 69:19–30.
2. Pak CYC, Peters P, Hurt G, et al. Is selective therapy of recurrent nephrolithiasis possible? Am J Med 1981; 71:615–622.
3. Frangos DN, Rous SN. Incidence and economic factors in urolithiasis. In: Rous SN, ed. Stone Disease: Diagnosis and Management. Orlando, FL: Grune & Stratton, 1987: 3–10.
4. Chulkaratana S, Van Reen R, Valyasevi A. Studies of bladder stone disease in Thailand. XV. Factors affecting the solubility of calcium oxalate. Invest Urol 1971; 9:246–250.
5. Prien EL, Prien EL Jr. Composition and structure of urinary stone. Am J Med 1968; 45:654–672.
6. Simmonds HA, Van Acker KJ, Cameron JS, et al. The identification of 2,8-dihydroxyadenine, a new component of urinary stones. Biochem J 1976; 157:485–487.
7. Vermeulen CW, Lyon ES, Fried FA. On the nature of the stone-forming process. J Urol 1965; 94:176–186.
8. Boyce WH. Organic matrix of human urinary concretions. Am J Med 1968; 45:673–683.

9. Howard JE, Thomas SW, Smith LH, et al. A urinary peptide with extraordinary inhibitory powers against biological "calcification" (deposition) of hydroxyapatite crystals. Trans Assoc Am Physicians 1966; 79:137–144.

10. Nancollas G. The kinetics of crystal growth and renal stone formation. In: Fleisch H, Robertson WG, Smith LH, et al., eds. Urolithiasis Research. New York: Plenum, 1976: 5–23.

11. Robertson WG, Peacock M, Nordin BEC. Activity products in stone-forming and nonstone-forming urine. Clin Sci 1968; 34:579–594.

12. Finlayson B. Calcium stones: some physical and clinical aspects. In: David D, ed. Calcium Metabolism in Renal Failure and Nephrolithiasis. New York: John Wiley & Sons, 1979: 337.

13. Pak CYC, Hayashi Y, Finlayson B, et al. Estimation of the state of saturation of brushite and calcium oxalate in urine: a comparison of three methods. J Lab Clin Med 1977; 89:891–901.

14. Pak CYC, Holt K. Nucleation and growth of brushite and calcium in urine of stone-formers. Metabolism 1976; 25:665–673.

15. Nicar MJ, Hill K, Pak CYC. A simple technique for the assessment of the propensity for the crystallization of calcium oxalate and brushite in urine from the increment in oxalate or calcium necessary to elicit precipitation. Metabolism 1983; 32:906–910.

16. Meyer JL, Smith LH. Growth of calcium oxalate crystals. II. Inhibition by natural urinary crystal growth inhibitors. Invest Urol 1975; 13:36–39.

17. Bisaz S, Felix R, Neiman W, et al. Quantitative determination of inhibitors of calcium phosphate precipitation in whole urine. Miner Electrolyte Metab 1978; 1:74.

18. Smith LH, Meyer JL, McCall JT. Chemical nature of crystal inhibitors isolated from human urine. In: Cifuentes L, Rapado A, Hodgkinson A, eds. Urinary Calculi: International Symposium on Renal Stone Research. Basel: S. Karger, 1973: 318.

19. Nakagawa Y, Kaiser ET, Coe FL. Isolation and characterization of calcium oxalate crystal growth inhibitors from human urine. Biochem Biophys Res Commun 1978; 84:1038–1044.

20. Bowyer RC, Brockis JG, McCulloch RK. Glycosaminoglycans as inhibitors of calcium oxalate crystal growth and aggregation. Clin Chim Acta 1979; 95:23–28.

21. Robertson WG, Peacock M, Nordin BEC. Inhibitors of the growth and aggregation of calcium oxalate crystals in vitro. Clin Chim Acta 1973; 43:31–37.

22. Kok DJ, Papapoulos SE, Bijvoet OLM. Excessive crystal agglomeration with low citrate excretion in recurrent stone-formers. Lancet 1986; 1:1056–1058.

23. Pak CYC, Holt K, Britton F, et al. Assessment of pathogenetic roles of uric acid, monopotassium urate, monoammonium urate and monosodium urate in hyperuricosuric calcium oxalate nephrolithiasis. Miner Electrolyte Metab 1980; 4:130–136.

24. Meyer JL, Bergert JH, Smith LH. Epitaxial relationship in urolithiasis: the calcium oxalate monohydrate–hydroxyapatite system. Clin Sci Mol Med 1975; 49:369–374.

25. Lonsdale K. Epitaxy as a growth factor in urinary calculi and gallstones. Nature 1968; 217:56–58.

26. Pak CYC. Idiopathic renal lithiasis: new developments in evaluation and treatment. In: Fleisch H, Robertson WG, Smith LH, et al., eds. Urolithiasis Research. New York: Plenum, 1976: 213–244.

27. Zerwekh JE, Hwang TIS, Poindexter J, et al. Modulation by calcium of the inhibitor activity of citrate, chondroitin sulfate and urinary glycoprotein against calcium oxalate crystallization. Kidney Int 1988; 33:1005–1008.

28. Strauss AL, Coe FL, Deutsch L, et al. Factors that predict relapse of calcium nephrolithiasis during treatment. Am J Med 1982; 71:17–24.

29. Pak CYC, Galosy RA. Propensity for spontaneous nucleation of calcium oxalate. Quantitative assessment by urinary FPR-APR discriminant score. Am J Med 1980; 69:681–689.

30. Yendt ER, Cohanim M. Prevention of calcium stones with thiazides. Kidney Int 1978; 13:397–409.

31. Finlayson B, Smith A. Stability of first dissociable proton of uric acid. J Chem Eng Data 1974; 19:94.

32. Coe FL. Hyperuricosuric calcium oxalate nephrolithiasis. Kidney Int 1978; 13:418–426.

33. Pak CYC, Waters O, Arnold L, et al. Mechanism for calcium urolithiasis among patients with hyperuricosuria: supersaturation of urine with respect to monosodium urate. J Clin Invest 1977; 59:426–432.

34. Robertson WG. Physical chemical aspects of calcium stone-formation in the urinary tract. In: Fleisch H, Robertson WG, Smith LH, eds. Urolithiasis Research. New York: Plenum, 1976: 25–39.

35. Pak CYC, Barilla DE, Holt K, et al. Effect of oral purine load and allopurinol on the crystallization of calcium salts in urine of patients with hyperuricosuric calcium urolithiasis. Am J Med 1978; 65:593–599.

36. Pak CYC, Holt K, Zerwekh JE. Attenuation by monosodium urate of the inhibitory effect of glycosaminoglycans on calcium nucleation. Invest Urol 1979; 17:138–140.

37. Zerwekh JE, Holt K, Pak CYC. Attenuation by the urate salts of the inhibitory effect of naturally occurring urinary macromolecules on calcium oxalate nucleation and crystal growth. Kidney Int 1983; 23:838–841.

38. Pak CYC, Nicar MJ, Northcutt C. The definition of the mechanism of hypercalciuria is necessary for the treatment of recurrent stone formers. Contrib Nephrol 1982; 33:136–151.

39. Nicar MJ, Hill K, Pak CYC. Inhibition by citrate of spontaneous precipitation of calcium oxalate, in vitro. J Bone Miner Res 1987; 2:215–220.

40. Kitamura T, Zerwekh JE, Pak CYC. Partial biochemical and physiochemical characterization of organic macromolecules in urine from patients with renal stones and control subjects. Kidney Int 1981; 21:379–386.

41. Griffith DP, Musher DM. Prevention of infected urinary stones by urease inhibition. Invest Urol 1973; 11:228–233.

42. Pak CYC, Fuller C. Assessment of cystine solubility in urine and heterogeneous nucleation between cystine and calcium salts. Invest Urol 1983; 129:1066–1070.

43. Pak CYC, Sakhaee K, Crowther C, et al. Evidence justifying a high fluid intake in treatment of nephrolithiasis. Ann Intern Med 1980; 93:36–39.

44. Henneman PH, Benedict PH, Forbes AP. Idiopathic hypercalciuria. N Engl J Med 1958; 259:801–807.

45. Pak CYC. Pathogenesis of hypercalciuria. In: Peck WA, ed. Bone and Mineral Research. Vol 4. New York: Elsevier, 1985: 303–334.

46. Pak CYC. Physiological basis for absorptive and renal hypercalciurias. Am J Physiol 1979; 237:F415–F423.

47. Brannan PG, Morawski S, Pak CYC, et al. Selective jejunal hyperabsorption of calcium in absorptive hypercalciuria. Am J Med 1979; 66:425–428.

48. Pak CYC, Nicar MJ, Krejs GJ. Intestinal absorption of calcium, magnesium, phosphate and oxalate: deviation from normal in idiopathic urolithiasis. In: Schwille PO, Smith LH, Robertson WG, et al., eds. Urolithiasis and Related Clinical Research. New York: Plenum, 1985: 127–133.

49. Zerwekh JE, Pak CYC, Kaplan RA, et al. Pathogenetic role of $1\alpha,25$-dihydroxyvitamin D in sarcoidosis and absorptive hypercalciuria: different response to prednisolone therapy. J Clin Endocrinol Metab 1980; 51:381–386.

50. Zerwekh JE, Pak CYC. Selective effects of thiazide therapy on serum $1\alpha,25$-dihydroxyvitamin D and intestinal calcium absorption in renal and absorptive hypercalciurias. Metabolism 1980; 29:13–17.

51. Barilla DE, Zerwekh JE, Pak CYC. A critical evaluation of the role of phosphate in the pathogenesis of absorptive hypercalciuria. Miner Electrolyte Metab 1979; 2:302–309.

52. Coe FL, Parks JH, Moore ES. Familial idiopathic hypercalciuria. N Engl J Med 1979; 300:337–340.

53. Pak CYC, McGuire J, Peterson R, et al. Familial absorptive hypercalciuria in a large kindred. J Urol 1981; 126:717–719.

54. Bushinsky DA, Johnston RB, Nalbantian CE, et al. Increased calcium absorption and retention without elevated serum $1,25(OH)_2D_3$ in genetically hypercalciuric rats. In: Abstract Program, The American Society of Nephrology 20th Annual Meeting, December 13–16, 1987, Washington, DC, 55:189A.

55. Pak CYC, Galosy RA. Fasting urinary calcium and adenosine $3',5'$-monophosphate: a discriminant analysis for the identification of renal and absorptive hypercalciuria. J Clin Endocrinol Metab 1979; 48:260–265.

56. Barilla DE, Townsend J, Pak CYC. An exaggerated augmentation of renal calcium excretion following oral glucose ingestion in patients with renal hypercalciuria. Invest Urol 1978; 15:486–488.

57. Sakhaee K, Nicar MJ, Brater DC, et al. Exaggerated natriuretic and calciuric response to hydrochlorothiazide in renal hypercalciuria but not in absorptive hypercalciuria. J Clin Endocrinol Metab 1985; 61:825–829.

58. Coe FL, Canterbury JM, Firpo JJ, et al. Evidence for secondary hyperparathyroidism in idiopathic hypercalciuria. J Clin Invest 1973; 52:134–142.

59. Lemann J, Piering WF, Lennon EJ. Possible role of carbohydrate-induced calciuria in calcium oxalate kidney-stone formation. N Engl J Med 1969; 280:232–237.

60. Muldowney FP, Freaney R, Moloney MF. Importance of dietary sodium in the hypercalciuria syndrome. Kidney Int 1982; 22:292–296.

61. Lawoyin S, Sismilich S, Browne R, et al. Bone mineral content in patients with primary hyperparathyroidism, osteoporosis, and calcium urolithiasis. Metabolism 1979; 28:1250–1254.

62. Pak CYC. Medical management of nephrolithiasis: update 1987. J Urol 1988; 140:461–467.

63. Garabedian M, Holick MF, DeLuca HF, et al. Control of 25-hydroxycholecalciferol metabolism by parathyroid glands. Proc Natl Acad Sci USA 1972; 69:1673.

64. Lloyd HM. Primary hyperparathyroidism: an analysis of the role of the parathyroid tumor. Medicine 1968; 47:53.

65. Broadus AE, Horst RL, Lang R, et al. The importance of circulating 1,25-dihydroxyvitamin D in the pathogenesis of hypercalciuria and renal-stone formation in primary hyperparathyroidism. N Engl J Med 1980; 302:421–426.

66. Patron P, Gardin J-P, Paillard M. Renal mass and reserve of vitamin D: determinants of plasma 1,25(OH)$_2$D$_3$ in primary hyperparathyroidism. Kidney Int 1987; 31:1174–1180.

67. Pak CYC, Nicar MJ, Peterson R, et al. A lack of unique pathophysiologic background for nephrolithiasis of primary hyperparathyroidism. J Clin Endocrinol Metab 1981; 53:536–542.

68. Smith LH, Werness PG, Lee KE, et al. Inhibitors of crystal growth and aggregation in calcium urolithiasis. Clin Res 1979; 26:727A.

69. Kaplan RA, Haussler MR, Deftos LJ, et al. The role of 1α,25-dihydroxyvitamin D in the mediation of intestinal hyperabsorption of calcium in primary hyperparathyroidism and absorptive hypercalciuria. J Clin Invest 1977; 59:756–760.

70. Bone HG III, Zerwekh J, Haussler MR, et al. Effect of parathyroidectomy on serum 1α,25-dihydroxyvitamin D and on intestinal calcium absorption in primary hyperparathyroidism. J Clin Endocrinol Metab 1979; 48:877–879.

71. Shen FH, Baylink DJ, Nielson RL, et al. Increased serum 1,25-dihydroxyvitamin D in idiopathic hypercalciuria. J Lab Clin Med 1977; 90:955–962.

72. Gray RW, Wilz DR, Caldas AE, et al. The importance of phosphate in regulating plasma 1,25-(OH)$_2$vitamin D levels in humans: studies in healthy subjects, in calcium-stone formers and in patients with primary hyperparathyroidism. J Clin Endocrinol Metab 1977; 45:299–306.

73. Bordier R, Ryckewart A, Gueris J, et al. On the pathogenesis of so-called idiopathic hypercalciuria. Am J Med 1977; 63:398–409.

74. Broadus AE, Erickson SB, Gertner JM, et al. An experimental human model of 1,25-dihydroxyvitamin D–mediated hypercalciuria. J Clin Endocrinol Metab 1984; 59:202–206.

75. Reynolds JJ, Holick MF, DuLuca HF. The role of vitamin D metabolites on bone resorption. Calcif Tissue Res 1973; 12:295–301.

76. Zerwekh JE, Sakhaee K, Pak CYC. Short term 1,25-dihydroxyvitamin D$_3$ administration raises serum osteocalcin in patients with postmenopausal osteoporosis. J Clin Endocrinol Metab 1985; 60:615–617.

77. Insogna KL, Broadus AE, Dreyer BE, et al. Elevated production rate of 1,25-dihydroxyvitamin D in patients with absorptive hypercalciuria. J Clin Endocrinol Metab 1985; 61:490–495.

78. Coe FL, Favus MJ, Crockett T, et al. Effects of low-calcium diet on urine calcium excretion, parathyroid function and serum 1,25-(OH)$_2$D$_3$ levels in patients with idiopathic hypercalciuria and in normal subjects. Am J Med 1982; 72:25–32.

79. Buck AC, Lote CJ, Sampson WF. The influence of renal prostaglandins on urinary calcium excretion in idiopathic urolithiasis. J Urol 1983; 129:421–426.

80. Lemann J Jr, Gray RW. Hypercalciuric kidney stone formers exhibit enhanced intestinal calcium absorption (Ca$_A$) despite only slightly elevated serum 1,25-(OH)$_2$-D concentrations. In: Abstract Program, The American Society of Nephrology 20th Annual Meeting, December 13–16, 1987, Washington, DC, 139:196A.

81. Coe FL, Kavalach AG. Hypercalciuria and hyperuricosuria in patients with calcium nephrolithiasis. N Engl J Med 1974; 291:1344–1350.

82. Breslau NA, Pak CYC. Lack of effect of salt intake on urinary uric acid excretion. J Urol 1983; 129:531–532.

83. Loffler W, Grobner W, Medina R, et al. Influence of dietary purines on pool size, turnover, and excretion of uric acid during balance conditions. Res Exp Med (Berl) 1982; 181:113–123.

84. Earnest DL, Williams HE, Admirand WH. A physicochemical basis for treatment of enteric hyperoxaluria. Trans Assoc Am Physicians 1975; 88:224–234.

85. Smith LH, Fromm H, Hofmann AF. Acquired hyperoxaluria, nephrolithiasis and intestinal disease: description of a syndrome. N Engl J Med 1972; 286:1371–1374.

86. Nicar MJ, Skurla C, Sakhaee K, et al. Low urinary citrate excretion in nephrolithiasis. Urology 1983; 21:8–14.

87. Simpson DP. Regulation of renal citrate metabolism by bicarbonate ion and pH: observations in tissue slices and mitochondria. J Clin Invest 1967; 16:225–238.

88. Morrissey JF, Ocha M, Lotspeich WD, et al. Citrate excretion in renal tubular acidosis. Ann Intern Med 1963; 55:159–166.

89. Nicar MJ, Peterson R, Pak CYC. Use of potassium citrate as potassium supplement during thiazide therapy of calcium nephrolithiasis. J Urol 1984; 131:430–433.

90. Preminger GM, Sakhaee K, Skurla C, et al. Prevention of recurrent calcium stone formation with potassium citrate therapy in patients with distal renal tubular acidosis. J Urol 1985; 134:20–23.

91. Pak CYC, Fuller C, Sakhaee K, et al. Long-term treatment of calcium nephrolithiasis with potassium citrate. J Urol 1985; 134:11–19.

92. Breslau NA, Brinkley L, Hill KD, et al. Relationship role of animal protein–rich diet to kidney stone formation and calcium metabolism. J Clin Endocrinol Metab 1988; 66:140–146.

93. Sakhaee K, Nigam S, Snell P, et al. Assessment of the pathogenetic role of physical exercise in renal stone formation. J Clin Endocrinol Metab 1987; 65:974–979.

94. Rudman D, Dedonis JL, Fountain MT, et al. Hypocitraturia in patients with gastrointestinal malabsorption. N Engl J Med 1980; 303:657–661.

95. Drach GW, Gaines J, Donovan J. Is magnesium metabolism related to

96. Pak CYC, Sakhaee K, Fuller C. Successful management of uric acid nephrolithiasis with potassium citrate. Kidney Int 1986; 30:422–428.

97. Yu TF. Uric acid nephrolithiasis. In: Kelly WN, Weiner IM, eds. Handbook of Experimental Pharmacology. Vol 51. New York: Springer-Verlag, 1978: 397–422.

98. Deren JJ, Porush JG, Levitt MF, et al. Nephrolithiasis as complication of ulcerative colitis and regional ileitis. Ann Intern Med 1962; 56:843–853.

99. Broadus A, Thier S. Metabolic basis of renal stone disease. N Engl J Med 1979; 300:839–845.

100. Dent CE, Rose GA. Amino acid metabolism in cystinuria. Q J Med 1951; 20:205–219.

101. Thier SO, Segal S. Cystinuria. In: Stanbury JB, Wyngaarden JB, Fredrickson DS, eds. The Metabolic Basis of Inherited Disease. New York: McGraw-Hill, 1972: 1504–1519.

102. Rosenberg LE, Downing S, Durant JL, et al. Cystinuria: biochemical evidence for three genetically distinct diseases. J Clin Invest 1966; 45:365–371.

103. Pak CYC, Skurla C, Harvey J. Graphic display of urinary risk factors for renal stone formation. J Urol 1985; 134:867–870.

104. Pak CYC, Kaplan RA, Bone H, et al. A simple test for the diagnosis of absorptive, resorptive and renal hypercalciurias. N Engl J Med 1975; 292:497–500.

105. Coe FL, Boro ES. Hypercalciuria and hyperuricosuria in patients with calcium nephrolithiasis. N Engl J Med 1974; 291:1344–1350.

106. Pak CYC. Medical management of nephrolithiasis. J Urol 1982; 128:1157–1164.

107. Kaplan RA, Snyder WH, Stewart A, et al. Metabolic effects of parathyroidectomy on asymptomatic primary hyperparathyroidism. J Clin Endocrinol Metab 1976; 42:415–426.

108. Pak CYC. Effect of parathyroidectomy on crystallization of calcium salts in urine of patients with primary hyperparathyroidism. Invest Urol 1979; 17:146–148.

109. Broadus AE, Magee JS, Mallette LE, et al. A detailed evaluation of oral phosphate therapy in selected patients with primary hyperparathyroidism. J Clin Endocrinol Metab 1983; 56:953–961.

110. Selby PL, Peacock M. Ethinyl estradiol and norethindrone in the treatment of primary hyperparathyroidism in postmenopausal women. N Engl J Med 1986; 314:1481–1485.

111. Pak CYC. Sodium cellulose phosphate: mechanism of action and effect on mineral metabolism. J Clin Pharmacol 1973; 13:15–27.

112. Pak CYC. A cautious use of sodium cellulose phosphate in the management of calcium nephrolithiasis. Invest Urol 1981; 19:187–190.

113. Hayashi Y, Kaplan RA, Pak CYC. Effect of sodium cellulose phosphate therapy on crystallization of calcium oxalate in urine. Metabolism 1975; 24:1273–1278.

114. Preminger GM, Pak CYC. Eventual attenuation of hypocalciuric response to hydrochlorothiazide in absorptive hypercalciuria. J Urol 1987; 137:1104–1109.

115. Pak CYC, Peterson R, Sakhaee K, et al. Correction of hypocitraturia and prevention of stone formation by combined thiazide and potassium citrate therapy in thiazide-unresponsive hypercalciuric nephrolithiasis. Am J Med 1985; 78:284–288.

116. Woelfel A, Kaplan RA, Pak CYC. Effect of hydrochlorothiazide therapy on crystallization of calcium oxalate in urine. Metabolism 1977; 26:201–205.

117. Ettinger B, Oldroyd NO, Sorge F. Triamterene nephrolithiasis. JAMA 1980; 244:2443–2445.

118. Leppla D, Browne R, Hill K, et al. Effect of amiloride with or without hydrochlorothiazide on urinary calcium and saturation of calcium salts. J Clin Endocrinol Metab 1983; 57:920–924.

119. Van Den Berg CJ, Kumar R, Wilson DM, et al. Orthophosphate therapy decreases urinary calcium excretion and serum 1,25-dihydroxyvitamin D concentrations in idiopathic hypercalciuria. J Clin Endocrinol Metab 1980; 51:998–1001.

120. Dudley FJ, Blackburn CRB. Extraskeletal calcification complicating oral neutral-phosphate therapy. Lancet 1970; 2:628–630.

121. Pak CYC, Peterson R. Successful treatment of hyperuricosuric calcium oxalate nephrolithiasis with potassium citrate. Arch Intern Med 1986; 146:863–868.

122. Barilla DE, Notz C, Kennedy D, et al. Renal oxalate excretion following oral oxalate loads in patients with ileal disease and with renal and absorptive hypercalciurias: effect of calcium and magnesium. Am J Med 1978; 64:576–585.

123. Harvey JA, Zobitz MM, Pak CYC. Calcium citrate: reduced propensity for the crystallization of calcium oxalate in urine resulting from induced hypercalciuria of calcium supplementation. J Clin Endocrinol Metab 1985; 61:1223–1225.

124. Kassirer JP, Berkman PM, Lawrenz DR, et al. The critical role of chloride in the correction of hypokalemic alkalosis in man. Am J Med 1965; 38:172–189.

125. Pak CYC, Fuller C. Idiopathic hypocitraturic calcium oxalate nephroli-

thiasis successfully treated with potassium citrate. Ann Intern Med 1986; 104:33–37.

126. Sakhaee K, Nicar M, Hill K, et al. Contrasting effects of potassium citrate and sodium citrate therapies on urinary chemistries and crystallization of stone-forming salt. Kidney Int 1983; 24:348–352.

127. Jaeger P, Portmann L, Saunders A, et al. Anticystinuric effects of glutamine and of dietary sodium restriction. N Engl J Med 1986; 315:1120–1123.

128. Perrett D. The metabolism and pharmacology of D-penicillamine in man. J Rheumatol 1981; 8(Suppl 7):41–50.

129. Halperin EC, Thier SO, Rosenberg LE. The use of D-penicillamine in cystinuria: efficacy and untoward reactions. Yale J Biol Med 1981; 54:439–446.

130. Pak CYC, Fuller C, Sakhaee K, et al. Management of cystine nephrolithiasis with alpha-mercaptopropionylglycine (Thiola). J Urol 1986; 136:1003–1008.

131. Griffith DP. Struvite stones. Kidney Int 1978; 13:372–382.

132. Williams JJ, Rodman JS, Peterson CM. A randomized double-blind study of acetohydroxamic acid in struvite nephrolithiasis. N Engl J Med 1984; 311:760–764.

133. Pak CYC, Smith LH, Resnick MI, et al. Dietary management of idiopathic calcium urolithiasis. J Urol 1984; 131:850–852.

30

MULTIPLE ENDOCRINE NEOPLASIA

Robert F. Gagel

INTRODUCTION

The multiple endocrine neoplasia (MEN) syndromes were described early in this century[1] and subsequently were classified into two broad categories, MEN type 1 (MEN 1) and MEN type 2 (MEN 2).[2–4] The MEN 2 syndrome has been further subcategorized into two variants called MEN 2A and MEN 2B (formerly MEN 3). Our understanding of the MEN syndromes has evolved through several phases. The first was the descriptive phase, in which the fully developed clinical syndromes and their genetic patterns were described.[2–7] The second involved the development of screening techniques to identify the syndromes before they could become significant clinical problems.[8–15] Early identification of the manifestations and improvements in management techniques have had a significant impact on the morbidity and mortality associated with these syndromes. We are now entering a third phase: elucidation of the genetic and molecular basis of these syndromes.[16–21] This chapter summarizes the current understanding of these disorders and attempts to provide a framework for understanding future developments.

MEN 1 and MEN 2 share certain characteristics. The first is the cell type involved in the neoplastic process. The usual tumor is composed of one or more specific polypeptide- and biogenic amine–producing cell types and has been given the acronym APUD, which stands for amine precursor uptake and decarboxylation.[22] The major tumors in these

two syndromes that are not composed of this cell type are the lipomas, associated with MEN 1,[5] and the mucosal neuromas and colonic polyps, associated with MEN 2B.[23–25] The APUD cell type is thought to derive embryologically from neuroectoderm and to have certain neuron-like properties. Although not all aspects of the APUD cell theory are widely accepted, this classification of cell types forms the basis for a useful unifying hypothesis for understanding the syndromes.

A second feature shared by these syndromes is the histological progression from hyperplasia to adenoma, and, in some cases, to carcinoma. Third, the development of hyperplasia is probably a multicentric process, with each focus of tumor derived from a single clone. This point has been proved for only one manifestation of these syndromes (medullary thyroid carcinoma[26]) but is likely to be true for other tumors as well.[27] Last, each of these syndromes has an autosomal dominant pattern of inheritance.

MULTIPLE ENDOCRINE NEOPLASIA, TYPE 1

The familial association of parathyroid, pancreatic islet, and pituitary hyperplasia or neoplasia is called MEN 1. Although there were earlier descriptions,[1] the syndrome was recognized as a clinical and genetic syndrome by Wermer in

1954[2] and was classified as an entity distinct from MEN 2 in 1968.[6] In previous years, patients presented with advanced manifestations of parathyroid, pancreatic islet, and pituitary neoplasia in the third and fourth decades of life. However, the use of family screening has resulted in earlier identification of hormonal syndromes. The most common mode of presentation for MEN 1 is within the context of an identified kindred; less frequently a newly ascertained individual with advanced disease may be the propositus of a new kindred, a previously unidentified member of a known kindred, or a new mutation.

Hyperparathyroidism

Hyperparathyroidism is the most common manifestation of MEN 1. Prospective screening of family members has shown that hypercalcemia (ionized or albumin-adjusted serum calcium) and abnormalities of parathyroid hormone secretion may appear as early as age 17,[10, 14, 28–32] and by age 40 almost all family members carrying the gene for MEN 1 are likely to be hypercalcemic.[10, 33] Hyperplasia of multiple parathyroid glands is the most common histological lesion observed in early MEN 1.[31–38] If, however, the disease is diagnosed late, adenomatous changes may be superimposed on a background of multiglandular parathyroid hyperplasia.[28, 29, 33, 39]

Several unique features of parathyroid hyperplasia associated with MEN 1 differentiate it from the more common syndrome of hyperparathyroidism caused by a parathyroid adenoma. First, the feedback relationship between the serum calcium level and parathyroid hormone secretion is different. In adenomatous parathyroid tissue, a supraphysiological extracellular calcium concentration of 1.2 to 1.4 mmol/L (4.8 to 5.6 mg/dL) is required to inhibit 50% of parathyroid hormone secretion, whereas a calcium concentration of only 1 mmol/L (4 mg/dL) is required to suppress similarly hyperplastic parathyroid tissue from MEN 1 patients.[40] Both of these set point values are higher than those for normal parathyroid tissue exposed chronically to a high extracellular calcium concentration.[40] An abnormality in the feedback relationship between the extracellular calcium concentration and parathyroid hormone synthesis and secretion may be one cause of the increased proliferation of parathyroid tissue, although additional factors are likely to be involved.[40, 41] A second difference between adenomatous disease and the hyperplasia associated with MEN 1 is the response to therapy. More than 85% of patients with adenomatous hyperparathyroidism have a long-term return of the serum calcium concentration to normal after surgical removal of a single adenoma.[42] Parathyroid surgery in MEN 1 results in an initial cure rate of approximately 75%, but recurrence of hypercalcemia in approximately half during a 10-y period.[34, 42–45] This result suggests that parathyroid growth in MEN 1 is a continuous and ongoing process. Third, a unique serum factor in patients with MEN 1 (possibly a transforming growth factor) may be able to stimulate endothelial cell growth in parathyroid glands.[46–49] Fourth, a parathyroid adenoma derives from a single cell type, whereas the parathyroid hyperplasia of MEN 1 is likely to result from expansion of multiple cell clones.[27]

The general features of hyperparathyroidism in MEN 1 include urolithiasis, parathyroid hormone–induced bone abnormalities, musculoskeletal complaints, and, with severe hypercalcemia, generalized weakness and alterations of mental status. These features are not different from those associated with other forms of hyperparathyroidism (see Chapter 27).

Several disorders other than MEN 1 should be considered in the differential diagnosis of familial hypercalcemia, including familial parathyroid hyperplasia,[50, 51] familial adenomatous hyperparathyroidism,[52] and familial hypocalciuric hypercalcemia.[53, 54] Diagnosis of these disorders is challenging and requires clinical information not only from the individual patient but also from other family members. The major feature separating MEN 1–associated hyperparathyroidism from other forms of familial parathyroid disease is the absence of pituitary and pancreatic manifestations in hyperparathyroidism not associated with MEN 1. Non–MEN 1 forms of familial hyperparathyroidism can be categorized into hyperplasia[38, 50, 51, 55–57] or adenomatous disease[58] on the basis of the histology of the parathyroid gland. Familial parathyroid hyperplasia is uncommon, and some families given this diagnosis later develop clear-cut manifestations of MEN 1. Familial hypocalciuric hypercalcemia is a distinct autosomal dominant disorder characterized by hypercalcemia and low urinary calcium excretion.[53, 54] Parathyroid hyperplasia and elevated serum parathyroid hormone concentrations may be present, but the hypercalcemia is not corrected by parathyroid gland resection. The diagnosis can usually be made by documenting hypercalcemia, a low urinary calcium/creatinine ratio, and similar biochemical abnormalities in other family members. A characteristic feature of familial hypocalciuric hypercalcemia is hypercalcemia from the time of birth,[53, 54] whereas MEN 1–associated hypercalcemia generally does not appear until the second decade of life.[10, 14] Other rare forms of hypercalcemia include hyperparathyroidism associated with MEN 2A[7, 59, 60] and the humoral hypercalcemia syndrome associated with a pancreatic islet cell tumor causing watery diarrhea.[61]

Surgery is the treatment of choice for hyperparathyroidism associated with MEN 1. The timing and the type of operative procedure remain controversial. Parathyroid surgery is definitely indicated in an MEN 1 patient with an albumin-adjusted serum calcium level higher than 3.0 mmol/L (12.0 mg/dL) or with clinical evidence of parathyroid hormone–induced bone disease or kidney stones and a documented diagnosis of primary hyperparathyroidism. As a result of prospective screening, however, affected family members may be identified with minimal elevations of serum calcium. The optimal management of such patients is not clear. Parathyroid surgery is indicated for MEN 1 patients with Zollinger-Ellison syndrome and mild hyperparathyroidism because return of serum calcium levels to normal may be associated with a lowering of serum gastrin level and of gastric acid secretion (Figs. 30–1 and 30–2).[15] Early surgery has been advocated in other minimally hypercalcemic MEN 1 patients both because of the suggestion of a causal relationship between hypercalcemia and elevation of serum gastrin[62, 63] and pancreatic polypeptide[64, 65–67] levels and because of the unproven contention that hypercalcemia stimulates growth of the pituitary and pancreatic manifestations of the syndrome. Arguments against early surgery include the high recurrence and/or persistence rate of hyperparathyroidism and the 10 to 25% incidence of hypoparathyroidism after surgery for hyperparathyroidism in patients with MEN 1.[34, 44] Postponement of surgery coupled with periodic assessment of the patient for several years may be a rational course of action in selected patients with minimal elevations of serum calcium.

The primary lesson from experience with parathyroid surgery in patients with MEN 1 is that cure is difficult and may require several operative procedures over an extended period. The standard surgical approach has been to remove three to three and one half parathyroid glands and to leave behind a mass of parathyroid tissue approximating that of normal subjects.[44] Because reoperation in these patients is likely, careful operative notes and marking of remaining parathyroid tissue with metal clips will enhance the likeli-

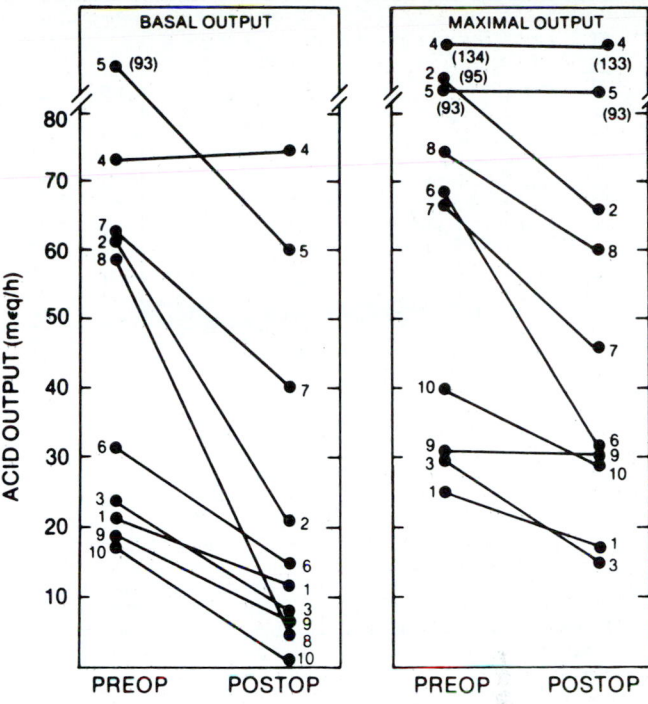

Figure 30–1. The basal gastric acid output *(left)* and maximal output *(right)* are shown before and after parathyroidectomy for 10 MEN 1 patients with primary hyperparathyroidism and Zollinger-Ellison syndrome. Basal gastric acid hypersecretion was defined as a level higher than 15 mmol/h (mEq/h) in patients without previous gastric surgery (patients 1, 2, and 4 to 10) or higher than 5 mmol/h in patients with previous gastric surgery (patient 3). Except for patient 4, all patients were normocalcemic after surgery. (From Norton JA, Cornelius MJ, Doppman JL, et al. Effect of parathyroidectomy in patients with hyperparathyroidism, Zollinger-Ellison syndrome, and multiple endocrine neoplasia type I: a prospective study. Surgery 1987; 102:958–966.)

hood of success in a subsequent parathyroid gland operation. The method of complete removal of parathyroid tissue from the neck and transplantation of small packets of tissue to the nondominant forearm has also been used for management of MEN 1–associated hyperparathyroidism. This technique does not necessarily prevent recurrent hyperparathyroidism (Fig. 30–3), but it does facilitate management. In one series approximately two thirds of MEN 1 patients developed recurrent hypercalcemia 7 to 75 mo after total parathyroidectomy and grafting of parathyroid tissue to the nondominant arm.[68] Recurrent hyperparathyroidism, however, can be managed by removal of individual islands of hyperplastic parathyroid tissue from the arm with the use of local anesthesia.[42, 68, 69] Another advantage appears to be

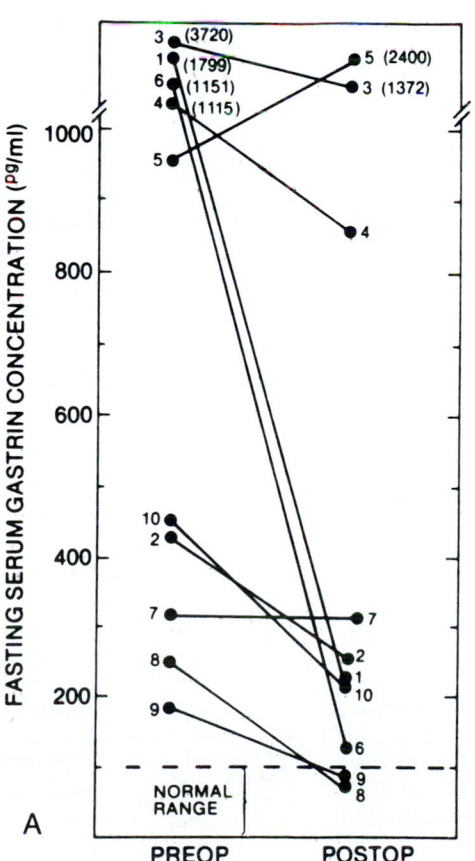

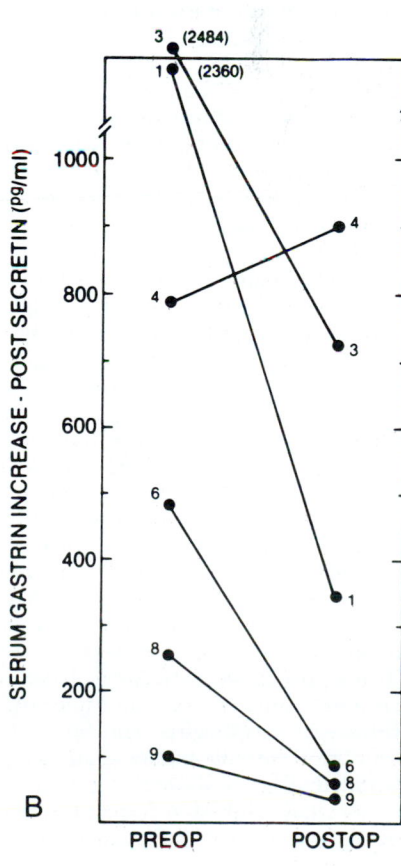

Figure 30–2. *A,* The fasting serum gastrin concentration before and after parathyroidectomy for 10 patients with primary hyperparathyroidism, Zollinger-Ellison syndrome, and MEN 1. The normal gastrin concentration is less than 48 pmol/L (100 pg/mL). Numbers in parentheses represent actual gastrin concentrations when higher than 475 pmol/L (1000 pg/mL). *B,* Serum gastrin increase after intravenous injection of 2 U/kg body weight secretin before and after parathyroidectomy for six of the same patients described in *A.* The response is considered to be positive if the serum gastrin increase is higher than 95 pmol/L (200 pg/mL). (From Norton JA, Cornelius MJ, Doppman JL, et al. Effect of parathyroidectomy in patients with hyperparathyroidism, Zollinger-Ellison syndrome, and multiple endocrine neoplasia type I: a prospective study. Surgery 1987; 102:958–966.)

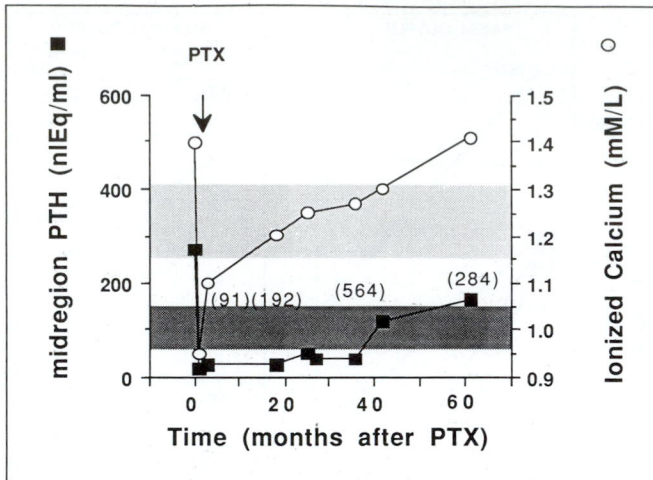

Figure 30–3. Serum ionized calcium and peripheral midregion parathyroid hormone (PTH) levels after total parathyroidectomy and graft of parathyroid tissue in a patient with MEN 1. After total parathyroidectomy (PTX) and grafting of parathyroid tissue to the nondominant forearm, the ionized calcium and parathyroid hormone levels fell to subnormal levels. Subsequent measurements demonstrated a continuous rise of the ionized calcium and peripheral parathyroid hormone levels (taken from the arm containing the transplant) over a 60-mo period, which necessitated removal of some of the grafted parathyroid tissue. The numbers in parentheses show selected parathyroid hormone values for blood taken from the brachial vein immediately proximal to the grafted parathyroid tissue. These results demonstrate continued secretion of parathyroid hormone by the graft in the presence of hypercalcemia. The upper, lighter shaded area shows the normal range for ionized calcium; the lower, darker shaded area shows the normal range for serum midregion parathyroid hormone. (Data kindly provided by L. E. Mallette, Baylor College of Medicine.)

the low incidence of permanent hypoparathyroidism. Graft function can be documented by measuring parathyroid hormone in venous blood obtained from a site proximal to the graft site and comparing it with a value obtained from a site distal to the graft (see Fig. 30–3).[68]

Pancreatic Islet Cell Tumors

Neoplasia of the pancreatic islet cells is the second most common manifestation of MEN 1 and eventually occurs in 80% of patients. The multicentric islet cell tumors produce hormonal manifestations and can undergo malignant transformation and metastasis. Although a pancreatic islet cell tumor is frequently identified by the clinical syndrome caused by a single hormone product, most of these tumors demonstrate hyperplasia of multiple cell types and produce several different peptides and biogenic amines.[70]

Increasing evidence that surgical cure is difficult[71, 72] and improved drugs for controlling the clinical manifestations of these syndromes[73, 74] have led many physicians to attempt pharmacological control of hormonal syndromes.

GASTRINOMA. Zollinger-Ellison syndrome (gastric acid hypersecretion caused by excessive production of gastrin) is the major cause of morbidity and mortality in patients with MEN 1. Increased gastrin production has been demonstrated in more than 60% of patients with MEN 1 and accounts for approximately a third of cases of Zollinger-Ellison syndrome.[5, 33] The clinical features of Zollinger-Ellison syndrome associated with MEN 1 include gastric acid hypersecretion, solitary or multiple peptic ulcers, diarrhea, refractory esophagitis, and an elevated serum gastrin concentration (usually higher than 171 pmol/L [300 pg/mL]).[74, 75] Confirmation of abnormal gastrin secretion can be obtained by a calcium infusion (calcium gluconate at a concentration of 4 mg elemental calcium/kg body weight/h for 3 h) (Fig.

30–4)[76] or a secretin test (intravenous injection of secretin 2 U/kg body weight) (see Fig. 30–2).[15, 76] The serum gastrin concentration in a patient with a gastrinoma should increase by more than 114 pmol/L (200 pg/mL), whereas the rise is minimal (usually less than 24 pmol/L [50 pg/mL]) in patients with other hypergastrinemic states such as retained gastric antrum, after massive small bowel resection, gastric outlet obstruction, hypercalcemia, or duodenal ulcer disease.[77]

Zollinger and Ellison recommended total gastrectomy to control the ulcer syndrome[78] because the multicentric nature of gastrinoma and the high incidence of hepatic metastases made surgical removal of all gastrin-producing tissue difficult. However, some patients can be cured by enucleation of a gastrinoma or by distal pancreatectomy. More extensive experience with surgical management of gastrinoma in patients with MEN 1 has confirmed a high recurrence rate,[71, 74, 79] but some surgeons still recommend selective removal of isolated tumors.[80] The introduction of H₂ receptor antagonists (cimetidine and ranitidine) has made it possible to perform a pharmacological gastrectomy. Doses of H₂ antagonists required for a therapeutic effect are usually higher than those for duodenal ulcer disease, and ranitidine is the preferred drug because of fewer side effects.[74] H^+,K^+-ATPase inhibitors promise even better control of gastric acid secretion.[81] Only a small percentage of patients treated with such drugs ultimately require total gastrectomy.[82] The somatostatin analogue octreotide inhibits both gastrin and gastric acid secretion[83] and in some patients lowers the requirements for H₂ receptor antagonists.[84] There is no convincing evidence the analogue has a beneficial effect on tumor growth, and it should be used only when H₂ receptor antagonists are ineffective or cause major side effects.

Total pancreatectomy to remove all gastrin-producing tissue has been advocated by some to decrease the recurrence and metastasis of gastrinoma in patients with MEN 1. The procedure may be curative and may prevent death from metastatic carcinoma[85] but should be avoided because the long-term effects of total pancreatectomy (pancreatic exocrine deficiency and diabetes mellitus) likely have a more adverse effect on the quality and length of life than Zollinger-Ellison syndrome itself.

INSULINOMA. Insulinoma is the second most common pancreatic islet cell tumor; about 35% of functional pancreatic neoplasms in MEN 1 are insulinomas. The clinical features do not differ from those associated with sporadic insulinoma, and the diagnosis is generally made by demonstrating fasting hypoglycemia with inappropriately elevated serum insulin and C peptide concentrations (see Chapter

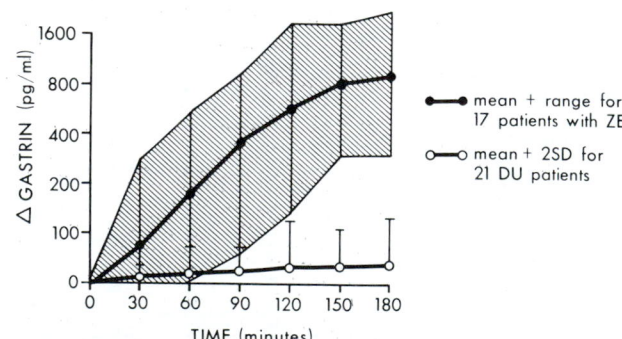

Figure 30–4. Gastrin response to intravenous infusion of calcium gluconate (4 mg elemental calcium/kg body weight/h for 3 h) in patients with Zollinger-Ellison (ZE) syndrome and in patients with duodenal ulcer (DU) unassociated with gastrinoma. To convert gastrin values to picomoles per liter, multiply by 0.48. (From Deveney CW, Deveney KS, Way LW. The Zollinger-Ellison syndrome—23 years later. Ann Surg 1978; 188:384–393.)

23). The insulinomas in MEN 1 are frequently multicentric (as many as 16 adenomas per pancreas) and malignant (25%).[33, 72, 86] Even when a single adenoma is found, it is likely that hyperplasia or microadenomatosis of insulin-producing cells is present elsewhere in the pancreas.

The primary treatment is surgical removal of insulin-producing tissue; there is no alternative form of long-term medical therapy. Preoperative evaluation should include computed tomography, magnetic resonance imaging,[87] or ultrasonography of the abdomen.[88] Despite improvements in imaging techniques the number of tumors found at surgery is usually underestimated.[72] Subtotal pancreatectomy (80% or more of the pancreas) is used for surgical management. At surgery it may be difficult to be certain that all insulin-producing tissue has been removed, and a variety of techniques including intraoperative ultrasonography[88] and monitoring of plasma glucose and insulin levels[89] have been used, with mixed success, to localize such tissue. Enucleation of a single adenoma in occasional patients has resulted in cure.[72] Surgical resection of metastatic insulinoma causing hypoglycemia is indicated, but reoperation for unidentified disease is less likely to be successful.[90] Hypoglycemia caused by unresectable metastatic insulinoma can be controlled with diazoxide;[90] chemotherapy (streptozocin or dacarbazine) may reduce the tumor size, but cure has not been reported.[91]

GLUCAGONOMA. The glucagonoma syndrome consists of hyperglycemia, a characteristic rash termed necrolytic migratory erythema, anorexia, glossitis, anemia, diarrhea, and venous thrombosis (see Chapter 32). It is not common in patients with MEN 1[92] despite the facts that plasma glucagon concentrations are elevated in more than half of MEN 1 patients[10, 93] and that large numbers of glucagon-positive cells are detectable in more than 30% of islet cell tumors.[10, 70, 93–96] The most common clinical finding associated with the glucagonoma syndrome in patients with MEN 1 is hyperglycemia; few patients exhibit the characteristic skin lesions.[97, 98] Glucagonomas are usually managed by surgical removal, although some patients respond to the somatostatin analogue octreotide.[73, 99]

THE WATERY DIARRHEA SYNDROME. The syndrome of watery diarrhea, hypokalemia, hypochlorhydria, and acidosis in MEN 1 (see Chapter 32) occurs in association with both pancreatic islet cell[61, 100] and carcinoid[101] tumors. Surgical removal of single or multiple tumors is the appropriate primary therapy. Streptozocin has been effective in reducing tumor size and the production of vasoactive intestinal peptide in some patients;[102] octreotide is effective for control of diarrheal symptoms in patients with unresectable or metastatic tumors.[73]

PANCREATIC POLYPEPTIDE. Serum concentrations of pancreatic polypeptide are frequently elevated in MEN 1 patients, and enhanced levels of serum pancreatic polypeptide after a standard meal test may be predictive for a pancreatic tumor in subjects with MEN 1.[66] Whether the elevated pancreatic polypeptide level is always related to a pancreatic tumor is not clear, because consistent elevations of pancreatic polypeptide levels have been reported in primary hyperparathyroidism.[67] The elevated concentrations of pancreatic polypeptide in MEN 1 do not appear to cause clinical manifestations.

Pituitary Adenomas

Pituitary tumors occur in more than half of patients with MEN 1.[5, 33] The tumors are multicentric, and excessive hormone production may cause galactorrhea, amenorrhea, acromegaly, or Cushing syndrome. At least two mechanisms appear to be involved in the formation of pituitary tumors. The first involves a local neoplastic transformation with clonal expansion of specific pituitary cell types. Genetic factors are thought to be the primary determinant of tumor development by this mechanism. The second mechanism is stimulation of specific pituitary cell growth by ectopic production of hypothalamic releasing hormones.

PROLACTINOMA. Prolactinomas are the most common pituitary tumor and the third most common manifestation of MEN 1.[10, 103] Prolactinomas in patients with MEN 1 are characteristically multicentric and may grow to be quite large.[104, 105] There is a significant recurrence rate after attempted surgical removal of these tumors, and dopamine agonists (bromocriptine or pergolide) have been tried for management. Although long-term experience with these agents is limited, bromocriptine has been used safely[106] and effectively[107, 108] for a decade or more (see Chapter 6). The major problems associated with bromocriptine therapy are poor long-term compliance and the side effects of nausea and hypotension, especially when the drug is used at higher doses.

GROWTH HORMONE–PRODUCING TUMORS AND GROWTH HORMONE–RELEASING HORMONE. Tumors that produce growth hormone are the second most common pituitary tumor in patients with MEN 1 (25% of pituitary adenomas).[5, 33] The clinical features of acromegaly in MEN 1 do not differ from those in sporadic acromegaly (see Chapter 6). There are at least two potential causes for increased growth hormone production in MEN 1. The first is the development of a multicentric pituitary tumor, presumably the result of the underlying lesion causing MEN 1. The second mechanism is the production of growth hormone–releasing hormone (GHRH) by pancreatic[5, 33, 95, 96, 109–111] or other endocrine tumors. The identification of the second mechanism provides an example of how the manifestation of the disease can be modified by production of a substance by one tissue (most commonly the pancreatic islets) that stimulates the growth of another tissue (the pituitary gland). Although GHRH-producing tumors are rare causes of both sporadic[112] and MEN 1–associated acromegaly, the serum GHRH level should be measured for evaluation of acromegaly in the MEN 1 patient.

The primary therapy for acromegaly in MEN 1 patients is transsphenoidal removal of the pituitary tumor or, when appropriate, removal of a GHRH-producing tumor. Although early surgery is indicated to prevent progression, many of these tumors are multicentric, and incomplete removal and recurrence of the disease are significant problems (see Chapter 6). Radiotherapy has been used to manage persistent or recurrent disease but is associated with long-term side effects of hypopituitarism and brain dysfunction.[113] Octreotide therapy is an effective alternative to radiation,[73] but there is little information about long-term efficacy.

CUSHING SYNDROME AND CORTICOTROPIN-RELEASING HORMONE. Cushing syndrome in patients with MEN 1 can be caused by a pituitary tumor producing corticotropin (ACTH, adrenocorticotropin),[33] by ectopic production of corticotropin by a carcinoid tumor,[114] or by ectopic production of corticotropin-releasing hormone.[115] Each of these disorders is rare. Treatment is directed toward surgical removal of the pituitary tumor or the source of the ectopic corticotropin or corticotropin-releasing hormone. In patients in whom pituitary surgery is not curative, radiation therapy to the pituitary, pharmacological inhibitors of steroid synthesis, or bilateral adrenalectomy may be indicated (see Chapters 6 and 9).

Carcinoid Tumors

Carcinoid tumors are uncommon in MEN patients.[33, 116] Carcinoid tumors are more common in MEN 1 (91%) than in MEN 2, are more likely to develop in the foregut (two thirds are in the thymus, lung, stomach, or duodenum), and are most likely to involve the thymus (men) or lung (women). About half of the carcinoids are either locally invasive or distantly metastatic, especially the thymic carcinoids. The usual clinical features of carcinoid syndrome (flushing, diarrhea, and bronchospasm) are not common,[114] although serotonin, calcitonin,[117] and corticotropin[114] may be produced. These tumors are generally removed surgically. The somatostatin analogue octreotide is an effective treatment for the rare MEN 1 patient with flushing and diarrhea.[73]

Miscellaneous Features of MEN 1

Subcutaneous and visceral lipomas occur in some patients. Whether they have a genetic or a hormonal basis is not known. There has also been a report of cutaneous leiomyomas associated with the MEN 1 syndrome.[118]

Family Screening

A rational screening program for MEN 1 must routinely identify gene carriers and be cost effective. The latter point is especially important because surveillance of an individual at risk may be needed for several decades. Experience in screening MEN families has shown that compliance with a *simple* and *regular* screening protocol is likely; overly complicated or erratic screening efforts are associated with a greater failure rate. Screening can be divided into two components: identification of the gene carrier state and management of the gene carrier. The optimal test for identification of the gene carrier state is an albumin-adjusted or ionized serum calcium measurement,[10, 14] which may be supplemented with a serum parathyroid hormone measurement. Measurement of serum prolactin improves the likelihood of early detection of gene carrier status[10] and, more important, allows identification of the occasional patient (or family) in whom prolactinoma is the initial manifestation.[119, 120] Measurement of serum gastrin slightly increases the yield of early identification of gene carrier status but is probably not cost effective. The frequency of testing can be as little as every 5 y,[10] although continuity of follow-up may be threatened by the long interval between testing. The identification of closely linked DNA markers for MEN 1 on chromosome 11 makes it possible to predict carrier status with greater than 95% certainty; use of such sequence polymorphisms to screen affected families may be possible.[16, 17]

Establishment of gene carrier status focuses attention on those family members likely to develop clinical disease. Prospective screening should then be directed to components of the syndrome, such parathyroid disease or pituitary tumors, for which early identification and treatment are likely to alter the clinical course. Periodic measurement of serum calcium and prolactin concentrations and biannual measurement of gastrin, growth hormone, and serum cortisol after an overnight dexamethasone suppression test (see Chapter 9) seem prudent. Imaging of the pituitary gland should be performed every 5 to 10 y or when hormone abnormalities are observed. Identification of pancreatic islet cell neoplasia before development of clinical symptoms of hormone excess seems less important because most investigators believe that operative intervention is not indicated for asymptomatic pancreatic neoplasia, although not all agree.[80, 85, 121]

MULTIPLE ENDOCRINE NEOPLASIA, TYPE 2A

In 1959 John Sipple was asked to see a hypertensive patient who subsequently died. At autopsy Sipple "was amazed when I saw large, bilateral pheochromocytomas and a 2 cm pale tan mass in each lobe of the thyroid gland and nodular enlargement of the only parathyroid gland we could find."[122] Sipple reported this case and reviewed five others from the literature;[123] the familial nature of the syndrome[6, 124] and the recognition of the thyroid tumor as medullary thyroid carcinoma were clarified by others.[125] Williams[126] reasoned that because medullary thyroid carcinoma was a malignancy of the C cells it might produce calcitonin. This concept led to the use of serum calcitonin measurements for early diagnosis of medullary thyroid carcinoma.[7, 13, 127, 128]

The clinical syndrome, as described by Sipple[4] and others,[6] consists of bilateral and multicentric medullary thyroid carcinoma, unilateral or bilateral pheochromocytoma, and, less commonly, parathyroid hyperplasia or adenomatosis. In the decade after Sipple's description, patients with this syndrome frequently presented with manifestations of a pheochromocytoma, a thyroid nodule, or hypercalcemia, or some combination of the three. Such clinical presentations are still observed, but at present the identification and routine screening of affected families make early thyroid C cell hyperplasia the most common initial presentation.[8, 9, 12, 102, 129-137] Pheochromocytomas are subsequently identified in about half of patients, and parathyroid abnormalities occur in 10 to 20%.[6, 7, 59, 138]

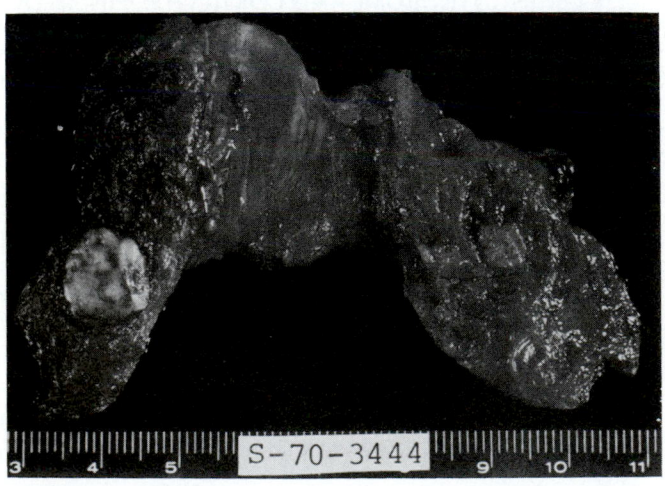

Figure 30–5. Bilateral medullary thyroid carcinoma in MEN 2A. Large bilateral foci of medullary thyroid carcinoma are located in each lobe of the thyroid gland.

Medullary Thyroid Carcinoma

Medullary thyroid carcinoma is a multicentric neoplasm of the parafollicular or C cell of the thyroid gland (Fig. 30–5). The earliest demonstrable abnormality in the thyroid gland of individuals with this syndrome is hyperplasia of C cells,[139, 140] followed by progression to nodular hyperplasia, microscopic medullary thyroid carcinoma, and finally frank medullary thyroid carcinoma (Fig. 30–6). These changes are multicentric, with the frequent occurrence of more than one type of histological lesion in one or both lobes of the thyroid.[141] The time required for progression through these several histological stages is not known, but the process may require one or more decades.[141] It is also not known at which histological stage metastasis occurs, but local lymph node metastasis is common when the tumor diameter is larger than 1 cm,[7, 11, 133, 135] whereas lymph node metastasis is rare in C cell hyperplasia.[9, 12, 13, 130, 137, 142, 143] Occasionally, foci of medullary thyroid carcinoma occur in extrathyroidal locations such as the thymus gland. Whether these lesions are primary or metastatic cannot be determined with certainty.

Total thyroidectomy is mandatory for treatment of medullary thyroid carcinoma in this syndrome. Abnormalities of the C cell are almost always bilateral and multicentric,[144] and, even if C cells remaining after surgery are not malignant initially, malignant transformation may occur later. If the tumor is large, there is a high likelihood of local nodal metastasis.[6, 7] Surgical removal of all central lymph nodes and selective removal of the lateral lymph nodes of the neck can result in cure of the disease, even in the presence of nodal metastasis.[7, 8, 60, 128, 134] Appropriate studies to exclude hyperparathyroidism and pheochromocytoma are mandatory; pheochromocytomas should be removed before thyroid surgery.

Reoperation for persistent medullary thyroid carcinoma has been attempted with overall poor results.[60, 145] However, one investigator has described return of the serum calcitonin level to normal after meticulous neck dissection in approximately a third of reoperated patients.[146] A major question confronting the physician contemplating reoperation is whether the tumor is located in the neck or whether distant metastases are present. Techniques that have been used with variable success for localizing the tumor include scanning with thallium[147] and [131I]metaiodobenzylguanidine[148–150] and venous catheterization for measurement of calcitonin in blood from specific anatomical locations.

Younger individuals diagnosed by prospective screening should have a total thyroidectomy.[12, 60, 137, 142] C cell hyperplasia or microscopic medullary thyroid carcinoma (see Fig. 30–6) without metastatic disease is the most common histological finding in these patients. Total regional node dissection is not mandatory, although random sampling of nodes is advisable.

TUMOR MARKERS ASSOCIATED WITH MEDULLARY THYROID CARCINOMA. Proteins produced by the normal C cell and by medullary thyroid carcinoma include calcitonin, calcitonin gene–related peptide,[151] somatostatin,[152] dihydroxyphenylalanine decarboxylase,[153] and chromogranin-A.[154] Genes that are not normally expressed in the C cell but that are expressed by medullary thyroid carcinoma include those for pro-opiomelanocortin, thyrotropin-releasing hormone,[155] gastrin-releasing peptide,[156] vasoactive intestinal peptide, neurotensin, substance P, carcinoembryonic antigen, histaminase,[157] and others.[158] Expression of these genes is of fundamental interest in the elucidation of factors regulating gene expression and the transformation process, but measurement of the products in serum yields little additional information beyond that provided by the measurement of calcitonin.

Pheochromocytoma

Adrenal chromaffin tissue in patients with MEN 2A undergoes the same type of histological progression as that observed for the C cell, including hyperplasia, diffuse expansion of the adrenal medulla, and pheochromocytoma. The usual finding is single or multiple pheochromocytomas, with a background of hyperplastic chromaffin tissue[159–161] (Fig. 30–7). The pheochromocytomas may be unilateral or bilateral, although if a tumor is present in one adrenal gland hyperplastic changes are likely in the contralateral gland. Invasion of the adrenal capsule by chromaffin cells is observed, but it is rare for these tumors to metastasize.[141, 159, 162]

The clinical syndrome caused by adrenomedullary disease has changed over the past two decades. Before prospective screening, patients frequently presented with large pheochromocytomas, hypertension, headaches, and cardiac arrhythmias. Sudden death secondary to a stroke or cardiac arrest was not uncommon. Routine screening of kindreds results in earlier identification of affected individuals. Early adrenomedullary abnormalities may cause intermittent

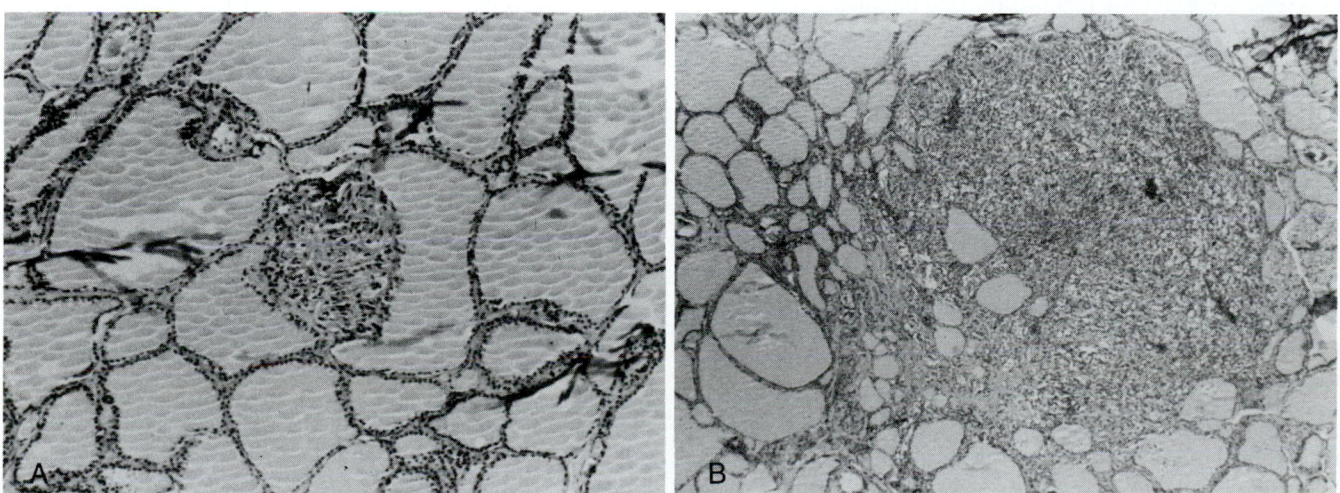

Figure 30–6. Progression of histological changes from C cell hyperplasia to medullary thyroid carcinoma. These sections were taken from a single thyroid lobe of a patient with hereditary medullary thyroid carcinoma and demonstrate the multicentric nature of this tumor. *A* shows nodular hyperplasia with containment of C cells within a thyroid follicle. Magnification × 250. *B* shows microscopic medullary thyroid carcinoma that is locally invasive. Magnification × 100.

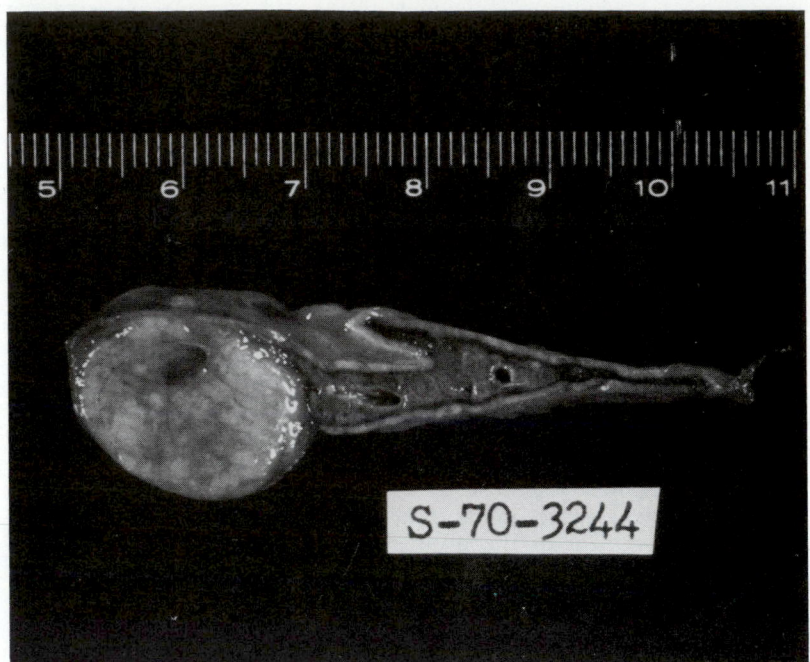

Figure 30–7. A pheochromocytoma set on a background of diffuse adrenomedullary hyperplasia in MEN 2A. In the normal adrenal gland the adrenal cortices are separated by a thin (less than 1 mm) band of adrenal medulla. In this pheochromocytoma there is diffuse expansion of the adrenal medulla.

headaches, palpitations, and nervousness; hypertension is uncommon.[8] Although deaths are fewer since the advent of prospective screening, vigilance is required for pregnant women, because of the possibility of death during labor[163, 164] and because of patients who are noncompliant with screening procedures.

Adrenomedullary abnormalities associated with MEN 2A produce distinctive biochemical features. Increased urinary excretion of epinephrine and an increased ratio of epinephrine to norepinephrine excretion in a 24-h urine sample are the first abnormalities noted[8, 165, 166] (Fig. 30–8). The goal of screening is to identify patients at this stage. Later in the course of the disease or with larger pheochromocytomas the 24-h excretion of epinephrine, norepinephrine, metanephrine, and normetanephrine metabolites is usually increased. Urinary vanillylmandelic acid excretion is usually normal early in the course of disease and is not useful for prospective screening.[131] Plasma catecholamine levels are rarely elevated early, although a provocative stimulus such as exercise may cause an abnormal release of epinephrine.[167] The increased production of epinephrine probably accounts for headaches, palpitations, nervousness, and the absence of hypertension.

The diagnosis of pheochromocytoma is confirmed by computed tomography or magnetic resonance imaging of the abdomen. Scanning with [131I]metaiodobenzylguanidine, a catecholamine analogue that is selectively concentrated in adrenal chromaffin tissue, is useful for confirming the presence of functioning intra-adrenal chromaffin tissue (Fig. 30–9) and the exclusion of the rare extra-adrenal pheochromocytoma.[168, 169] Increased [131I]metaiodobenzylguanidine uptake may be observed in adrenomedullary hyperplasia.[148] It is rarely necessary to perform adrenal angiography, and if it is performed, the patient should receive alpha- and beta-adrenergic antagonists during the procedure (see Chapter 10).

More than half of individuals with MEN 2A will develop unilateral or bilateral pheochromocytomas. In the rare family in which there is a documented history of adrenomedullary malignancy (fewer than 10 reported cases[169]), bilateral adrenalectomy is mandatory, preferably as soon as the diagnosis of gene carrier status is made.[160] There is a dichotomy of thought about how to manage the adrenal lesions in other MEN 2A kindreds. Most physicians remove only adrenal glands demonstrated to contain a pheochromocytoma.[8, 170, 171] If a unilateral pheochromocytoma is found, the contralateral adrenal gland is inspected at surgery and removed only if the gland is nodular or enlarged.[132] This selective approach may prevent or postpone the necessity for glucocorticoid and mineralocorticoid replacement. Because of the 50% likelihood that nonaffected adrenal glands will develop a pheochromocytoma within 10 y, other clinicians advocate a bilateral adrenalectomy at the time of first operation.[169, 172, 173] The major advantage of the latter approach is that the patient is subjected to the risk of a single surgical procedure; disadvantages include the necessity for glucocorticoid and mineralocorticoid replacement and the risks associated with adrenal insufficiency. Alpha- and beta-adrenergic antagonists should be administered before and during surgery (see Chapter 10). An anterior surgical approach should be used to allow inspection of both adrenal glands and to exclude the rare extra-adrenal pheochromocytoma.

Hyperparathyroidism

Hyperparathyroidism occurs in 10 to 20% of individuals with the mature form of the MEN 2A syndrome.[6, 7, 59, 60] The initial reports described the presence of either parathyroid hyperplasia or multiple parathyroid adenomas in association with hypercalcemia, urolithiasis, or osteitis fibrocystica. A careful review of the histology of these tumors has demonstrated occasional adenomatous formation with a background of parathyroid hyperplasia,[174] a finding that is analogous to that observed for C cell hyperplasia in the thyroid gland and chromaffin cell hyperplasia in the adrenal medulla. Hyperparathyroidism is almost never seen in patients thyroidectomized for early C cell abnormalities, although histological findings consistent with parathyroid hyperplasia have been observed.[8] Whether these patients will eventually develop hypercalcemia is unknown. Before development of hypercalcemia the earliest indication of abnormal parathyroid function is incomplete suppression of parathyroid function by a calcium infusion,[138] which implies a set point abnormality similar to that seen in patients with MEN 1.[40]

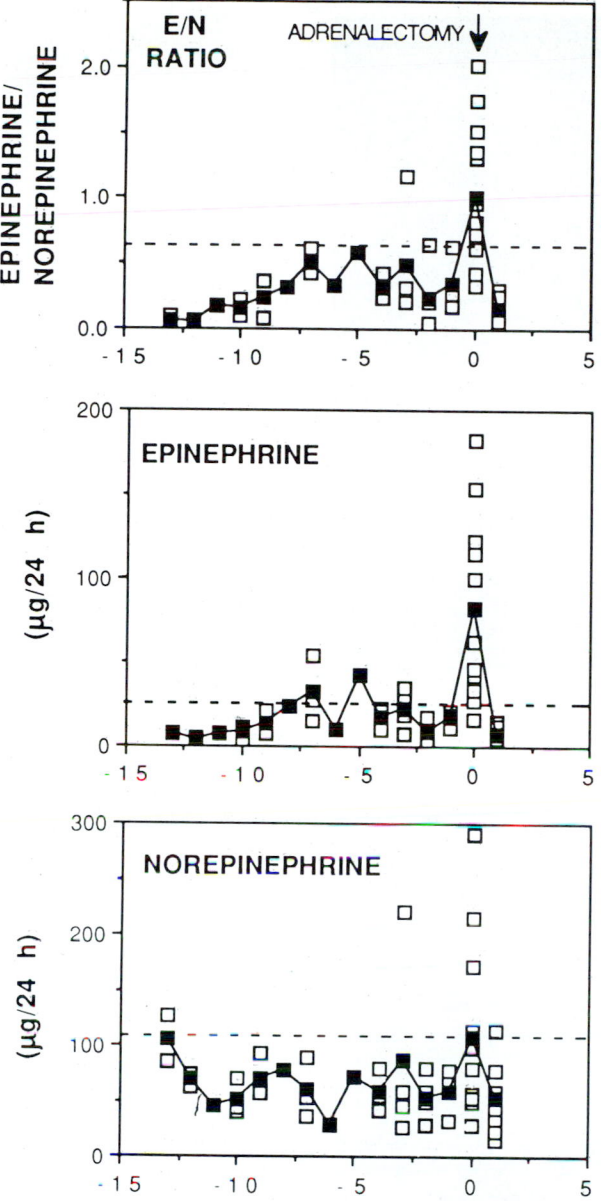

Figure 30–8. Results of 24-h urinary norepinephrine excretion, epinephrine excretion, and ratio of epinephrine to norepinephrine in 11 prospectively screened patients proved to have pheochromocytoma. Each open square indicates a value or the mean of two or more values for a patient, and each filled square, the mean for all the subjects in a particular year; the latter symbols are connected by a solid line. The dashed line shows the upper limit of normal. To convert epinephrine values to nanomoles, multiply by 5.458; to convert norepinephrine values to nanomoles, multiply by 5.911. (From Gagel RF, Tashjian AH Jr, Cummings T, et al. The clinical outcome of prospective screening for multiple endocrine neoplasia type 2a. An 18-year experience. Reprinted with permission from The New England Journal of Medicine, 318, 478–484, 1988.)

Surgical management of hyperparathyroidism is similar to that described for MEN 1.

Cutaneous Lichen Amyloidosis

Two families have been described in which MEN 2A was associated with a cutaneous form of lichen amyloidosis (Fig. 30–10). In the first, each individual with MEN 2A had a pruritic skin lesion over the scapular region of the upper back consisting of multiple infiltrated papules overlying a well-demarcated plaque.[175] In addition, three children at risk

for development of MEN 2A had the skin lesion. One of these children subsequently had an abnormal pentagastrin test. In the second family, three of five family members with MEN 2A had an identical skin lesion.[176] In the second kindred the skin lesion did not appear until after age 18 and increased in size over several decades, whereas in the first kindred the skin lesion was present early in life. In both families the histological picture was that of cutaneous lichen amyloidosis (deposition of amyloid at the juncture of the epidermis and dermis). Immunohistochemical staining of the amyloid for keratin but not calcitonin was observed in the second family, which indicates that the amyloid was likely of dermal origin and was not the result of deposition of calcitonin gene products from the thyroid carcinoma.[176]

Whether the two syndromes represent a contiguous gene syndrome (as has been suggested for MEN 2A and 2B) or result from a more complex abnormality is not clear. Nonetheless, it would seem prudent to screen patients with hereditary forms of cutaneous lichen amyloidosis for MEN 2A to determine the true incidence of this syndrome.

Family Screening

Screening for medullary thyroid carcinoma (Table 30–1) is performed by measurement of the serum calcitonin level before and 2, 5, and 10 min after the intravenous injection of pentagastrin (0.5 µg/kg body weight).[13, 177] The administration of calcium immediately before the pentagastrin injection enhances the sensitivity of the test,[177] although with the availability of more sensitive calcitonin assays this addition may be unnecessary. A positive test is one in which either the basal serum calcitonin concentration is elevated and is further increased by the administration of pentagastrin or one in which the basal value is normal but increases into the abnormal range after the administration of pentagastrin. It is important that the samples be analyzed with the most sensitive assay available; it is now possible to

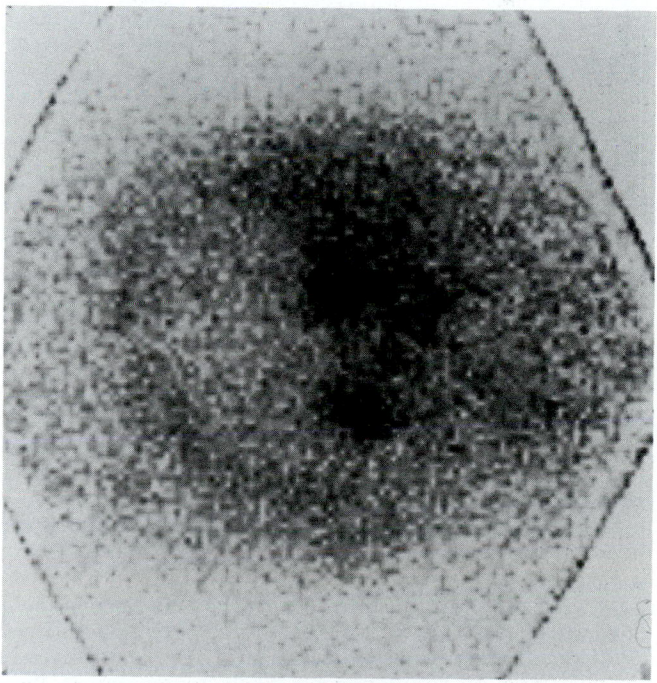

Figure 30–9. A positive radioactive iodine metaiodobenzylguanidine scan of a patient with MEN 2A and bilateral pheochromocytomas. A subtraction technique to remove hepatic and splenic background activity was used to enhance the image.

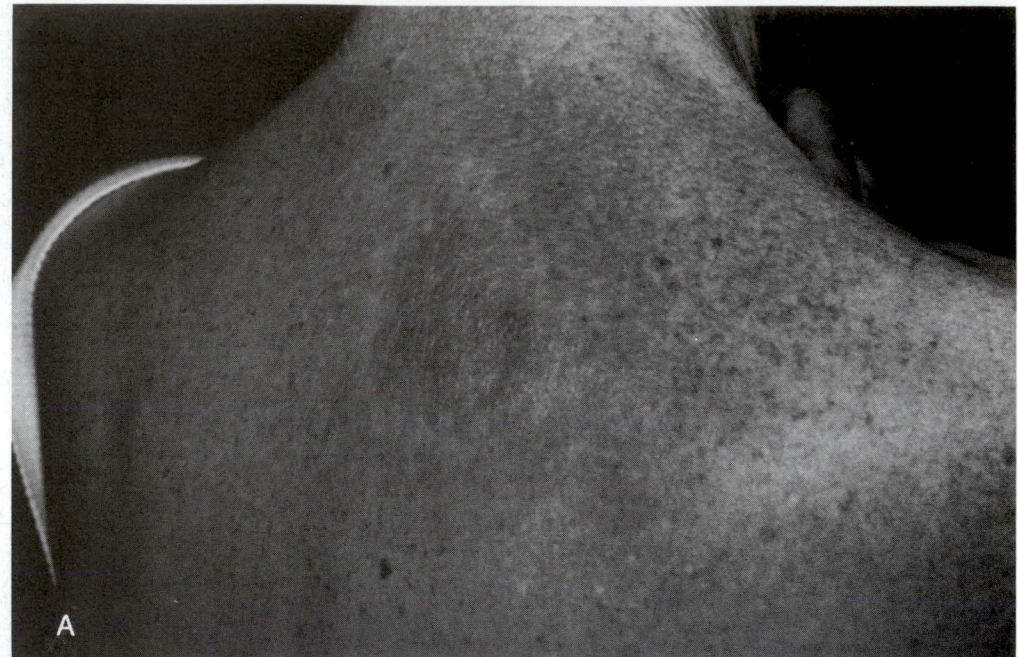

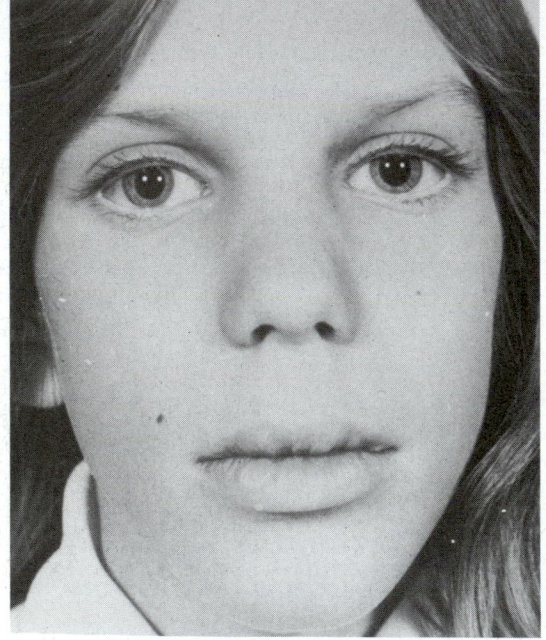

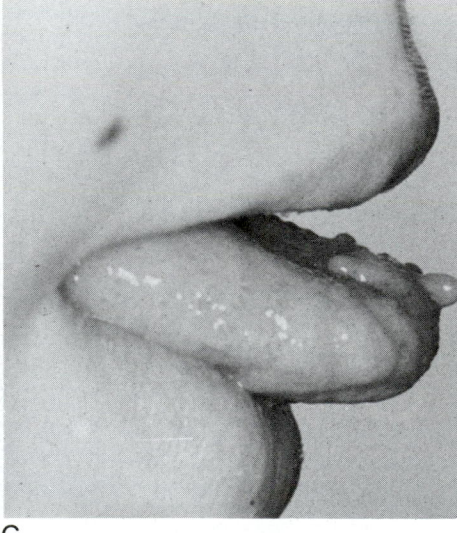

Figure 30–10. *A,* The characteristic clinical picture of cutaneous lichen amyloidosis associated with MEN 2A. The pruritic skin lesion may cover a small area or the entire right or left upper back, as shown in this patient. (From Gagel RF, Levy ML, Donovan DT, et al. Multiple endocrine neoplasia type 2A associated with cutaneous lichen amyloidosis. Ann Intern Med 1989; 111:802–806.)

B and *C,* Patient with MEN 2B demonstrating thick bumpy lips and eversion of upper eyelids *(B)* and neuromas on anterior third of tongue *(C).* (Reproduced with permission from Brown RS, Colle E, Tashjian AH Jr. The syndrome of multiple mucosal neuromas and medullary thyroid carcinoma in childhood. Importance of recognition of the phenotype for the early detection of malignancy. J Pediatr 1975; 86:77–83.)

routinely measure normal serum calcitonin levels (0.15 to 3 pmol/L [0.5 to 10 pg/mL]),[178–181] thereby making it possible to separate normal subjects from those with early C cell hyperplasia. Criteria that are useful for separation of normal from abnormal kindred members include a parent known to be affected and a consistently abnormal test result (two or more nonconsecutive test results that are abnormal).[8, 9]

A test result in which there is an elevation of the basal serum calcitonin level with no further increase after a provocative test can be difficult to interpret. Such a test result can be seen in association with C cell abnormalities, but this type of result is most likely to be caused by a nonspecific or false-positive increase of the serum calcitonin concentration[8, 182] or by production of calcitonin by a tumor other than medullary thyroid carcinoma (lung carcinoma, hepatoma, pheochromocytoma, pancreatic islet cell tumor, or benign liver disease). Separation of a false-positive test result from a true elevation of the serum calcitonin concentration can be made by a radioimmunoassay using a different polyclonal antiserum or a two-site immunoradiometric assay.[180, 181] Establishment of ectopic production of calcitonin by a tumor other than medullary thyroid carcinoma can be more difficult; however, such tumors frequently produce a high-molecular-weight form of unprocessed procalcitonin,[183] and release of immunoreactive calcitonin may not be increased by pentagastrin.

Screening should be offered to relatives of patients with MEN 2A and to relatives of individuals with medullary thyroid carcinoma who have features of hereditary medullary thyroid carcinoma. There are several reasons for such

TABLE 30–1. Screening for Multiple Endocrine Neoplasia

Syndrome	Test	Testing During Establishment of Gene Carrier Status		Testing After Establishment of Gene Carrier Status	
		Frequency	Age (y) at Testing	Frequency	Age (y) at Testing
MEN I	Ionized serum calcium*	Every 3–5 y	15–50	Every 3–5 y	20–50
	Serum prolactin†	Every 3–5 y	>15	Every 3–5 y	>15
	Serum gastrin‡			Every 3–5 y	>25
	Imaging of pituitary§			Every 5–10 y	20–60
MEN 2A	Pentagastrin test with serum calcitonin measurements at 0, 2, and 5 min‖	Yearly	1–35	1–2 y and then every 5 y#	Lifetime
	12- or 24-h urine test for epinephrine and norepinephrine**	Yearly	5–50	Yearly	5–60
	Ionized serum calcium*	Biyearly	20–40	Biyearly	Lifetime
MEN 2B	Pentagastrin test with serum calcitonin measurements at 0, 2, and 5 min††	Yearly	Birth–20	1–2 y and then every 5 y#	Lifetime
	12- or 24-h urine test for epinephrine and norepinephrine**	Yearly	5–50	Yearly	5–60

*This test could be serum ionized calcium or albumin-adjusted serum calcium.

†Hypercalcemia is generally the first manifestation of this syndrome and affects almost 100% of gene carriers by age 40. Therefore, screening for all manifestations including pituitary and pancreatic tumors can be discontinued or the frequency reduced if hypercalcemia is not observed by age 40.

‡Measurement of serum gastrin is indicated for all family members with symptoms consistent with Zollinger-Ellison syndrome at any age.

§The necessity for pituitary imaging studies is controversial, especially if measurements of prolactin, growth hormone, and cortisol are normal.

‖It may be difficult to perform a pentagastrin test in a 1-y-old child, but a two-point test (calcitonin measurements before and 3–5 min after pentagastrin injection) will provide maximal information.

#Medullary thyroid carcinoma will almost always be the first detectable manifestation of MEN 2. After total thyroidectomy for medullary thyroid carcinoma, a follow-up pentagastrin test should be performed at 1- to 2-y intervals for 5 y and then less frequently to detect tumor recurrence.

**Collection of a complete 24-h urine sample is difficult and a 12-h specimen will provide adequate sensitivity for screening purposes.

††Identification of the mucosal neuroma phenotype is frequently difficult at birth. For this reason all children born to a parent with the phenotype should be screened.

screening. First, reliance on family history alone systematically underestimates the true incidence of MEN 2A because the disease becomes clinically expressed in only about 60% by age 70.[184–186] Second, the new mutation rate for MEN 2A appears to be low, and therefore identification of a single MEN 2A case makes it likely that other family members will be identified. The fact that the disease appears to be benign in one generation should not deter screening efforts because the disease may assume a more virulent expression in a subsequent generation.[185] Although a physician's legal responsibility may end after immediate family members have been notified of the genetic nature of the disease, it is prudent to encourage patients to make even distant family members at risk aware of the nature of the disease. This notification has been done by giving pamphlets describing the syndrome to immediate family members for distribution to more distant relatives. In addition, an apparent case of sporadic medullary thyroid carcinoma may represent a familial form of the disease. Criteria for separation of hereditary from sporadic medullary thyroid carcinoma, including bilaterality and multicentricity of the hereditary form of the disease,[144] are not foolproof.[187] In many cases, screening of first-degree relatives is the only certain method for exclusion of hereditary disease.[185, 186] Development of the capacity to identify the MEN 2A gene or a closely linked genetic marker should make it easier to separate sporadic from familial disease.[18, 188]

Screening for medullary thyroid carcinoma in known kindreds should begin between ages 1 and 2 (see Table 30–1). C cell hyperplasia in MEN 2A has been reported as early as 20 mo, and microscopic medullary thyroid carcinoma has occurred at age 3;[12] metastasis in MEN 2A has been observed as early as age 6.[189] Performance of a pentagastrin test in a small child is challenging, but a modified test consisting of measurement of basal and 3- to 4-min values after pentagastrin administration provides useful information.

Widespread prospective screening has had an impact on the natural history of the syndrome. The mean age at diagnosis in prospectively screened kindreds is between ages 7 and 13, compared with a mean age of 33 when screening

first began in 1969.[184, 186] It is now possible to offer genetic counseling before childbearing, because more than 90% of cases are diagnosed before age 25.[184–186]

Because of the earlier age at diagnosis, more preneoplastic lesions of the thyroid (C cell hyperplasia) and a lower incidence of metastatic disease are present at the time of diagnosis. Whether prospective screening and early thyroidectomy are curative for the thyroid neoplasm is less clear. Although it is too early to draw firm conclusions, follow-up data from three groups (Table 30–2) indicate that approximately 90% of kindred members who were thyroidectomized for early disease have normal or nondetectable calcitonin values at mean follow-up periods ranging from 1 to 10 y.

The rapid progress in the identification of closely linked markers for MEN 2A has made it possible to use these markers for prediction of disease status with 90 to 98%

TABLE 30–2. Disease Status in Patients Thyroidectomized for Early Medullary Thyroid Carcinoma in MEN 2A

Group	n	Age (y)	Disease Status at Follow-up			Time Period of Follow-up (y)
			−	+	?	
Tufts and Harvard Universities	22	12	19	—	3	10
Mayo Clinic	15	7	14	1	—	?
Duke and Washington Universities	25		24	1	—	5.4
Totals	62		57	2	3	
% of total			92	3	5	

Data extracted from three large series with variable lengths of follow-up: Gagel RF, Tashjian AH Jr, Cummings T, et al. The clinical outcome of prospective screening for multiple endocrine neoplasia type 2a. An 18-year experience. N Engl J Med 1988; 318:478–484; Telander RL, Zimmerman D, van Heerden JA, et al. Results of early thyroidectomy for medullary thyroid carcinoma in children with multiple endocrine neoplasia type 2. J Pediatr Surg 1986; 21:1190–1194; and Wells SA Jr, Baylin SB, Leight GS, et al. The importance of early diagnosis in patients with hereditary medullary thyroid carcinoma. Ann Surg 1982; 195:595–599.

certainty.[190, 191] At present these techniques are used by investigators in conjunction with pentagastrin testing to be certain of gene carrier status before early thyroidectomy. The prospect of more closely linked markers for the identification of the disease gene within the next few years makes it likely that gene carrier status will be predicted with greater accuracy. It is not now clear exactly how to use this information, but it is likely that thyroidectomy will be recommended for gene carriers, even before pentagastrin test results become positive, because of the greater than 90% probability that gene carriers will develop medullary thyroid carcinoma.[185, 186] It is not likely that identification of gene carrier status will alter the management of hyperparathyroidism or pheochromocytoma in this syndrome, except in families with a history of malignant pheochromocytoma.

MULTIPLE ENDOCRINE NEOPLASIA, TYPE 2B

The association of medullary thyroid carcinoma and pheochromocytoma with multiple mucosal neuromas is termed MEN 2B. Documentation that MEN 2B is linked to the same area on chromosome 10 to which MEN 2A is mapped[192] suggests that MEN 2B is a more appropriate designation than MEN 3.[193] The hallmark of this syndrome is the presence of characteristic mucosal neuromas on the distal portion of the tongue (see Fig. 30–10), on the lips and subconjunctival areas, and throughout the gastrointestinal tract.[193–195] Affected corneal nerves may be identified by slit lamp examination, and enlarged nerves are frequently noted during neck or abdominal surgery. Ganglioneuromatosis of the gastrointestinal tract can cause obstruction, dilation of the colon, or a colic-like childhood syndrome with associated diarrhea[24, 196] and may be the first clinical manifestation of MEN 2B. Other features associated with this syndrome include a marfanoid habitus; pectus excavatum; slipped femoral epiphysis; and long, thin extremities.[193–195]

The presence of the mucosal neuroma phenotype is associated, in all reported cases, with bilateral and multicentric C cell hyperplasia and/or medullary thyroid carcinoma. The clinical course of patients with medullary thyroid carcinoma in this syndrome is more aggressive than that in MEN 2A; metastatic disease can occur in children younger than age 1 y,[12] and there is a shorter average survival time in patients with metastatic disease.[197] Less commonly, the disease may follow a more prolonged course, with survival into old age.[198, 199] MEN 2B is transmitted as an autosomal dominant trait,[200–202] but a large percentage of cases appear to represent new mutations. Unilateral or bilateral pheochromocytoma occurs in approximately half of individuals with this disorder[200–203] and is histologically similar to that in MEN 2A.

The identification of the mucosal neuroma phenotype in a child should alert the physician to the diagnosis of medullary thyroid carcinoma. Although it is important to confirm the diagnosis of C cell abnormalities by a provocative test for calcitonin release, the overwhelming likelihood of medullary thyroid carcinoma in such an individual makes it necessary to undertake thyroidectomy at the earliest possible age. It is not known whether such treatment is curative because experience is limited. The expressivity of the mucosal neuroma phenotype may be less than 100%. A case report in which a mother and one child had mucosal neuromas and medullary thyroid carcinoma and a second child

had medullary thyroid carcinoma but no evidence of the mucosal neuroma syndrome suggests this possibility.[204] Therefore, all children born to a parent expressing the phenotype, whether or not clinical evidence of ganglioneuromatosis is present, should be screened for medullary thyroid carcinoma. Routine screening (see Table 30–1) should not differ from that for MEN 2A except for the fact that hyperparathyroidism is rare in patients with MEN 2B.[200]

MULTIPLE ENDOCRINE NEOPLASIA OF MIXED TYPE

A number of hereditary MEN syndromes do not fit the MEN 1 or 2 categorization. These syndromes fall into four major categories. Overlap syndromes encompass one or more elements of either MEN 1 or 2, usually in a single patient. The majority of these cases likely represent the chance occurrence of an isolated tumor in a patient with one or the other MEN syndrome. A second type of syndrome is the familial occurrence of an unusual combination of endocrine organ neoplasia that does not fit either MEN 1 or 2 categorization. A third type of syndrome is an MEN 1 or 2 variant in which one manifestation predominates. Fourth, a few syndromes do not fit into any clear-cut pattern. Little is known about the molecular abnormalities in any of these disorders. It therefore seems most reasonable to chronicle these syndromes; an understanding of their pathogenesis awaits further developments.

OVERLAP SYNDROMES. Overlap syndromes in single patients include carcinoid and either MEN 1 or 2,[116] pituitary and adrenomedullary tumors with or without hyperparathyroidism,[205, 206] gastrinoma in an MEN 2 patient,[207] adenomatous polyposis coli and MEN 2B,[25] posterior pituitary tumor and MEN 1,[208] and prolactinoma in a patient with MEN 2A.[209]

FAMILIAL OCCURRENCE OF TWO OR MORE ENDOCRINE NEOPLASTIC DISORDERS. The association of pheochromocytoma and islet cell tumors can occur in familial[210–212] or nonfamilial patterns.[213–216] The association of von Hippel–Lindau disease, pheochromocytoma, and islet cell tumor has been described in one family, and other patients may have neurofibromatosis.[210] Neurofibromatosis with features of MEN 1 or 2[217] and neurofibromatosis in association with hyperparathyroidism have been reported,[218] although the infrequency of this association suggests a random occurrence. The von Hippel–Lindau and neurofibromatosis genes have been mapped to chromosomes 3 and 17, respectively, which makes it difficult to understand the connection between these two disorders and MEN 1 or 2.

MEN 1 OR 2 SYNDROMES IN WHICH A PARTICULAR MANIFESTATION PREDOMINATES. MEN 1 kindreds have been recognized in which prolactinoma[119, 120, 219] or insulinoma[47] is the predominant manifestation. Other families have been described in which other pituitary or pancreatic tumors predominate.[47] Whether these families represent true variants, result from variation in expressivity of a particular manifestation, or are a statistical aberration resulting from a small sample size is not clear. Variants of MEN 2A include familial medullary thyroid carcinoma[220] and familial pheochromocytoma.[221]

SYNDROMES THAT ARE DIFFICULT TO CATEGORIZE. A syndrome characterized by myxomas, spotty pigmentation, and generalized endocrine overactivity has been described in a single family. This syndrome appears to be transmitted as an autosomal dominant trait.[222]

GENETICS OF THE MULTIPLE ENDOCRINE NEOPLASIA SYNDROMES

At least one MEN syndrome (MEN 1) belongs to a group of heritable forms of neoplasia caused by deletion of a regulatory gene. Retinoblastoma (sporadic and familial) is the prototype for this type of malignancy. From an analysis of hereditary (bilateral) and nonhereditary (unilateral) retinoblastoma, Knudson[223, 224] proposed a "two-hit" theory for development of retinoblastoma and postulated that the first hit (or mutation) was inherited, whereas the second (mutation) occurred in somatic cells. Knudson's theory has been confirmed. Retinoblastoma in both its hereditary and nonhereditary forms results from deletion of a specific gene on chromosome 13. The retinoblastoma gene encodes a phosphoprotein and appears to function as a regulatory gene for growth of retinal cells.[225–229] In hereditary retinoblastoma the loss of one allele is inherited (the first hit), and the second is lost randomly via nondisjunction, nondisjunction reduplication, mitotic recombination, gene conversion, or point mutation–deletion (the second hit).[230] Retinal cells in which both copies of the gene are absent are likely to be transformed to the malignant state.

The MEN syndromes share many features with retinoblastoma. MEN is inherited as an autosomal dominant trait; the tumors in MEN, like hereditary retinoblastoma, are known to be polyclonal;[26] and the age at onset for medullary thyroid carcinoma and pheochromocytoma is similar to that observed for retinoblastoma.[231, 232] In MEN 1 families a deletional mechanism appears to be the basis for the syndrome. The MEN 1 gene has been mapped to the centromeric area of chromosome 11[16, 17] (Fig. 30–11). Studies of pancreatic islet tumors[17, 233–235] and parathyroid tumors[236, 237] from members of MEN 1 kindreds have demonstrated that the chromosome 11 allele inherited from the normal parent is lost, thereby indicating a mechanism similar to that in retinoblastoma.[17]

There is less evidence supporting a deletional mutation for MEN 2A or 2B. Studies with several families[18, 19, 20, 238–240] have linked MEN 2A to a locus near the centromere on chromosome 10 (see Fig. 30–11); attempts to demonstrate a deletion of genetic material in this region have been unsuccessful.[21, 241–244] MEN 2B has also been mapped to chromosome 10 by linkage analysis.[192] The significance of a previously described deletion on chromosome 20[245, 246] in MEN 2A and 2B is not clear and has not been observed for all kindreds.[247, 248]

Although studies to define the genetic lesion in the MEN syndromes are incomplete, certain conclusions can be drawn. The first is that MEN 1 and MEN 2 arise from different genetic lesions, thereby explaining the lack of clinical overlap between these two syndromes. A single genetic lesion may provide an explanation for the MEN 1 syndrome, but most investigators now believe that an inherited mutation on chromosome 10 coupled with other acquired genetic abnormalities is likely to be causative for the MEN 2A and 2B syndromes.[244] Second, at least two different genetic lesions can cause hyperparathyroidism, thereby explaining the differences in severity and age at onset for hyperparathyroidism in MEN 1 and MEN 2. Third, MEN 2A and 2B probably arise from similar genetic abnormalities or represent overlap syndromes, because both map to chromosome 10.

Animal models of MEN have been developed in transgenic mice by expression of known oncogenes.[249, 250] It is not clear how these model systems relate to human MEN, but these models or subsequent ones in which the specific genetic abnormality of MEN 1 or MEN 2 is expressed will serve as a starting point for understanding the molecular events causing neoplasia in these syndromes.

REFERENCES

1. Erdheim J. Zur normalen und pathologischen Histologie der Glandula Thyreoidea, Parathyreoidea und Hypophysis. Beitr Pathol Anat Allg Pathol 1903; 33:158–236.
2. Wermer P. Genetic aspects of adenomatosis of endocrine glands. Am J Med 1954; 16:363–371.
3. Underdahl LO, Woolner LB, Black BM. Multiple endocrine adenomas: report of 8 cases in which the parathyroids, pituitary and pancreatic islets were involved. J Clin Endocrinol 1953; 13:20–47.
4. Sipple JH. The association of pheochromocytoma with carcinoma of the thyroid gland. Am J Med 1961; 31:163–166.
5. Ballard HS, Frame B, Hartsock R. Familial multiple endocrine adenoma–peptic ulcer complex. Medicine 1964; 43:481–516.
6. Steiner AL, Goodman AD, Powers SR. Study of a kindred with pheochromocytoma, medullary carcinoma, hyperparathyroidism and Cushing's disease: multiple endocrine neoplasia, type 2. Medicine 1968; 47:371–409.
7. Melvin KEW, Tashjian AH Jr, Miller HH. Studies in familial (medullary) thyroid carcinoma. Recent Prog Horm Res 1972; 28:399–470.
8. Gagel RF, Tashjian AH Jr, Cummings T, et al. The clinical outcome of prospective screening for multiple endocrine neoplasia type 2a. An 18-year experience. N Engl J Med 1988; 318:478–484.
9. Graze K, Spiler IJ, Tashjian AH Jr, et al. Natural history of familial medullary thyroid carcinoma: effect of a program for early diagnosis. N Engl J Med 1978; 299:980–985.
10. Marx SJ, Vinik AI, Santen RJ, et al. Multiple endocrine neoplasia type I: assessment of laboratory tests to screen for the gene in a large kindred. Medicine 1986; 65:226–241.
11. Chong GC, Beahrs OH, Sizemore GW, et al. Medullary carcinoma of the thyroid gland. Cancer 1975; 35:695–704.
12. Telander RL, Zimmerman D, van Heerden JA, et al. Results of early thyroidectomy for medullary thyroid carcinoma in children with multiple endocrine neoplasia type 2. J Pediatr Surg 1986; 21:1190–1194.
13. Wells SA Jr, Ontjes DA, Cooper CW, et al. The early diagnosis of medullary carcinoma of the thyroid gland in patients with multiple endocrine neoplasia type II. Ann Surg 1975; 182:362–370.
14. Benson L, Ljunghall S, Akerstrom G, et al. Hyperparathyroidism presenting as the first lesion in multiple endocrine neoplasia type 1. Am J Med 1987; 82:731–737.
15. Norton JA, Cornelius MJ, Doppman JL, et al. Effect of parathyroidectomy in patients with hyperparathyroidism, Zollinger-Ellison syndrome, and multiple endocrine neoplasia type I: a prospective study. Surgery 1987; 102:958–966.
16. Bale S, Bale A, Stewart K, et al. Linkage analysis of multiple endocrine neoplasia type 1 with INT2 and other markers on chromosome 11. Genomics 1989; 4:320–322.
17. Larsson C, Skogseid B, Oberg K, et al. Multiple endocrine neoplasia type 1 gene maps to chromosome 11 and is lost in insulinoma. Nature 1988; 332:85–87.

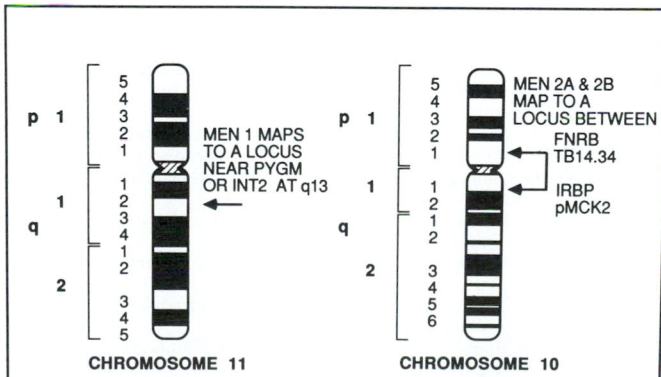

Figure 30–11. Schematic view of chromosomes 11 and 10 demonstrating the loci to which the MEN 1, 2A, and 2B genes have been mapped. PYGM (skeletal muscle glycogen phosphorylase), INT2, FNRB (beta subunit of the fibronectin receptor), TB14.34, IRBP (interstitial retinal-binding protein), and pMCK2 are DNA markers used to establish linkage and map the gene for each syndrome to a specific chromosome. MEN 1 has been tentatively mapped to 11q1 at a locus near PYGM or INT2. Flanking markers (shown on figure) have been identified for MEN 2A and 2B.

18. Simpson NE, Kidd KK, Goodfellow PJ, et al. Assignment of multiple endocrine neoplasia type 2A to chromosome 10 by linkage. Nature 1987; 328:528–530.

19. Mathew CG, Chin KS, Easton DF, et al. A linked genetic marker for multiple endocrine neoplasia type 2A on chromosome 10. Nature 1987; 328:527–528.

20. Sobol H, Salvetti A, Bonnardel C, et al. Screening multiple endocrine neoplasia type 2A families using DNA markers. Lancet 1988; 1:62.

21. Mathew CG, Smith BA, Thorpe K, et al. Deletion of genes on chromosome 1 in endocrine neoplasia. Nature 1987; 328:524–526.

22. Pearse A. Common cytochemical and ultrastructural characteristics of cells producing polypeptide hormones (the APUD series) and their relevance to thyroid and ultimobranchial C-cells and calcitonin. Proc R Soc Lond [Biol] 1968; 170:71–80.

23. Weidner N, Flanders DJ, Mitros FA. Mucosal ganglioneuromatosis associated with multiple colonic polyps. Am J Surg Pathol 1984; 8:779–786.

24. Khan AH, Desjardins JG, Youssef S, et al. Gastrointestinal manifestations of Sipple syndrome in children. J Pediatr Surg 1987; 22:719–723.

25. Perkins JT, Blackstone MO, Riddell RH. Adenomatous polyposis coli and multiple endocrine neoplasia type 2b. A pathogenetic relationship. Cancer 1985; 55:375–381.

26. Baylin SB, Gann DS, Hsu SH. Clonal origin of inherited medullary thyroid carcinoma and pheochromocytoma. Science 1976; 193:321–323.

27. Arnold A, Staunton CE, Kim HG, et al. Monoclonality and abnormal parathyroid hormone genes in parathyroid adenomas. N Engl J Med 1988; 318:658–662.

28. Jackson CE, Boonstra CE. The relationship of hereditary hyperparathyroidism to endocrine adenomatosis. Am J Med 1967; 43:727–734.

29. Jung RT, Grant AM, Davie M, et al. Multiple endocrine adenomatosis (type I) and familial hyperparathyroidism. Postgrad Med 1978; 54:92–94.

30. Johnson GJ, Summerskill WH, Anderson VE, et al. Clinical and genetic investigation of a large kindred with multiple endocrine adenomatosis. N Engl J Med 1967; 277:1379–1385.

31. Craven DE, Goodman D, Carter JH. Familial multiple endocrine adenomatosis. Multiple endocrine neoplasia, type I. Arch Intern Med 1972; 129:567–569.

32. Snyder N III, Scurry MT, Deiss WP. Five families with multiple endocrine adenomatosis. Ann Intern Med 1972; 76:53–58.

33. Eberle F, Grun R. Multiple endocrine neoplasia, type 1 (MEN I). Ergeb Inn Med Kinderheilkd 1981; 46:76–149.

34. Rizzoli R, Green J III, Marx SJ. Primary hyperparathyroidism in familial multiple endocrine neoplasia type I. Long-term follow-up of serum calcium levels after parathyroidectomy. Am J Med 1985; 78:467–474.

35. Marx SJ. Genetic defects in primary hyperparathyroidism. N Engl J Med 1988; 318:699–701 (editorial).

36. Marx SJ, Powell D, Shimkin PM, et al. Familial hyperparathyroidism. Ann Intern Med 1973; 78:371–377.

37. Marx SJ, Spiegel AM, Brown EM, et al. Family studies in patients with primary parathyroid hyperplasia. Am J Med 1977; 62:698–706.

38. Cutler RE, Reiss E, Ackerman LV. Familial hyperparathyroidism: a kindred involving eleven cases with a discussion of primary chief-cell hyperplasia. N Engl J Med 1964; 270:859–865.

39. Boey JH, Cooke TJ, Gilbert GM, et al. Occurrence of other endocrine tumours in primary hyperparathyroidism. Lancet 1975; 2:781–784.

40. Brown EM, LeBoff LM, Oetting M, et al. Secretory control in normal and abnormal parathyroid tissue. Recent Prog Horm Res 1987; 43:337–382.

41. Brown E, Gardner DG, Brennan MF, et al. Calcium-regulated parathyroid hormone release in primary hyperparathyroidism. Studies in vitro with dispersed parathyroid cells. Am J Med 1979; 66:923–931.

42. Niederle B, Roka R, Brennan MF. The transplantation of parathyroid tissue in man: development, indications, techniques and results. Endocr Rev 1982; 3:245–279.

43. Lamers CB, Froeling PG. Clinical significance of hyperparathyroidism in familial multiple endocrine adenomatosis type I (MEA I). Am J Med 1979; 66:422–424.

44. Prinz RA, Gamvros OI, Sellu D, et al. Subtotal parathyroidectomy for primary chief cell hyperplasia of the multiple endocrine neoplasia type I syndrome. Ann Surg 1981; 193:26–29.

45. van Heerden JA, Kent RB III, Sizemore GW, et al. Primary hyperparathyroidism in patients with multiple endocrine neoplasia syndromes. Surgical experience. Arch Surg 1983; 118:533–536.

46. Marx SJ, Sakaguchi K, Green J III, et al. Mitogenic activity on parathyroid cells in plasma from members of a large kindred with multiple endocrine neoplasia type 1. J Clin Endocrinol Metab 1988; 67:149–153.

47. Brandi ML, Marx SJ, Aurbach GD, et al. Familial multiple endocrine neoplasia type I: a new look at pathophysiology. Endocr Rev 1987; 8:391–405.

48. Brandi ML, Aurbach GD, Fitzpatrick LA, et al. Parathyroid mitogenic activity in plasma from patients with familial multiple endocrine neoplasia type 1. N Engl J Med 1986; 314:1287–1293.

49. Zimening MB, Brandi ML, deGrange DA, et al. Circulating fibroblast growth factor–like substance in familial multiple endocrine neoplasia type 1. J Clin Endocrinol Metab 1990; 70:149–154.

50. Goldsmith RE, Sizemore GW, Chen I, et al. Familial hyperparathyroidism: description of a large kindred with physiologic observations and a review of the literature. Ann Intern Med 1976; 84:36–43.

51. Sandler LM, Moncrieff MW. Familial hyperparathyroidism. Arch Dis Child 1980; 55:146–147.

52. Mallette L, Malini S, Rappaport M, et al. Familial cystic parathyroid adenomatosis. Ann Intern Med 1987; 107:54–60.

53. Marx SJ, Attie MF, Levine MA, et al. The hypocalciuric or benign variant of familial hypercalcemia: clinical and biochemical features in fifteen kindreds. Medicine 1981; 60:397–412.

54. Law WMJ, Heath H III. Familial benign hypercalcemia (hypocalciuric hypercalcemia). Clinical and pathogenetic studies in 21 families. Ann Intern Med 1985; 102:511–519.

55. Schachner SH, Riley TR, Old JW, et al. Familial hyperparathyroidism. Arch Intern Med 1966; 117:417–421.

56. Carey MC, Fitzgerald O. Hyperparathyroidism associated with chronic pancreatitis in a family. Gut 1968; 9:700–703.

57. Marsden P, Anderson J, Doyle D, et al. Familial hyperparathyroidism. Br Med J 1971; 3:87–90.

58. Kennett S, Pollick H. Jaw lesions in familial hyperparathyroidism. Oral Surg 1971; 31:502–510.

59. Keiser HR, Beaven MA, Doppman J, et al. Sipple's syndrome: medullary thyroid carcinoma, pheochromocytoma. Ann Intern Med 1973; 78:561–579.

60. Cance WG, Wells SA Jr. Multiple endocrine neoplasia type IIa. Curr Probl Surg 1985; 22:1–56.

61. Yamaguchi K, Abe K, Otsubo K, et al. The WDHA syndrome: clinical and laboratory data on 28 Japanese cases. Peptides 1984; 5:415–421.

62. Zaniewski M, Jordan PH Jr, Yip B, et al. Serum gastrin level is increased by chronic hypercalcemia of parathyroid or nonparathyroid origin. Arch Intern Med 1986; 146:478–482.

63. Wilson SD, Singh RB, Kalkhoff RK, et al. Does hyperparathyroidism cause hypergastrinemia? Surgery 1976; 80:2311–2317.

64. Friesen SR, Kimmel JR, Tomita T. Pancreatic polypeptide as screening marker for pancreatic polypeptide apudomas in multiple endocrinopathies. Am J Surg 1980; 139:61–72.

65. Lamers CB, Diemel J, Roeffen W. Serum levels of pancreatic polypeptide in Zollinger-Ellison syndrome and hyperparathyroidism from families with multiple endocrine adenomatosis type I. Digestion 1978; 18:297–302.

66. Skogseid B, Oberg K, Benson L, et al. A standardized meal stimulation test of the endocrine pancreas for early detection of pancreatic endocrine tumors in multiple endocrine neoplasia type 1 syndrome: five years experience. J Clin Endocrinol Metab 1987; 64:1233–1240.

67. Strodel WE, Vinik AI, Eckhauser FE, et al. Hyperparathyroidism and gastroenteropancreatic hormone levels. Surgery 1985; 98:1101–1106.

68. Mallette LE, Blevins T, Jordan PH, et al. Autogenous parathyroid grafts for generalized primary parathyroid hyperplasia: contrasting outcome in sporadic hyperplasia versus multiple endocrine neoplasia type I. Surgery 1987; 101:738–745.

69. Wells SA Jr, Ellis G, Gunnells J, et al. Parathyroid autotransplantation in primary parathyroid hyperplasia. N Engl J Med 1976; 195:57–62.

70. Pilato FP, D'Adda T, Banchini E, et al. Nonrandom expression of polypeptide hormones in pancreatic endocrine tumors. An immunohistochemical study in a case of multiple islet cell neoplasia. Cancer 1988; 61:1815–1820.

71. van Heerden JA, Smith SL, Miller LJ. Management of the Zollinger-Ellison syndrome in patients with multiple endocrine neoplasia type I. Surgery 1986; 100:971–977.

72. Rasbach DA, van Heerden JA, Telander RL, et al. Surgical management of hyperinsulinism in the multiple endocrine neoplasia, type 1 syndrome. Arch Surg 1985; 120:584–589.

73. Gorden P, Comi R, Maton P, et al. Somatostatin and somatostatin analogue (SMS 201–995) in treatment of hormone-secreting tumors of the pituitary and gastrointestinal tract and non-neoplastic diseases of the gut. Ann Intern Med 1989; 110:35–50.

74. Jensen RT, Maton PN, Gardner JD. Current management of Zollinger-Ellison syndrome. Drugs 1986; 32:188–196.

75. Zollinger RM. Gastrinoma: factors influencing prognosis. Surgery 1985; 97:49–54.

76. Deveney CW, Deveney KS, Way LW. The Zollinger-Ellison syndrome—23 years later. Ann Surg 1978; 188:384–393.

77. Lamers CB, Buis JT, van Tovgeren J. Secretin-stimulated serum gastrin levels in hyperparathyroid patients from families with multiple endocrine adenomatosis type I. Ann Intern Med 1977; 86:719–724.

78. Zollinger R, Ellison E. Primary peptic ulcerations of the jejunum associated with islet cell tumors of the pancreas. Ann Surg 1955; 142:709–728.

79. Jensen R, Doppman J, Gardner J. Gastrinoma. In: Gardner JD, Brooks FP, Lebenthal E, eds. The Endocrine Pancreas. New York: Raven, 1986: 729–745.

80. Ellison E, Carey L, Sparks J, et al. Early surgical treatment of gastrinoma. Am J Med 1987; 82:17–24.

81. Lambers CB, Lind T, Moberg S, et al. Omeprazole in Zollinger-Ellison syndrome. Effects of a single dose and of long-term treatment in patients resistant to histamine H₂-receptor antagonists. N Engl J Med 1984; 310:758–761.

82. Stabile BE, Ippoliti AF, Walsh JH, et al. Failure of histamine H₂-receptor antagonist therapy in Zollinger-Ellison syndrome. Am J Surg 1983; 145:17–23.

83. Gyr K, Whitehouse I, Beglinger C, et al. Human pharmacological effects of SMS 201–995 on gastric secretion. Scand J Gastroenterol 1986; 21(Suppl 119):96–102.

84. Kvols L, Buck M, Moertel C. Treatment of metastatic islet cell carcinoma with a somatostatin analogue (SMS 201–995). Ann Intern Med 1987; 107:162–168.

85. Tisell LE, Ahlman H, Jansson S, et al. Total pancreatectomy in the MEN-1 syndrome. Br J Surg 1988; 75:154–157.

86. Stefanini P, Carboni M, Patrassi N, et al. Beta-islet cell tumors of the pancreas: results of a study on 1,067 cases. Surgery 1974; 75:597–609.

87. Kolmannskog F, Schrumpf E, Valnes K. Computed tomography and angiography in pancreatic apudomas and cystadenomas. Acta Radiol [Diagn] (Stockh) 1982; 23:365–372.

88. Telander RL, Charboneau JW, Haymond MW. Intraoperative ultrasonography of the pancreas in children. J Pediatr Surg 1986; 21:262–266.

89. Tuft G, Edis A, Service F, et al. Plasma glucose monitoring during operation for insulinoma: a critical reappraisal. Surgery 1980; 88:519–526.

90. Stefanini P, Carboni M, Patrassi N, et al. The surgical treatment of occult insulinomas: a review of the problem. Br J Surg 1974; 61:1–4.

91. Kessenger A, Foley JF, Lemon HM. Therapy of malignant APUD cell tumors: effectiveness of DTIC. Cancer 1983; 51:790–794.

92. Croughs RJM, Hulsmans HAM, Israel DE, et al. Glucagonoma as part of the polyglandular adenoma syndrome. Am J Med 1972; 52:690–698.

93. Vance JE, Stoll RW, Kitabchi AE, et al. Familial nesidioblastosis as the predominant manifestation of multiple endocrine adenomatosis. Am J Med 1972; 52:211–227.

94. Bordi C, De Vita O, Pilato FP, et al. Multiple islet cell tumors with predominance of glucagon-producing cells and ulcer disease. Am J Clin Pathol 1987; 88:153–161.

95. Ramsay JA, Kovacs K, Asa SL, et al. Reversible sellar enlargement due to growth hormone–releasing hormone production by pancreatic endocrine tumors in a acromegalic patient with multiple endocrine neoplasia type I syndrome. Cancer 1988; 62:445–450.

96. Asa SL, Singer W, Kovacs K, et al. Pancreatic endocrine tumour producing growth hormone–releasing hormone associated with multiple endocrine neoplasia type I syndrome. Acta Endocrinol 1987; 115:331–337.

97. Ruttman E, Kloppel G, Bommer G, et al. Pancreatic glucagonoma with and without syndrome. Immunocytochemical study of 5 tumour cases and review of the literature. Virchows Arch [A] 1980; 388:51–67.

98. Stacpoole PW, Jaspan J, Kasselberg AG, et al. A familial glucagonoma syndrome: genetic, clinical and biochemical features. Am J Med 1981; 70:1017–1026.

99. Altimari A, Bhoopalam N, O'Dorsio T, et al. Use of a somatostatin analog (SMS 201–995) in the glucagonoma syndrome. Surgery 1986; 100:989–996.

100. Namihira Y, Achord JL, Subramony C. Multiple endocrine neoplasia, type 1, with pancreatic cholera. Am J Gastroenterol 1987; 82:794–797.

101. Lee CH, Ching KN, Lui WY, et al. Carcinoid tumor of the pancreas causing the diarrheogenic syndrome: report of a case combined with multiple endocrine neoplasia, type I. Surgery 1986; 99:123–129.

102. Gagel RF, Costanza ME, DeLellis RA, et al. Streptozotein-treated Verner-Morrison syndrome: plasma vasoactive intestinal peptide and tumor responses. Arch Intern Med 1976; 136:1429–1435.

103. Antunes JL, Housepian EM, Frantz AG, et al. Prolactin-secreting pituitary tumors. Ann Neurol 1977; 2:148–153.

104. Scheithauer BW, Horvath E, Kovacs K, et al. Plurihormonal pituitary adenomas. Semin Diagn Pathol 1986; 3:69–82.

105. Scheithauer BW, Laws ERJ, Kovacs K, et al. Pituitary adenomas of the multiple endocrine neoplasia type I syndrome. Semin Diagn Pathol 1987; 4:205–211.

106. Weil C. The safety of bromocriptine in long-term use: a review of the literature. Curr Med Res Opin 1986; 10:25–51.

107. Ferrari C, Crosignani PG. Medical treatment of hyperprolactinaemic disorders. Hum Reprod 1986; 1:507–514.

108. Fossati P, Dewailly D, Thomas DP, et al. Medical treatment of hyperprolactinemia. Horm Res 1985; 22:228–238.

109. Berger G, Trouillas J, Bloch B, et al. Multihormonal carcinoid tumor of the pancreas secreting growth hormone–releasing factor as a cause of acromegaly. Cancer 1984; 54:2097–2108.

110. Sano T, Yamasaki R, Saito H, et al. Growth hormone–releasing hormone (GHRH)–secreting pancreatic tumor in a patient with multiple endocrine neoplasia type I. Am J Surg Pathol 1987; 11:810–819.

111. Chadenas D, Pinsard D, Melliere D, et al. Endocrine pancreatic tumor secreting somatostatin and somatocrinin. Presse Med 1985; 14:2129–2134.

112. Thorner M, Frohman L, Leong D, et al. Extrahypothalamic growth-hormone–releasing factor (GRF) secretion is a rare cause of acromegaly: plasma GRF levels in 177 acromegaly patients. J Clin Endocrinol Metab 1984; 59:46–49.

113. Samaan NA, Schultz PN, Yang KP, et al. Endocrine complications after radiotherapy for tumors of the head and neck. J Lab Clin Med 1987; 109:364–372.

114. Amano S, Hazama F, Haebara H, et al. Ectopic ACTH-MSH producing carcinoid tumor with multiple endocrine hyperplasia in a child. Acta Pathol Jpn 1978; 28:721–730.

115. Hashimoto K, Suemaru S, Hattori T, et al. Multiple endocrine neoplasia with Cushing's syndrome due to paraganglioma producing corticotropin-releasing factor and adrenocorticotropin. Acta Endocrinol 1986; 113:189–195.

116. Duh QY, Hybarger CP, Geist R, et al. Carcinoids associated with multiple endocrine neoplasia syndromes. Am J Surg 1987; 154:142–148.

117. Samaan NA, Hickey RC, Bedner TD, et al. Hyperparathyroidism and carcinoid tumor. Ann Intern Med 1975; 82:205–207.

118. Burton JL, Hartog M. Multiple endocrine adenomatosis (type 1) with cutaneous leiomyomata and cysts of Moll. Br J Dermatol 1977; 15:74–75.

119. Hershon K, Kelley W, Shaw C, et al. Prolactinomas as part of the multiple endocrine neoplastic syndrome type 1. Am J Med 1983; 74:713–720.

120. Bear JC, Briones UR, Fahey JF, et al. Variant multiple endocrine neoplasia I (MEN I Burin): further studies and non-linkage to HLA. Hum Hered 1985; 35:15–20.

121. Thompson JC, Lewis BG, Wiener I, et al. The role of surgery in the Zollinger-Ellison syndrome. Ann Surg 1983; 197:594–607.

122. Sipple JH. Multiple endocrine neoplasia type 2 syndromes: historical perspectives. Henry Ford Hosp Med J 1984; 32:219–221.

123. Sipple JH. The association of pheochromocytoma with carcinoma of the thyroid gland. Am J Med 1961; 31:163–166.

124. Cushman P Jr. Familial endocrine tumors: report of two unrelated kindred affected with pheochromocytomas, one also with multiple thyroid carcinomas. Am J Med 1962; 32:352–360.

125. Hazard J, Hawk W, Crile GJ. Medullary (solid) carcinoma of the thyroid: a clinicopathologic entity. J Clin Endocrinol Metab 1959; 19:152–161.

126. Williams ED. A review of 17 cases of carcinoma of the thyroid and phaeochromocytoma. J Clin Pathol 1965; 18:288–292.

127. Melvin KEW, Miller HH, Tashjian AH Jr. Early diagnosis of medullary carcinoma of the thyroid gland by means of calcitonin assay. N Engl J Med 1971; 285:1115–1120.

128. Sizemore GW, Carney JA, Heath H III. Epidemiology of medullary carcinoma of the thyroid gland: a 5-year experience (1971–1976). Surg Clin North Am 1977; 57:633–645.

129. Baylin SB. The multiple endocrine neoplasia syndromes: implications for the study of inherited tumors. Semin Oncol 1978; 5:35–45.

130. Wells SA Jr, Baylin SB, Leight GS, et al. The importance of early diagnosis in patients with hereditary medullary thyroid carcinoma. Ann Surg 1982; 195:595–599.

131. Gagel RF, Melvin KE, Tashjian AH Jr, et al. Natural history of the familial medullary thyroid carcinoma-pheochromocytoma syndrome and the identification of preneoplastic stages by screening studies: a five-year report. Trans Assoc Am Physicians 1975; 88:177–191.

132. Gagel RF, Tashjian AH Jr, Cummings T, et al. Impact of prospective screening for multiple endocrine neoplasia type 2. Henry Ford Hosp Med J 1987; 35:94–98.

133. Sizemore GW, Heath H III, Carney JA. Multiple endocrine neoplasia type 2. Clin Endocrinol Metab 1980; 9:299–315.

134. Russell CF, van Heerden JA, Sizemore GW, et al. The surgical management of medullary thyroid carcinoma. Ann Surg 1983; 197:42–48.

135. Jackson CE, Talpos GB, Kambouris A, et al. The clinical course after definitive operation for medullary thyroid carcinoma. Surgery 1983; 94:995–1001.

136. Jackson CE, Norum RA, Talpos GB, et al. Clinical value of calcitonin and carcinoembryonic antigen doubling times in medullary thyroid carcinoma. Henry Ford Hosp Med J 1987; 35:120–121.

137. Block MA, Jackson CE, Tashjian AH Jr. Management of occult medullary thyroid carcinoma: evidenced only by serum calcitonin level elevations after apparently adequate neck operations. Arch Surg 1978; 113:368–372.

138. Heath H III, Sizemore GW, Carney JA. Preoperative diagnosis of occult parathyroid hyperplasia by calcium infusion in patients with multiple endocrine neoplasia, type 2a. J Clin Endocrinol Metab 1976; 43:428–435.

139. Wolfe HJ, Melvin KEW, Cervi-Skinner SJ, et al. C-cell hyperplasia preceding medullary thyroid carcinoma. N Engl J Med 1973; 289:437–441.

140. DeLellis RA, Dayal Y, Tischler AS, et al. Multiple endocrine neoplasia (MEN) syndromes: cellular origins and interrelationships. Int Rev Exp Pathol 1986; 28:163–215.

141. Wolfe HJ, DeLellis RA. Familial medullary thyroid carcinoma and C-cell hyperplasia. Clin Endocrinol Metab 1981; 10:351–365.

142. Leape LL, Miller HH, Graze K, et al. Total thyroidectomy for occult familial medullary carcinoma of the thyroid in children. J Pediatr Surg 1976; 11:831–837.

143. Baylin SB, Wells SA Jr. Management of hereditary medullary thyroid carcinoma. Clin Endocrinol Metab 1981; 10:367–378.

144. Block MA, Jackson CE, Greenawald KA, et al. Clinical characteristics distinguishing hereditary from sporadic medullary thyroid carcinoma. Arch Surg 1980; 115:142–148.

145. Samaan NA, Schultz PN, Hickey RC. Medullary thyroid carcinoma: prognosis of familial versus sporadic disease and the role of radiotherapy. J Clin Endocrinol Metab 1988; 67:801–805.

146. Tisell L, Hansson G, Jansson S, et al. Reoperation in the treatment of asymptomatic metastasizing medullary thyroid carcinoma. Surgery 1986; 99:60–66.

147. Talpos GB, Jackson CE, Froelich JW, et al. Localization of residual medullary thyroid cancer by thallium/technetium scintigraphy. Surgery 1985; 98:1189–1196.

148. Yobbagy JJ, Levatter R, Sisson JC, et al. Scintigraphic portrayal of the syndrome of multiple endocrine neoplasia type-2B. Clin Nucl Med 1988; 13:433–437.

149. Baulieu JL, Guilloteau D, Delisle MJ, et al. Radioiodinated meta-iodobenzylguanidine uptake in medullary thyroid cancer. A French cooperative study. Cancer 1987; 60:2189–2194.

150. Itoh H, Sugie K, Toyooka S, et al. Detection of metastatic medullary thyroid cancer with ^{131}I-MIBG scans in Sipple's syndrome. Eur J Nucl Med 1986; 11:502–504.

151. Cote GJ, Gould JA, Huang SC, et al. Studies of short-term secretion of peptides produced by alternative RNA processing. Mol Cell Endocrinol 1987; 53:211–219.

152. Gagel RF, Palmer WN, Leonhart K, et al. Somatostatin production by a human medullary thyroid carcinoma cell line. Endocrinology 1986; 118:1643–1651.

153. Atkins FL, Beaven MA, Keiser HR. Dopa decarboxylase in medullary carcinoma of the thyroid. N Engl J Med 1973; 289:545–548.

154. OConnor DT, Deftos LJ. Secretion of chromogranin A by peptide-producing endocrine neoplasms. N Engl J Med 1986; 314:1145–1151.

155. Sevarino K, Wu P, Jackson I, et al. Biosynthesis of thyrotropin releasing hormone by a rat medullary thyroid carcinoma cell line. J Biol Chem 1988; 263:620–623.

156. Yamaguchi K, Abe K, Adachi I, et al. Concomitant production of immunoreactive gastrin-releasing peptide and calcitonin in medullary carcinoma of the thyroid. Metabolism 1984; 33:724–727.

157. Baylin SB, Beaven MA, Buja LM, et al. Histaminase activity: a biochemical marker for medullary carcinoma of the thyroid. Am J Med 1972; 53:723–733.

158. Gagel RF. Tumor markers of medullary thyroid carcinoma. In: Fishman WH, ed. On Codevelopmental Markers: Biologic Diagnostic and Monitoring Aspects. Vol 1. New York: Academic, 1983: 222–239.

159. Carney JA, Sizemore GW, Sheps SG. Adrenal medullary disease in multiple endocrine neoplasia, type 2: pheochromocytoma and its precursors. Am J Clin Pathol 1976; 66:279–290.

160. Carney JA, Sizemore GW, Tyce GM. Bilateral adrenal medullary hyperplasia in multiple endocrine neoplasia, type 2: the precursor of bilateral pheochromocytoma. Mayo Clin Proc 1975; 50:3–10.

161. DeLellis RA, Wolfe HJ, Gagel RF, et al. Adrenal medullary hyperplasia. A morphometric analysis in patients with familial medullary thyroid carcinoma. Am J Pathol 1976; 83:177–196.

162. Webb TA, Sheps SG, Carney JA. Differences between sporadic pheochromocytoma and pheochromocytoma in multiple endocrine neoplasia, type 2. Am J Surg Pathol 1980; 4:121–126.

163. Moraca-Kvapilova L, Op de Coul AA, Merkus JM. Cerebral haemorrhage in a pregnant woman with a multiple endocrine neoplasia syndrome (type 2A or Sipple's syndrome). Eur J Obstet Gynecol Reprod Biol 1985; 20:257–263.

164. Chodankar CM, Abhyankar SC, Deodhar KP, et al. Sipple's syndrome (multiple endocrine neoplasia) in pregnancy—case report. Aust NZ J Obstet Gynaecol 1982; 22:243–244.

165. Takai S, Miyauchi A, Matsumoto H, et al. Multiple endocrine neoplasia type 2 syndromes in Japan. Henry Ford Hosp Med J 1984; 32:246–250.

166. Hamilton BP, Landsberg L, Levine RJ. Measurement of urinary epinephrine in screening for pheochromocytoma in multiple endocrine neoplasia type II. Am J Med 1978; 65:1027–1032.

167. Telenius BM, Adolfsson L, Berg B, et al. Catecholamine release after physical exercise. A new provocative test for early diagnosis of pheochromocytoma in multiple endocrine neoplasia type 2. Acta Med Scand 1987; 222:351–359.

168. Valk TW, Frager MS, Gross MD, et al. Spectrum of pheochromocytoma in multiple endocrine neoplasia. A scintigraphic portrayal using ^{131}I-metaiodobenzylguanidine. Ann Intern Med 1981; 94:762–767.

169. Sisson JC, Shapiro B, Beierwaltes WH. Scintigraphy with I-131 MIBG as an aid to the treatment of pheochromocytomas in patients with the multiple endocrine neoplasia type 2 syndromes. Henry Ford Hosp Med J 1984; 32:254–261.

170. Tibblin S, Dymling JF, Ingemansson S, et al. Unilateral versus bilateral adrenalectomy in multiple endocrine neoplasia IIA. World J Surg 1983; 7:201–208.

171. Jansson S, Tisell LE, Fjalling M, et al. Early diagnosis of and surgical strategy for adrenal medullary disease in MEN II gene carriers. Surgery 1988; 103:11–18.

172. van Heerden JA, Sizemore GW, Carney JA, et al. Surgical management of the adrenal glands in the multiple endocrine neoplasia type II syndrome. World J Surg 1984; 8:612–621.

173. Lips CJ, Minder WH, Leo JR, et al. Evidence of multicentric origin of the multiple endocrine neoplasia syndrome type 2a (Sipple's syndrome) in a large family in the Netherlands. Diagnostic and therapeutic implications. Am J Med 1978; 64:569–578.

174. Carney JA, Roth SI, Heath H III, et al. The parathyroid glands in multiple endocrine neoplasia type 2b. Am J Pathol 1980; 99:387–398.

175. Nunziata V, Giannattasio R, di Giovanni G, et al. Hereditary localized pruritus in affected members of a kindred with multiple endocrine neoplasia type 2A (Sipple's syndrome). Clin Endocrinol 1989; 30:57–63.

176. Gagel RF, Levy ML, Donovan DT, et al. Multiple endocrine neoplasia type 2a associated with cutaneous lichen amyloidosis. Ann Intern Med 1989; 111:802–806.

177. Wells SA Jr, Baylin SB, Linehan WM, et al. Provocative agents and the diagnosis of medullary carcinoma of the thyroid gland. Ann Surg 1978; 188:139–141.

178. Catherwood BD, Deftos LJ. General principles, problems and interpretation in the radioimmunoassay of calcitonin. Biomed Pharmacother 1984; 38:235–241.

179. Body JJ, Heath H III. Estimates of circulating monomeric calcitonin: physiological studies in normal and thyroidectomized man. J Clin Endocrinol Metab 1983; 57:897–903.

180. Motte P, Vauzelle P, Gardet P, et al. Construction and clinical validation of a sensitive and specific assay for serum mature calcitonin using monoclonal anti-peptide antibodies. Clin Chim Acta 1988; 174:35–54.

181. Seth R, Motte P, Kehely A, et al. A sensitive and specific two-site enzyme-immunoassay for human calcitonin using monoclonal antibodies. J Endocrinol 1988; 119:351–357.

182. Body J, Heath H III. "Nonspecific" increases in plasma immunoreactive calcitonin in healthy individuals: discrimination from medullary thyroid carcinoma by a new extraction technique. Clin Chem 1984; 30:511–514.

183. Ghillani P, Motte P, Bohuon C, et al. Monoclonal antipeptide antibodies as tools to dissect closely related gene products. A model using peptides encoded by the calcitonin gene. J Immunol 1988; 141:3156–3163.

184. Gagel RF, Jackson CE, Block MA, et al. Age-related probability of development of hereditary medullary thyroid carcinoma. J Pediatr 1982; 101:941–946.

185. Ponder BA, Ponder MA, Coffey R, et al. Risk estimation and screening in families of patients with medullary thyroid carcinoma. Lancet 1988; 1:397–401.

186. Easton DF, Ponder MA, Cummings T, et al. The clinical and screening age-at-onset distribution for the MEN-2 syndrome. Am J Hum Genet 1989; 44:208–215.

187. Ekblom M, Valimaki M, Pelkonen R, et al. Familial and sporadic medullary thyroid carcinoma: clinical and immunohistological findings. Q J Med 1987; 65:899–910.

188. Mathew CG, Chin KS, Easton DF, et al. A linked genetic marker for multiple endocrine neoplasia type 2A on chromosome 10. Nature 1987; 328:527–528.

189. Graham SM, Genel M, Touloukian RJ, et al. Provocative testing for occult medullary carcinoma of the thyroid: findings in seven children with multiple endocrine neoplasia type IIa. J Pediatr Surg 1987; 22:501–503.

190. Sobol H, Narod SA, Nakamura Y, et al. Screening for multiple endocrine neoplasia type 2a with DNA-polymorphism analysis. N Engl J Med 1989; 321:996–1001.

191. Gagel RF. The impact of gene mapping techniques on the diagnosis of multiple endocrine neoplasia type 2. Trends Endocrinol 1990; 2:19–25.

192. Norum RA, Lafreniere RG, O'Neal LW, et al. Linkage of multiple endocrine neoplasia type 2B (MEN2B) to chromosome 10 markers linked to MEN2A. Genomics 1990; 8:313–317.

193. Khairi MR, Dexter RN, Burzynski NJ, et al. Mucosal neuroma, pheochromocytoma and medullary thyroid carcinoma: multiple endocrine neoplasia type 3. Medicine 1975; 54:89–112.

194. Carney JA, Sizemore GW, Hayles AB. C-cell disease of the thyroid gland in multiple endocrine neoplasia, type 2b. Cancer 1979; 44:2173–2183.

195. Williams ED, Pollock DJ. Multiple mucosal neuromata with endocrine tumours: a syndrome allied to von Recklinghausen's disease. J Pathol Bacteriol 1966; 91:71–80.

196. Carney JA, Go VL, Sizemore GW, et al. Alimentary-tract ganglioneuromatosis. A major component of the syndrome of multiple endocrine neoplasia, type 2b. N Engl J Med 1976; 295:1287–1291.

197. Kakudo K, Carney JA, Sizemore GW. Medullary carcinoma of thyroid. Biologic behavior of the sporadic and familial neoplasm. Cancer 1985; 55:2818–2821.

198. O'Neal L. Multiple endocrine neoplasia, type IIb: medullary carcinoma of the thyroid, pheochromocytomas, neuromas, and ganglioneuromatosis. Res Med 1983; 1:7–16.

199. Carney JA, Sizemore GW, Hayles AB. Multiple endocrine neoplasia, type 2b. Pathobiol Annu 1978; 8:105–153.

200. Dyck PJ, Carney JA, Sizemore GW, et al. Multiple endocrine neoplasia, type 2b: phenotype recognition; neurological features and their pathological basis. Ann Neurol 1979; 6:302–314.

201. Hubner A, Holschneider AM. Multiple endocrine neoplasias in 3 generations. Langenbecks Arch Chir 1987; 372:747–750.

202. Aine E, Aine L, Huupponen T, et al. Visible corneal nerve fibers and neuromas of the conjunctiva—a syndrome of type-3 multiple endocrine adenomatosis in two generations. Graefes Arch Clin Exp Ophthalmol 1987; 225:213–216.

203. Norton JA, Froome LC, Farrell RE, et al. Multiple endocrine neoplasia type IIb: the most aggressive form of medullary thyroid carcinoma. Surg Clin North Am 1979; 59:109–118.

204. Sciubba JJ, D'Amico E, Attie JN. The occurrence of multiple endocrine neoplasia type IIb, in two children of an affected mother. J Oral Pathol 1987; 16:310–316.

205. Anderson RJ, Lufkin EG, Sizemore GW, et al. Acromegaly and pituitary adenoma with phaeochromocytoma: a variant of multiple endocrine neoplasia. Clin Endocrinol 1981; 14:605–612.

206. Tateishi R, Wada A, Ishiguro S, et al. Coexistence of bilateral pheochromocytoma and pancreatic islet cell tumor: report of a case and review of the literature. Cancer 1978; 42:2928–2934.

207. Cameron D, Spiro HM, Landsberg L. Zollinger-Ellison syndrome with multiple endocrine adenomatosis type II. N Engl J Med 1978; 299:152–153 (letter).

208. Tuch BE, Carter JN, Armellin GM, et al. The association of a tumour of the posterior pituitary gland with multiple endocrine neoplasia type 1. Aust NZ J Med 1982; 12:179–181.

209. Bertrand JH, Ritz P, Reznik Y, et al. Sipple's syndrome associated with a large prolactinoma. Clin Endocrinol 1987; 27:607–614.

210. Carney JA, Go VLW, Gordon H, et al. Familial pheochromocytoma and islet cell tumor of the pancreas. Am J Med 1980; 68:515–521.

211. Hull MT, Warfel KA, Muller J, et al. Familial islet cell tumors in von Hippel–Lindau's disease. Cancer 1979; 44:1523–1526.

212. Janson KL, Roberts JA, Varela M. Multiple endocrine adenomatosis: in support of the common origin theories. J Urol 1978; 119:161–165.

213. Probst A, Lotz M, Heitz P. von Hippel–Lindau's disease, syringomyelia and multiple endocrine tumors: a complex neuroendocrinopathy. Virchows Arch [A] 1978; 378:265–272.

214. Mori Y, Kiyohara H, Miki T, et al. Pheochromocytoma with prominent calcification and associated pancreatic islet cell tumor. J Urol 1977; 118:843–844.

215. Nathan DM, Daniels GH, Ridgway EC. Gastrinoma and phaeochromocytoma: is there a mixed multiple endocrine adenoma syndrome? Acta Endocrinol 1980; 93:91–93.

216. Zeller JR, Kauffman HM, Komorowski RA, et al. Bilateral pheochromocytoma and islet cell adenoma of the pancreas. Arch Surg 1982; 117:827–830.

217. Hansen OP, Hansen M, Hansen HH, et al. Multiple endocrine adenomatosis of mixed type. Acta Med Scand 1976; 200:327–331.

218. Chakrabarti S, Murugesan A, Arida EJ. The association of neurofibromatosis and hyperparathyroidism. Am J Surg 1979; 137:417–420.

219. Farid NR, Buehler S, Russell NA, et al. Prolactinomas in familial multiple endocrine neoplasia syndrome type I. Relationship to HLA and carcinoid tumors. Am J Med 1980; 69:874–880.

220. Farndon JR, Leight GS, Dilley WG, et al. Familial medullary thyroid carcinoma without associated endocrinopathies: a distinct clinical entity. Br J Surg 1986; 73:278–281.

221. Irvin GL, Fishman LM, Sher JA. Familial pheochromocytoma. Surgery 1983; 94:938–940.

222. Carney J, Gordon H, Carpenter P, et al. The complex of myxomas, spotty pigmentation, and endocrine overactivity. Medicine 1985; 64:270–283.

223. Knudson AJ. Mutation and cancer: statistical study of retinoblastoma. Proc Natl Acad Sci USA 1971; 68:820–823.

224. Knudson AG Jr. Genetics of human cancer. Genetics 1975; 79:305–316.

225. Friend S, Bernards R, Rogelj S, et al. A human DNA segment with properties of the gene that predisposes to retinoblastoma and osteosarcoma. Nature 1986; 323:643–646.

226. Lee WH, Bookstein R, Hong F, et al. Human retinoblastoma susceptibility gene: cloning, identification, and sequence. Science 1987; 235:1394–1399.

227. Fung YK, Murphree AL, T'Ang A, et al. Structural evidence for the authenticity of the human retinoblastoma gene. Science 1987; 236:1657–1661.

228. T'Ang A, Varley JM, Chakraborty S, et al. Structural rearrangement of the retinoblastoma gene in human breast carcinoma. Science 1988; 242:263–266.

229. Benedict WF, Fung YK, Murphree AL. The gene responsible for the development of retinoblastoma and osteosarcoma. Cancer 1988; 62:1691–1694.

230. Cavenee W. Identification of recessive mutations at human cancer loci. Birth Defects 1987; 23:93–107.

231. Jackson CE, Brock MA, Greenawald KA, et al. The two-mutational event in medullary thyroid carcinoma. Am J Hum Genet 1979; 31:704–710.

232. Cerny JC, Jackson CE, Talpos GB, et al. Pheochromocytoma in multiple endocrine neoplasia type II: an example of the two-hit theory of neoplasia. Surgery 1982; 92:849–852.

233. Yoshimoto K, Iizuka M, Iwahana H, et al. Loss of the same alleles of HRAS1 and D11S151 in two independent pancreatic cancers from a patient with multiple endocrine neoplasia type 1. Cancer Res 1989; 49:2716–2721.

234. Nakamura Y, Larsson C, Julier C, et al. Localization of the genetic defect in multiple endocrine neoplasia type 1 within a small region of chromosome 11. Am J Hum Genet 1989; 44:751–755.

235. Oberg K, Skogseid B, Eriksson B. Multiple endocrine neoplasia type 1 (MEN-1). Clinical, biochemical and genetical investigations. Acta Oncol 1989; 28:383–387.

236. Thakker RV, Bouloux P, Wooding C, et al. Association of parathyroid tumors in multiple endocrine neoplasia type 1 with loss of alleles on chromosome 11. N Engl J Med 1989; 321:218–224.

237. Friedman E, Sakaguchi K, Bale AE, et al. Clonality of parathyroid tumors in familial multiple endocrine neoplasia type 1. N Engl J Med 1989; 321:213–218.

238. Yamamoto M, Takai S, Miki T, et al. Close linkage of MEN2A with RBP3 locus in Japanese kindreds. Hum Genet 1989; 82:287–288.

239. Farrer LA, Castiglione CM, Kidd JR, et al. A linkage group of five DNA markers on human chromosome 10. Genomics 1988; 3:72–77.

240. Nakamura Y, Mathew CG, Sobol H, et al. Linked markers flanking the gene for multiple endocrine neoplasia type 2A. Genomics 1989; 5:199–203.

241. Landsvater R, Mathew C, Smith B, et al. Development of multiple endocrine neoplasia type 2a does not involve substantial deletions of chromosome 10. Genomics 1989; 4:246–250.

242. Myers S, Wu J, Goodfellow P, et al. A linkage map of the pericentric region of chromosome 10 including the locus for multiple endocrine neoplasia (MEN 2A). Genome 1988; 30:239.

243. Nelkin BD, Nakamura Y, White RW, et al. Low incidence of loss of chromosome 10 in sporadic and hereditary human medullary thyroid carcinoma. Cancer Res 1989; 49:4114–4119.

244. Nelkin BD, de Bustros AC, Mabry M, et al. The molecular biology of medullary thyroid carcinoma. A model for cancer development and progression. JAMA 1989; 261:3130–3135.

245. Babu VR, Van DDL, Jackson CE. Chromosome 20 deletion in human multiple endocrine neoplasia types 2A and 2B: a double-blind study. Proc Natl Acad Sci USA 1984; 8:2525–2528.

246. Butler MG, Rames LJ, Joseph GM. Cytogenetic studies of individuals from four kindreds with multiple endocrine neoplasia type II syndrome. Cancer Genet Cytogenet 1987; 28:253–260.

247. Krizman DB, Pathak S, Samaan NA, et al. Quantitative study of a proposed interstitial del (20p 12.2) in multiple endocrine neoplasia (MEN-II). Anticancer Res 1986; 6:191–194.

248. Wurster-Hill DH, Noll WW, Bircher LY, et al. A cytogenetic study of familial medullary carcinoma of the thyroid. Cancer Res 1986; 2:134–138.

249. Reynolds RK, Hoekzema GS, Vogel J, et al. Multiple endocrine neoplasia induced by the promiscuous expression of a viral oncogene. Proc Natl Acad Sci USA 1988; 85:3135–3139.

250. Murphy D, Bishop A, Rindi G, et al. Mice transgenic for a vasopressin-SV40 hybrid oncogene develop tumors of the endocrine pancreas and the anterior pituitary. A possible model for human multiple endocrine neoplasia type 1. Am J Pathol 1987; 129:552–566.

31

THE IMMUNOENDOCRINOPATHY SYNDROMES

George S. Eisenbarth and Richard A. Jackson

INTRODUCTION

In 1926 Schmidt described the clinical course and autopsy findings in two patients with "eine biglandulare Erkrankung" (a two-gland illness).[1] These patients died of adrenal insufficiency and were found at autopsy to have had a destructive lymphocytic infiltration of both thyroid and adrenal cortex. Schmidt concluded that (1) an absence of the adrenomedullary pressor substance (epinephrine) could not account for the hypotension and death associated with the adrenal insufficiency because the adrenal medullas of the patients were normal, and (2) a related pathological process resulted in lymphocytic infiltration and destruction of both the adrenal cortex and the thyroid.

The major syndrome discussed in this chapter has been known by various names: the Schmidt syndrome, the polyglandular failure syndrome, organ-specific autoimmune disease, polyendocrinopathy diabetes, and the autoimmune polyglandular syndrome type II. The diverse names reflect the large number of studies and case reports of this disorder. Each name has some deficiency, such as failure to reflect the fact that both hyperfunction and hypofunction of endocrine glands can occur or failure to recognize that nonendocrine illness such as pernicious anemia can be part of the syndrome. It has also become clear that there is more than one type of polyendocrinopathy. In this discussion a somewhat revised nomenclature of Neufeld and colleagues will be used for the more common disorders, namely, autoimmune polyglandular syndrome, type I and type II.[2] Additional immunoendocrinopathy syndromes will be identified by eponymic terms.[2, 3]

The major illnesses associated with type I and type II syndromes are given in Table 31–1, and the major differences between the syndromes are defined in Table 31–2. The disease associations and the inheritance pattern make it possible to detect additional components of these syndromes in patients before the appearance of serious manifestations and to make the diagnosis in some first-degree relatives with unrecognized disease.

AUTOIMMUNE POLYGLANDULAR SYNDROME TYPE II

Clinical Definition

Autoimmune polyglandular syndrome type II is the most common of the immunoendocrinopathy syndromes and is usually defined by the occurrence in the same individual of two or more of the following: primary adrenal insufficiency (Addison disease) (Fig. 31–1), hyperthyroidism (Graves disease) or primary hypothyroidism, insulin-dependent (type I) diabetes mellitus, primary hypogonadism, myasthenia gravis, and celiac disease. Vitiligo, alopecia, serositis, Parkinson disease, and pernicious anemia occur with increased frequency relative to the unaffected (general) population. The definition of the syndrome relies on the finding that if one of the component illnesses is present, an associated illness occurs more commonly than in the general population. Furthermore, circulating organ-specific autoantibodies are commonly present, even in the absence of overt clinical disease. The initial lesion and precipitating events that result in the syndrome are unknown, but im-

TABLE 31–1. Component Disorders of Type I and Type II Polyendocrine Autoimmune Syndromes

Type I	Type II
Adrenal insufficiency	Adrenal insufficiency[2, 3, 9]
Mucocutaneous candidiasis[2, 3, 9]	
Hypoparathyroidism[2, 3, 9]	"Geriatric" hypoparathyroidism[19]
Chronic active hepatitis[2, 3, 9]	
Graves disease[2, 3, 9]	Graves disease[2, 3, 9]
Hypothyroidism[2, 3, 9]	Hypothyroidism[2, 3, 9]
Pernicious anemia[17]	Pernicious anemia[17]
Insulin-dependent diabetes mellitus[2, 3, 9]	Insulin-dependent diabetes mellitus[2, 3, 9]
Vitiligo[73]	Vitiligo[18]
Malabsorption syndrome (? secondary to hypocalcemia[150])	Celiac disease[55]
Alopecia[151]	Alopecia[11, 154]
Hypophysitis[42–47]	Hypophysitis[42–47]
Primary hypogonadism[2, 3, 9]	Primary hypogonadism[2, 3, 9]
	Myasthenia gravis[11]
	Parkinson disease[53, 54]
Keratoconjunctivitis[152]	Serositis[149]

TABLE 31–2. Contrasting Features of Polyglandular Syndromes

Type I	Type II
Only siblings affected	Multiple generations affected
No HLA-DR association	HLA-DR3/HLA-DR4 association
Mucocutaneous candidiasis	No candidiasis
Destructive hypoparathyroidism	Rare hypoparathyroidism (antibody mediated)
Insulin-dependent diabetes mellitus > 4%	Insulin-dependent diabetes mellitus 50%

munogenetic and immunological similarities are present, with regard to both the time course and the pathogenesis of each of the component disorders.

For this group of organ-specific autoimmune diseases a human leukocyte antigen (HLA)–associated genetic predisposition coupled with additional genetic factors and an unknown triggering event (? environmental factor or factors or somatic "mutation") results in an autoimmune process that produces glandular destruction or hyperfunction.[3] The concept of progressive glandular destruction has long been accepted for autoimmune thyroid disease, and a similar progressive process precedes overt insulin-dependent diabetes mellitus. Multiple studies of first-degree relatives of patients with insulin-dependent diabetes have shown that development of a series of anti-islet antibodies (e.g., anti-insulin autoantibodies, anticytoplasmic islet cell antibodies, anti–glutamate decarboxylase [anti-64K] antibodies, and antibodies reacting with the secretory "pole" of rat insulinoma cells) precedes by years the development of overt diabetes.[4–7] In the majority of prediabetics a progressive decrease in insulin secretion[4] can be demonstrated that is temporally associated with the appearance of anti-islet antibodies; hypoinsulinemia in such genetic prediabetics is most apparent after the intravenous administration of glucose (Fig. 31–2). Progressive destruction of pancreatic beta cells results in overt diabetes; C peptide secretion eventually ceases, and few remaining beta cells can be identified in pathological specimens.

The chronic development of organ-specific autoimmunity necessitates endocrinological evaluation over time of patients and families with autoimmune polyglandular syndrome type II. In a family in which the syndrome has been documented, relatives should be advised of the early symptoms and signs of the principal component diseases. Even in the absence of early signs and symptoms, relatives at risk and patients with multiple disorders should be screened every 3 to 5 y, with measurement of fasting glucose levels, a sensitive thyrotropin assay, measurement of serum vitamin B_{12} levels, and, if any symptoms or signs that suggest adrenal insufficiency are present, assay of cosyntropin-stimulated cortisol levels. A careful history and physical examination should also be done. If available, assays of cytoplasmic islet cell antibodies and antiadrenal antibodies may be helpful. As many as 20 y may elapse between the onset of one endocrinopathy and the diagnosis of the next; thus individuals with idiopathic (autoimmune) adrenal insufficiency should be evaluated over time as just described because as many as 45% of all such patients eventually develop one or more associated endocrinopathies.[8] In contrast, patients who have isolated thyroid disease but no family history of autoimmune polyglandular syndrome type II have a low incidence of additional polyglandular involvement.[9]

Immunogenetics

Major component diseases of the type II polyglandular syndrome include (in order of decreasing prevalence) hyperthyroidism, atrophic thyroiditis, insulin-dependent diabetes mellitus, adrenal insufficiency, celiac disease, and myasthenia gravis. Each of these illnesses is associated with the antigens HLA-B8 and HLA-DR3,[3] and primary adrenal

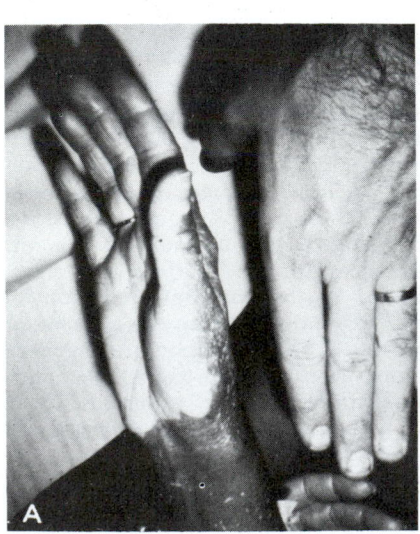
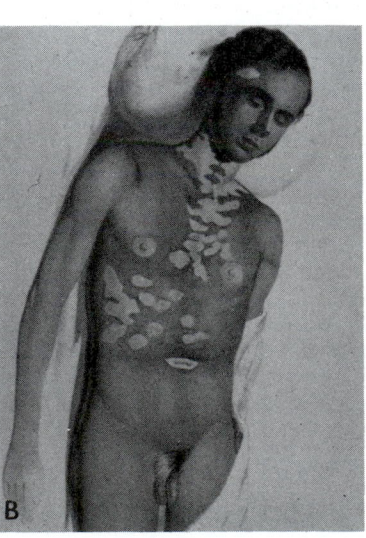

Figure 31–1. *A,* Hand of the proband of the family shown in Figure 31–3, with both hyperpigmentation of adrenal insufficiency and vitiligo, as contrasted with a normal hand. (Photograph courtesy of F. Neelon.) *B,* Reproduction of a plate from Addison's initial description of primary adrenal insufficiency (Addison disease). (From Addison T. On the Constitutional and Local Effects of Disease of the Supra-renal Capsules. London: Samuel Highley, 1855: plate XI.)

INTRAVENOUS GLUCOSE TOLERANCE TESTS   ORAL GLUCOSE TOLERANCE TESTS

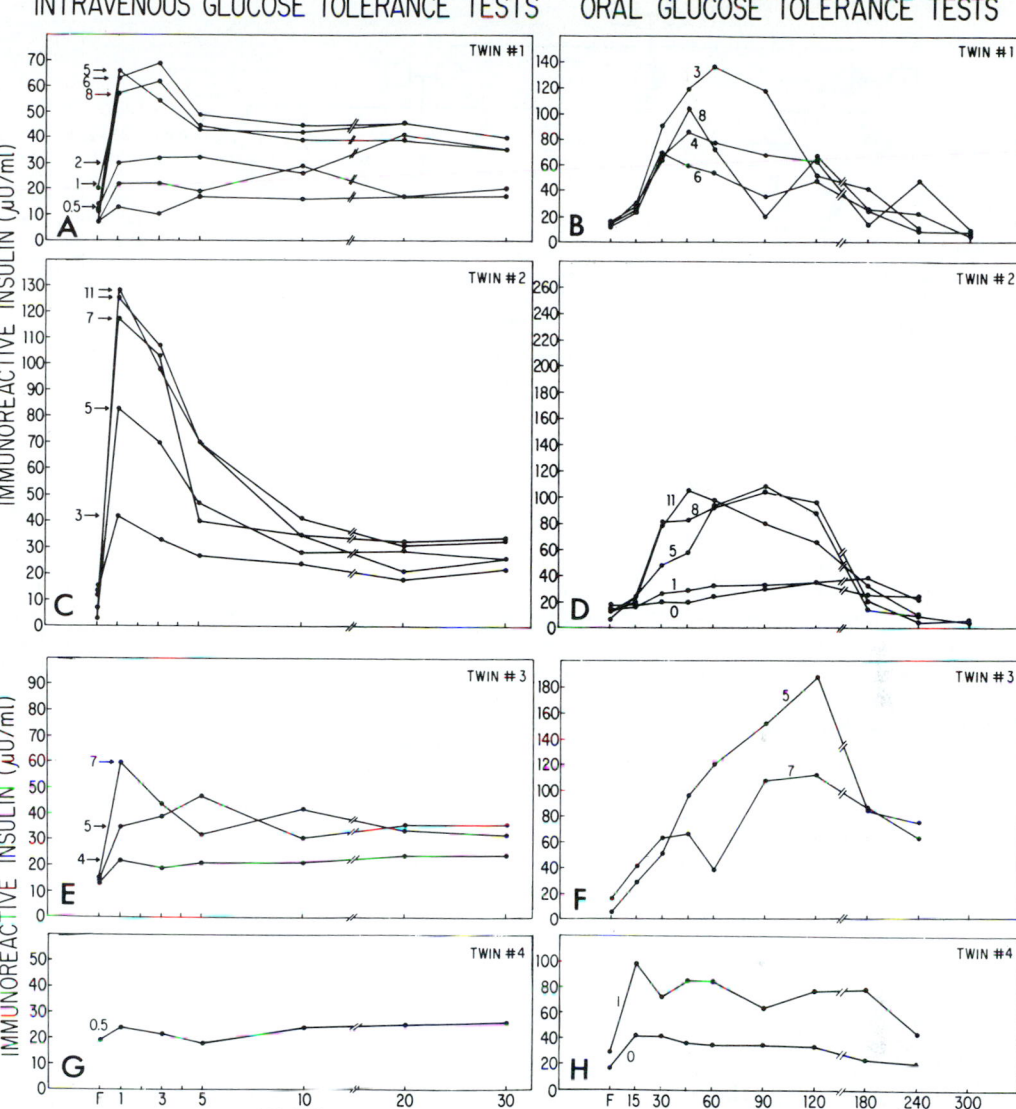

Figure 31–2. Insulin responses to intravenous and oral glucose in four monozygotic twins who developed insulin-dependent diabetes mellitus during prospective evaluation. The numbers adjacent to the curves indicate the number of years before the diagnosis of overt diabetes mellitus. The serum glucose level did not become abnormal even during oral glucose tolerance testing until the "acute" diagnosis of overt diabetes. (Reproduced, with permission, from Srikanta S, Ganda OP, Jackson RA, et al. Type I diabetes mellitus in monozygotic twins: chronic progressive beta cell dysfunction. Ann Intern Med 1983; 99:320–326.)

insufficiency, similar to insulin-dependent diabetes mellitus, is strongly associated with both HLA-DR3 and HLA-DR4.[10] In addition to this association with specific HLA markers, inheritance of disease within a given family usually (but not always) correlates with inheritance of a common HLA haplotype.[11–14] The inheritance of disease in three generations of a family in which all affected members share the same A1, B8 haplotype is schematized in Figure 31–3.[11] This family illustrates the fact that a susceptibility to the development of the polyendocrine syndrome, rather than a specific illness, is inherited. The proband had myasthenia gravis, adrenal insufficiency, hypothyroidism, premature ovarian failure, and vitiligo. The only family history of disease was of hyperthyroidism in a brother. When relatives were evaluated as part of an immunogenetic study, the mother and an aunt were found to have primary hypothyroidism, and both had had alopecia totalis since childhood. Another brother was hypothyroid and had primary testicular failure, and one niece had autoimmune thyroid disease. In one study of 10 families with this syndrome, one in seven relatives had unsuspected illness, most commonly autoimmune thyroid disease.[3]

Several disorders that occur in patients with the polyendocrine autoimmune syndrome are not associated with HLA-B8 or HLA-DR3 in population studies. These disorders include pernicious anemia,[15] goitrous thyroiditis,[16, 17] and vitiligo.[18] The association of vitiligo with adrenal insufficiency dates from Addison's initial description of the disease (see Fig. 31–1). These relatively common illnesses may have more than one pathogenic mechanism, one of which is associated with polyglandular failure.[3]

We have described several elderly patients with type II polyendocrine disease who had a distinct form of hypoparathyroidism, which, based on a small series of patients, may be termed *geriatric hypoparathyroidism*.[19] These elderly patients were distinct in that they had antibodies to the surface of parathyroid cells capable of suppressing parathyroid function and they had a self-limited course of antibody presence and hypoparathyroidism. Hypoparathyroidism frequently occurs in the type I polyendocrine syndrome but is rare with the type II syndrome. If hypocalcemia occurs in a patient with the type II syndrome, celiac disease may be a more likely diagnosis than primary hypoparathyroidism.

Other HLA-B8, HLA-DR3–associated autoimmune diseases are not thought to be classically associated disorders but probably should be considered part of the autoimmune polyglandular syndrome type II. These diseases include the Sjögren syndrome,[20] selective immunoglobulin A defi-

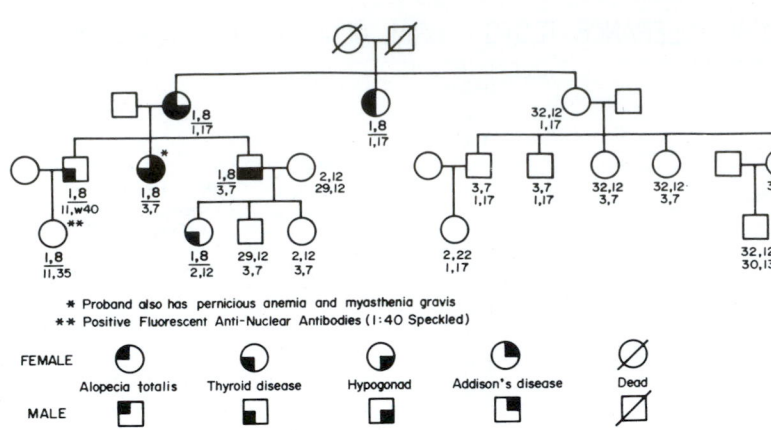

Figure 31–3. Results of HLA typing and clinical evaluation of a polyglandular kindred. Haplotypes, one above the other, were deduced from HLA typing and the pattern of inheritance. The occurrence of disease is as noted. An asterisk indicates the proband. (From Eisenbarth GS, Wilson P, Ward F, et al. HLA type and occurrence of disease in familial polyglandular failure. Reprinted with permission from The New England Journal of Medicine, 298, 92–94, 1978.)

ciency,[21, 22] juvenile dermatomyositis,[23] systemic lupus erythematosus,[24] chronic active hepatitis,[25–27] and dermatitis herpetiformis.[28, 29] Sjögren syndrome is associated with autoimmune thyroid disease,[30] and immunoglobulin A deficiency is associated with insulin-dependent diabetes mellitus and other endocrine diseases.[31–35] In addition to HLA-DR3–associated disorders, case reports also link polyendocrine autoimmunity with optic atrophy and lipodystrophy,[36] autoimmune thrombocytopenic purpura,[37–39] idiopathic diabetes insipidus with autoantibodies to vasopressin cells,[40] multiple endocrine neoplasia,[41] hypophysitis,[42–47] pseudolymphoma,[48] silent thyroiditis,[49] isolated corticotropin (ACTH, adrenocorticotropin) deficiency,[50, 51] pituitary tumors,[52] scleroderma,[12] and Parkinson disease.[53, 54]

The occurrence of one HLA-DR3–associated illness in a patient suggests that she or he may be genetically susceptible to other HLA-DR3–associated illnesses. In all the HLA-B8–associated diseases in white populations, HLA-DR3 is more strongly associated with disease than is HLA-B8. The HLA-B8 allele appears to be associated with these illnesses because it is nonrandomly associated with HLA-DR3 (linkage disequilibrium). Association of HLA alleles with each other and with disease can be complex. Celiac disease is strongly associated with insulin-dependent diabetes mellitus. One study of "random" small bowel biopsies of Finnish patients with insulin-dependent diabetes found that as many as 3% of these insulin-dependent diabetics had celiac disease.[55] Despite the association of both HLA-B8 and HLA-DR3 with insulin-dependent diabetes and celiac disease, celiac disease is associated primarily with chromosomes (termed *extended haplotypes*) containing HLA-B8 and HLA-DR3 and complement alleles S, C, 0, and 1, and with chromosomes lacking HLA-A1 and expressing the glyoxylase 1 or 2 allele. In insulin-dependent diabetes, the DR3-related disease–associated haplotype has HLA-A1 and glyoxylase 2 but not glyoxylase 1.[56] In the HLA region the extended haplotypes have deletions and duplications over almost a million base pairs[57] and appear to have been inherited as intact units of multiple alleles.

The HLA region has been extensively characterized.[58] Three class II genes (DP, DQ, DR, the immune response genes) are within the HLA region, as are the genes determining congenital adrenal hyperplasia, hemochromatosis, standard A and B transplantation antigens (class I genes), and complement molecules and tumor necrosis factor. Subclasses of human T lymphocytes react with antigen-presenting cells or target cells that express either class II (HLA-DP, HLA-DQ, and HLA-DR) or class I (HLA-A and HLA-B) molecules. For example, CD4-positive T cells (helper cells) react with antigen-presenting cells expressing class II molecules, whereas CD8-positive T cells (cytotoxic cells) react with target cells expressing class I molecules. Class II molecules (DP, DQ, DR) consist of two chains, an alpha chain and a beta chain. The beta chains of each class II molecule of different individuals differ in their amino acid sequence and are given numbers (also see Chapter 24). The crystallographic structure of a class I molecule (HLA-A, HLA-B, and HLA-C) has been defined, T cell receptor genes have been isolated, and the mechanism of generating immunological diversity has been described.[58, 59]

Class II molecules on the surface of antigen-presenting cells (predominantly lymphoid cells, although essentially any cell can be induced to express these molecules) function to bind peptides. The binding of peptides to these class II molecules can determine the immune response to a given antigen because the T cell receptor of CD4-positive T cells "sees" only antigen that is bound in the "cleft" of these molecules. Genetically determined differences in the linear sequence of class II molecules influence peptide binding and thereby alter antigen presentation and immune response.

In addition to a profound influence on T cell function by antigen presentation, expression of class II molecules at the level of the thymus can lead to the deletion of whole groups of T cells bearing families of related T cell receptors.[60] The unique T cell receptor of each clone of T cells is created by random genetic rearrangements. Whole families of variable region T cell receptor genes can be deleted, depending on the class II molecule expressed by an individual. This deletion of groups of T cells bearing specific families of T cell receptors may influence the development of autoimmunity.

An individual determined to be DR4-positive by standard HLA typing may have one of several different sequences at the DR beta and DQ beta loci. For example, a "DR4"-positive individual by standard antibody typing may express a sequence of DQ beta, DQ3.1, which has an aspartic acid at position 57 of the beta chain, or DQ3.2, which lacks aspartic acid at this position. In addition, the DR beta molecule may be any of several different subtypes: Dw4, Dw10, Dw13, Dw14, or Dw15. It has been reported that only DR4-positive individuals expressing the allele DQ3.2 and the allele Dw4 or Dw10 are at increased risk for developing diabetes mellitus (Fig. 31–4).[61] Other DR4-bearing haplotypes in white persons did not increase the risk of developing diabetes mellitus, and thus individuals who express DR4, DQ3.2 with Dw14, or DR4, DQ3.1 with Dw4 do not appear to have an increased vulnerability to this disease. Just as the class I allele B8 is associated with insulin-dependent diabetes mellitus because it is in linkage disequilibrium with DR3, the DR4 allele is associated with this disorder in large part because it is linked with a specific DQ allele (DQ3.2) and specific DR beta alleles Dw4 or Dw10.

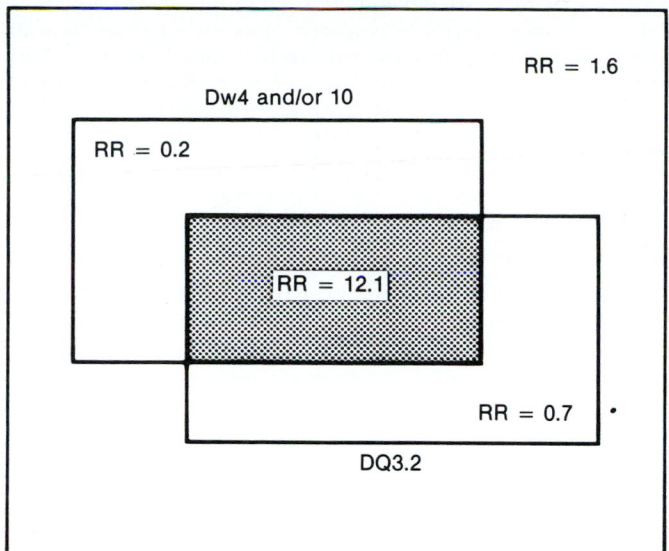

All DR4 Haplotypes

Figure 31–4. Venn diagram of relative risks for development of insulin-dependent diabetes mellitus in white patients, with DR4 divided by specific HLA-DQ and HLA-Dw4–defined haplotypes. Increased risk is conferred only by chromosomes expressing both DQ3.2 and Dw4 or Dw10. (From Sheehy MJ, Scharf SJ, Rose JR, et al. A diabetes-susceptible HLA haplotype is best defined by a combination of HLA-DR and DQ alleles. Reproduced from the Journal of Clinical Investigation, 1989, vol. 83, pp. 830–835 by copyright permission of the American Society for Clinical Investigation.)

Several human diabetes-associated DQ alleles, such as DQ3.2, lack an aspartic acid at position 57 of the beta chain, and even the nonobese diabetic (NOD) mouse (an animal model of insulin-dependent diabetes mellitus) lacks aspartic acid at position 57 in its analogous class II gene (termed I-A).[62, 63]

The specific genes that contribute to diabetes susceptibility on DR3-containing haplotypes are not well defined. It is likely that a gene or genes in linkage disequilibrium with HLA-DR3 (e.g., DP alleles or other genes within the HLA region such as the gene for tumor necrosis factor) contribute to the pathogenesis of the multiple autoimmune illnesses of the polyglandular autoimmune syndrome through an influence on immune function.

In human insulin-dependent diabetes mellitus at the time of onset of overt disease, but apparently not in the two animal models of this disease (NOD mouse and BB rat), class II antigens can be detected on beta cells.[64, 65] In thyroiditis and Graves disease, thyroid epithelial cells express such molecules. A combination of lymphokines can induce class II antigen expression and can enhance class I expression by almost all cells. Such antigenic changes of the target organ may contribute to the persistence of autoimmunity.

The genetic influence of the HLA region can only be a part of the pathogenesis of polyendocrine autoimmunity and is probably permissive. Indeed, HLA associations do not explain the various patterns of disease in different family members, the variation in the age at onset of the different disorders in a single affected individual, or the presence of only a 50% concordance for the respective diseases in monozygotic twins. The risk of identical twins developing insulin-dependent diabetes mellitus or Graves disease is greater than the risk of HLA-identical siblings developing these disorders, which suggests that, similar to animal models of diabetes (see later), a gene (or genes) outside the HLA region may contribute to disease susceptibility.

Organ-Specific Autoantibodies

The initial lesion of polyglandular syndrome type II and of its component illnesses is not known. Other chapters of this text detail immunological phenomena associated with the individual diseases. In each of these disorders, organ-specific autoantibodies are present. Some of these autoantibodies, such as the anti–acetylcholine receptor antibodies associated with myasthenia gravis, are specific disease markers and are also directly implicated in the pathophysiology of the disorder. For example, in the family shown schematically in Figure 31–3, only the proband with myasthenia gravis had antibodies that precipitated acetylcholine receptors. In contrast to the specificity and documented pathogenic role of anti–acetylcholine receptor antibodies, many of the organ-specific autoantibodies associated with other components of the syndrome, such as antithyroglobulin antibodies, thyroidal antimicrosomal antibodies, and anti–parietal cell antibodies, are present in the absence of clinically overt disease (and have a low positive predictive value for development of future disease).[66, 67] Such antibodies are also common in normal relatives of affected individuals, many of whom will not progress to overt disease.[67] Antithyroid antibodies reacting with thyroid peroxidase (antimicrosomal) and thyroglobulin are so frequent as to be of little predictive value for overt hypothyroidism, unless accompanied by subclinical elevations of thyrotropin. Antibodies to parietal cells and intrinsic factor are also found in a substantial number of normal individuals, but their presence correlates statistically with decreased gastric acid secretion and pernicious anemia.[68]

Anti–islet cell antibodies (ICAs) have been detected in the circulation of patients developing insulin-dependent diabetes mellitus (by using frozen sections of pancreas). Specific quantitative assays (>40 Juvenile Diabetes Foundation units of ICAs) have shown such antibodies to be present in 0.25% of the normal population. These normal individuals are at increased risk for development of diabetes. In the past 5 y, extensive studies of individuals with anti-ICAs have been undertaken.[69] Patients with type II polyendocrinopathy who express cytoplasmic ICAs appear to develop diabetes more slowly than ICA-positive first-degree relatives of insulin-dependent diabetics. Approximately 8% per year of ICA-positive first-degree relatives of such patients develop diabetes (Fig. 31–5), whereas the corresponding value for ICA-positive patients with polyendocrinopathy, who are on average older when screened, is approximately 2% per year. In families with a member who has insulin-dependent diabetes, approximately 1 of 50 first-degree relatives of the diabetic is antibody-positive. When autoantibodies are first detected, individuals may already be glucose intolerant or have partial loss of beta cell function, as determined by intravenous glucose tolerance testing.[4, 6] We have proposed a dual-parameter linear model[70] for prediction of time to onset of overt diabetes of ICA-positive relatives: years to diabetes = 2.5(1 + 3 min insulin on intravenous glucose tolerance testing)/(concentration of insulin autoantibodies). Insulin release during this test appears to reflect the amount of beta cell destruction, and the concentration of insulin autoantibodies the activity of the autoimmune process.[70] The slower rate of development of overt diabetes among ICA-positive patients with polyendocrinopathy[71] may reflect their older age, because older ICA-positive relatives usually have low titers of anti-insulin antibodies, different classes of ICA, and slower progression to diabetes.

Other autoantibodies associated with polyendocrine autoimmunity include thyroid-stimulating immunoglobulins,[72] antimelanocyte antibodies,[73] antiadrenal and antigonadal an-

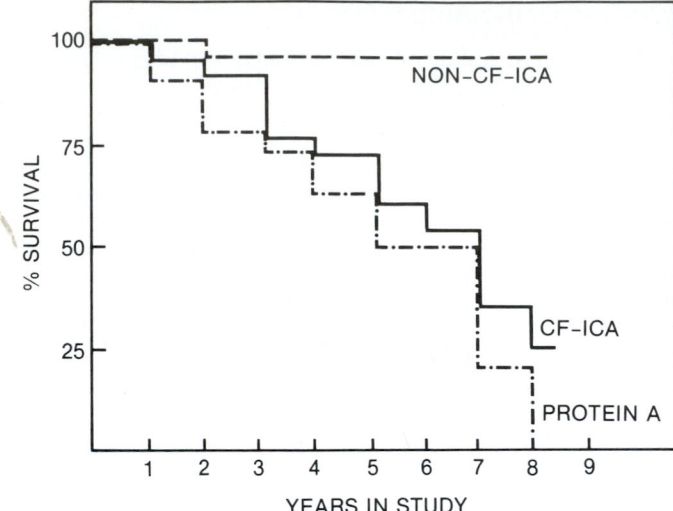

Figure 31–5. Life table analysis of progression to overt diabetes of ICA-positive relatives of the Barts-Windsor family (CF-ICA [complement fixing ICA-positive] and non–CF-ICA-positive) and the Joslin family (protein A; ICA-positive). With specific ICA assays (CF-ICA, protein A), a high proportion of relatives progress to diabetes. (From Jackson RA, Soeldner JS, Eisenbarth GS. Predicting insulin-dependent diabetes. Lancet 1988; 2:627 [letter].)

tibodies that react with frozen tissue sections, and antiadrenal antibodies that immunoprecipitate a 32-kd protein.[74, 75] In the polyendocrine autoimmune syndrome type I, antiadrenal cortical antibodies have been used to predict subsequent development of primary adrenal insufficiency.[76]

T Cell Abnormalities

Abnormalities of T lymphocytes in the type II syndrome include functional defects and alterations of cell-surface markers. The most consistent functional defect is a decrease in suppressor T cell activity.[77–79] Monoclonal antibodies to cell-surface antigens of T cells have been utilized to examine both resting and activated T cell populations in patients with the type II syndrome. Alterations in resting T cell populations are small. We have studied patients with insulin-dependent diabetes mellitus, hyperthyroidism, and polyglandular autoimmune syndrome type II by using several standard monoclonal antibodies to T lymphocytes, namely, CD3 (total T cells), CD4 (helper cells), CD8 (cytotoxic-suppressor cells), and CD7 (helper/concanavalin A–activated suppressor cells). We have not identified a characteristic abnormality of resting T cells.

However, studies of activated T cells that express the Ia or DR antigen reveal abnormalities in patients with a recent onset of insulin-dependent diabetes mellitus,[80, 81] hyperthyroidism,[82] premature menopause,[83] or polyglandular autoimmune syndrome type II. T cells, when stimulated to divide in vitro, acquire other cell-surface molecules in addition to the Ia or DR antigen, including the insulin receptor, the transferrin receptor, and the interleukin 2 receptor. The appearance of the interleukin 2 receptor on activated T cells has led to the study of immunotherapy directed at this receptor, either with monoclonal antibodies[84] or with a unique interleukin 2–diphtheria toxin conjugate produced by recombinant DNA technology. T cells that express many of these surface antigens are found in states associated with immune activation, such as tetanus toxoid immunization, Epstein-Barr virus infection, and sometimes systemic lupus erythematosus and rheumatoid arthritis. The increase in the numbers of Ia antigen–positive T cells in these disorders is probably the consequence of activation of the immune sys-

tem. Until markers of activated T cells with identifiable organ specificity are developed, such immunological markers should be considered as research tools rather than clinically useful assays. Support for this view comes from the observations that many ICA-negative relatives of diabetic patients (e.g., ICA twins[85]) and individuals with congenital rubella and trisomy-21,[86, 87] who have a relatively small risk of developing diabetes, also have T cells expressing Ia antigens.

The NOD Mouse and the BB Rat: Animal Models

The NOD mouse and the BB rat are inbred strains of animals in which insulin-dependent diabetes mellitus appears spontaneously. These animals develop hyperglycemia, hypoinsulinemia, and hyperketonemia. Diabetes mellitus, which is the consequence of lymphocytic infiltration of the islets with subsequent beta cell destruction, develops independent of the presence of infectious agents.[88, 89] Diabetes can be transferred by T lymphocytes of the BB rat and the NOD mouse, and in both animal models bone marrow cells injected into normal radiated recipient animals are sufficient to create the disease. These animal models suggest that the genes (including HLA class II genes) creating diabetes act at the level of bone marrow cells and not the target organ. In these two animal models, despite initial reports to the contrary, the target islet cells do not express readily detectable class II molecules.[65]

In both animal models a specific class II or immune response gene appears necessary but not sufficient for the development of diabetes.[90, 91] In the NOD mouse at least two autosomal recessive genes, as well as its unique (for mouse) class II gene, which lacks aspartic acid at position 57 of its I-A beta chain (analogous to the aspartic acid–deficient DQ allele in human diabetes), are essential for diabetes susceptibility.[92] Mice have two class II molecules, one analogous to the human DQ (i.e., I-A) and the other to the human DR (i.e., I-E). The NOD mouse has a deletion in the gene coding for its I-E alpha chain and therefore makes no I-E. Insulitis has been reported to be prevented in NOD mice by a transgenically introduced normal I-E alpha gene.[93] Thus it appears that in the NOD mouse diabetes susceptibility requires the absence of I-E and the presence of a unique I-A molecule. This finding in NOD mice may be analogous to the study by Sheehy and co-workers[61] of insulin-dependent diabetics in whom both a DQ allele (analogous to the I-A of the mouse) and a DR allele (analogous to the I-E of the mouse) were essential for disease susceptibility. In addition to developing diabetes, these animals develop lymphocytic thyroiditis, and the NOD mouse develops a form of Sjögren syndrome and other organ-specific autoantibodies similar to those in patients with the autoimmune polyglandular syndrome type II.

The pathogenesis of polyglandular autoimmunity in the BB rat has been linked to a dysfunction of T cells inherited as an autosomal recessive mutation.[94] The direct result of the mutation is severe T cell lymphopenia. Although the lymphopenia greatly accelerates the development of diabetes and thyroiditis, other factors (genetic or environmental) appear to determine the extent and specificity of organ involvement in the autoimmune process. Neither patients with the polyendocrine syndrome type II nor NOD mice have a profound T cell lymphopenia.

Multiple forms of immune suppression can prevent the development of diabetes in BB rats and NOD mice. Examples of this suppression are use of antilymphocyte globulin, neonatal thymectomy, and cyclosporine;[95] bone marrow transplantation;[96] and transfusion of whole blood.[97] Placing beta cells at rest with insulin can also prevent diabetes.[98]

Whether the success of immunotherapy in the BB rat and the NOD mouse will eventually be found to have a parallel in humans is unknown and is being studied in clinical trials. However, immunotherapies such as bone marrow transplantation and blood transfusions, which appear to work in the BB rat by transferring normal lymphocytes to severely immunodeficient animals,[88] are unlikely to be effective in human insulin-dependent diabetes because the transferred lymphocytes would be destroyed by a more normal immune system.

Therapy

Treatment of the individual diseases of the polyglandular syndrome is discussed in other chapters of this book. Therapeutic considerations related specifically to the type II syndrome include the following:

1. Levothyroxine therapy can precipitate a life-threatening addisonian crisis in a patient with untreated adrenal insufficiency and hypothyroidism. Thus it is necessary to evaluate adrenal function in all hypothyroid patients in whom the syndrome is suspected before the institution of levothyroxine therapy.

2. A decreasing insulin requirement in a patient with insulin-dependent diabetes mellitus can be one of the earliest indications of adrenal insufficiency, occurring before the development of hyperpigmentation or electrolyte abnormalities.

3. In patients with both adrenal insufficiency and primary hypothyroidism, thyroid function may improve after glucocorticoid replacement,[99] and in a similar manner ovulatory menstrual cycles can reappear in patients after hydrocortisone replacement therapy.[100]

4. Addisonian crisis that responds to mineralocorticoid therapy can occur in patients receiving high-dose glucocorticoids for inflammatory disease.[101]

5. In light of the long-term morbidity and mortality of insulin-dependent diabetes mellitus, novel approaches to therapy of diabetes are being studied. Immunotherapy for insulin-dependent diabetes has been tried almost exclusively in patients with overt hyperglycemia.[102–106] Limitations of such studies have been the toxicity of immunotherapeutic drugs and the severe degree of beta cell destruction at the time of diagnosis of diabetes. None of the initial immunotherapy trials has demonstrated a sufficient long-term clinical response, given known drug toxicities, to justify such therapy, except as part of a clinical research protocol aimed at improving such therapies. Toxic effects of cyclosporine include nephrotoxicity, hepatotoxicity, a falling hemoglobin level, hirsutism, gingival hyperplasia, hyperuricemia, and the extremely rare development of lymphoma. Complications of antilymphocyte globulin therapy include anaphylaxis, fever, rash, serum sickness, and occasional transient severe thrombocytopenia. Complications of azathioprine include myelosuppression. Glucocorticoids, depending on the amount given and dosage schedule, cause Cushing syndrome and appear to be ineffective in altering the clinical course if administered after overt diabetes has developed.

An interesting report suggests that intensive insulin therapy, delivered by Biostator, to place beta cells at rest followed by maintenance insulin therapy may preserve beta cell function for as long as a year.[105] Insulin therapy can prevent diabetes in NOD mice and BB rats.[98]

Follow-up of children treated with cyclosporine after the onset of insulin-dependent diabetes mellitus indicates that although 60% may be in a remission (free of insulin use) at 1 y, less than 10% maintain an insulin-free remission for 3 y, despite maintenance of significant C peptide secretion.[106, 107] Thus if the goal is long-term maintenance of a non–insulin-requiring remission, trials of immune treatment will have to target prediabetics, which makes the design of such trials more difficult and requires the expertise of specialty laboratories.

6. A number of studies have raised the real possibility that in addition to classic targets of autoimmunity, the autoimmunity associated with insulin-dependent diabetes mellitus and other endocrine autoimmune diseases may extend to "neuronal" tissues. Stiff-man syndrome in an insulin-dependent diabetic has been associated with antibodies to glutamate decarboxylase.[108] Parkinson disease has been associated with endocrine autoimmunity.[53, 54] Brown and coworkers[109] have discovered that more than 25% of insulin-dependent diabetics develop adrenomedullary fibrosis, at times in association with lymphocytic "invasion" of the adrenal medulla. In addition, a series of autoantibodies in patients with insulin-dependent diabetes react with adrenal medulla and with peripheral and autonomic nerves. One report links the presence of such antibodies with autonomic dysfunction.[110] Most patients with long-term insulin-dependent diabetes lose glucagon and adrenergic responses to hypoglycemia and are at high risk for insulin-induced hypoglycemia. Adrenomedullary fibrosis may be a pathological correlate of this hyporesponsiveness. Selected neuropathic syndromes associated with insulin-dependent diabetes can be so severe that clinical trials of immunotherapy in patients developing autonomic neuropathy will likely be considered.

AUTOIMMUNE POLYGLANDULAR SYNDROME TYPE I

Adrenal insufficiency associated with mucocutaneous candidiasis and hypoparathyroidism and aggregating in sibships defines the polyglandular syndrome type I, which is also known as the candidiasis endocrinopathy syndrome. The association of mucocutaneous candidiasis with glandular failure was recognized by Thorpe and Handley[111] in 1929, and more than 100 patients with idiopathic hypoparathyroidism and candidiasis have been reported.[112, 112a] In contrast to the type II syndrome, this syndrome is not HLA associated at a population level,[3, 10] nor does the disease correlate with HLA inheritance in several informative families.[3] Patients with adrenal insufficiency and the type I syndrome do not express an increase of HLA-DR3, HLA-DR4 antigens, whereas more than 95% of type II syndrome patients with adrenal insufficiency express HLA-DR3 or HLA-DR4.[10] Also in contrast to the type II syndrome, which characteristically involves multiple generations, this disease is limited to one generation of affected siblings.

The type I syndrome characteristically is recognized in early childhood, whereas the type II syndrome has a peak incidence in middle age (Fig. 31–6). Chronic mucocutaneous candidiasis is often first seen with accompanying hypoparathyroidism, followed by later development of adrenal insufficiency.[2] Decades may elapse between the diagnosis of one disease and the onset of the second in the same individual. Within a sibship, individuals may express only one of the three diseases. In addition to the classic triad of this syndrome, chronic active hepatitis (13%), malabsorption (22%), alopecia (32%), pernicious anemia (13%), gonadal failure (17%), and thyroid disease (11%) are significant problems. Insulin-dependent diabetes mellitus has been reported to occur in 4% of these patients, whereas 50% of the patients with the type II syndrome with adrenal insufficiency develop this disease. This 4% figure is probably an underestimate and may have resulted from the initial study of pediatric

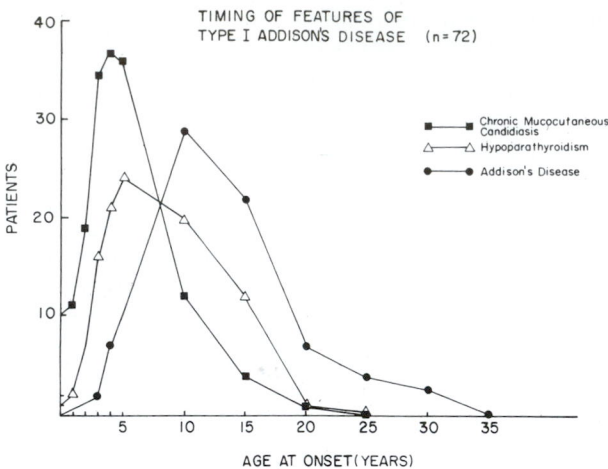

Figure 31–6. The age at onset of mucocutaneous candidiasis, hypoparathyroidism, and adrenal insufficiency in patients with autoimmune polyglandular syndrome type II. (From M Neufeld, NK Maclaren, RM Blizzard, Two types of autoimmune Addison's disease associated with different polyglandular autoimmune [PGA] syndromes, 60, 355–362, © by Williams & Wilkins, 1981.)

populations, in whom overt diabetes may develop at later ages.

The aggregation of the type I syndrome within sibships involving both males and females suggests an autosomal recessive inheritance. Antiadrenal and antiparathyroid antibodies have been reported.[113] The reason for the marked susceptibility to mucocutaneous candidiasis without systemic candidiasis is unknown. These patients have abnormalities of delayed hypersensitivity (in some patients to all stimuli and in others to candida),[114] and T cell abnormalities have been described.[115] Candidiasis developing in adults is rarely part of the type I syndrome but can be associated with immunological abnormalities accompanying thymomas.[116]

The treatment of adrenal insufficiency and hypoparathyroidism is the same as that discussed in Chapters 9 and 27, with the caveat that malabsorption may complicate treatment. Chronic active hepatitis is a particularly serious problem for many of these patients. The therapy of mucocutaneous candidiasis has been improved by the introduction of the orally active antifungal drug ketoconazole.[117, 118] Some patients have had long-term remissions after approximately a year of ketoconazole therapy, but in the majority of patients the disease relapses when the drug is discontinued or the dosage decreased. Relapse may also occur during therapy. Two potential hazards of ketoconazole therapy are its association with hepatitis and its inhibition of adrenal and gonadal steroid synthesis. Patients with the type I syndrome who are not known to have adrenal insufficiency and who are receiving ketoconazole should be carefully monitored for development of adrenal insufficiency. Despite these concerns, long-term ketoconazole therapy is the mainstay for mucocutaneous candidiasis.

ANTI–INSULIN RECEPTOR ANTIBODIES

In this rare (approximately 25 reported patients) disorder—also known as type B insulin resistance and acanthosis nigricans—insulin resistance is due to the presence of anti–insulin receptor antibodies.[119, 120] Approximately one third of patients with these antibodies have an associated autoimmune illness, such as systemic lupus erythematosus, Sjögren syndrome, and ataxia telangiectasia. Arthralgia, vitiligo, alopecia, and secondary amenorrhea have also been reported.[120] One patient had a daughter with hyperthyroidism and a granddaughter with systemic lupus erythematosus. Autoimmune thyroid disease has been described in two such patients, one with hypothyroidism and the other with antithyroid antibodies. Antinuclear antibodies and an elevated erythrocyte sedimentation rate, hyperglobulinemia, leukopenia, and hypocomplementemia are common.[121]

The major clinical manifestations relate to the anti–insulin receptor antibodies. Severe insulin resistance is profound, so that up to 175,000 U of insulin given intravenously per day may be ineffective in lowering the elevated glucose level. Despite hyperglycemia and marked insulin resistance, ketoacidosis is uncommon. The course of the diabetes is variable, and several patients have had spontaneous remissions. Other patients have had severe hypoglycemia (perhaps related to the insulin-like effects of anti–insulin receptor antibodies demonstrable in vitro).[121] The acanthosis nigricans (Fig. 31–7), which is due to hypertrophy and folding of otherwise histologically normal skin, appears to be related to the insulin-resistant state. Other forms of marked insulin resistance in the absence of antireceptor antibodies are also associated with acanthosis nigricans.[122]

POEMS SYNDROME

The components of this multisystem syndrome—also known as plasma cell dyscrasia with polyneuropathy, organomegaly, endocrinopathy, M protein, and skin changes—consist of diabetes mellitus (half the patients), primary gonadal failure (70% of the patients), plasma cell dyscrasia, sclerotic bone lesions, and neuropathy.[123–128] Patients usually present with severe progressive sensorimotor polyneuropathy, hepatosplenomegaly, lymphadenopathy, and hyperpigmentation. On evaluation they are found to have plasma cell dyscrasia and sclerotic bone lesions. The syndrome is assumed to be secondary to circulating immunoglobulins, but

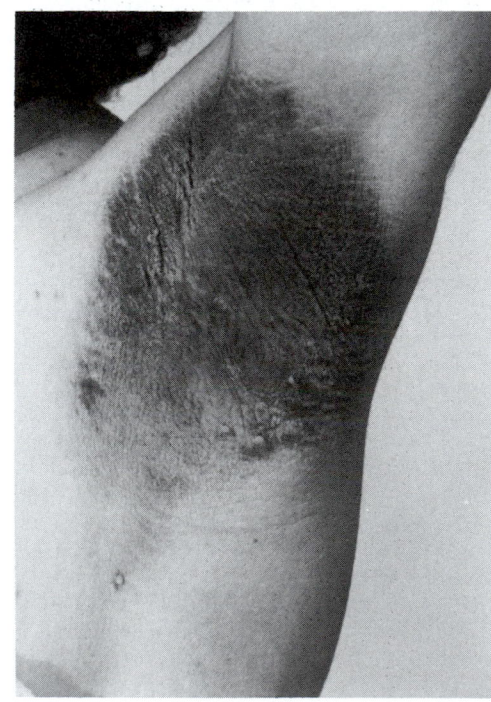

Figure 31–7. A patient with acanthosis nigricans and insulin resistance. (Photograph courtesy of Dr. R. Kahn.)

binding of antibody directly to involved tissues has not been demonstrated. The diabetes mellitus responds to small subcutaneous doses of insulin. The hypogonadism is associated with elevated plasma levels of follicle-stimulating hormone and luteinizing hormone. Temporary resolution of disease, including a return of the blood glucose level to normal, may occur after radiotherapy of localized plasma cell lesions of bone.

KEARNS-SAYRE SYNDROME

This rare syndrome—also known as oculocraniosomatic disease or oculocraniosomatic neuromuscular disease with ragged red fibers—is characterized by myopathic abnormalities leading to ophthalmoplegia and progressive weakness in association with several endocrine abnormalities, including hypoparathyroidism, primary gonadal failure, diabetes mellitus, and hypopituitarism.[129] These patients exhibit crystalline mitochondrial inclusions in muscle biopsy specimens, and such inclusions have also been observed in the cerebellum. The relationship between the mitochondrial disorders and endocrinological abnormalities is not known. Other abnormalities include retinitis pigmentosa and heart block. Antiparathyroid antibodies have not been described; however, antibodies to the anterior pituitary and striated muscle have been found, and the disease may have autoimmune components.

THYMIC TUMORS

The central role of the thymus in the ontogeny of cell-mediated immunity was recognized in 1961.[130–132] Soon after, DiGeorge described congenital aplasia of the thymus and parathyroid glands, both of which are derived from the third and fourth pharyngeal pouches.[133] These infants present with tetany secondary to hypocalcemia, severe infections with markedly suppressed T cell immunity, and normal humoral immunity.[134]

The thymus is a complex tissue with a specialized endocrine epithelium that synthesizes a variety of biologically active peptides involved in the control of T cell maturation. This epithelium is derived from the neural crest[134] and contains complex gangliosides that react with monoclonal antibody (A2B5) and tetanus toxin in a manner similar to that of pancreatic islets. The role of these biologically active peptides of the thymus has not been defined, but they may be trophic factors in T cell activation and increase in situations of primary failure of T cell activation, just as the levels of trophic hormones increase in primary endocrine failure.[135]

The illnesses associated with thymomas are similar to those in the autoimmune polyendocrine syndrome type II,[136] although the frequency of specific disorders is different. In one review of patients with thymoma, myasthenia gravis occurred in 44% of the patients, red blood cell aplasia in approximately 20%, hypoglobulinemia in 6%, autoimmune thyroid disease in 2%, and adrenal insufficiency in 1 of 423 patients. The frequency of autoimmune thyroid disease reported in patients with thymoma is probably an underestimate, given the frequency of unsuspected thyroid disease in patients with myasthenia gravis. Mucocutaneous candidiasis in adults is also associated with thymomas.[114] In the majority of the patients the thymomas are malignant,[137] but temporary remissions of the autoimmune disease can occur with resection of the tumor.

TRISOMY-21

Down syndrome, or trisomy-21, is associated with the development of insulin-dependent diabetes mellitus and thyroiditis.[138] We have observed one patient with a partial distal translocation "leading" to trisomy-21 and "associated" with adrenal insufficiency, celiac disease, hypothyroidism, and insulin-dependent diabetes.[139] Patients with trisomy-21 also have T cell abnormalities including increased Ia-positive T cells and a premature increase in the 3G5 age-related T cell subset.[140] It is not known whether the observed chromosomal abnormality influences the development of autoimmunity or whether part of the susceptibility to autoimmunity is associated with chromosomal disorders.[141] Organ-specific autoimmunity also occurs with gonadal dysgenesis.[142]

CONGENITAL RUBELLA

Patients with congenital rubella have almost a 20% risk of developing diabetes mellitus and a higher than normal risk of developing thyroiditis and hypothyroidism.[143] Those at highest risk for diabetes express diabetes-associated HLA-DR3 and HLA-DR4 alleles.[144] Rubella appears to be primarily associated with diabetes after fetal infection, and it is unknown whether the virus increases the probability of subsequent autoimmunity because it has permanent effects on the developing immune system.[87]

DIDMOAD SYNDROME

It is not known whether the DIDMOAD, or Wolfram, syndrome results from autoimmunity, but pathological and metabolic studies indicate that patients with this syndrome, similar to insulin-dependent diabetics, selectively lose beta cells from islets while retaining alpha and delta cells.[145] This syndrome is inherited in an autosomal recessive manner and consists of diabetes insipidus, diabetes mellitus, optic atrophy, and nerve deafness. The syndrome is not associated with HLA-DR3 or HLA-DR4 but may be associated with HLA-DR2.

CONCLUSION

Despite advances in basic immunology the initial lesion in the common autoimmune illnesses is not understood, and, indeed, multiple interacting abnormalities of more than one class of lymphocyte may be involved.[146, 147] The reason that most autoimmune illnesses are associated with specific HLA alleles is also not known. The crystal structure and mechanism by which the immune response is influenced by specific HLA alleles have been defined. It appears likely that at the level of bone marrow–derived cells, expression of specific HLA molecules focuses autoimmunity on specific normal target antigens such as insulin, the acetylcholine receptor, cytoplasmic islet antigens, thyroglobulin, and so on. Recall that transplantation of bone marrow–derived stem cells transfers susceptibility to diabetes in animal models. It should be stressed that polyendocrine autoimmune serology does not result from a few antibodies reacting with multiple organs but from a series of antibodies and immune responses reacting with different specific antigens. One can observe, in the same individual, autoantibodies directed at different organs appearing over time. However, with one organ a series of different antibodies may appear simultaneously, e.g., in insulin-dependent diabetes: anti-insulin, anti–glutamate decarboxylase, cytoplasmic islet cell antibodies; in Graves disease: antithyroid peroxidase (microsomal antigen), antithyroglobulin, antithyrotropin receptor. The highly specific immunoglobulin G antibodies that are characteristic of organ-specific autoantibodies are not similar to the multispecific low-affinity immunoglobulin M monoclonal antibodies produced by CD5-positive B lymphocyte hybridomas. Many of the latter antibodies react with more than a dozen different antigens.[148]

As with tests used for rheumatological disease in which the titer and specificity of assays for given antibodies are taken into account, clinically relevant information can now be obtained with selected autoantibody assays. These assays are beginning to be used to predict future disease and to diagnose the autoimmune form of a disorder (e.g., non–insulin-dependent vs. insulin-dependent diabetes).

Whether diabetes and other manifestations of autoimmunity will eventually be preventable by immunotherapy is not clear. The immune system may be amenable to regulation. Immunoregulation rather than immunosuppression is the eventual goal of therapy of autoimmune diseases. It is noteworthy that with current techniques more than a dozen types of immunotherapy and manipulations can prevent diabetes in the BB rat and the NOD mouse. The complexity of the immune system provides many opportunities for intervention but may also increase the hazards of such intervention.

Even though the pathogenesis is not understood and the drugs used for immunoregulation have serious side effects, recognition of the syndrome of HLA-B8, HLA-DR3–associated illnesses is clinically important. Fortunately, many of the illnesses such as hypothyroidism, adrenal insufficiency, and pernicious anemia are readily treatable. Early recognition also allows prevention of significant morbidity and mortality in polyendocrine autoimmune patients and, just as important, in relatives of patients with polyendocrine autoimmunity.

REFERENCES

1. Schmidt MB. Eine biglandulare Erkrankung (Nebennieren und Schilddruse bei Morbus Addisonni). Dtsch Pathol Ges 1926; 21:212–221.
2. Neufeld M, Maclaren NK, Blizzard RM. Two types of autoimmune Addison's disease associated with different polyglandular autoimmune (PGA) syndromes. Medicine 1981; 60:355–362.
3. Eisenbarth GS, Jackson RA. Immunogenetics of polyglandular failure and related diseases in HLA. In: Farid N, ed. Endocrine and Metabolic Disorders. New York: Academic, 1981: 235–264.
4. Eisenbarth GS. Type I diabetes mellitus. A chronic autoimmune disease. N Engl J Med 1986; 314:1360–1368.
5. Nakano K, Mordes JP, Handler ES, et al. Role of host immune system in BB/W rat. Predisposition to diabetes resides in bone marrow. Diabetes 1988; 37:520–525.
6. Maclaren NK. How, when and why to predict IDDM. Diabetes 1988; 37:1591–1594.
7. Bottazzo GF, Pujol-Borrel R, Gale E. Autoimmunity and type I diabetes: bringing the story up to date. Diabetes Annu 1987; 3:15–38.
8. Irvine WJ, Barnes EW. Addison's disease, ovarian failure and hypoparathyroidism. Clin Endocrinol 1975; 4:379–434.
9. Irvine WJ. Autoimmunity in endocrine disease. Recent Prog Horm Res 1980; 46:509–556.
10. Maclaren NK, Riley WJ. Inherited susceptibility to autoimmune Addison's disease is linked to human leukocyte antigens-DR3 and/or DR4 except when associated with type I autoimmune polyglandular syndrome. J Clin Endocrinol Metab 1986; 62:455–459.
11. Eisenbarth GS, Wilson P, Ward F, et al. HLA type and occurrence of disease in familial polyglandular failure. N Engl J Med 1978; 298:92–94.
12. Valenta LJ, Bull RW, Hackel E, et al. Correlation of the HLA-A1, B8 haplotypes with circulating autoantibodies in a family with increased incidence of autoimmune disease. Acta Endocrinol 1982; 100:143–149.
13. Riley WJ, Maclaren NK, Neufeld M. Adrenal autoantibodies and Addison's disease in insulin-dependent diabetes mellitus. J Pediatr 1980; 97:191–197.
14. Tucker WS, Niblack GD, McLean R, et al. Serositis with autoimmune endocrinopathy: clinical and immunogenetic features. Medicine 1987; 66:138–147.
15. van-den-Berg Loonen EM, Hillerman TC, Bins M, et al. Increased incidence of HLA DR2 in patients with pernicious anemia. Tissue Antigens 1982; 19:158–160.
16. Stenszky V, Valazs C, Kraszits E, et al. Association of goitrous thyroiditis with DR3 in eastern Hungary. J Immunogenet 1987; 14:143–148.
17. Petite J, Rosset N, Chapuis B, et al. Genetic factors predisposing to autoimmune diseases. Study of HLA antigens in a family with pernicious anemia and thyroid disease. Schweiz Med Wochenschr 1987; 117:2032–2037.
18. Peserica A, Rigon F, Semmenzoto G, et al. Vitiligo and polyglandular autoimmune disease with autoantibodies to melanin producing cells. Arch Dermatol 1981; 117:751–752.
19. Posillico JT, Wortsman J, Srikanta S, et al. Parathyroid cell surface autoantibodies that inhibit parathyroid hormone secretion from dispersed human parathyroid cells. Bone Miner Res 1986; 5:475–485.
20. Arnett FC, Goldstein R, Duvic M, et al. Major histocompatibility complex genes in systemic lupus erythematosus, Sjogren's syndrome and polymyositis. Am J Med 1988; 85:38–41.
21. Wilton AN, Cobain TJ, Dawkins RJ. Family studies of IgA deficiency. Immunogenetics 1985; 21:333–342.
22. Hoddinott S, Dornan J, Bearch JC, et al. Immunoglobulin levels, immunodeficiency and HLA in type I (insulin-dependent) diabetes mellitus. Diabetologia 1982; 23:326–329.
23. Sattar MA, Sughyer AA, Siboo R. Coexistence of rheumatoid arthritis, ankylosing spondylitis and dermatomyositis in a patient with diabetes mellitus and the associated linked HLA antigens. Br J Rheumatol 1988; 27:146–149.
24. Provost TT, Talal N, Bias W, et al. Ro(SS-A) positive Sjögren's/lupus erythematosus (SC/LE) overlap patients are associated with the HLA-DR3 and/or DRW6 phenotypes. J Invest Dermatol 1988; 91:369–371.
25. Kilby AE, Albertini RJ, Krawitt EL. HLA typing and autoantibodies in hepatitis B surface antigen negative chronic active hepatitis. Tissue Antigens 1986; 28:214–217.
26. MacKay IR, Tait BD. HLA association with chronic active hepatitis. In: Rose NR, Bigazzi PE, Warren NL, eds. Genetic Control of Autoimmune Disease. Amsterdam: Elsevier, 1978: 27–42.
27. Nouri A, Donaldson PT, Hegarty JE, et al. HLA A1-B8-DR3 and suppressor cell function in first degree relatives of patients with autoimmune chronic active hepatitis. J Hepatol 1985; 1:235–241.
28. Hitman GA, Niven MJ, Festenstein H, et al. HLA class II α gene polymorphisms in patients with insulin dependent diabetes, dermatitis herpetiformis and celiac disease. J Clin Invest 1987; 79:609–615.
29. Katz SI, Hertz KC, Rogentine GN, et al. HLA-B8 and dermatitis herpetiformis in patients with IgA deposits in skin. Arch Dermatol 1977; 113:155–156.
30. Ayala A, Canales ES, Karchmer S, et al. Premature ovarian failure and hypothyroidism associated with sicca syndrome. Obstet Gynecol 1979; 53:985–1019.
31. Hagen GA, Bolman RM, Frank JP. Atypical adrenal insufficiency with failure of the pituitary feedback receptor. Am J Med 1975; 59:882–888.
32. Smith WI, Rabin BS, Huellmantel A, et al. Immunopathology of juvenile onset diabetes mellitus. Diabetes 1978; 27:1092–1097.
33. Schwarz U, Lammie B, Six P, et al. Polyendocrine deficiency syndrome. Arch Intern Med 1980; 140:1247–1248.
34. Van Thiel DH, Smith WI Jr, Rabin BS, et al. A syndrome of immunoglobulin A deficiency, diabetes mellitus, malabsorption, a common HLA haplotype. Immunologic and genetic studies of forty-three family members. Ann Intern Med 1977; 86:10–19.
35. Stewart SR, Gershwin ME. The associations and relationships of congenital immune deficiency states and autoimmune phenomenon. Semin Arthritis Rheum 1979; 9:98–123.
36. Wilson WA, Sissons JGP, Morgan OS. Multiple autoimmune diseases with bilateral optic atrophy and lipodystrophy. Ann Intern Med 1978; 89:72–73.
37. Liechty RD. The thyrotoxicosis/thrombocytopenia connection. Surgery 1983; 94:966–968.
38. Porges A, Bussel J, Kimberly R, et al. Elevation of platelet associated antibody levels in patients with chronic idiopathic thrombocytopenia purpura expressing the B8 and/or DR3 allotypes. Tissue Antigens 1985; 26:132–137.
39. Remuzzi G, Livio M, Donati MB, et al. Myasthenia gravis, thrombocytopenia and HLA antigens. Ann Intern Med 1977; 87:250–251.
40. Scherbaum WA, Bottazzo GF. Autoantibodies to vasopressin cells in idiopathic diabetes insipidus: evidence for an autoimmune variant. Lancet 1983; 1:897–901.
41. Mershon JC, Dietrich JG. Hereditary Addison's disease and multiple endocrine adenomatosis in a kindred: autoimmune aspects. Ann Intern Med 1966; 65:252–258.
42. Flora S, Bottazzo GF, Doniach D. Immunofluorescence studies on

autoantibodies to steroid producing cells, and to germ line cells in endocrine disease and infertility. Clin Exp Immunol 1980; 39:97–111.

43. Pouplard A, Bottazzo GF, Doniach D, et al. Binding of human immunoglobulins to pituitary ACTH cells. Nature 1976; 261:142–144.

44. Bottazzo GF, Doniach D. Pituitary autoimmunity: a review. J R Soc Med 1978; 71:433–436.

45. Lack EE. Lymphoid "hypophysitis" with end organ insufficiency. Arch Pathol 1975; 99:215–219.

46. Goudie RB, Pinkerton PH. Anterior hypophysitis and Hashimoto's disease in a young woman. J Pathol Bacteriol 1957; 83:584–585.

47. Hume R, Roberts GH. Hypophysitis and hypopituitarism: a report of a case. Br Med J 1967; 2:548–550.

48. Snover DC, Filipovich AN, Dehner LP, et al. Pseudolymphoma: a case associated with primary immunodeficiency disease and polyglandular failure syndrome. Arch Pathol Lab Med 1981; 105:46–49.

49. Parker M, Klein I, Fishman LM, et al. Silent thyrotoxic thyroiditis in association with chronic adrenocortical insufficiency. Arch Intern Med 1981; 140:1108–1109.

50. Miller MJ, VanderHorst T. Isolated ACTH deficiency and primary hypothyroidism. Acta Endocrinol 1982; 99:573–576.

51. Kojima I, Nejima I, Ogata E. Isolated adrenocorticotropin deficiency associated with polyglandular failure. J Clin Endocrin Metab 1982; 54:182–186.

52. Aanderud S, Bassøe HH. A pituitary tumour with possible ACTH and TSH hypersecretion in a patient with Addison's disease and primary hypothyroidism. Acta Endocrinol 1980; 95:181–184.

53. Emile J, Pouplard A, Bossu Van Nieuwenhuyse C, et al. Maladie de Parkinson, dysautonomie et auto-anticorps dirigés contre les neurones sympathiques. Rev Neurol 1980; 136:221–233.

54. Brown FM, Freeman R, Tyler HR, et al. Polyglandular autoimmunity and Parkinson's disease. Clin Res 1989; 37:356A.

55. Savilahti E, Simell O, Koskimies S, et al. Celiac disease in insulin-dependent diabetes mellitus. J Pediatr 1986; 108:690–693.

56. Wescott MZ, Awdeh ZL, Yunis EJ, et al. Molecular analysis distinguishes two HLA-DR3 bearing major histocompatibility complex extended haplotypes. Immunogenetics 1987; 26:370–374.

57. Tokunaga K, Saueracher G, Kay PH, et al. Extensive deletions and insertions in different MHC supratypes detected by pulsed field gel electrophoresis. J Exp Med 1988; 168:933–940.

58. Brown WE. The HLA histocompatibility system in autoimmune states. Clin Lab Med 1988; 8:351–372.

59. Caccia N, Mak TW. T cell receptors. Am J Med 1988; 85:9–11.

60. Pullen AM, Kappler JW, Marrack P. Tolerance to self antigens shapes the T cell repertoire. Immunol Rev 1989; 107:125–139.

61. Sheehy MJ, Scharf SJ, Rose JR, et al. A diabetes-susceptible HLA haplotype is best defined by a combination of HLA-DR and DQ alleles. J Clin Invest 1989; 83:830–835.

62. Todd JA, Bell JI, McDevitt HO. HLA-DQ β gene contributes to susceptibility and resistance to insulin dependent diabetes mellitus. Nature 1987; 329:599–604.

63. Todd JA, Acha-Orbea H, Bell JI, et al. A molecular basis for MHC class II associated autoimmunity. Science 1988; 240:1003–1009.

64. Foulis AK, Farquharson MA, Meager A. Immunoreactive α-interferon in insulin-secreting β cells in type 1 diabetes mellitus. Lancet 1987; 2:1423–1427.

65. Pipeleers DG, In't Veld PA, Pipeleers-Marichal MA, et al. Presence of pancreatic hormones in islet cells with MHC-class II antigen expression. Diabetes 1987; 36:872–876.

66. Goldstein DE, Drash A, Gibbs J. Diabetes mellitus: the incidence of circulating antibodies against thyroid, gastric and adrenal tissue. J Pediatr 1970; 77:304–306.

67. Irvine WJ, Scarth L, Clarke BF, et al. Thyroid and gastric autoimmunity in patients with diabetes mellitus. Lancet 1970; 2:163–168.

68. Doniach D, Roitt IM. An evaluation of gastric and thyroid autoimmunity in relation to hematologic disorders. Semin Hematol 1964; 1:313–343.

69. Tarn AC, Thomas JM, Dean BM, et al. Predicting insulin-dependent diabetes. Diabetes 1988; 16:845–850.

70. Jackson RA, Vardi P, Herskowitz RD, et al. Dual parameter linear model for prediction of onset of type I diabetes in islet cell antibody positive relatives. Clin Res 1988; 36:585A.

71. Bosi E, Becker F, Schwarz G, et al. Natural history of pre-type I diabetes in polyendocrine patients with islet cell antibodies. Diabetes 1987; 36(Suppl 1):253A.

72. Mariotti S, Shiovato L, Vitti P, et al. Recent advances in the understanding of humoral and cellular mechanisms in thyroid autoimmune disorders. Clin Immunol Immunopathol 1989; 50:573–584.

73. Naughton GK, Eisenger M, Bystryn JC. Detection of antibodies to melanocytes in vitiligo by specific immunoprecipitation. J Invest Dermatol 1983; 81:540–542.

74. Atkinson MA, Lernmark A, Gerling I, et al. Adrenal cell surface autoantibodies in Addison's disease detected on a murine adrenocortical cell line. Endocr Soc Abstr 1987; 11A.

75. Bright GM, Blizzard RM, Kaiser DL, et al. Organ-specific autoantibodies in children with common endocrine diseases. J Pediatr 1982; 100:8–14.

76. Ahonen P, Miettinen A, Perheentup A. Adrenal and steroidal cell antibodies in patients with autoimmune polyglandular disease type I

77. Verghese MW, Ward FE, Eisenbarth GS. Lymphocyte suppressor activity in patients with polyglandular failure. Hum Immunol 1981; 3:173–179.

78. Jaworski MA, Colle E, Guttmann RD. Abnormal immunoregulation in patients with insulin-dependent diabetes mellitus and their healthy first degree relatives. Hum Immunol 1983; 7:25–34.

79. Horita M, Suzuki H, Onodera T, et al. Abnormalities of immunoregulatory T cell subsets in patients with insulin-dependent diabetes mellitus. J Immunol 1982; 129:1426–1429.

80. Jackson RA, Morris MA, Haynes BF, et al. Increased circulating Ia antigen bearing T cells in type I diabetes mellitus. N Engl J Med 1982; 306:785–788.

81. Alviggi L, Hoskins PJ, Pyke DA, et al. Pathogenesis of insulin dependent diabetes: a role for activated T lymphocytes. Lancet 1984; 1:4–6.

82. Jackson RA, Haynes BF, Burch WM, et al. Ia+ T cell in new onset Graves' disease. J Clin Endocrinol Metab 1984; 59:187–190.

83. Rabinowe SL, Ravnikar VA, Dib A, et al. Premature menopause: monoclonal antibody defined T cell lymphocyte abnormalities and anti-ovarian antibodies. Fertil Steril 1989; 51:450–454.

84. Kelly VE, Gaulton GN, Hattori M, et al. Anti–interleukin 2 receptor antibody suppresses murine diabetic insulitis and lupus nephritis. J Immunol 1988; 140:59–61.

85. Johnson C, Alviggi L, Millward BA, et al. Alterations in T lymphocytes in type I diabetes. Exploration of genetic influence in identical twins. Diabetes 1988; 37:1484–1488.

86. Rabinowe SL, Rubin L, George KL, et al. Trisomy 21 (Down's syndrome): autoimmunity, aging and monoclonal antibody defined T cell abnormalities. J Autoimmun 1989; 2:25–30.

87. Rabinowe SL, George KL, Laughlin R, et al. Congenital rubella: monoclonal antibody defined T cell abnormalities in young children. Am J Med 1986; 81:779–782.

88. Mordes JP, Handler ES, Burstein D, et al. Immunotherapy of the BB rat. In: Eisenbarth GS, ed. Immunotherapy of Diabetes and Selected Autoimmune Disorders. Boca Raton, FL: CRC Press 1989: 35–52.

89. Ikegami H, Yano N, Sato T, et al. Immunogenetics and immunopathogenesis of the NOD mouse. In: Eisenbarth GS, ed. Immunotherapy of Diabetes and Selected Autoimmune Disorders. Boca Raton, FL: CRC Press, 1989: 23–33.

90. Colle E, Guttmann RD, Fuks A, et al. Genetics of the spontaneous diabetic syndrome. Interaction of the MHC and non-MHC associated factors. Mol Biol Med 1986; 3:13–23.

91. Wicker LS, Miller BJ, Coker LZ, et al. Genetic control of diabetes and insulitis in the non-obese diabetic (NOD) mouse. J Exp Med 1987; 165:1639–1654.

92. Prochazka M, Leiter EH, Serreze DV, et al. Three recessive loci required for insulin-dependent diabetes in nonobese diabetic mice. Science 1987; 237:286–289.

93. Nishimoto H, Kikutani H, Yamamura K, et al. Prevention of autoimmune insulitis by expression of I-E molecules in NOD mice. Nature 1987; 328:432–434.

94. Greiner DL, Handler ES, Nakano K, et al. Absence of the RT6 T cell subset in diabetes-prone BB/W rats. J Immunol 1986; 136:148–151.

95. Like AA, Anthony M, Guberski DL, et al. Spontaneous diabetes mellitus in the BB/W rat. Effects of glucocorticoids, cyclosporin A and antiserum to rat lymphocytes. Diabetes 1983; 32:326–330.

96. Naji A, Silvers W, Bellgrau D, et al. Spontaneous diabetes in rats: destruction of islets is prevented by immunologic tolerance. Science 1983; 213:1390–1392.

97. Rossini AA, Mordes JP, Pelletier AM, et al. Transfusions of whole blood prevent spontaneous diabetes mellitus in the BB/W rat. Science 1983; 219:975–977.

98. Gotfredsen CF, Buschard K, Frandsen EK. Reduction of diabetes incidence of BB Wistar rats by early prophylactic insulin treatment of diabetes prone animals. Diabetologia 1985; 28:933–935.

99. Peterson HD, Bergman M. Cortisone-induced remission of hypothyroidism in Schmidt's syndrome. Acta Med Scand 1980; 208:125–127.

100. DeWailly D, Bourdelle-Hego MF, Pouplard BA, et al. Recovery of ovulatory menstrual cycles under hydrocortisone in two amenorrheic women with isolated corticotropin deficiency. Horm Res 1988; 29:14–16.

101. Jacobs TP, Whitlock RT, Edsall J, et al. Addisonian crisis while taking high-dose glucocorticoids. JAMA 1988; 260:2082–208.

102. Silverstein J, Maclaren N, Riley W, et al. Immunosuppression with azathioprine and prednisone in recent-onset insulin-dependent diabetes mellitus. N Engl J Med 1988; 319:599–604.

103. Feutren G, Assan G, Karsenty G, et al. Cyclosporine increased the rate and length of remissions in insulin dependent diabetes of recent onset. Results of a multicenter trial. Lancet 1986; 2:119–123.

104. Stiller CR, Laupacis A, Keown PA, et al. Cyclosporine: action, pharmacokinetics, and effect in the BB rat model. Metabolism 1983; 32(Suppl 1):69–72.

105. Shah SC, Malone JI, Simpson NE. A randomized trial of intensive insulin therapy in newly diagnosed insulin dependent diabetes mellitus. N Engl J Med 1989; 320:550–554.

106. Bougneres PF, Carel JC, Castano L, et al. Factors associated with early

remission of type I diabetes in children treated with cyclosporine. N Engl J Med 1988; 318:663–670.

107. Dupre J, Stiller CR, Gent M, et al. Effects of immunosuppression with cyclosporine in insulin dependent diabetes mellitus of recent onset: the Canadian open study at 44 months. Transplant Proc 1988; 20:184–192.

108. Solimena M, Folli F, Denis-Donini S, et al. Autoantibodies to glutamic acid decarboxylase in a patient with stiff-man syndrome, epilepsy, and type I diabetes mellitus. N Engl J Med 1988; 318:1012–1020.

109. Brown FM, Smith AM, Longway S, et al. Adrenal medullitis in type I diabetes. J Clin Endocrinol Metab 1990; 71:1491–1495.

110. Rabinowe SL, Brown FM, Watts M, et al. Anti-sympathetic ganglia antibodies and postural blood pressure in IDDM subjects of varying duration and patients at high risk of developing IDDM. Diabetes Care 1989; 12:1–6.

111. Thorpe ES, Handley HE. Chronic tetany and chronic mycelial stomatitis in a child aged four-and-one-half years. Am J Dis Child 1929; 38:328–338.

112. Wirfalt A. Genetic heterogeneity in autoimmune polyglandular failure. Acta Med Scand 1981; 210:7–13.

112a. Ahonen P, Sinikka M, Sipila I, et al. Clinical variation of autoimmune polyendocrinopathy-candidiasis-ectodermal dystrophy (APECED) in a series of 68 patients. N Engl J Med 1990; 322:1829–1836.

113. Blizzard RM, Chee D, Davis W. The incidence of parathyroid and other antibodies in the sera of patients with idiopathic hypoparathyroidism. Clin Exp Immunol 1966; 1:119–128.

114. Children RA, Meuwissen HJ, Quie PG, et al. The cellular immune defect in chronic mucocutaneous candidiasis. Lancet 1969; 1:1286–1288.

115. Eisenbarth GS, Wilson PW, Ward F, et al. The polyglandular failure syndrome: disease inheritance, HLA-type and immune function studies in patients and families. Ann Intern Med 1979; 91:528–533.

116. Kirkpatrick CH. Chronic mucocutaneous candidiasis. Eur J Clin Microbiol Infect Dis 1989; 8:448–456.

117. Petersen EA, Alling DW, Kirkpatrick CH. Treatment of chronic mucocutaneous candidiasis with ketoconazole. Ann Intern Med 1980; 93:791–795.

118. Horsburgh CR, Kirkpatrick CH. Long-term therapy of chronic mucocutaneous candidiasis with ketoconazole: experience with 21 patients. Am J Med 1983; 1(Suppl):23–29.

119. Kahn CR, Flier JS, Bar RS, et al. The syndromes of insulin resistance and acanthosis nigricans. N Engl J Med 1976; 294:739–745.

120. Kahn CR, Harrison LH. Insulin receptor autoantibodies. In: Rendle PJ, Steiner DF, Whelen SJ, eds. Carbohydrate Metabolism and Its Disorders. Vol IV. London: Academic, 1980: 279–330.

121. Flier JS, Bar RS, Muggeo M, et al. The evolving clinical course of patients with insulin receptor autoantibodies: spontaneous remission or receptor proliferation with hypoglycemia. J Clin Endocrinol Metab 1978; 47:985–995.

122. Moller DE, Flier JS. Detection of an alteration of the insulin receptor gene in a patient with insulin resistance, acanthosis nigricans, and polycystic ovary syndrome (type I insulin resistance). N Engl J Med 1989; 319:1526–1529.

123. Bardwich PA, Avaifler NJ, Gill GN, et al. Plasma cell dyscrasia with polyneuropathy, organomegaly, endocrinopathy, M protein and skin changes: the POEMS syndrome. Medicine 1980; 59:311–322.

124. Amiel JL, Machover D, Droz JP. Dyscrasie plasmocytaire avec artériopathie, polyneuropathie, syndrome endocrinien. Une maladie japonaise chez un italien. Ann Med Interne 1975; 126:745–749.

125. Imawari M, Akatsuka N, Ishabashi M, et al. Syndrome of plasma cell dyscrasia, polyneuropathy and endocrine disturbances. Ann Intern Med 1974; 81:490–493.

126. Iwashita H, Ohnishi A, Asada M, et al. Polyneuropathy, skin hyperpigmentation, edema and hypertrichosis in localized osteosclerotic myeloma. Neurology 1977; 27:675–681.

127. Meshkinpour H, Myung CG, Kramer LS. A unique multisystemic syndrome of unknown origin. Arch Intern Med 1977; 137:1719–1721.

128. Saihan EM, Burton JL, Heaton KW. A new syndrome with pigmentation, scleroderma, gynecomastia, Raynaud's phenomenon and peripheral neuropathy. Br J Dermatol 1978; 99:437–440.

129. Scully RE, ed. Case records of the Massachusetts General Hospital. Case 34-1987. N Engl J Med 1987; 317:493–502.

130. Miller JFAP. Immunological function of the thymus. Lancet 1961; 2:748–749.

131. Good RA, Dalmasso AP, Martinez C, et al. The role of the thymus in development of immunologic capacity in rabbits and mice. J Exp Med 1962; 116:773–796.

132. Jankovic BD, Waksman BH, Arnason BG. Role of the thymus in immune reactions in rats. J Exp Med 1962; 116:159–176.

133. Kretschmer R, Say B, Brown D, et al. Congenital aplasia of the thymus gland (DiGeorge's syndrome). N Engl J Med 1968; 279:1295–1301.

134. LeDouarin NM, Jotereau FV. Tracing of cells of the avian thymus through embryonic life in interspecific chimeras. J Exp Med 1975; 142:17–40.

135. Hersh EM, Reuben JM, Rios A, et al. Elevated serum thymosin α 1 levels associated with evidence of immune dysregulation in male homosexuals with a history of infectious diseases or Kaposi's sarcoma. N Engl J Med 1983; 308:45–46 (letter).

136. Combs RM. Malignant thymoma, hyperthyroidism and immune disorder. South Med J 1968; 61:337–341.

137. LeGolvan DP, Abell MR. Thymomas. Cancer 1977; 29:2142–2157.

138. Patterson D. The causes of Down syndrome. Sci Am 1987; 257(2):52–60.

139. Rabinowe SL, Ricker AT, Rubin IL, Korb BR, et al. Polyglandular autoimmunity associated with trisomy of chromosome 21. Clin Res 1987; 35:586A.

140. Rabinowe SL, Rubin TL, George KL, et al. Trisomy 21 (Down's syndrome): autoimmunity, aging and monoclonal antibody–defined T-cell abnormalities. J Autoimmun 1989; 2:25–30.

141. Fialkow PJ, Thuline HC, Hecth F, et al. Familial predisposition to thyroid disease in Down's syndrome: controlled immunochemical studies. Am J Hum Genet 1971; 23:67–85.

142. Fleming S, Cowell C, Bailey J, et al. Hashimoto's disease in Turner's syndrome. Clin Invest Med 1988; 11:243–246.

143. Clarke WL, Shaver KA, Bright GA, et al. Autoimmunity in congenital rubella syndrome. J Pediatr 1984; 104:370–373.

144. Rubenstein P, Walker ME, Fendun B, et al. The HLA system in congenital rubella patients with and without diabetes. Diabetes 1982; 31:1088–1091.

145. Karasik A, O'Hara C, Srikanta S, et al. Genetically programmed selective islet β cell loss in diabetes mellitus of Wolfram syndrome. Diabetes Care 1989; 12:135–138.

146. Berzofsky JA, Crase KB, Cornette JL, et al. Protein antigenic structures reorganized by T cells. Immunol Rev 1987; 98:9–52.

147. Strober W, James SP. The interleukins. Pediatr Res 1988; 24:549–557.

148. Nakamura M, Burastero SE, Ueki Y, et al. Probing the normal and autoimmune β repertoire with Epstein-Barr virus. Frequency of B cells producing monoreactive high affinity autoantibodies in patients with Hashimoto's disease and systemic lupus erythematosus. J Immunol 1988; 141:4165–4172.

149. Jordan SC, Bright GM, Pincus T. Serositis with autoimmune endocrinopathy: clinical and immunogenetic features. Medicine 1987; 66:138–147.

150. Heubi JE, Partin JC, Schubert WK. Hypocalcemia and steatorrhea—clues to etiology. Dig Dis Sci 1983; 28:124–128.

151. Stankler L, Bewsher PD. Chronic mucocutaneous candidiasis, endocrine deficiency and alopecia areata. Br J Dermatol 1972; 86:238–245.

152. Gass JD. The syndrome of keratoconjunctivitis, superficial moniliasis, idiopathic hypoparathyroidism and Addison's disease. Am J Ophthalmol 1962; 54:660–674.

153. Srikanta S, Ganda OP, Jackson RA, et al. Type I diabetes mellitus in monozygotic twins: chronic progressive β cell dysfunction. Ann Intern Med 1983; 99:320–326.

154. Hordinsky, MK, Hallgren H, Nelson D, et al. Familial alopecia areata. HLA antigens and autoantibody formation in an American family. Arch Dermatol 1984; 120:464–468.

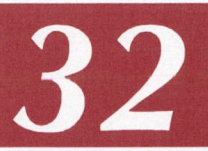

NON–INSULIN-SECRETING TUMORS OF THE GASTROENTEROPANCREATIC SYSTEM

Guenter J. Krejs

INTRODUCTION

In 1869 Langerhans described formations of "clear cells" in the pancreas that were subsequently termed the *islets of Langerhans*.[1] In 1938 Friedrich Feyrter discovered that *helle Zellen* (clear cells) are dispersed throughout the gastrointestinal tract as an endocrine (or neuroendocrine) system.[2] Sixteen different types of endocrine cells have now been functionally and/or morphologically characterized in the gastroenteropancreatic system[3, 4] (Table 32–1).

One functional characteristic of these cells became the basis for the APUD concept. That is, cells of the diffuse neuroendocrine system and the pancreatic islets share the capacity for amine precursor uptake and decarboxylation (APUD).[5, 6] A more useful classification of these endocrine cells is based on immunohistochemistry in combination with electron microscopy and in situ hybridization[7] (see Table 32–1). It is likely that all cells of the diffuse neuroendocrine system can give rise to endocrine tumors.

It is easy to understand that islet tumors may produce any of the peptides usually secreted by islet cells: insulin, glucagon, somatostatin (SRIF, somatotropin release–inhibiting factor), and pancreatic polypeptide (PP).[8] The presence of tumors that produce polypeptides other than those nor-

mally secreted by cells of the adult pancreas has been more difficult to understand. One possibility is that dedifferentiation to a pluripotent capacity allows these cells to produce any polypeptide. For instance, the adult pancreas does not produce gastrin, whereas gastrin-producing cells are found in the antrum of the stomach and the intestine. However, the fact that gastrin is not found in secretory granules of normal islet cells does not mean that the gene is not expressed. Many steps are necessary between the transcription of messenger RNA for gastrin and the packaging of gastrin-secretory granules. Normal pancreatic islet cells contain a high-molecular-weight progastrin, but post-translational modification of the molecule does not result in formation of biologically active gastrin.[9] Thus the tumor needs only to acquire the capacity to process the progastrin molecule appropriately to become gastrin-producing. The tools of molecular biology will make it possible to obtain additional insight into hormone production by endocrine tumors of the gastroenteropancreatic system.[10]

In the previous edition of this book the term *ectopic* was used for tumors that produce polypeptides not normally found in endocrine cells of the adult pancreas, namely gastrin, vasoactive intestinal peptide (VIP), peptide histidine-methionine (PHM), calcitonin, neurotensin, parathyroid hormone, corticotropin (ACTH, adrenocorticotropin), and

TABLE 32–1. Distribution of Human Gastroenteropancreatic Endocrine Cells*

Cell	Main Product	Pancreas	Stomach Fundus and Body	Antrum	Intestine Small Upper	Lower	Large
P/D₁	Unknown	f	+	+	+	f	f
EC	Serotonin + peptides	r	+	+	+	+	+
D	Somatostatin	+	+	+	+	f	f
B	Insulin	+					
PP(F/D₁)	Pancreatic polypeptide	+					
A	Glucagon	+	a				
X	Unknown		+				
ECL	Unknown		+				
G + IG	Gastrin			+	+	f	
CCK	Cholecystokinin				+	f	
S	Secretin				+	f	
GIP	Gastric inhibitory peptide				+	f	
Mo	Motilin				+	f	
N	Neurotensin				f	+	
L	Glicentin + PP-like peptide				f	+	+
VL	Unknown				+	+	

*f, few; r, rare; a, fetus and newborn: hybrid cells with both A and L cell granules.

From Solcia E, Capella C, Buffa R, et al. Endocrine cells of the digestive system. In: Johnson LR, ed. Physiology of the Gastrointestinal Tract. 2nd ed. New York: Raven, 1987: 111–130.

helodermin. However, the term ectopic is now considered to be inappropriate because production of a hormone by a tumor usually represents full expression of a particular gene that is only partially expressed in the normal cell from which the tumor originates[11] (also see Chapter 34).

Pancreatic endocrine tumors can also be a part of the syndrome multiple endocrine neoplasia type 1 (MEN 1), in which there is a hereditary predisposition to islet cell hyperplasia and islet cell tumor formation (see also Chapter 30). All islet cell tumors described in this chapter can occur in MEN 1. Most commonly, however, MEN 1 tumors of the gastrointestinal tract produce gastrin, VIP, or PP.[12, 13]

Pancreatic endocrine tumors may be composed of several different types of peptide-producing cells, and elevated levels of more than one peptide can be found in the plasma of such patients. The predominant type of cell and the predominant hormone produced define the clinical syndrome. On the other hand, 20 to 40% of islet cell tumors are nonfunctioning; that is, they do not release hormones into the circulation despite the presence of functioning endocrine cells on histological examination.[14, 15]

Endocrine tumors of the pancreas, like other endocrine tumors, may also secrete high-molecular-weight precursors of peptide hormones. These compounds usually have biological activity different from that of the native peptide, and the concentration of immunoreactive hormone may not correspond to the level of biological activity. For instance, in patients with gastrinoma large amounts of inactive progastrin circulate together with glycine-extended intermediates of gastrin, only some of which stimulate acid secretion and only some of which are detected by the COOH terminus–specific antisera used in conventional gastrin radioimmunoassays.[16] Thus clinical manifestations may be minimal despite a high plasma level of immunoactivity of a peptide and vice versa.

Endocrine tumors of the gastroenteropancreatic system are rare, with an incidence of 1 per 200,000 population per year. Gastrinomas are found in 1 per 2 million persons per year, VIPomas in 1 per 10 million per year, glucagonomas in 1 per 20 million per year, and somatostatinomas in 1 per 40 million per year.[17]

The several distinct endocrine syndromes will be described first (Table 32–2), and the features of diagnosis and treatment common to all endocrine tumors of the gastroen-

TABLE 32–2. Clinical Features of Endocrine Tumors of the Gastroenteropancreatic System*

Tumor Syndrome	Clinical Features	Diagnostic Features (Other Than Elevated Basal Plasma Peptide Concentration)
Glucagonoma	Necrolytic migratory erythema, mild diabetes, psychiatric disturbances, diarrhea, venous thrombosis	Excessive glucagon release after intravenous administration of tolbutamide
Somatostatinoma	Dyspepsia, diabetes, gallstones, steatorrhea, hypochlorhydria	Hyperglycemia without hyperketonemia; stool weight usually 400 to 800 g/d; stool fat 10 to 30 g/d
PPoma	None recognized (secretory diarrhea in three cases)	None known for pure PPoma
Gastrinoma	Severe peptic ulcer disease, secretory diarrhea	Serum gastrin level increases after intravenous administration of secretin; high basal and peak acid secretion; secretory diarrhea stops after omeprazole or H₂ receptor antagonist treatment
VIPoma	Large-volume secretory diarrhea, hypokalemia, metabolic acidosis, hypochlorhydria	Stool analysis of secretory diarrhea and fecal pH less than 8.0 on fasting (colonic bicarbonate secretion), plasma PHM level elevated in cases studied, occasionally cosecretion of calcitonin, PP, and helodermin
Calcitoninoma	Diarrhea	Secretory diarrhea while fasting, osmotic component while eating (decreased small bowel transit time)
GHRHoma	Acromegaly (long history)	Normal sella; negative head computed tomographic and negative resonance imaging scans; growth hormone release by endogenous GHRH (pituitary tumors respond)
Neurotensinoma	Esophageal reflux (in one case)	None known for pure neurotensin

*Excluding carcinoids (see Chapter 35) and insulinomas (see Chapter 23).

teropancreatic system will be discussed subsequently. Carcinoid tumors and insulinomas are discussed in Chapters 35 and 23, respectively.

TUMOR SYNDROMES

Glucagonoma

The pre-proglucagon gene on chromosome 2 encodes a polypeptide that gives rise in the pancreas to glucagon and in the intestinal wall and central nervous system to other products, originally known as enteroglucagon and now recognized to consist largely of glicentin, a 69-amino-acid peptide that includes the 29-amino-acid sequence of glucagon (Fig. 32–1).

The glucagonoma syndrome is often diagnosed by dermatologists because a characteristic rash, necrolytic migratory erythema, is frequently the major manifestation. Necrolytic migratory erythema is a figurate erythema with a moving edge that has the histological features of toxic epidermal necrolysis.[18–20] The lesions are found on the buttocks, groin, perineum, and thighs and commence as red patches that progress to form bullae and then break down and become encrusted, followed by healing and pigmentation.[21] The lesions tend to coalesce, often with extensive skin involvement and secondary infection.[22, 23] The determatological disorder may be a direct consequence of an elevated plasma glucagon level or an indirect effect secondary to lowered plasma amino acid levels or tissue zinc levels.[24, 25] The rash disappears promptly when the plasma glucagon level returns to normal after complete tumor resection.[22, 26] Glucagon excess causes increased hepatic conversion of amino acid nitrogen to urea nitrogen, resulting in decreased blood amino acid concentrations. Enhanced protein catabolism is associated with weight loss and decreased lean body mass.[27]

The glycogenolytic and gluconeogenic actions of glucagon result in mild hyperglycemia that can be treated by diet or the administration of oral hypoglycemic drugs. The levels of hyperglycemia and plasma glucagon are poorly correlated, possibly because of down-regulation of glucagon receptors but more likely because of the ability of intact beta cells to counteract the hyperglycemic effect of glucagon by releasing insulin.[25] Other manifestations include anorexia, glossitis, angular cheilitis, venous thrombosis, weight loss, anemia, and psychiatric disturbances such as depression. Diarrhea is prominent in some patients and is thought to result from the secretory effects of glucagon on the small bowel mucosa (reduction of absorption or enhancement of net secretion of water and electrolytes).[28]

Like most islet cell tumors, glucagonomas are slow-growing. Patients usually are middle-aged and have a long history of symptoms related to glucagon excess. The diagnosis is confirmed by documenting elevated plasma glucagon levels in the presence of a pancreatic mass. High plasma glucagon levels also occur in diabetes mellitus, pancreatitis, trauma, and a variety of other stresses such as burns and myocardial infarction. In consequence, diagnosis requires the presence of a tumor mass and the exclusion of other conditions known to elevate the plasma glucagon concentration. In patients with glucagonoma the plasma glicentin (enteroglucagon) concentration is also elevated,[29] and this may serve as an important disease marker. In enteroglucagonomas the plasma glicentin level is also high, but the serum glucagon level is normal.

Enteroglucagonoma

Glicentin (enteroglucagon) is produced by the L cells in the intestine (see Table 32–1 and Fig. 32–1). Three cases of so-called enteroglucagonoma have been described in which high tissue and plasma levels of enteroglucagon were associated with intestinal mucosal hyperplasia and giant intestinal

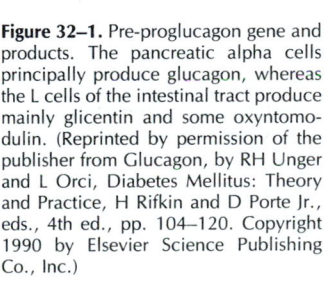

Figure 32–1. Pre-proglucagon gene and products. The pancreatic alpha cells principally produce glucagon, whereas the L cells of the intestinal tract produce mainly glicentin and some oxyntomodulin. (Reprinted by permission of the publisher from Glucagon, by RH Unger and L Orci, Diabetes Mellitus: Theory and Practice, H Rifkin and D Porte Jr., eds., 4th ed., pp. 104–120. Copyright 1990 by Elsevier Science Publishing Co., Inc.)

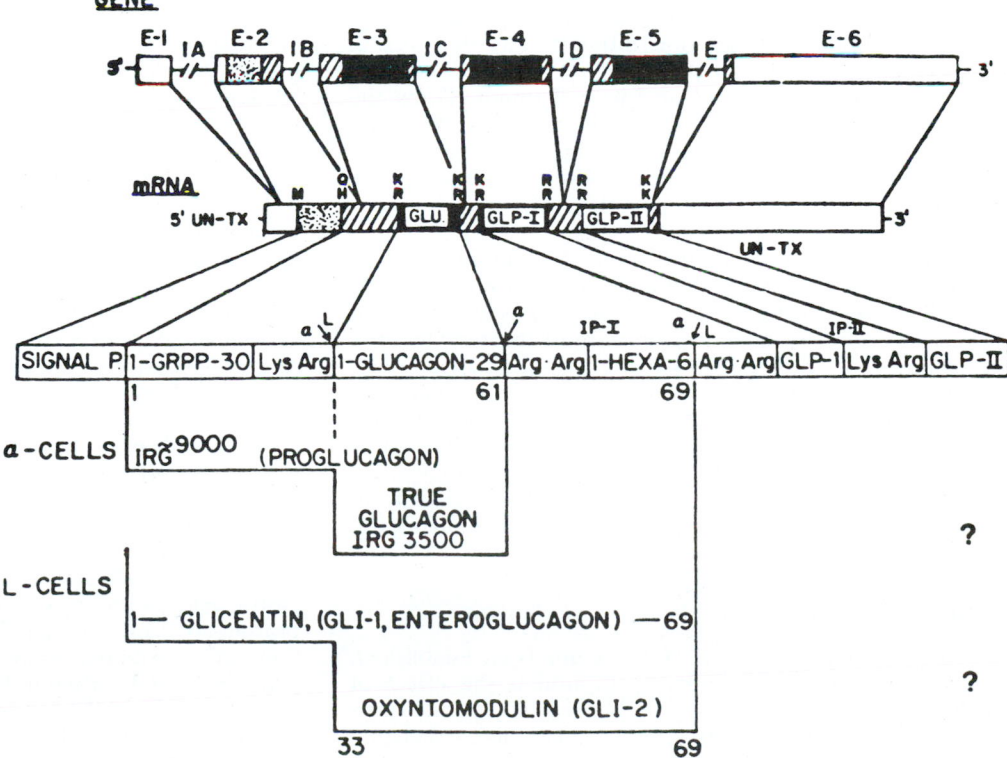

villi.[30] In one case the enteroglucagonoma was present in the kidney, and the intestinal abnormality disappeared after nephrectomy.[31] The second case was diagnosed when giant villi were seen in the duodenum by fiberoptic endoscopy. The third case was detected by computed tomographic scan of the abdomen, which showed enlarged folds and coarse mucosa in the small bowel.[33] In the second and third cases the enteroglucagonomas were located in the pancreas. In these cases the circulating hormone reacted with antibodies to glicentin but were not characterized at the molecular level.

Somatostatinoma

The somatostatinoma syndrome was first recognized in 1979.[34] A previous report of two somatostatinomas incidentally found at gallbladder surgery[35, 36] and study of the pharmacological actions of somatostatin allowed prediction of the clinical features of somatostatin excess.[37]

Somatostatin inhibits diverse endocrine functions in the anterior pituitary, pancreatic islets, gastrointestinal mucosa, thyroid follicle, and juxtaglomerular region of the kidney. Suppression of both insulin and glucagon causes mild diabetes mellitus, but hyperglycemia and hyperketonemia are not severe. Indeed, hyperglycemia usually responds to dietary management. Other features include cholelithiasis, steatorrhea, indigestion, and hypochlorhydria, which are all manifestations of the inhibitory actions of somatostatin on gastrointestinal function.[38] Approximately 25 cases of pancreatic somatostatinoma have been reported. Clinical manifestations include occasional hypoglycemia,[39, 40] flushing,[35] and Cushing syndrome.[41] The fact that somatostatinomas frequently contain subpopulations of other endocrine cells explains, at least in part, the variability in symptoms. Diarrhea, for instance, appears to be prominent in calcitonin-secreting somatostatinomas.[34, 42] The clinical manifestations may also be influenced by varying degrees of target organ resistance so that expected pharmacological effects of somatostatin are blunted. For instance, in two patients high somatostatin concentrations in plasma did not inhibit glucagon release.[34, 43] Variability of symptoms and the fact that the cardinal manifestations (dyspepsia, diabetes mellitus, cholelithiasis, diarrhea, steatorrhea, and hypochlorhydria) are common make recognition difficult. The diagnosis is usually dependent on identification of a pancreatic mass with histological features of an islet cell tumor. Often the diagnosis is suspected only when metastatic spread causes weight loss and other signs of malignant disease. Most patients with somatostatinomas have liver metastases at the time of diagnosis, but in retrospect the symptoms have been present for several years.[34]

Gastrointestinal somatostatinomas (mainly in the duodenal wall and ampulla of Vater) are histologically and clinically distinct from pancreatic somatostatinomas.[44–46] Histologically they are psammomatous tumors that tend to cause biliary tract or intestinal obstruction. Eight patients with neurofibromatosis type 1 have developed somatostatinoma of the papilla of Vater.[45, 47, 48] Because somatostatin is rarely released from gastrointestinal somatostatinomas, the somatostatinoma syndrome is not present. When combined calcium and pentagastrin are administered intravenously to such patients, however, a small rise in serum somatostatin concentration can be detected.[49]

Pancreatic Polypeptide–Producing Tumor

A physiological role for PP has not been established, but the capacity of the peptide to inhibit the effect of cholecystokinin may play a role in pancreatic exocrine function and gallbladder motility.[50] Patients with high circulating levels of PP do not display a characteristic clinical syndrome. In three patients a PP-containing pancreatic tumor (PPoma) or islet cell adenomatosis was associated with secretory diarrhea,[51–53] but PP is not an intestinal secretagogue in small bowel perfusion experiments.[54] In one patient a macular rash (distinct from necrolytic migratory erythema) disappeared with tumor treatment.[55] Because about half of pancreatic endocrine tumors contain PP, the peptide has been used as a marker for the diagnosis of pancreatic endocrine tumors and for monitoring the response to treatment.[56–59] PP has also been used to follow subjects at risk because of a family history of MEN 1.[60] Although in most patients an elevated basal plasma PP level is indicative of islet cell tumor, an exaggerated plasma PP response to meal stimulation can be indicative of the MEN 1 trait and islet cell hyperplasia.[13] The usefulness of PP as a marker of endocrine pancreatic tumors is limited because high plasma levels are present in patients with certain inflammatory diseases, renal failure, and laxative abuse.[56] Intravenous atropine lowers plasma levels when PP does not originate from a tumor.[58]

Gastrinoma

In 1955 Zollinger and Ellison[61] described a syndrome characterized by severe peptic ulcer disease that recurred after several surgical procedures, gastric hypersecretion, and the presence of a pancreatic endocrine tumor. The availability of a radioimmunoassay for gastrin makes the diagnosis straightforward, and cases are often recognized early in the course of disease. A basal serum gastrin level above 200 ng/L requires further assessment but is not specific for the gastrinoma syndrome, because the plasma gastrin level may be high in patients with atrophic gastritis and achlorhydria (pernicious anemia), antral gastrin-cell hyperplasia, retained antrum after a Billroth II partial gastrectomy, renal failure, pyloric stenosis, and short-bowel syndrome, as well as after vagotomy and during therapeutic achlorhydria induced by H_2 receptor antagonists and proton pump inhibitors.[62]

The rate of gastric acid secretion is high in patients with gastrinoma but may overlap with rates in patients with duodenal ulcer disease and in some healthy controls. About half of patients have a basal acid secretion rate of more than 15 mmol/h. A pattern of basal acid output equal to or greater than 60% of the peak acid output (after pentagastrin) is suggestive of gastrinoma, but about half of gastrinoma patients do not show this pattern.[62]

If serum gastrin elevation is moderate (200 to 1000 ng/L), a provocative test should be performed. The best provocative test is provided by the administration of intravenous secretin (2 U/kg body weight). In patients with gastrinoma, the serum gastrin level increases promptly (within 5 or 10 min), usually by more than 200 ng/L.[63] Measurement of the plasma level of progastrin, a high-molecular-weight precursor of gastrin, may also be useful in diagnosis of patients with the Zollinger-Ellison syndrome.[16]

Clinical features other than peptic ulcer include diarrhea and steatorrhea. Diarrhea is present in a third of patients and may precede peptic ulcer symptoms.[64] The major cause of diarrhea is the large amount of acidic fluid entering the jejunum.[65] In one patient studied by the author, the fluid of the proximal jejunum had a pH of 1.1, and 15 L of fluid was estimated from perfusion studies to enter the small bowel each day in the fasting state. Suppression of gastric acid secretion with H_2 receptor antagonists or omeprazole abolishes the diarrhea. High circulating concentrations of gastrin may play a minor direct role in causing diarrhea by reducing intestinal water and ion absorption.[66]

The traditional treatment for gastrinoma was total gastrectomy. However, H_2 receptor antagonists and omeprazole are now the first line of therapy. Surgery is still useful for tumor resection and with early diagnosis may allow a cure rate of 20%.[67] Vagotomy, once useful for reducing the required dosage of H_2 blockers,[68] has not been necessary since omeprazole became available.[69] The fact that gastrectomy is no longer performed in such patients has made it possible to study the effect of prolonged hypergastrinemia on enterochromaffin-like (ECL) cells of the stomach (see next section).

Gastric Carcinoids Caused by Hypergastrinemia

Rats given large doses of the proton pump inhibitor omeprazole for prolonged periods develop profound hypergastrinemia and gastric carcinoids.[70] These tumors arise from the ECL cells in the gastric mucosa (see Table 32–1). Other potent antisecretory agents (newer H_2 blockers) can also cause the tumor in rats.[71] The association of gastric carcinoids with hypergastrinemia in rats[72] is analogous to two situations in humans associated with hypergastrinemia: pernicious anemia and the Zollinger-Ellison syndrome. In both conditions ECL cell hyperplasia and gastric carcinoids occur but appear to be reversible;[71] metastases have not been observed. The prevalence of gastric carcinoids in patients with pernicous anemia appears to be about 5%.[73] Antrectomy has been suggested for patients with pernicious anemia who develop gastric carcinoids. In Zollinger-Ellison syndrome, gastric carcinoids appear to develop in patients in whom gastrinoma is a component of the MEN 1 syndrome rather than a sporadic disorder. In patients receiving long-term omeprazole therapy hypergastrinemia is less pronounced, and neither ECL cell hyperplasia nor carcinoid tumors have been found, even when carefully assessed by morphometry of the gastric mucosa.[74] Nevertheless, physicians treating patients with omeprazole should be aware of the possible association of hypergastrinemia with ECL cell hyperplasia and gastric carcinoids.

VIPoma

In 1957 Priest and Alexander[75] described a patient with islet cell tumor, severe watery diarrhea, and hypokalemia, and in 1958 Verner and Morrison[76] called attention to the syndrome of watery diarrhea, hypokalemia, and death resulting from renal failure in association with islet cell tumor. Synonyms for VIPoma include the Verner-Morrison syndrome, the watery diarrhea–hypokalemia–hypochlorhydria syndrome, and the pancreatic cholera syndrome.

The term *pancreatic cholera*, first used by Matsumoto and colleagues,[77] is appropriate because the diarrhea, as in Asiatic cholera, results from the intestinal secretion of fluid. However, some responsible tumors are outside the pancreas (neuroblastoma and ganglioneuroma in children). Bloom and colleagues[78] recognized that patients with this syndrome have elevated plasma levels and high tumor contents of VIP.

VIP was discovered by Said and Mutt[79] as a vasoactive substance and was considered to be a candidate gastrointestinal hormone by Grossman.[80] The peptide is also present in neurons of both the central and peripheral nervous systems,[81] where it functions as a neuromodulator.[82–84] The biological actions of VIP have been reviewed by Said.[85] VIP exerts profound effects on intestinal water and ion movement in experimental animals,[86] but it was not initially clear that VIP is the mediator of intestinal secretion and diarrhea in pancreatic cholera syndrome as opposed to being a marker of the disease.[87, 88] This uncertainty resulted from the fact that not all patients with islet cell tumors and diarrhea have

high plasma levels of VIP[89] and the finding that high plasma levels can occur in healthy controls[90] and in persons abusing laxatives.[91]

It is now established that VIP is the major mediator of pancreatic cholera. After removal of the tumors, diarrhea disappears as plasma VIP levels return to normal. Infusion of VIP intravenously during intestinal perfusion studies in healthy subjects changes the movement of water and ions from absorption to secretion.[92, 93] Finally, prolonged intravenous VIP infusion (10 h) in healthy subjects produces secretory diarrhea (mean 2.4 L/10 h) and causes metabolic acidosis, thus mimicking the clinical syndrome.[94]

Cosecretion of PHM occurs in patients with VIPomas. PHM concentrations are high in plasma, and both VIP and PHM are present in the same tumor cells as indicated by immunocytochemistry.[95] PHM has effects on intestinal mucosa similar to those of VIP but is 32 times less potent as a secretagogue than VIP.[96] Cosecretion of calcitonin (see later) and helodermin (personal communication, P. Robberecht) with VIP has also been observed.

The major clinical manifestation of VIPoma is large-volume secretory diarrhea, although many patients excrete less than 3 L of stool/d.[97] Because the diarrhea is secretory, stool water is isotonic with plasma, and diarrhea persists on fasting.[98] For practical purposes a stool volume of less than 700 mL/d excludes the syndrome.[99] Large amounts of potassium and bicarbonate are lost in the diarrheal stool, resulting in hypokalemia, acidosis, and volume depletion. In a few patients secretion of water and ions by the small intestine has been demonstrated directly by perfusion methods.[91, 100–102]

Achlorhydria or hypochlorhydria is often present. Of 43 patients reviewed by Verner and Morrison,[103] 14 had histamine-fast achlorhydria and 16 had hypochlorhydria. Because parietal cells in gastric mucosal biopsy specimens are normal even in achlorhydric patients and gastric hyposecretion can be corrected by resection of the VIPoma,[104] it is likely that the tumors release a gastric inhibitor. VIP infusion inhibits pentagastrin- and meal-stimulated acid secretion in the dog[105] but does not inhibit pentagastrin-induced acid secretion in acute experiments in humans.[106] Whether VIP affects meal-stimulated acid secretion in humans is not known.

Hypercalcemia occurs in half the cases,[103] but the mechanism is not clear. There appears to be a negative calcium balance with increased bone resorption.[107] Tetany is thought to be due to hypomagnesemia and may occur in the presence of hypercalcemia. Flushing is occasionally observed. Some patients have hypotension resulting from peripheral vasodilation, and severe hypertension may follow tumor removal.[108] These symptoms are compatible with the known cardiovascular effects of VIP.[109] Glucose intolerance occurs in about half of patients with the VIPoma syndrome. A direct diabetogenic effect of the secreted agent is suggested by the observation that operative manipulation of an islet cell VIPoma caused pronounced hyperglycemia in one patient.[110]

The average duration of symptoms before diagnosis is 3 y[111] and may range from 2 mo to 4 y.[112] Metastases (liver, lymph nodes) are present in half of patients at the time of diagnosis. Death results from renal failure or cardiac arrest caused by volume depletion and acidosis. The survival of patients with islet cell tumors used to be less than 1 y from the time of diagnosis. A better understanding of the pathophysiology has made possible more appropriate supportive treatment, and the introduction of cytotoxic chemotherapy has improved survival time. In our series of eight patients, two have survived 4 and 12 y without evidence of recurrent disease.

Pancreatic Calcitoninoma

Calcitonin has been found in a number of endocrine pancreatic tumors but usually not as the predominant peptide. It has been detected in tumors containing VIP,[110–113] somatostatin,[34, 42] PP,[114] motilin, gastric inhibitory polypeptide (also known as glucose-dependent insulinotropic polypeptide), neurotensin, and enkephalins.[115] Thus, like PP, calcitonin may be used as a marker peptide for the diagnosis of pancreatic endocrine malignancies.

Calcitonin infusion decreases transit time[116] and increases the secretion of water and electrolytes by the small bowel.[117] Thus diarrhea may be expected in these patients. However, only a third of the patients with calcitonin excess associated with medullary carcinoma of the thyroid have diarrhea (also see Chapter 30).

Neurotensinoma

Neurotensin can frequently be detected when pancreatic endocrine tumors are examined by immunocytochemistry and immunofluorescence.[118–120] However, no clear-cut syndrome has been attributed to a high plasma neurotensin level. In one patient neurotensin-secreting cells accounted for 80% of endocrine cells of a pancreatic tumor.[121] The patient had severe esophageal reflux, and it was suggested that a neurotensin-induced increase in enteric pressure was the cause. Additional cases of relatively pure neurotensinomas need to be studied before conclusions can be drawn. When both VIP and neurotensin are produced by pancreatic tumors, the symptoms are those of the pancreatic cholera syndrome.[122] Cosecretion of gastrin and neurotensin results in manifestations characteristic of Zollinger-Ellison syndrome.[122]

Parathyrinoma

Parathyroid hormone production by a pancreatic islet cell tumor is rare.[123] Evaluation of hypercalcemia in this setting may be difficult because the peptide released by the tumor may show molecular heterogeneity and may not be detected by standard radioimmunoassay.[8]

Corticotropinoma

Pancreatic corticotropinomas release corticotropin and result in Cushing syndrome (also see Chapters 6 and 9). Plasma cortisol and urinary 17-hydroxycorticosteroid levels are not suppressed by the high-dose dexamethasone suppression test.[8] These tumors may also secrete melanocyte-stimulating hormone and corticotropin-releasing hormone. Cushing syndrome resulting from ectopic corticotropin production is found in 5% of patients with the sporadic form of Zollinger-Ellison syndrome.[125]

GHRHoma

Release of growth hormone–releasing hormone (GHRH) from a pancreatic or gastrointestinal tumor stimulates the normal pituitary to excessive release of growth hormone. Patients develop acromegaly or gigantism. Such tumors were first recognized in 1982,[126, 127] and fewer than 10 cases have been described[128, 129] (also see Chapter 6). The sella is normal in size, and magnetic resonance imaging and computed tomographic scans of the pituitary are also normal. Growth hormone release in response to exogenous GHRH is blunted, whereas pituitary tumors that cause acromegaly respond normally. Several patients with this disorder have been successfully treated with the somatostatin analogue octreotide.[130]

MULTIPLE HORMONE–SECRETING TUMORS

Radioimmunoassay and immunohistochemical techniques demonstrate that more than half of pancreatic islet cell tumors produce more than one peptide.[131] Clinically, however, most patients with mixed pancreatic endocrine tumors have symptoms characteristic of single-hormone excess.[132] Some mixed tumors are "hormonally silent" and produce symptoms related only to tumor mass, metastases, or nonspecific signs of malignant disease (anemia, weight loss). When hormonal symptoms are produced, the immunocytochemical predominance of a certain cell type may not always correspond to the clinical picture. For instance, even when gastrin-secreting cells constitute only 10% of the cell population in a tumor, the secretion of gastrin may be sufficient to induce Zollinger-Ellison syndrome.[121]

Sometimes the clinical syndrome changes with time or after chemotherapy. A tumor may first present as an insulinoma but later show symptoms of glucagon or gastrin excess.[133, 134] Experimental evidence suggests that chemotherapy with streptozocin may precipitate such transformations.[135] In one case, transition from the Zollinger-Ellison syndrome to insulinoma was noted without detectable ultrastructural changes within the tumor itself.[136] Metastases of these mixed tumors may contain all cell types of the original tumor or only one or two of the original cell types.[137]

"CANDIDATE" TUMORS

Islet cell tumors and gastrointestinal tumors with predominant secretion of several gastrointestinal hormones have not been recognized. The following peptides may be considered for such candidate tumors: secretin, cholecystokinin, motilin, gastric inhibitory polypeptide, bombesin, enkephalin, and PYY (peptide P with NH_2-terminal and COOH-terminal tyrosines). If such tumors occur, they must be rare and cause mild symptoms. It is possible that some of the 20 to 40% of islet cell tumors that are usually classified as nonfunctional actually produce one or more of these hormones. Better assay techniques and increasing knowledge of the biological actions of regulatory peptides may allow recognition of such tumors and their associated syndromes in the future.

ISLET CELL HYPERPLASIA

Some of the endocrine syndromes related to pancreatic tumors have been described as resulting from islet cell hyperplasia rather than islet cell adenoma or carcinoma. For instance, Verner and Morrison's later series of patients with pancreatic cholera contained several patients without a pancreatic tumor, and it was deduced that a fifth of the cases were due to islet cell hyperplasia.[103] Likewise, in the Said series, 14% of the patients with the watery diarrhea syndrome were categorized as having islet cell hyperplasia.[138] On the other hand, Bloom and Polak[139] did not find elevated plasma VIP levels in any patient with islet cell hyperplasia, and J. Fahrenkrug (personal communication) believes that pancreatic cholera is rarely, if ever, due to islet cell hyperplasia. Many of the reports describing this entity are hard to interpret, because the diagnosis of islet cell hyperplasia is often poorly documented and morphometric data are lacking. Moreover, Chey and colleagues[140] described seven cases of pancreatic cholera syndrome and islet cell hyperplasia without elevated plasma VIP levels. PP cell hyperplasia and gastric inhibitory polypeptide cell hyperplasia have also been described in association with the watery diarrhea syndrome.[141]

The importance of islet cell hyperplasia in these disorders is unresolved, particularly when the possibility of subtotal pancreatectomy is considered in a patient with a high circulating concentration of a particular peptide but without pancreatic tumor. It is conceivable that islet cell hyperplasia is a premalignant condition, because patients with MEN 1 may demonstrate islet cell hyperplasia before the development of islet cell tumors.[13, 60]

GENERAL FEATURES

Diagnosis

Gut endocrine cell tumors are uncommon, occurring in about 1 per 200,000 population. The diagnosis is easy in the presence of characteristic signs and symptoms (e.g., rash in glucagonoma and intractable peptic ulcer in gastrinoma). However, some tumors cause nonspecific symptoms such as dyspepsia. Thus somatostatinomas may be found incidentally during gallbladder surgery. Other tumors may be diagnosed only during investigation of weight loss. Because these tumors grow slowly and are either benign or metastasize late, they are potentially curable. Early detection is highly desirable.

Radioimmunoassays for the various hormones secreted by these tumors are often diagnostic, particularly if plasma levels are very high, but not every assay is available in all laboratories. To send plasma samples to the appropriate laboratories, blood must be drawn in tubes containing ethylenediaminetetraacetic acid and aprotinin to inhibit serum peptidases (aprotinin, 0.5 mL [5000 kallikrein inactivator units] per 10 mL of blood). After immediate centrifugation, plasma is stored at $-25°C$ or lower until sent in the frozen state on dry ice. In screening for pancreatic endocrine tumors, we submit plasma samples for analysis of VIP, gastrin, calcitonin, somatostatin, PP, motilin, gastric inhibitory polypeptide, PHM, neurotensin, glucagon, and insulin. In some laboratories, a "gastrointestinal hormone profile" can be obtained with a single plasma sample.[142] Neuron-specific enolase and chromogranin A are also used by some as serum markers for endocrine tumors of the gastroenteropancreatic system, but experience is limited.[143, 144]

Tumor localization can usually be accomplished by use of an imaging technique such as sonography, computed tomographic scanning, angiography, and magnetic resonance imaging. If liver metastases are present, peritoneoscopic biopsy or biopsy guided by ultrasound or computed tomography can be used to obtain material for histological studies. For immunocytochemical studies, biopsy material should be fixed in Bouin solution. Aliquots of the biopsy material should also be frozen in liquid nitrogen to allow analysis of tissue extracts for various peptides. If the results of imaging procedures are negative, exploratory laparotomy may be necessary. Intraoperative sonography is superior to palpation of the pancreas in localizing small tumors. Selective venous sampling, although advocated by some investigators, is not recommended by the author because the procedure is difficult, and aberrant venous drainage of the tumor may lead to erroneous conclusions.[145]

Treatment

Total tumor resection is the first objective of therapy. Even in the presence of liver metastases, removal of the primary pancreatic tumor may sometimes be advisable. One of our patients with VIPoma was cured by removal of the primary tumor and, after chemotherapy, partial hepatectomy to remove the one area of tumor mass remaining in the liver. After successful resection of the primary pancreatic tumor, liver transplantation has been attempted in a few instances to remove the remaining tumor.[146] Metastatic tumor mass has also been reduced by hepatic artery embolization.[114]

Among chemotherapeutic drugs, streptozocin is highly effective, particularly in VIPomas.[147] 5-Fluorouracil and dacarbazine have also been used. Finally, drugs that modify the target organ response can render the patient asymptomatic for long periods despite continued slow tumor growth and elevated plasma peptide levels. Such regimens include use of antisecretory drugs for diarrhea in VIPoma or calcitoninoma syndrome[148] and omeprazole in Zollinger-Ellison syndrome.[69, 71]

Somatostatin inhibits the release of VIP from endocrine tumors in pancreatic cholera,[149] and octreotide, a long-acting somatostatin analogue, has been successfully used in a number of gastrointestinal endocrine syndromes including VIPomas,[150] glucagonomas,[29] and GHRHomas.[130] Administration of octreotide subcutaneously inhibits release (and formation) of hormones and other tumor products and thus prevents endocrine symptoms. Administration of the agent over longer periods of time may also cause tumor shrinkage.[151, 152] Öberg and co-workers have advocated the use of interferon in gut endocrine tumors, but experience is limited.[153, 154]

REFERENCES

1. Langerhans P. Über die mikroskopische Anatomie des Pankreas. Inaugural-Dissertation. Berlin: G. Lange, 1869.
2. Feyrter F. Über diffuse endokrine epitheliale Organe. In: Barth JA, ed. Leipzig: 1938.
3. Solcia E, Capella C, Buffa R, et al. Endocrine cells of the digestive system. In: Johnson LR, ed. Physiology of the Gastrointestinal Tract. 2nd ed. New York: Raven, 1987: 111–130.
4. Solcia E, Sessa F, Rindi G, et al. Classification and histogenesis of gastroenteropancreatic endocrine tumors. Eur J Clin Invest 1990; 20(Suppl 1):S72–S81.
5. Pearse AGE. Common cytochemical and ultrastructural characteristics of cells producing polypeptide hormones (the APUD series) and their relevance to thyroid ultimobranchial C cells and calcitonin. Proc R Soc Lond [Biol] 1968; 170:71–80.
6. Pearse AGE. The diffuse neuroendocrine system and the APUD concept: related "endocrine" peptides in brain, intestine, pituitary, placenta, and anuran cutaneous glands. Med Biol 1977; 55:115–125.
7. Rindi G, Solcia E, Polak JM. Transgenic mouse models and peptide producing endocrine tumours: morpho-functional aspects. In: Polak JM, ed. Regulatory Peptides. Basel: Birkhauser, 1989: 210–219.
8. Friesen SR. Tumors of the endocrine pancreas. N Engl J Med 1982; 306:580–590.
9. Bardam L. Gastrin in non-neoplastic pancreatic tissue from patients with and without gastrinoma. Scand J Gastroenterol (in press).
10. Rehfeld JF. Perspectives in the research of gut regulatory peptides. Eur J Clin Invest 1990; 20(Suppl 1):S91–S93.
11. Rehfeld JF, Lindhom J, Andersen BN, et al. Cholecystokinin and glucagonoma. N Engl J Med 1988; 318:122–123.
12. Hutcheon DF, Bayless TM, Cameron JL, et al. Hormone-mediated watery diarrhea in a family with multiple endocrine neoplasms. Ann Intern Med 1979; 90:932–934.
13. Friesen SR, Tomita T, Kimmel JR. Pancreatic polypeptide update: its roles in detection of the trait for multiple endocrine adenopathy syndrome, type I and pancreatic polypeptide–secreting tumors. Surgery 1983; 94:1028–1037.
14. Howard JM, Moss NH, Rhoades JE. Collective review: hyperinsulinism and islet cell tumors of the pancreas with 398 recorded tumors. Int Abstr Surg 1950; 90:417–455.
15. Broder LE, Carter SK. Pancreatic islet cell carcinoma. I. Clinical features of 52 patients. Ann Intern Med 1973; 79:101–107.
16. Bardram L. Progastrin in serum from Zollinger-Ellison patients. Gastroenterology 1990; 98, 1420–1426.
17. Krejs GJ. Gastrointestinal endocrine tumors. Am J Med 1987; 82(Suppl 5B):1–3.

18. Sweet RD. A dermatosis specifically associated with a tumour of pancreatic alpha cells. Br J Dermatol 1974; 90:301–308.
19. Wilkinson DS. Necrolytic migratory erythema with carcinoma of the pancreas. Trans St. John's Hosp Dermatol Soc 1973; 59:244–250.
20. Bloom SR, Polak JM. Glucagonoma syndrome. Am J Med 1987; 82(Suppl 5B):25–36.
21. Wood SM, Polak JM, Bloom SR. Gut hormone secreting tumours. Scand J Gastroenterol 1983; 18:165–179.
22. Binnick AN, Spencer SK, Dennison WL, et al. Glucagonoma syndrome. Report of two cases and literature review. Arch Dermatol 1977; 113:749–754.
23. Stacpoole PW. The glucagonoma syndrome: clinical features, diagnosis and treatment. Endocr Rev 1981; 2:347–361.
24. Mallinson CN, Bloom SR, Warin AP, et al. A glucagonoma syndrome. Lancet 1974; 2:1–5.
25. Wood SM, Polak JM, Bloom SR. Glucagonoma syndrome. In: Lefebvre PJ, ed. Handbook of Experimental Pharmacology. Vol 66. Part II. Glucagon. Stuttgart: Springer-Verlag, 1983: 411–430.
26. Higgins GA, Recant L, Fischman AB. The glucagonoma syndrome: surgically curable diabetes. Am J Surg 1979; 137:142–148.
27. Almdal TP, Heindorff H, Bardram L, et al. Increased amino acid clearance and urea synthesis in a patient with glucagonoma. Gut 1990; 31:946–948.
28. Hicks T, Turnberg LA. Influence of glucagon on the human jejunum. Gastroenterology 1974; 67:1114–1118.
29. Santangelo WC, Unger RH, Orci L, et al. Somatostatin analogue–induced remission of necrolytic migratory erythema without changes in plasma glucagon concentration. Pancreas 1986; 1:464–469.
30. Dowling RH. Update on intestinal adaptation. Triangle 1988; 27:149–164.
31. Gleeson MH, Bloom SR, Polak JM, et al. Endocrine tumour in kidney affecting small bowel structure, motility and absorptive function. Gut 1971; 12:773–782.
32. Stevens FM, Flanagan RW, O'Gorman D, et al. Glucagonoma syndrome demonstrating giant duodenal villi. Gut 1984; 25:784–791.
33. Jones B, Fishman EK, Bayless TM, et al. Villous hypertrophy of the small bowel in a patient with glucagonoma. J Comput Assist Tomogr 1983; 7:334–337.
34. Krejs GJ, Orci L, Conlon JM, et al. Somatostatinoma syndrome. Biochemical, morphologic and clinical features. N Engl J Med 1979; 301:285–292.
35. Larsson LI, Hirsch MA, Holst JJ, et al. Pancreatic somatostatinoma: clinical features and physiological implications. Lancet 1977; 1:666–668.
36. Ganda OP, Weir GC, Soeldner JS, et al. "Somatostatinoma": a somatostatin-containing tumor of the endocrine pancreas. N Engl J Med 1977; 296:963–967.
37. Unger RH. Somatostatinoma. N Engl J Med 1977; 296:998–1000.
38. Gerich JE, Patton GS. Somatostatin: physiology and clinical applications. Med Clin North Am 1978; 62:375–392.
39. Pipeleers D, Couturier E, Gepts W, et al. Five cases of somatostatinoma: clinical heterogeneity and diagnostic usefulness of basal and tolbutamide-induced hypersomatostatinemia. J Clin Endocrinol Metab 1983; 56:1236–1242.
40. Wright J, Abolfathi A, Penman E, et al. Pancreatic somatostatinoma presenting with hypoglycaemia. Clin Endocrinol 1980; 12:603–609.
41. Penman E, Lowry PJ, Wass JAH, et al. Molecular forms of somatostatinoma. Clin Endocrinol 1980; 12:611–620.
42. Galmiche JP, Chayvialle JA, Dubois PM, et al. Calcitonin-producing pancreatic somatostatinoma. Gastroenterology 1980; 78:1577–1583.
43. Jackson JA, Raju BU, Fachnie JD, et al. Malignant somatostatinoma presenting with diabetic ketoacidosis. Clin Endocrinol 1987; 26:609–621.
44. Kaneko H, Yanaihara N, Ito S, et al. Somatostatinoma of the duodenum. Cancer 1979; 44:2273–2279.
45. Dayal Y, Doos WG, O'Brien MJ, et al. Psammomatous somatostatinomas of the duodenum. Am J Surg Pathol 1983; 7:653–665.
46. Marcial MA, Pinkus GS, Skarin A, et al. Ampullary somatostatinoma: psammomatous variant of gastrointestinal carcinoid tumor: an immunohistochemical and ultrastructural study. Report of a case and review of the literature. Am J Clin Pathol 1983; 80:755–761.
47. Griffith DF, Williams GT, Williams ED. Multiple endocrine neoplasia associated with von Recklingshausen's disease. Br Med J 1983; 287:1341–1343.
48. Case 15–1989. Weekly clinicopathological conference. N Engl J Med 1989; 320:996–1004.
49. Budmiger H, Bühler H, Häcki W, et al. Comparative diagnostic value of the calcium-pentagastrin test versus the tolbutamide test in a patient with a somatostatinoma. Gastroenterology 1987; 92:800–804.
50. Schwartz TW. Pancreatic polypeptide: a hormone under vagal control. Gastroenterology 1983; 85:1411–1425.
51. Lundqvist G, Krause U, Larsson LI, et al. A pancreatic-polypeptide–producing tumour associated with the WDHA syndrome. Scand J Gastroenterol 1978; 13:715–718.
52. Tomita T, Kimmel JR, Friesen SR, et al. Pancreatic polypeptide cell hyperplasia with and without watery diarrhea syndrome. J Surg Oncol 1980; 14:11–20.

53. Hayes MM. Report of a pancreatic polypeptide–producing islet-cell tumor of the pancreas causing the watery diarrhea, hypokalemia, achlorhydria syndrome in a 55-year-old Zimbabwean African male. Cent Afr J Med 1980; 26:195–197.
54. Lewis DA, Gaginella TS, O'Dorisio TM. Effects of pancreatic polypeptide and vasoactive intestinal polypeptide on rat ileal and colonic water and electrolyte transport in vivo. Dig Dis Sci 1979; 24:625–630.
55. Choksi UA, Sellin RV, Hickey RC, et al. An unusual skin rash associated with a pancreatic polypeptide–producing tumor of the pancreas. Ann Intern Med 1988; 108:64–65.
56. Öberg K, Grimelius L, Lundqvist G, et al. Update on pancreatic polypeptide as a specific marker for endocrine tumours of the pancreas and gut. Acta Med Scand 1982; 210:145–152.
57. Larsson L-I, Sundler F, Hakanson R. Immunohistochemical localization of human pancreatic polypeptide to a population of islet cells. Cell Tissue Res 1975; 156:167–171.
58. Adrian TE, Uttenthal LO, Williams SJ, et al. Secretion of pancreatic polypeptide in patients with pancreatic endocrine tumors. N Engl J Med 1986; 315:287–291.
59. Polak JM, Adrian TE, Bryant MG, et al. Pancreatic polypeptide in insulinomas, gastrinomas, VIPomas and glucagonomas. Lancet 1976; 1:328–330.
60. Tomita T, Friesen SR, Kimmel JR, et al. Pancreatic polypeptide–secreting islet-cell tumors. A study of three cases. Am J Pathol 1983; 113:134–142.
61. Zollinger RM, Ellison EH. Primary peptic ulcerations of the jejunum associated with islet cell tumors of the pancreas. Ann Surg 1955; 142:709–728.
62. McGuigan JE. The Zollinger-Ellison syndrome. In: Sleisenger MH, Fordtran JS, eds. Gastrointestinal Disease: Pathophysiology, Diagnosis, and Management. 4th ed. Philadelphia: W. B. Saunders, 1989: 909–925.
63. McGuigan JE, Wolfe MM. Secretin injection test in the diagnosis of gastrinoma. Gastroenterology 1980; 79:1324–1331.
64. Bonfils S, Bernades P. Zollinger-Ellison syndrome: natural history and diagnosis. Clin Gastroenterol 1974; 3:539–557.
65. Rambaud JC, Modigliana R, Emonts P, et al. Fluid secretion in the duodenum and intestinal handling of water and electrolytes in Zollinger-Ellison syndrome. Dig Dis 1978; 23:1089–1097.
66. Wright HK, Hersh T, Floch MH, et al. Impaired intestinal absorption in the Zollinger-Ellison syndrome independent of gastric hypersecretion. Am J Surg 1970; 119:250–253.
67. Wolfe MM, Jensen RT. Zollinger-Ellison syndrome: current concepts in diagnosis and management. N Engl J Med 1987; 317:1200–1209.
68. Richardson CT, Peters MN, Feldman M, et al. Treatment of Zollinger-Ellison syndrome with vagotomy, exploratory laparotomy, and H₂-receptor antagonist. Gastroenterology 1985; 89:357–367.
69. Lamers CBHW, Lind T, Moberg S, et al. Omeprazole in Zollinger-Ellison syndrome: effects of a single dose and of long-term treatment in patients resistant to histamine H₂-receptor antagonists. N Engl J Med 1984; 310:758–761.
70. Carlsson E, Larsson H, Mattsson H, et al. Pharmacology and toxicology of omeprazole with special reference to the effects on the gastric mucosa. Scand J Gastroenterol 1986; 21(Suppl 118):31–38.
71. Maton PN, Lack EE, Collen MJ, et al. The effect of Zollinger-Ellison syndrome and omeprazole therapy on gastric oxyntic endocrine cells. Gastroenterology 1990; 99:943–950.
72. Hakanson R, Sundler F. Proposed mechanism of induction of gastric carcinoids: the gastrin hypothesis. Eur J Clin Invest 1990; 20(Suppl 1):S65–S71.
73. Borch K, Renvall H, Liedberg G. Gastric endocrine cell hyperplasia and carcinoid tumors in pernicious anemia. Gastroenterology 1985; 88:638–648.
74. Lamberts R, Creutzfeld W, Stöckman F, et al. Long-term omeprazole treatment in man: effects on gastric endocrine cell populations. Digestion 1988; 39:126–135.
75. Priest WM, Alexander MK. Islet cell tumor of the pancreas with peptic ulceration, diarrhoea, and hypokalaemia. Lancet 1957; 2:1145.
76. Verner JV, Morrison AB. Islet cell tumor and a syndrome of refractory watery diarrhea and hypokalemia. Am J Med 1958; 25:374–380.
77. Matsumoto KK, Peter JB, Schultze RG, et al. Watery diarrhea and hypokalemia associated with pancreatic islet cell adenoma. Gastroenterology 1966; 50:231–242.
78. Bloom SR, Polak JM, Pearse AGE. Vasoactive intestinal peptide and watery-diarrhoea syndrome. Lancet 1973; 2:14–16.
79. Said SI, Mutt V. Potent peripheral and splanchnic vasodilator peptide from normal gut. Nature 1970; 225:863–864.
80. Grossman M. Candidate hormones of the gut. Gastroenterology 1974; 67:730–755.
81. Pearse AGE. Peptides in brain and intestine. Nature 1976; 262:92–94.
82. Fahrenkrug J. Vasoactive intestinal polypeptide: measurement, distribution and putative neurotransmitter function. Digestion 1979; 19:149–169.
83. Said SI. Vasoactive intestinal polypeptide (VIP) as a neural peptide. In: Miyoshi A, Grossman M, eds. Gut Peptides: Secretion, Function and Clinical Aspects. Amsterdam: Elsevier/North-Holland, 1979: 268–273.

84. Bryant MG, Polak JM, Modlin I, et al. Possible dual role for vasoactive intestinal peptide as gastrointestinal hormone and neurotransmitter substance. Lancet 1976; 1:991–993.

85. Said SI. VIP overview. In: Bloom SR, Polak JM, eds. Gut Hormones. 2nd ed. Edinburgh: Churchill Livingstone, 1981: 379–384.

86. Krejs GJ. Effect of VIP infusion on water and electrolyte transport in the human intestine. In: Said SI, ed. Vasoactive Intestinal Peptide. New York: Raven, 1982: 193–200.

87. Unwin RJ, Calam J, Peart WS. VIPoma and watery diarrhea. N Engl J Med 1982; 307:377–378.

88. Ginsberg AL. The VIP controversy. Stephen R. Bloom vs. Jerry D. Gardner. Dig Dis 1978; 23:370–376.

89. Ebeid AM, Murray P, Hirsch H, et al. Radioimmunoassay of vasoactive intestinal peptide. J Surg Res 1976; 20:355–360.

90. Said SI, Faloona GR. Elevated plasma and tissue levels of vasoactive intestinal polypeptide in the watery-diarrhea syndrome due to pancreatic, bronchogenic and other tumors. N Engl J Med 1975; 293:155–160.

91. Krejs GJ, Walsh JH, Morawski SG, et al. Intractable diarrhea: intestinal perfusion studies and plasma VIP concentrations in patients with pancreatic cholera syndrome and surreptitious ingestion of laxatives and diuretics. Am J Dig Dis 1977; 22:280–292.

92. Krejs GJ, Fordtran JS. Effect of VIP infusion on water and ion transport in the human jejunum. Gastroenterology 1980; 78:722–727.

93. Krejs GJ. Peptidergic control of intestinal secretion—studies in man. In: Bloom SR, Polak JM, eds. Gut Hormones. 2nd ed. Edinburgh: Churchill Livingstone, 1981: 516–520.

94. Kane MG, O'Dorisio TM, Krejs GJ. Production of secretory diarrhea by intravenous infusion of vasoactive intestinal polypeptide. N Engl J Med 1983; 309:1482–1485.

95. Bloom SR, Christofides ND, Delamarter J, et al. Diarrhoea in VIPoma patients associated with cosecretion of a second active peptide (peptide histidine isoleucine) explained by single coding gene. Lancet 1983; 2:1163–1165.

96. Kane MG, Tatemoto K, Bloom SR, et al. Effect of PHI on water and ion movement in the canine jejunum in vivo. Dig Dis Sci 1984; 29(Suppl Aug):41S.

97. Rambaud JC, Matuchansky C. Diarrhea and digestive endocrine tumors. Clin Gastroenterol 1974; 3:657–669.

98. Krejs GJ, Fordtran JS. Physiology and pathophysiology of ion and water movement in the human intestine. In: Sleisenger M, Fordtran JS, eds. Gastrointestinal Disease. 2nd ed. Philadelphia: W. B. Saunders, 1978: 297–335.

99. Gardner JD. Plasma VIP in patients with watery diarrhea syndrome. Am J Dig Dis 1978; 23:370–373.

100. Krejs GJ, Hendler RS, Fordtran JS. Diagnostic and pathophysiologic studies in patients with chronic diarrhea. In: Field M, ed. Secretory Diarrhea. Bethesda: American Physiological Society, 1980: 141–151.

101. Rambaud JC, Modigliani R, Matuchansky C, et al. Pancreatic cholera: studies on tumoral secretions and pathophysiology of diarrhea. Gastroenterology 1975; 69:110–122.

102. Schmitt MG, Soergel KH, Hensley GT, et al. Watery diarrhea associated with pancreatic islet cell carcinoma. Gastroenterology 1975; 69:206–216.

103. Verner JV, Morrison AB. Endocrine pancreatic islet disease with diarrhea: report of a case due to diffuse hyperplasia of nonbeta islet tissue with a review of 54 additional cases. Arch Intern Med 1974; 133:492–500.

104. Anderson H, Dotevall G, Fagerberg G, et al. Pancreatic tumor with diarrhea, hypokalemia, and hypochlorhydria. Arch Chir Scand 1972; 138:102–107.

105. Escourrou J, Ebeid AM, Fischer JE. Vasoactive intestinal peptide associated inhibition of stimulated gastric secretion. II. Inhibition of pentagastrin-stimulated gastric secretion. Am J Surg 1980; 139:824–828.

106. Holm-Bentzen M, Christiansen J, Petersen B, et al. Infusion of vasoactive intestinal polypeptide in man: pharmacokinetics and effect on gastric acid secretion. Scand J Gastroenterol 1981; 16:429–432.

107. Kofstad J, Froyshov I, Gjone E, et al. Pancreatic tumor with intractable watery diarrhea, hypokalemia and hypercalcemia. Electrolyte balance studies. Scand J Gastroenterol 1967; 2:246–250.

108. Barraclough MA, Bloom SR. VIPoma of the pancreas. Observations on the diarrhea and circulatory disturbances. Arch Intern Med 1979; 139:467–471.

109. Frase LL, Gaffney FA, Lane LL, et al. Effect of VIP infusion on cardiovascular function in healthy subjects. Am J Cardiol 1987; 60:1356–1361.

110. Espiner EA, Beaven DW. Non-specific islet-cell tumour of the pancreas with diarrhoea. Q J Med 1962; 31:447–471.

111. Kraft AR, Tompkins RK, Zollinger R. Recognition and management of the diarrhea syndrome caused by nonbeta islet cell tumors of the pancreas. Am J Surg 1970; 119:163–170.

112. Krejs GJ. VIPoma syndrome. Am J Med 1987; 82(Suppl 5B):37–48.

113. Rambaud JC, Nisard A, Modigliani R, et al. Hypercalcitoninaemia in VIPomas. Lancet 1978; 1:220.

114. Manche A, Wood SM, Adrian TE, et al. Pancreatic polypeptide and calcitonin secretion from a pancreatic tumour—clinical improvement after hepatic artery embolization. Postgrad Med J 1983; 59:313–314.

115. Gutniak M, Rosenqvist U, Grimelius L, et al. Report on a patient with watery diarrhoea syndrome caused by a pancreatic tumour containing neurotensin, enkephalin and calcitonin. Acta Med Scand 1980; 208:95–100.

116. Williams ED. Medullary carcinoma of the thyroid. J Clin Pathol 1967; 20:395–398.

117. Gray TK, Bieberdorf FA, Fordtran JS. Thyrocalcitonin and the jejunal absorption of calcium, water, and electrolytes in normal subjects. J Clin Invest 1973; 52:3084–3088.

118. Theodorsson-Norheim E, Öberg K, Rosell S, et al. Neurotensinlike immunoreactivity in plasma and tumor tissue from patients with endocrine tumors of the pancreas and gut. Gastroenterology 1983; 85:881–889.

119. Rosell S, Rökaeus A, Theodorsson-Norheim E. The role of neurotensin in disease. Scand J Gastroenterol 1983; 18:59–67.

120. Shulkes A, Boden R, Cook I, et al. Characterization of a pancreatic tumor containing vasoactive intestinal peptide, neurotensin, and pancreatic polypeptide. J Clin Endocrinol Metab 1984; 58:41–48.

121. Feurle GE, Helmstaedter V, Tischbirek K, et al. A multihormonal tumor of the pancreas producing neurotensin. Dig Dis Sci 1981; 26:1125–1133.

122. Blackburn AM, Bryant MG, Adrian TE, et al. Pancreatic tumors produce neurotensin. J Clin Endocrinol Metab 1981; 52:820–822.

123. Friesen SR, Allen MS. Malignant hyperparathroidism of pancreatic and parathyroid origins. Bull Soc Int Chir 1975; 5:439–441.

124. O'Neal LW, Kipnis DM, Luse SA, et al. Secretion of various endocrine substances by ACTH-secreting tumors—gastrin, melanotropin, norepinephrine, serotonin, parathormone, vasopressin, glucagon. Cancer 1968; 21:1219–1232.

125. Maton PN, Gardner JD, Jensen RT. Cushing's syndrome in patients with the Zollinger-Ellison syndrome. N Engl J Med 1986; 315:1–5.

126. Rivier J, Spiess J, Thorner M, et al. Characterization of a growth hormone–releasing factor from a human pancreatic islet tumour. Nature 1982; 300:276–278.

127. Guillemin R, Brazeau P, Böhlen P, et al. Growth hormone–releasing factor from a human pancreatic tumor that caused acromegaly. Science 1982; 218:585–587.

128. Berger G, Tronillas, Bloch B, et al. Multihormonal carcinoid tumor of the pancreas secreting growth hormone–releasing factor as a cause of acromegaly. Cancer 1984; 54:2097–2108.

129. Donhuijsen K, Schulte HM, Schmidt U, et al. Akromegalie bei Wachstumshormon-Releasing-Hormon (GH-RH) produzierenden Pankreastumor: Klinik und Morphologie. Schweiz Med Wochenschr 1986; 116:615–621.

130. Maton PN, Gardner JD, Jensen RT. Use of long-acting somatostatin analog SMS201–995 in patients with pancreatic islet cell tumors. Dig Dis Sci 1989; 34(Suppl):S28–S39.

131. Owyang C, Go VL. Multiple hormone–secreting tumors of the gastrointestinal tract. In: Glass GBJ, ed. Gastrointestinal Hormones. New York: Raven, 1980: 741–748.

132. Belchetz PE, Brown CL, Makin HLJ, et al. ACTH, glucagon and gastrin production by a pancreatic islet cell carcinoma and its treatment. Clin Endocrinol 1973; 2:307–316.

133. D'Arcangues CM, Awoke S, Lawrence GD. Metastatic insulinoma with long survival and glucagonoma syndrome. Ann Intern Med 1984; 100:233–235.

134. Mordechai B, Burke M, Isakov A, et al. Insulinoma after streptozotocin therapy for metastatic gastrinoma: natural history or iatrogenic complication? J Clin Gastroenterol 1990; 12:579–580.

135. Yamagami T, Miwa A, Takasawa S, et al. Induction of rat pancreatic B-cell tumors by the combined administration of streptozotocin or alloxan and poly(adenosine diphosphate ribose) synthetase inhibitors. Cancer Res 1985; 45:1845–1849.

136. Hammar S, Sale G. Multiple hormone producing islet cell carcinomas of the pancreas. Hum Pathol 1975; 6:349–362.

137. Dunn PJS, Sheppard MC, Heath DA, et al. Recurrent insulinoma syndrome with metastatic glucagonoma. J Clin Pathol 1983; 36:1076–1080.

138. Said SI. Evidence for secretion of vasoactive intestinal peptide by tumours of pancreas, adrenal medulla, thyroid and lung: support for the unifying APUD concept. Clin Endocrinol 1976; 5(Suppl):201–204.

139. Bloom SR, Polak JM. VIP measurement in distinguishing Verner-Morrison syndrome and pseudo Verner-Morrison syndrome. Clin Endocrinol 1976; 5(Suppl):223–228.

140. Chey WY, Escoffery R, Chu TM. Verner-Morrison syndrome: clinical observation and search for origin of endocrine cell hyperplasia of the pancreas. Gastroenterology 1983; 84:1123 (abstract).

141. Kidd GS, Donowitz M, O'Dorisio T, et al. Mild chronic watery diarrhea–hypokalemia syndrome associated with pancreatic islet cell hyperplasia. Am J Med 1979; 66:883–888.

142. Bloom SR, Polak JM. Hormone profiles. In: Bloom SR, Polak JM, eds. Gut Hormones. 2nd ed. Edinburgh: Churchill Livingstone, 1981: 555–560.

143. Prinz RA, Bermes EW, Kimmel JR. Serum markers for pancreatic islet cell and intestinal carcinoid tumors: a comparison of neuron-specific enolase, β-human chorionic gonadotropin and pancreatic polypeptide. Surgery 1983; 94:1019–1023.

144. O'Connor DT, Deftos LJ. Secretion of chromogranin by peptide-producing endocrine neoplasias. N Engl J Med 1986; 314:1145–1151.

145. Kingham JGC, Dick R, Bloom SR, et al. VIPoma. Localization by percutaneous transhepatic portal venous sampling. Br Med J 1978; 2:1682–1683.

146. Koneru B, Cassavilla A, Bowman J, et al. Liver transplantation for malignant tumors. Gastroenterol Clin North Am 1988; 17:177–193.

147. Kahn CR, Levy AG, Gardner JD, et al. Pancreatic cholera: beneficial effects of treatment with streptozotocin. N Engl J Med 1975; 292:941–945.

148. Krejs GJ. Secretory diarrhea. In: Bayless TM, ed. Current Therapies in Gastroenterology and Liver Disease. Toronto: B. C. Decker, 1983: 255–259.

149. Krejs, GJ. Effect of somatostatin infusion on VIP-induced transport changes in the human jejunum. Regul Pept 1984; 5:271–276.

150. Santangelo WC, O'Dorisio TM, Kim JG, et al. Effect of synthetic somatostatin analogue on intestinal water and ion transport in pancreatic cholera syndrome. Ann Intern Med 1985; 103:363–367.

151. Kraenzlin ME, Ch'ng JC, Wood SM, et al. Long-term treatment of a VIPoma with somatostatin analogue resulting in remission of symptoms and possible shrinkage of metastases. Gastroenterology 1985; 88:185–187.

152. Santangelo WC, O'Dorisio TM, Kim JG, et al. VIPoma syndrome: effect of a synthetic somatostatin analogue. Scand J Gastroenterol 1989; 21(Suppl 119):87–190.

153. Öberg K, Lindström H, Alm G, et al. Successful treatment of therapy-resistant pancreatic cholera with human leucocyte interferon. Lancet 1985; 1:725–727.

154. Eriksson G, Alm G, Lundqvist G, et al. Treatment of malignant endocrine pancreatic tumours with human leucocyte interferon. Lancet 1986; 1:1307–1309.

33

ENDOCRINE-RESPONSIVE CANCERS OF HUMANS

Marc E. Lippman and Sandra M. Swain

INTRODUCTION

The fact that some human neoplasms are responsive to endocrine manipulation was recognized in the 19th century, but the role of hormones in the genesis and growth of cancer is still incompletely understood. The concept that a tumor may retain the growth-regulatory responses to hormones of the nonmalignant tissue from which it was derived is an oversimplification of the complex responses of clinical cancer to endocrine manipulations. Responses to some therapies occur for which no obvious physiological equivalent is yet known; in other cases concentrations of hormones employed vastly exceed normal levels and induce effects different from those seen with replacement doses.

Whether hormones play a role in carcinogenesis itself is uncertain. At least three types of action of hormones are potentially important in the development of a malignant tumor. First, both steroidal and nonsteroidal estrogens may be true carcinogens, capable of forming covalent links to DNA. This can result in mutations that eventually lead to heritable expression of the malignant phenotype. Second, hormones can function as promoters of the carcinogenic action of other carcinogens. Third, hormones may have a permissive action in allowing carcinogenic events to occur. Permissive and promotional roles for hormones often cannot be distinguished in clinical situations, such as the failure of prostatic cancer to occur in eunuchs or of endometrial or breast cancer to develop in women with gonadal dysgenesis. An experimental breast cancer induced by dimethylbenzanthracene in rats provides substantial insight into the process. Sexually mature females develop breast cancer when fed the carcinogen; however, dimethylbenzanthracene is ineffective if given before puberty or to males and is also ineffective if female animals are castrated shortly after administration of the carcinogen. Thus separate permissive and promotional effects of estrogens can be identified under some circumstances.

In this chapter we review the endocrine-responsive cancers of humans, restricting the focus to tumors known to respond to manipulation of the hormonal milieu. Breast cancer is discussed in depth, first, because the principles of endocrine therapy derived from the study of this disease may be applicable generally, and second, because the large volume of research in experimental and clinical mammary cancer illustrates the direction of research on endocrine involvement in cancer. Lymphoma and carcinomas of the prostate and uterine endometrium are also discussed, with emphasis on the basic endocrinology underlying carcinogenesis, tumor promotion, and therapy.

BREAST CANCER

Breast cancer is the leading cause of cancer deaths in women. As of 1989, there are about 130,000 new cases of breast cancer per year in the United States, and approximately one third of these are eventually fatal. The median age for the development of breast cancer is 59, and it is likely that even more women would die of metastatic disease if they survived long enough. The large number of women who eventually develop metastatic disease requires that therapy be improved.

Epidemiology

Epidemiological studies of breast cancer have provided information about genetic, chemical, viral, and hormonal factors.[1-3] The predictors of risk include sex, age, age at menarche and menopause, age at first pregnancy, geographic area of residence, dietary factors, family history of breast cancer (Table 33–1), and a variety of indicators related to steroid hormone concentrations in blood and urine. Many of these risk factors are interdependent, and most are probably related to endocrine status. Unfortunately, no risk factor, either alone or in combination (with the exception of certain rare high-risk kindreds), is sufficiently discriminatory to identify women in whom special therapeutic intervention is warranted. Nor is the absence of all risk factors sufficient to rule out breast cancer occurrence. Rather, these epidemiological factors suggest potentially alterable influences requiring further study.

The risk factors in which endocrine influences may be significant can be grouped under five headings: geographic variation, reproductive history, familial clustering, hormonal milieu, and miscellaneous.

Geographic Variation

There are striking variations in the rates of breast cancer in different areas of the world.[3] The incidence of breast cancer in women at age 50 is about six times higher in the United States than in Japan or Taiwan.[4] For older women the difference increases to nearly 20-fold. This difference was initially interpreted as evidence for a genetic basis for altered breast cancer risk, but the descendants of the Chinese who have lived in Hawaii for several generations have the same rate of breast cancer as the whites, and first- and second-generation Japanese in Hawaii have higher rates than women in Japan.[5] The incidence of breast cancer is now increasing in Japan, an increase that has occurred in association with important changes in diet, height, weight, and menstrual history.

The relationship of the incidence of breast cancer to age has different characteristics. In countries with a high incidence there is a continued increase with age, whereas in "low-risk" countries the rate of development of breast cancer decreases after menopause (Fig. 33–1). DeWaard[6] suggested that these data imply two different causes of breast cancer. Superimposed on the curve for incidence of breast cancer in countries of lower socioeconomic status is an additional

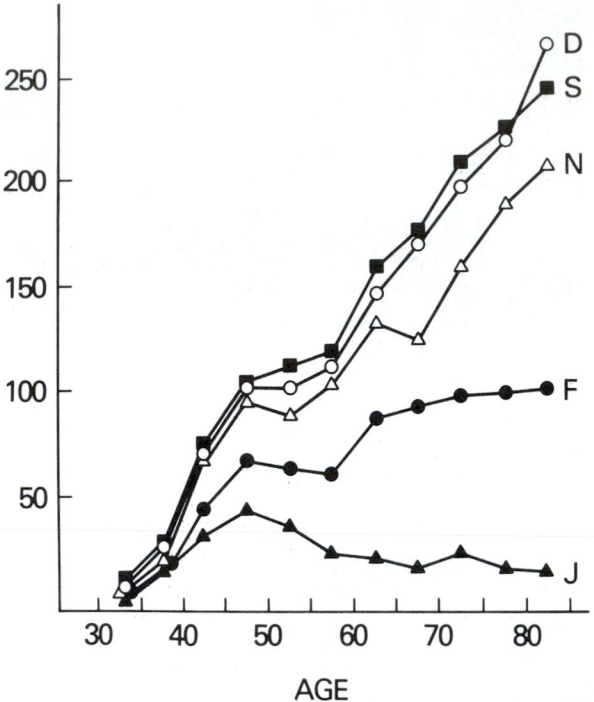

Figure 33–1. Incidence of breast cancer with age in countries with high and low cancer rates. D, Denmark; S, Sweden; N, Norway; F, Finland; J, Japan. The ordinate indicates incidence per 100,000 people. (From DeWaard F. The epidemiology of breast cancer: review and prospects. Int J Cancer 1969; 4:577–586.)

type of cancer risk related to factors generally associated with industrialization, such as increased food consumption, increased fat and meat intake, increased height, and higher rates of obesity. These suggestions are consistent with an impact of environmental change on altered cancer risk among Orientals.

Reproductive and Menstrual Histories

The reproductive and menstrual histories of women with breast cancer have been thoroughly studied. If one arbitrarily assigns a relative risk of 1 to nulliparous women, there is a nearly threefold alteration in the risk of breast cancer with parity, varying from 0.5 for women having their

TABLE 33–1. Risk Factors for Breast Cancer in Women

Factor	High Risk	Low Risk	Relative Risk
Age	Old age	Young age	>4
Country of residence	North America, northern Europe	Asia, Africa	>4
Socioeconomic class	Upper	Lower	2–4
Marital status	Never married	Ever married	1–2
Place of residence	Urban	Rural	1–2
Place of residence	Northern United States	Southern United States	1–2
Race	White	Black	1–2
Age at first birth	Older than 30	Younger than 20	2–4
Oophorectomy	No	Yes	2–4
Body build	Obese	Thin	2–4
Age at menarche	Early	Late	1–2
Age at menopause	Late	Early	1–2
Family history of premenopausal bilateral breast cancer	Yes	No	>4
History of cancer in one breast	Yes	No	>4
History of fibrocystic disease	Yes	No	2–4
Any first-degree relative with breast cancer	Yes	No	2–4
History of primary cancer in ovary or endometrium	Yes	No	2–4
Radiation to chest	Large doses	Minimal exposure	2–4
Alcohol use	Yes	No	1–2

Modified from Kelsey JL. Division of epidemiology of human breast cancer. Epidemiol Rev 1979; 1:74–109.

first child before age 20 to 1.4 for women giving birth to their first child after age 37. The protective effect of early age at the first pregnancy is maintained throughout life, even among women of age 75 and older.[7] Most data suggest that pregnancy at all ages leading to full-term live birth may be protective against breast cancer.[3]

The protective effect of early pregnancy may be due to either a permanent induced alteration in the mammary gland or a chronic postpartum alteration in circulating hormone levels. Study of this issue is critical because identification of the nature of the protection against breast cancer provided by early first delivery may allow prophylactic endocrine manipulations in young women. The protective effect is probably not due to lactation per se,[8, 9] although one study of women who nursed their babies on only one breast showed a significant reduction in breast cancer incidence on that side.[10]

Ovarian activity is a clear risk factor in breast cancer. Surgical menopause is protective against breast cancer in proportion to the reduction in years of menstrual life.[8] The age at menarche and the age at natural menopause are also risk factors in breast cancer, a longer menstrual life being associated with a higher risk of breast cancer.[11] This excess risk exists even in the elderly, a relation that is consistent with a long latent period for some human breast cancers. Ovarian estrogen is probably the causative factor, and the protective effects of early ovariectomy are negated by administration of estrogen.[12]

Pike and colleagues[13] have proposed that most of the geographic variation in breast cancer incidence can be understood by assigning different risk factors to menstrual life before the first full-term pregnancy and in the years thereafter.[13] In this construction, early menarche and menstrual life before first pregnancy are particularly weighted as risk factors. Because dietary practices are likely to influence height and weight and thereby the onset of menses (see Chapter 13), this is an attractive means of incorporating multiple risk factors into a unified hypothesis.

Family History

The family history is an important risk factor in breast cancer,[14] especially a family history of breast cancer and particularly if the cancer is bilateral or there is history of both male and female breast cancer.[15] Weak associations of breast cancer with human leukocyte antigens[16] and cerumen type[17] constitute additional evidence of genetic factors in the etiology. Genetic factors could be expressed at a variety of levels, including heritable alteration in the endocrine milieu. Comparisons of individuals known by family history to be at high risk for breast cancer with appropriate control groups have failed to identify familial hormone changes; that is, no significant differences were detected in prolactin, gonadotropin, estrone, estradiol, or estriol concentrations.[18, 19] Different results were obtained in similar studies of familial male breast cancer,[20] which suggests that genetic effects in women are mediated nonhormonally or that subtle changes in the endocrine milieu have not been appreciated. Pineal abnormalities may be important.[21, 22] For example, diminished nighttime peaks in serum melatonin concentration have been noted in some women with estrogen receptor–positive breast cancer.[23] Whether any single endocrine abnormality will explain a substantial part of the genetic differences in breast cancer risk is uncertain.

The Hormonal Milieu

The hormonal environment may influence the rate of progression of established cancer as well as the risk of its development. This concept has gained experimental support from studies of the induction of mammary cancer in rodents, in which a permissive or promotional role for estrogens can be clearly demonstrated. This phenomenon was first described by Lacassagne,[24] who noted that estrone administration can induce cancer in susceptible strains of mice. Demonstration of a role for estrogens in human breast cancer has not been clear-cut for several reasons, including inadequate methods of measurement; rapid fluctuations in the plasma concentrations of some hormones; variations in steroid metabolism in patients related to thyroid disease, nutrition, age, and abnormal liver function; and, most important, the probability that measurements at the time of development of clinical disease have little relevance to the hormonal milieu present during the initial stage of carcinogenesis some 5 to 15 y earlier.[25]

ESTROGENS. Because of the likelihood of a relationship of breast cancer to estrogen, urinary estrogen levels were measured by several groups, but no differences were identified between women with breast cancer and those in the normal population. These studies suffered from the fact that estrogens should have been measured at the beginning of carcinogenesis rather than at a later stage of clinical disease. Further, the wide fluctuations of estrogen levels during the menstrual cycle and the alterations in the rates of metabolism with disease and/or with drugs made interpretation difficult. Nevertheless, one review of this issue has concluded that hormonal patterns of high-risk groups of women do not differ from those of the normal population.[26]

An early hypothesis relating estrogens to cancer risk was that women with high urinary levels of estriol have a decreased risk for breast cancer because estriol is an estrogen antagonist.[27] For example, Japanese women (a low-risk group) have higher urinary estriol levels than do Australian women.[28] However, the hypothesis has been abandoned for the following reasons. First, estriol is an estrogen whose receptor-binding characteristics make it act as an antagonist only when it is given intermittently.[29] When given continuously, it is a potent estrogen that promotes mammary gland carcinogenesis in experimental systems and promotes growth of estrogen-responsive human breast cancer.[30] Second, urinary estriol has no clear relations to plasma estriol concentrations or production rates.[31] Further, the concentration ratio of estriol to estrone plus estradiol is not related to differences between estrogen blood levels and production rates in normal women or in women with breast cancer.

Studies of estrogen levels, sources, and production rates have also shown no differences between women with early breast cancer and a control population.[32] Similarly, plasma estrogen levels do not differ between these groups.[33]

However, several lines of investigation support the concept that abnormalities related to estrogen may contribute to the eventual development of breast cancer. Korenman[34] suggested that unopposed estrogen action is a major risk factor. Korenman's "estrogen window" hypothesis is based on five premises:

1. Human breast cancer is induced by carcinogens in a susceptible mammary gland.
2. Unopposed estrogen stimulation is the most favorable state for induction.
3. There is a long latency period between induction of tumor and clinical expression.
4. The duration of the estrogen window determines risk.
5. Inducibility declines with the establishment of normal ovulatory menses and becomes low during pregnancy.

These premises fit well with the epidemiological data of Pike and colleagues.[13] Brown[35] reviewed daily endocrine profiles in young women entering puberty during normal menstrual life and at menopause. These studies found multiple anovulatory cycles at both extremes of menstrual life and provided a theoretical basis for the estrogen window hypothesis.

Finally, Siiteri and colleagues[36] re-examined the role of serum estrogen concentrations in breast cancer. They found that although total serum estrogen concentrations may be normal in women with breast cancer, free estrogen concentrations may be high as a result of decreased plasma binding. The decreased binding results from a decrease in levels of testosterone-binding globulin (TeBG, sex hormone–binding globulin) or in some cases abnormal TeBG.

OTHER HORMONES. Bulbrook[38] has summarized studies dealing with discriminant functions based primarily on androgen excretion. Briefly, a higher urinary level of androgen metabolites is correlated with a greater likelihood of response of breast carcinoma to adrenalectomy or hypophysectomy.

In a prospective trial, urinary excretion of etiocholanolone (an androgen metabolite) was lower in women who subsequently developed breast cancer,[39] and in the same study women at high risk for breast cancer had the lowest plasma levels of androgens.[40] In other studies, urinary testosterone excretion[41] and plasma testosterone levels[42] were higher in women with early breast cancer. In still other studies, such discriminants appear to have had little validity.[43]

Most of the data regarding the hormonal milieu of breast cancer are related to hormones present in plasma or in urine. However, Adams and associates[44, 45] reported that human breast cancer tissue can metabolize dehydroepiandrosterone to androstenedione and possibly to estriol. Breast cancer tissue can also convert other androgens to estrogens. Thus the breast cancer cell has the potential to create its own microenvironment and thereby may defeat efforts to lower estradiol levels in surrounding medium. Some breast cancers can sulfurylate steroids, and the absence of the sulfokinase has been correlated with a lack of response to adrenalectomy. The fact that several androgen metabolites, including androstenediol, compete with estradiol for estrogen receptor[45] suggests a mechanism for relating androgen metabolism to the clinical response in hormonal therapy.

The role of prolactin in the etiology of human breast cancer remains enigmatic. Some investigators have reported abnormalities in prolactin levels in patients with breast cancer[46] as well as in their daughters.[47] Others have failed to detect significant abnormalities.[33] One review of the subject proposed that elevated prolactin levels may be associated with a risk for breast cancer, but whether causally or not remains to be determined.[48] As discussed later, however, there is no clear-cut evidence that a significant subset of established breast cancers is dependent on prolactin as a tropic hormone.

The incidence of abnormalities of thyroid function, usually goiter or hypothyroidism, has been reported to be increased in patients with breast cancer, but at least two critical reviews of this area have failed to support this contention.[3, 49]

Exogenous Hormones

Benign Breast Disease

Most benign breast diseases are not premalignant, but some benign abnormalities are associated with an increased risk (up to four times in one well-studied series) of developing breast cancer.[3, 50] Although other explanations are possible, benign and malignant forms of breast disease may share a common etiological factor(s) related to the endocrine milieu. There is evidence from both retrospective analyses[50–55] and prospective studies[56, 57] that oral contraceptives diminish the incidence of benign breast disease. Generally, such studies show a greater protective effect against cystic disease than against fibroadenoma. In addition, protection is greater in long-term users, a feature in favor of a causal relationship. A study conducted by the Royal College of General Practitioners[51] reported that the incidence of benign breast disease is inversely related to the amount of progestogen in the preparation. This relation was confirmed by surveys of women using noncontraceptive estrogen preparations, in whom no protection was demonstrated.[52, 57] Certain forms of benign breast disease, such as atypical lobular and ductal hyperplasia, are associated with a high likelihood of subsequent malignant disease,[58, 59] and the effects of oral contraceptives on women with these lesions have not been assessed. It should not be concluded, therefore, that the effectiveness of oral contraceptives in reducing benign breast disease is equivalent to a protection against breast cancer. In particular subsets of women with these conditions, estrogen use may increase the risk.

Danazol can induce objective and symptomatic improvement in most patients with benign breast disease.[60, 61] This drug is also useful in some instances in the management of advanced breast cancer.[62] It is conceivable that prolonged danazol administration may protect against breast cancer.

Breast Cancer

There was an increase in the incidence of breast cancer during the decade 1960 to 1970, a period in which the use of oral contraceptives and postmenopausal estrogens rose sharply.[63] Whether this increase in incidence was due to exogenous estrogens is unclear.[63, 64] Multiple retrospective case control studies have failed to reveal an increased risk of developing breast cancer among users of oral contraceptives.[50, 53, 65–67] However, several factors complicate the interpretation of these results. The time required for tumor promotion in humans is long, and there may not be sufficient experience to allow firm conclusions. Two studies of younger women showed a slightly higher relative risk ratio in those who had used oral contraceptives for more than 8 and 5 y, respectively,[68, 69] but the increase was not significant. Two other studies have failed to show an increase in risk with time.[53, 65] However, in one of these studies[65] oral contraceptive use increased the risk of breast cancer in three subsets of patients: nulliparous women, women who used the pill before the birth of the first child, and women with a history of benign breast disease. Some prospective trials of oral contraceptive use have not confirmed this relationship[55, 65] and, in fact, suggest a reduction in risk. Other prospective studies have suggested a small increase in breast cancer incidence in users of such contraceptives,[70, 71] most strikingly in young women (under age 32). Longer follow-up studies are required before the exact risk can be determined.

Of several retrospective analyses of women using estrogens after menopause, most do not show an association between use and risk of breast cancer.[57, 67–69] In one such study a relative risk ratio of 1.3 (of borderline statistical significance) was found for estrogen users.[72] The risk ratio was related to the duration of follow-up and doubled after 12 y of use. No follow-up study of oral contraceptive use of this duration is available. Another study suggested a dose-dependent increase in breast cancer incidence among users of menopausal estrogens.[73] The risk was greatest in women who took the largest amount but was not related to duration of use. Finally, as with oral contraceptives,[53] the risk increased sevenfold in women who developed benign breast disease after starting estrogen therapy.

Miscellaneous Factors

Alcohol intake is associated with an increased risk of breast cancer,[74] but it is unclear whether this is a causative or associative variable.[75] Exogenous radiation is also a risk factor for breast cancer, presumably through direct damage to DNA.

Hormone Receptors and Endocrine Therapy of Breast Cancer

That some human breast cancers might respond to endocrine manipulations has been appreciated since Beatson[76] induced tumor regressions in patients with bilateral oophorectomy. Patients who respond to endocrine therapy may not only experience palliation but also have longer survival than nonresponders. However, only about one third of unselected patients have objective tumor regressions. With the advent of effective chemotherapy regimens, a more precise selection of treatment modalities is necessary.

A variety of empirical clinical guidelines (disease-free interval, sites of involvement, and so forth) and a few biochemical tests (excretion of androgen metabolites, steroid sulfation) have been tried for the selection of patients with hormone-responsive tumors. Unfortunately, none of these approaches is reliable. However, developments in the field of hormone action have allowed more accurate selection of patients for hormone therapy.

The first step in the action of steroid hormones, including estrogen, is binding of the hormone to specific receptor proteins, which then function as transcriptional regulatory units (see Chapter 3). Functional receptor molecules are necessary for steroid hormone action,[77] and in animal systems regression of mammary cancer in response to endocrine ablation therapy also requires the presence of estrogen receptors.[78, 79] Likewise, human breast cancer samples were shown to take up and retain estrogen,[80, 81] and Jensen and colleagues[82] found specific estrogen-binding activity in human breast cancers and showed direct correlations between the presence of an estrogen receptor and the likelihood of response to endocrine therapy.

Comprehensive reviews of this field are available.[83, 84] In brief, about two thirds of primary cancers contain significant concentrations of estrogen receptor, and a somewhat smaller proportion of metastatic samples are positive for estrogen receptor. Tumors in premenopausal patients are less frequently estrogen receptor–positive and, when positive, contain lower concentrations of receptor, on the average, than those occurring after the menopause. These observations are only partially explained by the fact that the larger amounts of endogenous estrogen in the plasma of premenopausal women mask the binding sites. Overall there is a significant association between the presence of estrogen receptor and the likelihood of response to endocrine therapy. Predictive accuracy for the test is about 75%. Thus about 60% of the patients with estrogen receptor–positive tumors respond to endocrine therapy, whereas 95% of the 40% of patients with estrogen receptor–negative tumors do not respond. In general, the greater the estrogen receptor content of the tumor, the higher the response rate to endocrine therapy. Although estrogen receptor assays are useful in selecting therapy for patients with advanced disease, an even more valuable potential use of these tests is in selection of appropriate adjuvant regimens for patients with stage II (lymph node–positive) breast cancer at the time of

initial diagnosis. In this group correct selection of therapy is particularly important for two reasons. First, there is no adequate marker of response, the first indication of inadequate therapy being recurrence of tumors. Second, adjuvant endocrine therapy increases survival in some patients but may decrease survival in others.[85] Separation of responsive and unresponsive groups requires meticulous quality control and uniformity of assays.[86]

The response rate of tumors lacking estrogen receptors is low but not zero. Thus a single negative assay should be considered as only one component in the selection of appropriate therapy. There are several possible explanations for the appearance of an endocrine response in women with purportedly estrogen receptor–negative tumors. First, steroid receptors are labile proteins, and receptor activity may not be detected because of methodological artifacts. Common problems include incorrect handling and storage of samples. Second, the diagnosis of metastatic breast cancer may be based on observation of a few tumor cells infiltrating a nonmalignant tissue. A negative assay may result from insufficient sampling of malignant cells or inadvertent sampling of neighboring nonmalignant tissue. Third, various additive and ablative therapies in patients with breast cancer may act via mechanisms not involving estrogen receptors. Thus even in the absence of an estrogen receptor, some endocrine manipulations may cause a response. Fourth, breast tumors may be heterogeneous with respect to receptor status; a biopsy site that is estrogen receptor–negative may not be representative of other tumor deposits. Fifth, some assays may be falsely negative because most estrogen receptor analyses are performed under conditions that do not permit the detection of receptor sites occupied by endogenous hormone. Sixth, even in the absence of endogenous hormone, receptor sites may be localized to the nucleus[87] and thereby missed with standard methodologies. In view of these possibilities, it is surprising how rarely (about 5%) so-called estrogen receptor–negative tumors respond to endocrine therapy.

More surprising, and more common, is the failure of tumors containing estrogen receptor to respond to endocrine therapy. The usual explanation for this phenomenon is tumor cell heterogeneity. That is, a sufficient number of cells within the tumor sample contain receptor to give a positive assay result, while the majority (or the most malignant) are receptor-negative. If this is the case, one would anticipate a quantitative relationship between the amount of estrogen receptor and the likelihood of observing an endocrine response, a relation that has been reported.[88] It has also been demonstrated that tumor deposits contain a mixture of receptor-positive and receptor-negative cells.[89] Second, the presence of estrogen receptor may not explain the positive responses to all forms of endocrine therapy. If, for example, androgen administration were to induce tumor regression by a process involving interaction with androgen receptor, estrogen receptor–positive but androgen receptor–negative tumors might fail to respond to this endocrine therapy. Third, the presence of a receptor may suggest hormone-dependent breast cancer, but the endocrine therapy may not be adequate to effect a response. For example, pituitary ablation may be incomplete. Alternatively, alterations in more than one hormone may be required. About 10 to 15% of patients with metastatic breast cancer who fail to respond to oophorectomy do respond to a subsequent adrenalectomy. Presumably, at the time of oophorectomy these patients had hormone-dependent tumors that were estrogen receptor–positive but appeared to be hormone independent because of continued activity of the adrenal glands. Fourth, any step distal to the initial binding of hormone to receptor may be deranged in cancer cells.

Binding of hormone to receptor is only the first step in hormone action.[77]

Prediction of hormone dependence would be more reliable if a tumor were assessed for a hormone-inducible function, the induced response indicating adequate receptor and postreceptor function. The most useful of these tests is determination of the progesterone receptor level.[83, 84] In both normal uterus and malignant uterine and mammary tissue, progesterone receptor synthesis is regulated by estrogen acting through the estrogen receptor. Tumors lacking an estrogen receptor are rarely progesterone receptor–positive, whereas about two thirds of estrogen receptor–positive tumors are progesterone receptor–positive. Estrogen receptor–positive tumors lacking progesterone receptor respond to endocrine therapy only one third of the time (the same as the overall response rate seen in a cohort of unselected patients). The response rate to endocrine therapy in patients whose tumors contain both estrogen and progesterone receptors is in excess of 75%.

The responses that occur in women whose tumors are estrogen receptor–positive and progesterone receptor–negative can be explained on two bases. First, in premenopausal women during the later phase of the menstrual cycle and during pregnancy, endogenous progesterone may occupy receptor, translocate it to the nucleus, and obscure its detection.[90] Second, in some postmenopausal women with hormone-dependent tumors, estrogen concentrations may be insufficient to induce progesterone receptors.[91]

Despite many false-positive and false-negative results, steroid receptor studies in breast cancer are valuable. Table 33–2 summarizes the objective response rates to endocrine therapy as a function of estrogen and progesterone receptor status. In the majority of patients, the response to endocrine therapy can be predicted with reasonable accuracy.

Receptor determinations may also serve as prognostic guides. Patients with estrogen receptor–positive primary breast cancers have longer disease-free intervals than receptor-negative subjects, independent of other known prognostic variables including menopausal status, tumor size, histological grade, and axillary lymph node status.[92–96]

The development of specific monoclonal antibodies to the estrogen receptor protein allows detection of the receptor independent of the binding of labeled hormone.[97, 98] A plastic bead radioimmunoassay, using monoclonal antibodies, and methods using immunoperoxidase or immunofluorescence techniques provide a basis for the simple, efficient detection and localization of estrogen receptor in clinical samples.

TABLE 33–2. Response Rates to Endocrine Therapy as a Function of Steroid Hormone Receptor Status in Metastatic Breast Cancer

Estrogen Receptor Status	Progesterone Receptor Status	Approximate Objective Response Rate to Endocrine Therapy (%)
Positive	Positive	80
Positive	Negative	30
Negative	Positive	Not established
Negative	Negative	5

Management of Breast Cancer

The management of breast cancer can be divided into two phases: early-stage disease and advanced (metastatic) disease.

Early Breast Cancer

Nearly 90% of women with breast cancer present with apparently localized disease. A variety of surgical and radiotherapeutic options should be considered, and patients should be encouraged to consider all options available. An approach to patients with early breast cancer is shown in Table 33–3. All women with early breast cancer should have an estrogen receptor assay. Available data suggest that the estrogen receptor status of the primary cancer is maintained in metastases. Thus knowledge of the receptor status of the primary tumor permits assignment to the appropriate treatment category when metastases develop, even if there is no readily accessible tissue for biopsy. Measurements of other prognostic variables, such as S phase, ploidy, and amplification or overexpression of the proto-oncogene erb B-2 (HER-2), are also useful.

Therapy must be sufficient to control the disease, but attention to the cosmetic outcome is also desirable, so therapy should be individualized. In addition, staging should include assessment of axillary lymph node involvement. On the basis of this evaluation, adjuvant therapy may be considered, although its exact role in different subsets of patients remains to be defined.

Metastatic Breast Cancer

Although many patients with primary breast cancer remain free of disease after local therapy (with or without

TABLE 33–3. Management of Early-Stage Breast Cancer

Histological Status of Lymph Nodes	Estrogen Receptor Status	Recommended Therapy
Premenopausal patients		
Involved with tumor	Positive	Combination chemotherapy possibly with endocrine therapy
Involved with tumor	Negative	Combination chemotherapy
Negative	Positive	No therapy generally, unless other prognostic variables indicate
Negative	Negative	Combination chemotherapy
Postmenopausal patients		
Involved with tumor	Positive	Chemotherapy plus endocrine therapy
Involved with tumor	Negative	Combination chemotherapy
Negative	Positive	Endocrine therapy (tamoxifen)
Negative	Negative	Combination chemotherapy

All Patients

1. Adequate therapy for local control of disease
2. Histopathological evaluation of axillary lymph nodes
3. Analysis of estrogen and progesterone receptors in the primary tumor
4. Analysis of growth fraction, ploidy, and markers that are under investigation such as cathepsin D, erb B-2, and heat shock proteins

TABLE 33–4. Approach to Therapy for Patients with Metastatic Breast Cancer

	Premenopausal Patients		Postmenopausal Patients	
	ER positive	*ER negative*	*ER positive*	*ER negative*
First therapy	Castration or possibly antiestrogens Relapse: repeat ER assay	Combination chemotherapy	Antiestrogens Relapse: repeat ER assay	Combination chemotherapy
Second therapy	Endocrine therapy	Chemotherapy	Endocrine therapy	Chemotherapy
		All Patients		

1. Adequate staging of sites of involvement
2. Biopsy of accessible tumor for estrogen receptor (ER) and progesterone receptor
   or if not available
3. Receptor status of primary tumor

the addition of systemic adjuvant therapy), a substantial number of cancers eventually recur. At this time endocrine therapy may be attempted. As already mentioned, only about one third of unselected patients can be expected to achieve a response, but in women with appropriate steroid receptor and menopausal status, substantial improvement in response rates can be achieved. One approach to therapy for patients with metastatic cancer is outlined in Table 33–4. After assessment of receptor status, patients may be allocated to appropriate treatment regimens. A variety of factors must be weighed in such decision making, including prognostic variables such as sites of involvement and personal issues such as the impact of different treatments on lifestyle. There is substantial latitude in the choice of regimen because efficiency of individual regimens may still be in question.

Endocrine Therapy of Breast Cancer

Ablative Therapies

OOPHORECTOMY. Removal of the ovaries of premenopausal patients has been known for more than 90 y to be an effective treatment for some women with inoperable breast cancer.[76] The regression rate is 25 to 30%,[99, 100] and the median duration of remission is 9 mo. Assessment of absolute response rate and comparisons of different therapies are difficult because selection biases may strongly influence the apparent success of endocrine therapy. In addition to the presence of estrogen and progesterone receptors in a tumor sample, lack of visceral metastases, a long interval from local therapy to first recurrence, and a good response to previous endocrine therapy all tend to be correlated with a response to endocrine therapy. Surgical oophorectomy is the method of choice because radiation may require several weeks to be effective and incomplete destruction of the follicles has been reported.

It is important to document the ovarian status accurately before oophorectomy. A high plasma level of follicle-stimulating hormone (FSH) is a reliable indication of loss of follicles and consequent cessation of estradiol secretion. A low plasma estradiol level (<70 pmol/L [<20 pg/mL]) is also characteristic of cessation of ovarian function, but levels this low may also occur in patients with secondary amenorrhea. The vaginal smear is unreliable for distinguishing between secondary amenorrhea and cessation of ovarian function. In perimenopausal and postmenopausal patients, the regression rate after oophorectomy is below that of women with ovarian function.[101]

The role of oophorectomy as adjuvant therapy in the management of breast cancer is controversial.[102] Although the disease-free interval is prolonged, improvement in survival has not been demonstrated. Early information from a randomized comparison of five-drug chemotherapy with and without oophorectomy in estrogen receptor–positive premenopausal patients with axillary lymph node involvement

suggests a survival benefit for women receiving drugs in addition to oophorectomy, although statistical significance has not been reached (unpublished observations, S. Rivkin). In one important trial,[103] the addition of low daily doses of prednisone after oophorectomy led to improvement in survival in premenopausal women. The reason for this improved result is not clear; one possibility is suppression by glucocorticoids of the secretion of adrenal androgens that can serve as prohormones for extraglandular estrogen formation. The role of oophorectomy as first-line endocrine therapy in premenopausal patients is under reassessment.

ADRENALECTOMY AND HYPOPHYSECTOMY. Estrogens persist in the blood and urine after oophorectomy. The adrenal cortex may secrete a small amount of estrone,[104] but the principal source of estrogen after castration results from the transformation of androstenedione, secreted by the adrenal cortex, to estrone in extraglandular tissues.[105] It has been difficult to prove that the low concentrations of estradiol and estrone characteristic of menopause are sufficient to support the growth of endocrine-sensitive tumors. However, the demonstration that the absence of an estrogen receptor in tumor tissue predicts that adrenalectomy will fail to be beneficial is in accord with the view that these small amounts of estrogen may be important. Furthermore, when human breast cancer cells are maintained in continuous tissue culture, as little as 2 to 3×10^{-11} M estradiol is sufficient to stimulate protein synthesis.[106]

The mechanism of response to adrenalectomy appears to be removal of an additional source of estrogens, but the mechanism of response to hypophysectomy is less clear. Removal of corticotropin (ACTH, adrenocorticotropic hormone) is doubtless important because the incidence of response to adrenalectomy is quite low after hypophysectomy. Lowering of the prolactin level is not involved because equivalent response rates occur after pituitary stalk sectioning, which raises plasma prolactin levels. Furthermore, administration of drugs that lower prolactin concentration is ineffective in treating breast cancer. Other incompletely characterized hypothalamic and pituitary peptides may play roles in the regulation of tumor growth.[107]

There are several criteria for the selection of patients for adrenalectomy or hypophysectomy. First, if an estrogen receptor can be identified in the metastatic tissue, the chance of response is about 60%. Second, if the patient has responded to castration, the likelihood of a subsequent response to ablative surgery is more than 50%. Whether these criteria identify the same patients is not known, but it is likely. It is also likely that a longer disease-free interval is associated with higher remission rates. Functional adrenalectomy can now be achieved by medical means (see later). Comparisons of medical and surgical adrenalectomy suggest that response rates and duration are approximately equivalent.

The rates of response to adrenalectomy and hypophysectomy have been variously estimated to be equal or slightly in favor of hypophysectomy. The mean duration of remission tends to be longer after hypophysectomy (15 versus 8 mo).[108] Although these data suggest that hypophysectomy may offer some advantages, the choice of operation must usually be based on more pragmatic considerations, such as the sites of metastases and the age of the patient. The management of adrenal and pituitary insufficiency is discussed in Chapters 9 and 6, respectively. It is necessary here only to emphasize that the patient can be treated adequately after either procedure and, when a remission occurs, can often resume full activity.

Additive Therapies

ANDROGEN THERAPY. Lacassagne,[24] who was the first to show that estrogens promoted the development of mammary tumors in mice, found that the growth of these tumors could be inhibited by testosterone propionate. Androgen therapy of women with metastatic cancer was subsequently initiated. The mechanism by which androgens induce responses in women with breast cancer is unknown.[109] Some tumors have androgen receptors, but their role in mediating the response of the tumor to androgens has not been established.[110, 111] The Cooperative Breast Cancer Group surveyed the responses of 521 patients treated with testosterone propionate and reported an overall remission rate of 21% and a somewhat higher rate in postmenopausal women.[112] Within 1 y after menopause, the remission rate is less than 10%, and it is highest 5 y after menopause. Soft tissue metastases respond most favorably. The median period of remission is 8 mo. Any androgen, given in large amounts, produces about the same rate of regression. Long-acting preparations should be avoided so that therapy can be changed rapidly if necessary. The results of trials with androgens are summarized in refs. 112 and 113.

Attempts have been made to find effective steroids that are less androgenic than testosterone, which may produce severe and distressing virilization. A synthetic steroid, testolactone, has essentially no androgenic activity and has been reported to produce regression of disease,[114] suggesting that the antitumor effect is independent of androgenicity. Danazol is also effective in breast cancer and has minimal virilizing effects.[60–62, 115] Combined therapy using an antiestrogen, danazol, and aminoglutethimide improves the response rate compared with that with antiestrogen alone but does not benefit overall survival.[116] This is also the usual case when endocrine and chemotherapy are combined in advanced disease; that is, an improved initial response rate is not translated into improved survival.[117] However, in one randomized trial, tamoxifen together with androgen did lead to improved survival when compared with tamoxifen alone.[118]

ESTROGENS. Some patients with breast cancer paradoxically show tumor regression when treated with pharmacological doses of estrogens, but the response is not predictable; remission rates of 30 to 37% have been reported when estrogen is used as initial therapy.[119, 120] In a randomized trial, estrogen produced a 29% remission rate and androgen induced a 10% remission rate. The duration of response to estrogen is longer than that to androgen in most series. Estrogen responsiveness increases with years after menopause. As with androgen and the ablative procedures, the longer the disease-free interval, the higher the probability of response to estrogen. When estrogens are used in patients who have relapsed from other therapy, remission rates are low, the chances of response being less than 10%. Estrogen is generally ineffective after hypophysectomy or adrenalectomy.

The toxicity of estrogens, even at high doses, is moderate. Endometrial hyperplasia and breakthrough bleeding can usually be managed by giving a progestogen, followed by a short period of cessation of hormone therapy to permit sloughing of the endometrium. Salt and water retention, particularly in the elderly, may also occur. The most important side effect, however, is hypercalcemia, which can occur abruptly in any patient but is rare in subjects 10 y or more beyond the menopause. Hypercalcemia almost certainly results from direct stimulation of bone metastases and is managed by withdrawal of estrogen and hydration. Often, on gradual reinstitution of therapy, remission can be achieved without recurrence of hypercalcemia. Patients who develop hypercalcemia eventually have a higher response rate to endocrine therapy than patients who do not.

Response has rarely been recorded after withdrawal of estrogen or of androgen.[121] Thus new attempts at therapy should generally not be started until at least 2 mo after steroid administration has been stopped. Rapidly advancing disease, of course, is an exception to this suggestion.

PROGESTOGENS. Various progestogens, both C_{21}-steroids such as medroxyprogesterone and C_{19}-steroids such as norethindrone, have been used in patients with breast cancer. Their exact mechanism of action is unknown, but possibilities include blockade of a progesterone receptor, interference with estrogen receptor synthesis, androgen-like effects, or possibly effects on other tissues such as the immune system.[109] In general, remission rates are about 20%,[122] the same as those noted with androgens. The response to progestogens is not influenced by the response to castration, estrogen, or androgen. Thus progestogens may be given a trial in patients who fail to respond to other therapeutic modalities. In general, the drugs do not cause important side effects. The most troublesome side effects with medroxyprogesterone acetate are sweating and weight gain. Crona and colleagues[123] reported decreases in high-density lipoprotein cholesterol and apolipoprotein A-I levels with an increase in triglyceride levels in patients receiving 1000 mg medroxyprogesterone acetate weekly, suggesting that the risk of cardiovascular disease could be increased. Side effects with megestrol acetate include increased appetite, weight gain of 5 to 20 kg, abnormal liver function tests, thromboembolism, vaginal bleeding, hot flashes, fluid retention, nausea and vomiting, hypercalcemia and flare, and rash.[124, 125] Regression of soft tissue metastases appears to be more common than regression of bone metastases. Investigations in Italy using large doses of progestogens obtained response rates in the range 30 to 40% without significant toxicity.[126, 127] Randomized comparisons have suggested response rates similar to those with antiestrogen therapy. Failure to respond to the primary therapy is generally predictive of a minimal response to the second regimen.

ANTIPROGESTOGENS. Antiprogestational agents have also been tried for the treatment of hormone-dependent cancers such as breast carcinoma. Mifepristone is one such synthetic compound that has both antiprogestational and antiglucocorticoid effects.[128] Pretreatment of MCF-7 (breast cancer) cells with estradiol increases the inhibition seen with mifepristone.[129] There is one report of a clinical trial of mifepristone in the treatment of patients with metastatic breast cancer.[130] The dose used was 200 mg orally daily, and a response rate of 18% was achieved. The only toxicity reported was a decrease in serum potassium levels. Plasma concentrations of FSH, luteinizing hormone (LH), and prolactin were unchanged with treatment. Plasma cortisol concentrations were increased after 3 mo of treatment. Further clinical trials and research into the mechanisms of action are in progress.

LUTEINIZING HORMONE–RELEASING HORMONE ANALOGUES. Administration of a luteinizing hormone–releasing hormone (LHRH) analogue in a sustained or continuous manner causes inhibition of gonadal steroid hormone synthesis (see Chapter 12). Treatment of premenopausal women with LHRH agonists reduces plasma estradiol concentrations to levels seen in oophorectomized or postmenopausal women.[131–133] Furthermore, in premenopausal women treated with the LHRH agonist leuprolide, serum FSH and LH levels increase during the first 4 d of treatment and subsequently fall and remain persistently suppressed.[133] Plasma progesterone, estrone, estrone sulfate, and estradiol levels decrease to postmenopausal values. There is no change in levels of androstenedione, prolactin, or cortisol.

Buserelin in moderate doses also induces anovulation and a decrease in progesterone levels, but 60% of patients had transient elevation of estradiol levels with no change in FSH or LH,[134] so that high doses may be necessary to induce complete chemical castration. Furthermore, subcutaneous administration appears to be more effective than intranasal administration. Decreases in plasma LH, FSH, progesterone, and estradiol levels also occur in premenopausal women after treatment with goserelin.[135] Plasma progesterone levels are reduced after 2 wk and estradiol levels decrease after 4 to 6 wk of treatment.

Treatment of premenopausal women with breast cancer with LHRH agonists in two studies produced objective responses of 41%[134] and 44%.[133] This class of compounds may be useful as adjuvant therapy in the future. Side effects include hot flashes, nausea and vomiting, headache, dizziness, tumor flare, diarrhea, local reaction, irritability, hives, and severe polydipsia and (rarely) polyuria.[132–134] Also, amenorrhea is a physiological consequence of the therapy in all women.

GLUCOCORTICOIDS. Large doses of glucocorticoid (equivalent to 200 to 300 mg of hydrocortisone daily) can induce regression of metastatic breast cancer in 10 to 20% of patients.[136] Remissions are short-lived, but the rapid onset of action makes these agents useful in rapidly advancing disease. A response to glucocorticoids is not predictive of responses to other endocrine modalities. As mentioned previously, when combined with oophorectomy, glucocorticoids inhibit the synthesis of adrenal substrates for extraglandular aromatization and hence may improve survival for patients with early stages of breast cancer.[103] Glucocorticoids may also improve the response rate and survival time when combined with certain cytotoxic chemotherapeutic programs,[136] and they are of value in managing certain acute difficulties such as hypercalcemia and intracranial metastases.

ANTIESTROGENS. Substances that antagonize the action of estrogens are termed *antiestrogens*. (Also see Chapter 3.) Compounds that fit this definition include nonspecific inhibitors of protein and RNA synthesis. With the possible exception of certain weak, short-acting agonists, such as estriol, the compounds of current clinical relevance are derivatives of triphenylethylene and include nafoxidine, clomiphene, and tamoxifen. These agents compete with estradiol for binding to specific estrogen receptor sites. However, the biological activity is more complicated and cannot be explained in terms of this effect alone.[137] After binding to estrogen receptors, antiestrogens are thought to anchor these receptors to nuclear binding sites. It is not established whether these nuclear sites are identical with the nuclear sites occupied by estrogen-receptor complexes.

In addition to interactions with the specific estrogen binding sites, these agents interact with distinct antiestrogen binding sites.[138–140] Such sites have limited affinity for estrogens and do not translocate from cytoplasm to nucleus. The binding affinities of various antiestrogens with these binding sites correlate moderately well with antiestrogenic activity. In one study a loss of response to antiestrogens was associated with a decrease in number of antiestrogen binding sites.[141] Their role in the action of antiestrogens remains unknown.

Antiestrogens do not inhibit estrogen receptor synthesis or alter estrogen receptor degradation.[142] They do, however, induce conformational changes in the receptor that could lead to qualitatively or quantitatively altered RNA transcription and decreased cell proliferation.

Tamoxifen is a cell cycle phase–specific cytostatic and cytotoxic agent (depending on concentration) that acts during a specific 2- to 4-h time interval in mid-G_1 phase.[143] In the breast cancer cell line MCF-7 there are two populations of cells with different G_1 transit times, a rapidly cycling pool and a slowly cycling pool. Tamoxifen increases G_1 phase duration and appears to shift cells from the rapidly cycling to the slowly cycling pool. This increases overall cell cycle transit time, thereby decreasing the overall proliferation rates. A separate high-dose cytotoxic effect of tamoxifen occurs at a specific point in G_1 phase and results in an increase in the proportion of cells in G_1 and decrease in the proportion in S phase; the end result is cell death. The effects of tamoxifen at low concentrations can be reversed by estradiol, whereas effects at high concentrations cannot, which suggests that the effects at high concentrations are nonspecific. These findings suggest that tamoxifen controls a biochemical process critical in cell cycle regulation. It is not clear whether the in vitro tamoxifen concentrations at which these effects occur correlate with actual intratumor concentrations in patients given tamoxifen.

Tamoxifen can also stimulate hormone-dependent human breast cancer cells to secrete the polypeptide factor transforming growth factor β (TGF β).[144] (Also see Chapter 21.) This factor inhibits many epithelial cell lines, including breast carcinoma. Indeed, TGF β can also inhibit the growth of the estrogen receptor–negative breast cancer cell line MDA-MB-231.[144] Breast cancers contain mixtures of estrogen receptor–positive and –negative tumor cells. If TGF β has a paracrine effect on surrounding hormone-independent cells, it may make antiestrogens more effective in these tumors than would be expected on the basis of only blockade of estrogen action.

Whereas antiestrogens are useful in the management of postmenopausal breast cancer,[145–148] their role in premenopausal patients is unclear. Some premenopausal patients have apparently normal menstrual cycles during objective tumor regressions.[149] As already mentioned, antiestrogens are also weak estrogen agonists; for example, the vaginal epithelium of postmenopausal women usually shows an estrogenic effect. In addition, some women have a brief "flare" of tumor growth after the institution of antiestrogen therapy,[150] although this phenomenon has not been quantified.[151]

Antiestrogens induce a therapeutic response in about a third of men and women with breast cancer.[145–148] Thus the drugs are at least as efficacious as other forms of endocrine manipulation. A particular advantage of the antiestrogens is the paucity of toxicity. Tamoxifen administration is not associated with significant bone marrow, renal, hepatic, or central nervous system toxicity.

Patterson and colleagues[152] reviewed the treatment of nearly 3000 patients with antiestrogens in 45 separate studies. The overall response rate was 34%, with somewhat less than 7% achieving a complete remission. The range of response varied from 14 to 57%. In the absence of prior systemic therapy, 43% had an objective response to tamoxifen. Prior chemotherapy did not have a significant effect on the response to tamoxifen, whereas 59% of patients who had responded to prior endocrine therapy responded to tamoxifen. In contrast, only 21% of nonresponders to endocrine therapy improved with subsequent antiestrogen therapy. In a heavily pretreated cohort of women with advanced breast cancer, only 17% achieved an objective partial response or better.[118]

In the experience of Patterson and colleagues,[152] 56 of 180, or 31%, of premenopausal women (or at least women under age 50) had an objective response. This was similar to the results for women aged 51 to 60 (76 of 255, or 30%) or 61 to 70 (87 of 245, or 36%). Of note, 65 of 142 women over age 70, or 46%, responded to tamoxifen.

However, selection biases and different prognostic variables can result in highly variable outcomes. Visceral metastases, multiple sites of involvement, estrogen receptor negativity, the perimenopausal state, poor performance status, failure to respond to prior endocrine chemotherapy, and age less than 35 are factors in lower response rates to antiestrogen therapy.

There have been few comparisons of antiestrogen therapy with alternative endocrine therapies in younger women. However, in two studies[153, 154] antiestrogen therapy appeared to be equivalent to ovarian ablation. In one study,[153] a crossover design was used, and a 50% response rate occurred with the second therapy if the first had been successful. Second therapy failed uniformly if the first therapy had failed. The same results were seen whether castration or antiestrogen was used first.

If higher circulating estrogen concentrations were capable of overcoming the effects of antiestrogens, one would anticipate a dose-response effect. However, the relationship between the response and the dose is minimal. Of the patients who receive a total daily dose of 20 mg, 30% respond, and the response rate increases to 36% with 30 mg/d and to 40% with 40 mg/d. These differences are not significant. However, on occasion a second well-documented remission can occur after relapse when the dose is increased.[155]

The metabolism of tamoxifen has been studied extensively. The major metabolite was originally thought to be 4-hydroxytamoxifen[156] but now appears to be N-desmethyltamoxifen, a metabolite that is also present in the circulation of treated patients.[157] N-Desmethyltamoxifen reaches serum levels 1.2 to 1.8 times greater than those of tamoxifen.[158–160] The metabolites are excreted largely in the bile as conjugates.

4-Hydroxytamoxifen is also found at low levels in serum. 4-Hydroxytamoxifen binds to the estrogen receptor with an affinity 25 to 50 times that of tamoxifen and equal to that of estradiol.[160–162] N-Desmethyltamoxifen binds with an affinity less than 1% that of tamoxifen.[160] Therefore, although the blood levels of 4-hydroxytamoxifen are lower, the potency is 1250 times that of desmethyltamoxifen. This suggests that N-desmethyltamoxifen contributes little to the antiestrogenic properties of tamoxifen and that 4-hydroxytamoxifen exerts a significant antiestrogenic effect.

At a dose of 20 mg twice a day, tamoxifen levels range from 285 to 310 µg/L, N-desmethyltamoxifen levels from 462 to 481 µg/L, and 4-hydroxytamoxifen levels from 6 to 7 µg/L.[163–165] Tamoxifen doses of 10 mg twice a day yield serum levels of tamoxifen and its metabolites that are about half of those seen at the higher doses.[158, 165–167] The initial blood half-life of tamoxifen ranges from 4 to 14 h, and the secondary half-life is about 7 d.[165, 168–171] Thus it takes 16 wk to achieve a steady state.[171]

There is no or minimal change in levels of gonadotropin[159, 172, 173] or prolactin[159, 173] in premenopausal women treated with tamoxifen. However, estradiol and progesterone concentrations increase.[159] The increase in estrogen levels may be due to a direct stimulatory effect of tamoxifen on the ovary. Because the elevated estrogen levels do not cause a decrease in gonadotropin levels, tamoxifen may have a direct antiestrogenic effect on the hypothalamic-pituitary axis.

In postmenopausal women the elevated levels of both LH and FSH decrease with tamoxifen treatment but still are in the postmenopausal range in most studies,[174–179] with no change in one study.[180] Prolactin levels also decrease[175, 178] or remain unchanged.[176, 180]

Effects on vaginal cornification in postmenopausal women vary in different reports. Estrogens cause an increase in cellular maturity or an increase in karyopyknotic index (KPI). Boccardo et al.[181] treated postmenopausal women with tamoxifen and reported an increase in the KPI in two thirds of patients, no change in a tenth, and a decrease in a fourth. Increases in the KPI[182] and decreases in the KPI[183] have been observed in other studies.

Although prophylactic castration does not improve the long-term survival of women with stage I or stage II breast cancer, the advent of receptor analyses and the development of pharmacological means of ovarian ablation have rekindled interest in endocrine therapy. In a double-blind prospective randomized trial of 322 patients under the age of 70 y with stage I to stage III breast cancer whose primary treatment was radical mastectomy and postoperative radiation, adjuvant diethylstilbestrol (DES) was compared with tamoxifen or placebo administered for 2 y or more. Premenopausal patients were randomized to receive either placebo or tamoxifen; postmenopausal patients were randomized to receive placebo, tamoxifen, or DES. After a median 44 mo of observation, no significant difference in disease-free interval was apparent between placebo or tamoxifen treatment in premenopausal patients. In the postmenopausal group both adjuvant DES and tamoxifen prolonged the disease-free interval. The DES-treated patients had more severe side effects, necessitating withdrawal from therapy of 41% of the patients compared with 13% with severe side effects in the tamoxifen group.

A large prospective multicenter study compared adjuvant chemotherapy with melphalan and fluorouracil in the presence and absence of tamoxifen in 1861 stage II patients after radical or modified radical mastectomy.[184] Estrogen and progesterone receptor analyses were performed in the majority. Patients were stratified according to age ($\leq$49 y or $\geq$50 y) and axillary node status (one to three positive nodes or more than four positive nodes). Disease-free survival at 36 mo was better with melphalan, fluorouracil, and tamoxifen than with melphalan and fluorouracil for the entire population of patients (70% versus 61%, p = .001). This advantage of the three agents was the result of improvement in disease-free interval and survival in patients who were age 50 or older. In patients aged 49 or younger, especially those with four or more positive nodes, regardless of receptor status, melphalan, fluorouracil, and tamoxifen treatment was detrimental. The mechanism of this adverse effect is unknown.

PHARMACOLOGICAL INTERFERENCE WITH ADRENAL STEROIDOGENESIS. The fact that adrenalectomy and hypophysectomy are effective for some patients has prompted efforts to achieve similar results pharmacologically. It has long been appreciated that glucocorticoid administration can cause transient palliative responses in some patients with metastatic breast cancer. Although glucocorticoids may have direct inhibitory effects on cancer cells in tissue culture,[185] it is likely that suppression of adrenal androgen production and subsequent suppression of extraglandular estrogen synthesis play a major role in the therapeutic effect. The combined use of aminoglutethimide and dexamethasone was originally tried as a means of suppressing adrenal function.[186] Aminoglutethimide is a potent inhibitor of the conversion of cholesterol to pregnenolone,[187] but it also shortens the plasma half-life of dexamethasone, so that pituitary ACTH secretion resumes and overrides the adrenal blockade imposed by aminoglutethimide.[188] By substituting hydrocortisone (whose metabolism is not altered by aminoglutethimide), adequate adrenal suppression can be achieved in most patients.[189] Although the level of one adrenal androgen, dehydroepiandrosterone, decreased, that of androstenedione, another adrenal androgen that serves as the immediate precursor of estrone, increased. Because levels of estrone also fell rapidly, this finding suggested that aminoglutethimide might also block extraglandular aromatization. This possibility has been substantiated by in vitro measurements in which aminoglutethimide was shown to inhibit aromatization by human placenta.

The use of inhibitors of adrenal steroidogenesis is reviewed in ref. 190. Aminoglutethimide in combination with hydrocortisone causes decreases in plasma estrone and estradiol levels equivalent to those seen after surgical adrenalectomy. Furthermore, the response rate and duration of response in women with breast cancer appear to be equivalent after surgical adrenalectomy or treatment with aminoglutethimide.[191] Preliminary information suggests that medical adrenalectomy in combination with tamoxifen and danazol may be superior to either therapy alone.[116]

AROMATASE INHIBITION. There are two mechanisms for achieving blockade of aromatization.[192] Type I inhibitors act as substrates for the aromatase enzyme and bind to the active site of the enzyme. Some are competitive inhibitors, and some bind irreversibly to the enzyme, causing its inactivation (so-called suicide inhibition). The advantage of the latter type of inhibitor is that it is more specific and usually longer acting. An example of a type I inhibitor is 4-hydroxyandrostenedione.

Type II inhibitors interfere with steroid hydroxylations by binding to the cytochrome P-450 moiety of the aromatase enzyme and produce a different spectral pattern. These inhibitors are less specific because they inhibit hydroxylating enzymes involved in the biosynthesis of many steroids. Aminoglutethimide is an example of this type of inhibitor.

4-Hydroxyandrostenedione is up to 60 times more potent than aminoglutethimide in the inhibition of aromatase in a human placental preparation.[193-195]

Side effects of aminoglutethimide include lethargy in about 40% and ataxia in 10%.[192, 195-197] These soporific effects usually resolve over weeks. About a third of women develop a morbilliform, maculopapular rash, sometimes associated with fever. The rash is usually evanescent and does not necessitate cessation of therapy. The rash can rarely progress and cause desquamation. Other side effects include orthostatic hypotension, leg cramps, facial fullness, weight gain, cushingoid features, and nausea. Side effects make it necessary to discontinue therapy in approximately 5% of patients.[196, 198]

Hematological toxicity also occurs with aminoglutethimide.[122, 192, 197, 199-202] Thrombocytopenia occurs in about 4% of patients in different series.[192, 201, 202] In a review of 1345 patients treated with aminoglutethimide there was a 4% incidence of thrombocytopenia, a 1% incidence of leukopenia, and a 4% incidence of pancytopenia.[202] These effects usually occurred 3 to 7 wk after the beginning of therapy[199] and ameliorated within 3 wk after discontinuation of the drug. There have been case reports of death from septicemia caused by marrow aplasia.[199] Therefore, white blood cell and platelet counts should be done at weeks 4, 8, and 12 after starting therapy.

Attempts are being made to develop more effective and potent aromatase inhibitors. One such compound is 4-hydroxyandrostenedione.[193] It causes regression of dimethylbenzanthracine-induced mammary tumors in animal model systems,[203] inhibits extraglandular aromatization of androgens in rhesus monkeys,[204] inhibits the conversion of androstenedione to estrogens in human placenta and rat ovarian microsomes,[205] and has been reported to inhibit aromatization in human prostatic tissue.[206] 4-Hydroxyandrostenedione is 30 times more potent as an aromatase inhibitor than aminoglutethimide and 100 times more than testolactone.[194]

In 52 postmenopausal women with metastatic breast cancer the response rate to 4-hydroxyandrostenedione was 27%.[207] Half of these patients had had two or more previous endocrine therapies. The optimal dose and route of administration have not been determined.

Side effects with the use of intramuscular 4-hydroxyandrostenedione include sterile abscesses and painful lumps at the injection site.[207] Lethargy is common. Perioral edema occurred in one patient, and an anaphylactoid reaction has been reported.[207] Toxicity after oral administration includes rash, facial swelling, and leukopenia in one patient.[208] Hot flashes may also occur.[209]

Breast Cancer in Men

Although accounting for only about 1% of breast cancer cases, the disorder in men is commonly hormone dependent and provides certain distinct contrasts with the disorder in women.[210, 212] Known risk factors include exogenous estrogen exposure, enhanced endogenous estrogen formation (Klinefelter syndrome), radiation, family history of breast cancer, gynecomastia, and orchitis (also see Chapter 15). One of the most convincing arguments for a role of exogenous estrogen in the etiology of breast cancer was provided in a report of two 30-y-old trans-sexual men who developed breast cancer after castration and continuous estrogen use.[213] Breast cancers in men almost invariably contain estrogen receptor and are frequently positive for progesterone, glucocorticoid, and androgen receptors as well.[214] Although the survival rates in men and women at each stage of the disease are the same, a greater proportion of men present with advanced disease. Approximately two thirds of male patients respond to orchiectomy; this is twice the response rate to endocrine therapy in women with breast cancer.[212] Adrenalectomy and hypophysectomy are also frequently successful, even in patients who fail to respond to primary endocrine manipulations. In one study of 31 men with advanced breast cancer, treatment with tamoxifen caused a complete or partial response with minimal toxicity in 48%.[215] Antiestrogens may thus be the initial treatment of choice for men with breast cancer.

ENDOMETRIAL CANCER

Epidemiology

The uterine endometrium is under the control of two hormones, estradiol and progesterone. The identification of the specific uterine cytosolic receptor for estradiol in 1962[216] was an important milestone in the receptor era of endocrinology. As in the case of breast cancer, estrogen probably plays permissive, carcinogenic, and promotional roles in the development of endometrial cancer. The promotional activity of estrogens leading to expression of endometrial cancer is probably the most important.

Clinical, biological, and epidemiological data indicate that prolonged or unopposed estrogenic stimulation increases the risk of endometrial carcinoma. The longer the endometrium is stimulated, the greater the cancer risk, as shown by the association of endometrial carcinoma with the use of estrogens after menopause[217] and with late menopause. The increased incidence of endometrial cancer in women with estrogen-secreting tumors and the polycystic ovary syndrome[218] further suggests that progesterone-induced endometrial sloughing may be protective. A higher incidence of endometrial cancer is also seen with other ovarian abnormalities, such as stromal hyperplasia and persistent stromal thecal cells. In each case, estrogen secretion is not excessive but is continuous because ovulatory cycles with their accompanying progesterone secretory periods and subsequent endometrial sloughing do not occur. The occasional development of endometrial cancer in women with gonadal dysgenesis treated with estrogens alone is further evidence for this concept. A causal role for continued, unopposed estrogenic stimulus is also supported by the high incidence of pre-existing irregular menses in women with endometrial cancer.[218] The resumption of cyclic ovarian function in response to ovarian wedge resection in the polycystic ovary syndrome results in regression of endometrial hyperplasia; progesterone can also reverse estrogen-induced endometrial hyperplasia.[219]

Another risk factor for endometrial carcinoma (as for breast cancer) is obesity. In the premenopausal woman the association of anovulatory cycles and amenorrhea with obesity may be the physiological basis for the association. In the postmenopausal woman the etiological pathway is more clearly understood. After the menopause the predominant blood estrogen is estrone, derived almost entirely by formation in extraglandular tissues from androstenedione. The rate of this conversion increases with age[220] and weight.[221] Plasma estrogen concentrations increase with increasing weight.[222] Adipose tissue has the capacity to convert androgens to estrogens and constitutes the most important site of extraglandular estrogen formation. Plasma estrone production and concentrations are the same in women with endometrial cancer as in weight- and age-matched controls, but the higher incidence of obesity in the women with cancer means that as a group there is greater exposure to estrogen. The use of exogenous estrogen by postmenopausal women is also associated with an increased risk of endometrial cancer.[223] The relative risk factors for the development of endometrial cancer vary from 4:1 to 9:1, the higher figures occurring with longer use, as would be expected if the endometrium is maintained in a stimulated state for a longer period. Increased risk with increasing duration of exposure is a characteristic feature of tumor promoters in the two-step carcinogen promoter model for cancer induction. It was suggested that the risk of long-term exogenous estrogen use might be overestimated because of an increased likelihood of discovery of early endometrial cancer during the work-up of the vaginal bleeding that may accompany estrogen therapy.[223] This argument has been refuted by additional data and theoretical considerations.[217] In most studies of the use of estrogen in postmenopausal women, larger than physiological doses have been used and progestogen-induced withdrawal bleeding has not generally been part of the regimens. Attention to both of these factors would be expected to reduce the risk appreciably. The increased incidence of endometrial cancer has not been accompanied by a similar increase in the death rate from the disease, because estrogen use tends to be associated with a less aggressive form of endometrial cancer (see Chapter 12).

Endocrinology

The uterus is the best-studied estrogen-responsive tissue, and our understanding of the mechanism of action of estrogen has been derived largely from studies of animal uteri. The estrogen receptor content of the endometrium is highest in the proliferative phase and decreased in the luteal phase.[224–226] Administration of progestogen decreases estrogen receptor content.[226] Progesterone receptor capacity is highest at the time of the estradiol peak[224] and can be induced by estrogens. Estrogen receptor is present in most endometrial carcinomas, and the content of the receptor is inversely correlated with the degree of differentiation.[224] By contrast, cytosolic[224, 227] and nuclear progesterone receptor levels[228] are highest in well-differentiated cancer.[224] The uterine 17β-hydroxysteroid dehydrogenase enzyme that catalyzes the interconversion of estradiol and estrone is induced by progesterone[229] and can serve as an index of progestational effect.

The mechanism by which progestogen acts in endometrial cancer is incompletely understood. In the estrogen-primed uterus, progsterone causes specific maturational changes, followed by atrophy when progestogen administration is continued for long periods. After administration of progestogens to women with endometrial cancer, mitotic activity ceases, the glandular epithelium becomes more differentiated, and the ratio of cytoplasm to nucleus increases. Atrophy of the epithelium may also occur. These changes are similar to those of the normal endometrium during progestogen therapy. The fact that endometrial cancers contain progesterone receptors probably explains the therapeutic effect. Progestogen therapy also decreases estrogen receptor levels and increases the capacity of the endometrium to metabolize estradiol (see earlier). As with breast cancer, these tumors may be heterogeneous with respect to cell content of progesterone receptors, accounting for the variability of response.

Therapy

Kelly and Baker reported in 1961[230] that progestogens could cause regression in about a third of patients with metastatic endometrial cancer, an observation that has been confirmed in patients treated at many centers.[231] The response to therapy does not depend on the age of the patient, site of metastasis, or previous or concurrent therapy. However, women with slowly growing or more differentiated tumors respond better than those with more aggressive cancers. The duration of life after initiation of therapy was 27 mo in those who responded and only 7 mo in those who did not. It does not appear to matter which progestogen is used, but large doses seem to be necessary.[232] Progestogens that have been used include both the C_{21} 17-acetoxysteroids, such as medroxyprogesterone acetate and megestrol acetate, and C_{19}-steroids, such as norethindrone. Response is associated with presence of estrogen and progesterone receptors.[124]

The mechanism by which progestogens inhibit tumor growth is unknown. Several hypotheses have been postulated. First, they could have a direct cytotoxic effect on tumor cells, as has been shown in vitro in breast cancer cell lines.[129, 233] Second, the inhibition could be exerted endocrinologically by effects on the hypothalamic-pituitary-gonadal axis. Progestogens suppress basal and LHRH-simulated gonadotropin secretion and the secretion of cortisol, dehydroepiandrosterone, and estradiol in a dose-dependent manner.[234] Whether these hormonal changes affect tumor growth is unknown. Third, progestogens may decrease estrogen receptor levels and therefore the ability of the tumor to respond to endogenous estrogens. Progestogens bind weakly to other receptors, and their binding to androgen or glucocorticoid receptors may account for the tumor response. It is also proposed that progestogens may induce the formation of growth-inhibitory factors, inhibit the synthesis and secretion of estrogen-induced growth factors, or modulate other mitogens.

Finally, progestogens may decrease the mobility of membrane lipids and hence return membrane dynamics in tumor cells to normal.[235] Clearly, the mechanism of action by which progestogens inhibit tumor growth requires investigation.[236]

In view of the lack of effectiveness of chemotherapy in uterine cancer, a trial of progestogens is appropriate in any patient with metastatic disease. The remissions seen with progestogens are accompanied by essentially no toxicity. The response of pulmonary metastases may be better than that of bone metastases. Quantitative progesterone receptor determinations can be of value in selecting patients suitable for endocrine therapy.[237]

CARCINOMA OF THE PROSTATE

Epidemiology

Cancer of the prostate is the second most common cancer in men in the United States,[238] and more than 60% of the cases occur in men older than age 70. The death rate is higher in American black persons than in white, and American black men have an age-standardized incidence about six times that of Nigerian black men,[239] although incidences of latent carcinoma are the same.[240] A role of environmental factors in the etiology of clinical cancer of the prostate is further suggested by the finding that Japanese men living in Hawaii have a higher incidence of clinical cancer of the prostate than do men in Japan, although the incidence of latent carcinoma is the same.[241]

Endocrinology

The pioneering work of Huggins and associates[242–244] gave rise to the concept that prostatic cancer, like the normal prostate and the hyperplastic prostate, is androgen dependent. The demonstration that castration caused regression of prostatic cancer in men[244] initiated the era of hormonal management of cancer of the prostate.

In broad outlines, the mechanism of androgen action resembles that of estrogen (see Chapters 3 and 13); that is, the androgen is bound to a specific receptor protein and the hormone-receptor complex interacts with chromatin. The active intracellular androgen in the prostate is dihydrotestosterone, the 5α-reduced metabolite of testosterone.[245, 246] Plasma androgen levels are the same in men with prostatic cancer as in the normal population.[247]

Prolactin plays a role in prostatic growth in rodents. Hypophysectomy causes a more profound atrophy of the rat prostate than does castration, and endogenous prolactin may act synergistically with testosterone in maintaining the male mouse sexual accessory glands.[248] Injection of prolactin antiserum inhibits prostate growth in rabbits.[249] In addition, the prostate in some species has specific prolactin binding sites, and these receptors are androgen dependent.[250] However, a role for prolactin in the physiology of the human prostate has not been established.

In parallel with receptor studies in breast and endometrial cancers, attempts have been made to correlate the content of dihydrotestosterone receptor with response to therapy.[251] Sampling errors are only one of the several technical problems that have made these studies difficult. At any rate, as with endometrial cancer, predicting the clinical

response to endocrine therapy from evaluation of receptor levels is of less value than in breast cancer. Because no alternative therapies of proven value are available, virtually all symptomatic patients with prostate cancer receive a trial of endocrine therapy.

Therapy

Although the principles of therapy are simple, there is controversy about tactics. If, as proposed by Huggins,[242–244] it is necessary to decrease the plasma content of testicular androgens to a low level, surgical or "medical" orchiectomy should suffice; if total deprivation of adrenal and testicular androgen is necessary, additional steps may be required. Estrogen may have a direct inhibitory effect on the prostate in addition to its suppression of gonadotropin secretion by the pituitary. Thus a rationale may exist for the simultaneous use of orchiectomy and estrogen.

In large series of patients with metastatic disease,[252, 253] 3- and 5-y survival rates in treated patients with stage III or stage IV disease were better than those in untreated patients. The differences among castration, estrogen therapy, and combined treatment were not significant. Likewise, in a study using randomized assignments to therapeutic regimens, findings were similar with the three regimens.[254] High doses of DES (5 mg/d) are associated with increased mortality from cardiovascular disease.[254] Smaller doses of DES (1 mg/d) appear to be as effective as the 5-mg dose,[255] although plasma testosterone concentrations are not as completely suppressed;[256] at this dosage of DES there is no increase in cardiovascular mortality. DES does not improve the survival rates in stage I and stage II patients (carcinoma confined to the prostate). There is no evidence that one estrogen is better than another, although individual patients may have fewer side effects from one or another. When patients have responded to either estrogen or orchiectomy, subsequent use of the other modality is generally ineffective.

Remission of disease is usually defined as a lowering of the serum acid phosphatase level and relief of pain. One of the difficulties in evaluating therapy of prostate cancer is the problem of reproducibly defining the clinical response. Most patients have osteoblastic metastases, and definitions of tumor response are generally based on "soft" criteria such as acid phosphatase level, analgesia index, and performance status rather than objective tumor measurements. Because bone metastases are usually osteoblastic, sufficient remodeling to allow confirmation that remission has taken place may take several years. Nevertheless, regression rates after either orchiectomy or estrogen therapy have been reported to be 50 to 80%, varying with the grade and stage of the disease.[257] The average duration of remission is 15 mo, although occasional remissions may last more than 5 y.

Plasma concentrations of androstenedione and testosterone are measurable in some patients with prostatic cancer after orchiectomy.[258] Suppression of adrenal androgen production by exogenous glucocorticoids reduces these levels. Thus, some men, like some postmenopausal women with endometrial hyperplasia, may produce higher amounts of androstenedione or have a greater capacity for conversion of androstenedione to testosterone in extraglandular tissues than does the general population. Adrenal suppression may be beneficial in this group, but trials of glucocorticoid therapy have been inconclusive.

Because of residual androgen production by the adrenal cortex, adrenalectomy and hypophysectomy have also been tried in patients who have relapsed after primary therapy with estrogen or orchiectomy.[259–261] In none of the series was there a consistent decrease in the acid phosphatase level accompanying the decrease in pain, as occurs almost invariably after orchiectomy or estrogen therapy. Medical adrenalectomy using aminoglutethimide also does not cause clear-cut improvement.[262] Both types of approach may provide short-term clinical improvement but rarely produce objective evidence of regression of disease.[263]

Progestogens have been tried for treatment because they suppress plasma LH levels and can also act as antiandrogens, competing directly with androgens for binding to the prostatic androgen receptors. Remissions have been reported in response to cyproterone acetate, a progestational antiandrogen, when it was given before castration or estrogen therapy. The drug is ineffective after castration.[264] A nonsteroidal androgen agonist, flutamide, can also cause regression of disease in untreated patients and may be effective in patients who relapse after castration or estrogen therapy.[265, 266] A "pure" antiandrogen of this type should prove useful both therapeutically and as a probe for androgen dependence. LHRH analogues, with or without antiandrogens, can also induce responses with essentially no toxicity.[267, 268] These analogues inhibit LH secretion and thus cause medical castration (see Chapter 13).

More than 1600 LHRH agonists and antagonists have been synthesized.[269] Normally, LHRH is released in pulses, which leads to pulsatile release of LH and FSH. Constant infusions of exogenous LHRH[270] or intermittent high doses of LHRH analogues inhibit LH and FSH release. LHRH has also been reported to inhibit breast cancer cells directly in vitro in some[271–273] but not all studies.[274] There is no evidence for a direct action of LHRH in prostate.

In leuprolide therapy there is an initial fourfold rise in LH level and a twofold increase in testosterone level after the first dose; the levels return to normal within 72 to 80 h.[270] Gonadotropin levels become suppressed by 2 to 4 wk of therapy. Testosterone levels decrease by 95% 1 wk after treatment. After therapy for 1 to 2 y there is no escape from the androgen suppression, and no differences were noted in testosterone suppression with the 1-, 10-, and 20-mg doses of leuprolide. Similar results were obtained for men treated with buserelin subcutaneously, followed by chronic intranasal therapy.[275]

Smaller doses of LHRH analogues appear to be inadequate to achieve medical castration.[276] The oral bioavailability of LHRH analogues is very low because of proteolysis in the gastrointestinal tract.[277] Rectal administration also is ineffective.[277] Intravenously administered native LHRH has a half-life of 2 to 8 min for the fast phase and 15 to 60 min for the slower phase.[277] The intranasal route has also been used in attempts to make the administration more convenient. The bioavailability is only 1 to 2%, but lipophilic compounds are more effectively absorbed.[277]

Subcutaneous administration is the most widely used route. With this route absorption is rate-limiting and depends on injection volume, local blood flow, injection trauma, presence of capillaries and lymphatics, and proteolytic degradation at the injection site. The bioavailability of LHRH is 75 to 90% by this route. Administration of some analogues by this route is associated with depot-like effects.[277]

Once-monthly biodegradable depot formulations are under investigation. The formulation used for one of these preparations, goserelin, incorporates a rod of d,l-lactide-glycolide copolymer that releases drug for 28 d.[278, 279] This polymer degrades to lactic and glycolic acids.[280] Depot doses of goserelin of 3.6, 1.8, and 0.9 mg release about 120, 60, and 30 μg, respectively, of drug daily for approximately 28 d.[281] These doses decrease plasma testosterone levels to castration values in men by 2 to 3 wk with parallel decreases in plasma LH. These castration levels are maintained without escape for at least 18 mo. Subcutaneous injection of 3.6 mg of goserelin sustains amenorrhea in premenopausal women for 61 to 71 d after injection.[282] At 5 wk a rise in LH concentration was noted. This drug has a potency 100 to 200 times that of native LHRH.

The objective response rate with leuprolide (1.0 mg subcutaneously daily) in a large randomized study is 38%.[283] Labrie and associates[284] advocated the use of a combination of an LHRH agonist with an antiandrogen to achieve total androgen blockade. In a randomized study of 617 patients with stage D2 prostate cancer comparing leuprolide (1.0 mg subcutaneously) with leuprolide plus flutamide (250 mg orally three times a day), there was a 2.5-mo increase in progression-free survival in patients receiving the combination.[285] These studies suggest that a small benefit may be obtained with a combination, possibly because of more complete blockade of androgen action.

Side effects[286–292] of the administration of LHRH agonists in men include loss of libido in many and impotence in all, which is reversible after discontinuation. One study evaluated the testicular histology of men treated with LHRH agonists before orchiectomy and demonstrated peritubular thickening, a decreased number of Leydig cells, and fibrosis.[287] Side effects include hot flashes in a majority of men, gastrointestinal disturbances such as diarrhea, constipation, and indigestion, peripheral edema, weight gain, rash, gynecomastia, mastodynia, general allergic reactions, and exacerbation of tumor-related symptoms or disease flare, thought to be due to the initial gonadotropin release and temporary increase in plasma testosterone level. Local reactions and hematoma at the injection site also can occur.

Antiandrogens are also useful in prostate cancer. The most widely studied antiandrogen is cyproterone acetate, which is a steroidal antiandrogen. The relative binding affinity of cyproterone acetate to androgen receptor is 8, using testosterone as the standard at 100.[293] In several trials for the treatment of metastatic prostate carcinoma, doses of cyproterone acetate have ranged from 50 to 300 mg/d.[294, 295] The agent may also inhibit testosterone biosynthesis. Responses have been reported in 41 to 62% of patients no longer responding to other endocrine modalities. In prospective studies cyproterone acetate appears to be equivalent to DES in response rate and lower in toxicity.[296] Side effects include gynecomastia, loss of libido, and inhibition of spermatogenesis[297] and in women hirsutism and alopecia.[298] Levels of high-density lipoproteins decrease and levels of very-low-density lipoprotein triglyceride increase.[299]

Flutamide is a nonsteroidal compound that acts as a pure antiandrogen and blocks androgen binding to the androgen receptor competitively as an activated α-hydroxy metabolite.[297] It reduces prostate weight and the rate of DNA synthesis in the prostate in rats.[300] Plasma levels of LH rise because of inhibition of androgen feedback and cause a secondary increase in testosterone level. However, the levels of testosterone and dihydrotestosterone are reduced in androgen target tissues. The treatment of prostate cancer patients who had not had prior endocrine therapy with flutamide resulted in subjective improvement in 90% of patients in one study.[301] Toxicity of flutamide includes mastodynia, gynecomastia (36%), secretion of colostrum in males, hot flashes, decreased libido, loss of facial hair, decreased body hair, abnormal liver function tests, and abdominal discomfort.[297, 302, 303] Potency is maintained in most previously potent patients.[301]

LEUKEMIA AND LYMPHOMA

Glucocorticoids influence the growth, differentiation, and function of virtually every tissue and organ system of the body.[304] Among these diverse effects are inhibitory actions on lymphoid tissue, namely lymphocytopenia and thymic atrophy.[305, 306] Glucocorticoids can also kill some human leukemic lymphoblasts.[307] Nevertheless, several problems complicate their use. First, variable response rates occur in patients with different types of acute and chronic leukemia and lymphoma,[308] it has not been possible to identify prospective patients likely to benefit from glucocorticoid therapy. Second, clinical response to glucocorticoid therapy is frequently followed by relapse that is unresponsive to glucocorticoids.[309] Thus although the initial response rates in pediatric acute lymphoblastic leukemia are 45 to 65%, the rate of induction of a subsequent remission with glucocorticoids after primary relapse falls to 25%.

Glucocorticoid administration is also associated with many complications. These include immunosuppression with concomitant nosocomial infections, Cushing syndrome, diabetes mellitus, poor wound healing, psychosis, and other problems.[304, 310] Because most patients with leukemia die of infectious complications rather than the leukemia per se, glucocorticoid therapy may be a detriment to survival in some cases. This difficulty is amplified by the fact that most patients with leukemia and lymphoma are managed by combinations of drugs that include glucocorticoids along with cytotoxic agents. Thus potentially harmful components in the drug combination, such as the glucocorticoid, may be continued long after they have ceased to be of therapeutic benefit.

It would be of value to be able to predict when glucocorticoid therapy is indicated. One approach is to measure glucocorticoid sensitivity in vitro using a cytotoxic or inhibitory end point, but such methods have not proved useful. It is difficult to culture leukemia cells reliably and, furthermore, in vitro and in vivo effects of hormones may not be the same.

Because quantification of specific steroid receptors for estrogen was useful in predicting the response to endocrine therapy in breast disease,[311] glucocorticoid receptors have been studied in human leukemic and lymphoid cells.[312–314] Glucocorticoid receptors in normal peripheral blood lymphocytes and monocytes[315, 316] are similar to the glucocorticoid receptors in liver[317] and thymocytes.[318] Drugs that induce transformation of human lymphoid cells to blast cells, such as phytohemagglutinin or concanavalin A, increase intracellular glucocorticoid receptor activity.[314, 319, 320] Such lymphoblasts are similar morphologically and in glucocorticoid receptor content to human leukemic lymphoblasts.

Early studies of human acute lymphoblastic leukemia suggested that quantitative glucocorticoid receptor analyses would be clinically relevant.[321–324] Glucocorticoid receptors are demonstrable in lymphoblasts in most untreated patients with acute lymphoblastic leukemia, and there is good agreement between concentrations of glucocorticoids that saturate receptor sites and concentrations that inhibit cellular growth. Some data suggest that a reasonable correlation may exist between loss of glucocorticoid receptor activity and in vitro resistance to glucocorticoids.[322] Furthermore, the receptor contents of the various types of acute lymphoblastic leukemia of childhood differ, the so-called T cell leukemias having fewer receptors than in null cell leukemia.[323] The quantity of receptor in acute lymphoblastic leukemia correlates with the initial duration of remission,[324] a correlation that is independent of other prognostic factors such as cell type, initial white blood cell count, or sex. Thus, in acute lymphoblastic leukemia, a role for analysis of glucocorticoid receptors appears to have been established.

Glucocorticoid receptors are also present in acute myelogenous leukemia,[325, 326] chronic myelogenous leukemia in blast crisis,[326] chronic lymphocytic leukemia,[327–329] and the Sézary syndrome.[317] No correlations between receptor content and either clinical parameters or prognosis have been documented in any of these illnesses. However, Bloomfield and colleagues[330] have reported that quantitation of the glucocorticoid receptor can identify patients with non-Hodgkin lymphoma who will respond to single-agent glucocorticoid therapy.

Many chemotherapeutic protocols utilize pharmacological concentrations of glucocorticoid of drugs such as 1 g of prednisolone per square meter of body surface area. Plasma concentrations of drugs with these doses approach 1000 times those required to saturate receptor and induce killing of sensitive cells in vitro. However, with a once-daily dosage, 20 or more half-lives may elapse before the next dose of drug is administered, so there is a rationale for using such large doses. It is also possible that some effects of glucocorticoids may not involve the known receptors. There is no evidence, however, that such massive doses have any more benefit than conventional regimens.

Glucocorticoid effects at normal physiological levels are usually short-lived because most are cleared rapidly. Hydrocortisone, for example, has a plasma half-life of about 60 min and some other steroids are cleared from the plasma more rapidly.[331] (Also see Chapter 9.) The half-lives of some synthetic steroids in dog plasma are as follows: prednisone, 33 min; dexamethasone, 60 min; prednisolone, 60 to 71 min; 6α-methylprednisolone, 81 min; and triamcinolone, 116 min.[332] Hydrocortisone is extensively metabolized in a number of tissues, including liver.[333] The liver also activates certain 11-keto glucocorticoids such as cortisone and prednisone, which must be converted to 11-hydroxy metabolites to exert activity. Thus patients with compromised hepatic function may not respond to these agents because of decreased ability to convert to the 11β-hydroxy steroid by the 11-keto reductase system. Hyperthyroidism markedly shifts the equilibrium of this reaction in favor of the inactive oxidized forms, whereas hypothyroidism does the reverse.[334] Anorexia nervosa and other malnourished states influence equilibrium in a manner similar to the effect of hypothyroidism.[335] Drugs that induce hepatic enzymes, including barbiturates, phenytoin, and rifampin, may increase metabolism of glucocorticoids.[336]

MISCELLANEOUS

Ovarian Cancer

Ovarian cancer occurs at a higher rate in women with breast cancer[337] and in women with endometrial cancer.[338] Second-generation Japanese women in the United States have increased rates of ovarian cancer as well as of breast cancer,[339] and it is possible that the use of estrogen by postmenopausal women increases the risk of ovarian cancer.[340]

These data suggest an association between estrogen and ovarian cancers. Estrogen receptors are present in some cells in the ovary but not in normal ovarian epithelium, the site of origin of the common ovarian cancers. Nevertheless, progestogens have been reported to produce response rates of up to 38% in ovarian cancer,[341] and ovarian cancers may contain both progesterone and estrogen receptors.[342] Other groups have failed to substantiate high response rates with progestogens, and further study is needed before the hormonal dependence of ovarian cancer can be considered established.

Laryngeal Carcinoma

The larynx is a target organ for androgens, as evidenced by the hypertrophy of the vocal cords at puberty in the male, and androgen receptors are present in the human larynx and in epithelial cancers of the larynx.[343] Estrogen has been reported to produce remission in several patients with metastatic disease (personal communication, S. Saez); these findings are in accord with the concept that cancers derived from a tissue whose growth is normally stimulated by a hormone may regress after withdrawal of the hormone.

REFERENCES

1. MacMahon B, Cole P, Brown J. Etiology of human breast cancer: a review. J Natl Cancer Inst 1973; 50:21–36.
2. Miller AB. An overview of hormone-associated cancer. Cancer Res 1978; 38:3985–3990.
3. Kelsey JL. A review of the epidemiology of human breast cancer. Epidemiol Rev 1979; 1:74–109.
4. Doll R, Payne P, Waterhouse J, eds. Cancer Incidence in Five Continents. Berlin: Springer-Verlag, 1966.
5. Haenszel W, Kurihera M. Studies of Japanese migrants. I. Mortality from cancer and other diseases among Japanese in the United States. J Natl Cancer Inst 1968; 40:43–68.
6. DeWaard F. The epidemiology of breast cancer: review and prospects. Int J Cancer 1969; 4:577–586.
7. MacMahon B, Cole P, Lin TM. Age at first birth and breast cancer risk. Bull WHO 1970; 43:209–221.
8. MacMahon B, Feinleib M. Breast cancer in relation to nursing and menopausal history. J Natl Cancer Inst 1960; 24:733–753.
9. Abramson JH. Breastfeeding and breast cancer. A study of cases and matched controls in Jerusalem. Isr J Med Sci 1966; 2:457.
10. Ing R, Hoe JHC, Petrakis NL. Unilateral breast feeding and breast cancer. Lancet 1977; 2:124–127.
11. Yuasa S, MacMahon B. Lactation and reproductive histories of breast cancer patients in Tokyo, Japan. Bull WHO 1971; 42:195–204.
12. Hoover R, Gray LA, Cole P, et al. Menopausal estrogens and breast cancer. N Engl J Med 1976; 295:401–405.
13. Pike MC, Henderson BE, Casagrande JT. The epidemiology of breast cancer as it relates to menarche, pregnancy and menopause. In: Pike MC, Siiteri PK, Welsch CW, eds. Hormones and Breast Cancer. Cold Spring Harbor, NY: Cold Spring Harbor Laboratory 1981: 3–20.
14. Anderson DE. Breast cancer in families. Cancer 1977; 40:1855–1860.
15. Petrakis NL. Genetic factors in the etiology of breast cancer. Cancer 1977; 39:2709–2715.
16. Lynch HT, Thomas RJ, Terasaki PI, et al. HL-A in cancer family "N." Cancer 1975; 36:1315–1320.
17. Petrakis NL. Cerumen genetics and human breast cancer. Science 1971; 173:347–349.
18. Pike MC, Casagrande JF, Brown JB, et al. Comparison of urinary and plasma hormone levels in daughters of breast cancer patients and controls. J Natl Cancer Inst 1977; 59:1351–1355.
19. Fishman J, Fukershima D, O'Connor J, et al. Plasma hormone profile of young women at risk for familial breast cancer. Cancer Res 1978; 38:4006–4011.
20. Everson RB, Fraumeni JF, Wilson RE, et al. Familial male breast cancer. Lancet 1976; 1:9–12.
21. Cohen M, Lippman M, Chabner B: Role of pineal gland in aetiology and treatment of breast cancer. Lancet 1978; 2:814–816.
22. Tamarkin L, Cohen M, Roselle D, et al. Melatonin inhibition and pinealectomy enhancement of dimethylbenz(a)anthracene-induced mammary tumors in the rat. Cancer Res 1981; 41:4432–4436.
23. Tamarkin L, Danforth D, Lichter A, et al. Decreased nocturnal plasma melatonin peak in patients with estrogen receptor positive breast cancer. Science 1982; 216:1003–1005.
24. Lacassagne MA. Apparition de cancers de la mamelle chez la souris mâle, soumise à des injections de folliculine. CR Acad Sci 1932; 195:630–632.
25. Wallace RB, Sherman BM, Bean JA, et al. Menstrual cycle patterns and breast cancer risk factors. Cancer Res 1978; 38:4021–4024.
26. Zumoff B. Abnormal plasma hormone levels in women with breast cancer. In: Pike MC, Siiteri PK, Welsch CW, eds. Hormones and Breast Cancer. Cold Spring Harbor, NY: Cold Spring Harbor Laboratory 1981: 143–168.
27. Lemon HM, Wotiz HH, Parsons L, et al. Reduced estriol excretion in patients with breast cancer prior to endocrine therapy. JAMA 1966; 196:1128–1136.
28. MacMahon B, Cole P, Brown J, et al. Oestrogen profiles of Asian and North American women. Lancet 1971; 2:900–902.
29. Anderson JN. Estrogen-induced uterine responses and growth: relation-ship to receptor estrogen binding by uterine nuclei. Endocrinology 1975; 96:160–167.
30. Lippman ME, Monaco ME, Bolan G. Effects of estrone, estradiol and estriol on hormone-responsive human breast cancer in long-term tissue culture. Cancer Res 1977; 37:1901–1907.
31. Longcope C, Pratt JH. Relationship between urine and plasma estrogen ratios. Cancer Res 1978; 38:4025–4028.
32. Kirschner MA, Cohen FB, Ryan C. Androgen-estrogen production rates in postmenopausal women with breast cancer. Cancer Res 1978; 38:4029–4035.
33. Fishman J, Fukushima D, O'Connor J, et al. Plasma hormone profiles of young women at risk for familial breast cancer. Cancer Res 1978; 38:4006–4011.
34. Korenman SG. Reproductive endocrinology and breast cancer in women. In: Pike MC, Siiteri PK, Welsch CW, Eds. Hormones and Breast Cancer. Cold Spring Harbor, NY: Cold Spring Harbor Laboratory 1981: 71–82.
35. Brown JB. Hormone profiles in young women at risk of breast cancer: a study of ovarian function during thelarche, menarche and menopause and after childbirth. In: Pike MC, Siiteri PK, Welsch CW, eds. Hormones and Breast Cancer. Cold Spring Harbor, NY: Cold Spring Harbor Laboratory 1981: 33–54.
36. Siiteri PK, Hammond GL, Nisker JA. Increased availability of serum estrogens in breast cancer: a new hypothesis. In: Pike MC, Siiteri PK, Welsch CW, eds. Hormones and Breast Cancer. Cold Spring Harbor, NY: Cold Spring Harbor Laboratory 1981: 87–101.
37. Moore JM, Clark CMG, Bulbrook RD, et al. Serum concentrations of total and non–protein-bound estradiol in patients with breast cancer and in normal controls. Int J Cancer 1982; 29:17–21.
38. Bulbrook RD. Prediction of response of breast cancer to treatment. In: Holland JF, Frei E, eds. Cancer Medicine. Philadelphia: Lea & Febiger, 1973: 907–911.
39. Bulbrook RD, Hayward JL. Abnormal urinary steroid excretion and subsequent breast cancer. Lancet 1967; 2:519–521.
40. Wang DY, Moore JW, Thomas BS, et al. Plasma and urinary androgens in women with varying degrees of risk of breast cancer. Eur J Cancer 1979; 15:1269–1274.
41. Grattarola R, Secreto G, Recchione C. Androgens in breast cancer. III. Breast cancer recurrence years after mastectomy and increased androgenic activity. Am J Obstet Gynecol 1975; 121:169–172.
42. McFayden IJ, Prescott RJ, Groom RV, et al. Circulating hormone concentrations in women with breast cancer. Lancet 1976; 1:1100–1102.
43. Masnyk IJ, Silverman DT, Hankey BF. Prediction of response to adrenalectomy in the treatment of advanced breast cancer. J Natl Cancer Inst 1978; 60:271–278.
44. Adams JB, Wong MSF. Paraendocrine behaviour of human breast carcinoma: in vitro transformation of steroids to physiologically active hormones. J Endocrinol 1968; 41:41–52.
45. Adams JB, Archibald L, Clarke C. Adrenal dehydroepiandrosterone and human mammary cancer. Cancer Res 1978; 38:4036–4040.
46. Hill P, Wynder EL, Kumar J, et al. Prolactin levels in populations at risk for breast cancer. Cancer Res 1976; 36:4102–4106.
47. Levin PA, Malarkey WB. Daughters of women with breast cancer have elevated mean 24-hour prolactin (PRL) levels and a partial resistance of PRL to dopamine suppression. J Clin Endocrinol Metab 1981; 53:179–183.
48. Henderson BC, Pike MC. Prolactin—an important hormone in breast neoplasia? In: Pike MC, Siiteri PK, Welsch CW, eds. Hormones and Breast Cancer. Cold Spring Harbor, NY: Cold Spring Harbor Laboratory 1981: 115–127.
49. Bulbrook RD, Thomas BS, Fantl VE, et al. A prospective study of the relation between thyroid function and subsequent breast cancer. In: Pike MC, Siiteri PK, Welsch CW, eds. Hormones and Breast Cancer. Cold Spring Harbor, NY: Cold Spring Harbor Laboratory 1981: 131–140.
50. Kelsey JL, Holford TR, White C, et al. Oral contraceptives and breast disease. Am J Epidemiol 1978; 107:236–244.
51. Royal College of General Practitioners oral contraception studies. Effect on hypertension and benign breast disease of progestagen component of combined oral contraceptives. Lancet 1977; 1:624.
52. Nomura A, Comstock GW. Benign breast tumor and estrogenic hormones: a population-based retrospective study. Am J Epidemiol 1976; 103:439–444.
53. Paffenbarger RS, Fasal E, Simmons ME, et al. Cancer risk as related to the use of oral contraceptives during fertile years. Cancer 1977; 39:1887–1891.
54. Vessey MP, Doll R, Sutton PM. Oral contraceptives and breast neoplasia: a retrospective study. Br Med J 1972; 3:719–728.
55. Ravnihar B, Seigel DG, Lindtner J. An epidemiologic study of breast cancer and benign breast neoplasias in relation to the oral contraceptive and estrogen use. Eur J Cancer 1979; 15:395–405.
56. Ory H, Cole P, MacMahon B, et al. Oral contraceptives and reduced risk of benign breast diseases. N Engl J Med 1976; 294:419–422.
57. Boston Collaborative Drug Surveillance Programme. Oral contraceptives and venous thromboembolic disease, surgically confirmed, gallbladder disease, and breast tumours. Lancet 1973; 1:1399–1404.

58. Black MM, Barclay TH, Cutler SJ, et al. Association of atypical characteristics of benign breast lesions with subsequent risk of breast cancer. Cancer 1972; 29:338–343.
59. Dupont WD, Page DL. Risk factors for breast cancer in women with proliferative disease. N Engl J Med 1985; 312:146–151.
60. Mansel RE, Wisbey JR, Hughes LE. The use of danazol in the treatment of painful benign breast disease: preliminary results. Postgrad Med J 1979; 55:61–65.
61. Madanos AE, Farber M. Danazol. Ann Intern Med 1982; 96:625–630.
62. Coombes RC, Dearnaley D, Humphreys J, et al. Danazol treatment of advanced breast cancer. Cancer Treat Rep 1980; 64:1073–1976.
63. Armstrong B. Recent trends in breast cancer incidence and mortality in relation to changes in possible risk factors. Int J Cancer 1976; 17:204–211.
64. Vessey MP, Doll R, Jones K. Oral contraceptives and breast cancer. Progress report of an epidemiological study. Lancet 1975; 1:941–943.
65. Schlesselman JJ. Cancer of the breast and reproductive tract in relation to use of oral contraceptives. Contraception 1989; 40:1–38.
66. Henderson BE, Powell D, Rosario I, et al. An epidemiologic study of breast cancer. J Natl Cancer Inst 1974; 53:609–614.
67. Sartwell PE, Arthes FG, Tonascia JA. Exogenous hormones, reproductive history and breast cancer. J Natl Cancer Inst 1977; 59:1589–1592.
68. Casagrande J, Gerkins V, Henderson BE, et al. Brief communication: exogenous estrogens and breast cancer in women with natural menopause. J Natl Cancer Inst 1976; 56:839–841.
69. Craig TJ, Comstock GW, Geiser PB. Epidemiologic comparison of breast cancer patients with early and late onset of malignancy and general population controls. J Natl Cancer Inst 1974; 53:1577–1581.
70. Matthews PN, Millis RR, Hayward JL. Breast cancer in women who have taken contraceptive steroids. Br Med J 1981; 282:774–776.
71. Pike MC, Henderson BE, Casagrande JT, et al. Oral contraceptive use and early abortion as risk factors for breast cancer in young women. Br J Cancer 1981; 43:72–76.
72. Hoover R, Gray LA, Cole P, et al. Menopausal estrogens and breast cancer. N Engl J Med 1976; 295:401–405.
73. Brinton LA, Hoover RN, Szkio M, et al. Menopausal estrogen use and risk of breast cancer. Cancer 1981; 47:2517–2522.
74. Schatzkin A, Jones DY, Hoover RN, et al. Alcohol consumption and breast cancer in the epidemiologic follow-up study of the first national health and nutrition examination survey. N Engl J Med 1988; 316:1169–1180.
75. Lippman ME. Oncogenes and breast cancer. N Engl J Med 1988; 319:1281–1282.
76. Beatson GT. On the treatment of inoperable cases of carcinoma of the mamma: suggestions for a new method of treatment with illustrative cases. Lancet 1896; 2:162–165.
77. Grody WW, Schrader WT, O'Malley BW. Activation transformation and subunit structure of steroid hormone receptors. Endocr Rev 1982; 3:141–163.
78. McGuire WL, Julian JA, Chamness GC. A dissociation between ovarian dependent growth and estrogen sensitivity in mammary carcinoma. Endocrinology 1971; 89:969–973.
79. Terenius L. Parallelism between oestrogen binding capacity and hormone responsiveness of mammary tumours in GR/A mice. Eur J Cancer 1972; 8:55–58.
80. Folca PJ, Glascock RF, Irvine WT. Studies with tritium labelled hexoestrol in advanced breast cancer. Lancet 1962; 2:796–798.
81. Korenman SG, Dukes BA. Specific estrogen binding by the cytoplasm of human breast carcinoma. J Clin Endocrinol 1970; 30:639–645.
82. Jensen EV, DeSombre ER, Jungblut PP. Estrogen receptors in hormone responsive tissues and tumors. In: Wissler RV, Dao TL, Wood S, eds. Endogenous Factors Influencing Host Tumor Balance. Chicago: University of Chicago Press, 1967: 15–30.
83. Seibert K, Lippman ME: Hormone receptors in breast cancer. Clin Oncol 1982; 1:735–793.
84. Clark GM, McGuire WL. Progesterone receptors and human breast cancer. Breast Cancer Res Treat 1983; 3:157–163.
85. Fisher B, Redmond C, Brown A, et al. The influence of tumor estrogen and progesterone receptor levels on the response to tamoxifen and chemotherapy in primary breast cancer. J Clin Oncol 1983; 1:227–241.
86. Witliff JL, Fisher B, Durant JR. Establishment of uniformity in steroid receptor analysis used in cooperative trials of breast cancer treatment. In: Henningsen B, Linden F, Steichele C, eds. Recent Results in Cancer Research. Endocrine Treatment of Breast Cancer. New York: Springer-Verlag, 1980: 198–202.
87. Panko WB, MacLeod RM. Uncharged nuclear receptors for estrogen in breast cancer. Cancer Res 1978; 38:1948–1951.
88. McGuire WL. Steroid receptors in human breast cancer. Cancer Res 1978; 38:4289–4291.
89. Nenci I. Receptors and centriole pathways of steroid action in normal and neoplastic cells. Cancer Res 1978; 38:4204–4207.
90. Saez S, Martin PM, Chouvet CD. Estradiol and progesterone receptor levels in relation to plasma estrogen and progesterone levels. Cancer Res 1978; 38:3468–3478.
91. Degenshein GA, Bloom N, Ceccarelli F. Estrogen and progesterone receptor site studies as guides to the management of advanced breast cancer. Dis Breast 1977; 3:29–31.
92. Knight WA, Livingston RB, Gregory EJ, et al. Estrogen receptor as an independent prognostic factor for early recurrence in breast cancer. Cancer Res 1977; 37:4669–4671.
93. Maynard PV, Blamey RW, Elston CW, et al. Estrogen receptor assay in primary breast cancer and early recurrence of the disease. Cancer Res 1978; 38:4292–4296.
94. Allegra JC, Lippman ME, Simon R, et al. Association between steroid hormone receptor status and disease-free interval in breast cancer. Cancer Treat Rep 1979; 63:1271–1277.
95. Kinne DW, Ashikari R, Butler A. Estrogen receptor protein in breast cancer as a prediction of recurrence. Cancer 1981; 47:2364–2367.
96. Leake RE, Laing L, McArdle C, et al. Soluble and nuclear oestrogen receptor status in human breast cancer in relation to prognosis. Br J Cancer 1981; 43:59–66.
97. Greene GL, Nolan C, Engler JP, et al. Monoclonal antibodies to human estrogen receptor. Proc Natl Acad Sci USA 1982; 77:5115–5119.
98. Greene GL, Closs LE, Fleming H. Antibodies to estrogen receptor: immunochemical similarity of estrophilin from various mammalian species. Proc Natl Acad Sci USA 1977; 74:3681–3685.
99. Hall TC, Dederick MM, NeVinny HB, et al. Prognostic value of response of patients with breast cancer to therapeutic castration. Cancer Chemother Rep 1963; 31:47–48.
100. Lewison EF. Castration in the treatment of advanced breast cancer. Cancer 1965; 18:1558–1563.
101. Fracchia AA, Farrow JH, Miller TR, et al. Hypophysectomy as compared with adrenalectomy in the treatment of advanced carcinoma of the breast. Surg Gynecol Obstet 1969; 128:1226–1234.
102. Levine RM, Lippman ME. Breast cancer management: recent advances and recommendations. Adv Intern Med 1984; 29:215–224.
103. Meakin JW. Is there a place for adjuvant endocrine therapy of breast cancer? In: Henningsen B, Linder F, Steichele C, eds. Recent Results in Cancer Research. Endocrine Treatment of Breast Cancer. New York: Springer-Verlag, 1980: 178–184.
104. Longcope C. Metabolic clearance and blood production rates of estrogens in post-menopausal women. Am J Obstet Gynecol 1971; 111:778–781.
105. Grodin JM, Siiteri PK, MacDonald PC. Source of estrogen production in postmenopausal women. J Clin Endocrinol 1973; 36:207–214.
106. Aitken SC, Lippman ME. Steroid receptors in breast cancer. Arch Intern Med 1982; 142:363–366.
107. Schally AV, Reddin TW. Inhibition of cell growth by a hypothalamic peptide. Proc Natl Acad Sci USA 1982; 79:7014–7018.
108. Henderson IC, Canellos GP. Cancer of the breast: the past decade. N Engl J Med 1980; 302:17–30.
109. Davies P, Nicholson RI. How do androgens and progestins cause regression of breast cancer? Rev Endocr Related Cancer 1981; 10:19–25.
110. Allegra JC, Lippman ME, Thompson EB, et al. The distribution, frequency and quantitative analysis of estrogen, progesterone, androgen and glucocorticoid receptors in human breast cancer. Cancer Res 1979; 39:1447–1454.
111. Allegra JC, Lippman ME, Thompson EB, et al. Relationship between the progesterone, androgen and glucocorticoid receptor and response rate to endocrine therapy in metastatic breast cancer. Cancer Res 1979; 39:1973–1979.
112. Cooperative Breast Cancer Group. Testosterone propionate therapy in breast therapy. JAMA 1964; 188:1069–1074.
113. Johnston B, Novales ET. The use of valban (vinblastine sulfate) in metastatic carcinoma of the breast. Cancer Chemother Rep 1961; 12:109–112.
114. Goldenberg IS. Clinical trial of Δ^1-testololactone (NSC 23759), medroxy progesterone acetate (NSC 26386) and oxylone acetate (NSC 47438) in advanced female mammary cancer. Cancer 1969; 23:109–112.
115. Coombes RC, Dearnaley D, Humphreys J, et al. Danazol treatment of advanced breast cancer. Cancer Treat Rep 1980; 64:1073–1076.
116. Powles TJ, Gordon C, Coombes RC. Clinical trial of multiple endocrine therapy for metastatic and locally advanced breast cancer with tamoxifen-aminoglutethimide-danazol compared to tamoxifen used alone. Cancer Res 1982; 42:3458–3460.
117. Lippman ME. Efforts to combine endocrine and chemotherapy in the management of breast cancer: do two and two equal three? Breast Cancer Res Treat 1983; 3:117–127.
118. Tormey DC, Lippman ME, Edwards BK, et al. Evaluation of tamoxifen doses with and without fluoxymesterone in advanced breast cancer. Ann Intern Med 1983; 98:139–143.
119. Kennedy BJ. Hormone therapy in inoperable breast cancer. Cancer 1969; 24:1345–1349.
120. Kennedy BJ. Diethylstilbestrol versus testosterone propionate therapy in advanced breast cancer. Surg Gynecol Obstet 1965; 120:1246–1250.
121. Kaufman RJ, Escher GC. Rebound regression in advanced mammary carcinoma. Surg Gynecol Obstet 1961; 113:635–640.
122. Stoll BA. Progestin therapy of breast cancer: comparison of agents. Br Med J 1967; 3:338–341.

123. Crona N, Enk L, Samsioe G, et al. Medroxyprogesterone acetate (MPA) in adjuvant treatment of endometrial carcinoma—changes in serum lipoproteins. J Steroid Biochem 1983; Suppl 19:195–198.

124. Henderson IC. Endocrine therapy in metastatic breast cancer. In: Harris JR, Hellman S, Henderson IC, et al., eds. Breast Diseases. Philadelphia: J. B. Lippincott, 1987: 398–428.

125. Sikic BI, Scudder SA, Ballon SC, et al. High-dose megestrol acetate therapy of ovarian carcinoma: a phase II study by the Northern California oncology group. Semin Oncol 1986; 13:26–32.

126. Pannuti F, Martoni A, DiMarco AR, et al. Prospective, randomized clinical trial of two different high dosages of medroxyprogesterone acetate (MAP) in the treatment of metastatic breast cancer. Eur J Cancer 1979; 15:593–601.

127. Beretta G, Tabiadon D, Tedeschi L, et al. Hormonotherapy of advanced breast carcinoma: comparative evaluation of tamoxifen citrate versus medroxyprogesterone acetate. In: Iacobelli S, Lippman ME, Della Cona GR, eds. The Role of Tamoxifen in Breast Cancer. New York: Raven, 1982: 113–120.

128. Henderson D. Antiprogestational and antiglucocorticoid activities of some novel 11β-aryl substituted steroids. In: Furr BJA, Wakeling AE, eds. Pharmacological and Clinical Uses of Inhibitors of Hormone Secretion and Action. London: Bailliere Tindall, 1987: 184–211.

129. Vignon F, Bardon S, Chalbos D, et al. Antiproliferative effect of progestins and antiprogestins in human breast cancer cells. In: Klijn JGM, Paridaens R, Foekens JA, eds. Hormonal Manipulation of Cancer: Peptides, Growth Factors, and New (Anti) Steroidal Agents. New York: Raven, 1987: 47–54.

130. Maudelonde T, Romieu G, Ulmann A, et al. First clinical trial on the use of the antiprogestin RU486 in advanced breast cancer. In: Klijn JGM, Paridaens R, Foekens JA, eds. Hormonal Manipulation of Cancer: Peptides, Growth Factors, and New (Anti) Steroidal Agents. New York: Raven, 1987: 55–59.

131. Klijn JGM, de Jong FH. Long-term LHRH-agonist (buserelin) treatment in metastatic premenopausal breast cancer. In: Klijn JGM, Paridaens R, Foekens JA, eds. Hormonal Manipulation of Cancer: Peptides, Growth Factors, and New (Anti) Steroidal Agents. New York: Raven, 1987: 343–352.

132. Walker KJ, Turkes A, Williams MR, et al. Preliminary endocrinological evaluation of a sustained-release formulation of the LH-releasing hormone agonist D-Ser(But)6 Azgly10LHRH in premenopausal women with advanced breast cancer. J Endocrinol 1986; 111:349–353.

133. Harvey HA, Lipton A, Max DT, et al. Medical castration produced by the GnRH analogue leuprolide to treat metastatic breast cancer. J Clin Oncol 1985; 3:1068–1072.

134. Klijn JM, De Jong FH, Lamberts SJ, et al. LHRH-agonist treatment in clinical and experimental human breast cancer. J Steroid Biochem 1985; 23:867–873.

135. Nicholson RI, Walker KJ, Turkes A, et al. The British experience with LH-RH agonist Zoladex® (ICI 118630) in the treatment of breast cancer. In: Klijn JGM, Paridaens R, Foekens JA, eds. Hormonal Manipulation of Cancer: Peptides, Growth Factors, and New (Anti) Steroidal Agents. New York: Raven, 1987: 331–341.

136. Geiner NF, Donegan WL. Role and mechanism of corticosteroid therapy in breast cancer. Rev Endocr Related Cancer 1980; 6:5–11.

137. Sutherland RL, Jordan VC. Non-Steroidal Antioestrogens. Sydney: Academic, 1981.

138. Sutherland RL, Murphy LC, Foo MS, et al. High affinity anti-estrogen binding site distinct from the oestrogen receptor. Nature 1980; 288:273–275.

139. Murphy LC, Sutherland RL. Modifications in the aminoether side chain of clomiphene influence affinity for a specific antiestrogen binding site in MCF-7 cells cytosol. Biochem Biophys Res Commun 1981; 100:1353–1360.

140. Eckert RL, Katzenellenbogen BS. Physical properties of estrogen receptor complexes in MCF-7 human breast cancer cells. J Biol Chem 1982; 257:8840–8846.

141. Jozan S, Elalamy H, Bayard F. Étude du mecanisme d'action d'un antiestrogene du groupe triphényléthylène sur la croissance de la lignée cellulaire de cancer du sein human MCF-7 en culture. CR Acad Sci (Paris) 1981; 292:767–770.

142. Jordan VC. Biochemical pharmacology of antiestrogen action. Pharmacol Rev 1984; 36:245–276.

143. Sutherland RL, Reddel RR, Murphy LC, et al. Effects of antiestrogens on cell cycle progression. In: Jordan VC, ed. Estrogen/Antiestrogen Action and Breast Cancer Therapy. Madison: University of Wisconsin Press, 1986: 265–281.

144. Knabbe C, Lippman ME, Wakefield L, et al. Evidence that TGFβ is a hormonally regulated negative growth factor in human breast cancer. Cell 1987; 48:417–428.

145. Legha S, Muggia FM. Antiestrogens in the treatment of cancer. Ann Intern Med 1976; 84:751 (letter).

146. Mouridsen H, Palshof T, Patterson J. Tamoxifen in advanced breast cancer. Cancer Treat Rev 1978; 5:131–141.

147. Heel RC, Brogden RN, Speight TM. Tamoxifen—a review of its pharmacologic properties and therapeutic use in the treatment of breast cancer. Drugs 1978; 16:1–24.

148. Pearson OH, Manni A, Arafah BM. Antiestrogen treatment of breast cancer: an overview. Cancer Res 1982; 42:3424–3429.

149. Manni A, Trujillo J, Marshall JS, et al. Antiestrogen-induced remissions in stage IV breast cancer. Cancer Treat Rep 1976; 60:1445–1450.

150. McIntosh IH, Thynne GS. Tumour stimulation by anti-oestrogens. Br J Surg 1977; 64:900–901.

151. Tormey DC, Simon RM, Lippman ME, et al. Evaluation of tamoxifen dose in advanced breast cancer: a progress report. Cancer Treat Rep 1976; 60:1451–1459.

152. Patterson JS, Battersby LA, Edwards DG. Review of the clinical pharmacology and international experience with tamoxifen in advanced breast cancer. Rev Endocr Related Cancer 1982; 9:563–582.

153. Pritchard KI, Thomson DB, Myers RE. Tamoxifen therapy in premenopausal patients with metastatic breast cancer. Cancer Treat Rep 1980; 64:787–796.

154. Manni A, Pearson OH. Antiestrogen-induced remissions in premenopausal women with stage IV breast cancer: effects on ovarian function. Cancer Treat Rep 1980; 64:779–786.

155. Manni A, Arafah BM. Tamoxifen induced remission in breast cancer by escalating the dose to 40 mg daily after progression on 20 mg daily—a case report and review of the literature. Cancer 1981; 48:873–875.

156. Fromson JM, Pearson S, Bramah S. The metabolism of tamoxifen (I.C.I. 46,474). Part I: In laboratory animals. Xenobiotica 1973; 3:693–709.

157. Adam HK, Douglas EJ, Kemp KV. The metabolism of tamoxifen in humans. Biochem Pharmacol 1979; 27:145–147.

158. Furr BA, Jordan VC. The pharmacology and clinical uses of tamoxifen. Pharmacol Ther 1984; 25:127–205.

159. Lyman SD, Jordan VC. Metabolism of nonsteroidal antiestrogens. In: Jordan VC, ed. Estrogen/Antiestrogen Action and Breast Cancer Therapy. Madison: University of Wisconsin Press, 1986: 191–219.

160. Fabian C, Tilzer L, Sternson L. Comparative binding affinities of tamoxifen, 4-hydroxytamoxifen, and desmethyltamoxifen for estrogen receptors isolated from human breast carcinoma: correlation with blood levels in patients with metastatic breast cancer. Biopharmaceut Drug Dispos 1981; 2:281–390.

161. Nicholson RI, Syne JS, Daniel CP, et al. The binding of tamoxifen to oestrogen receptor proteins under equilibrium and non-equilibrium conditions. Eur J Cancer 1979; 15:317–329.

162. Wakeling AE, Slater SR. Estrogen-receptor binding and biologic activity of tamoxifen and its metabolites. Cancer Treat Rep 64:741–744.

163. Kemp JV, Adam HK, Wakeling AE, et al. Identification and biological activity of tamoxifen metabolites in human serum. Biochem Pharmacol 1983; 32:2045–2052.

164. Daniel P, Gaskell SJ, Bishop H, et al. Determination of tamoxifen and biologically active metabolites in human breast tumours and plasma. Eur J Cancer Clin Oncol 1981; 17:1183–1189.

165. Patterson JS, Settatree RS, Adam HK, et al. Serum concentration of tamoxifen and major metabolite during long-term Nolvadex® therapy, correlated with clinical response. In: Mouridsen HT, Palshoff T, eds. Breast Cancer—Experimental and Clinical Aspects. Oxford: Pergamon, 1980: 89–92.

166. Daniel CP, Gaskell SJ, Bishop H, et al. Determination of tamoxifen and a hydroxylated metabolite in plasma from patients with advanced breast cancer using gas chromatography—mass spectrometry. J Endocrinol 1979; 83:401–408.

167. Wilkinson PM, Ribiero GG, Adam HK, et al. Tamoxifen (Nolvadex®) therapy—rationale for loading dose followed by maintenance dose for patients with metastatic breast cancer. Cancer Chemother Pharmacol 1982; 10:33–35.

168. Fromson JM, Pearson S, Bramah S. The metabolism of tamoxifen (I.C.I. 46,474). Part II: In female patients. Xenobiotica 1973; 3:711–714.

169. Fabian C, Sternson L, Barnett M. Clinical pharmacology of tamoxifen in patients with breast cancer: comparison of traditional and loading dose schedules. Cancer Treat Rep 1980; 64:765–773.

170. Fabian C, Sternson L, El-Serafi M, et al. Clinical pharmacology of tamoxifen in patients with breast cancer: correlation with clinical data. Cancer 1981; 48:876–882.

171. Adam HK, Patterson JS, Kemp JV. Studies on the metabolism and pharmacokinetics of tamoxifen in normal volunteers. Cancer Treat Rep 1980; 64:761–764.

172. Sherman BM, Chapler FK, Crickard K, et al. Endocrine consequences of continuous antiestrogen therapy with tamoxifen in premenopausal women. J Clin Invest 1979; 64:398–404.

173. Paterson AG, Turkes A, Groom GV, et al. The effect of tamoxifen on plasma growth hormone and prolactin and postmenopausal women with advanced breast cancer. Eur J Cancer Clin Oncol 1983; 19:919–922.

174. Luciani L, Oriana S, Spatti G, et al. Hormonal and receptor status in postmenopausal women with endometrial carcinoma before and after treatment with tamoxifen. Tumori 1984; 70:189–192.

175. Jordan VC, Fritz NF, Tormey DC. Endocrine effects of adjuvant chemotherapy and long-term tamoxifen administration on node-positive patients with breast cancer. Cancer Res 1987; 47:624–630.

176. Bird CE, Masters V, Sterns EE, et al. Effects of tamoxifen on testosterone metabolism in postmenopausal women with breast cancer. Clin Invest Med 1985; 8:97–102.

177. Golder MP, Phillips MEA, Fahmy DR, et al. Plasma hormones in patients

with advanced breast cancer treated with tamoxifen. Eur J Cancer 1976; 12:719–723.

178. Helgason S, Wilking N, Carlstrom K, et al. A comparative study of the estrogenic effects of tamoxifen and 17β-estradiol in postmenopausal breast cancer patients. J Clin Endocrinol Metab 1982; 54:404–407.

179. Wilking N, Carlstrom K, Skoldefors H, et al. Effects of tamoxifen on the serum levels of oestrogens and adrenocortical steroids in postmenopausal breast cancer patients. Acta Chir Scand 1982; 148:345–349.

180. Szamel I, Vincze B, Hindy I, et al. Hormonal changes during a prolonged tamoxifen treatment in patients with advanced breast cancer. Oncology 1986; 43:7–11.

181. Boccardo F, Bruzzi P, Rubagotti A, et al. Estrogen-like action of tamoxifen on vaginal epithelium in breast cancer patients. Oncology 1981; 38:281–285.

182. Ferrazzi E, Cartei G, Mattarazzo R, et al. Oestrogen-like effect of tamoxifen on vaginal epithelium. Br Med J 1977; 1:1351–1352.

183. Estevez RA, Breier S, Kotliar M. Estudio preliminar con tamoxifen en cancer avanzado de mama. Proceedings, 12th International UICC Cancer Congress 1978: 78–79.

184. Fisher B, Redmond C, Brown A, et al. The influence of tumor estrogen and progesterone receptor levels on the response to tamoxifen and chemotherapy in primary breast cancer. J Clin Oncol 1983; 1:227–241.

185. Lippman ME, Bolan B, Huff K. The effects of glucocorticoids and progesterone on hormone-responsive human breast cancer in long-term tissue culture. Cancer Res 1976; 36:4602–4609.

186. Griffiths CT, Hall TC, Saba Z, et al. Preliminary trial of aminoglutethimide in breast cancer. Cancer 1973; 32:31–37.

187. Fishman LM, Liddle GW, Island DP, et al. Effects of amino-glutethimide on adrenal function in man. J Clin Endocrinol Metab 1967; 27:481–490.

188. Santen RJ, Lipton A, Kendall J. Successful medical adrenalectomy with amino-glutethimide. Role of altered drug metabolism. JAMA 1974; 230:1661–1665.

189. Santen RJ, Samojlik E, Lipton A, et al. Kinetic, hormonal and clinical studies with aminoglutethimide in breast cancer. Cancer 1977; 39:2948–2958.

190. Harvey HA, Lipton A, Sonfert RJ. Aromatase: new perspectives for breast cancer. Cancer Res 1982; 42:3267s–3468s.

191. Wells SA, Worsol TJ, Samojlik E, et al. Comparison of surgical adrenalectomy to medical adrenalectomy in patients with metastatic carcinoma of the breast. Cancer Res 1982; 42:3454s–3457s.

192. Brodie AM, Santen RJ. Aromatase in breast cancer and the role of aminoglutethimide and other aromatase inhibitors. CRC Crit Rev Hematol Oncol 1986; 5:361–396.

193. Brodie AMH, Wing LY, Dowsett M, et al. Inhibitors of the aromatase enzyme system: basic and clinical studies with 4-hydroxyandrostenedione. In: Jordan VC, ed. Estrogen/Antiestrogen Action and Breast Cancer Therapy. Madison: University of Wisconsin Press, 1986: 221–234.

194. Santen RJ, Rosen H, Osawa Y, et al. Additive effects of aminoglutethimide, testolactone and 4-hydroxyandrostenedione as inhibitors of aromatase. J Steroid Biochem 1984; 20:1239–1242.

195. Santen RJ. Suppression of estrogens with aminoglutethimide and hydrocortisone (medical adrenalectomy) as treatment of advanced breast carcinoma: a review. Breast Cancer Res Treat 1981; 1:183–202.

196. Powles TJ. The role of aromatase inhibitors in breast cancer. Semin Oncol 1984; 10:20–24.

197. Asbury RF, Bakemeier RF, Folsch E, et al. Treatment of metastatic breast cancer with aminoglutethimide. Cancer 1981; 47:1954–1958.

198. Santen RJ, Worgul TJ, Lipton A, et al. Aminoglutethimide as treatment of postmenopausal women with advanced breast carcinoma. Ann Intern Med 1982; 96:94–101.

199. Messeih AA, Lipton A, Stanten RJ, et al. Aminoglutethimide-induced hematologic toxicity: worldwide experience. Cancer Treat Rep 1985; 69:1003–1004.

200. Goz E, Sulkes A. Aminoglutethimide-induced leukopenia: a case report and review of the literature. Oncology 1984; 41:399–402.

201. Kampel LJ, Kurman MR. Severe leukopenia induced by aminoglutethimide. Cancer Treat Rep 1984; 68:1277–1281.

202. Young JA, Newcomer LN, Keller AM. Aminoglutethimide-induced bone marrow injury: report of a case and review of the literature. Cancer 1984; 54:1731–1733.

203. Wing LY, Garrett WM, Brodie AM. Effects of aromatase inhibitors, aminoglutethimide, and 4-hydroxyandrostenedione on cyclic rats and rats with 7,12-dimethylbenz(a)anthracene-induced mammary tumors. Cancer Res 1985; 45:2425–2428.

204. Brodie AM, Longcope C. Inhibition of peripheral aromatization by aromatase inhibitors, 4-hydroxy- and 4-acetyoxy-androstene-3,17-dione. Endocrinology 1980; 106:14–21.

205. Brodie AM, Schwarzel WC, Shaikh AA, et al. The effect of an aromatase inhibitor, 4-hydroxy-4-androstene-3,17-dione, on estrogen-dependent processes in reproduction and breast cancer. Endocrinology 1977; 100:1684–1695.

206. Stone NN, Fair WR, Fishman J. Estrogen formation in human prostatic tissue from patients with and without benign prostatic hyperplasia. Prostate 1986; 9:311–318.

207. Goss PE, Powles TJ, Dowsett M, et al. Treatment of advanced postmenopausal breast cancer with an aromatase inhibitor, 4-hydroxyandrostenedione: phase II report. Cancer Res 1986; 46:4823–4826.

208. Cunningham K, Powles TJ, Dowsett M, et al. Oral 4-hydroxyandrostenedione, a new endocrine treatment for disseminated breast cancer. Cancer Chemother Pharmacol 1987; 20:253–255.

209. Coombes RC, Goss P, Dowsett M, et al. 4-Hydroxyandrostenedione in treatment of postmenopausal patients with advanced breast cancer. Lancet 1984; 2:1237–1239.

210. Crichlow RW. Carcinoma of the male breast. Surg Gynecol Obstet 1972; 134:1011–1019.

211. Meyskins FL, Tormey EC, Nesfeld JP. Male breast cancer: a review. Cancer Treat Rev 1976; 3:83–93.

212. Everson RB, Lippman ME. Male breast cancer. In: McGuire WL, ed. Breast Cancer: Advances in Research and Treatment. Vol III. New York: Plenum, 1979: 239–267.

213. Symners WSC. Carcinoma of breast in trans-sexual individuals after surgical interference with the primary and secondary sex characteristics. Br Med J 1968; 2:83–85.

214. Everson RB, Lippman ME, Thompson EB, et al. Clinical correlations of steroid receptors and male breast cancer. Cancer Res 1980; 40:991–997.

215. Patterson JS, Battershy LA, Bach BK. Use of tamoxifen in advanced male breast cancer. Cancer Treat Rep 1980; 64:801–804.

216. Jensen EV, Jacobsen HI. Basic guides to the mechanism of estrogen action. Recent Prog Horm Res 1962; 18:387.

217. Antunes CMF, Stolley PD, Rosenshein NB, et al. Endometrial cancer and estrogen use (report of a large case-control study). N Engl J Med 1979; 300:9–13.

218. Nisker JA, Ramzy I, Collins JA. Adenocarcinoma of the endometrium and abnormal ovarian function in young women. Am J Obstet Gynecol 1978; 130:546–550.

219. Whitehead MI, Campbell SC, King RJ, et al. Oestrogen treatment and endometrial carcinoma. Br Med J 1977; 2:453–454.

220. Hensell DL, Grodin JM, Brenner PF, et al. Plasma precursors of estrogen. II. Correlation of the extent of conversion of plasma androstenedione to estrone with age. J Clin Endocrinol Metab 1974; 38:476–479.

221. MacDonald PC, Edman CD, Hemsell DL, et al. Effect of obesity on conversion of plasma androstenedione to estrone in postmenopausal women with and without endometrial cancer. Am J Obstet Gynecol 1978; 130:448–455.

222. Judd HL, Lucas WE, Yen SC. Serum 17β-estradiol and estrone levels in postmenopausal women with and without endometrial cancer. J Clin Endocrinol Metab 1976; 43:272–278.

223. Feinstein AR, Horowitz RI. A critique of the statistical evidence associating estrogens with endometrial cancer. Cancer Res 1978; 38:4001–4005.

224. Pollow K, Lubbert H, Boquoi E, et al. Characterization and comparison of receptors for 17β-estradiol and progesterone in human proliferative endometrium and endometrial carcinoma. Endocrinology 1975; 96:319–328.

225. Bayard F, Damilamo S, Robel P, et al. Cytoplasmic and nuclear estradiol and progesterone receptors in human endometrium. J Clin Endocrinol Metab 1978; 46:635–648.

226. King RJB, Dyer G, Collins WP, et al. Intracellular estradiol, estrone and estrogen receptor levels in endometria from postmenopausal women receiving estrogens and progestins. J Steroid Biochem 1980; 13:377–382.

227. Young PCM, Ehrlich CE, Cleary RE. Progesterone binding in human endometrial carcinomas. Am J Obstet Gynecol 1976; 125:353–360.

228. Feil PD, Mann WJ, Mortel R, et al. Nuclear progestin receptors in normal and malignant human endometrium. J Clin Endocrinol Metab 1979; 48:327–334.

229. Gurpide E, Gusberg SB, Tseng L. Estradiol binding and metabolism in human endometrial hyperplasia and adenocarcinoma. J Steroid Biochem 1976; 7:891–896.

230. Kelly RM, Baker WH. Progestational agents in the treatment of carcinoma of the endometrium. N Engl J Med 1961; 264:216–222.

231. Reifinstein EC Jr. Hydroxyprogesterone caproate therapy in advanced endometrial cancer. Cancer 1971; 27:485–502.

232. Malkasian GD Jr, Decker D, Mussey E, et al. Progesterone treatment of recurrent endometrial carcinoma. Am J Obstet Gynecol 1971; 110:15.

233. Allegra JC, Kiefer SM. Mechanisms of action of progestational agents. Semin Oncol 1985; 7:3–5.

234. Blossey HC, Wander HE, Koebberling J, et al. Pharmacokinetic and pharmacodynamic basis for the treatment of metastatic breast cancer with high-dose medroxyprogesterone acetate. Cancer 1984; 54:1208–1215.

235. Kauppila A, Janne O, Kujansuu E, et al. Treatment of advanced endometrial adenocarcinoma with a combined cytotoxic therapy. Cancer 1980; 46:2162–2167.

236. Silverberg E. Cancer statistics. Cancer 1982; 32:15–31.
237. Bojar H, Stuskchke M, Staib W. Effects of high-dose medroxyproges-terone acetate on plasma membrane lipid mobility. In: Bresciani F, ed. Progress in Cancer Research and Therapy. New York: Raven, 1984: 115–119.
238. Rochefort H. Biochemical basis of breast cancer treatment by androgens and progestins. In: Back N, Breiver GH, Eijsvoogel V, et al., eds. Hormones and Cancer. New York, Alan R. Liss, 1984: 79–95.
239. Kovi J, Heshmat MY. Incidence of cancer in Negroes in Washington, D.C., and other selected American cities. Am J Epidemiol 1972; 96:401–413.
240. Jackson MA, Ahluwalia BS, Herson J, et al. Characterization of prostatic carcinoma among blacks. A continuation report. Cancer Treat Rep 1977; 61:167–172.
241. Akazakis K, Stennerman GN. Comparative study of latent carcinoma of the prostate among Japanese in Japan and Hawaii. J Natl Cancer Inst 1973; 50:1137–1144.
242. Huggins C, Clark PJ. Quantitative studies of prostatic secretion. II. The effect of castration and of estrogen injection on the normal and on the hyperplastic prostate gland of dogs. J Exp Med 1940; 72:747–762.
243. Huggins C, Masina MH, Eichelberger L, et al. Quantitative studies of prostatic secretion. I. Characteristics of normal secretion. The influence of thyroid, suprarenal, and testis extirpation and androgen substitution of the prostatic output. J Exp Med 1939; 70:543–556.
244. Huggins C, Hodges CV. Studies on prostatic cancer. I. The effect of castration, of estrogen and of androgen injection on serum phosphatases in metastatic carcinoma of the prostate. Cancer Res 1941; 1:293–297.
245. Wilson JD. Recent studies on the mechanism of action of testosterone. N Engl J Med 1972; 287:1284–1291.
246. Baulieu EE, Lasnitzki I, Robel P. Metabolism of testosterone and action of metabolites on prostate glands grown in organ culture. Nature 1968; 219:1155–1156.
247. Hammond GL, Kontturi M, Vihko P, et al. Serum steroids in normal males and patients with prostatic diseases. Clin Endocrinol 1978; 9:113–121.
248. Peyre A, Ravault JP, Laporte P. Effet potentialisateur de la proactine endogène sur les effecteurs sexuels mâles soumis à la testostérone. C R Soc Biol (Paris) 1968; 162:1592–1595.
249. Asano M, Kanzaki S, Sekiguichi E, et al. Inhibition of prostatic growth in rabbits with antiovine prolactin serum. J Urol 1971; 106:248–252.
250. Aragona C, Bohnet HG, Friesen HG. Localization of prolactin binding in prostate and testis: the role of serum prolactin concentration on the testicular LH receptor. Acta Endocrinol 1977; 84:402.
251. Gustafsson J-A, Ekman P, Snochowski M, et al. Correlation between clinical response to hormone therapy and steroid receptor content in prostatic cancer. Cancer Res 1978; 38:4345–4348.
252. Nesbit RM, Baum WC. Endocrine control of prostatic carcinoma. JAMA 1950; 143:1317–1320.
253. Paulson DF. Multimodality therapy of prostate cancer. Urology 1981; 17(Suppl):53–56.
254. Byar DP. The Veterans Administration cooperative urological research group's studies of cancer of the prostate. Cancer 1973; 32:1126–1130.
255. Blackard CE. The Veterans Administration cooperative urological research group studies of the prostate: a review. Cancer Chemother Rep 1975; 59:225–232.
256. Shearer RJ, Hendry WF, Sommerville IF, et al. Plasma testosterone. An accurate monitor of hormone treatment in prostatic cancer. Br J Urol 1973; 45:668–677.
257. Blackard CE, Byer DF, Jordan WP. Orchiectomy for advanced prostatic carcinoma. Urology 1973; 1:553–562.
258. Sciarra F, Sorcini G, Di Silverio F, et al. Plasma testosterone and androstenedione after orchiectomy in prostatic adenocarcinoma. Clin Endocrinol 1973; 2:101–109.
259. Murphy P, Reynoso G, Schoonees R, et al. Hypophysectomy and adrenalectomy for disseminated prostatic carcinoma. J Urol 1971; 105:817–825.
260. Scott WV, Menon M, Walsh PC. Hormonal therapy of prostate cancer. Cancer 1980; 45:1929–1926.
261. Maddy JA, Winternitz WW, Norrell H. Cryohypophysectomy in the management of advanced prostatic cancer. Cancer 1971; 28:322–328.
262. Sanford EJ, Drago JR, Rohner TJ, et al. Aminoglutethimide medical adrenalectomy for advanced prostatic carcinoma. J Urol 1976; 115:170–174.
263. Silverberg GD. Hypophysectomy in the treatment of disseminated prostatic carcinoma. Cancer 1977; 39:1727–1731.
264. Rafla S, Johnson R. The treatment of advanced prostatic carcinoma with medroxyprogesterone. Curr Ther Res 1974; 16:261–267.
265. Airhart RA, Barnett TF, Sullivan JW, et al. Flutamide therapy for carcinoma of the prostate. South Med J 1978; 171:798–801.
266. Neri R, Florance K, Koziol P, et al. A biological profile of a non-steroidal antiandrogen, SCH13521 (4'-nitro-3'-trifluoromethyl-isobutyranilide). Endocrinology 1972; 91:427–437.
267. Ahmed SR, Brouman PJC, Shalet SM, et al. Treatment of advanced prostatic cancer with hormonal mechanisms. Lancet 1983; 1:415–419.
268. Tolis G, Ackman D, Stellos A. Tumour growth inhibition in patients with prostatic carcinoma treated with luteinising hormone–releasing hormone agonists. Proc Natl Acad Sci USA 1982; 79:1658–1662.
269. Gonzalez-Barcena D, Perez-Sanchez P, Ureta-Sanchez P, et al. Treatment of advanced prostatic carcinoma with D-Trp-6-LH-RH. Prostate 1985; 7:21–30.
270. Santen RJ, Manni A, Harvey H. Gonadotropin releasing hormone (GnRH) analogs for the treatment of breast and prostatic carcinoma. Breast Cancer Res Treat 1986; 7:129–145.
271. Foekens JA, Henkelman MS, Fukkinkk JF, et al. Combined effects of buserelin, estradiol and tamoxifen on the growth of MCF-7 human breast cancer cells in vitro. Biochem Biophys Res Commun 1986; 140:550–556.
272. Miller WR, Scott WN, Morris R, et al. Growth of human breast cancer cells inhibited by a luteinizing hormone–releasing hormone agonist. Nature 1985; 313:231–233.
273. Eidne KA, Flanagan CA, Millar RP. Gonadotropin-releasing hormone binding sites in human breast carcinoma. Science 1985; 229:989–991.
274. Wilding G, Chen M, Gelmann E, et al. LHRH agonists and human breast cancer cells. Nature 1987; 329:770.
275. Klijn JM, DeJong FH, Lamberts WJ, et al. LHRH-agonist treatment in metastatic prostate carcinoma. Eur J Clin Oncol 1984; 20:483–493.
276. Kerle D, Williams G, Ware H, et al. Failure of long term luteinising hormone releasing hormone treatment for prostatic cancer to suppress serum luteinising hormone and testosterone. Br Med J 1984; 289:468–469.
277. Handelsman DJ, Swerdloff RS. Pharmacokinetics of gonadotropin-releasing hormone and its analogs. Endocr Rev 1986; 7:95–105.
278. Furr BJA, Nicholson RI. Use of analogues of LHRH for treatment of cancer. J Reprod Fertil 1982; 64:529–539.
279. Furr BA, Hutchison FG. Biodegradable sustained release formulation of the LH-RH analogue "Zoladex" for the treatment of hormone-responsive tumors. In: Back N, Breiver GJ, Eijsvoogel V, et al., eds. EORTC Genitourinary Group Monograph 2. Part A: Therapeutic Principles in Metastatic Prostate Cancer. New York: Alan R. Liss, 1985: 143–153.
280. Beacock CJ, Buck AC, Zwinck R, et al. The treatment of metastatic prostatic cancer with the slow release LH-RH analogue Zoladex ICI 118630. Br J Urol 1987; 59:436–442.
281. Robinson MG, Denis L, Mahler C, et al. An LH-RH analogue (Zoladex) in the management of carcinoma of the prostate: a preliminary report comparing daily subcutaneous injection with monthly depot injections. Eur J Surg Oncol 1985; 11:159–165.
282. Thomas EJ, Jenkins J, Lenton EA, et al. Endocrine effects of goserelin, a new depot luteinising hormone releasing hormone agonist. Br Med J 1986; 293:1407–1409.
283. The Leuprolide Study Group. Leuprolide versus diethylstilbestrol for metastatic prostate cancer. N Engl J Med 1984; 311:1281–1286.
284. Labrie F, Dupont A, Giguere M, et al. Combination therapy with flutamide and castration (orchiectomy or LHRH agonist). The minimal endocrine therapy in both untreated and previously treated patients. J Steroid Biochem 1987; 27:525–532.
285. Crawford E, McLeod D, Dorr A, et al. Treatment of newly diagnosed stage D$_2$ prostate cancer with leuprolide and flutamide or leuprolide alone, phase III, intergroup study 0036. Proc Am Soc Clin Oncol 1988; 7:119 (abstract).
286. Mathe G, Schally AV, Comaru-Schally AM, et al. Phase II trial with D-Trp-6-LH-RH in prostatic carcinoma: comparison with other hormonal agents. Prostate 1986; 9:327–342.
287. Smith JA, Urry RL. Testicular histology after prolonged treatment with a gonadotropin-releasing hormone analogue. J Urol 1985; 133:612–614.
288. Peters CA, Walsh PC. The effect of nafarelin acetate, a luteinizing-hormone–releasing hormone agonist, on benign prostatic hyperplasia. N Engl J Med 1987; 317:599–604.
289. Kahan A, Delrieu F, Amor B, et al. Disease flare induced by D-Trp^6-LHRH analogue in patients with metastatic prostatic cancer. Lancet 1984; 1:971–972.
290. Murphy GP, Greco JM, Chin JL, et al. Zoladex (ICI 118,630): clinical trial of new luteinizing hormone–releasing hormone analog in metastatic prostatic carcinoma. Urology 1987; 29:185–190.
291. Jacobi GH, Wenderoth UK, Ehrenthal W, et al. Endocrine and clinical evaluation of 107 patients with advanced prostatic carcinoma under long term pernasal buserelin or intramuscular Decapeptyl depot treatment. In: Klijn JGM, Pariedens R, Foekens JA, eds. Hormonal Manipulation of Cancer: Peptides, Growth Factors, and New (Anti) Steroidal Agents. New York: Raven, 1987: 235–248.
292. Debruyne FMJ, Weil EHJ, del Mora F, et al. Clinical results with the depot preparation of Zoladex in prostate cancer. In: Klijn JGM, Parie-dens R, Foekens JA, eds. Hormonal Manipulation of Cancer: Peptides, Growth Factors, and New (Anti) Steroidal Agents. New York: Raven, 1987: 255–272.
293. Moguilewsky M, Fiet J, Tournemine C, et al. Pharmacology of an antiandrogen, Anandron®, used as an adjuvant therapy in the treatment of prostate cancer. J Steroid Biochem 1986; 24:139–146.

294. Tunn UW, Radlmaier A, Neumann F. Antiandrogens in cancer treatment. In: Stoll BA, ed. Endocrine Management of Cancer. Vol 2. Contemporary Therapy. New York: S. Karger, 1988: 43–56.

295. Frith RG, Phillipou G. 15-Hydroxycyproterone acetate and cyproterone acetate levels in plasma and urine. J Chromatogr 1985; 338:179–186.

296. De Voogt HH, EORTC-GU-Group. Cardiovascular side effects of diethylstilbestrol, cyproterone acetate, medroxyprogesterone acetate, and estramustine phosphate used for the treatment of advanced prostatic cancer: results from European Organization for Research and Treatment of Cancer—Trials 30761 and 30762. J Urol 1986; 135:303–307.

297. Rassmussen GH. Chemical control of androgen action. Annu Rep Med Chem 1986; 21:179–188.

298. Hammerstein J, Moltz L, Schwartz U. Antiandrogens in the treatment of acne and hirsutism. J Steroid Biochem 1983; 19:591–597.

299. Paisey RB, Kadow C, Bolton C, et al. Effects of cyproterone acetate and a long-acting LHRH analogue in serum lipoproteins in patients with carcinoma of the prostate. J R Soc Med 1986; 79:210–211.

300. Frohman LA. Disease of the anterior pituitary. In: Felig P, Baxter JD, Broodus AE, et al., eds. Endocrinology and Metabolism. 2nd ed. New York: McGraw-Hill, 1987:247–337.

301. Sogani PC, Vagaiwala MR, Whitmore WF. Experience with flutamide in patients with advanced prostatic cancer without prior endocrine therapy. Cancer 1984; 54:744–750.

302. Neri R, Kassem N. Biological and clinical properties of antiandrogens. In: Breciani F, ed. Progress in Cancer Research and Therapy. New York: Raven, 1984: 507–518.

303. Stoliar B, Albert DJ. SCH 13521 in the treatment of advanced carcinoma of the prostate. J Urol 1974; 111:803–807.

304. Thompson EB, Lippman ME. Mechanism of action of glucocorticoids. Metabolism 1974; 23:159–202.

305. Baxter JD, Forsham PH. Tissue effects of glucocorticoids. Am J Med 1972; 53:573–589.

306. Selye H. Studies on adaption. Endocrinology 1937; 21:169–188.

307. Claman HN. Corticoids and lymphoid cells. N Engl J Med 1972; 287:388–397.

308. Livingston RB, Carter SK, eds. Single Agents in Cancer Chemotherapy. New York: Plenum, 1970.

309. Vietti TJ, Sullivan MP, Berry DH, et al. The response of acute childhood leukemia to an initial and a second course of prednisone. J Pediatr 1965; 66:18–26.

310. Kjellstraad CM. Side effects of steroids and their treatment. Transplant Proc 1975; 7:123–129.

311. McGuire WL, ed. Estrogen Receptors in Human Breast Cancer. New York: Raven, 1975.

312. Schmidt TJ, Thompson EB. Glucocorticoid receptor function in lymphoma cells. In: Sharma RK, Criss WE, eds. Endocrine Control in Neoplasia. New York: Raven, 1978:263–290.

313. Lippman ME, Konior-Yarbro G, Leventhal BG. Clinical implications of glucocorticoid receptors in human leukemia. Cancer Res 1978; 38:4251–4256.

314. Crabtree GR, Smith KA, Munck A. Glucocorticoid receptors and sensitivity of isolated human leukemia and lymphoma cells. Cancer Res 1978; 38:4268–4272.

315. Neifeld JP, Lippman ME, Tormey DC. Steroid hormone receptors in normal human lymphocytes. Induction of glucocorticoid receptor activity by phytohemagglutinin stimulation. J Biol Chem 1977; 254:2972–2977.

316. Lippman ME, Barr R. Glucocorticoid receptors in purified subpopulations of human peripheral blood lymphocytes. J Immunol 1977; 118:1977–1981.

317. Thompson EB, Aviv D, Lippman ME. Variants of HTC cells with low tyrosine aminotransferase inducibility and apparently normal glucocorticoid receptors. Endocrinology 1977; 100:406–419.

318. Cidlowski JA, Munck A. Comparison of glucocorticoid receptor complex binding to nuclei and SNA cellulose. Biochim Biophys Acta 1978; 543:545–555.

319. Adler VV, Ioannesyants IA, Dmitreeva LA, et al. Action of dexamethasone on RNA synthesis in blood lymphocytes stimulated by phytohemagglutinin. Bull Exp Biol Med 1976; 81:850–855.

320. Smith KA, Crabtree GR, Kennedy SJ, et al. Glucocorticoid receptors and glucocorticoid sensitivity of mitogen stimulated and unstimulated human lymphocytes. Nature 1977; 267:523–526.

321. Lippman ME, Halterman R, Perry S, et al. Glucocorticoid binding proteins in human leukaemic lymphoblasts. Nature New Biol 1973; 242:157–158.

322. Lippman ME, Halterman R, Leventhal BG, et al. Glucocorticoid binding proteins in acute lymphoblastic leukemic blast cells. J Clin Invest 1973; 52:1715–1725.

323. Yarbro GS, Lippman ME, Johnson GE, et al. Glucocorticoid receptors in subpopulations of childhood acute lymphocytic leukemia. Cancer Res 1977; 37:2688–2695.

324. Lippman ME, Konior-Yarbro G, Leventhal BG. Clinical implications of glucocorticoid receptor in human leukemia. Cancer Res 1978; 38:4251–4256.

325. Lippman ME, Perry S, Thompson EB. Glucocorticoid binding proteins in myeloblasts of acute myelogenous leukemia. Am J Med 1975; 59:224–227.

326. Crabtree GR, Smith KA, Munck A. Glucocorticoid receptors and sensitivity of isolated human leukemia and lymphoma cells. Cancer Res 1978; 38:4268.

327. Gailiani S, Minowada J, Silvernail P, et al. Specific glucocorticoid binding in human hemopoietic cell lines and neoplastic tissue. Cancer Res 1978; 33:2653.

328. Homo F, Duval D, Meyer P, et al. Chronic lymphatic leukaemia: cellular effects of glucocorticoid in vitro. Br J Haematol 1978; 38:491–499.

329. Terenius L, Simonsson B, Nilsson K. Glucocorticoid receptors, DNA synthesis, membrane antigens and their relation to disease activity in chronic lymphatic leukemia. J Steroid Biochem 1976; 7:905–909.

330. Bloomfield C, Smith KA, Peterson BA, et al. In vitro glucocorticoid studies for predicting response to glucocorticoid therapy in adults with malignant lymphomas. Lancet 1980; 1:952–955.

331. Loriaux DL, Cutler GB Jr. Diseases of the adrenal glands. In: Kohler PO, ed. Basic Clinical Endocrinology. New York: John Wiley, 1981:167–238.

332. Fotherby K, James F. Metabolism of synthetic steroids. Adv Steroid Biochem Pharmacol 1972; 3:67–165.

333. Peterson RE. Metabolism of adrenal corticol steroids. In: Christy NP, ed. The Human Adrenal Cortex. New York: Harper & Row, 1971: 87.

334. Gordon GG, Southren AL. Thyroid-hormone effects on steroid-hormone metabolism. Bull NY Acad Med 1977; 53:241–259.

335. Boyar RM, Hellman LD, Roffwarg H, et al. Cortisol secretion and metabolism in anorexia nervosa. N Engl J Med 1977; 296:190–193.

336. Adrenals. In: McEvoy GK, ed. Drug Information 89. American Hospital Formulary Service Drug Information. New York: American Society of Hospital Pharmacists, 1989:1662–1685.

337. Schottenfeld D, Berg J. Incidence of multiple primary cancers. IV. Cancer of the female breast and genital organs. J Natl Cancer Inst 1971; 46:161–170.

338. Lynch HT, Krush AJ, Larsen AL, et al. Endometrial carcinoma: multiple primary malignancies, constitutional factors, and heredity. Am J Med Sci 1966; 252:381–390.

339. Haenszel W, Kurihara M. Studies of Japanese migrants. I. Mortality from cancer and other diseases among Japanese in the United States. J Natl Cancer Inst 1968; 40:42–68.

340. Hoover R, Gray LA, Fraumeni JF. Stilbestrol (diethylstilbestrol) and the risk of ovarian cancer. Lancet 1977; 2:533–534.

341. Tobias JS, Griffiths TC. Management of ovarian carcinoma: current concepts and future prospects. N Engl J Med 1976; 294:818–823.

342. Hamilton TC, Davies P, Griffiths K. Androgen and oestrogen binding in cytosols of human ovarian tumors. J Endocrinol 1981; 90:421–431.

343. Saez S, Martin PM, Gignoux B. Androgen receptors in normal mucosa and in epithelioma of human larynx and pharynx. In: Thompson EB, Lippman ME, eds. Steroid Receptors and the Management of Cancer. Boca Raton, FL: CRC Press, 1979: 205–214.

34

HUMORAL MANIFESTATIONS OF CANCER

William D. Odell and W. Scott Appleton

INTRODUCTION

In addition to manifestations caused by tumor mass or invasion, cancers can produce symptoms by means of humoral or hormonal products. The diversity of clinical presentation of humoral manifestations is enormous, including subtle and overt hormonal excess syndromes (e.g., Cushing syndrome and acromegaly), a wide range of neurological manifestations, and generalized symptoms such as anorexia and muscle weakness. In past years, humoral syndromes of cancer were thought to be rare, but with better understanding of the causes and improved diagnostic techniques it is now thought that most patients with cancer exhibit one or more humoral manifestations. The known causes of these syndromes are listed in Table 34–1, and the spectrum of the disorders is illustrated in Table 34–2.[1] Peptide hormones and hormone precursors are produced in small quantities by many normal tissues classically considered to be nonendocrine. When cancers develop in these tissues, they continue to produce these peptides, often in increased quantities. Some of these products have little or no effect, but others are biologically active and cause "ectopic hormonal syndromes" when secreted into the circulation. In short, these syndromes represent cancer-induced amplification of a property that is normally present in the cells from which the cancer originated,[1–3] and ectopic hormonal syndromes are not truly ectopic. In this chapter we discuss the pathogenesis of these syndromes.

HORMONE PRODUCTION AND HORMONE-LIKE SYNDROMES

Many hormones, hormonal fragments, and hormone precursors are produced by cancers (Table 34–3). With the exception of estrone and estradiol, these substances are all peptide or protein hormones. Some neoplasms can metabolize a steroid precursor to a bioactive steroid hormone (e.g., hepatomas may metabolize dehydroepiandrosterone to estrone and estradiol).[4] Malignant tumors derived from the adrenals, testes, ovaries, or thyroid often retain the capacity to synthesize and secrete steroid or thyroid hormones, but complete synthesis of steroid or thyroid hormones by nonendocrine cancers has not been described. Most cancers not associated with clinically recognizable syndromes also produce proteins "ectopically," but these proteins are not biologically active. In some instances they are either precursors or metabolites of protein hormones.

TABLE 34–1. Causes of Humoral Syndromes of Cancer

Production of protein hormone or hormone precursors
Metabolism of steroid hormone precursors
Stimulation of antibody production
Production of paracrine or autocrine substances (e.g., cytokines)
Increased susceptibility to viral infections

TABLE 34–2. Spectrum of Humoral Syndromes of Cancer

Humoral substances
  Protein hormones and hormone precursors
  Metabolism of steroids
Paraneoplastic syndromes of the nervous system
  Cerebellar syndromes
    Cerebellar cortical degeneration
    Myoclonic encephalopathy
  Subacute sensory neuropathy
  Visual paraneoplastic syndrome
  Limbic and bulbar encephalitis
  Multifocal leukoencephalopathy
  Skeletal muscle syndromes
    Polymyositis-dermatomyositis
    Carcinomatous neuromyopathy
  Myasthenic syndromes (e.g., Eaton-Lambert syndrome)
Miscellaneous syndromes
  Anorexia
  Fever
  Glomerular kidney disease
  Enzyme production (e.g., alkaline phosphatase, thymidine kinase)
  Fetal protein production (α-fetoprotein, carcinoembryonic antigen)
  Digital clubbing–pulmonary osteoarthropathy
  Hematological syndromes (e.g., idiopathic thrombocytopenic purpura)

Modified from Odell WD. Paraendocrine syndromes of cancer. Adv Intern Med 1989; 34:325–352.

TABLE 34–3. Hormones and Hormone Precursors Reported to Be Produced by Neoplasms

Pro-opiomelanocortin and related peptides
Corticotropin-releasing hormone
Chorionic gonadotropin and its subunits (alpha and beta)
Vasopressin
Growth factors (e.g., transforming growth factor β, epidermal growth factor, insulin-like growth factor II)
Parathyroid hormone–like protein
Erythropoietin
Eosinophilopoietin
Growth hormone
Growth hormone–releasing hormone
Prolactin
Gastrin
Gastrin-releasing peptide (and bombesin)
Secretin
Glucagon
Calcitonin
Renin
Vasoactive intestinal peptide
Somatostatin
Hypophosphatemia-producing factor
Estrone and estradiol

Corticotropin

Pro-opiomelanocortin (POMC) is a 31-kd glycoprotein precursor molecule that contains the sequences of lipotropin, melanocyte-stimulating hormone (MSH), the endorphins and enkephalins,[5] and corticotropin (ACTH, adrenocorticotropin) (Fig. 34–1). (Also see Chapter 6.) The smaller hormones are enzymatically cleaved from POMC during the process of secretion and, depending on the manner in which it is processed, the actual secretory products vary. For example, anterior pituitary cells secrete biologically active ACTH, which is a 39-amino-acid peptide hormone with a molecular mass of 4.5 kd. These cells can also store a smaller precursor than POMC, that is, a proACTH molecule. Intermediate-lobe cells process POMC to either MSH or a larger peptide, lipotropin, containing the MSH sequence. Brain neurons process POMC to form endorphins and enkephalins, which act as neurotransmitters and mediators of pain.

The association of Cushing syndrome with carcinoma was first recognized in 1928 and is now one of the best-understood ectopic hormonal syndromes.[6] In the 1960s Liddle and colleagues[7] characterized cancer-associated Cush-

ing syndrome in 88 patients and showed that primary and metastatic tumors contained large amounts of biologically active ACTH. Several hundred additional patients have since been reported.

The types of neoplasms associated with Cushing syndrome and their approximate frequency are summarized in Table 34–4. About half of such patients have carcinoma of the lung, predominantly oat cell or small round cell in type, and about a fifth have carcinoma of the thymus or pancreas. The remainder are patients with a wide array of carcinomas. Indeed, almost all types of carcinomas can cause ectopic ACTH secretion, but not all patients with these types of neoplasms have overt Cushing syndrome. For example, among patients with oat cell carcinoma, only 3% have clinical manifestations of ectopic ACTH production,[8] but approximately half have an elevated plasma cortisol level that is not suppressed by the administration of 8 mg of dexamethasone per day.

In addition, extracts of lung carcinomas of all histological types from patients without clinical manifestations of Cushing syndrome uniformly contain an ACTH-like material measurable by radioimmunoassay.[9–11] Odell and associates[2, 12, 13] showed that carcinomas of the lung and many

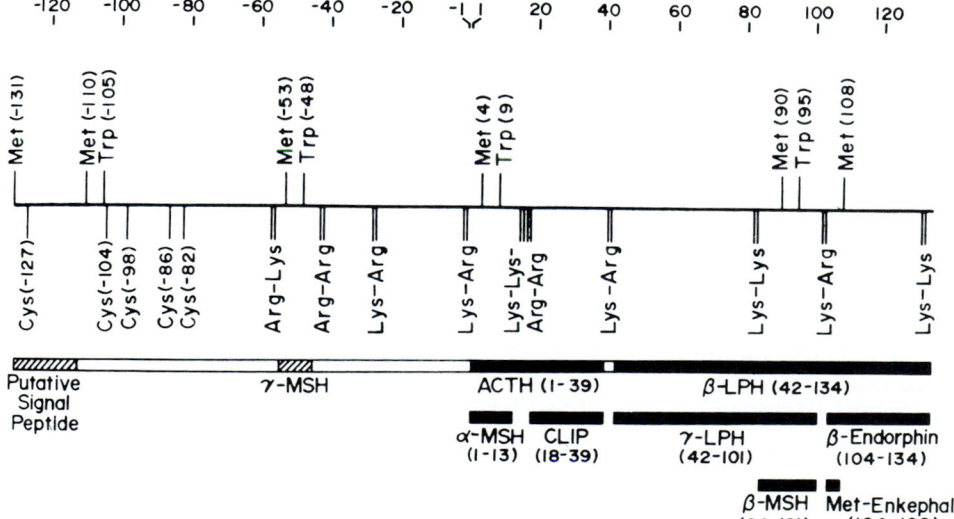

Figure 34–1. Schematic representation of the structure of bovine POMC. Characteristic amino acid residues are shown, and the positions of the methionine, tryptophan, and cysteine residues are given in parentheses. The location of the translation initiation site at the methionine residue at position −131 is assumed. Filled bars represent regions for which the amino acid sequence is known; open and striped bars represent regions for which the amino acid sequence has been predicted from the nucleotide sequence of precursor messenger RNA. Locations of known component peptides are shown by filled bars; amino acid numbers are given in parentheses. Locations of γ-MSH and the putative signal peptide are indicated by striped bars; the termini of these peptides are not definitive. (From Nakanishi S, Inoue A, Kita T, et al. Nucleotide sequence of cloned cDNA for bovine corticotropin–β-lipotropin precursor. Reprinted by permission from Nature, Vol. 278, pp. 423–427, Copyright © 1979 Macmillan Journals Limited.)

TABLE 34–4. Types of Neoplasms That Produce Biologically Active ACTH

Type of Neoplasm	Approximate Percentage of Cases
Carcinoma of the lung (predominantly small or oat cell)	50
Carcinoma of the thymus	10
Carcinoma of the pancreas (including carcinoid and islet cell)	10
Pheochromocytoma, neuroblastoma ganglioma, and paraganglioma	5
Medullary carcinoma of the thyroid	5
Bronchial adenoma and carcinoid	2
Miscellaneous carcinomas*	18

*For example, carcinoma of the ovary, prostate, breast, thyroid, kidney, salivary glands, testes, stomach, colon, gallbladder, esophagus, or appendix.

Modified from Odell WD. Paraendocrine syndromes of cancer. Adv Intern Med 1989; 34:325–352.

TABLE 34–5. ACTH Activity in Normal Tissues

Tissue	Immunoassay Potency (pg/mg protein)	Bioassay Potency (pg/mg protein)	
		Before Trypsin	After Trypsin
Colon	39	<2	24
Small intestine	37	<2	20
Liver	17	<2	12
Kidney	47	<2	8
Brain	278	99	30

Modified from Odell WD, Saito E. Protein hormone–like materials from normal and cancer cells—"ectopic" hormone production. Prog Clin Biol Res 1983; 132E:247–258.

carcinomas of diverse histological types commonly contain both ACTH-like activity and a lipotropin-like material (Fig. 34–2). Both of these immunoactive materials have molecular weights greater than that of standard ACTH. The ACTH-like material has little or no steroidogenic activity by in vitro bioassays and does not react in radioreceptor assays for ACTH. However, it can be converted to bioactive ACTH by incubation with trypsin.[10]

A 26-kd glycoprotein containing both MSH and ACTH immunoactivities can also be extracted from virtually all normal nonendocrine tissues of rats and humans.[3, 14–15a] Like the material extracted from cancers, this substance has no

detectable ACTH biological activity but can be converted to 4.5-kd biologically active ACTH by exposure to trypsin[3, 14, 15] (Table 34–5). This material is probably either POMC or another precursor form of ACTH (see Fig. 34–1). Although the sequence has not been reported, the POMC in normal tissues appears to be indistinguishable from the high-molecular-weight ACTH-like material extractable from most carcinomas. POMC messenger RNA is present in nonpituitary tissues in the rat, which adds further support to the concept that small amounts of POMC and related peptides are formed in peripheral tissues.[15b] Larger amounts of immunoreactive MSH, lipotropin, and ACTH are extractable from carcinomas than from normal tissues (see Fig. 34–2).

If one excludes patients with clinically recognizable symptoms of excess ACTH production, approximately three fourths of patients with lung cancer, independent of histo-

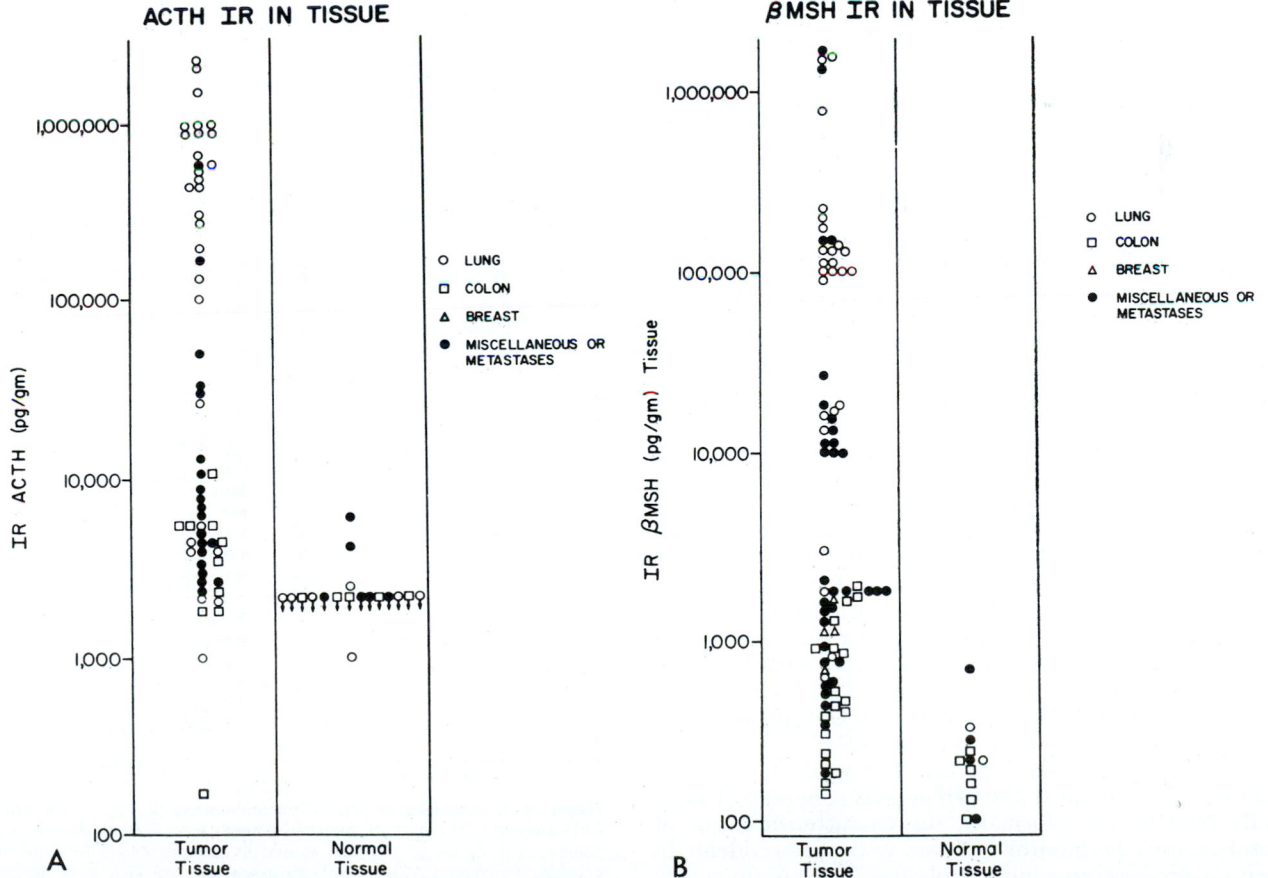

Figure 34–2. *A*, Immunoreactive ACTH (ACTH IR) in acetic acid extracts of various carcinomas and normal tissues. ACTH content is presented on a log scale. Symbols with arrows mean undetectable. *B*, Immunoreactive β-MSH (β-MSH IR) in acetic acid extracts of various carcinomas and normal tissues. β-MSH IR content is presented on a log scale. The peptide being measured in this system is β-lipotropin. To convert ACTH and MSH values to nanograms per kilogram, multiply by 1. (From Odell W, Wolfsen A, Yoshimoto Y, et al. Ectopic peptide synthesis: a universal concomitant of neoplasia. Trans Assoc Am Physicians 1977; 90:204–227.)

CANCER PLASMA

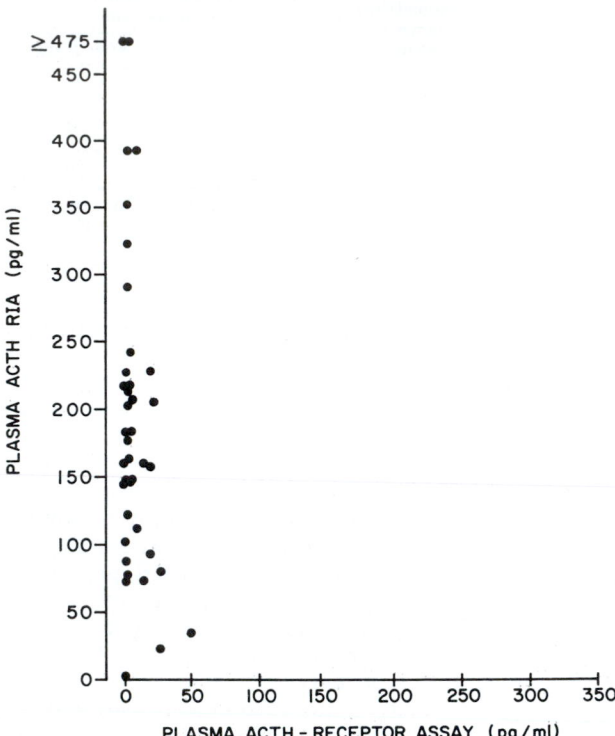

Figure 34–3. Concentration of plasma ACTH quantified by radioimmunoassay (ordinate) plotted against concentration quantified by radioreceptor assay (abscissa). Note that in these patients with carcinoma but no clinical evidence of ectopic ACTH syndrome, the level of radioimmunoassayable ACTH is elevated but that of radioreceptor-assayable ACTH is normal. The material being quantified by radioimmunoassay is probably POMC, which has little reaction in the radioreceptor assay. To convert ACTH values to nanograms per liter, multiply by 1. (From Odell W, Wolfsen A, Yoshimoto Y, et al. Ectopic peptide synthesis: a universal concomitant of neoplasia. Trans Assoc Am Physicians 1977; 90:204–227.)

tients with hypokalemia, muscle weakness, psychosis, increased pigmentation, edema, hypertension, or abnormal glucose tolerance should be suspected of having an ectopic ACTH syndrome. In patients with Cushing syndrome but without known cancer, ectopic ACTH production is suggested by any of the following: hypokalemia, a very high plasma cortisol level (>1000 nmol/L), a high plasma ACTH level (>36 pmol/L), markedly elevated 17-ketosteroid excretion, or high concentrations of plasma dehydroepiandrosterone sulfate.

In patients with Cushing syndrome associated with functioning adrenocortical tumors, blood ACTH concentrations are low or undetectable before dexamethasone administration. Therefore, further suppression of ACTH or plasma cortisol levels does not occur in these patients, in contrast to the suppression seen in Cushing disease. In most patients with ectopic ACTH syndrome, administration of dexamethasone (8 mg/d) also does not result in suppression of ACTH or plasma cortisol levels, but a small percentage of patients with ectopic ACTH production show suppression of both ACTH and cortisol levels with dexamethasone doses of 8 mg/d or higher. Such suppression occurs in approximately 50% of the patients with bronchial carcinoid and thymoma. This phenomenon could be explained if such tumors produce the hypothalamic peptide corticotropin-releasing hormone (CRH), which exerts its effect by stimulating pituitary secretion of ACTH, because glucocorticoids suppress CRH effects at the pituitary level. Rare patients with "ectopic ACTH syndrome" have tumors that contain both an ACTH-like and a CRH-like material.[20] CRH production by a medullary carcinoma of the thyroid can cause Cushing syndrome.[21] The CRH stimulation test can assist in distinguishing ectopic ACTH production from Cushing disease[22] (Fig. 34–4), but it may not distinguish ectopic CRH production from Cushing disease.

In summary, small amounts of proACTH and/or POMC are present in virtually all nonendocrine tissues including liver, kidney, lung, and heart. The same ACTH precursors

logical type, have an elevated plasma immunoreactive ACTH concentration and one third have an elevated plasma MSH-lipotropin level.[12, 13] However, none of the latter patients have increased levels of *biologically* active ACTH (Fig. 34–3).[2] Because the MSH sequence is contained within the structure of POMC and MSH per se is not secreted by the normal human pituitary,[16–18] the MSH-like materials in the serum of patients with carcinoma of the lung may represent cancer-produced POMC or lipotropin. Therefore, pigmentation in the ectopic ACTH syndrome would result from stimulation of melanin synthesis by lipotropin, ACTH, or other peptides containing the MSH sequence.

The ACTH concentrations in the blood of patients with cancer-associated ACTH production and Cushing syndrome are typically high. In contrast, patients with ACTH-producing pituitary tumors (Cushing disease) usually have ACTH concentrations in blood that are normal or slightly elevated. However, some patients with cancer-associated Cushing syndrome have minimally elevated blood ACTH levels and are difficult to distinguish from patients with Cushing disease.[19]

In patients whose cancers convert POMC to biologically active ACTH, typical signs of Cushing syndrome may be absent or subtle, because the carcinomas commonly have a rapidly fatal course. Normally, the characteristic signs of cortisol excess take months or years to become evident. In patients with slow-growing neoplasms, such as thymoma, bronchial carcinoid, pheochromocytoma, or medullary carcinoma of the thyroid, Cushing syndrome may be manifest months or years before tumor recognition. All cancer pa-

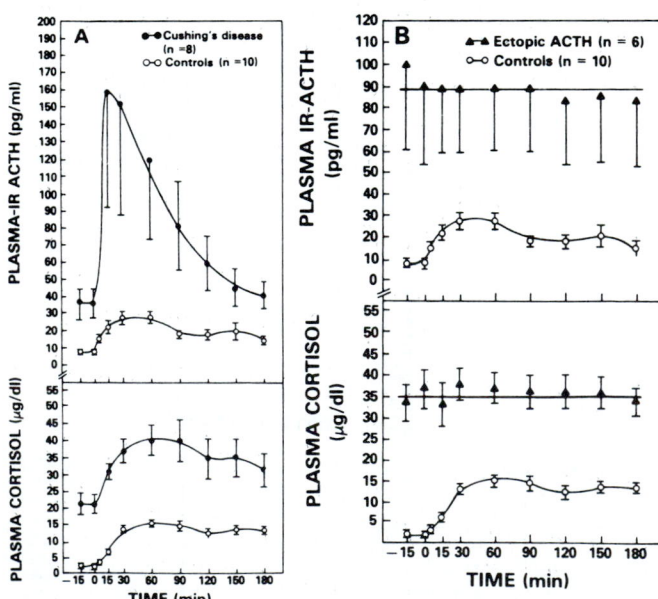

Figure 34–4. Responses of plasma immunoreactive (IR) ACTH and cortisol to CRH (means ± SE) in (A) 8 untreated patients with Cushing disease and (B) 6 patients with Cushing syndrome caused by ectopic ACTH secretion and 10 controls. To convert ACTH values to nanograms per liter, multiply by 1. To convert cortisol values to namomoles per liter, multiply by 27.6. (From Chrousos GP, Schulte HM, Oldfield EH, et al. The corticotropin-releasing factor stimulation test. An aid in the evaluation of patients with Cushing's syndrome. Reprinted with permission from The New England Journal of Medicine, 310, 622–626, 1984.)

are present in larger amounts in carcinomas, independent of histological type or tissue source. They are also present in blood of many patients with cancer but are biologically inactive and produce no symptoms. Occasional carcinomas convert these biologically inactive precursors to biologically active ACTH and secrete the active ACTH to produce ectopic ACTH syndrome.

Chorionic Gonadotropin

Chorionic gonadotropin (CG) is a glycoprotein of two peptide chains (alpha and beta) that are not covalently bound (Fig. 34–5). The alpha chain of CG is similar in amino acid sequence to the alpha chain of the other human glycoprotein hormones, such as thyrotropin, luteinizing hormone (LH), and follicle-stimulating hormone.[23] The beta chain of CG has 80% homology to the first 117 amino acid residues to the beta chain of LH and in addition possesses a 30-amino-acid, carbohydrate-rich tail at the COOH terminus.[24, 25] Neither the alpha nor the beta chains of the glycoproteins possess bioactivity, but the bioactivity of the intact molecule is determined by the beta chain.

It was originally thought that extrapituitary sources of gonadotropin were confined to primate placenta, the endometrial cusps of the pregnant mare, human neoplasms derived from the cytotrophoblast, and teratomas containing such cells.[26] Between 1949 and 1972 several patients were described with evidence of increased gonadotropin production and cancers that included malignant melanoma,[27] adrenocortical carcinoma,[28] undifferentiated carcinoma,[29] breast carcinoma,[30] renal carcinoma,[31] and carcinoma of the lung.[32-34] However, the assays used in these reports could not distinguish CG from LH. When a more specific radioimmunoassay for the beta chain was developed[35] and when patients with various neoplasms were studied,[36] it was found that 6 to 13% of all carcinomas are associated with increased plasma levels of a CG-like material.

Subsequently, a CG-like material was demonstrated in extracts of virtually all normal human tissues[2, 3, 37-40] including the pituitary[41, 42] (Fig. 34–6). It has been further characterized using the plant lectin concanavalin A.* Less than 10% of extrapituitary human chorionic gonadotropin (hCG)-like

---

*Concanavalin A and other plant lectins bind glycoproteins via their carbohydrate moieties. Each lectin has binding sites with carbohydrate specificity. Placental CG binds to concanavalin A because it is rich in the types of carbohydrate moieties that interact with concanavalin A.

---

material binds to concanavalin A (Table 34–6), whereas virtually all CG from normal placenta and from the blood of pregnant women binds to concanavalin A and can be eluted after addition of the carbohydrate competitor α-methylglucopyranoside.[3, 38, 39] Extracts of CG-like material from carcinomas have a wide range of concanavalin A–binding properties, from as low as that of extracts of normal tissue to as high as that of placental CG[43] (see Table 34–6). These findings indicate that the CG-like material in normal tissues either has a carbohydrate structure different from that of placental CG or has no carbohydrate. The absence of carbohydrate alters the bioactivity of the CG. For example, desialated CG has little biological potency because it is rapidly cleared from the circulation.[44,45] Desialated CG does react with CG receptors but also has decreased steroidogenic potency in vitro.[46, 47]

A CG-like material has been detected in blood from nonpregnant humans[48] and is secreted in a pulsatile fashion in parallel with LH.[49] This circulating CG is suppressed by estrogens and agonists by luteinizing hormone–releasing hormone (LHRH, also called gonadotropin-releasing hormone, GnRH) and is enhanced by LHRH itself.[49, 50] As a consequence, it has been postulated that the source of circulating CG-like material in normal individuals is the pituitary gland.[49] Human pituitary cells in culture secrete a CG-like material,[49a] and a previously uncharacterized pituitary cell immunostains for CG but not LH.[49b]

Certain aspects of CG metabolism are poorly understood. For example, analysis of the physical and immunological properties of the beta chain of CG produced by cells cultured from a cervical cancer indicated that two distinct forms of "ectopic" beta chain CG were produced. One is indistinguishable from the beta chain of placental CG, and the other lacks the COOH-terminal peptide (residues 116 to 145),[51] the portion that ordinarily distinguishes LH from CG (see Fig. 34–5). The molecular mass of normal liver CG is approximately 30 kd, consistent with the presence of little or no carbohydrate.[3] Furthermore, in in vitro Leydig cell bioassays, this material shows biological activity and also reacts in the COOH tail CG assay, which uses antisera directed against the unique COOH residues 116 to 145 of the beta chain of CG. Thus, all normal human tissues may synthesize the protein sequence of CG but not glycosylate it as richly as the placenta. The added carbohydrate residues protect the protein from rapid degradation and transform it into a hormone with patent bioactivity.

On the basis of the findings in normal tissues, it is not surprising that extracts of carcinomas contain CG, as tested in the beta chain CG radioimmunoassay, in the gonadotropin radioreceptor assay,[2, 3, 43] and by immunofluorescence techniques[52-54] (see Fig. 34–6). Because all cancers contain CG, the fact that only 6 to 13% of patients with cancer have detectable CG levels in blood must reflect some variable other than the capacity to produce CG. The fact that CG in cancer extracts exhibits variable concanavalin A binding indicates a variable carbohydrate content (or composition).

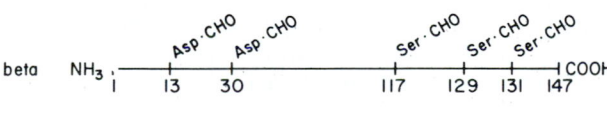

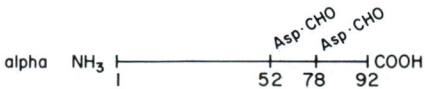

Figure 34–5. Human chorionic gonadotropin (hCG) structure shown schematically: the beta chain of placental hCG has 147 amino acids. Complex carbohydrate moieties are linked via asparagines at positions 13 and 30 and via serines at positions 117, 131, and 147. The beta chain of hCG is identical with that of human LH with the exception that the last 30 amino acids are not present in human LH. The alpha chain of hCG contains 92 amino acids and two asparagine-linked complex carbohydrate moieties. The hCG alpha differs from human LH alpha by a two-amino-acid inversion and a three-residue deletion at the NH₂ terminus. The carbohydrate moieties are made up of six different monosaccharides: D-mannose, N-acetylglucosamine, N-acetylgalactosamine, sialic acid, L-fucose, and D-galactose.

TABLE 34–6. Binding of Chorionic Gonadotropin to Concanavalin A

	Percent Bound (Mean ± SEM)	Range
Normal tissue (10)*†	6.1 ± 1.6	0.0–4.6
Cancer tissue (9)*	31.2 ± 9.1	4.0–86.0
Placenta (4)*	92.5 ± 0.9	90.1–94.0
Pregnant serum (3)*	100.0	
Cancer serum (8)*	54.7 ± 11.9	3.1–92.5

*Numbers in parentheses are numbers of patients studied.
†Extrapituitary tissue.

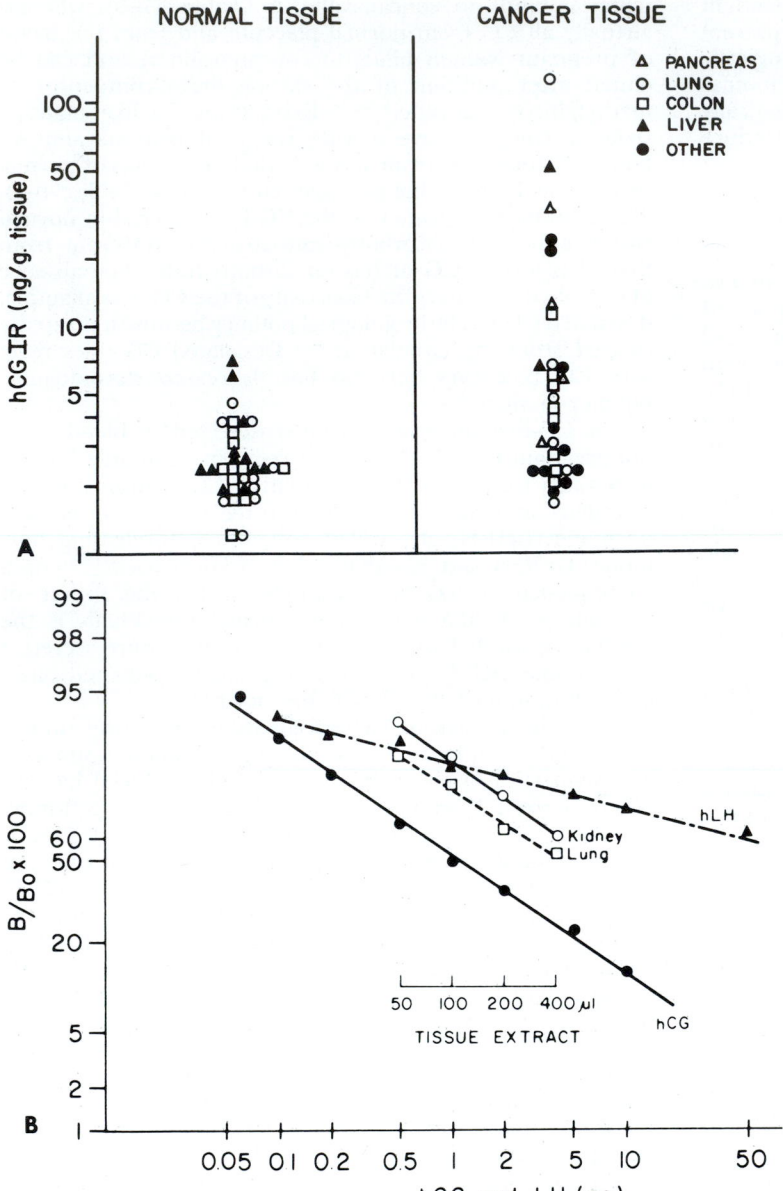

Figure 34–6. *A,* Human chorionic gonadotropin immunoreactivity (hCG IR) in acetic acid extracts of various carcinomas and normal tissues. hCG IR is presented on a log scale. (From Yoshimoto Y, Wolfsen AR, Odell WD. Glycosylation, a variable in the production of hCG by cancers. Am J Med 1979; 67:414–420.) *B,* Homologous hCG radioimmunoassay. Dose-response lines are shown for hCG reference preparation, for lung and kidney extracts, and for purified human LH. Results are shown as log dose of hCG standard or volume of lung or kidney extracts added per tube versus logit transformation of response. B_0, maximum ^{125}I counts bound with labeled hCG; B, counts bound in presence of labeled and unlabeled ligand. Purified human pituitary LH (LER-960) cross-reacted to 10% at the point of 80% of B/B_0, but did not show parallelism with hCG reference standard. (From Yoshimoto Y, Wolfsen AR, Hirose F, et al. Human chorionic gonadotropin–like material: presence in normal human tissues. Am J Obstet Gynecol 1979; 134:729–733.)

Therefore, the carcinomas associated with elevated blood CG levels probably glycosylate CG, increasing its half-time in the circulation. Thus an important variable is the level of glycosylation by the tumor cells.

In addition to the production of intact CG-like material, some tumors produce free alpha or beta subunits, and increased blood concentrations of free alpha chain may be more common than increased concentrations of intact CG. Weintraub and Rosen reported elaboration of the free beta chain of CG by an anaplastic pancreatic carcinoma[55] and elaboration of free alpha chains by a gastric carcinoid tumor.[56] Indeed, elevated serum concentrations of CG alpha chain can be found in a third of men with carcinoma of the lung, a fifth of men with gastric carcinoma, and a fifth of women with colon carcinoma.[2] Furthermore, elevated levels of CG have been reported in the blood of most patients with malignant pancreatic islet cell tumors but not in patients with benign islet cell tumors.[57]

In summary, small amounts of a CG-like material can be extracted from virtually all normal, nonendocrine tissues. A CG-like material is also present in small amounts in blood of normal humans and is probably secreted by the pituitary. In normal individuals this material appears to have little or no carbohydrate. In addition, a CG-like material is extractable from all carcinomas that are associated with increased quantities of CG in blood (so-called ectopic CG production). Carcinomas either produce greater amounts of this CG or glycosylate it, resulting in slower metabolism and enhanced biological activity.

Calcitonin

Calcitonin is normally produced by the parafollicular cells of the thyroid and is also a marker for medullary thyroid carcinoma that develops from these cells (see Chapters 8 and 30). Calcitonin is also produced ectopically by other carcinomas but typically causes no manifestations. The earliest reports of ectopic calcitonin production were by Milhaud and co-workers,[58] who described a carcinoid tumor that elaborated calcitonin, and Silva and colleagues,[59] who described hypercalcitoninemia in oat cell carcinoma of the

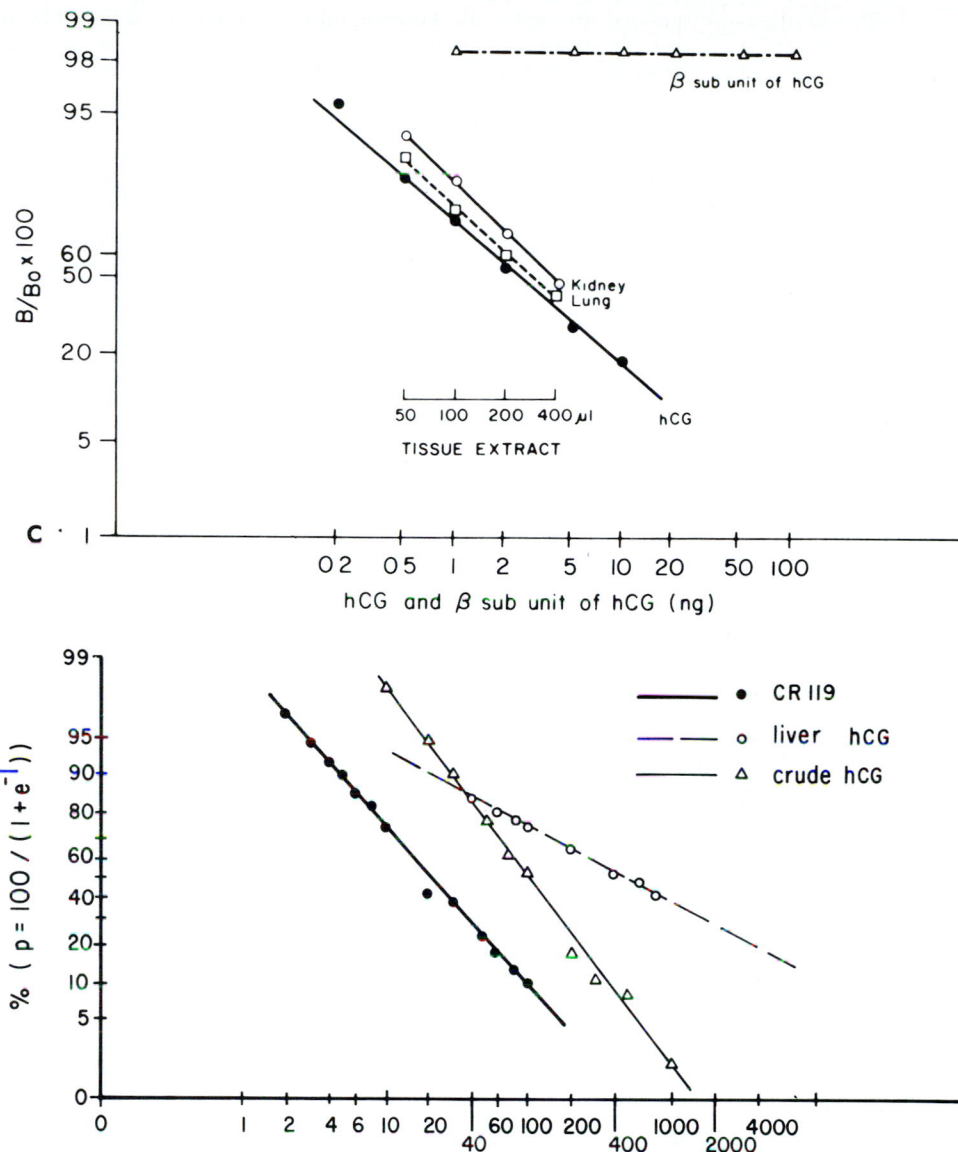

Figure 34–6 Continued C, Testicular LH-hCG radioreceptor assay. The amount of beta subunit of hCG or LH or the amount of tissue extract is plotted on the x axis. The y axis is plotted as in A and B. The beta subunit of hCG does not react in this assay. Human lung and kidney extracts produce dose-response curves parallel to that of purified hCG. (From Yoshimoto Y, Wolfsen A, Hirose F, et al. Human chorionic gonadotropin-like material: presence in normal human tissues. Am J Obstet Gynecol 1979; 134:729–733.) D, The COOH tail radioimmunoassay for hCG (believed to be specific for hCG). Liver hCG is a material extracted from human liver. The dose-response curve for liver hCG is not parallel to those of hCG in pregnancy (CR119 and crude hCG) and may be explained by a different carbohydrate composition or by differences in amino acid sequence. (From Odell WD, Saito F. Protein hormone–like materials from normal and cancer cells—"ectopic" hormone production. Prog Clin Biol Res 1983; 132E:247–258.)

lung. Patients with carcinoma of the lung and breast and elevated blood levels of calcitonin were then reported.[60, 61] Extracts of the breast carcinomas contained increased levels of immunoreactive calcitonin. Subsequently, 43 of 123 patients with carcinoma were found to have elevated plasma levels of calcitonin (>150 ng/L). These elevations were observed in 19 of 49 patients with carcinoma of the lung, 7 of 29 with colon cancer, 8 of 21 with breast cancer, 6 of 14 with pancreatic cancer, and 3 of 10 with gastric cancer.[62] In subsequent studies the frequency of elevated plasma calcitonin levels with malignant disease ranged from 35 to 60%.[60–62]

In some patients with nonthyroid tumors, the source of calcitonin might actually be the normal thyroid and not the tumor itself,[63] implying that the tumor could produce a substance that stimulates thyroid production of calcitonin. Alternatively, some factor only indirectly related to the tumor (e.g., stress or vitamin D metabolism by bone) might increase calcitonin production. Further studies will be required to ascertain whether increased production of calcitonin by the thyroid is common in nonthyroid cancers.

Vasopressin

The syndrome of hyponatremia, renal sodium loss, hypervolemia, and inappropriately high urine osmolality in patients with carcinoma was originally ascribed to sustained elaboration of vasopressin (AVP, also called antidiuretic hormone, ADH),[64] but the source of AVP was uncertain. In a further analysis of these patients, it was hypothesized that in some patients direct vagal stimulation by a lung carcinoma or the presence of brain metastases may cause pituitary hypersecretion of AVP or that the cancer itself could be the source.[65] Subsequently, an AVP-like material was demonstrated in tumor extracts from patients with carcinoma of the lung and the syndrome of inappropriate antidiuretic hormone (SIADH).[66, 67] In other cancer patients with inappropriate AVP secretion the AVP-like material in tumor extracts appeared to be identical with AVP by radioimmunoassay.[68] Subsequently, direct synthesis of AVP by lung cancer was demonstrated in vitro[69], and the AVP-like material was indistinguishable from AVP by bioassay, radioimmunoassay, and gel filtration.[70]

AVP and neurophysin are enzymatically cleaved into two separate products from the same precursor molecule, and neurophysin is present in tumor extracts associated with SIADH.[71] Elevated levels of neurophysins in plasma were also found in 11 of 26 patients with small cell carcinoma of the lung before therapy.[72]

The cancer most often associated with AVP production is cancer of the lung, commonly small cell or oat cell carcinoma. In one study 40% of patients with oat cell carcinoma had inappropriate AVP secretion.[73] Most carcinomas have not been studied for frequency of AVP elaboration, but squamous and anaplastic carcinomas of the lung, prostatic carcinoma,[74] carcinoma of the adrenal cortex,[75] and Hodgkin disease[76] can produce the syndrome. In one study 41% of patients with lung cancer of varied histological types and 43% of patients with carcinoma of the colon had inappropriately elevated levels of AVP and/or vasotocin.[2]

Many patients with elevated levels of AVP are not hyponatremic but might have developed the clinical syndrome if they had been water loaded. Indeed, Ginsberg and colleagues[77] reported that most patients with carcinoma extending beyond one hemithorax had abnormal water load test results, whereas only 4 of 11 patients with disease limited to one hemithorax had abnormal results.

Thus, in the absence of excess water intake, excess AVP may produce no symptoms. Furthermore, hyponatremia should be uncommon even when AVP is overproduced, provided thirst mechanisms are normally controlled. Thus to drink enough water to produce hyponatremia, patients with excess AVP levels must also have an abnormal thirst drive.

Erythropoietin

Polycythemia or erythrocytosis is common in patients with cancer, occurring in 3 to 12% of patients with hepatocellular carcinoma,[78] in 1 to 5% of patients with renal cell carcinoma,[79] and in most patients with renal carcinoma[79] (Table 34–7). However, the relation between increased levels of erythropoietin and erythrocytosis has been difficult to ascertain. By bioassay, erythropoietin levels are increased in virtually all patients with cancer and polycythemia.[80] Furthermore, extracts of tumor or renal cyst fluid usually contain greater amounts of erythropoietin than surrounding tissue.[80] In Wilms tumor, there is usually a correlation between tumor stage and plasma erythropoietin concentration,[81, 82] and several cell lines from human hepatic and renal cell carcinomas produce large amounts of erythropoietin in vitro.[83–85] In one study of patients with hepatocellular carcinoma, 15 of 65 had increased plasma erythropoietin levels by immunoassay, but only 4 had erythrocytosis.[86] Thus precursor of ineffective forms of erythropoietin may be produced that are immunologically reactive but lack biological activity.

Although the liver produces erythropoietin in the fetus,[87] the kidney is the predominant source of erythropoietin in adults.[88] Retention of the fetal secretory capacity by

TABLE 34–7. Tumors Associated with Erythrocytosis

Neoplasm	Approximate Percentage of Cases
Renal carcinomas	50
Cerebellar hemangioblastomas	20
Benign renal cysts and adenomas	15
Uterine fibroids	6
Miscellaneous*	9

*Hepatomas, adrenal carcinomas, virilizing ovarian neoplasms, lung carcinomas, thymomas, pheochromocytomas, paragangliomas, parotid fibrous histiocytomas.

neoplasms derived from those tissues is not surprising in the context of the current concepts of humoral syndromes of cancer (e.g., production of POMC and CG by both normal tissues and cancers from the same tissues).

Growth Hormone and Growth Hormone–Releasing Hormone

Acromegaly can also be associated with bronchial carcinoid or pancreatic tumors, and elevated serum growth hormone concentrations and the clinical syndrome of acromegaly may subside after removal of the tumor.[89–98] Because no therapy is directed to the hypothalamic-pituitary system, the cause must be related to the tumor.

One such patient, a 22-y-old woman with acromegaly, scoliosis, recurrent episodes of pneumonitis, and an enlarged sella turcica on x-ray examination, underwent hypophysectomy, and a histological diagnosis of eosinophilic adenoma was made.[94] However, serum growth hormone concentrations remained elevated. Because of recurrent episodes of pneumonia, a bronchial adenoma was suspected and diagnosed, and resection of the tumor caused growth hormone concentrations to fall to normal levels both before and after glucose loading. Extracts of the bronchial carcinoid contained a substance with growth hormone–releasing hormone (GHRH) activity, as assessed in vitro in a dispersed pituitary cell culture system. The authors concluded that the bronchial carcinoid elaborated a substance with growth hormone–releasing properties.

Subsequently, GHRH has been purified from tumors removed from several patients with this syndrome,[95–97] and the amino acid sequence of the hormone has been established.[98] GHRH is a 41-amino-acid protein normally produced by the hypothalamus and ectopically produced by rare neoplasms.

In some acromegalic patients, ectopic production of GHRH appears to induce a pituitary adenoma, but it appears unlikely that hypothalamic GHRH production is the cause of pituitary adenomas in most patients with acromegaly. Thorner and co-workers[99] assessed GHRH concentrations in 177 acromegalic patients and did not find any who had ectopic GHRH production as the cause. However, this possibility should be considered in patients with acromegaly and symptoms or findings suggesting an extrapituitary neoplasm.

In addition to ectopic GHRH production, growth hormone can be elaborated by neoplasms (e.g., lung tumors).[100–103] In one report,[104] growth hormone content was measured in tumor and normal tissue extracts by both radioreceptor assays and radioimmunoassays; high concentrations (over 10 ng/g tissue) were rare in normal tissues (e.g., 1 in 76 normal ovaries and none in two livers, four lungs, and four kidneys) but were common in primary or metastatic ovarian carcinomas. With both techniques, the highest concentrations were in breast cancer metastases and in cancer of the ovaries and skin. The lack of high levels of growth hormone in normal tissues has been confirmed,[105] but extracts of virtually all normal tissues contain small amounts of growth hormone, as assessed in both radioimmunoassays and radioreceptor assays. Thus production of growth hormone by tumors, like tumor production of POMC and other hormones, is the result of retention of the capacity of the normal tissue from which it arose.

Other Hypothalamic Neurosecretory Peptides

In addition to GHRH, CRH can also be produced by tumors (summarized in the earlier section on ACTH over-

TABLE 34–8. Types of Neoplasms Causing Hypoglycemia

Tumor Type	Approximate Percentage of Cases
Mesenchyma*	45
Hepatic carcinoma	23
Adrenal carcinoma	10
Gastrointestinal carcinoma†	8
Hematologic neoplasms	6
Miscellaneous	8

*Includes fibrosarcomas, mesotheliomas, neurofibromas, neurofibrosarcomas, spindle cell carcinomas, rhabdomyosarcomas, and leiomyosarcomas.
†Includes cholangiomas, gastric carcinomas, colon carcinomas, pancreatic carcinomas, and carcinoid tumors.
Modified from Odell WD. Paraendocrine syndromes of cancer. Adv Intern Med 1989; 34:325–352.

production). Production of somatostatin (SRIF, somatotropin release–inhibiting factor) occurred in 8 of 11 cell lines of small cell carcinoma.[106] To date, production of thyrotropin-releasing hormone or LHRH by tumors has not been reported.

Hypoglycemia-Producing Factors

In contrast to the tumors that cause most humoral syndromes, the neoplasms that produce hypoglycemia are usually mesenchymal tumors and include fibrosarcoma, neurofibroma, neurofibrosarcoma, spindle cell carcinoma, rhabdomyosarcoma, and leiomyosarcoma (Table 34–8). These neoplasms are usually quite large at the time hypoglycemia is noted, ranging from 800 to 10,000 g and averaging 2400 g in weight. Two thirds arise in the abdomen, in either peritoneal or retroperitoneal sites, and the remainder are in the thorax. The incidence is the same in males and females.*

Hypoglycemia associated with hepatic carcinomas can occur before diagnosis of the neoplasm, when liver function is normal or nearly normal. Thus the hypoglycemia cannot be caused simply by replacement of normal liver parenchyma by tumor and a decrease in hepatic glucose production. Furthermore, hypoglycemia is common in patients with primary hepatic neoplasms but rare in patients with metastatic carcinomas that infiltrate and replace much of the liver.

Hypoglycemia has also been described in association with malignant diseases of white blood cells.[108–110] In some instances, the hypoglycemia was an artifact because blood containing malignant cells was collected in tubes that permitted continued glucose utilization in vitro,[110] whereas in other cases, a true ectopic humoral syndrome appeared to exist.[108, 109]

The etiology of hypoglycemia in these various forms of malignant disease remains poorly understood. In 25 neoplasms associated with hypoglycemia, insulin-like activity could be demonstrated in all with an insulin bioassay (rat diaphragm and epididymal fat pad assays).[111] However, acid-alcohol extracts (used to extract insulin per se) exhibited less bioactivity than extracts made with saline solution, water, or buffer, and the extracts contained no insulin, as determined by radioimmunoassay.[111, 112] In addition, only rare patients have elevated plasma and tumor insulin levels in association with tumor hypoglycemia.[113–116]

Since the material extracted from tumors has insulin biological activity but fails to react in insulin radioimmunoassays, insulin-like growth factors (IGFs) have been implicated. For example, in studies using a radioreceptor assay, elevated plasma concentrations of a somatomedin-like or

IGF substance were demonstrated in five of seven patients with cancer and hypoglycemia.[117] In another study using a radioreceptor assay, 19 of 52 patients (37%) with tumor hypoglycemia had elevated IGF levels.[118] With a bioassay an elevated IGF II level was found in 10 of 14 patients with cancer-associated hypoglycemia.[119] In a 67-y-old woman with a large leiomyosarcoma and hypoglycemia, concentrations of IGF I (also called somatomedin-C) in both tumor and serum were low, tumor and serum levels of proIGF II were elevated, and tumor content of IGF II was elevated.[120] Removal of the tumor led to a decrease in serum proIGF II to undetectable levels and of IGF II to normal values (Fig. 34–7, Table 34–9). IGF II may cause hypoglycemia by a dual mechanism: increased glucose utilization as a consequence of insulin-like actions and inhibition of growth hormone secretion.[121] However, it has not been possible to show that production of IGF is a common cause of hypoglycemia. Two groups of investigators[122, 123] using both radioimmunoassays and radioreceptor assays for IGF I and IGF II were unable to demonstrate elevated IGF concentrations in serum from patients with this syndrome.

Differences in details of methodology may explain some of the discrepancies in published reports. More important, the same cancer-produced substance may not cause hypo-

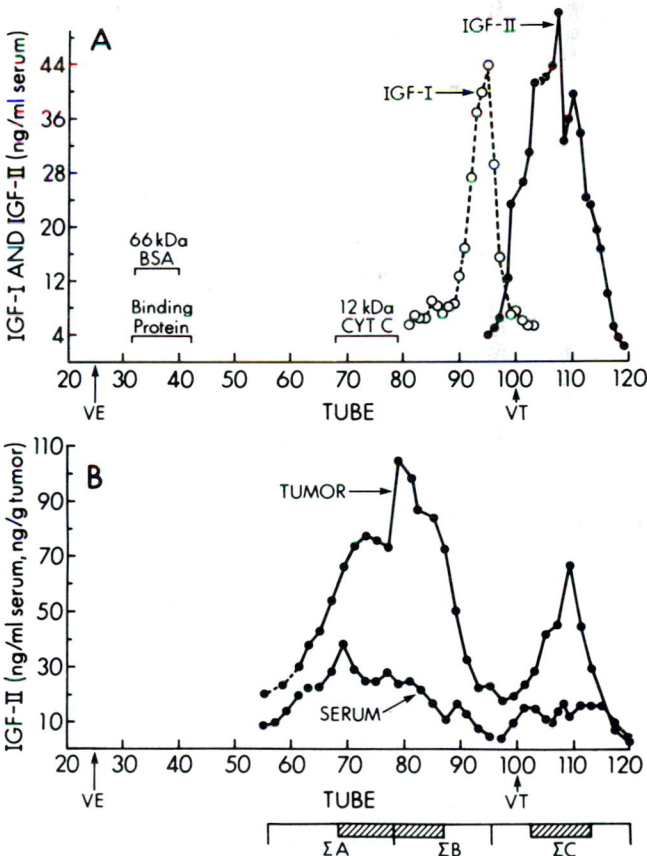

Figure 34–7. Identification of IGF II in serum and tumor extract from a 67-y-old woman with hypoglycemia caused by leiomyosarcoma. The concentrations of IGF I and IGF II were determined by specific radioimmunoassays. *A*, Elution positions of IGF I and IGF II and of bovine serum albumin (BSA) and cytochrome *c* (CYT C) as marker proteins. The column used was a BioGel P-60. *B*, Elution profile of IGF II activity in acetic acid extracts of tumor and acidified serum samples. IGF I concentrations in serum were low and IGF I was not detectable in tumor. The IGF II eluted in the position of lower-molecular-weight precursor forms of IGF II. To convert IGF II values (nanograms per gram or per milliliter) to micrograms per kilogram or per liter, multiply by 1. (From Daughaday WH, Emanuele MA, Brooks MH, et al. Synthesis and secretion of insulin-like growth factor II by a leiomyosarcoma with associated hypoglycemia. Reprinted with permission from The New England Journal of Medicine, 319, 1434–1440, 1988.)

*References to many case reports are given in earlier editions of this textbook.[107]

TABLE 34–9. Measurements of IGF I and IGF II Levels in Preoperative Serum and in Recurrent Tumor Obtained by Radioimmunoassay and Radioreceptor Assay*

	Radioimmunoassay		Radioreceptor Assay
	IGF I	IGF II†	IGF II
Serum (μg/L)			
Acid ethanol extraction	29	414	697
P-60 column			
HMW fraction A	—	534 (46)	—
HMW fraction B	—	273 (24)	—
LMW fraction C	—	342 (30)	—
Fraction A + B + C		1149	
Tumor (ng/g)			
Sep-Pak purified P-60 column	17.1	2100	—
Fraction A	—	1072 (37)	—
Pool A (tubes 67–77)	2.4	500	500
Fraction B	—	1172 (40)	—
Pool B (tubes 78–87)	2.1	850	808
Fraction C	—	682 (23)	—
Pool C (tubes 102–113)	1.5	280	512
Fraction A + B + C		2926	

*Serum measurements were made before the second operation. Other measurements were made on a portion of the tumor removed during the second operation. HMW, high molecular weight; LMW, low molecular weight.

†Numbers in parentheses are percentages.

From Daughaday WH, Emanuele MA, Brooks MH, et al. Synthesis and secretion of insulin-like growth factor II by a leiomyosarcoma with associated hypoglycemia. Reprinted with permission from The New England Journal of Medicine, 319, 1434–1440, 1988.

glycemia in every patient, and several IGFs and nonsuppressible insulin-like materials may be implicated. A fraction of such patients may have cancers that produce insulin itself. As with ACTH and CG, extracts of normal nonendocrine tissues may contain insulin.[124] It is not known whether normal nonendocrine tissues also contain IGF I or IGF II.

Hypercalcemia-Producing Factors

Neoplasms can produce hypercalcemia by at least four mechanisms (Table 34–10): (1) Solid tumors without evidence of bone metastases or with minimal metastatic disease can secrete proteins (e.g., parathyroid hormone–related protein [PTHRP]) that bind to the parathyroid hormone receptor. (2) Hematological malignancies can produce cytokines and possibly prostaglandins that act locally to mobilize bone calcium and phosphorus. Some such hematological malignancies hydroxylate 25-hydroxycholecalciferol (25-OHD) to 1,25-dihydroxycholecalciferol (1,25(OH)$_2$D), which causes vitamin D toxicity and hypercalcemia. (3) Rare solid tumors may secrete authentic parathyroid hormone. (4) Neoplasms with widespread bone metastases, typified by breast carcinoma, can cause hypercalcemia by enhancing bone resorption directly.

The association of hypercalcemia and solid tumors was one of the earliest described humoral manifestations of malignant disease. In 1924 Zondek and colleagues[125] described a man with hypercalcemia who at autopsy had normal parathyroids and carcinoma of the gallbladder. In 1936 Gutman and co-workers[126] reported a patient with hypophosphatemia, hypercalcemia, and a bronchogenic carcinoma. A possible cause of the hypercalcemia in such patients was first suggested by Albright,[127] who in describing a patient with renal cell carcinoma, hypercalcemia, and hypophosphatemia, pointed out that both hypercalcemia and hyperphosphatemia would be expected if bone metastases per se caused hypercalcemia and therefore postulated that the tumor must make a parathyroid hormone–like substance. At autopsy, no abnormalities were identified in the parathyroid glands.

Subsequently, evidence from early parathyroid hormone immunoassays supported the hypothesis that parathyroid hormone per se is a cause of cancer hypercalcemia.[128–132] However, in 1971 a patient with squamous cell carcinoma was described with hypercalcemia and hypophos-

phatemia but no detectable plasma parathyroid hormone by radioimmunoassay.[133] Furthermore, 11 other patients were described who had hypercalcemia, hypophosphatemia, and cancer and no demonstrable bone metastases but no parathyroid hormone detectable in either tumor extracts or blood.[134] However, all 11 tumor extracts caused bone resorption as indicated by in vitro calcium resorption from mouse calvarium. Furthermore, additional cancers that produce hypercalcemia have been studied and no parathyroid hormone messenger RNA was detected.[135] Therefore, it was concluded that a substance other than parathyroid hormone is elaborated by tumors that produce hypercalcemia.

Histologically, the bones of patients with cancer and hypercalcemia resemble those of patients with hyperparathyroidism, suggesting that the hypercalcemic factor has biological effects similar to those of parathyroid hormone. When a histocytochemical bioassay for parathyroid hormone was employed to evaluate cancer patients with hypercalcemia and increased nephrogenous cyclic AMP excretion, parathyroid hormone–like activity in the plasma was elevated in most.[136] Tumor extracts and cell-conditioned media also stimulate cyclic AMP production in vitro,[137] and the fact that similar effects are produced by media from cultured keratinocytes[138] suggests that this substance is also produced by normal cells.

TABLE 34–10. Types of Neoplasms Associated with Hypercalcemia

Type of Neoplasm	Approximate Percentage of Cases
Solid tumors	
Carcinoma of the lung	35
Carcinoma of the kidney	24
Carcinoma of the ovary	8
Miscellaneous carcinomas*	<2 each
Hematologic malignant neoplasms	
Multiple myeloma	7
T cell lymphoma	2
Other	1
Tumors with bone metastases	
Breast carcinoma	Not included in
Others	frequency estimates

*This includes almost any type of carcinoma (e.g., pancreas, urinary bladder, colon, prostate, penis, esophagus, parotid glands, testes, liver, stomach).

Modified from Odell WD. Paraendocrine syndromes of cancer. Adv Intern Med 1989; 34:325–352.

The proteins responsible have been purified, and partial amino acid sequences have been identified by five groups of investigators.[139–143] Subsequently, the cDNAs encoding a single gene have been cloned and shown to be expressed as three distinct proteins because of alternative splicing.[144, 145] The most abundant cDNA encodes a mature protein of 139 amino acids.[144] The sequence of amino acids 1 to 34 of this protein is similar to that of human parathyroid hormone, and this region is critical in receptor binding. Furthermore, the 139-amino-acid protein has biological effects similar to those of parathyroid hormone.[146] These PTHRPs are expressed in mammary tissues during lactation under control of prolactin[147, 147a] and in the human endocrine pancreas.[147b] PTHRP, which is present in several fetal tissues, promotes differentiation in some embryonal carcinoma cell lines[147c] and may play a role in calcium transport in the placenta.[147d]

In brief, hypercalcemia caused by solid tumors is commonly due to production of one or more proteins that bind to the parathyroid hormone receptor and have biological activities similar to those of parathyroid hormone. The failure of these proteins to react in parathyroid hormone immunoassays is due to the fact that the proteins are different throughout a large portion of their structure. The PTHRP level is increased in blood and/or tumor tissue in patients with hypercalcemia associated with cancer.[147e–147g] Some normal tissues express PTHRP, so elevated blood levels may not be diagnostic of cancer. For example, hypercalcemia in a woman with massive mammary hyperplasia was associated with PTHRP messenger RNA expression in breast tissue.[147h]

However, additional types of proteins may cause hypercalcemia in some patients with solid tumors. For example, not all patients with tumoral hypercalcemia have increased urinary cyclic AMP excretion.[137] In addition, some growth factors associated with neoplasms are powerful stimulators of bone resorption and may be the cause of hypercalcemia in occasional patients with solid tumors. For example, transforming growth factor α (TGF α), a 5-kd peptide, is more potent than parathyroid hormone in stimulating bone resorption,[148, 149] is produced by some carcinomas, and appears to be the cause of elevated calcium levels in two rat models of solid tumor hypercalcemia and in two human models of cancer hypercalcemia.[150] In one of the rat models (Leydig cell tumor) that produces TGF α, the increased bone resorption can be inhibited by antiserum to the TGF α receptor.

TGF β is larger than TGF α, is composed of two dimers, each with a molecular mass of 12.5 kd, and is produced by many normal tissues (e.g., platelets and bone cells) and many tumors. Like TGF α, it is more potent than parathyroid hormone in stimulating bone resorption.[149, 150] The Walker rat carcinosarcoma produces hypercalcemia via TGF β production.[151]

Production of authentic parathyroid hormone is a rare cause of tumor hypercalcemia; one such case was associated with a rearrangement of the parathyroid hormone gene.[151a]

Whatever the causes, hypercalcemia in cancer is relatively common.[152] In 200 consecutive patients with bronchogenic carcinoma, a tenth or more had hypercalcemia, the frequency depending on the type of cancer: 23% of patients with epidermoid carcinoma, 13% of those with large cell anaplastic carcinoma, and 2% of subjects with adenocarcinomas. Also, 14 of 20 patients with hypercalcemia did not have demonstrable metastases to bone.[152] In another series of 126 consecutive patients with hypercalcemia of malignancy, the median survival was only 30 d.[152a]

As with other hormones produced by cancer cells, nonparathyroid hypercalcemic factors are produced in small amounts by normal cells. Most solid tumors appear to cause hypercalcemia by increased production of these proteins that bind to the parathyroid hormone receptor. Other solid tumors may produce hypercalcemia by increased production of one or more growth factors.

Hematological malignancies can also cause hypercalcemia. For example, elevated serum calcium levels occur in 20 to 40% of patients with multiple myeloma.[150] In 1974 it was reported that a bone-resorbing substance produced by myeloma cells is similar to osteoclast-activating factor produced by normal activated leukocytes.[153] Osteoclast-activating factor activity consists of more than one substance, including lymphotoxin (produced by lymphocytes) and tumor necrosis factor (TNF) or cachectin (produced by monocytes).[154] Both lymphotoxin and TNF are potent stimulators of bone resorption in vitro.[150] Cultured myeloma cells secrete lymphotoxin, and this production may be related to the hypercalcemia caused by the myeloma.[155]

Additional factors have been implicated in causing hypercalcemia. More than half of patients with the type C virus-induced T cell lymphoma have hypercalcemia,[156, 157] and these tumors produce increased quantities of cytokines.[153] However, these patients have increased $1,25(OH)_2D$ concentrations in blood,[158, 159] and a teen-age boy has been reported with a large plasma cell granuloma, hypercalcemia, and increased blood levels of $1,25(OH)_2D$.[160] After tumor resection, $1,25(OH)_2D$ concentrations in blood returned to normal. Subsequently, plasma cell tumor homogenates were shown to synthesize $1,25(OH)_2D$. Hypercalcemia associated with increased blood $1,25(OH)_2D$ has also been reported in a patient with leiomyoblastoma[161] and in another with Hodgkin disease.[162] Patients with solid tumors and hypercalcemia do not have elevated blood $1,25(OH)_2D$ levels.

Metastases to bone may cause hypercalcemia by direct resorption of bone, and hyperparathyroidism and cancer in the same patient can produce cystic bone lesions that mimic metastases.[163] To differentiate hyperparathyroidism from cancer-induced hypercalcemia, the best current diagnostic procedure is the sandwich-type or immunometric parathyroid hormone assay. Over 90% of patients with hyperparathyroidism have elevated intact parathyroid hormone levels, whereas most patients with hypercalcemia caused by cancer have low or "normal" values.

Regardless of the mechanism by which neoplasms produce hypercalcemia, no therapy is entirely satisfactory.[164–166] Isotonic sodium chloride infused at a rate of 200 to 300 mL/h is often effective; higher infusion rates of 10 to 20 L/d have also been advocated, but such high rates require careful monitoring of the central venous pressure and frequent assessment for volume overload. If saline infusion does not lower the serum calcium levels, the administration of 40 to 60 mg of furosemide one to four times daily with adequate saline hydration is usually effective (also see Chapter 27). The patient should *not* be kept immobilized, and as much activity as practical should be encouraged. The next line of treatment includes calcitonin given twice daily, in combination with prednisone (40 to 60 mg/d).[166, 167] Calcitonin inhibits osteoclastic bone resorption. If calcitonin is effective, the response is rapid, but escape is common within a few days. Plicamycin usually lowers the serum calcium level in patients with cancer and probably acts by inhibiting osteoclast activity, but hematological toxicity often limits its use. Diphosphonates such as etidronate also inhibit osteoclast activity and are often effective in hypercalcemia of cancer.[166–168] The prolonged use of phosphorus in oral doses of 500 to 1500 mg several times per day may be useful in the long-term management of hypercalcemia caused by cancer but can lead to soft tissue calcification.

Hypocalcemia

Hypocalcemia is occasionally associated with cancer, for example, in patients with lung cancer,[169] prostatic carcinoma,[170] or chronic leukemia,[171] particularly after effective therapy. Hypocalcemia and hypophosphatemia also occur in patients with breast cancer and osseous metastases.[172, 173] Vitamin D deficiency and rapid bone formation were originally considered to be the most likely causes, but the syndrome was described before the relation of magnesium deficiency to parathyroid hormone secretion and action was recognized. In contrast to patients with *hypo*phosphatemia and hypocalcemia, six children with acute lymphoblastic leukemia developed *hyper*phosphatemia and hypocalcemia, possibly because hyperphosphatemia led to precipitation of calcium phosphate and hypocalcemia.[174] Some of the neoplasms associated with hypocalcemia and normal or low phosphate levels may produce excess calcitonin. However, calcitonin should not produce hyperphosphatemia, and hypocalcemia is not part of the thyroid medullary carcinoma syndrome in which levels of circulating calcitonin can be massive.

In summary, cancer-associated hypocalcemia is probably due to more than one cause. In hypocalcemia associated with hypophosphatemia, rapid bone calcification of unknown direct cause may be responsible. In hypocalcemia associated with hyperphosphatemia, dietary phosphate and a decrease in renal function may be the cause. It is not certain that the cancer is the direct cause of the hypocalcemia.

Hypophosphatemia

Hypophosphatemia with a normal serum calcium level has been described in approximately 50 patients with diverse neoplasms: pleomorphic sarcomas or mesenchymal neoplasms, giant cell tumors of bone, and prostatic carcinoma. This syndrome is associated with phosphaturia, glucosuria, and aminoaciduria (i.e., Fanconi syndrome). Blood parathyroid hormone and calcium concentrations are normal, and there is rapid reversal of urine and blood changes with tumor removal. These patients usually have muscle spasms and cramps or symptoms related to advanced osteomalacia.

In 1977 Drezner and Feinglos[175] reviewed published reports of the syndrome, summarized the clinical features, and described vitamin D metabolism in a woman with osteomalacia and a giant cell tumor of bone who had a normal plasma parathyroid hormone level. Serum 25-OHD concentrations were normal and $1,25(OH)_2D$ levels were low. Treatment with physiological amounts of calcitriol reversed the hypophosphatemia, which recurred when therapy was stopped. Resection of the tumor permanently abolished hypophosphatemia. These investigators postulated that the tumors elaborated a substance that inhibited 1-hydroxylation of 25-OHD. Similar findings were reported by Fukumoto and colleagues[176] who described a patient with a benign osteoblastoma of the tibia who responded partially to calcitriol and was cured by resection of the tumor. The defect is located in the proximal tubule of the nephron and is associated with aminoaciduria and glucosuria. Hypophosphatemia occurs in about a fifth of patients with prostatic carcinoma.[177] In one study, five such patients had renal phosphate wasting, normal 25-OHD levels, and low $1,25(OH)_2D$ levels.[177]

In 1988 Miyauchi and co-workers[178] reported a 54-y-old man with a hemangiopericytoma who had phosphaturia, glycosuria (with normal blood glucose level), and aminoaciduria. The serum phosphorus level was low and the alkaline phosphatase level was elevated. Resection of the tumor

resulted in an increase of serum phosphorus concentration to normal values, and bone pain subsided. This tumor was transplanted into nude mice, and the animals developed hypophosphatemia, increased urinary phosphorus excretion, and increased blood alkaline phosphatase concentration. In addition, tumor extracts inhibited 25-hydroxycholecalciferol 1α-hydroxylase activity in cultured kidney cells.

In summary, hypophosphatemia produced by mesenchymal tumors, prostatic carcinoma, and endodermal malignancy is associated with renal phosphate wasting and low $1,25(OH)_2D$ concentrations. The tumor also causes the Fanconi syndrome (glycosuria and aminoaciduria), but the mechanisms remain unknown.

PARANEOPLASTIC SYNDROMES OF THE NERVOUS SYSTEM

Paraneoplastic syndromes of the nervous system (see Table 34–2) are produced by at least two mechanisms: (1) stimulation of formation by the host of antibodies that cross-react with a host tissue resulting in alteration of structure or function or (2) viral infection of the nervous system, presumably because the tumor-bearing host has increased susceptibility.

Cerebellar Syndromes

Cerebellar degeneration can occur as a remote effect in patients with carcinomas of the lung, ovary, breast, uterus, stomach, colon, larynx, or fallopian tubes; Hodgkin, non-Hodgkin, and T cell lymphomas; malignant melanoma; and chondrosarcoma.[179, 180] In most patients the symptoms of cerebellar dysfunction are present months to years before the neoplasm is diagnosed. The cerebrospinal fluid is usually abnormal with increased concentrations of protein, gammaglobulin, and lymphocytes. This syndrome appears to be caused by tumor stimulation of the production of autoantibodies that cross-react with antigens in the cerebellum. In one patient with Hodgkin disease and cerebellar degeneration the serum contained antibodies that reacted with cerebellar Purkinje cells,[181] and the cerebrospinal fluid of one woman with this syndrome caused by ovarian carcinoma contained antibodies that bound to neonatal mouse cerebellum.[182] Additional patients with ovarian cancer and cerebellar degeneration have serum antibodies that react with Purkinje cells and with cells in the deep cerebellar nuclei.[183, 184] Additional patients with this syndrome include a 63-y-old man with a large chondrosarcoma and a 58-y-old woman with fallopian tube carcinoma, who had loss of cerebellar symptoms after resection of the tumor.[185]

In 1987 Dropcho and colleagues[186] cloned the cDNA for a brain protein identified by autoantibodies from a patient with this syndrome and a metastatic adenocarcinoma of unknown primary origin. A sequence of 18 nucleotides (six amino acids) repeated in tandem along the entire cDNA. Expression of this gene in normal tissues is largely restricted to brain tissue, but the gene is also expressed in cell lines from human cancers of neuroectodermal, renal, and pulmonary origin.

A second syndrome of cerebellar degeneration occurs in occasional children with neuroblastoma. The pathogenesis of this syndrome, termed *myoclonic encephalopathy*, is not known.[179]

In summary, cerebellar degeneration in patients with cancer appears to be due to tumor production of a protein (or proteins) that is normally restricted to brain tissue.

Resulting stimulation of antibody formation leads to neuronal damage and loss of cerebellar function.

Subacute Sensory Neuropathy

Subacute sensory neuropathy in patients with cancer causes progressive loss of sensory function, areflexia, and sensory ataxia. Motor function and other central nervous functions often remain intact as the debilitating sensory disorder progresses. The syndrome is associated with perivascular inflammatory cell infiltrates in dorsal root ganglia. Secondary to neuronal loss, degeneration of axons and demyelination of sensory nerves and dorsal posterior roots occur in the spinal cord. Most patients with this syndrome have small cell carcinoma of the lung. Four patients with small cell carcinoma and subacute sensory neuropathy had serum antibodies that reacted with nuclei of neurons.[187] The tumor antigen responsible for stimulating antibody production was a basic protein of 38 kd, and it was hypothesized that this syndrome was caused by an antibody directed against a tumor antigen that cross-reacts with a brain protein.

Furthermore, complement-fixing polyclonal immunoglobulin G from cancer patients with paraneoplastic nervous system disorders has been termed anti-Hu.[188, 189] Anti-Hu antibodies react with neuronal nuclei in the central nervous system, dorsal root, and trigeminal ganglia but do not react with non-neuronal nuclei and recognize nucleoprotein antigens with molecular masses of 35 to 40 kd.[189] Although these antibodies were initially thought to be a marker of small cell lung cancer and subacute sensory neuropathy, Graus and colleagues[189] reported anti-Hu was present in serum from a patient with subacute sensory neuropathy, dorsal root ganglionitis, and paraneoplastic encephalomyelitis. However, in 1988 Anderson and colleagues[190] reviewed the clinical, immunological, and pathological findings for 14 antibody-positive patients, all of whom had small cell carcinoma of the lung but varied clinical symptoms. Eight of the 14 patients had subacute sensory neuropathy, 2 had lower motor neuron weakness, 1 had autonomic neuropathy, 1 had cerebellar ataxia, 1 had myelopathy, and 1 had encephalomyelitis.

Considered together, these data suggest that anti-Hu is specific for small cell lung cancer with an associated paraneoplastic syndrome but that the manifestations of the antibody vary from patient to patient.

Visual Paraneoplastic Syndrome

This disorder has been described under several names, including visual paraneoplastic syndrome, photoreceptor degeneration, cancer-associated retinopathy, and paraneoplastic retinopathy. In 1976 Sawyer and colleagues[191] described a patient with metastatic oat cell carcinoma of the lung, night blindness, and visual hallucinations (e.g., shimmering, flickering, gold specks). Approximately 16 additional patients have since been reported. The majority[191–196] had small cell carcinoma of the lung, but patients with non–small cell cancer of the lung,[195] cervical cancer,[197] adenocarcinoma of the breast,[198] malignant melanoma,[199] and cancer of the uterine endometrium[200] have also been described. As with cerebellar cortical degeneration, symptoms may occur before the neoplasm is diagnosed.

Serum from two patients with this disorder contained antibodies that reacted with both the cancer cells and normal retina,[193] and some patients with visual paraneoplastic syndrome produce antibodies that react with retinal ganglion cells, photoreceptors, and small cell carcinoma.[192, 194] The antigens resemble proteins comprising a neurofilament triplet and are present in lung cancer. The serum of one patient with endometrial cancer of the uterus and this syndrome contained high titers (1:1000) of antibodies reacting with human retina and optic nerve.[200] Berson and Lessell[199] subsequently reported a man with acute onset of night blindness and visual hallucinations 3 y after a cutaneous malignant melanoma was resected. Several months after the onset of the visual symptoms, metastatic melanoma without ocular involvement was diagnosed, but serum from this patient was not examined for the presence of antibodies against the retina.

In summary, the visual paraneoplastic syndrome is probably caused by tumor stimulation of the production of antibodies that react against antigens shared by the tumor and retina and/or optic nerve. Interestingly, low titers of such antibodies may be present in normal serum.[201]

Limbic and Bulbar Encephalitis

These syndromes have been reported in a small number of patients[202] and the pathophysiology is unknown. Limbic encephalitis is characterized by subacute onset of dementia and loss of recent memory. Bulbar encephalitis or brain stem encephalitis is associated most frequently with lung cancer. Patients may present variably with dystonia, ophthalmoplegia, seizures, or central hypoventilation.[180]

Multifocal Leukoencephalopathy

Progressive multifocal leukoencephalopathy (PML) is an acute to subacute progressive disease that affects multiple areas of the central nervous system, most commonly the cerebrum, with alterations in cognitive functions, speech, movement, and sensation. Intellectual impairment and pyramidal tract changes occur in three fourths of patients. Pathological findings consist of multiple loci of demyelination with enlargement of oligodendroglial nuclei, loss of nuclear structure, and eosinophilic intranuclear inclusions. Astroglial proliferation occurs with bizarre transformation of nuclei, which resemble those of neoplastic cells. These microscopic findings are specific for PML.[202] PML is associated with lymphoreticular cancers and with lung cancers. It is not a humoral syndrome but is described here to complete the review of paraneoplastic syndromes of the nervous system. In 1965 Zu Rhein and Chou[203] demonstrated papovavirus-like particles in oligodendroglial cells by electron microscopy. The virus has been isolated and transmitted to animals.[204] PML has also been described in patients with severe systemic lupus erythematosus and in patients with acquired immunodeficiency syndrome.

Skeletal Muscle Syndromes

Polymyositis and dermatomyositis are related skeletal muscle disorders sometimes treated as a single entity. Both are characterized by proximal muscle weakness, inflammatory myopathy, and mononuclear cell infiltration in muscle. When the diagnostic criteria for polymyositis-dermatomyositis are not met, the term *carcinomatous neuromyopathy* is used. There have been many reports of an association between the development of these disorders and cancer, especially in patients older than age 40. This association occurs in patients with a wide variety of malignancies, including ovarian carcinoma,[205] Hodgkin disease,[206] and histiocytic lymphoma.[207] Because most patients have circulating antibodies against myosin or myoglobin, it has been speculated that a tumor antigen can elicit the production of antibodies that cross-react with a component of muscle tissue. Nevertheless, a cause-effect relationship has not been established. Barnes[208] reviewed 258 reported cases of dermatomyositis associated with malignancies and found that the diagnosis of cancer preceded the appearance of myopathy in a third. However, in 115 patients at the Mayo Clinc no difference was found between the incidence of cancer and the presence or absence of polymyositis-dermatomyositis.[209]

Myasthenic Syndromes

Myasthenic syndromes (e.g., Eaton-Lambert syndrome) are disorders of the neuromuscular junction caused by impaired release of acetylcholine from presynaptic nerve terminals. This diminished release appears to be caused by autoantibodies against presynaptic calcium channels.[210] Although this syndrome is associated with cancer, in particular bronchogenic carcinoma,[211] a causative relationship has not been established.

MISCELLANEOUS SYNDROMES

Table 34–2 also lists disorders usually thought to be produced by cancer as a humoral syndrome. For the most part, the agent (or agents) responsible for these syndromes remains speculative. When no mechanism is identified the association of these syndromes with cancer is based on less than rigorous data.

Anorexia

Anorexia may be an early symptom of cancer, particularly of carcinoma of the lung, hypernephroma, and carcinoma of the pancreas. A possible mediator of anorexia is TNF or cachectin. Starting from two seemingly unrelated points of view, investigators purified and determined the structure of a single protein with a spectrum of biological properties.

In 1975 Carswell and colleagues[212] reported that serum from endotoxin-treated animals previously infected with *Mycobacterium bovis* causes hemorrhagic necrosis of tumors in mice. The normal host tissue was not affected by the serum. The factor responsible, termed *tumor necrosis factor*, is cytotoxic against several transformed cell lines in vitro but not against normal cells. Shear and colleagues[213] isolated and partially purified TNF, a protein of 17 kd, with an isoelectric point of 5.3, and containing two cysteines in a disulfide bridge.[214]

Approaching another problem, Rouzer and Cerami[215] noted in 1980 that rabbits injected with *Trypanosoma brucei* manifest weight loss and wasting beyond the expected effects of the parasitic burden. During the later stages of this disease a profound lipemia develops, and when endotoxin-sensitive mice are given bacterial lipopolysaccharide, lipemia and suppression of lipoprotein lipase occur.[216] Endotoxin-resistant mice do not exhibit this response, but injection of serum from the endotoxin-sensitive animals produces lipemia and inhibition of lipoprotein lipase. The factor responsible for these effects is a product of macrophages from endotoxin-sensitive animals. This factor, cachectin, was purified from endotoxin-activated murine macrophages and shown to be a protein of 17 kd.[217] TNF and cachectin were found to be immunologically identical, to share bioactivities, and to have similar amino acid sequences.[218] The identity of the two substances was verified by sequence analysis.[219]

Cachectin/TNF is produced by macrophages as a prohormone that, like most prohormones, is biologically inactive[220] and is cleaved to the biologically active form. Glucocorticoids inhibit cachectin synthesis if they are applied to macrophages before activation. After injection of endotoxin, cachectin appears in the circulation within minutes, peaks in 2 h, and then rapidly disappears from plasma. Injections of cachectin produce many of the deleterious effects previously attributed to endotoxin and may produce profound anorexia. Cachectin is also a potent bone-resorbing substance.

Because anorexia and weight loss are common early symptoms in cancer, it is natural to ask whether cachectin/TNF may be produced by the tumor itself or as a host response to cancer.[221] In 1985 Aderka and colleagues[222] reported that TNF is produced by peripheral blood mononuclear cells of patients with cancer, and half of freshly obtained serum samples from cancer patients had detectable TNF as shown by enzyme-linked immunosorbent assay.[223] In contrast, only 1 of 32 samples (3%) from normal subjects and 7 of 39 samples (18%) from asymptomatic patients with cancer had detectable TNF. In addition, 69% of patients with ovarian cancer and 63% of patients with oat cell lung carcinoma had detectable TNF. However, several investigators[224–227] have reported that TNF is not detectable in patients with cancer and cachexia.

The explanation for these differences is uncertain, but several factors may be involved. (1) Balkwill and co-workers[223] emphasized the importance of fresh serum because cachectin/TNF may be labile. (2) Selby and colleagues[228] primarily studied lymphoma patients, whereas other types of patients were studied by Balkwill and co-workers.[223] (3) Balkwill and colleagues[223] used a simple monoclonal antibody in an equilibrium-type assay, whereas the assays of Socher and associates[224] and those of Selby and colleagues[227] react only with the intact molecule. (4) Nevertheless, Selby and co-workers[228] subsequently studied fresh samples from patients with small cell carcinoma and detected no TNF in these samples.

In summary, the hypothesis that cachectin/TNF production causes anorexia and weight loss in patients with cancer is attractive, but most published reports indicate that TNF is not detectable in these patients.

Fever

Fever can develop in tumor patients who lack evidence of any infection. For example, approximately 18% of patients with renal adenocarcinoma have fever,[229] and fever is common in Hodgkin disease in the absence of any infection. Fever could be caused by tumor stimulation of host white blood cell pyrogen production or by production of a pyrogen by the tumor. The pyrogen produced by various human tumor cell lines in vitro is similar to that produced by leukocytes.[230]

Glomerular Kidney Disease

On rare occasions, cancers cause glomerulonephritis and nephrotic syndrome.[231] In 1966 Lumeng and Moran[232] reported that removal of a carotid body tumor from a patient with nephrotic syndrome was associated with a remission of the renal findings, and in 1965 Rizzutto and co-workers[233] reported remission of nephrotic syndrome after removal of a pheochromocytoma. Arneil and associates[234] reported that treatment of two children with Wilms tumor by chemotherapy and radiation resulted in immune complex disposition nephritis.

Tumor Production of Enzymes or Fetal Proteins

Fetal proteins are normally produced during fetal development, and production is then suppressed during post-

TABLE 34–11. Serum α-Fetoprotein Levels in Patients with Cancer

Diagnosis	Number of Samples Assayed	Percentage of Values Over 40 μg/L
Hepatocellular carcinoma	130	72
Testicular teratocarcinoma	101	75
Pancreatic carcinoma	44	23
Gastric carcinoma	91	18
Colonic carcinoma	193	5
Bronchogenic carcinoma	150	7
Breast carcinoma	55	0
Nonhepatic benign lesions	300	0.3
Normal controls over 1 y of age	210	0

From Waldmann TA, McIntire KR. The use of a radioimmunoassay for alpha-fetoprotein in the diagnosis of malignancy. Cancer 1974; 34:1510–1515.

natal life. However, two such proteins are produced by a wide variety of cancers: carcinoembryonic antigen (CEA)[235] and α-fetoprotein (AFP).[236]

CEA is a glycoprotein of 200 kd produced by human colon carcinoma cells and is present in blood of almost all patients with this cancer. CEA can also be found in a wide variety of both benign and malignant human tumors and in association with nonmalignant conditions such as smoking, hepatic cirrhosis, inflammatory bowel disease, and pulmonary infections.[237]

AFP is an alpha-globulin of 70 kd and is normally synthesized by the endodermal cells of the liver and yolk sac of the fetus.[236] Maternal plasma AFP levels increase during pregnancy to peak by 12 to 15 wk and then fall to normal adult concentrations by about 6 to 12 mo after delivery. AFP is also produced by hepatic carcinomas and often by germ cell tumors such as teratocarcinomas. It is also produced by carcinomas of the pancreas, stomach, and colon[236] (Table 34–11).

In addition, some cancers produce increased quantities of enzymes that can be detected in blood as tumor markers but produce no clinical symptoms. Examples include alkaline phosphatase and thymidine kinase.

Digital Clubbing–Pulmonary Osteoarthropathy

Clubbing of the digits occurs in patients with a variety of malignant lung diseases, including primary lung carcinoma, mesothelioma, and metastatic cancer of the lung. It also occurs in patients with nonmalignant pulmonary diseases such as lung abscess, emphysema, interstitial pulmonary fibrosis, and pulmonary arteriovenous shunts. However, clubbing is unusual in patients with tuberculosis or pulmonary fungal infections. Clubbing often occurs in association with hypertrophic osteoarthropathy, periosteal new bone formation, long bone tenderness and pain, asymmetrical arthritis-like manifestations in joints, and increased thickness of soft tissues in distal arms and legs.[238] The cause of digital clubbing remains unknown, and, as stated previously, it is not specifically associated with cancer. It may be a humoral effect of lung tissue injured or modified by a benign or malignant tumor.

Hematological Syndromes

Idiopathic thrombocytopenic purpura (ITP), pure red blood cell aplasia, aplastic anemia, and other hematological syndromes occur in patients with a variety of carcinomas and cancers of the lymphoid system.[239–241] The association of ITP and cancer in 10 patients was reviewed by Kim and Boggs.[242] In most patients ITP either coincided with or

followed a diagnosis of cancer, and most patients had non-lymphoid malignancies. However, neither the presence of antiplatelet antibodies nor the cause of the syndrome was evaluated.

Subsequently, ITP has been reported in cancer patients with positive antiplatelet antibodies (e.g., two patients with multiple myeloma[243] and one patient with endometrial cancer[244]). However, it was not clear whether tumor development preceded antibody formation. ITP has been reported in one antibody-positive patient with a primary hepatic lymphoma.[245] Removal of the tumor restored the platelet count to normal.

In summary, many cancers are associated with hematological syndromes. Patients with cancer and ITP frequently have circulating antiplatelet antibodies, and an antigen on the surface of cancer cells may cause the formation of antibodies that could then cross-react with an antigen on the surface of platelets.

REFERENCES

1. Odell WD. Paraendocrine syndromes of cancer. Adv Intern Med 1989; 34:325–352.
2. Odell W, Wolfsen A, Yoshimoto Y, et al. Ectopic peptide synthesis: a universal concomitant of neoplasia. Trans Assoc Am Physicians 1977; 90:204–227.
3. Odell WD, Saito E. Protein hormone–like materials from normal and cancer cells—"ectopic" hormone production. In: Mirand EA, Hutchinson WB, Mihich E, eds. 13th International Cancer Congress. Part E: Cancer Management. New York: Alan R. Liss, 1983: 247–258.
4. Kew MC, Kirschner MA, Abrahams GE, et al. Mechanism of feminization in primary liver cancer. N Engl J Med 1977; 296:1084–1088.
5. Nakanishi S, Inoue A, Kita T, et al. Nucleotide sequence of cloned cDNA for bovine corticotropin–β-lipotropin precursor. Nature 1979; 278:423–427.
6. Brown WH. A case of pluriglandular syndrome: diabetes of bearded women. Lancet 1928; 2:1022–1023.
7. Liddle GW, Nicholson WE, Island DP, et al. Clinical and laboratory studies of ectopic humoral syndromes. Recent Prog Horm Res 1969; 25:283–314.
8. Kato Y, Ferguson TB, Bennett DE, et al. Oat cell carcinoma of the lung. A review of 138 cases. Cancer 1969; 23:517–524.
9. Ratcliffe JG, Knight RA, Besser GM, et al. Tumour and plasma ACTH concentrations in patients with and without the ectopic ACTH syndrome. Clin Endocrinol 1972; 1:27–44.
10. Gewirtz G, Yalow RS. Ectopic ACTH production in carcinoma of the lung. J Clin Invest 1974; 53:1022–1032.
11. Bloomfield GA, Holdaway IM, Corrin B, et al. Lung tumours and ACTH production. Clin Endocrinol 1977; 6:95–104.
12. Wolfsen AR, Odell WD. ProACTH: use for early detection of lung cancer. Am J Med 1979; 66:765–772.
13. Odell WD, Wolfsen AR, Bachelot I, et al. Ectopic production of lipotropin by cancer. Am J Med 1979; 66:631–638.
14. Saito E, Iwasa S, Odell WD. Widespread presence of large molecular weight adrenocorticotropin-like substances in normal rat extrapituitary tissues. Endocrinology 1983; 113:1010–1019.
15. Saito E, Odell WD. Corticotropin/lipotropin common precursor–like material in normal rat extrapituitary tissues. Proc Natl Acad Sci USA 1983; 80:3792–3796.
15a. Orwoll ES, Kendall JW. β-Endorphin and adrenocorticotropin in extrapituitary sites: gastrointestinal tract. Endocrinology 1980; 107:438–442.
15b. DeBold CR, Nicholson WE, Orth DN. Immunoreactive proopiomelanocortin (POMC) peptides and POMC-like messenger ribonucleic acid are present in many rat nonpituitary tissues. Endocrinology 1988; 66:2648–2657.
16. Bloomfield GA, Scott AP. β-Melanocyte stimulating hormone. Proc R Soc Med 1974; 67:748–749.
17. Bloomfield GA, Scott AP, Lowry PJ, et al. A reappraisal of human β MSH. Nature 1974; 252:492–493.
18. Bachelot I, Wolfsen AR, Odell WD. Pituitary and plasma lipotropins: demonstration of the artifactual nature of βMSH. J Clin Endocrinol Metab 1977; 44:939–946.
19. Howlett TA, Drury PL, Perry L, et al. Diagnosis and management of ACTH-dependent Cushing's syndrome: comparison of the features in ectopic and pituitary ACTH production. Clin Endocrinol 1986; 24:699–713.
20. Upton GV, Amatruda TT Jr. Evidence for the presence of tumor peptides with corticotropin-releasing-factor–like activity in the ectopic ACTH syndrome. N Engl J Med 1971; 285:419–424.

21. Belsky JL, Cuello B, Swanson LW, et al. Cushing's syndrome due to ectopic production of corticotropin-releasing factor. J Clin Endocrinol Metab 1985; 60:496–500.

22. Chrousos GP, Schulte HM, Oldfield EH, et al. The corticotropin-releasing factor stimulation test. An aid in the evaluation of patients with Cushing's syndrome. N Engl J Med 1984; 310:622–626.

23. Bellisario R, Carlsen RB, Bahl OP. Human chorionic gonadotropin. Linear amino acid sequence of the α subunit. J Biol Chem 1973; 248:6796–6809.

24. Papkoff H, Sairam MR, Farmer SW, et al. Studies on the structure and function of interstitial cell-stimulating hormone. Recent Prog Horm Res 1973; 29:563–590.

25. Canfield RE, Morgan FJ, Kammerman S, et al. Studies of human chorionic gonadotropin. Recent Prog Horm Res 1971; 27:121–164.

26. Odell WD, Hertz R, Lipsett MB, et al. Endocrine aspects of trophoblastic neoplasms. Clin Obstet Gynecol 1967; 10:290–302.

27. Li MC. Discussion of chemotherapy of choriocarcinoma and related trophoblastic tumors in women. Ann NY Acad Sci 1959; 80:280–284.

28. Chambers WL. Adrenal cortical carcinoma in a male with excess gonadotropin in the urine. J Clin Endocrinol Metab 1949; 9:451–456.

29. Matteini M. Su di un caso di ginecomastia (da displasia fibro-epiteliale) associata a tumore retroperitoneale a cellule indifferenziate (considerazioni sulla etiopatogenesi della ginecomastia). Rass Neurol Veget 1952; 9:252–271.

30. McArthur JW. Paraendocrine phenomena in obstetrics and gynecology. In: Meigs JV, Sturgis SH, eds. Progress in Gynecology. Vol 4. New York: Grune & Stratton, 1963: 146–172.

31. Case records of the Massachusetts General Hospital. Case 13–1972. N Engl J Med 1972; 286:713–719.

32. Fusco FD, Rosen SW. Gonadotropin-producing anaplastic large-cell carcinomas of the lung. N Engl J Med 1966; 275:507–515.

33. Faiman C, Colwell JA, Ryan RJ, et al. Gonadotropin secretion from a bronchogenic carcinoma. Demonstration by radioimmunoassay. N Engl J Med 1967; 277:1395–1399.

34. Rosen SW, Becker CE, Schlaff S, et al. Ectopic gonadotropin production before clinical recognition of bronchogenic carcinoma. N Engl J Med 1968; 279:640–641.

35. Vaitukaitis JL, Braunstein GD, Ross GT. A radioimmunoassay which specifically measures human chorionic gonadotropin in the presence of human luteinizing hormone. Am J Obstet Gynecol 1972; 113:751–758.

36. Braunstein GD, Vaitukaitis JL, Carbone PP, et al. Ectopic production of human chorionic gonadotrophin by neoplasms. Ann Intern Med 1973; 78:39–45.

37. Braunstein GD, Rasor J, Wade ME. Presence in normal human testes of a chorionic-gonadotropin–like substance distinct from human luteinizing hormone. N Engl J Med 1975; 293:1339–1343.

38. Yoshimoto Y, Wolfsen AR, Odell WD. Human chorionic gonadotropin–like substance in nonendocrine tissues of normal subjects. Science 1977; 197:575–577.

39. Yoshimoto Y, Wolfsen AR, Hirose F, et al. Human chorionic gonadotropin–like material: presence in normal human tissues. Am J Obstet Gynecol 1979; 134:729–733.

40. Braunstein GD, Kamdar V, Rasor J, et al. Widespread distribution of a chorionic gonadotropin–like substance in normal human tissues. J Clin Endocrinol Metab 1979; 49:917–925.

41. Chen H-C, Hodgen GD, Matsuura S, et al. Evidence for a gonadotropin from nonpregnant subjects that has physical, immunological, and biological similarities to human chorionic gonadotropin. Proc Natl Acad Sci USA 1976; 73:2885–2889.

42. Matsuura S, Ohashi M, Chen HC, et al. Physiochemical and immunological characterization of an hCG-like substance from human pituitary glands. Nature 1980; 286:740–741.

43. Yoshimoto Y, Wolfsen AR, Odell WD. Glycosylation, a variable in the production of hCG by cancers. Am J Med 1979; 67:414–420.

44. Van Hall EV, Vaitukaitis JL, Ross GT, et al. Immunological and biological activity of hCG following progressive desialylation. Endocrinology 1971; 88:456–464.

45. Tsuruhara T, Dufau ML, Hickman J, et al. Biological properties of hCG after removal of terminal sialic acid and galactose residues. Endocrinology 1972; 91:296–301.

46. Kalyan NK, Bahl OP. Role of carbohydrate in human chorionic gonadotropin. Effect of deglycosylation on the subunit interaction and on its in vitro and in vivo biological properties. J Biol Chem 1983; 258:67–74.

47. Thotakura NR, Bahl OP. Role of carbohydrate in human chorionic gonadotropin: deglycosylation uncouples hormone-receptor complex and adenylate cyclase system. Biochem Biophys Res Commun 1982; 108:399–405.

48. Borkowski A, Puttaert V, Gyling M, et al. Human chorionic gonadotropin–like substance in plasma of normal nonpregnant subjects and women with breast cancer. J Clin Endocrinol Metab 1984; 58:1171–1178.

49. Odell WD, Griffin J. Pulsatile secretion of human chorionic gonadotropin in normal adults. N Engl J Med 1987; 317:1688–1691.

49a. Odell WD, Griffin J, Bashey HM, et al. Secretion of chorionic gonadotropin by cultured human pituitary cells. J Clin Endocrinol Metab 1990; 71:1318–1321.

49b. Hammond E, Griffin J, Odell WD. A chorionic gonadotropin-secreting human pituitary cell. J Clin Endocrinol Metab 1991; 71:747–754.

50. Stenman U-H, Alfthan H, Ranta T, et al. Serum levels of human chorionic gonadotropin in nonpregnant women and men are modulated by gonadotropin-releasing hormone and sex steroids. J Clin Endocrinol Metab 1987; 64:730–736.

51. Cole LA, Birken S, Sutphen S, et al. Absence of the COOH-terminal peptide on ectopic human chorionic gonadotropin β-subunit (hCGβ). Endocrinology 1982; 110:2198–2200.

52. McManus LM, Naughton MA, Martinez-Hernandez A. Human chorionic gonadotropin in human neoplastic cells. Cancer Res 1976; 36:3476–3481.

53. Acevedo HF, Slifkin M, Pouchet GR, et al. Human chorionic gonadotropin in cancer cells. I. Identification in vitro and in vivo cancer cell systems. In: Nieburgs HR, ed. Detection and Prevention of Cancer. Part 2. Vol 1. New York: Marcel Dekker, 1978: 937–964.

54. Slifkin M, Acevedo HF, Pardo M, et al. Human chorionic gonadotropin in cancer cells. II. Ultrastructural localization. In: Nieburgs HR, ed. Detection and Prevention of Cancer. Part 2. Vol 1. New York: Marcel Dekker, 1978: 965–979.

55. Weintraub BD, Rosen SW. Ectopic production of the isolated beta subunit of human chorionic gonadotropin. J Clin Invest 1973; 52:3135–3142.

56. Rosen SW, Weintraub BD. Ectopic production of the isolated alpha subunit of the glycoprotein hormones. A quantitative marker in certain cases of cancer. N Engl J Med 1974; 290:1441–1447.

57. Kahn CR, Rosen SW, Weintraub BD, et al. Ectopic production of chorionic gonadotropin and its subunits by islet-cell tumors. A specific marker for malignancy. N Engl J Med 1977; 297:565–569.

58. Milhaud G, Calmettes C, Raymond JP, et al. Carcinoide sécrétant de la thyrocalcitonine. C R Acad Sci Ser D 1970; 18:2195–2198.

59. Silva OL, Becker KL, Primack A, et al. Ectopic production of calcitonin. Lancet 1973; 2:317.

60. Coombes RC, Hillyard C, Greenberg PB, et al. Plasma-immunoreactive-calcitonin in patients with non-thyroid tumours. Lancet 1974; 1:1080–1083.

61. Hillyard CJ, Coombes RC, Greenberg PB, et al. Calcitonin in breast and lung cancer. Clin Endocrinol 1976; 5:1–8.

62. Schwartz KE, Wolfsen AR, Forster B, et al. Calcitonin in nonthyroidal cancer. J Clin Endocrinol Metab 1979; 49:438–444.

63. Silva OL, Becker KL, Primack A, et al. Hypercalcitonemia in bronchogenic cancer. Evidence for thyroid origin of the hormone. JAMA 1975; 234:183–185.

64. Schwartz WB, Bennett W, Curelop S, et al. A syndrome of renal sodium loss and hyponatremia probably resulting from inappropriate secretion of antidiuretic hormone. Am J Med 1957; 23:529–542.

65. Bartter FC, Schwartz WB. The syndrome of inappropriate secretion of antidiuretic hormone. Am J Med 1967; 42:790–806.

66. Amatruda TT Jr, Mulrow PJ, Gallagher JC, et al. Carcinoma of the lung with inappropriate antidiuresis. Demonstration of antidiuretic-hormone–like activity in tumor extract. N Engl J Med 1963; 269:544–549.

67. Bower BF, Mason DM, Forsham PH. Measurement of antidiuretic activity (ADA) in plasma and tumor in carcinoma of the lung with inappropriate antidiuresis. Clin Res 1964; 12:121 (abstract).

68. Vorherr H, Massry SG, Utiger RD, et al. Antidiuretic principle in malignant tumor extracts from patients with inappropriate ADH syndrome. J Clin Endocrinol Metab 1968; 28:162–168.

69. George JM, Capen CC, Phillips AS. Biosynthesis of vasopressin in vitro and ultrastructure of a bronchogenic carcinoma. Patient with the syndrome of inappropriate secretion of antidiuretic hormone. J Clin Invest 1972; 51:141–148.

70. Hirata Y, Matsukura S, Imura H, et al. Two cases of multiple hormone-producing small cell carcinoma of the lung. Coexistence of tumor ADH, ACTH, and β-MSH. Cancer 1976; 38:2575–2582.

71. Hamilton BPM, Upton GV, Amatruda TT Jr. Evidence for the presence of neurophysin in tumors producing the syndrome of inappropriate antidiuresis. J Clin Endocrinol Metab 1972; 35:764–767.

72. North WG, LaRochelle FT Jr, Melton J, et al. Human neurophysins (HNPs) as potential tumor markers for small-cell carcinoma (SCC). Clin Res 1978; 26:536A (abstract).

73. Gilby ED, Rees LH, Bondy PK. Proceedings of the 6th International Symposium on Biology and Characterization of Human Tumours, Copenhagen, 1975. In: Davis W, Maltoni C, eds. Advances in Tumour Prevention, Detection and Characterization. Vol 3. New York: American Elsevier, 1976: 132.

74. Sellwood RA, Spencer J, Azzopardi JG, et al. Inappropriate secretion of antidiuretic hormone by carcinoma of the prostate. Br J Surg 1969; 56:933–935.

75. Falchuk KR. Inappropriate antidiuretic hormone–like syndrome associated with an adrenocortical carcinoma. Am J Med Sci 1973; 266:393–395.

76. Cassileth PA, Trotman BW. Inappropriate antidiuretic hormone in Hodgkin's disease. Am J Med Sci 1973; 265:233–235.

77. Ginsberg S, Comis R, Miller M. Syndrome of inappropriate antidiuretic

hormone secretion in oat cell carcinoma of the lung. Clin Res 1978; 26:435A (abstract).

78. Jacobson RJ, Lowenthal MN, Kew MC. Erythrocytosis in hepatocellular cancer. S Afr Med J 1978; 53:658–660.
79. Sufrin G, Mirand EA, Moore RH, et al. Hormones in renal cancer. J Urol 1977; 117:433–438.
80. Hammond D, Winnick S. Paraneoplastic erythrocytosis and ectopic erythropoietins. Ann NY Acad Sci 1974; 230:219–227.
81. Murphy GP, Allen JE, Staubitz WJ, et al. Erythropoietin levels in patients with Wilms' tumor. NY State J Med 1972; 72:487–489.
82. Murphy GP, Mirand EA, Staubitz WJ. The value of erythropoietin assay in the follow-up of Wilms' tumor patients. Oncology 1976; 33:154–156.
83. Sherwood JB, Shouval D. Continuous production of erythropoietin by an established human renal carcinoma cell line: development of the cell line. Proc Natl Acad Sci USA 1986; 83:165–169.
84. Nielsen OJ, Schuster SJ, Kaufman R, et al. Regulation of erythropoietin production in a human hepatoblastoma cell line. Blood 1987; 70:1904–1909.
85. Goldberg MA, Glass GA, Cunningham JM, et al. The regulated expression of erythropoietin by two human hepatoma cell lines. Proc Natl Acad Sci USA 1987; 84:7972–7976.
86. Kew MC, Fisher JW. Serum erythropoietin concentrations in patients with hepatocellular carcinoma. Cancer 1986; 58:2485–2488.
87. Zanjani ED, Poster J, Burlington H, et al. Liver as the primary site of erythropoietin formation in the fetus. J Lab Clin Med 1977; 89:640–644.
88. Jacobson LO, Goldwasser E, Fried W, et al. Role of the kidney in erythropoiesis. Nature 1957; 179:633–634.
89. Dabek JT. Bronchial carcinoid tumour with acromegaly in two patients. J Clin Endocrinol Metab 1974; 38:329–333.
90. Sönksen PH, Ayres AB, Braimbridge M, et al. Acromegaly caused by pulmonary carcinoid tumours. Clin Endocrinol 1976; 5:503–513.
91. Leveston SA, Lee Y-C, Jaffe BM, et al. Massive GH and ACTH hypersecretion associated with a metastatic carcinoid tumor. Endocr Soc Abstr 1978; 371.
92. Southren AL. Functioning metastatic bronchial carcinoid with elevated levels of serum and cerebrospinal fluid serotonin and pituitary adenoma. J Clin Endocrinol Metab 1960; 20:298–305.
93. Weiss L, Ingram M. Adenomatoid bronchial tumors. A consideration of the carcinoid tumors and the salivary tumors of the bronchial tree. Cancer 1961; 14:161–178.
94. Saeed uz Zafar M, Mellinger RC, Fine G, et al. Acromegaly associated with a bronchial carcinoid tumor: evidence for ectopic production of growth hormone-releasing activity. J Clin Endocrinol Metab 1979; 48:66–71.
95. Frohman LA, Szabo M, Berelowitz M, et al. Partial purification and characterization of a peptide with growth hormone–releasing activity from extrapituitary tumors in patients with acromegaly. J Clin Invest 1980; 65:43–54.
96. Melmed S, Ezrin C, Kovacs K, et al. Acromegaly due to secretion of growth hormone by an ectopic pancreatic islet-cell tumor. N Engl J Med 1985; 312:9–17.
97. Barkan AL, Shenker Y, Grekin RJ, et al. Acromegaly due to ectopic growth hormone (GH)–releasing hormone (GHRH) production: dynamic studies of GH and ectopic GHRH secretion. J Clin Endocrinol Metab 1986; 63:1057–1064.
98. Guillemin R, Brazeau P, Böhlen P, et al. Growth hormone-releasing factor from a human pancreatic tumor that caused acromegaly. Science 1982; 218:585–587.
99. Thorner MO, Frohman LA, Leong DA, et al. Extrahypothalamic growth-hormone–releasing factor (GRF) secretion is a rare cause of acromegaly: plasma GRF levels in 177 acromegalic patients. J Clin Endocrinol Metab 1984; 59:846–849.
100. Steiner H, Dahlbäck O, Waldenström J. Ectopic growth-hormone production and osteoarthropathy in carcinoma of the bronchus. Lancet 1968; 1:783–785.
101. Cameron DP, Burger HG, DeKretzer DM, et al. On the presence of immunoreactive growth hormone in a bronchogenic carcinoma. Aust Ann Med 1969; 18:143–146.
102. Sparagana M, Phillips G, Hoffman C, et al. Ectopic growth hormone syndrome associated with lung cancer. Metabolism 1971; 20:730–736.
103. Beck C, Burger HG. Evidence for the presence of immunoreactive growth hormone in cancers of the lung and stomach. Cancer 1972; 30:75–79.
104. Kaganowicz A, Farkouh NH, Frantz AG, et al. Ectopic human growth hormone in ovaries and breast cancer. J Clin Endocrinol Metab 1978; 48:5–8.
105. Kyle CV, Evans MC, Odell WD. Growth hormone–like material in normal human tissues. J Clin Endocrinol Metab 1981; 53:1138–1144.
106. Szabo M, Berelowitz M, Pettengill OS, et al. Ectopic production of somatostatin-like immuno- and bioactivity by cultured human pulmonary small cell carcinoma. J Clin Endocrinol Metab 1980; 51:978–987.
107. Odell WD. Humoral manifestations of nonendocrine neoplasms. In: Williams RH, ed. Textbook of Endocrinology. 4th ed. Philadelphia: W. B. Saunders, 1968: 1211–1222.
108. Collipp PJ. Hypoglycemia and leukemia. Pediatrics 1972; 49:788–790.

109. Buffet C, Bonnefond A, Mignon M, et al. Hypoglycémie au cours d'un lymphosarcome et d'un réticulosarcome. Nouv Presse Med 1974; 3:181–184.
110. Salomon J. Spurious hypoglycemia and hyperkalemia in myelomonocytic leukemia. Am J Med Sci 1974; 267:359–363.
111. Field JB, Keen H, Johnson P, et al. Insulinlike activity of nonpancreatic tumors associated with hypoglycemia. J Clin Endocrinol Metab 1963; 23:1229–1236.
112. Tranquada RE, Bender AB, Beigelman PM. Hypoglycemia associated with carcinoma of the cecum and syndrome of testicular feminization. N Engl J Med 1962; 266:1302–1306.
113. Smith NL, Janelli DE, Madariaga J, et al. Hypoglycemia and Hodgkin's disease with hyperinsulinemia. J Surg Oncol 1982; 19:27–30.
114. Lyall SS, Marieb NJ, Wise JK, et al. Hyperinsulinemic hypoglycemia associated with a neurofibrosarcoma. Arch Intern Med 1975; 135:865–867.
115. Shetty MR, Boghossian HM, Duffell D, et al. Tumor-induced hypoglycemia. A result of ectopic insulin production. Cancer 1982; 49:1920–1923.
116. Talstad I, Folling I, Boye NP. Hypoglycemia caused by an intrathoracic tumour. Acta Med Scand 1974; 196:347–351.
117. Megyesi K, Kahn CR, Roth J, et al. Hypoglycemia in association with extrapancreatic tumors: demonstration of elevated plasma NSILA-s by a new radioreceptor assay. J Clin Endocrinol Metab 1974; 38:931–934.
118. Gorden P, Hendricks CM, Kahn CR, et al. Hypoglycemia associated with non–islet-cell tumor and insulin-like growth factors. A study of the tumor types. N Engl J Med 1981; 305:1452–1455.
119. Daughaday WH, Trivedi B, Kapadia M. Measurement of insulin-like growth factor II by a specific radioreceptor assay in serum of normal individuals, patients with abnormal growth hormone secretion, and patients with tumor-associated hypoglycemia. J Clin Endocrinol Metab 1981; 53:289–294.
120. Daughaday WH, Emanuele MA, Brooks MH, et al. Synthesis and secretion of insulin-like growth factor II by a leiomyosarcoma with associated hypoglycemia. N Engl J Med 1988; 319:1434–1440.
121. Ron D, Powers AC, Pandian MR, et al. Increased insulin-like growth factor II production and consequent suppression of growth hormone secretion: a dual mechanism for tumor-induced hypoglycemia. J Clin Endocrinol Metab 1989; 68:701–706.
122. Froesch ER, Zapf J, Widmer U. Hypoglycemia associated with non–islet-cell tumor and insulin-like growth factors. N Engl J Med 1982; 306:1178–1179.
123. Widmer U, Zapf J, Froesch ER. Is extrapancreatic tumor hypoglycemia associated with elevated levels of insulin-like growth factor II? J Clin Endocrinol Metab 1982; 55:833–839.
124. Rosenzweig JL, Havrankova J, Lesniak MA, et al. Insulin is ubiquitous in extrapancreatic tissues of rats and humans. Proc Natl Acad Sci USA 1980; 77:572–576.
125. Zondek H, Petow H, Siebert W. Die Bedeutung der Calciumbestimmung im Blute für die Diagnose der Niereninsuffizienz. Z Klin Med 1924; 99:129–138.
126. Gutman AB, Tyson TL, Gutman EB. Serum calcium, inorganic phosphorus and phosphatase activity. Arch Intern Med 1936; 57:379–413.
127. Albright F. Case records of the Massachusetts General Hospital. Case 27461. N Engl J Med 1941; 225:789–791.
128. Tashjian AH Jr, Levine L, Munson PL. Immunochemical identification of parathyroid hormone in non-parathyroid neoplasms associated with hypercalcemia. J Exp Med 1964; 119:467–484.
129. Berson SA, Yalow RS. Parathyroid hormone in plasma in adenomatous hyperparathyroidism, uremia, and bronchogenic carcinoma. Science 1966; 154:907–909.
130. Sherwood LM, O'Riordan JLH, Aurbach GD, et al. Production of parathyroid hormone by nonparathyroid tumors. J Clin Endocrinol Metab 1967; 27:140–146.
131. Buckle RM, McMillan M, Mallinson C. Ectopic secretion of parathyroid hormone by a renal adenocarcinoma in a patient with hypercalcaemia. Br Med J 1970; 4:724–726.
132. Zidar BL, Shadduck RK, Winkelstein A, et al. Acute myeloblastic leukemia and hypercalcemia. A case of probable ectopic parathyroid hormone production. N Engl J Med 1976; 295:692–694.
133. Federman DD. Case records of the Massachusetts General Hospital. Case 15-1971. N Engl J Med 1971; 284:839–847.
134. Powell D, Singer FR, Murray TM, et al. Nonparathyroid humoral hypercalcemia in patients with neoplastic diseases. N Engl J Med 1973; 289:176–181.
135. Simpson EL, Mundy GR, D'Souza SM, et al. Absence of parathyroid hormone messenger RNA in nonparathyroid tumors associated with hypercalcemia. N Engl J Med 1983; 309:325–330.
136. Goltzman D, Stewart AF, Broadus AE. Malignancy-associated hypercalcemia: evaluation with a cytochemical bioassay for parathyroid hormone. J Clin Endocrinol Metab 1981; 53:899–904.
137. Stewart AF, Insogna KL, Goltzman D, et al. Identification of adenylate cyclase–stimulating activity and cytochemical glucose-6-phosphate dehydrogenase–stimulating activity in extracts of tumors from patients with humoral hypercalcemia of malignancy. Proc Natl Acad Sci USA 1983; 80:1454–1458.

138. Merendino JJ Jr, Insogna KL, Milstone LM, et al. A parathyroid hormone–like protein from cultured human keratinocytes. Science 1986; 231:388–390.

139. Burtis WJ, Wu T, Bunch C, et al. Identification of a novel 17,000-dalton parathyroid hormone–like adenylate cyclase-stimulating protein from a tumor associated with humoral hypercalcemia of malignancy. J Biol Chem 1987; 262:7151–7156.

140. Moseley JM, Kubota M, Diefenbach-Jagger H, et al. Parathyroid hormone–related protein purified from a human lung cancer cell line. Proc Natl Acad Sci USA 1987; 84:5048–5052.

141. Strewler GJ, Stern PH, Jacobs JW, et al. Parathyroid hormonelike protein from human renal carcinoma cells. Structural and functional homology with parathyroid hormone. J Clin Invest 1987; 80:1803–1807.

142. Suva LJ, Winslow GA, Wettenhall REH, et al. A parathyroid hormone–related protein implicated in malignant hypercalcemia: cloning and expression. Science 1987; 237:893–896.

143. Mangin M, Webb AC, Dreyer BE, et al. Identification of a cDNA encoding a parathyroid hormone–like peptide from a human tumor associated with humoral hypercalcemia of malignancy. Proc Natl Acad Sci USA 1988; 85:597–601.

144. Thiede MA, Strewler GJ, Nissenson RA, et al. Human renal carcinoma expresses two messages encoding a parathyroid hormone–like peptide: evidence for the alternative splicing of a single-copy gene. Proc Natl Acad Sci USA 1988; 85:4605–4609.

145. Mangin M, Ikeda K, Dreyer BE, et al. Two distinct tumor-derived, parathyroid hormone–like peptides result from alternative RNA processing. Endocr Soc Abstr 1988; 26.

146. Thorikay M, Kramer S, Reynolds FH, et al. Synthesis of a gene encoding parathyroid hormone–like protein-(1–141): purification and biological characterization of the expressed protein. Endocrinology 1989; 124:111–118.

147. Thiede MA, Rodan GA. Expression of a calcium-mobilizing parathyroid hormone-like peptide in lactating mammary tissue. Science 1988; 242:278–280.

147a. Thiede M. The mRNA encoding parathyroid hormone–like peptide is produced in mammary tissue in response to elevations in serum prolactin. Mol Endocrinol 1989; 3:1443–1447.

147b. Drucker DS, Asa SL, Henderson J, et al. The parathyroid hormone–like peptide gene is expressed in the normal and neoplastic human endocrine pancreas. Mol Endocrinol 1989; 3:1589–1595.

147c. Chan SDH, Strewler GJ, King KL, et al. Expression of a parathyroid hormone–like protein and its receptor during differentiation of embryonal carcinoma cells. Mol Endocrinol 1990; 4:638–646.

147d. Abbas SK, Pickard DW, Rodda CP, et al. Stimulation of ovine placental calcium transport by purified natural and recombinant parathyroid hormone–related protein (PTHrP) preparations. Q J Exp Physiol 1989; 74:549–552.

147e. Kao PC, Klee GG, Taylor RL, et al. Parathyroid hormone–related peptide in plasma of patients with hypercalcemia and cancer. Mayo Clin Proc 1990; 65:1399–1407.

147f. Burtis WJ, Brady TG, Orloff JS, et al. Immunochemical characterization of circulating parathyroid hormone–related protein in patients with humoral hypercalcemia of cancer. N Engl J Med 1990; 322:1106–1112.

147g. Heath DA, Senior PV, Varley JM, et al. Parathyroid-hormone–related protein in tumours associated with hypercalcaemia. Lancet 1990; 1:66–68.

147h. Khosla S, Van Heerden JA, Gharib H, et al. Parathyroid hormone–related protein and hypercalcemia secondary to massive mammary hyperplasia. Lancet 1990; 1:1157–1158.

148. Ibbotson KJ, D'Souza SM, Ng KW, et al. Tumor-derived growth factor increases bone resorption in a tumor associated with humoral hypercalcemia of malignancy. Science 1983; 221:1292–1294.

149. Mundy GR, Ibbotson KJ, D'Souza SM, et al. Evidence that transforming growth factor alpha production causes bone resorption and hypercalcemia in squamous cell carcinoma of the lung. Clin Res 1985; 33:573A (abstract).

150. Mundy GR. Pathogenesis of hypercalcaemia of malignancy. Clin Endocrinol 1985; 23:705–714.

151. D'Souza SM, Ibbotson KJ, Smith DD, et al. Production of a macromolecular bone-resorbing factor by the hypercalcemic variant of the Walker rat carcinosarcoma. Endocrinology 1984; 115:1746–1752.

151a. Nussbaum SR, Gaz RD, Arnold A. Hypercalcemia and ectopic secretion of parathyroid hormone by an ovarian carcinoma with rearrangement of the gene for parathyroid hormone. N Engl J Med 1990; 323:1324–1328.

152. Stewart AF, Horst R, Deftos LJ, et al. Biochemical evaluation of patients with cancer-associated hypercalcemia. Evidence for humoral and nonhumoral groups. N Engl J Med 1980; 303:1377–1383.

152a. Ralston SH, Gallacher SS, Patel U, et al. Cancer-associated hypercalcemia: morbidity and mortality. Ann Intern Med 1990; 112:499–504.

153. Mundy GR, Raisz LG, Cooper RA, et al. Evidence for the secretion of an osteoclast stimulating factor in myeloma. N Engl J Med 1974; 291:1041–1046.

154. Aggarwal BB, Henzel WJ, Moffat B, et al. Primary structure of human lymphotoxin derived from 1788 lymphoblastoid cell line. J Biol Chem 1985; 260:2334–2344.

155. Garrett IR, Durie BGM, Nedwin GE, et al. Production of lymphotoxin, a bone-resorbing cytokine, by cultured human myeloma cells. N Engl J Med 1987; 317:526–532.

156. Kinoshita K, Kamihira S, Ikeda S, et al. Clinical, hematologic, and pathologic features of leukemic T-cell lymphoma. Cancer 1982; 50:1554–1562.

157. Bunn PA Jr, Schechter GP, Jaffe E, et al. Clinical course of retrovirus-associated adult T-cell lymphoma in the United States. N Engl J Med 1983; 309:257–264.

158. Breslau NA, McGuire JL, Zerwekh JE, et al. Hypercalcemia associated with increased serum calcitriol levels in three patients with lymphoma. Ann Intern Med 1984; 100:1–7.

159. Rosenthal N, Insogna KL, Godsall JW, et al. Elevations in circulating 1,25-dihydroxyvitamin D in three patients with lymphoma-associated hypercalcemia. J Clin Endocrinol Metab 1985; 60:29–33.

160. Helikson MA, Havey AD, Zerwekh JE, et al. Plasma-cell granuloma producing calcitriol and hypercalcemia. Ann Intern Med 1986; 105:379–381.

161. Maislos M, Sobel R, Shany S. Leiomyoblastoma associated with intractable hypercalcemia and elevated 1,25-dihydroxycholecalciferol levels. Treatment by hepatic enzyme induction. Arch Intern Med 1985; 145:565–567.

162. Zaloga GP, Eil C, Medbery CA. Humoral hypercalcemia in Hodgkin's disease. Arch Intern Med 1985; 145:155–157.

163. Drezner MK, Lebovitz HE. Primary hyperparathyroidism in paraneoplastic hypercalcaemia. Lancet 1978; 1:1004–1006.

164. Mundy GR, Wilkinson R, Heath DA. Comparative study of available medical therapy for hypercalcemia of malignancy. Am J Med 1983; 74:421–432.

165. Stewart AF. Therapy of malignancy-associated hypercalcemia: 1983. Am J Med 1983; 74:475–480.

166. Stevenson JC. Current management of malignant hypercalcaemia. Drugs 1988; 36:229–238.

167. Binstock ML, Mundy GR. Effect of calcitonin and glucocorticoids in combination on the hypercalcemia of malignancy. Ann Intern Med 1980; 93:269–272.

168. Jung A. Comparison of two parenteral diphosphonates in hypercalcemia of malignancy. Am J Med 1982; 72:221–226.

169. Sackner MA, Spivack AP, Balian LJ. Hypocalcemia in the presence of osteoblastic metastases. N Engl J Med 1960; 262:173–176.

170. Ehrlich M, Goldstein M, Heinemann HO. Hypocalcemia, hypoparathyroidism, and osteoblastic metastases. Metabolism 1963; 12:516–526.

171. Schwarz G, Meiser J. Changes of the calcium phosphate metabolism in a case of osteoplastic metastases with hypocalcemia. Schweiz Med Wochenschr 1962; 92:1004–1006.

172. Ludwig GD. Hypocalcemia and hypophosphatemia accompanying osteoblastic osseous metastases: studies of calcium and phosphate metabolism and parathyroid function. Ann Intern Med 1962; 56:676–677 (abstract).

173. Hall TC, Griffiths CT, Petranek JR. Hypocalcemia—an unusual metabolic complication of breast cancer. N Engl J Med 1966; 275:1474–1477.

174. Zusman J, Brown DM, Nesbit ME. Hyperphosphatemia, hyperphosphaturia and hypocalcemia in acute lymphoblastic leukemia. N Engl J Med 1973; 289:1335–1340.

175. Drezner MK, Feinglos MN. Osteomalacia due to 1α,25-dihydroxycholecalciferol deficiency. Association with a giant cell tumor of bone. J Clin Invest 1977; 60:1046–1053.

176. Fukumoto Y, Tarui S, Tsukiyama K, et al. Tumor-induced vitamin D-resistant hypophosphatemic osteomalacia associated with proximal renal tubular dysfunction and 1,25-dihydroxyvitamin D deficiency. J Clin Endocrinol Metab 1979; 49:873–878.

177. Lyles KW, Berry WR, Haussler M, et al. Hypophosphatemic osteomalacia: association with prostatic carcinoma. Ann Intern Med 1980; 93:275–278.

178. Miyauchi A, Fukase M, Tsutsumi M, et al. Hemangiopericytoma-induced osteomalacia: tumor transplantation in nude mice causes hypophosphatemia and tumor extracts inhibit renal 25-hydroxyvitamin D 1-hydroxylase activity. J Clin Endocrinol Metab 1988; 67:46–53.

179. Palma G. Paraneoplastic syndromes of the nervous system. West J Med 1985; 142:787–796.

180. Henson RA, Urich H. The concept of paraneoplastic disorders. In: Henson RA, Urich H, eds. Cancer and the Nervous System: The Neurological Manifestations of Systemic Malignant Disease. Oxford: Blackwell Scientific, 1982: 311–313.

181. Trotter JL, Hendin BA, Osterland CK. Cerebellar degeneration with Hodgkin disease. An immunological study. Arch Neurol 1976; 33:660–661.

182. Steven MM, Mackay IR, Carnegie PR, et al. Cerebellar cortical degeneration with ovarian carcinoma. Postgrad Med J 1982; 58:47–51.

183. Greenlee JE, Brashear HR. Antibodies to cerebellar Purkinje cells in patients with paraneoplastic cerebellar degenerative and ovarian carcinoma. Ann Neurol 1983; 14:609–613.

184. Greenlee JE, Sun M. Immunofluorescent labeling of nonhuman cerebellar tissue with sera from patients with systemic cancer and paraneoplastic cerebellar degeneration. Acta Neuropathol 1985; 67:226–229.

185. Kearsley JH, Johnson P, Halmagyi GM. Paraneoplastic cerebellar disease. Remission with excision of the primary tumor. Arch Neurol 1985; 42:1208–1210.

186. Dropcho EJ, Chen YT, Posner JB, et al. Cloning of a brain protein identified by autoantibodies from a patient with paraneoplastic cerebellar degeneration. Proc Natl Acad Sci USA 1987; 84:4552–4556.

187. Graus F, Elkon KB, Cordon-Cardo C, et al. Sensory neuronopathy and small cell lung cancer. Antineuronal antibody that also reacts with the tumor. Am J Med 1986; 80:45–52.

188. Graus F, Cordon-Cardo C, Posner JB. Neuronal antinuclear antibody in sensory neuronopathy from lung cancer. Neurology 1985; 35:538–543.

189. Graus F, Elkon KB, Lloberes P, et al. Neuronal antinuclear antibody (anti-Hu) in paraneoplastic encephalomyelitis simulating acute polyneuritis. Acta Neurol Scand 1987; 75:249–252.

190. Anderson NE, Rosenblum MK, Graus F, et al. Autoantibodies in paraneoplastic syndromes associated with small-cell lung cancer. Neurology 1988; 38:1391–1398.

191. Sawyer RA, Selhorst JB, Zimmerman LE, et al. Blindness caused by photoreceptor degeneration as a remote effect of cancer. Am J Ophthalmol 1976; 81:606–613.

192. Kornguth SE, Klein R, Appen R, et al. Occurrence of anti-retinal ganglion cell antibodies in patients with small cell carcinoma of the lung. Cancer 1982; 50:1289–1293.

193. Grunwald GB, Klein R, Simmonds MA, et al. Autoimmune basis for visual paraneoplastic syndrome in patients with small-cell lung carcinoma. Lancet 1985; 1:658–661.

194. Kornguth SE, Kalinke T, Grunwald GB, et al. Anti-neurofilament antibodies in the sera of patients with small cell carcinoma of the lung and with visual paraneoplastic syndrome. Cancer Res 1986; 46:2588–2595.

195. Thirkill CE, Roth AM, Keltner JL. Cancer-associated retinopathy. Arch Ophthalmol 1987; 105:372–375.

196. Buchanan TAS, Gardiner TA, Archer DB. An ultrastructural study of retinal photoreceptor degeneration associated with bronchial carcinoma. Am J Ophthalmol 1984; 97:277–287.

197. Keltner JL, Roth AM, Chang RS. Photoreceptor degeneration. Possible autoimmune disorder. Arch Ophthalmol 1983; 101:564–569.

198. Klingele TG, Burde RM, Rappazzo JA, et al. Paraneoplastic retinopathy. J Clin Neuro Ophthalmol 1984; 4:239–245.

199. Berson EL, Lessell S. Paraneoplastic night blindness with malignant melanoma. Am J Ophthalmol 1988; 106:307–311.

200. Crofts JW, Bachynski BN, Odel JG. Visual paraneoplastic syndrome associated with undifferentiated endometrial carcinoma. Can J Ophthalmol 1988; 23:128–132.

201. Stefansson K, Marton LS, Dieperink ME, et al. Circulating autoantibodies to the 200,000-dalton protein of neurofilaments in the serum of healthy individuals. Science 1985; 228:1117–1119.

202. Smith FP, Posner J. Neurologic complications of cancer. In: Calabresi P, Schein PS, Rosenberg SA, eds. Medical Oncology. Basic Principles and Clinical Management of Cancer. New York: Macmillan, 1985:234–240.

203. Zu Rhein GM, Chou S-M. Particles resembling papova viruses in human cerebral demyelinating disease. Science 1965; 148:1477–1479.

204. Weiner LP, Herndon RM, Narayan O, et al. Isolation of virus related to SV40 from patients with progressive multifocal leukoencephalopathy. N Engl J Med 1972; 286:385–390.

205. Mordel N, Margalioth EJ, Harats N, et al. Concurrence of ovarian cancer and dermatomyositis. A report of two cases and literature review. J Reprod Med 1988; 33:649–655.

206. Dowsett RJ, Wong RL, Robert NJ, Abeles M. Dermatomyositis and Hodgkin's disease. Am J Med 1986; 80:719–723.

207. Yamamura T, Tsujimura M, Yoshikawa K, et al. True histiocytic lymphoma associated with dermatomyositis. Arch Dermatol 1987; 123:1272–1274.

208. Barnes BE. Dermatomyositis and malignancy. A review of the literature. Ann Intern Med 1976; 84:68–76.

209. Lakhanpal S, Melton LJ. Polymyositis-dermatomyositis and malignant lesions: does an association exist? Mayo Clin Proc 1986; 61:645–653.

210. Dropcho EJ, Stanton C, Oh SJ. Neuronal antinuclear antibodies in a patient with Lambert-Eaton myasthenic syndrome and small-cell lung carcinoma. Neurology 1989; 39:249–251.

211. Shirabe T, Hirokawa M, Yasuda T, et al. An autopsy case of carcinoma of the lung associated with subacute cerebellar degeneration and Eaton-Lamber syndrome. Kawasaki Med J 1981; 7:177–188.

212. Carswell EA, Old LJ, Kassel RL, et al. An endotoxin-induced serum factor that causes necrosis of tumors. Proc Natl Acad Sci USA 1975; 72:3666–3670.

213. Shear MJ, Turner FC, Perrault A, et al. Chemical treatment of tumors. V. Isolation of the hemorrhage-producing fraction from Serratia marcescens (Bacillus prodigiosus) culture filtrate. J Natl Cancer Inst 1943; 4:81–97.

214. Aggarwal BB, Kohr WJ, Hass PE, et al. Human tumor necrosis factor. Production, purification, and characterization. J Biol Chem 1985; 260:2345–2354.

215. Rouzer CA, Cerami A. Hypertriglyceridemia associated with Trypanosoma brucei infection in rabbits: role of defective triglyceride removal. Mol Biochem Parasitol 1980; 2:31–38.

216. Kawakami M, Cerami A. Studies of endotoxin-induced decrease in lipoprotein lipase activity. J Exp Med 1981; 154:631–639.

217. Beutler B, Mahoney J, Le Trang N, et al. Purification of cachectin, a lipoprotein lipase–suppressing hormone secreted by endotoxin-induced RAW 264.7 cells. J Exp Med 1985; 161:984–995.

218. Beutler B, Greenwald D, Hulmes JD, et al. Identity of tumour necrosis factor and the macrophage-secreted factor cachectin. Nature 1985; 316:552–554.

219. Caput D, Beutler B, Hartog K, et al. Identification of a common nucleotide sequence in the 3′-untranslated region of mRNA molecules specifying inflammatory mediators. Proc Natl Acad Sci USA 1986; 83:1670–1674.

220. Beutler B, Cerami A. Cachectin: more than a tumor necrosis factor. N Engl J Med 1987; 316:379–385.

221. Cerami A, Tracey KJ, Lowry SF, et al. Cachectin: a pluripotent hormone released during the host response to invasion. Recent Prog Horm Res 1987; 43:99–112.

222. Aderka D, Fisher S, Levo Y, et al. Cachectin/tumour-necrosis-factor production by cancer patients. Lancet 1985; 2:1190.

223. Balkwill F, Osborne R, Burke F, et al. Evidence for tumour necrosis factor/cachectin production in cancer. Lancet 1987; 2:1229–1232.

224. Socher SH, Martinez D, Craig JB, et al. Tumor necrosis factor not detectable in patients with clinical cancer cachexia. J Natl Cancer Inst 1988; 80:595–598.

225. Scuderi P, Sterling KE, Lam KS, et al. Raised serum levels of tumour necrosis factor in parasitic infections. Lancet 1986; 2:1364–1365.

226. Waage A, Espevik T, Lamvik J. Detection of tumour necrosis factor–like cytotoxicity in serum from patients with septicaemia but not from untreated cancer patients. Scand J Immunol 1986; 24:739–743.

227. Selby PJ, Hobbs S, Viner C, et al. Tumour necrosis factor in man: clinical and biological observations. Br J Cancer 1987; 56:803–808.

228. Selby PJ, Hobbs S, Viner C, et al. Endogenous tumour necrosis factor in cancer patients. Lancet 1988; 1:483.

229. Laski ME, Vugrin D. Paraneoplastic syndromes in hypernephroma. Semin Nephrol 1987; 7:123–130.

230. Bernheim HA, Block LH, Atkins E. Fever: pathogenesis, pathophysiology, and purpose. Ann Intern Med 1979; 91:261–270.

231. Glassock RJ, Friedler RM, Massry SG. Kidney and electrolyte disturbances in neoplastic diseases. Contrib Nephrol 1977; 7:2–41.

232. Lumeng J, Moran JF. Carotid body tumor associated with mild membranous glomerulonephritis. Ann Intern Med 1966; 65:1266–1270.

233. Rizzutto VJ, Mazzara JT, Grace WJ. Pheochromocytoma with nephrotic syndrome. Am J Cardiol 1965; 16:432–437.

234. Arneil GC, Harris F, Emmanuel IG, et al. Nephritis in two children after irradiation and chemotherapy for nephroblastoma. Lancet 1974; 1:960–963.

235. Krupey J, Gold P, Freedman SO. Purification and characterization of carcinoembryonic antigens of the human digestive system. Nature 1967; 215:67–68.

236. Waldmann TA, McIntire KR. The use of a radioimmunoassay for alpha-fetoprotein in the diagnosis of malignancy. Cancer 1974; 34:1510–1515.

237. Holyoke ED, Schein PS. Paraneoplastic phenomena. A. Tumor markers. In: Calabresi P, Schein PS, Rosenberg SA, eds. Medical Oncology. Basic Principles and Clinical Management of Cancer. New York: Macmillan, 1985: 178–188.

238. DeGowin RL. Hypertrophic osteoarthropathy. In: DeGowin RL, ed. DeGowin & DeGowin's Bedside Diagnostic Examination. 5th ed. New York: Macmillan, 1987: 650.

239. Klimberg I, Drylie DM. Renal cell carcinoma and idiopathic thrombocytopenic purpura. Urology 1984; 23:293–296.

240. Murphy WG, Allan NC, Perry DJ, et al. Hodgkin's disease presenting as idiopathic thrombocytopenic purpura. Postgrad Med J 1984; 60:614–615.

241. Milnes JP, Goorney BP, Wallington TB. Pure red cell aplasia and thymoma associated with high levels of the suppressor/cytotoxic T lymphocyte subset. Br Med J 1984; 289:1333–1334.

242. Kim HD, Boggs DR. A syndrome resembling idiopathic thrombocytopenic purpura in 10 patients with diverse forms of cancer. Am J Med 1979; 67:371–377.

243. Verdirame JD, Feagler JR, Commers JR. Multiple myeloma associated with immune thrombocytopenic purpura. Cancer 1985; 56:1199–1200.

244. Furie B. Case records of the Massachusetts General Hospital. Case 8-1988. N Engl J Med 1988; 318:500–508.

245. Aghai E, Quitt M, Lurie M, et al. Primary hepatic lymphoma presenting as symptomatic immune thrombocytopenic purpura. Cancer 1987; 60:2308–2311.

35

DISORDERS OF VASODILATOR HORMONES: THE CARCINOID SYNDROME AND MASTOCYTOSIS

L. Jackson Roberts II and John A. Oates

Two syndromes are associated with the release of excessive quantities of vasodilatory mediators into the circulation: the carcinoid syndrome and mastocytosis. Some of the manifestations, such as cutaneous flushing and diarrhea, are similar, and vasodilator hormones contribute prominently to the clinical syndrome in each. However, there are differences in clinical presentation and hormonal mediation.

CARCINOID SYNDROME

The term *carcinoid syndrome* refers to the various humoral manifestations that occur in patients with carcinoid tumors. The term carcinoid was first applied to these tumors by Oberndorfer in 1907 because, although they resembled carcinoma histologically, they followed a more benign clinical course than most other malignancies.[1] It was subsequently recognized that the tumors can invade locally and give rise to distant metastases.

The occurrence of flushing, bronchoconstriction, gastrointestinal hypermotility, and cardiac disease in association with carcinoid tumors eluded recognition until reported by Thorson and colleagues in 1954.[2] The findings that 5-hydroxytryptamine (serotonin) could be isolated from carcinoid tumors[3] and that patients with malignant carcinoid syndrome excrete increased quantities of the serotonin metabolite 5-hydroxyindoleacetic acid (5-HIAA)[4] led to speculation that the humoral manifestations of the carcinoid syndrome could be attributed to the overproduction of serotonin by these tumors. However, serotonin is not the sole mediator of the clinical syndrome, and other agents play a role in the different clinical characteristics of affected patients.

Pathology and Embryology

Enterochromaffin cells give a yellow-brown reaction after chromate fixation. They are distributed in the tissues derived from the primitive gut. Enterochromaffin cells in the intestine are the Kulchitsky cells in the crypts of Lieberkühn. Carcinoid tumors were shown to arise from the enterochromaffin cells by demonstration that both tumor cells and Kulchitsky cells reduce silver salts (argentaffin reaction); thus the term *argentaffinoma* has been used to describe carcinoid tumors.[5]

Polypeptide-secreting endocrine cells in the pituitary, thyroid, lung, pancreas, and gastrointestinal tract share a number of common cytochemical and ultrastructural characteristics. Pearse[6, 7] originally developed the concept of the APUD system—*amine precursor uptake and decarboxylation*—because of the ability of these cells to take up and decarboxylate amino acid precursors of biogenic amines such as serotonin and catecholamines. Included in this system are the enterochromaffin cells that give rise to carcinoid tumors. It has been proposed that this system of cells has a common embryonic origin from the neuronal ectoderm.[7–9] Related cells are also found in the adrenal medulla, sympathetic ganglia, paraganglia, and chemoreceptor system. By virtue of the apparent common embryonic ancestry of these cells, a unique concept of dysplasia of neuronal ectoderm has been proposed to explain the occurrence of multiple endocrine adenomatosis and the multipotentiality of neoplastic cells derived from this system to produce a variety of peptide hormones.[9]

Consistent with the above-mentioned concept, histological similarities among carcinoid tumors, islet cell tumors, and medullary carcinoma of the thyroid have been recognized.[10-12] Furthermore, carcinoid tumors may coexist with other endocrine tumors, and tumors that appear morphologically to be carcinoids may produce gastrin, calcitonin, insulin, vasoactive intestinal peptide, catecholamines, and corticotropin (ACTH, adrenocorticotropin).[13-22] Common embryonic ancestry may also explain the not infrequent occurrence of more than one primary carcinoid tumor in a single patient.[23-25] However, in most instances carcinoid tumors do not occur in association with other endocrine neoplasms, and they usually do not secrete hormones normally produced by cells other than enterochromaffin cells.

Clinical, biochemical, histological, and cytochemical heterogeneity of carcinoid tumors may be related to the site of origin.[26, 27] One classification is based on whether the tumor arose from the embryonic foregut (bronchus, stomach, pancreas), midgut (mid-duodenum to midtransverse colon), or hindgut (descending colon and rectum).[27] As mentioned previously, some carcinoid tumors reduce silver salts;[2, 28] most carcinoid tumors arising from the embryonic midgut are argentaffin-positive. Some tumors do not spontaneously reduce silver salts, although nuclear silver staining can be observed if a reducing substance is added after exposure to silver solutions. Such cells have been termed *argyrophilic*.[28] Carcinoid tumors arising from the embryonic foregut are commonly argentaffin-negative but argyrophilic-positive. In contrast, carcinoid tumors derived from the embryonic hindgut are usually both argentaffin-negative and argyrophilic-negative.[26]

Biochemical features also distinguish carcinoid tumors from different sites of origin. Isolation of serotonin from carcinoid tumors was first reported in 1953.[3] The biosynthesis of serotonin and its metabolic degradation are outlined in Figure 35–1. Overproduction of serotonin in association with carcinoid tumors was documented by demonstration of increased urinary excretion of 5-HIAA (see earlier).[5] Characteristically, carcinoid tumors arising from the embryonic midgut secrete serotonin, and patients with these tumors have elevated urinary excretion of 5-HIAA. Carcinoid tumors arising from the foregut, however, frequently have low activity of L-amino acid decarboxylase, which converts 5-hydroxytryptophan to serotonin.[29-31] Thus these tumors usually secrete primarily 5-hydroxytryptophan. Tumors arising from the midgut may secrete 5-hydroxytryptophan in addition to serotonin.[32] After 5-hydroxytryptophan is secreted, it is converted to serotonin and its metabolites by other tissues in the body. Therefore, although foregut carcinoid tumors usually do not directly secrete large quantities of serotonin, elevated urinary 5-HIAA levels are found in patients with these tumors. In contrast, carcinoid tumors arising from the embryonic hindgut usually do not secrete large amounts of either 5-hydroxytryptophan or serotonin, and patients with these tumors do not have elevated urinary excretion of 5-HIAA.[27, 32]

Incidence and Natural Course

Carcinoid tumors are relatively common. Carcinoids in the small intestine are found in about 1 of 150 patients at autopsy[23] and in the appendix in approximately 1 of 300 appendectomies.[33] Rectal carcinoids occur in about 1 of 2500 proctoscopic examinations.[34] However, the majority are localized and have no evidence of metastasis. The average age of patients is approximately 50, and there is no sexual predominance.[24, 25, 33, 35]

The most common site of carcinoid tumors is the appendix, followed by the ileum, rectum, and other sites in the gastrointestinal tract.[24, 25, 35, 36] Appendiceal carcinoids are usually found incidentally during appendectomy, have a low malignant potential, and rarely metastasize.[33] Rectal carcinoids also have a low malignant potential and are commonly discovered incidentally during proctoscopic examination.[34, 37] For both appendiceal and rectal carcinoids, the occurrence of metastases is related to the size of the primary lesion, in that tumors less than 2 cm in diameter metastasize rarely.[33, 34, 37]

Carcinoid tumors arising from locations other than the appendix and rectum are associated with a higher frequency of metastasis.[24, 25, 33, 35, 36] They initially invade surrounding tissues and spread to regional lymph nodes before distant metastasis occurs. Carcinoids commonly metastasize to the liver, and frequently this is the only site of distant metastasis even when the liver is extensively infiltrated. Extrahepatic metastasis to tissues such as bone occurs occasionally.

As a group, carcinoid tumors grow relatively slowly. Patients may live for many years, and the overall prognosis and survival rates are generally favorable in comparison with other neoplasms.[33] Because of the low incidence of metastasis of appendiceal carcinoids, the 5-y survival rate of patients

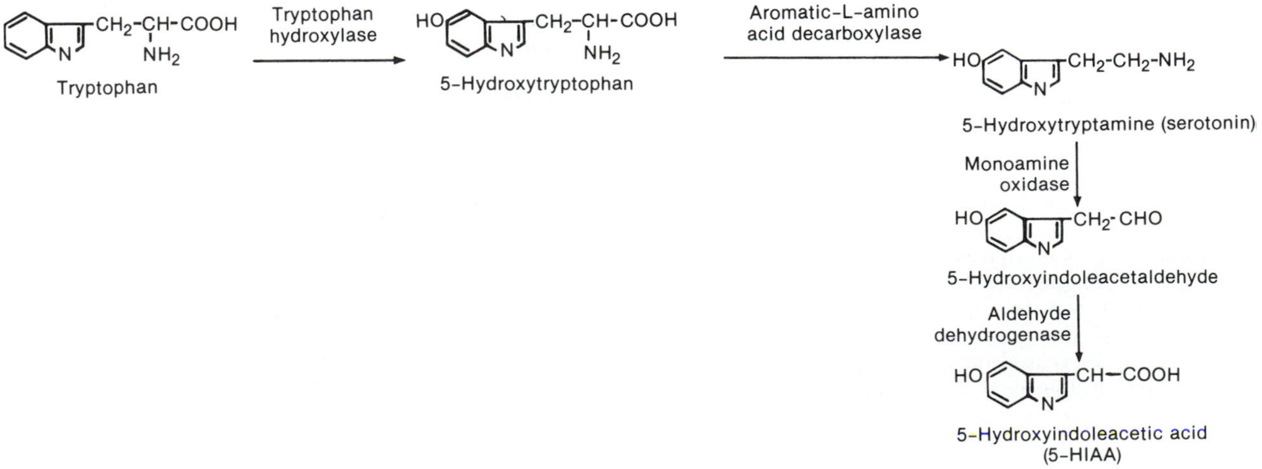

Figure 35–1. Biosysnthesis and metabolism of 5-hydroxytryptamine (serotonin).

with these tumors is approximately 99%. Patients with rectal and lung carcinoids also have a favorable prognosis, with a 5-y survival rate of about 80 to 90%. Patients with carcinoids in the small intestine have survival rates of approximately 50%. The prognosis associated with these tumors varies with the extent of metastasis evident at the time of diagnosis. For example, rectal carcinoids with only local invasion are associated with a greater than 90% 5-y survival rate, which decreases to approximately 45% in the presence of regional metastasis and to about 10% if distant metastasis is present at the time of diagnosis.[24, 25, 33]

Nonendocrine Symptoms

Recognition of nonendocrine symptoms early in the course of disease enhances the likelihood of diagnosis before distant metastasis or endocrine manifestations have occurred. Bronchial carcinoid tumors, like other lung tumors, may be associated with respiratory complaints such as cough, dyspnea, and hemoptysis, which lead to roentgenological examination and bronchoscopy. Rectal carcinoids are usually asymptomatic in the absence of advanced disease.[34, 37] Patients with carcinoids in the small intestine frequently have symptoms for long periods before the diagnosis is made. In this group of patients, early diagnosis can lead to cure by surgical resection of the localized tumor. The most common symptoms and signs of an intestinal carcinoid are abdominal pain, intermittent obstruction, and a palpable abdominal mass, each of which occurs in nearly 50% of patients.[23] Obstruction usually occurs after invasion of the mesentery, which causes a fibroblastic reaction with scarring and matting of loops of small bowel that in turn can produce a mass and intermittently obstruct the intestine. The clinical picture of recurrent intermittent intestinal obstruction should raise the suspicion of carcinoid tumor. Because this process is extraluminal, results of roentgenological examination are normal about half the time.

Hormonal Aspects

GENERAL COMMENTS. The term carcinoid syndrome has been used to describe the humoral manifestations of carcinoid tumors: flushing, bronchoconstriction, gastrointestinal hypermotility, and cardiac disease.[3] Most patients with carcinoid tumors do not develop the syndrome. The frequency of the humoral manifestations varies with the site of origin of the tumor; they are most common with tumors originating in the small intestine and proximal colon. Of patients with small intestinal and proximal colonic carcinoids, 40 to 50% experience the syndrome. It occurs less frequently in patients with bronchial carcinoids, is rarely seen in association with appendiceal carcinoids, and does not occur in patients with rectal carcinoids, even when the rectal carcinoid is in an advanced stage and has metastasized.[23, 24, 33, 34, 37, 38]

The development of the carcinoid syndrome is also a function of total tumor mass and extent of metastasis. It does not occur in patients in whom only a small tumor burden is present. Patients with the full-blown syndrome almost invariably have hepatic metastases.[24] The association with hepatic metastases may be due to efficient inactivation by the liver of hormones released from abdominal tumor into the portal circulation. In contrast, venous drainage from metastatic tumor in the liver goes directly into the systemic circulation and bypasses hepatic inactivation. Consistent with this concept is the fact that the tumors most likely to be associated with the carcinoid syndrome in the absence of hepatic metastasis are ovarian teratoma and bronchial carcinoids, which release mediators directly into the systemic rather than the portal circulation.

CLINICAL FEATURES OF CARCINOID SYNDROME. As noted, the major features of the carcinoid syndrome are paroxysms of flushing, diarrhea, bronchospasm, and cardiac disease.[3] Some patients experience all of these, whereas others lack one or more components.

Flushing. A hallmark of the carcinoid syndrome is paroxysmal flushing manifested by transient episodes of erythema that are usually limited to the face, the neck, and the upper trunk. Patients usually experience a sensation of warmth during flushing and sometimes note palpitations. Occasionally, flushing can be more intense, with cutaneous erythema spreading over the entire body. In such cases dizziness may result from a fall in blood pressure. Severe attacks of flushing can rarely be accompanied by shock and syncope. When patients experience flushing over a long period, a constant facial erythema or plethora may develop, with a cyanotic hue and persistent cutaneous telangiectasia. Such changes can be striking.[39]

The distribution of the flush in patients with the carcinoid syndrome does not usually differ from that occurring in patients with mastocytosis. Although severe flushing and hypotension can occur in patients with the carcinoid syndrome, most episodes are brief (1 or 2 min or less) without dizziness or palpitations.[24] These episodes are merely an embarrassment or a nuisance. In contrast, patients with mastocytosis tend to experience more severe and prolonged flushing accompanied by dizziness or frank syncope.

Flushing usually occurs spontaneously in patients with the carcinoid syndrome in the absence of any evident precipitating cause, but some patients note factors that seem to evoke attacks, such as physical exertion, emotional upset, eating, alcohol ingestion, or heat.[24, 39] Similar factors operate in patients with mastocytosis, with the exception of eating, which rarely provokes flushing in this condition.

Diarrhea. Diarrhea is a common feature of the carcinoid syndrome and can vary from as few as 2 to as many as 30 stools a day. In most patients it is a discomfort and an annoyance but not disabling. Occasionally, voluminous diarrhea may be associated with malabsorption and fluid and electrolyte imbalance. The diarrhea is frequently accompanied by abdominal cramping.

In many patients it is difficult to be certain whether diarrhea and other abdominal symptoms are a result of intestinal hypermotility from stimulation of intestinal smooth muscle by mediators released from the tumor or whether they are a consequence of mechanical factors. The latter include intermittent intestinal obstruction, diminished vascular perfusion, and impaired lymphatic drainage from invasion of the mesentery by tumor and the associated desmoplastic reaction. In addition, many patients have undergone partial surgical resection of small intestine, which can result in the short-bowel syndrome or diarrhea from malabsorption of bile salts after ileal resection. Both endocrine and mechanical factors may contribute to the diarrhea and abdominal symptoms in many patients.

Pulmonary Manifestations. Paroxysms of bronchospasm occur in a small fraction of patients, almost always developing in association with attacks of flushing and resulting from the release of a bronchoconstricting mediator or mediators from the tumor.

Cardiac Manifestations. A unique endocrine effect of carcinoid tumors is the development of plaque-like thickenings on the endocardium of the cardiac valve leaflets, atria, and ventricles in about 20% of patients.[24] Deposition of this fibrous material is also found frequently in the superior and inferior venae cavae, coronary sinus, and pulmonary artery. The aorta and other arterial blood vessels are less commonly involved.[40–42] The right side of the heart is affected predominantly, but left-sided heart involvement, usually of lesser functional consequence, may occur.[41]

Histologically, the plaque-like thickenings in the endocardium consist of smooth muscle and myofibroblast-like cells embedded in a stroma that is rich in mucopolysaccharides, basement membrane–like material, collagen fibrils, and microfibrils. Elastic fibers are missing. An inflammatory reaction is absent, and the plaques are covered by an intact layer of endothelium.[42]

Thickening of mural and valvular endocardium distorts the architecture of the valves and commonly results in pulmonic stenosis and tricuspid insufficiency. When tricuspid insufficiency is severe, right-sided congestive heart failure can result, which contributes in a major way to mortality. Rarely, the left side of the heart is sufficiently involved to produce murmurs of the mitral valve or left-sided congestive heart failure.

Variants of Carcinoid Syndrome

The manifestations just outlined are most characteristic of the syndrome in patients with tumors arising from the small intestine. The syndrome associated with tumors arising from the stomach has several distinguishing features.[31] Gastric carcinoids usually secrete 5-hydroxytryptophan rather than serotonin and usually also secrete histamine, which is uncommon for tumors of midgut origin. The cutaneous flushing in such patients usually consists of patchy serpiginous areas of cutaneous erythema with sharply delineated borders rather than the more typical diffuse cutaneous erythema that is characteristic of patients with carcinoids in the small intestine. Diarrhea and cardiac disease are less common in patients with gastric carcinoids. Patients with gastric carcinoids may experience flushing after ingestion of food and have a high incidence of peptic ulcer disease, possibly related to the release of histamine by the tumors.

The syndrome associated with bronchial carcinoids also frequently has distinctive characteristics. Flushing tends to be prolonged (sometimes lasting days), severe, and associated with tremulousness, bronchospasm, profuse lacrimation, nasal congestion, periorbital edema, and explosive diarrhea. With such severe attacks, marked hypotension is frequent.[43] Differences in the therapeutic aspects of the syndrome associated with bronchial carcinoid tumors are discussed under Treatment.

Mediators of Carcinoid Syndrome

Serotonin may be a primary mediator of the diarrhea associated with the carcinoid syndrome. Infusions of serotonin in humans cause an increase in intestinal motility,[44] and treatment with serotonin antagonists such as methysergide and cyproheptadine usually reduces the severity of diarrhea.[45–48] Similar attenuation of diarrhea is seen after administration of *p*-chlorophenylalanine, which inhibits serotonin biosynthesis by blocking tryptophan hydroxylase.[49–51]

Serotonin is not an important mediator of the flushing. First, some patients experience flushing with only modestly elevated urinary excretion of 5-HIAA, whereas some patients with marked increases in 5-HIAA excretion do not have flushing.[24] Second, serotonin may or may not be released into the circulation during flushing.[52] Third, intravenous infusion of serotonin does not produce a flush similar to the flush in patients with the carcinoid syndrome.[52]

Other potential mediators of the carcinoid flush include bradykinin, prostaglandins, histamine, and tachykinins. Bradykinin is released in some patients during flushing,[53, 54] but the absence of detectable bradykinin release in other patients indicates that it is not a universal mediator of the flush.[54, 55] Although a role for prostaglandins has been considered, we have not found overproduction of prostaglandin E_2, a vasodilator, in patients with the carcinoid syndrome. Moreover, treatment of patients with inhibitors of prostaglandin biosynthesis does not ameliorate attacks of flushing. It therefore seems unlikely that prostaglandins participate in the flushing.

In patients with carcinoid syndrome associated with tumors arising from the midgut, vasoactive peptides called tachykinins are believed to be mediators of the flushing. Tachykinins are a family of structurally related peptides that possess a common COOH-terminal sequence and exert similar biological activities such as vasodilation and contraction of various types of smooth muscle.[56–60] These peptides include substance P, substance K (neurokinin A), and neuropeptide K (an extended form of substance K). Two precursors of these tachykinins, α- and β-pre-protachykinin, are derived from a single gene. These peptides are stored in carcinoid tumors and are present in elevated concentrations in plasma from patients with carcinoid syndrome.[61–69] Documentation that these peptides are linked to the manifestations of the carcinoid syndrome will contribute significantly to our understanding of the pathophysiology of this syndrome.

Gastric carcinoid tumors usually secrete histamine, and affected patients generally have increased urinary excretion of histamine.[31] In contrast, midgut carcinoid tumors produce histamine uncommonly. Treatment of such patients with histamine H_1 receptor antagonists generally fails to abolish episodes of flushing, which suggests that histamine is not the sole mediator of flushing associated with gastric carcinoids. However, flushing in a patient with the gastric carcinoid syndrome was ameliorated with combined administration of H_1 and H_2 receptor antagonists, whereas neither of these given singly prevented attacks.[70] We have observed similar results in another patient with gastric carcinoid syndrome who responded to treatment with H_1 and H_2 receptor antagonists. These results indicate that histamine is secreted by many gastric carcinoid tumors, and in these patients histamine can be the primary mediator of the flushing.

Serotonin may play an important role in the cardiac manifestations. There is a correlation between urinary 5-HIAA levels and carcinoid cardiac disease,[24] and significant cardiac involvement is usually limited to patients with markedly increased levels of urinary 5-HIAA. Conversely, cardiac disease is uncommon in patients with gastric carcinoids that secrete 5-hydroxytryptophan instead of serotonin, which thus spares the heart from exposure to high concentrations of serotonin released directly by the tumor. Attempts to reproduce the cardiac lesion in experimental animals by administration of serotonin have produced inconsistent results.[71–75] In some but not all studies, prolonged administration of serotonin has caused endocardial fibrosis. When present, the fibrosis appeared similar to, but not identical with, that in human carcinoid cardiac lesions. Such differences may arise from species variation or from the fact that it is difficult to reproduce the carcinoid syndrome completely, such as the duration of exposure of the heart to circulating serotonin. Other factors may act in concert with serotonin in producing the cardiac lesion. For example, in one study hepatic damage and tryptophan deficiency were required before chronic administration of serotonin produced endocardial fibrosis in guinea pigs.[75]

Pharmacological Aspects

Flushing in patients with the carcinoid syndrome can be evoked by administration of a variety of pharmacological agents: epinephrine, norepinephrine, isoproterenol, and dopamine.[76–78] Phentolamine prevents flushing in response to epinephrine, norepinephrine, and dopamine,[77, 78] but propranolol does not block flushing in response to epinephrine.[78]

The fact that ingestion of food precipitates flushing in some patients raised the possibility that this response may be due to the release during eating of gastrointestinal hormones, which in turn evoke the release of vasoactive mediators from carcinoid tumors. Low doses of the synthetic analogue of gastrin, pentagastrin, consistently provoked flushing in three patients,[70, 79] and the synthetic COOH-terminal octapeptide of cholecystokinin elicited a flush in one patient.

Somatostatin (SRIF, somatotropin release–inhibiting factor) inhibits the release and action of a number of gastrointestinal hormones[80] and prevents pentagastrin-evoked flushing.[79] Furthermore, somatostatin appears to exert this effect by inhibiting the release of mediators from the tumor.[81, 82] Somatostatin also inhibits the diarrhea and the bronchoconstriction associated with the carcinoid syndrome.[82–84] Whether carcinoid tumors are under constant tonic stimulation by gastrointestinal hormones that are normally inhibited by somatostatin or whether somatostatin exerts a direct inhibitory effect independent of an influence on gastrointestinal hormonal stimulation cannot be determined. In support of the latter possibility is the finding that somatostatin also reversed hypotension after surgical manipulation of a carcinoid tumor in one patient.[85] Whether somatostatin is capable of inhibiting catecholamine-induced flushing has not been examined.

Diagnostic Considerations

In patients with flushing and other manifestations of the carcinoid syndrome, the diagnosis can be established by measuring the urinary excretion of 5-HIAA because it is invariably elevated under these circumstances. In most laboratories the upper limit for the urinary excretion of 5-HIAA is approximately 50 μmol/d (10 mg/d). In patients with the carcinoid syndrome, the magnitude of elevation of urinary 5-HIAA can range from 50 to 3000 μmol/d (10 to 600 mg/d). As mentioned, the degree of elevation in 5-HIAA levels does not always correlate with the severity of flushing. As also noted earlier, patients with the gastric carcinoid syndrome also have increased urinary excretion of 5-HIAA, even though the tumors secrete 5-hydroxytryptophan rather than serotonin. This increase occurs because the 5-hydroxytryptophan released from these tumors is converted to serotonin in other tissues and is subsequently metabolized to 5-HIAA.

A variety of foods and drugs can interfere with the laboratory determination of urinary 5-HIAA (Table 35–1).[86] It is likely that other drugs also interfere. Therefore, when urine is to be collected for 5-HIAA determination, patients must avoid the ingestion of foods listed in Table 35–1 and (when possible) the use of known interfering drugs and any other nonessential drugs.

In a patient with features of the syndrome and urinary 5-HIAA excretion greater than 150 μmol/d (30 mg/d) from collections that avoid interfering substances, the diagnosis is reasonably secure. If 5-HIAA excretion is in the range of 50 to 150 μmol/d (10 to 30 mg/d), additional diagnostic considerations emerge. Intestinal obstruction and other diseases of the small bowel such as nontropical sprue can release sufficient serotonin to cause modest elevations of 5-HIAA, normally less than 130 μmol/d (25 mg/d). Therefore, when the urinary excretion of 5-HIAA is less than 150 μmol/d (30 mg/d), definitive evidence for the presence of a carcinoid

TABLE 35–1. Factors Interfering with Determination of Urinary 5-HIAA

Factors Producing False-Positive Results	
Foods	
Avocados	Pineapples
Bananas	Plums
Eggplants	Walnuts
Drugs	
Acetaminophen	Mephenesin
Acetanilide	Methamphetamine
Caffeine	Methocarbamol
Fluorouracil	Methysergide maleate
Guaifenesin	Phenacetin
Lugol solution	Phenmetrazine
Melphalan	Reserpine
Factors Producing False-Negative Results	
Drugs	
Corticotropin	Methenamine mandelate
p-Chlorophenylalanine	Methyldopa
Chlorpromazine	Monoamine oxidase inhibitors
Heparin	Phenothiazine
Imipramine	Promethazine
Isoniazid	

tumor should be sought, and the distinction from mastocytosis should be addressed. Differentiation from mastocytosis is aided by provocative tests. Whereas epinephrine effectively reverses flushing in patients with mastocytosis, it provokes flushing in patients with the carcinoid syndrome. This differential response can be used as an aid to distinguish the two disorders. A 1 μg/mL solution of epinephrine in normal saline is administered by intravenous bolus beginning with an initial dose of 0.05 μg. The dose is doubled at intervals of 10 min until flushing appears or a maximum of 6.4 μg is given. When flushing occurs, it usually begins within 60 s after the epinephrine is administered and dissipates after 3 or 4 min. If it does occur, it is important to repeat the same, or next higher, dose of epinephrine to make certain that the flush was not spontaneous but was in fact induced by the epinephrine. It is also important to begin with 0.05 μg and not administer doses greater than double the minimal threshold dose that provokes flushing. Larger doses of epinephrine can cause potentially dangerous tachycardia and hypotension. The epinephrine test is not useful for patients suspected of having carcinoid tumors in whom spontaneous episodes of flushing do not occur, because epinephrine usually does not evoke flushing in such patients.[87]

In patients with carcinoid tumors who lack symptoms of the carcinoid syndrome but may experience other symptoms such as intestinal obstruction, which leads to evaluation and the finding of a tumor, diagnosis is made by histological examination of biopsied or resected tumor.

Treatment

Treatment of carcinoid tumors and the carcinoid syndrome has two aims: (1) reduction of tumor mass and (2) control of the disabling symptoms. There is an additional therapeutic aspect to consider in all patients with urinary 5-HIAA levels that are grossly elevated (>500 μmol/d [>100 mg/d]). Tryptophan is an essential amino acid. Normally, about 1% of tryptophan turnover in the body is converted to serotonin, and the remaining 99% is utilized for the synthesis of protein and niacin. In patients with serotonin-secreting carcinoid tumors, as much as 60% of the available tryptophan may be diverted for the synthesis of serotonin, which results in protein and niacin deficiency.[39] Although dietary supplementation with large quantities of tryptophan may be hazardous because it leads to enhanced production of serotonin,[31] it is advisable to treat all patients with supplemental niacin to prevent the development of pellagra.

THERAPEUTIC APPROACHES TO REDUCE TUMOR MASS. As a general principle of surgical treatment, the attempt should be made to remove all visible tumor at the time of operation, because many of these tumors have only invaded surrounding tissue or metastasized to local or regional lymph nodes. Removal of these involved tissues may result in a cure. Even if this is not possible, palliation may be achieved by tumor debulking including the resection of portions of the liver in which metastases are localized. Frequently this renders patients free of symptoms for extended periods.[23] Although the maximal amount of tumor should be removed in these patients, as much small intestine as possible should be preserved to prevent the short-bowel syndrome.

During surgery a massive mediator release can result in a carcinoid crisis. The hazards and precautions required preoperatively, intraoperatively, and postoperatively and the treatment of complications have been reviewed.[88–90] As discussed, somatostatin prevents flushing, diarrhea, and bronchospasm. Successful treatment of hypotension associated with carcinoid crisis during surgery has been reported with somatostatin and the synthetic somatostatin analogue octreotide.[85, 91] Therefore, somatostatin should be available for infusion during surgery in patients with the carcinoid syndrome.

Another treatment modality is surgical resection of hepatic metastases and either ligation or percutaneous embolization of the hepatic artery.[92, 93] The objective is to diminish the bulk of tumor in the liver, which is usually responsible for the carcinoid syndrome. Symptomatic improvement or amelioration of symptoms may be achieved with these procedures in most patients. Surgical resection of hepatic tumor is most effective when metastases are primarily confined to a single lobe. In some patients, one or a few large solitary metastatic nodules can be wedge resected or removed by subsegmental resection of the liver. In patients with more diffuse metastatic involvement confined primarily to one lobe, a total lobectomy is required.

In patients with diffuse metastases involving both lobes of the liver, the hepatic artery can be ligated or embolized by means of a percutaneous catheter.[92, 93] These procedures seem to be associated with relatively few major complications. One advantage of hepatic artery ligation over embolization is that the primary tumor can be removed at the time of surgery. On the other hand, embolization can be repeated without the risk of a major surgical procedure.[92] The mean duration of response is approximately 3 y after surgical resection of hepatic metastases and up to a year for hepatic artery ligation or embolization. Hepatic artery occlusion followed by chemotherapy with doxorubicin and streptozocin appears to be more effective than either treatment used singly.[94] With the combined approach, a response rate of 86% has been achieved, and the median duration of response appears to be longer than 2 y.

A variety of chemotherapeutic regimens have been investigated for patients with inoperable metastatic carcinoid tumors.[92, 95–97] Unfortunately, none is associated with a good response; the average duration of remission is usually less than 1 y. The most effective regimens appear to be streptozocin combined with fluorouracil, which is associated with an objective response (more than 50% regression of tumor) of about 33%,[97] and methotrexate combined with cyclophosphamide, which is associated with an objective response of approximately 55%. In treating patients with severe manifestations of the carcinoid syndrome, initiation of chemotherapy should be undertaken with doses of drugs below what are normally used because rapid lysis of tumor can cause massive release of mediators (carcinoid crisis) that can cause death.[95, 97] If low doses of the chemotherapeutic agents

do not exacerbate the carcinoid syndrome, the dosages should be escalated as tolerance permits. A major drawback of both streptozocin plus fluorouracil and methotrexate plus cyclophosphamide is toxicity. Fluorouracil alone is not usually associated with substantial toxicity and is well tolerated by most patients. Although it less commonly produces an objective response than combination drug therapy, consideration may be given to an initial trial with this agent alone because of its relatively low toxicity. One protocol is to give 400 mg/m^2/d of fluorouracil for 5 d and to repeat this in 6 wk. Six weeks after the second 5-d course, a maintenance dose of 500 mg/m^2 once weekly should be begun. Response should be monitored by computed tomography, ultrasonography, and/or radioisotope scanning for evidence of reduction in tumor mass such as metastatic lesions in the liver. Also, determinations of urinary excretion of 5-HIAA during periods when tumor lysis is not active provide an additional marker of response.[97]

Treatment with human leukocyte interferon and the somatostatin analogue octreotide has resulted in objective evidence of regression and/or stabilization of tumor growth in some patients.[94, 98, 99] This therapy has also been associated with reduction in the severity of the hormonal manifestations of the carcinoid syndrome. Furthermore, patients treated with octreotide have increased survival compared with patients treated with chemotherapy.[94] These early results are encouraging.

Two patients with metastatic carcinoid tumors have been treated with the antiestrogen tamoxifen.[100, 101] Both experienced amelioration of symptoms, and in one there was a reduction in urinary excretion of 5-HIAA and in the size of hepatic metastases and retroperitoneal lymph nodes. These limited observations indicate a need for additional studies of the use of tamoxifen.

PHARMACOLOGICAL THERAPY. Pharmacological therapy aimed at inhibiting the production or effects of mediators released by the tumor may assist in controlling manifestations of the syndrome. Antiserotonin agents such as methysergide and cyproheptadine can ameliorate the diarrhea. For long-term therapy, cyproheptadine is preferred to methysergide because of the potentially serious retroperitoneal, cardiac, and pulmonary fibrosis associated with the latter.[102] Commonly used antidiarrheal agents such as loperamide and diphenoxylate can also be helpful.

The flushing associated with gastric carcinoid tumors appears to be mediated primarily by histamine and can be controlled by treatment with combined histamine H$_1$ and H$_2$ receptor antagonists.[70] Attempts to control flushing associated with carcinoid tumors of midgut origin by use of antiserotonin agents, antihistamines, and inhibitors of prostaglandin biosynthesis have not been effective.

A synthetic long-acting analogue of somatostatin (octreotide) has proved to be of considerable value in the treatment of carcinoid syndrome.[94, 99, 103] The self-administration of the drug by subcutaneous injection every 8 h results in marked or complete relief of flushing and diarrhea in approximately 90 and 75% of patients, respectively. Amelioration of these clinical manifestations is also accompanied by a marked reduction in the urinary excretion of 5-HIAA. The most troublesome side effects are hypoglycemia and steatorrhea, both of which are reversible and rarely severe enough to limit treatment.

Carcinoid syndrome associated with bronchial carcinoid tumors has distinctive features and is treated differently.[43] Many patients experience amelioration of symptoms with glucocorticoids or phenothiazines. The mechanism by which these drugs exert a beneficial effect is unclear.

Cardiac disease can be one of the most serious complications of the carcinoid syndrome and can be responsible for death. Unfortunately, there is no known means to reverse or halt the progression of the endocardial fibrosis. In patients with severe valvular lesions and intractable cardiac failure, surgical replacement of damaged cardiac valves has been undertaken with mixed results.[104–106] This surgery is associated with technical problems because of the marked fibrosis of the endocardium.

MASTOCYTOSIS AND OTHER DISORDERS OF SYSTEMIC MAST CELL ACTIVATION

The mast cell was described in 1877 by Paul Erhlich. Although the origin of mast cells remains unclear, they are distributed in almost all organs[107] and contain a variety of mediators including histamine, heparin, numerous enzymes, leukocyte chemotactic factors, and prostaglandin D_2 (PGD_2).[108, 109] Mast cells can be activated to release these mediators by immunoglobulin E–dependent mechanisms (via surface-bound immunoglobulin E receptors) and by a variety of non–immunoglobulin E–mediated stimuli.[107–114] Although their function remains speculative, mast cells play a role in immediate hypersensitivity reactions.

Several disorders are characterized by systemic activation of mast cells by non–immunoglobulin E–dependent mechanisms, with attendant release of mediators. The archetypical disorder of this type is mastocytosis, a disease characterized by mast cell proliferation. In 1869 Nettleship described a patient with pigmented cutaneous lesions that became urticarial on stroking and called the condition urticaria pigmentosa. Unna subsequently reported finding excessive numbers of mast cells in urticaria pigmentosa. The disorder was initially thought to be limited to skin, but it can be associated with mast cell proliferation in other organs (systemic mastocytosis). The etiology of the proliferation is unknown, and there may be more than a single cause. For example, whereas most cases of mastocytosis do not appear to have any clear-cut hereditary basis, an inheritable form of the disease has been described.[115–117] The latter may be more common than previously recognized.[118]

Symptoms are primarily attributed to paroxysms of mediator release from the mast cells. In addition, some patients without definitive evidence of increased mast cell proliferation exhibit a syndrome virtually indistinguishable from that in patients with the typical disorder.[118] Although increased mast cell proliferation is not evident in such patients with current methods of histological examination, episodic systemic release of excessive quantities of mast cell mediators occurs. Such patients have a syndrome of systemic mast cell activation distinct from the typical mastocytosis that is characterized by excessive proliferation of mast cells in body tissues.

Pathophysiology

The clinical symptoms exhibited by patients with systemic mastocytosis or mast cell activation syndrome are due primarily to the episodic release of mast cell mediators. Prominent among the systemic manifestations is vasodilation manifested by flushing, tachycardia, and occasionally hypotension. Increased intestinal motility can result in abdominal cramping and sometimes nausea, vomiting, and diarrhea. Thus the syndrome resembles that exhibited by patients with the carcinoid syndrome.

Histamine is a potent vasodilator that also causes contraction of gastrointestinal smooth muscle.[119] Histamine is rapidly metabolized in vivo, as outlined in Figure 35–2. Only a small fraction (2 to 3%) of histamine released into the circulation is excreted into the urine unmetabolized. The major urinary metabolite is methylimidazoleacetic acid. Because histamine is released from mast cells and because overproduction of histamine occurs in patients with systemic mastocytosis, it was thought that the humoral symptoms of mastocytosis are attributable to this agent. However, except for a few reports of improvement in diarrhea by histamine H_2 receptor antagonist therapy,[120–122] antihistamine therapy alone usually does not relieve the symptoms. In particular, life-threatening episodes of vasodilatory shock in some patients are not preventable with antihistamine therapy, even with high doses of both H_1 and H_2 receptor antagonists.[123] This experience suggests that histamine is not the sole mediator responsible for symptoms in mastocytosis, in particular the vasodilatory episodes.

In this regard, the discovery of overproduction of the prostaglandin PGD_2 in patients with mastocytosis has contributed importantly to our understanding of the pathophysiology of the disease.[123] PGD_2 is metabolized rapidly in vivo (Fig. 35–3). The major initial pathway involves reduction of the prostane ring keto group at C-11 by an 11-ketoreductase enzyme. This reaction yields the product $9\alpha,11\beta$-prostaglandin F_2 ($9\alpha,11\beta$-PGF_2). $9\alpha,11\beta$-PGF_2 and PGD_2 are further metabolized by dehydrogenation of the C-15 hydroxyl group, reduction of the Δ^{13}-double bond, beta-oxidation, and omega-oxidation, yielding a series of metabolites that are excreted into the urine. Metabolites with a PGF ring are excreted in greater abundance than are PGD-ring me-

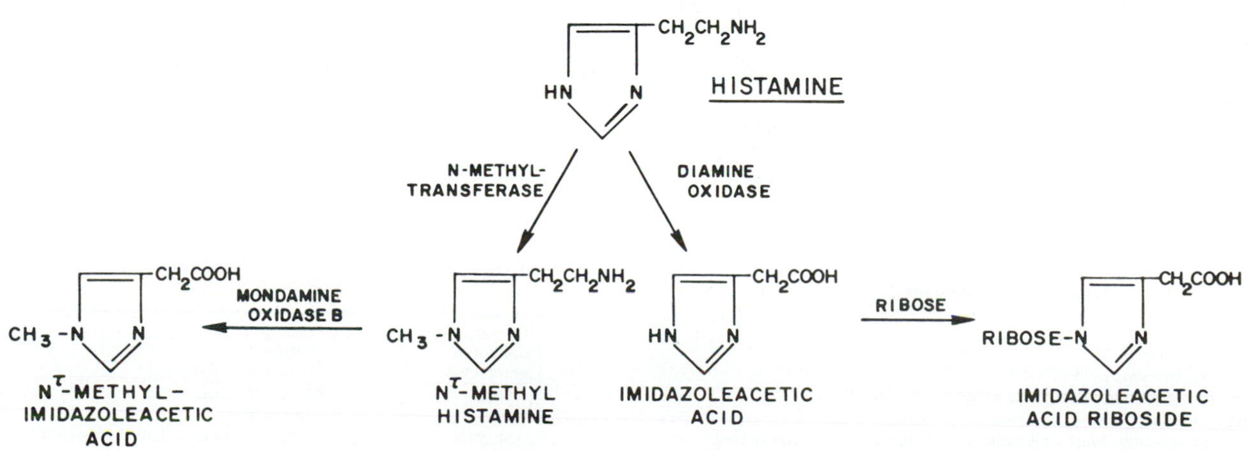

Figure 35–2. Metabolism of histamine.

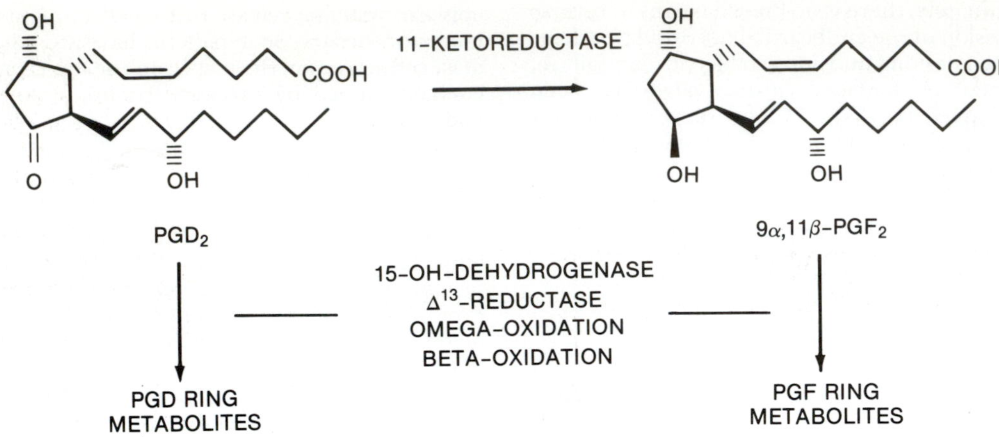

Figure 35–3. Metabolism of PGD_2.

tabolites. Infusion of PGD_2 into animals is associated with marked systemic hypotension and increases in pulmonary artery pressure.[124] Infusion of PGD_2 causes flushing.[125] The possibility that PGD_2 is an important mediator in mastocytosis is supported by studies demonstrating amelioration of symptoms by inhibitors of prostaglandin biosynthesis. In summary, histamine and PGD_2 are both likely to be mediators of the symptoms.

Clinical Syndromes

As just noted, two broad categories of mast cell disorders can be distinguished: those involving mast cell infiltration of various tissues and organs and those in which evidence of proliferation of mast cells is lacking. Heterogeneity exists within each of the categories as to symptoms and signs and severity of symptoms.

CLASSIFICATION. A classification of mast cell activation disorders is given in Table 35–2. The symptoms are protean and can involve almost every organ system. Certain symptoms may be prominent and severe in some patients but minor or absent in others. It is rare for a single patient to experience all the symptoms known to be associated with the disease. In general, patients with mastocytosis limited to cutaneous involvement experience symptoms localized to the skin, whereas patients with systemic proliferation or systemic mast cell activation syndrome experience systemic symptoms. Because of the various combinations and different severity of symptoms, the clinical presentation can be diverse and can mimic a variety of unrelated medical disorders. For these reasons, mast cell activation disorders often go unrecognized and lead to erroneous diagnoses.[118, 126] This problem

seems particularly true in patients who do not have urticaria pigmentosa as a cutaneous clue.[118]

SYMPTOMS. The symptoms are attributed almost entirely to the release of secretory products and only rarely to the physical effects of increased mast cell number. Release of mast cell mediators may be consistently increased, but mast cells can be triggered by largely unknown factors to release increased quantities of mediators episodically. For this reason, symptoms associated with the disease are paroxysmal in nature and frequently referred to as "attacks" by patients. After attacks of moderate to marked severity, patients characteristically experience profound lethargy and prostration that may last for hours or days. This postattack prostration can be useful in differentiating syncope related to mastocytosis from that related to other causes such as cardiac arrhythmia in which return of consciousness is not associated with extreme prostration. After the postattack lethargy subsides, many patients notice an improvement in symptoms and a feeling of general well-being for several days. This phenomenon may be explained by a depletion of mediators during a severe attack, and a few days are required to replenish mediators or precursors of mediators. Although the frequency of attacks in most patients is rather constant, some experience periods of months without attacks and periods in which attacks may occur almost daily. The duration of attacks varies from 1 or 2 min to as long as 2 h. Paroxysms lasting several hours are unusual. In general, milder attacks are shorter than severe attacks.

Symptoms are given in Table 35–3. The prevalence of these symptoms has been compiled from reports of patients with mastocytosis and urticaria pigmentosa and does not include subjects without urticaria pigmentosa or those with systemic mast cell activation syndromes. Until data can be compiled from all groups of patients, it is preferable to discuss the prevalence of symptoms in general terms such as common or uncommon.

A history of flushing is the most important clinical clue. Flushing almost invariably is experienced by patients with

---

TABLE 35–2. Classification of Mast Cell Activation Disorders

Mast Cell Infiltrative Disorders
  Localized Mastocytosis
    Cutaneous
      Without visible lesions
      With 1- to 2-mm erythematous or acneiform papular lesions
      Urticaria pigmentosa
      Telangiectasia macularis eruptiva perstans
      Nodular
      Bullous
    Solitary mastocytoma
  Systemic Mastocytosis
    Mast cell infiltration of multiple organs
    Mast cell leukemia
Syndromes of Systemic Mast Cell Activation Without Evident Increased Mast Cell Proliferation

---

TABLE 35–3. Symptoms of Mastocytosis and Systemic Mast Cell Activation

Flushing	Pruritus
Palpitations	Diarrhea
Lightheadedness	Nausea and vomiting
Syncope	Chronic fatigue
Dyspnea	Paresthesias
Chest pain	Central nervous system dysfunction
Headache	

systemic symptoms, occurs predominantly in the face and upper trunk (flush area), and usually is diffuse rather than mottled or patchy. Occasionally, patients do not realize that they are flushed, do not spontaneously complain of flushing, and may even deny it. However, in most it is possible to elicit a history of feeling hot during attacks. Because other symptoms may be more severe, some patients do not volunteer a history of flushing until this is elicited by careful questioning. Flushing also may not be evident when a severe attack is accompanied by a fall in systemic blood pressure of sufficient magnitude to prevent the filling of dilated cutaneous blood vessels. This effect is important because the lack of a flushed appearance in a patient with unexplained shock should not lead one to exclude the possibility of massive mast cell mediator release. In such patients, however, flushing usually develops as the attack is resolving and the blood pressure rises. A flushed appearance of the skin can also be noted in patients who do not experience systemic symptoms and appear to have mastocytosis limited to skin. In this situation, however, cutaneous vasodilation does not result from high circulating concentrations of vasodilating mast cell mediators but from the local release of these mediators in the skin. The appearance of flushed skin in these patients is usually not limited to the face and upper trunk and may be mottled and patchy rather than diffuse.

Palpitations are common during episodes of flushing; with severe flushing tachycardias of more than 150 beats/min may occur. Tachycardia is predominantly a secondary baroreceptor response to systemic vasodilation, although histamine may contribute directly through a positive chronotropic effect on the heart.[127]

Lightheadedness and a feeling of faintness occur during severe attacks of flushing accompanied by systemic vasodilation and a fall in blood pressure. Characteristically, this lightheadedness improves when the patient assumes the supine position. Blood pressure can fall precipitously and result in shock and syncope that may be life-threatening. Fortunately, the hypotension usually is not prolonged and thus rarely progresses to refractory vascular collapse or death.[123] Onset of attacks may be rapid and result in syncope or near-syncope in less than a minute. Such a rapid onset may be dangerous, as when the patient is driving a car. Occasionally, syncope may develop so rapidly that antecedent flushing is not appreciated even though it is present during milder episodes. After syncope some patients exhibit amnesia for symptoms and events occurring before the syncopal episode as a result of cerebral ischemia. In summary, the failure to elicit a history of flushing before syncopal episodes does not exclude the possibility of mastocytosis.

Headaches are common and are usually, but not always, bilateral and throbbing in nature. Many patients experience chronic headaches, whereas others have headaches only during an attack of flushing. Headache probably results from dilation of cranial vessels.

Dyspnea is common during episodes of intense flushing. Interestingly, however, it is not accompanied by subjective or auscultatory wheezing. The mechanisms underlying the dyspnea remain unclear.

Chest pain is also frequent during attacks. Although usually mild, it may be severe and the presenting complaint. It is not likely to be of coronary origin because it can occur in young patients and because electrocardiograms taken during the chest pain fail to reveal evidence of cardiac ischemia. Thus the origin of the chest pain remains speculative.

Many patients experience intermittent mild pruritus. Severe chronic pruritus is unusual but does occur. In some patients, pruritus occurs only after hot showers.

Diarrhea is usually intermittent and not severe. Patients may experience one or two loose stools 1 d a week. Other patients who do not have even mild diarrhea between attacks can develop explosive diarrhea during or after severe episodes of flushing. This pattern can be valuable diagnostically because severe diarrhea does not characteristically accompany syncope from causes other than mastocytosis, although it can occur during attacks in patients with the carcinoid syndrome. Many patients experience abdominal cramps in the absence of diarrhea during severe attacks of flushing. Chronic diarrhea is uncommon with mastocytosis and seems to occur predominantly in patients with severe systemic disease involving extensive mast cell infiltration of multiple organs.

Nausea is frequent during severe attacks of flushing, but vomiting is unusual. Nausea and vomiting between attacks are most likely unrelated to mastocytosis.

Chronic fatigue is a common complaint and may be severe. Although the fatigue can wax and wane in severity, it is typically chronic.

Paresthesias may occur, usually during or at the beginning of episodes of flushing, and can involve the entire body. They have been described as a "creeping crawling" sensation in the skin. The pathogenesis is unknown.

Abnormalities in central nervous system function include emotional lability and cognitive dysfunction.[128, 129] Another complaint is periodic forgetfulness.

The Hypertensive Variant. In one variant of the clinical syndrome patients experience the same symptoms just described, but these patients exhibit elevations in blood pressure, sometimes of a marked degree, rather than a fall in blood pressure during episodes of systemic mast cell activation. These patients also appear flushed, and for reasons that are unclear, they may also experience syncope, even though they are not hypotensive. Many of these patients are thought to have a pheochromocytoma, even though patients with pheochromocytoma do not flush.

The pathogenesis of the increase in blood pressure is not known but may be related to quantitative differences in the metabolism of PGD_2 in that PGD_2, which is a vasodilator, is initially metabolized to $9\alpha,11\beta$-PGF_2, which elevates blood pressure in animals.[130] Regardless of the etiology of the hypertension, these patients also respond to the acute and chronic therapy described later.

SIGNS. ***Cutaneous Signs.*** The signs of cutaneous involvement are varied. In the past it was thought that most patients (99%) with mastocytosis had urticaria pigmentosa.[131] The appearance of the skin of a patient with urticaria pigmentosa is depicted in Figure 35–4. The lesions are small, slightly pigmented, and maculopapular; they become urticarial when rubbed. Biopsy reveals increased numbers of mast cells. Mastocytosis can occur without urticaria pigmentosa.[118] Patients with lesions of urticaria pigmentosa are more easily diagnosed, but the diagnosis cannot be excluded because of the absence of classic lesions in the skin.

The appearance of urticaria after stroking has been termed Darier sign. However, almost all patients with mastocytosis, including those without visible lesions, also demonstrate a wheal-and-flare response in apparently uninvolved areas when the skin is stroked with a blunt instrument. Although the flare response develops rapidly, the whealing usually takes several minutes to develop after stroking.

We have described in patients with mastocytosis without urticaria pigmentosa and in patients with systemic mast cell activation syndromes the occurrence of small, 1- to 2-mm, red, papular or acneiform lesions with a surrounding erythematous base (Fig. 35–5).[118] These cutaneous lesions do

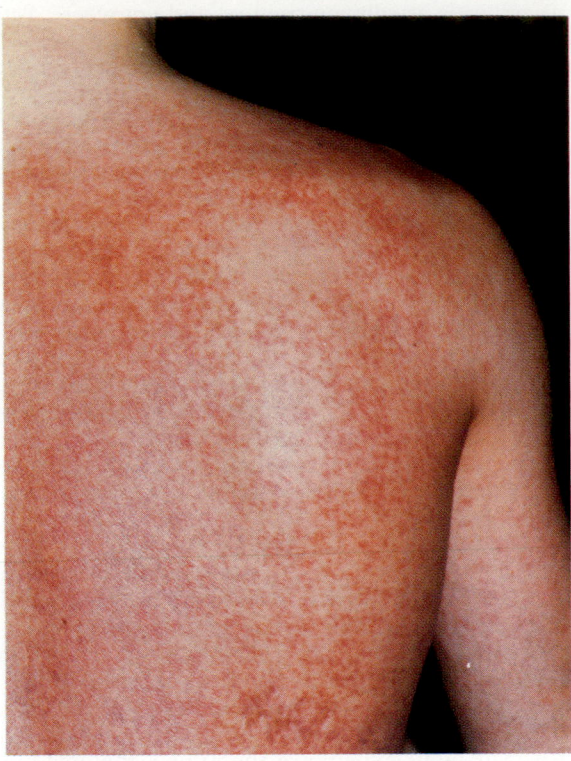

Figure 35–4. Cutaneous lesions of urticaria pigmentosa.

not persist but appear intermittently. Biopsy does not reveal excessive mast cells in the lesions. The whitish material in the acneiform lesions is not purulent but appears to be a fibrous exudate. These lesions may be pruritic.

In addition to the cutaneous signs of mastocytosis, an adult form of cutaneous mastocytosis has been termed *telangiectasia macularis eruptiva perstans*.[132] Such patients have erythematous skin and persistent telangiectasias that are presumed to result from chronic vasodilation secondary to the release of mast cell mediators in the skin.

Two additional forms of cutaneous mastocytosis in children are manifested by bullous or nodular lesions.[132] Such lesions may range from a few millimeters to several centimeters in diameter. At times, the bullous type is hemorrhagic. Both bullous and nodular lesions can occasionally be intermixed with typical lesions of urticaria pigmentosa.

Solitary mastocytomas occur almost exclusively in children[132] and are single, isolated tumors. The size can range up to 3 or 4 cm in diameter; histologically they consist of a dense infiltration of mast cells. Mastocytomas usually respond favorably to surgical removal, without recurrence.

Systemic Signs. The signs of systemic mastocytosis can occur in various combinations and with variable severity. Organ enlargement such as hepatomegaly and splenomegaly may occur as a result of dense infiltration of mast cells.[107, 126, 131, 132] The high incidence of hepatosplenomegaly in some series may be due to the fact that such patients are diagnosed more frequently than those with milder forms of the disease. In patients with systemic mast cell activation without increased mast cell proliferation, hepatosplenomegaly is not seen.

Osseous involvement can be manifested by either osteoporosis or osteosclerosis.[107, 126, 132, 133] Both forms of bone disease can occur in the same patient, but radiologically evident bone disease is probably uncommon. Explanations for the occurrence of both osteoporosis and osteosclerosis in patients with mastocytosis remain speculative.[134] Increased proliferation of mast cells in the bone marrow can be diffuse or can involve focal, granuloma-like lesions.[126, 132]

Radiological signs of gastrointestinal mastocytosis have also been described.[107, 132, 135–139] In some patients, small, evanescent, 1- to 3-mm, nodular mucosal filling defects can be seen, usually in the jejunum but on occasion also in the ileum, the stomach, and the large bowel.[135–138] The mucosal nodules do not appear to be focal accumulations of mast cells but are analogous to papular urticaria. With endoscopy, only small mucosal urticarial-like lesions are seen, and biopsy of the lesions does not demonstrate focal mast cell accumulation.[135–138] The radiological findings can be subtle and easily overlooked, and special precautions should be taken during the examination to differentiate small, mobile air bubbles from the fixed, nodular filling defects in the mucosa. Less specific radiological signs such as gastric hypersecretion and increased transit time of contrast media through the small intestine may also be noted. Furthermore, diffuse thickening of the bowel wall can at times be demonstrated radiologically, usually in patients with severe abnormal mast cell proliferation. In contrast to the mucosal nodules, mast cell infiltration of the lamina propria is usually found with bowel wall thickening.[135]

Peripheral blood abnormalities are largely nonspecific.[132] With marked mast cell infiltration of the bone marrow, anemia is common, and varying degrees of leukocytosis may be present. Eosinophilia, usually of a slight degree, is found in about 10% of patients. Although the cause of eosinophilia is not entirely clear, the release of eosinophil chemotactic factor of anaphylaxis may play a role.

A rare but specific peripheral blood abnormality is mast cell leukemia. This condition develops in a small percentage of patients with systemic mastocytosis and appears to be associated with a more grave prognosis than that for patients with systemic mastocytosis who lack mast cells in the peripheral circulation.[107, 132]

Provoking Factors

NONPHARMACOLOGICAL FACTORS. More often than not, patients spontaneously experience the sudden onset of flushing that is temporally unassociated with an identifiable inciting cause. Little is known regarding nonimmunological endogenous factors that cause the sudden, synchronous systemic activation of mast cells in patients with mastocytosis.

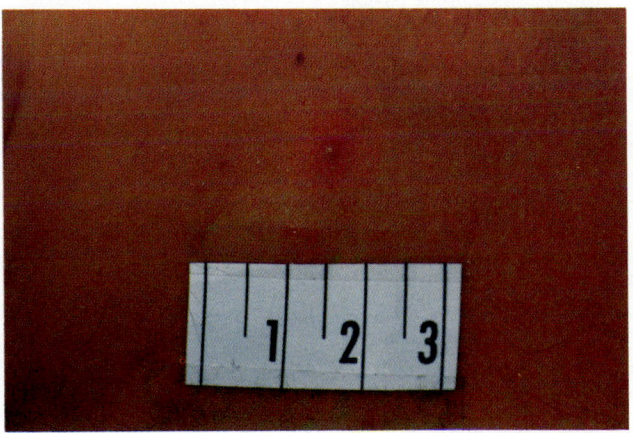

Figure 35–5. Acneiform cutaneous lesions found in some patients with mastocytosis and the syndrome of systemic mast cell activation.

However, many patients can identify factors or situations that may precipitate attacks; the most common are physical exertion, heat, and emotional anxiety.[107, 123] How these factors lead to mast cell activation is unclear. In women, symptoms of mastocytosis may increase just before the onset of menses, which suggests a possible influence of gonadal hormones on mast cell activation.

PHARMACOLOGICAL PROVOKING AGENTS. Several pharmacological agents can cause mast cell activation. For obvious reasons, these drugs should be avoided or used with caution (beginning with minuscule doses) in patients known to have a mast cell disorder. The narcotic analgesics[107] are one class of drugs that can produce severe adverse reactions. These drugs include meperidine, morphine, and codeine. Intradermal injection of meperidine into normal volunteers elicits a typical wheal-and-flare reaction. The authors have used intravenous butorphanol for analgesia in several patients with mastocytosis without producing untoward reactions. However, we have administered this drug only if there is absence of a local reaction after intradermal injection and then beginning with small initial doses. Agents known to produce occasional anaphylactoid reactions and histamine release such as dextran and radiological contrast dyes should also be avoided if possible.[140, 141] Alcohol ingestion can also evoke flushing in some patients;[107] the reaction to alcohol may not be consistent or reproducible.

Surgical management of patients with mastocytosis can be hazardous because drugs used during surgery and anesthesia can evoke potentially fatal reactions.[142] However, with appropriate precautions, patients with mastocytosis can undergo surgery without adverse effects.[143, 144]

Beta-adrenergic receptor antagonists are contraindicated. Indeed, beta-receptor agonists effectively inhibit mast cell degranulation in vitro and, as discussed later, epinephrine is effective in reversing severe attacks of flushing and hypotension.[145] During attacks there is substantial release of endogenous epinephrine from the adrenal medulla, which may serve to attenuate the severity of the attack. Therefore, beta-receptor antagonists may be expected to prevent the beneficial effects of endogenous epinephrine release and would also render the attacks refractory to pharmacological treatment with epinephrine. Furthermore, because cholinergic and alpha-adrenergic agonists can potentiate mast cell mediator release,[146] administration of these agents should probably be avoided. The antihypertensive drug clonidine can evoke mast cell mediator release in vitro, presumably through its action as an alpha-adrenergic receptor agonist.[147]

PROVOCATION BY NONSTEROIDAL ANTI-INFLAMMATORY DRUGS. In a subset of patients with mast cell activation disorders, attacks are evoked by aspirin and other nonsteroidal anti-inflammatory drugs.[107] It is important to recognize this group because the attacks triggered by such drugs can be severe and even fatal. This phenomenon has been termed *aspirin hypersensitivity*. Patients exhibiting these reactions can react to minuscule doses of these drugs, even as low as 10 to 20 mg of aspirin. Aspirin hypersensitivity occurs in 5 to 10% of patients with asthma, in whom ingestion of these agents evokes severe bronchospasm.[148, 149] In a similar percentage of patients with mastocytosis, ingestion of these drugs can evoke massive mast cell mediator release that can culminate in shock and death. Unlike the case in asthmatic patients, bronchospasm is not a prominent feature. The mechanisms involved are unclear. It is unlikely that they are due to allergic reactions because these patients react similarly to all nonsteroidal anti-inflammatory drugs, despite their dissimilar structures. Because a common property shared by all these drugs is an ability to inhibit prostaglandin biosynthesis, it is generally accepted that the reactions are triggered by inhibition of prostaglandin production. Inhibition of PGD_2 production within the mast cell itself does not appear to be the triggering event.[150] Often a clear history of provocation by nonsteroidal anti-inflammatory drugs is absent, which requires cautious testing to identify the problem. Such provocative testing should be conducted only by physicians with experience in managing the severe reactions that may ensue.

Natural Course and Prognosis

The natural course of mastocytosis is variable and unpredictable. One general predictor, however, is related to the age at the time of onset of the disease. When mastocytosis appears during infancy, the disease regresses spontaneously and disappears before adulthood in approximately half of cases. However, when onset is during adulthood, the disorder rarely, if ever, spontaneously disappears. In part, the prognosis is determined by whether there is systemic involvement. In cutaneous mastocytosis, symptoms are usually limited to the skin, and the prognosis is favorable. However, the disease may initially appear limited to the skin and subsequently progress to systemic involvement.[132] Some patients with the systemic form may experience only mild symptoms that do not increase in severity over time. In others the disease follows an unrelenting course of increasing severity, and in rare instances it may be fatal. Death usually occurs as a consequence of the massive release of mast cell mediators. However, advances in understanding of mast cell mediators, in particular the role of PGD_2, have led to more effective therapy for the systemic attacks resulting from mediator release (see later). Whether the natural course of the disorder and overall prognosis differ in patients with abnormal mast cell proliferation compared with those with the syndrome of systemic mast cell activation is not known.

Diagnostic Evaluation

In patients without visible urticaria pigmentosa, the diagnosis probably will not be made unless it is suspected on the basis of clinical symptoms. Indeed, in most cases the results of physical examination and routine laboratory and radiological tests are normal. The diagnosis initially involves the recognition of a compatible clinical syndrome. Mimicking diseases such as the carcinoid syndrome must be excluded. Histological evidence of increased proliferation of mast cells is sought to distinguish mastocytosis from systemic mast cell activation. The levels of mast cell mediators are measured; if mediators are not found to be chronically present, episodic release of mediators is assessed after attacks of flushing. Finally, the clinical response to treatment directed at preventing the effects of mast cell mediators is evaluated.

BIOCHEMICAL INDICATORS OF MAST CELL ACTIVATION DISORDERS. During mast cell activation, increased quantities of mast cell secretory products are released, including histamine, PGD_2, tryptase, and heparin. Thus quantitative analysis of these products and their metabolites can provide biochemical evidence of systemic mast cell activation.

Determination of histamine levels in plasma is most valuable when blood is obtained during an acute episode of flushing. For a more integrated assessment of endogenous production, the 24-h urinary excretion of histamine should be determined. However, 24-h urinary excretion of histamine in patients with the mast cell activation syndrome may be normal during quiescent periods. In such patients, an increased amount of histamine is released into urine for approximately 4 h after an attack of flushing.

Patients who do not have elevated urinary histamine levels may have increased urinary excretion of the histamine metabolites methylhistamine and methylimidazolacetic acid.[151] Thus quantification of histamine metabolites may be a more sensitive index of overproduction of histamine. Unfortunately, assays for these metabolites are available in only a few laboratories. Levels of urinary histamine and histamine metabolites are also influenced by diet.[152] Dietary histidine can be decarboxylated in vivo to histamine, so foods such as cheese, spinach, eggplant, and chicken liver that contain large quantities of histamine and foods with high histidine content (meat) can artifactually increase the urinary excretion of histamine and its metabolites.[153] Thus it is advisable to quantify the urinary excretion of these compounds under controlled dietary conditions.

Another problem with determination of histamine in urine and plasma concerns the accuracy and reliability of analytical methods.[154] The most widely used methods are radioenzymatic and fluorometric assays that at times can be inaccurate. As assayed by methods using gas chromatography–mass spectrometry,[155] normal individuals rarely excrete more than 50 μg/24 h. Unfortunately, until existing methods are improved or the more accurate gas chromatographic methods become more generally available, some caution must be exercised regarding quantification and interpretation of histamine levels in patients with suspected mastocytosis.

A second approach to assess the release of excessive quantities of mast cell mediators is measurement of endogenous production of PGD_2, which can be assessed by quantifying the urinary metabolite of PGD 9α-hydroxy-11,15-dioxo-2,3,18,19-tetranorprost-5-ene-1,20-dioic acid.[156] Up to 150-fold increases in endogenous production of PGD_2 have been found in patients with mastocytosis.[118, 123] Unfortunately, this assay is available only as a research procedure.

Increased quantities of the granule-associated enzyme tryptase are present in plasma during anaphylaxis and in some patients with systemic mastocytosis.[157] Peak concentrations occur approximately 1 to 2 h after mastocyte activation.[158] Tryptase can be measured by radioimmunoassay in some laboratories.

During severe attacks it may be possible to obtain indirect semiquantitative evidence of release of excessive quantities of heparin in patients with mastocytosis. Namely, the partial thromboplastin time may be prolonged during severe attacks.[159, 160] Correction of prolonged partial thromboplastin time by protamine provides evidence that the defect in coagulation is a result of increased circulating heparin.

HISTOLOGICAL EVALUATION. Histological examination is useful for distinguishing patients with mast cell infiltrative disease from those with systemic mast cell activation. The most accessible sites for demonstration of increased proliferation of mast cells are the skin and the bone marrow. When any tissue is obtained for this purpose, the pathologist must be informed that mastocytosis is suspected; unless the tissue sample is examined specifically for mast cells with stains such as toluidine blue, it is not possible to distinguish mast cells from other cells.

Biopsy of urticaria pigmentosa lesions demonstrates sheets of mast cells too numerous to count microscopically.[132] Urticaria pigmentosa is thus easily recognized histopathologically. The interpretation of skin biopsy samples from patients without the lesions of urticaria pigmentosa is more difficult. Rigid criteria for interpretation of such samples have not been established. More than 30 mast cells per high-power field suggests mast cell proliferation, but this finding in isolation is not sufficient to establish a diagnosis with certainty.[161] Clinically uninvolved skin from patients with urticaria pigmentosa may not clearly demonstrate abnormal mast cell proliferation. Similarly, in patients with cutaneous mastocytosis without urticaria pigmentosa the skin may not

be homogeneously involved. Thus a normal skin biopsy result in a patient suspected of having mastocytosis does not necessarily exclude the diagnosis.

Bone marrow examination can also be useful, but criteria for determining mildly to moderately increased mast cell proliferation in the bone marrow have not been established. Also, as with skin, a single sample may not be representative of the entire bone marrow. In patients with severe attacks, a bone marrow biopsy should be performed only after therapeutic doses of antihistamines and a prostaglandin biosynthesis inhibitor have been given to minimize the effects of activation of mast cells in the bone marrow that result from the procedure.

RADIOLOGICAL AND OTHER LABORATORY TESTS. Radioisotopic scans of the liver, spleen, and bone are of little value unless the physical examination suggests hepatosplenomegaly or regular x-ray examination suggests osteoporosis or osteosclerosis. Modest eosinophilia may be present in a small percentage of patients. In all patients with suspected mastocytosis, the 24-h excretion of 5-HIAA should be quantified to exclude the carcinoid syndrome. Urinary excretion of 5-HIAA is not elevated even in patients with severe mastocytosis. On rare occasions, patients with mastocytosis experience angioneurotic edema, and if this does occur, levels of C1 esterase inhibitor and C4 should be measured.

All patients should undergo radiological examination of the stomach and small bowel, for two reasons. First, small mucosal nodules and nonspecific abnormalities such as bowel wall thickening may be seen. Second, such examination can exclude the presence of peptic ulcer disease because most patients are treated with potentially ulcerogenic, nonsteroidal anti-inflammatory drugs.

INCIDENCE OF SYSTEMIC INVOLVEMENT IN PATIENTS WITH CUTANEOUS MASTOCYTOSIS. It was previously thought that patients with cutaneous mastocytosis uncommonly had systemic involvement. This erroneous assumption may be due to a failure to evaluate patients adequately for evidence of systemic disease, especially patients without severe systemic symptoms. Rigorous histological evaluation of the bone marrow and careful assessment of histamine production by quantifying the urinary excretion of histamine metabolites have revealed that half of adult patients with urticaria pigmentosa have systemic involvement.[162]

Treatment

Pharmacological interventions can prevent the recurrence of severe attacks and reverse acute episodes. The most life-threatening aspect of mastocytosis and the systemic mast cell activation syndrome is the severe attack associated with hypotension that can culminate in shock, syncope, and death. The ability to prevent these attacks with pharmacological therapy has improved the overall prognosis.

TREATMENT OF THE ACUTE HYPOTENSIVE EPISODE. As in the treatment of allergic anaphylaxis, epinephrine is effective in reversing the hypotension associated with mast cell mediator release.[145] Doses of epinephrine that are effective in reversing marked hypotension associated with mastocytosis cause only modest elevations in blood pressure and pulse rate in normal volunteers.[163] This result suggests that the mechanism by which epinephrine exerts its effect is not linked solely to its direct pressor effects. Rather, epinephrine may act predominantly by inhibiting mast cell mediator release.[145] This possibility is supported by demonstration in vitro that beta-receptor agonists inhibit mast cell mediator release from sensitized lung.[164]

Patients with severe flushing and hypotension should be given epinephrine either subcutaneously or intravenously. The subcutaneous injection of 300 μg usually effectively reverses hypotension, but the action may be short-lived owing to rapid absorption and metabolic inactivation of the drug. Thus maintenance of the effect of epinephrine is best achieved by continuous intravenous infusion at a rate of 2 to 10 μg/min. Beginning with an initial dose of 4 μg/min, the dose can be subsequently adjusted depending on the response. After return of blood pressure to normal and resolution of other symptoms, the dose of epinephrine should be reduced by increments of about 1 μg/min at ½-h intervals until discontinued or until the requirement for continued infusion becomes apparent with return of flushing and other manifestations.

As mentioned previously, a subset of patients experience marked elevation in blood pressure rather than hypotension during episodes of systemic mast cell activation. It is interesting that administration of epinephrine to these patients results in a lowering of the blood pressure to near-normal levels. This response supports the assumption that the increase in blood pressure is linked to mast cell mediator release, possibly involving $9\alpha,11\beta$-PGF_2, as discussed previously.

It is advisable to instruct patients who have experienced severe attacks to self-administer epinephrine as outpatients, in case an attack occurs when medical help is not immediately available. Outpatient use of epinephrine can be in the form of subcutaneous injection or inhalation. EpiPen (Center Laboratories) and Ana-Kit (Miles Pharmaceutical) are commercially available, predosed syringes for subcutaneous injection designed to deliver 300 μg of epinephrine. A more convenient means of administration of smaller doses is by inhalation. Another advantage of the use of such inhalers is that repeated doses can be given if symptoms recur.

CHRONIC THERAPY. Chronic therapy for the disease is designed to reduce the quantity and effects of mediator release. Antihistamine therapy combined with inhibition of prostaglandin biosynthesis effectively prevents recurrent episodes of severe vasodilation and improves other symptoms such as dyspnea, diarrhea, headache, fatigue, and pruritus.[118, 123] Blockade of both histamine H_1 and H_2 receptors is required to prevent the vasodilator effects of histamine.[165] Thus an H_1 receptor antagonist such as chlorpheniramine (16 to 32 mg daily) or doxepin (5 to 20 mg daily)[166] should be given in combination with an H_2 receptor antagonist such as ranitidine (300 mg daily). For patients with refractory pruritus, higher doses of doxepin may be required, up to 100 mg daily.

Inhibition of prostaglandin biosynthesis is accomplished by administration of nonsteroidal anti-inflammatory drugs that inhibit the cyclooxygenase enzyme responsible for the initial conversion of arachidonic acid to the endoperoxide intermediates prostaglandin G_2 and prostaglandin H_2. Although numerous nonsteroidal anti-inflammatory drugs are available, there are advantages in the use of aspirin. Aspirin is less expensive, and therapy can be monitored with plasma salicylate determinations, whereas blood level measurements of other nonsteroidal anti-inflammatory drugs are not generally available. Determination of drug levels is of value because interindividual variation in absorption and metabolism can cause differences in plasma levels in individuals given the same amounts of drug.[167] Documentation that an effective blood level of drug is achieved is of value in the treatment of recurrent episodes of life-threatening hypotension. In our experience, plasma salicylate levels in the range of 1.5 to 2 μmol/L (20 to 30 mg/dL) 4 to 5 h after a dose are required to prevent the recurrence of severe episodes of vasodilation. In most adult patients, the dose of aspirin required to achieve a plasma salicylate level in this range is 3.9 to 5.2 g/d. Failure to achieve adequate plasma salicylate levels is usually associated with continuing symptoms. If

salicylates are not well tolerated, another nonsteroidal anti-inflammatory drug such as piroxicam or naproxen may be substituted.

As discussed earlier, about 5% of patients with mastocytosis or the systemic mast cell activation syndrome are aspirin hypersensitive. In these patients, ingestion of minuscule doses of aspirin or other nonsteroidal anti-inflammatory drugs can evoke potentially lethal vasodilatory shock. Therefore, initiation of aspirin therapy must be undertaken with caution. Because aspirin is generally considered to be a trivial drug that can be taken casually, some patients with aspirin-evoked systemic mast cell mediator release do not give a clear history of aspirin provocation. Accordingly, it is prudent to initiate aspirin therapy in all such patients under careful observation. The initial dose should be small, 20 mg or less if attacks have been severe. Reactions to aspirin usually occur between 30 min and 3 h after ingestion, and if no adverse effects are seen the dose can be doubled at 3-h intervals. Severe reactions to aspirin associated with hypotension may be treated with intravenous epinephrine, as discussed earlier. Patients with aspirin-evoked mast cell activation should be instructed in the avoidance of all nonsteroidal anti-inflammatory drugs; they probably should also avoid the ingestion of tartrazine (FD&C Yellow No. 5), as well as acetaminophen, which in some patients may evoke reactions.

Treatment of patients with aspirin-evoked mast cell activation disorders involves administration of antihistamines and self-administration of epinephrine to abort severe attacks. Other approaches to the treatment of such patients are experimental at present. Isolated reports have suggested that oral administration of cromolyn sodium may be effective for controlling diarrhea in patients with mastocytosis,[168, 169] and a single study has reported amelioration of systemic symptoms of mastocytosis in some patients.[128] However, the efficacy of this drug is not established.

Although treatment of patients with systemic mastocytosis with oral glucocorticoids is not effective for ameliorating symptoms of systemic mast cell activation, potent topical glucocorticoids under occlusion can be helpful in the treatment of urticaria pigmentosa.[170] It is interesting that topical glucocorticoids may induce a prolonged resolution of urticaria pigmentosa lesions associated with a marked reduction in the number of lesional mast cells.

REFERENCES

1. Oberndorfer S. Uber die "kleinen Dumdarn-Carcinome." Verh Dtsch Ges Pathol 1907; 11:113–116.
2. Thorson G, Bjork G, Bjorkmann G, et al. Malignant carcinoid of the small intestine with metastasis to liver, valvular disease of the right side of the heart (pulmonary stenosis and tricuspid regurgitation without septal defects), peripheral vasomotor symptoms, bronchoconstriction, and an unusual type of cyanosis. Am Heart J 1954; 47:795–817.
3. Lembeck F. 5-Hydroxytryptamine in a carcinoid tumor. Nature 1953; 172:910–911.
4. Page IH, Corcoran AC, Udenfriend S, et al. Argentaffinoma as an endocrine tumour. Lancet 1955; 1:198–199.
5. Masson P. Carcinoid (argentaffin-cell tumors) and nerve hyperplasia of appendicular mucosa. Am J Pathol 1928; 4:181–212.
6. Pearse AGE. Common cytochemical and ultrastructural characteristics of cells producing polypeptide hormones (the APUD series) and their relevance to thyroid and ultimobronchial C cells and calcitonin. Proc R Soc Biol 1968; 170:71–80.
7. Pearse AGE. The cytochemistry and ultrastructure of polypeptide hormone–producing cells of the APUD series and the embryologic, physiologic, and pathologic implications of the concept. J Histochem Cytochem 1969; 17:303–313.
8. Pearse AGE, Polak JM. Neural crest origin of the endocrine polypeptide (APUD) cells of the gastrointestinal tract and pancreas. Gut 1971; 12:783–788.
9. Weichert RF III. The neural ectodermal origin of the peptide-secreting endocrine glands. Am J Med 1970; 49:232–241.

10. Ibaney ML, Cole VW, Russell WO, et al. Solid carcinoma of the thyroid gland. Analysis of 53 cases. Cancer 1967; 20:706–723.
11. Weichert RF III, Roth LM, Harkin JC. Carcinoid-islet cell tumor of the duodenum and associated multiple carcinoid tumors of the ileum. Cancer 1971; 27:910–918.
12. Horvath E, Kovacs K, Ross RC. Medullary cancer of the thyroid gland and its possible relations to carcinoids. Virchows Arch [A] 1972; 356:281–292.
13. Pearse AGE, Polak JM, Heath CM. Polypeptide hormone production by "carcinoid" apudomas and their relevant cytochemistry. Virchows Arch [B] 1974; 16:95–109.
14. Friesen SR, Hermreck AS, Mantz FA Jr. Glucagon, gastrin, and carcinoid tumors of the duodenum, pancreas, and stomach: polypeptide "apudomas" of the foregut. Am J Surg 1974; 127:90–101.
15. Williams ED, Celestrin LR. The association of bronchial carcinoid and pluriglandular adenomatosis. Thorax 1962; 17:120–127.
16. Warner RRP, Blanstein AS. Coexistence of pheochromocytoma and carcinoid syndrome produced by metastatic carcinoid of the ileum. Mt Sinai J Med 1970; 37:536–548.
17. Thompson JC, Hirose FM, Lemmi CAE, et al. Zollinger-Ellison syndrome in a patient with multiple carcinoid–islet cell tumors of the duodenum. Am J Surg 1968; 115:177–184.
18. Samaan NA, Hickey RC, Bedner TD, et al. Hyperparathyroidism and carcinoid tumor. Ann Intern Med 1975; 82:205–207.
19. Goedert M, Ottern U, Suda K, et al. Dopamine, norepinephrine, and serotonin production by an intestinal carcinoid tumor. Cancer 1980; 45:104–107.
20. Sönksen PH, Ayres AB, Braimbridge M, et al. Acromegaly caused by pulmonary carcinoid tumours. Clin Endocrinol 1976; 5:503–513.
21. Smith PM. Successful treatment of Cushing's syndrome secondary to an argentaffinoma by bilateral adrenalectomy. Proc R Soc Med 1965; 58:573–575.
22. Yang K, Ulich T, Cheng L, et al. The neuroendocrine products of intestinal carcinoids. Cancer 1983; 51:1918–1926.
23. Moertel CG, Sauer WG, Dockerty MB, et al. Life history of the carcinoid tumor of the small intestine. Cancer 1961; 14:901–912.
24. Davis Z, Moertel CG, McIlrath DC. The malignant carcinoid syndrome. Surg Gynecol Obstet 1973; 137:637–644.
25. Godwin JD. Carcinoid tumors. An analysis of 2837 cases. Cancer 1975; 36:560–569.
26. Black WC. Enterochromaffin cell types and corresponding carcinoid tumors. Lab Invest 1968; 19:473–486.
27. Williams ED, Sandler M. The classification of carcinoid tumours. Lancet 1963; 1:238–239.
28. Lillie RD, Glenner GG. Histochemical reactions in carcinoid tumors of the human gastrointestinal tract. Am J Pathol 1960; 36:623–651.
29. Sandler M, Snow PDJ. An atypical carcinoid tumour secreting 5-hydroxytryptophan. Lancet 1958; 1:137–138.
30. Sandler M, Scheuer PJ, Watt PJ. 5-Hydroxytryptophan-secreting bronchial carcinoid tumour. Lancet 1961; 2:1067–1069.
31. Oates JA, Sjoerdsma A. A unique syndrome associated with secretion of 5-hydroxytryptophan by metastatic gastric carcinoids. Am J Med 1962; 32:333–344.
32. Feldman JM. Serotonin metabolism in patients with carcinoid tumors: incidence of 5-hydroxytryptophan-secreting tumors. Gastroenterology 1978; 75:1109–1114.
33. Moertel CG, Dockerty MB, Judd ES. Carcinoid tumors of the vermiform appendix. Cancer 1968; 21:270–278.
34. Caldarola VT, Jackman RJ, Moertel CG, et al. Carcinoid tumors of the rectum. Am J Surg 1964; 107:844–849.
35. Van Sickle DG. Carcinoid tumors. Analysis of 61 cases, including 11 cases of carcinoid syndrome. Cleve Clin Q 1972; 39:79–86.
36. MacDonald RA. A study of 356 carcinoids of the gastrointestinal tract. Am J Med 1956; 21:867–878.
37. Peskins GW, Orloff MJ. A clinical study of 25 patients with carcinoid tumors of the rectum. Surg Gynecol Obstet 1959; 109:673–682.
38. Smith RA. Bronchial carcinoid tumors. Thorax 1969; 24:43–50.
39. Sjoerdsma A, Terry LL, Udenfriend S. Malignant carcinoid. A new metabolic disorder. Arch Intern Med 1957; 99:1009–1012.
40. MacDonald RA, Robbins SL. Pathology of the heart in the carcinoid syndrome. Arch Pathol 1957; 63:103–112.
41. Roberts WC, Sjoerdsma A. The cardiac disease associated with the carcinoid syndrome (carcinoid heart disease). Am J Med 1964; 36:5–34.
42. Ferraus VJ, Roberts WC. The carcinoid endocardial plaque. An ultrastructural study. Hum Pathol 1976; 7:387–409.
43. Melmon KL, Sjoerdsma A, Mason DT. Distinctive clinical and therapeutic aspects of the syndrome associated with bronchial carcinoid tumors. Am J Med 1965; 39:568–581.
44. Haverback BJ, Davidson JD. Serotonin and the gastrointestinal tract. Gastroenterology 1958; 35:570–578.
45. Peart WS, Robertson JIS. The effect of a serotonin antagonist (UML 491) in carcinoid disease. Lancet 1961; 2:1172–1174.
46. Vroom FQ, Brown RE, Dempsey H, et al. Studies on several possible antiserotonin compounds in a patient with the functioning carcinoid syndrome. Ann Intern Med 1962; 56:941–945.
47. Melmon KL, Sjoerdsma A, Oates JA, et al. Treatment of malabsorption and diarrhea of the carcinoid syndrome with methysergide. Gastroenterology 1965; 48:18–24.
48. Oates JA, Butler JC. Pharmacologic and endocrine aspects of carcinoid syndrome. Adv Pharmacol 1967; 5:109–128.
49. Jequier E, Lovenberg W, Sjoerdsma A. Tryptophan hydroxylase inhibition: mechanism by which p-chlorophenylalanine depletes rat brain serotonin. Mol Pharmacol 1967; 3:274–278.
50. Engelman K, Lovenberg W, Sjoerdsma A. Inhibition of serotonin synthesis by para-chlorophenylalanine in patients with the carcinoid syndrome. N Engl J Med 1967; 277:1103–1108.
51. Satterlee WG, Serpick A, Bianchine JR. The carcinoid syndrome: chronic treatment with para-chlorophenylalanine. Ann Intern Med 1970; 72:919–921.
52. Robertson JIS, Peart WS, Andrews TM. The mechanism of facial flushes in the carcinoid syndrome. Q J Med 1962; 31:103–123.
53. Oates JA, Melmon K, Sjoerdsma A, et al. Release of a kinin peptide in the carcinoid syndrome. Lancet 1964; 1:514–517.
54. Oates JA, Pettinger WA, Doctor RB. Evidence for the release of bradykinin in carcinoid syndrome. J Clin Invest 1966; 45:173–178.
55. Gardner B, Dollinger M, Silen W. Studies of the carcinoid syndrome: its relationship to serotonin, bradykinin, and histamine. Surgery 1967; 61:846–852.
56. Erspamer V. The tachykinin peptide family. Trends Neurosci 1981; 4:267–269.
57. Nawa H, Doteuchi M, Igano K, et al. Substance K: a novel mammalian tachykinin that differs from substance P in its pharmacological profile. Life Sci 1984; 34:1153–1160.
58. Hunter JC, Miaggio JE. Pharmacologic characterization of a novel tachykinin isolated from mammalian spinal cord. Eur J Pharmacol 1984; 97:159–160.
59. Tatemoto K, Lundberg JM, Jormvall H, et al. Neuropeptide K: isolation, structure and biological activities of a novel brain tachykinin. Biochem Biophys Res Commun 1985; 128:947–953.
60. Duner H, Pernow B. Circulatory studies on substance P in man. Acta Physiol Scand 1960; 49:261–266.
61. Wilander E, Grinelius L, Portela-Gomes G, et al. Substance P and enteroglucagon-like immunoreactivity in argentaffin and argyrophil midgut carcinoid tumors. Scand J Gastroenterol 1979; 14(Suppl 53):19–25.
62. Hakanson R, Bengmark S, Brodin E, et al. Substance P–like immunoreactivity in intestinal carcinoid tumors. In: von Euler US, Pernow B, eds. Substance P. New York: Raven 1977: 55–58.
63. Skrabanek P, Dervan P, Cannon D, et al. Substance P in ovarian carcinoid. J Clin Pathol 1980; 33:160–162.
64. Ratzenhofer M, Gamse R, Hofler H, et al. Substance P in an argentaffin carcinoid of the caecum: biochemical and biological characterization. Virchows Arch [A] 1981; 392:21–31.
65. Alumets J, Hakanson R, Ingemansson S, et al. Substance P and 5-HT in granules isolated from an intestinal carcinoid. Histochemistry 1977; 52:217–222.
66. Roth KA, Makk G, Beck O, et al. Isolation and characterization of substance P, substance P 5-11, and substance K from two metastatic ileal carcinoids. Regul Pept 1985; 12:185–199.
67. Conlon JM, Deacon CF, Richter G, et al. Measurement and partial characterization of the multiple forms of neurokinin A–like immunoreactivity in carcinoid tumors. Regul Pept 1986; 13:183–196.
68. Emson PC, Gilbert RFT, Martensson H, et al. Elevated concentrations of substance P and 5-HT in plasma in patients with carcinoid tumors. Cancer 1984; 54:715–718.
69. Theodorsson-Norheim E, Norheim I, Oberg K, et al. Neuropeptide K: a major tachykinin in plasma and tumor tissues from carcinoid patients. Biochem Biophys Res Commun 1987; 131:77–83.
70. Roberts LJ II, Marney SR Jr, Oates JA. Blockade of the flush associated with metastatic gastric carcinoid by combined histamine H_1 and receptor antagonists: evidence for an important role of H_2 receptors in human vasculature. N Engl J Med 1979; 300:236–238.
71. MacDonald RA, Robbins SL, Mallory GK. Morphologic effects of serotonin (5-hydroxytryptamine). Arch Pathol 1958; 65:369–377.
72. Gottlieb LS, Broitman SA, Vitale JJ, et al. Failure of endogenous serotonin to produce lesions of the carcinoid syndrome. Arch Pathol 1960; 69:77–81.
73. Tammes AR. Exogenous serotonin administered to rats with liver damage. Arch Pathol 1965; 79:626–628.
74. McKinney B, Crawford MA. Fibrosis in guinea pig heart produced by plantain diet. Lancet 1965; 2:880–882.
75. Spatz M. Pathogenetic studies of experimentally induced heart lesions and their relation to the carcinoid syndrome. Lab Invest 1964; 13:288–300.
76. Peart WS, Robertson JIS, Andrews TM. Facial flushing produced in patients with carcinoid syndrome by intravenous adrenaline and noradrenaline. Lancet 1959; 2:715–716.
77. Levine RJ, Sjoerdsma A. Pressor amines and the carcinoid flush. Ann Intern Med 1963; 58:818–828.
78. Adamson AR, Peart WS, Grahame-Smith DG, et al. Pharmacological blockade of carcinoid flushing provoked by catecholamines and alcohol. Lancet 1969; 2:293–296.
79. Frolich JC, Bloomgarden ZT, Oates JA, et al. The carcinoid flush.

Provocation by pentagastrin and inhibition by somatostatin. N Engl J Med 1978; 299:1055–1057.

80. Schlegel W, Raptis S, Dollinger HC, et al. Inhibitors of secretin, pancreozymin and gastric release and their biological activities by somatostatin. In: Bonfils S, Fromageot P, Rosselin G, et al, eds. First International Symposium on Hormonal Receptors in Digestive Tract Physiology. INSERM Symposium No. 3. Amsterdam: Elsevier/North-Holland, 1977: 361–367.

81. Roberts LJ II, Bloomgarden ZT, Marney SR Jr, et al. Histamine release from a gastric carcinoid: provocation by pentagastrin and inhibition by somatostatin. Gastroenterology 1983; 84:272–275.

82. Dharmsathaphorne K, Sherwin RS, Cataland S, et al. Somatostatin inhibits diarrhea in the carcinoid syndrome. Ann Intern Med 1980; 92:68–69.

83. Davis GR, Camp RC, Raskin P, et al. Effect of somatostatin infusion on jejunal water and electrolyte transport in a patient with secretory diarrhea due to malignant carcinoid syndrome. Gastroenterology 1980; 78:346–349.

84. Klapdor R. Effects of somatostatin on bronchial constriction in a patient with carcinoid syndrome. N Engl J Med 1980; 302:464.

85. Thulin L, Samnegård H, Tydén G, et al. Efficacy of somatostatin in a patient with carcinoid syndrome. Lancet 1978; 2:43 (letter).

86. Fischbach FT. A Manual of Laboratory Diagnostic Tests. Philadelphia: J. B. Lippincott, 1984: 160–162.

87. Levine RJ, Elsas LJ, Duvall CP, et al. Malignant carcinoid tumors with and without flushing. JAMA 1963; 186:905–907.

88. Mason RA, Steane PA. Carcinoid syndrome: its relevance to the anaesthetist. Anaesthesia 1976; 31:228–242.

89. Mason RA, Steane PA. Anaesthesia for a patient with carcinoid syndrome. Anaesthesia 1976; 31:243–246.

90. Miller R, Patel AU, Warner RRP, et al. Anaesthesia for the carcinoid syndrome: a report of nine cases. Can Anaesth Soc J 1978; 25:240–244.

91. Marsh HM, Martin JK, Kvols LK, et al. Carcinoid crisis during anesthesia: successful treatment with a somatostatin analogue. Anesthesiology 1987; 66:90–91.

92. Melia WM, Nunnerley HB, Johnson PF, et al. Use of arterial devascularization and cytotoxic drugs in 30 patients with the carcinoid syndrome. Br J Cancer 1982; 46:331–339.

93. Martin JK, Moertel CG, Adson MA, et al. Surgical treatment of functioning metastatic carcinoid tumors. Arch Surg 1983; 118:537–542.

94. Moertel CG. Progress and hope in the treatment of gastrointestinal cancer. In: Fortner JG, Rhoads JE, eds. Accomplishments in Cancer Research 1987. Philadelphia: J. B. Lippincott, 1988: 295–317.

95. Mengel CE, Shaffer RD. The carcinoid syndrome. In: Holland JF, Frei E III, eds. Cancer Medicine. Philadelphia: Lea & Febiger, 1973: 1584–1594.

96. Legha SS, Valdivieso M, Nelson RS, et al. Chemotherapy for metastatic carcinoid tumors: experiences with 32 patients and a review of the literature. Cancer Treat 1977; 61:1699–1703.

97. Moertel CG, Hanley JA. Combination chemotherapy trials in metastatic carcinoid tumor and the malignant carcinoid syndrome. Cancer Clin Trials 1979; 2:327–334.

98. Oberg K, Norheim I, Lind E, et al. Treatment of malignant carcinoid tumors with human leukocyte interferon: long term results. Cancer Treat Rep 1986; 70:1297–1304.

99. Kvols LK, Moertel CG, O'Connell MJ, et al. Treatment of the malignant carcinoid syndrome. Evaluation of a long-acting somatostatin analogue. N Engl J Med 1986; 315:663–666.

100. Stathopoulos GP, Karvountzis GG, Yiotis J. Tamoxifen in carcinoid syndrome. N Engl J Med 1981; 305:52 (letter).

101. Meyers CF, Ershler WB, Tannenbaum MA, et al. Tamoxifen and carcinoid tumor. Ann Intern Med 1982; 98:383.

102. Graham JR. Cardiac and pulmonary fibrosis during methysergide therapy for headache. Am J Med Sci 1967; 254:1–12.

103. Oates JA. The carcinoid syndrome. N Engl J Med 1986; 315:702–704.

104. Wright PW, Mulder DG. Carcinoid heart disease: report of a case treated by open heart surgery. Am J Cardiol 1963; 12:864–868.

105. Aroesty JM, De Weese JA, Hoffman MJ, et al. Carcinoid heart disease. Successful repair of the valvular tissues under cardiopulmonary bypass. Circulation 1966; 34:105–110.

106. Carpena C, Kay JH, Mendey AM, et al. Carcinoid heart disease. Surgery for tricuspid and pulmonary valve lesions. Am J Cardiol 1973; 32:229–233.

107. Selye H. The Mast Cells. Washington: Butterworth, 1965.

108. Roberts LJ II, Lewis RA, Oates JA, et al. Prostaglandin, thromboxane, and 12-hydroxy-5,8,10,14-eicosatetraenoic acid production by ionophore-stimulated rat serosal mast cells. Biochim Biophys Acta 1979; 575:185–192.

109. Lewis RA, Soter NA, Diamond PT, et al. Prostaglandin D_2 generation after activation of rat and human mast cells with anti-IgE. J Immunol 1982; 129:1627–1631.

110. Coleman JW, Godfrey RC. The number and affinity of IgE receptors on dispersed human lung mast cells. Immunology 1981; 44:859–863.

111. Ishizaka T. Analysis of triggering events in mast cells for immunoglobulin E mediated histamine release. J Allergy Clin Immunol 1981; 67:90–96.

112. Schwartz LB, Austen KF, Wasserman SI. Immunologic release of β-hexosaminidase and β-glucuronidase from purified rat serosal mast cells. J Immunol 1979; 123:1445–1450.

113. Yurt RW, Leid RW Jr, Spragg J, et al. Immunologic release of heparin from purified rat peritoneal mast cells. J Immunol 1977; 118:1201–1207.

114. Sullivan TJ, Parker CW. Pharmacologic modulation of inflammatory mediator release by rat mast cells. Am J Pathol 1976; 85:437–463.

115. Gross BG, Hashimoto K. Hereditary urticaria pigmentosa. Arch Dermatol 1964; 90:401–403.

116. Shaw JM. Genetic aspects of urticaria pigmentosa. Arch Dermatol 1968; 97:137–138.

117. James MP, Eady RAJ. Familial urticaria pigmentosa with giant mast cell granules. Arch Dermatol 1981; 117:713–718.

118. Roberts LJ II, Fields JP, Oates JA. Mastocytosis without urticaria pigmentosa: a frequently unrecognized cause of recurrent syncope. Trans Assoc Am Physicians 1982; 95:36–41.

119. Douglas WM. Histamine and 5-hydroxytryptamine (serotonin) and their antagonists. In: Gilman AG, Goodman LS, Gilman A, eds. Goodman and Gilman's The Pharmacological Basis of Therapeutics. 6th ed. New York: Macmillan, 1980: 609–619.

120. Achord JL, Langford H. The effect of cimetidine and propantheline on the symptoms of a patient with systemic mastocytosis. Am J Med 1980; 69:610–614.

121. Bredfeldt JE, O'Laughlin JC, Durham JB, et al. Malabsorption and gastric hyperacidity in systemic mastocytosis. Am J Gastroenterol 1980; 74:133–137.

122. Hirschowitz BI, Groarke JF. Effect of cimetidine on gastric hypersecretion and diarrhea in systemic mastocytosis. Ann Intern Med 1979; 90:769–771.

123. Roberts LJ II, Sweetman BJ, Lewis RA, et al. Increased production of prostaglandin D_2 in patients with systemic mastocytosis. N Engl J Med 1980; 303:1400–1404.

124. Wasserman MA, DuCharme DW, Griffin RL, et al. Bronchopulmonary and cardiovascular effects of prostaglandin D_2 in the dog. Prostaglandins 1977; 13:255–269.

125. Heavey DJ, Lumley P, Barrow SE, et al. Effects of intravenous infusions of prostaglandin D_2 in man. Prostaglandins 1984; 28:755–767.

126. Webb TA, Li C-Y, Yam LT. Systemic mast cell disease: a clinical hematopathologic study of 26 cases. Cancer 1982; 49:927–938.

127. Grund VR, Hunninghake DB. Inhibition of histamine-stimulated increases in heart rate in man with the H_2-histamine receptor antagonist cimetidine. J Clin Pharmacol 1981; 21:87–91.

128. Soter NA, Austen KF, Wasserman SI. Oral disodium cromoglycate in the treatment of systemic mastocytosis. N Engl J Med 1979; 301:465–469.

129. Rodgers MP, Bloomingdale K, Murrawski BJ, et al. Mixed organic brain syndrome as a manifestation of systemic mastocytosis. Psychosom Med 1986; 48:437–447.

130. Liston TE, Roberts LJ II. Transformation of prostaglandin D_2 to 9α,11β-(15S)-trihydroxyprosta-(5Z,13E)-dien-1-oic acid (9α,11β-prostaglandin F_2): a unique biologically active prostaglandin produced enzymatically in vivo in humans. Proc Natl Acad Sci USA 1985; 82:6030–6034.

131. Demis DJ. The mastocytosis syndrome: clinical and biological studies. Ann Intern Med 1963; 59:194–206.

132. Sagher F, Even-Paz Z. Mastocytosis and the Mast Cell. Chicago: Year Book Medical, 1967.

133. Sostre MS, Handler HL. Bony lesions in systemic mastocytosis. Arch Dermatol 1977; 113:1245–1247.

134. Cryer PI, Kissane JM. Osteopenia. Clinicopathologic conference. Am J Med 1980; 69:915–922.

135. Clemett AR, Fishbone G, Levine RJ, et al. Gastrointestinal lesions in mastocytosis. AJR 1968; 103:405–412.

136. Janower ML. Mastocytosis of the gastrointestinal tract. Acta Radiol 1962; 57:489–493.

137. Robbins AH, Schimmel EM, Rao KC. Gastrointestinal mastocytosis: radiologic alterations after ethanol ingestion. AJR 1972; 115:297–299.

138. Ammann RW, Vetter D, Deyhle P, et al. Gastrointestinal involvement in systemic mastocytosis. Gut 1976; 17:107–112.

139. Scott BB, Hardy GJ, Losowsky MS. Involvement of the small intestine in systemic mast cell disease. Gut 1975; 16:918–924.

140. Ansell G. Adverse reactions to contrast agents. Invest Radiol 1970; 5:374–391.

141. Seidel G, Groppe G, Meyer-Burgdorff HC. Contrast media as histamine liberators in man. Agents Actions 1974; 4:143–150.

142. Fisher MM, More DG. The epidemiology and clinical features of anaphylactic reactions in anaesthesia. Anaesth Intensive Care 1981; 9:226–234.

143. Scott HW, Parris WCV, Sandidge PC, et al. Hazards in operative management of patients with systemic mastocytosis. Ann Surg 1983; 197:507–514.

144. Parris WCV, Sandidge PC, Petrinely G. Anesthetic management of mastocytosis. Anesthesiol Rev 1981; 8:32–35.

145. Turk J, Oates JA, Roberts LJ II. Intervention with epinephrine in hypotension associated with mastocytosis. J Allergy Clin Immunol 1983; 71:189–192.

146. Kaliner M, Orange RP, Austen KF. Immunological release of histamine and slow reacting substance of anaphylaxis from human lung. IV. Enhancement by cholinergic and alpha adrenergic stimulation. J Exp Med 1972; 136:556–567.

147. Lakdawala AD, Dadkar NK, Dohadwalla AN. Actions of clonidine on the mast cells of rats. J Pharm Pharmacol 1980; 32:790–791.

148. Abrishami MA, Thomas J. Aspirin intolerance—a review. Ann Allergy 1977; 39:28–37.

149. Settipane GA. Adverse reactions to aspirin and related drugs. Arch Intern Med 1981; 141:328–332.

150. Roberts LJ II, Oates JA. Evidence against a role of mast cell cyclooxygenase inhibition in aspirin hypersensitivity reactions. Clin Res 1983; 31:165A.

151. Keyzer JJ, deMonchy JGR, van Doormaal JJ, et al. Improved diagnosis of mastocytosis by measurement of urinary histamine metabolites. N Engl J Med 1983; 309:1603–1605.

152. Granerus G. Effects of oral histamine, histidine, and diet on urinary excretion of histamine, methylhistamine, and 1-methyl-4-imidazole-acetic acid in man. Scand J Clin Lab Invest 1968; 22(Suppl 104):49–58.

153. Feldman JM. Histaminuria from histamine-rich foods. Arch Intern Med 1983; 143:2099–2102.

154. Gleich GJ, Hull WM. Measurement of histamine: a quality control study. J Allergy Clin Immunol 1980; 66:295–298.

155. Roberts LJ II, Oates JA. Accurate and efficient method for quantification of urinary histamine by gas chromatography negative ion chemical ionization mass spectrometry. Anal Biochem 1984; 136:258–263.

156. Roberts LJ II. Quantification of the PGD$_2$ urinary metabolite 9α-hydroxy-11,15-dioxo-2,3,18,19-tetranorprost-5-ene-1,20-dioic acid by stable isotope dilution mass spectrometric assay. Methods Enzymol 1982; 86:559–570.

157. Schwartz LB, Metcalf, DD, Miller JJ, et al. Tryptase levels as an indicator of mast cell activation in systemic anaphylaxis and mastocytosis. N Engl J Med 1987; 316:1622–1626.

158. Schwartz LB, Yunginger JW, Miller J, et al. Time course of apppearance and disappearance of human mast cell tryptase in the circulation after anaphylaxis. J Clin Invest 1989; 83:1551–1555.

159. Campbell EW Jr, Hector D, Gossain V. Heparin activity in systemic mastocytosis. Ann Intern Med 1979; 90:940–941.

160. Guillet GY, Dore N, Maleville J. Heparin liberation in urticaria pigmentosa. Arch Dermatol 1982; 118:532–533.

161. Meyers J. Diagnosis: urticaria pigmentosa. Arch Dermatol 1960; 81:161–162.

162. Ridell B, Olafsson JH, Roupe G, et al. The bone marrow in urticaria pigmentosa and systemic mastocytosis. Arch Dermatol 1986; 122:422–427.

163. FitzGerald GA, Barnes P, Hamilton CA, et al. Circulating adrenaline and blood pressure: the metabolic effects and kinetics of infused adrenaline in man. Eur J Clin Invest 1980; 10:401–406.

164. Ishizaka T, Ishizaka K, Orange RP, et al. Pharmacologic inhibition of the antigen-induced release of histamine and slow reacting substance of anaphylaxis (SRS-A) from monkey lung tissues mediated by human IgE. J Immunol 1971; 106:1267–1273.

165. Roberts LJ II, Marney SR Jr, Oates JA. Blockade of the flush associated with a metastatic gastric carcinoid by combined histamine H$_1$ and H$_2$ receptor antagonists: evidence for an important role of H$_2$ receptors in human vasculature. N Engl J Med 1979; 300:236–238.

166. Sullivan TJ. Pharmacologic modulation of the whealing response to histamine in human skin: identification of doxepin as a potent in vivo inhibitor. J Allergy Clin Immunol 1982; 69:260–267.

167. Rane A, Oelz O, Frolich JC, et al. Relationship between plasma concentration of indomethacin and its effect on prostaglandin synthesis and platelet aggregation in man. Clin Pharmacol Ther 1978; 23:658–668.

168. Dolovich J, Punthakee ND, MacMillan AB, et al. Systemic mastocytosis: control of lifelong diarrhea by ingested disodium cromoglycate. Can Med Assoc J 1974; 111:684–685.

169. Zachariae H, Herlin T, Larsen PO. Oral disodium cromoglycate in mastocytosis. Acta Derm Venereol (Stockh) 1981; 61:272–273.

170. Barton J, Lavker RM, Schechter NM, et al. Treatment of urticaria pigmentosa with corticosteroids. Arch Dermatol 1985; 121:1516–1523.

ASSESSMENT OF ENDOCRINE FUNCTION

36

RADIOIMMUNOASSAY OF HORMONES

Rosalyn S. Yalow

INTRODUCTION

The development of radioimmunoassay[1-5] during the late 1950s and the 1960s coincided with a period of great advances in the chemistry of peptide hormones. During this time, highly purified preparations of many peptide hormones first became available to investigators. The fact that hormones sufficiently pure for labeling with radioactive isotopes and in adequate supply for immunization could be obtained was an essential element in the development of radioimmunoassay techniques. In turn, radioimmunoassay provided the sensitivity, specificity, and reliability that made possible studies of in vivo hormonal regulation that otherwise would not have been possible. The synergistic interaction between advances in the biochemistry of hormones and investigations with radioimmunoassay resulted in an information explosion in endocrinology.

The primary emphasis in this chapter is on the development of in-house assays. Laboratories are increasingly dependent on commercial kits for which the details concerning sensitivity, specificity, and quality control should be provided by the supplier. Nonetheless, familiarity with problems and pitfalls in radioimmunoassay methodology should be of value when interpreting results with kit assays.

RADIOIMMUNOASSAY PRINCIPLE

The basis of radioimmunoassay is competitive inhibition of the binding of labeled hormone to antibody by unlabeled hormone contained in standards or in unknown samples

(Fig. 36–1). It should be appreciated that there is no requirement in radioimmunoassay for biological or chemical identity between standards and unknowns. All that is required for a properly validated radioimmunoassay is that the unknown be *immunochemically* identical with the standards. A necessary but insufficient condition for ensuring a properly validated radioimmunoassay is superposability of a dilution curve of the unknown sample along a dilution curve of standards. However, as will be seen later, an assay may give useful clinical information even though it cannot be completely validated.

A typical radioimmunoassay is performed by the simultaneous preparation of standard and unknown mixtures in test tubes. To these tubes are added fixed amounts of radiolabeled antigen and antibody. After an appropriate reaction time, antibody-bound (B) and unbound (F) labeled antigens are separated by any of a variety of techniques. The method commonly used in our laboratory for plotting a standard curve and determining the hormone concentration in an unknown sample is illustrated in Figure 36–2. A variety of other modes of plotting the data have been used for the standard curve. These include, among others, the percentage of the tracer bound or the ratio of the percentage bound to that percentage bound in the absence of unlabeled hormone as a function of hormone concentration. Linearity of the standard curve is sometimes approached by the use of logarithmic or semilogarithmic plotting.

REAGENTS

From the competing reactions shown in Figure 36–1 it is evident that two reagents are required to perform an

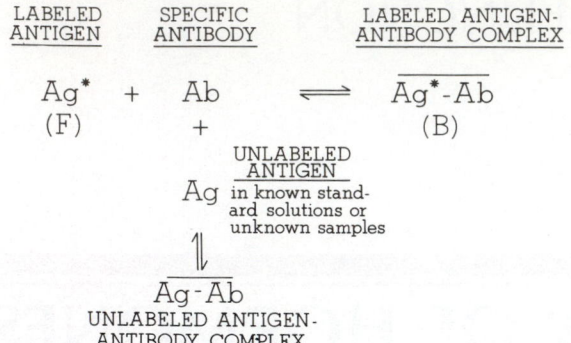

LABELED   SPECIFIC   LABELED ANTIGEN-
ANTIGEN   ANTIBODY   ANTIBODY COMPLEX

$$Ag^* + Ab \rightleftharpoons \overline{Ag^*\text{-}Ab}$$
(F)   (B)

+

UNLABELED
ANTIGEN
Ag in known stand-
ard solutions or
unknown samples

$$\Uparrow$$

$$\overline{Ag\text{-}Ab}$$
UNLABELED ANTIGEN-
ANTIBODY COMPLEX

Figure 36–1. Competing reactions that form the basis of radioimmunoassay.

assay: labeled antigen and specific antibody. Furthermore, it is necessary to provide a method for distinguishing between antibody-bound and free labeled antigen.

SPECIFIC ANTIBODY. Most peptide hormones are satisfactorily immunogenic in a variety of experimental animals when the hormone is administered as an emulsion in Freund adjuvant. We have generally used commercial or low-purity hormone preparations to take advantage of the possible slight denaturation of such preparations, which renders the hormones more "foreign" and thereby enhances their antigenicity. We have used a preparation containing as little as 0.5% gastrin to prepare antisera suitable for radioimmunoassay of gastrin.[6] There appears to be little or no advantage to immunizing with highly purified antigens, because contaminants are not likely to lead to immunological reactions that interfere with the assay. The labeled antigen must, of course, be highly purified to avoid interaction of labeled contaminants with nonspecific antibody.

Peptides of low molecular weight or nonpeptide substances that are not themselves antigenic may be rendered so by coupling them to a large protein. A variety of methods may be used to bind the small molecules to immunogenic carriers.[7–10] Because the presence of other immunological reactions does not interfere with the reaction between labeled antigen and its specific antibody, immunization with several unrelated antigens can be performed simultaneously. The concentration, sensitivity, and specificity of antibodies directed toward the various antigens appear to be unrelated. Because the probability of obtaining a satisfactory antiserum increases with the number of animals immunized, multiple-antigen immunization is advantageous for reducing the number of animals to be immunized and bled by a factor equal to the number of antigens used simultaneously.

Antibody concentration usually increases with repeated immunization, generally reaching a plateau after three to five doses of antigen. On occasion, antibody concentrations may fall after repeated regular immunizations.[6] In general the animals should then have an immunization-free interval of 3 to 6 mo, after which reimmunization usually results in an enhanced antibody response.

The production of a satisfactory antiserum remains more of an imprecise art than a science. Although numerous papers have described specialized procedures for immunization, there is no general agreement concerning the most suitable animal species or the optimal technique for producing the best antiserum for each of the diverse substances for which radioimmunoassay has been described. The use of large animals for immunization permits harvesting of large volumes of antiserum. However, the degree of foreignness may be a more important factor in the choice of a suitable animal for preparation of antisera for peptide hormones. Because guinea pig hormones such as insulin,[11] glucagon,[12]

vasoactive intestinal peptide,[13] gastrin,[14] and even cholecystokinin COOH-terminal octapeptide[15] differ from the corresponding peptides of Old World mammals, the guinea pig has proved to be an extremely useful animal for antibody production. Thus a single guinea pig immunized with commercial porcine insulin and glucagon has provided sera useful at dilutions of 3×10^6 for assay of insulin and 3×10^5 for assay of glucagon. Because the chinchilla, like the guinea pig, is a New World hystricomorph, and because several of its peptides, like those of the guinea pig, differ from the usual mammalian peptides,[16, 17] it is predicted that the chinchilla will also prove to be a most satisfactory animal for production of antisera to a variety of peptides.

There is considerable interest in the use of monoclonal antibodies for radioimmunoassay. This method permits production of large amounts of monospecific antibody. However, the sensitivity obtained with the use of such antisera is generally less than that obtainable by proper selection among the heterogeneous antisera produced by traditional immunization. The reason for this difference is that selection of the monoclonal antibodies generally yields those having equilibrium constants (K) for the reaction of antigen with antibody that are intermediate between those with high and low constants. When the usual heterogeneous antiserum is used, it is diluted sufficiently so that only antibody binding sites with the highest equilibrium constants, and hence the highest sensitivities, are able to bind the antigen. If optimal sensitivity is not required, the use of monoclonal antibodies may be advantageous.

LABELED ANTIGEN. It is obvious that it is inadvisable for the assay to use an amount of labeled tracer antigen whose immunochemical concentration is large compared

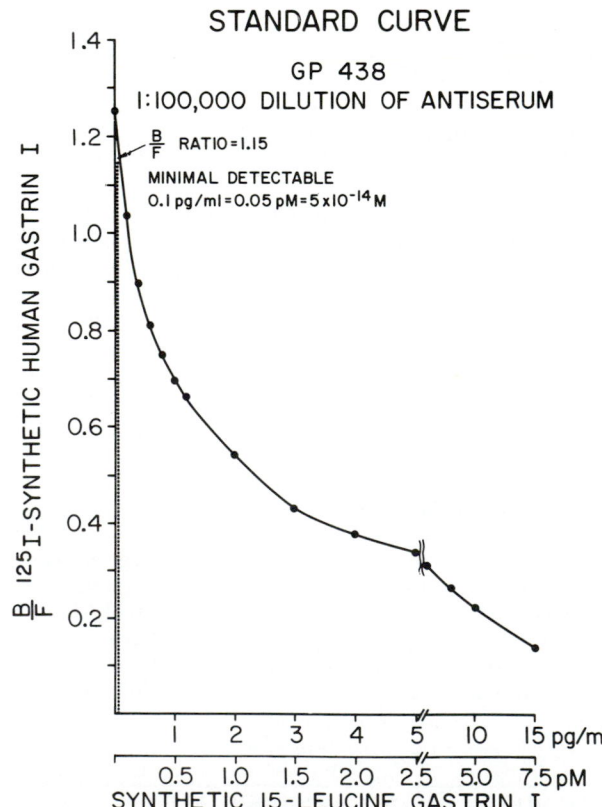

STANDARD CURVE

GP 438
1:100,000 DILUTION OF ANTISERUM

$\dfrac{B}{F}$ RATIO = 1.15

MINIMAL DETECTABLE
0.1 pg/ml = 0.05 pM = 5×10^{-14} M

(y-axis) $\dfrac{B}{F}$ ^{125}I-SYNTHETIC HUMAN GASTRIN I

(x-axis) 1   2   3   4   5   10   15 pg/ml
0.5   1.0   1.5   2.0   2.5   5.0   7.5 pM
SYNTHETIC I5-LEUCINE GASTRIN I

Figure 36–2. Standard curve for detection of gastrin by radioimmunoassay. Note that as little as 0.2 pg gastrin/mL incubation mixture (0.1 pmol/L) is readily detectable. (From Yalow RS. Radioimmunoassay: a probe for the fine structure of biologic systems. In: Les Prix Nobel En 1977. Stockholm: Nobel Foundation, 1978: 243–264.)

with the concentration of unlabeled antigen in the unknown. The use of a tracer of 10 fmol/L (10×10^{-12} M) to measure a hormone concentration of 1 fmol/L (1×10^{-12} M) would mean that a random 5% uncertainty in the tracer would produce a 50% uncertainty in the hormone concentration.

Calculations based on considerations of fractional decay rate demonstrate that when there is a requirement for high specific activity, ^{125}I is the radionuclide of choice. Radioiodine can readily be substituted onto a tyrosyl or histidyl residue by using a variety of procedures. The chloramine-T technique for oxidation of the radioiodide[18] is most commonly used. With minor modifications[19] it has proved to be completely satisfactory for all assays developed in our laboratory. It is advisable to avoid iodination procedures that take place below pH 7. In an acidic state, the radioiodide is converted to radioiodine, some of which volatilizes and may contribute to contamination of the laboratory or the persons therein. For peptide hormones that do not contain a suitable tyrosyl or histidyl residue for iodination, the Bolton-Hunter reagent is commonly used.[20] This preiodinated acylating reagent is readily condensed with free amino groups of peptides such as the epsilon-amino side chains of lysine or the NH_2-terminal amino group. This reagent is also useful if the tyrosine in the peptide is sulfated and hence does not readily iodinate, or if the tyrosyl residue is in the antigenic site and the presence of an added iodine atom would diminish the reaction of antigen with antibody, thus decreasing the sensitivity of the assay. Use of the Bolton-Hunter reagent may also be desirable if the peptide does not tolerate even the gentle oxidation associated with the chloramine-T reaction because the reagent is preiodinated before coupling.

The specific activity of a ^{125}I-labeled antigen may be increased by increasing the number of radioiodine substitutions. However, the more highly iodinated preparations generally show diminished immunoreactivity as well as increased susceptibility to radiation damage.[19] The latter appears to arise from radiation self-damage within the molecule, a damage we have designated as *decay catastrophe*.[19] When a radioactive atom undergoes decay, it is likely that the rest of the molecule is altered and perhaps even completely dissociated. If the molecule contains two or more radioactive atoms, decay of the first results in production of labeled molecular fragments or free radioiodide. As a result, the radioactivity is no longer associated with unaltered molecules, and damage is said to have occurred. For maximal stability and immunoreactivity, it is therefore preferable for the labeled molecule to contain only one radioiodine atom.

It must be appreciated that iodination at an average of one radioiodine atom per molecule does not mean that all or even the major fraction of the radioactivity is incorporated into molecules containing one radioactive atom. For instance, iodination of insulin in aqueous solution results in the same distribution of iodine atoms, independent of experimental method and dependent only on the average iodine number. On basis of the assumptions that an average of one iodine atom per molecule or less iodination will occur only at the two A chain tyrosyl residues, that there is equal probability of iodinating each residue, and that the presence of an iodine on a tyrosyl residue is nondirecting for subsequent iodination, Monte Carlo simulation has been used to calculate the theoretical distribution of iodine atoms in labeled insulin preparations containing an average of one iodine atom or less per molecule.[21] The theoretical analysis indicates that at an average of only 0.8 radioiodine atom per molecule, approximately half of the radioactivity is in other than monoiodoinsulin. Thus purification methods that separate on the basis of charge, such as starch gel electrophoresis or ion-exchange chromatography, are required to obtain mon-

oiodoinsulin. Similar considerations obtain in the preparation of other monoiodopeptides.

For nonpeptide hormones and drugs that are generally present at much higher concentrations in plasma than are the peptide hormones, the experimental requirements for labeled antigens with high specific activity are much less stringent than those for the peptide hormones. For these assays, ^{3}H-labeled tracers prepared and purified in commercial laboratories have frequently been used. ^{3}H-labeled antigens are usually identical with the unlabeled antigen except that, because of the limited shelf life of some preparations, some altered products may appear. Most commercial kits for assay of these substances use ^{125}I-coupled tracers, to avoid the use of liquid scintillation counters needed for the detection of [3]H.

Although the radioisotopic label has been most commonly used in the application of radioimmunoassay in endocrinology, there has been increasing interest in the use of nonradioactive ligands such as enzymes and fluorescent and chemiluminescent substances as labels in virology and pharmacology.[22]

SEPARATION METHODS. The classic immunological method for separation of antibody-bound from free antigen was based on spontaneous precipitation of antigen-antibody complexes. However, radioimmunoassay is generally used because of its high potential sensitivity. This requires that the molar concentration of the reagents be so low that spontaneous precipitation does not occur and the antigen-antibody complexes remain soluble, and a wide variety of methods have been used to effect separation of antibody-bound and free antigen.[23]

The methods in most common use include (1) precipitation of antigen-antibody complexes with a second antibody directed against the antibody complex (double antibody); (2) the use of organic solvents or salting out to precipitate complexes; (3) adsorption or complexing of antibody to solid-phase material; and (4) adsorption of free antigen to solid-phase material such as cellulose, charcoal, silicates, or ion-exchange resins.

The double-antibody method is generally the method of choice for developing new radioimmunoassay procedures. However, the cost of the second antibody may make this method prohibitively expensive when thousands of samples are to be analyzed. The aqueous polyethylene glycol method[24] for precipitation of antigen-antibody complexes may be used after an assay has been validated with the double-antibody methodology. The adsorption or complexing of antibody to solid-phase material has the advantage of being a generally applicable method and is frequently used in commercial kits. However, it has the disadvantage that because of possible chemical alterations in the antibody molecule introduced by coupling procedure or because of steric hindrance, the assays using solid-phase techniques are generally somewhat less sensitive than assays with the same antiserum when it is not complexed.

For routine procedures we have generally preferred a method dependent on adsorption of free antigen to solid-phase material;[25] it is usually the least expensive and is quite generally applicable. Certain common principles apply to all antigen-adsorbent techniques. A given mass of adsorbent is usually more effective if the total surface area is increased, i.e., if the adsorbing particles are made smaller. Both free antigen and antigen-antibody complexes may be adsorbed if there is insufficient carrier protein to compete successfully against binding of the complexes. Thus trace amounts of antibody as well as the free antigen may be adsorbed to materials such as charcoal, cellulose, and silicate, unless the concentration of plasma or other protein in the incubation mixture is sufficiently high to saturate the binding sites for gamma-globulin. In general the antigen adsorption methods are most satisfactory for small antigens, those with molecular sizes of 30 kd or less. The greater affinity of the adsorbent for the smaller substances in the presence of plasma proteins permits their near-total adsorption, even in the presence of virtually undiluted plasma or high concentrations of other proteins.

The fact that a large number of different methods of separation of antibody-bound from free labeled hormone have been used is a consequence of the variety of chemical properties of the now hundreds of substances for which radioimmunoassay has been employed, as well as of the experimental predilections of the many independent laboratories that have developed such procedures.

The use of a radioisotopic label requires some type of separation system. However, the use of a variety of nonisotopic labels has permitted the development of homogeneous assays that do not require the separation of antibody-bound from free antigen.[22] In these assays particular attention should be paid to substances in plasma that may interfere in a nonspecific fashion with the action of the enzyme or the fluorescence or luminescence of the system.

VALIDATION

Radioimmunoassay differs from traditional bioassay in that it is an immunochemical procedure that is not affected by biological variability of the test system or by the presence of other substances that might inhibit or enhance biological action. The measurement depends only on the interaction of chemical agents in accordance with the law of mass action. However, nonspecific factors do interfere in chemical reactions, and cross-reacting prohormones, molecular fragments, and related hormonal antigens may alter the specificity of the immune reaction.

Necessary conditions for establishing the validity of any assay procedure for a substance such as a peptide hormone require that hormone added to the fluid to be assayed be recovered quantitatively and that the hormone not be detectable in body fluids such as plasma at an appropriate interval after all secreting tissue is extirpated. It was once thought that a single organ was the source of each peptide hormone, but it is now generally appreciated that many peptides are synthesized in more than one site in the body. For instance, not only are a variety of peptides synthesized both in the brain and in the gut, but it is now apparent that the enkephalins, previously demonstrated to be derived from a β-endorphin precursor in the pituitary,[26] are also derived from an unrelated precursor in the adrenal medulla.[27] Techniques other than organ extirpation may then be required to prepare hormone-free plasma or tissue extracts.

A necessary condition for proper validation of a radioimmunoassay is that the apparent hormone content of an unknown sample be independent of the dilution at which it is assayed. Thus the observed concentrations in the unknown sample must decrease linearly with dilution, or alternatively, a dilution curve of the unknown sample must be superposable on a dilution curve of the standard substance over a wide concentration range, i.e., at least 100-fold or more. Experimental errors often obscure the lack of superposability when the concentration range is too small. A logarithmic dose-response plot is generally less sensitive to dissimilarity of standards and unknowns than is a linear plot.

Superposability is a necessary but insufficient condition to ensure immunochemical identity of standards and unknowns. However, lack of superposability means that the assay lacks quantitative validity even though it may be useful clinically if carefully interpreted.[28] Nonsuperposability of dilution curves of standards and unknowns can arise from chemical interference with the antigen-antibody reaction; from degradation of labeled and unlabeled antigen and/or antibody; or from a variety of immunological factors including the use of heterologous hormonal standards, the heterogeneity of immunologically related hormones of the same species, and the presence of precursors or metabolites in addition to the usual hormonal forms.

NONHORMONAL EFFECTS

EFFECTS OF pH, IONIC ENVIRONMENT, AND TEMPERATURE ON IMMUNE REACTION. Nonspecific factors such as changes in pH, ionic strength and chemical nature of buffering solutions, and the presence or absence of a variety of anticoagulants or protective agents can have profound effects on the reaction of antigen with antibody.[19] The question must be addressed as to whether one can predict in a systematic way how these nonspecific factors may influence the immune reaction.

The equilibrium constant for the reaction of antigen with antibody is generally higher at 4°C than at room temperature.[29] Thus dissociation of antigen-antibody complexes may occur if mixtures are incubated at 4°C and then free and antibody-bound labeled antigens are separated at room temperature. Because the dissociation depends on the time during which the sample is at room temperature, which may not be identical for standards and unknowns, errors can be introduced into the results. More sensitive assays are obtained by incubation at 4°C. However, low temperature decreases the rates of association and dissociation. If a less sensitive assay is acceptable, incubation at room temperature or even in a water bath at 37°C permits a more rapid assay.

Since the first demonstration of the effect of pH on the reaction of insulin with antibody,[30] it has been commonly accepted that radioimmunoassay systems for peptide hormones do not exhibit significant pH dependency in the range from 7 to 8.5.[19] In the earlier study,[30] insulin dissociated from antibody at or below pH 5, and its binding to antibody was maximal and constant between pH 7 and 9. However, we have demonstrated[31] that, for some peptide hormones such as secretin and for some radioimmunoassay systems, optimal sensitivity is obtained at pH 5 and that the sensitivity is enhanced at a pH as low as 4 in 20 mmol/L (0.02 M) acetate buffer compared with that obtainable in 20 mmol/L (0.02 M) barbital buffer (pH 8.6). This study[31] showed that there was no predictable effect of pH and ionic strength on the immune reaction. The effects depend on the particular hormone, the particular antiserum used, and the buffer.

EFFECT OF DEGRADATION OF LABELED ANTIGEN AND/OR ANTIBODY. Many peptide hormones are subject to proteolytic damage by enzymes in blood and other biological fluids. Differential damage of the labeled antigen in standards and unknowns decreases the reliability of a radioimmunoassay procedure and, depending on the extent of damage, may completely invalidate the results. When a specific adsorbent method is used for separation of free from antibody-bound labeled antigen, a control mixture containing the labeled antigen and either the unknown sample or the diluent used for standards but without antiserum is used to evaluate the differential damage occurring during the incubation period. The incubation damage is then evaluated by the failure of the damaged labeled antigen to be adsorbed by the specific adsorbent.[19] Charcoal is widely used for this purpose and is quite useful for detection of alterations that result in nonspecific binding of damaged labeled antigen to serum proteins, as is often the case when there is no extensive damage. However, this method does have some disadvantages. When there is extensive proteolytic destruction of the labeled hormone, small radiolabeled peptides and iodotyrosines are produced. These adsorb to charcoal to some extent and appear to give a satisfactory control reading. However, they do not react with antibody, and the lowered fraction of radioactivity found in the antibody-bound form is falsely interpretable as related to a higher hormone concentration. Other adsorbents such as talc, silicate, and ion-exchange resins that are more discriminating than charcoal may not adsorb the small peptides and iodotyrosines, and their use may be more revealing of damage to the labeled antigen than is possible with charcoal.

The only certain method for ensuring integrity of the labeled antigen is demonstration of its ability to bind to antibody at the end of the incubation period. Excess antibody is usually used for this evaluation, even though it may fail to reveal subtle alterations in immunoreactivity. When the double-antibody method is used for separation of the labeled immune complexes, damaged labeled antigen that does not bind to the first antibody is not precipitable by the second antibody and appears in the supernatant along with free labeled antigen. If during the incubation period either labeled antigen or antibody is destroyed, immune precipitation is reduced, and the reduction is often interpreted erroneously as being due to high hormone content.

The assumption that degradation of antibody during incubation is unlikely to occur unless there is simultaneous degradation of antigen during incubation is often but not always valid. For instance, trypsin or trypsin-like enzymes in the incubation mixture would destroy antibody but not radioiodine-labeled heptadecapeptide gastrin, because the latter does not contain lysine or arginine residues. Although this is a rare problem in peptide hormone assays, it may be of greater concern in assay of nonpeptide hormones in body fluids.

USEFUL STRATEGIES FOR DEALING WITH NONSPECIFIC EFFECTS. It is generally desirable for standards and unknowns to have the same milieu during the incubation period. Thus if acid-alcohol extracts are to be assayed, either the same volume of acid-alcohol must be added to standards as is used in the unknown sample or it must be demonstrated that the volume of acid-alcohol used does not affect the standard curve. Similarly, incubation tubes of standards and unknowns should contain the same amounts of protective agents, anticoagulants, salts, proteins, and so forth.

Perhaps the most subtle type of nonspecific effect to guard against is unsuspected destruction of labeled antigen and/or antibody. It was earlier shown[32] that apparently high concentrations of gastrin and insulin in gastric and duodenal secretions as determined by radioimmunoassay were due to artifacts caused by the presence of proteolytic enzymes not inactivated before assay. If the peptide hormone in the unknown fluid can tolerate boiling, this method is perhaps the simplest to inactivate such enzymes. However, simple boiling is not always effective. In a study on the radioimmunoassay artifacts in tissue extracts and plasma,[33] we demonstrated that all authentic forms of corticotropin (ACTH, adrenocorticotropin) were adsorbable to and could be eluted from precipitated silica (QUSO G32) (Fig. 36–3). However, the apparent immunoreactivities in extracts of human pancreas made in boiling acid (see Fig. 36–3, *lower right*) or extracts of antrum, duodenum, or pancreas made in boiling water (Table 36–1) were not adsorbed by silica.

Silica adsorption is a simple, inexpensive technique for demonstrating the presence of authentic ACTH and also a variety of other peptide hormones. Affinity chromatography should prove to be equally satisfactory, although the cost of the reagents is greater and the procedure is technically more difficult in that it requires coupling of antibody to the matrix. More recently we have made use of octadecylsilyl cartridges (C_{18} Sep-Pak cartridges purchased from Waters Associates) to extract insulin and other peptide hormones from plasma and tissue extracts.[34] This method permits preparation of hormone-free plasma for standard curves. Furthermore, the

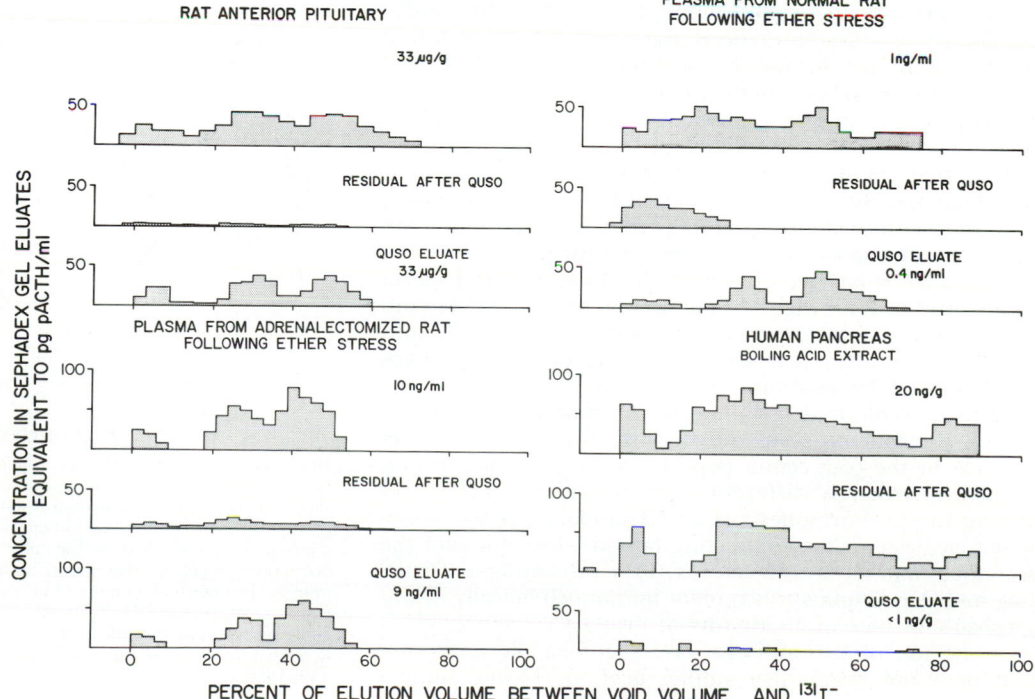

SEPHADEX G50 FILTRATION PATTERNS OF IMMUNOREACTIVITY

Figure 36–3. The effect of adsorption to and elution from precipitated silica (QUSO) on the patterns of immunoreactivity in an extract of rat pituitary, plasma from ether-stressed adrenalectomized and normal rats, and a boiled acid extract of a human pancreas. The volume applied to the column depended on the hormone content of the extract or plasma. Thus only 0.1 mL of adrenalectomized rat plasma was applied but 1.0 mL of normal rat plasma was fractionated. (From Moldow RL, Yalow RS. Artifacts in the radioimmunoassay of ACTH in tissue extracts and plasma. Horm Metab Res 1980; 12:105–110.)

TABLE 36–1. Adsorption to and Elution from Precipitated Silica (QUSO) of Apparent Immunoreactive ACTH (ng/g) Extracted from Tissue in Boiling Water

Tissue	In Extract	Residual After QUSO	Eluted from QUSO
Rat			
Hypothalamus	15	ND*	15
Antrum	4	4	ND
Duodenum	8	7	ND
Human			
Hypothalamus	10	ND	10
Pancreas	6	7	ND
Antrum	5	5	ND
Duodenum	9	8	ND

*ND, not detected (<1 ng/g).

From Moldow RL, Yalow RS. Artifacts in the radioimmunoassay of ACTH in tissue extracts and plasma. Horm Metab Res 1980; 12:105–110.

peptide hormone can readily be extracted from the cartridge in concentrated form, usually free of nonspecific interfering substances. The authenticity of the peptide hormone being assayed can then be verified by Sephadex gel elution or other fractionation techniques.

In summary, a number of different kinds of studies are required to establish whether nonspecific phenomena interfere in such radioimmunoassay systems.

HORMONAL CROSS-REACTIVITY

The factors that interfere with the chemical reaction in a nonspecific fashion can and should be avoided. However, problems relating to hormonal cross-reactivity cannot always be dealt with so simply. These problems include, among others, choice of an appropriate standard when a suitable reference preparation is not available from the species whose endogenous hormone is to be measured; the presence of immunologically related but different hormones; and the heterogeneity of hormonal forms.

HETEROLOGOUS HORMONE STANDARDS. The primary structures of many hormonal peptides have diverged during the course of evolution. The species differences resulting from these mutations are most likely to be found in regions of the hormone not essential for its biological activity. However, because the immunogenicity of exogenous hormone from another species is likely to depend on the foreignness, i.e., the regions of difference, it is not unexpected that immunological and biological potencies of a hormone may differ among different species. Furthermore, immunochemical identity among peptides may require more than identification of the primary structure of a molecule. For instance, it has been reported that hog, dog, and sperm whale insulins have identical amino acid sequences[11] but are distinguishable immunochemically with some, not all, antisera.[35, 36] The differences among these insulins can perhaps be explained by assuming that the configuration of the insulin molecule is determined at the time of its synthesis via its proinsulin precursor. Because the amino acid sequences of the connecting peptides of dog and hog proinsulins are strikingly different,[37] conformational differences among the prohormones are understandable. If the subsequent cleavage of the connecting peptide does not alter the secondary and tertiary structures of the remaining molecule, hog and dog insulins will remain immunochemically distinguishable in spite of an identity of primary structure.

The use of two antisera, one a guinea pig antiserum that does not distinguish among beef, pork, and human insulins and the other a human antiserum obtained from an insulin-resistant diabetic subject that does distinguish among the three insulins, has made possible differentiation between human insulin and animal insulins in cases of accidental insulin administration,[38] murder,[39] and child abuse.[40] The method of analysis is shown in Figure 36–4. This same technique has been used to demonstrate that insulin in the cord blood of a neonate whose mother was an insulin-requiring diabetic was a mixture of beef insulin that had crossed the placental barrier while bound to antibody and human insulin from the fetal pancreas.[41]

One cannot predict among which hormones and among which species mutational changes have occurred that drastically affect immunological and even biological characteristics of a peptide hormone. There are numerous examples of marked divergence of biological and immunological potencies. For instance, bovine and other animal growth hormones are not active in promoting growth in primates because of significant chemical differences between growth hormones from primates and those from other species.[42] Marked immunological differences are also noted in that only primate growth hormones, but not those of other animal species, react significantly with antisera against human growth hormone.[4] Human growth hormone is biologically active in the dog[43] and rat[44] but does not react in immunoassay systems for the animal growth hormones.[45] It was initially thought that, in primates, growth hormone and prolactin were the same hormone because all pituitary preparations that possessed lactogenic activity contained growth hormone.[46] However, primate prolactin was subsequently identified by the demonstration that both monkey[47] and human[48] pituitary glands incubated in vitro synthesize and secrete proteins that can be measured in a sheep prolactin assay system. In fact, the first prolactin radioimmunoassay with sufficient sensitivity to measure human prolactin used labeled monkey prolactin purified by affinity chromatography and an anti–sheep prolactin serum.[49] Thus two pituitary peptides that are as closely related as growth hormone and prolactin manifest marked differences in the species specificities of their biological and immunological properties.

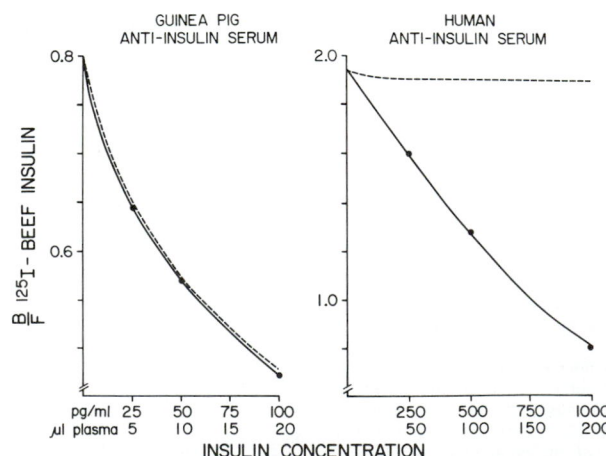

Figure 36–4. Standard curves for insulin assay of plasma from a hypoglycemic patient. Solid lines show standard curves for bovine insulin, and broken lines show standard curves for human insulin. Circles denote dilutions of patient's plasma. *Left,* Bovine insulin and human insulin cross-react almost identically in a guinea pig antiserum assay; the curve of dilutions of plasma is superposed on both curves. *Right,* Human insulin hardly cross-reacts with human antiserum to insulin. The pattern of dilutions of plasma can be superposed only on the bovine curve. (From Bauman WA, Yalow RS. Differential diagnosis between endogenous and exogenous insulin reduced refractory hypoglycemia in a non-diabetic patient. Reprinted, by permission from The New England Journal of Medicine, 303; 198–199, 1980.)

The use of a heterologous radioimmunoassay may or may not be practical. If a dilution curve of the unknown is not superposable on a dilution curve of heterologous hormone standards, the assay of the unknown will certainly not have quantitative validity. Under those circumstances it is probably advisable to use crude tissue extracts or biological fluids containing as high a concentration of the material as the known samples. However, evaluation of the true absolute concentration does require preparation of a suitable reference standard from the appropriate species.

IMMUNOLOGICALLY RELATED BUT DIFFERENT HORMONES. Consideration must be given to the possibility that plasma or tissue extracts may contain a biologically different substance that is nevertheless immunologically cross-reacting. In the assay for growth hormone, it was noted that the hormone concentration decreased linearly with dilution in plasma obtained from cord blood, acromegalic patients, and stimulated control subjects, but not in plasma obtained from pregnant women.[50, 51] The interfering substance in the pregnant women was human placental lactogen (hPL, also called human chorionic somatomammotropin, hCS), which is of placental origin and resembles growth hormone but is neither biologically nor immunologically identical with it. The synthesis by the placenta and other tissues of additional hormones (e.g., chorionic gonadotropin) that have biological and immunological properties similar to those of pituitary hormones may also render nonspecific the assays for the glycoproteins in the plasmas of pregnant women.

Problems of nonspecificity must also be considered and evaluated whenever pairs of hormones share common amino acid sequences that might result in immunological and/or biological cross-reactivity. Such systems include, among others, gastrin and cholecystokinin, which share the same COOH-terminal pentapeptide; ACTH and melanocyte-stimulating hormones, which have similar NH_2-terminal sequences; and lipotropin, which contains within it the complete structure of β-melanocyte-stimulating hormone.[52]

HETEROGENEITY OF PEPTIDE HORMONES. It is now clear, largely on the basis of studies involving radioimmunoassay, that many, if not all, peptide hormones are found in more than one form in plasma and in glandular and other tissue extracts. These forms may or may not have biological activity and may represent either precursor(s) or metabolic product(s) of the well-known, well-characterized, biologically active hormone. Such heterogeneity complicates the interpretation of hormone concentrations as measured by radioimmunoassay. However, recognition of the problem has opened new vistas in our understanding of the paths of synthesis and metabolism of the peptide hormones.

It is indeed fortunate that the first radioimmunoassay was described for insulin. The 6-kd peptide with full biological activity is the predominant form in the circulation of virtually all subjects in the stimulated state. Only in patients with insulinoma[53] or in those with a rare genetic abnormality that prevents cleavage of the C peptide[54, 55] does the prohormone appear to predominate. However, there are several assays of other hormones in which the usual biologically active form is not predominant. In this section, three examples will be considered: the parathyroid hormone (PTH) assay, which is complicated by the presence of a biologically inactive metabolic fragment; the gastrin assay, which is complicated by the presence of a biologically active precursor; and the assay for ectopic ACTH production, which is complicated by the presence of a biologically inactive precursor.

Parathyroid Hormone. Immunochemical heterogeneity was first shown for PTH when it was observed that a constant factor could be used to superpose a plasma dilution curve on a curve of standards obtained from a normal parathyroid gland for two antisera, but this factor resulted in discrepant results when a third antiserum was used (Fig. 36–5).[56] Furthermore, the disappearance rate of plasma immunoreactivity after parathyroidectomy was more rapid when measured with one specific antiserum (C329). The nature of the hormonal forms responsible for the observed heterogeneity of plasma and tissue PTH was subsequently elucidated.[28] One antiserum (273) sees intact PTH and a biologically inactive COOH-terminal fragment as immunochemically similar; antiserum C329 is an NH_2-terminal antiserum that cross-reacts primarily with intact PTH in plasma, because there have been no reports demonstrating the existence of a biologically active NH_2-terminal fragment in the circulation. Because of the longer turnover time of the COOH-terminal fragment compared with intact hormone, its concentration in plasma is generally higher than that of intact hormone. Therefore most laboratories use a COOH-terminal assay for the diagnosis of primary hyperparathyroidism, as it permits the use of less sensitive antisera for

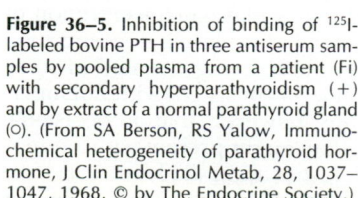

Figure 36–5. Inhibition of binding of ^{125}I-labeled bovine PTH in three antiserum samples by pooled plasma from a patient (Fi) with secondary hyperparathyroidism (+) and by extract of a normal parathyroid gland (o). (From SA Berson, RS Yalow, Immunochemical heterogeneity of parathyroid hormone, J Clin Endocrinol Metab, 28, 1037–1047, 1968, © by The Endocrine Society.)

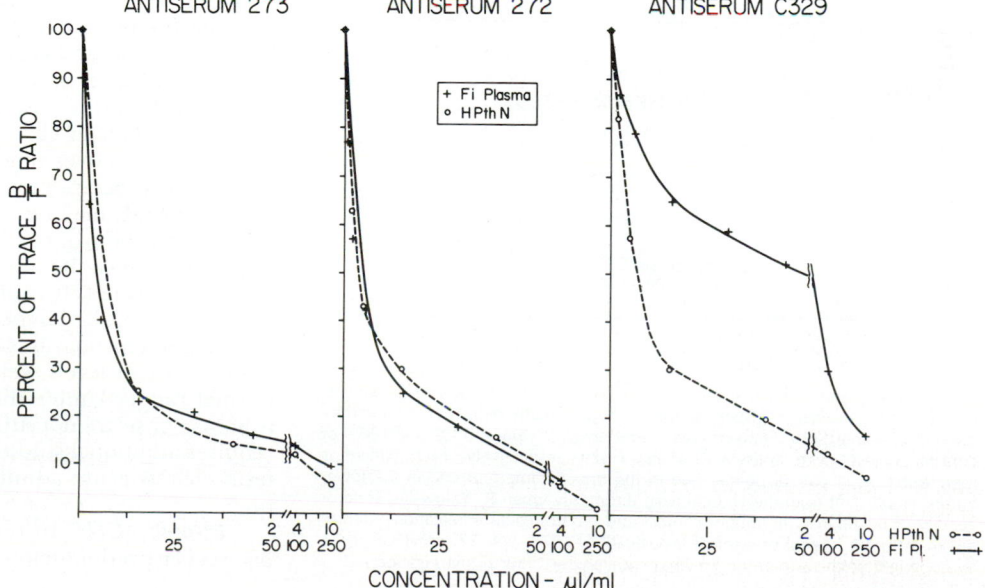

diagnostic differentiation (Fig. 36–6). However, the turnover time of the fragment in uremia is prolonged as much as 50 times normal.[57] Therefore marked elevations of immunoreactivity as measured in the COOH-terminal assay are found even in the absence of secondary hyperparathyroidism in uremic patients.

Even now, a quarter century after the first description of a PTH assay,[3] it remains a test seldom properly validated because of the differences between standards and unknowns and the consequent difficulty in interpretation. It is not surprising that discrepancies are found among the same samples sent to different laboratories.[58]

A high-sensitivity, two-site immunoradiometric assay has been described for human PTH that appears to be specific for the intact (1–84) peptide.[59] This assay depends on the preparation of goat antisera to PTH and their subsequent purification on affinity columns. Thus one purified antiserum directed to PTH(1–34) and another directed to PTH(39–84) are available. To perform the assay the anti-PTH(39–84) antiserum is immobilized on plastic beads. The unknowns or the PTH(1–84) standards in hormone-free plasma are then added, followed by addition of ^{125}I-labeled anti-PTH(1–34). The assay depends on intact hormone binding to the COOH-terminal–immobilized antiserum and its capturing the ^{125}I-labeled antibody directed against the NH$_2$-terminal PTH. This assay is reported to have the sensitivity to distinguish among primary hyperparathyroidism, normal function, and the hypercalcemia of malignancy.[59] In this report serum samples from uremic patients were not studied. However, various PTH fragments (1–34, 39–68, 53–84, 44–68, and 39–84) appeared not to interfere in the assay.[59] We have compared PTH concentrations in the plasma of dialysis patients as determined with a commercial kit assay using this methodology with an in-house NH$_2$-terminal PTH assay (Fig. 36–7). The relatively good agreement between the two assays suggests the absence in uremic plasma of substances that interfere nonspecifically in

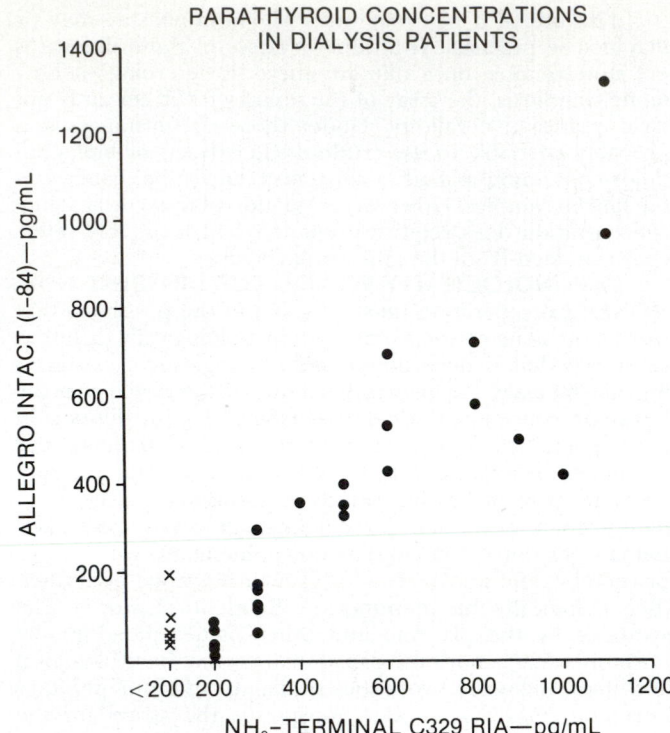

Figure 36–7. PTH concentrations in the plasma of patients with end-stage renal disease as determined by using the Allegro kit assay and an in-house assay specific for NH$_2$-terminal portion of PTH molecule. The points shown as (X) were measurable in the Allegro assay but not in the C329 assay.

the PTH assays. The two-site immunoradiometric assay appears to be more useful for determination of the concentrations of intact PTH in serum than the assays previously described.

Gastrin. The predominant form of gastrin in plasma in the fasted state of normal subjects and of hypersecretors such as patients with Zollinger-Ellison syndrome or pernicious anemia is generally, but not always, a 34-amino-acid peptide (G34),[60, 61] not the 17-amino-acid peptide (G17) initially extracted and purified from the antrum by Gregory and colleagues.[62] Both hormonal forms are stimulated by feeding in normal subjects and in patients with pernicious anemia (Fig. 36–8). The infusion of equimolar amounts of G34 and G17 results in about the same acid response in the dog, but the plasma levels of G34 during such infusions are four times higher because of a fourfold slower turnover time. Knowledge of the hormonal form(s) of circulating gastrin is therefore essential for interpretation of radioimmunoassay data in clinical situations. If it is assumed that the relative turnover times in humans are similar to those in dogs, it must be appreciated that a plasma concentration of 50 pg G17/mL may be as potent as a plasma concentration of 200 pg G34/mL, the latter value being deemed in some laboratories to be the minimal level consistent with Zollinger-Ellison syndrome. It is obvious, however, that an occasional patient with marked hyperacidity might present with a tumor that secretes primarily G17 rather than G34 but still have plasma gastrin levels well within what is believed to be the normal range. Under those circumstances, plasma concentrations per se are not sufficient for diagnosis. Discrimination requires additional studies using the appropriate stimulation tests such as acute administration of calcium salts or secretin.[63]

Ectopic ACTH. In normal human subjects the usual 1–39 ACTH predominates in the pituitary and in the plasma

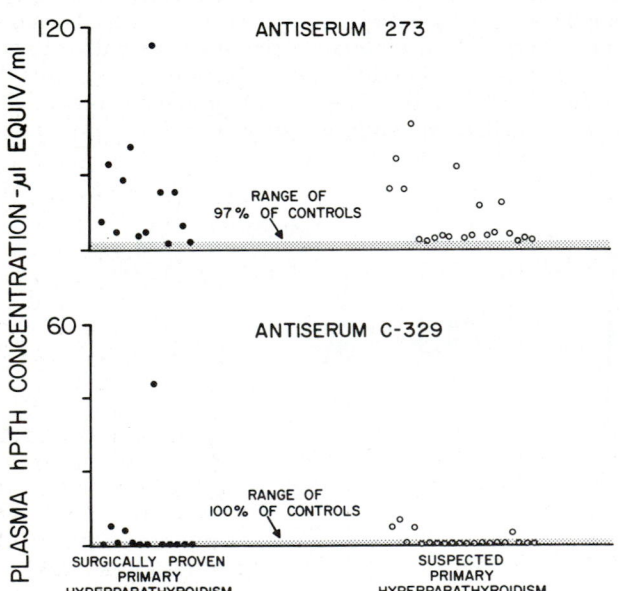

Figure 36–6. Immunoreactive human PTH concentration in plasma of patients with surgically proven or suspected primary hyperparathyroidism as measured by antisera 273 and C329. Stippled areas show range of values for 97 and 100% of control subjects with antisera 273 and C329, respectively. Each patient is represented by a pair of points, one in the upper frame and one in the lower frame, equidistant from the vertical axis. (From Silverman R, Yalow RS. Heterogeneity of parathyroid hormone: clinical and physiological implications. Reproduced from the Journal of Clinical Investigation, 1973, vol. 52, pp. 1958–1971 by copyright permission of the American Society for Clinical Investigation.)

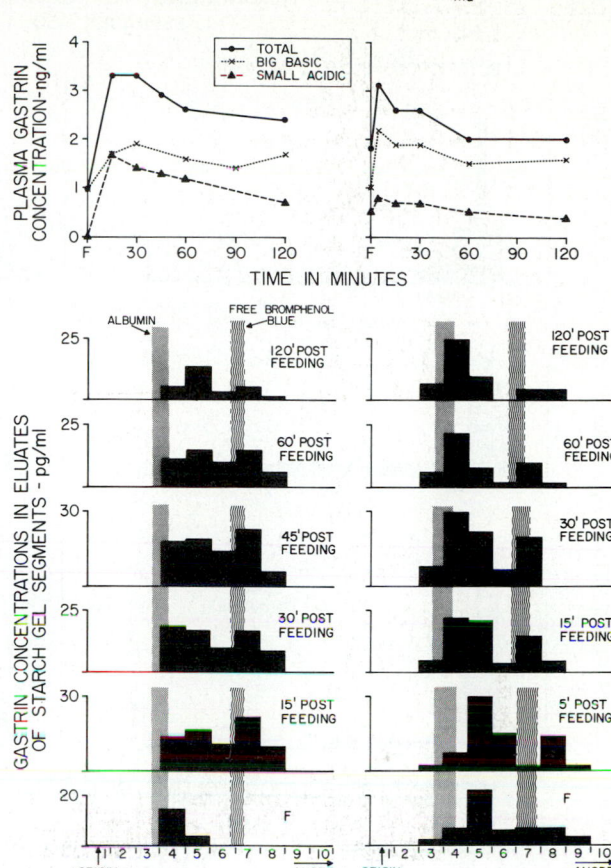

Figure 36–8. Effects of feeding on concentrations of two immunoreactive plasma gastrin components in two patients with pernicious anemia. (From Yalow RS, Berson SA. Further studies on the nature of immunoreactive gastrin in human plasma. Gastroenterology 1971; 60:203–214. © 1971, The Williams & Wilkins Co., Baltimore.)

after pituitary stimulation. However, in patients with ectopic Cushing syndrome, the predominant form in plasma was often "big ACTH," a component that eluted in the void volume on Sephadex G-50 gel filtration (Fig. 36–9).[64] Big ACTH has been given a variety of new names, among them pro-opiomelanocortin. Its biological activity is less than 4% that of the 1–39 peptide.[65] It is frequently elevated in patients with bronchogenic carcinoma and in those with chronic obstructive pulmonary disease but without invasive carcinoma.[65] The finding of the precursor form of ACTH in a smoking dog with atypical histological changes but not invasive carcinoma[65] suggests that ectopic ACTH production may occur at the stage of squamous metaplasia. Thus the finding of elevated plasma ACTH or the apparent absence of its diurnal rhythm may or may not be clinically useful in the management of patients who are heavy smokers.

RADIOIMMUNOASSAY VERSUS BIOASSAY

In the first major description[2] of the radioimmunoassay of insulin and its application to what is now known as non–insulin-dependent diabetes mellitus, reasons were given for the apparent discrepancies sometimes observed between concentrations of radioimmunoassayable insulin and those of biologically active insulin. Levels of immunoassayable insulin appeared to be higher in non–insulin-dependent diabetes mellitus, but the patients failed to respond with an appropriate lowering of blood glucose levels. Four possibilities were then considered: (1) abnormal tissues with a high

threshold for the action of insulin; (2) an abnormal insulin that acts poorly with respect to hormone activity in vivo but reacts well immunologically in vitro; (3) an abnormally rapid inactivation of hormonally active sites but not of immunologically active sites on the insulin molecules; and (4) the presence of insulin antagonists. The apparent insulin insensitivity associated with this disorder was subsequently confirmed by many investigators and the circulating immunoassayable insulin was shown to be predominantly the biologically active 6-kd peptide. As assays were described for other peptide hormones, it became evident that radioimmunoassay levels may appear to exceed levels obtained by bioassay because of the presence of multiple molecular forms of the peptide, often with diminished biological compared with immunological activity.[23, 28, 64, 65] However, the opposite type of discrepancy may also occur. It has been shown that the ratio of biological luteinizing hormone (measured by the rat interstitial cell testosterone assay) to immunological luteinizing hormone is higher than 1 and varies as a function of sex, age, physiological state, and other factors.[66–69] The ratio averages about 1.5 during a normal menstrual cycle,[66] and it is considerably higher in postmenopausal women and in men.[68, 69] In these several papers[66–69] there was no attempt to fractionate the sera so as to determine whether there was more than one molecular form of the hormone with different ratios, nor was consideration given to the possibility that there may be another hormone present that could potentiate the biological effectiveness of luteinizing hormone in the rat interstitial cell testosterone assay. Such interactions are well known in other bioassay systems. For example, stimulation of amylase release from dispersed acini from guinea pig pancreas[70] can be effected both by cholecystokinin octapeptide[15] and by vasoactive intestinal peptide.[71] If both

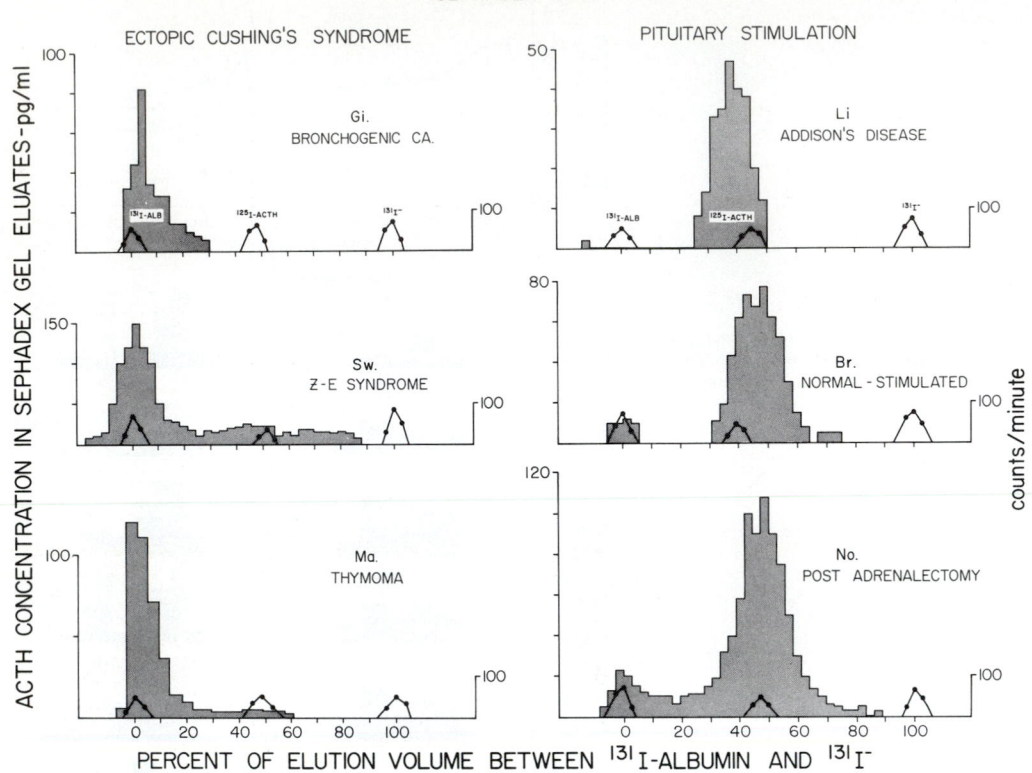

IMMUNOREACTIVE PLASMA ACTH
SEPHADEX G50

Figure 36–9. Distribution of immunoreactive ACTH in plasma of patients with ectopic Cushing syndrome *(left)* and in plasma of patients after pituitary stimulation *(right)*. (From Gewirtz G, Yalow RS. Ectopic ACTH production in carcinoma of the lung. Reproduced from the Journal of Clinical Investigation, 1974, vol. 53, pp. 1022–1032 by copyright permission of the American Society for Clinical Investigation.)

cholecystokinin octapeptide and vasoactive intestinal peptide were present in a biological fluid at equimolar concentrations, the apparent ratio of biological activity (stimulated amylase release) to immunological activity of either peptide would be higher than 1. It must be appreciated that biological activity in vivo can be enhanced by the presence of substances other than the one presumably being assayed. For instance, it is known that several peptides enhance and other peptides suppress pancreatic secretion of water and bicarbonate.[72] Thus in any bioassay system in which multiple peptides interact, it is essential that the possible presence of the other substances be considered. Whenever the ratio of biological to immunological activity is less than or more than 1, the existence of factors other than the specific molecular form of the peptide to be assayed must be evaluated.

CONCLUSIONS

A brief review of the technical aspects of radioimmunoassay has been presented, with emphasis on some of the pitfalls. The approach has been quite general and applicable to those assays in which reagents are prepared in a research laboratory or those in which the reagents are commercially supplied separately or in kit form. Wherever possible, the problem of quality control is often best solved by clinical rather than chemical control, e.g., by the use of appropriate stimulation or suppression tests. Although radioimmunoassay permits the simple and expeditious determination of a large number of clinical parameters of health and disease, its use in a casual manner without insight into the pitfalls can be destructive of its important role in clinical medicine. Similar pitfalls must also be considered in the use of bioassay systems.

REFERENCES

1. Yalow RS, Berson SA. Assay of plasma insulin in human subjects by immunological methods. Nature 1959; 184:1648–1649.
2. Yalow RS, Berson SA. Immunoassay of endogenous plasma insulin in man. J Clin Invest 1960; 39:1157–1175.
3. Berson SA, Yalow RS, Aurbach GD, et al. Immunoassay of bovine and human parathyroid hormone. Proc Natl Acad Sci USA 1963; 49:613–617.
4. Glick SM, Roth J, Yalow RS, et al. Immunoassay of human growth hormone in plasma. Nature 1963; 199:784–787.
5. Yalow RS, Glick SM, Roth J, et al. Radioimmunoassay of human plasma ACTH. J Clin Endocrinol Metab 1964; 24:1219–1225.
6. Yalow RS, Berson SA. Radioimmunoassay of gastrin. Gastroenterology 1970; 58:1–14.
7. Goodfriend TL, Levine L, Fasman GD. Antibodies to bradykinin and angiotensin: a use of carbodiimides in immunology. Science 1964; 144:1344–1346.
8. Talamo PC, Haber E, Austen KF. Antibody to bradykinin: effect of carrier and method of coupling on specificity and affinity. J Immunol 1968; 101:333–341.
9. Richards FM, Knowles JB. Glutaraldehyde as a protein cross-linking reagent. J Mol Biol 1968; 37:231–233 (letter).
10. Erlanger BF, Beiser S. Antibodies specific for ribonucleosides and ribonucleotides and their reaction with DNA. Proc Natl Acad Sci USA 1964; 52:68–74.
11. Smith LF. Species variation in the amino acid sequence of insulin. Am J Med 1966; 40:662–666.
12. Huang CG, Eng J, Pan YCE, et al. Guinea pig glucagon differs from other mammalian glucagons. Diabetes 1986; 35:508–512.
13. Eng J, Du BH, Raufman JP, et al. Purification and amino acid sequences of dog, goat and guinea pig VIP. Peptides 1986; 7:17–20.
14. Bonato C, Eng J, Pan YCE, et al. Guinea pig "little" gastrin is a hexadecapeptide. Life Sci 1985; 37:2563–2568.
15. Zhou ZZ, Eng J, Pan YCE, et al. Unique cholecystokinin peptides isolated from guinea pig intestine. Peptides 1985; 6:337–341.
16. Fan ZW, Eng J, Miedel M, et al. Cholecystokinin octapeptides purified from chinchilla and chicken brains. Brain Res Bull 1987; 18:757–760.
17. Shinomura Y, Eng J, Yalow RS. Chinchilla "big" and "little" gastrins. Biochem Biophys Res Commun 1987; 143:7–14.
18. Hunter WM, Greenwood FC. Preparation of iodine-131 labelled human growth hormone of high specific activity. Nature 1962; 194:495–496.
19. Berson SA, Yalow RS. General radioimmunoassay. In: Berson SA, Yalow

RS, eds. Methods in Investigative and Diagnostic Endocrinology. Part I. Amsterdam: North-Holland Publishing, 1973: 84–120.

20. Bolton AE, Hunter WM. The labelling of proteins to high specific radioactivities by conjugation to a ^{125}I-containing acylating agent. Biochem J 1973; 133:529–538.

21. Schneider BS, Straus E, Yalow RS. Some considerations in the preparation of radioiodoinsulin for radioimmunoassay and receptor assay. Diabetes 1976; 25:260–267.

22. Collins WP. Alternative Immunoassays. New York: John Wiley & Sons, 1985.

23. Yalow RS. Radioimmunoassay methodology: applications to problems of heterogeneity of peptide hormones. Pharmacol Rev 1973; 25:161–178.

24. Desbuquois B, Aurbach GD. Use of polyethylene glycol to separate free and antibody-bound peptide hormones in radioimmunoassays. J Clin Endocrinol Metab 1971; 33:732–738.

25. Yalow RS, Berson SA. Separation techniques—antigen adsorption. In: Berson SA, Yalow RS, eds. Methods in Investigative and Diagnostic Endocrinology. Part I. Amsterdam: North-Holland Publishing, 1973: 120–125.

26. Hughes J, Smith TW, Kosterlitz HW, et al. Identification of two related pentapeptides from the brain with potent opiate agonist activity. Nature 1975; 258:577–579.

27. Stern AS, Jones BN, Shively JE, et al. Two adrenal opioid polypeptides: proposed intermediates in the processing of proenkephalin. Proc Natl Acad Sci USA 1981; 78:1962–1966.

28. Silverman R, Yalow RS. Heterogeneity of parathyroid hormone: clinical and physiological implications. J Clin Invest 1973; 52:1958–1971.

29. Berson SA, Yalow RS. Quantitative aspects of reaction between insulin and insulin-binding antibody. J Clin Invest 1959; 38:1996–2016.

30. Grodsky GM, Peng CT, Forsham PH. Effect of modification of insulin on specific binding in insulin-resistant sera. Arch Biochem Biophys 1959; 81:264–272.

31. Kajubi SK, Yang RK, Li HR, et al. Differential effects of nonspecific factors in several radioimmunoassay systems. Ligand Q 1981; 4:63–66.

32. Straus E, Yalow RS. Artifacts in the radioimmunoassay of peptide hormones in gastric and duodenal secretions. J Lab Clin Med 1976; 87:292–298.

33. Moldow RL, Yalow RS. Artifacts in the radioimmunoassay of ACTH in tissue extracts and plasma. Horm Metab Res 1980; 12:105–110.

34. Eng J, Yalow RS. Evidence against extrapancreatic insulin synthesis. Proc Natl Acad Sci USA 1981; 78:4576–4578.

35. Berson SA, Yalow RS. Immunochemical distinction between insulins with identical amino acid sequences from different mammalian species (pork and sperm whale insulins). Nature 1961; 191:1392–1393.

36. Berson SA, Yalow RS. Insulin in blood and insulin antibodies. Am J Med 1966; 40:676–690.

37. Peterson JD, Nehrlich S, Oyer PE, et al. Determination of the amino acid sequence of the monkey, sheep, and dog proinsulin C-peptides by a semimicro Edman degradation procedure. J Biol Chem 1972; 247:4866–4871.

38. Bauman WA, Yalow RS. Differential diagnosis between endogenous and exogenous insulin induced refractory hypoglycemia in a nondiabetic patient. N Engl J Med 1980; 303:198–199.

39. Bauman WA, Yalow RS. Insulin as a lethal weapon. J Forensic Sci 1981; 26:594–598.

40. Bauman WA, Yalow RS. Child abuse: parenteral insulin administration. J Pediatr 1981; 99:588–591.

41. Bauman WA, Yalow RS. Transplacental passage of insulin complexed to antibody. Proc Natl Acad Sci USA 1981; 78:4588–4590.

42. Knobil E, Hotchkiss J. Growth hormone. Annu Rev Physiol 1964; 26:47–74.

43. Raben MS, Hollenberg CH. Growth hormone and the mobilization of fatty acids. Ciba Found Colloq Endocrinol [Proc] 1960; 13:89–105.

44. Li CH. Comparative biochemical endocrinology of pituitary growth hormone. Acta Endocrinol Suppl 1960; 50:75–81.

45. Tashijian AH Jr, Levine L, Wilhelmi AE. Use of complement fixation for the quantitative estimation of growth hormone and as a method for examining its structure. In: Pecile A, Muller E, eds. Growth Hormone. Amsterdam: Excerpta Medica, 1968: 70–83.

46. Lyons WR, Li CH, Ahwad N, et al. Mammotrophic effects of human hypophysial growth hormone preparations in animals and man. In: Pecile A, Muller E, eds. Growth Hormone. Amsterdam: Excerpta Medica, 1968: 349–363.

47. Friesen H, Guyda H. Biosynthesis of monkey growth hormone and prolactin in vitro. Endocrinology 1971; 88:1353–1362.

48. Hwang P, Friesen H, Hardy J, et al. Biosynthesis of human growth hormone and prolactin by normal pituitary glands and pituitary adenomas. J Clin Endocrinol Metab 1971; 33:1–7.

49. Hwang P, Guyda H, Friesen H. A radioimmunoassay for human prolactin. Proc Natl Acad Sci USA 1971; 68:1902–1906.

50. Greenwood FC, Hunter WM, Klopper A. Assay of human growth hormone in pregnancy at parturition and in lactation: detection of a growth-hormone–like substance from the placenta. Br Med J 1964; 1:22–24.

51. Glick SM, Roth J, Yalow RS, et al. Regulation of growth hormone secretion. Recent Prog Horm Res 1965; 21:241–283.

52. Crétien M. Lipotropins. In: Berson SA, Yalow RS, eds. Methods in Investigative and Diagnostic Endocrinology. Part II. Amsterdam, North-Holland Publishing, 1973: 617–632.

53. Goldsmith SJ, Yalow RS, Berson SA. Significance of human plasma insulin Sephadex fractions. Diabetes 1969; 18:834–839.

54. Gabbay KH, Bergenstal RM, Wolff J, et al. Familial hyperproinsulinemia: partial characterization of circulating proinsulin-like material. Proc Natl Acad Sci USA 1979; 76:2881–2885.

55. Robbins DC, Blix PM, Rubenstein AH, et al. Hereditary variation in insulin gene products: identification of a human proinsulin variant at Arg^{65}. Nature 1981; 291:679–681.

56. Berson SA, Yalow RS. Immunochemical heterogeneity of parathyroid hormone in plasma. J Clin Endocrinol 1968; 28:1037–1047.

57. Yalow RS. Significance of the heterogeneity of parathyroid hormone. Excerpta Med Int Congr Ser 1977; 421:308–312.

58. Raisz LG, Yajnik CH, Bockman RS, et al. Comparison of commercially available parathyroid hormone immunoassays in the differential diagnosis of hypercalcemia due to primary hyperparathyroidism or malignancy. Ann Intern Med 1979; 91:739–740.

59. Nussbaum SR, Zahradnik RJ, Lavigne JR, et al. Highly sensitive two-site immunoradiometric assay of parathyrin, and its clinical utility in evaluating patients with hypercalcemia. Clin Chem 1987; 33:1364–1367.

60. Yalow RS, Berson SA. Size and charge distinctions between endogenous human plasma gastrin in peripheral blood and heptadecapeptide gastrins. Gastroenterology 1970; 58:609–615.

61. Yalow RS, Berson SA. Further studies on the nature of immunoreactive gastrin in human plasma. Gastroenterology 1971; 60:203–214.

62. Gregory RA, Tracy HJ, Grossman MI. Isolation of two gastrins from human antral mucosa. Nature 1966; 209:583.

63. Straus E, Yalow RS. Differential diagnosis of hypergastrinemia. In: Thompson JC, ed. Gastrointestinal Hormones. Austin: University of Texas Press, 1975: 99–113.

64. Gewirtz R, Yalow RS. Ectopic ACTH production in carcinoma of the lung. J Clin Invest 1974; 53:1022–1032.

65. Gewirtz G, Schneider B, Krieger DT, et al. Big ACTH: conversion to biologically active ACTH by trypsin. J Clin Endocrinol Metab 1974; 38:227–230.

66. Dufau ML, Pock R, Neubauer A, et al. In vitro bioassay of LH in human serum: the interstitial cell testosterone (RICT) assay. J Clin Endocrinol Metab 1976; 42:958–969.

67. Dufau ML, Beitins IZ, McArthur JW, et al. Effects of luteinizing hormone releasing hormone (LHRH) upon bioactive and immunoactive serum LH levels in normal subjects. J Clin Endocrinol Metab 1976; 43:658–667.

68. Dufau ML, Veldhuis JD, Fraioli F, et al. Mode of secretion of bioactive luteinizing hormone in man. J Clin Endocrinol Metab 1983; 57:993–1000.

69. Warner BA, Dufau ML, Santen RJ. Effects of aging and illness on the pituitary testicular axis in men: qualitative as well as quantitative changes in luteinizing hormone. J Clin Endocrinol Metab 1985; 60:263–268.

70. Peikin SR, Rottman AJ, Batzri S, et al. Kinetics of amylase released by dispersed acini prepared from guinea pig pancreas. Am J Physiol 1978; 235:E743–E749.

71. Raufman JP, Eng J, Du BH, et al. Comparison of mammalian VIP bioactivities in dispersed acini from guinea pig pancreas. Regul Peptides 1986; 14:93–97.

72. Chey WY. Gastrointestinal hormones and pancreatic, biliary, and intestinal secretions. In: Glass GBJ, ed. Gastrointestinal Hormones. New York: Raven, 1980: 565–586.

37

RADIORECEPTOR AND OTHER FUNCTIONAL HORMONE ASSAYS

Phillip Gorden and Bruce D. Weintraub

INTRODUCTION

The science of endocrinology was originally based on in vivo bioassays, which involved the injection of test material into an animal, with measurement of a target gland response, such as growth or steroidogenesis. These assays were and are used to measure hormones extracted in large quantities from glands, and certain hormones—growth hormone (GH), follicle-stimulating hormone (FSH), luteinizing hormone (LH), and thyrotropin (TSH)—are still standardized in units defined by in vivo bioassays. However, despite the fact that the ideal test for a hormone is the measurement of the end result of action of the hormone in target tissues, most bioassays lack the precision, sensitivity, and specificity to measure the low concentration of hormones in plasma and other biological fluids.

The introduction of immunoassay techniques overcame most of these problems. Radioimmunoassays have been developed for essentially all the polypeptide, steroid, and thyronine hormones and usually have appropriate sensitivity, precision, convenience, and specificity to measure levels in unextracted biological fluids. Because of these advantages, radioimmunoassay and nonradioactive immunoassays are the most widely used techniques for measuring hormone concentrations (see Chapter 36).

In some cases, however, other types of hormone assays based on functional parameters provide additional insight into endocrine physiology. Such functional assays include radioreceptor assays, which utilize only one function of a hormone (namely, the capacity to combine with hormone receptor sites), and bioassays based on measurements of more complicated end results of hormone action, most often utilizing in vitro techniques.

In this chapter we review the general principles and applications of radioreceptor assay. In addition, we consider bioassays that exploit cellular responses to hormone binding. The use of radioreceptor techniques to characterize binding properties of receptors in peripheral tissues is considered under the general topic of hormone action (Chapters 3 and 4).

RADIORECEPTOR ASSAYS

Radioreceptor assays measure the interaction of ligand with specific receptor sites on cells or subcellular constituents. Radioreceptor assay was first introduced for corticotropin (ACTH, adrenocorticotropin),[1, 2] and assays have subsequently been developed for most polypeptide and steroid hormones. In contrast to radioimmunoassays, in which specificity is determined by sites on the hormone that are recognized by antibodies prepared from immunized animals, specificity in the radioreceptor assay is determined by binding to a biological receptor that mediates the action of the hormone. Such assays are of importance in three types of situations. First, they supplement radioimmunoassays by providing additional indices of biological activity, as, for example, in distinguishing stereoisomers of catecholamines and in distinguishing weak from active hormones, such as proinsulin from insulin. Second, they are useful for measuring hormonally active substances for which radioimmunoassay techniques are not readily available; e.g., dexamethasone and prednisone can be estimated in plasma by measuring the displacement of radioactive ligand from the glucocorticoid receptor. This technique is also used in the search for unknown hormones that may bind to candidate receptor molecules. Third, radioreceptor assays provide insights into endocrine disorders that involve autoantibodies to hormone receptors.

General Techniques

MATERIALS. Radioreceptor assays utilize principles first developed for radioimmunoassays. Initially, the tissues selected for binding studies were typical target tissues for the hormone. Examples include Leydig cells or granulosa cells for gonadotropins,[3] thyroid cells for TSH,[4] liver or fat cells for insulin,[5–7] and adrenal cells for corticotropin.[1, 2, 8] Theoretically, whole organs or pieces of freshly isolated tissue might be used, but in practice they are usually unsatisfactory. Single-cell preparations or purified plasma membranes are most frequently used. Crude membrane fractions are sometimes used, but more highly purified preparations provide greater specificity.

In addition to typical target tissues, nontarget tissues may possess specific binding sites for different ligands. Cultured human lymphocytes have specific receptors for insulin,[9, 10] human growth hormone (hGH),[11, 12] and calcitonin.[13] These cells grow in an isolated form in suspension culture and are especially convenient for radioreceptor studies.

LABELED LIGAND. When an appropriate isolated cell or membrane fraction has been prepared and a suitable incubation buffer formulated, the next ingredient for the assay is the labeled ligand. For peptide and protein hormones, material with high specific activity can usually be prepared by iodination, usually with [125]I. For radioreceptor assay the iodinated preparation must retain biological activity. During the early phase of development of radioreceptor techniques, it was necessary to verify the biological activity of the labeled species by separation of the labeled molecules on ion-exchange columns and demonstration of biological activity in bioassays.[1, 14] At present, biologically active labeled ligands are prepared by stoichiometric iodinations with low concentrations of an oxidizing agent such as chloramine-T[15] or lactoperoxidase.[16] In some instances, high-performance liquid chromatography is used for further purification of the labeled material.[17] With these techniques the loss of biological activity is less common.

INCUBATION CONDITIONS. Several features of the incubation conditions deserve special comment. First, the amount of binding for most radioreceptor assays is less than that for radioimmunoassay; therefore, every effort must be made to maximize binding. For example, the binding of insulin to membrane receptors is pH dependent. Maximal binding occurs between pH 7.8 and 8, and the buffer must therefore be suitable for maintaining this pH range for prolonged periods. Second, biological fluids often contain enzymes that degrade the ligand, the receptor, or both. Protease inhibitors and low-temperature incubations can be utilized to combat these problems. The sensitivity of radioreceptor assays is usually somewhat lower than that of radioimmunoassays; the concentration of reactants, i.e., re-

ceptor and labeled ligand, must be adjusted in an analogous fashion to immunoassay to achieve maximal sensitivity. Separation of the receptor-bound and free ligand is usually carried out by centrifugation at low temperature.

For measurement of the concentration of an unknown, a standard curve is constructed so that at the end of the incubation the ratio of bound to free (B/F) ligand can be derived and the concentration of unknown calculated from the plot of B/F vs. total unlabeled hormone concentration (analogous to radioimmunoassay) (Fig. 37–1). As with radioimmunoassay, derivations of the B/F plot can be used for specific purposes.[18, 19]

VALIDATION. The general principles of validation for radioreceptor assays are the same as those for radioimmunoassay, bioassay, or any other type of hormone assay. One advantage of radioreceptor techniques, like other radioligand assays, is their inherent precision. Precision does not guarantee validity or accuracy but is a requirement for assay validity. Because the number of sample replicates is usually limited, it is important that intra-assay variation be small if accuracy is to be provided. This requirement is particularly relevant to radioreceptor assay because in most methods the receptor is not solubilized but is in an insoluble form, such as in membranes or cells. Thus aggregation, sedimentation, or other factors that cause a nonuniform distribution of receptor among assay tubes may cause poor precision. Nevertheless, conditions can usually be devised to provide precision and accuracy.

Other hormones, antibodies, and unidentified factors in biological fluids may affect receptor assays even more than radioimmunoassays. Antibodies and other hormone-binding proteins may compete with the receptor for tracer binding. In addition, pH, ionic strength, anticoagulants, proteases, and poorly characterized serum "inhibitors" may directly damage tracer or inhibit tracer binding to receptor or impair assay validity. Although such effects can be minimized by dilutions of serum, the requirements of sensitivity may not permit such dilution (see Table 37–1 for further details of validation).

In radioimmunoassay it is usually possible to establish validity by using unfractionated serum at a final dilution of 1:5 to 1:20, but this practice is not generally feasible for radioreceptor assay. Considerations of specificity and sensitivity usually require that the hormone or antibody be partially purified and concentrated before assay. The more specific the purification method, the less chance that cross-

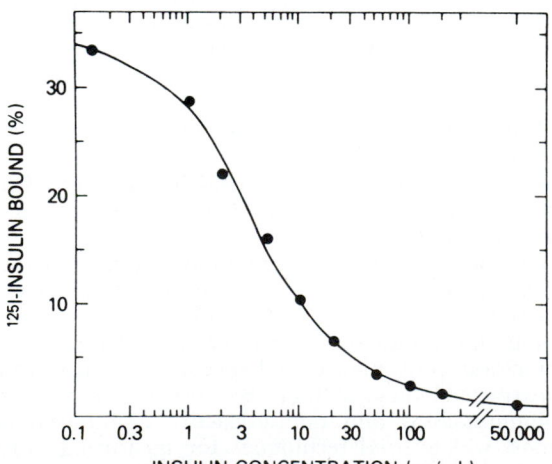

Figure 37–1. Typical standard curve for a radioreceptor assay. In this case the percentage of ^{125}I-insulin bound (vertical axis) to cultured human lymphocytes is plotted as a function of unlabeled insulin concentration. To convert insulin values to picomoles per liter, multiply by 0.1722.

TABLE 37–1. Criteria for Validation of Radioreceptor Assay

Appropriate specificity and precision
Agreement with in vitro bioassay
Agreement with known physiology of hormone
Concentration of hormone in sample independent of initial dilution (i.e., parallelism of dose-response curve with standard hormone)
Quantitative recovery of hormone added to sample
No evidence of cross-reactivity, nonspecific serum interference, proteolysis, binding proteins
Agreement of assays in crude vs. purified samples

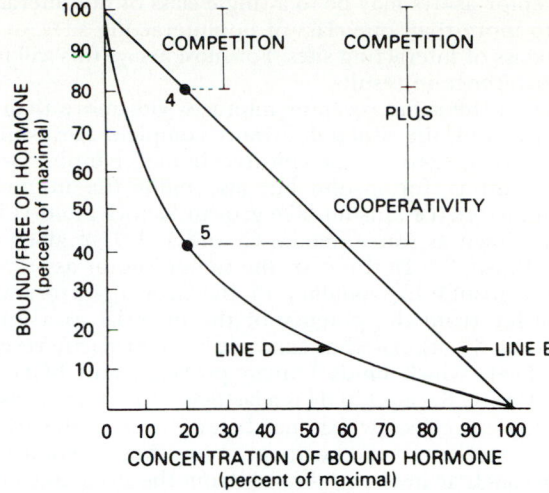

Figure 37–2. Analysis of the binding isotherm of ^{125}I-insulin to cultured human lymphocytes. Line E represents fall in the B/F ratio, at 20% receptor occupancy, that would be produced by competition alone. Line D represents the actual reduction in the B/F ratio at the same receptor occupancy produced by competition plus negative cooperativity (accelerated dissociation of bound ligand in the presence of increasing receptor occupancy by unlabeled ligand). (From Eastman RC, Lesniak MA, Roth J, et al. Regulation of receptor by homologous hormone enhances sensitivity and broadens scope of radioreceptor assay for human growth hormone. J Clin Endocrinol Metab 1979; 49:262–267.)

reactants or interfering substances will affect the subsequent receptor assay. A number of such purification methods are given in Table 37–2, of which the most specific is affinity chromatography.[20]

DETERMINANTS OF SENSITIVITY. The interaction between a hormone and its receptor is largely determined by the affinity of the receptor for the ligand and is therefore governed by the laws of mass action. The higher the affinity constant (K), the greater the sensitivity of the system.[6] In general, the affinity constant for the radioreceptor assay should be within an order of magnitude of the concentration of the hormone to be measured. Specific binding refers to the binding that is displaced competitively by unlabeled hormone. Radioactivity that remains bound to cells in the presence of a high concentration of unlabeled hormone is referred to as nonspecific (a more accurate term is low-affinity binding; specificity can be determined only by analogue studies; see later). Nonspecific binding is usually subtracted from total binding to give specific binding. The decrease in the B/F ratio with increasing ligand concentration is a function of competitive inhibition of binding of unlabeled ligand with the labeled ligand—analogous to the interaction of a hormone and an antibody.

For some radioreceptor systems, factors other than affinity affect binding. For example, the dissociation rate of insulin from its receptor is a function of receptor occupancy; this dissociation is referred to operationally as negative cooperativity (although the molecular mechanism of this effect is unclear).[21] Thus the drop in the B/F ratio of ^{125}I-insulin as a function of increasing amounts of unlabeled insulin bound to its receptor is a function of both competition and accelerated dissociation of the negative cooperativity type (Fig. 37–2).[22]

Another mechanism that influences radioreceptor assays with whole cells is down-regulation. For instance, low concentrations of hGH ($\sim 10^{-10}$ M) will lead to the loss of cell-surface binding of ^{125}I-hGH in cultured human lymphocytes. This loss of cell-surface receptors is due to internalization of the receptor, not to competition.[23] Regulation of receptor number can alter the sensitivity of the system (Fig. 37–3).[22, 24, 25]

RECEPTOR SPECIFICITY. The key element in the radioreceptor assay is specificity. Operationally, receptors are defined on the basis of binding specificity for a particular ligand. Because receptor preparations may be obtained from

target tissues, nontarget tissues, isolated plasma membranes, and solubilized membrane preparations, each system must be validated by comparing the ability of compounds of known biological activity to compete for binding sites. For example, more than 50 naturally occurring or synthetic insulins have been compared for their abilities to stimulate a biological effect and to compete for binding to cell-surface receptors; binding and biological activity correlate closely. Similar studies have been carried out for other polypeptide hormones, hypothalamic releasing hormones, and catecholamines.

The minimal requirement for a receptor system for polypeptide hormones is that the system be saturable, i.e., that there be a finite number of sites. Radioreceptors for catecholamines must also be stereospecific.[26] Binding in ra-

TABLE 37–2. Techniques Commonly Used for Purification of Labeled or Unlabeled Hormones in Receptor Assay

Gel filtration
Ion-exchange chromatography
Gel electrophoresis
Hydrophobic chromatography
High-performance liquid chromatography
Affinity chromatography with the following ligands
  Insoluble receptors on tissues or cells
  Immobilized antibodies
  Immobilized lectins

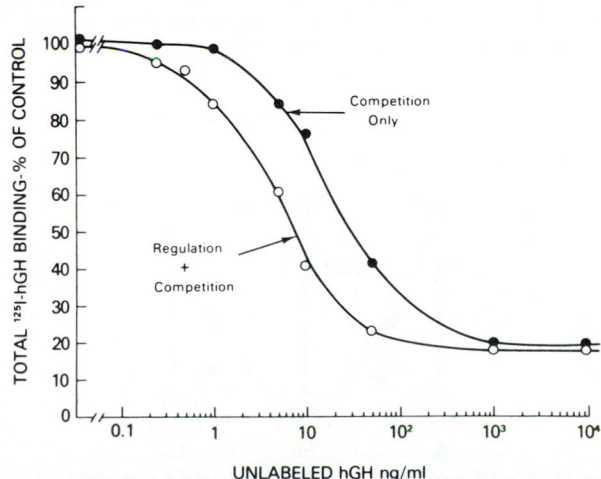

Figure 37–3. Standard curve of ^{125}I-hGH binding to cultured human lymphocytes. The combination of down-regulation and competition makes the curve steeper and hence more sensitive. (From Eastman RC, Lesniak MA, Roth J, et al. Regulation of receptor by homologous hormone enhances sensitivity and broadens scope of radioreceptor assay for human growth hormone. J Clin Endocrinol Metab 1979; 49:262–267.)

dioreceptor assays may be to a single class of noninteracting sites, to more than one class of noninteracting sites, or to a single class of interacting sites. For most assays this will make little difference in results.

When the same receptor interacts with more than one class of ligand, the situation is more complex. For example, the insulin receptor of the cultured human lymphocyte has a high affinity for insulin but also binds the insulin-like growth factors (i.e., insulin-like growth factors I and II [IGF I, also known as somatomedin-C; and IGF II]), albeit with lower affinity.[27-31] In this case, the radioreceptor assay measures the insulin-like potency of the growth factor, which may differ from the potency of the material as a growth factor (Fig. 37–4). Another example is the prolactin receptor of rat liver, which binds human prolactin and hGH with equal affinity. Because hGH is a lactogen, this assay measures the lactogenic effect, which may be unrelated to the growth-promoting effect of the hormone.[32] In other receptor preparations such as liver membranes from the pregnant rabbit, growth hormone receptors show little interaction with prolactin.[33] The cultured human lymphocyte offers still another advantage in this regard because it does not react with prolactin or with nonhuman growth hormones (Fig. 37–5).[34] In other instances variation among species in receptor concentration of the same tissue has been exploited to enhance IGF I and IGF II receptor concentration in different placental tissues.[35]

An even more complex situation exists when multiple receptors for the same or unrelated ligands are present on the same cell (see Fig. 37–4). For example, the rat liver contains receptors for insulin and IGF II; the human fibroblast contains receptors for insulin, IGF I, and IGF II. The growth factors interact with the insulin receptor with such low affinity that radioreceptor assay is not practical with the insulin receptor. On the other hand, the growth factors react with high affinity to their own receptors, and this property has been exploited to create a growth factor assay with liver membrane preparations.[27] This type of nonspecificity provides a major advantage for the radioreceptor assay. In this case one is identifying the effect of a hormone rather than a specific hormone. Both insulin and proinsulin interact with the growth factor receptors. Preliminary separation of these various factors, therefore, may be necessary before radioreceptor assay. Furthermore, the insulin-like growth factors circulate in plasma primarily bound to high-molecular-weight proteins. Thus acidification combined with gel filtration may be necessary to free the ligand before assay.[30, 31]

The TSH receptor offers another example of a special

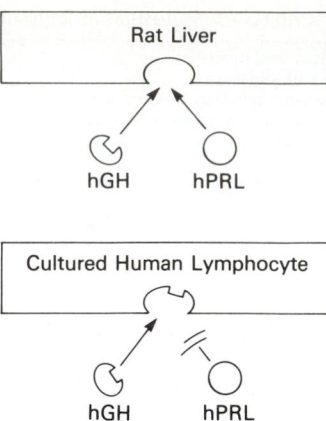

Figure 37–5. An example of one receptor with equal affinity for two different ligands (rat liver) and a second receptor on a different cell type that recognizes only one of these ligands (cultured human lymphocyte). The latter provides a more specific assay for hGH. hPRL, human prolactin.

situation. TSH binding sites are present in thyroid, testes, fat cells, plasma membranes, and lymphocytes. Specificity for these receptor preparations should be relatively similar. However, specificity in thyroid membranes varies, depending on the conditions of isolation and of the incubation. Thus under certain conditions of assay other glycoproteins such as the alpha and beta subunits of TSH, LH, and human chorionic gonadotropin (hCG); immunoglobulins; thyroglobulin; cholera toxin; and gangliosides cross-react in the assay.[36]

The interaction of LH and hCG, when present in high concentrations, with the TSH receptor is consistent with the structural homology among these hormones: there is complete homology of the amino acid sequence of the alpha subunits and partial homology among the unique beta subunits.[37] Moreover, certain patients with trophoblastic neoplasms such as choriocarcinoma develop clinical hyperthyroidism that appears to be caused by the high concentrations of hCG,[38, 39] amounts that are in excess of those present during normal pregnancy. Thus the cross-reactivity of hCG and LH in the TSH receptor assay appears to be another example of specificity spillover.[40]

In summary, a single receptor may bind more than one ligand, and the same ligand may bind to more than one receptor. It is sometimes possible to simplify an assay by finding a tissue with a single receptor, i.e., the IGF II receptor in human placenta,[41] or by establishing appropriate incubation conditions for a receptor that improve specificity.

HETEROLOGOUS EFFECTS. A decrease in the B/F ratio of a given labeled hormone as a function of increasing ligand concentration superficially suggests competitive binding interaction. However, this can be misleading in some circumstances. For instance, phorbol esters decrease epidermal growth factor binding to its specific receptors in several cell types[42] and insulin binding to insulin receptors on cultured lymphocytes and monocytes.[43, 44] Initially, it was thought that the phorbol esters competitively inhibit the binding of epidermal growth factor to its receptor; however, phorbol ester binds to its own specific receptor, and this hormone-receptor complex in turn decreases epidermal growth factor binding in a regulatory fashion.

Another heterologous effect is represented by the transforming growth factors. Transforming growth factor α is essentially equipotent to epidermal growth factor in competing for binding to the epidermal growth factor receptor. Both of these growth factors have the same biological effects in many cell types.[45]

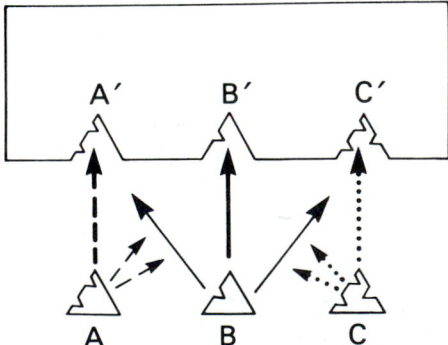

Figure 37–4. In a family of related peptides, each ligand A, B, and C binds with high affinity to its respective receptor A', B', and C'. In addition, each ligand can bind to a related receptor but with a lower affinity. For example, ligand B preferentially binds to its receptor B'; at high concentrations B can also bind to related receptors, A' and C', but the affinity of ligand B for A' and C' receptors is decreased. This example is relevant to cross-specificity of insulin and insulin-like growth factors on cells. (For further discussion, see Chapter 4.)

These types of heterologous effects may be exploited in radioreceptor assays, provided the underlying nature of the interaction is understood.

RELATION TO BIOLOGICAL ACTIONS. Under certain conditions, the radioreceptor assay estimates the biological activity of a hormone more closely than does the radioimmunoassay. Furthermore, the radioreceptor assay is usually simpler to perform and has greater sensitivity than bioassay, so that it can be applied to the low hormone concentrations in plasma.

Binding of a polypeptide hormone to its cell-surface receptor is the first step in the action of the hormone. The radioreceptor assay measures the affinity of the ligand for its receptor and may reflect the effects of cooperativity and down-regulation (see earlier). After binding, the hormone-receptor complex must transduce a further signal. Intrinsic activity refers to those properties of the ligand once bound to its receptor that are necessary to elicit a biological signal (Fig. 37–6).

AGONIST AND ANTAGONIST. The catecholamines illustrate the relationship of binding affinity to intrinsic activity. Catecholamines bind to specific alpha- and beta-adrenergic receptors on the surface of cells. In contrast to polypeptide hormones, they bind in a stereospecific fashion, as noted previously. Most of the early studies of catecholamine binding were specific in the sense that they were competitive and saturable but were nonspecific in regard to stereospecificity.[26] In fact, the first stereospecific studies were carried out with antagonists. These compounds have high affinity for the receptor but little or no intrinsic hormonal activity. Thus an agonist is a compound with variable affinity and full intrinsic activity, and an antagonist is a compound with variable affinity and little intrinsic activity. A partial agonist is a compound that both exerts a biological signal (a weak agonist) and inhibits binding (i.e., has relatively high affinity).

Discrepancy between radioreceptor assays and in vitro bioassays can also occur when abnormal hormones are formed. The TSH from a euthyroid patient had normal receptor-binding properties but decreased activity in an in vitro bioassay.[46] Heterogenous forms of mouse and bovine TSH also exhibit dissociation between receptor binding and biological activity.[47] Furthermore, certain chemical modifications produce molecules with normal receptor binding but decreased biological activity, similar to the naturally occurring forms just described. Most chemical modifications decrease both receptor binding and biological activity.[5, 6, 48]

To summarize, the radioreceptor assay measures only the first step in the biological cascade (see Fig. 37–6). The

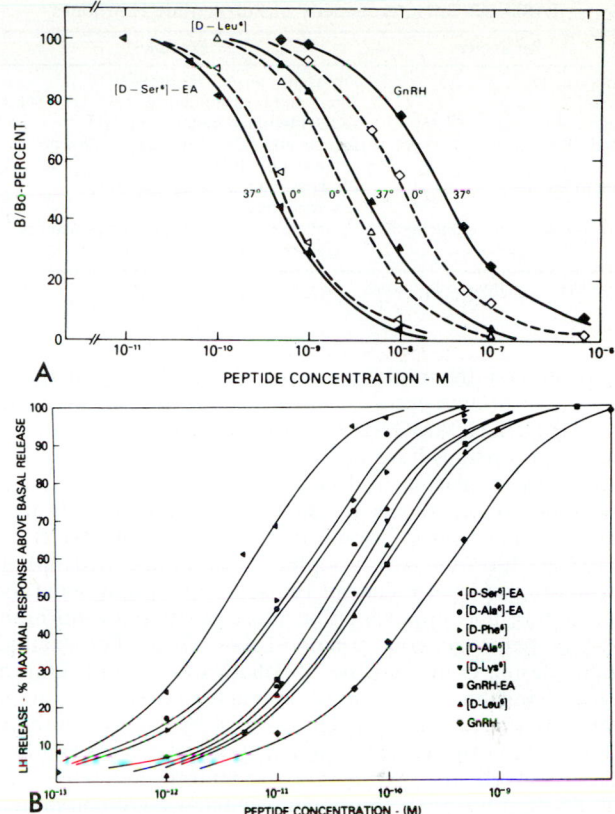

A

B

Figure 37–7. Effects of different LHRH analogues. *A*, Radioreceptor assay. *B*, Bioassay. (From Loumaye E, Naor Z, Catt KJ. Binding affinity and biological activity of gonadotropin-releasing hormone agonists in isolated pituitary cells. Endocrinology 1982; 111:730–736.)

assay estimates biological activity only if the ligand is known from independent assessment to have full intrinsic activity.

IN VITRO VS. IN VIVO ASSAYS. Radioreceptor assays are in vitro tests and under most circumstances provide information similar to that provided by in vitro bioassays. In vivo bioassays may differ, however, in that these assays are influenced by the metabolism of the ligand as well as by its affinity and intrinsic activity. For instance, proinsulin has only ~2 to 4% of the biological activity of insulin in vitro, but in vivo this compound has ~20% of the activity of insulin owing to its prolonged half-life in the circulation.

Applications

PEPTIDE HORMONE: STRUCTURE-FUNCTION RELATIONSHIPS. Radioreceptor assay is especially useful for studies of structure-function relationships. Either small or large concentrations of a given preparation can be assayed to estimate potential biological activity. Synthetic analogues of a hormone can be assayed to relate specific structural features influencing receptor-binding properties; these assays may include measurement of the affinity of the ligand for receptor and of its ability to induce negative cooperativity and/or receptor regulation.

The radioreceptor assay is of particular use in the study of structure-function relationships of synthetic analogues of peptide hormones. For example, the affinity of binding of analogues of luteinizing hormone–releasing hormone (LHRH, also called gonadotropin-releasing hormone, GnRH) can be determined by receptor assay. In this way, analogues with higher affinity than the naturally occurring LHRH were identified (Fig. 37–7).[49] A superagonist can also

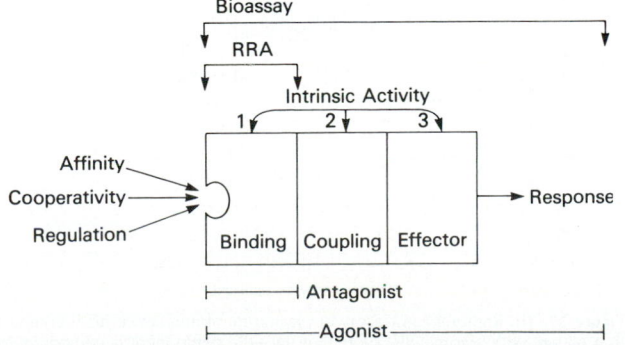

Figure 37–6. An example of the binding component of a receptor and its coupling and effector units. All actions must go through the binding component. Arrows at the top represent portions of system measured by bioassay and radioreceptor assay (RRA). At the bottom, various parts of system affected by agonists and antagonists are shown.

TABLE 37–3. Heterogeneity of Polypeptide Hormones

Parameter	Examples*
Prohormones	Proinsulin, proACTH, proPTH
Subunits	Alpha and beta subunits of TSH, LH, FSH, CG
Fragments	COOH-terminal fragment of PTH
Aggregates	Dimers and other aggregates of growth hormone, prolactin
Protein bound	Binding proteins for vasopressin, somatomedins
Post-translational modifications	Variations in carbohydrate composition of glycoprotein hormones

*PTH, parathyroid hormone; CG, chorionic gonadotropin.

be produced by modification of the molecule so that its lifetime on the receptor or in the circulation is prolonged.

PEPTIDE HORMONE: HETEROGENEITY IN PLASMA. Radioreceptor assays have been especially helpful for studying hormones in plasma and other body fluids. Total plasma hormone concentration is usually measured directly in diluted plasma by radioimmunoassay. When plasma is subjected to filtration over Sephadex columns, hydrophobic chromatography, or charge or isoelectric point separation techniques, it is apparent that most polypeptide hormones exist in heterogeneous forms (Table 37–3). For example, when plasma is filtered over Sephadex G-50 and immunoreactive insulin is measured in each eluted fraction, the major plasma component elutes in the region of authentic 6-kd insulin. In addition, higher-molecular-mass immunoreactive insulin components are distinguished (Figs. 37–8 and 37–9). One of the higher-molecular-weight components is a biosynthetic precursor of insulin, proinsulin. When the insulin-like component is measured by radioreceptor assay and radioimmunoassay, the two activities are approximately equal; however, the proinsulin-like component is less than one fifth as active in the radioreceptor assay as in the radioimmunoassay.[50, 51] In addition, mutant insulins have been described in which the insulin moiety has less than 15% of the activity in a receptor assay as in an immunoassay.[52, 53]

Similarly, when plasma is filtered over Sephadex G-100 and hGH immunoreactivity is measured in each fraction, a major peak elutes as a 22-kd protein, but additional high-molecular-mass components are seen (Fig. 37–10).[54–57] The higher-molecular-mass components are less well defined

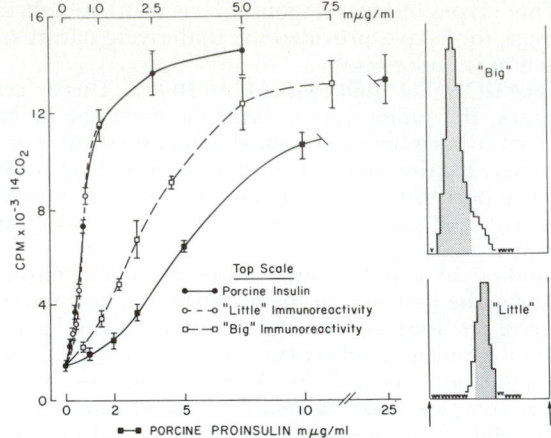

Figure 37–9. Bioassay of plasma immunoreactive insulin. "Big" refers to the proinsulin-like component (PLC) fraction of Figure 37–8, and "little" refers to the insulin-like component (ILC) of Figure 37–8. Note that the little fraction is equipotent to the insulin standard, whereas the big fraction is less potent than insulin but somewhat more potent than the proinsulin standard. (From Gorden P, Freychet P, Nankin H. A unique form of circulating insulin in human islet cell carcinoma. J Clin Endocrinol Metab 1971; 33:983–987. © 1971, The Endocrine Society.)

than for insulin, but they exhibit decreased radioreceptor activity.[58] This high-molecular-weight component probably consists of oligomeric forms of hGH and a bound form of hGH. The binding protein appears to be a secreted form of the hGH receptor.[59–61] When only the major peak is considered there is a higher ratio of radioreceptor to radioimmunoassay activity in plasma from acromegalic patients than from normal subjects.[55] Discrepancies between radioreceptor assays and radioimmunoassays can thus be due to different affinities of precursor and product hormones, mixtures of hormones of different origin, or post-translational modifications of a single protein.[62, 63]

STEROID HORMONES. Although there are receptor assays for several steroid hormones including androgens and vitamin D, these assays are used infrequently. Two exceptions, however, are relevant. An assay to measure total glucocorticoid activity utilizes pituitary tumor cells and [^{3}H]dexamethasone. Because dexamethasone does not bind

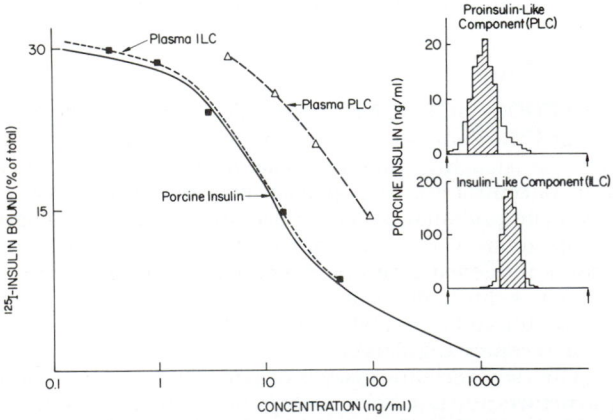

Figure 37–8. Radioreceptor assay of plasma insulin separated into insulin-like component (ILC) and proinsulin-like component (PLC) fractions by Sephadex G-50 gel filtration. The former fraction is equipotent to insulin standards; the latter is much less reactive. To convert insulin values to picomoles per liter, multiply by 0.1722. (From Gavin JR III, Kahn CR, Gorden P, et al. Radioreceptor assay of insulin: comparison of plasma and pancreatic insulins and proinsulins. J Clin Endocrinol Metab 1975; 41:438–445. © 1975, The Endocrine Society.)

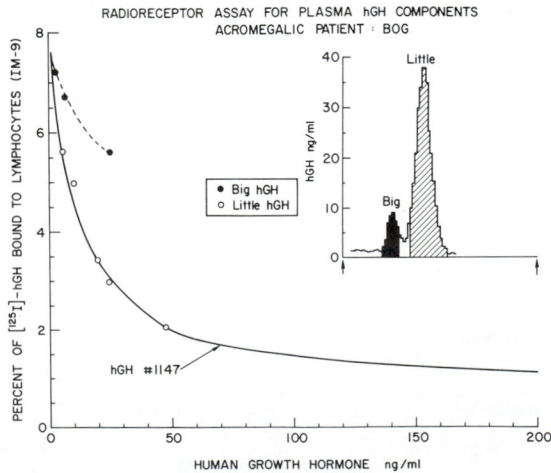

Figure 37–10. Radioreceptor assay of plasma immunoreactive hGH components in a patient with acromegaly. Note that the little component is equipotent to the growth hormone standard, whereas the big component is less reactive. (From Gorden P, Lesniak MA, Hendricks CM, et al. "Big" growth hormone components from human plasma: decreased reactivity demonstrated by radioreceptor assay. Science 1973; 182:829–831. Copyright 1973 by the American Association for the Advancement of Science.)

well to plasma proteins, competition for [³H]dexamethasone binding to the receptor is a measure of total glucocorticoid activity.[64] This technique is of use in monitoring blood levels of pharmacological glucocorticoids for which no radioimmunoassay is available.

A similar approach, with rat kidney receptors, has been used to screen for "mineralocorticoid" activity in hypertensive patients.[65] With this technique, elevated mineralocorticoid activity was found in serum from patients with primary aldosteronism but not in serum from other patients with low-renin essential hypertension. The failure of this type of functional assay to detect an unknown form of mineralocorticoid suggests that low-renin essential hypertension is not due to mineralocorticoid excess.[66]

OPIATE RECEPTORS. The presence of receptors for the opiate alkaloids in brain tissues suggested that endogenous ligands for these receptors existed within the central nervous system. It was then verified that endogenous ligands do indeed interact with these binding sites in a specific manner. This result represents one of the most powerful aspects of radioreceptor technique, i.e., the discovery of biologically active substances that bind to known or candidate receptor molecules.

The endogenous opioids are peptides known as endorphins and enkephalins and are derived from the higher-molecular-weight biosynthetic precursor pro-opiomelanocortin, which itself can react with both opioid and corticotropin receptors.[67-69] (See also Chapters 3 and 4.)

AUTOANTIBODIES TO HORMONE RECEPTORS. The radioreceptor assay measures an activity, not a specific structure. Thus molecules such as antibodies that are structurally unrelated to hormones may interact with hormone receptors and be detected and quantitated by this technique. For example, autoantibodies have been detected in several disease states (Table 37–4). These immunoglobulins are not reactive in immunoassays but do interact with cell-surface receptors.

Autoantibodies to hormone receptors may be recognized in two ways. If the autoantibody is directed against the binding site for a polypeptide hormone, the ligand is detected in a typical competition assay. For instance, autoantibodies to the insulin receptor[70] and the TSII receptor[71, 72] are detected by competitive inhibition of binding of the labeled polypeptide hormone by the specific immunoglobulin. On the other hand, some immunoglobulins do not interact at the level of the binding site and thus may go undetected in a radioreceptor assay. In this case, the autoantibody may be directed against some other component of the receptor, as is true for the antibody to the acetylcholine receptor in myasthenia gravis,[73] which does not inhibit binding but can be detected by immunoprecipitation (Fig. 37–11).[74, 75]

Radioreceptor assays have been developed specifically for antibodies to hormone receptors. An assay for detection of antibodies to the insulin receptor uses a small concentration of ¹²⁵I-insulin incubated with a detergent-solubilized

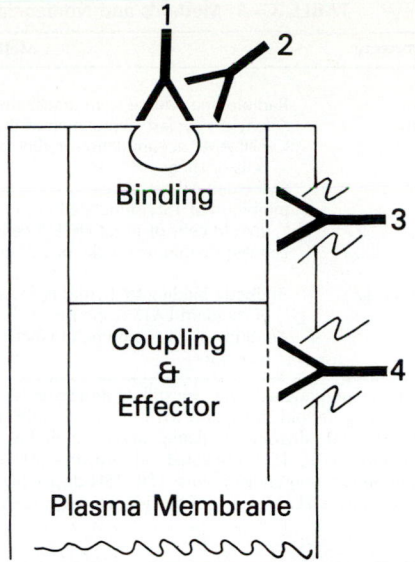

Figure 37–11. An example of binding of antireceptor antibodies to various components of the receptor. Examples 1 and 2 represent immunoglobulins that interact with the hormone binding site and will compete with the hormone for binding in a radioreceptor assay. Examples 3 and 4 represent antibodies that bind to different components of system to immunoprecipitate the receptor or to activate biological activity. Broken lines represent detergent-solubilized systems that may react with immunoglobulins that could not penetrate the membrane of intact cells.

tissue, such as placenta, that contains insulin receptors.[74] The receptor-insulin complex serves as the tracer, and the antireceptor antibody immunoprecipitates the ligand-receptor complex. Other techniques have used direct iodination of purified insulin receptor.[75] Under these conditions, appropriate controls must be performed to detect anti-insulin antibodies also.

TSH Receptor. Autoantibodies to the TSH receptor have been carefully studied (Table 37–5). (Also see Chapter 8.) The first indirect evidence of autoantibodies to the TSH receptor was provided by the discovery of a thyroid stimulator, apparently different from TSH, in the serum of patients with Graves disease.[76] This substance was termed *long-acting thyroid stimulator* (LATS) because its peak of stimulating activity (16 to 24 h after injection) occurred later than that of TSH (about 2 to 5 h). LATS activity was originally measured by a guinea pig bioassay[76] and subsequently by a variety of in vivo bioassay methods,[77] the most popular of which assessed the release of ¹²⁵I label from thyroid into the blood of mice whose endogenous TSH had been suppressed by thyroxine.[78] This assay is important historically but was subject to considerable interassay variation and a variety of technical artifacts.[79] Most important, the assay gave positive results in only a fraction (less than 20% in unselected series) of patients with Graves disease, presumably because only a small percentage of patients had high enough titers of LATS to cross-react in the heterologous mouse assay.[80]

LATS is a 7S gamma-globulin,[81] the activity of which is associated with antibodies directed against a thyroid antigen.[82] In a modification of the LATS assay, the so-called LATS protector assay,[83] a known positive LATS serum is bioassayed after preincubation with human thyroid tissue containing enough thyroid antigen to neutralize the standard thyroid-stimulating immunoglobulin. Serum from Graves patients and from other unknown samples is tested for ability to bind to the human thyroid antigen and "protect" the LATS serum from neutralization. Thus a serum with

TABLE 37–4. Diseases Associated with Autoantibodies to Cell-Surface Hormone Receptors

Disease/Dysfunction	Receptor	Functional Consequence
Hyperthyroidism or hypothyroidism	TSH	Agonist or antagonist
Myasthenia gravis	Acetylcholine	Antagonist
Infertility/premature menopause	FSH, LH	Antagonist
Asthma	Beta-adrenergic	Antagonist
Diabetes or hypoglycemia	Insulin	Agonist or antagonist

TABLE 37–5. Methods and Nomenclature for the Measurement of Autoantibodies to the TSH Receptor*†

Type of Assay	Methods	Nomenclature	Selected References
Bioassay			
In vivo	Radioiodine release from mouse thyroid	LATS, MTS	78, 162, 163
In vitro	Adenylate cyclase stimulation in thyroid membranes	HTACS	141
	Cyclic AMP accumulation, iodide trapping, or T_3 release in thyroid cells or slices	TSAb, TSI	142, 143
	Cytochemical bioassay	TSAb, TSI	92
	Inhibition of TSH-stimulated cyclic AMP or iodide trapping in primary thyroid cells or in rat FRTL-5 cells	TSII	98
	Labeled thymidine uptake or cell growth in FRTL-5 cells	TSGAb (stimulatory), TGII (inhibitory)	95, 99
Receptor assay	Antibody binding to thyroid homogenate prevents expected inhibition of standard LATS response	LATS protector	83
	Antibody inhibits binding of labeled TSH to membranes or solubilized receptors	TBI, TBIAb, TBII, TDI	71

*Certain of these antibody activities are still controversial (see text).

†LATS, long-acting thyroid stimulator; MTS, mouse thyroid stimulator; HTACS, human thyroidal adenylate cyclase stimulator; T_3, triiodothyronine; TSAb, thyroid-stimulating antibody; TSI, thyroid-stimulating immunoglobulins; TSII, TSH-stimulated cyclic AMP response–inhibitory immunoglobulins; TGSAb, thyroid growth–stimulatory antibodies; TGII, TSH-stimulated cell growth–inhibitory immunoglobulins; TBI, TSH-binding inhibition; TBIAb, TSH-binding inhibitory antibodies; TBII, thyroid-binding inhibitory immunoglobulins; TDI, TSH-displacing immunoglobulins.

Modified from Davies TF. Diseases of the TSH receptor. Clin Endocrinol Metab 1983; 12:79–100.

LATS protector activity would cause a significant response in the subsequent mouse bioassay. This method is more sensitive than the direct LATS assay, presumably because the serum being tested is preincubated with homologous human tissue. However, the assay is cumbersome and has been used in few laboratories. Moreover, the test is actually a receptor assay rather than a bioassay and, as discussed later, certain Graves antibodies bind to the TSH receptor (and thus protect LATS from neutralization) without themselves having agonistic activity.

The next advance was the development of direct radioreceptor assays for Graves immunoglobulins. Partially purified immunoglobulin fractions were tested for the ability to inhibit the binding of labeled bovine TSH to thyroid cells,[84] membranes,[71, 72] and solubilized receptors.[85] The assays were often performed under conditions of physiological pH and temperature and NaCl concentration of 50 mmol/L or higher, which favor binding to the high-affinity receptor. However, certain variants of the assay used lower concentrations of NaCl that promote less specific interactions with the low-affinity sites. In some instances, normal immunoglobulin G[86] and possibly other globulins may cause false-positive responses. This is relevant because the usual purification method with ammonium sulfate precipitation may yield immunoglobulin G contaminated with many other proteins. Thus it is preferable to use more specific methods in immunoglobulin G purification.[87]

A variant of the receptor assay utilizes fat cells rather than thyroid membranes as the source of the TSH receptor.[88] Both TSH and antibodies from Graves patients stimulate adipose tissue,[89] and such tissue contains high-affinity TSH receptors.[90] It was reasoned that adipose membranes would not contain other thyroidal antigens to which antibodies in Graves disease might be directed and would thus yield a more specific assay. This approach has not been examined critically in a large series.

Several in vitro bioassays have utilized the stimulation of cyclic AMP, adenylate cyclase, or thyroid hormone release from human thyroid slices, membranes, or dispersed cells in primary culture (see Table 37–5). Other variants of the bioassay utilize nonhuman thyroid tissue or cells,[91] including the cytochemical bioassay that has been used in only a few centers.[92] The most important advance in this field has been the development of the FRTL-5 thyroid cell strain.[93] Although these cells do not organify iodide or produce thyroid hormones, they maintain some differentiated thyroid cell functions including cyclic AMP production, iodide trapping

or efflux, and TSH-dependent cell growth.[94] The last effect can be estimated by measuring the incorporation of [³H]thymidine into DNA, although such labeling techniques are subject to various caveats and may not always correlate with unlabeled DNA synthesis or with increase in cell number. Because of the convenience and reproducibility of assays with these cells, a number of reports have examined the effects of immunoglobulins from patients with Graves and other thyroid diseases on various differentiated functions.[95–99] Such assays have revealed considerable variability of antibodies in stimulating various functions (i.e., dissociations among cyclic AMP production, iodide trapping, and stimulation of growth).

All the modern radioreceptor and in vitro bioassays provide higher sensitivity for Graves serum than did the LATS assay. The frequency of positive responses in the receptor assay ranges between 54 and 100% in various series,[100] whereas most of the in vitro bioassays are in the range of 80 to 90% positive.[101] However, many of these are small series that are subject to the bias of patient selection. For example, patients with pretibial myxedema or malignant exophthalmos tend to have the highest titers in all assays, and those with "euthyroid" Graves disease tend to have the lowest titers. The specificity of most assays for Graves immunoglobulin G is generally good, but certain of the methods, including the radioreceptor assay and cytochemical bioassays, have given positive results in other forms of thyroid disease including autoimmune thyroiditis, subacute thyroiditis, multinodular goiter, and thyroid carcinoma.[102]

The clinical application of these assays is considered in detail in Chapter 8. In brief, as a marker for Graves disease, both receptor assays and in vitro bioassays are useful. Although the correlation between receptor-binding activity and bioactivity of individual sera is good, there are many reported discordances.[103] These discrepancies have been attributed to antibodies that bind to the receptor but are not agonistic (in some cases, even antagonistic) or to antibodies that perturb the interaction of labeled TSH without actually being directed at the receptor site. Nonetheless, both types of assays are useful for predicting relapse and remission in hyperthyroid patients and for predicting the development of neonatal hyperthyroidism.[104]

Antagonistic or blocking antibodies may cause hypothyroidism in a variety of clinical states. Such antibodies have been identified in patients with congenital hypothyroidism, idiopathic primary myxedema, goiters, and atrophic autoimmune thyroiditis.[97–99] Moreover, new types of stimulating antibodies have been described, including growth-promoting antibodies in the serum of certain patients with goitrous disease.[95] Other antibodies that stimulate collagen synthesis in human fibroblasts seem to correlate with the presence of exophthalmos in Graves patients.[96]

The recognition of multiple types of TSH receptor antibodies in various autoimmune thyroid diseases may help to explain the diverse features of these syndromes. Moreover, serum from individual patients with Graves disease has heterogeneous populations of both stimulatory and blocking antibodies,[98] and the ratio of these two classes can change temporally such as during antithyroid drug therapy.[97] However, the non-TSH receptor antibodies may account for the dominant clinical effect even in the presence of antibodies to the TSH receptor. Thus a patient with cytotoxic, organ-specific antibodies destructive of thyroid cell function would develop hypothyroidism even if there were a dominant population of thyroid-stimulating antibodies in the serum. Finally, the increased number of antibody activities now recognized in patients with Graves disease has led to a confusing increase in the terms and abbreviations used in this field (see Table 37–5). At this time there is general agreement about the importance of thyroid-stimulating immunoglobulins as the cause of Graves hyperthyroidism. However, the physiological roles of inhibiting antibodies as a major cause of hypothyroidism, and of growth-stimulating antibodies as a major cause of goiter remain controversial.

Insulin Receptor. The assays and caveats described in detail for autoantibodies to the TSH receptor apply to assays for autoantibodies to the insulin receptor. Insulin receptor autoantibodies are detected in vitro in three ways: (1) a typical binding inhibition assay in cultured human lymphocytes in which the autoantibody competitively inhibits ^{125}I-insulin binding,[70] (2) immunoprecipitation assays in which the autoantibody immunoprecipitates the receptor,[74, 75] and (3) demonstration of a direct insulin-like effect similar to any other nonsuppressible insulin-like activity. In this third type of assay, specificity must be determined by additional steps such as purification of the immunoglobulin.[105]

The best detection methods depend on the nature of the antibody and the specific component of the receptor-effector system to which it is targeted (see Fig. 37–11). The metabolic state induced by autoantibodies to the insulin receptor is variable; both hypoglycemia or, more commonly, insulin resistance and hyperglycemia have been described.[105, 106] All autoantibodies thus far studied mimic the action of insulin in vitro, and most inhibit insulin binding regardless of the metabolic state of the patients (Fig. 37–12).[105] Because these antibodies are polyclonal, however, subfractions may manifest different properties.[107]

IN VITRO BIOASSAYS

Most hormones were initially identified by bioassays involving the injection of preparations into groups of normal animals or animals prepared in a manner yielding a maximal endocrine response. Not only are such in vivo bioassays of historical interest, they are still used in the assay and standardization of many hormones, especially those not available in a completely purified form. Examples of such bioassays include the mouse hypoglycemia test for insulin, rat tibial growth response for growth hormone, pigeon crop sac assay for prolactin, rat ovarian weight response for gonadotropins, release of labeled thyroidal iodide into mouse blood for TSH, and so on. However, in vivo bioassays are usually insensitive, not completely specific, expensive, and imprecise,

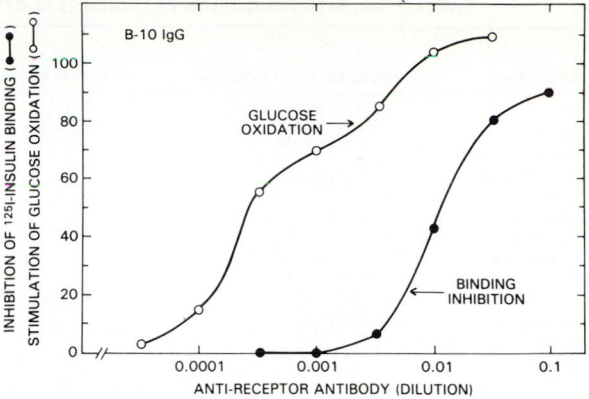

Figure 37–12. Relationship of the insulin-like activity of an anti-insulin receptor antibody to its binding inhibitory effects in rat adipocytes. (From Dons RF, Havlik R, Taylor SI, et al. Clinical disorders associated with autoantibodies to the insulin receptor. Reproduced from The Journal of Clinical Investigation, 1983, vol. 72, pp. 1072–1080 by copyright permission of the American Society for Clinical Investigation.)

yielding values with broad confidence limits. Thus most bioassays developed in recent years have been in vitro, involving the incubation of endocrine tissues, membranes, primary cultures of dispersed cells, or permanent cell lines in a partially or completely defined culture medium.

General Techniques

In vitro bioassays may be classified in terms of the nature of the hormone response (Table 37–6). These bioassays measure proximal responses, the most popular of which is the stimulation of cyclic AMP or adenylate cyclase in tissues, cells, or membranes. Other assays involve responses distal to the second messenger, such as the steroidogenic response to LH and hCG and the release of labeled thyroidal iodine for TSH.[78] Another response is a mitogenic response, such as the stimulation of cell growth in a permanent lymphoid cell line by prolactin,[108–110] or in the rat FRTL-5 cell line by TSH.[94] Finally, the most sensitive bioassays are cytochemical responses measured by microdensitometry, such as the enhancement by TSH of penetration of 2-naphthylamide into thyroid lysosomes,[111] or stimulation of glucose-6-phosphate dehydrogenase activity in chondrocytes by parathyroid hormone.[112]

The most widely used in vitro bioassays measure proximal responses such as the increase of cyclic AMP or the stimulation of adenylate cyclase because these responses are applicable to a wide variety of endocrine tissues. Distal responses must be individualized for each hormone. They have become increasingly important with the discovery of second messengers in addition to cyclic AMP (e.g., calcium ion). To illustrate, dissociations have been reported between the cyclic AMP and steroidogenic responses to certain forms of chorionic gonadotropin (CG).[113] Dissociations have also been observed between the cyclic AMP response and the iodide-trapping response to TSH in rat thyroid FRTL-5 cells.[114] Mitogenic responses are applicable in only a few instances in which permanent endocrine-responsive cell lines are available. Because such lines are transformed and are usually selected for the hormone response, one must be cautious in attributing the same mitogenic response to the hormone in vivo. Finally, cytochemical assays are technically difficult, and the dose-response curves are often shallow, which predisposes to a low index of precision.[111]

VALIDATION. The validation of in vitro bioassays is generally similar to that of receptor assays (see earlier). In

TABLE 37–6. Selected References to Studies of Receptor Assays and In Vitro Bioassays for Polypeptide Hormones

Hormone	Receptor Assay Response	In Vitro Bioassay*			
		Proximal Response	Distal Response	Mitogenic Response	Cytochemical Response
Insulin	+ (5, 6, 25)	+ (179)	+ (165–167)	–	–
Parathyroid hormone	+ (168, 169)	+ (170, 171)	+ (172)	–	+ (173)
Growth hormone	+ (12, 22, 24, 25, 33)	–	–	–	–
Prolactin	+ (32)	–	–	+ (108, 109)	–
Corticotropin	+ (2, 8)	–	+ (174, 175)	–	–
LH, chorionic gonadotropin	+ (176)	–	+ (3)	–	–
FSH	+ (135)	–	+ (118)	–	–
TSH	+ (71, 72)	+ (114, 141–143)	+ (114, 139, 140)	+ (94)	+ (92)
Thyrotropin-releasing hormone	+ (177)	–	+ (178)	–	–

*Some form of in vitro bioassay exists for essentially every hormone; those listed are selected on the basis of practical utility. + means that an assay is available; – means that an assay is not available.

contrast to radioreceptor and other radioligand assays, all bioassays are subject to more serious problems regarding the specificity of the endocrine response. Most endocrine tissues respond to stimulatory substances such as toxins, prostaglandins, cations, mitogens, and many other substances in biological fluids. Certain of these substances may act in a synergistic way with the stimulatory effect of the hormone.[115] The same tissue may also respond to inhibitory substances in the sample. Therefore, the endocrine response to a sample may represent the balance of the stimulatory and the inhibitory substances present. For example, the purification of certain stimulatory hypothalamic hormones was made difficult by the presence in the same fractions of inhibitory substances that blunted the response of in vitro bioassays.[116]

Because of these inherent problems of specificity, it is essential that all bioassays, especially those involving unfractionated serum, be validated. One of the most powerful techniques is to examine the endocrine response in vitro before and after the addition of excess antihormone antibody. If the antibody-hormone complex is no longer active, all activity should be eliminated. However, when such a test was applied to the insulin-like activity of serum, it was found that only a fraction of this activity could be neutralized by anti-insulin antibodies.[31] This finding led to the discovery of additional insulin-like growth factors in serum. By contrast, in the mitogenic assay for prolactin[108, 109] and in the in vitro bioassay for gonadotropins,[3] most of the activity is eliminated after addition of antihormone serum.

As noted for radioreceptor assay, it often is not possible to establish a valid bioassay by using unfractionated serum. Again, considerations of sensitivity and specificity usually require that the hormone be partially purified and concentrated before assay. The same purification methods (see Table 37–2) used in receptor assay are applicable in bioassay; affinity chromatography is the most powerful single-step method. For example, in various bioassays for TSH, it was necessary to purify serum by a column of agarose-bound antibody to TSH alpha or beta subunits before a valid assay could be established.[114, 117] Certain bioassays for FSH and TSH require only partial purification of the hormone from serum by polyethylene glycol extraction.[114, 118]

Certain in vitro bioassays have not been adequately validated. Thus cytochemical bioassays generally use unfractionated serum, albeit at a high dilution, and it is not clear whether other factors in serum can influence the technique. Although the relative lack of specificity poses problems in validation, it can also be an advantage in the discovery of new endocrine stimulators and inhibitors.

Applications

GONADOTROPINS. Early in vivo bioassays of gonadotropins were of limited sensitivity, specificity, and precision. Although not applicable to the measurement of hormone in unfractionated serum, they could be used with concentrates of urine. The methods included measurements of the response of rat ovary, rat ventral prostate, and mouse uterus.[119] The last two are indirect bioassays because the changes in the uterus and prostate are caused by gonadal steroids secreted in response to gonadotropins.

Subsequently, Dufau and associates[3] developed a sensitive and precise bioassay for LH and CG that is capable of measuring the hormones in small volumes of human and animal serum. The method measures testosterone synthesis by dispersed rat Leydig cells in respone to gonadotropic stimulation in vitro. Purified human, ovine, bovine, porcine, rat, and rabbit LH, purified human and equine CG, and unpurified LH and CG in human, rat, and monkey serum all yield parallel dose-response curves. Thus the method has permitted cross-species comparison of the intrinsic biological activity of native and modified gonadotropins, without being affected by differences in metabolic clearance that influence in vivo gonadotropin bioassays. Sensitivity is equal to or higher than that of radioimmunoassay, with detection limits of 50 mIU/mL for human menopausal gonadotropin and 20 mIU/mL for CG. Such sensitivity is greater than that of the gonadotropin radioreceptor assay or the in vitro adenylate cyclase response (see Table 37–6).

The specificity of this assay has been validated by the demonstration that the response to human gonadotropins and serum samples is abolished by incubation with antisera to LH or CG. However, unlike certain specific radioimmunoassays using the beta subunit of CG, the in vitro bioassay is incapable of distinguishing between CG and LH, because the two hormones act through a common receptor. The assay has been used to detect previously unknown gonadotropins, such as a potent activity in pregnant rat serum that is presumably rat CG.[120]

This in vitro bioassay has been used to demonstrate physiological regulation of the qualitative as well as quantitative aspects of LH production.[121] Qualitative features of the molecule were measured as a bioactive to immunoactive (B/I) ratio of LH in human, rat, and monkey serum. The B/I ratios in human male serum were 2 to 4, with maximal values of 4 to 6 being coincident with the peak of LH pulses, which suggests regulation by LHRH.[121] The B/I ratios in young women are close to 1 but are increased in the late follicular phase by administration of LHRH. Postmenopausal women and patients with gonadal dysgenesis had higher B/I ratios than did cycling women, but the ratios in such women could be reduced by prolonged estrogen therapy.[122] Moreover, the B/I ratio for LH in the serum of prepubertal boys was near 1 and increased after the onset of testicular androgen secretion.[123]

There have been a number of additional studies showing altered B/I ratios in the serum of patients with nonorganic male impotence,[124] as well as patients treated with LHRH agonists.[125] Of particular interest are reports that patients with prostatic cancer treated with an LHRH agonist and antiandrogen show a marked decrease in the B/I ratio of serum LH.[126, 127] Moreover, the close parallelism between serum testosterone and bioactive LH levels has led these groups to conclude that the decreased LH bioactivity is principally, if not exclusively, responsible for the inhibition of testicular androgen secretion.

In vitro FSH bioassays have also been developed (see Table 37–6) that permit measurement of activity in small amounts of human serum.[118] As previously noted for LH, the FSH B/I ratios vary among men, among pre- and postmenopausal women, in various pathological conditions, and after various endocrine therapies, including LHRH agonists and antagonists.[118, 128–134] Moreover, after LHRH antagonist therapy in hypogonadal women, interesting serum FSH isoforms have been observed that bind to gonadal receptors but are devoid of bioactivity.[135] Such forms block standard FSH action in ovarian cells, analogous to previously described naturally occurring TSH antagonists[136] (see later).

These data indicate that LHRH, gonadal steroids, and possibly other factors can modulate the biological activity of serum LH in a manner not reflected by radioimmunoassay. The chemical basis of these qualitative changes has not been clearly defined and could reflect differences in gonadotropin biosynthesis, intracellular processing, secretion, or metabolic clearance in different physiological states. Such changes may be related to glycosylation and possibly other post-translational modifications of gonadotropin. Many lines of evidence suggest that glycosylation of LH can be specifically regulated by LHRH[137] and that carbohydrate residues play a major role in the expression of its biological activity.[113] Because glycosylation is important at a postreceptor step, its effects are not reflected in gonadotropin receptor assays. Thus in vitro bioassays are necessary to elucidate the physiology and pathophysiology of glycoprotein hormones and possibly other polypeptide hormones that undergo extensive post-translational modification.

THYROTROPIN. The earliest in vivo TSH bioassays were of limited sensitivity and precision and not applicable to the measurement of hormone in unfractionated normal serum. They included the stimulation of colloid droplet formation in guinea pig thyroid, assessment of hind limb growth in a tadpole whose metamorphosis had been arrested by starvation, measurement of ^{131}I or ^{32}P uptake into mouse or chick thyroid, and measurement of release of labeled iodine from thyroid into guinea pig or mouse blood.[138] Subsequent sensitive in vitro bioassays involved assessment of ^{131}I release from prelabeled guinea pig thyroid slices[139] or intact mouse thyroid glands,[140] cytochemical bioassay,[92] and measurement of cyclic AMP accumulation or adenylate cyclase activity in thyroid membranes,[141] slices,[142] and cells.[143] Although the cytochemical bioassay is capable of measuring normal or even suppressed TSH in unfractionated serum, it is technically difficult, and it has not been established that the assay is unaffected by other stimulators and inhibitors in unfractionated serum.

The most widely used bioassays utilize the stimulation of thyroid cyclic AMP or adenylate cyclase activity. The stimulation of cyclic AMP accumulation in fresh human thyroid gland slices (obtained at surgery for thyroid nodules) has been employed by several groups.[144] Unfortunately, frozen tissue cannot be used, and there is considerable interassay variation. Cultured monolayers of thyroid cells have been utilized after the enzymatic dispersion of thyroid glands.[145] Unlike slices, these cells can be cryopreserved in liquid nitrogen, which allows for a more convenient assay[146] with less interassay variation. Moreover, by use of an extremely sensitive immunoassay for cyclic AMP, a relatively small number of cells (10^4 to 10^5) are needed per assay. Alternatively, the direct measurement of adenylate cyclase activity in human thyroid membranes provides a precise assay and is convenient because the membranes may be stored for long periods at $-70°C$.[147] Although the assay is not as sensitive as the direct cyclic AMP methods, sensitivity can be enhanced by addition of the GTP analogue 5'-guanylylimidodiphosphate (Gpp(NH)P) to the incubation.[148]

As mentioned in the previous section concerning antibodies to the TSH receptor, the rat FRTL-5 thyroid cell line provides a convenient and precise new assay system. Moreover, multiple end points can be studied, including cyclic AMP production, iodide trapping, and stimulation of cell growth.[94] Unfortunately, such methods still require purification and concentration of TSH from serum before assay, and recovery of immunoactive TSH is not always complete.[114, 149]

The most important application of the TSH bioassay is in measurement of autoantibodies to the TSH receptor. In addition, the adenylate cyclase assay has been used to characterize the biological activity of heterogeneous forms of human, mouse, and bovine TSH purified by immunoaffinity or gel chromatography.[117] Interestingly, certain naturally occurring forms of immunoreactive TSH, including an unusual high-molecular-weight human TSH, have normal receptor-binding properties but poor in vitro biological activity.[46] Although not completely characterized, these forms interact with lectins in a manner different from that of normally bioactive forms of TSH, which suggests differences in carbohydrate composition.[47] The adenylate cyclase assay has been used also to demonstrate that such weak agonists behave as competitive antagonists to standard TSH.[47] Asialo-CG was shown to be a competitive antagonist to TSH in a similar bioassay.[150]

Some TSH bioassays have shown decreased B/I ratios in certain patients with hypothalamic hypothyroidism.[151, 152] When some of these patients had long-term treatment with thyrotropin-releasing hormone, the B/I ratio increased, associated with an increase in thyroid hormone concentrations.[152] These observations are similar to increased B/I ratios of secreted TSH noted in vitro when rat pituitary explants were stimulated by thyrotropin-releasing hormone.[153] Increased B/I ratios were noted in certain patients with primary hypothyroidism, with a general correlation between the degree of hypothyroidism and the elevation of the ratio.[149] Increased B/I ratios have also been observed in hyperthyroid or euthyroid patients with TSH-producing tumors and have decreased after pituitary surgery.[114, 154] As noted previously for antibodies to the TSH receptor, certain dissociations have been seen between the cyclic AMP response and the iodide-trapping response for certain forms of TSH.[114]

As for changes in B/I ratios for gonadotropins, the molecular basis of changes in TSH activity is not known. However, it is clear that carbohydrate residues play a major role in the expression of the biological activity of TSH[155] and that changes in thyroid hormone levels,[156] as well as administration of thyrotropin-releasing hormone,[153] definitely change the glycosylation pattern of secreted TSH in the rodent. Moreover, during ontogeny[157] and after paraventricular nuclear ablation[158] in the rat, when there are major changes in hypothalamic and thyroid hormones, several changes in TSH glycosylation have been observed. Such changes include the branching pattern of complex oligosaccharides as well as the degree of sialylation and sulfation of each branch.[157, 159] Thus it seems likely (with the caveats mentioned in the next section) that at least some of the altered TSH B/I ratios in humans result from altered glycosylation. Unfortunately, it has not been possible to purify human serum TSH and directly determine its carbohydrate structure.

Interpretation of Ratios of Bioactive to Immunoactive Hormone

A change in the B/I ratios of thyrotropin, gonadotropins, or other hormones does not necessarily prove alteration in intrinsic bioactivity of the hormone. It is possible that the immunological activity of this ratio may also vary, although most polyclonal antisera are relatively insensitive to minor structural modifications, including near-total chemical or enzymatic deglycosylation.[114, 155] Such altered immunoreactivity may be more of a problem with certain monoclonal antibodies developed to specific epitopes that are used in new sandwich immunoassays. Unfortunately, assay of immunoactivity is the only available technique to estimate the mass of the hormone in serum, and it is usually not feasible to purify the hormone from serum to estimate mass by more rigorous chemical methods.

Other factors may influence absolute B/I ratios, including the particular standards used, molecules that mimic or synergize with the hormone, and molecules that inhibit hormone action.[115] Such factors may be estimated by adding known amounts of standard hormone to the serum sample and determining if the expected total activity (endogenous plus exogenous) is recovered. Finally, all of the above-mentioned bioassays involve brief continuous administration to animal cells in vitro. It is completely unknown how the same hormone would act in vivo in humans under the physiological conditions of chronic pulsatile secretion. As pointed out previously, in vivo assays are influenced by the metabolic clearance rate of the hormone as well as by complex factors related to desensitization. Clear differences between in vitro and in vivo activity have been observed for several hormones. Moreover, the metabolic clearance rates of both gonadotropins[160] and TSH[161] are prolonged when the hormone is derived from gonadectomized and thyroidectomized animals, respectively, and infused into normal animals. Such decreased clearance rates appear related to increased sialylation as well as increased carbohydrate branching of the glycoprotein hormones after target organ ablation[156] and could provide an important mechanism for enhanced in vivo bioactivity that is not reflected by in vitro bioassays.

CONCLUSIONS AND FUTURE DIRECTIONS

Although radioimmunoassay is likely to remain standard for most hormones in clinical endocrinology, radioreceptor assays and bioassays provide information not always attainable with immune techniques. They thus continue to be important to both investigators and clinicians.

In the future we can expect the development of many new receptor assays for hormones. With the cloning of the cDNAs for hormone receptors, it should be possible to produce large amounts of pure receptors. Such synthetic receptors could be used to develop novel assays with improved sensitivity and specificity. Similarly, application of these receptors may involve the same nonradioactive methods now proliferating in the field of immunoassay. Moreover, site-directed mutagenesis could provide a method to develop receptor assays of different affinity and specificity, not present in natural receptors. Such developments may provide a receptor assay able to distinguish agonists from antagonists, which is not currently possible for any such assay. Similarly, new in vitro assays may utilize second messenger systems or distal hormone actions. Also, new in vivo assays must ultimately be developed to duplicate endogenous serum hormone patterns of diurnal variation and pulsatile secretion over extended periods.

REFERENCES

1. Lefkowitz RJ, Roth J, Pricer W, et al. ACTH receptors in the adrenal: specific binding of ACTH-^{125}I and its relation to adenyl cyclase. Proc Natl Acad Sci USA 1970; 65:745–752.
2. Lefkowitz RJ, Roth J, Pastan I. Radioreceptor assay of ACTH: a new approach to assay of polypeptide hormones in plasma. Science 1970; 170:633–635.
3. Dufau ML, Pock R, Neubauer A, et al. In vitro bioassay of LH in human serum: the rat interstitial cell testosterone (RICT) assay. J Clin Endocrinol Metab 1976; 42:958–969.
4. Pastan I, Roth J, Macchia V. Binding of hormone to tissue: the first step in polypeptide hormone action. Proc Natl Acad Sci USA 1966; 56:1802–1809.
5. Freychet P, Roth J, Neville DM Jr. Insulin receptors in the liver: specific binding of [^{125}I]insulin to the plasma membrane and its relation to insulin bioactivity. Proc Natl Acad Sci USA 1971; 68:1833–1837.
6. Kahn CR. Membrane receptors for hormones and neurotransmitters. J Cell Biol 1976; 70:261–286.
7. Cuatrecasas P. Insulin-receptor interactions in adipose tissue cells: direct measurement and properties. Proc Natl Acad Sci USA 1971; 68:1264–1268.
8. Wolfsen AR, McIntyre HB, Odell WD. Adrenocorticotropin measurement by competitive binding receptor assay. J Clin Endocrinol Metab 1972; 34:684–689.
9. Gavin JR III, Gorden P, Roth J, et al. Characteristics of the human lymphocyte insulin receptor. J Biol Chem 1973; 248:2202–2207.
10. De Meyts P. Insulin and growth hormone receptors in human cultured lymphocytes and peripheral blood monocytes. In: Blecher M, ed. Methods in Receptor Research. New York: Marcel Dekker, 1976: 301–383.
11. Lesniak MA, Gorden P, Roth J, et al. Binding of ^{125}I-hGH to specific receptors in human cultured lymphocytes: characterization of the interaction and a sensitive radioreceptor assay. J Biol Chem 1974; 249:1661–1667.
12. Lesniak MA, Roth J, Gorden P, et al. Human growth hormone radioreceptor assay using cultured human lymphocytes. Nature 1973; 241:20–22.
13. Marx SJ, Aurbach GD, Gavin JR III, et al. Calcitonin receptors on cultured human lymphocytes. J Biol Chem 1974; 249:6812–6816.
14. Freychet P, Roth J, Neville DM Jr. Monoiodoinsulin: demonstration of its biological activity and binding to fat cells and liver membranes. Biochem Biophys Res Commun 1971; 43:400–408.
15. Roth J. Methods for assessing immunologic and biologic properties of iodinated peptide hormones. Methods Enzymol 1975; 37:223–233.
16. Thorell JI, Johansson BG. Enzymatic iodination of polypeptides with I[125] to high specific activity. Biochim Biophys Acta 1971; 251:363–369.
17. Frank BH, Peavy DE, Hooker CS, et al. Receptor binding properties of monoiodotyrosyl insulin isomers purified by high performance liquid chromatography. Diabetes 1983; 32:705–711.
18. Rodbard D, Guardabasso V, Munson PJ. Statistical aspects of radioimmunoassay. In: Patrono C, Peskar BA, eds. Handbook of Experimental Pharmacology. Vol 82. Berlin: Springer-Verlag, 1987: 193–212.
19. Munson PJ, Rodbard D. LIGAND: a versatile computerized approach for characterization of ligand-binding systems. Anal Biochem 1980; 107:220–239.
20. Weintraub BD. Concentration and purification of human chorionic somato-mammotropin (HCS) by affinity chromatography: application to radioimmunoassay. Biochem Biophys Res Commun 1970; 39:83–89.
21. De Meyts P, Bianco AR, Roth J. Site-site interactions among insulin receptors: characterization of the negative cooperativity. J Biol Chem 1976; 251:1877–1888.
22. Eastman RC, Lesniak MA, Roth J, et al. Regulation of receptor by homologous hormone enhances sensitivity and broadens scope of radioreceptor assay for human growth hormone. J Clin Endocrinol Metab 1979; 49:262–267.

23. Barazzone P, Lesniak MA, Gorden P, et al. Binding, internalization, and lysosomal association of ^{125}I-human growth hormone in cultured human lymphocytes: a quantitative morphological and biochemical study. J Cell Biol 1980; 87:360–369.
24. Rosenfeld RG, Hintz RL. Modulation of homologous receptor concentrations: a sensitive radioassay for human growth hormone in acromegalic, newborn, and stimulated plasma. J Clin Endocrinol Metab 1980; 50:62–69.
25. Gavin JR III, Trivedi B, Daughaday WH. Homologous IM-9 lymphocyte radioreceptor and receptor modulation assays for human serum growth hormone. J Clin Endocrinol Metab 1982; 55:133–139.
26. Williams LTW, Lefkowitz RJ. Adrenergic Pharmacology. New York: Raven, 1978.
27. Megyesi K, Kahn CR, Roth J, et al. The NSILA-s receptor in liver plasma membranes. Characterization and comparison with the insulin receptor. J Biol Chem 1975; 250:8990–8996.
28. Rechler MM, Zapf J, Nissley SP, et al. Interactions of insulin-like growth factors I and II and multiplication-stimulating activity with receptors and serum carrier proteins. Endocrinology 1980; 107:1451–1459.
29. Rechler MM, Nissley SP, King GL, et al. Multiplication stimulating activity (MSA) from the BRL 3A rat liver cell line: relation to human somatomedins and insulin. J Supramol Struct 1981; 15:253–386.
30. Axelrod L, Ron D. Insulin-like growth factor II and the riddle of tumor-induced hypoglycemia. N Engl J Med 1988; 319:1477–1479.
31. Froesch ER, Zapf J, Humbel RE. Insulin-like activity, IGF I and II, and the somatomedins. In: Ellenberg M, Rifkin H, eds. Diabetes Mellitus, Theory and Practice. 3rd ed. New Hyde Park, NY: Medical Examination Publication, 1983: 179–201.
32. Shiu RPC, Kelly PA, Friesen HG. Radioreceptor assay for prolactin and other lactogenic hormones. Science 1973; 180:968–971.
33. Tsushima T, Friesen HG. Radioreceptor assay for growth hormone. J Clin Endocrinol Metab 1973; 37:334–337.
34. Lesniak MA, Gorden P, Roth J. Reactivity of non-primate growth hormones and prolactins with human growth hormone receptors on cultured human lymphocytes. J Clin Endocrinol Metab 1977; 44:838–849.
35. van Buul-Offers S, Hoogerbrugge CM, de Poorter TL. The bovine placenta: a specific radioreceptor assay for both insulin-like growth factor I and insulin-like growth factor II. Acta Endocrinol 1988; 118:306–313.
36. Pekonen F, Weintraub BD. Thyrotropin receptors on bovine thyroid membranes: two types with different affinities and specificites. Endocrinology 1979; 105:352–359.
37. Pierce JG, Parsons TF. Glycoprotein hormones: structure and function. Annu Rev Biochem 1981; 50:465–495.
38. Nisula BC, Morgan FJ, Canfield RE. Evidence that chorionic gonadotropin has intrinsic thyrotropin activity. Biochem Biophys Res Commun 1974; 59:86–91.
39. Pekonen F, Weintraub BD. Interaction of crude and pure chorionic gonadotropin with the thyrotropin receptor. J Clin Endocrinol Metab 1980; 50:280–285.
40. Fradkin JE, Eastman RC, Lesniak MA, et al. Specificity spillover at the hormone receptor—exploring its role in human disease. N Eng J Med 1989; 320:640–645.
41. Daughaday WH, Mariz IK, Trivedi B. A preferential binding site for insulin-like growth factor II in human and rat placental membranes. J Clin Endocrinol Metab 1981; 53:282–288.
42. Lee LS, Weinstein IB. Studies on the mechanism by which a tumor promoter inhibits binding of epidermal growth factor to cellular receptors. Carcinogenesis 1980; 1:669–679.
43. Grunberger G, Gorden P. Affinity alteration of the insulin receptor induced by a phorbol ester. Am J Physiol 1982; 243:E319–E324.
44. Thomopoulos P, Testa U, Gourdin MF, et al. Inhibition of insulin receptor binding by phorbol esters. Eur J Biochem 1982; 129:389–393.
45. Marquardt H, Hunkapiller MW, Hood LE, et al. Rat transforming growth factor type I: structure and relation to epidermal growth factor. Science 1984; 223:1079–1082.
46. Spitz IM, Le Roith DL, Hirsch H, et al. Increased high-molecular-weight thyrotropin with impaired biologic activity in a euthyroid man. N Engl J Med 1981; 304:278–282.
47. Joshi LR, Weintraub BD. Naturally occurring forms of thyrotropin with low bioactivity and altered carbohydrate content act as competitive antagonists to more bioactive forms. Endocrinology 1983; 113:2145–2154.
48. King GL, Kahn CR. Non-parallel evolution of metabolic and growth-promoting functions of insulin. Nature 1981; 292:644–646.
49. Loumaye E, Naor Z, Catt KJ. Binding affinity and biological activity of gonadotropin-releasing hormone agonists in isolated pituitary cells. Endocrinology 1982; 111:730–736.
50. Gavin JR III, Kahn CR, Gorden P, et al. Radioreceptor assay of insulin: comparison of plasma and pancreatic insulins and proinsulins. J Clin Endocrinol Metab 1975; 41:438–445.
51. Gorden P, Freychet P, Nankin H. A unique form of circulating insulin in human islet cell carcinoma. J Clin Endocrinol Metab 1971; 33:983–987.
52. Iwamoto Y, Sakura H, Ishii Y, et al. A new case of abnormal insulinemia

with diabetes. Reduced insulin values determined by radioreceptor assay. Diabetes 1986; 35:1237–1242.
53. Gruppuso PA, Frank BH, Schwartz R. Binding of proinsulin and proinsulin conversion intermediates to human placental insulin-like growth factor I receptors. J Clin Endocrinol Metab 1988; 67:194–197.
54. Goodman AD, Tanenbaum R, Rabinowitz D. Existence of two forms of immunoreactive growth hormone in human plasma. J Clin Endocrinol Metab 1972; 35:868–878.
55. Gorden P, Lesniak MA, Hendricks CM, et al. Evidence for higher proportion of "little" growth hormone with increased radioreceptor activity in acromegalic plasma. J Clin Endocrinol Metab 1976; 43:364–373.
56. Baumann G, MacCart JC, Amburn K. The molecular nature of circulating growth hormone in normal and acromegalic man: evidence for a principal and minor molecular forms. J Clin Endocrinol Metab 1983; 56:946–952.
57. Stolar MW, Amburn K, Baumann G. Plasma "big" and "big-big" growth hormone (GH) in man: an oligomeric series composed of structurally diverse GH monomers. J Clin Endocrinol Metab 1984; 59:212–218.
58. Gorden P, Lesniak MA, Hendricks CM, et al. "Big" growth hormone components from human plasma: decreased reactivity demonstrated by radioreceptor assay. Science 1973; 182:829–831.
59. Baumann G, Stolar MW, Amburn K, et al. A specific growth hormone–binding protein in human plasma: initial characterization. J Clin Endocrinol Metab 1986; 62:134–139.
60. Herington AC, Ymer S, Stevenson J. Identification and characterization of specific binding proteins for growth hormone in normal human sera. J Clin Invest 1986; 77:1817–1823.
61. Leung DW, Spencer SA, Cachianes G, et al. Growth hormone receptor and serum binding protein: purification, cloning and expression. Nature 1987; 330:537–543.
62. Pavlakis GN, Hizuka N, Gorden P, et al. Expression of two human growth hormone genes in monkey cells infected by simian virus 40 recombinants. Proc Natl Acad Sci USA 1981; 78:7398–7402.
63. Hizuka N, Hendricks CM, Pavlakis GN, et al. Properties of human growth hormone polypeptides: purified from pituitary extracts and synthesized in monkey kidney cells and bacteria. J Clin Endocrinol Metab 1982; 55:545–550.
64. Lan NC, Baxter JD. A radioreceptor assay for direct measurement of plasma free glucocorticoid activity. J Clin Endocrinol Metab 1982; 55:516–523.
65. Baxter JD, Schambelan M, Matulich DT, et al. Aldosterone receptors and the evaluation of plasma mineralocorticoid activity in normal and hypertensive states. J Clin Invest 1976; 58:579–589.
66. Ulick S, Land M, Chu MD. 18-Oxocortisol, a naturally occurring mineralocorticoid agonist. Endocrinology 1983; 113:2320–2322.
67. Grossman A, Clement-Jones V. Opiate receptors: enkephalins and endorphins. Clin Endocrinol Metab 1983; 12:31–56.
68. Krieger DT. The multiple faces of pro-opiomelanocortin, a prototype precursor molecule. Clin Res 1983; 31:342–353.
69. Quirion R, Gaudreau P. Strategies in neuropeptide receptor binding research. Neurosci Biobehav Rev 1985, 9:413–420.
70. Flier JS, Kahn CR, Roth J, et al. Antibodies that impair insulin receptor binding in an unusual diabetic syndrome with severe insulin resistance. Science 1975; 190:63–65.
71. Smith BR, Hall R. Thyroid stimulating immunoglobulins in Graves' disease. Lancet 1974; 2:427–431.
72. Manley SW, Bourbe JR, Hauber RW. The thyrotropin receptor in guinea pig thyroid homogenate: interaction with the long acting thyroid stimulator. J Endocrinol 1974; 61:437–445.
73. Blecher M, Bar RS. Acetylcholine receptors: myasthenia gravis. In: Blecher M, Bar RS, eds. Receptors and Human Disease. Baltimore: Williams & Wilkins, 1981:237–257.
74. Harrison LC, Flier JS, Itin A, et al. Radioimmunoassay of the insulin receptor: a new probe of receptor structure and function. Science 1979; 203:544–547.
75. Boden G, Fujita-Yamaguchi Y, Shimoyama R, et al. Nonbinding inhibitory antiinsulin receptor antibodies: a new type of autoantibodies in human diabetes. J Clin Invest 1988; 81:1971–1978.
76. Adams DD, Purves HD. Abnormal response in assay of thyrotropin. Proc Univ Otago Med Sch 1956; 34:11–12.
77. McKenzie JM. Delayed thyroid response to serum from thyrotoxic patients. Endocrinology 1958; 62:865–868.
78. McKenzie JM, Williamson A. Experience with the bio-assay of the long-acting thyroid stimulator. J Clin Endocrinol Metab 1966; 26:518–566.
79. Florsheim WH, Williams AD, Schönbaum E. On the mechanism of the McKenzie bioassay. Endocrinology 1970; 87:881–888.
80. Zakarija M, McKenzie JM. Zoological specificity of human thyroid-stimulating antibody. J Clin Endocrinol Metab 1978; 47:249–254.
81. Adams DD, Kennedy TH. Association of long acting thyroid stimulator with the gamma globulin fraction of serum. Proc Univ Otago Med Sch 1962; 40:6–7.
82. Smith BR, Munro DS. The nature of the interaction between thyroid stimulating gamma globulin (long acting thyroid stimulator) and thyroid tissue. Biochim Biophys Acta 1970; 208:285–289.
83. Adams DD, Kennedy TH. Occurrence in thyrotoxicosis of a gamma

globulin which protects LATS from neutralization by an extract of thyroid gland. J Clin Endocrinol Metab 1967; 27:173–177.

84. Fayet G, Verrier B, Giraud A, et al. Effect of long-acting thyroid stimulator on the reorganization into follicles of isolated thyroid cells and on the binding of radioiodinated thyrotropin to reassociated cells. FEBS Lett 1973; 32:299–302.

85. Petersen VB, Dawes PJD, Smith BR, et al. The interaction of thyroid stimulating antibodies with solubilized human thyrotropin receptors. FEBS Lett 1977; 83:63–69.

86. Borges M, Ingbar JC, Endo K, et al. A new method for assessing the thyrotropin binding inhibitory activity in the immunoglobulins and whole serum of patients with Graves' disease. J Clin Endocrinol Metab 1982; 54:552–558.

87. Carayon P, Adler G, Roulier R, et al. Heterogeneity of the Graves' immunoglobulins directed toward the thyrotropin receptor–adenylate cyclase system. J Clin Endocrinol Metab 1983; 56:1202–1208.

88. Endo K, Amir SM, Ingbar SH. Development and evaluation of a method for the partial purification of immunoglobulins specific for Graves' disease. J Clin Endocrinol Metab 1981; 52:1113–1123.

89. Hart IR, McKenzie JM. Comparison of the effects of thyrotropin and the long-acting thyroid stimulator on guinea pig adipose tissue. Endocrinology 1971; 88:26–30.

90. Teng CS, Smith BR, Anderson J, et al. Comparison of thyrotropin receptors in membranes prepared from fat and thyroid tissue. Biochem Biophys Res Commun 1975; 66:836–841.

91. Vitti P, Rotella CM, Valente WA, et al. Characterization of the optimal stimulatory effects of Graves' monoclonal and serum immunoglobulin G on adenosine 3′,5′-monophosphate production in FRTL-5 thyroid cells: a potential clinical assay. J Clin Endocrinol Metab 1983; 57:782–791.

92. Peterson VB, Smith BR, Hall R. A study of thyroid stimulating activity in human serum with the highly sensitive cytochemical bioassay. J Clin Endocrinol Metab 1975; 96:199–202.

93. Ambesi-Impiombato FS, Parks LAM, Coon HG. Culture of hormone-dependent epithelial cells from rat thyroids. Proc Natl Acad Sci USA 1980; 77:3455–3459.

94. Valente WA, Vitti P, Kohn LD, et al. The relationship of growth and adenylate cyclase activity in cultured thyroid cells: separate bioeffects of thyrotropin. Endocrinology 1983; 112:71–79.

95. Medeiros-Neto GA, Halpern A, Cozzi ZS, et al. Thyroid growth immunoglobulins in large multinodular endemic goiters: effect of iodized oil. J Clin Endocrinol Metab 1986; 63:644–650.

96. Rotella CM, Zonefrati R, Toccafondi R, et al. Ability of monoclonal antibodies to the thyrotropin receptor to increase collagen synthesis in human fibroblasts: an assay which appears to measure exophthalmogenic immunoglobulins in Graves' sera. J Clin Endocrinol Metab 1986; 62:357–367.

97. Tamai H, Hirota Y, Kasagi K, et al. The mechanism of spontaneous hypothyroidism in patients with Graves' disease after antithyroid drug treatment. J Clin Endocrinol Metab 1987; 64:718–722.

98. Takasu N, Yamada T, Katakura M, et al. Evidence for thyrotropin (TSH)–blocking activity in goitrous Hashimoto's thyroiditis with assays measuring inhibition of TSH receptor binding and TSH-stimulated thyroid adenosine 3′,5′-monophosphate responses/cell growth by immunoglobulins. J Clin Endocrinol Metab 1987; 65:239–245.

99. Iida Y, Konishi J, Kasagi K, et al. Inhibition of thyrotropin-induced growth of rat thyroid cells, FRTL-5, by immunoglobulin G from patients with primary myxedema. J Clin Endocrinol Metab 1987; 64:124–130.

100. Endo K, Kasagi K, Konishi J, et al. Detection and properties of TSH-binding inhibitor immunoglobulins in patients with Graves' disease and Hashimoto's thyroiditis. J Clin Endocrinol Metab 1978; 46:734–739.

101. Zakarija M, McKenzie JM, Banovac K. Clinical significance of assay of thyroid-stimulating antibody in Graves' disease. Ann Intern Med 1980; 93:28–32.

102. McKenzie JM, Zakarija M. LATS in Graves' disease. Recent Prog Horm Res 1977; 33:29–57.

103. Sugenoya A, Kidd A, Row VV, et al. Correlation between thyrotropin-displacing activity and human thyroid-stimulating activity by immunoglobulins from patients with Graves' disease and other thyroid disorders. J Clin Endocrinol Metab 1979; 48:398–402.

104. Teng CS, Tong TC, Hutchison JH, et al. Thyroid stimulating immunoglobulins in neonatal Graves' disease. Arch Dis Child 1980; 55:894–895.

105. Dons RF, Havlik R, Taylor SI, et al. Clinical disorders associated with autoantibodies to the insulin receptor. J Clin Invest 1983; 72:1072–1080.

106. Taylor SI, Grunberger G, Marcus-Samuels B, et al. Hypoglycemia associated with antibodies to the insulin receptor. N Engl J Med 1982; 307:1422–1426.

107. De Pirro R, Roth RA, Rossetti L, et al. Characterization of the serum from a patient with insulin resistance and hypoglycemia: evidence for multiple populations of insulin receptor antibodies with different receptor binding and insulin-mimicking activities. Diabetes 1984; 33:301–304.

108. Tanaka T, Shiu RPC, Gout PW, et al. A new sensitive and specific bioassay for lactogenic hormones: measurement of prolactin and growth

hormone in human serum. J Clin Endocrinol Metab 1980; 51:1058–1063.

109. Friesen HG, Shiu RPC, Robertson MC, et al. Studies of prolactin and prolactin receptors using the Nb$_2$ node lymphoma cells. In: Motta M, Zanisi M, Piva F, eds. Pituitary Hormones and Related Peptides. Serono Symposium No. 49. London: Academic, 1982: 101–115.

110. Tokuhiro E, Dean HJ, Friesen HG, et al. Comparative study of serum human growth hormone measurement with Nb$_2$ lymphoma cell bioassay, IM-9 receptor modulation assay, and radioimmunoassay in children with disorders of growth. J Clin Endocrinol Metab 1984; 58:549–554.

111. Bitensky L, Alaghband-Zadeh J, Chayen J. Studies on thyroid stimulating hormone and the long-acting thyroid stimulating hormone. Clin Endocrinol 1974; 3:363–374.

112. Bradbeer JN, Dunham J, Fischer JA, et al. The metatarsal cytochemical bioassay of parathyroid hormone: validation, specificity, and application to the study of pseudohypoparathyroidism type I. J Clin Endocrinol Metab 1988; 67:1237–1243.

113. Moyle WR, Bahl OP, März L. Role of the carbohydrate of human chorionic gonadotropin in the mechanism of hormone action. J Biol Chem 1975; 250:9163–9169.

114. Nissim M, Lee KO, Petrick PA, et al. A sensitive thyrotropin (TSH) bioassay based on iodide uptake in rat FRTL-5 thyroid cells: comparison with the adenosine 3′,5′-monophosphate response to human serum TSH and enzymatically deglycosylated bovine and human TSH. Endocrinology 1987; 121:1278–1287.

115. Robertson WR, Lambert A, Loveridge N. The role of modern bioassays in clinical endocrinology. Clin Endocrinol 1987; 27:259–278.

116. Brazeau P, Vale W, Burgus R, et al. Hypothalamic polypeptide that inhibits the secretion of immunoreactive pituitary growth hormone. Science 1973; 179:77–79.

117. Pekonen F, Williams DM, Weintraub BD. Purification of thyrotropin and other glycoprotein hormones by immunoaffinity chromatography. Endocrinology 1980; 106:1327–1332.

118. Jia XC, Kessel B, Yen SSC, et al. Serum bioactive follicle-stimulating hormone during the human menstrual cycle and in hyper- and hypogonadotropic states: application of a sensitive granulosa cell aromatase bioassay. J Clin Endocrinol Metab 1986; 62:1243–1249.

119. Licht P, Popkoff H, Farmer SW, et al. Evolution of gonadotropin structure and function. Recent Prog Horm Res 1977; 33:169–248.

120. Blank MS, Dufau ML, Friesen HG. Demonstration of potent, gonadotropin-like biological activity in the serum of rats during midpregnancy. Life Sci 1979; 25:1023–1028.

121. Dufau ML, Beitins IZ, McArthur JW, et al. Effects of luteinizing hormone releasing hormone upon bioactive and immunoreactive serum LH levels in normal subjects. J Clin Endocrinol Metab 1976; 43:658–667.

122. Lucky AW, Rebar RW, Rosenfield RL, et al. Reduction of the potency of luteinizing hormone by estrogen. N Engl J Med 1979; 300:1034–1036.

123. Lucky AW, Rich BH, Rosenfield RL, et al. LH bioactivity increases more than immunoreactivity during puberty. J Pediatr 1980; 97:205–213.

124. Fabbri A, Jannini EA, Ulisse S, et al. Low serum bioactive luteinizing hormone in nonorganic male impotence: possible relationship with altered gonadotropin-releasing hormone pulsatility. J Clin Endocrinol Metab 1988; 67:867–875.

125. Spratt DI, Finkelstein JS, Badger TM, et al. Bio- and immunoactive luteinizing hormone responses to low doses of gonadotropin-releasing hormone (GnRH): dose-response curves in GnRH-deficient men. J Clin Endocrinol Metab 1986; 63:143–150.

126. St. Arnaud R, LaChance R, Dupont A, et al. Serum luteinizing hormone (LH) biological activity in castrated patients with cancer of the prostate receiving a pure antiandrogen and in estrogen-pretreated patients treated with an LH-releasing hormone agonist and antiandrogen. J Clin Endocrinol Metab 1986; 63:297–302.

127. St. Arnaud R, LaChance R, Kelly SJ, et al. Loss of luteinizing hormone bioactivity in patients with prostatic cancer treated with an LHRH agonist and a pure antiandrogen. Clin Endocrinol 1986; 24:21–30.

128. Dahl KD, Pavlou SN, Kovacs WJ, et al. The changing ratio of serum bioactive to immunoreactive follicle-stimulating hormone in normal men following treatment with a potent gonadotropin releasing hormone antagonist. J Clin Endocrinol Metab 1986; 63:792–794.

129. Tenover JS, Dahl KD, Hsueh AJW, et al. Serum bioactive and immunoreactive follicle-stimulating hormone levels and the response to clomiphene in healthy young and elderly men. J Clin Endocrinol Metab 1987; 64:1103–1107.

130. Padmanabhan V, Lang LL, Sonstein J, et al. Modulation of serum follicle-stimulating hormone bioactivity and isoform distribution by estrogenic steroids in normal women and in gonadal dysgenesis. J Clin Endocrinol Metab 1988; 67:465–473.

131. Padmanabhan V, Kelch RP, Sonstein J, et al. Bioactive follicle-stimulating hormone responses to intravenous gonadotropin-releasing hormone in boys with idiopathic hypogonadotropic hypogonadism. J Clin Endocrinol Metab 1988; 67:793–800.

132. Huhtaniemi IT, Dahl KD, Rannikko S, et al. Serum bioactive and immunoreactive follicle-stimulating hormone in prostatic cancer patients

during gonadotropin-releasing hormone agonist treatment and after orchidectomy. J Clin Endocrinol Metab 1988; 66:308–313.

133. Kessel B, Dahl KD, Kazer RR, et al. The dependency of bioactive follicle-stimulating hormone secretion on gonadotropin-releasing hormone in hypogonadal and cycling women. J Clin Endocrinol Metab 1988; 66:361–366.

134. Pavlou SN, Dahl KD, Wakefield G, et al. Maintenance of the ratio of bioactive to immunoreactive follicle-stimulating hormone in normal men during chronic luteinizing hormone–releasing hormone agonist administration. J Clin Endocrinol Metab 1988; 66:1005–1009.

135. Dahl KD, Bicsak TA, Hsueh AJW. Naturally occurring antihormones: secretion of FSH antagonists by women treated with a GnRH analog. Science 1988; 239:72–74.

136. Joshi LR, Weintraub BD. Naturally occurring forms of thyrotropin with low bioactivity and altered carbohydrate content act as competitive antagonists to more bioactive forms. Endocrinology 1983; 113:2145–2154.

137. Liu TC, Jackson GL, Gorski J. Effects of synthetic gonadotropin-releasing hormone on incorporation of radioactive glucosamine and amino acids into luteinizing hormone and total protein by rat pituitaries in vitro. Endocrinology 1976; 98:151–163.

138. Condliffe PG, Weintraub BD. Pituitary thyroid-stimulating hormone and other thyroid-stimulating substances. In: Gray CH, James VHT, eds. Hormones in Blood. Vol 3. London: Academic, 1979: 499–574.

139. El Kabir DJ. Assay of thyrotropic hormone in blood. Nature 1962; 194:688–689.

140. Brown J, Munro DS. A new in vitro assay for thyroid-stimulating hormone. J Endocrinol 1967; 38:439–449.

141. Yamashita K, Field JB. Effects of long acting thyroid stimulator on TSH stimulation of adenyl cyclase activity in thyroid plasma membranes. J Clin Invest 1972; 51:463–472.

142. Knox AJS, Von Westarp C, Row VV, et al. The use of cryopreserved human thyroid tissue for the in vitro assay of thyroid stimulators. Cryobiology 1977; 14:543–548.

143. Hinds WE, Rapoport B, Filetti S, et al. Thyroid stimulating immunoglobulin bioassay using cultured human thyroid cells. J Clin Endocrinol Metab 1981; 52:1204–1210.

144. Onaya T, Kotani M, Yamada T, et al. New in vitro tests to detect the thyroid stimulator in sera from hyperthyroid patients by measuring colloid droplet formation and cyclic AMP in human thyroid slices. J Clin Endocrinol Metab 1973; 36:859–866.

145. Stockle G, Wahl R, Seif FJ. Micromethod of human thyrocyte cultures for detection of thyroid stimulating antibodies and thyrotropin. Acta Endocrinol 1981; 97:369–373.

146. Rapoport B, Filetti S, Takai N, et al. Studies on the cyclic AMP response to thyroid stimulating immunoglobulin (TSI) and thyrotropin (TSH) in human thyroid cell monolayers. Metabolism 1982; 31:1159–1167.

147. Carayon P, Guibout M, Lissitzky S. The interaction of radioiodinated thyrotropin with human plasma membranes from normal and diseased thyroid glands. Ann Endocrinol (Paris) 1979; 40:211–227.

148. Pekonen F, Carayon P, Amr S, et al. Heterogeneous forms of thyroid-stimulating hormone in mouse thyrotropic tumor and serum: differences in receptor binding and adenylate cyclase–stimulating activity. Horm Metab Res 1981; 13:617–620.

149. Dahlberg PA, Petrick PA, Nissim M, et al. Intrinsic bioactivity of thyrotropin in human serum is inversely correlated with thyroid hormone concentrations. J Clin Invest 1987; 79:1388–1394.

150. Carayon P, Amr S, Nisula B. A competitive antagonist of thyrotropin: asialo-choriogonadotropin. Biochem Biophys Res Commun 1980; 97:69–74.

151. Faglia G, Bitensky L, Pinchera A, et al. Thyrotropin secretion in patients with central hypothyroidism: evidence for reduced biological activity of immunoreactive thyrotropin. J Clin Endocrinol Metab 1979; 48:989–998.

152. Beck-Peccoz P, Amr S, Menezes-Ferreira MM, et al. Decreased receptor binding of biologically inactive thyrotropin in central hypothyroidism. N Engl J Med 1985; 312:1085–1090.

153. Gesundheit N, Fink DL, Silverman LA, et al. Effect of thyrotropin-releasing hormone on the carbohydrate structure of secreted mouse thyrotropin: analysis by lectin chromatography. J Biol Chem 1987; 262:5197–5203.

154. Beck-Peccoz P, Piscitelli G, Amr S, et al. Endocrine, biochemical and morphological studies of a pituitary adenoma secreting GH, TSH and α-subunit: evidence for secretion of TSH with increased bioactivity. J Clin Endocrinol Metab 1986; 62:704–711.

155. Amr S, Menezes-Ferreira M, Shimohigashi Y, et al. Activities of deglycosylated thyrotropin at the thyroid membrane receptor–adenylate cyclase system. J Endocrinol Invest 1985; 8:537–541.

156. DeCherney GS, Gesundheit N, Gyves PW, et al. Alterations in the sialylation and sulfation of secreted mouse thyrotropin in primary hypothyroidism. Biochem Biophys Res Commun 1989; 159:744–762.

157. Gyves PW, Gesundheit N, Stannard BS, et al. Alterations in the glycosylation of secreted mouse thyrotropin during ontogenesis: analysis of sialylated and sulfated oligosaccharides. J Biol Chem 1989; 264:6104–6110.

158. Taylor T, Gesundheit N, Gyves PW, et al. Hypothalamic hypothyroidism caused by lesions in rat paraventricular nuclei alters the carbohydrate structure of secreted TSH. Endocrinology 1988; 122:283–290.

159. Gesundheit N, Gyves PW, DeCherney GS, et al. Characterization and charge distribution of the asparagine-linked oligosaccharides on secreted mouse thyrotropin and free alpha subunits. Endocrinology 1989; 124:2967–2977.

160. Peckham WD, Knobil E. The effects of ovariectomy, estrogen replacement, and neuraminidase treatment on the properties of the adenohypophysial glycoprotein hormones of the rhesus monkey. Endocrinology 1976; 98:1054–1060.

161. Constant RB, Weintraub BD. Differences in the metabolic clearance of pituitary and serum thyrotropin (TSH) derived from euthyroid and hypothyroid rats: effects of chemical deglycosylation of pituitary TSH. Endocrinology 1986; 119:2720–2727.

162. McKenzie JM. Studies on the thyroid activator of hyperthyroidism. J Clin Endocrinol Metab 1961; 21:635–642.

163. Dorrington KJ, Munro DS. The long acting thyroid stimulator. Clin Pharmacol Ther 1967; 7:788–806.

164. Davies TF. Diseases of the TSH receptor. Clin Endocrinol Metab 1983; 12:79–100.

165. Rodbell M. Metabolism of isolated fat cells. I. Effects of hormones on glucose metabolism and lipolysis. J Biol Chem 1964; 239:375–380.

166. Kahn CR, Baird K, Flier JS, et al. Effects of autoantibodies to the insulin receptor on isolated adipocytes. Studies of insulin binding and insulin action. J Clin Invest 1977; 60:1094–1106.

167. Moody AJ, Stan MA, Stan M, et al. A simple free fat cell bioassay for insulin. Horm Metab Res 1974; 6:12–16.

168. Nissenson RA, Arnaud CP. Properties of the parathyroid hormone receptor–adenylate cyclase system in chicken renal plasma membranes. J Biol Chem 1979; 254:1469–1475.

169. Rizzoli RE, Somerman M, Murray TM, et al. Binding of radioiodinated parathyroid hormone to cloned bone cells. Endocrinology 1983; 113:1832–1838.

170. Nissenson RA, Abbott SR, Teitelbaum AP, et al. Endogenous biologically active human parathyroid hormone: measurement by a guanyl nucleotide–amplified renal adenylate cyclase assay. J Clin Endocrinol Metab 1981; 52:840–846.

171. Lindall AW, Elting J, Ellis J, et al. Estimation of biologically active intact parathyroid hormone in normal and hyperparathyroid sera by sequential N-terminal immunoextraction and midregion radioimmunoassay. J Clin Endocrinol 1983; 57:1007–1014.

172. Stern PH, Krieger NS. Comparison of fetal rat limb bones and neonatal mouse calvaria: effects of parathyroid hormone and 1,25-dihydroxyvitamin D3. Calcif Tissue Res 1983; 35:172–176.

173. Chambers DJ, Zanelli JM, Parsons JA, et al. A sensitive bioassay of parathyroid hormone in plasma. Clin Endocrinol 1978; 9:375–379.

174. Simonian MH, Gill GN. Regulation of the fetal human adrenal cortex: effects of adrenocorticotropin on growth and function of monolayer cultures of fetal and definitive zone cells. Endocrinology 1981; 108:1769–1779.

175. Rainey WE, Hornsby PJ, Shay JW. Morphological correlates of adrenocorticotropin-stimulated steroidogenesis in cultured adrenocortical cells: differences between bovine and human adrenal cells. Endocrinology 1983; 113:48–54.

176. Dufau ML, Catt KJ. Gonadotropin receptors and regulation of steroidogenesis in the testis and ovary. Vitam Horm 1978; 36:461–592.

177. Gershengorn MC. Bihormonal regulation of the thyrotropin-releasing hormone receptor in mouse pituitary thyrotropic tumor cells in culture. J Clin Invest 1978; 62:937–943.

178. Vale W, Grant G, Amoss M, et al. Culture of enzymatically dispersed anterior pituitary cells: functional validation of a method. Endocrinology 1972; 91:562–572.

179. Kasuga M, Zick Y, Blithe DL, et al. Insulin stimulates tyrosine phosphorylation of the insulin receptor in a cell-free system. Nature 1982; 298:667–669.

38

DYNAMIC TESTS OF ENDOCRINE FUNCTION

James E. Griffin

INTRODUCTION

The development of techniques for the measurement of hormones in biological fluids has made it possible to assess endocrine function in quantitative terms in both health and disease. Indeed, many endocrine disorders can be diagnosed by measurements of hormone levels in plasma or urine (see Chapters 36 and 37). However, measurement of individual hormones does not always allow separation of the normal and the abnormal. The broad normal range for some plasma hormone concentrations makes the interpretation of values in individuals unreliable if the previous normal value for the person is unknown. For example, a serum thyroxine (T_4) concentration that is at the upper limits of a normal population may be associated with hyperthyroidism in a person whose usual concentration is in the low-normal range. In addition, there are subtle degrees of endocrine organ dysfunction that can be compensated for under basal conditions. Thus the cortisol levels in plasma and the cortisol secretion rates can be normal in patients with partial adrenocortical insufficiency as the result of increased secretion of corticotropin (ACTH, adrenocorticotropin). Likewise, in early hyperfunctioning states such as Cushing disease, the initial evidence of abnormality may be only a blunting of the normal diurnal variation in hormone secretion, which is indicative of a subtle regulatory disorder. Furthermore, in the recovery phase of many endocrine illnesses (e.g., after partial hypophysectomy for a pituitary tumor or in a patient who has been receiving temporary glucocorticoid replacement), basal hormone levels do not necessarily provide insight into the ultimate needs for hormone replacement.

Thus the new methodologies made it possible to identify advanced or florid disease states in a simple fashion, and they also made it possible to design approaches for the recognition of more subtle degrees of endocrine dysfunction. Three general types of functional tests are useful in assessing partial abnormalities of endocrine control mechanisms: serial

hormone measurements, measurement of hormone pairs, and dynamic tests of endocrine reserve and endocrine feedback control. These tests are of major importance in the assessment of clinical problems, but, like all other diagnostic procedures, they are influenced by a variety of factors that may complicate interpretation. The purpose of this chapter is to review briefly the various types of functional endocrine tests and to describe some of the problems in their interpretation.

SERIAL HORMONE MEASUREMENTS

In some instances the variation in hormone secretion is not the result of any obvious rhythmicity, such as pulsatile secretion or an inherent circadian rhythm (see Chapter 1), but is instead the consequence of poorly understood waxing and waning of disease processes. For this reason, repeated measurements of calcium levels and of parathyroid hormone (PTH) levels over long periods may be required to allow the diagnosis of hyperparathyroidism to be made. Other conditions such as Cushing syndrome may also show a waxing/waning pattern with time. In other instances, variability in endocrine function is a result of diurnal variations in hormone secretion. For example, early in puberty luteinizing hormone (LH) is secreted predominantly during sleep,[1] and documentation of such nocturnal surges can be the first evidence that a child is entering a normal but delayed puberty. As noted earlier, loss of the normal diurnal rhythm of cortisol secretion may be an early indication of Cushing disease.[2]

Diurnal and sleep-associated changes in hormone release vary widely in normal persons. Most published values are means obtained from large groups, and normal individuals may deviate widely from these norms. Furthermore, diurnal rhythmicity is altered by a variety of factors including disturbed sleep patterns, drugs (particularly drugs with effects on the central nervous system), psychiatric disease, and stress. The demonstration of normal diurnal variability may be good evidence of normal function but its absence does not necessarily indicate primary endocrine disease. Rather, abnormal diurnal variation is an indication of a need for additional diagnostic studies.

Other examples of the importance of serial measurements of hormone concentrations are the temporary increases in plasma cortisol[3] and decreases in plasma testosterone[4] that may be associated with heavy alcohol ingestion. Both cortisol and testosterone levels usually return to normal after cessation of ethanol abuse.

MEASUREMENT OF HORMONE PAIRS

Because virtually every hormone system is under regulatory feedback control (notable exceptions being placental hormones and the formation of androgens in normal women and of estrogens in normal men) (see Chapter 1), measurement of both arms of a critical hormone pair (e.g., T_4 and thyrotropin [TSH], calcium and PTH, testosterone and LH) may provide insight not available from individual values (Fig. 38–1). Indeed, this paradigm is central to the assessment of endocrine status. For example, because the normal range of plasma T_4 encompasses more than a doubling, the level in a given individual could decrease by half and still be within the normal range. However, a low-normal T_4 concentration coupled with an elevated plasma TSH level indicates early, compensated thyroid failure. Likewise, a high-normal serum PTH level in a patient with a simultaneous serum calcium value of 2.7 mmol/L (11.0 mg/dL) has a completely different implication from that of the same PTH value in a patient with a serum calcium value of 2.0 mmol/L (8.0 mg/dL). Basically, the measurement of hormone pairs allows assessment of the effects of a hormone on its regulatory control mechanism.

Other possible outcomes of measuring both members of a hormone pair are also depicted in Figure 38–1. The finding of low levels of both members of the hormone pair indicates the primary problem to be deficiency of the trophic hormone (pituitary insufficiency in the case of TSH and T_4; hypoparathyroidism in the case of calcium and PTH). High levels of the target endocrine hormone coupled with low levels of the trophic hormone suggest autonomous secretion of the target endocrine organ (typical thyrotoxicosis results in suppression of TSH secretion, and hyperfunctioning adrenal adenomas inhibit ACTH secretion). The finding of elevated levels of both members of a hormone pair is compatible with several disease mechanisms. Autonomous secretion of a trophic hormone can arise either at the normal site or at an ectopic location; for example, Cushing syndrome can result either from secretion of pituitary ACTH or from the secretion of ACTH from lung tumors. Alternatively, releasing factors may be secreted from tumors in peripheral organs and cause hypersecretion of pituitary hormones, as, for example, the acromegaly that results from the ectopic secretion of growth hormone–releasing factor(s). On the other hand, the combined elevation of trophic and target endocrine gland hormone concentrations can be due to resistance to the action of the target endocrine gland hormone. Such resistance can be either inherited, as in the case of defects in the androgen receptor that cause resistance to the action of the hormone and result in elevated plasma levels of both LH and testosterone, or acquired, as in the case of the insulin resistance of obesity that may lead to both hyperinsulinism and hyperglycemia. In some instances, insight into whether autonomous trophic hormone secretion or resistance to hormone action is more likely can be deduced on clinical grounds, because hormone resistance is usually associated with evidence of hormone deficiency, whereas autonomous hyperfunction is usually associated with evidence of hormone excess. It is also helpful to know the frequency of autonomous trophic hormone secretion versus resistance to target gland hormone action. Glucocorticoid resistance is exceedingly rare, so that elevation of ACTH and cortisol values generally means autonomous secretion of ACTH, whereas androgen resistance is more likely than a pituitary tumor to be the explanation for simultaneous elevation of LH and testosterone concentrations. An elevation of TSH and T_4 values may indicate either autonomous secretion of TSH or resistance to the action of T_4; however, neither condition is common.[5]

There are two main limitations to the usefulness of the assessment of such hormone pairs. One is that valid assays are not available for every situation. Some hormones are difficult to assay, notably arginine vasopressin (AVP, also called antidiuretic hormone, ADH) and ACTH. Another problem is that trophic hormone secretion is subject to complex regulatory control; for example, starvation, malnutrition, and even strenuous exercise can suppress gonadotropin secretion and lead to anovulation. As with diurnal variation, demonstration of normal concentrations of hormone pairs is generally more definitive than the finding of abnormalities. Finally, in mild or early disease states—e.g., particularly those states involving subtle disturbance of feedback regulation, as in early Cushing disease—even assessment of hormone pairs may not provide adequate information.

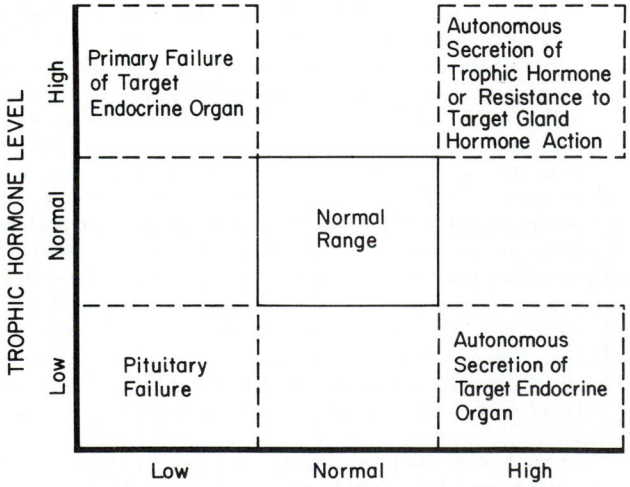

Figure 38–1. Alteration in trophic and target organ hormone pairs and their interpretation (e.g., TSH and T_4). (Adapted from Hershman JM. Endocrine Pathophysiology: A Patient-Oriented Approach. 2nd ed. Philadelphia: Lea & Febiger, 1982.)

DYNAMIC ENDOCRINE TESTS

Dynamic endocrine tests provide additional information to that obtained from measurements of single hormones or of trophic–target gland hormone pairs. Such tests are based on either the stimulation or the suppression of endogenous hormone production.

The ultimate functional test of endocrine status is demonstration of a normal response in target tissues to physiological or stressful stimulation of hormone secretion in vivo. For example, the fact that the urine can be maximally concentrated in response to water deprivation implies that the osmolality-sensing mechanism in the hypothalamus, the secretion of vasopressin, the receptor for vasopressin, and postreceptor events in the action of the hormone in the kidney are all normal. However, when such a test is abnormal it provides little insight into the responsible mechanism, and other functional tests must be done to discern the cause.

STIMULATION TESTS. Stimulation tests are utilized most often when hypofunction of an endocrine organ is suspected and are designed to perturb the endogenous control mechanisms so as to assess the reserve capacity to form and secrete hormone. This assessment is done in either of two general ways. A trophic hormone can be administered to test the capacity of the target organ to increase hormone production. The trophic hormone can be a hypothalamic-releasing factor such as thyrotropin-releasing hormone (TRH) or a substitute for a pituitary hormone (cosyntropin for ACTH or chorionic gonadotropin for LH). In each instance the capacity of the target organ is assessed by measuring the increment in the plasma hormone, in these examples TSH, cortisol, or testosterone. Alternatively, a stimulatory test may be performed by causing an increase in the secretion of an endogenous trophic hormone or stimulatory factor and measuring the effect of the procedure on a target hormone. For example, metyrapone is given to block a late enzymatic step in cortisol synthesis, and the ability of the pituitary to respond with increased ACTH secretion is assessed by measuring the subsequent increase in adrenal steroidogenesis. Similarly, clomiphene citrate exerts an antiestrogenic effect at the level of the hypothalamus and consequently causes an increase in gonadotropin secretion because of decreased negative feedback that can be followed by ovulation and/or increased formation of gonadal steroids. Stimulation tests in which endogenous trophic hormone secretion is altered actually assess the overall capacity of the hypothalamic-pituitary–target organ axis to respond to challenge.

Examples of some commonly used stimulation tests are given in Table 38–1. As stated earlier, most are applicable to the delineation of suspected hypofunction and utilize exogenous hormones, physiological stimuli, or metabolic blocking agents to enhance endogenous hormone synthesis. However, a stimulation test is occasionally useful in suspected hyperfunction of endocrine organs. For example, the demonstration of an exaggerated calcitonin secretion after administration of pentagastrin or calcium helps to identify subjects with thyroid C cell hyperplasia or medullary carcinoma of the thyroid. One stimulation test is useful in assessing potential hormone resistance, namely, measurement of the increase in cyclic AMP and phosphate excretion in urine after administration of PTH. The response is blunted or absent in patients with PTH resistance (pseudohypoparathyroidism) but normal in patients with hypoparathyroidism related to PTH deficiency. Likewise, the lack of increase in urine osmolality after injection of aqueous vasopressin may indicate vasopressin resistance. Tests to assess resistance to other hormones would be helpful.

SUPPRESSION TESTS. Suppression tests are utilized when endocrine hyperfunction is suspected and are designed to determine whether negative feedback control is intact. A hormone or other regulatory substance is administered, and the inhibition of endogenous hormone secretion is assessed. Glucocorticoid (dexamethasone) is given to persons with suspected Cushing syndrome to assess the capacity to inhibit ACTH secretion and thus cortisol production by the adrenal.

TABLE 38–1. Some Commonly Used Stimulation Tests in Endocrine Diagnosis

Organ System	Stimulus	Response Measured*
Hypothalamic-pituitary	Hypoglycemia	Growth hormone and ACTH (cortisol)
	Metyrapone	ACTH (cortisol and 11-deoxycortisol)
	Levodopa	Growth hormone
	Arginine	Growth hormone
	Clomiphene citrate	Gonadotropins
	Exercise	Growth hormone
	Water deprivation	Vasopressin (urine concentration)
Pituitary	TRH	TSH and prolactin
	Luteinizing hormone–releasing hormone	Gonadotropins
	Corticotropin-releasing hormone	ACTH (cortisol)
	Growth hormone–releasing hormone	Growth hormone
Thyroid	TSH	Thyroid uptake of radioactive iodine
	Pentagastrin	Calcitonin
	Calcium	Calcitonin
Adrenals	Cosyntropin	Cortisol
	Metyrapone	Cortisol and 11-deoxycortisol
	Upright posture	Renin and aldosterone
Gonads	Human chorionic gonadotropin	Testosterone and testosterone precursors
Pancreatic islets	Glucose	Glucose tolerance and insulin release
Parathyroid	PTH	Cyclic AMP and phosphate excretion
	Edetate	Calcium
Water balance	Vasopressin	Urine concentration
Calcium metabolism	Calcium load	Urine calcium

*Plasma or serum levels unless urine is stated.

Likewise, thyroid hormones may be administered to determine the capacity to inhibit TSH production and inhibit the uptake of radioactive iodine by the thyroid gland. Failure to suppress in these tests indicates the presence either of autonomous secretion of the target endocrine gland hormone or of the secretion of trophic hormones (from the pituitary or ectopic sites) that is not under normal regulatory control. Other suppression tests use glucose to evaluate suspected growth hormone excess or saline to assess excess aldosterone secretion. Examples of commonly used suppression tests in endocrine diagnosis are given in Table 38–2. As in the case of the stimulation tests, they use either exogenous hormones or known regulatory factors to attempt to inhibit endogenous hormone production.

INTERPRETATION OF FUNCTIONAL TESTS. The dynamic endocrine tests just described provide useful information under a variety of circumstances. They are usually the best measure of subtle endocrine dysfunction. For example, when basal cortisol secretion is normal in patients with partial adrenocortical insufficiency, documentation that cortisol secretion does not rise after cosyntropin administra-

TABLE 38–2. Some Commonly Used Suppression Tests in Endocrine Diagnosis

Organ System	Stimulus	Response Measured
Hypothalamic-pituitary	Glucose	Growth hormone
	Dexamethasone	ACTH or cortisol
Thyroid	T$_4$	Thyroid uptake of radioactive iodine
Adrenal	Dexamethasone	Cortisol
	Saline	Renin and aldosterone
	Clonidine	Plasma norepinephrine
Pancreatic islets	Fasting	Glucose and insulin

tion can establish the diagnosis. A second major use of dynamic tests is to determine the site of the pathogenetic defect. For example, hypogonadism related to a deficiency of gonadotropins may be a consequence of pituitary failure or of inadequate secretion of luteinizing hormone–releasing hormone (LHRH) from the hypothalamus. Stimulation testing may help to localize the defect in that increases in LH secretion after LHRH administration suggest that the pituitary is not at fault. Dynamic testing can also serve to localize the nature of abnormality in Cushing syndrome in that patients with pituitary hypersecretion of ACTH usually have suppression of cortisol production in response to high-dose dexamethasone, whereas most individuals with adrenal tumors or ectopic secretion of ACTH do not.

General Considerations. The central problem in interpreting the results of dynamic endocrine tests is that, for most such tests, the range of so-called normal responses has not been adequately defined in suitable numbers of control subjects and, in particular, in control subjects with other diseases. For example, athletes who are highly physically trained have demonstrated increased responses of ACTH and cortisol after administration of corticotropin-releasing hormone.[6] In addition, a variety of other factors influence the responses to such functional tests. Changes with age in response to a test, a requirement for repeated stimulation to elicit a normal response, and the need to appreciate an inherent rhythmicity or response characteristics of a pathological process are important considerations during interpretation. Stimulation of plasma testosterone by human chorionic gonadotropin may increase from little or no effect to normal with repetition of the stimulation test in some underandrogenized young boys.[7] At the other end of the age spectrum, the magnitude of the TSH response to TRH stimulation decreases in men over age 60[8] but is not decreased in older women.[9] Likewise, the growth hormone response to growth hormone–releasing hormone is greater in premenopausal women than in age-matched men but is lower in elderly individuals of both sexes.[10] Repetitive stimulation, or a "priming" effect, may be required to produce a normal glucocorticoid response after ACTH stimulation in some patients with long-standing secondary adrenal insufficiency.[11] Thus, although most persons respond to 2 or

3 d of ACTH infusion, some patients with panhypopituitarism do not have a normal response even after 5 d of stimulation.[11] In a similar manner, men with severe hypogonadotropic hypogonadism related to presumed hypothalamic disease may have a subnormal LH response to an initial bolus dose of LHRH but respond normally to a bolus dose after a week of daily infusions of LHRH.[12] Such a protocol may allow the distinction between hypothalamic and pituitary hypogonadism (Fig. 38–2).[12] Occasionally, reliable dynamic tests of endocrine function are misleading owing to unusual patterns of response of the specific endocrinopathy. Rare patients with pituitary-dependent Cushing syndrome may have an atypical response to dexamethasone suppression as a result of periodic hormonogenesis; in these individuals an increase in cortisol production follows dexamethasone administration because of an inherent rhythmicity in the secretion of cortisol.[13] In addition, a few patients with insulinoma do not demonstrate inappropriately elevated levels of plasma insulin during a 72-h fast but require a stimulus for insulin secretion to confirm the diagnosis.[14]

Even if dynamic test results are abnormal with apparent autonomous function, it cannot be assumed that progressive disease is present or that surgical intervention is necessarily warranted. For example, long-standing thyroidal[15] or gonadal[16] insufficiency can cause pituitary enlargement, but the enlargement regresses with appropriate hormone replacement. Similarly, men with long-standing untreated Klinefelter syndrome may not exhibit normal suppressibility of plasma LH during initial therapy with testosterone. However, after testosterone has been administered in sufficient doses for a prolonged period, the plasma LH level does suppress to normal.[17] Another example of problems in interpretation of endocrine autonomy is the autonomously functioning thyroid nodule.[18] Study of a large group of such patients demonstrated toxicity (hyperthyroidism) in less than one fifth and found progression to toxicity in those initially nontoxic in less than one tenth.[18]

The final note of caution concerning specific characteristics of given endocrine disorders and their impact on dynamic endocrine testing is the recognition that subtle syndromes of hormone resistance must be considered in the interpretation of endocrine tests. Failure to do so may result

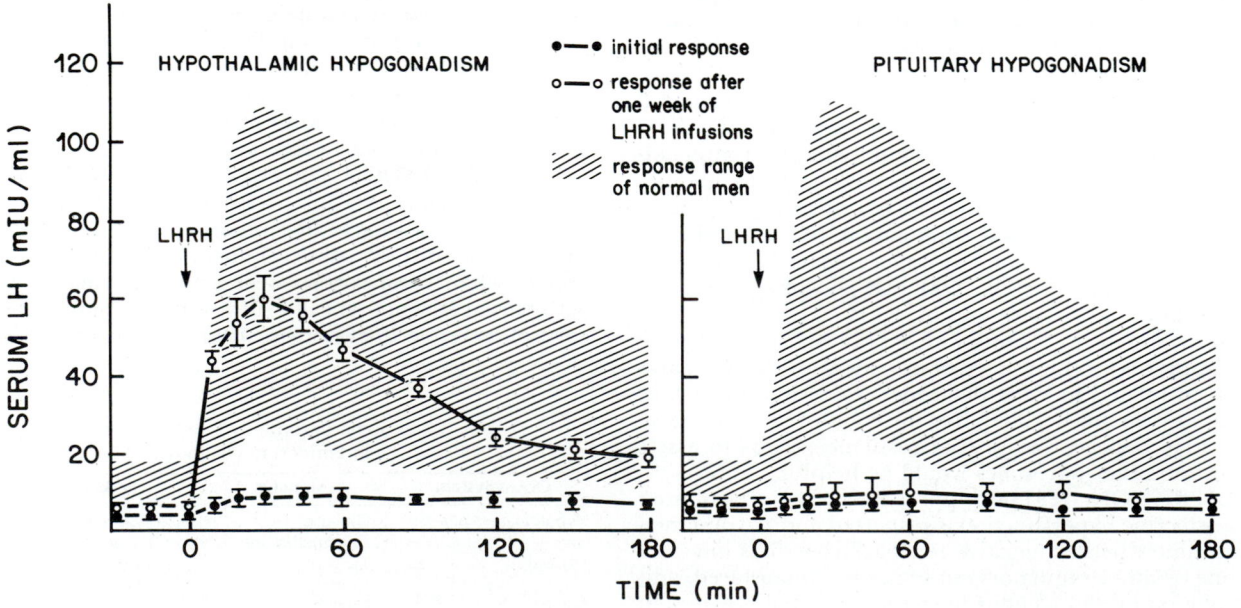

Figure 38–2. Mean serum LH responses of 10 men with hypogonadotropic hypogonadism to a 250-μg intravenous bolus dose of LHRH before and after daily infusions (500 μg over 4 h) of LHRH for 1 wk. Five men had presumed hypothalamic disease and five had presumed pituitary disease. (From Snyder PJ, Rudenstein RS, Gardner DF, et al. Repetitive infusion of gonadotropin-releasing hormone distinguishes hypothalamic from pituitary hypogonadism. J Clin Endocrinol Metab 1979; 48:864–868. © 1979, The Endocrine Society.)

in erroneous diagnoses and inappropriate treatment. Perhaps the best example of this is thyroid hormone resistance.[19] Patients with generalized thyroid hormone resistance typically present with a goiter, and on evaluation they are found to have elevated plasma thyroid hormone levels. A diagnosis of Graves disease is frequently made.[20] Although an elevated and nonsuppressible radioactive iodine uptake is consistent with such a diagnosis, the patients do not have symptoms of thyrotoxicosis. The finding of a normal ultrasensitive TSH is a clue that thyrotoxicosis is not present. Because the condition is rarely considered, many patients with thyroid hormone resistance undergo ablative thyroid procedures. The possibility of other poorly recognized or as-yet undefined forms of subtle hormone resistance must be kept in mind when interpreting all dynamic endocrine test results.

Other Disease States. Disease states that may cause difficulty in interpreting dynamic endocrine tests can be grouped into the categories of coexisting endocrinopathies, systemic medical diseases, and psychiatric disease.

The main endocrine disorders to consider are hypothyroidism, thyrotoxicosis, and Cushing syndrome, all of which may cause impaired growth hormone responsiveness to one or more of the usual stimuli.[21–23] Patients with hypo- or hyperthyroidism may also have abnormal responses in tests of pituitary ACTH reserve with metyrapone.[24–26] The mechanism of the abnormal response to metyrapone appears to be delayed turnover of glucocorticoids in hypothyroidism, and accelerated turnover of glucocorticoids in hyperthyroidism.[27] Patients with adrenal insufficiency related to ACTH deficiency may have an impaired growth hormone response to provocative stimuli that returns to normal after glucocorticoid replacement.[28]

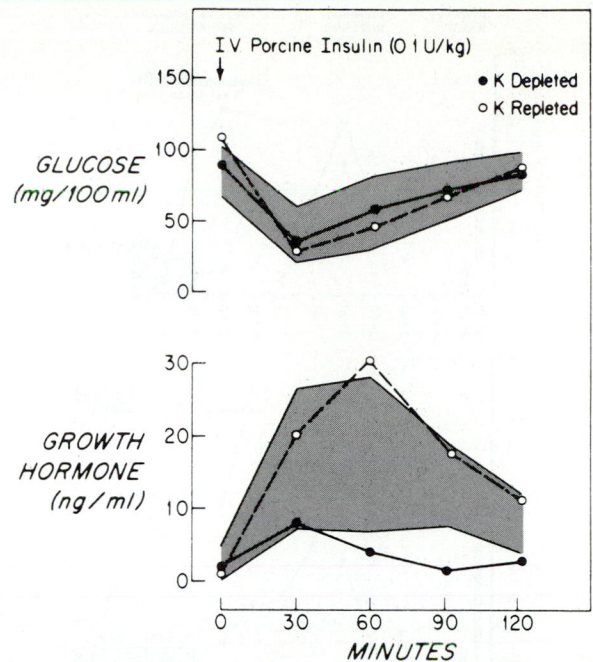

Figure 38–4. Glucose and growth hormone responses during intravenous insulin tolerance tests performed when a patient was potassium depleted (K depleted) and again after potassium repletion (K repleted). Shaded areas represent values for 10 control subjects (mean ± 1 SD). To convert glucose values to nanomoles per liter, multiply by 0.05551. (From Podolsky S, Melby JC. Improvement of growth hormone response to stimulation in primary aldosteronism with correction of potassium deficiency. Metabolism 1976; 25:1027–1032. By permission.)

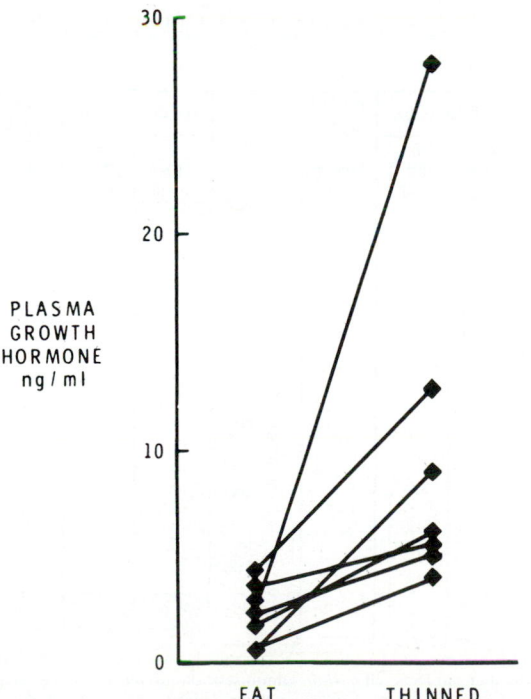

PEAK RESPONSE OF OBESE MALE SUBJECTS TO AN ARGININE INFUSION

Figure 38–3. Peak plasma growth hormone level during an arginine infusion test. Each symbol represents the peak level in an individual patient, with the solid line connecting the values in an individual before and after weight reduction. (From El-Khodary AZ, Ball MF, Stein B, et al. Effect of weight loss on the growth hormone response to arginine infusion in obesity. J Clin Endocrinol Metab 1971; 32:42–51. © 1971, The Endocrine Society.)

Problems in interpretation of dynamic endocrine test results may also be caused by obesity, malnutrition, chronic renal failure, cirrhosis, and hyperkalemia. The response of growth hormone to insulin-induced hypoglycemia, arginine infusion, and levodopa may be blunted in the presence of obesity.[29–31] After a return to ideal body weight, the response of growth hormone to arginine infusion improves in most persons (Fig. 38–3).[30] In contrast to obese patients, patients with severe protein-calorie malnutrition,[32] chronic renal failure,[33] or cirrhosis of the liver[34] tend to have elevated basal growth hormone values, with either a lack of suppression or a paradoxical increase after a glucose load. Renal disease without renal failure can impair urinary concentrating ability and lead to an abnormal water deprivation test result in spite of normal vasopressin release and renal receptors for the hormone. Hypokalemia related to primary aldosteronism has been reported to blunt the growth hormone response to insulin-induced hypoglycemia; the response returns to normal after potassium repletion (Fig. 38–4).[35]

A number of psychiatric disorders are associated with abnormal dynamic endocrine test results in the absence of a specific endocrine disorder. The most frequently incriminated psychiatric disease is depression. The growth hormone response to levodopa is often reduced in depressed patients.[36] More frequently, patients with severe primary depression have an impaired suppression of plasma cortisol after administration of dexamethasone, which may return to normal after treatment of the depression (Fig. 38–5).[37] Elevated total serum T_4 concentrations and free T_4 indices are encountered in almost one fifth of patients with acute psychiatric disorders in the absence of persistent laboratory or clinical evidence of thyrotoxicosis.[38] Furthermore, TSH responsiveness to TRH stimulation is unreliable in evaluating for thyroid disease because a blunted or absent response occurs in about one fourth of all psychiatric patients without

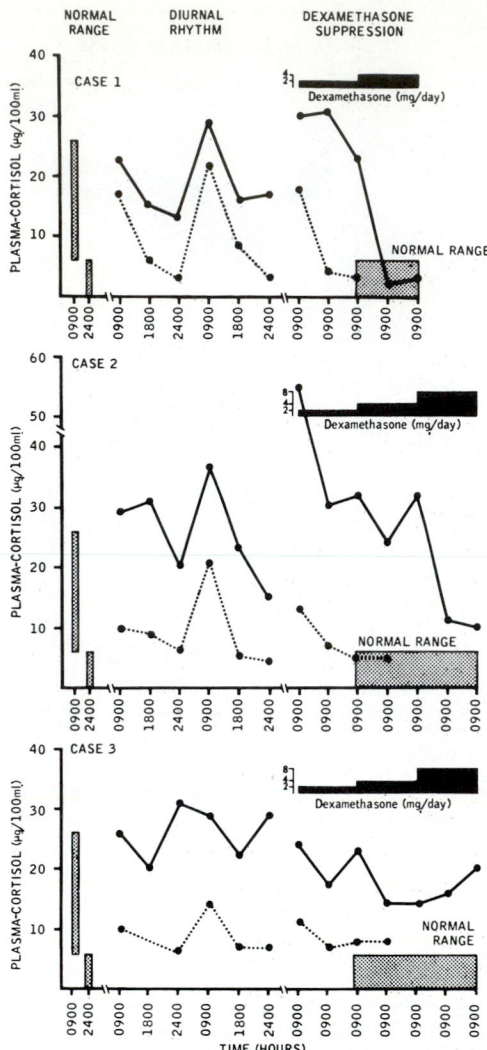

Figure 38–5. Diurnal rhythm and dexamethasone suppression of plasma cortisol before (•————•) and after (· · · · ·) treatment in three patients with severe depression. To convert plasma cortisol values to nanomoles per liter, multiply by 27.59. (From Butler PWP, Besser GM. Pituitary-adrenal function in severe depressive illness. Lancet 1968; 1:1234–1236.)

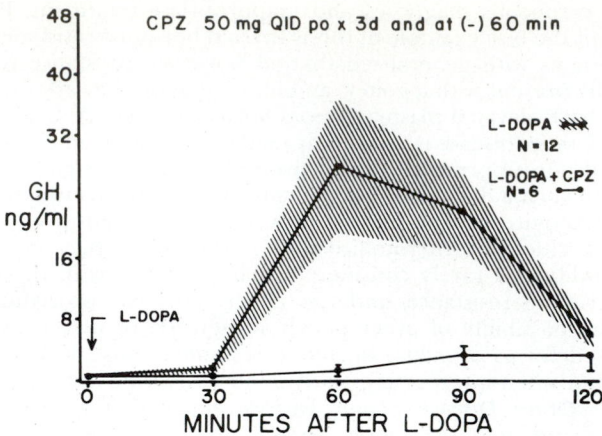

Figure 38–6. Mean growth hormone (GH) responses in subjects who ingested 1.0 g of levodopa (L-dopa) alone and then received chlorpromazine (CPZ) for 3 d before repeating the levodopa dose. The shaded area and bars represent ±1 SEM. (From Mims RB, Scott CL, Modebe O, et al. Inhibition of L-dopa–induced growth hormone stimulation by pyridoxine and chlorpromazine. J Clin Endocrinol Metab 1975; 40:256–259. © 1975, The Endocrine Society.)

enhance hepatic conjugation of metyrapone, which results in decreased free metyrapone concentrations in plasma.[47] Phenytoin therapy also results in decreased levels of unconjugated metyrapone and thus impairs the increase in plasma 11-deoxycortisol and ACTH (Fig. 38–7).[48] Increasing the plasma level of unconjugated metyrapone, either by giving a large oral dose (see Fig. 38–7) or by administering the drug intravenously, compensates for the accelerated metabolism.[48]

Chronic phenytoin therapy also accelerates the metabolism of dexamethasone and hence may result in low (and ineffective) plasma levels of the hormone. As a result, decreased suppression of plasma cortisol occurs in normal persons[49] and presumably also in patients with Cushing syndrome. Studies involving administration of radioactive

thyroid disease, especially in those with unipolar or bipolar depression.[38]

Drugs. Drugs may interfere with endocrine dynamic tests by altering the responsiveness of growth hormone to stimuli, by making the metyrapone test unreliable, by invalidating the dexamethasone suppression test, or by impairing the TSH response to TRH.

Glucocorticoids in pharmacological doses,[39] progestogens,[40] theophylline,[41] and chlorpromazine (Fig. 38–6)[42] all impair the growth hormone response to the usual stimuli. In contrast, estrogen therapy[43] and enhanced endogenous cholinergic tone related to pyridostigmine administration[44] increase the growth hormone response to insulin-induced hypoglycemia and to growth hormone–releasing hormone, respectively.

Estrogens and phenytoin are associated with impaired responsiveness of the pituitary-adrenal axis to metyrapone stimulation.[45–48] The effect of estrogens on metyrapone responsiveness may occur either as a result of increased endogenous estrogens (pregnancy)[45] or in response to the exogenous estrogens ethinyl estradiol[46] and mestranol.[47] Although the mechanism for the impaired response in normal pregnancy is unknown, the synthetic estrogens appear to

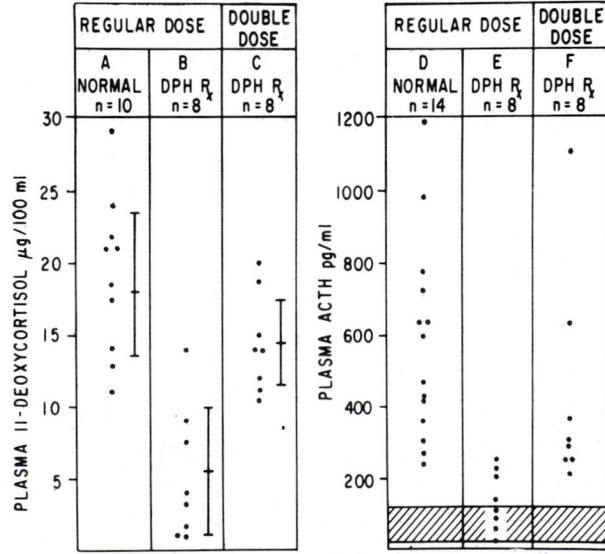

Figure 38–7. Plasma levels of 11-deoxycortisol and ACTH in normal and phenytoin-treated subjects after oral administration of metyrapone (regular or double dose). The cross-hatched area is the normal range for the 8 AM plasma ACTH assay. Bars show the mean ±1 SD. To convert 11-deoxycortisol values to nanomoles per liter, multiply by 28.86. To convert ACTH values to picomoles per liter, multiply by 0.2202. (From Meikle AW, Jubiz W, Matsukura S, et al. Effect of diphenylhydantoin on the metabolism of metyrapone and release of ACTH in man. J Clin Endocrinol Metab 1969; 29:1553–1558. © 1969, The Endocrine Society.)

dexamethasone demonstrate higher total and conjugated urinary metabolites of the drug in patients receiving phenytoin during the first 4 h after dexamethasone administration.[49] In addition, chronic ethanol excess may result in impaired suppression of plasma cortisol levels after dexamethasone. Other drugs have been reported to be associated with false-positive and false-negative dexamethasone suppression test results.[50] Barbiturates, narcotics, high-dose estrogen contraceptives, and carbamazepine may enhance dexamethasone metabolism and result in failure of suppression of plasma cortisol.[50] Stimulants such as cocaine and amphetamines, high-dose benzodiazepines, and nonsteroidal anti-inflammatory drugs have been reported to be associated with normal cortisol suppression in individuals with disease.[50]

Phenytoin,[51] levodopa,[52] dopamine,[53] and aspirin in large doses[54] all impair the response of TSH to TRH injection. Phenytoin enhances the cellular uptake and metabolism of T_4, which leads to lower free T_4 levels. The observation that phenytoin therapy in the usual doses results in a 50% decrease in the integrated TSH response to TRH casts doubt on the reliability of normal basal TSH levels to confirm euthyroidism in patients with decreased T_4 who are receiving phenytoin.[51] Chronic levodopa therapy results in profound inhibition of the TSH response to TRH (Fig. 38–8),[52] and a dopamine infusion begun only 5 min before TRH injection results in a 50% decrease in peak TSH levels.[53] Therapy with aspirin (900 mg four times daily) results in significant suppression of the TSH response to TRH, unrelated to effects on inhibition of prostaglandin synthesis.[54] The mechanism for the aspirin effect may be displacement of thyroid hormones from thyroid-binding globulin.[54]

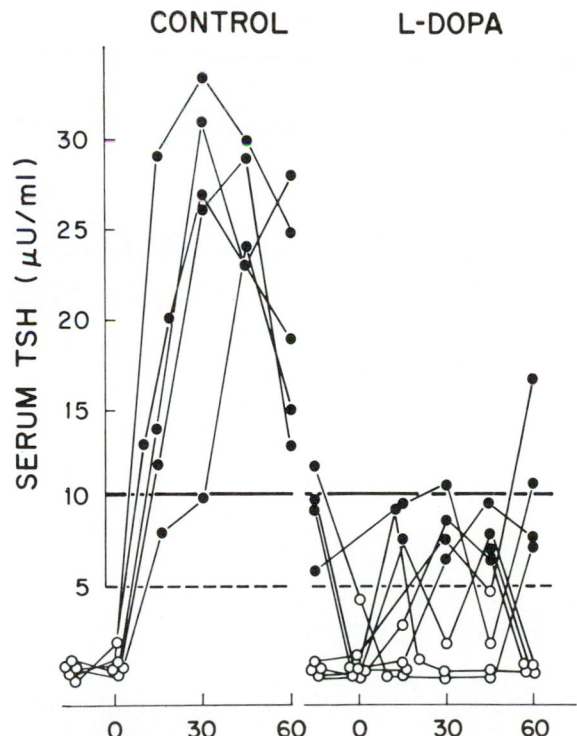

Figure 38–8. Effect of levodopa (L-dopa) on the response of serum TSH to TRH stimulation. The abscissa represents time in minutes after the injection of TRH. Normal unstimulated values for serum TSH are less than 10 μU/mL. Values less than 5 μU/mL are indicated by open circles in view of less accuracy, which is due to the limits of detectability in the assay. (From Spaulding SW, Burrow GN, Donabedian R, et al. L-Dopa suppression of thyrotropin releasing hormone response in man. J Clin Endocrinol Metab 1972; 35:182–185. © 1972, The Endocrine Society.)

REFERENCES

1. Boyar RM, Rosenfeld RS, Kapen S, et al. Human puberty. Simultaneous augmented secretion of luteinizing hormone and testosterone during sleep. J Clin Invest 1974; 54:609–618.
2. Knapp MS, Keane PM, Wright JG. Circadian rhythm of plasma 11-hydroxycorticosteroids in depressive illness, congestive heart failure, and Cushing's syndrome. Br Med J 1967; 2:27–30.
3. Lamberts SWJ, Klijn JGM, de Jong FH, et al. Hormone secretion in alcohol-induced pseudo-Cushing's syndrome. JAMA 1979; 242:1640–1643.
4. Gordon GG, Altman K, Southren AL, et al. Effect of alcohol (ethanol) administration on sex-hormone metabolism in normal men. N Engl J Med 1976; 295:793–797.
5. Weintraub BD, Gershengorn MC, Kourides IA, et al. Inappropriate secretion of thyroid-stimulating hormone. Ann Intern Med 1981; 95:339–351.
6. Luger A, Deuster P, Kyle SB, et al. Acute hypothalamic-pituitary-adrenal responses to the stress of treadmill exercise. N Engl J Med 1987; 316:1309–1316.
7. Allen TD, Griffin JE. Endocrine studies in patients with advanced hypospadias. J Urol 1984; 131:310–314.
8. Snyder PJ, Utiger RD. Response to thyrotropin releasing hormone (TRH) in normal man. J Clin Endocrinol Metab 1972; 34:380–385.
9. Snyder PJ, Utiger RD. Thyrotropin response to thyrotropin releasing hormone in normal females over forty. J Clin Endocrinol Metab 1972; 34:1096–1098.
10. Lang I, Guntram S, Pietschmann P, et al. Effects of sex and age on growth hormone response to growth hormone–releasing hormone in healthy individuals. J Clin Endocrinol Metab 1987; 65:535–540.
11. Chakmakjian ZH, Nelson DH, Bethune JE. Adrenocortical failure in panhypopituitarism. J Clin Endocrinol Metab 1968; 28:259–265.
12. Snyder PJ, Rudenstein RS, Gardner DF, et al. Repetitive infusion of gonadotropin-releasing hormone distinguishes hypothalamic from pituitary hypogonadism. J Clin Endocrinol Metab 1979; 48:864–868.
13. Brown RD, Van Loon GR, Orth DN, et al. Cushing's disease with periodic hormonogenesis: one explanation for paradoxical response to dexamethasone. J Clin Endocrinol Metab 1973; 36:445–451.
14. Rayfield EJ, Pulini M, Golub A, et al. Nonautonomous function of a pancreatic insulinoma. J Clin Endocrinol Metab 1976; 43:1307–1311.
15. Samaan NA, Osborne BM, MacKay B, et al. Endocrine and morphologic studies of pituitary adenomas secondary to primary hypothyroidism. J Clin Endocrinol Metab 1977; 45:903–911.
16. Samaan NA, Stepanas AV, Danziger J, et al. Reactive pituitary abnormalities in patients with Klinefelter's and Turner's syndromes. Arch Intern Med 1979; 139:198–201.
17. Caminos-Torres R, Ma L, Snyder PJ. Testosterone-induced inhibition of the LH and FSH responses to gonadotropin-releasing hormone occurs slowly. J Clin Endocrinol Metab 1977; 44:1142–1153.
18. Hamburger JI. Evolution of toxicity in solitary nontoxic autonomously functioning thyroid nodules. J Clin Endocrinol Metab 1980; 50:1089–1093.
19. Refetoff S. Syndromes of thyroid hormone resistance. Am J Physiol 1982; 243:E88–E98.
20. Bantle JP, Seeling S, Mariash CN, et al. Resistance to thyroid hormones: a disorder frequently confused with Graves' disease. Arch Intern Med 1982; 142:1867–1871.
21. Iwatsubo H, Omori K, Okada Y, et al. Human growth hormone secretion in primary hypothyroidism before and after treatment. J Clin Endocrinol Metab 1967; 27:1751–1754.
22. Burgess JA, Smith BR, Merimee TJ. Growth hormone in thyrotoxicosis: effect of insulin-induced hypoglycemia. J Clin Endocrinol Metab 1966; 26:1257–1260.
23. Krieger DT. Lack of responsiveness of L-dopa in Cushing's disease. J Clin Endocrinol Metab 1973; 36:277–284.
24. Gold EM, Kent JR, Forsham PH. Clinical use of a new diagnostic agent, methopyrapone (SU-4885), in pituitary and adrenocortical disorders. Ann Intern Med 1961; 54:175–188.
25. Brownie AC, Sprunt JG. Metopirone in the assessment of pituitary-adrenal function. Lancet 1962; 1:773–778.
26. Kaplan NM. Methopyrapone test in primary hypothyroidism. J Clin Endocrinol Metab 1965; 25:146–148.
27. Cushman P Jr. Hypothalamic-pituitary-adrenal function in thyroid disorders: effects of methopyrapone infusion on plasma corticosteroids. Metabolism 1968; 17:263–270.
28. Giustina A, Romanelli G, Candrina R, et al. Growth hormone deficiency in patients with idiopathic adrenocorticotropin deficiency resolves during glucocorticoid replacement. J Clin Endocrinol Metab 1989; 68:120–124.
29. Beck P, Koumans JHT, Winterling CA, et al. Studies of insulin and growth hormone secretion in human obesity. J Lab Clin Med 1964; 64:654–667.
30. El-Khodary AZ, Ball MF, Stein B, et al. Effect of weight loss on the growth hormone response to arginine infusion in obesity. J Clin Endocrinol Metab 1971; 32:42–51.

31. Fingerhut M, Krieger DT. Plasma growth hormone response to L-dopa in obese subjects. Metabolism 1974; 23:267–271.
32. Smith SR, Edgar PJ, Pozefsky T, et al. Growth hormone in adults with protein-calorie malnutrition. J Clin Endocrinol Metab 1974; 39:53–62.
33. Samaan NA, Freeman RM. Growth hormone levels in severe renal failure. Metabolism 1970; 19:102–113.
34. Conn HO, Daughaday WH. Cirrhosis and diabetes. V. Serum human growth hormone levels in Laennec's cirrhosis. J Lab Clin Med 1970; 76:678–688.
35. Podolsky S, Melby JC. Improvement of growth hormone response to stimulation in primary aldosteronism with correction of potassium deficiency. Metabolism 1976; 25:1027–1032.
36. Sachar EJ, Mushrush G, Perlow M, et al. Growth hormone responses to L-dopa in depressed patients. Science 1972; 178:1304–1305.
37. Butler PWP, Besser GM. Pituitary-adrenal function in severe depressive illness. Lancet 1968; 1:1234–1236.
38. Spratt DI, Pont A, Miller MB, et al. Hyperthyroxinemia in patients with acute psychiatric disorders. Am J Med 1982; 73:41–48.
39. Hartog M, Gaafar MA, Fraser R. Effect of corticosteroids on serum growth hormone. Lancet 1964; 2:376–378.
40. Lawrence AM, Kirsteins L. Progestins in the medical management of active acromegaly. J Clin Endocrinol Metab 1970; 30:646–652.
41. Losa M, Huss R, König A, et al. Theophylline blunts the GH-response to growth hormone releasing hormone in normal subjects. Acta Endocrinol 1986; 112:473–480.
42. Mims RB, Scott CL, Modebe O, et al. Inhibition of L-dopa–induced growth hormone stimulation by pyridoxine and chlorpromazine. J Clin Endocrinol Metab 1975; 40:256–259.
43. Spellacy WN, Carlson KL, Schade SL. Human growth hormone levels in normal subjects receiving an oral contraceptive. JAMA 1967; 202:451–454.
44. Penalva A, Muruais C, Casanueva FF, et al. Effect of enhancement of endogenous cholinergic tone with pyridostigmine on the dose-response relationships of growth hormone (GH)–releasing hormone–induced GH secretion in normal subjects. J Clin Endocrinol Metab 1990; 70:324–327.
45. Beck P, Eaton CJ, Young IS, et al. Metyrapone response in pregnancy. Am J Obstet Gynecol 1968; 100:327–330.
46. Sprunt JG, Rutherford ER, Nelson DH. The impaired response to metyrapone in patients taking oestrogen. Acta Endocrinol 1968; 59:447–453.
47. Meikle AW, Jubiz W, Matsukura S, et al. Effect of estrogen on the metabolism of metyrapone and release of ACTH. J Clin Endocrinol Metab 1970; 30:259–263.
48. Meikle AW, Jubiz W, Matsukura S, et al. Effect of diphenylhydantoin on the metabolism of metyrapone and release of ACTH in man. J Clin Endocrinol Metab 1969; 29:1553–1558.
49. Jubiz W, Meikle AW, Levinson RA, et al. Effect of diphenylhydantoin on the metabolism of dexamethasone: mechanism of the abnormal dexamethasone suppression in humans. N Engl J Med 1970; 283:11–14.
50. Burch EA Jr, Goldschmidt TJ, Schwartz BD. Drug intake and the dexamethasone suppression test. J Clin Psychiatry 1986; 47:144–146.
51. Surks MI, Ordene KW, Mann DN, et al. Diphenylhydantoin inhibits the thyrotropin response to thyrotropin-releasing hormone in man and rat. J Clin Endocrinol Metab 1983; 56:940–945.
52. Spaulding SW, Burrow GN, Donabedian R, et al. L-Dopa suppression of thyrotropin releasing hormone response in man. J Clin Endocrinol Metab 1972; 35:182–185.
53. Burrow GN, May PB, Spaulding SW, et al. TRH and dopamine interactions affecting pituitary hormone secretion. J Clin Endocrinol Metab 1977; 45:65–72.
54. Ramey JN, Burrow GN, Spaulding SW, et al. The effect of aspirin and indomethacin on the TRH response in man. J Clin Endocrinol Metab 1976; 43:107–114.

INDEX

Note: Page numbers in *italics* refer to illustrations; page numbers followed by a t refer to tables.

REFERENCE VALUES

In preparing the book and the reference values, the editors have taken into account the fact that the system of international units (Système International d'Unités, SI) is used in all medical and scientific journals and in most clinical laboratories throughout the world. However, in the United States most clinical laboratories continue to report values in conventional units. Therefore, in the book and in the reference values we use both systems. *In the text, values in SI units appear first and conventional units appear in parentheses after the SI units.* The exception to this dual approach is when the numbers remain the same but the terminology changes (e.g., mmol/L for meq/L in the case of sodium or IU/L for mIU/mL in the case of luteinizing hormone). Most conversions from one system to the other can be made as follows:

$$mmol/L = \frac{mg/dL \times 10}{atomic\ or\ molecular\ weight} \quad or \quad mg/dL = \frac{mmol/L \times atomic\ or\ molecular\ weight}{10}$$

Conversion of mEq/L to mmol is made by dividing mEq/L by the valence of the molecule. For the convenience of the reader, factors for converting conventional to SI units are included (see Young DS. Implementation of SI units for clinical laboratory data. Ann Intern Med 106:114–128, 1987). *Please note that the conversion factors are valid only when the conventional units are exactly as specified.* The reference values are meant to be used only as general guidelines because actual values vary among laboratories. Unless indicated otherwise, an overnight fast is assumed.

Measure	SI	Conventional (C)	Conversion Factor (CF) $C \times CF = SI$
Acetoacetate, plasma	<100 µmol/L	<1.0 mg/dL	97.95
Adrenal steroids, plasma			
Aldosterone, supine, saline suppression	<220 pmol/L	<8 ng/dL	27.74
Cortisol			
8 AM	220–660 nmol/L	8–24 µg/dL	27.59
4 PM	50–410 nmol/L	2–15 µg/dL	27.59
Overnight dexamethasone suppression	<140 nmol/L	<5 µg/dL	27.59
Dehydroepiandrosterone (DHEA)	0.6–70 nmol/L	0.2–20 µg/L	3.467
Dehydroepiandrosterone sulfate (DHEAS)	5.4–9.2 µmol/L	820–3380 ng/mL	0.002714
11-Deoxycortisol (compound S)	<60 nmol/L	<2 µg/dL	28.86
17α-Hydroxyprogesterone			
Women	1–13 nmol/L	0.3–4.2 µg/L	3.026
Men	1.5–7.5 nmol/L	0.5–2.5 µg/L	3.026
Adrenal steroids, urinary excretion			
Aldosterone	15–70 nmol/d	5–26 µg/d	2.774
Cortisol, free	30–300 nmol/d	10–100 µg/d	2.759
17-Hydroxycorticosteroids	5.5–28 µmol/d	2–10 mg/d	2.759
17-Ketosteroids			
Women	14–52 µmol/d	4–15 mg/d	3.467
Men	22–88 µmol/d	7–25 mg/d	3.467
Ammonia (as NH_3), venous whole blood	6–45 µmol/L	10–80 µg/dL	0.5872
Angiotensin II, plasma, 8 AM	10–30 ng/L	10–30 pg/mL	1.0
Arginine vasopressin (AVP), plasma, random fluid intake	2.3–7.4 pmol/L	2.5–8 ng/L	0.92
Bicarbonate, serum	18–23 mmol/L	18–23 mEq/L	1.0
Calciferols (see vitamin D)			
Calcitonin, serum	<50 ng/L	<50 pg/mL	1.0
Calcium			
Ionized serum	1–1.5 mmol/L	4–4.6 mg/dL	0.2495
Total serum	2.2–2.6 mmol/L	9–10.5 mg/dL	0.2495
β-Carotene, serum	0.9–4.6 µmol/L	50–250 µg/dL	0.01863
Catecholamines, plasma			
Epinephrine, basal supine	170–520 pmol/L	30–95 pg/mL	5.458
Norepinephrine, basal supine	0.3–2.8 nmol/L	15–475 pg/mL	0.005911
Catecholamines, urinary			
Epinephrine	<275 nmol/d	<50 µg/d	5.458
Normetanephrine	0–11 µmol/d	0–2.0 mg/d	5.458
Total catecholamines (as norepinephrine)	<675 nmol/d	<120 µg/d	5.911
Vanillylmandelic acid (VMA)	<35 µmol/d	<68 mg/d	5.046
Chloride, serum	98—106 mmol/L	98–106 mEq/L	1.0
Cholesterol, plasma			
Total cholesterol			
Desirable	<5.20 mmol/L	<200 mg/dL	0.02586
Borderline high	5.2–6.18 mmol/L	200–239 mg/dL	0.02586
High	≥6.21 mmol/L	≥240 mg/dL	0.02586
High-density lipoprotein (HDL) cholesterol			
Desirable	≥1.29 mmol/L	≥50 mg/dL	0.02586
Borderline high	0.9–1.27 mmol/L	36–49 mg/dL	0.02586
High	≤0.91 mmol/L	≤35 mg/dL	0.02586
Low-density lipoprotein (LDL) cholesterol			
Desirable	<3.36 mmol/L	<130 mg/dL	0.02586
Borderline high	3.39–4.11 mmol/L	131–159 mg/dL	0.02586
High	≥4.14 mmol/L	≥160 mg/dL	0.02586
Corticotropin (ACTH), plasma	4–22 pmol/L	20–100 pg/mL	0.2202
C peptide, plasma	0.5–2 µg/L	0.5–2 ng/mL	1.0
Creatinine, serum	<133 µmol/L	<1.5 mg/dL	88.40
Fatty acids, nonesterified or free (FFA), plasma	<0.7 mmol/L	<18 mg/dL	0.03906
Gastrin, serum	<120 ng/L	<120 pg/mL	1.0
Glucagon, plasma	50–100 ng/L	50–100 pg/mL	1.0
Glucose, plasma			
Overnight fast, normal	4.2–6.4 mmol/L	75–115 mg/dL	0.05551
Overnight fast, diabetes mellitus	7.8 mmol/L	>140 mg/dL	0.05551
72-h fast, normal men	>2.8 mmol/L	>50 mg/dL	0.05551
72-h fast, normal women	>2.2 mmol/L	>40 mg/dL	0.05551